OXFORD TEXTBOOK OF
MEDICINE

OXFORD MEDICAL PUBLICATIONS

OXFORD TEXTBOOK OF MEDICINE

THIRD EDITION

VOLUME 2
Sections 11–17 and Index

Edited by

D. J. Weatherall

Regius Professor of Medicine, University of Oxford;
Honorary Director, Institute of Molecular Medicine, Oxford

J. G. G. Ledingham

Clinical Professor and May Reader in Medicine,
Nuffield Department of Clinical Medicine, University of Oxford

D. A. Warrell

Professor of Tropical Medicine and Infectious Diseases,
Nuffield Department of Clinical Medicine, University of Oxford

Oxford   New York   Tokyo
OXFORD UNIVERSITY PRESS
1996

Oxford University Press, Walton Street, Oxford OX2 6DP

Oxford   New York
Athens   Auckland   Bangkok   Bombay
Calcutta   Cape Town   Dar es Salaam   Delhi
Florence   Hong Kong   Istanbul   Karachi
Kuala Lumpur   Madras   Madrid   Melbourne
Mexico City   Nairobi   Paris   Singapore
Taipei   Tokyo   Toronto
and associated companies in
Berlin Ibadan

Oxford is a trade mark of Oxford University Press

Published in the United States
by Oxford University Press Inc., New York

First published 1983
Second edition 1987
Third edition 1996

A catalogue record for this book is available from the British Library

Library of Congress Cataloging in Publication Data
(Data Available)

ISBN 0 19 262140 8 (Three volume set)
ISBN 0 19 262706 6 (vol 1)
ISBN 0 19 262707 4 (vol 2)
ISBN 0 19 262708 2 (vol 3)
Available as a three volume set only

Typeset by University Graphics Inc, New Jersey, USA
Printed in the United States of America

Preface to the Third Edition

As the third edition of the *Oxford Textbook of Medicine* begins to see the light of day, medical textbooks are having a bad press in Great Britain. The stimulus to the recent resurgence of the age-old argument about the educational value, or lack of it, of textbooks was a presentation to a House of Lords Select Committee that suggested that many patients are losing their lives because doctors rely on information obtained from outdated texts and clinical teaching based on archaic practice.

In the preface to the first edition of the *Textbook* we discussed the late Professor Mitchell's similarly jaundiced views on the value of medical textbooks. He had suggested that they were likely to suffer the same fate as dinosaurs in that their very weight would preclude survival (it is not just the medical sciences that need constant revision; this view of the reason for the extinction of the dinosaurs may also have to be modified!). He went on to say that textbooks were already out of date before they were published, and hence, as well as being a health hazard due to their weight, were of limited educational value to their readers. However, having had a few more years to ponder further on Professor Mitchell's forecasts, we remain largely unrepentant.

A number of factors have combined greatly to increase the complexity of medical practice over the relatively short timespan since this *Textbook* was first published. There has been a major revolution in the basic biological sciences that has enormous implications for clinical practice in the future. In the richer countries the mean age of the population has risen dramatically and hence the pattern of disease has become much more complex and multifactorial. The populations of the developing countries continue to expand and, if anything, malnutrition and infectious disease present an even more frightening problem than they did fifteen years ago. And the remarkable achievements of the basic biomedical sciences combined with the inability of the richer countries to contain the costs of health care, and the poorer ones to provide it, are raising many new ethical problems for doctors.

Set against this complex and rapidly changing scene what should be the objective of a textbook of medicine? Clearly, no student or practitioner can own a library of monographs and journals that covers the whole of internal medicine. One important function is to provide a sound basic account of the many disorders that comprise internal medicine and thus give the background to more recent advances that are best sought in specialist journals. Furthermore, as well as the greater complexity of the diseases of the richer countries, the increasing ease of international travel and the movements of massive refugee populations round the world mean that internal medicine today is truly global; diseases that once were restricted to tropical climates or particular countries can turn up in hospitals or consulting rooms anywhere in the world. It is clear, therefore, that some basic textbooks that give students and doctors a 'way in' to the literature on the bulk of the diseases that they are likely to encounter, common or rare, are still required. With this background in mind we have added a number of new chapters and topics to this edition and have had many of the previous ones completely rewritten. We have expanded some of the background chapters on the basic sciences, particularly for students and doctors in countries in which access to current literature in these fields is limited. We have introduced new sections on medical ethics, clinical trials and evidence-based medicine, forensic medicine, and related topics that are an important part of the modern medical scene. As in previous editions, we have attempted to provide a global view of internal medicine rather than describe it as it is seen in day-to-day practice in the richer industrialized countries. And because of the increasing evidence of the clinical value of the management of cancer by specialists in the field we have included a new section on clinical oncology as a background to the descriptions of malignant disease in individual sections.

We are well aware that parts of this book will rapidly date and hence it is important that students and practitioners continue to augment their reading with up-to-date journals, and refresh themselves by regular visits to postgraduate meetings. Information systems and related technology are rapidly changing the face of communication in medicine and readers should avail themselves of every opportunity of learning the complexities and potentials of this rapidly evolving branch of practice.

As before we are particularly grateful to those of our colleagues who helped in the planning of particular sections: Dr J.A. Vale (poisoning by drugs and chemicals); Dr E. Hodgson and Professor J.M. Harrington (occupational and environmental health and safety); Dr R.W.E. Watts (metabolic disorders); Professor Alan McGregor (endocrine disorders); Professor C. Redman (medical disorders of pregnancy); Dr Derek Jewell, Dr Margaret Bassendine, and Professor Sir Leslie Turnberg (gastroenterology); Professor Stuart Cobbe (cardiovascular disorders); Drs Julian Hopkin and Donald Lane (respiratory medicine); Professor M.W. Adler (sexually-transmitted diseases and sexual health); Professor Paul Dieppe (rheumatology); Professors John Goldman and Sam Machin (disorders of the blood); Drs J. Strang, I. Glass, and M. Farrell (alcohol and drug-related problems); Professor J. Newsom-Davis (neurology and disorders of voluntary muscle). The section on Psychiatry was organized and edited by Professor Michael Gelder.

We wish to thank Dr Irene Butcher who has edited this edition of the *Textbook*; her forbearance with its editors, some of its more errant authors, and Oxford University Press has, at times, bordered on the saintly. We also thank Mrs Pam Herridge for invaluable editorial work. Finally, we are particularly grateful to our personal secretaries who have stayed the course with us through yet another phase of this saga, Mrs Janet Watt, Mrs Maureen Stacey, and Miss Eunice Berry.

Oxford
April 1995

D.J. WEATHERALL
J.G.G. LEDINGHAM
D.A. WARRELL

Summary of Contents

Volume 1

Section 1   On being a patient   1

Section 2   On modern scientific medicine   5

Section 3   The spectrum of disease and clinical
            practice   33

Section 4   Medical relevance of molecular and
            cell biology and genetics   55

Section 5   Immune mechanisms in health and
            disease   139

Section 6   Clinical oncology   189

Section 7   Infection   263

Section 8   Chemical and physical injuries and
            environmental and occupational
            diseases   1041

Section 9   Principles of clinical pharmacology
            and drug therapy   1235

Section 10 Nutrition   1265

Volume 2

Section 11 Metabolic disorders   1333

Section 12 Endocrine disorders   1551

Section 13 Medical disorders in pregnancy   1721

Section 14 Gastroenterology   1817

Section 15 Cardiovascular disease   2141

Section 16 Intensive care   2561

Section 17 Respiratory medicine   2589

Volume 3

Section 18 Rheumatology   2941

Section 19 Disorders of the skeleton   3053

Section 20 Nephrology   3099

Section 21 Sexually-transmitted diseases and
            sexual health   3363

Section 22 Disorders of the blood   3373

Section 23 Diseases of the skin   3703

Section 24 Neurology   3813

Section 25 Disorders of voluntary muscles   4137

Section 26 The eye in general medicine   4177

Section 27 Psychiatry in medicine   4201

Section 28 Alcohol and drug-related problems   4261

Section 29 Forensic medicine   4307

Section 30 Sports medicine   4319

Section 31 Medicine in old age   4331

Section 32 Terminal illness   4347

Section 33 Reference intervals for biochemical
            data   4361

Contents

Volume 1

Preface

Contents

Contributors

Plates to Volume 1

Section 1   On being a patient *C. Clothier*   1

Section 2   On modern scientific medicine   5

2.1   Scientific method and the art of healing *D.J. Weatherall*   7
2.2   Medical ethics *G.R. Dunstan*   10
2.3   Evaulation of clinical method *D.L. Sackett*   15
2.4   Large-scale randomized evidence: trials and overviews
       R. Collins, R. Peto, R. Gray, and S. Parish   21

Section 3   The spectrum of disease and clinical
practice   33

3.1   The diseases of gods: some newer threats to health
       M. King and C.M. Elliott   35
3.2   Health and sickness in the community *M.J. Goldacre
       and M.P. Vessey*   39
3.3   Primary care *G.H. Fowler*   46
3.4   Health care in developing countries *H. Annett and
       A. Cassels*   51

Section 4   Medical relevance of molecular and
cell biology and genetics   55

4.1   Molecular biology and medicine *D.J. Weatherall*   57
4.2   Medical applications of cell biology   68

       4.2.1   Introduction *D.J. Weatherall*   68
       4.2.2   Cell biology of organelles and the endomembrane
                system *D.J.T. Vaux*   68
       4.2.3   The mononuclear phagocyte system and tissue
                homeostasis *S. Gordon*   84
       4.2.4   Cytokines *S. Keshav*   95
4.3   Genetic factors in disease *M.E. Pembrey*   100

Section 5   Immune mechanisms in health and
disease   139

5.1   Principles of immunology *A.J. McMichael*   141
5.2   Immune mechanisms of disease *J.I. Bell and
       R.E. O'Hehir*   154
5.3   Immunodeficiency *A.D.B. Webster*   166
5.4   Complement and disease *H.M. Chapel*   175
5.5   Principles of transplantation immunology *P.J. Morris*   182

Section 6   Clinical oncology   189

6.1   General characteristics of neoplasia *H. Harris*   191
6.2   Epidemiology of cancer *R. Doll and R. Peto*   197
6.3   Growth factors and oncogenes *W.J. Gullick*   222
6.4   Tumour immunology *P.C.L. Beverley*   226
6.5   Medical imaging in oncology *S.J. Golding*   234
6.6   Cancer: clinical features and management *R.L. Souhami*   240
6.7   Role of radiotherapy in the treatment of cancer
       A. Horwich   253
6.8   New approaches to cancer therapy *A.L. Harris and
       J. Carmichael*   258

Section 7   Infection   263

7.1   Clinical approach to the patient with suspected
       infection *H.P. Lambert*   265
7.2   Biology of pathogenic micro-organisms   268

       7.2.1   Introduction to the diversity of bacterial
                pathogens *P.J. Sansonetti*   268
       7.2.2   Molecular taxonomy of bacterial pathogens
                P.J. Sansonetti   272
7.3   The host's response to infection *B.M. Greenwood*   275
7.4   Epidemiology and public health *R.T. Mayon-White*   285
7.5   Physiological changes in infected patients *P.A. Murphy*   290
7.6   Antimicrobial therapy *P.G. Davey*   295
7.7   Immunization *D. Isaacs and E.R. Moxon*   315
7.8   Travel and expedition medicine *C.P. Conlon and
       D.A. Warrell*   322
7.9   Nosocomial infection *D.W.M. Crook and I.C.G.
       Bowler*   327
7.10   Viruses   333

       7.10.1   Respiratory tract viruses *D. Isaacs*   333
       Herpes viruses   341
       7.10.2   Herpes simplex virus infections *T.E.A. Peto
                and B.E. Juel-Jensen*   341
       7.10.3   Varicella-zoster infections: chickenpox and
                zoster *T.E.A. Peto and B.E. Juel-Jensen*   346
       7.10.4   Epstein-Barr virus *M.A. Epstein and
                D.H. Crawford*   352
       7.10.5   Human infections cause by simian
                herpesviruses *L.E. Chapman and
                C.J. Peters*   357
       7.10.6   Cytomegalovirus *S. Stagno*   359
       7.10.7   Human herpesviruses 6 *P.E. Pellett and
                J.A. Stewart*   364
       Poxviruses   365
       7.10.8   Poxviruses *G.L. Smith*   365
       7.10.9   Orf *T.E.A. Peto and B.E. Juel-Jensen*   369
       7.10.10   Molluscum contagiosum *T.E.A. Peto and
                B.E. Juel-Jensen*   371

Paramyxoviruses 372

    7.10.11   Mumps: epidemic parotitis *B.K. Rima and A.B. Christie* 372

    7.10.12   Measles *H.C. Whittle and P. Aaby* 375

7.10.13 Enteroviruses *N.R. Grist and E.J. Bell* 381

7.10.14 Viruses in diarrhoea and vomiting *C.R. Madeley* 390

7.10.15 Rhabdoviruses: rabies and rabies-related viruses *M.J. Warrell and D.A. Warrell* 394

7.10.16 Colorado tick fever and other arthropod-borne reoviruses *M.J. Warrell and D.A. Warrell* 406

Togaviruses 407

    7.10.17   Alphaviruses *D.I.H. Simpson* 407

    7.10.18   Rubella *S. Logan and P. Tookey* 409

    7.10.19   Flaviviruses *T.P. Monath* 412

    7.10.20   Dengue haemorrhagic fever *Suchitra Nimmanitya and M.J. Cardosa* 419

7.10.21 Bunyaviridae *J.S. Porterfield and J.W. LeDuc* 423

7.10.22 Arenaviruses *S. Fisher-Hoch and J.B. McCormick* 429

7.10.23 Filoviruses: Marburg and Ebola fevers *D.I.H. Simpson* 439

7.10.24 Papovaviruses *K.V. Shah* 443

7.10.25 Parvoviruses *J.R. Pattison* 447

7.10.26 Viral hepatitis *A.J. Zuckerman and J.N. Zuckerman* 448

7.10.27 Viruses and cancer *R.A. Weiss* 460

Retroviruses 463

    7.10.28   Human immunodeficiency viruses *R.A. Weiss* 463

    7.10.29   HIV infection and AIDS *I.V.D. Weller, C.P. Conlon, and T.E.A. Peto* 467

    7.10.30   Human immunodeficiency virus in the developing world *C.F. Gilks* 483

    7.10.31   HTLV-I and -II associated diseases *C.R.M. Bangham and S. Nightingale* 489

7.11 Bacteria 493

7.11.1   Diphtheria *A.B. Christie and Tran Tinh Hien* 493

Streptococci 497

    7.11.2   Pathogenic streptococci *G. Colman* 497

    7.11.3   Pneumococcal infection *B.M. Greenwood* 511

    7.11.4   Staphylococci *S.J. Eykyn* 523

7.11.5 Meningococcal infection *B.M. Greenwood* 533

7.11.6 *Neisseria gonorrhoeae* *D. Barlow and C.A. Ison* 544

Enteropathogenic bacteria 550

    7.11.7   Enterobacteria and miscellaneous enteropathogenic and food-poisoning bacteria *M.B. Skirrow* 550

    7.11.8   Typhoid and paratyphoid fevers *J. Richens* 560

    7.11.9   Rhinoscleroma *J. Richens* 568

7.11.10 Anaerobic bacteria *S.J. Eykyn* 569

7.11.11 Cholera *C.C.J. Carpenter* 576

7.11.12 *Haemophilus influenzae* *E.R. Moxon* 580

7.11.13 *Haemophilus ducreyi* and chancroid *A.R. Ronald* 584

7.11.14 Bordetella *C.C. Linnemann Jr.* 587

7.11.15 Melioidosis and glanders *D.A.B. Dance* 590

7.11.16 Plague *T. Butler* 595

7.11.17 Yersiniosis, pasteurellosis, and tularaemia 599

    (a) Tularaemia *A.D. Pearson* 599

    (b) Pasteurellosis *A.D. Pearson* 606

    (c) Yersiniosis *A.D. Pearson* 608

7.11.18 Anthrax *A.B. Christie and P.C.B. Turnbull* 612

7.11.19 Brucellosis *M.M. Madkour* 619

7.11.20 Tetanus *F.E. Udwadia* 624

7.11.21 Botulism, gas gangrene, and clostridial gastrointestinal infections *H.E. Larson* 630

Tuberculosis and its problems in developing countries 638

    7.11.22   Tuberculosis *P.D.O. Davies, D.J. Girling, and J.M. Grange* 638

    7.11.23   Particular problems of tuberculosis in developing countries *C.G. Uragoda* 661

7.11.24 Disease caused by environmental mycobacteria *J.M. Grange, D.J. Girling, and P.D.O. Davies* 664

7.11.25 Leprosy (Hansen's disease, hanseniasis) *M.F.R. Waters* 667

7.11.26 *Mycobacterium ulcerans* infection *M.F.R. Waters* 679

7.11.27 Actinomycoses *K.P. Schaal* 680

7.11.28 Nocardiosis *R.J. Hay* 686

7.11.29 Rat bite fevers *D.A. Warrell* 687

Spirochaetes 689

    7.11.30   Lyme disease *W. Burgdorfer and T.G. Schwan* 689

    7.11.31   Other Borrelia infections *D.A. Warrell* 692

    7.11.32   Leptospirosis *V. Sitprija* 698

    7.11.33   Non-venereal treponemes: yaws, endemic syphilis, and pinta *P.L. Perine* 703

    7.11.34   Syphilis *D.J.M. Wright and G.W. Csonka* 706

7.11.35 Listeria and listeriosis *P.J. Wilkinson* 720

7.11.36 Legionellosis and legionnaires' disease *J.B. Kurtz and J.T. Macfarlane* 722

Rickettsial diseases 728

    7.11.37   Rickettsial diseases including the ehrlichioses *D.H. Walker* 728

    7.11.38   Scrub typhus *Kyaw Win and G. Watt* 739

    7.11.39   *Coxiella burnetii* infections (Q fever) *T.J. Marrie* 742

    7.11.40   Cat scratch disease, bacillary angiomatosis, and trench fever *B.A. Perkins* 744

Chlamydial infections and lymphogranuloma venereum 748

    7.11.41   Chlamydial infections *D. Taylor-Robinson, D.C.W. Mabey, and J.D. Trehearne* 748

    7.11.42   Lymphogranuloma venereum *P.L. Perrine* 759

7.11.43 Mycoplasmas *D. Taylor-Robinson* 762

7.11.44 Bartonellosis *E.A. Llanos-Cuentas, C. Maguiña-Vargas, and D.A. Warrell* 773

7.11.45 Donovanosis (granuloma inguinale) *J. Richens* 776

7.11.46 'Newer' and lesser known bacteria causing infection in humans *J. Paul* 778

7.12 Fungal infections (mycoses) 797

7.12.1   Fungal infections *R.J. Hay and D.W.R. Mackenzie* 797

7.12.2   Coccidioidomycosis *J.R. Graybill* 812

7.12.3   Chromoblastomycosis *M.A.H. Bayles* 813

7.12.4   Paracoccidioidomycosis *M.A.S. Yasuda*   814

7.12.5   *Pneumocystis carinii J.M. Hopkin*   820

7.13   Protozoa   825

7.13.1   Amoebiasis *R. Knight*   825

7.13.2   Malaria *D. Bradley, C.I. Newbold, and D.A. Warrell*   835

7.13.3   Babesia *T.K. Ruebush*   863

7.13.4   Toxoplasmosis *J. Couvreur and P. Thulliez*   865

7.13.5   Cryptosporidium and cryptosporidiosis *D.P. Casemore and D.A. Warrell*   869

7.13.6   Cyclospora *D.P. Casemore*   876

7.13.7   Sarcocystosis *V. Zaman*   877

7.13.8   Giardiasis, balantidiasis, isosporiasis, and microsporidiosis *M.F. Heyworth*   878

7.13.9   *Blastocystis hominis V. Zaman*   887

7.13.10   African trypanosomiasis *D.H. Smith*   888

7.13.11   American trypanosomiasis *P.D. Marsden*   895

7.13.12   Leishmaniasis *A.D.M. Bryceson*   899

7.13.13   Trichomoniasis *J.P. Ackers*   907

7.14   Nematodes (roundworms)   911

7.14.1   General principles of filarial infections and diseases *B.O.L. Duke*   911

7.14.2   Lymphatic filariasis *B.A. Southgate*   919

7.14.3   Guinea-worm disease: human dracunculiasis *M.M. Kliks*   924

7.14.4   Strongyloidiasis, hookworm, and other gut strongyloid nematodes *R. Knight*   928

7.14.5   Nematode infections of lesser importance *D.I. Grove*   933

7.14.6   Other gut nematodes *V. Zaman*   936

7.14.7   Toxocariasis and visceral larval migrans *V. Zaman*   944

7.14.8   Angiostrongyliasis *Sompone Punyagupta*   945

7.14.9   Gnathostomiasis *Pravan Suntharasamai*   949

7.15   Cestodes (tapeworms)   955

7.15.1   Hydatid disease *A.J. Radford*   955

7.15.2   Gut cestodes *R. Knight*   959

7.15.3   Cysticercosis *D. Overbosch*   964

7.15.4   Diphyllobothriasis and sparganosis *Seung-Yull Cho*   969

7.16   Trematodes (flukes)   970

7.16.1   Schistosomiasis *A.E. Butterworth and J.E.P. Thomas*   970

7.16.2   Liver fluke diseases of man *Swangjai Pungpak and Danai Bunnag*   981

7.16.3   Lung flukes (paragonimiasis) *Sirivan Vanijanonta*   988

7.16.4   Intestinal trematodiasis *Khanying Tranakchit Harinasuta and Prayong Radomyos*   992

7.17   Non-venomous arthropods *A.J. Radford and J. Paul*   1000

7.18   Pentastomiasis (porocephalosis) *D.A. Warrell*   1012

7.19   Infectious disease syndromes   1015

7.19.1   Fever of unknown origin *D.T. Durack*   1015

7.19.2   Septicaemia *P.A. Murphy*   1020

7.19.3   Infection in the immunocompromised host *J. Cohen*   1027

7.19.4   Chronic fatigue syndrome (postviral fatigue syndrome and myalgic encephalomyelitis) *M. Sharpe*   1035

Section 8   Chemical and physical injuries and environmental and occupational diseases   1041

8.1   Poisoning (Section Editor *J.A. Vale*)   1043

8.1.1   Introduction and epidemiology *T.J. Meredith, J.A. Vale, and A.T. Proudfoot*   1043

8.1.2   Clinical and metabolic features and general principles of management *A.T. Proudfoot, J.A. Vale, and T.J. Meredith*   1044

8.2   Poisoning by drugs (Section Editor *J.A. Vale*)   1051

8.2.1   Poisoning caused by analgesic drugs *T.J. Meredith, J.A. Vale, and A.T. Proudfoot*   1051

8.2.2   Poisoning from antidepressants, hypnotics, antihistamines, anticonvulsants, and antiparkinsonian drugs *A.T. Proudfoot, J.A. Vale, and T.J. Meredith*   1058

8.2.3   Poisoning from cardiovascular drugs *J.A. Vale, A.T. Proudfoot, and T.J. Meredith*   1062

8.2.4   Poisoning caused by respiratory drugs *A.T. Proudfoot, J.A. Vale, and T.J. Meredith*   1067

8.2.5   Poisoning caused by drugs acting on the gastrointestinal system *J.A. Vale, A.T. Proudfoot, and T.J. Meredith*   1069

8.2.6   Poisoning by haematinics and vitamins *A.T. Proudfoot, J.A. Vale, and T.J. Meredith*   1070

8.2.7   Poisoning by endocrine drugs *A.T. Proudfoot, J.A. Vale, and T.J. Meredith*   1071

8.2.8   Poisoning from antimicrobials *A.T. Proudfoot, J.A. Vale, and T.J. Meredith*   1072

8.2.9   Poisoning from cinchona alkaloids and other antimalarials *P.A. Winstanley*   1072

8.2.10   Poisoning from drugs of abuse *A.T. Proudfoot, J.A. Vale, and T.J. Meredith*   1074

8.2.11   Poisoning due to miscellaneous drugs *J.A. Vale, A.T. Proudfoot, and T.J. Meredith*   1077

8.3   Poisoning by chemicals (Section Editor *J.A. Vale*)   1078

8.3.1   Poisoning from household products *T.J. Meredith, J.A. Vale, and A.T. Proudfoot*   1078

8.3.2   Poisoning by alcohols and glycols *J.A. Vale, A.T. Proudfoot, and T.J. Meredith*   1079

8.3.3   Poisoning from hydrocarbons and chlorofluorocarbons, and volatile substance abuse *J.A. Vale, A.T. Proudfoot, and T.J. Meredith*   1083

8.3.4   Poisoning by inhalational agents *J.A. Vale, A.T. Proudfoot, and T.J. Meredith*   1093

8.3.5   Poisoning due to corrosive substances *T.J. Meredith, J.A. Vale, and A.T. Proudfoot*   1102

8.3.6   Poisoning from metals *Tar-Ching Aw and J.A. Vale*   1105

8.3.7   Poisoning in conflict *R.L. Maynard and T.C. Marrs*   1115

8.3.8   Pesticides *A.T. Proudfoot and J.A. Vale*   1120

8.4   Venoms, toxins, and poisons of animals and plants   1124

8.4.1   Injuries, envenoming, poisoning, and allergic reactions caused by animals *D.A. Warrell*   1124

8.4.2   Poisonous plants and fungi *M.R. Cooper and A.W. Johnson*   1151

8.5   Occupational and environmental health and safety (Section Editors *J.M. Harrington and E.S. Hodgson*)   1160

8.5.1   General introduction *E.S. Hodgson and
        J.M. Harrington*   1160
8.5.2   The investigation of occupational disease
        J.M. Harrington and E.S. Hodgson   1162
8.5.3   The main occupational diseases   1164
        (a) Occupational dermatology *I. Foulds*   1164
        (b) Occupational cancer *J.M. Harrington*   1165
        (c) Musculoskeletal disorders *R.W. Jubb*   1168
        (d) Neurological disorders *E.L. Baker*   1169
        (e) Cardiovascular system *J.M. Harrington*   1169
        (f) Genitourinary system *J.M. Harrington*   1171
        (g) Gastrointestinal tract *E.S. Hodgson*   1171
        (h) The haemopoietic system *E.S. Hodgson*   1172
        (i) Infections *E.S. Hodgson*   1173
        (j) Reproductive system *E. McCloy*   1173
        (k) Neuropsychological disorders *A. Spurgeon*   1174
8.5.4   Occupational safety *R.T. Booth*   1174
8.5.5   Environmental factors and disease   1180
        (a) Heat *W.R. Keatinge*   1180
        (b) Drug-induced increases of body temperature
            W.I. Cranston   1181
        (c) Cold, drowning, and seasonal mortality
            W.R. Keatinge   1182
        (d) Diseases of high terrestrial altitudes
            D. Rennie   1185
        (e) Aerospace medicine *J.A.C. Hopkirk and
            D.M. Denison*   1193
        (f) Diving medicine *D.M. Denison*   1204
        (g) Lightning and electric shock *B.A. Pruitt and
            A.D. Mason*   1211

        (h) Podoconiosis (non-filarial endemic
            elephantiasis of the lower legs) *A.A. Adish,
            and E.W. Price*   1215
        (i) Radiation *R.J. Berry*   1217
        (j) Noise *R.C. Williams*   1223
        (k) Vibration *Tar-Ching Aw*   1225
        (l) Air pollution *J.G. Ayres*   1227
        (m) Environmental disasters *P.J. Baxter*   1232

**Section 9   Principles of clinical pharmacology
and drug therapy** *J.K. Aronson and N.J. White*   1235

Section 10   Nutrition   1265

10.1   Introduction *R. Smith and W.P.T. James*   1267
10.2   Biochemical background *R. Smith and
       D.H. Williamson*   1271
10.3   Severe malnutrition *M.H.N. Golden*   1278
10.4   Eating disorders *C.G. Fairburn*   1296
10.5   Obesity *J.S. Garrow*   1301
10.6   Special nutritional problems and the use of enteral and
       parenteral nutrition *M. Elia*   1314
10.7   Diseases of overnourished societies and the need for
       dietary change *J.I. Mann*   1326

Index

Volume 2

Preface

Contents

Contributors

Plates to Volume 2

Section 11   Metabolic disorders   1333

11.1   The inborn errors of metabolism: general aspects
       R.W.E. Watts   1335

11.2   Disorders of carbohydrate metabolism other than
       diabetes mellitus and hypoglycaemia   1339

   11.2.1   Glycogen storage diseases *T.M. Cox*   1339

   11.2.2   Inborn errors of fructose metabolism
       T.M. Cox   1345

   11.2.3   Disorders of galactose metabolism *T.M. Cox* 1349

11.3   Inborn errors of amino acid and organic acid
       metabolism *D.P. Brenton*   1352

11.4   Disorders of purine and pyrimidine metabolism
       G. Nuki   1376

11.5   Porphyrin metabolism and the porphyrias
       *K.E.L. McColl, S. Dover, E. Fitzsimons, and
       M.R. Moore*   1388

11.6   Lipid and lipoprotein disorders *P.N. Durrington*   1399

11.7   Trace metal disorders *C.A. Seymour*   1415

11.8   Lysosomal storage diseases *R.W.E. Watts*   1426

11.9   Peroxisomal disorders *R.B.H. Schutgens and
       R.J.A. Wanders*   1438

11.10   Disorders of oxalate metabolism *R.W.E. Watts*   1444

11.11   Diabetes mellitus *J.I. Bell and T.D.R. Hockaday*   1448

11.12   Hypoglycaemia *R.C. Turner*   1505

11.13   Amyloid, familial Mediterranean fever, and acute
        phase response   1512

   11.13.1   Amyloidosis *M.B. Pepys*   1512

   11.13.2   Recurrent polyserositis (familial
        Mediterranean fever, periodic disease)
        M. Eliakim   1525

   11.13.3   The acute phase response and C-reactive
        protein *M.B. Pepys*   1527

11.14   Disturbances of acid-base homeostasis *R.D. Cohen
        and H.F. Woods*   1533

11.15 α_1-Antitrypsin deficiency *R.W. Carrell and
        D.A. Lomas*   1545

11.16   Metabolic effects of accidental injury and surgery
        R. Smith   1548

Section 12   Endocrine disorders   1551

12.1   Principles of hormone action *J.L. Jameson*   1553

12.2   Anterior pituitary disorders *M.O. Thorner*   1573

12.3   The posterior pituitary *P.H. Baylis*   1599

12.4   The thyroid gland and disorders of thyroid function
       A.M. McGregor   1603

12.5   Thyroid cancer *M. Sheppard*   1618

12.6   Disorders of calcium metabolism *J.A. Kanis*   1622

12.7   The adrenal   1639

   12.7.1   Adrenocortical diseases *C.R.W. Edwards*   1639

   12.7.2   Congenital adrenal hyperplasia *I.A. Hughes*   1664

12.8   The reproductive system   1669

   12.8.1   The ovary *H.S. Jacobs*   1669

   12.8.2   Disorders of male reproduction *F.C.W. Wu*   1679

   12.8.3   The breast *H.S. Jacobs*   1687

12.9   Disorders of development   1689

   12.9.1   Normal and abnormal sexual differentiation
        M.O. Savage   1689

   12.9.2   Normal growth and its disorders *M.A. Preece*   1695

   12.9.3   Puberty *R.J.M. Ross and M.O. Savage*   1700

12.10   Non-diabetic pancreatic endocrine disorders and
        multiple endocrine neoplasia *P.J. Hammond and
        S.R. Bloom*   1703

12.11   Endocrine manifestations of non-endocrine disease
        J.A.H. Wass   1711

Section 13   Medical disorders in pregnancy   1721

13.1   Benefits and risks of oral contraceptives *M.P. Vessey*   1723

13.2   Hypertension in pregnancy *C.W.G. Redman*   1726

13.3   Renal disease in pregnancy *C.W.G. Redman and
       J.G.G. Ledingham*   1733

13.4   Heart disease in pregnancy *J.C. Forfar*   1735

13.5   Thromboembolism in pregnancy *M. de Swiet*   1741

13.6   Chest diseases in pregnancy *M. de Swiet*   1744

13.7   Endocrine disease in pregnancy *A.M. McGregor*   1747

13.8   Diabetes in pregnancy *M.D.G. Gillmer*   1752

13.9   Blood disorders in pregnancy *E.A. Letsky*   1758

13.10   Neurological disease in pregnancy *G.G. Lennox*   1766

13.11   Nutrition in pregnancy *D.M. Campbell*   1769

13.12   Infection in pregnancy   1775

   13.12.1   Viral infections in pregnancy *J.E. Banatvala*   1775

   13.12.2   Bacterial, fungal, and protozoal infections in
        pregnancy and the newborn *H.R. Gamsu*   1784

13.13   Liver and gastrointestinal disease in pregnancy
        E.A. Fagan   1796

13.14   The skin in pregnancy *F. Wojnarowska*   1804

13.15   Malignant disease in pregnancy *P.A. Philip and
        A.L. Harris*   1806

13.16   Prescribing in pregnancy *P.C. Rubin*   1809

13.17   Benefits and risks of hormone therapy *J.C. Stevenson*   1813

Section 14   Gastroenterology   1817

14.1   Introduction *D.P. Jewell*   1819

14.2   Symptomatology of gastrointestinal disease   1819

   14.2.1   Dysphagia and other symptoms in
        oesophageal disease *J. Dent*   1819

   14.2.2   Vomiting *D.P. Jewell*   1821

   14.2.3   Abdominal pain *D.P. Jewell*   1822

   14.2.4   Diarrhoea *L.A. Turnberg*   1823

14.2.5   Constipation *D.G. Thompson*   1825
14.2.6   Gastrointestinal bleeding *D.P. Jewell*   1827

14.3   Methods for investigation of gastrointestinal diseases   1829

14.3.1   Endoscopy *D.P. Jewell*   1829
14.3.2   Radiology *D.J. Nolan and E.W.L. Fletcher*   1830

14.4   Immune disorders of the gastrointestinal tract
M.R. Haeney   1836

14.5   The mouth and salivary glands *T. Lehner*   1846

14.6   Diseases of the oesophagus *J. Dent*   1865

14.7   Peptic ulceration *J.J. Misiewicz and R.E. Pounder*   1877

14.8   Hormones and the gastrointestinal tract
P.J. Hammond, S.R. Bloom, and J.M. Polak   1891

14.9   Malabsorption   1899

14.9.1   Mechanisms of intestinal absorption
J.R.F. Walters   1899
14.9.2   Investigation and differential diagnosis of
malabsorption *M.S. Losowsky*   1904
14.9.3   Small-bowel bacterial overgrowth *S. Pereira
and R.H. Dowling*   1911
14.9.4   Coeliac disease *D.P. Jewell*   1916
14.9.5   Disaccharidase deficiency *T.M. Cox*   1920
14.9.6   Whipple's disease *H.J.F. Hodgson*   1923
14.9.7   Short gut syndrome *H.J.F. Hodgson*   1925
14.9.8   Enteropathy-associated T-cell lymphoma
P.G. Isaacson   1927
14.9.9   Malabsorption in the tropics *M.J.G. Farthing*   1930

14.10   Crohn's disease *D.P. Jewell*   1936

14.11   Ulcerative colitis *D.P. Jewell*   1943

14.12   Disorders of motility *D.L. Wingate*   1951

14.13   Functional bowel disease and irritable bowel
syndrome *D.G. Thompson*   1965

14.14   Colonic diverticular disease *N.J.McC. Mortensen and
M. Kettlewell*   1969

14.15   Congenital abnormalities of the gastrointestinal tract
V.M. Wright and J.A. Walker-Smith   1972

14.16   Tumours of the gastrointestinal tract *M.L. Clark,
I.C. Talbot, and C.B. Williams*   1980

14.17   Vascular and collagen disorders *G. Neale*   1994

14.18   Gastrointestinal infections *C.P. Conlon*   2001

14.19   The peritoneum, omentum, and appendix *M. Irving*   2007

14.20   Computed tomography and magnetic resonance
imaging of the liver and pancreas *R. Dick*   2012

14.21   Congenital disorders of the biliary tract and pancreas
J.A. Summerfield   2014

14.22   Hereditary disease of the liver and pancreas
C.A. Seymour   2017

14.23   Diseases of the pancreas   2027

14.23.1   Acute pancreatitis *C.W. Imrie*   2027
14.23.2   Chronic pancreatitis *P.P. Toskes*   2034
14.23.3   Tumours of the pancreas *R.C.G. Russell*   2040

14.24   Diseases of the gallbladder and biliary tree
J.A. Summerfield   2045

14.25   Jaundice *E. Elias*   2054

14.26   Clinical features of viral hepatitis *H.C. Thomas*   2061

14.27   Autoimmune liver disease   2069

14.27.1   Autoimmune hepatitis *P.J. Johnson and
A.L.W.F. Eddleston*   2069

14.27.2   Primary biliary cirrhosis *M.F. Bassendine*   2074
14.27.3   Primary sclerosing cholangitis
R.W. Chapman   2077

14.28   Alcoholic liver disease *O.F.W. James*   2080

14.29   Cirrhosis, portal hypertension, and ascites *N. McIntyre
and A.K. Burroughs*   2085

14.30   Hepatocellular failure *E.A. Jones*   2100

14.31   Liver transplantation *R. Williams*   2111

14.32   Liver tumours *I.M. Murray-Lyon*   2115

14.33   Hepatic granulomas *G.M. Dusheiko*   2120

14.34   Drugs and liver damage *J. Neuberger*   2124

14.35   The liver in systemic disease *J. Neuberger*   2130

14.36   Miscellaneous disorders of the gastrointestinal tract
and liver *D.P. Jewell*   2136

Section 15   Cardiovascular disease   2141

15.1   Physiological considerations: biochemistry and
cellular physiology of heart muscle *P.A. Poole-Wilson
and P.H. Sugden*   2143

15.2   Clinical physiology of the normal heart
D.E.L. Wilcken   2152

15.3   Symptoms of cardiac disease   2162

15.3.1   Breathlessness *S.W. Davies and D. Lipkin*   2162
15.3.2   Chest pain *A.H. Henderson*   2165
15.3.3   Oedema *J.D. Firth and J.G.G. Ledingham*   2169
15.3.4   Fatigue *S.W. Davies and D. Lipkin*   2171
15.3.5   Syncope and palpitation *R. Sutton*   2173
15.3.6   Cardiac cachexia *W.L. Morrison*   2176

15.4   The clinical assessment of cardiovascular function   2177

15.4.1   Chest radiography in heart disease
M.B. Rubens   2177
15.4.2   The electrocardiogram *D.J. Rowlands*   2182
15.4.3   Doppler echocardiography *I.A. Simpson*   2200
15.4.4   Nuclear techniques *D.J. Rowlands and
H.J. Testa*   2204
15.4.5   Magnetic resonance and computed X-ray
tomography *S.R. Underwood and
P.F. Ludman*   2212
15.4.6   Cardiac catheterization *R.H. Swanton*   2220
15.4.7   Exercise testing *K. Dawkins*   2225

15.5   The syndrome of heart failure *A.J.S. Coats and
P.A. Poole-Wilson*   2228

15.6   The treatment of heart failure   2238

15.6.1   Diuretics *J.G.G. Ledingham and
A.E.G. Raine*   2238
15.6.2   Digitalis *D.A. Chamberlain*   2241
15.6.3   Vasodilators *J.H. Dargie*   2246
15.6.4   Catecholamines and the sympathetic nervous
system *J.C. Forfar*   2253

15.7   Cardiac transplantation *J.H. Dark*   2255

15.8   Cardiac arrhythmias   2259

15.8.1   Cardiac arrhythmias *S.M. Cobbe and
A.C. Rankin*   2259
15.8.2   Pacemakers *R. Sutton*   2285

15.9   Atheroma, the vessel wall, and thrombosis   2289

15.9.1   The pathogenesis of atherosclerosis *J. Scott*   2289
15.9.2   Vascular endothelium, its physiology and
pathophysiology *P. Vallance*   2295

15.9.3   Haemostatic variables in ischaemic heart
         disease *T.W. Meade*   2300
15.10 Ischaemic heart disease   2305
       15.10.1 Epidemiology and prevention *M.G. Marmot
                and J.I. Mann*   2305
       15.10.2 The pathophysiology of ischaemic heart
                disease *M.J. Davies*   2318
       15.10.3 Angina and unstable angina *R.H. Swanton*   2321
       15.10.4 Myocardial infarction *P. Sleight*   2331
       15.10.5 Coronary angioplasty *D.P. de Bono*   2349
       15.10.6 Coronary artery bypass grafting *T. Treasure*   2353
       15.10.7 Vocational aspects of coronary artery disease
                M. Joy   2356
15.11 Peripheral arterial disease *P.J. Morris*   2362
15.12 Cholesterol embolism *C.R.K. Dudley*   2375
15.13 Takayasu's disease *K. Ishikawa*   2377
15.14 The cardiomyopathies   2380
       15.14.1 The cardiomyopathies, myocarditis, and
                specific heart muscle disorders
                W.J. McKenna   2380
       15.14.2 HIV-related heart muscle disease *N.A. Boon*   2394
       15.14.3 The hypereosinophilic syndrome and the
                heart *C.J.F. Spry*   2396
15.15 Congenital heart disease in adolescents and adults
       J. Somerville   2398
15.16 The cardiac aspects of rheumatic fever *J.M. Neutze*   2432
15.17 Infective endocarditis *B. Gribbin and D.W.M. Crook*   2436
15.18 Valve disease *D.G. Gibson*   2451
15.19 Cardiac myxoma *T.A. Traill*   2472
15.20 Pericardial disease *D.G. Gibson*   2474
15.21 Cardiovascular syphilis *B. Gribbin and D.W.M. Crook*   2482
15.22 The pulmonary circulation in health and disease
       J.S. Prichard   2484
15.23 Pulmonary oedema *J.S. Prichard*   2495
15.24 pulmonary hypertension *J.S. Prichard*   2505
15.25 Cor pulmonale *J.S. Prichard*   2515
15.26 Pulmonary embolism *J.G.G. Ledingham and
       D.J. Weatherall*   2522
15.27 Essential hypertension *J.D. Swales*   2527
15.28 Secondary hypertension   2544
       15.28.1 Renal and renovascular hypertension
                A.E.G. Raine and J.G.G. Ledingham   2544
       15.28.2 Phaeochromocytoma *M. Brown*   2553
       15.28.3 Coarctation of the aorta as a cause of
                secondary hypertension in the adult
                N.A. Boon   2557
15.29 Lymphoedema *J.G.G. Ledingham*   2559

Section 16   Intensive care *R.D. Bradley and
D.F. Treacher*   2561

Section 17   Respiratory medicine *(Section
Editors J.M. Hopkin and D.J. Lane)*   2589

17.1   Introduction *J.M. Hopkin and D.J. Lane*   2591
17.2   Structure and function   2593

17.2.1   Functional anatomy of the lung *E.R. Weibel
         and C.R. Taylor*   2593
17.2.2   The upper respiratory tract *J.R. Stradling*   2609
17.3   Lung defences and responses   2612
       17.3.1   Non-immune defence mechanisms of the
                lung *C. Haslett*   2612
       17.3.2   Inflammation and the lung *C. Haslett*   2616
17.4   Pathophysiology of lung disease *P.D. Wagner*   2628
17.5   The clinical presentation of chest diseases *D.J. Lane*   2642
17.6   Investigation of respiratory disease   2652
       17.6.1   Thoracic imaging *D.M. Hansell*   2652
       17.6.2   Tests of ventilatory mechanics *N.B. Pride*   2666
       17.6.3   Microbiological methods in the diagnosis of
                respiratory infections *D.W.M. Crook and
                T.E.A. Peto*   2675
       17.6.4   Diagnostic bronchoscopy and tissue biopsy
                M.F. Muers   2678
       17.6.5   Histopathology and cytology in diagnosis of
                lung disease *M.S. Dunnill*   2685
17.7   Respiratory infection   2691
       17.7.1   Upper respiratory tract infection
                J.M. Hopkin   2691
       17.7.2   Acute lower respiratory tract infections
                J.T. Macfarlane   2692
       17.7.3   Suppurative pulmonary and pleural
                infections *J.M. Hopkin*   2704
       17.7.4   Chronic specific infections *J.M. Hopkin*   2707
       17.7.5   Respiratory infection in the
                immunosuppressed *J.M. Hopkin*   2708
17.8   The upper respiratory tract   2714
       17.8.1   Allergic rhinitis ('hay fever') *S.R. Durham*   2714
       17.8.2   Upper airways obstruction *J.R. Stradling*   2719
17.9   Airways disease   2724
       17.9.1   Asthma   2724
                (a) Basic mechanisms and pathophysiology
                    A.J. Frew and S.T. Holgate   2724
                (b) Clinical features and management
                    D.J. Lane   2729
                (c) Occupational asthma *A.J. Newman
                    Taylor*   2742
       17.9.2   Cystic fibrosis *D.J. Lane*   2746
       17.9.3   Bronchiectasis *R.A. Stockley*   2755
       17.9.4   Chronic obstructive pulmonary disease
                N.B. Pride and R.A. Stockley   2766
17.10 Diffuse parenchymal lung disease   2779
       17.10.1 Introduction *R.M. du Bois*   2779
       17.10.2 Cryptogenic fibrosing alveolitis
                R.M. du Bois   2786
       17.10.3 Bronchiolitis obliterans *J.M. Hopkin*   2795
       17.10.4 The lung in collagen-vascular diseases
                R.A. Shaw   2796
       17.10.5 Pulmonary vasculitis and granulomatosis
                D.J. Lane and J.M. Hopkin   2800
       17.10.6 Pulmonary haemorrhagic disorders
                D.J. Lane   2803
       17.10.7 Pulmonary eosinophilia *D.J. Lane*   2804
       17.10.8 Lymphocytic infiltrations of the lung
                D.J. Hendrick   2806

17.10.9   Extrinsic allergic alveolitis *D.J. Hendrick*   2809
17.10.10   Sarcoidosis *P.R. Studdy*   2817
17.10.11   Pulmonary histiocytosis X (eosinophilic granuloma of the lung) and lymphangiomatosis *R.J. Shaw*   2832
17.10.12   Pulmonary alveolar proteinosis *D.J. Hendrick*   2833
17.10.13   Pulmonary amyloidosis *D.J. Hendrick*   2835
17.10.14   Lipoid (lipid) pneumonia *D.J. Hendrick*   2837
17.10.15   Pulmonary alveolar microlithiasis *D.J. Hendrick*   2838
17.10.16   Pneumoconioses *A. Seaton*   2839
17.10.17   Toxic gases and fumes *J.M. Hopkin*   2847
17.10.18   Radiation pneumonitis *J.M. Hopkin*   2848
17.10.19   Drug-induced lung disease *G.J. Gibson*   2848
17.10.20   Adult respiratory distress syndrome *C. Garrard and P. Foëx*   2852
17.10.21   Lung disorders in genetic syndromes *R.A. Shaw and D.J. Hendrick*   2861
17.11   Pleural disease *M.K. Benson*   2863
17.12   Disorders of the thoracic cage and diaphragm *J.M. Shneerson*   2872

17.13   Neoplastic disorders   2879
17.13.1   Tumours of the lung   2879
           (a) Lung cancer *S.G. Spiro*   2879
           (b) Pulmonary metastases *S.G. Spiro*   2893
17.13.2   Pleural tumours *M.K. Benson*   2893
17.13.3   Mediastinal tumours and cysts *M.K. Benson*   2895
17.14   Respiratory failure   2901
17.14.1   Definition and causes *J. Moxham*   2901
17.14.2   Sleep-related disorders of breathing *J.R. Stradling*   2906
17.14.3   The management of respiratory failure   2918
           (a) Acute respiratory failure: intensive care *C. Garrard*   2918
           (b) Chronic respiratory failure *J. Moxham*   2925
17.14.4   Lung and heart-lung transplantation *T.W. Higenbottam*   2933

Index

Volume 3

Preface

Contents

Contributors

Plates to Volume 3

Section 18   Rheumatology (*Section Editor P. Dieppe*)   2941

18.1   Introduction *P. Dieppe*   2943
18.2   Clinical presentation and diagnosis *P.T. Dawes*   2944
18.3   Use and abuse of investigations *P. Creamer and P. Dieppe*   2947
18.4   Rheumatoid arthritis *B.P. Wordsworth*   2953
18.5   Seronegative spondarthropathies *C.J. Eastmond*   2965
18.6   Osteoarthritis *C.W. Hutton*   2975
18.7   Crystal-related arthropathies *M. Doherty*   2983
18.8   Back pain and periarticular disease *I. Haslock*   2992
18.9   Septic arthritis *M.H. Seifert*   2998
18.10 Miscellaneous conditions *B. Hazleman*   3003
18.11 Connective tissue disorders and vasculitis   3008

        18.11.1   Introduction *C.M. Black and D.G.I. Scott*   3008
        18.11.2   Small-vessel vasculitis *C.M. Lockwood*   3010
        18.11.3   Systemic lupus erythematosus and related disorders *M.L. Snaith and D.A. Isenberg*   3017
        18.11.4   Systemic sclerosis *C.M. Black*   3027
        18.11.5   Sjögren's syndrome *P.J.W. Venables*   3036
        18.11.6   Polymyositis and dermatomyositis *J. Walton*   3038
        18.11.7   Polymyalgia rheumatica and giant-cell arteritis *A.G. Mowat*   3039
        18.11.8   Behçet's disease *T. Lehner*   3043
        18.11.9   Kawasaki disease *Tomisaku Kawasaki*   3047
        18.11.10 Cryoglobulinaemia *S.A. Misbah*   3050

Section 19   Disorders of the skeleton *R. Smith*   3053

Section 20   Nephrology   3099

20.1   Clinical physiology of the kidney: tests of renal function and structure *K.M. Bannister and M.F. Field*   3101
20.2   Water and electrolyte metabolism   3116

        20.2.1   Water and sodium homeostasis and their disorders *P.H. Baylis*   3116
        20.2.2   Idiopathic oedema of women *J.G.G. Ledingham*   3126
        20.2.3   Disorders of potassium metabolism *J.G.G. Ledingham*   3127

20.3   Common presentations of renal disease *J.S. Cameron*   3136
20.4   Primary renal glomerular diseases   3149

        20.4.1   IgA nephropathy, Henoch-Schönlein purpura, and thin membrane nephropathy *A.R. Clarkson, A.J. Woodroffe, and A.C. Thomas*   3149

        20.4.2   Idiopathic glomerulonephritis *D. Adu*   3153
        20.4.3   Rapidly progressive glomerulonephritis and antiglomerular basement membrane disease *C.D. Pusey and A.J. Rees*   3162
20.5   Renal manifestations of systemic disease   3167

        20.5.1   Diabetic nephropathy *E. Ritz, D. Fliser, and M. Siebels*   3167
        20.5.2   Infections and associated nephropathies *D.G. Williams and D. Adu*   3173
        20.5.3   Amyloid, myeloma, light chain deposition disease, fibrillary glomerulonephritis, and cryoglobulinaemia *J.-P. Grünfeld*   3179
        20.5.4   Renal manifestations of malignant disease *A.M. Davison*   3183
        20.5.5   Sarcoidosis and the kidney *A.M. Davison*   3186
        20.5.6   Rheumatological disorders and the kidney: systemic lupus erythematosus, mixed connective tissue disease, scleroderma, Sjögren's syndrome, and rheumatoid arthritis *J.S. Cameron and D.G. Williams*   3187
        20.5.7   Sickle-cell disease *G.R. Serjeant*   3194
20.6   Haemolytic uraemic syndrome *G.H. Neild*   3196
20.7   Clinical aspects of inherited renal disorders *J.-P. Grünfeld*   3202
20.8   Urinary tract infection, pyelonephritis, reflux nephropathy, and papillary necrosis   3205

        20.8.1   Urinary tract infection *R.R. Bailey*   3205
        20.8.2   Vesicoureteric reflux and reflux nephropathy *R.R. Bailey*   3214
20.9   Other interstitial nephritides   3221

        20.9.1   Kidney disease from analgesics and non-steroidal anti-inflammatory drugs *J.H. Stewart*   3221
        20.9.2   Gout, purines, and interstitial nephritis *J.S. Cameron and H.A. Simmonds*   3224
        20.9.3   Hypercalcaemic nephropathy *R.W.E. Watts*   3227
        20.9.4   Balkan (endemic) nephropathy and irradiation nephritis *A.W. Asscher*   3229
20.10 Urinary-tract obstruction *L.R.I. Baker*   3232
20.11 Hypertension: its effects on the kidney *A.E.G. Raine*   3247
20.12 Urinary stone disease (urolithiasis) *R.W.E. Watts*   3251
20.13 Toxic nephropathy *B.T. Emmerson*   3258
20.14 Drugs and the kidney *D.J.S. Carmichael*   3268
20.15 Genitourinary tuberculosis *L.R.I. Baker*   3275
20.16 Acute renal failure *J.D. Firth and C.G. Winearls*   3279
20.17 Chronic renal failure and its treatment   3294

        20.17.1 Chronic renal failure *A.M. El Nahas and C.G. Winearls*   3294
        20.17.2 Replacement therapy by dialysis *R. Gokal*   3306
        20.17.3 Renal transplantation *P.J. Ratcliffe and D.W.R. Gray*   3313
20.18 Renal bone disease *J.A. Kanis*   3322
20.19 Renal tubular disorders *J. Cunningham*   3330

        20.19.1 The renal tubular acidoses *R.D. Cohen*   3338

Section 21 Sexually-transmitted diseases and sexual health (*Section Editor M.W. Adler*) 3343

21.1   Sexually-transmitted diseases and sexual health *M.W. Adler and A. Meheus* 3345
21.2   Sexual behaviour *A.M. Johnson* 3349
21.3   Genital herpes *A. Mindel* 3351
21.4   Vaginal discharge *J. Schwebke and S.L. Hillier* 3353
21.5   Pelvic inflammatory disease *L. Weström* 3357
21.6   Infections and other medical problems in homosexual men *A. McMillan* 3360
21.7   Genital warts *J.D. Oriel* 3366
21.8   Cervical cancer and other cancers caused by sexually transmitted infections *V. Beral* 3369

Section 22 Disorders of the blood 3373

22.1   Introduction *D.J. Weatherall* 3375
22.2   Haemopoietic stem cells 3381

22.2.1   Stem cells and haematopoiesis *C.A. Sieff and D.G. Nathan* 3381
22.2.2   Stem-cell disorders *D.C. Linch* 3390

22.3   The leukaemias and other disorders of haemopoietic stem cells 3393

22.3.1   Cell and molecular biology of leukaemia *M.F. Greaves* 3393
22.3.2   The classification of leukaemias *D. Catovsky* 3399
22.3.3   Acute myeloblastic leukaemia *A.J. Barrett* 3404
22.3.4   Acute lymphoblastic leukaemia *I.A.G. Roberts* 3410
22.3.5   Chronic myeloid leukaemia *J. Goldman* 3415
22.3.6   Chronic lymphocytic leukaemia and other leukaemias of mature B and T cells *D. Catovsky* 3419
22.3.7   Myelodysplastic syndromes *D. Catovsky* 3425
22.3.8   Polycythaemia vera *D.J. Weatherall* 3431
22.3.9   Myelosclerosis *D.J. Weatherall* 3434
22.3.10 Primary thrombocythaemia *D.J. Weatherall* 3439
22.3.11 Aplastic anaemia and other causes of bone marrow failure *E.C. Gordon-Smith* 3441
22.3.12 Paroxysmal nocturnal haemoglobinuria *J.V. Dacie and L. Luzzatto* 3449

22.4   The red cell 3452

22.4.1   Erythropoiesis and the normal red cell *D.J. Weatherall* 3452
22.4.2   Anaemia: pathophysiology, classification, and clinical features *D.J. Weatherall* 3457
22.4.3   Anaemia as a world health problem *A.F. Fleming* 3462
22.4.4   Iron metabolism and its disorders *M.J. Pippard* 3470
22.4.5   Normochromic, normocytic anaemia *D.J. Weatherall* 3482
22.4.6   Megaloblastic anaemia and miscellaneous deficiency anaemias *A.V. Hoffbrand* 3484
22.4.7   Disorders of the synthesis or function of haemoglobin *D.J. Weatherall* 3500
22.4.8   Other anaemias resulting from defective red cell maturation *D.J. Weatherall* 3521

22.4.9   Haemolytic anaemia: the mechanisms and consequences of a shortened red cell survival *D.J. Weatherall* 3524
22.4.10 Genetic disorders of the red-cell membrane *S.W. Eber and S.E. Lux* 3527
22.4.11 Haemolysis due to red-cell enzyme deficiencies *E.C. Gordon-Smith and D.J. Weatherall* 3533
22.4.12 Glucose 6-phosphate dehydrogenase (G6PD) deficiency *L. Luzzatto* 3537
22.4.13 Acquired haemolytic anaemia *E.C. Gordon-Smith and M. Contreras* 3541
22.4.14 The relative and secondary polycythaemias *D.J. Weatherall* 3551

22.5   The white cells and lymphoproliferative disorders 3555

22.5.1   Leucocytes in health and disease *A.J. Thrasher and A.W. Segal* 3555
22.5.2   Introduction to the lymphoproliferative disorders *C. Bunch and K.C. Gatter* 3561
22.5.3   The lymphomas *C. Bunch and K.C. Gatter* 3568
22.5.4   The spleen and its disorders *S.M. Lewis and D. Swirsky* 3587
22.5.5   Myeloma and other paraproteinaemias *F.J. Giles and B.G.M. Durie* 3597
22.5.6   The histiocytoses *V. Broadbent and J. Pritchard* 3606
22.5.7   The hypereosinophilic syndrome *C.J.F. Spry* 3610

22.6   Haemostasis and thrombosis 3613

22.6.1   The biology of haemostasis and thrombosis *I.J. Mackie* 3613
22.6.2   Introduction to disorders of haemostasis and coagulation *S.J. Machin and I.J. Mackie* 3627
22.6.3   Purpura *S.J. Machin* 3630
22.6.4   The pathogenesis of genetic disorders of coagulation *I. Peake* 3637
22.6.5   Clinical features and management of hereditary disorders of haemostasis *G.F. Savidge* 3642
22.6.6   Acquired coagulation disorders *B.J. Hunt* 3653
22.6.7   Thrombotic disease *M. Greaves and D.A. Taberner* 3661

22.7   The blood in systemic disease *D.J. Weatherall* 3676
22.8   Blood replacement 3687

22.8.1   Blood transfusion *H.H. Gunson and V.J. Martlew* 3687
22.8.2   Marrow transplantation *C. Bunch* 3696

Section 23 Diseases of the skin *T.J. Ryan* 3703

Section 24 Neurology 3813

24.1   Introduction *J. Newsom-Davis and M. Donaghy* 3815
24.2   Investigation 3816

24.2.1   Principles of neuroradiology *I. Isherwood and A. Jackson* 3816
24.2.2   Electroencephalography *B.B. MacGillivray* 3829
24.2.3   Evoked potentials *A.M. Halliday* 3831

24.2.4 Investigation of central motor pathways: magnetic brain stimulation *K.R. Mills* 3836

24.2.5 Electrophysiological investigation of the peripheral nervous system *J. Payan* 3839

24.2.6 Lumbar puncture *R.A. Fishman* 3842

24.3 Organization and features of dysfunction 3845

24.3.1 Disturbances of higher cerebral function *J.M. Oxbury and S.M. Oxbury* 3845

24.3.2 The motor and sensory systems, midbrain, and brain-stem *W.B. Matthews* 3856

24.3.3 Subcortical structures—the cerebellum, thalamus, and basal ganglia *N.P. Quinn* 3859

24.3.4 Visual pathways *R.W. Ross Russell* 3863

24.3.5 The eighth cranial nerve *P. Rudge* 3869

24.3.6 Other cranial nerves *P.K. Thomas* 3876

24.3.7 The autonomic nervous system *R. Bannister* 3881

24.3.8 Respiratory problems in neurological disease *J. Newsom-Davis* 3887

24.3.9 Spinal cord *W.B. Matthews* 3891

24.3.10 Spinal cord injury and the management of paraplegia *D.J. Grundy* 3895

24.3.11 Disorders of the spinal nerve roots *R.S. Maurice-Williams* 3902

24.4 Disorders of consciousness 3909

24.4.1 Epilepsy in later childhood and adult life *A.P. Hopkins* 3909

24.4.2 Syncope *L.D. Blumhardt* 3925

24.4.3 Narcolepsy and related sleep disorders *C.D. Marsden* 3927

24.4.4 Coma *M.J.G. Harrison* 3930

24.4.5 Brain death and the vegetative state *B. Jennett* 3933

24.5 Pain: pathophysiology and treatment *J.W. Scadding* 3936

24.6 Cerebrovascular disease *C.P. Warlow* 3946

24.7 Dementia 3965

24.7.1 Introduction *J.R. Hodges* 3965

24.7.2 Alzheimer's disease *M.N. Rossor* 3971

24.7.3 Pick's disease (focal lobar atrophy) *J.R. Hodges* 3974

24.7.4 Prion diseases *J. Collinge* 3977

24.7.5 Kuru *M.P. Alpers* 3981

24.8 Inherited disorders *P.K. Thomas* 3984

24.9 Demyelinating disorders of the central nervous system *D.A.S. Compston* 3989

24.10 Movement disorders *C.D. Marsden* 3998

24.11 Headache *J.M.S. Pearce* 4022

24.12 Intracranial tumours *P.J. Teddy* 4029

24.13 Benign intracranial hypertension *N.F. Lawton* 4040

24.14 Head injuries *G.M. Teasdale* 4044

24.15 Clinical presentation of infections of the nervous system 4050

24.15.1 Bacterial meningitis *D.W.M. Crook, Prida Phuapradit, and D.A. Warrell* 4050

24.15.2 Viral infections of the central nervous system *D.A. Warrell and P.G.E. Kennedy* 4064

24.15.3 Neurological manifestations of infection with human immunodeficiency virus type 1 *R.K.H. Petty and P.G.E. Kennedy* 4075

24.15.4 Intracranial abscess *P.J. Teddy* 4081

24.15.5 Neurosyphilis *R.J. Greenwood* 4083

24.16 The motor neurone diseases *M. Donaghy* 4087

24.17 Peripheral neuropathy *P.K. Thomas* 4091

24.17.1 The POEMS syndrome *J.G.G. Ledingham* 4104

24.18 Developmental abnormalities of the nervous system *D. Gardner-Medwin* 4105

24.19 Metabolic and deficiency disorders of the nervous system *C.D. Marsden* 4123

24.20 Neurological disorders due to physical agents *C.D. Marsden* 4128

24.21 Neurological complications of systemic diseases *M.J.G. Harrison* 4129

Section 25 Disorders of voluntary muscles 4137

25.1 Introduction *J. Walton* 4139

25.2 The muscular dystrophies *J. Walton* 4145

25.3 The floppy infant syndrome *J. Walton* 4150

25.4 Myotonic disorders *J. Walton* 4151

25.5 Inflammatory myopathies *J. Walton* 4154

25.6 Miscellaneous disorders *J. Walton* 4159

25.7 Disorders of neuromuscular transmission *J. Newsom-Davis* 4160

25.8 Metabolic and endocrine myopathies *D. Hilton-Jones* 4165

25.9 Mitochondrial myopathies and encephalomyopathies *A.E. Harding* 4171

25.10 Tropical pyomyositis (tropical myositis) *D.A. Warrell* 4174

Section 26 The eye in general medicine
P. Frith

4177

Section 27 Psychiatry in medicine (Section Editor M.G. Gelder)

4201

27.1 Introduction *M.G. Gelder* 4203

27.2 Psychiatric disorders as they concern the physician 4204

27.2.1 Reactions to stressful events *M.G. Gelder* 4204

27.2.2 Anxiety and obsessional disorders *M.G. Gelder* 4205

27.2.3 Psychiatric conditions with physical complaints *M.G. Gelder* 4208

27.2.4 Dissociative disorder *M.G. Gelder* 4209

27.2.5 Malingering and factitious disorders *M.G. Gelder* 4211

27.2.6 Personality and its disorders *M.G. Gelder* 4211

27.2.7 Eating disorders *C.G. Fairburn* 4212

27.2.8 Affective disorders *D.H. Gath* 4218

27.2.9 Schizophrenia *M.G. Gelder* 4221

27.2.10 Organic (cognitive) mental disorders *R.A. Mayou* 4223

27.2.11 Mental disorders of old age *R.J. Jacoby* 4228

27.2.12 The patient who has attempted suicide *H.G. Morgan* 4228

27.3 The relationship between psychiatric disorders and physical illness 4231

27.3.1   Complications of drug use, particularly
         injecting drug use *C. Bass*   4231
27.3.2   Emotional reactions in the dying and the
         bereaved *R.A. Mayou*   4233
27.3.3   Specific conditions giving rise to mental
         disorder *W.A. Lishman*   4236
27.3.4   Sexual problems associated with physical
         illness *K.E. Hawton*   4243

27.4   Aspects of treatment   4247

27.4.1   Psychopharmacology in medical practice
         P.J. Cowen   4247
27.4.2   Psychological treatment in medical practice
         M.G. Gelder   4254
27.4.3   Psychiatric emergencies *R.A. Mayou*   4256

Section 28   Alcohol and drug-related problems
(Section Editors J. Strang, I.B. Crome, and
M. Farrell)   4261

28.1   Assessment and diagnosis   4263

28.1.1   Drug problems as every doctor's business
         G. Edwards   4263
28.1.2   Assessing substance use and misuse *M. Farrell,*
         I.B. Crome, and J. Strang   4265
28.1.3   Diagnoses and classifications: substance
         problems and dependence—what is the
         difference? *I.B. Crome*   4267

28.2   Brief interventions for prevention   4270

28.2.1   Screening and brief intervention *P.D. Anderson* 4270
28.2.2   Harm reduction *J. Strang and M. Farrell*   4275
28.2.3   Physical complications   4276
         (a) Physical complications of alcohol misuse
             T.J. Peters   4276
         (b) Physical complications of drug misuse
             D.A. Hawkins   4278

28.3   Problems and crises for the clinician   4281

28.3.1   Complications of drug use, particularly
         injecting drug use *R.P. Brettle*   4281
28.3.2   The management of substance-related problems
         in a general ward *M. Farrell, I.B. Crome, and*
         J. Strang   4286
28.3.3   Drugs and the law *J. Strang*   4288
28.3.4   Management of withdrawal syndromes
         A.R. Johns   4290
28.3.5   Drug misusers and addicts in accident and
         emergency *A.H. Ghodse and G.S. Tregenza*   4294
28.3.6   The pregnant drug abuser *C. Gerada*   4297
28.3.7   Management of pain in the drug abuser
         A.C. de C. Williams and M. Gossop   4300
28.3.8   Caring for the HIV-positive drug user *J. Strang*
         and M. Farrell   4302
28.3.9   The needs of the alcohol/drug user in custody
         A. Maden   4304

Section 29   Forensic medicine *B. Knight*   4307

Section 30   Sports medicine *A. Young*   4319

Section 31   Medicine in old age *F.I. Caird and*
J. Grimley Evans   4331

Section 32   Terminal illness *M.J. Baines*   4347

Section 33   Reference intervals for biochemical
data *A.M. Giles and P. Holloway*   4361

Index

Contributors

P. AABY
Senior Researcher, Statens Seruminstitut, Copenhagen, Denmark
7.10.2 Measles

J.P. ACKERS
Senior Lecturer, Department of Medical Parasitology, London School of Hygiene and Tropical Medicine, London, UK
7.13.13 Trichomoniasis

A.A. ADISH
% McGill Community Health Project, Addis Ababa, Ethiopia
8.5.5(h) Podoconiosis (non-filarial endemic elephantiasis of the lower legs)

M.W. ADLER
Professor of Genito-Urinary Medicine, Academic Department of Genito-Urinary Medicine, University College London Medical School, UK
21.1 Sexually transmitted diseases and sexual health

D. ADU
Consultant Nephrologist, Queen Elizabeth Hospital, Birmingham, UK
20.4.2 Idiopathic glomerulonephritis
20.5.2 Infections and associated nephropathies

M.P. ALPERS
Director, Papua New Guinea Institute of Medical Research, Goroka, Papua New Guinea
24.7.5 Kuru

P.D. ANDERSON
Consultant, World Health Organization Regional Office for Europe, Copenhagen, Denmark
28.2.1 Alcohol and drug-related problems: screening and brief intervention

H. ANNETT
Head, Health Department, Secretariat de Son Altesse l'Aga Khan, Aiglemont, Gouvieux, France
3.4 Health care in developing countries

J.K. ARONSON
Clinical Reader in Clinical Pharmacology, University of Oxford; Honorary Consultant Physician, Anglia and Oxfordshire Health Authority, Oxford, UK
9 Principles of clinical pharmacology and drug therapy

A.W. ASSCHER
Principal, St George's Hospital Medical School, University of London, UK
20.9.4 Balkan (endemic) nephropathy and irradiation nephritis

TAR-CHING AW
Senior Lecturer in Occupational Medicine, Institute of Occupational Health, University of Birmingham, UK
8.3.6 Poisoning from metals
8.5.5(k) Environmental factors and disease: vibration

J.G. AYRES
Consultant Respiratory Physician, Heartlands Hospital, Birmingham, UK
8.5.5(l) Environmental factors and disease: air pollution

R.R. BAILEY
Nephrologist, Christchurch Hospital, New Zealand
20.8.1 Urinary tract infection
20.8.2 Vesicoureteric reflux and reflux nephropathy

M.J. BAINES
Consultant Physician, St Christopher's Hospice, London, UK
32 Terminal illness

E.L. BAKER
Centers for Disease Control and Prevention, Atlanta, Georgia, USA
8.5.3(d) The main occupational diseases: neurological disorders

L.R.I. BAKER
Consultant Physician and Nephrologist, St Bartholomew's Hospital, London, UK
20.10 Urinary-tract obstruction
20.15 Genitourinary tuberculosis

J.E. BANATVALA
Professor of Clinical Virology, United Medical and Dental Schools of Guy's and St Thomas's Hospital, St Thomas's Campus, London, UK
13.12.1 Viral infections in pregnancy

C.R.M. BANGHAM
Consultant Virologist, John Radcliffe Hospital, Oxford, UK
7.10.31 HTLV-I and -II associated diseases

SIR ROGER BANNISTER
Honorary Consultant Neurologist, The National Hospital for Neurology and Neurosurgery, London, and Oxford Regional and District Health Authority, UK
24.3.7 The autonomic nervous system

K.M. BANNISTER
Senior Consultant, Renal Unit and Department of Nuclear Medicine, Royal Adelaide Hospital, South Australia
20.1 Clinical physiology of the kidney: tests of renal function and structure

D. BARLOW
Consultant Physician, Department of Genitourinary Medicine, St Thomas's Hospital, London, UK
7.11.6 Neisseria gonorrhoeae

A.J. BARRETT
Chief, Bone Marrow Transplant Unit, National Heart, Lung, and Blood Institute, National Institutes of Health, Bethesda, Maryland, USA
22.3.3 Acute myeloblastic leukaemia

C. BASS

Consultant in Liaison Psychiatry, John Radcliffe Hospital, Oxford, UK
27.3.1 Psychological factors and the presentation and course of illness

M.F. BASSENDINE

Professor of Hepatology, Department of Medicine, The Medical School, University of Newcastle; Consultant Physician, Freeman Hospital, Newcastle upon Tyne, UK
14.27.2 Primary biliary cirrhosis

P.J. BAXTER

Consultant Occupational Physician, University of Cambridge and Addenbrooke's Hospital, Cambridge, UK
8.5.5(m) Environmental factors and disease: environmental disasters

M.A.H. BAYLES

Senior Specialist and Senior Lecturer, Department of Dermatology, King Edward VIII Hospital and Medical School, University of Natal, Durban, South Africa
7.12.3 Chromoblastomycosis

P.H. BAYLIS

Professor of Experimental Medicine, University of Newcastle upon Tyne; Consultant Physician, Royal Victoria Infirmary, Newcastle upon Tyne, UK
12.3 The posterior pituitary
20.2.1 Water and sodium homeostasis and their disorders

J.I. BELL

Nuffield Professor of Clinical Medicine, John Radcliffe Hospital, University of Oxford; Consultant Physician in General Medicine, Oxford Radcliffe NHS Trust, UK
5.2 Immune mechanisms of disease
11.11 Diabetes mellitus

E.J. BELL*

Regional Virus Laboratory, Ruchill Hospital, Glasgow, UK
7.10.13 Enteroviruses

M.K. BENSON

Consultant Chest Physician, Osler Chest Unit, The Churchill Hospital, Oxford, UK
17.11 Pleural disease
17.13.2 Pleural tumours
17.13.3 Mediastinal tumours and cysts

V. BERAL

Director, Imperial Cancer Research Fund's Cancer Epidemiology Unit, Oxford, UK
21.8 Cervical cancer and other cancers caused by sexually transmitted infections

R.J. BERRY

Director, Westlakes Research Institute, Moor Row, Cumbria, UK
8.5.5(i) Environmental factors and disease: radiation

---

* It is with regret that we report the deaths of those authors marked with an asterisk. Although their deaths occurred between the appearance of the second edition and preparation of the third edition, much of their contribution to the former has been incorporated into this edition, with appropriate updating from their coauthors.

P.C.L. BEVERLEY

Professor of Tumour Immunology and Staff Member of the Imperial Cancer Research Fund, University College London Medical School, UK
6.4 Tumour immunology

C.M. BLACK

Professor of Rheumatology, Royal Free Hospital and School of Medicine, University of London, UK
18.11.1 Connective tissue disorders and vasculitis—introduction
18.11.4 Systemic sclerosis

S.R. BLOOM

Professor of Endocrinology, Royal Postgraduate Medical School, Hammersmith Hospital, London, UK
12.10 Non-diabetic pancreatic endocrine disorders and multiple endocrine neoplasia
14.8 Hormones and the gastrointestinal tract

L.D. BLUMHARDT

Professor of Clinical Neurology, University of Nottingham; Consultant Neurologist, University Hospital, Queen's Medical Centre, Nottingham, UK
24.4.2 Syncope

N.A. BOON

Consultant Cardiologist, Royal Infirmary of Edinburgh, UK
15.14.2 HIV-related heart muscle disease
15.28.3 Coarctation of the aorta as a cause of secondary hypertension in the adult

R.T. BOOTH

Professor of Safety and Health, Health and Safety Unit, Aston University, Birmingham, UK
8.5.4 Occupational safety

I.C.G. BOWLER

Consultant Microbiologist, Oxford Regional Public Health Laboratory, John Radcliffe Hospital, Oxford, UK
7.9 Nosocomial infection

D. BRADLEY

Professor of Tropical Hygiene, London School of Hygiene and Tropical Medicine, University of London, UK
7.13.2 Malaria

R.D. BRADLEY

Emeritus Professor of Intensive Care Medicine, St Thomas's Hospital, London, UK
16 Intensive care

D.P. BRENTON

Reader in Inherited Metabolic Diseases, Department of Medicine, University of College London School of Medicine, UK
11.3 Inborn errors of amino acid and organic acid metabolism

R.P. BRETTLE

Consultant Physician and Part-time Senior Lecturer, Regional Infectious Disease Unit, City Hospital, Edinburgh, UK
28.3.1 Complications of drug use, particularly injecting drug use

V. BROADBENT
Consultant Paediatric Oncologist, Addenbrooke's Hospital, Cambridge, UK
22.5.6 The histiocytoses

M. BROWN
Professor of Clinical Pharmacology, University of Cambridge; Honorary Consultant Physician, Addenbrooke's Hospital, Cambridge, UK
15.28.2 Phaeochromocytoma

A.D.M. BRYCESON
Consultant Physician, Hospital for Tropical Diseases, London
7.13.12 Leishmaniasis

C. BUNCH
Medical Director, Oxford Radcliffe Hospital NHS Trust, John Radcliffe Hospital, Oxford, UK
22.5.2 Introduction to the lymphoproliferative disorders
22.5.3 The lymphomas
22.8.2 Marrow transplantation

DANAI BUNNAG
Professor Emeritus, Clinical Tropical Medicine, Mahidol University, Bangkok, Thailand
7.16.2 Liver fluke diseases of humans

W. BURGDORFER
Scientist Emeritus, Laboratory of Vectors and Pathogens, National Institutes of Health, Rocky Mountain Laboratories, Hamilton, Montana, USA
7.11.30 Lyme disease

A.K. BURROUGHS
Consultant Physician and Hepatologist, Liver Transplantation and Hepato-biliary Medicine, Royal Free Hospital, London, UK
14.29 Cirrhosis, portal hypertension, and ascites

T. BUTLER
Professor of Internal Medicine and of Microbiology and Immunology, Texas Technical University, Health Sciences Center; Attending Physician, University Medical Center, Lubbock, USA
7.11.6 Plague

A.E. BUTTERWORTH
Medical Research Council External Scientific Staff and Honorary Professor of Medical Parasitology, Department of Pathology, University of Cambridge, UK
7.16.1 Schistosomiasis

F.I. CAIRD
Formerly David Cargill Professor of Geriatric Medicine, University of Glasgow, UK
31 Medicine in old age

J.S. CAMERON
Professor of Renal Medicine, United Medical and Dental Schools, Guy's Campus, London, UK
20.3 Common presentations of renal disease
20.5.6 Rheumatological disorders and the kidney
20.9.2 Gout, purines, and interstitial nephritis

D.M. CAMPBELL
Senior Lecturer in Obstetrics and Gynaecology and Reproductive Physiology, University of Aberdeen, UK
13.11 Nutrition in pregnancy

M.J. CARDOSA
Lecturer, School of Pharmaceutical Sciences, Universiti Sains Malaysia, Penang, Malaysia
7.10.20 Dengue haemorrhagic fever

D.J.S. CARMICHAEL
Consultant Nephrologist, Southend Health Care NHS Trust, Essex, UK
20.14 Drugs and the kidney

J. CARMICHAEL
J.B. Cochrane Professor of Clinical Oncology, University of Nottingham, UK
6.8. New approaches to cancer therapy

C.C.J. CARPENTER
Professor of Medicine, Brown University, Providence, Rhode Island, USA
7.11.11 Cholera

R.W. CARRELL
Professor of Haematology, University of Cambridge, Addenbrooke's Hospital, Cambridge, UK
11.15 α_1-Antitrypsin deficiency

D.P. CASEMORE
Clinical Scientist, PHLS Cryptosporidium Reference Unit, Glan Clwyd District General Hospital, Bodelwyddan, Clwyd, UK
7.13.5 Cryptosporidium and cryptosporidiosis
7.13.6 Cyclospora

A. CASSELS
Independent Health Systems Development Consultant, Chilham, Canterbury, Kent, UK
3.4 Health care in developing countries

D. CATOVSKY
Professor of Haematology, Institute of Cancer Research and Royal Marsden Hospital, London, UK
22.3.2 The classification of leukaemia
22.3.6 Chronic lymphocytic leukaemia and other leukaemias of mature B and T cells
22.3.7 Myelodysplastic syndromes

D.A. CHAMBERLAIN
Consultant Cardiologist, Royal Sussex County Hospital, Brighton: Senior Visiting Research Fellow, University of Sussex, UK
15.6.2 Digitalis

H.M. CHAPEL
Consultant Immunologist and Senior Clinical Lecturer, John Radcliffe Hospital, Oxford, UK
5.4 Complement and disease

L.E. CHAPMAN

Supervising Medical Epidemiologist, Division of Viral and Rickettsial Diseases, National Center for Infectious Diseases, Center for Disease Control, Atlanta, Georgia, USA
7.10.5 Human infections caused by simian herpesviruses

R.W. CHAPMAN

Consultant Gastroenterologist, John Radcliffe Hospital, Oxford, UK
14.27.3 Primary sclerosing cholangitis

SEUNG-YULL CHO

Professor of Parasitology, College of Medicine, Chung-Ang University, Seoul, Korea
7.15.4 Diphyllobothriasis and sparganosis

A.B. CHRISTIE*

Honorary Consultant, Fazakerley Hospital, Liverpool, UK
7.10.11 Mumps: epidemic parotitis
7.11.1 Diphtheria
7.11.18 Anthrax

M.L. CLARK

Senior Lecturer, St Bartholomew's Hospital Medical College, London, UK
14.16 Tumours of the gastrointestinal tract

A.R. CLARKSON

Associate Professor of Medicine, University of Adelaide; Director, Renal Unit, Royal Adelaide Hospital, Australia
20.4.1 IgA nephropathy, Henoch-Schönlein purpura, and thin membrane nephropathy

SIR CECIL CLOTHIER

Formerly Parliamentary Commissioner for Administration and Health Service Commissioner for England and Wales, and Scotland
1 On being a patient

A.J.S. COATS

Senior Lecturer and Honorary Consultant Cardiologist, Royal Brompton Hospital, London, UK
15.5 The syndrome of heart failure

S.M. COBBE

Professor of Medical Cardiology, University of Glasgow, Glasgow Royal Infirmary, UK
15.8.1 Cardiac arrhythmias

J. COHEN

Professor of Infectious Diseases and Bacteriology, Royal Postgraduate Medical School, Hammersmith Hospital, London, UK
7.19.3 Infection in the immunocompromised host

R.D. COHEN

Professor of Medicine, The London Hospital Medical College, University of London, UK
11.14 Disturbances of acid-base homeostasis
20.19.1 The renal tubular acidoses

---

* It is with regret that we report the deaths of those authors marked with an asterisk. Although their deaths occurred between the appearance of the second edition and preparation of the third edition, much of their contribution to the former has been incorporated into this edition, with appropriate updating from their coauthors.

J. COLLINGE

Wellcome Senior Research Fellow in the Clinical Sciences and Honorary Consultant in Neurology and Molecular Genetics, St Mary's Hospital Medical School, Imperial College London, UK
24.7.4 Prion diseases

R. COLLINS

British Heart Foundation Research Fellow and Co-ordinator, Clinical Trial Service Unit, Nuffield Department of Clinical Medicine, University of Oxford, UK
2.4 Large-scale randomized evidence: trials and overviews

G. COLMAN

Formerly Consultant Microbiologist, Division of Hospital Infection, Central Public Health Laboratory, Colindale, London, UK
7.11.2 Pathogenic streptococci

D.A.S. COMPSTON

Professor of Neurology, University of Cambridge, UK
24.9 Demyelinating disorders of the central nervous system

C.P. CONLON

Consultant Physician, Infectious Diseases Unit, Nuffield Department of Medicine, John Radcliffe Hospital, Oxford, UK
7.8 Travel and expedition medicine
7.10.29 HIV infection and AIDS
14.18 Gastrointestinal infections

M. CONTRERAS

Chief Executive and Medical Director, North London Blood Transfusion Centre, London, UK
22.4.13 Acquired haemolytic anaemia

M.R. COOPER

Formerly Commonwealth Bureau of Animal Health, Central Veterinary Laboratory, Addlestone, Surrey, UK
8.4.2 Poisonous plants and fungi

J. COUVREUR

Associate Professor of Paediatrics, Hôpital Trousseau, Paris, France
7.13.4 Toxoplasmosis

P.J. COWEN

Medical Research Council Clinical Scientist, University Department of Psychiatry, Littlemore Hospital, Oxford, UK
27.4.1 Psychopharmacology in medical practice

T.M. COX

Professor of Medicine, University of Cambridge, and Honorary Consultant Physician, Addenbrooke's Hospital, Cambridge, UK
11.2.1 Glycogen storage diseases
11.2.2 Inborn errors of fructose metabolism
11.2.3 Disorders of galactose metabolism
14.9.5 Disaccharidase deficiency

W.I. CRANSTON

Emeritus Professor of Medicine, United Medical and Dental Schools, St Thomas's Hospital, London, UK
8.5.5(b) Environmental factors and disease: drug-induced increases of body temperature

D.H. CRAWFORD

Professor of Microbiology, London School of Hygiene and Tropical Medicine, UK
7.10.4 The Epstein-Barr virus

P. CREAMER

Senior Registrar in Rheumatology, Bristol Royal Infirmary, UK
18.3 Rheumatology: use and abuse of investigations

I.B. CROME

Consultant Psychiatrist, Keele, Staffordshire, UK
28.1.2 Assessing substance use and misuse
28.1.3 Diagnoses and classifications: substance problems and dependence—what is the difference?
28.3.2 The management of substance-related problems in a general ward

D.W.M. CROOK

Consultant Microbiologist, Public Health Laboratory, John Radcliffe Hospital, Oxford, UK
7.9 Nosocomial infection
15.17 Infective endocarditis
15.21 Cardiovascular syphilis
17.6.3 Microbiological methods in the diagnosis of respiratory infections
24.15.1 Bacterial meningitis

G.W. CSONKA

Consultant Physician in Genitourinary Medicine (retired), Charing Cross Hospital, London, UK
7.11.34 Syphilis

J. CUNNINGHAM

Consultant Physician and Honorary Senior Lecturer in Nephrology, Royal London Hospital and Medical College, London, UK
20.19 Renal tubular disorders

SIR JOHN DACIE

Emeritus Professor of Haematology, Royal Postgraduate Medical School, University of London, UK
22.3.12 Paroxysmal nocturnal haemoglobinuria

D.A.B. DANCE

Director/Consultant Microbiologist, Public Health Laboratory, Derriford Hospital, Plymouth, Devon, UK
7.11.15 Melioidosis and glanders

J.H. DARGIE

Consultant Cardiologist, Western Infirmary, Glasgow, UK
15.6.3 Vasodilators

J.H. DARK

Consultant Cardiothoracic Surgeon, Freeman Hospital, Newcastle upon Tyne, UK
15.7 Cardiac transplantation

P.G. DAVEY

Reader in Clinical Pharmacology and Infectious Diseases, Ninewells Hospital and Medical School, Dundee, UK
7.6 Antimicrobial chemotherapy

M.J. DAVIES

BHF Professor of Cardiovascular Pathology, St George's Hospital Medical School, University of London, UK
15.10.2 The pathology of ischaemic heart disease

S.W. DAVIES

Consultant Cardiologist, The Royal Brompton Hospital, London, UK
15.3.1 Breathlessness
15.3.4 Fatigue

P.D.O DAVIES

Consultant Respiratory Physician, Cardiothoracic Centre and Aintree Hospital NHS Trust, Liverpool, UK
7.11.22 Tuberculosis
7.11.24 Disease caused by environmental bacteria

A.M. DAVISON

Consultant Renal Physician, St James's University Hospital, Leeds, UK
20.5.4 Renal manifestations of malignant disease
20.5.5 Sarcoid and the kidney

P.T. DAWES

Consultant Rheumatologist, Staffordshire Rheumatology Centre; Senior Lecturer, University of Keele, Staffordshire, UK
18.2 Rheumatology: clinical presentation and diagnosis

K. DAWKINS

Consultant Cardiologist and Clinical Services Manager, Wessex Cardiothoracic Centre, Southampton General Hospital, UK
15.4.7 Exercise testing

D.P. DE BONO

British Heart Foundation Professor of Cardiology, University of Leicester Medical School, UK
15.10.5 Coronary angioplasty

M. DE SWIET

Consultant Physician, Queen Charlotte's Hospital for Women and University College Hospital, London and Northwick Park Hospital, Harrow, Middlesex, UK
13.5 Thromboembolism in pregnancy
13.6 Chest diseases in pregnancy

D.M. DENISON

Professor and Director, Lung Function Unit, Royal Bromptom Hospital, London, UK
8.5.5(e) Environmental factors and disease: aerospace medicine
8.5.5(f) Environmental factors and disease: diving medicine

J. DENT

Gastroenterology Unit, Royal Adelaide Hospital, South Australia
14.2.1 Dysphagia and other symptoms in oesophageal disease
14.6 Diseases of the oesophagus

R. DICK

Consultant Radiologist, Royal Free Hospital Trust, London, UK
14.20.1 Computed tomography and magnetic resonance imaging of the liver and pancreas

P. DIEPPE

ARC Professor of Rheumatology, Bristol University, UK
18.1 Rheumatology: introduction
18.3 Rheumatology: use and abuse of investigations

M. DOHERTY

Reader in Rheumatology, University of Nottingham Medical School, Rheumatology Unit, City Hospital, Nottingham, UK
18.7 Crystal-related arthropathies

SIR RICHARD DOLL

Honorary Consultant, Imperial Cancer Research Fund, Radcliffe Infirmary, Oxford, UK
6.2. Epidemiology of cancer

M. DONAGHY

Clinical Reader in Neurology, University of Oxford; Consultant Neurologist, Radcliffe Infirmary, Oxford, UK
24.1 Neurology: introduction
24.16 The motor neurone diseases

S. DOVER

Senior Registrar in Medicine and Gastroenterology, Fazakerley Hospital, Liverpool, UK
11.5 Porphyrin metabolism and the porphyrias

R.H. DOWLING

Professor of Gastroenterology, United Medical Schools of St Thomas's and Guy's Hospitals, Guy's Campus, London, UK
14.9.3 Small-bowel bacterial overgrowth

R.M. DU BOIS

Consultant Physician, Royal Brompton Hospital and Honorary Senior Lecturer, National Heart and Lung Institute, London, UK
17.10.1 Alveolar and interstitial disease: introduction
17.10.2 Cryptogenic fibrosing alveolitis

C.R.K. DUDLEY

Consultant Nephrologist, The Richard Bright Renal Unit, Southmead Hospital, Bristol, UK
15.12 Cholesterol embolism

B.O.L. DUKE

River Blindness Foundation, Lancaster, UK
7.14.1 General principles of filarial infections and diseases

M.S. DUNNILL

Fellow of Merton College, Sometime Consultant Histopathologist, John Radcliffe Hospital, Oxford, UK
17.6.5 Histopathology and cytology in diagnosis of lung disease

G.R. DUNSTAN

Professor Emeritus of Moral and Social Theology, University of London; Honorary Research Fellow, University of Exeter, UK
2.2. Medical ethics

D.T. DURACK

Consulting Professor of Medicine, Duke University Medical Center, Durham, North Carolina, USA
7.19.1 Fever of unknown origin

S.R. DURHAM

Senior Lecturer and Honorary Consultant Physician, Royal Brompton Hospital, London, UK
17.8.1 Allergic rhinitis ('hay fever')

B.G.M. DURIE

Division of Hematology/Oncology, Department of Medicine, Cedars-Sinai Medical Center, Los Angeles, California, USA
22.5.5 Myeloma and other paraproteinaemias

P.N. DURRINGTON

Reader in Medicine, University of Manchester Department of Medicine, Manchester Royal Infirmary, Chester, UK
11.6 Lipid and lipoprotein disorders

G.M. DUSHEIKO

Reader in Medicine, Royal Free Hospital and School of Medicine, London, UK
14.33 Hepatic granulomas

C.J. EASTMOND

Consultant Physician, Department of Rheumatology, Aberdeen Royal Infirmary, UK
18.5 Seronegative spondarthropathies

S. EBER

Professor of Paediatrics, Universitäts-Kinderklinik, Göttingen, Germany
22.4.10 Genetic disorders of the red cell membrane

A.L.W.F. EDDLESTON

Professor of Liver Immunology and Dean of Clinical Medicine, King's College School of Medicine and Dentistry, London, UK
14.27.1 Autoimmune hepatitis

C.R.W. EDWARDS

Professor of Clinical Medicine, University of Edinburgh, UK
12.7.1 Adrenocortical diseases

G. EDWARDS

Emeritus Professor of Addiction Behaviour, National Addiction Centre, University of London, UK
28.1.1 Drug problems as every doctor's business

A.M. EL NAHAS

Consultant Renal Physician, Sheffield Kidney Institute, Northern General Hospital, Shefffield, UK
20.17.1 Chronic renal failure

M. ELIA

Head of Clinical Nutrition Group, MRC, Dunn Clinical Nutrition Centre; Honorary Consultant Physician, Addenbrooke's Hospital, Cambridge, UK
10.6 Special nutritional problems and the use of enteral and parenteral nutrition

M. ELIAKIM

Professor of Internal Medicine; Chairman, Department of Medicine, Bikur Cholim Hospital, Jerusalem, Israel
11.13.2 Recurrent polyserositis (familial Mediterranean fever, periodic disease)

E. ELIAS

Consultant Physician, Liver Unit, Queen Elizabeth Hospital, Birmingham, UK
14.25 Jaundice

C.M. ELLIOTT

Dean of Trinity Hall, Cambridge, UK
3.1 The diseases of gods: some newer threats to health

B.T. EMMERSON

Professor of Medicine, University of Queensland and Consultant Physician, Princess Alexandra Hospital, Brisbane, Australia
20.13 Toxic nephropathy

SIR ANTHONY EPSTEIN

Professor Emeritus of Pathology, University of Bristol; Fellow of Wolfson College, Oxford, UK
7.10.4 The Epstein–Barr virus

S.J. EYKYN

Reader (Honorary Consultant) in Clinical Microbiology, United Medical and Dental Schools, St Thomas's Hospital, London, UK
7.11.4 Staphylococci
7.11.4 Anaerobic bacteria

E.A. FAGAN

Senior Lecturer in Medicine, Royal Free Hospital School of Medicine and University College London Medical School, London
13.13 Liver and gastrointestinal disease in pregnancy

C.G. FAIRBURN

Wellcome Trust Senior Lecturer, Department of Psychiatry, University of Oxford, UK
10.4 Eating disorders
27.2.7 Psychiatric disorders as they concern the physician: eating disorders

M. FARRELL

Senior Lecturer/Consultant Psychiatrist, National Addiction Centre, the Maudsley Hospital, London, UK
28.1.2 Assessing substance use and misuse
28.2.2 Harm reduction
28.3.2 The management of substance-related problems in a general ward
28.3.8 Caring for the HIV-positive drug user

M.J.G. FARTHING

Professor of Gastroenterology and Honorary Consultant Physician, St Bartholomew's Hospital, London, UK
14.9.9 Malabsorption in the tropics

M.F. FIELD

Associate Professor of Medicine, University of Sydney, Concord Hospital, New South Wales, Australia
20.1 Clinical physiology of the kidney: tests of renal function and structure

J.D. FIRTH

Wellcome Fellow, Honorary Consultant Physician, Oxford, UK
15.3.3 Oedema
20.16 Acute renal failure

S. FISHER-HOCH

Department of Pathology, Aga Khan Hospital Medical School, Karachi, Pakistan
7.10.22 Arenaviruses

R.A. FISHMAN

Professor of Neurology, University of California, San Francisco, USA
24.2.6 Lumbar puncture

E. FITZSIMONS

Consultant and Senior Lecturer in Haematology, Monklands Hospital, Airdrie and Western Infirmary, Glasgow, UK
11.5 Porphyrin metabolism and the porphyrias

A.F. FLEMING

Professor of Haematology at Baragwanath Hospital, Soweto School of Pathology of the South African Institute for Medical Research and the University of the Witwatersrand, Soweto, South Africa
22.4.3 Anaemia as a world health problem

E.W.L. FLETCHER

Consultant Radiologist, John Radcliffe Hospital, Oxford, UK
14.3.2 Methods for investigation of gastrointestinal diseases: radiology

D. FLISER

Physician, Department of Internal Medicine, Division of Nephrology, University of Heidelberg, Germany
20.5.1 Diabetic nephropathy

P. FOËX

Nuffield Professor of Anaesthetics, University of Oxford, Radcliffe Infirmary, Oxford, UK
17.10.20 Adult respiratory distress syndrome

J.C. FORFAR

Consultant Physician, John Radcliffe Hospital, Oxford, UK
13.4 Heart disease in pregnancy
15.6.4 Catecholamines and the sympathetic nervous system

I. FOULDS

Senior Lecturer, Occupational Dermatology, Institute of Occupational Health, University of Birmingham, UK
8.5.3(a) Occupational dermatology

G.H. FOWLER

Reader in General Practice, University of Oxford; Honorary Director, Imperial Cancer Research Fund General Practice Research Group, Oxford, UK
3.3 Primary care

A.J. FREW

Senior Lecturer in Medicine, University Medicine, University of Southampton, UK
17.9.1(a) Asthma: basic mechanisms and pathophysiology

P. FRITH

Consultant Medical Ophthalmologist, University College Hospitals, London, UK
26 The eye in general medicine

H.R. GAMSU

Professor of Neonatology, King's College Hospital School of Medicine and Dentistry, University of London, UK
13.12.2 Bacterial, fungal, and protozoal infections in pregnancy and the newborn

D. GARDNER-MEDWIN

Consultant Paediatric Neurologist, Newcastle General Hospital, Newcastle upon Tyne, UK
24.18 Developmental abnormalities of the nervous system

C. GARRARD

Consultant Physician in Intensive Care, John Radcliffe Hospital, Oxford, UK
17.10.20 Adult respiratory distress syndrome
17.14.3(a) Acute respiratory failure: intensive care

J.S. GARROW

Professor of Human Nutrition, St Bartholomew's Hospital Medical College, University of London, UK
10.5 Obesity

D.H. GATH
Clinical Reader in Psychiatry, University Department of Psychiatry, Warneford Hospital, Oxford, UK
27.2.8 Affective disorders

K.C. GATTER
University Lecturer in Pathology, Department of Cellular Science, John Radcliffe Hospital, Oxford, UK
22.5.2 Introduction to the lymphoproliferative disorders
22.5.3 The lymphomas

M.G. Gelder
Handley Professor of Psychiatry, University of Oxford, UK
27.1 Psychiatry in medicine: introduction
27.2.1 Reactions to stressful events
27.2.2 Anxiety and obsessional disorders
27.2.3 Psychiatric conditions with physical complaints
27.2.4 Dissociative disorder
27.2.5 Malingering and factitious disorders
27.2.6 Personality and its disorders
27.2.9 Schizophrenia
27.4.2 Psychological treatment in medical practice

C. GERADA
Principal in General Practice, Hurley Clinic, Kennington, London, UK
28.3.6 The pregnancy drug abuser

A.H. GHODSE
Professor of Psychiatry and Director, Centre for Addiction Studies, St George's Hospital Medical School, University of London, UK
28.3.5 Drug misusers and addicts in accident and emergency

C.J. GIBSON
Professor of Respiratory Medicine, University of Newcastle upon Tyne and Consultant Physician, Freeman Hospital, Newcastle upon Tyne, UK
17.10.19 Drug-induced lung disease

D.G. GIBSON
Consultant Cardiologist, Royal Brompton Hospital, London, UK
15.18 Valve disease
15.20 Pericardial disease

A.M. GILES
Medical Laboratory Scientific Officer, Department of Clinical Biochemistry, John Radcliffe Hospital, Oxford, UK
33 Reference intervals for biochemical data

F.J. GILES
Assistant Professor, University of California at Los Angeles; Director, Myeloma Research and Treatment Center, Bone Marrow Transplantation Unit, Cedars-Sinai Medical Center, Los Angeles, California, USA
22.5.5 Myeloma and other paraproteinaemias

C.F. GILKS
Senior Lecturer and Consultant Physician, Liverpool School of Tropical Medicine, Liverpool, UK
7.10.30 Human immunodeficiency virus in the developing world

M.D.G. GILLMER
Honorary Lecturer, Nuffield Department of Obstetrics and Gynaecology, University of Oxford and Consultant Obstetrician and Gynaecologist, John Radcliffe Hospital, Oxford, UK
13.8 Diabetes in pregnancy

D.J. GIRLING
Clinical Coordinator, MRC Cancer Trials Office, Cambridge, UK
7.11.22 Tuberculosis
7.11.24 Disease caused by environmental mycobacteria

R. GOKAL
Consultant Nephrologist and Honarary Lecturer, Manchester Royal Infirmary, UK
20.17.2 Replacement therapy by dialysis

M.J. GOLDACRE
Consultant in Public Health Medicine, Anglia and Oxford Regional Health Authority, and Honorary Senior Clinical Lecturer in Public Health, University of Oxford, UK
3.2 Health and sickness in the community

M.H.N GOLDEN
Professor of Medicine (Nutrition), University of Aberdeen, UK
10.3 Severe malnutrition

S.J. GOLDING
Lecturer in Radiology, University of Oxford, UK
6.5 Medical imaging in oncology

J. GOLDMAN
Professor of Leukaemia Biology, Royal Postgraduate Medical School, Hammersmith Hospital, London, UK
22.3.5 Chronic myeloid leukaemia

S. GORDON
Glaxo Professor of Cellular Pathology, Sir William Dunn School of Pathology, University of Oxford, UK
4.2.3 The mononuclear phagocyte system and tissue homeostasis

E.C. GORDON-SMITH
Professor of Haematology, St George's Hospital Medical School, University of London, UK
22.3.11 Aplastic anaemia and other causes of bone marrow failure
22.4.11 Haemolysis due to red-cell enzyme deficiencies
22.4.13 Acquired haemolytic anaemia

M. GOSSOP
Head of Research, Drug Dependence Unit, National Addiction Centre, The Maudsley Hospital, London, UK
28.3.7 Management of pain in the drug abuser

J.M. GRANGE
Reader in Clinical Microbiology, National Heart and Lung Institute, University of London, UK
7.11.22 Tuberculosis
7.11.24 Disease caused by environmental mycobacteria

R. GRAY
Senior Research Fellow, Clinical Trial Service Unit, Nuffield Department of Clinical Medicine, University of Oxford, UK
2.4 Large-scale randomized evidence: trials and overviews

D.W.R. GRAY
Reader in Transplantation and Consultant Surgeon, Nuffield Department of Surgery, University of Oxford, UK
20.17.3 Renal transplantation

J.R. GRAYBILL

Professor of Medicine, University of Texas Health Science Center, San Antonio, USA
7.12.2 Coccidioidomycosis

M.F. GREAVES

Professor of Cell Biology and Director, Leukaemia Research Fund Centre at the Institute for Cancer Research, London, UK
22.3.1 Cell and molecular biology of leukaemia

M. GREAVES

Reader in Haematology, Central Sheffield University Hospital, UK
22.6.7 Thrombotic disease

B.M. GREENWOOD

Director, MRC Laboratories, Fajara, The Gambia
7.3 The host's response to infection
7.11.3 Pneumococcal infection
7.11.5 Meningococcal infection

R.J. GREENWOOD

Consultant Neurologist, St Bartholomew's and The National Hospitals for Neurology and Neurosurgery, London, UK
24.15.5 Neurosyphilis

B. GRIBBIN

Consultant Cardiologist, The John Radcliffe Hospital, Oxford, UK
15.17 Infective endocarditis
15.21 Cardiovascular syphilis

J. GRIMLEY EVANS

Professor of Clinical Geratology, University of Oxford, UK
31 Medicine in old age

N.R. GRIST

Emeritus Professor of Infectious Diseases, University of Glasgow; formerly Consultant Virologist, Head of Regional Virus Laboratory, Ruchill, Glasgow, UK
7.10.13 Enteroviruses

D.I. GROVE

Director of Clinical Microbiology and Infectious Diseases, The Queen Elizabeth Hospital, Woodville, South Australia
7.14.5 Nematode infections of lesser importance

D.J. GRUNDY

Consultant in Spinal Injuries, The Duke of Cornwall Spinal Treatment Centre, Salisbury District Hospital, UK
24.3.10 Spinal cord injury and the management of paraplegia

J.-P. GRÜNFELD

Professor of Nephrology, Necker Medical School, University René Descartes, Necker Hospital, Paris, France
20.5.3 Amyloid, myeloma, light chain deposition disease, fibrillary glomerulonephritis and cryoglobulinaemia
20.7 Clinical aspects of inherited renal disorders

W.J. GULLICK

Principal Scientist, Imperial Cancer Research Fund, Hammersmith Hospital, London, UK
6.3 Growth factors and oncogenes

H.H. GUNSON

Medical Director, National Blood Authority, Manchester, UK
22.8.1 Blood transfusion

M.R. HAENEY

Consultant Immunologist, Salford General Hospitals Trust, Salford, UK
14.4 Immune disorders of the gastrointestinal tract

A.M. HALLIDAY

Formerly Consultant in Clinical Neurophysiology, National Hospital for Neurology and Neurosurgery, London; Member of the External Staff of the Medical Research Council, UK
24.2.3 Evoked potentials

P.J. HAMMOND

Senior Registrar, St James's University Hospital, Leeds, West Yorkshire, UK
12.10 Non-diabetic pancreatic endocrine disorders and multiple endocrine neoplasia
14.8 Hormones and the gastrointestinal tract

D.M. HANSELL

Consultant Radiologist, Royal Brompton Hospital, London, UK
17.6.1 Thoracic imaging

A.E. HARDING

Professor of Clinical Neurology, Institute of Neurology; Consultant Neurologist, National Hospital for Neurology and Neurosurgery, London, UK
25.9 Mitochondrial myopathies and encephalomyopathies

KHUNYING TRANAKCHIT HARINASUTA

Professor of Tropical Medicine and Consultant, Faculty of Tropical Medicine, Mahidol University, Bangkok, Thailand
7.16.4 Intestinal trematodiasis

J.M. HARRINGTON

Professor of Occupational Health, University of Birmingham, UK
8.5.1 Occupational and environmental health and safety: general introduction
8.5.2 The investigation of occupational disease
8.5.3 The main occupational diseases. (b) Occupational cancer. (e) Cardiovascular system. (f) Genitourinary system

A.L. HARRIS

Imperial Cancer Research Fund Professor of Clinical Oncology, University of Oxford, ICRF Clinical Oncology Unit, Churchill Hospital, Oxford, UK
6.8 New approaches to cancer therapy
13.15 Malignant disease in pregnancy

SIR HENRY HARRIS

Regius Professor of Medicine Emeritus, University of Oxford
6.1 General characteristics of neoplasia

M.J.G. HARRISON

Professor in Clinical Neurology, University College London Medical School; Consultant Neurologist, Middlesex Hospital and the National Hospital, London, UK
24.4.4 Coma
24.21 Neurological complications of systemic diseases

C. HASLETT

Professor of Respiratory Medicine, Edinburgh University and Honorary Consultant Physician, Royal Infirmary, Edinburgh, UK
17.3.1 Non-immune defence mechanisms of the lung
17.3.2 Inflammation and the lung

I. HASLOCK

Consultant Rheumatologist, South Tees Acute Hospitals Trust; Visiting Professor of Clinical Bio-engineering, University of Durham, UK
18.8 Back pain and periarticular disease

D.A. HAWKINS

Consultant Physician in Genitourinary Medicine, Chelsea and Westminster Hospital, London, UK
28.2.3(b) Physical complications of drug abuse

K.E. HAWTON

Consultant Psychiatrist, University Department of Psychiatry, Warneford Hospital, Oxford, UK
27.3.4 Sexual problems associated with physical illness

R.J. HAY

Mary Dunhill Professor of Cutaneous Medicine, United Medical and Dental Schools, Guy's Hospital, London, UK
7.11.28 Nocardiosis
7.12.1 Fungal infections

B. HAZLEMAN

Consultant Rheumatologist, Addenbrooke's Hospital, Cambridge, UK
18.10 Miscellaneous conditions

A.H. HENDERSON

Professor of Cardiology, University of Wales College of Medicine, Cardiff, UK
15.3.2 Chest pain

D.J. HENDRICK

Consultant Physician and Honorary Senior Lecturer, Newcastle General Hospital, University of Newcastle upon Tyne, UK
17.10.8 Lymphocytic infiltrations of the lung
17.10.9 Extrinsic allergic alveolitis
17.10.12 Pulmonary alveolar proteinosis
17.10.13 Pulmonary amyloidosis
17.10.14 Lipoid (lipid) pneumonia
17.10.15 Pulmonary alveolar microlithiasis
17.10.21 Lung disorders in genetic syndromes

M.F. HEYWORTH

Associate Professor of Medicine, University of California; Staff Physician, Veterans Affairs Medical Center, San Francisco, USA
7.13.8 Giardiasis, balantidiasis, isosporiasis, and microsporidiosis

TRAN TINH HIEN

Clinical Research Unit, Centre for Tropical Diseases (Cho Quan Hospital), Ho Chi Minh City, Vietnam
7.11.1 Diphtheria

T.W. HIGENBOTTAM

Consultant Physician and Respiratory Physiologist, Papworth and Addenbrooke's Hospitals, Cambridge, UK
17.14.4 Lung and heart-lung transplantation

S.L. HILLIER

Research Associate Professor of Obstetrics and Gynecology, University of Washington, Seattle, USA
21.4 Vaginal discharge

D. HILTON-JONES

Consultant Neurologist, Radcliffe Infirmary, Oxford, and Milton Keynes General Hospital, UK
25.8 Metabolic and endocrine myopathies

T.D.R. HOCKADAY

Honorary Consultant Physician, Radcliffe Infirmary, Oxford, UK
11.11 Diabetes mellitus

J.R. HODGES

University Lecturer and Consultant Neurologist, University of Cambridge Clinical School, Addenbrooke's Hospital, Cambridge, UK
24.7.1 Dementia: introduction
24.7.3 Pick's disease (focal lobar atrophy)

H.J.F. HODGSON

Professor of Gastroenterology, Royal Postgraduate Medical School, London, UK
14.9.6 Whipple's disease
14.9.7 Short gut syndrome

E.S. HODGSON

Occupational Health Physician and Lecturer in Occupational Health, University of Oxford: Honorary Consultant Occupational Physician, Radcliffe Hospital, Oxford, UK
8.5.1 Occupational and environmental health and safety: general introduction
8.5.2 The investigation of occupational medicine
8.5.3 The main occupational diseases: (g) Gastrointestinal tract; (h) The haematopoietic system; (i) Infections

A.V. HOFFBRAND

Professor of Haematology, Royal Free Hospital, London, UK
22.4.6 Megaloblastic anaemia and miscellaneous deficiency anaemias

S.T. HOLGATE

MRC Clinical Professor of Immunopharmacology, Southampton General Hospital, UK
17.9.1(a) Asthma: basic mechanisms and pathophysiology

P. HOLLOWAY

Clinical Lecturer and Senior Registrar, Department of Clinical Biochemistry, John Radcliffe Hospital, Oxford, UK
33 Reference intervals for biochemical data

J.M. HOPKIN

Consultant Physician, John Radcliffe Hospital, UK
7.12.5 Pneumocystis carinii
17.1 Respiratory medicine: introduction
17.7.1 Upper respiratory tract infection
17.7.3 Suppurative pulmonary and pleural infections
17.7.4 Chronic specific infections
17.7.5 Respiratory infection in the immunosuppressed
17.10.3 Bronchiolitis obliterans
17.10.5 Pulmonary vasculitis and granulomatosis
17.10.17 Toxic gases and fumes
17.10.18 Radiation pneumonitis

A.P. HOPKINS

Director of the Research Unit, Royal College of Physicians: Consultant Neurologist, Royal Hospital NHS Trust, London, UK
24.4.1 Epilepsy in later childhood and adult life

J.A.C. HOPKIRK

Consultant Physician, King Edward VII Hospital, Midhurst, West Sussex, UK
8.5.5(e) Environmental factors and disease: aerospace medicine

A. HORWICH

Professor of Radiotherapy, Institute of Cancer Research, London University; Consultant in Clinical Oncology, Royal Marsden Hospital, London, UK
6.7 Role of radiotherapy in the treatment of cancer

I.A. HUGHES

Professor of Paediatrics, University of Cambridge, UK
12.7.3 Congenital adrenal hyperplasia

B.J. HUNT

Consultant/Honorary Senior Lecturer in Haematology, St Thomas's Hospital; Honorary Senior Lecturer in Cardiothoracic Surgery at The National Heart and Lung Hospital, London, UK
22.6.6 Acquired coagulation disorders

C.W. HUTTON

Consultant Rheumatologist, Mount Gould Hospital, Plymouth, UK
18.6 Osteoarthritis

C.W. IMRIE

Honorary Senior Lecturer, University of Glasgow; Consultant Surgeon, Royal Infirmary, Glasgow, UK
14.23.1 Acute pancreatitis

M. IRVING

Professor of Surgery, Hope Hospital (University of Manchester School of Medicine), Salford, UK
14.19 The peritoneum, omentum, and appendix

D. ISAACS

Head of Department of Immunology and Infectious Diseases, Royal Alexandra Hospital for Children, Sydney: Associate Professor, University of Sydney, Australia
7.7 Immunization
7.10.1 Respiratory tract viruses

P.G. ISAACSON

Professor of Morbid Anatomy, University College London Medical School, London, UK
14.9.8 Enteropathy-associated T-cell lymphoma

D.A. ISENBERG

Professor of Rheumatology, Bloomsbury Rheumatology Unit, The Middlesex Hospital, London, UK
18.11.3 Systemic lupus erythematosus and related disorders

I. ISHERWOOD

Emeritus Professor of Diagnostic Radiology, University of Manchester, UK
24.2.1. Principles of neuroradiology

K. ISHIKAWA

Director, Department of Internal Medicine, Higashi Nagahara Hospital, Osaka, Japan
15.13 Takayasu's disease

C.A. ISON

Lecturer in Medical Microbiology, St Mary's Hospital Medical School, London, UK
7.11.6 Neisseria gonorrhoeae

A. JACKSON

Senior Lecturer in Neuroradiology, University of Manchester, UK
24.2.1 Principles of neuroradiology

H.S. JACOBS

Professor of Reproductive Endocrinology, University College London Medical School; Consultant Physician, The Middlesex Hospital, London, UK
12.8.1 The ovary
12.8.3 The breast

R.J. JACOBY

Clinical Reader in Old Age Psychiatry, University of Oxford, UK
27.2.11 Mental disorders of old age

O.F.W. JAMES

Professor of Geriatric Medicine, University of Newcastle upon Tyne, UK
14.28 Alcoholic liver disease

W.P.T. JAMES

Professor and Director, Rowett Research Institute, Aberdeen, UK
10.1 Nutrition: introduction

J.L. JAMESON

C.F. Kettering Professor of Medicine, Northwestern University School of Medicine, Chicago, Illinois, USA
12.1 Principles of hormone action

B. JENNETT

Emeritus Professor of Neurosurgery, Institute of Neurological Science, Glasgow, UK
24.4.5 Brain death and the vegetative state

D.P. JEWELL

Consultant Physician, John Radcliffe Hospital; Clinical Lecturer, University of Oxford, UK
14.1 Gastroenterology: introduction
14.2.2 Vomiting
14.2.3 Abdominal pain
14.2.6 Gastrointestinal bleeding
14.3.1 Endoscopy
14.9.4 Coeliac disease
14.10 Crohn's disease
14.11 Ulcerative colitis
14.36 Miscellaneous disorders of the gastrointestinal tract and liver

A.R. JOHNS

Senior Lecturer, Division of Psychiatry of Addictive Behaviour, St George's Hospital Medical School, University of London, UK
28.3.4 Management of withdrawal syndromes

A.M. JOHNSON

Reader in Epidemiology, Academic Department of Genito-urinary Medicine, University College London Medical School, UK
21.2 Sexual behavior

A.W. JOHNSON

Formerly Commonwealth Bureau of Animal Health, Central Veterinary Laboratory, Addlestone, Surrey, UK
8.4.2 Poisonous animals and plants

P.J. JOHNSON
Institute of Liver Studies, King's College School of Medicine and Dentistry, London, UK
14.27.1 Autoimmune hepatitis

E.A. JONES
Chief of Hepatology, Department of Gastrointestinal and Liver Diseases, Academic Medical Centre, Amsterdam, The Netherlands
14.30 Hepatocellular failure

M. JOY
Consultant Cardiologist, St Peter's District General Hospital, Chertsey, Surrey, UK
15.10.7 Vocational aspects of coronary artery disease

R.W. JUBB
Consultant Rheumatologist, Selly Oak Hospital, Birmingham, UK
8.5.3(c) The main occupational diseases: musculoskeletal disorders

B.E. JUEL-JENSEN
Honorary Consultant Physician, Nuffield Department of Clinical Medicine, John Radcliffe, Hospital, Oxford, UK
7.10.2 Herpes simplex virus infections
7.10.3 Varicella-zoster virus infections: chickenpox and zoster
7.10.9 Orf
7.10.10 Molluscum contagiosum

J.A. KANIS
Professor in Human Metabolism and Clinical Biochemistry, University of Sheffield Medical School, UK
12.6 Disorders of calcium metabolism
20.18 Renal bone disease

TOMISAKU KAWASAKI
Director, Japan Kawasaki Disease Research Center, Tokyo, Japan
18.11.10 Kawasaki disease

W.R. KEATINGE
Professor of Physiology, Queen Mary and Westfield College, University of London
8.5.5 Environmental factors and disease: (a) heat; (c) Cold, drowning, and seasonal mortality

P.G.E. KENNEDY
Burton Professor of Neurology, University of Glasgow, UK
24.15.2 Acute viral infections of the central nervous system
24.15.3 Neurological manifestations of infections with human immunodeficiency virus type 1

S. KESHAV
Research Fellow, Sir William Dunn School of Pathology, University of Oxford, UK
4.2.4 Cytokines

M. KETTLEWELL
Consultant Surgeon, Oxford Radcliffe Trust; Fellow, Green College, Oxford, UK
14.14 Colonic diverticular disease

M. KING
Honorary Research Fellow, University of Leeds, UK
3.1 The diseases of gods: some newer threats to health

M.M. KLIKS
President and Director of Research, CTS Foundation, Honolulu, Hawaii, USA
7.14.3 Guinea-worm disease: human dracunculiasis

B. KNIGHT
Professor of Forensic Pathology, University of Wales College of Medicine, Cardiff, Wales, UK
29 Forensic medicine

R. KNIGHT
Associate Professor of Parasitology, Department of Medical Microbiology, Faculty of Medicine, Unity of Nairobi, Kenya
7.13.1 Amoebiasis
7.14.4 Strongyloidiasis, hookworm, and other gut cestodes
7.15.1 Gut cestodes

J.B. KURTZ
Consultant Virologist, John Radcliffe Hospital, Oxford, UK
7.11.36 Legionellosis and legionnaires' disease

H.P. LAMBERT
Emeritus Professor of Microbial Diseases, St George's Hospital Medical School, London; Visiting Professor, London School of Hygiene and Tropical Medicine, UK
7.1 Clinical approach to the patient with suspected infection

D.J. LANE
Consultant Chest Physician, Oxford Radcliffe Hospital, The Churchill, Oxford
17.1 Respiratory medicine: introduction
17.5 The clinical presentation of chest diseases
17.9.2 Cystic fibrosis
17.9.1(b) Asthma: clinical features and management
17.10.5 Pulmonary vasculitis and granulomatosis
17.10.6 Pulmonary haemorrhagic disorders
17.10.7 Pulmonary eosinophilia

H.E. LARSON
Consultant in Infectious Disease and General Medicine, Southborough, Massachusetts, USA
7.11.21 Botulism, gas gangrene, and clostridial gastrointestinal infections

N.F. LAWTON
Consultant Neurologist, Wessex Neurological Centre, Southampton General Hospital; Honorary Senior Lecturer, University of Southampton, UK
24.13 Benign intracranial hypertension

J.G.G. LEDINGHAM
May Reader in Medicine and Honorary Consultant Physician, John Radcliffe Hospital, Oxford, UK
13.3 Renal disease in pregnancy
15.3.3 Oedema
15.6.1 Diuretics
15.26 Pulmonary embolism
15.28.1 Renal and renovascular hypertension
15.29 Lymphoedema
20.20.2 Idiopathic oedema of women
20.20.3 Disorders of potassium metabolism
24.17.1 The POEMS syndrome

J.W. LeDUC
Medical Officer, Division of Communicable Diseases, World Health Organization, Geneva, Switzerland
7.10.21 Bunyaviridae

T. LEHNER

Head of Division of Immunology, United Medical and Dental Schools of Guy's and St Thomas's Hospital, Guy's Hospital, London
14.5 The mouth and salivary glands
18.11.8 Behçet's disease

G.G. LENNOX

Senior Lecturer in Clinical Neurology, University of Nottingham Medical School, UK
13.10 Neurological disease in pregnancy

E.A. LETSKY

Consultant Haematologist, Queen Charlotte's and Chelsea Hospitals, London, UK
13.9 Blood disorders in pregnancy

S.M. LEWIS

Emeritus Reader in Haematology, University of London; Senior Research Fellow, Department of Haematology, Royal Postgraduate Medical School, London, UK
22.5.4 The spleen and its disorders

D.C. LINCH

Professor of Haematology, University College London, UK
22.2.2 Stem-cell disorders

C.C. LINNEMANN JR.

Professor, Departments of Medicine and Pathology and Laboratory Medicine, University of Cincinnati, Ohio, USA
7.11.14 Bordetella

D. LIPKIN

Consultant Cardiologist, The Royal Free Hospital, London, UK
15.3.1 Breathlessness
15.3.4 Fatigue

W.A. LISHMAN

Emeritus Professor of Neuropsychiatry, Institute of Psychiatry, London, UK
27.3.3 Specific conditions giving rise to mental disorder

A. LLANOS-CUENTAS

Professor of Medicine and Public Health, Universidad Peruana Cayetano Heredia; Senior Research Assistant at Instituto de Medicina Tropical 'Alexander von Humboldt', Lima, Peru
7.11.45 Bartonellosis

C.M. LOCKWOOD

Wellcome Reader in the School of Clinical Medicine, Addenbrooke's Hospital, Cambridge, UK
18.11.3 Small-vessel vasculitis

S. LOGAN

Senior Lecturer in Paediatric Epidemiology, Institute of Child Health, London, UK
7.10.18 Rubella

D.A. LOMAS

Lecturer in Medicine/Honorary Consultant Respiratory Physician, University of Cambridge, UK
11.5.α_1-Antitrypsin deficiency

M.S. LOSOWSKY

Professor of Medicine and Dean of the Faculty of Medicine, University of Leeds, UK
14.9.2 Investigation and differential diagnosis of malabsorption

P.F. LUDMAN

Senior Registrar in Cardiology, Papworth Hospital NHS Trust, Papworth Everard, Cambridgeshire, UK
15.4.5 Magnetic resonance and computed X-ray tomography

S.E. LUX

Professor of Pediatrics, Harvard Medical School; Chief, Division of Hematology/Oncology, Children's Hospital, Boston, Massachusetts, USA
22.4.10 Genetic disorders of the red-cell membrane

L. LUZZATTO

Professor of Haematology, Royal Postgraduate Medical School, Hammersmith Hospital, London, UK
22.3.12 Paroxysmal nocturnal haemoglobinuria
22.4.12 Glucose 6-phosphate dehydrogenase (G6PD) deficiency

D.C.W. MABEY

Professor of Communicable Diseases, London School of Hygiene and Tropical Medicine, UK
7.11.42 Chlamydial infections

J.T. MacFARLANE

Consultant Physician in General and Respiratory Medicine, City Hospital, Nottingham; Clinical Teacher, University of Nottingham, UK
7.11.36 Legionellosis and legionnaires' disease
17.7.2 Acute lower respiratory tract infections

B.B. MacGILLIVRAY

Physician in charge, Department of Clinical Neurophysiology, Royal Free Hospital; Consultant in Clinical Neurophysiology, National Hospitals for Neurology and Neurosurgery, London, UK
24.2.2 Electroencephalography

S.J. MACHIN

Professor of Haematology, University College London, UK
22.6.2 Introduction to disorders of haemostasis and coagulation
22.6.3 Purpura

D.W.R. MacKENZIE

Visiting Professor of Medical Mycology, London School of Hygiene and Tropical Medicine, UK
7.12.1 Fungal infections (mycoses)

I.J. MACKIE

Non-Clinical Lecturer in Haematology, University College London, UK
22.6.1 The biology of haemostasis and thrombosis
22.6.2 Introduction to disorders of haemostasis and coagulation

C.R. MADELEY

Professor of Clinical Virology, University of Newcastle upon Tyne, UK
7.10.14 Viruses in diarrhoea and vomiting

A. MADEN

Senior Lecturer in Forensic Psychiatry, The Institute of Psychiatry, London, UK
28.3.9 The needs of the alcohol/drug user in custody

M.M. MADKOUR
Consultant Physician, Military Hospital, Riyadh, Saudi Arabia
7.11.19 Brucellosis

C. MAGUIÑA-VARGAS
Professor of Medicine, Cayetano Heredia Peruvian University; Physician, Instituto Nacional de Salud; President, Instituto de Medicina Tropical 'Alexander von Humboldt', Lima, Peru
7.11.45 Bartonellosis

J.I. MANN
Professor in Human Nutrition and Medicine, University of Otago, Dunedin, New Zealand
10.7 Diseases of overnourished societies and the need for dietary change
15.10.1 Ischaemic heart disease: epidemiology and prevention

M.G. MARMOT
Professor of Epidemiology and Public Health, University College London, UK
15.10.1 Ischaemic heart disease; epidemiology and prevention

T.J. MARRIE
Professor of Medicine and Associate Professor of Microbiology, Dalhousie University; Active Staff Physician, Victoria General Hospital, Halifax, Nova Scotia, Canada
7.11.39 Coxiella burnetti infections (Q fever)

T.C. MARRS
Senior Medical Officer, Department of Health, London, UK
8.3.7 Poisoning by conflict

P.D. MARSDEN
Professor of Medicine, University of Brasilia, Brazil
7.13.11 American trypanosomiasis

C.D. MARSDEN
Professor and Head of Neurology, Institute of Neurology and the National Hospital for Neurology and Neurosurgery, London, UK
24.4.3 Narcolepsy and related sleep disorders
24.10 Movement disorders
24.19 Metabolic and deficiency disorders of the nervous system
24.20 Neurological disorders due to physical agents

V.J. MARTLEW
Chief Executive and Medical Director, National Blood Service: Mersey and North Wales, Liverpool, UK
22.8.1 Blood transfusion

A.D. MASON
Chief, Laboratory Division, US Army Institute of Surgical Research, Fort Sam Houston, Texas, USA
8.5.5(g) Environmental factors and disease: lightning and electric shock

W.B. MATTHEWS
Professor Emeritus of Clinical Neurology, University of Oxford, UK
24.3.2 The motor and sensory systems, midbrain, and brain-stem
24.3.9 Spinal cord

R.S. MAURICE-WILLIAMS
Consultant Neurosurgeon, The Royal Free Hospital, London, UK
24.3.11 Disorders of the spinal nerve roots

R.L. MAYNARD
Senior Medical Officer, Department of Health, UK
8.3.7 Poisoning in conflict

R.T. MAYON-WHITE
Consultant in Communicable Disease Control, Oxfordshire Health Authority, Oxford, UK
7.4 Epidemiology and public health

R.A. MAYOU
Clinical Reader in Psychiatry and Honorary Consultant, Warneford Hospital, Oxford, UK
27.2.10 Organic (cognitive) mental disorders
27.3.2 Emotional reactions in the bereaved and dying
27.4.3 Psychiatric emergencies

E. McCLOY
Medical Adviser to the Civil Service; Director, Civil Service Occupational Health Service, Edinburgh, UK
8.5.3 The main occupational diseases: reproductive system

K.E.L. McCOLL
Professor of Gastroenterology, University Department of Medicine and Therapeutics, Western Infirmary, Glasgow, UK
11.5 Porphyrin metabolism and the porphyrias

J.B. McCORMICK
Center for Bacterial and Mycotic Diseases, Centers for Disease Control, Atlanta, Georgia, USA
7.10.22 Arenaviruses

A.M. McGREGOR
Professor of Medicine, King's College School of Medicine, London, UK
12.4 The thyroid gland and disorders of thyroid function
13.7 Endocrine disease in pregnancy

N. McINTYRE
Professor of Medicine, Royal Free Hospital School of Medicine, London, UK
14.29 Cirrhosis, portal hypertension, and ascites

W.J. McKENNA
Professor of Cardiac Medicine, St George's Hospital Medical School, London, UK
15.14.1 The cardiomyopathies, myocarditis, and specific heart muscle disorders

A.J. McMICHAEL
MRC Clinical Research Professor of Immunology, Nuffield Department of Medicine, Institute of Molecular Medicine, Oxford, UK
5.1. Principles of immunology

A. McMILLAN
Consultant Physician, Department of Genito-urinary Medicine, Edinburgh Royal Infirmary, UK
21.6 Infections and other medical problems in homosexual men

T.W. MEADE
Director of MRC Epidemiology and Medical Care Unit and Professor of Epidemiology, Medical College of St Bartholomew's Hospital, London, UK
15.9.3 Haemostatic variables in ischaemic heart disease

A. MEHEUS
Professor of Epidemiology and Community Medicine, University of Antwerp, Belgium
21.1 Sexually transmitted diseases and sexual health

T.J. MEREDITH

Professor of Medicine and Pathology, School of Medicine, Vanderbilt University and Director, Center for Clinical Toxicology, Vanderbilt University Medical Center, Nashville, Tennessee, USA
8.1.1 Poisoning: introduction and epidemiology
8.1.2 Poisoning: clinical and metabolic features and general principles of management
8.2.1 Poisoning caused by analgesic drugs
8.2.2 Poisoning from antidepressants, hypnotics, antihistamines, anticonvulsants, and antiparkinsonian drugs
8.2.3 Poisoning from cardiovascular drugs
8.2.4 Poisoning caused by respiratory drugs
8.2.5 Poisoning caused by drugs acting on the gastrointestinal system
8.2.6 Poisoning by haematinics and vitamins
8.2.7 Poisoning by endocrine drugs
8.2.8 Poisoning from antimicrobials
8.2.10 Poisoning from drugs of abuse
8.2.11 Poisoning due to miscellaneous drugs
8.3.1 Poisoning from household products
8.3.2 Poisoning by alcohols and glycols
8.3.3 Poisoning by hydrocarbons and chlorofluorocarbons
8.3.4 Poisoning by inhalational agents
8.3.5 Poisoning due to corrosive substances

K.R. MILLS

University Lecturer and Consultant in Clinical Neurophysiology, The Radcliffe Infirmary, Oxford, UK
24.2.4 Investigation of central motor pathways: magnetic brain stimulation

A. MINDEL

Professor of Sexual Health Medicine, Universities of Sydney and New South Wales, Sydney, Australia
21.3 Genital herpes

S.A. MISBAH

Consultant Immunologist, Leeds General Infirmary; Senior Clinical Lecturer in Immunology, University of Leeds, UK
18.11.10 Cryoglobulinaemia

J.J. MISIEWICZ

Consultant Physician and Joint Director, Department of Gastroenterology and Nutrition, Central Middlesex Hospital, London, UK
14.7 Peptic ulceration

T.P. MONATH

Chief, Virology Division, USAMRIDD, Fort Detrick, Frederick, Maryland, USA
7.10.19 Flaviviruses

M.R. MOORE

Professor of Medicine, National Research Centre for Environmental Toxicology, University of Queensland, Australia
11.5 Porphyrin metabolism and the porphyrias

H.G. MORGAN

Professor of Mental Health, University of Bristol, Avon, UK
27.2.12 The patient who has attempted suicide

P.J. MORRIS

Nuffield Professor of Surgery and Director of the Oxford Transplant Centre, University of Oxford, John Radcliffe Hospital, Oxford, UK
5.5 Principles of transplantation immunology
15.11 Peripheral arterial disease

W.L. MORRISON

Consultant Cardiologist, Cardiothoracic Centre, Liverpool, UK
15.3.6 Cardiac cachexia

N.J.McC. MORTENSEN

Consultant Surgeon and Clinical Reader in Colorectal Surgery, John Radcliffe Hospital, Oxford, UK
14.14 Colonic diverticular disease

A.G. MOWAT

Honorary Senior Clinical Lecturer in Rheumatology, Oxford University; Consultant Rheumatologist, Nuffield Orthopaedic Centre, Oxford, UK
18.11.7 Polymyalgia rheumatica and giant-cell arteritis

J. MOXHAM

Professor of Thoracic Medicine, King's College Hospital, London, UK
17.14.1 Respiratory failure: definition and causes
17.14.3(b) Chronic respiratory failure

E.R. MOXON

Action Research Professor of Paediatrics, University of Oxford, UK
7.7 Immunization
7.11.12 Haemophilus influenzae

M.F. MUERS

Consultant Physician, Respiratory Unit, Regional Cardiothoracic Centre, Killingbeck Hospital, Leeds, UK
17.6.4 Diagnostic bronchoscopy and tissue biopsy

P.A. MURPHY

Professor of Medicine, Johns Hopkins University School of Medicine, Baltimore, Maryland, USA
7.5 Physiological changes in infected patients
7.19.2 Septicaemia

I.M. MURRAY-LYON

Consultant Gastroenterologist, Charing Cross Hospital, London, UK
14.32 Liver tumours

D.G. NATHAN

Robert A. Stranahan Professor of Pediatrics, Harvard Medical School, Boston, Massachusetts, USA
22.2.1 Stem cells and haematopoiesis

G. NEALE

Consultant Physician, Addenbrooke's Hospital, Cambridge, UK
14.17 Vascular and collagen disorders

G.H. NEILD

Professor of Nephrology, Institute of Urology and Nephrology, University College London Medical School, UK
20.6 Haemolytic uraemic syndrome

J. NEUBERGER

Consultant Physician, Queen Elizabeth Hospital, Birmingham, UK
14.34 Drugs and liver damage
14.35 The liver in systemic disease

J.M. NEUTZE

Chairman, Department of Cardiology, Green Lane Hospital, Auckland, New Zealand
15.16 The cardiac aspects of rheumatic fever

C.I. NEWBOLD

University Lecturer, University of Oxford, UK
7.13.2 Malaria

A.J. NEWMAN TAYLOR

Professor of Occupational and Environmental Medicine, National Heart and Lung Institute and Consultant Physician, Royal Brompton Hospital, London, UK
17.9.13 Occupational asthma

J. NEWSOM-DAVIS

Professor of Clinical Neurology, University of Oxford, Radcliffe Infirmary, Oxford, UK
24.1 Neurology: introduction
24.3.8 Respiratory problems in neurological disease
25.7 Disorders of neuromuscular transmission

S. NIGHTINGALE

Consultant Neurologist, Midland Centre for Neurosurgery and Neurology, West Midlands, UK
7.10.31 HTLV-I and -II associated diseases

SUCHITRA NIMMANNITYA

Consultant Paediatrician, Children's Hospital, Bangkok, Thailand
7.10.20 Dengue haemorrhagic fever

D.J. NOLAN

Consultant Radiologist, John Radcliffe Hospital, Oxford, UK
14.3.2 Methods for investigation of gastrointestinal disease: radiology

G. NUKI

Professor of Rheumatology, Department of Medicine, University of Edinburgh; Consultant Rheumatologist, Western General Hospital and Royal Infirmary of Edinburgh, UK
11.5 Disorders of purine and pyrimidine metabolism

R.E. O'HEHIR

Academic Head of Allergy and Clinical Immunology, St Mary's Hospital Medical School, London, UK
5.2 Immune mechanisms of disease

J.D. ORIEL

Formerly Consultant Physician in Genito-Urinary Medicine, University College Hospital, London, UK
21.7 Genital warts

D. OVERBOSCH

Consultant Physician, Department of Internal Medicine and Imported Tropical Medicine, Red Cross Hospital, The Hague, The Netherlands
7.15.3 Cysticercosis

S.M. OXBURY

Consultant Clinical Neuropsychologist, Radcliffe Infirmary, Oxford, UK
24.3.1 Disturbances of higher cerebral function

J.M. OXBURY

Consultant Neurologist, Radcliffe Infirmary, Oxford, UK
24.3.1 Disturbances of higher cerebral function

S. PARISH

Senior Research Fellow, Clinical Trial Service Unit, Nuffield Department of Clinical Medicine, University of Oxford, UK
2.4 Large-scale randomized evidence: trials and overviews

J.R. PATTISON

Professor of Medical Microbiology, University College London Medical School, UK
7.10.25 Parvoviruses

J. PAUL

Senior Registrar, Public Health Laboratory, John Radcliffe Hospital, Oxford, UK
7.11.46 'Newer' and lesser known bacteria causing infection in humans
7.17 Non-venomous arthropods

J. PAYAN

Consultant in Clinical Neurophysiology to Guy's and King's College Hospitals and the Hospital for Sick Children, London, UK
24.2.5 Electrophysiological investigation of the peripheral nervous system

I. PEAKE

Professor of Molecular Medicine, University of Sheffield, UK
22.6.4 The pathogenesis of genetic disorders of coagulation

J.M.S. PEARCE

Honorary Consultant Neurologist, Hull Royal Infirmary, Hull, UK
24.11 Headache

A.D. PEARSON

Senior Lecturer in Microbiology and Public Health Medicine; Clinical Director, Infection Control Department, St Thomas's Hospital, London, UK
7.11.17(a) Tularaemia (b) Pasteurellosis. (c) Yersiniosis

P.E. PELLETT

Chief, Herpesvirus Section, Centers for Disease Control and Prevention, Atlanta, Georgia, USA
7.10.7 Human herpesvirus 6

M.E. PEMBREY

Professor of Paediatric Genetics, Institute of Child Health, University of London, UK
4.3 Genetic factors in disease

M.B. PEPYS

Professor of Immunological Medicine, Royal Postgraduate Medical School, Hammersmith Hospital, London, UK
11.13.1 Amyloidosis
11.13.3 The acute phase response and C-reactive protein

S. PEREIRA

Research Fellow in Gastroenterology, United Medical Schools of St Thomas's and Guy's Hospitals, Guy's Campus, London, UK
14.9.3 Small-bowel bacterial overgrowth

B.A. PERKINS

Medical Epidemiologist, Childhood and Respiratory Diseases Branch, Centers for Disease Control and Prevention, Atlanta, Georgia, USA
7.11.41 Cat scratch disease, bacillary angiomatosis, and trench fever

P.L. PERRINE

Professor of Epidemiology, School of Public and Community Medicine, University of Washington, Seattle, USA
7.11.33 Non-venereal treponemes: yaws, endemic syphilis, and pinta
7.11.43 Lymphogranuloma venereum

C.J. PETERS

Chief, Special Pathogens Branch, Centers for Disease Control and Prevention, Atlanta, Georgia, USA
7.10.5 Human infections caused by simian herpesviruses

T.J. PETERS

Professor of Clinical Biochemistry, King's College; Consultant Physician and Chemical Pathologist, King's College Hospital, London, UK
28.2.3(a) Physical complications of alcohol misuse

R. PETO

Professor of Medical Statistics and Epidemiology, ICRF Cancer Studies Unit, Radcliffe Infirmary, Oxford, UK
2.4 Large-scale randomized evidence: trials and overviews
6.2 Epidemiology of cancer

T.E.A. PETO

Consultant Physician, Infectious Diseases, John Radcliffe Hospital, Oxford, UK
7.10.2 Herpes simplex virus infections
7.10.3 Varicella-zoster infections: chickenpox and zoster
7.10.9 Orf
7.10.10 Molluscum contagiosum
7.10.29 HIV infection and AIDS
17.6.3 Microbiological methods in the diagnosis of respiratory infections

R.K.H. PETTY

Lecturer in Neurology and Neurovirology, Institute of Neurological Sciences, University of Glasgow, UK
24.15.3 Neurological manifestations of infection with human immunodeficiency virus type 1

P.A. PHILIP

Senior Registrar in Medical Oncology, ICRF Clinical Oncology Unit, Churchill Hospital, Oxford, UK
13.15 Malignant disease in pregnancy

PRIDA PHUAPRADIT

Professor of Neurology, Division of Neurology, Department of Medicine, Ramathibodi Hospital, Mahidol University, Bangkok, Thailand
24.15 Bacterial meningitis

M.J. PIPPARD

Professor of Haematology, Ninewells Hospital and Medical School, University of Dundee, UK
22.4.4 Iron metabolism and its disorders

J.M. POLAK

Professor of Endocrine Pathology, Royal Postgraduate Medical School, Hammersmith Hospital, London, UK
14.8 Hormones and the gastrointestinal tract

P.A. POOLE-WILSON

Professor of Cardiology, National Heart and Lung Institute; Honorary Physician, Royal Brompton Hospital, London, UK
15.1 Cardiovascular disease: physiological considerations: biochemistry and cellular physiology of heart muscle
15.5 The treatment of heart failure

J.S. PORTERFIELD

Formerly Reader in Bacteriology, Sir William Dunn School of Pathology, University of Oxford, UK
7.10.21 Bunyaviridae

R.E. POUNDER

Professor of Medicine, Royal Free Hospital School of Medicine, University of London, UK
14.7 Peptic ulceration

M.A. PREECE

Professor of Child Health and Growth, Institute of Child Health, University of London, UK
12.9.2 Normal growth and its disorders

E.W. PRICE*

Research Fellow, Department of Clinical and Tropical Medicine, London School of Hygiene and Tropical Medicine, London, UK
8.5.5(h) Podoconiosis (non-filarial endemic elephantiasis of the lower legs)

J.S. PRICHARD

Professor of Medicine, St James's Hospital, Dublin, Eire
15.22.7 The pulmonary circulation in health and disease
15.23 Pulmonary oedema
15.24 Pulmonary hypertension
15.25 Cor pulmonale

N.B. PRIDE

Professor of Respiratory Medicine, Royal Postgraduate Medical School, Hammersmith Hospital, London, UK
17.6.2 Tests of ventilatory mechanics
17.9.4 Chronic obstructive pulmonary disease

J. PRITCHARD

Senior Lecturer in Paediatric Oncology, Institute of Child Health and Consultant, Hospital for Sick Children, Great Ormond Street, London, UK
22.5.6 The histiocytoses

A.T. PROUDFOOT

Consultant Physician, Royal Infirmary of Edinburgh NHS Trust; Director, Scottish, Poisons Information Bureau, Edinburgh, UK
8.1 Poisoning: introduction and epidemiology
8.1.2 Poisoning: clinical and metabolic features and general principles of management
8.2.1 Poisoning caused by analgesic drugs
8.2.2 Poisoning from antidepressants, hypnotics, antihistamines, anticonvulsants, and antiparkinsonian drugs
8.2.3 Poisoning from cardiovascular drugs
8.2.4 Poisoning caused by respiratory drugs
8.2.5 Poisoning caused by drugs acting on the gastrointestinal system
8.2.6 Poisoning by haematinics and vitamins
8.2.7 Poisoning by endocrine drugs
8.2.8 Poisoning from antimicrobials
8.2.10 Poisoning from drugs of abuse
8.2.11 Poisoning due to miscellaneous drugs
8.3.1 Poisoning from household products
8.3.2 Poisoning by alcohols and glycols
8.3.3 Poisoning from hydrocarbons and chlorofluorocarbons
8.3.4 Poisoning by inhalational agents
8.3.5 Poisoning due to corrosive substances
8.3.8 Pesticides

---

* It is with regret that we report the deaths of those authors marked with an asterisk. Although their deaths occurred between the appearance of the second edition and preparation of the third edition, much of their contribution to the former has been incorporated into this edition, with appropriate updating from their coauthors.

B.A. PRUITT

Commander and Director, US Army Institute of Surgical Research, Fort Sam Houston, Texas, USA

8.5.5(g) Environmental factors and disease: lightning and electric shock

SWANGJAI PUNGPAK

Associate Professor of Clinical Tropical Medicine, Mahidol University, Bangkok, Thailand

7.16.2 Liver fluke diseases in man

SOMPONE PUNYAGUPTA

President and Chairman, Department of Medicine, Vichaiyut Hospital, Bangkok, Thailand

7.14.8 Angiostrongyliasis

C.D. PUSEY

Reader in Renal Medicine, Royal Postgraduate Medical School, Hammersmith Hospital, London, UK

20.4.3 Rapidly progressive glomerulonephritis and antiglomerular basement membrane disease

N.P. QUINN

Reader in Clinical Neurology, Institute of Neurology, London, UK

24.3.3 Subcortical structures—the cerebellum, thalamus, and basal ganglia

A.J. RADFORD

Professor of Primary Health Care, Flinders University of South Australia

7.15.1 Hydatid disease
7.17 Non-venomous arthropods

PRAYONG RADOMYOS

Associate Professor of Parasitology, Bangkok School of Tropical Medicine, Faculty of Tropical Medicine, Mahidol University, Bangkok, Thailand

7.16.4 Intestinal trematodiasis

A.E.G. RAINE

Professor of Renal Medicine, St Bartholomew's Hospital Medical College, London, UK

15.6.1 Diuretics
15.28.1 Renal and renovascular hypertension
20.11 Hypertension: its effects on the kidney

A.C. RANKIN

Senior Lecturer in Medical Cardiology, Glasgow Royal Infirmary, UK

15.8.1 Cardiac arrhythmias

P.J. RATCLIFFE

University Lecturer and Honorary Consultant Physician, Nuffield Department of Medicine, Oxford, UK

20.17.3 Renal transplantation

C.W.G. REDMAN

Professor of Obstetric Medicine, Nuffield Department of Obstetrics and Gynaecology, John Radcliffe Hospital, Oxford, UK

13.2 Hypertension in pregnancy
13.3 Renal disease in pregnancy

A.J. REES

Regius Professor of Medicine, University of Aberdeen; Honorary Consultant Physician, Aberdeen Royal Hospitals, UK

20.4.3 Rapidly progressive glomerulonephritis and antiglomerular basement membrane disease

D. RENNIE

Professor of Medicine, Institute for Health Policy Studies, University of California, San Francisco, USA

8.5.5(d) Environmental factors and disease: diseases of high terrestrial altitudes

J. RICHENS

Clinical Lecturer, University College London Medical School, UK

7.11.8 Typhoid and paratyphoid fevers
7.11.9 Rhinoscleroma
7.11.45 Donovanosis (granuloma inguinale)

B.K. RIMA

Professor of Molecular Biology, School of Biology and Biochemistry, The Queen's University of Belfast, UK

7.10.11 Mumps: epidemic parotitis

E. RITZ

Professor of Medicine and Head of the Division of Nephrology, Ruperto Carola University of Heidelberg, Germany

20.5.1 Diabetic nephropathy

I.A.G. ROBERTS

Senior Lecturer and Honorary Consultant in Haematology, Royal Postgraduate Medical School, Hammersmith Hospital, London, UK

22.3.4 Acute lymphoblastic leukaemia

A.R. RONALD

Associate Dean, Research University of Manitoba; Director of Infectious Diseases, St Boniface Hospital, Winnipeg, Canada

7.11.13 Haemophilus ducreyi and chancroid

R.J.M. ROSS

Senior Lecturer in Endocrinology, Northern General Hospital, Sheffield, UK

12.9.3 Puberty

R.W. ROSS RUSSELL

Consultant Physician, St Thomas's Hospital, National Hospital of Neurology and Neurosurgery, and Moorfields Eye Hospital, London, UK

24.3.4 Visual pathways

M.N. ROSSOR

Consultant Neurologist, National Hospital for Neurology and Neurosurgery and St Mary's Hospital, London, UK

24.7.2 Alzheimer's disease

D.J. ROWLANDS

Consultant Cardiologist, Royal Infirmary, Manchester, UK

15.4.2 The electrocardiogram
15.4.4 Nuclear techniques

M.B. RUBENS

Consultant Radiologist, Royal Brompton Hospital, London and Honorary Senior Lecturer, National Heart and Lung Institute, University of London, UK

15.4.1 Chest radiography in heart disease

P.C. RUBIN

Professor of Therapeutics, University of Nottingham; Consultant Physician, University Hospital, Birmingham, UK

13.16 Prescribing in pregnancy

P. RUDGE

Consultant Neurologist, National Hospital for Neurology and Neurosurgery, London, UK
24.3.5 The eighth cranial nerve

T.K. RUEBUSH

Chief, Malaria Section, Division of Parasitic Diseases, Centers for Disease Control and Prevention, Atlanta, Georgia, USA
7.13.3 Babesia

R.C.G. RUSSELL

Consultant Surgeon, The Middlesex Hospital, London, UK
14.23.3 Tumours of the pancreas

T.J. RYAN

Clinical Professor of Dermatology, Oxford Radcliffe Trust, UK
23 Diseases of the skin

D.L. SACKETT

Professor of Clinical Epidemiology and Director, Centre for Evidence-Based Medicine, University of Oxford, UK
2.3 Evaluation of clinical method

P.J. SANSONETTI

Professeur à l'Institut Pasteur, Chef de l'Unite de Pathogenie Microbienne Moleculaire and INSERM U389, Institut Pasteur, Paris, France
7.2.1 Introduction to the diversity of bacterial pathogens
7.2.2 Molecular taxonomy of bacterial pathogens

M.O. SAVAGE

Reader in Paediatric Endocrinology, St Bartholomew's Hospital, London, UK
12.9.1 Normal and abnormal sexual differentiation
12.9.3 Puberty

G.F. SAVIDGE

Director, Haemophilia Reference Centre, St Thomas's Hospital, London, UK
22.6.5 Clinical features and management of the hereditary disorders of haemostasis

J.W. SCADDING

Consultant Neurologist, The National Hospital for Neurology and Neurosurgery, London, UK
24.5 Pain: pathophysiology and treatment

K.P. SCHAAL

Professor and Director, Institutes of Medical Microbiology and Immunology, University of Bonn, Germany
7.11.27 Actinomycoses

R.B.H. SCHUTGENS

Associate Professor and Clinical Chemist, Department of Paediatrics, University of Amsterdam, The Netherlands
11.9 Peroxisomal disorders

T.G. SCHWAN

Acting Head, Arthropod-borne Diseases Section, Laboratory of Vectors and Pathogens, National Institutes of Health, Rocky Mountain Laboratories, Hamilton, Montana, USA
7.11.30 Lyme disease

J. SCHWEBKE

Assistant Professor of Medicine, University of Alabama at Birmingham, USA
21.4 Vaginal discharge

J. SCOTT

Professor of Medicine, Royal Postgraduate Medical School, Hammersmith Hospital, London, UK
15.9.1 The pathogenesis of atherosclerosis

D.G.I. SCOTT

Consultant Rheumatologist, Norfolk and Norwich Health Care Trust, UK
18.11.1 Connective tissue diseases: introduction

A. SEATON

Professor of Environmental and Occupational Medicine, University of Aberdeen Medical School, UK
17.10.16 Pneumoconioses

A.W. SEGAL

Charles Dent Professor of Medicine, The Rayne Institute, University College London Medical School, UK
22.5.1 Leucocytes in health and disease

M.H. SEIFERT

Consultant Rheumatologist and Honorary Clinical Senior Lecturer in Medicine, St Mary's Hospital Medical School, London, UK
18.9 Septic arthritis

G.R. SERJEANT

Director, MRC Laboratories (Jamaica), University of the West Indies, Kingston, Jamaica
20.5.7 Renal manifestations of systemic disease: sickle-cell disease

C.A. SEYMOUR

Professor of Clinical Biochemistry and Metabolism and Honorary Consultant Physician, St George's Hospital Medical School, University of London, UK
11.7 Trace metal disorders
14.22 Hereditary disease of the liver and pancreas

K.V. SHAH

Professor of Immunology and Infectious Diseases, Johns Hopkins University School of Hygiene and Public Health, Baltimore, Maryland, USA
7.10.24 Papovaviruses

M. SHARPE

Clinical Tutor in Psychiatry, Oxford University, UK
7.19.4 Chronic fatigue syndrome (postviral fatigue syndrome and myalgic encephalomyelitis)

R.J. SHAW

Senior Lecturer and Consultant Physician in Respiratory Medicine, St Mary's Hospital Medical School, London, UK
17.10.4 The lung in collagen–vascular diseases
17.10.11 Pulmonary histiocytosis X (eosinophilic granuloma of the lung) and lymphangiomatosis
17.10.21 Lung disorders in genetic syndromes

M.C. SHEPPARD

Professor of Medicine, University of Birmingham, UK
12.5 Thyroid cancer

J.M. SHNEERSON

Director, Respiratory Support and Sleep Centre, Papworth Hospital, Cambridge, UK

17.12 Disorders of the thoracic cage and diaphragm

M. SIEBELS

Department of Internal Medicine, Division of Nephrology, University of Heidelberg, Germany

20.5.1 Diabetic nephropathy

C.A. SIEFF

Associate Professor in Pediatrics, Harvard Medical School and Dana Farber Cancer Institute; Senior Associate in Medicine, Children's Hospital, Boston, Massachusetts, USA

22.2.1 Stem cells and haematopoiesis

H.A. SIMMONDS

Senior Lecturer, Purine Research Laboratory, United Medical Schools of Guy's and St Thomas's Hospitals, London Bridge, UK

20.9.2 Gout, purines, and interstitial nephritis

I.A. SIMPSON

Consultant Cardiologist, Southampton General Hospital, UK

15.4.3 Doppler echocardiography

D.I.H. SIMPSON

Professor of Microbiology, Department of Microbiology and Immunology, Queen's University of Belfast, UK

7.10.17 Alphaviruses
7.10.23 Filoviruses: Marburg and Ebola fevers

V. SITPRIJA

Professor and Chairman, Department of Medicine, Chulalongkorn University; Director of Queen Saovabha Memorial Institute, Thai Red Cross, Bangkok, Thailand

7.11.32 Leptospirosis

M.B. SKIRROW

Honorary Emeritus Consultant Microbiologist, Public Health Laboratory, Gloucester Royal Hospital, UK

7.11.7 Enterobacteria and miscellaneous enteropathogenic and food-poisoning bacteria

P. SLEIGHT

Field Marshal Alexander Professor Emeritus of Cardiovascular Medicine, John Radcliffe Hospital, Oxford, UK

15.10.4 Myocardial infarction

R. SMITH

Consultant Physician and Consultant in Metabolic Medicine, John Radcliffe Hospital and Nuffield Orthopaedic Centre, Oxford, UK

10.1 Nutrition: introduction
10.2 Nutrition: biochemical background
11.6 Metabolic effects of accidental injury and surgery
19 Disorders of the skeleton

G.L. SMITH

Reader in Bacteriology, Sir William Dunn School of Pathology, University of Oxford, UK

7.10.8 Poxviruses

D.H. SMITH

Senior Lecturer and Honorary Consultant Physician in Tropical Medicine; Head of Division of Tropical Medicine, Liverpool School of Tropical Medicine, UK

7.13.10 Human African trypanosomiasis

M.L. SNAITH

Senior Lecturer in Rheumatic Diseases, Section of Rheumatology, University of Sheffield Medical School, UK

18.11.3 Systemic lupus erythematosus and related disorders

J. SOMERVILLE

Consultant Physician for Congenital Diseases, Cardiology Directorate, Royal Brompton Hospital, London, UK

15.15 Congenital heart disease in adolescents and adults

R.L. SOUHAMI

Kathleen Ferrier Professor of Clinical Oncology, University College London Medical School, UK

6.6 Cancer: clinical features and management

B.A. SOUTHGATE

Senior Lecturer in Tropical Disease Epidemiology, London School of Hygiene and Tropical Medicine, University of London, UK

7.14.2 Lymphatic filariasis

S.G. SPIRO

Consultant Physician, University College Hospitals London Trust, UK

17.13.1(a) Lung cancer. (b) Pulmonary metastases

C.J.F. SPRY

B.H.F. Professor of Cardiovascular Immunology, St George's Hospital Medical School, University of London, UK

15.4.3 The hypereosinophilic syndrome and the heart
22.5.7 The white cells and lymphoproliferative disorders: the hypereosinophilic syndrome

A. SPURGEON

Lecturer in Occupational Health Psychology, Institute of Occupational Health, University of Birmingham, UK

8.5.3(k) The main occupational disorders: neuropsychological disorders

S. STAGNO

Katharine Reynolds Ireland Professor and Chairman, Department of Pediatrics, University of Alabama, Birmingham, USA

7.10.6 Cytomegalovirus

J.C. STEVENSON

Director, Wynn Institute for Metabolic Research; Honorary Senior Lecturer, National Heart and Lung Institute, University of London; Honorary Consultant Physician, Royal Brompton Hospital, London, UK

13.17 Benefits and risks of hormone therapy

J.A. STEWART

Chief, Clinical Virology Section, Centers for Disease Control and Prevention, Atlanta, Georgia, USA

7.10.7 Human herpesvirus 6

J.H. STEWART

Professor in Medicine and Associate Dean, Western Clinical School, University of Sydney, Australia

20.9.1 Kidney disease from analgesics and non-steroidal anti-inflammatory drugs

R.A. STOCKLEY

Reader in Respiratory Medicine, Queen Elizabeth Hospital, Edgbaston, Birmingham, UK

17.9.3 Bronchiectasis
17.9.4 Chronic obstructive pulmonary disease

J.R. STRADLING

Consultant Physician, Oxford Radcliffe Trust (Churchill), Oxford, UK
17.2.2 The upper respiratory tract
17.8.2 Upper airways obstruction
17.14.2 Sleep-related disorders of breathing

J. STRANG

Professor and Director, Addiction Research Unit, National Addiction Centre, The Maudsley/Institute of Psychiatry, London, UK
28 Alcohol and drug-related problems: introduction
28.1.2 Assessing substance use and misuse
28.2.2 Harm reduction
28.3.2 The management of substance-related problems in a general ward
28.3.3 Drugs and the law
28.3.8 Caring for the HIV-positive drug user

P.R. STUDDY

Consultant Physician, Harefield Hospital NHS Trust and Mount Vernon and Watford Hospitals Trust, Hertfordshire, UK
17.10.10 Sarcoidosis

P.H. SUGDEN

Reader in Biochemistry, Department of Cardiac Medicine, National Heart and Lung Institute, University of London, UK
15.1 Cardiovascular disease: physiological considerations: biochemistry and cellular physiology of heart muscle

J.A. SUMMERFIELD

Professor of Experimental Medicine, St Mary's Hospital Medical School, Imperial College London, UK
14.21 Congenital disorders of the biliary tract and pancreas
14.24 Diseases of the gallbladder and biliary tree

PRAVAN SUNTHARASAMAI

Associate Professor, Department of Clinical Tropical Medicine, Mahidol University, Bangkok, Thailand
7.14.9 Gnathostomiasis

R. SUTTON

Consultant Cardiologist and Director of Pacing and Electrophysiology, Royal Brompton Hospital, London, UK
15.3.5 Syncope and palpitation
15.8.2 Pacemakers

J.D. SWALES

Professor of Medicine, University of Leicester, UK
15.27 Essential hypertension

R.H. SWANTON

Consultant Cardiologist, University College London, UK
15.4.6 Cardiac catheterization
15.10.3 Angina and unstable angina

D.M. SWIRSKY

Senior Lecturer in Haematology, Royal Postgraduate Medical School; Honorary Consultant, Hospital, London, UK
22.5.4 The spleen and its disorders

D.A. TABERNER

Clinical Director, Thrombosis Reference Centre, University Hospital of South Manchester, UK
22.6.7 Thrombotic disease

I.C. TALBOT

Consultant Pathologist, St Mark's Hospital, London, UK
14.16 Tumours of the gastrointestinal tract

C.R. TAYLOR

Charles P. Lyman Professor of Biology, Harvard University, Cambridge, Massachusetts, USA
17.2.1 Functional anatomy of the human lung

D. TAYLOR-ROBINSON

Professor of Genitourinary Microbiology and Medicine, St Mary's Hospital Medical School, Paddington, London, UK
7.11.41 Chlamydial infections
7.11.43 Mycoplasmas

G.M. TEASDALE

Professor of Neurosurgery, Institute of Neurological Sciences, University of Glasgow, UK
24.14 Head injuries

P.J. TEDDY

Consultant Neurosurgeon, The Radcliffe Infirmary, Oxford, UK
24.12 Intracranial tumours
24.15.4 Intracranial abscess

H.J. TESTA

Consultant in Nuclear Medicine, Royal Infirmary, Manchester, UK
15.4.4 The clinical assessment of cardiovascular function: nuclear techniques

A.C. THOMAS

Senior Specialist and Consultant in Tissue Pathology, Institute of Medical and Veterinary Science, Adelaide, South Australia
20.4.1 IgA nephropathy, Henoch-Schönlein purpura, and thin membrane nephropathy

P.K. THOMAS

Emeritus Professor of Neurology, Royal Free Hospital School of Medicine and Institute of Neurology, London, UK
24.3.6 Neurology: organization and features of dysfunction; other cranial nerves
24.8 Neurology: inherited disorders
24.17 Peripheral neuropathy

H.C. THOMAS

Professor of Medicine, St Mary's Hospital Medical School, Imperial College of Science, Technology and Medicine; Consultant Physician and Hepatologist, St Mary's Hospital, London, UK
14.26 Clinical features of viral hepatitis

J.E.P. THOMAS

Formerly Professor of Medicine, University of Zimbabwe, Harare, Zimbabwe
7.16.1 Schistosomiasis

D.G. THOMPSON

Senior Lecturer in Medicine and Consultant Physician, Hope Hospital, Salford, UK
14.2.5 Constipation
14.13 Functional bowel disease and irritable bowel syndrome

M.O. THORNER

Kenneth R. Crispell Professor of Medicine; Chief, Division of Endocrinology and Metabolism, University of Virginia School of Medicine, Charlottesville, USA
12.2 Anterior pituitary disorders

A.J. THRASHER
Honorary Lecturer and Wellcome Training Fellow, University College London Medical School, UK
22.5.1 Leucocytes in health and disease

P. THULLIEZ
Head, Laboratoire de la Toxoplasmose, Institut de Puériculture de Paris, France
7.13.4 Toxoplasmosis

P. TOOKEY
Research Fellow, Department of Epidemiology and Biostatistics, Institute of Child Health, London, UK
7.10.18 Rubella

P.P. TOSKES
Professor and Associate Chairman for Clinical Affairs; Director, Division of Gastroenterology, Hepatology and Nutrition, Department of Medicine, University of Florida College of Medicine, Gainsville, USA
14.23.2 Chronic pancreatitis

T.A. TRAILL
Associate Professor of Medicine, Johns Hopkins University School of Medicine, Baltimore, Maryland, USA
15.19 Cardiac myxoma

D.F. TREACHER
Consultant Physician, Department of Intensive Care, St Thomas's Hospital, London, UK
16 Intensive care

T. TREASURE
Consultant Cardiothoracic Surgeon, St George's Hospital, London, UK
15.10.6 Coronary artery bypass grafting

G.S. TREGENZA
Associate Specialist, Division of Addictive Behavior, St George's Hospital Medical School, University of London, UK
28.3.5 Drug misusers and addicts in accident and emergency

J.D. TREHARNE
Reader in Virology, Institute of Ophthalmology, University of London, UK
7.11.41 Chlamydial infections

SIR LESLIE TURNBERG
Section of Gastroenterology, Hope Hospital, Salford, Lancashire, UK
14.2.4 Diarrhoea

P.C.B. TURNBULL
Head, Anthrax Section, Centre for Applied Microbiology and Research, Porton Down, Salisbury, Wiltshire, UK
7.11.18 Anthrax

R.C. TURNER
Clinical Reader, Nuffield Department of Clinical Medicine, Diabetes Research Laboratories, Radcliffe Infirmary, Oxford, UK
11.12 Hypoglycaemia

F.E. UDWADIA
Emeritus Professor of Medicine, Grant Medical College and J.J. Group of Hospitals; Consultant Physician, Breach Candy Hospital and Parsee General Hospital, Bombay, India
7.11.20 Tetanus

S.R. UNDERWOOD
Senior Lecturer in Cardiac Imaging, National Heart and Lung Institute; Honorary Consultant, Royal Brompton Hospital NHS Trust, London, UK
15.4.5 Magnetic resonance and computed X-ray tomography

C.G. URAGODA
Physician, Chest Hospital, Welisera; Course Director of Clinical Studies, Postgraduate Institute of Medicine, University of Colombo, Sri Lanka
7.11.23 Particular problems of tuberculosis in developing countries

J.A. VALE
Director, National Poisons Information Service (Birmingham Centre), West Midlands Poisons Unit, City Road Hospital, Birmingham; Senior Clinical Lecturer, University of Birmingham, UK
8.1.1 Poisoning: introduction and epidemiology
8.1.2 Poisoning: clinical and metabolic features and general principles of management
8.2.1 Poisoning caused by analgesic drugs
8.2.2 Poisoning from antidepressants, hypnotics, antihistamines, anticonvulsants, and antiparkinsonian drugs
8.2.3 Poisoning from cardiovascular drugs
8.2.4 Poisoning caused by respiratory drugs
8.2.5 Poisoning caused by drugs acting on the gastrointestinal system
8.2.6 Poisoning by haematinics and vitamins
8.2.7 Poisoning by endocrine drugs
8.2.8 Poisoning from antimicrobials
8.2.10 Poisoning from drugs of abuse
8.2.11 Poisoning due to miscellaneous drugs
8.3.1 Poisoning from household products
8.3.2 Poisoning from alcohols and glycols
8.3.3 Poisoning from hydrocarbons and chlorofluorocarbons, and volatile substance abuse
8.3.4 Poisoning by inhalational agents
8.3.5 Poisoning due to corrosive substances
8.3.6 Poisoning from metals
8.3.8 Pesticides

P. VALLANCE
Senior Lecturer and Honorary Consultant in Clinical Pharmacology, St George's Hospital Medical School, London, UK
15.9.2 Vascular endothelium, its physiology and pathophysiology

SIRIVAN VANIJANONTA
Associate Professor, Head, Department of Clinical Tropical Medicine, Faculty of Tropical Medicine, Mahidol University, Bangkok, Thailand
7.16.3 Lung flukes (paragonimiasis)

D.J.T. VAUX
Lecturer in Experimental Pathology, Sir William Dunn School of Pathology, University of Oxford, UK
4.2.2 Cell biology of organelles and the endomembrane system

P.J.W. VENABLES
Reader in Rheumatology, Charing Cross and Westminster Medical School; Consultant Rheumatologist; Charing Cross Hospital, London, UK
18.11.5 Sjögren's syndrome

M.P. VESSEY
Professor of Public Health, Department of Public Health and Primary Care, University of Oxford, UK
3.2 Health and sickness in the community
13.1 Benefits and risks of oral contraceptives

P.D. WAGNER
Professor of Medicine, University of California San Diego, La Jolla, California, USA
17.4 Pathophysiology of lung disease

D.H. WALKER
Professor and Chairman, Department of Pathology, University of Texas Medical Branch at Galveston, USA
7.11.37 Rickettsial diseases including the ehrlichioses

J.A. WALKER-SMITH
Professor of Paediatric Gastroenterology, Medical College of St Bartholomew's Hospital and Queen Elizabeth Hospital for Children, London, UK
14.15 Congenital abnormalities of the gastrointestinal tract

J.R.F WALTERS
Senior Lecturer, Gastroenterology Unit, Royal Postgraduate Medical School, Hammersmith Hospital, London, UK
14.9.1 Mechanisms of intestinal absorption

LORD WALTON OF DETCHANT
President, World Federation of Neurology; Former Professor of Neurology, University of Newcastle on Tyne; Honorary Consultant Neurologist, Oxford, UK
18.11.6 Polymyositis and dermatomyositis
25.1 Disorders of voluntary muscle: introduction
25.2 The muscular dystrophies
25.3 The floppy infant syndrome
25.4 Myotonic disorders
25.5 Inflammatory myopathies
25.6 Miscellaneous disorders (of voluntary muscle)

R.J.A. WANDERS
Senior Biochemist and Associate Professor, University Hospital Amsterdam, Academic Medical Centre, Amsterdam, The Netherlands
11.9 Peroxisomal disorders

C.P. WARLOW
Professor of Medical Neurology, University of Edinburgh, UK
24.6 Cerebrovascular disease

D.A. WARRELL
Professor of Tropical Medicine and Infectious Diseases, University of Oxford
7.8 Travel and expedition medicine
7.10.15 Rhabdoviruses: rabies and rabies-related viruses
7.10.16 Colorado tick fever and other arthropod-borne reoviruses
7.11.29 Rat bite fevers
7.11.31 Other Borrelia infections

7.11.44 Bartonellosis
7.13.2 Malaria
7.13.5 Cryptosporidium and cryptosporidiosis
7.18 Pentastomiasis (porocephalosis)
8.4.1 Injuries, envenoming, poisoning, and allergic reactions caused by animals
24.15.1 Bacterial meningitis
24.15.2 Acute viral infections of the central nervous system
25.10 Tropical pyomyositis (tropical myositis)

M.J. WARRELL
Clinical Virologist, Centre for Tropical Medicine and Infectious Diseases, John Radcliffe Hospital, Oxford, UK
7.10.15 Rhabdoviruses: rabies and rabies-related viruses
7.10.16 Colorado tick fever and other arthropod-borne reoviruses

J.A.H. WASS
Professor of Clinical Endocrinology, St Bartholomew's Hospital Medical College, London, UK
12.11 Endocrine manifestations of non-endocrine disease

M.F.R. WATERS
Consultant Leprologist, Hospital for Tropical Diseases, London; sometime Member of the Medical Research Council External Scientific Staff, Middlesex Hospital, London, UK
7.11.25 Leprosy (Hansen's disease, hanseniasis)
7.11.26 Mycobacterium ulcerans infection

G. WATT
Chief, Department of Medicine, AFRIMS, Bangkok, Thailand
7.11.38 Scrub typhus

R.W.E. WATTS
Royal Postgraduate Medical School Visting Professor and Honorary Consultant Physician, Hammersmith Hospital, London, UK
11.1 The inborn errors of metabolism: general aspects
11.8 Lysosomal storage diseases
11.10 Disorders of oxalate metabolism
20.9.3 Hypercalcaemic nephropathy
20.12.2 Urinary stone disease (urolithiasis)

SIR DAVID WEATHERALL
Regius Professor of Medicine and Honorary Director of the Institute of Molecular Medicine, University of Oxford, UK
2.1.2 Scientific method and the art of healing
4.1 Molecular biology and medicine
4.2.1 Medical applications of cell biology: introduction
15.26 Pulmonary embolism
22.1 Disorders of the blood: introduction
22.3.8 Polycythaemia vera
22.3.9 Myelosclerosis
22.3.10 Primary thrombocythaemia
22.4.1 Erythropoiesis and the normal red cell
22.4.2 Anaemia: pathophysiology, classification, and clinical features
22.4.5 Normochromic, normocytic anaemia
22.4.7 Disorders of the synthesis or function of haemoglobin
22.4.8 Other anaemias resulting from defective red cell maturation
22.4.9 Haemolytic anaemia: the mechanisms and consequences of a shortened red cell
22.4.11 Haemolysis due to red-cell enzyme deficiencies
22.4.14 The relative and secondary polycythaemias
22.7 The blood in systemic disease

A.D.B. WEBSTER

MRC Immunodeficiency Research Group, Royal Free Hospital Medical School, London, UK
5.3 Immunodeficiency

E.R. WEIBEL

Professor of Anatomy Emeritus, University of Bern, Switzerland
17.2.1 Functional anatomy of the lung

R.A. WEISS

Professor of Viral Oncology, Institute of Cancer Research, London, UK
7.10.27 Viruses and cancer
7.10.28 Human immunodeficiency viruses

I.V.D. WELLER

Professor and Head of the Academic Department of Genitourinary Medicine, University College London Medical School, UK
7.10.29 HIV infection and AIDS

L. WESTRÖM

Associate Professor of Obstetrics and Gynaecology, University of Lund, Sweden
21.5 Pelvic inflammatory disease

N.J. WHITE

Director, Wellcome-Mahidol University, Oxford Tropical Medicine Research Programme, Faculty of Tropical Medicine, Mahidol University, Bangkok, Thailand
9 Principles of clinical pharmacology and drug therapy

H.C. WHITTLE

Deputy Director, Medical Research Council Laboratories, The Gambia, West Africa
7.10.12 Measles

D.E.L. WILCKEN

Consultant Physician, The Prince Henry and Prince of Wales Hospitals, Sydney, Australia
15.2 Clinical physiology of the normal heart

P.J. WILKINSON

Consultant Medical Microbiologist and Director, Public Health Laboratory, University Hospital, Nottingham, UK
7.11.35 Listeria and listeriosis

D.G. WILLAMS

Professor of Medicine, United Medical and Dental Schools of Guy's and St Thomas's Hospitals, University of London, UK
20.5.2 Infections and associated nephropathies
20.5.6 Rheumatological disorders and the kidney

R.C. WILLIAMS

Chief Medical Officer, GKN plc, Redditch, Worcestershire, UK
8.5.5(j) Environmental factors and disease: noise

A.C. de C. WILLIAMS

Consultant Clinical Psychologist, INPUT Pain Management Unit, St Thomas's Hospital, London, UK
28.3.7 Management of pain in the drug abuser

R. WILLIAMS

Director, Institute of Liver Studies and Consultant Physician, King's College Hospital, London, UK
14.31 Liver transplantation

C.B. WILLIAMS

Consultant Physician in Gastrointestinal Endoscopy, St Mark's Hospital, Northwick Park, London, UK
14.16 Tumours of the gastrointestinal tract

D.H. WILLIAMSON

Medical Research Council, External Scientific Staff, Nuffield Department of Clinical Medicine, Oxford University, UK
10.2 Biochemical background

BRIGADIER GENERAL KYAW WIN

Director and Consultant Physician, Directorate of Medical Services, Ministry of Defence, Union of Myanmar
7.11.38 Scrub typhus

C.G. WINEARLS

Consultant Nephrologist, Churchill Hospital, Oxford, UK
20.16 Acute renal failure
20.17.1 Chronic renal failure

D.L. WINGATE

Professor of Gastrointestinal Science, London Hospital Medical College, University of London, UK
14.12 Disorders of motility

P.A. WINSTANLEY

Senior Lecturer in Clinical Pharmacology, Department of Pharmacology and Therapeutics, University of Liverpool, UK
8.2.9 Poisoning from cinchona alkaloids and other antimalarials

F. WOJNAROWSKA

Consultant Dermatologist and Senior Clinical Lecturer, Churchill Hospital, Oxford, UK
13.14 The skin in pregnancy

A.J. WOODROFFE

Renal Physician, Royal Adelaide Hospital, Australia
20.4.1 IgA nephropathy, Henoch-Schönlein purpura, and thin membrane nephropathy

H.F. WOODS

Sir George Franklin Professor of Medicine, University of Sheffield, UK
11.14 Disturbances of acid-base homeostasis

B.P. WORDSWORTH

Clinical Reader in Rheumatology, Nuffield Department of Clinical Medicine, University of Oxford, UK
18.4 Rheumatoid arthritis

V.M. WRIGHT

Consultant Paediatric Surgeon, Queen Elizabeth Hospital for Children and University College London Hospitals, London, UK
14.15 Congenital abnormalities of the gastrointestinal tract

D.J.M. WRIGHT

Reader in Medical Microbiology, Charing Cross and Westminster Medical School, London, UK
7.11.34 Syphilis

F.C.W. WU

Senior Lecturer, Department of Medicine, University of Manchester, UK
12.8.2 Disorders of male reproduction

M.A.S. YASUDA

Associate Professor, Department of Infectious and Parasitic Diseases, São Paulo University School of Medicine (USP), Brazil
7.12.4 Paracoccidioidomycosis

A. YOUNG

Professor of Geriatric Medicine, Royal Free Hospital School of Medicine, London, UK
30 Sports medicine

V. ZAMAN

Professor of Microbiology, Aga Khan University, Karachi, Pakistan
7.13.7 Sarcocystosis
7.13.9 Blastocystis hominis
7.14.6 Other gut nematodes
7.14.7 Toxocariasis and visceral larval migrans

A.J. ZUCKERMAN

Dean and Professor of Medical Microbiology and Director of the World Health Organization Collaborating Centre for Reference and Research on Viral Diseases, Royal Free Hospital School of Medicine, London, UK
7.10.26 Viral hepatitis

J.N. ZUCKERMAN

Clinical Research Fellow, Royal Free Hospital School of Medicine, London, UK
7.10.26 Viral hepatitis

Plates for Section 11
CHAPTER 11.6

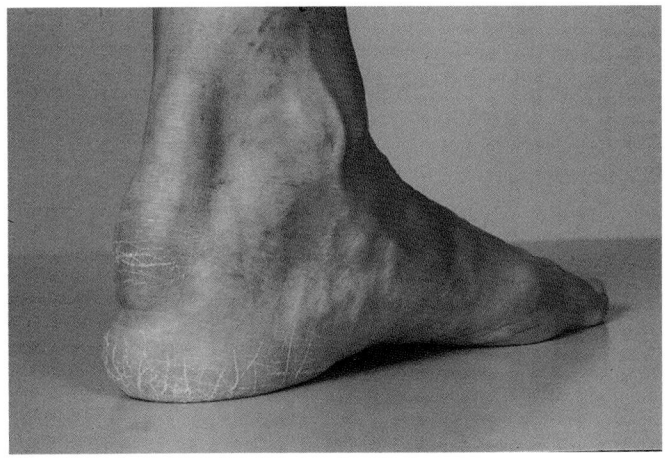

Plate 1 Achilles tendon xanthoma (heterozygous familial hypercholesterolaemia).

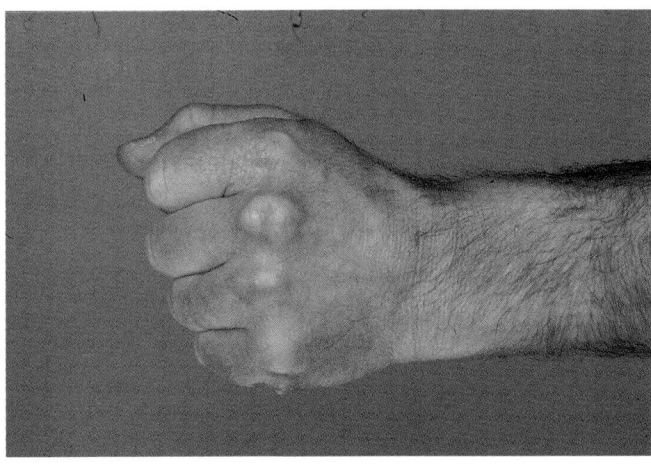

Plate 2 Tendon xanthomata on the dorsum of a hand (heterozygous familial hypercholesterolaemia).

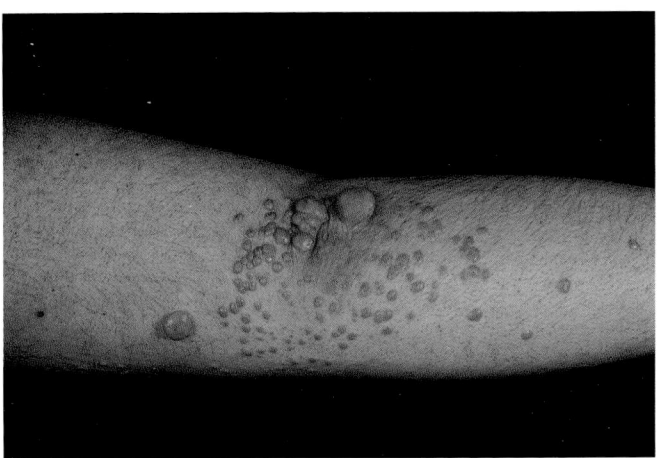

Plate 3 Eruptive and tuberose xanthomata on an arm (type III hyperlipoproteinaemia with marked hypertriglyceridaemia).

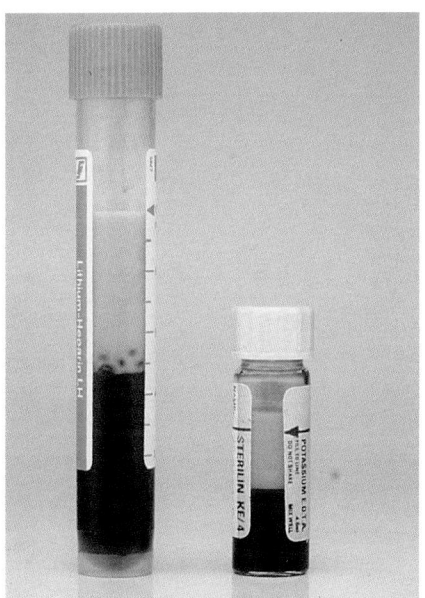

Plate 4 Milky plasma indicating marked hypertriglyceridaemia (blood samples from a patient with acute abdominal pain).

CHAPTER 11.7

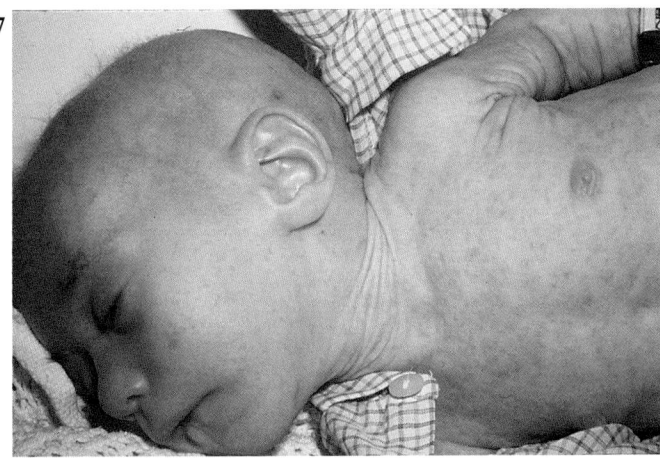

Plate 1 Appearance of Menkes disease.

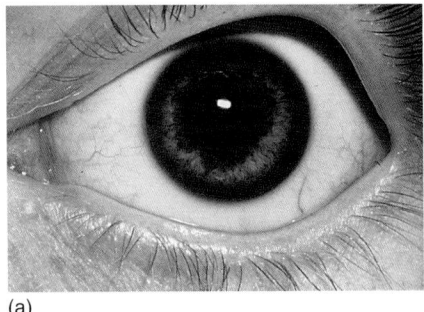
(a)

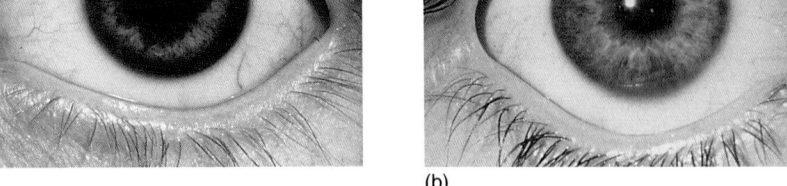

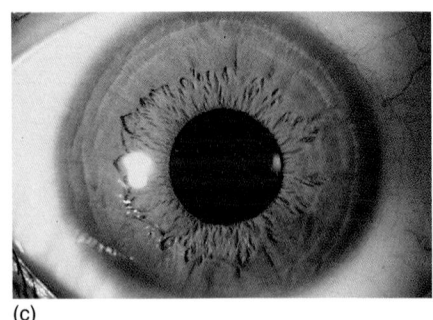
(b)

(c)

Plate 2 Kayser–Fleischer rings.

Plates For Section 12
CHAPTER 12.8.1

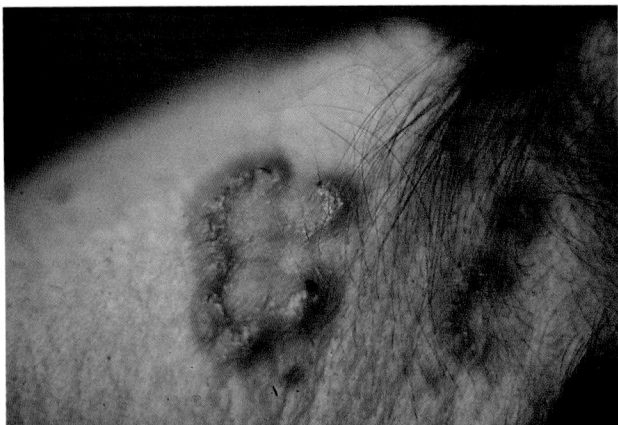

Plate 3 Penicillamine dermatopathy.

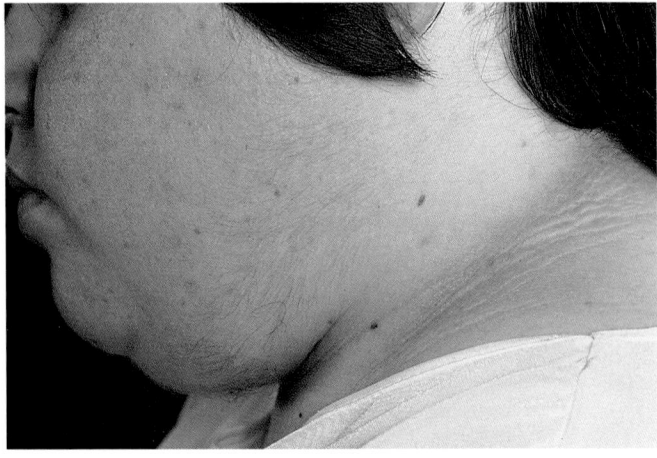

Plate 1 Acanthosis nigricans in a young woman with polycystic ovary syndrome.

CHAPTER 12.10

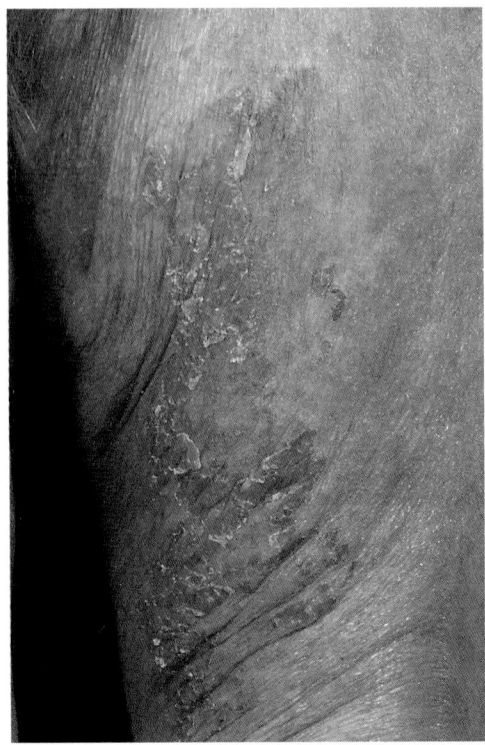

(a)

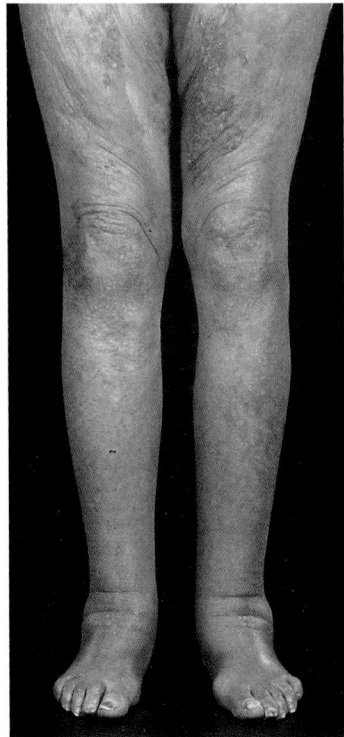

(b)

Plate 1 (a) Necrolytic migratory erythema in a patient with the glucagonoma syndrome. (b) Pigmentation in healed areas.

Plates for Section 13
CHAPTER 13.14

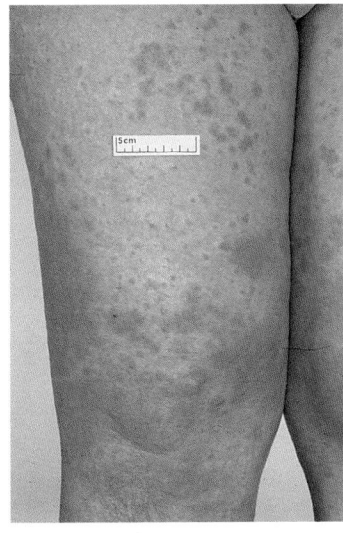

Plate 1 Polymorphic eruption of pregnancy: urticated papules and plaques on the thigh.

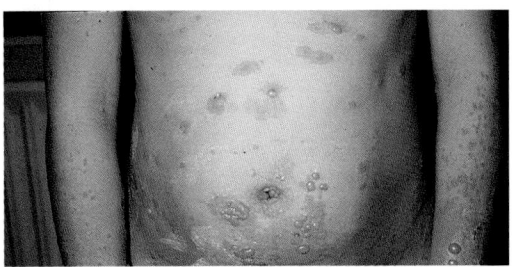

Plate 2 Pemphigoid gestationis: urticated papules and plaques and blisters, (reproduced with permission from Charles-Holmes and Black 1990).

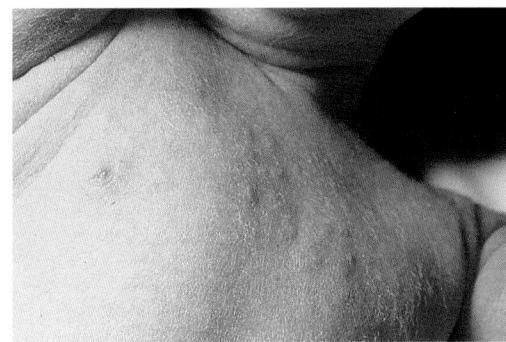

Plate 3 Pemphigoid gestationis: urticated papules in the neonate (reproduced with permission from Charles-Holmes and Black 1990).

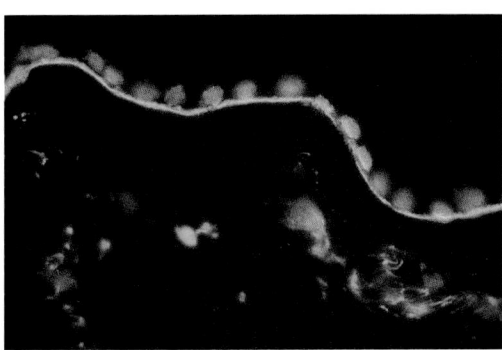

Plate 4 Pemphigoid gestationis: linear deposition of C3 at the amnion basement membrane zone as demonstrated by immunofluorescence. The nuclei are counterstained with propidium iodide. (Provided by B.S. Bhogal and M.M. Black, St John's Institute of Dermatology, St Thomas's Hospital, London.)

Plates for Section 14
CHAPTER 14.16

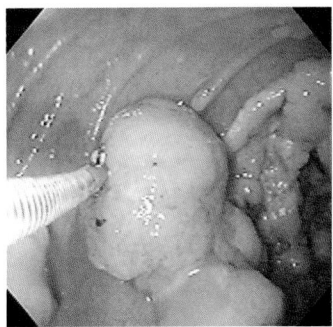

Plate 1 Duodenal adenomatous polyps in familial adenomatous polyposis.

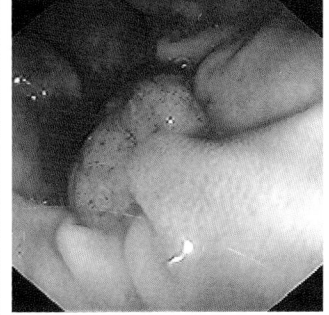

Plate 2 Stalked (pedunculated) benign adenoma in the colon.

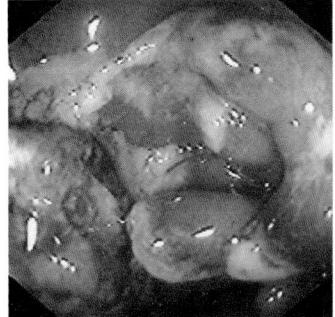

Plate 3 Multiple, inflamed-looking polyps in 'cap polyposis' of the distal sigmoid colon.

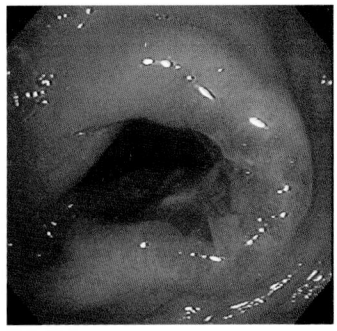

Plate 4 Tell-tale ulceration at the distal margin of a malignant stricture of the colon; note the raised edge of normal undermined mucosa.

CHAPTER 14.27.1

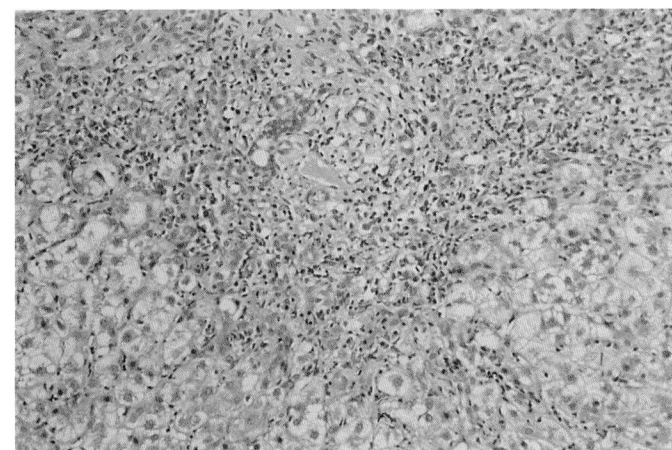

Plate 1 Section of liver biopsy from a patient with autoimmune hepatitis showing features of chronic active hepatitis, with dense lymphoplasmacytic infiltrate of the portal tract spreading into the periportal area with piecemeal necrosis of periportal hepatocytes and rosetting of regenerating liver cells.

Plates for Section 15
CHAPTER 15.4.3

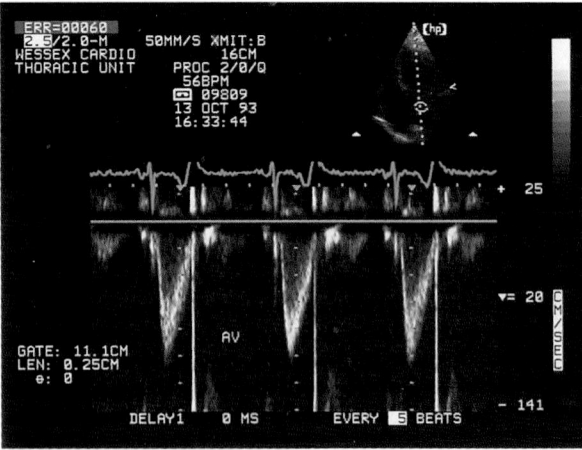

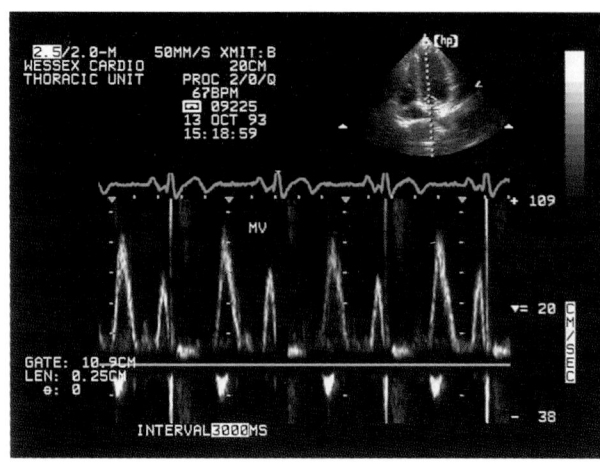

Plate 1 Spectral pulsed wave Doppler recording of normal aortic valve flow. Velocity information is seen during systole displayed below the zero velocity line. This indicates that flow is directed away from the ultrasound transducer which is located at the cardiac apex. The peak velocity is just over 1 m/s. Note that there is a rapid acceleration of flow in early systole with a narrow band on the spectral display, indicating laminar flow. The deceleration of flow in late systole is associated with a broader spectral signal indicating there is a wider range of velocities occurring at any given time. The bright thin line at end systole is due to aortic valve closure.

Plate 2 Spectral pulsed wave Doppler recording of normal mitral valve flow. Note the M-shaped appearance of normal mitral flow due to the initial peak velocity due to ventricular filling in early diastole and a second late diastolic peak resulting from atrial contraction. Unlike Plate 1, the spectral velocity information is above the zero velocity line, indicating flow towards the ultrasound transducer from the left atrium to the left ventricle. The peak velocity, occurring in early diastole is 0.9 m/s. Note also the narrow band of velocities throughout diastole indicating organized, laminar flow across the normal mitral valve.

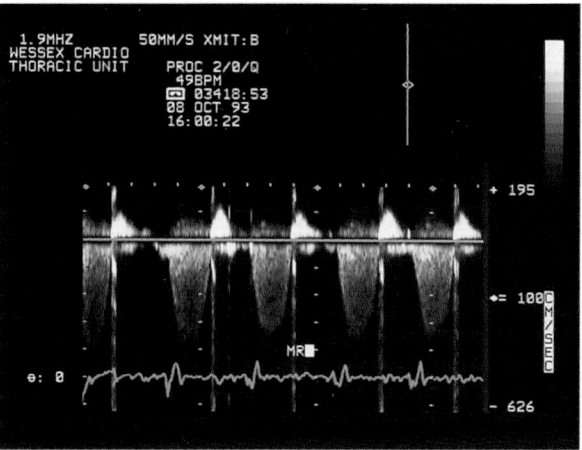

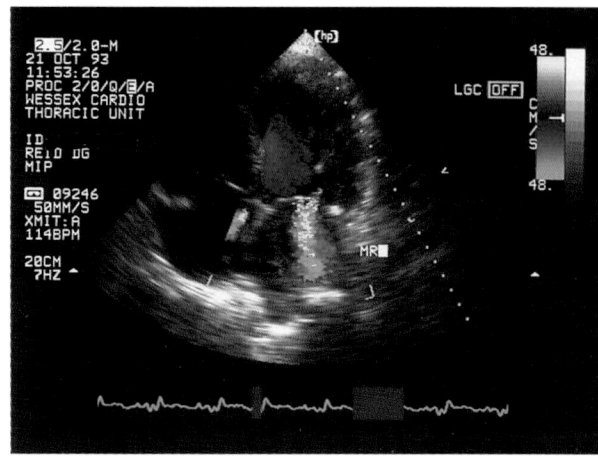

Plate 3 Spectral continuous wave Doppler recording of mitral regurgitation. The high velocity jet throughout systole is characteristic of mitral regurgitation. Here the signal is obtained from the cardiac apex and results in a display below the zero velocity line as flow is away from the ultrasound transducer into the left atrium. The peak velocity is around 4 m/s. Note the more intense signal of mitral inflow above the line with a peak velocity of around 1 m/s with the loss of the secondary peak due to the presence of atrial fibrillation.

Plate 4 Colour Doppler flow map image of mitral regurgitation visualized from the apical four-chamber view at the cardiac apex. The multicoloured jet is seen centrally in the left atrium originating at the level of the mitral valve. The variation in colour encoding is a function of the high velocity and turbulent nature of the regurgitant jet.

CHAPTER 15.13

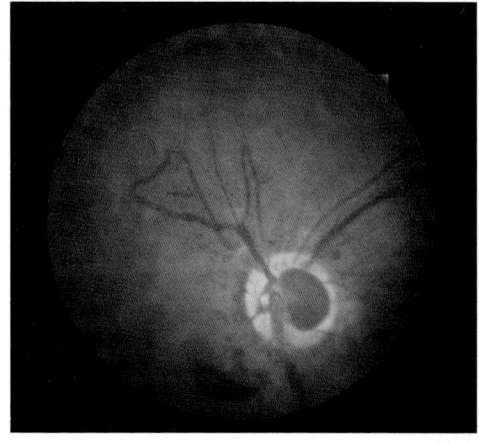

Plate 1 Fundus photograph of the left eye of a 32-year-old Japanese woman with Takayasu's disease in group III, but with inflammation suppressed by corticosteroid therapy. Note arteriovenous anastomoses (very severe Takayasu's retinopathy) on and around the disc and preretinal haemorrhages (reproduced from Ishikawa (1978), by permission of the American Heart Association, Inc.).

Section 11 *Metabolic disorders*

11.1	*The inborn errors of metabolism: general aspects*	1335
11.2	*Disorders of carbohydrate metabolism other than diabetes mellitus and hypoglycaemia*	1339
	11.2.1 Glycogen storage diseases	1339
	11.2.2 Inborn errors of fructose metabolism	1345
	11.2.3 Disorders of galactose metabolism	1349
11.3	*Inborn errors of amino acid and organic acid metabolism*	1352
11.4	*Disorders of purine and pyrimidine metabolism*	1376
11.5	*Porphyrin metabolism and the porphyrias*	1388
11.6	*Lipid and lipoprotein disorders*	1399
11.7	*Trace metal disorders*	1415
11.8	*Lysosomal storage diseases*	1426
11.9	*Peroxisomal disorders*	1438
11.10	*Disorders of oxalate metabolism*	1444
11.11	*Diabetes mellitus*	1448
11.12	*Hypoglycaemia*	1505
11.13	*Amyloid, familial Mediterranean fever, and acute phase response*	1512
	11.13.1 Amyloidosis	1512
	11.13.2 Recurrent polyserositis (familial Mediterranean fever, periodic disease)	1525
	11.13.3 The acute phase response and C-reactive protein	1527
11.14	*Disturbances of acid-base homeostasis*	1533
11.15	*α_1-Antitrypsin deficiency*	1545
11.16	*Metabolic effects of accidental injury and surgery*	1548

11.1 The inborn errors of metabolism: general aspects

R. W. E. WATTS

There are between three and four thousand known unifactorially inherited diseases (that is, familial diseases), the inheritance of which can be described as being autosomal recessive, autosomal dominant, sex-linked recessive, or sex-linked dominant. Inheritance of this type is sometimes referred to as Mendelian and results from mutations in the nuclear deoxyribonucleic acid (DNA). A small number of mitochondrial proteins have their structures encoded in the mitochondrial DNA. This genetic information is passed on from generation to generation in a non-Mendelian manner, being transmitted only through the female line. This arises because the spermatozoal cytoplasm, including its mitochondria, is entirely lost at fertilization. Lebar's optic atrophy shows such maternal transmission and is due to a mitochondrial mutation. Both the Mendelian and the mitochondrially inherited diseases all stem from single mutations within a cistron (the functional unit of DNA) which directs the synthesis of a single specific polypeptide. Among these inherited diseases, there are some (the inborn errors of metabolism) in which the mutation affects a protein with a metabolic function such that a characteristic clinical and biochemical pattern (phenotype) results, and in which the metabolic lesion (defective enzyme or enzyme activator protein) can be identified. The deficient, or occasionally overactive, enzyme catalytic activity leads to the phenotype by causing either lack of a metabolic product or the accumulation of intermediary metabolites, or by the opening up of alternative metabolic pathways. In some cases, the abnormal protein is a carrier responsible for translocating metabolites either across the cell plasma membrane or across the limiting membranes of subcellular organelles. Classic cystinuria, in which there is defective transport of cystine, lysine, ornithine, arginine, and homoarginine across the cells lining the proximal convoluted tubule of the kidney and the small intestine epithelium is an example of defective transport across plasma membranes. Cystinosis (cystine storage disease, Lignac's disease) is an example of a disease in which there is defective transport across a subcellular membrane, in this case, the lysosomal membrane, so that cystine produced by proteolysis within the lysosomes cannot pass out into the cytosol. Except for Salla disease, in which N-acetylneuraminic acid (sialic acid) cannot be transported out of the lysosomes, the other lysosomal storage diseases are due to deficient catalytic activity of lysosomal enzymes so that undegraded macromolecules, for example glycosaminoglycans (mucopolysaccharides) accumulate in these subcellular organelles. Inborn errors of metabolism due to enzyme deficiencies located in peroxisomes (Table 1) and mitochondria (Table 2) are also known. The processes whereby enzyme proteins move about within cells, from their site of synthesis on the rough endoplasmic reticulum to their final locations within specific organelles, may be defective. Thus, in one variant of GM_2 gangliosidosis (Tay-Sachs disease),* there is defective post-translational processing of the α-chain of β-N-acetylhexosaminidase (hexosaminidase-A). This prevents the enzyme migrating normally from the endoplasmic reticulum, where it is glycosylated, to the Golgi apparatus for phosphorylation of its mannosyl residue and

* The term GM_2-gangliosidosis is derived from the non-systematic chemical nomenclature introduced for the sialoglycosphingolipids (gangliosides). 'G' stands for ganglioside, 'M' indicates that the compound is monosialylated, and the arabic numeral indicates the position of the compound relative to the other gangliosides as separated in Svennerholm's (1963) thin layer chromatographic system.

Table 1 *Peroxisomal diseases*

Zellweger syndrome (absent peroxisomal membranes)
Pseudo-Zellweger syndrome
Adrenoleukodystrophy
Pseudoneonatal adrenoleukodystrophy
Acatalasia
Infantile Refsum's disease
Refsum's disease (classic form)
Hyperpipecolic acidaemia
X-linked adrenoleukodystrophy
Chondrodysplasia punctatum rhizomelia
Primary hyperoxaluria type I

Table 2 *The main groups and clinical manifestations of diseases due to mitochondrial dysfunction*

Disease group	Clinical manifestations
Defects of fatty acid oxidation	Hypoglycaemia
	Hepatic dysfunction
	Cardiac failure
	Myopathy
	Sudden infant death
Respiratory chain disorders	Lactic acidosis
	Encephalopathy
	Hypotonia
	Poor feeding
	Failure to thrive
	Convulsions

The structure of only a minority of the mitochondrial enzymes is encoded in mitochondrial DNA, causing the corresponding diseases to be transmitted purely through the female line.

hence to lysosomes and the exterior of the cell. Another example of disordered intracellular enzyme trafficking relates to those patients with primary hyperoxaluria type I, in whom a mutationally induced alteration in the conformation of the amino terminus of the alanine:glyoxylate aminotransferase molecule causes it to be targeted to mitochondria instead of to its normal peroxisomal location.

HETEROGENEITY IN THE INBORN ERRORS OF METABOLISM

The individual inborn errors of metabolism are defined on the basis of the phenotype, including the specific enzyme lesion, and by their unifactorial (Mendelian) pattern of inheritance. Close study of any particular inborn error of metabolism reveals unexpected heterogeneity. This is due to: (1) multiple allelism; (2) mutations at different gene loci affecting the structure of different polypeptide chains in a single enzyme protein; (3) mutations at different gene loci affecting different proteins with similar catalytic functions; (4) differences in the overall genetic background against which the single mutation acts; and (5) environmental factors.

CLINICAL POINTERS TOWARDS A DIAGNOSIS OF AN INBORN ERROR OF METABOLISM

Although the symptoms of metabolic disease may appear vague and protean, and an inherited disease cannot be diagnosed in the absence of an appropriate family history, some clinical settings suggest the presence of an inborn error of metabolism (Table 3). In taking the family history, special inquiries should be made about affected sibs, possible parental consanguinity, paternity, miscarriages, perinatal deaths, abortions, about the sexes of possibly affected relatives and their placement on the maternal or paternal side of the family, and the ethnic and geographic origins of the parents.

GENERAL APPROACHES TO THE TREATMENT OF INBORN ERRORS OF METABOLISM

The treatments available for the individual inborn errors of metabolism cover a wide range and may need to be specially developed for individual patients. However, the principles involved can be broadly classified as in Table 4. Palliative surgical and other measures may be needed to deal with specific complications (for example corneal grafting to restore vision in patients with corneal clouding due to one of the mucopolysaccharidoses). Consideration should also be given to meeting the educational and social needs of these patients, as well as to optimizing their overall clinical state and correcting the biochemical parameters. The successful management of patients with inborn errors of metabolism requires a multidisciplinary approach which utilizes the special skills of dietitians, social workers, educationalists, and occupational therapists, as well as those of physicians, surgeons, biochemists, and geneticists. It is particularly important to plan for the handover of specialist care from the paediatrician to the most appropriate adult physician when follow-up in a paediatric department becomes inappropriate. The perfect outcome is to achieve a physically and mentally normal adult who is capable of begetting normal children. Unfortunately the nature of many of the inborn errors of metabolism mitigates against the attainment of this ideal, so that treatment has to aim at optimizing the child's potential in all its physical, mental, and social aspects. Treatment and support also have to be extended to the parents and siblings who, if not overtly affected themselves, may be carriers of the abnormal gene concerned and require appropriate advice about the genetic and other aspects of the disease.

The ability to clone human genes into bacteria and yeasts, which can then produce large amounts of the human gene product, may widen the horizons for treatment by enzyme administration in the future. The development of macrophage-targeted β-glucocerebrosidase enzyme replacement therapy for Gaucher disease (glucosylceramidase deficiency) is a notable recent development in this field.

Attempts to utilize transplanted fibroblasts and amniotic cells as a source for enzyme replacement therapy have not proved to be successful.

Bone marrow transplantation has been used for the treatment of two groups of inherited metabolic disorders: (1) those in which it is desired to replace a particular type of non-functioning bone marrow cell by its normally functioning counterpart; and (2) those in which an attempt has been made to utilize the fact that the bone marrow produces 50 to 100 g of polymorphonuclear leucocytes per day and that these cells exocytose (release) their lysosomal enzymes for uptake by enzyme-deficient cells in the body tissues generally. This strategy has been more successful with the first group of diseases, which includes disorders of neutrophil function (e.g. cyclic neutropenia), functional abnormalities of lymphocytes, and osteopetrosis. The beneficial effect of the last disease is due to the introduction of normal osteoclast precursors. The results in the second group of diseases, namely those in which the white cell lineage derived from the transplanted bone marrow is used to supply normal enzyme to enzyme deficient tissues, has been less successful. The longest studies have been with Hurler disease (mucopolysaccharidosis IH, i.e. mucopolysaccharidosis type I, the Hurler clinical variant

Table 3 *Clinical presentation which, in the absence of acquired or other congenital causes, suggest an inborn error of metabolism*

Unexplained acute neonatal illness and/or failure to thrive in early infancy. (Marked muscle hypotonia, recurrent fits, comas, acidosis and vomiting, especially if withholding milk feeds causes temporary improvement, are especially suggestive)

Developmental slowing and arrest followed by retrogression

Developmental slowing and arrest leading to unexplained mental handicap

Unusual physiognomy, multiple skeletal deformities with developmental delay and retrogression

Multiple skeletal deformities alone (dysostosis multiplex especially suggests a lysosomal storage disease)

Gross visceromegaly

Specific dietary intolerances

Haemolytic anaemia

Unusual body odour[a]

Urolithiasis

Cataracts in early life[b]

Dislocation of the optic lens[c]

Persistent jaundice and hepatic cirrhosis in infancy

Abnormal cutaneous photosensitivity

Hypopigmentation

Abnormal drug sensitivity

A history of recurrent perinatal deaths and/or stillbirths

Hydrops fetalis in the absence of blood group incompatibility between mother and fetus (red cell enzyme defects)

[a]Examples are: phenylketonuria (mousy, musty), branched-chain ketoacidosis (maple syrup), methionine malabsorption (oast house, dry celery), isovaleric acidaemia (sweaty feet), methylaminuria (stale fish), multiple carboxylase deficiency (tom cat's urine), Hawkinsinuria (swimming pool).

[b]Examples are: Fabry's disease, galactosaemia, galactokinase deficiency, Lowe's syndrome, mannosidosis, osteogenesis imperfecta, Refsum's disease, Wilson's disease.

[c]Examples are: Ehlers–Danlos syndrome, homocystinuria, hyperlysinuria, Marfan's syndrome, sulphite oxidase deficiency.

as opposed to the Scheie and intermediate Hurler/Scheie clinical variants), where there has been some clinical improvement, but the skeletal deformities have not been corrected; and the long-term results in terms of neurological function remain to be fully assessed.

The greatly improved long-term results of liver transplantation for hepatic failure have encouraged its application as a sophisticated form of enzyme replacement therapy in patients with inborn errors of metabolism. From the point of view of enzyme replacement, liver transplantation has the advantage that the enzyme is introduced in the correct organ, the correct cell with its correct subcellular location (mitochondrial, lysosomal, or cytosolic) and correctly orientated with respect to its substrate and other enzymes with which it must act in concert. Tables 5 and 6 summarize some recent experience and possible future developments in this area. In this context, liver transplantation can also be regarded as a form of gene replacement therapy in that the donor liver contains the normal gene which will direct the synthesis of a normal enzyme protein.

Table 4 *General approaches to the treatment of inborn errors of metabolism*

Method	Examples
Restriction of a dietary subtrate which cannot be metabolized	Phenylalanine restriction in phenylketonuria Protein restriction in the hyperammonaemias Elimination of galactose in galactosaemia
Avoidance of specific hazards	Ultraviolet radiation (congenital erythropoietic and variegate porphyrias, and in albinism) Ionizing radiation in the DNA repair enzyme defects (xeroderma pigmentosum, ataxia telangiectasia) Infections (agammaglobinaemia) Medications (oestrogens, barbiturates, etc. in acute intermittent porphyria)
Replacement of a missing metabolic product	Orotic aciduria: treatment by uridine which is metabolized to uridylic acid Hartnup disease: nicotinic acid to control skin manifestations
Removal of a toxic metabolite	Haemodialysis and peritoneal dialysis as temporary treatment of an acute metabolic crisis due to a diffusible toxic metabolite, and to correct certain secondary biochemical abnormalities quickly Either specific chemical detoxication (e.g. penicillamine in Wilson's disease) or solubilization (e.g. penicillamine in cystinuria)
Pharmacological doses of a cofactor (only some cases of each disease respond)	Propionic acidaemia: biotin Homocystinuria: pyridoxine Primary hyperoxaluria (Type I): pyridoxine Methylmalonic acidaemia: vitamin B_{12}
Replacement of a missing gene product	Adenosine diaminase deficiency Gaucher disease: β-glucocerebrosidase Haemophilia: clotting factor VIII
Bone marrow transplantation	Adenosine deaminase deficiency
Liver transplantation	Hereditary tyrosinaemia (type I)-antitrypsin deficiency Primary hyperoxaluria (Type I) (see also Tables 5 and 6
Gene replacement	None so far

The examples chosen are situations in which either the proposed treatment is established or in which it can be recommended as elective therapy even though the results of long-term evaluation are still awaited.

Treatment by gene replacement using retroviral vectors to introduce the desired DNA sequence into the patient's explanted haemopoietic stem cell genome, these genetically corrected cells being cultured and then returned to the patient's circulation, may have some potential in diseases where the expression of the metabolic lesion in the haemopoietic system determines the phenotype, or in those situations where genetically corrected migratory cells of haemopoietic origin (e.g. polymorphonuclear leucocytes) can deliver normal enzyme to the enzyme-deficient tissues. Although somatic cell gene therapy, possibly using viral vectors to introduce desired DNA sequences into other cell types, may prove to be practicable in the future, the prospect of correcting inherited defects in the germ cell line at the clinical level remains remote.

SCREENING FOR INBORN ERRORS OF METABOLISM

The realization that very early diagnosis is essential in order to achieve good results in the treatment of some inborn errors of metabolism such as phenylketonuria and galactosaemia has stimulated interest in the possibility of examining either whole populations or selected groups of predisposed individuals for the biochemical differences, which characterize particular inherited metabolic diseases. Diagnosis is needed at a stage which is not only presymptomatic but which precedes the onset of self-perpetuating secondary pathological changes.

Screening programmes should be established only for treatable or preventable diseases, and the consistency of the association of the proposed biochemical or other marker and the serious clinical phenotype

must have been proved beyond any doubt. There must be a reliable and robust analytical method suitable for use with a sample of blood or urine, which can be obtained without distressing either the parents or the baby. The possibility that metabolic screening will bring to light previously unrecognized variants, which are either mild and do not require treatment, or which by virtue of a fundamentally different biochemical lesion will resist the currently established therapies, has to be borne in mind. Phenylketonuria illustrates these problems. Here, beside classic phenylketonuria, whole population screening has identified both the clinically unimportant, essential (mild) hyperphenylalaninaemia, and the devastatingly serious, but treatable, inborn errors of tetrahydrobiopterin synthesis, which produce the 'malignant' hyperphenylalaninaemia syndrome.

Screening for inborn errors of metabolism may be either non-selective (i.e. the whole population) or selective. The latter, which includes carrier detection studies, aims to cover only part of the population, which may be defined on clinical, genetic, ethnic, or geographical grounds. Screening for phenylketonuria and congenital hypothyroidism are the only, generally practised, neonatal whole population screening procedures for this group of disorders, although some authorities propose the inclusion of galactosaemia and congenital adrenal hyperplasia (21-hydroxylase deficiency).

A precise cost–benefit analysis to define the disease incidence which merits whole population screening is impracticable but there is a general consensus that this should be at least similar to that of phenylketonuria in Caucasians (between 1:6000 and 1:12 000). Cystic fibrosis has an incidence of 1:2500 in Caucasians and would merit neonatal whole pop-

Table 5 *Inborn errors of metabolism which have been treated by liver transplantation*

Aetiological metabolic lesion in the liver, damage to which determines the prognosis
α₁-antitrypsin deficiency
Wilson's disease
Hereditary tyrosinaemia (type I)
Galactosaemia
Glycogen storage diseases types 1a and 4
Byler syndrome
Alagille's disease
Reye's syndrome
Aetiological metabolic lesion in the liver, the prognosis being determined by secondary damage to other organs
Primary hyperoxaluria type I (has been combined with renal transplantation)
Primary hypercholesterolaemia (has been combined with cardiac transplantation)
Crigler–Najjar syndrome type I
Haemophilia A
Haemophilia B
Homozygous protein C deficiency
Urea cycle disorders
Aetiological metabolic lesion in the extrahepatic organs producing liver damage
Protoporphyria
Diseases in which the liver and extrahepatic organs both share and express the metabolic lesion and its pathophysiological effects
Cystic fibrosis
Niemann–Pick disease
Sea blue histiocyte syndrome
Sanfilippo syndrome (mucopolysaccharidosis type 3)

Data from Cohen, O'Grady, Mowat, and Williams, 1989.

Table 6 *Inborn errors of metabolism which are potential candidates for treatment by liver transplantation*

Aetiological metabolic lesion in the liver, damage to which determines the prognosis
Glycogen storage diseases type 0 and 3
Hereditary fructose intolerance
Trihydroxycoprostatic (THCA) syndrome
Fatty acid acyltransferase deficiency
Aetiological metabolic lesion in the liver, the prognosis being determined by secondary damage to other organs
Disorders of lactate/pyruvate metabolism
Diseases in which the liver and extrahepatic organs both share and express the metabolic lesion and its pathophysiological effects
Wolman disease
Gaucher disease

Data from Cohen, O'Grady, Mowat, and Williams, 1989.

ulation screening on this basis. However, the available tests are not of proven value for whole population screening, although they may be helpful in the selective screening of the family members of known cases. The measurement of the trypsin activity of a spot of blood collected onto filter paper is widely used. The 'sweat test' (measurement of the sodium content of sweat) remains the most reliable diagnostic procedure for cystic fibrosis. However, it is not suitable for use in neonates and it is too cumbersome to employ in screening beyond a patient's immediate family. Four different mutations account for about 85 per cent of cases of cystic fibrosis and the identification of these, after *in vitro* DNA amplification (the polymerase chain reaction (PCR), is being increasingly used for the diagnosis of both the affected homozygotes and the heterozygous carriers of the mutant gene. The mutational change in the DNA structure is detected either by the presence or absence of a restriction endonuclease site, or by probing with another primer that hybridizes with only one of the alleles. An appreciable proportion of the so-called homozygotes are in fact proving to be doubly heterozygous for two different mutations in the same gene. The number of inborn metabolic errors in which the affected individuals and the heterozygous carriers can be identified by such molecular genetic analysis is increasing rapidly. It includes such numerically important diseases as sickle cell anaemia, β-thalassaemia, haemophilia, Duchenne muscular dystrophy, and phenylketonuria, as well as some rarer but devastating conditions such as the Lesch–Nyhan syndrome.

PRENATAL DIAGNOSIS

The procedures used in prenatal diagnosis are: (1) direct examination of the fetus by ultrasonography and fetoscopy; (2) chemical analysis of amniotic fluid; (3) biochemical and cytological analysis of cultured amniotic cells (amniocytes) obtained by amniocentesis at the fifteenth or sixteenth week of pregnancy; (4) DNA analysis on uncultured amniocytes; (5) karyotypic enzymological and DNA analysis of chorionic villi obtained by biopsy at the eighth to tenth week of pregnancy; (6) biochemical studies on tissue obtained by biopsy on the fetus *in utero*.

CARRIER STATE DIAGNOSIS

In relation to the study of inherited diseases, a carrier is defined as: 'An individual, who possesses, in the heterozygous state, the gene determining an inherited disorder, and who is essentially healthy at the time of study' (Harper, 1988). This includes individuals carrying the gene for a recessive disorder, one that does not express itself in the heterozygous state (e.g. phenylketonuria), and those who are carrying the gene for a dominant disorder, one that does express itself in the heterozygous state, but in which symptoms occur in later life (e.g. Huntington's chorea (Huntington's disease).

The general approaches to carrier state diagnosis are: (1) the detection of minor clinical, radiological, and clinicopathological abnormalities; (2) the demonstration of levels of enzyme activity in tissue which are intermediate between those observed in individuals homozygous for the abnormal and the normal forms of the enzyme respectively; (3) the demonstration of intermediate levels of a characteristic metabolite in an accessible body fluid; (4) the demonstration of mosaicism with respect to the product of the mutant x-linked gene in the case of sex-linked recessive disorders; and (5) direct gene analysis using either a specific gene probe or a linked restriction fragment length polymorphism (RFLP).

IN VITRO FERTILIZATION AND THE INBORN ERRORS OF METABOLISM

The human embryo produced by *in vitro* fertilization can be biopsied at a very early stage of development (e.g. at the eight cell stage). A single cell is removed and examined for the DNA mutation responsible for the disease which the parents are known to be carrying. This enables only fertilized ova which do not carry the mutant gene to be implanted.

ANIMAL GENETIC MODELS OF SOME INBORN ERRORS OF METABOLISM WHICH OCCUR IN MAN

Animal genetic models of the inborn errors of metabolism can be useful in the early stages of investigating new approaches to treatment before attempting to transfer these to man. It is also possible to investigate the pathophysiology of the diseases at different stages of their evolution more easily, rapidly, and predictably than if one has to rely entirely on the *ad hoc* availability of clinical and pathological material. The wider availability of these models could accelerate progress in this area. However, it has to be borne in mind that although the enzyme deficiency is the same in human and animal species, the exact abnormality at the genomic and molecular level will almost certainly be different. Animal models have been used particularly in the study of some of the lysosomal storage diseases.

REFERENCES

Akhurst, R.J. (1989). Prospects for gene therapy now and in the future. *Journal of Inherited Metabolic Disease*, **12,** Supplement 1, 191–201.

Barton, N.W. et al. (1991). Replacement therapy for inherited enzyme deficiency-macrophage targeted glucocerebrosidase for Gaucher's disease. *The New England Journal of Medicine*, **324,** 1464–70.

Besley, G.T.N., Young, E.P., Fensom, A.H., and Cooper, A. (1991). First trimester diagnosis of inherited disease: experience in the U.K. *Journal of Inherited Metabolic Disease*, **14,** 128–33.

Brenton, D.P. (Ed.) (1992). Review issue. Mitochondrial DNA and associated disorders; the X chromosome. *Journal of Inherited Metabolic Disease*, **15,** 437–688.

British Medical Association. (1992). *Our genetic future: a report by the BMA on the scientific basis and social and ethical consequences of gene isolation, analysis and therapy*. British Medical Association, London.

Burdelski, M., Rodeck, B., Latta, A., Brodell, J., Ringe, B., and Pichmayr, R. (1991). Treatment of inherited metabolic disorders by liver transplantation. *Journal of Inherited Metabolic Disease* **14,** 604–618.

Carman, W.F. (1991). The polymerase chain reaction. *Quarterly Journal of Medicine*, **78,** 195–203.

Cohen, A., O'Grady, J., Mowat, A., and Williams, R. (1989). Liver trans- plantation for metabolic disorders. *Ballieres Clinical Gastroenterology*, **3,** 767–786.

Desnick, R.S. (1991). *The treatment of genetic disease*, Churchill Livingstone, New York.

Firth, H.V., Boyd, P.A., Chamberlain, P., MacKenzie, I.Z., Lindenbaum, R.H., and Huson, S.M. (1991). Severe limb abnormalities after chorion villus sampling at 56–66 days gestation. *Lancet*, **337,** 762–763.

Friedman, T. (1991). Approaches to human gene therapy. In *Inborn errors of metabolism* (ed. J. Shaub, F. van Hoof, and H.L. Vis), pp. 275–82. Nestlé Nutrition Workshop Series, Vol. 24, Nestec Ltd., Vevey/Raven Press Ltd, New York.

Harper, P.S. (1988). *Practical genetic counselling*. Wright, Bristol.

Hobbs, J.R. (1991). Displacement bone marrow transplantation can correct some inborn errors of metabolism. In *Inborn errors of metabolism* (ed. J. Shaub, F. van Hoof, and H.L. Vis). pp. 223–47. Nestlé Nutrition Workshop Series, Vol. 24, Nestec Ltd., Vevey/Raven Press Ltd, New York.

Krivic, W., and Paul, N.W. (eds) (1986). *Bone marrow transplantation for treatment of lysosomal storage diseases*. March of Dimes Birth Defects Foundation. Birth Defects Original Article Series, Vol. 22, No. 1. Alan R. Liss Inc., New York.

McKusick, V.A. (1990). *Mendelian inheritance in man. Catalogues of autosomal dominant, autosomal recessive and x-linked phenotypes*, (9th edn). The Johns Hopkins University Press, Baltimore.

Medical Research Council Working Party on the Evaluation of Chorion Villus Sampling (1991). Medical Research Council European Trial of chorion villus sampling. *Lancet*, **337,** 1491–9.

Terrenoire, G. (1992). Huntington's disease and the ethnics of genetic prediction. *Journal of Medical Ethics*, **18,** 79–85.

Watts, R.W.E. and Gibbs, D.A. (1986). Animal genetic models of some inborn errors of metabolism which occur in man. In *Lysosomal storage diseases, biochemical and clinical aspects*, (ed. R.W.E. Watts and D.A. Gibbs), pp. 235–6. Taylor and Francis, London.

Williamson, R. (1992). Testing for Huntington's disease. Early clinical studies suggest uptake is low. *British Medical Journal*, **304,** 1585–6.

11.2 Disorders of carbohydrate metabolism other than diabetes mellitus and hypoglycaemia

11.2.1 Glycogen storage diseases

T. M. COX

Glycogen, the main energy store in liver and muscle, contains polymerized α-D-glucose units anchored covalently at their reducing termini to a small protein, glycogenin. The structure of glycogen is elaborate: its many-branched macromolecular tree is linked by α-1,4 glycosidic bonds with α-1,6 bonds at the branch points. These branch points are arranged in several tiers with increasingly long outer chains that terminate in non-reducing glucose residues. Glycogen is configured for compact storage of glucose in a form that has an insignificant osmotic effect and that allows the outer chains access to enzymes of biosynthesis and degradation.

The polymerized structures of liver and muscle glycogen can be seen with the electron microscope: liver glycogen consists mainly of α aggregates or rosettes of smaller particles (β-particles) that are found in muscle cytoplasm. Each β-particle contains up to 60 000 glucose residues but despite its size the glycogen molecule undergoes remodelling as a result of constant breakdown and synthesis. Defects in the enzymatic steps for the synthesis, utilization, or degradation of glycogen lead to its pathological storage. Accumulation of glycogen may be generalized or involve certain tissues selectively; the glycogen may have a normal or aberrant structure.

Glycogen metabolism

The individual enzymatic steps for the formation and breakdown of glycogen are summarized in Fig. 1.

Glycogen synthesis

The immediate precursor for glycogen synthesis is uridine diphosphoglucose that is formed from glucose 1-phosphate by UDP glucose pyrophosphorylase. This enzyme has a high affinity for its substrates and is abundant – no deficiencies have been recorded. In contrast, glycogen synthase is a highly regulated enzyme complex that exists in distinct isoforms in muscle and liver: the enzyme catalyses the transfer of UDP glucose units to glucose residues already covalently attached to a tyrosine residue of glycogenin, which acts as a primer. The tyrosine glucosyl transferase activity has not been identified but the glycogenin adduct possesses an intrinsic glucosyltransferase activity. Initially one molecule each of glycogen synthase and glycogenin occur as a complex in each β-glycogen particle. After elongation, branching of the molecule is catalysed by amylo (1,4 → 1,6) transglucosidase, 'branching enzyme'.

Glycogen synthase is subject to phosphorylation control that inhibits its activity: this inhibition is overcome by the allosteric activator, glucose 6-phosphate. The phosphorylation of at least nine serine residues is brought about by protein kinases. Glucagon and adrenaline, while stimulating phosphorylase via phosphorylase kinase, inhibit glycogen synthase indirectly by maintaining protein phosphatase I in its inactive configuration. Insulin stimulates glycogen synthase by promoting its dephosphorylation through the action of this same phosphatase: protein phosphatase I is activated by a cascade of protein kinases whose phosphorylation is initiated by the insulin receptor tyrosine kinase. Inherited deficiency of glycogen synthase activity is associated with reduced storage of liver glycogen and fasting hypoglycaemia. Branching enzyme activity is essential for the formation of the compact spherical molecules of glycogen especially in liver. It transfers a minimum of six α-1,4-linked glucose units from the distal ends of glycogen chains to a 1,6 position on the same or a neighbouring chain. Deficiency of branching enzyme leads to the accumulation of abnormal molecules that are partially resistant to degradation.

Glycogen breakdown

Glycogen is degraded by three enzymes: phosphorylase, debranching enzyme, and acid α-glucosidase. Phosphorylase brings about the sequential release of glucose units from the α-1,4-linked chains of glycogen to liberate glucose 1-phosphate. After conversion to glucose 6-

phosphate by phosphoglucomutase, free glucose is formed by the action of glucose 6-phosphatase. Debranching enzyme possesses transferase and α-1,6 glucosidase activities. When phosphorylase has degraded glycogen chains to within four α-1,4 glucosyl units of an α-1,6 linkage, three glucose residues are transferred to the end of another chain by the glycosyltransferase activity. Debranching enzyme then hydrolyses the remaining α-1,6 bond to release free glucose using its amylo-1,6-glucosidase activity. Debranching enzyme also cleaves the unique glucosyl–tyrosine linkage that anchors the terminal reducing glucose unit to glycogenin. Deficiency of debranching enzyme leads to the storage of glycogen that possesses short outer chains, 'limit dextrin'.

The main product of glycogen breakdown in muscle and liver is glucose 1-phosphate, which is produced by the sequential action of phosphorylase on α-1,4 glycosidic bonds. Glucose 1-phosphate is a key intermediate of glycolysis, gluconeogenesis, glycogenolysis, and the pentose phosphate pathway but, by virtue of phosphoglucomutase, the hepatic glucose 6-phosphatase system is the predominant metabolic source of blood glucose. Glucose 6-phosphatase exists as a multicomponent complex in the endoplasmic reticulum of hepatocytes and, to a lesser extent, renal tubular cells – it is not found in muscle. The system contains glucose 6-phosphatase, several proteins that facilitate transport of glucose, glucose 6-phosphate, and phosphate, as well as other stabilizing and regulatory moieties. Several genetic defects in this compartmentalized system are recognized to affect overall glucose 6-phosphatase activity: they are associated with severe hypoglycaemia, metabolic acidosis, and hepatic disease.

Glucose 6-phosphate obtained from the breakdown of glycogen in

Fig. 1 The synthesis and degradation of glycogen.

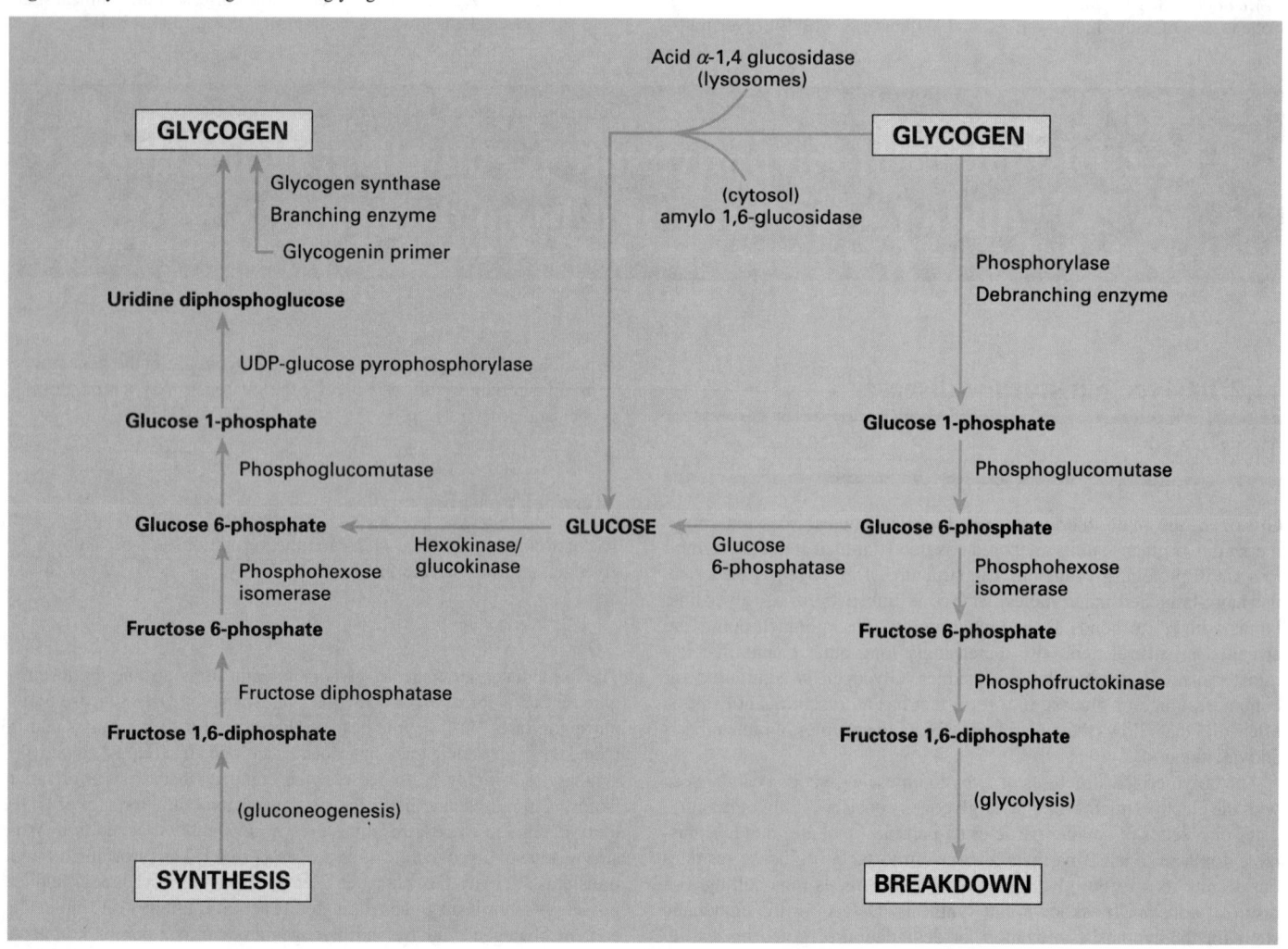

skeletal muscle is used directly in glycolysis. Defects of muscle phosphorylase lead to a defective supply of adenosine triphosphate (ATP), especially during ischaemic exercise. There is a failure of conversion of glycogen to lactate, and exercise-induced muscle cramps reflect mild muscle necrosis with increased accumulation of glycogen. Phosphofructokinase-1 catalyses an irreversible step in the glycolytic pathway and is a key regulatory enzyme. Inherited defects that render it inactive or affect its positive allosteric regulation by the effectors AMP and fructose 2,6-diphosphate resemble muscle phosphorylase deficiency. Because deficiency of phosphofructokinase affects the metabolism of endogenous glycogen as well as carbon units derived from extracellular glucose, the symptoms of phosphofructokinase-1 deficiency are more severe and of earlier onset than muscle phosphorylase deficiency. As expected, glucose 6-phosphate, fructose 6-phosphate, and glycogen, accumulate in the muscle cells.

Breakdown of glycogen in liver and skeletal muscle is brought about by the concerted activities of phosphorylase and debranching enzyme in the cytoplasm. Phosphorylase is activated by phosphorylation in response to hormonal or neural stimulation – a complex process that is mediated by phosphorylase kinases. Phosphorylase kinase is a multisubunit protein with regulatory, catalytic, and calcium-binding subunits that are encoded on separate genes. Separate isoforms are found in liver and muscle. The final common pathways for the regulation of phosphorylase kinase involve protein kinase A (cAMP-dependent protein kinase), calcium and kinase activation of calmodulin, and protein phosphatases 1 and 2A. Another enzyme, acid α-1,4-glucosidase, has an important role in the metabolism of glycogen. This lysosomal hydrolase is present in all cells except erythrocytes and, although it has no relation to glycolysis, its deficiency causes a generalized disorder in which muscle disease, especially of the heart, is usually severe. Deficiency of acid α-glucosidase is associated with rapidly progressive cardiac hypertrophy with hepatic enlargement and generalized muscle weakness. Skeletal muscle symptoms may be prominent in patients with the infantile or late-onset forms of this condition, but disease progression is usually rapid. Acid α-1,4 glucosidase deficiency was the first inborn lysosomal disease to be clearly recognized and represents a prototype for the other storage diseases: intracellular vesicles containing glycogen represent lysosomes distended by an undegradable substrate that accumulates as a result of autophagy. The accumulation of glycogen in lysosomes indicates that glycogen fragments are constantly being synthesized and taken up for degradation.

Diagnosis of glycogen storage disease

Affecting the liver

The diagnosis may be suspected in infants and children with hepatomegaly, growth retardation, and hypoglycaemia, which is not invariable. A previous biopsy might have indicated glycogen deposition. In many cases a glucagon stimulation test (20 µg/kg intramuscularly) fails to induce the normal (> 2 mmol/l) rise in blood glucose, but, for prognosis, future antenatal diagnosis and to direct treatment, definitive diagnosis by biopsy is warranted. Direct assay of liver tissue for glycogen and fat content as well as enzymatic analysis is desirable. Histochemical and electron microscopic study of glycogen structure provides useful additional information. Where possible, open wedge-biopsy of the liver should be carried out to obtain sufficient material for diagnosis and ensure haemostasis under direct vision. However, the procedure is hazardous for young infants with acidosis or bleeding tendency and close attention should be given to prevention of hypoglycaemia.

A particular difficulty arises in the diagnosis of certain variants of Type I glycogen storage disease. The glucose 6-phosphatase system is uniquely incorporated into the endoplasmic reticulum: latency of its membrane-bound components renders diagnosis of specific lesions affecting transport of substrates or products impossible when frozen tissue is thawed for analysis. Type 1B glycogen storage disease (in which glucose 6-phosphate translocation is defective) is an example where study of fresh tissue is essential for establishing a diagnosis, since analysis of freeze-thawed material disrupts the integrity of the microsomal enzyme system and, by rendering it permeable to glucose 6-phosphate, overcomes the biochemical lesion. Thus, where defects of glycogen storage are suspected, it is essential to seek the prior advice of a laboratory that is competent to carry out the appropriate investigations using fresh and deep-frozen biopsy material.

In muscle

Forearm exercise tests are useful for detecting defects in skeletal muscles that interfere with the metabolic pathway from glucose and glycogen to lactate. In the absence of oxygen, glycolysis is the sole means by which ATP may be generated and glucosyl units derived from glycogen, rather than glucose obtained from the plasma, is the preferred energy source. Defects in glycolysis (glycogenosis type VII and other enzyme deficiencies) cause similar symptoms. Exercise-induced cramps may occur in the purine pathway disorder, myoadenylate deaminase deficiency, which may be also diagnosed safely by exercise testing. Unlike the earlier test devised by McArdle (1951) these provocative tests do not induce rhabdomyolysis accompanied by raised creatine kinase activity in the serum with acute myoglobinuric renal failure – features in the history that may indicate muscle glycogenosis.

After 30 min rest, blood is taken from the antecubital vein of the non-exercising arm and a small sphygmomanometer cuff placed around the other wrist is inflated to 200 mmHg. A second standard cuff around the upper arm to be tested is inflated to mean arterial pressure and the patient squeezes as powerfully as possible 120 times over 2 min. Immediately afterwards, the second cuff is inflated to 200 mmHg. Blood is drawn through a needle placed in the antecubital vein of the exercising arm 2 min after completing the exercise and the upper cuff is released. To complete the test, five further samples are drawn at 1-min intervals. The samples are transported rapidly to the laboratory for analysis of lactate and ammonia. Reduced or absent generation of lactate is characteristic of glycogenolytic and glycolytic defects that affect muscle; in contrast, plasma levels of ammonia (as well as inosine and hypoxanthine) increase greatly in patients with glycogenosis types III, V, and VIII. These abnormalities reflect excessive degradation of purines that occurs in the exercising muscles of patients in whom there is a disturbance of ATP generation. Measurement of ammonia release as well as lactate production also adds discriminatory value to the exercise test, as it controls for low levels of lactate release that result merely from inadequate exercise during performance of the test. The test also may identify myoadenylate kinase deficiency: in such patients lactate production is normal but failure to utilize the purine cycle to conserve intracellular nucleotides and provide alternative substrates for energy production, is shown by the failure of venous ammonia concentrations to rise.

Pompe's disease is a generalized disorder that predominantly affects skeletal and cardiac muscle. Carbohydrate metabolism is otherwise normal and phosphorylysis of cytosolic glycogen in the liver is sufficient to maintain euglycaemia. The diagnosis may be suspected on the basis of cardiac and liver enlargement in an infant with respiratory distress and hypotonia. Macroglossia is frequent and the electrocardiogram shows left axis deviation, a short P-R interval and broad QRS complexes. Myopathic changes – occasionally with pseudomyotonic discharges – are observed on electromyography and the diagnosis is revealed by biopsy, which shows vacuolar myopathy: massive deposits of glycogen in and between myofibrils. Under the electron microscope, free and lysosomal α-glycogen particles are observed. Enzymatic deficiency of acid α-1,4-glucosidase is readily confirmed in cultured amniocytes and all tissues except erythrocytes.

Definitive diagnosis of muscle glycogenoses depends on biopsy with histochemical, ultrastructural, and biochemical analyses. Biopsy should be carried out after liaison with the laboratory so that, if necessary, tissue can be stored frozen for further study and enzymatic analysis. Biopsy and electromyography may be needed to differentiate suspected glycogen storage diseases from other myopathies including Duchenne's dystrophy, Kugelberg–Welander disease, dystrophia myotonica, and mitochondrial and secondary disorders of muscle such as polymyositis.

Individual glycogen storage diseases

The main features of these disorders are surveyed and summarized in Table 1. Brief accounts of selected conditions are set out below.

von Gierke's disease

Glucose formation from glycogen and gluconeogenesis is defective and affected infants develop hypoglycaemia on fasting or as a result of intercurrent infection or other stress. The liver is enlarged at birth. It contains excess glycogen and shows gross infiltration with fat but cirrhosis and portal hypertension are rare. In contrast, growth retardation often combined with obesity, is common. The kidneys are enlarged by glycogen deposition. Progressive focal glomerulosclerosis and proximal tubular failure with a secondary Fanconi syndrome may also occur. Stress and starvation provoke acidotic attacks with marked lactic acidaemia. Poor metabolic control causes growth arrest; hyperuricaemia and gout; marked hypertriglyceridaemia and hypercholesterolaemia with raised very low density lipoprotein (VLDL) and normal low density lipoprotein (LDL) cholesterol concentrations in the plasma (skin and retinal xanthomas accompany these findings) and prolonged bleeding time related to an acquired von Willebrand-like defect affecting the platelet. Patients with defects of the glucose 6-phosphate translocase system (type 1B) are prone to bacterial infection: there is neutropenia and neutrophil migration and chemotaxis are impaired. These patients may develop episodes of severe diarrhoea in association with granulomatous infiltration of the colonic mucosa. Partial deficiencies of the glucose 6-phosphatase system lead to variable clinical expression and subtypes of Type I glycogen storage disease have been convincingly demonstrated in patients presenting with glucagon-unresponsive hypoglycaemia with or without liver enlargement in adult life. Adult patients or children with uncontrolled disease develop hepatic adenomas; frank hepatocellular carcinomata occur.

METABOLIC DISTURBANCE

Hypoglycaemia in von Gierke's disease is often asymptomatic and tolerance of it improves with increasing age. Residual production of glucose probably occurs by lysosomal hydrolysis of glycogen and recycling through the glycogen synthase–debranching enzyme pathway, but metabolic adaptation of the brain, which can use lactate as an alternative substrate, is very important. Hypertriglyceridaemia is induced by increased provision of reduced nictotinamide adenine dinucleotide (NADH) and reduced nicotinamide adenine dinucleotide phosphate (NADPH), glycerol and acetyl-coenzyme A (CoA) because of enhanced flux through glycolysis and underutilization of gluconeogenic precursors. Malonyl-coenzyme A, derived from acetyl-coenzyme A, inhibits the carnitine acyltransferase system and blocks the oxidation of fatty acids; thus ketosis does not occur. Lactic acidaemia results from stimulation of glycolysis at the level of phosphofructokinase by high concentrations of glucose 6-phosphate (and hence fructose 6-phosphate). Lactate cannot be recycled in the liver to form new glucose and lactic acidosis results. Lactate competes with urate for excretory pathways in the kidney and thus contributes to the hyperuricaemia. Uric acid is also overproduced in the liver: it arises from degradation of purine nucleotides by adenosine monophosphate (AMP) deaminase. The deaminase is activated when the concentration of free phosphate falls as a result of sequestration in sugar phosphate esters.

TREATMENT

The main objective is to maintain euglycaemia: most of the other metabolic abnormalities are thereby corrected and the prognosis improves.

In infants normoglycaemia is maintained throughout 24 h by intravenous alimentation at 0.25 to 0.5 g/kg.h and, later, by continuous nasogastric administration at night with glucose supplements at intervals of 1 to 2 h during the day. These intensive regimens correct acidosis, hyperuricaemia, and hyperlipidaemia; they also promote normal development and allow catch-up growth to occur in stunted infants and children. After growth in later childhood and in adult patients, metabolic control can be maintained by the use of raw corn starch that serves as a source of glucose slowly released by hydrolysis. 1 to 2 g/kg is given orally every 4 to 6 h as a suspension in water.

In Type Ib glycogen storage disease it is vital to avoid intercurrent infection, and prophylactic antimicrobial drugs may therefore be necessary. Patients with Type Ia disease may require treatment for their bleeding tendency. The bleeding diathesis is associated with a qualitative defect of platelet function, prolonged bleeding time and reduced factor VIIIc and vW factor activities. These abnormalities and the haemorrhagic tendency respond to administration of 1-deamino-8-D-arginine vasopressin (DDAVP) at 0.3 μg/kg infused in 50 ml of saline over 30 min intravenously. Correction of the bleeding disorder lasts for several hours and is useful for the treatment of bleeding after trauma or surgery.

Failure of metabolic control in Type I glycogen storage disease appears to be associated with tissue complications: hepatic adenomata or malignant transformation, renal disease due to hyperfiltration, focal glomerulosclerosis, and postinfective scarring. Lately, an inflammatory disorder of the colon, resembling granulomatous colitis, has been recognized in Type Ib disease. Long-term follow-up care with monitoring of biochemical parameters of kidney function and periodic ultrasonic examination of the liver is necessary. Continuing failure of growth, enlarging hepatic adenomata or progressive renal failure raise the question of organ transplantation. Several successful renal, as well as hepatic, allografts have been carried out in this condition using 1-deamino-8-D-arginine vasopressin infusions to control haemorrhagic manifestations. However, as regression of most complications, including hepatic adenomata, can be achieved by strict dietary measures, transplantation should be reserved for patients in whom nutritional treatment has failed. Survival into adult life (and parenthood) can be now expected.

Type II glycogen storage disease

Pompe's disease is usually a rapidly-progressive disorder with effects on the heart, skeletal muscle, and nervous system. Affected children usually die within the first year or two of life and no measures other than supportive therapy are beneficial. Given that enzyme-replacement therapy is theoretically possible for lysosomal storage diseases, administration of purified acid α-1,4 glucosidase has been attempted. Neither this approach nor bone marrow transplantation appear so far to be beneficial.

Type III glycogen storage disease

The clinical manifestations of Forbes-Cori's disease resemble Type I glycogenosis, especially in infants, who present with hypoglycaemia, short stature, and hepatomegaly. Mild progressive myopathy, occasionally with signs of hypertrophic cardiomyopathy, may occur. Generally the signs of liver disease regress during maturation and myopathy improves also with nutritional therapy as outlined for von Gierke's disease. Protein supplements, which may provide additional sources of energy, appear to benefit the muscle disorder.

Table 1 *Diseases of glycogen storage*

Designation number	Enzymatic defect	Affected tissues	Principal manifestations	Diagnostic tissue
von Gierke's disease (Cori Type I)	Glucose-6-phosphatase[a]	Liver, kidney	Usually severe: liver and kidney enlargement Hypoglycaemia, acidosis, bleeding tendency, growth failure, hyperlipidaemia, hyperuricaemia	Liver Intestinal mucosa
Pompe's disease (Type II)	Acid α-1,4-glucosidase (lysosomal)	Generalized especially heart, muscles and liver.	Usually severe: adult cases recognized hypotonia, cardiomegaly, weakness, and arrhythmias Mild cases respond to high-protein diet	Liver, muscle, myocardium, fibroblasts leucocytes, amniotic fluid cells
Forbes–Cori disease or limit dextrinosis (Type III)	Debranching enzyme	Liver and usually muscle[b]	Often mild: hepatomegaly, hypoglycaemia, progressive muscle weakness in adults. Ketosis – lactic acidosis and hyperuricaemia absent	Liver, (muscle), fibroblasts, amniotic fluid cells
Andersen's disease or amylopectinosis (Type IV)	Branching enzyme	Liver.[b] Rare variant, polyglucosan disease, affects peripheral nerves[b]	Severe: hepatosplenomegaly in infancy; death from cirrhosis and portal hypertension. Polyglucosan variant affects adults	Liver, leucocytes, (peripheral nerves)
McArdle's disease (Type V)	Muscle phosphorylase	Skeletal muscle	Exercise-induced muscle cramps	Muscle (lactate production absent)
Hers' disease (Type VI)	Liver phosphorylase	Liver	Moderate to severe hepatomegaly with hypoglycaemia in childhood	Liver, leucocytes
Tarui's disease (Type VII)	Muscle phosphofructokinase	Muscle, red cells	Marked weakness and stiffness after exertion, haemolytic anaemia (Glucose 6-phosphate and fructose 6-phosphate also accumulate)	Erythrocyte, muscle (Lactate production absent)
Type VIII	Unknown	Liver, brain	Very rare. Hepatomegaly. Progressive neural degeneration and death in childhood	Liver/brain
Type IX	Phosphorylase b kinase	Liver	Mild hepatomegaly. Variable hypoglycaemia. Sex-linked and autosomal recessive forms.	Liver, leucocytes
Type O	Glycogen synthase	Liver	Very rare. Severe fasting hypoglycaemia: seizures before feeds. Failure of glucagon response. Reduced or absent glycogen	Liver
	Phosphoglucoisomerase	Red cells	Very rare. Haemolytic anaemia. Excess glycogen in liver and erythrocytes	Red cells
	Lactate dehydrogenase	Muscle	Resembles McArdle's disease. Very rare.	Muscle
	Phosphoglycerate kinase	Muscle	Resembles McArdle's disease. Very rare.	Muscle
	Lactate dehydrogenase	Muscle	Resembles McArdle's disease. Very rare.	Muscle

[a]Designations beyond Type V are extensions of Cori's classification; beyond Type VII they are controversial.

[b]Several defects described in components of the glucose-6-phosphatase system (see text). NB. Enzyme activity may be normal in tissue after freeze-thawing.

[c]Abnormal glycogen structure – total glycogen concentration may be normal.

Type IV glycogen storage disease

Deficiency of branching enzyme in Anderson's disease gives rise to the deposition of an abnormal glycogen in many tissues. Severe inflammation occurs in the liver, resulting in cirrhosis, with splenomegaly due to portal hypertension. This fatal disorder is characterized by failure to thrive, hepatosplenomegaly, jaundice, and hypotonia. Diagnosis is based on the appearances of the liver biopsy and abnormal glycogen structure shown by histochemical and biochemical analysis. Deficiency of branching enzyme is demonstrable in leucocytes. No definitive therapy is available but a few patients have survived hepatic transplantation without the development of neuromuscular or cardiac complications in up to 7 years after the procedure. Generally the prognosis is poor; most patients die before the age of 4 years with liver failure, variceal bleeding, and intercurrent infection.

Type V glycogen storage disease

This disorder is characterized by the late onset of muscle fatigue and cramps during adolescence or early adult life. Hepatomegaly is absent. Strenuous exercise may induce episodic myoglobinuria and biochemical evidence of rhabdomyolysis. Occasionally acute myoglobinuric renal failure may result. Muscle biopsy may show abnormal muscle fibres with necrosis, atrophy, and hypertrophied fibres alongside. The course of this disease is benign; ingestion of glucose or pre-exercise administration of glucagon may partially ameliorate the symptoms but avoidance of strenuous exercise is advisable.

Type VI glycogen storage disease and phosphorylase b kinase deficiency

These disorders cause hepatomegaly, intermittent hypoglycaemia, and markedly increased liver glycogen content. Although many polypeptides constitute the intact phosphorylase b kinase complex (encoded on autosomes and the X-chromosome), glycogen mobilization is usually only partially defective. X-linked phosphorylase b kinase deficiency is the most frequent variant and is associated with growth retardation, mild ketosis, and hyperlipidaemia in childhood. The symptoms improve with age and the disorder is compatible with a normal life expectancy. Cirrhosis of the liver is very rare and the incompleteness of the defect is shown by almost normal hyperglycaemic responses to glucagon administration. Rare autosomal variants of phosphorylase kinase deficiency affecting liver and muscle or restricted to skeletal or cardiac muscle have been documented. These subtypes are associated with hypotonia or cardiac failure, respectively. Treatment of liver phosphorylase or kinase deficiency with frequent feeding to avoid hypoglycaemia may be needed but the general prognosis is good so that intensive nutritional therapy is rarely indicated. No specific treatment for the isolated cardiac form of kinase deficiency is known but if the diagnosis can be established, cardiac transplantation could be considered.

Type VII glycogen storage disease

This disorder, which is most frequent in patients of Japanese or Russian Ashkenazi ancestry, closely resembles Type V muscle glycogenosis but severe symptoms usually come to light in childhood. There may be hyperuricaemia which is aggravated by exercise. Deficiency of red cell phosphofructokinase leads to chronic haemolysis. Decreased 2,3-diphosphoglycerate synthesis resulting from the metabolic block has been noted and probably contributes to exercise-induced symptoms by reducing oxygen delivery. No specific therapy for this disorder is known – in contrast to McArdle's disease, glucagon or glucose infusions do not improve exercise tolerance. Indeed, carbohydrate-rich meals aggravate the symptoms, presumably by diminishing the concentration of non-esterified fatty acids in plasma, which serve as the alternative source of muscle energy production. Several very rare variants of phosphofructokinase deficiency are known: a severe infantile form with progressive and fatal myopathy and a late-onset form which causes fixed muscle weakness in middle-aged subjects are both clearly recognized.

Glycogen synthase deficiency

Deficiency of glycogen synthase is very rare and causes deficiency of glycogen formation in the liver. It is, therefore, a disorder of storage rather than a true glycogenosis. The condition causes severe interprandial hypoglycaemia. Biopsy examination of the liver shows fatty infiltration and depletion of glycogen: uridine diphosphate-pyrophosphorylase, phosphorylase, glucose 6-phosphatase activities are normal but glycogen synthase is absent. Glucose polymers and uncooked cornstarch are effective therapy.

FURTHER READING

Burchell, A. (1992). The molecular basis of the type I glycogen storage diseases. *BioEssays*, **14**, 395–400.

Cabello, A., Benlloch, T., Franch, O., Feliü, J.F., and Ricoy, J.R. (1981). Glycogen storage disease in skeletal muscle. Morphological, ultrastructural and biochemical aspects in 10 cases. *Acta Neuropathologica (Basel)*, **Suppl. VII**, 297–300.

Chen, Y-T., Cornblath, M., and Sidbury, J.B. (1984). Cornstarch therapy in type I glycogen-storage disease. *New England Journal of Medicine*, **310**, 171–5.

Chen, Y-T., Coleman, R.A., Scheinman, J.I., Kolbeck, P.C., and Sidbury, J.B. (1988). Renal disease in type I glycogen storage disease. *New England Journal of Medicine*, **318**, 7–11.

Chen, Y-T. and Burchell, A. (1994). Glycogen storage disease In: *The metabolic basis of inherited disease* (ed. C.R. Scriver, A.L. Beaudet, W.S. Sly, and D. Valle), (7th edn.) McGraw-Hill, New York. (in press).

de Barsy, T. and Hers, H-G. (1990). Normal metabolism and disorders of carbohydrate metabolism. *Baillière's Clinical Endocrinology and Metabolism*, **4**, 499–522.

Fernandes, J. et al. (1988). Glycogen storage disease: recommendations for treatment. *European Journal of Paediatrics*, **147**, 226–8.

Kono, N. et al. (1984). Metabolic basis of improved exercise tolerance: muscle phosphorylase deficiency after glucagon administration. *Neurology*, **34**, 1471–6.

Malatack, J.J. et al. (1983). Liver transplantation for type I glycogen storage disease. *Lancet*, **i**, 1073–5.

Marti, G.E., Rick, M.E., Sidbury, J., and Gralnick, H.R. (1986). DDAVP infusion in five patients with type Ia glycogen storage disease and associated correction of prolonged bleeding times. *Blood*, **68**, 180–4.

McArdle, B. (1951). Myopathy due to a defect in muscle glycogen breakdown. *Clinical Science*, **10**, 13–33.

Parker, P., Burr, I., Slonim, A., Ghishan, F.K., and Greene, H. (1981). Regression of hepatic adenomas in type Ia glycogen storage disease with dietary therapy. *Gastroenterology*, **81**, 534–6.

Pears, J.S., Jung, R.T., Hopwood, D., Waddell, I.D., and Burchell, A. (1992). Glycogen storage disease diagnosed in adults. *Quarterly Journal of Medicine*, **82**, 207–2.

Selby, R., Starzl, T.E., Yunis, E., Brown, B.I., Kendall, R.S., and Tzakis, A. (1991). Liver transplantation for type IV glycogen storage disease. *New England Journal of Medicine*, **324**, 39–42.

Shin, Y.S. (1990). Diagnosis of glycogen storage disease. *Journal Inherited Metabolic Disease*, **13**, 419–434.

Williams, J.C. (1986). Nutritional goals in glycogen storage disease. *New England Journal of Medicine*, **314**, 709–10.

Wolfsdorf, J.I., Rudlin, C.R., and Cirgler, J.F. (1990). Physical growth and development of children with type I glycogen-storage disease: comparison of the effects of long-term use of dextrose and uncooked cornstarch. *American Journal of Clinical Nutrition*, **52**, 1051–7.

11.2.2 Inborn errors of fructose metabolism

T. M. COX

Three inborn errors of fructose metabolism are recognized: (1) essential or benign fructosuria due to fructokinase deficiency; (2) fructose-1,6-diphosphatase deficiency; and (3) hereditary fructose intolerance (fructosaemia). There are discussed in relation to the overall metabolism of fructose.

Metabolism of fructose

Phosphorylated forms of fructose are critical intermediates in the glycolytic and gluconeogenic pathways of metabolism in all cells. Fructose is also an important component of the diet: it occurs as a free monosaccharide in fruit, nuts, honey, and some vegetables. Free fructose is released from sucrose in the gut lumen by sucrase–isomaltase in the brush-border membrane of the mucosal epithelium. Finally, the sugar alcohol, sorbitol (a constituent of medicines and tablets, as well as some foods for diabetics), is converted quantitatively to fructose in the liver and intestine. Most individuals in developed countries ingest 50 to 150 g fructose equivalents daily in the diet.

The pathways of fructose metabolism are summarized in Fig. 1. Fructose is absorbed rapidly by a carrier mechanism that facilitates transport across the intestinal epithelium. It is then conveyed via the portal bloodstream to the liver, where it is assimilated. The jejunal mucosa and proximal tubule of the kidney are subsidiary sites of fructose metabolism. Assimilation of fructose depends on the concerted activities of the enzymes ketohexokinase (fructokinase), aldolase B, and triokinase, which are expressed specifically in these tissues. Uptake of fructose occurs independently of insulin and its incorporation into intermediary metabolism bypasses regulation of glycolysis at the level of phosphofructokinase-1. For these reasons solutions of fructose or sorbitol have been advocated for parenteral nutrition. However, the occurrence of lactic acidosis, hyperuricaemia and other serious consequences have led to their withdrawal from hyperalimentation regimens.

Fructokinase rapidly phosphorylates fructose at the 1-carbon position.

This enzyme has a high affinity for its substrates and the intestinal mucosa and liver rapidly convert fructose to fructose 1-phosphate: in other tissues the capacity of hexokinase to phosphorylate fructose at the 6-carbon position is limited. Similarly, the fate of fructose 1-phosphate in the fructose-metabolizing tissues is dependent on a specific isozyme of aldolase, aldolase B. This has activity towards fructose 1-phosphate than does its ubiquitous counterpart, aldolase A, the natural substrate of which is fructose 1,6-diphosphate. Cleavage of fructose 1-phosphate generates glyceraldehyde and dihydroxyacetone phosphate. These trioses enter the intermediary pools of carbohydrate metabolism and, as a result of triokinase activity, glyceraldehyde is phosphorylated so that the two triose phosphates may be condensed by aldolase A to form the glycolytic and gluconeogenic intermediate, fructose 1,6-diphosphate.

Gluconeogenesis from triose phosphates, lactate, glycerol, amino acids, and Krebs' cycle intermediates such as oxaloacetate, requires reversal of the committed reactions of glycolysis. It is the enzyme fructose 1,6-diphosphatase that releases the glucose precursor fructose-6-phosphate from fructose-1,6-diphosphate. Thus, when the remaining reactions of glycolysis are reversed, exogenous fructose provides a source of glucose or glycogen. Fructose 1,6-diphosphatase is active in the liver, kidney, and intestine and is a key enzyme for gluconeogenesis.

Essential (benign) fructosuria

This is a rare disorder (estimated frequency 1 in 130 000) of little clinical consequence. The abnormality is transmitted as an autosomal recessive condition and manifests itself by the presence of a reducing sugar in the blood and urine, especially after meals rich in fructose. The abnormality results from deficiency of fructokinase activity in the liver and intestine, significantly reducing the capacity to assimilate this sugar. Fructose metabolism occurs slowly in essential fructosuria as a result of conversion to fructose 6-phosphate by hexokinase in adipose tissue and muscle, but while plasma concentrations remain high postprandially, large amounts of fructose appear in the urine. Essential fructosuria may be confused with diabetes mellitus if the nature of the mellituria is not defined but with the use of glucose oxidase strips in preference to the older chemical methods for urinalysis, this is now unlikely. No treatment beyond recognition and explanation appears to be necessary.

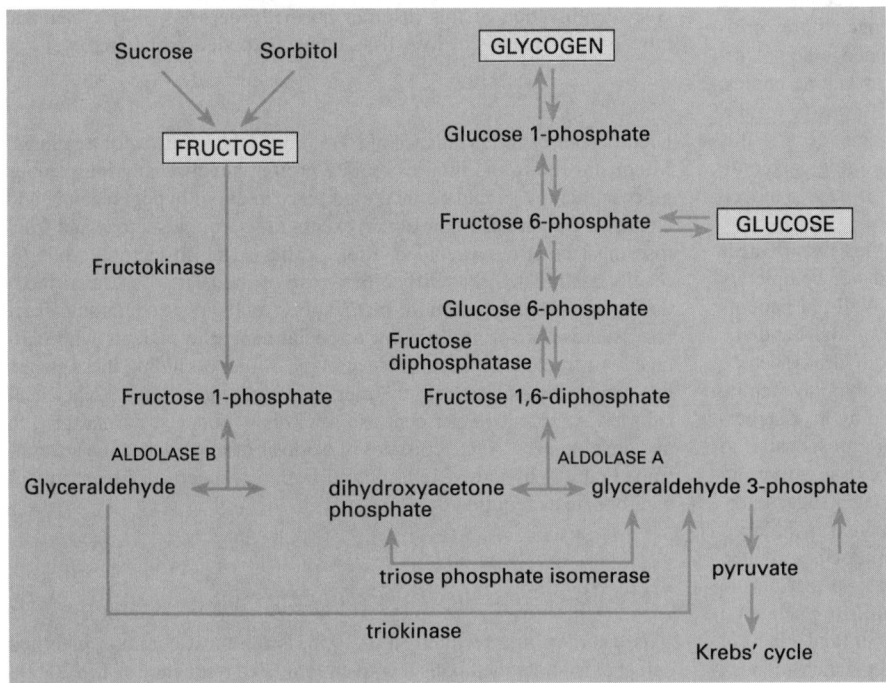

Fig. 1 Fructose metabolism.

Fructose diphosphatase deficiency

Description

This very rare, recessively-inherited disorder presents with hypoglycaemia, ketosis, and lactic acidosis in early infancy. Fewer than 30 cases have been reported since the original description in 1970. Severe, sometimes fatal, acidosis is associated with infection and starvation and most cases have presented within the first few days of life or in the neonatal period. Onset during the first year of life is the rule.

In newborn infants, the severe metabolic disturbance shows itself by acidotic hyperventilation, which may be accompanied by irritability, disturbed consciousness, or coma. The unusual combination of ketonaemia, lactic acidaemia, and hypoglycaemia is induced by fasting, administration of fructose, sorbitol, and glycerol, and by ingestion of a diet rich in fat. Episodes in the neonatal period respond well to infusions of glucose and bicarbonate but, after an interval, further attacks occur, often provoked by intercurrent infection. Lethargy accompanied by hyperventilation is followed abruptly by prostration, coma, and seizures. Investigations reveal hypoglycaemia, ketosis, and profound lactic acidosis; there is hyperuricaemia, amino aciduria, and ketonuria. If the infant survives, hepatomegaly due to fatty infiltration may be detected but overt clinical disturbances of hepatic or renal tubular function are not seen. The untreated disease is associated with growth retardation.

The first infant that is affected by fructose diphosphatase deficiency in a given pedigree may succumb before the diagnosis is established, and in any case fares worse than siblings for whom the appropriate diet and prompt control of the condition are instituted. The response to treatment is favourable, however, and fructose diphosphatase deficiency is ultimately compatible with a benign course and with normal growth and development.

Metabolic defect

Deficiency of fructose 1,6-diphosphatase causes failure of gluconeogenesis in the liver—although the abnormality may be detected in intestinal mucosa, kidney and in cultured mononuclear cells from peripheral blood. The muscle isozyme of fructose 1,6-diphosphatase is not affected.

Between meals blood glucose is maintained by glucogenolysis and hence the onset of disturbed metabolism in fructose diphosphatase deficiency depends on the availability of hepatic glycogen. Febrile illnesses accelerate consumption of liver glycogen and the accompanying anorexia with or without vomiting may deplete glycogen stores critically. Acidosis results from the accumulation of gluconeogenic precursors including lactate, pyruvate, and alanine as well as ketone bodies, which cannot be utilized. Hypoglycaemia, that is unresponsive to glucagon and associated with exhaustion of glycogen stores, occurs: this does not respond to normal gluconeogenic substrates (e.g. glycerol, amino acid solutions, dihydroxyacetone, sorbitol, or fructose) indeed administration of these aggravates the disorder.

The pathogenesis of hypoglycaemia and accompanying disturbances in fructose diphosphatase deficiency is complex and not completely explained by exhaustion of hepatic glycogen stores. Well-fed patients have a normal response to glucagon but are intolerant of high-fat diets, as well as of fructose, sorbitol, alanine, glycerol, and dihydroxyacetone administration. Challenge with these nutrients induces hypoglycaemia, hyperuricaemia, and hypophosphataemia, accompanied by an exaggerated rise in blood lactate. The hypoglycaemia is then unresponsive to glucagon, indicating a secondary inhibition of phosphorylase activity in the liver. This results from the build-up of phosphorylated sugar intermediates that cannot be further metabolized in the context of reduced intracellular free inorganic phosphate. Adenosine deaminase is activated primarily because of reduced phosphate concentrations, so that purine nucleotides are broken down to uric acid. Failure to utilize glucogenic amino acids and metabolites such as dihydroxyacetone and glycerol appears to stimulate triglyceride formation in the liver which induces

steatosis. Unlike hereditary fructose intolerance (see below) high concentrations of fructose-1-phosphate do not occur and profound disturbances of blood coagulation or hepatic or renal tubule function with progressive structural damage are absent in fructose diphosphatase deficiency. Similarly, aversion to foods that aggravate the disorder does not develop in affected infants and children; this may be explained by the absence of pain and abdominal symptoms in the condition.

Diagnosis

The importance of establishing the diagnosis of fructose diphosphatase deficiency cannot be overemphasised: proper dietary control and protocols for institution of appropriate therapy depend upon recognition of the complex disturbance that underlies this disease.

Fructose diphosphatase deficiency should be considered in otherwise normal infants who develop unexplained severe acidosis or hypoglycaemia associated with episodes of infection. The combination of ketosis and lactic acidosis with hypoglycaemia is highly suggestive of a disorder affecting the gluconeogenic pathway, including deficiency of glucose 6-phosphatase, pyruvate carboxylase, pyruvate dehydrogenase, and phosphoenolpyruvate carboxykinase. The absence of abdominal distress, haemolysis, jaundice, coagulopathy, and disturbances of the proximal renal tubule differentiate the condition from hereditary fructose intolerance, tyrosinosis, and Wilson's disease. Confusion may arise with disorders associated with secondary defects in gluconeogenesis, especially the Reye's-like syndrome seen with deficiencies of long-, medium- and short-chain acyl coenzyme A dehydrogenase activities, as well as defects of carnitine metabolism. Organic acidaemias are also readily distinguished by biochemical screening protocols.

Provocative tests by starvation and by using infusions of fructose, sorbitol or glycerol should be avoided in the acutely-ill infant or child with suspected deficiency of fructose-1,6-diphosphatase. Definitive diagnosis is dependent on demonstration of selectively decreased fructose diphosphatase activity in samples of tissue. Most frequently the enzymatic defect will be identified by biochemical assay of a liver biopsy specimen, which allows other metabolic disorders and gluconeogenic defects to be confidently excluded. The defect may also be demonstrated in biopsy samples of jejunal mucosa, and in cultured lymphocytes and monocyte-derived macrophages obtained from peripheral blood. However, the presence of fructose-1,6-diphosphatase in these tissues is metabolically inconsequential and, although useful for confirmation of the diagnosis where it is strongly suspected, in practice decisive identification of this disorder normally depends on a systematic biochemical analysis of liver tissue by an experienced laboratory.

Treatment

Dietary control and avoidance of starvation is the mainstay of treatment. Minor infections and injuries require prompt attention and intravenous glucose therapy should be instituted early to avoid hypoglycaemia and acidosis. The diet should exclude excess fat; sorbitol, sucrose and fructose must be strictly avoided. Breast milk is rich in lactose, which is readily assimilated, but difficulties arise on transfer to artificial feeds during weaning. In addition, medications and syrups containing fructose, sucrose or sorbitol present a special danger to patients with deficiency of fructose diphosphatase activity. A diet excluding these sugars but containing 56 per cent calories as carbohydrate with 32 per cent calories as fat and 12 per cent as protein has produced normal growth and development. Acute episodes of acidosis or hypoglycaemia are controlled rapidly by intravenous administration of glucose with or without bicarbonate as required.

Hereditary fructose intolerance (fructosaemia)

This disorder, first recognized in 1956, is the most common inherited defect of fructose metabolism with an estimated frequency of 1 in 20 000 births. The condition is transmitted as an autosomal recessive abnormality and, although it manifests itself first in early infancy, the effects of clinical disease may not be recognized until late childhood or adult life. Provided the diagnosis is made before visceral damage occurs, hereditary fructose intolerance responds completely to an exclusion diet.

The cardinal features of the illness are vomiting, diarrhoea, abdominal pain, and hypoglycaemia, which are induced by consumption of foods, drinks, or medicines that contain fructose or the related sugars, sucrose or sorbitol. There is a generalized metabolic disturbance with lactic acidosis, hyperuricaemia, and hyperphosphataemia. Hypoglycaemia causes trembling, irritability, and cognitive impairment. Attacks are associated with pallor, sweating, and, when severe, loss of consciousness sometimes accompanied by generalized seizures. These episodes usually occur within 30 min of feeds that contain large quantities of fructose or sucrose. Continued ingestion of noxious sugars is associated with renal tubular disease, liver damage with jaundice, and defective blood coagulation. There is failure to thrive and growth retardation. Persistent exposure to fructose in infants leads to structural liver injury with cirrhosis, amino aciduria, coagulopathy, and coma leading to death. The infant is first exposed to the offending sugars at weaning or upon transfer from breast milk to artificial feeds: survival is dependent on recognition of the effects of fruit and sugar by the mother or, especially in older infants, by vomiting or forcible rejection of food.

In infants that survive the stormy period of weaning, a strong aversion to sweet-tasting foods, vegetables and fruits develops. This usually affords protection against the worst effects of fructose and sucrose, but abdominal symptoms with bouts of tremulousness, irritability, and altered consciousness due to hypoglycaemia usually continue. It has become clear that many cases escape diagnosis in infancy and childhood but the risk of illness, related to dietary indiscretion, remains throughout life. Characteristically these patients show a striking reduction in or absence of dental caries.

Recently, a syndrome of chronic sugar intoxication has been recognized in older children and adolescents with hereditary fructose intolerance. General lack of vigour and developmental retardation are prominent features. Hypoglycaemia, though obvious after heavy fructose loading, may be insignificant after chronic low-level exposure in older children. Similarly, tests of hepatic and renal function may be only mildly abnormal. Persistent ingestion of fructose and sucrose is toxic to the kidney and liver, so that renal tubular acidosis (occasionally with calculi) as well as hepatosplenomegaly are frequently detectable in the younger patients. Severe growth retardation may be accompanied by rachitic bone disease that complicates the Fanconi-like syndrome of proximal renal tubular disturbance. Growth retardation responds to dietary treatment and is usually accompanied by regression of the other disease manifestations.

Provided that organ failure and serious tissue injury do not supervene, patients with hereditary fructose intolerance recover rapidly when the offending sugars are completely withdrawn. Children that survive by acquiring the protective pattern of eating behaviour avoid foods that they associate with abdominal symptoms. The aversion extends to most sweet-tasting articles of food and drink as well as fruits and vegetables—it remains lifelong and consumption of fructose is usually reduced to less than 5 g daily. It has been shown that normal growth and development can be secured in children if less than 40 mg/kg fructose equivalents are ingested daily.

Metabolic defect

Hereditary fructose intolerance is caused by a deficiency of aldolase B in the liver, small intestine, and proximal renal tubule. These tissues suffer injury as a result of persistent exposure to fructose in patients affected by the disorder. In the absence of fructose 1-phosphate splitting activity of aldolase B, the intracellular pool of inorganic phosphate is depleted. Studies *in vivo* by ^{31}P magnetic resonance spectroscopy show that 80 per cent of hepatic free phosphate is sequestered as sugar phos-

phates after infusion of small quantities of fructose (250 mg/kg body weight). The secondary metabolic disturbances are initiated by the accumulation of fructose 1-phosphate in a milieu where free inorganic phosphate is reduced: there is competitive inhibition of aldolase A and inhibition of phosphorylase activity so that glycogenolysis and gluconeogenesis are impaired. Thus challenge with fructose leads to hypophosphataemia and hypoglycaemia that is refractory to glucagon or infusion of gluconeogenic metabolites such as glycerol or dihydroxyacetone. During challenge with fructose, high concentrations of fructose 1-phosphate cause feedback inhibition of fructokinase, thereby limiting the incorporation of fructose in the liver. As a result, fructosaemia occurs and when the concentration exceeds about 2 mmol/l in peripheral blood, fructosuria becomes apparent. Although assimilation of fructose by the specialized pathway is blocked, only a small fraction of the fructose load is recovered in the urine. Studies show that 80 to 90 per cent of the fructose is taken up under these circumstances by adipose tissue and muscle, where it can be alternatively metabolized by phosphorylation to fructose 6-phosphate.

Electrolytic disturbances occur during challenge with fructose. Hypokalaemia results from acute renal impairment with defective urinary acidification. There is a defect of proximal tubule function with bicarbonate wasting and acidosis. Occasionally, acute flaccid weakness due to hypokalaemia accompanies the other effects of fructose exposure. In patients with hereditary fructose intolerance, administration of fructose reproducibly increases serum magnesium concentrations. This is probably explained by the breakdown of magnesium–adenosine triphosphate complexes, releasing intracellular magnesium ions as a result of nucleotide degradation by adenosine deaminase. Significant ingestion of fructose is thus also accompanied by marked hyperuricaemia in patients with hereditary fructose intolerance.

Pathology and molecular genetics

Chronic ingestion of fructose in hereditary fructose intolerance causes hepatic injury: there is diffuse fatty change and increased glycogen deposition. Hepatocyte necrosis with intralobular and periportal fibrosis occurs and fully developed cirrhosis results from continued exposure to fructose. After acute experimental challenge, electron microscopy has shown irregular electron-dense material surrounded by membraneous structures, suggesting a florid lysosomal reaction to intracellular deposits of fructose 1-phosphate. Fatal administration of fructose or sorbitol parenterally is associated with the abrupt onset of hepatorenal failure associated with bleeding. Histological examination shows hepatic necrosis in these cases. Loss of cellular functions, for example in the proximal renal tubule, is probably caused by depletion of adenosine triphosphate resulting from the arrested metabolism of fructose by the specialized pathway. The source of the severe abdominal pain that follows ingestion of fructose is unknown, but stimulation of visceral afferent nerves by local release of purine nucleotides or lactate may be responsible.

The genetic basis of aldolase B deficiency has been studied intensively. Several point mutations affecting the function of the enzyme are sufficiently widespread in patients of European origin to merit diagnostic investigation. One particular mutation, Ala^{149}→Pro, which disrupts residues in a substrate-binding domain of aldolase B, is prevalent in Europe. This mutation accounts for most alleles responsible for intolerance of fructose.

Diagnosis

In infancy and childhood, hereditary fructose intolerance most characteristically causes persistent vomiting with failure to thrive, acidosis, hypoglycaemia, and jaundice. Clearly in very young infants there is a wide differential diagnosis, but fructose intolerance may be indicated by the nutritional history and feeding difficulties. The presence of reducing sugar in the urine may indicate that fructosuria and amino acids may also be present. Older children and adults report food aversion and may show a striking absence of dental caries. If fructose intolerance is considered, then sucrose, sorbitol, and fructose should be excluded completely before definitive tests can be carried out. Striking improvement, suggestive of hereditary fructose intolerance may be seen within a few days but the differential diagnosis includes pyloric stenosis, galactosaemia, hepatitis, renal tubular disease, Wilson's disease, and tyrosinosis.

The intravenous fructose tolerance test is the bench mark for diagnosis: 0.25 g/kg (0.2 g/kg in infants) of D+ fructose is infused as a 20 per cent solution over a few minutes and blood samples for potassium ions, magnesium ions, phosphate ions, and glucose are taken at regular intervals over 2 h. Epigastric and loin pain accompany the infusion, and hypoglycaemic coma may occur. The hypoglycaemia does not respond to glucagon and glucose for parenteral injection should be available. The test should be carried out under controlled conditions with medical personnel at hand: oral challenge with fructose or sucrose may produce severe pain and shock and is best avoided. Responses differ between individuals and hypoglycaemia is usually milder in adults but typical responses in hereditary fructose intolerance and a control subject are depicted in Fig. 2.

Aldolase B deficiency may be demonstrated by enzymatic analysis of biopsy samples obtained from the liver or small intestinal mucosa. Biochemical assay of fructaldolases characteristically demonstrates reduced or absent fructose-1-phosphate cleavage activity with a partial deficiency of fructose-1,6-diphosphate aldolase. Fructaldolase deficiency may accompany other parenchymal disease of the liver and these assays may be of limited value in the acutely ill or jaundiced patient.

Recently, direct diagnosis of hereditary fructose intolerance has been

Fig. 2 (a) Intravenous fructose tolerance tests in a woman aged 39 with hereditary fructose intolerance proven by fructaldolase essay and DNA analysis and (b) an age- and sex-matched control subject with alcohol-related episodic hypoglycaemia.

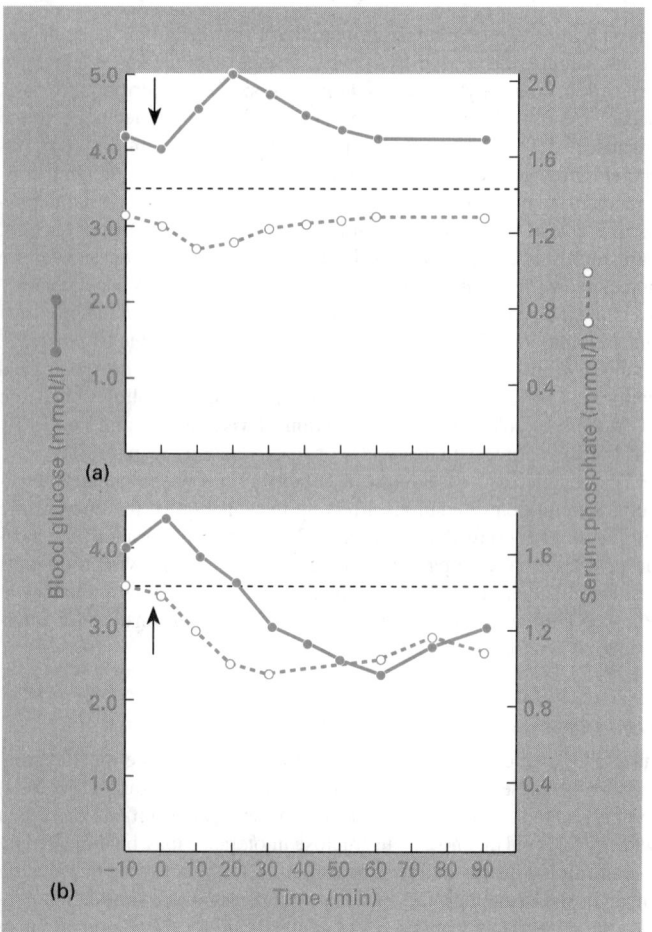

Table 1 *Food items not allowed for patients with hereditary fructose intolerance and fructose diphosphatase deficiency*

Table sugar
Fruit sugar, all fruit and fruit products, including tomatoes
Sorbitol
Honey, syrup, treacle, molasses
Diabetic foods
Chocolate, sherbet
Preserves, jams, and marmalade
Frankfurters, honey-roast, and sweet-cured ham
Processed cheese spreads
Cream and cottage cheese with chives, pineapple, etc.
Flavoured milks and yoghurts
Wheatgerm, brown rice, bran
Breakfast cereals
Coffee essence, powdered milk
Carbonated sweet drinks
Allspice, nuts, coconut, carob, peanut butter
Mayonnaise, pickles, salad dressings, sauces
Some potatoes (especially stored, new potatoes)
Most legumes

Further information is provided in the references.

possible in European patients: examination of aldolase B genes for the presence of common mutations responsible for the disease in this population can be carried out by laboratories that specialize in the molecular analysis of genomic DNA. The ability to identify disease alleles by analysis of minute samples of blood or tissue may be beneficial for the investigation of infants with this disorder and, eventually, for postnatal screening before dietary exposure occurs.

Treatment

Dietary treatment of fructose intolerance alleviates the disorder but requires almost complete exclusion of sucrose, fructose and sorbitol. Daily consumption of sugar should be reduced to less than 40 mg of fructose equivalents per kilogram body weight (i.e. 2–3 g for an adult) in order to reverse the disease manifestations and establish normal development in affected children. The ubiquity of fructose and its cogeners in the Western diet presents serious difficulties. Adult patients have usually restricted their consumption of fructose to less than 20 g daily and the source of the residual sugar may be difficult to establish. For this reason, the advice of an experienced dietitian should be sought (Table 1). Particular care needs to be taken with sugar-coated pills and, especially, liquid medications for paediatric use, as large amounts of fructose, sucrose, and sorbitol are frequently present. Occasionally patients are unable to tolerate certain foods that are permitted on their diet sheets—in doubtful cases it is advisable to avoid the offending item or to have it analysed. Patients with hereditary fructose intolerance may lack folic acid and vitamin C. Vitamin supplements are recommended, especially during pregnancy but, as with other medicines, care has to be taken to avoid harmful sugars contained in the preparation: Ketovite®; (Paines and Byrne, Ltd., Surrey, England) is a satisfactory source of these vitamins.

REFERENCES

Baker, L., and Wingrad, A.I. (1970). Fasting hypoglycaemia and metabolic acidosis associated with deficiency of fructose-1,6-diphosphatase deficiency. *Lancet*, **ii**, 13–16.

Bell, L. and Sherwood, W.G. (1987). Current practices and improved recommendations for treating hereditary fructose intolerance. *Journal of the American Dietetic Association*, **87**, 721–8.

Chambers, R.A. and Pratt, R.T.C. (1956). Idiosyncrasy to fructose. *Lancet*, **ii**, 340.

Cox, T.M. (1988). Hereditary fructose intolerance. *Quarterly Journal of Medicine*, **68**, 585–94.

Cox, T.M. (1994). Aldolase B and fructose intolerance. *Journal of the Federation of American Societies for Experimental Biology*, **8**, 62–71.

Gitzelmann, R., Steinmann, B., and Van den Berghe, G. (1989). Disorders of fructose metabolism. In *The metabolic basis of inherited disease* (6th edn), (ed C.R. Scriber, A.L. Beaudet, W.S. Sly, and D. Valle), pp. 399–424. McGraw-Hill, New York.

Greenwood, J. (1989). Sugar content of liquid prescription medicines. *Pharmaceutical Journal*, **243**, 553–7.

Oberhaensli, R.D., Rajagopalan, B., Taylor, D.J., Leonard, J.V., and Radda, G.K. (1987). Study of hereditary fructose intolerance by use of ³¹P magnetic resonance spectroscopy. *Lancet*, **ii**, 931–4.

Odièvre, M., Gentil, C., Gantier, M., and Alagille, D. (1978). Hereditary fructose intolerance in childhood. Diagnosis, management and course in 55 patients. *American Journal of Diseases of Childhood*, **132**, 605–8.

Pagliara, A.S., Karl, I.E., Keating, J.P., Brown, B.I., and Kipnis, D.M. (1972). Hepatic fructose-1,6-diphosphatase deficiency. A cause of lactic acidosis and hypoglycaemia in infancy. *Journal of Clinical Investigation*, **51**, 2115–23.

Sachs, B., Sternfeld, L., and Kraus, G. (1942). Essential fructosuria: its pathophysiology. *American Journal of Diseases of Childhood*, **63**, 252.

11.2.3 Disorders of galactose metabolism

T. M. COX

Galactose is derived from lactose in the diet by the action of the mucosal disaccharidase lactase in the small intestine. After absorption, galactose serves as a source of glucose and is a component of many membrane glycoproteins and glycolipids. Complex galactosylated lipids are abundant in nervous tissue.

The conversion of galactose to glucose involves reactions that lead to the formation of glucose 1-phosphate, which can enter the main pathways of carbohydrate metabolism, directly (Fig. 1). The first step

Fig. 1 Galactose metabolism.

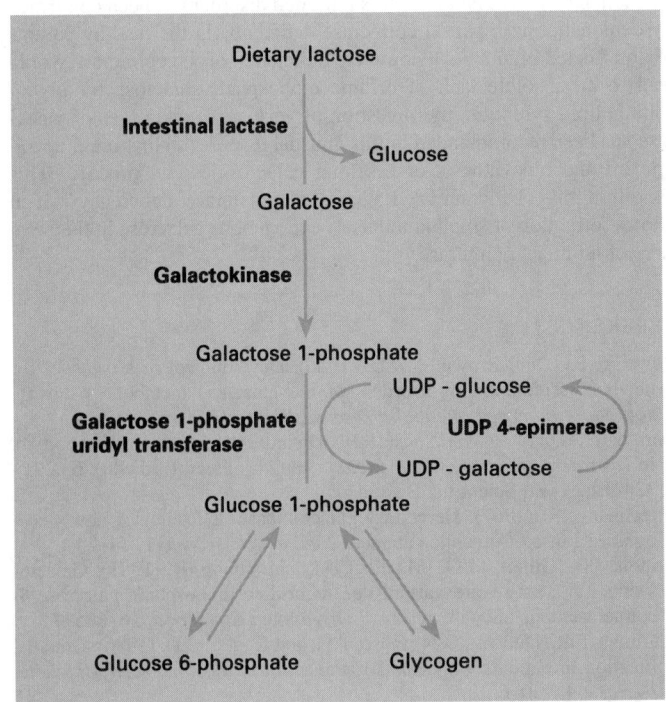

involves phosphorylation to form galactose 1-phosphate, which is converted to glucose 1-phosphate and uridine diphosphate-galactose after reaction with the nucleoside diphosphate sugar uridine diphosphoglucose. Uridine diphosphoglucose is regenerated by the action of uridine diphosphate-galactose-4-epimerase. Enzymatic defects in the interconversion of these metabolites lead to increased blood and tissue concentrations of galactose, especially after meals containing milk or dairy products. Three inborn errors of galactose metabolism are recognized: (1) galactokinase deficiency; (2) galactose 1-phosphate uridyl transferase deficiency; and (3) uridine diphosphate-4-epimerase deficiency.

Galactokinase deficiency: 'galactose diabetes'

Failure to phosphorylate galactose at the 1-carbon position in the liver and other tissues impairs its clearance from the blood so that the free sugar and its metabolites, galactonic acid and galactitol; appear in the urine. Homozygous deficiency of galactokinase occurs with an approximate frequency of 1 in 100 000 live births.

Clinical features

Precocious formation of cataracts in infants and children is characteristic and some heterozygotes appear to develop cataracts before the age of 40 years. When blood concentrations are high, galactose is taken up by the lens and converted to the end-product galactitol by the action of aldose reductase: subsequent toxic or osmotic effects lead to swelling and irreversible damage to lens fibres. Patients with galactokinase deficiency persistently excrete reducing sugar in their urine but, apart from possible confusion with diabetes mellitus, this has no apparent significance.

Diagnosis and treatment

Galactokinase deficiency should be suspected in infants or children with cataracts and reducing sugar should be sought in the urine. This sugar will not react with glucose oxidase test strips. Definitive diagnosis by enzymatic assay of galactokinase in erythrocytes or cultured fibroblasts differentiates the disorder from classic galactosaemia. Treatment with a strict lactose–galactose exclusion diet prevents cataract formation.

Galactose 1-phosphate uridyl transferase deficiency: galactosaemia

Unlike individuals in whom galactokinase is deficient, when patients who lack uridyl transferase deficiency ingest lactose, there is a significant rise in intracellular galactose 1-phosphate, as well as blood galactose concentration. The severe consequences of classical galactosaemia thus result from the toxic effects of galactose 1-phosphate principally in cells of the liver, proximal renal tubule, and brain. Although the exact mechanism of toxicity is unknown, as in hereditary fructose intolerance, the accumulated metabolite probably inhibits other enzymatic reactions involving phosphorylated intermediates and may lead to purine nucleotide depletion.

Clinical and pathological features

The affected infant appears normal at birth but vomiting or diarrhoea, jaundice, and hepatomegaly usually occur in the first few weeks. There is failure to gain weight, subcutaneous bruising, and progressive enlargement of the liver. Cataracts may be apparent at 1 month of age, by which time abdominal distension with ascites has developed. Mental retardation does not become manifest until later in the first year of life and varies greatly in severity. Many patients suffering from galactosaemia develop severe infections with *Escherichia coli* during the neonatal period, and Gram-negative bacterial sepsis may represent a significant diagnostic indicator of this disorder in young infants.

Occasional patients with galactosaemia remain asymptomatic while ingesting milk but gradually fail to gain weight. Such patients may come to light in childhood, or even adult life, because of varying degrees of mental retardation and cataracts. Hepatomegaly and intermittent galactosuria are usually present and often there is a history of feeding difficulties with institution of reduced milk intake and modified formula feeds during the neonatal period.

The neurological manifestations of classical galactosaemia are highly variable but despite prompt institution of dietary therapy, a degree of mental retardation is common in affected children and adults. Characteristic learning difficulties in mathematics and spatial relationships with behavioural deficits have been observed. It appears that the galactose-free diet fails to confer benefit on mental development when instituted beyond the age of 2 years. In follow-up studies of galactosaemic children and adults, a range of neurological deficits including seizures, apraxia, extrapyramidal disorders, and cerebellar signs have been documentated despite strict dietary measures.

Serum tests of liver function are non-specifically deranged: histological examination shows lobular fibrosis, fatty change, bile ductular proliferation, and progression to frank cirrhosis. Involvement of the proximal renal tubule is shown by generalized aminoaciduria and occasionally a full-blown Fanconi syndrome with vacuolation of tubular epithelial cells. Histological examination of the brain shows non-specific signs of injury with gliosis and Purkinje cell loss in the cerebellum. Follow-up studies of female patients with galactosaemia has shown a high incidence of gonadal failure with ovarian atrophy: although this complication appears to be more common in patients in whom dietary therapy was delayed, no clear cause-and-effect relationship has been established. No evidence of gonadal failure has been found in male patients.

Genetic studies

Galactosaemia is transmitted as an autosomal recessive trait with an overall estimated frequency of 1 in 62 000. In black patients from the United States a relatively mild disorder has been reported that is probably due to an unstable enzyme variant; uridyl transferase activity is absent from their red cells but amounts to some 10 per cent of normal in samples of liver and small intestinal tissue. Individuals with the Duarte variant possess about half-normal enzyme activity in erythrocytes but remain asymptomatic.

The human galactosyl-1-phosphate uridyl transferase gene maps to human chromosome 9p13 and encodes a protein of molecular weight 43 000 Da. Molecular analysis of the transferase gene indicates that most patients with classical galactosaemia harbour mis-sense type mutations. Several other variant transferase enzymes have been described but the significance of any individual mutation for diagnostic purposes has not yet been established.

Diagnosis

Galactosaemia may be suspected in an infant with growth failure, cataracts, liver disease, aminoaciduria, mental retardation, and especially where reducing sugar is present in the urine. The occurrence of unexplained bacterial sepsis, especially if due to *E. coli* infection in a newborn infant, may also indicate the presence of galactosaemia.

Definitive diagnosis is mandatory and relies on the determination of galactose 1-phosphate uridyl transferase activity in red cells or leucocytes by means of a specific enzymatic assay. Reliable testing for heterozygotes can be carried out in the parents of a child that has died before the diagnosis has been confirmed and, in some parts of the world, neonatal screening for elevated blood galactose and galactose 1-phosphate concentrations is carried out routinely.

Treatment

Without strict dietary treatment, most patients with galactosaemia die in early infancy, although some may survive with liver disease and mental retardation beyond childhood. The course of galactosaemia is altered strikingly upon withdrawal of lactose (and galactose). However, lactose is present in many non-dairy foods and advice from an experienced dietician as well as meticulous attention to detail, is required to eliminate it completely. In infants, soybean milks or commercial casein hydrolysates 'Nutramigen' are used as milk substitutes and therapy is monitored by periodic assay of red cell galactose 1-phosphate concentrations. Despite reports that galactose may be reintroduced as the patient develops, lifelong strict adherence to the exclusion diet should be advocated. In subsequent pregnancies of heterozygous mothers who have had affected children there is evidence that premature cataracts can be avoided in the fetus if the intake of lactose is restricted.

Prognosis

The acute manifestations of galactosaemia and growth failure respond quickly to dietary therapy and cataract formation is prevented. Unfortunately a proportion of patients have significant neurological deficits despite prompt and conscientious treatment. The presence of ovarian failure and elevated galactose 1-phosphate concentrations in patients apparently ingesting no lactose or galactose raises the possibility that an endogenous pathway of galactose 1-phosphate formation from pyrophosphorlysis of uridine diphosphate-galactose may occur. This may also explain the late emergence of neurological disease in treated patients. Long-term follow-up and periodic neuropsychiatric, as well as physical, monitoring is recommended.

Uridine diphosphate 4-epimerase deficiency

Epimerase deficiency is very rare but may be identified during screening for classic galactosaemia. In most cases no symptoms attributable to galactosaemia are apparent and follow-up studies have confirmed the usually benign nature of this anomaly. However, a few cases of marked deficiency of uridine diphosphate-4-epimerase have been discovered in patients otherwise manifesting the classic features of galactosaemia. The autosomal recessive nature of this inherited disorder has been confirmed by demonstrating a partial epimerase deficiency in the healthy parents of an affected infant. As a complete deficiency of the epimerase would lead to an absolute lack of uridine diphosphate-galactose for glycosphingolipid synthesis, the ingestion of very small quantities of galactose has been recommended in this unusual disorder so that brain development and biosynthesis of essential galactosides can proceed. This condition may be contrasted with the transferase deficiency which allows formation of small amounts of endogenous galactose in the presence of an intact epimerase.

REFERENCES

Bowring, F.G. and Brown, A.R.D. (1986). Development of a protocol for newborn screening for disorders of the galactose metabolic pathway. *Journal of Inherited Metabolic Disease*, **9**, 99–104.

Cornblath, M. and Schwartz, R. (1991). Disorders of galactose: metabolism. In *Disorders of Carbohydrate Metabolism in Infancy*, (3rd edn), pp.295–324. Blackwell Scientific, Boston.

Gitzelmann, R. (1967). Hereditary galactokinase deficiency; a newly-recognized cause of juvenile cataracts. *Pediatric Research*, **1**, 14–23.

Holton, J.B., Gillett, M.G., MacFaul, R., and Young, R. (1981). Galactosaemia. A new severe variant due to uridine diphosphate galactose-4-epimerase deficiency. *Archives of Diseases in Childhood*, **56**, 885–7.

Kaufman, F.R., Donnell, G.N., Rose, T.F., and Kogut, M.D. (1986). Gonadal function in patients with galactosaemia. *Journal of Inherited Metabolic Disease*, **9**, 140–6.

Segal, S. (1989). Disorders of galactose metabolism. In *The metabolic basis of inherited disease* (ed C.R. Scriver, A.L. Beaudet, W.S. Sly, and D. Valle), (6th edn), pp. 453–80. McGraw-Hill, New York.

Waggoner, D.D., Buist, N.R.M., and Donnell, G.N. (1990). Long-term prognosis in galactosaemia: results of a survey of 350 cases. *Journal of Inherited Metabolic Disease*, **13**, 802–18.

Pentosuria

Pentosuria is caused by the excessive renal excretion of L-xylulose: this has no clinical significance except that it may lead to the incorrect diagnosis of diabetes mellitus should tests for reducing sugar be carried out on the urine. Xylulose does not react with urinary test strips based on the glucose oxidase method.

Pentosuria is a rare autosomal recessive trait but its frequency in Ashkenazi Jews may be as high as 0.05 per cent. It is caused by enzymatic deficiency of L-xylulose reductase in the oxidative pathway of glucuronate metabolism and 1 to 4 g of xylulose and L-arabitol appear continuously in the urine: output is greatly enhanced by ingestion of glucuronic acid or drugs that are excreted as glucuronides.

REFERENCES

Hiatt, H.H. (1978). Pentosuria. In *The metabolic basis of inherited disease*, (ed J.B. Stanbury, J.B. Wyngaarden and D.S. Fredrickson), (4th edn), p 110. McGraw-Hill, New York.

Inborn errors of pyruvate metabolism

Pyruvate dehydrogenase

Deficiency of pyruvate dehydrogenase is the most common cause of lactic acidosis in newborn infants and children, but it is also associated with neurodegenerative syndromes in later life. Pyruvate dehydrogenase exists as a multi-enzyme complex representing the products of ten distinct genes. However, defects in one subunit of pyruvate dehydrogenase itself (E1α) account for most patients so far investigated, although defects in dihydrolipoyl dehydrogenase (E3) are also described.

Biochemical defect

The pyruvate dehydrogenase complex catalyses the conversion of pyruvate to acetyl coenzyme A within mitochondria and operates at about 10, 40, and 70 per cent of capacity in the liver, heart, and brain, respectively. Three main activities are associated in the complex: (1) pyruvate dehydrogenase, a thiamine-dependent moiety (E1); (2) dihydrolipoyl transacetylase (E2); and (3) dihydrolipoyl dehydrogenase (E3). Also associated are a pyruvate dehydrogenase-specific kinase and phosphatase (both involved in overall metabolic regulation of the complex) and an essential lipoic acid moiety.

The accumulated pyruvate may either be reduced to lactate or transaminated to alanine so that hyperalaninaemia and varying degrees of lactic acidaemia occur. Very rare defects in dihydrolipoyl dehydrogenase are associated with deficiency of branched-chain keto acid dehydrogenase. Failure to carry out oxidative reactions in regions of the cortex and midbrain causes neuronal death and deficiency of 4-carbon intermediates may critically impair neurotransmitter synthesis.

Clinical features and prognosis

Severe deficiency of pyruvate dehydrogenase affects intrauterine development and causes marked acidosis (blood lactate > 10 mmol/l) at birth with early death. Many victims do not show clinically significant metabolic acidosis and come to light because of intrauterine growth failure, neonatal hypotonia asphyxia, and feeding difficulty. In those with neurological manifestations, blood lactate concentrations do not exceed 10 mmol/l. Should feeding by gavage be instituted, there is a protracted course with failure of neurological development, microcephaly, quadriplegia, seizures, and blindness. Intermittent cerebellar ataxia or torsion dystonia has been recorded and choreoathetoid movements occur. Involuntary eye movements in children are associated with a progressively deteriorating course. In a few patients, hereditary spinocerebellar degeneration appearing in early adult life has been attributed to deficiency of pyruvate dehydrogenase, but the relationship to Friedreich's ataxia is controversial. In patients who present with severe acidosis at birth, subacute necrotizing encephalomyelopathy of the the Leigh's type has been confirmed at necropsy and deficiency of pyruvate dehydrogenase activity has been demonstrated.

Genetics

The most common cause of pyruvate dehydrogenase deficiency is due to a defect in the E1α subunit—a protein encoded on the X chromosome. Although the disease is characteristically more severe in males, manifestations in the heterozygous female are frequent and probably reflect the low functional reserve of the enzyme complex in the brain. Neonatal lactic acidosis is more frequent in males. An auxiliary gene for the E1α subunit is localized to the long arm of chromosome 4 but is expressed only during spermatogenesis in the testis; its presence, however, indicates the critical need for activity of the complex in nearly all tissues. Causal mutations in the E1α gene on the X chromosome have been described—most appear to be short deletions or duplications and at present are not generally applicable for diagnosis. However, analysis of X chromosome inactivation patterns by determination of methylation status has proved useful for the evaluation of enzymatic assays of fibroblasts obtained from obligate carriers or female patients in whom the diagnosis is suspected.

Diagnosis and treatment

The diagnosis is suspected from the presence of severe acidosis at birth. It may also emerge during the investigation of neurological deficits, especially where they are associated with intrauterine growth failure. Routine screening of urine samples for organic acids may identify excessive pyruvate, lactate, and alanine excretion. In patients without clinically evident acidosis, cerebral disease is accompanied by striking elevations of lactate and pyruvate in the cerebrospinal fluid.

Neuroradiological procedures, including cerebral ultrasonography and computized tomography, reveal ventricular dilatation and cerebral atrophy. Pathological examination of previously affected siblings shows shrinkage of gyri, with involvement of the medulla shown by loss or hypoplasia of the pyramids. The pathological features of Wernicke's encephalopathy may be present. The corpus callosum may be absent. Definitive diagnosis, however, depends on enzymatic assay in skin fibroblasts.

Institution of a high fat, low carbohydrate, ketogenic diet may ameliorate the biochemical abnormalities but given the degree of neurological impairment that is normally present at diagnosis, little clinical improvement can be expected. Therapeutic responses to administration of high-dose thiamine have been reported in patients with partial enzymatic deficiency, notably where ataxia and abnormal eye movements reminiscent of Wernicke's encephalopathy were conspicuous. In rare patients with the autosomally recessive condition due to dihydrolipoyl dehydrogenase deficiency, oral administration of lipoic acid has been reported to correct the organic acidaemia with clinical improvement.

Pyruvate carboxylase deficiency

Inborn defects in pyruvate carboxylase, a key gluconeogeneic enzyme, cause hypoglycaemia or profound metabolic acidosis with neurological disease. The manifestations of this latter syndrome closely resemble those caused by deficiencies of pyruvate dehydrogenase activity. A severe form, associated with hyperammonaemia and citrullinaemia is also recognized, particularly in patients of French descent.

Metabolic defect

Pyruvate decarboxylase is a biotin-dependent enzyme that catalyses the first step in the formation of oxaloacetate from pyruvate and is activated allosterically by acetyl coenzyme A. Thus, hypoglycaemia would be expected only after glycogen stores had been depleted. Krebs' cycle intermediates may become depleted so that there is insufficient synthesis of neurotransmitters. There may also be a reduced supply of aspartate for the arginosuccinate synthase reaction of the urea cycle.

Clinical features

Patients with severe deficiency of pyruvate carboxylase may present with the Leigh syndrome (necrotizing encephalomyopathy with lactate/pyruvate acidosis) or hypotonia and neurological retardation. The presence of ataxia and abnormal ocular movements in life suggest the occurrence of midbrain disease resembling Wernicke's encephalopathy. Hypoglycaemia occurs during intercurrent infection or during starvation and acidosis, requiring bicarbonate therapy, occurs frequently. The most severe form, originally reported from France, progresses rapidly with evidence of liver damage, hyperammonaemia, and citrullinaemia.

Genetics

This disorder is transmitted as an autosomal recessive trait. In severely affected patients with hyperammonaemia, pyruvate carboxylase protein and its messenger ribonucleic acid (mRNA) are absent in the liver. In other patients a partially inactive variant enzyme is detectable.

Diagnosis and treatment

The condition is suspected when acidosis and neurological disease occur in infants, especially in the presence of hypoglycaemia. Specific diagnosis requires enzymatic assay in fibroblasts and this can be used for carrier detection. Disorders of pyruvate metabolism may be mimicked biochemically by mitochondrial diseases and acquired deficiencies of thiamine or biotin. Biotin therapy has been disappointing in pyruvate carboxylase deficiency but occasional responses to high-dose lipoic acid and thiamine treatment, which may stimulate the pyruvate metabolism by the dehydrogenase complex, have been recorded.

Therapy

Episodes of acidosis are treated with intravenous sodium bicarbonate and glucose may be required for hypoglycaemia. There is evidence that ketogenic diets containing 50 per cent fat and 20 per cent carbohydrate ameliorate the biochemical disturbance and delay the onset of neurological disease: in some patients administration of glutamate and aspartate, that may act as a source of oxaloacetate, appear to have been beneficial.

REFERENCES

Brown, G.K. et al. (1988). Cerebral lactic acidosis: defects in pyruvate metabolism with profound brain damage and minimal systemic acidosis. *European Journal of Pediatrics*, **147**, 10–14.

Brown, G.K., Brown, R.M., Scholem, R.D. Kirby, D.M., and Dahl H-H.M. (1989). The clinical and biochemical spectrum of human pyruvate dehydrogenase deficiency. *Annals of the New York Academy of Sciences*, **573**, 360–8.

Brown, G.K. (1992). Pyruvate dehydrogenase E1α deficiency. *Journal of Inherited Metabolic Disease*, **15**, 625–33.

Hinman, L.M., Shen, K-F.R., Baker, A.C., Kim, Y.T., and Blass, J.P. (1989). Deficiency of pyruvate dehydrogenase complex in Leigh's disease fibroblasts: an abnormality in lipoamide dehydrogenase affecting PDHC activation. *Neurology*, **39**, 70–5.

Robinson, B.H. et al. (1987). The French and North American phenotypes of pyruvate carboxylase deficiency. *American Journal of Human Genetics*, **40**, 50–9.

11.3 Inborn errors of amino acid and organic acid metabolism

D. P. BRENTON

Introduction

An overview of amino acid metabolism and genetic defects

Man depends upon dietary protein as a source of amino acids, some of which he cannot synthesis, and all of which are used very economically. Stool nitrogen losses are only about 1 g/day and bacterial protein accounts for much of this. Renal conservation of amino acids is extremely effective with low clearance values (Table 1). Amino acids taken in excess of requirement are not stored but used for energy. After the removal of the amino group for conversion to ammonia and urea (Fig. 1), the carbon skeletons degrade to major metabolic intermediates such as acetyl coenzyme A, acetoacetyl coenzyme A, pyruvate, or to citric acid cycle intermediates (Fig. 2) via individual amino acid pathways. Amino acids are referred to as glucogenic when their carbon skeletons degrade to intermediates used in gluconeogenesis, and ketogenic when their degradation products can form ketone bodies. Degradative enzymes frequently have important coenzymes and inherited defects of catabolism may be due to defects of the apoenzymes or their vitamin coenzymes. Table 2 offers a biochemical classification of the genetic defects of amino acid metabolism. A clinical classification would have more practical value but is difficult because of the non-specific nature of many clinical features, e.g. mental retardation.

Table 1 *Plasma amino acid values, excretion, and clearances in young adult males and females (author's data). Cystine expressed as 0.5 mol (molecular weight = 120)*

Amino acid	Plasma μmol/l range	Mean	Excretion μmol/ min (mean)	Clearance (ml/min/1.73 m²) (mean)
Taurine	65–179	100	0.54	5.8
Aspartic	17–51	36	0.04	1.3
Threonine	111–236	143	0.09	0.7
Serine	114–210	159	0.20	1.4
Glutamic	73–296	182	0.29	0.1
Glutamine	332–652	441	0.02	0.7
Glycine	180–311	246	0.64	2.6
Alanine	212–407	325	0.16	0.5
½ Cystine	14–38	26	0.04	2.0
Valine	152–270	217	0.03	0.2
Methionine	13–41	24	0.01	0.5
Isoleucine	47–78	66	0.01	0.2
Leucine	83–163	129	0.05	0.4
Tyrosine	33–79	62	0.05	0.9
Phenylalanine	54–78	64	0.05	0.8
Histidine	88–128	92	0.44	4.2
Ornithine	92–194	130	0.02	0.1
Lysine	91–170	122	0.05	0.4
Arginine	27–91	57	0.05	0.9

Fig. 2 Amino acids as a source of energy. The multiple entry points to the citric acid cycle for the metabolites of carbon chain catabolism.

Fig. 1 The urea cycle functions partly in the mitochondrion and partly in the cytosol. Carbamyl phosphate, if it accumulates, may be diverted to orotic acid synthesis. Asterisked enzymes are: 1, carbamyl phosphate synthetase; 2, ornithine transcarbamylase; 3, argininosuccinate synthetase; 4, argininosuccinate lyase; and 5, arginase.

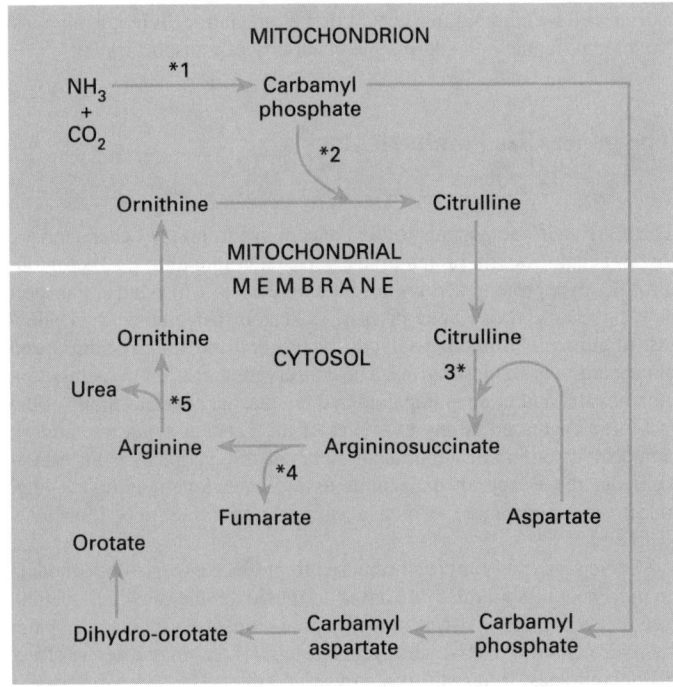

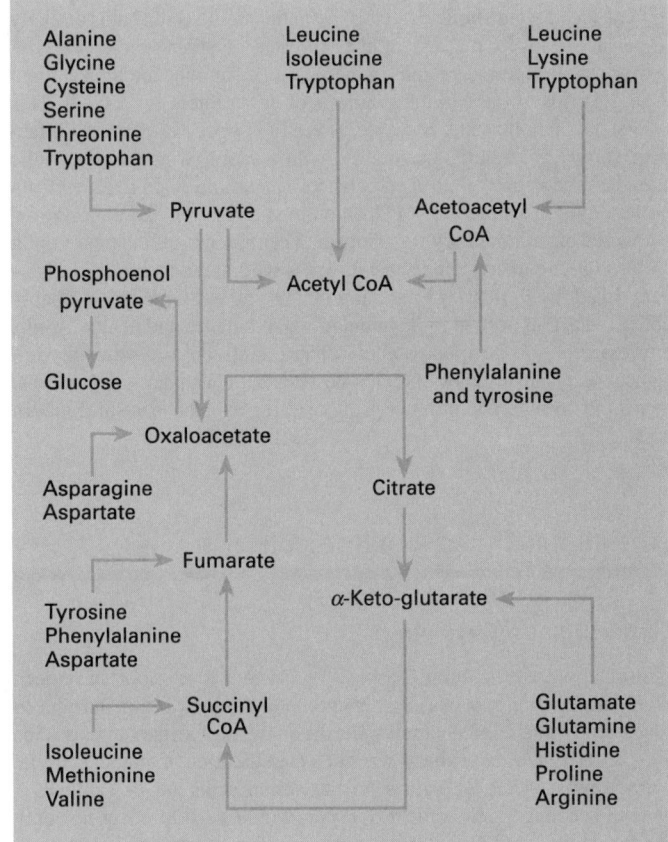

Table 2 *A biochemical classification of amino acid disorders*

The defects of amino acid transport
  intestinal and renal
  across cellular membranes

Defects of the amino group metabolism
  primary urea cycle defects
  secondary interference of urea cycle function

Defects of carbon chain metabolism
  those close to the parent amino acid with raised amino acid
    concentrations but mild or no acidosis
  those further down the pathway with organic acid
    accumulation and acidosis
  those at the end of the degradative pathways which may also
    involve catabolism of carbohydrates or fats

Defects primarily of major vitamin coenzymes
  pyridoxine
  vitamin B_{12}
  biotin
  biopterins

Nitrogen balance and dietary treatment

Some biochemical defects respond well to vitamin (coenzyme) supplementation and others are treated by diet. Generalized moderate protein restriction is a usual approach to urea cycle defects and one or two other diseases, but very specific restriction of one or two amino acids applies crucially to a small number of essential amino acid disorders. Rose and colleagues, 30 years ago, defined the eight essential amino acids in adults (Table 3) and the minimum daily requirements for sustaining nitrogen balance. This also requires an additional intake of 'non-essential' amino acid nitrogen and an adequate calorie intake. Histidine and taurine may be essential in the neonate. Dietary restriction can be used to treat specific metabolic defects of essential amino acids but is unlikely to be successful for non-essential amino acid disorders.

Almost all ingested protein in the infant (recommended intake about 2 g/kg/day) is utilized in the synthesis of new protein for growth. This persistent anabolic state, however, is easily upset by intercurrent infection, starvation, trauma, or surgery, with a rapid swing to a catabolic situation and negative nitrogen balance. The amino acids released from protein hydrolysis increase the load on urea formation and their normal pathways of intermediary metabolism. This renders infants and young children prone to frequent clinical illness with some amino acid disorders. In adults an intake of natural protein of 60 to 80 g/day is probably about twice that needed to maintain nitrogen balance and health. Adults are less prone to become catabolic than infants but the same circumstances may nevertheless precipitate it. Insulin and growth hormone have both been used to produce positive nitrogen balance in some inborn errors.

Amino acid transport defects

General pathophysiology

Historically, the renal tubular aspects of amino acid transport have been of major importance because paper chromatography was first introduced successfully into clinical practice for the analysis of urinary amino acids by C. E. Dent (1948). Table 4 sets out a classification of amino aciduria. Normal renal clearance values for the amino acids are in Table 1. A general account of amino acid transport would need to cover not only the renal tubule but the intestinal mucosa, the placenta, the blood-brain

Table 3 *The essential amino acids in man with recommended dietary intakes*

	Infants (mg/kg/day)	Adults (mg/kg/day)
Leucine	161	14.0
Isoleucine	70	10.0
Valine	93	10.0
Methionine*	58	13.0
Phenylalanine*	125	14.0
Threonine	87	7.0
Lysine	103	12.0
Tryptophan	17	3.5
Histidine	28	Not essential

*Requirements are lowered by the inclusion in the diet of cystine or tyrosine, respectively.

Table 4 *A classification of aminoaciduria*

Overflow aminoaciduria (secondary to high plasma amino acid concentrations)

generalized	increased plasma concentrations of many amino acids, e.g. acute liver necrosis or amino acid infusions
specific	increased plasma concentration of one or a few amino acids

Renal aminoaciduria (with normal plasma amino acid concentrations)

generalized	the Fanconi syndrome; early premature infants
specific	(i) basic aminoaciduria with or without cystine; lysinuric protein intolerance; cystinuria
	(ii) neutral aminoaciduria; the Hartnup syndrome
	(iii) glycine iminoaciduria; the normal neonatal pattern; genetic iminoglycinuria

barrier, cell membranes in a host of tissues and intracellular membranes. No attempt is made to address the generality of transport issues.

The generalized aminoacidurias

The Fanconi syndrome. General aspects

There are four components to the Fanconi syndrome: (1) characteristic low molecular weight proteinuria, e.g. α_1-microglobulin, β_2-microglobulin, β_1-glycoprotein, and retinol binding protein; (2) tubular transport defects; (3) metabolic bone disease, rickets, or osteomalacia; (4) slow loss of glomerular function. Glycosuria, generalized amino aciduria, and phosphaturia are a classic triad. The conservation of sodium, potassium, bicarbonate, and urate is impaired and the plasma concentrations of the last three decreased. Many examples of the Fanconi syndrome are not primarily disorders of amino acid metabolism (cystinosis is an exception) but the effects of exogenous toxins or endogenous toxins (e.g. galactose 1-phosphate), which accumulate in other genetic defects (Table 5).

Maleic acid (maleate) has been used to produce experimental models of the Fanconi syndrome, as have 4-pentenoate and succinyl acetone (see below). Maleate affects mitochondrial oxidation processes, impairs 1α-hydroxylation of 25-hydroxycholecalciferol and may directly affect cell membranes. It has still not proved possible to be sure whether the

Table 5 *The inherited causes of the Fanconi syndrome. Acquired causes are due to heavy metals, drugs, dysproteinaemias, and some immunological disorders of the kidney*

Idiopathic
Cystinosis
Hereditary fructose intolerance
Tyrosinaemia type I
Galactosaemia
Glycogen storage disease type I
Oculocerebrorenal syndrome of Lowe
Wilson's disease
Cytochrome *c* oxidoreductase deficiency

Fanconi syndrome should be regarded as a disorder of proximal or distal tubule, or both; whether efflux from cell to lumen is more important than reabsorption defects and whether all causes of the syndrome act through some final undefined common mechanism. Experimentally, maleate lowers intracellular concentrations of amino acids and sugars predominantly by increasing efflux. The general role of impaired energy production is suggested by new reports of tubular defects in mitochondrial disorders, for example cytochrome *c* oxidoreductase deficiency and the Kearns–Sayre syndrome.

The dominantly inherited Fanconi syndrome

This disorder, of unknown cause, characteristically presents in the second to fourth decade and slowly evolves into late adult life when renal failure may be advanced (Fig. 3). The clinical presentation is commonly with rickets or osteomalacia, which require treatment with calcitriol. Potassium, sodium bicarbonate, and phosphate supplements may also be needed.

The oculocerebrorenal syndrome of Lowe

This is an X-linked disease characterized by dwarfism, very profound mental retardation, and blindness secondary to cataracts, microphthalmos, and glaucoma. The tubular defect includes proteinuria, rickets but not usually glycosuria, the amino aciduria with relative sparing of the branched chain amino acids. The gene is on the long arm of the X chromosome and probably codes for inositol polyphosphate-5-phosphatase.

Cystinosis
Clinical

Cystinosis results from defective carrier-mediated transport of cystine through the lysosomal membrane, which may rupture due to cystine crystallization in hexagonal or rectangular forms causing cell damage. In the proximal renal tubule this leads to the Fanconi syndrome. In the severe infantile form clinical presentation occurs after a few months of life with polyuria, thirst, salt and water depletion, hypokalaemia, and proximal renal tubular acidosis. Poor feeding and failure to thrive are characteristic. Hypophosphataemia and impaired 1-hydroxylation of 25-hydroxycholecalciferol contribute to florid rickets.

Photophobia develops with the accumulation of cystine crystals in the cornea and retinopathy. Hypothyroidism is common and renal failure develops leading to death by 10 years of age. Growth is invariably impaired even before kidney transplantation and the associated steroid immunosuppression. Sexual development is late. Intelligence is normal. In transplanted patients retinopathy and visual loss may progress and central nervous system changes may occur. Cystine crystals are not seen here, but tissue cystine concentrations are very elevated. Cortical atrophy occurs in some and memory defects have been described with frank neurological features in a few. The spectrum of organ defects is likely to widen in long-term postrenal transplant survivors.

Variant forms

A benign adult form presents with photophobia due to corneal crystals. There may also be crystals in the bone marrow and leucocytes but the kidney is spared and life expectation is normal. An intermediate form is like the classic infantile form but presents in late childhood or early adult life. Renal involvement and renal failure occur.

Biochemistry

It is probable that all tissues accumulate cystine, but not equally, and some (e.g. muscle and brain) never seem to develop crystals. Crystals occur in the tissues with the highest cystine concentrations, increasing with age to values several hundred times normal. Cultured fibroblasts and leucocytes have values 50 to 100 times normal, but cultured lymphoid cells are only 4 to 5 times normal. Leucocyte cystine content is higher in the intermediate than the benign form, and highest in the severe classic infantile form. The intralysosomal cystine originates from proteins catabolized within the lysosome and extracellular cystine transported into the cell. Cystine egress from the lysosome is defective. The

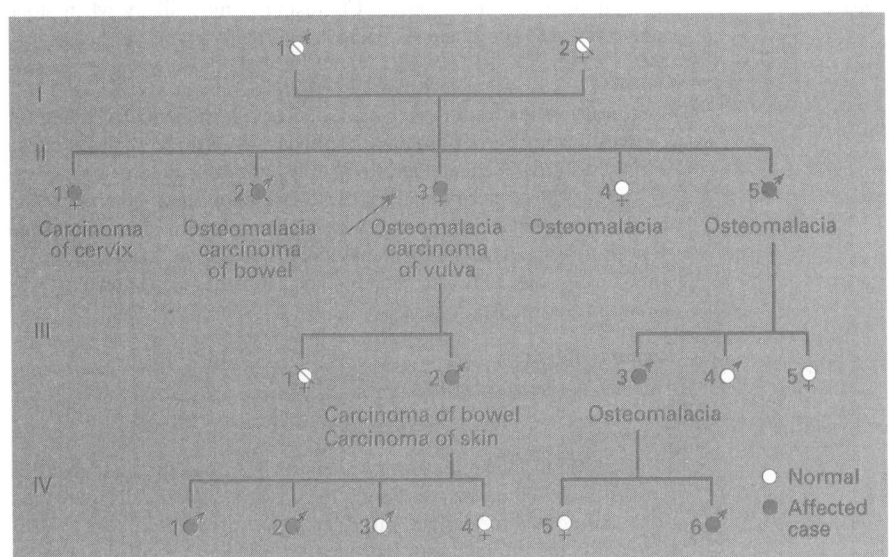

Fig. 3 Pedigree of dominantly inherited Fanconi syndrome. (From Brenton et al. (1981). with permission).

carrier is not shared by other amino acids, which have other lysosomal transport systems.

Diagnosis

This is based on the clinical features, the Fanconi syndrome, and the cystine crystals. In the cornea these can be seen with a hand lens or a slit lamp in an older child but in infancy they are best seen in bone marrow aspirates (Fig. 4) fixed in alcohol and examined under polarized light. Analysis of peripheral leucocytes for their cystine content is possible in only a few laboratories.

Genetics

The disease is an autosomal recessive. The incidence is about 1 in 200 000 live births. A higher incidence has been reported from parts of France. Heterozygotes are clinically normal but have raised leucocyte cystine concentrations. There is no described chromosomal localization for the defective gene.

Prenatal diagnosis

This has been successfully achieved using cultured amniocytes and measuring ^{35}S cystine uptake, or by direct analysis of chorionic villus samples for cystine content.

Treatment

Resuscitation with intravenous fluids, if required, is followed by free access to water and oral supplementation with sodium bicarbonate and potassium chloride. Citrate salts may be preferred. Treatment is adjusted to maintain normal hydration and normal plasma concentrations of potassium and bicarbonate.

The rickets requires treatment with calcitriol 0.25 µg daily, increasing as required as the child grows. Phosphate supplementation may help to heal the bone disease.

An agent that has proved effective, in vitro and in vivo, at reducing cystine load is cysteamine. As it has an offensive taste and odour, the more acceptable phosphocysteamine and cysteamine bitartrate are under trial as alternatives. Oral cysteamine, given in divided doses, depletes leucocyte cystine and gives better growth and better preservation of renal function. Cysteamine eye drops have been used in very young children to clear corneal crystals. The role of cysteamine in preventing the consequences of cystine accumulation in non-renal tissues after transplantation is under study.

Fig. 4 Cystine crystals in the marrow of a child with cystinosis. × 2200. Partially polarized light. (By courtesy of Dr B. Lake, The Hospital for Sick Children, Great Ormond Street, London and with the permission of W. Heinemann Medical Books.)

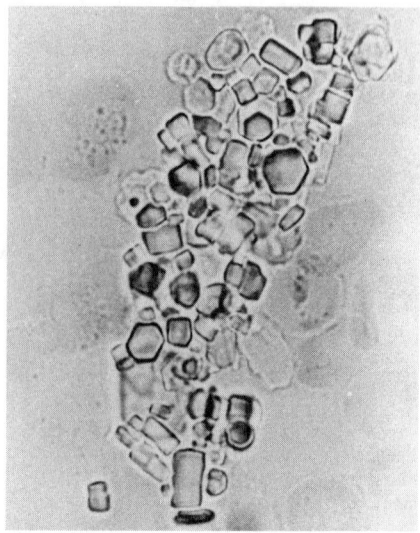

Dialysis and renal transplantation is required for renal failure. Transplanted kidneys do not accumulate cystine.

Thyroxine is needed for hypothyroidism. Growth hormone increases height but has been reported to hasten the need for renal replacement. Plasma carnitine concentrations are often low and can be increased to normal by the use of supplements, but this may not help any muscular weakness.

Specific aminoacidurias

The recognition of genetic disorders characterized by the excretion of a specific group of amino acids stimulated research into amino acid transport. Major clinical problems are found in cystinuria and lysinuric protein intolerance

Cystinuria

Clinical

Cystine stone formation in the kidneys and its attendant complications of pain, haematuria, renal obstruction, and infection is the classic clinical presentation. Only 1 to 2 per cent of all renal stones in adult life are cystine stones but the proportion is higher in childhood. The stones may have grown to large staghorn calculi before diagnosis. They are radio-opaque.

Biochemistry

Cystine has a solubility of 400 mg/l at neutral pH and excretion varies from 400 to 1200 mg/day in affected individuals, with increased excretion of lysine (up to 2 g/day), ornithine, and arginine, and impaired intestinal absorption of the free amino acids. All are absorbed as dipeptides in combination with another amino acid outside the group. There is no deficiency of any amino acid and no urea cycle defect. The faecal and urinary excretion of diamines such as putrescine and cadaverine result from the action of intestinal bacteria on unabsorbed lysine and arginine. Experimental work indicates that the renal transport defect in cystinuria affects a low Km system in the brush border shared by the four amino acids. Other transport systems for cystine and the dibasic amino acids exist. Cystine excretion can exceed glomerular filtration rate, implying the possibility of tubular secretion.

Diagnosis

Diagnosis requires an amino acid chromatogram and quantitation of cystine excretion. Calcium containing stones have been observed in cystinuria – possibly because infection predisposes to deposition of calcium salts on small cystine deposits. Confusion is most likely when stone analysis is used for diagnosis without a chromatogram.

Genetics

Cystinuria results from three mutant alleles at a single locus coding for a group specific carrier protein. Combinations of these alleles produce slightly different renal and intestinal transport abnormalities. Some heterozygotes have normal amino acid excretion and others excrete increased amounts of lysine and cystine, although insufficient for cystine stone formation. The chromosomal localization is not known. There is some linkage data to favour chromosome 2 which is also known to carry an amino acid transport gene.

Prenatal diagnosis

This has not been described.

Treatment

The daily fluid intake must not be less than 3 l/day in adults and this must include 500 ml before retiring to bed with a nocturnal rise to pass urine and drink a further 500 ml. Keeping the urine dilute over the 24-h period is the difficult part, but may be sufficient treatment for those without stones.

Reduced protein intake diminishes cystine excretion but this is not much used in treatment. Cystine is much more soluble at alkaline pH (> 7.5). Use of sodium bicarbonate is limited by the large doses (6 g/day or more) needed to raise urine pH significantly. These are contraindicated in hypertension or renal failure. In addition, alkaline urine may dispose to the precipitation of calcium salts.

Penicillamine treatment produces the much more soluble disulphide – half cystine and half penicillamine and an overall reduction of cystine excretion greater than can be accounted for by disulphide formation. The effective dose (1 to 3 g/day) should reduce the free cystine excretion to around 200 mg/day if stones are to dissolve. It is usual to start at a dose of 125 mg/day and increase over several weeks to full dose. The side-effects include blood dyscrasias, rash with arthralgia, fever, and lymphadenopathy. Patients on penicillamine need blood counts every 2 weeks initially and then monthly. Regular urinalysis is needed. Proteinuria is common and above 2 g/day may necessitate stopping penicillamine, as do blood dyscrasias or other severe reactions. Penicillamine is a helpful preventive treatment in recurrent stone formers at lower doses. Large doses are reserved for trying to dissolve large calculi, which may take 1 to 2 years. It is usually well tolerated in cystinuria.

Sulphydryl compounds with similar side-effects (e.g. mercaptopropionylglycine), have been used in some countries in place of penicillamine but are not available in the United Kingdom. Captopril is a sulphydryl compound which forms a disulphide with cystine. Reports of decreased cystine excretion related to treatment with captopril have not been confirmed and no therapeutic use has yet been established. Similarly, decreasing sodium intake and excretion reduces cystine excretion but a therapeutic role has not been accepted.

Cystine stones are not easily broken by lithotripsy. Percutaneous removal may have its place for smaller stones, particularly in those who cannot take penicillamine and who are unable to regulate their drinking adequately.

Lysinuric protein intolerance

Clinical

Defective ornithine, lysine, and arginine transport affect the renal tubule and intestine with only minor defects of cystine transport. Stones do not form. There is genuine evidence of amino acid deficiency. At weaning, vomiting and diarrhoea begin. Failure to thrive and poor appetite are common with poor growth. Occasional intermittent hyperammonaemic encephalopathy occurs. Osteoporosis is an important part of the clinical picture, with vertebral collapse. Interstitial lung disease causes breathlessness, cough, fever and reduced arterial P_{O_2}. Intellect is normal or mildly impaired. Pregnancy is associated with haemorrhage during labour.

Biochemistry

Plasma concentrations of arginine, ornithine, and lysine are low but citrulline, alanine, and glutamine are increased. Renal clearance values for lysine are 20 to 30 times normal and renal losses may be up to 1 g/day. Less marked increases of orthinine and arginine excretion are found but cystine increases are minor.

Plasma lysine values fail to rise after oral lysine loads or the ingestion of lysyl peptides. Intracellular peptide hydrolysis liberates lysine, which cannot be transported across the basolateral membrane, the site of the transport defect. There is also evidence of a transport defect in cultured fibroblasts but not in red cells. A deficiency of intramitochondrial ornithine due to a transport defect across the mitochondrial membrane may impair the urea cycle, causing hyperammonaemia and orotic aciduria (see below).

Genetics

The disease is an autosomal recessive with a relatively high incidence in Finland (1 in 60 000) compared to the rest of the world. Chromosomal localization of the gene is not known.

Prenatal diagnosis

This has not been described.

Treatment

Hyperammonaemia can be largely prevented by a low protein diet. However, adequate calorie intake is difficult to sustain in infancy and appetite often remains poor. Protein restriction does not correct lysine deficiency and oral lysine supplementation causes diarrhoea. Oral citrulline (2.5 to 8.5 g/day), absorbed via a different transport system, corrects ornithine and arginine deficiency and lowers plasma ammonia by priming the urea cycle. Acute hyperammonaemic crises are managed with intravenous (IV) glucose and intravenous or oral sodium benzoate or phenylbutyrate (see below). Citrulline treatment should be maintained but intravenous citrulline is not readily available. Intravenous ornithine and arginine have been tried.

In the attempt to overcome lysine deficiency, which may be a factor in the osteoporosis and other problems, ε-N-acetyl lysine has been tried. Plasma lysine concentrations rise but there is no agreement on its use, and cost and availability are said to be a problem.

The cause of the serious interstitial pneumonia is not clear. It has not apparently responded to antibiotics given for the possibility of pneumocystis infection. A successful treatment with prednisolone has been reported.

Neutral aminoaciduria: the Hartnup syndrome

This is an autosomal recessive disorder of neutral amino acid transport across the luminal brush border membrane of kidney and intestine. It does not involve cystine and the basic amino acids, the acidic acids, glycine, or the iminoacids (see Fig. 3). Clinical effects include a light-sensitive rash on exposed skin, cerebellar ataxia, and mental disturbance. Most patients with this disorder remain normal, however. Affected individuals may respond to nicotinamide, but this does not change the amino acid transport defect. The relative deficiency of nicotinamide is attributed to the losses of the precursor amino acid tryptophan and its impaired intestinal absorption. Bacterial action on unabsorbed tryptophan generates indoles, which appear in the stools and urine and are characteristic of the disorder.

Familial renal iminoglycinuria

The excretion of glycine, proline, and hydroxyproline is raised in the Fanconi syndrome and in the inborn errors of proline or hydroxyproline metabolism when plasma concentration of these amino acids are raised. Transient raised excretion of the three amino acids is usual in neonates, which reflects the ontogeny of one shared transport system. Genetic iminoglycinuria is an autosomal recessive defect of another transport system. The evidence supports several allelic mutations in the genetic defect with some heterozygotes having raised glycine excretion and some normal amino acid excretion. Familial iminoglycinuria is the consequence of a well worked out transport defect which is clinically harmless.

The γ-glutamyl cycle

A possible amino acid transport system

Six enzyme-catalysed reactions link the steps for the synthesis of glutathione and its metabolism (Fig. 5). Glutathione is believed to be transported to the cell membrane, where its antioxidant properties may be important in preventing lipid peroxidation. Tissues with low γ-glutamyl transpeptidase levels in the cell membrane transport glutathione into the body fluids and circulation. Some is filtered at the glomerulus. γ-Glutamyl transpeptidase, bound to the cell membrane of transport epithelia such as the choroid plexus, ciliary body, nephron, and jejunum has been assigned a role in the membrane transport of amino acids via the formation of γ-glutamyl–amino-acid peptides, which is quite different from free amino acid transport. The peptides are cleaved by γ-glutamyl cyclotransferase to free the transported amino acid and the γ-glutamyl moiety, which cyclizes to 5-oxoproline (pyroglutamic acid). Cystine is among the amino acids transported in this way and one function of the cycle may be to conserve cystine and indirectly cysteine. There is no suggestion of any defect in the cycle in cystinuria. The inherited defects of the γ-glutamyl cycle are summarized in Table 6. Some of the links between biochemical defects and clinical manifestations are tentative.

Defects of the urea cycle

Amino acids taken in excess of synthetic need are catabolized and the amino group effectively converted to urea. Hyperammonaemia is one of the major metabolic abnormalities in urea cycle defects but not unique to them (Table 7).

The formation of urea

Nearly all waste nitrogen disposal – 10 to 12 g/day – is in the form of urea synthesized in the liver from ammonium ions (NH_4^+) and the α-amino nitrogen of aspartic acid (see Fig. 1). The ammonium nitrogen is incorporated into the first committed synthetic step to urea formation – the production of carbamyl phosphate for which N-acetyl glutamine is believed to be regulatory. The α-amino nitrogen of aspartic acid comes from many amino acids during their transamination reactions with oxaloacetic acid. It is incorporated during the formation of argininosuccinic acid. Ornithine nitrogen is not incorporated into urea. Bicarbonate provides the carbon moiety of urea but this is not generally regarded as important in acid:base balance.

The source of ammonium ions (NH_4^+) for the generation of carbamyl phosphate is less clear. Glutamine synthesized in skeletal muscle is extensively taken up by the intestine. Glutamine nitrogen is released into the portal blood as alanine, ammonium ions, and citrulline. Apart from these urea precursors, ammonium ions are released into the renal

Fig. 5 The γ-glutamyl cycle synthesizes glutathione and may play a role in amino acid transport. Asterisked enzymes are: 1, glutathione synthetase; 2, γ-glutamyl-cysteine synthetase; and 3, 5-oxoprolinase.

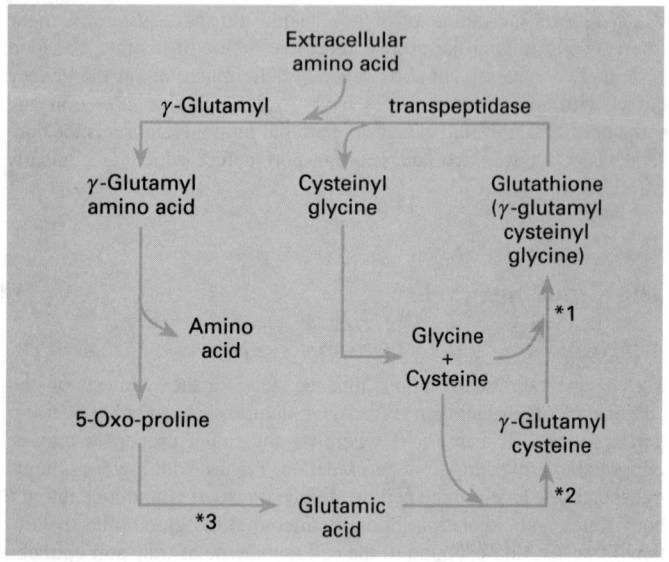

vein by the action of renal glutaminase on glutamine. The generation of ammonium ions within the liver had been attributed to the deamination of glutamate by glutamate dehydrogenase. Transamination reactions involving glutamate are probably more important in linking glutamate to the urea cycle. Within the liver a number of other amino acids are deaminated and may be a source of ammonium for urea synthesis.

The extrahepatic urea cycle enzymes

The urea cycle synthesizes arginine but it has been noted that hepatic transplantation for urea cycle defects does not correct previously low plasma concentrations of citrulline and arginine. The intestine also can synthesize citrulline with the mitochondrial parts of the cycle. Other tissues contain only some of the urea cycle enzymes. Citrulline transported to a variety of tissues with the cytosolic components of the cycle can be used to synthesize arginine via argininosuccinic acid. This extrahepatic synthesis of arginine may be crucial to the body's needs.

The inherited defects of the urea cycle

Four of five inherited defects of the urea cycle (see Fig. 1) have common clinical features but arginase deficiency is different. The abbreviations CPSD, OTCD, ASD, ALD, and AD stand for deficiencies of carbamyl phosphate synthetase, ornithine transcarbamylase, argininosuccinic acid synthetase, argininosuccinic acid lyase, and arginase, respectively. Quite separately the activity of carbamyl phosphate synthetase can be impaired by a rare genetic defect in N-acetylglutamine formation which is not considered here.

Clinical features of carbamyl phosphate synthetase deficiency, ornithine transcarbamylase deficiency, arginosuccinic acid synthetase deficiency, argininosuccinic acid lyase deficiency

The neonatal presentation of these conditions are identical. After a brief normal period of 24 to 72 h, poor feeding, lethargy, and vomiting presage the descent to unresponsiveness and hyperammonaemic coma. Argininosuccinic acid lyase deficiency may be less acute and severe than carbamyl phosphate synthetase deficiency, ornithine transcarbamylase deficiency, or argininosuccinic acid synthetase deficiency because argininosuccinic acid excreted at the glomerular filtration rate (there being no tubular reabsorption) is a means of nitrogen excretion, and hyperammonaemia tends to be less severe. In males, ornithine transcarbamylase deficiency is usually fatal, but survival in the other conditions more likely. Survivors may suffer intellectual impairment and other neurological damage. Only one of the four is X-linked and female heterozygotes for ornithine transcarbamylase deficiency may sometimes present in the neonatal period, presumably because of preponderant inactivation of the X chromosome with a normal gene.

Later presentations come in two broad clinical forms. Mental retardation and epilepsy without any clear neonatal history are well described in argininosuccinic acid lyase deficiency and also in carbamyl phosphate synthetase deficiency, ornithine transcarbamylase deficiency, and argininosuccinic acid synthetase deficiency. Children with argininosuccinic acid lyase deficiency may also show the hair defect of trichorrhexis nodosa, which is not shared by the other urea cycle defects. Another late presentation is with intermittent encephalopathy. This is seen in ornithine transcarbamylase deficiency carrier females, including presentation in the puerperium after a symptomless pregnancy and hemizygous ornithine transcarbamylase-deficient males who have presented in late childhood or teenage years. Death has been recorded in these late onset encephalopathies. Carbamyl phosphate synthetase deficiency and argininosuccinic acid synthetase deficiency may also present this way.

Clinical features of arginase deficiency

There is a progressive spastic quadriparesis, most marked in the legs, with psychomotor retardation, epilepsy, and poor growth. Obvious man-

Table 6 *Genetic defects of the γ-glutamyl cycle*

Enzyme deficiency	Clinical effects	Biochemical abnormalities
Glutathione synthetase		
(i) generalized deficiency	Neonatal acidosis	Large excretion 5-oxoproline
	Haemolysis; variable central nervous system effects	(pyroglutamic aciduria)
	Mental retardation	
(ii) red cell deficiency	Haemolysis only	No urinary defect
γ-Glutamylcysteine synthetase	Haemolysis; spinocerebellar degeneration; myopathy	Generalized aminoaciduria
γ-Glutamyl transpeptidase	Mental retardation	Raised plasma concentration and urine excretion of glutathione
5-Oxoprolinase	Variable from no effect to enterocolitis and renal stones	Moderate increases of 5-oxoproline excretion

Table 7 *Causes of hyperammonaemia*

Urea cycle defects
Transport defects of intermediates of the urea cycle
  lysinuric protein intolerance
  hyperornithinaemia-hyperammonaemia-
  homocitrillinuria syndrome
Organic acidurias
  branched chain organic acid defects
  propionic acidaemia and methylmalonic acidaemia
  pyruvate carboxylase or dehydrogenase deficiencies
  multiple carboxylase deficiencies
  glutaric aciduria type II
  acyl coenzyme A dehydrogenase deficiencies
Drugs
  valproate encephalopathy
  Reye's syndrome
Liver disorders
  cirrhosis of variable aetiology
  portal systemic shunts
Transient neonatal hyperammonaemia

ifestations present in early childhood. Hyperammonaemic coma occurs but hyperammonaemia is less marked than in the other disorders.

Biochemistry

These defects are summarized in Table 8. Hyperammonaemia is preceded by raised plasma alanine and glutamine concentrations and may be accompanied by a rise in transaminases and prolongation of the prothrombin time. The raised excretion of orotic acid in some defects is possibly caused by the accumulation of carbamyl phosphate, which is directed to pyrimidine synthesis (see Fig. 1).

Experimental hyperammonaemia in primates initially causes decreased activity, lethargy, and vomiting, and then hyperventilation and respiratory alkalosis, which have also been recorded in man. Seizures and coma follow with progressive rise of intracranial pressure and cerebral oedema. The astrocytes, which occupy a one-quarter to one-third of brain volume, exhibit marked swelling and mitochondrial change. High astrocyte glutamine concentrations may act osmotically to cause cerebral oedema. Many metabolic changes in hyperammonaemia could be secondary to cerebral oedema. Glutamine concentrations ten times normal have been recorded in the cerebrospinal fluid in ornithine transcarbamylase deficiency and argininosuccinic acid lyase deficiency. Other amino acid abnormalities in the cerebrospinal fluid have been described in arginase deficiency. An early effect of hyperammonaemia on amino acid transport across the blood–brain barrier has been described, with tryptophan transport being regarded as particularly important.

Diagnosis

The biochemical defects are diagnostically important (see Table 8). Carbamyl phosphate synthetase deficiency can only be diagnosed when hyperammonaemia is not associated with the biochemical changes of the other urea cycle defects, although a low plasma citrulline value gives a clue. Other causes of hyperammonaemia must be excluded (see Table 7), which requires urinary organic acid analysis, consideration of Reye's syndrome, and acute valproate encephalopathy. Confirmatory enzyme assays on liver biopsy samples may be needed in carbamyl phosphate synthetase deficiency and ornithine transcarbamylase deficiency. Liver function and clotting tests should be checked.

Genetics

With the exception of ornithine transcarbamylase deficiency, the diseases are autosomal recessives. The gene for carbamyl phosphate synthetase is on the short arm of chromosome 2. Inherited deficiency is rare. The enzyme protein may be targeted to the mitochondria by a leader peptide and the mature enzyme constitutes a relatively high proportion of mitochondrial protein. The gene for ornithine transcarbamylase is on the short arm of the X chromosome and its product targeted to mitochondria in a manner similar to carbamyl phosphate synthetase. Functional catalytic trimers form within the mitochondrial matrix. Ornithine transcarbamylase deficiency is associated with a variety of gene defects both deletions and point mutations, a number of which have been worked out in detail.

Argininosuccinic acid synthetase, argininosuccinic acid lyase, and arginase are cytoplasmic enzymes. Argininosuccinic acid synthetase catalyses the synthesis of argininosuccinic acid (ASA) from citrulline and aspartic acid, requires adenosine triphosphate and magnesium ions, and functions as a tetramer of about 185 000 Da. The gene is on the long arm of chromosome 9. Argininosuccinic acid lyase which cleaves ASA functions as a tetramer of about 173 000 Da and the coding gene is on the short arm of chromosome 7. Fibroblast studies of argininosuccinic acid lyase indicate that cross-reacting material is usually present and correlates poorly with residual enzyme activity. There are multiple complementation groups and, by implication, multiple alleles at the structural gene locus.

Hepatic arginase, a tetramer of around 107 000 Da, cleaving arginine to urea and ornithine, has a locus on the long arm of chromosome 6.

Antenatal diagnosis

A restriction fragment length polymorphism has been helpful in carbamyl phosphate synthetase deficiency, with fetal liver biopsy and enzyme assay the only alternatives. Antenatal diagnosis in ornithine transcarbamylase deficiency is complex. If the mother is known to be a carrier from pedigree analysis or biochemical testing, three approaches are possible: (1) if the mutation is known within the family then direct examination of the fetal genotype is possible using appropriate probes, but

Table 8 *A general approach to the biochemical disturbances in the urea cycle defects*

	Normal	CPSD	OTCD	ASD	ALD	AD
Plasma ammonia	15–40	Up to 25×	Up to 25×	Up to 10–15×	Up to 10×	Up to 2–3×
glutamine	350–650	2–3×	2–3×	2–3×	2–3×	2×
alanine	200–400	2–3×	2–3×	2–3×	2–3×	2×
citrulline	10–30	Low	Low	up to 200×	Increased	Normal
arginine	30–90	Low	Low	Low	Low	Up to 15×
argininosuccinate	Not detectable	None	None	None	400–600	None
Urine orotic acid	2–6	Not increased	Increased	Increased	Increased	Increased
Urine amino acids	—	—	—	Citrulline	ASA	Arginine/ cystine lysine

AD, arginase deficiency; ALD, argininosuccinic acid lyase deficiency; ASD, argininosuccinic acid synthetase deficiency; CPSD, carbamyl phosphate synthetase deficiency; OTCD, ornithine transcarbamylase deficiency. Normal plasma values μmol/l. Urine orotic acid mg/day.

this occurs in a minority of cases; (2) if a restriction fragment polymorphism is linked to the mutant gene in the family then this approach may be possible; (3) if no such information is available then sexing the fetus followed by fetal liver biopsy and enzyme assay in the male is the only approach left. Antenatal diagnosis for argininosuccinic acid synthetase deficiency is also difficult. The enzyme can be assayed in amniocytes and placental villus material, but it is more reliable to culture amniocytes with radioactive citrulline and measure the incorporation of the radioactive products into cell protein. Amniotic fluid citrulline concentrations may help. There is no molecular approach in argininosuccinic acid lyase deficiency but analysis of amniotic fluid for ASA or enzyme assay on cultured amniocytes has been used successfully. Arginase deficiency has been detected on fetal red cells and a number of mutations have now been identified.

Heterozygote detection in ornithine transcarbamylase deficiency

Because of its X-linked inheritance carrier detection is particularly important. Pedigree analysis including DNA studies where necessary, or investigation of frank symptomatic episodes may settle the issue. The symptomless female can be a problem, however. Protein loading with serial measurements of plasma ammonia and urinary orotic acid may reveal the biochemical defect but may also cause serious symptoms. Allopurinol causes a greater excretion of orotic acid and orotidine in carrier females than in normals and forms the basis of an acceptable safe test of heterozygosity. It may fail to identify some carriers.

Treatment and prognosis

The management of acute encephalopathy involves reducing the need to synthesize urea. Dietary protein is stopped and endogenous protein breakdown suppressed by a high oral carbohydrate intake or using intravenous 10 to 20 per cent dextrose and insulin if needed to control blood glucose concentrations. The blood ammonia is lowered in the neonatal period by peritoneal dialysis or haemodialysis (more effective). Slower methods useful in carbamyl phosphate synthetase deficiency and ornithine transcarbamylase deficiency include the use of intravenous or oral sodium benzoate, which is excreted as its glycine conjugate, hippuric acid, so raising nitrogen excretion. More effective is the oral use of sodium phenylacetate (or better sodium phenylbutyrate), which is excreted as phenyl acetylglutamine. Few physicians have experience in the use of these compounds which are not licensed drugs. Third, in argininosuccinic acid synthetase and argininosuccinic acid lyase deficiencies, oral or intravenous arginine is an urgent and important therapy to remedy deficiency. In argininosuccinic acid lyase deficiency in particular, plasma ammonia levels fall when arginine is administered. The prognosis for severe neonatal illness is poor (see above).

Maintenance treatment of all urea cycle defects (including arginase deficiency) between encephalopathic episodes involves protein restric-

tion to the minimum required for growth and development and supplementation with arginine in argininosuccinic acid synthetase deficiency and argininosuccinic acid lyase deficiency. The continuous use of sodium benzoate or sodium phenylbutyrate in carbamyl phosphate synthetase deficiency and ornithine transcarbamylase deficiency is a more difficult issue, especially with regard to potential long-term toxicity, but should diminish abnormal plasma ammonia concentrations. Late onset forms of the urea cycle diseases carry a better prognosis, but arginase deficiency seems relentlessly progressive. Babies with argininosuccinic acid lyase deficiency picked up by neonatal screening but who have not developed early clinical illness, are reported to develop with normal IQ on large arginine supplements and a low protein intake. Others do less well and generally urea cycle defects have a poor prognosis.

Valproate should be avoided in the treatment of seizures in urea cycle defects and ornithine transcarbamylase carriers because it may precipitate coma.

Liver transplantation remains a possibility and has sometimes been carried out for urea cycle defects.

The disorders of carbon chain metabolism

Introduction

The classification in Table 1 is a useful approach, but many different catabolic pathways and associated clinical abnormalities necessitates separate consideration of individual amino acids (or groups of them) with their relevant vitamin coenzymes. Pyridoxine, because of its central and varied roles, is considered separately below. The relatively 'nonspecific' nature of some biochemical abnormalities is stressed again.

Pyridoxine

Pyridoxal phosphate is the coenzyme in amino acid transaminations, decarboxylations, and deaminations. Considerable molecular detail of its role in transamination has been worked out. It is also the coenzyme in the synthesis and breakdown of cystathionine in the trans-sulphuration pathway. The normal dietary pyridoxine intake is 2 to 3 mg/day but a number of diseases respond to doses of 10 to 500 mg/day. These include deficiencies of ornithine aminotransferase, cystathionine synthase, cystathionase, hyperoxaluria due to peroxisomal glyoxylate aminotransferase deficiency, and some neonates with seizures considered due to defective glutamine decarboxylase, the enzyme which generates GABA (see later).

'Non-specific' biochemical defects

The multiple causes of hyperammonaemia have been listed (see Table 15). Elevations of plasma glycine may also be non-specific and not necessarily a result of primary enzyme defects in glycine metabolism. Glutamine and alanine increases in plasma are common in the early stages of ammonia accumulation. Hypoglycaemia is frequent in the organic acidurias as well as in specific defects of gluconeogenesis or glycogen metabolism. Alanine concentrations rise in lactic acidosis.

Defects of ornithine metabolism

Ornithine is a non-protein amino acid upon which the synthesis of urea takes place (see Fig. 1) and which is regenerated once the urea moiety is split off. It is also produced when arginine reacts with glycine to produce guanidinoacetate the precursor of creatine. Ornithine-δ-amino transferase produces glutamic semialdehyde, which cyclizes to pyrroline-5-carboxyllic acid, which is also produced from proline. The decarboxylation of ornithine produces the diamine putrescine.

Deficiency of ornithine-δ-aminotransferase: Gyrate atrophy

Clinical

The major abnormality is an atrophy of choroid and retina, beginning as a small yellowish spot and increasing to a circular lesion edged with pigment giving an 'atypical retinitis pigmentosa' appearance. Children present with myopia and decreased night vision progressing to blindness in middle life. Cataracts also develop but optic discs, cornea, and iris remain normal. A few patients develop mild proximal muscle weakness. Microscopic abnormalities of skeletal muscle fibres are found.

Biochemistry

Plasma ornithine values range from 400 to 1000 μmol/l (normal 75 μmol/l) with high concentrations in CSF and aqueous humor. 400 to 900 mg/day is excreted with increased amounts of arginine and lysine (competitive inhibition of reabsorption). The lactam of ornithine also appears in the urine.

The activity of ornithine-δ-aminotransferase is low in liver and skeletal muscle. Most affected patients have less than 1 per cent of normal activity in fibroblasts. Some have values up to 5 to 6 per cent and some enzyme-deficient lines show marked increase of activity with very high concentrations of pyridoxal phosphate.

Diagnosis

The clinical picture and the amino acid defects are adequate means of diagnosis. Enzyme assays can be used to confirm it.

Genetics

It is an autosomal recessive with the highest incidence in Finland, (where it may be as high as 1 in 50 000). There are several mutants, as evidenced by complementation studies. The gene has been mapped to chromosome 10. Two pseudogenes exist on the X chromosome. Different mis-sense mutations have been described in pyridoxine responsive and non-responsive forms. Splicing defects have also been described.

Treatment

There are no reports of clinical improvement but deterioration may be slower in patients whose plasma ornithine levels fall with pyridoxine treatment (500 mg/day or less). Low arginine diets may reduce ornithine concentrations and lysine has been given to augment renal ornithine excretion. Creatine has been given and has been reported to improve muscle histology, but ocular deterioration continues. Local proline deficiency in the retina has been suggested as a cause of the retinal degeneration. Proline supplementation does not stop disease progression.

Hyperornithinaemia with hyperammonaemia and homocitrillinuria

Clinical

This is sometimes referred to as the HHH syndrome. Intermittent hyperammonaemic encephalopathy with vomiting, drowsiness, and coma may date back to infancy, or patients may present much later. Impairment of IQ from low normal to more severe retardation, with epilepsy and frank neurological features, is another form of presentation. Growth tends to be poor. There are no eye defects.

Biochemistry

Intermittent hyperammonaemia, with plasma ornithine values three to ten times normal and increased excretion of orotic acid are believed to result from impaired transport of ornithine into the mitochondria which leads to the accumulation of carbamylphosphate. This increases orotic acid formation and the production of homocitrulline by the transcarbamoylation of lysine.

Genetics

Nothing is known except it is almost certainly an autosomal recessive disease.

Treatment

Moderate protein reduction (1 g/kg/day) reduces plasma ammonia and ornithine concentration. Ornithine supplementation may then lower plasma ammonia further by raising intracellular ornithine concentrations, which may induce entry of more ornithine into the mitochondria. In adult presenting siblings, treatment with citrulline and sodium phenylbutyrate has decreased plasma ammonia, increased plasma ornithine, and relieved episodic confusional episodes.

Defects of phenylalanine metabolism

The importance of tetrahydrobiopterin

The hyperphenylalaninaemias are a group of disorders characterized by defective hydroxylation of phenylalanine to tyrosine and plasma phenylalanine values above the normal fasting range of 40 to 80 μmol/litre. An adult phenylalanine intake is about 3 to 4 g/day, one-quarter of which is incorporated into protein and three-quarters hydroxylated to tyrosine (Fig. 6). Adults need about 1 g/day, but in classic severe phenylketonuria (PKU) health is maintained on half this. Transamination to phenylpyruvic acid and decarboxylation to phenylethylamine assume much greater importance in phenylketonuria because they occur only at elevated phenylalanine concentrations.

Classic phenylketonuria

Clinical

Phenylalanine values are higher than 1000 μmol/l (sometimes much higher). Untreated, phenylketonuria almost invariably causes severe mental retardation, with IQ values only occasionally above 60, and most often well below. Inexplicably, a few patients have normal IQ values despite the biochemical defect; some female patients have been discovered only because of abnormalities in their offspring (see below). Both microcephaly and epilepsy are common. About one in 20 untreated patients develop neurological problems in adult life, usually spastic paraparesis but sometimes extrapyramidal features. Pigmentary deficiency in the iris and hair are features of the untreated disease and so is eczema.

Milder variants

Mutations with greater residual enzyme activity produce phenylalanine values of 300 to 1000 μmol/l. Those over 400 μmol/l should be treated. Some were not with variable outcome for IQ.

Biochemistry

Plasma phenylalanine concentrations are elevated to 20 to 60 times, being highest in babies. Phenyl pyruvic acid which is converted to phenyl lactic acid, phenylacetic acid, and phenylacetyl glutamine accumulates with phenylethylamine. The ketone phenylpyruvic acid in the urine gives the disease its name and a green colour in the ferric chloride test. The defective enzyme phenylalanine hydroxylase, which requires tetrahydrobiopterin as a cofactor, has been found only in the liver in man. It has never been found in brain of any species. Phenylalanine hydroxylase may be tetrameric or trimeric with units of molecular weight between 50 000 and 60 000.

Pathology

The pathology of phenylketonuria is not clear. Phenylalanine itself is probably the damaging agent but there is controversy on the mechanism. High phenylalanine concentrations are associated with impaired brain growth and probably fewer nerve cells. Phenylalanine inhibits an enzyme important in sulphation of myelin intermediates and myelin formation is abnormal. Transport of other amino acids is reduced at the blood–brain barrier and at the placenta by high phenylalanine concentrations in animal experiments. In addition, many *in vitro* biochemical processes (e.g. protein synthesis) are impaired by high phenylalanine concentrations. Patients with classic phenylketonuria also have low cerebrospinal fluid concentrations of homovanillic acid and 5-hydroxyindoleacetic acid, indicative of possible deficiency of the neurotransmitters dopamine, noradrenaline, and 5-hydroxytryptamine. Dietary treatment restores normal concentrations in the cerebrospinal fluid.

Fig. 6 The metabolism of phenylalanine and tyrosine and the role of tetrahydrobiopterin. The asterisked enzymes are: 1, phenylalanine hydroxylase; 2, tyrosine hydroxylase; 3, dihydrobiopterin reductase; 4, tyrosine amino transferase; 5, homogentisic acid oxidase; 6, fumaryl acetoacetate hydrolyase; and 7, tryptophan hydroxylase.

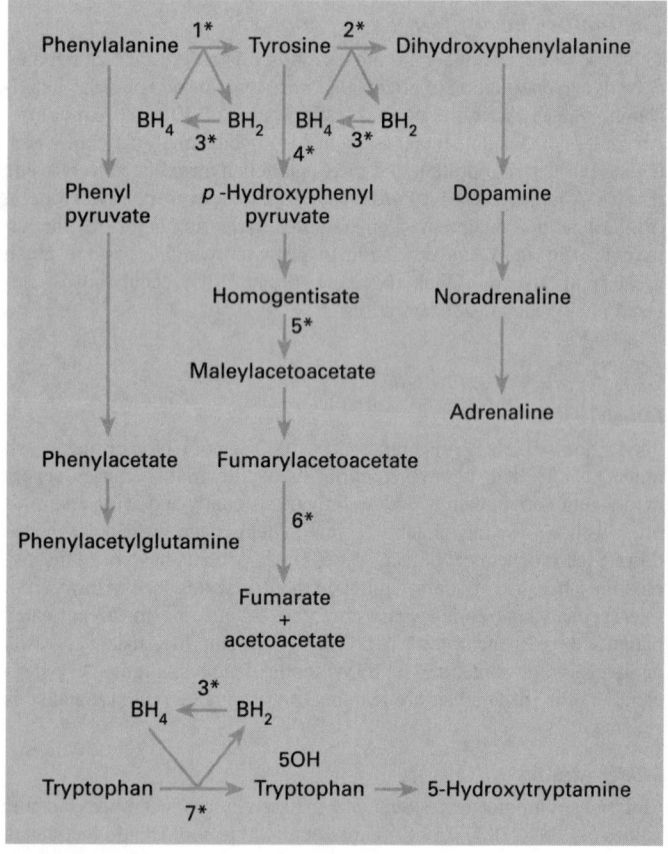

Diagnosis

All newborns in the United Kingdom are screened for raised phenylalanine values on about the seventh day of life, usually by Guthrie's bacterial inhibition assay. Some centres use one-dimensional chromatography. Phenylalanine values greater than 240 μmol/l are rechecked and, if confirmed, are investigated. Raised phenylalanine values are seen in the important variants due to defects in tetrahydrobiopterin synthesis and these must be excluded as they require specific treatment. Transient neonatal hyperphenylalaninaemia is probably less common now that cow's milk, with its relatively high protein content, is used less in infancy, but it must be distinguished from permanent forms.

Genetics

The disease is an autosomal recessive whose incidence in Western countries is 1 in 8000 to 12 000 live births. It is rare in Finland and Japan. One in 50 people carry a mutant gene. These include splicing mutations, deletions, and mis-sense mutations. The location on chromosome 12 has been confirmed. The majority of patients are compound heterozygotes rather than being homozygous for a single mutation. Residual enzyme activity in liver biopsies has correlated fairly well with *in vivo* studies on the conversion of deuterated phenylalanine to tyrosine and there is growing information on which genotypes cause the most severe functional defects in the enzyme.

Antenatal diagnosis

Restriction fragment polymorphisms in linkage disequilibrium with these mutations have been useful in some families for antenatal diagnosis. Patient demand for antenatal diagnosis has been relatively low.

Treatment

Natural protein intake is reduced to provide just what is necessary for growth and development while keeping the plasma phenylalanine between 120 and 360 μmol/l using the Guthrie test or other technique for regular monitoring. These are lower phenylalanine values than were once recommended because outcome in terms of IQ is closely related to the control of abnormally high values. Persistently low values may also adversely affect outcome. Despite normal or near normal IQ results, subtler neuropsychological defects have been described in well treated phenylketonuria patients and may be very important scholastically.

In infancy, milk restriction with supplements is relatively easy. Later it is necessary to introduce other foods on an exchange basis using tables that define the weight of the food containing 1 g of protein (roughly 50 mg phenylalanine). Fruits and some vegetables very low in protein are allowed freely. Adults with classic phenylketonuria tolerate only three to four exchanges, which provide about the same amount of phenylalanine as the free foods. These diets are supplemented with phenylalanine-free amino acid mixtures, minerals, and vitamins.

Regression of IQ when diets were stopped in later childhood has led to continuation of dietary treatment into the teenage years. Patients generally have not suffered when diets have stopped at 15 or 16 years of age. However, there is no follow-up of a substantial number with respect to IQ change who have been off diet for 10 years or more, and there is concern about possible neurological deterioration.

High plasma phenylalanine concentrations may produce a pharmacological impairment of mental function revealed by psychological tests in short term studies, which improve when concentrations fall. Long term damage to intellect or neurological function is another issue. A small number of patients in adult life have developed spastic paraparesis, epilepsy, or extrapyramidal features. All these have cerebral MRI changes, as does an appreciable proportion of those without such manifestations. Together with the known neurotransmitter defects there is a genuine concern for the long term welfare of patients. Diet for life is restricting and costs £7000 to £8000 annually for the diet alone. There is an urgent need for more information.

Table 9 *The incidence of abnormalities in the offspring of phenylketonuric mothers*

	Maternal phenylalanine concentration mg/100 ml ($\times$ 60 = μmol/l)			
	20	16–19	11–15	3–10
Mental retardation	92 (172)	73 (37)	22 (23)	21 (29)
Microcephaly	73 (138)	68 (44)	35 (23)	24 (21)
Congenital heart disease	12 (225)	15 (46)	6 (33)	0 (44)
Birth weight < 2500 g	40 (89)	52 (33)	56 (9)	13 (16)

Percentage figures with sample size in parentheses (from Lenke, R.L. and Levy, H.L. (1980), with permission from *New England Journal of Medicine*). **303**, 1202–8.

Maternal phenylketonuria

The retrospective review of Lenke and Levy in 1983 did a lot to emphasize the adverse fetal effects of maternal hyperphenylalaninaemia (Table 9). Experience in other centres with large clinics broadly supports these figures. Microcephaly and congenital heart disease in the offspring of mothers returning to diet at the seventh or eighth week emphasizes the need for preconception diet. This is the best policy. Even if starting diet very early in the first trimester (5 to 6 weeks) lowers the incidence of impaired brain development, an increased risk certainly remains to brain and heart.

The ratio of fetal to maternal phenylalanine plasma levels is around 1.5 to 1.7 because of active placental transport. Maternal values should be controlled at between 100 and 300 μmol/l, which requires very careful monitoring twice weekly. Some values will rise above this in the critical first trimester when tolerance is very low and nausea restricts calorie intake. Dietary tolerance in the mother increases from about week 18 due to increased requirement for growth by the fetus and uterus, but also probably because phenylalanine hydroxylase in the fetal liver can be detected early in the second trimester (Fig. 7). There is already clear evidence that lower maternal phenylalanine values result in neonates of higher birth weight and larger head circumference.

Fig. 7 Diet for a phenylketonuric mother illustrating the marked rise in phenylalanine tolerance in the second half of the pregnancy. (From Brenton and Haseler (1990). with permission of Springer-Verlag.)

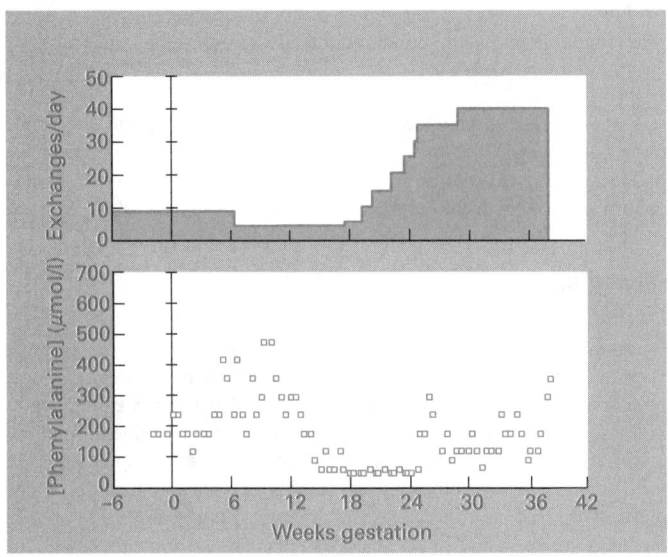

Defects of biopterin metabolism

In the hydroxylation of phenylalanine the cofactor tetrahydrobiopterin (BH$_4$) is consumed and must be regenerated. A deficiency of tetrahydrobiopterin adversely affects the function not only of phenylalanine hydroxylase, but also of tyrosine hydroxylase and tryptophan hydroxylase (Fig. 7). Tyrosine hydroxylation is needed for the synthesis of noradrenaline and dopamine, and tryptophan hydroxylation for the production of 5-hydroxytryptamine. Tetrahydrobiopterin is therefore crucial to the production of neurotransmitters. The supply of this coenzyme is impaired in several enzyme defects. All produce hyperphenylalaninaemia, which may not be marked, and all produce progressive neurological disability despite a low phenylalanine diet. About 1 to 2 per cent of newborns with abnormally raised phenylalanine values have a deficiency of tetrahydrobiopterin.

Dihydropteridine reductase deficiency

Clinical

Progressive neurological deterioration occurs with psychomotor retardation, epilepsy, pyramidal, and extrapyramidal features, especially the latter. Calcification occurs in the cerebral hemispheres.

Biochemistry

Plasma phenylalanine values are elevated. The enzyme dihydropteridine reductase (DHPR) is a tetramer of four units, each 25 000 Da. It has a wide tissue distribution.

Diagnosis

The most reliable test is an enzyme assay on red cells. It can be carried out on dried blood spots. Oral loading tests with tetrahydrobiopterin may be useful as the plasma phenylalanine may then fall but, as it is not regenerated when enzyme is deficient, the results may be equivocal. Urinary biopterin analyses are needed in the differential diagnosis of these defects.

Genetics and prenatal diagnosis

The disease is an autosomal recessive and the enzyme assay can be carried out on cultured amniocytes. There are cross-reacting material-positive and -negative forms and different mutations have been described.

Treatment

A low phenylalanine diet is combined with the administration of L-dopa, 5-hydroxytryptophan, and, in some cases, folinic acid. Early treatment has been reported to give good results.

Guanosine triphosphate cyclohydrolase deficiency and 6-pyruvoyltetrahydrobiopterin synthase deficiency

The clinical features are similar to those of dihydropteridine reductase deficiency. Intermittent hyperthermia has been described. All urinary biopterin and neopterin values are low in the cyclohydrolase deficiency whereas 6-pyruvoyltetrahydrobiopterin deficiency has high neopterin values and low biopterin values. Tetrahydrobiopterin is used in treatment because, in the presence of dihydropteridine reductase, it can be regenerated from dihydrobiopterin. However, the clinical outcome is not assured and there is concern that tetrahydrobiopterin does not easily enter the central nervous system. Treatment, therefore, is also being attempted with low phenylalanine diet, L-dopa, and in addition, 5-hydroxytryptamine. From reports on Saudi Arabian families with a high incidence of 6-pyruvoyltetrahydrobiopterin synthase deficiency, tetrahydrobiopterin is said to produce a good outcome if started very early in life.

Disorders of tyrosine metabolism

The steps in tyrosine metabolism starting with the rate-limiting step – the conversion to p-hydroxyphenyl pyruvic acid by tyrosine aminotransferase – are outlined in Fig. 6. They are the means of production of the catecholamines, dopamine, and the principal pigments of hair and skin. Diagnosing a specific disorder of tyrosine metabolism needs consideration of the non-specific elevations of plasma tyrosine and methionine seen in liver disorders of various aetiologies and the frequency of transient neonatal tyrosinaemia.

Neonatal tyrosinaemia

An increase of plasma tyrosine concentration and excretion of tyrosine and phenolic acids was commonly seen in premature infants given cow's milk feeds. Lower protein infant feeds approximating to breast milk have reduced the incidence greatly. Transient deficiency of p-hydroxyphenylpyruvate oxidase is considered the unproven cause and appears to be harmless. It responds to reducing any high protein intake and sometimes to ascorbic acid. A repeat tyrosine measurement is indicated to exclude other persistent causes of a raised tyrosine.

Tyrosinaemia type I

Clinical

An acute presentation occurs in the early weeks of life with failure to thrive, vomiting, hepatomegaly, fever, oedema, and epistaxis. Death from hepatic failure occurs within the first year. A milder more chronic presentation is compatible with survival for several years with chronic liver disease, a renal tubular Fanconi syndrome with hypophosphataemic rickets, and sometimes abdominal pain and neuropathy suggestive of acute porphyria (see below). Hypertrophic obstructive cardiomyopathy has been described. One-third of patients progress to hepatocellular carcinoma of the liver.

Biochemistry

Deficiency of fumarylacetoacetate hydrolyase (FAH; see Fig. 6) is the cause. A raised plasma tyrosine (and often a raised methionine) result. Succinyl acetone is excreted, formed from fumarylacetoacetate, which also inhibits porphobilinogen synthesis so that δ-amino laevulinic acid (ALA) increases in the urine. Human fumarylacetoacetate hydrolyase is a dimer with a monomer molecular weight of 43 000. Activity is found in liver, kidney, fibroblasts, lymphocytes, and amniocytes.

Diagnosis

Raised plasma tyrosine, succinyl acetone and δ-aminolaevulinic acid excretion and a Fanconi syndrome are the biochemical markers. Fumarylacetoacetate hydrolyase can be assayed in lymphocytes or fibroblasts. It is non-specifically depressed in the liver in a variety of liver diseases. A pseudodeficiency gene in the general population causes low 'in vitro' assay results for fumarylacetoacetate hydrolyase but no clinical illness. Untreated plasma tyrosine values in proven tyrosinaemia type I may be normal, creating another diagnostic problem. Liver function tests are abnormal.

Genetics

The disease is an autosomal recessive. The acute neonatal form lacks immunologically detectable enzyme protein in contrast to the more chronic form. The fumarylacetoacetate hydrolyase gene has been localized to chromosome 15 and a variety of mutations identified.

Prenatal diagnosis and carrier detection

The measurement of succinyl acetone in amniotic fluid and fumarylacetoacetate hydrolyase in cultured amniocytes or chorionic villus samples form the basis of prenatal diagnosis. In approximately 5 per cent of families one parent carries both a true mutant allele and the pseudogene, which lowers the parental enzyme activity into the homozygous disease state and causes confusion in prenatal diagnosis. The pseudogene also makes the detection of carriers less certain.

Treatment

Restricted intake of tyrosine and phenylalanine may reduce the excretion of succinyl acetone and produce regression of the Fanconi tubular defects. Rickets may require treatment however. The liver disease is not cured. The risk of hepatocellular carcinoma remains. Liver transplantation is the treatment of choice for some, which may also improve renal function, although some succinyl acetone continues to be excreted (presumably by renal tissue). In the more chronic form of the disease, transplant timing is immensely problematic. Neither α-fetoprotein nor ultrasound are totally reliable at detecting early malignant change. After liver transplantation the future is uncertain. Chronic renal failure has occurred. Therapeutic trials are in progress using a metabolic inhibitor blocking the pathway before homogentisic acid which reduces the production of more toxic metabolites.

Tyrosinaemia type II

Clinical

The corneal erosions and dendritic ulcers may form within a few months of birth with later scarring, nystagmus, and glaucoma. Corneal transplants can be valuable. The skin lesions may begin after the eye lesions with blistering, painful palms and soles, and hyperkeratosis. Tongue changes have been described. Mental retardation is an inconstant feature but language defects may be more common with possible impaired co-ordination and self-mutilation. The pathology is considered secondary to the deposition of tyrosine crystals in cells precipitating an inflammatory response.

Biochemistry

Tyrosine aminotransferase (TAT), which is deficient catalyses the formation of p-hydroxyphenylpyruvic acid (see Fig. 8) and requires pyridoxal phosphate and α-ketobutyrate. It is a liver enzyme, absent from brain, heart, or kidney, with a subunit size of 49 000 which forms dimers. The enzyme is synthesized rapidly, induced by steroids, and has a short half-life. The gene has been mapped to chromosome 16.

Plasma tyrosine values reach 20 times normal (normal 40 to 100 μmol/l) in younger patients and 10 times normal in others. There is increased excretion of tyrosine, N-acetyl tyrosine, and tyramine; there is no Fanconi syndrome. Excreted phenolic acids come from phenylalanine or tyrosine metabolized at high concentrations by other enzymes.

Diagnosis

The clinical features and amino acid analyses are usually sufficient.

Treatment

A low tyrosine and phenylalanine diet has been used to produce rapid improvement of skin and eye manifestations. There is little information on the neurological results of treatment and little on the degree of dietary control needed to sustain clinical improvement.

Alcaptonuria

Clinical

Presentation in infancy occurs only if discoloration of the urine is noticed. It is usually normal when passed, but darkens on standing (more rapidly at alkaline pH) to deep brown or almost black. Back pain begins in the second and third decade with increasing stiffness due to intervertebral disc degeneration. Involvement of the hips, knees, and shoulders follows. Greyish discoloration of cartilage is seen in the pinna, and pigment is deposited in the sclera. Abnormal pigmentation is seen in the heart valves and pigmented stones are common in the prostate. Discoloration of cartilage, tendons, and ligaments is more orange when seen

Table 10 *A classification of albinism according to whether the hair bulbs have tyrosinase activity (positive) or not (negative)*

	Oculocutaneous tyrosinase −ve	Oculocutaneous tyrosinase +ve	Ocular
Hair colour	White	White Yellow tan	Normal
Skin colour	Pink	White No tan	Normal
Pigmented naevi	0	+	+
Risk of skin cancer	+++	+++	Normal
Eye colour	Grey to blue	Blue to yellow brown	Normal range
Fundal pigment	0	0	0
		+	+
Photophobia	+++	++	+++
Nystagmus	+++	++	+++
Visual acuity	Severely impaired	Impaired	Impaired
Genetics	AR	AR	X-linked or AR

AR, autosomal recessive.

microscopically (ochronosis). The prognosis for the joints is poor. By the fifth decade the lumbar spine is likely to be rigid and other joints will be seriously affected.

Pathology

The pigment is assumed to be a polymer derived from homogentisic acid after enzymatic conversion to the corresponding quinone (homogentisic acid polyphenol oxidase). Virchow described the internally pigmented cartilages including the larynx, tracheal rings, and ribs. The joint cartilages become thinned and fragmented. The intervertebral discs calcify.

Biochemistry

Homogentisic acid oxidase contains ferrous iron and several -SH groups. Molecular oxygen is consumed in splitting the ring to convert homogentisic acid to maleylacetoacetic acid. Homogentisic acid produces a false positive for glucose in the 'clinitest' reaction but the reaction mixture quickly darkens because of the alkaline pH. There is no reaction with glucose in standard dip-stick tests for glucose. Affected individuals excrete 4 to 8 g of homogentisic acid per day.

Diagnosis

In the presence of the clinical symptoms simple urine tests virtually make the diagnosis secure. The homogentisic acid can be demonstrated on thin layer chromatography and quantitated by gas liquid chromatography or high pressure liquid chromatography.

Genetics

It is an autosomal recessive with an incidence of only 1 in 200 000 but small populations of very high incidence exist, especially in Czechoslovakia. The gene has not been localized.

Antenatal diagnosis

This has not been required.

Treatment

The amount of homogentisic acid produced is decreased by a low protein diet. It is very probable that specifically designed low phenylalanine and tyrosine diets would lower the production still further. There seems to be no demand for such a restricting diet to deal with an arthritis which begins only in adult life and progresses slowly over many years. Ascorbic acid may slow the rate of oxidation of homogentisic acid to pigment precursors but there are no data on its clinical usefulness.

Albinism

Tyrosinase deficiency in melanocytes prevents the conversion of *p*-hydroxyphenylalanine acid to dihydroxyphenylalanine and thence to dopaquinone, the precursor for pigment formation in the skin, the iris, the fundus, and the inner ear. The absence of pigment is the characteristic of the group of disorders referred to together as albinism. It is a complex group of ten or more types. The manifestations are primarily in the skin and eye.

The three main types are compared in Table 10. However, two points worth noting are: (1) oculocutaneous albinism may also occur in association with a bleeding tendency – the Hermansky Pudlak syndrome; and (2) in association with the leucocyte killing defect – the Chédiak–Higashi syndrome. Ocular albinism, too, in some genetic forms, occurs in association with nerve deafness.

Oculocutaneous albinism is characterized by structural optic tract defects. All the fibres at the optic chiasma cross over so there are no ipsilateral fibres and no binocular vision. The geniculate bodies and the radiation onwards to the cortex are also structurally abnormal. The inner ear lacks pigment that is normally said to be protective against noise trauma. The predisposition to squamous carcinoma of the skin is important. Further details are in Table 10.

Disorders of sulphur amino acid metabolism

The trans-sulphuration pathway transfers the sulphur of methionine, to serine to produce cysteine (Fig. 8). Methionine adenosyltransferase, with widely distributed isoenzyme forms, produces *S*-adenosylmethionine, the donor in a variety of methylation reactions. In creatine formation alone adult males may utilize more methyl groups than provided by dietary methionine. *S*-Adenosyl homocysteine is cleaved to homocysteine, the sulphhydryl compound in reversible equilibrium with its disulphide homocystine. Half of the homocysteine formed goes through the trans-sulphuration pathway and the other half takes a methyl group from betaine (betaine methyltransferase) or 5-methyltetrahydrofolic acid (methionine synthase). The latter is a cobalamin-dependent enzyme which is functionally impaired in defects of vitamin B_{12} metabolism. The remethylation of homocysteine is also impaired if the activity of the reductase that generates 5-methyltetrahydrofolate (5-MTF) is inadequate.

When accumulation of homocystine results from defects of homocysteine remethylation plasma methionine concentrations are low. They are high when homocystine accumulates from impaired activity of cystathionine synthase, which forms the thioether cystathionine, an intermediate subsequently cleaved to produce the sulphydryl compound cysteine. Further metabolism of cysteine produces inorganic sulphate for excretion.

Cystathionine synthase (CS) deficiency

Clinical

The classic clinical features in the older child and adult are mental retardation, lens dislocation, a thrombotic tendency, and skeletal abnormalities. Mental retardation, affecting two-thirds is sometimes gross but more commonly IQ values are around 65. Others are in the normal range with a few high values. Pyridoxine (B₆) responsive patients (see below) have generally higher IQ values than non-responsive patients. Seizures affect about one-fifth and a few patients show extrapyramidal features, sometimes with severe involuntary movements. Psychiatric disturbances have been described but an increased frequency of schizophrenia is unproven.

Lens dislocation is acquired, usually in the preschool years, but later dislocation is well recognized especially in pyridoxine-responsive patients, and a few have not developed it even in adult life. Monocular and binocular blindness has been relatively frequent due to secondary glaucoma, staphyloma formation, buphthalmos, and retinal detachment.

The skeletal abnormalities include osteoporosis and spontaneous crush vertebral fractures. The common abnormalities seen in Marfan's syndrome – high arched palate, pectus excavatum or carinatum, genu valgum, pes cavus or planus, scoliosis – are all well recognized in homocystinuria. Arachnodactyly is less common and the fingers not infrequently (and elbows occasionally) show mild flexion contractures. Skeletal disproportion with a crown pubis length less than the pubis heel length is usual. (Fig. 9).

Pathology

Thromboembolism is a major cause of morbidity and the main cause of the relatively high premature mortality. Thromboses have been described in a wide variety of arteries and veins, cerebral, coronary, mesenteric, renal, and peripheral. About 50 per cent are in peripheral veins with associated pulmonary emboli in many. Postoperative and postpartum thrombotic risks are high. Premature atheromatous vascular degeneration has been described and arterial aneurysm formation.

Homocysteine may interfere with cross-linking in collagen. Degeneration of zonular fibres around the lens causes the lens dislocation but these fibres are not collagen. The recent work on fibrillin in Marfan's syndrome suggests that defects in this protein may be important in cystathionine synthase deficiency. There is still no accepted explanation for the relationship of homocystine/homocysteine to endothelial damage, platelet abnormalities, thromboses, and vascular change. Heterozygotes for the enzyme defect may be disposed to premature vascular disease and thrombosis. Finally, although the cerebral hemispheres normally have a high concentration of cystathionine, which is reduced in cystathionine synthase deficiency, this is not considered a cause of the mental deficiency, and neither does diffuse vascular disease seem relevant to this problem.

Biochemistry

Elevated plasma methionine values between 100 and 500 μmol/l (sometimes higher) are seen with homocystine values of 50 to 200 μmol/l (Fig. 8). Free homocysteine can only be measured by special techniques but is lower than homocystine. More homocysteine circulates bound to plasma proteins. A mixed disulphide (half homocysteine, half cysteine) is always present at concentrations somewhat below homocystine. The urinary excretion of homocystine is usually 250 to 1000 μmol/day, which accounts for only about 10 to 20 per cent of ingested methionine sulphur. The active cystathionine synthase apoenzyme which requires pyridoxal phosphate, is a tetramer of 63kDa units found predominantly in liver but also in brain and intestinal mucosa. Much lower levels of activity can be found in cultured fibroblasts and stimulated lymphocytes. Residual hepatic activity of 1 to 2 per cent occurs in affected patients, this may increase two to four-fold in pyridoxine-responsive cases. In some patients higher residual activities up to 9 to 10 per cent have been

Fig. 8 The trans-sulphuration pathway from methionine to cysteine is shown on the right and the remethylation of homocysteine on the left. Asterisked enzymes are: 1, cystathionine synthase; 2, methylene tetrahydrofolate reductase, 3, methionine synthase; and 4, betaine methyl transferase.

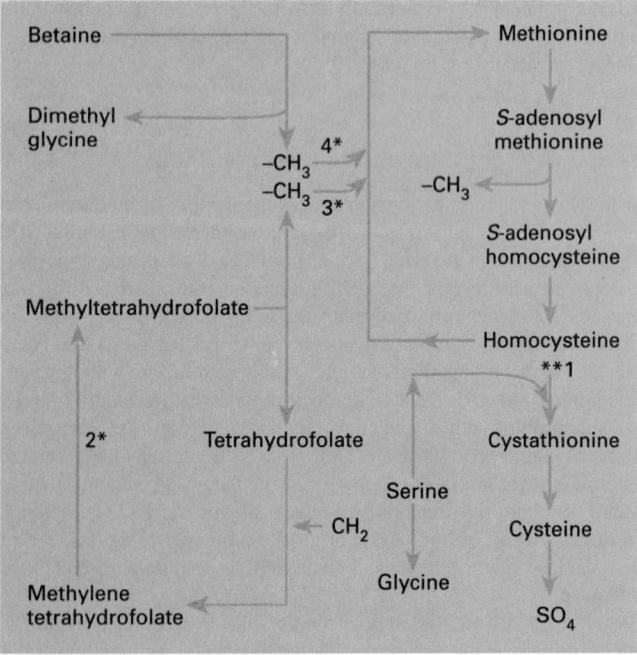

Fig. 9 Child with cystathionine synthase deficiency. Note the kyphosis and short trunk.

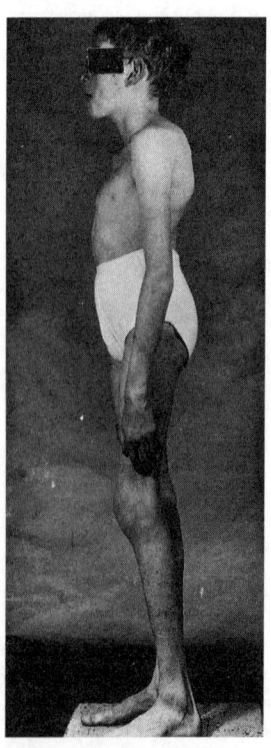

found. Heterozygotes have 25 to 45 per cent of normal activity. *In vitro* responsiveness to pyridoxal phosphate can also be detected in cultured fibroblasts.

Diagnosis

The urine gives a positive nitroprusside test (it is also positive in cystinuria). The amino acid defects are diagnostic if the plasma is deproteinized promptly to minimize homocystine binding to protein. Plasma methionine concentrations are usually well above the normal values of 15 to 30 μmol/l and homocystine is not present in normal plasma.

Genetics

The disease is an autosomal recessive with a birth incidence of about 1 in 40 000. The gene is on chromosome 21 with 15 mutations already described.

Antenatal diagnosis

This has so far rested on enzyme assays on cultured amniotic cells. It is likely that work on the mutant gene will supersede this.

Treatment

Oral pyridoxine may rapidly reduce methionine and homocystine to near normal values. It is the first treatment to try using 150 to 300 mg/l in the older child or adult and reducing the dose if a response is achieved. Very large sustained doses (1000 mg/day or more) in adults cause peripheral neuropathy. A very low protein diet with a system of exchanges is appropriate for those not responding to pyridoxine and requires a methionine-free amino acid supplement, minerals, and vitamins. Biochemical control may only be achieved in older children and adults on protein intakes of 5 to 10 g/day. Cystine supplementation of diets should be considered in patients partially responsive to pyridoxine. Both folic acid (5 to 10 mg/day) and betaine (up to 6 g/day) can further reduce plasma homocystine levels but may produce large elevations of plasma methionine. Low red cell folate values occur and even megaloblastic anaemia. Low serum vitamin B_{12} values have also been found.

Defects of homocysteine remethylation

Two defects have been described: (1) a deficiency of methylene tetrahydrofolate reductase (MTR); and (2) a deficiency of methionine synthase (methyltetrahydrofolate homocysteine methyltransferase). The latter requires methylcobalamin as coenzyme.

Methylene tetrahydrofolate reductase deficiency

Clinical

Neurological features predominate with psychomotor retardation, seizures, abnormalities of gait, and psychiatric disturbance. Presentation occurs from early to late childhood. The risk of vascular disease is high.

Pathology

At autopsy dilated ventricles and low brain weight have been seen; thromboses may be present in arteries and veins. Demyelination occurs and the changes may resemble the classic findings of subacute combined degeneration seen in vitamin B_{12} deficiency. Calcification of the basal ganglia occurs.

Biochemistry

Plasma methionine concentrations are below normal and plasma homocystine concentrations in the range 20 to 200 μmol/l with an excretion of 15 to 600 μmol/day.

Diagnosis

Homocystine is easily missed at low concentrations but is the important clue. The enzyme can be assayed in liver or fibroblasts.

Genetics and prenatal diagnosis

It is an autosomal recessive and enzyme assays on cultured amniocytes have been used for prenatal diagnosis. Several mutations are already described.

Treatment

Betaine in large doses lowers plasma homocystine and raises plasma methionine. Other treatments tried alone or in combination include folinic acid, vitamin B_{12}, pyridoxine, and methionine. Some have suggested a 'cocktail' of all these treatments. It is difficult to be sure of clinical success.

Methionine synthase deficiency

The enzyme transfers a methyl group from methyltetrahydrofolate to homocysteine. Methyl cobalamin is the required coenzyme. This metabolic step may be impaired by an apoenzyme defect or defects in cobalamin metabolism, some of which limit only the formation of methyl cobalamin. Other cobalamin defects are considered under methyl malonic acidaemia.

Clinical

The characteristic findings are developmental delay and megaloblastic anaemia, but the onset may be in later in childhood with dementia and spasticity. Retinal degeneration, cardiac defects, and haemolysis have been described.

Biochemistry and diagnosis

The findings include low plasma methionine and raised homocystine in plasma and urine. Methylmalonic acid should be measured in urine to exclude other cobalamin defects (see methylmalonic aciduria). Methione synthase can be assayed in liver or fibroblasts and antenatal diagnosis has been carried out on cultured amniocytes.

Treatment

This may involve large doses of hydroxycobalamin with betaine and possibly folinic acid.

Other defects of sulphur amino acid metabolism

Among several known defects, cystathioninuria due to cystathionase deficiency is probably clinically harmless. Cystathionine in excess of 1 g/day may be excreted at clearance values close to the glomerular filtration rate.

Methionine adenosyl transferase deficiency causes raised plasma methionine levels (up to 1200 μmol/l; normal 15 to 30 μmol/l) which seems to be harmless. The enzyme defect is partial.

Neither of these defects is considered further but sulphite oxidase deficiency is clinically important.

Sulphite oxidase deficiency

Most cases are due to abnormalities of the molybdenum cofactor, which therefore affects the action also of xanthine oxidase and aldehyde oxidase.

Clinical

Lens dislocation occurs, with severe neurological abnormalities, delayed psychomotor development, and xanthinuria. The neurological defects include seizures and axial hypotonia with increased limb tone. The disease is fatal.

Biochemistry

Sulphite concentrations are raised and sulphite is excreted in the urine. Direct reaction in the body between sulphite and cysteine yield *S-*

sulphocysteine. Plasma urate levels are low and urine xanthine is increased when the disease is due to cofactor abnormalities but not if the defect is in the apoenzyme of sulphite oxidase.

Diagnosis

There is a dipstick test for sulphite which must be applied to fresh urine. S-Sulphocysteine can be detected on an amino acid analyser. Sulphite oxidase can be measured in fibroblasts or liver.

Genetics and prenatal diagnosis

It is an autosomal recessive. Prenatal diagnosis has been carried out on cultured amniocytes by enzyme assay.

Treatment

No effective treatment is known. Some damage may be prenatal. Measures that could be considered include diets low in methionine and cystine. Penicillamine might lower sulphite concentrations by binding with it. The nature of the molybdenum containing cofactor is not well enough understood to be a useful therapeutic approach.

Defects of glycine metabolism

Folate and activated 1-carbon units

Tetrahydrofolate carries 1-carbon units – methyl, methylene, methenyl, formyl, or forminino – bonded to the N-5 or N-10 nitrogen atoms and the units are interconvertible. One carbon units are donated from the tetrahydrofolate derivatives in a variety of syntheses. New 1-carbon units are accepted by tetrahydrofolate in degradative reactions, of which the most important is the conversion of serine to glycine. As serine can be formed from 3-phosphoglycerate, carbohydrates are the ultimate source of 1-carbon units (Fig. 10).

The glycine cleavage system

This system, which generates methylene tetrahydrofolate from carbon-2 of glycine, and carbon dioxide from carbon-1, consists of four mitochondrial proteins. The P protein is a decarboxylase requiring pyridoxal phosphate. The heat-resistant H protein contains lipoic acid and carries the aminomethyl moiety. Both proteins are needed to generate carbon dioxide from the carbon-1 of glycine. The T protein requires tetrahydrofolate and produces methylene tetrahydrofolate from carbon-2 of glycine. The fourth protein (L protein) is needed to transfer hydrogen from the lipoic acid moiety of the H protein to nictotinamide adenine diphosphate. Reversal of the sequence synthesizes glycine. Glycine can be converted to glyoxylate and to δ-aminolaevulinic acid for porphyrin synthesis.

Fig. 10 Reversible glycine cleavage to carbon dioxide and water is illustrated together with reversible interconversion of serine and glycine. These reactions also serve to generate 1-carbon units. 3-Phosphoglycerate (glycolysis) is the ultimate source.

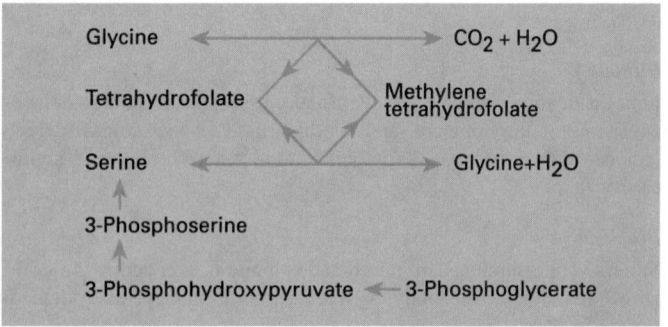

Non-ketotic hyperglycinaemia

Clinical

Twenty-four to 48 h after birth, lethargy, convulsions, anorexia, poor feeding, and vomiting progress to coma and unresponsiveness. Apnoea may require ventilation at least temporarily. The mortality at this stage is high. Intellectual development does not occur in survivors, seizures persist, and tendon reflexes are increased. Microcephaly, poor head control, profound retardation, and a picture of spastic cerebral palsy result.

There is a later childhood form presenting with spastic paraparesis, clonus and extensor plantar responses with modestly raised plasma and cerebrospinal fluid glycine values. Optic atrophy with cerebellar signs has also been described.

Biochemistry

The defect is in the glycine cleavage system with plasma glycine values of 600 to 1200 μmol/l. Normal values for cerebrospinal fluid levels of glycine are around 4–5 μmol/l, the cerebrospinal fluid plasma ratio being around 0.02. Cerebrospinal fluid values 20 times this are seen in patients, raising the cerebrospinal fluid:plasma ratio to between 0.07 and 0.30. Large quantities of glycine appear in the urine, as much as 2 g/day. This is not accompanied by proline or hydroxyproline.

Diagnosis

This rests on the analysis of plasma and cerebrospinal fluid for glycine concentrations. Few people can assay the enzymes.

Genetics

The variant forms are autosomal recessives. The P protein is absent in classic phenotypes. T protein defects have been found in different phenotypes and H protein defects in later onset degenerative forms. Hyperglycinaemia seems to be commoner in Japan and Finland. Different mutations in these two populations affect the P protein.

Antenatal diagnosis

The enzyme system is unstable and not present in fibroblasts or cultured amniotic cells. Chorionic villi are being used for enzyme assay in prenatal diagnosis combined with amniotic fluid glycine:serine ratios.

Treatment

This is very unsatisfactory. Some central nervous system damage may be prenatal. Plasma glycine levels can be lowered by exchange transfusion or peritoneal dialysis but without clinical improvement. Low protein diets have only a limited effect on decreasing plasma glycine concentrations. Supplying '1-carbon units' in the form of methionine or N-formyltetrahydrofolate has not helped. The combination of sodium benzoate and diazepines, which compete for glycine receptors in the central nervous system has lowered plasma and cerebrospinal fluid levels of glycine and reduced seizures without clearly improving prognosis. Strychnine, known to block glycine receptors, was initially reported to be therapeutically useful, but this finding was not supported subsequently. A favourable clinical response to tryptophan therapy has been reported and attributed to the tryptophan metabolite kynurenic acid, which may block the excitatory action of glycine at the N-methyl-D-aspartate (NMDA) receptor. Another NMDA receptor blocker dextromethorphan has had variable therapeutic success.

Defects in branched chain amino acid metabolism

Leucine, isoleucine, and valine

These essential amino acids, with a branched carbon chain structure, collectively make up 10 to 15 per cent of animal protein and are catabolized by transamination to the corresponding keto acids, 2-keto-isocaproic, 2-keto-3-methylvaleric and 2-keto-isovaleric acids (Fig. 11). In all tissues except the liver aminotransferase activity exceeds α-ketode-hydrogenase activity. Peripheral tissues, notably muscle, predominantly transaminate but the keto acids are largely transported back to the liver for subsequent metabolism.

Branched chain α-keto dehydrogenase (BCKD): the role of thiamine

The oxidative decarboxylation of branched chain keto acids is analogous to the oxidative decarboxylation of pyruvate and α-ketoglutarate to acetyl coenzyme A and succinyl coenzyme A, respectively. All are three subunit mitochondrial enzymes, the first part of which – E_1 – uses thiamine pyrophosphate as coenzyme. The thiamine moiety is crucial to the decarboxylase function of branched chain α-keto dehydrogenase (E_1) and the release of carbon dioxide. Branched chain α-keto dehydrogenase (E_2) is the core protein of the complex, the acyl transferase that generates acyl coenzyme A while its lipoate moiety is reduced. The third part (E_3) regenerates the oxidized lipoate and is actually shared by all three dehydrogenase complexes. Branched chain α-keto dehydrogenase (E_1) is active in a dephosphorylated form and inactivated by phosphorylation, which provides a control mechanism. Branched chain ketoaciduria (BCKA) (maple syrup urine disease) arises from defects in the branched chain α-keto dehydrogenase complex. Some patients have a thiamine responsive form of this disease (see below).

Branched chain ketoaciduria (BCKA)

Clinical

In the classic disease the baby is well for 2 to 3 days and then poor feeding and sleepiness progress to coma and apnoea. Vomiting is inconstant. The mortality is high and survivors show dystonia, psychomotor retardation, and other neurological abnormalities.

Milder forms of the disease are described, sometimes with later presentation and intermittent forms where patients may be biochemically normal between attacks but succumb during intercurrent infection or illness or excessive protein intake.

Pathology

Myelin abnormalities that occur in patients dying of branched chain ketoaciduria are also found in Poll-Hereford calves with the same genetic defect, and in other experimental animal models.

Biochemistry

In the acute stage, hypoglycaemia and hyperammonaemia may occur. Leucine values may be as high as 4000 to 5000 μmol/l. Isoleucine and valine are also much increased in plasma and urine. (See Table 1 for normal values.) The three keto acids cause mild metabolic acidosis and the sweetish smell in urine of maple syrup. Residual enzyme activity in fibroblasts is 1 to 2 per cent for the classic severe disease but 20 to 40 per cent of normal in mild variants.

Diagnosis

The plasma amino acids and urine keto acids are diagnostic. Delays of 2 to 3 days in diagnosis may cause permanent brain damage.

Genetics

This is an autosomal recessive disorder. Screening is possible by bacterial assay but the disease is too rare to justify the cost. The incidence is about 1 in 120 000 in Europe but 1 in 200 000 in most of the United States, although an incidence of more than 1 in 1000 has been recorded in a Mennonite community. As the E_1 component of the branched chain α-keto dehydrogenase is subdivided further into $E_{1\alpha}$ and $E_{1\beta}$, at least four genes code for the complex, plus two genes for the controlling phosphatase and kinase. Enzyme assays and immunological and complementation studies have already revealed genetic defects in $E_{1\alpha}$, $E_{1\beta}$, and E_2 in different families. The Mennonite mutation is an asparagine substitution for tyrosine in the $E_{1\alpha}$ subunit.

Prenatal diagnosis

This has been based on enzyme assays in cultured amniocytes or chorionic villus samples.

Treatment

A high calorie intake, given parenterally as 10 to 20 per cent dextrose if necessary, is needed to suppress nitrogen catabolism in the acutely ill. An amino acid mixture excluding leucine, isoleucine, and valine can be introduced by nasogastric tube to provide 2 g protein/kg/day. Normal protein sources (milk, etc.) are omitted until the branched chain amino acid concentrations fall towards normal. Both exchange transfusion and peritoneal dialysis have been used to speed biochemical recovery. Hypoglycaemia, sepsis, and hypotension need intensive care and monitoring. Dietary treatment is lifelong but needs frequent adjustments. The aim is to keep plasma leucine, isoleucine, and valine concentrations about twice their normal values (see Table 1). Coma carries a poor prognosis for subsequent central nervous system development and function. The incidence of impaired intellect and neurological handicap is high and special schooling will be necessary.

Responsiveness to thiamine has also been described in a few patients (10 to 20 mg/day). It is claimed that large doses up to 500 mg/day improve some cases of classic branched chain ketoaciduria. In vitro evidence indicates that the $E_{1\alpha}$ subunit is stabilized by thiamine supplements, which may saturate all subunits. An increase in enzyme activity has even been described in normal subjects on thiamine treatment.

Other defects of branched chain amino acid metabolism

Rare cases of defective deamination have been described causing isolated hypervalinaemia or hyperleucinaemia–isoleucinaemia, indicating either separate amino transferases in man or different mutations affecting different substrate binding sites in a common enzyme.

Fig. 11 Branched chain amino acid metabolism. Transamination produces the keto acids (top) all of which are metabolized by the branched chain α-keto dehydrogenase complex (asterisked) 1. 2, Propionyl coenzyme A carboxylase; and 3, methylmalonyl coenzyme A mutase.

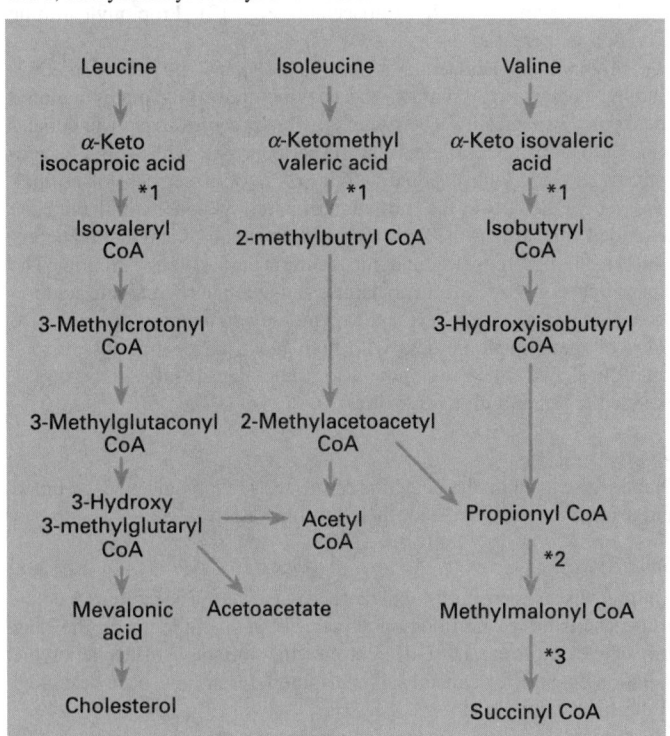

Table 11 *Some less common branched chain organic acidurias not covered in the text. Patients have been described with normal activities of the two asterisked enzymes but the organic acid pattern of enzyme deficiency and clinical illness*

Deficient enzyme	Clinical	Blood/urine metabolites	Treatment
3-Methylcrotonyl CoA carboxylase	Vomiting, acidosis, hypoglycaemic coma	3-Methylcrotonyl glycine, 3-hydroxy isovalerate	Protein restriction, no biotin response
3-Methyl glutaconyl CoA hydratase*	Neurodegeneration, hypotonia, optic atrophy	3-Methyl glutaconate, 3-hydroxy isovalerate 3-methyl glutarate	Protein restriction
3-Hydroxy-3-methyl* glutaryl CoA lyase*	Vomiting, hypotonia, lethargy, coma, hypoglycaemia and raised ammonia, Reye's type presentation	3-Methyl glutaconate, 3-hydroxy 3-methyl glutarate	Protein restriction, high carbohydrate intake
Mevalonate kinase	Failure to thrive, hepatosplenomegaly, anaemia and death	Mevalonate	None
2-Methyl aceto acetyl CoA thiolase	Acidosis, ketosis, vomiting, coma	2-Methyl acetoacetate, 2-methyl 3-hydroxybutyrate	Protein restriction
3-Hydroxyisobutyryl CoA deacylase	Malformations and death	Carboxypropyl cysteine	None

CoA, coenzyme A.

The organic acidaemias in branched chain amino acid metabolism

The catabolic steps outlined in Fig. 11 illustrate the formation of isovaleric acid, propionic acid, and methylmalonic acid, each of which accumulates in one of the three more common organic acidaemias. In the further metabolism of two of these acids there are important vitamin coenzymes – biotin for priopionyl coenzyme A carboxylase and cobalamin for methylmalonyl coenzyme A mutase. Biotin metabolism is considered under multiple carboxylase deficiency later and cobalamin metabolism immediately below. Less common branched chain organic acidaemias are listed in Table 11.

Vitamin B₁₂ metabolism

Vitamin B_{12} has a complex metabolism but is required in only two metabolic steps – the remethylation of homocysteine to methionine and the conversion of methylmalonyl coenzyme A to succinyl coenzyme A. An outline of cobalamin metabolism in the body is shown in Fig. 12. In the cytosol hydroxycobalamin may become the coenzyme methyl cobalamin, which is required by methionine synthase, or be transported into the mitochondria to be metabolized to adenosyl cobalamin, the coenzyme of methylmalonyl coenzyme A mutase.

Isovaleric, propionic and methylmalonic acidaemias

Clinical

One to several days after a normal pregnancy and delivery the child stops feeding. Respiratory problems ensue with varying tonal change both axial hypotonia and episodes of generalized hypertonia and myoclonic jerking. Apnoea, coma, and death supervene. Characteristically the child is acidotic, possibly ketotic, and non-specific increases of ammonia and glycine may occur. Both hypoglycaemia and hyperglycaemia have been described, the latter causing confusion with diabetic ketoacidosis. Hypocalcaemia is also found.

A more chronic form of these diseases is recognized, with anorexia, failure to thrive, psychomotor retardation, hypotonia, and weakness. Cardiomyopathy has been reported.

The intermittent clinical forms present as recurrent attacks of encephalopathy and ataxia with normality between attacks. Changes in blood glucose may again be confusing (see above). Acute attacks may be followed by neurological abnormalities of pyramidal or extrapyramidal nature. Leucopenia and thrombocytopenia sometimes occur.

Biochemistry

Isovaleric acidaemia is due to a deficiency of isovaleryl coenzyme A dehydrogenase and characterized by the excretion in the urine of isovaleric acid, isovalerylglycine, 3-hydroxy isovaleric acid, and isovalerylcarnitine.

Isolated propionic acidaemia is due to a deficiency of the apoenzyme for propionyl CoA coenzyme A carboxylase, a biotin-requiring enzyme. The enzyme converts proprionyl coenzyme A to methylmalonyl coenzyme A. Characteristically, plasma and urine propionate values are raised with the formation of methylcitrate from the condensation of propionyl coenzyme A with oxaloacetate (Fig. 13). Propionylcarnitine excretion is increased.

Methylmalonic acidaemia is due to deficient activity of methylmalonyl coenzyme A mutase, the enzyme converting methylmalonyl coenzyme A to succinyl coenzyme A, which requires adenosyl cobalamin. Two apoenzyme defects are described, one with virtually zero activity and one with residual activity of 2 to 75 per cent of normal. Two genetic defects in the formation of adenosyl cobalamin have been described. One affects the formation of both adenosyl and methyl cobalamin, resulting in methylmalonic aciduria and homocystinuria. The other affects only adenosyl cobalamin, and only methylmalonic aciduria occurs. Patients with severe apoenzyme defects excrete up to 5 to 6 g/day of methylmalonic acid with high blood concentrations up to 6 mmol/litre (Fig. 14). Propionate also accumulates in the blood and is excreted together with methylcitrate.

Diagnosis

Diagnosis rests upon the detection of the relevant organic acids in blood and urine, their conjugates or their carnitine esters.

Genetics

All three diseases are autosomal recessive. Isovaleryl coenzyme A dehydrogenase is a four-unit homopolymer with a single locus on the long arm of chromosome 15. Different enzyme variants cause phenotypic variation but severe neonatal and intermittent forms have been described in the same family.

Propionyl coenzyme A carboxylase has the subunit structure α_6/β_6.

Fig. 12 Naturally occurring cobalamin is converted in the cytosol to methyl cobalamin, or by successive valency reductions of the cobalt moiety within the mitchondria adenosyl cobalamin is eventually formed.

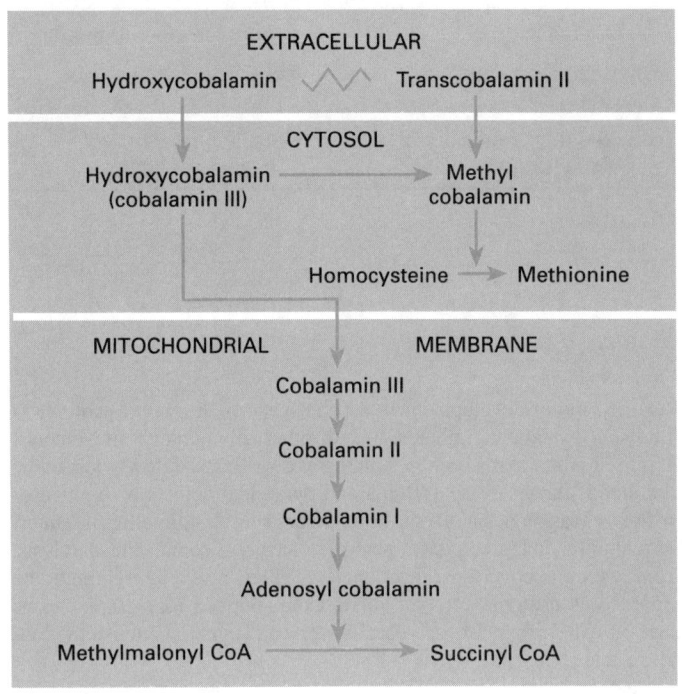

Fig. 13 Neonatal propionic acidaemia with hyperammonaemia raised plasma methylcitrate levels and low levels of citrate (μmol/l). Treated by diet, exchange transfusion, and peritoneal dialysis. (From Brenton and Krywawych, unpublished data.)

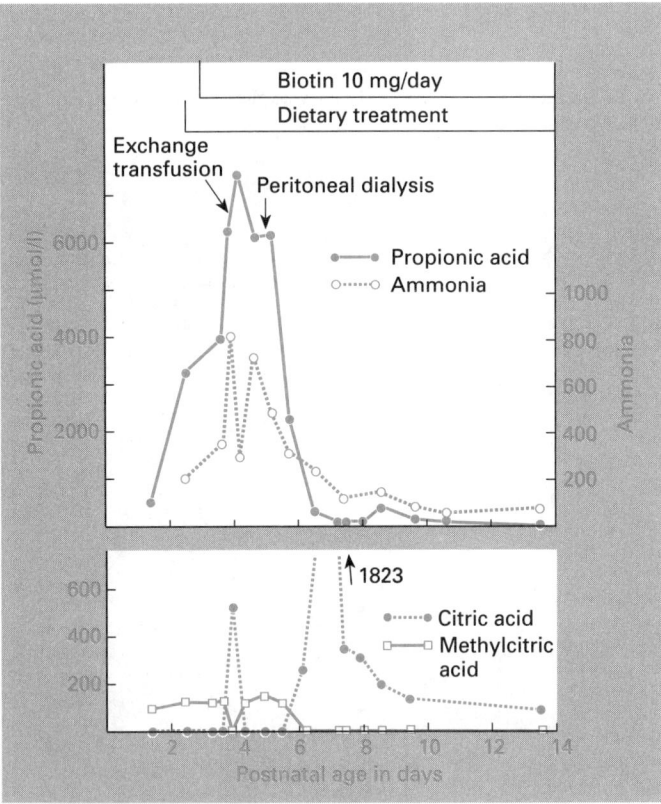

The α subunit gene is on chromosome 13 and the β subunit gene is on chromosome 3. Defects in the α chain (which binds the biotin) are associated with 50 per cent enzyme activity in heterozygotes and 1 to 5 per cent activity in homozygotes. Homozygous β chain defects are similarly severe but heterozygotes have near normal activity. β chains are produced in half-normal amounts. β chains are normally produced in excess of α chains.

Methyl malonyl coenzyme A mutase is a dimer of subunit size 75 000 with adenosyl cobalamin bound to each subunit. The gene locus is on chromosome 6. The mutant mutase with no residual enzyme activity has no detectable enzyme protein, either because none is made or because it is highly unstable.

There is now considerable information on the causal mutations in all three diseases.

Prenatal diagnosis

Isovaleric acid in amniotic fluid is measured reliably by stable isotope dilution analysis, and isovaleryl coenzyme A dehydrogenase can be measured in cultured amniocytes. For propionic acidaemia the measurement of methylcitrate in amniotic fluid and enzyme assay in cultured amniocytes has been used. Similar approaches to prenatal diagnosis in isolated methylmalonic aciduria have used the measurement of methylmalonate acid in amniotic fluid and enzyme assays or studies of adenosyl vitamin B_{12} metabolism in cultured amniocytes.

Treatment

In the severe neonatal form of these diseases the initial treatment is concerned with: (1) removal of toxic organic acids by exchange transfusion. Because urinary excretion of propionate is poor this may be followed in propionic acidaemia by peritoneal dialysis; and (2) encouraging anabolism by the provision of calories as 10 to 20 per cent glucose and electrolyte solutions intravenously with or without insulin. Enteral feeding should be started by nasogastric tube as soon as possible (after 24 to 48 h), initially this should be with protein-free feeds, but soon changing to a low protein feed (0.5 g/kg/day) and later increasing to tolerance and supplemented with amino acid mixtures that omit the amino acids whose metabolism is impaired. The requirements of these

Fig. 14 Plasma concentrations of methylmalonate (a dicarboxylic acid) and bicarbonate in an affected teenage girl indicating that the acidosis is due almost entirely to the methymalonate. (From Brenton and Krywawych, unpublished data.)

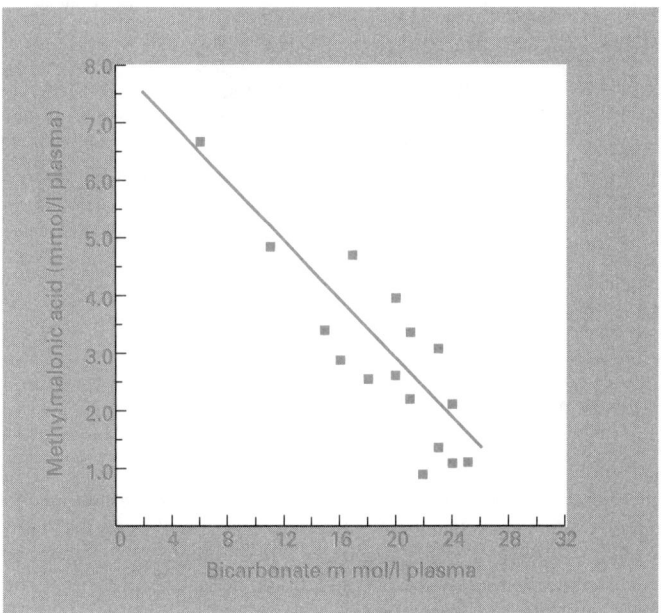

Table 12 *Defects of γ-aminobutyric acid metabolism. The asterisk indicates that deficiency of glutamic acid decarboxylase has not been proven*

Deficient enzyme	Clinical	Blood/urine metabolites	Treatment
Glutamic acid decarboxylase*	Seizures	No abnormality	Pyridoxine 10–100 mg/day
GABA transaminase	Psychomotor retardation, increased growth	Increased plasma and CSF GABA	No pyridoxine response reported
Succinic semialdehyde dehydrogenase	Mental retardation, cerebellar dysfunction	Increased 4-hydroxybutyrate in blood, urine and CSF	None but ? neurology improves with age

CSF, cerebrospinal fluid; GABA, γ-aminobutyric acid.

amino acids for growth are provided by the natural protein, whose intake must be adjusted accordingly. L-Glycine supplements of 0.25 to 0.5 g/kg/day are helpful in isovaleric acidaemia because it increases the formation of the non-toxic isovalerylglycine. L-Carnitine 100 mg/kg/day may help in all three diseases by replenishing carnitine and increasing the excretion of non-toxic carnitine acyl esters. Both insulin and growth hormone have been tried to produce positive nitrogen balance and hasten recovery in catabolic states.

No true *in vivo* responsiveness to biotin has been demonstrated in isolated propionic acidaemia. However, *in vivo* response to hydroxy cobalamin therapy in methylmalonic acidaemia occurs and should be tested in all such patients and continued long term if response occurs. Diet is needed long term in all three disorders; this is relatively easy in isovaleric acidaemia where a low protein diet may suffice. A low protein diet may also suffice in some patients with methylmalonic acidaemia, combined with regular oral sodium bicarbonate to control residual acidosis. Patients with propionic acidaemia are more difficult to manage and require a low protein diet with supplements of amino acids more frequently. Chronic nasogastric feeding may be needed for anorexia. Oral metronizanole may reduce propionate production in the intestine by gut bacteria in propionic and methylmalonic acidaemia but therapeutic usefulness is not yet clear. Similarly, the use of L-carnitine on a chronic basis may help in all diseases but it is not proven.

Disorders of γ-aminobutyric acid (GABA) metabolism

γ-Aminobutyric acid is formed from glutamate in the brain by the cytosolic enzyme glutamate decarboxylase, which requires pyridoxal phosphate. Pyridoxine-dependent seizures in neonates is postulated to be due to this enzyme deficiency, which is difficult to prove because other tissues have a genetically different mitochondrial glutamate decarboxylase. Glutamate can be regenerated from γ-aminobutyric acid by transamination with ketoglutarate (γ-aminobutyric acid transaminase), which is also pyridoxal phosphate-dependent. The other product is succinic semialdehyde, which is dehydrogenated to succinate, which enters the citric acid cycle. Deficiency of succinic semialdehyde dehydrogenase leads to the excretion of 4-hydroxybutyric acid. Some more details of disordered γ-aminobutyric acid metabolism are given in Table 12.

Defects of lysine metabolism

Lysine catabolism

The main pathway is via saccharopine to acetyl coenzyme A (Fig. 15) and others less important. Glutaryl coenzyme A dehydrogenase catalyses the conversion of glutaryl coenzyme A to crotonyl coenzyme A and its defects are serious disorders. Other lysine degradation defects are of uncertain clinical consequence.

Glutaric aciduria type I

Clinical

Retarded motor development in the first year of life with hypotonia is followed by ataxia, athetosis, and other involuntary movements. Acquired motor skills such as walking and writing are slowly lost in the childhood years. Severe dystonia and pyramidal defects with extensor or flexor spasms occur. Dysarthria renders speech unintelligible. Intercurrent infection precipitates acidosis, seizures, coma, and paralysis, from which recovery is incomplete. The overall picture might be regarded as dystonic cerebral palsy. Computerized tomography scans have revealed progressive cerebral atrophy and hyperlucency of the caudate nucleus.

Biochemistry

Glutaryl coenzyme A dehydrogenase deficiency causes an accumulation of glutaryl coenzyme A (also derived from tryotophan degradation), increasing glutaric acid concentrations in plasma and urine, and increasing concentrations of 3-hydroxyglutarate and glutaconic acid. These are all inhibitors of glutamic acid decarboxylase, which may explain the low γ-aminobutyric acid concentrations in the central nervous system. Glutaryl carnitine is excreted in the urine even when free glutaric acid is absent. Systemic acidosis occurs in acute attacks with ketosis and hypoglycaemia.

Fig. 15 The metabolism of lysine. The enzyme glutaryl coenzyme A dehydrogenase is asterisked.

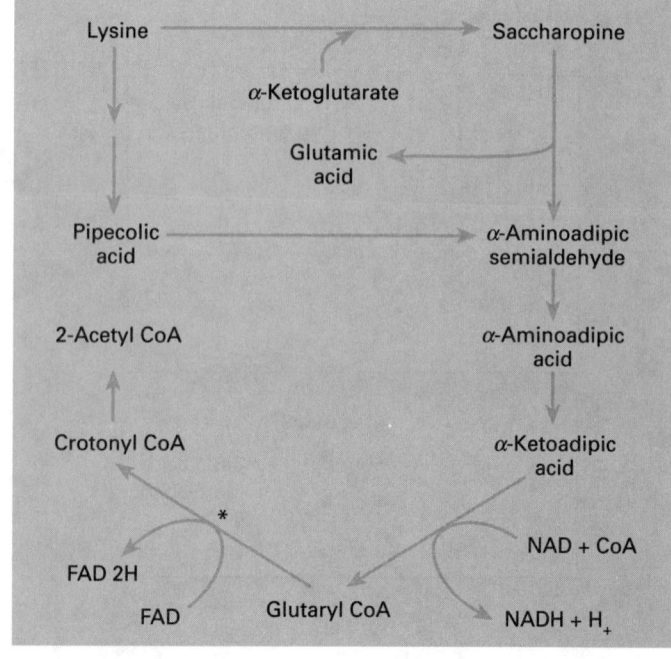

Diagnosis

This cause of progressive dystonic cerebral palsy is usually indicated by the organic acids in plasma and urine. Sometimes the organic acids have not been detected, particularly between acute attacks. Enzyme assays on leucocytes or fibroblasts are then indicated.

Prenatal diagnosis

This has been carried out by finding glutaric acid in the amniotic fluid and enzyme assay on cultured amniocytes.

Genetics

The disease is an autosomal recessive. Varying residual enzyme activity and several different mutations have been described.

Treatment

Low protein diets reduce glutaric acid excretion. Carnitine supplementation corrects low plasma levels which are secondary to losses from glutaryl carnitine excretion. Riboflavin has been reported to diminish glutaric acid excretion in some patients, the treatment rationale being that increased flavine adenine dinucleotide might stabilize the enzyme. Baclofen has also been studied because it activates γ-aminobutyric acid receptors. No treatment has proved of any clinical benefit.

Defects in the final stages of carbon chain metabolism

Biotin dependent carboxylation

Biotin is important in transferring a 1-carbon unit (carbon dioxide) to acceptor molecules. Defects in biotin metabolism disturb the function of four enzymes – pyruvate carboxylase, acetyl-coenzyme A carboxylase, propionyl coenzyme A carboxylase, and 3-methylcrotonyl coenzyme A carboxylase (Fig. 16). These apoenzymes are converted to holoenzymes by the attachment of biotin, which needs the catalytic activity of an enzyme holocarboxylase synthetase (Fig. 17). When the holoenzymes are themselves biologically degraded the biotin is initially released still attached to lysine peptides. The enzyme biotinidase frees biotin from these peptides. It also liberates dietary biotin from proteins in the gastrointestinal tract. In its absence biotin peptides are excreted, dietary biotin is not absorbed, and biotin deficiency occurs. Biotinidase is widely distributed.

Electron transport and the acyl coenzyme A dehydrogenases

The electrons accumulating during oxidation in the citric acid cycle are carried by reduced nicotinamide adenine dinucleotide and reduced flavine adenine dinucleotide, to be transferred along the electron transporting chain to molecular oxygen, with the generation of adenosine triphosphate and water. Transfer from reduced nicotinamide adenine dinucleotide takes place sequentially across four multienzyme complexes (I–IV), which are part of the structure of the inner mitochondrial membrane. The flavin-containing acyl coenzyme A dehydrogenases transfer electrons differently to an intermediate electron transferring flavoprotein (ETF) and from there to ubiquinone catalysed by the enzyme electron transferring flavoprotein ubiquinone oxidoreductase (Fig. 18).

Defects at this level affect not only amino acid catabolism but fatty acid oxidation, and the organic acid defects are complex. The affected acyl coenzyme A dehydrogenases include glutaryl coenzyme A dehydrogenase and defects in electron transport at this point in metabolism are labelled glutaric aciduria type II.

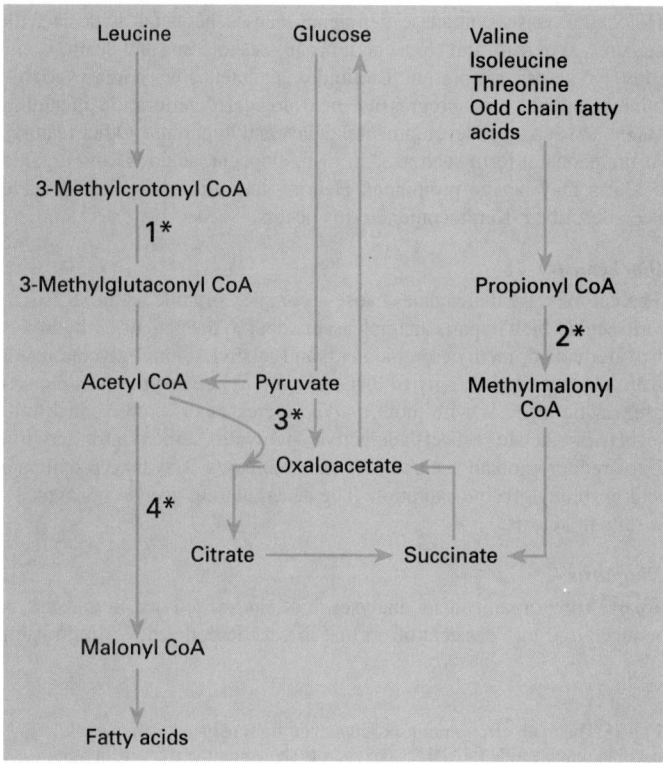

Fig. 16 Important carboxylases in amino acid metabolism. Asterisked enzymes are: 1, 3-methylcrotonyl coenzyme A carboxylase; 2, propionyl coenzyme A carboxylase; 3, pyruvate carboxylase; and 4, acetyl coenzyme A carboxylase.

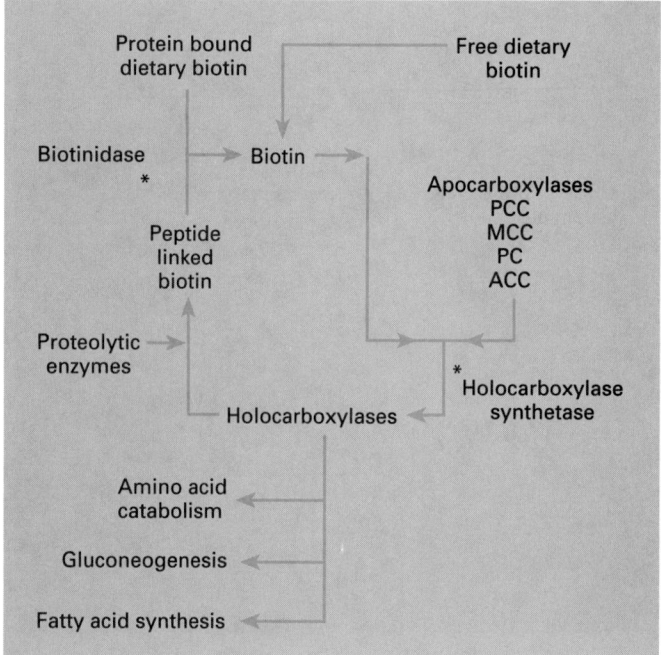

Fig. 17 The metabolism of biotin. MCC (3-methylcrotonyl coenzyme A) and PCC (propionyl coenzyme A carboxylase) are important in amino acid catabolism, and PC (pyruvate carboxylase) is important in gluconeogenesis, and ACC (acetyl coenzyme A carboxylase) in fatty acid synthesis. Important enzymes are asterisked.

Multiple carboxylase deficiency

Clinical

Holocarboxylase synthetase deficiency causes neonatal acidosis with seizures, skin rash, and alopecia; it progresses to coma and death. Vomiting and ketosis are present. Biotinidase deficiency has a more variable clinical picture with progressive neurological deterioration including ataxia and seizures, developmental delay, and hypotonia. Other features of the neonatal form such as skin rash, alopecia, acidosis, and organic aciduria may not be prominent. Hearing loss and optic atrophy have been described. Keratoconjunctivitis occurs.

Biochemistry

The carboxylase deficiencies cause a complex organic aciduria. Isovaleric acid (which imparts an unpleasant odour to the patient), 3-hydroxy-isovaleric acid, methylcrotonic acid, and methylcrotonyl glycine result from the impaired activity of 3-methylcrotonyl coenzyme A carboxylase. Lactic acidosis with more marked increases in cerebrospinal fluid levels of lactate reflects defective pyruvate carboxylase activity. Impaired propionate metabolism also increases 3-hydroxypropionate and propionylglycine excretion. The accumulating acetyl coenzyme A results in ketosis.

Diagnosis

Apart from organic acid analyses biotinidase activity in plasma is reduced to 0 to 5 per cent of normal in genetic deficiency. Biotin itself

Fig. 18 The main electron transporting chain from reduced nicotinamide adenine dinucleotide (NADH) to oxygen is shown on the right, with other entry points for the flow of electrons coming from the left. ETF, electron transporting flavoprotein; FADH$_2$, reduced flavin adenine dinucleotide; QH$_2$, reduced ubiquinone.

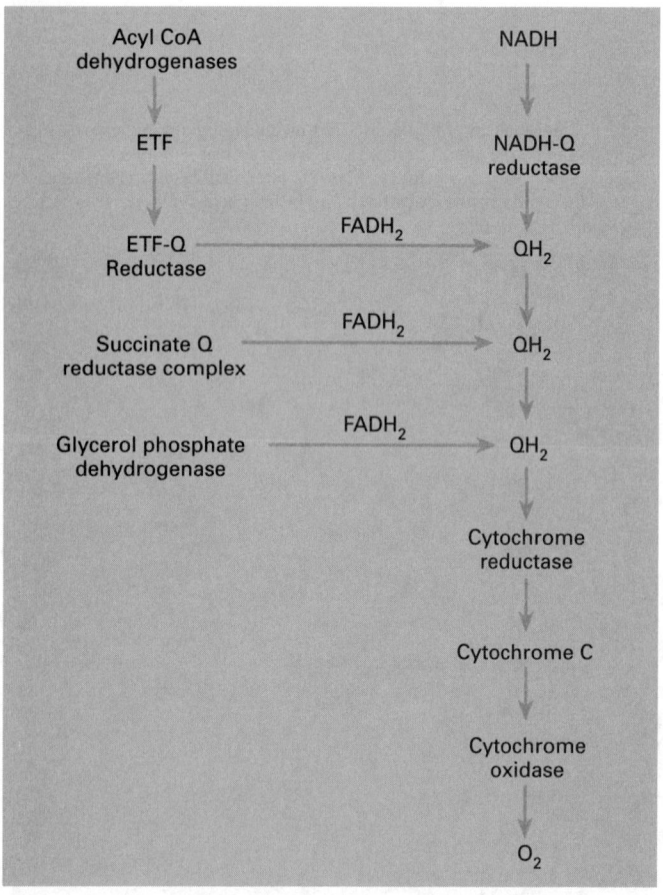

can be measured in plasma and urine. The assay of holocarboxylase synthetase is difficult and possible only in a few places. The therapeutic response to biotin does not distinguish between the two defects.

Genetics

Both are recessive disorders and biotinidase deficiency seems to be more common than holocarboxylase synthetase deficiency. The gene for the latter has been assigned to chromosone 21 and several mutations described.

Prenatal diagnosis

This is only required in holocarboxylase synthetase deficiency and depends on amniotic fluid analysis for organic acids and enzyme assay in cultured amniotic cells.

Treatment

Biotinidase deficiency responds well to 5 to 10 mg/day of oral biotin. Deficiency develops in a few days if biotin is stopped. Pre-existing neurological damage may not reverse. Most patients with holocarboxylase deficiency respond well to 10 mg daily, but larger doses may be needed and some have not fully responded to doses as high as 100 mg/day.

Glutaric acidaemia type II

Clinical

The most severe neonatal presentation, with associated congenital abnormalities, often leads to premature birth, metabolic acidosis, hypoglycaemia, hepatomegaly, and hypotonia. Severe cystic dysplasia of the kidneys is common; the kidneys may be palpable. Other defects include facial dysmorphism, 'rocker-bottom' feet, anterior abdominal wall defects, and defects of the external genitalia. Death usually occurs in the first week of life. Some affected neonates, without congenital defects, have the other clinical abnormalities of metabolic acidosis, hypoglycaemia, hypotonia, and hepatomegaly. The prognosis remains poor, with death in the early days or weeks of life, often with severe cardiomyopathy.

Milder forms presenting after the neonatal period, or survivors of early illness, may suffer recurrent encephalopathic episodes similar to Reye's syndrome. Cases with a predominantly late clinical presentation of lipid storage myopathy are described. Adult presentation has been recorded. From their predominant organic acid pattern, some of these clinically milder patients are given the diagnosis of ethylmalonic–adipicaciduria.

Biochemistry

Glutaric aciduria type II is due to deficiency of electron transferring flavoprotein or electron transferring flavoprotein-ubiquinone oxido-reductase, the latter causing the severest neonatal form with congenital defects. The flavin-containing acyl coenzyme A dehydrogenases affected include glutaryl coenzyme A dehydrogenase, isovaleryl coenzyme A dehydrogenase, the long, medium and short chain dehydrogenases used in fatty acid oxidation and the dehydrogenases involved in sarcosine synthesis and breakdown. The organic acids found in urine as a consequence include short chain acids – isovaleric, 3-hydroxy isovaleric, glutaric, 2-hydroxyglutaric – the ω-oxidation products of medium chain fatty acids – adipic, suberic and sebacic acids – ethylmalonic acid, 5-hydroxy hexanoic acid, and glycine conjugates of a variety of these. Carnitine concentrations in plasma are low and a range of acyl carnitines are found in urine and increased by carnitine therapy. Hypoglycaemia is very common.

Diagnosis

The florid organic acid pattern in severe patients is characteristic but in those more mildly affected it is less marked. Hepatomegaly and hypo-

Table 13 *Some well-recognized genetic amino acid defects not described in the text*

Enzyme defect	Clinical	Blood/urine metabolites	Treatment
Carnosinaemia Serum carnosinase	Uncertain. Mental retardation, myoclonic seizures	Excretion of β-alanyl-L-histidine (carnosine) and β-alanyl-1-methyl-L-histidine (anserine)	None
Hyperiminodipeptiduria Prolidase	Chronic dermatitis with skin ulcers. Mental retardation. Frequent infections	Excretion of glycyl proline and other imino peptides	Ascorbic acid. Locally to ulcers cream containing glycine and proline, value uncertain
Sarcosinaemia Sarcosine dehydrogenase	Probably none. Original patients mentally retarded	Increased plasma and urine sarcosine (N-methylglycine)	None
Histidinaemia Histidase	Usually none. Low IQ and CNS abnormalities	Raised plasma histidine	None, but if symptoms low protein diet
Familial hyperlysinaemia α-amino adipic semialdehyde synthase	Usually none	Plasma lysine raised 6–7 × normal saccharopin excretion in some	Probably none
Hyperprolinaemia type I Proline oxidase	Usually none	Plasma proline raised 3–5 × normal. Increased excretion proline, hydroxyproline and glycine	None
Hyperprolinaemia type II Δ-pyrroline-5-carboxylic acid dehydrogenase	Mental retardation and seizures but many asymptomatic	Plasma proline raised 10 × normal. Increased excretion proline, hydroxyproline and glycine	None
Hydroxyprolinaemia Hydroxyproline oxidase	None	Plasma hydroxyproline raised 10–50 ×	None

glycaemia in older patients raise the diagnosis of glycogen storage diseases, but ketonaemia does not occur in glutaric aciduria type II. Electron transferring flavoprotein and electron transferring flavoprotein-ubiquinone oxidoreductase can be assayed in some centres using cultured fibroblasts.

Genetics

Both of the basic defects are autotomal recessive with assays of electron transferring flavoprotein and the electron transferring flavoprotein-ubiquinone oxidoreductase showing variable residual activity. The electron transferring flavoprotein protein has α and β subunits. The relevant genes have been localized to chromosomes 15 and 19 and mutations in both described.

Prenatal diagnosis

This has been carried out using amniotic fluid analysis and cultured amniocytes for electron transferring flavoprotein and oxidoreductase assays.

Treatment

Nothing has influenced severe early cases. Diets low in fats and protein reduce organic acid accumulation in milder cases and carnitine supplements increase the formation of the less toxic carnitine acyl esters. Oral riboflavin 100 to 300 mg/day has apparently been beneficial in some older patients, perhaps by stabilizing electron transferring flavoprotein or the oxidoreductase.

Other defects of amino acid metabolism

Many are not covered in the text. Table 13 gives details of some of them.

REFERENCES

Specialized texts

Fernandes, J., Saudubray, J-M., and Tada, K. (1990). *Inborn metabolic diseases. Diagnosis and treatment.* Springer-Verlag, Berlin.

Scriver C.R., Beaudet A.L., Sly W.S., and Valle, D. (Ed.) (1989). *The metabolic basis of inherited disease*, (6th edn). McGraw-Hill, New York.

Review articles

Adamson, M.D., Andersson, H.C., and Gahl, W.A. (1989). Cystinosis. *Seminars in Nephrology*, **9**, 147–61.

Kvittingen, E.A. (1991). Tyrosinaemia Type I – an update. *Journal of Inherited Metabolic Disease*, **14**, 554–62.

Milliner, D.A. (1990). Cystinuria. *Endocrinology and Metabolism Clinics of North America*, **19**, 889–907.

Saudubray, J-M. et al. (1989). Clinical approach to inherited metabolic disease in the neonatal period: a 20-year survey. *Journal of Inherited Metabolic Disease*, **12**, Supplement 1, 25–42.

Schneider, J.A., Jatz, B., and Nellis, R.B. (1990). Update on nephropathic cystinosis. *Pediatric Nephrology*, **4**, 645–53.

Smith, I. (1993). Phenylketonuria due to phenylalanine hydroxylase deficiency: an unfolding story. Report of the MRC Working Party on P.K.U. *British Medical Journal*, **306**, 115–19.

Smith, I. (1993). Recommendations on the dietary management of phenylketonuria. Report of the MRC Working Party on PKU. *Archives of Diseases in Childhood*, **68**, 426–7.

Stephens, A.D. (1989). Cystinuria and its treatment, 25 years experience at St Bartholomew's Hospital. *Journal of Inherited Metabolic Disease*, **12**, 197–209.

Wolf, B. and Heard, G.S. (1991). Biotinidase deficiency. *Advances in Pediatrics*, **38**, 1–21.

Original articles

Attree, O. et al. (1992). The Lowe's oculocerebrorenal gene encodes a protein highly homologous to inositol polyphosphate-5-phosphatase. *Nature*, **358**, 239–42.

Brenton D.P., Isenberg D.A., Cusworth D.C., Garrod R., Kaywaroych S., and Stamp T.C.B. (1981). The adult presenting idiopathic Fanconi syndrome. *Journal of Inherited Metabolic Diseases*, **4**, 211–15

Brenton D.P. and Itaseler M.E. (1990). Maternal phenylketonuria. In *Inborn metabolic diseases, diagnosis and treatment*. (ed J. Fernandes, J.-M. Sanderbray, and K. Tada) pp. 175–82. Springer-Verlag. Berlin.

Brody, L.C. et al. (1992). Ornithine delta amino transferase mutations in gyrate atrophy, allelic heterogeneity and functional consequences. *Journal of Biological Chemistry*, **267**, 3302–7.

Charnos, L.R., Bernadine, I., Rader, D., Hoeg, J.N., and Gahl, W.A. (1991). Clinical and laboratory findings in the oculo-cerebro-renal syndrome of Lowe with special reference to growth and function. *New England Journal of Medicine*, **324**, 1318–25.

Dent C.E. (1948). A study of the behaviour of some sixty amino acids and other ninhydrin-reacting substances on phenol-collidine filter paper chromatograms with notes as to the occurrence of some of them in biological fluids. *Biochemical Journal*, **43**, 169–80.

Dhondt, J.L. (1991). Strategy for the screening of tetrahydrobiopterin deficiency among hyperphenylalaninaemic patients: 15 years experience. *Journal of Inherited Metabolic Disease*, **14**, 117–27.

Haworth, J.C. et al. (1991). Phenotypic variability in glutaric aciduria type I: Report of 14 cases in five Canadian Indian kindreds. *Journal of Pediatrics*, **118**, 52–8.

Kaplan, P. et al. (1991). Intellectual outcome in children with Maple Syrup urine disease. *Journal of Pediatrics*, **119**, 46–50.

Lenke R.L. and Levy H.L. (1980). Maternal phenylketonuria and hyperphenylalaninemia. *New England Journal of Medicine*, **303**, 1202–8.

Maestri, N.E., Hauser, E.R., Bartholomew, D., and Brusilow, S.W. (1991). Prospective treatment of urea cycle disorders. *Journal of Pediatrics*, **119**, 923–8.

Norden, A.G., Fulcher, L.M., Lapsley, M., and Flynn, F.V. (1991). Excretion of β_2 glycoprotein (apolipoprotein H) in renal tubular disease. *Clinical Chemistry*, **37**,(1), 74–7.

Paradis, K. et al. (1990). Liver transplantation for hereditory Tyrosinaemia: The Quebec experience. *American Journal of Human Genetics*, **47**, 338–42.

Rose, W.C., Wixon R.L., Lockhart H.B. and Lambert F.G. (1955). The amino acid requirements of man. XV The valine requirement. Summary and final observations. *Journal of Biological Chemistry*, **217**, 987.

Tada K. and Kure S. (1993). Non-ketotic hyperglycinaemia: molecular lesions, diagnosis and pathophysiology. *Journal of Inherited Metabolic Disease*, **16**, 691–703.

Tuchman, M., Knopman, D.S., and Shih, V.E. (1990). Episodic hyperammonaemia in adult siblings with hyperornithinaemia, hyperammonaemia and homocitrillinuria syndrome. *Archives of Neurology*, **47**, 1134–7.

Tuchman, M. and Holzknecht, R.A. (1991). Heterogeneity of patients with late onset ornithine transcarbamylase deficiency. *Clinical and Investigative Medicine*, **14**, 320–4.

Widhalm, K. et al. (1992). Long term follow up of 12 patients with the late onset variant of argininosuccinic acid lyase deficiency. *Pediatrics*, **89**, 1182–4.

11.4 Disorders of purine and pyrimidine metabolism

G. NUKI

Ribonucleotides and deoxyribonucleotides are the monomeric building blocks from which nucleic acids (RNA and DNA) are constructed. Each nucleotide consists of a heterocyclic ring derived from a purine or pyrimidine base to which a pentose sugar and phosphate group have been added. Purine and pyrimidine nucleotides, nucleosides, and bases are key substrates, cofactors, and regulatory molecules in almost every branch of human metabolism, and ATP and other purine nucleotides provide the energy needed for many metabolic processes. Purines and pyrimidines are required for transcription, translation, and protein synthesis. Purine compounds play an essential physiological role in membrane signal transduction and as neurotransmitters, vasodilators, and mediators of platelet aggregation and hormone action. Not surprisingly, disorders of purine and pyrimidine metabolism are associated with a wide range of human disease.

Gout (see also Chapter 18.7)

Gout is the term used to describe a group of metabolic disorders in which clinical problems result from tissue deposition of crystals of monosodium urate monohydrate from hyperuricaemic body fluids. Major clinical manifestations include:

(1) acute inflammatory arthritis, tenosynovitis, bursitis, or cellulitis;

(2) chronic, erosive, deforming arthritis associated with periarticular and subcutaneous urate deposits (tophi);

(3) nephrolithiasis and urolithiasis;

(4) chronic renal disease and hypertension.

Hyperuricaemia alone is not sufficient for the development of clinical disease. Tissue deposition of crystals of monosodium urate and resulting clinical symptoms and signs of gout usually only follow prolonged elevation of serum urate. Hyperuricaemia can result from increased purine intake, turnover, or production; from decreased urate elimination by the kidneys, or from a combination of these.

EPIDEMIOLOGY

Gouty arthritis occurs predominantly in postpubertal males and is seldom seen in women before the menopause. The self-reported prevalence of gout, which is approximately double that found in studies that include a medical examination, increases with age from 2.4/1000 in men aged 18 to 44 to 34.4/1000 in men aged 45 to 64. The 2-year incidence of gout was found to be 3.2/1000 for men and 0.5/1000 for women in the Framingham study. There is evidence that the prevalence of gout has increased more than threefold in the past 10 years in the United States, where it is now the most common cause of inflammatory arthritis in men over the age of 40. In addition to male gender, risk factors include obesity, alcohol consumption, occupational and environmental lead exposure, hypertension, renal insufficiency, the use of diuretic drugs, and a family history of gout. All these risk factors are mediated through increases in serum and tissue urate levels. The incidence of gout by serum urate levels in men is shown in Table 1. Current epidemiological studies define gout using preliminary criteria of the American College of Rheumatology (Table 2). The presence of six of the 11 criteria has a specificity of 93 per cent in differentiating gout from pseudogout, with an overall sensitivity of 85 per cent.

Table 1 *Incidence of gout by uric acid level in men*

Serum uric acid (mg/dl)	5-year cumulative incidence (%)	Incidence (per 1000 person years)
<6	0.5	0.8
6–6.9	0.6	0.9
7–7.9	2.0	4.1
9–9.9	9.8	43.2
>10	30.5	70.2

(Campion *et al.* 1987)

Table 2 *American College of Rheumatology survey criteria for acute gouty arthritis*

More than one attack of acute arthritis
Maximum inflammation develops within 1 day
Oligoarthritis attack
Redness observed over joints
First metatarsophalangeal joint painful or swollen (podagra)
Unilateral first metatarsophalangeal joint attack
Unilateral tarsal joint attack
Tophus (proven or suspected)
Hyperuricaemia
Asymmetrical swelling within a joint on radiography
Complete termination of an attack

(Wallace *et al.* 1977)

SERUM URATE LEVELS

Serum urate concentrations are distributed in the community as a continuous variable (Fig. 1). Mean values are higher in men than in women and the sex-specific distribution curve is broader for males than females, with skewing to the higher end of the scale in both sexes. Serum levels rise in boys at puberty and then remain virtually unchanged throughout adult life. In girls the pubertal rise is smaller and the serum level only approaches that of males after the menopause (Fig. 2).

Epidemiological studies demonstrate significant variations of serum urate levels in different ethnic groups. The Maoris of New Zealand and the Polynesians of the Western Pacific, for example, have high levels. Although some polygenic control of serum urate levels is well established, environmental factors are also important. Members of the Chinese community in Taiwan have lower serum urate levels than those in Malaysia or British Columbia; Filipinos resident in the United States have higher serum urate levels than those in the Philippine Islands; and urban South African Negroes have significantly higher levels than those in rural communities. These differences within ethnic groups result from a less than average capacity to increase the renal excretion of urate when the purine load is increased. The association of high serum urate levels with high purine and protein intake, alcohol consumption, weight, body bulk, and social class suggest that in most communities environmental factors are the major determinants of the serum urate—the associates of hyperuricaemia are the associates of plenty.

HYPERURICAEMIA

Serum is saturated with monosodium urate at a concentration of 7 mg/100 ml (0.42 mmol/l) but much higher concentrations of urate may remain in stable supersaturated solution for long periods. A majority of subjects with hyperuricaemia are asymptomatic. Hyperuricaemia is arbitrarily defined as a serum urate level greater than 2 standard deviations from the mean—7 mg/100 ml (0.42 mmol/l) for adult males and 6 mg/100 ml (0.36 mmol/l) for females in communities in the United Kingdom and United States.

URIC ACID METABOLISM

Uric acid is the end product of purine metabolism in humans and some higher apes. These species lack the enzyme uricase which degrades uric acid to allantoin in the majority of mammals.

Plasma and tissue urates are derived from the catabolism of purine nucleotides synthesized *de novo* and from dietary purines. The miscible pool of urate in normal individuals ranges from 0.9 to 1.6 g, of which about 60 per cent is replenished daily from the catabolism of newly synthesized purines. Two-thirds of the urate formed each day is eliminated by the kidney and one-third via the gastrointestinal tract (Fig. 3).

PURINE NUCLEOTIDE SYNTHESIS

Purine synthesis in mammalian cells is regulated by a balanced interaction of a number of biochemical pathways (Fig. 4). The *de novo* path-

Fig. 1 Distribution of serum urate values in male and female populations of Tecumseh, Michigan, 1959–60. (Reproduced from Mikkleson *et al.* (1965) with permission.)

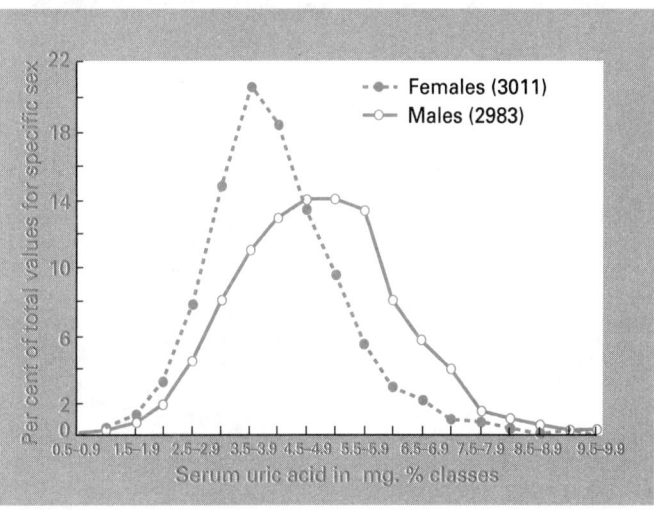

Fig. 2 Sex- and age-specific mean serum urate values in the population of Tecumseh, Michigan, 1959–60. (Reproduced from Mikkleson *et al.* (1965) with permission.)

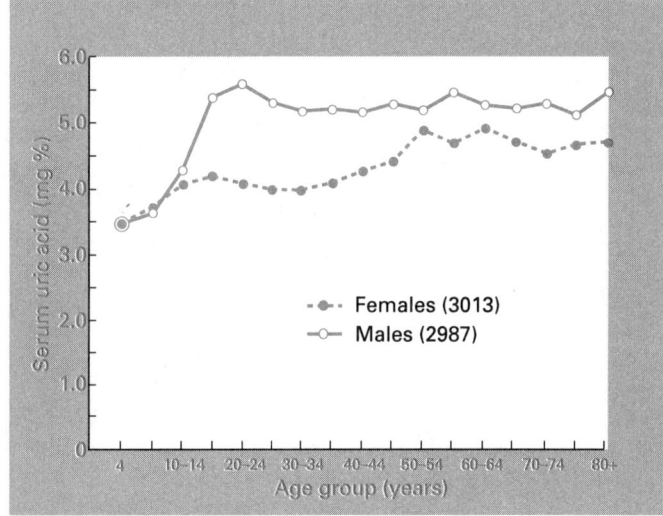

Fig. 3 The uric acid pool; origins and disposal in normal man.

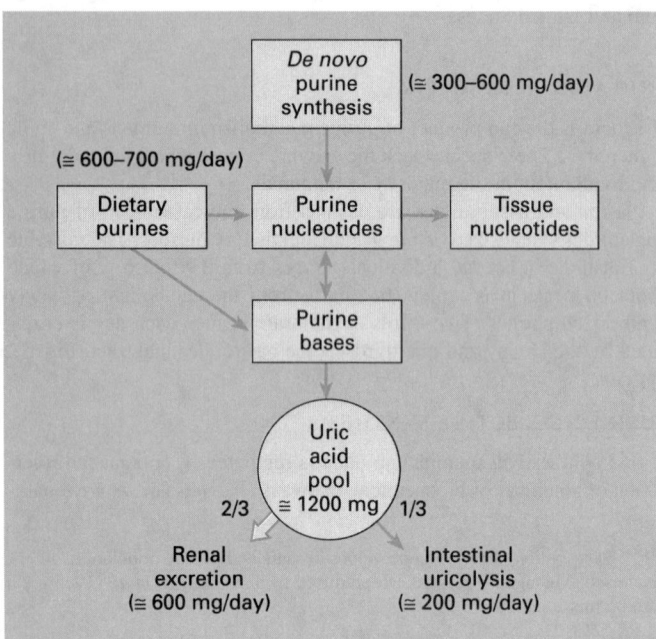

way of purine biosynthesis consists of a series of 10 enzymatic reactions in which glutamine, glycine, carbon dioxide, aspartate, and one-carbon formyl derivatives of folate are added to the ribose moiety of phosphoribosyl pyrophosphate (PP-ribose-P) to form inosinic acid (IMP). Adenosine monophosphate (AMP) and guanosine monophosphate (GMP) are each formed from inosinic acid by two enzymatic steps before phosphorylation to their respective di- and triphosphates. Alternatively, the nucleotide monophosphates can also be synthesized by phosphorylation of purine bases by phosphoribosyl transferase enzymes reacting with PP-ribose-P, and AMP can be formed by phosphorylation of adenosine by adenosine kinase. *In vitro* studies of PP-ribose-P amidotransferase, the first enzyme in the *de novo* pathway of purine synthesis, show it to have allosteric properties that one might associate with a rate-limiting enzyme, and have provided a molecular model for the mechanism whereby the rate of purine synthesis is regulated. The enzyme exists in two forms; a catalytically inactive dimer and an active monomer. PP-ribose-P converts the larger form of the enzyme to the active monomer while purine nucleotide monophosphates have the opposite effect. A good deal of evidence suggests that PP-ribose-P, which is present in cells at limiting concentrations, is the major regulator of the rate of *de novo* purine synthesis in clinical situations associated with increased or decreased purine production.

The purine nucleotide monophosphates are degraded to nucleosides by 5′-nucleotidase. Adenosine is deaminated by the enzyme adenosine deaminase and inosine and guanosine are dephosphorylated to purine bases by nucleoside phosphorylase. Guanine and hypoxanthine are converted to xanthine by guanase and xanthine oxidase and the latter enzyme is also responsible for the final oxidation of xanthine to uric acid.

Fig. 4 Pathways of purine metabolism in humans. ADA, adenosine deaminase; APRT, adenine phosphoribosyl transferase; HGPRT, hypoxanthine-guanine phosphoribosyl transferase; NP, nucleoside phosphorylase; 5′-NP, 5′ nucleotidase; PAT, phosphoribosyl pyrophosphate amidotransferase; PPRPS, phosphoribosyl pyrophosphate synthetase; XO, xanthine oxidase. (Reproduced from Nuki, (1979) with permission.)

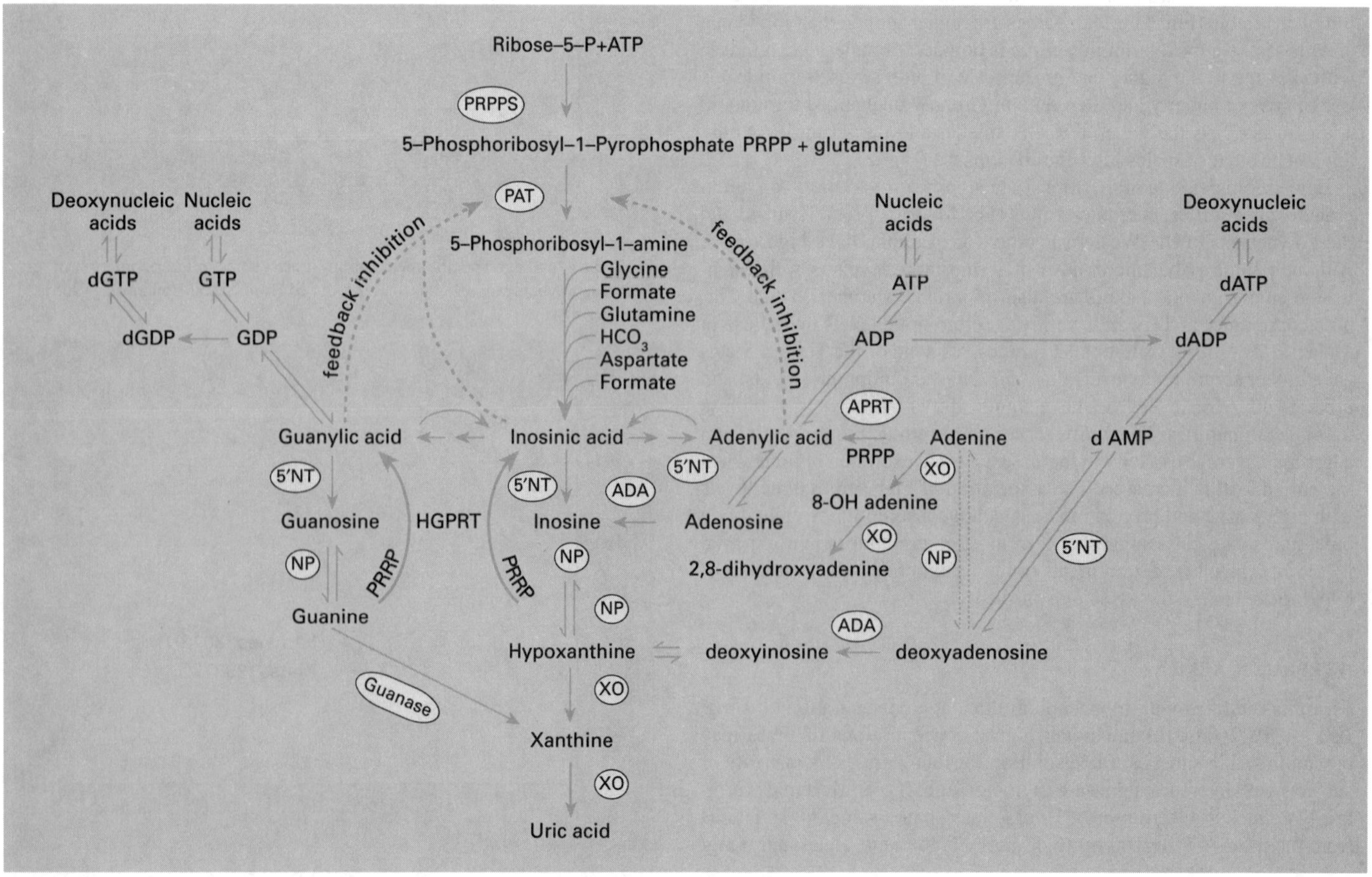

Ribose–5–P+ATP

(PRPPS)

5–Phosphoribosyl–1–Pyrophosphate PRPP + glutamine

(PAT)

Deoxynucleic acids	Nucleic acids		Nucleic acids	Deoxynucleic acids
dGTP	GTP	5–Phosphoribosyl–1–amine	ATP	dATP
dGDP ←	GDP	Glycine / Formate / Glutamine / HCO₃ / Aspartate / Formate	ADP →	dADP

feedback inhibition ⟶ ⟵ feedback inhibition

Guanylic acid ← ← Inosinic acid → → Adenylic acid   Adenine   d AMP

(5′NT)   (5′NT) (ADA)   (5′NT)   PRPP   (XO)

Guanosine   HGPRT   Inosine ←   Adenosine   8-OH adenine

(NP)   PRRP   PRRP   (NP)   2,8-dihydroxyadenine   (XO)   (NP)   (5′NT)

Guanine

Hypoxanthine ⇌ deoxyinosine ← deoxyadenosine

(NP)   (ADA)

(Guanase)   (XO)

Xanthine

(XO)

Uric acid

URIC ACID EXCRETION

Uric acid excreted in the urine is derived from both endogenous purine production and dietary purines (Fig. 3). On an unrestricted diet, uric acid excretion in the urine can exceed 1000 mg/day, each gram of dietary nucleic acid contributing 115 to 150 mg of urinary uric acid. Although 100 to 200 mg of uric acid are secreted daily into the gastrointestinal tract, where it is degraded by bacterial uricolysis, an approximate estimate of uric acid synthesis can be made by measuring uric acid excreted in the urine on an isocaloric purine-free diet. Twenty-four hour urine excretion of more than 600 mg (3.6 mmol) of uric acid on a 2600 calcium, 70 g protein, purine-free diet or 10 mg/kg body weight/day on a low-purine diet strongly suggests an increase in *de novo* purine synthesis or increased turnover of cellular purine nucleotides. Accurate assessment of the rate of *de novo* purine synthesis requires measurement of ^{14}C-isotopically labelled glycine into urine uric acid with simultaneous administration of ^{15}N-labelled uric acid to correct for extrarenal disposal of urate.

Renal handling of uric acid has four components; glomerular filtration, proximal tubular reabsorption, tubular secretion, and post-secretory reabsorption (Fig. 5). Glomerular ultrafiltration is complete as there is no significant protein binding of urate *in vivo*. Proximal tubular reabsorption occurs by an active transport mechanism closely linked to, or identical with, the tubular reabsorption of sodium. Evidence for active secretion comes from inherited and pharmacologically induced tubular defects in which urate clearance can exceed inulin clearance. The paradoxical effect of high- and low-dose aspirin on uric acid excretion can be explained by differential effects on active secretion and reabsorption. Low-dose aspirin blocks urate secretion with consequent hyperuricaemia while high-dose therapy also blocks reabsorption and results in a net increase in uric acid excretion. Postsecretory reabsorption of urate is suggested by the fact that pre-treatment with probenecid, which inhibits tubular reabsorption of urate, prevents the decrease in uric acid excretion that normally follows administration of low-dosage aspirin or pyrazinamide.

Renal clearance of urate in normal subjects ranges from 6 to 9 ml/min, which is less than one-tenth of inulin or creatinine clearance.

PATHOGENESIS OF HYPERURICAEMIA

The concentration of urate in body fluids depends on a balance between purine synthesis plus ingestion and uric acid elimination (Fig. 3). Hyperuricaemia may be the result of increased urate production, decreased renal excretion, or a combination of both mechanisms. Decrease in

Fig. 5 Four-component model for the renal handling of urate in the human kidney. Numerical values indicate hypothetical orders of magnitude of the transport processes. (After Rieselbach and Steele (1974).)

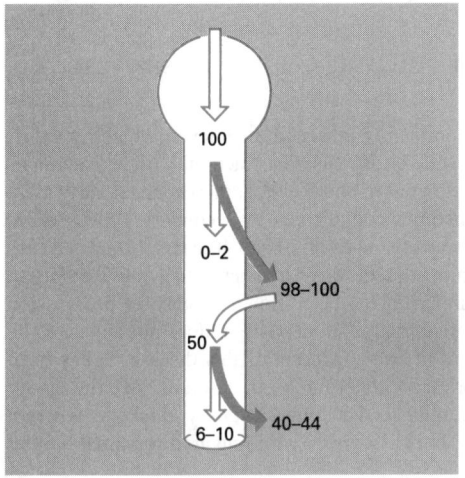

extrarenal elimination of uric acid in the gut has not been shown to be a cause of hyperuricaemia. Dietary ingestion of purine can be an important contributing factor, and there is evidence to suggest that gout and hyperuricaemia are much more frequent in affluent than in malnourished populations. To a large extent, however, the normal kidney is able to increase uric acid excretion in response to a dietary purine load.

In 75 to 90 per cent of patients with gout, hyperuricaemia is associated with impairment of fractional excretion of uric acid. Uric acid clearance is significantly reduced (mean 3.6 ml/min) while creatinine clearance is normal. Theoretically this decrease in uric acid clearance could result from a decreased filtered load, increased urate reabsorption, or decreased urate secretion. As urate does not bind plasma proteins significantly, one or both of the latter mechanisms must be operative.

Secondary hyperuricaemia and gout may, however, be a consequence of a variety of factors that influence renal blood flow, tubular reabsorption, and secretion of uric acid (Table 3).

Increased uric acid production and excretion are found in 10 to 15 per cent of patients with gout. In the majority of these patients the basis for increased synthesis of purines is unknown, but in a few there is evidence of a specific, inherited purine enzyme defect. In approximately 10 per cent of patients with gout seen in a hospital setting, hyperuricaemia results from increased turnover of preformed purines, and in a few, accelerated *de novo* purine synthesis may be a secondary subordinate manifestation of an inherited enzyme defect (Table 3).

PATHOGENESIS OF CRYSTAL INFLAMMATION

This complex subject, the clinical features of gout, and its management are described in Chapter 18.7.

UROLITHIASIS (SEE ALSO CHAPTER 20.12)

In the United Kingdom uric acid stones account for 5 per cent of all renal calculi and 10 per cent of patients with gout have a history of renal colic. In Israel, uric acid calculi are responsible for 40 per cent of cases of nephrolithiasis and 75 per cent of patients with primary gout develop renal calculus disease. Urine uric acid concentration is the most important aetiological factor and in temperate climates this is mainly determined by urate production and purine ingestion. The prevalence of renal stones in patients with primary gout is 20 per cent in patients excreting up to 200 mg of uric acid/24 h and 50 per cent in those excreting more than 1100 mg/day. In addition to dehydration, primary purine overproduction, increased turnover of purines, and excessive purine ingestion, uric acid calculi may be associated with defects in tubular reabsorption of uric acid, uricosuric drug therapy, chronic diarrhoeal diseases, and ileostomy, the last as a result of lowered urine pH. Although the incidence of urolithiasis is increased threefold in persons with asymptomatic hyperuricaemia, only 20 per cent of uric acid stone formers are hyperuricaemic.

Calcium oxalate stone formation is also increased thirtyfold in patients with gout and hyperuricosuria is common in non-gouty calcium stone formers. Uric acid crystals themselves may act as epitaxial nucleation sites for calcium oxalate stone formation. It is also possible that colloidal uric acid adsorbs urinary glycosaminoglycans which normally act as endogenous inhibitors of stone formation.

ACUTE URIC ACID NEPHROPATHY

Acute renal failure may result from sudden precipitation of un-ionized crystals of uric acid in the renal collecting ducts and ureters. This form of acute obstructive uropathy occurs most often when ill, dehydrated, acidotic patients with leukaemia or lymphoma are treated with cytotoxic drugs. It has also been recorded following epilepsy, severe muscular exercise, and in patients with gout and grossly increased synthesis of purines *de novo*. The diagnosis is suggested by finding crystals of uric acid and a uric acid:creatinine ratio greater than 1.0 in the residual

Table 3 *Causes of hyperuricaemia and gout*

Decreased uric acid excretion		Increased uric acid production	
Primary	Secondary	Primary	Secondary

Decrease in fractional urate excretion
Idiopathic
Familial juvenile gouty nephropathy
	Reduction in functional renal mass
	  Chronic renal disease
	
	Reduction in glomerular filtration
	  Volume depletion
	  Nephrogenic diabetes insipidus
	
	Reduction in fractional urate clearance
	  Hypertension
	  Hyperparathyroidism
	  Sickle-cell anaemia
	  Myxoedema
	  Bartter's syndrome
	  Congenital chloride losing enteropathy
	  Down's syndrome
	  Chronic beryllium poisoning
	  Lead nephropathy
	  Cystinuria
	  Sarcoidosis
	  Increased levels of organic acids (e.g. exercise, starvation, alcohol, ketoacidosis)
	  Drug administration (e.g. diuretics, low-dose salicylates, pyrazinamide ethambutol, angiotension)
		Increased purine synthesis *de novo*
		Idiopathic
		Specific enzyme defects:
		  1 HGPRT deficiency (partial);
		  2 PRPP synthetase overactivity;
		  3 ribose-5-phosphate overproduction;
		  4 AMP-deaminase deficiency
			Increased purine synthesis *de novo*
			Specific enzyme defects:
			  1 HGPRT deficiency (complete) Lesch–Nyhan syndrome;
			  2 glucose-6-phosphatase deficiency (GSD type I);
			  3 myogenic (GSD types III, V, and VII);
			  4 hereditary fructose intolerance (aldolase B deficiency)
			
			Increased turnover of preformed purines
			  Myeloproliferative disorders, e.g. polycythaemia rubra vera, granulocytic leukaemia
			  Lymphoproliferative disorders, e.g. lymphomas, myeloma, lymphocytic leukaemia
			  Waldenström's macroglobulinaemia
			  Infectious mononucleosis
			  Carcinomatosis
			  Chronic haemolytic anaemia
			  Secondary polycythaemia
			  Gaucher's disease
			  Severe exfoliative psoriasis

GSD, glycogen storage disease; HGPRT, hypoxanthine-guanine phosphoribosyl transferase; PPRP, phosphoribosyl pyrophosphate.

urine of an oliguric patient with renal failure. The problem is entirely preventable by ensuring high fluid intake and the administration of bicarbonate to render the urine alkaline, and/or the prophylactic administration of allopurinol to prevent the sudden rise in uric acid which follows cellular destruction during chemotherapy.

CHRONIC RENAL DISEASE (SEE ALSO SECTION 20)

In the past decade the pathogenesis and very existence of chronic urate nephropathy as an important clinical entity have been critically re-examined. Earlier studies suggested that clinically significant, progressive, chronic renal disease was an important complication of untreated tophaceous gout, and that renal failure accounted for 20 to 25 per cent of deaths in these patients. The pathogenesis of this chronic urate nephropathy was complex and poorly defined. It appeared that the initial lesion may have been crystal-induced damage to the tubular epithelium of the loop of Henle and adjacent interstitial tissue, and this was later complicated by tubular obstruction, tophus formation, hypertensive damage, glomerulosclerosis, and secondary pyelonephritis. It is now apparent that this form of progressive renal failure is largely limited to patients with inherited abnormalities of purine metabolism leading to primary purine overproduction, rare forms of inherited renal disease, chronic lead intoxication, and some other types of pre-existing nephropathy.

Mild intermittent proteinuria is found in 20 to 30 per cent of patients

with gout, but the minor progression of renal insufficiency that occurs in the majority of subjects with gout is largely age-related and overall life expectancy is not reduced. Significant renal disease is a very rare complication of hyperuricaemia in the absence of recurrent gouty arthritis. When faced with a patient with renal insufficiency and hyperuricaemia it can, however, be extremely difficult to ascertain whether the raised serum urate is a cause or a consequence of renal failure.

FAMILIAL JUVENILE GOUTY NEPHROPATHY (SEE ALSO SECTION 20)

This is an autosomal dominantly inherited disorder in which hyperuricaemia is associated with a decrease in fractional urate clearance. Patients may present with gout in childhood, adolescence, or early adult life. Renal failure, sometimes complicated by secondary hypertension, usually supervenes between the ages of 20 and 40 years. Renal biopsies are characterized by a non-specific interstitial nephritis without evidence of urate deposition. Allopurinol has been shown to delay the progression of renal damage, although renal urate deposition does not appear to be an important element in the pathogenesis of this disease. It has been postulated that the primary abnormality in familial juvenile gouty nephropathy may be similar to that found in gouty chickens, where a defective urate transporter is associated with impaired proximal tubular urate secretion.

POLYCYSTIC RENAL DISEASE

Hyperuricaemia and gouty arthritis may preceed the development of renal failure in patients with polycystic kidney disease, and about one-third of patients with polycystic renal disease develop gouty arthritis. The basis for this association may be abnormal tubular reabsorption of urate, and similar mechanisms may account for the increase in gout and hyperuricaemia seen in patients with medullary sponge kidney and cystinuria.

LEAD NEPHROPATHY

The association between gout and chronic lead poisoning (saturnine gout) was a major problem in previous centuries as a result of contamination of wine and other beverages by lead-containing glass bottles or lead glazed pottery and stoneware. An outbreak of 'saturnine gout' occurred again in Queensland, Australia in the 1960s as a result of ingestion of lead-containing paint by children, and it continues to be an important cause of gout in the south-eastern United States, where illicit moonshine alcohol contaminated from the soldered truck radiators used as stills, is the source of the lead. The possibility of chronic lead intoxication should be considered in all patients presenting with gout and chronic renal failure.

OTHER CLINICAL ASSOCIATIONS

Gout and hyperuricaemia are often associated with obesity, heavy alcohol intake, hyperlipoproteinaemia, impaired glucose tolerance, and ischaemic heart disease in men but not in women.

Obesity may be the major linking factor. Men with gout are on average 15 to 20 per cent overweight, and the prevalence of hyperuricaemia in the community rises from 3 per cent in those whose weight is on the 20th percentile to 11 per cent in those above the 80th percentile.

Hypertriglyceridaemia occurs in more than 75 per cent of patients with gout, and hyperuricaemia in a similar proportion of individuals with hypertriglyceridaemia. The pattern is most commonly one of type IV hyperlipoproteinaemia with elevated pre-β, very low density lipoproteins, and normal levels of serum cholesterol, but types IIa and IIb are also observed and apolipoprotein B levels are frequently elevated. Non-gouty family members are not affected and heavy alcohol intake and obesity are both predisposing factors.

Hypertension occurs in 25 to 50 per cent of patients with gout, while hyperuricaemia is a feature in one-third of untreated hypertensive patients and two-thirds of those receiving anti-hypertensive drug therapy. Impaired glucose tolerance and ischaemic heart disease are associated with gout and obesity rather than with asymptomatic hyperuricaemia and there is no good evidence to suggest that hyperuricaemia alone is a risk factor for diabetes mellitus or myocardial infarction.

In women the clinical stereotype is often one of a lean and abstemious postmenopausal woman with mild renal insufficiency, who has received diuretic drugs for many years. Polyarticular involvement is more common and hypertriglyceridaemia is not a feature.

ASYMPTOMATIC HYPERURICAEMIA

Although hyperuricaemia may be associated with hypertension, atherosclerosis, ischaemic heart disease, and renal insufficiency, there is no evidence to suggest that the raised serum urate itself is a direct cause of any of these. Since the majority of hyperuricaemic individuals never develop gout or renal complications there is no indication to treat asymptomatic hyperuricaemia unless the serum urate is very high (>0.8 mmol/l) and the urine uric acid excretion very great (>7.2 mmol/24 h). In the majority of persons with asymptomatic hyperuricaemia, it is reasonable to exclude a history, family history, and clinical evidence of gout, search for a secondary cause of the hyperuricaemia, and monitor the blood pressure and renal function annually.

Inborn errors of purine metabolism

Hypoxanthine-guanine phosphoribosyl transferase

This enzyme catalyses the reactions:

$$\text{Hypoxanthine} + \text{PP-ribose-P} \xrightarrow{\text{Mg}^{2+}} \text{Inosine-5'-phosphate} + \text{PPi}$$

$$\text{Guanine} + \text{PP-ribose-P} \xrightarrow{\text{Mg}^{2+}} \text{Inosine-5'-phosphate} + \text{PPi}$$

Lesch–Nyhan syndrome

Severe cellular deficiency of the purine salvage enzyme hypoxanthine-guanine phosphoribosyl transferase (HPRT) is associated with primary purine overproduction, hyperuricaemia, and gout, together with a neurological syndrome comprising choreoathetosis, spasticity, a variable degree of mental deficiency, and a striking behavioural disturbance characterized by self-mutilation (Fig. 6).

Clinical expression of disease is virtually limited to males. Babies appear normal at birth but mothers may observe the presence of orange crystals in the diapers. Occasional vomiting and hypotonia is followed by a delay in motor development at the age of 3 to 4 months. The characteristic pyramidal and extrapyramidal signs which eventually progress to severe spasticity and choreoathetosis are seldom apparent before 1 year and the compulsive behavioral disturbance can commence at any time between the ages of 2 and 16 years. Episodes of involuntary and occasionally unilateral self-mutilation come and go without any clear relationship to endogenous or environmental factors. These episodes are often associated with agitation and anxiety which can be partially relieved by physical restraint to prevent finger biting. In some cases self-mutilation of the lips can only be prevented by extraction of

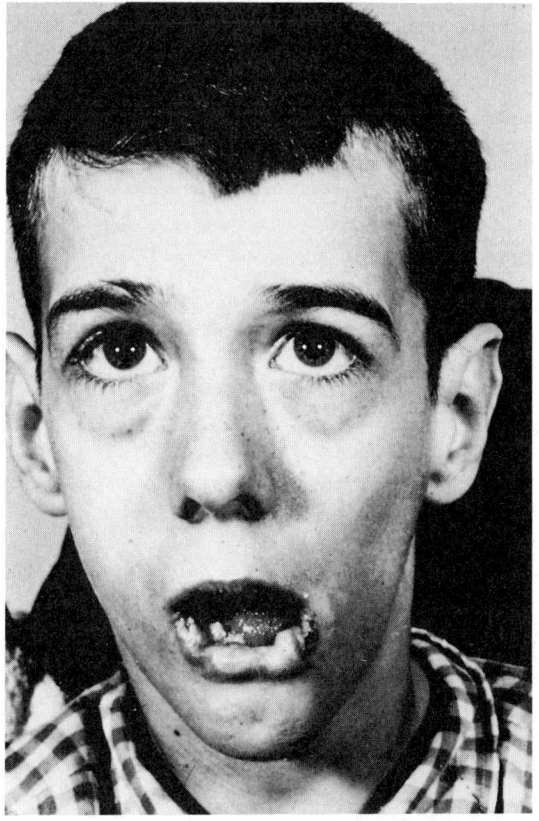

Fig. 6 Boy with Lesch-Nyhan syndrome showing evidence of self-mutilation of lips (By courtesy of Dr J.E. Seegmiller).

teeth. Aggression towards others may take the form of hitting, spitting, biting, and abusive language, typically accompanied by a smile and an apology. The majority of boys affected are mentally retarded with an IQ in the range 40 to 65, but the severity of the behavioural disturbance is unrelated to the degree of mental deficiency.

Haematuria and renal colic may occur during the first decade of life but gouty arthritis and tophi seldom develop before puberty. A macro-cytic or frankly megaloblastic anaemia is an occasional feature. Death from infection or renal failure commonly occurs between the ages of 20 and 30 years.

BIOCHEMICAL FINDINGS

Grossly accelerated production of uric acid results in greatly increased urine uric acid excretion (0.15–0.75 mmol/kg/24 h) and a characteris-tically high urine uric acid:creatinine ratio (Fig. 7). The serum urate is usually, but not invariably, raised, in the range 0.42 to 0.9 mmol/l.

Lesch–Nyhan syndrome is characterized by raised concentrations of phosphoribosyl pyrophosphate (PP-ribose-P) and severe deficiency of HPRT in red cell lysates. Complete or nearly complete deficiency of the enzyme is also found in leucocytes, cultured fibroblasts, amniotic fluid cells, and other tissues such as liver and brain. Associated biochemical abnormalities include increased activity of adenine phosphoribosyl transferase, inosine monophosphate dehydrogenase, and the pyrimidine enzymes orotate phosphoribosyl transferase and orotidine 5′-phosphate decarboxylase. Concentrations of the pyrimidine nucleotides UDP, UTP, and CTP are increased in HPRT-deficient lymphoblasts and fibro-blasts, but steady-state purine nucleotide concentrations are not reduced as might be expected. It seems probable that accelerated *de novo* purine biosynthesis *in vivo* is primarily due to the effect of increased avail-ability of PP-ribose-P on the rate-limiting amido transferase enzyme rather than decreased feedback inhibition by purine nucleotides.

The biochemical basis for the neurological dysfunction in Lesch–Nyhan syndrome remains uncertain. Morphological abnormalities have not been detected in postmortem studies of the brain. As neuronal cells are able to synthesize purine nucleotides *de novo* it seems reasonable to assume that accumulation of purine metabolites, rather than deficiency of purine nucleotides, interferes in some way with neurotransmitter function in the brain-stem. The demonstration of decreases in dopamine,

homovanillic acid, dopa decarboxylase, and tyrosine hydroxylase activ-ity in the dopamine-terminal-rich regions of the putamen and the caudate nucleus suggest that there may be secondary abnormalities of terminal arborization of dopaminergic neurones.

HPRT-deficient mice (the first mouse model engineered by use of enzyme-deficient embryonic stem cells) do not exhibit abnormal neu-rological behavior, but this can be induced following administration of amphetamine or the administration of the adenine phosphoribosyl trans-ferase inhibitor, 9-ethyl adenine, suggesting that adenine phosphoribosyl transferase is important for purine salvage in mouse brain in a way that it is not in the human brain. However mice with both HPRT and APRT deficiency do not self-mutilate.

The biochemical basis for the megaloblastic anaemia also remains unclear. In isolated cases the anaemia has been shown to respond to adenine rather than to folic acid.

GENETICS—PRENATAL DETECTION AND PREVENTION

Lesch–Nyhan syndrome is an X-linked disorder which is only fully expressed in males. Asymptomatic carrier females can be detected by hair root analysis or by finding HPRT-positive and HPRT-negative pop-ulations of cells in fibroblast cultures from skin biopsies using an auto-radiographic technique, incidentally providing confirmation of the Lyon hypothesis of random inactivation of the X chromosome. Using these techniques, only four out of 47 mothers were homozygous normal, sug-gesting a lower than expected ratio of new to established mutations. Culture of amniotic fluid cells following amniocentesis allows the detec-tion of affected males *in utero* and preventive therapeutic abortion.

Biochemical studies of normal human HPRT have revealed a variety of electrophoretic HPRT variants. Although much of the electrophoretic heterogeneity appears to be the result of post-translational modification, there is evidence of true genetic heterogeneity in cells from patients with the disease. In the majority of cases of Lesch–Nyhan syndrome, complete absence of catalytic enzyme activity is associated with absence of protein cross-reacting with antibody to normal enzyme (CRM-neg-ative mutants) but CRM-positive mutants with absent catalytic activity have also been detected, providing good evidence of structural gene mutations. Amino acid sequencing shows that there is a whole spectrum of mutations at the HPRT locus, resulting in cells with varying amounts of residual enzyme activity and HPRT with altered substrate affinities. Indeed, the level of HPRT activity in red cells from some patients with Lesch–Nyhan syndrome overlaps the range of activities seen in some families with gout and overproduction of purines alone. Heterozygote carriers can have subtle subclinical alterations in purine metabolism with modest increases in the rates of *de novo* purine biosynthesis, increases in uric acid excretion, and occasionally asymptomatic hyperuricaemia.

Following the cloning of human HPRT cDNA, more than 50 HPRT mutants have been characterized at the DNA and mRNA level. Four independent mutational events representing three unique base substitu-tions have been described within the codon for Arg 51 and a single base substitution has been found within the codon for Ala 50. Approximately 40 per cent of HPRT point mutations are estimated to occur in exon-3 within two regions. This work has contributed to the development of earlier and more reliable methods for antenatal diagnosis using DNA analysis, and a better understanding of the molecular defects underlying this disorder.

TREATMENT

Treatment with allopurinol is mandatory in all affected subjects. Serum and urine uric acid levels are effectively lowered by inhibition of xan-thine oxidase, but total purine excretion is not reduced when allopurinol is given to patients with Lesch–Nyhan syndrome as it is in other patients with gout and purine overproduction. Nevertheless gouty arthritis, urate stone formation, and urate nephropathy can be effectively prevented and the possibility of xanthine stone formation is minimized by ensuring adequate hydration and urine flow. Hypouricaemic drug therapy does

Fig. 7 Ratio of uric acid to creatinine concentrations (expressed as milligrams/ 100 ml) in urine samples from patients with Lesch-Nyhan syndrome and gout with partial HPRT deficiency. (Reproduced from Kaufman *et al.* (1968) with permission.)

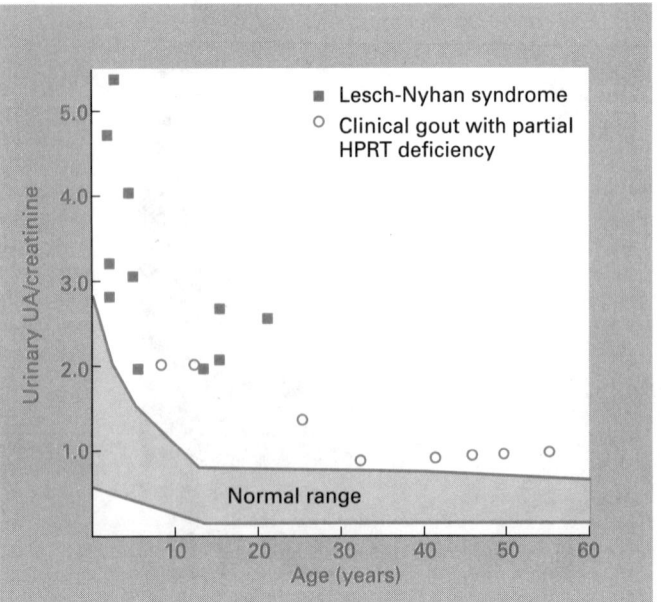

not, however, influence the neurological manifestations or the behavioural disturbance. Diazepam, haloperidol, and other sedatives can be helpful in managing the extrapyramidal movements, but tooth extraction and physical restraint with splints and bandages are often required to control the compulsive self-mutilation.

Partial HPRT deficiency

Severe familial X-linked gout with minor or absent neurological features may be associated with partial deficiency of HPRT.

These patients usually present with uric acid calculi or gouty arthritis in adolescence or adult life. In about 25 per cent there is a mild neurological disturbance. In some families this resembles a *forme fruste* of Lesch–Nyhan syndrome with disorders of movement and compulsive behaviour. In others there has been a history of convulsions, mental retardation, and a spinocerebellar syndrome. As in the Lesch–Nyhan syndrome, macrocytosis and megaloblastic marrow changes may be observed.

BIOCHEMICAL FINDINGS AND GENETICS

Serum uric acid levels are high and there is evidence of primary purine overproduction with urine uric acid excretion usually in excess of 5 mmol/24 h and a uric acid:creatinine ratio greater than 0.75 unless renal insufficiency has already supervened. HPRT activity in erythrocyte lysates is usually in the range 0.01 to 30 per cent of normal, with similar levels of residual enzyme activity in individuals from the same family. Identical phenotypes have, however, been reported where red blood cell HPRT was undetectable or apparently normal. In the latter instances structural gene mutations led to subtle abnormalities of HPRT protein with an altered K_M for PP-ribose-P in one case and abnormal sensitivity to feedback inhibition by purine nucleotides in the other. These cases illustrate how the clinical features of disease associated with HPRT deficiency cannot be reliably predicted from simple assays of erythrocyte HPRT alone. Phenotypic expression is, however, always similar within each family; typical Lesch–Nyhan syndrome and X-linked gout without neurological features never occur in related patients.

As in Lesch–Nyhan syndrome, intracellular concentrations of PP-ribose-P and pyrimidine nucleotides are increased and there is increased activity of adenine phosphoribosyl transferase, inosine monophosphate dehydrogenase, orotate phosphoribosyl transferase, and orotidine 5'-phosphate decarboxylase in erythrocyte lysates.

Also as in Lesch–Nyhan syndrome, there is genetic heterogeneity. Most of the mutations are associated with normal mRNA and immunologically detectable catalytically defective HPRT. Point mutations in genomic DNA have been identified by allele-specific polymerase chain reaction.

Carrier detection of heterozygotes is as for Lesch–Nyhan syndrome but amniocentesis, prenatal detection, and preventive abortion are not justified. Treatment is with allopurinol.

Adenine phosphoribosyl transferase (APRT)

$$\text{Adenine} + \text{PP-ribose-P} \xrightarrow{\text{Mg}^{2+}} \text{Adenosine 5'-phosphate} + \text{PPi}$$

Severe homozygous deficiency of APRT is associated with the formation of renal calculi of 2,8-dihydroxyadenine. While most cases present in early childhood with or without acute renal failure, some remain free from symptoms of renal lithiasis until middle age. This rare autosomal recessive disorder is not associated with primary purine overproduction, hyperuricaemia, or gout, although the renal calculi are invariably mistaken for uric acid stones if only standard laboratory methods of stone analysis are used. Their true identity can be established by X-ray diffraction and infrared and ultraviolet spectroscopy. Homozygous APRT deficiency is characterized by increased urinary excretion of polyamine-derived adenine and its metabolites 8-hydroxyadenine and 2,8-dihy-

droxyadenine, formed by the action of xanthine oxidase. Renal stone formation in this condition can be successfully prevented by administration of the xanthine oxidase inhibitor allopurinol, but care must be taken to reduce the dose in patients with renal failure.

Heterozygous APRT deficiency is a rather common trait. As many as 1 per cent of the normal population may be heterozygotes with partial APRT deficiency, and 8 to 45 per cent of normal enzyme activity in erythrocyte lysates. Partial APRT deficiency does not usually appear to be associated with clinical metabolic disease, but 2,8-dihydroxyadenine urine lithiasis has recently been described in Japanese patients with partial deficiency of APRT.

Phosphoribosyl pyrophosphate synthetase (PPRPS)

$$\text{Ribose-5-phosphate} + \text{ATP} \xrightarrow{\text{Mg}^{2+}\ \text{Pi}} \text{PP-ribose-P} + \text{AMP}$$

A number of families have been described in which X-linked gout and severe primary purine overproduction are associated with structural enzyme mutations resulting in superactive PP-ribose-P synthetase (PPRPS). In some, increased enzyme activity is associated with abnormal resistance to feedback inhibitors while in others superactive PPRPS appears to be associated with an increased V_{max} or affinity for ribose-5-phosphate.

Affected males develop uric acid lithiasis or gouty arthritis in childhood or early adult life. Hyperuricaemia is often severe and in the range 0.5 to 1 mmol/l, with urine uric acid excretion of 5 to 15 mmol/24 h. Heterozygotes remain asymptomatic, although clinical investigation shows them to have evidence of increased purine synthesis *de novo*.

In some families the disorder presents in childhood with associated neurological features such as motor and mental retardation, ataxia, hypotonia, and disturbed development of speech. Polyneuropathy, intracerebral calcifications, and dysmorphic facial features have also been described, and in one family deafness was an associated clinical feature both in affected males and their heterozygous mothers.

Heterozygotes can be identified by studies in cultured skin fibroblasts but amniocentesis, prenatal diagnosis, and preventive abortion are not justified in this condition.

The hyperuricaemia, primary purine overproduction, and uricosuria can be controlled well with allopurinol.

Glucose-6-phosphatase

$$\text{Glucose-6-phosphate} + \text{H}_2\text{O} \rightarrow \text{Glucose} + \text{Pi}$$

Severe deficiency of glucose-6-phosphatase (glycogen storage disease type I, von Gierke's disease) is associated with marked hyperuricaemia from infancy (see Chapter 11.2.1). Gouty arthritis may become a problem before the age of 10 years, and chronic tophaceous gout with renal involvement can be a major cause of morbidity in those lucky enough to survive to adult life, unless preventive measures are taken.

Children with this condition have a characteristic appearance. They are pale, with chubby cheeks, stunted growth, and a large protuberant abdomen due to massive hepatomegaly. Severe and recurrent hypoglycaemia may result in convulsions or insidious and progressive mental retardation. Epistaxis and other bleeding phenomena may be a consequence of abnormal platelet function. Xanthomata frequently develop over the buttocks and extensor surfaces of the extremities and need to be distinguished from tophi.

BIOCHEMICAL FINDINGS AND DIAGNOSIS

In the absence of glucose-6-phosphatase the liver is unable to generate glucose from glycogen stores of glycogenic precursors. Glycogen accumulates in the liver and kidneys but not the heart or skeletal muscles. Maintenance of blood sugar in these patients is entirely dependent on regular feeding and absorption of glucose from the gut. Recurrent hypoglycaemia is accompanied by increased lipolysis, glycogenolysis, and gluconeogenesis with elevation of serum levels of lactate, pyruvate, free fatty acids, glycerol, cholesterol, triglycerides, phospholipids, and urate.

Renal clearance of uric acid is decreased but the urine uric acid:creatinine ratio is frequently greater than 0.75 and glycine incorporation into urine uric acid is increased. Thus hyperuricaemia is a consequence of both decreased urate excretion secondary to competitive inhibition of renal tubular urate secretion by lactate and excessive purine synthesis *de novo*. It has been suggested that the accelerated purine synthesis which occurs in these patients may result from increased availability of phosphoribosyl pyrophosphate following shunting of metabolites through the pentose phosphate pathway, but more recent evidence points to accelerated purine degradation following recurrent glycogenolysis and depletion of ATP. Glucose-6-phosphatase deficiency can usually be distinguished from glycogen storage disease type III (debrancher enzyme deficiency) by an exaggerated increase in lactic acid and a failure to mount a glucose response to injections of glucagon or galactose. Definitive diagnosis is made by direct assay of the enzyme, which is confined to liver, intestinal mucosa, and renal tissue. A less severe form of the disease is characterized by absence of hypoglycaemia and partial deficiency of glucose-6-phosphatase.

Patients with glucose-6-phosphate translocase deficiency (glycogen storage disease (GSD type Ib) present with clinical and biochemical features suggestive of von Gierke's disease with the addition of an increased susceptibility to infections associated with neutropenia and impairment of neutrophil migration. Liver glucose-6-phosphatase activity appears to be normal in conventional *in vitro* assays following freezing and detergent extraction but is defective in fresh liver tissue.

Myogenic hyperuricaemia

Hyperuricaemia, particularly following exercise, is also a feature of glycogen storage disease with primary muscle involvement (debranching enzyme deficiency (GSD type III), myophosphorylase deficiency (GSD type V), and phosphofructokinase deficiency (GSD type VII)). In each of these disorders hyperuricaemia results from excessive degradation of muscle ATP following exercise because of lack of carbohydrate substrates necessary for the synthesis of muscle ATP.

Fructose intolerance (see also Chapter 11.2.2)

Fructose ingestion and infusion are associated with hyperuricaemia, accelerated purine synthesis, and catabolism in normal subjects, and hyperuricaemia is a feature in patients with hereditary fructose intolerance. The finding of clinical gout in three out of nine subjects with heterozygous deficiency of aldolase B, identified by magnetic resonance spectroscopy, has led to the suggestion that this relatively common genetic trait (1/250 in Great Britain) could be responsible for a significant proportion of cases of familial gout. Fructose-induced hyperuricaemia is associated with degradation of liver adenine nucleotides and increased cellular concentrations of PP-ribose-P.

Adenylosuccinase

SAICA-ribotide $\rightarrow$ AICA-ribotide + fumarate
Adenylosuccinic acid $\rightarrow$ AMP + fumaric acid

Adenylosuccinase deficiency has recently been associated with an infantile autistic syndrome characterized by the presence of succinyl purines in the plasma, urine, and cerebrospinal fluid. Psychomotor retardation occurs before the age of 2 years and autism, axial hypotonia, and normal tendon reflexes are characteristic. Self-mutilation can also be a feature and there is evidence of cerebellar hypoplasia on computerized tomographic (CT) scanning. The diagnosis is suggested by the finding of aspartic acid and glycine in body fluids and confirmed by the identification of succinyl adenosine and SAICA riboside by high-performance liquid chromatography. Tissue studies show partial enzyme deficiency in the liver, kidney, and muscle, as well as lymphocytes and fibroblasts but not red cells. Adenylosuccinase deficiency is associated with a secondary increase in purine nucleotide synthesis and/or a decrease in degradation. It is inherited as an autosomal recessive. Patients with growth retardation have been shown to benefit from the administration of adenine (10 mg/kg/day) together with allopurinol.

Adenylate deaminase

AMP $\rightarrow$ IMP + NH$_3$

Gross deficiency of myoadenylate deaminase has recently been associated with a syndrome of muscular weakness and muscle cramps following exercise. Symptoms begin in early childhood. Physical and neurological abnormalities are limited to some decrease in muscle mass, hypotonia, and a little muscle weakness. Laboratory abnormalities include a modest rise in creatine phosphokinase in some but not all patients, non-specific abnormalities of the electromyogram, absence of ammonia in venous blood following exercise, and a complete absence of the enzyme on histochemical analysis of the muscle biopsy. The condition is inherited as an autosomal recessive.

Biochemical studies suggest that AMP deaminase deficiency leads to reduced entry of adenine nucleotides into the purine nucleotide cycle during exercise, with resultant impairment of muscle function.

Patients are advised to avoid vigorous exercise to prevent rhabdomyolysis, and administration of oral ribose (2–60 g/day) has been found to be beneficial in some, but not all cases.

A regulatory mutation of liver AMP deaminase has been suggested as a possible cause of primary gout and overproduction of uric acid; and this has been substantiated in a single patient.

Erythrocyte AMP deaminase deficiency is a relatively common autosomal recessive trait in Japan, Korea, and Taiwan, which is not associated with disease.

Xanthine oxidase

Hypoxanthine + H$_2$O + O$_2$ $\rightarrow$ Xanthine + H$_2$O$_2$
Xanthine + H$_2$O + O$_2$ $\rightarrow$ Uric acid + H$_2$O$_2$

Hereditary xanthinuria is a rare autosomal recessive disorder in which severe deficiency of xanthine oxidase is associated with hypouricaemia and excessive urinary excretion of xanthine and hypoxanthine.

Some persons affected appear to remain free from symptoms throughout their lives, the condition only being detected by finding a low serum urate on routine biochemical testing. In others the formation of xanthine calculi has been associated with renal colic, a mild myopathy, and crystal synovitis.

Plasma uric acid levels are usually less than 1 mg/100 ml and urinary uric acid excretion is less than 50 mg/24 h. Plasma oxypurines are correspondingly raised in the range 0.1 to 1.0 mg/100 ml and urine oxypurine excretion may be as high as 500 mg/24 h. Assays of hepatic or intestinal xanthine oxidase usually show no detectable activity but cases with as much as 10 per cent (liver) and 25 per cent (intestine) residual activity have been recorded.

Not all patients with xanthine stones have xanthine oxidase deficiency or even increased oxypurine excretion.

Treatment is usually restricted to maintaining a high fluid intake. Since xanthine solubility increases at higher pH, oral administration of alkali can be considered in recurrent stone formers but care must be taken. Allopurinol should be considered in those patients with residual enzyme activity, as hypoxanthine is significantly more soluble than xanthine.

Table 4 *Causes of hypouricaemia*

Decreased production of uric acid	Increased excretion of uric acid

Purine enzyme defects
  Xanthine oxidase
  PP-ribose-P synthetase
  Purine nucleoside phosphorylase
	Isolated defects in renal tubular handling
	  Idiopathic (Dalmatian dog mutation)
	  Malignant diseases
	  Hepatic diseases

Severe hepatic disease
 	
Acute intermittent porphyria
 	
Drugs
  Allopurinol
	Generalized defects in renal tubular transport (Fanconi syndrome)
	  Idiopathic
	  Wilson's disease
	  Carcinoma of bronchus
	  Multiple myeloma
	  Lymphomas
	  Hepatic disease and alcoholism
	  Hyperparathyroidism
	  Heavy metal poisoning
	  Cystinosis
	  Galactosaemia
	  Hereditary fructose intolerance

	Drugs
	Uricosuric agents (e.g. probenecid, sulphinpyrazone, benzbromarone)
	  Radiographic contrast agents
	  NSAID with uricosuric properties (e.g. phenylbutazone, azapropazone, high-dose aspirin)
	  Oestrogens
	  Glyceryl guaiacholate
	  Coumarin anticoagulants
	  Outdated tetracycline

OTHER CAUSES OF HYPOURICAEMIA

Hypouricaemia may be associated with reduction in uric acid formation in patients with deficiencies of PP-ribose-P synthetase and purine nucleoside phosphorylase as well in hereditary xanthinuria, allopurinol therapy, and severe hepatic disease. More commonly, however, hypouricaemia results from increased excretion, which may be associated with isolated or more generalized defects of renal tubular transport, and particularly with drug therapy of various kinds (Table 4).

Inborn errors of purine metabolism in immunodeficiency (see also Chapter 5.3)

A number of immunodeficiency disorders appear to be a direct consequence of inherited defects in purine metabolism.

Adenosine deaminase

$$\text{Adenosine} \rightarrow \text{Inosine} + NH_3$$

In about half the patients with the autosomal recessive form of severe combined immunodeficiency, the enzyme adenosine deaminase is absent.

Affected babies usually come to medical attention soon after birth, with diarrhoea, chest infections, and failure to thrive. Some infants present with lymphopaenia and hypogammaglobulinaemia with low or absent T and B lymphocytes, while others initially have normal immunoglobulins and a normal or increased percentage of B lymphocytes. T lymphocytes, and especially T suppressor cells, appear to be particularly vulnerable, possibly because these cells require expansion of their effector population for functional expression. In about a third of cases there are multiple radiological abnormalities including fraying of the long bones, abnormally thick growth arrest lines, and chondro-osseous dys-

plasia affecting the costochondral junctions. In a few there are additional abnormalities, such as renal tubular acidosis, choreoathetosis, spasticity, and the development of fine sparse hair.

BIOCHEMICAL FINDINGS

Adenosine deaminase deficiency is associated with the accumulation and excretion of deoxyadenosine as well as adenosine. Intracellular dATP, a potent inhibitor of ribonucleotide reductase, is markedly elevated in erythrocytes and T lymphoid cells but not in B cells. Initially, this differential toxicity for T and B cells was attributed to the relative deficiency of ecto 5'-nucleotidase in T cells, but it now seems intrinsically unlikely that this ecto enzyme can be serving such an important regulatory role. More recent work suggests that deoxyadenosine inhibits DNA polymerization. The resultant accumulation of DNA strand-breaks triggers poly ADP ribose synthesis and lethal NAD depletion. Deoxyadenosine is also a 'suicide' inactivator of *S*-adenosylhomocysteine hydrolase which catalyses the synthesis of *S*-adenosylhomocysteine from adenosine and L-homocysteine and is a key enzyme for numerous methylation reactions.

The prognosis in untreated adenosine deaminase deficiency severe combined immunodeficiency is very poor, death due to infection usually occurring in the first year of life.

TREATMENT

Until recently the treatment of choice was marrow transplantation if a histocompatible donor was available. Enzyme replacement therapy with repeated red blood cell transfusions can provide transient clinical benefit, while more sustained protection follows the administration of polyethylene glycol modified bovine adenosine deaminase. Very recently severe combined immunodeficiency associated with adenosine deaminase deficiency has been successfully treated by gene transfer; the first example of successful somatic cell gene therapy in man.

Purine nucleoside phosphorylase

Inosine + Pi → Hypoxanthine + ribose-1-P

Inherited purine nucleoside phosphorylase deficiency is associated with isolated T-cell immune deficiency. These children present with recurrent upper and lower respiratory tract infections, usually during the first year of life. Susceptibility is particularly to virus infections such as varicella, vaccinia, or cytomegalovirus. The tonsils are small or absent and lymph-nodes are deficient in thymic-dependent areas. Circulating lymphocyte counts are usually very low, with a low percentage of T lymphocytes and depressed or absent responsiveness to mitogen-induced transformation. Serum immunoglobulin levels and antibody responses to pneumococcal polysaccharide and keyhole limpet haemocyanin are typically increased in these children and the occasional finding of monoclonal IgG paraprotein strongly suggests that the changes in antibody production are secondary to T-cell defects. Autoimmune haemolytic anaemia, megaloblastic bone marrow, and spastic tetraplegia have been occasional associations.

BIOCHEMICAL FINDINGS

Purine nucleoside phosphorylase deficiency is associated with the accumulation and excretion of deoxyguanosine and deoxyinosine as well as guanosine and inosine. Paradoxically there is massive purine overproduction and excretion, although all patients are severely hypouricaemic. Erythrocyte concentrations of dGTP are markedly raised in purine nucleoside phosphorylase deficient cells. T cells but not B cells appear to be susceptible to deoxyguanosine toxicity, probably as a result of accumulation of dGTP, inhibition of ribonucleotide reductase, impairment of DNA synthesis, and eventually cell death.

TREATMENT

The prognosis in children with purine nucleoside phosphorylase deficiency is often much better than that in severe combined immunodeficiency with adenosine deaminase deficiency. Since some children have remained healthy and free from viral infection until the age of 6 years, high-risk procedures such as marrow transplantation are currently not thought to be justified in all cases. Conservative treatment with gammaglobulin replacement with later attempts at enzyme replacement with red cell transfusions in children with recurrent infections are the current approach to management.

5'-Nucleotidase

Adenylic acid → Adenosine + Pi

Deficiency of the ecto enzyme 5'-nucleotidase is found in some patients with X-linked and 'acquired' adult onset hypogammaglobulinaemia. There is no evidence that the enzyme deficiency causes the immunodeficiency in either case. It is currently thought much more likely simply to reflect an arrested stage of lymphocyte development in these patients.

Inborn errors of pyrimidine metabolism

There are three major pathways of pyrimidine metabolism in man, analogous to the pathways of purine metabolism; *de novo* synthesis, salvage, and degradation (Fig. 8).

Pyrimidine biosynthesis

The *de novo* pathway of pyrimidine biosynthesis in mammalian cells consists of a series of six enzymatic reactions coded for by three structural genes which lead to the formation of orotic acid, orotidine monophosphate (OMP) and uridine monophosphate (UMP). Cytidine monophosphate (CMP) and thymidine monophosphate (TMP) are derived from UMP by a series of enzymatic steps before phosphorylation to their respective di- and triphosphates and synthesis of RNA and DNA.

UMP and TMP are also synthesized by the salvage enzymes uridine kinase, thymidine kinase, and uracil phosphoribosyl transferase.

The pyrimidine nucleotide monophosphates are degraded to the nucleosides cytidine, uridine, and thymidine by 5'-nucleotidase. Cytidine is deaminated to uridine, and uridine and thymidine are further degraded to the pyrimidine bases uracil and thymine by pyrimidine nucleoside phosphorylase. Further catabolism leads to the formation of β-alanine and β-aminoisobutyrate and metabolic incorporation in the citric acid cycle.

UMP synthase

Orotate phosphoribosyl transferase (OPRT) and orotidine monophosphate decarboxylase (ODC) constitute the single bifunctional enzyme UMP synthase.

Orotic acid + PP-ribose-P → OMP + PPi

OMP → UMP + CO$_2$

Hereditary orotic aciduria is an autosomal recessive disorder associated with homozygous deficiency of UMP synthase. Massive overproduction of orotic acid results from loss of feedback inhibition of the rate-limiting enzyme, carbamyl phosphate synthetase II, by pyrimidine nucleotides, and deficiency of pyrimidine nucleotides is associated with inhibition of cell division, megaloblastic anaemia, and retardation of growth and development.

The disease presents soon after birth with a hypochromic, megaloblastic anaemia which is resistant to haematinics. If the diagnosis is

Fig. 8 Pathways of pyrimidine metabolism in humans. CPS, carbamyl phosphate synthetase II; OPRT, orotate phosphoribosyl transferase; ODC, orotidine monophosphate decarboxylase (OPRT + ODC form UMP synthase); 5'-NT, pyrimidine 5'-nucleotidase; NP, pyrimidine nucleoside phosphorylase; DHPD, dihydropyrimidine dehydrogenase; UK, uridine kinase; UPRT, uracil phosphoribosyl transferase; TK, thymidine kinase.

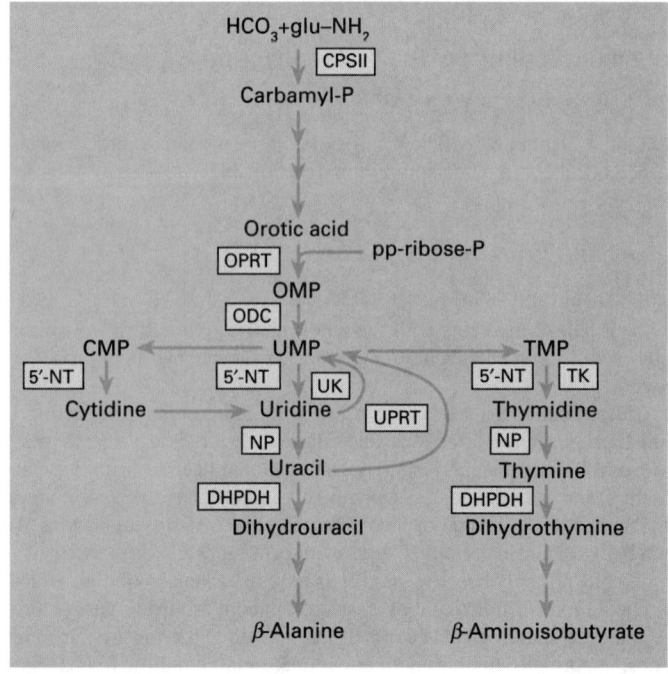

delayed, the disorder is associated with retardation of growth and psychomotor development. Urinary orotic acid excretion is increased 200–1000-fold (1–1.5 mg/24 h) and orotic acid crystalluria may follow dehydration. Other clinical features have included strabismus, cardiac malformations, and increased susceptibility to infections.

The diagnosis can be confirmed by red blood cell enzyme assays which show low but detectable levels of OPRT and ODC (hereditary orotic aciduria type I) or ODC alone (hereditary orotic aciduria type II). Kinetic studies of the fibroblast enzyme have suggested structural gene mutations. Northern blot and S1 nuclease assays have shown normal levels of stable mRNA in the enzyme-deficient cells. Treatment is with uridine (100–150 mg/kg/day) which is converted to UMP by uridine kinase (Fig. 8). The haematological response to treatment is prompt and consistent but some patients have been left with neurological impairment, possibly because of delay in commencing therapy.

Orotic aciduria is also found in patients with urea cycle defects, lysinuric protein intolerance, PP-ribose-P synthetase deficiency, and deficiency of purine nucleoside phosphorylase. Mild increases in urine orotic acid also occur in normal pregnancy and in patients receiving treatment with allopurinol.

Dihydropyrimidine dehydrogenase (DHPDH)

$$\text{Uracil} \rightarrow \text{Dihydrouracil}$$
$$\text{NADP} \quad \text{NADPH}$$
$$\text{Thymine} \rightarrow \text{Dihydrothymine}$$

Homozygous deficiency of DHPDH leads to the accummulation of uracil and thymine in body fluids.

Affected children may present with hypertonia, hyperreflexia, and mental deficiency, or with epilepsy and autistic features. Others have remained asymptomatic until adult life and then presented with severe toxic side-effects (pancytopaenia, stomatitis, diarrhoea, and neurological symptoms) following cancer chemotherapy with 5-fluorouracil, which is normally metabolized by the same enzyme.

Uracil and thymine are elevated in plasma and cerebrospinal fluid, and urinary excretion of the pyrimidine bases is greatly increased in patients with DHPDH deficiency (uracil, 2–10 mmol/g creatinine; thymine, 2–7 mmol/g creatinine). The disorder is characterized by a complete absence of enzyme activity in white blood cells, liver, and fibroblasts.

There is no effective treatment for this condition and the prognosis for life is very variable.

Pyrimidine-5′-nucleotidase

$$\text{UTP} \rightarrow \text{UDP} \rightarrow \text{UMP}$$
$$\text{CTP} \rightarrow \text{CDP} \rightarrow \text{CMP}$$

Homozygous deficiency of erythrocyte pyrimidine-5′-nucleotidase is associated with an hereditary form of non-spherocytic haemolytic anaemia with basophilic stippling of red blood cells.

Patients present with a mild or moderate well-compensated anaemia, usually associated with splenomegaly.

Red blood cell concentrations of uridine and cytidine ribonucleotides are markedly increased and erythrocyte enzyme activity varies from 0 to 30 per cent of normal.

Pending the development of a safe inhibitor of orotate transport, there is no effective therapy for this condition. Treatment with allopurinol is associated with inhibition of UMP synthase, increased salvage of orotate, and increased intracellular concentrations of pyrimidine nucleotides.

Lead poisoning can be associated with a haemolytic anaemia and acquired deficiency of erythrocyte pyrimidine-5′-nucleotidase (see Section 8).

REFERENCES

Gout

Cameron, J.S. *et al.* (1993). Gout, uric acid and purine metabolism in paediatric nephrology. *Nephron,* **7**, 105–18.

Campion *et al.* (1987). *American Journal of Medicine* **84**, 421–6.

Emmerson, B.T. (1991). Identification of the causes of persistent hyperuricaemia. *Lancet* **337**, 1461–3.

Henderson, J.F. (1972). *Regulation of Purine Biosynthesis,* ACS Monograph 170. American Chemical Society, Washington.

Holmes, E.W., Wyngaarden, J.B., and Kelley, W.N. (1973). Human glutamine phosphoribosyl phosphate amidotransferase: two molecular forms interconvertible by purine ribonucleotides and phosphoribosyl pyrophosphate. *Journal of Biological Chemistry* **248**, 6035–40.

Mikkleson, W.H., Dodge, H.I., and Valkenburg, H. (1965). The distribution of plasma uric acid values in a population unselected as to gout and hyperuricaemia. *American Journal of Medicine,* **39**, 242–51.

Nuki, G. (1979). Crystal, arthritis and connective tissue. In *Advanced Medicine Symposium* **15**, (eds P.S. Harper and J.R. Muir) pp. 138–57. Pitman Medical, Tunbridge Wells.

Rieselbach, R.E. and Steele, T.H. (1974). Influence of the kidney upon urate homeostasis in health and disease. *American Journal of Medicine,* **56**, 665–75.

Roubenoff, R., *et al.* (1991). Incidence and risk factors for gout in white men. *American Journal of Medicine,* **266**, 3004–7.

Seegmiller, J.E., *et al.* (1990). Fructose-induced aberration of metabolism in familial gout identified by ³¹P magnetic resonance spectroscopy. *Proceedings of the National Academy of Sciences USA* **87**, 8326–30.

Sperling, O. (1989). Hereditary renal hypouricaemia. In *The metabolic basis of inherited disease,* (ed. C.R. Scriver *et al.*), (6th edn), p. 2605. McGraw Hill, New York.

Terkeltaub, R.A. (1993). Gout and mechanisms of crystal induced inflammation. *Current Opinion in Rheumatology,* **5**, 510–16.

Wallace, S.L., Robinson, H., and Masi, A.T. (1977). Preliminary criteria for the classification of the acute arthritis of primary gout. *Arthritis and Rheumatism* **20**, 895–900.

Hypoxanthine-guanine phosphoribosyl transferase

Emmerson, B.T. and Thompson, L. (1973). The spectrum of hypoxanthine-guanine phosphoribosyl transferase deficiency. *Quarterly Journal of Medicine* **42**, 423–31.

Kaufman, J.M., Greene, M.L., and Seegmiller, J.E. (1968). Urine uric acid to creatinine ratio: a screening test for inherited disorders of purine metabolism. *Journal of Pediatrics,* **73**, 583–92.

Kelley, W.N., *et al.* (1969). Hypoxanthine-guanine phosphoribosyl transferase deficiency in gout. *Annals of Internal Medicine* **70**, 155–206.

Lesch, M., and Nyhan, W.L. (1964). A familial disorder of uric acid and central nervous system dysfunction. *American Journal of Medicine* **36**, 561–70.

Lloyd, K.G., *et al.* (1981). Biochemical evidence of dysfunction of brain neurotransmitters in the Lesch–Nyhan syndrome. *New England Journal of Medicine* **305**, 1106–11.

Sculley, D.G., Dawson, P.A. Emmerson, B.T., and Gordon, R.B. (1992). A review of the molecular basis of hypoxanthine-guanine phosphoribosyl transferase [HPRT] deficiency. *Human Genetics,* **90**, 195–207.

Seegmiller, J.E., Rosenbloom, F.M., and Kelley, W.E. (1967). Enzyme defect associated with a sex-linked human neurological disorder and excessive purine synthesis. *Science* **155**, 1682–4.

Stout, J.T. and Caskey, C.T. (1989). Hypoxanthine phosphoribosyl transferase deficiency: the Lesch–Nyhan syndrome and gouty arthritis. In *The metabolic basis of inherited disease,* (ed. C.R. Scriver *et al.*), (6th edn), pp. 1007–28. McGraw Hill, New York.

Tarle, S.A., *et al.* (1991). Determination of the mutations responsible for the Lesch–Nyhan syndrome in seventeen subjects. *Genomics* **10**, 499–513.

Wilson, J.M., *et al.* (1986). A molecular survey of hypoxanthine-guanine phosphoribosyl transferase deficiency in man. *Journal of Clinical Investigation* **77**, 188–95.

Adenine phosphoribosyl transferase

Kamatani, M., Hakoda, M., Otsuka, S., Yoshikawa, H., and Kashiwazaki, S. (1992). Only 3 mutations account for almost all defective alleles causing adenine phosphoribosyl transferase deficiency in Japanese patients. *Journal of Clinical Investigation,* **90**, 130–5.

Simmonds, H.A., Sahota, A.S., and Van Acker, K.J. (1989). Adenine phosphoribosyl transferase deficiency and 2,8-dihydroxyadenine lithiasis. In *The metabolic basis of inherited disease,* (ed. C.R. Scriver *et al.*), (6th edn), pp. 1029–44.

Phosphoribosyl pyrophosphate synthetase

Becker, M.A., *et al.* (1986). Phosphoribosyl pyrophosphate synthetase superactivity. *Arthritis and Rheumatism* **29**, 880–8.
Becker, M.A., *et al.* (1988). Inherited superactivity of phosphoribosyl pyrophosphate synthetase: association of uric acid overproduction and sensineural deafness. *American Journal of Medicine* **85**, 383–90.
Roessler, B.J., Nosal, J.M., Smith, P.R., *et al.* (1993). Human X-linked phosphoribosyl pyrophosphate superactivity is associated with distinct point mutations in the PRPS1 gene. *Journal of Biological Chemistry,* **268**, 26476–81.

Glucose-6-phosphatase

Greene, H.L., *et al.* (1978). ATP depletion, a possible role in the pathogenesis of hyperuricaemia in glycogen storage disease type 1. *Journal of Clinical Investigation* **62**, 321–8.
Tada, K., *et al.* (1985). Glycogen storage disease type 1B: a new model of genetic disorders involving the transport system of intracellular membrane. *Biochemical Medicine* **33**, 215–22.

Adenylosuccinase

Jaeken, J., *et al.* (1988). Adenylosuccinase deficiency: an inborn error or purine nucleotide synthesis. *European Journal of Pediatrics* **148**, 126–31.
Stone, R.L., Aimi, J., Barshop, B.A. *et al.* (1992). A mutation in adenylosuccinate lyase associated with mental retardation and autistic features. *Nature Genetics,* **1**, 59–63.

Adenylate deaminase

Sabina, R.L., Swain, J.L., and Holmes, E.W. (1989). Myoadenylate deaminase deficiency. In *The metabolic basis of inherited disease,* (ed. C.R. Scriver *et al.*), (6th edn), pp. 1077–84. McGraw Hill, New York.

Xanthine oxidase

Holmes, E.W. and Wyngaarden, J.B. (1989). Hereditary xanthinuria. In *The metabolic basis of inherited disease,* (ed. C.R. Scriver *et al.*), (6th edn), pp. 1085–94. McGraw Hill, New York.

Hypouricaemia

Sperling, O. (1989). Hereditary renal hypouricaemia. In *The metabolic basis of inherited disease,* (ed. C.R. Scriver *et al.*), (6th edn), pp. 2605. McGraw Hill, New York.
Sperling, O. (1991). Urate deposition and stone formation in the kidney in renal hypouricaemia. In *Urate deposition in man and its clinical consequences,* (ed. U. Gresser, and N. Zollner), pp. 65–77. Springer Verlag, Berlin.

Disorders of purine metabolism associated with immunodeficiency

Kredich, N.M. and Hershfield, M.S. (1989). Immunodeficiency diseases caused by adenosine deaminase deficiency and purine nucleoside phosphorylase deficiency. In *The metabolic basis of inherited disease,* (ed. C.R. Scriver *et al.*), (6th edn), pp. 1045–75. McGraw Hill, New York.
Hershfield, M.S., *et al.* (1987). Treatment of adenosine deaminase deficiency with polyethylene glycol-modified adenosine deaminase. *New England Journal of Medicine* **316**, 589.

Inborn errors of pyrimidine metabolism

Suttle, D.P., Becroft, D.M.O., and Webster, D.R. (1989). Hereditary orotic aciduria and other disorders of pyrimidine metabolism. In *The metabolic basis of inherited disease,* (ed. C.R. Scriver *et al.*), (6th edn), pp. 1095–126. McGraw Hill, New York.

11.5 Porphyrin metabolism and the porphyrias

K. E. L. McColl, S. Dover, E. Fitzsimons, and M. R. Moore

Porphyrin biosynthesis is one of the essential biochemical processes in the great majority of life-forms. In plants, the porphyrin molecule is combined with magnesium to form chlorophyll and thus allows photosynthesis. In animals, the porphyrin molecule is combined with iron to form haem, which plays a central role in controlling the body's oxidation and reduction processes. The porphyrias are inherited disorders involving the biochemical pathway of porphyrin haem biosynthesis. Though comparatively rare, they may mimic many other common conditions. Porphyrin metabolism may also be disturbed in a variety of other disease processes including iron deficiency, alcohol excess, lead poisoning, and hereditary tyrosinaemia.

Classification

Clinically, the porphyrias can be divided into the acute porphyrias (acute intermittent porphyria, variegate porphyria, hereditary coproporphyria) and the non-acute porphyrias (porphyria cutanea tarda (PCT), erythropoietic protoporphyria, and congenital porphyria) (Fig. 1). The acute porphyrias present with severe attacks of neurovisceral dysfunction associated with the overproduction and increased urinary excretion of the porphyrin precursors δ-aminolaevulinic acid (ALA) and porphobilinogen (PBG). Patients with variegate porphyria and hereditary copro-

Fig. 1 Classification of the main types of porphyria.

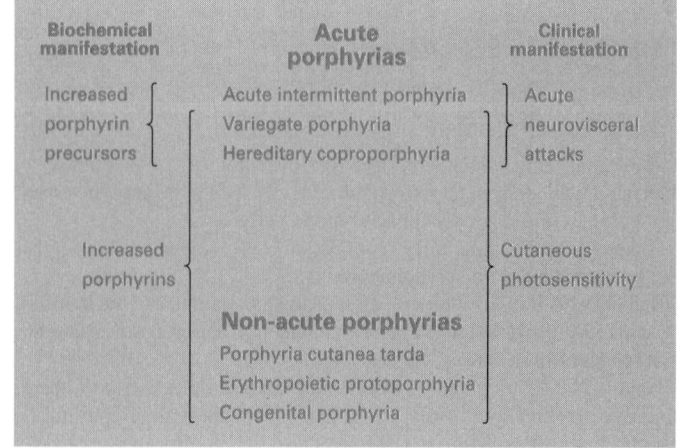

porphyria patients may, in addition, experience cutaneous photosensitivity associated with the overproduction of porphyrins. In the non-acute porphyrias there is only overproduction of porphyrins and not of porphyrin precursors and, therefore, patients only present with cutaneous photosensitivity.

Biochemistry

Haem biosynthesis is one of the essential pathways of life and occurs in all metabolically active cells. It is most active in erythropoietic tissue, where it is required for haemoglobin synthesis, and in hepatic tissue, where the haem forms the basis of various haem-containing enzymes such as cytochrome P-450, catalase, peroxidases, and tryptophan pyrrolase. The control of haem biosynthesis has been most fully documented in hepatic tissue (Fig. 2). The process starts with the condensation of glycine and succinyl coenzyme A to form δ-aminolaevulinic acid under the control of the mitochondrial enzyme δ-aminolaevulinic acid synthase. A series of enzymes then controls the conversion of δ-aminolaevulinic acid to porphobilinogen and then to the various porphyrins. Finally, iron is inserted into protoporphyrin by the enzyme ferrochelatase to form haem. The rate of the pathway is regulated by the activity of the initial enzyme δ-aminolaevulinic acid synthase, which is under negative feedback control by haem.

The various porphyrias are due to deficiencies of individual enzymes in the pathway of haem biosynthesis. The enzyme deficiency impairs the production of the end product haem and there is a compensatory increase in activity of the initial and rate-controlling enzyme δ-aminolaevulinic acid synthase. As a consequence of this, there is overproduction and increased excretion of the haem precursors formed prior to the enzyme defect. The porphyrin precursors δ-aminolaevulinic acid and porphobilinogen are excreted in the urine, whereas the porphyrins are mainly excreted in the faeces via the bile. The pattern of overproduction and increased excretion of porphyrins and porphyrin precursors in the different porphyrias is therefore determined by the site of the enzymic

defect. In the acute porphyrias there is overproduction of all the porphyrins and porphyrin precursors formed proximal to the enzyme defect. However, in the non-acute porphyrias there is overproduction of all porphyrins formed prior to the enzyme defect, but no overproduction of porphyrin precursors. The reason for the lack of overproduction of porphyrin precursors in the non-acute porphyrias is unclear, but may be due to a compensatory increase in the activity of the enzyme porphobilinogen deaminase in addition to increased activity of δ-aminolaevulinic acid synthase. The pattern of overproduction and excretion of porphyrins and porphyrin precursors in the various porphyrias is shown in Table 1.

Though haem biosynthesis occurs in all metabolically active cells, the overproduction of porphyrins and their precursors in the different porphyrias is mainly hepatic or erythropoietic in origin. In the acute porphyrias and in porphyria cutanea tarda, the liver is the main source of overproduction, in congenital porphyria the marrow is the main source, and in erythropoietic protoporphyria porphyrins are overproduced by both the liver and marrow.

Molecular biology

During the past 5 years, complementary DNA (cDNA) clones have been obtained for eight of the nine enzymes of haem biosynthesis and the structures of the corresponding genes have been determined. These advances are transforming our knowledge of haem biosynthesis and are certain to improve both understanding of the pathogenesis of the porphyrias and methods for identification of carriers of the genes for these disorders. The enzymes of the biosynthetic pathway have all now been mapped to specific chromosomes (Table 2).

Recent studies have examined the nature of the genetic mutations leading to the enzyme deficiencies in the various porphyrias. Most of this work had concentrated on the genetic basis of the reduced activity of porphobilinogen deaminase in acute intermittent porphyria. These studies have shown marked heterogeneity of mutations. Most are single base changes on exons 10 and 12, and include substitutions and dele-

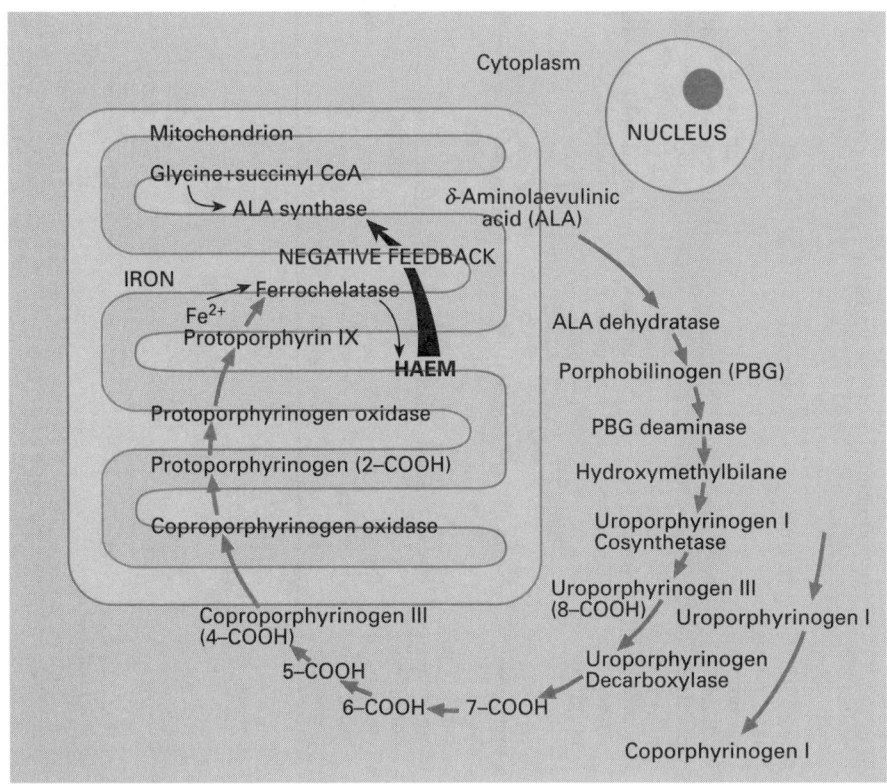

Fig. 2 Haem biosynthesis within the cell. This figure shows how haem is synthesized from the precursors glycine and succinyl CoA and the different compartmentation of the stages of the pathway in the mitochondrion and in the cytoplasm. Control of the pathway is maintained by haem acting by negative feedback on ALA synthase. Any of the series I isomer porphyrins synthesized will be excreted. The biosynthetic intermediate is the porphyrinogen and not the porphyrin.

Table 1 *Normal values and abnormal porphyrin and precursor patterns in the porphyrias*

	Erythrocyte proto-porphyrin	Erythrocyte copro-porphyrin	Urinary ALA	Urinary porphobilinogen	Urinary uro-porphyrin	Urinary copro-porphyrin	Faecal X porphyrin	Faecal proto-porphyrin	Faecal copro-porphyrin
Normal levels	0–50 µg/dl cells	0–4.2 µg/dl cells	0–5.3 mg per day	0–3.6 mg per day	0–41 µg per day	0–280 µg per day	0–15 µg per g dry wt	0–113 µg per g dry wt	0–50 µg per g dry wt
SI units	0–900 nmol/l	0–64 nmol/l	0–40 µmol per day	0–16 µmol per day	0–49 nmol per day	0–432 nmol per day	—	0–200 nmol per g dry weight	0–76 nmol per g dry weight
Acute intermittent porphyria	Normal	Normal	Raised—very high in attack	Raised—very high in attack	Usually raised	Sometimes raised	Normal	Sometimes raised	Sometimes raised
Variegate porphyria	Normal	Normal	Raised in attack	Raised in attack	Sometimes raised	Sometimes raised	Raised very high in attack	Raised	Raised
Hereditary coproporphyria	Normal	Sometimes raised in attack	Raised only in attack	Raised only in attack	Sometimes raised in attack	Usually raised—always raised in attack	Sometimes raised especially in photosensitive cases	Usually normal	Raised
Cutaneous hepatic porphyria	Normal	Normal	Normal	Normal	Raised—very high in attack	Slightly raised	Raised	Raised in remission	Raised in remission
Congenital porphyria	Usually raised	Usually raised	Usually normal	Usually normal	Raised	Sometimes raised	Normal	Sometimes raised	Raised
Erythropoietic protoporphyria	Raised—usually very high	Sometimes slightly raised	Normal	Normal	Normal	Normal	Normal	Usually raised	Normal

Table 2 *Details of the enzymes which are defective in the different forms of porphyrias and related disorders and their chromosomal location*

Names (abbreviation) (synonyms)	Chromosomal location	Related porphyria or other disease
5-Aminolaevulinate synthase (ALA.S)	3p21	
Erythroid ALA-synthase (eALA.S)	Xp11.2	X-linked sideroblastic anaemia
ALA dehydratase (ALAD) (porphobilinogen (PBG) synthase)	9q34	Plumboporphyria
PBG deaminase (PBGD and ePBGD) (hydroxymethylbilane synthase) (uroporphyrinogen I synthase)	11q23	Acute intermittent porphyria
Uroporphyrinogen cosynthase (URO COS)	10q26	Congenital porphyria
Uroporphyrinogen decarboxylase (UROD)	1p34	Porphyria cutanea tarda Hepatoerythropoietic porphyria
Coproporphyrinogen oxidase (COPRO O) (coproporphyrinogenase)	9	Hereditary coproporphyria
Protoporphyrinogen oxidase (PROTO O)	14	Variegate porphyria
Ferrochelatase (FERRO C) (haem synthase)	18q21.3	Erythropoietic protoporphyria

tions. These have resulted in amino acid substitution, splicing defects, and premature insertion of stop codons. It had been hoped that identification of the genetic basis of the various porphyrias would facilitate screening for the various diseases but the marked genetic heterogeneity characterizing each of the porphyrias makes this unlikely.

Prevalence

The prevalence of the various forms of porphyria varies widely from country to country. In the United Kingdom this has not been definitely established. In Scotland, 1 person in 50 000 has some form of porphyria, with a predominance of acute intermittent porphyria and porphyria cutanea tarda. In South Africa the prevalent form of the disease is variegate porphyria, with a possible incidence of 1 in 1000 in the white population, whilst the Bantu population suffers mainly from porphyria cutanea tarda.

The acute porphyrias

The acute porphyrias (acute intermittent porphyria, hereditary coproporphyria, and variegate porphyria), and occasionally plumboporphyria, present with intermittent attacks of neurovisceral dysfunction, which may be precipitated by various drugs and other exogenous factors. Patients with variegate porphyria or hereditary coproporphyria may, in addition, develop photosensitive skin lesions. Each of the acute porphyrias is characterized by overproduction and increased urinary excretion of the porphyrin precursors δ-aminolaevulinic acid and porphobilinogen. In variegate porphyria and hereditary coproporphyria there is also overproduction of porphyrins that produce the cutaneous photosensitivity.

Acute intermittent porphyria

This is the most common and most severe form of the acute porphyrias. Though the genetic trait is inherited in an autosomal dominant fashion, manifest disease is more common in females, with a female : male ratio of around 5 : 1. This is probably due to hormonal fluctuations precipitating clinical attacks. The highest incidence of onset of symptoms is between puberty and 30 years of age and attacks are most common in the third decade. In one-third of reported cases there is no family history; the condition probably having remained latent or unidentified for several generations.

The frequency and severity of attacks vary considerably from patient to patient. In a proportion, the disease remains latent throughout life, even in the presence of precipitating factors. Other patients experience frequent and sometimes life-endangering attacks even in the absence of extrinsic precipitating factors.

UNDERLYING BIOCHEMICAL DISORDER

The basic defect in acute intermittent porphyria is partial deficiency of the enzyme porphobilinogen deaminse. As a result, there is excess formation and urinary excretion of the porphyrin precursors δ-aminolaevulinic acid and porphobilinogen, which are formed prior to the enzyme defect. There is also increased excretion of uroporphyrin in the urine. Excretion of these haem precursors is always increased during clinical attacks but may be either normal or increased during clinical remission (see Table 2).

FEATURES OF THE PORPHYRIC ATTACK

The prevalence of symptoms and physical signs in patients presenting with an acute porphyric attack is shown in Fig. 3.

Gastrointestinal manifestations

Abdominal pain is the most frequent complaint, occurring in 95 per cent of attacks of acute porphyria. It is often very severe, requiring parenteral narcotic analgesics. The pain is usually felt diffusely over the abdomen and often radiates round the back. Abdominal examination may be normal or reveal mild generalized tenderness, sometimes associated with a degree of muscle guarding. Bowel sounds are normal. Anorexia usually occurs and there is often associated nausea and vomiting. Some patients develop marked delayed gastric emptying and a succussion splash may be elicited. Constipation is usually present. Abdominal radiographs are usually normal though in some patients dilatation of the colon may be seen.

Patients presenting with their first attack may be misdiagnosed as suffering from an acute abdomen. Unnecessary anaesthetic and laparotomy may result in a fatal outcome.

Neuropathy

Neuropathy may be the presenting feature and complicates more than 50 per cent of porphyric attacks. Motor involvement is most common but paraesthesia may also occur. The paralysis usually starts peripherally and then spreads proximally; however, in some patients shoulder girdle involvement may be the first manifestation. The neuropathy may progress rapidly, resulting in respiratory embarrassment.

Psychiatric manifestations

Psychiatric manifestations are also a common feature of the porphyric attack and may result in a patient being misdiagnosed as suffering from a primary psychiatric disorder. Agitation, mania, depression, hallucinations, and schizophrenic-like behaviour may occur. Psychiatric manifestations may persist between attacks.

Autonomic dysfunction

Tachycardia and hypertension disproportionate to the pain are usually present. Other manifestations of autonomic dysfunction, such as profuse sweating, pallor, and pyrexia, may occur. Severe hyponatraemia due to inappropriate secretion of antidiuretic hormone complicates a proportion of attacks and sometimes presents with convulsions or deterioration in conscious level following commencement of intravenous fluids.

DIAGNOSIS OF ACUTE PORPHYRIC ATTACK

The most important factor in determining a satisfactory outcome for a patient presenting in acute porphyric crisis is early diagnosis. The disorder should be considered in any patient presenting with unexplained abdominal pain. A helpful clue to the diagnosis is the passage of dark urine due to the excessive excretion of haem precursors. If the urine is left standing in the light, the discoloration becomes more pronounced. The diagnosis is confirmed by demonstrating excess porphobilinogen in the urine. A useful side room test for excess porphobilinogen is to add an equal volume of Ehrlich's aldehyde reagent to the patient's urine. This causes a red discoloration that remains in the upper aqueous layer following the further addition of chloroform.

RELATIONSHIP BETWEEN BIOCHEMICAL DISORDER AND CLINICAL FEATURES OF THE PORPHYRIC ATTACK

All the clinical features of the attack of acute porphyria can be explained by neurological dysfunction affecting the central, peripheral, and autonomic nervous systems. The abdominal pain, vomiting, and constipation are all thought to be the result of dysfunction of the autonomic control of the gastrointestinal tract. The mechanism by which the abnormal haem biosynthesis results in the functional structural alterations of the nervous system remains to be elucidated.

FACTORS WHICH MAY PRECIPITATE ACUTE PORPHYRIA

Various factors may precipitate attacks of acute porphyria in subjects with the genetic trait and great care must be taken to prevent exposure to them:

    (1) drugs
    (2) alcohol
    (3) fasting
    (4) hormones
    (5) infection

Drugs are the most common precipitating agents. A list of drugs believed to be unsafe in patients with acute porphyria is given in Appendix 1 and a list of drugs thought to be safe in Appendix 2.

Other factors that may trigger attacks include alcohol ingestion, reduced caloric intake due to fasting or dieting, and infection. Hormones are also important. Attacks are more common in females and rarely occur before puberty or after the menopause. Pregnancy and oral contraceptives may also precipitate attacks and some women experience regular attacks commencing in the week prior to the onset of menstruation.

MANAGEMENT OF THE ACUTE ATTACK

An attack of acute porphyria still carries a significant mortality. A successful outcome largely depends on early diagnosis, removal of precipitating factors, and provision of intensive supportive therapy. In addition, correcting the underlying biochemical disorder by the administration of haem may speed recovery.

Nutrition

Steps should be taken to ensure that the patient has an adequate carbohydrate intake. In mild attacks, this may be done by ensuring an adequate oral intake of glucose polymer drinks, such as Caloreen (Roussel) or Hycal (Beecham Products). In more severe cases, 2 litres of 20 per cent dextrose should be infused every 24 h into a large peripheral vein or via a central line.

Control of pain

For severe pain, pethidine, morphine, or diamorphine may be required. There is a danger of addiction in patients experiencing frequent attacks and who require large amounts of narcotic analgesics; every

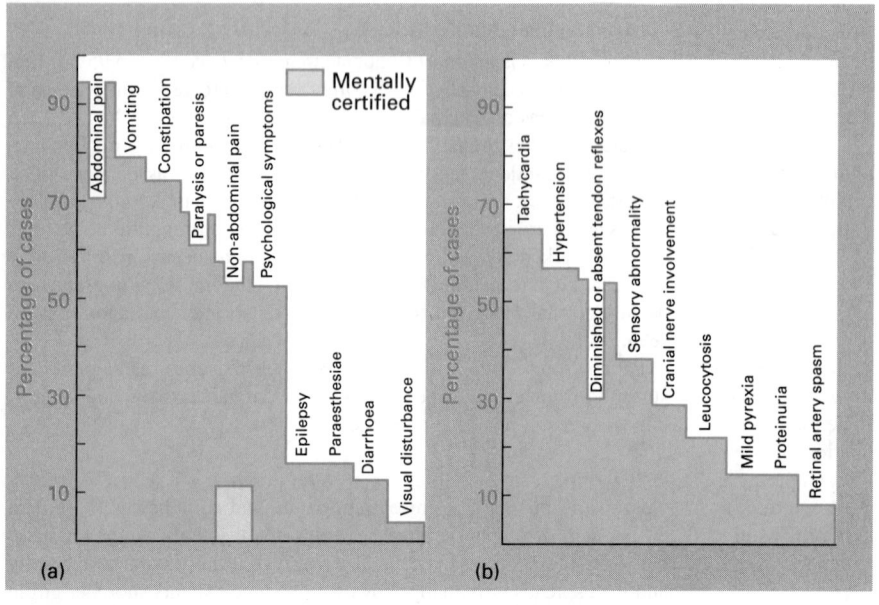

Fig. 3 (a) Prevalence of symptoms, and (b) incidence of physical signs, blood, and urine findings in 50 cases of acute intermittent porphyria.

attempt should be made to withdraw all narcotic drugs between attacks.

In a few unfortunate patients the pain is refractory to even very large doses of intravenous narcotic analgesics, and signs of respiratory and cardiovascular system depression appear before pain relief is obtained. Some of our patients report that the only time the pain goes away is when they are asleep. This observation may be used to advantage by encouraging sleep for several hours by combining chloropromazine or promazine with the analgesics and leaving the patients relatively undisturbed in a darkened room.

Some patients continue to complain of chronic abdominal pain unaccompanied by any other symptom between attacks. This can be very difficult to manage and the risk of narcotic addiction in these patients is high. Although, in some cases, a psychological element may be a factor, in others the pain is clearly genuine and presumably a manifestation of residual neurological damage.

Tachycardia and hypertension

These are features of the majority of attacks. They are thought to be the result of sympathetic overactivity and should be controlled with propranolol. The dose should be titrated against its effect on the cardiovascular system and frequently a very large dose is required. Pulse and blood pressure should be closely monitored as they tend to be labile and a marked postural effect is commonly seen.

Convulsions

These are not infrequent at the peak of an attack. Their onset may be a sign of hyponatraemia due to inappropriate antidiuretic hormone secretion and plasma osmolality and electrolyte values should be checked. If hyponatraemia is the underlying cause it should be corrected by fluid restriction. Convulsions occurring during the attack usually settle as the attack resolves and therefore therapy should be aimed at treating the underlying disease process. Some patients, however, continue to suffer convulsions outside the acute attack. As all the commonly employed anticonvulsants are porphyrinogenic, management of chronic epilepsy in porphyric patients is extremely difficult.

Neuropathy

All patients should be examined regularly for evidence of developing peripheral neuropathy. This may progress rapidly leading to quadriplegia and bulbar and ventilatory paralysis. When signs of peripheral neuropathy are present the expiratory peak flow rate should be monitored regularly. If there is any reduction in this, blood gases should be checked and the patient nursed in an Intensive Care Unit with facilities for assisted ventilation. Even in patients in whom there is widespread paralysis requiring assisted ventilation for many months, good functional recovery can still be expected. The usual attention should be given to splinting of the joints and appropriate physiotherapy in the paralysed patient.

Haematin therapy

It is possible to improve the underlying biochemical disturbance by the administration of the end product of the haem biosynthetic pathway. Haem preparations administered in this way bind to haemopexin and albumin in the plasma and are taking up by the liver. They supplement the depleted intracellular free haem pool, thus suppressing activity of the initial and rate-controlling enzyme of the pathway δ-aminolaevulinic acid synthase and thereby reducing the overproduction of porphyrins and the precursors formed prior to the enzyme block. The administration of haem preparations results in a marked and consistent reduction in porphyrin precursor excretion (Fig. 4). The most suitable haem preparation for the treatment of acute porphyria is haem arginate (Normosang, Leiras) as it is stable when stored in solution.

The clinical response to haem therapy is more difficult to assess. There has only been one placebo-controlled trial of haem arginate therapy and it did not show a statistically significant benefit for the active

therapy though there was a trend in favour of it. The lack of significant effect, however, may be due to the small numbers studied and variability of severity of attacks. The overall impression is that the marked improvement of biochemistry is accompanied by a significant, though less dramatic, clinical response.

Haem arginate is administered in a dose of 3 mg/kg/day for 3 or 4 days. It is given intravenously over 15 min by slow-running infusion. In some patients the treatment results in phlebitis around the injection site. It also causes slight prolongation of the prothrombin time and should be avoided in any patient with a coagulopathy.

Recent studies have demonstrated that the biochemical remission induced by haematin therapy can be prolonged by the coadministration of tin–protoporphyrin, which inhibits the breakdown of haem by haem oxygenase. Whether this increases the clinical benefit of haematin therapy has yet to be established. A significant side-effect of tin–protoporphyrin is cutaneous photosensitivity, which may persist for several weeks. For this reason it may not be suitable for use in any of the porphyrias in which cutaneous photosensitivity is a feature of the disease itself.

PREVENTION OF ATTACKS

Patients who have experienced a clinical attack of porphyria should be carefully counselled concerning the avoidance of precipitating factors. They should be given a booklet indicating which drugs are safe and which are unsafe to take. It is also important to ensure that their family doctor is fully informed about the disease and given advice about prescribing drugs. In addition, they should wear a bracelet or necklace indicating that they have porphyria.

Some women experience regular attacks in the week prior to the onset of menstruation. The use of the contraceptive pill to suppress ovulation and prevent these attacks cannot be recommended as all forms of contraceptive pill may, themselves, trigger attacks. We, and others, have found some benefit from treating these patients with the long-acting analogue of luteinizing hormone releasing hormone, Buserilin, which can be administered nasally. This therapy may cause osteoporosis and bone density should be closely monitored.

Pregnancy may precipitate attacks of acute porphyria with attacks being most common in early pregnancy and during the puerperium. When attacks occur during pregnancy they should be treated in the usual manner. No information is available concerning the effects of haem arginate on the fetus. The vast majority of patients with acute porphyria

Fig. 4 Effect of intravenous administration of haem arginate on the urinary excretion of δ-aminolaevulinic acid (ALA) in four patients in a clinical attack of acute intermittent porphyria.

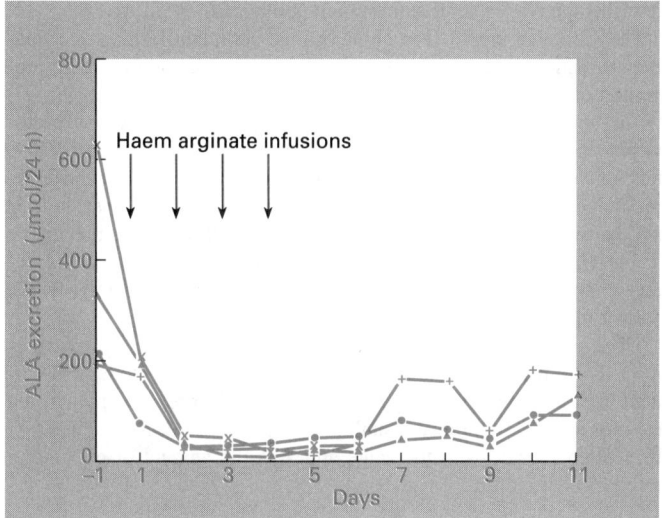

tolerate pregnancy well with a successful outcome for mother and child. However, patients experiencing frequent and severe attacks should probably be advised not to become pregnant until the porphyric process is more quiescent.

SURGERY AND ANAESTHETICS

Provided the appropriate precautions are taken, most patients with acute porphyria can tolerate surgery and general anaesthesia. Patients with acute porphyria have undergone such major surgery as coronary artery bypass grafts, hip replacement, and cholecystectomy without any complications. Care must be taken in selecting safe anaesthetic agents. Atropine and morphine may be used as premedication. Intravenous ketamine has been found to be a safe alternative to thiopentone as an anaesthetic-inducing agent. Cyclopropane and ether are safe inhalation agents in respect of the porphyria but they suffer the disadvantage of being potentially explosive and inducing postoperative vomiting. Nitrous oxide used in conjunction with intravenous narcotics may be a more acceptable alternative. Suxamethonium and D-tubocurarine can be used as muscle relaxants and diamorphine, morphine, pethidine or fentanyl are suitable narcotics for controlling postoperative pain. In some situations, epidural anaesthesia may be preferable to general anaesthesia, in which case bupivincaine is the local anaesthetic of choice. To prevent an attack being induced by fasting, an intravenous infusion of dextrose should be commenced prior to surgery and continued until the patient is able to take an adequate diet.

LONG-TERM COMPLICATIONS

A small proportion of patients with acute porphyria develop chronic hypertension. In addition, a small minority develop chronic renal failure and may require renal transplantation. The cause of the renal failure is not clear but may be partly related to hypertension and therefore patients with a history of porphyria should have their blood pressure monitored.

SCREENING OF RELATIVES

Blood relatives should be screened for latent disease in order that they can be advised about necessary precautions if positive. Urinalysis will only pick up 50 per cent of latent cases of acute intermittent porphyria and, therefore, analysis of the activity of porphobilinogen deaminase in erythrocytes be performed.

Variegate porphyria and hereditary coproporphyria

These may present clinically with attacks identical to those seen in acute intermittent porphyria. They are provoked by the same precipitating factors and patients should be managed in exactly the same way as described above for acute intermittent porphyria.

They are also inherited in an autosomal dominant fashion and relatives should be screened for the condition and given advice about prevention of attacks.

The underlying defect in variegate porphyria is deficiency of protoporphyrinogen oxidase activity and in hereditary coproporphyria it is deficiency of coproporphyrinogen oxidase activity. The site of the enzymic defects in these two forms of acute porphyria means that there is marked overproduction of porphyrins as well as of porphyrin precursors (Table 1). For this reason patients with variegate porphyria and hereditary coproporphyria may experience cutaneous phtosensitivity, which is most marked in sunny climates (Fig. 5).

There is no specific treatment for the skin photosensitivity occurring in variegate porphyrin and hereditary coproporphyria, although β-carotene treatment has been suggested as useful. Barrier creams may be used for avoidance of excess sunlight advised. The dermatological features often subside with the acute attack as the amount of circulating porphyrin is reduced.

Chester porphyria

An unusual form of acute porphyria has recently been described in which there is deficiency of both porphobilinogen deaminase and protoporphyrinogen oxidase. In some of the patients the excretion pattern and clinical manifestation is identical to acute intermittent porphyria whereas others resemble variegate porphyria.

Plumboporphyria or δ-aminolaevulinic acid dehydratase deficiency porphyria

A further type of porphyria has been described in which the biochemical presentation is of excess urinary excretion of δ-aminolaevulinic acid analogous to that found in lead poisoning, although blood lead levels are normal. The activity of δ-aminolaevulinic acid dehydratase is depressed. This genetic trait is inherited as an autosomal dominant. In the few cases described to date, in Germany and in the United States, acute features are similar to those of acute intermittent porphyria. All clinically manifest cases have been homozygotes.

The non-acute porphyrias

Porphyria cutanea tarda

Otherwise called cutaneous hepatic porphyria or symptomatic porphyria, this is predominantly an acquired disease, but there may be some genetic predisposition. A familial pattern is evident in a few patients, with the disorder being inherited as an autosomal dominant. The biochemical abnormality lies in hepatic uroporphyrinogen decarboxylase. Diagnosis, once again, is by the analysis of the porphyrin excretion pattern in which the dominant finding is an increased urinary uroporphyrin excretion (Table 1). The urinary porphyrin precursors δ-aminolaevulinic acid and porphobilinogen are never elevated.

Fig. 5 Bullous eruption which developed over the exposed skin of a woman with hereditary coproporphyria after sunbathing.

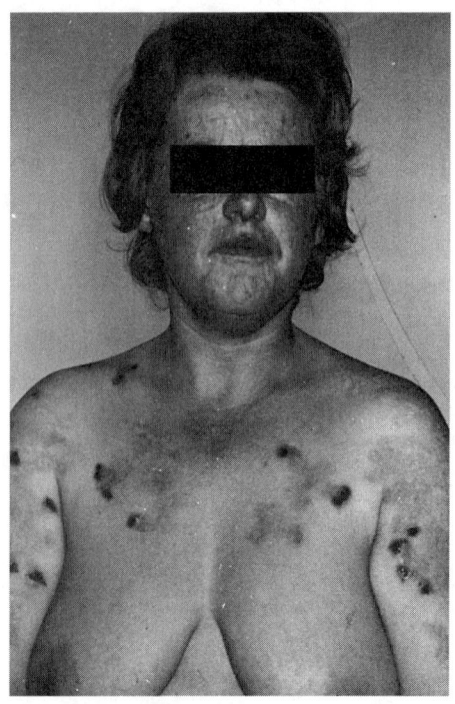

CUTANEOUS MANIFESTATIONS

The most striking and consistent clinical feature of porphyria cutanea tarda is bullous dermatosis on exposure to sunlight. The lesions are encountered on exposed areas such as the scalp, face, neck, and backs of the forearms and hands. They usually start with erythema, and progress to vesicles that become confluent to form bullae. Haemorrhage may occur into the bullae, which heal, leaving scars. Pruritus is often troublesome. There may be local pitting oedema at the site of the skin lesion. Increased fragility of the skin is an important feature and in less severe cases may be the only clinical sign. Hyperpigmentation is common and women often complain of hirsutism. Histological examination of the skin shows gross hyaline swelling in the walls of the capillaries in the upper curium of the bullae. Monochromator studies demonstrate that light of about the same wavelength as that absorbed by the porphyrin molecule (400 nm) will cause skin lesions in the porphyric patient.

UNDERLYING HEPATIC DISEASE

In addition to the cutaneous signs there may be evidence of hepatic disease both clinically and biochemically. Hepatomegaly is particularly common when alcohol has an aetiological role. Several other laboratory tests may be helpful. Liver function tests in nearly all cases are abnormal, including elevated bilirubin concentration and alkaline phosphatase, and serum transminase activities. Serum iron and transferrin saturation are usually increased, and there may be an accelerated plasma iron turnover with early uptake of radioactive iron by the liver. Histological examination of the liver reveals features that reflect the whole spectrum of alcoholic liver disease, although occasionally liver damage is minimal and non-specific. Siderosis almost invariably occurs and an underlying active chronic hepatitis may rarely be present. There is a 25 per cent incidence of diabetes mellitus, and some association with systemic lupus erythematosus and chronic active hepatitis.

EXOGENOUS PRECIPITATING FACTORS

Alcohol is the most important aetiological factor in porphyria cutanea tarda. More than 90 per cent of patients admit to excessive alcohol consumption. Oestrogenic steroids are also implicated in some cases. An outbreak that occurred in south-east Turkey in 1956 was traced to seed wheat dressed with the fungicide hexachlorobenzene. There was evidence of liver damage as well as photosensitivity and a number of patients died, especially children under 15 years. Some of the survivors were reviewed 20 years after exposure and still had skin manifestations of porphyria. Abnormal porphyrin excretion can be demonstrated in animals given dietary hexachlorobenzene. More recently, other polychlorinated hydrocarbons have been implicated in production of this toxic form of porphyria cutanea tarda. A neoplastic subgroup includes a similar condition secondary to benign or malignant primary liver tumour.

MANAGEMENT

The clinical features are reduced and even reversed by withdrawal of the offending agent. Alcohol, in particular, should be avoided. Correction of iron overload by venesection brings about clinical remission. Weekly venesection of 500 ml is carried out until clinical remission occurs or until the haemoglobin level falls below 12 g/dl. A rising urinary uroporphyrin level is a useful index of the requirement for further venesection before clinical symptoms become manifest. Treatment may be required for the underlying liver disease, e.g. active chronic hepatitis. Chloroquine may also be of value in the treatment of porphyria cutanea tarda. A small dose of 125 mg twice weekly results in increased urinary excretion of uroporphyrin with an associated fall in plasma and tissue levels and symptomatic improvement. The precise mechanism of its action is not clear but it probably forms complexes with uroporphyrin which are more readily cleared by the kidney.

Congenital porphyria

Although extremely rare, congenital porphyria, also known as erythropoietic porphyria or Gunther's disease, was the first porphyria to be described by Schultz in 1874. Since then, less than 100 cases have been reported. Solar sensitivity is the most striking symptom but systemic effects may also be severe. The disorder is inherited in a Mendelian autosomal recessive manner. There is evidence that the defect lies at the level of uroporphyrinogen cosynthetase in the biosynthetic pathway. Boys and girls are equally affected and symptoms usually begin during the first few years of life, although the disease can occasionally present in middle age.

CUTANEOUS MANIFESTATIONS

The skin reaction to sunlight is more severe than that of porphyria cutanea tarda. Pruritus and erythema are the initial features, followed by vesicle and bullous formation. The bullae rupture, leaving ulcers that frequently harbour secondary infection. Eventually the ulcers heal leaving scars. The severity of the lesions varies considerably but the result in most cases is devastating. Dystrophic changes in the nails may cause them to curl and drop off. Scarring of the skin on the hand may produce a claw-shaped deformity; lenticular scarring may lead to blindness. Hypertrichosis may be seen on the face, arms, and legs. Eyebrows and eyelashes may become thick and long. Pigmentation may be marked. The teeth become brownish-pink (erythrodontia) due to their high porphyrin content.

HAEMATOLOGICAL PROBLEMS

In addition to these integumentary lesions, a number of patients also develop anaemia and splenomegaly. The anaemia is caused by ineffective erythropoiesis with shortened red cell survival. The bone marrow reveals normoblastic hyperplasia; a proportion of erythrocyte precursors fluoresce red in ultraviolet light due to high porphyrin content. The peripheral blood film shows a normocytic normochromic anaemia with polychromasia. There is usually a moderate reticulocytosis with Howell–Jolly bodies; leucopenia and thrombocytopenia may occur when the spleen is large. Splenectomy may improve the anaemia and can reduce the degree of photosensitization.

MANAGEMENT

Treatment with chloroquine has been shown to be helpful in this disease, reducing erythrocyte fragility and diminishing the photosensitization. Patients with congenital porphyria have a much shortened life expectancy. Bone marrow transplantation should be considered in severe cases as it theoretically offers the chance of a cure.

Erythropoietic protoporphyria

Although not described until 1961, this form of erythropoietic porphyria, also known as erythrohepatic protoporphyria, is much more common than congenital porphyria. It is inherited as an autosomal dominant and symptoms may occur at any age, including infancy and childhood. Ferrochelatase activity is reduced in peripheral blood, liver, bone marrow, and skin. Diagnosis can be made by demonstrating fluorescence in a proportion of red cells (fluorocytes) in the peripheral blood and confirmed by measurement of greatly increased erythrocyte and faecal protoporphyrin (Table 1).

CUTANEOUS MANIFESTATIONS

The clinical features are mainly cutaneous with pruritic urticarial swelling and redness of the skin on exposure to sunlight. The most distressing symptom is a burning sensation of the affected parts, which may be unbearable. There may also be an eczematous skin reaction with scarring.

HEPATIC PROBLEMS

Systemic manifestations are not usually severe, but hepatic involvement can occur. There is evidence that protoporphyrin is hepatotoxic and that its deposition in the liver can lead to fatal liver failure from a process similar to active chronic hepatitis with cirrhosis. Liver function tests should be monitored in all patients and liver biopsy performed on the first sign of disturbance. There is also a tendency to the formation of protoporphyrin-containing gallstones.

MANAGEMENT

β-Carotene taken orally is an effective protective measure against the solar sensitivity. This may produce the side-effect of some yellowing of the skin (carotenaemia) after prolonged treatment, which may be made cosmetically acceptable by concurrent ingestion of canthaxanthin. The mode of action of β-carotene involves quenching of activated porphyrin triplet states, but it does not affect the biochemical pattern of the disease. Retardation of the progress of the liver lesions may be attempted by interruption of the enterohepatic circulation of protoporphyrin by bile salt sequestering agents such as cholestyramine. This reduces plasma protoporphyrin levels and thus diminishes the exposure of the liver cells to excessive protoporphyrin. Liver failure occasionally develops and should be treated with liver transplantation.

Other diseases associated with abnormal porphyrin metabolism

Increased excretion of circulating porphyrins is found in a number of other diseases, either because the synthesis of haem is disturbed or because the mechanism of excretion is abnormal. The most important of these are lead poisoning, iron-deficiency anaemia, and alcohol ingestion, although there is a heterogenous group of other diseases in which porphyrin metabolism is deranged.

Lead poisoning

It has been known for some time that patients suffering from lead poisoning have accumulation of protoporphyrin in the erythrocytes and increased urinary excretion of δ-aminolaevulinic acid and coproporphyrin. The elevated protoporphyrin chelated by zinc is retained in the erythrocyte, which may explain the absence of photosensitivity. This accumulation of porphyrins and precursors is due to the inhibition by lead of the haem biosynthetic enzymes: δ-aminolaevulinic acid dehydratase, coproporphyrinogen oxidase, and ferrochelatase. An increase in the activity of the rate-controlling enzyme δ-aminolaevulinic acid synthase results.

Many of the clinical manifestations of lead poisoning may be the result of altered haem biosynthesis. The anaemia of lead poisoning is due in part to the depressant effect of the lead on haem biosynthesis, though haemolysis and depression of globin synthesis are also important. The abdominal pain, constipation, and peripheral neuropathy that occur in lead poisoning are also seen in acute attacks of hepatic porphyria. Alterations in porphyrin metabolism have provided a useful means of detecting and assessing the severity of lead exposure and poisoning. The diminution in activity of erythrocyte δ-aminolaevulinic acid dehydratase and elevated erythrocyte protoporphyrin levels are the most sensitive measures although others, such as raised urinary δ-aminolaevulinic acid and coproporphyrin, are more frequently used. For screening purposes, portable front-surface fluorimeters have been developed for the rapid determination of protoporphyrin in whole blood.

Iron-deficiency anaemia

It has been recognized for some time that in iron-deficiency anaemia there is a marked accumulation of protoporphyrin in erythrocytes where insufficient iron is available for incorporation into haem. This rarely reaches the level found in erythropoietic protoporphyria. There have been a number of conflicting reports regarding alterations of other porphyrins and precursors. The measurement of erythrocyte protoporphyrin is a useful diagnostic procedure in the investigation of anaemia. It may be raised in latent iron deficiency before changes appear in peripheral blood. It is also helpful when serum iron and ferritin levels are misleading after patients have started iron therapy. Measurement of protoporphyrin concentration may be helpful in differentiating iron deficiency from β-thalassaemia in which erythrocyte protoporphyrin levels are normal.

Alcohol

The association between ethanol ingestion and alterations in porphyrin metabolism was first noted in 1935 when it was found that a subject generally doubled his urinary coproporphyrin excretion after drinking 1 litre of beer or 90 ml of cognac. Chronic alcoholics have an increased urinary excretion of coproporphyrin, mainly isomer 3, but normal urinary excretion of uroporphyrin, δ-aminolaevulinic acid, and porphobilinogen. Ethanol has been shown to alter the activities of a number of the enzymes of haem biosynthesis. Administration of ethanol to rats inhibits activity of δ-aminolaevulinic acid dehydratase and ferrochelatase and results in increased activity of δ-aminolaevulinic acid synthase in hepatic tissue. In humans, acute and chronic ethanol ingestion markedly depresses the activity of δ-aminolaevulinic acid dehydratase in peripheral blood. Ethanol administration to normal subjects results in increased activity of leucocyte δ-aminolaevulinic acid synthase and erythrocyte porphobilinogen deaminase, the two rate-controlling enzymes of the pathway. The activities of each of the other four enzymes is depressed. Ferrochelatase, the enzyme which inserts iron into protoporphyrin to form haem, shows the most marked depression, and in alcoholism there is prolonged depression of uroporphyrinogen decarboxylase, which provides a rationale for the role of ethanol in the aetiology of porphyria cutanea tarda. The alterations in haem biosynthesis may also be relevant to ethanol-induced sideroblastic anaemia. In this condition, there is accumulation of non-haem iron in the mitochondria of blood cell precursors and of protoporphyrin and coproporphyrin in erythrocytes, which may be explained by the marked depression of ferrochelatase activity. Patients with ethanol-related sideroblastic anaemia have been noted to have increased activity of δ-amino laevulinic acid synthase in bone marrow.

Other conditions

Abnormalities of haem biosynthesis have been reported in a variety of other haematological conditions including several forms of sideroblastic anaemia. In hereditary tyrosinaemia excess urinary δ-aminolaevulinic acid is excreted because δ-aminolaevulinic acid dehydratase is inhibited by succinyl acetone and, like the acute porphyria and lead poisoning, this disease is associated with neurobehavioural disturbance. In liver disease there may be increased urinary excretion of coproporphyrin predominantly the I isomer. In the Dubin–Johnson syndrome the ratio of coproporphyrin isomer I to isomer 3 is markedly increased in the urine (> 80 per cent) possibly as a result of deficiency of hepatic uroporphyrinogen III cosynthase and increased activity of porphobilinogen deaminase. In Rotor syndrome total urinary excretion of coproporphyrin is markedly increased and consists predominantly of coproporphyrin isomer I. In the unconjugated hyperbilirubinaemia of Gilbert's syndrome depressed activity of protoporphyrinogen oxidase and increased activity of δ-aminolaevulinic acid synthase has been noted in peripheral leucocytes. Increased urinary excretion of porphyrin-like substances has been found in a varying proportion of psychiatric patients not having porphyria. The association between this biochemical finding and the psychiatric disorder is not known, although the monopyrrole, haemopyrrole lactam, is excreted in excess in urine in both acute intermittent porphyria and schizophrenia.

REFERENCES

Anderson, K.E., Spitu, I.M., Bardin, C.W. and Kappas, A. (1990). A gonadotrophin releasing hormone analogue prevents cyclical attacks of porphyria. *Archives of Internal Medicine*, **150**, 1469–74.

Brodie, M.J., Moore, M.R., Thompson, G.G., Goldberg, A. and Low, R.A.L. (1977). Pregnancy and the acute porphyrias. *British Journal of Obstetrics and Gynaecology*, **84**, 726–31.

Herrick, A.L., McColl, K.E.L., Moore, M.R., Cook, A. and Goldberg, A. (1989). Controlled trial of haem arginate in acute hepatic porphyria. *Lancet*, **June 10**, 1295–7.

Herrick, A.L., McColl, K.E.L., Wallace, A.M., Moore, M.R., Goldberg, A. (1990). LHRH analogue treatment for the prevention of premenstrual attacks of acute porphyria. *Quarterly Journal of Medicine*, **New Series 75, 276**, 355–63.

Lamon, J.L., Frykholm, B.C., Hess, R.A., Tschudy, D.P. (1979). Haematin therapy for acute porphyria. *Medicine*, **58**, 252–69.

McColl, K.E.L., Moore, M.R., Thompson, G.G. and Goldberg, A. (1981). Treatment with haematin in acute hepatic porphyria. *Quarterly Journal of Medicine*, **New Series L, 198,** 161–74.

McColl, K.E.L., Moore, M.R., Thompson G.G., and Goldberg A. (1982). Screening for latent acute intermittent porphyria: the value of measuring both leucocyte and aminolaevulinic acid synthase and erythrocyte uroporphyrinogen-L-synthase activities. *Journal of Medical Genetics*, **19** no. 4, 271–6.

McColl, K.E.L., Wallace, A.M., Moore, M.R., Thompson, G.G. and Goldberg, A. (1982). Alterations in haem biosynthesis during the female menstrual cycle: studies in normal subjects and patients with acute intermittent porphyria. *Clinical Science*, **62**, 183–91.

McColl, K.E.L., Moore, M.R., Thompson, G.G. and Goldberg, A. (1985). Chester porphyria: biochemical studies of a new form of acute porphyria. *Lancet*, **12**, 796–8.

Meyer, U.A., Strand, L.J., Doss, M., Rees, A.C. and Marver, H.S. (1992). Intermittent acute porphyrika – demonstration of a genetic defect in porphobilinogen metabolism. *New England Journal of Medicine*, **286**, 1277–86.

Mgone, C.S., Langon, N.G., Moore, M.R., and Connor, J.M. (1992). Detection of seven point mutations in the porphobilinogen deaminase gene in patients with acute intermittent porphyria by direct sequencing of in vitro couplified cDNA. *Human Genetics*, **90**, 12–16.

Moore, M.R. and McColl, K.E.L. (1987). Drugs and the acute porphyrias. *Bollettino dell' Istituto Dermatologico S. Gallicano*, **13**, 151–8.

Parikh, R.K., and Moore, M.R. (1978). The effects of certain anaesthetic agents on the activity of rat hepatic delta aminolaevulinate synthase. *British Journal of Anaesthesia*, **50**, 1099–103.

Watson, C.J., Dhar, G.J., Bossemaier, I., Cardinal, R. and Petryka, Z.J. (1973). Effect of haematin in acute porphyric relapse. *Annals of Internal Medicine*, **79**, 80–92.

Yeung Laiwah, A.C., Moore, M.R., Goldberg, A. (1987). Pathogenesis of acute porphyria. *Quarterly Journal of Medicine*, **63**, 377–92.

Appendix 1: Drugs that are unsafe for use in acute porphyria

These drugs have been classified as 'unsafe' because all have been shown to be porphyrinogenic in animals or *in vitro* systems, or to have been associated with acute attacks in humans.

   () Drugs in parentheses are those in which there is conflicting experimental evidence of porphyrinogenicity – some positive, some negative.

   * Those marked in **bold** with an asterisk have been associated with acute attacks of porphyria.

Alcuronium
*Alphaxolone:A
   Alphadolone
Alprazolam
Aluminium preparations
Amidopyrine
Aminoglutethimide
Aminophylline
Amiodarone
(Amitriptyline)
(Amphetamines)
*Amylobarbitone
Antipyrine
Auranofin
Aurothiomalate
Azapropazone

Baclofen
*Barbiturates
*Bemegride
Bendrofluazide
Benoxaprofen
Benzbromarone
(Benzylthiouracil)
Bromocriptine
Busulphan

Captopril
*Carbamazepine
*Carbromal

*Carisoprodol
(Cefuroxime)
(Cephalexin)
(Cephalosporins)
(Cephradine)
(Chlorambucil)
*Chloramphenicol
*Chlordiazepoxide
Chlormezanone
Chloroform
*Chlorpropamide
(Cimetidine)
Cinnarizine
Clemastine
(Clobazam)
(Clomipramine HCl)
(Clonazepam)
Clonidine HCL
Clorazepate
Cocaine
(Colistin)
(Co-Trimoxazole)
Cyclophosphamide
Cycloserine
Cyclosporin

Danazol
Dapsone
Dexfenfluramine

Dextropropoxyphene
Diazepam
*Dichloralphenazone
Diclofenac Na
Diethylpropion
Dihydralazine
*Dihydroergotamine
Diltiazem
*Dimenhydrinate
*Diphenhydramine
(Dothiepin HCl)
Doxycycline
(Dydrogesterone)

Econazole nitrate
*Enalapril
Enflurane
*Ergot compounds
Ergometrine maleate
Ergotamine tartrate
*Erythromycin
Ethamsylate
*Ethanol
Ethionamide
Ethosuximide
Etidocaine
Etomidate

Fenfluramine
*Flucloxacillin

*Flufenamic acid
Flunitrazepam
Flupenthixol
Flurazepam
*Frusemide

*Glutethimide
Glipizide
Gramicidin
*Griseofulvin

(Haloperidol)
*Halothane
*Hydantoins
Hydralazine
*Hydrochlorothiazide
*Hydroxyzine
Hyoscine

*Imipramine
Iproniazid
Isometheptene mucate
(Isoniazid)

Ketoconazole

Lignocaine
*Lisinopril
Lofepramine
Loprazolam
Loxapine
Lysuride maleate

Maprotiline HCl
Mebeverine HCl
(Mefenamic acid)
Megestrol acetate
Mepivacaine
*Meprobamate
Mercaptopurine
Mercury compounds
Mestranol
(Metapramine HCl)
Methamphetamine
Methohexitone
Methotrexate
Methoxyflurane
Methsuximide
*Methyl dopa
*Methyl sulphonal
*Methyprylone
Methysergide
*Metoclopramide
Metyrapone
Mianserin HCl
Miconazole
(Mifepristone)
Minoxidil

Nalidixic acid
Natamycin

(Nandrolone)
(Nicergoline)
*Nifedipine
*Nikethamide
Nitrazepam
(Nitrofurantoin)
Nordazepam
Norethynodrel
(Nortriptyline)
Novobiocin

*Oral contraceptives
*Orphenadrine
(Oxazepam)
Oxybutynin HCl
Oxycodone
*Oxymetazoline
Oxyphenbutazone
Oxytetracycline

Paramethadione
*Pentazocine
Perhexiline
Phenacetin
Phenelzine
*Phenobarbitone
Phenoxybenzamine
Phensuximide
(Phenylbutazone)

Phenylhydrazine
*Phenytoin
*Piroxicam
*Pivampicillin
Prenylamine
*Prilocaine
*Primidone
(Probenecid)
*Progesterone
Promethazine
(Propanidid)
*Pyrazinamide
Pyrrocaine

Quinalbarbitone

Rifampicin

Simvastatin
Sodium aurothiomalate
Sodium oxybate
(Sodium valproate)
Spironolactone
Stanozolol
Succinimides
Sulphacetamide
*Sulphadimidine
Sulphadoxine
Sulphamethoxazole

*Sulphasalazine
Sulphonylureas
Sulphinpyrazone
Sulpiride
Sulthiame
Sultopride

Tamoxifen
*Terfenadine
Tetrazepam
*Theophylline
*Thiopentone
Thioridazine
Tilidate
Tinidazole
Tolazamide
Tolbutamide
Tranylcypromine
Trazodone HCl
Trimethoprim
(Trimipramine)
Troxidone

Valpromide
Veralipride
*Verapamil
Viloxazine HCl

Zuclopenthixol

Appendix 2: Drugs thought to be safe for use in acute porphyria

Each drug in parentheses () has had conflicting evidence of experimental porphyrinogenicity. Occasionally positive, but mainly negative – none of the drugs in this list has been associated with human porphyric attacks.

α-Tocopheryl-
    acetate
Acetazolamide
Acetylcholine
Actinomycin D
Acyclovir
Adrenaline
Alclofenac
Allopurinol
Amethocaine
Amiloride
Aminocaproic acid
Aminoglycosides
Amoxycillin
Amphotericin
Ampicillin
Ascorbic acid
Aspirin
Atenolol
Atropine
Azathioprine

β-Carotene
Beclomethasone
Benzhexol HCl
Biguanides
(Bromazepam)
Bromides
Bumetanide
Bupivacaine
Buprenorphine

Buserelin
Butacaine SO$_4$

Canthaxanthen
Carbimazole
(Carpipramine HCl)
Chloral hydrate
(Chlormethiazole)
(Chloroquine)
(Chlorothiazide)
Chlorpheniramine
Chlorpromazine
Ciprofloxacin
Cisplatin
Clavulanic acid
Clofibrate
Clomiphene citrate
Cloxacillin
Co-codamol
Codeine phosphate
Colchicine
(Corticosteroids)
Corticotrophin (ACTH)
Coumarins
Cyclizine
Cyclopenthiazide
Cyclopropane
(Cyproterone acetate)
Danthron
Desferrioxamine
Dexamethasone
(Dextromoramide)

Dextrose
Diamorphine
Diazoxide
Dicyclomine HCl
Diflunisal
Digoxin
Dihydrocodeine
Dimercaprol
Dimethicone
Dinoprost
Diphenoxylate HCl
Dipyridamole
(Disopyramide)
Domperidone
Doxorubicin HCl
Droperidol

Ethacrynic acid
Ethambutol
(Ethinyl oestradiol)
Ethoheptazine citrate
Etoposide

Famotidine
Fenbrufen
(Fenofibrate)
Fenoprofen
Fentanyl
Flucytosine
Flumazenil
Flurbiprofen
(Fluvoxamine maleate)
Folic acid

Fructose
Fusidic acid

Gentamicin
Glucagon
Glucose
Glyceryl trinitrate
Guanethidine

(Haloperidol)
Heparin
Hexamine
(Hydrocortisone)

Ibuprofen
Indomethacin
Insulin
Iron

(Ketamine)
Ketoprofen
Ketotifen

Labetalol
Lithium salts
Loperamide
(Lorazepam)

(Mebendazole)
Mecamylamine
Meclofenoxate HCl
Mefloquine HCl
(Melphalan)
Mequitazine
Metformin

Methadone
(Methotrimeprazine)
Methylphenidate
Methyluracil
Metoprolol
(Metronidazole)
Mianserin
(Midazolam)
Minaprine HCl
Minaxolone
Morphine

Nadolol
(Naproxen sodium)
Nefopam HCl
Neostigmine
Nitrous oxide
Norfloxacin

Ofloxacin
Oxybuprocaine
(Oxyphenbutazone)
Oxytocin

(Pancuronium bromide)
Paracetamol

Paraldehyde
Penicillamine
Penicillin
Pentolinium
Pethidine
Phenformin
Phenoperidine
Phentolamine mesylate
Piracetam
Pirbuterol
Pirenzepine
Pizotifen
(Prazosin)
(Prednisolone)
Primaquine
Procainamide HCl
Procaine
Prochlorperazine
Proguanil HCl
Promazine
Propantheline Br
Propofol
Propranolol

Propylthiouracil
(Proxymetacaine)
Pseudoephedrine HCl
Pyridoxine
(Pyrimethamine)

Quinidine
Quinine

(Ranitidine)
Reserpine
Resorcinol

Salbutamol
Senna
Sodium bromide
Sodium Ca EDTA
Sodium fusidate
Sorbitol
Streptomycin
Sulindac
Sulfadoxine
Suxamethonium

Temazepam

Tetracaine
(Tetracyclines)
Thiouracils
Thyroxine
Ticarcillin
Tienilic acid
Timolol maleate
Tranexamic acid
Triacetyloleandomycin
Triamterene
Triazolam
(Trichlormethiazide)
Trifluoperazine
Trimetazidine HCl
Tubocurarine

Vancomycin
(Vincristine)
Vitamins

Warfarin sodium

Zidovudine
Zinc preparations (topical)

Note

While very great care has been taken in the compilation of this list and the drug information is given in the belief that it is correct at the time of publication, all information contained herein and opinions expressed must be taken as information and opinions given for general guidance only.

The authors hereby disclaim for themselves, the Porphyrias Service, the University of Glasgow, and the Greater Glasgow Health Board, all responsibility for any misstatement or for the consequences to any person of any person acting in reliance on any statement or opinion contained herein.

Medical practitioners and patients must make their own decisions in the circumstances of the particular case about therapy appropriate in any case of acute porphyria.

DRUG NAMES GIVEN HEREIN ARE APPROVED NAMES, NOT TRADE OR COMMON NAMES

11.6 Lipid and lipoprotein disorders

P. N. DURRINGTON

Lipids are a heterogeneous group of substances, distinguished by their low solubility in water and their high solubility in a mixture of chloroform and methanol (2:1 v/v) and commonly in other non-polar (organic) solvents. The difference between an oil or fat is determined by the melting point. Lipids are essential as energy stores and respiratory substrates, as structural components of cells, as vitamins, as hormones, for the protection of internal organs, for heat conservation, for digestion, and for lactation. Lipoproteins are macromolecular complexes of lipid and protein, major roles of which are to transport lipids through the vascular and extravascular body fluids and as components of milk. The proteins present in the lipoproteins include apolipoproteins and enzymes. Increases in levels of a circulating lipoprotein are termed hyperlipoproteinaemia, and decreases, hypolipoproteinaemia. Disturbances of the composition of the circulating lipoproteins are described as dyslipoproteinaemia.

The greater part of this section will deal with the hyperlipoproteinaemias relevant to atherosclerosis, because that is the context in which lipid disorders most commonly present to clinicians, but it is undoubtedly the case that in the future they will be found to have wider involvement in disease processes.

Lipid physiology

Triglycerides (triacylglycerols)

These are formed by the esterification of glycerol with fatty acids, which have a hydrocarbon group attached to a carboxyl group. Generally the hydrocarbon part is present in a long chain. Naturally occurring fatty acids usually have even numbers of carbon atoms, most of them linked by single bonds; but some contain double bonds. Those with double bonds are termed unsaturated, whereas those with only single bonds are the saturated fatty acids. Fatty acids with one double bond are termed monounsaturated and those with more, polyunsaturated. Each double bond creates the possibility of two stereoisomers according to whether the hydrogen atoms of the —CH = CH— are both on the same side of the double bond (cis-) or on the opposite sides (trans-). Naturally occurring fatty acids are mostly cis-isomers. Trans-isomers are, however, present in the milk of ruminants, such as the cow, and in some margarines.

Triglycerides in adipose tissue provide our principal energy store. The body of a 70 kg man of ideal body weight contains some 15 kg of stored triglycerides, representing 135 000 Cal (560 000 J) of energy which would permit survival during total starvation for up to 3 months (compare this to 225 mg of glycogen, representing only 900 Cal (3800 J)). Obesity represents an excess of stored fat and it is unfortunately the case for those wishing to slim that considerable and very prolonged dietary energy restriction is necessary to lose weight, given the large amount of energy stored in fat. Each gram of triglyceride produces 9 cal (38 J) of energy, whereas the same mass of carbohydrate or protein only produces 4 cals (17 J), and the latter are more difficult to store because they require an aqueous environment. Thus a muscle or liver cell can only store a minute amount of glycogen. The adipocyte, on the other hand, contains a droplet of hydrophobic triglyceride surrounded by only a tiny rim of cytoplasm: probably 85 per cent of the adipocyte is triglyceride. Thus each gram of adipose tissue yields almost 8 cals (33 J) of energy, whereas tissues containing cells packed to capacity with glycogen would not even approach a yield of 1 cal (4.2 J) for each gram.

For other organs to utilize the energy in adipose tissue the stored triglyceride must first be hydrolysed to give its constituent glycerol and non-esterified fatty acids, a process known as lipolysis. This is accomplished by adipose tissue lipase, an intracellular enzyme, which is inhibited by insulin (not to be confused with lipoprotein lipase, an extracellular enzyme located on the vascular endothelium of fat and muscle and which is activated by insulin (see below)).

$$
\begin{array}{c}
\text{H}_2\text{COOCR} \\
| \\
\text{RCOOCH} \\
| \\
\text{H}_2\text{COOCR}
\end{array}
\quad + 3\text{H}_2\text{O}
\quad
\xrightarrow[\text{lipase}]{\substack{\text{intracellular} \\ \text{adipose tissue}}}
\quad
\begin{array}{c}
\text{CH}_2\text{OH} \\
| \\
\text{HOCH} \\
| \\
\text{CH}_2\text{OH}
\end{array}
\quad + 3\text{RCOOH}
$$

Triglyceride   Glycerol   non-esterified
                                                      fatty acids

The products of lipolysis are released into the circulation. The non-esterified fatty acids become bound to albumin. Normally their circulating concentration is 300 to 800 μmol/l (8–23 mg/dl), but this falls when insulin is secreted following a meal and rises in starvation when insulin secretion is low. Their importance as a system for transporting lipid energy should not be underestimated, even at low concentrations, since their half-life in the circulation is only 2 to 3 min and their turnover is thus 100 to 200 g/day, even more in starvation and in diabetes.

Non-esterified fatty acids can be oxidized to acetyl-CoA by some tissues, such as muscle and liver, and then entered into the Krebs (carboxylic acid) cycle. Other tissues, which in the fed state rely on glucose as an oxidative substrate, cannot directly utilize non-esterified fatty acids. During starvation these tissues are supplied with water-soluble ketone bodies (acetone, acetoacetate, β-hydroxybutyrate), which the liver produces by partial oxidization (β-oxidation) of non-esterified fatty acids transported to it from adipose tissue. These ketone bodies, which can readily be entered into the Krebs cycle by tissues lacking the ability to oxidize fatty acids, constitute the second system for the transport of lipid energy. They are vital for survival when dietary energy is at a premium, but are also the cause of diabetic ketoacidosis when the insulin production is insufficient to suppress the flux of non-esterified fatty acids from adipose tissue, so that the production of ketone bodies takes place at a faster rate than they can be respired. The amount of insulin required to decrease blood glucose increases in the presence of high levels of circulating non-esterified fatty acids. The higher flux of non-esterified fatty acids out of adipose tissue in diabetes thus contributes to insulin resistance. In the case of non-insulin-dependent diabetes a high rate of release of non-esterified fatty acids may have predated the development of hyperglycaemia by many years, because obesity, which is a common antecedent of this type of diabetes, is itself associated with an increased flux of non-esterified fatty acids through the circulation and with insulin resistance.

Phospholipids

These also have at least one fatty acyl group esterified to an alcohol and one phosphate group linked both to the alcohol and to another organic compound. The glycerolipids have glycerol as the alcohol. Examples of these are phosphatidylcholine (lecithin) and lysophosphatidylcholine (lysolecithin). Another abundant class of phospholipids are the sphingolipids, such as sphingyomyelin. Phospholipids are essential components of cell membranes and, because of the great diversity of their physical properties permitted by their structure, are responsible for much of the diversity of membrane structure.

Cholesterol

Cholesterol is also an essential component of cell membranes, where it allows the phospholipid molecules to pack more closely, increasing membrane rigidity. It is also a precursor for the synthesis of steroid hormones, vitamin D, and bile acids. It is present in arterial fatty streaks and in atheromatous plaques (see below).

Cholesterol is an alcohol and may be unesterified as free cholesterol or esterified with a fatty acyl group (Fig. 1).

Lipoprotein physiology

LIPOPROTEIN STRUCTURE

The general structure of lipoprotein molecules is globular (Fig. 2). The physicochemical considerations, which govern the arrangement of their constituents, are similar to those involved in the formation of mixed micelles in the lumen of the intestine. Thus, within the outer part of the lipoprotein are found the more polar lipids, namely the phospholipids and free cholesterol, with their charged groups pointing out towards the water molecules. In physical terms, however, the role of bile salts, which are also in the outer layer in the mixed micelle, is assumed by proteins, so that the surface of a lipoprotein structurally resembles the outer half of a cell membrane. Within the core of the lipoprotein particle are the more hydrophobic lipids, the esterified cholesterol and triglycerides. These form a central droplet, to which are anchored, by their hydrophobic regions, the surface-coating molecules, phospholipids, free cholesterol, and proteins. The exception to this general structure is the newly formed or nascent high density lipoprotein (HDL), which lacks the central lipid droplet and appears to exist as a disc-like bilayer, consisting largely of phospholipids and proteins.

The protein components of lipoproteins are the apolipoproteins, a group of proteins of immense structural diversity, some of which have a largely structural role and others of which are major metabolic regulators. In addition, enzymes are found as components of lipoproteins. The leading example is lecithin: cholesterol acyltransferase which is located on the HDLs, which are also its site of action.

Fig. 1 The structure of free cholesterol and cholesteryl ester.

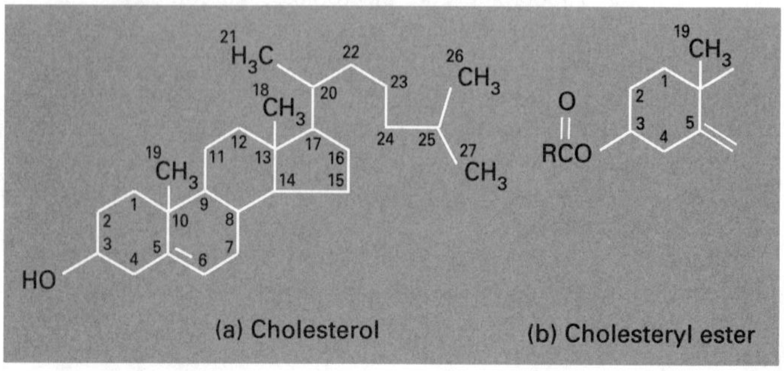

(a) Cholesterol   (b) Cholesteryl ester

LIPID TRANSPORT FROM LIVER AND GUT TO PERIPHERAL TISSUES

The products of fat digestion (fatty acids, monoglycerides, lysolecithin, and free cholesterol) enter the enterocytes from the mixed micelles. They are re-esterified in the smooth endoplasmic reticulum of these cells. Long-chain fatty acids (> 14C) are esterified with monoglycerides to form triglycerides and with lysolecithin to form lecithin. Free cholesterol is esterified by the enzyme, acyl-CoA: cholesterol O-acyltransferase.

The triglycerides, phospholipids, and cholesteryl esters are then combined with an apolipoprotein, known as apo B_{48}, in the enterocyte. The lipoproteins thus formed are secreted into the lymph (chyle) and are termed chylomicrons. They are large (diameter > 75 nm; density < 950 g/l) and are rich in triglycerides, but contain only relatively small amounts of protein (Fig. 3). They travel through the lacteals to join lymph from other parts of the body and enter the blood circulation via the thoracic duct. In addition to cholesterol absorbed from the diet, the chylomicrons may also receive cholesterol that has been newly synthesized in the gut or transferred from other lipoproteins present in the lymph and plasma. The newly secreted, or nascent, chylomicrons receive C apolipoproteins from HDL, which in that respect appears to act as a circulating reservoir, since later in the course of the metabolism of the chylomicron, the C apolipoproteins are transferred back to the HDL pool. The chylomicrons also receive apolipoprotein E (apo E), although the manner in which they do so is unclear. Unlike other apo-lipoproteins, which are synthesized either in the liver or the gut, or both, apo E is exceptional in that it is synthesized (and perhaps secreted) by a large number of tissues: liver, brain, spleen, kidney, lungs, and adrenal gland.

Once the chylomicron has acquired the apolipoprotein, apo CII, it is capable of activating the enzyme, lipoprotein lipase (Fig. 4(a). This enzyme is located on the vascular endothelium of tissues with a high requirement for triglycerides, such as skeletal and cardiac muscle (for energy), adipose tissue (for storage), and lactating mammary gland (for milk). Lipoprotein lipase releases triglycerides from the core of the chylomicron by hydrolysing them to fatty acids and glycerol, which are taken up by the tissues locally. In this way the circulating chylomicron becomes progressively smaller. Its triglyceride content decreases and it becomes relatively richer in cholesterol and protein. As the core shrinks, its surface materials (phospholipids, free cholesterol, C apolipoproteins) become too crowded and they are transferred to HDL. The cholesteryl ester-enriched, triglyceride-depleted product of chylomicron metabolism is known as the chylomicron remnant. The apo B_{48}, present from the time of assembly, remains tightly anchored to the core throughout. The apo E also remains and regions of its structure are exposed, permitting chylomicron remnant catabolism via the 'remnant receptor' of the liver and also the low density lipoprotein (LDL) receptors (also

Fig. 2 Lipoprotein structure. The most hydrophobic lipids (triglycerides, cholesteryl esters) form a central droplet-like core, which is surrounded by more polar lipids (phospholipids, free cholesterol) at the water interface. Apolipoproteins are anchored by their more hydrophobic regions, with their more polar regions often exposed to the surface. (Reproduced from Durrington 1994, with permission.)

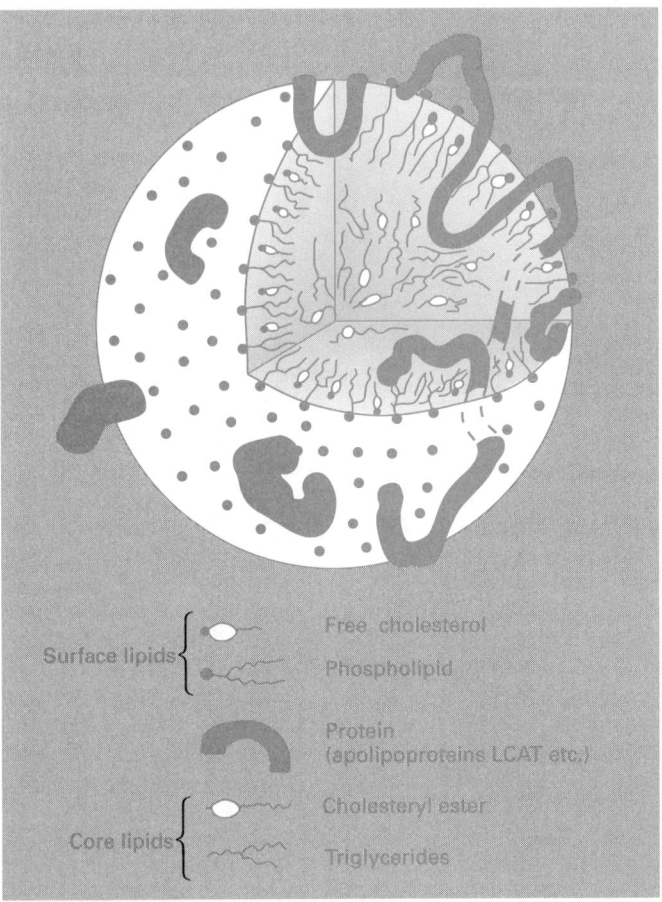

Fig. 3 The spectrum of plasma lipoprotein particles according to their hydrated density, molecular mass, molecular diameter, relative concentration, lipid composition, and apolipoprotein composition. (Reproduced from Durrington 1994, with permission.)

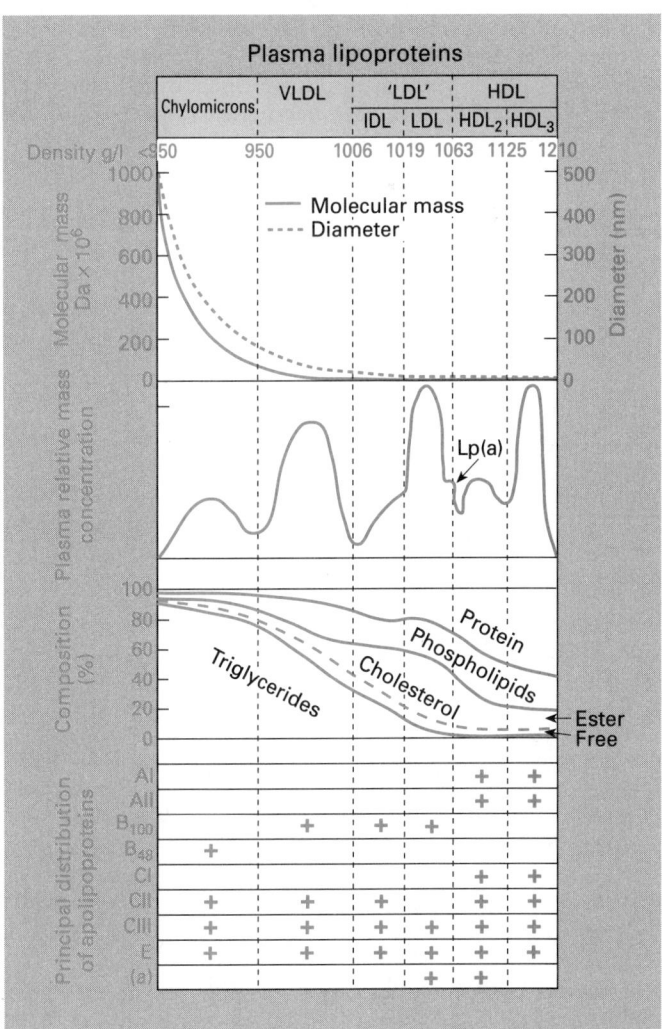

called apo B$_{100}$/E receptors), which can be expressed by virtually every cell in the body, including the liver. It is possible that apo E is inhibited from binding to its receptors earlier in the metabolism of chylomicrons, because its receptor-binding domain is blocked by the apolipoprotein, apo CIII. Remnants are largely removed from the circulation by the liver. Although the clearance of these particles via the LDL receptor is theoretically possible, this route is not likely to contribute greatly to remnant uptake in the adult, since the binding affinity of the hepatic apo E receptor for apo E is greater and the remnant particles must compete for binding at the LDL receptor with LDL, the particle concentration of which is much higher that of the chylomicron remnants (even more so in the tissue fluid than in the plasma). Also the LDL receptor is rapidly down-regulated by the lysosomal release of free cholesterol into the cell, which follows the entry of lipoprotein–receptor complexes into the cell, whereas expression of the remnant clearance pathway is unaffected by entry of cholesterol into the liver.

The liver itself secretes a triglyceride-rich lipoprotein known as very low density lipoprotein (VLDL). Teleologically, this allows the supply of triglycerides to tissues in the fasting state as well as postprandially. VLDL particles are somewhat smaller than the chylomicrons (diameter 30–45 nm; density < 1006 g/l). Once secreted they undergo exactly the same sequence of changes as chylomicrons; that is the acquisition of apolipoproteins and the progressive removal of triglycerides from their core by the enzyme, lipoprotein lipase. However, some additional transformations are involved in their metabolism in the human. In man, the liver, unlike the gut, does not esterify cholesterol before its secretion. This is different from the situation in species such as the rat. In the human, most of the cholesterol released from the liver each day into the circulation is secreted in the VLDL as free cholesterol, and it undergoes esterification in the circulation. Free cholesterol is transferred to HDL along a concentration gradient. There it is esterified by the action of the enzyme, lecithin:cholesterol acyl transferase, which esterifies the hydroxyl group in the 3-position of cholesterol to a fatty acyl group.

This it selectively removes from the 2-position of lecithin to give lyso-lecithin. The fatty acyl group in this position is generally unsaturated and the cholesteryl esters thus formed are frequently cholesteryl oleate or cholesteryl linoleate. Familial deficiency of lecithin:cholesterol acyl-transferase is a very rare disorder, in which HDL fails to mature, and circulating free cholesterol levels increase. It leads to anaemia, corneal opacities, proteinuria, and renal failure.

Esterified cholesterol on HDL is transferred back to VLDL. This cannot take place by simple diffusion, because cholesteryl ester is intensely hydrophobic and because the concentration gradient is unfavourable. A special protein called cholesteryl ester transfer protein, or lipid transfer protein, is present in plasma, which transports cholesteryl ester from HDL to VLDL. It does this in exchange for triglycerides in VLDL and thus also contributes to the removal of core triglycerides from VLDL. The major mechanism for the removal of triglycerides from VLDL is, however, lipolysis catalysed by lipoprotein lipase.

Another major difference between VLDL and chylomicrons is that the apolipoprotein B produced by the liver in man is not apo B$_{48}$, but is almost entirely apo B$_{100}$. As in the case of chylomicrons, the quantum of apo B packaged in the VLDL remains tightly associated with the particle until its final catabolism and its amount does not vary after secretion. It is probable that each molecule of VLDL contains one molecule of apo B$_{100}$. The apo B$_{100}$ produced in the liver contains the protein sequence necessary to bind to the LDL receptors, whereas that produced by the gut, although derived from the same gene, does not, due to a process of 'gene editing', which stops the ribosome translating the messenger RNA before the receptor-binding sequence, producing an apo B with 48 per cent of the molecular mass of that from the liver.

The circulating VLDL particles become progressively smaller as their core is removed by lipolysis and surface materials are transferred to HDL. In normal man most of the VLDL is converted to smaller LDL particles through the intermediary of a lipoprotein known as intermediate density lipoprotein (IDL). This has a density of 1006–1019 g/l and

Fig. 4 Metabolism of (a) triglyceride-rich lipoproteins secreted by the gut and liver; and (b) hepatic triglyceride-rich lipoproteins and lipoproteins transporting cholesterol to and from the tissues.

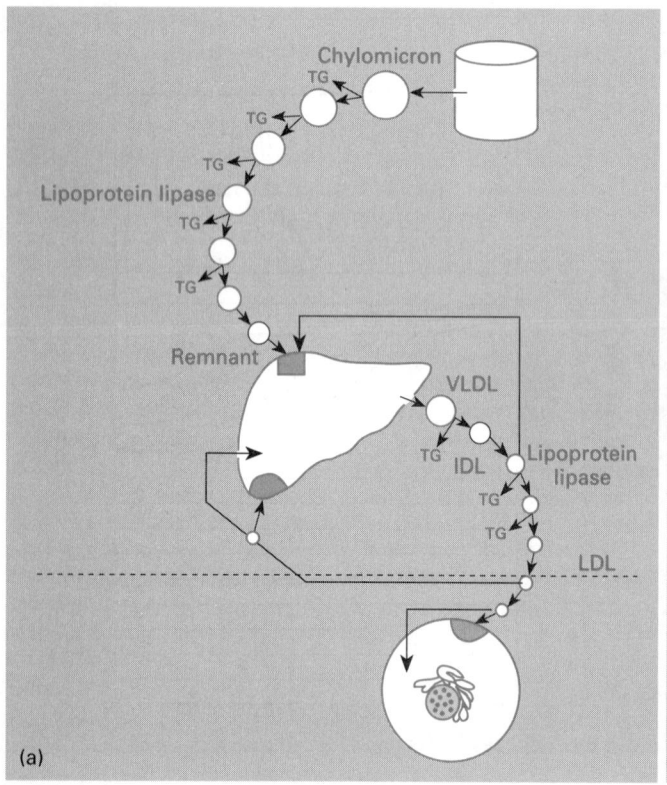
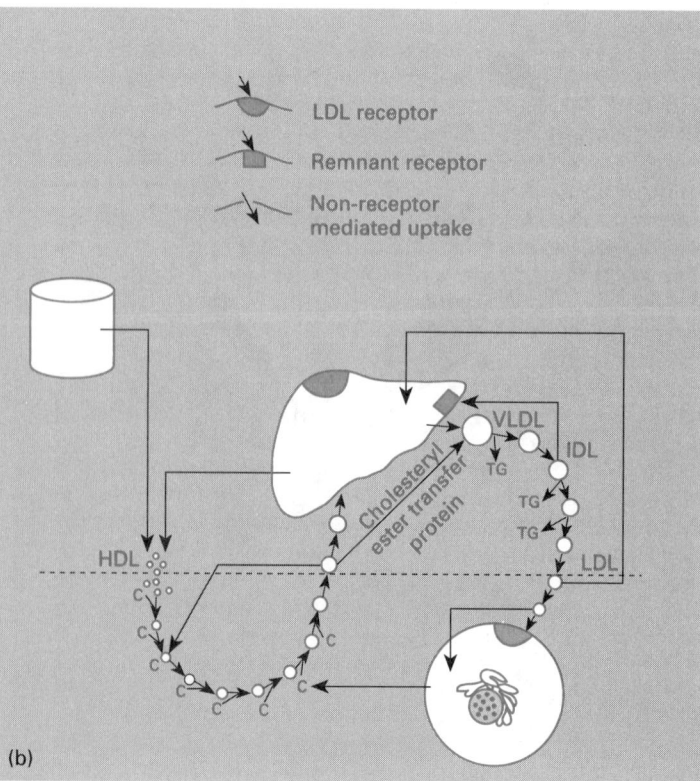

possesses apo E. In this latter respect it is similar to chylomicron remnants. In some species, such as the rat, it is largely removed by the hepatic remnant receptor, and LDL formation is thus bypassed. The enzyme, hepatic lipase, may be important in the conversion of IDL to LDL.

In man, LDL particles, which are relatively enriched in cholesterol, but are small enough (diameter 18–25 nm; density 1019–1063 g/l) to cross the vascular endothelium and enter the tissue fluid, serve to deliver cholesterol to the tissues. Their concentration in the extracellular fluid is probably about 10 per cent of that in the plasma. Cells require cholesterol for membrane repair and growth and, in the case of specialized tissues such as the adrenal gland, gonads, and skin, as a precursor for steroid hormone and vitamin D synthesis. LDL is able to enter cells by two routes making a major contribution to its catabolism: one which is regulated according to the cholesterol requirement of each individual cell, and one which appears to depend almost entirely on the extracellular concentrations of LDL.

The first of these two routes is by a cell-surface receptor, which specifically binds lipoproteins that contain apolipoprotein B_{100} or E. This is the LDL receptor. As mentioned previously, the receptor, although capable of binding apo E-containing lipoproteins, in practice usually binds largely to the apo B_{100}-containing lipoproteins of which LDL is the most widely distributed. After binding, the LDL–receptor complex is internalized within the cell, where it undergoes lysosomal degradation. Its apo B is hydrolysed to its constituent amino acids, and its cholesteryl ester is hydrolysed to free cholesterol. The release of this free cholesterol is the signal by which the cellular cholesterol content is precisely regulated by three co-ordinated reactions. First the enzyme, which is rate-limiting for cholesterol biosysthesis (3-hydroxy, 3- methylglutaryl CoA reductase), is repressed, thus effectively centralizing cholesteryl biosynthesis to organs such as the liver and gut. Secondly, the synthesis of the LDL receptor itself is suppressed. Thirdly, acyl-CoA:cholesterol O-acyltransferase is activated so that any cholesterol that is surplus to immediate requirements can be converted to cholesteryl ester, which, because of its hydrophobic nature, forms into droplets within the cytoplasm and is thus conveniently stored. The effect of the lysosomal release of free cholesterol on the expression of the LDL receptor contrasts with its effect on the hepatic remnant receptor, which is not subject to any similar down-regulatory process. Free cholesterol released by lysosomal digestion of cholesteryl ester-rich, apo E-containing lipoproteins entering the hepatocyte via the remnant receptor does not influence its own expression; it will, nevertheless, down-regulate the hepatic LDL receptors. Defective LDL uptake by the LDL receptor is the basis of familial hypercholesterolaemia (see below).

The other quantitatively important mechanism by which LDL cholesterol may enter cells is by a non-receptor-mediated pathway: LDL binds to cell membranes at sites other than those where the LDL receptors are located and some of it passes through the membrane by pinocytosis. HDL is able to compete with LDL for this type of cell-membrane association. The absence of a receptor means that the 'binding' is of low affinity and thus, at low concentrations, LDL entry by this route may have little significance. However, unlike receptor-mediated entry, non-receptor-mediated LDL uptake, is not saturable, but continues to increase with increasing extracellular LDL concentrations. When LDL levels are relatively high, entry of cholesterol into the cells by this route may thus assume greater quantitative importance than that via the LDL receptor, which will be both saturated and down-regulated. This appears to be the situation in the typical adult consuming a high fat diet in Britain, whose LDL cholesterol is high relative to most animal species and in whom only about one-third of LDL is catabolized by receptors and two-thirds by non-receptor-mediated pathways. In hypercholesterolaemia, even more is catabolized via the non-receptor pathway (four-fifths in patients heterozygous for familial hypercholesterolaemia, virtually all in homozygotes, see below).

LDL may also be removed from the circulation by a number of receptors other than the classical LDL receptor. Probably these are responsible

for the catabolism of only relatively minor amounts of LDL, but two such receptors present on the macrophage have excited considerable interest, because they may lie at the heart of atherogenesis. They are the beta-VLDL receptor, a modified LDL receptor, which allows the uptake of the beta-VLDL from patients with type III hyperlipoproteinaemia (see below), and the acetyl-LDL receptor, which permits the uptake of modified LDL by macrophages. Uptake at both these receptors is so rapid *in vitro* that foam cells resembling those in arterial fatty streaks are formed. On the other hand, uptake of unmodified LDL by the macrophage via the LDL receptor is too slow for foam cell formation. Modifications, which permit LDL uptake at the acetyl-LDL receptor include acetylation (hence its name) but also oxidation, which may occur *in vivo* and is of potential relevance to atherogenesis (see below).

Lipoprotein (a)

Lipoprotein (a) (Lp(a)) is a lipoprotein first identified as a result of blood transfusion reactions occurring due to genetic variation in its antigenicity. Its precise location in the LDL and HDL_2 also varies from individual to individual, as does its serum concentration. It may be undetectable in some people or present at concentrations equalling those of LDL in others. The protein moiety of Lp(a) like that of LDL contains apo B_{100}, but, in addition, apolipoprotein (a) (apo(a)) is also present. This is a huge homologue of plasminogen, in which part of the plasminogen protein sequence (the kringle 4 domain) is repeated many times. The number of these repeats, which is determined at a genetic locus adjacent to the plasminogen gene, determines the molecular mass of apo (a), and individuals expressing polymorphisms with fewer kringle 4 repeats have the highest serum concentrations of Lp(a). Lp(a) is associated with the risk of coronary heart disease in people of European origin, particularly when serum cholesterol levels are also raised and when there is a family history of premature coronary heart disease. It does not possess fibrinolytic activity, because of a mutation of its activation site. It has, therefore, been suggested that it may interfere with thrombolysis. Furthermore because Lp(a) binds to a wide variety of cells and connective tissue matrices, it is retained in the arterial wall longer than LDL and is thus more likely to undergo oxidative modification and macrophage uptake, leading to atheroma (see below).

TRANSPORT OF CHOLESTEROL FROM TISSUES BACK TO LIVER

In the human, cholesterol is transported out of the gut and liver in quantities which greatly exceed its peripheral catabolism (largely as a result of conversion to steroid hormones and skin loss in sebum). Therefore, except when the requirement for membrane synthesis is high, for example during growth or active tissue repair, the greater part of the cholesterol transported to the tissues (if it is not to accumulate there) must be returned to the liver for elimination in the bile, or for reassembly into lipoproteins. The return of cholesterol from the tissues to the liver is termed 'reverse cholesterol transport'. It is less well understood than the pathways by which cholesterol reaches the tissues, but it may well be critical to the development of atheroma. HDL has many features that make it very likely that it is intimately involved in the reverse transport process.

The precursors of plasma HDL (nascent HDL) are probably disc-shaped bilayers composed largely of protein and phospholipid secreted mainly by the gut and liver (Fig. 4(b)). These are converted to the spherical, mature form of HDL by the action of lecithin:cholesterol acyltransferase. HDL components are also derived from surplus material (phospholipids, free cholesterol, and apoproteins) of triglyceride-rich lipoproteins released during lipolysis. Apolipoproteins AI and AII, which are the major apolipoproteins of HDL, and apolipoprotein E have been identified in nascent HDL. Other apolipoproteins and the bulk of its lipid are acquired as it circulates through the vascular and other extracellular fluids. In this respect the transformation of HDL from its lipid-poor precursor to a relatively lipid-rich molecule is the opposite of that undergone by the other lipoproteins following their secretion.

HDL is a small particle compared with the other lipoproteins (diameter 5–12 nm; density 1063–1210 g/l) and easily crosses the vascular endothelium, so that its concentration in the tissue fluids is much closer to its intravascular concentration than is the case for LDL. Because the serum HDL cholesterol concentration is only about one-quarter that of the LDL, it is often wrongly assumed that its particle concentration is lower. In fact, the particle concentrations of HDL and LDL in human plasma are often similar, and in the tissue fluids there are several times as many HDL molecules as those of other lipoproteins unless the capillary endothelium is fenestrated. Generally, therefore, cells are in contact with higher concentrations of HDL molecules than of any other lipoprotein. In man, unlike the rat, HDL serves no function in transporting cholesterol to cells.

Recently it has been suggested that cells express receptors for HDL, particularly HDL_3, which might permit the transfer of cholesterol out of the cell. Passage across the cell membrane may not simply depend on receptors, however, since free cholesterol can cross by diffusion. Factors regulating the balance between intracellular cholesterol esterification and free cholesterol (activities of acyl-CoA:cholesterol O acyltransferase and cholesterol esterase) and free cholesterol may also therefore be important. Apo E synthesized within certain cells may also be instrumental in transporting cholesterol out on to HDL. Once outside the cell, free cholesterol must be re-esterified in order that it can be transported in any quantity in the core of lipoproteins. Therefore, whether or not HDL is involved as the initial acceptor molecule, cholesterol must at some stage on its return journey to the liver reside on HDL, because it is the site of lecithin:cholesterol acyltransferase activity. However, once cholesterol has been esterified and packed into the core of HDL, simple clearance of the whole lipoprotein particle by the liver is not the route by which most cholesterol is returned to it. This is because LDL equivalent to 1500 mg of cholesterol is produced each day, whereas the rate of catabolism of the HDL apolipoproteins AI and AII would permit less than 200 mg of HDL cholesterol to be returned each day. Therefore:

(1) the liver must be capable of selectively removing cholesterol from HDL and then returning the particle to the circulation with most of its apolipoproteins intact, or

(2) the cholesterol in HDL must be transferred to another lipoprotein class which is capable of being cleared in quantity by the liver, or

(3) a class of HDL, which contains little apo AI or AII, must be cleared by the liver at a much greater rate than the bulk of HDL.

In support of (1), there is some evidence that hepatic lipase might act on the phospholipid envelope of HDL during its passage through hepatic sinusoids, and release the cholesteryl ester contained in its core, and that some hepatic trapping or even a receptor-mediated mechanism might enhance the process. On the other hand, in support of (2) there is a well-established mechanism for the transfer of cholesteryl ester from HDL to VLDL through the agency of cholesteryl ester transfer protein. Once on VLDL, the conversion of this lipoprotein to IDL and then LDL means that the cholesteryl ester can then arrive at the liver via remnant receptors, LDL receptors, or by the non-receptor-mediated route for LDL uptake. Evidence for pathway (3), the return of cholesterol to the liver from HDL by a rapidly metabolized form of HDL present at low concentration in serum, is at present largely lacking in man, although it is possible that binding of the subclass of HDL containing apo E to hepatic remnant receptors permits the return of some cholesterol to the liver.

It is incorrect to regard HDL as a single homogeneous species, since it is known to be a mixture of particles differing in size, in lipid and apolipoprotein composition, and in function. Two peaks are seen in the analytical ultracentrifuge, the less dense of which is designated HDL_2 ($d = 1063$–1125 g/l) and the more dense, HDL_3 ($d = 1125$–1210 g/l).

HDL_3 may be converted to HDL_2 by the acquisition of cholesterol, HDL_3 thus being a precursor of HDL_2. Whereas antisera to apo AI precipitate virtually all of HDL, antisera to AII do not, suggesting that some molecules of HDL contain AI and AII, whereas others contain AI only. The AI-only HDL molecules, which predominate in HDL_2, may arise from different metabolic channels than do the AI/AII particles. Apo E-containing HDL, as has previously been mentioned, may also have a different metabolic fate. Furthermore, HDL may contain other molecular species with overlapping density ranges, such as Lp(a). HDL thus represents a rather heterogeneous entity.

Disorders produced by raised levels of lipoproteins

Coronary heart disease incidence varies enormously in different parts of the world. Those countries with a Northern European culture (and in particular diet) have the highest rates, and places such as China, Japan, and rural Africa the lowest. Mediterranean countries are intermediate. There are, of course, many differences between these countries, but the one that relates most closely to coronary heart disease is the median cholesterol of the middle-aged male population. Of considerable interest is that in a country such as Japan, where the average serum cholesterol is low, other coronary risk factors do not seem to operate. Thus in Japan coronary heart disease is comparatively uncommon, even in cigarette smokers and people with diabetes and hypertension.

Within populations there is an exponential relationship between serum cholesterol and the incidence of coronary heart disease (Fig. 5). This depends on the LDL cholesterol which comprises some 70 to 80 per cent total cholesterol in men and a little less in women. The greater part of the rest of the cholesterol in serum is on HDL, and the concentration of this HDL cholesterol is inversely related to the likelihood of developing coronary heart disease.

Fig. 5 Probability of 50-year-old men developing coronary heart disease each year as a function of serum cholesterol concentration, in the absence and in the presence of increasing numbers of risk factors. (Data from Kannel *et al.* 1973.)

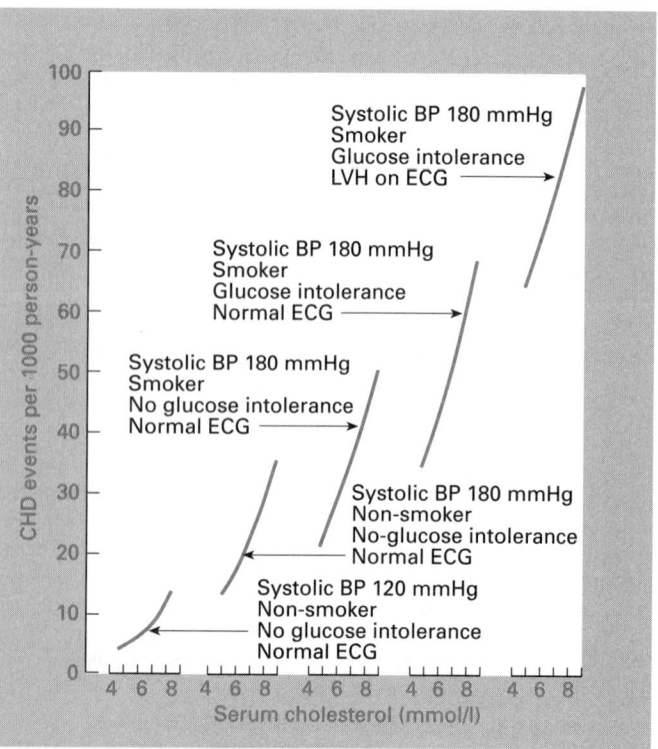

In populations in which death from coronary heart disease is common, fatty streaks are evident in the arteries, such as the aorta, of men dying in their late teens of causes unrelated to cardiovascular disease. This was seen dramatically in American casualties in the Korean and Vietnam wars. The fatty streak is the precursor of atheroma (see Section 15). The epidemiological and histopathological evidence implicating LDL in atherogenesis seems overwhelming. Yet in tissue culture LDL uptake by macrophages or smooth muscle cells proves disappointingly slow and foam cells are not formed. Recently, the probable answer to this conundrum was discovered when it was found that the macrophage has a receptor, which will allow the rapid uptake of LDL to form foam cells, if the LDL has undergone some chemical modification. The receptor is known as the acetyl-LDL receptor (after the first experimental chemical modification leading to its discovery) or the scavenger receptor. It is thought likely that the chemical modification leading to LDL uptake in human atherogenesis is oxidation of the polyunsaturated fatty acyl groups of phospholipids of LDL which has crossed the arterial endothelium to enter the subintimal space. The lipid peroxides so formed break down to lysophospholipids and aldehydes, which directly damage the apo B of the LDL, which can then bind to the scavenger receptor. The same substances are directly cytotoxic and may further damage the overlying arterial endothelium, increasing its permeability, and the oxidatively modified LDL itself is chemotactic to blood monocytes (from which arterial wall macrophages are derived) and may thus aid recruitment of more of these cells into the lesion.

In addition to uptake of LDL through the scavenger receptor, macrophages can also take up aggregated LDL to become foam cells by phagocytosis, and LDL–antibody complexes via Fc receptors. Other lipoproteins can also be taken up to form foam cells. In particular, the beta-VLDL (a mixture of chylomicron remnants and IDL), which accumulates in the circulation in type III hyperlipoproteinaemias (see below), is rapidly taken up by a macrophage receptor.

Triglyceride-rich lipoproteins can also be taken up by macrophages by phagocytosis to form foam cells, although because of their large size these would not be expected to cross the vascular endothelium unless it is fenestrated. Thus in extreme hypertriglyceridaemia lipid-engorged macrophages are present in the reticuloendothelial system. They are found, for example, on bone marrow biopsy, and are the cause of the hepatosplenomegaly associated with extreme hypertriglyceridaemia. When hypertriglyceridaemia occurs in association with elevated levels of LDL cholesterol, it increases the likelihood of atheroma developing still further, perhaps because this combination is associated with low serum HDL cholesterol, perhaps because of an increase in circulating IDL and delayed clearance of chylomicron remnants, perhaps because it is associated with smaller LDL particles, which are more readily oxidized, or perhaps because there are associated increases in the coagulability of blood due to increased plasma fibrinogen levels and factor VII activity. When, however, triglyceride-rich lipoproteins are increased without any increase in LDL, as in familial lipoprotein lipase deficiency (see below), there appears to be no increase in atheroma risk. There is, however, an increased likelihood of acute pancreatitis in all types of severe hypertriglyceridaemia both primary and secondary, particularly when serum triglyceride levels exceed 20 to 30 mmol/l (2000–3000 mg/dl). The cause of this is not known for certain, but may be because of direct damage to the pancreas by fatty acids released as a result of lipolysis due to pancreatic lipase leaking into pancreatic capillaries, or pancreatic damage due to the products of lipid peroxidation, both of which would be enhanced when increased concentrations of large triglyceride-rich lipoproteins move sluggishly through the pancreatic microcirculation.

Normal serum lipid concentrations

Whereas the average serum concentrations of most substances, for example sodium or fasting glucose, are much the same in all parts of the world, cholesterol displays considerable variation. In Britain the median serum cholesterol for a middle-aged man is 6.1 mmol/l and deaths from coronary heart disease comprise around 40 per cent of total mortality at this age. In China the average for men of middle age is 2 mmol/l less, and coronary heart disease accounts for less than 5 per cent of their deaths.

Conventionally, the normal range for a variable in a particular population is chosen to include values between the 2.5 and 97.5 percentiles, or sometimes the 1 and 99 percentile, on the assumption that 19 out of 20 of the population, or 49 out of 50, respectively, are normal. To be rational, the implication in a medical context must also be that those people in the normal range are healthy. In the case of cholesterol, which is clearly linked to coronary heart disease, the healthy range must therefore be that of a society in which coronary heart disease is uncommon, such as China or Japan. This has led the National Institute of Health in the United States of America and the European Atherosclerosis Society to define healthy limits for serum cholesterol based on the risk of coronary heart disease. Thus an optimal serum cholesterol is 5.2 mmol/l (200 mg/dl) or less. A level of 6.3 mmol/l (250 mg/dl) (at the 75th percentile in the United States) is considered to indicate 'moderate risk' and 6.7 mmol/l (270 mg/dl), which is the 90th percentile in the United States, 'high risk'. Some caution is required in using this concept. The risk of fatal coronary heart disease in an American middle-aged male population whose serum cholesterol is 5 mmol/litre (200 mg/dl) over the next 6 years is about 6 in 1000. At 6 mmol/l (250 mg/dl) it is about doubled, but that is only 10 in 1000, and at 7 mmol/l (270 mg/dl) it is still less than 15 in 1000. Thus although these levels may be of great importance for public health initiatives aimed at reducing the cholesterol level in societies in which the risk of coronary heart disease is high, the clinician must be wary about overtreating men with cholesterol at these levels, if it is their only risk factor for coronary heart disease. The risk conferred by a particular level of cholesterol increases considerably when it is combined with another risk factor and this may considerably increase the benefits of treatment (Fig. 5). This is why there can be no single cholesterol level which demands a particular therapeutic response: the cholesterol value must always be viewed in the context of an individual's overall cardiovascular risk (see below).

An upper limit of normality for fasting serum triglycerides is often regarded as 2.2 mmol/l (200 mg/dl). This is close to the 90th percentile for men and the 95th percentile for women. For serum HDL cholesterol a lower limit of normality of 0.9 mmol/l (35 mg/dl) is frequently quoted, which is close to the 10th percentile for men and between the 5th and the 10th percentile for women.

The Fredrickson/WHO classification

The concentration of four classes of serum lipoproteins when elevated can be regarded as pathological. These are chylomicrons, VLDL, LDL, and beta-VLDL. The hyperlipoproteinaemias can be classified according to which of them is increased (Table 1).

The Fredrickson/WHO classification causes great confusion, largely because it is difficult to remember and is frequently wrongly regarded as a diagnostic classification when it is simply a way of reporting which of the serum lipoproteins are elevated. It is usually sufficient to remember that when cholesterol alone is elevated there is a type IIa hyperlipoproteinaemia. When both cholesterol and triglycerides are elevated the hyperlipoproteinaemia is generally type IIb, but occasionally it is type V (the serum will look milky if it is) and rarely type III. Type I is extraordinarily rare. An isolated increase in fasting serum triglycerides almost invariably signifies type IV hyperlipoproteinaemia.

All hospital laboratories, in addition to measuring cholesterol and triglyceride levels, should also measure HDL cholesterol in patients whose overall cardiovascular risk is being critically assessed when treatment of their hyperlipoproteinaemia with drugs is under consideration. Particularly in women, an elevated level of cholesterol may result from

Table 1 *The Fredrickson/WHO classification of hyperlipoproteinaemia*

Type	Lipoprotein increased	Lipids increased
I	Chylomicrons	Triglycerides
IIa	LDL	Cholesterol
IIb	LDL and VLDL	Cholesterol and triglycerides
III	beta-VLDL (= IDL + chylomicron remnants)	Cholesterol and triglycerides
IV	VLDL	Triglycerides
V	Chylomicrons and VLDL	Cholesterol and triglycerides

a relatively high HDL cholesterol concentration and thus not signify any increased risk of coronary heart disease. High serum HDL cholesterol does not have a Fredrickson/WHO class, but as evidence suggests it is associated with longevity, it cannot be regarded as hyperlipoproteinaemia in the pathological sense. It is low HDL cholesterol which is associated with an increased cardiovascular risk, particularly if total serum cholesterol and triglycerides are also elevated.

Primary hyperlipoproteinaemias

Primary hyperlipoproteinaemias in which there is hypercholesterolaemia (type IIa)

Serum cholesterol levels exceeding 6.5 mmol/l are common in adults in Britain and much of Europe, the United States, Australia, and New Zealand. In Britain, for example, 25 to 30 per cent of middle-aged people have levels exceeding this, and the proportion in the United States is at least 10 per cent. Most of this hypercholesterolaemia does not represent the effect of any single cause, but is due to some combination of dietary fat, obesity, and individual susceptibility to develop hypercholesterolaemia. This susceptibility is partly genetic, probably involving more than one gene, and this common type of hypercholesterolaemia is usually referred to as polygenic hypercholesterolaemia. At the very top end of the cholesterol distribution are to be found individuals who have the less common monogenic condition, familial hypercholesterolaemia.

FAMILIAL HYPERCHOLESTEROLAEMIA

Heterozygous familial hypercholesterolaemia

Familial hypercholesterolaemia is a dominantly inherited. The heterozygous form of the condition affects about 1 in 500 people in Britain and the United States, making it the most common genetic disorder in these countries. In some populations, such as the Lebanese Christians, the Afrikaner and Cape-coloured peoples of South Africa, and French Canadians, it is considerably more common. This is because such people have descended from a relatively small number of early settlers, a few of whom by chance had familial hypercholesterolaemia. This is known as a founder effect. In yet other populations, such as Africans who have not intermingled with Europeans, familial hypercholesterolaemia is rare.

Typically, the serum cholesterol in adult heterozygotes is 9 to 11 mmol/l (350–450 mg/dl). The condition is expressed regardless of diet or age, and elevated cholesterol levels are present throughout childhood. The lipoprotein phenotype is usually IIa, but occasionally there is a moderate increase in fasting serum triglycerides to produce a IIb pattern. There is a tendency for HDL cholesterol to be at the lower end of the range, particularly if triglycerides are elevated.

The clinical hallmark of familial hypercholesterolaemia is the presence of tendon xanthomata. These appear in heterozygotes from the age of 20 onwards. The most common sites for tendon xanthomata are in the tendons overlying the knuckles and in the Achilles tendons (Plates 1, 2). Less commonly, they may also be found in the extensor hallucis longus and triceps tendons, and occasionally others. It is also common to find subperiosteal xanthomata on the upper tibia where the patellar tendon inserts. The skin overlying tendon xanthomata is of normal colour and they do not appear yellow. The cholesteryl ester deposits are deep within the tendons. Tendon xanthomata feel hard because they are fibrotic. Indeed, it is not uncommon for those in the Achilles tendons to become inflamed from time to time, sometimes presenting as chronic Achilles tenosynovitis. More generalized tendinitis may follow rapid therapeutic reduction in serum cholesterol levels. Tendon xanthomata occur in only two disorders apart from familial hypercholesterolaemia and these are so rare as not to pose any diagnostic difficulty. They are cerebrotendinous xanthomatosis, in which plasma cholestanol is elevated and deposited in tendons, and phytosterolaemia (beta sitosterolaemia), in which there is abnormal intestinal absorption of plant sterols, which are then deposited in tendons.

Corneal arcus is also a frequent occurrence in familial hypercholesterolaemia. When it occurs in adolescence or early adulthood, it is more likely to be associated with familial hypercholesterolaemia than corneal arcus occurring in middle age or later. It is, however, not uncommon to encounter patients with familial hypercholesterolaemia who have florid tendon xanthomata, but no arcus. It is thus not a very valuable physical sign. Xanthelasmata palpebrarum, although occurring with greater frequency and at a younger age in familial hypercholesterolaemia, affect only a minority of heterozygotes. Xanthelasmata are not specific for any particular type of hypercholesterolaemia and occur in polygenic hypercholesterolaemia, pregnancy, primary bilary cirrhosis, and hypothyroidism. They are also common in middle-aged women, often overweight, with no very marked increase in serum cholesterol, if any. They may run in families apparently independently of hypercholesterolaemia.

Identifying familial hypercholesterolaemia heterozygotes as early as possible is important, because of their risk of coronary heart disease. Untreated, over half of affected men die before the age of 60 years. It is not uncommon for men to have their first myocardial infarction or develop angina in their thirties and occasionally even earlier. Some 15 per cent of women with familial hypercholesterolaemia die of coronary heart disease before the age of 60 years and the majority have symptomatic coronary disease by that age. Perhaps as many as 10 per cent of women have some evidence of cardiac ischaemia before their menopause. However, whereas it is exceptional for a man with familial hypercholesterolaemia to live to 70 without symptomatic coronary heart disease, almost a quarter of women do so. This accounts in large part for the reason why a family history of premature coronary heart disease is absent in as many as one-quarter of patients discovered to have familial hypercholesterolaemia on screening, or in men who are discovered to have familial hypercholesterolaemia when they present with a heart attack in early life: the condition has been inherited from their mother, who has herself not yet developed coronary symptoms. The majority of people with familial hypercholesterolaemia are not overweight and do not have risk factors for coronary heart disease other than hypercholesterolaemia and a family history of the premature disease. Those without a family history of premature coronary heart disease (approximately 25 per cent) will be missed in screening programmes for risk factors for coronary heart disease, in which cholesterol is only measured selectively.

Those patients with familial hypercholesterolaemia who develop coronary heart disease particularly early often come from families in which the affected members have all tended to develop coronary heart disease early. This may be because other genetic factors in the family predispose to coronary heart disease. Thus low serum HDL cholesterol and increased fasting triglycerides are associated with a worse prognosis. Serum lipoprotein (a) is increased in familial hypercholesterolaemia and any familial tendency to run a high level of Lp(a) is exacerbated in those members who also have familial hypercholesterolaemia. The apo E_4

genotype (see below) is also associated with more aggressive atheroma in familial hypercholesterolaemia. A knowledge of the average age at which affected members of a family developed coronary heart disease may be helpful in planning how actively to treat boys and young adult women.

There is a increased risk of atheroma in other parts of the arterial tree in heterozygous familial hypercholesterolaemia, but this is strikingly less so than in the coronary arteries. Some heterozygotes have aortic systolic cardiac murmurs due to deposits of atheroma in the aortic root, sometimes involving the aortic cusps.

Homozygous familial hypercholesterolaemia

Most cases of homozygous familial hypercholesterolaemia occur in societes in which consanguineous marriages and heterozygous familial hypercholesterolaemia are frequent. The chance of marriage between unrelated heterozygotes, meeting by chance in countries such as the United Kingdom or United States of America is 1 in 500[2], and each of their children would stand a 1 in 4 chance of being homozygotes. Assuming no adverse effect on the survival of the conceptus, an incidence of homozygous familial hypercholesterolaemia of 1 in 10^6 births would be predicted. It is thus a rare condition under these circumstances.

Clinically, homozygous familial hypercholesterolaemia is characterized by the development of cutaneous xanthomata in childhood. These may be present in the first year of life or may not develop until late childhood. They are typically orange-yellow, subcutaneous, planar xanthomata, occurring on the buttocks, antecubital fossae, and the hands, frequently in the webs between the fingers. Tuberose subcutaneous xanthomata on the knees, elbows, and knuckles are also a feature. Serum cholesterol is typically greater than 15 mmol/l (600 mg/dl). Myocardial infarction and angina frequently occur in childhood, sometimes even in infancy. Atheromatous deposits at the aortic root, invariably present by puberty, are so marked as to produce significant aortic stenosis, which contributes to the risk of sudden death. Death before the age of 30, and often considerably younger, was the rule before the advent of plasmapheresis and similar techniques for the extracorporeal removal of LDL (see below).

Polyarthritis, predominantly affecting the ankles, knees, wrists, and proximal interphalangeal joints, is common in homozygotes for familial hypercholesterolaemia.

The metabolic defect in familial hypercholesterolaemia

In familial hypercholesterolaemia there is decreased catabolism of LDL so that it remains for longer in the circulation. Normally the plasma half-life of LDL is 2.5 to 3 days, whereas in familial hypercholesterolaemia heterozygotes it is 4.5 to 5 days, and even longer in homozygotes. The molecular defect which causes this has been elucidated following the discovery of the LDL receptor (see above) by Goldstein and Brown in 1973, for which they received the Nobel Prize for Medicine in 1985. The gene encoding the LDL receptor protein is located on chromosome 19. Heterozygotes express only about half the LDL receptors of a normal person. Homozygotes have between none and 25 per cent of normal receptor activity. The mutations in the LDL receptor gene produce either receptors with no binding activity (receptor negative; because the receptor is not synthesized, is not transported to the cell surface, or, if it gets there, cannot be internalized after binding to LDL) or because, although the mutation allows some LDL to be bound and to enter the cell, this occurs only slowly because the binding site is abnormal (receptor defective). Some 200 mutations have been described and undoubtedly more exist. In Afrikaners or French Canadians far fewer mutations are associated with familial hypercholesterolaemia. For example, three mutations account for 90 per cent of familial hypercholesterolaemia in Afrikaners. In societies such as Britain and the United States, however, the most frequent of these mutations is likely to occur in no more than 3 to 4 per cent of patients with familial hypercholesterolaemia. This means that the prospect of developing a DNA test for this condition in most countries is unrealistic. It also means that only in populations with a small number of mutations, or where intermarriage is common, are clinical homozygotes truly homozygous in the sense that both their LDL gene mutations are identical. Most will be mixed heterozygotes. For clinical purposes it is reasonable to label as homozygotes patients who have the clinical syndrome. However, it is instructive to realize that some of the heterogeneity of the severity of the syndrome relates to the nature of the two LDL mutations present. Thus the worst prognosis is associated with inheritance of two receptor-negative mutations, and the best is with two receptor-defective mutations. The type of receptor mutation in heterozygotes is also probably of some importance, but here it is blurred against a background of other acquired or genetic factors, which can find expression over a much longer time than in homozygotes.

A small proportion (3 per cent) of patients, who clinically have the same features as heterozygotes for familial hypercholesterolaemia, do not have an LDL receptor defect, but a mutation of apolipoprotein B in which glutamine is substituted for arginine at amino acid residue 3500, which is part of the LDL receptor binding domain. This disorder has been termed familial defective apo B_{100}. It probably has a frequency of 1 in 500 to 600 in Britain and the United States, but only the minority of affected individuals have tendon xanthomata and typically the serum cholesterol associated with it is around 8.0 mmol/l (310 mg/dl), which is less than in most heterozygotes for familial hypercholesterolaemia.

COMMON OR POLYGENIC HYPERCHOLESTEROLAEMIA

When a diagnosis of familial hypercholesterolaemia can be made, either because hypercholesterolaemia is present in childhood or an adult has the clinical features of the syndrome, a reasonably accurate estimate of clinical risk can be made and appropriate therapy given. In Britain, however, familial hypercholesterolaemia probably accounts for no more than 3 per cent of men dying of coronary heart disease before the age of 60. There is overlap between the range of LDL cholesterol levels encountered in familial hypercholesterolaemia and those due to the commoner, polygenic hypercholesterolaemia. Epidemiological studies have not included sufficient numbers of people with particularly high cholesterol levels to be certain, but it is probable that the risk in familial hypercholesterolaemia is greater than in polygenic hypercholesterolaemia. This may be because in the familial condition the hypercholesterolaemia has been present since birth, whereas polygenic hypercholesterolaemia is frequently not fully developed until the third or fourth decade. Furthermore familial hypercholesterolaemia, unlike many other types of hypercholesterolaemia, is associated with increased serum concentrations of Lp(a).

Estimates of how much different levels of cholesterol contribute to the overall cumulative male mortality from coronary heart disease by the age of 60 years are given in Table 2. The majority of such premature deaths come from the middle part of the cholesterol distribution, and therefore it has been argued that if a significant reduction in the incidence of coronary heart disease is to be achieved in countries such as the United Kingdom, efforts to lower cholesterol cannot simply be confined to those individuals whose plasma cholesterols lie at the upper end of the distribution. Nevertheless because the number of people in the middle range is so huge (the vast majority of whom are not at increased risk of premature coronary heart disease), a different strategy must be applied to reducing their cholesterol from that applied to those in the upper part of the cholesterol distribution. This is the 'low-risk' or 'population' strategy, which aims to lower serum cholesterol by public health measures aimed at encouraging the adoption of a lower fat diet and avoidance of obesity. Some patients from the middle range of cholesterol are, however, at much greater individual risk from their cholesterol level than the majority, because they have other risk factors for coronary heart disease which much increase their susceptibility. Probably the most potent of these is that the individual already has coronary heart disease. In middle-aged myocardial infarction survivors, serum cholesterol is an important indicator of cardiac prognosis (Fig. 6(a)), ranking after left ventricular function, but ahead of most of the other risk factors

Table 2 *Estimates of the proportion of men in the United Kingdom dying before the age of 60 years from coronary heart disease (CHD) according to their serum cholesterol and whether they have the familial hypercholesterolaemia (FH) clinical syndrome* (Durrington 1994)

Serum cholesterol (mmol/l)	Risk of death before the age of 60 (per 1000)	Percentage of UK male population with these cholesterol levels	Percentage of UK male population dying before the age of 60 from CHD with these cholesterol levels
< 5	25	10	0.25
5–6	30	35	1.05
6–7	43	40	1.72
7–8	55	10	0.55
8–9	74	4	0.30
> 9	130	1	0.13
Heterozygous FH	500	0.2	0.1
Total			4.1

Death up to 60 in men is chosen because of limited data about cholesterol in older age groups and in women and about morbidity. The combined CHD death and non-fatal symptomatic CHD rate is probably two to three times that of CHD death.

for coronary heart disease. Lipoproteins are also the most important risk factors for occlusion of coronary artery bypass grafts after the initial postoperative period. In people, who have not yet developed coronary heart disease, the effect of risk factors such as cigarette smoking, hypertension, and diabetes is also to increase the risk from any given level of cholesterol (Fig. 5). A family history of coronary heart disease at an early age in a first-degree relative also increases the likelihood of coronary heart disease, and part of this effect is independent of other risk factors for coronary heart disease. The combination of all these factors with a relatively modestly increased serum cholesterol level can increase individual risk substantially to a level where clinical intervention is as justified as it is with more marked elevations in serum cholesterol. This

Fig. 6 (a) The risk of subsequent fatal myocardial infarction in survivors of myocardial infarction according to their serum cholesterol concentration (data from Pekkanan *et al.* 1990). (b) The likelihood of developing coronary heart disease in patients with moderately raised serum cholesterol concentrations (on average 6.9 mmol/l) is increased when serum triglyceride levels are also raised and HDL cholesterol concentrations decreased (data from Manninen *et al.* 1989).

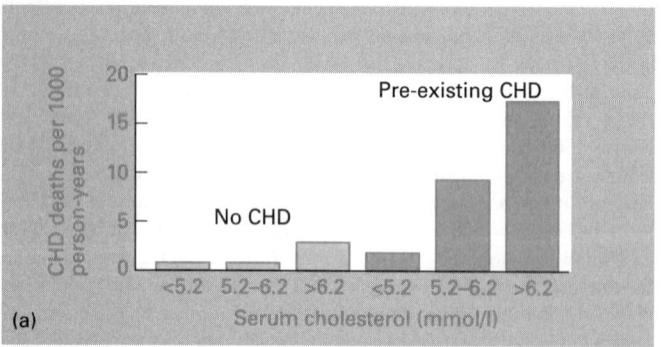

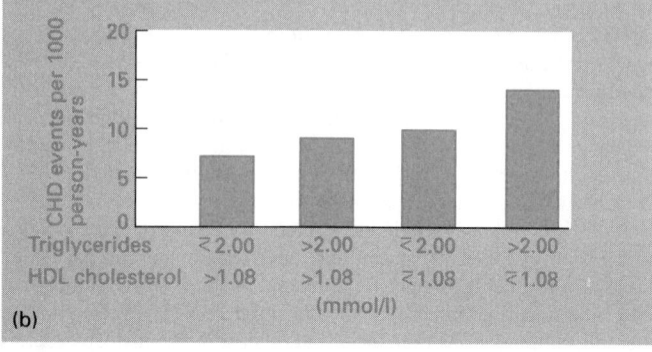

is the 'high-risk' or clinical approach to prevention of coronary heart disease.

Metabolic defect in polygenic hypercholesterolaemia

In polygenic hypercholesterolaemia there is generally overproduction of VLDL by the liver. If this is rapidly converted to LDL there is no increase in serum triglyceride levels. The LDL receptor mechanism is probably overloaded in many individuals and in any case appears to catabolize only about one-third of LDL, so that the build-up of cholesterol in most patients is not due to any defect in the LDL receptor, but the inability of non-receptor-mediated catabolism to cope without a rise in the serum cholesterol concentration. Obesity and a high fat diet (particularly saturated fat) are probably the major reasons for the enormous differences in the prevalence of polygenic hypercholesterolaemia in different parts of the world. Undoubtedly, however, individual responses to diet vary tremendously and there is probably a complex interplay between dietetic and genetic factors in the genesis of polygenic hypercholesterolaemia. The rise in cholesterol with age, which occurs in both men and women until the climacteric, seems less evident in societies where the cholesterol level is, for dietetic reasons, lower. There is an impression that dietary modification aimed at lowering cholesterol in middle age in societies where serum cholesterol is high does not reduce it to the extent that might be anticipated from populations habitually consuming such a diet. Whether this is simply a matter of non-compliance with diet or represents some permanent change in metabolism caused by a high fat diet in early life is at present uncertain.

Primary hyperlipoproteinaemias in which there is hypercholesterolaemia combined with hypertriglyceridaemia

TYPE III HYPERLIPOPROTEINAEMIA

Type III hyperlipoproteinaemia has several synonyms: broad beta disease, floating beta disease, dysbetalipoproteinaemia, and remnant removal disease. It is rare, probably occurring in fewer than 1 in 5000 people. Type III hyperlipoproteinaemia has the distinction of being the first clinical syndrome associated with hyperlipoproteinaemia to be described (by Addison and Gull in 1851).

Type III hyperlipoproteinaemia is due to the presence in the circulation of increased amounts of chylomicron remnants and IDL, often collectively termed beta-VLDL. This is the result of decreased clearance of these lipoproteins at the hepatic remnant (or apo E) receptor. There is an increase in both the serum cholesterol and fasting triglyceride concentrations. Typical levels are 7 to 12 mmol/l (270–470 mg/dl) for cholesterol and 5 to 20 mmol/l (450–1800 mg/dl) for triglycerides. Often the molar concentrations of cholesterol and triglycerides are similar, and this may be a clue that a patient has type III. Occasionally the condition is associated with marked hypertriglyceridaemia due to overwhelming chylomicronaemia.

Xanthomata are present in more than half of the patients who have the type III lipoprotein phenotype. Characteristic of the condition are striate palmar xanthomata and tuberoeruptive xanthomata. Striate palmar xanthomata may simply be an orange-yellow discoloration within the creases of the skin of the palms of the hands. They may, however, be more florid and appear as raised, seed-like lesions (sometimes even larger) in the skin creases of the palms, fingers, and flexor surfaces of the wrists. Tuberoeruptive xanthomata are raised yellow lesions, usually on the elbows and knees (Plate 3). They may be nodular or cauliflower like, often surrounded by smaller satellites. Sometimes they may be found over other tuberosities, such as the heels and dorsum of the interphalangeal joints of the fingers. They resolve entirely with successful treatment.

Type III hyperlipoproteinaemia is rare in women before the menopause, perhaps because hepatic remnant particle uptake is enhanced by oestrogen. It is also rare in childhood, but has a definite incidence in men by early adulthood. Type III hyperlipoproteinaemia is generally an autosomal recessive condition with variable penetrance. In all cases there appears to be a mutation or polymorphism of the apo E gene, which impairs the receptor binding of apo E. The commonest is a polymorphism, called apo E_2, in which cysteine is substituted for arginine at position 158 of the amino acid sequence. At least 90 per cent of patients with type III hyperlipoproteinaemia are homozygous for E_2. More often than not, however, apolipoprotein E_2 homozygosity, which is present in around 1 per cent of the population, does not itself impose such a severe strain on lipoprotein metabolism that hyperlipoproteinaemia develops: its combination with some other disorder, leading to overproduction of VLDL or some additional catabolic defect, is required. This explains the association of type III hyperlipoproteinaemia with diabetes and hypothyroidism. More often, however, the additional stimulus to hyperlipoproteinaemia is obesity or the coinheritance of a polygenic tendency to hypertriglyceridaemia. Rarer mutations of apo E have been described, which behave clinically similarly to apo E_2 homozygosity. More severe is a mutation leading to apo E deficiency, which in homozygotes does not require other factors for the expression of the type III phenotype. Heterozygous apo E deficiency finds little clinical expression, but, interestingly, mutations directly involving the receptor-binding domain of apo E (amino acids 124–150) produce the type III phenotype even in heterozygotes (dominant expression), implying that such mutations are a greater handicap to receptor clearance than mutations in which one gene is not producing apo E.

Type III undoubtedly causes accelerated atherosclerosis in the coronary, femoral, and tibial arteries. Intermittent claudication occurs at least as frequently as coronary heart disease and the incidence of the latter is about the same as that in familial hypercholesterolaemia. It is of considerable interest that in familial hypercholesterolaemia peripheral arterial disease is uncommon relative to coronary heart disease, indicating that the leg arteries are much more susceptible to the larger lipoprotein particles in type III.

In the presence of typical xanthomata, the diagnosis of type III hyperlipoproteinaemia is not difficult. When these are absent the diagnosis must be made in the laboratory. Type IIb or V hyperlipoproteinaemia can give similar serum lipid levels. Lipoprotein electrophoresis is still available in some hospital laboratories and, when it clearly shows separate pre-beta (VLDL) and beta (LDL) bands, is useful in establishing type IIb rather than III hyperlipoproteinaemia. Frequently, however, the classical broad beta band associated with type III hyperlipoproteinaemia cannot be distinguished from a smear stretching from the origin into the pre-beta and sometimes beta region in the more severe IIb or type V phenotype. However, polyacrylamide isoelectric focusing, available in many specialized centres, can identify apolipoprotein E_2 homozygosity and this, in the presence of hyperlipidaemia, makes type III virtually

certain. Rarely, the apo E mutation does not affect the electrical charge of apo E, or affects only one gene so that apo E_2 homozygosity is not found. The only way then to confirm the diagnosis is to send plasma to a centre that can provide ultracentrifugation to identify the cholesterol-rich VLDL (beta-VLDL) typical of type III. It is also important in these circumstances to exclude paraproteinaemia, which can produce both hyper- and hypolipoproteinaemia and can mimic type III.

TYPE IIB HYPERLIPOPROTEINAEMIA

The common lipoprotein phenotype associated with a combined increase in serum cholesterol and triglycerides is IIb. In the majority of people with this, in whom it is primary, the cause is probably best regarded as a polygenic tendency exacerbated by acquired nutritional factors, such as obesity. A few patients will have tendon xanthomata, indicating familial hypercholesterolaemia (see above). The great majority will not. Cardiovascular risk is greater for any given level of cholesterol when the serum triglyceride concentration is also elevated (Fig. 6(b)). Often the HDL is low, which further compounds the risk. Some authorities believe that there is a specific syndrome, in which there is a combined increase in serum cholesterol and triglycerides and greatly increased coronary risk. They term this familial combined hyperlipidaemia. In this, multiple lipoprotein phenotypes occur in different family members: some IIa, some IIb, some IV, or occasionally even V. It is more than probable that what is being observed is the genetic tendency for hypercholesterolaemia and hypertriglyceridaemia running in the same family to combine in some members and not in others, and that when this occurs in a family susceptible to coronary disease a particularly high premature mortality ensues. However, until the arguments about whether familial combined hyperlipidaemia is a distinct genetic entity are resolved the message, for practical purposes, is that hypertriglyceridaemia (especially when HDL cholesterol is low) is an additional factor increasing the risk of hypercholesterolaemia, and that when these are combined with a family history of premature coronary heart disease the outlook is bleak unless the condition is detected and treated.

Primary hyperlipidaemias in which hypertriglyceridaemia predominates

SEVERE HYPERTRIGLYCERIDAEMIA (TYPES I AND V)

Diagnosis and underlying mechanism

In any circumstance in which the serum triglycerides exceed 11 mmol/l (1000 mg/dl) chylomicrons in addition to VLDL will be major contributors to the hyperlipidaemia, even when the patient is fasting. This is because in the circulation both chylomicrons and VLDL compete for the same clearance mechanism (lipoprotein lipase). The lipoprotein phenotype is usually type V. This severe hypertriglyceridaemia generally ensues when an increase in hepatic VLDL production either familial or secondary to, for example, obesity, diabetes, alcohol, or oestrogen administration is associated with decreased triglyceride clearance, which again may be genetic or acquired, for example hypothyroidism, β-blockade, or diabellitus (diabetes can cause both an overproduction of VLDL and decreased lipoprotein lipase activity). With the clearance mechanism already overloaded with VLDL, the rise in serum triglyceride levels when chylomicrons enter the circulation following a fatty meal may be tumultuous and they may spend days rather than hours in the circulation. The serum takes on the appearance of milk and triglyceride levels may exceed 100 mmol/l (9000 mg/dl). Thus a patient, who might otherwise have a fasting serum triglyceride level of 5 mmol/l, can, with the injudicious use of alcohol or the development of diabetes, achieve extraordinarily high serum triglyceride levels. Overall the frequency of severe hypertriglyceridaemia (> 11 mmol/l (1000 mg/dl)) is probably no more than 1 in 1000 in adults and less in children.

Rarely, severe hypertriglyceridaemia is caused by familial lipoprotein lipase deficiency, a genetic deficiency in lipoprotein lipase activity. This is inherited as an autosomal recessive trait. Usually it is due to mutation in the lipoprotein lipase gene, leading to defective function or production, but occasionally it is due to a genetic deficiency of apolipoprotein CII, the activator of lipoprotein lipase. In familial lipoprotein lipase deficiency severe hypertriglyceridaemia may be encountered in childhood. Occasionally, in children and young adults presenting for the first time, it produces type I hyperlipoproteinaemia, in which only serum chylomicron levels are elevated. It is not known why the VLDL is not also raised, but with advancing age the increase in both VLDL and chylomicrons, which might be expected if lipoprotein lipase is ineffective, becomes the rule.

Physical signs in severe hypertriglyceridaemia

Tuberoeruptive xanthomata are characteristic of extreme hypertriglyceridaemia. These appear as yellow papules on the extensor surfaces of the arms and legs, buttocks, and back. Often there is hepatosplenomegaly. Liver imaging shows the liver to be fatty, and bone marrow biopsy may reveal macrophages engorged with lipid droplets (foam cells). Because the triglyceride-rich lipoprotein may interfere with the determination of transaminases, giving spuriously high values, liver disease, in particular alcoholic liver disease, may be difficult to exclude, other than by the prompt resolution of the syndrome when a low-fat diet is instituted. Other features include lipaemia retinalis (pallor of the optic fundus, with both the retinal veins and arteries appearing white).

Complications of severe hypertriglyceridaemia

Atheroma is not a complication of familial lipoprotein lipase deficiency, but it does complicate severe hypertriglyceridaemia in which there is lipoprotein lipase activity, albeit diminished. It is difficult to make a precise estimate of the risk from the hyperlipidaemia *per se* because it is so frequently associated with insulin resistance or frank diabetes, which are themselves risk factors for atherosclerosis. If these are included as part of the syndrome, both coronary heart disease and peripheral arterial disease are common. The reason for the complete absence of lipoprotein lipase removing the risk of atheroma is not known with certainty, but it may be because the incidence of diabetes is not increased in familial lipoprotein lipase deficiency, because fibrinogen and factor VII activity are not increased, or because the conversion of VLDL and chylomicrons to the atherogenic IDL and remnant lipoproteins, respectively, is impaired in the absence of lipoprotein lipase.

Although atheroma is not directly due to the high levels of triglyceride-rich lipoproteins, other complications are. Acute pancreatitis may occur when serum triglyceride levels exceed 20 to 30 mmol/l (2000–3000 mg/dl) (see above). The presentation of acute pancreatitis is similar to that from other causes (see Chapter 14.23.1). However, the diagnosis may not be confirmed by detecting increased serum amylase activity, because falsely low values may be encountered due to interference by triglyceride-rich lipoproteins in the laboratory method. All laboratories should inspect serum for milkiness before reporting normal or only moderately raised serum amylase activity in patients with severe abdominal pain (Plate 4). Clinicians may otherwise wrongly exclude the diagnosis of acute pancreatitis, in favour, for example, of perforated peptic ulcer. Some patients do not develop acute pancreatitis, even when serum triglyceride levels exceed 100 mmol/l (9000 mg/dl). Others, who are more susceptible, experience recurring acute episodes. Chronic pancreatitis is not a feature of the condition. Generally the pain subsides within a few hours or days of commencing nasogastric aspiration and intravenous fluids with nothing taken by mouth. Occasionally, if such treatment is delayed, pseudocysts may develop.

Recurrent abdominal pain, not typical of pancreatitis, sometimes occurs in patients prone to marked hypertriglyceridaemia. It may mimic irritable bowel syndrome. Severe abdominal pain may also sometimes be the result of splenic infarction.

Pseudohyponatraemia is another complication of extreme hypertriglyceridaemia, which may lead to serious consequences, if unrecognized.

Spuriously low serum sodium values are reported, because much of the volume of the serum aliquot on which the sodium measurement is made is occupied by lipoproteins as opposed to water. When the serum triglycerides exceed 40 to 50 mmol/l (3500–4500 mg/dl) the concentration of sodium in the aqueous phase (and thus the serum osmolality) may be normal while spurious serum sodium levels of 120 to 130 mmol/l are being reported. The hazard is that these will be misinterpreted by the clinician and a patient already seriously ill with pancreatitis, or occasionally uncontrolled diabetes, will be made more so by infusion of large volumes of isotonic saline or, worse, hypertonic saline.

Focal neurological syndromes such as hemiparesis, memory loss, and loss of mental concentration may complicate extreme hypertriglyceridaemia, perhaps because of ischaemia due to sluggish microcirculation caused by the high concentrations of chylomicrons in the blood. Paraesthesiae, especially in the feet, may also be an occasional feature, even in the absence of diabetes. Sicca syndrome and polyarthritis have also been described, but undoubtedly the commonest articular association is gout (see below).

MODERATE HYPERTRIGLYCERIDAEMIA (TYPE IV)

Raised fasting serum triglyceride levels in the range 2.2 to 5.0 mmol/l (200–450 mg/dl) in the absence of an elevated cholesterol level are commonly encountered, principally the result of obesity. Diabetes and an excess of alcohol are other important causes. Sometimes hypertriglyceridaemia is present in a fit, non-obese person with none of these factors. Family studies may then reveal similar increases in relatives, when the condition is called familial as opposed to sporadic hypertriglyceridaemia. In univariate analysis, epidemiological studies show that the triglyceride level is associated with the risk of coronary heart disease, but there is little evidence that the triglyceride level itself is causal and much of the association might be because of associated low levels of HDL, raised cholesterol, or glucose intolerance.

Hypertriglyceridaemia increases the risk of any associated increase in serum cholesterol (Fig. 6(b)), but present evidence would not favour its treatment in the absence of hypercholesterolaemia as a means of coronary heart disease prevention. Occasionally, levels of 5 mmol/l (450 mg/dl) or less must be treated, if they occur in patients prone to periodic exacerbations associated with acute pancreatitis. Generally, levels exceeding 10 mmol/l justify therapy, but for levels between 5 and 10 mmol/l clinical judgement must apply. In diabetes, evidence that serum triglycerides are an independent risk factor for coronary heart disease in the view of some authorities justifies specific lipid-lowering therapy at lower levels than in non diabetics after improvements in diet and glycaemic control have been exhausted as a means of decreasing triglyceride levels.

Secondary hyperlipoproteinaemias

Secondary hyperlipoproteinaemias are those which are caused by another primary disorder (Table 3). When a disease that has hyperlipidaemia as a complication occurs in an individual who has a primary hyperliproteinaemia, the two frequently synergize to produce marked hyperliproteinaemia. This means that in societies in which polygenic hyperlipoproteinaemia in prevalent, secondary hyperlipoproteinaemia will have most impact. The best-known example of this is diabetes mellitus, which in Japan is only rarely complicated by coronary heart disease, whereas in the United Kingdom and the United States, coronary heart disease is the most common cause of premature death in diabetics.

Diabetes mellitus

The dominant hyperlipidaemia in diabetes is hypertriglyceridaemia. This is more likely to be associated with hypercholesterolaemia and with

Table 3 *The more common causes of secondary hyperlipoproteinaemia*

Endocrine	Diabetes mellitus
	Thyroid disease
	Pregnancy
Nutritional	Obesity
	Alcohol excess
	Anorexia nervosa
Renal disease	Nephrotic syndrome
	Chronic renal failure
Drugs	β-adrenoreceptor blockers
	Thiazide diuretics
	Steroid hormones
	Microsomal enzyme-inducing agents
	Retinoic acid derivatives
Hepatic disease	Cholestasis
	Hepatocellular dysfunction
	Cholelithiasis
Immunoglobulin excess	Paraproteinaemia
Hyperuricaemia	

decreased HDL cholesterol in type 2 diabetes. Despite this, the risks of coronary heart disease and peripheral arterial disease are increased in both types 1 and 2 diabetes. This may be because in both disorders the hypertriglyceridaemia results not simply from an increase in VLDL, but also from an increase in IDL and a small triglyceride-rich, cholesterol-depleted LDL particle. Since neither of these may contribute greatly to an increase in lipids, the term dyslipoproteinaemia is particularly aptly applied in diabetes. Also, plasma fibrinogen levels, which are increased in both types of diabetes relate to serum triglyceride levels. Although lipoprotein abnormalities in type 1 diabetes may be less frequent than in type 2, the risk of coronary heart disease in type 1 is more often compounded by the presence of proteinuria. In diabetes uncomplicated by proteinuria, the risk of coronary heart disease is about two to three times (Fig. 5) that of non-diabetic people of a similar age. Proteinuria increases the risk by as much as 40 times. This may stem partly from hypertension and an exacerbation of the dyslipoproteinaemia, which accompany the development of proteinuria. However, the increase in risk is greater than can be explained in this way (see Chapter 11.11) and may result because the proteinuria reflects a generalized increase in the permeability of arterial endothelium, enhancing the entry of macromolecules into the subintima and thus accelerating atherogenesis (see above).

The increased blood glucose in diabetes mellitus results from insulin resistance, insulin deficiency, or both. Insulin resistance may be present in non-diabetic, usually obese, people who are still able to secrete sufficient insulin to maintain control of blood sugar, but in such people there is often hypertriglyceridaemia with low HDL cholesterol and hypercholesterolaemia, hypertension and increased risk of coronary heart disease. This syndrome is often referred to as the insulin resistance syndrome (syndrome X) or chronic cardiovascular risk syndrome. Clearly, it has features in common with familial combined hyperlipidaemia and also with diabetes. Indeed, a proportion of people with the condition ultimately develop diabetes, sometimes not until after they have already developed coronary heart disease. This may be part of the reason why glycaemic control in diabetes seems to have little impact in preventing its atheromatous complications.

Diabetic women, particularly those with type 2 disease, tend to have a distribution of adipose tissue resembling that of obese men, being mostly around the abdomen and waist, rather than the more female pattern which involves the buttocks and thighs, but leaves the waist relatively small. The relative protection from coronary heart disease which most women have, even those with familial hypercholesterolaemia, is largely lost by diabetic women, and it has been suggested that this may

result from this androgenization. Many women with a similar body habitus, but who have not yet developed diabetes, are insulin resistant, hypertensive, have hyperlipidaemia, and have an associated increased risk of coronary heart disease.

Other secondary hyperlipoproteinaemias

Obesity is a potent cause of hyperlipidaemia and has most impact in people with glucose intolerance. In its own right obesity predominantly causes hypertriglyceridaemia (usually type IV), but, there is no form of primary hyperlipidaemia that it will not exacerbate. It frequently therefore accompanies hypercholesterolaemia as well as hypertriglyceridaemia. The exception appears to be familial hypercholesterolaemia, which is not associated with obesity. Alcoholic beverages, particularly wine and beer, are energy rich and may be a cause of obesity. Alcohol itself also causes hypertriglyceridaemia. Weight loss is generally associated with decreases in serum cholesterol and triglyceride levels. Anorexia nervosa is paradoxical in that it may be associated with quite marked elevations of serum cholesterol.

In hypothyroidism, serum LDL cholesterol and, less frequently, serum triglycerides are raised. HDL levels tend to be increased. There is decreased receptor-mediated LDL catabolism and lipoprotein lipase activity may be decreased. Hypothyroidism should always be considered in the diagnosis of hyperlipidaemia, and it is particularly important to exclude it when marked hyperlipidaemia occurs in women and in diabetic patients.

Renal disease is becoming an important cause of secondary hyperlipidaemia in clinical practice, because improvements in long-term renal management are now exposing coronary heart disease as the major cause of premature death in many renal disorders. In nephrotic syndrome the major lipoprotein disorder is a rise in serum LDL cholesterol. In chronic renal failure hypertriglyceridaemia is produced by an increase in both VLDL and in LDL triglycerides. Haemodialysis, chronic ambulatory peritoneal dialysis, and high-energy diets exacerbate the hyperlipidaemia. Following renal transplantation, many of the lipoprotein abnormalities resolve if good renal function is established, but corticosteroid therapy, weight gain, antihypertensive therapy, and perhaps cyclosporin treatment mean that even then hyperlipidaemia persists in about one-quarter of patients. Lp(a) is markedly elevated in renal disease, even after transplantation.

Drugs are a common cause of hyperlipidaemia. β-Blockers without intrinsic sympathomimetic activity raise triglycerides and lower HDL cholesterol. Thiazide diuretics tend to increase both cholesterol and triglycerides. These effects may be relatively small in people whose serum lipids are not elevated at the outset, but in patients with hypertriglyceridaemia or with diabetes they may be substantial. Oestrogens tend to raise serum triglycerides, but will often lower LDL cholesterol after the menopause. They also raise serum HDL. Androgens have the opposite effect, decreasing triglycerides, raising LDL cholesterol, and lowering HDL. They may contribute to premature cardiac death in athletes unwise enough to use them in training. Glucocorticoids increase serum LDL cholesterol and triglycerides and often HDL cholesterol. Retinoic acid derivatives used in the management of skin disorders cause hypertriglyceridaemia. Phenytoin and phenobarbitone raise serum HDL cholesterol.

Cholestatic liver diseases, such as primary biliary cirrhosis, produce hypercholesterolaemia. This is not due to an increase in apo B-containing LDL, but to an abnormal lipoprotein, designated lipoprotein X (LpX), produced largely as the result of reflux of biliary phospholipids into the circulation. Xanthelasmata are common in biliary obstruction and other xanthomata occasionally develop. In the later phase of chronic biliary obstruction, when secondary biliary cirrhosis and hepatocellular disease sets in, hepatic lipid biosynthesis plummets and the hyperlipidaemia of biliary obstruction resolves. Hepatocellular diseases may be associated with moderate hypertriglyceridaemia, probably because of

Table 4 *Dietary fatty acids and their sources*

Saturated	Myristic Palmitic Stearic	Pork, beef, sheep fat, and dairy products
Monounsaturated	Oleic	Olive oil, rapeseed oil
Polyunsaturated	Linoleic	Sunflower, safflower, corn, soyabean oil
	Eicosapentaenoic Docosahexaenoic	Fish oil

All can contribute to obesity. Saturated fats lead to raised cholesterol and triglyceride levels. Oleic acid and linoleic acid decrease LDL cholesterol and often triglycerides. Oleic acid is widely distributed in foods rich in saturated fats, but these sources are not helpful in a diet designed to decrease saturated fat intake. Fish oil decreases triglycerides, but does not decrease LDL cholesterol.

impaired hepatic lipoprotein clearance. HDL concentrations are markedly decreased and lecithin:cholesterol acyltransferase activity is low. Some authorities believe that this defect in cholesterol esterification contributes to the complications of liver failure.

Hyperuricaemia is present in as many as half the men with hypertriglyceridaemia. It may lead to gout, particularly if such patients are receiving diuretic therapy. The association of hypertriglyceridaemia and hyperuricaemia appears to be more common than can be entirely explained by the coincidence of common aetiological factors, such as obesity and high alcohol consumption. Yet they are not causally related, because specifically lowering one does not usually decrease the other. They must therefore have some unknown antecedent in common.

Management of hyperlipoproteinaemia

Clinical trials have established beyond all question of doubt that reduction in serum cholesterol decreases both coronary morbidity and mortality. Doubt exists about whether dietary or drug therapy decrease total mortality by as much as would be anticipated from the decrease in deaths from coronary heart disease and thus whether it increases deaths from non-cardiac causes, such as neoplasms and trauma. The arguments and counterarguments for this are many and complex, and beyond the scope of this section. An important practical point is that the trials that have raised the possibility that cholesterol lowering is of not overall benefit, have been conducted in people whose overall risk of coronary heart disease was below the level clinicians should be treating. Overall benefit was achieved in those trials in which participants were at high risk of coronary heart disease, in particular because they had established coronary heart disease, or higher cholesterol levels, and in which substantial decreases in cholesterol had been achieved. The essential point to grasp in management is that the decision to treat hyperlipidaemia is not based simply on any particular cholesterol value, but on an assessment of individual risk of coronary heart disease. For instance, a 35-year-old man with a cholesterol level of 9.00 mmol/l and no other risk factors, has a risk of coronary heart disease similar to that of a man of the same age, who has a serum cholesterol concentration of only 6.5 mmol/l, but who is a smoker with moderate hypertension.

Against the background of the knowledge that decreasing serum cholesterol reduces morbidity and mortality due to coronary heart disease, it is sensible to select for treatment those patients with a very high overall probability of dying prematurely of this disease. If the balance of risk suggests that they are not, they will be exposed to any possible ill-effects of such treatment with no likelihood of benefit. The identification of patients with gross hypercholesterolaemia and of those with more modest increases in serum cholesterol combined with multiple risk factors, a bad family history, or established coronary heart disease (Figs 5, 6 (a,b)) allows the targeting of cholesterol-lowering management to high-risk individuals, who can benefit.

DIETARY MANAGEMENT

It is generally agreed that dietary advice should be given to people whose serum cholesterol exceeds the optimal level of 5.2 mmol/l (200 mg/dl). It would, however, be hard to justify the use of medical or dietetic resources for this purpose in a country, such as the United Kingdom, where 85 per cent of middle-aged people have cholesterol levels exceeding this level. Thus, except in the case of the patient with established atherosclerotic disease or diabetes mellitus, dietetic or medical supervision beyond the provision of a diet sheet is not reasonable at levels of cholesterol of less than 6.5 mmol/l. It is particularly important to remember that cigarette smoking is a greater cause of ill-health than are minor elevations of serum cholesterol, and advice to stop smoking should be reiterated whenever a medical consultation occurs.

The principal aims of a cholesterol-lowering diet are to reduce obesity by a decrease in dietary energy intake and to decrease saturated fat consumption. Fat is a major source of dietary energy and the reduction in its intake should be the main objective of any weight-reducing diet. In the non-obese, dietary advice should focus on decreasing saturated fat to below 10 per cent of dietary energy intake and substituting it with a mixture of unrefined carbohydrate and monounsaturated and polyunsaturated fats (Table 4). Polyunsaturates should not be the only fats to replace saturated fat, because it is not certain that in large amounts they do not have harmful long-term effects. Increasingly, oils rich in the monounsaturated oleic acid, present in the diet of Mediterranean people as olive oil since time immemorial, are being encouraged by nutritionists as substitutes for saturated fat. Fibre is frequently advised as part of a cholesterol-lowering diet. Mucilaginous fibre in fruit, vegetables, and oats may have a small hypocholesterolaemic effect. Dietary cholesterol itself, although featuring prominently on food labels, usually has little influence on serum cholesterol levels. Avoiding coffee is probably pointless. Some authorities believe that the epidemological evidence indicating that alcohol is protective against coronary heart disease is strong enough to justify encouraging moderate indulgence (red wine finds particular favour in view of the lower risk of coronary heart disease in southern as opposed to northern Europe). However, alcoholic beverages can lead to obesity and to exacerbation of hypertriglyceridaemia (see above) and a trial of abstinence should be considered in the patient with hyperlipidaemia suspected of overindulgence.

This cholesterol-lowering diet does not need to be modified for treatment of moderate hypertriglyceridaemia and is also suitable for the management of diabetes. Carbohydrate-restricted diets are no longer in general use for either of these purposes. One exception to the value of this general lipid-lowering diet is the patient with severe hypertriglyceridaemia. In such patients it is necessary to limit the production of chylomicrons and so any fat in the diet must be avoided. Often a 25 to 30 g low-fat diet (in which, if the patient is not obese, carbohydrate is substituted to maintain dietary energy intake) can be employed, but occasionally even lower fat intakes must be achieved. Lipid-lowering drugs are frequently ineffective in patients with severe hypertriglyceridaemia, whereas diet is particularly effective. Admission to a specialized centre with experienced dietetic services is often necessary.

DRUG THERAPY OF HYPERLIPIDAEMIA

The indication for drug therapy is not the failure of serum cholesterol to decrease below some arbitrary level despite dietary treatment in all patients. There are people with levels as high as 8 mmol/l (310 mg/dl) whose risk of coronary heart disease is not sufficiently high to justify the use of lipid-lowering drugs. The following categories may be considered for lipid-lowering drugs:

Patients with established coronary heart disease or other significant atherosclerotic disease

There is general agreement that secondary prevention trials provide evidence of overall benefit for lipid-lowering treatment. Trials using coronary angiographic evidence of atheroma regression with lipid-lowering therapy have also been successful. Lipid-lowering drugs are indicated therefore in patients with coronary heart disease (including those who have undergone coronary surgery or angioplasty) should their cholesterol level persist above 5.2 mmol/l (200 mg/dl) (LDL cholesterol > 3.4 mmol/l (130 mg/dl)) despite diet. It is probably reasonable to extend this policy to patients with peripheral arterial, aortic, or significant carotid atherosclerosis, because there are angiographic studies to demonstrate favourable effects of lipid-lowering therapy on femoral and carotid atheroma and because this type of disease is closely associated with risk of coronary heart disease.

Familial hypercholesterolaemia and type III hyperlipoproteinaemia

The high risk of coronary heart disease and the known metabolic defects in these conditions justifies the use of lipid-lowering drug therapy. Few patients with familial hypercholesterolaemia will achieve a reduction of serum cholesterol to 6.5 mmol/l with diet alone. Many patients with type III hyperlipoproteinaemia can, however, control their condition with diet. Often when their cholesterol is 6.5 mmol/l, their triglyceride levels are still elevated, indicating that significant beta-VLDL is still present in the circulation. The indication for drug therapy should therefore probably be at around 6.00 mmol/l in this group.

Diabetes mellitus

Reduction of the high risk of coronary heart disease and peripheral arterial disease should be an essential part of diabetic management. The low rate of coronary heart disease in diabetic patients in countries where cholesterol levels are generally low justifies the use of lipid-lowering therapy alongside prompt treatment of hypertension and cessation of smoking in diabetes management. Both men and women with diabetes should have equal consideration for lipid-lowering therapy. Diet (particularly the avoidance of obesity) and improvements in glycaemic control can improve serum lipid levels dramatically. Lipid-lowering drugs are indicated if a cholesterol level above 6.5 mmol/l persists. Some authorities would choose a lower starting point, say 6.0 mmol/l, particularly in the presence of raised triglyceride levels, a frequent occurrence.

Multiple risk factors

The risk of coronary heart disease in some patients with additional adverse factors, whose serum cholesterol remains elevated despite diet, justifies the use of lipid-lowering drugs. Just how high the risk needs to be, and how it can be determined with any degree of exactitude, is a persisting problem for the clinician. Recommendations for treatment, for example from the United States National Institutes of Health and from the European Atherosclerosis Society, could undoubtedly be over-interpreted, so that patients who would not stand to benefit might be prescribed drugs inappropriately. The decision should be made depending on individual circumstances. The case is stronger in men whose cholesterol persists above 6.5 mmol/l than in women. This, combined with hypertension or a bad family history (coronary heart disease in either parent before 60 years old), or perhaps a long smoking history, may justify the use of lipid-lowering treatment in men. Two of these factors would be required in most women. The finding of raised triglycerides and a low HDL cholesterol in combination with raised cholesterol also militates in favour of drug therapy when other risk factors for coronary heart disease are present. It is always important to seek evidence of existing coronary heart disease, since, if present, this makes the clinical decision to start lipid-lowering therapy easier, and, of course, may require investigation in its own right.

Markedly elevated cholesterol with no other risk factors and no clearly identifiable genetic syndrome

Many people fall into this category, and it is important to remember that they are not at sufficiently high risk of coronary heart disease to justify lipid-lowering drug therapy unless serum cholesterol is at least 8.0 mmol/l despite diet. Even then, many women do not require such therapy because they have relatively high HDL cholesterol, and it is not my practice to introduce it in the absence of risk factors in women unless the total cholesterol : HDL cholesterol ratio exceeds 7 and total cholesterol exceeds 8 mmol/l. If women do come into this category when they are peri- or postmenopausal, the possibility of prescribing hormone replacement therapy should be considered, particularly if the menopause is surgical or spontaneously premature, or if there are also menopausal symptoms. Hormone replacement therapy often decreases LDL cholesterol and may increase HDL cholesterol. Although the effect of this therapy is generally beneficial in preventing coronary heart disease, care should be exercised in patients with hypertension (because of its mineralocorticoid properties) and in patients with established coronary heart disease (because of its possible thrombogenic effects). In men, in whom high levels of HDL are less commonly encountered, it is reasonable to advocate lipid-lowering therapy if the total cholesterol exceeds 8 (or the LDL cholesterol is greater than 6 mmol/l) and probably at somewhat lower levels if serum triglyceride levels are also raised.

Lipid-modifying drugs

Before patients are considered for lipid-lowering drugs, diet should have been instituted. No major therapeutic decision, such as the decision to introduce a particularly restrictive diet or lipid-modifying drug therapy, should be taken as the result of a single cholesterol determination, because this will be influenced both by biological and by laboratory variation. A laboratory result for cholesterol is generally within ± 10 per cent of the true mean value, but may occasionally fluctuate more widely. Increasingly, portable or 'on-site' cholesterol analyses are being used in an attempt to make cholesterol measurement as immediate for the clinician as that of blood pressure. This has some advantages, but it must be remembered that such tests may be more expensive than those performed in the laboratory, will be less accurate unless performed by someone who is trained and regularly uses the instrument, and the method may be calibrated differently from that used in a hospital laboratory.

Non-fasting cholesterol levels are satisfactory for the management of patients responding to simple dietary measures, but for those in whom drug therapy is under consideration, at least two, and preferably three, fasting determinations of cholesterol, triglycerides, and HDL cholesterol are necessary (serum cholesterol and HDL cholesterol levels are not affected by meals, but serum triglyceride levels are). Knowledge of the HDL and triglyceride levels is essential at this stage because abnormal values for these would be an additional factor in favour of lipid-lowering drug therapy, and because their concentration may influence the choice of drug. Fasting blood glucose and serum creatinine and transaminases should also be measured, and urine should be tested for protein. Serum thyroxine should be measured if there is any suspicion of hypothyroidism and some authorities advocate its measurement in all patients whose serum cholesterol exceeds 8 mmol/l (310 mg/dl) even if hypothyroidism is not clinically evident.

Bile-acid sequestrating agents (cholestyramine and colestipol) are indicated in the treatment of hypercholesterolaemia in the absence of hypertriglyceridaemia, which they may exacerbate. A dose (two sachets) is best taken well soaked in fruit juice before breakfast. In larger, more frequent doses these agents often cause nausea, heartburn, and constipation. However, in patients with moderate hypercholesterolaemia their value as monotherapy in small doses should not be overlooked. Some patients with more severe hypercholesterolaemia will tolerate larger doses. In children and women of child-bearing potential, who have heterozygous familial hypercholesterolaemia and in whom drug therapy may be justified because of a particularly adverse family history, the author is reluctant to turn to other agents.

In patients whose hypercholesterolaemia is combined with hypertriglyceridaemia, the fibrate drugs (bezafibrate, ciprofibrate, fenofibrate, gemfibrozil) are first-line therapy. Fibrate drugs may be tried as sole therapy in patients with moderate hypercholesterolaemia, who do not respond to, or cannot tolerate, bile-acid sequestrating agents. They are also often highly effective in type III hyperlipoproteinaemia and useful in primary type V hyperlipoproteinaemia and in the dyslipoproteinaemia of diabetes mellitus. Neither bezafibrate nor gemfibrozil are very effective in lowering LDL cholesterol, most of their cholesterol-lowering effect being due to a decrease in VLDL cholesterol. Fenofibrate and ciprofibrate are more effective at lowering LDL cholesterol. All the fibrate drugs raise HDL cholesterol. They may all be used in diabetes mellitus, but must be avoided in patients with disturbed hepatic or renal function. They potentiate anticoagulants. They may be used in combination with bile-acid sequestrating agents in the management of combined hypercholesterolaemia and hypertriglyceridaemia.

Increasing use is being made of 3-hydroxy-3-methylglutaryl-CoA reductase inhibitor (statin) drugs (fluvastatin, lovastatin, pravastatin, and simvastatin). The agents are often effective, even in marked hypercholesterolaemia, as monotherapy, although advantage may be taken of their synergism with bile-acid sequestrating agents, by prescribing two sachets in the morning with an evening dose of statin. Statins have a small triglyceride-lowering effect as well as potent cholesterol-lowering properties. Their use in combination with fibrate drugs requires strict clinical supervision, because there is a risk that myositis may ensue. There is a small incidence of this occurring spontaneously in patients on statins and creatine kinase levels should be monitored. Cyclosporin also increases the risk of myositis, and care must be taken if statins are used after cardiac or renal transplantation. Although bile-acid sequestrating agents can be used to lower cholesterol in patients with renal diseases (in whom fibrates are contraindicated), their use is limited because they may exacerbate accompanying hypertriglyceridaemia and because patients who are receiving multiple drug regimes frequently find these agents intolerable. Statins may therefore be particularly valuable in this group of patients.

Nicotinic acid (niacin) can be used to lower serum cholesterol and triglyceride levels. The effective dose is usually associated with unpleasant flushing. This can be minimized if aspirin is taken before the nicotinic acid. There are also many other side-effects and liver function must be monitored. Nicotinic acid has not found great therapeutic favour outside the United States, but it is enjoying renewed interest because, unlike other lipid-lowering drugs, it is effective in lowering serum Lp(a). Acipimox, an analogue, has a similar spectrum of action to the fibrate drugs and causes less flushing. Probucol is a cholesterol-lowering drug, which lowers HDL cholesterol more markedly than LDL. Despite its undoubted antioxidant properties, it requires further clinical evaluation before it can be regarded as beneficial in its overall action. Oily fish (e.g. mackerel, herring, salmon) may be important in the dietary treatment of hyperlipidaemia, but fish oil pharmacological preparations, despite their triglyceride-lowering properties, do not lower LDL cholesterol and even exacerbate diabetic hyperlipidaemia. The evidence that oily fish are beneficial after coronary surgery or myocardial infarction may not relate to their effects on lipid metabolism.

Non-pharmacological lipid-lowering treatment

In addition to pharmacological agents and diet, extracorporeal removal of LDL is available in many centres for severe hypercholesterolaemia, usually homozygous familial hypercholesterolaemia in which it improves survival. Plasmapheresis or LDL apheresis, using systems that absorb LDL, are the two methods employed. Plasmapheresis and most LDL apheresis methods also lower serum Lp(a). They must be repeated every 2 to 4 weeks. Occasionally, patients with homozygous familial hypercholesterolaemia have also been treated with liver transplantation to provide an organ with normally functioning LDL receptors. Partial ileal bypass surgery has been used to treat heterozygous familial hypercholesterolaemia (it is ineffective in homozygotes), but with the advent of more effective lipid-lowering drugs this is now only exceptionally necessary.

Hypolipoproteinaemia

Hypolipoproteinaemia is increasing as a clinical problem, because more cases are being discovered as a result of population screening for high cholesterol. People who have had a low serum cholesterol level all their lives do not seem to be at any disadvantage unless the decrease is profound, as in abetalipoproteinaemia. Indeed, their relative freedom from cardiovascular disease may lead to longevity. When the condition is discovered for the first time it is often difficult, however, to be sure that the low cholesterol is not due to an acquired disease, such as malignancy (for example colonic or prostatic neoplasms, leukaemia, reticulosis, or myeloma) or malabsorption (due, for example, to a short bowel, blind-loop syndrome, coeliac disease, pancreatic exocrine insufficiency, or giardiasis).

Some people with serum cholesterol levels around 1.0 to 3.5 mmol/l (40 to 140 mg/dl) will have heterozygous familial hypobetalipoproteinaemia, which is an autosomal dominant condition in which a truncated apo B mutation occurs. The condition is benign. However, homozygous hypoapobetalipoproteinaemia and another condition, abetalipoproteinaemia (inherited as an autosomal recessive; site of mutation unknown, but not the apo B gene itself), which produce more profound hypocholesterolaemia, are associated with retinitis pigmentosa, unusually shaped erythrocytes (acanthocytes), a syndrome resembling Friedreich's ataxia (preventable with fat-soluble vitamin administration), steatorrhoea (which can create diagnostic confusion with other causes of malabsorption leading to secondary hypocholesterolaemia), and fatty liver.

Analphalipoproteinaemia (Tangier disease) is a very rare disorder associated with virtually absent HDL, reduced LDL cholesteryl ester, and cholesteryl ester deposition throughout the body, leading to enlarged orange-yellow tonsils and adenoids, lymph node enlargement, hepatosphenomegaly, bone marrow infiltration (thrombocytopenia), orange-brown spots on the rectal mucosa, neuropathy, and corneal cloudiness. A less severe form of this disorder (fish-eye disease) has been described. In another disorder, combined deficiency of the apolipoproteins AI and CIII due to a DNA rearrangement affecting the transcription of both their genes, which are clustered together on chromosome 11, leads to markedly decreased serum HDL levels, accelerated atherosclerosis, and corneal opacities. Some authorities believe that a much more common genetic HDL deficiency is the cause of HDL cholesterol levels in the lower 10 per cent of the frequency distribution. Evidence for this contention is incomplete.

REFERENCES

Assmann, G., Schmitz, G., and Brewer, H.B. (1989). Familial high density lipoprotein deficiency: Tangier disease. In *The metabolic basis of inherited disease*, (6th edn), (Ed. C.R. Scriver, A.L. Beaudet, W.S. Sly, D. Valle) pp. 1267–82. McGraw-Hill, New York.

Brown, M.S. and Goldstein, J.L. (1992). Koch's postulates for cholesterol. *Cell*, **71**, 187–8.

Brunzell, J.D. (1989). Familial lipoprotein lipase deficiency and other causes of the chylomicronaemia syndrome. In *The metabolic basis of inherited disease*, (6th edn), (ed: C.R. Scriver, A.L. Beaudet, W.S. Sly, and D. Valle) 1165–80.

Durrington, P.N. (1994). *Hyperlipidaemia. Diagnosis and management*, (2nd edn). Butterworth Heinemann, London.

Durrington, P.N. (1992). Hyperlipidaemia: should we treat patients? Should we treat populations? What treatment should we use? *Recent Advances in Cardiology* **11**, 47–71.

European Atherosclerosis Society (1992). Prevention of coronary heart disease: scientific background and new clinical guidelines. *Nutrition, Metabolism and Cardiovascular Diseases*, **2**, 113–56.

Expert Panel on Detection, Elevation and Treatment of High Blood Cholesterol in Adults (Adult Treatment Panel II). (1993). Summary of Second Report of the National Cholesterol Education Program (NCEP). *Journal of the American Medical Association*, **269**, 3015–23.

Goldstein, J.L. and Brown, M.S. (1989). Familial hypercholesterolaemia. In *The metabolic basis of inherited disease*, (6th edn), (C.R. Scriver, A.L. Beaudet, W.S. Sly, and D. Valle), pp. 1215–50. McGraw-Hill, New York.

Grundy, S.M. (1987). Dietary therapy of hyperlipidaemia. *Baillière's Clinical Endocrinology and Metabolism*, **1**, 667–98.

Holme, I. (1990). An analysis of randomised trials evaluating the effect of cholesterol reduction on total mortality and coronary heart disease incidence. *Circulation* **82**, 1916–24.

Kane, J.P. and Havel, R.J. (1989). Disorders of the biogenesis and secretion of lipoproteins containing the beta apolipoproteins. In *The metabolic basis of inherited disease*, (6th edn), (ed. C.R. Scriver, A.L. Beaudet, W.S. Sly, and D. Valle), pp. 1139–64. McGraw-Hill, New York.

Kannel, W.B., Gordon, T., and McGee, D. (1973). The Framingham Study. An epidemiological investigation of cardiovascular disease. Section 28: The probability of developing certain cardiovascular diseases in eight years at specific values of some characteristics. Publication 74–618, US Department of Health Education and Welfare. Government Printing Office, Washington DC.

Karathanasis, S.K. (1992). Lipoprotein metabolism in high-density lipoproteins. In *Molecular genetics of coronary artery disease*, (ed. A.J. Lusis, J.I. Rotter, and R.S. Sparkes), pp. 140–71. Karger, Basel.

Law, M.R., Thompson, S.G., and Wald, N.J. (1994). Assessing possible hazards of reducing serum cholesterol. *British Medical Journal*, **308**, 373–9.

Law, M.R., Wald, N.J., and Thompson, S.G. (1994). By how much and how quickly does reduction in serum cholesterol concentration lower risk of ischaemic heart disease? *British Medical Journal*, **308**, 367–73.

Mahley, R.W. and Rall, S.C. (1989). Type III hyperlipoproteinaemia (dysbetalipoproteinaemia): the role of apolipoprotein E in normal and abnormal lipoprotein metabolism. In *The metabolic basis of inherited disease*, (6th edn) (ed. C.R. Scriver, A.L. Beaudet, W.S. Sly, and D. Valle), pp. 1195–213.

Mahley, R.W., Weisgraber, K.H., Inneranty, T.L., and Rall, S.C. (1991). Genetic defects in lipoprotein metabolism. Elevation of atherogenic lipoproteins caused by impaired catabolism. *Journal of the American Medical Association*, **265**, 78–83.

Manninen, V., Huttunen, J.K., Tenkanen, L., Heinonen, O.P., Manttari, M., and Frick, M.H. (1989). High density lipoprotein cholesterol as a risk factor for coronary heart disease in the Helsinki Heart Study. In *High density lipoproteins and atherosclerosis II*, (ed. N.E. Miller). Excerpta Medica, Amsterdam.

MBewu, A.D. and Durrington, P.N. (1990). Lipoprotein (a): structure, properties and possible involvement in thrombogenesis and atherogenesis. *Atherosclerosis* **85**, 1–14.

Norum, K.R., Gjone, E., and Glomset, J.A. (1989). Familial lecithin: cholesterol acyltransferase deficiency, including Fish Eye disease. In *The metabolic basis of inherited disease*, (6th edn), (ed. C.R. Scriver, A.L. Beaudet, W.S. Sly, and D. Valle), pp. 1181–94. McGraw-Hill, New York.

Pekkanen, J., *et al.* (1990). Ten-year mortality from cardiovascular disease in relation to cholesterol level among men with and without preexisting cardiovascular disease *New England Journal of Medicine* **322**, 1700–7.

Rossouw, J.E., Lewis, B., and Rifkind, B.M. (1990). The value of lowering cholesterol after myocardial infarction. *New England Journal of Medicine* **323**, 1112–19.

Scandinavian Simvastatin Survival Study Group. (1994). Randomised trial of cholesterol lowering in 4444 patients with coronary heart disease: the Scandinavian Simvastatin Survival Study (4S). *Lancet,* **344**, 1383–89.

Schumaker, V. and Lambertas, A. (1992). Lipoprotein metabolism: chylomicrons, very-low density lipoproteins and low density lipoproteins. In *Molecular genetics of coronary artery disease*, (ed. A.J. Lusis, J.I. Rotter, and R.S. Sparkes), pp. 98–139.

Steinberg, D., Parthasarathy, S., Carew, T., Khoo, J.C., and Witztum, J.L. (1989). Beyond cholesterol. Modifications of low-density lipoproteins that increase its atherogenicity. *New England Journal of Medicine* **320**, 915–24.

Taskinen, M.R. (1990). Hyperlipidaemia in diabetes. *Baillière's Clinical Endocrinology and Metabolism*, **4**, 743–75.

Woolf, N. (1988). Morphological changes in atherosclerosis and the effects of hyperlipidaemia on the artery wall. *Atherosclerosis Reviews* Volume 18. Hypocholesterolemia. Clinical and Therapeutic Implications (ed. J. Stokes and M. Mancini). Rower Press, New York.

11.7 Trace metal disorders

C. A. SEYMOUR

Trace elements in the body

By convention, trace elements are present in amounts less than 0.005 per cent of body weight (Table 1).

About 15 trace elements are known to be essential for health and have various roles in cells and tissues of the body. Deficiency and toxicity states are often insidious, with the former being particularly important in the developing fetus or neonate. Gastrointestinal absorption, on the one hand, and excretion in urine and bile, on the other, are the mechanisms by which concentrations of trace elements are normally regulated.

The process of absorption of iron from the intestine, which regulates body iron content, is a good model for a number of other trace metals (see Chapter 22.4.4). Absorbed iron is bound to different proteins, for example transferrin, and is then in a rapidly exchangeable pool in equilibrium with ferritin, in which iron is stored and from which it is more slowly exchanged (Fig. 1). Transfer of iron to plasma transferrin is rapid, whereas its passage in the reverse direction is slow. Iron absorption also affects intestinal transport of other chemically related metals (zinc, copper, cobalt, and manganese) by competition depending on their affinity for mucosal transferrin. Absorption of cobalt and manganese is increased in states of iron deficiency and a high dietary intake of these metals may inhibit iron absorption.

The other regulatory site in trace metal homeostasis is via excretion in the bile (cf. copper and zinc). Genetic defects in transport systems

Table 1 *Trace elements: elements present in amounts less than 0.005 per cent of body weight*

Essential	Less essential	Toxic	No functional/ toxic effects
Copper	Arsenic	Cadmium	Barium
Iodine	Cobalt	Lead	Bromine
Iron	Chromium	Mercury	Gold
(Magnesium)	Fluoride	Plutonium	Rubidium
Manganese	Molybdenum		Silver
Selenium	Nickel		
Zinc	Silicon		
	Tin		
	Vanadium		

(cf. iron in haemochromatosis and copper in Wilson's and Menkes diseases) as well as hepatobiliary disease can be expected to cause deficiency or toxicity of trace metals in the body.

Various roles for trace metals are outlined in Table 2. It is notable that both deficiency and toxicity of certain trace elements (iron, copper, selenium, and cadmium) may interact with hormonal and cell-mediated immune responses, as well as being cofactors for bacterial growth. This may result in the spread of bacterial and viral infections.

Trace elements and cell damage

Cell and tissue injury and death are often mediated by the presence or incomplete removal of free radicals produced by the cellular reduction of oxygen to water. Oxygen-derived free radicals are produced by tissues of all living organisms by redox, chain, and enzyme reactions. Incomplete removal from the cell of these chemically active molecules may lead to lysosomal, microsomal, and peroxisomal membrane damage, as well as interaction with polyunsaturated fatty acids which may also trigger a further series of damaging reactions. Trace elements such as copper, zinc, manganese, selenium, and cobalt are essential to the function of free-radical scavenging enzymes, as well as to mitochondrial and ATP-generating enzyme systems. Thus many trace elements have a protective role in cell and tissue damage because of involvement in free-radical scavenging antioxidant activities.

Fig. 1 Schematic diagram of iron uptake and release from a cell.

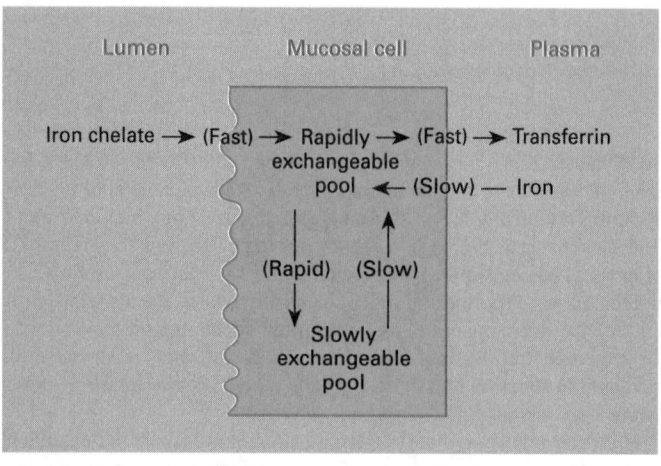

Trace metal disorders

Copper

Copper is ubiquitous in nature and in relative excess in most diets. It is a prosthetic element of many metalloenzymes playing a vital role in mitochondrial energy generation, melanin formation, and cross-linking of collagen and elastin. Acquired copper deficiency is rare because of the efficiency of the liver in maintaining body copper homeostasis. Excretion of copper into bile is dependent on its incorporation into caeruloplasmin (copper-binding protein); toxic accumulation is infrequent and arises only with genetic defects in these homeostatic mechanisms (cf. Wilson's disease and Menkes disease). In Wilson's disease, the liver is the site of the metabolic defect and is the organ most affected by accumulated copper. Other acquired liver conditions in which there is cholestasis, or when significant damage has occurred to bile canaliculi, may also result in copper accumulation and damage to hepatocytes (cf. Indian childhood cirrhosis and primary biliary cirrhosis).

Copper homeostasis

Total body copper is in the range of 50 to 150 mg, of which some 8 per cent is found in the liver. High concentrations are also found in the brain, kidney, heart, and bone. Neonatal and fetal liver tissue tolerates much higher quantities than does adult liver, the copper is probably stored in this major site within lysosomes in association with metallothionein.

About 2 to 5 mg of copper is absorbed from the diet each day, and is transported loosely bound to albumin, this moiety accounting for about 10 per cent of circulating copper. Net uptake of copper (around 40–60 per cent) reflects its differential binding to low molecular weight ligands present in saliva, gastric, and duodenal juice, and high molecular weight ligands present in bile. The regulatory mechanisms involved in intestinal copper transport are still unknown, although binding occurs to two cytosolic proteins, one similar to superoxide dismutase, and the other metallothionein. Although metallothionein and active transport of copper–amino acid complexes are involved in absorption, there is no evidence that overall copper homeostasis is controlled at the intestinal site.

Maintenance of copper homeostasis depends uniquely on its excretion in bile, with around 1.5 to 1.7 mg excreted daily; some (*c.* 0.7 µg/day) is excreted in urine. Gastrointestinal secretions contain small amounts of copper but, because of their volume, probably account for a significant amount of luminal copper. Any interruption in the secretion of bile, such as cholestasis induced in experimental animals by bile-duct ligation, or disease such as primary biliary cirrhosis or biliary atresia, leads to copper accumulation in the liver, and subsequently in other tissues as the liver becomes cirrhotic. In bile, copper is bound to low and high molecular weight complexes, and intestinal reabsorption of biliary copper is negligible.

Copper deficiency

Copper deficiency may occur as genetic and acquired forms, although both are rare.

Acquired form

The acquired form may occur in malnourished children, adults with severe malabsorption syndromes, in patients on regular total parenteral nutrition, or in patients regularly taking chelating agents (penicillamine) as treatment for rheumatoid arthritis.

The diagnosis rests on low serum copper measurements associated with reduced serum caeruloplasmin, hypochromic microcytic anaemia, and evidence of bone demineralization.

Genetic form—Menkes disease

DEFINITION

Menkes disease, or steely hair syndrome, was first described in 1961. Menkes emphasized its X-linked inheritance, although subsequently two girls have been described with the condition.

It is an X-linked cause of copper deficiency, the abnormal gene having been cloned to the long arm of the X chromosome. Full-length complementary DNA sequences have predicted the production of a protein of 1500 amino acids, containing six transmembrane domains with database homology with members of a cation-transporting p-type ATPase protein subfamily, which is involved in copper transport.

Copper is an essential component of a number of key enzyme systems (for example lysyl oxidase, superoxide dismutase, cytochrome oxidase, and dopamine β-hydroxylase) and many symptoms of Menkes disease can be explained by deficiency of these enzymes. In Menkes disease most tissues (except the liver) have increased copper concentrations, and cultured fibroblasts show defective copper efflux, suggesting that intracellular transport of copper is defective.

The predicted structure of Menkes disease protein contains phosphorylating and phosphatase domains as well as a cation channel. The N-terminus, containing six 23-residue repeats, each containing a Cys–X–X–Cys motif, is involved in copper binding. Abnormality of such a protein could account for defects in other copper-transporting disease (cf. Wilson's disease) attributable to a defect in a related liver-specific transporting protein.

CLINICAL FEATURES

Symptoms first occur between 6 weeks and 6 months of age, the major signs being poor growth, mental retardation, and hair abnormality.

The disorder can present early as premature birth, and episodes of hypothermia may occur within the first few days or weeks. Some babies develop normally until 3 months, but many are ill and inactive from birth. The disease is progressive, culminating in death by the age of 3 years.

Classical characteristics are an abnormal facial appearance (Plate 1) with flaccid skin typical of cutis laxa, defective pigmentation (grey colour) of skin and lightly pigmented hair, due to reduced copper control of tyrosinase involved in melanin synthesis. Typically the hair shaft is twisted to give pili torti, where the hair stands at right angles to scalp, and is termed 'steely hair' or, with reference to the hair shaft, 'kinky' hair syndrome. This arises because of deficiency of disulphide bonding in keratin with excess free disulphide bonds, which occurs later in keratin maturation. Abnormalities of major arteries occur, giving thickened, tortuous vessels due to abnormal elastin fibres, which are not cross-linked because this process is dependent on the copper-containing enzyme, lysyl oxidase.

Progressive focal cerebral and cerebellar degeneration are also typical of the disorder, with associated convulsions and mental retardation.

DIAGNOSIS

The clinical features are diagnostic of Menkes disease. In addition, circulating levels of copper and caeruloplasmin are markedly reduced, as is hepatic copper concentration. Liver histology is usually normal but copper-containing enzymes such as mitochondrial cytochrome oxidase

Table 2 *Clinical features and treatment of some trace metal disorders*
(a) Trace metal toxicity

Element	Metabolic role	Organ/tissue affected	Disorder	Clinical features	Specific treatment
Copper	Free radical scavenging enzymes Mitochondria Collagen synthesis	Red cells Liver CNS-basal ganglia	**Primary** Wilson's disease	Haemolysis, anaemia Hepatitis, cirrhosis CNS: Kayser-Fleischer rings Dysarthria, tremor Parkinsonian-like Osteoarthritis Renal tubular acidosis	Chelation: Penicillamine Trientine Ammonium thiomolybdate Zinc acetate (normally adjunct to other chelators) Liver transplantation
			Indian childhood cirrhosis	Jaundice Hepatitis and cirrhosis	Liver transplantation
			Biliary atresia	Jaundice Hepatitis and cirrhosis	Liver transplantation
			Secondary Primary biliary cirrhosis Sclerosing cholangitis Chronic acute hepatitis	Jaundice ⎱ Hepatitis and cirrhosis ⎰	Ursodeoxycholic acid Liver transplantation
Iron	Haemoglobin Iron stores Red cell formation	Red cells Liver Spleen Bone marrow Endocrine agents	**Primary** Genetic haemochromatosis	Cirrhosis Hypersplenism Diabetes Osteoarthritis	Phlebotomy Chelation: desferrioxamine
			Secondary Thalassaemias Alcoholic cirrhosis Porphyria cutanea tarda Sideroblastic anaemia	Cirrhosis Hypersplenism	Chelation: desferrioxamine + phlebotomy

Table 2 (*cont.*)
(b) Trace metal deficiency

Element	Metabolic role	Organ/tissue affected	Disorder	Clinical features	Specific treatment
Coppper	As Table 2(a)	Hair Skin CNS development	**Primary** Menke's disease **Secondary** TPN Nutritional deficiency	Neonatal death, Kinky, steely hair Cutis laxis, dermatitis CNS degeneration Anaemia, neutropenia Bone changes secondary to reduced cross-linking elastin/collagen Skin/skeletal abnormalities Aortic aneurysm Abnormal lung development	Copper replacement (copper histidine)
Iron	As Table 2(a)	Bone marrow Red cells Skin, hair, nails	**Primary** Iron deficiency **Secondary** Iron deficiency	Anaemia (microcytic) Ischaemic effects on organs/ tissues	Iron supplement Ascorbic acid (low dose)
Manganese	Mitochondrial function Mucopoly- saccharide synthesis	CNS Skeletal	**Primary** Manganese deficiency *in utero* **Secondary** TPN Nutritional deficiency	Early neonatal death CNS: Irreversible ataxia Inner ear otolith abnormality Skeletal: anomalous inner ear calcification	Manganese replacement
Selenium	Free radical scavenging enzymes (glutathione peroxidase)	Muscle Skeletal	Keshan disease Kashin-Beck disease	Congestive cardiomyopathy Osteoarthropathy Muscle weakness/pain	Sodium selenite replacement
Zinc	?	Skin CNS Gastrointestinal system Reproductive system	**Primary** Acrodermatitis enteropathica Sickle-cell disease **Secondary** Gastrointestinal tract Crohn's disease Malabsorption syndromes Liver disease	Growth retardation Congenital malformation Chromsome aberration Alopecia CNS Mental lethargy Emotional disorder Convulsions Gastrointestinal tract Weight loss/anorexia Diarrhoea Skin Bullous/pustular dermatitis Increased infections Impaired wound healing Oligospermia	Zinc replacement Zinc sulphate Zinc acetate

are reduced. Skin fibroblasts from these patients show a reduced copper uptake.

Identification of the gene on the X chromosome now allows specific diagnosis on chorionic villus biopsy material, where in the past confirmation of the diagnosis rested on the increased copper concentration of these biopsies.

BASIC DEFECT

In Menkes disease (and in the animal model—mottled mouse) there is defective copper transport in the placenta and intestine due to an abnormal copper-transporting protein. In the majority of patients recently studied, an 8.5 kb mRNA has been shown to be either qualitatively or quantitatively abnormal, due to a number of deletions in the gene, some of which were non-overlapping.

The primary defect produces abnormal copper concentrations in intestinal mucosa, kidney, placenta, and testis. Defective transport within the mucosal cell or across the serosal surface may account for the 20 per cent reduction in intestinal absorption of copper.

MANAGEMENT

Copper replacement by intravenous therapy can correct the skin, hair, and pigmentation abnormalities, but the neurological damage appears to be irreversible. However, now that the condition can be reliably detected *in utero*, early replacement with copper histidine given daily, may be a more promising approach.

CUTIS LAXIS

This is an X-linked Ehlers–Danlos syndrome, diagnosed in childhood or early adult life (see Sections 19 and 23). The clinical features include generalized skin, joint, and bladder laxity, and recurrent urinary-tract infections. The cause is as yet unknown, but may relate to a closely linked gene involved in copper transport.

Copper overload or toxicity

Copper toxicity has been well documented to occur naturally in animals (the Bedlington terrier, Domenican toad (*Bufo marinus*), and the mute swan (*Cygnus olor*)), and in experimental animals given copper or in acquired copper toxicity in sheep. In all of these, copper accumulates in the liver. Chronic copper toxicity in man occurs in two major forms:

(1) the primary inherited form, in which copper accumulates in and damages the liver, later the nervous system and other tissues, giving rise to the clinical entity of hepatolenticular degeneration, or Wilson's disease;

(2) the secondary form, which arises because of an acquired defect. In this form, copper accumulates as a consequence of chronic cholestasis, either congenital (biliary atresia or Indian childhood cirrhosis) or acquired (primary biliary cirrhosis) conditions. Amounts of hepatic copper may then be similar to those in found Wilson's disease, but some damage has always preceded the excessive amounts of liver copper. In chronic active hepatitis, smaller amounts of accumulated copper exacerbate preceding hepatocyte injury.

Wilson's disease

In 1912, Samuel Kinnier Wilson first described a copper toxic condition as a neurological disorder (progressive lenticular degeneration) which was usually fatal. Although a neurologist, he noted that severe motor and mental disturbances were always associated with liver cirrhosis and suggested that the 'morbid agent', now known to be copper, was a 'toxin associated with the cirrhosis'.

DEFINITION

Wilson's disease, or hepatolenticular degeneration, is an autosomal recessively inherited disorder due to an abnormal gene located on chromosome 13. Pathognomonic features of the disease include hepatic copper accumulation (>25 µg/g dry weight) in association with reduced or absent circulating caeruloplasmin (< 200 mg/dl), and reduction in biliary excretion of copper (< 1.5 mg/day). These defects result in copper accumulation in the body, initially within hepatocytes and then, as damage leads to cirrhosis and portal hypertension, increasing copper in the circulation deposits in the central nervous system, eye, kidneys, and other organs. If untreated, the disorder results in cirrhosis and extensive central nervous system damage, with a fatal outcome within a few years of onset of the symptoms. Chelating therapy prevents progression of the disease and may also reverse some neurological and the eye abnormalities.

INCIDENCE

Although previously considered one of the rare inborn errors of metabolism, Wilson's disease has a prevalence of 1 in 30 000 with a carrier frequency of 1 in 90. The abnormal gene is present in all racial groups studied so far and a higher incidence has been noted in Arabs, natives of southern Italy, Jews of Eastern Europe, Japanese, Chinese, and Indians, as well as in communes with a high rate of consanguineous marriages. There is no known HLA association.

GENETICS

Bearn (1953) was the first to provide evidence in an extended family study, for an autosomal recessive mode of inheritance. Subsequently, the demonstration of a linkage between the locus for Wilson's disease and the esterase D enzyme localized the gene mutation to chromosome 13. More recently, DNA restriction length polymorphism studies have further localized the position to 13q14–q21. Identification of the Menkes disease gene mutation, coding for a transporter protein, has raised the possibility that the abnormal gene of Wilson's disease may code for a defective liver-specific copper transporter protein. Using strategies for positional cloning, a candidate gene for Wilson's disease has been recently assigned to 13q14–21. Expression studies of this gene reveal a 7.5 kb transcript which is expressed strongly in the liver, kidney, and placenta and weakly in heart, brain, lung, muscle, and pancreas. Mutation analysis has also revealed four disease-specific mutations (two transversions and two frameshift mutations) affecting different domains of the putative protein. These correlate with distinct Wilson disease haplotypes.

A 1411 amino acid protein has been predicted from the cDNA sequence obtained by Cox *et al.* which, as a cation-transporting P-type ATPase, has close homology with the predicted protein product of the Menkes disease gene. These proteins additionally share similarity with caeruloplasmin in having six potential copper-binding motifs.

The link with reduced or absent plasma caeruloplasmin is still uncertain, since the caeruloplasmin gene has been mapped to chromosome 3q25. However, mRNA for caeruloplasmin is reduced in Wilson's disease patients, but not sufficiently to account for the variable reduction in plasma caeruloplasmin. In addition, the presence of intracellular caeruloplasmin, even when plasma caeruloplasmin levels are reduced or absent, suggests that the critical defect is likely to be post-translational.

Detection of gene carriers in families is now possible by development of several highly polymorphic microsatellite markers tightly linked and in linkage disequilibrium with the Wilson's disease locus, if one affected sibling and parents are available for genotyping. Using PCR for detection of these markers, haplotypes associated with the defective gene can be detected even if only traces of DNA are available, and the carrier status of siblings can be determined. In contrast, carrier data by mutation analysis would be difficult because of allelic heterogeneity.

CLINICAL FEATURES

Wilson's disease may be clinically undetectable until 5 years of age. However, during this period copper accumulates in the liver without clinical signs, and excess copper in red cells may present as chronic haemolytic anaemia or an episode of acute haemolysis.

In 90 per cent of patients, the disease presents with juvenile hepatic disease or with neurological/psychiatric manifestations. About 40 per cent of patients present with a spectrum of liver disease, from acute to chronic hepatitis, or with abnormal liver function tests without clinical findings. Copper initially accumulates in the hepatic cytosol, then, as saturation occurs, in mitochondria and eventually in lysosomes prior to biliary excretion, while some copper is released to the circulation bound to caeruloplasmin. If this redistribution occurs rapidly, patients may develop fulminant hepatic failure or intravascular haemolysis. It has been shown clearly that copper accumulation in, and damage to, mitochondria precedes the accumulation in hepatic lysosomes and leads to cirrhosis. Continued extrahepatic redistribution increases as portal hypertension and shunting of blood from liver occurs. At this stage neurological, psychiatric, ophthalmological, and renal damage occurs due to increasing copper deposition.

CLINICAL PRESENTATIONS

Haematological

Presentation with non-spherocytic, Coombs-negative intravascular haemolysis may occur in 10 to 15 per cent of patients with Wilson's disease. Severe haemolysis may also accompany fulminant hepatitis.

Hepatic (see also Section 14)

Before puberty, symptoms and signs of mild hepatic dysfunction are common, and if they coincide with abdominal pain and haemolysis, Wilson's disease should be suspected. Some 10 per cent of patients with Wilson's disease have pigment gallstones, suggesting previous episodes of haemolysis.

The more usual presentation is with chronic liver damage progressing to cirrhosis. In the early stages, patients are vaguely unwell, but later develop more specific features of liver dysfunction such as nausea, easy bleeding, fluid retention, and jaundice. Portal hypertension develops, with progressive hepatic insufficiency with splenomegaly, gastro-oesophageal varices, and ascites. Patients are often investigated incorrectly for other causes of splenomegaly, such as idiopathic thrombocytopenic purpura. Around 1 to 30 per cent of patients present with a picture of chronic active hepatitis, when the diagnosis of Wilson's disease may be missed since plasma caeruloplasmin levels may increase to within the normal range, along with secretion of acute phase reacting proteins. A minority of patients present with fulminant hepatitis and encephalopathy, sometimes just after starting chelating therapy. In these the prognosis is poor unless the liver is transplanted. It is notable that hepatocellular carcinoma is rare in the cirrhosis of Wilson's disease, unlike the situation in haemochromatosis.

Neurological (see also Section 24)

Symptoms may be diverse and present between the ages of 14 and 40 years. In all patients, some degree of liver damage, usually cirrhosis, is present. The neurological symptoms may be acute or chronic in onset and may be rapidly progressive.

A common presentation is with the insidious onset of dysarthria and deteriorating physical performance at school (handwriting, for example) and with increasing tremor (rest, intention, and postural). Early physical signs include flexion-extension tremor of hands, becoming a parkinsonian 'batswing' or intention type; orolaryngeal dysphagia and sialorrhoea are associated with hypokinesia; abnormal movements become more obvious, with grimacing and choreiform movements. Later features include spasticity, rigidity of limbs and neck muscles, and convulsions. Cognitive and sensory functions are usually preserved at least until a very late stage.

Psychiatric

About 60 per cent of patients with neurological features also show evidence of behavioural or psychiatric disorders caused by excess cerebral copper. These may present with a fall off in intellectual ability at school and/or with truancy and trouble with authorities. These are important to recognize, since failure to do so may place these individuals in mental health care rather than that of a neurologist or metabolic physician.

Ophthalmic

Kayser–Fleischer rings (Plate 2) are usually pathognomonic of Wilson's disease, but similar appearances have been noted in cryptogenic cirrhosis and with prolonged cholestasis. They are due to deposition of copper in the limbus of the cornea and appear brown in a grey blue iris, or grey in a brown eye. They are best seen by standing behind the patient and by asking the patient to look downwards, or by slit-lamp examination. Rarely, the posterior membrane of the lens is involved, producing the appearance of a sunflower cataract (see Section 26).

Renal

Renal tubular acidosis due to damage by copper in proximal and/or distal tubules is not uncommon. Osteomalacia and rickets may occur as a result of tubular loss of phosphate. Aminoaciduria and nephrocalcinosis may also occur.

Joints

Skeletal abnormalities, particularly early osteoarthritis of the spine (Scheuermann's disease), is not uncommon, but polyarthritis as well as hypermobile joints and chondromalacia patellae are also recognized features.

Skin

The skin may be hyperpigmented in Wilson's disease, appearing slightly grey with a bluish appearance of the lanulae of the nails.

Cardiac

Cardiac abnormalities have been noted rarely, with cardiac hypertrophy (but not cardiomyopathy) associated with interstitial fibrosis, small-vessel sclerosis, and perivascular myocarditis, which may lead to congestive cardiac failure.

Endocrine disturbances

Endocrine disturbances are mainly due to liver dysfunction, with gynaecomastia in men and menstrual disturbance in women, with some infertility. It is notable that most women conceive easily once they have been treated and excess copper removed.

PATHOLOGY

Histological changes vary with the amount of copper accumulated.

Liver

The liver is most affected, although in neonates it may appear normal despite increased amounts of hepatic copper. The neonatal liver can tolerate 6 to 8 times the copper concentration tolerated by the adult liver.

The precise sequence of hepatocyte change is not certain and there may be few changes in liver lobular structure in the asymptomatic patient. Early changes are evident on liver biopsy even in the asymptomatic patient, with pericellular fatty droplet infiltration of cytoplasm and 'glycogen' degeneration of the nuclei, with copper distributed diffusely in the cytoplasm.

Concurrently, or preceding these changes, mitochondrial, microsomal, and peroxisomal abnormalities are seen. Some of the lipid is contained within lysosomes. Progression from fatty infiltration to cirrhosis occurs at variable rates; either patients develop inflammatory changes indistinguishable from chronic active hepatitis, or cirrhosis may develop with little inflammatory infiltrate. Once cirrhosis has occurred, the ultrastructural changes are not specific for Wilson's disease except that more copper is found within pericanulicular lysosomes (about 25 per cent) than in any other intracellular compartment. Despite increased hepatic copper content, histochemical stains for copper (rubeanic acid) or copper-associated protein (orcein) are of little value in diagnosis and do not correlate well with the degree of copper overload.

Brain

Pathological effects of copper are widespread but non-specific except for cystic changes in the region of the internal capsule, which can be detected by computed tomography or nuclear magnetic resonance scans.

Cornea

Copper is deposited in Descemet's membrane (Plate 2).

Kidney

Copper accumulates in the renal cortex and may account for generalized proximal tubular dysfunction or Fanconi syndrome and aminoaciduria or glycosuria.

Bone

A wide variety of bone lesions have been described in Wilson's disease, due to the toxic effect of copper on chondroblasts and on collagen formation.

DIAGNOSIS

General investigations

The majority of patients with Wilson's disease have Kayser–Fleischer rings and low plasma caeruloplasmin concentrations. Haematological and biochemical investigations to detect anaemia, haemolysis, and disturbed hepatocellular function are all important in screening patients presenting with features compatible with the disease.

Specific investigations

These are necessary to confirm the diagnosis of Wilson's disease and in monitoring the effects of treatment (Table 3).

Serum caeruloplasmin

This can be measured enzymatically by radial immunodiffusion or by reverse passive haemagglutination. The activity and concentration of this glycoprotein is reduced or absent (< 25 mg/dl) in 95 per cent of patients with Wilson's disease. There is overlap of caeruloplasmin levels in those with Wilson's disease, in obligate heterozygotes, and in normal subjects in the lower range of normal distribution. Non-caeruloplasmin copper is loosely bound to albumin or amino acids (5–12 μg/dl) and is increased in untreated Wilson's disease.

Urine copper

Twenty-four hour urinary excretion of copper is always increased in untreated Wilson's disease (>70–100 μg/day), although this may also occur in other liver diseases, such as chronic active hepatitis and primary biliary cirrhosis. Special care is needed when collecting the urine samples to avoid contamination. Measurement of urinary copper excretion is also important in monitoring the effects of chelating therapy, where, early in treatment, urine levels may rise to 2000 μg/day and fall to less than 100 μg/day as the copper overload is reduced.

Liver copper concentration

In normal individuals, the copper concentration varies between 15 and 55 μg/g dry weight of liver and can be measured by spectrophotometric

Table 3 *Normal and Wilson's disease parameters*

	Normal	Wilson's disease
Serum		
Caeruloplasmin (mg/dl)	25–40	< 25
Copper (μmol/l)	11–24	3–10
Urine		
Copper (μg/24 h)		
untreated	< 40	100–1000
treated (penicillamine)	100–600	1500–3000
Hepatic copper		
(μg/g dry weight)	15–55	250–3000

assay, by atomic absorption spectrophotometry, or by neutron activation analysis. In untreated patients, the level of hepatic copper is greater than 250 μg/g dry weight, and in heterozygotes the concentration range is between 55 and 250 μg/g dry weight. Increased hepatic copper occurs in secondary copper overload, such as Indian childhood cirrhosis, primary biliary cirrhosis, sclerosing cholangitis, and chronic active hepatitis, but can be readily distinguished from Wilson's disease on clinical, biochemical, and histological grounds.

Radio-copper studies

Measurement of the incorporation of radiocopper into caeruloplasmin is helpful in distinguishing patients with suspected Wilson's disease when diagnosis is uncertain, for example when caeruloplasmin levels are normal, or when liver biopsy is contraindicated. Measurement of incorporation of orally administered radiocopper into caeruloplasmin at 1, 2, 3, and 48 h distinguishes clearly between normal patients and those with Wilson's disease, in whom little or no radiocopper is incorporated into newly synthesized caeruloplasmin.

BASIC DEFECT

Several hypotheses have been advanced to explain the primary defect of failure of biliary excretion of copper. Only recently has the link been made between this defect and reduced plasma caeruloplasmin (Fig. 2).

The clinical sequelae of Wilson's disease arise from accumulation of copper in various body organs. It is now clear that the liver in Wilson's disease produces caeruloplasmin and that the defect in this glycoprotein must be post-translational. Evidence of reduced amounts of hepatic mRNA for caeruloplasmin has not yet been linked to the underlying metabolic defect. The recent demonstration that there are different molecular forms of caeruloplasmin, a 132 kDa form found in plasma and a 125 kDa form in bile which is reduced or absent in Wilson's disease, lends further support for a post-translational abnormality. It also suggests that caeruloplasmin may play more than a secondary role in the underlying metabolic defect. It is known that reabsorption of biliary copper from the intestine in Wilson's disease is not increased.

The localization of the defect in copper homeostasis to the biliary tract may be the result of the liver synthesizing a high-affinity copper-binding protein or of a deficiency in synthesis of a biliary copper-binding protein. The latter possibility is supported by the reduced amounts of the 125 kDa caeruloplasmin in bile and liver in Wilson's disease. Sternlieb has suggested that there is also an abnormality of hepatic lysosomes, known to participate in intracellular processing and excretion of copper to bile.

Since the metabolism of copper in the liver of neonates is similar to that of patients with untreated Wilson's disease, it has been suggested that a mutation in a 'controller' gene is responsible for repression of normal copper metabolism in the fetus and that Wilson's disease results from a failure to switch from the positive balance in the fetus and neonate to the normal balance of the adult. With the recent identification of the Menkes gene mutation, it is also possible that the Wilson's disease gene codes for an altered specific membrane copper transporter.

PATHOGENESIS OF THE LIVER LESION

Copper, in free ionic form, is toxic to hepatocytes in man and animals. Although the retained copper accumulates in lysosomes, there is no evidence that copper-filled lysosomes are fragile. Indeed, this copper is not in a form to catalyse free radicals which could damage the lysosomal membrane. In contrast, copper-containing mitochondria are more fragile, and it is likely that the mechanism of copper-induced hepatocyte damage is due to mitochondrial damage, reducing oxidative phosphorylation. It is possible that the low molecular weight form of caeruloplasmin may not be able to bind to 'abnormal' lysosomal or plasma membranes, or that after binding the 'transporting system' is defective.

MANAGEMENT

Walshe (1956) was the first to show how effective D-penicillamine (dimethylcysteine) was in removing copper from patients with Wilson's disease. The optimum time for treatment is in the early stages, and all patients with Wilson's disease should be treated even if asymptomatic. Treatment must be lifelong, unless patients have had a liver transplant. A majority of symptomatic patients improve or have an almost complete resolution of their symptoms. Non-compliant patients who discontinue treatment may relapse rapidly and die.

The management of Wilson's disease also involves the general care of a patient with liver disease and possibly anaemia, and investigation of the family and siblings of the propositus, as well as specific therapy.

Chelating agents

Use of a low-copper diet and copper chelating agents is essential to induce a state of negative copper balance. D-penicillamine is still the drug of first choice, although triethylene tetramine and ammonium thiomolybdate (so successful in copper-toxic sheep) can be alternatives. Divided daily doses of penicillamine range from 500 mg to 2 g, depending on the response. Larger doses are required initially and should be reduced as urinary copper excretion falls. Progress can be monitored by clinical improvement, 24-h urine copper and serum copper measurements, blood and platelet counts, and urinalysis for protein and aminoaciduria, in addition to clinical examination and slit-lamp examination of the cornea.

Triethylene tetramine dihydrochloride (trientine), given orally in divided daily doses of 750 mg to 2 g, can be used when penicillamine is not tolerated or causes side-effects such as renal damage, bone marrow suppression, or rarely a systemic lupus syndrome. As copper is mobilized from different body pools, trientine causes a rise in the serum-free copper concentration.

Oral zinc is a third agent used in the treatment of copper toxicosis. Zinc may act by promoting gastrointestinal excretion of copper by inhibiting copper absorption in a competitive way, or by inducing synthesis of metallothioneins within the enterocyte and hepatocyte which would bind copper to form mercaptides. Copper would then remain as a complex within the enterocyte, to be excreted in faeces as cells turn over or to be transferred to the portal circulation.

Zinc (150 mg) is given orally either as the sulphate or the acetate form in divided doses 1 h before meals. There is still some doubt as to whether zinc can be used alone as therapy for Wilson's disease or only as an adjunct to chelating agents. There is evidence that using zinc concurrently with penicillamine may reduce treatment-induced fulminant hepatic failure.

Liver transplantation

This is an attractive option for treatment of Wilson's disease since it corrects the metabolic defect in the liver. With limited resources, however, it is reserved for young patients with severe hepatic and neurological damage (for example acute hepatitis or fulminant hepatic failure). Patients who have had liver transplants no longer need chelating therapy, and at least two case reports have claimed complete reversal of extensive neurological impairment after transplantation. In fulminant hepatic failure, a prognostic index based on prothrombin time, bilirubin, and transaminase determines whether the patient is suitable for transplantation (see Chapter 14.31).

Screening of family members

This is an essential part of management of any patient with Wilson's disease. Screening of children should be after 3 years of age. It should

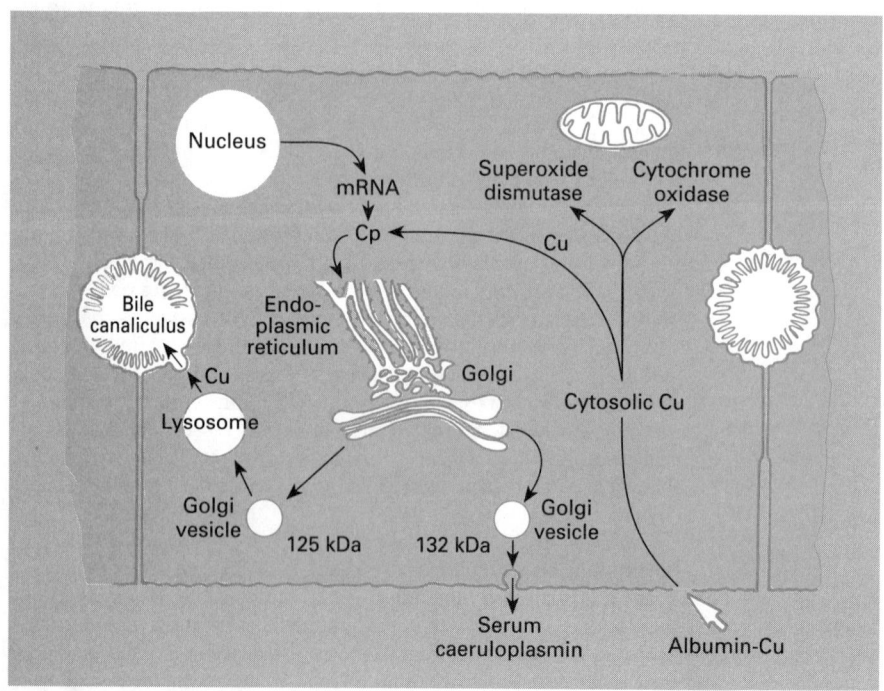

Fig. 2 Caeruloplasmin secretion and excretion in a normal hepatocyte indicating different molecular forms. White arrow shows site of defect in Wilson's disease.

Table 4 *Clinical features of zinc deficiency*

Mild	Moderate	Severe
Oligospermia	Growth retardation	Bullous/pustular dermatitis
Weight loss	Hypogonadism	Keratitis
↑ Hyperammonaemia	Skin changes	Alopecia
	Anorexia	Diarrhoea
	Mental lethargy	Weight loss
	↓ Wound healing	Emotional disorder
	Neurosensory disorders	↑ Infections
	Taste abnormalities	Fatal if untreated
	Abnormal dark adaptation	

include a careful history, clinical examination, and slit-lamp examination of the eyes, liver function tests and assay of the serum caeruloplasmin level. If the results of these are suggestive of Wilson's disease, liver biopsy and quantitative measurement of hepatic copper should follow. It is as important not to miss a homozygote as to treat a heterozygote with lifelong therapy.

Women with cirrhosis due to copper toxicity have an increased risk of infertility, abortion, stillbirth, and premature delivery. Conversely, once chelation therapy has reduced the copper overload, successful pregnancies occur and both major chelating agents do not appear to harm the fetus or cause fetal copper deficiency.

Side-effects of therapy

Adverse effects of penicillamine are not uncommon. In the first few weeks of therapy, 20 per cent of patients may develop hypersensitivity with a maculopapular rash, lymphadenopathy, granulocytopenia, and thrombocytopenia. In these situations, the drug should be discontinued immediately, and when re-introduced it should be at much lower dose (0.25 g/day) and with steroid cover. A nephrotic syndrome may occur in as many as 3 to 7 per cent. Much rarer are reports of a Goodpasture-like syndrome or drug-related systemic lupus erythematosus.

Skin lesions are not uncommon with long-term chelation therapy, and patients may develop lax skin due to inhibition of elastin and collagen cross-linking in the subcutaneous tissues. The rarest form is elastosis perforans serpiginosa (Plate 3). Trientine has been used much less, but has also been associated with rashes and systemic lupus erythematosus nephritis. The major problem with zinc therapy is gastrointestinal intolerance, which may inhibit iron absorption, causing a microcytic anaemia; it may also alter phagocytic activity against bacteria and affect lipoprotein metabolism.

PROGNOSIS

Early diagnosis and chelation therapy is the only way to ensure a good prognosis in Wilson's disease. Poor progress is more likely in patients with severe liver damage, including acute fulminant hepatic failure, and acute neurological disease and dystonia. In addition, in the presence of cirrhosis, even when copper-depleted, risks of variceal bleeding and intercurrent infections remain. Prognosis is best in the asymptomatic individuals who are detected early, often by the meticulous screening of families of index cases.

Chronic cholestatic syndromes

Intra- and extrahepatic obstruction to bile excretion will also affect copper excretion and cause its accumulation in the liver. Liver damage due to congenital or acquired abnormalities precedes the copper retention, which increases with the duration of cholestasis and exacerbates hepatocyte damage.

Iron

Abnormalities of iron metabolism and associated clinical features are described elsewhere (Chapter 22.4.4).

Zinc

Zinc is an essential trace element required for RNA and DNA synthesis and for the function of some 200 metalloenzymes. Its importance for human health has been noted over the past 25 years, particularly in relation to zinc deficiency, which is prevalent worldwide. Zinc deficiency is associated with protein malnutrition which is common in populations of low income or those eating cereal proteins high in phosphate and phytate. It becomes manifest quickly in individuals with increased requirements, such as growing infants, children, and pregnant women.

About 20 to 30 per cent (12–15 mg/day) of zinc is absorbed in the duodenum, where it competes with iron for binding to mucosal sites. Absorption is also reduced by calcium, phytate, and fibre. Daily losses occur through the gastrointestinal tract (1.2 mg/day) with less in urine and insensible losses. The clinical spectrum of zinc deficiency varies from severe to mild, as shown in Table 4. Prenatal zinc deficiency has a particularly rapid effect on the fetus, causing intrauterine death or low birth weight. Congenital malfunction and hyperplasia of the oesophagal mucosa are also particularly common. Persistent zinc deficiency causes postnatal behavioural problems and the low zinc content of tissues may cause chromosomal aberrations and decreased synthesis of DNA and proteins, such as pulmonary surfactant and pancreatic proteins.

METABOLIC EFFECTS OF ZINC

Zinc is found in a number of organs (liver, kidney, bone, retina, prostate, and muscle). It is carried in plasma mainly bound to albumin, but other proteins such as caeruloplasmin and α_2-macroglobulin also have a strong affinity for zinc.

Zinc has a major enzymatic function; around 70 metalloenzymes require this element but not all are sensitive to zinc deficiency. It appears that alkaline phosphatase in bone, carboxypeptidase in pancreas, and deoxythymidine kinase in connective tissue are among the sensitive forms.

Zinc also interacts with iron, copper, calcium, lead, and cadmium, competing with these trace elements for binding sites. Thus zinc can be used as an antisickling agent, because of its antagonistic affect on red cell calcium, and to alleviate toxic effects of cadmium and copper (see above).

Certain hormones, thymosin, somatomedin, and testosterone, are zinc dependent, which may account for some of the hormonal abnormalities arising with zinc deficiency. It has a well-defined role in inhibiting histamine release from mast cells, and has other anti-inflammatory actions on phagocytic cells and platelets as well as interfering in cell-mediated immunity (zinc is essential for T-cell function), thus predisposing zinc-deficient individuals to infection. Zinc ions are also protective against free-radical injury, although the mechanism is uncertain.

Zinc is now known to have a specific role in the nucleus of cells, where it stabilizes native RNA, promotes catalytic activity of RNA polymerases, and is essential for the function of at least two of the chromatin proteins involved in transcription. Zinc deficiency appears to alter chromatin to a more compact form which is far more accessible to hydrolytic enzymes. An essential part of gene expression is binding of a regulatory protein to the recognition sequence of an appropriate gene and it now seems that a commonly used structural motif for DNA recognition is the 'zinc finger'. Putative 'zinc fingers' are present in the structures of many regulatory proteins.

CLINICAL FEATURES

The clinical features of zinc deficiency are summarized in Table 4.

DIAGNOSIS

Body zinc status can be assessed by measurement of zinc in body fluids (plasma and urine), although in severe deficiency white cell or platelet zinc concentrations probably give a more accurate assessment of body depletion and stores. A zinc tolerance test (using oral challenge of 200 mg zinc sulphate) is useful in detecting abnormalities of absorption, but will not distinguish between a malabsorption state causing zinc deficiency or one where malabsorption is caused by the zinc deficiency (cf. acrodermatitis enteropathica). Measurement of the activity of zinc-dependent enzymes may also be helpful in assessing the degree of zinc deficiency, as may measurements of serum thymulin and plasma metal-lothionein concentrations.

TREATMENT

Zinc replacement can be given as the sulphate or acetate form, the former causing less gastrointestinal upset. The nutritional requirement for zinc is in the order of 10 to 15 mg/day. Zinc is absorbed more efficiently as a salt than from the normal diet, zinc replacement is normally as zinc sulphate 30 to 150 mg/day taken orally. More rarely, zinc deficiency in association with hepatic cirrhosis, and particularly hepatic encephalopathy, can respond to zinc (one mechanism for the latter may be an improved enzymatic conversion of ammonia to urea). Replacement should be with oral zinc acetate, 600 mg/day in divided doses.

Selenium

Selenium is an essential element for key free-radical scavenging enzymes such as glutathione peroxidase, which reduce hydrogen peroxide and a range of lipid peroxides which could potentially damage cell membranes. It is absorbed from the gastrointestinal tract as a water-soluble complex in a process which is not regulated. Selenium is normally excreted in urine via direct methylation, the normal route with standard dietary intake. In toxic situations, a differently methylated metabolite is excreted. Selenium concentrations are highest in the liver and kidneys, perhaps reflecting their role as organs of storage and excretion.

Selenium and disease states

Selenium deficiency is associated with two human diseases which occur in the East, particularly in China.

Keshan disease

This is a cardiomyopathy where multifocal necrosis and fibrosis of the myocardium occurs, presenting with muscle weakness and myalgia.

This condition is improved by administration of sodium selenite. It is still unknown whether this condition is due entirely to selenium deficiency and whether this interacts with a genetic deficiency of a selenium-dependent enzyme (glutathione peroxidase), or whether interaction with a virus component occurs. Some protection has been claimed for prophylactic dosing with 150 μg/day of selenium, given as seleno-methionine.

Kashimbeck disease

This is an endemic osteoarthropathy occurring in East Asia and China. It is characterized by chronic osteoarthrosis affecting fingers, toes, and long bones and is found in children aged between 5 and 12 years. It is a progressive disorder which results in deformity and growth retardation. Some improvement has been noted with sodium selenite treatment.

The standard replacement dose of selenium is difficult to assess, since daily recommended intake is between 50 and 200 μg for an adult, and for the pre-term infant, a minimum requirement of 1 μg/kg/day has been suggested. Supplementation of total parenteral nutrition fluids to supply selenium at a level of 1 μg/kg/day is recommended. Thus a normal daily intake of 100 μg in total parenteral nutrition fluids is needed to maintain levels at about 100 ng/ml. Selenium is usually replaced in the form of selenious acid, and a dosage of 100 μg/day is administered intravenously for 21 to 31 days in order to reverse any symptoms of selenium deficiency.

Selenium toxicity is rare and occurs in parts of America where there is a high content of selenium in the soil. The major clinical features are alopecia and nail deformities. Selenium overload due to hyperalimentation is covered in Section 10.

Chromium

This is an essential element in carbohydrate and lipid metabolism, where deficiency due to insufficient intake results in clinical features indistinguishable from those of non-insulin-dependent diabetes and associated vascular disease. It is absorbed from the diet, by a mechanism similar to that of iron uptake, in very small amounts (1 p.p.m.) and is excreted through the kidneys at a rate that is increased by exercise, physical trauma, and diets high in refined sugars.

Chromium may also have a role in nucleic acid function, since trace amounts are bound to DNA, RNA, and nuclear proteins. In vitro evidence suggests that chromium enhances RNA synthesis by binding to DNA and increasing the number of initiation sites. Its precise role in glucose metabolism is unclear, but evidence suggests that chromium may increase the expression of insulin receptors and thus have a role to play in hyperglycaemia in both insulin-dependent and non-insulin-dependent diabetes mellitus.

Manganese

The liver and pancreas contain the highest concentrations of this element. It is absorbed in constant amounts from the duodenum, which are increased in cirrhotic or iron-deficient patients. This may be due, in part, to an increase in transport binding proteins which participate in a carrier-mediated transport of iron and manganese. Manganese absorption, like that of zinc, is reduced by the presence of phytates, calcium, and phosphates in the diet. Once absorbed, it is transported bound to α_2-macro-globulin in the portal circulation and is taken up by the liver and excreted in bile. This, like copper, appears to be a site for regulating body manganese. It also interacts with iron metabolism in that a proportion is bound to transferrin and released in circulation for uptake by other tissues.

Manganese is an essential component of several proteins/enzymes involved in intermediary metabolism (arginase and pyruvate carboxylase), in free-radical scavenging (Mn-superoxide dismutase), and in transport proteins (calmodulin-dependent protein phosphatases). It may also be involved in glucose homeostasis and in intracellular function, perhaps participating in second-messenger interactions (phosphorylation, dephosphorylation cascades), and signal transduction systems coupled to specific receptors. It also affects calcium fluxes across cell membranes in excitable and other tissues (liver and pancreas), playing a role in intracellular calcium fluxes in mitochondria.

Manganese deficiency may be associated with joint disease (congenital dislocation of the hips) and osteoarthritis, but the mechanisms are not certain.

Other trace metal toxicity syndromes

Aluminium toxicity deserves a brief mention but is covered more fully elsewhere (see Chapter 8.3.6). Aluminium has no recognized physiological role in the human body and thus even small amounts may cause disease. Its absorption is similar to that of iron, and it comes from water, additives, and contamination by utensils and containers. Foods such as herbs and leaves contain small quantities, but processed foods contain very little (less than 5 μg/g). Most adults absorb around 1 to 10 mg/day and can cope with this by excretion in urine.

Toxicity may arise from contamination of food, the use of aluminium containing antacids and phosphate binders, or in parenteral solutions used in dialysis treatment of renal failure. Although neurotoxicity of aluminium was well known in animals to cause bulbar palsy, tremor, spasticity, and spinal cord changes, the first description of aluminium toxicity in man was in patients with chronic renal failure (see Chapter 20.17.1). High amounts of aluminium in dialysate fluids have been associated with anaemia, encephalopathy, and a particular form of metabolic bone disease resembling osteomalacia. Use of reverse osmosis and deionization to remove aluminium has largely removed this problem. The aluminium can also be chelated with desferroxamine. Environmental exposure to aluminium has given rise to similar problems.

A good example of acute aluminium poisoning occurred when 20 tons of concentrated aluminium sulphate were discharged into the treated water reservoir of Lowermoor Water Treatment Works, North Cornwall, UK, contaminating the water supply. The initial toxic symptoms were gastrointestinal disturbances, skin rashes, and mouth ulcers. Long-term effects on brain, bones, and joints, such as have been reported with aluminium toxicity in renal dialysis, were thought to be unlikely. Two government reports (in January 1989 and November 1991) concerning the water pollution at Lowermoor found that there was no evidence to suggest that aluminium exposure in the contaminated water caused any of the long-term effects and, in particular, there was no evidence for causation of Alzheimer's disease or other forms of dementing illness, despite suggestions in the literature linking chronic exposure to aluminium with Alzheimer's disease (see below). The reports, however, did highlight certain features about aluminium which were important for environmental exposure. Aluminium is a major component of dust, and analysis of integuments such as hair and skin are therefore likely to be contaminated. In contrast, its presence in serum is in very small amounts, with levels less than 10 μg/ml, and bulk bone aluminium is in the order of 1.5 to 13.3 μg/g. Aluminium salts can cause hypersensitivity reactions, but only when given by injection or in relation to the work place, not by oral ingestion.

Aluminium salts may deposit in bone, and around 30 to 80 mg may accumulate in the human body during a lifetime, half of which will be found in bone since this is a protective mechanism, removing aluminium from circulation when the levels become elevated. This explains the occurrence of osteomalacia-like disease in patients exposed to aluminium during dialysis treatment for chronic renal failure.

Postmortem reports on the brains of patients with renal failure exposed to chronically increased levels of aluminium in dialysis fluid have shown the effects of chronic aluminium poisoning on the brain.

Aluminium enters the brain at a slow rate by an iron-uptake system (transferrin-related transport), accumulating in the cortex and hippocampus, which are selectively vulnerable to Alzheimer's disease. In some patients with renal failure and prolonged exposure to high blood aluminium, β-amyloid protein is deposited in the brain as lesions which may be precursors of senile plaques, one of the major neuropathological features of Alzheimer's disease (Chapter 24.7.2); but no neurofibrillary tangles, the other hallmark of this disease, have been found. In addition, miners exposed over years to inhalation of aluminium particles to reduce silicotic lung disease, showed a dose-related declining cognitive function, and treatment with desferroxamine, removing the aluminium, slowed the progress of this disorder.

In summary, the reports suggest that there was some circumstantial evidence that exposure to aluminium over a prolonged period could contribute to the age-related decline in cognitive function, or could accelerate the deposition of β-amyloid protein, but that there was no evidence that brief toxic exposure to aluminium, as occurred during the Lowermoor incident, would have harmful consequences.

The precise mechanism of cellular toxicity is not known. Cognitive defects resulting from impaired neuronal function may arise because of effects of aluminium on second-messenger systems (DNA, kinases, cyclic AMP, phosphoinositides) which also affect the cytoskeleton and could cause neuronal dysfunction.

REFERENCES

Wilson's disease

Bearn, A.G. (1960). A genetic analysis of 30 families with Wilson's disease. *Annals of Human Genetics* 24, 33–43.

Bull, P.C., Thomas, G.R., Rommens, J.M., Forbes, J.R., and Cox, D.W. (1993). The Wilson's disease gene is a putative copper-transporting P-type ATPase similar to Menkes gene. *Nature*, 5, 327–37.

Dening, T.R. The neuropsychiatry of Wilson's disease: a review. *International Journal of Psychiatry in Medicine* 21, 135–48.

Houwen, R.H., et al. (1991). Isolation and regional localisation of 25 anonymous DNA probes on a chromosome 13 hybrid panel. *Cytogenetics and Cell Genetics* 57, 87–90.

Houwen, R.H.J., Roberts, E.A., Thomas, G.R., and Cox, D.W. (1993). DNA markers for the diagnosis of Wilson's disease. *Journal of Hepatology*, 17, 269–76.

McClain, C.J. (1991). Trace metals in liver disease. *Seminars in Liver Disease* 11, 321–39.

Sternlieb, I. (1990). Perspectives on Wilson's disease. *Hepatology* 12, 1234–9.

Stewart, E.A., White, A., Tomfohrde, J., et al. (1993). Polymorphic microsatellites and Wilson's disease (WD). *American Journal of Human Genetics*, 53, 864–73.

Tanzi, R.E., et al. (1993). The Wilson's disease gene is a copper-transporting ATPase with homology to the Menkes disease gene. *Nature*, 5, 344–50.

Walshe, J.M. and Yealland M. (1993). Chelation treatment of neurological Wilson's disease. *Quarterly Journal of Medicine* 86, 197–204.

Wilson, S.A.K. (1912). Progressive lenticular degeneration. A familial nervous disease associated with cirrhosis of the liver. *Brain* 34, 295–507.

Yarze, J.C., Martin, P., Munoz, S.J., and Friedman L.S. (1992). Wilson's disease: current status. *American Journal of Medicine* 92, 643–54.

Yang, F., et al. (1986). Characterisation, mapping and expression of the human caeruloplasmin gene. *Proceedings of the National Academy of Sciences USA* 83, 3257–61.

Yuzbasiyan-Gurkan V., Johnson V., and Brewer, G.J. (1991). Diagnosis and characterisation of presymptomatic patients with Wilson's disease and the use of molecular genetics to aid in diagnosis. *Journal of Laboratory and Clinical Medicine* 118, 458–565.

Menkes disease

Davies, K. (1993). Cloning the Menkes disease gene. *Nature*, 361, 98.

Gerdes, A.M., et al. (1990). Clinical expression of Menkes syndrome in females. *Clinical Genetics* 38, 452–9.

Menkes, J.H., Alter, M., Steigleder, G.K., Weakley, D.R., and Jung, J.H. (1962). A sex linked recessive disorder with retardation of growth, peculiar hair, focal cerebral and cerebellar degeneration. *Pediatrics* **29**, 764–99.

Tonnesen, T. and Horn, N. (1989). Prenatal and postnatal diagnosis of Menkes disease, an inherited disorder of copper metabolism. *Journal of Inherited Metabolic Disease* **12**, 207–14.

Vulpe, C., Levinson, B., Whitney, S., Packman, S., and Gitschier, J. (1993). Isolation of a candidate gene for Menkes disease is evidence that it encodes a copper-transporting ATPase. *Nature*, **3**, 7–13.

Zinc

Prasad, A.S. (1988). Clinical spectrum and diagnostic aspects of human zinc deficiency. In *Essential and toxic trace elements in human health and disease*, (ed. A.S. Prasad), pp. 3–53. A.R. Liss, New York.

Vallee, B.L. and Falchuk, (1983). Genetic expression and zinc. In *Biological aspects of metals and metal related diseases*, (ed. B. Sarker), Ch. 1–15. Raven Press, New York.

Selenium

Chen, X., Yang, G., Chen, J., Wen, Z., and Ge, K. (1980). Studies on the relations of selenium and Keshan disease. *Biological Trace Element Research* **2**, 91–107.

Diplock, A.T. and Chaudhry F.A. (1988). The relationship of selenium biochemistry to selenium-responsive disease in man. In *Essential and toxic trace elements in human health and disease*, (ed. A.S. Prasad), pp. 211–26. A.R. Liss, New York.

Simmer, K. and Thompson, R.P.H. (1990). Trace elements. In *The metabolic and molecular basis of acquired disease*, (ed. R.D. Cohen, B. Lewis, K.G.M.M. Alberti, and A.M. Denman), Vol. 1, pp.670–83. Baillère Tindall, London.

Aluminium

Brem, A.S., DiMario, C., and Levy, D.L. (1989). Perceived aluminium-related disease in a dialysis population. *Archives of Internal Medicine* **149**, 2541–4.

Cannata, J.B. and Domingo, J.L. (1989). Aluminium toxicity in mammals: a minireview. *Veterinary and Human Toxicology* **31**, 577–83.

Clayton, B. (1989). *Water pollution at Lowermoor, Cornwall*. Report of the Lowermoor Incident Health Advisory Group. Cornwall and Isles of Scilly District Health Authority, Truro.

Clayton, B. (1991). *Water pollution at Lowermoor, Cornwall*. Second report of the Lowermoor Incident Health Advisory Group, pp. 1–51. HMSO, London.

Cooke, K. and Gould, M.H. (1991). The health effects of aluminium – a review. *Journal of the Royal Society of Health* **111**, 163–8.

Eastwood, J.B., Levin, G.E., Pazianaz, M., Taylor, A.P., Denton, J., and Freemont, A.J. (1990). Aluminium deposition in bone after contamination of drinking water supply. *Lancet* **336**, 462–4.

Rifat, S.L., Eastwood, M.R., Crapper McLachlan, D.R., and Corey, P.N. (1990). Effect of exposure of miners to aluminium powder. *Lancet* **336**, 1162–5.

Van der Voet, G.B. (1992). Intestinal absorption of aluminium. In *Aluminium in biology and medicine*, pp. 107–122. Ciba Foundation, London.

11.8 Lysosomal storage diseases

R.W.E. WATTS

Lysosomes are subcellular organelles containing hydrolases with low optimum pH values ('acid hydrolases'), which catalyse the degredation of macromolecules. The macromolecules are either derived from the metabolic turnover of structural cellular components or have entered the cell by endocytosis. The products of this macromolecular degradation process leave the lysosomes by specific eflux processes. In most of the lysosomal storage diseases an inborn error of metabolism affects a specific lysosomal enzyme so that either undegraded or partial degraded macromolecules accumulate in the lysosomes. The engorged lysosomes distort the internal architecture of the cell, disturb its function, and inhibit the activities of other lysosomal enzymes, so that macromolecules other than those related to the primary enzyme deficiency also accumulate.

Cystinosis (cystine storage disease) and Salla disease (*N*-acetylneuraminic (sialic) acid storage disease) are due to metabolic lesions involving the specific efflux processes whereby these two low molecular weight products of macromolecule metabolism leave the lysosome.

Lysosomal enzymes are glycoproteins that are subject to exocytosis and reuptake by endocytosis. The protein moieties are synthesized on the rough endoplasmic reticulum and the oligosaccharide side chains are added in the Golgi apparatus. The addition of a terminal mannose 6-phosphate residue is necessary if the enzyme molecule is to be correctly routed into the lysosomes, and if it is to be available for receptor-mediated reuptake from the interstitial fluid. This mannose 6-phosphate residue is referred to as the enzyme's recognition marker.

Sphingolipidoses

The sphingolipid molecule contains a hydrophobic portion ceramide (*N*-acylsphingosine) and either a hydrophilic mono- or oligosaccharide chain in the case of the gangliosides, or phosphorylcholine in the case of sphingomyelin. The galactose residues are sulphated in the sulphatides. The sphingolipids are degraded by a series of lysosomal hydrolases and deficiencies of the individual enzymes cause the degradation products, which are characteristic of each disease (Fig. 1, Table 1), to accumulate intralysosomally. The different diseases and different variants of the same disease have characteristic organ distribution patterns of the abnormal storage products. The diseases in which there is an abnormal sphingolipid accumulation in the neuronal cells of the central nervous system, and therefore in the ganglion cells of the retina also, show retinal degeneration, which is particularly apparent at the macula, causing pallor of this part of the retina with a central red area (the cherry-red spot); pigmentary retinal changes are also found in some cases. The cherry-red spot is a useful clinical pointer to the sphingolipidoses with neuronal involvement.

Except for Fabry disease, which is inherited in a sex-linked recessive manner, the sphingolipidoses are all autosomal recessive disorders.

FARBER'S DISEASE (CERAMIDASE DEFICIENCY)

A hoarse cry, painful swollen joints with periarticular nodules, and pulmonary infiltrations developing in a previously healthy infant between

2 and 4 months of age suggest this diagnosis. The macular region of the retina appears grey with a cherry-red centre. The disease exists in severe and mild forms and death is usually due to pulmonary involvement. Most cases develop severe mental handicap. The heart valves are usually thickened. Hepatosplenomegaly and generalized lymphadenopathy are inconstant features.

NIEMANN–PICK DISEASE (SPHINGOMYELIN LIPIDOSIS: SPHINGOMYELINASE DEFICIENCY)

There are five phenotypic variants: (1) Type A, the acute neuropathic form; (2) Type B, the chronic form without neurological involvement; (3) Type C, the chronic neuropathic form; (4) Type D, the Nova Scotia variant and; (5) Type E, the adult non-neuropathic form. They all show abnormal lipid (sphingomyelin) storage in the reticuloendothelial macrophages. The abnormal cells in the sternal marrow and sometimes in the circulation (monocytes) are 50 to 90 μm in diameter and look foamy. Niemann–Pick disease is one of the causes of the sea-blue histiocyte phenomenon.

Type A is the most common variety. Hepatosplenomegaly, lymphadenopathy, and neurological retrogression with epileptic attacks begin during the first 6 to 12 months of life, and most patients die before the

age of 2 years. About half the cases have the cherry-red spot appearance at the macular. Type B patients develop hepatosplenomegaly and pulmonary infiltration with sphingomyelin-laden histiocytes, but there is no neurological involvement. Type C patients show psychomotor delay and retrogression during early childhood and die in later childhood and adolescence. Hepatosplenomegaly is less marked in this variant than in Types A and B. Type D patients resemble those with the chronic neuropathic variant but they have been shown to share a common ancestry arising in Western Nova Scotia. Type E patients present in adult life with moderate hepatosplenomegaly, but no neurological involvement. Some late presenting cases have shown mild cerebellar ataxia and the cherry-red spot at the macula.

GAUCHER DISEASE (GLUCOCEREBROSIDOSIS, GLUCOCEREBROSIDASE DEFICIENCY)

There are three clinical types of Gaucher disease: Type 1, chronic non-neuronopathic (adult); Type 2, acute neuronopathic (infantile) and; Type 3, subacute neuronopathic (juvenile). All types of patients have hepatosplenomegaly and large (20 to 100 μm in diameter) glucocerebroside-containing reticuloendothelial histiocytes (Gaucher cells) in the bone marrow. These cells have a crumpled-silk appearance in the usual

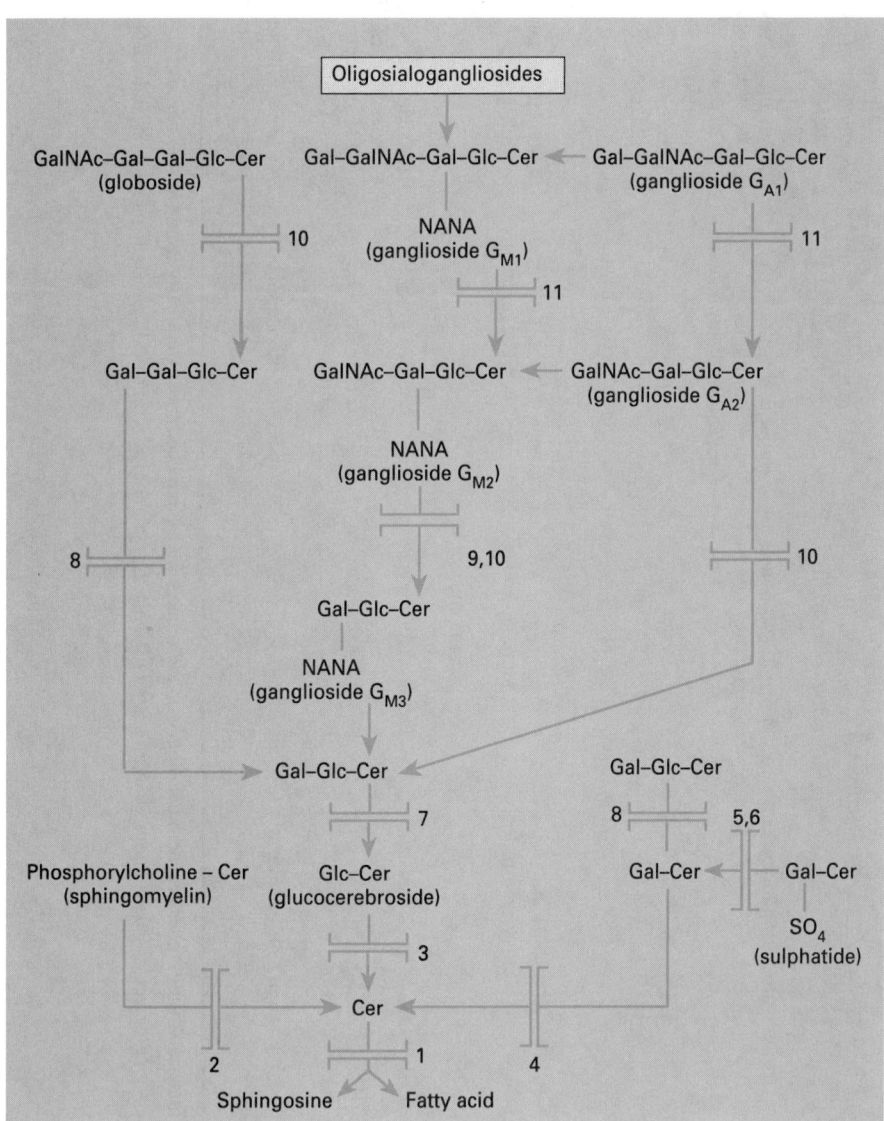

Fig. 1 Sphingolipid catabolism and the abbreviated structures of the sphingolipids which accumulate in the sphingolipidoses. The numerals indicate the metabolic blocks in the individual sphingolipidoses and correspond to those used in Table 1. Oligosialogangliosides are gangliosides with either 2, or 3, N-acetylneuraminic acid residues per molecule as opposed to the monosialogangliosides (G_M series) and asialogangliosides (G_A series). Cer, ceramide; Glc, glucose; Gal, galactose; GalNAc, N-acetylgalactosamine; NANA, N-acetylneuraminic acid (sialic acid). G_{M3} gangliosidosis is due to reduced activity of the transferase which converts the G_M series gangliosides to the more highly sialylated G_D and G_T series (oligosialogangliosides). (Redrawn from Watts, R.W.E and Gibbs, D.A. (1986). *Lysosomal storage diseases: Biochemical and clinical aspects*. Taylor and Francis, London.)

Table 1 *The sphingolipidoses*

No. in Fig. 1	Systematic name	Eponymous and/or other generally used name	Main storage compound	Enzyme deficiency	Biochemical diagnosis	Chromosome assignment
1	Ceramidosis	Farber disease	Ceramide	Ceramidase (EC 3.5.1.23)	Ceramide in skin nodules. Enzyme in leucocytes, fibroblasts	Not assigned
2	Sphingomyelinosis	Niemann–Pick disease	Sphingomyelin	Sphingomyelinase (EC 3.1.4.12)	Enzyme in leucocytes, fibroblasts	17
3	Glucocerebrosidosis	Gaucher disease	Glucocerebroside	β-Glucocerebrosidase (EC 3.2.1.45)	Glucocerebroside in liver erythrocytes. Enzyme in leucocytes, fibroblasts	1q21
4	Galactocerebrosidosis	Krabbé disease Globoid cell leukodystrophy	Galactocerebroside	Galactocerebroside β-galactosidase (EC 3.2.1.46)	Enzyme in serum, leucocytes, fibroblasts	17
5	Sulphatidosis	Metachromatic leukodystrophy	Cerebroside sulphates	Arylsulphatases A (cerebroside sulphatase) (EC 3.1.6.1)	Enzyme in leucocytes, fibroblasts, hair bulbs, plasma	22q13.31→q ter
6	Mucosulphatidosis	Multiple sulphatase deficiency syndrome	Cerebroside sulphates Steroid sulphates	Arylsulphatases A, B, C and steroid sulphatase (?sulphate receptor protein)	Enzymes in leucocytes, fibroblasts, urine. Dermatan and heparan sulphates in urine	22q13.31→q ter / Not assigned
7	Lactosylceramidosis	–	Lactosylceramide	Ceramide-lactoside β-galactosidase	Enzyme in fibroblasts. Lactosyl-ceramide in erythrocytes, plasma, bone marrow, urine sediment	Not assigned
8	α-Galactosyl-lactosylceramidosis	Fabry disease, Anderson–Fabry disease Angiokeratoma corporis diffusum	α-Galactosyl-lactosylceramide	α-Galactosidase A (EC 3.2.1.22)	Enzyme in leucocytes, hair bulbs, fibroblasts, tissue biopsy. Trihexoside in urine deposit	Xq22
9	G_{M2}-gangliosidosis type A_oB_H	Tay-Sachs disease	Ganglioside G_{M2}	β-D-Hexosaminidase A (α-subunit) (EC 3.2.1.30)	Enzymes in leucocytes, fibroblasts, plasma	15q25→q25.1
10	G_{M2}-gangliosidosis type A_oB_o	Sandhoff disease	Ganglioside G_{M2} Globoside	β-D-Hexosaminidases A and B (β-subunit) (EC 3.2.1.30)	Enzymes in leucocytes, fibroblasts, plasma	5q13
11	G_{M1}-gangliosidosis	–	Ganglioside G_{M1}	G_{M1} ganglioside β-galactosidase (EC 3.2.1.23)	Enzymes in leucocytes, fibroblasts, urine	3p14→cen

The materials listed under biochemical diagnosis are those which have been most frequently used for this purpose.

The enzyme defect is usually more generally demonstrable. Enzymological prenatal diagnosis is usually possible using either amniocytes or chorionic villus samples.

stained preparations. Increased amounts of glucocerebroside occur in the plasma and erythrocytes.

Type I is the most common and has an especially high incidence in Ashkenazi Jews (1 : 2,500 births), it may present with hepatosplenomegaly in childhood, although the main disabilities occur later. The spleen and liver become very large and the spleen may undergo torsion and infarction. Grey–brown pigmentation of the forehead, hands, and pretibial region is characteristic. Wedge-shaped yellow–brown discoloration of subconjunctival areas (pingueculae) develop in the region of the corneoscleral junction. Bone growth and mineralization are deficient and the skeletal manifestations such as pain, pathological fractures, bone infarcts, and avascular necrosis of the femoral heads may dominate the clinical picture. It is sometimes relatively mild and confined to the Ehrlenmeyer flask-like expansion of the lower end of the femur. Anaemia is due to a combination of bone marrow replacement, hypersplenism, and haemorrhage associated with thrombocytopenia. The serum level of non-prostatic acid phosphatases is increased.

Thrombocytopenia, hypersplenism, recurrent painful splenic infarction, and abdominal discomfort due to a greatly enlarged spleen are indications for splenomegaly. Enzyme replacement therapy with macrophage-targeted glucocerebrosidase is a promising approach to treatment. Haematological improvement, reduction in the hepatosplenomegaly, and improvement in the skeletal lesions have been documented. Treatment with disodium pamidronate (a second generation bisphosphonate) reduces bone resorption, improves calcium balance, and maintains or improves bone density in both the axial and peripheral skeleton. Bone marrow transplantation is indicated in patients in whom infiltration of the bone marrow presents the main threat to life.

Patients with acute neuronopathic (Type II) Gaucher disease have hepatosplenomegaly, and show developmental delay and retrogression by age 6 months. There are fits, focal neurological signs, and pulmonary infections due to infiltration of the lung parenchyma by Gaucher cells. These patients die in the first year of life. The subacute neuropathic (Type III) cases present in later childhood and may survive into adult life with a variable degree of intellectual impairment, focal neurological manifestations, and seizures, as well as the systemic manifestations of the disease.

KRABBE'S DISEASE (GLOBOID CELL LEUKODYSTROPHY: GALACTOSYL CERAMIDE LIPIDOSIS)

Many of these patients present with progressive neurological degeneration between 3 and 9 months of age and die before 3 years. Developmental delay and retrogression, optic atrophy, deafness, and progressive long tract signs are prominent features. A few cases present later in childhood and run a slower but equally fatal course. The white matter of the central nervous system contains large PAS-positive, sometimes multinucleate, cells. These globoid cells are rich in galactosylceramide, which accumulates behind the metabolic block (see Fig. 1). They are mesodermal, not modified neuroglia, and are a specific histiocytic response to galactosylceramide. The white matter shows very extensive demyelination and astrocytic gliosis.

METACHROMATIC LEUKODYSTROPHY (SULPHATIDOSIS)

The three clinical types of metachromatic leukodystrophy are defined by the age of onset of symptoms and their evolution. The late infantile type (incidence about 1 : 40 000) usually presents with increasing flaccid paresis, lack of co-ordination, and hyporeflexia between the ages of 1 and 4 years. A few patients pass through a phase of spastic paraplegia or diplegia. Psychomotor retrogression progresses until the patients reach a bedridden vegetative state, having lost all contact with their surroundings. Optic atrophy, with a grey discoloration and a cherry-red spot at the macula, are characteristic ophthalmoscopic findings. The juvenile form (incidence about 1 : 160 000) presents in later childhood and adolescence, with greater emphasis on intellectual deterioration;

emotional disorders are early symptoms, and locomotor disturbances, including dystonia, begin somewhat later. Adult patients present with psychosis and dementia, followed by progressive loss of motor functions and seizures, and die in early middle life. Metachromatic deposits are demonstrable in sural nerve biopsy specimens, and the conduction velocity in peripheral nerves is reduced.

There have been unsuccessful attempts to treat metachromatic leukodystrophy by displacement bone marrow transplantation.

MULTIPLE SULPHATASE DEFICIENCY (MUCOSULPHATIDOSIS)

The clinical course of these patients resembles that of late infantile metachromatic leukodystrophy, except that features reminiscent of the mucopolysaccharidoses are added. Thus, the facies is coarse and Hurler disease-like, the liver and spleen are enlarged, the skeleton shows dysostosis multiplex, and there is icthyosis (as in steroid sulphatase deficiency). The urine contains dermatan and heparan sulphates.

LACTOSYLCERAMIDOSIS

The few reported cases of this rare condition have shown psychomotor delay and retrogression beginning at about 2 years. There is marked muscle hypotonia, ataxia, and tremor with optic atrophy, and progressive neurological damage leads to death within about a year of presentation. The liver, spleen, and lymph nodes are enlarged. There are no skeletal abnormalities but the cells of the reticuloendothelial system contain fine lipid droplets and these can be demonstrated in a bone marrow aspirate.

FABRY DISEASE (ANDERSON–FABRY DISEASE; GLYCOSPHINGOLIPID LIPIDOSIS, CERAMIDE TRIHEXODISOSIS)

Fabry disease is inherited in an X-linked recessive manner. The male hemizygotes therefore show the full syndrome and the heterozygous female carriers either show the disease in a mild form or are asymptomatic.

The clinical manifestations are mainly due to intralysosomal deposits of α-galactosyl-lactosyl-ceramide (trihexoside) in the endothelial, perithelial, and smooth muscle cells of the blood vessels, and in the histiocytic cells of the reticuloendothial system. The crystalline trihexoside is birefringent with a characteristic Maltese cross appearance. Deposits are prominent in the epithelial cells of the cornea, the glomeruli and tubules of the kidney, the myocardium, the ganglion cells of the autonomic nervous system, and the Schwann cells of peripheral nerves. The abnormal cells in the kidney look foamy. Intra- and extracellular trihexoside is present in the urinary centrifuged deposit.

Attacks of severe burning pain and paraesthesiae in the extremities may be the presenting feature in childhood and adolescence. Heat, cold, and physical exertion may precipitate the attacks, which may be accompanied by fever. Episodes of nausea, vomiting and abdominal pain, Raynaud phenomenon, and musculoarticular pains may also occur. The cutaneous lesions (angiokeratoma corporis diffusum) usually appear in childhood or around puberty and their number increases with the passage of time. They are bright red to blue–black telangiectases, which may be flat or slightly raised and scaly, and are most numerous on the lower trunk and thighs. Small numbers of these lesions are usually present elsewhere, including the buccal mucosa and conjunctiva.

The eyes show corneal and lens opacities, and aneurysmal dilatation of small thin-walled retinal venules. The corneal dystrophy begins as a diffuse haziness in the subepithelial layer, which in more advanced cases acquires the appearance of whorled streaks extending from the centre to the periphery of the cornea. Chloroquine and amiodarone cause identical corneal lesions.

The trihexoside deposits in the walls of the coronary arteries predispose to ischaemic heart disease, and the heart valves are distorted by infiltration with trihexoside-laden histiocytes and secondary fibrosis. Pulmonary infiltration and avascular necrosis of bone are other complications.

The hemizygous males die in the fourth or fifth decade from renal failure, cerebrovascular disease, myocardial infarction, or cardiac failure. The heterozygous carrier females may have any of the manifestations that occur in the affected males but to a lesser degree. The characteristic renal histological appearances on renal biopsy are seen in the heterozygous females, and they may die of renal or cardiovascular disease due to the abnormal trihexoside deposition. Careful examination of the eyes often shows corneal changes in otherwise unaffected female carriers.

The angiokeratoma have to be distinguished from Campbell de Morgan spots (senile angioma), which are usually brighter red in colour on the upper trunk and less numerous, and angiokeratomas of the scrotum (Fordyce), which are common in older men. The lesions of Osler–Weber–Rendu disease (congenital haemorrhagic telangiectasia) are brighter red, less grouped, and occur chiefly around the mouth, nose, lips, and on the fingers. Angiokeratoma identical to those of Fabry's disease have been reported in fucosidosis.

Reports that a grafted kidney supplied a therapeutically useful amount of the missing enzyme as well as relieving the uraemia have not been confirmed. However, the results of preliminary studies suggest that Fabry disease may be amenable to enzyme replacement therapy with exogenously administered α-galactosidase when sufficiently large amounts of genetically engineered enzyme are available for long-term clinical trials.

THE G_{M2}-GANGLIODOSES

There are two isoenzymes (A and B) of the hexosaminidase which catalyse the conversion of G_{M2}- to G_{M3}-ganglioside,[1] G_{A2}-ganglioside to lactosylceramide (Gal-Glc-Cer), and globoside to α-galactosyl-lactosyl-ceramide (Gal-Gal-Glc-Cer) (see Fig. 1). Severe deficiency of both isoenzymes causes Sandhoff's disease, and a severe deficiency of isoenzyme-A causes Tay-Sachs disease. Less severe deficiencies of hexosaminidase-A are associated with the juvenile and adult variants of G_{M2}-gangliosidosis. These four disorders are genetically distinct.

Tay-Sachs disease (infantile G_{M2} gangliosidosis)

The incidence is approximately 1 : 2000 in Ashkenazi Jews. Progressive generalized motor weakness begins at about 6 months of age, and there is rapid psychomotor regression with seizures, blindness, and deafness between 12 and 18 months. The child lapses into a vegetative state with decerebrate rigidity and increasing severe fits and dies before it is 3 years old. The cherry-red spot appearance of the macula is often present early in the evolution of the disease, and the head enlarges abnormally rapidly due to neuronal ganglioside accumulation and cerebral gliosis. A doll-like facies, pale skin and the startle reaction (a flexion of the arms and extension of the legs in response to a sudden sound) are classic although non-specific features of patients in the late stages of the disease. Microscopically, the neuronal cells of the central and autonomic nervous system contain large amounts of ganglioside G_{M2}, which is arranged as laminated masses within engorged lysosomes. These appearances in the autonomic nervous system can be demonstrated by a rectal biopsy.

Sandhoff's disease

This cannot be distinguished from very rapidly evolving Tay-Sachs disease either clinically or on histopathological grounds. There are, how-

ever, minor differences in the proportion of the different gangliosides in the brain and other tissue.

Juvenile G_{M2} gangliosidosis

This presents between 2 and 6 years of age with ataxia, loss of speech, progressive spasticity, dystonia, posturing, and seizures. Blindness occurs late, although optic atrophy, retinitis pigmentosa, and the macula cherry-red spot have been reported. The patients die in later childhood or in their teens.

Adult G_{M2} gangliosidosis

This presents with slowly progressive difficulty in walking, muscular atrophy, lack of co-ordination, dystonia, and dysarthria. Intellect and vision are not affected.

THE G_{M1}-GANGLIOSIDOSES (GENERALIZED GANGLIOSIDOSES)

Undegraded gangliosidoses (G_{M1} and G_{A1}) accumulate in the parenchymal and reticuloendothelial cells of the viscera as well as in neurones, hence the term generalized gangliosidoses. The abnormal ganglioside storage impairs the degradation of the mycopolysaccharides and some tissues also contain a keratan sulphate-like glycosaminoglycan. The cells of the visceral organs look foamy.

Infantile G_{M1}-gangliosidosis

Psychomotor retardation, poor muscle tone, and oedema are obvious from the first weeks of life. Sucking and swallowing are poor, there are frequent seizures, the patient passes into a state of decerebrate rigidity with blindness, deafness, and spastic quadriplegia and dies before the age of 2 years. The main physical features are a coarse physiognomy, frontal bossing, depressed nasal bridge, low-set ears, gum hyertrophy, macroglossia, clear corneae, and often a cherry-red spot at the macula. Head size increases abnormally rapidly but to a lesser degree than in Tay-Sachs disease. Hepatosplenomegaly is usually evident by the time the child is a few months old, and dysostosis multiplex develops.

Juvenile G_{M1}-gangliosidosis

Symptoms begin between 6 and 20 months but these patients rarely survive beyond 10 years. Psychomotor delay is often apparent by the end of the first year, and is followed by retrogression. Ataxias, squints, generalized muscle weakness, lack of co-ordination, spasticity, and sometimes blindness develop. The facial features are not coarsened, the retina and macula appear normal, hepatosplenomegaly is rare and dystosis multiplex is minimal. The changes in the neurones are identical with these in the infantile type. The bone marrow contains foamy-looking histiocytes and there is usually some visceral histiocytosis.

Adult G_{M1}-gangliosidosis

This presents with progressive cerebellar dysarthria and ataxia, accompanied by progressive spaciticity and mild intellectual impairment.

G_{M3}-GANGLIOSIDOSIS

No clinical phenotype associated with a failure to convert G_{M3}-ganglioside to glucocerebroside (Fig. 1) due to ganglioside neuraminidase deficiency has yet been identified. This enzyme is distinct from the neuraminidase, deficiency of which causes mucopolidosis I (sialidosis). Failure to convert G_{M3} ganglioside to G_{M2} ganglioside due to G_{M3}-UDP-GalNAc transferase deficiency has been reported and ascribed to an acquired cause. There was progressive failure of neurological functions from birth, macroglossia, and a coarse facies. There were no gross intraneuronal deposits of gangliosides but the proportion of G_{M3} relative to the longer chain gangliosides and the more highly sialylated homologues was abnormally high.

---

[1] The Svennerholm notation for the gangliosides is built up as follows: G, ganglioside; M, monosialo-; D, diasialo-; T, trisialo-; A, asialo-. The arabic numerals indicate the sequence of migration on thin-layer chromatograms.

Mucopolysaccharidoses

The mucopolysaccharidoses are a group of seven inborn errors of metabolism in which the activity of one of the exoglycosidases which catalyse the sequential removal of individual carbohydrate groups from the mucopolysaccharides (glycosaminoglycans) is deficient. They have a combined incidence of about 1 : 10 000 births and their nomenclature, biochemistry, genetics, and main clinical features are summarized in Table 2. Formerly, Hurler and Hunter diseases were not differentiated from one another and were called gargoylism because of their characteristic facies. The mucopolysaccharidoses are all inherited as autosomal recessives, except Hunter disease, which is a sex-linked recessive. The term dysostosis multiplex is now used specifically for the skeletal changes demonstrated radiologically in this group of disorders. The term lipochondodystrophy, which was formerly used because it was thought that the stored material was a lipid, has been abandoned. The primary abnormal storage products are carbohydrate polymers. These produce secondary changes in lysosomal function, including some impairment of ganglioside turnover. The tissue deposits of highly sulphated mucopolysaccharides stain metachromatically.

Mucopolysaccharide deposits in relation to the meninges can cause hydrocephalus, spinal cord compression, arachnoid cysts, and radiculopathies. These complications arise in all of the mucopolysaccharidoses irrespective of whether the neuronal and glial cells are primarily affected by intracellular mucopolysaccharide deposits or not.

Leucocytes contain mucopolysaccharide inclusion bodies (Alder–Reilly bodies) in all of the mucopolysaccharidoses. Except in Morquio disease (mucopolysaccharidosis IV), the accumulation of sulphated mucopolysaccharides in cultured fibroblasts can be demonstrated by studying the uptake and release of $^{35}SO_4$ by the cells in vitro. The cross-correction of the enzyme-deficient cells is demonstrated by growing them in tissue culture medium in which normal cells, or cells from a patient with another lysosomal storage disease, have been grown. The precise enzymological diagnosis is made on either leucocytes or cultured fibroblasts and prenatal diagnosis on either cultured amniotic cells or chorionic villus samples.

HURLER DISEASE (MUCOPOLYSACCHARIDOSIS I H)

The skin, soft tissue, and subcutaneous cartilages are thickened and stiff, the nasal bridge is depressed, there is a wide vertical bony ridge in the centre of the forehead and some degree of macrocephaly (Fig. 2). Upper respiratory obstruction with mouth breathing and chronic upper respiratory tract infection are prominent features. The gums are hyperplastic and the teeth widely spaced and poorly formed. The eyes show corneal clouding, and there is combined sensorineural and conductive deafness. The hair becomes stiff and straight, the eyebrows bushy and hypertrichosis develops.The diagnosis is usually suggested at age 6 to 12 months by the association of psychomotor delay and the developing facial appearance. Corneal clouding and loss of the normal lumbar lordosis are other early signs. Dwarfing is usually evident 2 or 3 years of age and the children die before they are 10 years old, having shown profound psychomotor regression. Other prominent clinical features are hepatosplenomegaly, progressive joint stiffness, and contractures; the latter affect the terminal interphalangeal joints and radio-ulnar joints early and there is a dorsolumbar kyphosis. Figures 3 to 7 show the bone changes, some of these are visible radiologically during the first weeks of life.

Complicating hydrocephalus due to mucopolysaccharide deposits in the meninges and interference with the circulation of cerebrospinal fluid or with its absorption through the arachnoid granulations may accelerate the neurological deterioration. Blindness is due to the combined effects of corneal clouding, retinal degeneration, damage to the visual pathways, cerebral infiltration, hydrocephalus, and glaucoma. The latter may develop acutely due to mucopolysaccharide deposits in the cells lining the trabecular meshwork of the iridocorneal angle.

HUNTER DISEASE (MUCOPOLYSACCHARIDOSIS II)

Although this disease usually follows a slower course than Hurler disease, cases of the severe variant cannot be distinguished from Hurler disease on clinical grounds except for the almost universal absence of corneal clouding. Patients with the genetically distinct mild variant may survive beyond the age of 30 and have either low or near normal intelligence. Most cases die in childhood or in their teens. Occasional female patients with Hunter disease are due either to translocation of a piece of the X-chromosome bearing the mutant gene for iduronosulphate–sulphatase on to an autosome or to the presence of the mutation in a patient with the X-O karyotype (Turner syndrome) or to a mating between a patient with Hunter disease and a heterozygous female carrier of the mutant gene.

SANFILIPPO DISEASE (MUCOPOLYSACCHARIDOSIS III)

The four biochemically distinct types are indistinguishable from one another clinically. The patients show severe mental deterioration with hyperkinetic behaviour but few somatic abnormalities. They usually die before the end of the second decade. Accelerated physical growth and abundant coarse scalp hair in the presence of the other features may be a useful diagnostic pointer. The routine qualitative tests for abnormal mucopolysacchariduria sometimes become negative in older children with Sanfilippo disease.

MORQUIO DISEASE (MUCOPOLYSACCHARIDOSIS IV)

Severe skeletal deformities dominate the clinical picture and growth virtually stops after about 6 years of age. The development of the vertebral bodies is grossly disordered, producing flat, anteriorly beaked vertebrae, kyphoscoliosis, a lumbodorsal gibbus, and hypoplasia of the odontoid process. Spinal cord compression is a frequent complication. Other features are deafness, pectus carinatum with flaring of the lower ribs, fine corneal opacities, a broad mouth with widely spaced teeth, cardiac valvular lesions especially aortic incompetence, moderate hepatosplenomegaly, and hypermobility of the joints. Intellect is normal and the facies is not Hurler-like.

The metabolic lesions prevent the normal degradation of keratan sulphate, which is a constituent of cartilage, the nucleus pulposus and cornea. The disease evolves more slowly in Type B than in Type A cases. Cardiorespiratory complications (restrictive ventilatory defect due to the thoracic deformity, collapse of the trachea, left ventricular failure due to the valvular lesions and pulmonary infections, and cervical cord compression) are potentially fatal.

The amount of keratan sulphate excreted decreases in older patients and may be missed with routine screening procedures. Patients with G_{M1}-gangliosidosis and Kniest dysplasia also excrete keratan sulphate but they are easily differentiated from Morquio disease on clinical and radiological grounds.

MAROTEAUX–LAMY DISEASE (MUCOPOLYSACCHARIDOSIS VI)

Skeletal, corneal, and cardiac involvement, and hepatosplenomegaly are prominent features. The facies resembles that in Hurler disease. Phenotypically mild, intermediate, and severe variants have been described. The degree of intellectual impairment is variable.

SCHEIE DISEASE (MUCOPOLYSACCHARIDOSIS I S)

Scheie disease is a clinically mild phenotype due to a mutation at the α-iduronidase locus allelic with that which causes Hurler disease. The patients are mainly incapacitated by the arthropathy but they may develop cardiac valvular lesions and glaucoma. Mucopolysaccharide deposits in the meninges cause hydrocephalus, cervical myelopathy,

Table 2 *The mucopolysaccharidoses*

McKusick's classification	Eponymous name	Enzyme deficiency	Excreted glycosaminoglycans	Organs mainly affected	Facial appearance	Chromosome assignment
IH	Hurler	α-L-iduronidase (EC 3.2.1.76)	Dermatan sulphate Heparan sulphate	Central nervous system Skeleton Viscera	Classic Hurler appearance	22pter→q11
IS	Scheie	α-L-iduronidase (EC 3.2.1.76)	Dermatan sulphate Heparan sulphate	Skeleton (mild relative to Hurler) Viscera (mild relative to Hurler)	Coarse features ± (Not specifically Hurler-like)	22pter→q11
IH/S	Hurler/Scheie	α-L-iduronidase (EC 3.2.1.76)	Dermatan sulphate Heparan sulphate	Phenotype intermediate between Hurler and Scheie diseases	Coarse features ± (Not specifically Hurler-like)	22pter→q11
II	Hunter	Iduronate sulphate sulphatase	Dermatan sulphate Heparan sulphate	Central nervous system Skeleton Viscera Mild and severe phenotypes reported	Micrognathism Hurler-like	Xq28
III A	Sanfilippo A	Heparan N-sulphatase	Heparan sulphate	Central nervous system	Not characteristic	Not assigned
III B	Sanfilippo B	N-acetyl-α-D-glucosaminidase (EC 3.2.1.50)	Heparan sulphate	Central nervous system	Not characteristic	Not assigned
III C	Sanfilippo C	Acetyl-CoA:α-glucosaminide N-acetyltransferase	Heparan sulphate	Central nervous system	Not characteristic	?14 ?21
III D	Sanfilippo D	N-acetylglucosamine 6-sulphate sulphatase	Heparan sulphate	Central nervous system	Not characteristic	12q14
IV A	Morquio A	N-acetylgalactosamine 6-sulphate sulphatase	Keratan sulphate	Skeleton	Not characteristic	Not assigned
IV B	Morquio B	β-galactosidase	Keratan sulphate	Skeleton	Not characteristic	3pter→p21
V*	—	—	—	—	—	—
VI	Maroteaux–Lamy	N-acetylgalactosamire 4-sulphatase (Aryl sulphatase B) (EC 3.1.6.1)	Dermatan sulphate	Skeleton Mild and severe phenotypes reported	Hurler-like	5q12→q13
VII	—	β-glucuronidase (EC 3.2.1.31)	Dermatan sulphate Heparan sulphate	Central nervous system Skeleton Viscera	Hurler-like	7q11→q21

*Originally Scheie disease which was reclassified as Mucopolysaccharidosis IS when the enzyme defect was shown to be the same as that in Hurler disease. The possibility that Hurler and Scheie diseases are due to allelic mutations and that the intermediate Hurler/Scheie phenotype (mucopolysaccharidosis IH/S) is due to double heterozygosity for the allelic mutations concerned has been widely proposed. The Hurler/Scheie phenotype could also be due to homozygosity for a third allelic mutation at the same gene locus.

Fig. 2 The typical facies of a patient with Hurler disease.

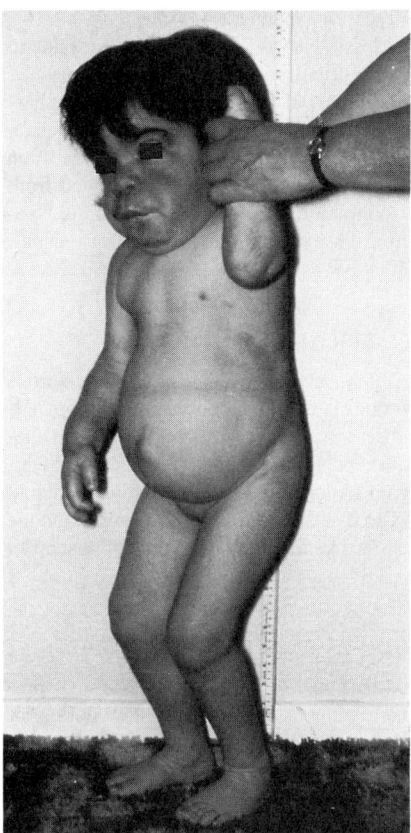

Fig. 3 Dysostosis multiplex. The skull in a case of Hurler disease (female, age 13 months). Premature fusion of the sagittal suture produces dolichocephaly. The pituitary fossa is J-shaped or shoe-shaped, with a large recess extending under the anterior clinoid processes. The normal markings on the skull vault are reduced due to thickening of the meninges. The occipital suture is widened, other radiological signs of hydrocephalus may occur as the disease progresses. The teeth are irregularly placed.

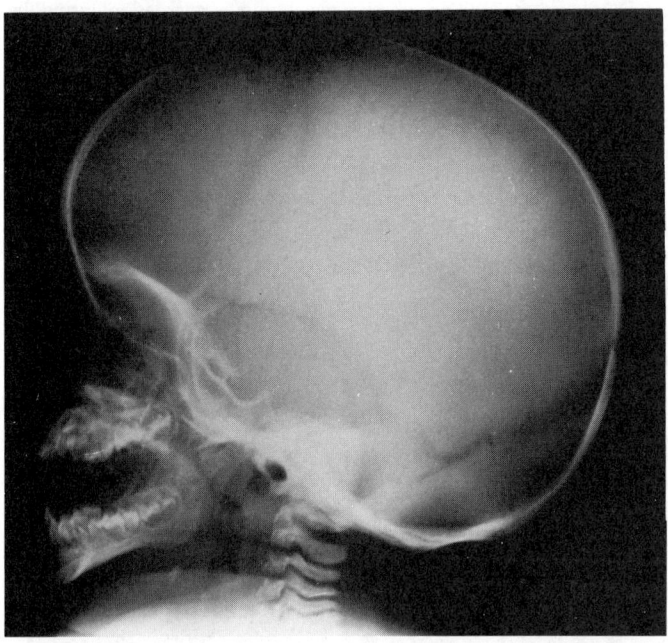

Fig. 4 Dysostosis multiplex. The spine in a case of Hurler disease (female, age 13 months) showing oval vertebral bodies, anterior inferior beaking of the lumbar vertebrae and elongation of the vertebral pedicles. The loss of the normal lumbar curvature is noteworthy.

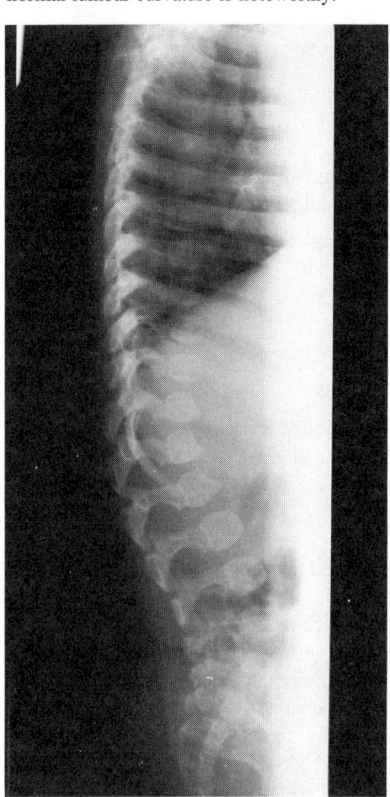

Fig. 5 Dysostosis multiplex. The chest in a case of Hurler disease (male, age 7 years). The ribs appear to lie more horizontally than normal, their anterior ends are expanded, and they are constricted posteriorly so that they assume a paddle shape. The clavicles are hypoplastic.

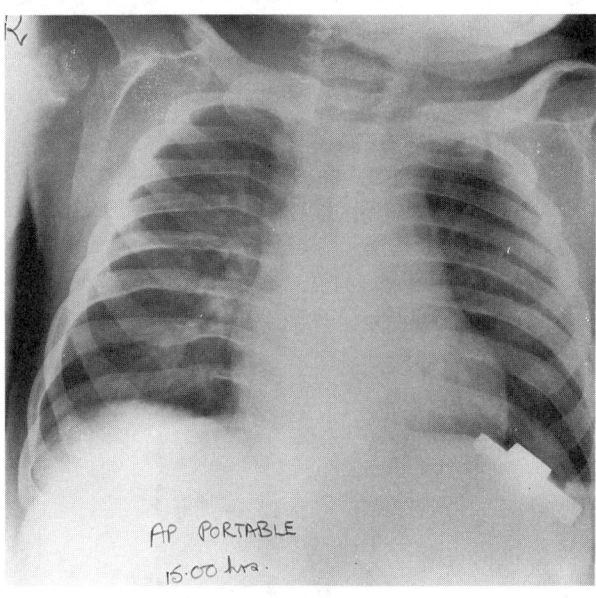

radiculopathy, and arachnoid cysts. Nerve entrapment syndromes are also a well recognized neurological complication. Mental handicap is not a feature.

HURLER–SCHEIE DISEASE (MUCOPOLYSACCHARIDOSIS I H/S)

This phenotype is intermediate in severity between Hurler and Scheie diseases. The patients may be homozygous for a third allelic mutation or they may be heterozygous for both Hurler and Scheie disease. They usually present in childhood with joint involvement, the degree of mental handicap, if any, is variable, and they are liable to have the same neurological, cardiac and ocular complications as patients with both Hurler and Scheie diseases.

β-GLUCURONIDASE DEFICIENCY (MUCOPOLYSACCHARIDOSIS VII)

These patients have the clinical features of Hurler disease but the degree of mucopolysacchariduria is relatively slight.

Mucolipidoses

The term mucolipidosis was introduced to encompass a group of patients with clinical features that were a mixture of those encountered in the sphingolipidoses and the mucopolysaccharidoses and who did not have abnormal mucopolysacchariduria. It now includes patients with: (1) neuraminidase (sialidase) deficiency, termed Mucolipidoses I and IV; (2) two groups of patients with deficiency of uridine diphosphate-*N*-acetylglucosamine : lysosomal enzyme precursor *N*-acetylglucosamine phosphate transferase who are termed Mucolipidoses II (I-cell disease) and III (pseudo-Hurler polydystrophy), respectively (Tables 3 and 4). Pre-

natal diagnosis is possible in all four conditions but carrier state diagnosis only appears possible in Mucolipidosis I. All of the mucolipidoses are inherited in an autosomal recessive manner.

Mucolipidoses I and IV are classic lysosomal storage diseases due to deficiency of an enzyme which normally degrades a macromolecule. The metabolic lesion in Mucolipidoses II and III blocks the phosphorylation of the terminal mannose residue of the oligosaccharide side chain of the lysosomal hydrolases. This deprives them of the recognition marker, mannose 6-phosphate, which enables them to be guided from their site of synthesis on the rough endoplasmic reticulum to the lysosomes, and to be taken up from an extracellular location by receptor mediated pinocytosis.

MUCOLIPIDOSIS II (I-CELL DISEASE)

This disease was first recognized as an entity because of the numerous inclusions seen in cultured fibroblasts on phase contrast microscopy ('I-cell' disease–'inclusion cell' disease). A severe Hurler disease-like phenotype is present in infancy except that corneal clouding and hepatosplenomegaly are mild and gum hypertrophy is particularly prominent relative to the other features. The dysostosis multiplex is severe and the patients usually die during the first 5 years of life. Prenatal but not carrier state diagnosis is possible.

MUCOLIPIDOSIS III (PSEUDO-HURLER POLYDYSTROPHY)

These patients usually present at 4 to 5 years of age because of progressive arthropathy. Their intelligence is usually in the low normal or mildly handicapped range and they develop dysostosis multiplex, spinal deformities, atlantoaxial subluxation, nerve entrapment syndromes, cardiac valvular lesions and corneal clouding in later childhood. Visceromegaly is not a prominent feature. Cultured fibroblasts show I-cell type inclusions. Prenatal but not carrier state diagnosis is possible.

THE NEURAMINIDASE (SIALIDASE) DEFICIENCIES

Mucolipidosis I, deficient neuraminidase activity with respect to glycoprotein substrate, is referred to with the other glycoproteinoses. Mucolipidosis IV, in which the catalytic activity of the enzyme with respect to cleavage of neuraminyl residues from gangliosides G_{M3} and G_{D3} is deficient, presents with progressive psychomotor retardation during the first 2 years of life. The patients usually die in later childhood. The

Fig. 6 Dysostosis multiplex. The hands in the case of Hurler disease (female, age 8 years). Bone remodelling is very abnormal with marked undertubulation. The proximal phalanges show the bullet-shaped appearance, proximal tapering of the metacarpals is marked and the fingers are curved radially. Ossification is delayed and disordered, the lower end of the radius is expanded, the radial and ulna metaphyses are slanted and tilt towards each other.

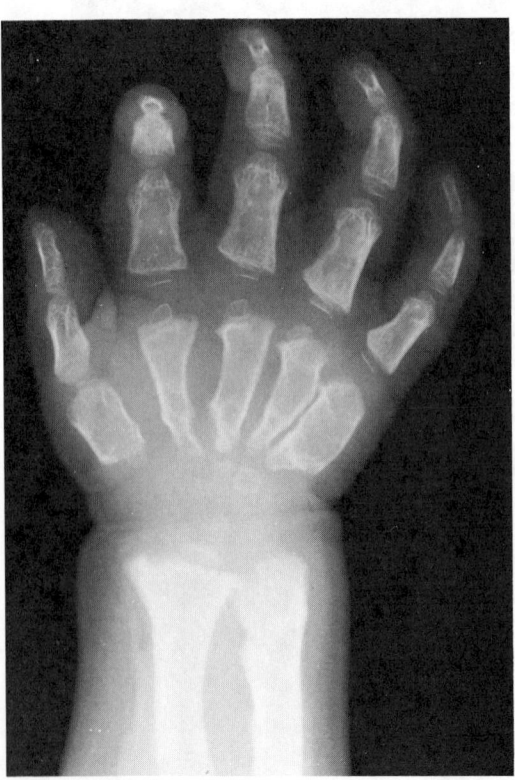

Fig. 7 Dysostosis multiplex. The pelvis in a case of Hurler disease (female, aged 7 years). The triradiate cartilage and ischiopubic synchondroses are widened. The femoral heads are hypoplastic and uncovered due to hypoplasia of the supra-acetabular part of the ilium. The wings of the ilia are flared and there is a marked coxa valga deformity.

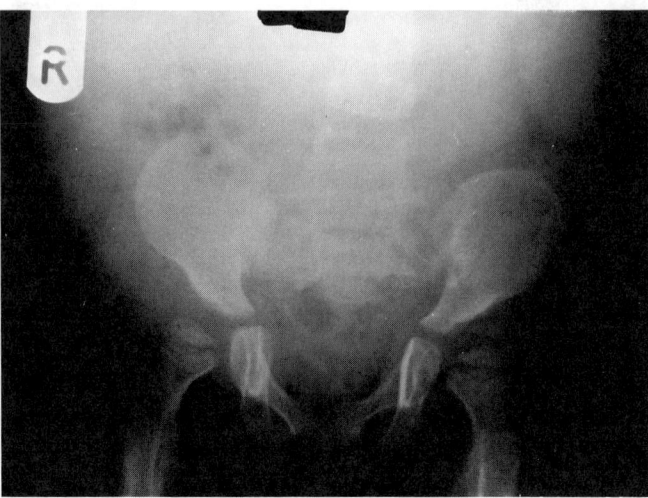

Table 3 *The mucolipidoses*

Mucolipidosis number	Alternative name	Metabolic lesion	Clinical features
I	Sialidosis	Deficient neuraminidase (sialidase EC 3.2.1.18) activity with respect to glycoprotein substrates	Two clinical types: 1. Normosomatic, myoclonus and ''cherry red spot'' appearance of the macula lutea 2. Dysmorphic, resembles Hurler disease
II	I-cell disease	Failure to phosphorylate terminal mannosyl residues of the glycoprotein lysosomal hydrolases due to deficiency of uridine-*N*-acetylglucosamine: lysosomal enzyme precursor *N*-acetyl-glucosamine phosphate transferase. This deprives these enzymes of their recognition markers for transfer from the rough endoplasmic reticulum into the lysosomes and for receptor-mediated pinocytic uptake into cells	Resembles very early onset Hurler disease
III	Pseudo-Hurler polydystrophy	As for mucolipidosis II	Resembles either intermediate severity Maroteaux–Lamy disease, or some cases of Scheie disease
IV	Berman's disease	Deficient neuraminidase activity with respect to ganglioside substrates (GM$_3$ and GD$_{1a}$)	Progressive neurological deterioration beginning in infancy. Hypotonia, pyramidal and extrapyramidal signs. Corneal clouding. No visceromegaly. Not dysmorphic

Table 4 *The mucolipidoses, glycoproteinoses, acid lipase deficiencies, and glycogenosis Type II: nomenclature, enzyme deficiencies, and chromosome assignments*

Systemic or more commonly used name	Eponymous or other alternative name	Enzyme deficiency	Chromosome assignment
Mucolipidosis I	Sialidosis	Neuraminidase (EC 3.2.1.18) with respect to glycoprotein substrates	Not assigned
Mucolipidosis II	I-cell disease	UDP-GlcNAC:glycoprotein GlcNAc-1-phosphotransferase	4q21→q23
Mucolipidosis III	Pseudo-Hurler polydystrophy	UDP-GlcNAC:glycoprotein GlcNAc-1-phosphotransferase	4q21→q23
Mucolipidosis IV	–	Neuraminidase (EC 3.2.1.18) with respect to ganglioside substrates	Not assigned
Fucosidosis	–	α-Fucosidase (EC 3.2.1.51)	1p34
Mannosidosis	–	α-Mannosidase (EC 3.2.1.24)	19p13.2→q12
Aspartylglycosaminuria	–	1-Aspartamido-β-*N*-acetyl-glucosamine amidohydrolase (EC 3.2.2.11)	4q21→4qter
–	Wolman's disease	Acid lipase (EC 3.1.1.3)	10q25
Cholesteryl ester storage disease	–	Acid lipase (EC 3.1.1.3)	10q25
Glycogenosis II	Pompé disease	α-1,4-glucosidase (EC 3.2.1.20)	17q23

neurological picture includes muscle hypotonia, truncal ataxia, and the signs of an upper motor neurone lesion. Corneal clouding is marked and appears early. There is neither visceromegaly nor dysostosis multiplex.

Glycoproteinoses

The glycoproteinoses are a group of four autosomal recessively inherited inborn errors of metabolism in which the metabolic lesion causes faulty degradation of the oligosaccharide side chains of glycoproteins.

SIALIDOSIS (MUCOLIPIDOSIS I): THE CHERRY-RED SPOT/MYOCLONUS SYNDROME

Sialidosis is due to the deficiency of the *N*-acetylneuraminic hydrolase, which cleaves sialic acid from oligosaccharides, glycoproteins, and glucolipids. The urine contains large amounts of sialic-acid-rich oligosaccharides. The patients are divided into Type 1 and Type 2 according to the absence or presence of dysmorphic features and mental deterioration. Infantile (onset at or below 1 year of age) and juvenile (onset at 8 to 15 years) variants of Type 2 are recognized. The Type 1 patients present at between 8 and 15 years with visual failure and action myoclonus, and have the cherry-red spot at the macula. They appear normal, and have normal or near normal intelligence. In Type 2 patients, the features and skeletal abnormalities resmembe those of Hurler disease. These patients also have spasticity and ataxia, as well as the cherry-red spot at the macula and myoclonus. Seizures may occur in both types. Visceromegaly is rare except in the infantile variant of Type 2. Vacuolated mononuclear cells ('foam cells') are seen in the blood and/or bone marrow in most cases.

Sialidosis can be diagnosed prenatally and in the carrier state.

ASPARTYLGLYCOSAMINURIA

Aspartylglycosaminuria is due to deficiency of aspartylglucosaminidase, which catalyses the hydrolysis of the linkage between asparagine and N-acetylglucosamine splitting the carbohydrate from the polypeptide chain of glycoproteins. The patients excrete large amounts of aspartylglucosamine in their urine. Most of the reported patients have been Finnish. They present with psychomotor delay at about 1 to 5 years and become severely retarded with some degree of motor incoordination. Coarse facial features, optic lens opacities, mild dysostosis multiplex, hypermobile joints, short stature, and cardiac systolic murmurs are other features. Hepatosplenomegaly is not a characteristic finding. Aspartylglucosaminuria can be diagnosed prenatally and in the carrier state.

MANNOSIDOSIS

Mannosidosis is due to deficiency of α-mannosidase, which cleaves terminal mannosyl residues form the carbohydrate moieties of glycoproteins. Characteristic mannose-rich oligosaccharides are excreted in the urine and accumulate in the cells of the brain, viscera, and connective tissues. The more severely affected patients, who present at 3 to 12 months, die in childhood. Less severely affected patients present at 1 to 4 years and die as young adults. The main clinical features are psychomotor delay, the development of severe mental handicap, coarsened facial features, hepatosplenomegaly, posterior 'spoke-like' cataracts, deafness, and dysostosis multiplex. Clinically the patients resemble Hurler disease more or less closely. Prenatal and carrier state diagnoses are possible.

FUCOSIDOSIS

Fucosidosis is due to deficiency of α-fucosidase, which cleaves terminal fucosyl residues from the oligosaccharide side chains of the glycoproteins. The external appearances, visceromegaly and skeletal changes resemble those seen in Hurler disease. Severe and mild variants are recognized. Psychomotor delay and regression evolve rapidly in the former group, who also show increased sweat sodium and chloride and die in early or mid-childhood. The mild cases have angiokeratomata resembling those seen in Fabry disease, there is less neurological damage, normal sweat salinity, and they survive longer. The erythrocyte and saliva Lewis blood group antigen (Le^a and Le^b) titres are raised and the abnormal tissue glycoconjugates have Lewis blood group acitivty. These findings reflect the failure to cleave fucosyl residues from glycoproteins. Heterozygotes for the abnormal gene causing fucosidosis can be identified and prenatal diagnosis is possible.

Salla disease and infantile sialic acid storage disease

Salla disease, named after the region in Northern Finland from whence most of the early patients came, is characterized by the excretion of large amounts of free sialic acid in the urine. Few cases have been reported in non-Finnish people. Psychomotor delay becomes apparent towards the end of the first year and most cases become severely handicapped mentally. Dysarthria, dyspraxia, abnormal tendon reflexes, ataxia, and athetosis are common features. Life expectancy seems not

to be greatly reduced. The basic biochemical defect is failure to transport sialic acid (N-acetylneuraminic acid) derived from the breakdown of sialic-acid-containing glycoconjugates out of the lysosomes. The inheritance is autosomal recessive.

Infantile free sialic acid storage disease (ISSD) is a severe variant of Salla disease in which the patients are more severely affected and present earlier. Ascites, hepatosplenomegaly, and a coarse facies may be apparent at birth. These infants fail to thrive, show gross developmental delay, usually hyper-reflexia and die in the first years of life.

Prenatal diagnosis has been achieved in both Salla disease and infantile free sialic acid storage disease, although this appears to be more reliable in the latter. The free sialic acid content of amniocytes was diagnostic for both Salla disease and infantile free sialic acid storage disease, but the free sialic acid content of amniotic fluid was only diagnostic for the latter. The election microscopic appearances of chorionic villi (abnormal lysosomal storage) are diagnostic for infantile free sialic acid storage disease.

There is no specific treatment for either Salla disease or infantile free sialic acid storage disease.

Acid cholesteryl ester hydrolase (lysosomal acid lipase) deficiency (Wolman's disease and cholesteryl ester storage disease)

Wolman's disease and cholesteryl ester storage disease are due to allelic mutations. There are two isoenzymes of lysosomal acid lipase, only one of these, the 'A' isoenzyme is lacking in Wolman's disease and cholesteryl ester storage disease. Lysosomal acid lipase catalyses the hydrolysis of low density lipoprotein-bound cholesteryl esters and triacyl glycerides but not phospholipids. The liberated cholesterol is transferred to cellular membranes where it: (1) suppresses the activity of 3-hydroxyl-3-methylglutaryl-coenzyme A reductase (HMGA reductase), which regulates the rate of cholesterol synthesis; (2) reduces low density lipoprotein receptor synthesis and hence suppresses further transport of low density lipoprotein-cholesteryl esters into the cell; (3) stimulates fatty acyl coenzyme A: cholesterol acyltransferase (ACAT), which catalyses cholesterol re-esterification with oleic (9 : 10) and other C$_{14}$ to C$_{18}$ saturated and monounsaturated fatty acids as opposed to the linoleic acid (9 : 10, 12 : 13) with which cholesterol is esterified when it enters the cell. Therefore, failure to liberate cholesterol from low density lipoprotein-bound cholesteryl esters in lysosomal acid lipase deficiency will secondarily augment cholesterol synthesis, the uptake of more low density lipoprotein-bound cholesteryl esters, and the esterification of newly synthesized cholesterol.

Lysosomal acid lipase deficiency can be demonstrated in leucocytes, fibroblasts, and amniotic cells.

Wolman's disease

This is the clinically more severe phenotype presenting in the first weeks of life with vomiting, diarrhoea, failure to thrive, hepatosplenomegaly, and intestinal malabsorption with marked adrenal gland enlargement and calcification.

Except for psychomotor delay and regression, symptoms related specifically to the nervous system are unusual. The infants usually die before the age of 6 months. Lysosomes distended with triglycerides and cholesteryl esters are found in leucocytes, and the parenchymal, reticuloendothelial, and vascular endothelial cells of most organs, including the central and autonomic nervous systems.

Cholesteryl ester storage disease

This follows a more benign course and may not be detected until adult life. There are widespread intralysosomal cholesteryl ester and triglyceride deposits, although hepatomegaly may be the only clinical abnormality. Hypercholesterolaemia is common and there may be severe premature atherosclerosis. No specific treatment is available.

The main differential diagnoses of cholesteryl ester storage diseases are: (1) Tangier disease (familial high density lipoprotein deficiency); (2) familial lecithin cholesterol acyl transferase deficiency; (3) neutral lipid storage disease and; (4) type I glycogen storage disease.

Other lysosomal storage diseases

Cystinosis (cystine storage disease) and Pompe's disease (type II glycogen storage disease, α-glucosidase deficiency) are reviewed with the inborn errors of amino acid metabolism and the glycogen storage diseases respectively.

Lysosomal acid phosphatase deficiency is a rare cause of failure to thrive and death in the first weeks or months of life. It is inherited as an autosomal recessive.

Inborn errors of metabolism with non-lysosomal storage of phytanic acid, β-sitosterol, and cholestanol

Phytanic acid storage disease (Refsum's disease)

Refsum's disease is an autosomal recessively inherited disease in which the long chain aliphatic alcohol phytol, which is a component of chlorophyll, cannot be degraded beyond the stage of the corresponding acid, phytanic acid, because the peroxisomal enzyme, phytanic acid 2-hydroxylase, is deficient. Phytanic acid accumulates in the plasma, blood cells, and tissues. The peripheral nerves show segmental demyelination with hypertrophy due to concentric Schwann cell proliferation. Symptoms begin in the second decade and the course may be either relapsing or steadily progressive. The main abnormalities are: mixed motor and sensory polyneuropathy, cerebellar ataxia, pigmentary degeneration of the retina with failing night vision (retinitis pigmentosa), pupillary abnormalities, nerve deafness, anosmia, ichthyosis, cardiomyopathy, and epiphyseal dysplasia (short fourth metatarsal, syndactyly, hammer toe, pes cavus, osteochondritis dessicans).

The cerebrospinal fluid protein level is raised without a pleocytosis. A chlorophyll-free diet may produce clinical improvement and it should be begun as early in life as possible because established demyelinating lesions are irreversible. Plasmapheresis is useful in the initial stages in order to reduce the body burden of phytanic acid as quickly as possible, the low levels then being maintained by dietary restriction.

Although the heterozygous carriers for Refsum's disease can be identified by their 50 per cent oxidation rate for phytanic acid in cultured fibroblasts, they are asymptomatic and do not accumulate phytanic acid.

Some degree of phytanic acid accumulation also occurs in some of the other peroxisomal enzyme deficiency diseases.

Grossly impaired oxidation of phytanic acid can be demonstrated in skin fibroblasts from patients with Refsum's disease and in those with global peroxisomal enzyme deficiencies (e.g. Zellweger syndrome).

Phytosterolaemia (sitosterolaemia; sitosterol storage disease)

These patients present in childhood or early adult life with tendon and subcutaneous xanthomata. There is hypercholesterolaemia in about half the cases. Other inconsistent manifestations include xanthelasma, corneal arcus, premature atherosclerosis, haemolysis associated with abnormally shaped spherostomatocytic erythrocytes, hypersplenism, abnormal platelets, and arthropathy. There is hyperabsorption of a wide range of plant and shell-fish sterols which include β-sitosterol, stigmasterol, and campestanol. These are all closely related to cholesterol and, like cholesterol, their esterification is catalysed by lecithin : cholesterol acyl-

transferase. Some of the absorbed sterols (e.g. β-sitosterol) are normally converted to bile acids and this process may also be defective in β-sitosterolaemia. It has also been proposed that the presence of plant sterol in lipoproteins may affect the binding of cholesterol. The plant sterols become widely distributed in the body although unesterified cholesterol is the main constituent of the xanthomata. Histologically, the xanthomata resemble those seen in familial hypercholesterolaemia and cererbrotendinous xanthomatosis. The available data are compatible with autosomal recessive transmission. Plant sterols should be excluded from the diet and cholestyramine administered in order to bind bile acids in the gastrointestinal tract. This accelerates the synthesis of bile acids and accelerates the metabolism of the absorbed plant sterols.

Cholesterol storage disease (cerebrotendinous xanthomatosis)

Cerebrotendinous xanthomatosis is an autosomal recessively inherited inborn error of metabolism due to deficiency of the hepatic mitochondrial enzyme which catalyses the hydroxylation of cholestanol (5,6-dihydrocholesterol). This reaction is on the pathway of bile acid (cholic and deoxycholic acids) synthesis. This metabolic lesion reduces the feedback inhibition of the rate-limiting enzyme cholesterol 7α-hydroxylase and thereby accelerates the synthetic pathway via cholesterol and cholestanol. The patients present in childhood or early adult life with tendon xanthomata, progressive mental handicap, and disseminated neurological lesions due to xanthomata in the brain with associated demyelination, premature atherosclerosis, and cataracts. There are granulomata (xanthomata) in most organs, and these contain cholesterol and cholestanol. The plasma concentration of cholestanol is elevated but cholesterol and other lipid concentrations are usually normal. Treatment with chenodeoxycholic acid which inhibits bile acid synthesis reduces the plasma cholestanol concentration. This approach offers the prospect of arresting or preventing xanthoma formation and cerebral damage.

REFERENCES

Brady, R.O. and Barranger, J.A. (eds) (1985). *The molecular basis of storage disorders.* Academic Press, New York.

Callahan, J.W. and Lowden, J.A. (eds) (1981). *Lysosomes and lysosomal disorders.* Raven Press, New York.

Cox, T.M. (1993). Gaucher's disease: a brand leader. *Lancet*, **342**, 694–5.

Desnick, R.J. (Ed.) (1991). *Treatment of genetic diseases.* Churchill Livingstone Inc., New York.

Desnick, R.J., Gatt, S., and Grabowski, G.A. (eds) (1982). Gaucher disease: a century of delineation and research. Proceedings of the First International Symposium on Gaucher disease held in New York City, July 22–24th, 1981. *Progress in Clinical and Biological Research*, **95**, Alan R. Liss Inc., New York.

Durand, P. (1987). Recent progress of lysosomal diseases. *Enzyme*, **38**, 256–61.

Durand, P. and O'Brien, J.S. (eds) (1982). *Genetic errors of glycoprotein metabolism.* Edi-ermes, Milan and Springer-Verlag, Berlin, Heidelberg, New York (1982).

Lancet (1986). Lysosomal storage diseases (Editorial). *Lancet*, **328**, 898–899.

Hopwood, J.J. and Morris, C.P. (1990). The mucopolysaccharidoses. Diagnosis, molecular genetics and treatment. *Molecular Biology and Medicine*, **7**, 381–404.

Krivit, W. and Paul, N.W. (eds), (1991). *Bone marrow transplantation for lysosomal storage diseases.* March of Dimes Birth Defects Foundation, Birth Defects Original Article Series, Volume 22, No. 1. Alan R. Liss Inc., New York.

Mistry, P.K., Smith, S.J., Ali, M., Hatton, C.S.R., McIntyre, N., and Cox, T.M. (1992). Genetic diagnosis of Gaucher's disease. *Lancet*, **339**, 889–92.

Neufeld, E.F. (1991). Lysosomal storage diseases. *Annual Review of Biochemistry*, **60**, 257–80.

Scriver, C.R., Beaudet, A.L., Sly, W.S. and Valle, D. (eds) (1989). *The metabolic basis of inherited disease.* 6th edn, Volume 2. McGraw-Hill Information Sciences Company, Philadelphia. This comprehensive reference work covers most of the conditions described in this chapter.

Watts, R.W.E. and Gibbs, D.A. (1986). *Lysosomal storage diseases: Biochemical and clinical aspects.* Taylor and Francis, London and Philadelphia.

11.9 Peroxisomal disorders

R. B. H. Schutgens and R. J. A. Wanders

In recent years a growing number of genetic disorders that result from an impairment of one or more metabolic functions catalysed by peroxisomes (microbodies) have been recognized. As a group they are called the peroxisomal disorders.

Peroxisomes

Peroxisomes are cellular organelles present in every human cell except for the mature erythrocyte.

In addition to peroxisomes in liver and kidney, smaller peroxisomes (microperoxisomes) are present in other cell types, including cultured cells. Microperoxisomes seem to have essentially the same enzyme content and functions as the larger peroxisomes in liver and kidney, except for several oxidases that are absent in fibroblasts.

It is now well established that peroxisomes, like mitochondria and chloroplasts, arise by growth and division of pre-existing peroxisomes, rather than by budding from the endoplasmic reticulum. Unlike mitochondria and chloroplasts, peroxisomes contain no DNA, so that all peroxisomal proteins must be coded for by nuclear genes. During the past few years, the genes for a larger number of peroxisomal proteins have been cloned and characterized.

All peroxisomal proteins investigated so far, including soluble matrix proteins and integral membrane proteins are synthesized on free ribosomes and are imported post-translationally into peroxisomes. One of the most common topogenic signals that control the import of proteins into peroxisomes is a SKL (serine—leucine–lysine) sequence at the carboxy terminus of the protein.

Biochemistry

Functions of peroxisomes, including peroxisomal oxidation and respiration, are summarized in Table 1. The pathway is based upon the formation of hydrogen peroxide by a collection of oxidases and the decomposition of the hydrogen peroxide by catalase. Among the oxidases identified are D-aminoacid oxidase, L-α-hydroxyacid oxidase A and B, acyl-coenzyme A oxidases, glutaryl-coenzyme A oxidase, polyamine oxidase, pipecolic acid oxidase, oxalate oxidase, trihydroxycholestanoyl-coenzyme A oxidase, and pristanoyl-coenzyme A oxidase.

Ethanol catabolism via catalase may be significant if substrates such as fatty acids are available to generate hydrogen peroxide inside the peroxisome.

Another major function of peroxisomes is the β-oxidation of a distinct set of substrates that mostly cannot be handled by the mitochondrial β-oxidation system. The enzymic organization of this pathway is given in Fig. 1.

Since acyl-coenzyme As rather than free fatty acids are the true substrates for β-oxidation, conversion to coenzyme A-esters is the first obligatory step in the catabolism of fatty acids. This is brought about by a variety of acyl-coenzyme A synthetases, which differ with respect

Table 1 *Functions of peroxisomes mammalian cells*

Catabolic functions
Hydrogen peroxide-based cellular respiration
β-Oxidation of:
    long chain fatty acids (C_{16}–C_{22}; saturated/unsaturated)
    very long chain fatty acids (C_{22}–C_{26}; saturated/unsaturated)
    branched chain fatty acids
    prostaglandins
    xenobiotics with an acyl side-chain
L-Pipecolic acid oxidation
Purine catabolism
Polyamine catabolism

Anabolic functions
Ether–lipid biosynthesis*
Cholesterol biosynthesis
Bile acid biosynthesis*
Dolichol biosynthesis
Glyoxylate transamination

*Only part of this pathway is localized in peroxisomes.

to their substrate specificity. Next to a long-chain acyl-coenzyme A synthetase, peroxisomes – at least in liver – also contain a second acyl-coenzyme A synthetase, which preferentially activates very long chain ($> C_{22}$) fatty acids (VLCFAs) such as tetracosanoic ($C_{24:0}$) and hexacosanoic ($C_{26:0}$) acid respectively. Similar activity has been detected in the endoplasmic reticulum, but not in mitochondria. There is evidence suggesting obligatory coupling between activation of very long chain fatty acids on the peroxisomal membrane and their subsequent β-oxidation within the peroxisome.

Peroxisomal β-oxidation proceeds via successive steps of dehydrogenation, hydration, dehydrogenation, and thiolytic cleavage. The enzymes involved are distinct from their mitochondrial counterparts. The first step in the β-oxidation of fatty acids is catalysed by acyl-coenzyme A oxidases yielding hydrogen peroxide. Short chain acyl-coenzyme A esters are not suitable substrates for the acyl-coenzyme A oxidases. There is a separate oxidase in peroxisomes catalysing the first step in the oxidation of trihydroxycholestanoyl-coenzyme A, an intermediate in the biosynthesis of cholic acid. This enzyme is expressed in liver only.

The next two reaction in the peroxisomal β-oxidation are catalysed by a multifunctional protein, which, apart from enoyl-coenzyme A hydratase and L-3-hydroxyacyl-coenzyme A dehydrogenase activities, may also harbour a $\triangle^3$-*cis*-$\triangle^2$-trans-enoyl-coenzyme A isomerase activity. This enzyme was once known as bifunctional protein.

The last reaction in the peroxisomal β-oxidation is catalysed by 3-oxoacyl-coenzyme A thiolases. Apart from the enzymes directly involved in β-oxidation, peroxisomes also contain the auxiliary enzymes required for the degradation of unsaturated fatty acids. In addition, peroxisomes have been implicated in the β-oxidation of dicarboxylic acids, prostaglandins and xenobiotics with an acyl side-chain.

Peroxisomes also play an essential role in the pathway of glycero–ether bond formation. The biosynthesis of ether-linked phosphoglycerides like plasmalogen starts with the acylation of dihydroxyacetone phosphate, catalysed by the peroxisomal enzyme acyl-coenzyme A: dihydroxy acetone phosphate (DHAP) acyltransferase (DHAP-AT).

Subsequently, alkyl-dihydroxy acetone phosphate synthase, the peroxisomal enzyme responsible for the glycero–ether bond formation, replaces the acyl moiety in acyl-dihydroxy acetone phosphate by a long chain alcohol, generating alkyl-dihydroxy acetone phosphate that is subsequently translocated to the cytoplasm for the final steps in plasmalogen biosynthesis. Plasmalogens are widely distributed in mammalian cell membranes. They are particularly abundant in brain. Plasmalogens probably protect animal cell membranes against damage by reactive oxygen species such as singlet oxygen.

In humans, glyoxylate can be metabolized in liver by conversion to glycine in a reaction catalysed by the peroxisomal enzyme alanine: glyoxylate aminotransferase. In this way glyoxylate enters the gluconeogenic pathway.

Mammalian peroxisomes have recently been implicated as a site of cholesterol biosynthesis. The physiological and quantitative significance of this putative peroxisomal pathway for cholesterol synthesis is not yet clear.

Peroxisomes in the liver play an essential role in the biosynthesis of bile acids.

Recent studies suggest that *in vivo* the peroxisomal membrane acts as a true permeability barrier towards peroxisomal substrates and/or products and that specific carrier systems mediate the transport of substrates and products over the peroxisomal membrane.

Fig. 1 Enzymic organization of the peroxisomal pathway in the degradation of very long chain fatty acids (VLCFA) and trihydroxycholestanoic acid (THCA)

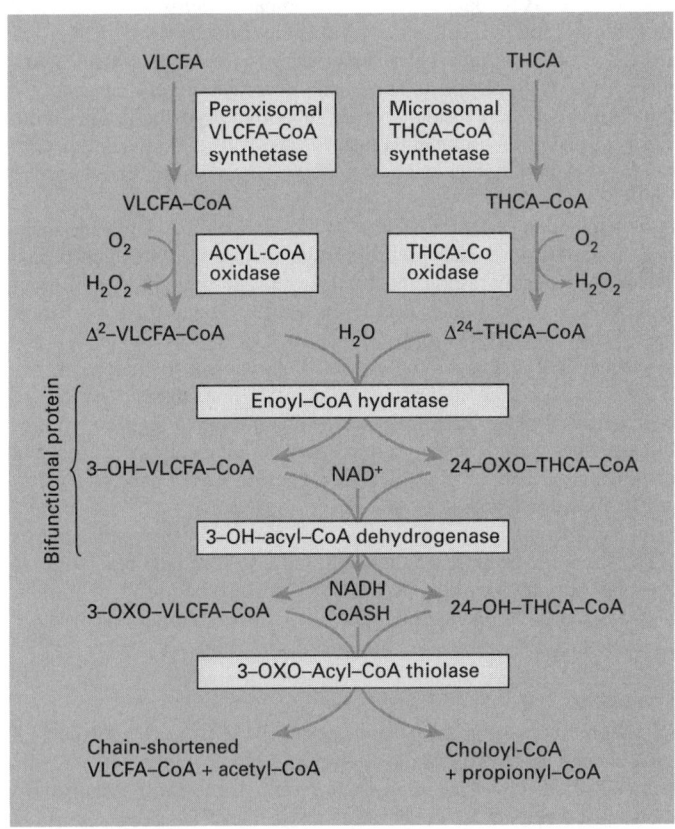

Classification of peroxisomal disorders

A tentative classification of the peroxisomal disorders is presented in Table 2. Three major subgroups are recognized.

Group A includes the disorders with a deficiency of a single peroxisomal enzyme activity in which normal peroxisomal structures are found in morphological and cytochemical studies of tissues and cultured cells.

One can subdivide this subgroup into two classes: (1) the disorders of peroxisomal β-oxidation; and (2) other disorders. Major representatives of this subgroup are X-linked adrenoleukodystrophy and its variants, primary hyperoxaluria type I, and acatalasaemia. Other disorders are listed in Table 2.

Group B includes disorders with normal peroxisomal structures – at least in fibroblasts – in which multiple peroxisomal enzyme activities are deficient.

The rhizomelic type of chondrodysplasia punctata and a rare disorder called Zellweger-like syndrome belong to this subgroup.

Group C includes the disorders of peroxisome biogenesis in which functional peroxisomes are absent or strongly reduced in number in all cell-types studied due to a defect at the level of the biogenesis of peroxisomes.

Analyses with specific antibodies raised against the different peroxisomal integral membrane proteins have shown that empty peroxisomal membrane structures ('ghosts') are present in the cells of these patients. Zellweger syndrome, the neonatal type of adrenoleukodystrophy and the infantile type of Refsum disease belong to this subgroup.

ADRENOLEUKODYSTROPHY/ADRENOMYELONEUROPATHY (ALD/AMN)

Clinical characteristics

Adrenoleukodystrophy

This is a relatively common X-linked recessive disorder with a remarkable phenotypic variation. The disorder affects mainly the nervous system white matter and the adrenal cortex.

Moser and his co-workers list at least six phenotypes in man based upon criteria such as age of onset of neurological symptoms and site of main pathological involvement, which can be cerebrum, spinal cord, peripheral nerve, or, in the absence of neurological involvement, the adrenal gland.

Childhood adrenoleukodystrophy

This is the most serious variant, usually presenting in young boys at about 6 to 8 years of age, whose progress in earlier years has appeared completely normal. The course of the disease is then rapidly progressive, starting from behavioural disturbances, abnormal gait and central nervous system abnormalities and culminating within a few years in adrenal dysfunction, blindness, quadriplegia, and vegetative state. In most patients the location in the brain of MRI abnormal white matter signals is the parieto-occipital region. Patients usually die within 4 years of the onset of clinical symptoms.

Adrenomyeloneuropathy

The most common form of adrenoleukodystrophy manifests later and is characterized by slowly progressive spastic paraparesis, impaired vibration sense in the most distal aspects of the lower extremities, sphincter disturbances, and varying degrees of sexual dysfunction. The mean age of onset that has been reported is about 28 years, with a range from 14 to 60 years. About 70 per cent of adrenomyeloneuropathy patients have primary adrenal insufficiency, evidenced by overt adrenal insufficiency or impaired cortisol responsiveness to adrenocorticotrophic hormone in the presence of elevated baseline adrenocorticotrophic hormone levels; 20 per cent also have low testosterone levels.

Table 2 *Classification of peroxisomal disorders*

A. *Disorders with a deficiency of a single peroxisomal enzyme activity; peroxisomes present*
  1. Disorders of peroxisomal β-oxidation
     X-linked adrenoleukodystrophy and variants
     trihydroxycholestanoyl-coenzyme A oxidase deficiency
     acyl-coenzyme A oxidase deficiency (pseudoneonatal adrenoleukodystrophy)
     bi (tri) functional protein deficiency
     peroxisomal thiolase deficiency (pseudo-Zellweger)
  2. Other disorders
     acatalasaemia
     hyperoxaluria type I
     glutaryl-coenzyme A oxidase deficiency
     dihydroxyacetone phosphate acyltransferase deficiency

B. *Disorders with a deficiency of multiple peroxisomal enzyme activities; peroxisomes present in fibroblasts*
  rhizomelic chondrodysplasia punctata
  Zellweger-like syndrome

C. *Disorders with a general deficiency of peroxisomal functions (disorders of peroxisome biogenesis)*
  No functional peroxisomes
  Zellweger (cerebrohepatorenal) syndrome
  neonatal adrenoleukodystrophy
  Infantile Refsum disease

Table 3 *Main biochemical characteristics of peroxisomal disorders*

	X-linked ALD	RCDP	Zellweger
Plasma			
very long chain fatty acids	↑	n	↑↑
abnormal bile acid intermediates	n	n	↑↑
phytanic acid	n	↑↑	↑
Platelets			
DHAP-AT activity	n	↓	↓↓
Erythrocytes			
plasmalogens	n	↓↓	↓/n
Fibroblasts/amniocytes			
DHAP-AT activity	n	↓	↓
de novo plasmalogen biosynthesis	n	↓↓	↓
plasmalogens	n	↓↓	↓
very long chain fatty acids	↑	n	↑↑
phytanic acid α-oxidation	n	↓↓	↓

ALD, adrenoleukodystrophy; DHAP-AT, dihydroxyacetone phosphate acyltransferase; RCDP, rhizomelic chondrodysplasia punctata. n, normal; ↑↑ greatly elevated; ↑ elevated; ↓↓ greatly decreased; ↓ decreased.

Other variants

An 'Addison's-only' form of adrenoleukodystrophy was only recognized recently. Some of the patients also have subtle abnormalities that are revealed only by detailed neurological examination or MRI. All are at risk of developing overt neurological symptoms later.

Identification of Addison's disease due to adrenoleukodystrophy is important because of the need for genetic counselling and specific, dietary treatment.

The adolescent cerebral form resembles the childhood cerebral syndrome except for the later onset. The adult cerebral form is a rapidly progressive disorder that may present as a psychosis or dementing illness in the third decade of life.

Approximately 15 per cent of the female heterozygotes for adrenoleukodystrophy develop moderately severe spastic paraparesis. In principle, the neurological findings in women resemble those in adrenomyeloneuropathy patients but are of later onset and somewhat milder. Somatosensory evoked responses are abnormal in virtually all of the symptomatic heterozygotes. A diagnosis of multiple sclerosis is often considered in symptomatic carriers for X-linked adrenoleukodystrophy.

X-linked adrenoleukodystrophy is an entirely different disorder compared with the autosomal-recessive neonatal adrenoleukodystrophy disease that belongs to the classification subgroup C.

Biochemical characteristics

The principal biochemical abnormality in X-linked adrenoleukodystrophy is the abnormal accumulation of very long chain ($> C_{22}$) fatty acids in blood and all cell-types studied, including cultured cells such as skin fibroblasts and amniotic fluid cells. (Table 3). This is caused by an impaired capacity to degrade them via the peroxisomal β-oxidation system. The defect involves the deficient activity of the peroxisomal very long chain acyl-coenzyme A synthetase (ligase). This enzyme normally activates the very long chain fatty acids at the peroxisomal membrane. Very long chain fatty acids originate from dietary sources and endogenously from chain elongation of long chain fatty acids.

Recently a putative ALD gene has been identified. The amino acid sequence of the ALD protein (ALDP) deduced showed significant homology to the peroxisomal membrane protein PMP 70, belonging to the 'ATP-binding cassette' superfamily of transporters. ALDP is a peroxisomal membrane protein. No immune response with a monoclonal antibody against ALDP is detectable in tissues of most X-linked adrenoleukodystrophy patients.

ALD/AMN is probably caused by an impaired peroxisomal transport process resulting in a deficiency of the peroxisomal VLCFA/CoA synthetase. Mutations have been characterized in different exons of the adrenoleukodystrophy gene. There is no clear relation between genotype and phenotype. These results strongly support the hypothesis that a modifier gene and/or environmental factors are involved in modulating clinical expression of adrenoleukodystrophy. The gene has been mapped to Xq28.

Accumulation of saturated very long chain fatty acids in central nervous system white matter precedes inflammatory mediated demyelination and is probably responsible for neurological symptoms. Highly elevated very long chain fatty acid levels are also found in adrenocortical cells, Schwann cells, and in Leydig cells.

Biochemical diagnosis of X-linked adrenoleukodystrophy hemizygotes is based upon demonstration of a characteristic pattern of increased very long chain fatty acid levels in plasma, erythrocytes, or cultured fibroblasts. These techniques also permit identification of about 85 per cent of heterozygotes. DNA diagnostics can be used to identify nearly all heterozygotes.

Prenatal diagnosis of affected males is achieved by the demonstration of increased levels of very long chain fatty acids in cultured chorionic fibroblasts or amniocytes; DNA analysis can also be useful. A complication is the great phenotypic variability of the disorder, even within the same kindred.

Treatment

Adrenal hormone supplementation is essential in correcting the adrenal insufficiency in adrenoleukodystrophy patient but does not alter the course of the neurological disease. In recent years several groups have shown that dietary treatment based on restriction of very long chain fatty acids and oral addition of the monounsaturated fatty acids oleic acid

($C_{18:1}$) and erucic acid ($C_{22:1}$) can correct the very long chain fatty acid levels in the plasma of X-linked adrenoleukodystrophy patients within several weeks. This is probably the result of competition between the monounsaturated erucic acid and the saturated counterpart behenic acid ($C_{22:0}$) for chain elongation in the endogenous synthesis of very long chain fatty acids.

Unfortunately the results of this dietary therapy are as yet not very encouraging for patients affected by the childhood cerebral type in whom there are already overt neurological signs. The clinical outcome of this therapy in adrenomyeloneuropathy patients, presymptomatic patients, and heterozygotes is the subject of prospective therapeutic trials in several clinics.

Bone marrow transplantation has been performed in about 25 childhood adrenoleukodystrophy patients. It has been relatively successful, especially when given to boys who are still free, or nearly free, of neurological disease. Because at this stage it is not possible to predict whether a mildly affected boy with the biochemical defect is destined to develop the fatal childhood form this approach is complicated.

ACYL-COENZYME A OXIDASE DEFICIENCY (PSEUDONEONATAL ADRENOLEUKODYSTROPHY), BIFUNCTIONAL PROTEIN DEFICIENCY, PEROXISOMAL 3-OXO-ACYL-COENZYME A THIOLASE DEFICIENCY (PSEUDO-ZELLWEGER SYNDROME)

The clinical characteristics of these relatively rare disorders of early childhood often resemble those in Zellweger syndrome or in the neonatal type of adrenoleukodystrophy.

Biochemical characteristics

Biochemical diagnosis is based on the finding of highly elevated levels of the very long chain fatty acids in tissues, blood(cells) and body fluids from patients in combination with normal peroxisomal structures in tissues and cultured cells. Plasmalogen metabolism is normal.

No accumulation of di- and trihydroxycholestanoic acid is found in the plasma of patients affected by acyl-coenzyme A oxidase deficiency. This is in line with the current view of specific tri(di)hydroxycholestanoyl-coenzyme A oxidase activity different from acyl-coenzyme A oxidase (Fig. 1).

In patients with either a bifunctional protein deficiency or a peroxisomal thiolase deficiency, highly elevated plasma levels of tri(di)hydroxycholestanoic acids are found.

In some patients, immunoblot studies can be helpful for the diagnosis by detection of the absence of one of the specific peroxisomal enzyme proteins. In others, immunoblot studies reveal no abnormality and complementation studies or detailed enzymatic studies are necessary to identify the enzymic defect.

Prenatal diagnosis is done by analysing the profile of the very long chain fatty acids in cultured chorionic villus fibroblasts or in cultured amniotic fluid cells. Immunoblot studies with a specific antiserum can be useful in some families.

Treatment

No effective treatment for these disorders is available. Treatment with dietary restriction of fat and oral supplementation with glycerol-trioleate and glycerol trierucate can result in lowering of the plasma $C_{24:0}$ and $C_{26:0}$ levels but can also result in very high (possibly toxic) $C_{22:1}$ levels.

ACATALASAEMIA/HYPOCATALASAEMIA

Pathophysiology

Acatalasaemia is a rare autosomal recessive inborn error of metabolism in which the homozygotes have extremely low or even undetectable levels of catalase activity in erythrocytes. Other tissues may display variable levels of enzyme deficiency. Normally, the highest catalase activities in mammals are found in erythrocytes, liver, kidney, and phagocytic cells. In liver, catalase is present within peroxisomes in which it plays an essential role in oxidation reactions.

Catalase is part of a cluster of antioxidant enzymes which normally act to protect cells against oxygen free radicals (O_2^-). Detoxification of these radicals by superoxide dismutase generates H_2O_2. In addition, O_2^- and H_2O_2 may also arise from stimulated phagocytes, γ-and ultraviolet radiation, and oxidative processes. Catalase has a rather low affinity for hydrogen peroxide when it acts in the catalitic mode. In this reaction catalase catalyses the reaction $2H_2O_2 \rightarrow H_2O + O_2$.

However, the enzyme has a substantial higher substrate affinity when acting peroxidatically according to the equation $H_2O_2 + X(H_2) \rightarrow 2H_2O + X$ in which X is a hydrogen donor like ethanol, formate, or reduced pyridine nucleotides. Next to the reduced glutathione/glutation peroxidase system, catalase probably does play a part in the clearance of H_2O_2 *in vivo* thus protecting cells against oxidant challenge.

Acatalasaemia has a worldwide distribution but it has been particularly studied in Japan, Switzerland, and Israel. It is genetically heterogeneous as judged by the levels of residual catalase activity in erythrocytes, tissues and cultured cells and by the biochemical and electrophoretic properties of the enzyme.

In general, acatalasaemia is a relatively benign disease without neurological involvement. In some younger Japanese patients it is associated with ulcerating, often gangrenous, oral lesions (Takahara disease) but has no other serious manifestations. None of the Swiss acatalaemics had oral gangrene or any other health problem related to the deficiency. Heterogeneity in the severity of catalase deficiency at the tissue level, dietary factors, and differences in oral flora are important factors.

Treatment

Surgical treatment with excursion of any necrotic areas and antimicrobial therapy is followed by satisfactory healing in severely affected cases.

PRIMARY HYPEROXALURIA TYPE I

Patients usually present during the second decade of life with recurrent calcium oxalate nephrolithiasis and nephrocalcinosis due to the deficiency of the peroxisomal enzyme alanine : glyoxylate aminotransferase in liver. However, others suffer from an acute neonatal type with rapid progression of kidney insufficiency and early death. There is no neurological involvement in this peroxisomal disease.

The disorder is described in detail in Chapter 11.10.

DIHYDROXYACETONE PHOSPHATE ACYLTRANSFERASE DEFICIENCY

Several young children have recently been described showing all the clinical features of the rhizomelic type of chondrodysplasia punctata (RCDP), including craniofacial abnormalities, hypotonia, cataracts, and pronounced rhizomelic shortening (especially of the upper extremities), in which only an isolated deficiency of the peroxisomal enzyme acyl-coenzyme A : dihydroxyacetone phosphate acyltransferase (DHAP-AT) has been detectable. In contrast to the rhizomelic type of chondrodysplasia punctata the metabolism of phytanic acid is normal in these patients. All patients identified so far have died in the first year of life.

Prenatal diagnosis should be possible by measuring the dihydroxyacetone phosphate acyltransferase activity in chorionic villus cells or amniocytes.

RHIZOMELIC CHONDRODYSPLASIA PUNCTATA

Chondrodysplasia punctata refers to a heterogeneous group of bone dysplasias in which non-specific punctate epiphyseal and extra-epiphyseal calcifications can be found in radiological studies. Two major types are the rhizomelic type with an autosomal recessive mode of inheritance and the autosomal dominant Conradi–Hünermann type. Abnormal peroxisomal functions have only been found in the rhizomelic form.

Clinical characteristics

Rhizomelic chondrodysplasia punctata patients have a typical facial appearance (Fig. 2), a striking symmetrical shortening of the proximal limbs, severely disturbed endochondral bone formation and coronal clefts of vertebral bodies of the spine, and severe psychomotor retardation. Most patients have ichthyosis and cataracts. They can survive until the second decade of life.

Biochemical characteristics

The biochemical abnormalities in rhizomelic chondrodysplasia punctata include deficiency of the two peroxisomal enzymes essential for the *de novo* plasmalogen biosynthesis, dihydroxyacetone phosphate acyltransferase and especially alkyl-dihydroxyacetone phosphate synthase, a deficiency of phytanic acid oxidase and a defect in the maturation of the peroxisomal 3-oxoacyl-coenzyme A thiolase enzyme protein. The residual dihydroxyacetone phosphate acyltransferase activity in fibroblasts and platelets can be relatively high, approaching low normal range.

Peroxisomes are present in fibroblasts as demonstrated by the finding of catalase activity in the organelle in patients. It is not yet clear whether the peroxisome structure is normal in the liver of rhizomelic chondroplasia punctata patients.

Biochemical diagnosis of rhizomelic chondrodysplasia punctata is based on the finding of decreased plasmalogen levels, in erythrocyte membranes, elevated plasma phytanic acid levels, the finding of precursor (44hDa) peroxisomal rhiolase in fibroblasts, and normal profiles of the plasma very long chain fatty acids and bile acids respectively (Table 3). In cultured cells, the *de novo* plasmalogen biosynthesis is strongly impaired, the phytanic acid oxidase activity is deficient, and the plasmalogen level is very low.

The multiple biochemical abnormalities in rhizomelic chondrodysplasia punctata are presumably due to one underlying biochemical defect probably at the level of an impairment of the post-translational import of several newly synthesized proteins into peroxisomes.

Prenatal diagnosis for rhizomelic chondrodysplasia punctata has been

Fig. 2 The craniofacial characteristics of a rhizomelic chondrodysplasia punctata patient. (By courtesy of Dr B. Jaume, Palma de Mallorca, Spain.)

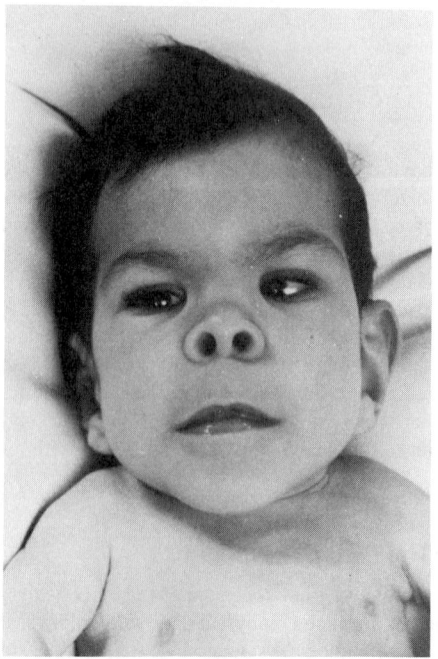

performed by measuring one or more of the specific parameters in cultured chorionic villous fibroblasts or in cultured amniocytes.

Treatment

No effective treatment for rhizomelic chondrodysplasia punctata is available. Prognosis is very poor. Survival can be into the second decade of life.

ZELLWEGER-LIKE SYNDROME

Only two patients have been described with a clinical presentation indistinguishable from classical Zellweger syndrome, but showing abundant peroxisomes in liver. The peroxisomal β-oxidation enzyme proteins in liver were found to be deficient upon immunoblotting and the dihydroxyacetone phosphate acyltransferase activity was also deficient.

Patients exhibited biochemical abnormalities related to an impaired peroxisomal β-oxidation and a defective plasmalogen metabolism.

ZELLWEGER SYNDROME

Clinical characteristics

Zellweger syndrome is an autosomal recessive inborn error of peroxisome metabolism with a worldwide distribution. Some phenotypic variability has been found.

The main clinical characteristics of the classic syndrome are summarized in Table 4.

The clinical presentation is dominated by the typical craniofacial dysmorphism exemplified by the presence of a high forehead, large fontanelles, shallow orbital ridges, low/broad nasal bridge, epicanthus, high arched palate, external ear deformities, micrognathia, redundant folding of the neck, severe hypotonia, abnormal reflexes, epileptic seizures, severe psychomotor retardation, ocular abnormalities, and renal cysts (Fig. 3). In the neonatal period a prolonged icterus with elevated transaminases is frequently found, while hepatomegaly develops during the first months of life, reflecting progressive hepatic fibrosis.

Radiological examination demonstrates stippled scimitar-shaped calcifications of the patellae in about 75 per cent of the patients.

Pathological investigations in Zellweger patients have revealed a great number of abnormalities in various organs, most notably in the brain, liver, and kidney. Neuronal migration disturbances are already present *in utero*.

Most patients die within the first 6 months of life; some survive beyond the neonatal period.

Biochemical characteristics

Patients with Zellweger syndrome lack functional peroxisomes in liver, kidney, and all other cell types. The organelle is not demonstrable by electron microscopy or by electron microscopic cytochemistry for catalase.

Recent immunofluorimetric studies in cultured fibroblasts from Zellweger patients have shown that some of the peroxisomal integral membrane proteins are present in those cells in unusual, largely empty membrane structures. That these peroxisomal 'ghosts' are in fact peroxisomal membranes being degraded in autophagosomes cannot yet be excluded.

It is likely that all peroxisomal enzyme proteins are synthesized normally in the cells of Zellweger patients, but most of them are degraded rapidly in the cytosol post-translationally, as no peroxisome structures are present for import and protection of the newly synthesized enzyme proteins.

A few enzyme proteins, like catalase and alanine : glyoxylate aminotransferase, escape rapid degradation in the cytosol and are still functionally active, although they are present in the cytosol and not in the peroxisomes.

Secondary to the defective biogenesis of peroxisomes, patients show a characteristic set of biochemical abnormalities. These include impaired plasmalogen biosynthesis, defective peroxisomal β-oxidation system,

Table 4 *Main clinical characteristics in Zellweger syndrome*

Psychomotor retardation
Hypotonia
Craniofacial dysmorphia
Hyporeflexia, areflexia
Seizures
Impaired hearing
Hepatomegaly
Nystagmus
Cataract
Retinitis pigmentosa
Renal cysts
Chondrodysplasia calcificans
Cryptorchidism/cliteromegaly

and defective metabolism of phytanic acid and L-pipecolic acid, resulting in characteristic abnormalities in plasma, urine, tissues, and in cultured cells of the patients (Table 3).

Diagnostic tests include fractionation of very long chain fatty acids and bile acids in plasma, quantification of plasma levels of phytanic acid and L-pipecolic acid, measurement of the dihydroxyacetone phosphate acyltransferase activity in platelets and fibroblasts, analyses of the *de novo* plasmalogen biosynthesis and the very long chain fatty acids in cultured cells, and analysis of the intracellular localization of catalase in cultured cells.

Heterozygote detection is not possible with these biochemical procedures, probably reflecting the fact that all these biochemical abnormalities in Zellweger syndrome are secondary phenomena to an as yet unidentified primary defect at the level of the biogenesis of peroxisomes.

Prenatal diagnosis can be performed in pregnancies at recurrent risk for Zellweger syndrome by measuring the dihydroxyacetone phosphate acyltransferase activity in chorionic biopsy material or in cultured amniocytes or chorionic fibroblasts, by immunoblot studies in chorionic villous cells, by measuring the *de novo* plasmalogen biosynthesis in cultured chorionic villous cells or amniocytes and by the fractionation of the very long chain fatty acids in cultured chorionic villous cells or amniocytes.

NEONATAL ADRENOLEUKODYSTROPHY

Clinical characteristics

Zellweger syndrome and neonatal adrenoleukodystrophy resemble one another in their principal clinical and biochemical characteristics, although differences have been reported. Neonatal adrenoleukodystrophy is a slightly less severe illness. Facial dysmorphia is less frequent in neonatal adrenoleukodystrophy; glomerulocystic disease of the kidney and chondrodysplasia punctata are absent.

The neuronal and grey matter changes in neonatal adrenoleukodystrophy are less consistent and less severe compared to Zellweger syndrome. Most neonatal adrenoleukodystrophy patients show a widespread sudanophilic leukodystrophy, often associated with perivascular accumulation of lymphocytes as found in X-linked adrenoleukodystrophy.

Biochemical characteristics

Peroxisomes are either scarce and much smaller than in control liver, or are completely absent in neonatal adrenoleukodystrophy patients. As a result of the deficiency of peroxisomes, the same set of biochemical abnormalities is found in neonatal adrenoleukodystrophy and in Zellweger syndrome (Table 3).

INFANTILE REFSUM DISEASE

Clinical characteristics

The infantile Refsum disease category includes the most mildly involved patients with disordered peroxisomal biogenesis. Distinct abnormalities are absent in the neonatal period. Most patients survive the first decade of life and show some psychomotor development. All have sensorineural hearing loss and pigmentary degeneration of the retina. Patients usually have moderately dysmorphic features and hypoplastic adrenals. Renal cortical cysts and chondrodysplasia punctata are absent.

Biochemical characteristics

Peroxisomes are absent or seriously diminished in number in this disorder resulting in essentially the same set of biochemical abnormalities as seen in Zellweger syndrome.

Complementation analyses with cultured fibroblasts from patients belonging to the peroxisome deficiency category (subgroup C) have revealed a remarkable genetic heterogeneity. In these studies cultured fibroblasts from different patients are fused and the resulting multinucleated cells are studied for complementation. These studies have revealed the existence of at least nine different complementation groups within this category, indicating that mutations in many different genes result in a defect in peroxisome biogenesis.

REFERENCES

Bosch, v.d. H., Schutgens, R.B.H., Wanders, R.J.A., and Tager, J.M. (1992). Biochemistry of peroxisomes. *Annual Review of Biochemistry*, **61**, 157–97.

Clayton, P.T. (1991). Inborn errors of bile acid metabolism. *Journal of Inherited Metabolic Disease*, **14**, 478–497.

Eaton, J.W. (1989). Acatalasemia. In *The metabolic basis of inherited disease* (eds C.R. Scriver, A.L. Beaudet, W.S. Sly., and D. Valle) (6th edn), pp. 1551–62. McGraw Hill, New York.

Hiltunen, J.A. (1991). Peroxisomes and β-oxidation of long-chain unsaturated carboxylic acids. *Scandinavian Journal of Laboratory Investigation*, **51**, Suppl., 33–46.

Kelley, R.I. et al. (1986). Neonatal adrenoleukodystrophy: new cases, biochemical studies and differentiation from Zellweger and related peroxisomal polydystrophy syndromes. *American Journal of Medical Genetics*, **23**, 869–901.

Lazarow, P.B. and Moser, H.S. (1989). Disorders of peroxisome biogenesis. In *The metabolic basis of inherited disease* (eds C.R. Scriver, A.L. Beaudet, W.S. Sly., and D. Valle), (6th edn), pp. 1479–510. McGraw Hill, New York.

Moser, H.W. and Moser, A.B. (1989). Adrenoleukodystrophy. In *The metabolic basis of inherited disease*, (eds C.R. Scriver, A.L. Beaudet, W.S. Sly., and D. Valle), (6th edn), pp. 1511–33. McGraw Hill, New York.

Moser, H.W., Moser, A.B., Naidu, S., and Bergin, A. (1991). Clinical aspects of adrenoleukodystrophy and adrenomyeloneuropathy. *Developmental Neuroscience*, **13**, 254–61.

Fig. 3 The craniofacial characteristics of a Zellweger patient. (By courtesy of Dr A. Oberle, Göppingen, Germany.)

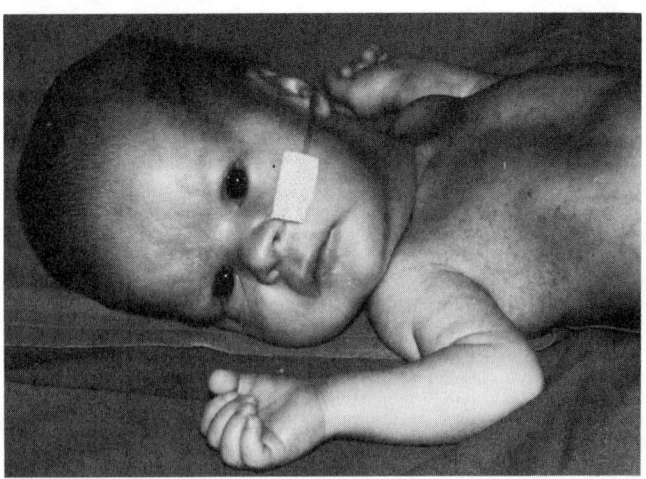

Moser, H.W. et al. (1992). Adrenoleukodystrophy: Phenotypic variability and implications for therapy. *Journal of Inherited Metabolic Disease*, **15**, 645–64.

Mosser, J., Douar, A.M., Sarde, C.O. *et al.* (1993). Putative X-linked adrenoleukodystrophy gene shares unexpected homology with ABC transporters. *Nature*, **361**, 726–30.

Powers, J.M., Liu Y., Moser, A.B., and Moser, H.W. (1992). The inflammatory myelinopathy of adreno-leuko dystrophy: cells, effector molecules, and pathogenetic implications. *Journal of Neuropathology and Experimental Neurology*, **51**, 630–43.

Rizzo, W.B., Leshner, R.T., Odone, A., and Dammann, A.L. (1989). Dietary erucic acid therapy for X-linked adrenoleukodystrophy. *Neurology*, **30**, 1415–22.

Sarde, S.D., Mosser, J., Kioschis, P., *et al.* (1994). Gene organisation of the adrenoleukodystrophy gene. *Genomics*, **22**, 13–20.

Schutgens, R.B.H., Heymans, H.S.A., Wanders, R.J.A., and van den Bosch, H. (1986). Peroxisomal disorders: a newly recognized group of genetic diseases. *European Journal of Pediatrics*, **144**, 430–40.

Shimozawa, N., Tsukamoto, T., Suzuki, Y., *et al.* (1992). A human gene responsible for Zellweger syndrome that affects peroxisome assembly. *Science*, **255**, 1132–4.

Singh, I., Greame, H., Johnson, M.B., and Brown III, F.R. (1988). Peroxisomal disorders. *American Journal of Diseases in Children*, **142**, 1297–1301.

Wanders, R.J.A., Heymans, H.S.A., Schutgens, R.B.H., Barth, P.G., van den Bosch, H., and Tager, J.M. (1988). Peroxisomal disorders in neurology. *Journal of the Neurological Sciences*, **88**, 1–39.

Wanders, R.J.A. et al. (1990). The inborn errors of peroxisomal β-oxidation. A Review. *Journal of Inherited Metabolic Disease*, **13**, 4–36.

11.10 Disorders of oxalate metabolism

R. W. E. WATTS

The oxalate anion is metabolically inert in man and its overall metabolism can be represented by a single compartment model (Fig. 1) in which the oxalate metabolic pool is somewhat larger than the extracellular fluid volume. The normal plasma oxalate concentration is 1 to 3 μmol/l and shows a circadian rhythm, being lowest in the morning and highest in the evening with superimposed postprandial rises. The urinary excretion of oxalate does not normally exceed 450 μmol/24 h in adults. The results in children are similar if they are adjusted to a standard body surface area (1.73 m^2). Adult levels of excretion are reached when the child is about 14 years old. The urinary excretion of oxalate also rises during the waking hours and shows seasonal variations related to a dietary oxalate and calcium intake and the effects of vitamin D supply on the latter. The oxalate in the plasma and tissues is of both dietary and biosynthetic origin. The following foods and beverages have particularly high oxalate contents:

(1) beans
(2) beetroot
(3) celery
(4) chocolate
(5) cocoa
(6) nuts
(7) rhubarb
(8) strawberries
(9) tea

The only proven and clinically important biosynthetic sources of oxalate in man are glycine via the glyoxylate anion, and the C_1–C_2 fragment of ascorbate.

Glycollate, hydroxyproline, serine, and the side chains of the aromatic amino acids and have been shown to be minor metabolic precursors of

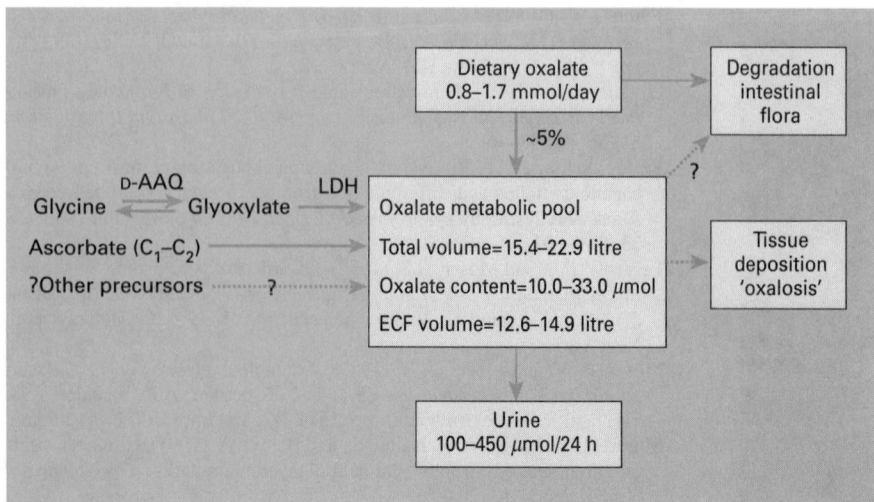

Fig. 1 The one compartment model of oxalate metabolism in man. The numerical values relate to adults and the data for the oxalate metabolic pool have been normalized to a body surface area of 1.73 m^2. The proportion of the dietary oxalate, which is absorbed, depends on whether it is ingested in an ionizable form and on the calcium content of the intestinal tract. AGT, alanine : glyoxylate aminotransferase (EC 2.6.1.44); D-AAO, D-amino acid oxidase (glycine oxidase, EC 1.4.3.3); LDH, Lactate dehydrogenase (EC 1.1.1.27).

Oxalobacter formigenes is an example of a gut commensal which degrades oxalate. The metabolic pathway from glycine to oxalate is a minor component (not more than 1 per cent) of the total metabolic turnover of glycine. Except for carbon atoms 1 and 2 of ascorbate, the importance of other putative metabolic precursors of oxalate (e.g. the aliphatic side-chains of phenylalanine and tryptophan) is unproven in man and they are not important clinically. The system is normally in equilibrium and there is no tendency for oxalate to be deposited in the tissues. Perturbation of the system with expansion of the oxalate metabolic pool occurs in renal failure and when there is either overproduction or over-absorption. Overt oxalosis only occurs when renal failure is combined with one of these other pathophysiological factors.

oxalate in experimental animals. Negligible amounts of oxalate appear to be derived from carbohydrates and polyols (e.g. xylitol) under normal dietary conditions. The claim that the artificial sweetening agent, diethylene glycol, is converted to oxalate in man has not been confirmed. The absorption of oxalate from the small intestine involves both an active carrier mediated transport system with oxalate–chloride exchange and passive diffusion. It is greatly influenced by the calcium ion concentration in the gut lumen, being reduced when this is high and vice versa.

The kidney handles the oxalate ion by 100 per cent filtration at the glomerulus, tubular secretion involving active tubular transport into the lumen, and passive back-diffusion into the peritubular capillaries. The ratio (oxalate clearance) glomerular filtration rate is normally about 1.2, indicating net tubular secretion. Apart from acute oxalic acid poisoning, diseases attributable to oxalate occur when calcium oxalate stones form in the urinary tract and when this salt crystallizes in either the renal parenchyma (calcium oxalate nephrocalcinosis) or in other tissues (oxalosis). The disorders of oxalate metabolism are due to either overproduction or excessive absorption of oxalate. Reduced renal excretion of oxalate does not cause oxalosis unless one of these other pathophysiological processes is also operating. Conversely, increased oxalate biosynthesis and hyperabsorption do not cause oxalosis unless recurrent oxalate urolithiasis and nephrocalcinosis have impaired renal function to the point where there is superadded oxalate retention. The risk of oxalosis developing, as judged by rapidly rising plasma oxalate concentrations and expansion of the oxalate metabolic pool, is greatly increased when the glomerular filtration rate decreases to about 25 ml/min/1.73 ms². Hyperoxaluria is the hallmark of the disorders of oxalate metabolism; Table 1 lists its causes.

Primary hyperoxaluria type I

BIOCHEMISTRY

Primary hyperoxaluria type I (PHI) is due to autosomal recessively inherited deficient activity of hepatic peroxisomal alanine : glyoxylate aminotransferase (AGT; EC 2.6.1.44) (see Chapter 11.9). This enzyme appears to be confined to the liver and Fig. 2 shows the location of the metabolic lesion with some related metabolic reactions. There are four genetic variants of primary hyperoxaluria type I as shown in Table 2. The group of patients in whom the enzyme is mislocated, being mitochondrial and not peroxisomal, is of particular interest. This defect is attributed to a mutation that alters the peptide leader sequence that guides the enzyme from its site of synthesis on the rough endoplasmic reticulum to the correct organelle. It is present in about one-third of primary hyperoxaluria type I patients with residual enzyme catalytic activity and appears to be unique among the inborn errors of metabolism.

Table 1 *The hyperoxalurias*

Primary

Type I	Hyperoxaluria due to hepatic peroxisomal alanine : glyoxylate aminotransferase (AGT; EC 2.6.1.44) deficiency. Associated with hyperglycollic aciduria in about 75% of cases
Type II	Hyperoxaluria due to glyoxylate reductase (D-glycerate dehydrogenase, EC 1.1.1.29) deficiency. Always associated with L-glyceric aciduria
Type III	Hyperoxaluria due to intestinal hyperabsorption (primary absorptive hyperoxaluria). Not associated with any other abnormal organic aciduria

Secondary
Enteric
  jejunoileal ileal bypass
  small intestine reaction
  blind loops
  diffuse disease of the small intestine (e.g. Crohn's disease)
  chronic pancreatic and biliary tract disease
Oxalata ingestion (acute poisoning)
Excessive intake of ascorbic acid
Ethylene glycol poisoning
Adverse reaction of methoxyfluorane inhalation
Adverse reaction to xylitol infusion
Glycine irrigation (after transurethral prostatectomy)
Aspergillus infection
Pyridoxine (vitamin B₆) deficiency

The chromosomal assignment of the alanine : glyoxylate aminotransferase gene is 2q36–37. The coding region of about 10 kilobase pairs is organized into 11 exons and 10 introns. The gene has been sequenced and several different mutations identified. Most attention has been paid to explaining the misrouting phenomenon. It appears that the critical mutations affect the conformation (shape) of the amino terminus peptide sequence of the protein molecule in such a way that it becomes more alpha-helical, therefore more like the recognition sequence of a true mitochondrial protein and is recognized as such by specific receptor sites on the mitochondrial membrane.

PATHOLOGY

In the early stages, the pathological findings are confined to the kidney and comprise a variable degree of hydrocalycosis and hydronephrosis

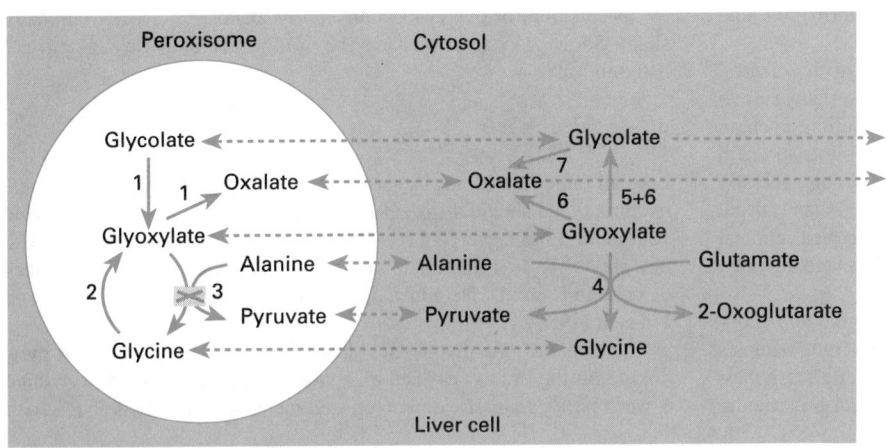

Fig. 2 The site of the metabolic lesion in primary hyperoxaluria type I (reaction 3 in this diagram). The outer rectangle represents the plasma membrane of the hepatocyte and the circle represents the membrane of a peroxisome. The solid arrows show enzyme-catalysed metabolic pathways and the broken arrows indicate diffusion pathways. The enzymes catalysing the reactions are: 1, glycollate oxidase (L-2 hydroxyacid oxidase; EC 1.1.3.1); 2, glycine oxidase (D-amino acid oxidase; EC 1.4.3.3); 3, alanine : glyoxylate aminotransferase (serine : pyruvate aminotransferase, EC 2.6.1.44); 4, (glutamate : glyoxylate aminotransferase EC 2.6.1.4); 5, glyoxylate reductase (D-glycerate dehydrogenase, EC 1.1.1.26); 6, lactate dehydrogenase (EC 1.1.1.27); 7, glycollate dehydrogenase (EC 1.1.1.79). Glyoxylate reductase is the site of the metabolic lesion in type II primary hyperoxaluria. (Reproduced with permission from the *Journal of Inherited Metabolic Disease* vol. 12, p. 214. Copyright © Society for the Study of Inborn Errors of metabolism and Kluwer Academic Publishers 1989.)

Table 2 *Genetic heterogeneity in primary hyperoxaluria type I*

Pyridoxine responsive and non-responsive variants
Residual catalytic activity present or absent
Immunologically demonstrable enzyme present (CRM$^+$) or absent (CRM$^-$)
Alanine : glyoxylate aminotransferase mislocated into mitochondria as opposed to its normal location in peroxisomes

Table 3 *The clinical grading of patients with primary hyperoxaluria*

	Grade					
	1	2	3	4	5	6
Passage of stones	−	+	± *	± *	± *	± *
Stones/nephrocalcinosis on imaging	−	−	+	± *	± *	± *
Stone removal procedure	−	−	−	+	± *	± *
Impaired overall renal function	−	−	−	−	+	+
Renal support or replacement	−	−	−	−	−	+

*usually present.

with multiple calculi. Interstitial deposits of calcium oxalate, which mainly form later, cause severe renal fibrosis and shrinkage, and the kidney feels tough and gritty when incised. The changes of renal hypertension and chronic interstitial nephritis are often present, and the renal tubules may be blocked by aggregates of calcium oxalate crystals, particularly if the terminal illness has been associated with a hypotensive-oliguric episode. The characteristic rosette-like calcium oxalate monohydrate crystals are highly birefringent and easily recognized under a polarizing microscope. Their full extent will only be observed if unfixed tissues are examined or if non-aqueous fixatives are used, but they are usually sufficiently insoluble for some to remain and be apparent after routine fixation in formol–saline. They are found most extensively in the myocardium, tunica media of muscular arteries and arterioles, the rete testes, and at sites of rapid bone turnover. Careful examination reveals a few crystals associated with the arterial supply of all organs and tissues. Similar deposits have been found intra-axonally in peripheral nerves.

CLINICAL ASPECTS

Patients usually present with recurrent urolithiasis during the first decade and, if untreated, die in uraemia before they are 20 years old. The terminal phase of rapidly progressing uraemia and oliguria usually lasts at most only a few months and is associated with dense calcium oxalate nephrocalcinosis and with the development of oxalosis. Intracardiac conduction defects, including complete heart block, may develop during the terminal illness. Ischaemic lesions occur on the extremities, particularly in the pulps of the fingers and toes, and are attributable to the extensive crystallization of calcium oxalate in the walls of small arteries and arterioles. Progressive peripheral neuropathy and mononeuritis multiplex are associated with calcium oxalate deposition within axons as well as in the wall of the vasa nervorum. These vascular and neurological manifestations, as well as a wider range of oxalotic features, occur particularly in patients in whom the terminal renal failure has been treated by standard haemodialysis, by peritoneal dialysis, or by an unsuccessfull renal transplantation. The additional manifestations include livedo reticularis, subcutaneous calcinosis which may ulcerate, retinal changes (white flecks, exudates, infarcts, yellow crystalline deposits especially along the courses of the renal arteries, black 'geographic' lesions at the macula), dilated cardiomyopathy, synovitis and a painful osteodystrophy with dense osteosclerosis, deformation, and stress fractures (especially in the vertebrae).

A few cases present during the first months of life with seizures, advanced renal failure and dense nephrocalcinosis, but few if any calculi (the infantile type). Another small group (the adult type) follow a benign course, presenting in adult life and surviving into the fourth and fifth decade with only occasional stone formation. This last group generally has less grossly elevated levels of urinary oxalate excretion than is usual in the clinical group (juvenile type), which follows a typical clinical pattern. However, the amount of oxalate excreted and the age at which renal failure develops are not very closely correlated.

A few patients present with severe uraemia and may give no history of urolithiasis. Others present with symptoms arising from oxalosis rather than renal disease, involving principally the heart, arteries, bones, and nerves. The severity of the overall clinical picture for a particular patient can be expressed in terms of a six-point scale (Table 3). Considering this in relation to the patient's age, pyridoxine responsiveness and the plasma and urine oxalate concentrations gives a clinical guide to prognosis.

Although the metabolic lesion of primary hyperoxaluria type I is located in the peroxisome, it does not share any of the features of the other peroxisomal diseases, such as Zellweger's syndrome, adrenoleukodystrophy, and rhizomelic chondrodysplasia punctata. Similarly, the patients in whom alanine : glyoxylate aminotransferase has been misrouted into mitochondria do not show evidence of mitochondrial dysfunction (impaired fatty acid oxidation and disorders of respiratory chain function).

DIAGNOSIS

Primary hyperoxaluria type I should be considered in any child with urinary stones or nephrocalcinosis and in adults with recurrent calcium oxalate stones for which no alternative explanation has been found, especially if the clinical history extends back into childhood. The presence of calcium oxalate crystals in the urinary centrifuged deposit is not a specific diagnostic sign; 24-h urinary oxalate excretion is more helpful. About 75 per cent of patients have an associated hyperglycollic aciduria. The definitive diagnosis is made by assaying alanine : glyoxylate aminotransferase activity on a percutaneous needle biopsy of the liver, which can also be examined by immunoelectron microscopy to establish whether the enzyme protein is present and its intracellular location. Liver biopsies have been used for prenatal diagnosis as early as the seventeenth week of pregnancy. The plasma oxalate concentration should be determined when the patient is first evaluated and subsequently as a guide to prognosis. A progressively rising plasma oxalate concentration indicates an increasing risk of oxalosis developing. In renal failure not due to hyperoxaluria there is a linear regression relationship between plasma oxalate and creatinine, and a plasma oxalate value that is high for the corresponding creatinine level is a valuable pointer to oxalate overproduction (or overabsorption). Early oxalosis is usually clinically silent. Some procedures that may be used to detect and evaluate it are listed in Table 4.

TREATMENT

Like all patients with urinary stone disease, those with primary hyperoxaluria type I should drink sufficient fluid to maintain a measured urine volume of 3 litres every 24 h, with proportionately less in children. The diet should be low in oxalate and calcium and have minimum intakes of vitamin C and D. Details of such a diet were published by Watts and Mansell (1988).

The effect of pharmacological doses (150 to 1000 mg/day) of pyridoxine on the urinary oxalate excretion should be assessed over three 1-week periods – pretreatment, on-treatment, and post-treatment – with

Table 4 *Diagnosis of oxalosis*

Skeletal muscle biopsy: small arteries and arterioles

Bone marrow biopsy: sternal aspiration, iliac crest trephine

Soft tissue radiographs of hands

Skeleton
   Radiographs
   [^{99}Tc^m] medronate
   computerized tomography scanning
   bone density measurements

Joint aspiration

Arteriography

Peripheral nerve conduction

Heart
   electrocardiography
   ambulatory monitoring
   nuclear techniques to evaluate ejection fraction and
     myocardial function
   cardiac muscle biopsy

assays of urinary oxalate and creatinine (a check for completeness of urine collection) on each 24-h urine collection. If the urinary oxalate decreases appreciably, pyridoxine should be continued indefinitely. A favourable response can probably be anticipated in between about 10 per cent and 30 per cent of cases.

Orthophosphates (e.g. Phosphate-Sandoz®) equivalent to 2 g of elemental phosphorus per day and magnesium oxide or hydroxide (e.g. 200 mg magnesium oxide) are recommended as non-specific inhibitors of crystal growth and aggregation, as in other forms of recurrent urinary stone disease. The doses used should be sufficient to produce a material increase in the urinary excretion of either phosphate or magnesium.

Patients who are pyridoxine resistant ultimately require orthotopic liver transplantation to correct the metabolic lesion, and renal transplantation if they are approaching endstage renal disease. Ideally, planning for liver transplantation should begin when the glomerular filtration rate falls to below 20 per cent of the mean predicted normal value to minimize oxalosis and reduce the risk of oxalate deposition in the grafted kidney. After a successful liver transplant, the hyperglycollic aciduria returns to normal immediately, the plasma oxalate value normalizes over the course of a few weeks or months, and the urinary oxalate excretion returns to normal over the course of one or more years, depending on the size of the oxalate deposits that are gradually mobilized from the tissues.

Should endstage renal failure occur before liver transplantation, neither haemodialysis nor peritoneal dialysis can keep up with the rate of oxalate production, but either treatment may limit further deposition of oxalate pending transplantation. These palliative measures should be instituted early and carried out more vigorously then in other forms of renal failure, that is, as intensively as the patient can tolerate.

A renal transplant performed while the glomerular filtration rate is in the 15 to 20 ml/min/ms^2 range can 'buy time', during which liver transplantation can be organized, but the long-term prognosis for such a grafted kidney is almost always very poor.

TREATMENT OF THE URINARY STONES

Surgical intervention should be the minimum necessary to relieve obstruction and every effort should be made to avoid removing functioning renal tissue. Close follow-up is essential, with regular radiological and/or ultrasonographic assessment. Patients who have previously passed stones often do so with little pain and unsuspected collections of stones may be found in the lower ureter on a routine abdominal radiograph. Every effort should be made to encourage the stones to pass spontaneously before resorting to open surgery, because further obstructive episodes and surgical intervention are inevitable. Nephroscopic lithotomy, endoscopic lithotripsy with ultrasonic, electrohydraulic and laser techniques, as well as extracorporeal shock-wave lithotripsy, which produces relatively little damage to functioning kidney tissue, can be used to deal with asymptomatic stones and with obstructive uropathy as soon as it is diagnosed. If these techniques are available then early stone removal or disruption can be recommended in order to avoid obstructive uropathy later. The effect of these procedures on overall renal function and plasma oxalate concentration should be monitored. It is possible that nephrocalcinotic kidneys may be more easily damaged by shockwaves than normal or purely fibrotic kidneys.

Primary hyperoxaluria type II

Primary hyperoxaluria type II is due to autosomal recessively inherited deficiency of glyoxylate reductase (D-glycerate dehydrogenase; EC 1.1.1.26). This enzyme is cytosolic, widely distributed and the enzymological diagnosis can be made on peripheral blood leucocytes. The hyperoxaluria is accompanied by L-glyceric aciduria. The clinical features, complications, and pathological findings are the same as those of primary hyperoxaluria type I. There have been no reports of the possible biochemical and genetic heterogeniety of this disease. Table 5 summarizes and contrasts the treatments that are available for the three types of primary hyperoxaluria. Enzyme replacement by organ transplantation has not been attempted in type II, although if the liver proved to contain the major part of the total body's glyoxylate reductase activity liver transplantation might be beneficial. The expression of the enzyme in leucocytes suggests that bone marrow transplantation from a fully histocompatible sibling might also be a therapeutic option.

Primary hyperoxaluria type III

Patients with primary hyperoxaluria type III do not have an associated hyperglycollic or L-glyceric aciduria and have, therefore, to be distinguished from the approximately 25 per cent of type I patients with isolated hyperoxaluria. The diagnosis of primary hyperoxaluria type III rests on: firm evidence of normal intestinal anatomy and absorptive function; the demonstration of excessive oxalate absorption (this may be difficult to establish by the available ^{14}C-labelled oxalate absorption and/or oxalate loading tests); normal hepatic alanine : glyoxylate aminotransferase levels. The urinary oxalate excretion (usually 1 to 2 mmol/24 h) is similar to that in some patients with type I and type II, and type III patients are at risk of urinary stones, renal failure, and oxalosis. The metabolic lesion has not been identified precisely, but it might involve an oxalate–chloride exchanger in the small intestine. It has been reported that thiazides reduce the urinary oxalate excretion in type III. As in secondary hyperoxaluria due to diffuse small intestinal disease, treatment is by a low oxalate diet with oxalate binding agents such as cholestyramine, and calcium ions (given as calcium carbonate). A marine hydrocolloid preparation (Ox-absorb®) has recently been developed as an intestinal oxalate binding therapeutic agent.

Enteric hyperoxaluria

Enteric hyperoxaluria is an uncommon but potentially serious complication of the diseases listed in Table 1. It can cause extensive urolithiasis with nephrocalcinosis and renal failure. Expansion of the oxalate pool has been demonstrated and there is the same potential for oxalosis developing as in the primary hyperoxalurias. Treatment depends upon reducing dietary oxalate intake, the use of oxalate binding agents, and correcting the steatorrhoea.

Table 5 *The relevance of different treatment modalities to the different types of primary hyperoxaluria*

	Type I	Type II	Type III
Diet			
low oxalate	+	+	+
low calcium	+	+	−
low vitamin C	+	+	+
low vitamin D	+	+	+
Hydration	+	+	+
Inhibition of crystal growth (administration of MgO, Mg(OH)$_2$ or orthophosphate)	+	+	+
Oxalate binding agents	−	−	+
Thiazides	−	−	+
Pyridoxine	+	−	−
Dialysis	+	+	+
Renal transplantation	+	+	+
Hepatic transplantation	+	−	−

Reproduced from Watts and Mansell (1988).

REFERENCES

Rose, G.A. (ed.) (1988). *Oxalate metabolism in relation to urinary stone disease*. Springer-Verlag, Berlin.

Scheinman, J.I. (1991). Primary hyperoxaluria: therapeutic strategies for the 90s. Editorial Review. *Kidney International*, **40**, 389–99.

Watts, R.W.E. (1990). Treatment of renal failure in the primary hyperoxalurias. *Nephron*, **56**, 1–5.

Watts, R.W.E. (1992). Alanine:glyoxylate aminotransferase deficiency: biochemical and molecular genetic lessons from the study of a human disease. *Advances in Enzyme Regulation*, **32**, 309–27.

Watts, R.W.E. and Mansell, W.A. (1988). Primary hyperoxaluria. In *Oxalate metabolism in relation to urinary stone disease* (ed. G.A. Rose). Springer-Verlag, London.

Watts, R.W.E., and Mansell, M.A. (1990). Oxalate, livers and kidneys. Combined renal and hepatic transplants transform the outlook in primary hyperoxaluria type I. *British Medical Journal*, **301**, 772–3.

Watts, R.W.E., Danpure, C.J., De Pauw, L., Toussaint, C. and the European Study Group on Transplantation in Primary Hyperoxaluria Type I (1991). Combined liver-kidney and isolated liver transplantations for primary hyperoxaluria type I: the European Experience. *Nephrology Dialysis Transplantation*, **6**, 502–11.

Watts, R.W.E. *et al.* (1991). Combined hepatic and renal transplantation in primary hyperoxaluria type I: clinical report of 9 cases. *American Journal of Medicine*, **90**, 179–88.

Watts, R.W.E., Veall, N., and Purkiss P. (1983). Sequential studies of oxalate dynamics in primary hyperoxaluria. *Clinical Science*, **65**, 627–33.

Yent, E.R. and Cohanim, M. (1986). Absorptive hyperoxaluria: a new clinical entity–successful treatment with hydrochlorothiazide. *Clinical and Investigative Medicine*, **9**, 44–50.

11.11 Diabetes mellitus

J. I. Bell and T. D. R. Hockaday

Introduction

Definition

Diabetes mellitus is a state of chronic hyperglycaemia, classically associated with symptoms of excessive thirst, increased urine volume, and, if severe enough, weight loss. Over time, particular types of tissue damage may develop in the affected patients. It can be produced by several different disease processes, for as well as types I and II, the two forms commonly found in the United Kingdom, type III occurs in the tropics. Also, in addition to these 'primary' forms of the disease, diabetes may be secondary to other diseases such as pancreatitis (acute or chronic), haemochromatosis, and a number of endocrine disorders producing excessive levels of cortisol (Cushing's syndrome), growth hormone (acromegaly), glucagon (glucagonoma), or adrenalin (phaeochromocytoma).

The term 'diabetes' was originally introduced to describe the clinical symptoms associated with unduly high glucose levels. Diagnostic emphasis then shifted to the glucose levels themselves, and in addition to 'diabetes' a milder level of hyperglycaemia, denoted 'impaired glucose tolerance', has been defined by the World Health Organization (WHO) (Table 1). However, it is difficult to produce a single binding definition because of the different aetiologies and varying severity and manifestations of diabetes. The fundamental defect occurs in insulin secretion and/or action. In the classical young onset form of the disorder, there is near-total insulin deficiency, with inevitable widespread metabolic changes. In the older age onset form, there is diminished and/or delayed insulin secretion in response to glucose combined with varying degrees of diminished effectiveness of circulating insulin. When there is associated obesity, insulin resistance predominates. Therefore diabetes can be defined as a state of diminished insulin action due to its decreased availability or effectiveness in varying combinations.

Arguments can be advanced in favour of the term impaired glucose tolerance rather than the nearest previous term of ·'chemical diabetes', used to distinguish clear-cut hyperglycaemia without clinical symptoms or signs from more severe hyperglycaemia with symptoms and/or signs.

Table 1 *Degrees of hyperglycaemia*

Mild	Moderate	Severe
Impaired glucose and insulin control (sophisticated tests necessary)	Impaired glucose tolerance (WHO) (temporary or permanent)	Diabetes mellitus (WHO) (temporary or permanent)
	Chemical diabetes	Clinical diabetes
		Liability to retinopathy and nephropathy
	Increased risk of ischaemic heart disease	More pronounced risk of ischaemic heart disease

However, impaired glucose tolerance is a mild version of the diabetic defect, whether progressive or not, although 2 to 5 per cent of those so classified progress to 'diabetic' (WHO) glucose levels annually. Hence, although few subjects with impaired glucose tolerance initially show the most typical of the various forms of diabetic tissue damage (small blood vessel lesions or microangiopathy), many do so later as they progress to higher glucose levels.

Diagnosis

Diagnosis depends on measurement of glucose levels, usefully in the urine but crucially in the blood. Glucose tolerance testing was introduced when the measurement of blood glucose was much less accurate and reproducible than it is today. It involves measuring the rise and subsequent fall of blood glucose values after drinking 75 g of glucose dissolved in water within 10 min. The test is best done with a little flavouring (for example lemon juice) added to the glucose drink and a small drink of water alone afterwards. Traditionally, venous or capillary blood glucose is measured every 30 min from the start of the drink for 2 to 2.5 h (the defining glucose values vary according to which type of blood is used). The 2 h value is generally the most informative, and the test is often performed with just initial overnight fasting and the 2 h values. Indeed, with the more precise blood glucose measurements now available, the fasting value alone is very predictive of glucose tolerance. However, the handling of a metabolic load involves processes additional to those maintaining the fasting near 'steady state' equilibrium, particularly when there is a high level of insensitivity (resistance) to the hypoglycaemic action of insulin, resulting in blood insulin concentrations which are particularly high, for example in pregnancy. Bacterial and viral infections also cause insulin insensitivity, and so there is little point in performing diagnostic tests during or soon after an infection, unless the symptoms of diabetes are clear cut, when the random or fasting glucose level will be notably raised and diagnostic in itself.

The WHO has suggested that in a symptomatic patient a random plasma glucose value of 11.1 mmol/l (200 mg/dl) or more is diagnostic (Table 2). This is also adequate for the asymptomatic patient if found on more than one occasion (and not due to an obvious hyperglycaemic stimulus such as glucose infusion in a surgical patient!). If random glucose estimates show lower degrees of hyperglycaemia estimation of fasting glucose levels or an oral glucose tolerance test may be used. The defining glucose levels are given in Table 2.

The differences between plasma and whole-blood glucose concentrations, and between capillary and venous levels, are too often ignored. Whole-blood values are about 10 to 15 per cent lower than those of plasma, and capillary values are 7 per cent higher than venous values in the fasting state and 8 per cent higher after a glucose load. These differences are important because clinical laboratories may use venous plasma whereas bedside monitoring techniques use capillary whole blood or plasma.

The term impaired glucose tolerance was probably substituted for 'chemical diabetes' in an attempt to remove the possible stigma, and probable insurance consequences, of a diagnosis of diabetes. At that time it was also believed that clinically apparent microangiopathy was an essential component of true diabetes, at least after the disease had been present for some time. This neglected the apparent absence of such lesions in a minority of long-term frankly hyperglycaemic diabetic patients, as well as the evolution of many subjects with initial impaired glucose tolerance into diabetics with time. It should also be noted that many patients who fall within the lower part of the diabetic range (as defined by the WHO) are also only 'chemical diabetics' in the sense that they have no symptoms and no evidence of diabetic tissue damage on examination.

The control of blood glucose levels, like that of blood pressure or weight, fluctuates from time to time. Glucose levels vary with nutritional state and are raised by infection, sterile inflammation, psychological upset, and medicaments such as oral glucocorticoids or thiazide-type diuretics, although to what extent the latter is due to any associated change in potassium distribution is not clear—adrenergic β-blockers also impair glucose tolerance.

Emphasis on the term diabetes rather than hyperglycaemia has led epidemiologists to mishandle this risk factor for accelerated arteriosclerosis. They tend to score subjects as plus or minus for 'diabetes' or sometimes also for 'impaired glucose tolerance'. With blood pressure or plasma cholesterol concentrations, the straightforward terms hypertension and hypercholesterolaemia have been adopted, and risk is analysed in terms of the blood pressure reading or the plasma cholesterol concentration. Such an approach, using the blood glucose level, would be much more appropriate for hyperglycaemics, although the level of insulin, or an insulin-like molecule, might also need to be incorporated.

Table 1 lists some of the terms discussed above and the ways in which they interrelate. It also indicates that the glucose levels necessary to act over time to produce diabetic microangiopathy are higher than those necessary to produce macroangiopathy, which is expressed as accelerated arteriosclerosis. Microangiopathy, which is potentially present anywhere in the body, may also contribute to diabetic neuropathy. Table 3 lists these important types of diabetic tissue damage as well as the widespread accelerated loss of elasticity of collagen throughout the body, perhaps because of its non-enzymatic glycosylation, and the increased risk of cataract. These last two lesions occur in the general population with ageing and, for instance, may be more frequent among non-diabetics aged 80 than among diabetics aged 40. However, at any given age, these lesions will be found more commonly among diabetics than non-diabetics.

These different types of tissue damage may interact, for instance in the aetiology of diabetic foot ulcers to which poor arterial supply (macroangiopathy), diseased small blood vessels (microangiopathy), loss of feeling from sensory neuropathy, and disordered regulation of blood flow in small vessels owing to autonomic neuropathy all contribute, together with abnormality of the connective tissue collagen. Similarly, in the ischaemic heart disease of diabetes, abnormal cardiac collagen, autonomic neuropathy, and microangiopathy of the vasa vasorum may all add to the effects of the dominant lesion of coronary arteriosclerosis.

Table 2 *Diagnostic glucose values for diabetes in oral glucose tolerance tests*

	Fasting (mmol)		2 h postglucose (mmol)
Diabetes mellitus			
Venous whole blood	>6.7	*and/or*	>10.0
Capillary whole blood	>6.7	*and/or*	>11.1
Venous plasma	>7.8	*and/or*	>11.1
Impaired glucose tolerance			
Venous whole blood	<6.7	*and*	>6.7 ≤ 10.0
Capillary whole blood	<6.7	*and*	>7.8 ≤ 11.1
Venous plasma	<7.8	*and*	>7.8 ≤ 11.1
Normal			
Venous whole blood	<6.7	*and*	<6.7
Capillary whole blood	<6.7	*and*	<7.8
Venous plasma	<7.8	*and*	<7.8

All for 75 g oral glucose load in 250–350 ml water, or 1.75 g/kg ideal body weight for children to a maximum of 75 g. Values are for a specific enzymatic glucose assay.

Adapted from the *Report of the WHO Study Group on Diabetes Mellitus, 1985.*

Table 3 *Types of diabetic tissue damage*

Microangiopathy (particularly retina, kidneys)
Macroangiopathy (accelerated arteriosclerosis (distally), e.g. ischaemic heart disease, cerebrovascular disease, intermittent claudication or gangrene of feet)
Neuropathy (autonomic, sensory, motor)
Ocular cataracts
Inelastic collagen (e.g. Dupuytren's contractures)

The disease processes of diabetes

There are at least three different disease processes contributing to the primary diabetic state, in addition to the various causes of secondary diabetes. Type III diabetes appears to be confined to those born in the tropics, particularly India and East Africa, and is very rare among those who later leave these areas. The destruction of the pancreatic islets of Langerhans in type III disease seems to be the result of an initially exocrine pancreatic lesion caused by multiple small calculi in the finer branches of the pancreatic duct; the whole process is known as tropical fibrocalculous disease. Thus, although clearly distinct in the exact lesion, it has similarities with diabetes secondary to acute or chronic pancreatitis in developed countries.

Type I diabetes (once termed juvenile-type onset diabetes) is the result of an autoimmune destruction of the islets of Langerhans. It typically presents before 30 years, but can occur at any age. It generally causes a very substantial destruction of the total capacity of the islet β-cells to secrete insulin. Islet-cell antibodies are usually found in the plasma for a period of 1–2 years after diagnosis, but in a minority (perhaps 20 per cent) these may persist for the remainder of the patient's life. Members of this subgroup, sometimes called type Ib, are particularly liable to suffer other autoimmune diseases or conditions believed to involve disturbed immune mechanisms, for example coeliac disease or rheumatoid arthritis.

Most type I patients are 'insulin dependent' because of the severe degree of β-cell destruction. This term, again defined by WHO, implies that without insulin injection they will become ketoacidotic within days or a few weeks, lapse into coma, and die. The hyperketonaemia occurs because of excessive flux of fatty acids to the liver from adipose tissue, leading to overproduction of ketone bodies (acetoacetate and 3-hydroxybutyrate). These spill over into the urine, causing an excessive loss of cations because they are relatively strong acids. The loss of potassium may be particularly important because one of insulin's actions is to promote passage of potassium from extracellular fluid into cells.

Type II diabetes lacks associations such as the circulating islet antibodies found early in type I or the presence of particular forms of the HLA system coded for on chromosome 6. Hence a variety of disease processes may give rise to the 'type II' syndrome. Some patients with maturity-type onset diabetes of the young have a variety of abnormalities of the glucokinase gene, which is important in the metabolism of glucose in both hepatic and pancreatic β-cells. A few others with mild type II features secrete an abnormal insulin of reduced potency through an inherited error. However, there is also a growing consensus that the pathogenesis of the majority of type II patients may stem from deficient fetal nutrition, probably more often resulting from placental deficiencies than from maternal malnutrition. Somehow this appears to affect the development of β-cell function, so that there is a predisposition to secrete an unduly large proportion of proinsulin or products of its catabolism before insulin itself is reached, and there is probably additional insensitivity to insulin which may be related to changes in muscular metabolism or altered adipose tissue composition. Perhaps because of the abnormality in the insulin production chain or chronic elevated glucose levels, a very insoluble polymer derived from amylin forms between the β-cells. This amyloid deposit may well contribute to the islet destruction but is probably not the only mechanism of β-cell glucotoxicity in this condition.

The details of this general hypothesis may well change with time, but it is essentially based on the demonstration of increased risk of ischaemic heart disease, hypertension, hyperlipidaemia, and impaired glucose tolerance or diabetes around the age of 60 years in those with a small birth weight. Such importance of fetal development calls into question the extent of the genetic contribution to the very strong concordance of type II diabetes among identical twins. The marked tendency of type II diabetic patients to obesity may also stem from a maladaptation to reduced energy supply during very early growth. This may explain the paradox that obesity is more common in members of social classes IV and V who are usually less well off.

Classification

Two main methods of classification have appeared in recent years. The first separates type I primary diabetes from types II and III and secondary diabetes, while the second separates insulin-dependent diabetes (IDDM) from non-insulin-dependent diabetes (NIDDM) (see Table 4).

These classifications have different aims, or at least are based on different aspects of the problem, for otherwise it is insidiously easy to

Table 4 *Simplified classification of diabetes mellitus and kindred states*

Type	Alternative name	Clinical characteristics	Aetiological features
Ia	Insulin-dependent diabetes (IDDM) Juvenile onset diabetes Ketosis-prone diabetes	In early phase retain some endogenous insulin secretion and may have honeymoon phase Later have no endogenous insulin Develop ketoacidosis when insulin withdrawn or with stress states Mostly young, often markedly thin at diagnosis	(i) Association with HLA types (e.g. DR3, DR4) (ii) Generally cytoplasmic and complement-fixing islet cell antibody positive at diagnosis but later becomes negative
Ib	As for type Ia	Higher percentage of females and older age of onset than type Ia	Also: (i) Close association with other autoimmune endocrinopathies (ii) Persistent islet cell antibodies (iii) Presumed autoimmune aetiology
II (non-obese)	Non-insulin-dependent diabetes (NIDDM) Maturity onset diabetes of the young, now non-insulin-dependent known as diabetes of the young	Always measurable insulin present Tendency to insulin resistance Ketosis not provoked by insulin withdrawal but may become ketoacidotic with severe illness Onset usual above age of 40	(i) Heterogeneous aetiologies (ii) Familial aggregation (iii) Environmental factors
II (obese)	As for type II (non-obese)	Hyperinsulinaemic and insulin resistant Rarely if ever ketotic	(i) Related to obesity (ii) Glucose tolerance often normal after weight loss (iii) Probably different aetiology from type II (non-obese)
III	Malnutrition-related diabetes Tropical diabetes J-type K-type Z-type	Often underweight with history of malnutrition Mostly restricted to tropical countries and non-Caucasians May have severe insulin resistance Often associated with exocrine malfunction and pancreatic fibrocalculous disease Endogenous insulin secretion intermediate between types I and II	Alcohol may be important Malnutrition and cassava consumption also implicated (Z-type)
Other types— Secondary diabetes Pancreatic disease		Pancreatectomized subjects are insulin dependent	Chronic pancreatitis Pancreatic calcification Pancreatectomy

equate, for instance, type I diabetes with IDDM. Indeed, some patients fall into both these categories, but others belong to one only. The type I–type II classification attempts to assign a pathogenetic mechanism, to which the patient will be subject all his or her life once it has started. The two mechanisms may not be mutually exclusive. People can be afflicted very severely or very mildly by either. Examples of the different degrees of severity with which type I diabetes may affect subjects are a classic ketoacidosis-prone young patient dependent upon daily injections of insulin to prevent the development of ketoacidosis within the next 3 to 4 days and, much less commonly, a type I subject (also afflicted by autoimmune damage to his islet cells) with mildly raised fasting plasma glucose but no glycosuria. However, the serum of the latter subject may well be positive for islet-cell antibodies, he may have the leucocyte histocompatibility factors associated with an increased risk of type I diabetes, and he may have a first-degree relative with full-blown disease. This second subject is not a diabetic, although he may well become so in the future. If the disease becomes more severe, his fasting

and postprandial glucose levels could increase to diabetic levels but, for a time at least, his condition might be adequately managed by dietary advice with or without added sulphonylurea treatment. At this stage he would not be liable to ketoacidosis and so would be classified as having NIDDM.

Conversely, the IDDM–NIDDM classification applies to the metabolic state of a subject at one instant, and can change with time. Thus the second subject described above could well progress from NIDDM to IDDM as his disease worsens. During this progression there could be a phase when he remains without risk of ketoacidosis although his medical advisors recommend treatment by insulin. He would then be in the not uncommon state of a subject with NIDDM who is treated with insulin. This conjunction is much more common among type II patients, where the proportion recommended to receive insulin treatment varies considerably from country to country (and from clinic to clinic). It is clear cut whether patients are or are not insulin-treated, but there can be considerable doubt as to whether or not they have IDDM because the

Table 4 (*cont.*)

Type	Alternative name	Clinical characteristics	Aetiological features
Hormonal		Obvious signs of steroid excess	(i) Corticosteroid excess (exogenous or endogenous)
		Associated with skin rash	(ii) Glucagonomas
		Diabetes mild	(iii) Acromegaly
		Obvious signs and symptoms of excess of particular hormone	(iv) Thyrotoxicosis
			(v) Phaeochromocytoma
			(vi) ?Hypothalamic lesions
Drug-induced			(i) Diuretics
			(ii) Catecholaminergic agents, e.g., salbutamol
Insulin receptor abnormalities			(i) Congenital lipodystrophy
			(ii) Associated with acanthosis nigricans
			(iii) Autoimmune insulin receptor antibodies
Genetic syndromes			Glycogen storage disease
			Ataxia telangietasia
			DIDMOAD syndrome
			Huntingdon's chorea
			Laurence–Moon–Biedl syndrome
			Werner's syndrome
			Prader–Willi syndrome
Impaired glucose tolerance	Asymptomatic diabetes	Increased risk of macrovascular disease and of later diabetes	Mild glucose intolerance from any cause (see Table 2)
	Borderline diabetes	Likely to be obese	
	Chemical diabetes		
	Latent diabetes		
	Subclinical diabetes		
Gestational diabetes		Diagnosis as for IGT or more severe forms of glucose intolerance	Pregnancy; normal glucose tolerance test beforehand but may have been abnormal in previous pregnancy
Potential abnormality of glucose tolerance	Prediabetes	Strong family history Mother of big baby	

Adapted from National Diabetes Data Group, 1979, *Diabetes* **28,** 1039–57, from where further details may be obtained.

basic test for insulin dependency is rarely applied (i.e., observation after withdrawal of insulin treatment from a subject thought to be dependent on it). The IDDM classification usually depends upon the patient's past history (Table 4), and the WHO Committees have analysed insulin dependence according to the development of ketoacidosis (or death from this condition) in the absence of insulin treatment and have not considered whether the patient's glycaemic control is dependent upon exogenous insulin. This narrowing of the concept of dependence to grossly disturbed lipid metabolism suggests that use of the IDDM classification will gradually disappear. IDDM probably describes a particular severity of reduced β-cell mass, often accompanied by weight loss.

The clinical characteristics and markers for types I and II diabetes are given in Table 4. None are absolute, and there is much debate as to whether most type II patients have the same pathogenetic aetiology. There is also argument as to whether maturity onset diabetes of the young is a separate entity, or a modification of common type II diabetes which is unusually severe and has a younger onset. The natural history of the condition often does not resemble that of 'usual' type II diabetes. There is a general impression that, despite the early onset, hyperglycaemia does not increase as rapidly as might be expected from the assumed severity. Perhaps because of persistence of relatively mild hyperglycaemia, patients with maturity-type onset diabetes of the young are tradionally relatively immune from microangiopathic and neuropathic tissue damage, but do develop these conditions with increasing duration

of disease. Some patients with maturity-type onset diabetes of the young have an abnormality of the glucokinase gene, but this abnormality is not found in most of these patients. Other rare subsets depend on genetically dependent flaws in insulin synthesis, which result in the production of weakly active insulin, or inherited abnormalities of the insulin receptor.

There are at least two different clinical manifestations of type III diabetes in tropical areas where malnutrition is rife. One is the well-characterized 'tropical calcific pancreatic diabetes', found in India, parts of Africa, and South America, which is often, but not necessarily, associated with poverty and malnutrition in youth. The aetiological factors, which are probably dietary, have not been discovered, nor has the precise reason for the fluctuating insulin dependence of these patients. A separate question is whether other aspects of malnutrition cause poor islet-cell development and hence failure of function in early adult life. A recent survey in Tanzania found no clear association of diabetes with a specific body mass index, but did find, particularly in men, that the prevalence of impaired glucose tolerance was greater in shorter subjects and those with lower body mass index. It is not clear whether this result is an artefact of using the same oral load of glucose (75 g) for every subject, or whether those with impaired glucose tolerance are liable to progress to true diabetes.

Direct toxicity from cyanogens is an unproven cause of β-cell damage, although undercooked yams and overchewed betel nuts have been suspected as specific agents.

Table 4 gives a simplified version of the classification of diabetes published by the American National Diabetes Data Group in 1979. It lists types I–III and the causes of secondary diabetes. The latter include a number of inherited syndromes, ranging from DIDMOAD (diabetes insipidus, diabetes mellitus, optic atrophy, and deafness) via the progeria of Werner's syndrome to the obesity usual in both the Laurence–Moon–Biedl and Prader–Willi syndromes. It is suspected that in conditions with abnormal connective tissue (for example Werner's syndrome and ataxia telangiectasia) there may be abnormalities involving interaction between insulin and insulin-like growth factors and/or their receptors. Diabetes (usually IDDM) may also accompany the various mitochondrial myopathy syndromes, as may a variety of other endocrine defects.

Diabetes, or often just impaired glucose tolerance, has been associated with a variety of neurological or muscular diseases (for example motor neurone disease and dystrophia myotonica), at least when they are severe. This may well be a consequence of the associated marked muscular wasting.

Presenting features

Diabetes may be diagnosed where symptoms lead to measurement of blood glucose concentrations, while both diabetes and impaired glucose tolerance may be diagnosed through the finding of high glucose levels on screening tests. Again, in the absence of high glucose levels, pathognomic types of tissue damage, such as background diabetic retinopathy, or associated clinical findings, such as cardiac infarction or cataract, may lead to detection of hyperglycaemia.

The classic symptoms of hyperglycaemia are polyuria, thirst, weight loss, and lassitude. Although thirst and polyuria can have other explanations, diabetes mellitus is the most common and the presence of either of these features should always lead at least to a urine test for glucose. Weight loss may be severe in patients with IDDM, and in type II diabetes it is often substantial even though the patient is still obese. Pruritus vulvae is a frequent symptom in women, even without development of a full-blown candidial rash in the perineum. Balanitis, sometimes causing paraphimosis, is much less common but can be severe. Other non-specific symptoms commonly reported are the appearance or exacerbation of cramp in the calves or feet, and tingling in the fingers rather than the feet, where it will predominate as peripheral sensory neuropathy develops years later. Some patients complain of a loss of appetite, but others develop a craving, particularly for sweet foods. Occasionally, crystallized glucose can be seen as white spots on the shoes of elderly males. Patients are often relatively constipated, and develop a mild (or occasionally severe) change in lens refraction which causes visual blurring.

Pathogenesis

Type I diabetes mellitus

IMMUNE MECHANISMS

It is widely accepted that type I diabetes results from immunologically mediated damage to the β-cells in the pancreas. This process may occur over many years and probably results from environmental insults in genetically susceptible individuals. The evidence has been obtained from a variety of observations.

Lymphocyte infiltration of islets, suggesting involvement of the immune system, has been seen in post-mortem material occasionally obtained early in the disease. Most type I patients have circulating autoantibodies to β-cell antigens, including insulin and glutamic acid decarboxylase, as well as anti-islet-cell antibodies. Similarly, lymphocyte subsets in peripheral blood are distorted in patients with type I diabetes, again indicative of an active immune response. At a genetic level, the observation that HLA alleles are implicated in the disease has provided further strong evidence that these molecules are responsible for activating the immune response to specific peptides (and hence are labelled immune response genes).

Animal models also provide evidence for an immunological role in the disease. The non-obese diabetes (NOD) mouse and the BB Worcester rat both spontaneously develop immunologically mediated islet-cell destruction. Both models have many similarities to human type I diabetes, although the lymphocyte infiltrate in animal models is much more extensive than in humans. The disease can be spread between NOD mice by transferring groups of CD4 and CD8 lymphocytes, so establishing a central role for the immune sytem.

The destruction of pancreatic β-cells may result from either a normal immune response to a pathogen trophic for such tissue or an aberrant immune response to self-antigens. There has been much speculation about the role of a viral pathogen which is responsible, directly or indirectly, for islet damage. Seasonal variation in frequency and young age of onset are consistent with a viral pathogen. Coxsackie virus and mumps virus are two candidates, but many others, including retroviruses, have been implicated. However, the exact nature of such infectious pathogens has not yet been been defined. Because of the potentially long natural history of β-cell damage (up to 10 years), observations at the time of endstage β-cell failure are unlikely to reveal useful information about an initiating role of such infectious pathogens.

GENETIC SUSCEPTIBILITY

Susceptibility to type I diabetes has a substantial genetic component. The disease runs in families, with sibling risk of developing the disease substantially greater than in the normal population (6 per cent versus 0.4 per cent), but the pattern of inheritance is complex. Twin studies suggest that approximately one-third of disease susceptibility is genetic. However, these studies do not consider contributions from somatic genetic events that may differ in twins, including T-cell receptor and immunoglobulin genes, nor do they account for shared environment, perhaps particularly intrauterine or immediately postnatal.

The complex pattern of inheritance, the relatively high frequency of non-familial disease, and the increasingly rapid reduction in risk for first-, second-, and third-degree relatives all suggest that multiple loci are involved. Two loci encoding susceptibility have been defined, HLA and insulin (INS), although together these account for no more than 30 per cent of total genetic susceptibility. HLA has by far the largest effect defined to date, with the risk to siblings rising to 12 per cent if they are HLA identical. Of the 15-fold increase in relative risk in siblings, approximately 25 per cent is accounted for by HLA alone. INS contributes less to the genetic susceptibility; in some populations this effect is predominant in individuals with HLA DR4.

HLA was originally implicated in diabetes susceptibility with HLA-B locus alleles (B8 and B15). These were subsequently shown to be in strong linkage disequilibrium with alleles in the class II region that mediated disease susceptibility. Approximately 90 per cent of Caucasian type I diabetics carry either HLA DR3 or DR4 specificities compared with 45 per cent of the general population. There is a pronounced heterozygous effect, whereby DR3 and DR4 heterozygotes have an increased susceptibility compared with DR3,3 or DR4,4 homozygotes. Other HLA haplotypes (DR1, DR8, and DR5) also have a more modest susceptibility to the disease. Disease protection is provided by the HLA-DR2 haplotype.

The identification of the precise molecular basis of HLA-mediated susceptibility has been hampered by strong linkage disequilibrium across the region. Evidence of a role for HLA-DQ molecules was provided by the correlation between the disease and HLA-DQ sequences at position 57 of the β-chain. This correlation, as well as similar correlations with α-chain sequences, provides evidence that the structural context of the DQ binding site usually dictates the HLA-mediated disease susceptibility. However, this correlation is not valid in all ethnic populations. Other evidence demonstrates an important role for HLA-

DR alleles in determining susceptibility for disease. HLA-DR and HLA-DQ effects together account for the majority of HLA-mediated disease susceptibility.

The INS locus on chromosome 11p is also associated with disease susceptibility. This locus is flanked on the upstream side by a multiple repeat of 14 base pairs. Variations in the length of this repeat correlate with disease susceptibility. The shorter repeats are associated with the disease, and this region has recently been shown to be linked to familial disease. The short and long repeat classes are in tight linkage disequilibrium with a set with 10 single-base-pair polymorphisms within and adjacent to the INS locus. The mechanism of this disease susceptibility has not been clearly defined, but it is likely that one or more of these polymorphisms contributes to disease susceptibility through variations in INS gene regulation.

EPIDEMIOLOGY

The world-wide incidence of type I diabetes varies greatly. In some Scandinavian countries it is as high as 35 per 100 000 per year, while in countries such as Japan it is only 2 per 100 000 per year. The disease is predominantly one of white Caucasian populations and is relatively rare in both oriental and black populations. Accurate data for the incidence of the disease in Africa is unavailable, but the disease is probably extremely rare in this population with a risk of less than 3 per 100 000 per year. Wide variations also exist within Europe, with extremely high incidences seen in Finland, Sweden, Denmark, Norway, and the United Kingdom, and much lower incidences in France and Italy. An environmental factor which varies with latitude has been suggested to explain this north–south gradient, but several dramatic exceptions argue strongly against this incidence gradient. Incidence figures in Sardinia appear to be very high and similar to those in Scandinavia, while the incidence in Iceland is closer to the usual Mediterranean figures. Estonia provides an interesting anomaly, for the incidence of diabetes in this population, which is ethnically extremely similar to the Finns, is approximately one-third of that seen in Finland. Although these detailed incidence figures argue against a gradient of disease from north to south in Europe, they are not easily explained by either genetic or environmental factors alone. In some cases (Sardinia) the difference in incidence appears to be consistent with a variation in ethnic factors, particularly HLA alleles. In other situations (Iceland), the genetic variation does not easily account for the dramatic differences with other Scandinavian countries, but suggestions concerning an environmental toxin (nitrosamines from smoked fish) have not been substantiated.

The incidence of type I diabetes may be increasing. Increases have been noted in Scotland, Norway, and Denmark in northern Europe, but not observed in studies from North America or from Poland, Sweden, and Finland. The disease is slightly more common in males than in females, and several studies have reported seasonal variation in the incidence which is greater during the winter months.

Migration studies suggest that environmental factors play a substantial role in the geographical variation of disease incidence. Studies of Japanese in America, Ashkenazi Jews in Canada, and Asians in the United Kingdom have all suggested that the incidence in populations at low risk of the disease will rise if they enter a region with a relatively high incidence. This provides some evidence for an environmental factor which contributes substantially to these variations in disease incidence.

ENVIRONMENTAL FACTORS

Despite clear evidence of a genetic component to disease susceptibility, twin data suggest strongly that the majority of susceptibility must be environmental. Several broad themes dominate the literature relating to environmental factors of type I diabetes, but no individual contributor has yet been identified. Viruses have often been suggested to be implicated in the disease, largely because they can damage β cells in animals. However, the evidence that viruses are involved in human diabetes is extremely sparse. Three viruses have been implicated in direct damage to pancreatic β-cells in man. Mumps virus has shown some tropism for pancreatic β cells, and similarly Coxsackie virus can damage β cells in mice. Cytomegalovirus has recently been implicated in both type II and type I diabetes, but reproducible evidence is still lacking. Perhaps the only viral infection with a definite link to IDDM is congenital rubella. Type I diabetes is increased in individuals who have suffered from congenital rubella, as are other autoimmune disorders such as thyroid disease and Addison's disease. Rubella-associated diabetes is found predominantly in populations with the same HLA susceptibility alleles as non-rubella-associated diabetes and is associated with the same immunological abnormalities.

Toxins have been suggested as another general class of environmental factors involved in type I diabetes. Again, the evidence for their contribution is unconvincing. N-Nitroso derivatives are known to destroy β-cells, and some have been directly implicated in both neurotoxicity and diabetes after fatal poisoning. Nitrates and nitroso compounds in the diet have also been suggested to have a role in disease pathogenesis but the data to support this hypothesis are weak.

The third major environmental factor which has been repeatedly implicated in disease susceptibility is exposure to cow's milk in early life. It has been suggested that the rising incidence of the disease may correlate with the declining prevalence of breast-feeding. However, this is inconsistent with the rather patchy evidence for increasing incidence of type I diabetes and an overall reduction in breast-feeding broadly throughout the Western world. This hypothesis has been suggested repeatedly, but to date the best data have been provided by Karjalainen and colleagues who have demonstrated that patients with type I diabetes have antibodies to cow's milk albumin that react to a β-cell surface protein.

Type II diabetes mellitus

There are many mechanisms underlying the development of type II diabetes which is far more common than type I. The apparent prevalence varies with the thoroughness of testing in a given population, and particularly with the proportion of the elderly that are tested. When the WHO glycaemic definition is used for the condition, it may be as high as 40–50 per cent in some populations of Polynesian–Micronesian stock, whether on affluent Pacific islands (for example Nauru) or in reservations in Arizona (Pima Indians). The prevalence in the United Kingdom was once believed to be 2 per cent of the population, but recent studies suggest values of 8 to 12 per cent, depending on ethnic mix. Patients typically present clinically between 50 and 65 years of age, but may be as young as 15 to 20 years or of any age above 65.

There are four major hypotheses (not mutually exclusive) for the pathogenesis.

Genetic

Evidence for genetic influence is based on familial incidence, supported by identical twin studies, with concordance varying from below 60 per cent to above 85 per cent, although the interpretation of these results is questionable (see below). A substantial number of genetic abnormalities have been linked with type II diabetes, involving genes with products of metabolic importance (for example glucokinase variants, glycogen synthetase variants) or hormonal importance (for example, abnormal insulin, gross increase in the proinsulin to insulin ratio), or genes with an unknown product, (for example mitochondrial DNA deletions and duplications). The last category often show maternal inheritance. The mitochondrial defects may be more common than yet realized because there is more mutant mitochondrial DNA in muscle, which is a relatively non-dividing tissue, than in peripheral blood cells, but the latter have been studied much more. Clinically, the diabetes associated with mitochondrial DNA abnormalities may be linked with myopathy or deafness.

These genetic defects may not be a good model for the disease affecting the majority of Type II patients because their hyperglycaemia often presents at a relatively young age but is relatively non-progressive. Again, many of these patients are not obese, unlike the majority of type II patients. It is tempting to extrapolate from recent discoveries to believe that a multitude of defects at a variety of genetic loci may account for only 10–15 per cent of classical type II patients, but for a very much larger proportion of those who are not and have not been overweight.

If there is a genetic cause for the common overweight majority, it would seem to be multifactorial. The only clue at present comes from tentative links between a lipoprotein locus abnormality and the conjunction of glucose intolerance, hypertension, and some types of hyperlipidaemia (syndrome X) which occurs more often than the chance concurrence of these three common abnormalities.

Adaptation to early environment

If the genetic structure is important, so is the expression of those genes. Animal studies have shown that the adult phenotype is strongly affected by nutritional and other intrauterine factors, as well as by the postnatal environment. The great majority of cell divisions occur in the early days of an organism, and habitual patterns of gene expression or physiological function may be established according to the environment at that time. These considerations accord with the observations of Barker and colleagues that hyperglycaemia (diabetes and impaired glucose tolerance) at the age of about 60 years is more common in those with lower birthweights (adjusted for delivery date) provided that an allowance is made for an increase at the high birthweight end of the proportional relationship because the babies of diabetic mothers are often heavy (this is seen particularly in a population where diabetes is common, such as Pima Indians). Further study has shown that low birthweight (or low weight at the age of 1 year) is associated with both lower insulin and 32–33 split proinsulin levels, particularly during an oral glucose tolerance test, and decreased insulin sensitivity. Therefore, not surprisingly, hyperglycaemia is most common when there was a low weight at birth or at 1 year and obesity as an adult, with the decreased sensitivity that the latter alone causes. It is possible that those who have adapted metabolically to prenatal and perinatal deprivation are more liable to the ill effects of excess food in adult life. The causes of lower birthweight are unclear, but it may be due to deprivation from maternal malnutrition, or anaemia, poor placental function, or constitutional factors.

Pancreatic amyloid

In 1901 Opie observed a hyaline material in post-mortem histological preparations of pancreatic islets from diabetic patients, and later this was also seen in material from elderly subjects not diagnosed as diabetic but whose glycaemic status was not known. The protein responsible, which was later realized to be an amyloid deposit (with β-pleated polypeptide folding), has been identified and named 'amylin' or 'islet amyloid polypeptide'. The material lies outside the surviving β-cells of the morbid islet and may be concentrated near the islet's small blood vessels. It has been recognized both to lie also within lysosomes of β-cells and to damage β-cells where its spiky projections abut them. Amylin is secreted from β-cells together with insulin. It has been detected in plasma, but at levels about two orders of magnitude below those at which disturbed muscle metabolism with insulin insensitivity has been reported in animals following its injection. There is stronger evidence that it has a paracrine influence within the islets, inhibiting insulin secretion. The amylin of mammalian species which can develop amyloid deposits in their islets and maturity-type onset hyperglycaemia is less soluble than that of species (rat, mouse) which do not. The hypothesis is that if amylin is secreted to excess (or differs in fine structure), it may polymerize in the intercellular spaces of the islets. It is not known whether this is directly affected by glucose levels. Amylin is a vasodilator with similarities to calcitonin-gene-related polypeptide, and therefore could influence islet blood flow. It remains to be demonstrated whether islet amyloid deposits are primary or secondary influences in β-cell failure in type II diabetes.

β-Cell overstimulation

When β-cells are strongly stimulated for any length of time they secrete more proinsulin (intact and split) per unit insulin secreted. It has been suggested that this disturbance, possibly allied to a constitutional abnormality in the cellular processing of proinsulin, damages β-cells. The overstimulation is ascribed to the excess food intake that must have occurred during the development of obesity in typical type II patients. The crucial question is whether obesity precedes glucose/insulin disturbance in type II diabetes or whether the basic abnormality itself generates obesity.

GENETICS

Candidate genes that might contribute to either insulin resistance or insulin deficiency have been studied. In both cases functional mutations have been identified that account for the disease phenotype in a small number of patients. It is likely that the major genes, accounting for larger subsets of the population, remain to be identified. The disease displays substantial genetic heterogeneity, and hence characterization of some of the genetic factors responsible for the common form of the disease is likely to be extremely difficult.

The existence of ethnic populations with an extremely high prevalence of the disease (Pima Indians or Nauruans) suggests that genetic polymorphisms may have been selected in these populations to allow them to have adapted to survive more effectively during earlier periods of prolonged starvation. Subsequent exposure of such populations to Western diets might leave them at a substantial metabolic disadvantage in coping with the high-carbohydrate high-fat diets of the developed world. Therefore the high incidence of obesity and type II diabetes in the developing world might be accounted for by the prevalence of genetic polymorphisms that are relatively rare in Western populations.

The first mutations to be associated with type II diabetes were those of the insulin receptor gene, which was an obvious candidate to explain some of the insulin resistance syndromes. Several specific syndromes exist where extreme insulin resistance is evident. Leprechaunism is a congenital disorder associated with glucose intolerance and extremely high insulin levels. The Rabson–Mendenhall syndrome is associated with insulin resistance, acanthosis nigricans, ectodermal abnormalities (teeth and nails), and pineal hyperplasia. Type A insulin resistance, which is a syndrome consisting of insulin resistance, acanthosis nigricans and hyperandrogenism, is most common in females. These patients all have impaired glucose tolerance associated with hyperinsulinaemia. All these syndromes are associated with mutations in the insulin receptor gene including non-sense mutations, deletions, splicing defects, and single-base-pair substitutions. They may result in defects in receptor synthesis, receptor transport, insulin binding, transmembrane signalling, or receptor recycling. In some cases these mutations correlate specifically with the type and severity of insulin resistance seen.

Severe forms of insulin resistance are associated with homozygocity for insulin receptor mutations, but heterozygous patients occasionally have more modest degrees of insulin resistance consistent with a diagnosis of type II diabetes. The frequency of insulin receptor mutations in the population is unknown. Based on the incidence of leprechaunism, at least 0.1 per cent of the population are heterozygous for insulin receptor mutations, and this figure may be as much as 10 times higher. However, even this higher figure suggests that insulin receptor mutations are more important in the rare syndromes of severe insulin resistance than in the more common forms of type II diabetes.

Patterns of type II diabetes that are consistent with a dominant mode of inheritance have been know to exist since the description of maturity onset diabetes of the young. This disorder is characterized by early onset of mild hyperglycaemia and is found in families, where it appears to be associated with a single gene defect. Large family pedigrees where 50 per cent of siblings are affected with glucose intolerance at an early age and where one parent is also affected have been useful in identifying other genetic factors in diabetes. The first such localization was obtained in a large pedigree where linkage to the regions surrounding the adenine deaminase locus on chromosome 20 was identified. Subsequent studies have established that this locus is likely to be important in only a small subset of pedigrees with maturity-type onset diabetes of the young. However, the glucokinase locus has been shown to be an important genetic susceptibility factor in approximately half such pedigrees. The mutations in glucokinase cluster round the active side of the molecule where glucose is bound. They are found predominantly in pedigrees with maturity-type onset diabetes of the young, but occasionally families with more conventional type II diabetes have been shown to have such mutations, and association studies have suggested that mutations may be associated with the disease in black and Creole populations. It is difficult to estimate the overall contribution of glucokinase mutations to type II diabetes, but they are unlikely to account for more than 1 per cent of the disease.

A further genetic susceptibility factor has been defined in mitochondrial DNA. The combination of diabetes and deafness has been found to be associated with an A to G mutation in position 3243 of leucine tRNA. This mutation appears to interfere with the synthesis of leucine tRNA and also with its ability to bind a transcription termination factor. Recent studies have looked for this mutation in a large set of families and found it to be common, particularly in families with some evidence of sensory hearing disturbance. The role of this mutation in the more common type II diabetes has not yet been established.

These initial efforts to characterize genetic factors in type II diabetes have identified a number of rare genetic factors which contribute to the disease. In all cases the inheritance pattern of these defects has been simple, but despite this there appears to be substantial heterogeneity in the mechanisms by which glucose intolerance can be produced. The challenge for the future will be to characterize genetic factors that contribute to larger sets of type II patients.

Metabolic basis of diabetes mellitus

Intermediary metabolism

The intermediary metabolism of carbohydrate, fat, and protein substrates is disturbed in diabetes. The osmotic diuresis of glycosuria carries sodium, potassium, calcium, and magnesium out of the body, so that mineral balance is also disturbed. However, the cationic loss is much greater if ketonuria is present because acetoacetate and 3-hydroxybutyrate are relatively strong acids for organic compounds, with $pK = 5.5$.

Hence 1 mole of ketoacid will be accompanied by 1 mole of monovalent cation even at maximal urinary acidity.

Carbohydrate metabolites

The organs most closely involved in blood glucose control are the liver, the pancreas, and muscle. Disease of any of these may impair glucose tolerance, but sustained glycaemic elevation always implies some failure of insulin secretion. The main action of insulin in this respect is the inhibition of hepatic glucose release and effectively of gluconeogenesis.

The liver (Fig. 1) takes up excess glucose from the gut as a meal is digested and stores it as glycogen or uses the resulting acetyl-CoA not only for oxidation but also for fatty acid synthesis. This increases hepatic triacylglycerides and other lipids, and these will later be released as low density lipoproteins and cholesterol esters. When blood glucose drops, perhaps particularly in the systemic hepatic artery blood, the liver releases glucose, in the short term by glycogenolysis to glucose-6-phosphate and hence glucose, but in the longer term from gluconeogenesis and the sparing of hepatic carbohydrate by using triacylglycerides as the principal source of hepatic acetyl-CoA for energy. The substrates for gluconeogenesis are lactate, glycerol, and amino acids. Lactate comes principally from skeletal and cardiac muscle and from the gut. It is released during any muscular sprinting, when the work rate exceeds the available oxygen and hence anaerobic metabolism supports activity. However, it may also be released, perhaps initally as pyruvate, whenever the rate of glucose uptake is very high. Glycerol is released from adipose tissue during lipolysis, while amino acids leave muscle during fasting. Indeed, alanine can be considered as 'aminated lactate', taken up by muscle in the digestive phase in excess of its structural needs and released later to be deaminated in the liver. The amino acids fall into two main groups, glucogenic (for example alanine, glutamate, aspartate) and the ketogenic (for example valine, leucine), depending upon whether the carbon skeleton remaining after deamination is converted into 3-C pyruvate or a 4-C ketoacid. A general rule is that during fasting the plasma levels of the essential amino acids, and some of their corresponding ketoacids, rise because they undergo relatively little deamination in the liver. However, the level of the essential amino acids falls, despite increased peripheral release, because of increased hepatic uptake. These changes are not totally the result of the low insulin concentration of the fasting phase. When there is gross insulin deficiency, net protein degradation in muscle increases markedly and the plasma concentration of all the amino acids rises.

Hepatic gluconeogenesis occurs from phospho-enol-pyruvate, generated via malate but not directly from acetyl-CoA. Hence non-esterified

Fig. 1 Main metabolic shifts in the absorbtive postprandial and the basal states, with principal actions of insulin marked, *inhibitory, **stimulatory. TAG (triacylglycerides) subdivided as (C) chylomicra, (RC) remnant chylomicra; and (LP) lipoproteins, especially LDL and VLDL. NEFA, non-esterified fatty acids.

	Gut		Liver		Adipose tissue		Muscle	
	In	Out	In	Out	In	Out	In	Out
Post prandial		Glucose	Glucose		TAG(C)**	TAG(RC)	Glucose**	Lactate
		TAG(C)	NEFA	TAG(LP)	NEFA		NEFA	
		Amino acids**	Amino acids**		Glucose**		Amino acids**	
		Lactate	Lactate					
Basal	NEFA		Lactate	Glucose*		NEFA*	NEFA	Amino acids*
	Glucose		Glycerol*	TAG(LP)		Glycerol*	Glucose**	Lactate
			Amino acids*					

fatty acids are not net substrates for gluconeogenesis, while the 3C compounds just discussed are.

The glycaemic level is also affected by the rate of glucose removal in the periphery. This may be either insulin independent or insulin-dependent; uptake due to non-basal cellular work will not be considered. Insulin-independent uptake can be divided into two categories: uptake into insulin-insensitive tissue, and that component of increased uptake into insulin-sensitive tissue that results from hyperglycaemia rather than hyperinsulinaemia. This last division is artificial because glucose entry into muscle or adipose tissue is always the resultant of a glucose–insulin pair of values, as well as the many other factors that affect insulin sensitivity. Thus, in health a high glucose concentration should be accompanied by a high insulin level. However, in a typical inadequately controlled but not acutely ill diabetic patient, the rate of peripheral glucose disposal is approximately normal because the increased uptake due to hyperglycaemia balances the effects of reduced insulin action. Insulin can be regarded as an agent that facilitates glucose entry into the sensitive tissues at any glucose level. However, its potential for effective action is much less when blood glucose is either very high or very low than it is around the usual levels of 3.5–6 mmol/l because of the steep rise of insulin levels over that range of the dose–response curve (Fig. 2).

The rate of glucose disposal is also affected by the plasma levels of non-esterified fatty acids in that the cellular uptake of these acids depends on their plasma concentration in a surprisingly direct way and

Fig. 2 Dose–response curve of plasma glucose and insulin secretion.

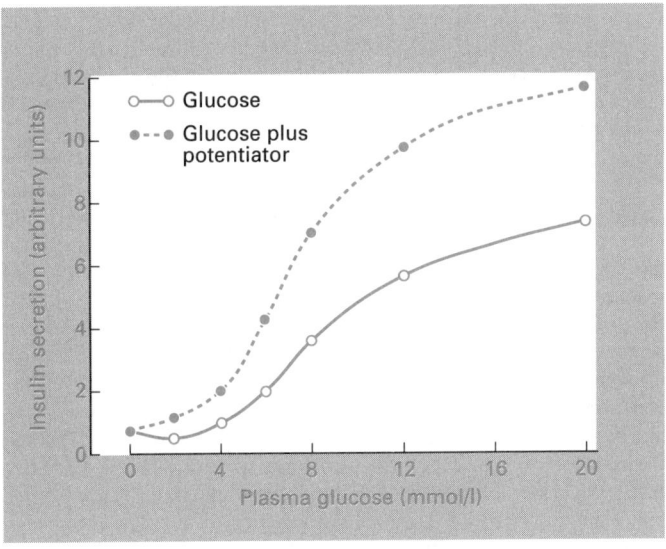

Fig. 3 Glucose fatty-acid cycle, blood phase. 1. Uptake of glucose by muscle and adipose tissue. 2. Release of fatty acids from adipose tissue to plasma albumin. 3. Formation of ketone bodies from fatty acids by liver. 4. Uptake of fatty acids and ketone bodies by muscle.

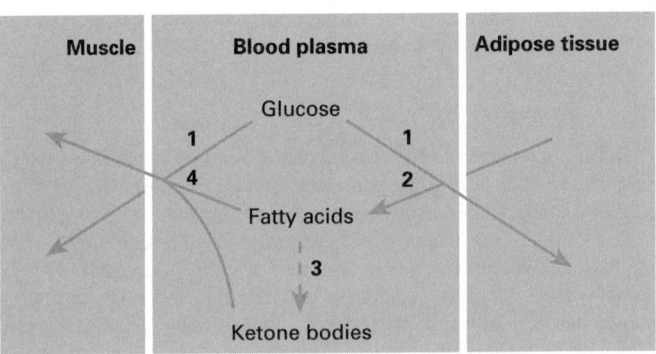

Table 5 *Clinical consequences of increasing degrees of insulin deficiency*

| Degrees of insulin deficiency | Maintained metabolism | | | Clinical consequences |
	Carbohydrate	Protein	Fat	
Mild	−	+	+	Glycosuria, thirst, weight steady
Moderate	−	−	+	Weight loss
Severe	−	−	−	Ketosis

inhibits the uptake of glucose. These properties are the basis of the glucose–fatty acids cycle (Fig. 3).

The low insulin levels of the fasting state allow a steady release of glucose to sustain normoglycaemia. However, they also allow steady release of non-esterified fatty acids from adipose tissue via hormone-sensitive lipase activity, and in the fasting resting state these acids are the main body fuel with the respiratory quotient RQ around 0.7. Any sudden increased activity will be supported by muscle glycogen, which has the great advantage over non-esterified fatty acids of degradation yielding anaerobic energy. Hence in the fasting state increased gluconeogenesis, and hence hepatic glucose release, are necessary to sustain exercise, particularly the capacity to sprint. Intramuscular lipolysis of triacylglycerides may also be useful. A plasma insulin concentration of only 10–20 mU/l is necessary for the effective restraint of adipose tissue lipolysis and hepatic glucose release, in contrast with the 100–200 mU/l required for the maximum optimal uptake of glucose by skeletal muscle.

The clinical consequences of increasing degrees of insulin deficiency crudely illustrate the different sensitivities of some of these actions (Table 5).

Lipid metabolites

Fatty acids are synthesized from acetyl-CoA in the liver and so triacylglycerides can be formed from glucose there. However, the cellular triacylglyceride fatty acids in adipose tissue come from the plasma non-esterified fatty acids via lipoprotein-lipase-determined intravascular lipolysis. It is only the glycerol moiety of the triacylglycerides which comes, apparently entirely, from dihydroxyacetone phosphate at the triose phosphate level via adipocyte glucose metabolism. Insulin will promote supply of the necessary glucose, as will hyperglycaemia.

Lipids are mostly transported in blood as particles varying in size from chylomicra to high density lipoprotein (HDL) cholesterol (Table 6). As they decrease in size, they correspondingly increase in both specific gravity, from less than 0.95 to 1.21, and generally in phospholipid, cholesterol, and protein contents as a percentage of total lipoprotein, but they decrease in triglyceride. Chylomicra travel from the gut via the thoracic duct and so differ from most absorbed nutrients in not having an obligatory first path through the liver before exposure to the adipose tissue, which is their main degradation site. Depending upon the activity of the adipose tissue and its degree of stimulation by insulin, the resulting remnant chylomicra particles undergo some reduction in triglyceride. The very low density lipoprotein (VLDL) particles arise from the liver and carry triglyceride, cholesterol, and phospholipid, which are synthesized there, to the periphery. As the VLDL particles are progressively depleted of lipid throughout the circulation, they form the main source of low density lipoprotein (LDL). Remnant chylomicra and partially degraded VLDL particles are distinguished by their apoprotein composition, but it is uncertain whether particles of the two types, which are of approximately similar lipid composition, are metabolized very differently or not. High plasma LDL cholesterol and high VLDL triglyceride concentrations favour accelerated arteriosclerosis, as do low HDL cholesterol levels.

Table 6 *Transportation of lipids in blood*

	Mean diameter (nm)	Density (g/ml)	Electrophoretic or mobility	Percentage			Estimated percentage cholesterol	Lipoprotein as percentage of total
				TAG	PHLI	CHOL		
Chylomicra	100–1000	<0.95	Origin	88	9	3	46	1–2
VLDL	43	0.95 ≤ 1.006	Pre-β	56	19	17	57	10
IDL*	27	1.006–1.019 ⎤	β	32	27	41	66	18
LDL	22	1.019–1.063 ⎦		7	28	59	70	25
HDL2	9.5	1.063–1.125 ⎤	α	6	42	43	74	40
HDL3	6.5	1.125–1.21 ⎦		7	41	38	81	55
Lp(a)	26	1.051–1.082	Pre-β	—	—	—	—	—

TAG, triacylglycerides; PHLI, phospholipids; CHOL, cholesterol

*Also termed VLDL remnants.

HDL particles form a completely different family and are distinguished by high apo-A protein content. With time in the circulation they show progressively increasing esterification of their cholesterol, partly because they are involved in removal of cholesterol esters in the reticuloendothelial system whose presence predisposes to the development of arteriosclerosis. HDL particles also receive apo-C as it leaves the LDL particles. Another marker of accelerated arteriosclerotic disease is a high Lp(a) plasma concentration. Originating in the liver, the plasma concentration of Lp(a) varies from virtually zero to 100 mg/dl. Its function is unknown but it is present in notably high levels in approximately 10 per cent of the population who have an associated high risk of cardiovascular disease.

Insulin is an important agent in lipid metabolism because it activates adipose tissue lipoprotein lipase and inhibits adipocyte-hormone-sensitive lipase. Deficient insulin action has two effects on the adipose tissue: first, impaired degradation of both chylomicra and VLDL particles with an increase in the remnant chylomicra and large VLDL particles: second, through decreased inhibition of hormone-sensitive lipase, there is an increased flux of non-esterified fatty acids to the liver as a potential source of hepatic cell triacylglyceride, and of both VLDL and ketone bodies leaving the liver. Hence diabetics show high VLDL levels, and less abnormality in cholesterol concentrations than in triglyceride concentrations. However, HDL cholesterol levels are reduced but, like the raised VLDL levels, they return towards normal with improved glycaemic control. LDL levels are usually normal, although they tend to increase with gross hyperglycaemia.

When there is a rapid oxidative cleavage of fatty acids within the hepatic cell cytoplasm, the acetyl-CoA produced must enter the mitochondrion via the carnitine shuttle for the reaction to proceed. Glucagon favours the necessary formation of acylcarnitine and also decreases malonyl-CoA, which inhibits an enzyme of the carnitine shuttle reactions. Fatty acids themselves are powerful inhibitors of malonyl-CoA formation, and so insulin deficiency and glucagon excess provide the conditions for a very high rate of formation of acetyl-CoA within the mitochondria. It can either condense with oxaloacetate to yield citrate, and so enter the tricarboxylic acid (TCA) cycle, or react with CoA to form acetoacetyl-CoA. The latter is transformed to hydroxymethylglutaryl-CoA which can either yield acetoacetate and 3-hydroxybutyrate or be the basis for synthesis of cholesterol, dolichols, and ubiquinones via mevalonate.

The mitochondrial membrane is also crossed by malate in another shuttle important in gluconeogenesis. This compound, which is part of the TCA cycle within the mitochondrion, passes out to the cytoplasm to yield phospho-enol-pyruvate and so enter the anabolic limb of the glycolytic pathway.

The ketone bodies are normal metabolites, although they are not oxidizable in the liver which lacks thiolase. They normally circulate at a combined blood level of about 0.1 mmol/l, compared with the level of 10 mmol/l which is not uncommon in ketoacidosis. They are available as fuels for most tissues, including muscle, but have a particular role as substrates for the neurosystem, which otherwise has an obligatory requirement for glucose. On fasting, ketone bodies are increasingly used in the brain.

Metabolic regulation

The control of metabolic processes is fourfold. Direct mass action considerations are always important but these are modified by the following three possible actions on particular metabolic steps. First, synthetic and degradative processes may be predominantly conducted by separate enzymes even though one or more of them may theoretically catalyse the reverse process. Thus the conversion of glucose-6-phosphate to glycogen depends primarily upon the glycogen synthetase enzyme complex which promotes conversion of glucose-1-phosphate to glycogen, while the reverse conversion of glycogen to glucose-1-phosphate is brought about via the phosphorylase enzyme complex. Second, the enzymes responsible for certain key processes are influenced by some of the metabolites involved in the reactions. Such allosteric effects are important for pyruvate oxidase, which controls the generation of acetyl-CoA from pyruvate and hence the entry of carbohydrate into the oxidative final common path of the TCA cycle, fructose-1,6-diphosphatase which acts upon the diphosphate ester high in the glycolytic chain to convert it to the monophosphate which is then cleaved to two triose phosphates, and citrate synthetase which catalyses the reaction between acetyl-CoA and oxaloacetate at the entry to the carboxylic acid cycle. For example the ratio of CoA to acetyl-CoA enhances pyruvate oxidase activity, while the ratio of ATP to ADP negatively influences it. Sometimes minor alternative pathways produce allosterically important compounds such as fructose-bis-phosphate which influences fructose-1,6-diphosphatase. On other occasions the divergent compound (for example 2,3-diphosphoglycerate produced as an alternative to the more usual 1,3-diphosphate) is of allosteric importance in an unrelated reaction, in this case increasing the binding of oxygen to the haem metalloprotein complex of erythrocyte haemoglobin. Finally, enzyme activity may be influenced by hormonal action, for instance adrenaline on phosphorylase or insulin on adipose tissue lipases.

Insulin biosynthesis

Insulin is synthesized in the β-cells of the islets of Langerhans which comprise 1–3 per cent of the pancreatic mass and are probably derived from the ectoderm. The estimated number of islets varies from 100 000 to 2 500 000. They contain not only the insulin-secreting β-cells (approximately half the cells), but also α-cells (glucagon), D-cells (somatostatin), PP-cells (pancreatic polypeptide), and other less well-defined neuroendocrine cells. The islets have a rich sympathetic, para-

Table 7 *Stimulators and inhibitors of insulin secretion*

	Mechanism	Glucose required
Stimulators		
Glucose	?Glucoreceptor	
	?Metabolite	
	±Calcium shifts	
Glucagon	↑ Cyclic AMP	+
Gut hormones (GIP)	↑ Cyclic AMP	+
β-Adrenergic agents	↑ Cyclic AMP	+
Prostaglandins	↑ Cyclic AMP	+
Leucine	?Membrane effect	−
	?Metabolite	
Other amino acids (arginine)	?	+
Fatty acids	?	−
Ketone bodies	?	−
Acetylcholine	?Ca^{2-} shifts	−
Vagal stimulation		
Inhibitors		
α-Adrenergic agents	↓ Cyclic AMP	−
Sympathetic nerve stimulation		
Dopamine	?Ca^{2-} shifts	−
Serotonin	?Ca^{2-} shifts	−
Somatostatin	?	

sympathetic, and peptidergic nerve supply, and many active substances have been identified in them. Some are neurotransmitters, either peptidergic (thyrotropic hormone) or non-peptidergic (serotonin), while peptides other than insulin (galinin, amylin) may be secreted by β-cells.

Insulin is synthesized initially on the rough endoplasmic reticulum as a large precursor, preproinsulin, of molecular weight 11 500 Da. This has a very short half-life, for it is split almost immediately to yield a long polypeptide chain, proinsulin, of molecular weight 9000 Da, which is held in an overlapping circle by two disulphide bridges. At the Golgi apparatus the proinsulin is packed into granules surrounded by a single membrane layer. The connecting or C-peptide part of the molecule is then split off, but not always cleanly; indeed, an appreciable amount of 32–33 split proinsulin is found in plasma. The characteristic double chain of insulin, C-peptide, and such split products remain in the granule, where a small amount of proinsulin is also found. The β-cell granules migrate via the microtubular–microfilamentary system from the Golgi apparatus to the cell surface where the vesicular membrane fuses with the outer cell membrane to discharge C-peptide in a 1:1 ratio with insulin together with small amounts of proinsulin and its split products. Perhaps 10–15 per cent of insulin leaves the cell via another constitutive pathway which does not involve a secretory granule and in which the ratio of proinsulin (intact or split) to insulin may not be the same as in the secretory pathway.

When a β-cell has not been strongly stimulated for some time, there are many secretory vesicles close to the cell membrane at its secretory pole. Discharge of these can permit a large first-phase secretion in response to a strong stimulus. When the cell is continuously stimulated it takes 90 to 120 min for newly synthesized preproinsulin to yield secreted insulin; meanwhile secretion is sustained by degradation of preproinsulin which has already been formed and movement of the products to the secretory surface. Such new synthesis presumably underlies the observations that, with time, β-cells respond more strongly to a given raised level of glucose than early in this prolonged second phase of secretion. Such persistent hyperglycaemia also increases the β-cell insulin response to other secretagogues, for example isoprenaline or gastrointestinal peptide.

The A chain of insulin has 21 amino acids and the B chain has 30 amino acids, with the two cystine disulphide bridges linking them at the A7–B7 and A20–B19 positions. The A chain has a further internal disulphide link between its 6 and 11 positions.

The insulins of different species show remarkably similarities. Human and porcine insulin differ only in the B30 amino acid (threonine in man, alanine in pig) while bovine insulin differs only at the A8, A9, and B30 positions. In the β-cell, insulin occurs mostly in hexamers bound to zinc, but it is almost certainly monomeric after release into the circulation.

Insulin secretion

The exact mechanism of action of the different insulin secretagogues has not been established. Glucose is the prime stimulus and acts via generation of ATP, certainly through oxidative metabolism of the hexose, but possibly also via an active receptor on the cell surface. Other related metabolites that seem particularly active in evoking secretion are glyceraldehyde phosphate and fructose-2,6-biphosphate as well as the branch chain amino acids and corresponding ketoacids. Stimulation leads to an increased outward flux of potassium through the voltage-sensitive potassium channel. This flux activates an inward movement of calcium to increase its cytosolic concentration which may also be raised by purely intracellular mechanisms. A variety of substances, for example gastrointestinal peptide and some prostaglandins, although not themselves strong stimuli to insulin secretion, potentiate the action of glucose or other direct stimuli (Table 7). They are known to raise the level of intracellular cyclic AMP and this may act more strongly on the partitioning of intracellular calcium than on the voltage-sensitive potassium channel.

The stimulatory action of sulphonylurea drugs depends on their binding to the voltage-sensitive potassium channel at a point distinct from ATP, with consequent activation of the channel. β-Adrenergic agents probably also act through the cyclic AMP mechanism, but both the stimulatory acetylcholine and the inhibitory agents dopamine and serotonin probably act more directly on the cytoplasmic calcium level. Another important inhibitory agent is somatostatin which is secreted by the islet D-cells. It inhibits the action of many endocrine cells, for example secretion of growth hormone from the pituitary and glucagon from the pancreatic α-cells. There are probably other important paracrine influences within the islets, as yet little understood, because glucagon promotes insulin secretion, insulin may promote glucagon secretion, and somatostatin inhibits both.

Neural regulation of insulin secretion is active *in vivo,* with vagal stimulation, adrenergic activity on balance inhibitory, and effects from other neurotransmitters. Vagal discharge is probably responsible for the cephalic pre-first phase of insulin secretion which occurs when a meal is seen or smelt and before any food has been ingested. This is a small effect, but may be important with natural meals because the arrival of some insulin in the liver ahead of the main ingested load of metabolites is likely to be beneficial in the control of systemic blood glucose concentrations, perhaps by early inhibition of gluconeogenesis and hepatic glucose release. Recently there has been interest in the central regulation of insulin secretion by the hypothalamus, with the ventrolateral nucleus stimulating the parasympathetic innervation. It is conceivable that such hypothalamically induced hyperinsulinaemia could promote obesity in

humans, possibly via increase in appetite. However, there are many stimulatory factors in the hypothalamic region which act to increase food intake in animals, and so far the place of hyperinsulinaemia has not been defined although there have been suggestive experiments in monkeys with insulin injected into the cerebrospinal fluid.

Secretion occurs in two phases. The first is fast, probably resulting from the release of granules which have already been formed that are situated near the cell surface. If the stimulus is sustained, there is a subsequent slower second phase of secretion in which much of the insulin is newly synthesized. Attempts have been made to relate the two phases of insulin secretion to morphological compartments with small and large storage pools, but their exact identity remains uncertain. In humans the two phases are not seen clearly unless a constant stimulus is applied, as with a constant glucose infusion. Early in type II diabetes there is usually some diminution in the first phase and a slight delay in

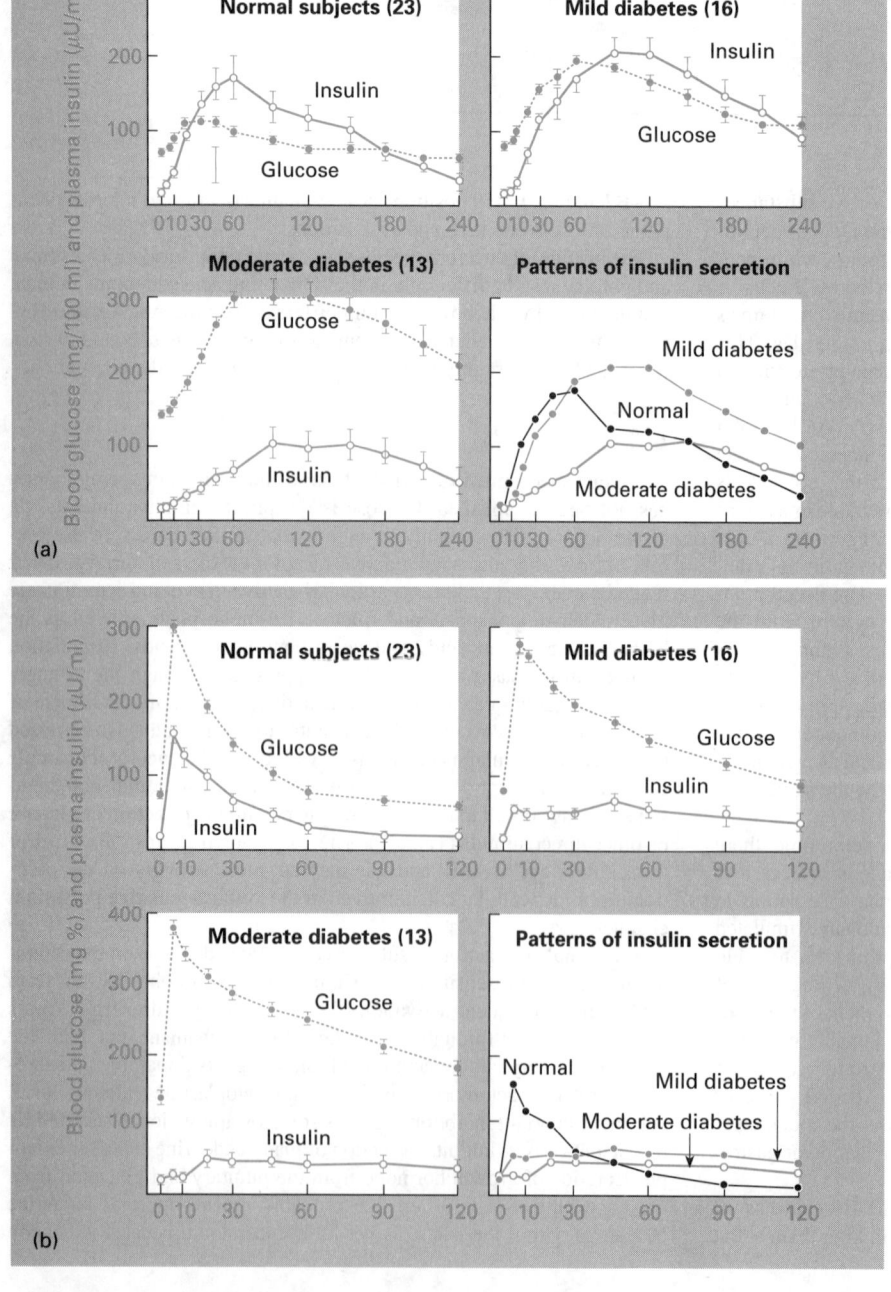

Fig. 4 (a) Oral glucose tolerance test (1.75 g/kg body weight), showing blood glucose and plasma insulin values for 4 h in non-diabetic healthy subjects and 'mild' and 'moderate' diabetics (fasting blood glucose below 11 mM). (b) Intravenous glucose tolerance tests (0.5 g/kg body weight injected over 5 min) for 2 h in the same people as in (a). (Reproduced from Seltzer *et al.* (1967) *Journal of Clinical Investigation* **46,** 323, with permission.)

a sustained second phase. At the same time there may be a normal response to a non-glucose stimulus such as arginine. In type I and more severe type II diabetes, the first phase is generally entirely absent, and in type I the second phase is greatly diminished and eventually disappears altogether. Some of these features are illustrated in Figs. 4 and 5 which show the plasma insulin and glucose concentrations at sequential points throughout glucose tolerance tests.

Insulin secretion *in vivo* is controlled by a finely integrated combination of the metabolic, hormonal, and neural mechanisms. In response to eating the earliest rise in insulin secretion precedes ingestion and is mediated by cephalic vagal stimulation. This is followed by release of gut hormones and absorption of glucose, which together cause a steady rise of insulin levels to peak after 45–60 min. Absorbed amino acids have a synergistic effect with that of glucose. There may also be an additional effect from amino-acid-stimulated glucagon secretion, although this will be counteracted by the action of glucose on the α-cells and will only be of major importance with a pure protein meal. As food absorption is completed, the stimulus to insulin secretion falls and plasma levels return to baseline after 2–3 hours.

In the fasting state basal insulin secretion is maintained in part by the plasma glucose concentration and in part by neuroregulation. In addition, as levels of non-esterified fatty acids and ketone bodies rise, there will be a slight increase in insulin secretion which serves to damp down lipolysis. Basal insulin secretion is crucial to the restraint of catabolism. It is normally phasic with a cycle length of about 13 min and a variability of 20 per cent of the mean value from trough to peak. Neither the mechanism nor the consequences of this pattern are fully understood, but a given amount of insulin has a greater effect if infused phasically rather than at a steady rate. Phasic secretion allows a higher concentration of insulin to reach the far end of each hepatic sinusoid intermittently. It would require perhaps twice the secretory rate to achieve this concentration constantly because about half the insulin reaching the liver is cleared in one passage.

From the pancreas insulin reaches the liver via the portal vein at a concentration three to ten times that in the systemic circulation. Insulin is degraded in the kidney as well as being excreted in the urine. About 40 per cent of the insulin is extracted in a single passage through the kidney, while smaller amounts are removed in the lung and by muscle. The half-life of insulin in the circulation is 4–5 min with a metabolic clearance rate of 1.2–1.4 l/min and an apparent distribution space of approximately 10–13 l in people of average build.

C-peptide is secreted in equimolar amounts with insulin. Its practical importance is twofold. First, it is not metabolized by the liver so that measurement in peripheral blood gives a better index of pancreatic β-cell function than does peripheral insulin measurement, with the reservation that, since C-peptide has a half-life of 20–35 min in the circulation, it cannot be used to follow short-term changes in insulin secretion. It is degraded and excreted by the kidney, and its use to assess insulin secretion requires precise analysis of its renal handling in any individual case. Its measurement is useful to check insulin secretion in the basal state or to analysis the response to eating a standard meal. However, it can never give all the information obtainable from measurements of venous insulin. C-peptide measurement is particularly useful for assessing endogenous insulin secretion in insulin-treated diabetics, where either exogenous insulin cross-reacts with the human insulin assay or insulin antibodies interfere.

Table 8 gives typical values of the circulating concentrations of insulin and its related molecules in systemic venous blood, both after overnight fasting and in response to an oral glucose tolerance test.

The insulin receptor

Considerable controversy still surrounds the mechanism of action of insulin. However, the first step now seems clear. Insulin binds to specific cell-surface receptors in insulin-sensitive tissues, including fat, muscle, liver, and brain. Binding to circulating white cells and red blood cells

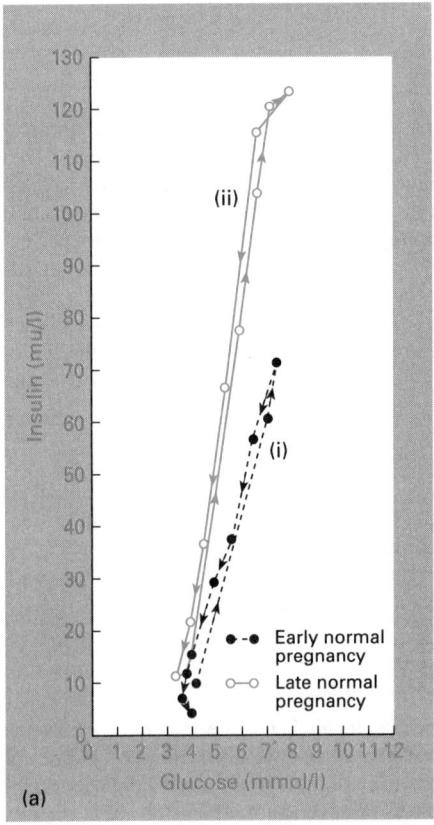

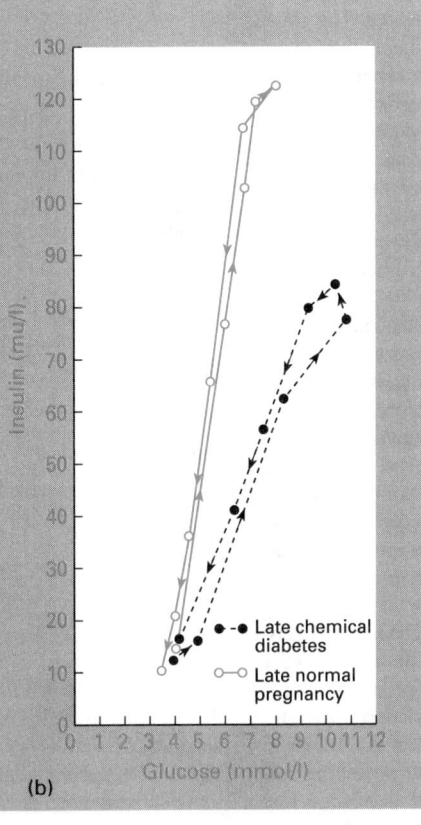

Fig. 5 (a) Plots of insulin and glucose values at sequential time points during oral glucose tolerance tests in non-diabetic women (i) early —O—▶—O— and (ii) late -O--▶--O- in pregnancy. The figures show the increased insulin secretion late in pregnancy (because of both increased resistance to insulin's action and increased β cell activity) but maintained glucose control. (b) As in (a), but here the late normal women (--O--▶--O--) are compared to some gestational diabetics, equally late in pregnancy (--●--▶--●--). The reduced insulin secretion, and impaired efficiency of return to the starting point are seen, especially from the slow and poorly directed 'turn-round'.

Table 8 *Plasma concentration of insulin and its precursors in normal subjects and those with glucose intolerance, all non-obese (approximate values for both fasting levels and those from an oral glucose tolerance test)*

	Normal subjects			IGT subjects		
	Fasting	Peak	Peak time (min)	Fasting	Peak	Peak time (min)
Insulin						
Immunoreactive						
mU/l	6	50	30	7	52	90
pmol/l	40	340	30	50	365	120
'True' 2 site immunoradiometric (pm/l)	35	300	30	40	310	90–120
C-peptide (pmol/l)	500	1800	60	550	2000	120
Proinsulin (pmol/l)	4	14	120	6	23	120
32–33 split proinsulin	3	7	120	3	18	120
Glucose (mmol/l)	4.5	8.5	60	6	10	90

can also be demonstrated, and other tissues responsive to insulin include peripheral nerve, smooth muscle, large arteries, skin, cartilage, bone, fibroblasts, leucocytes, and seminal vesicles.

The receptor is postulated to be a symmetric tetrameric complex of glycoproteins with a molecular weight of approximately 350 to 400 kDa. It comprises two subunits, each of 125 kDa, and two smaller subunits, each of 90 kDa, with disulphide linkages between them. However, there is still argument about subunit size, particularly in different tissues. There is also evidence for subunit specialization of function.

In both the intact cell and membrane preparations the receptor displays 'negative co-operativity', a form of feedback control in which the affinity of unoccupied receptors for insulin decreases with increasing number of occupied receptors. Insulin receptors also show the phenomenon of down-regulation in number in the presence of hyperinsulinaemia, with the converse that in hypoinsulinaemic states, such as untreated insulin-deficient diabetes, the number of receptors increases. The classical example of down-regulation is obesity. If such patients diet, there is an immediate increase in affinity followed by a slower increase in receptor number. This regulation of receptor number may be a protective mechanism in obesity due to hyperphagia, when the resultant reduced response to insulin would limit triglyceride synthesis and deposition. However, a vicious circle can result, with more and more insulin secreted to overcome the fall in receptor number and activity. This can impose an unusually high work-load on the secretion of insulin by β-cells, and there are indications that a persistently high work-load can lead to cellular failure and damage.

Another feature is that maximal insulin action on the fat cell, for example, can be obtained with only 10 per cent of the receptors occupied, giving rise to the concept of spare receptors. It is possible that *in vivo* these receptors are either buried within the cell membrane or inaccessible to insulin because of morphological relations between the cells.

After binding of insulin, the insulin receptor complex is internalized as a vesicle. The vesicle fuses with lysosomes in which both insulin and the receptor are degraded, although some internalized receptors seem to be recycled to the cell membrane. In addition, new receptors are synthesized within the cell and then inserted into the cell membrane.

Although the binding of insulin to its receptor is now well characterized, the subsequent steps in its action are less certain. The receptor acts as a protein kinase which is inactive when unoccupied but activated by the binding of insulin. This results in autophosphorylation of a tyrosine residue, which may be linked to the further phosphorylation of neighbouring proteins. This latter may be the vital link with the hormone's cellular action, although autophosphorylation may be necessary for receptor clustering in the cell membrane and subsequent internalization

of the receptor complex; it is also possible that the internalized receptor complex could be active as a kinase. Initially it was postulated that insulin acted through decreasing cyclic AMP via an effect on adenyl cyclase. This action and possible action through release of a small peptide from the cell membrane are no longer believed. However, other intermediaries, such as Ca^{2+} and other known organic secondary intracellular messengers, could exist after the phosphorylation step. Some further steps are essential as the final action often occurs via the dephosphorylation of a particular enzyme. Any hypothesis must explain changes in the transport of substances such as glucose, aminoacids, and potassium. The increase in glucose transport is (at least partly) secondary to mobilization of glucose transporters from the Golgi apparatus which are inserted into the cell membrane. This process could be controlled by any of the putative second messengers or phosphorylated enzyme–protein complexes within the cytoplasm.

Assay of insulin

Insulin was one of the first hormones to be measured by radio-immunoassay in which the sensitivity of isotopic work was combined with the specificity of immune mechanisms to give a major advance in accuracy of measurement. An insulin antibody detects all those compounds in plasma containing the epitope against which the antibody reacts. Several such compounds may be present in the plasma, depending on the properties of the particular antibody employed. These include some of the insulin precursor molecules already described. The presence of such compounds together with breakdown products also carrying the appropriate epitope may result in overestimation of the amount of insulin present.

Insulin has been detected in lymph as well as plasma. Thoracic duct lymph is particularly rich in insulin as it contains lymph from the pancreas itself as well as several other organs. The modelling of interactions between insulin and glucose is made more precise by using the concentrations of insulin in hind-limb lymph from experimental animals rather than in plasma. This is a reminder that it is insulin in the tissue fluids rather than in the plasma that acts on cells.

Importance of metabolic control

The two main aims of therapy for diabetics are to relieve symptoms secondary to either hyperglycaemia or hypoglycaemia and to prevent the long-term complications from tissue damage. (Table 9). The second aim is much more difficult to achieve and there is still no unanimous

Table 9 *The chronic complications of diabetes*

Complication	Possible causes
Macroangiopathy (arteriosclerosis, myocardial disease)	Hyperglycaemia Hyperlipidaemia Hyperinsulinaemia Smoking ?Increased growth hormone levels ?Platelet and other vascular factors
Microangiopathy (retinopathy, nephropathy, capillary basement membrane thickening)	Hyperglycaemia Protein (basement membrane) glycosylation Hormonal factors (e.g. growth hormone) Insulin deficiency
Neuropathy	Hyperglycaemia Sorbitol accumulation Deficient myoinositol Myelin glycosylation
Diabetic cataract	Hyperglycaemia Sorbitol accumulation Protein glycosylation
Collagen change	Glycosylation

view on the best approach to the problem, but adequate control of glycaemia is agreed to be crucial.

The consensus view is that optimal control of glycaemia will prevent or delay the onset of tissue damage, although it should be recognized that the aetiologies of tissue damage are different in detail for the different forms. Thus small blood vessel disease (microangiopathy) may be related to hyperglycaemia through protein glycosylation and other metabolic disturbances, and perhaps also to insulin deficiency, while macroangiopathy may depend upon blood pressure, smoking, and lipid levels as well as glucose and insulin levels and disease of the vasa vasorum. Neuropathy may be associated with myelin or myoinositol abnormalities, as well as with glucose and insulin disturbances, again acting partly via abnormalities of the vasa nervorum. Different aspects of metabolism may need to be controlled to prevent the individual complications. It is possible that protein glycosylation will present a unifying theme, but there is little direct evidence of this yet.

The term 'diabetic control' is confusing. It should mean such control of the total condition that would avoid both present symptoms and future tissue damage, and so should refer to measures to control the plasma lipids, for instance, as well as glucose concentration. Control of the latter alone should be termed glycaemic control. Although it is impossible to determine whether a patient is persistently normoglycaemic, as blood glucose levels cannot be determined continuously, assessment of glycaemic control has become easier through blood glucose assay in the home and measurement of glycosylation of haemoglobin or plasma proteins (see below). However, hyperglycaemia is only one facet of diabetes since insulin has a broad effect on metabolism.

Three lines of evidence now favour tight control of the blood glucose as the best approach to the prevention of chronic tissue damage: epidemiological studies, animal studies, and a few prospective studies of patients. Observations in Oxford (Massachusetts), Bedford, (United Kingdom), Athens, and Arizona (among Pima Indians) have shown a close association between the blood glucose levels 2 h after a glucose load and the risk of developing retinopathy. There appears to be a cut-off point at approximately 11 mmol/1 (200 mg/dl) below which retinopathy develops infrequently. This corresponds very approximately to a fasting glycaemia of 7.5 mmol/1. The studies in Bedford and Massachusetts also showed an association between the risk of cardiovascular disease and blood glucose, but with less hyperglycaemia necessary to establish the increased risk than in the case of retinopathy. A lower rate

of complications in patients treated with multiple injections than in patients treated with a single daily injection of insulin was reported in Malmö, Sweden, in the 1930s, with the inference that control was better in the former group. In addition, of 14 retrospective studies undertaken in the 1950s and 1960s, four showed no relation of glucose to complications, whilst the other 10 all provided some evidence that improved control slowed the development of retinal or renal glomerular changes. Taken together, most epidemiological evidence suggests that improved glycaemic control and/or improved control of plasma insulin can prevent or delay the development of neuropathic and microangiopathic lesions in type I diabetics.

Two prospective observational studies (on insulin-treated patients in Brussels and on NIDDM patients in Oxford, United Kingdom) have clearly shown relationships between glycaemic levels, the liability to develop retinopathy, neuropathy, and proteinuria, and an increased earlier mortality.

Comparison of good versus poor control of glycaemia over 5 years in dogs with experimental diabetes has revealed frequent development of background retinopathy in the group with poor control but little evidence of this in the group with good control.

Two large studies of NIDDM patients in the United Kingdom and IDDM patients in the United States, both prospective from diagnosis, were started in the 1980s. The former should report during the next 2–3 years and was designed to randomize patients between different therapeutic approaches rather than the different glucose levels obtained by different applications of the same agent as used in the American study. Therefore the United Kingdom study should tell us whether lower glucose levels are associated with diet alone or with diet combined with insulin, a sulphonylurea, or metformin in the obese. This study should also provide evidence as to whether the amount of tissue damage at a given overall glycaemic level is different with different therapies, but its evidence on the relationship between glycaemia and tissue damage will be no stronger than that from prospective non-randomized studies.

The American DCCT (Diabetes Control and Complications Trial) study of IDDM patients has recently provided direct proof that tighter glycaemic control reduces the development of retinopathy, neuropathy, and nephropathy during the earlier years from diagnosis. Patients were randomized either within a year of diagnosis or about 5 years later to their usual therapy (diet, exercise, and insulin) or an intensified insulin regimen (multiple subcutaneous injections or continuous subcutaneous insulin infusion). The latter regimen was successful in achieving lower glycaemia and was also associated with a significant reduction (40–60 per cent) in the development of tissue damage, including retinal appearance, urinary albumin, and neuropathic features. Reservations about this study include concern that the features that differed between the groups were not of such a severity as to cause disability, although all are established as precursors of probable symptomatic deterioration. The intensive regimen was also associated with a threefold increase in severe hypoglycaemic episodes. It was also admitted that it would not be easy to provide to the population at large the level of advice, surveillance, and support given to the intensive group.

Both the duration and degree of hyperglycaemia have been found to be important in the context of the risk of developing diabetic tissue damage. Thus the following relationship can be proposed:

$$\text{time} \propto \text{average glycaemia} = k \text{ [tissue damage]}$$

Clearly, the hypothetical constant k may range from near zero to a very high value. The lower level refers to patients who have maintained markedly raised glucose levels for decades but none the less are free from clinically evident tissue damage. The higher values account for those who come within the usual targets for good glycaemic control but nevertheless have developed pronounced tissue damage.

Perhaps some 10 per cent of IDDM patients have a k value approaching zero. It has been known for many years that long-lived survivors with IDDM, going 40 years from diagnosis without clinical tissue damage or surviving for 50 years, are characterized by three features: they are not obese or overweight, they have blood pressure on the low side of normal, and they have long-lived non-diabetic relatives.

This emphasizes that other factors, probably genetic, in addition to hyperglycaemia are important in determining diabetic tissue damage. Relationships between blood pressure and liability to neuropathy or retinopathy, and to survival, have been found in many studies.

Pirart has suggested that diabetic macroangiopathic lesions, such as ischaemic heart disease or peripheral vascular disease, have little relationship to glycaemia, although the latter condition was substantially estimated from urine glucose assay. Other studies have found an increase in macroangiopathic lesions with increased glucose levels, but the added risk appears at lower levels than the threshold for retinopathy discussed above. Subjects with impaired glucose tolerance show markedly increased liability to ischaemic heart disease, but not to the extent of known diabetics. This may reflect duration rather than severity of hyperglycaemia. Overall, studies have not shown such a clear relationship between glycaemia and liability to cardiac damage as has been found for retinopathy and nephropathy.

A study of diabetics with proteinuria in Denmark showed that they have a 10 times greater rate of death from cardiac disease than those without proteinuria, and there is also evidence of a similar risk for those with microalbuminuria compared with those with normal urinary albumin secretion. Proteinuria and microalbuminuria are generally due to microangiopathic lesions, whereas cardiac infarction is believed to be a consequence of macroangiopathy of the coronary arteries. If the glycaemic relationship with the tissue lesion is different for micro- and macroangiopathy, what is the link here? It may be disease of the vasa vasorum. Pathologists have occasionally observed proliferative neovascularization of the vasa vasorum deep to sclerotic plaques in coronary artery walls. These new vessels may bleed to initiate vascular obstruction. Similarly, lesions of the vasa nervorum undoubtedly contribute to diabetic neuropathy, but to an uncertain extent.

The link between renal and other microangiopathic lesions is less of a problem. Increased glomerular vascular permeability to albumin may be just a special case of a general increase in the permeability of the microvasculature revealed by the demonstration that albumin labelled with radio-iodine escapes more quickly from the circulation of diabetics than from that of non-diabetics.

Thickening of the capillary and precapillary basement membranes is an important morphological change in the development of diabetic microangiopathy. In the glomeruli the basement membrane is not thickened until 18 to 36 months after diagnosis in typical type I diabetic patients, but thickening increases with further time from diagnosis. In animals the degree of thickening is proportional to the degree of hyperglycaemia.

Accelerated damage

One more set of observations needs to be described before a hypothetical scheme for the development of diabetic damage can be presented, as in Fig. 6. There are two phases in the development of lesions in both the retina and the kidney. Background retinopathy accumulates according to the duration and degree of hyperglycaemia (Fig. 7) and causes relatively little damage to vision. It is only when proliferative changes occur that retinal haemorrhage becomes serious and vision is threatened. Similarly, microalbuminuria and proteinuria are more likely the greater the hyperglycaemic exposure, but renal failure only occurs when glomerular fusion drops to a critically low level. Unfortunately, intense glycaemic control does not drastically change the advance of either severe background or preproliferative retinopathy, nor does it slow the rate of decrease of the glomerular filtration rate, once these abnormalities are present. Indeed, excessively rapid return to normoglycaemia can apparently provoke second-phase damage for a short period. Hence there seems to be an early phase which depends on the degree of hyperglycaemic exposure and individual susceptibility, and a later phase in which damage progresses relatively independently of hyperglycaemia.

The scheme illustrated in Fig. 6 is hypothetical. It is based on the concept of an initial period of hyperglycaemic damage, however mediated, resulting in thickening of the basement membrane and an increase in permeability. In the second phase what is filtered through the altered capillary wall appears to become critical, with the filtration pressure and plasma composition now the determinants of future damage. Following Landis's pioneering direct determinations of capillary pressure, Tooke found that diabetic patients have higher mean capillary pressures in their extremities than non-diabetics, and that this increase in pressure was present quite early after diagnosis of diabetes. A higher local capillary pressure could be one factor making diabetics more susceptible to serious tissue damage, provided that there is marked hyperglycaemic exposure. Doubtless, capillary permeability is also important outside diabetes; for example some hypertensive patients develop a higher level of microalbuminuria than others with equally raised blood pressure.

Practical consequences

Glycaemic control which is as near normal as possible should be instituted immediately after diagnosis and then maintained except under the following conditions.

Fig. 6 Hypothetical schematic scheme of two-phase development of microangiopathic (and probably other forms of) diabetic tissue damage. It does not preclude some influence of hyperglycaemia on the second phase of development.

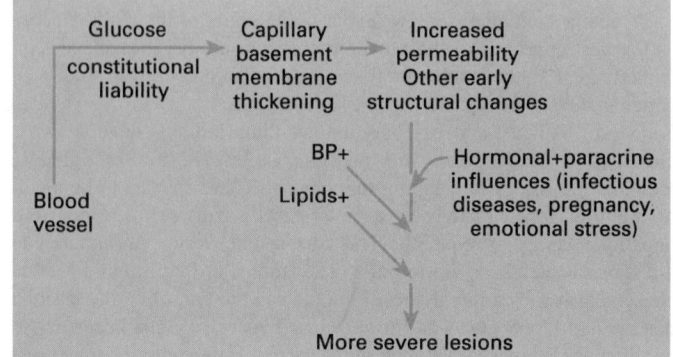

1. Concomitant hypoglycaemic attacks seem more dangerous than the risk of future tissue damage.

2. A severe degree of microangiopathic tissue damage has already occurred, in which case other approaches, such as control of hypertension, may become relatively more important. However, any relaxation of glycaemic control will depend on how difficult or restrictive it is to achieve tight control and how patchy the tissue damage is believed to be, i.e. how much relatively undamaged tissue is still present.

3. If, after 20 or 30 years of relatively high glycaemic levels because of a failure or absence of strict prescription, there is virtually no clinically evident diabetic tissue damage, the weighting assigned to the risks of hypoglycaemia should be greatly increased against the small advantage that might accrue from meticulous avoidance of significant hyperglycaemia.

Treatment of diabetes mellitus

Aims of therapy

The management of a diabetic patient is not aimed solely at glycaemic control. Various aspects requiring assessment and control are shown in Tables 10 and 11. The aims of treatment have been varied according to an arbitrary division of patients into three categories, ranging from those in whom symptomatic relief alone seems the most appropriate or only attainable goal to those in whom an attempt at maximal prophylaxis against future tissue damage seems desirable and possible. This assessment depends on a 'therapeutic contract' established between the medical adviser and the particular patient. It is hoped that the contract will increasingly be reached after full discussion with the patient. Sometimes, however, the doctor will supply much of the initiative in deciding on the targets, but with every consideration of clues from the patient. The contract should never be assumed to be permanent, as patients may move from one category into another, or merely within the wide range of the large middle category which embraces all those who, while finding it impossible to comply with every aspect of currently recommended ideal treatment, none the less are keen to maintain good health as long as possible, and are willing to suffer some inconvenience to do so.

Diet

Dietary treatment is a difficult issue in diabetes. In type II diabetes, obesity is such a common contribution to the relative pancreatic failure, through the associated increase in insulin resistance, that successful management depends essentially on dietary treatment to reduce it. It is not known why it is so difficult to achieve lasting weight reduction in these patients. It is probable that a tendency to obesity is one component inherent in the basic abnormality or very early adaptations to it. This view is strengthened by the even greater weights previously reached by many of these patients years before they present as diabetic and still obese. Indeed, the larger is the decrease at diagnosis from their highest remembered weight, the more likely are hypoglycaemic agents to be prescribed in the first year after diagnosis. An understanding of the whole weight trajectory of these patients would greatly increase our insight into type II diabetes. It is not known whether the obesity comes after a demonstrable abnormality in insulin secretion or precedes it.

In type I diabetes less fundamental ignorance was once complicated by excessive attention to wrong approaches, and two different fallacies became widespread. The first arose from the controversy, particularly active around 1920, as to whether diabetes was a disorder of total metabolism or just of carbohydrate. Allen's arguments for the former view were swept aside with the increased emphasis placed on plasma glucose concentrations which followed the discovery of insulin, and emphasis on a low carbohydrate diet became widespread. There were two good reasons to doubt its validity: first, diabetics in Africa or India often show sustained good control of glucose levels despite following the high carbohydrate diets traditional in those regions; second, since a low carbohydrate diet was likely to be high in fat, it might contribute to the hyperlipidaemia seen in some diabetic patients, particularly with only moderately controlled glycaemia, perhaps contributing substantially to the development of macroangiopathy. Good clinical studies around 1930 indicated that even in the West high carbohydrate diets were compatible with successful glucose control, but low carbohydrate diets were seriously questioned only with the renewed interest in natural or high fibre diets that arose in Africa and from the American 'green revolution'. Experiments by Anderson in America, and by Jenkins and by Mann in Oxford, then showed that a high carbohydrate diet, avoiding excess of quickly absorbed forms, achieved at least as good glycaemic control in diabetics as did the traditional 'low carbohydrate' regime. Indeed, slightly better results were often obtained.

The second fallacy came from the emphasis on chemical analysis of food 'on the shelf' without any thought as to how it was dealt with in the body. This may have been because the analysis was so crude as to deal only in 'carbohydrate', 'protein', and 'fat', so that, for instance, any form of carbohydrate was presented as equivalent to any other. Consequently, diets were based on building blocks of 10 g portions of carbohydrate. Many patients, and some of their advisers, had more sense in practice than to believe that 10 g of carbohydrate as table sugar was really equivalent to 10 g of carbohydrate taken as legumes, but that was the theoretical position in much dietary instruction. Investigators in continental Europe showed a more sensible approach than those in the United Kingdom and America, listing 'bread portions', 'milk portions', 'fruit portions', etc. separately.

Eventually it was realized that what mattered was the effect of the food on the blood glucose of the recipient, and that this would be greatly influenced by the speed of its passage through and digestion within the gut, all determining the rate at which the nutrients were absorbed from the gut into the blood. Two main lines of experiment contributed to this understanding.

First, around 1970 Kinsell showed that diabetic patients had a smaller rise in blood glucose when a 50 g glucose load was taken together with a liquid fat and protein meal than when it was taken alone. This was not a simple phenomenon, as in different patients the lower glucose levels with more nutrient were accompanied by either higher or lower plasma insulin concentrations, probably depending upon the β-cell responsiveness to amino acids. Obviously, the important consideration is the effect on the blood glucose of a food when it is taken as part of a meal and not merely ingested alone. This involves both the effect on its absorption of the other foods with which the substance in question is taken, and its own effect in speeding or slowing the absorption of those other foods. How a particular food is cooked can affect its rate of absorption, which is clearly illustrated by the greater rise in blood glucose when the juice from a particular weight of apples is drunk than when the apples are taken as a purée, which is greater again than if the apples are eaten raw.

Second, studies in which dietary fibre was added to meals showed lower blood glucose rises and lower insulin concentrations in both normal and diabetic subjects owing to a delay but not an overall decrease in absorption. This effect may also be useful in preventing both hypoglycaemia in insulin-treated diabetics and reactive hypoglycaemia in non-diabetics. The delayed absorption may be because of slower gastric emptying, slower enzymatic digestion of these foods, or directly from the more viscous alimentary contents which reduce the stirring caused at the gut surface by the pumping movement of the villi. There may also be changes in the response of the gastrointestinal hormones to different meals.

When different fibres were examined, the viscosity of their standard solutions in water correlated strongly with the reduction in glycaemia; the viscous fibres (for example pectins from fruits or galactomannans from legumes) were more effective than the fibrous fibres (for example bran). This was confirmed by other studies which have shown a lack of

Table 10 *Aims of management of patients with diabetes mellitus*

Factor	Aim of therapy		
	Optimal management	Compromised prophylaxis	Symptomatic management
Blood glucose	Fasting: below 6.5 mmol/l usually 2 h postprandial: below 9 mmol/l usually	Fasting: <8 mmol/l usually 2 h postprandial: <11 mmol/l usually	Under 12 mmol/l
Glycosylated haemoglobin	Within normal range of local laboratory (mean ±2 SD)	Mean ±4 SD	Neglect
Glycosuria	Absent (if normal renal threshold)	Fasting: absent postprandial ≤0.25%	<1%
Plasma cholesterol	<6.5 mmol/l	<7.5 mmol/l	Neglect
Plasma triglyceride (fasting)	<2.0 mmol/l	<3.5 mmol/l	Neglect
Blood pressure, upper limits (mmHg)	<50 years* >50 years*	<50 years* > 50 years*	As for general population, or neglect unless renal or cardiovascular disease
Systolic	145 160	155 165	
Diastolic	80 90	85 95	
Tobacco	None	<5 cigarettes/daily No limit pipe	<20 cigarettes/daily No limit pipe
Obesity (body mass index)	<27.0 kg/m²	<30.0 kg/m²	<33.0 kg/m²
Exercise	Walk for at least 30 min 4 days weekly (or alternatives)	Active job *or* walk for at least 30 min once weekly (or alternative)	As wished
Alcohol	Not >2 units/day usual Not >4 units/day special	Not >4 units/day usual Not >6 units/day special	As wished, up to social limits
Dietary modifications	High carbohydrate (>45–50% total calories) High 'viscous' fibre diet Low fat (<35% total calories) Increased unsaturated fats (P:M:S = 2:2:3) Limited 'quick' carbohydrate, only at meal end 6 intakes daily Limit calories according to BMI and exertion	Ample carbohydrate (>45% total calories) High fibre diet, some 'viscous' Limit fat (<35% total calories) Increased unsaturated fats (P:M:S = 1:1:2) Limited 'quick' carbohydrate 6 intakes daily Limit calories according to BMI and exertion	Limit calories according to BMI
Expectation of hypoglycaemia	Mild symptoms if meal delayed or unusual exercise without extra food	Only if exceptional exertion or starvation	Avoid

*Values require more precise adjustment acording to actual age.

association between the reduction in hyperglycaemia produced by a fibre and its effect on stool bulk.

The delayed absorption is accompanied by earlier satiety, increased feelings of epigastric fullness, and abdominal distention with borborygmi together with increased rectal flatus and looser bulkier stools. When a European eats rural African food, such abdominal symptoms lessen greatly within 3 months. Concentrations of some viscous fibres are available (for example, Guar gum from the cluster bean of India, already used in the food trade as a thickener for gravy), but some people find much viscous fibre repugnant because of its 'slimy' or 'gummy' feel, and this revulsion is not easily lost with time. Unfortunately, 'mouth feel' is also associated with the physical property of viscosity, so that the most effective fibre concentrates are likely to be unpalatable to many people.

An increase in the viscous fibre content of the diet can be achieved by one of two methods. First, natural foods which are rich in these substances can be made predominant constituents of the diet, and in practice this means a high legume content because galactomannans are their main storage carbohydrate. The pectins of cell walls (particularly fruits) form another major group, and to some extent galactomannans and pectins have additive qualities. The other approach is pharmacological, either by taking concentrates of viscous fibre as capsules or, more usually, by adding them to meals or incorporating them into particular foods, for example soups or crispbreads.

Such addition of viscous fibres is of most effect in improving postprandial glycaemia, while an increase in total dietary carbohydrate is effective primarily in reducing overnight glucose levels and those well away from a meal. To obtain the best results from these two dietary changes, quickly absorbed simple sugars should be limited in amount and taken late in a meal, and the overall level of glycaemia should be reasonably controlled. Usefully, viscous fibres are also effective in lowering cholesterol levels.

There is still much scope for improved understanding of the interreactions between different foods, and for observation as to which foods, combined in a meal, give the lowest glucose responses (Fig. 7). This can be predicted to some extent from studies of single foods (Table 12). Some other values for the glycaemic index of single foods should be noted to emphasize particular points. Both white and wholemeal bread, usually made from wheat, have the same value (72 per cent), but wholegrain wheat bread is lower, while wholegrain rye bread is lower still (42 per cent). Wholemeal bread contains rather more dietary fibre than white bread, but it is the metabolically neutral 'fibrous' fibre. Mashed potatoes have a similar glycaemic index to wholemeal bread, but white rice has a lower value (60 per cent) and pasta has an even lower value

Table 11 *Hypoglycaemic treatment and its monitoring for diabetic patients according to use of insulin and therapeutic aim.*

| Type of patient | Aim of therapy | | |
	Optimal management	Compromised prophylaxis	Symptomatic management
Insulin-dependent			
Mode of insulin treatment	At least two, often three, perhaps four SC injections daily *or* continuous SC pump with preprandial boosts.	One or two SC injections daily	One SC injection daily if adequate
Mode of monitoring	2 × 5/day BG profile weekly 2 BG tests daily on other days 2 Urine tests 4 days a week	2 BG tests on 4 days weekly *or* 2 BG tests on 2 days and 2 urine tests on 5 days	4 BG tests weekly *or* 2 urine tests 4 days a week
Non-insulin dependent (even if insulin treated)			
Hypoglycaemic treatment	Insulin (1 or 2 SC injections daily) if oral hypoglycaemics inadequate. Oral hypoglycaemics if diet alone inadequate	As for 'optimal'	Insulin only if acceptable, and probably once daily Oral hypoglycaemics as required
Mode of monitoring	1 × 5/day BG profile weekly 2 BG tests daily or other days 2 Urine tests on 4 days/week	2 BG tests thrice weekly *or* 2 BG tests on 1 day and 2 urine tests on 5 days weekly	4 BG tests weekly *or* 2 urine tests on 4 days a week

(48 per cent). This is because the starches in these three foods have different branching structures and so are digested at different rates by the alimetary enzymes. Wholegrain bread has a lower value because the natural grain husks are removed in the gut rather than during milling. A superficially surprising value is that of about 55 per cent for Mars Bar confectionery, which is probably due to the caramelization of some of the carbohydrate, something viscous in the pale foamy layer, use of sucrose rather than glucose, and fat in the chocolate. Indeed, a Mars Bar is a mixture of foods, unlike the constituents of Table 12. This emphasizes the importance of studying real meals and not single foods. With regard to the above values, bread is often eaten with butter or margarine while olive oil is added to pasta.

The importance of the effect on the metabolic response of the delay in gastric emptying caused by fat is unknown. It is probably one reason why recommendations for the percentage of total dietary calories that should be derived from fat will settle nearer to 35 per cent than the value of 30 per cent that has been suggested recently. However, the type of fat is also important (see below).

In general, foods ingested in a more natural state are likely to be more slowly absorbed, as digestion has to break down cell walls and other natural components. 'Lente' carbohydrate (to match prolonged acting insulins) is obtained from 'spansuled' food, and nature often provides such 'spansule' coatings. However, preparation of food for the table in lightly cooked form is often more time-consuming than using the convenience foods widely marketed today. Of course, raw food may be the easiest to serve, but it takes longer to chew and may be judged less tasty.

Timing is important. Glucose peaks will be avoided if meals are eaten slowly, and small frequent meals are more suitable than a few large ones for any type of diabetic (but particularly those treated with insulin).

Many natural foods contain small quantities of specific components, some of which have major effects on the metabolic responses. Thus soya beans (Fig. 7) contain an inhibitor of the starch-digesting enzymes.

Although dietary fibre has been defined as those carbohydrates (non-starch polysaccharides, celluloses, hemicelluloses) and lignins that are not digested by enzymes in the human gut, this refers only to those enzymes secreted as far as the ileum. The appendix may be a vestigial caecum, but a substantial amount of bacterial fermentation of fibre and other unabsorbed food occurs in the colon. Hydrogen and methane are formed, but so are the nutrients acetic acid, propionic acid, and butyric

acid. The last of these may be important to the health of the colonic mucosa but is not widely available in the body, absorbed propionate is nearly all extracted and metabolized in the liver, but enough acetate may be absorbed from a high fibre diet to exceed its uptake by the liver from portal venous blood and contribute to the systemic plasma acetate level. Acetate is also released from the liver, seemingly in excess in diabetics whose blood level of perhaps 0.2 mmol (rising with hyperglycaemia) is higher than that of normal subjects (*c.* 0.05 mmol). Acetate acts metabolically as a non-esterified fatty acid.

Another consideration is that the diet of a diabetic must contain all the beneficial factors that are necessary for non-diabetics, such as vitamins and minerals. It has been realized that fruits and vegetables contain valuable compounds that may act as antioxidants and help to remove free radicals. Whatever their action, the presence of these compounds in the diet is associated with a reduction in both coronary arteriosclerosis and cancer. Thus the amount of fruit currently recommended is greater than might be expected from a consideration of its content of simple sugars alone. Some of the compounds had already been identified as vitamins even though their antioxidant role was not initially recognized; these include β-carotene (vitamin A) and α-tocopherol (vitamin E). Others, such as anthrocyanins present in the juice from red grapes and thus present in red wine, have been identified more recently. Although not essential to maintain life, in trace quantities they appear to be of benefit in delaying the onset of disease.

Before considering practical dietary advice for diabetics, it is important to realize the different targets likely to be addressed in different studies. The patient is interested in long-term health and long-term glycaemic and lipaemic control as guides to this. The measurements made on test diets range from the blood glucose levels after a single ingestion (ranging from an artificially liquidized preparation to a normally mixed meal), to the fasting glucose level the day after a given regime, to the level of glycated HbA_{1c} or fractional lipids after several weeks on a diet. Much attention is given to ensuring weight stability during such studies because of its effect on insulin sensitivity, but a key question about any dietary regimen followed during normal life is its effect on weight over months and years. This question is particularly relevant to sucrose; 5–10 g of table sugar (glycaemic index 60 per cent because of its fructose content) taken even twice daily towards the end of meals, in place of the less quickly digested carbohydrate, does not impair glycaemic control over a period of weeks. However, apart from any effect on plasma triglycerides, which is not important in this amount, it is unknown whether such an intake increases the desire for sweet foods with possible increases in the intake of other carbohydrate-rich foods and/or weight.

Another example of the differences between single meal and more realistic long-term studies is provided by the improved glycaemic tolerance to meals that is seen with normal subjects or relatively mildly affected NIDDM patients if a small glucose load is taken 30 min before eating. This activates the β-cell insulin secretory mechanisms so that they are more potent in their reaction to the meal, with consequent improved glucose control subsequently. However, subjects on this regimen would be expected to gain weight over a period of months with ultimately adverse effects on glycaemic control.

THERAPEUTIC CONSIDERATIONS

The most important nutritional approach to a typical type II diabetic is to restrict caloric intake, although energy expenditure is also important in the regulation of body weight. There is some evidence that moderate physical activity reduces appetite and intake, at least in relation to need, compared with really low levels of activity. Again, insulin sensitivity is believed to be increased if muscle replaces adipose tissue.

Fig. 7 Rise in blood glucose concentrations in six healthy volunteers after meals containing 50 g carbohydrate as wholemeal bread or lentils (top) or wholemeal bread and/or soya beans (bottom). (Reproduced from Jenkins. (1980). *British Medical Journal*, **281**, 16, with permission.)

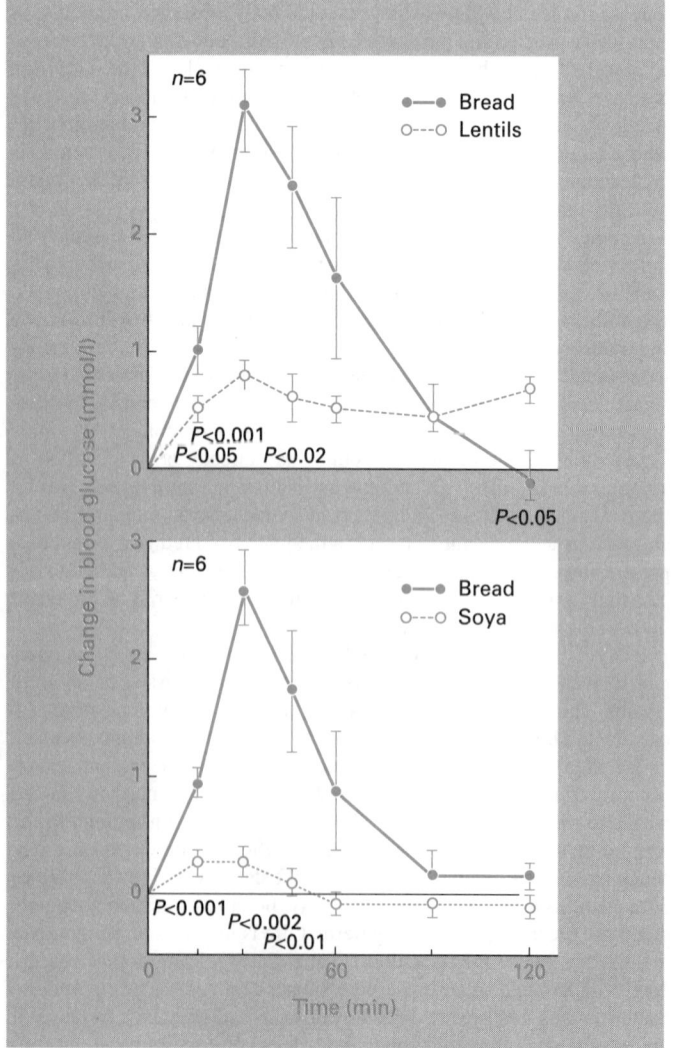

Table 12 *Increases in blood glucose after ingestion by non-diabetics of food portions of equal carbohydrate content expressed as a percentage of the increase after ingestion of 50 g of glucose in aqueous solution*

Food	Blood glucose increase $\pm$SD (%)
Apples	62 $\pm$ 9
Orange juice	46 $\pm$ 6
Bananas	62 $\pm$ 9
Soya beans	15 $\pm$ 5
Lentils	29 $\pm$ 3
Kidney beans	29 $\pm$ 8
Haricot beans	31 $\pm$ 6
Peas (black-eye)	33 $\pm$ 4
Peas (marrowfat)	47 $\pm$ 3
Porridge oats	49 $\pm$ 8
All-Bran®	51 $\pm$ 5
Cornflakes	80 $\pm$ 6
Oatmeal biscuits	54 $\pm$ 4
Ryvita®	69 $\pm$ 10

The regulation of caloric intake by those tending to obesity is extremely important (Chapter 10.5). The possibility of weight loss seems to depend principally on the strength of motivation. While long-term health aspirations can contribute to this, the good opinions won from mentors or intimates by success seem to be more important. Limitation of caloric intake by the potentially fat is unlikely to be achieved by the overtired, frustrated, or miserable. The use of fibre to augment stool bulk, and so lessen constipation, in those on a low calorie diet can be helpful.

Dietitians should always be aiming to reduce the liability of diabetics to arteriosclerosis, and since this results from the interaction of several risk factors they should give advice on both restriction of sodium intake to reduce the risk of hypertension and measures to regulate the blood lipids. Diabetics are probably no more liable to hypercholesterolaemia than non-diabetics, but when there is a deficiency of effective insulin action they certainly have increased liability to hypertriglyceridaemia. It is essential to recognize the importance of smoking as a risk factor for arteriosclerosis and of the beneficial effects of physical exercise in preventing its development.

The particular disease process that has produced diabetes is probably of little importance with regard to the dietary advice given. However, dietary advice will vary depending on whether or not the patient is treated with insulin. Subcutaneous injections of insulin do not mimic adequately the normal pancreatic response to eating, and such injections also pass into the systemic circulation rather than straight to the liver. Whether the patient is insulin-dependent or non-insulin-dependent, or whether their diabetes is type I or type II, is relatively unimportant with regard to dietary advice compared with the substantial difference in the timing rather than the content of meals according to whether or not a patient is being treated with insulin. The action of oral sulphonylurea tablets seems to be much less dependent on the exact time at which they are taken, but none the less it seems sensible that the quicker-acting types, such as tolbutamide, should be taken about 30 min before meals. Such a regimen is unnecessary for long-acting agents such as chlorpropamide.

Dietary advice may need to be amended in the presence of renal failure. It may be necessary to reduce dietary protein (Section 20.17). Any reduction in protein should not be compensated mainly by fat, as could occur from the 'low carbohydrate' fallacy; many nephropaths die from ischaemic heart disease. It has also been argued that at early stages of renal damage, evidenced by microalbuminuria, progression of the renal lesion may be reduced by a marked decrease in dietary protein to about 0.6 g/kg body weight. There is no doubt that the albumin in the urine can be reduced in this way, but any real effect of protein reduction on the retardation of the rate of loss of renal function is uncertain.

PRACTICAL ADVICE

The important aspects are as follows.

1. The diet should provide the calorie intake that will both support necessary activity and, where appropriate, normal growth and bring the patient's weight to the correct value. For most type II diabetics this means weight loss. Restricted intake is crucial and requires much motivation. Exercise can be a useful adjunct. Each insulin-taking diabetic must work out the right balance between extra food intake and extra exercise. As a general rule walking for an hour would be expected to increase carbohydrate requirements by about 20 g, while more active exercise such as playing tennis or football may require at least 40 g of carbohydrate per hour. This is best taken as extra food at a preceding meal, but small amounts may be taken as quickly absorbed carbohydrate just before the exercise or halfway through it.

2. Food should be spread out throughout the day, and those taking conventional insulin therapy should have three main meals and three snacks. The latter are necessary because of the relatively slow absorption of insulin from subcutaneous tissue. Older patients who wake regularly during the night may have a small intake then.

3. Meals should consist of foods that are slowly digested and absorbed, with particular reference to slowly absorbed carbohydrate and increased fibre content, particularly of the more viscous type. Simple sugars (glucose, sucrose) should be confined to small amounts taken with meals (for example 5–10 g). This must not be allowed to increase total intake. The only exceptions are treatment of hypoglycaemia and illness, particularly gastrointestinal, when simple sugars in easily digestible form may be added to drinks to supplement a greatly reduced total food intake.

4. The carbohydrate content of the diet should provide 50 to 55 per cent of the total calories, although in individual meals this can vary as widely as from 30 to 60 per cent.

5. Patients should be thoroughly instructed in both the calorie and carbohydrate content of their food, with particular emphasis on the high calorie content of fatty foods. They should also aim at a ratio of polyunsaturated to mono-unsaturated to saturated fatty acids of around 2:2:3, and be advised to restrict intake of eggs to a maximum of eight a week, to limit the consumption of hard cheese, and to keep the intake of other high cholesterol foods such as shellfish at a modest level. Fat should not contribute more than 35 per cent to total calorie intake.

6. The need for a regular pattern of feeding should be stressed in insulin-dependent diabetics who are on fixed insulin regimens. In some patients appropriate advice can be given on varying the timing of insulin injection to match altered meal times. This is socially important for young diabetics, and is a major advantage for those on continuous insulin infusion or repeated subcutaneous injections of quick-acting insulin against a background of long-acting insulin.

Three specimen diets, with calorie contents of 1000, 1500, and 2500 kcal, are given in Table 13, which also includes the carbohydrate content of each meal. The aim is for the diabetic to eat normally but to watch timing and total quantity. Approximately 1000–1200 kcal/day should be advised when the body mass index exceeds 30.0 kg/m², 1500 kcal/day for a body mass index of 27.5–29.9 kcal/day, and 2000 or more for a body mass index of less than 27.5 kcal/day, but the optimum amount will depend on exercise, muscularity, and height.

ETHANOL

There is no reason why diabetics should not enjoy alcoholic drinks in sensible moderation. The weekly intake should probably not exceed 21 equivalents for men or 14 for women (one equivalent is a single measure of spirits, a small glass of wine, or a half-pint of beer), although recent data suggest that a slightly higher intake may be acceptable. Diabetics should also spread their weekly intake evenly around three equivalents per day for men or two for women. There is a tendency to neglect the caloric content of alcoholic drinks when analysing diets. The carbohydrate in sweet wines or liqueurs is quickly absorbed, which means that these should be avoided, as should sugar-containing mixers such as tonic water (which can be obtained in low calorie form). Ethanol differs from other foods in many respects. It is a potent inhibitor of gluconeogenesis and may be responsible for hypoglycaemia after 2 to 3 h if it is taken without food or 4 to 8 h after a small meal if it is taken in excess. The effect of real excess may persist even until lunchtime the following day. The mental effects of ethanol can be confused with those of hypoglycaemia, and so it is always important to measure the blood glucose in a diabetic suspected of being drunk and to smell the breath or measure plasma ethanol in a diabetic suspected of suffering from hypoglycaemia. Heavy ethanol intake can cause peripheral neuropathy and so compound the symptoms and signs of diabetic nerve damage. Alcoholic flushing is greatly increased by chlorpropamide, and to a lesser extent by some other sulphonylureas, and may be a reason for the severe limitation of the enjoyment of a modest alcohol intake.

Sulphonylureas

Although sulphonylureas are the most widely used oral hypoglycaemic agents, their place in diabetic treatment is far from established. They act in two different ways. First, they sensitize the β-cell to the stimulatory effect of glucose and other agents on insulin secretion, causing a leftward shift in the dose–response curve of insulin secretion against glucose concentration which may be maintained for years. They also increase the ratio of intact to 32–33 split proinsulin in plasma, as do several secretory stimuli. The metabolism of glucose within pancreatic β-cells generates ATP which binds with a receptor on cell-membrane voltage-dependent potassium channels to favour a potassium efflux. Such an efflux stimulates a change in adjacent calcium channels, and the resulting influx of calcium leads, through a series of reactions, to insulin secretion from the cell. The sulphonylureas bind at a different site from ATP to this same voltage-dependent potassium channel with an avidity proportional to their potency as hypoglycaemic agents. Sulphonylureas bind similarly to some neurones, particularly of the substantia nigra, but the significance of this has yet to be assessed.

The sulphonylureas do not affect blood glucose in pancreatectomized animals, but there is evidence that their effect on intact animals is not solely due to the extra insulin secreted; they may up-regulate insulin receptors, increasing their number and so magnifying the effect of the available insulin. The hypoglycaemic effectiveness of these drugs often decreases with time. It is possible that the insulin receptor action is relatively short lasting. The effective β-cell mass is also likely to decrease with time, at least in some patients. The main argument about the use of sulphonylurea drugs is the extent to which they can be replaced by proper dieting, or indeed interfere with this. Dieting can be extremely successful in reducing glucose levels quickly, and long-term weight loss alone always improves glucose tolerance, often to a degree that makes sulphonylureas superfluous. However, in practice there are limitations to dietary treatment, particularly in the more hyperglycaemic type II diabetics, and sulphonylureas can then be a real aid in glucose control. They probably interfere with dietary effort because a close approach to normoglycaemia stimulates appetite and particularly because a large initial dose may be persisted with long after it is no longer necessary.

The report of the American University Group Diabetes Program,

Table 13 *Menus for three specimen diets*

Meal	1000 kcal	CHO (g)	1500 kcal	CHO (g)	2500 kcal	CHO (g)
Breakfast	Fresh orange segments One Weetabix® with skimmed milk (130 ml) Wholemeal toast: one slice with margarine Tea with skimmed milk (20 ml)	40	Fresh grapefruit, half Small bowl All-Bran® with skimmed milk (150 ml) Wholemeal toast: one slice with margarine Tea with skimmed milk (20 ml)	38	Large bowl Puffed Wheat® with milk (150 ml) (or medium helping Puffed Wheat® + one banana) Wholemeal toast: one slice with baked beans One glass of milk (150 ml)	73
Mid-morning	Tea with skimmed milk (20 ml)	1	Tea with skimmed milk (20 ml) One apple	12	Tuna and cucumber sandwiches from two slices wholemeal bread Tea with milk (20 ml)	30
Lunch	Butter beans, sweetcorn, and ham salad Lemon juice dressing One apple Tea with skimmed milk (20 ml)	37	Tuna and cucumber sandwiches from two slices wholemeal bread One small banana and a small carton of natural yoghurt Tea with skimmed milk (20 ml)	53	Beef and bean hot pot Rice and pineapple condé Low calorie squash	81
Mid-afternoon	Coffee with skimmed milk (40 ml)	2	Coffee with skimmed milk (40 ml) One wholewheat cracker biscuit	10	One wholewheat fruit scone Coffee with milk (40 ml) One apple	29
Evening meal	Lean roast lamb: two slices Sugar-free mint sauce Garden peas and carrots One large jacket potato Stewed pear with cinnamon Low-calorie squash	42	Red bean and lamb casserole One large jacket potato Runner beans Fresh fruit jelly Diabetic squash	86	Vegetable and pasta soup Red bean and cheese flan Red cabbage salad with yoghurt dressing Orange fruit jelly Coffee with milk (40 ml)	90
Bedtime	Skimmed milk as tea/ hot milk/coffee (40 ml) Two rye crispbreads (Ryvita®)	15	Skimmed milk as coffee/hot milk (50 ml) One digestive biscuit	13	One tall glass unsweetened fruit juice (or one glass milk) Two digestive biscuits	39
Total Percentage of total calories from carbohydrate		137 55%		212 57%		342 55%

which implied an excessive risk of cardiovascular deaths in diabetics if they had been treated with a fixed dose of tolbutamide (500 mg three times daily) together with their diet, has deterred treatment with sulphonylureas. The concern aroused has been largely dissipated with greater understanding of the imperfections of this trial and how the data may be more clearly interpreted. There has also been a lack of confirmation of any such risk from tolbutamide or other sulphonylureas in a number of other, albeit smaller, studies. The United Kingdom prospective study should provide important data in this regard.

TOXIC EFFECTS

The sulphonylureas can cause a wide range of allergic reactions, particularly on the skin. Some compounds are particularly associated with rare but severe bone marrow depression. This has most often been reported in those given more than 500 mg of chlorpropamide daily, a dose that would rarely be exceeded today. All can produce hypoglycaemia, rarely severe enough to cause unconsciousness. This can happen spontaneously, but is particularly likely to occur under special circum-

Table 14 *Major oral hypoglycaemic agents available in the United Kingdom*

	Daily dose range (mg)	t_{max} (h)	t_i (h)	No. of daily doses	Site of metabolism
Sulphonylurea					
Acetohexamide	250–1500	1–2	1.3–4.5	1–3	Liver
Chlorpropamide	100–500	1–7	33–43	1	Most excreted unchanged in urine
Glibenclamide	2.5–20	1–2	6–10	1–3	Liver
Glibornuride	12.5–75	2–4	8–9	1–2	Liver
Gliclazide	80–240	4–8	10–12	1–3	95% liver
Glipizide	2.5–30	0.5–2	3–7	2–3	90–95% excreted unchanged
Gliquidone	30–180	2–3	—	1–3	95% liver-metabolites excreted in bile
Glymidine	500–2000	1–2	5–8	1–2	?
Tolazamide	100–1000		7	1–3	Liver
Tolbutamide	1000–3000	3–4	7	2–3	Liver
Biguanide					
Metformin	500–1700	2–4	12–20	1–3	Excreted unchanged in urine

stances, for example in synergy with β-adrenergic blocking agents or monoamine oxidase inhibitors, when displaced from binding plasma proteins by another drug (for instance dicoumarins or salicylates), or in the neonate if the agent was unwisely administered to the pregnant mother within a few days of delivery. The risk is generally greater for longer-acting agents, and is enhanced by hepatic or renal disease which affects the usual elimination of the drug and so increases its plasma concentration. This may be one mechanism underlying the risk of severe and prolonged nocturnal hypoglycaemia in some elderly persons given long-acting preparations.

ADMINISTRATION

The commonly used sulphonylureas are listed in Table 14. Many patients prefer a long-acting agent such as chlorpropamide, or sometimes glibornuride, even though more effective glucose control and higher insulin levels may be achieved by shorter-acting drugs, such as glibenclamide or glipizide, which are more frequently administered. Although there is no advantage in adding a second sulphonylurea when a maximum dose of one has already been prescribed, it is reasonable to supplement a small dose of a long-acting agent with a quick-acting drug, for instance before a large evening meal or regularly before breakfast in those with a marked morning hyperglycaemic surge.

Particular agents may have special advantages, although the well-established drugs chlorpropamide and tolbutamide are usually as effective as any of the more expensive second-generation drugs. Gliquidone may be more suitable in the presence of renal impairment, as it is mostly metabolized in the liver with excretion of its metabolites in the bile. Glymidine is chemically a sulphapyrimidine rather than a sulphonylurea and so may be acceptable when sensitivity to a sulphonylurea proves to be a group phenomenon rather than a more specific response.

Indications for sulphonylurea prescription will depend mostly on the ability of a type II diabetic to initiate and sustain dietary effort, and in the physician's aim of glucose control. Although neither the mechanism nor time course of continuing β-cell deterioration in type II diabetes are understood, this will be a major cause of secondary failure of these agents. Increased insulin resistance with time can also contribute to secondary failure. Sulphonylureas are relatively contraindicated in young thin type I patients, particularly if they are ketotic. Nevertheless some slow-onset type I diabetics can achieve adequate glucose control on sulphonylureas without insulin for many years. However, recognition of type I disease (for example by a positive islet-cell antibody test) or evidence of deficient insulin secretion should increase the readiness to transfer to insulin should glucose control become borderline. In some centres the choice between sulphonylurea and insulin treatment is based

on the maximal C-peptide secretory response to a stimulus such as glucagon, or even the response to a sulphonylurea itself. However, glucose levels, perhaps particularly when assessed by glycated haemoglobin, may be almost as useful, especially if combined with fasting insulin and ketone body measurements or, more crudely, with the body weight.

Most diabetics requiring sulphonylureas are prescribed them within a year of diagnosis, but there is a continuing tail of secondary dietary failures. About 30 per cent of those on sulphonylureas will be transferred to insulin treatment within 4 years. The change tends to be made earlier now, with increasingly strict criteria for acceptable glycaemic control. There is no recognized benefit from combining insulin and sulphonylurea therapy. The sulphonylurea may decrease the required dose of insulin, but this is neither significantly cheaper nor of help in glycaemic control.

Although the issue is not clear cut the sulphonylureas probably have no specific effect in reducing the rate of long-term deterioration of blood glucose homeostasis in type II diabetics with mild hyperglycaemia.

Biguanides

Biguanides, which are believed to act by reducing the efficiency of ion exchange across membranes, decrease the efficiency of cellular metabolism. Both hepatic gluconeogenesis and the yield of chemical energy from peripheral utilization of glucose are decreased, with a resulting fall in blood glucose. Doubtless the same properties underlie the toxic effects that these agents may cause, ranging from generalized lassitude and vague muscular discomfort via increased intestinal motor activity to the serious complication of lactic acidosis. Lactic acidosis, although rare, is particularly liable to occur with phenformin therapy; hence this agent is no longer available in many countries, including the United Kingdom. Lactic acidosis is more likely when there has been an acute reduction in hepatic blood flow, for example after myocardial infarction, pulmonary embolus, or Gram-negative septicaemia, but is also predisposed to by excess alcohol intake or leukaemia. Since the biguanides are largely eliminated by the kidney, renal impairment is another contraindication to their use.

The risk of lactic acidosis is least, and indeed is extremely small, with metformin (Table 14), but the dose should probably not exceed 500 mg three times daily or 850 mg twice daily. It is best taken during or after meals and introduced gradually to reduce the risk of dyspepsia. A reasonable regimen is to prescribe 500 mg daily for a week and then 500 mg twice daily with a delay of at least a week before any further increase.

Traditionally, the principal role of biguanides in treatment is synergistic to a sulphonylurea when this, together with dietary advice, has failed to produce satisfactory glucose control. Such a state is often an indication for transfer to insulin, but combined sulphonylurea–biguanide therapy is a useful method of attempting continued oral treatment, particularly if symptomatic relief rather than strict glycaemic control is the aim (Table 11). The biguanides remain active after months or years of therapy, and their efficacy shows little dependence on the residual effective β-cell mass. They are gradually being considered more often for initial drive therapy. Further information from the United Kingdom Prospective Study should define their role more clearly. It is not advantageous to combine biguanides with insulin treatment.

The use of biguanides has been particularly advocated in the treatment of persistently and severely obese diabetics. However, their use may favour weight loss because of anorexia rather than minimal malabsorption, and there is little evidence that sulphonylureas are specifically fattening, although any agent improving glucose control may be associated with weight gain in a diabetic. However, it is reasonable to use a biguanide alone in the obese diabetic refractory to dietary therapy who gains weight on sulphonylureas.

Other oral hypoglycaemic agents

No other oral hypoglycaemic agent is widely used in Europe or North America in the treatment of diabetes. Certain herbal preparations, for example kerala, are widely used in India and are weakly hypoglycaemic, and onion extract is also weakly active. Other agents can be grouped as follows.

1. Specific hypoglycaemic agents of no practical advantage, including dichloroacetate and demethylpyrazole. The former may also cause hyperketonaemia.
2. Widely used pharmaceuticals with a weak hypoglycaemic action. The salicylates are a special case with a variety of potential actions, including interference with prostaglandin metabolism as well as displacement of sulphonylureas from their binding proteins.
3. Enhancing sulphonylurea activity: phenylbutazone and dicoumarols also displace sulphonylureas from their plasma-binding proteins; monoamine oxidase inhibitors potentiate sulphonylureas, particularly in depressives.
4. Some drugs developed to treat hyperlipidaemia also have mild hypoglycaemic effects in patients with NIDDM. These include acipimox, which inhibits release of non-esterified fatty acids from adipose tissue and so might be predicted from the glucose–fatty acid cycle to lower glucose levels, and bezafibrate which, like the sulphonylureas, should not be combined with monoamine oxidase inhibitors.

Reduction of tissue damage

The various processes involved in the development of diabetic tissue damage have already been discussed. Apart from the need for tight glycaemic control and attention to other risk factors for arteriosclerotic disease, various drug therapies have been suggested.

ALDOSE REDUCTASE INHIBITORS

Finding an effective agent with acceptable side-effects has proved more difficult than was initially expected. Sorbinil was withdrawn because of rash, fever, and lymphadenopathy. Ponalrestat was a less active enzyme inhibitor than had been hoped. Tolrestat is the only agent still undergoing large-scale trials against microangiopathic and neuropathic tissue damage, but already its potency has been questioned. There is as yet no convincing evidence that any of these agents are beneficial in humans; at best they may very slightly decrease the deterioration in conduction velocity in peripheral nerve fibres but not to a clinically useful extent. They may have been prescribed too late, but there is nothing yet to warrant their long-term prophylactic use beyond theoretical considera-

tion and results in some experimental animals. However, the possible importance of this approach has been increased by a preliminary report of higher erythrocyte aldose reductase per unit haemoglobin in patients with NIDDM who had developed retinopathy more than 10 years after diagnosis.

AMINOGUANIDINE

Animal studies have shown that aminoguanidine interferes with the development of advanced glycosylation end-products and the consequent cross-linking of protein chains. Its use has not progressed beyond the treatment of experimental diabetes in small laboratory animals in which regional albumin clearance was reduced in some parts of the body but albuminuria was not decreased. It has also diminished experimental diabetic retinopathy and decreased its acceleration by hypertension, with less microthrombus formation, less deposition of protein with a positive reaction to periodic acid–Schiff reagent, and fewer acellular capillaries. More recent derivatives show similar general effects without the inhibition of diamine oxidase and nitric oxide synthetase exhibited by the parent compound.

POLYUNSATURATED FATTY ACIDS (OMEGA W-6)

Because of their potential importance as precursors of prostaglandins and thromboxanes, the N6 series of polyunsaturated fatty acids are important nutrients and potential therapeutic agents. Steps in the conversion of linolenate to arachidonate may be deficient in diabetic patients, and so D-linolenate could be useful therapy. It has been tried (as evening primrose oil), particularly against diabetic neuropathy. There is uncertain evidence of prevention of slowing of nerve conduction but, again, no clear evidence of clinical efficacy. More general polyunsaturated fatty acid supplements have decreased the development of diabetic retinopathy, particularly of the advanced type, but the benefit could be limited to those with hyperglycaemia of a level unacceptable by present standards. It is also uncertain whether the fatty acids act merely via vasodilatation or by metabolic effects.

Insulin

The aim of insulin therapy will vary from patient to patient. There are two main targets, which are not mutually exclusive: present well-being and future health. To achieve the latter, glycaemia needs to be kept close to normal. This should be possible without excessive administration of insulin, and so exercise and dietary discipline are necessary to maintain normal sensitivity to insulin. The current inevitably inappropriate route of insulin injection into the systemic, not the portal, circulation may prevent total normalization of intermediary metabolism even when glucose levels are virtually normal, although this does not appear to be the case in some species.

Such metabolic near-normalization requires a highly motivated and educated patient. At present it is the best that can be offered to a recently diagnosed diabetic still substantially free from tissue damage. This intensity of care may be inappropriate under the following circumstances: when prognosis in a diabetic is limited by another disease (for example carcinoma), when some incapacity (for example blindness in the elderly) makes the routine excessively demanding compared with the likely benefits, and when diabetic tissue damage in crucial organs has already developed to a degree that dominates the prognosis for morbidity and mortality and cannot be reversed by improved glycaemia control.

TYPES OF INSULIN AVAILABLE

The various insulin preparations have three main characteristics—species of origin, purity, and duration of action (Table 15)—to these may be added concentration, now fixed in the United Kingdom at 100 IU/ml.

Table 15 *Main types of therapeutic insulins*

Species	Bovine
	Porcine
	Human
Purity	Conventional
	Single peak
	Highly purified
Duration of action	Short
	Intermediate
	Long

Species

Insulin was first isolated from bovine pancreas in 1922, and shortly afterwards it was also extracted from porcine pancreas. Since then bovine and porcine insulins have been the mainstays of therapy. Recently, synthetic human insulin has become available. Human insulin differs from porcine insulin only at the amino acid in position 30 of the β-chain. Bovine insulin differs at two other sites—amino acids 8 and 10 of the α-chain. Human insulin is currently produced by one of two methods. The first is chemical substitution of the B30 amino acid of porcine insulin. The second involves DNA coding of *Escherichia coli* to produce separately the α- and β-chains of human insulin which are then combined *in vitro*. Earlier DNA production of proinsulin with subsequent cleavage has been abandoned.

The potency of the three insulins is very similar. So far no convincing clinical difference has been shown between human and porcine insulins *in vivo* except for a small difference in solubility, which leads to slightly quicker absorption of the human preparations. Acute experiments with bovine insulin show that it acts similarly to human and pork insulin, but it is increasingly used less frequently because of its greater antigenicity, although in this respect purity is probably more important than the species of origin of the preparation. Other insulins have been prepared, (for example fish insulin) but in general they have not been used therapeutically.

Purity

For many years insulin was prepared by acid–ethanol extraction of porcine or bovine pancreas followed by a series of isoelectric precipitations and recrystallizations. The resulting aqueous preparation was mainly insulin, but also contained small amounts of other pancreatic hormones, such as glucagon, pancreatic, and vasoactive intestinal polypeptides, as well as insulin dimers and degradation products, and significant amounts of proinsulin (1–4 per cent). In the last 20 years, purer preparations have become available. Thus, with gel filtration chromatography to remove most of the contaminants, the proinsulin content can be reduced to less than 50 ppm. However, significant amounts of desamido-insulin, arginyl insulins, and insulin ethylesters remain. These insulins are the so-called 'single-peak' or purified insulins, available now as Hypurin insulins. Further purification has been achieved by ion-exchange chromatography of the single-peak insulins. This yields 'highly purified' (so-called monocomponent or 'rarely immunogenic') insulins which contain less than 10 ppm proinsulin and insignificant amounts of other contaminants.

The significance of purity will be discussed below as an aspect of complications of insulin therapy, but a basic rule is that the less pure the preparation the greater is the antigenicity. Antibodies to insulin have been recognized for nearly 30 years in the plasma of insulin-treated diabetics. The antigenicity resides mainly in non-insulin insulin-like molecules, either natural or degraded, particularly proinsulin. Substances that prolong the action of insulin (for example protamine and zinc), also appear to increase antigenicity, perhaps acting as adjuvants. Originally the species of origin was thought to be a major factor, but highly purified bovine and porcine insulins are much less antigenic than less pure preparations. However, even in highly purified preparations

bovine insulin is slightly more antigenic than porcine insulin. Human preparations are slightly less antigenic still, but purity or local change after injection are still the most important determinants of antigenicity.

Are insulin antibodies clinically significant? One effect could be to retard the action of quick-acting insulins, with a later sustained release which may be unwanted. Such changes may be detrimental if precise glycaemic control is required, but are inconsequential if only background insulin therapy is the aim and allowance is made for the delay by injecting insulin earlier before a meal. Insulin doses are on average less in patients with low antibody titres, which is certainly an economic and possibly a clinical advantage, for with antibodies present relative hyperinsulinaemia would be expected late in the anticipated phase of action. Production of insulin antibodies may also shorten the honeymoon phase of low (or absent) insulin requirement often seen early in the course of type I diabetes. Insulin antibodies cross the placenta and may increase hypoglycaemia in the neonates of diabetic mothers. The suggestion that insulin antibodies are implicated in the development of diabetic tissue damage, particularly retinopathy and nephropathy, has not been substantiated, and indeed there was never evidence of this from humans and only indirectly from animals. Indeed, non-insulin-treated type II diabetics develop tissue damage which is qualitatively indistinguishable from that present in insulin-treated diabetics. Antibodies against insulin are found in diabetics never treated with it but at much lower levels than in those routinely treated by subcutaneous injection.

It is also questionable whether the antibodies formed to the non-insulin components of old-fashioned insulin preparations have any clinical significance. Thus antibodies to glucagon, vasoactive intestinal peptide, and somatostatin have been detected, but they have not been shown to be harmful.

Duration of action and pharmacokinetics

The other main properties of available insulins are speed and duration of action, and time of peak action. Broadly, insulins given subcutaneously can be divided into short-acting, intermediate, and long-acting preparations (Table 16), although experimental ultrafast preparations have recently been tested to try to mimic the rapid initial secretion normally occurring at the start of or early in a meal.

The duration of action depends on the site of injection. Insulin injected intravenously has a half-life in the plasma of 4–5 min and an effective half-life of 20 min. Thus if intravenous insulin is used, it must be infused continuously to produce a sustained effect. This is pertinent to the therapy of diabetics in ketoacidosis or undergoing surgery. Only short-acting insulins should be used intravenously, as the longer-acting insulins are particulate and carry a theoretical risk of embolism. Insulin may also be given intramuscularly, when the half-life of crystalline (short-acting) insulin is approximately 2 h. However, in day-to-day therapeutic use insulin is given subcutaneously, with a plasma half-life for the quick-acting preparations of 2 to 4 h in diabetics already treated with insulin but less in normal subjects. The onset of action varies from 15 to 60 min, with peak effects at 2 to 6 h and some effect for up to 8 hours, although this may exceed 12 h in patients with high antibody levels. It is probably correct to include Semitard as a short-acting insulin, although it has a somewhat slower action than the neutral insulins. It is a crystalline zinc suspension popular as a twice-daily preparation in children, but is unsuitable in totally insulin-deficient patients as it rarely acts for the required 12 to 14 h.

Absorption of insulin from subcutaneous sites is variable both within and between subjects. This makes it necessary to individualize therapy, but even then the same dose of insulin may have quite different effects on different days in the same patient. Some of the main factors affecting absorption are shown in Table 17. The effect of the type of insulin has been discussed already. The species of origin may also have an effect: human insulin preparations seem to be absorbed more rapidly than porcine insulin, which in turn is absorbed more rapidly than bovine insulin. This may reflect differences in solubility; small changes can be clinically significant.

Table 16 *Some insulin preparations available in the United Kingdom*

Type of insulin	Species	Purity	Retarding agent	Action (hours), after SC injection		
				Initial	Maximum	Total
Short-acting						
Actrapid	Human	+++	—	0.5	2–4	6–8
Human Velosulin	Human (from pig)	+++	—	0.3	2–4	6–8
Humulin S	Human	+++	—	0.3	2–4	6–8
Hypurin Neutral	Bovine	++	—	0.5–1	2–4	6–8
Velosulin	Porcine	+++	—	0.4	2–4	6–8
Intermediate						
Human Insulatard	Human	+++	Protamine	1–2	2–8	14–18
Human Monotard	Human	+++	Zinc	1–2	4–12	14–16
Humulin I	Human	+++	Protamine	1–2	2–8	14–18
Humulin Lente	Human	+++	Zinc	1–2	2–12	16–20
Human Protophane	Human	+++	Protamine	1–2	2–8	14–18
Hypurin Isophane	Bovine	++	Protamine	1–2	5–8	18
Insulatard	Porcine	+++	Protamine	1–2	2–8	16–18
Hypurin Lente	Bovine	++	Zinc	1–2	6–10	20–26
Lentard	30% porcine 70% bovine	+++	Zinc	1–3	6–12	20–26
Semitard	Porcine	+++	Zinc	1–2	4–8	10–16
Long-acting						
Human Ultratard	Human	+++	Zinc	2	8–16	30–40
Humulin Zn	Human	+++	Protamine + zinc	3	8–12	30–40
Hypurin Protamine Zinc	Bovine	++	Protamine + zinc	3	8–12	30–40
Ultratard	Bovine	+++	Zinc	3	10–30	60–80
Biphasic (or mixed)						
Human Actraphane	Human	+++	Protamine	0.4	2–10	20–24
Human Initard 50/50	Human	+++	Protamine	0.3	3–7	20–24
Human Mixtard 30/70	Human (from pig)	+++	Protamine	0.3	4–10	20–24
Humulin M1	Human	+++	Protamine	0.5–1	2–9	14–18
Humulin M4	Human	+++	Protamine	0.3–0.5	1–8	14–16
Initard 50/50	Pig	+++	Protamine	0.3	3–8	20–24
Mixtard 30/70	Pig	+++	Protamine	0.3	4–9	22–26
Pen mix 10/90	Human	+++	Protamine	0.5	2–12	20–24
Pen mix 50/50	Human	+++	Protamine	0.3	2–12	20–24
Rapitard	25% pig + 75% bovine	+++	Zinc	1	4–12	20–22

++ = purified insulin, +++ = highly purified insulin.

†Only some examples from some ranges are given.

Table 17 *Factors influencing the rate of absorption of insulin*

Type of insulin
?pH
Species
Concentration
Anatomical site (abdomen > arm > thigh)
Depth of injection
Local blood flow, as from exercise, massage, and skin
  temperature
Interaction with antibodies
?Local degradation

A more important influence on the rate of absorption is the tissue blood flow, and this varies with ambient temperature and site of injection. Absorption is quicker from the abdomen than from the arm, which in turn is quicker than from the thigh. A consistent approach should be taught to the patient. Depth of injection is also important—shallow injections are absorbed more rapidly than deeper ones, provided that the former are not intradermal and the latter are not intramuscular, which is all too easily achieved by vertical injections in thin people, particularly in the arm, unless short needles are used. Exercise, particularly of the injected part, as well as massage or hot baths, can also speed absorption to a clinically important degree. Emotional state also affects subcutaneous blood flow, as may other neuroendocrine changes. Finally, insulin may be sequestered locally by antibodies resulting in delayed absorption.

Such variations in absorption rate also apply to the intermediate and long-acting insulins. Indeed, the variability between and within patients is then greater. There are several intermediate preparations. Either protamine or zinc are used as retarding agents. The duration of action varies from 16 to 30 h with peak effect at 5 to 12 h. The duration of action is usually less than 24 h, and so these preparations must be used twice daily to provide total insulin replacement. The tard and lente insulins (mixtures of amorphous and crystalline zinc insulin) depend on zinc, whilst protamine is used for the isophane insulins. Both these agents may increase the antigenicity of insulin.

The long-acting insulins (protamine, zinc, and ultralente type insulins) have a broad peak of maximum effect and a duration of action of up to 3 days. They can be used to give a constant background of insulin but they require familiarity for easy use. Because of the long half-life several days may be required to achieve stability unless a large loading dose is given; correspondingly, if too much is given the patient may be at risk

Table 18 *Regimens for insulin therapy in diabetic patients*

Regimen	Patient group

1. Once daily
Monotard or Lente
Quick-acting plus Lente or
isophane type: Actrapid +
    Monotard
    Velosulin + Insulatard
Ultratard or Humulin Zn
	Elderly patients requiring symptomatic relief
	Non-obese type II diabetics, uncontrolled on oral agents
	Older type I patients with significant residual insulin
	    secretion*

2. Twice daily Intermediate insulin Short-acting + intermediate insulin* (e.g. Actrapid or Velosulin + Monotard or Insulatard, Ultratard once daily with Actrapid (12 h apart)	New type I diabetics Type I diabetics Pregnant diabetics

3. Three times daily
Short-acting + intermediate
insulin* with breakfast, short-
acting before evening meal,
intermediate at bedtime
Short-acting insulin* three times
daily + intermediate or long-
acting before evening meal
	Type I diabetics with morning hyperglycaemia and/or
	    nocturnal hypoglycaemia
	Labile diabetics; diabetics requiring near-perfect
	    glycaemic control

*Short-acting insulins lose some of their rapid action when mixed with insulin zinc suspensions.

of hypoglycaemia for several days. It must be emphasized that the human ultralente preparation is considerably shorter-acting than the more antigenic bovine ultralente insulin, and in some patients may not last adequately even for 24 h.

Mixed insulin preparations are also available (Table 16). These are useful when less than optimal control is sought or when mixing insulins proves difficult, but they prevent a patient from flexibly altering his insulin regimen according to glucose levels.

Routine use of insulins

If the patient is simply to be kept asymptomatic, then a once-daily regimen can be used (Table 18). Commonly this would be achieved with a single dose of an intermediate insulin of the lente or isophane type. The latter in particular carries little risk of nocturnal hypoglycaemia, an important consideration in some elderly patients. It may be necessary to add a short-acting insulin if there is severe post-breakfast hyperglycaemia.

Once-daily therapy may also be successful in type II diabetics who are not controlled satisfactorily by oral agents by using, for example, a mixture of short-acting and intermediate insulins. In such cases fasting blood glucose is the best index of the adequacy of glycaemic control. If there is persistent fasting hyperglycaemia, an additional evening injection may be required. Ultratard insulin injected once daily has also been suggested as an alternative (or adjuvant) to sulphonylurea therapy in type II diabetics, but if insulin treatment is decided upon, it is best to optimize this as sulphonylureas give no added advantage.

Most type I diabetics require two or three injections of insulin daily, as one aim of therapy is to reproduce the natural peak levels of insulin during and after meals with basal concentrations preprandially. The pharmacokinetics of insulin makes this difficult, if not impossible, to achieve when patients lack endogenous insulin secretion. The absorption of even short-acting insulin from subcutaneous tissue is slower than the physiological pancreatic responses to a meal. More important, circulating levels do not return to baseline sufficiently quickly. However, some of these disadvantages can be countered by appropriate dietary adjustments. Thus a small breakfast, with the carbohydrate mostly slowly absorbed, followed by an equivalent carbohydrate load 2 h later as a snack can match the profile from a short-acting insulin injection given in the morning. Similar dietary adjustments can be made at other times of the day.

The majority of patients can be dealt with satisfactorily using a twice-daily mixture of short-acting and intermediate insulins. Velosulin or Actrapid with Insulatard or Humulin insulins, for instance, can give excellent control, but some supplementary quick-acting insulin is usually required. Otherwise there is not a clear insulin peak at lunchtime, but this can be compensated for by a light lunch and a small mid-afternoon snack. Guidelines for modifying twice-daily insulin therapy are shown in Table 19.

The day is usually divided into unequal portions with respect to insulin injections; the morning injection may be at 7 a.m. and that before the evening meal be between 5.30 and 6.30 p.m, with the latter covering the larger nocturnal fraction of the 24 h period. Many patients on twice-daily therapy have morning hyperglycaemia, which correlates with the low levels of insulin circulating at that time. However, if additional intermediate insulin is given in the early evening, there may be nocturnal hypoglycaemia. Hence a longer-acting insulin is required in the evening, or the evening meal should be later, or a different insulin regimen is required. One successful manoeuvre is to give short-acting insulin alone before the evening meal and an intermediate insulin at bedtime.

Another pattern is the twice-daily or thrice-daily injection of short-acting insulin against a background of long-acting insulin (Ultratard or Humulin Zn). Frequent, even four times daily, injections of short-acting insulin may be particularly helpful for labile diabetics, those with early rapidly advancing tissue damage in whom excellent glycaemic control is the aim, the pregnant diabetic who is not perfectly controlled on thrice-daily therapy, or the diabetic requiring maximum flexibility in life-style. In these patients, therapy can be altered frequently depending on glucose levels and approaching events. The most popular version of this technique is to use thrice-daily quick-acting highly purified insulin injections before each meal, with additional intermediate or long-acting insulin before the evening meal.

The introduction of readily portable multidose pen injectors has been a help to many patients in increasing the flexibility of insulin administration when they are away from home. The pens also have the great

Table 19 *Guide to modification of twice-daily (short-acting and intermediate) insulin regimen*

	Pre-breakfast	Prelunch	Pre-evening meal	Bedtime
Persistent hyperglycaemia (>10 mmol/l) or glycosuria (>0.5%)	↑ Evening* intermediate 2–4 units	↑ Morning short-acting 2–4 units or decrease† breakfast or mid-morning snack	↑ Morning intermediate 2–4 units or decrease† afternoon snack	↑ Evening short-acting 2–4 units or decrease† evening snack
Persistent hypoglycaemia Symptomatic or BG <4 mmol/l	↓ Evening intermediate 2–4 units	↓ Morning short-acting 2–4 units or †increase mid–morning carbohydrate	↓ Morning intermediate 2–4 units or †increase afternoon carbohydrate	↓ Evening short-acting 2–4 units or †increase evening meal carbohydrate

BG, blood glucose

*This may result in nocturnal hypoglycaemia in which case the evening intermediate insulin should be moved to bedtime

†Carbohydrate should be increased or decreased in approximately 10 g amounts.

advantage of carrying the insulin for many injections in cartridges, thus obviating the necessity to draw up each insulin dose. For this reason they are popular with patients with a constant regimen who are injecting at home. However, the pens prevent flexible mixing of insulins, and hence many mixtures are now commercially available and a single patient may have more than one pen in his armoury.

There have been great advances in needle technology in recent years, and some needles are narrower than those used a few years ago. These needles are popular.

Most syringes are now made of plastic. When they were introduced it was implied that they could only be used once. This seems quite unnecessary and, provided that a proper standard of domestic cleanliness is applied, a syringe can be used for a week (some have lasted for a year). In those with a needle attached, it is usually the sharpness of the needle that leads to a change, perhaps after six or more injections.

There are many commercially available insulins (Table 16). It is probably best for the doctor to become conversant with the use of a few insulin preparations rather than to attempt to command the whole range, although he or she will need to know of others when caring for a patient already controlled on one of them. If a patient is well controlled by porcine rather than human or less pure preparations, there would seem to be no need for change.

When change is made from one type of insulin to another care should be taken, particularly when the change is from less pure to more pure preparations, for instance from bovine or porcine to human. If the daily dose has been modest (less than 0.7 units/kg body weight), the same amount of the new preparation may be correct, but the new preparation may be more potent. Therefore it is prudent to reduce the dose on transfer by 20 per cent if the daily total is more than 0.9 units/kg body weight and by 10 per cent if it is less. The dose can readily be adjusted upwards depending on blood glucose measurements which should be performed more frequently than usual at such a time of change.

PRACTICAL ASPECTS OF INSULIN THERAPY

Emphasis should be placed on the correct injection technique at the start of insulin therapy. Simple problems such as air bubbles in the syringe can substantially affect the amount of insulin injected. Neutral short-acting and isophane-type insulins can be mixed in the same syringe. The insulin used in the smaller dose should be drawn up first. Injections are considerably less traumatic if finer rather than blunter needles are used.

The rotation of injection sites should also be taught. This can be used to advantage if rapidly absorbing sites, such as the abdomen or arm, are used in the morning and more slowly absorbing sites, such as the thigh or buttocks, in the evening when more prolonged action is required. The initial delay in the absorption of insulin administered subcutaneously

should also be allowed for. If the insulin is given 30 min before eating, the upstroke of the resulting plasma insulin profile usually closely matches the physiological rise, but in some patients the interval between injection and eating may need to be 40 to 45 min to obtain the best glucose control. In general, when patients are first started on insulin they should be advised to inject 20 min before eating, with the interval increased if necessary as indicated by blood glucose tests 90 to 150 min after the meal. It is also important that a different injection site be used for each of at least 20 consecutive injections, because repeated injections in one place predispose to lipohypertrophy.

Initial dosage of insulin

When a patient is started on insulin, the two main indices of the required total daily dose are the prevailing blood glucose and the height and weight. Other factors involved include the degree of insulin resistance and the degree of apprehension, which may affect insulin sensitivity. However, apprehension may also decrease subcutaneous blood flow and delay the absorption of the initial injections.

Two main strategies can be employed in deciding the initial dose of insulin. One is deliberate administation of a small dose. The response can then be a help in the calculation of succeeding doses. The second approach is to calculate the expected dose from formulae based on the body mass index and the glucose level. The disadvantage here is that the formulae are derived statistically from the effects of insulin on an inhomogeneous population. The recommended doses are the means of a range of effective doses, and in a small proportion of patients a dose that is only 80 per cent of that given by the formula may be correct. Therefore some patients are liable to suffer hypoglycaemia if the formulae are adhered to rigidly.

A compromise between the two approaches is probably best. If a formula is used, it is wise to start with doses that are about 80 per cent of those calculated. If no formula is available, the patient should start on a total daily dose of 0.5 units/kg body weight, initially using a relatively rapidly acting insulin. The requirement a few days after the start of therapy is usually less than that needed to control the initial hyperglycaemia. If the patient is obese and succeeds in losing weight, the insulin doses will need to fall *pari passu*. Some patients avoid food excessively around the time of diagnosis and may need rather more insulin a week or so after the initiation of treatment as they settle down to a more appropriate calorie intake.

Complications of insulin therapy

The complications of insulin therapy are listed in Table 20. Hypoglycaemia is by far the most common and results from inadequate matching of insulin to diet and activity or the use of an inappropriate regimen. The probable time for an attack of hypoglycaemia is often predictable,

Table 20 *Complications of insulin therapy*

Hypoglycaemia
Antibody formation—?impaired control, transplacental transfer
Lipoatrophy
Lipohypertrophy
Local allergy
Generalized allergy
Insulin resistance
Insulin oedema
Sepsis

for instance late morning or late afternoon in patients taking mixed insulins twice daily. If an attack cannot be explained by some uncompensated departure from routine, the insulin dose and/or diet should be modified the next day to prevent recurrence. Apart from the unpleasantness of the attacks, a disadvantage of frequent hypoglycaemia is weight gain because of the extra carbohydrate taken to combat the attacks. Hypoglycaemia is generally correctly recognized by patients, but long-standing and/or older diabetics may lose their typical warning symptoms. The family and work-mates of a diabetic should be instructed in both the symptoms and signs of hypoglycaemia and in the action to be taken.

The second most common complication of insulin therapy is lipodystrophy, either atrophy or hypertrophy. The loss of fat at sites of insulin injection is described as lipoatrophy. It is much less common now than it was a few years ago when 25 to 75 per cent of patients treated with insulins were likely to show signs of it. At present it is most common in countries where less pure insulins are used. It may be due to immunogenic components of conventional insulin preparations which lead to the formation of either immune complexes or IgE antibody which binds locally and so stimulates lipolysis. Lipoatrophy is rare in patients who use highly purified insulins, confirming that it is caused by impurities in the older preparations. It is treated by injecting a purer insulin into the centre or edge of the atrophic area until this fills. If patients also have local allergy (see below), this may need to be treated before the lipoatrophy responds to therapy.

Lipohypertrophy is commoner than lipoatrophy in countries where most patients are treated with highly purified insulins. It is due to repeated injection at the same site, which is particularly common in children, and presumably results from continued lipid synthesis in response to a high local concentration of insulin. It is prevented by proper rotation of injection sites, and disappears with time if the patient stops injecting into the affected area. Patients are often loathe to do this, as injection into these fatty lumps is smooth and relatively painless. A further problem is that insulin absorption from these relatively avascular areas may be delayed.

Insulin allergy, either local or general, is a rare complication. The local form comprises pruritic, erythematous, indurated, and occasionally painful lesions subsequent to insulin injection. There are three distinct types. The commonest is a biphasic IgE-dependent reaction called the late-phase reaction. Arthus-type or delayed reactions also occur. Insulin impurities and the retarding agents zinc and protamine have all been implicated as causative agents. The incidence is much decreased in populations using predominantly highly purified insulins. The first step in treatment is to ensure that the lesions are not due to faulty technique, for example intradermal injection. Skin testing with different insulins, including zinc-free preparations, can then be used to find a non-reactive preparation. Oral antihistamines may also be useful. Local steroid therapy may be necessary, and the appropriate steroid can be mixed with the insulin before injection, for example 1 mg of prednisolone per millilitre of insulin preparation. Generalized allergy is extremely rare and presents classically. The antigen is usually insulin itself, and the β-chain of all commonly used insulins induces the response. The allergy responds to conventional desensitization regimens based on frequent injections starting with a very small dose.

Occasionally, insulin injection produces septic lesions. If these are recurrent, they are usually due to faulty injection technique, but occasionally the patient may be a staphylococcal carrier or have impaired antibacterial defences.

Insulin therapy is affected by the formation of insulin antibodies. High titres are more common with conventional insulins, but may still occur even with highly purified human insulin. Caucasians who carry HLA-B15, HLA-CW3, and HLA-DR4 are more likely to develop antibodies those who carry HLA-B8 or HLA-DR3. Insulin resistance is a relatively uncommon complication of insulin therapy in type I diabetics in the United Kingdom. It is not clear whether it depends upon altered immunity. Before insulins of high purity were available, it was much more common and most cases were due to high levels of antibodies. At that time it was defined as a daily insulin dose of more than 200 units. More usefully, insulin resistance can now be defined as a daily intake of more than 1.5 units/kg body weight, which is about twice the usual level necessary for full insulin replacement therapy. Obesity is its most common non-immunological cause. Treatment of this is obvious but difficult, and depends on restabilizing the patient on a lower food intake balanced by a lower insulin dose. The two should be instituted together, because the reduced requirement for insulin will occur well before any obvious weight loss. In the case of immunologically based resistance, the insulin preparation should be changed to highly purified human insulin. Failing this, systemic prednisolone may be useful, but only when the resistance is severe because of its own diabetogenic properties and other side-effects. Other forms of insulin resistance include antireceptor antibodies or elevated levels of counter-regulatory hormones.

Pseudo-insulin resistance has been recognized among patients who are overtreated with insulin, hence becoming hypoglycaemic and thus eating excessively in response, only to become hyperglycaemic and so have their insulin dose increased. Hepatomegaly is a rare clinical feature. Somogyi emphasized this clinical picture in his accounts of reduction of 24 hour urinary glucose after the total insulin dose was lowered. A dramatic improvement in glycaemic level and stability can be obtained by drastic reduction of the insulin dose and appropriate dietary advice.

Insulin oedema is rare but is extremely troublesome when it does occur. It is seen when proper glycaemic control is achieved in markedly hyperglycaemic and underweight diabetics. Marked pitting oedema may develop within 3 to 4 days of the start of insulin therapy but resolves spontaneously usually 5 to 10 days later. Occasionally the condition is so severe that pulmonary oedema occurs. The cause is unknown though there is certainly accompanying sodium retention; the plasma albumin concentration is usually normal.

Alternative methods of insulin delivery

In view of the moderate glycaemic control that is achieved in most insulin-dependent diabetics, better methods of insulin therapy have been sought (Table 21). Modern thinner and sharper needles have been more successful than jet injectors in decreasing the discomfort of injection. Otherwise the main aims have been to speed up the slow insulin absorption that occurs with conventional injection and to seek a system that will respond to ambient blood glucose by automatic provision of an appropriate insulin dose, for example via an insulin infusion pump. These pumps deliver soluble insulin subcutaneously using a fine cannula with a needle inserted under the skin which is resited every 24 to 48 h. A background infusion is given at a predetermined rate (0.5–1.2 units/ h on average). Extra boluses are delivered as desired at mealtimes, using an override switch or a manual drive. Most systems are simple syringe pumps, and the newer generation are reasonably small. Much more sophisticated programmable pumps with long-lasting insulin reservoirs are also available, but seem unnecessary for extracorporeal use. Pumps or open-loop devices should only be used in conjunction with appropriate patient education and self-monitoring (see below). Their untutored use has resulted in disaster due to hypoglycaemia and ketoacidosis. A minority of patients have found them very helpful in improving glycaemic control, but the majority who have tested them have found that

Table 21 *Alternative methods of insulin delivery in the treatment of diabetes*

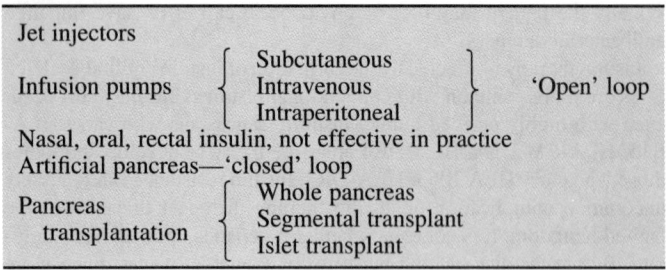

they are a physical nuisance and provide no advantage in achieving good control of blood sugar.

Pumps can also be used to deliver insulin intravenously or intraperitoneally. The intravenous route has been used occasionally in patients with brittle diabetes, but the risks of septicaemia and thrombosis are considerable even though the technique works well and is the only route whereby normal plasma insulin profiles can be reproduced accurately. Wider use is under consideration, but if the intravenous route is to be used it is logical to implant the pump to reduce the possibility of infection. This has been done in over 100 patients but alterations in the infusion rate remain a problem. A potentially more useful route for insulin delivery is via the peritoneal cavity, mimicking secretion from the pancreas into the portal venous system. With subcutaneous or intravenous therapy either the peripheral tissues receive the correct amount of insulin and less than usual reaches the liver, or the liver receives the correct amount and there is peripheral hyperinsulinaemia. Current data reveal raised peripheral insulin concentrations in insulin-treated diabetics with consequent constant reduction in lipolysis as well as other biochemical abnormalities even if the patient is normoglycaemic. More important is the possibility that hyperinsulinaemia increases the deposition and synthesis of lipid in arterial walls, potentially worsening macrovascular disease. Increased deposition of triglyceride in arteries has been shown experimentally with artificially produced peripheral hyperinsulinaemia.

Peritoneal insulin is used routinely in diabetics undergoing chronic ambulatory peritoneal dialysis. Intraperitoneal infusion from either external or implanted pumps also results in good glycaemic control with less peripheral hyperinsulinaemia. Other attempts to deliver insulin to the portal vein have used the gastrointestinal tract. Insulin given by mouth has been protected from proteolytic degradation by inclusion within liposomes, but unfortunately only a variable small number of these are absorbed. Rectal insulin suppositories are better absorbed, but this approach is unreliable and has little aesthetic appeal; it is also uncertain what fraction of absorbed insulin actually passes into the portal circulation. Recently, insulin has been given intranasally. A hypoglycaemic effect has been found, but it is of no practical value. None of these methods will be adopted as long as the absorbed fraction of the administered insulin remains very small, because a slight change in that fraction will result in a large alteration in the absolute amount of insulin entering the body.

Two major new developments are under way. The first aims at the production of an artificial endocrine pancreas comprising a glucose sensor, a small computer programmed to respond to both absolute levels of, and changes in, glucose concentration, and an insulin infusion pump directed by the computer. Effective systems are available, but they are large, expensive, and extracorporeal. It is hoped that they can be miniaturized, but the outstanding problem is the lack of a glucose sensor which is reliable and can function for a lengthy period *in vivo*. Partial advance may come from a 'needle' sensor which can be inserted subcutaneously and connected to an insulin pump outside the body, but even then there are very variable relationships between general glycaemia and the glucose concentration at a particular subcutaneous site.

Pancreatic transplantation has been successfully achieved, particularly with segmental grafts, but with poor long-term endocrine function. Most patients have received simultaneous pancreatic and renal transplants, which probably does not provide a fair assessment of the technique. Autologous islet transplants have been used more successfully in patients made diabetic by total pancreatectomy for chronic pancreatitis. Several have been independent of insulin for up to 3 years, although it is possible that there may be functioning islets in small amounts of remaining pancreas. Overall results from pancreatic and islet transplantation indicate that much more work is necessary. Rejection problems are considerable, although cyclosporin A has provided some improvement. Islet cell transplants with or without a protective porous membrane are also under continued testing, but still face many problems.

Exercise

Exercise affects glycaemic levels and so is a major factor influencing day-to-day food and insulin requirements. The diabetic should expect to be able to enjoy both exercise itself and its beneficial effects on health as much as anyone else. It can be harnessed as a tool for glycaemic control, particularly in non-insulin-treated patients in whom replacement of adipose tissue by muscle will increase the sensitivity to the insulin that they do secrete. In non-diabetics, the consumption of glucose and other fuels increases rapidly on exercise. Muscle glucose utilization increases independently of variations in insulin levels, provided that basal amounts of insulin are present. There is a parallel increase in hepatic glucose production, resulting from associated increases in glucagon and catecholamine secretion, and often a slight drop in insulin levels. Consequently, plasma glucose levels alter little. Several of these responses are absent in type I diabetics, so that in the well-controlled diabetic glucose levels fall and hypoglycaemia may result unless treatment is modified. This is particularly true in the overinsulinized diabetic. Paradoxically, in the poorly controlled diabetic (blood glucose above 12 mmol/l) blood glucose rises with exercise because of insulinopenia. Muscle glucose uptake does not increase normally, but hepatic glucose production increases supranormally. There may also be a profound increase in ketone body levels—a magnification of the normal postexercise ketosis. There is also increased insulin absorption from subcutaneous injection sites during exercise, particularly if the injection has been made into the exercising limb, probably because of increased blood flow.

Management will vary with the individual. In the mildly overweight subject it is probably wisest to decrease insulin before planned exercise; for example less intermediate insulin should be given in the morning if afternoon exercise is anticipated. The lean diabetic should take extra carbohydrate before commencing exercise and more may be necessary during prolonged exercise. It is also sensible to inject insulin into a nonexercising part of the body on the day of exercise. Hypoglycaemia may occur several hours after exercise, and patients with autonomic neuropathy may have both diminished exercise capacity and a highly abnormal metabolic response. This is best avoided by starting exercise with optimum metabolic control.

A fall in blood glucose with exercise resulting from fuel consumption, also occurs in type II diabetics. There may be a reduced catecholamine response, particularly in those with autonomic neuropathy or in the obese, which reduces the normal compensatory increase in hepatic glucose production.

Exercise can make a major contribution to glycaemic control. The obese type II diabetic may lose little weight even with intense exercise, but this will depend on how zealously dietary advice is followed, and indeed whether exercise affects appetite and food intake. The extra carbohydrate required by insulin-treated patients during exercise varies considerably from person to person, but may be surprisingly large, particularly if the exercise is prolonged and takes place outdoors in cold surroundings. If exercise is to last only 1 to 2 h, a rough and ready rule is to take 20 g of fairly quickly absorbed carbohydrate before exercise and hourly during exercise. If exercise is prolonged and strenuous, again remembering the potential effect of cold, 40 g of carbohydrate per hour may well be needed, at least half of which should be in a quick-acting form.

Education

Diabetics who know little or nothing about their disease are unlikely to maintain good day-to-day control. Self-management should be the watchword for both type I and type II patients.

A good understanding of dietary needs is important for all diabetics, who should also be well informed about the effects of exercise and alcohol and the means of self-monitoring glucose levels (see below). The patient requiring insulin not only must be taught injection technique and appropriate adjustment of dose, but should also be given guidelines on balancing insulin dose and diet to meet changes in health and lifestyle. A well-taught patient can generally cope well and will know when to seek professional help, provided that the necessary confidence has been instilled. In the elderly or long-standing diabetic, education in care of the feet is mandatory, as is advice on possible means by which the risks of cardiovascular disease may be reduced.

Diabetics can be taught in many ways. The least satisfactory is a personal interview with a physician if this is unduly brief or occurs only at the time of diagnosis. Simple booklets, films, and audiovisual aids are likely to be more helpful, but frequent reinforcement is necessary. A team of teaching nurses and dietitians may well make the greatest impact, and group teaching is often successful; a phone-in service is often useful. Crucial factors are kindness and patience from the teachers, and repetition of material which must be expressed in an appropriate manner for the particular audience. Little information is available as to the best means of educating patients, although any system is likely to reduce both acute admissions and the development of chronic foot disease. It is essential that each professional group responsible for the care of diabetic patients has a commitment to the need to teach self-care. Local circumstances and the competence of individual patients will influence the exact approaches selected.

Monitoring of therapy

Testing of urine for glucose has been the cornerstone of the assessment of metabolic control for over 50 years. The introduction of methods for home measurement of blood glucose has permitted much closer glycaemic control. Body weight is another excellent, if crude, overall index of progress. The available means of monitoring control, and others which may be used more in the future, are listed in Table 22.

Urinary glucose

Measurement of urinary glucose gives only limited information. The renal threshold for glucose varies between 7 and 12 mmol/l. In general, if results are positive, blood glucose values are at least twice normal. If tests are negative, there is no indication whether blood glucose is at the low or high end of the normal range. However, unlike a spot blood glucose test, the reading is a result of control over several hours. If short-term information is needed, a second-void specimen is tested; this technique is too troublesome for routine use and depends on the assumption that the volume of residual urine is very small.

Passing a test strip through the urine stream is the quickest and easiest of all urinary glucose tests. Glucose-specific methods such as Diastix and Diabur are preferable. Despite the inadequacies of urine testing, a patient who is persistently aglycosuric and free of hypoglycaemic symptoms may well be satisfactorily controlled.

When control is more erratic, a method (Diabur test strips) which measures up to 5 g of glucose per 100 ml urine is useful in indicating

Table 22 *Biochemical methods for monitoring effectiveness of therapy and metabolic control in diabetes*

Clinical methods	
Urine glucose	Solid state strip tests
	24 h collection or random
Urine ketones	Solid state strip tests
Blood glucose	Random clinic measurement
	Timed post-prandial
	Fasting
	In-hospital profile
	Home blood glucose monitoring
Glycosylated protein	Haemoglobin
	Albumin
	Fructosamine
Blood lipids	Cholesterol (total, HDL)
	Trigylceride
Experimental methods	
Blood metabolites	Lactate, pyruvate
	Ketone bodies, glycerol, fatty acids
Free insulin	Diurnal profiles
Flux measurements	Glucose turnover and recycling
	Ketone bodies

the degree of glycosuria. More crudely, urine diluted 1:1 with water can be tested approximately. There is also some benefit from periodic 24 h quantitative measurement of urinary glucose. This is more useful than spot testing, since the confounding effects of change in the rate of urine flow on concentration are reduced by the longer collection period.

Urinary ketones

The routine measurement of urinary ketones is not necessary in the majority of type I diabetics or in any type II diabetics. The test is useful for home monitoring of labile ketosis-prone diabetics and can serve as a guide to increased insulin need or a call for medical assistance. The available methods measure only acetone and acetoacetate and not the quantitatively important 3-hydroxybutyrate. Because of this and limited sensitivity, blood ketones may be elevated by a factor of 10–20 before the urinary test is positive. A high urinary concentration interferes to a practically important extent with the interaction of glucose with Diastix, which should therefore never be relied on in a sick patient suspected of ketoacidosis (Ketodiastix or Ketodiabur should be used instead).

Urinary protein

Chemical measurement of urinary protein using sulphosalicyclic acid was replaced long ago by 'strip' colorimetric dip methods, such as Albustix, with a threshold sensitivity of about 200 mg/dl. Persistent albuminuria at this level, in the absence of sustained infection, is crucial evidence of nephropathy and a poor prognosis. Hence more sensitive methods have been developed to measure smaller amounts of urinary albumin (microalbuminuria). Radio-immunoassay is not yet widely employed in clinical practice because of its novelty and expense, and is likely to be supplanted in routine practice by the cheaper and quicker, but much less quantitatively precise, immunoturbimetric method. The concentration of albumin varies substantially with urinary dilution, so that either a timed urine collection is made or the urinary creatinine concentration is measured simultaneously and the albumin-to-creatinine ratio is calculated. Exercise can increase urinary albumin in the absence of nephropathy, so that analysis is best performed on a timed overnight urine collection or a spot urine passed on rising from sleep. The thresholds for abnormality may still be too high, but are currently taken as about 20–30 μg/min for the mean of three timed specimens or 2–3 mg/mmol for the albumin-to-creatinine ratio from three early morning specimens.

Blood glucose

There are many different approaches to the use of blood glucose measurement to assess or control diabetes. It is of little value to measure this routinely at a diabetic clinic, generally at a random time, as patients may alter their behaviour just before a clinic appointment, be stricter with dietary compliance for the few preceding days, or indeed miss meals in order to lower their blood glucose. Conversely, a wait of 1 to 2 h in a busy clinic may cause an adrenergic hyperglycaemic response.

Fasting and timed post-prandial glucose measurements may be more useful, particularly in the type II diabetic, but the same strictures apply with regard to unusual behaviour on clinic days. There is an arguable case for not measuring blood glucose routinely in diabetic clinics, but only if arrangements are made to obtain more useful information.

The estimation of fasting blood glucose is useful in assessing control in type II diabetics. It reflects overall glycaemic control accurately but is limited in usefulness if performed only two or three times per year.

In insulin-treated type I diabetics, a single blood glucose level may give a misleading impression of glycaemic control, even on the day of measurement. Thus, with twice-daily therapy, there may be a two- to fourfold difference between blood glucose levels measured 2 h after breakfast and those measured in the late morning or late afternoon. The only useful way to use this approach to assess control in such patients is to obtain a blood glucose profile with measurements before and after each main meal. This can be done on a day clinic basis and is useful in the investigation of problem patients, but this method may be invalid if it provides a poor reflection of normal life.

Home blood glucose monitoring has revolutionized the assessment of blood glucose fluctuations, particularly in insulin-dependent diabetics. It has enabled insulin and dietary therapy to be adjusted by the patient, as well as providing a useful educational guide.

There are two main forms of home blood glucose monitoring. In one, blood from a finger-prick is collected on impregnated filter paper in containers which are delivered to the hospital laboratory or health centre for later measurement. This is useful for assessing control, but is not immediate enough for true self-management by the diabetic. The second and more commonly employed method of home blood glucose monitoring uses test strips whose colour can be read visually, so that there is no need to issue all patients with meters. However, meters are useful if greater accuracy is required, during initial education, to reduce observer bias, or for colour-blind patients. The various methods available are shown in Table 23 and now include non-colorimetric methods, for an electric current generated on the test strip determines the numerical display on the meter. Patients use small lances (Monolets) with or without an additional spring-loaded device (Autolets or Autoclix) to draw blood, and many are prepared to do this 10 to 12 times each week. Indeed, approximately two-thirds of patients prefer home blood glucose monitoring to routine daily urine testing. The frequency of home blood glucose monitoring varies between centres and patients. One common protocol is for the patient to measure blood glucose before and after each main meal and at bedtime on one weekday and one weekend day each week, with fasting and bedtime samples on the other days. Alternatively, tests are performed four times daily on two or three days per week with intermittent urine testing. Such frequent testing is unnecessary in type II diabetics, for whom periodic fasting and postprandial sampling is adequate.

The accuracy of measurements performed by patients has been questioned. Provided that the initial instructions are adequate and are then followed, results obtained by patients are at least as accurate as those of tests performed by hospital staff and are certainly accurate enough

Table 23 *Methods of home blood glucose monitoring*

1. Methods not giving immediate results
    Blood collection into containers
    Blood collection on to filter paper
2. Methods giving immediate colorimetric results
    Solid state test strips
    (a) Visual methods
    (b) Methods using meter and appropriate test strips
3. Methods giving immediate non-colorimetric result

Table 24 *Indications for home blood glucose monitoring*

Routine testing
All type I diabetics in whom precise control is desired
Younger type II diabetics
Patients with abnormal renal thresholds
Patient preference

Intensive testing
Labile and brittle diabetics
Pregnant diabetics
Problem solving, e.g. nocturnal hypoglycaemia
In association with intensive therapy, e.g. pumps, multiple injection regimens
Patient education

for clinical purposes. The educational benefits derived may also lead to improved overall control. However, not all patients are prepared to monitor blood glucose themselves. Present indications are shown in Table 24. The more cautious have surmised that more vigorous attempts to achieve good glycaemic control could lead to a catastrophic increase in hypoglycaemia. Home blood glucose monitoring has shown that this is not the case in the United Kingdom and indeed can reassure patients that they are not on the verge of hypoglycaemia. Home blood glucose monitoring is a *sine qua non* when intensive therapy is contemplated, for example subcutaneous insulin infusion, and allows all hypoglycaemic therapies to be used to their maximum potential.

Glycated haemoglobin

Measurement of glycated protein can provide useful evidence of overall glycaemic control. Haemoglobin A has been observed to be glycated post-translationally and non-enzymatically at the terminal valine of the β- chain. This produces haemoglobin A1c. There are two further minor glycation fractions, haemoglobin A1a and haemoglobin A1b. Together these three fractions are referred to as glycated haemoglobin. It is important to be accurate in describing the analytical method used, for glycated haemoglobin A1 (all three types) is present in rather larger quantities than the somewhat more relevant haemoglobin A1c. The former is assessed by chromogenic reactions, such as that with thiobarbaturic acid, while the latter is assessed by isoelectric focusing. Electrophoretic methods can give either value, but that generally used gives haemoglobin A1. Assay values should never be used without knowing the mean and standard deviation of the particular laboratory method concerned for a population found to be normal by simultaneous blood glucose measurement. Many then take the mean plus two standard deviations as indicating the limit between overall normoglycaemia and hyperglycaemia.

The percentage of haemoglobin A that is glycated is directly proportional to the time that the red cells have been exposed to glucose and the glucose concentrations. Measurement of the glycated haemoglobin fraction gives an integrated picture of the mean blood glucose level during half the average life-span of the red blood cells, i.e. 60 days. It is important that the stable irreversibly glycated form, resulting from an

Amadori condensation, is separated from the unstable intermediate formed reversibly via a Schiff base condensation which is present in relatively large amounts shortly after meals. The result depends approximately on the arithmetic means of the varying blood glucose levels over 60 days.

The result will be unduly low for a given blood glucose level if the life-span of the red blood cell is appreciably shortened, and this must be taken into account in patients with haemolytic anaemias or other conditions when the red-cell survival is significantly shortened by chronic sepsis, rheumatoid arthritis, or chronic blood loss.

Depending upon the exact method used, another source of error arises from the similar reactions between free amino groups of amino acids on the side-chains of haemoglobin and other compounds condensing with these non-enzymatically. Two examples are urea, which carbamylates the valine amino groups, and acetaldehyde, derived from ethanol, which also condenses with the amino groups. Although the plasma levels of acetaldehyde are probably always very low (at least compared with urea or glucose), acetaldehyde reacts avidly with the amino group so that formation of the condensation product is not negligible in those drinking 30 or more units of ethanol per week. These condensation compounds may move electrophoretically in very similar ways to glycated haemoglobin and may also react in the colorimetric assays, but they do not show up in tests based on the electroendosmosis technique.

The colorimetric methods can be automated and so may be much cheaper than the other tests, but they are less reliable and more likely to be affected by interfering substances such as uric acid or large amounts of vitamin C. The costs of more accurate measurements of glycated haemoglobin have resulted in an increase in the consideration given to other techniques, such as colorimetric measurements of serum fructosamine which represents the glycated component of all the plasma proteins. These proteins have a variety of half-lives in the circulation, but albumin with a half-life of 8 days is dominant. If this method is used, the result is best expressed per unit of albumin, but the albumin half-life may change substantially with a variety of physiological and pathophysiological events. Therefore fructosamine measurements have not been widely adopted.

Glycated haemoglobin gives a derived notion of the mean glucose levels over the preceding weeks, and it is possible for a normal or minimally raised value to be obtained from patients suffering frequent and dangerous episodes of hypoglycaemia if these are balanced by other episodes of excessive hyperglycaemia. The assay is of particular value in assessing those patients who give overoptimistic reports of the results of their home assessment of glucose levels and explain away high glucose levels on the day of the clinic visit by intercurrent infection or some other transient upset. However, a patient with a high value may have taken the necessary corrective measures a few days previously, and this should be allowed for.

Protein glycation and advanced glycation end-products

Excessive glycoprotein formation was once suggested as a cause of diabetic tissue damage, particularly the thickening of the basement membrane of very small blood vessels. Since then there has been a great advance in the understanding of the importance of the carbohydrate cloud or shell that surrounds many proteins, with some of the links made by compounds such as the dolichols derived from hydroxymethyl-glutaryl-CoA. There has also been a greatly increased appreciation of how widespread is non-enzymatic glycation of the free amino groups on protein side-chains. The subject has been particularly advanced by the appreciation and utilization of the glycation of haemoglobin. An increase in the protein glycation of collagen and the ocular lens proteins in diabetics was recognized in 1981. It has also been established that, at any given age, patients with diabetes have much greater glycation than normal subjects and that this depends on the duration of diagnosed diabetes. However, elderly normal subjects may have more glycation than young diabetics. This relationship between the amount of glycation and age, as between diabetics and non-diabetics, is similar to that for certain types of tissue damage including ocular cataract or collagen changes in the hand (for example Dupuytren's contracture and flexion deformity of the proximal metacarpophalangeal joint of the fifth finger). This is the basis of the old maxim of diabetes as 'accelerated ageing'.

Blood lipids

Blood lipid concentrations are important relative to the risk of macrovascular disease. Abnormally high levels must be corrected by improved glycaemic control and/or dietary advice or the use of hypolipidaemic agents (Chapter 11.6).

Experimental methods

Experimental methods of assessing therapy are listed in Table 22. These emphasize the restricted nature of current metabolic monitoring, despite the major analytical advances in recent years. If one aim of therapy is to produce more normal patterns of circulating insulin concentrations, these should be measured *pari passu* with blood glucose. This is technically difficult in insulin-treated patients if insulin antibodies are present, but an approximation can be achieved using preprecipitation of antibody–insulin complexes. This has proved invaluable in the investigation of insulin pharmacokinetics and has also confirmed the supposition that there is peripheral hyperinsulinaemia in conventionally treated diabetics, but probably unduly low insulin levels in the portal vein. Measurement of fasting insulin concentrations is useful for detecting hyperinsulinaemia in non-insulin-treated diabetics. The patient's β-cell capacity to secrete insulin and sensitivity to its hypoglycaemic effect, albeit as a percentage of a somewhat arbitrary normal level, can be calculated approximately from the fasting glucose and insulin levels. Calculations from oral glucose tolerance tests can be used similarly.

There is no reason to believe that raised blood levels of metabolites such as lactate or ketone bodies, which oscillate widely in health, contribute directly to diabetic tissue damage. Mild fasting hyperketonaemia at diagnosis (for example above 0.3 mmol/l) makes the need for insulin treatment within the next few months more likely. Lactate levels are often high during conventional insulin therapy, probably because of an excess of peripheral insulin, but they are also raised after ingesting ethanol or in patients treated with biguanides. In neither case is the rise excessive, but the combination of biguanides with excess ethanol can approach the threshold for acidosis.

As circulating substrate concentrations may be normal even though the flux in and out of cells is grossly elevated or depressed, methods for measuring the rates of appearance and disappearance of glucose, ketone bodies, and other substances have been developed. They have shown abnormalities of flux despite normal concentrations of circulating substrates. The relevance of such findings to the future clinical management of diabetic patients is unknown, but they illustrate the need to continue to seek better methods of assessing management.

Diabetic tissue damage

Diabetics are prone to many varieties of tissue damage (Table 9). This is most common in those with the highest concentrations of blood glucose, although the extent of the damage to an individual depends on the interaction of such hyperglycaemia with other factors which probably differ with different lesions. Identification of the genetic or biochemical factors which allow tissue damage in the presence of hyperglycaemia in some, but not all, patients may in time allow rigid glycaemic control to be applied selectively only to susceptible subjects, but that ideal has not been achieved yet.

A useful generalization is that development of microangiopathic lesions requires higher sustained glucose levels than those associated with an increased risk of macroangiopathy. Even so, glycaemic control must always be extremely rigorous by the standards pertaining even a few years ago. The proper target now appears to be to achieve blood glucose values below 7 mmol/l fasting and a maximum of 10–11 mmol/l throughout the day. Alternatively, the results of the American Diet Study may be considered. Reduction in the mean value for haemoglobin Alc from 9 to 1 per cent decreased the development of significant retinopathy in the primary prevention cohort by 75 per cent (from 36 to 9 per cent of subjects after 7 years) while in the secondary prevention cohort (recruited a mean of 9 years after diagnosis and with at least minimal retinopathy already present) significant deterioration in retinopathic appearance was reduced by 55 per cent (from 40 to 18 per cent of subjects after 7 years). Approximately similar reductions were seen in nephropathy as judged by microalbuminuria or clinical grade albuminuria, and in neuropathy (vibration sensitivity, autonomic fibre tests).

The development of tissue damage follows certain clinical patterns. Thus diabetic nephropathy which is severe enough to cause renal failure in a type I patient occurs mainly in individuals under the age of 50 who have had diabetes diagnosed less than 30 years previously. However, foot ulceration, particularly if mainly ischaemic in origin, is rare under the age of 45 years but is increasingly common thereafter, up to at least age 70. This is predominantly a lesion of type II diabetics. Visual disturbance in this group is more likely to be due to cataract or exudative retinopathy than to proliferative retinopathy, which is found mainly in type I diabetics, often accompanying nephropathy. Such differences may explain the trough in age-corrected diabetic mortality seen between the ages of 45 and 55 years, at which stage the more vulnerable type I diabetics will have died whereas little damage will yet have developed in type II diabetics.

It is difficult to give an accurate quantitative description of the complications of diabetes because there has not yet been a conclusive long-term cohort study to assess prevalence and incidence, and because of interacting factors, for example the factor determining the much greater frequency of peripheral vascular disease in European or North American diabetics than among the Japanese who, in contrast, have a relatively greater liability to develop severe retinopathy.

There has been an improvement in the prognosis of diabetic patients in the last 20 years. This has been well documented in Scandinavia and cannot be explained purely by improved care of such problems as myocardial infarction, peripheral vascular disease, or developing retinopathy. It probably reflects improved glycaemic control, as well as better and more active antihypertensive and hypolipidaemic treatment. Older data indicate the average expectation of life of a type I diabetic diagnosed younger than 30 years to be 29 years, with only half of them reaching the age of 50. A third of such patients had severe renal failure, although several of these died from coronary artery disease which altogether accounted for at least half the group. Expectation is now at least 35 years, with over 60 per cent reaching the age of 50.

The mortality rate of type I diabetics is about five times greater than that of the general population, with the relative risk being greater the younger the patient. It is difficult to state an exact rate for type II diabetics as this depends on accurate detection, which is a particular problem in studies undertaken before the definition of impaired glucose tolerance came into use. Estimates range upwards from the increased mortality of around 40 per cent recorded in the most widely based study which was carried out in Birmingham in the United Kingdom and recently confirmed in Oxford. Insurance company figures indicate values nearer 300 per cent, but these are not unbiased. Whatever the precise figures, the risk is larger the younger the patient. The relative risk of macroangiopathic problems is also always greater than that of mortality. Foot ulceration is a much greater cause of morbidity than in the general population, as macroangiopathy (such as cardiac infarction or cerebrovascular accident) is of death.

A recent study of deaths of diabetics aged under 50 showed that the great majority occurred above age 40, mostly from cardiac infarction but also from renal failure in the long-term type I diabetic. However, some 15 per cent were the result of acute metabolic derangement, either hyperglycaemic or hypoglycaemic (Table 25).

Table 25 *Principal causes of death in diabetics*

	Joslin Clinic 1966–1968	United Kingdom survey of deaths in diabetics under 50 years old (via death certificate)
Cardiovascular		
Cardiac causes (%)	54.6	35
Cerebral (%)	10.0	7
Other (%)	1.6	+—
Renal (%)	8.0	17
(Diabetic nephropathy (%))	(6.0)	
Infections (%)	5.9	2
Cancer (%)	12.8	7
Hepatic cirrhosis (%)	1.5	2
Hyperglycaemic coma (%)	1.0	16
Hypoglycaemia (%)	0.7	4
Suicide (%)	0.3	+—
Others (%)	3.6	10
Respiratory (%)		5
Chronic neurological (%)		3

Microangiopathy

Microvascular disease is the most serious form of tissue damage seen in diabetic populations. The two most serious forms of microangiopathy lead to diabetic retinal disease and diabetic nephropathy. Microvascular changes elsewhere probably contribute to both diabetic neuropathy and diabetic foot disease. It has been frequently suggested that poor glucose control is a major cause of microangiopathy. The Diabetes Control and Complications Trial has provided firm evidence that tight glycaemic control has a significant impact on the frequency of microvascular disease in type I diabetics but does not resolve the exact place of such intensive therapy in patients with type II diabetes. Individuals with type II diabetes may suffer problems associated with intensive insulin therapy, for example the weight gain likely to be associated with high doses of insulin and the risk of hypoglycaemic complications in those patients with macrovascular disease.

Given the evidence that hyperglycaemia may account for many of the microvascular complications seen in diabetes, it is possible to identify potential metabolic mechanisms that might contribute to pathogenesis. The aldose reductase pathway is responsible for the conversion of glucose to sorbitol, leading to the subsequent conversion of sorbitol to fructose by sorbitol dehyrogenase. Animal data suggest that aldose reductase inhibitors may reduce albuminuria and may also lower the glomerular filtration rate, which is often elevated in early diabetes, to the normal level. However, convincing human data on the benefit of these inhibitors is difficult to find. Excessive activity of the sorbitol pathway may have multiple effects leading to tissue damage. It has been suggested that tissue damage arose because of the capacity of increased sorbitol to produce osmotic effects. However, there is little evidence for this; sorbitol levels are never in excess of 2 mmol/l even after profound hyperglycaemia. Mechanisms are more likely to involve either an impairment of myoinositol uptake or alterations in diacyglycerol production. Thus the evidence that the sorbitol pathway is involved in diabetic tissue damage remains indirect and aldose reductase inhibitors have been ineffective in treating human populations.

A second mechanism which might be responsible for some forms of tissue damage is the oxidative stress that occurs at the time of glucose metabolism. Reactive oxygen can modify both lipids and proteins, and the oxidated modification of glycoproteins has been implicated in both atherosclerosis and diabetic nephropathy.

Glucose can also form Schiff bases directly with proteins and, through a non-enzymatic reaction related to glucose concentrations, convert them to Amordori products. Chemical reactions can then also lead to advanced glycation end-products and the accumulation of these is increased in diabetes. In animal models, inhibition of advanced glycation end-products limits basement membrane thickening. It has been suggested that the glycation of amino groups can alter the rate at which free radicals are produced, potentially adding to tissue damage.

The *de novo* synthesis of diacylglycerol leading to protein kinase C has been suggested as having a role in microvascular disease in diabetics. Protein kinase C has many functions within the cell, and dissecting exactly the mechanism by which increased diacylglycerol synthesis might lead to complications has proved difficult. One of the many functions of protein kinase C is the activation of phospholipase A2 which may alter prostaglandin synthesis in the diabetic kidney. This may in turn account for some of the effects such as hyperfiltration seen in diabetic nephropathy.

Despite the interest in metabolic events leading to diabetic tissue damage and a variety of candidate mechanisms for this process, little convincing data for human populations have been produced to support the role of any single pathway, and it is likely that multiple events are responsible for the ensuing tissue damage.

Diabetic nephropathy

The risk of nephropathy in type I diabetics appears to be 30–40 per cent and similar figures are probably applicable to type II patients. The mechanism of diabetic nephropathy remains uncertain, although clear data are available to suggest that there is a significant inherited component to susceptibility to this form of tissue damage. This subject is discussed further in Section 20.

Diabetic eye disease

Twenty to thirty years ago diabetic eye disease was the main cause of blindness in the United Kingdom between the ages of 20 and 65 years. It is largely due to diabetic retinopathy or cataract. Other less frequent causes are glaucoma associated with rubeosis iridis and thrombotic occlusion of the retinal vein or artery. The prevalence of open-angle glaucoma is probably increased in diabetics. This subject is discussed further in Section 26.

DIABETIC RETINOPATHY

Diabetic retinopathy almost certainly has a multifactorial pathogenesis. There are changes in the endothelial cells, thickening of the capillary basement membranes, and a decreased number of intramural pericytes, together with tissue hypoxia and increased retinal blood flow. All these, together with increased permeability of the blood–retina barrier (measurable in one respect by fluorescein leakage), are the most likely factors underlying the occurrence of haemorrhages, exudates, and oedema.

Somehow the retinal changes lead to blockage of capillaries and arterioles with reduced blood flow and non-perfusion of certain areas. The veins draining such areas may become uneven in diameter and show increased tortuosity, while vessels close to the non-perfused area show abnormal permeability with a risk of development of surrounding oedema and fatty deposits (the basis of retinal exudates). New blood vessels develop at the margins of such areas. There is little risk of serious visual loss from peripheral neovascularization or from small degrees of neovascularization which are not associated with previous haemorrhage, but marked neovascularization (particularly on or very close to the optic disc) is associated with rapidly advancing retinopathy. The stimulus for such neovascularization (perhaps a vascular growth factor) is believed to arise from ischaemic retina and presumably reaches the affected vessels by diffusion.

Retinopathy can be divided into three types:

(1) simple 'background' retinopathy which is harmless in itself and is often present without substantial alteration for many years, but is nearly always observed before either of the two other vision-threatening types of retinopathy;

(2) proliferative retinopathy which is associated with neovascularization, vitreous haemorrhage, fibrous overgrowth, retinitis proliferans, and retinal detachment;

(3) exudative retinopathy which only threatens vision severely when the macula lutea is involved by either oedema or exudates.

Simple retinopathy

This has a number of ophthalmoscopic features ranging from small red dots (microaneurysms or dot haemorrhages) to much larger, although still usually regular, red 'blot haemorrhages'. There may also be small areas of exudate, either cottonwool spots (prognostically worrying, as these indicate areas of retinal ischaemia) or small 'fatty' exudates, either circular or crescent-shaped and usually slightly yellow in colour. There may be an increase in the size and tortuosity of the veins.

There are many data which associate an increased risk of retinopathy with higher blood glucose values, and the recent DCCT American study of type I diabetics has proved that lower glucose levels are associated with less retinopathy. In a randomized trial between poor and moderately good glucose control by insulin of experimental diabetes in dogs, Engerman and Bloodworth have shown that those with the higher glucose values (who had received less insulin) had marked retinopathy after 5 years, while the others showed little. More recently, Engerman has obtained experimental confirmation of a long-standing clinical observation that the imposition of tighter glycaemic control after a period of loose control (2.5 years in his dogs) gives little advantage over higher glucose levels throughout. This emphasizes the progressive tendency of established retinopathy, and shows that the momentum to deterioration may be established relatively early and then be relatively resistant to close glycaemic control. This accords with the increase in visible retinopathy, particularly cottonwool exudates, seen in patients with established background retinopathy brought rapidly to normoglycaemia by continuous subcutaneous infusion. This degeneration is transient, and tight glycaemic control carries no ill effects after 2 or 3 years (and indeed may have some benefit). However, the real aim is to prevent substantial amounts of retinopathy from ever developing by ensuring that there is adequate glycaemic control throughout. Various studies indicate an almost continuous relationship between glycaemic control and the prevalence of background retinopathy such that a fasting plasma glucose level of 6 mmol/l, a mean glucose level of 8.5 mmol/l, or a glycated haemoglobin A1c value of 7.5 per cent (upper limit of normal range is 6.0 per cent) should markedly restrain the development of background retinopathy, while a haemoglobin A1c value below 8 per cent (enzyme immunoassay method with normal range 2.9–4.8 per cent should markedly restrict the development of proliferative retinopathy (Fig. 8).

Proliferative retinopathy

This is dominated by neovascularization and evidence of preretinal, usually vitreous, haemorrhage. Neovascularization is recognized by an increased density of fine arteriolar elements arranged in a disorganized fashion, as in a crazy lattice. Such areas are often smaller than a quarter of the optic disc, but may be larger and are often widespread throughout the retina. They are particularly likely to be seen close to the disc or even on it. Vitreous haemorrhages vary widely in size, but are rarely as small as a typical subhyaloid haemorrhage, as seen in subarachnoid haemorrhage. They usually resolve over 2 to 4 months, with complete remission even if the initial loss of vision was complete. However, any single haemorrhage, and particularly repeated haemorrhages, may become 'organized', with forward spread of fibrous elements, often as a sheet running at right angles to the retina. This is liable both to cause a retinal detachment and to be a source of further vitreous haemorrhage, as the vessels growing forward over these fibrous sheets are particularly fragile.

No single feature of diabetic proliferative retinopathy is unique, but the evolution of retinal change is characteristic. However, similar features are seen in hypertensive retinopathy and in the reaction to ischaemic areas of retina as are present after fat embolus, in sickle-cell disease, after venous occlusion, and in the hyperviscosity syndrome.

Hypertension exacerbates background and proliferative retinopathy, but smoking is believed to exacerbate only the latter. There have been claims that increased ocular tension may retard the development of retinopathy, but this is unproven.

Exudative retinopathy

This may present as either macular oedema or macular exudates or, much less seriously for vision, with exudates away from the macula. Of the serious forms of retinopathy, macular oedema is the most difficult to recognize ophthalmoscopically, and so any deterioration of visual acuity in a diabetic should be taken seriously until the cause is determined with reference to a specialist ophthalmologist if required. The retina shows a glazed appearance, with some diminution of vascular calibre and number, which is not necessarily accompanied by any obvious focal feature such as haemorrhage or exudate. Exudates are particularly liable to occur as crescents just lateral to the macula, but they may be sited anywhere. They should be distinguished from the usually smaller and highly refractile cholesterol deposits in the walls of vessels, particularly where they bifurcate. These obviously indicate vascular change but are usually less directly related to visual disturbance. Fluorescein angiography may be particularly helpful in assessing the probable course of oedema or exudates by indicating the nature of the vascular pattern close to them and whether there is markedly increased permeability. This can be particularly helpful in deciding whether to coagulate vessels believed to be responsible for the formation of perimacular exudates. While exudative retinopathy is usually accompanied by background haemorrhagic lesions, when exudates occur alone the patient often has clinical features more typically linked with macro- rather than microangiopathy (for example in a male with only mildly raised glucose levels but relatively high insulin levels).

MANAGEMENT

The corrected visual acuity should be assessed in each eye separately in every diabetic 1 to 3 months from diagnosis to allow the temporary, but not uncommon, refractile disturbance (due to rapid onset of hyperglycaemia) to settle. The fundi should be examined after pupillary dilation because about a third of abnormalities are missed in examination through undilated pupils. Non-mydriatic fundal cameras are not as satisfactory although they provide a permanent record when satisfactory pictures are obtained and are obviously better than inadequate ophthalmoscopy. In patients aged under 40 years, checks should be carried out at intervals of 2 years until 10 years after diagnosis when annual checks should start. Annual review is wise in all those diagnosed over the age of 40 years. Some 4 per cent of diabetics have clinically observable retinopathy at diagnosis, and some 15 per cent on retinal photography, and nearly all these are type II patients aged at least 50 years old. Younger patients are more prone to develop proliferative retinopathy, and older patients to show exudative changes with insidious visual disturbance from macular exudate or oedema. A minority (perhaps 10–15 per cent of type I patients) can be diabetic for 40 or 50 years without any ophthalmoscopic sign of retinopathy. Background retinopathy commonly develops 10 to 20 years after the disease is recognized, but often never progresses to threaten vision. Minor ophthalmoscopic features (such as microaneurysms) may disappear, but this does not always indicate improvement for fluorescein angiography may show reduced perfusion. However, even fluorescein examination often shows that the deterioration ceases spontaneously. Proliferative retinopathy may become much worse during pregnancy, but such deterioration usually regresses substantially after delivery unless an irreversible lesion has occurred, for example organization of a vitreous haemorrhage.

It is not known how background retinopathy evolves into a vision-threatening form, and although this is related to blood glucose levels, these are not the sole cause. The deterioration must involve individual constitution (as indicated by identical twin studies), and physical stress (for example infection), hormonal stress (for example pregnancy), or emotional stress may be temporarily implicated.

The crux of management is that any drop in a patient's visual acuity (of one eye tested separately) that cannot be explained by any examination that the carer is competent to perform must cause referral of the patient to an appropriate expert. Treatment performed relatively early is

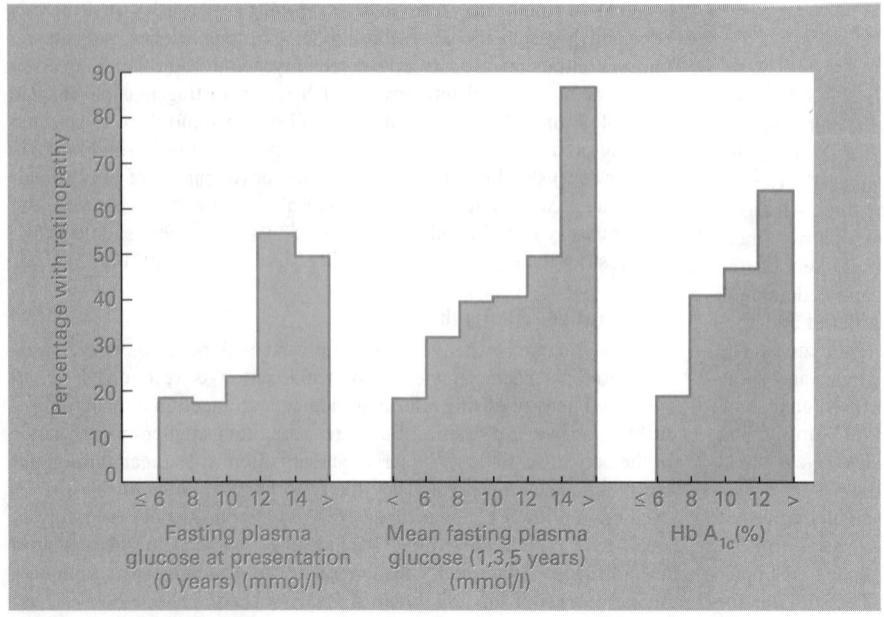

Fig. 8 Effects of control of blood glucose on diabetic retinopathy 7 to 9 years after diagnosis of NIDDM patients.

more effective than treatment at a late and almost irreversible stage. It is not known at present whether photocoagulation can be beneficial at the stage of mild background retinopathy, but probably the main demand is for improved glycaemic control.

TREATMENT

Blood glucose must be controlled as closely as possible.

1. The fasting blood glucose may need to be consistently below 7 mmol/l and the post-prandial blood glucose value below 9 mmol/l if the risk of retinopathy is to be reduced substantially. Such a target requires much work by both the patient and his advisors, but it is achievable by some type I diabetics with careful monitoring and flexible use of insulin and diet. It should be achieved by many type II diabetics, at least for a period of several years, if they follow the necessary dietary advice.

2. Attention must be paid to contributory factors such as blood pressure and hyperlipidaemia. High lipid levels are likely to increase the liability to retinal exudates, although this has not been shown directly, and they will certainly affect both viscosity and liability to blood coagulation or aggregation.

3. The retina can be photocoagulated by either xenon or argon arcs. The former gives a larger lesion and is absorbed deeper in the retina than the argon beam, which is absorbed by intravascular haemoglobin. Hence a xenon arc may be preferable for widespread peripheral ablation, while an argon beam is certainly better for accurate coagulation of small vessels from which a vitreous haemorrhage may occur and for destroying that part of the retina that may serve as the source of the putative vasoproliferative factor discussed above. The treatment is paradoxical in that it mimics the disease by reducing blood flow by blocking vessels, but its specific aims are both to attack selectively vessels particularly likely to cause retinal haemorrhage and to reduce overproduction of the postulated vaso-active factors. The aim is to preserve the function of the crucial central retinal areas, even if this involves destruction of less important peripheral regions. Photocoagulation has been shown to be effective in randomized controlled trials in both the United States and the United Kingdom. Its use was associated with a decrease of some 60 per cent over the following 5 years in the incidence of blindness both in patients with severe proliferative retinopathy and when perimacular lesions threatened function. In untreated eyes of this second group, loss of vision was not always associated with progression of the macular lesion but sometimes with associated proliferative complications. Once retinitis proliferans has become established, or retinal detachment has occurred, or large exudates have developed close to the macula, treatment has no effect. Similarly, and as with high levels of proteinuria in diabetic nephropathy, it is probable that improved glycaemic control will no longer retard deterioration once substantial retinopathy is established.

4. Vitrectomy has been developed as a treatment for blindness due to unresolved vitreous haemorrhage and as a treatment of retinal detachment subsequent to vitreous haemorrhage. Therefore specialist opinion may well be required before diabetics who have been blind in one eye for as long as 5 years are considered to have irreversible loss of sight.

5. Pituitary ablation has been used in the past to prevent the production of growth hormone and perhaps prolactin, although the exact role of diminished gonadotrophin secretion (with secondary changes in sex steroid levels) was never fully elucidated. Hypophysectomy is followed by a decrease in capillary fragility, as tested on small blood vessels in the skin by suction; this may be secondary to changes in catecholamine levels, although recent animal studies show that the permeability of newly formed small vessels is decreased by gonadectomy. In two small studies hypophysectomy was found to be beneficial against severe proliferative retinopathy, but it is unsuitable for patients aged over 40 years. It also requires the patient to cope with the subsequent increased insulin sensitivity, and is only feasible when there is unusually well-preserved renal function despite severe retinopathy. Nowadays photocoagulation is almost always the treatment of choice, as hypophysectomy produces so much endocrine disturbance.

OCULAR CATARACT

As with some other types of tissue damage, there is both a specific 'diabetic' lesion and an increased incidence of a severe, common, but non-specific lesion.

The metabolic or 'snowflake' cataract of poorly controlled juvenile diabetics is much less common than in the past. It may be seen at first diagnosis of type I diabetes, but more often after a few years of poor glycaemic control. It may be very severe, causing blindness within a few days, but it can be reversed by early successful blood glucose control. Such a cataract can be extracted if it progresses, but this is very rarely necessary.

The common accelerated 'senile' cataract, which leads to a disproportionate frequency of diabetics among those operated on for cataract, is very different. The overall prevalence of cataract seems no higher among diabetics than non-diabetics, but the former develop it earlier. On average, diabetics presenting for cataract extraction are 5 years younger than non-diabetics. If a cataract starts, it extends more rapidly and interferes more with vision among diabetics. Around 50 per cent of diabetics diagnosed more than 20 years previously have some lens opacity visible on examination, while the frequency of cataract extraction among diabetics is perhaps six times that in the general population. Operative results are almost as good in diabetics as in non-diabetics, although particular care must be taken to guard against infection. Lens opacities are more common in diabetic women than in men, and women show a faster progression of cataract.

Mild lens opacities may disappear during a period of tight glucose control but cataracts usually develop slowly until extraction is required. With a dense cataract it is always difficult to know whether diabetic retinopathy may have developed during its maturation. However, retinopathy accounts for blindness after extraction in only one-third of retinopaths from whom a lens is removed.

Although it is hoped that a medical treatment of cataract will be developed, surgery still remains the only effective method. Lens implantation is now common, with less call for the very strong lenses required previously. Another major change is that patients are now discharged on the same day as or the day after operation.

Despite the sugar alcohol (sorbitol) hypothesis for cataract formation, no effective enzyme inhibitor treatment has been developed for humans although in experimental animals an inhibitor has been found to reduce lens opacities in experimental galactosaemia in which dulcitol, the corresponding sugar alcohol, accumulates. The failure of treatment to date may be because it has not been started early enough or because the enzyme inhibitors used in the current therapies are not sufficiently potent. However, it is also possible that the sorbitol hypothesis does not apply to accelerated 'senile' cataract even if it is valid for the 'rare' snowflake cataract. Protein glycation or some other mechanism may be the explanation.

OTHER ABNORMALITIES

When there is marked hypertriglyceridaemia from any cause, but most commonly associated with ketoacidosis, the retinal arteries appear creamy. This lipaemia retinalis usually resolves within a few days with usual metabolic treatment and is not itself dangerous.

Hyaline asterosis, i.e. a snowstorm appearance in the vitreous humour, is another unusual appearance which may cause concern. Surprisingly, vision is not obscured. It is debatable whether the condition is more common in diabetics than in non-diabetics.

Rubeosis iridis is caused by proliferative microangiopathy of the iris and is usually seen only in patients with severe retinopathy. The lesion may interfere with normal drainage of aqueous humour from the anterior chamber and can lead to acute glaucoma and blindness if untreated.

Retinal artery or venous thrombosis does not seem to be particularly associated with diabetic retinopathy although, as with other vascular disorders, it may be more commoner among diabetics than in the general population.

Neuropathy

Diabetic peripheral neuropathy affects the axonal processes of somatic and autonomic neurones. It is debatable whether there is also primary neuropathy within the central nervous system. An increased liability to cerebral and presumably spinal arterial disease is widely accepted, as is the possibility of damage due to hypoglycaemia, particularly to certain layers of the cerebral cortex.

Peripheral neuropathy is both common and symptomatic, but it is more often annoying rather than life-threatening. It contributes to much of the foot ulceration of diabetics and is the cause of the uncommon Charcot's neuroarthropathy. Autonomic neuropathy is also essentially a nuisance initially, but later causes major morbidity and may even result in fatal complications. Thus, although severe postural hypotension is uncommon, disorders in the motility of stomach, large bowel, or urinary bladder can all be distressing, and predispose to infection or malnutrition, as well as carrying a poor prognosis. Impotence is particularly distressing.

The most important factor in the development of neuropathy is probably the duration of diabetes. The time since diabetes was diagnosed is usually the only index of this that is available, although other features may be used as weighting factors, for example the duration of typical symptoms at diagnosis or the fall in weight at that time from its highest remembered value. In diabetics aged 40 years or more, who have been diagnosed for at least 20 years, it is uncommon for there to be no evidence of peripheral neuropathy even though it may have little effect on the patient. The frequency of excruciating dysaesthesiae has been estimated at 3 per cent, that of incapacitating proximal neuropathy in at least one leg at 7 per cent, that of feet so numb that they are at real risk of traumatic ulceration at 24 per cent, that of diabetic bowel disturbance at 28 per cent, and that of impotence (males only) at 40 per cent. In contrast, at any one time each clinic will usually contain only two or three patients with severe postural hypotension, and urinary retention severe enough for operation is rare.

Some of the electrical properties of peripheral nerves, especially their conduction velocity, are altered by diabetes. Treatment, at least of newly diagnosed type I diabetics, can produce substantial improvement within 3 to 4 weeks although normality is not restored. Recent studies of large-fibre peripheral neuropathy in the legs have shown a positive correlation between glycaemic control over 5 years and the average degree of deterioration in vibration sense. This applied across a range of mean fasting glucose of 5–12 mmol/l. However, glucose levels are not the only factor contributing to the neuropathy; for example women are less affected than men. Impairment already present at diagnosis of type II patients is strongly correlated with that persisting 3 to 5 years later.

The pathogenesis of diabetic neuropathy is multiple. In addition to vascular lesions and segmental demyelination, there are abnormalities of both axoplasmic transport and the mechanism generating the action current, and perhaps also of the nodal membranes. One hypothesis proposed to explain Schwann cell and myelin abnormalities is an excessive entry of glucose into the glucose 6-phosphate pathway, with a resulting increase in sorbitol. This sugar alcohol largely remains where it is formed, for example within the ocular lens or Schwann cell. The high sorbitol content of the peripheral nerves of diabetics is not in doubt, and one argument for the involvement of sorbitol is slightly improved peripheral nerve conduction in animals with experimental diabetes given aldose reductase. Lens opacities in animals can also be partially reversed by such an inhibitor. The sorbitol excess hypothesis may be better stated in terms of inositol deficiency, for the former leads to the latter. Inositol is essential for phosphoinositide synthesis and the formation of diacylglycerol, which is an important activator of protein kinase C. Increased glycosylation of myelin is another potential pathogenetic process.

CLASSIFICATION (Table 26)

1. Somatic sensory neuropathy involves both large fibres, such as those serving the modalities of joint position and vibration and contributing to that of touch, and small fibres, which serve as pain and temperature sensors as well as contributing to touch. This type of neuropathy is almost always largely symmetrical and affects both the arms and the legs, but the latter predominantly. It is responsible for the loss of tendon jerks, first at the ankles.

2. Mononeuropathy can result from pressure palsy or from a vascular accident to a nerve. Both motor and sensory nerves are unduly vulnerable to pressure in diabetics. Occasionally, clinical episodes occur that suggest a stroke affecting a peripheral nerve, with excruciating short-lived pain followed by interrupted nerve function, but more commonly the onset is insidious. If biopsy or postmortem specimens are examined microscopically, obstruction of the vasa nervorum is common in this condition, particularly with either femoral neuropathy or palsy of cranial nerve III. Mononeuropathy may be multiple, giving the clinical picture of mononeuritis multiplex, with interruption of more than one peripheral nerve trunk, otherwise seen in disorders such as polyarteritis nodosa or sarcoidosis.

3. Motor neuropathy affects proximal nerves asymmetrically and usually involves part of the femoral plexus. Some clinicians believe that this is a special example of mononeuropathy, but it may be too widespread to make this likely. Motor neuropathy accompanies somatic sensory neuropathy, but is less obtrusive. It reduces nerve conduction velocity and may partially impair muscle function.

4. Autonomic neuropathy affects small afferent and efferent unmedullated fibres. Sweat tests often reveal its presence earlier than somatic sensory loss is apparent. The defect often has a more patchy distribution than somatic sensory neuropathy.

CLINICAL FEATURES AND MANAGEMENT

Peripheral sensory neuropathy

Large-fibre disease is clinically demonstrable as decreased appreciation of vibration (at a frequency of 128 Hz) or loss of ankle jerks even after reinforcement. More importantly to the patient, it underlies loss of joint position sense. It is uncommon for this to be severe enough to interfere with walking, but occasionally it produces a pseudotabetic picture. Postural loss also contributes to the gross disorganization of the small joints of the foot in Charcot's neuroarthropathy, but loss of pain is probably even more important. Large-fibre neuropathy also contributes to numb feet, with the feeling early on that the subject is walking on a bed of feathers or a thick-pile carpet, and later a total loss of appreciation of the underlying surface so that vision becomes unusually important in maintaining the gait.

Small-fibre damage causes loss of normal sensibility to pain, clinically demonstrated by pinprick. Curiously some patients will show

Table 26 *Diabetic neuropathies*

Type	Structure involved	Main parts affected
Radiculopathy	Nerve root	
Mononeuropathy	Mixed spinal or cranial nerve	Single dermatome
	Nerve terminal	Arm, leg, cranial nerves III, IV, VI, X, XII
Polyneuropathy	Sensory and motor fibres	Feet
Amyotrophy	Motor fibres	Quadriceps, gluteal muscles, hamstrings
	?Ventral ham cells	
Autonomic neuropathy	Sympathetic ganglia and fibres	Cardiovascular
		Gastrointestinal
		Bladder
		Impotence

impairment of this with little evidence of large-fibre neuropathy while others show the reverse, although commonly both modalities are affected. Small-fibre neuropathy probably underlies the troublesome dysaesthesiae of diabetics, which range from feelings of numbness or compression via bizarre sensations of warmth or cold to the common tingling, pricking, or diffuse irritability. In a few the discomfort is excruciating and they are totally incapacitated, spending hours sitting with their feet either in bowls of cold water or raised high against a wall. This indicates a contribution to the symptoms from the local blood flow, which may well be affected by accompanying autonomic neuropathy.

Small fibre neuropathy also reduces or abolishes temperature sensation. This is rarely clinically important, except for the increased risk of burns or frost-bite. The former requires the usually more normal hand to be used as a tester, while the latter, exaggerated if there is poor circulation, requires warm, well-fitting clothing and general caution.

Most dysaesthesiae become more obtrusive as the patient settles for sleep or later in the night, and hence interfere severely with rest. The most successful management consists in a combination of simple sedation or analgesia, although the latter alone is rarely very effective, with identification of exacerbating physical factors. These probably involve an interaction between the neuropathy and the peripheral circulation, for there is often significant arteriovenous shunting and impaired microcirculation. Many find relief by sleeping with their feet exposed, but others are helped more by bedsocks. Again, several are helped by raising the foot of the bed on blocks, while in others raising the head is more successful. There is no fixed relationship between which manoeuvre will be successful and the presence or absence of foot pulses, except that an erythromelalgic picture with retained and even bounding peripheral pulses, and a reddish-blue but often cool foot is more likely to be helped by cool surroundings and foot elevation. As with any chronic sensory upset, it is important to prevent the patient from becoming unduly attentive to the sensation. Any successful distraction may be helpful. The patients may be depressed, whether as cause or effect. Antidepressant drugs may then relieve the symptoms, while improvement in disadvantageous social factors can also be important.

One comforting aspect of the prognosis is that, as the neuropathy worsens and the foot becomes more numb, the dysaesthesiae lessen. However, the advice classically given to all diabetics to take good care of their feet then becomes critically important; they must both wear well-fitting shoes and avoid unnecessary trauma to the feet. Even more important, they should inspect otherwise invisible parts of the foot each evening to ensure absence of any break in the skin or consequent infection. If their vision is impaired, they must ask relatives or friends to do this for them. Advice on foot care is often only given to young diabetics at diagnosis, when both the nerves and circulation to the feet are excellent, so that it is often forgotten or disregarded when it is really needed.

The hands are only rarely seriously involved clinically, although paraesthesiae of recent onset are more common at diagnosis in the hands than the feet. Diabetics are possibly more liable than others to nocturnal or early morning tingling of the fingers, but otherwise dysaesthesiae in the hands are rare. Uncommonly, diabetics may develop a painful swollen hand with discoloured clammy skin, altogether suggestive of rheumatoid arthritis (diabetic cheiroarthropathy). However, the typical joint deformities are absent, while muscle wasting is more localized than the generalized involvement in relation to every severely affected joint of the rheumatoid. Such hands may suggest the causalgic syndrome and are presumably due to neuropathy, not least of the vasomotor nerves. Sympathectomy is not a successful treatment of this or other forms of diabetic dysaesthesiae.

Femoral neuropathy (proximal motor neuropathy)

This is typically of rapid onset and is very rare in young type I diabetics. In diabetics aged over 50 years it usually causes weakness at the hip and knee, but seldom affects those on insulin treatment. It develops within a few days or sometimes more suddenly. Within weeks or months the other leg is often affected, but one is usually substantially worse. The thighs may be uncomfortable or even intensely painful. There may or may not be accompanying peripheral sensorimotor neuropathy. The lesion can be severe enough to prevent walking, even with a supporting frame. Rising from a chair or climbing stairs is often severely affected. However, there is excellent long-term prognosis, for within 12 to 24 months the patient is usually walking again, albeit with one or two sticks, because a substantial but mostly incomplete recovery is the rule. In the same way patients usually recover substantially from external ophthalmoplegia, so that one can confidently expect loss of diplopia in 3 to 9 months.

The affected muscles waste and uncommonly fasiculate. The tendon jerk is lost or retained as a flicker. There is no reason to believe that forced or excessive exercise speeds recovery. However, passive movement is essential to preserve the neighbouring joints, and some practice in voluntary effort is almost certainly a help. It is very rare for the proximal shoulder muscles to be affected, and when these are involved in a diabetic it may well be a coincidence of diabetes with neuralgic amyotrophy. More widespread and even entirely distal motor lesions may be seen along with marked weight loss. This is sometimes termed 'diabetic cachexia' and may be severe enough to provoke an overzealous search for malignancy. These lesions may represent pressure palsies of vulnerable nerves. This condition is usually seen in insulin-dependent type I patients, sometimes quite soon after diagnosis.

Diabetic mononeuropathy

The typical pressure mononeuropathies occur in the median nerve in the carpal tunnel, the lateral popliteal nerve just below the knee, the cervical spinal roots as they pass through the spinal foramina, and the first thoracic root if a cervical rib (or corresponding fibrous structure) is present. However, sometimes the lesion probably results from a vascular accident to a peripheral or cranial nerve. Its onset is then sudden and occasionally, when the nerve has a substantial somatic sensory component, is accompanied by a severe lancinating pain of very short duration. The cranial nerves most often affected are the oculomotor nerves, particularly III or VI, but mononeuritides of the hypoglossal and recurrent laryngeal nerves, and an intercostal nerve, have been described in diabetics. More than one of these lesions may occur in a single patient, who may even have symptoms from both simultaneously.

Autonomic neuropathy

This can affect nerves anywhere in the body. It is uncertain whether it most affects the longest nerves, as do somatic sensory lesions. The degree of autonomic neuropathy of vasomotor nerves, for example in the feet, is uncertain. The main clinical pictures due to diabetic autonomic neuropathy are as follows.

Postural hypotension

This is rare but can be dramatic, with syncope and collapse on standing at its worst. The effect of a given degree of venous vasomotor failure will vary with circumstances. Thus, if there has been a spell of heavy glycosuria with loss of sodium and water, the circulating blood volume may have dropped and postural hypotension be more likely. A similar exacerbation may occur 30 min to 2 h after subcutaneous injection of insulin owing to increased transcapillary passage of albumin, again with a reduction in circulating blood volume although by no more than 5 per cent. This is asymptomatic when autonomic function is normal. The vasodilatation that occurs during hot weather or a febrile illness may exacerbate the symptoms similarly, as may a temporary disturbance caused by spinal herpes zoster.

Treatment is by simple management. For example, the patient should change slowly from a lying to a sitting position by sitting on the edge of the bed and exercising the legs for a minute before standing. This is particularly necessary if patients wake at night to pass urine. Sitting on the lavatory during and after micturition may prevent associated syncope. Glycosuric natriuresis should be avoided. Otherwise treatment is as described under chronic autonomic failure. Elastic bandages or antigravity suits must be applied with caution if there is impairment of the arterial supply to the feet.

Impotence

Diabetics may become impotent insidiously or suddenly through failure of the autonomic functions controlling erection. The role of the peptidergic nervous system in all these autonomic lesions is still unknown, but a marked deficiency in tissue concentration of vasoactive intestinal peptide has been shown in impotence. It is uncertain whether this is closely related to mechanisms including endothelium-derived relaxing factor (nitric oxide), but locally acting vasomotor transmitters are almost certainly involved. Libido is normal, and there is often other evidence of autonomic neuropathy. Again, there is often accompanying somatic sensory neuropathy, but autonomic neuropathy may be present without clinical evidence of this. The cremasteric or bulbocavernous reflexes may be tested; their absence certainly supports the diagnosis of organic neuropathic impotence but their presence by no means excludes it.

The differential diagnosis is from behavioural, psychic, or functional impotence and other organic causes, of which the most important are pelvic arteriosclerosis and endocrine disease of either the testes or the pituitary. Occasionally the endocrine disease may be part of an autoimmune syndrome with the islets of Langerhans and either the pituitary or testes affected. More often it is a coincidence of a more common unrelated disease, for example Klinefelter's syndrome or pituitary tumour, with the diabetes.

Impotence of higher central nervous origin is common, and may stem from emotional disturbance from the diagnosis of diabetes itself either because this has diminished self-image or because the patient has heard that the disease may produce impotence. Onset of type I diabetes of any severity may cause a temporary organic impotence because of general weakness and the catabolic state, and this may be confused with long-term disability. Balanitis at the time of diagnosis or later may also lead to undue anxiety over erection and intercourse, which may also occur in the husbands of diabetics with pruritus vulvae. Later in the disease a temporary period of impotence, from intercurrent disease, exacerbation of hyperglycaemia, or functional causes, may be made permanent by overwhelming anxiety. Impotence occasionally arises from a horror that any children may develop diabetes.

A careful history is important in management, regarding both erections other than with the spouse and possible causes of emotional upset in either the marriage or the patient. Much depends upon the attitude of the partner, and it is important that she should not confuse a temporary or even long-lasting period of impotence with loss of affection. Marriage guidance counselling should be freely recommended. However, to help clarify the situation the plasma prolactin concentration should first be determined to exclude hyperprolactinaemia as a rare cause, and other endocrine tests should be performed if there are suggestive features.

Nocturnal penile plethysmography records expansion of the base of the penis during sleep, as normally happens during the recurrent phases of rapid eye movement sleep. If a normal tracing is seen, this gives good evidence of an adequate neurovascular mechanism and allows substantial reassurance, particularly by showing the tracing to the patient.

Effective treatment of organic impotence is now more possible than in the past, but both the effective methods depend upon a reasonable arterial supply to the penis, so that if the impotence is due to arterial insufficiency rather than neuropathy these simpler treatments are unlikely to work. Pelvic angiography may then be considered, with consideration of arterial surgery, but the affected vessels may be too small for this to be possible. Angioplasty, including by laser beam, has yet to be evaluated. The likelihood of pelvic arterial disease is increased if arteriosclerosis is manifest elsewhere, particularly when intermittent claudication affects the thighs or buttocks rather than the calves.

The two methods adopted with the more common impotence of autonomic neuropathy are application of a partial vacuum, using a plastic cylinder surrounding the penis and a hand-operated extractor pump, or self-injection of a smooth-muscle relaxant (papaverine) or, less usually, an α-adrenergic blocker (for example phentolamine) into the corpora cavernosa. The second method requires careful education of the patient and trial as to the correct dose. The risks of priapism, thrombosis, or a corpora cavernosal infection must be set against the possible nuisance of the rubber ring at the base of the shaft required to maintain the vacuum-induced erection. The wisdom of all such manoeuvres greatly depends upon the individuals concerned, and careful understanding of their needs is essential. It is wise to include the patient's partner at some stage in the necessary advice and counselling. Diabetic autonomic neuropathy is sometimes the cause of retrograde ejaculation.

There is conflicting evidence regarding the existence of any comparable abnormalities in female diabetics, but certainly nothing as disabling as male impotence has been described.

Diabetic diarrhoea

This is usually intermittent, occurring for a few days and then possibly disappearing for weeks or months, but gradually increasing in frequency as the condition worsens. The motions are typically watery with mucus and only small amounts of faecal material, but the first one or two motions of a cluster may be fairly normal. Typically, diarrhoea begins in the early morning with up to 10 further motions during the day, and it often settles by evening. However, a burst of diarrhoea may begin at any time, and in some there is undue frequency of defaecation soon after meals. Doubtless there may be an emotional contribution, and sometimes the condition mimics the irritable bowel syndrome. There is rarely pain, but there may be abdominal distention. It is rare for particular foods to precipitate attacks.

Differential diagnosis includes the irritable bowel syndrome or other more serious organic causes of diarrhoea, but particularly pancreatic steatorrhoea; diabetes may be the presenting feature of chronic pancreatitis. Also, many patients with type I diabetes eventually show deficient pancreatic exocrine function, and although it is rare for this to progress severely enough to produce clinical steatorrhoea, it may cause some malabsorption. Malabsorption usually causes weight loss, which autonomic diarrhoea does not. There is an increased prevalence of gluten enteropathy among type I diabetics.

The pathogenesis may depend upon incomplete digestion in an abnormal upper alimentary tract, altered bowel flora, or motor disturbance of the colon. The exact roles of the parasympathetic, sympathetic, and peptidergic nervous systems are uncertain, as is the possibility of disturbance in gastrointestinal hormonal production and response.

Codeine is usually an effective treatment, but this should become the main prop only if there is not a good response to a 5 day course of a broad-spectrum antibiotic such as metronidazole, neomycin, a cephalosporin, or tetracyline. Another course should be equally successful on recurrence, which often follows a few months later. Increased dietary bulk is usually helpful.

If there is marked gastroparesis, treatment should be proffered. At its worst diabetic gastroparesis can produce a gastric stagnation that is almost as severe as pyloric stenosis, and can cause intermittent vomiting or a succussion splash on examination. However, it is usually asymptomatic except for feelings of upper abdominal distension after meals. It probably leads to diabetic diarrhoea as a result of the production of irritant compounds in the sluggishly moving contents of the dilated viscera. It causes erratic glucose control in that the rate of absorption of meals becomes unpredictable. Breath hydrogen studies may indicate abnormal flora of colonic origin in the small bowel, and culture of duodenal aspirates may also reveal abnormal flora. Direct gastric motility studies are also useful.

Treatment of gastroparesis is by cisapride (10 mg twice or three times daily) or by metoclopramide in the same dose, or by cholinergic or anticholinesterase drugs. The last-mentioned drugs may relieve many of the visceral effects of diabetic autonomic neuropathy but usually only partially or when it is mild; they also have side-effects, particularly on visual focusing and salivation.

Severe gastroparesis has a grave prognosis (50 per cent mortality within 2 years in one early study, which probably gave an exaggerated picture). The danger is mostly through an association with other severe manifestations of diabetic tissue damage but perhaps also through cardiac autonomic disturbance.

Sluggish motility of the gall bladder in long-standing diabetes may contribute to either gallstone formation or impaired digestion. Any evidence of pancreatic steatorrhoea should be followed by a trial of pancreatic enzymes given with meals which, if improving digestion, often also considerably increases the possibility of adequate glycaemic control.

Urinary retention

This may result from impaired urinary bladder motility. Treatment is by education in facilitating micturation by abdominal straining and by trial of anticholinesterase or cholinergic agents, with only secondary consideration of self-catheterization which increases the risk of urinary tract infection. Surgery to the bladder neck can relieve retention, but often only at the risk of dribbling incontinence. Electrical devices to stimulate bladder contractility are disappointing; sooner or later the device may fail, and there is always a risk of infection at the prosthetic site.

Gustatory sweating

Rarely, on starting a meal, a diabetic has diffuse sweating and reddening of the face and blush area. The sweating may be so profuse that it is both uncomfortable and embarrassing, and this may turn the patient into a recluse. Particular foods, such as cheese, may precipitate attacks in some.

Pupillary reflexes

These may be sluggish or absent.

Cardiac autonomic disturbance

It is difficult to know how serious this is. Electrocardiograph studies show frequent failure of the normal cardiac acceleration with deep breathing, standing, or mental arithmetic, and a plethora of manoeuvres have been used to illustrate this. Simple clinical tests include measurement of the R–R interval on the ECG during sleep or on slow deep breathing, or determining the ratio of the R–R interval on standing to that when lying down. Thus the ratio of the R–R interval at the 30th beat after standing compared with that at the 15th beat should be 1.0 or more. The more severe the abnormality, the more likely are other forms of autonomic neuropathy to be present. Patients often have a moderate resting tachycardia, presumably due to vagal neuropathy, but such a finding is not rare in elderly non-diabetics, particularly if there is cardiomyopathy. Indeed, the usual response for age-matched non-diabetics should always be clearly established for any of these tests. This condition may contribute to postural hypotension.

It is not known whether autonomic neuropathy contributes to sudden death from cardiac dysrhythmia either independently of or following cardiac infarction. There is strong circumstantial evidence that patients with marked cardioneuropathy are at risk of sudden death from cardiorespiratory arrest following anaesthesia. Some patients have a long Q–T_c interval on the ECG, and this is a worrying prognostic feature. Diabetic patients with neuropathy should be watched particularly carefully as an anaesthetic wears off, with the necessary equipment for resuscitation at hand until they have regained normal alertness. Aspiration from a paretic stomach, or perhaps autonomic disturbance of more purely respiratory reflexes, is also a particular postoperative risk.

Collagen disturbance

This is a relatively recently recognized form of diabetic tissue damage. It may result from increased glycation of collagen, with consequent change in its physical properties. Skin collagen is abnormal in diabetics. Few clinical consequences are obvious, but Dupuytren's contracture is more frequently found in diabetics than others. This is more true of men than women, but in women surprisingly soft fibrous cords may be felt causing deformity of the metacarpophalangeal joints. A tendency to slight flexion of the hand is often seen, even in quite young diabetics of several years' standing. Certainly, failure to press one palm completely against another or closely to oppose the palmar surfaces of the fifth digits is not uncommon even in adolescent type I diabetics, and is frequent among older patients. This is due to a change in collagen, perhaps particularly in periarticular membranes and ligaments, and may be associated with a waxy appearance of the skin. Thickening of the knuckle-pads of the first interphalageal joint is also common. The foot may also be affected, as shown particularly in the hammer toe deformity.

It is unknown how much collagen disturbance contributes to diabetic dermopathy, which presents mainly as trivial pigmented macules found particularly on the shins and usually regarded as the result of past trauma. These areas neither ulcerate nor cause discomfort. They are sometimes called hockey stick marks. Secondly, there is the curious blistering that can occur in diabetics through accumulation of serous fluid in a split in the epidermis, similar to what may occur in non-diabetics after deep coma from intoxication. In diabetics the blisters may be precipitated by exposure to cold or wet, but sometimes occur without obvious cause. The sterile fluid within them may be mildly bloodstained. The lesions are best treated conservatively, but if the blister is large the fluid should be aspirated with a thin needle. Even then the pierced overlying skin is best left in place, at least until some repair of the base of the blister has occurred, when the overlying and then dead skin should be removed with scissors. The only indication to remove the overlying skin straight away is an infection of the contained fluid, but this is rare. The lesion should be covered, usually with a dry dressing initially, but once the dead skin has been removed, Vaseline gauze is better.

A third type of diabetic skin lesion is necrobiosis lipoidica diabeticorum. This presents as painless areas, usually on the anterior aspects of the lower leg and typically 2 to 8 cm long. Although red at first, established lesions are yellowish in colour, often with slightly raised edges. Rarely, they become infected and then they are slow to heal, with difficulty in removing all infection. They persist for many years, typically in type I diabetics between 15 and 40 years old. Curiously, similar lesions are seen in non-diabetics, where their genesis is unknown. On biopsy in diabetics, microangiopathy is nearly always found in the underlying dermis.

Granuloma annulare is commoner among diabetics than in the general population, although the reason is unknown. Diabetics are also unduly liable to certain skin infections, particularly by fungi. These include Candida which, in addition to the well-recognized vulvovaginitis, is seen in particular in the webs of the fingers and toes and which, as angular stomatitis may also readily involve the nail-plates, particularly of the toes. As with other fungi these infections are all much more likely if there is poor glycaemic control; otherwise, treatment is with topical antifungal agents or sometimes, when there is a reservoir of colonic Candida which may make vulvular infection persistent, oral nystatin may be required. Nail-plate infections by dermatophytes, giving ony-chomycosis, are more common. Although trivial in themselves, the resulting nail dystrophy may make proper care of the nails more difficult for the patient with consequent damage to surrounding skin and the possibility of bacterial infection. Also, fungal infections may cause fis-suring, providing an entry for bacterial infection, and the oxygen demand of either infection can precipate gangrene in a foot with com-promised circulation. Tinea pedis should be aggressively managed in patients with poor circulation. Treatment of dermatophytosis is by oral griseofulvin or ketoconazole. The third fungal infection is by phyco-mycetes, which should always be suspected if a diabetic ulcer is unduly slow to heal. Diagnosis of all these fungi is by microscopic recognition of hyphae or sometimes by culture. Occasionally, diabetics with gross hyperglycaemia, often complicated by ketosis, may develop a rare but very serious deep mycotic infection with mucormycosis. This typically involves the linings of the nasopharynx where black crusting or pus is seen on the turbinates, nasal septum, or pallet. Infection may spread to the nasal sinuses or the orbit. Treatment is by aggressive debridement of necrotic tissue and intravenous amphotericin. The frequent yellowing of the nails of diabetics is not usually the result of dermatophytosis. It probably results from glycation; while the keratin of the epidermis is present for only about a month before being shed, that of the nail-plate may be present for more than a year. As with other features of glycation, it is also seen among elderly non-diabetics.

Diabetic foot disease

Different types of diabetic tissue damage interact and combine in the feet, giving a wide variety of lesions ranging from relatively harmless dysaesthesiae to fulminating infections and widespread ulceration. Ulcers or ischaemic or dead tissue can develop in the absence of appre-ciable neuropathy, but never without some circulatory disturbance. However, this may be slight, with neuropathy the main cause of the lesion. Reduction in blood flow may be the consequence of macro- or microangiopathy. There may also be a contribution from autonomic neu-ropathy which, when combined with microangiopathy, results in a dis-turbed pattern of blood flow. Collagen change is one cause of the ham-mer-toe type of deformity that is so common among diabetics, with hyperextension at the metacarpophalangeal joints. This causes excessive pressure on the skin beneath the metacarpal heads and excessive flexion at the first interphalangeal joints, so that shoes put undue pressure on the dorsal aspect. Finally, the leucocytes of hyperglycaemic patients have reduced anti-infective activity.

Infections of painless traumatic abrasions of neuropathic feet have the best prognosis. They occur particularly after trauma to the sole, which becomes progressively infected to an extent that would be impossible if there were normal sensation. The poor eyesight of elderly diabetics exac-erbates this problem. The spreading infection may cause acute local vascular damage as a result of endarteritis obliterans, which leads to cell death and faster spread of the infection, resulting in wet gangrene. This contrasts with the dry gangrene that occurs with ischaemia of uninfected tissue, although such dead tissue may be secondarily infected to produce a common wet state. Infarction of the toes may be due to thrombosis, for instance of the deep plantar arch or its prime branches. Less com-monly it is due to an embolus, either of thrombus from the atrium of a fibrillating heart or of grumous material discharged from an arterioscle-rotic ulcer of the abdominal aorta or more distal large vessel. Another serious lesion is the Charcot neuroarthropathic foot, which is grossly distorted, usually at the tarsal level, but remarkably painless, although sometimes there is discomfort as the distorted foot causes traumatic ulceration of the skin.

Preventive management is as important as correct treatment of estab-lished lesions. While medical and nursing staff, as well as patients, should know the principles of this, chiropodists and their assistants are likely to be the key agents. The main aim is to prevent excessive pressure on particular areas of skin. Corns and callosities, or even areas of exces-sive keratinization on the soles or heels, may warn of this. Static foot-prints can be of help in identifying individual risk sites, while in feet particularly at risk because of impaired circulation or gross sensory loss, pressure measurements during walking can be made using specialized equipment.

The time to recommend diabetics to inspect their feet regularly is when they begin to show evidence of impaired sensation or disturbed peripheral blood flow. If the diabetic cannot see his feet properly, some-one else must look at them at least weekly or, if there is marked loss of pinprick sensation, thrice weekly.

The principles of treatment are the same for every type of ulcer, even if different aspects become more important with some than with others. They are based on the elimination of infection by draining pus or remov-ing infected bone, by removing dead tissue likely to provide a focus for infection, and by using antibiotics if necessary. Healing is speeded by encouraging the greatest possible blood flow, and protecting the foot from trauma.

TREATMENT OF DIABETIC FOOT DISEASE

Debridement

This must be thorough, extensive, and readily repeated. The aim is to remove all dead tissue and to prevent pseudohealing by secondary inten-tion. Drainage of infection must be ensured by opening out narrow sinuses into deep-lying pus, as well as saucerizing more superficial lesions. Radiographic evidence of bony infection is an immediate indi-cation for amputation of such tissue, for however successful conserva-tive management of osteomyelitis may be in the young and healthy, antibiotics alone do not succeed in diabetic feet. The bony infection will always persist and break out again later, whatever resolution of the soft tissue infection may have occurred. It may be difficult radiologically to distinguish avascular necrosis from early osteomyelitis, and so another radiograph a few days later may be needed for certainty. Magnetic res-onance imaging is likely to give more helpful results than plain radi-ography. Thermal scanning and radio-isotope imaging have too coarse a focus and produce too many false positives to replace repeated radi-ography. Undue haste in amputation should be avoided, but equally such a focus of infection should be removed as quickly as possible. The debrided tissue should be packed firmly with ribbon gauze soaked in a solution such as half-strength saline, and only when primary healing is well established should drier dressings be contemplated. As healing pro-ceeds, it is wise to test its integrity by gentle probing; this may easily reveal that granulation tissue from secondary healing conceals residual spreading infection.

Antibiotics

Local antibiotic application is generally avoided, as in time it is too liable to cause local skin sensitivity and further reduce the health of skin already compromised by vascular and neuropathic damage. Culture of pathogens from the surface of otherwise well-healing lesions is not an indication for systemic antibiotics. However, they should be used if the infection invades surrounding tissue, and particularly if there is gener-alized disorder such as fever or deterioration in glucose control. The choice of agent should be guided by culture of either the local lesion or blood when infection is widespread. Any bone removed at operative debridement should be carefully cultured as persistent infection may depend upon subperiosteal foci of infection, only detected by drilling bone lying close to an ulcer floor. If a Staphylococcus has been found, then it is best to prescribe both flucloxacillin and fucidic acid, as the latter seems useful in preventing emergence of resistant strains. Often a more broad-based antibiotic may be required, such as one of the cephalosporins or amoxycillin. The most difficult organisms to treat are Pseudomonas and Proteus, and their elimination usually depends on successful local therapy, which may include antiseptics such as iodine soaks or acriflavin. If there is excessive granulation tissue, and while awaiting debridement, lotions such as acerbin may help. Care should be taken to prevent the lesion from becoming either too wet or too dry; absorbent dressings may be of help.

Pain relief

This should be effective and repeated, as pain is vasoconstrictive.

Immobilization

Initially this is achieved by bed rest, but as soon as possible the patient should sit out if this does not cause pressure on the lesion. He or she should also walk once the affected part can be immobilized by a lightweight plaster cast, which can have suitably placed gaps to spare the lesion from pressure and is often split to allow effective dressings. Patients lying too long in bed to heal a toe ulcer can develop a dangerous ulcer of either heel. It is a disaster if the contralateral heel ulcerates in this way during recovery from a below-knee amputation; careful inspection and nursing are essential.

Immobilization by rest and then a suitable cast is the only treatment, other than improved glycaemic control, known to improve the Charcot lesion.

Improved vascular supply

Before any substantial amputation of tissue, vascular repair to improve the blood supply should be considered. This does not apply if at least one of the two ankle pulses is palpable or Doppler ultrasound measurements indicate appreciable flow there. Vascular surgery does not as yet tackle blocks distal to the arterial trifurcation just below the knee. Hence a palpable popliteal artery also makes successful vascular repair unlikely, although this is becoming less absolute a rule as vascular techniques improve. If there is evidence of obstruction above the knee, angiography should always be considered. In perhaps 10 to 15 per cent of patients likely to undergo a mid-tarsal or more severe amputation, there may be a substantial proximal obstruction which is local enough for worthwhile vascular surgery. The disappointment is that lesions in the iliac and more distal large arteries are often so widespread in diabetics that they are beyond the scope of effective vascular surgery. Lumbar sympathectomy may relieve the pain from a diabetic foot, and occasionally aid healing. The improved blood flow is probably only temporary. Pain relief may depend more on interruption of afferent fibres. There would seem little point in this manoeuvre when there is widespread evidence of autonomic neuropathy.

Anaemia should be treated, if necessary, by a transfusion of packed cells, and any oedema from coincident heart failure should be appropriately managed. Elevation of an oedematous foot can reduce swelling, but may also reduce arterial perfusion if this is severely compromised.

Smoking

The patient should not smoke because of its ill effects on the peripheral circulation.

Glycaemic control

The control of glucose levels should be as strict as possible, and blood glucose levels above 10 mmol/l must be avoided, as they are associated with impaired function of the leucocytes, both polymorphonuclear and mononuclear. This degree of glucose control should not be achieved by excessive restriction of food intake in someone with tissues to heal and an infection to combat. Insulin will often be required in those not previously receiving it, even if only temporarily. Its anabolic effect may be an advantage, but there is no evidence that it is helpful as a local dressing.

Amputation

The indications for amputation are as follows.

Life-threatening infection

This is now rare because of the use of antibiotics, but is still occasionally necessary particularly if there is surgical crepitus or air within the tissues, revealed by radiography, indicating a gas-forming organism. The three most likely organisms to be found are anaerobic Streptococci, gas-forming Coliforms, or Clostridia. There must be extensive debridement to allow good access of oxygen to the tissues and effective antibiotics are required, certainly including penicillins for the first and third organisms and clostridial antitoxin if Clostridia is believed to be the culprit.

Removal of dead tissue (including osteomyelitic bone)

The only exceptions are the very ill or very old, who are not thought able to withstand the physical or psychological shock of the amputation, or if one or two toes have undergone dry gangrene when it may be best to leave them to wither and slowly separate spontaneously, when the bare area exposed to possible infection will be much smaller than after surgery.

Intractable pain

This is rarely a problem with infections, but sometimes results from dry gangrene or severe ischaemia.

Lifestyle needs

These range from the inability of a wage-earner to have the long period of rest sometimes necessary for conservative management, to undue boredom and deterioration of personality in an old person excessively confined, whether in hospital or the home, through the immobility necessary to attempt healing. This is less common with use of lightweight splints.

Nibbling amputations should be avoided wherever possible. The strain of successive anaesthetics in an elderly and infected patient may be lethal, as removal of a toe is followed successively by amputation of a metatarsal, a mid-tarsal operation, and finally a below-knee amputation. It is much better to go to the latter first, if it really seems likely that this will eventually be necessary. It is usually important to be relatively radical where the small bones of the forefoot are concerned, and cosmetic considerations for the elderly to conserve the phalanges of a toe whose metatarsal has mostly been removed are misplaced. The difficulty arises with the decision between a mid-tarsal amputation and an amputation a little below the knee, for the latter means that there will be no heel to walk on. Unfortunately, the amount of background diabetic tissue damage in these patients nearly always prevents success of Syme's amputation at the ankle.

Some patients may not be best served by a prolonged period in hospital to achieve healing or by surgery; a return home with a discharging sinus is always an option. A low grade infection controlled by long-term antibiotics may be preferable to an amputation at knee level.

Diabetic macroangiopathy

DIABETIC HEART DISEASE

Several different processes contribute to diabetic heart disease. Most damage to the cardiac tissue is a consequence of accelerated coronary artery disease. Although abnormalities in the plasma lipids and the increased liability to hypertension among diabetics account for much of this, the diabetic state itself, and indeed that of impaired glucose tolerance, is associated with this process, perhaps through increased micro-angiopathy of the vasa vasorum and perhaps through changes in vessel wall collagen and other changes also produced by protein glycation. Structural narrowing of the lumen may then be worsened by thrombus formation on the endothelial lining, while the resulting increase in hyp-oxia may increase fibrosis, eventually with further vascular narrowing. In general, diabetics have increased plasma concentrations of some coa-gulative factors, for example fibrinogen and von Willebrand's factor, and their platelets have an increased sensitivity to aggregatory stimuli. The endothelium is also abnormal in its functional metabolism with regard to nitric oxide, plasminogen activator and its inhibition, and platelet-derived factors.

The increase in fibrosis and the change in the nature of the connective tissue act outside the coronary circulation to reduce the contractile power of the ventricular walls. Whether or not these changes result from increased glycation, the myocardium becomes increasingly rigid, so that on the one hand the end diastolic filling pressure is higher than usual and on the other a given amount of contractile force generated by the myocardium diminishes the cardiac lumen less; overall there is likely to be a decrease in stroke volume. The first evidence of diabetic heart disease often comes from flattening or inversion of the T waves over the left ventricular leads on the ECG. This may develop in the absence of angina pectoris or any clinical episode suggestive of infarction, and it may not worsen greatly in an exercise tolerance test. It probably reflects increased fibrosis and loss of elasticity of the left ventricular wall. Therefore patients suffer two different clinical problems.

First, they experience all the features of ischaemic heart disease. A greater proportion of cardiac infarcts seem painless in patients with dia-betes than in non-diabetics, with perhaps 15 to 20 per cent of painless infarcts in the former compared with 5 to 8 per cent in the latter. Painless angina is obviously a contradiction in terms, but it is probable that the symptoms from ischaemic heart muscle may also be less in diabetics. Therefore the ECG record of a diabetic obtained during an exercise tolerance test is just as important as his or her symptoms.

It is not known why diabetics are relatively free from such cardiac symptoms, although it may result from neuropathy of afferent fibres, which are not usually tested in investigations of diabetic cardiac auto-nomic neuropathy. The relationship with the 'sudden death' syndrome among diabetics is also uncertain. A long Q–T interval in the ECG is associated with such deaths, and patients showing this feature should be monitored for at least 12, and preferably 24, h after operation or at any other time of increased risk.

Secondly, diabetics can develop heart failure in the absence of cor-onary heart disease. This diabetic cardiomyopathy responds to conven-tional treatment, in which angiotensin-converting enzyme inhibitors may be particularly useful.

Heart disease is the major cause of death among both type I and type II diabetics, and ultimately is likely to affect about 60 per cent of patients. Thus the avoidance of smoking is a particularly important fea-ture of diabetic management. The diabetic state also makes normaliza-tion of lipids and blood pressure more important than among the general population.

The management of ischaemic heart disease among diabetics differs little from that generally employed. The minor disadvantages of β block-ers for diabetics do not prevent the use of selective agents such as aten-olol. The hypoglycaemic action of aspirin when combined with sul-phonylureas is so slight that this should never prevent its use. Coronary angiography is more likely to show multiple lesions with a tendency to be relatively distal in the arterial tree, but many patients are suitable for arterial bypass or angioplasty.

The 1 month mortality after cardiac infarction is increased some two- to threefold among diabetics. This is partly because they suffer larger infarcts on average, but may also be because of an increased liability to fatal dysrhythmias, particularly 8 to 12 days after infarction. Patients treated by sulphonylureas seem to be more vulnerable than those given insulin or managed by diet alone. The infarct precipitates a phase of hyperglycaemia for 1 to 3 days, and short-acting insulins should be used as supplements to usual therapy, aiming at control of the blood sugar to between 8 and 12 mmol/l.

HYPERTENSION IN DIABETICS

The accelerated change in connective tissue in diabetics, with increased fibrosis and loss of elasticity, is particularly important in the develop-ment of systolic hypertension. Diastolic hypertension is also increased among diabetics, sometimes as a consequence of renal disease, some-times by coincidence, and sometimes as one of the features comprising early malnutrition adaptation syndrome. Much thought has been given to whether hypertension or renal disease comes first among diabetics. For type I patients, the evidence from microalbuminuria suggests mild renal involvement first; for many type II patients the two appear to develop in parallel. Constitutional factors are bound to be important, and a possible marker of the risk of hypertension is an increased eryth-rocyte sodium–lithium exchange mechanism. It has been argued that this is only a marker of increased activity of the sodium–hydrogen anti-port, which has been linked to increased cellular growth and so perhaps to hyperplasia of arteriolar walls.

Poorly controlled hypertension may accelerate the rate of progress of both diabetic nephropathy and retinopathy. Therefore antihypertensive treatment must be particularly meticulous in diabetics. In general, the preferred antihypertensive agents are the angiotensin-converting enzyme inhibitors, the α-adrenergic antagonists and the calcium-channel block-ers. A combination of the last with one of the first two will often be necessary if one of them alone is inadequate. The thiazide diuretics and related drugs tend to impair glucose tolerance as well as elevate blood lipids, and β-blockers also raise the lipid levels as well as impairing insulin secretion.

Special problems

Infection

Diabetics with poor glycaemic control are particularly prone to devel-oping severe bacterial or fungal infections. A classical presentation of diabetes is with recurrent infection, such as boils or abscesses, or fungal infections such as candida. Approximately half the cases of ketoacidosis in known diabetics are due to infection. In the late 1920s 20 per cent of deaths in diabetics were due to infection; with the development of che-motherapy and antibiotics this figure had already dropped to 5 per cent by the 1960s. There are three aspects of the problem: first, the effect of infection on metabolism; second, the increased liability to serious infec-tions in hyperglycaemic diabetics; third, those infections which occur specifically with much increased frequency in diabetics.

METABOLIC EFFECTS OF INFECTION

Infections, particularly bacterial, lead to a clearly defined stress response, marked particularly by increased secretion of cortisol, gluca-gon, and catecholamines. Together, these increase insulin resistance and blood glucose concentration and, in the absence of a normal insulin response, they also increase ketogenesis. In the type II diabetic there may be a temporary need for exogenous insulin, and in the type I patient insulin requirements may rise dramatically. Infected patients often stop eating and may mistakenly decrease their insulin, although at least as much or even more insulin is usually needed. Home glucose monitoring, either of blood or urine, should be used to guide insulin therapy during such illness, and urine ketones should be checked repeatedly. Patients should receive clear instructions for the action to be taken, particularly if they are type I diabetics.

The two basic principles are as follows: first, even when no food is being taken the daily dose of insulin should be as much as or more than usual; second, if the diabetic is too ill to carry out his own urine or blood tests it is more important than ever that they are done by someone else. Every effort should be made to maintain a reasonable calorie intake, if necessary purely in liquid form, for example lemon squash with 20 g of sucrose, glucose, or honey every 2 h, or Ribena or Lucozade, or milk with added sucrose. If food intake is likely to be erratic, it may be easier to rely on several injections per day of quick-acting soluble insulins, but this does not take into account the increase in the basal insulin requirement. Hence those on Ultratard and Actrapid should increase the Ultratard dose by some 20 per cent and decrease the Actrapid by about the same number of units initially, but the latter should be divided between three injections instead of the usual one or two. It may be better for patients on twice-daily mixtures of medium- and short-acting insulins to move 10 per cent of the medium morning insulin to the evening injection, and split their total quick-acting dose into three, as with the Ultratard patients. Blood tests will then indicate whether adjustments, up or down, are necessary in the total daily dose. As the infection clears, the increase in insulin probably needed if food intake was maintained should be omitted once satisfactory glucose levels are approached.

HOST DEFENCES AGAINST INFECTION IN DIABETES

The normal response to infection is complex, including immunological responses as well as the mobilization and action of phagocytic cells, particularly polymorphonuclear leucocytes. The four steps in the normal functioning of polymorphonuclear leucocytes are chemotaxis in response to bacterial products, adherence of the polymorphonuclear leucocyte to endothelium at the site of invasion, phagocytosis involving opsonins, and microbicidal activity. Components of the complement system are involved in the first three steps.

Chemotaxis and phagocytosis have long been known to be defective in both hyperglycaemic and ketoacidotic diabetics, and more recently it has been shown that the microbicidal activity of polymorphonuclear leucocytes may also be impaired. However, there is no evidence to suggest any defect in the response to infection in diabetics with good glycaemic control. No defect has been found in the complement system or in opsonin production and function, even in ketoacidotic diabetics. This suggests strongly that the intrinsic properties of the polymorphonuclear leucocytes are altered and function is impaired by poor glycaemic control. Abnormalities are consistently found when fasting blood glucose levels exceed 10 mmol/l.

It is probable that the abnormalities are secondary to impairment of the sustained energy production required for normal polymorphonuclear leucocyte function. Polymorphonuclear leucocytes are freely permeable to glucose, but thereafter there are several insulin-dependent steps including glucose phosphorylation, glycogen synthesis, and pyruvate formation. Diabetic granulocytes have diminished glycogen content and this may be critical in limiting maximal energy production. Mononuclear leucocytes show comparable defects in their different functions.

Thus there is good *in vivo* and *in vitro* evidence for impaired host resistance to infection in the poorly controlled diabetic. This should be taken as a strong indication for rigorous glycaemic control in any diabetic patient with an infection.

SPECIFIC INFECTIONS IN DIABETES

Some of the infections proved or suggested to be particularly associated with diabetes are shown in Table 27. The most common are urinary tract infections, particularly in females. The prevalence of bacteriuria has been found to be three times higher in diabetic than non-diabetic women. Poor glycaemic control is not the only factor; abnormal bladder function from autonomic neuropathy can also be important. Pyelonephritis, perinephric abscesses, and papillary necrosis are also associated with diabetes, particularly when there has been poor glycaemic control. Presumably, impaired motor function of a viscus, secondary to autonomic neuropathy, is one reason for the increased liability to cholecystitis

Table 27 *Infections associated with diabetes mellitus*

Urinary tract infections* (females): cystitis, pyelonephritis, perinephric abscess*, acute papillary necrosis*, fungal urinary tract infection
Mucocutaneous candidiasis
Furunculosis (staphylococcus)
Gram-negative pneumonia, staphylococcal pneumonia*
Tuberculosis*
Foot-ulcer-related infections*
Cryptococcosis, histoplasmosis, blastomycosis, coccidioidomycosis
Rhinocerebral mucormycosis*
Malignant otitis external*
Cholecystitis*
Influenza*

*Proven associations; the remainder are possible or suggested associations.

among diabetics, together with altered cholesterol and bile salt metabolism.

For many years an association between tuberculosis and diabetes mellitus has been suspected, with a greater incidence in poorly controlled diabetics. Prior to good antituberculous therapy and the emphasis on good glycaemic control, 5 per cent of diabetic deaths were due to tuberculosis and the combined diagnosis was almost invariably fatal. It is still a scourge in some parts of the world.

Fungal infections are also frequently associated with poorly controlled diabetes. *Candida albicans* is the most common agent, particularly in females who present with vaginal or vulval candidiasis. Candidial infections of the bladder and skin are also found. Other fungal infections are rarer but can be catastrophic, such as rhinocerebral mucormycosis. Most of the fungal infections are directly related to both impaired host defences and increased fungal growth in high glucose media.

Cutaneous infections are more common in poorly controlled diabetics. Staphylococcal infections predominate but respond well to therapy if the diabetes is brought under control. The rare but severe malignant otitis externa due to *Pseudomonas aeruginosa* should probably be included in this group.

Infected foot lesions are extremely common in diabetics, and have already been described in detail.

TREATMENT OF INFECTIONS

In most cases infections in diabetics respond to standard therapy, provided that the glucose levels are simultaneously brought under good control. The essentials of therapy are as described for the diabetic foot. It is always essential to remove dead tissue and ensure proper drainage of infection, for example removing a tooth when there is troublesome infection at its root. As glycaemic control is often poor because of the infection, non-insulin treated diabetics with chronic infections may need insulin for a period which may be as long as several months. Insulin-treated diabetics will generally require increased doses of insulin. Infections which respond less well to therapy are those in which there are added complicating factors, such as bladder dysfunction with some urinary tract infections or circulatory impairment with foot ulcers.

Anaesthesia and surgery

A diabetic has a 50 per cent risk of requiring surgery at some time. Although there are no recent comprehensive figures, surgical procedures probably carry both increased morbidity and mortality compared with those performed on non-diabetics. Coincident cardiovascular disease and obesity increase perioperative morbidity, as does neurological impairment, particularly autonomic neuropathy. Although many of the important factors cannot be modified, there is a need for straightforward therapeutic guidelines. Examples are given below.

METABOLIC RESPONSE TO ANAESTHESIA AND SURGERY

Anaesthesia provokes a stress response which was greater with the older anaesthetic agents; however, even with modern anaesthetics there is generally an increase in secretion of cortisol and catecholamines, although halothane does not increase catecholamines. These effects are only avoided by spinal anaesthesia, provided that it is not accompanied by excessive hypotension. Therefore there will be an initial decrease in insulin secretion, in those still capable of producing it, and an increase in insulin resistance. However, the effects of anaesthesia are small when compared with the metabolic upset of the surgery itself.

Surgery has long been known to cause a major catabolic response. There is an immediate neuroendocrine response with release of ACTH, cortisol, catecholamines, and growth hormone. Noradrenaline increases, particularly peroperatively, with adrenaline rising later. Glucagon secretion also increases, primarily as a result of the rise in noradrenaline secretion. Insulin levels may fall owing to inhibition by catecholamines and other factors, with a loss of responsiveness to glucose. The end result is hyperglycaemia, with the rise in blood glucose proportional to the severity of surgery. This is primarily due to increased gluconeogenesis. During and after surgery the mobilization of lipids is less than would be expected, particularly in fasting patients. This is probably because insulin levels rise postoperatively in response to the hyperglycaemia and suppress lipolysis, despite levels inadequate to control the hyperglycaemia. Thus there is a dependence on glucose for oxidative metabolism, and so an increased utilization of amino acid for gluconeogenesis. The increase in cortisol also increases protein catabolism.

These changes will be exaggerated in the non-insulin-treated diabetic, where insulin secretion is already compromised and insulin resistance is present. Thus severe hyperglycaemia and increased protein losses are likely. In the untreated insulin-dependent diabetic the endocrine changes will lead to severe hyperglycaemia and ketoacidosis, as well as disturbances of electrolyte metabolism and major loss of protein. The rise in blood glucose levels may not be very large if glucose solutions are not infused, but this may be because of incipient starvation and is compatible with impending severe ketoacidosis.

Management of insulin-treated diabetics undergoing surgery

A guideline to pre-, per-, and postoperative management is shown in Table 28.

For major procedures in particular, patients should be admitted to hospital 2 or 3 days preoperatively to enable optimal glycaemic control to be established. Long-acting insulins should be stopped and the patient stabilized on twice-daily mixtures of short- and intermediate-acting insulins; alternatively, a thrice-daily regimen containing some intermediate-acting insulin can be used if glycaemic control is initially very poor. Blood glucose should be monitored frequently at the bedside so that dose adjustments can be made rapidly.

Details of preoperative management should be agreed with the anaesthetist. Whenever possible, surgery should be scheduled early in the day. On the morning of the operation insulin and food should be omitted, unless the procedure is scheduled after 3 p.m. when breakfast should be taken covered by a short-acting insulin. An intravenous infusion of 10 per cent glucose, insulin, and potassium should be set up, but if the operation is delayed for more than 2 h, blood glucose should again be measured and the insulin content of the infusate adjusted accordingly (Table 29). A persistent high glucose level (above 13 mmol/l) should lead to consideration of postponement of surgery or delaying it until late in the day. During lengthy operations (more than 1.5 h) blood glucose should again be measured in the theatre, and it should always be checked in the recovery room.

Table 28 *The management of insulin-treated diabetics during surgery*

Preoperative
1. Admit to hospital 2–3 days before operation
2. Stop long-acting insulins and stabilize on either twice-daily short-acting and intermediate insulins or thrice-daily short-acting insulin with intermediate insulin in the evening
3. Monitor blood glucose (bedside methods) before and after each main meal and at bedtime
4. Aim to maintain fasting blood glucose <8 mmol/l, and other values between 4 and 10 mmol/l
5. Check urea, electrolytes, and renal, cardiovascular, and neurological systems

Perioperative
1. Schedule operation for early in the day
2. Check fasting glucose. If ≥13 mmol/l, delay operation
3. Omit morning insulin and breakfast
4. Start infusion of glucose–insulin–potassium (see Table 29) as early as possible and at least 1 h preoperatively
5. If operation delayed more than 2 h from onset of infusion, recheck blood glucose and adjust infusion if necessary
6. Recheck blood glucose at end of operation (and during lengthy operations) and modify regimen if necessary
7. Check K^+ as in point 6

Postoperative
1. Check glucose every 2–4 h and K^+ every 6 h, then twice daily
2. Continue infusion until first meal taken; restart SC insulin at preoperative dose 1 h before infusion stopped
3. Consider total parenteral or gastrointestinal nutrition if oral refeeding not recommenced within 48 h

SC, subcutaneous.

Table 29 *Insulin infusion regimen for pre-, per- and postoperative management of diabetes during surgery*

1. Add 15 units short-acting insulin (soluble) + 10 mmol KCl to 500 ml 10% glucose (dextrose)
2. Run 25–50 ml through infusion tubing before attaching to patient
3. Infuse at 100 ml/h

(If there is need to limit fluids, use double amounts of insulin and KCl in 20% glucose and infuse at 50 ml/h)

If blood glucose >10 mmol/l increase insulin by 4 units/500 ml; check blood glucose 2 h later; increase by further 4 unit increments as necessary

If blood glucose <5 >3 mmol/l decrease insulin by 4 units/500 ml; check blood glucose 2 h later; decrease by further 4 unit decrements as necessary (if glucose <3 mmol/l, stop insulin for 1 h)

Plasma potassium should be rechecked postoperatively and blood glucose should be measured by strip every 2 to 4 h, with appropriate changes in the infusion regimen. Few changes are usually necessary if the defined aim is to maintain blood glucose between 5 and 10 mmol/l. The infusion should be continued until the first meal has been taken, when the subcutaneous insulin regimen may be reinstituted. Subcutaneous insulin should be given at least 1 h before the infusion is discontinued because of its relatively slow absorption and the rapid decay in plasma insulin level once the infusion has stopped.

There are several ways in which the insulin can be given. The safest method is to put it directly into the bag or bottle of intravenous dextrose. In this case variations in infusion rate will affect all components equally,

Table 30 *The management of non-insulin-treated diabetics during surgery*

Minor operations	
Diet-treated	If BG ≤10 mmol/l treat as non-diabetic
	If BG >10 mmol/l treat with insulin infusion regimen during operation
Oral agent treated	1. Stop biguanides and long-acting sulphonylureas 2–3 days preoperatively
	Stabilize on diet alone or short-acting sulphonylureas
	2. If BG ≤10 mmol/l on day of operation treat as non-diabetic
	If BG >10 mmol/l treat with insulin infusion regimen during operation
Major operations	
Diet-treated	Admit to hospital 2 days before operation
	1. If BG ≤7 mmol/l, treat as type I diabetic on day of surgery
	2. If BG >7 mmol/l treat with short-acting insulin three times daily preoperatively; treat as type I diabetic on day of surgery
Oral agent treated	1. Stop all oral agents 2 days preoperatively
	2. Treat with short-acting insulin three times daily
	3. Treat as type I diabetic on day of surgery
Postoperative management	
	1. Minor surgery: recommence usual therapy with first meal
	2. Major surgery: Convert to SC insulin two times daily with first oral feeding; recommence oral agent or diet-alone therapy 24–48 h later

BG, blood glucose; SC, subcutaneous.

and wide glycaemic swings are less likely. Some give insulin by pump because absorption of insulin to tubing is less from concentrated solutions, but in practice this is not a problem.

Insulin resistance is common, and is most severe during and following cardiopulmonary bypass surgery. In this case the standard glucose–insulin–potassium infusion should be used preoperatively, but insulin alone should be infused during surgery when as much as 20 units/h may be needed, with the amount being determined by frequent glucose monitoring. A combined glucose–insulin infusion should be restarted at the end of the operation, but insulin requirements will continue to be high for the next 24 h.

Other infusions (saline or blood) are often required during surgery. They should be given through separate lines in amounts dictated by clinical need. If metabolic requirements result in potential fluid overload, half the volume of 20 per cent dextrose can be used instead of the 10 per cent preparation.

Day admissions for minor procedures present a separate problem. They should not be encouraged for insulin-treated patients, but may be tolerated because of lack of beds. There are two approaches, but in both patients should come to the hospital early in the day, omitting their usual insulin and breakfast. Blood glucose should then be checked. If it is less than 13 mmol/l, the patient can go immediately to theatre and return to the day ward to be given insulin and breakfast as usual. Blood glucose can be checked once more, and the patient can return home in the late afternoon.

The alternative is to start an infusion on admission, and this will apply to all patients with fasting blood glucose above 13 mmol/l. The infusion is then continued until the first postoperative meal when short-acting insulin is given. Usual therapy is reinstituted with the evening meal, after which the patient may return home.

Management of non-insulin-treated diabetics undergoing surgery (Table 30)

The general principles of management are as for insulin-treated diabetics, but treatment is simpler for well-controlled patients undergoing minor procedures.

Diet-treated patients who are well controlled (fasting blood glucose concentration below 10 mmol/l) can be treated in the same way as non-diabetics. Similarly, in the case of well-controlled patients taking a short-acting oral hypoglycaemic agent, this should be omitted on the day of operation and the patient treated as a non-diabetic. Oral therapy should then be reinstituted when the ability to eat is restored.

Biguanides and long-acting sulphonylureas should be stopped for at least 3 days before major surgery and the patient restabilized on short-acting sulphonylureas. Patients undergoing minor surgery who are poorly controlled should be treated like insulin-treated patients with a glucose–insulin–potassium infusion on the day of surgery. The infusion can be stopped at the time of the first meal and sulphonylurea therapy recommenced.

Even with major surgery, patients on short-acting sulphonylureas with fasting glucose concentration below 7 mmol/l can continue such treatment until the morning of surgery, when sulphonylureas should be omitted and infusion therapy started as for insulin-treated diabetics. If patients are poorly controlled preoperatively (fasting glucose levels above 8 mmol/l, random blood glucose above 12 mmol/l), they should be stabilized on insulin, best given as a highly purified short-acting type before each meal. They should then be treated as insulin-treated diabetics.

Blood glucose monitoring both pre- and postoperatively should be performed every 2 to 4 h, as for insulin-treated diabetics. After major surgery it is probably safest to use thrice-daily insulin therapy for 1 or 2 days when refeeding begins before attempting reconversion to sulphonylureas or therapy with diet alone. These patients are particularly at risk of cardiovascular illness and meticulous attention should be paid to potassium, fluid balance, and myocardial function.

Emergency surgery in diabetes

Two to five per cent of operations on diabetics can be classified as emergencies, usually because of infection. In nearly all cases there is some metabolic disturbance and sometimes frank ketoacidosis. The trap of abdominal pain consequent to the ketoacidosis in younger patients, which disappears with rehydration and insulin therapy, must be emphasized. One important guide is that if vomiting precedes abdominal pain, the latter is more likely to be due to ketoacidosis, and vice versa.

The first priority is to assess glycaemic and acid–base status. While results are awaited a saline infusion should be started and nasogastric suction applied where appropriate. If moderate or severe ketoacidosis is confirmed, the operation should be delayed for 4 to 5 h if possible whilst rehydration and standard therapy for ketoacidosis is applied (see below). After reasonable metabolic correction, surgery can be performed safely using the glucose–insulin–potassium regimen. Similarly, with less severe hyperglycaemia and ketosis the glucose–insulin infusion can be used throughout. In all such cases hourly blood glucose monitoring is desirable. It must be stressed that both metabolic decompensation and infection will cause insulin resistance and a higher insulin infusion rate will be required (0.5–0.8 units/g glucose compared with the usual 0.3 units/g). If extra fluids are required these should be given through a separate line. Good glycaemic control should be sought postoperatively to aid healing, particularly if infection was a precipitating factor.

Brittle diabetes

A small proportion of type I diabetics are unstable and difficult to control. These are referred to variously as 'labile' or 'brittle' diabetics. The terms are used loosely, and some paediatricians claim that all children with diabetes are brittle. In practice only about 1 to 2 per cent of diabetics fall into this category. A useful working definition of a brittle diabetic is one whose life is constantly disrupted by episodes of hypoglycaemia or hyperglycaemia, whatever their cause. The causes of brittle diabetes fall into five main groups: therapeutic errors, intercurrent illness, accessible emotional causes, self-induced (or carer-induced), and unknown aetiology.

The most common category is that of therapeutic error by either the physician or the patient. For example attempts to achieve morning normoglycaemia in a totally insulin-deficient patient by once-daily therapy can cause repeated severe hypoglycaemia in the late afternoon or evening. Similarly, nocturnal hypoglycaemia can be produced by overenthusiastic increases in intermediate insulin in the late afternoon. When this is absorbed relatively rapidly, which is increasingly likely with purified and human insulins, both unduly high peak insulins between midnight and 3 a.m. and unduly low insulin levels before breakfast are found. This is associated with nocturnal hypoglycaemia, possibly leading to extra food intake, and early morning hyperglycaemia. Improper or imperfect dietary advice can also result in wide glycaemic fluctuations from day to day. Equally, the patient can generate the brittle state by erratic exercise and lack of dietary compliance. Somogyi described the not infrequent phenomenon of reduction in overall glycosuria by lowering the dose of insulin, and characterized the patients in whom this was likely to occur as those liable to occasional clinical hypoglycaemia and in whom otherwise glycosuria was likely to be either absent or very heavy. This could well be because even chemical, but clinically silent, hypoglycaemia can provoke increased food intake. Later suggestions that an undetected period of hypoglycaemia can trigger a counter-regulatory response, with subsequent hyperglycaemia, glycosuria, and ketonuria have been much debated. Often the reduction in total insulin dose is only effective when accompanied by some reorganization of the insulin regimen or sometimes the dietary disposition.

The second main cause of brittle diabetes is intercurrent illness. This can be subdivided broadly into infections, endocrine disorders, and pancreatic disease. The most common occult infective cause worldwide is probably tuberculosis, but other infections can have equally severe effects on glycaemic stability. The brittle diabetes always resolves with cure of the infection. Endocrine causes include hyperthyroidism, Addison's disease, and hypopituitarism. Again, treatment resolves the diabetic problem. Amongst pancreatic causes are pancreatectomy, which is predictable from the lack of pancreatic glucagon, chronic pancreatitis, which is not uncommon and may present insidiously, and, more obviously, any pancreatic steatorrhoea.

The third and fourth causes may well be linked. Home disturbances and family conflict may cause glycaemic instability. It is not certain how much of this is due to a neuroendocrine disturbance of metabolism and how much to manipulative behaviour. Whatever the cause, this type of brittle diabetes is not uncommon in adolescence, may disappear spontaneously when the psychosocial problems resolve, or may occasionally respond to psychotherapy or family group therapy. The liability to premenstrual hyperglycaemia, most marked in adolescence and sometimes episodic monthly before menarche, certainly has an endocrine basis. It may be complicated later by emotional factors and it is not well understood overall.

The fourth group is the most difficult to deal with and is estimated to have a prevalence of one per 1000–2000 type I diabetics in the United Kingdom. It is perhaps not as heterogeneous a group as was originally thought. The majority of such patients are female aged between 14 and 26 years, and the onset is soon after menarche. They are all mildly overweight, which may be secondary to overeating in response to intermittent hypoglycaemia. However, their brittle state is reflected more in recurrent ketoacidosis. The majority require large subcutaneous doses of insulin with considerable day-to-day variation in requirement. Many have sluggish insulin absorption from subcutaneous injection, and this is often an intermittent defect, possibly due to markedly varied subcutaneous blood flow. They respond well to intravenous insulin, but their requirements are slightly higher than normal. They also show persistent metabolic abnormalities which are consistent with adrenergic overactivity, although circulating catecholamine levels are normal. There is an accelerated glycaemic response to insulin withdrawal.

Few are diagnosed as psychotic, but closer analysis by measurement of plasma insulin concentrations has shown that a notable proportion are producing the situation by contrived manipulation. There may also be evidence of manipulation by the carer, whether a parent or nurse (Munchausen's syndrome by proxy). The key questions are as follows.

1. Does insulin, whether administered by the patient, the carer, or the nurse, appear in the plasma as expected?
2. Does a given insulin dose affect plasma glucose as expected, and consistently, at times when nutrient intake is closely controlled?

It may be necessary to rephrase the latter question in terms of a given plasma insulin level rather than administered dose. Although sophisticated manipulative patients may produce alarming metabolic swings, they usually ensure that help is available in time to provide proper therapy. One frequent feature is that introduction of new techniques of insulin administration are followed by a period of relative stability until a manipulative patient has worked out what is happening. Thus automatic insulin pumps, surgically implanted subcutaneously and supplying insulin intravenously at a rate which can be changed by a magnet (kept by a doctor or nurse), may so impress or baffle such patients that adequate glycaemic control is achieved for days or weeks. Sometimes such improved glycaemic control breaks a vicious circle and the restored physical well-being is so welcome that a return to conventional treatment may eventually be successful. These patients often have appealing and winning personalities. They are expert at manipulating their carers to allow them unsupervised freedom in measuring their glucose levels, in deciding, preparing, or measuring their insulin dose, or in unrecorded access to food.

By definition one cannot describe the last group. The two analytical approaches mentioned above should help in diagnosis of abnormalities such as fluctuating levels of antibodies against the insulin receptors.

Adolescence

There are probably only two features of diabetes particular to adolescence: unusually large daily variations in energy output and variability in the nature and timing of meals, and a generally increased inner turmoil, both emotional and hormonal. But perhaps the marked anabolism of growth disturbs metabolism more than is realized. Otherwise the problems are no more than an intensification of many factors that contribute to unstable diabetes at any age. Much of the problem reflects the difficulties in self-discipline in members of this age group as they seek self-determination.

Adolescent patients are often very interested and highly motivated in their care, but equally are readily discouraged by apparent lack of technical skill or failure of involvement with what each sees as a unique individual problem. This is a period of care when time must be taken to explain the details of therapeutic regimens, often previously understood by their parents rather than themselves. They also seek greater flexibility, and successful withdrawal of previous maxims can only be based on understanding of the principles that produced them and the technical adjustments that can allow variation from day to day to meet altered states of exercise, timing and nature of meals, or emotions. Flexibility does not mean lack of firmness in therapeutic advice; smoking should be discouraged even more firmly than with non-diabetic adolescents.

Some girls experience particular problems around menarche. Either during the first few menstrual cycles, or at approximately monthly intervals before onset of menstruation, rapid deterioration in glycaemic control may occur, sometimes even into ketoacidosis. So far no convincing hormonal explanation has been advanced, nor has the absorbability of subcutaneous injected insulin at these times been properly examined. It remains a clinically important but usually relatively short-lived conundrum. Prescription of oral contraceptives (low oestrogen) for a few months sometimes helps. Rapid response with extra insulin to incipient loss of control is also very important.

Another special problem is that of cessation of upward growth. If the large energy intake necessary for growth continues after it has ceased, a correspondingly large dose of insulin may become customary. This sustains the food intake at a time when it would have fallen in the healthy self-regulating adolescent. Obesity then develops, and a conflict of interests and guilt may develop if good advice is not given regarding coincident reduction of food intake and insulin dose. The onset of the growth spurt early in puberty poses the opposite problems; failure to increase caloric intake as necessary to fuel the initial spurt can result in well-controlled glycaemia but failure in growth.

Coma in diabetics

Comas in diabetics can be grouped as in Table 31.

Hypoglycaemic coma (see Chapter 11.12)

Hypoglycaemia occurs frequently in diabetics treated with insulin. At least one-third of insulin-treated patients suffer an episode severe enough to cause loss of consciousness at some time, 10 per cent have such coma annually, and, at some stage, 3 per cent suffer recurrent attacks so frequently as to be incapacitating. Hypoglycaemia also occurs in those taking sulphonylureas; however, true coma is uncommon in these patients except when there is some synergistic action between the sulphonylureas and another drug (for example monoamine oxidase inhibitors), or when a long-acting sulphonylurea accumulates (for example gross chlorpropamide overdosage), or in a new-born baby whose diabetic mother has been unwisely treated with chlorpropamide (which crosses the placenta).

DIAGNOSIS

Usually there are three important points in the history, if this can be obtained from a friend or bystander. In the case of iatrogenic hypoglycaemia these are as follows: the patient is a known diabetic, probably on insulin; the patient is nearly always completely normal as little as 15 or 30 min before the onset of the stupor; there may have been a phase

Table 31 *Coma in diabetics*

Abnormal glycaemia
Hypoglycaemic
Hyperglycaemic: (i) ketoacidotic; (ii) non-ketoacidotic

Other metabolic comas consequent upon the diabetic state
Uraemic coma, with or without glycaemic upset
Lactic acidosis, with or without glycaemic upset
Alcoholic coma, with possible abnormalities in 'ketone bodies', lactate, or glucose

Non-metabolic coma
For example, subarachnoid haemorrhage

of typical symptomatic hypoglycaemia or of abnormal behavior, usually mild confusion and sluggish speech, but occasionally wild and aggressive. This third phase is by no means constant as hypoglycaemia may occur with remarkable rapidity, particularly when the patient has reached the well-recognized phase in diabetes when there is no longer awareness of the premonitory symptoms of hypoglycaemia. This is more likely the longer a patient has been on insulin treatment. However, it may be induced temporarily by recurrent hypoglycaemia against a background of tight control, but can then be restored by deliberate relaxation of control for 1 to 2 weeks.

On examination of the stuporose or comatose patient, the diagnostically important points are negative, i.e. the patient is not dehydrated, hyperventilating, or ketotic. The most important evidence is of insulin injection sites, whether in the form of needle marks or local change in subcutaneous fat. There may be non-specific helpful physical signs, such as symmetrically dilated pupils (which react normally to light) and tachycardia, but a drenching sweat is often the most useful. The body temperature tends to be low, and there can be marked heat loss during the phase of falling central temperature. The condition clearly has to be distinguished from non-metabolic comas; the neck is not stiff, but the plantar reflexes may be upgoing. A rapid measurement of the blood glucose is essential in any undiagnosed comatose patient.

Hypoglycaemic episodes are more likely to occur several hours after the last meal or after unusual physical exertion without compensatory intake of extra food. However, attacks do not always occur classically. Sometimes they occur inexplicably within 1 to 2 h of an insulin injection, and it is probable that occasionally subcutaneous insulin is absorbed more rapidly than usual into the circulation, perhaps through damage to local blood vessels at the time of injection.

Self-administered insulin overdosage must always be remembered as a further possibility, as must simple errors in the preparation of the insulin dose. Some patients are particularly prone to hypoglycaemia through loss of normal counter-regulation (loss of both glucagon and catecholamine responses). They can be identified on testing with standard doses of intravenous insulin under close observation. Tight glycaemic control should not be attempted in these patients.

PATHOGENESIS

There has been much recent interest in hypoglycaemia because of both unjustified concern that human insulin had unique properties in this regard and the stricter aims of glycaemic control adopted with the knowledge that this retards or prevents the development of diabetic tissue damage.

Different people have different hypoglycaemic thresholds for neuroglycopenia, and the effective hypoglycaemic level alters in the same patient under different circumstances. This threshold is affected by the rate of glycaemic fall (the faster, the higher), by the size of the fall (the bigger, the higher), and by the habitual glycaemic levels for 36 to 60 h (the higher, the higher the threshold). There is a marked tendency for 'hypoglycaemic unawareness' to develop in patients with increasing duration of diabetes, particularly if they are treated with insulin. The cause of this is uncertain, although developing autonomic neuropathy with failure of normal catecholamine release may be implicated, as may increasing α-cell damage with failure of glucagon release, but neither of these is a constant feature of these unaware patients. The condition is probably the result of a combination of reduced afferent detection and reduced efferent expression of counter-regulatory mechanisms. Hypoglycaemia leads to a release of cortisol and growth hormone as well as catecholamines and glucagon, with the last two almost always secreted before the first two. The glycaemic threshold for such hormonal responses varies between different patients, usually over a range from 2.6 to 3.8 mmol/l, but when blood glucose has fallen rapidly from high levels adrenergic symptoms may appear even at 5.0 mmol/l.

An important clinical point is that the threshold concept is more appropriate for mild relatively early symptoms of hypoglycaemia than for loss of consciousness or other gross neuronal deficiency.

SYMPTOMS

Each individual usually maintains a fairly constant pattern in the evolution and occurrence of the many possible symptoms of hypoglycaemia. These can be divided into two categories. The first is consequent on neuroglycopaenia, with defective function of the central nervous system. It includes visual blurring, a feeling of uncertainty as to what is happening and then increasing ignorance of this, intense hunger, and a throbbing headache. The second group probably stems from increased catecholamine release as a counter-regulation against impending hypoglycaemia. It includes palpitation (a fast regular beat), paraesthesiae in the fingers or lips, a feeling of impending doom, fine muscular tremor, and excessive sweating which is due to cholinergic fibres, albeit of the sympathetic nervous system.

Onlookers may note sweating and increasing pallor as well as curious mannerisms such as stroking the back of the head or yawning. Also, some patients wake during the night feeling unduly warm when mildly hypoglycaemic. As hypoglycaemia develops, diabetics are very likely to resist advice to take sugar from onlookers who believe that the patient is becoming hypoglycaemic and great firmness may be needed by relatives or friends to achieve intake of quickly absorbed carbohydrate.

The frequency of undetected nocturnal hypoglycaemia is difficult to assess, but a value below 2.0 mmol/l probably occurs at least annually in a third of insulin-treated patients. Patients sometimes wake in the morning with grossly disturbed bedclothes, or even lying on the floor, without any memory of upset during the night. Alternatively, a throbbing headache may be the only residue. Again, hypoglycaemia may precipitate epilepsy, either by day or by night, but this is rare and not always realized during sleep. Anticonvulsants do not seem to protect against epilepsy which occurs as a complication of diabetic hypoglycaemia, although they are not less effective in diabetics who also have idiopathic epilepsy; the avoidance of hypoglycaemia is an important consideration in these latter patients.

Patients have a considerable capacity to recover from neuroglycopenia spontaneously, but it is still possible that it contributes to an unknown extent to unexplained nocturnal deaths of diabetics.

The amount of cumulative brain damage that results from recurrent hypoglycaemia is difficult to assess, but most studies indicate mild impairment of higher mental function in any insulin-treated patients suffering over 5 to 10 years two or three attacks annually, which are severe enough to require help from others.

TREATMENT

Prevention is better than cure. It is easy for a diabetic to take some oral sucrose or glucose, in solid or liquid form, at a time when there are early symptoms or signs of hypoglycaemia, but once the mental state has altered significantly this may be difficult. It is vital that no quantity of fluid be put into the mouth of a patient who is so comatose that he or she cannot swallow properly. A patient in such a state requires urgent medical help so that an intravenous injection of concentrated glucose solution can be given, usually 20 ml of 50 per cent glucose initially. The alternative treatment is by intramuscular injection of 1 mg glucagon by a relative or other carer. This may increase the blood glucose sufficiently to allow oral glucose to be given. However, it does not help some comatose patients (presumably those with little liver glycogen left for mobilization) and it is often less effective than intravenous glucose. Consequently, while it has a real place in the management of the stuporose, it should never be allowed to delay the call for help that will lead to the administration of intravenous glucose. It has the great advantage of providing independence to the family unit, and whenever possible a family member should be trained in glucagon injection.

After the administration of intravenous glucose, the patient usually opens his or her eyes and takes notice within a minute or two, but then may lapse back into stupor or sleep. If there has been no substantial response to the first injection within 5 min, a further intravenous injection of 20 ml of 50 per cent glucose should be given. There is no point in increasing the dose of 50 per cent glucose further, but if the patient still does not respond a continuous intravenous infusion of 5 per cent glucose in water (or 4 per cent glucose in N/5 saline) should be started. The blood glucose should be checked by glucose oxidase strips and confirmed in the laboratory.

If consciousness is still clearly abnormal after an hour, further treatment should be considered. There is no objective evidence that high dose glucocorticoid treatment or any other measure against cerebral oedema is beneficial, but equally none that they do harm, although the steroids will increase the insulin dose required in management over the next 24 to 48 h. Many physicians use such agents.

After glycaemic recovery from a severe attack a patient may be best managed either by continuous intravenous insulin (if an intravenous infusion is running for other reasons) or by frequent injections of small doses of short-acting insulin. The routine daily dose of insulin should be decreased by at least 4 units when it is resumed unless there is some other obvious explanation for the hypoglycaemic episode.

Hyperglycaemic comas

The majority of patients with major hyperglycaemia are not comatose as defined neurologically, but confused or stuporose. Type I diabetics generally suffer ketoacidotic hyperglycaemia, while type II diabetics may present with or without ketosis. In the United Kingdom as many as 70 deaths occur annually from hyperglycaemic coma in those under 50 years old, and the mortality rate in this condition increases with age to approximately 50 per cent in those aged over 70. These emergencies occur perhaps once in 200 patients each year, but as particular patients may contribute several of these emergencies, rather fewer patients are affected annually. Ketoacidosis is relatively common in girls around menarche who may suffer repeated attacks at intervals of 1 or 2 months.

The mortality from ketoacidosis remains as high as 3 to 10 per cent in hospitals that admit all the emergencies from particular localities. If individual factors are examined for their correlation with high mortality, age is the most important. However, when the interaction between factors is considered, associated illnesses (such as overwhelming infection, cardiac infarction, and pulmonary embolism) are dominant; the elderly are more likely to present with coma accompanied (and very likely precipitated) by such associated conditions. The depth and duration of coma are also prognostic factors. As a general guide to therapy the clinical state of the patient is of greater prognostic influence than their plasma biochemistry. Indeed, the blood urea concentration is a more important guide than the blood glucose, the blood ketones, the plasma bicarbonate, or the arterial pH, as it reflects the adequacy of the renal circulation as well as the metabolic disturbance.

The biochemical feature most related to the depth of unconsciousness is plasma osmolality; the blood glucose concentration and the degree of

Table 32 *Differential diagnosis of coma in diabetics*

	Blood glucose* (mmol/l)	Plasma ketones†	Dehydration	Hyperventilation	Blood pressure
Hypoglycaemic coma	≤2	0	0	0	Normal
Severe diabetic ketoacidosis	>13	+ to +++	+++	+++	Normal or low
Hyperglycaemic hyperosmolar non-ketotic coma	>13	0 to +	++++	0	Normal or low
Lactic acidosis	Variable	0 to +	0 to +	+++	Low
Non-metabolic comas	Normal to high	0 to +	0 to +	0 to +	Variable

*Assessed with Visidex or BM-Glycemie 20-800 R.

†Assessed with Ketostix.

acidosis or ketosis correlate poorly with unconsciousness. Certainly patients can walk about with blood glucose values as high as those that may accompany coma. In experimental diabetes the fall in cerebral oxygen uptake also correlates with the depth of coma.

The onset of severe ketoacidosis is linked indirectly to depletion of total body water, sodium, and potassium, and no doubt major changes in the intracellular electrolyte state. The final catastrophe may depend upon a switch from fat to protein to provide the alternative fuel to carbohydrate, or upon the steadily increasing loss of total body water and electrolytes. Because of either the circulatory or metabolic disturbance, or one of the common precipitating causes, the levels of the anti-insulin, catabolic, and hyperglycaemic hormones increase markedly to magnify the crisis.

There is probably no fundamental difference between ketoacidotic and non-ketotic comas. The latter occur in older patients and there tends to be less severe insulin deficiency. One crucial difference may be defective renal function in the older patients, so that more water and electrolytes are lost when there is severe persistent glycosuria. There may also be differences in the size and effectiveness of the counter-regulatory hormonal and autonomic nervous responses.

KETOACIDOTIC HYPERGLYCAEMIC COMA

The three cardinal clinical features of ketoacidotic hyperglycaemic coma found on examination are signs of extracellular volume and intracellular water depletion ('dehydration'), air hunger with an increased depth and rate of breathing, and ketosis. Many clinicians can identify the last of these by the typical sickly sweet smell on the breath, but 20 per cent cannot detect this usefully and the sensitivity of the remaining 80 per cent varies greatly. Hence every medical student should establish his or her own sensitivity to this odour. The degree of ketosis can also be readily assessed either by testing the urine (often not available in dehydrated and comatose patients) or by centrifuging heparinized blood and testing the clear supernatant with Ketostix or Ketodiabur.

When a history is available this varies from several weeks to a few days, and is often shorter in those already on insulin treatment. There may be weight loss, fatigue, excessive thirst, and polydipsia with polyuria. Other typical symptoms of developing hyperglycaemia may also be present. However, even in patients with previously unrecognized hyperglycaemia the history may be as short as 3 to 4 days, while occasionally excessive physical activity precipitates ketoacidosis in someone already severely hyperglycaemic from marked insulin deficiency. Other cardinal features are anorexia or vomiting, with or without diarrhoea. The onset of vomiting is always a threatening symptom and is particularly useful as a warning in those already known to be diabetic. An uncommon but well-recognized complicating symptom is of abdominal pain, which is particularly likely to occur in younger patients as a dull persistent severe discomfort often affecting the whole abdomen but usually centred on the umbilicus. It may cause unjustified suspicions of an abdominal emergency.

On examination, in addition to the three cardinal clinical features mentioned above, the patient is likely to show signs of weight loss, with rapid pulse of low volume and low systolic pressure, particularly if previously undiagnosed. There may be postural hypotension, certainly because of the dehydration and decreased total body sodium, and perhaps because of temporary autonomic neuropathy which may also contribute to the vomiting and diarrhoea. Significant postural hypotension in a markedly hyperglycaemic and ketonuric young patient, however alert and physically active, should always indicate the need for immediate parenteral fluid treatment. It is most unusual to find evidence of pathognomic tissue damage in newly diagnosed patients, but there may be symptoms and signs of a precipitating condition, for example infection (bronchopneumonia or an infected foot ulcer in a known diabetic), in any patient. Infection of the urinary tract or other inaccessible sites, for example ischiorectal, dental, or perinephric abscess, should be sought.

DIFFERENTIAL DIAGNOSIS

Table 32 shows guidelines for differential diagnosis. The main problems are as follows.

Any other illness with overventilation

These conditions are usually due to acidosis (for example uraemic or lactic acidosis) and may or may not be complicated by hyperglycaemia. Hyperventilation from salicylate overdosage is a potential problem, but the most confusing picture is Claude Bernard's 'piqure' diabetes which is a short-lived hyperglycaemia from a lesion in the region of the fourth ventricle. It probably results from massive discharge of the sympathetic division of the autonomic nervous system. The accompanying hyperventilation is due to irritation of pathways involved in respiration, and such overbreathing (as with excess salicylate) produces a respiratory alkalosis rather than the usual metabolic acidosis.

Determination of the arterial pH is decisive, as the plasma venous bicarbonate concentration will be low in both instances. Patients with such fourth-ventricle lesions (for example subarachnoid haemorrhage) may have mild ketonaemia because of reduced food intake and a degree of hypermetabolism (possibly with fever), and their conscious state will also be disturbed. The hyperglycaemia of piqure diabetes settles spontaneously in 6 to 12 h, and unless the glucose concentration is watched carefully unnecessary insulin treatment can cause a rapid swing to hypoglycaemia. The fall in glucose is unaccompanied by any improvement in consciousness, unlike the situation in classical diabetes. Hypoglycaemia then further worsens central nervous function.

Fourth-ventricle lesions are often accompanied by neck stiffness, but a degree of this (meningism rather than true meningitis) may occur in ketoacidosis as a facet of a general irritability present in about 5 per cent of stuporose patients. If there is doubt, a lumbar puncture (after checking for the absence of papilloedema) will differentiate, or a small intravenous injection of diazepam (for example 2 mg) may be given to see if this relaxes the neck as it settles the restlessness of a ketoacidotic.

Table 33 *Management of diabetic hyperglycaemic comas*

Initial assessment	
Clinical examination	Hydration, respiration, pulse, blood pressure, consciousness, signs of infection
Biochemical	Bedside: glucose, ketone body test strips, ECG Laboratory: glucose, Na^+, K^+, urea arterial pH, Po_2
Treatment Fluid	1 litre of 150 mmol/l saline in 30 min; 1 l/h for next 2 h, then 0.5 l/h until 5–7 l given in total, when give 500 ml 2–4 hourly, but change to 4% glucose in 30 mmol/l saline, 500 ml every 4 h, when blood glucose 10–15 mmol/l. If plasma Na^+ >150 mmol/l use hypotonic saline after early isotonic saline. Consider use of central venous catheterization
Insulin	IV regimen. 6 unit IV bolus, then 6 units/hour continuously IV; change to 2–4 units/h continuous IV when dextrose infusion commenced; change to SC with first meal IM regimen; 20 units IM (or 10 ml IM/10 units IV) initially, then 6 units every hour; change to 6 units every 2 h or 12 units SC every 4 h when dextrose infusion commenced
Potassium	Start at 13–20 mmol/l/hour in saline just after first insulin; adjust rate according to plasma values (26 mmol/h if plasma K^+ 3–4 mmol/l, 39 mmol/h if K^+ < 3 mmol/l, 10 mmol/h if K^+ 5–6 mmol/l, stop IV potassium if plasma K^+ >6 mmol/l)
Bicarbonate	Give 100 mmol + 20 mmol KCl in 20–40 min if pH <7.0; repeat after 60–90 min if pH still <7.0 Give 50 mmol + 10 mmol KCl if pH <7.1 but >7.0 or if patient distressed by hyperventilation

IV, intravenous; SC, subcutaneous; IM, intramuscular.

Certain physical signs may be unexpectedly absent during ketoacidosis. Thus, even if there is a pyogenic infection, there is usually no fever until insulin treatment has been given for 6 to 12 h. Indeed, some patients may be hypothermic initially. Again, perhaps owing to gross dehydration, classical signs of consolidation in patients with lobar pneumonia may not be elicited even though the radiograph shows lung shadows. The blood leucocyte count is of no help in assessing the likelihood of an infection, for the metabolic disturbance itself can cause a severe (95 per cent) polymorphonuclear leucocytosis of up to 30×10^9/l.

Non-ketotic hyperglycaemic states

Of the previously mentioned ketoacidotic features, only dehydration is present. This is not uncommon in many elderly patients, and so glucose levels should be checked in any stuporose or even confused patient, particularly if old. This is best done by one of the rapid bedside methods of blood glucose estimation. Unilateral signs of central nervous system abnormality do not exclude the diagnosis, for if a metabolic disturbance coincides with asymmetry of cerebral blood flow (even when this itself causes no problems) focal neurological signs may be present.

One may note, too, that many ketoacidotic patients are markedly hyperosmolar. The differences in management depend upon the levels of acidity and plasma sodium.

INVESTIGATION

The pretreatment state must be determined both for diagnostic purposes and to allow accurate assessment of the response to treatment. Blood urea, plasma sodium and potassium, and arterial pH should all be measured in addition to glucose and ketones. Arterial pH measurement is usually accompanied by measurement of arterial po_2, and in perhaps 20 per cent of patients this is surprisingly low initially, even below 8 torr; the hypoxia is not associated with the usual degree of cyanosis because of a shift of the dissociation curve of oxyhaemoglobin to the left (i.e.

oxyhaemoglobin dissociates less readily to release oxygen to the tissues). The haematocrit may provide a guide to dehydration, but chronic infection or uraemia will affect the premorbid value. The clinical states of the patient must be observed initially and regularly, with heart rate, blood pressure, respiratory rate, and level of consciousness being recorded. It is also useful to note the discrepancy between the warmth of the centre (for example abdominal wall temperature) and the periphery (big toe or tip of nose) as a guide to impaired peripheral circulation from reduced blood volume and the general illness.

Blood glucose and potassium levels should be reassessed 1 hour after the start of insulin treatment and, unless the clinical course is convincingly satisfactory, arterial pH and blood urea should be remeasured 3 hours after start of treatment together with glucose and potassium. These latter two should also be measured after 5 hours. Crucial targets are normality of the plasma potassium concentration and the level of blood glucose (about 12 mmol/l) at which glucose should be added to the intravenous infusion.

TREATMENT

Treatment is summarized in Tables 33 and 34.

Metabolic

Fluid

The basis of treatment is the provision of water, sodium, insulin, and potassium. Water and sodium are the most important as restoration of an adequate circulation is the pre-eminent need. Despite a greater loss (usually) of water than of sodium, the correct replacement fluid is 'physiologically normal' saline (0.9 per cent) and this should be given rapidly, for example 0.5 l in the first 20 min and 2.5 l in the next 3 h, with infusion of 500 ml hourly thereafter to a total of about 5 litres (or until a normal circulation is present and obvious clinical features of dehydration have disappeared). The use of hypotonic sodium chloride is indicated only when there is marked hypernatraemia, for example an initial

Table 34 *General measures in the treatment of diabetic hyperglycaemic coma*

1. Nasogastric tube in unconscious patients
2. Continuous venous pressure line in patients with cardiovascular disease
3. Plasma or plasma expanders in persistent hypotension
4. Low dose subcutaneous heparin in comatose, obese, or severely hyperosmolar patients, provided that there is no contraindication
5. Antibiotics if infection detected or suspected
6. ECG; cardiac monitor as guide to K$^+$ therapy
7. Bladder catheterization if prolonged failure to pass urine
8. Frequent monitoring of pulse, blood pressure, respiration, conscious state

plasma sodium concentration of 150 mmol/l or higher, and even then not initially (see below).

Once insulin has been administered the plasma sodium rises because water moves intracellularly together with glucose and potassium. There is abnormal water balance of the central nervous system in ketoacidosis, with undue liability to oedema. Hence the osmolality of the extracellular fluid should be kept relatively high, which is benefit of physiologically 'normal' saline. Most patients with ketoacidosis have a low plasma sodium concentration on admission as an osmolar compensation for hyperglycaemia, and so a sodium concentration of 145 mmol/l, still within the normal range, represents a marked excess loss of water over sodium. If the plasma sodium concentration exceeds 149 mmol/l, half-normal physiological saline should be infused after 2 litres of normal saline to prevent undue hypernatraemia. The mechanisms that underlie this are poorly understood, but hypernatraemia is particularly liable to occur in non-ketotic patients and can cause cerebral irritation. The initial 2 litres are still of 'normal' saline because the first priority is always to achieve an adequate circulation (which requires a reasonable plasma volume). Indeed, if the blood pressure is unduly low (below 90 mmHg systolic) and/or the peripheral circulation is little improved 2 hours after start of treatment, a plasma expander should be infused (or, sometimes even better, whole blood). If the plasma expander affects blood grouping, this must be established first just in case an operation becomes necessary (rare but possible, particularly if deep-seated infection needs drainage).

Insulin

The necessary actions of insulin in diabetic ketoacidosis are to inhibit inappropriate gluconeogenesis and excessive adipose tissue lipolysis. Relatively low concentrations of insulin are adequate for this, for example 30–40 mU/l which is half the normal maximum peripheral insulin concentration during an oral glucose tolerance test and about a quarter of the insulin concentration necessary to achieve maximum glucose and potassium uptake in the forearm at normal blood glucose levels. However, insulin concentrations of 60–80 mU/l are the aim during treatment of ketoacidotic hyperglycaemic coma; because of the high glucose concentrations the maximum uptake of glucose by peripheral tissues can then be achieved, with a decrease in blood glucose of 3–5 mmol/l/h.

Insulin can be administered either by hourly intramuscular injection or by continuous intravenous infusion. Every institute should choose the method which suits its facilities best. The aim is continuous entry into the blood of small but adequate amounts of insulin.

Intramuscular regimen An initial injection of 20 IU of short-acting insulin should be followed by a further 6 IU hourly. It is important that the injections are intramuscular and not subcutaneous, because absorption of insulin from the poorly perfused subcutaneous site is slow. If blood glucose has not dropped by 5 mmol/l after 2 h, a change to the intravenous route is indicated together with reassessment of fluid status.

Intravenous After an initial bolus of 6 IU of crystalline insulin the same amount (6 IU) is infused hourly. In children the loading dose is 0.1 IU/kg with 0.1 IU/kg/hour subsequently. This is best given by a pump with insulin joining the giving set from a separate line, but if this facility is unavailable insulin can be added to an ordinary giving set (or Metriset). Again, a Y-connection is best so that the rate of insulin administration is independent of that of the bulk of intravenous fluid. Absorption of insulin to the walls of syringes or tubing occurs but is not a clinical problem. It is always vital to check that insulin is given in an amount adequate to produce the expected rate of fall of blood glucose (between 3 and 5 mmol/l/h). The recommended rate of insulin administration should be doubled if glucose falls by less than 5 mmol/l in the first 2 h. The rate of fall is remarkably constant in individual patients, and allows a rough and ready prediction of when intravenous glucose should be infused, which is at a blood glucose between 10 and 15 mmol/l. This serves both to provide necessary fuel to a starving patient and further to reduce the chances of cerebral oedema. The intravenous glucose is best given as 500 ml of 4 per cent dextrose in 0.18 per cent saline (one-fifth normal) every 4 h.

Insulin can be continued by continuous intravenous infusion at 2–4 IU/h. If the intramuscular route has been used, the injections may be changed to 6 IU every 2 h; alternatively subcutaneous injections of 12 IU insulin can be given every 4 h. The intravenous route should be used only as long as it is necessary to give intravenous fluids on other grounds. Ingestion of nutrients should be encouraged as soon as possible, beginning with small quantities of simple fluids.

Potassium The details of potassium replacement treatment remain surprisingly contentious. Many regard the greater attention to this as one of the more important developments in the treatment of diabetic ketoacidosis. The reasons for more active potassium infusion, advanced at least 15 years ago, are still valid. Patients in diabetic ketoacidosis have a total body deficit of potassium averaging 500 mmol and sometimes more than twice this. A major action of insulin is to increase tissue potassium uptake. Therefore once insulin treatment has been started, it is safe to infuse potassium provided that both the potassium and the insulin will reach the tissues. Thus the only contraindication to early potassium supplementation is a grossly inadequate circulation, such that potassium added to a small circulating blood volume does not reach enough cells for its uptake to be increased effectively by insulin. It is also only in patients with such an inadequate circulation that there is a real risk of acute renal tubular necrosis, with the possibility of prolonged anuria or gross oliguria. Obviously this makes ill-judged potassium administration potentially dangerous, but this is much less so now that peritoneal dialysis and haemodialysis are more widely available.

Even though a quarter of the patients admitted with diabetic ketoacidosis have a plasma potassium concentration above the normal range, potassium should be given once saline infusion and insulin treatment have started; in other words, a few minutes after intravenous insulin and about 10 min after intramuscular insulin, with the exceptions noted above. Blood should be sent for plasma potassium assay before insulin is given. In the first hour 10–13 mmol/l potassium chloride can be given safely, by which time the initial potassium concentration should be available. At this stage another sample should be sent for potassium assay, as the change over the first hour helps greatly in the prediction of future doses, which can be altered accordingly. With resalination and insulin treatment plasma potassium may fall fast, particularly from high values. Thus a drop from 6.4 to 5.2 mmol/l may occur in the first hour, even though 13 mmol/l potassium were given. If plasma potassium is between 3 and 4 mmol/l the rate of intravenous infusion can be increased to 26 mmol/l/hour, while if it is below 3 mmol/l at least 39 mmol/l/h should be given.

Patients particularly liable to have a low initial plasma potassium concentration in diabetic ketoacidosis are the newly diagnosed, when the period of kaliuresis is likely to have been considerably longer than in those already on insulin, and patients treated with a thiazide or similar diuretic, as the usual urinary potassium loss with these agents will be magnified by the osmotic diuresis of heavy glycosuria. Such patients may require 400–600 mmol of potassium in the first 12 h of treatment.

Plasma potassium should certainly be measured 1 h and 5 h after the start of treatment, as well as initially and, if there is any doubt about its concentration, 3 h after the start of treatment. The ECG is a useful, albeit indirect, guide to potassium status, with particular reference to the T waves, whose inversion implies a low plasma potassium. However, the T waves can also be influenced by acidosis, and so they are an uncertain guide to absolute potassium levels although a useful index of change. Potassium is usually given intravenously as the chloride salt, but may also be partly administered as a hydrogen phosphate salt.

Potassium should be started orally as soon as fluids are taken, initially as potassium-rich fluids such as meat soups, fruit juice, or even milk, and later as more definite supplements when solids are being taken.

Urinary potassium losses may remain large during the first 12 to 24 h despite the deficit of total potassium, perhaps because of intracellular deficits in renal tubular cells. As expected, patients with lower initial potassium concentrations conserve most added potassium.

Particular attention must also be paid to potassium replacement when intravenous bicarbonate is given (see below).

Bicarbonate There is good reason for this also to be a contentious aspect of treatment. The advantages of bicarbonate infusion are reduction in metabolic acidosis and consequent relief of distressing hyperventilation (air hunger) in a conscious patient. If acidaemia is severe (pH < 7.0), tissue function may be impaired with a negative inotropic effect on the heart, analogous peripheral vasodilatation, and depression of the central nervous system. However, bicarbonate infusion also has the disadvantages of hypokalaemia, with possible consequent cardiac dysrhythmia, and a leftward shift in the dissociation curve of oxyhaemoglobin so that oxygen less readily reaches the tissues. Perhaps surprisingly, the dissociation curve is approximately normal on admission of ketoacidotic patients, despite the marked acidosis which, by the Bohr effect, would be expected to have moved the curve to the right. However, the right shift is approximately balanced by decreased red-cell 2,3-diphosphoglycerate. If the metabolic acidosis is rapidly corrected, the curve will shift to the left as the 2,3-diphosphoglycerate deficit persists for 24 to 72 h after treatment starts. In addition, after bicarbonate infusion a metabolic alkalosis often appears as ketonaemia disappears. This is rarely severe enough to disturb health, but it shows that the amount of bicarbonate needed is often less than that given.

Ketosis disappears through oxidation of the ketone bodies in the periphery, coincident with inhibition of their further formation in the liver once insulin has checked the typical excessive lipolysis. The drop in concentration of these organic acids is faster than the rise in bicarbonate concentration of the plasma, and usually a mild hyperchloraemic acidosis occurs for a short while during replacement therapy.

Therefore bicarbonate should not be given as long as the peripheral circulation is grossly restricted, for it will almost certainly reduce oxygen delivery to the periphery. However, once sufficient saline has been given to restore a reasonable circulation, 100 mmol sodium bicarbonate should be given over 20 min if pH is below 7.0, and 50 mmol in the same time if it is between 7.1 and 7.0. Such bicarbonate should be accompanied by an extra 20 mmol of potassium chloride per 100 mmol of bicarbonate. Arterial pH should be measured 60–90 min later to decide whether more bicarbonate is needed (with the amount judged similarly).

Oxygen Approximately one-fifth of patients have an arterial pO_2 below 8 torr. If this is coincident with any leftward shift of the dissociation curve of oxyhaemoglobin it may help to administer oxygen via a facemask, initially at 100 per cent, which is stopped for 10 min before arterial blood is taken for pH and pO_2 determination. If pO_2 is still low, 28 per cent oxygen is continued until the peripheral circulation has improved substantially.

Management of hyperosmolar hyperglycaemic non-ketotic coma

The patient should be treated in similar fashion to the more classical ketoacidotic case. However, the following special points should be noted

1. Approximately half such patients are normo- or hypernatraemic, so that hypotonic fluid replacement may be necessary during treatment but not initially. In general, total fluid requirements are likely to be greater (but so is the risk of cardiac failure).
2. There is an increased likelihood of thrombotic events, so that prophylactic anticoagulation should be seriously considered.
3. Bicarbonate replacement is obviously unnecessary, and smaller amounts of potassium are required than in ketoacidotic patients. A replacement rate of 10–13 mmol/h is probably adequate.
4. Blood glucose levels are likely to be extremely high, so that restoration of normoglycaemia will take many hours, but, as with ketoacidotic patients, too great a fall of glucose levels could be harmful because of the effects of osmotic disequilibrium on the central nervous system.

GENERAL MANAGEMENT

An unconscious patient should be nursed semiprone until a thin nasogastric tube has been passed and any gastric content aspirated. Frequently this is of large volume, and if vomited by an unconscious patient aspiration of the acid liquid will produce a severe chemical pneumonitis, possibly with a fatal outcome. If aspiration occurs, anti-inflammatory doses of glucocorticoid should be given even though this will probably increase the need for insulin. Thus the nasogastric tube should be passed as soon as possible after admission in the unconscious patient.

Urethral catheterization is sometimes recommended early in management, for instance if no urine has been passed after 4 to 6 h of treatment, but it is not surprising if a hypotensive and severely dehydrated patient does not void urine in this time. Catheterization of devitalized tissues readily introduces infection. Hence it may be an advantage to delay catheterization unless, of course, there is clinical evidence of distressing bladder distension. If oliguria persists 6 to 8 h after the start of intravenous fluids, 80 mg of frusemide intravenously may be helpful.

Although some advocate central venous catherization for the majority, it is probably better confined to patients in whom there is real suspicion of cardiac embarrassment, as when intravenous fluid is rapidly administered to those with known cardiac disease, or to the aged. If there is any suspicion of deterioration from fluid infusion, a central line should be inserted but, as with any other catheter, it should be removed as soon as it becomes unnecessary in order to reduce the risk of infection. Failure of the heart rate to decrease during treatment can indicate cardiac insufficiency, but another cause may be the uncommon deterioration in pulmonary function that can occur 4 to 8 h after treatment starts. This is associated with a radiographic appearance like that of pulmonary oedema and a marked drop in arterial pO_2. Medium or coarse crepitations are heard over the lung fields, quite unlike the fine moist crepitations of left-sided heart failure. If the condition is severe enough to warrant artificial ventilation, pulmonary compliance is very low. The cause of such stiff lungs is uncertain, but they may result from interstitial pulmonary oedema or, alternatively, from a disseminated intravascular coagulation affecting particularly the lungs. The possibility of interstitial oedema has led to arguments about whether it is the osmotic or the oncotic pressure of the plasma that matters in this state, and whether colloids should be infused as well as crystalloids. This only seems important in the more severe patients, but reinforces the advice given above to add a plasma expander intravenously if the circulation has not improved after 2 to 3 h of crystalloids.

Rarely, ketoacidosis is associated with disseminated intravascular coagulation of clinical significance. Clinically, evidence of vascular occlusion and/or excessive bruising or spontaneous bleeding should suggest this possibility, which is diagnosed by the conjunction of low platelet count, reduced plasma fibrinogen, and increased amounts of fibrinogen degradation products.

ECG should always be recorded early in management in case an acute (and possibly painless) cardiac infarction has precipitated the metabolic emergency. It is an advantage to repeat the recording frequently or, ideally, for the patient to be on an ECG monitor.

Routine anticoagulation has been suggested for diabetics with metabolic emergencies. It is probably wiser to confine their prophylactic use to high risk patients, such as those in deep coma, those with a known history of venous thrombosis, the very obese, and the very hyperosmolar. Subcutaneous heparin injections should not be started until 4 to 6 h after admission, which will allow some time for clinical assessment of any predisposing or precipitating factors, some of which might contraindicate routine coagulation.

While routine use of antibiotics has been suggested, prescription on more positive grounds is probably preferable. When diabetes newly presents as a metabolic emergency and there is a history of steadily increasing severity, infection is rarely a precipitating cause. Also, bacterial infection is rarely present in known diabetics who present after 2 or 3 days of vomiting (with or without accompanying diarrhoea), particularly if admission has been precipitated by marked reduction in their usual insulin dose. However, infection, for example an ischiorectal abscess or a relatively small foot ulcer at the mouth of a sinus leading to a deeper collection of pus, should be sought avidly. As mentioned previously, the body temperature or white blood cell count and certain physical signs (particularly abdominal pain and guarding) are all potentially misleading in ketoacidosis. The management of a suspected 'acute abdomen' may not be as difficult as the differential diagnosis in the early state. Whether or not there is intraperitoneal infection, conservative treatment by intravenous fluids and insulin, together with gastric aspiration, is best for at least the first 4 to 6 h. If the illness is purely metabolic, there should then be substantial improvement in the signs on physical examination of the abdomen; if peritonitis is present, a fever is then likely to have appeared and the patient's condition will probably have worsened rather than improved as expected. Surgery, for however good a cause, is dangerous in the presence of severe ketoacidosis, which should be dealt with first. With current antibiotics, intravenous fluids, and gastric aspiration, little will be lost on the surgical side by such delay but a great deal will be gained medically. If antibiotics are to be given, blood, urine, and throat swabs should first be taken for culture.

Routine observations include the usual nursing observations of pulse and respiration rate, level of consciousness, temperature, and blood pressure. These are the most important guides to the success of treatment in that they report the patient's organ functions directly; metabolic measurements only predict what they are likely to become in the coming hours.

Occasionally the metabolic reports give strange results, such as a plasma sodium concentration under 110 mmol/l, and this should raise suspicion of gross lipaemia which may be missed if the plasma is not looked at after centrifugation. A clinical clue to this may be lipaemia retinalis, in which the small retinal vessels are yellow. The high chylomicra count may occupy as much as 30 per cent of the plasma volume and so distort the biochemical reports. Taking blood proximal to an intravenous infusion may also falsify the picture, as may finger-prick blood testing from fingers on which glucose solutions have dried (the latter is particularly important in hypoglycaemic patients when 50 per cent glucose may have been spilt).

Organization of therapy

There have been substantial changes in the pattern of care of diagnosed diabetics in the United Kingdom in recent years. Home blood glucose testing has allowed a drive towards increased self-care by well-informed

Table 35 *Routine for annual review*

Visual acuity
Fundoscopy through dilated pupils

Microalbuminuria
Plasma creatinine

Vibration sense, peripheral sensation. Foot examination
Autonomic examination: R–R interval on provocation
Cardiac examination, resting ECG
Foot pulses
Blood pressure (lying and standing)
Total cholesterol
HDL cholesterol
Triglycerides (using fed values for screening, enquire for fatty meal)

Doppler ultrasound

Weight

and well-monitored patients. Health professionals play a vital role in education, primarily of the patient but importantly of one another. Fewer patients attend hospital clinics than in the past. This is entirely justified if they receive equivalent or better care in health centre 'miniclinics' or in the home from doctors and specialist nursing advisors. However, access to specialist knowledge and experience must be maintained, in the same way as it is available from consultants to younger doctors working in hospital clinics. The benefits to the patient of reduced travelling time and usually shorter waiting time must not be counter-balanced by a lower standard of care, and so this must be carefully monitored. The best interactions between hospital specialist consultants and general practitioners have probably still to be established.

The diabetic clinic

In the United Kingdom care was once centred on the hospital-based diabetic clinic, all too often understaffed for its work-load. Individual doctors might have been required to see 20 to 30 patients in a single clinic (one every 5–6 min). In such a setting it was possible for general practitioners to see clinic care, wrongly, as all-embracing, so that they restricted themselves to issuing repeat prescriptions.

Hospital clinics should now be staffed by registered doctors who have received training in the speciality, and the staffing level should be sufficient to allow at least 15 min per patient. Each patient should generally see the same doctor on successive visits, at least throughout 1 year. Each visit should include educational reinforcement. Glycosylated haemoglobin assay should be routinely available. Patients should be screened for complications, possibly through special annual review clinics. Features that should be investigated in such a clinic are listed in Table 35. A dietitian should be in attendance and should have his or her own clinic on a separate occasion when the advice given at the diabetic clinic can be reinforced and extended. A chiropodist should also be present for advice on remedial footwear and preventive foot education. The presence of a teaching nurse as an integral part of the clinic is a major advantage. He or she can both teach practical aspects of therapy (home blood glucose monitoring, injection technique, urine testing) and provide general advice on self-management. The provision of simple brochures may also be helpful. Video films are best organized as a separate activity, with time for discussion afterwards. However, the major requirement is for consistent continued care, which requires a great deal of time.

In centres responsible for many diabetics it is advantageous to have separate clinics for separate functions: a pregnancy clinic shared with

an obstetrician, a pre-pregnancy clinic for 'super-control', and an adolescent clinic. Even separating clinics into 'routine' and 'problem' sessions may be helpful. Use of a day unit for more detailed investigation
and for further education is another advantage, as are clinics held at
special times, for instance in the evening.

Despite the increasing costs of health care and decreased provision
relative to what is potentially available, such preventive measures are
very likely to be cost effective in the long run. Some centres make
arrangements for 24 h advice to be available by telephone, but this
requires discipline in both the patients and their doctors. There should
be more ready access for most type I patients as well as those in whom
problems are detected at the annual review.

Shared care

In the care of patients attending a conventional diabetic clinic, the role
of the general practitioner can become diminished, so that he or she is
often involved only when emergencies occur. There is no reason in this
context why general practitioners should not take on the regular care of
most of their diabetic patients. The clinic can then concentrate on particular problems. Care can be shared with the hospital clinic to a greater
or lesser degree depending on whether or not the disease is behaving in
an uncomplicated way. A 'shared care' card is useful with joint care.
This system is clearly sensible, but it requires sustained interest from
both hospital and family doctors.

Miniclinics

An alternative to shared care is the establishment of small clinics outside
the main centre. This can be done in local hospitals or health centres.
The clinics are staffed by general practitioners with periodic visits from
the consultant diabetologist. If a prevalence of diabetes of 4 to 8 per
cent is accepted, a group practice of 10 000 patients will include more
than 400 diabetics, which is more than enough to have a monthly diabetic clinic, even excluding the most elderly. Open access to hospital
investigations, an ophthalmologist, the dietitian, and chiropody services
is essential, together with provision of appropriate educational materials.
The advantage of this system is the increased attention given to the
individual patient, continuity of care, and knowledge of family
background.

Diabetes nurse

Over the years there has been a steady increase in the number of nurses
with a special responsibility for diabetes. They play an essential role in
total diabetic care, as is now recognized by the Royal College of Nursing
in the United Kingdom. The diabetes nurse is generally attached to a
specific clinic and/or community district. He or she has several distinct
roles including (1) teaching the practical and theoretical aspects of diabetes in the clinic, (2) coordinating the care of diabetic patients in different parts of the hospital, advising on their therapy, and teaching them
and their families where necessary, (3) following new patients and
patients with specific problems into their homes in liaison with district
nurses, and (4) working with community health services and with
patients in the community. The domiciliary aspect is particularly important in that problems may be unravelled which have their roots in home
circumstances and which might not be revealed during a busy diabetic
clinic. It is widely recognized that patients communicate more freely
with nurses than with doctors, and that trained nurses often communicate
more effectively with patients.

Diabetes education centres

The concept of and need for formal education centres in diabetes has
been slow to develop in the United Kingdom compared with the United
States and mainland Europe. Such a centre should be available to every
diabetic patient, whether it be based in a hospital or in general practice.
Coherent teaching programmes can be organized for new patients and
their families, and as reinforcement for old patients, with different programmes for type I and type II diabetics, and for young and old patients.
Both group and individual teaching can be useful. There is much scope
for audiovisual aids. Such a scheme should include evaluation and audit
to ensure that the objectives initially established are met.

The exact structure of such centres and their relation to the diabetic
clinic will depend on local circumstances and resources. At the simplest
level one teaching nurse in a single room can have a great effect. The
minimum requirement for a large health district is probably three or four
staff who also serve as diabetic nurses in the clinic and community. The
centre should include a phone-in service for patients and families, which
can have a major effect on both patient health and clinic work-load.

The diabetic record

In most hospitals the notes of diabetic patients form part of the overall
medical records system, can be disorganized, and therefore offer little
help to the physician. There are three possible solutions to this problem.
The first is to have separate diabetic records. This has the disadvantage
that the records, although less voluminous, may still be disorganized
and difficulties may arise when patients are admitted or seen with non-
diabetic problems. The second solution is to have a flowsheet at the
front of the notes which records all major events, in-patient admissions,
the dose of antidiabetic and other therapeutic agents, diet, weight, and
indices of control, and when appropriate indicates when physical examinations and interviews were performed (i.e. eyes, feet, blood pressure,
neurological, chiropodist, and dietitian). This is certainly preferable to
the usual 'random' notes but requires adequate staff to complete these
details. The best approach is to introduce a computerized records system.
In the past most of these schemes have been unduly complicated, requiring main-frame computers and a computer programmer. At best they
have been used to run appointment systems, to identify defaulters, and
to provide research information. Nowadays clinic microcomputers can
provide a summary of each patient seen, ask appropriate questions of
the clinician, and receive new information typed in directly. Such interactive systems are being developed; they should be relatively simple
and inexpensive, and could prove a major advance in patient care. Their
initiation may require extra staff and expenditure but, once running, they
should potentiate clinic and community care.

REFERENCES

Alberti, K.G.M.M. and Johnston, D.G. (1992). Secondary diabetes. *Bailli-
ère's Clinical Endocrinology and Metabolism*, **6** (4).
Alberti, K.G.M.M. and Krall, L.P. (ed.) (1988). *The diabetes annual*, Vol.
4. Elsevier, Amsterdam.
Hales, C.N. and Barker, D.J.P. (1993) *Fetal and infant origins of adult dis-
ease*, pp. 241–72. British Medical Journal, London.
Jovanovic, L. and Peterson, C.M. (ed.) (1985). Nutrition and diabetes. In:
Contemporary Issues in Clinical Nutrition, Vol. **8**. Liss, New York.
Kahn, C.R. and Weir, G.C. (1994). *Joslin's diabetes mellitus* (13th edn.).
Lea and Febiger, Philadelphia.
Karam, J.H. (ed.) (1992) Diabetes mellitus: perspectives on therapy. *Clinics
in Endocrinology and Metabolism*, **21** (2).
Leslie, R.D.G. (ed.) (1989) Diabetes. *British Medical Bulletin*, **45** (1).
Mann, J.I., Pyrälä, K., and Teucher, A. (ed.) (1983). *Diabetes in epidemio-
logical perspective*. Churchill Livingston, Edinburgh.
Mogensen, C.E. and Standl, E. (ed.) (1989). *Prevention and treatment of
diabetic late complications*. de Gruyter, Berlin.
Rifkin, H., Colwell, J.A., and Taylor, S.I. (1991). *Diabetes 1991, Interna-
tional Congress Series No. 1000*. Excerpta Medica, Amsterdam.
Taskinen, M.-R. (1990). Hyperlipidaemia in diabetes. In D.J. Betteridge
(ed.), *Lipid and Lipoprotein Disorders, Baillière's Clinical Endocrinology and Metabolism*, **4** (4).
West, K.M. (1978). *Epidemiology of diabetes and its vascular lesions*.
Elsevier, New York.

11.12 Hypoglycaemia

R. C. TURNER

Hypoglycaemia is an uncommon cause of symptoms in adults, apart from diabetic patients on insulin or sulphonylurea therapy. Any curious attack, in which a low plasma glucose concentration is found, should be investigated as some of the causes of hypoglycaemia can be life-threatening, yet are readily treatable.

Physiology of glucose control

Glucose enters the circulation either by absorption from the gut or, when fasting, by hepatic glucose efflux. This is initially derived from glycogen stores and then predominantly via gluconeogenesis from certain amino acids, such as alanine, and carbohydrate substrates, such as glycerol and lactate. Although the kidney is capable of gluconeogenesis, insufficient glucose is produced to affect plasma glucose concentrations. The liver thus has a predominant role in regulating the plasma glucose concentration. During a meal, hepatic glucose production is inhibited both by raised plasma insulin levels and by the raised plasma glucose concentrations. If following a meal, the plasma glucose concentration falls below the normal fasting level, the resultant decrease in plasma insulin allows increased hepatic glucose efflux, raising the plasma glucose concentration towards the normal level. Thus in the fasting state, the concentration of plasma glucose and insulin are closely regulated in a negative feedback loop between the liver and islet β-cells.

The liver is unable to produce normal glucose efflux in the absence of cortisol or growth hormone, and the presence of glucagon may be even more important. A protein meal stimulates glucagon as well as insulin secretion, and the glucagon probably prevents insulin-induced hypoglycaemia that would occur if protein were not accompanied by carbohydrate. The role of glucagon is apparent from a somatostatin infusion in man, that inhibits both insulin and glucagon production and induces hypoglycaemia. Fasting plasma glucagon concentrations increase in response to hypoglycaemia and other stresses in man, as do those of cortisol, growth hormone, and adrenaline. The plasma glucagon rise after birth may be particularly important in preventing neonatal hypoglycaemia, and its lack may contribute to the neonatal hypoglycaemia sometimes found in infants of diabetic mothers.

Insulin is the major hormone regulating fuel supply and is the only known physiological hormone to directly lower the plasma glucose. Other insulin-like peptides are present in plasma, and their biological activity in vitro on muscle or adipose tissues is not completely abolished by addition of insulin antiserum. This remaining activity is termed non-suppressible insulin-like activity (NSILA). These peptides are growth promoting and, when assayed in vitro, they were termed somatomedins. There are two major fractions, an ethanol-precipitated protein (NSILA-p) and soluble fraction (NSILA-s). The NSILA-s has been purified and consists of pro-insulin-related peptides, called insulin-like growth factors, ILGF-I and ILGF-II. ILGF-I is primarily produced by the liver and is stimulated by growth hormone production. Control of ILGF-II secretion is less well defined. The peptides are thought to be primarily growth factors rather than being concerned with fuel supply. In plasma both ILGF-I and ILGF-II are bound to specific binding proteins.

STARVATION

In the first 24 h of a fast, hepatic glucose efflux is primarily from glycogenolysis, but this provides only about 600 kcal in non-obese subjects. Thereafter, gluconeogenesis has a major role. As the plasma glucose concentration falls from the normal level of approximately 4.5 mmol/l to 3.5 mmol/l, the plasma insulin decreases from approximately 5 to 3 mU/l. This not only allows gluconeogenesis to proceed, but also allows free fatty acid flux from adipose tissue to the liver, where β-oxidation to form acetyl CoA and ketone bodies provides the energy needed for gluconeogenesis. The increased free fatty acids and ketone bodies are preferentially utilized by muscle, and markedly decrease the glucose requirement of the body. The ketone bodies are also utilized by the brain which, however, still needs glucose to provide approximately 50 per cent of its energy requirements. After a 30-h fast, normal women have a lower fasting plasma glucose (3.5 ± 0.2 mmol/l) than men (4.0 ± 0.2 mmol/l).

In a prolonged fast, a new steady state is reached in which the fasting plasma glucose concentration falls to approximately 2 to 3 mmol/l, with a low plasma insulin concentration and high plasma free fatty acid and ketone body concentrations. In some patients the plasma glucose concentration falls to 1 mmol/l, but it is not associated with symptoms of hypoglycaemia until very low levels are produced, because of the alternative ketone body substrate supply for the brain.

Pathological hypoglycaemia

Spontaneous hypoglycaemia can usually be divided into two main categories:

1. Fasting hypoglycaemia only occurs after several hours without food. Symptoms can occur during the night, on waking, or after a longer fast, sometimes precipitated by exercise. Fasting hypoglycaemia always indicates an identifiable underlying disease.
2. Reactive or postprandial hypoglycaemia occurs 2 to 5 h after meals. Patients with reactive hypoglycaemia never have hypoglycaemia during a fast, although occasionally patients with fasting hypoglycaemia may have a reactive component. Reactive hypoglycaemia usually occurs in the absence of organic disease.

CLINICAL FEATURES

Hypoglycaemic symptoms are unusual unless the plasma glucose falls to less than 2.5 mmol/l. However, the threshold varies from person to person. Patients with prolonged hypoglycaemia (from an insulinoma, for example, or a diabetic patient chronically overtreated with insulin), have a lower threshold, and can have a plasma glucose of 1 mmol/l for several hours without symptoms. At the other extreme, a diabetic who has had prolonged hyperglycaemia may get adrenergic symptoms if the plasma glucose concentration is rapidly lowered towards the normal level.

Adrenergic symptoms

Adrenergic symptoms usually predominate, particularly when the plasma glucose falls rapidly, as in reactive hypoglycaemia. Adrenaline is secreted (together with the other counter-regulatory hormones including glucagon, growth hormone, and cortisol) and induces pallor, sweating, tremor, and palpitation.

Neuroglycopenic symptoms

These occur when the brain has insufficient glucose. Lack of glucose may induce poor concentration, slow movements, dysarthria, double vision, tingling around the mouth, transient strokes, fits, and coma in a variety of combinations. Each patient may have a characteristic group of symptoms which he or she can recognize. The features may resemble ethanol intoxication. Poor judgement and inco-ordination can be especially dangerous if the patient is driving, swimming, or near to dangerous machinery.

Neuroglycopenic symptoms predominate when chronic hypoglycaemia occurs, since the threshold to adrenergic symptoms is then lowered. Examples are overtreated insulin-dependent diabetic patients and patients with insulinomas.

TREATMENT OF ACUTE HYPOGLYCAEMIA

If a patient is unconscious and unable to take glucose by mouth, 20 to 50 ml of 50 g/dl glucose is given intravenously into a large vein and repeated as necessary. The administering needle should not be withdrawn from the vein immediately, as pressure on the vein to secure homeostasis maintains the glucose in the vein and can cause venous thrombosis. There should either be a pause before withdrawing the needle from the vein, or an intravenous injection of saline following the glucose infusion. If, after intravenous glucose, the patient remains unconscious for longer than 30 min in spite of normoglycaemia, it is possible that secondary cerebral oedema may have occurred; mannitol or high-dose dexamethasone therapy, for example 5 mg 6 hourly, then sometimes appears to expedite recovery.

If a patient is unconscious, and intravenous glucose or a suitable vein is not available, 1 mg glucagon can be given intramuscularly. This is a sufficient dose; larger doses increase the likelihood of inducing nausea and vomiting. Glucagon increases hepatic glucose efflux, so that the patient becomes semiconscious after 10 to 15 min, allowing oral glucose to be given. The glucagon effect will wear off after about 30 min, so giving additional food on waking is mandatory. Glucagon is not effective when there is hepatic dysfunction, as in ethanol-induced hypoglycaemia when hepatic glycogen is depleted. Glucagon should not be given to a patient with an insulinoma, as it may stimulate more insulin secretion and induce greater hypoglycaemia.

PREVENTION OF HYPOGLYCAEMIA

If medical therapy of an intractable condition is indicated, frequent (3–4 hourly) small meals and snacks are essential. A high fibre content is particularly appropriate for the pre-bed meal, and a snack at 3 a.m. Therapy with an α-glucosidase inhibitor, such as acarbose or miglitol, delays absorption of disaccharides and starch from the jejunum. When these drugs are used, a subsequent hypoglycaemia has to be treated with glucose and not sucrose. The dose needs to be kept below that which hinders the ileal as well as the jejunal enzyme, to prevent carbohydrate transfer to the colon where bacteria can digest the carbohydrate and cause flatulence.

SEQUELAE OF HYPOGLYCAEMIA

Short-duration hypoglycaemia does not produce obvious, permanent neurological sequelae, which are rarely apparent after hypoglycaemic coma of less than 4 h duration. Occasionally, normal recovery occurs in patients who have been unconscious for more than 24 h, although they may be drowsy and confused for several days. Nevertheless, prognosis for recovery of cerebral function deteriorates with increasing duration of coma. Animal studies suggest that brain damage is more likely if hypoglycaemia is accompanied by hypoxaemia or hypotension. Cerebral oedema may be a secondary factor and mannitol or high-dose dexamethasone therapy sometimes appears to expedite recovery. Prolonged severe hypoglycaemia can lead to cortical atrophy and prolonged coma or dementia, but seldom causes death unless complicated by fits or inha-

lation of vomit. The degree to which multiple, short-duration hypoglycaemic comas can cause insidious brain damage is uncertain, but clinically apparent neurological deterioration is only recognized in those patients who, for some reason, have experienced in the order of hundreds of events.

Fasting hypoglycaemia

Diagnosis

Anybody with an unexplained 'funny turn' or transient stroke should promptly have blood glucose measurement with a glucose-oxidase strip, to exclude hypoglycaemia. The results are semiquantitative, and if the result is 'low' (< 4.0 mmol/l), blood samples should be taken for laboratory assay of glucose and insulin. A fasting plasma glucose of less than 3.5 mmol/l is likely to be pathological. If a patient is recovering from a hypoglycaemic episode, in part due to secretion of adrenergic and other stress hormones, by the time a blood sample is taken, a level of 4 to 5 mmol/l may be found. Thus a normal value after an attack may not exclude an episode of hypoglycaemia. Different laboratories have different assays and normal ranges, and this makes definition difficult.

Table 1 lists the differential diagnosis, and details of specific diseases are given below. A history to define fasting or reactive hypoglycaemia is very important. In adults most of the causes of fasting hypoglycaemia, other than insulinoma can be recognized clinically by history and examination. Liver disease, Addison's disease, or hypopituitarism are usually clinically obvious. An extrapancreatic tumour is usually large, and either palpable or easily seen on radiography. Ethanol-induced hypoglycaemia only occurs in patients who have had a prolonged fast, and can usually be excluded by the history. Thus, an adult who does have fasting hypoglycaemia, and who is otherwise well, will usually have an insulinoma, or be self-administering insulin or a sulphonylurea. Other possibilities are primary adrenocorticotropic hormone (ACTH) or growth hormone deficiency, an occult sarcoma, or autoimmune anti-insulin or anti-insulin receptor antibodies.

Any disease or drug that inhibits glycogenolysis or gluconeogenesis may lead to fasting hypoglycaemia. They can be divided conveniently into categories:

(1) excess insulin-like activity;
(2) non-insulin-induced hepatic dysfunction.

The plasma insulin during spontaneous hypoglycaemia is the key investigation, and measurement of plasma 3-hydroxybutyrate is also helpful. The 3-hydroxybutyrate can be assayed on the plasma sample taken for insulin.

Excess insulin or insulin-like activity (for example ILGF-II, or insulin receptor antibodies) inhibit both hepatic glucose and ketone-body production, so patients do not have ketonuria, ketosis, or raised 3-hydroxybutyrate levels. Ketonaemia is a feature of starvation or ethanol-induced hypoglycaemia, since the low plasma insulin levels secondary to the hypoglycaemia allow free fatty acid release and ketone-body production. Insulinomas might be expected to give a high insulin and low 3-hydroxybutyrate level after an overnight fast, but a normal 3-hydroxybutyrate level is usually found. The insulin immunoassay can be used to detect the presence of insulin antibodies, from self-administration of bovine or porcine insulin or autoimmunity.

Insulinomas

There is a low incidence of insulinomas (approximately 4/million/year) but it is the most common cause of fasting hypoglycaemia in non-diabetic subjects admitted to hospital for investigation of their hypoglycaemia. The tumours are semi-autonomous and maintain insulin secretion in the presence of hypoglycaemia, which suppresses normal β-cell function. The persistent basal insulin secretion by insulinomas inhibits hepatic glucose efflux and thus causes hypoglycaemia. Insulinomas can occur at any age, the median being in the sixth decade. The aetiology

Table 1 *The differential diagnosis and investigation appropriate to either fasting hypoglycaemia or postprandial hypoglycaemia in adults*

Fasting attacks
  Exclude clinically
    Hypopituitarism
    Addison's disease
    Ethanol ingestion after a fast
    Cirrhosis of the liver and acute hepatic failure
    Sarcoma (including chest radiography, plain abdomen
      radiography)
    Availability of insulin/sulphonylurea for self-administration
    Severe heart failure or renal failure
    Septicaemia, e.g. shigellosis or malaria
    Aspirin, β-blocker, pentamidine, or other drugs
    Any autoimmune disease, including thyrotoxicosis treated
      by methimazole
    Surgical removal of phaeochromocytoma
  Investigations
    No ketonaemia during hypoglycaemia
      Insulinoma
        Inordinately raised plasma insulin and C-peptide
        during hypoglycaemia:
          during spontaneous episode
            after an overnight fast
          insulin suppression test with C-peptide assay
            during prolonged fast
        Fasting plasma proinsulin
      Self-administration of sulphonylurea
        Investigation results as for insulinoma
        Tablets in patient's possession
        Plasma sulphonylurea assay
      Self-administration of insulin
        Available insulin supply
        Insulin antibodies
        During 'spontaneous' hypoglycaemia, low plasma C-
        peptide with high plasma insulin
      Autoimmune insulin antibodies
        Detected with immunoassay
        During 'spontaneous' hypoglycaemia, low plasma C-
        peptide with high plasma insulin
      Autoimmune insulin receptor antibodies
        Hypoglycaemia with low plasma insulin and C-peptide
        Send plasma for insulin receptor-binding studies
      Sarcoma hepatoma, or other solid tumour
        Hypoglycaemia with low plasma insulin and C-peptide
        Send plasma for ILGF-II assay
    Often ketonaemia during hypoglycaemia
      Pituitary/adrenal failure
        Plasma cortisol and growth hormone during
        hypoglycaemia
        Pituitary stimulation tests
        ACTH response to corticotropin-releasing factor
        Synacthen test (6 days' administration for isolated
        ACTH deficiency)
      Ethanol
        Plasma ethanol during hypoglycaemia
Postprandial attacks
  Exclude clinically
    Gastric surgery
    Mild diabetes
    Think of possibility of fasting hypoglycaemia
  Investigations
    Extended oral glucose tolerance test with either capillary
      blood or 'arterialized' venous samples from the back of
      a warm hand.
    Home blood glucose sampling with memory meter or filter
      paper blots and a diary

ACTH, adrenocorticotropic hormone.

is usually unknown, although when associated with multiple endocrine neoplasia (see below) the inherited tendency is mediated by a deletion of part of chromosome 11q. In sporadic insulinomas, deletions of both alleles of the retinoblastoma gene have been reported.

Patients characteristically present with drowsiness on waking, which is relieved by a sweet drink or breakfast. They may present to a neurologist, because of confusional states or 'funny turns' (including paraesthesiae, diplopia, faintness, light headedness, fits, or an apparent stroke that is secondary to hypoglycaemia). Symptoms can occur several hours after a meal, particularly associated with exercise, for example prior to lunch after a busy morning's shopping. The tumours grow very slowly, and patients have often had symptoms for several years. Nevertheless, cognitive impairment is very unusual. Most patients have no change in weight, but a few find symptoms can be prevented by frequent meals and become obese. There are no abnormal physical signs when the patient is normoglycaemic.

The tumours are usually small, 0.5 to 5 cm diameter, and occur in any part of the pancreas. Ectopic insulinomas rarely, if ever, occur. The tumours can be well or poorly differentiated histologically, often secreting more proinsulin than insulin. They respond subnormally to meals, and blood glucose after a meal or an oral glucose tolerance test may paradoxically be moderately high (for example 10 mmol/l). Although immunostaining may show a few other islet cells containing glucagon, somatostatin, gastrin, ACTH, or other hormones, it is rare for these to be secreted or to cause symptoms, even in the 5 to 10 per cent of insulinomas which are malignant.

The diagnosis or exclusion of an insulinoma is needed in any patient with suspected fasting hypoglycaemia. Insulinomas are primarily diagnosed by a suppression test, as are other diseases caused by excessive hormone secretion, (for example the glucose tolerance test in acromegaly, and the dexamethasone test for Cushing's disease). Normally, hypoglycaemia inhibits insulin secretion, the plasma insulin level being less than 1.5 mU/l for a fasting plasma glucose of less than 2 mmol/l (normal range 3–13 mU/l at normal fasting plasma glucose concentrations). The possible investigations are:

Overnight fasting plasma glucose and insulin measurements

Patients with insulinomas in effect do their own suppression tests, as 90 per cent of the patients have marked hypoglycaemia after just an overnight fast. Their plasma insulin concentration, which induced the hypoglycaemia, is inordinately high in relation to the normal plasma glucose/insulin relationship (Fig. 1). If the fasting plasma glucose is below 2.5 mmol/l, a plasma insulin concentration greater than 5 mU/l is diagnostic. Values greater than 3 mU/l are suggestive and indicate an additional suppression test.

Overnight plasma pro-insulin measurement

A high proportion of pro-insulin is secreted by insulinomata. Its diminished biological effect, compared with insulin, means that patients with normal fasting plasma glucose concentrations still have inordinately high pro-insulin concentrations. Thus, the ideal screening test is measurement of one or two fasting samples for pro-insulin. However, pro-insulin assays are not widely available.

Additional suppression tests, when required

The 10 per cent of patients with insulinomas who have normal fasting plasma glucose concentrations need to be distinguished from the more common situation of the patient with a 'funny turn' in whom an insulinoma needs to be excluded. In making a diagnosis of an insulinoma it is essential to demonstrate:

    (1) spontaneous hypoglycaemia;
    (2) inordinately high insulin secretion during hypoglycaemia.

Admission for 2 day fast

This test is time-consuming and uncomfortable for patients, and is rarely needed now that dynamic tests are available. It is usually not needed in patients with insulinomas as after an overnight fast they already have hypoglycaemia. During the fast, it is important to maintain exercise to try to induce hypoglycaemia. Blood samples are taken every 6 h for insulin, C-peptide and laboratory glucose assay, and are monitored promptly with a meter. If hypoglycaemia, below 2.5 mmol/l, occurs at any time during the fast, an additional blood sample should be taken for glucose, insulin, C-peptide, cortisol, growth hormone, and 3-hydroxy-butyrate assay. A plasma or urine sample for sulphonylurea assay may be indicated. After a 72-h fast, normal subjects have a plasma C-peptide concentration below 0.1 nmol/l, whereas in those with insulinomas it exceeds 0.2 nmol/l when the fasting glucose levels are less than 2.8 mmol/l.

The plasma for C-peptide assay has to be kept at 4°C, and frozen at −20°C as soon as possible, because it is susceptible to degradation if blood or plasma is kept at room temperature, whereas insulin and pro-insulin are remarkably stable, even at room temperature. Once hypo-glycaemia has been induced, a blood sample should be taken 30 min later for cortisol and growth hormone assay, as a test of pituitary/adrenal function.

If a dynamic test (see below) suggests an insulinoma, but spontaneous hypoglycaemia has not been documented, a fast is required. A fast is also needed if a dynamic suppression test is normal, but the clinical suspicion of hypoglycaemia is sufficiently high that one needs to exclude rare causes such as autoimmune hypoglycaemia or isolated ACTH or growth hormone deficiency.

Dynamic suppression test

Insulin is administered over a 2-h period to induce hypoglycaemia, (for example, 0.05 U/kg/h intravenously) and plasma C-peptide, which is secreted on an equimolar basis with each insulin molecule, is measured to monitor endogenous β-cell secretion. An intravenous cannula should be used to ensure venous access in the unlikely event of a fit. When the

Fig. 1 Inordinately raised fasting plasma insulin concentrations after an overnight fast in 31 patients with insulinomas (each shown as a black square). The dark shaded area is the normal fasting plasma glucose and insulin range, and the lighter area the normal suppression of plasma human insulin in response to hypoglycaemia. The majority of patients with insulinomas have a diagnostic high plasma insulin during their spontaneous hypoglycaemia. Those with normal fasting plasma glucose fail to suppress their plasma insulin to below 1.5 mU/l during a hypoglycaemic suppression test. (Adapted from Turner, R.C. (1976). Hypoglycaemia: Proceedings of the European Symposium, Rome. *Hormone and Metabolic Research* **6**, 40.)

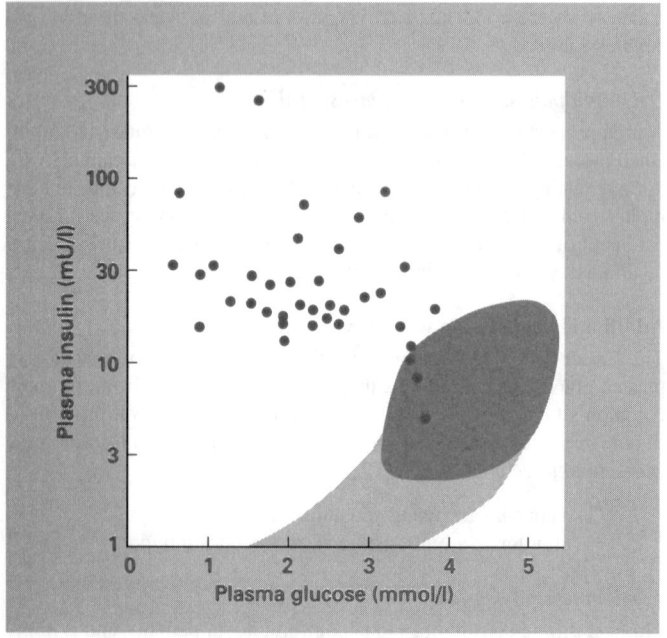

plasma glucose is below 2.5 mmol/l, the test can be terminated. At that glucose level, the plasma C-peptide should suppress to below 50 per cent of the basal level and to less than 150 pmol/l.

Stimulation tests

Measurement of the blood glucose response to intravenous tolbutamide or glucagon is no longer recommended as they give both false positive and negative results. They can provoke acute hypoglycaemia which is difficult to control in patients with insulinomas, and suppression tests with insulin are more efficient and predictable. The calcium infusion test has been recommended, but gives false positive and negative results in the same way as do other stimulation tests.

LOCALIZATION AND EXCISION OF INSULINOMAS

Abdominal ultrasound and CT scan only detect large tumours and are usually not helpful. MRI is more sensitive but might not detect small tumours. As with other gut endocrine tumours, insulinomas have somatostatin receptors. Tumours of diameter 3 mm can be detected with a gamma camera following intravenous labelled octreotide. Specificity and sensitivity have not yet been assessed, but the test is likely to become a major localization procedure. The need for accurate preoperative localization has been reduced by the efficiency of intraoperative ultrasound and it is reasonable to proceed directly to surgery if this technique is available.

Alternative preoperative localization techniques are more invasive. Endoscopic ultrasonography can detect small tumours, particularly in the head of the pancreas. Coeliac axis angiography used to be the only method. It can localize an adenoma in 60 to 70 per cent of patients, with additional superior mesenteric artery angiography required for adeno-mas in the uncinate lobe of the head of the pancreas. When the tumour is visible on angiography, it is usually large enough to be found easily at operation. It is doubtful whether angiography is now ever warranted in view of radiation exposure, potential morbidity, and the availability of alternative methods such as octreotide scanning and intraoperative ultrasound.

Percutaneous transhepatic cannulation of the portal vein for multiple blood sampling of effluent from the pancreas in the portal, splenic, and superior mesenteric veins is only needed if there has been a failed oper-ation and other investigations have been inconclusive. High localized plasma insulin concentrations indicate the position of the tumour, but many venous samples are needed to confirm localization. In a normal subject, the pulsatility of basal insulin secretion provides variable levels that may imply a tumour. The test should only be done in patients in whom a suppression test has confirmed the diagnosis, since the insulin secretion from the rest of the pancreas is suppressed by chronic hypo-glycaemia, and this aids localization. In addition, it is advantageous if the blood glucose is low–normal (around 3–5 mmol/l) during the inves-tigation to assist inhibition of secretion from the normal pancreas.

Surgical therapy and intraoperative ultrasound

Surgical excision of the tumour is the main therapy for fit patients. The majority of insulinomas can be palpated at operation, even if they were not detected preoperatively, although mobilization of the pancreas may be required. The use of direct operative ultrasonography is of great assis-tance in locating a tumour, which appears as a dense area with a sur-rounding non-reflective halo. These tumours can then usually be pal-pated, although occasionally can only be detected by ultrasonography. The insulinoma can then be enucleated, with care being taken not to damage the exocrine pancreatic duct in the posterior part of the pancreas.

During an operation, repeated measurement of the plasma glucose concentration, with a rise following excision of the tumour, has been suggested to be helpful in confirming excision of a tumour. A lack of rise after excision of one tumour might indicate that other tumours are still present. However, these techniques are not completely reliable, par-ticularly if the anaesthetist has to give blood or other glucose-containing fluid. It can take 30 to 60 min for the plasma glucose to rise after excision, and the technique is probably only indicated if multiple tumours have been found. A 'Biostater', which infuses glucose to maintain a particular plasma glucose level, has been used to demonstrate a decrease in glucose requirement on excision of a tumour, but this is mainly of experimental interest.

If an insulinoma cannot be found, distal pancreatectomy should not be undertaken, as the tumour is most likely to be hidden in the head of the pancreas. Biopsy of the tip of the pancreas to exclude β-cell hyperplasia or nesidioblastosis should be performed. Then the abdomen should be closed and the patient referred to a centre that undertakes endoscopic ultrasonography or labelled octreotide scanning.

MEDICAL TREATMENT

Hypoglycaemic attacks can usually be prevented by frequent fibre-containing meals, including taking a meal during the night if necessary. Somatostatin infusion, (up to 300 μg/day), with physiological glucagon replacement, can be used in the short term if attacks are very severe. Octreotide injections are often unsuccessful, as suppression of glucagon and growth hormone secretion can aggravate the hypoglycaemia. Diazoxide therapy, 150–800 mg/day, will relieve symptoms in about 50 per cent of patients. However, it may induce nausea, rashes, and, in women, hirsutism. Sodium retention can be counteracted with a thiazide diuretic. Despite its limitations, medical treatment may be preferable to an operation in the elderly, or in other patients in whom surgery is undesirable.

MULTIPLE ENDOCRINE NEUROPLASIA

(See also Chapter 12.10)

It is unusual for insulinomas to be part of a multiple endocrine neoplasia (MEN) type 1 syndrome, but measurement of plasma calcium to detect hyperparathyroidism is indicated, particularly if there is a family or personal history of other endocrine neoplasia. If MEN 1 is present, there is a greater chance of multiple adenomata or malignancy. MEN 1 is due to deletion of part of chromosome 11q. This has also been found in some sporadic cases of insulinoma, suggesting that some may have undiagnosed MEN 1.

β-CELL HYPERPLASIA

There have been a few reports of β-cell hyperplasia or β-cell adenomatosis as a cause of hypoglycaemia in adults. Most are poorly documented and depend on a non-quantitative, subjective interpretation of islet size. Many of these patients have probably had an occult insulinoma, but diffuse islet abnormality can occur rarely in adults.

MALIGNANT INSULINOMAS

These account for 5 to 10 per cent of insulinomas, and often such patients already have hepatic metastases at presentation. The undifferentiated tumour usually is inefficient at secreting insulin, and large hepatic or lymph node metastases are present before the tumour bulk is sufficient to induce enough insulin secretion to produce symptoms. It is rare for the tumours to secrete other peptides giving symptoms, although 75 per cent secrete β-choriogonadotrophin. These tumours occasionally induce symptoms from the secretion of ACTH, gastrin, vasoactive intestinal polypeptide, or the mediators of the carcinoid syndrome.

Diazoxide and somatostatin, given by intravenous infusion or subcutaneous injections of octreotide, are usually of little benefit. 'Debulking' by surgical excision of large hepatic metastases, or by infarcting them by selective application of thrombin gel via a catheter positioned from the femoral artery into the coeliac axis, can give relief of symptoms for several months.

Streptozotocin, particularly combined with 5-fluorouracil, can dramatically decrease the size of the tumour and its deposits, and temporarily relieve persistent hypoglycaemia. Relapse usually occurs within a year, but some patients are free of symptoms for 2 or 3 years. Strep-

tozotocin can cause renal failure, and the dose has to be titrated carefully, for example 500 mg/m² streptozotocin and 400 mg/m² 5-fluorouracil intravenously given on alternate days for 10 days, stopping the course if albuminuria or hepatic or bone marrow dysfunction occur. The course can be repeated every 2 to 3 months for 3 to 4 courses, with a 6 month wait to assess the effect or side-effects. Mithramycin, carboplatin, cyclophosphamide, and α-interferon have also been used.

Death eventually ensues from uncontrollable hypoglycaemia or from metastases, but the tumours sometimes grow slowly. When other therapy fails, patients can become dependent on a continuous glucose infusion through a central intravenous catheter. The management of such patients can be complex.

Factitious hypoglycaemia

This can occur when a patient surreptitiously takes either insulin or a sulphonylurea drug. If a doctor, nurse, or ancillary hospital worker has hypoglycaemia, it is usually self-induced. A secondary gain to the patient is usually not obvious, and other hysterical or psychiatric symptoms may not be apparent. The patients usually deny self-administration and are remarkably plausible.

SELF-ADMINISTRATION OF INSULIN

Until recently, insulin self-administration has usually been readily apparent, because impure insulin preparations have induced insulin antibodies, which can be detected with a suitable modification of the insulin immunoassay. The availability of pure pork and human insulins, which are seldom immunogenic, will make the detection of self-administration more difficult. If a blood sample is taken when the patient has a hypoglycaemic episode, the presence of immunoreactive insulin in the absence of immunoreactive C-peptide, confirms the exogenous origin of the insulin. One patient, who took a large, suicidal dose of insulin, was successfully and appropriately treated by excision of the adipose tissue at the site of injection!

SELF-MEDICATION WITH SULPHONYLUREA

This presents exactly like an insulinoma with similar lack of suppression of insulin or C-peptide in response to hypoglycaemia. These patients are usually detected only because of clinical suspicion leading to the finding of sulphonylurea tablets in the patient's possession. The wide variety of sulphonylurea drugs available makes the detection of sulphonylurea in plasma or urine difficult, although immunoassays for individual sulphonylurea drugs are provided by several manufacturers. If an overdose of sulphonylurea has been taken, therapy with diazoxide or somatostatin is feasible.

Sarcoma, hepatoma, and other tumours

Fasting hypoglycaemia can occur with low-grade malignancy tumours of many cell types, the most common being retroperitoneal fibrosarcoma and mesothelioma. The tumours are large, usually weighing 2 to 4 kg, the smallest recorded being 310 g. The syndrome can also arise from some epithelial cell tumours, such as malignant hepatoma, cholangioma, and adrenocortical tumours. The tumours are usually obvious either on palpation of the abdomen or on chest or abdomen radiography, CT scan, or MRI.

Patients with mesotheliomata or sarcomata do not have ketosis, since hypoglycaemia is caused by excess secretion of an insulin-like growth factor, ILGF-II. The patients have low–normal concentrations of ILGF-I. Increased expression of the mRNA for ILGF-II in the tumour may be an oncogenic factor that induced the tumour to develop. The tumour can secrete a large precursor, a proinsulin-like peptide, pro-ILGF-II, and a specific immunoassay for the first 21 amino acids of the E-domain can be diagnostic. The peptide circulates predominantly with ILGF binding proteins as a small, 50 kDa complex rather than as the usual 150 kDa complex, and this increases its bioavailability through the capillaries.

The hypoglycaemia is resistant to treatment other than taking regular, fibre-containing meals, which may need to be given throughout the day and night; eventually intravenous glucose infusion may be necessary.

Operative removal of a tumour stops the hypoglycaemia, but recurrence of the tumour is common even if the lesion was reported histologically to be benign.

Autoimmune hypoglycaemia

INSULIN RECEPTOR ANTIBODIES

Patients with insulin receptor antibodies usually present with a rare variant of insulin-resistant diabetes, because these antibodies bind with insulin receptors and displace the binding of insulin. However, sometimes the antibodies activate the receptor and cause an insulin-like effect and fasting hypoglycaemia. This is analogous to Graves' disease, in which thyroid stimulating hormone receptor antibodies may stimulate the thyroid gland. Autoimmune hypoglycaemia is much less common and similarly tends to occur in middle-aged women, but can occur in either sex at any age. Such antibodies can be detected by assaying the patient's plasma or serum for antibody binding to insulin receptors. The insulin receptors on the patient's red cells may be occupied by antibody and unable to bind labelled insulin *in vitro*. The hypoglycaemia is resistant to treatment except by plasmapheresis and immune suppression, including prednisolone therapy. The condition often remits spontaneously and can transmute to the production of predominantly blocking antibodies, giving rise to insulin-resistant diabetes.

INSULIN ANTIBODIES

The autoimmune production of antibodies to insulin can lead to the accumulation of antibody-bound insulin in the circulation, which dissociates to maintain higher-than-normal free insulin levels h after a meal. Hypoglycaemia occurs either 5 to 7 hours after a meal, or many hours later as fasting hypoglycaemia. The C-peptide concentrations can then be low, even though insulin levels are high. The condition may be more common in Japanese patients, particularly in those treated for thyrotoxicosis with antithyroid drugs containing an -SH group. Patients often, but not invariably, have other autoimmune disease and have the HLA-DR4 antigen. The antibodies are usually polyclonal but can be monoclonal. If symptoms are not controlled by frequent meals and α-glucosidase inhibitors, immunosuppression with prednisolone, or even plasmapheresis, may be needed.

Acute infections

SEPTICAEMIA

Hypoglycaemia occasionally occurs with severe infections. Affected patients are usually children or the elderly. Gram-negative septicaemia is the most common cause; in particular, hypoglycaemia from Shigella dysentery. Infections with streptococci or *Haemophilus influenzae* also can occur. The pathophysiology is unclear, but may be due to a combination of acute calorie deprivation, high metabolic demands from fever, and hepatic dysfunction. Accompanying medication, such as β-blockers or calcium antagonists, can reduce hepatic glucose efflux. Preceding cirrhosis or renal failure may make a patient susceptible. Ketonuria is not found, and production of cytokines, such as tumour necrosis factor or interleukin-6, has been postulated to stimulate insulin production, but direct evidence for this is lacking.

MENINGOCOCCAL INFECTION

Hypoglycaemia may accompany hypotension and indicate adrenal failure from Waterhouse-Friderichsen syndrome.

MALARIA

Hypoglycaemia can occur with fulminant *Plasmodium falciparum* infection, and this may be the cause of coma rather than the usual direct effects of parasitaemia on cerebral blood flow and function. Hypoglycaemia is usually caused by hyperinsulinaemia stimulated by quinine therapy. Hypoglycaemia can be found in milder infections in pregnancy, partly because of the greater glucose demand of the fetus and partly because the β-cells may be more responsive to quinine. Large amounts of glucose may be needed to prevent hypoglycaemia. Suppression of insulin secretion by somatostatin is an alternative therapy.

Hypoglycaemia can also occur without quinine therapy and is then probably due to the mechanisms described under septicaemia.

Ethanol-induced hypoglycaemia

The oxidation of ethanol in the liver reduces the NAD^+ to NADH (nicotinamide adenine dinucleotide), and the altered redox potential means that gluconeogenesis from lactate is no longer possible. Glycogenolysis is not affected, so ethanol has little effect on plasma glucose concentration in those who are eating meals and have glycogen stores. However, after a 24-h fast, when the glycogen is depleted, ethanol consumption causes marked hypoglycaemia. As hypoglycaemia is due to decreased hepatic glucose efflux accompanied by low plasma insulin concentrations, these patients characteristically have ketonuria and raised plasma ketone-body levels. In rats, the effect is maximal with a plasma ethanol concentration of 10 mmol/l, half the legal driving limit in the United Kingdom. Ethanol-induced hypoglycaemia is usually only seen in alcoholics who drink and do not eat. It is important to consider hypoglycaemia as a cause of drowsiness and unruly behaviour in alcoholics who require medical attention in the casualty department or in police stations.

Children, with their greater proportional turnover of fuel supply, can have ethanol-induced hypoglycaemia after a few hours without food, for example children taking wine at wedding receptions, sometimes with fatal consequences. In the wider world, except for preterminal starvation, ethanol is probably the most common cause of fasting hypoglycaemia.

Severe liver disease

Only gross liver disease is severe enough to deplete hepatic glucose efflux and induce hypoglycaemia. Hypoglycaemia is more a feature of acute hepatic coma than of uncomplicated cirrhosis or other liver disease. When hypoglycaemia does occur in cirrhosis, interaction with ethanol or drug therapy is usually a feature (see below). Hypoglycaemia associated with a hepatoma is discussed above.

Endstage renal failure

Hypoglycaemia can occur following intraperitoneal dialysis, when it may follow termination of the high glucose concentration-containing peritoneal infusion, which has stimulated insulin secretion and decreased glucagon secretion. Hypoglycaemia can also occur in endstage renal failure *per se* and should be suspected if there is a change of mental or neurological status. It is often a marker of multisystem failure, including hepatic failure. Acute calorie deprivation and drugs, such as ethanol, β-blockers, salicylates, or disopyramide are often implicated; hypoglycaemia rarely occurs in uncomplicated renal failure.

Heart failure

Hypoglycaemia in elderly patients with severe heart failure is well recognized. It is usually due to a combination of fasting, ethanol, certain drugs (see below), and possibly hepatic congestion.

Cortisol deficiency

Patients with deficiency of cortisol production from Addison's disease, pan-hypopituitarism, or isolated ACTH deficiency, have slightly low fasting plasma glucose concentrations. Frank hypoglycaemia may be precipitated by exercise but usually only develops after missing meals. Patients presenting with persistent vomiting are particularly at risk from hypoglycaemia. Hypoglycaemia may be provoked by ethanol in the absence of the usual 24-h fast needed to deplete liver glycogen. Half the patients with this condition present with fasting hypoglycaemia that clinically mimics an insulinoma. It is important to treat the hypoglycaemia with hydrocortisone as well as with glucose.

Patients with Addison's or hypopituitary disease can usually be diagnosed because of associated symptoms and signs. The characteristic findings are of a low plasma glucose accompanied by a low insulin, but without gross ketonuria. Plasma cortisol measurements, as with any spontaneous hypoglycaemia of unidentified origin, are of considerable value. The diagnosis is made by lack of an ACTH or cortisol response to hypoglycaemia or corticotrophin releasing factor. Isolated ACTH deficiency is rare and can be difficult to detect without specific investigation. It is autoimmune in origin, but other autoimmune diseases may not be apparent.

Growth hormone deficiency

Isolated growth hormone deficiency occasionally induces hypoglycaemia, but it is even less common than isolated ACTH deficiency. Hypoglycaemia also occurs in Laron dwarfism, in which a defect of ILGF-I production is associated with high plasma growth hormone levels.

Pregnancy

The metabolic demands of the fetus mean that even with short periods of fuel deprivation there is accelerated starvation, with the plasma glucose reducing to 3 mmol/l and resultant moderate ketonaemia. It is rare to develop symptomatic hypoglycaemia. Placental lactogen may have developed evolutionarily as a protective mechanism. Nevertheless, illness in pregnancy causing acute calorie deprivation sometimes induces hypoglycaemia, which may be aggravated by the use of β_2-adrenoreceptor agonists given to retard premature labour.

Drugs

Salicylates and non-selective β-blockers sometimes induce hypoglycaemia even when given in normal pharmacological doses, particularly in children and in the elderly when illness prevents feeding. The cause is uncertain, but they may both directly prevent hepatic glucose efflux. Salicylate may also enhance insulin secretion. This effect of salicytate is distinct from Reye's syndrome, which is an idiosyncratic response to aspirin in children, leading to acute liver failure and encephalopathy. Drugs for treating arrhythmia, particularly disopyramide, have also been implicated. Hypoglycaemia due to quinine has been mentioned above.

HIV PATIENTS AND PENTAMIDINE THERAPY OF *PNEUMOCYSTIS CARINII* INFECTION.

Pentamidine induces β-cell death and subsequent release of stored insulin to induce hypoglycaemia. Hypoglycaemia is common following intravenous pentamidine and can also occur after inhalation of a pentamidine aerosol.

Reactive postprandial hypoglycaemia

The timing of the symptoms in relation to meals is an important feature in the differential diagnosis.

Alimentary hypoglycaemia

Several operations (such as partial gastrectomy and pyloroplasty) can give rise to rapid gastric emptying, with brisk absorption of glucose and prompt release of enteric insulin-stimulating hormones. These induce greater than normal insulin release, which can induce hypoglycaemia 1.5 to 3 h after a meal. These need to be distinguished from the 'dumping' syndrome 30 min after a meal, which is probably induced by increased secretion of gastroenteric peptides such as neurotensin, vaso-

active intestinal polypeptide, and motilin, and is not related to hypoglycaemia.

All forms of reactive hypoglycaemia are likely to benefit from therapy with an α-glucosidase inhibitor, such as acarbose or miglitol (see above).

Incipient diabetes

Patients with diabetes, usually of maturity-onset type with near-normal fasting plasma glucose levels, occasionally present with postprandial hypoglycaemia 3 to 5 h after a meal. An initial subnormal insulin response to a meal leads to hypoglycaemia which may eventually stimulate sufficient insulin release to produce reactive hypoglycaemia. The symptoms disappear as β-cell function decreases and fasting hypoglycaemia ensues.

Idiopathic reactive hypoglycaemia

This is the most frequently diagnosed form of postprandial hypoglycaemia in the United States, whereas it is uncommon in the United Kingdom. Patients are often of an anxious disposition, and the possibility that non-specific symptoms may be due to hypoglycaemia seems in some patients to aggravate their symptoms. The 'diagnosis' is often made on a suggestive history and is 'confirmed' by a 5 h oral glucose tolerance test. The condition is markedly overdiagnosed because use of venous blood samples taken from the cubital fossa during an oral glucose test can spuriously indicate hypoglycaemia. Glucose uptake by forearm muscle can give a venous plasma glucose concentration of 2 mmol/l when the arterial glucose concentration is normal at 4 mmol/l. It is not unusual for the venous plasma glucose level to fall to 2.5 to 3.0 mmol/l (44–52 mg/100 ml), between 90 and 150 min after a glucose tolerance test, and such levels are often overinterpreted. Thus, postprandial hypoglycaemia should only be confirmed by taking plasma glucose levels after a normal meal or an oral glucose tolerance test by arterialized blood from a vein on the back of a warmed hand or from finger-tip or ear-lobe capillary blood samples. The diagnosis should only be made when proven low arterialized glucose levels are accompanied by symptoms that improve as the plasma glucose rises.

Patients in whom this condition is suspected, with a low plasma glucose level during a glucose tolerance test, do not usually show abnormal low glucose concentrations after taking mixed meals. Confirmation of low blood glucose levels at the time of symptoms may be achieved by the patient putting blood on a special filter paper for laboratory testing, or by use of home blood-glucose monitoring with a memory meter. A parallel diary of symptoms is helpful.

The few patients who show true reactive hypoglycaemia are usually underweight or of normal weight. Some have been reported to have a greater than normal initial insulin response to meals. One patient has been reported to have abnormal hepatic glucose 6-phosphatase activity.

The plasma insulin or proinsulin concentration measured during a reactive hypoglycaemic episode may still be raised from secretion induced by a previous meal, and the diagnostic criteria for insulinomas that apply to fasting hypoglycaemia should not be applied to postprandial hypoglycaemia.

Hypoglycaemia in childhood

Several rare enzyme defects present in childhood, such as type 1 glycogen storage disease and galactosaemia. These are not diagnostic problems that present as hypoglycaemia alone. Neonatal hypoglycaemia can occur in small-for-date babies or in the babies of diabetic mothers. Apart from unusual diseases, such as aspirin-induced Reye's syndrome, there are two major causes of hypoglycaemia in infancy.

NESIDIOBLASTOSIS

This is a rare condition, causing persistent hypoglycaemia in the neonate, and occasionally presenting at up to 6 months of age. A developmental abnormality of the pancreas features a large number of duct overgrowths associated with β-cells which are not in the normal islet formation (i.e. the 'nest' which provides the 'nesidio-' description). A defect of the paracrine effect of D cells producing somatostatin has been suggested as a cause for the increased insulin secretion. The diagnosis is made from persistent hypoglycaemia without ketonuria and inappropriately raised plasma insulin levels. It is very important to maintain the baby's plasma glucose concentration during diagnosis, to prevent long-term brain damage and mental retardation. A glucose infusion is required. An infusion of somatostatin can ameliorate hypoglycaemia while surgery is being planned. The hypoglycaemia seldom responds to glucagon or diazoxide. At operation no insulinoma is found and the diagnosis is confirmed by the pathology of the excised pancreas. Usually a 95 per cent or 100 per cent pancreatectomy is required, with institution of insulin and exocrine pancreas replacement.

KETOTIC HYPOGLYCAEMIA

This is the most common form of hypoglycaemia in infancy, usually occurring in boys aged between 1 and 8 years, who were often small-for-date when born. A defect in glucose delivery can be due to several causes, including hepatic glycogen synthetase deficiency, impaired release of gluconeogenic amino acid from muscles, or decreased adrenergic stimulation of the liver. Children present with drowsiness or fits, either after a period without food, often induced by an intercurrent illness, or by unusual exercise. The name arises from the ketosis secondary to the low plasma insulin induced by the low plasma glucose. Attacks usually disappear in adult life, probably because of the proportionately lower glucose turnover in adults than in children.

LEUCINE-SENSITIVE HYPOGLYCAEMIA

This probably relates to patients with nesidioblastosis or hypoglycaemia due to insulinoma and is not a specific entity.

REFERENCES

Arem, R. (1989). Hypoglycaemia associated with renal failure. *Endocrinology and Metabolism Clinics of North America* **18**, 103–21.

Battershill, P.E. and Clissold, S.P. (1989). Octreotide: A review of its pharmacodynamic and pharmacokinetic properties, and therapeutic potential in conditions associated with excessive peptide secretion. *Drugs* **38**, 658–702.

Brightbill, T.C., Templeton, E.O., Sperling, D., and Mooney, L.P. (1992). Insulinoma: detection by intraoperative ultrasonography. *Journal of Clinical Ultrasound* **20**, 615–16.

Burch, H.B., Clement, S., Sokol, M.S. and Landry, F. (1992). Reactive hypoglycaemic coma due to insulin autoimmune syndrome: case report and literature review. *American Journal of Medicine* **92**, 681–5.

Daughaday, W.H. and Trivedi, B. (1992). Measurement of derivatives of proinsulin-like growth factor-II in serum by a radioummunoassay directed against the E-domain in normal subjects and patients with non-islet cell tumour hypoglycaemia. *Journal of Clinical Endocrinology and Metabolism* **75**, 110–15.

Eriksson, B., et al. (1990). Neuroendocrine pancreatic tumours: clinical presentation, biochemical and histopathological findings in 84 patients. *Journal of Internal Medicine* **228**, 103–13.

Haymond, M.W. (1989). Hypoglycaemia in infants and children. *Endocrinology and Metabolism Clinics of North America* **18**, 211–52.

Hofeldt, F.D. (1989). Reactive hypoglycaemia. *Endocrinology and Metabolism Clinic of North America* **18**, 185–201.

Palardy, J. et al. (1989). Blood glucose measurements during symptomatic episodes in patients with suspected postprandial hypoglycaemia. *New England Journal of Medicine* **321**, 1421–5.

Palazzo, L., Roseau, G. and Salmeron, M. (1992). Endoscopic ultrasonography in the preoperative localisation of pancreatic endocrine tumours. *Endoscopy* **24**, 350–3.

Patel, P., O'Rahilly, S., Buckle, V., Nakamura, Y., Turner, R.C. and Wainscoat, J.S. (1990). Chromosome 11 allele loss in sporadic insulinoma. *Journal of Clinical Pathology* **43**, 377–78.

Romijn, J.A., Godfried, M.H., Wortel, C. and Sauerwein, H.P. (1990). Hypoglycaemia, hormones and cytokines in fatal meningococcal septicemia. *Journal of Endocrinological Investigation* **13**, 743–7.

Seltzer, H.S. (1989) Drug-induced hypoglycaemia. A review of 1418 cases. *Endocrinology and Metabolism Clinics of North America* **18**, 163–83.

Service, F.J., McMahon, M.M., O'Brien, P.C., and Ballard, D.J. (1991). Functioning insulinoma—incidence, recurrence, and long-term survival of patients: a 60 year study. *Mayo Clinic Proceedings* **66**, 711–19.

Taylor, S.I., Barbetti, F., Accili, D., Roth, J. and Gorden, P. (1989). Syndromes of autoimmunity and hypoglycaemia. Autoantibodies directed against insulin and its receptor. *Endocrinology and Metabolism Clinics of North America* **18**, 123–43.

Uchigata, Y., et al. (1992). Strong association of insulin autoimmune syndrome with HLA-DR4. *Lancet* **339**, 393–4.

Yamamoto, T., Fukuyama, J., Hasegawa, K. and Sigiura, M. (1992). Isolated corticotropin deficiency in adults. Report of 10 cases and review of literature. *Archives of Internal Medicine* **152**, 1705–12.

11.13 Amyloid, familial Mediterranean fever, and acute phase response

11.13.1 Amyloidosis

M.B. Pepys

Introduction

Amyloidosis is a disorder of protein metabolism, which may be either acquired or hereditary, characterized by extracellular deposition of abnormal protein fibrils. Many different proteins can form amyloid fibrils (Tables 1, 2). In addition, the deposits contain glycosaminoglycans, some of which are tightly associated with the fibrils, and also a non-fibrillar plasma glycoprotein, amyloid P component (AP). Small focal, clinically silent, amyloid deposits in the brain, heart, seminal vesicles, and joints are a universal accompaniment of ageing. However, systemic or significant local amyloid deposits usually accumulate progressively, disrupting the structure and function of affected tissues and leading inexorably to organ failure and death. No treatment yet exists which specifically causes resolution, but intervention which reduces availability of the protein precursors of amyloid fibrils may lead to regression.

Clinical amyloidosis

Introduction

Clinically significant amyloidosis is not rare. Amyloid deposits in the brain and cerebral blood vessels are a central part of the pathology of

Table 1 *Acquired amyloidosis syndromes*

Clinical syndrome	Fibril protein
Systemic AL amyloidosis, associated with immunocyte dyscrasia, myeloma, monoclonal gammopathy, occult dyscrasia	AL fibrils derived from monoclonal immunoglobulin light chains
Local nodular AL amyloidosis (skin, respiratory tract, urogenital tract, etc.) associated with focal immunocyte dyscrasia	AL fibrils derived from monoclonal immunoglobulin light chains
Reactive systemic AA amyloidosis, associated with chronic active diseases	AA fibrils derived from serum amyloid A protein (SAA)
Senile systemic amyloidosis	Transthyretin derived from plasma transthyretin
Focal senile amyloidosis:	
atria of the heart	Atrial natriuretic peptide
brain	β-protein
joints	Not known
seminal vesicles	Seminal vesicle exocrine protein
prostrate	β_2-microglobulin
Non-familial Alzheimer's disease, Down's syndrome	β-protein derived from β-amyloid protein precursor (APP)
Sporadic cerebral amyloid angiography	β-protein derived from β-amyloid precursor protein (APP)
Inclusion body myositis	β-protein derived from β-amyloid precursor protein (APP)
Sporadic Creutzfeldt–Jakob disease, kuru (transmissible spongiform encephalopathies, prion diseases)	Prion protein derived from prion protein precursor
Type II diabetes mellitus	Islet amyloid polypeptide (IAPP), amylin, derived from its precursor protein
Endocrine amyloidosis, associated with APUDomas	Peptide hormones or fragments thereof (e.g. precalcitonin in medullary carcinoma of thyroid)
Haemodialysis-associated amyloidosis; localized to osteoarticular tissues or systemic	β_2-microglobulin derived from high plasma levels
Primary localized cutaneous amyloid (macular, papular)	? Keratin-derived
Ocular amyloid (cornea, conjunctiva)	Not known
Orbital amyloid	Not known

Alzheimer's disease, which is the fourth most common cause of death in the Western world, whilst amyloid is present in the islets of Langerhans of the pancreas in all patients with type II, maturity onset, diabetes mellitus. Amyloid deposition in the bones, joints, and periarticular structures eventually affects most patients who are on long-term haemodialysis for endstage renal failure and is the most frequent cause of serious morbidity among the approximately 500 000 such individuals worldwide. Systemic amyloidosis complicating myeloma and other B cell dyscrasias, or chronic infections and inflammatory diseases, is very important because of the difficulty, which is often still experienced, in making the diagnosis, its poor prognosis, and the increasing availability of effective treatments. Hereditary amyloidosis is very rare, except in a few geographic foci, but its diversity is remarkable. Its importance derives both from its poor clinical prognosis and from its value as a model for understanding the pathogenesis of amyloid deposition.

Although there are some correlations between fibril protein type and clinical manifestations, there are also many forms of acquired and hereditary amyloidosis in which there is little or no concordance between the fibril protein, or the genotype of its precursor, and the clinical phenotype. There are evidently genetic and/or environmental factors, which are distinct from the amyloid fibril protein itself, which determine whether, when, and where clinically significant amyloid deposits form. The nature of these important determinants of amyloidogenesis is obscure.

Reactive systemic, AA, amyloidosis

ASSOCIATED CONDITIONS

Amyloid A protein (AA) amyloidosis occurs in association with chronic inflammatory disorders, chronic local or systemic microbial infections, and malignant neoplasms. In Western Europe and the United States the most frequent predisposing conditions are rheumatic and connective tissue diseases (Table 3). Amyloidosis complicates up to 10 per cent of cases of rheumatoid arthritis and juvenile rheumatoid arthritis (JRA), although for reasons that are not clear the incidence is lower in the United States than in Europe. Amyloidosis is exceptionally rare in systemic lupus erythematosus, and in ulcerative colitis in contrast to Crohn's disease. Tuberculosis and leprosy are important causes of AA amyloidosis, particularly in the major endemic areas. Chronic osteomyelitis, bronchiectasis, chronically infected burns and decubitus ulcers as well as the chronic pyelonephritis of paraplegic patients are other well recognized associations (Table 3). Hodgkin's disease and renal carcinoma, which often cause fever, other systemic symptoms, and a major acute phase response, are the malignancies most commonly associated with systemic AA amyloid.

CLINICAL FEATURES

AA amyloid involves the viscera but may be widely distributed without causing clinical symptoms. It most commonly presents with non-selec-

Table 2 *Hereditary amyloidosis syndromes*

Clinical syndrome	Fibril protein
Predominant peripheral nerve involvement, familial amyloid polyneuropathy. Autosomal dominant	Transthyretin genetic variants (most commonly Met30, but over 30 others described)
Predominant peripheral nerve involvement, familial amyloid polyneuropathy. Autosomal dominant	Apolipoprotein AI *N*-terminal fragment of genetic variant Arg26
Predominant cranial nerve involvement with lattice corneal dystrophy. Autosomal dominant	Gelsolin, fragment of genetic variant Asn187 or Tyr187
Non-neuropathic, prominent visceral involvement (Ostertag-type) Autosomal dominant	Apolipoprotein, *N*-terminal fragment of genetic variant Arg26 or Arg60
Non-neuropathic, prominent visceral involvement (Ostertag-type) Autosomal dominant	Lysozyme genetic variant Thr56 or His67
Non-neuropathic, prominent visceral involvement (Ostertag-type) Autosomal dominant	Fibrinogen α-chain genetic variant Val526 or Leu554
Predominant cardiac involvement, no clinical neuropathy. Autosomal dominant	Transthyretin genetic variants Thr45, Ala60, Ser84, Met111, Ile122
Hereditary cerebral haemorrhage with amyloidosis (cerebral amyloid angiopathy). Autosomal dominant Icelandic type (major asymptomatic systemic amyloid also present) Dutch type	Cystatin C, fragment of genetic variant Glu68 β-protein derived from genetic variant β-amyloid precursor protein Gln693
Familial Alzheimer's disease	β-protein derived from genetic variant β-amyloid precursor protein Ile717, Phe717 or Gly717
Familial dementia – probable Alzheimer's disease	β-protein derived from genetic variant β-amyloid precursor protein Asn670, Leu671
Familial Creutzfeldt–Jakob disease, Gerstmann–Sträussler–Scheinker syndrome (hereditary spongiform encephalopathies, prion diseases)	Prion protein derived from genetic variants of prion protein precursor protein 51–91 insert, Leu102, Val117, Asn178, Lys200
Familial Mediterranean fever, prominent renal involvement. Autosomal recessive	AA derived from SAA
Muckle–Well's syndrome, nephropathy, deafness, urticaria, limb pain	AA derived from SAA
Cardiomyopathy with persistent atrial standstill	Not known
Cutaneous deposits (bullous, papular, pustulodermal)	Not known

tive proteinuria due to glomerular deposition, and may cause nephrotic syndrome before terminating in endstage renal failure. Haematuria, isolated tubular defects, nephrogenic diabetes insipidus, and diffuse renal calcification occur rarely. Kidney size is usually normal, but may be enlarged, or, in advanced cases, reduced. Endstage chronic renal failure is the cause of death in 40 to 60 per cent of cases but acute renal failure may be precipitated by hypotension and/or salt and water depletion following surgery, excessive use of diuretics, or intercurrent infection, and may be associated with renal vein thrombosis. The second most common presentation is with organomegaly, e.g. hepatosplenomegaly or thyroid enlargement. It may occur in either the presence or absence of overt renal abnormality, but in any case deposits are almost invariably widespread at the time of presentation. Involvement of the heart and gastrointestinal tract is frequent, though in neither case does it commonly cause functional impairment.

AA amyloidosis may become clinically evident early in the course of associated disease, but the incidence increases with duration of the primary condition. The mean duration of chronic rheumatic diseases such as rheumatoid arthritis, ankylosing spondylitis, or juvenile rheumatoid arthritis before amyloid is diagnosed is 12 to 14 years, though it can present much sooner. For most patients the prognosis is closely related to the presence of renal involvement, found in 70 per cent or more, and is poor. Fifty per cent of patients with AA amyloid die within 5 years of the amyloid being diagnosed. By 15 years a further 25 per cent are dead, but the remainder, including those who do not have significant renal impairment and some in whom the renal lesion is static or even regresses, clearly have a better prognosis. Availability of chronic hemodialysis and transplantation prevents early death from uraemia *per se*, but the extensive amyloid deposition in extrarenal tissues causes the prognosis in these patients to be less favourable than in others with endstage renal failure.

Table 3 *Conditions associated with reactive systemic (AA) amyloidosis*

Chronic inflammatory disorders
rheumatoid arthritis
juvenile chronic arthritis
ankylosing spondylitis
psoriasis and psoriatic arthropathy
Reiter's syndrome
adult Still's disease
Behçet's syndrome
Crohn's disease
Chronic microbial infections
leprosy
tuberculosis
bronchiectasis
decubitus ulcers
chronic pyelonephritis in paraplegics
osteomyelitis
Whipple's disease
Malignant neoplasms
Hodgkin's disease
renal carcinoma
carcinomas of gut, lung, urogenital tract
basal cell carcinoma
hairy cell leukaemia

Amyloidosis associated with immunocyte dyscrasia, AL amyloidosis

ASSOCIATED CONDITIONS

Almost any dyscrasia of cells of the B lymphocyte lineage, including multiple myeloma, malignant lymphomas and macroglobulinaemia, and 'benign' monoclonal gammopathy, may be complicated by immunoglobulin light chain (AL) amyloidosis. In some cases deposition of AL amyloid may be the only evidence of the dyscrasia. Amyloid occurs in up to 15 per cent of cases of myeloma and in a lower proportion of other malignant B cell and plasma cell disorders. The incidence in 'benign' monoclonal gammopathy is probably around 5 to 10 per cent. Most patients with AL amyloid have Bence Jones protein in the urine and, because the AL fibril proteins are derived from immunoglobulin light chains, it should be possible to detect either a monoclonal paraprotein or free light chains in serum or urine of all patients. However, some patients present with amyloid in the absence of detectable abnormal protein in serum or urine. The finding of immunoglobulin gene rearrangement in bone marrow samples, or even peripheral blood, sometimes confirms a monoclonal gammopathy in the absence of protein abnormality apart from the amyloid. If there is no previous predisposing inflammatory condition or family history of amyloidosis, it is likely that such apparently 'primary' cases of amyloidosis are related to an immunocyte dyscrasia and that analysis of the fibrils will show them to be AL in type. Sometimes the paraprotein manifests after presentation and diagnosis of the amyloid, and subnormal levels of some or all serum immunoglobulins or increased numbers of marrow plasma cells may provide less direct clues to the underlying aetiology.

CLINICAL FEATURES

AL amyloid usually occurs over the age of 50, but may be seen in young adults. It is more common in men than in women, and in Caucasians than in non-Caucasians. The clinical manifestations are protean, as any tissue may be involved. Uraemia, heart failure, or other effects of the amyloid usually cause death within a year of diagnosis. Patients with myeloma complicated by amyloid have a significantly worse prognosis than those with myeloma alone.

The heart is affected in 90 per cent of AL patients, in 30 per cent of whom cardiac dysfunction is the presenting feature and in up to 50 per cent of whom it is fatal. Restrictive cardiomyopathy with signs and symptoms of right ventricular failure and arrhythmias due to involvement of the conducting system are most common. Sensitivity to digoxin may cause fatal arrhythmias. Renal AL amyloid has the same manifestations as renal AA amyloid, but the prognosis is even worse. Gut involvement may cause motility disturbances (often secondary to autonomic neuropathy), malabsorption, perforation, haemorrhage, or obstruction. Macroglossia is quite frequent and is almost pathognomonic. Hyposplenism sometimes occurs in both AA and AL amyloidosis. Painful sensory polyneuropathy with early loss of pain and temperature sensation followed later by motor deficits is seen in 10 to 20 per cent of cases and carpal tunnel syndrome in 20 per cent. Autonomic neuropathy leading to orthostatic hypotension, impotence, and gastrointestinal disturbances may occur alone or together with the peripheral neuropathy. Skin involvement takes the form of papules, nodules, and plaques usually on the face and upper trunk, and involvement of dermal blood vessels results in purpura occurring either spontaneously or after minimal trauma and is very common. Articular amyloid usually occurs in association with myeloma and may mimic acute polyarticular rheumatoid arthritis affecting large joints, or it may present as asymmetrical arthritis affecting the hip or shoulder. Infiltration of the glenohumeral articulation occasionally produces the characteristic 'shoulder pad' sign. A rare but serious manifestation of AL amyloid is an acquired bleeding diathesis that may be associated with deficiency of factor X and sometimes also factor IX, or with increased fibrinolysis. It does not occur in AA amyloidosis, although in both AL and AA disease there may be serious bleeding in the absence of any identifiable factor deficiency.

Senile amyloidosis

Some amyloid is present in all autopsies on individuals over 80 years of age but it is not known whether this contributes to the ageing process or whether it is an epiphenomenon that becomes clinically important only when it is extensive.

SENILE SYSTEMIC AMYLOIDOSIS

Up to 25 per cent of old people have microscopic, clinically silent systemic deposits of transthyretin (TTR) amyloid involving the heart and blood vessel walls, smooth and striated muscle, fat tissue, renal papillae, and alveolar walls. In contrast to most other forms of systemic amyloidosis, including hereditary transthyretin amyloid caused by point mutations in the transthyretin gene, the spleen and renal glomeruli are rarely affected. The brain is not involved. Occasionally more extensive deposits in the heart, affecting ventricles and atria and situated in the interstitium and vessel walls, cause significant impairment of cardiac function and may be fatal. The transthyretin involved is probably usually of the normal wild-type but cases with transthyretin variants have been described which may be hereditary.

SENILE FOCAL AMYLOIDOSIS

Microscopic and clinically silent amyloid deposits of different fibril types, localized to particular tissues, are very commonly present in old people. Deposits of β-protein (see below) as amyloid in cerebral blood vessels and intracerebral plaques seen in 'normal' elderly brains may or may not be the harbinger of Alzheimer's disease, had the patient survived long enough. Amyloid deposits are present in most osteoarthritic joints at surgery or autopsy, usually in close association with calcium pyrophosphate deposits, affecting the articular cartilage and joint cap-

Table 4 *Cerebral amyloidosis*

Age-related amyloid angiopathy with or without intracerebral
    deposits
Hereditary amyloid angiopathy of meningeal and cortical
    vessels associated with cerebral haemorrhage: (a) Icelandic
    type; (b) Dutch type
Hereditary amyloid angiopathy affecting the entire central
    nervous system
Alzheimer's disease: sporadic, familial or associated with
    Down's syndrome
Cerebral amyloid associated with prion disease:
    sporadic spongiform encephalopathy: Creutzfeldt–Jakob
        disease
    familial prion disease: familial Creutzfeldt–Jakob disease.
        Gerstmann–Sträussler–Scheinker disease and atypical
        familial prion disease
    prion disease in animals
Familial oculoleptomeningeal amyloidosis

sule. However neither the clinical significance of this age-associated articular amyloid nor its biochemical nature are known. The corpora amylacea of the prostate are composed of β_2-microglobulin amyloid fibrils. Amyloid in the seminal vesicles is derived from an as yet unidentified exocrine secretary product of the vesicle cells. Isolated deposits of cardiac atrial amyloid consist of atrial natriuretic peptide.

Cerebral amyloidosis

INTRODUCTION

The brain is a very common and important site of amyloid deposition (Table 4), although interestingly, and perhaps because of the blood–brain barrier, it is never affected in any form of acquired systemic visceral amyloidosis. In familial amyloid polyneuropathy due to the transthyretin Met30 variant, cerebrovascular amyloid has been reported, but intracerebral deposits and clinical brain involvement have not. The common and major forms of brain amyloid are likewise confined to the brain and cerebral blood vessels with the single exception of cystatin C amyloid in hereditary cerebral haemorrhage with amyloidosis, Icelandic type, in which there are major though clinically silent systemic deposits.

ALZHEIMER'S DISEASE

By far the most frequent and important type of amyloid in the brain is that related to Alzheimer's disease, which is the most common cause of dementia and affects about 3 million individuals in the United States and a corresponding proportion of other Western populations. It is generally a disease of the elderly and its prevalence is therefore increasing. The clinical differential diagnosis of senile dementia and the positive identification of Alzheimer's disease are difficult and often of limited precision in life. However, there is currently an overwhelming consensus that intracerebral and cerebrovascular amyloid deposits are hallmarks of the neuropathological diagnosis. The vast majority of cases of Alzheimer's disease are sporadic but there are also families with an autosomal dominant pattern of inheritance. The gene(s) responsible are not known in most of these kindreds but point mutations in the gene for the precursor protein of the amyloidogenic β-protein, which forms the cerebral amyloid fibrils, have lately been identified in at least nine different families. Although neither the cause nor the pathogenesis of Alzheimer's disease are known, and there has been much controversy about the importance of amyloid, the concordance between dementia and inheritance of amyloid precursor protein (APP) mutations unequivocally places this molecule at the heart of at least one pathogenetic mechanism. Nevertheless it remains unclear whether or how the β-protein fragment

per se, or the amyloid fibrils that it forms, contribute to the neuronal dysfunction damage which underlie the dementia.

β-Protein amyloid is present in the cerebral vessel walls and as the core of the 'senile' or neuritic plaques in the white matter. A further neuropathological hallmark of Alzheimer's is the neurofibrillary tangle located intracellularly within neuronal cell bodies and processes. These tangles have a characteristic ultrastructural morphology of paired helical filaments and although they bind Congo red and then give the pathognomonic green birefringence of amyloid when viewed in polarized light, they differ structurally from all other known amyloid fibrils. There has been controversy over whether paired helical filaments contain β-protein and also other neurofilament materials but their main constituent is an abnormally phosphorylated form of the normal neurofilament protein, *tau*.

The degree of dementia in Alzheimer's correlates poorly with the extent of amyloid angiopathy and plaques, though somewhat better with the number of tangles. Nevertheless the fact that patients with Alzheimer's disease caused by APP mutations have exactly the same neuropathology as sporadic cases, including tangles, argues strongly that the APP and β-protein pathway can be of primary pathogenetic significance. Furthermore, all individuals with Down's syndrome (trisomy 21) develop clinically and neuropathologically typical Alzheimer's disease if they live into their fourth decade, that is at a much earlier age than normals. As APP is encoded by a gene on chromosome 21, it seems that excessive gene dose with wild-type APP can have the same effect as the APP variants in familial Alzheimer's.

In addition to the amyloid deposits composed of β-protein in the brains of patients with Alzheimer's disease and Down's syndrome, there are much more extensive 'amorphous' deposits of β-protein throughout the brain. These do not contain amyloid fibrils and therefore do not stain with Congo red, and are detectable only by immunohistochemical staining. Their significance is unknown. They apparently precede the appearance of amyloid but are not necessarily the precursor of it because they are present in areas, such as the cerebellum, in which amyloid of β-protein type is never seen.

SENILE CEREBRAL AMYLOIDOSIS AND AMYLOID ANGIOPATHY

The cerebral blood vessels contain amyloid, consisting of β-protein, in up to 60 per cent of aged brains of non-demented individuals and there may also be focal intracerebral amyloid plaques of the same fibril type. These deposits are usually clinically silent and may or may not be harbingers of Alzheimer's disease, had the patients survived long enough. Sometimes the amyloid angiopathy is more extensive and it is a rare but important cause of cerebral haemorrhage and stroke, to be distinguished from atherosclerotic cerebrovascular disease.

HEREDITARY CEREBRAL HAEMORRHAGE WITH AMYLOIDOSIS; HEREDITARY CEREBRAL AMYLOID ANGIOPATHY

Icelandic type

Cerebrovascular amyloid deposits composed of a fragment of a genetic variant of cystatin C are responsible for recurrent major cerebral haemorrhages starting in early adult life in members of families originating in Western Iceland. There is autosomal dominant inheritance and appreciable but clinically silent amyloid deposits are present in the spleen, lymph nodes, and skin. There is no extravascular amyloid in the brain and the neurological deficits of patients who survive are compatible with their cerebrovascular pathology. Multi-infarct dementia is common.

Dutch type

In families originating in a small region on the Dutch coast the autosomal dominant inheritance of recurrent normotensive cerebral hemorrhages starting in middle age, is due to deposition of a genetic variant of β-protein as cerebrovascular amyloid. There are also 'amorphous' β-protein deposits in the brain and early senile plaques, without congophilic amyloid cores. Multi-infarct dementia occurs in survivors but some patients become demented in the absence of stroke. Amyloid outside the brain has not been reported.

CEREBRAL AMYLOID ASSOCIATED WITH PRION DISEASE

The neuropathology of a group of progressive, invariably fatal spongiform encephalopathies which are transmissible, and in some cases are hereditary, sometimes includes intracerebral amyloid plaques and amyloid cerebral angiopathy. These diseases, sporadic and familial Creutzfeldt–Jakob disease, the familial Gerstmann–Sträussler–Scheinker syndrome, and kuru are caused by prions, and are closely related to the animal diseases scrapie of sheep and goats; transmissible encephalopathy of mink, elk, and male deer; and bovine spongiform encephalopathy. The significance of amyloid *per se* in these disorders is not clear, because it may not be present, and in bovine spongiform encephalopathy, which is apparently a result of transmission of ovine scrapie to cattle, it has never been reported. When scrapie or its human counterparts are transmitted to experimental animals by inoculation of affected brain tissue the development of intracerebral amyloid depends on the strain of infectious agent and the genetic background of the recipient. Even when amyloid is present in the brain it is not seen elsewhere (e.g., in the spleen), although the latter is a rich source of the infective agent. However, when the infective agent is exhaustively and highly purified from brain or spleen it forms typical congophilic amyloid fibrils, composed of an extremely proteinase resistant subunit which is the prion, PrP, and when typical amyloid deposits are present in affected brains they immunostain with antiprion antibodies. The amyloid is thus directly related to the cause of the encephalopathy but is evidently not necessary for expression of disease. This is a different situation from the extracerebral amyloidoses and from cystatin C and non-hereditary cerebral amyloid angiopathies, in which the damaging effects of amyloid deposition are, as far as is known, the actual and only cause of disease.

Hereditary systemic amyloidosis

FAMILIAL AMYLOID POLYNEUROPATHY

Familial amyloid polyneuropathy is an autosomal dominant syndrome with onset at any time from the second to the seventh decade, characterized by progressive peripheral and autonomic neuropathy and varying degrees of visceral involvement affecting especially the vitreous of the eye, the heart, kidneys, thyroid, and adrenals. There are usually amyloid deposits throughout the body involving blood vessel walls as well as the connective tissue matrix and the pathology is due to these deposits. Apart from major foci in Portugal, Japan, and Sweden, familial amyloid polyneuropathy has been reported in most ethnic groups throughout the world. There is considerable variation in the age of onset, rate of progression, and involvement of different systems, although within families the pattern is usually quite consistent. There is remorseless progression and the disorder is invariably fatal. Death results from the effects and complications of peripheral and/or autonomic neuropathy, or from cardiac or renal failure.

Familial amyloid polyneuropathy is caused by mutations in the gene for the plasma protein transthyretin, formerly known as prealbumin, the most frequent of which causes Met for Val substitution at position 30 in the mature protein, but 35 other amyloidogenic mutations have been described. There is no correlation between the underlying mutation and the clinical phenotype, which is evidently determined by other genetic and possibly also environmental factors. Furthermore the transthyretin mutations are not always penetrant, asymptomatic Met30 homozygotes over the age of 60 having been reported. One kindred with familial amyloid polyneuropathy due to a mutation in the apolipoprotein AI (apoAI) gene has also been reported.

FAMILIAL AMYLOID POLYNEUROPATHY WITH PREDOMINANT CRANIAL NEUROPATHY

Originally described in Finland but now reported in other ethnic groups, this autosomal dominant hereditary amyloidosis presents in adult life with cranial neuropathy, lattice corneal dystrophy, and distal peripheral neuropathy. There may be skin, renal, and cardiac manifestations and microscopic amyloid deposits are widely distributed in connective tissue and blood vessel walls, although life expectancy approaches normal. The mutant gene responsible encodes a variant of the actin-modulating protein, gelsolin. Individuals homozygous for the mutation have severe renal amyloidosis in addition to the usual neuropathy.

NON-NEUROPATHIC SYSTEMIC AMYLOIDOSIS, OSTERTAG TYPE

In this rare autosomal dominant syndrome of major systemic amyloidosis without clinical evidence of neuropathy, the patterns of organ involvement and overall clinical phenotype vary between families. The kidneys are often most severely affected leading to hypertension and renal failure, but the heart, spleen, liver, bowel, connective tissue, and exocrine glands, may all be involved. There is inexorable progression to death or organ failure requiring transplantation. Clinical presentation is usually in early adulthood though in a few kindreds it may be as late as the sixth decade. The amyloid proteins identified so far are genetic variants of apolipoprotein AI, lysozyme, and the α-chain of fibrinogen.

CARDIAC AMYLOIDOSIS

Cardiac amyloidosis, without other systemic involvement or neuropathy, progressing inexorably to death, is associated with transthyretin gene mutations (see Table 1). In a large Danish family with autosomal dominant transthyretin Met111 cardiac amyloid, deposition starts only in adult life a few years before the clinical presentation, despite presence of the variant transthyretin from birth.

FAMILIAL MEDITERRANEAN FEVER

Familial Mediterranean fever is an autosomal recessive disorder of unknown mechanism, characterized by recurrent episodes of fever, abdominal pain, pleurisy or arthritis, which predominantly affects non-Ashkenazi Jews, Armenians, Anatolian Turks, and Levantine Arabs. In Sephardi Jews of North African origin, and in the other ethnic groups except Armenians and to a lesser extent Askenazi Jews, untreated familial Mediterranean fever is eventually complicated in a high proportion of cases by typical systemic AA amyloidosis. Furthermore, a subset of familial Mediterranean fever patients may present with AA amyloidosis before they have experienced any clinical attacks of the inflammatory disease. It is not clear why this should occur but it is possible that they may have been mounting an acute phase response to subclinical manifestations of the underlying familial Mediterranean fever. The absence of amyloid in Armenians and the lower incidence in Ashkenazis is another illustration of the unknown genetic factors, other than the fibril protein itself, which determine clinical amyloidosis. The gene causing familial Mediterranean fever is on the short arm of chromosome 16 but has not yet been identified.

HAEMODIALYSIS-ASSOCIATED AMYLOIDOSIS

Almost all patients with endstage renal failure who are maintained on haemodialysis for more than 5 years develop amyloid deposits composed of β_2-microglobulin. These deposits are predominantly osteoarticular and are associated with carpal tunnel syndrome, large joint pain and stiffness, soft tissue masses, bone cysts, and pathological fractures. Renal tubular amyloid concretions may also form. The serious clinical problems associated with β_2-microglobulin amyloidosis constitute the major morbidity in long-term dialysis patients. Furthermore, in some such patients more extensive deposition occurs, most commonly in the spleen but also in other organs, and a few cases of death associated with systemic β_2-microglobulin amyloid have been reported. The β_2-microglobulin is derived from the high plasma concentrations, which develop in renal insufficiency and which are not cleared by dialysis. This type of amyloid also occurs in patients on continuous ambulatory peritoneal dialysis and has even been reported in a patient with chronic renal failure who had never been dialysed.

ENDOCRINE AMYLOIDOSIS

Many tumours of APUD cells which produce peptide hormones have amyloid deposits in their stroma. These are probably composed of the hormone peptides and in the case of medullary carcinoma of the thyroid the fibril subunits are derived from procalcitonin. In insulinomas the amyloid fibril protein is a novel peptide first identified in that site and subsequently shown to be the fibril protein in the amyloid of the islets of Langerhans in type II, maturity onset, diabetes. This peptide is called islet amyloid polypeptide, and also amylin, and shows appreciable homology with calcitonin gene-related peptide. Islet amyloid polypeptide amyloid is an almost universal feature of the pancreatic islets in type II diabetes and becomes more extensive with increasing duration and severity of the disease. Although it is not clear whether the amyloid itself is initially responsible for the metabolic defect in this form of diabetes, it seems likely that progressive amyloid deposition leading to islet destruction subsequently does contribute to the pathogenesis. The possible hormonal or other role of islet amyloid polypeptide itself, which is produced by the islet B cells, is also not yet clear.

RARE LOCALIZED AMYLOIDOSIS SYNDROMES

Amyloid deposits localized to the skin occur in both acquired and hereditary forms. Primary localized cutaneous amyloidosis presents in adult life as macular or papular lesions, the fibrils of which may be derived from keratin. Hereditary cutaneous amyloid lesions are rare, of unknown fibril type and sometimes associated with other, non-amyloid, multisystem disorders. Amyloid deposits in the eye cause local problems in the cornea (corneal lattice dystrophy) or conjunctiva, whilst orbital amyloid presents as mass lesions which can disrupt eye movement and the structure of the orbit. In one such case the fibril protein has been identified as a fragment of IgG heavy chain but otherwise the proteins involved in these non-hereditary conditions have not been characterized.

Localized foci of AL amyloid can occur anywhere in the body, in the absence of systemic AL amyloidosis, the most common sites being the skin, upper airways and respiratory tract, and the urogenital tract. They may be associated with a local plasmacytoma or B cell lymphoma producing a monoclonal immunoglobulin, but often the cells, which must be present to produce the amyloidogenic protein, are rather inconspicuous. The clinical problems caused by these space-occupying amyloidomas are usually cured by surgical resection, but this is not always possible.

Amyloid fibrils

Regardless of their very diverse protein subunits, amyloid fibrils of different types are remarkably similar: straight, rigid, non-branching, of indeterminate length and 10 to 15 nm in diameter. They are insoluble in physiological solutions, relatively resistant to proteolysis, and bind Congo red dye producing pathognomonic green birefringence when viewed in polarized light. X-ray diffraction and infrared spectroscopy studies of all different amyloid fibrils, including synthetic fibrils formed *in vitro*, indicate the presence of β-sheet structure, and many proteins that are precursors of amyloid fibrils are rich in β-sheet secondary structure. This led to the concept that amyloid fibrils consist exclusively of stacks of anti-parallel β-pleated sheets arranged with their long axes perpendicular to the long axis of the fibril, resembling the structure

proposed for silk, which, like amyloid, is proteinase resistant. Congo red binding and birefringence have also been ascribed to the presence of the repeating β-sheet motif. However, the precise molecular interactions between the dye and amyloid fibrils have not been elucidated, and the structure of neither silk nor any amyloid fibril is known because none of these fibrillar proteins forms single crystals suitable for high resolution X-ray diffraction analysis. There is a well-established relationship between increasing β-sheet structure and decreased protein solubility associated with aggregation and precipitation, so that the general evidence of β-sheets may be a consequence of the insolubility of the fibrils. On the other hand fibrillar morphology *per se* does not require β-sheet structure, and the X-ray diffraction pattern suggesting a shared repeating structure in different amyloid fibrils may derive from similar intermolecular packing motifs rather than shared secondary structure. Indeed, given the remarkable sequence diversity among amyloid fibril proteins, it is inherently more likely that the ultimate uniformity of the fibrils reflects a common packing mechanism.

Amyloid fibril proteins and their precursors

AL

AL proteins are derived from the *N*-terminal region of monoclonal immunoglobulin light chains and consist of the whole or part of the variable (V_L) domain. Intact light chains may rarely be found, and the molecular weight therefore varies between about 8000 and 30 000. The light chain of the monoclonal paraprotein is either identical to, or clearly the precursor of, AL isolated from the amyloid deposits.

AL is more commonly derived from λ chains than from κ chains, despite the fact that κ chains predominate among both normal immunoglobulins and the paraprotein products of immunocyte dyscrasias. A new λ chain subgroup, λ_{VI}, was identified first as an AL protein in two cases of immunocyte dyscrasia-associated amyloidosis before it had been recognized in any other form, and it has subsequently been observed in many more cases of AL amyloidosis. Furthermore, there is increasing evidence from sequence analyses of Bence Jones proteins of both κ and λ type from patients with AL amyloidosis, and of AL proteins themselves, that these polypeptides contain unique amino acid replacements or insertions compared to non-amyloid monoclonal light chains. In some cases these changes involve replacement of hydrophilic framework residues by hydrophobic residues, changes likely to promote aggregation and insolubilization, and in others the monoclonal light chains from amyloid patients have been demonstrated directly to have decreased solubility and a greater propensity for precipitation than control non-amyloid proteins. The inherent 'amyloidogenicity' of particular monoclonal light chains has been elegantly confirmed in an *in vivo* model in which isolated Bence Jones proteins are injected into mice. Animals receiving light chains from AL amyloid patients developed typical amyloid deposits composed of the human protein whereas animals receiving light chains from myeloma patients without amyloid did not.

AA

The AA protein is a single non-glycosylated polypeptide chain usually of mass ~ 8000 Da and containing 76 residues corresponding to the *N*-terminal portion of the 104 residue serum amyloid A protein (SAA). Smaller and larger AA fragments, even some whole serum amyloid A molecules, have also been reported in AA fibrils. SAA is an apolipoprotein of high density lipoprotein particles and is the polymorphic product of a set of genes located on the short arm of chromosome 11. SAA is highly conserved in evolution and is a major acute phase reactant in all species in which it has been studied. Most of the SAA in plasma is produced by hepatocytes in which the synthesis is under transcriptional regulation by cytokines, especially interleukin 1(IL-1), interleukin 6 (IL-6), and tumour necrosis factor, acting via nuclear factor κB-like and possibly other transcription factors. After secretion it rapidly associated with high density lipoproteins from which it displaces apolipoprotein AI. The circulating concentration can rise from normal levels of up to 3 mg/l to over 1000 mg/l within 24 to 48 h of an acute stimulus, whilst with ongoing chronic inflammation the level may remain persistently high. Certain isoforms of SAA, the products of different genes, are predominantly synthesized elsewhere in the body, by macrophages, adipocytes, and certain other cells. Although they also associate with high density lipoproteins, their acute phase synthesis is stimulated differently and they presumably have different functions. There is also a closely related family of high density lipoprotein trace apoproteins which are not acute phase reactants and which have been designated 'constitutive SAAs', although they do not form amyloid.

Circulating SAA is the precursor of amyloid fibril AA protein, from which it is derived by proteolytic cleavage. Such cleavage can be produced by macrophages and by a variety of proteinases but since further cleavage of AA is readily demonstrable in vitro it is not clear why the AA peptide persists in amyloid. Furthermore, it is not known whether in the process of AA fibrillogenesis, cleavage of SAA occurs before and/or after aggregation of monomers. Persistent overproduction of SAA causing sustained high circulating levels is a necessary condition for deposition of AA amyloid but it is not known why only some individuals in this state get amyloid. In mice, only SAA2, one of the three major isoforms of murine serum amyloid A, is the precursor of AA in amyloid fibrils, but in man there is no association between expression of particular isoforms and amyloidogenesis.

The normal functions of SAA are not known, although modulating effects on reverse cholesterol transport and on lipid functions in the microenvironment of inflammatory foci have been proposed. A protein, homologous with SAA, produced by rabbit fibroblasts has been reported to act as an autocrine stimulator of collagenase production in vitro. Other reports of potent cell regulatory functions of isolated denatured delipidated SAA have yet to be confirmed with physiological preparations of SAA-rich high density lipoproteins. Regardless of its physiological role the behaviour of SAA as an exquisitely sensitive acute phase protein with an enormous dynamic range makes it an extremely valuable empirical clinical marker. It can be used to monitor objectively the extent and activity of infective, inflammatory, necrotic, and neoplastic disease. Furthermore, routine monitoring of SAA should be an integral part of the management of all patients with AA amyloid or disorders predisposing to it, as control of the primary inflammatory process in order to reduce SAA production is essential if amyloidosis is to be halted, enabled to regress, or prevented. Automated immunoassay systems for SAA are becoming available and a World Health Organization International Reference Standard for SAA Immunoassay is currently being evaluated.

TRANSTHYRETIN

Transthyretin, formerly known as prealbumin, is a normal non-glycosylated plasma protein, with a relative molecular mass of 54 980. It is composed of four identical non-covalently associated subunits each of 127 amino acids. It is produced by hepatocytes and the choroid plexus and is a significant negative acute phase protein. Each tetrameric molecule is able to bind a single thyroxine or tri-odothyronine molecule and up to 15 per cent of circulating thyroid hormone is transported in this way. Transthyretin also forms a 1 : 1 molecular complex with retinol-binding protein, which transports vitamin A.

Transthyretin is encoded by a single copy gene but is appreciably polymorphic and over 40 different point mutations encoding single residue substitutions have been identified so far. Normal wild-type transthyretin is an inherently amyloidogenic protein which forms the fibrils in senile systemic amyloidosis, and in vitro exposure to reduced pH is sufficient to generate transthyretin amyloid fibrils from the pure protein. Of the variant forms of transthyretin, 36 have been associated with hereditary amyloidosis. Transgenic mice expressing human transthyretin Met30 in the liver develop extensive systemic amyloidosis, though even when the transgene is expressed in the choroid plexus and transthyretin

amyloid is deposited in the meninges and choroid plexus, no amyloid deposits have yet been reported in the peripheral nerves.

Individuals heterozygous for transthyretin mutations have a mixture of wild-type and variant transthyretin monomers in their circulating transthyretin, and if they develop amyloidosis both forms are often present although the variant may predominate in the amyloid fibrils. Although fragments of transthyretin, usually cleaved around residue 49, are commonly present, intact transthyretin subunits are also found and fibrillogenesis does not depend on an initial proteolytic step.

β-PROTEIN

The fibril protein in the intracerebral and cerebrovascular amyloid of Alzheimer's disease, Down's syndrome and hereditary amyloid angiopathy of Dutch type is a 39–43 residue sequence derived by proteolysis from a high molecular weight precursor protein, the so-called amyloid precursor protein (APP), encoded on the long arm of chromosome 21. Several isoforms of APP are generated by alternative splicing of transcripts from the 19 exon gene, and yielding major forms: APP695, APP751, and APP770. These are each single-chain, multidomain glycoproteins with the carboxy-terminal 47 residues within the cytoplasm, a 25-residue membrane-spanning region, and the rest of the molecule lying extracellularly. APP751 and APP770 contain a 56-residue Kunitz-type serine proteinase inhibitor domain encoded by exon 7. Following glycosylation and membrane insertion, APPs are cleaved extracellularly by so-called APP secretase activity, close to the transmembrane sequence, releasing, in the case of the isoforms containing the proteinase inhibitor domain, a molecule known as proteinase nexin II, which avidly binds factor XIa, trypsin, and chymotrypsin as well as epidermal growth factor-binding protein and the γ subunit of nerve growth factor. Although mRNA encoding APP695, which lacks the proteinase inhibitor domain, is the predominant species found in brain, whereas mRNA for APP751 is the most abundant in other tissues, 85 per cent of secreted APP in the brain is proteinase nexin II. Interestingly, APP secreted by a glial cell line is substantially glycosylated with chondroitin sulphate glycosaminoglycan chains. APP also undergoes high affinity interactions with heparan sulphate. These observations suggest that APP may have important functions in cell adhesion, cell migration and modulation of growth factor activities. APP proteinase nexin II is present in and released by platelets and probably functions in the clotting cascade.

The amyloidogenic β-protein, encoded by parts of exons 16 and 17, corresponds to the part of the APP sequence which extends from within the cell membrane into the extracellular space. Secretase cleavage of APP to release the soluble form cannot therefore generate the intact β-protein itself, or larger fragments containing it. However, there is an alternative processing pathway for APP, in which it is taken up whole by lysosomes and cleaved to yield fragments that do contain the whole β-protein sequence. Furthermore, it has lately been demonstrated that APP cleaved at the N-terminus of β-protein and also free soluble β-protein itself are normally produced by cell lines and by mixed brain cells in culture and are present in the cerebrospinal fluid. They must be produced by a secretase pathway different from that previously reported. However, the source of the β-protein in the intracerebral amorphous deposits and of that which aggregates as amyloid fibrils in the brain and cerebral blood vessels is still not known. Likewise the mechanism by which mutations leading to amino acid substitutions at position 717, outside the β-protein sequence, cause β-protein amyloidosis remains obscure. Intriguingly, it has recently been reported that cultured cells expressing APP cDNA encoding the double substitution Lys for Asn 595, Met for Leu 596, which is responsible for hereditary Alzheimer's disease in a Swedish family, produce 6 to 8 times more β-protein than cells expressing wild-type APP. Increased abundance of the respective amyloid fibril precursor may thus be a unifying theme between familial Alzheimer's disease caused by APP mutations, trisomy 21 in Down's syndrome, and many forms of extracerebral amyloidosis. On the other hand the substitution at residue 693, corresponding to 22 in β-protein, which causes the Dutch-type of hereditary amyloid angiopathy, apparently promotes fibrillogenesis *in vitro* and may be analogous to the other types of hereditary amyloid in which variant proteins are inherently less soluble *in vitro* and are deposited as amyloid fibrils in the tissues. In any case even peptides with the normal wild-type sequence of β-protein are relatively insoluble and readily converted to amyloid-like fibrils *in vitro*.

CYSTATIN C

Cystatin C (formerly called γ-trace) is an inhibitor of cysteine proteinases, including cathepsins B, H, and L, is encoded by a gene on chromosome 20 and consists of a single non-glycosylated polypeptide chain of 120 residues. It is present in all major human biological fluids at concentrations compatible with a significant physiological role in proteinase inhibition. The normal concentration in cerebrospinal fluid is 6.5 mg/l (range 2.7 to 13.7, $n = 34$), but is much lower (2.7 mg/l, range 1.0 to 4.7, $n = 9$) in patients with the Icelandic type of hereditary cerebral amyloid angiopathy in whom fragments of the Gln 68 genetic variant of cystatin C form the amyloid fibrils. This reduced concentration is useful diagnostically and is evident even in presymptomatic carriers of the cystatin C gene mutation. The point mutation that causes the disease encodes a Gln for Leu substitution in the mature protein and the amyloid fibril protein consists of the C-terminal 110 residues of the variant. This amino-terminally truncated form is not detectable in the cerebrospinal fluid of affected patients, suggesting that cleavage takes place either in close proximity to fibril deposition or is a postfibrillogenic event. Fibril formation *in vitro* by variant cystatin C or fragments of it has not been reported, but by analogy with other types of hereditary amyloidosis caused by single residue substitutions it is likely that the variant is inherently fibrillogenic. It is not known whether cerebral haemorrhage in cystatin C amyloidosis is caused simply by the damaging effects of vascular amyloid deposition or whether deficiency in inhibitory capacity for cysteinase proteinases also plays a part.

GELSOLIN

Gelsolin (relative molecular mass ∼ 90 000) is a widely distributed cytoplasmic protein which binds actin monomers, nucleates actin filament growth and severs actin filaments. Alternative transcriptional initiation and message processing from a single gene on chromosome 9 are responsible for synthesis of a secreted form of gelsolin (relative molecular mass ∼ 93 000), which circulates in the plasma at a concentration of about 200 mg/l. Its function in the blood is not known but may be related to clearance of actin filaments released by dying cells.

In the Finnish type of hereditary amyloidosis the amyloid fibril protein is a 71-residue fragment of variant gelsolin with Asn substituted for Asp at position 15, corresponding to residue 187 of the mature molecule, and the same mutation has been discovered in affected kindreds from different ethnic backgrounds. In one Danish family with the same phenotype there is a different mutation at the same nucleotide, predicting a Tyr for Asp substitution at residue 187. Synthetic peptides including the Asn for Asp187 substitution are much less soluble *in vitro* than the wild-type sequence and readily form amyloid fibrils *in vitro*.

APOLIPOPROTEIN AI

Apolipoprotein AI is the most abundant apolipoprotein of high density lipoprotein particles and participates in their central function of reverse cholesterol transport from the periphery to the liver. Variants of apolipoprotein AI are extremely rare and only two of them, Arg26 and Arg60, have been associated with amyloidosis, but in the few affected families identified hitherto all carriers of the corresponding mutation have developed clinical amyloidosis. Interestingly both these amyloidogenic substitutions produce Arg–Arg doublets and in the case of Arg60 the triplet Lys–Arg–Arg, but whether this is of pathogenetic significance is not

known. The amyloid fibril protein has been fully characterized only in one individual, with the Arg60 variant, and consisted of the intact N-terminal portion of the variant molecule up to residues 88–94. Similar length fragments were found in a case with the Arg26 variant. It is not known whether these fragments are normally produced or whether they are cleaved from apolipoprotein AI as a result of the amino acid substitution, but in any case the variant sequence is presumably predisposed to aggregate as fibrils.

LYSOZYME

Lysozyme (EC 3.2.1.17) is the classic bacteriolytic enzyme of external secretions, discovered by Fleming in 1922. It is also present at high concentration within articular cartilage and in the granules of polymorphs, and is the major secreted product of macrophages. Lysozymes are present in most organisms in which they have been sought, although their physiological role is not always clear. The complete structures of hen egg white and human lysozymes are known to atomic resolution and their catalytic mechanism, epitopes, folding and other aspects of structure–function relationship have been analysed exhaustively. This contrasts with the absence of detailed three-dimensional structural information on all other amyloid fibril proteins and their precursors except transthyretin and β₂-microglobulin. Lysozyme, unlike transthyretin and β₂-microglobulin, is not inherently amyloidogenic, and may therefore become a particularly valuable model for investigation of amyloid fibrillogenesis. There is only one copy of the lysozyme gene in the human genome and no polymorphism or mutations in the coding region have been reported hitherto, nor is any disease other than amyloidosis associated with lysozyme. The mutations which cause amyloid produce substitution of Thr for Ile56 in one family and His for Asp67 in the other. These dramatic changes in residues which are extremely conserved throughout the lysozyme and related α-lactalbumin protein families are likely to be of major structural significance.

ISLET AMYLOID POLYPEPTIDE

Islet amyloid polypeptide (IAPP, amylin) is a 37-residue molecule encoded by a gene on chromosome 12 and with 46 per cent sequence homology to the neuropeptide, calcitonin gene-related peptide (CGRP). Islet amyloid polypeptide is produced in the β cells of the pancreatic islets of Langerhans and is stored in and released from their secretory granules together with insulin. It has been reported to modulate insulin release, and to induce peripheral insulin resistance, vasodilatation and lowering of plasma calcium but neither its physiological role nor its contribution to diabetes are yet known.

Amyloidogenicity of islet amyloid polypeptide depends on the amino acid sequence between residues 20–29, as shown by *in vitro* fibrillogenesis with synthetic peptides. The synthetic decapeptide IAPP20–29 and even the hexapeptide IAPP25–29, Gly–Ala–Ile–Leu–Ser–Ser, form amyloid-like fibrils *in vitro*, whereas other islet amyloid polypeptide fragments do not. There is also a correlation between conservation of this sequence and deposition of islet amyloid polypeptide amyloid in the islets of diabetic animals of different species. However, the role of the amyloid in diabetogenesis remains to be established. In the degu, a South American rodent, spontaneous diabetes is associated with islet amyloid composed of insulin, and xenogeneic insulin can also form amyloid in man at sites of repeated therapeutic insulin injections.

β₂-MICROGLOBULIN

β₂-Microglobulin is a non-glycosylated, non-polymorphic single chain protein of 99 residues with a single intrachain disulphide bridge (relative molecular mass 11 815) encoded by a single gene on chromosome 15. It becomes non-covalently associated with the heavy chain of major histocompatibility class I antigens and is required for transport and expression of the complex at the cell surface. Amino acid sequence-homology places β₂-microglobulin in the superfamily including immunoglobulins, T cell receptor α and β chains, Thy 1, major histocompatibility class I and II molecules, secretory component, etc. Its three-dimensional structure is a typical β-barrel with two antiparallel pleated sheets comprising three and four strands respectively, and closely resembles an immunoglobulin domain.

β_2-Microglobulin is produced by lymphoid and a variety of other cells in which it stabilizes the structure and function of class I antigens at the cell surface. When these complexes are shed by cleavage of the heavy chain at the cell surface, free β_2-microglobulin is released. The circulating concentration of β_2-microglobulin is 1 to 2 mg/l and the protein is rapidly cleared by glomerular filtration and then catabolized in the proximal renal tubule. Impairment of renal function is associated with retention of β_2-microglobulin and increased circulating levels because there is no other site for its catabolism. Daily production of β_2-microglobulin is about 200 mg and in endstage renal failure patients on haemodialysis, plasma β_2-microglobulin levels rise to and remain at levels of about 40 to 70 mg/l. Isolated unaltered β_2-microglobulin can form amyloid-like fibrils itself *in vitro*, and most studies of *ex vivo* β_2-microglobulin fibrils show the whole intact molecule to be the major subunit, although fragments and altered forms of β_2-microglobulin have also been reported.

Glycosaminoglycans

Amyloidotic organs contain more glycosaminoglycans than normal tissues and at least some of this is a tightly bound, integral part of the amyloid fibrils. These fibril-associated glycosaminoglycans are heparan sulphate and dermatan sulphate in all forms of amyloid which have been investigated. Fibrils isolated by water extraction and separated from other tissue components contain 1 to 2 per cent by weight of glycosaminoglycan, none of which is covalently associated with the fibril protein. Interestingly, in systemic AA and AL amyloidosis, the only forms in which this has been studied so far, there is marked restriction of the heterogeneity of the glycosaminoglycan chains, suggesting that particular subclasses of heparan and dermatan sulphates are involved. Immunohistochemical studies demonstrate the presence of proteoglycan core proteins in all amyloid deposits, and that these are closely related to fibrils at the ultrastructural level. However, in isolated fibril preparations much of the glycosaminoglycan material is free carbohydrate chains and it is not yet clear whether this represents aberrant glycosaminoglycan metabolism related to amyloidosis or is just an artefact of postmortem core protein degradation.

The significance of glycosaminoglycans in amyloid remains unclear, but their universal presence, intimate relationship with the fibrils and restricted heterogeneity all suggest that they may be important. Glycosaminoglycans are known to participate in the organization of some normal structural proteins into fibrils and they may have comparable fibrillogenic effects on certain amyloid fibril precursor proteins. Furthermore the glycosaminoglycans on amyloid fibrils may be ligands to which serum amyloid P component, another universal constituent of amyloid deposits, binds.

Amyloid P component, and serum amyloid P component

Amyloid deposits in all different forms of the disease, both in man and in animals, contain the non-fibrillar glycoprotein amyloid P component (AP). Amyloid P component is identical to and derived from the normal circulating plasma protein, serum amyloid P component (SAP), a member of the pentraxin protein family which includes C-reactive protein (CRP). SAP consists of ten identical non-covalently associated subunits, each with a molecular mass of 25 462 Da, which are non-covalently associated in two pentameric disc-like rings interacting face-to-face. SAP is a calcium-dependent ligand binding protein, the best defined specificity of which is for the 4,6-cyclic pyruvate acetal of β-D-galactose. It is therefore a lectin, but it also binds avidly and specifically to DNA, to chromatin, to glycosaminoglycans, particularly heparan and dermatan sulphates, and to all known types of amyloid fibrils. Aggregated, but not native, SAP also binds specifically to C4-binding protein and fibronectin from plasma, although SAP is not complexed with any other protein in the circulation. In addition to being a plasma protein, SAP is also a normal constituent of certain extracellular matrix structures. It is covalently associated with collagen and/or other matrix components in the *lamina rara interna* of the human glomerular basement membrane and is present on the microfibrillar mantle of elastin fibres throughout the body.

The normal function of SAP is not known, nor its role, if any, in the pathogenesis of amyloidosis. However, no deficiency of SAP has been described and it has been stably conserved in evolution. There is a single copy of its gene on chromosome 1, and although there are reports of variation in a single amino acid residue, Ser or Pro82, mass spectrometric analyses of an extensive series of SAP preparations revealed only Ser82. There is thus no significant polymorphism of the amino acid sequence, and furthermore the single biantennary oligosaccharide chain attached to Asn32 is the most invariant glycan of any known glycoprotein. This all suggests that SAP is likely to have important physiological function(s). The interaction with DNA, to which SAP is the single serum protein to undergo specific calcium-dependent binding, and with chromatin, are of particular interest in this regard. In binding to native long chromatin, SAP selectively and completely displaces histone H1, thereby solubilizing the chromatin. Coupled with the fact that SAP from whole serum also binds specifically to chromatin within normal nuclei, and that SAP binds *in vivo* to extracellular deposits of chromatin, these observations suggest that SAP may participate in the *in vivo* handling of chromatin released by dead cells.

SAP is only produced by hepatocytes and its plasma concentration is tightly regulated (women: mean 24 mg/l, SD 8, range 8 to 55, $n = 274$; men: mean 32 mg/l, SD 7, range 12 to 50, $n = 226$). The value remains normal even during massive deposition of SAP into amyloid, indicating that even though SAP is not a major acute phase protein, unlike its close homologue C-reactive protein, the rate of synthesis and secretion can be remarkably increased. The normal plasma half-life of SAP is 24 h, and in the absence of amyloid it is taken up and catabolized by hepatocytes. Persistence of SAP in the circulation is absolutely dependent on intactness of its oligosaccharide, loss of the terminal sialic acid residues of which is associated with extremely rapid uptake and catabolism in the liver.

The three-dimensional structure of SAP has lately been solved to atomic resolution. The tertiary fold of the subunit is dominated by antiparallel β-sheets, forming a flattened β-barrel with jellyroll topology and a core of hydrophobic side-chains. On one side of the jellyroll there is a short helix sitting above the Cys36–Cys95 disulphide bridge and adjacent to the Asn32 glycosylation site. The calcium binding site on the other side of the subunit consists of two loops co-ordinating two calcium ions 4 Å apart. Remarkably, the arrangement of β-strands in the SAP subunit is very similar to the subunit fold of concanavalin A and pea lectin, despite absence of sequence homology with these plant proteins. The SAP structure, with relatively short and tightly hydrogen bonded loops joining the β-strands, also fits with the known resistance of SAP to digestion by proteinase. Despite some claims to the contrary, SAP is probably not itself a proteinase inhibitor; however its own inherent resistance to degradation could well be of importance in amyloid deposits *in vivo* and once associated with fibrils in the tissues SAP/amyloid P is completely insusceptible to catabolism.

Other proteins in amyloid deposits

A number of plasma proteins, other than the fibril proteins themselves and SAP, have been detected immunohistochemically in some amyloid deposits. These include α_1-antichymotrypsin, some complement components, apolipoprotein E, and various extracellular matrix or basement membrane proteins. The significance of these findings and their role, if any, in pathogenesis of amyloid deposition or its effects remain to be determined.

Diagnosis and monitoring of amyloidosis

Introduction

Until recently amyloidosis was an exclusively histological diagnosis, and green birefringence of deposits stained with Congo red and viewed in polarized light remains the gold standard. Furthermore, immunohistochemical staining of amyloid-containing tissue is the simplest method for identifying the amyloid fibril type. However, biopsies provide extremely small samples and therefore can never provide information on the extent, localization, progression or regression of amyloid deposits. A major advance in clinical amyloidosis has been the development of radiolabelled SAP as a specific tracer for amyloid. Combined scintigraphic imaging and metabolic analysis using labelled SAP have provided a wealth of new information on the natural history of many different forms of amyloid and their response to treatment (see above).

Histochemical diagnosis of amyloid

BIOPSY

Amyloid may be an incidental finding on biopsy of the kidneys, liver, heart, bowel, peripheral nerve, lymph node, skin, thyroid, or bone marrow. When amyloidosis is suspected clinically, biopsy of rectum or subcutaneous fat is the least invasive. Amyloid is present in these sites in more than 90 per cent of cases of systemic AA or AL. Alternatively, a clinically affected tissue may be biopsied directly. Fixation in neutral buffered formalin and wax embedding are satisfactory, although most staining reactions are best examined on cryostat sections of fresh-frozen tissue.

CONGO RED AND OTHER HISTOCHEMICAL STAINS

Many cotton dyes, fluorochromes, and metachromatic stains have been used, but Congo red staining, and its resultant green birefringence when viewed with high intensity polarized light, is the pathognomonic histochemical test for amyloidosis. The stain is unstable and must be freshly prepared every 2 months or less. Section thickness of 5 to 10 μm and inclusion in every staining run of a positive control tissue containing modest amounts of amyloid are critical.

IMMUNOHISTOCHEMISTRY

Although many amyloid fibril proteins can be identified immunohistochemically, the demonstration of amyloidogenic proteins in tissues does not, on its own, establish the presence of amyloid. Congo red staining and green birefringence are always required and immunostaining may then enable the amyloid to be classified. Antibodies to serum amyloid A protein are commercially available and always stain AA deposits, similarly with anti-β_2-microglobulin antisera and haemodialysis-associated amyloid. In AL amyloid the deposits are stainable with standard antisera to κ or λ in only about half of all cases, probably because the light-chain fragment in the fibrils is usually the N-terminal variable domain, which is largely unique for each monoclonal protein. Immunohistochemical staining of transthyretin, β-protein, and prion protein amyloids may require pretreatment of sections with formic acid or alkaline guanidine or deglycosylation.

ELECTRON MICROSCOPY

Amyloid fibrils cannot always be convincingly identified ultrastructurally, and electron microscopy alone is not sufficient to confirm the diagnosis of amyloidosis.

Problems of histological diagnosis

The tissue sample must be adequate (for example, the inclusion of submucosal vessels in a rectal biopsy specimen), and failure to find amyloid does not exclude the diagnosis. The unavoidable problem of sampling error means that biopsy cannot reveal the extent or distribution of amyloid. Experience with Congo red staining is required if clinically important false-negative and false-positive results are to be avoided. Immunohistochemical staining requires positive and negative controls, including demonstration of specificity of staining by absorption of positive antisera with isolated pure antigens.

Non-histological investigations

Two-dimensional echocardiography showing small, concentrically hypertrophied ventricles, generally impaired contraction, dilated atria, homogeneously echogenic valves, and 'sparkling' echodensity of ventricular walls can be diagnostic of cardiac amyloidosis. However, some of the signs may be absent despite histologically confirmed involvement. Imaging after injection of isotope-labelled calcium-seeking tracers has poor sensitivity and specificity and is of no clinical use.

In cases of known or suspected hereditary amyloidosis the gene defect must be characterized. If amyloidotic tissue is available the fibril protein may be known and the corresponding gene can then be studied; but if no tissue containing amyloid is available, screening of the genes for known amyloidogenic proteins must be undertaken.

Biochemical and immunochemical screening tests for the presence in the plasma of amyloidogenic variant protein products of mutant genes also exist, for example for transthyretin Met 30 and apolipoprotein AI Arg26 and Arg60, but molecular genetic analysis of DNA is probably easier to perform and is most direct. Ultimately, however, regardless of the DNA results, it is essential to identify directly in the amyloid the presence of the respective protein.

Serum amyloid P component as a specific tracer in amyloidosis

The universal presence in amyloid deposits of AP, derived from circulating SAP, suggested the use of radioisotope-labelled SAP as a diagnostic tracer in amyloidosis. No localization or retention of labelled SAP occurs in healthy subjects or in patients with diseases other than amyloidosis (Fig. 1(a)). Radio-iodinated SAP has a short half-life (24 h) in the plasma and is rapidly catabolized with complete excretion of the iodinated breakdown products in the urine. However, in patients with amyloidosis, the tracer rapidly and specifically localizes to the deposits, in proportion to the quantity of amyloid present, and persists there without breakdown or modification (Fig. 1(b,c)). For clinical purposes, highly purified SAP is isolated from the plasma of single accredited donors and is oxidatively iodinated under conditions that preserve its function intact. The medium-energy, short half-life, pure gamma emitter ^{123}I is used for scintigraphic imaging, and the long half-life isotope ^{125}I is used for metabolic studies. The doses of radioactivity administered (less than 4 mSv) are well within accepted safety limits. More than 1000 studies have been completed without any adverse effects in more than 400 patients and 120 controls. In addition to high resolution scintigraphs, the uptake of tracer into various organs can be precisely quantified and, together with highly reproducible metabolic data on the plasma clearance and whole body retention of activity, the progression or regression of amyloid can be monitored serially and quantitatively.

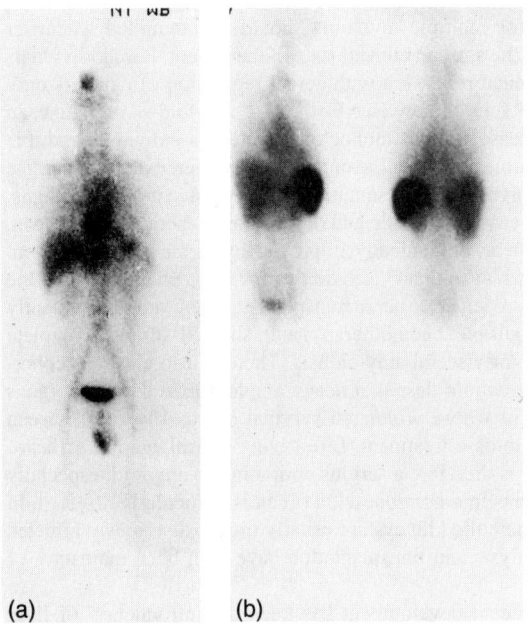 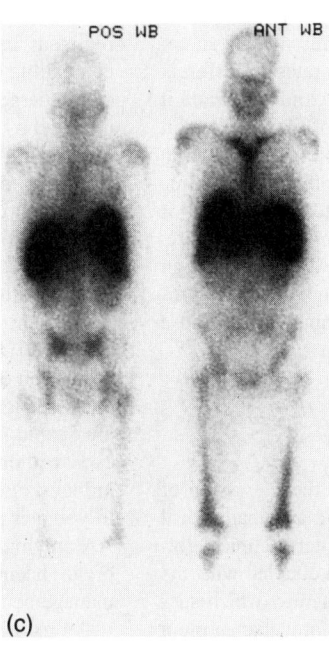

(a)   (b)   (c)

Fig. 1 Whole body scintigraphs 24 h after intravenous injection of ^{123}I-labelled human SAP. (a) Anterior view of normal control subject showing distribution of residual tracer in the blood pool and radioactive breakdown products in urine in the bladder; note the absence of localization or retention of tracer anywhere in the body. (b) Posterior (left) and anterior (right) views of patient with juvenile chronic arthritis complicated by AA amyloidosis. There is uptake of tracer in the spleen, kidneys, and adrenal glands, a typical distribution of AA amyloid in which the spleen is involved in 100 per cent of cases, kidneys in 75 per cent, and adrenals in 40 per cent. Note the reduced blood pool and bladder signal compared to (a). This patient, whose amyloid was diagnosed by renal biopsy 15 years ago when nephrotic syndrome developed, and who was then treated with chlorambucil, had been in complete remission for 10 years during which there had been no acute phase response. At the time of this scan there was no biochemical abnormality in blood or urine, despite the very appreciable amyloid deposits, illustrating the discordance between presence of amyloid and clinical effects. (c) Posterior (left) and anterior (right) views of patient with monoclonal gammopathy complicated by extensive AL amyloidosis. There is uptake and retention of tracer in the liver, spleen, kidneys, bone marrow, and soft tissues around the shoulder. This scintigraphic pattern of amyloid distribution revealed is pathognomonic for AL amyloidosis; bone marrow uptake has not been seen in any other type. Note the complete absence of blood pool or bladder signal resulting from complete uptake of the tracer dose into the substantial amyloid deposits.

Study no.	1	2	3	4

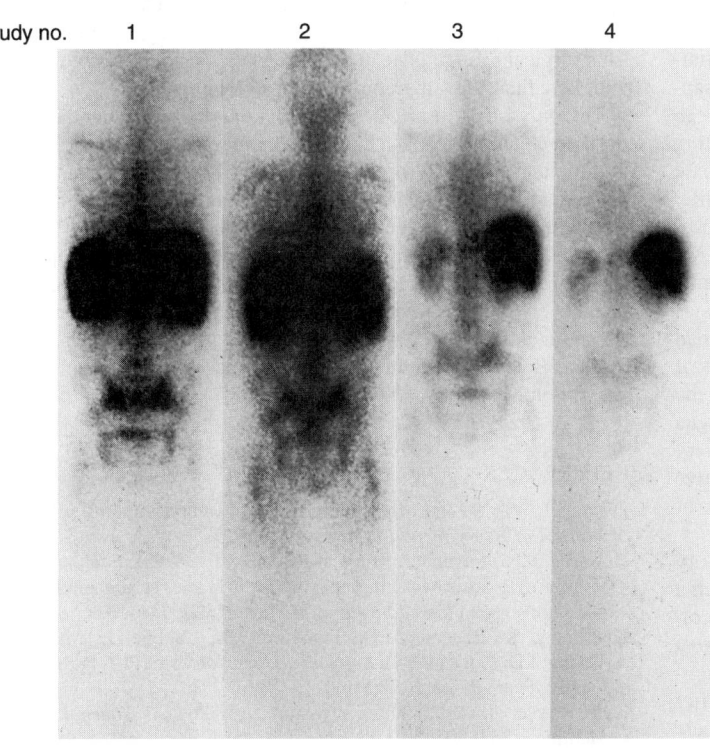

Date	November 1989	April 1990	June 1990	January 1991
		6	8	14

Fig. 2 Serial posterior whole body ^{123}I-SAP scintigraphs of a man with AL amyloidosis complicating benign monoclonal gammopathy. At presentation, scan 1, there was uptake in the spleen, liver, and bone marrow, obscuring any possible renal signal. Chemotherapy was given before the second scan, which shows increased spleen uptake, reduced liver uptake, and some renal uptake, but no change in total amyloid load determined by measurements of the clearance and retention of the tracer (not shown). Subsequently he suffered from recurrent splenic infarction and splenectomy was performed. Thereafter, in scan 3, there was increased tracer uptake in liver although a notably lower total amyloid load. Six months later, in scan 4, liver and kidney uptake, plasma clearance and whole body retention of tracer were all reduced, indicating regression of amyloid. Clinically he was much improved and still remains well.

Important observations regarding amyloid (which have been made for the first time *in vivo*) include the following: the different distribution of amyloid in different forms of the disease; amyloid in anatomic sites not available for biopsy (adrenals, spleen); major systemic deposits in forms of amyloid previously thought to be organ-limited; a poor correlation between the quantity of amyloid present in a given organ and the level of organ dysfunction; a non-homogeneous distribution of amyloid within individual organs; and evidence for rapid progression and sometimes regression of amyloid deposits with different rates in different organs (Fig. 2). Examples of major regression of amyloidosis, when it has been possible to reduce or eliminate the supply of fibril precursor, are very encouraging. Labelled SAP makes a valuable contribution to the diagnosis and management of patients with systemic amyloidosis, and although it is still a specialized tool of restricted availability, it should become more accessible and widely used in the near future. Encouragingly, it has lately been possible to label SAP with $^{99}Tc^m$, an inexpensive and universally available gamma emitting isotope, to produce a tracer which gives images of quality comparable to those obtained with radioiodine.

Management of amyloidosis

No treatment exists as yet which specifically causes the regression of amyloid deposits, and the prognosis of both systemic and many local forms of amyloidosis remains grave. However, long-term clinical follow-up studies of several different forms of amyloid coupled with the results of serial labelled SAP studies, indicate that therapy which succeeds in cutting off the supply of the amyloid fibril precursor protein results in major regression of existing deposits in some cases. This has now been documented in AA, AL, and β_2-microglobulin amyloidosis, and in familial amyloid polyneuropathy due to the Met30 variant.

It has long been known that eradication of chronic infection in patients with secondary AA amyloidosis was sometimes followed by recovery of normal function in organs, such as the kidney, previously damaged by amyloid. Apparent regression of AL amyloid with reduction in organomegaly and improved function has also been documented in individuals with monoclonal gammopathy whose B cell or plasma cell clones responded well to cytotoxic drug therapy. However, recent studies with labelled SAP have shown actual diminution and even disappearance of visceral amyloidosis of both AA and AL type. This has been clearest with chlorambucil treatment in AA amyloidosis complicating juvenile rheumatoid arthritis (Still's disease). Although this cytotoxic drug causes infertility and may increase risks of malignancy in later life, it effectively controls inflammation and suppresses the acute phase production of serum amyloid A, reduces proteinuria caused by renal AA amyloid, and may greatly improve survival. SAP scans demonstrate major reduction in amyloid load in many such patients over periods as short as 12 to 30 months, although in some individuals the amyloid load just remains static instead of increasing (see Fig. 1(b)). Indeed one of the most telling findings to emerge from use of labelled SAP is the discrepancy between quantity of amyloid present and the resulting organ dysfunction. Measurement of 'target' organ function is therefore a very poor index of the amount of amyloid and a correspondingly ineffective means of monitoring treatment aimed at promoting resolution of amyloid.

Familial Mediterranean fever is a unique example of an inflammatory disease of unknown aetiology complicated by AA amyloid for which a specific and effective treatment exists. Uninterrupted prophylactic colchicine prevents the symptoms of familial Mediterranean fever in most patients, and in all, even those whose symptoms persist despite compliance, it prevents development of amyloidosis. Furthermore, even after appearance of amyloid, colchicine, probably by suppressing the acute phase response of SAA, has beneficial effects. Colchicine has also been given to patients with most other forms of amyloid, although there is little or no rational basis for this. No appreciable benefit has been reported except in a few cases of AA disease secondary to chronic rheumatic inflammation. However, given that colchicine does suppress the acute phase response in experimental animals there are grounds for further investigation of its value in AA amyloidosis in general.

In AL amyloid the aim of treatment is to suppress the abnormal clone and this is usually difficult to achieve or to sustain. However, the drug regimens used for multiple myeloma should be attempted whenever compatible with the age and clinical state of the patient. Rare individuals can undergo clinical remission with actual regression of deposits documented by SAP scintigraphy (see Fig. 2). AL amyloid is, of course, an idiosyncratic disease, as each monoclonal protein is individual and it is therefore impossible to predict the outcome. However, extensive cardiac and/or renal involvement at presentation are very grave prognostic signs. Although the disease is systemic and deposits are generally widespread, the outcome can be dramatically improved by organ transplantation. This permits survival so that cytotoxic therapy has a chance to act. One AL patient who received a heart transplant 9 years ago subsequently responded to multiple chemotherapy and showed almost complete regression of major visceral amyloidosis. There is also clearly a cohort of AL patients in whom despite a heavy amyloid load the vital organs are spared, and in whom prolonged survival (10 to 15 years) is seen even without cytotoxic treatment. Life-saving transplantation of heart, kidneys, or liver is therefore a serious option in AL amyloid, especially in younger patients in whom one vital organ is particularly affected. In AA amyloid, where the kidneys are usually the most seriously affected organ, haemodialysis and transplantation have long been mainstays of management.

An exciting recent development has been the introduction of liver transplantation as treatment for familial amyloid polyneuropathy caused by transthyretin gene mutations. Although transthyretin is produced in the choroid plexus as well as the liver, liver transplantation leads to rapid and complete disappearance of the variant transthyretin from the plasma. Furthermore, the usual inexorable progression of the disease has been halted in all liver transplant recipients and most have shown some improvement, especially in symptoms related to autonomic neuropathy. In those with significant visceral amyloidosis, demonstrable by SAP scintigraphy, there has also been marked regression of amyloid. This surgical form of gene therapy thus holds much promise for patients with hereditary transthyretin-related amyloidosis.

The only other form of amyloidosis in which the abundance of the fibril precursor protein can be sharply reduced is β_2-microglobulin amyloidosis in haemodialysis patients. Successful renal transplantation lowers β_2-microglobulin plasma concentrations immediately and is associated with rapid improvement of osteoarticular symptoms. Preliminary observations suggest that the β_2-microglobulin amyloid deposits can also regress. Unfortunately, however, in the vast majority of dialysis patients in whom β_2-microglobulin has accumulated, there are medical, social, or political reasons which deny them transplantation. Attempts to clear β_2-microglobulin effectively by haemodiafiltration or *ex vivo* absorption have not yet been successful.

REFERENCES

Duchen, L.W. (1992). Current status review: cerebral amyloid. *International Journal of Experimental Pathology*, **73**, 535–50.

Hawkins, P.N., Lavender, J.P., and Pepys, M.B. (1990). Evaluation of systemic amyloidosis by scintigraphy with ^{123}I-labeled serum amyloid P component. *New England Journal of Medicine*, **323**, 508–13.

Kisilevsky, R. Benson, M.D., Frangione, B., Gauldie, J., Muckle, T.J., Young, I.D. (eds). (1994). *Amyloid and amyloidosis 1993*. Parthenon Publishing, Pearl River, New York.

Kyle, R.A. et al. (1992) Minisymposium: Amyloidosis. *Journal of Internal Medicine*, **232**, 507–34.

Natvig, J.B., Førre, Ø., Husby, G., Husebekk, A., Skogen, B., Sletten, K. and Westermark, P. (eds) (1990). *Amyloid and amyloidosis 1990*. Kluwer Academic Publishers, Dordrecht.

11.13.2 Recurrent polyserositis (familial Mediterranean fever, periodic disease)

M. ELIAKIM

Recurrent polyserositis is a genetic disorder characterized by bouts of abdominal pain and fever. Pleurisy and arthritis, affecting one or more joints, occur in more than half the cases. The disease exhibits a preference for Jews of any ethnic group. It is frequently familial and is inherited by Arabs, Armenians, and Turks but may affect subjects recessive autosomal transmission. Prognosis is generally good, but some patients develop amyloidosis with nephropathy which is usually fatal.

HISTORY

The first thorough description of recurrent polyserositis was provided by Siegal in 1945. Rachmilewitz and Ehrenfeld described the first cases in Israel in 1946. In 1948, Reimann, Cattan, and Mamou published additional cases under the designation 'periodic disease'. In 1952, Mamou identified the renal lesion as amyloidosis. Extensive studies on various aspects of the disease were reported later by Heller and his co-workers. The effect of colchicine on the symptoms was reported independently by Goldfinder in 1972 and Eliakim and Licht in 1973. Large series of patients have been published from Israel, France, the United States, and Russia.

NOMENCLATURE

The nomenclature of recurrent polyserositis is subject to controversy. The term 'familial Mediterranean fever' has been used widely, although it fails to convey the recurrent character of the disorder and the symptoms due to serosal inflammation. The disease is not limited to the Mediterranean region any more than are thalassaemia and brucellosis, the latter also known as Mediterranean fever. The term 'familial' is inadequate, since many other hereditary disorders with familial clustering are not referred to as 'familial'. Periodic disease implies recurrence at regular intervals and a close relationship to other periodic disorders. In fact, the paroxysms of recurrent polyserositis occur usually at irregular intervals. The term 'recurrent polyserositis' is preferable and will be employed herein, because it seems to convey most closely the main characteristics of the disease.

RACIAL AND ETHNIC DISTRIBUTION

Recurrent polyserositis occurs predominantly in Jews, Armenians, Arabs, and Turks. However, it has been reported in subjects of many other nationalities and races. More than 90 per cent of the Jewish patients are of either Sephardic or Iraqi origin. Sephardic Jews are those whose ancestors left Spain in the fifteenth century and were dispersed over various North African, Middle Eastern, and South American countries, while Iraqi Jews are descendants of the Babylonian Jews exiled to Mesopotamia about 2600 years ago. Most of the Sephardic patients originate from North African countries.

MODE OF INHERITANCE

Recurrent polyserositis is inherited by recessive autosomal transmission. The incidence of multiple familial occurrence varies between 20 and 40 per cent in families reported in different series. The disease usually occurs in several members of one generation. The actual incidence in families with healthy parents has been reported to be 18 per cent, and that in families with one affected parent, 36 per cent. With full penetrance, the expected figures would have to be 25 and 50 per cent respectively. The lower figures observed can be explained by incomplete pen-

etrance of the gene, or alternatively, by later appearance of the disease in some of the children. The disease is slightly more prevalent in males (1.7 to 1.0). The male predominance has not been explained adequately, but may be accounted for by the milder form of disease leading to undiagnosed cases in females. Partial penetrance in females is an alternative explanation. The frequency of the gene in Sephardic and Iraqi Jews has been calculated to be 1 in 45 and the homozygous incidence 1 in 2000. The respective figures for the Armenian population in Lebanon are 1 in 32 and 1 in 1000. The HLA system has been studied in a smaller number of subjects but no associations have been found. Recently, the gene that causes recurrent polyserositis in non-Ashkenazi Jews has been located in the short arm of chromosome 16.

PATHOLOGY

The underlying pathological lesion in recurrent polyserositis is hyperaemia and an acute non-bacterial inflammatory reaction, affecting mainly the serous membranes. Adhesions, when present, are thin and mechanical ileus is extremely rare. Microscopically, the picture is that of non-specific inflammation. The most striking finding is marked hyperaemia and a cellular infiltrate consisting of varying proportions of neutrophils, lymphocytes, monocytes, and, sometimes, plasma cells and eosinophils. The picture is different from the ordinary inflammation observed in appendicitis and cholecystitis in that it is not as purulent. The reaction seems to originate in the serosa and may not reach the mucosa. The inflammatory exudate concentrates around the venules and arterioles, some of which have thickened walls. In the synovia, pannus formation and extensive intra-articular damage may occur. Ultrastructural studies of synovial biopsies have shown that the most prominent vascular change is thickening of the basement membrane, which is organized in many concentric, closely arranged layers, separated by a less dense ground substance (Fig. 1). It has been suggested that reduplication of the basement membrane is due to repeated episodes of cell death and regeneration, each lamina representing the residue of one cell generation.

Fig. 1 Electron microscopic picture of a synovial blood vessel with a pericyte (P) and cell processes in between the many basement membrane layers. (Reproduced from Eliakim, M. *et al.* (1981). *Recurrent polyserositis (familial Mediterranean fever, periodic disease)*. Elsevier/North Holland Biomedical Press., Amsterdam, by permission.)

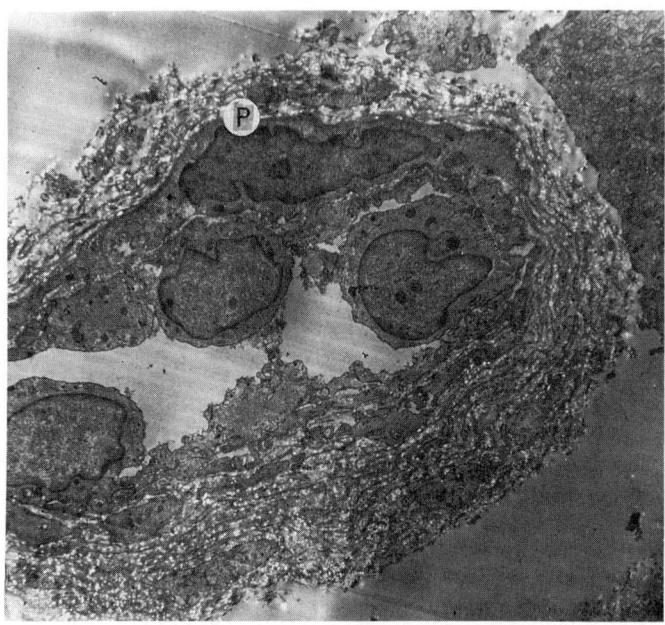

AETIOLOGY AND PATHOGENESIS

The aetiology of recurrent polyserositis is unknown. The blood vessels seem to be the primary target organ of the disease process. This is indicated by the ultrastructural changes in the vessels, as well as by the systemic manifestations of the disease, the fleeting character of the symptoms, the appearance of transient haematuria, electrocardiographic and electroencephalographic abnormalities, and the occasional development of permanent vascular damage. The pathogenesis of the vascular lesion is, however, obscure. Most authors tend to relate recurrent polyserositis to the 'collagen' disorders. The similarity between the former and systemic lupus erythematosus is sometimes striking. The incidence of atopic allergy, rheumatic fever, glomerulonephritis. Schönlein–Henoch purpura, and periarteritis nodosa is higher in recurrent polyserositis than in the general population. High serum immunoglobulin levels, circulating immune complexes, and lymphocytotoxins have been demonstrated in patients suffering from the disease. Results of additional immunological studies are still controversial. Although the pathogenesis of recurrent polyserositis is not clear, several facts seem to be established: the genetic nature of the disease, the involvement of the vascular system, and the presence of immunological disturbances.

Recently, it has been suggested that C5a-inhibitor deficiency in joint and peritoneal fluids from patients with recurrent polyserositis may have a role in the pathogenesis of the attacks. This inhibitor antagonizes the chemotactic activity of C5a and its deficiency may result in severe inflammatory attacks following the accidental release of C5a.

CLINICAL MANIFESTATIONS

The symptoms start in the first decade of life in about 50 per cent of the cases and before the age of 20 years in at least 80 per cent. Only 1 per cent of the patients may manifest the first symptoms after the age of 40 years, a fact of importance in the differential diagnosis. Almost all patients have attacks of abdominal pain, often originating in one area, but spreading over the whole abdomen within a few hours. The temperature rises to 38 to 40 °C with tachycardia, and about one-quarter of the patients report a chill. The attack usually reaches its peak in 12 h. The clinical picture is that of acute peritonitis, manifested by exquisite abdominal tenderness, involuntary rigidity, rebound tenderness, and diminished peristalsis. Constipation is the rule and vomiting is frequent. The patients frequently flex their thighs and lie motionless to relieve the pain. Surprisingly, however, instead of developing into classical peritonitis which terminates in shock and death, the crisis resolves spontaneously and is usually over within 24 to 48 h. The temperature returns to normal after a variable period of 12 h to 3 days and the pain subsides gradually. The attacks recur, usually at irregular periods of several days to several months. Spontaneous remissions may last years. The severity of the pain varies from mild discomfort to that in severe generalized peritonitis. Mild attacks may be afebrile. In pregnant women, the attacks usually abate spontaneously after the second trimester. After the first attacks, many patients avoid visits to the emergency wards because they fear aggressive treatment. In fact, they learn to caution their physicians against performing unnecessary surgery and request symptomatic relief of pain.

Pleurisy

More than 50 per cent have chest pain due to pleurisy. Pain in the chest is sharp and stabbing, localized in the lower part, more frequently on the right than on the left, and radiating to the abdomen and the shoulders. Patients with stethalgia splint their respiratory excursions, deeper breath sounds causing much pain. Suppression of breath sounds over the affected side is usual but pleural friction is exceptional. A small effusion is occasionally detected in the costophrenic angle.

Arthritis

Arthritis is another common manifestation of the disease, its incidence varying between 24 and 84 per cent in various reported series (mean 55

per cent). Sephardic Jews seem to be affected more frequently than patients of other ethnic origins. Several clinical forms have been identified. Rheumatic fever is more common in patients with recurrent polyserositis and has to be differentiated from the clinical forms typical of the disease. Most patients manifest an asymmetric, non-destructive mono- or oligoarthritis affecting the large joints. The knees and ankles are affected about three times more often than the hips, shoulders, feet, and wrists. Involvement of small joints is very rare. The affected joint becomes painful and swollen but local redness and heat are not pronounced and may be absent. The synovial fluid is usually turbid but it forms a good mucin clot. The white count ranges between 15 000 and 30 000 polymorphonuclears per mm³ and the fluid is always sterile. The symptoms intensify during the first 24 to 48 h but may last as long as a week. Usually, one, or mostly two, large joints are affected at a time. However, when the attacks are frequent, involvement of one joint may start before the symptoms from the previous joint have subsided, and the impression of migratory arthritis is created. The clue to the differential diagnosis may lie in the temperature curve, which shows high peaks lasting 1 to 3 days. In about 5 per cent of the cases, the acute attack fails to resolve and the symptoms may persist several weeks or even months before they abate with no residual damage. About 2 per cent of the patients develop a chronic destructive mono- or oligoarthritis affecting most frequently the hip or the knee. Permanent organic damage results from one protracted attack or from repeated short attacks. Marked X abnormalities shown by radiography and functional disability may result and surgical treatment may be necessary. Recently, sacroiliitis, frequently asymptomatic, has been described in a considerable number of patients. The radiographic changes include loss of cortical definition, sclerosis with or without bone erosion, and fusion of the joints.

Skin rash

Skin rash occurs in 10 to 20 per cent of the cases. The typical lesion resembles erysipelas, which appears invariably over the extensor surfaces of the legs below he knees, over the ankle joints, or the dorsum of the foot. The skin becomes bright-red, hot, swollen, and painful. The rash is usually unilateral and its border may or may not be sharply defined. It resembles cellulitis and frequently prompts initiation of antibiotic therapy. Fever and arthralgia or arthritis are frequently present. The symptoms intensify rapidly and then fade within 2 to 3 days without any therapy. On biopsy the epidermis shows mild acanthosis and hyperkeratosis, while the dermis contains an inflammatory exudate consisting of polymorphonuclear cells, lymphocytes, and some histiocytes concentrated mainly around the blood vessels. Nodular rashes, Schönlein–Henoch purpura, and urticaria are also encountered.

OTHER MANIFESTATIONS

Attacks of pericarditis appear occasionally and severe headache may occur during attacks. Transient electrocardiographic signs of myopericarditis and non-specific electroencephalographic abnormalities have been observed during paroxysms. Severe myalgia has been reported and muscle atrophy adjacent to affected joints is not infrequent. Numerous attacks in children may lead to growth retardation. Colloid bodies are often found in the eye grounds and the spleen is palpable in more than one-third of the patients.

LABORATORY INVESTIGATIONS

There are no specific laboratory criteria for the diagnosis of recurrent polyserositis. The urine may show transient microscopic haematuria during attacks. Persistent albuminuria is due to renal amyloidosis or, more rarely, glomerulonephritis. The white blood count usually rises to 12 000 to 18 000 per mm³ during attacks and the differential count remains normal or shows mild neutrophilia. Persistent leucocytosis is frequent in the presence of amyloidosis. The red cell count is normal but mild anaemia may occur. The erythrocyte sedimentation rate, rises during attacks, usually to between 40 and 60 mm after 1 h and the plasma fibrinogen level to more than 5 g/l. Other serum protein changes include inversion of the albumin–globulin ratio, a rise in alpha-2 and, less consistently, gammaglobulin and a rise in IgG, IgA, and IgM. Liver function tests are normal, although a mild and transient hyperbilirubinaemia has been reported. Bacteriological and serological examinations of blood, throat, urine, stool, peritoneal and joint exudates reveal no abnormal findings. The Rose–Waaler and latex globulin fixation tests are negative, and antinuclear factor and lupus erythematosus cells are not found.

AMYLOIDOSIS

This is the most important complication of recurrent polyserositis and its incidence varies between 0 and 27 per cent in various reported series. Amyloidosis occurs more frequently in Sephardic Jews and Turks and is rare in non-Sephardic Jews and Armenians. Patients who develop amyloidosis have a higher familial incidence, more frequent joint involvement, and skin rashes. The first sign of amyloidosis is massive albuminuria. Within several years, the clinical picture of complete nephrotic syndrome and advancing renal failure develops. Renal vein thrombosis is a frequent complication, signalled by a rapid decline of renal function. Unless treated, the patients will die within 3 to 13 years. Most patients are subjected to haemodialysis and renal transplantation. Rectal biopsy will confirm the diagnosis in 70 per cent of the cases. On autopsy, amyloid deposits are found in the kidneys, intestines, adrenals, heart, ovaries, pancreas, and muscles. In most organs the deposition is perivascular. Recently, the complete amino acid sequence of the amyloid has been identified as the A component characteristic of amyloidosis secondary to chronic-inflammatory diseases. A marked decrease in new cases of amyloidosis seems to have occurred since the advent of colchicine therapy. Genetic factors probably explain the greater incidence of amyloidosis in Sephardic Jews. In fact a form of familial amyloidosis occurs in this ethnic group in the absence of symptoms of recurrent polyserositis.

DIFFERENTIAL DIAGNOSIS

During the initial attacks, most patients are erroneously diagnosed as suffering from appendicitis or cholecystitis. Explorative laparotomy is performed so frequently as to constitute a characteristic anamnestic detail. It is important that cholecystitis, diverticulitis, pancreatitis, and perforation of peptic ulcer are unlikely to occur before the age of 30. Helpful hints in the differential diagnosis are the early fall of the temperature, the history of previous attacks, a positive family history, and the ethnic origin of the patient. A high plasma fibrinogen and a normal amylase are of additional help. Recurrent pleurisy may occasionally simulate pulmonary embolism. Joint attacks are frequently misdiagnosed as septic arthritis. The main feature of the arthritic attacks in recurrent polyserositis is their episodic occurrence, starting during childhood or adolescence. The temperature curve is typical, the leucocyte count in the synovial fluid rarely exceeds 30 000 per mm³, and the fluid is always sterile. The destructive form of arthritis may be mistaken for juvenile rheumatoid arthritis or tuberculous arthritis but the diagnosis should present no difficulties. The association of fever, arthritis, splenomegaly, and skin rashes may suggest the diagnosis of systemic lupus erythematosus. However, accepted criteria for this disease will not be met, in particular, the lupus erythematosus cell and antinuclear factor tests are always negative and the leucocyte count is usually high. In cases of doubt, a therapeutic trial with colchicine is indicated. Indeed, suppression of attacks is the only reliable diagnostic test.

TREATMENT

Since 1972, colchicine has been established as the only effective treatment of recurrent polyserositis. A daily dose of 1.0 to 1.5 mg will pre-

vent the attacks in 95 per cent of the cases. Short courses of colchicine taken at the onset of attacks have been reported to suppress the symptoms but continuous therapy is more reliable. The mechanism of the action of colchicine is not definitively established. Patients on colchicine manifest diminished polymorphonuclear chemotaxis both *in vitro* and *in vivo*. It seems, therefore, that a failure to amplify the inflammatory reaction and to generate a normal response to inflammation may account for the suppression of attacks. Chromosome studies have revealed no abnormalities after 4 years of treatment. Pregnancy is no longer considered a contraindication for continuing colchicine therapy. Caution should be exercised in the treatment of children.

PROGNOSIS

Most authors regard recurrent polyserositis as a relatively benign disease which does not affect the life expectancy of the patients, unless amyloidosis appears. Children are frequently physically underdeveloped because of the recurrent fever, nausea, and vomiting. Colchicine therapy seems to provide, for the first time, relief of much suffering for many patients, and opens a new horizon as a potential drug for the prevention of amyloidosis. The prognosis of patients with amyloidosis on chronic dialysis seems to be similar to that of patients with renal failure due to other causes.

REFERENCES

Eliakim, M., Levy, M., and Ehrenfeld, M. (1981). *Recurrent polyserositis (familial Mediterranean fever, periodic disease)*. Elsevier/North Holland Biomedical Press, Amsterdam.

Levy, M. and Eliakim, M. (1977). Long-term colchicine prophylaxis in familial Mediterranean fever. *British Medical Journal* **ii,** 808.

Mazner, Y. and Brzezinski, A. (1984). C5a-inhibitor deficiency in peritoneal-fluids from patients with familial mediterranean fever. *New England Journal Medicine.* **311,** 287–90.

Pras, E., *et al.* (1993). Mapping of a gene causing familial Mediterranean fever to the short arm of chromosome 16. *New England Journal of Medicine* **326,** 1509–13.

Reimann, H.A., (1963). *Periodic diseases*. Blackwell Scientific Publications, Oxford.

Schwabe, A.D. and Peters, R. (1974). Familial mediterranean fever in Armenians. Analysis of 100 cases. *Medicine* **53,** 453–62.

Siegal, S. (1964). Familial paroxysmal polyserositis. *American Journal of Medicine* **36,** 893–918.

Sohar, E., Gafni, J. and Heller, H. (1967). Familial Mediterranean fever. *American Journal of Medicine* **43,** 227–53.

11.13.3 The acute phase response and C-reactive protein

M. B. PEPYS

The acute phase response

Trauma, tissue necrosis, microbial infection, and acute exacerbations of inflammatory diseases induce a complex series of non-specific responses including fever, leucocytosis, catabolism of muscle proteins, and the greatly increased *de novo* synthesis and secretion, principally by the liver, of a number of plasma proteins. This latter phenomenon is known as the acute phase response and the major human acute phase proteins, the plasma levels of which increase significantly, are listed in Table 1. In contrast the concentrations of a few plasma proteins, of which albumin is the most notable, typically decrease (Table 1). The response persists in individuals with chronic infections or inflammatory disorders and in those with malignant neoplasia, especially when it is extensive

Table 1 *Plasma protein concentrations in the acute phase response*

	Increased	Decreased
Proteinase inhibitors	α_1-Antitrypsin α_1-Antichymotrypsin	Inter α-antitrypsin
Coagulation proteins	Fibrinogen Prothrombin Factor VIII Plasminogen	
Complement proteins	C1s C2, B C3, C4, C5 C56 C1 INH	Properdin
Transport proteins	Haptoglobin Haemopexin Caeruloplasmin	

Miscellaneous	C-reactive protein
	Serum amyloid A
	  protein
	Fibronectin
	α_1-Acid glycoprotein
	Gc globulin
		Albumin
		Transthyretin
		  (prealbumin)
		High-density
		lipoprotein
		Low-density
		lipoprotein

and metastatic. Indeed the acute phase response generally is sustained even with the most severe illness and, provided there is not complete hepatocellular failure, it is maintained until death. Together with the fact that all endothermic animals mount similar responses, this strongly suggests that it may have survival value. Increased availability of proteinase inhibitors, complement, clotting, and transport proteins presumably enhances host resistance, minimizes tissue injury, and promotes regeneration and repair. On the other hand, high levels of some acute phase proteins may be damaging, for example, sustained increased production of serum amyloid A protein (SAA) can lead to the deposition of AA-type amyloidosis, a serious and usually fatal condition.

Most acute phase proteins are synthesized by hepatocytes, in which their transcription is controlled by cytokines including interleukin 1 (IL-1), interleukin 6 (IL-6), tumour necrosis factor, and leucocyte inhibiting factor. The circulating concentrations of complement proteins and clotting factors increase by up to 50 to 100 per cent whereas some of the proteinase inhibitors and α_1-acid glycoprotein can increase three to five fold. C-reactive protein (CRP) and serum amyloid A protein are unique in that their concentrations can change by more than three orders of magnitude. Furthermore, in contrast to most other acute phase proteins for which there are wide variations in consumption, clearance and catabolic rates, the plasma half-life and fractional catabolic rate of C-reactive protein is constant under virtually all conditions. Its plasma level is therefore determined only by its synthesis rate which objectively reflects the presence, extent and activity of disease.

C-reactive protein

C-reactive protein belongs to the pentraxin family of proteins, the other member of which is serum amyloid P component, and consists of five identical non-glycosylated subunits, encoded by a single gene on chromosome 1. The monomers, each of molecular mass 23 027, are non-covalently associated in a very stable disc-like configuration with cyclic pentameric symmetry, which is notably resistant to proteolysis. In the presence of calcium, C-reactive protein undergoes specific ligand-binding to phosphocholine in autologous phospholipids and microbial polysaccharides. Complexed or aggregated C-reactive protein efficiently activates the classical complement pathway and can thereby opsonize

ligands for phagocytosis. C-reactive protein neutralizes the potent inflammatory mediator, platelet-activating factor (PAF) which contains phosphocholine and has down-regulatory effects on polymorph function. C-reactive protein may thus contribute to host defence, modulation of inflammation and lipid metabolism but, since no polymorphism or deficiency of C-reactive protein has yet been described, its functions *in vivo* are not definitely known.

The median normal circulating concentration of C-reactive protein is 0.8 mg/l and the interquartile range is 0.3 to 1.7 mg/l. Normal levels may be as low as 0.07 mg/l and among apparently healthy individuals 90 per cent have less than 3 mg/l and 99 per cent less than 10 mg/l. Higher values are abnormal and indicate the presence of organic disease.

C-reactive protein is synthesized exclusively in the liver and is secreted in increased amounts within about 6 h of an acute stimulus such as elective surgery or myocardial infarction. Thereafter the plasma level can double at least every 8 h, reaching a peak after about 50 h. With a sustained stimulus values as high as 500 mg/l are seen. After effective treatment or cessation of the stimulus the value can fall almost as rapidly as the 19-h plasma half-life of labelled exogenous C-reactive protein. However if the stimulus persists, so does the C-reactive protein response, and very high serum values can be maintained for prolonged periods.

Clinical applications of measurement of serum C-reactive protein

Introduction

The C-reactive protein response is non-specific and can therefore never be precisely diagnostic but there are important differential patterns in certain diseases (see below). Also, C-reactive protein production *per se* is not suppressed or modified by any drugs or other therapies currently in use, unless these affect the underlying pathological process which has provoked the acute phase reaction. The only condition that interferes with the 'normal' C-reactive protein response is severe hepatocellular impairment. C-reactive protein levels thus usually provide an objective index of the presence and activity of disease and of response to treatment. By virtue of its speed and extended dynamic range, the C-reactive protein response yields valuable information which, when interpreted at the bedside together with all other available clinical and laboratory results, can contribute significantly to management of a wide range of conditions.

Conditions associated with major elevation of serum C-reactive protein concentration

The conditions in Table 2 are associated with increased C-reactive protein production, usually reflecting closely the extent and activity of disease.

INFECTION

Most systemic microbial infections are associated with high levels of serum C-reactive protein and, although the peak values attained in different patients cover a wide range, serial assays in individual subjects usually show an excellent correlation between the serum C-reactive protein concentration, the severity of disease and its response to treatment (Table 3). Acute systemic Gram-positive and Gram-negative bacterial infections are among the most potent stimuli for C-reactive protein production. Systemic fungal infections occurring in immunodeficient hosts are also associated with high C-reactive protein values, whereas the levels in chronic bacterial infections such as tuberculosis and leprosy are usually rather lower, though nevertheless still markedly raised. Uncomplicated viral infections, particularly meningitis, may induce no or only a very modest response. Clinical infections with rhinoviruses,

Table 2 *C-reactive protein response in disease; conditions associated with major elevation of serum C-reactive protein concentration*

Infections	
Allergic complications of infections	Rheumatic fever
	Erythema nodosum leprosum
Inflammatory disease	Rheumatoid arthritis
	Juvenile chronic arthritis
	Ankylosing spondylitis
	Psoriatic arthritis
	Systemic vasculitis
	Polymyalgia rheumatica
	Reiter's disease
	Crohn's disease
	Familial Mediterranean fever
Allograft rejection	Renal transplantation
Malignant neoplasia	Lymphoma, Hodgkin's carcinoma, sarcoma
Necrosis	Myocardial infarction
	Tumour embolization
	Acute pancreatitis
Trauma	Surgery
	Burns
	Fractures

Table 3 *Measurement of serum C-reactive protein concentration in infectious disease*

Bacteraemia and septicaemia in children and adults
Bacteraemia and septicaemia in neonates
Bacterial and other infections in immunosuppressed patients
Deep fungal infections
Meningitis viral < tuberculosis < bacterial
Bacterial infections after major elective surgery or other invasive procedures
Infective relapse after abdominal surgery for sepsis
Peritonitis in patients on chronic ambulatory peritoneal dialysis
Acute appendicitis (differential diagnosis)
Evaluation of antibiotic therapy for female pelvic infection
Laryngotracheitis/pharyngitis/epiglottitis in children
Chorioamnionitis after premature rupture of membranes
Disseminated vs. localized gonococcal infection
Infection precipitating sickle-cell crisis

adenoviruses, or influenza are associated with minor C-reactive protein elevation in a proportion of individuals, though this may reflect secondary bacterial infection. However, systemic cytomegalovirus or Herpes simplex infections in immunosuppressed patients do cause major C-reactive protein responses. Little is known about the C-reactive protein response to metazoan parasitic infestation in otherwise healthy subjects but malaria, especially with *Plasmodium falciparum*, is associated with high C-reactive protein values as are pneumocystis and toxoplasma infections in immunodeficient patients.

Minor or localized low-grade infection may not stimulate C-reactive protein production appreciably but the major C-reactive protein response in acute, serious bacterial infection is almost invariable and is present at all ages from premature neonates to the elderly. It also occurs in patients who are immunosuppressed either by primary diseases such as leukaemia, lymphoma or other malignancy, AIDS, or by treatment with cytotoxic drugs, corticosteroids, or irradiation. This is of particular importance in the very young, in the old, in compromised hosts, and in any other types of patients in whom the usual clinical signs and symptoms of infection, including fever and neutrophil leucocytosis, may be masked or lacking (Fig. 1). Furthermore, at the onset of bacterial infec-

tion, especially in patients who are otherwise well following elective surgery or myocardial infarction, the C-reactive protein response frequently precedes clinical symptoms, including fever, by up to 24 to 48 h.

Once infection is diagnosed or suspected and antimicrobial treatment has been commenced, frequent monitoring of the serum C-reactive protein concentration provides an objective means of assessing the response which is often not available in any other way. Appropriate and effective therapy is associated with a rapid exponential fall in C-reactive protein level, with a half-life of around 24 h; occurrence of this pattern is an encouraging prognostic sign (Fig. 2). Normalization of the C-reactive protein usually corresponds to clinical cure of the infection and may thus be used to determine the necessary duration of antimicrobial therapy. On the other hand, especially in neutropenic or immunodeficient patients, persistent elevation of C-reactive protein at the end of a course of antibiotics often presages relapse or recurrence of infection.

When bacterial infection is complicated by abscess formation or for any other reason is less readily eradicated by antimicrobial drugs, the serum C-reactive protein concentration may remain elevated or may fall linearly rather than exponentially during treatment. Such a pattern should raise questions regarding dosage of the drugs, sensitivity of the organism and/or stimulate a diagnostic search both for localized pus and for other underlying non-infective pathology such as malignancy. Indeed, in the absence of one of the chronic idiopathic inflammatory conditions that are known to be associated with high C-reactive protein

Fig. 1 A 69-year-old diabetic man was admitted with a 3-day history of confusion, cough, and incontinence of urine. There was clinical and radiological evidence of a left-sided pneumonia and although both the temperature and white cell count remained normal, the serum C-reactive protein was high (119 mg/l), confirming the suspicion of infection. Following treatment with amoxycillin 250 mg thrice daily the C-reactive protein level fell rapidly, in a characteristic exponential manner, and he made a speedy recovery with return of continence and improved mental state.

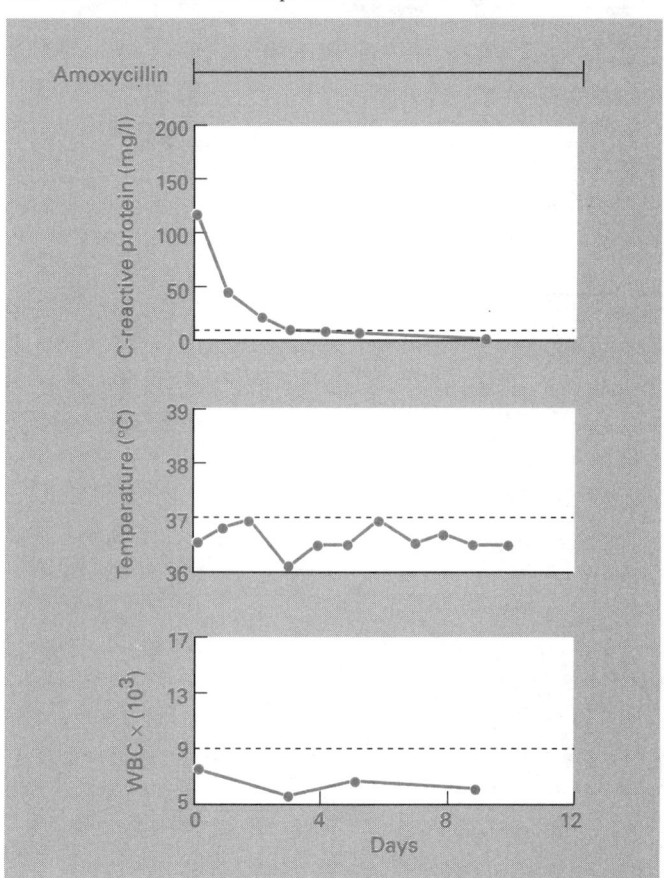

levels (see below), the persistence of a raised serum C-reactive protein concentration is usually a grave prognostic sign, indicating the presence of either uncontrolled infection and/or other serious pathology. However, with alteration in antimicrobial drug regimen or the evacuation of pus or elimination of other pathology, the rapid fall in C-reactive protein which may then be observed is an encouraging objective sign of clinical improvement (see Fig. 2).

In bacterial meningitis the serum C-reactive protein levels at presentation are much higher than in aseptic or proven viral meningitis, in which C-reactive protein concentrations are within the normal range or only very slightly raised. Intermediate C-reactive protein values are seen in tuberculous meningitis.

INFLAMMATORY DISEASE

Most of the chronic inflammatory diseases of unknown aetiology (see Table 2), with the notable exceptions described below (Table 4), are associated with high C-reactive protein values when they are active or in relapse. Serial measurements of C-reactive protein in individuals with any of these diseases generally reflect the extent and activity of their condition as determined by clinical examination and other laboratory

Fig. 2 An 86-year-old woman had been refusing food and drink for 6 weeks. She was dehydrated but rehydration in hospital failed to improve her mental state. She was paranoid and refused nursing and medical care. Paraphrenia was diagnosed and deterioration continued. A C-reactive protein of 130 mg/l and a white cell count of 13.5×10^9/l were then found. Chest radiograph, normal on admission, now showed a cavitating lesion from which 150 ml of pus was aspirated. Intravenous ampicillin reduced neither the C-reactive protein nor white cell count prompting a change of therapy to gentamicin and metronidazole. *Strep. equinus* was finally identified in the pus and treatment was changed to benzylpenicillin alone. The C-reactive protein then fell exponentially but rather slowly. The patient's clinical and mental state gradually improved and she was eventually discharged.

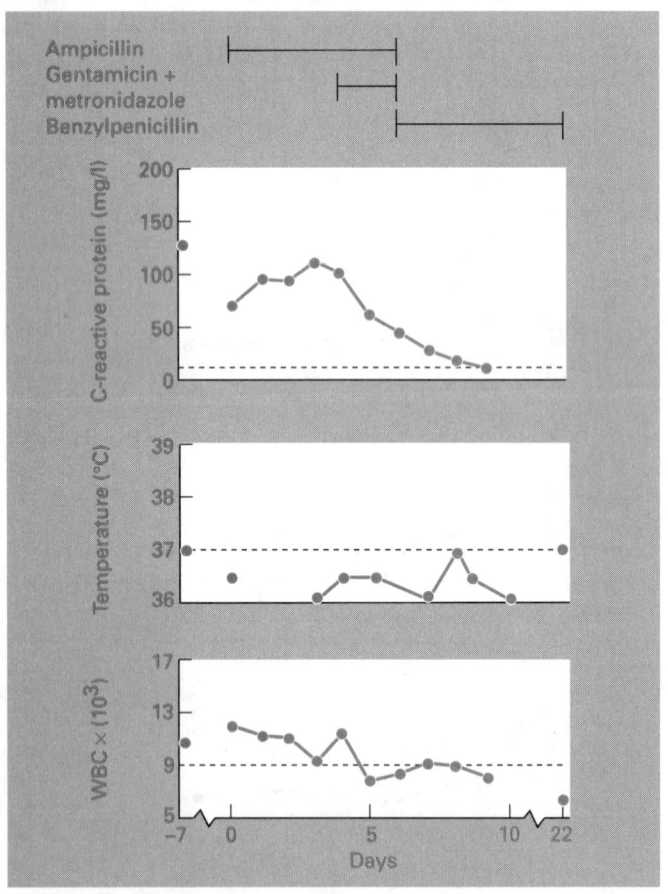

Table 4 *C-reactive protein response in disease; conditions associated with minor elevation of serum C-reactive protein concentration*

Systemic lupus erythematosus
Systemic sclerosis
Dermatomyositis
Ulcerative colitis
Leukaemia
Graft-versus-host disease (GVHD)

tests. As the pathology in many of these patients, (for example with systemic vasculitis or Crohn's disease) is relatively inaccessible to direct examination, the serum C-reactive protein value provides the best available objective index of disease activity (Fig. 3). Furthermore, the presence or absence of a C-reactive protein response can distinguish between symptoms or organ dysfunction which are due to currently active inflammatory activity or just to the consequences of fibrosis and scarring from previous episodes. This can be of great importance when treatment involves the use of steroids and other powerful and hazardous immunosuppressive, cytotoxic, and anti-inflammatory drugs. It permits precise titration of dosages required and may help to avoid excessive or unnecessary use.

Induction of clinical remission and control of the underlying disease process is associated with prompt normalization of the C-reactive protein. However, C-reactive protein also becomes abnormal with intercurrent infection, a common complication of some of these disorders and their treatments, and this serves to focus diagnostic attention often before the infection has become too severe or even before it is clinically evident. Monitoring the C-reactive protein response to antimicrobial therapy can then help to confirm the diagnosis and the efficacy of therapy. Persistent elevation of the C-reactive protein after eradication of infection may indicate relapse of the underlying inflammatory disease, requiring additional anti-inflammatory treatment.

ALLOGRAFT REJECTION

Rejection episodes following renal allografting, whether from living or cadaver donors, are almost invariably associated with increased production of C-reactive protein. Regular monitoring of serum C-reactive protein levels from the immediate postoperative period can therefore assist in appropriate management, provided that the possibility that intercurrent causes of an acute phase response, particularly infection, are borne in mind. Failure of the C-reactive protein response to the surgical trauma of grafting to subside in the usual way indicates the possibility of early acute rejection. Following return of the serum C-reactive protein concentration to normal postoperatively, a second rise may antedate any other clinical or laboratory evidence of rejection by 1 to 2 days. Successful antirejection therapy is associated with return of the C-reactive protein to normal, whereas persistence even of a modest elevation of C-reactive protein concentration may suggest on-going chronic rejection and may be abolished only by graftectomy. These interpretations of the C-reactive protein response can only be attempted in the light of full clinical information especially regarding the possible presence of intercurrent infection.

MALIGNANCY

Most malignant tumours, especially when they are extensive and metastatic, induce an acute phase response. This is particularly so with those neoplasms which cause systemic symptoms such as fever and weight loss, for example, Hodgkin's disease (stage B) and renal carcinoma, but raised C-reactive protein levels are seen with many others. In some studies, notably of prostatic carcinoma and bladder carcinoma, the C-reactive protein level at presentation has been found to correlate with the overall tumour load and also with the prognosis, being higher for a given mass of tumour in those patients who subsequently fare worse. The C-reactive protein may also correlate better with progress and regression of tumour than other more specific tumour markers. However, given the non-specific nature of the acute phase response and the limited number of studies performed so far, a definite role for C-reactive protein measurements in the management of cancer patients, other than in cases of intercurrent infection, has not yet been established.

NECROSIS

Myocardial infarction

Myocardial infarction is invariably associated with a major C-reactive protein response, as is elective embolization leading to necrosis of tumours in the liver and elsewhere. The peak level of C-reactive protein occurs about 50 h after the onset of pain in myocardial infarction and correlates closely with the peak serum level of the cardiac isoenzyme creatine kinase MB. In patients who recover uneventfully, the C-reactive protein falls rapidly towards normal in the usual exponential fashion. However, complications such as persistent dysrhythmias, heart failure, further infarction, aneurysm formation, intercurrent infection, thromboembolism, or postinfarction syndrome, are associated with either persistently raised C-reactive protein levels or secondary elevation after the initial decrease. Patients with unstable angina who present with a normal C-reactive protein value generally settle on medical treatment but those

Fig. 3 A 26-year-old man with pancolonic Crohn's disease. He was admitted with severe exacerbation; temperature 38°C; pulse, 110 beats/min; 16 stools per day; haematocrit, 41.5 per cent, leucocytes 13.8 × 10⁹/l. Rectal mucosa severely inflamed with histiocytic granulomata on biopsy. Rapid improvement with oral and rectal prednisolone, ampicillin, and metronidazole, with complete clinical and histological remission on day 11. Relapse 5 months later responded promptly to a short course of oral and rectal prednisolone. C-reactive protein and ESR were both high during the initial exacerbation. The rapid response to treatment was paralleled by a prompt fall in C-reactive protein, whereas the ESR responded more slowly. Despite clinical remission and a normal ESR, the C-reactive protein remained slightly elevated suggesting persistent low-grade inflammatory activity, and it rose further during a subsequent relapse when the ESR did not change. (Reproduced from Fagan, E. A., *et al.* (1982). Serum levels of C-reactive protein in Crohn's disease and ulcerative colitis. *European Journal of Clinical Investigation* **12**, 351–9, with permission.)

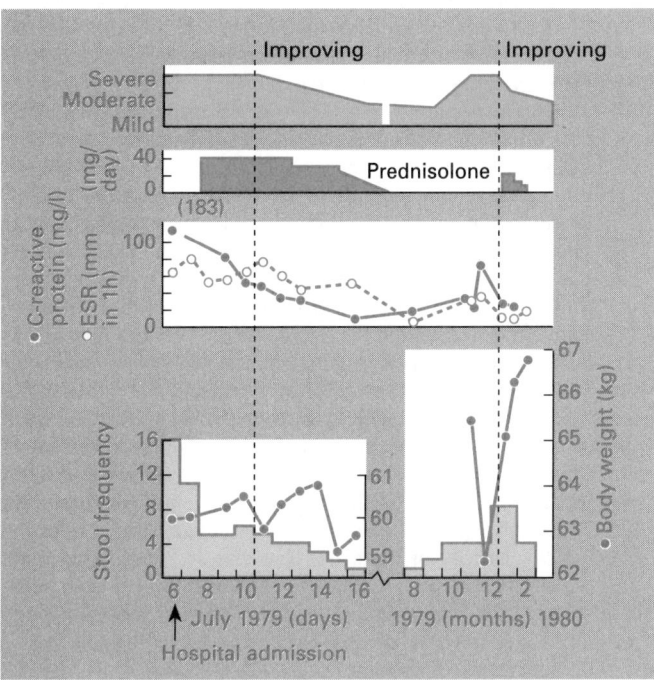

with raised levels mostly proceed to infarction or require urgent angioplasty or bypass surgery. Stable angina without infarction and invasive investigation, such as coronary arteriography, do not stimulate C-reactive protein production, whereas some other causes of chest pain such as pulmonary embolism, pleurisy, or pericarditis are usually associated with raised C-reactive protein levels. Routine assays of C-reactive protein after infarction or in patients with chest pain may thus assist in diagnosis, in prognosis, and in the recognition and management of complications, including iatrogenic infection associated with invasive cardiovascular monitoring.

Serum C-reactive protein levels closely reflect the severity and progress of acute pancreatitis, providing a better guide to intra-abdominal events than other markers such as leucocyte counts, erythrocyte sedimentation rate, temperature, and the plasma concentrations of antiproteinases. A C-reactive protein concentration greater than 100 mg/l at the end of the first week of illness is associated with a more prolonged subsequent course and a higher risk of the development of a pancreatic collection. Serial C-reactive protein measurements, therefore, can serve as a useful guide to the need for appropriate imaging techniques and finally to confirm resolution before discharge from hospital.

TRAUMA

The C-reactive protein concentration always rises after significant trauma, surgery or burns, peaking after about 2 days and then falling towards normal with recovery and healing. Infections or other tissue-damaging complications alter this 'normal' pattern of C-reactive protein response and the failure of the C-reactive protein to continue falling or the appearance of a second peak may precede clinical evidence of intercurrent infection by 1 to 2 days.

Conditions associated with minor elevation of serum C-reactive protein concentrations

Despite unequivocal evidence of active inflammation and/or tissue damage the conditions listed in Table 4 are usually associated with only minor elevations of the serum C-reactive protein concentration, and in many cases it remains normal in the face of severe disease. The difference in this respect between, for example systemic lupus erythematosus (SLE) and rheumatoid arthritis, or ulcerative colitis and Crohn's disease, is very striking. However, intercurrent microbial infection provokes a major C-reactive protein response in all these conditions so that although C-reactive protein measurements cannot be used to monitor the activity of these diseases *per se* they are valuable in testing for the presence and managing the treatment of infection. The mechanism of the apparently selective failure of the acute phase response of C-reactive protein (and also of serum amyloid A protein) is not known. The inbred mouse strain that develops genetically determined autoimmune lupus-like disease behaves just like human systemic lupus erythematosus patients with respect to its acute phase responses and there may thus be a genetic basis for the phenomenon.

Pyrexia is common in systemic lupus erythematosus and may be caused by microbial infection or by activity of the lupus itself. Both systemic lupus erythematosus and its treatment predispose to infection, and steroids and immunosuppressives can mask the usual symptoms and signs of infection. Furthermore, infection can trigger exacerbations of the lupus. This is a serious clinical situation and infection is the most common cause of death in patients with systemic lupus erythematosus. C-reactive protein values of 60 mg/l or more are rare in systemic lupus erythematosus in the absence of infection whilst levels below 60 mg/l are seen in patients with documented infection only when it is rather mild and often localized, for example, to the skin or lower urinary tract. Differential diagnosis and management of fever in systemic lupus erythematosus are thus considerably improved by the measurement of serum C-reactive protein concentration (Fig. 4), always interpreted, of course, in the light of the overall picture.

The C-reactive protein response in acute and chronic leukaemia is usually modest or absent, even during induction therapy when there is massive death of leukaemic cells, although these patients still mount a normal acute phase response to microbial infection. Since febrile episodes in leukaemia must always be treated initially as infective, C-reactive protein measurements are most useful for assessment of response and duration of antimicrobial treatment.

Although there may sometimes be a modest increase in serum C-reactive protein concentration in bone marrow transplant recipients who are suffering episodes of either acute or chronic graft-versus-host disease, usually there is little response. The reason for this difference from renal allograft rejection is not known. The immunosuppressive treatments used to prevent bone marrow rejection and to control graft-versus-host disease naturally render the patients very susceptible to intercurrent infection and, particularly in the case of bacterial infections, this is associated with high levels of C-reactive protein. C-reactive protein monitoring can therefore play a valuable role in management in the post-transplant period.

Table 5 *Clinical applications of measurement of serum C-reactive protein concentration*

Screening for organic disease	
Monitoring of extent and activity of disease:	Infection
	Inflammation
	Malignancy
	Necrosis
Detection and management of intercurrent infection	

Clinical interpretation of serum C-reactive protein measurements

The C-reactive protein response is not specific and C-reactive protein measurements on their own can never be diagnostic of any particular condition. The C-reactive protein value must be interpreted at the bedside in the light of all other available clinical and laboratory information. Provided this is done it can make a most useful contribution to overall assessment of the patient and determination of the best management. These applications fall into three main categories (Table 5):

1. *Screening for organic disease.* C-reactive protein production is a very sensitive index of organic disease. A normal C-reactive protein makes many otherwise possible diagnoses very unlikely and is a reassuring finding. Those serious conditions which only stimulate C-reactive protein production weakly if at all, for example, systemic lupus erythematosus, ulcerative colitis, or leukaemia, are all readily recognized by clinical examination or other simple investigations. A raised C-reactive protein is unequivocal evidence of active disease, though this may not necessarily be the cause of the complaint for which the patient presented. Such a finding, in the absence of other obvious abnormality, warrants a repeat C-reactive protein assay after a few days when a trivial cause will have resolved. Further investigation of a persistently raised C-reactive protein level will then depend on the severity of the complaint and other clinical findings.

2. *Monitoring the extent and activity of disease.* Once the diagnosis is established in any disease that causes major elevation of the C-reactive protein, serial measurements reflect activity and response to treatment and can be used for monitoring. However, they can only be interpreted provided other possible intercurrent causes of an acute phase response, particularly infections, are excluded.

3. *Detection and management of intercurrent infection.* C-reactive protein production is a very sensitive response to most forms of infection and a raised level is thus a useful guide to the possible presence of infection in otherwise normal subjects or individuals with a primary condition which predisposes to infection. In disorders which themselves elevate the C-reactive protein concentration the decision as to whether infection is present or not must depend on clinical examination and other laboratory tests and the role of C-reactive protein testing is then to demonstrate rapidly and objectively whether there is a response to whatever treatment is used. Appropriate and effective antimicrobial therapy of infection is always associated with a prompt fall in the C-reactive protein whilst persistent C-reactive protein elevation indicates continuing infection and/or activity of the underlying disease. There is no other objective test which yields this sort of information so accurately, and changes in results of clinical examination and tests of organ function usually lag hours or days behind the C-reactive protein response.

Fig. 4 A 12-year-old girl with a 3-year history of SLE; recurrent febrile episodes, polyarthritis, cutaneous vasculitis, and episodes of asymptomatic bacteriuria. Intermittent treatment with prednisolone, azathioprine, and plasma exchange. Serum C-reactive protein was only marginally elevated throughout but ESR was persistently raised. Fever recurred with diarrhoea and abdominal pain. All microbial cultures were negative except for growth of *E. coli* from the urine. Despite oral cephalexin and prednisolone her condition deteriorated with severe neutropenia, probably due to azathioprine. C-reactive protein rose from 36 to 101 and then 137 mg/l, and at this stage her blood culture grew *E. coli*. Intravenous antibiotics were given and the serum C-reactive protein level fell rapidly, but there was little clinical improvement. Active SLE appeared then to be the sole cause of the fever and this was confirmed by the development of a diffuse vasculitic rash and polyarthritis. Three pulse doses of methylprednisolone were given intravenously on successive days and produced a dramatic improvement in her clinical state with resolution of the fever. This case illustrates (i) the differential response of the C-reactive protein to fever resulting from activity of SLE alone and fever due to bacterial infection; (ii) the rapid response of the C-reactive protein both to the onset and to the effective treatment of serious bacterial infection; (iii) the failure of ESR measurements to provide any useful information in this complex and rapidly evolving clinical situation. (Reproduced from Pepys, M. B., Langham, J. G., and de Beer, F. C. (1982). C-reactive protein in SLE. *Clinics in Rheumatic Diseases*, **8**, 91–103, with permission.)

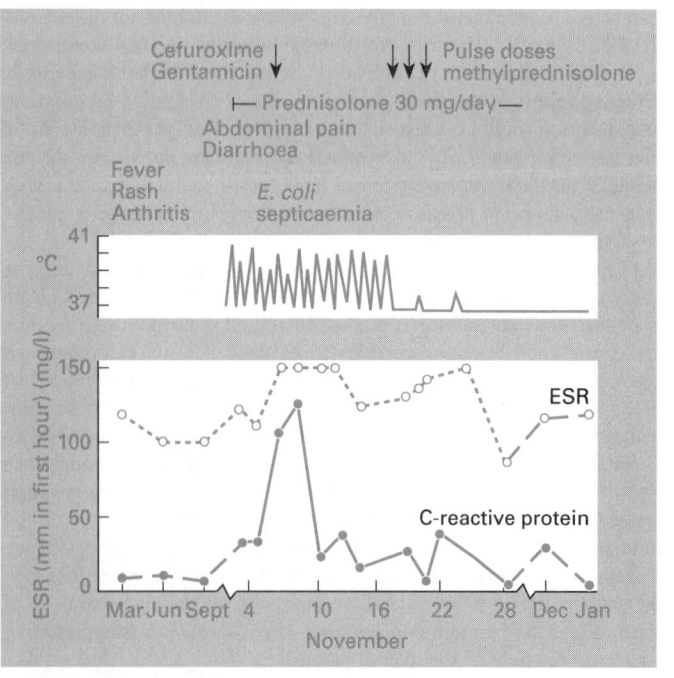

C-reactive protein and body temperature

Fever and the acute phase response are both aspects of the systemic response to disease, mediated by cytokines. C-reactive protein measurements are important complements to the use of temperature charts in clinical practice, as C-reactive protein production is not affected by either drugs or environmental factors, which may influence thermoregulation. The precise numerical value of the C-reactive protein concentration and its changes with time reflect much more accurately than the temperature the intensity of the underlying stimulus. Furthermore, there is often a C-reactive protein response in the absence of fever, especially in neonates and the elderly though also in many chronic inflammatory conditions.

C-reactive protein or erythrocyte sedimentation rate?

The erythrocyte sedimentation rate (ESR) is another index of the acute phase response, especially reflecting concentrations of fibrinogen and the α-globulins, but also those of immunoglobulins that are not acute phase reactants. These proteins all have half-lives of days to weeks. The rate of change of the erythrocyte sedimentation rate is thus very much slower than that of the C-reactive protein level and it rarely reflects precisely the clinical status of the patient at the actual time of testing. Furthermore, the erythrocyte sedimentation rate is greatly affected by the number and morphology of the red cells, and there is a significant diurnal variation in erythrocyte sedimentation rate, depending on food intake, which is not seen in the C-reactive protein. The dynamic range of the erythrocyte sedimentation rate is also much less than that of C-reactive protein and at a purely technical level the precision and reproducibility of erythrocyte sedimentation rate measurements are poor compared to immunoassays of C-reactive protein.

In all clinical situations which have been carefully evaluated, including acute and chronic bacterial infections and chronic remittent inflammatory diseases, such as Crohn's disease, rheumatoid arthritis, other inflammatory arthropathies, and the systemic vasculitides, frequent prospective measurements of C-reactive protein reflect disease activity more closely than do measurements of the erythrocyte sedimentation rate. Rapid precise C-reactive protein immunoassays are generally available. However, the erythrocyte sedimentation rate remains a useful test for the detection of paraproteinaemias which often do not provoke an acute phase response.

Serum amyloid A protein

Serum amyloid A protein is an apolipoprotein of high-density lipoprotein particles which is a marked acute phase reactant. It is described in detail in the section on amyloidosis. Like C-reactive protein, serum amyloid A protein is synthesized in the liver and its concentration rises from normal levels of about 2 mg/l as much as 1000 times in the acute phase response. Serum amyloid A protein has been less studied than C-reactive protein, but reliable immunoassays are now becoming available and may provide additional clinically useful information. Serum amyloid A protein production is certainly exquisitely sensitive and may respond differently from C-reactive protein in some conditions, such as allograft rejection. Also, sustained high circulating levels of serum amyloid A protein are the precursor of AA protein which is deposited as amyloid fibrils in chronic inflammatory diseases. Therapy adequate to suppress the serum amyloid A protein response, monitored by quantitative assays for serum amyloid A protein, has been shown to halt amyloid deposition and allow it to regress.

REFERENCES

Liuzzo, G., Biasucci, L.M., Gallimore, J.R., et al. (1994). The prognostic value of C-reactive protein and serum amyloid A protein in severe unstable angina. New England Journal of Medicine, 331, 417–24.
Pepys, M.B. (1981). C-reactive protein fifty years on. Lancet, i, 653–6.
Pepys, M.B., and Baltz, M.L. (1983). Acute phase proteins with special reference to C-reactive protein and related proteins and serum amyloid A protein. Advances in Immunology, 34, 141–212.
Vigushin, D.M., Pepys, M.B., and Hawkins, P.N. (1993). Metabolic and scintigraphic studies of radioiodinated human C-reactive protein in health and disease. Journal of Clinical Investigation, 91, 1351–7.

11.14 Disturbances of acid–base homeostasis

R. D. COHEN and H. F. WOODS

The normal acid burden

In resting humans arterial blood pH (pH_a) is normally tightly maintained between 7.36 and 7.42, as a result of control of arterial partial pressure of carbon dioxide ($Paco_2$) and plasma bicarbonate between the limits 4.7 to 5.7 kPa and 24 to 30 mmol/l, respectively. Intracellular pH is also controlled and varies between tissues within the range 6.3 to 7.4, depending on prevailing physiological circumstances, though lysosomes are very acid (pH 5). Most physiological and clinical disturbances shift, or tend to shift, pH in the acid direction, and are due to the accumulation in the body fluids of hydrogen ions (H^+) derived from metabolism. Table 1 shows the approximate order of magnitude of the various sources of endogenous acid in moles of hydrogen ions per day in a resting normal human.

The many extracellular and intracellular buffers, notably haemoglobin, other proteins, bicarbonate, and phosphate, play a transient role in counteracting pH changes but normally the acid burdens listed in Table 1 are quantitatively eliminated in the middle or long term. They have been grouped into three classes according to the mode of elimination. It may be seen that carbon dioxide derived from cellular respiration is much the largest potential generator of hydrogen ions, the burden from lactic and other organic acid production and urea synthesis being approximately ten times less and that derived from the metabolism of sulphur- and phosphorus-containing compounds is a further order of

Table 1 *Production and elimination of hydrogen ions*

Class		Daily production (mol)	Source	Excreted in breath	Metabolic removal possible	Normal organ of elimination
I	CO_2	15	Tissue respiration	+	−	Lungs
II	*Organic acids and urea synthesis*					
	Lactic	1.2	Muscle, brain erythrocytes, skin, etc.	−	+	Liver (50%), kidneys, heart
	Hydroxybutyric and acetoacetic	0.6*	Liver	−	+	Many tissues (not liver)
	Free fatty acids (FFA)	0.7	Adipose tissue	−	+	Most tissues
	H^+ generated during urea synthesis	1.1†	Liver	−	+	Most tissues (see text) small fraction in urine
III	*'Fixed acids'*					
	Sulphuric		Dietary sulphur-containing amino acids	−	−	Urinary excretion (partly)
	Phosphoric	0.1	Organic phosphate metabolism	−	−	

The daily production rates for the organic acids are calculated from results obtained in resting 70 kg man after an overnight fast, and are proportioned up to 24 h values.

*Because of ingestion of food during daytime and consequent suppression of FFA and ketone body production, the values for these acids may be considerable overestimates.

†On 100 g protein diet.

magnitude lower. The modes of elimination of these three types of acid are also shown in Table 1. Disposal of carbon dioxide is dependent on adequate respiratory function. The metabolism of sulphur-containing amino acids in the diet eventually results in the production of sulphuric acid, and phosphoric acid may be derived from many sources. Both of these acids are non-volatile and excretion of hydrogen ions from these sources may occur in the urine, virtually entirely in combination with urinary buffer.

The organic acids (Table 1) have pK values much less than blood pH and are, therefore, present in blood as the organic acid anions rather than as the undissociated acid, the equivalent amount of hydrogen ions, which was formed at the site of production of these acids, having titrated blood bicarbonate and other buffers. The organic acid anions (lactate, 3-hydroxybutyrate, acetoacetate, and fatty acids) are non-volatile but may be eliminated by metabolism. Figure 1 shows an example of the general principle that when these organic acid anions are metabolized to electroneutral products (e.g. glucose, or carbon dioxide and water), hydrogen ions are consumed and the bicarbonate is regenerated. Hydro-

gen ions from organic acids can also be eliminated by the urinary route referred to above, but this is under normal circumstances a much slower process than the metabolic route. In the case of the ketone bodies, for which the renal threshold is quite low, substantial amounts can be lost in the urine when their plasma concentration is elevated. Although maximally acid urine (pH 4.5) results in about half of the urinary ketone body excretion being as the undissociated acid, the remaining free anion moiety in fact represents loss of potential alkali from the body, since by escaping into the urine it eludes eventual metabolism to bicarbonate.

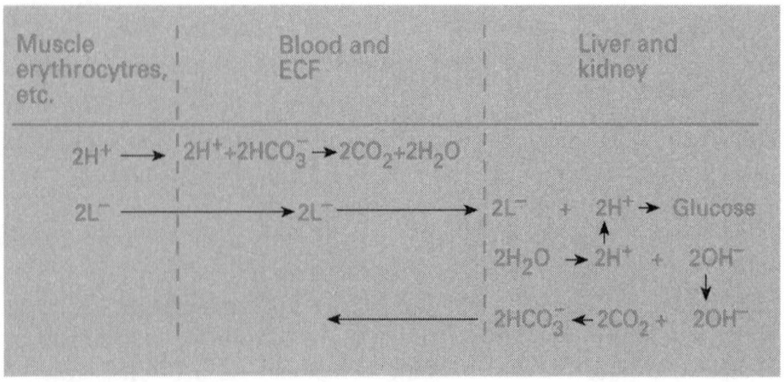

Some comment is needed on the rather unconventional appearance in Table 1 of urea synthesis as a source of acid burden. Each mole of urea synthesis results in the production of two moles of hydrogen ions, as follows:

$$CO_2 + 2NH_4^+ \rightarrow CO(NH_2)_2 + H_2O + 2H^+$$

A person consuming 100 g of protein daily produces approximately 1.1 moles of hydrogen ions during the conversion of most of the protein nitrogen into urea. Atkinson and Camien have pointed out that this concentration of hydrogen ions is almost exactly neutralized by the bicarbonate (HCO_3^-) produced from the metabolism of the carbon skeletons of the amino acid residues of the original proteins. There is, in fact, a slight excess under ordinary dietary conditions of dibasic over dicarboxylic amino acid residues; by conversion of the nitrogen of the excess dibasic acids into urea this would tend to lead to acidosis.

However, the kidneys, either by excreting hydrogen ions buffered as dihydrogen phosphate or by excreting the excess nitrogen as the ammonium ion (NH_4^+), can normally prevent this occurring. The more nitrogen excreted as ammonium ions, the less is available for urea synthesis and concomitant hydrogen ion production and there is correspondingly less neutralization of bicarbonate produced from the carbon skeletons of the amino acids; the tendency to acidosis due to protein metabolism is thus countered. It should be noted that ammonium ion excretion in the urine does not directly eliminate hydrogen ions; this is contrary to the classical view, which states that ammonia, derived in the kidney from glutamine, buffers secreted hydrogen ions as follows:

$$NH_3 + H^+ \rightarrow NH_4^+$$

Fig. 1 A scheme, using lactate conversion to glucose as an example, showing how the conversion of an organic acid of low pK to an electroneutral substance consumes H^+ and regenerates HCO_3^-. The lactate ion is shown as L^-.

As Oliver and Bourke have pointed out, this is unlikely to be correct, as ammonium derived from the hydrolysis of glutamine is already in the ammonium ion form and therefore cannot buffer hydrogen ions. This reinterpretation is not academic, because in addition to viewing renal ammonium excretion primarily as a modulator of availability of nitrogen for urea synthesis and accompanying hydrogen ion production, rather than a direct vehicle for hydrogen ion excretion, it suggests that disturbances of urea synthesis could play a substantial role in disorders of acid–base status (see below).

Despite the large quantitative differences in the burden due to the three classes of acid in Table 1, their correct elimination is in a sense equally important, for no class is able substantially to use a disposal route normally associated with another class. The distinction lies in the potential rate at which the clinical state may become critical when a disposal route is deranged. Thus it has been calculated that total failure of elimination of carbon dioxide would result in critically severe acidosis in 30 min. Observations in clinical lactic acidosis suggest that elimination of the lactate removal mechanisms would take several hours to produce a lethal acidosis; in acute renal failure several days may elapse before acidosis becomes a major problem.

Normally the production and elimination of each class of acid are balanced. The homeostasis of arterial blood pH that this balance provides is given quantitative expression in the classic Henderson–Hasselbalch equation:

$$pH = 6.1 + \log_{10} \{[HCO_3-]/0.225 \times Pa_{CO_2}\}$$

where Pa_{CO_2} is the partial pressure of arterial carbon dioxide expressed in kiloPascals (kPa). The constancy of arterial bicarbonate ions (HCO_3^-) is maintained by the removal of class II and III acids and by ureogenesis (see above) and that of the partial pressure of arterial carbon dioxide by the lungs, thereby fixing arterial blood pH within a narrow normal range.

Definitions

The terminology of acid–base disturbances has always been confused. Here we use the terms acidaemia and alkalaemia simply to indicate that the arterial blood pH is lower or higher than the normal range, respectively. The term acidosis is used to encompass both the situation where the arterial blood pH is low, and also that in which, although arterial blood pH is normal, the nature of the responsible disturbance is such that if compensatory mechanisms had not operated, arterial blood pH would be low. An equivalent definition applies to alkalosis. Most acid–base disturbances are due to imbalance of production and removal of hydrogen ions derived from the endogenous sources classified in Table 1. However, some are due to ingestion or infusion of excessive amounts of acids or bases (particularly bicarbonate). When the primary disturbance is related to abnormal carbon dioxide elimination, the acidosis or alkalosis is termed 'respiratory'. All other primary disturbances (i.e. those due to disturbances of class II and III acid production or removal or of ureogenesis), are termed 'metabolic' or 'non-respiratory'. The term 'primary' is used to contrast with 'secondary' disturbances, which are compensatory in nature. Thus metabolic acidosis is compensated for by hyperventilation due to stimulation of the respiratory centre, and consequently the arterial partial pressure of carbon dioxide is lowered; respiratory acidosis is compensated for by metabolic events which result in elevation of plasma bicarbonate.

The diagnosis of acid–base disturbances

The clinical manifestations of acid–base disturbances are described later. They are rather non-specific and may not be evident until the disturbance is quite severe. Thus, although clinical features may provide the first indication of a disturbance of acid–base homeostasis, accurate characterization, both qualitatively and quantitatively, requires laboratory investigation. Measurement of pH and partial pressure of carbon dioxide

on arterial, or arterialized venous blood is the most definitive procedure. Additional useful information may be obtained from measurement of plasma sodium, potassium, chloride, and bicarbonate, and subsequent calculation of the anion gap.

Measurement of pH_a and Pa_{CO_2}

Blood gas analysers measure pH and partial pressure of carbon dioxide and calculate bicarbonate from the Henderson–Hasselbalch equation. Interpretation of the results is best achieved by the use of an acid–base diagram, which has arterial blood pH on one axis and arterial partial pressure of carbon dioxide in the other. Diagrams which use the concentration of arterial bicarbonate ions $[HCO_3^-]_a$ instead of either arterial blood pH and arterial partial pressure of carbon dioxide are less suitable, as arterial bicarbonate ion concentration is calculated from arterial blood pH and partial pressure of carbon dioxide and is not only affected by the errors in both the latter measurements, but also by the fact that pK_a in the Henderson–Hasselbalch equation is subject to some poorly understood variations in blood from severely ill patients.

The acid–base diagram shown in Fig. 2 has bands drawn in to show the range of expected response to uncomplicated acid-base disorders. The shaded square represents the approximate limits of arterial blood pH and arterial partial pressure of carbon dioxide in normal individuals. Thus a patient with uncomplicated metabolic acidosis will have values lying in the band marked metabolic in the region to the left and above the shaded area; the metabolic band is in fact the envelope of measurements of arterial blood pH and partial pressure of carbon dioxide from patients recorded in the literature with completely uncomplicated metabolic acidosis or alkalosis. The band marked acute respiratory is the 95 per cent confidence range of values obtained in normal individuals voluntarily hyperventilating or breathing air/carbon dioxide mixtures for short periods of time. Since, after a few days of carbon dioxide retention in respiratory acidosis, an increase in plasma bicarbonate produces substantial or complete compensation, the response expected in chronic respiratory acidosis is different from the acute response, the presence of the extra bicarbonate reducing the fall in pH for a given rise in arterial partial pressure of carbon dioxide.

Fig. 2 For explanation see text. P_{CO_2} = partial pressure of carbon dioxide.

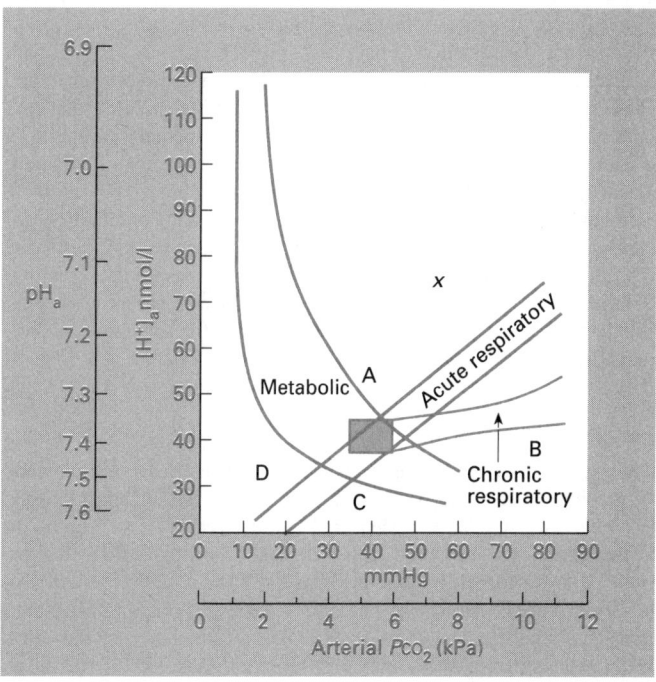

Figure 2 therefore also includes the uncomplicated response to chronic respiratory acidosis. It may be seen that the band for metabolic alkalosis (to the right of and below the shaded region) is rather restricted, extending only a short distance along the partial pressure of carbon dioxide axis. This is because compensation by hypoventilation for metabolic alkalosis is often, but by no means invariably poor, perhaps because hypoxia sets a limit to compensating hypoventilation and also possibly because a number of conditions in which metabolic alkalosis is a feature may be associated with intracellular acidosis, which could stimulate the respiratory centre. Marked hypercapnia is, however, occasionally seen in metabolic alkalosis.

The arterial blood pH and arterial partial pressure of carbon dioxide measurements in some patients will not fall within any of the defined bands shown in Fig. 2. Such patients have a mixture of acid–base disorders. Thus a patient whose arterial blood pH and partial pressure of carbon dioxide is represented by the point 'x' has mixed respiratory and metabolic acidosis (e.g. a patient with an exacerbation of chronic bronchitis and coexistent diabetic ketoacidosis). It may be noted that a disturbance lying in sectors A or C results from the combination of two primary acid–base conditions; in sectors B and D one of the two disturbances could be compensatory for the other. The diagram not only permits the diagnosis of acid–base disorders, but by serially plotting results the course of an individual patient's disturbance and its response to treatment may be closely followed.

Contemporary acid–base analytical equipment usually also provides at least two further acid–base variables if the haemoglobin concentration is also known. These are the 'standard bicarbonate' and the 'base excess' or 'base deficit' variables. The standard bicarbonate represents what the plasma bicarbonate would be if the blood had a normal arterial partial pressure of carbon dioxide (5.33 kPa, 40 mmHg) rather than its actual value. Standard bicarbonate was introduced in an attempt to provide a measurement which was independent of respiratory disturbance and thus to provide an estimate of underlying pure metabolic disturbance. 'Base deficit' represents the amount of alkali in mmol required to restore the pH of 1 litre of the patient's blood in vitro to normal at partial pressure of carbon dioxide 5.33 kPa and might at first sight be considered a quantitative measure of metabolic acidosis. Unfortunately the titration curve of blood in vitro is different from when it is circulating in vivo, since in the latter situation the interstitial and intracellular fluids are in equilibrium with blood and may gain or lose bicarbonate from it; in addition their buffering capacity differs from that of blood. These considerations detract from the usefulness of base excess or deficit as a guide either to diagnosis or therapy. Further difficulties arise from ambiguities in the interpretation of base excess or deficit. Thus a patient with chronic respiratory acidosis will have a high standard bicarbonate and a base excess due to compensatory renal retention of bicarbonate. It could be said, therefore, that this patient has simultaneously a respiratory acidosis and a metabolic alkalosis, as a base excess indicates the latter. This way of regarding the situation, which is quite widely adopted, seems to us confusing, and is not compatible with the definitions of acidosis and alkalosis we have given, which are intended to indicate the direction of the primary disturbance. For these reasons we prefer the use of the acid–base diagram shown in Fig. 2, which is based entirely on directly measured variables and is not subject to the difficulties associated with the derived variables described above.

Use of the anion gap

The main electrolytes routinely measured in plasma are sodium ions (Na^+), chloride ions (Cl^-), potassium ions (K^+), and bicarbonate ions (HCO_3^-). The sum of the measured cations ($Na^+ + K^+$) normally exceeds that of the measured anions by about 14 mmol/litre (reference range 10 to 18 mmol/l). This difference is known as the 'anion gap' and is attributable largely to negatively charged proteins but also to phosphate, sulphate, and some organic acids. Calculation of the anion gap is principally of value in the differential diagnosis of metabolic acidosis and in following the progress of therapy. Metabolic acidoses

may be divided broadly into those with normal and those with high anion gap.

METABOLIC ACIDOSES WITH NORMAL ANION GAP

These are due to the direct loss of bicarbonate from the body, either through the gut (e.g. diarrhoea, pancreatic fistulae, ureterosigmoidostomy) or through the kidney (e.g. renal tubular acidosis, acetazolamide therapy) or, rarely to the ingestion or infusion of hydrochloric acid or substances effectively giving rise to it (e.g. ammonium chloride, arginine hydrochloride). When bicarbonate is lost more chloride is retained by the renal tubules; thus low plasma bicarbonate is accompanied by hyperchloraemia and the anion gap remains unaltered. In the case of hydrochloric acid intake bicarbonate is titrated and replaced by chloride.

METABOLIC ACIDOSES WITH HIGH ANION GAP

These are due to the ingestion or endogenous generation of acids, usually organic, whose anions are not routinely measured. Plasma bicarbonate is titrated and the anion gap is now widened by the presence of these unmeasured anions. The principal causes are ketoacidosis, lactic acidosis, uraemic acidosis, and poisoning by salicylates. In uraemic acidosis the anion gap seldom exceeds 28 mmol/l, but considerably higher values may be found in severe lactic acidosis and ketoacidosis. It should be noted that there are causes of raised anion gap other than metabolic acidosis, for example therapy with sodium salts of relatively strong acids (e.g. lactate, acetate) and high-dose sodium carbenicillin therapy, and respiratory or metabolic alkalosis.

Causes of acid–base disturbance

In surveying the spectrum of causation of acid–base disorders, by far the most diverse problems of aetiology and classification arise in metabolic acidosis. Table 2 classifies those conditions associated with high anion gap metabolic acidosis and attempts to divide them into those in which the predominant unmeasured anion is lactate, ketoacids or other often less well-defined acid anions. The term 'ketoacid' is loosely used to refer both to a ketoacid itself (e.g. acetoacetic acid) and its reduced derivative (e.g. 3-hydroxybutyrate). It may be seen from Table 2 that high anion gap acidosis is often due to a mixture of acids, but where possible the predominant acid has been indicated in italic type. It is often the case that the acid anions actually identified in plasma can only account for a part, often minor, of the acidosis and this has been shown by an asterisk. The common form of uraemic acidosis is the best example of this. Table 3 metabolic acidoses with normal anion gap classifies according to whether they are due to gut or renal bicarbonate loss, or to ingestion or infusion of acidifying agents.

Metabolic alkalosis (Table 4) is due either to ingestion or infusion of excessive alkali in circumstances (e.g. poor renal function) when it cannot be excreted, or to loss of acid, either from the stomach as in pyloric stenosis, or in secretion of an inappropriately acid urine. Most of the causes of the latter occurrence are related to the complex disturbances occurring in potassium and chloride deficiency (see Chapter 20.2.3). The metabolic alkalosis not infrequently seen in fulminant hepatic failure has not been explained; however, it now appears possible that it is due to failure of urea synthesis, and consequent failure to neutralize bicarbonate derived from metabolism of the carbon skeletons of amino acids (see above).

Respiratory acidoses, presented in Table 5 are due to problems at one or more of three levels, namely, the lungs and airways, the neuromuscular and mechanical aspects of respiration, and the central nervous system.

Respiratory alkalosis (Table 6) is nearly always due to some form of stimulus to the respiratory centre, whether it be psychogenic, reflex, chemically induced or due to a local lesion; the exception is deliberate or inadvertent hyperventilation during anaesthesia or other occasions when assisted ventilation is used.

Table 2 *High anion gap metabolic acidoses*

(i)	*Predominant ketoacidosis*	*Associated serum acid anions**
	Diabetic ketoacidosis	*3-hydroxybutyrate*, acetoacetate, lactate
	Starvation ketoacidosis	*3-hydroxybutyrate*, acetoacetate, lactate
	Alcoholic ketoacidosis	*3-hydroxybutyrate*, acetoacetate, lactate
	Ketotic hypoglycaemia ofchildhood	*3-hydroxybutyrate*, acetoacetate, lactate
(ii)	*Predominant lactic acidosis Type A lactic acidosis*	
	Exercise	*Lactate*
	Postepileptic	*Lactate*
	Shock (traumatic,haemorrhagic, cardiogenic, septic)	*Lactate*
	Severe hypoxia.	*Lactate*
	Type B lactic acidosis	
	Biguanide-associated(phenformin, buformin, metformin)	*Lactate*, 3-hydroxybutyrate
	Ethanol-associated	*Lactate*, 3-hydroxybutyrate
	Following recovery from diabetic ketoacidosis	*Lactate*
	Fructose, sorbitol, or xylitol infusion	*Lactate*
	Other poorly characterized acquired lactic acidoses	*Lactate*
	Severe liver disease	*Lactate*
	Leukaemia and reticulosis	*Lactate*
	Paracetamol poisoning	*Lactate*
	Thiamine deficiency	*Lactate*
	Type I glycogenosis	*Lactate*
	Hepatic fructose 1,6-diphosphatase deficiency	*Lactate*
	Lactic acidosis associated with metabolic myopathies	*Lactate*
	Pyruvate carboxylase deficiency	*Lactate*
	Other poorly characterized hereditary lactic acidoses	*Lactate*
	D(−) lactic acidosis due to lactobacillus ingestion	*Lactate*
(iii)	*Conditions with imperfectly defined source of acidoses*	
	Uraemic acidosis	Phosphate, sulphate, etc.
	Salicylate poisoning (acidotic phase)	Salicylate lactate, ketoacids
	Methanol poisoning	*Formate, lactate*
	Ethylene glycol poisoning	Lactate, glycolate, oxalate
	Paraldehyde poisoning	?
	Reye's syndrome	Lactate
	Jamaican vomiting sickness (ackee poisoning)	?
	Glutaric aciduria Type II	Lactate, free fatty acids
	Ethylmalonic-adipic aciduria	?
	Propionyl CoA carboxylase deficiency	Higher ketoacids, propionic acid
	Methylmalonic aciduria	Ketoacids (including higher ones), lactate, methylmalonate
	β-Ketothiolase deficiency	Methylhydroxybutyrate, methylacetoacetate

*The predominant acid anion is shown in italics.

Except when otherwise stated, lactate refers to the L(+)isomer.

Tables 2 to 6 illustrate both the wide range of aetiology and the major causes of acid–base disturbances; they are not intended to be comprehensive.

The consequences of acid–base disturbances

The effect of acid–base disturbances on physiological and biochemical mechanisms are widespread. We limit ourselves here to a brief description of those currently known, or thought to have clinical relevance.

Respiratory effects

Both metabolic acidosis and acute respiratory acidosis induced by breathing high partial pressure of carbon dioxide gas mixtures result in hyperventilation. Deep sighing respiration (Kussmaul breathing) is a familiar sign of metabolic acidosis. The degree of hyperventilation achieved in given clinical circumstances is dependent on complex factors which are related both to the magnitude and the rate of development of the acid–base disturbance. pH control of ventilation is determined both by the pH perceived by the carotid and aortic body chemoreceptors

Table 3 *Normal anion gap metabolic acidoses*

(i) *Gastrointestinal bicarbonate loss*
     Diarrhoea
     Pancreatic fistula

(ii) *Ureteroenterostomy*

(iii) *Renal causes*
     Renal tubular acidosis (RTA)
       (a) *Gradient distal type, Type I RTA)*
            Primary $\begin{cases}\text{transient, in infancy}\\\text{permanent (childhood or adult)}\end{cases}$
            Secondary
              In hypergammaglobulinaemia and some
                 autoimmune states
              Amphotericin B therapy
              Vitamin D intoxication
              Hyperthyroidism
              Carnitine palmitoyl transferase (Type I)
                 deficiency
       (b) *Bicarbonate wastage (proximal type, Type II
            RTA)*
            Primary $\begin{cases}\text{isolated}\\\text{as part of idiopathic Fanconi}\end{cases}$
            syndrome
            Secondary
              Hyperthyroidism
              Vitamin D deficiency
              Uraemia (occasionally)
              Dysproteinaemic states (myeloma, Sjögren's
                 syndrome)
              Heavy metal poisoning (cadmium, mercury)
              Outdated tetracycline
              Renal transplant rejection
              Hereditary disorders (e.g. cystinosis,
                 Wilson's disease, hereditary fructose
                 intolerance, galactosaemia, Lowe's
                 syndrome)
              Acetazolamide treatment
       (c) *Type IV RTA (hyperkalaemic)*
            Hypoaldosteronism, aldosterone insensitivity
            Types I and II pseudohypoaldosteronism
            Hyporeninaemia
            Diabetes
            Pyelonephritis
            Potassium sparing diuretics
            Angiotensin converting enzyme inhibitors
            Non-steroidal anti-inflammatory drugs.
            As part of moderate renal insufficiency

(iv) *Ingestion or infusion of acidifying agents*
     Ammonium chloride
     Arginine hydrochloride, hydrochloric acid
     Intravenous feeding with solutions containing excess
     cationic aminoacids

(v) *Rapid intravenous hydration* (dilutional acidosis)

Table 4 *Causes of metabolic alkalosis*

Ingestion or infusion of alkali in excess of excretory ability
     Milk–akali syndrome
     'Alkaline overshoot' during therapy of high anion gap
        acidoses
     Forced alkaline diuresis therapy of salicylate and barbiturate
        poisoning

Loss of acid inappropriately (gastric or renal routes)
     Pyloric stenosis, self-induced persistent vomiting
     Potassium depletion (other than in tubular
        acidosis)
     Chloride depletion $\Big\}$ Frequently
     Hyperaldosteronism   associated

'Contraction alkalosis'
     Rapid diuresis

?Failure of ureogenesis
     Fulminant hepatic failure

Table 5 *Causes of respiratory acidosis*

1 *Structural and mechanical pulmonary disease*
   Chronic obstructive airways disease
   Severe asthma (uncommonly)
   Large airway obstruction

2 *Neuromuscular and mechanical problems*
   Acute ascending polyneuritis (Guillian-Barré)
   Poliomyelitis
   Acute porphyria
   Myasthenia gravis
   Motor neurone disease
   Muscular dystrophies
   Traumatic 'flail chest'
   Ankylosing spondylitis
   Severe kyphoscoliosis
   Gross obesity, often in association with sleep aponea
   Muscle relaxant drugs

3 *Respiratory centre disorders*
   Organic disease affecting respiratory centre
   Numerous respiratory centre depressant drugs
     e.g. opiates, barbiturates, benzodiazepines, anaesthetic
        agents
   Respiratory arrest

Table 6 *Causes of respiratory alkalosis*

Spontaneous or psychogenic hyperventilation
Reflex hyperventilation (e.g. in pulmonary disease and
   pulmonary embolism)
Other stimuli to respiratory centre
   (a) Via chemoreceptors
          Low inspired oxygen concentration (e.g. high altitude)
          Alveolo-capillary diffusion block
          Right to left shunt
          Carbon monoxide poisoning
   (b) Via drugs or metabolites
          Salicylate poisoning
          Acute liver failure
   (c) After recovery from metabolic acidosis
   (d) Local lesion affecting centre
          Overventilation during anaesthesia or other assisted
             ventilation

and also by chemoreceptors in the medulla which appear to monitor the pH of brain extracellular fluid (ECF). In the steady–state brain extracellular fluid pH is closely similar to that of cerebrospinal fluid (CSF). Sudden development of metabolic acidosis, resulting in low arterial blood pH and plasma bicarbonate, induces hyperventilation by stimulating the carotid and aortic body chemoreceptors and arterial partial pressure of carbon dioxide is thus lowered. However, the first effect on brain extracellular fluid pH is to raise it. This is because brain extracellular fluid partial pressure of carbon dioxide is lowered, since because carbon dioxide is rapidly equilibrated across the blood–brain barrier. In contrast, it takes many hours for the brain extracellular fluid bicarbonate concentration to fall in response to the lowering of plasma bicarbonate because active and passive movement of bicarbonate across the barrier is very much slower than that of carbon dioxide. The temporary alkalinization of brain extracellular fluid pH in the presence of systemic metabolic acidosis somewhat offsets the ventilatory drive provided by the peripheral chemoreceptors. In the longerterm, brain extracellular fluid and cerebrospinal fluid pH are tightly controlled and their initial high pH in acute metabolic acidosis is eventually restored to normal or slightly below normal. This removes the partial inhibition of ventilatory response and the degree of hyperventilation increases. Though clinical circumstances usually prevent the observation of this sequence of events, the opposite effect, namely the persistence of hyperventilation after restoration of normal arterial pH during the therapy of metabolic acidosis is commonly seen. In this situation systemic alkalinization has suppressed the peripheral chemoreceptors, raising partial pressure of carbon dioxide and thus causing paradoxical acidification of brain extracellular fluid and cerebrospinal fluid. Over 24 h may elapse before the resulting persisting hyperventilation ceases. In acute and chronic respiratory acidosis the ventilatory manifestations of phased events equivalent to those seen in metabolic acid-base disorders are seldom given full expression, because the respiratory disease usually prevents this. In chronic CO_2 retention direct depression of the respiratory centre occurs, and the respiratory response to increments of arterial partial pressure of carbon dioxide becomes progressively lost, ventilation becoming increasingly dependent upon hypoxic drive.

Cardiovascular effects

ON THE HEART

It is generally agreed that acidosis has adverse effects on cardiac contractility (negative inotropism) and alkalosis smaller but opposite effects. The negative inotropic effects are particularly related to changes in cardiac intracellular pH and are experimentally found to be rather greater in acute respiratory than in acute metabolic acidosis in the presence of the same extracellular pH. The negative inotropic effect of acidosis is due to a combination of mechanisms connected with excitation–contraction coupling and energy supply; amongst other effects, acidosis inhibits the inward slow calcium current during the action potential and the release of calcium from sarcoplasmic reticulum, and depresses glycolysis. In the rat, progressive metabolic acidosis induced by oral feeding of ammonium chloride results in a fall of cardiac output due to both bradycardia and to negative inotropy, with consequent hypotension and decreased renal and hepatic blood flow. This sequence of events may provide a model for the circulatory collapse, which is often seen to occur in patients after some hours of severe metabolic acidosis not primarily due to shock.

Although mild to moderate acidosis has often not been associated with negative inotropic effects in the intact animal this appears to be due to the protective effect of catecholamine release, which is increased in acidosis. The adrenergic stimulation of contractility is sufficient to overcome the negative effects of mild to moderate acidosis, but in more severe acidosis this protection breaks down. Patients receiving blocking drugs are thus potentially more susceptible to the negative inotropic effects of acidosis.

ON THE PERIPHERAL VASCULATURE

Cerebral arterioles are very sensitive to the pH of brain extracellular fluid, being dilated when this falls and constricted by increases. The cerebrovascular resistance is therefore subject to similar phased responses to different types of acute acid–base disturbances as is ventilation, due to the differential time response of brain extracellular fluid, partial pressure of carbon dioxide, and bicarbonate to acute systemic changes. Dilatation is also the response of most systemic arterioles to acidosis, although this response may be modified or offset completely by catecholamine effects. The peripheral veins, however, constrict in acidosis, resulting in a shift of blood from the peripheral capacitance vessels to the central circulation. This effect has been demonstrated during treatment of the dehydration and acidosis associated with cholera.

Effects on intermediary carbohydrate metabolism

In all tissues in which observations have been made, glycolysis is inhibited by acidosis and stimulated by alkalosis, due to the effects of intracellular pH on phosphofructokinase, a rate-limiting enzyme of glycolysis. Respiratory alkalosis might, therefore, be expected to raise blood lactate, but in normal individuals the effect is very small, no doubt due to removal of lactate by the liver. However, in the presence of severe liver disease gross elevation of blood lactate may be seen in association with respiratory alkalosis and the increased production of lactic acid may partially compensate for the alkalosis.

Animal studies have shown that hepatic gluconeogenesis from lactate is inhibited by severe acidosis due to an effect on the step between pyruvate and oxaloacetate. This phenomenon could be responsible for perpetuating and worsening lactic acidosis. It may be partially offset by the effects of the increased catecholamine levels seen in lactic acidosis due to shock.

Effects on blood oxygen uptake and delivery

One of the factors determining pulmonary oxygen uptake and tissue oxygen delivery is the position of the blood oxygen dissociation curve with respect to the ordinate (the oxygen saturation) and abscissa (the partial pressure of oxygen; Po_2). Right shifts of this curve improve unloading of oxygen in the tissues, but, in the presence of low inspired oxygen concentration or pulmonary disease, impair oxygen uptake in the lungs; left shifts have the opposite effect. The position of the curve is determined by three ligands capable of interacting with the haemoglobin molecule, namely, hydrogen ions, carbon dioxide, and 2,3-bisphosphoglycerate (2,3-BPG). Increases in the concentration of any of these result in a shift to the right. The effects of changes in extracellular hydrogen ions (Bohr effect) and carbon dioxide are immediate and operate through changes in intraerythrocytic hydrogen ions and carbon dioxide. In addition, an increase in intraerythrocytic hydrogen ions (i.e. fall in pH) inhibits the synthesis of 2,3-bisphosphoglycerate and encourages its breakdown. Opposite effects occur in alkalosis. These reactions are, however, very slow in comparison with the immediate Bohr effect.

The effect of these differences in time scale on oxygen delivery during the course of acid–base disturbances may be exemplified by the changes occurring during the development (over a few hours) and treatment of acute metabolic acidosis. Initially the acute acidosis causes a right shift and hence improved oxygen delivery. After several hours the 2,3-bisphosphoglycerate level falls, thus restoring the position of the curve approximately to normal. If the patient is now rapidly treated with alkalinizing solution, the Bohr effect results in an immediate shift to the left; it may be many hours, even up to 2 to 3 days, before 2,3-bisphosphoglycerate concentrations are restored. The sudden deterioration in oxygen delivery caused by alkalinization could have adverse clinical effects unless the effect of shift in the curve is counteracted by other factors—such as increase in tissue blood flow.

Effects on the nervous system

The effects of acid–base disturbances on the central nervous system are a result of many factors, including changes in cerebral blood flow and oxygen dissociation (see above) and other mechanisms less well characterized. Severe acidosis is frequently associated with a variety of degrees of impairment of consciousness, varying from mild drowsiness to coma. The degree of disturbance is not closely related to systemic pH, and the mechanism is not understood. Attempts to relate this effect of acidosis to cerebrospinal fluid pH have proved unsuccessful.

The excitability of neuromuscular tissues is in general increased by alkalosis and decreased by acidosis. Tetany is a common feature of respiratory alkalosis, and may also be seen when a chronic metabolic acidosis is corrected in a patient with low plasma calcium, a combination of events which may occur in renal failure. The effect has been attributed to increased protein binding of plasma calcium but it is very doubtful whether this is sufficient quantitatively to account for the phenomenon. Epileptic attacks in those prone to them are precipitated by alkalosis and suppressed by acidosis.

Effects on potassium homeostasis

Acute acidosis results in a shift of potassium out of the intracellular compartment into the extracellular fluid. Hyperkalaemia is thus often seen in the acidosis of renal failure, untreated diabetic ketoacidosis, and in acute respiratory failure. The mechanism is unclear, a number of factors in addition to extracellular pH also being involved. Alkaline therapy in such patients causes shift of potassium back into cells. As substantial amounts of potassium may be lost through the kidneys during the period of hyperkalaemia, the body may be potassium depleted even in the presence of hyperkalaemia and alkali therapy may result in serious hypokalaemia. This is a well-known hazard in the treatment of diabetic ketoacidosis and is even more dangerous in renal tubular acidosis, when, because of prior potassium depletion, plasma potassium may be very low even in the severely acidotic patient. Such patients should be treated with potassium salts before alkalinization, or at least concomitantly. Treating the acidosis first may result in cardiac arrest due to further fall of plasma potassium.

Chronic metabolic alkalosis is frequently accompanied by potassium depletion, due to distal tubular potassium secretion uninhibited by competition for secretion with hydrogen ions. The increased tubular potassium secretion is further enhanced by the chloride depletion, which is frequently present in chronic metabolic alkalosis (see below).

Effects on the kidney

The kidney is a major organ of acid–base control and many of its responses to acid–base disturbances are therefore geared to their correction. Acidosis causes a marked increase in renal gluconeogenesis, primarily due to increased activity of the relevant rate-limiting enzyme, phosphoenolpyruvate carboxykinase. The increased gluconeogenesis is thought to be causally linked with the increase of renal ammoniagenesis which is a crucial part of the renal response to acidosis. The mechanism of this link is still under debate. The ammoniagenic response to acidosis also depends on an adequate supply of ammonium precursors to the kidney, and an intact ammonium production mechanism within the tubular cells. The main precursor of renal ammonium is glutamine and substantial changes take place in glutamine metabolism in acidosis. Glutamine release from liver and skeletal muscle is increased and disposal of glutamine nitrogen is shifted away from urea production in the liver to ammonium excretion in the kidney. This is due not only to the stimulatory effects of acidosis on renal ammoniagenesis, but also to direct inhibition of urea production, thus, as indicated earlier, tending to counteract the acidosis. In addition to the above mechanisms for increasing ammoniagenesis, chronic acidosis also results in the increased activity of renal glutaminase, the critical enzyme of ammoniagenesis.

Most textbooks of physiology state that the kidneys are capable during acidosis of increasing their effective acid secretion from a typical normal value of 100 mmol/day to about 500 mmol/day. This assertion, however, is based on calculating the daily urinary acid excretion as:

$$(\text{Titratable acid} + \text{ammonium} - \text{bicarbonate}) \text{ excretion}$$

Here 'titratable acid' refers mainly to hydrogen ions carried in phosphate buffer and is typically, in millimolar terms, about 25 to 30 per cent of the ammonium excretion. Bicarbonate excretion is normally small except in alkaline urine. During acidosis, further titration of the phosphate buffer produces a modest increment in effective hydrogen ion excretion, but ammonium excretion may increase five-fold or more, and it is this latter effect which has largely given rise to the quoted values for total hydrogen ion excretion during acidosis. But, if, as indicated above, it is incorrect to regard the ammonia/ammonium system as a urinary buffer, then the classic explanation of the renal response to acidosis must be incorrect. The alternative view, which we believe likely to be correct, is that the increased ammonium excretion in acidosis results in diversion of nitrogenous substrate from urea synthesis, and consequent counteraction of acidosis by the mechanism described earlier. The ability of the kidney to excrete ammonium and thereby activate this mechanism depends on its ability to lower the urinary pH to the normal minimum of 4.5 to 5.3, as well as upon the adaptive mechanisms described in the previous paragraph.

In alkalosis other than that due to potassium chloride, and extracellular volume depletion, large quantities of bicarbonate are excreted in the urine, the maximum pH of which is about 8.

Effects on bone

It has been shown that bone acts as a buffer in chronic metabolic acidosis, in that leaching out of a calcium carbonate phase in bone and exchange of extracellular phosphate for carbonate within the apatite crystal result in the neutralization of hydrogen ions. The first of these mechanisms gives rise to a negative calcium balance in chronic metabolic acidosis and in chronic uraemic acidotic subjects it has been shown that calcium balance can be restored by treatment with sodium bicarbonate. Although chronic experimental metabolic acidosis in rats leads to osteoporosis, renal tubular acidosis and the acidosis of ureterosigmoidostomy in humans lead to osteomalacia, which can be corrected by alkali therapy alone.

Effects on leucocytes

Severe acidosis is often associated with marked leucocytosis, unrelated to the presence of infection. Blood leucocyte counts of up to $60000/\text{mm}^3$ have been recorded in lactic acidosis and high values are also common in diabetic ketoacidosis. It has been suggested that this phenomenon may be partly specifically due to the acidosis and not merely an indication of stress.

Effects on the distribution of metabolites and drugs

When weak acids and bases are distributed between body compartments by non-ionic diffusion, pH differences between the two compartments will determine their relative concentrations in these compartments. Weak bases are concentrated in the more acid ones, and weak acids in the more alkaline compartments. Examples of physiological metabolites thus affected are ammonia (weak base) and urobilinogen (weak acid). The urinary excretion of ammonium is thus markedly increased in acid urine and that of urobilinogen decreased. The distribution of ammonium between blood and cerebrospinal fluid is partly determined by the blood–cerebrospinal fluid pH difference. Examples of drugs exhibiting this behaviour are salicylates and phenobarbitone, which are both weak acids; use of the pH dependence of distribution is made in the therapy of salicylate and phenobarbitone poisoning by forced alkaline diuresis.

Major syndromes of metabolic acidosis

(For renal tubular acidosis see Section 20)

Uraemic acidosis

Metabolic acidosis of varying degree is a classical feature of both acute and chronic renal failure and has traditionally been attributed to failure of the kidneys to excrete hydrogen ions derived from 'fixed acids' – class III acids of Table 1. The remaining nephrons are usually able to lower the urinary pH to the normal minimum value, but occasionally failure of proximal bicarbonate reabsorption prevents achievement of the minimum urinary pH until the plasma bicarbonate has been substantially lowered, and, if the primary condition giving rise to the overall glomerulotubular failure has principally affected the renal papilla, some intrinsic acidification defect may exist. However, the fact that acidification is usually normal means that the phosphate buffers in the urine can be fully titrated; titratable acid excretion is therefore commonly normal in the steady state, even though phosphate excretion often has to be maintained by a high plasma phosphate and secondary hyperparathyroidism. The excretion of ammonium is, however, low, presumably both because of loss of glutaminase containing proximal tubules and because the supply of glutamine is curtailed by impairment of renal blood flow. The classic explanation of the acidosis of renal failure has therefore been that the diminished supply of ammonia lowers the ability of the tubular contents to buffer secreted hydrogen ions and that the minimum pH of the urine is therefore attained before the normal content of buffered hydrogen ion is achieved.

However, if as indicated earlier in this section, the ammonium cannot act as a urinary buffer, an alternative explanation has to be sought for the acidosis of uraemia. Atkinson and Camien have suggested that the nitrogen which, in renal insufficiency fails to be excreted as ammonium, is diverted to the liver where it is converted into the urea, with hydrogen ion production as a result (see above). The acidosis of acute or chronic generalized renal failure is therefore due to overproduction of urea, not to failure of excretion of hydrogen ions in the urine as ammonium ions. As indicated above, the elevation of anion gap in uraemic acidosis is usually relatively modest, and the unmeasured anions have not been well characterized, but include minor contributions from phosphate and sulphate. When there is an element of proximal bicarbonate wastage, the anion gap may not be grossly raised, and chloride may be reabsorbed instead of bicarbonate, giving rise to moderate hyperchloraemia.

Diabetic ketoacidosis

The pathogenesis of hyperglycaemic ketotic diabetic coma is described in detail elsewhere (see Chapter 11.11). Only the acid–base disturbance will be discussed here. Though the acidosis has been conventionally regarded as being due mainly to overproduction of ketoacids by the liver, recent evidence has suggested that, although the anions of ketoacids are indeed generated in the liver, the hydrogen ions are wholly or partly derived from other tissues.

Diabetic ketoacidosis has usually been regarded as a classic high anion gap metabolic acidosis in which extracellular bicarbonate has been simply titrated by the ketoacids. If this were the case, the fall in plasma bicarbonate should roughly equal the rise in anion gap and the plasma concentration of ketoacids. However, Adrogué and colleagues have shown that, whilst under some conditions this is true, the situation is frequently more complex. Patients who present in ketoacidosis with relatively well-preserved renal function tended to have an elevation of anion gap which is much less than the fall in bicarbonate. This appears to be due to the loss of large quantities of ketoacid anions in the urine and concomitant retention of chloride to maintain electroneutrality. This process leads to hyperchloraemia which, together with the urinary loss of ketones, results in a relatively low elevation of anion gap compared with the bicarbonate deficit. On the other hand, patients who have relatively poor renal function on admission, because of dehydration, lose much smaller quantities of ketoacid anions in the urine and present with a more classical high anion gap metabolic acidosis.

The total ketone body concentration in blood in the well-controlled fed diabetic patient attending a diabetic clinic is about 0.1 mmol/l. In diabetic ketoacidosis the concentration is often above 10 mmol/l and can rise as high as 30 mmol/l. Though there are many mild cases, some of the severest acidoses observed in clinical practice may be seen in diabetic ketoacidosis, with arterial pH values as low as 6.8 being not uncommon. The minimum possible urinary pH is achieved (4.5 to 5.3). At the lower of these urine pH values about half the urinary ketoacids are undissociated and some hydrogen ions are lost in this way.

With insulin and fluid therapy (see below), metabolism of the ketones via oxidation generates alkali returning the blood and tissue pH to normal over the course of several hours. Those patients who have presented with a near classic high anion gap acidosis tend to recover their plasma bicarbonate concentration more rapidly on treatment, since they have lost less ketoacid anions in the urine and therefore less potential alkali than those presenting with relatively normal anion gaps.

The clinical picture of diabetic ketoacidosis may be complicated in several ways. Volume depletion caused by fluid loss via an osmotic diuresis or vomiting may compromise renal function. Complex acid–base changes can occur during treatment. Metabolic alkalosis can follow ketoacidosis when vomiting has been severe and when excessive amounts of bicarbonate have been infused to treat the acidaemia. In such circumstances, although arterial blood pH may initially be returned to normal, the quantity of acid anions in the form of ketone bodies remains high as does the anion gap. When the ketone bodies are metabolized during treatment metabolic alkalosis ensues.

Another accompanying abnormality may be of lactic acidosis, either developing during therapy, or playing a major role in the pathogenesis of the presenting acidosis. During the therapy of diabetic ketoacidosis, if the blood sugar is falling satisfactorily and the blood ketone concentration is also decreasing, the persistence of a severe metabolic acidosis should alert the clinician to the possibility of supervening lactic acidosis. This is a relatively rare event, but much more common (in 5 to 10 per cent of cases of diabetic ketoacidosis) is a significant contribution to the initial metabolic acidosis by the accumulation of lactic acid to concentrations of 5 mmol/l or above. This occurs particularly when there is shock or hypoxia or infection as an underlying condition. In most cases these concentrations fall with successful treatment of ketoacidosis but may, on occasions, rise further late in the progress of the disease.

Lactic acidosis

NATURE AND CLASSIFICATION

In a normal person, the concentration of lactate in venous blood varies within the narrow limits of 0.6 to 1.2 mmol/l. It is relatively low after fasting and rises after meals, but the homeostatic mechanisms are such as to maintain the concentration within the limits defined above. The main exception to this is severe physical exercise where the concentration may rise to 10 mmol/l or above, rapidly returning to normal on cessation of exercise. Lactic acid has a pK of 3.86 and thus over the physiological range of pH is virtually completely dissociated, so that the generation of the lactate ion in body tissues is accompanied by a similar amount of hydrogen ion.

Regulation of lactate metabolism may be disturbed in such a way as to cause the accumulation of lactic acid. These conditions can be divided into two groups: (1) hyperlactataemia, in which there is raised lactate concentration without changes in blood pH, and (2) lactic acidosis, when the rise in lactate concentration and the accompanying hydrogen ion accumulation is sufficient to lower the blood pH. Many definitions of lactic acidosis exist, and a working definition is that lactic acidosis is characterized by a persistently raised blood lactate concentration together with a lowered blood pH. The acidosis is seldom significant unless blood lactate exceeds 5 mmol/l. Cases of lactic acidosis fall into two groups. In Type A lactic acidosis, which is the most common, the patients have signs of poor tissue perfusion with or without hypoxia. Patients with haemorrhagic shock or a severe myocardial infarct and left ventricular failure provide good examples of this type. The type B patients, however, do not have signs of tissue hypoxia or underperfusion except as a secondary and late event. The type B cases can be further subclassified into those occurring as a result of the administration of certain drugs, chemicals and toxic compounds, and those in which the patient has an inherited metabolic defect which results in lactate accumulation (a detailed classification is given in Table 2). Many of the causes listed in this table are rare, being the subject of single case reports. The vast majority of information has been collected from the study of either patients with shock (type A) or those associated with biguanide therapy – usually phenformin (type B). The condition has been almost exclusively confined to the accumulation of the natural L(+) isomer of lactic acid. Although humans have the capacity to metabolize the D-isomer, it is not a product of normal metabolism, but a small amount is ingested in food and produced by bacterial metabolism in the gut. A few cases of D-lactic acidosis in humans have been described due to excessive D-lactic acid production in the gut, related to the presence of an unusual distribution of bacterial flora commonly associated with short gut syndromes.

The clinical presentation in type B lactic acidosis is fairly uniform, the patients having the following collection of symptoms listed in order of frequency: hyperventilation or dyspnoea, stupor or coma, vomiting, drowsiness, and abdominal pain. The onset of symptoms and signs is usually rapid with development of the acidosis over the course of a few hours accompanied by a deterioration in the level of consciousness which varies from mild confusion to coma and may, in the early stages, be accompanied by profound lethargy. Although by definition there is initially no clinical evidence of poor tissue perfusion or hypoxia, patients with severe type B lactic acidosis commonly become shocked after a few hours.

Although these symptoms and signs are not specific, some indication that lactic acidosis may be present can be obtained from general clinical assessment and biochemical tests. Lactic acidosis has been described in association with many disorders but most frequently with diabetes mellitus (especially in association with biguanide therapy), liver disease, renal impairment, acute pancreatitis, bacterial infections, septicaemia, leukaemia and lymphoma. Although the reported cases may reflect the experience and specialty of the reporting author rather than the true incidence, the associations listed above may alert the clinician to the possibility of lactic acid accumulation as a cause of a metabolic acidosis. An indication that the metabolic acidosis is due to the accumulation of organic acids may be obtained by the finding of a high anion gap. The definitive diagnosis depends on the identification of lactate as the organic anion causing the acidosis. The measurement of lactate in blood is simple, rapid, and specific through the use of enzymatic spectrophotometric micromethods. In patients with hyperglycaemic ketotic diabetic coma a substantial contribution to the metabolic acidosis can be made by lactate, and, occasionally, while the patient may not have a very raised blood lactate concentration at presentation, lactic acidosis may develop during the course of treatment (see above).

PATHOGENESIS

Disturbances of lactate homeostasis sufficient to cause an acidosis must be due to: (1) an increased lactate production; (2) impaired lactate utilization; or (3) a combination of these two processes.

Up to 70 per cent of the total daily lactate production of about 1.2 mol/24 h/70 kg body weight in resting humans is taken up by the liver. Many patients with liver disease have an elevated resting blood lactate concentration and their ability to dispose of an exogenous lactate load is impaired. Some 30 to 40 per cent of patients with lactate acidosis have evidence of liver disease and thus many explanations of the pathogenesis of lactic acidosis have centred upon the liver. Although hyperlactataemia is a common finding in patients with liver disease, only a few develop lactic acidosis. The hyperlactataemia in liver disease can be explained by impaired utilization but before lactic acidosis can

develop the extent of the impairment must be severe or increased production must be present. There was no doubt that use of the antidiabetic biguanide phenformin resulted in an unacceptably high incidence of type B lactic acidosis. The drug has been shown to both increase lactate production in the splanchnic bed and decrease hepatic lactate uptake. Increased peripheral production of lactic acid may also be involved. Phenformin has now been withdrawn, but another biguanide, metformin, is still widely used. The incidence of lactic acidosis during metformin therapy is an order of magnitude less than for phenformin, but occasional severe and fatal cases are still seen, nearly always in patients with renal insufficiency. Metformin should not be administered to such patients, or to those at particular risk of suffering a decrease in renal function during intercurrent illness.

Increased lactate production is probably the main contributing factor in type A lactic acidosis but impaired utilization is also involved. The latter factor may be a result of impaired blood flow and energy supply in those tissues usually removing lactate and both animal and human experimental data show that organs which usually remove lactate may produce lactate in the presence of shock. Infusion of fructose, sorbitol, or xylitol have all been associated with lactic acidosis in humans and during fructose infusion the liver becomes a site of net lactate production because a major portion of the infused substrate is metabolized to lactate at a rate which is greater than the removal capacity of the extrahepatic tissues. In the cases described in association with malignant disease, the increased lactate production consequent upon the high glycolytic capacity of malignant tissue is probably important.

Overall the prognosis of lactic acidosis is poor, the mortality being very high in type A cases where their survival is clearly related to the blood lactate concentration on presentation. A blood lactate concentration of 9 mmol/l or greater is accompanied by a mortality of 80 per cent or greater. In the type B cases, the mortality is substantial, depending on the aetiology, but lower than in type A cases. There is some evidence that since the withdrawal of phenformin in most countries, the incidence of type B cases has fallen and the prognosis improved.

Acidosis associated with alcohol (ethanol) ingestion

In normal subjects, relatively modest ethanol ingestion after a 12 to 24 h period without adequate food intake may result in quite severe hypoglycaemia. Because of the poor or absent calorie intake, liver glycogen reserves have fallen to a low level and maintenance of blood glucose depends solely on gluconeogenesis from lactate and other substrate. Ethanol inhibits gluconeogenesis by diversion of NAD^+ for its own metabolism; lactate therefore accumulates and a significant though usually mild lactic acidosis may be seen. Administration of glucose and refeeding is all that is needed to deal with this situation, but it should be stressed that the hypoglycaemic element of this syndrome may be dangerously severe.

In chronic alcoholics, many of whom have significant hepatic damage, a range of acid–base disorders may be seen. In alcoholic ketosis, there is a history of a longer period of heavy alcohol ingestion, culminating in a few days of severe vomiting, and (usually) cessation of alcohol intake for that reason. A few of these patients have significant acidosis due to ketoacid accumulation, but in others, metabolic alkalosis is seen, presumably because the ketoacidosis is outweighed by the effects of vomiting. Whatever the acid–base disturbance in alcoholic ketosis, administration of glucose and rehydration is usually adequate to deal with the metabolic disturbance. Occasionally, particularly when alcohol intake has not been stopped, moderate or severe lactic acidosis occurs, presumably related both to liver damage, the direct effect of ethanol on gluconeogenesis, and other intercurrent factors such as gastrointestinal haemorrhage. Finally, alcoholic intake may precipitate hepatic encephalopathy in those prone; respiratory alkalosis is commonly seen in these patients, due, it is suggested, to direct stimulation of the respiratory centre by ammonium and amines responsible for encephalopathy.

Methanol-induced acidosis

(See also Section 8)

A severe metabolic acidosis of somewhat delayed onset is a characteristic feature of methanol poisoning. Formic and lactic acids are responsible for the acidosis. Formic acid is generated as a result of the metabolism of methanol via formaldehyde and has been shown to accumulate in blood in large quantities but the extent of accumulation may not always account for the whole of the increase in anion gap in poisoned patients. In some cases, substantially raised blood lactate concentrations may be found. Lactate may accumulate because of the inhibition of gluconeogenesis from lactate by methanol or the effect of formaldehyde in inhibiting oxidative phosphorylation.

Salicylate poisoning

(See also Section 8)

The initial acid–base abnormality in cases of salicylate poisoning is a respiratory alkalosis secondary to direct stimulation of the respiratory centre. Children, however, rapidly develop metabolic acidosis, and in adults metabolic acidosis may occur as a later event. The metabolic acidosis is thought to be secondary to the effects of salicylate upon intermediary metabolism, particularly its action in uncoupling oxidative phosphorylation and inhibiting lactate disposal via gluconeogenesis; the acids responsible are the salicylate itself, the ketoacids acetoacetate and 3-hydroxybutyrate, and lactate.

Principles of treatment of acid–base disorders

In general the mainstay of treatment is to eliminate the primary cause of the disorder, the acid–base control mechanisms then restoring the normal situation in due course. However, it may be necessary to make a direct attempt to restore normality and this is more often the case in respiratory and metabolic acidosis than in the alkaloses. The treatment of respiratory failure is dealt with elsewhere (Section 17).

Acute metabolic acidosis

In deciding whether to treat acute metabolic acidosis the main difficulty is in assessing the relative risks of treatment against the advantages. The main potential advantages are improvement in cardiac performance, redistribution of blood volume away from the central circulation, correction of hyperkalaemia, restoration of hepatic lactate removal, and alleviation of distressing hyperventilation. Disadvantages lie in adverse effects on the oxygen dissociation curve, and, in the case of lactic and ketoacidosis, the production of 'alkaline overshoot' due to metabolism of the organic acids after the arterial blood pH has been normalized.

Major controversies have arisen in the past decade concerning the use of sodium bicarbonate as an alkalinizing agent in acute metabolic acidosis. It has become clear that the value of such therapy depends very much on the cause of the metabolic acidosis and also on the particular circumstances of individual patients. There are a few situations in which sodium bicarbonate is clearly beneficial, and these are summarized below.

1. *Metabolic acidosis in severe renal failure.* Sodium bicarbonate here may correct hyperkalaemia by inducing shift of potassium into the cellular compartment. It may also relieve distressing hyperventilation and may make time for definitive renal support therapy to be introduced. If the patient is already fluid-overloaded, the bicarbonate should be administered intravenously as a hypertonic solution (8.4 per cent; 1 mmol/ml). If the patient is dehydrated the isotonic solution (1.4 per cent) should be given.

2. *In severe diarrhoea (cholera).* It has been shown in patients with cholera and metabolic acidosis due to dehydration and alkali loss that sodium bicarbonate is superior to sodium chloride. These patients have severe peripheral venoconstriction, displacing their blood volume towards the lungs. The administration of sodium chloride may thus induce pulmonary oedema before the volume depletion has been corrected. Sodium bicarbonate appears to relieve the peripheral venoconstruction and full replacement is thus made less hazardous.

3. *In exacerbations of renal tubular acidosis.* Sodium bicarbonate is of clear value in this situation, but it is of the utmost importance to correct hypokalaemia before alkali therapy, or at least in conjunction with it, and with frequent monitoring of plasma potassium. If this is not done, systemic alkalinization may further worsen the hypokalaemia, with potentially fatal results.

It is in the treatment of lactic acidosis, particularly type A, and in diabetic ketoacidosis that the uncertainty of the value of bicarbonate therapy principally lies. In a number of animal models of lactic acidosis, treatment with bicarbonate has been shown to produce less favourable haemodynamic and metabolic results than equivalent amounts of sodium chloride. In the only available randomized cross-over trial of sodium bicarbonate versus sodium chloride in critically ill patients with lactic acidosis due to shock, there was no advantage of one therapy over the other and increases in cardiac output were transient.

The theoretical basis for the failure of sodium bicarbonate to produce the expected improvement is based on the probability that alterations in intracellular pH in various organs are more important determinants of the functional changes seen in metabolic acidosis than is the lowered extracellular pH. This has been shown experimentally to be true for both inotropic effects and hepatic lactate disposal. When sodium bicarbonate is infused, it titrates acid, with elevation of partial pressure of carbon dioxide. As partial pressure of carbon dioxide traverses cell membranes more rapidly than bicarbonate, cells may be acidified by bicarbonate infusion even though extracellular pH is elevated. It is, however, generally very difficult to predict cell pH changes from changes in extracellular pH, partial pressure of carbon dioxide, and bicarbonate as many factors other than partial pressure of carbon dioxide affect cell pH, and these factors vary between organs.

Considerable interest has been shown in the observation that in circulatory insufficiency the partial pressure of carbon dioxide of mixed venous blood may be much greater than in arterial blood, which is often normal. On occasion, bicarbonate therapy exaggerates this difference. It has therefore been inferred that bicarbonate therapy must be acidifying the tissues by the mechanism outlined above. However, consideration of the mechanisms responsible for the elevated mixed partial pressure of carbon dioxide suggest that only if arterial partial pressure of carbon dioxide is raised by bicarbonate therapy is cellular acidification likely to occur. Whether arterial partial pressure of carbon dioxide is elevated by bicarbonate therapy depends on numerous factors, including cardiac output, ventilation, the dead space to total volume ratio and, in particular, the rate of administration of bicarbonate. It is the authors' view that if raised arterial partial pressure of carbon dioxide were the only reason for the doubt about bicarbonate, this could simply be obviated by administering it more slowly than in the customary rapid infusion protocols.

The following practical guidance to therapy is empirical and largely based on current practice rather than proper trials:

1. *Diabetic ketoacidosis.* In this condition, it is generally accepted that provided arterial blood pH is not below 7.0, bicarbonate treatment is not indicated. Rehydration and insulin therapy result in improved renal function, a fall in ketone body production and increase in ketone body metabolism, all of which contribute to the correction of the acidosis. When arterial blood pH is less than 7.0, many give just sufficient bicar-

bonate to bring arterial blood pH above 7.0, with careful attention to changes in plasma potassium, but there is no evidence which indicates this is better than rehydration and insulin alone. If bicarbonate is given, it is essential that it should be isotonic (1.4 per cent). To give hypertonic bicarbonate would merely exacerbate the already present hyperosmolality. The amount required only seldom exceeds 0.5 to 1 litre, given intravenously over 60 to 90 min. More bicarbonate creates an 'alkaline' overshoot, as the metabolism of ketone bodies itself generates bicarbonate.

2. *Lactic acidosis*. By far the most common dilemma is in type A lactic acidosis, i.e. in shock. Of paramount importance is the correction of hypovolaemia and cardiogenic and other factors which are the primary causes of the condition. Such correction will relieve tissue anaerobism and promote intracellular metabolism of the lactate ion, with consequent alkalinization and regeneration of bicarbonate. Whether the administration of exogenous bicarbonate can trigger or hasten this process is uncertain, and the only trial which addresses this question in anything like a satisfactory fashion offers no support for this idea. Nevertheless, the possibility of bicarbonate helping in some circumstances cannot be ruled out. If it is given, it should be given relatively slowly, as the isotonic solution unless there is a fluid overload problem, and probably only sufficient to raise arterial blood pH to a 'safe' level (e.g. 7.1 to 7.2). It is particularly in the situation of circulatory insufficiency when the effect of rapid blood alkalinization on the haemoglobin oxygen dissociation curve might be deleterious, since the impaired oxygen release to the tissues cannot be compensated for by an increase in blood flow.

In the special case of the acidosis of cardiac arrest – which is a complex situation in which tissue acidosis is contributed to by accumulation of metabolic carbon dioxide, lactic acid and hydrolysis of adenosine triphosphate (ATP) – the previous priority given to infusion of sodium bicarbonate has disappeared, because of lack of evidence of efficacy and use of alkaline overshoot when lactate is metabolised on restoration of circulation. Hypertonic sodium bicarbonate is now only recommended as a secondary treatment after prolonged arrest.

The amount of alkali therapy, if given, should be determined by an iterative process of administration of a relatively small quantity (e.g. 80 mmol), followed by reassessment of the clinical condition and arterial blood pH, and partial pressure of carbon dioxide with the aid of serial plots on Fig. 2 before repeating the cycle. Attempts to calculate the amount of alkali needed from the 'base excess' have little validity both for reasons outlined earlier and, because the primary cause of proton accumulation may still be operative, such estimates can in no way replace the need for repeated clinical and biochemical monitoring.

There has been considerable interest in the possible use of alkalinizing agents other than sodium bicarbonate. Of these alternative alkalinizing agents, sodium lactate has the disadvantage that lactate has to be metabolized before the alkalinizing effect occurs and in some patients lactate metabolism is impaired. Trishydroxyaminomethane (THAM) has the theoretical advantages of dealing with intracellular as well as extracellular acidosis, and does not involve the administration of a sodium load. However, hypoglycaemia and adverse effects on the renal tubules are possible complications of its use and its place in the treatment of acidosis is uncertain. It has recently been suggested that an equivalent mixture of sodium bicarbonate and sodium carbonic ('carbicarb') would have advantages over sodium bicarbonate, because the infusion of this mixture is accompanied by little if any rise in partial pressure of carbon dioxide. Though 'carbicarb' compares favourably with sodium bicar-

bonate in some animal models of metabolic acidosis, it does not in others. At the time of writing, it has not been demonstrated to have important advantages in clinical metabolic acidosis. Another agent for treating lactic acidosis is sodium dichloroacetate, which increases the metabolism of lactate and results in cell alkalinization. However, a recent multicentre trial of sodium dichloroacetate in patients with lactic acidosis, most of whom were receiving pressor or inotropic therapy, showed no haemodynamic or survival advantage of the drug over a sodium chloride-treated control group, despite reducing blood lactate levels and slightly increasing arterial pH.

Chronic metabolic acidosis

Chronic acidosis is mainly seen in chronically uraemic subjects. Here oral bicarbonate may be helpful in the severe cases. It may improve well being and increase tolerance and there is evidence that it protects against the osteomalacic component of renal osteodystrophy and the negative nitrogen balances which may be seen in these patients. It may usefully constitute part of the treatment in patients with chronic renal failure and renal salt wasting due to chronic renal failure. The use of bicarbonate in the maintenance therapy of renal tubular acidosis is discussed in Section 20.19.

Metabolic alkalosis

It is seldom necessary to treat metabolic alkalosis by direct attempts at acidification. However, occasions arise when a severe metabolic alkalosis unrelated to potassium and chloride deficiency may need treating because of tetany or suspected effects in the cerebral circulation. In such rare instances oral ammonium chloride or intravenous infusion of arginine hydrochloride may be indicated.

REFERENCES

Adrogué, H.J., Wilson, H., Boyd, A.E., Suki, W.N. and Eknoyan, G. (1982). Plasma acid-base patterns in diabetic ketoacidosis. *New England Journal of Medicine*, **307**, 1603–10.

Arieff, A.I. (1991). Indications for use of bicarbonate in patients with metabolic acidosis. *British Journal of Anaesthesia*, **67**, 165–77.

Atkinson, D.E. and Camien, M.N. (1982). The role of urea synthesis in the removal of metabolic bicarbonate and the regulation of blood pH. *Current topics in cellular regulation*, pp. 261–302. Academic Press, London.

Campbell, E.J.M. (1984). Hydrogen ion (acid–base) regulation. In *Clinical physiology*, (5th edn), (ed E.J.M. Campbell, C.J. Dickinson, J.D.H. Slater, C.R.W. Edwards and E.K. Sikora). Blackwell Scientific Publications, Oxford.

Cohen, R.D. (1991). Roles of the liver and kidney in acid-base regulation and its disorders. *British Journal of Anaesthesia*, **67**(1), 54–164.

Cohen, R.D. and Woods, H.F. (1976). *Clinical and biochemical aspects of lactic acidosis*. Blackwell Scientific Publications, Oxford.

Cooper, D.J., Walley, K.R., Wiggs, B.R., Russell, J.A. (1990). Bicarbonate does not improve haemodynamics in critically ill patients who have lactic acidosis. *Annals of Internal Medicine*, **112**, 492–8.

Emmett, M. and Narins, R.G. (1977). Clinical use of the anion gap. *Medicine* (Baltimore), **56**, 38–54.

Hindman, B.J. (1990). Sodium bicarbonate in the treatment of subtypes of acute lactic acidosis: physiological considerations. *Anesthesiology*, **72**, 1064–76.

Mitchell, J.H., Wildenthal, K. and Johnson, R.C. (1972). The effects of acid–base disturbance on cardiovascular and pulmonary function. *Kidney International*, **1**, 375–89.

Oliver, J. and Bourke, E. (1975). Adaptations in urea and ammonium excretion in metabolic acidosis in the rat: a reinterpretation. *Clinical Science and Molecular Medicine*, **48**, 515–20.

11.15 α₁-Antitrypsin deficiency

R. W. CARRELL and D. A. LOMAS

Introduction

People of European descent are particularly prone to disease arising from a genetic deficiency of the plasma protein α_1-antitrypsin. This is a 394-amino acid, 52 kDa, acute phase glycoprotein synthesized by the liver and by macrophages and present in the plasma at a concentration of 1.5 to 3.5 g/l. It functions as an inhibitor of a range of proteolytic enzymes but its primary role is to inhibit the enzyme neutrophil elastase. Activated neutrophil leucocytes release elastase to break down connective tissue at sites of inflammation. This breakdown is limited by the antielastase activity of α_1-antitrypsin but if the plasma concentration of this protein falls below 40 per cent of normal, as in genetic deficiency, then unimpeded tissue destruction may ensue. The most vulnerable tissue is the elastic connective tissue of the lung and clinically the major consequence of α_1-antitrypsin deficiency is the premature onset of emphysema. This association between the deficiency of a protease inhibitor and the loss of lung elasticity has drawn attention to the way in which other factors, particularly cigarette smoking, contribute to the onset of emphysema.

Structure and function

SERPIN SUPERFAMILY

α_1-Antitrypsin is the archetype of the serine protease inhibitor, or serpin, superfamily, members of which have closely related structures and functions. These inhibitors control the various inflammatory cascades, including coagulation (antithrombin), complement activation (C1-inhibitor) and fibrinolysis (α_2-antiplasmin). A surprising member of the family is angiotensinogen, which retains the same overall structure as the other members of the family but has lost its function as a protease inhibitor.

MOLECULAR FUNCTION AND REACTIVE CENTRE

α_1-Antitrypsin functions by presenting its reactive centre methionine residue on an exposed loop of the molecule such that it forms an ideal substrate for the enzyme neutrophil elastase (Fig. 1). The exact fit between enzyme and inhibitor causes them to form a tightly bound 1 : 1 complex, which inhibits the enzyme and allows it to be eliminated from the circulation. A reduction in the activity of antitrypsin may result from genetic deficiency, from oxidation of the methionine residue or from cleavage of the reactive centre loop.

Genetic deficiency

α_1-Antitrypsin is subject to genetic variation resulting from mutations in the 12.2 kb, 7-exon gene at q31–31.2 on chromosome 14. Over 75 allelic variants have been reported and classified using the Pi (protease inhibitor) nomenclature, which assesses antitrypsin mobility in isoelectric focusing analysis. Mutations are inherited by simple Mendelian trait; the normal genotype is designated PiMM, a heterozygote for the Z gene is PiMZ and a homozygote is PiZZ.

DEFICIENCY

The medically interesting variants are those associated with deficiency: namely the S and Z mutants and the uncommon Null (non-production) gene. Most important are the S and Z variants of α_1-antitrypsin, which are commonly found in Europeans. About 6 per cent of people of Northern European descent are heterozygotes for the S variant (PiMS) and 3 to 4 per cent for the Z variant (PiMZ).

Each of the deficiency genes results in a characteristic decrease in the plasma concentration of α_1-antitrypsin; the S variant forms 60 per cent of the normal M concentration and the Z variant 15 per cent. The critical level for health is a plasma concentration of at least 40 per cent of normal and therefore, the common heterozygote states MZ (60 per cent) and MS (80 per cent), and the S homozygote (60 per cent) do not pose a threat to health. However the ZZ homozygote (15 per cent) and the SZ heterozygote (40 per cent) do predispose to emphysema.

In summary, 1 in 10 Northern Europeans is a carrier of a deficiency gene and 1 in 2500 has the PiZZ genotype which predisposes to disease. A greater number again are PiSZ heterozygotes which results in 'at risk' plasma levels of α_1-antitrypsin.

MOLECULAR PATHOLOGY OF S AND Z VARIANTS

The S and Z variants of α_1-antitrypsin are both due to single amino acid replacements. In the S variant there is a substitution of a valine residue for the glutamic acid at position 264; this amino acid forms a stabilizing salt bridge in the molecule and the mutation results in misfolding with increased turnover of the newly synthesized protein and lower plasma levels. The Z abnormality differs from the S in that it affects secretion rather than synthesis. The gene is normally translated but 85 per cent of the Z antitrypsin is retained within the endoplasmic reticulum, with only 15 per cent entering the circulation. The Z mutation results from the substitution of a positively charged lysine for a negatively charged glutamic acid residue at position 342 at the base of the reactive centre loop (Fig. 1). This mutation distorts the relationship between the loop and the β-pleated (A) sheet that forms the major feature of the molecule. The consequent perturbation in structure allows the reactive centre loop of one antitrypsin molecule to lock into the A sheet of a second to form fibril-like loop-sheet polymers. The formation of these polymers is temperature and concentration dependent and localized to the endoplasmic reticulum of the hepatocyte (Fig. 2(a)). These chains of polymers become interwoven to form the insoluble aggregates which are the hallmark of antitrypsin liver disease (Fig. 2(b)).

Oxidation and inactivation

The need for an exact fit between enzyme and inhibitor provides a molecular explanation for the causative relationship between cigarette

Fig. 1 α_1-Antitrypsin: inactivation by oxidation of the reactive centre methionine residue or by cleavage of the reactive centre loop.

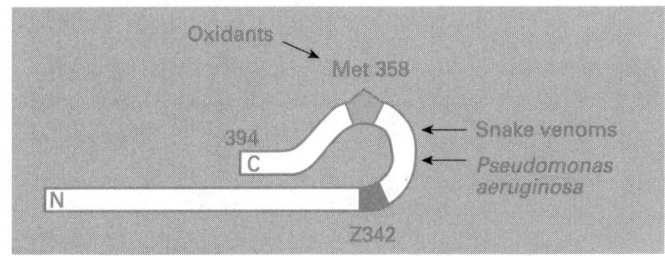

smoking and emphysema. The reactive centre of methionine of α_1-antitrypsin is readily oxidized to the much larger methionine sulphoxide, with a consequent loss of function as an inhibitor of elastase. Thus the oxidants released by stimulated neutrophils can oxidize the key methionine residue and switch off the activity of α_1-antitrypsin. Normally this switch mechanism is advantageous in allowing elastase activity to continue in the immediate vicinity of an inflammatory focus. However, it becomes disadvantageous when there is chronic and excessive leucocyte activity, as occurs in the lungs of a heavy smoker.

Cleavage and inactivation

The presence of the exposed molecular loop of antitrypsin renders it vulnerable to inactivation by other proteases such as those contained in snake venoms. The damaging effects of pulmonary infection with *Pseudomonas aeruginosa* is similarly explained by the secretion of a protease that specifically cleaves the exposed loop of α_1-antitrypsin allowing fulminant damage to lung connective tissue (Fig. 1).

Fig. 2 Electron microscopy (20 000 × magnification) of a hepatocyte from a Z homozygote showing a massive inclusion (arrow) in the endoplasmic reticulum. (b) Electron microscopy (222 000 × magnification) of Z antitrypsin loop-sheet polymers *in vitro* (inset and arrowed) and isolated from a patient undergoing liver transplantation for Z antitrypsin cirrhosis. The *in vitro* material is negatively stained with uranyl acetate whilst the hepatic inclusions are highlighted with platinum rotary shadowing.

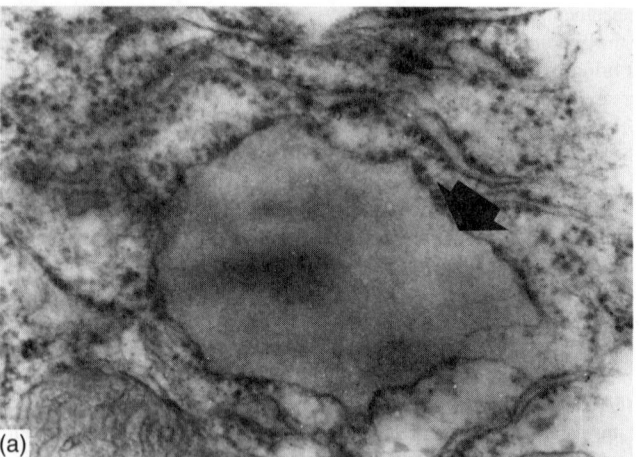

(a)

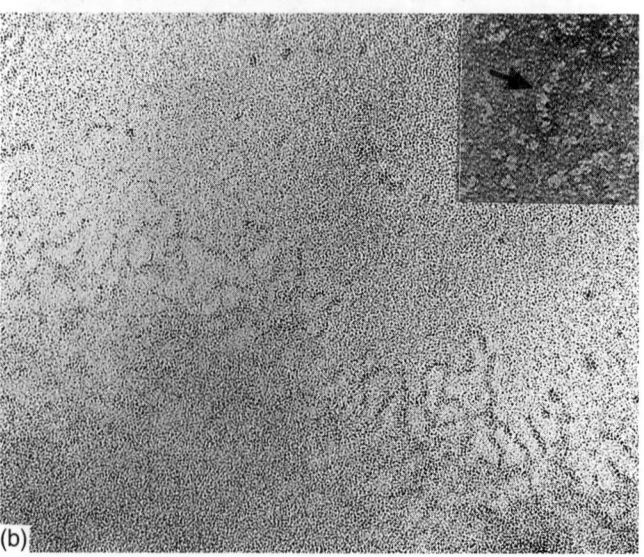

(b)

Clinical features

α_1-ANTITRYPSIN DEFICIENCY AND EMPHYSEMA

The association between α_1-antitrypsin deficiency and the development of premature panlobular emphysema was first described by Laurell and Eriksson in 1963. Patients usually present with increasing dyspnoea and weight loss, with cor pulmonale and polycythaemia occurring late in the course of the disease. Chest radiographs typically show bilateral basal emphysema with paucity and pruning of the basal pulmonary vessels. Upper lobe vascularization is relatively normal. Ventilation perfusion radioisotope scans and angiography also show abnormalities with a lower zone distribution. Lung function tests are typical for emphysema with a reduced forced expiratory volume/forced vital capacity (FEV_1/FVC) ratio and low gas transfer factor.

The association of α_1-antitrypsin with the development of premature emphysema has led to the wider conclusion that emphysema results from an imbalance between proteases and antiproteases within the lung. Undoubtedly the situation is more complex than a simple balance between elastase and α_1-antitrypsin, both in terms of the numbers of enzymes and inhibitors involved, and the contribution of other mechanisms. Nevertheless, the elastase-α_1-antitrypsin balance clearly illustrates the processes involved in the development of emphysema and the interplay between the environmental and genetic factors that determine its onset.

Decline in lung function in health and disease

As with other tissues, there is a decline in the elasticity of the lungs with increasing age. Clinically the most convenient measure of elasticity is the forced expiratory volume in 1 second (FEV_1), which is approximately 3500 ml in young adults. After the age of 30 years in healthy non-smokers, the forced expiratory volume decreases by 35 ml/year, although there is considerable individual variation. By old age, most people will have an appreciable loss of lung elasticity but only occasionally in the non-smoker will this be clinically apparent. The loss of forced expiratory volume is accelerated to 80 ml/year in the ZZ antitrypsin homozygote. As a consequence there is a hastened but still variable onset of emphysema. Most PiZZ non-smokers are free from dyspnoea up to the age of 50 years with an average age of death from respiratory disease being 67 years. Again there is considerable individual variation and, particularly in women, there is a good likelihood of a full life span without significant respiratory impairment. The outlook, however, is poor for the ZZ antitrypsin homozygote who is a heavy smoker as the loss in forced expiratory volume increases to as much as 300 ml/year. The onset of dyspnoea occurs around the age of 30 years with death from respiratory disease by the age of 50 years.

Smoking and oxidation

The heavy smoker has a large increase in the leucocyte population of the lungs with the secretion of proteolytic enzymes by macrophages as well as by neutrophils. Stimulation of the neutrophils results in the release of oxygen radicals which, together with the free radicals from the tobacco smoke, can oxidize and inactivate α_1-antitrypsin. If these threats are added to the weakened defence of a genetic deficiency of α_1-antitrypsin, the premature breakdown of elastic connective tissue and the early onset of emphysema are inevitable.

LIVER DISEASE

Z α_1-antitrypsin liver disease is characterized by the accumulation of the abnormal antitrypsin as diastase-resistant periodic acid-Schiff positive inclusions in the periportal cells. This insoluble material accumulates within the endoplasmic reticulum of hepatocytes (see Fig. 2) stimulating a massive increase in cellular degradative activity. The PiMZ and SZ individuals are able to degrade much of the abnormal antitrypsin, but not the Z homozygote, in whom aggregation overwhelms the degradative process resulting in antitrypsin accumulation, hepatocellular damage and cell death. The accumulation of antitrypsin within hepatocytes is also seen with two other rare mutations, antitrypsin S_{iiyama} (53 phenylalanine $\rightarrow$ serine) and M_{malton} (52 phenylalanine deletion). Both of these point mutations result in perturbations of antitrypsin structure, which favour loop-sheet polymer formation. The observation that polymer formation is temperature and concentration dependent accounts for the variation in the number and density of liver inclusions between individuals. Antitrypsin is an acute phase protein and, as such, undergoes a manifold increase in production during even minor illnesses. At these times there may also be temperature increases of up to 41°C and the combined effects of the increase in protein concentration and temperature favour rapid polymerization which leads to inclusion formation and liver disease.

Neonatal jaundice and juvenile cirrhosis

Eighty per cent of ZZ antitrypsin homozygote infants show biochemical evidence of hepatocellular damage in the first year of life. One in ten develops neonatal hepatitis which presents as cholestatic jaundice and 6 per cent develop clinical evidence of liver disease without jaundice. These symptoms usually resolve by the second year but 10 to 15 per cent of patients with cholestatic jaundice progress to a juvenile cirrhosis. The reasons for this variable progression are not known; intercurrent illness will certainly contribute but other hormonal and genetic factors may also be involved. Juvenile cirrhosis is three times more common in boys than girls and the likelihood of juvenile cirrhosis may be increased if there is a history of a Z homozygote sibling having developed liver disease. The overall risk of death from liver disease in PiZZ children during childhood is 2 to 3 per cent.

Adult liver disease

All PiZZ individuals have slowly progressive hepatic damage which is often subclinical and only evident as a minor degree of portal fibrosis. However up to 50 per cent of ZZ antitrypsin homozygotes eventually present with clinically evident cirrhosis and occasionally with hepatocellular carcinoma. The presence of Z α_1-antitrypsin deficiency including the heterozygous PiMZ and PiSZ should always be considered before making the diagnosis of cryptogenic cirrhosis.

ASSOCIATED CONDITIONS

α_1-Antitrypsin deficiency is associated with an increased incidence of bronchiectasis, glomerulonephritis and panniculitis and a likely association with inflammatory bowel disease. There is also a considerably increased incidence in both heterozygotes (PiMZ) and homozygotes (PiZZ) of antineutrophil cytoplasm antibodies (c-ANCA) with consequent risk of Wegener's granulomatosis.

Diagnosis

The severe genetic deficiency of α_1-antitrypsin is readily diagnosed by the virtual absence of the α_1-antitrypsin band on protein electrophoresis. The deficiency is then assigned a Pi phenotype according to the migration of the protein on an isoelectric focusing gel. Most cases are detected in this way, as an incidental finding, but in some areas the systematic identification of homozygotes is achieved by neonatal blood-spot testing.

Treatment

The treatment of α_1-antitrypsin deficiency depends largely on the avoidance of stimuli causing repeated pulmonary inflammation – primarily smoking. The lung disease is a result of a deficiency in the antielastase screen. This may be rectified biochemically by intravenous infusions of α_1-antitrypsin and trials have now demonstrated the feasibility of maintaining long-term plasma replacement therapy. This approach has a sound physiological basis but the assessment of the protective effect of replacement therapy has been handicapped by the lack of a properly controlled trial and it may be another decade until firm conclusions can be reached as to its value. There is a good theoretical reason for short-term intravenous supplementation at times of stress such as respiratory infections but this too requires further evaluation.

All Z homozygotes have some liver damage and, as such, would be wise to avoid alcohol abuse. The deduction that loop-sheet polymerization of α_1-antitrypsin complicates the acute phase response highlights the importance of antipyretic agents in infants with PiZZ antitrypsin deficiency. Although this has yet to be proven by clinical trials there is anecdotal evidence that these intercurrent illnesses account for the variation in progression of liver disease in infants. Moreover there is good reason to believe that conservative treatments to lessen pyrexia and the inflammatory response will be of value in reducing α_1-antitrypsin aggregation within hepatocytes and hence liver disease. PiZZ homozygotes should be monitored for the persistence of hyperbilirubinemia as this along with deteriorating results of coagulation studies indicate the need for liver transplantation. Parents with a child with severe Z α_1-antitrypsin liver disease require genetic counselling although the likelihood of similar severe liver damage in a subsequent Z homozygote sibling is less than 5 per cent.

The panniculitis associated with α_1-antitrypsin deficiency usually responds to dapsone 100 to 150 mg daily for 2 to 4 weeks but occasionally necessitates the administration of intravenous α_1-antitrypsin replacement therapy.

REFERENCES

Carrell, R.W., Whisstock, J., and Lomas, D.A. (1994). Conformational changes in serpins and the mechanism of α_1-antitrypsin deficiency. *American Journal of Respiratory and Critical Care Medicine*, **150**, S171–6.

Ibarguen, E., Gross, C.R., Savik, S.K. and Sharp, H.L. (1990). Liver disease in alpha-1-antitrypsin deficiency: prognostic indicators. *Journal of Pediatrics*, **117**, 864–70.

Larsson, C. (1978). Natural history and life expectancy in severe α_1-antitrypsin PiZ. *Acta Medica Scandinavica*, **204**, 345–52.

Laurell, C.-B. and Erikson, S. (1963). The electrophoretic α_1-globin pattern of serum in α_1-antitrypsin deficiency. *Scandinavian Journal of Clinical and Laboratory Investigation*, **15**, 132–40.

Lomas, D.A., Evans, D.Ll., Finch, J.T. and Carrell, R.W. (1992). The mechanism of Z α_1-antitrypsin accumulation in the liver. *Nature*, **357**, 605–607.

Sveger, T. (1988). The natural history of liver disease in α_1-antitrypsin deficient children. *Acta Paediatrica Scandinavica*, **77**, 847–51.

11.16 Metabolic effects of accidental injury and surgery

R. SMITH

Accidental injury is the major cause of death in young people in the Western world, and elective surgery an everyday occurrence. Both produce a spectrum of biochemical change. Modern elective surgery is often so small an insult to the body that its metabolic effects are insignificant; in contrast, multiple injuries cause a widespread metabolic upset, some elements of which are directed towards survival. This metabolic response to injury is the result of many sequential processes.

The first, and the most important, is the effect of the injury itself, which produces powerful afferent stimuli of pain, blood loss, volume depletion, and tissue damage. Secondly is the neuroendocrine response to these stimuli, leading to the production of readily utilizable metabolic fuels, such as glucose, fatty acids, and ketone bodies. Thirdly is variable food deprivation, leading to a reduction in the intake of nitrogen and energy-providing substrates; and fourthly is immobility, which may be prolonged and which leads to loss of muscle and skeletal mass. To these can be added the metabolic effects of sepsis and burns.

Severe injury and complicated surgery lead to complex nutritional deficiencies which require prevention and correction (see Section 10), and although the biochemical effects of injury are not simply those of starvation, they have similarities (Table 1). Severe injury is characterized by an increase in circulating catecholamines and cortisol, by initial hyperglycaemia, and by a greater eventual loss of muscle-derived protein and nitrogen than in starvation alone. In total starvation, weight loss will be more rapid than in uncomplicated injury, but it will be most severe where injury and starvation are combined.

The biochemical effects of injury are related both to its severity and nature; and increase in the following order: elective surgery, multiple injuries, sepsis and burns. In humans the phases originally proposed by Cuthbertson (Fig. 1) are less easy to define than in animals. In the immediate 'ebb' phase the organism is reacting to the injury; rapid neuroendocrine changes occur as the body tries to survive, and there is an equally rapid mobilization of body fuels; in the experimental animal temperature and energy production fall, and severe injury may overwhelm the homeostatic defences so that necrobiosis and death ensue. In man the thermoregulatory response varies and is influenced by the ambient temperature. In survivors this early phase is followed by a 'flow' phase in which biochemical processes accelerate and energy production, metabolic rate, and temperature increase, leading to eventual recovery with catabolism giving way to anabolism and tissue repair.

The length of these phases varies according to many factors, particularly the severity of injury, and some attempt has been made to relate the early biochemical changes to the subsequent outcome. These biochemical changes are begun and orchestrated by the complex neuroendocrine response to injury.

Neuroendocrine response to injury

The neuroendocrine response is complex; again this problem has been more fully studied in experimental animals than in injured humans. Those components mobilizing metabolic fuels include increased activity of the sympathetic nervous system, increased secretion of hypothalamic hormones which stimulate adrenocorticotrophic hormone (ACTH) production by the anterior pituitary, and the release of vasopressin from the posterior pituitary. Stimulation of the sympathetic nervous system increases adrenaline (epinephrine) and glucagon secretion and sup-

Table 1 *Similarities and differences between the effects of injury and starvation*

	Total starvation	Injury	Starvation and injury
Weight loss	++	+	+++
Nitrogen loss	+	++	+++
Blood glucose	↓	↑	
Blood alanine	↓	↓	↓
Blood BCAA[a]	↑	↑	↑
Endocrine response			
Catecholamine	↓	↑	↑
Cortisol	↓	↕	↕
Insulin	↓	↓ (early)	↓
Metabolic rate	↓	↑	↑
Ketonaemia	++	Variable	Variable
Water and sodium	Early loss	Retention	Retention
Potassium loss	+	++	+++

[a]BCAA; branched chain amino acids—leucine, isoleucine, and valine.

presses that of insulin; release of vasopressin has its main influence on salt and water balance, but may have other biochemical effects; and the increased secretion of ACTH produces a wide range of metabolic effects through enhanced corticosteroid secretion.

The effect of trauma on the hypothalamopituitary axis varies with the type of injury. It seems that ACTH is released in response to all noxious stimuli. Acute injury may also stimulate the production of endorphins, prolactin, vasopressin, and intermediate lobe peptides. Interestingly, vasopressin release is increased by only some forms of injury. The production of other pituitary hormones, such as growth hormone, thyrotrophins, and gonadotrophins, may also be variably affected. In prolonged stress with continuing production of ACTH, gonadotrophin production is inhibited.

The pituitary responses to injury result from changes in the hypothalamus, and most require connections with other parts of the nervous system. The ways in which the production of vasopressin and ACTH are controlled and stimulated by injury differ.

Vasopressin secretion is stimulated by an increase in osmolality (detected by hypothalamic osmoreceptors) or by a reduction in blood volume as produced by haemorrhage (detected by volume and stretch baroreceptors in the atria and carotid sinuses). Emotional trauma, exercise, anaesthetics, and visceral manipulation during operation are also recognized causes.

The control of ACTH secretion is complicated. It is certainly influenced by corticotrophin releasing factors, but also by vasopressin, which may act synergistically with corticotrophin releasing factors. The effects of these two substances do not fully account for those of crude hypothalamic extracts, so there are probably other unidentified components. Together they stimulate the production of pro-piomelanocortin (POMC), the common precursor for ACTH and other peptides which are secreted into the bloodstream. The main metabolic effect of ACTH is through the production of glucocorticoids. Whether glucocorticoids exert a mainly permissive role, allowing the normal physiological response to stress to occur, or whether they have more direct metabolic actions is debated. They also combine with many other neuronal and hormonal factors to control the production of corticotrophin releasing factors and of ACTH itself.

Thermoregulation after injury

There are undoubted changes in heat production and heat loss after injury, which are most marked after extensive burns. Their cause is debated. In addition to the widespread changes in fuel utilization, there are important alterations in hypothalamic thermoregulation. Insight into these processes in injured man has come from the use of mobile calorimeters. Contrary to the data from animal work, there is no clear evidence of a reduction of basal metabolic rate. Indeed, studies on patients undergoing elective surgery show that the metabolic rate tends to increase rather than decrease in the first 24 h postoperatively. There is, however, an inhibition of thermoregulation and failure of shivering, despite a fall in whole-body temperature. In the later response to injury (in the 'flow' phase) there is an increase in core temperature and also in basal metabolic rate. This increase, only moderate after multiple fractures, is more marked after head injury, and is greatest after extensive burns. The large increase in evaporative water loss from the burned surface is compensated for by an increase in heat production, but the two events are not closely related. In the absence of burns the increase in heat production after injury may be prolonged and may lead to marked weight loss; it could be due to increased protein breakdown, but this does not provide a complete explanation.

Water and electrolytes

The secretion of aldosterone, cortisol, and vasopressin are all increased after injury. There is usually a retention of water in excess of sodium, and a dilutional hyponatremia which may be associated with potassium deficiency. This relatively simple picture is often complicated by fluid and blood loss and their intravenous replacement. If the effects of injury are prolonged and recovery is delayed, body composition may alter considerably, with an increase in water relative to both lean body mass and body weight, and a continuing loss of intracellular electrolytes such as magnesium, potassium, and zinc. The causes of these changes are not fully understood. In practice it is important to remember that after surgery or injury hyponatraemia rarely means sodium deficiency, and that during recovery from such insults body composition can no longer be regarded as normal.

Fig. 1 A diagram of the phases of response to injury in man. The time scale is variable and the phases merge into each other. Fuel mobilization and the neuroendocrine response may begin in anticipation of injury. (Modified from Barton *et al.* 1990.)

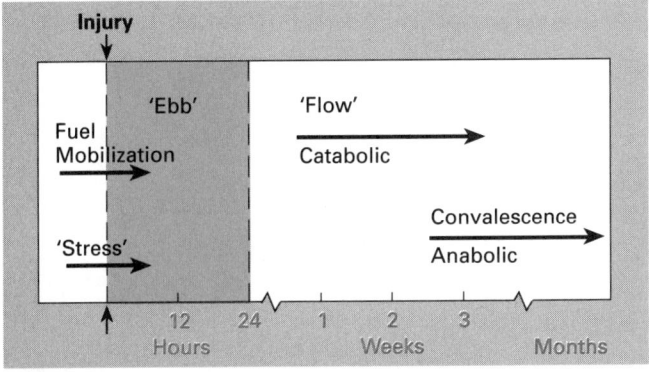

Glycogen and fat

The earliest metabolic result of the neuroendocrine responses of the hypothalamic pituitary axis and of the sympathetic nervous system to noxious stimuli is the mobilization of body fuels by the breakdown of glycogen (from liver and muscle) and fats (triacylglycerols). Because of its immediacy, this occurs in the 'ebb' phase. The production of glucose from the amino acids of muscle protein, associated with negative nitrogen balance, is a later event (in the 'flow' phase).

Mobilization of glycogen results mainly from the marked increase in catecholamines, an increase in glucagon, and a deficiency of insulin relative to the hyperglycaemia produced by injury. The main contribution to glucose comes from hepatic glycogen.

After injury there is an increase in the concentration of free fatty acids and glycerol derived from triacylglycerol stores. Lipolysis is stimulated mainly by the increase in catecholamines, although many other hormones (glucagon, ACTH, growth hormone) may also stimulate lipolysis at a sufficiently high concentration. The rate of lipolysis is high in all severities of injury, but the ketone body levels are variable. The hepatic conversion of free fatty acids to ketone bodies depends particularly on the ratio between glucagon and insulin, and is increased when this ratio is also increased. Some studies of accidentally injured subjects suggest that after severe injury the ketone body levels do not increase as much as after less severe trauma (and certainly not to the level associated with starvation alone). Whether this is related to the injury or to the individual is not established. Furthermore, in those who do not develop hyperketonaemia subsequent protein breakdown and gluconeogenesis may be increased compared with hyperketonaemic subjects.

Substrate turnover

The immediate neuroendocrine response to injury produces an excess of readily available energy from glycogen and fat. Teleologically this is wasteful unless the energy can be utilized. However, despite hyperglycaemia there is good evidence of a reduced uptake of glucose in early injury, whereas the uptake of free fatty acids is probably increased. The response to sepsis is similar in some respects to that of injury; however, most studies have been done in experimental endotoxaemia in animals and not in humans.

In the flow phase of injury the carbohydrate fuels have been utilized, and energy is derived from fat and protein (see below). There is hypermetabolism and increased nitrogen excretion. The relative contribution of fuels to this increased metabolism is related to the available nutritional source. However, protein contributes less than 20 per cent to the metabolic rate even under the most catabolic conditions. Where large amounts of glucose are given (as in parenteral nutrition, see Section 10) the effects are complex and unexpected.

In the normal uninjured person the administration of large amounts of glucose leads to net lipogenesis, but this does not occur after injury. The infusion of glucose after injury does not completely suppress hepatic glucose production, and the respiratory quotient does not rise above 1.0, which implies continuing oxidation of fat. There is a large increase in oxygen consumption and in metabolic rate. These changes may be due to persistent sympathetic overactivity. A major problem is the fate of the infused glucose, especially since storage as glycogen is impaired in both injured and septic patients.

Protein metabolism

A major deleterious effect of injury is loss of body protein, mainly from skeletal muscle, which begins soon after injury and leads to a negative nitrogen balance which is maximal on the second or third post-traumatic day. The negative nitrogen balance is proportional to the severity of the injury and is accentuated and prolonged by sepsis, burns, and immobility.

Nitrogen loss is most marked after severe injury in a previously fit young adult. It is reduced in the elderly and also by an increase in the external temperature to the thermoneutral zone (28–32°C). Its extent is not always appreciated; the loss of 15 g of nitrogen/day (which is not unusual, especially when surgery and semistarvation are combined) is equivalent to nearly 100 g of protein, much of it from skeletal muscle.

Nitrogen loss depends on the balance between synthesis of protein from amino acids and protein catabolism. Since the approach to treatment of nitrogen loss depends on its cause, much work has been done to identify the relative contribution to this of changes in protein synthesis and breakdown. In some conditions both synthesis and breakdown may alter in the same direction (that is, both reduced in starvation, both increased in exercise-induced hypertrophy); but after injury the changes are very diverse and depend on its severity and on nutritional state. After mild injury, synthesis and breakdown both appear to be depressed and both increase with severity of injury, although the increase in breakdown is more marked. Therefore at some stage, which depends on the initial nutritional status, breakdown exceeds synthesis. Such results are derived from measurements of whole-body protein turnover by methods which are often controversial. In general, it seems that for skeletal muscle synthesis is primarily controlled, whereas for liver and other gastrointestinal proteins the processes of breakdown are under physiological and pathological control.

More direct measurements have now been made on the protein-containing tissues, particularly voluntary muscle, although most results come from studies of experimental injury in animals, and they are as variable as those on whole-body protein turnover. In humans cachexia and muscle wasting diseases both appear to reduce muscle protein synthesis, and synthesis and breakdown of muscle are both decreased in patients having surgical operations. In severe injury and in sepsis there is evidence of both increased synthesis and breakdown (measured by 3-methylhistidine). After burns, 3-methylhistidine excretion is also considerably increased; this is likely to be due to direct muscle damage.

Parenteral nutrition can lessen the fall in synthetic rate after injury, and claims have been made that the branched-chain amino acids (leucine, isoleucine, and valine) also have specific effects on protein synthesis.

Important changes occur in the circulating concentrations of amino acids after injury. That of alanine, a major precursor for gluconeogenesis tends to fall after the first day; in contrast, the concentration of the branched-chain amino acids may remain considerably increased, and is highest after severe injuries where hyperketonaemia does not develop. The reason for these changes is not clear.

Injury also has interesting effects on plasma protein concentrations. Many of these, such as albumin, transferrin, and prealbumin fall, whereas others, the 'acute phase' plasma proteins (C reactive protein, fibrinogen, for example) increase. This acute phase protein response may directly result from tissue damage. The suggestion that this response is turned on by macrophages which produce interleukin-1 seems unlikely. Recent work points to the likely importance of other cytokines, such as interleukin-6 and tumour necrosis factor.

Whatever the cause there seems little doubt about the deleterious effects of prolonged protein loss. Apart from loss of weight, of muscle tissue, and of muscle strength, there is delayed healing of wounds, sus-ceptibility to infection, and hypoproteinaemic oedema. Importantly, continuing loss of nitrogen appears to increase the mortality rate.

Immobility

The mass of both the skeleton and of voluntary muscle appears to depend on the mechanical forces to which they are subjected, but the underlying mechanisms are largely unknown. Most patients are immobilized after injury. After a minor operation, such as a hernia repair, this may be of no significance, but after the multiple fractures of a road traffic accident immobility produces widespread effects. In the skeleton (see Section 19) there is a fall in the rate of new bone formation and an apparent increase in bone resorption, providing a striking example of 'uncoupling' of these two processes. It is not known how bone cells perceive mechanical stimuli; *in vivo* these cells are likely to be the osteocytes or osteoblasts. The muscles of immobilized limbs rapidly waste; again it is not clear whether this is due to a failure of synthesis or an increase in myofibrillar breakdown, or both. Neither skeletal nor muscular wasting can be satisfactorily prevented or reversed until mobility is restored; and for this reason it is very difficult to maintain muscle mass, whatever form of nutrition is used, in the immobile patient.

Sepsis and burns

Sepsis is a common complication of injury, but its metabolic effects are poorly understood. It is known to increase nitrogen loss and 3-methylhistidine excretion and to worsen prognosis. Myofibrillar breakdown rate is increased. The most extreme post-traumatic biochemical and endocrine changes occur in the burned patient. In addition to the injury itself there is excessive fluid loss from the damaged surfaces and an increase in metabolic rate. The energy requirements are high and may be difficult to satisfy.

Tissue repair and recovery

The repair of tissue begins at the time of injury with the control of haemorrhage and the production of local hormones leading to cell migration, with eventual fibroblast proliferation, scar formation, and fracture repair. The factors that initiate, control, and terminate repair processes are, however, largely unknown. There is similar ignorance about the detailed control of whole-body recovery, although an increase in mobility, return of appetite, and sufficient sleep appear to be basic requirements.

REFERENCES

Barton, R.N. (ed.) (1985). Trauma and its metabolic problems. *British Medical Bulletin* **41,** (no. 3).

Barton, R.N., Frayn, K.N. and Little, R.A. (1990). Trauma, burns and surgery. in *The metabolic and molecular basis of acquired disease*, (1st edn), (ed. R.D. Cohen, K.G.M.M. Alberti, and A.M. Denman), pp. 684–717. Baillière Tindall, London.

Davies, J.W.L. (1982). *Physiological responses to burning injury*. Academic Press, London.

Frayn, K.N. (1986). Hormonal control of metabolism in trauma and sepsis. *Clinical Endocrinology* **24,** 577–99.

Section 12 *Endocrine disorders*

12.1   *Principles of hormone action*   1553

12.2   *Anterior pituitary disorders*   1573

12.3   *The posterior pituitary*   1599

12.4   *The thyroid gland and disorders of thyroid function*   1603

12.5   *Thyroid cancer*   1618

12.6   *Disorders of calcium metabolism*   1622

12.7   *The adrenal*   1639

     12.7.1   Adrenocortical diseases   1639
     12.7.2   Congenital adrenal hyperplasia   1664

12.8   *The reproductive system*   1669

     12.8.1   The ovary   1669
     12.8.2   Disorders of male reproduction   1679
     12.8.3   The breast   1687

12.9   *Disorders of development*   1689

     12.9.1   Normal and abnormal sexual differentiation   1689
     12.9.2   Normal growth and its disorders   1695
     12.9.3   Puberty   1700

12.10   *Non-diabetic pancreatic endocrine disorders and multiple endocrine neoplasia*   1703

12.11   *Endocrine manifestations of non-endocrine disease*   1711

12.1 Principles of hormone action

J. L. JAMESON

Historical perspectives

Most current concepts in endocrinology have evolved during the past century. Although some of the effects of castration had been recognized since ancient times, Berthold is usually credited with using the model of castration as the first recorded experiment in endocrinology. In 1849, he demonstrated that castration of a cock caused regression of secondary sexual characteristics and mating behaviour. Transplantation of the testes into the abdominal cavity restored these features, proving a role for the gonads in sexual development. By the turn of the century, the clinical manifestations of a number of endocrine diseases were described, along with their probable association with glandular dysfunction. Among these disorders were the first descriptions of acromegaly and its association with tumours of the pituitary gland, a detailed account of myxoedema and its treatment with thyroid extracts, recognition that adrenal extracts could treat Addison's disease, and an association between pressor attacks and adrenal tumours. These and other observations firmly established the presence of glandular disorders, although the physiological basis for these diseases was poorly understood at the time. For example, acromegaly was initially thought to be caused by pituitary hypofunction rather than overactivity.

In 1902, Bayliss and Starling described the effects of 'secretin', a substance from the duodenal mucosa that caused marked pancreatic secretion when injected into the bloodstream of experimental animals. This result laid the foundation for the concept of a secreted hormone. There followed a number of efforts to isolate and synthesize hormones. Early successes included the isolation of adrenaline, thyroxine, and adrenal steroids. The identification of these hormones was facilitated by the fact that methods in organic chemistry were available for characterization and synthesis of relatively small compounds. Identification of insulin in 1922 by Banting and Best represented a major advance, not only for its ultimate clinical use as a treatment for diabetes, but also because it represented the successful isolation of a peptide hormone.

Over the next 50 years, many other peptide hormones were isolated, sequenced, and their physiological functions described. Important principles were established, including the concept of hypothalamic–pituitary control of multiple glands and the principle of feedback regulation by hormones produced in target glands. These principles of endocrinology established the basis for many current stimulation and suppression tests of endocrine function.

In the 1960s, the conceptual framework for mechanisms of hormone action was outlined. For peptide hormones, Sutherland established the idea of a second messenger system in which the hormone binds to a membrane receptor, thereby activating intracellular second messenger pathways such as cAMP. For steroid and thyroid hormones, Tata established the concept of hormone action at the nuclear level, whereby receptors mediated alterations in gene expression that were followed later by changes in protein levels. The development of the radio-immunoassay by Berson and Yalow in 1963 revolutionized endocrine physiology and diagnosis by allowing accurate measurements of minute circulating levels of hormones. Radio-immunoassays and related assays are now used routinely for almost all hormone measurements and have replaced many less sensitive chemical methods and bioassays.

Important advances in approaches to treatment have accompanied improvements in the understanding of endocrine diseases. Strategies for hormonal replacements have been refined together with improvements in surgery for endocrine tumours. Trans-sphenoidal techniques for pituitary tumours and the ability to resect parathyroid, adrenal, and other endocrine tumours represent a crucial aspect of the management of hormone excess syndromes. In addition to hormonal replacements, important medical therapies that have been developed include the use of radioactive iodine and antithyroid drugs for hyperthyroidism, bromocriptine for prolactinomas and acromegaly, oral hypoglycaemics for diabetes, gonadal steroids as contraceptives, and somatostatin analogues for acromegaly and tumours of the gastrointestinal tract.

In recent years, there have been rapid advances in our understanding of endocrinology based upon the tools of molecular genetics. DNA sequences encoding hormones such as somatostatin, growth hormone, insulin, and chorionic gonadotrophin were among the first genes cloned in humans. Recombinant DNA techniques are now used routinely to identify new hormones, their receptors, and to help elucidate their functions. Currently, the genetic basis of a wide array of endocrine disorders is being elucidated based upon molecular biological approaches.

Definition of endocrinology

Endocrinology encompasses the study of glands and the hormones that they produce. The phrase, endocrine, can be traced to Starling and his classic contrast of hormones that were secreted internally (endocrine) versus those that are secreted externally (exocrine) into lumina such as the gastrointestinal tract. The word 'hormone' is derived from a Greek phrase meaning 'to set in motion'. This name remains appropriate as all hormones elicit dynamic responses at a subcellular level as well as in terms of whole-animal physiology. Indeed, endocrinology has evolved into a discipline that is primarily concerned with dynamic physiological responses to hormones and feedback relationships that control various hormonal axes (e.g. hypothalamic–pituitary–adrenal axis).

Endocrinology is ultimately a form of communication between cells and different organs. The form of communication can involve peptide hormones or growth factors, derivatives of amino acids such as neurotransmitters or thyroxine, or derivatives of cholesterol such as steroids. As our understanding of these communications has advanced, the traditional lines of division that separate different physiological disciplines have become blurred. For example, the nervous system and endocrine system are intimately connected. The brain produces a vast array of peptide hormones and exerts critical input via the hypothalamus to control pituitary hormone secretion. The peripheral nervous system also modulates hormonal responses by the adrenal medulla and the pancreatic islets. Neuroendocrinology is rapidly becoming a separate discipline, reflecting the complexity of the interactions between the nervous and endocrine systems. Similarly, there are complex interactions between the immune system and the endocrine system. Hormones such as glucocorticoids are powerful immunosuppressants and there is accumulating evidence that many immune cells produce peptide hormones such adrenocorticotrophic hormone (ACTH). Cytokines and interleukins have profound effects on hormone secretion in glands such as the pituitary, adrenal, and gonads, and may play an important role in the process of embryonic implantation. Some of the most common diseases in endocrinology, such as autoimmune thyroid disease and type I diabetes mellitus, are caused by alterations in immune surveillance and tolerance. A variety of other less common diseases, such as polyglandular failure, adrenal insufficiency, lymphocytic hypophysitis, and others, also have an immunological basis. Given the interface between immunology and endocrinology, there is a growing discipline focused on immunoendocrinology. Two areas that are making rapid strides in this field include HLA genotyping in autoimmune endocrine diseases and the use of transgenic models whereby selective alterations in the immune system (e.g. altered expression of cytokines or MHC class I and II) allow investigation of the immune basis of endocrine diseases.

In general, the principles of hormone action can be applied readily to the physiology of other subspecialties. For example, hormones play a crucial role in maintenance of blood pressure, intravascular volume, and peripheral resistance in the cardiovascular system. The heart is the primary source of the peptide, atrial natriuretic factor, and vasoactive substances such as catecholamines, angiotensin II, endothelin, and endothelium-derived relaxing factor (nitric oxide) are involved in dynamic changes in vascular tone in addition to their many roles in other tissues. The gastrointestinal tract is a remarkably rich source of peptide hormones, such as cholecystokinin, gastrin, secretin, vasoactive intestinal peptide among many others. Many gastrointestinal hormones are also produced in the central nervous system, where their functional roles are poorly understood. The kidney is the primary source of erythropoietin, a circulating hormone that stimulates erythropoiesis. The kidney is also integrally involved in the renin–angiotensin axis and is a primary target of several hormones, including parathyroid hormone and mineralocorticoids. In the haematological system, a number of colony-stimulating growth factors, such as G-CSF and GM-CSF, have been identified. Interestingly, the receptors for these cytokines are members of a superfamily that includes the growth hormone receptor. As in therapy with erythropoietin, treatment with these naturally occurring cytokines shares many similarities with hormonal treatment paradigms, even though the disorders being managed are outside the traditional boundaries of endocrinology. It is apparent that hormones and growth factors play an important functional role in all organ systems. Although endocrinologists may not always be involved in the management or administration of hormones that are specific to the cardiovascular or haematological systems, the principles of endocrinology apply in these cases, emphasizing their importance across many disciplines.

Nature of hormones

Hormones can be divided generally into those that are based on amino acids or peptides and those that are derived from steroids. Hormones such as dopamine and catecholamines are derived from amino acids and reflect the close relationship between the endocrine system and neurotransmitters. Other small peptides such as thyrotrophin releasing hormone, gonadotrophin releasing hormone, and somatostatin are often considered to be neurohormones because they are produced by neurones or cells derived from neuroendocrine lineage, but they circulate in a manner that is more characteristic of hormones than neurotransmitters. Larger peptides such as parathyroid hormone, insulin, or luteinizing hormone are characteristic of circulating hormones. For the most part, amino acid derivatives and peptide hormones interact with membrane receptors on the cell surface. After binding to membrane receptors, hormones are often internalized, although it is unclear whether they play any further role after transport inside the cell.

A second general class of hormones is synthesized from cholesterol precursors or from other lipid-soluble substances obtained in the diet. Derivatives of cholesterol include steroid hormones such as progesterone, cortisol, and testosterone. Hormones such as vitamin D and retinoic acid are derived, for the most part, from dietary sources but can also be generated by additional pathways. Unlike peptide hormones, steroids, vitamin D, and retinoids are lipid soluble and act by crossing the plasma membrane to interact with intracellular receptors. Thyroid hormone, although produced by modifications of tyrosines in thyroglobulin, is generally classified with the steroid hormones because of its lipophilic nature and the fact that it binds to nuclear receptors.

Hormone binding proteins

Many hormones circulate in association with serum binding proteins. For example, T_4 (thyroxine) and T_3 (tri-iodothyronine) are bound to thyroxine-binding globulin, albumin, and thyroxine-binding prealbumin. Cortisol is bound to cortisol-binding globulin, while oestrogens and androgens are bound to sex-hormone-binding globulin. The primary role of the serum binding proteins is to provide a reservoir of hormone that would otherwise be cleared from the circulation rapidly. The interactions of hormones with the binding proteins are relatively weak in comparison with those of their receptors. This allows the hormones to have rapid on and off rates of combination with the binding proteins so that new equilibria can be established quickly. Although a variety of binding-protein abnormalities have been defined, these have few clinical consequences apart from creating diagnostic problems. For example, thyroxine-binding globulin deficiency can greatly reduce total thyroid hormone levels, even though free concentrations of T_4 and T_3 are normal. Hormonal perturbations in binding protein levels can cause a variety of diagnostic problems. For example, increased oestrogen levels in pregnancy, or in association with the use of oral contraceptives, stimulate thyroxine-binding globulin levels, raising the concentrations of total T_4 and T_3. Again, the free hormone and thyroid stimulating hormone levels are normal, indicating that the intact feedback loop responds to this change by re-establishing equilibrium. A guiding principle is that free hormone concentrations dictate hormonal responsiveness. This concept is readily understood when viewed from the perspective of high-affinity hormone–receptor interactions for which only free hormone is able to bind and thereby elicit a biological response. This feature of hormone action provides the basis for attempts to measure free hormone concentrations whenever possible.

In contrast to circulating hormones for which binding proteins do not appear to play a crucial functional role, the situation is less clear for proteins that bind growth factors. A large family of proteins bind insulin-like growth factor I, again emphasizing the importance of measuring free hormone concentrations. However, some of these insulin-like growth factor binding proteins appear to inhibit the action of insulin-like growth factor I, whereas others may facilitate its action. Consequently, within a given target tissue, the composition of insulin-like growth factor binding proteins may play an important role as modulators of insulin-like growth factor I activity. Likewise, follistatin has been identified as a binding protein for activin and to a lesser degree, inhibin. Because activin and inhibin themselves have opposing actions, the presence of follistatin might serve to further alter the relative impact of the two hormones. Growth hormone provides an unusual situation because its binding protein is derived by cleavage and release of the extracellular binding domain of the growth hormone receptor. Thus, growth hormone can circulate bound to its native receptor target site. Whether the circulating form of the growth hormone binding protein is capable of modifying growth hormone action remains to be determined.

Hormone interactions with receptors

Receptors for hormones are divided into membrane and nuclear receptors. As illustrated in Fig. 1, hormones that bind to membrane receptors act in combination with membrane-associated effector proteins to activate second messenger signalling pathways. The second messengers, whether cAMP, calcium, diacylglycerol, or others, stimulate a cascade of kinases which then act upon target substrates on the membrane, in the cytoplasm, or in the nucleus. Hormones that act through nuclear receptors diffuse, or are pumped, across the plasma membrane into the cytoplasm. Some nuclear receptors, such as the glucocorticoid or progesterone receptors, bind hormones in the cytoplasm before undergoing translocation into the nucleus by a process that probably involves dissociation of heat-shock and other chaperone proteins. Other receptors in this family, such as the thyroid hormone receptor, bind hormone in the nucleus without a separate hormone-induced translocation step. In the nucleus, these receptors interact with DNA target sites either to stimulate or repress the expression of specific genes. Consequently, most of the cellular actions of nuclear receptors are mediated by changes in levels of mRNA which, in turn, alter levels of enzymes, hormones, or other proteins.

Regardless of the class of receptors, certain principles apply generally to hormone–receptor interactions. Hormones bind to receptors with high affinity and specificity, to allow appropriate physiological responses. Hormone–receptor interactions are described in terms of equilibrium reactions. Low concentrations of free hormone (usually 10^{-12}–10^{-9} mol) rapidly associate and dissociate from receptors in a bimolecular reaction. The occupancy of the receptor at any given moment is a function primarily of the hormone concentration and the affinity of the receptor for the hormone. The binding characteristics of a receptor can be determined by performing Scatchard plots, an analysis that allows determination of affinity constants (K_a) and receptor number. Most receptors have affinity constants which are appropriate for circulating levels of hormones, allowing responses over a dynamic range of physiological concentrations of hormone. Receptor numbers vary greatly in different target tissues, providing one of the major determinants of specific cellular responses to widely circulating hormones. For example, adrenocorticotrophic hormone receptors are located almost exclusively in the adrenal cortex, and luteinizing hormone receptors are formed only in the gonads. In contrast, insulin receptors are widely distributed, reflecting the need for insulin-induced metabolic responses in most tissues.

Receptor specificity is a reflection of highly variable affinities of receptors for structurally related molecules. Although similar in structure, thyroid stimulating hormone, luteinizing hormone, and follicle stimulating hormone are highly selective for their individual receptors. Similarly, progesterone, oestrogen, and testosterone exhibit no physiologically significant cross-reactivity among their receptors. There are important exceptions to these examples of specificity. Parathyroid hormone (PTH) and parathyroid hormone related peptide appear to share a common receptor, accounting for similar physiological concomitants of their actions. Insulin and insulin-like growth factors I and II also cross-react to some degree with one anothers' receptors. In malignancies that overproduce insulin-like growth factor II, one can see hypoglycaemia as a consequence of inappropriate stimulation of insulin or insulin-like growth factor I receptors by insulin-like growth factor II.

Hormone and receptor families

A striking feature of hormones is that they often occur as groups of proteins or steroids that are structurally related (Table 1). For example, the glycoprotein hormones, thyroid stimulating hormone, follicle stimulating hormone, luteinizing hormone and chorionic gonadotrophin, represent a family that shares many structural features in common even though their physiological roles are quite different. Each of the glycoprotein hormones are heterodimeric proteins that contain an identical α-subunit, and distinct, but structurally related β-subunits. When their protein sequences are aligned, it is apparent that certain structural features in the β-subunits, such as the locations of cysteines that form disulphide bridges, have been highly conserved. Consequently, the overall three-dimensional architecture of the β-subunits has been conserved with sequences in the peptide loops that span the disulphide bridges providing specificity to the proteins. The subtle, but distinct differences in the glycoprotein hormone β-subunits allows them to recognize different receptors and consequently to induce specific biological responses. After the genes for the glycoprotein hormone β-subunits were cloned, it was apparent that the similarities in protein structure were also reflected at the genetic level. Each of the β-subunit genes has the same number of exons and the locations of the intervening introns is identical. These observations suggest that this family of genes and their encoded proteins arose from a common ancestral gene, probably by gene duplication and subsequent divergence to attain a new biological function.

Fig. 1 Mechanisms of membrane and nuclear receptor action. Hormones act through two major types of receptors that are activated on the cell membrane or in the nucleus. (Left) Hormone binding to membrane receptors induces coupling to intracellular effectors such as G-proteins and kinases, which stimulate one or more second messenger pathways to activate protein kinases. These then cause phosphorylation of target proteins in the cytoplasm and the nucleus. (Right) Other hormones pass through the plasma membrane to bind to intracellular receptors and are then translocated to the nucleus; still others bind to receptors located in the nucleus which act by either stimulating or repressing gene transcription (see text).

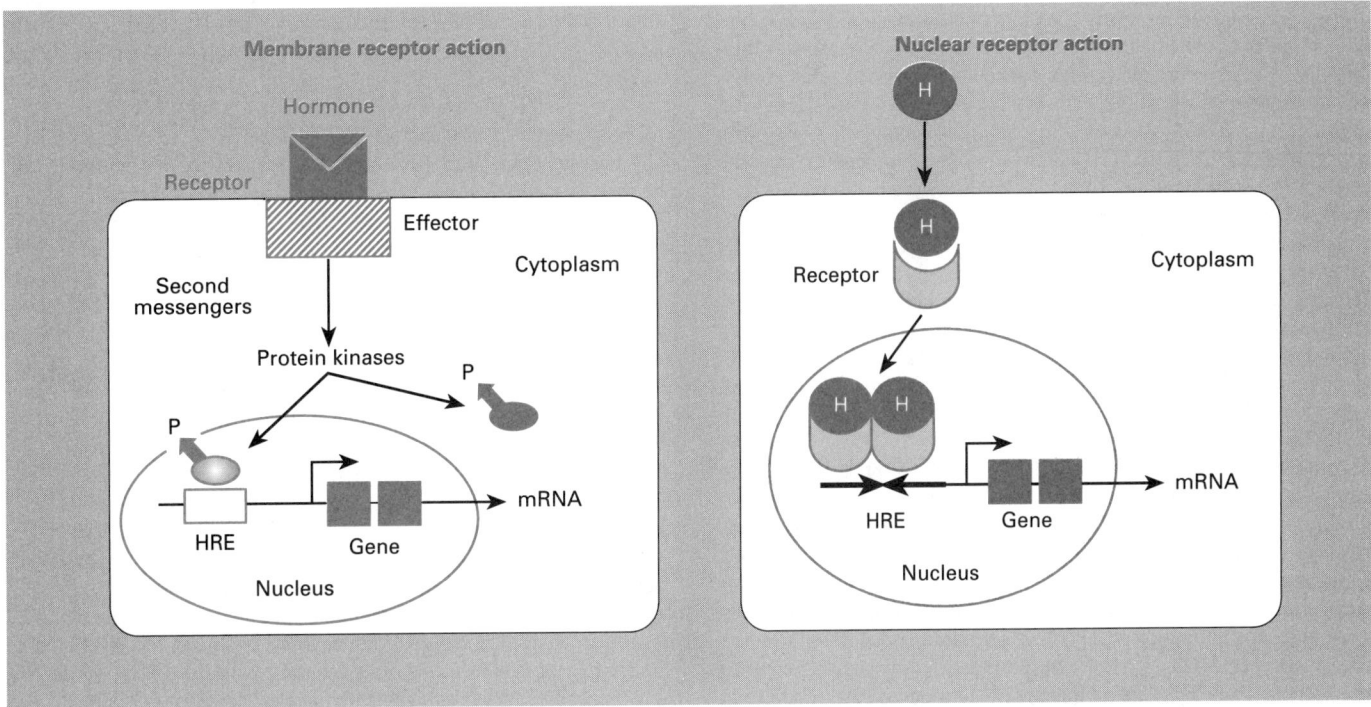

Table 1 *Examples of hormone and receptor families*

Hormone family	Receptor family
TSH, FSH, LH, CG	TSH-R, FSH-R, LH/CG-R
GH, CS, PRL	GH-R, PRL-R, cytokine receptors
ACTH	ACTH-R
PTH, PTH-RP	PTH-R, Calcitonin-R
Calcitonin, CGRP	Calcitonin-R, PTH-R
Vasopressin, oxytocin	Vasopressin-R, oxytocin-R
Glucagon, GLP, secretin, VIP, PACAP, GRF	Glucagon-R, GLP-R, secretin-R, VIP-R, PACAP-R, GRF-R
Somatostatin	Somatostatin-R 1–5
Insulin, IGF-I, IGF-II	Insulin-R, IGF I-R, IGF II-R
Activin A,B, inhibin A,B, TGFβ, MIS	Activin-R I,II, TGFβ-R I,II, MIS-R
Glucocorticoid, mineralocorticoid, progesterone, androgen, oestrogen	GR, MR, PR, AR, ER
Thyroid hormone, retinoids, vitamin D	TR α,β,γ, RAR α,β,γ, RXR α,β,γ, VDR
Dopamine	Dopamine-R 1–5
Noradrenaline, adrenaline	α Adren-R 1,2, β Adren-R 1,2

Receptors for the different hormones are denoted by capital 'R'. The peptide hormones, peptide hormone receptors, and nuclear hormone receptors shown in this table have been cloned. There is biochemical evidence for additional receptors not indicated and other hormone families are not shown because of space limitations.

Abbreviations include: TSH, thyroid stimulating hormone; FSH, follicle stimulating hormone; LH, luteinizing hormone; CG, chorionic gonadotrophin; GH, growth hormone; CS, chorionic somatomammotrophin; PRL, prolactin; ACTH, adrenocorticotrophin; PTH, parathyroid hormone; PTH-RP, parathyroid-related peptide; CGRP, calcitonin gene related peptide; GLP, glucagon related peptide; VIP, vasoactive intestinal peptide; PACAP, pituitary adenylyl cyclase activating peptide; GRF, growth hormone releasing factor; IGF, insulin-like growth factor; TGF, transforming growth factor; MIS, müllerian inhibiting substance; GR, glucocorticoid receptor; MR, mineralocorticoid receptor; PR, progesterone receptor; AR, androgen receptor; ER, (o)estrogen receptor; TR, thyroid hormone receptor; RAR, retinoic acid receptor; RXR, retinoid X receptor; VDR, vitamin D receptor.

Co-evolution of specific hormone receptors is of equal importance if a newly acquired gene is to confer a biological advantage. In the case of the glycoprotein hormones, there has apparently been parallel evolution of a family of receptors that are capable of recognizing specific differences in the hormones. Not surprisingly, there is considerable homology in the primary protein sequence of the glycoprotein hormone receptors. Domain swapping experiments in which the hormone-binding extracellular regions of the luteinizing hormone and thyroid stimulating hormone receptors are exchanged, demonstrate that the specificity for hormone binding can be localized to areas of sequence divergence in the receptors.

The structural features of the glycoprotein hormones and their receptors are not the only important components of their evolutionary relationships. The glycoprotein hormone receptors appear to share similar second messenger signalling pathways, specifically coupling to Gsα resulting in activation of adenylyl cyclase. Ultimately, the ability of a particular target tissue to respond to a hormone is conferred by the genetic regulatory elements which dictate that thyroid stimulating hormone receptors will be expressed in the thyroid gland and that luteinizing hormone and follicle stimulating hormone receptors will be expressed in specific cells in the gonads. Therefore, promoter regulatory elements have also evolved to allow appropriate cell-specific expression of the receptors.

Similarly, the hormone genes have evolved in a manner that allows expression in different cell types and in response to distinct positive and negative inputs. For example, thyroid stimulating hormone is expressed in pituitary thyrotropes where it is regulated positively by thyrotropin releasing hormone and negatively by T_4 and T_3. Follicle stimulating hormone and luteinizing hormone are expressed in pituitary gonadotropes where they are regulated in a positive manner by pulsatile gonadotrophin releasing hormone and negatively by gonadal steroids. Chorionic gonadotrophin represents an apparent exception to the rule of coevolution of hormones and receptors. Evolutionary dating based upon DNA sequence homology reveals that chorionic gonadotrophin is the newest member of the glycoprotein hormone family, having evolved very recently from an ancestral luteinizing hormone β gene. Consistent with this idea, chorionic gonadotrophin is only found in primates, suggesting that the gene duplication occurred after the divergence of mammals. Interestingly, luteinizing hormone and chorionic gonadotrophin (like parathyroid hormone and parathyroid hormone related peptide) still share a single luteinizing hormone/chorionic gonadotrophin receptor.

The evolutionary relationships described for the glycoprotein hormones also hold for most other hormones. In the case of the growth hormone, chorionic somatomammotrophin, and prolactin family, there is a parallel group of specific receptors which are members of a larger superfamily of cytokine receptors such as those that bind colony-stimulating factors. Given this evolutionary foundation, it is sometimes possible to derive structural information more rapidly, based upon comparisons with another well-characterized family member. These relationships sometimes provide important insights into pathways of receptor signalling as well.

The molecules of insulin and insulin-like growth factors I and II have long been recognized to share structural similarities, particularly when the precursor forms of the proteins are compared. However, unlike the high degree of receptor specificity exhibited by the glycoprotein hormones, the members of the insulin/insulin-like growth factor family show a moderate degree of receptor cross-talk. For example, high concentrations of insulin bind to the insulin-like growth factor I receptor, where they may cause some of the biological effects that are seen in states of insulin resistance. Similarly, high concentrations of insulin-like growth factor II that occur in certain malignancies can cause hypoglycaemia, in part due to cross-talk with the insulin or insulin-like growth factor I receptors. Because the insulin and insulin-like growth factor I receptors are dimers; heterodimers may be able to form, although the biological role for such hybrid receptors is not well understood.

Based upon the specificity for DNA sequences, the nuclear receptor family can be subdivided into steroid receptors (glucocorticoid, mineralocorticoid, androgen and progesterone receptors) and receptors that bind oestrogen, thyroid hormone, retinoic acid, or vitamin D. Isolation of similar receptor molecules from species ranging from *Drosophila* spp. to *Homo sapiens* reveals that this family has been evolving across broad stretches of evolutionary time. Certain functional domains, such as the zinc-finger motifs, are most highly conserved, although subtle modifications result in DNA sequence selectivity. The hormone-binding domains of the nuclear receptors are more variable, allowing a diverse array of small ligands to activate receptor responses in a highly specific manner. This feature is particularly well illustrated for the steroid receptors, which share nearly identical DNA binding domains and consensus DNA target sequences. For these receptors, the presence or absence of a given receptor and exposure of the cell to a particular hormone, such as glucocorticoid or progesterone, provides the major determinants of hormonal responsiveness. For the highly related glucocorticoid and mineralocorticoid receptors, the issue of specific responses to different hormones is even more tenuous, because the mineralocorticoid receptor also binds glucocorticoids with high affinity. In this case, renal tubular cells involved in mineralocorticoid responses have developed an enzymatic step (11β-hydroxysteroid dehydrogenase) to inactivate glucocorticoids, thereby preventing substantial cross-talk by glucocorticoids at the receptor level. Under conditions of very high glucocorticoid concentrations, such as occur in Cushing's syndrome, the pathway for glucocorticoid degradation at the local cellular level can become overwhelmed, and the mineralocorticoid effects (sodium retention; potassium wasting) of glucocorticoids can be seen. Moreover, inhibition of 11β-hydroxysteroid dehydrogenase by liquorice or related compounds can occasionally cause hypertension by mimicking hyperaldosteronism.

Gene transcription, protein biosynthesis, and hormone secretion

Endocrine genes share structural features with many other genes, but are notable in their requirements for exquisite regulatory control by other hormones. The structure of a prototypical endocrine gene and the cellular pathways that lead to hormone biosynthesis are depicted in Fig. 2. It is convenient to consider the gene separately in terms of its promoter regulatory elements and the structural elements that encode its protein products. The promoter is located in the upstream 5′ flanking region of the gene and contains regulatory DNA elements and sequences that specify the location of transcriptional initiation. At the 3′ end of the gene, there are regulatory sequences involved in transcriptional termination, and, in some instances, hormone- or tissue-specific regulatory elements may also reside downstream of the gene or in introns.

The regulatory components of the promoter consist of an array of modular DNA elements, such as hormone response elements, tissue-specific elements, and second messenger response elements, in addition to sequences that are required for basal transcription (see Fig. 3). These regulatory DNA elements function by binding to specific transcription factors that can be classified into three groups:

1. Enhancer binding proteins;
2. General transcription factors; and
3. Transcriptional activating factors.

Fig. 2 Pathways of hormone gene expression and biosynthesis. Biosynthetic pathways are illustrated, beginning with gene expression (left) and mRNA processing in the nucleus, continuing with mRNA translation into proteins which are then processed through a series of post-translational steps (right). In the example shown, the gene is divided into exons (A, B, C) that are separated by two introns. Untranslated sequences are represented as white boxes, signal sequence as a black box, and mature prohormone as stippled boxes. After transcription of the gene, mRNA is processed in the nucleus where introns are spliced out and polyadenylation occurs. Messenger RNA is then transferred to ribosomes for translation in the rough endoplasmic reticulum. Specific codons such as AUG and UGA provide signals for translational initiation and termination, respectively. After translation of the preprohormone, the signal sequence directs translocation across a membrane and is removed. Additional proteolytic processing may then convert prohormones to one or more mature peptides. A variety of post-translational modifications such as amidation, phosphorylation, or glycosylation can also occur during or after hormone translocation from the endoplasmic reticulum through the Golgi, and ultimately into secretory granules.

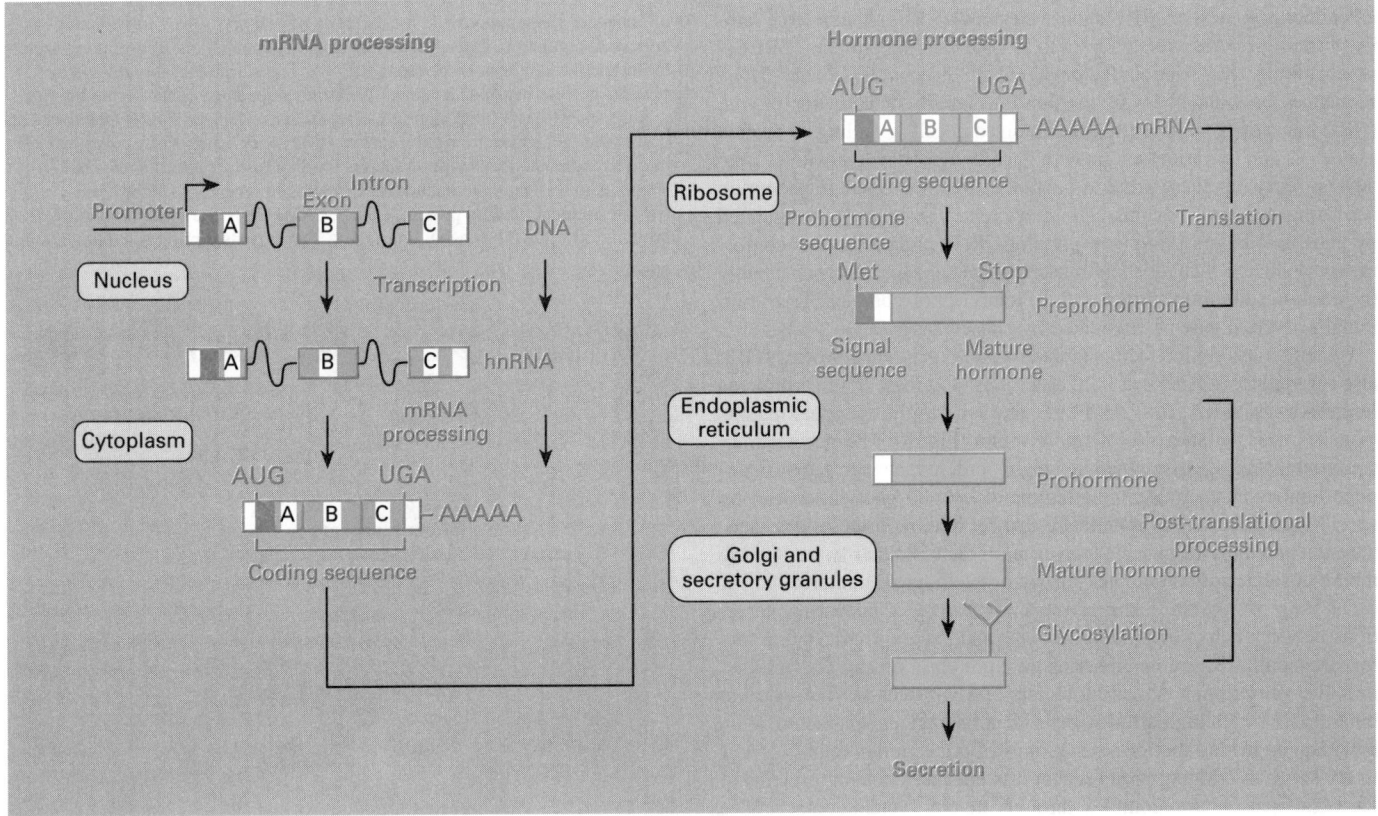

Table 2 *Families of transcription factors involved in the control of endocrine genes*

Transcription factor families	Signalling pathways
CREB/ATF	Protein kinase A; calcium; MAP kinase
C/EBP	Calcium; cell differentiation
Jun	ERK; protein kinase C; MAP kinase; Jun kinase
Fos/Fra	ERK; protein kinase C
Pou/Homeo	Cell-specificity; cell differentiation
Helix–loop–helix	Cell-specificity; cell differentiation
Nuclear receptors	Steroids, thyroid hormone, retinoids, vitamin D

Abbreviations: CREB, cAMP response element binding protein; ATF, activating transcription factor; C/EBP, CAAT box/enhancer-binding protein; Fra, Fos-related antigen; ERK, extracellular signal-regulated kinase; MAP, mitogen activated pathway.

Enhancer binding proteins typically interact with DNA sequences within several hundred base pairs of the transcriptional initiation site, but they sometimes bind to sites that are several kilobases removed from the promoter. Enhancer binding proteins are bipartite, having a DNA binding domain and separate domains that are involved in protein–protein contacts and transcriptional activation. The enhancer binding proteins include transcription factors with a broad range of regulatory functions (Table 2). As described above, nuclear receptors are representative of enhancer proteins for which separate DNA and transcription activating domains have been well characterized. Other regulatory proteins include tissue-specific factors such as Pit-1, a homeodomain class (related to homeobox genes involved in Drosophila embryonic development) of transcription factor that is expressed specifically in somatotropes, lactotropes, and thyrotropes. Pit-1 is involved in differentiation of these cells as well as transcription of the growth hormone and prolactin genes. As described below, mutations in the Pit-1 gene cause deficiencies of growth hormone, prolactin, and thyroid stimulating hormone, probably because these cell lineages do not develop normally in its absence. One or more second messenger signal response sequences, such as cAMP, calcium, and protein kinase C response elements, are found in almost all endocrine genes. cAMP response elements (CREs) bind a large family of transcription factors referred to as CRE-binding proteins (CREBs) or activating transcription factors (ATFs). Structurally related DNA sequences bind members of the Jun/Fos family of activator protein (ARI) transcription factors that are involved in cell signalling by protein kinase C and a variety of growth factor signalling pathways. Like nuclear receptors, these proteins contain distinct DNA and transcription activating domains. For this class of factors, transcription is regulated by phosphorylation. Phosphorylation of CREB protein induces conformational changes that result in transcriptional enhancement, presumably by recruiting additional proteins to the transcription complex. Transcriptional activation may be attenuated by phosphatases.

General transcription factors include the TATA binding protein (TBP, also referred to as TFIID) as well as a series of at least 20 other proteins referred to as TFIIA, B, C, E, F, etc. that bind to the proximal regions of genes near the start site of transcription (Fig. 3). The general transcription factors are assembled in a highly ordered manner that provides opportunities at many steps for regulation by phosphorylation and by specific combinations of proteins. Enhancer binding proteins can facilitate the assembly of general transcription factors either by stabilizing the basal transcription complex through protein–protein interactions or by altering nucleosome phasing, causing removal of histones. Interactions between enhancer binding proteins and general transcription factors frequently require members of the third class of transcription factors, the transcription activating factors (TAFs). Because TAFs do not bind to DNA with high affinity, their identification and characterization have lagged behind that of other groups of transcription factors. TAFs likely serve as bridging proteins that link enhancer binding proteins to the basal transcription complex through protein–protein contacts. The

complex array of different transcription factors that bind to the promoter provides an important means for regulatory control. Somewhat analagous to the genetic code, it is not really necessary for every gene to bind unique proteins to achieve specific patterns of expression or regulatory control. Rather, specific combinations of transcription factors may result in unique properties that are not necessarily applicable to another gene.

Fig. 3 Transcriptional regulation of an endocrine gene. A typical promoter is illustrated schematically and is divided into a group of basal promoter elements and enhancer elements. Basal promoter elements often contain regulatory sequences that are found in many other genes, including an initiator (INR) near the transcriptional start site adjacent to a TATA box that is a recognition site for TATA-binding protein (TBP). Other common basal elements include CAAT box sequences and the GC-rich SP1 site. Variable combinations of these and other basal elements confer specificity. Enhancer elements are frequently targets for dynamic regulation and are often relatively independent of orientation and precise location. Enhancer elements shown here include: a hormone response element (HRE) which is a target for nuclear receptors; an AP1 site which binds members of the Jun/Fos transcription factor family; a tissue-specific element (TSE) which is involved in cell-specific expression; and a cyclic AMP response element (CRE) which interacts with members of the CREB/ATF transcription factor family. Different combinations of enhancer elements provide for diversity of cell-specific expression and hormonal regulation. These regulatory DNA elements bind transcription factors to initiate the synthesis of messenger RNA. Transcriptional initiation is an ordered process in which a series of limiting steps must occur before the final recruitment of basal transcription factors such as TBP and TFIIB (see text) can bring other general transcription factors (GTFs) including RNA polymerase II into the complex. Transcription factors binding to their specific response elements in this example include: ER, oestrogen receptor; TSEB, tissue-specific element binding protein; CREB, cAMP response element binding protein; CBF, CAAT box binding factor; TAFs, transcription activating factors.

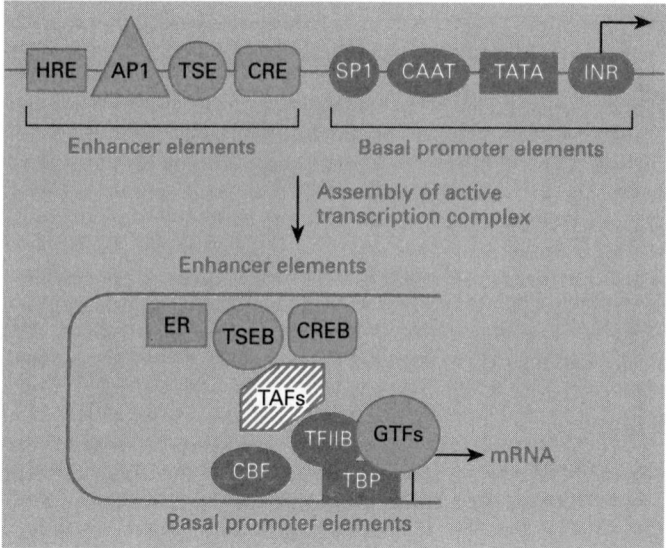

The structural gene is divided into exons and introns (Fig. 2). After transcription of nascent mRNA, exons are spliced together to form mRNA that is processed further by the addition of a 5′ cap and 100–250 adenine residues (polyadenylation) at the 3′ end of the mRNA. RNA processing provides several opportunities for regulatory steps. In some genes, alternate exon splicing allows substitution of some exons for others, or splicing out and removal of particular exons. In this manner, the protein that is ultimately produced can have blocks of sequences that are variable, depending upon which exons are included in the mRNA. In the calcitonin gene, alternate splicing allows production of either calcitonin or calcitonin gene related peptide. In this case, alternate splicing occurs in a tissue-specific manner such that calcitonin gene related peptide is produced preferentially in brain whereas calcitonin is produced in the C-cells of the thyroid. There are many other examples of alternate processing of hormone genes and receptors. In cases such as the thyroid hormone receptor α gene, alternate splicing results in the production of either a normal receptor protein or a variant that cannot bind hormone (c-erbA α II) because a critical region of the hormone-binding domain has been substituted with a different exon. There is growing evidence that exons represent separate functional domains that provide genetic modules that can be shuffled to provide diversity and new functions in evolutionarily related genes.

In the cytoplasm, mRNA levels can be regulated at the post-transcriptional level by proteins that selectively induce RNA degradation or stability. Regulatory sequences that control mRNA stability are often located in the 3′ untranslated sequence of the mRNA. Current evidence suggests that much of the control of RNA stability may take place at the level of the ribosome and possibly in conjunction with protein translation. Messenger RNA is translated by ribosomes where translational efficiency provides an additional level of regulation. Much of the control of insulin biosynthesis, for example, occurs at the translational level in response to elevated glucose or amino acids.

In the case of secretory proteins and membrane receptors that ultimately reside in the extracellular environment, a signal sequence at the aminoterminus of the protein directs translocation of the protein across the endoplasmic reticulum where the signal sequence is then cleaved. Hormones that are destined to be secreted are completely translocated across the membrane. Proteins, such as receptors, that will remain on the cell surface are inserted into the membrane with stretches of hydrophobic amino acids remaining within the confines of the lipid bilayer. After or during translocation, proteins are subjected to a variety of post-translational modifications. Polypeptide hormones in particular are frequently cleaved into smaller functional peptides. Classic examples include the cleavage of proinsulin to insulin by removal of the internal C peptide, and conversion of the parathyroid hormone precursor to parathyroid hormone by removal of its carboxyterminus. In addition to these examples which yield a single bioactive peptide, there are many examples of polypeptide hormones that give rise to multiple functioning peptides. For example, pro-opiomelanocortin is variably cleaved by endopeptidases to yield adrenocorticotrophic hormone, melanocyte stimulating hormone (α, β, γ), β-endorphin, and lipocortin (β, γ). Proglucagon is similarly cleaved to result in glucagon, glicentin, oxytomodulin, and several glucagon-like peptides (GLP I, II). Other examples of post-translational modifications include amidation, particularly of neuropeptides, and glycosylation. There is great heterogeneity in carbohydrate chains. Some of the carbohydrate heterogeneity reflects the composition of glycosyltransferases in selected cell types. In other cases, heterogeneity within a cell type (e.g. luteinizing hormone v. follicle stimulating hormone) is specified by the primary amino acid sequence of the protein. Glycosylation of secreted hormones such as the glycoprotein hormones (luteinizing hormone, follicle stimulating hormone, thyroid stimulating hormone, and human chorionic gonadotrophin) can affect circulating half-life as well as biological activity. Glycosylation of membrane receptors can affect protein conformation as well as inter-

Fig. 4 Structures of membrane and nuclear receptors. A seven transmembrane spanning receptor is depicted at the left. The amino-terminal (NH₂) end is located extracellularly and contains sequences involved in high-affinity binding of peptide hormones. Hormones also bind to receptor sequences within and adjacent to the lipid bilayer. Seven discrete stretches of hydrophobic amino acids are shown in the lipid bilayer (stippled) and are connected by intra-and extracellular loops of amino acids. It is likely that the hydrophobic 'barrels' in the lipid bilayer are circularized when viewed from above. The intracellular loops and carboxy-terminal tail (COOH) are involved in coupling to G-proteins and in intracellular signalling. Phosphorylation of the cytoplasmic tail and interactions with cellular proteins such as arrestin modulate receptor signalling, desensitization, and recycling. The structure of a nuclear receptor is illustrated at the right. Nuclear receptors contain several modular domains that are highly conserved in different members of the family. The DNA binding domain contains cysteine-rich zinc fingers that bind to specific DNA recognition sites. Hormones bind to the carboxy-terminus of the receptor, which is also involved in receptor dimerization and in transcriptional activation. The amino-terminal domain of the nuclear receptors is the most variable and is also involved in transcriptional regulation.

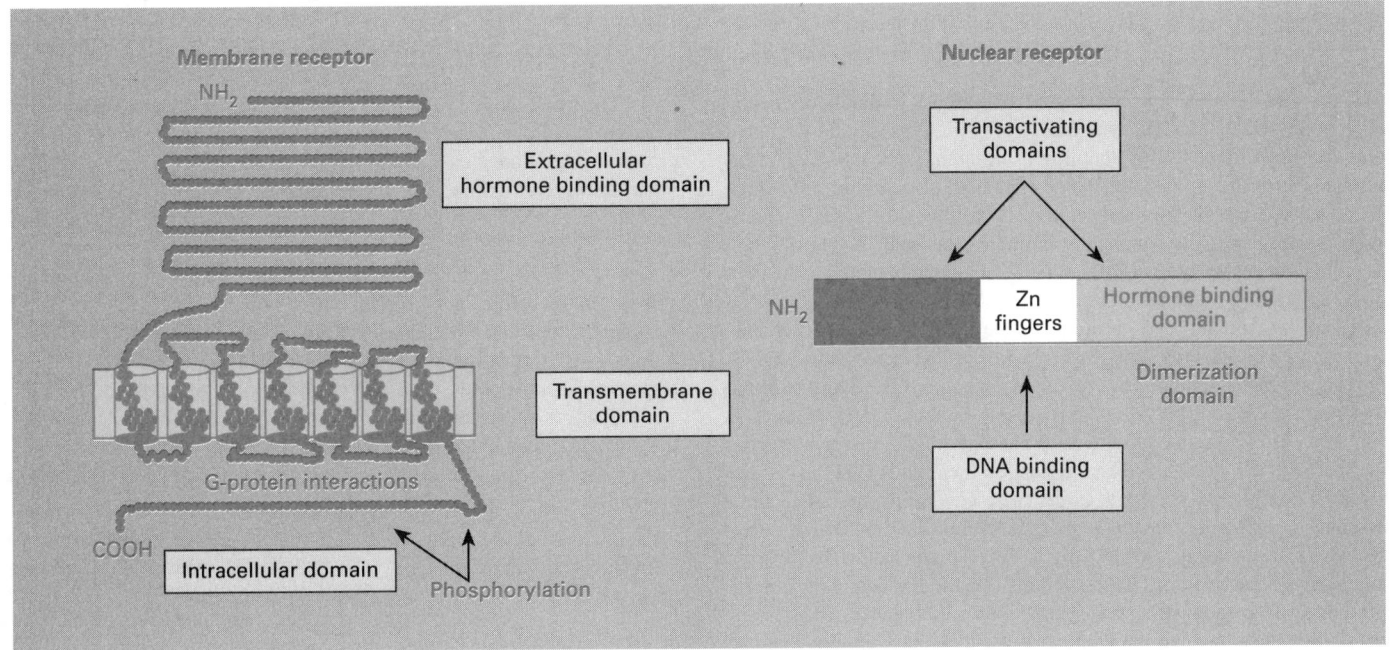

Table 3 *Examples of membrane receptor signalling pathways*

Receptors	Effectors	Signalling pathways
β-Adrenergic LH, FSH, TSH Glucagon PTH ACTH GRF	Gsα, adenylate cyclase Ca^{2+} channels	Stimulation of cAMP, protein kinase A Calmodulin, Ca^{2+} dependent kinases
α-Adrenergic Somatostatin	Giα	Inhibition of cAMP
TRH, GnRH GH, Prl Insulin EGF, NGF ANP	Gq, G_{11} JAK Tyrosine kinases, IRS-1 Tyrosine kinases, ras Guanylate cyclase	Phospholipase C, protein kinase C, voltage-dependent Ca^{2+} channels Tyrosine kinases MAP kinases, PtdIns-3-kinases, RSK Raf, MAP kinases, RSK Increased cGMP, cGMP-dependent protein kinase

LH, luteinizing hormone; FSH, follicle stimulating hormone; TSH, thyroid stimulating hormone; PTH, parathyroid hormone; ACTH, adrenocorticotrophic hormone; GRF, growth hormone releasing factor; TRH, thyrotrophin releasing hormone; GnRH, gonadotrophin releasing hormone; GH, growth hormone; Prl, prolactin; JAK, Janus kinase; IRS, insulin receptor substrate; MAP, mitogen activated pathway; PtdIns, phosphatidyl inositol; RSK, ribosomal S6 kinase; EGF, epidermal growth factor; NGF, nerve growth factor; ANP, atrial natriuretic peptide.

actions with ligands. Phosphorylation of proteins also represents a pervasive post-translational mechanism for modulating the activity of enzymes and receptor pathways (see below).

Structure and signalling by membrane receptors

Membrane receptors can be divided into several major groups, although the diversity observed sometimes defies discrete categorization. A large class of membrane receptors is comprised of the G protein-coupled, seven transmembrane spanning family of receptors. This group of receptors is characterized by the presence of seven separate hydrophobic domains that are embedded within the lipid bilayer (Fig. 4). Hormone binding domains are positioned on the extracellular side of the receptor. For small hormones such as catecholamines and thyrotropin releasing hormone, high-affinity binding occurs to residues that lie within the transmembrane domain of the receptor. Larger hormones such as gonadotrophins have high-affinity contact sites with the extracellular region of the receptor, but also make contact with residues within the transmembrane domain. This class of receptors is typically coupled to one or more G-proteins which make contact with intracellular domains of the receptor.

G-proteins are so named because of their ability to bind the guanine nucleotides, GTP and GDP. The family of G-proteins is quite large and provides great diversity for coupling to different receptors. G-proteins form a heterotrimeric complex that is composed of α, β, and γ subunits. The G-protein complex transduces signals from the receptor to enzymes such as adenylate cyclase and phospholipase C, as well as channels such as voltage-dependent calcium channels. The α-subunit contains the guanine nucleotide binding site. The β and γ-subunits are usually associated with one another and serve to modulate the activity of the α-subunit as well as probably having independent actions on effector pathways. G-protein activity is regulated by a cycle that involves GTP hydrolysis and dynamic interactions between the α-subunit and a complex of the βγ-subunits. After hormone binding to the receptor, GDP dissociates from the inactive αβγ complex. The Gα-subunit then binds GTP and it dissociates from the βγ complex. Under these conditions, the Gα-subunit assumes an activated state that allows signal transduction. GTP hydroysis to GDP by an intrinsic GTPase in the Gsα-subunit causes inactivation and allows reassociation of the subunit with the βγ complex. The G-protein cycle of activation and inactivation is subject to a variety of regulatory steps that can modulate activity, including proteins that can enhance or inhibit GTPase activity. As described below, a variety of

disease states can result from mutations that alter the activity of G-proteins. Mutations that allow GTP binding, but eliminate GTPase activity, result in a constitutively activated state that causes altered cell growth and neoplasia.

There are more than a dozen isoforms of the Gα-subunit. Some of these are referred to as Gsα because they are stimulatory for adenylate cyclase. Others are inhibitory for adenylate cyclase and are referred to as Giα1, Giα2, etc. The diversity of G-proteins allows a large array of potential combinations of receptor–G-protein–enzyme complexes to be formed within any given cell. It also allows receptors to interact with different G-protein isoforms in various tissues. The receptor specificities for individual G-proteins and the specificities of G-proteins for different enzymatic isoforms is only beginning to be elucidated (Table 3).

Activation of adenylate cyclase by Gsα has been particularly well studied (Fig. 5). Adenylate cyclase converts ATP to the second messenger, cyclic AMP. There are four isoforms of adenylate cyclase and it has a structure that resembles transporters such as the product of the cystic fibrosis gene. It is unclear whether adenylate cyclase also serves as a transporter. Production of cAMP initiates a well-characterized cascade of enzymatic steps. Binding of cAMP to the regulatory subunit of protein kinase A causes dissociation of the regulatory and catalytic subunits. The free catalytic subunit of protein kinase A then phosphorylates a variety of cellular targets on serines or threonines that reside in specific protein recognition sites. Continuing the theme of regulatory diversity, there are several isoforms of the regulatory and catalytic subunits of protein kinase A that are differentially expressed in various tissues and under different physiological conditions. Cellular targets for protein kinase A include structural components of the cytoskeleton, membrane and nuclear receptors, metabolic enzymes, mitochondrial enzymes, transcription factors, and other kinases. Consequently, stimulation of protein kinase A is a proximal step that leads to a wide array of cellular responses. In most cases, the effect of phosphorylation is to induce allosteric changes in protein conformation. In enzymes, these conformational changes can either activate or inhibit enzyme activity. Phosphorylation of transcription factors such as cAMP response element binding protein by protein kinase A induces transcriptional activation. Mechanisms that modulate cAMP-stimulated pathways are also important for integrating other cellular signalling pathways. Phosphodiesterase can deactivate cAMP, and a variety of specific phosphatases can terminate protein kinase A stimulated events by removing phosphate groups. One of the central unresolved questions in cellular signalling is how a ubiquitous second messenger such as cAMP can elicit specific cellular responses. It is likely that the diversity of isoforms at each step in the signalling cascade in combination with the ability for 'cross-talk' between different signalling pathways provides an important mechanism for generating unique responses.

Although many members of the seven transmembrane family of receptors utilize cAMP as a signalling pathway, other receptors in this class, such as the thyrotrophin releasing hormone and gonadotrophin releasing hormone receptor use different pathways (Fig. 5). In these cases, the receptors couple to Gq or G_{11} isoforms, endowing them with the capability to activate a distinct group of enzymes and channels. Phospholipase C is one of the important enzymes that is activated by gonadotrophin releasing hormone and thyrotrophin releasing hormone. Phospholipase C stimulates phosphotidyl inositol turnover, resulting in the production of several metabolites including diacylglycerol and inositol triphosphate. Diacylglycerol activates protein kinase C by a mechanism that is mimicked by tumour promoters such as phorbol esters. Inositol triphosphate increases calcium concentrations by binding to inositol triphosphate receptors and opening intracellular calcium channels.

Fig. 5 Cellular pathways of membrane receptor signalling. Membrane receptors (R_1, R_2, R_3, R_4) are illustrated with their second messenger and protein kinase pathways. R_1 receptors are typified by members of the seven transmembrane family of receptors that couple to Gsα and stimulate adenylate cyclase. cAMP activates protein kinase A (PKA) which phosphorylates specific proteins on serine and threonine residues. R_2 receptors selectively activate a variety of kinases including ras, raf, and proximal components of the MAP (mitogen activated protein) kinase pathway such as MEK (MAPK or ERK, extracellular signal-regulated kinase). The MAP kinase pathway can also be activated by G-proteins such as Giα$_2$. The RSK (ribosomal S6 kinases) and other kinases not shown are also activated by tyrosine receptor kinase pathways. The MAP kinases are activated by phosphorylation of threonine and tyrosine residues requiring enzymes with dual specificity or activation of two different classes of kinases. R_3 receptors activate guanylate cyclase which in turn activates cGMP dependent protein kinases (G-kinases) that are homologous to protein kinase A. R_4 type receptors are coupled to Gq or G_{11} and activate the enzyme phospholipase C to produce diacylglycerol (DAG), an activator of protein kinase C (PKC), and inositol triphosphate (IP$_3$), which increases the concentration of intracellular calcium. Increased intracellular calcium facilitates DAG stimulation of PKC and also activates calmodulin, which activates calmodulin dependent kinases (CAM kinase) and other cellular proteins. There are multiple isoforms of most of the illustrated components including G-proteins, adenylate cyclases, phospholipases, and various kinases. There are also many interactions among pathways reflecting phosphorylation as one of the primary means for regulating the system. Important roles for phosphodiesterases and phosphatases as mechanisms for terminating the activated pathways are not shown.

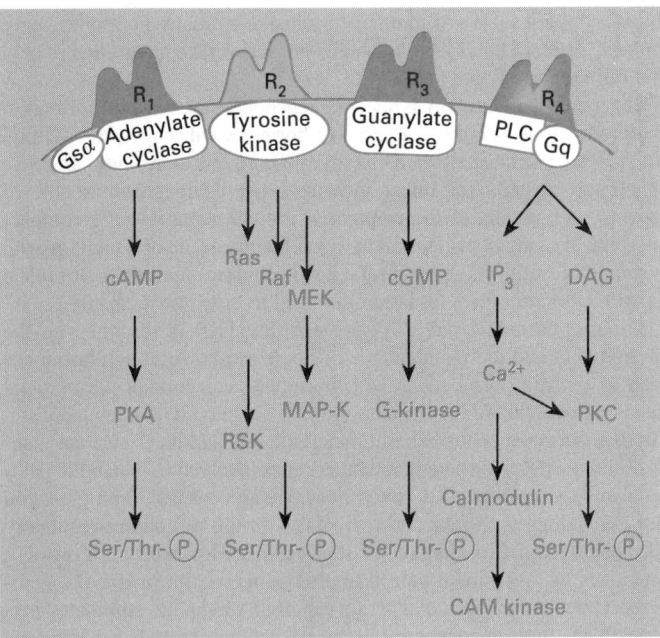

Ca^{2+} facilitates diacylglycerol activation of protein kinase C, allowing the distinct arms of the phospholipase C pathway to converge on this enzyme. There are several protein kinase C isoforms that differ in tissue distribution, and in their ability to undergo depletion and desensitization after agonist stimulation. Inositol triphosphate stimulation of Ca^{2+} also results in activation of calmodulin, a protein with several acceptor sites for Ca^{2+}. The Ca^{2+}–calmodulin complex activates an array of calmodulin-dependent kinases. Most of the calmodulin-dependent kinases are cytoplasmic and are involved processes such as muscle contraction, neuronal signalling, and metabolic enzyme pathways. However, some are nuclear and may be involved in calcium-dependent gene transcription.

The tyrosine kinase class of receptors also represents a large and diverse family that transduces signals for hormones and growth factors (Table 3). This group includes receptors for insulin, and a variety of growth factors such as epidermal growth factor, nerve growth factor, platelet-derived growth factor, and fibroblast growth factor (FGF). The extracellular ligand-binding domains of these receptors contain cysteine-rich domains that create highly structured binding sites for proteins. Some of these receptors are monomeric (e.g. epidermal growth factor), whereas others (e.g. platelet-derived growth factor) form dimers. The cytoplasmic domains of the tyrosine kinase receptors contain ATP binding sites as well as target sites for tyrosine phosphorylation. This class of receptors can undergo autophosphorylation and, through domains first identified in the Src oncogene (SH$_2$, SH$_3$), the receptors are coupled to a variety of adaptor proteins and enzymes to transduce specific signals. Some of the enzymatic steps distal to tyrosine kinase receptors have now been identified. A protein referred to as insulin receptor substrate-1 has been recognized as a proximal target for insulin receptor signalling and appears to be a key intermediary that links the insulin receptor to distal signalling pathways. A similar role has been proposed for Janus-associated kinase-2 (JAK-2), which is a proximal target of the growth hormone receptor. Another member of the GTP-binding group of proteins, ras p21, is an important effector for some growth factor receptors. The three ras proteins (N-ras, K-ras, H-ras) are activated by GTP and inactivated by GTP hydrolysis in a pathway that is reminiscent of G-protein cycling. The parallels between the two systems also extend to neoplastic diseases in which ras mutations that inhibit GTP hydrolysis have been found to contribute to cellular transformation because of constitutive ras signalling. A role for ras in growth factor signalling has been provided by using ras inhibitors (dominant negative mutants of ras) that block some of the effects of growth factors, such as NGF and nerve growth factor and epidermal growth factor. Tyrosine kinases also activate a pathway that converges at the level of the mitogen activated pathway (MAP) kinases. Raf-1 (MAP kinase kinase kinase) activates MEK (MAP or ERK kinase, MAP kinase kinase) which in turn activates several isoforms of MAP kinase. As their name implies, the MAP kinases are involved in cell proliferation in addition to other cellular processes that are activated by growth factors. MAP kinases phosphorylate a number of transcription factors including myc, CAAT box/enhancer binding protein-β, activating transcription factor-2, Elk-1, and Jun. The MAP kinases also activate the ribosomal S6 kinase class of kinases as well as phosphatases such as protein phosphatase 1.

Structure and action of nuclear receptors

The binding characteristics and structures of nuclear receptors were defined later than those for the membrane receptors. Most of the nuclear receptors have been cloned in recent years, providing a wealth of information about their structure and function. When the sequences of the oestrogen, glucocorticoid, and progesterone receptors were first identified, it was recognized that the receptors were homologous and shared certain structural features with the v-*erb*A oncogene which later proved to be the viral counterpart of c-erbA, the thyroid hormone receptor. This family of nuclear receptors has now grown to have nearly 100 members, many of which are still classified as orphan receptors because their ligands, if any exist, remain to be identified.

The most highly conserved region of the nuclear receptors is in the DNA binding domain. This region of the receptor contains a series of cysteines which chelate zinc, to form two so-called zinc fingers (Fig. 4). X-ray crystallography and mutagenesis studies demonstrate that the receptor contacts with specific DNA sequences are made by amino acids at the base of the first zinc finger. Almost all nuclear receptors bind to DNA as dimers. Consequently, each monomer recognizes an individual DNA sequence that is referred to as a 'half-site' of a hormone response element (Fig. 6). The second zinc finger and portions of the first finger are involved in receptor dimerization and help to define the spacing between the 'half-sites' of hormone response elements (Fig. 6). Because nuclear receptor recognition of specific DNA sequences in target genes is one of the major determinants of their biological activity, the zinc-finger motifs involved in DNA recognition and response element spacing are highly specific for different receptors. The receptors that bind steroids, such as glucocorticoid, oestrogen, progesterone, and androgen receptors, bind to DNA as homodimers. The steroid receptor HREs are typically palindromic, reflecting the twofold symmetry of the homodimer at the DNA level. The thyroid, retinoid, and vitamin D receptors also bind to DNA as homodimers, although most of their hormone response elements are arranged as direct repeats rather than in a palindromic orientation. This latter group of receptors also binds to DNA as heterodimers with accessory proteins such as the retinoid X receptors.

Fig. 6 Nuclear receptor interactions with response elements. Nuclear receptors that bind steroids include the oestrogen receptor (ER), glucocorticoid receptor (GR), progesterone receptor (PR), androgen receptor (AR), and mineralocorticoid receptor (MR). They bind to target hormone response elements (HREs) in DNA as homodimers. The HREs for the steroid receptors are typically palindromic, reflecting the twofold symmetry of the homodimer. The HRE 'half-sites' (arrows) differ in primary sequence and spacing (designated by n's). The ER half site (AGGTCA) is distinct from the recognition sites for the GR, but the recognition sites for the GR, AR, and PR are similar or identical. The non-steroid receptors include the vitamin D receptor (VDR), the thyroid hormone receptor (TR), the retinoic acid receptor (RAR), as well as several 'orphan' receptors (not shown) for which ligands do not exist or are still being characterized. This class of receptors binds to their HREs as homodimers or as heterodimers with accessory proteins such as the retinoic acid X receptor (RXR). The heterodimers for VDR, TR, and RAR recognize direct repeats of similar half-sites (AGGTCA) that are spaced by 3, 4, or 5 nucleotides, respectively. Amino acid sequences in the nuclear receptor DNA-binding domains that are involved in binding to half-sites and in spacing between receptor monomers have now been characterized by mutagenesis and structural studies. Subtle differences in the amino acid sequences of the receptors confer specificity for different HREs.

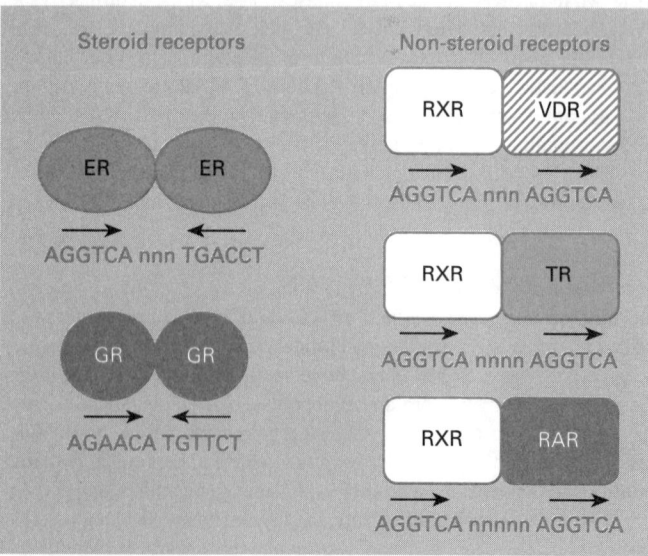

When the heterodimers bind to direct repeats, different dimerization contacts in the zinc fingers are used and provide the primary determinants of hormone response element specificity. In this case, the primary DNA sequence of the hormone response element half-site is similar or identical for different receptors but the spacing between the half-sites is variable. For example, vitamin D, thyroid, and retinoid receptors recognize direct repeat half-sites that are spaced by 3, 4, and 5 nucleotides, respectively.

The hormone-binding domain of the nuclear receptors is located in the carboxy-terminal region of the protein. This region of the nuclear receptors also contains other functional domains, including nuclear localization signals and binding sites for chaperone proteins such as heat-shock proteins. Hydrophobic surfaces in the carboxy-terminus are also involved in dimerization with appropriate protein partners.

The fact that nuclear receptors are also transcription factors has led to intensive investigation of the mechanisms by which they activate or repress gene transcription. The nuclear receptors are directed to DNA via their DNA-binding domains. In some cases, such as the oestrogen, progesterone, and glucocorticoid receptors, hormone binding is a prerequisite for DNA binding. Members of the thyroid hormone receptor subfamily bind to DNA in the absence of ligand binding. For all nuclear receptors, hormone binding induces conformational changes in the carboxy-terminus, an event which triggers transcriptional activation. Exactly how the activated receptor stimulates transcription remains somewhat obscure. However, transcriptional activating domains have been localized by mutagenesis studies. There appear to be distinct transcriptional activating domains located in the carboxy-terminal and in the amino-terminal regions of the receptors. The transcriptional activating domains have been demonstrated to interact with components of the basal transcription complex, such as TFIIB, providing a likely molecular basis for enhancement of transcription (see below). How the same receptor can alternatively cause transcriptional repression is less clear. There is accumulating evidence that hormone-induced repression is mediated by receptor inhibition of positively acting transcription factors.

Functions of hormones

The physiological roles for traditional hormones can be divided into three major areas:

(1) growth and differentiation;
(2) maintenance of homeostasis; and
(3) reproduction.

These categories are not mutually exclusive as many hormones serve multiple roles and many biological responses require integration of several different hormonal pathways.

The process of growth is clearly dependent upon many hormones. Children who are deficient in growth hormone will have short stature. But, it is also well established that thyroid hormone deficiency can cause an abrupt cessation in linear growth. Most well-studied models of growth, such as that of the epiphyseal growth plate, reveal a complex interplay of many hormones and growth factors, some of which (growth hormone, insulin-like growth factor I, thyroid hormone) stimulate growth, whereas others (sex steroids) lead to epiphyseal closure.

Multiple hormonal pathways are also involved in responses to the environment and the maintenance of homeostasis. Although hormones such as thyroid hormone, growth hormone, and cortisol play crucial roles in growth and development, they are also involved in metabolism. Thyroid hormone controls basal metabolic rate and its effects are manifest in most tissues where it activates genes involved in metabolic pathways and thermogenesis. Growth hormone and cortisol, with glucagon and adrenaline, are often considered as a group of counter-regulatory hormones that act to raise blood sugar levels. However, each of these hormones has additional selective effects on specific metabolic pathways. Glucagon and adrenaline act rapidly. Adrenaline stimulates glycogenolysis and gluconeogenesis by its actions through β-adrenergic receptors which activate cAMP pathways. Glucagon acts predominantly on the liver to initiate glycolysis of stored glycogen, as well as activating multiple enzymatic pathways involved in gluconeogenesis and ketogenesis. Growth hormone stimulates growth in large measure via insulin-like growth factor I, but it also exerts specific metabolic effects, including lipolysis and the conversion of glucose and amino acids into protein. Cortisol acts through nuclear receptors and exerts its effects by changes at the level of gene expression. Consequently, its metabolic actions are also longer term. Cortisol is gluconeogenic and permissive for the actions of other hormones. In Cushing's syndrome, muscle wasting and redistribution of fat leading to centripetal obesity are the result of the metabolic consequences of long-term cortisol excess.

Insulin is the primary hormone involved in metabolic responses to meals and mobilization of nutrients in response to caloric deprivation. It is secreted rapidly in response to meals and is released particularly in response to absorbed glucose and amino acids. Secreted insulin causes a series of shifts in metabolic pathways, with a net effect of enhancing glucose uptake by cells and the stimulation of pathways that allow energy storage. It enhances glycogen synthesis, lipogenesis, and protein biosynthesis. It also inhibits gluconeogenesis, lipolysis, and protein breakdown. Insulin action is readily monitored by changes in circulating glucose levels. When there are metabolic demands, suppression of insulin secretion activates an opposing cascade causing glycogenolysis, protein degradation, and lipolysis.

Other aspects of homeostasis, such as fluid and electrolyte balance, are also under strict hormonal control. Vasopressin, secreted by the posterior pituitary acts upon receptors in the distal collecting tubules of the kidney to restrict free water excretion. Osmoreceptors in the hypothalamus sense serum tonicity and control vasopressin release such that serum osmolality is controlled within a remarkably narrow range (281–287 mosmol/kg).

The renin–angiotensin axis is involved in blood pressure control at several different levels. Agents such as angiotensin II are potent vasoconstrictors and there is evidence for a locally acting renin–angiotensin system that contributes to the control of vascular resistance. In addition, by stimulating aldosterone production by the adrenal cortex, angiotensin II can influence longer-term mineralocorticoid effects, resulting in sodium retention, volume expansion, and potassium excretion. The serum potassium concentration also has an important role in the control of aldosterone production.

Serum calcium concentrations are controlled by parathyroid hormone, which acts upon several target organs to increase calcium levels. Parathyroid hormone causes calcium release from bone where it activates osteoclasts that have access to readily mobilized calcium stores. Parathyroid hormone also enhances calcium absorption from the gastrointestinal tract and in the kidney, where it also stimulates conversion of 25-hydroxyvitamin D to its more active metabolite, 1,25-dihydroxyvitamin D. Vitamin D facilitates the actions of parathyroid hormone by enhancing absorption of calcium from the gastrointestinal tract and its mobilization from bone. Calcitonin opposes many of the actions of parathyroid hormone and acts to lower serum calcium. Although administration of calcitonin is sometimes used in the management of hypercalcaemia, it plays a secondary role in the physiological control of serum calcium.

The third major group of hormonal actions is involved in the control of reproduction. Many of the hormonal events involved in reproduction actually occur very early in development. During fetal development, a number of hormones influence sexual differentiation. In the absence of the influence of Y-chromosomal genes, the female phenotype develops. In the male, expression of the testis determining factor results in a cascade of events that leads to testicular development, regression of müllerian structures under the influence of müllerian inhibiting substance, and development of wolffian ducts. Testis determining factor has now been localized on the Y chromosome and it encodes a DNA-binding protein that activates a series of other genes involved in sexual differentiation. Müllerian inhibiting substance has also been characterized and

is a member of a family of hormones that includes the transforming growth factor-β, inhibin, and activin. After development of the testis, testosterone and its derivative, dihydrotestosterone, cause further development and differentiation of the external genitalia.

Puberty is the next major stage in sexual development, when the hypothalamic–pituitary–gonadal axis becomes reactivated after a period of relative dormancy during early childhood. Puberty is heralded by nocturnal pulses of luteinizing hormone and follicle stimulating hormone, driven by gonadotrophin releasing hormone. As the hypothalamic–pituitary–gonadal axis matures, the pulsatile pattern of gonadotrophin secretion becomes more regular and continues throughout the day. The gonadotrophins stimulate further maturation of the gonads. In males, testicular growth is accompanied by increased testosterone secretion from Leydig cells, resulting in virilization and the development of secondary sexual characteristics. In females, ovarian production of oestrogen and progesterone induces secondary sexual features and provides feedback to the hypothalamus and pituitary, resulting in menstrual cycles. The hormonal changes that occur during the 28-day menstrual cycle represent one of the most remarkable examples of highly co-ordinated endocrine systems. In the early follicular phase, pulsatile secretion of luteinizing hormone and follicle stimulating hormone cause progressive maturation of the ovarian follicle. The resulting gradual increase in oestrogen and progesterone lead to increased pituitary sensitivity to gonadotrophin releasing hormone, which, combined with a sudden acceleration of gonadotrophin releasing hormone secretion, causes the luteinizing hormone surge and rupture of the mature follicle. A number of hormones in addition to gonadotropins and sex steroids are involved in the reproductive system. Inhibin and activin have important roles in the regulation of follicle stimulating hormone and likely have local effects in the gonads. Other growth factors, such as epidermal growth factor and insulin-like growth factor I also modulate responsiveness to gonadotrophins. In females, the menopause is the final stage of reproductive development. Menopause is often preceded by several years of irregular menses, followed by more complete ovarian senescence when the capacity for steroid synthesis declines. In the absence of gonadal hormones, gonadotrophins are elevated, reflecting decreased feedback inhibition.

Integrated hormonal responses

Responses to environmental changes represent one of the primary functions of the endocrine system. In addition to the hormonal pathways involved in the maintenance of homeostasis, there are a number of adaptive responses that involve the endocrine system. Typically, these responses involve many hormones and their integrated effects can result in a much more pronounced effect than is seen with any one hormone alone. The stress response is a good example of an integrated hormonal system. Depending upon the severity of a given stress and whether it is acute or chronic, a wide array of endocrine pathways can be activated. In severe acute stress such as trauma or shock, the sympathetic nervous system is activated and release of catecholamines results in increased cardiac output and primes the musculoskeletal system for appropriate responses. Catecholamines also increase mean blood pressure and cause the release of glucose. In the central nervous system, multiple stress-induced pathways converge on the hypothalamus, resulting in the release of several hormones including vasopressin and corticotrophin releasing factor (CRF). Pituitary hormones including adrenocorticotrophic hormone, growth hormone, and prolactin are also secreted in response to stress. Vasopressin serves to increase vascular resistance as well as conserving free water at the level of the kidney. Adrenocorticotrophic hormone increases serum cortisol, which acts on many organs as an adaptation to stress. Cortisol helps to sustain blood pressure and reduces inflammatory responses. In conjunction with other hormones, cortisol elevates blood glucose levels. In patients with adrenal insufficiency, the requirement for increased levels of cortisol in the presence of trauma or infection is illustrated by manifestations of cortisol deficiency that are evident when only standard replacement doses of the hormone are administered.

Many other processes such as bone growth, lactation, and metabolic enzyme pathways require input from many hormones to occur effectively. At a cellular level, the requirement for many hormones reflects distinct pathways for modulating cellular responses. Although free water clearance is primarily controlled by vasopressin, cortisol and thyroxine are also important for preparing the renal tubular cell for the effects of vasopressin. During pregnancy, the increased production of prolactin in combination with placental lactogen and placentally derived steroids, including oestrogen and progesterone, is required to prepare the breast for lactation. Oestrogens induce the production of progesterone receptors, allowing increased responsivity to the hormone. In addition to these and other hormones involved in lactation, the nervous system and oxytocin are involved in the suckling response and milk release.

Fig. 7 Positive and negative feedback regulation in an endocrine axis. The hypothalamic–pituitary–thyroid axis is illustrated to represent a typical example of feedback regulatory pathways. Hypothalamic thyrotrophin releasing hormone (TRH) is produced by neurones that surround the third ventricle and terminate at the median eminence where TRH is released into the portal circulation to stimulate thyroid stimulating hormone (TSH) secretion by the pituitary gland. TSH stimulates the biosynthesis and secretion of thyroid hormones (T_4/T_3) from the thyroid gland; these cause feedback inhibition at the pituitary and hypothalamus. Because the pituitary integrates both positive and negative regulation, it establishes a setpoint for TSH and, consequently, thyroid hormones.

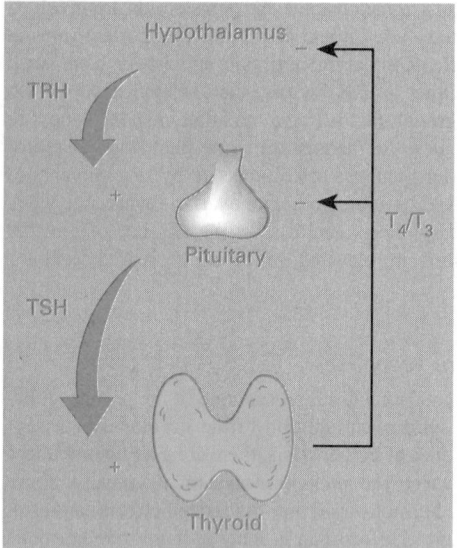

Concept of feedback regulatory systems

The concept of negative feedback control represents a fundamental tenet of endocrinology. Each of the major hypothalamic–pituitary hormone axes are governed by negative feedback, which serves to maintain hormone levels within a very narrow range. Examples include feedback of thyroid hormones on the thyrotrophin releasing hormone–thyroid stimulating hormone axis, cortisol on the corticotrophin releasing hormone–adrenocorticotrophic hormone axis, and gonadal steroids on the gonadotrophin releasing hormone–luteinizing hormone/follicle stimulating hormone axis and insulin-like growth factor I on the growth hormone releasing factor–growth hormone axis. A representative feedback loop is illustrated by the hypothalamic–pituitary–thyroid axis (Fig. 7). Hypothalamic thyrotrophin releasing hormone stimulates thyroid stimulating hormone secretion from the pituitary. Thyroid stimulating hormone increases thyroid hormone secretion which, in turn, suppresses hypothalamic thyrotrophin releasing hormone as well as pituitary thyroid stimulating hormone. A typical regulatory loop therefore has both positive (TRH, TSH) and negative (T_4, T_3) components, allowing a high degree of fine tuning of hormone levels. In this case, the pituitary gland integrates positive thyrotrophin releasing hormone signals and negative effects of thyroid hormone. Ultimately, the pituitary acts as a sensor for circulating free thyroid hormone, which binds to its nuclear receptors to modulate gene transcription—in this case, the thyroid stimulating hormone α and β genes. These principles of feedback regulation are important not only for understanding endocrine physiology, but because they provide strategies for sensitive assessments of endocrine gland function. For example, a thyrotrophin releasing hormone stimulation test provides a very sensitive assessment of the presence of autonomous, excess production of T_3. In this case, tonic feedback suppression by thyroid hormone prevents thyroid stimulating hormone secretion in response to exogenous thyrotrophin releasing hormone.

In addition to these examples of classic endocrine systems in which hormones are released by one gland and travel through the circulation to act on another, several other types of more local regulatory pathways are now recognized (Fig. 8). Paracrine regulation refers to factors that are released by one cell and act upon a nearby cell in the same tissue. Paracrine regulation is well illustrated in the pancreatic islets, in which secretion of somatostatin by the δ cells can inhibit secretion of insulin from the β cells. Autocrine regulation refers to production of a factor that acts upon the same cell in which the factor is produced. This type of control is difficult to document, but it probably applies to a number of growth factors, including, for example, production of activin by pituitary gonadotrophs. In this case, locally produced activin can act to stimulate production of follicle stimulating hormone by the gonadotroph cell. Finally, it is likely that there are hormonal feedback loops that can

Fig. 8 Pathways of hormone action. Endocrine hormones are secreted from one gland and enter the circulation to act on a different target gland. Paracrine hormones or growth factors are produced by one cell but act locally on an adjacent cell. Autocrine action is similar to that of paracrine, except that a growth factor acts upon the same cell that produced it. Intracrine action suggests that some hormones act upon intracellular receptors of the same cells in which they are produced.

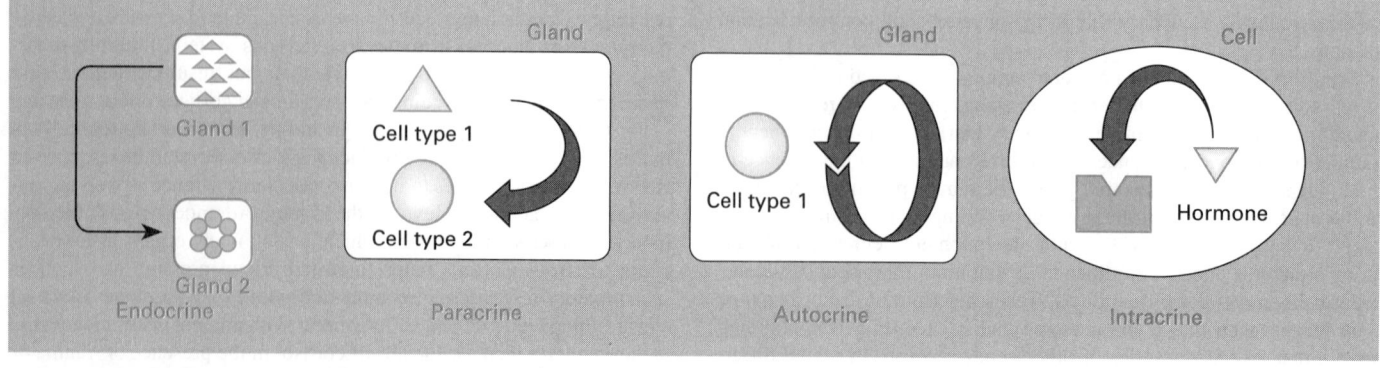

even occur within cells. These pathways would be somewhat analogous to the regulatory pathways that control enzymes, except that hormones and their receptors would be involved rather than allosteric interactions of enzyme substrates or products.

Regulatory pathways can also be influenced by the anatomical relationships of hormones and their target organs. For example, a rich vascular network connects the hypothalamus and pituitary gland. This relationship allows the pituitary gland to be exposed to relatively high concentrations of hypothalamic hormones. Moreover, the waveforms of hypothalamic secretion can be transmitted directly to the pituitary gland with minimal diffusion, allowing very discrete pulses of hormones such as gonadotrophin releasing hormone to be delivered. Another important anatomical relationship concerns the connection of the pancreas to the gastrointestinal tract and the liver. The pancreatic islets are critically positioned to receive signals from absorbed nutrients and to release insulin into the portal circulation such that the liver is the proximal recipient of secreted insulin. In the testis, local production of high concentrations of testosterone are important for spermatogenesis.

Hormonal rhythms

The feedback regulatory systems described above are superimposed upon hormonal rhythms that are used for adaptation to the environment. The seasonal changes and the daily occurrence of the light–dark cycle are but two of many environmental events which have major impacts on hormonal rhythms. Many hormonal pathways appear to be entrained upon the circadian cycle, causing highly reproducible fluctuations that occur approximately every 24 h. For example, the hypothalamic–pituitary–adrenal axis demonstrates characteristic peaks of cortisol production in the early morning with a nadir in the late afternoon and evening. Recognition of the occurrence of these rhythms has practical importance in terms of endocrine investigation and treatment. For example, testing for CRF response is most sensitive when performed in the late evening when adrenocorticotrophic hormone and cortisol levels are low. Moreover, the hypothalamic–pituitary–adrenal axis is more susceptible to suppression by glucocorticoids administered at night in comparison with the morning.

In addition to the CRF–adrenocorticotrophic hormone system, other hypothalamic–pituitary regulatory pathways can be shown to exhibit diurnal rhythms. These can be altered most profoundly by light–dark cycles, but in many cases also by sleep, stress, exercise, or by meals. The early pubertal surges of luteinizing hormone occur at night and usually in association with sleep. Nocturnal surges of growth hormone secretion are also characteristic and account in part for the dawn phenomenon which refers to a state of relative resistance to insulin that can be seen in diabetics. The nocturnal increase in vasopressin allows diminished excretion of free water during sleep.

A number of other endocrine rhythms do not appear to be linked to circadian cycles. One of the most carefully studied is the pulsatile secretion of luteinizing hormone and follicle stimulating hormone which reflects pulsatile secretion of hypothalamic gonadotrophin releasing hormone. In women, the pulse frequency of gonadotrophin releasing hormone varies during the menstrual cycle from those that occur about every 90 min in the follicular phase to a slower pulse frequency of one pulse every 2 to 3 h in the luteal phase. The gonadotrophin releasing hormone–luteinizing hormone/follicle stimulating hormone pathway is exquisitely sensitive to pulse frequency and it has been shown that the intermittent pulses of gonadotrophin releasing hormone are required to maintain pituitary sensitivity to this hormone. Continuous exposure to gonadotrophin releasing hormone actually causes pituitary desensitization, a phenomenon which forms the basis for using long-acting gonadotrophin releasing hormone superagonists to treat central precocious puberty or to create a state of 'medical castration' for the management of prostate cancer.

Insulin also exhibits rapid (about every 10 min) secretory pulses that appear to be entrained to changes in circulating glucose concentrations. These small, rapid secretory bursts of insulin are superimposed upon larger pulses of insulin that occur about every hour and in response to meals. Defects in the ability of the islet cell to sense changes in glucose probably represents one of the early alterations in certain forms of type 2 diabetes mellitus (e.g. maturity-onset diabetes of the young). Like the gonadotroph cell in the reproductive axis, the 'set-point' of the B cell may also be influenced by its hormonal milieu.

Certain hormonal rhythms such as the menstrual cycle occur on a much longer time scale (28 days). The pattern of the menstrual cycle is coupled to cycles of follicular development in the ovary. As the numbers and state of differentiation of granulosa and thecal cells change, their responsiveness to pituitary luteinizing hormone and follicle stimulating hormone is altered. As follicular development progresses, levels of gonadal steroids and inhibin feedback to the hypothalamus and pituitary to modulate luteinizing hormone and follicle stimulating hormone secretion. Consequently, hormonal rhythms of the menstrual cycle are comprised of a set of rapidly secreted pulses of gonadotrophins superimposed upon a changing population of target cells in the ovary which have an inherent developmental cycle of about 28 days in humans. There is tremendous variability in reproductive cycles in different species of animals, representing remarkable adaptation to specific environmental demands. Seasonal breeding species of sheep and deer, for example, exhibit reproductive cycles that are co-ordinated with the lengths of light–dark cycles to allow breeding during a season such that gestation terminates during favourable climatic conditions.

Because many hormones are released in a pulsatile manner and in a rhythmic fashion, it is important to be aware of the characteristics of secretion when attempting to relate serum hormone measurements to normal values. Clearly, luteinizing hormone values will vary widely from the nadir of a pulse to the peak of a pulse. In addition, an luteinizing hormone determination at the midcycle gonadotrophin surge will be much greater than one determined in the early follicular phase. Similar considerations apply for determinations of growth hormone pulses or for measurements of serum cortisol at different times of the day. Strategies for determining accurately hormone concentrations in the context of a given physiological state have been intensively investigated in endocrinology. At one end of the spectrum, frequent blood sampling (every 10 min) over several hours allows one to generate detailed pulse contours and estimates of pulse frequency, amplitude, and mean serum hormone concentration. Although this approach is useful as an investigative tool, it is rarely practical in a clinical setting. In some instances, 24 hour urine collections for free cortisol, for example, allow determination of an 'integrated' measurement of hormone production over a typical diurnal cycle of the hypothalamic–pituitary–adrenal axis. In the case of growth hormone, it is possible for some purposes to use insulin-like growth factor I as a biological marker of growth hormone action. Circulating insulin-like growth factor I, produced primarily by the liver, fluctuates less than growth hormone, although its levels can be altered independently by nutritional state or by sex steroids. Nevertheless, when taken in association with other clinical criteria, insulin-like growth factor I provides a measure of growth hormone action that reflects multiple peaks of growth hormone secretion, many of which may have occurred during the night. Measurement of haemoglobin A1C represents another example of an integrated assay. It reflects mean glucose concentrations in a manner that is insensitive to hourly fluctuations, thereby providing a more reliable index of long-term (weeks to months) control of blood sugar.

Often, one must interpret endocrine data only in the context of an array of other hormonal results. For example, parathyroid hormone levels are typically assessed in combination with serum calcium concentrations. A high serum calcium level in association with elevated parathyroid hormone is suggestive of hyperparathyroidism, whereas a suppressed parathyroid hormone level in this situation is more likely to be caused by some other disorder such as hypercalcaemia of malignancy. Similarly, one expects the thyroid stimulating hormone level to be elevated when T_4 and T_3 concentrations are low, reflecting loss of feedback inhibition. When this is not the case, it is important to consider other abnormalities in the hormonal axis. These might include secondary hypothyroidism with a defect at the level of the pituitary. Alternatively, an abnormality in thyroxine binding globulin could cause low total T_4 and T_3 even though the free concentrations of hormone are normal, resulting in appropriate feedback inhibition at the pituitary level. Additional tests would then be required to assess these and other potential explanations for unexpected ratios in hormonal feedback relationships.

Mechanisms of endocrine disease

For the most part, endocrine diseases can be divided into conditions of hormone excess, hormone deficiency, and hormone resistance (Table 4). Most disorders that cause overproduction are caused by the neoplastic growth of endocrine cells. However, autoimmune disorders, such as Graves' disease can also cause hormone overproduction by virtue of antibody interactions with membrane receptors. Most examples of hormone deficiency states can be attributed to glandular destruction whether caused by autoimmunity, or by infection, inflammation, infarction, haemorrhage, or tumour infiltrate. Iatrogenic causes of endocrine hyperfunction and hypofunction are relatively common. Glucocorticoid therapy is a frequent cause of Cushing's syndrome and hypothyroidism often occurs in conjunction with radio-iodine or surgical therapy of Graves' disease or thyroid carcinoma. Most examples of hormone resistance are due to inherited defects in membrane receptors, nuclear receptors, or in the pathways that transduce receptor signals. As described in more detail below, inherited defects can also cause endocrine hyperfunction (e.g. multiple endocrine neoplasia syndromes) or hypofunction (e.g. 21-hydroxylase deficiency).

Endocrine hyperfunction: pathophysiology of endocrine neoplasia

Neoplastic causes of hormone excess include benign adenomas, hyperplasia, malignant endocrine tumours, and ectopic sources of hormone production (Table 5). In addition, the multiple endocrine neoplasia (MEN) I and II syndromes represent a special case of endocrine neoplasia in which the predisposition to tumourigenesis is inherited in an autosomal dominant manner. Most endocrine tumours are benign and well differentiated. Examples include the majority of pituitary, thyroid, adrenal, and parathyroid adenomas. Benign endocrine tumours often retain the capacity to produce hormones, perhaps reflecting the fact that they remain relatively well differentiated and still have intact pathways for hormone biosynthesis and secretion. In fact, tumour de-differentiation is sometimes associated with loss of hormone production. Autopsy series have revealed a surprisingly high prevalence (10–25 per cent) of nodules in the pituitary, thyroid, and adrenal glands, which in most cases are clinically silent. This observation emphasizes the fact that most of these benign tumours acquire clinical significance only when they produce hormones above a threshold level. Autonomously functioning thyroid nodules (hot nodules) only cause hyperthyroidism when they secrete an amount of thyroid hormone that first causes complete suppression of thyroid stimulating hormone and then exceeds the level of thyroid hormone that is normally secreted. Similar circumstances apply to functioning adrenal nodules which cause hypercortisolism in the setting of adrenocorticotrophic hormone suppression.

The functional properties of pituitary tumours have been subjected to particularly careful study because of the availability of sensitive stimulation and suppression tests. Many pituitary tumours appear to have relatively subtle defects in their 'set-points' for feedback regulation. For example, Cushing's disease is caused by a corticotroph adenoma which secretes adrenocorticotrophic hormone (ACTH). The altered feedback inhibition of ACTH secretion by the tumour cells is readily observed in

Table 4 *Pathophysiological causes of endocrine dysfunction*

Hyperfunction
  Neoplastic
    benign
    malignant
    ectopic
    multiple endocrine neoplasia
  Autoimmune
  Iatrogenic
  Inflammatory

Hypofunction
  Autoimmune
  Iatrogenic
  Infectious
  Hormone mutations
  Enzyme defects
  Vitamin deficiency

Hormone resistance
  Receptor mutations
  Signalling pathway mutations
  Postreceptor

the dexamethasone suppression test. When low, but pharmacological doses of dexamethasone (0.5 mg every 6 h) are administered, ACTH secretion by the corticotroph tumour is minimally decreased, whereas normal corticotrophs are suppressed by this treatment. However, when a higher dose of dexamethasone (2 mg every 6 h) is given, ACTH production by the tumour cells is also suppressed. In contrast, most tumours that produce ACTH ectopically are poorly suppressed even by high doses of dexamethasone, presumably because they lack some aspect of the inhibitory pathways that exist in corticotroph tumours. Cortisol-producing tumours of the adrenal gland are also unaffected by high doses of dexamethasone as ACTH levels are already suppressed and the adrenal tumour produces cortisol in an ACTH-independent manner. Thus, the altered set-point for hormone regulation provides a useful clinical tool for the differential diagnosis of Cushing's syndrome. Similar defects in set-points are seen in other endocrine tumours such as parathyroid adenomas in which the dose–response curve for calcium-induced inhibition of parathyroid hormone secretion is shifted to the right. Although the tumour cells are less sensitive to feedback inhibition, the fact that partial inhibition is retained is probably important for restraining tumour growth. This point is illustrated by the occasional occurrence of Nelson's syndrome after adrenalectomy for Cushing's disease.

Although most hormone-producing endocrine tumours are benign, malignant tumours can also account for hormone excess syndromes. For example, adrenal carcinomas may be recognized because of hirsutism or Cushing's syndrome, reflecting excess steroid production. Many carcinoid and islet cell tumours are detected after metastases have already occurred. In other glands, the transition from a benign to malignant state is unusual, but nevertheless occurs. For example, parathyroid carcinomas, pituitary carcinomas, and malignant phaeochromocytomas can produce clinical syndromes that closely resemble those of their more benign counterparts. For these groups of endocrine tumours, the distinction between benign and malignant cannot always be made reliably based upon the histological appearance of the cells, and is usually based upon evidence of invasion of normal tissue or the presence of metastases. Thyroid carcinomas, although relatively common, are rarely associated with excess production of thyroid hormone. As mentioned above, this may reflect the loss of differentiated cellular function during the progression from a benign to malignant state.

Tumours that produce hormones ectopically represent a heterogeneous category of neoplasms that can cause hormone excess. Paramount among these are lung carcinomas that produce vasopressin (causing syn-

Table 5 *Genetic causes of endocrine dysfunction*

Site of mutation	Disorder	Inheritance	Mutation
Hyperfunction			
Genetic causes of neoplasia			
TSH receptor	Thyroid adenomas	S	P
Ras p21	Thyroid adenomas and cancer	S	P
Gsα	Acromegaly, thyroid autonomy	S	P
Gsα	McCune–Albright	S	P
Giα	Ovary, adrenal, thyroid tumours	S	P
p53	Anaplastic thyroid cancer	S	D,P
Retinoblastoma	Parathyroid	S	D,P
PRAD-1 (cyclin D1)	Parathyroid adenomas	S	Trans
PTC (papillary thyroid carcinoma)	Papillary thyroid cancer	S	Trans
MEN I (multiple endocrine neoplasia I)	Neoplasia: pituitary, pancreas, parathyroid	AD	Chrom 11
MEN II (ret mutations)	Neoplasia: parathyroid, phaeochromocytoma, medullary thyroid carcinoma	AD	P
MEN IIb (ret mutations)	MEN II and neurofibromas	AD	?P
Hypofunction			
Hormone mutations			
Insulin	Hyperproinsulinaemia	AD	P
Growth hormone	Dwarfism	AR	D, P
Parathyroid hormone	Hypoparathyroidism	AD	P
Thyroid stimulating hormone	Hypothyroidism	AR	D, P
Thyroglobulin	Hypothyroidism; goitre	AR	P
Luteinizing hormone	Hypogonadism	AR	P
Follicle stimulating hormone	Hypogonadism	AR	P
Vasopressin/neurophysin II	Central diabetes insipidus	AD	P
Enzyme mutations			
Thyroid peroxidase	Goitre, hypothyroidism	AR	P
21-hydroxylase	CAH	AR	P,D
17α-hydroxylase	Androgen deficiency, hypertension	AR	P
11β-hydroxylase	Androgen excess, hypertension	AR	P
3β-hydroxysteroid dehydrogenase	Androgen excess, often lethal	AR	?
5α-reductase type 2	Male pseudohermaphroditism	AR	D,P
Aldosterone synthetase	Glucocorticoid remediable hypertension	AD	D,Trans
VLC fatty acid CoA synthetase	Adrenoleucodystrophy	XL	D
Cell development/migration			
Kallmann syndrome	Hypogonadotropic hypogonadism	XL,AR,AD	D,P,Trans
Transcription factors			
SRY	XY female	YL	P,Trans
Pit-1	GH,PRL,TSH deficiency	AR,AD	D,P
Hormone resistance			
Membrane receptor mutations			
Insulin receptor	Insulin resistance	AR,AD	P
Growth hormone receptor	Laron dwarfism	AR	P
Vasopressin V_2 receptor	Nephrogenic diabetes insipidus	XL	P
Thyroid stimulating hormone receptor	TSH resistance	AR	P
Calcium sensing receptor	Familial hypocalciuric hypercalcaemia	AR	P
Signalling pathway mutations			
Gsα	Albright hereditary osteodystrophy	AD,S	P
Nuclear receptor mutations			
Vitamin D	Vitamin D resistance	AR	P
Thyroid hormone	Thyroid hormone resistance	AD,AR	P,D
Glucocorticoid	Glucocorticoid resistance	AD	P
Androgen	Androgen resistance	XL	P,D
Oestrogen	Oestrogen resistance	AR	P

GH, growth hormone; PRL, prolactin; TSH, thyroid stimulating hormone; SRY, sex reversed Y; CAH, congenital adrenal hyperplasia; AD, autosomal dominant; AR, autosomal recessive; S, somatic cell mutation; XL, X-linked; YL, Y-linked; Trans, Translocation; D, deletion; P, point mutation; ?, unknown.

drome of inappropriate ADH secretion), parathyroid hormone related peptide (causing hypercalcaemia of malignancy), and ACTH (causing an ectopic form of Cushing's syndrome).

The causes of hypercalcaemia of malignancy include excess production of parathyroid hormone related protein, production of locally acting cytokines that cause bone resorption, and excess synthesis of 1,25-dihydroxyvitamin D. Ectopic production of parathyroid hormone itself is rare, but has been well-documented in several case reports, one of which involved a gene rearrangement such that the parathyroid hormone gene was brought under the control of regulatory elements that caused its overexpression in the ovary, thereby accounting for hyperparathyroidism with an ovarian source for parathyroid hormone. Parathyroid hormone related protein elicits biological effects that closely resemble those of parathyroid hormone, including high calcium, and low phosphate concentrations in plasma, together with increased urinary cAMP. The similar biological effects of parathyroid hormone and parathyroid hormone related peptide are now understood, in that the hormones bind to a common receptor. Although the parathyroid hormone and parathyroid hormone related peptide proteins are structurally similar, particularly at the amino-terminal end that is involved in receptor binding, there are sufficient differences in sequence to allow the development of specific immunoassays. Consequently, in the appropriate clinical setting, patients with elevated calcium and suppressed parathyroid hormone are suspected of having humoral hypercalcaemia of malignancy, and this can often be confirmed by measurements of parathyroid hormone related peptide. Some malignancies may not show elevated parathyroid hormone related peptide levels because other cytokines such as interleukin-6 (IL-6), IL-α or β, tumour necrosis factor-α, (TNF α), or others may cause osteoclastic resorption. In certain lymphomas or in granulomatous diseases such as sarcoidosis, increased 1α-hydroxylase activity can result in increased conversion of 25-hydroxyvitamin D to its more active metabolite, 1,25-dihydroxyvitamin D.

The multiple endocrine neoplasia syndromes (MEN I, MEN IIa, MEN IIb) represent some of the few well-characterized inherited diseases that predispose to neoplasia. The MEN syndromes are each inherited in an autosomal dominant manner, although the gene defects in MEN I and II are clearly distinct. Major advances in the understanding and management of the MEN syndromes have occurred in conjunction with identification of the genetic basis for these disorders. In the case of MEN I, genetic linkage studies have localized a candidate gene on the long arm of chromosome 11 (11q13). Although the MEN I gene has not been cloned, speculation on its function has centred on its role as a possible tumour suppressor gene. Tumour tissue from patients with MEN I has been shown to exhibit loss of heterozygosity at the MEN I locus. In this situation, it is suggested that the inherited (presumably defective) MEN I allele remains and that somatic loss of the normal MEN I gene represents a 'second hit' at the suppressor gene locus, thereby leading to tumorigenesis. This scenario is analogous to the two-hit model for loss of retinoblastoma gene function, a well-characterized example of a tumour suppressor gene. Cloning of the MEN I gene will clarify how it leads to neoplasia and should provide a specific genetic test for predisposition to MEN I.

The MEN II gene has been localized to the long arm of chromosome 10. Unlike MEN I, loss of heterozygosity is not seen in tumours from patients with MEN II, suggesting that a different pathophysiology exists for MEN II. In MEN II, affected individuals often have thyroid C-cell hyperplasia in childhood before the development of medullary thyroid carcinoma. This observation is consistent with a pathophysiology in which the MEN II gene predisposes to hyperplastic growth with a second and perhaps distinct somatic mutation leading to tumorigenesis and clonal proliferation of tumour cells. Recently, mutations in the ret proto-oncogene, a putative tyrosine kinase receptor, have been identified as the probable cause of MEN IIa. In several MEN II kindreds, distinct ret mutations were found in a cluster of cysteines located at the juncture of the extracellular and transmembrane domains of the protein. The functional effects of these mutations are not currently understood, but

it is likely that they activate signalling pathways involved in the proliferation of neuroendocrine cells. Identification of MEN II gene carriers is particularly significant because of the importance of early diagnosis of medullary thyroid carcinoma or phaeochromocytoma. In the future, screening for ret mutations may allow high-risk individuals to be selected for more intense endocrine screening.

Theories of tumourigenesis and clonality in endocrine neoplasia

An increasing body of evidence suggests that similar mechanisms of tumorigenesis may underlie the neoplastic transformation of cells in different tissues. This 'universal' theory of tumourigenesis holds that cellular transformation is the consequence of an accumulation of mutational events that ultimately leads to altered cell growth and clonal expansion of a neoplastic cell.

Implicit in the foregoing model of tumourigenesis is the concept that somatic mutations lead to a clonal expansion of a progenitor cell that harbours the mutation. Monoclonal tumours are contrasted with polyclonal tumours or hyperplasia in which proliferation might be caused by exposure of a group of cells to a growth factor, for example (Fig. 9). The concept of clonality is important because it implies the presence of an underlying mutation that either provides a growth advantage to the precursor tumour cell or prevents the cells from reaching terminal differentiation and senescence. These mutations could take the form of gene rearrangements, activating mutations in oncogenes such as *ras*, or loss of the function of a tumour suppressor gene such as *Rb*. The distinction between monoclonal and polyclonal events is not mutually exclusive. For example, a somatic mutation (a clonal event) could cause overproduction of a growth factor that results in polyclonal expansion of a group of cells. It is also possible that chronic overstimulation that leads to hyperplasia could somehow predispose to somatic mutations that would cause secondary monoclonal expansion. As noted above, in MEN II, there is clear hyperplasia of thyroid C cells prior to the development of medullary thyroid carcinoma. Other examples of autonomous hyperplastic growth include CRF-induced Cushing's disease, nesidioblastosis, and in micronodular adrenal hyperplasia.

The phenomenon of hyperplasia leading to tumourigenesis is, however, rare in most other endocrine tumors. Almost all pituitary, thyroid, and parathyroid tumors are monoclonal in origin. Because of X-chromosome inactivation in females (Lyon hypothesis), it is possible to determine whether tumours have arisen from a single cell, in which case all tumour cells show the same pattern of X-inactivation. Alternatively, multiple cell origin would result in random inactivation of paternal and maternal X chromosomes. This approach reveals that a single X chromosome is inactivated in most parathyroid, thyroid, and pituitary tum-

Fig. 9 Clonality of tumours. Origins of endocrine or other tumours are illustrated as being monoclonal or polyclonal. Monoclonal tumours arise from a single cell as a consequence of a somatic mutation. Polyclonal tumours have multiple cell origin reflecting either germ-line inheritance of a mutation or exposure to trophic factors that cause hyperplasia.

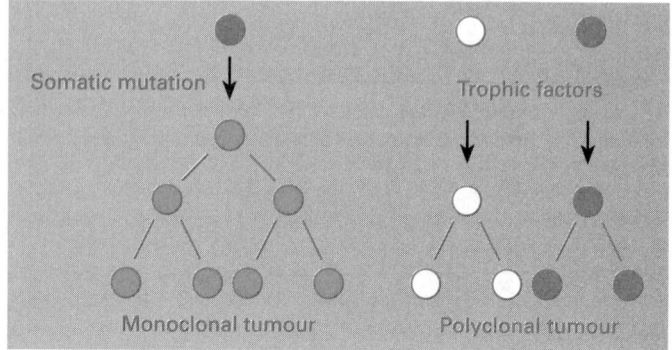

ours, consistent with monoclonality. A second line of evidence for clonal origin is that gene rearrangements or chromosomal losses are often seen in the entire population of tumour cells, suggesting that these defects either contribute to tumourigenesis or were fortuitously present in the original tumour cells. In either case, these alterations also support a model of monoclonal expansion.

Signalling pathway mutations in endocrine neoplasia

Given the probable monoclonal origin of most endocrine tumours, it is reasonable to try to identify the somatic mutations that lead to clonal expansion (Table 5). This issue is of particular interest in endocrine tumours where the somatic mutations might be predicted to involve hormone signalling pathways or to at least preserve the differentiated phenotype of the endocrine cell such that hormone biosynthesis is preserved.

For many peptide hormone receptors, signals are transduced via G-proteins. As described above, G-proteins are GTPases that are active when GTP is bound and inactivated after GTP hydrolysis to GDP. Mutations in G-proteins have been described in several different types of endocrine neoplasia. Mutations in the Gsα-subunit were first identified in somatotroph adenomas, either at codon 201 or 227. Each of these mutations inhibits GTP hydrolysis and thereby causes constitutive activation of the Gsα-subunit. Activation of Gsα in this cell type stimulates adenylate cyclase, leading to elevated cAMP levels, a situation that mimics growth hormone releasing factor stimulation. As a result, the Gsα mutation causes excess growth hormone secretion and probably contributes to abnormal cell growth as cAMP is known to cause proliferation of somatotroph cells. Mutations in Gsα are found in approximately 35 to 40 per cent of somatotroph adenomas. Predictably, the biochemical characteristics of tumours with and without Gsα mutations are distinguishable *in vitro* in that tumours with mutations have high basal levels of cAMP which are not stimulated further after treatment with growth hormone releasing factor. However, *in vivo*, it is unclear whether the Gsα mutation results in tumours with substantially different biological behaviour than tumours without the mutation. Tumours with Gsα mutations tend to be sightly smaller in size, but growth hormone and insulin-like growth factor I levels are similar in tumours with and without mutations. The Gsα mutations that cause acromegaly are clearly somatic rather than inherited, since the mutation is not seen in other tissues. Gsα mutations have also been identified in autonomous thyroid adenomas, and mutations in other G-proteins (e.g. the Gi2-subunit) have been found in adrenal and ovarian tumours.

It is interesting to note that Gsα mutations identical to those described in somatotroph adenomas also cause the McCune–Albright syndrome. In McCune–Albright syndrome, the mutations occur early in development such that the tissue distribution of the mutation is broad rather than being restricted to somatotroph cells. Nevertheless, patients with McCune–Albright syndrome are predisposed to somatotroph adenomas along with the more typical clinical features of polyostotic fibrous dysplasia, autonomous ovarian function, *café au lait* spots, and autonomous thyroid or adrenal nodules. These clinical features are caused by the presence of Gsα mutations in each of these tissues. The variable clinical phenotype that is seen in McCune–Albright syndrome is thought to result in part from the time during development when the Gsα mutation arises, thereby leading to different degrees of mosaicism. In view of these findings, it may be reasonable to consider the effects of Gsα mutations in terms of a spectrum. At one end is McCune–Albright syndrome in which mutations occur early in development causing multiple tissues to be affected. At the other end of the spectrum, Gsα mutations that occur in fully developed tissues may lead to thyroid, pituitary, or adrenal nodules without other manifestations of McCune–Albright syndrome.

The ras protein is structurally related to the G-protein family and is also a GTPase. Ras proteins modulate cell growth and differentiation. Somatic mutations in the three *ras* genes have been identified in a number of different human malignancies, including tumours of the endocrine

system. Analogous to Gsα, mutations at two specific loci in *ras* (codons 12/13, codon 61) convert it into an oncogene by inhibiting its GTPase activity. *ras* mutations occur in approximately 30 per cent of thyroid tumours, but appear to be uncommon in other endocrine tumours that have been examined.

A novel mechanism for tumourigenesis has been provided by studies of oncogene defects in parathyroid adenomas. Based upon precedents for gene rearrangements in haematological malignancies, a subset of parathyroid tumours has been found to contain rearrangements of the parathyroid hormone gene. The translocation involves an intrachromosomal rearrangement on chromosome 11. The parathyroid hormone promoter becomes fused to a member of the cyclin D family. The fusion gene is referred to as PRAD for parathyroid adenomatosis. The cyclins regulate progress through the cell cycle and it is likely that overexpression of cyclin D1 from the highly active parathyroid hormone promoter causes altered growth regulation. This particular somatic rearrangement is an interesting example of how monoclonal expansion could occur, because the mutation involves a gene that is directly involved in cell proliferation. In addition to playing a role in the development of a subset of parathyroid adenomas, there is emerging evidence that cyclin D1 may be involved in the development of some breast tumours and lymphomas.

As summarized above, endocrine neoplasms, while not necessarily representing the most aggressive forms of cancer, are providing important models for identification of new oncogenes, as well as delineation of the steps involved in the progression of tumours from the benign to the malignant phenotype. The thyroid gland provides a relatively good model for multistep tumourigenesis because of the well-characterized histological subtypes and extensive clinical information concerning risk factors and prognosis. A hypothetical model for thyroid tumourigenesis is summarized in Fig. 10, incorporating identified mutations as well as steps that are likely to be involved in the progression from the benign to the malignant state. In this model, exogenous hormones and growth factors are viewed as agents which could initiate hyperplasia, predisposing to mutations or possibly contributing to cell growth after the occurrence of a mutation. Mutations in the thyroid stimulating hormone receptor would activate pathways for cell proliferation, but now in the absence of exogenous thyroid stimulating hormone. Moreover, because these mutations are somatic, they would be expected to cause clonal proliferation rather than a hyperplastic response. One step further in the signalling pathway, Gsα mutations have been described in some thyroid tumours, particularly nodules with autonomous production of thyroid hormone. By analogy with the Gsα mutations in somatotroph pituitary adenomas, constitutive activation of the adenylate cyclase pathway mimics the effects of thyroid stimulating hormone, stimulating production of cAMP and proliferation of thyroid follicular cells. *ras* mutations are seen in benign as well as malignant thyroid tumours and there is not a clear predilection for papillary versus follicular cancers. Thus, *ras* mutations do not appear to be sufficient for transformation, but they may contribute to abnormal growth control in combination with other somatic mutations. The exact signalling pathways activated by ras remain to be identified, but probably include the mitogen activated pathway (MAP) kinase and nuclear transcription factors such as Jun. Additional defects in the kinase pathways themselves are theoretical candidates for other oncogenes. A gene rearrangement has been described in papillary carcinomas that appears to be relatively specific for this type of tumour. This rearrangement involves an intrachromosomal inversion on the long arm of chromosome 10 that is analogous the rearrangement between parathyroid hormone and cyclin D1. The result of the inversion is that part of a gene encoding a putative tyrosine kinase (ret) is brought under the control of a new promoter, presumably altering its pattern and/or level of expression. The rearranged oncogene is referred to as *PTC* for papillary thyroid carcinoma and is observed in approximately 20 per cent of papillary carcinomas. As noted above, mutations in *ret* have also been identified in patients with MEN IIa, indicating that this oncogene can be activated in several different ways. The exact signalling pathway activated by ret also remains poorly defined. Other mutations must also be capable of causing transformation to the papillary tumour phenotype as most tumours do not contain the rearranged *PTC* oncogene. Studies of loss of heterozygosity, presumably involving tumour suppressor genes have revealed deletions on several different chromosomes, particularly in association with follicular carcinomas. Not surprisingly, anaplastic carcinomas have accumulated the largest array of oncogene 'hits', including a high prevalence of mutations in the p53 tumour suppressor gene. Thus, thyroid tumourigenesis is not unlike the situation that is evolving with other well-studied models such as colon and lung carcinomas, in which a stepwise accumulation of different mutations is associated with more invasive tumour types. Additional studies may clarify whether specific types of mutations are correlated with characteristic histological appearances. Ultimately, it is hoped that characterization of oncogene mutations in the thyroid and other types of endocrine tumours will provide biological markers of diagnostic and prognostic value.

Autoimmune causes of endocrine hyperfunction

Autoimmune-induced overproduction of hormones can almost always be attributed to the presence of circulating antibodies that can bind to membrane receptors. A classic example of this phenomenon is illustrated by Graves' disease. Initially described as long-acting thyroid stimulators, the antibodies in Graves' disease are only part of a complex autoimmune syndrome with components of cell-mediated and humoral immunity. There is often lymphocytic infiltration of the thyroid gland in Graves' disease. Other targets of the autoimmune process can include the connective tissue and fat of the orbits, leading to ophthalmopathy, and the skin, leading to infiltrative dermopathy such as pretibial myxoedema. The antibodies in Graves' disease are directed at the thyroid stimulating hormone (TSH) receptor as well as a panoply of other thyroid antigens, including other membrane proteins and the microsomal enzyme, thyroid peroxidase. The anti-TSH receptor antibodies include thyroid stimulating immunoglobulins as well as TSH-binding inhibitory immunoglobulins. The thyroid stimulating immunoglobulins can be detected in bioassays based upon their ability to stimulate thyroid stimulating hormone receptor activation of adenylate cyclase, thereby mimicking thyroid stimulating hormone action. The TSH-binding inhibitory immunoglobulins are detected based upon their ability to block the binding of radiolabelled thyroid stimulating hormone to its receptor. Although there is not a strict correlation between the composition and titres of these antibodies and the severity of hyperthyroidism, it is clear that the antibodies cause thyroid overactivity *in vivo* as well as *in vitro*.

The causes of autoimmunity in Graves' disease are not well understood. There is often a strong family history of thyroid autoimmunity that can include Hashimoto's thyroiditis as well as Graves' disease. Autoimmune thyroid disease is about 10 times more common in women than in men. Studies of HLA haplotypes have provided evidence for several subtypes that occur with increased frequency in various ethnic populations. Presumably, these associations with the HLA locus reflect some defect in immune surveillance which, in association with other genetic factors or tissue injury, predispose to development of autoimmunity.

Aside from Graves' disease, other examples of autoimmune stimulation of hormone pathways are rare. Particularly in association with other autoimmune diseases such as idiopathic thrombocytopenic purpura, one occasionally sees antibodies directed against other membrane receptors. For example, antibody stimulation of the insulin receptor is a rare cause of hypoglycaemia that can simulate excessive production of insulin.

Endocrine hypofunction: autoimmune causes of hormone deficiency

Endocrine tissues are relatively common targets for autoimmunity. There is evidence for subclinical levels of autoimmunity against thyroid, adrenal, and islet specimens in many individuals who have no clinical evidence for hormone deficiency. The significance of these low levels of antibodies is unclear, but suggests that autoimmune endocrine diseases may represent a spectrum that becomes clinically significant when sufficient tissue destruction has occurred to preclude compensatory hormonal responses.

As discussed above, autoimmune thyroid disease encompasses disorders that can result in stimulation of thyroid hormone secretion or deficiency of thyroid hormone. Occasionally, this spectrum of immunological processes can be seen in the same patient who may begin with Graves disease and progress to thyroid gland destruction and hypothyroidism, even in the absence of radioactive iodine or surgical intervention. These features, in combination with the variable presentation of autoimmune thyroid disease in different members of the same family, emphasize the complexity of the autoimmune process. Autoimmune causes of hypothyroidism can be divided into goitrous and atrophic forms. The goitrous form of autoimmune thyroid disease is also called Hashimoto's thyroiditis, which is typified by lymphocytic infiltration and high circulating anti-thyroid antibodies. In Hashimoto's thyroiditis, antibodies may be goitrogenic, causing thyroid cell proliferation without

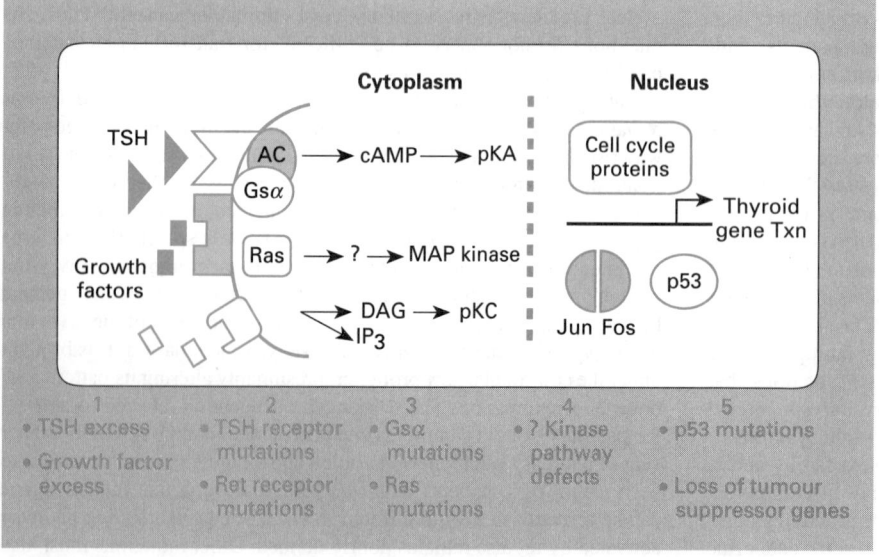

Fig. 10 Mutations that cause thyroid neoplasia. A theoretical model for thyroid neoplasia is illustrated as an example of multistep carcinogenesis as it applies to endocrine tumours. Cellular pathways that are sites for potential mutations are divided into five groups. Details concerning specific types of mutations are discussed in the text. AC, adenylate cyclase; DAG, diacylglycerol; IP3, inositol phosphate 3; pKC, protein kinase C; pKA, protein kinase A; MAP kinase, mitogen activated pathway kinase.

resulting in stimulation of the thyroid stimulating hormone receptor. The presence of thyroid stimulating hormone receptor blocking immuno-globulins may account in part for the relative degree of hypothyroidism despite the presence of increased levels of thyroid stimulating hormone. Additional cellular defects in iodide trapping or other steps in hormone biosynthesis may also contribute to hypothyroidism. Immune-mediated production of cytokines may also stimulate thyroid growth. In later stages, it is not uncommon to see progressive destruction of the thyroid gland, ultimately resulting in conversion of the goitre to an atrophic thyroid gland. Hypothyroidism associated with an atrophic thyroid gland can also be seen without a goitrous stage if the autoimmune process is highly destructive or if antibodies effectively block thyroid stimulating hormone or other growth factors in the thyroid.

The role of autoimmunity in type 1 diabetes is of great interest. Studies as early as 1910 demonstrated lymphocytic infiltrates in the pancreatic islets of individuals with the recent onset of diabetes. It has subsequently been demonstrated that lymphocytes from children with insulin-dependent diabetes mellitus adhere to islets, and that most have circulating antibodies that react with islet specimens. Together, it is likely that these immune-mediated processes lead to islet destruction, although it is unclear whether the circulating antibodies that are detected by current methods are markers that react to damaged tissue or whether they play a causative role in the disease. There is reason to suspect an important role for infection or other environmental agents that cause islet damage in the onset of insulin-dependent diabetes mellitus. The onset of the condition often coincides with, or closely follows, a variety of viral infections. Whether these infections initiate the autoimmune process, unmask compromised β-cell function, or cause direct destruction of the islets is an area of ongoing investigation. It is possible that all three mechanisms may apply in different instances. Genetic predisposition appears to be encoded by genes in the major histocompatibility locus. HLA markers such as DR3 and DR4 are seen with increased frequency in individuals with insulin-dependent diabetes mellitus and there is growing evidence for altered expression of class II MHC antigens in insulin-containing cells. Transgenic models with specific alterations in immune pathways are likely to clarify the interactions between the immune system and environmental agents in the pathogenesis of type 1 diabetes. In contrast to type 1 diabetes, type 2 diabetes is not accompanied by autoimmune destruction of the islets. In fact, islet cell mass is preserved or even increased in type 2 non-insulin-dependent diabetes, emphasizing the role for defective insulin secretion and/or action in this disorder.

There are two major types of polyglandular autoimmune syndromes. Type I polyglandular failure is characterized primarily by adrenal insufficiency, mucocutaneous candidiasis, hypoparathyroidism, and an array of other endocrine and non-endocrine disorders which occur with variable frequency. The type I syndrome usually presents in childhood. The immunological basis for the type I remains elusive. Type II polyglandular failure shares the high prevalence of adrenal insufficiency, but differs from the type I syndrome in that common features include autoimmune thyroid disease and insulin-dependent diabetes mellitus. The onset of type II polyglandular failure is usually later than in type I, occurring primarily in adults. There is a strong association of the type II syndrome with HLA-DR3 and HLA-DR4 and the disorder tends to occur in many generations, consistent with an important role for genetics in the disease. Autoimmune adrenal insufficiency also occurs as an isolated disease. Unlike many other autoimmune diseases, it is more common in males than females.

Hormone deficiencies caused by mutations and enzyme defects

Genetic mutations have now been defined for a number of endocrine deficiency syndromes (Table 5). Mutations in hormones themselves, however, are a relatively uncommon cause for endocrine dysfunction.

For example, growth hormone deficiency can be caused by deletions or mutations in the growth hormone gene, but more often it is caused by a hypothalamic defect. Growth hormone gene mutations are usually associated with an autosomal recessive form of growth hormone deficiency. Evolutionary duplication of the growth hormone genes appears to enhance the probability of gene deletions because of unequal recombination of homologous sequences during meiosis. Examples of unequal crossover leading to gene deletions or rearrangements are also seen in other gene clusters, such as the 21-hydroxylase locus and the aldosterone synthetase locus.

Mutations in preproinsulin prevent processing of the precursor molecule or result in biologically inactive insulin. A mutation in the signal sequence of parathyroid hormone causes hypoparathyroidism, even when only one of the two parathyroid hormone genes is affected, probably because this mutation interferes with the transport of other cellular proteins, including the normal parathyroid hormone protein. Mutations in the vasopressin gene appear to be somewhat analogous to the parathyroid hormone mutation. An autosomal dominant form of diabetes insipidus is caused by one of several heterozygous mutations in neurophysin, the precursor protein for vasopressin. The fact that the amino acid substitutions occur in the carboxy-terminal carrier protein as well as in vasopressin itself suggests that abnormalities in protein processing may result in cellular toxicity or inhibition of processing of the remaining normal vasopressin gene.

Homozygous mutations in the thyroid stimulating hormone, follicle stimulating hormone, and luteinizing hormone β-subunits have been described and provide important insights into the structure–function relationships of this family of hormones. In the thyroid stimulating hormone β-gene, several mutations involve large deletions or frameshift mutations such that little or no hormone is produced. However, one of the thyroid stimulating hormone β-mutations involves an amino acid that is required for heterodimerization with the α-subunit and thereby defines a critical region of the dimerization interface. Premature truncation of the follicle stimulating hormone β-subunit has been identified, eliminating a region required for protein folding and receptor binding. A mutation in the luteinizing hormone β-subunit results in a hormone that still dimerizes with the α-subunit and retains immunoreactivity in serum. However, the luteinizing hormone β-mutation results in a biologically inactive hormone because it prevents binding of luteinizing hormone to its receptor. Because of the reliance on immunoassays for most endocrine testing, this type of defect is important to recognize because it might otherwise be interpreted as primary hypogonadism.

Remarkably, mutations in transcription factors have already been identified, even though they have only been characterized and cloned very recently. Not surprisingly, some of the transcription factor mutations involve developmental pathways. Mutations in the testis determining factor gene provide a dramatic example of one these developmental mutations. The testis determining factor gene was located by examining rare cases of phenotypic females with an XY genotype. Mutations in a testis determining factor gene (also referred to as SRY for sex reversed Y) have now been identified in XY females but not in their fathers. Although these and other data indicate that SRY is a critical early gene for determination of male sex, it is likely that it is only one of several developmental switches that initiate a cascade of sex-specific gene expression. Mutations in another transcription factor, Pit-1, have been identified in patients with specific deficits of growth hormone, prolactin, and thyroid stimulating hormone. Pit-1 is a member of the POU-homeodomain class of transcription factors and is known to have an important role in the regulation of cell-specific expression of the growth hormone and prolactin genes. Interestingly, different Pit-1 mutations result in an autosomal recessive or dominant inheritance pattern, suggesting that distinct mutations have markedly different effects on Pit-1 function. It is likely that the recessive mutation involves an inactivated form of Pit-1, whereas the dominant disorder may involve a dominant negative type of mutation analogous to that for mutations in the thyroid hormone receptor (see below).

Kallmann syndrome, or idiopathic hypogonadotropic hypogonadism associated with anosmia, is an inherited disorder that is caused by gonadotrophin releasing hormone deficiency. Several different inheritance patterns have been described, including autosomal recessive, X-linked, and autosomal dominant with incomplete penetrance. In contrast to an animal model of this disorder (the hypogonadal mouse) in which there is a gonadotrophin releasing hormone gene deletion, deficiency of this hormone in humans is not caused by defects in the gonadotrophin releasing hormone gene. Instead, Kallmann syndrome (at least the X-linked form) is caused by mutations in an X-chromosomal gene referred to as KAL. The KAL gene encodes a protein that is involved in the migration of the gonadotrophin releasing hormone-producing neurones along a path that leads to the hypothalamus as well as to the olfactory tract. These observations provide another example of endocrine deficiency on the basis of a developmental abnormality, and might account for some of the phenotypic variants, in that different extents of neuronal migration could lead to isolated anosmia, gonadotrophin releasing hormone deficiency, or both.

Because a number of enzymatic steps are required for steroid hormone biosynthesis and metabolism, it is not surprising that a number of genetic defects occur in these pathways. Deficiency of 21-hydroxylase is the most common cause of congenital adrenal hyperplasia. As a result of impaired cortisol production, excess adrenocorticotrophic hormone is secreted, leading to stimulation of the adrenal gland and the overproduction of precursor steroids, including adrenal androgens. Deficiency of 21-hydoxylase encompasses a broad phenotypic spectrum. In females affected with the classic form of the disease, hypersecretion of adrenal androgens during fetal development causes ambiguous external genitalia, whereas in males the classic form is usually recognized because of severe salt wasting caused by enzymatic defects in the mineralocorticoid and glucocorticoid pathways. In the non-classic form, prenatal virilization does not occur, but there is virilization of variable severity postnatally. The inheritance of congenital adrenal hyperplasia is autosomal recessive. Heterozygotes are typically unaffected clinically and are detected only by hormonal or genetic testing. The classic form of the disease is due to large deletions or severe mutations of both 21-hydroxylase genes, whereas the non-classic form of the disease is caused by one of several combinations of severe and mild mutations. Thus, the variability in clinical phenotype appears to be the consequence of a high degree of heterogeneity at the genetic level. The 21-hydroxylase locus is on the short arm of chromosome 6, adjacent to the HLA locus, explaining previous findings that HLA typing was useful for predicting the risk of the disease. Large deletions and rearrangements occur in about 10 to 20 per cent of cases, probably caused in many cases by unequal crossover between the two 21-hydroxylase genes, A and B. The 21-hydroxylase B gene is functional whereas the 21A gene contains a number of inactivating mutations. Many of the point mutations that occur in the 21B gene may result from the phenomenon of gene conversion in which sequences from the adjacent 21A gene are substituted for sequences in 21B.

Mutations in the 11β-hydroxylase and 17α-hydroxylase genes are also classified under congenital adrenal hyperplasia because impaired production of cortisol causes elevation of adrenocorticotrophic hormone and, consequently, adrenal stimulation. Mutations in 11β-hydroxylase cause androgen excess and virilization, but are distinguished clinically from 21-hydroxylase mutations by mineralocorticoid excess, which causes hypertension in about two-thirds of patients. Defects in 17α-hydroxylase cause sex-steroid deficiency, with overproduction of mineralocorticoids, resulting in hypertension and hypokalaemia.

Glucocorticoid remediable aldosteronism represents another adrenal enzyme defect that causes hypertension. It is characterized by high levels of abnormal adrenal steroids 18-oxocortisol and 18-hydroxycortisol with a variable degree of hyperaldosteronism. The genes encoding aldosterone synthetase and steroid 11β-hydroxylase are normally arranged in tandem on chromosome 8q. These two genes are 95 per cent identical, predisposing to gene duplication and the formation of a fusion gene that contains the regulatory regions of 11β-hydroxylase and the coding sequence of aldosterone synthetase. Consequently, aldosterone synthetase is subjected to an abnormal pattern of expression in the adrenocorticotrophic hormone dependent zone of the adrenal gland, resulting in overproduction of mineralocorticoids. Administration of glucocorticoids suppresses adrenocorticotrophic hormone production, causing reduction in the inappropriate production of mineralocorticoids.

Defects in the enzyme 5α-reductase result in a complex phenotype of male pseudohermaphroditism. 5α-Reductase causes conversion of testosterone to dihydrotestosterone, an androgen that has an important role in development of male external genitalia. Males with 5α-reductase deficiency are born with ambiguous genitalia characterized as pseudovaginal perineoscrotal hypospadias. At puberty, they undergo masculinization with good muscle development and enlargement of the phallus. As with 21-hydroxylase deficiency, a number of different sites in the enzyme are mutated in different patients.

Hormone resistance syndromes

Most examples of hormone resistance are caused by mutations that occur in receptor or postreceptor steps of hormone action (Table 5). Exceptions to the mutational causes of hormone resistance include forms of functional resistance. In type 2 diabetes mellitus, tissues become resistant to endogenous and exogenous insulin. In this case, insulin resistance is partially reversible with weight loss and improvements in metabolic control. The cellular mechanisms for this form of postreceptor resistance remain obscure. Other examples of physiological resistance include homologous desensitization in which a hormone downregulates its own receptor or postreceptor pathways (e.g. continuous exposure to gonadotrophin releasing hormone). There are also situations in which a relative form of resistance reflects the permissive effects of co-operative hormonal processes. Progesterone cannot mediate its effects in the absence of oestrogen induction of progesterone receptors. Thyroid hormone and glucocorticoids exert permissive effects for other hormones in the liver and kidney.

RESISTANCE CAUSED BY MEMBRANE RECEPTOR MUTATIONS

An increasing number of membrane receptor mutations have been described in recent years (Table 5). In Laron-type dwarfism, a variety of different point mutations have been identified in the growth hormone receptor. Mutations in the insulin receptor have been characterized extensively in patients with severe insulin resistance. Multiple mis-sense and non-sense mutations have been described in different regions of the insulin receptor. Some of the insulin receptor mutations alter its ability to bind insulin, whereas others affect receptor signalling, stability, or recycling. Estimates of the frequency of insulin receptor mutations suggest that they are a rare cause of diabetes. An X-linked form of vasopressin resistance has now been attributed to mutations in the vasopressin 2 (V_2) receptor. Like most other disorders, vasopressin receptor mutations include a wide array of different mutants, suggesting that because the disorder does not significantly alter viability, spontaneous mutations have arisen independently to result in similar clinical phenotypes.

SIGNALLING PATHWAY RESISTANCE

As noted above, mutations in second messenger signalling pathways that occur in neoplasia cause constitutive activation. Distinct mutations in the Gsα-subunit can also cause inactivation, resulting in pseudohypoparathyroidism or Albright hereditary osteodystrophy. The latter is characterized by short stature, obesity, and skeletal abnormalities. Resistance to several Gsα protein-coupled hormones, such as parathyroid hormone, thyroid stimulating hormone, luteinizing hormone, and follicle stimulating hormone, is characteristic. Albright hereditary osteo-dystrophy is inherited in an autosomal dominant manner, suggesting that the heterozygous deficiency in Gsα is sufficient to cause the disease and that other variables dictate its clinical expression. Variable phenotypes of hormone resistance are seen with different Gsα mutations, but also within families with the same mutation.

RESISTANCE CAUSED BY NUCLEAR RECEPTOR MUTATIONS

A relatively large number of defects have now been described in nuclear receptors. The syndrome of resistance to thyroid hormone is representative of nuclear receptor resistance syndromes, but also illustrates some unique aspects of a disease that is inherited in a dominant manner. Resistance to thyroid hormone is characterized by elevated circulating levels of free thyroid hormone, inappropriately normal or increased levels of thyroid stimulating hormone, and the relative absence of clinical manifestations of thyrotoxicosis. The mutant receptors bind thyroxine with reduced affinity. Consequently, their ability to modulate target gene expression is impaired. Because the affected individuals still have a normal β receptor allele and two normal thyroid hormone receptor α alleles, the mutant receptor has been proposed to inhibit the activity of normal receptors. In support of this concept, the receptor mutants have been shown to block the action of the wild-type receptors in transient gene expression assays, probably by binding to DNA target sites where the mutant receptors function as antagonists.

Syndromes of androgen resistance represent one of the more common and well-studied receptor defects. These disorders exhibit sex-linked transmission, consistent with the location of the androgen receptor on the X chromosome. One of the striking features of this syndrome is its broad phenotypic spectrum that includes, at one end, complete testicular feminization, and, at the other end, men with subtle defects in virilization. Many mutations in the androgen receptor result in premature termination, although gene deletions and single amino acid substitutions have also been found. Some of the milder mutations have relatively subtle effects on receptor stability.

Hypocalcaemic vitamin D resistant rickets is a rare inherited form of rickets that is unresponsive to treatment with 1,25-dihydroxyvitamin D. The disease has a recessive pattern of inheritance. A variety of mutations have been identified in different kindreds, including amino acid substitutions in the zinc-finger DNA binding domains as well as nonsense mutations that cause premature termination. The naturally occurring mutations in the vitamin D receptor have provided insights into the biological role of vitamin D in skin differentiation, hair growth, and lymphocyte function.

In familial glucocorticoid resistance, serum concentrations of cortisol are elevated without the characteristic clinical manifestations of glucocorticoid excess. Adrenocorticotrophic hormone levels are inappropriately increased, indicating reduced feedback inhibition at the level of the hypothalamic–pituitary axis. Because adrenocorticotrophic hormone also stimulates adrenal androgens and mineralocorticoids, precocious puberty and hypertension can comprise features of this syndrome. An autosomal co-dominant mode of inheritance has been suggested in view of the fact that heterozygotes are mildly affected. By analogy with mutations in the ligand-binding domain of the thyroid hormone receptor, it is possible that the mutant GR (glucocorticoid receptor) can function in a dominant negative manner to block the activity of the normal receptor.

A mutation has also been described in the oestrogen receptor. In the hemozygous state, this mutation caused oestrogen resistance. One of the more prominent clinical manifestations of oestrogen resistance was the failure of epiphyseal closure, resulting in tall stature. Importantly, this condition suggests that androgen effects on the epiphyseal plate may occur by aromatization to oestrogens. Oestrogen and progesterone receptor variants and mutations have been described in breast cancers, although a role in pathogenesis has not been clearly defined.

REFERENCES

Braverman, L.E. and Utiger, R.D. (ed.) (1991). *Werner and Ingbar's The thyroid*, (6th edn). J.B. Lippincott, Philadelphia.

Darnell, J., *et al.* (1990). *Molecular biology of the cell*, (2nd edn). W.H. Freeman, New York.

DeGroot, L.J., *et al.* (ed.) (1994). *Endocrinology*, (3rd edn). W.B. Saunders, Philadelphia.

Felig, P., *et al.* (ed.) (1987). *Endocrinology and metabolism*, (2nd edn). McGraw-Hill, New York.

Lewin, B. (1990). *Genes IV*. Oxford University Press, Oxford.

Medvei, V.C. (1982). *A history of endocrinology*. MTP Press, Lancaster, UK.

Watson, J.D., *et al.* (1987). *Molecular biology of the gene*, (4th edn). Benjamin/Cummings, Menlo Park, CA.

Wilson, J.D. and Foster, D.W. (ed.) (1992). *Williams textbook of endocrinology*, (8th edn). W.B. Saunders, Philadelphia.

Yen, S.S.C. and Jaffe, R.B. (ed.) (1991) *Reproductive endocrinology*, (3rd edn). W.B. Saunders, Philadelphia.

12.2 Anterior pituitary disorders

M. O. THORNER

INTRODUCTION

The anterior pituitary gland is the source of at least six hormones which regulate growth, development, and function of the thyroid gland, adrenal cortex, gonads, and breast. Such regulation involves integration of signals from the brain, and feedback effects of peripheral hormones. Several pituitary hormones also target multiple peripheral non-endocrine tissues. Disorders of pituitary function may produce selective overstimulation of target glands (for example the adrenal in Cushing's disease) or result in pituitary hormone deficiency, which may or may not be selective. Due to its anatomical location in the sella turcica, expanding lesions of the pituitary may give rise to visual disturbances, cavernous sinus syndrome(s), and headaches.

Over the past 30 years the hormones of the hypothalamus and pituitary have been isolated, characterized, and sequenced, and their physiological role determined. The importance of regulation of anterior pituitary function by secretion of hypothalamic hormones into the hypothalamo-hypophyseal portal circulation, is well established. Precision in diagnosis and management in patients suffering from pituitary diseases has been revolutionized by the development of sensitive, specific, and reliable immunoassays for pituitary hormones and those secreted by its target glands. Magnetic resonance imaging (MRI) and computer assisted tomographic scanning (CT) now allow precise evaluation of the anatomy of the hypothalamus, pituitary, and surrounding structures. Immunocytochemistry, electron microscopy, and *in situ* hybridization have permitted the identification of different pituitary cell types and the development of a logical framework for classification of pituitary tumours. Modern molecular biological techniques probably will elucidate further the pathogenesis of pituitary disease.

Advances have been made in treatment of hypothalamic and pituitary disease with the development of synthetic replacement therapy, for pituitary hormones, those of its target glands, and, most recently, of the hypothalamus. Trans-sphenoidal pituitary microsurgery has made operative intervention safer, simpler and more effective, and medical therapy is successful in controlling certain types of pituitary tumours, avoiding the need for surgery in many patients.

PITUITARY EMBRYOLOGY AND ANATOMY

The pituitary is derived from two sources. The epithelial portion, which includes the pars distalis, intermediate lobe, and the pars tuberalis, originates from evagination of the stomodeal ectoderm, Rathke's pouch. The neural portion, which includes the infundibulum, the neural stalk, and the posterior lobe, arises in the saccus infundibuli, a part of the diencephalon. It is clear that the hormone-producing cells can develop without hypothalamic stimulation. This reflects the intrinsic property of cellular maturation and is exemplified in anencephaly when all adenohypophysial cell types, with the exception of corticotrophes, develop normally and are capable of hormone synthesis and release despite the absence of hypothalamic tissue.

The pituitary is located in the sella turcica (Fig. 1), is protected by the sphenoid bone which surrounds it bilaterally and inferiorly and is covered by the dura, a dense layer of connective tissue which lines the sella turcica. Superiorly it is covered by the diaphragma sellae which has a 5 mm wide central opening which is penetrated by the hypophyseal stalk. In some subjects this opening is much wider, and is thought to allow transmission of pulsations of the cerebrospinal fluid pressure, leading to the development of the 'empty sella syndrome', or cisternal herniation.

The pituitary measures 13 mm transversely, 9 mm anteroposteriorly, and 6 mm vertically. Its weight is approximately 100 mg, somewhat more in women than in men; it enlarges during pregnancy and may weigh 0.9–1.0 g.

Several structures may be affected by an enlarged pituitary gland. The lateral walls of the sella are close to the cavernous sinuses containing the internal carotid arteries, the oculomotor (III), trochlear (IV), and abducens (VI) nerves, and V_1 and V_2 divisions of the trigeminal (V) nerve. The sphenoid sinus lies anteriorly and inferiorly to the pituitary and is separated from it by the inferior portion of the sella, a thin layer of bone. When a pituitary tumour enlarges, the thin bone is resorbed and may be eroded, allowing extension into the sphenoid sinus. The optic chiasm lies directly above the diaphragma sellae, in front of the hypophyseal stalk; suprasellar growth of a pituitary tumour may compress the chiasm giving rise to visual compromise. The tuber cinereum of the hypothalamus and the third ventricle of the brain lie above the roof of the sella. Space-occupying lesions arising in or above the pitu-

itary may compress and compromise the tuber cinereum, causing hypothalamic/hypophyseal dysfunction which is usually manifest as hypopituitarism associated with mild hyperprolactinaemia.

The blood supply to the pituitary is complex and plays an important role in its regulation by the hypothalamus. It receives blood from paired arteries: the superior and two inferior hypophysial vessels which originate from the internal carotid arteries. The hypothalamic hormones are produced in neurones which originate in various parts of the hypothalamus and terminate at the infundibulum. There they permeate through fenestrations in capillaries to enter the portal circulation. The portal veins, or portal vessels, consist of a confluence of capillaries. High concentrations of hypothalamic hormones are present in the portal blood, which transports the hormones to the capillaries in the anterior pituitary. The portal circulation provides approximately 80 to 90 per cent of the blood supply to the anterior lobe. The remaining 10 to 20 per cent of the blood supply to the pituitary is provided by arterial blood from superior hypophysial arteries.

The neurohypophysis receives its blood supply from the inferior hypophysial arteries. Venous blood leaves the pituitary through adjacent venous sinuses to enter the internal jugular veins bilaterally.

Unidirectional blood flow, from the hypothalamus to the anterior pituitary, has been assumed, but under certain circumstances, this may be reversed to produce ultrashort loop feedback by pituitary hormones on several hypothalamic centres. The posterior lobe is important in the regulation of the local circulation since it can direct blood to the adenohypophysis, the hypothalamus, or the systemic circulation.

The anterior lobe has no direct innervation except for a few sympathetic nerve fibres which spread to the anterior lobe along blood vessels. Hypothalamic regulation is exerted via the neurohormonal link, the hypothalamic regulatory peptides reaching the pituitary via the portal vessels.

Hypothalamic–pituitary regulation

Each pituitary hormone is regulated by substances which are synthesized in the hypothalamus and transported from the median eminence to the anterior pituitary via the hypothalamic–pituitary portal circulation. These hypothalamic regulatory hormones bind to specific high-affinity cell membrane receptors of the particular pituitary cell type to regulate pituitary hormone secretion. With the possible exception of prolactin, all anterior pituitary hormones are also regulated by the hormones secreted by their target glands. A normal endocrine state is therefore maintained by interaction and integration of signals from the brain and the periphery which tightly regulate the pituitary function. When a target gland fails, negative feedback is reduced, augmenting secretion of the trophic hypothalamic hormone, as well as reducing secretion of any tonic hypothalamic inhibiting hormone, negative feedback occurring at both pituitary and hypothalamic levels. Additionally, 'short loop' feed-

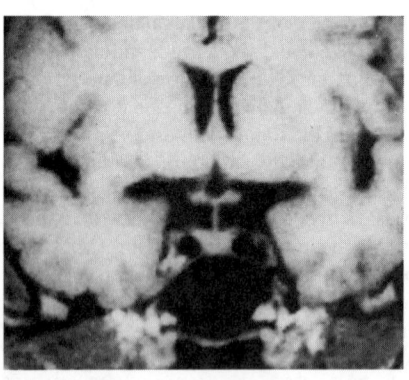
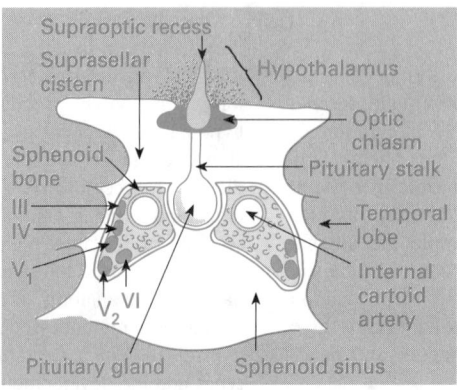

Fig. 1 MRI scan (left) and diagram (right) of the normal pituitary fossa. The pituitary gland is bordered laterally by the cavernous sinus which contains the internal carotid artery and cranial nerves III, IV, V_1, V_2, and VI. The optic chiasm lies immediately above the pituitary gland and is separated from it by a cerebrospinal fluid-filled cistern. Note the location of the sphenoid sinus and temporal lobes. (Modified and reproduced with permission from Lechan, R.M. (1987). Neuroendocrinology of pituitary hormone regulation. *Endocrinology and Metabolism Clinics of North America*, **16**, 475–502.)

Diagram labels: Supraoptic recess; Suprasellar cistern; Hypothalamus; Sphenoid bone; III; IV; V_1; V_2; VI; Pituitary gland; Optic chiasm; Pituitary stalk; Temporal lobe; Internal cartoid artery; Sphenoid sinus

back, in which pituitary hormones are probably transported back to the hypothalamus, reduces further secretion by reducing hypothalamic stimulation (Fig. 2).

All anterior pituitary hormones are secreted in a pulsatile fashion, so that accurate assessment of function often requires more than one measurement.

Anterior pituitary ontogeny

Immunohistochemical studies indicate that five phenotypically distinct cell types appear during anterior pituitary ontogeny in a stereotypical order. Expression of the α-glycoprotein subunit prior to the formation of Rathke's pouch defines the onset of pituitary organogenesis. The apparent order of initial appearance of phenotypically distinct cell types is: corticotrophs, producing pro-opiomelanocortin (POMC); thyrotrophs, producing thyroid stimulating hormone (TSH); gonadotrophs, producing luteinizing hormone (LH) and follicle stimulating hormone (FSH); somatotrophs, producing growth hormone (GH); and lactotrophs, producing prolactin. The coexpression of GH and prolactin in precursor cells prior to the appearance of the mature lactotroph cell and in a subpopulation of mature anterior pituitary cells suggest that prolactin and GH genes are regulated by related factors.

The role of transcription factors in the ontogeny of the pituitary and in pituitary tumorigenesis, and the molecular defects that have been described in human pituitary tumours, are discussed in detail in Section 6. The vast majority of pituitary tumours are monoclonal in origin.

Hormones

Corticotrophin (ACTH)

Adrenocorticotrophin (ACTH) stimulates the adrenal cortex to secrete cortisol, adrenal androgens, and mineralocorticoids. Pituitary ACTH

Fig. 2 Schematic representation of the hypothalamic–pituitary–target gland axis. Hypothalamic hormones regulate pituitary hormone secretion which in turn stimulates target gland hormone production. Peripheral hormones feed back on the hypothalamus and pituitary to modulate secretion in a classical negative fashion. For example, hypothalamic thyroid releasing hormone (TRH) stimulates pituitary release of thyroid stimulating hormone (TSH) which stimulates thyroidal hormone release. Thyroid hormones inhibit TRH and TSH in the hypothalamus and pituitary, respectively. (Modified and reproduced with permission from Reichlin, S. (1987). Neuroendocrine control of pituitary function. In: *Clinical endocrinology: an illustrated text* (ed. G.M. Besser and A.G. Cudworth) pp. 1.1–1.14. J.B. Lippincott, Philadelphia.)

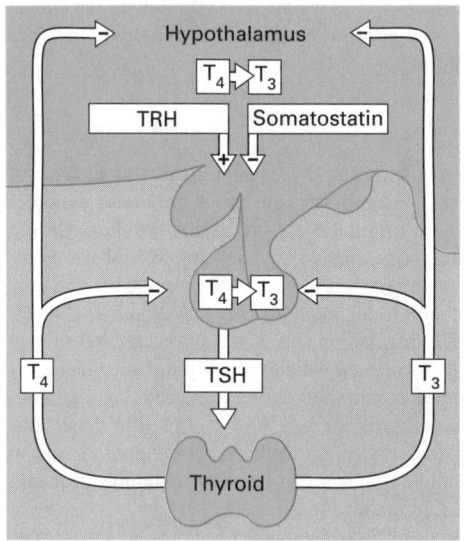

secretion is regulated by hypothalamic corticotrophin releasing hormone (CRH) and vasopressin (AVP), both of which stimulate ACTH secretion. Cortisol exerts negative feedback on AVP, CRH, and ACTH secretion; additionally, ACTH acts via a 'short loop' feedback to suppress CRH secretion.

ACTH, a 39 amino acid peptide, is synthesized as part of a large precursor molecule, pro-opiomelanocortin (POMC; 241 amino acids). POMC undergoes considerable post-translational processing including glycosylation, enzymatic cleavage and phosphorylation, N-terminal acetylation, and C-terminal amidation of certain cleaved peptides. In the human anterior pituitary gland POMC is enzymatically cleaved at dibasic amino acids, predominantly into β-lipotrophin, ACTH, joining peptide, and an amino-terminal peptide. In the intermediate lobe (vestigial except in fetal life and at the end of pregnancy), ACTH is cleaved into melanocyte stimulating hormone (α-MSH) ($ACTH_{1-13}$) and corticotrophin-like peptide ($ACTH_{8-39}$), and β-lipotrophin into lipotrophin (LPH) and β-endorphin.

The first 18 amino acids of ACTH have full biological activity and the first 24 amino acids are identical across species. Synthetic $ACTH_{(1-24)}$ has a longer half-life than does native $ACTH_{(1-18)}$ and is useful in clinical investigation.

Because these peptides are derived from the same precursor molecule, they are secreted in equimolar amounts, but circulating concentrations do not vary in tandem because their half-lives are different. Since the half-life of β-lipotrophin is longer than that of ACTH, the β-LPH/ACTH ratio is increased after hydrocortisone administration, which inhibits secretion of both ACTH and β-LPH. Concentrations of β-LPH are also increased in renal failure because of slower metabolic clearance. The hyperpigmentation observed in ACTH hypersecretory states and in uraemia is not a result of secretion of intermediate lobe peptides; rather is it dependent on the MSH-like activity of β-LPH and ACTH.

CORTICOTROPH CELLS AND ACTH CONTENT

Corticotroph cells reside primarily in the median wedge, comprising some 10 per cent of the cells there. The human pituitary contains approximately 250 μg of ACTH.

REGULATION OF SECRETION

To stimulate ACTH secretion, CRH binds to high-affinity receptors on corticotrophs stimulates the accumulation of cAMP and activates protein kinase A, resulting in rapid release of ACTH and related peptides and in increased POMC gene transcription and synthesis. Exogenous CRH also stimulates ACTH and cortisol secretion, the magnitude of the response depending on the time of day and the prevailing level of circulating glucocorticoids; for instance, the cortisol response is greater in the afternoon than in the morning. Exogenous glucocorticoids inhibit both the ACTH and cortisol responses to CRH, whereas metyrapone, by reducing cortisol secretion, enhances them. Arginine vasopressin (AVP) alone is a weak secretagogue for ACTH, but it acts synergistically with CRH to stimulate ACTH release.

ACTH SECRETION

ACTH is secreted in bursts, which stimulate sharp increases in plasma cortisol concentrations. These secretory bursts increase in frequency after 3 to 5 h of sleep and are maximal in the last hours before awakening and the hour thereafter. The overall circadian rhythm of ACTH secretion is regulated by a number of factors, one of the most important being light. Blind people have a free-running ACTH rhythm of about 25 h, but in normal subjects, ACTH concentrations decline through the morning, reaching a nadir in the evening. This rhythm is established after the first year of life, with an acrophase shift to 3 h earlier in the elderly. The rhythm is resilient, but is disrupted by a major time shift, as occurs with transmeridian jet travel. Physical stress, for example, trauma, major surgery, fever, hypoglycaemia, and burn injury, activates the hypothalamic–pituitary–adrenal axis by increasing both ACTH and cortisol secretion. Hypoglycaemia and fever both activate the hypothalamic–pituitary axis; the former by direct action at the basomedial hypothalamus while the latter has indirect effects through the release of interleukins 1, 2, and 6. These act predominantly in the hypothalamus to release CRH. Increased cortisol secretion also occurs during psychological stress, for instance in anticipation of physical activity, during mental activity, and in patients with anorexia nervosa and depression, but not in schizophrenia or chronic anxiety. Glucocorticoids act at multiple sites to inhibit ACTH secretion by inhibiting the ACTH response to CRH by way of inhibition of POMC gene transcription and synthesis, and inhibition of CRH and AVP synthesis and release in the hypothalamus.

ACTH ACTIONS

The actions of ACTH at the adrenal are mediated through specific high-affinity cell membrane receptors. Activation of adenylate cyclase, leading to accumulation of intracellular cAMP, increases protein kinase A activity, and phosphorylation of a number of important proteins, leading to increased synthesis and secretion of cortisol, only small amounts of which are stored in the adrenal.

ACTH has both acute and prolonged actions. The acute effects, which occur within minutes, are stimulation of the initial and rate-limiting step of conversion of cholesterol to pregnenolone. In addition, the supply of free cholesterol ester is increased. The prolonged effects promote maintenance of the adrenal size (and growth) by increasing protein synthesis, including the enzymes involved in steroidogenesis. In Nelson's syndrome and in Addison's disease, circulating ACTH concentrations are extremely high; pigmentation of the skin in those conditions is then probably dependent on the effects of ACTH and β-LPH on melanocytes.

Prolactin–growth hormone family

Based on their homologies and chromosomal segregation, the prolactin–growth hormone family may be divided into prolactin and growth hormone (GH) subfamilies. A single prolactin gene appears on chromosome 6. The human growth hormone subfamily is better characterized and consists of five members, all located on a 78 kilobase section of chromosome 17. They include the normal GH gene, a GH variant gene, two expressed chorionic somatomammotrophin genes, and an incompletely characterized chorionic somatomammotrophin-like gene, which is thought not to be expressed, (i.e. a pseudogene). The GH-variant gene codes for a protein different from GH by 13 amino acids. The genes in this GH subfamily all have greater amino acid and nucleotide homology among each other than with prolactin.

PROLACTIN STRUCTURE

Human prolactin consists of 199 amino acids and has three disulphide intramolecular bonds. Only 16 per cent of the amino acids of prolactin are homologous with those of GH.

LACTOTROPH CELL AND PITUITARY PROLACTIN CONTENT

The lactotroph cell has a wide distribution throughout the pars distalis and constitutes from 10 per cent of the cells in men, to 30 per cent, in multiparous women. The normal pituitary contains 100 microgram of prolactin, some 50 times less than the content of GH; the pituitary prolactin pool therefore turns over more rapidly than does that of GH.

REGULATION OF PROLACTIN SECRETION

Prolactin is synthesized by the human anterior pituitary from the 5th week of gestation. Its secretion varies under different physiological conditions. Like all anterior pituitary hormones, it is secreted in an episodic manner, regulated by hypothalamic dopamine, and by various prolactin releasing factors (PRF). Prolactin is unique among anterior pituitary hormones in that it is under tonic hypothalamic inhibition by dopamine produced by tubero-infundibular dopamine neurones. Dopamine acts by stimulating the lactotrophe D2 receptor which inhibits adenylate cyclase, and thereby inhibits both prolactin release and synthesis. The putative prolactin releasing factors include thyrotrophin releasing hormone (TRH), vasoactive intestinal peptide (VIP), and PHM-27, a peptide with structural homology to VIP; the physiological significance of these factors in man is unknown. VIP is produced in the anterior pituitary cells and has been proposed to act as an autocrine or paracrine hormone, regulating prolactin secretion. If large quantities of VIP were to be secreted in the anterior pituitary and normal lactotrophs be responsive, it is possible that disorders of pituitary VIP secretion may produce hyperprolactinaemia, lactotroph hyperplasia, or adenoma formation.

Normal base-line serum prolactin concentrations are < 20 μg/l in adults; in men they are usually < 10 μg/l. Circulating levels are lowest at midday, with a modest increase during the afternoon. Marked increases in concentration occur shortly after the onset of sleep, whenever that takes place, but peak levels are seen during the middle to end of the night.

Prolactin synthesis is also regulated by direct effects of oestrogen on prolactin gene expression. Concentrations are higher in normal premenopausal women than in men, and they rise during menarche in girls, and during pregnancy in both the mother and the fetus. Fetal prolactin probably originates from the fetal pituitary, in contrast to that of amniotic fluid which originates from decidual cells. Maximal amniotic fluid prolactin levels are 100-fold higher than those of fetal or maternal blood and occur at mid-trimester, in contrast to maximal serum levels which are observed at term in both the fetus and mother. The decidual prolactin, which is also produced by decidualized endometrial cells from days 22 to 28 of the menstrual cycle, is not under tonic dopaminergic inhibition, but is instead stimulated by progesterone. Following delivery, maternal prolactin concentrations decline into the normal range over the course of the first 3 months if breast feeding does not occur. With suckling, maternal prolactin rises, with the greatest response just after delivery. If breast feeding is intermittently supplemented with bottle feeding the suckling-induced prolactin increase wanes, although normal prolactin levels are sufficient to sustain established lactation. Prolactin levels increase in women during sexual stimulation of the nipple, during orgasm, and in both men and women in response to stress.

Hyperprolactinaemia occurs with any disruption of the hypothalamus, the hypothalamo/hypophyseal stalk, or administration of drugs which interfere with dopamine synthesis or action. In some patients with primary hypothyroidism there may be mild hyperprolactinaemia due to increased hypothalamic TRH secretion. Thyroid hormone replacement, although it lowers TSH concentrations rapidly, may require months for prolactin to decline to normal.

ACTIONS OF PROLACTIN

Prolactin acts through specific receptors present in many tissues, including the liver, ovary, testis, and prostate, but the main site of action is the mammary gland, where it initiates and maintains lactation. During pregnancy the breast undergoes considerable development of the secretory apparatus through an interaction of several hormones. Insulin, cortisol, and thyroid hormone are all required, but the stimuli for development are oestrogen and progesterone, as well as prolactin and several placental mammotrophic hormones, which probably include GH (or its placental variant). Lactation is inhibited during pregnancy by high concentrations of oestrogen and progesterone. The rapid fall in concentrations of these after delivery enables prolactin to act unopposed, and to initiate lactation. Dopamine agonists can be used to inhibit prolactin secretion, and thereby lactation, after delivery.

The physiological functions of prolactin at other sites is poorly characterized, but it is known to regulate dopamine turnover and affect gonadotrophin secretion in the hypothalamus; both the hyperprolactinaemia, of pregnancy and lactation, and pathological hyperprolactinaemia are associated with suppression of the hypothalamic–pituitary–gonadal axis. This is likely to be due to prolactin-mediated inhibition of pulsatile gonadotrophin releasing hormone (GnRH) secretion, resulting in disorganized gonadotrophin secretion and dysregulation of gonadal function.

GROWTH HORMONE STRUCTURE

Human GH is a non-glycosylated, single-chain, 191 amino acid, 22 kDa protein with two intramolecular disulphide bonds. Approximately 75 per cent of pituitary GH is in this form and some 5 to 10 per cent in a 20 kDa form, the latter produced by alternate splicing of the mRNA that deletes the codons for amino acids 32 to 46 from the RNA. Growth hormone is present in several different forms in the anterior pituitary.

SOMATOTROPH CELL AND PITUITARY GROWTH HORMONE CONTENT

The somatotroph cells, which secrete GH, make up about 50 per cent of the hormone-producing adenohypophyseal cells and occupy the lateral wings. They are remarkably stable and their number, morphology, and immunoreactivity are unchanged by age or by various diseases. The human adenohypophysis contains 5 to 10 mg of GH, synthesized and stored in somatotrophs; GH in the secretory granules accounts for as much as 30 per cent of the protein in these cells.

GROWTH HORMONE VARIANTS, GROWTH HORMONE RECEPTOR, AND GROWTH HORMONE BINDING PROTEIN

Human GH circulates in several forms, including a 22 kDa, a 20 kDa form, and at least one acidic form. Additionally, a mixture of GH oligomers (up to pentamer) can also be detected in peripheral blood.

The proportions of GH variants in the circulation are broadly similar to those in the pituitary, except that the 20 kDa form and oligomeric forms are more predominant in the circulation, due to slower metabolic clearance rates.

Growth hormone receptor

The cDNA of the human GH receptor encodes 638 amino acids and has homology with the prolactin receptor. In the middle of the protein there is a sequence of 24 hydrophobic amino acids representing the transmembrane domain, dividing the molecule into extracellular and intracytoplasmic domains of approximately equal size. The translated molecular weight of the receptor is 70 kDa, which is smaller than the originally isolated receptor (130 kDa), the difference being accounted for largely by glycosylation. Abnormalities in the cDNA encoding this GH-receptor found in many children with Laron dwarfism (GH resistance syndrome) lend evidence that this is the biologically important receptor.

Growth hormone binding protein

When radiolabelled monomeric GH is incubated with human plasma, two high molecular weight forms result. This is accounted for by the presence of a binding protein, which is identical to the extracellular domain of the human GH receptor. The absence of binding protein in the plasma of Laron dwarfs, in whom there is a functional deficiency of the GH receptor, supports a relationship between the GH-binding protein and receptor.

Forty-five per cent of 22 kDa GH and 25 per cent of 20 kDa GH are complexed with the binding proteins, the high-affinity binding protein accounting for 85 per cent of this binding. When circulating GH concentrations are consistently above 10 to 20 µg/l, a progressively smaller proportion is linked to the binding protein. Protein-bound GH is metab-

olized differently than monomeric GH; it persists 10 times longer in plasma and its volume of distribution is twice the intravascular compartment, while that of monomeric GH is the extracellular space. These two factors may enhance the biological activity of the bound hormone, but are countered by the competition for binding between receptors and circulating protein.

The plasma concentrations of the binding proteins appear to remain fairly constant with wide variability among individuals. Levels are low prenatally and at birth, increasing markedly during the first year of life; those of the high-affinity protein increase throughout childhood.

REGULATION OF GROWTH HORMONE SECRETION

Growth hormone is secreted in a pulsatile fashion, regulated by two hypothalamic regulatory hormones, growth hormone releasing hormone (GHRH) and somatostatin (SRIF). GHRH is necessary for GH synthesis, increasing transcription of GH messenger RNA within minutes by increasing cyclic AMP. Somatostatin appears to be particularly important in the timing and amplitude of GH pulses but has no effect on synthesis.

Figure 3 illustrates this regulation of GH secretion. The somatotroph is also regulated by negative feedback at the pituitary itself by circulating insulin-like growth factor (IGF-I) and by 'short loop' feedback on the hypothalamus by GH.

Growth hormone appears in fetal serum at approximately the end of the first trimester and increases rapidly thereafter to reach a peak of 100 to 150 µg/l at about 20 weeks of gestation, but it is not thought to be essential for normal intrauterine development and growth. Mean GH levels subsequently decrease to about 30 µg/l in cord serum and con-

Fig. 3 Schematic illustration of regulation of serum growth hormone (GH) secretion. GH is secreted in a pulsatile fashion under the co-ordinate regulation by hypothalamic somatostatin (SS) and growth hormone releasing hormone (GHRH). GH acts on multiple tissues to regulate metabolic functions and growth. Peripheral tissues produce insulin like growth factor-I (IGF-I) which is both secreted into the circulation and acts as a paracrine factor. Circulating and hypothalamic or pituitary-derived IGF-I may also inhibit GH secretion at the pituitary and/or hypothalamic levels. GH also regulates its own secretion by 'short-loop' feedback. Oestrogen stimulates GH secretion in humans; the mechanism of action is unclear, but it may act either to inhibit the action of GH peripherally or stimulate GH secretion at the hypothalamic level. (Reproduced with permission from Thorner, M.O., Vance, M.L., Horvath, E., and Kovacs, K. (1992). The anterior pituitary. In: *Williams Textbook of Endocrinology*, 8th edition, (ed. J.D. Wilson and D.W. Foster) p. 231. W.B. Saunders, Philadelphia.)

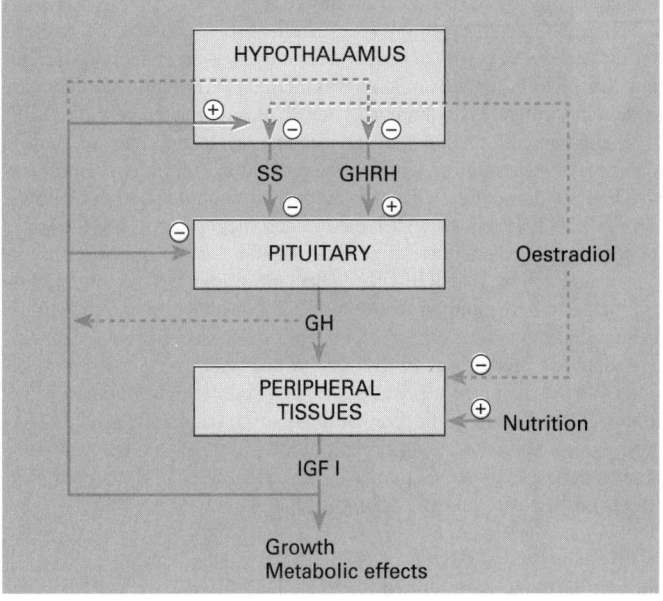

tinue to fall during the early postnatal months. The amount of GH secreted is greatest during adolescence and decreases with age. Premenopausal women have higher rates of production than do young men.

The pattern of GH secretion is dependent upon a number of factors, including stage of development, nutritional state, sleep stage, stress, and exercise. Increased secretion during puberty suggests that gonadal steroids, particularly oestradiol, are important regulators. Secretion is enhanced by sleep, with levels highest during slow-wave sleep and lowest during rapid eye movement (REM) sleep. A number of neurogenic, metabolic, and hormonal influences also affect GH secretion, albeit transiently. For example, hyperglycaemia in normal subjects acutely suppresses GH secretion, while in poorly controlled type 1 diabetics, GH levels are increased. Similarly, although acute increases in free fatty acid concentrations inhibit GH release, fatty acid levels are increased during starvation when GH secretion is augmented. Growth hormone secretion is augmented in fasting, anorexia nervosa, insulin-dependent diabetes mellitus, and hepatic cirrhosis. Certain amino acids, particularly arginine and leucine, also stimulate GH secretion. In contrast, its secretion is suppressed in obesity.

While exercise, stress, and some neurogenic factors stimulate GH secretion, emotional deprivation can inhibit its release in children and lead to diminished linear growth. Central α-adrenergic agonists (for instance clonidine) stimulate GH secretion, and β-antagonists augment the efficacy of various GH stimuli. Dopamine agonists stimulate dopamine receptors and thereby GH secretion in normal subjects. Acetylcholine agonists also stimulate, while agents which lower acetylcholine tone suppress GH release. Stimulation of GH by sleep, dopamine agonists, α-adrenergic agonists, glucagon, and by amino acids is inhibited by cholinergic muscarinic blocking drugs. These agents are considered to act at the level of hypothalamus or the median eminence. GH secretory responses to a number of stimuli are augmented after pretreatment with oestrogens (e.g. diethylstilbestrol 3 mg/day for 3 days). The role of serotonin in human GH secretion is unclear. Endogenous or exogenous opiates probably do not directly influence GH secretion, but nalorphine and an enkephalin analogue (DAMME, FK33824) stimulate GH secretion through naloxone-sensitive mechanisms. The pharmacological agent, growth hormone-releasing peptide (GHRP), developed from an enkephalin series of peptides, is a potent GH releasing agent, whose mechanism of action is unknown.

GROWTH HORMONE ACTIONS

There are two theories regarding the actions of GH; the GH hypothesis and the somatomedin hypothesis. It is clear that there are direct actions of GH, as well those mediated through IGF-I.

The somatomedin hypothesis came from observations that growth and mitotic activity of cartilage *in vivo* were crucially dependent on GH, but that direct addition of GH *in vitro* was ineffective. Essential components present in serum are now known to be two closely related peptides, IGF-I (or somatomedin C) and IGF-II. Each is a single-chain peptide with a high degree of homology with human proinsulin. Serum concentrations of IGF-I are markedly elevated in acromegaly and reduced in GH deficiency; IGF-II levels are unaffected in acromegaly and only modestly reduced in GH deficiency, suggesting that IGF-I is the important mediator of GH action; that IGF-I feeds back to inhibit GH secretion lends support to this hypothesis. The site of IGF-I production and the significance of circulating levels are the subject of controversy.

A dual effector model of GH action has been proposed, based on studies of its action in a preadipocyte cell line. It first stimulates precursor cells to undergo differentiation, and somatomedins then act as mitogens to stimulate clonal growth of the differentiated cells. Locally produced IGF-I, under GH regulation, contributes to the stimulatory effects of GH, particularly on longitudinal growth.

Growth hormone action *in vivo*

Growth hormone is described as 'anabolic', 'lipolytic', and 'diabetogenic', and its administration produces alterations in carbohydrate and lipid utilization. When administered to GH-deficient children it produces positive nitrogen balance, decreased urea production, redistributed body fat, and reduced carbohydrate utilization without development of diabetes. These effects may also occur in normal subjects and have led to the experimental use of GH in attempting to reverse some of the metabolic changes associated with ageing and catabolic illness.

Glycoprotein hormone family

The three anterior pituitary glycoprotein hormones are thyroid stimulating hormone (thyrotrophin; TSH), luteinizing hormone (lutrophin; LH), and follicle stimulating hormone (follitrophin; FSH). Each consists of two non-covalently bound subunits: the α-subunit is common to all three hormones, while the β-component is unique for each hormone and confers biological specificity. All subunits are synthesized as separate peptides from distinct mRNAs. There is considerable microheterogeneity of the carbohydrate constituents of the individual hormones, which leads to heterogeneity in receptor affinity, biological potency, and metabolic clearance.

The α-subunit peptide is more abundant than the unique β-subunits. Free serum α-subunits are secreted and are present in concentrations equivalent to those of combined TSH, LH, and FSH. Free serum β-subunit concentrations are much lower and are usually close to the level of detectability in conventional assays.

The α-subunits are approximately 20 to 22 kDa in molecular weight, have 92 amino acid residues, and contain two N-linked carbohydrate groups. The TSH β-subunit is approximately 18 kDa, consists of 110 amino acids, and contains one N-linked complex carbohydrate. Both TSH α- and β-subunits are negatively regulated by thyroid hormone. Thyroid hormone receptors bind to the 5′ flanking regions of α- and TSH β-subunit genes; which thyroid hormone receptor, and whether it acts directly or by interacting with transacting factors, remains to be elucidated.

THYROTROPH CELLS AND TSH CONTENT

Thyrotroph cells are the least common anterior pituitary cell type (about 5 per cent) and are located in the anteromedial portion of the gland.

REGULATION OF TSH SECRETION

Secretion of TSH is regulated both by hypothalamic and circulating thyroid hormones. The hypothalamic tripeptide, TRH, stimulates thyrotrophin release. If the hypothalamic pituitary stalk is interrupted, secondary hypothyroidism develops and TSH secretion is reduced, but not absent. While somatostatin and dopamine can inhibit TSH secretion, it is not clear whether this inhibitory mechanism is an important physiological regulator of thyrotrophin. It is likely that they regulate the circadian rhythm of TSH, since it is preserved in humans during constant TRH infusions.

Thyrotrophin secretion is regulated principally by feedback by thyroid hormones, which act at the hypothalamic level to inhibit TRH synthesis as well as at the pituitary to inhibit TSH secretion. Intracellular tri-iodothyronine (T_3) in thyrotroph cells regulates TSH secretion, although plasma thyroxine (T_4) levels correlate better with TSH levels than do tri-iodothyronine levels in normal subjects and in hypothyroid patients. In contrast, in hypothyroid patients receiving thyroxine hormone replacement, the serum tri-iodothyronine level correlates better with suppression of TSH levels than does serum thyroxine. The recently developed immunoradiometric TSH assays are more sensitive and have fewer cross-reacting substances. These assays can distinguish between normal and low TSH levels, which was often not possible with previous techniques.

Thyrotrophin is secreted in a pulsatile fashion, with low-amplitude peaks, and in a circadian fashion. Levels may rise before the levels of T_4 and T_3 decline below the normal range; in hypothalamic/pituitary disease the TSH level may be in the 'normal' range but be inappropriately low for the circulating concentration of thyroid hormone.

TRH administration has been used as a diagnostic test for TSH reserve; to amplify the TSH signal, to distinguish between low, normal, and high TSH levels, and to assess feedback inhibition by peripheral thyroid hormone levels. Figure 4 illustrates the TSH responses to TRH in normal subjects, patients with primary hypothyroidism, and pituitary and hypothalamic hypothyroidism. Patients with thyrotoxicosis had no response to TRH, reflecting enhanced negative feedback by thyroid hormone. The need for this test to exclude hyperthyroidism largely has been eliminated with the development of the sensitive immunoradiometric TSH assay. However, there are still two areas in which it may be helpful. In the patient with elevated thyroid hormone levels and detectable 'normal' TSH levels, the absence of a TSH response is compatible with either hyperthyroidism or a thyrotrope adenoma (see below), while a positive response may suggest pituitary resistance to thyroid hormone. TRH is also administered to distinguish between pituitary and hypothalamic hypothyroidism in which the peripheral thyroid hormone level is low and TSH is normal or low. If there is adequate TSH response to TRH, the abnormality is most likely hypothalamic in origin; in this case the 60 min TSH level is often greater than that of the 20 min response. An absent TSH response to TRH more likely reflects pituitary failure, often associated with other pituitary hormone deficiencies.

TSH ACTIONS (SEE ALSO CHAPTER 12.4)

TSH binds to specific thyroid cell plasma membrane receptors.

The TSH receptor also binds human thyroid stimulating immunoglobulins (TSIG). After TSH is bound to its receptor, it activates adenylate cyclase which increases intracellular cyclic AMP to activate protein kinase A, leading to phosphorylation of specific proteins which regulate the thyroid cells. TSH regulates both synthesis and secretion of thyroid hormones.

Gonadotrophins

LH β-, FSH β-, AND HCG β-SUBUNITS:

Both LH β- and FSH β-subunits are composed of 115 amino acids and have two carbohydrate side-chains. The structure of the β-subunit of LH is similar to that of human chorionic gonadotrophin (hCG) except for an additional 32 amino acids and additional carbohydrate residues on the carboxyl end of the β-subunit of hCG. A terminal sialic acid is frequently present on the carbohydrate side-chains of hCG β and FSH β. Sialic acid is not necessary for receptor binding but decreases the metabolic clearance of these hormones in contrast to TSH and LH (which do not have sialic acid side-chains).

PITUITARY LH AND FSH CONTENT

The content of gonadotrophins is low in the pituitaries of prepubertal children. In men and in menstruating women, the pituitary contains approximately 700 IU of LH and 200 IU of FSH. After menopause, the content of pituitary LH rises approximately two- to threefold, but there is no change in FSH content, although both LH and FSH are synthesized in the gonadotroph cell. hCG is present in small amounts in the pituitary.

REGULATION OF LH AND FSH SECRETION

Secretion from gonadotroph cells is regulated by the integration of the GnRH signal and feedback effects of gonadal steroids and peptides (e.g. inhibin). GnRH interacts with a membrane receptor to regulate both LH and FSH release and synthesis. GnRH is necessary for gonadotroph function; gonadal steroids and peptides are ineffective alone in stimulating release. However, once GnRH is secreted, the effects of gonadal steroids and inhibin are demonstrable.

Oestradiol

Oestradiol inhibits GnRH secretion from the hypothalamus. Its negative effects on pituitary gonadotrophin secretion appear to modulate GnRH action at the pituitary level rather than directly affecting transcription of mRNA for the subunits. It can also act in a positive manner, which may be a result of both direct effects at the pituitary level, for example to increase transcription of LH β-subunit mRNA synthesis, and at the hypothalamus to enhance GnRH secretion.

Progesterone regulates gonadotrophin secretion at the hypothalamus by slowing the GnRH pulse generator; thus, during the luteal phase of the menstrual cycle the LH pulse frequency is decreased.

Androgens suppress GnRH secretion by the hypothalamus, an effect best exemplified in patients with testicular feminization syndrome with an androgen receptor defect. In these patients the mean LH levels are elevated and the number of LH secretory episodes per 24 h are increased. Gonadotrophins are not suppressed by elevated endogenous testosterone levels nor by exogenous administration of androgens in these patients.

GnRH is essential for gonadotrophin secretion, and the timing of GnRH delivery is crucial for the regulation of LH and FSH secretion. The frequency and the amplitude of GnRH pulses are important in differentially regulating LH and FSH secretion. Both LH and FSH pulse secretion are maintained with one GnRH pulse per hour, while higher GnRH pulse frequencies initially increase the frequency of LH pulses and the basal LH concentrations. In contrast, when the GnRH pulse frequency is decreased to once every 3 h, FSH secretion is preferentially stimulated. Removal of hypothalamic influence results in a progressive decline in mRNA levels for α-, LHβ-, and FSHβ-subunits.

Gonadal peptides

Peptides produced in the gonad have important feedback effects on gonadotrophin secretion, and possibly other pituitary hormones. Inhibin plays an important and complex role in the regulation of FSH secretion. Gonadal secretion of inhibin is regulated by gonadotrophins, growth factors, and by gonadal steroids. Gonadectomy is followed by increased FSH secretion, indicating that the gonad produces factors which inhibit FSH secretion. Gonadal steroids (in physiological concentrations) are

Fig. 4 Serum TSH changes after TRH administration in normal subjects (shaded area) and in patients with primary hypothyroidism, hypothalamic disease, and pituitary hypothyroidism. Patients with hypothalamic disease may have a delayed TSH response to TRH. (Modified and reproduced with permission from Utiger, R.D. (1986)). Tests of the thyroregulatory mechanisms. In: *The thyroid* 5th edn. (ed. S.H. Ingbar and L.E. Braverman, p. 516. J.B. Lippincott, Philadelphia.)

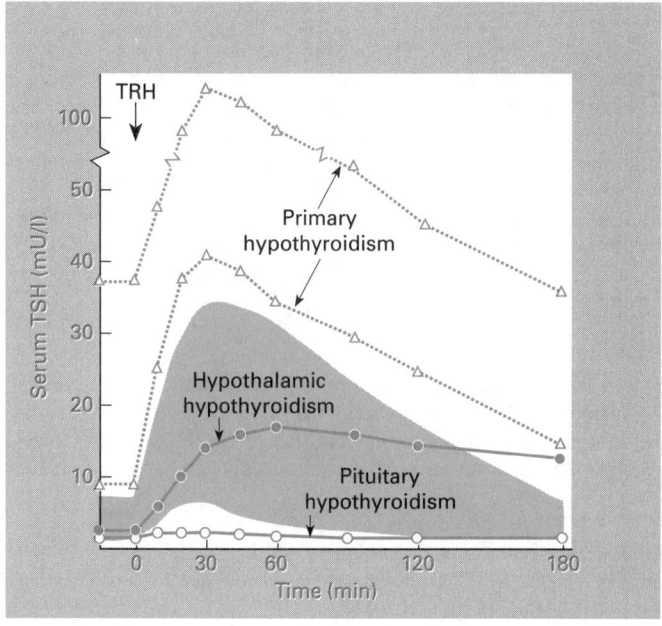

effective in lowering LH levels to those observed in the intact individual, but those of FSH remain elevated.

Inhibin is a member of a large family of glycoprotein hormones and growth factors that include müllerian inhibiting substance, transforming growth factor-β, an erythroid differentiation factor, and an insect protein that plays an important role in cellular differentiation. It is synthesized by Sertoli cells of the testis, granulosa cells of the ovary, the placenta, pituitary gonadotrophs, and the brain. It is possible therefore that inhibin regulates GnRH and gonadotrophin secretion not only as a gonadal feedback hormone, but by local production and as an autocrine or paracrine factor.

Activin is a hetero- or homodimer of the inhibin β-subunit (βA and βB). It stimulates FSH synthesis and secretion. Follistatin is a single-chain glycosylated polypeptide produced in the ovary. It is not a member of the inhibin family, but it selectively decreases levels of FSH β mRNA, and inhibits FSH secretion *in vitro*, as does inhibin. Follistatin action is thought to be due to its ability to bind activin and thus prevent its action.

LH AND FSH SECRETION

The two principal functions of the gonads in men and women are to produce sex steroids and gametes. These activities are precisely regulated by co-ordinated secretion of LH and FSH, which are controlled by hypothalamic GnRH secretion and feedback effects of gonadal steroids and peptides. These hormones are also responsible for the timing and control of pubertal development. Some reduction in gonadal function in men may occur with ageing, which may be centrally mediated. This differs from the primary ovarian failure of female menopause, which is associated with a three- to 15-fold increase in production rates of FSH and LH.

The regulation of LH and FSH secretion is unique in that the pulsatile pattern of gonadotrophin and GnRH secretion are necessary for normal gonadal stimulation. Kallmann's syndrome is the result either of a disordered GnRH secretion or of a deficiency of GnRH neuronal development or migration. Pulsatile administration of GnRH reverses hypothalamic hypogonadism. Long-acting GnRH agonist analogues can be administered to simulate continuous administration. This initially increases gonadotrophin secretion, but within 14 days inhibits it with resultant cessation of gonadal function. This therapy is used to reverse gonadotrophin-dependent precocious puberty, to inhibit ovarian function, for example in endometriosis, and to treat metastatic prostatic cancer ('medical gonadectomy'). Effective GnRH antagonists have been developed and are likely to replace the GnRH agonists in the future, having the advantage of immediate suppression, of gonadotrophin secretion.

Gonadal development is regulated by gonadotrophin secretion. Prior to puberty, the release of FSH is greater than that of LH; this is reversed at puberty. The pubertal response to GnRH probably reflects hormonal input, rather than the stage of development. The reason for the preferential release of LH to FSH or vice versa is uncertain, but may reflect inhibin secretion. It is likely that the major restraint on GnRH secretion originates in the central nervous system. The development of the human hypothalamo-pituitary gonadotrophin–gonadal axis may be divided into five stages: fetal, early infancy, late infancy, late prepubertal period, and puberty.

Fetal

By day 80 of gestation the mediobasal hypothalamic GnRH neurones are operative and stimulate pulsatile LH and FSH secretion. From day 100 to 150 of gestation there is unrestrained GnRH secretion. Development of negative sex steroid feedback occurs by day 150 of gestation.

Early infancy

At term, the secretion of GnRH is low. During the first few days after delivery plasma hCG, α-subunit, and placental steroid concentrations decline in both sexes, and testosterone declines in the male. Hypothalamic GnRH pulsatile secretion is highly functional by 12 days of age and prominent FSH and LH episodic discharges occur until approximately 6 months of age in boys and 12 months of age in girls. Transient increases in testosterone and oestradiol occur in boys and girls, respectively.

Late infancy and childhood

A proposed intrinsic CNS inhibition of hypothalamic GnRH secretion becomes functional, and by 4 years of age inhibition of GnRH is maximal. The negative feedback of LH and FSH secretion is highly sensitive to gonadal steroids (low set point). GnRH pulsatile secretion is inhibited and the amplitude and frequency of GnRH discharges are low, with resultant minimal secretion of FSH, LH, and gonadal steroids.

Late prepubertal period

Coincidentally, the intrinsic CNS inhibitory influences and the sensitivity of the hypothalamus and pituitary to gonadal steroids decrease, resulting in an increased set point and a resultant increased amplitude and frequency of GnRH pulses. Initially these pulses are most prominent during sleep. There is an increase in gonadotroph sensitivity to GnRH, increased secretion of FSH and LH, and increased gonadal responsiveness to FSH and LH, with resultant increase in gonadal hormone secretions.

Puberty

A further decrease occurs in both the CNS restraint of the hypothalamic 'GnRH pulse generator' and the sensitivity of negative feedback by gonadal steroids. The prominent sleep-associated increase in episodic secretion of GnRH gradually changes to the adult pattern of one pulse approximately every 90 min; the pulsatile pattern of LH follows this GnRH pattern. Progressive development of secondary sex characteristics occurs and spermatogenesis is initiated in boys. In girls, at mid- to late puberty, the capacity for oestrogen positive feedback develops and this culminates in a midcycle LH surge and ovulation.

Menstrual cycle

The minimum requirements for the complicated changes in gonadotrophin secretion during the menstrual cycle can be generated by the pituitary under invariant pulsatile GnRH stimulation (e.g. GnRH pump therapy at one fixed dose administered hourly for the full cycle of 28 days). This suggests that the feedback effects of gonadal steroids and peptides can occur at the pituitary level. Although this minimum requirement is definite, it is likely that under physiological conditions, there are other levels of regulation, including the hypothalamus. During the menstrual cycle changes occur in the frequency, amplitude, and mass of GnRH bursts secreted into the portal circulation.

Characteristic changes in the serum concentrations of LH and FSH occur in the normal menstrual cycle. Figure 5 shows gonadotrophin, 17-OH progesterone, progesterone, and basal body temperature changes during the human menstrual cycle synchronized around the day of the midcycle preovulatory peak. LH levels rise slightly during the follicular phase, peak at the time of the midcycle surge and then decline during the luteal phase of the cycle. The serum FSH concentration begins to rise during the late luteal phase, increases during early follicular phase of the next cycle and declines just before the midcycle FSH surge. This midcycle FSH surge is more modest than that of LH. FSH levels then decline during the luteal phase to increase again prior to the next menses. Studies of gonadotrophin secretion conducted by frequent sampling over a 24 h period have demonstrated that the frequency of LH peaks varies with different phases of the menstrual cycle. The greatest number of LH peaks occurs during the late follicular phase, and the fewest during the luteal phase of the cycle, with an intermediate number during the early follicular phase.

LH AND FSH ACTIONS

LH is primarily responsible for the regulation of sex steroid production by Leydig cells of the testis and the ovarian follicles. The preovulatory LH surge observed in women produces rupture of the follicle and luteinization. FSH stimulates gametogenesis; in the male it also stimulates Sertoli cells which have an important role in spermatogenesis. In the female FSH is important for follicular development. FSH also stimulates the production of LH receptors.

Pituitary diseases

Pituitary tumours account for 10 to 20 per cent of intracranial tumours, and are usually classified as microadenomas (diameter < 10 mm) or macroadenomas (diameter>10 mm). The patient with a pituitary tumour presents with symptoms of a mass lesion, or with endocrine dysfunction, or symptoms of both. Endocrine dysfunction may comprise hyperfunction or hypofunction, or a combination of the two.

Clinical manifestations

PITUITARY MASS

The symptoms of a sellar mass (Fig. 6) include headache or symptoms secondary to compression of intracranial nerves: visual field disturbances, ophthalmoplegia, and, occasionally, compression of the first or second branch of the trigeminal nerve, giving rise to facial pain. The extent of the abnormality depends upon the size of the tumour and its anatomical position. Thus, microadenomas may be asymptomatic except

for producing endocrine dysfunction. A macroadenoma which extends inferiorly may also be asymptomatic other than headache, while a superior extension with abutment of the optic chiasm may produce visual field defects. Bitemporal hemianopia is the classic finding, but any visual disturbance can occur, depending on the extent of suprasellar extension and the location of the optic chiasm, whether pre-fixed or post-fixed. A pituitary tumour can produce diminished visual acuity, scotoma, quadrantic defects, and total blindness of one or both eyes. The fibres of the optic nerve course along a precise path, depending on their site of origin in the retina. Those from the temporal halves of the retina (for nasal vision) do not cross, but course posteriorly along the ipsilateral optic tract. Those from the nasal half (for temporal vision) cross in the chiasm and course posteriorly along the contralateral optic tract. Even when bitemporal hemianopia is present it is often asymmetrical.

Headache from pituitary tumour can be variable and is often non-specific. While it may be occipital, retrorbital pain or bitemporal headaches are more typical, which are sometimes worse on awakening and generally improve over the course of the day, and are often ameliorated by analgesics. Very large pituitary tumours or a suprasellar hypothalamic tumour (for example, craniopharyngioma) may extend sufficiently superiorly or posteriorly to compress either the foramen of Munro or the aqueduct of Sylvius. The former leads to obstruction of the lateral

Fig. 6 Various symptoms of a pituitary tumour in addition to hypopituitarism. Headaches are only rarely caused by hydrocephalus. Visual field defects caused by extension of the tumour are readily plotted using the Goldmann perimeter. (Modified and reproduced with permission from Wass, J.A.H. (1987). Hypopituitarism. In: *Clinical endocrinology: an illustrated text* (ed. G.M. Besser and A.G. Cudworth) pp. 2.1–2.14 J.B. Lippincott, Philadelphia.)

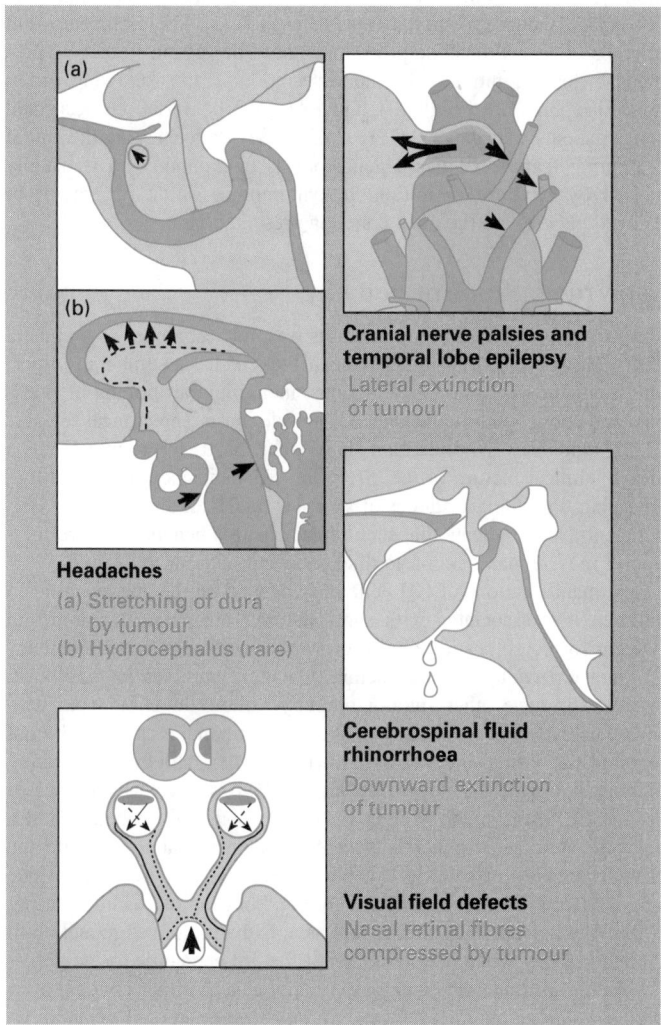

Cranial nerve palsies and temporal lobe epilepsy
Lateral extinction of tumour

Headaches
(a) Stretching of dura by tumour
(b) Hydrocephalus (rare)

Cerebrospinal fluid rhinorrhoea
Downward extinction of tumour

Visual field defects
Nasal retinal fibres compressed by tumour

Fig. 5 Mean daily plasma FSH, LH, progesterone, and 17-OH progesterone concentrations and basal body temperature during 16 presumptively ovulatory cycles from 15 young women. (Modified and reproduced with permission from Ross, G.T., Cargiu, C.M., Lipsett, *et al.* (1970). Pituitary and gonadal hormones in women during spontaneous and induced ovulatory cycles. *Recent Progress in Hormone Research*, **26**, 1–62.)

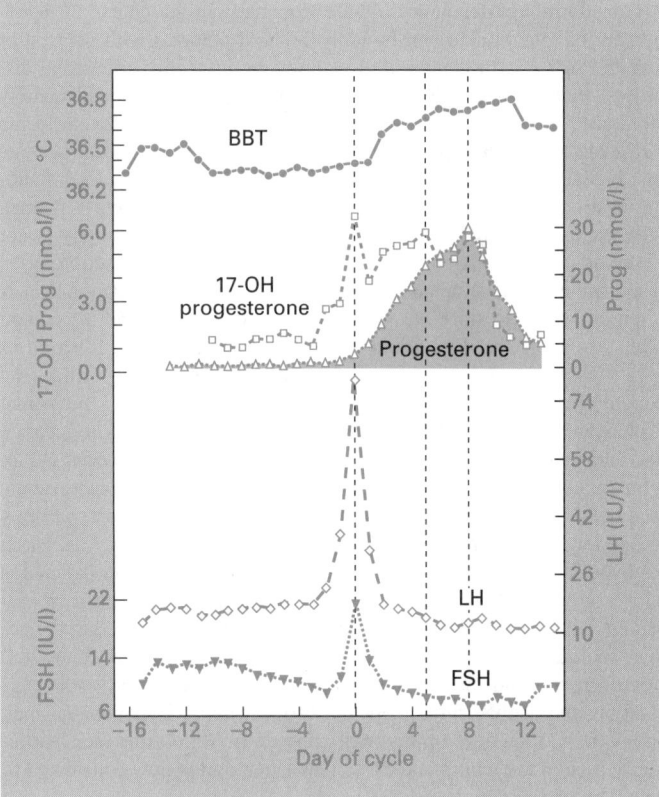

ventricles and later to obstruction of the cerebrospinal fluid flow from the third ventricle to the fourth. This leads to hydrocephalus, involving the lateral ventricles or the lateral and third ventricles, respectively. Extensive lateral extension may produce dysfunction of the third, fourth, the first and second divisions of the fifth (V_1 and V_2), and the sixth cranial nerves.

Patients with macroadenomas usually have marked symptoms from the mass lesion, although occasionally large tumours are discovered incidentally during evaluation for another medical complaint and there may be no signs or symptoms. Visual disturbance occurs during the course of illness in about 60 per cent of patients with macroadenomas. If the tumour extends inferiorly, the patient may have no symptoms or may develop sphenoid sinusitis, producing pain. Rare complications include CSF rhinorrhoea (the fluid discharged contains glucose) or recurrent meningitis from erosion of the sella turcica and loss of the barrier between CSF and the exterior. Giant tumours may extend into the temporal lobes, causing temporal lobe epilepsy, and occasionally can extend to the cerebral peduncles and give rise to motor and/or sensory disturbances.

MANIFESTATIONS OF ANTERIOR PITUITARY HORMONE DEFICIENCIES

Total or selective hypopituitarism may occur in patients with pituitary adenomas, with parasellar diseases (see below), in those who have had pituitary surgery or radiation (including cranial radiation for intracranial malignancies), or following head injury. Deficiency of any or all of the six major hormones secreted by the pituitary can occur. The most common symptom in both men and women is cessation of gonadal function. Secondary hypogonadism may result from LH and FSH deficiency, but may also occur with hyperprolactinaemia. The classic finding is progressive loss of pituitary hormone secretion in the following order: gonadotrophin (LH, FSH), GH, TSH, ACTH, but, variations occur and some patients may have ACTH and/or TSH deficiency as the initial presenting feature. Prolactin deficiency is uncommon and is usually caused by pituitary infarction. In children, cessation of growth or delayed puberty are the most common presentations.

GROWTH HORMONE DEFICIENCY

Until recently GH deficiency in adults was not recognized as a clinical entity. However, recent studies indicate that GH has a number of important modulatory physiological actions, including partitioning of nutrients and energy and maintenance of muscle mass. The clinical features of GH deficiency syndrome are shown in Table 1. In the mid 1990s a clearer clinical picture of the effects of GH deficiency in the adult is emerging. Preliminary studies of short-term GH administration to GH-deficient adults indicate that such replacement is beneficial for restoration of muscle mass, skin-fold thickness, and nutrient utilization.

The manifestations of GH deficiency depend on the age of onset. In children it is associated with short stature, relatively good nutrition (weight for height), and reduced growth velocity. Neonatal deficiency is characterized by hypoglycaemia, which is particularly marked in infants who have other anterior pituitary failure, but may occur with severe isolated GH deficiency. Growth hormone is apparently not required for normal intrauterine growth. Affected children are usually of normal weight and length at birth, but growth velocity decreases during the first 2 years. Weight is normal for length or height and a delay in bone age frequently occurs. It is important to measure the growth velocity, as well as the height and weight percentiles, since height reflects only the cumulative growth. For example, a child starting at the 70th percentile at birth would have had a prolonged reduction in growth velocity when observed later at the 3rd percentile for height.

Growth hormone deficiency in children can be either congenital or acquired. Idiopathic GH deficiency is most often a result of hypotha-

Table 1 *Clinical features of adult GH deficiency syndrome*

Mixed truncal and generalized adiposity
Increased waist : hip ratio
Reduced strength and exercise capacity
Thin, dry skin; cool peripheries; poor venous access
Cold intolerance
Impaired psychological well-being:
poor general health
impaired emotional reaction
depressed mood
impaired self-control
anxiety
reduced vitality and energy
increased social isolation

Modified and reproduced with permission from Cuneo *et al.* (1992).

lamic GHRH deficiency, while GH gene mutations are rare. Other congenital causes include deficiency associated with various developmental abnormalities, including pituitary aplasia or hypoplasia, and midline brain abnormalities. Acquired causes include tumours of the hypothalamus or pituitary, other intracranial tumours (optic nerve glioma, for example), hypopituitarism secondary to cranial irradiation (now a common cause in many children who are long-term survivors after radiation therapy for leukaemia), head injury (including injury at birth), or infection/inflammation. Growth hormone deficiency may also occur in the setting of severe psychosocial deprivation.

GONADOTROPHIN DEFICIENCY

Gonadotrophin deficiency results from either a pituitary defect or the lack of hypothalamic GnRH stimulation of the gonadotrophe. It may be due to hypothalamic disease, disease of the pituitary stalk, or a functional abnormality as occurs with hyperprolactinaemia, anorexia nervosa, secondary adrenal insufficiency, or secondary hypothyroidism.

Gonadotrophin deficiency often occurs early in the course of development of hypopituitarism. In adolescents, it presents with delayed or arrested puberty. In women it is manifest by infertility, menstrual disorders, or amenorrhoea. The low gonadotrophin levels do not adequately stimulate the ovaries, resulting in low serum oestradiol levels in the range of the follicular phase of the menstrual cycle. Hypooestrogenaemia is often associated with lack of libido and dyspareunia; long-standing oestrogen deficiency produces breast atrophy. However, in women who are hypogonadal from hyperprolactinaemia, breast atrophy is not observed. Long-standing oestrogen deficiency of any aetiology is responsible for development of osteopenia. In men, hypogonadism is often undiagnosed since the syndrome develops slowly and the patient often discounts the diminished libido and impotence as a function of 'age'. Hypogonadism is often diagnosed retrospectively when the patient presents with the symptoms of a mass lesion. Even if the patient is unaware of deficiencies, his partner may often provide a more accurate and objective assessment of the onset of sexual dysfunction. As in women, gonadotrophin deficiency may result from hyperprolactinaemia (see below). Low gonadotrophin concentrations result in serum testosterone levels in the prepubertal range and testicular size may decrease; testicular consistency may be soft. Acquired gonadotrophin deficiency is a rare cause of male infertility. Spermatogenesis is often well preserved and the significant semen analysis abnormality is a reduced ejaculate volume, which is a function of the testosterone concentration. Beard growth and muscle bulk may also be reduced, and with long-standing hypogonadism osteopenia also develops. Hypogonadal men and women often develop fine wrinkling of the skin of the face, particularly around the mouth and eyes. This latter sign is now considered to be a sign of GH deficiency.

THYROTROPHIN DEFICIENCY

Secondary hypothyroidism usually occurs relatively late in the development of hypopituitarism and is usually characterized by failure to thrive, weight gain, lack of energy, cold intolerance, and constipation. The degree of hypothyroidism depends upon the duration of thyrotrophin deficiency, but is rarely as profound as the myxoedema of primary hypothyroidism.

CORTICOTROPHIN DEFICIENCY

Secondary adrenal failure may occur as an isolated deficiency, or may occur late in the course of the development of panhypopituitarism. The symptoms are essentially the same as those of Addison's disease, but differ in two important respects. Secondary adrenal insufficiency results from lack of ACTH stimulation of the adrenal. Therefore, only the adrenal steroids, which are under predominant corticotrophin regulation, are affected. These include absence of cortisol and adrenal androgen secretion. Mineralocorticoid secretion, primarily regulated by renin and angiotensin, is preserved, although it may not be optimal. Because of preserved mineralocorticoid secretion, these patients may not experience an adrenal crisis. More commonly the symptoms are of malaise, loss of energy, anorexia, and weight loss. Postural hypotension and orthostatic dizziness may be present. These patients are often misdiagnosed as malingerers. Women tend to lose secondary sexual hair and libido, while men have preserved secondary sexual hair unless there is coexistent gonadotrophin deficiency. In contrast to patients with Addison's disease, these patients have a pale and sometimes slightly sallow complexion; since corticotrophin levels are low they are not hyperpigmented. Severe cortisol deficiency may result in hypoglycaemia and hyponatraemia; hyperkalaemia usually occurs only with the aldosterone deficiency of primary adrenal disease. These patients, particularly those with panhypopituitarism, may deteriorate gradually and a relatively trivial illness may precipitate circulatory collapse, coma, or a hypoglycaemia-induced seizure. Adrenal insufficiency, regardless of the cause, is a medical emergency.

Morphological classification of pituitary adenomas

Pituitary tumours are no longer classified by their tinctural qualities. Instead classification is based on their immunocytochemical staining and electron microscopic appearances. Table 2 shows the functional morphological classification of pituitary adenomas and their prevalence in unselected surgical specimens.

Application of immunohistochemical testing has led to discovery of plurihormonality in pituitary adenomas.

Evaluation of suspected pituitary disease

Therapy for a pituitary tumour is dictated by its type and the extent of growth. The evaluation of the patient with such a tumour should determine:

(1) Presence and type of hormone hypersecretion;
(2) Any hormonal deficiencies and need for replacement therapy;
(3) Presence of any visual abnormalities;
(4) Pituitary anatomy including presence of extrasellar extension.

All of these areas need to be evaluated prior to treatment.

ASSESSMENT OF HYPOTHALAMIC PITUITARY FUNCTION

A number of factors need to be considered. These include:

(1) Interpreting the level of the pituitary hormone in relation to the level of the target hormone;

Table 2 *Prevalence of pituitary adenoma types in unselected surgical material (1960 cases)*

	Prevalence (%)
Prolactin producing adenoma	26.2
Null cell adenoma, including oncocytoma	25.5
Growth hormone producing adenoma	14.1
Corticotroph adenoma	10.0
Gonadotroph adenoma	9.3
Growth hormone and prolactin producing adenoma	6.6
Silent corticotroph adenoma, subtypes I, II, III	5.3
Unclassified adenoma	2.0
Thyrotroph adenoma	1.0

Frequency is based on careful electron microscopic analysis. Many adenomas contain more than one hormone by immunocytochemistry. To date, the frequency of plurihormonal adenomas is not clarified. (Data kindly provided by K. Kovacs, St Michael's Hospital, Toronto, Canada.)

(2) Pulsatile secretion of anterior pituitary hormones;
(3) Specific factors that affect the concentration of each of the pituitary hormones (for example, time of day, stress, fed or fasting, asleep or awake, stage of development).

In general, screening for hyperfunction and hypofunction can usually be achieved by taking a history, performing a physical examination, and drawing a single basal blood sample for assessment of pituitary and target organ hormone levels. More subtle abnormalities require more sophisticated studies.

In Table 3 are listed the hypothalamic and pituitary hormones and the target gland hormones. Each laboratory should provide a normal range of values for each test.

Interpretation of hormone concentrations requires consideration of several issues. Currently, hormone concentrations are measured by radioimmunoassay or by immunoradiometric assay. Radiometric assays are now being replaced by chemiluminescence assays. These have two major advantages: that they do not require use of radioisotopes and have greater sensitivity.

PLASMA ACTH

Plasma ACTH should probably be measured only in the evaluation of adrenal failure or Cushing's syndrome. Because of the short half-life of plasma ACTH, the sample must be collected into a cold syringe, placed in an EDTA tube, immediately centrifuged at 4 °C, and the plasma frozen immediately. If these precautions are not followed the peptide will be degraded, producing uninterpretable results. In addition, ACTH secretion is pulsatile, with a circadian rhythm, and it increases during stress. Results must therefore be interpreted with knowledge of time of sample collection, whether it was drawn from an indwelling cannula (in place for at least 2 h), whether the patient was stressed, and whether exogenous synthetic glucocorticoids were administered. A simultaneously obtained plasma cortisol sample is necessary to interpret the appropriateness of the plasma ACTH concentration. Practically, much information is obtained from a plasma cortisol measurement alone. Since ACTH is the prime regulator of cortisol secretion, the plasma cortisol is an index of hypothalamic–pituitary–adrenal function. An 8 a.m. cortisol between 10 and 20 µg/dl effectively excludes adrenal insufficiency, although it does not assess ACTH reserve.

SERUM THYROTROPHIN

Ultrasensitive immunoradiometric assays have greatly improved the utility of TSH assays, which now distinguish between low, normal, and high levels and have decreased the need for dynamic function tests,

Table 3 *Relationship between hypothalamic and pituitary hormones, target glands, and feedback hormones*

Hypothalamic hormone	Pituitary hormone	Target gland	Feedback hormone
TRH	TSH	Thyroid	T_4 and T_3
GnRH	LH	Gonad	Oestradiol (E2) (women), testosterone (T) (men)
	FSH	Gonad	Inhibin, and ? E2 and T
SS	GH	Multiple	IGF-I
DA	PRL	Breast	?
CRH	ACTH	Adrenal	Cortisol
AVP	ACTH	Adrenal	Cortisol
GHRH	GH	Multiple	IGF-I

Reproduced with permission from Thorner *et al.* (1992).

particularly the TRH test. If the TSH concentration is in the normal range, in association with normal serum thyroid hormone levels, the patient is euthyroid and requires no further testing. If the serum thyroid hormone levels are low, and the TSH level is normal (but inappropriately low for the prevailing thyroid hormone levels) or low, the patient has secondary thyroid failure. Distinction between pituitary and hypothalamic failure can be attempted by administering TRH, but in long-standing thyrotrophin deficiency of hypothalamic aetiology, a single dose of TRH may not stimulate intrinsically normal, but quiescent, thyrotrophs.

SERUM GROWTH HORMONE

Growth hormone is secreted in a pulsatile fashion and values in a normal subject may vary from undetectable to levels which may exceed 40 µg/l. Its secretion is affected by ingestion of food; it is suppressed by hyperglycaemia and is stimulated by amino acids and hypoglycaemia. Stages III and IV of sleep, or slow-wave sleep, are associated with increased GH secretion, particularly in young adults and children. For these reasons, a random serum GH measurement is usually not helpful. To evaluate GH deficiency a stimulation test is required (Table 4). A suppression test is employed, for example the oral glucose tolerance test, if GH hypersecretion is suspected. Since the bursts of spontaneous GH secretion may occur at any time of day, timing of the sample is not helpful. Similarly GH, like ACTH and prolactin, is a stress hormone and secretion increases in response to psychogenic or physical stress or to pain. The serum IGF-I provides an overall index of GH secretion and is particularly useful as a screening test for acromegaly. Since GH secretion is influenced by nutritional status, fasting for 24 h increases its secretion. Growth hormone secretion is also increased in type 1 diabetes mellitus, in anorexia nervosa, and in hepatic failure, and is reduced in obesity. Secretion increases during puberty and is then greater in girls than in boys; this increase is accompanied by an increase in the serum IGF-I concentration. During pregnancy, GH secretion is progressively suppressed by the human GH variant secreted by the placenta which presumably feeds back on the maternal hypothalamus and pituitary to suppress GH secretion. However, serum IGF-I concentrations are increased, indicating a biological effect of the variant GH.

SERUM LH AND FSH

Serum LH and FSH are secreted in a pulsatile fashion. In men the levels of these hormones, despite their pulsatile secretion pattern, are within a fairly narrow range; marked abnormalities of secretion are therefore easily diagnosed from a single blood sample, particularly when interpreted with the clinical findings, simultaneous testosterone levels, and possibly semen analysis.

In women the situation is more complex because of the marked changes in gonadotrophin secretion during different phases of the menstrual cycle. Clinically, measurement of serum LH and FSH in a woman who is not taking an oral contraceptive and who has regular menstrual

Table 4 *Provocative tests of GH secretion*

1. Insulin, 0.15 U/kg body weight, causes a peak GH response in 45–60 min. A physician should be in attendance. Severe hypoglycaemic symptoms should be reversed with intravenous glucose
2. Arginine hydrochloride, 0.5 g/kg body weight in normal saline, is administered intravenously over 30 min. GH peak occurs at 45–60 min
3. Levodopa (>30 kg body weight; 500 mg; 15–30 kg; 250 mg; < 15 kg; 125 mg) is given orally. Transient nausea is common and vomiting may occur. Side-effects are minimized if patient is kept supine in a quiet room. Peak GH response usually occurs between 45 and 90 min
4. Glucagon, 1 mg, is given intramuscularly. Peak GH usually occurs 2–3 hours later. Nausea and vomiting may result

Reproduced with permission from Thorner *et al.* (1992).

cycles almost begs the question; a normal menstrual cycle with documentation of a normal luteal phase serum progesterone concentration effectively excludes significant gonadotrophin dysfunction. In amenorrhoeic women it is important to measure the serum LH and FSH concentrations, and simultaneous serum 17β-oestradiol, prolactin, and choriogonadotrophin (hCG) concentrations. In this manner, the following diagnoses can be made positively:

(1) Primary ovarian failure with the resultant increase in LH and FSH (FSH > LH) with usually prolactin normal or low;

(2) Hyperprolactinaemia, with an elevated prolactin, normal or follicular phase LH, FSH, and 17β-oestradiol levels;

(3) Pregnancy with a positive hCG test, normal or high prolactin; high LH (if hCG cross-reacts in the assay), and high 17β-oestradiol.

SERUM PROLACTIN

Prolactin is also secreted in a pulsatile fashion. It is increased in the early hours of the morning, particularly just before awakening. It is a stress hormone and its levels rise in response to psychological and physical stress, including pain. Levels also rise in response to nipple stimulation and may increase during sexual intercourse. Prolactin secretion is increased in response to oestrogens, and during pregnancy it may increase to levels of 3600 to 9000 mIU/l (200–500 µg/l).

Clinically, a random prolactin, drawn by venepuncture, is useful if the level is normal, or if the level is markedly elevated. If the concentration is greater than 4500 mIU/l (250 µg/l), it is almost certainly diagnostic of a prolactinoma, and further measurements are unnecessary. However, if the level is mildly elevated (for example, 450 mIU/l (25 µg/l)), this is likely to reflect the stress of venepuncture or of the physical examination, including examination of the breasts. In this situation, it is necessary to repeat the measurement once or twice. Alternatively, samples can be obtained from an indwelling venous cannula after a rest period of 2 h; samples should be obtained at 20 min intervals over the ensuing 2 h. If the prior elevation was a result of stress, results obtained with this procedure are usually normal. Although prolactin concentrations vary during the day, with lower levels observed in the afternoon, the time of day is not critical.

DYNAMIC TESTS OF PITUITARY FUNCTION

The combined anterior pituitary test

Simultaneous administration of four hypothalamic releasing hormones with measurement of target pituitary hormone concentrations permits assessment of pituitary reserve without need for admission to hospital.

Rationale

Pituitary hormone responses depend upon the presence of specific pituitary cell type(s), the previous exposure of these cells to endogenous hypothalamic hormones which 'prime' them, enabling them to respond to the exogenous hormones, and the feedback effects of target cell hormone(s) on the hypothalamus and pituitary.

Indication

The combined anterior pituitary test is a screening test in suspected pituitary dysfunction. If there is a clinical indication of a deficiency, definitive testing is performed, for example insulin hypoglycaemia or metyrapone administration for suspected ACTH deficiency. The combined anterior pituitary test may be useful in assessing pituitary function after pituitary surgery or radiation.

The four hypothalamic hormones are administered intravenously (sequentially) over 20 seconds. The doses are: GnRH, 100 μg; TRH, 200 μg; CRH, 1 μg/kg; and GHRH, 1 μg/kg. The normal pituitary hormone response ranges have been established by Sheldon and colleagues. Over 300 patients with various hypothalamic–pituitary diseases were studied before and/or after therapy. These studies indicate that useful information is obtained from samples drawn at − 30, 0, 15, 30, 60, 90, and 120 min for measurement of ACTH, TSH, LH, FSH, GH, and prolactin. Results can be interpreted only in light of the circulating levels of the target gland hormones. Baseline samples are obtained at 08.00 h for cortisol, thyroxine, T_3 resin uptake, oestradiol (amenorrhoeic women), testosterone (men), and IGF-I.

Results from administration of the hypothalamic hormones may be of limited use, but if the pituitary hormone response is normal, in the setting of an appropriate peripheral target hormone level, then pituitary reserve is likely to be normal. The combined anterior pituitary test is useful to amplify the abnormalities; thus, if the TSH level is low, together with low peripheral thyroxine levels, there is a high probability of secondary hypothyroidism; an absent TSH response to TRH confirms the suspicion. An absent response to a hypothalamic hormone may be a result of absent or dysfunctional pituitary cells or because of increased negative feedback by the peripheral hormone. An example of the latter situation is an absent TSH response to TRH in thyrotoxicosis. An absent or diminished pituitary response may also result from a lack of priming because of insufficient exposure to the hypothalamic hormone (for example isolated gonadotrophin deficiency, which in most instances results from GnRH deficiency). The administration of CRH may also be useful in distinguishing between ectopic ACTH production and Cushing's disease. However, there are exceptions, and differentiating between these two conditions still remains difficult. Over 70 per cent of presumed GH-deficient children have an increase of serum GH to greater than 7 μg/l when GHRH is administered. In those who do not, an adequate GH response may occur after repeated GHRH injections. Thus, a single injection of GHRH is not particularly useful to identify the aetiology of GH deficiency, which is most commonly a result of hypothalamic GHRH deficiency. However, a deficient GH response to GHRH makes a diagnosis of GH deficiency very likely.

The combined anterior pituitary test is useful to document the presence of a functional specific cell type in the anterior pituitary. It does not diagnose hypopituitarism or hyperpituitarism, but may aid in defining pituitary function, for example, following pituitary surgery, pituitary or cranial radiation, or pituitary infarction before administering chronic replacement therapy. Patients receiving chronic hormone replacement therapy may also be reassessed after short-term hormone withdrawal for documentation of the extent of hypopituitarism.

Insulin tolerance test

The insulin tolerance test is the most widely used test to determine ACTH and GH reserve.

Rational

Insulin-induced hypoglycaemia activates hypothalamic neurones to stimulate pituitary secretion of corticotrophin, GH, and prolactin.

Indication

To test ACTH and GH reserve in a patient suspected of having hypothalamic/pituitary dysfunction.

Test procedure

If the test is performed by knowledgeable, well-trained, and experienced personnel in a properly equipped unit, this is a very effective and safe test. The contraindications to the insulin tolerance test are: 08.00 h basal plasma cortisol less than 5 μg/dl, history of a seizure disorder, altered mental status, or ischaemic heart disease. If the 08.00 h plasma cortisol is less than 5 μg/dl the patient has adrenal failure and requires a test to distinguish primary from secondary adrenal failure, for example a plasma corticotrophin measured simultaneously with plasma cortisol and a short ACTH (Synacthen®) test followed by a 48 h ACTH (Synacthen®) infusion. Hypoglycaemia may precipitate fits in a patient with a seizure disorder or myocardial infarction in a patient with ischaemic heart disease. An alternative test such as metyrapone administration should be performed in such patients.

The test must be performed only when a physician is present. Before insulin administration, a recent history, physical examination, and ECG must be performed and interpreted and the 08.00 h plasma cortisol of greater than 5 μg/dl documented. The test and symptoms of hypoglycaemia must be explained in detail to the patient, who should have fasted from midnight, but may have taken water *ad libitum*. A heparin-lock venous cannula is placed about 1 h prior to commencement of the test, which should take place in the morning. Blood is drawn for blood glucose, plasma cortisol (and, if indicated, for corticotrophin), prolactin, and GH at − 30, 0, 30, 45, 60, and 90 min. At 0 min, 0.15 units/kg of soluble or Actrapid® insulin is injected intravenously. Pulse rate, blood pressure, and clinical observations are made at the times of blood sampling. During the initial 30 min after the injection there are often no symptoms, but between 30 and 45 min sweating, tachycardia, drowsiness, and hunger usually occur. If there are no signs of hypoglycaemia and the blood glucose has not fallen to less than 2.2 mmol/l (40 mg/dl), a second dose of insulin, 0.3 units/kg, is administered. In the event of adverse effects (e.g. a fit) the hypoglycaemia is reversed with intravenous glucose, and 1 mg dexamethasone administered intravenously. Sampling should continue until the end of the test since it is likely that the hypothalamic–pituitary–adrenal axis will have been activated. In patients known to have insulin resistance (e.g. acromegaly) a dose of 0.3 U/kg may be used initially. However, if doubt exists, it is safer to start with the standard dose and then double it. There is no point repeating the same dose because it is unlikely to induce hypoglycaemia if it was initially unsuccessful.

Interpretation

Clinical signs of hypoglycaemia and a blood glucose of less than 2.2 mmol/l (40 mg/dl) are required for the ACTH and GH levels to be interpretable. If these two criteria are fulfilled, the plasma cortisol should rise to greater than 580 nmol/l (21 μg/dl) and GH should increase to above 10 (in children) and 3 (in adults) μg/l. If these levels are not achieved, then the patient has ACTH and/or GH deficiency.

Oral glucose tolerance test

Rationale

Growth hormone secretion is inhibited by acute hyperglycaemia. The test is performed to diagnose or exclude acromegaly.

Indication

Suspected acromegaly and to determine glucose tolerance.

Test procedure

The patient fasts from midnight and is allowed to take water *ad libitum*. A heparin-lock cannula is placed in a forearm vein 1 h before the test. Blood samples for blood glucose and serum GH are obtained at − 30, 0, 30, 60, 90, and 120 min. Glucose (75 g) is dissolved in iced orange- or lemon-flavoured water and given to the patient immediately after the 0 minute blood sample is obtained.

Interpretation

If sensitive immunoradiometric assays are used, serum GH should decrease to less than 1 μg (2 mU/l) after oral glucose ingestion. These criteria have been established for 50 g, 75 g, and 100 g glucose doses. In routinely used GH radioimmunoassays, a normal GH response to oral glucose ingestion is said to decrease to less than 2 μg/l.

The development of ultrasensitive chemiluminescence GH assays which measure GH concentrations as low as 0.002 μg/l will probably lead to re-evaluation of the normal GH response to oral glucose. In a study by the author, GH levels in response to 100 g oral glucose were significantly lower in normal young men than in women (mean GH concentrations 0.029 v. 0.23 μg/l). Therefore, the new criteria using this assay are: suppression of GH to < 0.06 μg/l in men and to < 0.71 μg/l in women.

In acromegaly, serum GH concentrations may be unchanged, partially lowered, or may increase paradoxically.

PITUITARY IMAGING

The skull radiograph, hypocycloidal sellar tomography, cerebral arteriography, and pneumoencephalography were once used to assess pituitary gland anatomy. For direct visualization of the gland and its relationship to surrounding structures, these techniques are limited. Additionally, arteriography and pneumoencephalography are invasive and associated with some risk and discomfort for the patient. Computerized tomography (CT) and magnetic resonance imaging (MRI) techniques are excellent non-invasive methods to image directly the pituitary gland and, with respect to MRI, the structures surrounding the pituitary gland. Currently, the evaluation of a patient with suspected pituitary or hypothalamic disease is best performed with an MRI or CT scan (Table 5). Since pituitary enlargement may occur without enlargement of the sella, a normal skull radiograph or sellar tomograms do not exclude a pituitary mass. Thus, unless specific visualization of the bone anatomy surrounding the pituitary gland is required, a skull radiograph or sellar tomograms have little value in assessing pituitary anatomy. Cerebral angiography may occasionally be required in some patients prior to surgical intervention, but has no place in the initial evaluation of such patients unless there are no facilities for MRI or CT. MRI is superior to CT because the optic chiasm is easily visualized and can be distinguished from the diaphragma sellae, vascular structures (including aneurysms) can be seen and any lateral tumour extension can be delineated; it also requires no radiation.

Pituitary mass

Although both CT and MRI scans can effectively identify a large pituitary tumour, the MRI scan can better delineate the full extent of the

Table 5 *Anatomical evaluation of hypothalamic–pituitary disease*

Skull radiograph	No value
CT scan	High resolution, direct coronals
	1.5 mm sections through pituitary
	Contrast enhancement
MRI scan	First choice
	Images relationship of optic chiasm to diaphragma sellae
	Distinguishes aneurysms, lateral tumour extension
	Images cavernous sinus
	No contrast or radiation

tumour and its relationship to the surrounding structures, and more accurately identify small lesions (Fig. 7). A comparison of patients with a surgically proven microadenoma demonstrated that the MRI scan detected the microadenoma and its correct location in 100 per cent of cases; but only 50 per cent of cases were detected on CT scans. A pituitary microadenoma on MRI scan may range from 1.5 to 10 mm in diameter and is round and hypointense in relation to the normal gland on T_1-weighted images; lesions, best demonstrated on coronal images, give a higher signal on T_2-weighted scans. Deviation of the infundibulum away from the side of the tumour may be observed. Macroadenomas (>10 mm) tend to have signal characteristics that are similar to those of the normal gland, but may contain cystic or haemorrhagic areas. Intravenous administration of gadolinium-diethylenetriamine penta-acetic acid (Gd-DTPA) produces prompt enhancement of the normal pituitary which is maximal after approximately 30 min; adenomas enhance more slowly and persistently than the normal gland. The use of Gd-DTPA and coronal images increases the probability of identifying a small lesion and should be used in all studies in which a pituitary tumour is suspected. MRI may also successfully identify a non-pituitary intrasellar mass such as a meningioma or internal carotid artery aneurysm. MRI is currently the most sensitive method to identify a microadenoma, but very small tumours may not be detectable. This is particularly true for patients with Cushing's disease where only 83 per cent of the tumours are detectable by MRI.

NEURO-OPHTHALMOLOGICAL EVALUATION

The assessment of the anatomical relationship between a pituitary mass and the optic chiasm has been greatly improved by the use of the MRI scan. A distinct separation between the tumour and the optic chiasm and absence of invasion into the cavernous sinus can be shown using MRI, but imaging with a CT scan cannot provide this information.

Visual acuity and visual fields should be assessed at the initial examination, most commonly by use of a Snellen chart or card and estimation of visual fields by confrontation. Confrontation testing with a red coloured object (e.g. tip of a pen) may reveal subtle visual field loss. A normal clinical examination does not exclude abnormalities which are only detectable using perimetry. In patients with visual symptoms or evidence of optic chiasm compression on MRI or CT scan, the extent of visual field compromise must be documented using automated perimetry.

Permanent loss of vision or visual field defect(s) usually results from long-standing nerve compression, but the relationship between duration of compression and permanency of damage is not known. If vision from one eye is normal, the patient may fail to notice any abnormality or describe the vision as dim or foggy. Vision is usually lost gradually, except in the case of significant haemorrhage into the tumour (pituitary apoplexy), when it may be sudden with loss of central vision and development of bitemporal field defects, ophthalmoplegia, and changes in mental function.

Visual acuity may range from 20/20 to near or complete blindness.

Loss of perception of colour, particularly red, and a decreased pupillary light reaction may accompany decreased visual acuity. If the optic nerve has been compromised for 6 weeks or more optic disc pallor may be present and occurs in 30 to 70 per cent of patients with large tumours.

Ophthalmoplegia, the result of lateral extension of the tumour is less common. Involvement of the cavernous sinus occurs in up to 15 per cent of patients, but is clinically apparent in only a minority of these. Symptoms include diplopia and/or ptosis or altered facial sensation. Depending on the degree of cavernous sinus invasion, cranial nerves III, IV, VI, and the V_1 and V_2 divisions of V may be impaired, most commonly the third nerve.

Successful decompression of the optic nerves and chiasm, either by surgical resection or shrinkage of the tumour by medical therapies, is often accompanied by marked improvement in visual function, usually occurring within hours or days of surgery continuing thereafter for some months. Visual abnormalities may worsen in some 4 to 10 per cent after surgical decompression. The transsphenoidal approach carries the least risk of such deterioration. The prognosis is best in those with a short history and absence of clinical evidence of optic atrophy.

Hormone replacement therapy

Replacement therapy usually consists of administration of the hormones produced by the target gland rather than of the deficient pituitary product. Exceptions are the use of GH for GH deficiency, gonadotrophin therapy for induction of ovulation in women, and treatment of infertility in men, as well as desmopressin for treatment of diabetes insipidus. GH therapy may in future be replaced by analogues of GHRH which selectively stimulate pulsatile GH secretion analogous to the administration of GnRH instead of exogenous gonadotrophins to treat delayed puberty and many cases of hypogonadotrophic hypogonadism.

Thyroid hormone replacement should not be given until the hypothalamic–pituitary–adrenal axis has been assessed since in a cortisol deficient subject it may precipitate an adrenal crisis.

MEDICALERT BRACELET

Every patient receiving adrenal, posterior pituitary, and/or thyroid hormone replacement therapy should have and wear an identifying necklace or bracelet in the event of an emergency.

CORTISOL DEFICIENCY

Cortisol deficiency is usually treated by oral administration of 20 mg hydrocortisone on awakening and 10 mg at 6 p.m. This is the simplest method to simulate crudely the circadian rhythm of cortisol secretion. Some patients require an additional 10 mg at lunch time, while others, particularly very small patients, may require a lower dose of 10 mg on awakening and 5 mg at 6 p.m. Alternatively, synthetic glucocorticoids may be used; prednisone, 5 mg on awakening and 2.5 mg at 6 p.m., or dexamethasone, 0.5 mg on awakening. The appropriate dose is usually determined clinically; measurement of plasma cortisol concentrations through the day may be helpful, but urinary free cortisol levels are not. During stress, whether psychological or physical, fever, and during illness, the dose should be increased to an equivalent of hydrocortisone 20 mg every 6 to 8 h. More severe illness may require intravenous administration of hydrocortisone in a dose of 100 mg intravenously every 4 h. It is often more convenient to administer dexamethasone either intravenously or intramuscularly at a dose of 1 mg every 12 h, a regimen which is frequently used in patients undergoing surgery.

THYROID HORMONE DEFICIENCY

Thyroid hormone deficiency is treated with L-thyroxine; 0.075 to 0.15 mg once daily. The dose is adjusted according to the clinical response but measurement of the serum tri-iodothyronine level aiming at the middle or upper part of the normal range can also be helpful. Measurement of serum TSH is of no value in patients with hypothalamic/pituitary hypothyroidism.

GONADAL STEROIDS

Gonadal steroids are required for hypogonadal patients in whom hyperprolactinaemia is not the cause, and for patients who do not desire fertility.

Testosterone enanthate for hypogonadal men is usually given intramuscularly, 200 mg every 2 weeks or 300 mg every 3 weeks. It is advisable to begin with a low dose (50 mg every 2 weeks, for example) to avoid breast tenderness, gynaecomastia, or excessive and painful erections. This can then be doubled every 2 weeks until the patient is receiving a full dose.

There are numerous regimens for oestrogen replacement in hypogonadal women. It is given to improve sense of well being, to maintain sexual function (libido and vaginal lubrication), and to prevent bone loss. If the uterus has not been removed, oestrogens are administered cyclically with appropriate progestogens; a convenient choice is a low dose (containing 30 μg ethinyl oestradiol) oral contraceptive preparation. These are readily available, are conveniently packaged, and do not require the patient to remember when to take the progestogen and when to stop the tablets. Alternatively, oestrogen can be given for 3 weeks

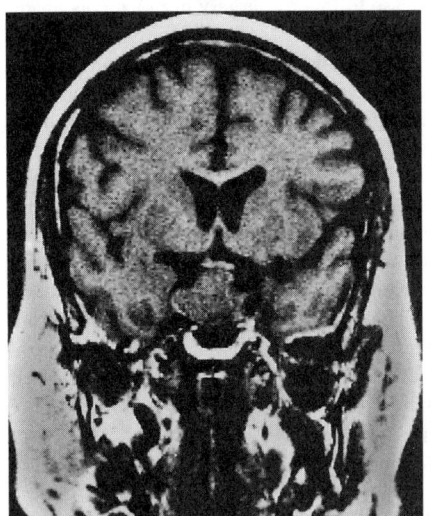
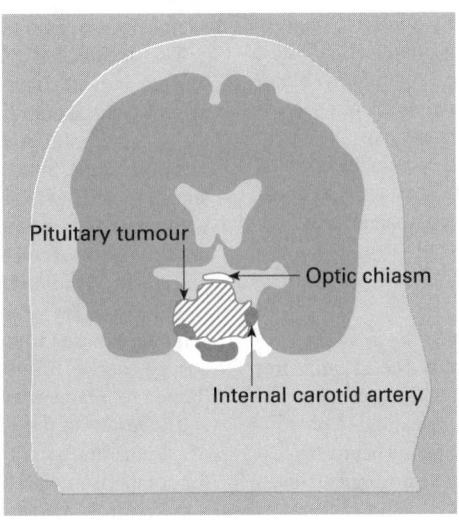

Fig. 7 Coronal MRI scan and schematic drawing demonstrating a large pituitary tumour extending laterally into both cavernous sinuses and superiorly abutting the optic chiasm. (Reproduced with permission from Thorner et al. (1992).)

out of four and a small dose of progestogen administered for the third week; for instance conjugated oestrogen 0.625 mg daily for 3 weeks together with medroxyprogesterone acetate 5 mg or 10 mg daily for the last 7 or 10 days.

GONADOTROPHINS AND GnRH

Gonadotrophins and GnRH are administered to initiate puberty and to restore fertility (see Section 12.8).

GROWTH HORMONE

Recombinant DNA-produced preparations of natural sequence GH are now available, and are given subcutaneously to GH deficient children once daily at a dose of 0.045 mg/kg/day (0.3 mg/kg/week), resulting in accelerated linear growth in the first year (catch-up growth) and maintenance of normal growth rates in subsequent years. GH is not normally replaced in GH-deficient adults, although trials of its efficacy are currently under way.

GROWTH HORMONE RELEASING HORMONE

Growth hormone releasing hormone has been administered in GH-deficient children, given once or twice daily and by pulsatile subcutaneous administration. Results are encouraging but further experience is needed to determine whether chronic GHRH treatment is equivalent to, or has advantages over, the use of GH.

VASOPRESSIN

In patients with diabetes insipidus from hypothalamic or pituitary disease, the drug of choice is desmopressin, which is 1000 times more potent than vasopressin in increasing distal tubular water reabsorption and has 1000 times less vasopressor activity. It is administered by nasal spray, 10 μg given once or twice daily. If nasal insufflation is inappropriate, for instance after trans-sphenoidal surgery, subcutaneous administration, 1 or 2 μg every 12 or 24 h, is an alternative.

Pituitary surgery

Large pituitary tumours were once approached transcranially. Modern pituitary trans-sphenoidal surgery allows clearer distinction between tumour and normal tissue, much increasing the chances of selective removal to leave the normal gland intact and functional. Decompression of the pituitary fossa from below, also allows a recurrence to extend inferiorly instead of laterally or superiorly. Other advantages include lack of disturbance of the brain, absence of external scars and of requirement to shave the head. Trans-sphenoidal surgery is often well-tolerated by the elderly or frail patient who might not survive a craniotomy. Major contraindications to this approach include anatomical problems, such as lack of pneumatization of the sphenoid sinus or hyperostosis; the extent and localization of the suprasellar extension which precludes removal from below; and ambiguity regarding the type of lesion, such as aneurysm or meningioma, which cannot be resected trans-sphenoidally.

INDICATIONS FOR PITUITARY SURGERY

Pituitary apoplexy

Minor haemorrhage into a pituitary tumour probably occurs quite frequently and may be clinically insignificant; many such cases are probably not diagnosed. However, a severe haemorrhage leading to prostration, visual disturbance, profound headache, and coma is a neurosurgical emergency. If sudden visual compromise occurs, neurosurgical intervention is mandatory.

Pituitary tumour

Therapy is indicated if pituitary tumours hypersecrete or if they are large enough to produce mass effects. With the exception of prolactin-secreting adenomas, most authorities recommend transsphenoidal surgery as the first intervention. Extirpation of the tumour in theory, and often in practice, cures the endocrine disturbance and allows decompression of any involved structures such as the optic chiasm and cavernous sinus.

Failure of other therapies

Patients who have undergone previous failed therapies are candidates for surgery, for example, children with Cushing's disease or adults with acromegaly not cured by pituitary radiation. Patients with a prolactinoma in whom the 'tumour' continues to grow also may require surgery even if prolactin levels have returned to normal. Situations arise when there are two lesions, for example a prolactinoma and a meningioma. Intolerance to bromocriptine or other dopamine agonists is another indication for surgery. Additionally, prolactinomas are not always fully responsive to treatment with dopamine agonists. Surgery is then often helpful in reducing the bulk of the tumour allowing a better response to medical therapy.

RESULTS OF PITUITARY SURGERY

The results of surgery are usually good, particularly in patients with suprasellar extension and visual abnormalities. Improvement in visual field abnormalities occurs in over 80 per cent of such patients, progression of visual disturbance is arrested in 16 per cent but there is deterioration in 4 per cent. The endocrine results of pituitary surgery are discussed below. Important considerations for optimal results include: (1) the experience and expertise of the neurosurgeon; (2) the size of the tumour; (3) tumour invasion of bone; and (4) previous therapy.

There are few complications of pituitary surgery, but, every operation carries a risk, which is lowest in patients with microadenomas and highest in patients who have had previous therapy (for example, recurrent or persistent tumour). The incidence of postoperative hypopituitarism is 3 per cent in patients with microadenomas but increases with invasiveness of the tumour.

Pituitary radiation

This was once the only available treatment for many patients with pituitary tumours. It usually prevented further tumour growth and eventually resulted in a reduction in hormone hypersecretion. However, these responses were rarely prompt and hypopituitarism, either total or partial, was a common sequel. Currently, pituitary radiation is administered only to patients with residual disease following surgery or in patients unable to undergo surgical resection.

The techniques used include conventional supervoltage therapy, yttrium implantation, stereotactic radiosurgery with alpha particles or proton beam therapy, or a single high dose of focused radiation from the gamma knife unit. The choice is made according to the size and location of the tumour (proximity to the optic chiasm and cavernous sinus) and the available resources. Conventional supervoltage therapy is the approach most commonly used, administered in daily fractions 5 days per week over 4 or 5 weeks. Yttrium implantation involves surgical placement of radioactive yttrium-90 seeds into the pituitary and is now used in very few centres. Alpha particle and proton beam radiotherapy can only be used to treat small tumours and require a cyclotron for the energy source. Focused radiation using the gamma knife unit is also limited to treatment of small tumours and is not widely available.

The results of these treatments are broadly similar, with the exception of gamma knife unit therapy in which there is inadequate information for comparison with other techniques. Most studies have demonstrated that very few patients have progression of disease after radiotherapy.

Partial reduction in hormone hypersecretion may occur within 3 to 6 months of therapy, but a complete response requires at least 5 years, and more often is delayed until 10 years after treatment.

Hypopituitarism is an expected consequence of radiotherapy; it may be partial or complete and can develop at any time after treatment. In one study, 50 per cent of patients treated with conventional supervoltage radiation developed hypopituitarism within 26 months of therapy. Other series indicate that at least one-third of patients develop pituitary deficiencies within 2 to 3 years, the incidence increasing with length of follow-up. Any patient treated with pituitary radiation must therefore be closely followed in order to detect and treat the earliest signs of pituitary failure.

Other complications of radiotherapy include damage to the optic chiasm, and/or optic nerve(s) or other cranial nerves with consequent visual loss or ophthalmoplegia, vascular damage, resulting cerebral ischemia, seizures and development of a pituitary or brain malignancy. The incidence of these complications varies between centres and the type of radiation administered. Complications of radiotherapy occur more frequently in patients who have received prior surgery.

Pituitary tumours

Prolactinoma

Hyperprolactinaemia, the result of excessive prolactin production by the lactotropes, is the most common anterior pituitary disorder encountered in clinical medicine.

The natural history of the development and progression of a prolactinoma is not precisely known, but the majority of these tumours grow slowly, usually over years. Autopsy studies have suggested that 23 to 27 per cent of the general population may have an asymptomatic microadenoma. Serial observations of untreated patients with a microadenoma indicate that a minority have a significant increase in serum prolactin and or in tumour size, while in the majority there is a decrease in serum prolactin concentrations over time.

AETIOLOGY

This is unknown, although several theories have been proposed. There is no association between oral contraceptive use and development of prolactinomas which probably arise *de novo* and are not a result of hypothalamic dysfunction. Analyses of tumour DNA indicate a monoclonal origin.

CLINICAL FEATURES

The clinical presentation varies according to the patient's age and sex, the duration of hyperprolactinaemia and, if present, the size of the tumour. Men and postmenopausal women usually come to medical attention because of symptoms of a pituitary mass, such as headache and disturbances of vision. Table 6 illustrates the common clinical features, among which hypogonadism is almost invariable. Women of reproductive age commonly seek medical attention because of delayed menarche, disturbance of menstrual function, or infertility. Galactorrhoea is present in 30 to 80 per cent of these women, a symptom which is less common in those with long-standing amenorrhoea, an observation which probably reflects prolonged oestrogen deficiency. Other features of oestrogen deficiency include decreased libido, vaginal dryness, and dyspareunia. In the majority of premenopausal women the cause of hyperprolactinaemia is a microadenoma.

In men, hypogonadism may be complete or partial, producing decreased libido, complete or partial impotence and/or infertility. Many hyperprolactinaemic men report 'normal' sexual function and realize there was dysfunction only after successful treatment. When hypogonadism has been long-standing, beard and body hair may be decreased

Table 6 *Symptoms associated with hyperprolactinaemia*

Women	Men	Men and postmenopausal women
Galactorrhoea (30–80%) Menstrual irregularity Infertility	Galactorrhoea (< 30%) Impotence	Visual field abnormalities Headache Extraocular muscle weakness Anterior pituitary malfunction

A variable incidence of galactorrhoea is reported in different studies. Reproduced with permission from Thorner, M.O. (1987). Hyperprolactinaemia. In: *Clinical Endocrinology*, (ed. G.M. Besser and A.G. Cudworth) 2nd edition, p. 4.3 Wolfe Publishing.

and the testes are usually soft but of normal size (>12 ml volume). Galactorrhoea occurs in 14 to 33 per cent of affected men, but its presence may require vigorous breast manipulation; gynaecomastia is uncommon. In those with arrested puberty, a female body habitus may be evident and the testes are usually small (< 12 ml volume) and soft. Symptoms other than decreased libido (which affects 83 per cent) include adiposity (69 per cent), apathy (63 per cent) and headache (63 per cent). Although in the majority of men seeking treatment for sexual dysfunction the cause is psychogenic, some 8 per cent have hyperprolactinaemia, emphasizing the importance of measuring the serum prolactin concentration in such patients.

A pituitary tumour may be found coincidentally when a CT or MRI scan is obtained because of head trauma or for evaluation of headaches. A less common presentation is that of severe headache and/or prostration secondary to haemorrhage into a previously undiagnosed pituitary tumour (see above).

COMPLICATIONS

A tumour which extends beyond the confines of the sella turcica most commonly produces headache and visual abnormalities. The classic presentation is with a bitemporal hemianopia from compression of the optic chiasm by a tumour which has extended superiorly. Lateral extension into the cavernous sinus causes impaired oculomotor function involving the cranial nerves III, IV, VI, and the V_1 and V_2 divisions of V, either singly or in combination. Occasionally, very large tumours may extend into the temporal lobe of the brain, increasing the risk of fits.

Compression of normal pituitary tissue by a large tumour may result in disturbance of secretion of other pituitary hormones, resulting in GH, ACTH, LH, FSH, or TSH deficiency, singly or in combination. The most common deficiency in patients with large prolactinomas is most probably that of GH, but this has not been systematically studied. Hyperprolactinaemia is associated with impaired pulsatile gonadotrophin (LH, FSH) release, probably by alteration of hypothalamic GnRH secretion. Gonadal insufficiency or failure results from altered pituitary LH and FSH release and is reversible with reduction of prolactin secretion. Both men and women with chronic hyperprolactinaemia have decreased bone density, when compared with age-matched normal subjects.

ENDOCRINE EVALUATION

Any patient with a suspected or documented pituitary tumour requires full investigation of pituitary function. In the case of hyperprolactinaemia a full drug history is important since a number of medications may produce hyperprolactinaemia (see Table 7.). A single prolactin measurement may be sufficient to diagnose a prolactinoma if the value is sufficiently elevated, for example greater than 3600 mIU/l (200 μg/l).

Table 7 *Causes of hyperprolactinaemia*

Hypothalamic disease
  Tumour, e.g. metastases, craniopharyngioma, germinoma,
    cyst, glioma, hamartoma
  Infiltrative disease, e.g. sarcoidosis, tuberculosis,
    histiocytosis X, granuloma
  Pseudotumor cerebri
  Cranial radiation
Pituitary disease
  Prolactinoma
  Acromegaly
  Cushing's disease
  Pituitary stalk section
  Empty sella syndrome
  Other tumours, e.g. metastases, non-secretory, gonadotroph
    adenoma, meningioma
  Intrasellar germinoma
  Infiltrative disease, e.g. sarcoidosis, giant cell granuloma,
    tuberculosis
Drugs
  Dopamine receptor antagonists, e.g. chlorpromazine,
    fluphenazine, fluorperazine, haloperidol, perphenazine,
    promazine, domperidone, metoclopramide, sulpiride
  Other drugs
    Antihypertensives, e.g. alpha methyldopa, reserpine,
      verapamil
    Oestrogens
    Opiates
    Cimetidine
Primary hypothyroidism
Chronic renal failure
Cirrhosis
Neurogenic, e.g. breast manipulation, chest wall lesions, spinal
  cord lesions
Stress, e.g. physical, psychological
Idiopathic

Reproduced with permission from Thorner *et al.* (1992).

Since prolactin is secreted in a pulsatile fashion and in response to breast manipulation, a mildly increased concentration of 400 to 1200 mIU/l (20–60 μg/l) may reflect these factors; it is prudent therefore to obtain several measurements before making the diagnosis of true hyperprolactinaemia. A morning cortisol concentration may be used to screen for adrenal function, but a normal value does not assess hypothalamic–pituitary reserve and a stimulatory test such as insulin-induced hypoglycaemia or metyrapone administration is necessary to determine if the hypothalamic–pituitary–adrenal axis is functionally intact. Induction of hypoglycaemia can also be used to determine GH reserve. Additional helpful studies include measurement of plasma testosterone (in men) and oestradiol (in women).

A raised serum prolactin must be interpreted in conjunction with MRI or CT scanning of the pituitary to determine whether the hyperprolactinaemia is a result of a prolactinoma or is a secondary phenomenon. A prolactin concentration of 3600 mIU/l (200 μg/l) or greater, in the presence of a macroadenoma (>10 mm), is most likely caused by a prolactinoma. Conversely, a prolactin concentration of less than 3600 mIU/l (200 μg/l) in the setting of a large pituitary tumour is most likely to be caused by compression of the pituitary stalk, resulting in interference with dopamine transport from the hypothalamus to the gland. This distinction is particularly important in selecting appropriate therapy, since dopamine agonists will reduce serum prolactin in both instances, but will not shrink the tumour which has caused secondary hyperprolactinaemia. Prolactin-secreting microadenomas do not usually increase prolactin concentrations beyond 3600 mIU/l (200 μg/l). Hyperprolactinaemia can also be caused by non-pituitary intracranial lesions.

Craniopharyngiomas, meningiomas, ectopic pinealomas, metastatic tumours or third ventricle tumours do not usually increase prolactin concentrations above 2000 mIU/l (100 μgs/l).

AIMS OF TREATMENT

Treatment should reduce hormonal hypersecretion to normal, reduce tumour size, correct visual and/or cranial nerve abnormalities, restore any abnormal pituitary function, and, if possible, avoid the need for chronic hormonal replacement therapy. Ideal results cannot always be achieved, particularly in the presence of very large tumours.

Successful treatment of a prolactinoma is most often and easily accomplished with administration of a dopamine agonist drug, but there may be an additional need for surgery and/or radiotherapy in some cases.

MEDICAL THERAPY

The effectiveness of dopamine agonist drugs in lowering serum prolactin concentrations, reducing tumour size, improving visual field and cranial nerve abnormalities, and restoring gonadal function has been well demonstrated, although the degree of response is variable. Bromocriptine has been shown to lower serum prolactin to normal in 64 to 100 per cent, to improve galactorrhoea in 57 to 100 per cent, and to return menses and ovulation to normal in 57 to 100 per cent of patients. The results of treatment in patients with macroadenomas are similar to those with microadenomas, except that in some with large tumours, a longer time is required to lower the serum prolactin to normal.

Reduction in tumour size with improvement in visual abnormalities usually occurs before the serum prolactin returns fully to normal. Some 76 to 100 per cent of patients can expect a reduction in tumour size, and visual field defects improve in 90 per cent, often before any demonstrable decrease in tumour size assessed by CT or MRI, emphasizing the importance of careful monitoring of vision and visual fields in these patients.

The usual dose of bromocriptine is 2.5 mg three times daily. When prolactin concentrations have been reduced to normal, the dose may be reduced to 2.5 mg twice daily and continued suppression may be expected with this reduced dose. Some patients have been given larger doses (e.g. 20–30 mg/day) in resistant cases but there is no conclusive evidence that these larger doses are any more effective than is the standard regimen, and they are certainly more costly.

Other currently available dopamine agonists include lisuride, pergolide, metergoline, and a non-ergot preparation, CV 205-502. These drugs act by direct stimulation of pituitary cell membrane dopamine receptors (DA 2) to inhibit prolactin secretion. A single 2.5 mg dose of bromocriptine suppresses serum prolactin for up to 14 h and the effect may persist up to 24 h in some patients. The most common side-effects of dopamine agonists are nausea and orthostatic hypotension which occur commonly on initiation of treatment and can be minimized by beginning with a small dose, given with food, increasing gradually over 1 to 2 weeks. Less common side-effects include headache, fatigue, nasal stuffiness, abdominal cramping, and constipation. Despite taking it with food, some patients have intolerance to bromocriptine. Hallucinations and psychosis have also been observed; the incidence of psychosis was 1.3 per cent in one study of 600 patients, the symptoms including auditory hallucinations, delusions, and mood changes that abated when the dopamine agonist was discontinued. Concomitant alcohol ingestion may exacerbate the symptoms of nausea and abdominal discomfort. Patients usually develop a tolerance to the drug, however, and there is no loss of effectiveness in suppression of prolactin secretion.

Most patients require long-term treatment, and withdrawal usually results in recurrent hyperprolactinaemia and re-expansion of the tumour. It is occasionally possible to stop treatment in a patient with a microadenoma or no demonstrable tumour. Whether or not this reflects spontaneous infarction of the tumour is not known.

Pregnancy in women with hyperprolactinaemia

Suppression of prolactin to normal and resumption of ovulatory menses occurs in 80 to 90 per cent of hyperprolactinaemic women during bromocriptine therapy. Fertility in these patients is identical to that of other women of the same age. A recommendation for women attempting to become pregnant is that barrier contraception should be used until the patient has had two or three regular cycles, so that cycle length can be determined. After discontinuation of mechanical contraception, a serum β-human chorionic gonadotrophin (β-hCG) measurement is obtained to confirm pregnancy as soon as there is a delay in expected menses. This regimen allows for early diagnosis of pregnancy so that dopamine agonist therapy can be discontinued. Bromocriptine is not associated with an increased risk of multiple pregnancies, spontaneous abortion, ectopic pregnancy, trophoblastic disease, or congenital malformation. Complications related to tumour expansion during pregnancy may occur, particularly in women with macroadenomas. Clinically significant enlargement has been estimated to occur in 1.4 per cent of women with microadenomas and approximately 16 per cent of those with macroadenomas, but these are almost certainly overestimates due to observer bias. The incidence in microadenomas is probably less than 1 per cent and may even be less than 0.1 per cent. When significant tumour enlargement has occurred, options include surgical resection, high-dose steroid treatment, and/or reinstitution of bromocriptine. Bromocriptine is effective and is the most benign therapy. Patients with macroadenomas treated with bromocriptine continuously during pregnancy do not have tumour-related complications, and bromocriptine is effective in resolving headache and improving vision in those treated after the tumour has expanded. Given the risk of tumour expansion, a full ophthalmological examination should be undertaken before pregnancy and throughout its course.

After cyclic menses have been restored, the need for contraception in those not desiring pregnancy should be addressed. The use of a low-dose oestrogen-containing oral contraceptive is a reasonable regimen, as long as dopamine agonist treatment is continued.

Men with prolactinomas

Men treated with a dopamine agonist have improvement in libido and potency. Some note marked improvement in function early in treatment, before the testosterone concentration becomes normal. The semen analysis can be expected to improve with lowering of prolactin to normal and restoration of normal pulsatile gonadotropin (LH, FSH) secretion.

Resistance to dopamine agonist therapy

A few patients have a partial response or no response to this therapy, probably dependent on the number and affinity of dopamine receptors in the tumour. Surgically resected adenomas from bromocriptine-responsive patients have been shown to have twice the number of dopamine receptors and approximately 50 per cent greater binding affinity for dopamine than did adenomas from bromocriptine-resistant patients. This may explain tumour growth during bromocriptine therapy, loss of responsiveness, and possibly metastatic progression of some tumours. Fortunately, resistance to bromocriptine is an uncommon event, but patients should be closely monitored during medical therapy. Failure to respond leads to consideration of surgical resection.

SURGICAL THERAPY

Transsphenoidal resection of the adenoma is the most frequently employed approach and is associated with better results and less morbidity than is craniotomy. Although surgical resection offers the potential cure, this is only accomplished in a minority of patients with large tumours and is associated with a definite risk of recurrence in all patients. The surgical results are dependent on the skill and experience of the surgeon. Patients with microadenomas (< 10 mm) treated surgically at centres where the procedure is frequently performed have a normal postoperative serum prolactin concentration in 60 to 80 per cent of cases, while in patients with macroadenomas (>10 mm) this is achieved in 0 to 40 per cent of patients. The most important factors predictive of successful surgery are the preoperative serum prolactin concentration and the tumour size.

Recurrence rates in patients with a microadenoma range from 10 to 50 per cent for up to 5 years of follow-up and from 0 to 91 per cent of those with a macroadenoma followed for up to 5 years.

RADIATION THERAPY

Pituitary radiation is rarely used as primary treatment of a prolactinoma. Although it is effective in preventing further growth or expansion of the tumour, it is much less effective in promoting a prompt reduction of the serum prolactin concentration.

Acromegaly

The estimated prevalence of acromegaly is 38 to 69 per million, with an annual incidence of 3 to 3.3 per million. The percentage of acromegalics in pituitary surgical series is about 15 per cent. It is seen with equal frequency in men and women, and may occur at any age, but is diagnosed most frequently in the fourth and fifth decades of life. When it occurs prior to puberty, gigantism develops; this is an extremely rare syndrome and it accounts for less than 5 per cent of acromegalics. In about 6 per cent of patients, acromegaly may occur as a part of multiple endocrine neoplasia type 1 syndrome.

AETIOLOGY

In over 99 per cent of cases, acromegaly results from a primary pituitary adenoma, but in a very few, less than 1 per cent, it results from excessive production of GHRH which causes somatotroph hyperplasia and possibly tumour formation. GHRH secretion occurs in gangliocytomata (eutopic; either hypothalamic or pituitary) or peripheral tumours (ectopic). One case of ectopic GH secretion by a pancreatic islet cell tumour has been described.

Most evidence suggests that acromegaly due to somatotroph adenoma is a primary pituitary disease. Morphological examination of somatotroph adenomas reveals a circumscribed tumour; the remaining pituitary is normal without evidence of somatotroph hyperplasia. Additionally, after successful removal of the tumour and reduction of GH to normal, recurrence is rare.

Point mutations in α_s, the GTP-binding subunit of the stimulatory regulator of adenyl cyclase (G_s), has been found in about half of somatotroph tumours, demonstrating that adenylate cyclase is constitutively activated. Somatotroph tumours are monoclonal in origin.

CLINICAL FEATURES

Patients with acromegaly have a gradual progression of symptoms and signs, so that the diagnosis is often delayed for as many as 15 to 20 years. The symptoms usually begin insidiously and anatomical changes develop gradually and go unnoticed until complications develop. Symptoms and signs may be a result of: (1) the pituitary tumour mass; (2) hypopituitarism; (3) excessive GH secretion; or (4) a combination of features (Table 8).

The tumour mass may produce headaches and/or visual disturbances, including a visual field defect or diplopia from ophthalmoplegia. Hypopituitarism may occur if the tumour is very large; gonadal dysfunction is more common than hypothyroidism and secondary adrenal insufficiency. The symptoms and signs of excessive secretion of GH are the most common presentation, gigantism before puberty and acromegaly after it. Acromegaly is characterized by thickening and oiliness of the

Table 8 *Clinical features and complications of acromegaly*

Enlarged hands, feet, head, tongue, vocal cords
Skin: hyperhidrosis, greasiness, skin tags, acne
Increased interdental spaces, malocclusion
Mass effects:
    headache, visual field defects, cranial nerve palsies
Osteoarthritis, arthralgias
Carpal tunnel syndrome
Organomegaly
Hypertension
Cardiomyopathy
Neuropathy
Impaired glucose tolerance, diabetes mellitus
Renal calculi
Gonadal dysfunction

skin, particularly of the face. Facial changes include thick lips, exaggerated nasolabial folds, thickening of the scalp, giving rise to the development of deep folds, which are visible on skull radiograph or CT scan—cutis verticis gyrata. Acanthosis nigricans may also occur. The vocal cords thicken which, in conjunction with sinus enlargement, results in a deep and resonant voice. The overall appearance and a deep voice give acromegalic women a rather masculinized appearance often associated with mild hirsutism. The hands and feet enlarge; rings become tighter, cannot be removed and may have to be cut off. The increased hand and finger size (requiring larger gloves) may cause difficulty with performing fine tasks such as picking up a pin from the floor. Increased foot size is manifested particularly by an increase in the shoe width. An increase in both soft tissue and skull mass leads to increased head, and therefore, hat size. The calvarium of the skull thickens; hyperostosis frontalis is common and frontal sinuses expand resulting in protrusion of the brows ('frontal bossing'). The zygomatic arch enlarges to produce prominence of the cheek bones and relative hollowness of the temporal fossae, particularly evident after successful treatment when the soft tissues regress. The mandible grows in length and breadth, which leads to protrusion of the lower jaw, malocclusion, and development of temporomandibular arthritis. The changes in the lower jaw and the temporomandibular arthritis are sometimes the particular feature leading to the diagnosis of acromegaly.

Joint pain from accelerated osteoarthrosis may also be a presenting symptom and may be misdiagnosed without recognition of the underlying acromegaly. In addition to changes in the soft tissues, there may be thickening of the shafts of the metacarpals, metatarsals, and phalanges, and of the articular cartilages. Tufting of the ends of the terminal phalanges develops with exostoses of the bones of the hands and feet.

Arthralgia is present in 62 to 75 per cent of acromegalic patients and demonstrable arthropathy is present in 16 to 62 per cent. Between 10 and 40 per cent of patients have joint disease severe enough to limit daily activities. The knees, hips (main weight bearing joints), and shoulders are most frequently affected, while elbows and ankles are relatively spared. The spine may also be affected, with the lumbosacral region most commonly involved. The initial symptoms are of joint stiffness, particularly of the hands; this may reflect the increase of subcutaneous tissue which is reversible with reduction of circulating GH concentration.

Early in the course of the disease, joint spaces are increased secondary to cartilage proliferation. The synovial and periarticular swelling produces joint swelling without effusion. Weight bearing on proliferating cartilage in joints leads to ulceration and development of osteoarthritis. Cartilage degeneration, characterized by joint pain, is irreversible. This is often sufficiently disabling as to require artificial joint replacement. The arthropathy is often severe at the time of diagnosis and is usually irreversible, unless the disease is treated before destruction of the articular cartilage.

Backache is common, especially when associated with dorsal kypho-

sis. Disc spaces are increased and anterior osteophytes are common. Spinal mobility is normal or increased since the discs are resilient and paraspinal ligaments become hypertrophied and lax.

Patients with acromegaly often develop a characteristic barrel chest, caused by a combination of the changes in the vertebrae and the ribs.

High levels of GH are associated with excessive sweating, particularly of the face, head, hands, and feet; hyperhidrosis may be the presenting symptom. The increase in soft tissue mass may produce median nerve compression and carpal tunnel syndrome, which is a very common presentation of acromegaly.

Galactorrhoea is common in acromegalic women, but is rare in men. Hyperprolactinaemia occurs in up to 40 per cent of acromegalics but in its absence galactorrhoea is idiopathic or the result of the lactogenic effects of GH. Between 32 and 87 per cent of acromegalic women under the age of 45 years have menstrual abnormalities and decreased libido, and 27 to 46 per cent of acromegalic men are impotent; these features probably relate to the high frequency of hyperprolactinaemia and the lactogenic effects of GH.

Other features of acromegaly include enlargement of the thyroid, sometimes with palpable nodules. Other organs increase in size. The skin, particularly of the palms of the hands and soles of the feet, is often moist. Multiple skin tags are frequently present and correlate with the occurrence of colonic polyps.

COMPLICATIONS

Metabolic and endocrine

Hypersecretion of growth hormone induces insulin resistance and glucose intolerance, which occurs in 29 to 45 per cent of cases; clinical diabetes mellitus is present in 10 to 20 per cent. The excessive GH secretion in non-diabetic acromegalics is associated with an exaggerated insulin response to intravenous glucose. In those with impaired glucose tolerance or diabetes mellitus, the insulin response is decreased or delayed. The higher the GH levels the more likely is diabetes, but the HLA phenotype, a family history of diabetes, and duration of acromegaly do not appear particularly to influence its development.

Hypertriglyceridaemia occurs in 19 to 44 per cent of acromegalic patients. There is a positive correlation between the serum insulin response to glucose and in increased serum triglyceride concentrations. Hepatic triglyceride lipase and lipoprotein lipase activities are decreased in acromegaly. The activity of these enzymes rises following successful lowering of GH levels. No consistent abnormalities of cholesterol have been observed.

Respiratory

Pulmonary complications of acromegaly account for some of the increased risk of premature mortality in this disease. A threefold increase in respiratory deaths occurred in the study of morbidity and mortality reported by Wright and colleagues, probably dependent on associated narrowing of the airway. Exacerbation of upper airway narrowing during an upper respiratory tract infection may result in acute dyspnoea and stridor. Difficult intubation during induction of anaesthesia and airway obstruction from an enlarged tongue following extubation are not uncommon. These risks of anesthaesia are avoidable by proper preparation, use of fibreoptic laryngoscopy, and careful monitoring. Many acromegalic patients suffer from the obstructive sleep apnoea syndrome. A prevalence of 38 per cent has been reported, with men more commonly affected than women. Both the prolapse of an enlarged tongue and the inspiratory collapse of the hypopharynx have been implicated in the pathogenesis of this disorder. Cure of acromegaly does not necessarily correct sleep apnoea.

Cardiovascular

Acromegaly is associated with an increased prevalence of death from cardiovascular causes, hypertension, and cardiomyopathy. Indeed, cardiovascular disease is the most common cause of death in acromegalics.

Since these patients often have hypertension and/or diabetes it is difficult to determine whether the cardiac disease is secondary to these disorders or due to a specific effect of GH; there is controversy as to whether a specific acromegalic cardiomyopathy exists. No specific pathological findings have been demonstrated at autopsy, at which myocardial hypertrophy has been reported in 93 per cent, interstitial fibrosis of the myocardium in 85 per cent, and lymphomononuclear myocarditis in 59 per cent of 27 cases. Echocardiography has shown cardiac enlargement, usually with an increase of left ventricular mass, in 80 per cent of patients, findings apparently independent of hypertension or known ischaemic heart disease. Impaired left ventricular function is present in some, but not all patients. The severity of these abnormalities does not consistently correlate with GH levels, but the duration of the disease may be a more important determinant. After restoration of normal GH levels the cardiac abnormalities may persist in some patients, while in others there may be significant improvement.

Hypertension occurs in 18 to 41 per cent of acromegalics. Its pathophysiology is poorly understood. Sodium retention, extracellular fluid volume expansion, and suppression of the renin/angiotensin/aldosterone system occurs, but in both hypertensive and normotensive acromegalic patients. Overactivity of the sympathetic nervous system has been suggested as a possible aetiologic factor. Hypertension has been associated with higher mean GH concentrations and prolonged duration of acromegaly; it is usually mild and uncomplicated and is treated with conventional antihypertensive medications. Rarely, the hypertension may result from other endocrine causes, such as phaeochromocytoma, primary hyperparathyroidism, or an aldosterone-secreting adenoma.

Calcium and bone metabolism

In acromegaly serum 1,25-dihydroxyvitamin D concentrations are increased, while 25-hydroxyvitamin D levels are low and serum parathyroid hormone and calcitonin levels are normal. The increase in 1,25-dihydroxyvitamin D concentrations occurs as a result of GH stimulation of renal 1α-hydroxylase activity. The net effect is an increase in intestinal calcium absorption and hypercalciuria; serum calcium levels are normal unless coincidental hyperparathyroidism is present. Growth hormone increases tubular phosphate reabsorption with resultant hyperphosphataemia in approximately 50 per cent of acromegalics. Urolithiasis occurs in 6 to 12.5 per cent. Acromegaly is associated with increased bone turnover. Bone density in acromegalics is increased; osteoporosis does not occur unless hypogonadism is also present.

Neuromuscular

Although acromegalics have a very muscular appearance they are often weak. The precise cause of this weakness is unknown; a myopathic process has been suggested.

The bony changes of the vertebral column may cause nerve root compression at the vertebral foramina, giving rise to lumbar radiculopathy. Spinal stenosis and an amyotrophic-like syndrome may occur. Carpal tunnel syndrome occurs in 35 to 45 per cent of patients.

Colonic polyps and malignancies

A recent prospective study identified an increased incidence of colonic polyps in acromegalic patients. Although several retrospective studies have suggested increased incidence of gastrointestinal malignancies, a survey of mortality in 194 acromegalic patients did not reveal an increased mortality from malignant neoplasms, a finding confirmed by other studies on prevalence of malignant disease in acromegaly.

BIOCHEMICAL EVALUATION

The clinical diagnosis of acromegaly is confirmed by biochemical tests which should be performed before imaging studies are undertaken.

Serum IGF-I concentration

The serum IGF-I concentration is the best screening test for acromegaly; an elevated value suggests excessive GH secretion, except during pregnancy or puberty when IGF-I levels are appropriately increased. Serum IGF-I levels are increased in acromegaly compared with age- and sex-matched normal subjects and vary minimally, thus providing a reliable index of GH secretion during the previous 24 h period. The circulating IGF-I concentration also correlates with the 24 h integrated serum GH level when GH is measured at frequent intervals (every 5–20 min). Reliability of IGF-I assays is variable, so that proper interpretation of results requires knowledge of the assay used, for instance whether or not the serum has been pretreated to remove the various binding proteins. The predominant IGF-I binding protein, IGF-BP3, is positively regulated by GH and may well be a further useful marker of GH secretion. Serum IGF-I should be used as an initial screen, as an index of disease activity, and to assess efficacy of therapy.

Oral glucose tolerance test

The definitive test to diagnose acromegaly is failure of serum GH to decrease to less than 2 µg/l after ingestion of glucose (see above).

Other tests that have been proposed to diagnose acromegaly include administration of TRH, GnRH, L-DOPA, and other dopamine agonists which produce different (paradoxical) effects in acromegalic patients compared with normal subjects. These responses are not as uniform as is the abnormal response to oral glucose, and therefore are not routinely used.

Administration of the two physiological hypothalamic regulators of GH secretion, somatostatin and GH-releasing hormone (GHRH) does not discriminate between normal and excessive GH secretion.

Insulin-induced hypoglycaemia is used in acromegalic patients to evaluate the hypothalamic–pituitary–adrenal axis. Patients with acromegaly have insulin resistance and frequently require higher doses of insulin to decrease the blood glucose to interpretable levels. Until the degree of insulin resistance is known, however, the usual intravenous dose of regular insulin, 0.15 U/kg, is administered. If there is insufficient reduction in serum glucose or absence of hypoglycaemic symptoms within 45 min, a second dose of insulin, 0.3 U/kg, is administered. If, after another 45 min, the response is inadequate, the dose is again increased, to 0.6 U/kg. Results are interpretable when the blood glucose has decreased to below 2.2 mmol/l (40 mg/dl) with associated hypoglycaemic symptoms.

The differential diagnosis of acromegaly includes a primary pituitary adenoma, either a micro- or macroadenoma, and GH hypersecretion from a hyperplastic pituitary gland which is hyperstimulated by eutopic (hypothalamic tumour) or ectopic (peripheral tumour) GHRH. There is only one documented case of acromegaly caused by ectopic GH secretion from a pancreatic tumour. Over 99 per cent of acromegalics have a primary pituitary tumour. Since initial therapy is directed to the primary lesion, it is important to make the correct diagnosis. Unfortunately, radiological studies cannot distinguish between an enlarged pituitary with an adenoma and an enlarged hyperplastic gland. To date, no patient with hypothalamic acromegaly from a GHRH-secreting hypothalamic tumour has been diagnosed antemortem, but there have been retrospective diagnoses of extension of hypothalamic gangliocytoma neurones into the pituitary, producing surrounding somatotroph hyperplasia. Theoretically, a mass lesion in the hypothalamus in association with acromegaly presumes eutopic GHRH secretion by a hypothalamic tumour. Ectopic GHRH secretion is more common than eutopic, but very few cases of ectopic GHRH production have been diagnosed prospectively. Ectopic GHRH secretion should be suspected in a patient with acromegaly and elevated circulating GHRH levels. Plasma GHRH levels in normal subjects are less than 100 ng/l; in contrast, patients with acromegaly from ectopic GHRH secretion have plasma GHRH levels in the µg/l range. Thus, when a patient has an elevated GHRH level, a search for a peripheral or hypothalamic tumour should be carried out. However, since GHRH may be secreted in a pulsatile fashion even by tumours, a normal GHRH or only modestly elevated GHRH level may not exclude ectopic GHRH secretion. The most likely peripheral sites are the pancreas, lung, thymus, adrenal (in association with phaeochromocytoma), or gastrointestinal tract, but occasionally, no ectopic source can be found.

AIMS OF TREATMENT

The ideal response to treatment should be the return of normal GH secretion; abatement of clinical symptoms and signs; reversal of tumour mass effects; and preservation of other anterior pituitary function. In practice cure is defined as a reduction in the serum IGF-I to normal for age and sex and a normal GH response to oral glucose.

SURGICAL THERAPY

The preferred surgical approach is the trans-sphenoidal route. The surgical outcome is dependent on the size of the tumour and the expertise of the neurosurgical team. The presence of an intrasellar microadenoma (< 10 mm diameter) offers the greatest possibility for a surgical cure. Results are less good for macroadenomas (>10 mm diameter), particularly when there is suprasellar extension or extension into the cavernous sinus, although a substantial reduction in tumour mass and immediate improvement in visual abnormalities, headaches, and symptoms of excessive GH are to be expected.

Trans-sphenoidal surgery achieves a basal postoperative GH concentration of less than 5 µg/l in approximately 60 per cent of patients in the best centres. While a basal serum GH of less than 5 µg/l may be indicative of successful surgery, dynamic studies, particularly the oral glucose tolerance test, are a more accurate method to evaluate postoperative GH secretion.

The serum IGF-I concentration should be measured before and after surgery. Although GH concentrations decline rapidly after tumour removal, the serum IGF-I does not decrease immediately. Clearance of IGF-I, complexed with a binding protein, may require several days and thus does not reflect the immediate change in circulating GH concentrations. Even if all tests of GH secretion are normal postoperatively, some patients relapse, emphasizing the need for careful follow-up and monitoring. The precise incidence of recurrence is not known, but probably ranges from 0 to 13 per cent over 2 to 3.5 years.

Surgical mortality is rare. Particular care with intubation and extubation must be taken since airway obstruction from an enlarged tongue is a risk. Permanent diabetes insipidus follows surgery in 1 to 9 per cent of patients.

RADIATION THERAPY

Currently, pituitary radiation is most frequently administered in patients with persistent disease following surgery. Limitations of radiotherapy include its inability to effect a prompt reduction in tumour size or in hormone hypersecretion.

MEDICAL THERAPY

Bromocriptine reduces GH concentrations in acromegalic patients. A majority of patients have improvement in clinical symptoms (70–90 per cent) and a reduction in GH concentrations during chronic bromocriptine treatment (approximately 70 per cent), but reduction of serum GH to less than 5 µg/l occurs in only a minority. Other effects of bromocriptine include reduction in urinary hydroxyproline excretion, improvement in diabetic control or glucose intolerance, resolution of hyperprolactinaemia (if present), and improvement in visual field abnormalities. A larger dose of bromocriptine is required to treat acromegaly than to treat hyperprolactinaemia; usually 10 to 20 mg per day (or higher) in divided doses, 4 times per day. A small dose should be used initially, with a gradual increase to minimize side-effects.

Although suppression of GH secretion in response to bromocriptine is incomplete, this drug is useful for symptomatic treatment of patients with residual postoperative disease or until radiation therapy can become effective.

Somatostatin analogue

Somatostatin (SRIF) is a 14 amino acid cyclic peptide which is present in the brain, hypothalamus, pancreas, and in the gastrointestinal tract. In the hypothalamus, somatostatin inhibits GH release and, in conjunction with GHRH, produces episodic GH release. Intravenous administration of somatostatin produces a prompt reduction in serum GH concentrations in normal subjects and in patients with acromegaly. After cessation of the infusion, there is a rapid rise in serum GH, and a rebound hypersecretion in some acromegalics. Somatostatin must be administered by continuous intravenous infusion because its half-life is less than 3 min, thus making this peptide impractical for clinical use. Octreotide, an 8 amino acid cyclic peptide analogue of somatostatin, has a serum half-life of approximately 90 min and suppresses GH release for up to 8 h in normal subjects and in acromegalic patients. This peptide, administered subcutaneously, is 20-fold more suppressive of GH release than is the native peptide, and is 22 times more suppressive of GH release than of insulin release. Despite its greater selectivity for GH, insulin release is decreased for approximately 3 h after administration, and postprandial hyperglycaemia may occur.

Octreotide has been used in clinical trials to treat acromegaly and other hypersecretory endocrine tumours since 1984. Several studies in a limited number of acromegalic patients, usually treated briefly, indicate that most patients have improvement in symptoms and signs of disease and a reduction in serum GH and IGF-I concentrations. A small number of patients have had a reduction in pituitary tumour size. Reduction in serum GH concentrations occurs within an hour of administration, with continued suppression for 6 to 8 h in most patients; partial inhibition of insulin release is usually observed for less than 3 h after administration. While some patients have suppression of GH and IGF-I concentrations to normal, others have only a partial suppression of GH release. This heterogeneity of response is most likely dependent upon the density of somatostatin receptors on the adenoma and the binding affinity for octreotide.

The recommended octreotide dose is 100 µg every 8 h, but, some patients have adequate GH suppression with 100 µg/day, and others require as much as 1500 µg/day in divided doses. Some patients have a better response to continuous subcutaneous octreotide infusion than with intermittent injections. A good clinical response occurs in 70 to 88 per cent of patients; however, a mean 24 h GH concentration less than 5 µg/l is achieved in only about 50 per cent of patients. IGF-I concentrations are normalized in 45 to 68 per cent of patients. Additionally, a small number of patients have greater GH suppression with the combination of octreotide and bromocriptine. The precise dose and frequency of administration should be adjusted according to the patient's response and preference.

Octreotide inhibits gallbladder contractility and this may facilitate formation of gallstones. The incidence of gallstone formation or sludge during octreotide therapy is about 20 per cent. Since postprandial gallbladder motility is decreased by octreotide, a potential method of decreasing the risk of gallstone formation is administration of the drug 2 to 3 h after meals.

Ectopic GHRH secretion

Acromegaly secondary to somatotroph stimulation by a tumour secreting GHRH occurs in less than 1 per cent of patients. If an ectopic GHRH-secreting tumour is identified, surgical resection is curative provided there are no metastases. Patients with metastatic disease are responsive to octreotide therapy, with subsequent lowering of circulating GHRH and GH concentrations.

PROGNOSIS

There are no studies which demonstrate that treatment of acromegaly leads to a reduction in the increased morbidity and premature mortality associated with this condition. However, *a priori*, one would predict that reversal of the adverse metabolic effects of excessive GH secretion would be likely to prevent progression of the disease. Reversal of such changes as soft tissue swelling, and restoration of normal glucose tolerance might be expected to favour a return to a normal prognosis in terms of morbidity and premature mortality. Increased awareness of the symptoms and signs of acromegaly, easier diagnosis, modern transsphenoidal pituitary microsurgery (which has shown that the smaller the tumour at the time of operation the better the outcome), and the use of radiotherapy and medical therapies all suggest that patients with acromegaly are more likely to be cured today than in the past.

Cushing's disease

Cushing's syndrome, referred to as Cushing's disease when it is caused by an adenoma of the corticotroph cells of the anterior pituitary, or more rarely by corticotroph hyperplasia, is discussed in Chapter 12.7.1.

Nelson's syndrome

Nelson's syndrome is the result of the development of an aggressive ACTH-secreting pituitary adenoma in patients who have undergone bilateral adrenalectomy for Cushing's disease. These patients develop symptoms of a mass, including headaches, visual field defects, and external ophthalmoplegia. The very high ACTH levels cause hyperpigmentation in the distribution of that seen in Addison's disease. Since the patient initially had a pituitary tumour secreting ACTH, this syndrome presumably represents acceleration of the tumour growth by the removal of the negative feedback of excessive cortisol from the adrenal glands. The estimated incidence of Nelson's syndrome varies from 10 to 50 per cent. Some studies, but not all, suggest that this syndrome is preventable by external pituitary irradiation prior to or at the time of adrenalectomy.

The condition is suspected from the characteristic history and physical findings. Plasma ACTH levels are extremely high, often ranging from 220 pmol/l (1000 pg/ml) to 2202 pmol/l (10 000 pg/ml) or higher. However, the level of ACTH does not accurately reflect the size or aggressiveness of the tumour, the presence of which tumour is confirmed by CT scan or MRI scan. In contrast to the tumours of Cushing's disease, these are usually macroadenomata.

Once the diagnosis of Nelson's syndrome is made, the treatment should be aggressive, as these tumours are locally invasive and grow rapidly. Pituitary surgery by the trans-sphenoidal route is the preferred treatment. Pituitary irradiation is useful in the treatment of those with residual tumour after surgery. The ACTH secretion by the tumour is responsive to endogenous CRH and AVP. Thus, by optimizing negative feedback to the hypothalamus by both using a long-acting glucocorticoid and by judicious timing of its administration to reverse the normal glucocorticoid rhythm, hypothalamic stimulation of the tumour can be minimized; a suggested regimen is dexamethasone 0.5 mg on retiring. This approach has not been fully evaluated but it seems logical and is used by several groups.

Glycoprotein-producing adenomata

Glycoprotein adenomata produce LH, FSH, TSH or the α-subunit, alone or in combination, which may or may not result in increased serum concentrations. When serum hormone concentrations are normal, glycoprotein hormone production may be detectable by *in vitro* studies, such as radioimmunoassay of medium from pituitary tumour cell cultures, detection of specific mRNAs, or immunocytochemical staining of surgical specimens. Using *in vitro* techniques and serum hormone measurements it has been found that glycoprotein-producing adenomata may occur as frequently as in 24 per cent of surgical specimens. The aetiology of these tumours is unknown and they appear to arise spontaneously without an identifiable cause. One hypothesis on the origin of those secreting FSH is that gonadotroph hyperplasia develops into an

adenoma in the setting of primary gonadal failure; Another is that increased FSH production results from a 'non-secretory' adenoma that impairs secretion of LH, but not of FSH. These theories do not adequately explain the clinical and biochemical features associated with a gonadotroph-producing tumour; for instance, the gonadal failure of female menopause is not associated with an increase in the incidence of this tumour.

Patients with glycoprotein-producing adenomas most commonly come to medical attention with symptoms and/or signs of a mass lesion, unless the product is TSH, when the presenting features are those of hyperthyroidism. The majority of cases are diagnosed in middle-aged men (mean age 55 years) with symptoms of headache, visual disturbance, and acquired hypogonadism. These tumours appear to be uncommon in women of reproductive age but the precise prevalence in postmenopausal women is unknown since serum LH and FSH concentrations may be appropriately increased. Mild hyperprolactinaemia (< 1800 mIU/l (100 μg/l)) may be present, perhaps resulting from stalk compression. Affected men often have a subnormal serum testosterone concentration associated with low, normal, or increased LH and FSH concentrations. The reasons for hypogonadism are unclear but have been attributed to depression of secretion of bioactive LH, secretion of abnormally glycosylated gonadotrophins, or to an abnormal pulsatile pattern of gonadotrophin secretion.

Thyrotroph adenoma

The thyroid stimulating hormone (TSH) adenoma is the least common type of pituitary tumour, representing less than 1 per cent of cases, and the only glycoprotein tumour producing a characteristic clinical syndrome. Common clinical features include symptoms referable to the pituitary mass lesion and/or hyperthyroidism with goitre. The tumour also frequently secretes free α-subunit, so that a molar ratio of α-subunit to TSH of greater than 1 is helpful in distinguishing a TSH-secreting adenoma from other forms of hyperthyroidism. Other secretory products of thyrotroph adenomas include GH or prolactin. The diagnosis of acromegaly or hyperprolactinaemia may then only be evident when the patient seeks medical care for symptoms of hyperthyroidism. Increased concentrations of T_3 and T_4 are then associated with inappropriately normal or an elevated serum TSH concentrations. Sensitive TSH assays distinguish between normal and suppressed values, allowing easier diagnosis of a TSH secreting adenoma. Serum TSH concentrations may be markedly increased; but values of less than 10 mU/l occur in 30 per cent of patients with a TSH secreting adenoma. It is in these cases that measurement of the serum α-subunit is particularly helpful. This assay also helps to exclude the syndrome of pituitary resistance to thyroid hormone in which serum concentrations of TSH (but not those of the α-subunit) are inappropriately increased in the setting of hyperthyroxinaemia. Administration of TRH may also help distinguish between these rare conditions. TRH given to patients with TSH-secreting tumours does not increase TSH, whereas the response in pituitary resistance to thyroid hormone is often exaggerated.

The ideal treatment of a TSH-secreting adenoma is surgical resection, but complete resection may not be possible and there may be a need for postoperative irradiation. Preliminary reports indicate that treatment with octreotide, may then lower serum TSH concentrations, allowing a return to euthyroidism, but antithyroid drugs have to be used in some cases.

Gonadotroph adenoma

Gonadotroph adenomata are identified by either increased serum LH, FSH, and/or α-subunit concentrations or by *in vitro* studies, including immunocytochemistry, electron microscopy, or tumour cell culture studies.

The precise prevalence of gonadotroph adenomata is unknown. In a series of 139 men with untreated macroadenomas reported by Snyder, 24 per cent were gonadotroph tumours; 17 per cent had hypersecretion of FSH, either alone or in combination with LH α-, LH β-, and FSH β-subunits, and 7 per cent had hypersecretion of only the α-subunit. The majority of these men, 87 per cent, presented with visual impairment indicative of a large tumour. Other series of surgical specimens report a lower prevalence of gonadotroph adenomata (< 5 per cent).

The glycoprotein hormone most commonly secreted is FSH, which elutes by gel filtration chromatography as intact FSH. This may be accompanied by an increase in circulating α-subunit concentrations, which also occurs in association with tumours producing the LH β-subunit. Hypersecretion of intact LH occurs less commonly than does secretion of intact FSH or free FSH β- or α-subunits, and an apparent increase in serum LH may also be the result of assay cross-reactivity with free α-subunit or LH β; gel filtration chromatography is necessary for precise identification of the secretory product. In the majority of men with this kind of adenoma the serum testosterone concentration is either normal or below normal, since intact LH is not being produced. Hormone measurements then show inappropriately normal serum LH concentrations in the setting of reduced testosterone production; but when intact LH is produced, the serum testosterone concentration is above normal.

Administration of TRH may be helpful in diagnosis, since approximately 50 per cent of patients with a gonadotroph adenoma have an increase in LH or FSH after TRH stimulation. The FSH and LH responses to exogenous GnRH are variable; approximately 50 per cent of patients with an FSH-secreting tumour have an increase in serum FSH concentrations, an increase in serum LH occurs less frequently.

Gonadotroph adenomata are most commonly diagnosed in middle-aged men. It is not known if these tumours truly occur more frequently in men or whether they are more difficult to diagnose in women, for instance in the case of a postmenopausal woman with a pituitary tumour in whom increased LH and FSH levels are attributed to the menopause. The distinction between a non-secretory adenoma and a gonadotroph adenoma may then not be possible clinically or biochemically and may only be decided by electron microscopic or immunocytochemical studies of the excised tumour.

Diagnostic difficulty arises in men when the serum testosterone is below normal and the serum immunoreactive LH is increased from increased free α-subunit or LH β secretion with assay cross-reactivity; this pattern may then erroneously suggest the diagnosis of primary gonadal failure. The possibility of a gonadotroph tumour, should always be considered in such a case if there is a history of headache or change in vision, when MRI or CT of the pituitary is indicated.

The initial treatment of a gonadotroph tumour is surgical resection, particularly if visual function is abnormal. Trans-sphenoidal surgery improves vision in the majority and may correct hormonal hypersecretion, hypogonadism, and the abnormal gonadotrophin response to TRH. Persistent hormonal hypersecretion and the presence of residual tumour may require postoperative pituitary radiation treatment.

Medical treatment of gonadotroph adenomata has involved the use of bromocriptine, octreotide, and more recently, long-acting GnRH agonist and antagonist analogues. Medical treatment of gonadotroph adenomata is not established, but it is used in an attempt to reduce hormone hypersecretion and tumour size after unsuccessful surgery, or while awaiting the full effects of pituitary radiation. Since efficacy has not been determined in a suitably large number of patients, close and careful medical evaluations are necessary.

Non-secretory adenoma

A non-secretory or non-functioning pituitary tumour, sometimes called a chromophobe adenoma, is characterized by the absence of any particular clinical syndrome and the absence of detectable increased serum hormone concentrations. Pituitary tumours have been classified as non-secretory in 25 to 30 per cent of cases. However, on morphological examination, these apparently non-secreting tumours often contain secre-tory granules, suggesting hormone synthesis and storage. Immunocytochemical and electron microscopic studies have identified many of them as gonadotroph, α-subunit, or corticotroph tumours and immunocytochemistry and molecular biological techniques have revealed combinations including hCG α, LH β, FSH α, TSH β, and ACTH. The absence of increased serum hormone concentrations in such cases has been attributed to abnormal post-translational processing or the lack of specific glycoprotein subunit assays. With increased use of specific glycoprotein subunit assays, it is anticipated that more presumed non-functioning lesions will come to be identified as glycoprotein-producing tumours.

The majority of patients are diagnosed with symptoms of a macroadenoma (headache, visual disturbance) or symptoms of hypopituitarism such as adrenal insufficiency, hypothyroidism and, more commonly, hypogonadism. These tumours occur most commonly in men and in postmenopausal women. A mild or moderate elevation of serum prolactin < 1800 mIU/l (< 100 μg/l) often occurs and is thought to reflect stalk compression.

Pretreatment evaluation to determine hormone hypersecretion should include measurement of serum prolactin, IGF-I, LH, FSH, TSH and α-subunit, and when assays are available, LH β-, FSH β-, and TSH β-subunit concentrations. The need for hormone replacement, particularly of cortisol and thyroxine, should be assessed by measuring basal thyroxine, cortisol and testosterone (men) concentrations. A normal morning cortisol concentration is not sufficient to exclude impairment of the hypothalamic–pituitary–adrenal axis; an insulin-induced hypoglycaemia or metyrapone test is required for accurate assessment. An ophthalmological examination should include fundoscopy, ocular motility determination, visual acuity, and quantitative assessment of visual fields with Goldmann, Octopus, or Humphries perimetry. The precise anatomy of the tumour is best assessed by a gadolinium-enhanced MRI scan or coronal CT scan with contrast.

The treatment for a non-secretory tumour is surgical excision, usually via the trans-sphenoidal approach. Residual tumour is usually treated with postoperative conventional supervoltage radiation. If the patient is unable to undergo surgery or the tumour is asymptomatic and intrasellar (uncommon) and vision is normal, pituitary radiation with careful monitoring of pituitary function, tumour size, and vision is an alternative. The response to pituitary radiation is similar to that of other pituitary tumours; prompt reduction in tumour size is rare but additional growth may be inhibited.

Medical treatment with the dopamine agonist drugs has been used in a small number of patients. Non-secretory tumours do possess high-affinity membrane-bound dopamine receptors, but they are fewer in number than in prolactin-secreting tumours, so that this approach is mostly unsuccessful, but worth a trial in those unfit for or unwilling to accept surgery.

The postoperative management is the same as that of any patient undergoing pituitary surgery and should include regular assessment of the visual system and the need for hormone replacement, as well as MRI or CT examinations within a month of surgery and at 6 and 12 months. If no tumour is visible on the postoperative and the 6 and 12 month scans, it is still sensible to repeat them at yearly intervals.

Non-pituitary sellar masses

A number of lesions occur in the region of the hypothalamus and pituitary that are not pituitary tumours. These include craniopharyngioma, hypophysitis, apoplexy, aneurysm, Rathke's pouch cyst, arachnoid cyst, germinoma, chordoma, optic nerve glioma, reticulosis, meningioma, and secondary deposits. Only the first four will be discussed, as the management of the others follows standard medical lines. It is important to make the correct diagnosis since therapy is often quite different. Specifically, the trans-sphenoidal approach can be disastrous for some lesions, such as an internal carotid artery aneurysm. The advent of modern imaging techniques has greatly facilitated the accurate diagnosis prior to therapeutic intervention.

Craniopharyngioma

A craniopharyngioma, or Rathke's pouch tumour, arises from embryonic squamous cell rests which persist after the upward migration of stomodeal epithelium to the anterior pituitary. Since a tumour may arise from any position along the craniopharyngioma canal, it may be intrasellar or extrasellar. The tumour is usually well encapsulated and composed of cystic and solid components. The cysts may be multiloculated and contain dark brown, oily fluid. These tumours may occur at any age, but are most common in children, accounting for 5 to 10 per cent of primary brain tumours in children. Approximately one-quarter are diagnosed after the age of 40 years.

CLINICAL PRESENTATION

Children are usually diagnosed because of growth failure or with symptoms of increased intracranial pressure (headache, vomiting, somnolence). Sixty per cent of children have been reported to have had visual disturbances, and growth retardation was present in the majority. In adults, 80 per cent presented with complaints of visual disturbance while 93 per cent had visual abnormalities on examination. Disturbance of intellectual function which may cause dementia has been reported in approximately 30 per cent of adults.

A prospective study of endocrine function in 20 patients with craniopharyngioma (six adults, 14 children and adolescents) revealed some degree of hypopituitarism in most. Growth hormone and gonadotrophin deficiency were most common, occurring in 19 of 20. Sixty-five per cent had secondary hypothyroidism and half had corticotrophin deficiency; none had diabetes insipidus, which occurs more commonly after surgical resection of the tumour.

Craniopharyngiomas are characteristically suprasellar. They may extend inferiorly into the sella turcica causing destruction of bony margins of the sella and dorsum sellae. They may also extend superiorly into the third ventricle, producing hydrocephalus from block at the foramen of Monro. The CT scan appearance may be helpful in suggesting the diagnosis pre-operatively. Calcification of the tumour occurs in 70 to 90 per cent of children and 40 to 60 per cent of adults and is detectable on a CT scan, but not on an MRI scan. The solid portion of the tumour may enhance on CT scan after administration of intravenous contrast. The high cholesterol content of cyst fluid produces a characteristic MRI signal which may also aid in the diagnosis.

The primary treatment of a craniopharyngioma is surgical resection. Surgery is associated with considerable morbidity and mortality, usually from the standard surgical approach (craniotomy) and from diabetes insipidus and other hypothalamic–pituitary dysfunction. Recurrence is a definite risk. Since these tumours are relatively radioresistant and grow slowly, it is difficult to assess the efficacy of radiotherapy.

With the use of CT and MRI scans to evaluate patients with complaints referable to the cranium, more relatively asymptomatic patients with a craniopharyngioma are being diagnosed. These patients present a therapeutic dilemma since a craniotomy is associated with substantial risks. If the patient is asymptomatic, an argument can be made for an anticipatory approach with careful follow-up, including a repeat imaging study at 6 months or 1 year. The interval between scans may be doubled if there has been no increase in tumour size.

Lymphocytic hypophysitis

This is a rare pituitary disorder of lymphocytic infiltration of the pituitary gland associated with complete or partial hypopituitarism, a pituitary mass, and occurrence exclusively in women, often during pregnancy or in the postpartum period. A maternal death rate of approximately 50 per cent, most likely due to unrecognized secondary adrenal failure, emphasizes the need for consideration of this diagnosis in a pregnant or postpartum woman with symptoms of headache, visual disturbance, weakness, and fatigue.

Lymphocytic hypophysitis was first described in an autopsy specimen in 1962; fewer than 30 cases have been reported subsequently. Most of them were in the second or third trimester of pregnancy or up to 7 months postpartum. The clinical presentation was of symptoms and signs of pituitary dysfunction, frequently hypocortisolism, and of a pituitary mass. Pituitary deficiencies have included ACTH, TSH, LH, FSH, and vasopressin, either alone or in combination; an increased serum prolactin occurred in 50 per cent. The most common symptoms and signs of the mass were headache in the majority and visual field loss in 32 per cent. In those patients who underwent imaging studies, suprasellar extension of the mass was present in 64 per cent. Although the majority of women had permanent destruction of all or part of the pituitary and required chronic hormone replacement therapy, a report of one patient who had transient hypopituitarism of 12 months' duration suggests that total pituitary destruction may not always occur. These patients should therefore probably be evaluated at regular intervals to determine the necessity for continued hormone replacement.

The aetiology of lymphocytic hypophysitis is unknown, but several studies have suggested an autoimmune cause. Antipituitary antibodies were present in the sera of some women and others had other autoimmune endocrine disorders, including thyroiditis and adrenalitis. Another proposed aetiology is virus-induced autoimmune destruction of the gland as suggested by studies in animals. The common association with pregnancy has been attributed to increased exposure to pituitary antigens or changes in maternal immunological status.

Although the diagnosis may be suspected in a pregnant or postpartum woman with the typical clinical features, confirmation resides in surgical biopsy and histological examination of the tissue. Diffuse infiltration with lymphocytes and plasma cells, some areas of follicles with germinal centres and destruction of normal pituitary cells are the characteristic morphological changes on light and electron microscopy. Immunoperoxidase staining is positive for all pituitary cell types which remain intact. The differential diagnosis of light microscopic findings includes sarcoidosis, syphilis, tuberculosis, granulomatous hypophysitis, and postpartum haemorrhagic infarction. Examination of the specimen with electron microscopy is helpful to demonstrate the characteristic interdigitation of lymphocytes and pituitary cells, fusion of lysosomes and secretory granules, and swollen mitochondria indicative of oncocytic transformation. Evidence of vascular injury or immune complex deposition was not present in the cases examined with electron microscopy.

Suprasellar germinoma (ectopic pinealoma)

This highly malignant tumour has no sex preponderance and appears to have an increased prevalence in Japan. It has been diagnosed in patients aged between 6 and 41 years, but is very rare over the age of 30 years. This tumour is of hypothalamic origin and is curable by radiotherapy. It is vital that the correct diagnosis is made, thus avoiding an unnecessary and likely destructive operation.

The tumour may originate in the ventral region of the hypothalamus, in association with a pineal tumour (either metastatic or multifocal origin), in the anterior third ventricle or, more rarely, in the pituitary fossa, and mimics a pituitary tumour. Because of rapid growth and large size it often compresses the optic nerves and chiasm and extends inferiorly into the pituitary and sella. Extension into the third ventricle produces hydrocephalus.

CLINICAL PRESENTATION

The most common initial symptom is diabetes insipidus, which occurs in 50 per cent of patients. Other symptoms include visual disturbance, symptoms of increased intracranial pressure (headaches, nausea, vomiting) and obesity. At the time of diagnosis, diabetes insipidus is present in 83 per cent, visual disturbance in 78 per cent, headache in 50 per cent, and endocrine abnormalities, including growth retardation in 39 per cent and hypogonadism in 17 per cent of cases. Other systemic symptoms include anorexia in 28 per cent and nausea and vomiting in 11 per cent of cases, which likely reflect hydrocephalus, electrolyte disturbances, and/or secondary adrenal or thyroid failure. This tumour is malignant, often multifocal and may metastasize not only within CNS, but extracranially, and also outside the CNS. For these reasons, staging is very important.

The radiological appearances are not distinctive. Usually a large mass is observed in the third ventricle which extends superiorly and inferiorly. It may enhance with intravenous contrast on CT scan. A suprasellar germinoma should be considered if hypothalamic mass is present, particularly if diabetes insipidus is present. This is an unusual presentation for either a pituitary tumour or for a craniopharyngioma.

In addition to performing the same tests as in a patient with a pituitary tumour, a number of other studies are necessary. Serum β-hCG should be measured and if elevated is suggestive of a germinoma. If the level is undetectable, germinoma is not excluded and a cerebrospinal fluid sample should be obtained for cytological examination and measurement of glucose, protein, β-hCG and alpha-fetoprotein. Expected results are malignant cells, elevated serum protein, and increased concentrations of hCG and alpha-fetoprotein. This is sufficient to make the diagnosis which is confirmed by the rapid reduction in the size of the lesion with as little as 5 Gy of radiation.

THERAPY

The first step is to correct any hormonal deficiencies. If there is likely to be a delay in obtaining the results, glucocorticoid and thyroid hormone replacement should be given; these can always be discontinued if the results are normal. Diabetes insipidus should be promptly treated with desmopressin. If the thirst centre is intact and if the patient is alert, he/she will usually be able to drink an adequate amount of fluid, but loss of thirst does occur and leads to great difficulty in maintaining water balance.

Because of the location of this tumour and its propensity to metastasize in the central nervous system, surgery is not likely to effect a cure. It may be required to relieve hydrocephalus, but the risk of seeding tumour cells must be considered and it should be only performed if high-dose steroids and radiation therapy have failed. Any surgery of the hypothalamus can potentially damage remaining hypothalamic centres. If the diagnosis is uncertain, a therapeutic trial of 5 Gy may be administered. If within 14 days the tumour decreases in size, the diagnosis is confirmed since other types of masses are not that sensitive to radiation therapy. A full course of radiation therapy to the whole brain and spinal cord is then recommended. If there is evidence of peripheral metastases, chemotherapy may also be indicated.

Pituitary apoplexy

Pituitary apoplexy is classically defined as an acute, life-threatening infarction of the pituitary gland. Haemorrhagic infarction most commonly occurs in the presence of a pituitary tumour but may also occur spontaneously in a normal gland, after obstetric haemorrhage (Sheehan's syndrome), in the setting of increased intracranial pressure or systemic anticoagulation therapy. Other predisposing factors include diabetes mellitus, bleeding disorders, following pituitary radiation, pneumoencephalography, carotid angiography, mechanical ventilation, trauma, and upper respiratory infection. Sheehan's syndrome may result from occlusive arterial spasm of the arteries supplying the anterior lobe and infundibulum. After a period of complete ischaemia, revascularization and vascular congestion with thrombosis of the anterior lobe is observed.

Pituitary infarction usually produces anterior pituitary dysfunction which may be permanent or transient, with the degree of impairment being dependent upon the amount of tissue destruction. Hormone deficiencies include GH (88 per cent), gonadotrophins (58–76 per cent), and corticotrophin (66 per cent). Secondary hypothyroidism occurs in 42 to 53 per cent and abnormal prolactin secretion is present in 67 to 100 per cent. Diabetes insipidus is uncommon, occurring in only 2 to 3 per cent of patients. The precise incidence of pituitary infarction and haemorrhage is unknown. In unselected autopsy studies, infarction of more than 25 per cent of the gland was present in 1 to 3 per cent of specimens. The frequency of apoplexy in patients with a known pituitary tumour was 17 per cent in one series of 560 patients undergoing pituitary surgery; 8 per cent had no clinical symptoms of haemorrhage. Imaging studies of patients with a known pituitary tumour using CT and MRI scans indicate that intratumoural haemorrhage can occur without clinical evidence of apoplexy. Of 12 patients with radiographically proven haemorrhage only three had clinical evidence of apoplexy. The pattern of tumour growth, the size of the tumour, and the amount of haemorrhage and oedema within the gland determine the clinical symptomatology. Infarction with haemorrhage and oedema may cause rapid expansion of the lesion with compression of surrounding structures and abnormal neurological function. In a conscious patient, the initial symptom is usually a severe retro-orbital headache which is frequently accompanied by nausea and vomiting. Extravasation of blood or necrotic tissue into the subarachnoid space may cause meningeal irritation, fever, alteration of consciousness, or coma. Superior expansion produces compression of the optic chiasm and/or optic nerve(s) with development of visual field loss and/or decreased visual acuity. Lateral expansion into the cavernous sinus produces cranial nerve dysfunction which may include cranial nerves III, IV, VI, and the first division of cranial nerve V. The most common abnormality is unilateral involvement of the third cranial nerve with ophthalmoplegia (impaired medial and downward gaze), diplopia, ptosis, and mydriasis. If expansion causes mechanical compression of the carotid siphon against the anterior clinoid process, hemispheric dysfunction, including seizures and hemiplegia, may result. Hemispheric dysfunction may also occur with vasospasm secondary to irritation from subarachnoid haemorrhage.

Clinical evaluation of a patient with a sudden change in sensorium, headache, ophthalmoplegic or visual loss, or prostration should include an immediate imaging study of the pituitary area and orbits, either a non-contrast enhanced CT scan or an MRI scan. If a CT scan is chosen, thin sections (1.5 mm) through the pituitary in the coronal plane are optimal to identify the lesion; an unenhanced scan is necessary to identify haemorrhage, but intravenous contrast may be administered after initial images are obtained. Increased intensity, signifying haemorrhage, is observed on a T_1-weighted MRI scan. A CT scan may be superior to visualize intratumoural haemorrhage within the first few days of the event, but an MRI scan is more sensitive in detecting and following the haemorrhage in the subacute stage.

If pituitary apoplexy is suspected, the patient should be presumed to have anterior pituitary insufficiency and treated accordingly. Blood should be obtained for measurement of serum cortisol and thyroxine, and glucocorticoid treatment should be instituted immediately. The dose must be adequate for the stress of the illness and presumptive cerebral oedema (for example dexamethasone 2 mg every 6 hours). If there are significant visual deficits or altered sensorium, neurosurgical intervention may be required. Immediate surgical decompression of the haemorrhage and tumour affords the opportunity for recovery of visual deficits and alleviation of increased intracranial pressure. After recovery from surgery the patient should undergo a complete endocrinological evaluation to determine the nature and degree of residual hormone deficits. Since these may be transient, re-evaluation is sensible several months after the event.

Surgical decompression may not be necessary in the setting of normal sensorium and visual function. The patient should be in hospital, treated with glucocorticoid replacement, and needs serial ophthalmological and imaging examinations. With modern imaging techniques, careful assessment of the visual system, surgical decompression as indicated, and prompt hormone replacement treatment, the previous high mortality from pituitary gland apoplexy should be reduced.

REFERENCES

Bengtsson, B.A., Eden, S., Ernest, I., Oden, A., and Sjogren, B. (1988). Epidemiology and long-term survival in acromegaly. A study of 166 cases diagnosed between 1955–1984. *Acta Medica Scandinavica* **223**, 327–35.

Burrow, G.N., Wortzman, G., Rewcastle, N.B., Holgate, R.C., and Kovacs, K. (1991). Microadenomas of the pituitary and abnormal sellar tomograms in an unselected autopsy series. *New England Journal of Medicine* **304**, 156–8.

Cuneo, R.C., Salomon, F., McGauley, G.A., and Sonksen, P.H. (1992). The growth hormone deficiency syndrome in adults. *Clinical Endocrinology* **37**, 387–97.

Ezzat, S., *et al.* (1992). Octreotide treatment of acromegaly: multicenter controlled studies. *Annals of Internal Medicine* **117**, 711–18.

Halberg, F.E. and Sheline, G.E. (1987). Radiotherapy of pituitary tumors. [Review]. *Endocrinology and Metabolism Clinics of North America* **16**, 667–84.

Howlett, T.A., Drury, P.L., Perry, L., Doniach, I., Rees, L.H., and Besser, G.M. (1986). Diagnosis and management of ACTH-dependent Cushing's syndrome. *Clinical Endocrinology* **24**, 699–713.

Jameson, J.L., *et al.* (1987). Glycoprotein hormone genes are expressed in clinically nonfunctioning pituitary adenomas. *Journal of Clinical Investigation* **80**, 1472–8.

Kovacs, K. and Horvath, E. (1986). Tumors of the pituitary gland. In *Atlas of tumor pathology*, Fascicle 21, 2nd series, pp. 1–264. Armed Forces Institute of Pathology, USA.

Laws, E.R., Jr (1987). Pituitary surgery. [Review]. *Endocrinology and Metabolism Clinics of North America* **16**, 647–65.

Laws, E.R., Jr (1987). Craniopharyngiomas: diagnosis and treatment. In *Tumors of the cranial base: diagnosis and treatment*, (ed. L.N. Sekhar and V.L. Schramm, Jr), pp. 347–72. Future Publishing Company.

Lechan, R.M. (1987). Neuroendocrinology of pituitary hormone regulation. *Endocrinology and Metabolism Clinics of North America* **16**, 475–502.

Liuzzi, A., *et al.* (1985). Low doses of dopamine agonists in the long-term treatment of macroprolactinomas. *New England Journal of Medicine* **313**, 656–9.

McGrail, K.M., Beyerl, B.D., Black, P.M., Klibanski, A., and Zervas, N.T. (1987). Lymphocytic adenohypophysitis of pregnancy with complete recovery. *Neurosurgery* **20**, 791–3.

Melmed, S., Braunstein, G.D., Horvath, E., Ezrin, C., and Kovacs, K. (1983). Pathophysiology of acromegaly. [Review]. *Endocrine Reviews* **4**, 271–90.

Molitch, M.E., *et al.* (1985). Bromocriptine as primary therapy for prolactin-secreting macroadenomas: results of a prospective multicenter study. *Journal of Clinical Endocrinology and Metabolism* **60**, 698–705.

Neuwelt, E.A., Frenkel, E.P., and Smith, R.G. (1980). Suprasellar germinomas (ectopic pinealomas): aspects of immunological characterization and successful chemotherapeutic responses in recurrent disease. *Neurosurgery* **7**, 352–8.

Orth, D.N. (1992). The adrenal cortex. In *Williams Textbook of Endocrinology*, (8th edn), (ed. J.D. Wilson and D.W. Foster), pp. 489–620. W.B. Saunders Company.

Reichlin, S. (1987). Neuroendocrine control of pituitary function. In *Clinical endocrinology: an illustrated text*, (ed. G.M. Besser and A.G. Cudworth), pp. 1.1–1.14. J.B. Lippincott, Philadelphia.

Ross, G.T., *et al.* (1970). Pituitary and gonadal hormones in women during spontaneous and induced ovulatory cycles. *Recent Progress in Hormone Research* **26**, 1–62.

Sheldon, W.R., Jr, *et al.* (1985). Rapid sequential intravenous administration of four hypothalamic releasing hormones as a combined anterior pituitary function test in normal subjects. *Journal of Clinical Endocrinology and Metabolism* **60**, 623–30.

Snyder, P.J. (1985). Gonadotroph cell adenomas of the pituitary. [Review]. *Endocrine Reviews* **6**, 552–63.

Thorner, M.O., Vance, M.L., Kovacs, K., and Horvath, E. (1992). The anterior pituitary. In *Williams textbook of endocrinology*, (8th edn), (ed. J.D. Wilson and D.W. Foster), pp. 221–310. W.B. Saunders.

Utiger, R.D. (1986). Tests of thyroregulatory mechanisms. In *The thyroid* 5th edn., (ed. S.H. Ingbar and L.E. Braverman). J.B. Lippincott, Philadelphia.

Vance, M.L., and Harris, A.G. (1991). Long-term treatment of 189 acromegalic patients with the somatostatin analog octreotide. Results of the International Multicenter Acromegaly Study Group. *Archives of Internal Medicine*, **151**, 1573–8.

Wass, J.A.H. (1987). Hypopituitarism. In *Clinical endocrinology: an illustrated text*, (ed. G.M. Besser and A.G. Cudworth), pp. 2.1–2.14. J.B. Lippincott, Philadelphia.

Witte, R.J., Mark, L.P., and Haughton, V.M. (1993). Imaging of the pituitary and hypothalamus. In *Atlas of endocrine imaging*, (ed. G.M. Besser and M.O. Thorner), pp. 79–112. Wolfe Publishing.

12.3 The posterior pituitary

P. H. BAYLIS

Neuroanatomy of the posterior pituitary

The two major peptides secreted by the posterior pituitary are arginine vasopressin, the antidiuretic hormone of most mammals including man, and oxytocin. Both are synthesized principally in magnocellular neurones of the supraoptic and paraventricular nuclei of the hypothalamus (Fig. 1). Neuronal pathways from these nuclei pass to:

(1) the posterior pituitary;
(2) the median eminence of the hypothalamus;
(3) the brain-stem and spinal cord;
(4) the floor of the third ventricle; and
(5) throughout the brain substance.

Afferent sensory tracts to the nuclei control peptide synthesis and secretion. Osmotically sensitive cells in the organum vasculosum of the lamina terminalis (OVLT), the putative osmoreceptor, situated in the anterior hypothalamus, transmit information mainly to the supraoptic nucleus. Arginine vasopressin secretion is also influenced by baroregulatory afferents from the great vessels in the chest and heart, and oxytocin by sensory input from the nipples and female genital tract.

Chemistry of arginine vasopressin and oxytocin

Both arginine vasopressin and oxytocin are nonapeptides. Their genes are located on chromosome 20, only a few kilobases apart, and, interestingly, are transcribed in opposing directions (Fig. 2). Three exons encode the large precursor molecule which contains signal peptide, nonapeptide with its specific neurophysin (the carrier protein within the neuronal tracts), and, for arginine vasopressin, a glycoprotein moiety. Following synthesis in the cell bodies of the hypothalamic nuclei, the precursors are processed as they migrate along the tracts to secrete arginine vasopressin or oxytocin separate from their specific neurophysins into the systemic circulation from the posterior pituitary, or into the portal blood from the median eminence to influence anterior pituitary function.

The molecular weights of arginine vasopressin and oxytocin are 1084 and 1007 Da, respectively. Both circulate unbound to proteins and have short half-lives of the order of 5 to 15 min. Arginine vasopressin is metabolized principally in the liver and kidneys, and oxytocin in the uterus, liver, and kidneys.

Arginine vasopressin

Physiology

CONTROL OF ARGININE VASOPRESSIN SECRETION

The principal determinant of arginine vasopressin secretion is blood osmolality, which is sensed in the region of the OVLT. There is an exquisitely sensitive linear relationship between increasing plasma osmolality and arginine vasopressin release (Fig. 3(a)). Hyperosmolality induced by sodium chloride is a more potent stimulus to arginine vasopressin secretion than other solutes. As the concentration of arginine vasopressin in the plasma rises, renal water excretion is reduced, thus lowering plasma osmolality, a mechanism which maintains plasma osmolality within the narrow range of 284 to 295 mosmol/kg.

Reductions in blood pressure and/or volume stimulate arginine vasopressin release in an exponential manner, which can result in a massive release of this hormone following severe acute hypotension. Baroreceptors in the carotid arteries, aorta, heart, and great veins mediate the pressure/volume changes via the vagus and glossopharyngeal nerves, the brain-stem nuclei, and hypothalamus. Nausea and/or emesis are also potent stimuli of arginine vasopressin secretion.

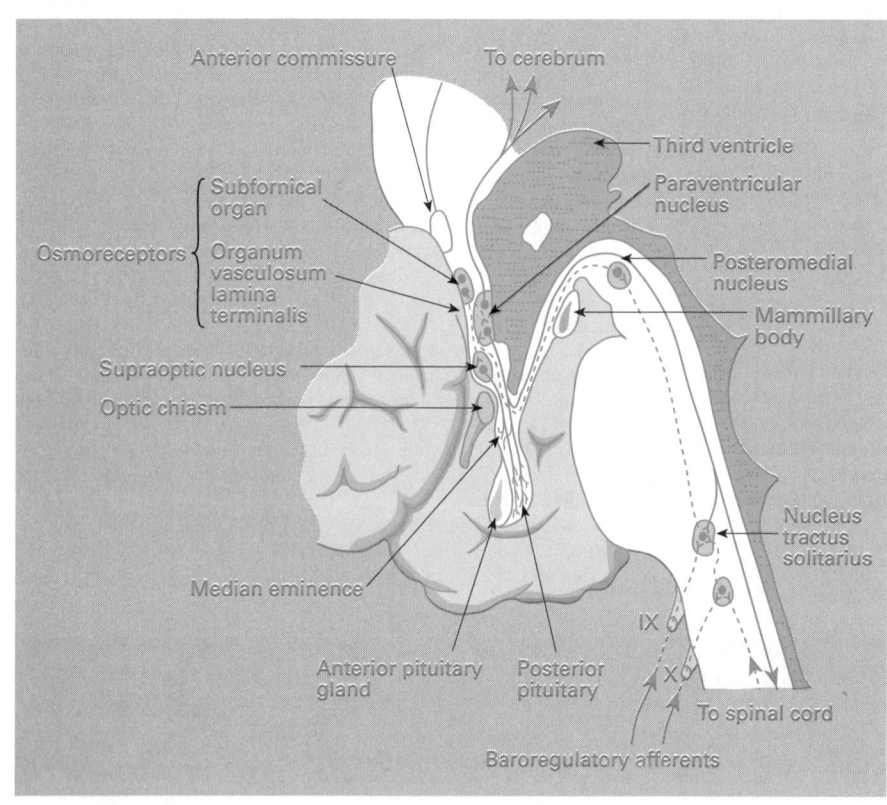

Fig. 1 Schematic representation of the posterior pituitary, supraoptic, and paraventricular nuclei, and surrounding neuroanatomical structures. Major efferent pathways (———) pass to the posterior pituitary, the median eminence, floor of the third ventricle, brain-stem, spinal cord, and brain substance. Afferent sensory pathways (----) arise from the osmoreceptors and brain-stem nuclei. IX and X, glossopharyngeal and vagus nerves).

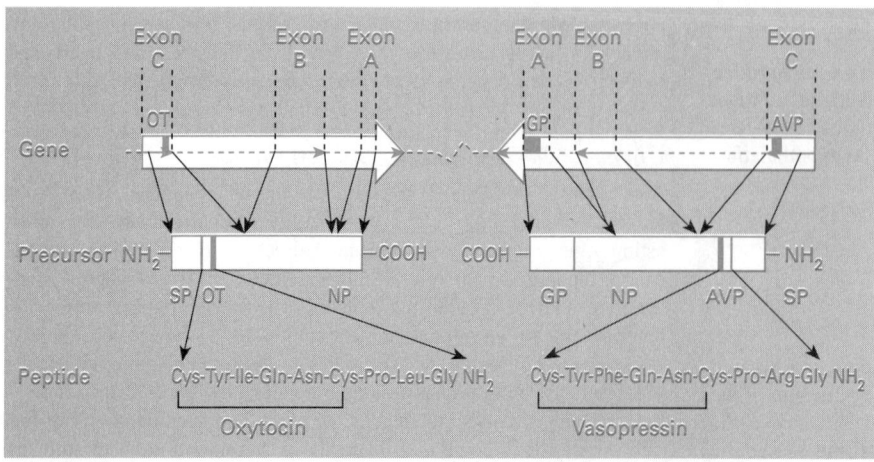

Fig. 2 Diagram of oxytocin and arginine vasopressin genes on chromosome 20, precursor molecules and structures. SP, signal peptide; NP, neurophysin; GP, glycoprotein moiety. (Reproduced by permission of Dr W.S. Young.)

ACTIONS OF ARGININE VASOPRESSIN

The main renal action of arginine vasopressin is the reduction of solute-free water excretion. Its effect is mediated by the V_2 receptor coupled to adenylate cyclase in the distal collecting tubular cell. Arginine vasopressin opens water channels in the cells to allow water to flow from the hypotonic luminal fluid into the hypertonic renal interstitium, thus concentrating urine. As the level of arginine vasopressin in the plasma rises, so the urine is concentrated (Fig. 3(b)), but at concentrations greater than about 4 pmol/l no further urinary concentration occurs in man.

At high plasma concentrations arginine vasopressin contracts the smooth muscle of blood vessels, the gut, and renal tract, binding to the V_{1a} receptor which activates the inositol phosphate pathways.

Arginine vasopressin in the hypothalamopituitary portal circulation acts synergistically with corticotrophin releasing factor to stimulate adrenocorticophin release from the anterior pituitary gland (V_{1b} receptor).

THIRST

In addition to a normal arginine vasopressin osmoregulatory system and a healthy kidney responsive to this hormone, normal water homeostasis is dependent on a thirst mechanism. This is particularly evident when the body continues to lose water despite maximal urine concentration when a mechanism to increase fluid intake is essential. The osmoregulatory control of thirst appreciation is similar to that of arginine vasopressin secretion. Thirst osmoreceptors, probably distinct from arginine vasopressin osmoreceptors, are sited in the anterior hypothalamus.

Disorders of arginine vasopressin secretion

DEFICIENCY OF ARGININE VASOPRESSIN

Cranial diabetes insipidus is defined as a disorder of urinary concentration which results from decreased secretion of osmoregulated arginine vasopressin. Patients develop polyuria (urine volumes 3–20 l/24 h) and polydipsia. They rely upon an intact thirst mechanism and adequate fluid to maintain water homeostasis. Destruction of at least 80 per cent of the hypothalamic neurones is necessary before symptoms appear. The causes of cranial diabetes insipidus are given in Table 1. The familial causes are very rare, some of which are due to point mutations in the arginine vasopressin gene. At least 30 per cent of all cases are idiopathic.

Diagnosis of cranial diabetes insipidus

Three pathogenetic mechanisms are responsible for the symptoms of polyuria and polydipsia:

(1) vasopressin deficiency;
(2) renal resistance to the antidiuretic action of vasopressin; and
(3) increased drinking or primary polydipsia (see Chapter 20.2.1).

The fluid deprivation test is the most commonly used investigation to distinguish the three types of disorders, although confusing results from the test occur frequently.

Confirmation of polyuria (urine output greater than 3 l/24 h) is wise prior to performing the fluid deprivation test (Table 2). Patients who fail to concentrate urine to above 750 mosmol/kg after dehydration, but do so following desmopressin, have cranial diabetes insipidus. Unfortunately, many patients with this disorder have equivocal results. A definitive diagnosis of cranial diabetes insipidus can be made by infusing 5 per cent hypertonic saline to increase plasma osmolality. Subnormal plasma arginine vasopressin values confirm the diagnosis (Fig. 3(a)). The other causes of polyuria can be differentiated by arginine vasopressin measurements (Fig. 3(a,b)).

Alternatively, a carefully supervised therapeutic trial of desmopressin will establish a diagnosis of cranial diabetes insipidus, with such a patient improving symptomatically and remaining normonatraemic (see Chapter 20.2.1).

Treatment of cranial diabetes insipidus

Desmopressin (DDAVP®) is the treatment of choice. It is administered orally (100–600 μg daily in divided doses), intranasally at a dose of 5 to 40 μg once to three times daily, or parenterally up to 4 μg daily. Desmopressin is a long-acting synthetic analogue of arginine vasopressin with no pressor activity and twice the antidiuretic action of the natural hormone. Hyponatraemia is the only significant adverse effect due to overdosage. Lysine vasopressin is rarely given as it has a short period of duration (4 h) and possesses pressor activity that can lead to renal or intestinal colic. There is no place for the oral agents, chlorpropamide, thiazides, clofibrate, or carbamazepine in the treatment of cranial diabetes insipidus.

SYNDROME OF INAPPROPRIATE ANTIDIURESIS

The commonest cause of normovolaemic hyponatraemia is the syndrome of antidiuresis (SIAD), due to posterior pituitary or ectopic secretion of arginine vasopressin in the majority of instances. Arginine vaso-

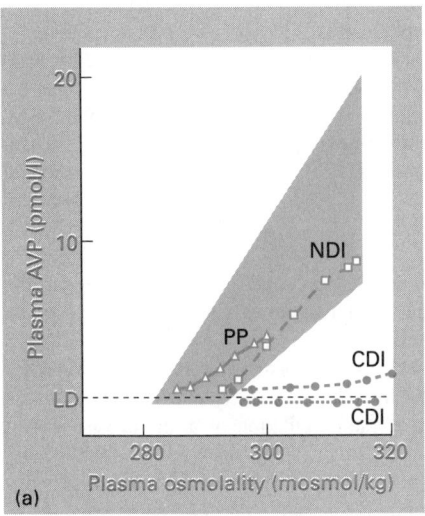

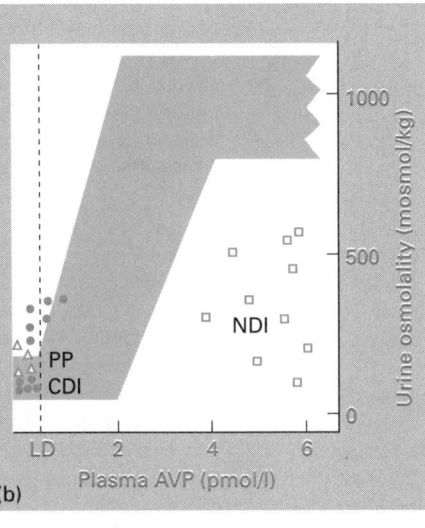

Fig. 3 (a) Relationship between plasma arginine vasopressin (AVP) and osmolality after infusion with hypertonic saline. Shaded area represents the normal response, patients with cranial diabetes insipidus (CDI, ●——●), nephrogenic diabetes insipidus (NDI, ■——■), and primary polydipsia (PP, ▲——▲). (b) Relationship between urine osmolality and plasma arginine vasopressin after dehydration. Shaded area represents the normal response, CDI (●), NDI (■), PP (▲). LD, limit of detection of the arginine vasopressin assay.

Table 1 *Causes of cranial diabetes insipidus*

Familial
Dominant (rarely recessive) inheritance
DIDMOAD syndrome[a]
Acquired
Idiopathic
Trauma (neurosurgery, head injury)
Tumour (craniopharyngioma, large pituitary tumour, dysgerminoma, metastasis to hypothalamus, pinealoma)
Granuloma (sarcoidosis, histiocytosis X, eosinophilic granuloma)
Infection (meningitis, encephalitis)
Vascular (aneurysm, infarction, sickle-cell anaemia, Sheehan's syndrome)

[a]DIDMOAD; diabetes insipidus, diabetes mellitus, optic atrophy, deafness.

Table 2 *Fluid deprivation test*

Preparation of patient
Fluid intake encouraged during the night before the test
Light breakfast—no tea, coffee, alcohol, smoking for 12 h before or during the test
Constant supervision of the patient throughout the test.
Response to dehydration
No fluid for up to 8 h—dry snacks allowed
Patient weighed hourly—stop test if there is a 5% loss of initial body weight.
Urine samples hourly—measure volume and osmolality
Blood drawn hourly—measure plasma osmolality (and plasma arginine vasopressin if possible)
Response to exogenous vasopressin
After dehydration, administer desmopressin (DDAVP®) 4 μg intramuscularly
Urine samples at 3, 5, and 16 h after desmopressin—measure volume and osmolality
Blood drawn at 5 and 16 h—measure plasma osmolality
Patient allowed to eat and drink up to twice the urine volume passed during dehydration

Table 3 *Cardinal features of the syndrome of inappropriate antidiuresis*

Hyponatraemia with appropriately low plasma osmolality
Urine osmolality greater than plasma osmolality
Persistent excessive renal sodium excretion
Absence of hypotension, hypovolaemia, and oedema-forming states
Normal renal and adrenal function

Table 4 *Some causes of the syndrome of inappropriate antidiuresis*

Malignant disease	Central nervous system disorders
Carcinoma	Meningitis encephalitis
Lymphoma	Head injury
Leukaemia	Brain tumour, abscess
Thymoma	Subarachnoid haemorrhage
Sarcoma	Cerebral thrombosis
Mesothelioma	Guillain–Barré syndrome
Chest disorders	Miscellaneous
Pneumonia	Drugs: arginine vasopressin,
Tuberculosis	chlorpropamide,
Empyema	carbamazepine, cytotoxics,
Asthma	oxytocin
Pneumothorax	Porphyria
Positive-pressure ventilation	ACTH deficiency
	Acute psychosis
	Idiopathic

pressin secretion is persistent and inappropriate in relation to the normal physiological mechanisms that regulate its release.

SIAD presents with hyponatraemia, defined as serum sodium less than 130 mmol/l. Moderate chronic hyponatraemia (serum sodium 120–130 mmol/l) is usually asymptomatic, but clinical features became increasingly severe as the serum sodium approaches 100 mmol/l. They range from mild anorexia and nausea, through symptoms of drowsiness, cramps, and confusion, to convulsions, coma, and death. Rapid falls in serum sodium lead to clinical features at higher absolute sodium values.

Diagnosis of SIAD

Most causes of hypo-osmolar hyponatraemia are associated with detectable or elevated concentrations of arginine vasopressin in the plasma (for classification and causes of hyponatraemia see Chapter 20.2.1). A diagnosis of SIAD should only be made if the criteria established by Bartter and Schwartz (1967) are fulfilled (Table 3). Although detectable plasma arginine vasopressin is consistent with the diagnosis of SIAD it is not in itself diagnostic.

A large number of conditions and drugs have been purported to cause this syndrome, some of which are given in Table 4.

Osmoregulatory studies on patients with SIAD have indicated two common patterns of arginine vasopressin secretion. The first shows erratic release of arginine vasopressin with dissociation between plasma osmolality and the hormone, the second indicates arginine vasopressin secretion with increasing plasma osmolality but occurring around a lower absolute plasma osmolality, i.e. a shift to the left of the normal relationship (Fig. 3(a)).

Treatment of SIAD

The underlying cause should be treated whenever possible (Table 4). Mild chronic asymptomatic hyponatraemia (serum sodium greater than 120 mmol/l) does not necessarily require specific therapy. If hyponatraemia is life-threatening or associated with significant clinical features, therapy is appropriate. Fluid restriction to about 500 ml/24 h remains the traditional approach. Drugs (for example, phenytoin) to suppress neurohypophyseal arginine vasopressin secretion have met with limited success. The antidiuretic action of arginine vasopressin may be blunted by democlocycline (600–1200 mg daily) or the more toxic and less reliable lithium; both induce nephrogenic diabetes insipidus. A specific V_2 antagonist effacious in man has yet to be designed. Infusion of hypertonic saline to increase serum sodium in chronic hyponatraemia is dangerous, and may cause demyelination.

Whatever method is used to raise serum sodium in chronic hyponatraemia it is essential that the rate of increase is no greater than 0.5 mmol/l/h or 12 mmol/l/24 h. Rapid correction can lead to osmotic demyelination in central pontine and/or extrapontine structures. Neurological sequelae or death occur up to 4 days after correction of hyponatraemia.

THIRST DEFICIENCY

Hypodipsia or adipsia is an uncommon condition due to damage to the anterior hypothalamic thirst osmoreceptors, which leads to chronic hypernatraemia (serum sodium greater than 150 mmol/l). Causes include vascular lesions (such as haemorrhage from an anterior communicating artery aneurysm), hypothalamic metastatic or granulomatous disease, or trauma. Defective osmoregulation of arginine vasopressin may also occur.

A complete osmoreceptor defect leads to intra- and extracellular dehydration causing life-threatening hypernatraemia (serum sodium up to 190 mmol/l). Slow rehydration is vital to avoid cerebral oedema, convulsions, and death. Long-term therapy is difficult but requires forced fluid intake of 2 to 3 l/24h to maintain constant body weight.

In 'essential' hypernatraemia, osmoregulation of thirst and arginine vasopressin secretion is maintained around plasma osmolalities higher than normal, i.e. a shift to the right (Fig. 3(a)). Hypernatraemia is discussed in greater detail in Chapter 20.2.1.

Oxytocin

The oxytocin gene is on chromosome 20 close to the arginine vasopressin gene. It is a nonapeptide similar to arginine vasopressin with a molecular weight of 1007 Da (Fig. 2). Like arginine vasopressin, it is synthesized in the supraoptic and paraventricular nuclei, moves by axonal flow along neuronal tracts to the median eminence, posterior pituitary, brain-stem, spinal cord, and brain.

CONTROL OF OXYTOCIN SECRETION

The precise physiological control of oxytocin release is poorly defined. Stimulation of the nipple leads to oxytocin secretion and milk ejection of the lactating breast (the suckling reflex), which is probably mediated by spinothalamic afferent fibres. The Ferguson reflex, release of oxytocin following cervical distension of the pregnant uterus, may initiate parturition.

ACTIONS OF OXYTOCIN

The effects of oxytocin are confined mainly to pregnancy and the postpartum period. In addition to contraction of myoepithelial cells surrounding breast ducts, oxytocin stimulates contraction of the uterine myometrium, binding to specific oxytocin receptors. During pregnancy, the numbers of uterine oxytocin receptors increase, and the placenta secretes an enzyme, oxytocinase, which degrades avidly circulating oxytocin and arginine vasopressin. It is unlikely that oxytocin is the sole initiator of labour, but plasma oxytocin concentrations increase substantially during the final stages of labour, to expel the placenta and maintain uterine contraction.

There are no significant physiological actions of oxytocin in men or non-pregnant, non-lactating women. Even in pregnancy the role of oxytocin does not appear to be essential, as patients with posterior pituitary hormone deficiency have normal pregnancy, labour, and lactation. No disorders of oxytocin deficiency or excess have been described, despite the occurrence of some tumours synthesizing and releasing oxytocin ectopically.

CLINICAL USE OF OXYTOCIN

Infusion of oxytocin in increasing doses is used routinely to initiate and maintain labour. A significant adverse effect can occur when high doses are administered with large volumes of intravenous fluid, which causes rapid profound hyponatraemia, leading to convulsions. This is due to low-affinity binding of oxytocin to the arginine vasopressin V_2 renal receptor, resulting in antidiuresis.

REFERENCES

Bartter, F.C. and Schwartz, W.B. (1967). The syndrome of inappropriate secretion of antidiuretic hormone. *American Journal of Medicine* **42**, 790–806.
Baylis, P.H. (1992). Disorders of water balance. In *Clinical endocrinology*, (ed. A. Grossman), pp. 238–52.
Pickering, B.T. (1989). Oxytocin and its neurophysin. In *Endocrinology*, (ed. L.J. DeGroot), pp. 230–9.
Sterns, R.H., Riggo, J., and Schochet, S.S. (1986). Osmotic demyelination syndrome following correction of hyponatraemia. *New England Journal of Medicine* **314**, 1535–42.
Verbalis, J.G. (1992). Hyponatraemia: endocrinologic causes and consequences of therapy. *Trends in Endocrinology and Metabolism* **3**, 1–7.
Young, W.S. (1992). Expression of the oxytocin and vasopressin genes. *Journal of Neuroendocrinology* **4**, 527–40.

12.4 The thyroid gland and disorders of thyroid function

A. M. McGREGOR

Embryological development

Thyroid tissue is confined to the vertebrates and is the first endocrine glandular tissue to appear in mammalian development. In humans the thyroid gland arises from two distinct regions of the endodermal pharynx. The median anlage arises from the midline of the anterior pharyngeal floor between branchial arches 1 and 2 and is visible by day 17 of gestation. In contrast, the two lateral anlage (ultimobranchial bodies) develop as caudal projections from the fourth or fifth pharyngeal pouches. The growth and descent of the median anlage is accompanied by the development of a stalk (thyroglossal duct) which keeps it attached to its pharyngeal floor origin. The subsequent obliteration of the lumen of the duct is associated with lateral expansion of the anlage and the beginnings of the formation of the characteristic bi-lobed structure of the thyroid. Simultaneously with the descent of the medial anlage, the ultimobranchial bodies separate from the pharyngeal pouches and fuse with the lateral parts of the medial anlage. Degeneration of the attachments of the ultimobranchial bodies to their pharyngeal origins is accompanied by proliferation of medial anlage cells which surround the tissues of the lateral anlage. This association between the medial and lateral anlage is complete by the ninth week of gestation, at which stage the thyroid has its characteristic shape. The contribution of the lateral anlage tissues to the formation of functioning thyroid tissue is minimal and their main contribution is in the provision of parafollicular calcitonin-secreting (C) cells.

Structure

The thyroid gland consists of two lobes connected by an isthmus, with the adult normal gland in an iodine replete population weighing 15–20 g. The gland is attached to the anterior and lateral aspects of the trachea by loose connective tissue such that the isthmus lies just below the cricoid cartilage. The recurrent laryngeal nerves lie in the grooves between the lateral lobes and the trachea and the lateral extent of the thyroid lobes are marked by the carotid sheaths and sternocleidomastoid muscles. The well-vascularized gland is supplied by the superior and inferior thyroid arteries on each side. The gland has both adrenergic and cholinergic innervation.

The basic functional unit of the thyroid gland is the follicle (Fig. 1).

These hollow, spherical structures ranging in size from 15 to 500 μm in diameter are surrounded by a basement membrane. The wall of the unit is made up of a single layer of thyroid follicular cells, which are cuboidal when quiescent. The lumen of the follicle contains the proteinaceous colloid which is normally the major constituent of the thyroid mass and serves as the primary site of storage of thyroglobulin secreted by the thyroid follicular cells. The rich capillary network surrounding the follicles and the high blood flow through the gland ensure easy access of thyroid hormone to the circulation. Interspersed between the thyroid follicles are the parafollicular C cells which secrete calcitonin.

Function

Iodine metabolism

Uniquely amongst the endocrine glands the thyroid not only maintains a large store of preformed hormone but in addition requires iodide for hormone synthesis. Adequate dietary intake of iodide is therefore essential (Fig. 2). Although mechanisms for conserving iodine exist, in situations of iodine deficiency they are not always capable of preventing depletion of iodine stores. The major sources of dietary iodide are both food and water and when natural levels of iodide are insufficient the iodination of water or food products, such as bread and salt, ensure adequate intake. Medications, diagnostic agents, and dietary supplements are also potential sources of iodine. Iodine intake varies widely across the world. In western Europe a level of 200 μg/day is considered optimal, although the range of iodine intake in adults across areas of the world in which iodine deficiency is not severe enough to impair thyroid hormonogenesis is from 50 to 1000 μg/day. Iodine is almost completely absorbed in the gastrointestinal tract where it enters the inorganic iodide pool in the extracellular fluid. Provided renal function is normal, inorganic iodide is rapidly cleared from the extracellular fluid with a half-life of about 2 h. Besides dietary iodide, a small contribution to the extracellular fluid iodide pool is made by iodide released following the deiodination of thyroid hormones in peripheral tissues and the leak of inorganic iodide from the thyroid gland. Iodide clearance from the extracellular pool is via the thyroid and the kidney. The thyroid is able to

regulate the amount of iodide it clears, taking up only as much as is required for hormone synthesis. In so doing it is able to buffer itself against marked changes in dietary iodide intake, taking up relatively less from the extracellular pool when iodide is ingested in excess and relatively more when intake declines. The major iodine pool in the body is the organic component synthesized by the thyroid follicular cell and stored as iodinated thyroglobulin in the colloid within the follicular lumen. When dietary iodine intake is in the range of 500 μg daily an equivalent amount will be cleared into the urine over the same period in its inorganic form. On this intake the removal of iodide from the extracellular pool by the thyroid ensures the maintenance of a thyroid pool of iodine of about 8000 μg which turns over slowly at about 1 per cent/day. From this pool the thyroid secretes about 75 μg of organic iodine per day in the form of the thyroid hormones, predominantly thyroxine (T_4) with a small amount of triiodothyronine (T_3), and this intravascular pool of thyroid hormones contains about 600 μg of iodine. Cellular uptake of thyroid hormones is of the order of 75 μg of iodine per day, of which about 60 μg re-enters the extracellular fluid iodide pool following intracellular deiodination of the thyroid hormones, and the remainder of the iodine is excreted in the faeces.

Thyroid hormone synthesis and secretion

Synthesis of adequate quantities of thyroid hormone necessitates more rapid entry of iodide into thyroid follicular cells than is possible by passive diffusion from the extracellular fluid. A poorly characterized (trapping) mechanism ensures that sufficient iodide substrate is available for hormone formation. This process is enhanced by thyroid stimulating hormone, thyrotropin (TSH) and is responsive to the glandular content of organic iodine. The mechanism for concentrating iodide is shared by the other monovalent anions perchlorate and pertechnetate. Glandular tissue in the salivary glands and gastric mucosa, tissues of endodermal origin, have a similar capacity for concentrating iodide.

Once iodide is trapped within the thyroid follicular cell it is rapidly oxidized in the presence of hydrogen peroxide by the enzyme thyroid peroxidase, a 933 amino acid, membrane bound, glycosylated, haem-containing protein. Oxidation is followed by the incorporation of the resulting reactive intermediate into the tyrosine residues of thyroglobulin (iodide organification). Thyroid peroxidase, which is central to this

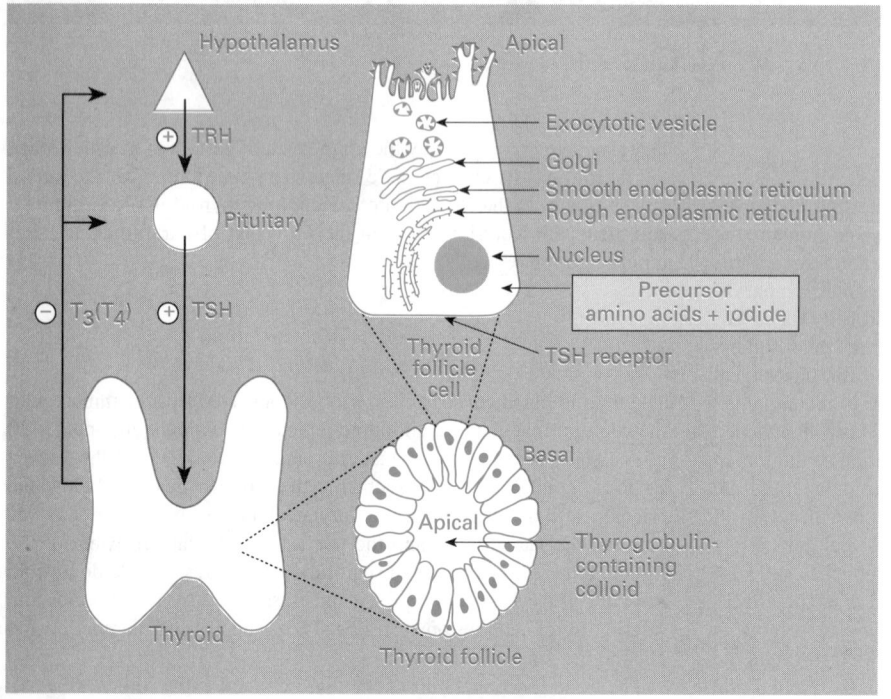

Fig. 1 The basic functional unit of the thyroid gland is the thyroid follicle which is involved in the synthesis and storage of thyroglobulin and its iodination to form thyroid hormones. These processes are closely regulated by interaction between the thyroid and the hypothalamic–pituitary axis.

process, is predominantly localized on the apical border of the thyroid cell and this location suggests that it is at this interface between the follicular cell apical surface and the colloid that organification occurs.

Oxidation and organification of iodide result in the formation of hormonally inactive iodotyrosines (monoiodotyrosine and diiodotyrosine). The coupling of these iodinated tyrosines leads to the formation of the hormonally active iodothyronines T_4 and T_3. The synthesis of T_4 results from the fusion of two molecules of diiodotyrosine, whereas the formation of T_3 results from the coupling of a molecule of monoiodotyrosine with one of diiodotyrosine. Thyroid peroxidase plays a key role in thyroid hormone biosynthesis, not only in the catalysis of the iodination of tyrosyl residues in thyroglobulin but also in the coupling of iodotyrosyl residues in thyroglobulin to form T_4 and T_3.

Thyroglobulin, the main precursor of thyroid hormones is a large glycoprotein molecule present in the follicular luminal colloid in multiple forms, with the most prevalent and the major source of thyroid hormone being the 19S molecule with a molecular size of 660 kDa. The sites in the molecule for thyroid hormone formation have been identified. There are approximately three to four T_4 molecules per mole of human thyroglobulin under conditions of normal iodination, but only one in five molecules of human thyroglobulin contains a T_3 residue. Thyroglobulin synthesis in the thyroid follicular cell is the same as that for other glycoproteins. Following transcription and processing of thyroglobulin mRNA and its ribosomal translation, the resulting polypeptide chain is extruded into the endoplasmic reticulum and glycosylated during transport to the Golgi apparatus. Packaging of the thyroglobulin into exocytotic vesicles in the Golgi apparatus then allows the transport of the protein in these vesicles, which also contain membrane-bound thyroid peroxidase, to the apical surface of the follicular cell, where the contents are released into the colloid-containing follicular lumen. The process of thyroglobulin biosynthesis and exocytosis is regulated by TSH.

For thyroid hormone to be secreted into the circulation, thyroglobulin from the large colloid reservoir needs to re-enter the thyroid follicular cell where it undergoes proteolytic cleavage with the release of T_4 and T_3, which leave the thyroid follicular cell at its basal surface to enter the capillary circulation. This process is activated by TSH with the formation of pseudopodia induced on the apical surface of the follicular

Fig. 2 Iodine metabolism in a healthy subject ingesting 500 μg of iodine daily.

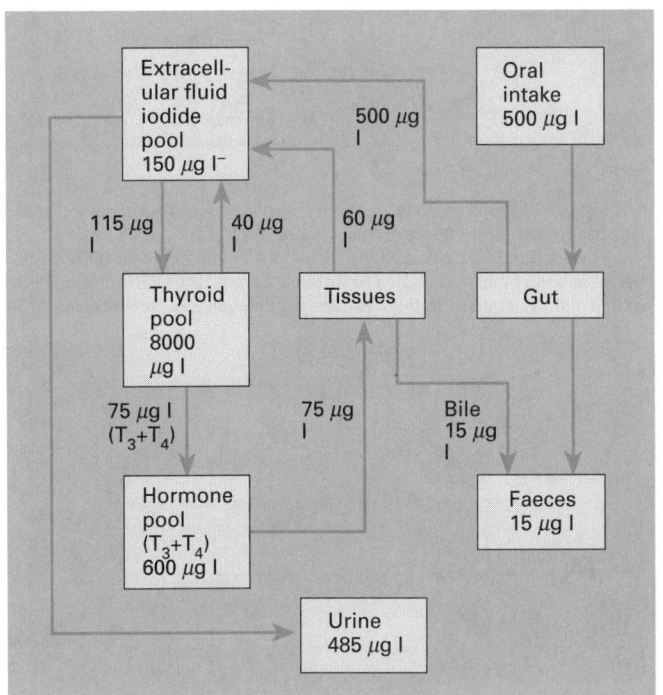

Table 1 *Situations that impair T_4 to T_3 conversion*

Physiological
    Fetal/early neonate
Pathological
    Fasting/malnutrition
    Severe systemic illness
    Hepatic or renal impairment
    Trauma
    Postoperative hypercatabolic state
Pharmacological
    Propylthiouracil
    Glucocorticoids
    Propranolol
    Amiodarone
    Iodinated radiographic contrast media

cells which engulf colloid to produce colloid-containing endocytotic vesicles within the follicular cell. The subsequent fusion of enzyme-containing lysosomes with these droplets leads to the hydrolysis of thyroglobulin and the liberation of the iodotyrosines from the thyroglobulin.

Thyroid hormone transport and metabolism

Of the iodothyronines circulating in the plasma, T_4 is the most abundant and is the only one that arises solely by direct secretion from the thyroid gland. Very little T_3 is secreted, with most of it in the plasma being derived from the peripheral conversion of T_4 as a result of enzymatic monodeiodination. Of the remaining iodothyronines and their derivatives, of importance is reverse T_3, which is generated almost entirely in the peripheral tissues from T_4. Within the circulation, T_4 and T_3 are reversibly bound to a variety of proteins synthesized by the liver including thyroxine-binding globulin, thyroxine-binding prealbumin, transthyretin, and, to a smaller extent, by albumin. Of the thyroid hormones present in the plasma, only about 0.04 per cent of T_4 and 0.4 per cent of T_3 circulate in the unbound state (free). Of the binding proteins, thyroxine-binding globulin is responsible for the transport of about 75 per cent of T_4. With alterations in binding protein concentration or in the ability of binding proteins to bind thyroid hormones, the concentration of protein-bound thyroid hormones will clearly alter (see Table 3).

The most important pathway for the metabolism of T_4 is its conversion to the biologically active hormone T_3. The remaining deiodination reactions of T_4 and of T_3 all lead to the generation of inactive products. Three enzymes catalyse the deiodination of iodothyronines in man. These are the selenoenzyme 5′-deiodinase type I (5′DI), the type II 5′-iodothyronine deiodinase (5′DII), and the 5-, or inner ring, deiodinase type III (5DIII). These enzymes are expressed in particular tissues, major sites being the liver, kidney, thyroid, and pituitary for the 5′DI enzyme; the pituitary, brain, placenta, and keratinocytes for the 5′DII, and the placenta, brain, and epidermis for 5DIII. The 5′DI and 5′DII enzymes activate the prohormone T_4 to form T_3, with the T_3 formed by 5′DI catalysis entering the plasma, whereas that formed from 5′DII catalysis largely remains within the tissue in which it is produced. In the brain, T_3 production from the action of 5′DII is the major source, accounting for up to 80 per cent of the T_3 found in neuronal nuclei. The 5DIII enzyme inactivates T_4 to reverse T_3 or T_3 to 3,3′-diiodothyronine. Up to 90 per cent of T_3 production results from the monodeiodination of T_4 to T_3, which utilizes up to 40 per cent of the secreted T_4. Virtually all of the reverse T_3 (95 per cent) is produced by the monodeiodination of T_4 and this represents a further 40 per cent of the T_4 secreted by the thyroid gland. The remaining 20 per cent of secreted T_4 is excreted in the faeces or urine, either free or conjugated. A number of factors impair the peripheral conversion of T_4 to T_3 (Table 1) and will clearly impair the supply of T_3 to tissues which do not have the capacity for intracellular T_4 to T_3 conversion.

The fractional rate of turnover of T_4 in the periphery is normally about 10 per cent/day (half-life 6.7 days). This relatively slow rate is a reflection of the predominant extent to which T_4 is bound. The kinetics of T_3 metabolism contrast greatly with those of T_4 (Table 2). T_3 is cleared rapidly from the plasma because of its widespread distribution and rapid cellular metabolism. Its fractional turnover rate is about 60 per cent/day (half-life 0.75 days).

Regulation of thyroid function

Thyroid hormone synthesis and secretion are closely regulated by extra-thyroidal (TSH) and intrathyroidal mechanisms. The thyroid participates with the hypothalamus and pituitary in a classical feedback control system (see Fig. 1). Fluctuations in hormone secretion are prevented in part by the large intraglandular store of hormone which buffers the effects of acute increases or decreases in hormone synthesis. Autoregulatory mechanisms within the gland maintain the constancy of the intraglandular hormone pool.

TSH is the major regulator of thyroid structure and function. Its secretion, in turn, is regulated by thyrotropin releasing hormone (TRH) from the hypothalamus which stimulates the pituitary thyrotroph to release and later synthesize TSH. It is at this level in the feedback system that thyroid hormones act to inhibit function. TRH is a tripeptide synthesized by the peptidergic neurones in the supraoptic and paraventricular nuclei of the hypothalamus, and is transported from them and stored in the median eminence. Thereafter TRH enters the hypophyseal portal venous system to act on the pituitary thyrotrophs to release TSH. Although TRH and thyroid hormones are the major regulators of TSH secretion, somatostatin, dopamine, and pharmacological doses of glucocorticoids impair the release of TSH in response to TRH.

TSH is a glycoprotein hormone secreted by thyrotroph cells of the anterior pituitary. It is composed of a 14 kDa α-subunit in common with luteinizing hormone, follicle stimulating hormone and human chorionic gonadotropin, and a specific β-subunit. It is secreted in both 1 to 2 hourly pulses and with a circadian rhythm which is characterized by a nocturnal surge which precedes the onset of sleep. By binding to the TSH receptor on the thyroid follicular cells (one of the family of seven-transmembrane spanning G-protein linked receptors), TSH activates thyroid function, predominantly through adenylate cyclase. A number of key elements of thyroid cell function have been demonstrated to be responsive to TSH stimulation; these include iodide transport with both acute and delayed effects, iodide organification, the release of thyroglobulin from exocytotic vesicles into the follicular lumen, increased pseudopod formation on the apical cell border allowing endocytosis of colloid, lysosome maturation and interaction with the endocytotic vesicle, thyroid hormone secretion, and, with chronic stimulation, hyperplasia and thyroid growth.

Autoregulatory control mechanisms are assumed to be at work when the level of TSH remains constant. In situations of TSH deficiency, variations in dietary iodine intake continue to influence iodide transport. The influence of iodine on the rate of thyroid hormone synthesis is determined by the amount and duration of administration of iodine. With increasing doses of iodide given acutely, the initial increase in the organification of iodine is then followed by a decrease. This decreasing yield of organic iodine, despite increasing dosage of iodide, is termed the acute Wolff–Chaikoff effect. As a result, synthesis of hormonally active iodothyronine is abolished and overproduction of thyroid hormone is prevented. Chronic repeated lower dose iodide administration allows 'escape' from this process, thus preventing the development of goitrous hypothyroidism. Pharmacological doses of iodine will, in addition, rapidly inhibit thyroid hormone release. This acute effect occurs much more rapidly than is seen with the Wolff–Chaikoff effect and the mechanism remains uncertain.

Despite the well-recognized and abundant adrenergic nerve fibre supply to the thyroid, the contribution that catecholamines make to thyroid hormone production is less well defined.

Table 2 *Comparison of T_3 and T_4 in a euthyroid human*

	T_3	T_4
Production rate (nmol/day)	34	100
Relative metabolic potency	1	0.3
Body pool (nmol)	71	1023
Serum concentration		
Total (nmol/l)	1.2–2.8	70–150
Free (pmol/l)	3–9	9–25
Fraction of total hormone in free form ($\times 10^{-2}$)	0.3	0.02
Half-life (days)	0.75	7.0

Thyroid hormone action

With the demonstration in the early 1970s of high-affinity nuclear receptors for T_3, it became clear that the cellular site of action for thyroid hormones is within the nucleus (Fig. 3). Since then the discovery of multiple thyroid hormone receptor isoforms (Fig. 4) and the characterization at the molecular level of their structure and function have greatly clarified the mode of action of thyroid hormones and, in addition, allowed the elucidation of mechanisms that result in clinical syndromes of thyroid hormone resistance. The thyroid hormone receptors, which have been named α and β, map to human chromosomes 17 and 3, respectively, and are cellular homologues of the viral oncogene v-*erbA*. They belong to a family of similar cell-protein receptors, which include

Fig. 3 Thyroid hormone action.

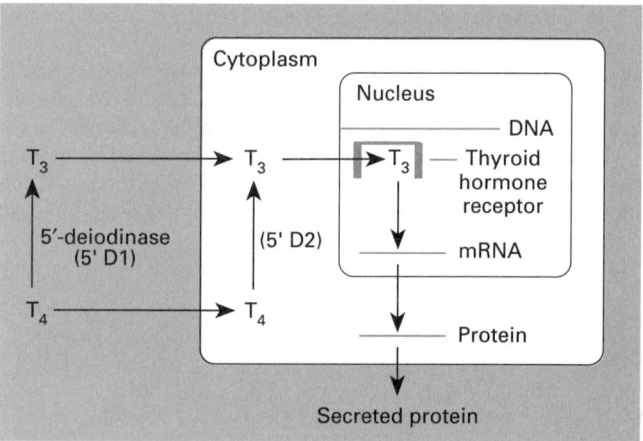

Fig. 4 Thyroid hormone receptor isoforms. The two thyroid hormone receptor (TR) genes (α and β) express two major isoforms (1 and 2). They exhibit considerable homology, particularly in their DNA binding domain (DBD) and T_3 ligand/binding domain (LBD). The different carboxyl (COOH) terminal of TRα2 prevents T_3 binding so this TR does not function as a true receptor.

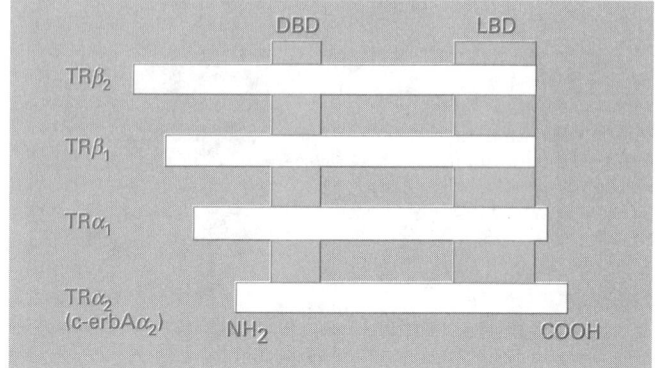

the glucocorticoid, mineralocorticoid, oestrogen, androgen, progesterone, vitamin D, and retinoic acid receptors. All possess a well-conserved DNA-binding domain and a hormone-binding domain. Two peptide loops (zinc fingers) which project from the surface of the protein in the DNA-binding domain interact with specific DNA response elements, and it is through this interaction that thyroid hormones coupled to their receptor regulate gene function. Several thyroid hormone receptor (TR) isoforms are produced by alternative splicing, with the principal TRβ isoforms being β-1 and β-2 and those for the TRα gene being α-1 and α-2. TRα-2 does not function as a true thyroid hormone receptor. The most highly regulated TR isoform is the TRβ-2 which is expressed only in the pituitary gland and in selective areas of the central nervous system. Unlike TRβ-2, mRNAs encoding the TRα-1, α-2 and β-1 isoforms are expressed in virtually all tissues, although they have characteristic distributions. TRα-1 is particularly abundant in skeletal muscle and brown fat, TRα-2 in the brain, and TRβ-1 is more homogeneously distributed but high levels are detectable in the brain, liver, and kidney. The relative expression of the TR genes varies during different stages of embryonic and postnatal development and is regulated by thyroid hormones. It seems increasingly likely that all thyroid hormone-dependent processes are initiated by the interaction of thyroid hormone with the nuclear receptor and the subsequent interaction of the thyroid hormone–thyroid hormone receptor complex with the DNA sequence of the thyroid hormone response element (Fig. 5). In this context thyroid hormones influence a number of metabolic processes by their action on a variety of enzymes; the metabolism of substrates, vitamins, and minerals; the secretion and degradation rates of virtually all other hormones and the response of their target tissues to them. They stimulate calorigenesis (as reflected in increased oxygen consumption), protein synthesis, all aspects of carbohydrate and lipid metabolism, increasing the demands for coenzymes and the vitamins from which they are derived, and in so doing have an impact on every tissue and organ system in the body. In this context, therefore, it is hardly surprising that the deleterious effects of over- or underproduction of thyroid hormones should be so protean.

Laboratory investigation of structure and function

Assessment of a patient with suspected thyroid disease is designed to answer two specific questions: (1) is the patient making too much, too little, or adequate amounts of thyroid hormone; and (2) what is the cause of the underlying disorder?

Thyroid hormones

The techniques of measurement of thyroid hormones have moved through several eras, which began with the measurement of iodine con-

Table 3 *Situations in which the binding of T_4 by thyroxine-binding globulin is impaired*

Increased binding	Decreased binding
Genetic	Genetic
Pregnancy	Androgens
Neonate	Anabolic steroids
Oestrogens	Glucocorticoids
Tamoxifen	Acromegaly
Hepatitis, cirrhosis	Nephrotic syndrome
Perphenazine	Severe systemic illness
Opiates	Protein malnutrition
Acute intermittent porphyria	

tent of serum protein (protein bound iodine) as an indirect measure of serum content of T_4, evolved to competitive binding assays that use the displacement of T_4 from thyroxine-binding globulin, which, in turn, have been replaced by improved immunoassays using highly specific antibodies to T_4. Similar immunoassay methods have been developed for the measurement of total serum T_3. Using such assay systems it is possible to establish normal ranges for circulating thyroid hormones; these are 70 to 150 nmol/l for total T_4 and 1.2 to 2.8 nmol/l for total T_3. Total T_4 discriminates well between hyperthyroidism, hypothyroidism, and the euthyroid state, but total T_3 measurements, in contrast, are of little value in the investigation of patients suspected of being hypothyroid because in this condition the levels of total T_3 are often within the normal range. They may, however, be of value in patients suspected of being hyperthyroid, when they may rise before changes in total T_4 levels are detectable. Since these hormone measurements reflect the concentrations of protein-bound hormone in the blood, they will vary with alterations in thyroid hormone binding protein concentrations (Table 3). In order to overcome these problems, tests designed to measure the concentrations of free thyroid hormone levels have been developed. The reference method against which all other methods have been assessed is that of equilibrium dialysis. In this assay plasma is dialysed against buffer so that only free hormone enters the dialysis fluid and a measurement in the dialysis fluid after an incubation period of about 12 h provides an indication of the 'true' free hormone concentration in the plasma as measured by radio-immunoassay. The cumbersome nature of this assay methodology has not permitted its development for routine use. Currently available assays for the assessment of free thyroid hormone which are capable of automation and therefore of handling large numbers of samples are based either on analogue methodology or methods using two-step or labelled antibody immunoassays.

In analogue methods an antibody to thyroid hormone is added to the sample in conjunction with a labelled derivative of the thyroid hormone being measured (analogue) that is able to bind to the antibody but not to the plasma-binding proteins. Competition between the free hormone in the sample and the analogue for binding to the antibody allows measurement of a free thyroid hormone level. This approach has not been without problems. Many of the commercially available analogues bind to albumin so that in situations in which the concentration and binding capacity of albumin is abnormal, free thyroid hormone levels will likewise be abnormal. Low levels of albumin will be associated with lower apparent levels of free hormones. Genetic variants of both albumin and prealbumin will also give rise to problems in interpreting free thyroid hormone levels in analogue-based methods of assessment.

In two-step immunoassays, initial extraction of the free thyroid hormone from the sample using a thyroid hormone antibody coated on to the assay tube is followed, after washing of the tube, by measurement of the free thyroid hormone concentration by quantitation of the amount of binding of labelled thyroid hormone to the remaining unoccupied sites on the antibody. Such methodology is not interfered with by changes in albumin concentration or the presence of autoantibodies to

Fig. 5 Diagrammatic representation of gene activation through interaction of the thyroid hormone receptor (TR)–thyroid hormone (T3) complex with the DNA sequence of the thyroid hormone response element (TRE). Depending on the target gene, thyroid hormone receptor auxillary proteins (TRAP) interact with the T_3–TR complex to augment their binding to the TRE and either enhance or inhibit gene activation.

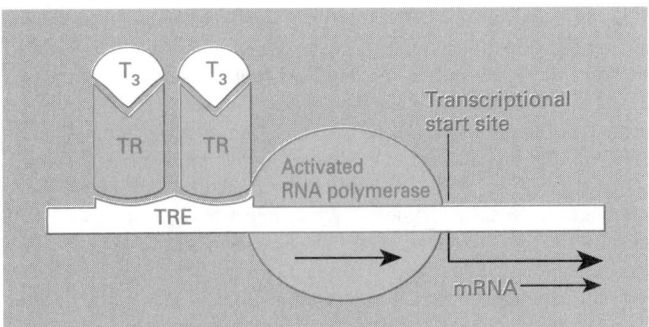

thyroid hormones. Normal ranges for free thyroid hormones using such assay systems are 9 to 25 pmol/l for free T_4 and 3 to 9 pmol/l for free T_3. Although radio-immunoassays are available for the measurement of reverse T_3, its measurement is rarely required.

Thyroglobulin

Thyroglobulin is present at low levels (up to 30 pmol/l) in the circulation of normal individuals. Measurement of thyroglobulin in most available assays is difficult in the presence of circulating thyroglobulin autoantibodies. The major clinical value of measurements of serum thyroglobulin concentration is in the management of patients with differentiated thyroid carcinoma (see Chapter 12.5).

Thyroid gland iodine metabolism

The only means of measuring thyroid function directly is by the use of a tracer dose of a radioactive isotope of iodine and measurement of its fractional uptake by the gland. Following the administration of an oral preparation of radiolabelled iodine, a γ-scintillation counter is used to measure radioactivity over the area of the thyroid 24 h later, when the tracer uptake is near maximum. In patients with hyperthyroidism, uptake is likely to be higher much earlier and an additional measurement is therefore performed at 6 h. Variations in dietary iodine intake will determine the normal range of the radioactive iodine uptake within a given population. High values do not always indicate thyroid hormone overproduction and caution is required in interpreting the result.

The efficiency of thyroid organification is examined using the discharge of radioactive iodine from the thyroid in response to the administration of potassium perchlorate. Two to three hours after an oral dose of radio-iodine, 0.5 g of potassium perchlorate is given orally in solution and its effect on radioactive iodine uptake is assessed. In subjects with a normal organification mechanism no further uptake of radio-iodine by the thyroid occurs and less than 5 per cent of the accumulated iodide is discharged during the succeeding hour. Where an iodide organification defect exists, diffusion of iodine out of the thyroid continues and this is seen as an increased discharge of radioactivity from the thyroid gland.

Thyroid imaging

Radionuclide scanning is based on the principle that isotopically labelled materials accumulate differentially in thyroid tissue and the detection and quantification of this information is transformed into a visual display. This allows the localization of functioning and non-functioning thyroid tissue. A number of isotopes of iodine and $^{99}Tc^m$ pertechnetate have been used. Because pertechnetate is not organified following concentration by the thyroid gland, it diffuses rapidly out of the thyroid and this, together with its short physical half-life (6 h), makes the radiation delivered to the thyroid, by a standard dose, very low and allows imaging 20–30 min after the dose has been given. An important consideration when using pertechnetate is that some tumours of the thyroid appear to be functioning when examined by pertechnetate but are cold with radio-iodine. Improvements in scanning apparatus and in particular the development of the pinhole collimated gamma-camera (scintillation), make it possible to scan the whole thyroid without moving the camera. This method provides more rapid scanning of increased resolution.

Ultrasonography of the normal thyroid produces a pattern of sparse, fine echos in the paratracheal region. It is possible to demonstrate diffuse or localized enlargement of the gland and provide objective assessments of change in size. The sensitivity of the technique allows detection of nodules which are not clinically palpable. When these nodules are solitary the significance of their detection in this way is as yet unresolved. The major role of ultrasonography is in the differentiation of cystic from solid lesions in the thyroid and when a solitary nodule can be shown to be purely cystic this considerably reduces the likelihood of it being malignant.

The demonstration by radio-isotope scanning of a solitary cold nodule, which is then shown by ultrasonography to be solid, demands further investigation. The use in this setting of fine-needle aspiration biopsy coupled with cytological examination provides a simple, safe, and rapid means for diagnosis and significantly reduces the need for referral for surgical investigation and removal.

Hypothalamic–pituitary–thyroid axis

There has been a dramatic improvement in the sensitivity of assay systems for the measurement of plasma TSH. First-generation radio-immunoassays with detection limits of 1.0 mU/l were replaced by immunometric assays with detection limits of 0.1 ml/l in the second generation, and now third-generation immunometric assays allow the measurement of TSH levels of 0.01 mU/l. The use of such assays not only allows the diagnosis of primary hypothyroidism to be made with confidence, but now symptomatic hyperthyroidism can also be shown to be accompanied almost without exception by TSH levels below 0.01 mU/l. Using these sensitive third-generation assays, it is also possible to discriminate between hypothyroidism of thyroid origin and that due to diseases of the hypothalamic–pituitary axis. The need to perform TRH infusion tests or thyroid suppression tests has now become almost non-existent. The technology for immunometric assays is based on the use of two monoclonal antibodies directed at separate epitopes on the TSH molecule, with one antibody bound to a solid phase and the other to a detectable marker, usually a radio-isotope but more recently an enzyme or a chemiluminescent agent. The signal generated is proportional to the amount of TSH in the serum. As a result, the assay is specific, highly sensitive, and rapid. Patients with TSH levels above 5.0 mU/l are likely to have primary hypothyroidism. With third-generation immunometric assays, symptomatic hyperthyroidism is almost invariably present when TSH levels below 0.01 mU/l are recorded. Since immunometric assays commonly use mouse-derived monoclonal antibodies for the assay of TSH it is important to be aware of the uncommon, but possible, presence in the patients' sera of endogenous antibodies to mouse immunoglobulin, which may produce a spuriously high TSH result in normal individuals and an apparently normal result in patients who are hyperthyroid. Difficulties also arise in the group of patients in whom TSH levels lie between 0.01 mU/l and 0.1 mU/l, in whom there is no clinical evidence of hyperthyroidism. These patients may have conditions such as euthyroid multinodular goitre, ophthalmic Graves' disease, or a solitary autonomous nodule. In rare patients in whom mild clinical evidence of hyperthyroidism is accompanied by a modest elevation in TSH confirmed by a different assay technique, the failure of the TSH to respond to TRH administration suggests a TSH-producing tumour. A disproportionate increase in the concentration of the TSH α-subunit as compared with the β-subunit provides further evidence of a likely pituitary tumour.

The assessment of the basal TSH level and its increase 20 min after the intravenous administration of 200 μg of TRH (the TRH stimulation test), was once used to establish both intrinsic TSH secretory reserve and the extent to which this was inhibited by thyroid hormones. The increased sensitivity of assays for TSH has largely replaced this test, which now has a limited role. In patients with hypothyroidism of thyroid origin (primary hypothyroidism) an increased basal serum TSH level in conjunction with clinical evidence of hypothyroidism and low free thyroid hormone levels makes the TRH test unnecessary. In contrast, in patients in whom there is clinical evidence of hypothyroidism with low plasma concentrations of T_4, the absence of an increase in basal serum TSH level suggests damage to the hypothalamic–pituitary axis (secondary hypothyroidism); then an absent, subnormal, or delayed response to TRH confirms such a diagnosis. When hyperthyroidism is suspected clinically and free thyroid hormone levels are equivocal, a sensitive TSH measurement may lie between 0.01 and 0.1 mU/l. The TSH response to TRH may then be subnormal or absent, and this is seen particularly in patients with solitary autonomous nodules, euthyroid Graves' disease

Table 4 *Autoantigens in autoimmune thyroid disease*

	Thyroglobulin	Thyroid peroxidase	Thyroid stimulating hormone receptor
Protein	Iodinated glycoprotein	Haemoprotein enzyme	G-binding protein-linked receptor
Glycosylated	+	+	+
Function	Biosynthetic precursor of T_3 and T_4	Catalyses iodination and coupling of tyrosine to yield T_3 and T_4	Receptor for TSH
Thyroid location	Follicular lumen Circulation	Membrane-bound cell surface (apical) Exo/endocytotic vesicles	Membrane-bound cell surface (basal)
Molecular weight	660 000	105 000; 110 000	86 000
Amino acids	2748	TPO-1 933; TPO-2 876 Alternatively spliced products	764 (excludes 20aa signal sequence)
Regions	–		
extracellular	–	842 (TPO-1)	418
transmembrane	–	29	265 (seven transmembrane domains)
intracellular	–	62	81
Chromosome location	8	2	14
Homologies	Acetylcholinesterase	Myeloperoxidase	LH/hCG, FSH receptors

FSH, follicle stimulating hormone; hCG, human chorionic gonadotrophin; LH, luteinizing hormone; TSH, thyroid stimulating hormone.

with ophthalmopathy, patients with treated hyperthyroid Graves' disease and some of their relatives, a significant number of patients with multinodular goitre, and many patients receiving replacement or suppressive therapy with exogenous thyroid hormone. In this grey area, clinical judgement ultimately determines the appropriate management.

Peripheral effects of thyroid hormones

In theory a good test of whether a patient's tissues are being exposed to too much or too little thyroid hormone would not be a measurement of circulating hormone concentrations but rather a measure of the direct effects of thyroid hormones on peripheral tissues. Unfortunately no simple, reproducible, specific, and sensitive test of such effects is available. Such a measure, would be of particular value in patients without clinical and biochemical evidence of hyperthyroidism but in whom a subnormal TSH or an absent TSH response to TRH suggests subnormal thyroid function. In this group of patients two subgroups can be discriminated: those in whom the decision concerns whether or not treatment of subclinical hypothyroidism might result in benefit, and, in contrast, those on replacement thyroxine in whom concerns about over treatment could then be more directly addressed. Further groups of patients in whom such an approach might contribute to management are those presenting with mild hypothyroidism in whom biochemical parameters have not been decisively helpful, others with thyroid hormone resistance, and those with non-thyroidal illness (the sick euthyroid syndrome). In these settings the best established and validated (but also most cumbersome) investigation is the basal metabolic rate; the calorigenic effect of thyroid hormones increases energy expenditure and heat production. Since heat production cannot be measured directly, the test measures oxygen consumption converted into an energy equivalent and then related to body surface area. Other tests make use of the relationship between muscle relaxation after a contraction and thyroid status by measuring the speed of relaxation of the Achilles tendon reflex, which is prolonged in hypothyroidism and shortened in hyperthyroidism. Tests of myocardial contractility have also been developed and the best validated is the measurement of the interval between the initiation of the QRS complex on the electrocardiogram and the arrival of the pulse wave in the brachial artery at diastolic pressure (QKd). This is shortened in hyperthyroidism and prolonged in hypothyroidism. All three of these measures are altered by a number of non-thyroidal states, so that they can only be interpreted with circumspection. The serum cholesterol is usually elevated in hypothyroidism and decreased in hyperthyroidism and the serum creatinine phosphokinase may be increased in the hypothyroid state. It is suggested that absent serum sex hormone binding globulin and absent serum ferritin responses to administered thyroxine are likely to be associated with generalized resistance to thyroid hormone.

Thyroid autoantibodies

In areas of the world where iodine intake is adequate the commonest cause of altered thyroid function is autoimmune thyroid disease. This group of diseases spans a spectrum which ranges from clinically and biochemically overt hyperthyroidism to clinically and biochemically overt hypothyroidism. Within the spectrum are included euthyroid situations such as euthyroid Graves' disease with ophthalmopathy, transient syndromes of altered thyroid function such as occur in the postpartum period (postpartum thyroid dysfunction), and transient syndromes of altered thyroid function in neonates. The commonest cause of hyperthyroidism is Graves' disease which is due to antibodies which bind to the thyroid follicular cell TSH receptor and stimulate thyroid function (TSH receptor antibodies). Goitrous (Hashimoto's thyroiditis) and atrophic (primary myxoedema) thyroiditis are the commonest causes of hypothyroidism in areas of adequate iodine intake. Thyroid destruction in these diseases is predominantly the result of cell-mediated mechanisms, but antibodies to the thyroid biosynthetic enzyme thyroid peroxidase, and antibodies that bind the TSH receptor without stimulating it, and thus block receptor occupancy by TSH (TSH receptor blocking antibodies), may well have a role in contributing to their pathogenesis. It seems highly unlikely, particularly in humans, that antibodies to thyroglobulin have any role in the pathogenesis of autoimmune thyroid disease. All three of the putative target autoantigens have been characterized at the molecular level (Table 4).

THYROGLOBULIN ANTIBODIES

These autoantibodies were the first to be recognized in autoimmune thyroid diseases. The original haemogglutination assays have now been replaced by more sensitive and specific enzyme-linked and radio-immunoassays. The enzyme-linked assay reveals antibody in 80 per cent of patients with autoimmune thyroiditis, irrespective of whether it is goitrous or atrophic, and in some 35 per cent of patients with newly diagnosed hyperthyroid Graves' disease.

THYROID PEROXIDASE ANTIBODIES

The molecular characterization of thyroid peroxidase has led to the recognition that almost all of the microsomal antigenic determinants recognized by autoantibodies in patients with autoimmune thyroid disorders are directed towards this enzyme. Molecular biology has also led to an appropriate improvement in the sensitivity and specificity of assay systems for these antibodies, having progressed from haemogglutination techniques to enzyme-linked and radio-immunoassays which now use affinity purified or recombinant thyroid peroxidase. These modern assay systems reveal peroxidase antibodies in almost all those with autoimmune thyroid disease at some stage in the disease process.

THYROID STIMULATING HORMONE RECEPTOR ANTIBODIES

Historically, difficulties in measuring this antibody activity, either because of problems in obtaining sufficiently pure TSH receptor or because of the need to use cumbersome biological assays, has meant that measurement has been largely a research tool in a few specialized laboratories. The molecular characterization of the TSH receptor is already leading to larger quantities of pure receptor or the development of assay systems in which recombinant TSH receptor preparations are being used in immunoassays or in transfected cells in bioassays for the measurement either of the quantitative or functional assessment of this antibody activity. There are now two distinct approaches to the assay of these antibodies. In the radioreceptor technique, antibody activity is measured by the degree of inhibition of the binding of radiolabelled TSH to preparations of thyroid membrane or of purified TSH receptors. This method gives no indication of the functional nature of the antibody. The other techniques involve an assessment of the biological activity of TSH measured by the ability of the antibodies to stimulate thyroid cells by binding to TSH receptors on a variety of preparations, including primary cell cultures, cell lines (FRTL5 rat cells), or cells transfected with the human recombinant TSH receptor; the measurement of cell activation is then most easily assessed by the generation cAMP. TSH receptor antibodies are present in all patients with hyperthyroid Graves' disease prior to treatment. Other systems allow the detection of antibodies that block function. These can be shown by their pre-incubation with thyroid cells, resulting in inhibition of the subsequent binding of TSH to these cells and therefore of the resultant stimulation of cAMP production.

All three of these types of antibody measurement provide evidence of autoimmune disease. Since antibodies to thyroid peroxidase are present in almost all patients with such disorders they provide all the information needed by the clinician suspecting altered thyroid function to be due to autoimmune disease. Easier access to measurements of TSH receptor antibody activity will provide information on the pathogenesis of atrophic thyroiditis in patients with primary myxoedema, among whom this antibody activity may contribute to the development of thyroid failure in up to 30 per cent of patients. Of greater importance is the recognition that since TSH receptor antibodies, which are predominantly of the IgG1 subclass of immunoglobulins, cross the placenta, babies born to mothers with high enough levels of this antibody activity are at risk of either developing transient neonatal hyper- or hypothyroidism, depending on the type of antibody in the maternal circulation and its passage across the placenta. The ability to measure this antibody activity easily in the third trimester of pregnancy provides paediatricians caring for the neonate in the postpartum period with early warning of potential alteration in thyroid function in the offspring.

Disorders of the thyroid

Introduction

Patients presenting with disorders of the thyroid may present with symptoms which relate to hyperthyroidism, hypothyroidism, to enlargement of the gland, and/or to the complications of Graves' disease such as ophthalmopathy or, more rarely, of dermopathy (pretibial myxoedema). Local symptoms include pain or compression of adjacent structures. A careful history and physical examination allow assessment both of the

functional state of the gland and of its size, consistency, position, and relationship to adjacent structures. Evidence of possible exposure to ionizing radiation, of iodide ingestion in the form of food preparations, such as those derived from seaweed, or of iodine-containing medications, such as amiodarone, is of considerable importance. Other agents (e.g. lithium carbonate) may affect thyroid function other than by way of iodine content. In large areas of the world low dietary iodide intake is common and leads to iodine deficiency goitre (endemic goitre). A family history of goitre, altered thyroid function, and a personal and family history of other organ-specific autoimmune diseases may be helpful, since the autoimmune thyroid diseases occur more commonly in association with the other organ-specific autoimmune diseases in both patients and their families. Of particular importance are histories of insulin-dependent diabetes, pernicious anaemia, vitiligo, and myasthenia gravis.

Examination of the neck in order to assess the thyroid should be performed while standing behind the patient and palpating with the fingertips of both hands. Having identified the cricoid cartilage, the isthmus of the thyroid should be identifiable just below it. The extent of the thyroid gland is then assessed by determining the lower borders of the lateral lobes and the rest of the outline of the gland. This process can be enhanced by inviting the patient to swallow sips of water at regular intervals during the procedure with the physician palpating the gland as it moves up and down in the neck in response to swallowing. It is important not only to assess the size and consistency of the gland but also the presence or absence of nodules within it. The normal thyroid is more difficult to feel in the male. A record should be made of the size of the gland, its consistency, the presence or absence of nodules, whether the enlargement is diffuse or nodular and the size of individual nodules. The thyroid may be tender or, rarely, exceedingly painful to touch. A search should be made of the neck for enlarged local lymph nodes. Auscultation over the thyroid in patients with hyperthyroidism may, as a result of the increased vascularity of the gland, produce an audible bruit. A thyroglossal cyst is a midline structure attached to the base of the tongue, which on protrusion of the tongue moves upwards. Transillumination of large nodules within the thyroid may allow the discrimination between a solid and cystic mass. If palpation of the neck fails to reveal a thyroid gland in the expected position there may be a retrosternal goitre; elevation of the arms above the head may then cause venous obstruction by further compromising the thoracic inlet so causing facial congestion and in addition respiratory distress (Pemberton's sign). Displacement of the trachea and inspiratory stridor may also be signs indicating compression of the trachea by retrosternal goitre or of a goitre extending retrosternally. Hoarseness of the voice requires consideration of possible involvement of the recurrent laryngeal nerve, most usually by a malignant thyroid lesion.

Thyroid hormone excess

Thyrotoxicosis is the clinical syndrome that results when tissues are exposed to high levels of circulating thyroid hormone. In most instances this situation arises as a result of hyperactivity of the thyroid gland (hyperthyroidism). Rarely the syndrome is due to other causes, such as the excessive ingestion of thyroid hormone, but since these are so uncommon the terms hyperthyroidism and thyrotoxicosis are used interchangeably. A number of conditions lead to the development of hyperthyroidism (Table 5). The prevalence of this disorder is approximately 20 per 1000 in females and 2 per 1000 in males. The presentation of the disease depends on its severity, duration, aetiology, age of the patient, and the presence or absence of disease in other organs. It may present gradually, which is usual, or acutely.

PRESENTATION

Patients can present with a wide variety of symptoms and accompanying physical signs (Table 6). Confirmation of the diagnosis requires laboratory assessment. Hyperthyroidism is indicated by elevated concentrations of free or total T_4 and T_3 in the presence of an undetectable level of TSH. Uncommonly, T_3 values are elevated despite normal T_4 values (T3 toxicosis). In interpreting the results of thyroid function tests a number of considerations need to be borne in mind (see above). The presence of thyroid autoantibodies in conjunction with a diffuse goitre, and evidence of increased uptake in an isotope scan makes the cause of the hyperthyroidism almost certainly due to Graves' disease. A radioisotope scan also allows the demonstration of a solitary toxic nodule or of a toxic mutlinodular goitre. In these last two situations thyroid autoantibodies will not be detected. These three disease states make up over 95 per cent of all cases of hyperthyroidism presenting in a specialized endocrine clinic in the United Kingdom.

GRAVES' DISEASE

Graves' disease is the most common cause of hyperthyroidism (75 per cent of all cases in the United Kingdom). The disease is characterized by a diffusely enlarged thyroid gland, hyperthyroidism, ophthalmopathy (Table 7), and, uncommonly, dermopathy (pretibial myxoedema). The exact aetiology of the condition remains unknown, but it is an organ-specific autoimmune disease with a strong familial predisposition, occurring much more commonly in females and with a peak incidence between the ages of 20 and 40 years. It is associated with other organ-specific autoimmune diseases and is characterized by associations with particular major histocompatibility complex (HLA) antigens, with different associations being reported for different racial groups. Lymphocytic infiltration of the thyroid gland is a hallmark of the autoimmune process. The disease is assumed to be multifactorial in origin, with perhaps an infectious insult leading to its development in genetically susceptible individuals. In addition to a possible infectious aetiology, a number of environmental factors clearly influence the development of the disease, including iodine ingestion. If there is uncertainty about the nature of these precipitating factors, the pathogenetic process finally leading to hyperthyroidism is no longer in doubt. This depends on the presence of antibodies directed against the thyroid follicular cell surface membrane TSH receptor; they are usually of the IgG1 subclass and in binding to the TSH receptor activate the adenylate cyclase system, and thus stimulate thyroid function *in vitro* and *in vivo*. The levels of antibody correlate with thyroid function, and in humans the innoculation *in vivo* with purified antibody preparations leads to increased thyroid activation; and, in the offspring of mothers with high levels of antibodies, passage of these antibodies across the placenta leads to transient neonatal hyperthyroidism.

TOXIC MULTINODULAR GOITRE

Hyperthyroidism in this setting usually occurs in an older age group with a long-standing multinodular goitre. Hyperthyroidism may be precipitated by the administration of iodides. The gland itself is characterized by structural and functional heterogeneity and functional autonomy. Thyroid hormone overproduction is usually much less marked than occurs in Graves' disease, so that the clinical presentation is less dramatic. Although thyroid function tests will allow the demonstration of definite biochemical hyperthyroidism, a subgroup of patients with TSH levels between 0.01 and 0.1 mU/l are defined as having thyroid autonomy without hyperthyroidism.

TOXIC SOLITARY ADENOMA

Less than 2 per cent of patients presenting with hyperthyroidism are found to have a solitary toxic adenoma as the cause. Unlike toxic multinodular goitres, these solitary nodules occur in a younger age group, usually in patients in their 30s and 40s. The disorders is usually caused by a single palpable nodule. Laboratory investigation depends on the stage of the disease. At first the only evidence of abnormality may be borderline suppression of the serum TSH level. Later a thyroid scan will demonstrate localization of radio-isotope to the nodule, with suppression

Table 5 *Causes of hyperthyroidism*

Common
Graves' disease (diffuse toxic goitre)
Toxic multinodular goitre
Toxic solitary adenoma
Thyroiditis
sub-acute, viral, de Quervain's
silent, painless
postpartum
Uncommon
Hyperthyroid phase of Hashimoto's thyroiditis
Neonatal hyperthyroidism
Iodine-induced
Thyrotoxicosis factitia
Hydatidiform mole, choriocarcinoma
TSH-secreting pituitary adenoma
Metastatic thyroid carcinoma (follicular)
Struma ovarii (thyroid-tissue-containing teratoma)

Table 6 *Clinical features associated with hyperthyroidism*

General	Neuromuscular
Heat intolerance	Fatiguability
Sweating	Restlessness
Fatigue	Muscle weakness—proximal
Apathy	Choreoathetosis
Tremor	Hypokalaemic periodic
Diffuse goitre*	paralysis
Nodular goitre	Myasthenia gravis*
Cardiovascular	Psychiatric
Palpitation	Irritability
Dyspnoea	Nervousness
Angina	Agitation
Tachycardia	Emotional lability
Atrial fibrillation	Psychosis
Heart failure	Dermatological
Gastrointestinal	Pruritus
Weight loss despite	Palmar erythema
↑ appetite	Pretibial myxoedema*
Diarrhoea, steatorrhoea	Hair thinning
Vomiting	Onycholysis
	Vitiligo*
Genitourinary	Acropachy*
Polyuria and	
polydipsia	Ocular
Amenorrhoea	Lid lag/lid retraction
Infertility	Ophthalmopathy*

*Symptoms and signs which may occur in patients with Graves' disease

Table 7 *American Thyroid Association abridged classification of the eye changes (ophthalmopathy) associated with Graves' disease*

Class	Definition*
0	No physical symptoms or signs
1	Only signs (upper lid retraction, stare, lid lag, proptosis to 22 mm)
2	Soft tissue involvement (symptoms and signs)
3	Proptosis > 22 mm
4	Extraocular muscle involvement
5	Corneal involvement
6	Sight loss (optic nerve involvement)

*Initial letters of the definitions provide a useful mnemonic 'NO SPECS'.

of uptake by the surrounding normal thyroid. Plasma concentrations of T_3 and T_4 will be increased. Histologically these lesions are almost always benign follicular adenomas.

THYROIDITIS

Subacute thyroiditis, also known as granulomatous giant cell or de Quervain's thyroiditis, is due to a viral infection of the thyroid gland, often following an upper respiratory infection. The disease is uncommon and may be mistakenly diagnosed as pharyngitis. Mononuclear cell infiltration of follicles with follicular disruption and loss of colloid are characteristic and may be confused with autoimmune thyroiditis. In contrast to the classical autoimmune histology is the presence of multinucleate giant cells. Colloid may be present within these or leak into the interstitium. The follicular changes progress to granuloma formation. Follicular destruction leads to the release of the preformed hormone, often with clinical and biochemical evidence of hyperthyroidism. The radioactive iodine uptake is low and new thyroid hormone synthesis is impaired.

Once stores of preformed hormone are depleted, clinical and biochemical evidence of hypothyroidism may follow. Ultimately thyroid function returns to normal. Associated with the changes occurring in the thyroid the characteristic clinical presentation is with pain in the thyroid which may be accompanied by a fever. The pain may be excruciating and some enlargement of the gland occurs. The erythrocyte sedimentation rate is markedly elevated during the active phase of the disease.

Hyperthyroidism may also occur in painless or so-called 'silent' thyroiditis, when biopsy reveals histological evidence of lymphocytic rather than of subacute thyroiditis; it is important to remember, however, that subacute thyroiditis can also be painless. As with the subacute viral disease, silent thyroiditis is associated with a markedly decreased radioactive iodine uptake in the absence of excess iodide intake and with a transient hyperthyroid phase followed by a period of transient hypothyroidism. The thyroid may be enlarged during the disease but is not tender to touch. The disease is almost certainly autoimmune in origin, with the characteristic lymphocytic infiltration of the gland, the presence of antithyroid antibodies and HLA associations (at least in the postpartum variant of this syndrome) similar to those observed in autoimmune thyroid disease.

OTHER CAUSES OF THYROID HORMONE EXCESS

A hydatidiform mole or a choriocarcinoma can stimulate thyroid function as a result of the high levels of human chorionic gonadotropin secreted by the tumour. Clinical and biochemical evidence of thyroid overactivity in conjunction with a normal or elevated level of TSH suggest the possibility of a TSH-secreting pituitary adenoma. Although these patients may have a diffuse, hyperfunctioning goitre, the absence of any features of autoimmune thyroid disease, the presence of a mass in the pituitary fossa, the elevated concentration of free TSH α-subunits, and the failure of TSH to respond to TRH suggest the likelihood of a tumour secreting TSH. In a rarer group of patients, biochemical evidence of hyperthyroidism is due to resistance to thyroid hormone and is associated, if anything, with tissue deficiency rather than excess of thyroid hormone; this problem is addressed later. The ingestion of iodine can lead to iodine-induced hyperthyroidism, particularly in patients with autonomously functioning thyroid nodules. Assessment of radioactive iodine uptake will demonstrate this to be low and urinary iodine excretion is greatly increased. Less commonly, even normal individuals given large doses of iodine may develop iodine-induced hyperthyroidism.

Epidemics of exogenous thyrotoxicosis can occur when large quantities of animal thyroid tissue, for example from beef, are used in the preparation of hamburgers. The surreptitious ingestion of excessive quantities of thyroid hormone (thyrotoxicosis factitia) characteristically occurs in individuals with an underlying psychiatric background and usually with some medical knowledge and access to such preparations.

Table 8 *Causes of euthyroid hyperthyroxinaemia*

Increased thyroxine-binding globulin concentration
Familial dysalbuminaemic hyperthyroxinaemia
Increased T_4 binding to thyroxine-binding prealbumin or anti-T_4 antibodies
Thyroid hormone resistance
Non-thyroidal illness (sick euthyroid)
Acute psychiatric illness
Hyperemesis gravidarum
Medication, e.g. amiodarone
Exogenous T_4 administration

In both of the latter situations, a radioactive iodine uptake assessment of the thyroid shows absence or reduced uptake of the isotope.

It is important to be aware of situations in which T_4 levels are elevated in the absence of clinical evidence of hyperthyroidism (Table 8).

TREATMENT

Despite the considerable progress that has been made in understanding the pathogenesis of Graves' disease, little change has been made in the standard methods long available for management of the disease. These are still directed towards controlling the hyperthyroidism either by inhibiting thyroid hormone synthesis and release by means of antithyroid drugs or by reducing the bulk of the thyroid tissue which is overproducing thyroid hormone, by either partial thyroidectomy or radioiodine administration.

Antithyroid drugs

The major group of drugs used for the treatment of hyperthyroidism are the thionamides. Carbimazole is the most widely used of these compounds in the United Kingdom whereas in the United States propylthiouracil or methimazole, the active metabolite of carbimazole, are the agents of choice. They all inhibit both oxidation and organification, thus leading to a state of intrathyroidal iodine deficiency and inhibition of thyroid hormone synthesis. In addition, propylthiouracil inhibits the conversion of T_4 to T_3 in the periphery. All these compounds are weakly immunosuppressive and this effect may contribute to the control of Graves' disease by reducing the levels of TSH receptor antibodies. Carbimazole is usually begun at a dose of 40 mg daily and this can be given as two 20 mg tablets once daily. Since these agents inhibit the synthesis but not the release of thyroid hormone, a reduction in secretion does not occur immediately but only after glandular stores have been depleted. Patients begin to feel better and there is improvement in thyroid function by 4 to 8 weeks after commencing therapy. Subsequent management is either by 'titration' of the dose of carbimazole against the clinical and biochemical response, which requires fairly frequent reassessment of the patient; alternatively a blocking and replacement regimen can be used, in which carbimazole is maintained at a dose of 40 mg once daily with thyroxine (50–150 µg/day) being added once thyroid function is under control. There is evidence to suggest that maintaining a high dose of carbimazole in this way may contribute to controlling the disease by having the greatest effect on the autoimmune process, in addition to its effects on thyroid hormone synthesis. Importantly, once a patient is stabilized on such a regimen the need for regular follow-up is considerably decreased. Traditionally in Europe, patients presenting with the first episode of hyperthyroid Graves' disease under the age of 40 years have been treated with a course of antithyroid drugs. Following such treatment with carbimazole in a blocking and replacement regimen for 6 to 12 months, between a third and half the patients achieve lasting remission. Factors that predict the likelihood of long-term remission at the end of a course of drug therapy are a small goitre, a decrease in goitre size during treatment, a normal serum TSH level and disappearance of TSH receptor antibody activity from the serum. Patterns of subsequent management of those who relapse are changing; in Europe in particular, and in the United Kingdom to a lesser extent, partial thyroidectomy was once the treatment of choice for those under the age of 40, particularly if there were concerns about ophthalmopathy or if the patient had a large goitre. There is now more widespread use of radio-iodine, irrespective of the patient's age, as has been long-standing common practice in the United States.

All the thionamides produce similar side-effects. The most common is an itchy maculopapular skin rash, occurring in up to 5 per cent of patients. Although it may settle spontaneously, should this fail to occur it is worth trying to switch from carbimazole to propylthiouracil or vice versa. Other less common adverse reactions include arthralgia, myalgia, neuritis, hepatitis, thrombocytopenia, nausea and vomiting, lymphadenopathy, and fever. All of these may resolve spontaneously or after changing treatment to another thionamide, but it is often better to proceed to surgery or radio-iodine treatment. The most important ill-effect of these agents is agranulocytosis, which is seen in less than 1 per cent of patients. It tends to occur early in the course of treatment and is accompanied by fever, sore throat, mouth ulcers, and other evidence of infection. Patients should be advised of this rare but serious complication and, should these symptoms develop, they should discontinue the drug immediately and seek medical advice urgently. Agranulocytosis occurs rapidly but recovers provided that the drug is stopped quickly. Any patient who has developed this complication should not be treated with a thionamide again.

Partial thyroidectomy

Surgery is exceedingly effective in relieving hyperthyroidism. In the hands of a skilled thyroid surgeon mortality and morbidity is exceedingly low. Patients should be made euthyroid prior to surgery and this can be achieved by the use of carbimazole for at least 2 to 3 months before the operation and by the addition of Lugol's solution (0.1–0.3 ml three times a day) for 10 days immediately prior to the operation. One-year follow-up figures suggest that 80 per cent of patients are euthyroid, about 15 per cent have developed hypothyroidism, and 5 per cent have relapsed. Less than 1 per cent develop hypoparathyroidism or damage to the recurrent laryngeal nerve. With longer follow-up, up to half the patients may go on to develop hypothyroidism, particularly those who had high levels of antithyroid peroxidase antibody prior to treatment. Transient hypothyroidism following surgery is not uncommon and thyroxine replacement should be withheld until the physician is confident that the patient is indeed permanently hypothyroid. The only other important complication of surgery is bleeding into the operative site and, although this is exceedingly rare, it can be rapidly fatal because of asphyxia if not recognized and treated urgently.

Radio-iodine

Radio-iodine is simple and cheap and achieves the same ends as does surgery without the costs and complications associated with partial thyroidectomy. It achieves its effect via the radiation-induced destruction of thyroid follicular cells. An acute inflammatory response in the thyroid with follicular cell death is followed by fibrosis, vascular narrowing, and lymphocytic infiltration. The principal long-term consequence of radio-iodine therapy is hypothyroidism, which occurs in most patients despite all efforts to titrate the dose against various parameters of thyroid function, size, or iodine uptake. Historically the major concern was that this therapy might lead to thyroid malignancy, leukaemia, or teratogenic effects. Long-term follow up over a number of years has failed to provide any evidence that there is any increased risk of any of these three possible side-effects. It is against this background that the move, particularly in the United States, has been to reduce the age limit for giving radio-iodine from 40, so that in some centres radio-iodine is now used for children and adolescents. Side-effects from the administration of radio-iodine are minimal and uncommon. Transient soreness over the thyroid may occur. Ill effects of radiation to the parathyroids, particularly at higher dosage, has rarely been reported to lead to clinically overt

hypoparathyroidism. In patients with severe hyperthyroidism, thyrotoxic crisis has been reported to occur following radio-iodine, so glandular hormone stores of such patients should be depleted by administration of antithyroid drugs for several weeks before radio-iodine. Carbimazole should be withdrawn 5 days before the dose of radio-iodine, and can be given again a few days after it, if indicated. Pregnancy is an absolute contraindication to radio-iodine, and should be avoided until 6 months after the last dose, because of the effects on the fetal thyroid. With the failure to develop measures for determining the appropriate dose of radio-iodine in the United Kingdom, doses are now given on a fairly arbitrary basis in a range between about 185 and 555 MBq orally. Good control of thyroid function is unlikely for some 2 to 3 months after the dose, so it is often necessary to prescribe carbimazole or a β-blocker for this short time. Failure to control the disease with a first dose of radio-iodine may require the administration of a second one 6 months later. Long-term follow-up is essential because of the ultimate development of hypothyroidism in almost all patients. An alternative approach, which has the advantage of making such follow-up unnecessary, is to seek to achieve thyroid ablation initially with a large enough dose of radio-iodine to ensure that hypothyroidism is induced early. Patients can then be treated with thyroxine replacement and need not be followed thereafter.

β-Blockers

These agents are effective in resolving some of the peripheral manifestations of hyperthyroidism such as tremor, palpitation, sweating, and tachycardia. They work rapidly if an adequate dose is given. Although they are not a main-line therapy for patients with hyperthyroidism, they may serve as a useful adjunct at the start of treatment with thionamides or following radio-iodine, i.e. in situations where they may help to control peripheral manifestations of hyperthyroidism before antithyroid treatment becomes effective. Propranolol can be used in a dose of 40 to 80 mg by mouth every 8 h. It is clearly contraindicated in patients with asthma or with congestive cardiac failure.

The management of hyperthyroidism without the features of Graves' disease varies with the cause of the hyperthyroidism. In those with toxic multinodular goitre the only indication for antithyroid drugs is the presence of severe hyperthyroidism, when the disease is best controlled with antithyroid drugs before definitive treatment is administered. The treatment of choice is radio-iodine and when antithyroid drugs have been used, these should be stopped 5 days before the radio-iodine is given. Larger doses of radio-iodine may need to be given than those used in Graves' disease (555–1100 MBq). Surgery is indicated in patients with large goitres, particularly in those in whom there is concern about obstructive features or where it is feared that these might develop following radio-iodine treatment. In patients with solitary toxic adenomas the treatment of choice is again radio-iodine, with the same alternative available as for a toxic multinodular goitre if the disease is severe or the nodule particularly large. Unlike the situation in patients with multinodular goitres, doses of radio-iodine similar to those used in Graves' disease are often adequate. The ultimate risk of hypothyroidism in patients with nodular goitres following radio-iodine is much lower than that in Graves' disease.

In patients with subacute thyroiditis, aspirin may be all that is required to control the symptoms, although in more severe cases glucocorticoids may be of benefit. Neither of these two therapies influences the disease process. Uncommonly, antithyroid drugs may be indicated if the hyperthyroid phase induces marked clinical disease. In patients with molar pregnancies, the treatment is to remove the lesion, and the same applies to pituitary tumours secreting TSH. Iodine-induced hyperthyroidism is often difficult to manage. Even after discontinuation of the exogenous source of iodide, if this is possible (and it may not be, for example in patients taking amiodarone), the uptake of radio-iodine by the thyroid gland remains low and usually not sufficient for a conventional dose to be effective in controlling the hyperthyroidism. Control may be achieved with large doses of antithyroid drugs given for 6 to 9 months. It has also been suggested that the addition of 750 mg of sodium perchlorate, which inhibits the thyroid iodide trap, in combination with an antithyroid drug, results in a more rapid control of the hyperthyroidism.

THYROTOXIC CRISIS

Thyrotoxic crisis or thyroid storm is a rare but serious complication most commonly occurring in patients with Graves' disease, when it is a manifestation of the severity of the hyperthyroidism. Its onset is often abrupt and it occurs in patients whose hyperthyroidism has either been treated inadequately or not at all. Often it is precipitated by factors such as infection, trauma, following radio-iodine treatment, and childbirth. The patient is markedly hypermetabolic, with fever, profuse sweating, and marked tachycardia, which may progress to congestive cardiac failure and pulmonary oedema. The patient is restless with a marked tremor and may develop delirium or frank psychosis; further progression to coma may result. Nausea, vomiting, and abdominal pain are often present, as is hypotension. Unrecognized, the condition is fatal. The aim of treatment is to control the hyperthyroidism and the underlying cause of the precipitated crisis. In controlling the severe hyperthyroidism there is a need both to inhibit hormone synthesis and release and to block adrenergically mediated effects of thyroid hormones. Large doses of carbimazole (up to 60 mg a day, if necessary by nasograstric tube) should be used, and propylthiouracil at doses of 300 to 400 mg every 4 h may be preferable because of its additional effects in inhibiting the peripheral conversion of T_4 to T_3. In the absence of evidence of cardiac insufficiency, propranolol at doses up to 80 mg every 6 h can be given orally. The most urgent requirement is to administer iodine in order to block acutely the release of thyroid hormones from the thyroid. This is best given after the administration of the antithyroid drug, so that the latter is present to inhibit the synthesis of new thyroid hormone from the iodine load. Lugol's solution is given at a dose of 5 drops every 6 h. Additionally, large doses of dexamethasone (2 mg orally every 6 h) are given, both to provide glucocorticoids in a time of crisis and because dexamethasone inhibits hormone release from the thyroid and the peripheral conversion of T_4 to T_3. Coupled with these medications, correction of hydration and of any other metabolic anomalies is essential. Separate manoeuvres may need to be directed at lowering the body temperature, although salicylates should be avoided because, by competing with thyroid hormones for sites on binding proteins, they increase the free hormone concentration.

GRAVES' OPHTHALMOPATHY

Patients with Graves' disease frequently develop ophthalmopathy, which usually occurs within 12 months of the onset of their hyperthyroidism but less commonly may precede or accompany the onset of the disease. On rarer occasions, it is seen in patients who have never been clinically hyperthyroid and even in some who present with hypothyroidism. The pathogenesis remains uncertain. Some observations suggest that it is mediated by an autoimmune process directed primarily at the orbital extraocular muscles. The presence and severity of the eye disease both appear to be associated with cigarette smoking. Patients present with a number of symptoms, including pain, watering of the eyes, photophobia, and blurred or double vision. A variety of physical signs are associated with the disease, including proptosis, lid retraction and lid lag, periorbital oedema, extraocular muscle functional impairment, conjuctival oedema and injection, exposure keratitis, which may lead to corneal ulceration, visual field defects, impaired visual acuity, and papilloedema. When there is doubt about the diagnosis, ultrasound or a CT of the orbits reveals the characteristic enlargement of the extraocular muscles, with the medial and inferior rectus being those most usually involved by the process. Since hypothyroidism has an adverse effect on ophthalmopathy, management of hyperthyroid Graves' disease should be designed to ensure that hypothyroidism does not develop and, if it does, is recognized early and treated appropriately. In most patients symptoms of ophthalmopathy are mild and require no treatment, beyond

Table 9 *Causes of hypothyroidism*

Primary
    Lymphocytic (autoimmune) thyroiditis
        Hashimoto's (goitrous) thyroiditis
        Atrophic thyroiditis; primary myxoedema
        Postpartum thyroid dysfunction
        Silent, painless thyroiditis
    Iatrogenic (for hyperthyroidism)
        Post-radio-iodine
        Following partial thyroidectomy
        Antithyroid drugs
    Non-thyroidal medication
        Lithium
        Amiodarone
    Iodine excess
    Iodine deficiency (endemic goitre)
    Congenital (sporadic)
        Thyroid agenesis
        Thyroid maldescent
        Dyshormonogenesis
    Riedel's thyroiditis
Secondary
        Hypothalamic–pituitary disease/damage
Peripheral resistance to thyroid hormone

advice about wearing protective glasses against bright lights, wind, or cold air. Elevation of the head of the bed at night and the use of conjunctival lubricants such as 1 per cent methylcellulose may be of benefit if there is incomplete closure of the eyelids when sleeping. When the disease progresses, the major therapies are designed either to reduce the volume of the orbital soft tissues medically or to expand the space within which the soft tissues and the globes sit, by surgically decompressing the orbit. High-dose steroids, with or without cyclosporin, have been effective in controlling the disease but both these medications carry with them significant side-effects. Dexamethasone, 4 mg 6 hourly initially, reducing by 4 mg every 48 h until the total daily dose is 4 mg is a reasonable regimen during the first week. Thereafter transfer on to prednisolone and its very gradual reduction is necessary. The addition of cyclosporin may improve results; the standard starting dose is 10 mg/kg body weight continued for some 3 to 10 months. External radiation to the orbits in conjunction with corticosteroids is more effective than radiotherapy alone, and is particularly effective in treating relatively acute disease. Where glucocorticoids alone or in conjunction with external radiation fail to halt the progression of the disease, and particularly if loss of vision is threatened, due to damage to the cornea or the optic nerve, orbital decompression is the only alternative. A number of different surgical approaches are used. Although this procedure will relieve the acute situation and allow considerable regression of proptosis, once the disease process settles there is often a need for surgical correction of the resulting extraocular muscle dysfunction.

Thyroid hormone deficiency

Hypothyroidism is the clinical presentation which results from structural or functional abnormalities of the thyroid leading to thyroid hormone deficiency. The causes of hypothyroidism (Table 9) can be classified into those resulting from thyroid disease (primary hypothyroidism) or those resulting from disease of the hypothalamic–pituitary axis (secondary hypothyroidism). The onset may be insidious and the symptoms and signs reflect the fact that thyroid hormone deficiency affects every tissue in the body (Table 10).

PRESENTATION

In the newborn presenting with sporadic cretinism, hypothyroidism may be difficult to detect by clinical examination. An increased birth weight

Table 10 *Clinical features associated with hypothyroidism in the adult*

General	Mental state
Lethargy	Mental slowing
Easy fatiguability	Inability to concentrate
Weight gain	Poor memory
Cold intolerance	Hypersomnolence
Pallor or yellow skin	Depression
Goitre	Psychosis (myxoedema
Hyperlipidaemia	madness)
Puffy face and hands	
	Neuromuscular
Cardiovascular	Weakness
Angina	Muscle cramps
Bradycardia	Paraesthesiae
Cardiac failure	Hoarseness
Pleural effusion	Deafness
Pericardial effusion	Cerebellar ataxia
Low voltage complexes	Delayed reflexes
(ECG)	Entrapment neuropathies
Gastrointestinal	Haematological
Constipation	Anaemia-iron or folate
Ascites	deficiency
Ileus	Pernicious anaemia
Genitourinary	Dermatological
Water retention	Dry skin
Menorrhagia	Vitiligo
Infertility	Alopecia
Hyperprolactinaemia	Erythema ab igne

ECG, electrocardiogram.

due to postmaturity, hypothermia, delay in the passage of meconium, persistence of neonatal jaundice, poor feeding, hoarse cry, umbilical hernia, and marked retardation of bone maturation if present, are characteristic in the newborn of hypothyroidism. In children, hypothyroidism is characterized by retarded growth and evidence of mental retardation. In the adolescent precocious puberty may occur and there may be enlargement of the sella turcica in addition to short stature. In adults common features of hypothyroidism include tiredness, lethargy, weight gain, constipation, cold intolerance, muscle cramps, menstrual irregularities, cold dry skin, husky voice, and slow relaxing reflexes (Table 10). In patients with primary hypothyroidism a reduction in the total and free thyroxine level is accompanied by an increase in the serum TSH. Measurement of serum total or free T_3 levels are usually of little help in making the diagnosis since these are often within the normal range at a time when the serum T_4 concentration is decreased. In this context it is important to remember that there may be low levels of T_3 in euthyroid patients when they are seriously ill with non-thyroidal systemic illness (see below). In patients with secondary hypothyroidism with low levels of total or free T_4, the TSH level may be decreased or normal or only slightly elevated.

PRIMARY HYPOTHYROIDISM

Previous treatment for hyperthyroidism with either radio-iodine or by partial thyroidectomy, cannot be overemphasized as a common cause of primary hypothyroidism.

Hypothyroidism with or without development of a goitre may follow the chronic ingestion of iodine in either organic or inorganic form. Similarly, a number of non-iodine-containing compounds may lead to hypothyroidism, with or without goitre formation, including lithium, which decreases thyroid hormone synthesis.

Sporadic hypothyroidism

Hypothyroidism is detected in 1 in 3500 to 4500 births and results primarily from developmental defects in the thyroid, such that there is

either a complete absence of thyroid tissue or failure of the gland to descend properly during embryological development. Less commonly, the condition may be due to a genetically determined defect in hormone biosynthesis, or to hypothalamic–pituitary disease. Because of the difficulty in making the diagnosis of hypothyroidism clinically in the newborn period, and the disastrous consequences on the intellectual development of the child if the condition is not recognized early, neonatal screening programmes are now well established and have largely eliminated the problem of failure to recognize the condition early on clinical grounds. Cretinism (mental retardation, short stature, a characteristic facial appearance, and often deaf mutism and pyramidal tract signs) is now preventable. Early introduction of thyroid hormone replacement has now been shown to result in normal development and intellect.

Lymphocytic thyroiditis

In areas of the world where iodine intake is adequate, autoimmune lymphocytic thyroiditis is the commonest cause of hypothyroidism. It is more common in women than men, and occurs particularly in the age group between 30 and 50 years. There is often a family history of autoimmune thyroid disease, or of other organ-specific autoimmune diseases in the patient or in his or her relatives. The two major variants of lymphocytic thyroiditis are distinguished most easily by the presence or absence of a goitre. Patients with Hashimoto's thyroiditis have enlargement of the thyroid, whereas those with idiopathic or primary myxoedema (atrophic thyroiditis) have no goitre. In the presence of biochemical evidence of hypothyroidism, the demonstration of circulating autoantibodies to thyroglobulin and thyroid peroxidase make autoimmune lymphocytic thyroiditis the likely cause. There is also a small subpopulation of patients with primary myxoedema in whom antibodies which bind to the TSH receptor block its activation (TSH receptor blocking antibodies), thereby probably playing an important role in the development of impaired thyroid function.

Lymphocytic thyroiditis is uncommonly associated with pain and tenderness of the thyroid gland; differentiation from subacute thyroiditis is helped by the demonstration of high levels of thyroid autoantibodies in the former and an elevated erythrocyte sedimentation rate in the latter. Riedel's thyroiditis, predominantly seen in middle-aged women, may uncommonly be associated with low levels of thyroid autoantibodies. The aetiology is unknown. Biopsy of the thyroid reveals extensive fibrosis which often extends into adjacent structures. Fibrosis elsewhere, particularly retroperitoneally, may also be seen. The enlarged thyroid is rock-hard and symptoms result from the local fibrotic invasion of surrounding structures.

Endemic goitre and cretinism

Endemic goitre occurs in areas of environmental iodine deficiency and may afflict as many as 200 million people throughout the world. It is particularly prevalent in mountainous areas. Most individuals with endemic goitre are not hypothyroid and this may be because of the increased synthesis of T_3 at the expense of T_4. The incidence and severity of endemic goitre and the biochemical state of the individual depend primarily on the degree of iodine deficiency. Iodine supplementation, either in the form of iodine-enriched table salt, injections of iodized oil, or the introduction of iodine to communal drinking water, reduces the incidence of endemic goitre.

Endemic cretinism develops in the offspring of mothers living in severe endemic goitre areas of the world. The mother usually has a goitre and the child with endemic cretinism may present with either hypothyroidism, a neurological deficit, or a combination of the two.

Thyroid hormone biosynthetic defects

A number of rare inherited disorders of thyroid hormone biosynthesis may lead to goitrous hypothyroidism. Most of the defects appear to be inherited as autosomal recessive conditions. Although the goitre may be present at birth, it more commonly appears several year later. Five specific defects in the pathway of hormone synthesis have been identified (Table 11).

Table 11 *Major defects and clinical features in patients with dyshormonogenetic goitres*

Defect	Inheritance	Abnormality	Clinical features	Diagnosis	Treatment
Iodide transport defect	AR	Thyroid unable to concentrate iodide from circulation Complete or partial	Goitre, hypothyroid	Low RAIU	High-dose iodine therapy or thyroxine
Organification defects	AR	Deficiency or abnormality of TPO Unknown defect in iodination (Pendred's syndrome) Abnormality of Tg	Goitre and hypothyroid Congenital sensorineural deafness in Pendred's syndrome Rarely mental handicap	Positive perchlorate discharge test	Thyroxine therapy if hypothyroid Surgery if large goitre
Coupling defect	AR	Limited ability to convert MIT and DIT into T_3 and T_4	Goitre, hypothyroid, occasional mental handicap	Normal RAIU Negative perchlorate discharge Low ratio of intrathyroidal iodothyronines to iodotyrosines	Thyroxine
Dehalogenase deficiency	AR	Absent breakdown of uncoupled iodotyrosines, resulting in iodine loss	Goitre, hypothyroid, mental handicap	Large amounts of labelled MIT and DIT in serum after RAIU	Thyroxine or iodide
Thyroglobulin defect	AR	Heterogeneous group of inborn errors in Tg synthesis resulting in presence of abnormal circulating iodoproteins	Goitre, variable hypothyroidism, or mental handicap	Low butanol-extractable iodide RAIU (indicates abnormal iodoprotein)	Thyroxine

AR, autosomal recessive; RAIU, radioactive iodine uptake; TPO, thyroid peroxidase; Tg, thyroglobulin; MIT, monoiodotyrosine; DIT, diiodotyrosine.

HYPOTHALAMIC–PITUITARY DISEASE

In patients presenting with secondary hypothyroidism, the commonest causes are postpartum pituitary necrosis (Sheehan's syndrome) or tumours of the pituitary or adjacent structures. In the latter group craniopharyngiomas are particulary common. Postpartum pituitary necrosis is characterized by a history of heavy bleeding and/or shock following delivery and necessitating blood transfusion, followed thereafter by failure to lactate, amenorrhoea, and loss of libido and of pubic hair. It is important to be aware of the possibility of deficiencies in other pituitary hormones. In other patients with lesions in the pituitary or surrounding area, symptoms and signs of raised intercranial pressure or visual field defects are suggestive. Radiology may demonstrate an enlarged pituitary fossa and CT or MRI scanning may help to localize and define the mass. In the investigation of patients with secondary hypothyroidism, consideration needs to be given to the possible deficiencies of other pituitary hormones.

TREATMENT

Patients with symptomatic hypothyroidism require treatment with thyroxine. A dose of 100 to 150 μg/day is effective in most patients; this can be taken as a single daily dose since the half-life of the drug is long (7 days). Symptomatic improvement occurs within 2 to 3 weeks of beginning treatment, although it may take several weeks longer before the serum TSH returns into the normal range. Replacement doses of thyroxine should aim ultimately to achieve TSH values within the normal range, and serum T_4 values towards the upper end of the normal range. Considerable concern has been focused in the past few years on the possibility that overreplacement with thyroxine, particularly in women, may be associated with reducing bone density. Occasional patients require more thyroxine than might be expected and this may reflect normal variations in absorption. Rarely the diagnosis of coeliac disease is made in patients requiring suprapharmacological doses of thyroxine because of their malabsorption. The dose of thyroxine may need to be increased in some patients during pregnancy.

Particular care is needed in beginning treatment in the elderly and in those with a history of heart disease. In patients with coronary artery disease low levels of circulating thyroid hormone may protect the heart against increased demands that would otherwise result in increasing angina. In such patients appropriate therapy for their coronary artery disease should be considered before beginning thyroxine. When thyroxine is given it should be begun at a low dose (25 μg daily or on alternate days) and be increased cautiously every 4 weeks until euthyroidism is achieved.

MYXOEDEMA COMA

Myxoedema coma is an uncommon complication of long-standing hypothyroidism and is typically seen in the elderly, often precipitated by severe infection, therapy with sedative agents, or by inadequate heating during cold weather. It is has a high mortality. It is characteristically associated with depression of the level of consciousness, and hypothermia. Alveolar hypoventilation leading to carbon dioxide retention and a dilutional hyponatremia are often seen. Early recognition of the condition and its management are essential. The latter is complicated by the sluggish circulation and hypometabolism. General supportive measures include intravenous fluids, antibiotics, ventilation, and slow rewarming. Thyroid hormone replacement is best given as an intravenous bolus of 100 microgram of T_3, because of its rapid action. Thereafter a reasonable dose is 20 μg three times a day. It is worth covering the initial treatment period with hydrocortisone (100 mg daily) to protect against the possibility of associated adrenocortical insufficiency.

Simple, non-toxic goitre

Simple or non-toxic goitre is diagnosed when thyroid enlargement is not associated with altered function and is not due to an inflammatory or neoplastic process. It is not usually seen in an area of endemic goitre. The pathogenesis of this condition remains uncertain. In the majority of patients, TSH levels are not elevated, and claims that there may be thyroid growth stimulating immunoglobulins have not been substantiated. These goitres occur much more commonly in women and particularly at puberty and during pregnancy. Patients present usually because of thyroid enlargement and the effects of this. Thyroid function tests are normal, although the serum thyroglobulin concentration is often raised. Thyroid autoantibodies are negative. In managing the condition, thyroid hormone has been advocated in patients in whom there is biochemical evidence of a detectable or mildly raised TSH. The dose of thyroxine used in such a trial should not induce hyperthyroidism. Usually such measures fail to reduce the size of the goitre and if there are associated symptoms, particularly obstructive ones, surgery may be required. Postoperative replacement therapy should be given to reduce the likelihood or recurrence of the goitre.

Non-thyroidal illness

In patients who are severely ill, alterations, primarily in the transport and peripheral metabolism of thyroid hormones, induce changes in thyroid function, the physiological significance of which remain uncertain but the consequences of which make the interpretation of tests of thyroid function difficult. In this situation, the serum T_3 concentration is reduced, often markedly so, and this is accompanied (were it measured) by an increase in the concentration of reverse T_3. These changes result from a reduction in 5'-monodeiodination of T_4 and reverse T_3. Although alterations in the binding of thyroid hormones to their binding proteins occur in this situation, there is not, as might be expected, a normal or increased level of free T_3 because of the marked reduction in total T_3, so that usually the free T_3 concentration is also reduced. The more severe the illness, the lower will be the serum T_3 concentration. In early illness there may be no change in the total or free T_4 concentration, but both of these levels decline with progression of the non-thyroidal illness. The TSH level in this group of patients is characteristically retained within the normal range. The interpretation of thyroid function tests in this group of patients may be further complicated by medication given during their severe illness. Of particular importance are glucocorticoids, which reduce TSH secretion from the pituitary and, therefore, reduce thyroid hormone secretion.

Management of patients in this situation has been shown not to be improved by the administration of thyroid hormone. As and when the patient recovers, there is a recovery in thyroid function, usually preceded by a small rebound in TSH secretion, so that serum TSH levels may be mildly elevated until thyroid hormone levels have returned to the normal range.

In patients with acute psychiatric illness, particularly schizophrenics, serum total and free T_4 concentrations are frequently noted to be elevated. These changes, if present, precede the introduction of medication and there is often an absent TSH response to TRH, although usually with a sensitive assay the basal TSH remains detectable. If the TSH is suppressed, there may be concern that the patient is hyperthyroid, but again these changes in thyroid function return to normal without intervention with antithyroid medication once the patient's psychiatric illness is brought under control.

Resistance to thyroid hormones

In adult patients with goitre, or children and adolescents with short stature, hyperactivity, or learning disabilities, thyroid function tests may demonstrate elevations of total and free T_4 and T_3 in the presence of a non-suppressed serum TSH. Having excluded the possibilities of alter-

Table 12 *Thyroid hormone resistance; possible mechanisms to explain the phenomenon*

Structurally abnormal hormone
Reduced accessibility of hormone to tissue due to binding/ interaction with another substance
Cell membrane defect
Impaired metabolism of a hormone precursor
Defective receptor for hormone
Postreceptor abnormalities

Hormone resistance represents a situation in which inappropriately elevated levels of hormone occur in a setting in which the accompanying biological/clinical manifestations are inappropriate.

ations of thyroid hormone binding proteins, drugs, or intercurrent illness as causes of the elevated levels of thyroid hormone, the possibility of resistance to thyroid hormone needs to be considered. Despite the elevated levels of thyroid hormones, these patients are not clinically hyperthyroid. A number of mechanisms may underlie such cases (Table 12). The lack of sensitive and specific measures of the peripheral effects of thyroid hormones on target tissues, makes it exceedingly difficult to determine whether, in the face of elevated levels of serum thyroid hormones, there is in fact evidence of deficiency of thyroid hormone action at the target tissue. To date, two major subgroups of patients with evidence of thyroid hormone resistance have been defined by defects at the level of the thyroid hormone receptor. Most such patients have generalized tissue resistance to thyroid hormone, but there is a smaller group in whom resistance is confined to the pituitary. This last condition is characterized by evidence of hypermetabolism and, in addition, is more commonly sporadic. In the generalized syndrome, the pattern of inheritance is autosomal dominant in the majority of families described. Variability in the clinical manifestations among affected members suggests that the syndrome encompasses a wide variety of defects at various stages in the process of thyroid hormone action. Once it is suspected, diagnosis is aided by tests that measure the effects of doses of T_3 on concentrations of serum sex hormone binding globulin, ferritin, cholesterol, triglycerides, and creatinine phosphokinase. In addition, assessment of the sleeping pulse rate, the basal metabolic rate, echocardiography, and deep tendon relaxation time may all help to demonstrate evidence of peripheral tissue hypothyroidism.

With the cloning of the nuclear T_3 receptor, a number of different point mutations in the thyroid hormone receptor β-gene have been identified in various families with the generalized syndrome. These mutations result in substitutions of a single amino acid in the T_3-binding domain. The ability to identify these mutations provides a means for potential prenatal diagnosis and appropriate counselling, and this is of particular importance in families where there is evidence of growth and mental retardation. In the majority, however, an increase in the endogenous supply of thyroid hormone adequately compensates for the degree of tissue resistance to thyroid hormone. Therefore, in these patients, identification of the cause of their abnormal thyroid function is necessary so they are not treated erroneously in the future as individuals with hyperthyroidism, but there is no requirement for treatment with thyroid hormone.

REFERENCES

Berry, M.J. and Larsen, P.R. (1992). The role of selenium in thyroid hormone action. *Endocrine Reviews* **13**, 207–19.

Boyages, S.C. and Halpern, J.-P. (1993). Endemic cretinism: Toward a unifying hypothesis. *Thyroid* **3**, 59–69.

Braverman, L.E. and Utiger, R.D. (1991). *Werner and Ingbar's The Thyroid*, (6th edn). J.B. Lippincott, Philadelphia.

Lazar, M.A. (1993). Thyroid hormone receptors: multiple forms, multiple possibilities. *Endocrine Reviews* **14**, 184–193.

McGregor, A.M. (1992). Autoimmunity in the thyroid – can the molecular revolution contribute to our understanding? *Quarterly Journal of Medicine (New Series)* **82**, 1–13.

Nicoloff, J.T. and Spencer, C.A. (1990). The use and misuse of sensitive thyrotropin assays. *Journal of Clinical Endocrinology and Metabolism* **71**, 553–8.

Refetoff, S., Weiss, R.E., and Usala, S.J. (1993). The syndromes of resistance to thyroid hormone. *Endocrine Reviews* **14**, 348–99.

Weetman, A.P. (1992). Thyroid-associated ophthalmopathy. *Autoimmunity* **12**, 215–22.

12.5 Thyroid cancer

M. C. Sheppard

Prevalence

Although thyroid cancers are by far the most common endocrine gland malignancies, clinically apparent thyroid cancer is a relatively rare disease. In the United Kingdom, thyroid cancer accounts for less than 0.5 per cent of new malignancies and less than 0.5 per cent of cancer deaths, while in the United States the annual incidence is approximately 40 per 1 million people, and the annual death rate about 4 per million. In contrast, the prevalence of thyroid nodules is considerable. The Whickham survey, carried out in the north-east of England, reported that thyroid enlargement was present in up to 10 per cent of the population, being four times more common in females than males. Similarly, the Framingham study in the United States found that 4.2 per cent of the surveyed population had a thyroid nodule. The presence of nodular thyroid disease may be even more common than suggested by such epidemiological surveys, since in postmortem studies up to 50 per cent of the population are found to have either single or multiple nodules, many of which are very small. Furthermore, recent ultrasound studies have revealed discrete nodules in up to 50 per cent of the population beyond the fifth decade of life. Thyroid cancer is reported to occur in approximately 10 per cent of thyroid nodules which have been selected for surgery on clinical grounds, although the risk of malignancy is lower in multinodular goitre than in solitary nodules, with a reported malignancy rate of between 4 and 10 per cent. Cancer rates are probably much lower in small nodules such as those noted incidentally at ultrasound scanning or autopsy.

Aetiological factors

While ^{131}I given as treatment for hyperthyroidism or as a thyroid-scanning agent is not associated with an increased risk of thyroid cancer, carefully conducted epidemiological studies have confirmed a relationship between radiation and thyroid nodules and neoplasms. These data are derived from the previous practice of treating a wide range of benign conditions during childhood with external irradiation of the head and neck (including thymic enlargement, tinea capitis, and tonsilitis), as well as from studies of exposed individuals in the Marshall Islands and at Hiroshima. The risk of developing thyroid nodules and thyroid cancer is greater for women and is inversely related to the age at which radiation exposure occurs. Almost all cancers are well differentiated, nearly all being papillary in type. The principal question that arises when a thyroid nodule is discovered in a patient exposed to radiation is whether the patient should undergo thyroidectomy. A high proportion (30–40 per cent) of patients with nodules after radiation are found to have thyroid cancer at the time of surgery. Either surgery should be performed for most palpable thyroid nodules or be selective following fine-needle aspiration.

Another environmental risk is iodine deficiency, probably operating through the action of thyroid stimulating hormone, but Graves' disease does not appear to increase risk to any degree; the stimulating immu-noglobulin responsible for enhanced growth and function does not seem to be a significant mitogen.

Normal and neoplastic thyroid tissues express a variety of proto-oncogenes, growth factors, and growth factor receptors. Mutated forms of the H-*ras*, K-*ras*, and N-*ras* oncogenes are found in thyroid neoplasms; benign and malignant tumours have the same mutations, but the abnormalities are more frequent in the cancers. Therefore, these mutations will not be of diagnostic use but may have a role as prognostic factors. Whereas *ras* mutations are found in most thyroid tumour phenotypes, a novel oncogene unique to papillary thyroid cancer (*ptc*) has been reported, which has been identified as a mutation of the *ret* proto-oncogene (of unknown cellular function). An intriguing observation is that the *ptc* oncogene is located in the region of the gene for multiple endocrine neoplasia type 2A, a condition associated with medullary thyroid cancer.

Clinical presentation

Most patients present with an otherwise asymptomatic nodule noticed by themselves, or the nodule is detected on routine physical examination. A family history of goitre or thyroid dysfunction usually suggests a benign disorder; if, however, this includes medullary thyroid carcinoma, phaeochromocytoma, or the multiple endocrine neoplasia syndrome, thyroid cancer should be considered. Age is important because nodular thyroid disease is uncommon in childhood and its presence should be viewed with suspicion. Similarly there appears to be a greater risk of malignancy in nodules developing over the age of 60. Thyroid cancers usually develop over a period of weeks or months and a particularly important feature is whether the thyroid nodule developed or increased in size while the patient was on suppressive doses of thyroid hormones. The development of local symptoms such as dysphagia, dysphonia, dyspnoea, and haemoptysis may suggest oesophageal or tracheal involvement by a thyroid cancer, although such symptoms may occur in association with a benign goitre, especially if multinodular. Local pain in the neck or pain radiating to the jaw or ear may occur. The physical characteristics are, on the whole, poor predictors of malignancy, although some features, such as the presence of lymph nodes or obvious fixation to local structures may be of greater value in pointing to a diagnosis. Patients may present with advanced disease with evidence of metastases to lungs, bone, or liver, and in some cases without clinically obvious thyroid pathology. Well-differentiated follicular carcinoma causing thyrotoxicosis is a very rare entity.

Laboratory tests

In general there is no laboratory test of value in distinguishing benign from malignant lesions of the thyroid. It is, none the less, important to assess thyroid function in patients presenting with nodular thyroid disease because the presence of hyperthyroidism is rarely associated with malignancy. Conversely, it is important to exclude hypothyroidism,

Table 1 *Thyroglobulin levels in thyroid cancer*

Thyroglobulin (μg/l)	Cancer state	
	Off T$_4$ (T$_3$)	On T$_4$ (T$_3$)
< 5	Absent	Absent
5–35	(Ambiguous)	Present (or non-compliance with taking T$_4$)
35–50	? Present	Present
50–100	Present, possible metastases	
> 100	Present, metastases, probably lung or bone	

The normal range for thyroglobulin is 1–35 μ/l with considerable overlap between euthyroid, hyper- and hypothyroid individuals and patients with benign or malignant goitre. Thyroglobulin cannot therefore be used in the diagnosis of thyroid disease.

which if secondary to Hashimoto's thyroiditis, may be associated with the presence of a firm goitre, raising the clinical suspicion of malignancy. The presence of positive thyroid autoantibodies may also be helpful in this situation, although there appears to be an increased risk of lymphoma in Hashimoto's thyroiditis. Serum thyroglobulin concentrations are often elevated in patients with differentiated thyroid cancers (Table 1); however, they are also elevated in a variety of other thyroid disorders, including endemic goitre, multinodular goitre, benign adenoma, Graves' disease, and Hashimoto's thyroiditis. Measurement of serum thyroglobulin is of no use therefore in the differential diagnosis of thyroid carcinoma at presentation.

Imaging tests

Neither isotope nor ultrasound scanning techniques have sufficient diagnostic accuracy to be used as single investigations on which to base management decisions.

TECHNETIUM SCANNING

Technetium (^{99}Tc^m)-pertechnetate is now the most widely used thyroid imaging agent. Although Tc^m is concentrated within the thyroid, it is not incorporated into thyroglobulin, unlike iodide. Normally there is uniform tracer uptake throughout both lobes. A solitary thyroid nodule can usefully be characterized by either reduced or enhanced uptake compared with that of the surrounding normal thyroid tissue. Hypofunctioning (cold) nodules are most frequently associated with thyroid cancer. While the great majority of solitary thyroid nodules are hypofunctioning, only 20 per cent of solitary hypofunctioning nodules are cancers, the remaining 80 per cent being benign lesions, including cysts, colloid nodules, adenomas, degenerative nodules, and thyroiditis. Hypofunctioning lesions warrant further investigation, usually biopsy. The incidence of cancer in a cold nodule within a multinodular goitre is lower than in a solitary nodule, but the risk of cancer in such lesions is still sufficiently high that needle biopsy is warranted for hypofunctioning lesions that are dominant, hard, or rapidly growing. Autonomously functioning (hot) thyroid nodules are so rarely malignant that neither biopsy nor surgical removal is indicated.

IODINE SCANNING

Multiple radio-isotopes of iodine are available (and permit tracer studies of the entire metabolic pathway of iodine), but only ^{131}I and ^{123}I are clinically useful. Radio-iodine is given by mouth as sodium iodide.

Table 2 *Thyroid malignancy*

Papillary carcinoma
Follicular carcinoma
Hürthle cell carcinoma
Anaplastic carcinoma
Lymphoma
Medullary carcinoma
Metastasis

Imaging doses are now most frequently given in the form of capsules to reduce radiation exposure to the technical staff. Imaging is usually performed 18 to 24 h after administration, at which time the majority of radioactivity within the thyroid is present as radio-iodotyrosine residues on thyroglobulin, reflecting hormonogenesis. The imaging patterns for radio-iodine scanning of the thyroid are similar to those of Tc^m, in that nodules demonstrating radio-iodine uptake greater than that of surrounding tissue are almost invariably benign. Hypofunctioning nodules carry a higher risk of malignancy, although most are benign. The disadvantages of iodine scanning are the expense of the isotope and the inconvenience and possible loss of income to the patient because of the necessity of two visits. There are no clear clinical advantages.

ULTRASOUND

High-resolution images of the thyroid may be obtained using ultrasonography. In the imaging of thyroid nodules this technique is most often used to determine whether the lesion is cystic or solid and whether it is solitary. True cysts of the thyroid are benign. However, they are uncommon and most large nodules contain areas of cystic or haemorrhagic degeneration. Although solitary nodules pose a greater risk for malignancy than multiple nodules, the finding of additional nodules does not eliminate the potential for malignancy or the need for further evaluation. The detection of small nodules in up to 50 per cent of the population older than 60 is not of proven advantage, given the low incidence of thyroid cancer and its frequent benign outcome.

Needle biopsy

A major advance in the assessment of thyroid nodules that might be malignant is the development of reliable fine-needle aspiration cytology. In the presence of an experienced cytopathologist, fine-needle aspiration has largely replaced radio-isotope and ultrasound imaging in the preoperative evaluation of most patients with thyroid nodules. The ability to make a diagnosis preoperatively allows one to select patients for thyroidectomy more accurately. It also expedites definitive treatment, allows the planning of a procedure in advance of surgery, and facilitates counselling of patients. Risks associated with fine-needle aspiration are few, but false negative results can be generated by sampling error. The histopathological patterns of thyroid cancers are shown in Table 2.

Fine-needle aspiration is useful in the initial assessment, but cannot reliably distinguish between a follicular adenoma and a follicular carcinoma. A patient with a thyroid nodule should be evaluated with recognized risk factors in mind. It remains to be seen whether new techniques such as DNA amplification combined with gene analysis, flow cytometry with chromosome ploidy analysis, or cell cycle analysis can be combined with traditional cytology to improve diagnostic accuracy.

Papillary thyroid carcinoma

Papillary thyroid carcinoma is the most frequently diagnosed malignant thyroid tumour; in 25 retrospective analyses of 12 855 treated cases of differentiated thyroid cancer from North and South America, Japan, and Europe, papillary thyroid carcinoma comprised 50 to 89 per cent of these cases (average, 74 per cent). Papillary thyroid carcinoma and follicular cancer are more common in women (3:1) and although occurring at all ages, are rarest in childhood. Papillary cancers are most frequent in the third and fourth decades, whereas follicular cancers tend to occur in older individuals.

Papillary cancers are locally invasive, rarely encapsulated, and may have areas of cystic degeneration. They often appear multifocal, small foci being scattered elsewhere in the gland. Colloid may be present but is usually absent. Some papillary cancers are small (< 1 cm in diameter) and are often referred to as occult. At the other extreme is the diffuse papillary type, often sclerosing, which infiltrates the whole thyroid; it usually occurs in children and young adults. The presence of small papillary cancers has been demonstrated in 6 to 13 per cent of autopsied American patients and 36 per cent in Finland. These occult papillary tumours rarely undergo transition to clinically evident carcinomas.

The two most controversial topics in the management of papillary thyroid carcinoma are the extent of thyroid surgery that is optimal and the indications for postoperative radio-iodine therapy. Surgery is the primary mode of treatment and unless there is clear evidence of contra-lateral disease or of metastasis, simple lobectomy is the preferred option. Those advocating near-total thyroidectomy do so because papillary cancers are often multifocal and follow-up is rendered easier. Patients in whom lymph nodes are involved require removal of these but block dissection is usually unwarranted. There is no consensus with regard to the use of ^{131}I in patients with small, solitary lesions, but radio-iodine has a clear role in the management of residual disease or established metastases. Some authorities recommend ^{131}I ablation for nearly all patients with papillary cancer, others reserving this treatment for only a few very high-risk patients. In those most commonly affected, that is aged between 20 and 40 years, papillary cancer is a relatively benign condition, with 10- to 20-year recurrence rates of 5 to 10 per cent, and death rates of 2 to 5 per cent. Metastases, if present, are usually to cervical lymph nodes; because local treatment (surgery or ^{131}I administration) is effective, the prognosis is not adversely affected. Unfortunately, in individuals aged over 40 years, papillary cancers often progress by slowly invading local structures.

Follicular thyroid carcinoma

Follicular thyroid carcinoma is a relatively uncommon malignancy, accounting for about 15 per cent of all thyroid cancers. Although most radiation-related thyroid cancers have papillary histology, follicular thyroid carcinoma has also been associated with radiation. Other epidemiological factors associated with the development of follicular thyroid carcinoma include relative iodine deficiency and endemic goitre, suggesting a possible role for thyroid stimulating hormone as a promoter. The diagnosis of follicular thyroid carcinoma is generally made during the evaluation of a solitary non-functioning thyroid nodule. In approximately 15 per cent of patients, distant metastases are already present when the tumour in the neck is diagnosed. In contrast to papillary cancer, in which cervical adenopathy is relatively common at presentation (25–30 per cent) follicular thyroid carcinoma only occasionally involves regional nodes. Distant metastases ultimately develop in approximately 20 per cent of patients with follicular thyroid carcinoma. The most common sites of involvement are lung and bone.

Appearances of follicular cancers range from almost normal-looking follicles to sheets of cells with only an occasional follicle; the tumours are not multifocal. One of the most difficult distinctions in thyroid pathology is the differentiation between benign follicular adenomas and encapsulated low-grade or minimally invasive follicular carcinomas. In view of the histological difficulties in distinguishing follicular adenomas from encapsulated carcinomas, cytological examination cannot replace surgery in this situation. Thus most cytopathologists consider follicular neoplasms to be suspicious, although a small minority prove to be truly malignant when examined histologically. While controversy surrounds the appropriate extent of surgery in patients with small papillary tumours, preponderant opinion appears to be that total thyroidectomy is the

procedure of choice in follicular thyroid carcinoma. Unfortunately, prospective data are not available; studies showing that total thyroidectomy improves survival are retrospective and conflicting, and they have often included patients with papillary carcinoma, making interpretation of data more difficult. Because of these uncertainties, most authorities recommend total thyroidectomy, despite its higher morbidity.

Although controversy surrounds the role of routine remnant ablation in papillary thyroid carcinoma, it is accepted practice in follicular thyroid carcinoma because of the more aggressive behaviour of the latter. Nevertheless, only few data show that routine remnant ablation in follicular thyroid carcinoma is of benefit, either in preventing recurrences or in prolonging life. Most endocrinologists recommend total body scanning using 5 to 10 mCi of [131]I 6 to 8 weeks after total thyroidectomy. If significant uptake is noted in the thyroid bed, ablation of these remnants is usually performed. Such ablation may destroy microscopic tumour left behind at the time of surgery and will simplify radioiodine therapy by removing all functioning tissue so that the serum thyroid stimulating hormone will rise to maximal levels, enhancing visualization and treatment of possible distant metastases with radio-iodine.

The prognosis is poor in metastatic follicular thyroid carcinoma, with 5- and 10-year mortality rates of about 60 and 80 per cent, respectively. Radio-iodine is the mainstay of treatment. Several studies of metastatic spread of differentiated thyroid cancer have shown that survival is improved in patients treated with radio-iodine, compared with those in whom treatment cannot be given because the tumour fails to concentrate the radio-isotope. Poor prognostic features include older age, greater degrees of invasiveness, distant metastases, and possibly an abnormal chromosomal number (aneuploidy) within tumour tissue.

Hürthle cell carcinoma

Hürthle cell carcinoma is an uncommon form of thyroid neoplasm, comprising about 3 to 6 per cent of all differentiated thyroid cancers. Hürthle cells (also known as oxyphil or Askanazy cells) are large polygonal cells with pleomorphic hyperchromatic nuclei and eosinophilic granular cytoplasm. Most malignant Hürthle cell tumours are considered to be variants of follicular carcinoma. Hürthle cell carcinoma is primarily a disease of adults, and most patients are diagnosed in the fourth to seventh decade. As with other thyroid malignancies, there is a predominance of this lesion in women. Hürthle cell carcinoma is associated with previous head and neck irradiation. As in the case of follicular carcinomas, cervical lymphadenopathy is infrequent but distant metastatic disease is present in 10 to 15 per cent of patients at the time of the initial diagnosis of tumour in the neck. The most common metastatic sites are lung and bone. Pathological distinction between benign and malignant Hürthle cell tumours may be extremely difficult and requires demonstration of vascular, or full-thickness, capsular invasion in a surgical specimen. Hürthle cells are commonly found in benign thyroid disorders. Because these cytological features are difficult to interpret, fine-needle aspiration biopsy is of limited use in the diagnosis of Hürthle cell nodules. Surgical resection of lesions where cytology reveals the presence of Hürthle cells is commonly recommended, total thyroidectomy being the treatment of choice for patients with histologically malignant lesions. Patients with apparently benign Hürthle cell tumours may be treated with lobectomy. Radioactive iodine is generally ineffective in the treatment of metastatic Hürthle cell carcinoma because of a lack of uptake of ^{131}I by the metastases. Hürthle cell carcinoma is a relatively aggressive thyroid tumour and is associated with a 5-year mortality rate of about 80 per cent. Major adverse prognostic factors include extensive tumour load and inadequate initial surgery. DNA aneuploidy in histologically malignant lesions also correlates with decreased survival.

Anaplastic carcinoma

Anaplastic carcinoma is rare and accounts for 5 to 14 per cent of primary malignant thyroid neoplasms. In contrast to papillary and follicular thyroid carcinoma, anaplastic carcinoma is very aggressive, with a 5-year survival rate of 7 per cent and a mean survival period of 6 months from diagnosis. The peak incidence of the disease is in the seventh decade of life. Anaplastic carcinoma is characterized by rapid growth of a mass in the neck that was not present before, or by a rapid growth in a pre-existing thyroid tumour. On physical examination the thyroid or neck mass is usually firm or hard and fixed to the underlying structures. The skin overlying the tumour may also undergo necrosis. Enlargement of the neck lymph nodes may occur early. Large anaplastic carcinomas almost always encroach on the trachea, but to varying degrees. Severe respiratory obstruction may occur. Frequently the tumour is fixed to the larynx and nearby major vessels. Because of infiltration into these structures, the mass does not move with swallowing. Vocal chord paralysis can occur, as well as obstruction of the superior vena cava. Coexistence of well-differentiated carcinoma and anaplastic carcinoma has been reported in a number of cases. Anaplastic thyroid carcinoma is very resistant to any form of therapy and is rarely cured. The best survival results have been obtained with a combination of surgery, external irradiation, and chemotherapy. Whenever possible, although opportunities are rare, a total or near total thyroidectomy with resection of positive lymph nodes should be done. Neither radioactive iodine nor thyroid hormone treatment significantly alters the course of the disease. There is no consensus on the selection of chemotherapeutic regimens.

Lymphomas

Lymphoma may affect the thyroid primarily, or may involve the gland as part of a systemic disease. Thyroid lymphomas are uncommon, accounting for only 1 to 2 per cent of all thyroid malignancies. It rarely occurs under the age of 40 years and has a female predominance of approximately 4:1. Patients usually present with a short history of enlargement of the thyroid gland. On palpation, the gland is often firm and may appear to be fixed to adjacent tissues. Regional lymph nodes may be enlarged because of lymphoma involvement. The majority of patients are euthyroid although some are hypothyroid secondary to auto-immune thyroiditis. Follow-up studies have estimated that the relative risk of thyroid lymphoma in patients with autoimmune thyroiditis is 60 to 80 times greater than in controls. The nature of this relationship is unknown.

Fine- and large-needle aspiration biopsies are the initial procedures of choice in attempting to confirm the diagnosis. The vast majority of thyroid lymphomas are non-Hodgkin's in type. Non-involved areas of thyroid tissue may be normal or altered by a concomitant autoimmune thyroiditis. Radiotherapy alone appears to be an excellent treatment for disease limited to the thyroid, with or without cervical lymphadenopathy. Results for patients with mediastinal extension treated by radiotherapy alone are unsatisfactory, and therefore the addition of combination chemotherapy is indicated.

Follow-up evaluation

All patients require suppressive thyroxine therapy following definitive treatment for differentiated thyroid cancer (usually 200 µg/day). The degree of suppression of serum thyroid stimulating hormone concentration needed to minimize tumour recurrence rates is as yet unclear but most clinicians would aim for a serum thyroid stimulating hormone measurement below the limit of the assay. Following radio-ablation of

the thyroid, patients should have a total body radio-iodine scan at 6 to 12 months to document successful ablation, but the optimal frequency of subsequent scans is uncertain. It is essential to withdraw thyroid hormone therapy prior to such investigation. Serum thyroglobulin measurement is a valuable tumour marker. Patients with known differentiated papillary or follicular thyroid cancers who have undergone definitive treatment have normal or undetectable serum thyroglobulin concentrations in the absence of residual tumour, but elevated levels in the presence of metastases or recurrence. It has become widely accepted that it is no longer necessary in the follow-up of thyroid cancer to perform frequent, routine neck or whole-body radio-iodine scans after withdrawal of suppressive thyroid hormone treatment. Stopping the patient's replacement thyroid therapy makes them miserably ill. It is possible instead to measure serum thyroglobulin at regular intervals, often while thyroxine treatment is continued, and to perform radio-iodine scans only when the thyroglobulin result is above a level defined for each assay, or where there is clinical evidence suggesting recurrence.

Prognosis

The goal of the long-term management after primary surgical treatment of thyroid cancer is to minimize the morbidity and mortality of the disease, while also minimizing the morbidity of the diagnostic and therapeutic medical interventions to which the patients are subjected. Prolonged survival is common even in those few patients who ultimately succumb to their malignancy; prospective therapeutic studies are thus difficult to design.

Medullary thyroid carcinoma

This arises from the parafollicular or C cells of the thyroid and constitutes about 3 to 5 per cent of all thyroid cancers. These tumours secrete calcitonin which provides a useful diagnostic criterion and a marker to monitor response or relapse after treatment. In cases of doubt, calcitonin secretion may be enhanced by infusion of calcium, pentagastrin, or ingestion of alcohol. Medullary carcinoma forms part of the multiple endocrine neoplasia type 2 syndrome. Genetic and biochemical tests are likely to be complementary, both being useful until the actual genetic defect in multiple endocrine neoplasia type 2A (lying in chromosome 10) is identified.

REFERENCES

DeGroot, L.J., Kaplan, E.L., McCormick, M. and Straus, F.H. (1990). Natural history, treatment, and course of papillary thyroid carcinoma. *Journal of Clinical Endocrinology and Metabolism*, **71**, 414–24.

Franklyn, J.A. and Sheppard, M.C. (1988). Thyroid nodules and thyroid cancer—diagnostic aspects. *Balliere's Clinical Endocrinology and Metabolism*, **2**.

Hay, I.D. (1989). Prognostic factors in thyroid carcinoma. *Thyroid n Today*, **12**.

Kaplan, M.M., ed. (1990). Thyroid carcinoma. *Endocrinology and Metabolism Clinics of North America.* **19**.

Samaan, N.A., *et al.* 1992. The results of different modalities of treatment of well differentiated thyroid carcinoma: a retrospective review of 1599 patients. *Journal of Clinical Endocrinology and Metabolism*, **75**, 714–20.

Sheppard, M.C. (1986). Serum thyroglobulin and thyroid cancer. *Quarterly Journal of Medicine*, **59**, 429–33.

12.6 Disorders of calcium metabolism

J. A. KANIS

Introduction

There has been a rapid growth in our understanding of the biochemistry, metabolism, and actions of the calcium regulating hormones, clarifying the pathophysiology of several disorders and leading to the identification of several new syndromes. There are still large gaps in our understanding of hormone action, particularly on the skeleton, and very little is known about the local control of skeletal growth and remodelling.

This chapter reviews the common disorders of plasma calcium homeostasis, but there are inevitably overlaps with disorders of skeletal metabolism since the skeleton is the major reservoir of extracellular calcium. Detailed discussion of disorders of the skeleton are found in Section 19. Reference should be made to Chapter 20.18 for details of renal bone disease.

Distribution and function of calcium

FUNCTION OF CALCIUM

Calcium and phosphate are widely distributed throughout living tissue. The great majority of calcium and phosphate is found in bone, and the ability of the skeleton to turn over calcium and phosphate is essential for growth, the prevention and healing of fractures, and skeletal remodelling in response to physiological and pathological stresses. During skeletal growth and remodelling of bone, there is a bidirectional flux of calcium between bone and the extracellular fluid compartment. The skeleton can also provide substantial amounts of buffers, such as phosphate and carbonate, to the extracellular fluid, for example in acidosis, but at the risk of inducing metabolic bone disease.

The extracellular fluid concentration of calcium is critical to maintain normal neuromuscular activity, and a fall in plasma calcium concentration results in tetany and convulsions. Also, a rise in extracellular fluid calcium levels has many adverse effects, including delayed neuromuscular conduction and muscle paralysis.

The two major functions for calcium, the maintenance of the skeleton and the maintenance of extracellular fluid calcium concentrations, are closely related and disorders of the one may induce disorders of the other. This is commonly but not invariably the case. For example, in primary hyperparathyroidism, skeletal disease and disturbed plasma calcium homeostasis commonly coexist. On the other hand, in Paget's disease, where bone turnover is characteristically increased, plasma calcium is usually normal.

The total amount of calcium within soft tissues is similar to that found in the extracellular fluid (approximately 25 mmol). However, cytosol calcium concentrations are 100 to 1000 times lower than extracellular concentrations. Within cells, mitochondria are capable of accumulating large amounts of calcium against electrochemical gradients, to an extent that mitochondrial deposits of insoluble calcium phosphate can form. The activation of many different types of cells by hormones or pharmacological agents is now thought to be accompanied by changes in intracellular calcium concentrations, derived from the extracellular fluid or from mitochondria. Hormonal activation, enzyme activity, membrane function, and cell division are all important roles for intracellular calcium. Calcium is also essential for neurotransmitter release as well as for the release of hormones and other secretory products.

Table 1 *Distribution of plasma calcium*

Ultrafilterable calcium (53%)	
Ionized calcium	47%
Complexed calcium	
Phosphate	1.5%
Citrate	1.5%
HCO_3, etc.	3%
Protein-bound calcium (47%)	
Albumin	37%
Globulin	10%
Total plasma calcium (2.12–2.6 mmol/l)	100%

PLASMA CALCIUM

The concentration of plasma calcium in health is maintained within a very narrow range, varying by less than 5 to 10 per cent, despite the large movements of calcium across gut, bone, kidney, and other tissues. Several hormones, including parathyroid hormone and calcitriol (1,25-dihydroxyvitamin D_3; $1,25(OH)_2D_3$), regulate the ionized fraction of plasma calcium (approximately 50 per cent of total plasma calcium; Table 1) by modulating calcium fluxes to and from the extracellular fluid. In turn, the secretion rates for these hormones are regulated in part by the calcium concentration of the extracellular fluid, thereby completing a negative feedback loop.

Changes in plasma calcium are usually due to changes in the total amount of calcium in the extracellular fluid, since there is a free distribution of ionized calcium throughout the extracellular fluid compartment. Within the plasma compartment, however, approximately half of the calcium is bound to proteins, mainly albumin, and the binding is pH dependent. Major changes in plasma protein concentrations, the presence of abnormal proteins, and large shifts in extracellular hydrogen ion concentration can therefore affect the amount of calcium that is bound to protein, so that the estimation of total plasma calcium may not accurately reflect the ionized calcium concentration. These changes in protein binding have some important clinical consequences. Thus, the paraesthesiae seen in patients with hyperventilation syndrome are associated with a decreased ionized calcium concentration due to alkalosis, but total plasma calcium is normal. Also, the infusion of alkalis into patients with long-standing metabolic acidosis (for example, those with chronic renal failure) may precipitate hypocalcaemic convulsions due to a decrease in ionized calcium, without changing the total plasma calcium.

In the absence of severe acidosis or alkalosis, the major factor influencing the amount of calcium found is the quantity of albumin present, since the proportion of calcium which is bound varies little. Failure to account for protein binding may result in the erroneous diagnosis of hypercalcaemia in conditions where increased concentrations or abnormal plasma proteins are found, for example, dehydration, prolonged venostasis, and myeloma. Also, in hypoproteinaemic states, such as disseminated carcinoma or chronic renal failure, total plasma calcium may be low, though ionized calcium is normal. Similarly, in such disorders total plasma calcium may be normal and mask true hypercalcaemia.

Since the ionized plasma calcium is the physiologically relevant fraction, ideally this should be measured, but the present methods are often unreliable and not widely available. Many formulae have been proposed for predicting the ionized calcium from the total plasma calcium, or 'correcting' the total plasma calcium to a normal protein value. These methods depend on the concurrent measurement of total proteins, albumin, or specific gravity of plasma. None is entirely satisfactory but a widely used simple adjustment factor for plasma calcium is to subtract from the total plasma calcium 0.02 mmol/l for every 1 g/l that the plasma albumin exceeds 40 g/l, provided the sample is withdrawn without venostasis. A similar addition is made when the plasma albumin is less than 40 g/l. Many laboratories now report 'corrected' plasma calcium or 'ionized' plasma calcium, but it should be realized that these are at best a guide to the ionized calcium concentration.

A small proportion of total plasma calcium is complexed with cations such as phosphate, citrate, and bicarbonate (see Table 1). The calcium that is normally filtered by the kidney includes this complexed calcium as well as ionized calcium. In several disorders the proportion of complexed, ultrafilterable calcium is increased (that is disorders of acid–base, phosphate, and citrate metabolism).

DISTRIBUTION OF CALCIUM AND PHOSPHATE

Most of the total body calcium and phosphate resides in bone (99 and 88 per cent, respectively). The concentration of calcium is low in most soft tissues, but 12 to 15 per cent of phosphorus lies outside the skeleton as inorganic and organic phosphates, such as nucleic acids, nucleotides, phospholipids, and phosphorylated metabolites. Extracellular concentrations, and probably intracellular concentrations, of phosphate vary much more than those of calcium, particularly in response to circadian rhythms, growth, and meals. The measurement of plasma phosphate is a valuable adjunct in the diagnosis of disturbances of plasma calcium homeostasis, but it is important to recognize that high values occur after food and that plasma phosphate in childhood is commonly higher than in adults.

PRINCIPLES OF REGULATION OF PLASMA CALCIUM

The total amount of calcium in the extracellular fluid, and hence its concentration, is dependent upon movements of calcium to and from the extracellular fluid. The major fluxes occur across the gut, bone, and kidneys. The relative sizes of these fluxes determine their potential in plasma calcium homeostasis (Fig. 1).

There is a significant exchange of calcium between extracellular fluid and bone. Studies with radio-isotopes in normal human adults show that between 1 and 2 per cent of total body calcium is exchanged over a few days. This represents 1000 or 2000 mmol, which is a substantial amount considering that the extracellular fluid contains somewhat less than 20 mmol as ionized calcium. This exchangeable pool may therefore be very important in plasma calcium homeostasis, although how these large movements of calcium between body fluids, cells, and surfaces of bone are subject to metabolic regulation is controversial.

These large and rapid fluxes should be distinguished from the movements of calcium that occur in bone as a result of mineralization and bone resorption. Bone resorption is defined as the complete removal of bone mineral and matrix, and is a result of osteoclast activity which occurs in adults during physiological remodelling. This accounts for only a fraction of the total calcium exchange between extracellular fluid and bone, the remainder occurring across the large surface area of osteocytes and their canaliculi without synthesis or destruction of bone matrix. Approximately 10 per cent of the adult skeleton is thought to be renewed each year by remodelling activity, although this is not uniformly distributed throughout the skeleton and, for example, trabecular bone has a faster turnover than cortical bone. This means that disturbances of bone turnover commonly have greater and earlier effects at trabecular than at cortical sites.

Calcium is lost from the body by urinary and intestinal excretion, and to a lesser extent in sweat, and enters by intestinal absorption and renal tubular reabsorption of glomerular filtrate. The true intestinal absorption of calcium is greater than the net absorption because some calcium is returned to the gut lumen in biliary, pancreatic, and intestinal secretions. Thus, from an average daily dietary intake of 25 mmol, approximately 10 mmol is absorbed. This is offset by intestinal secretion amounting to approximately 5 mmol daily, leaving a net transport into the extracellular fluid pool of 5 mmol. Apparent and real fluxes across the gut can be measured by tracer and balance studies, some of which are used in specialized clinical practice.

The kidney is a major site for calcium excretion. A large amount of calcium is filtered (see Fig. 1), but most of this is reabsorbed, leaving only some 5 mmol for urinary excretion. Several hormones, particularly parathyroid hormone, alter renal tubular reabsorption and, since the fluxes to and from the extracellular fluid compartment are large, this means that small changes in tubular reabsorption have profound effects on the extracellular fluid concentration of calcium. This has led to the view that the kidney is a major site for plasma calcium regulation. Calcium is also lost from the body in sweat, but these losses are small. However, losses can be as high as 8 mmol daily under extreme conditions where sweat production is increased, for example fever and in tropical climates.

In mature adults who are neither gaining nor losing calcium, bone and soft tissues contribute neither a net gain nor a loss of calcium to the extracellular fluid; the amount of bone resorbed exactly matches the amount formed. Also, the total amount of calcium absorbed by the gut matches the urinary excretion. Because plasma and intracellular calcium levels are controlled within a narrow range, changes in bone mass are reflected as changes in the external balance for calcium. For example, during growth, when there is a net daily gain of calcium which is incorporated into the skeleton, plasma and intracellular concentrations of calcium are normal. In the long term, therefore, the total body balance of calcium reflects exactly the skeletal balance for calcium (in this case positive calcium balance). Mineral losses begin at middle age (negative balance). Between the age of 25 and 45 the body should be neither gaining nor losing calcium, so that inflow and outflow of calcium are matched.

The transport of calcium between the extracellular fluid and bone, gut and kidneys is continually changing and is regulated by a variety of

Fig. 1 Major fluxes of calcium (mmol/day) in a healthy adult. Exchange of calcium in the extracellular fluid occurs across bone, gut, and the kidneys. The net balance for calcium equals the net absorption minus the losses of calcium in faeces and urine, which in a healthy adult is zero. The major fluxes of calcium are regulated by the regulating hormones. Parathyroid hormone (PTH) increases renal tubular reabsorption of calcium and bone resorption, calcitonin inhibits bone resorption, and vitamin D augments intestinal absorption of calcium. The precise role of vitamin D in augmenting bone resorption and mineralization *in vivo* is unclear (1 mmol = 40 mg calcium).

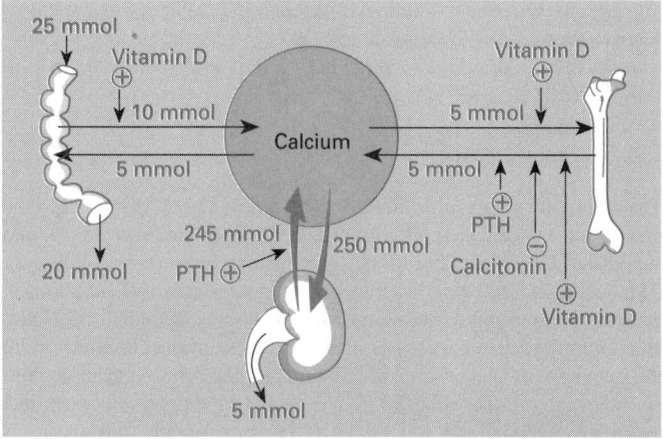

factors, including several hormones (see Fig. 1). These hormones can be subdivided into 'controlling hormones' and 'influencing hormones'. The controlling group are the major regulating hormones of plasma calcium, comprising parathyroid hormone (PTH), calcitonin, and vitamin D metabolites, and the production of each is altered in response to changes in ionized calcium concentrations. The influencing hormones are those hormones such as thyroid hormone, growth hormone, and adrenal and gonadal steroids which have effects on calcium metabolism, but the secretion of which is determined primarily by factors other than changes in plasma calcium.

Major regulating hormones

Parathyroid hormone

In the circulation, PTH consists of several polypeptide fragments which are degraded in the liver, kidneys, and skeleton. The major stimulus to the secretion of PTH is a fall in the ionized fraction of plasma calcium. The biological actions of PTH at a variety of target organs serve to increase plasma calcium and thus there exists an efficient negative feedback hormonal loop.

In humans there are usually four parathyroid glands, two embedded in the superior poles of the thyroid and two in the inferior poles. There is considerable individual variation, both in the site and the number of parathyroid glands. Parathyroid tissue is occasionally found in the mediastinum. Each gland, approximately the size of a match head, comprises chief cells, with clear cytoplasm and larger oxyphil cells.

PTH is released from the parathyroid glands as a single peptide chain containing 84 amino acids (molecular weight 5500). In common with several other peptide hormones, PTH is synthesized as a prohormone which contains an additional six amino acids at its amino-terminal end. A further precursor form, pre-pro-PTH, containing a total of 150 amino acids has been identified in studies in vitro. The site of synthesis of the precursor hormone is the rough endoplasmic reticulum of the chief cells. The function of the oxyphil cells is unknown. The precursor forms of PTH are probably converted to the 84 amino acid polypeptide before secretion from the gland in secretory granules.

Only the first 32 to 34 amino acids, reading from the amino-terminal end, are necessary for biological activity. There is evidence that cleavage occurs naturally, partly in the liver, to produce a short amino-terminal fragment with biological activity and a larger inactive carboxy-terminal fragment. This cleavage may be necessary for PTH to act on bone. There are also many less well-characterized circulating fragments of PTH. The liver and kidney are important sites for degradation. For example, the C-terminal fragment normally cleared by the kidney may be increased in chronic renal failure, although the circulating levels of biologically active PTH may be normal. This causes some problems in the interpretation of radio-immunoassay results, particularly in patients with renal impairment, since the C-terminal fragment is the major component measured in many assay systems. Sensitive assays for the intact PTH molecule have been developed but are not yet universally available in clinical practice.

SECRETION OF PTH

The major physiological stimulus to the secretion of PTH is a fall in the plasma ionized calcium concentration. A rise in plasma ionized calcium suppresses PTH secretion. Many other factors are known to influence PTH secretion, including β-adrenergic agonists, vitamin D metabolites, growth hormone and somatostatin, vitamin A, prostaglandins, prolactin, aluminium, and divalent cations such as magnesium and strontium. With the exception of magnesium and aluminium, the physiological or clinical relevance of these factors is uncertain. In the presence of chronic hypomagnesaemia, the release of PTH from parathyroid tissue is impaired, and this, together with an impaired target organ response

to PTH, accounts for the hypocalcaemia occasionally observed in magnesium deficiency.

ACTIONS OF PTH

The target organ actions of PTH include effects on bone, kidney, and indirectly on gut. PTH acts on the proximal and distal tubules of the kidney to increase the renal tubular reabsorption of calcium and to depress the tubular reabsorption of phosphate. This leads to a rise in plasma calcium and fall in plasma phosphate. Inhibition of proximal tubular reabsorption of phosphate appears to be mediated by cyclic AMP as a result of activation of adenylate cyclase in the renal cortex. PTH also decreases the proximal renal tubular reabsorption of bicarbonate which leads to increased excretion of bicarbonate ions and to a hyperchloraemic acidosis. A mild metabolic acidosis is commonly seen in primary and secondary hyperparathyroidism, whereas in hypoparathyroidism a metabolic alkalosis is observed. Alkalosis may also be observed when the secretion of PTH is suppressed, for example by hypercalcaemia due to malignant disease affecting the skeleton. In this example the alkalosis is also partly due to the release of buffer from bone. It is possible that the acidosis induced by PTH augments calcium release from bone.

PTH has a further important effect on the kidney, to stimulate the 1α-hydroxylase enzyme responsible for the production of 1,25-dihydroxy-vitamin D_3 (calcitriol) from calcifidiol. This potent metabolite of vitamin D increases calcium absorption from the gut and possibly releases calcium from the bone. Thus, the various effects of PTH on the kidney and gut appear, either directly or indirectly, to increase the extracellular fluid concentration of calcium. Other effects of PTH on the kidney include decreased proximal tubular reabsorption of sodium and increased amino acid excretion.

The major effect of PTH on bone is to increase bone resorption, by increasing the activity and numbers of osteoclasts. Since mature osteoclasts do not appear to have receptors for PTH this action is likely to be indirect. Both primary and secondary hyperparathyroidism can be associated with obvious radiographic and histological evidence of increased bone resorption. There is evidence, however, that PTH also increases bone formation, suggesting that the major effect of PTH on the skeleton is to increase bone turnover.

There is a great deal of controversy as to whether PTH (and indeed calcitonin) affects the rapid exchange of calcium that occurs between the extracellular fluid and bone and soft tissue. This rapid transfer appears to be important in determining the set-point of plasma calcium.

Calcitonin

Calcitonin is a peptide hormone containing 32 amino acid residues with a disulphide bond between cystine residues in positions 1 and 7. A major stimulus to its secretion is an increase in the serum concentration of calcium. Many of its actions serve to lower serum calcium.

Calcitonin is produced from the parafollicular (C-cells) of the thyroid in man, but is derived embryologically from the ultimobranchial body seen in lower vertebrate species. The entire amino acid sequence is essential for biological activity. There are several differences in amino acid composition of the calcitonins from different species and this is associated with different potencies. Surprisingly, the salmon hormone resembles the human more than other mammalian calcitonins and it is more potent in man than the human hormone itself. The site of calcitonin secretion is not exclusive to thyroid tissue. C-cells are derived embryologically from the APUD cell series of the neural crest. Extrathyroidal sites for calcitonin production have been demonstrated in the thymus, adrenal, and the pars intermedia of the pituitary gland.

Many agents are known to affect the secretion of calcitonin in addition to calcium. These include gastrointestinal hormones, such as glucagon and gastrin, β-adrenergic agents, and whisky. Since an obvious action of calcitonin is to inhibit osteoclast numbers and activity, and thereby lower plasma calcium, it is widely believed that calcitonin is a calcium-regulating hormone with a negative feedback loop provided by plasma calcium. Thus, calcitonin can be seen to have actions opposite to those of parathyroid hormone with respect to the maintenance of plasma calcium.

The physiological role of calcitonin is, however, unclear. In addition to inhibiting bone resorption, it decreases renal tubular reabsorption of calcium, sodium, phosphate, magnesium, potassium, and some other ions. Calcitonin also inhibits the secretion of several gastrointestinal hormones including gastrin, cholecystokinin, insulin, and glucagon. Whether or not these multiple effects are physiological or pharmacological is still uncertain. One difficulty of ascribing any physiological role for calcitonin is that calcitonin deficiency (total thyroidectomy) or excess (medullary carcinoma of the thyroid) are associated with only minor disturbances in skeletal or calcium homeostasis.

A further difficulty in assessing the role of calcitonin arises from conflicting radio-immunoassay data. As in the case of PTH, calcitonin circulates in heterogeneous form and many of the forms measured have uncertain biological significance. The assay for calcitonin is important in the diagnosis of medullary carcinoma of the thyroid, and for the detection of family members with the disease in a presymptomatic form.

The major clinical interest in calcitonin is its pharmacological use as an inhibitor of bone resorption and turnover for the treatment of osteoporosis, Paget's disease, and of hypercalcaemia associated with increased bone resorption.

Vitamin D

In humans vitamin D_3 (cholecalciferol) is derived from the diet and from the skin by ultraviolet irradiation of 7-dehydrocholesterol. Vitamin D_2 (calciferol) is a product originally derived from the ultraviolet irradiation of plant sterols and is used to supplement the diet, particularly in margarine. In most respects these vitamin Ds are comparable in their metabolism and their actions.

Following the photochemical conversion of 7-dehydrocholesterol to vitamin D, it is transported in plasma bound to a specific α-globulin (vitamin D binding protein). Vitamin D is fat soluble and absorbed primarily from the duodenum and jejunum into the lymphatic circulation.

A large amount of the vitamin may be stored in adipose and muscle tissues.

Before exerting biological effects, vitamin D undergoes a series of further metabolic conversions (Fig. 2). The first step involves its conversion in liver to a 25-hydroxylated derivative. The 25-hydroxyvitamin D (25-OHD; calcifidiol) so formed is the major circulating vitamin D metabolite and is commonly measured to provide an index of vitamin D nutrition. Serum values of calcifidiol less than 5 ng/ml (12.5 nmol/l) occur in privational vitamin D deficiency. There is a marked seasonal variation in its serum concentration, with a peak in late summer and a trough in late winter, reflecting exposure to ultraviolet irradiation. In northern Europe, serum values in winter commonly approach those associated with vitamin D deficiency states, suggesting that both sunlight and dietary intake may be of crucial importance in maintaining vitamin D nutrition. A proportion of the calcifidiol formed is secreted into the intestinal lumen, some of which may be available for reabsorption. The physiological importance of this enterohepatic circulation is controversial, but it could contribute to losses of vitamin D in malabsorption syndromes and liver disease.

The next step in the metabolism of vitamin D is its further hydroxylation, mainly in the kidney to calcitriol (1,25-dihydroxyvitamin D_3), secalciferol (24,25(OH)$_2$D$_3$) or 25,26(OH)$_2$D$_3$. The kidney is the major, if not sole, site for 1α-hydroxylation, apart from the placenta and decidua, a factor which is of considerable importance in the pathogenesis of vitamin D resistance in renal failure. The renal metabolism of calcitriol is closely regulated, and its production is favoured under conditions of vitamin D, calcium, or phosphate deficiency. Production of calcitriol is also augmented by a variety of hormones, including PTH, oestradiol, prolactin, and growth hormone, but it is unclear whether or not all these are direct effects. The rise in calcitriol concentrations during pregnancy are partly due to increased synthesis of vitamin D binding protein.

The kidney is a major site for production of secalciferol. In many experimental systems its production is favoured under conditions which inhibit synthesis of calcitriol, such that a reciprocal relationship is commonly observed between their respective production rates. Under conditions of vitamin D, calcium, or phosphate repletion, it is the major circulating dihydroxymetabolite. A variety of observations suggest that this metabolite may have a physiological role in cartilage, bone, or para-

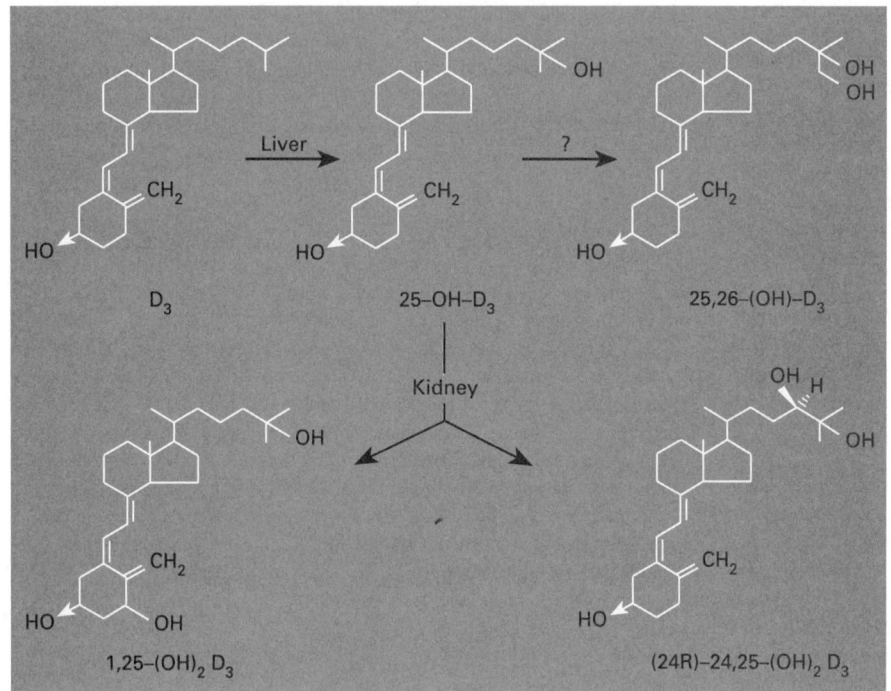

Fig. 2 Steps in the metabolism of vitamin D. The site of synthesis of 25-hydroxyvitamin D_3 (calcidiol) is in the liver. The active form of vitamin D (1,25(OH)$_2$D$_3$; calcitriol) is made in the kidney and placenta. Secalciferol (24,25(OH)$_2$D$_3$) is synthesized in several tissues, but the kidney is probably the major site. The site of synthesis and function of 25,26(OH)$_2$D$_3$ is unknown.

thyroid homeostasis. Many other vitamin D metabolites have been identified in serum. Some appear to have biological activity but their metabolic function, if any, is unclear.

Calcitriol has a serum half-life measured in hours and a normal plasma concentration of approximately 30 pg/ml in adults. Higher concentrations are observed in growing children and during late pregnancy and lactation. Serum values of calcifidiol and secalciferol are 1000-fold and 100-fold greater than those of calcitriol, and both metabolites have a long biological half-life in the circulation, perhaps related to their greater affinity for the vitamin D binding protein. Despite these differences in serum concentrations, calcitriol is considered the active form of vitamin D because it is so much more potent than other derivatives in exerting actions on the target organs.

ACTIONS OF VITAMIN D

The principal effects of calcitriol on calcium metabolism are to increase intestinal absorption of calcium and phosphate and to increase resorption of bone mineral and matrix. Although lack of vitamin D in humans is associated with defective mineralization of cartilage and bone, the question of whether or not vitamin D and its metabolites directly increase mineralization of bone is unsettled. There is also surprisingly little evidence that physiological amounts of calcitriol or of any other vitamin D metabolite increase bone resorption, although increased bone resorption is well documented in vitamin D toxicity. From a teleological viewpoint, the action of calcitriol can be thought of as increasing the availability of calcium and phosphate for mineralization. Alternatively, its function may be to maintain extracellular concentrations of calcium and phosphate in concert with PTH. Calcitriol can be considered to be a hormone in the sense that its production from endocrine tissue (the kidney) is controlled by the calcium and phosphate status of the individual, and that the action of this hormone reverses the stimulus to its secretion.

Receptors for calcitriol have been found in many other tissues apart from bone and gut. These include skin, breast, salivary, and parathyroid tissue. Their physiological significance may be in the differentiation of tissues, and in the case of parathyroid tissue there is pharmacological evidence that calcitriol also decreases the synthesis of parathyroid hormone.

A striking weakness of skeletal muscles, particularly of the pelvic and shoulder girdles, are well-described features of vitamin D deficiency. Moreover, myopathy improves rapidly following treatment with vitamin D or one of its metabolites. The mechanisms whereby vitamin D produces an effect on muscle function is unknown but it may involve calcium transfer across the sarcoplasmic reticulum or modifications in the metabolism of troponin C. It is notable that severe phosphate deficiency induced by dietary deprivation or by hyperparathyroidism is associated with muscle weakness, suggesting that the effects of vitamin D deficiency could be mediated by way of hypophosphataemia or changes in intracellular phosphate. However, in the inherited tubular disorder, hypophosphataemic osteomalacia, muscle weakness is characteristically absent even though there is profound hypophosphataemia. There are several other poorly understood trophic effects of vitamin D, particularly on cellular differentiation, endocrine secretion, growth, the maintenance of intestinal mucosa, and on the maturation of collagen and cartilage.

Other hormones

The hormones PTH, calcitonin, and calcitriol are all found under physiological conditions, and their secretion might be expected to exert continuous influences on bone. But, since they are regulated by changes in extracellular concentrations of calcium or phosphate, the physiological role of these hormones seem less important for skeletal homeostasis itself than for plasma calcium homeostasis. Other factors must maintain the integrity of the skeleton in health and under various conditions of stress. Many of these factors are reviewed in Section 19, but a summary of their effects is relevant in the consideration of plasma calcium homeostasis, since disorders of their metabolism commonly induce changes in plasma calcium.

GROWTH HORMONE

Growth hormone is best known for its effects on the growth of cartilage, an effect which is probably brought about indirectly by growth hormone-dependent production of somatomedins. There are several somatomedins, not all of which are dependent on the growth hormone. Growth hormone also causes a rise of plasma phosphate by increasing the renal tubular reabsorption of phosphate. Growth hormone excess or deficiency is associated with obvious abnormalities in skeletal growth. In acromegaly there is increased periosteal apposition of bone, but there is no convincing evidence for the widely expressed view that acromegaly causes osteoporosis. Changes in growth hormone secretion have very little effect on plasma calcium and the occasional finding of hypercalcaemia in acromegalic patients should alert one to the possibility of coexisting primary hyperparathyroidism (pluriglandular syndrome). Hypercalciuria is more common and may be related to increased synthesis of calcitriol.

THYROID HORMONES

Deficiency of thyroid hormones early in life produce the well-known skeletal abnormalities of cretinism. Before skeletal maturity, thyrotoxicosis may increase skeletal growth. In the adult, thyrotoxicosis is associated with hypercalciuria, hypophosphataemia, augmented bone turnover, and occasionally hypercalcaemia, probably due to direct effects of thyroid hormones on bone.

ADRENAL STEROIDS

The most important effect of glucocorticoids on the skeleton is to regulate growth. Their action on calcium metabolism is complex and probably involves effects on many target tissues in addition to effects on the metabolism and action of other hormones, including calcitriol. In the adult, adrenal insufficiency is not associated with skeletal abnormalities, but is occasionally accompanied by hypercalcaemia. This is probably due to haemoconcentration and to increased renal tubular reabsorption of calcium because of extracellular volume depletion. Chronic glucocorticoid excess can induce osteoporosis, but the mechanisms are far from clear. The ability of corticosteroids to decrease plasma calcium in some forms of hypercalcaemia has been used for many years as a diagnostic aid (see below), but once again the mechanism of action is uncertain. One effect of corticosteroids is to suppress the secretion of osteoclast-activating factors and prostaglandins, both of which may have direct effects on bone to increase bone resorption.

SEX STEROIDS

Characteristic growth abnormalities are associated with deficiencies of either male or female sex hormones, which appear to play a crucial role in epiphyseal closure and in the growth spurts seen before this event. They may also influence the amount of calcium present in the skeleton at the time of maturity. In adults, the effects of oestrogens are of particular interest because of the loss of bone that occurs in women after the menopause. Administration of oestrogen may prevent this loss. Oestrogen administration also lowers plasma calcium, an effect more marked in postmenopausal women with hyperparathyroidism or hypercalcaemia from carcinoma of the breast. It is interesting that hypercalcaemia is also occasionally seen with the use of tamoxifen, an oestrogen inhibitor, when used in the treatment of carcinoma of the breast.

GASTROINTESTINAL HORMONES

(See also Section 14.)

There are many interactions between calcium-regulating and gastrointestinal hormones. The relationships between gastrin and calcitonin secretion have been described earlier. Calcium and parathyroid hormone also influence gastrin secretion, which is increased in hyperparathyroidism, due to the stimulation of gastrin secretion by calcium. Among other gastrointestinal hormones, large doses of glucagon may induce hypocalcaemia by inhibiting bone resorption, either directly or by stimulating the secretion of calcitonin. Secretion may cause hypercalcaemia, perhaps by stimulating parathyroid hormone release. Insulin is an important hormone for skeletal growth and diabetics often have diminished skeletal mass; it is one of the few endocrine hormones shown to stimulate specifically bone collagen synthesis *in vitro*.

OSTEOCLAST ACTIVATING FACTORS

Osteoclast activating factor was thought to be a single bone-resorbing agent derived from mononuclear leucocytes. It is now clear that several factors derived from leucocytes are potent bone-resorbing agents. These include lymphotoxin, tumour necrosis factors, and interleukin-1α and -1β. Their physiological importance is unknown, but the production of leucocyte-derived factors is increased in haematological neoplasias and may be responsible for the hypercalcaemia and bone loss seen in myeloma, which is characteristically sensitive to treatment with corticosteroids. Other factors have been identified which may be important in the activation of osteoclasts in solid tumours. These include the prostaglandins and procathapsin D. In addition, transforming growth factors and the PTH-related protein are causes of generalized bone resorption (see below).

Sites of calcium regulation

With the exception of the pregnant or lactating female, the major fluxes of calcium to and from the extracellular fluid occur across the intestinal mucosa, bone, and kidneys. The following pages describe the extent to which these fluxes are controlled by hormonal agents and the influence they have on plasma calcium.

INTESTINE

Unlike the fluxes of calcium between the extracellular fluid, bone, and kidneys, intestinal absorption of calcium is episodic and is dependent on an adequate supply of calcium delivered in an available form to the intestinal mucosa. The availability of calcium for absorption depends on many dietary factors. For example, excess phosphorus, lipids, and phytates bind calcium and render it unavailable for absorption. The influx of calcium depends both on active transport and diffusion processes. Absorption occurs throughout the length of the small intestine and to a lesser extent in the colon. The major site for active transport is the duodenum and upper part of the jejunum. However, because the duodenum is relatively short compared to the entire length of the gastrointestinal tract, more calcium is probably absorbed at the sites distal to the duodenum at normal dietary intakes than within the duodenum itself.

At very low intakes of calcium, net absorption may be negative since endogenous faecal calcium secretion may exceed the amount absorbed. In malabsorption syndromes the endogenous faecal calcium may appear to rise, but this does not necessarily mean that calcium secreted in the digestive juices is increased, since the rise is probably due to malabsorption of digestive-juice calcium.

Humans are able to adapt to variations in dietary intake of calcium so that net absorption remains relatively constant over a fairly wide range of intake, probably regulated by calcitriol. The biochemical mechanisms involved in active calcium transport have been partially identified. Calcitriol stimulates the synthesis of a calcium-binding protein (calbindin) in addition to an intestinal alkaline phosphatase, by a mechanism similar to that described for many other steroid hormones. This involves the translocation of calcitriol plus its receptor protein to the nucleus to stimulate the synthesis of messenger RNA and new protein synthesis.

There is good evidence that calcium and phosphate can be absorbed separately from each other, though calcitriol has independent effects to enhance the absorption of each. Unlike the absorption of calcium, which appears to be closely regulated, the proportion of the dietary phosphate absorbed does not vary much with increasing intake but remains relatively constant at approximately 80 per cent of the dietary intake over a wide range of intake. This explains in part the fluctuations in plasma phosphate seen after a meal and underlines the need to study phosphate metabolism under controlled conditions.

A variety of tests are available to study calcium and phosphate absorption, including metabolic balance and the use of tracer techniques. These are generally available only to a few centres. A 24-h urine collection for calcium provides an indirect index of absorption, provided it is assumed or known that the net flux of calcium across bone is zero. The expression of excretion as a ratio of creatinine excretion standardizes somewhat for variations in body weight and for incomplete urine collections.

Increased intestinal absorption of calcium is found in pregnancy, during lactation, and in several disease states, including hyperparathyroidism, sarcoidosis, and idiopathic hypercalciuria due to increased production of calcitriol. Conversely, malabsorption of calcium is often caused by low levels of calcitriol, for example in hypoparathyroidism, vitamin D deficiency states, and in chronic renal failure. Calcium malabsorption is also seen in untreated coeliac disease where a target tissue for calcitriol has been destroyed.

KIDNEYS

The fluxes of calcium across the kidneys are much greater than those across the gut. Renal tubular reabsorption of calcium in the kidneys is a very complex process and the total amount reabsorbed is the result of several mechanisms in various parts of the nephron. The total amount of calcium reabsorbed can be estimated by subtracting the amount of calcium excreted by the kidneys from the filtered load. The filterable calcium is approximately 60 per cent of total plasma calcium, and the filtered load represents the product of the glomerular filtration rate and the filterable calcium (approximately 200–250 mmol/day).

In health there is a curvilinear relationship between plasma calcium (an index of filtered load) and renal excretion. The renal excretion may be expressed per unit of glomerular filtration rate to take account of variations in this rate (Fig. 3). Any value below the line depicting the normal relationship would indicate an increase in the net tubular reabsorption of calcium, and values above the lines denote decreased tubular reabsorption. A high value for renal calcium excretion indicates an increase in the filtered load (gut or bone derived) or a low glomerular filtration rate. When calcium excretion is measured in the fasting state, this will reflect more closely calcium derived from skeletal sources. An important corollary is that the estimation of urinary calcium excretion does not give information concerning renal tubular reabsorption unless the filtered load is also known. Some normal ranges for these values are shown in Table 2.

The assessment of renal tubular reabsorption in this way has several limitations in clinical practice since ultrafilterable calcium is rarely measured, and its derivation from total plasma calcium may be difficult in disorders of acid–base metabolism, dysproteinaemia, and renal damage. In health, approximately 97 per cent of the calcium filtered by the kidney is reabsorbed. Many hormones influence renal tubular reabsorption, of which PTH is probably the most important. In mild primary hyperparathyroidism, the hypercalcaemia is due mainly to increased renal tubular reabsorption. Conversely, in hypoparathyroidism the fasting renal excretion is commonly normal. The low plasma calcium is therefore due to decreased renal tubular reabsorption of calcium.

Plasma phosphate varies more than plasma calcium and its concentration is set mainly by the kidney. Unlike serum calcium, the vast majority of inorganic phosphate is ultrafilterable (90 per cent). The measurement of renal tubular reabsorption of phosphate may be used in clinical investigation, for example in the diagnosis of hyperparathyroidism. There are several methods available to calculate phosphate reabsorption; the best is probably an estimation of TmP/GFR (tubular maximum for phosphate reabsorption). This examines the relationship between filtered load and renal excretion which, like that for calcium reabsorption, is curvilinear at physiological concentrations. A nomogram has been produced for deriving this measurement (Fig. 4). Phosphate reabsorption is increased by growth hormone, in hypoparathyroidism, and in phosphate deprivation. It is low in several inherited or acquired renal tubular disorders, and may also be influenced by drugs such as corticosteroids.

Both calcium and phosphate excretion are influenced by other factors, notably sodium excretion, extracellular fluid volume expansion, and by the administration of diuretics. Infusion of sodium chloride increases the excretion of both calcium and phosphate, an effect which contributes to its value in the treatment of hypercalcaemia.

The biochemical mechanisms of transport of calcium and phosphate have not been elucidated, but the action of PTH on the kidneys is known to produce an increase in cortical adenylate cyclase activity, which increases tubular cell and urine concentrations of cyclic AMP. It is not known whether this increase in cyclic AMP is the cause of the subsequent changes in phosphate and calcium transport.

BONE

The major organic component of bone matrix is type I collagen, but other constituents may have considerable importance. The metabolism of the organic component of bone is reviewed in Section 19. Measurements of mineral turnover and the indirect indices of bone matrix turnover are considered here.

The processes of bone formation, its mineralization, and resorption are closely coupled but do not occur in the same anatomical site at the

Fig. 3 Relationship between urinary calcium excretion (expressed as mg/100 ml of glomerular filtrate) and serum calcium in health and disorders of parathyroid function. The solid and dashed lines denote the mean values (+ 2 SD) obtained in normal subjects during calcium infusions. The shaded area represents the normal basal range. Patients with primary hyperparathyroidism (−) lie to the right of the line describing normal subjects, indicating increased renal tubular reabsorption for calcium. In contrast, patients with hypoparathyroidism lie to the left of the normal line, indicating decreased renal tubular reabsorption for calcium. Note that the determination of calcium excretion alone (without concurrent measurement of serum calcium) does not give information concerning renal tubular reabsorption for calcium. Note also that hypoparathyroid patients, not infused with calcium, and many hyperparathyroid patients, have normal values of calcium excretion. (From Nordin, B.E.C. and Peacock, M. (1969).)

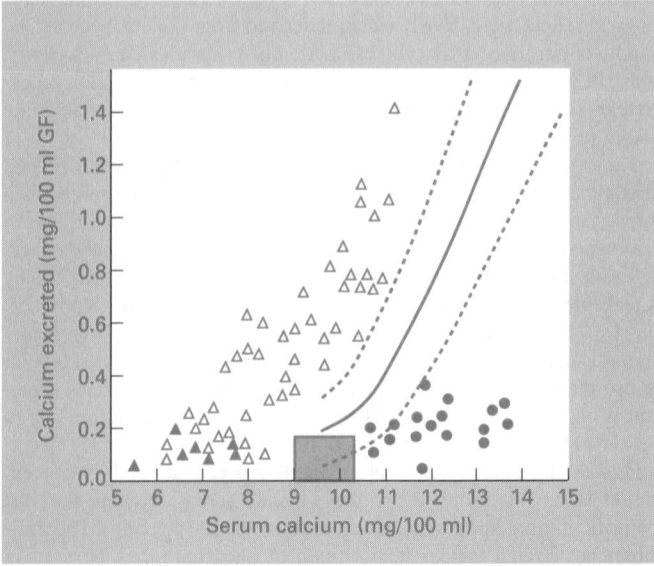

Table 2 *Typical normal adult ranges for some simple biochemical measurements used in the investigation of patients with disorders of calcium homeostasis*

Measurement	Units	Reference range
Plasma		
Total calcium	mmol/l	2.12–2.60
Ionized calcium	mmol/l	1.10–1.35
Fasting inorganic phosphate	mmol/l	0.6–1.5
Urine		
Calcium	mmol/24 h	M 2.5–10
	mmol/24 h	F 2.5–9.0
Phosphate	mmol/24 h	16–32
Total hydroxyproline	μmol/24 h	M 55–250
	μmol/24 h	F 75–430
Fasting urine		
Calcium/creatinine ratio	mmol/mmol	0.10–0.32
Calcium excretion	mmol/l GF	0.04
TmP/GFR	mmol/l	0.8–1.35
Total hydroxyproline/ creatinine	μmol/mmol	<40

M or F denotes sex; TmP/GFR, tubular maximum for phosphate reabsorption; GF, glomerular filtrate.

Fig. 4 Nomogram for the derivation of TmP/GFR (estimate of phosphate reabsorption) from simultaneous measurements of tubular reabsorption (TRP) or the ratio of the clearance of phosphate to the clearance of creatinine (CPO$_4$/Creat) and plasma phosphate (PO$_4$). TRP can be calculated from the concentrations of phosphate and creatinine in plasma; the urine volume is not required:

$$\frac{\text{Phosphate clearance}}{\text{Creatinine clearance}} = \frac{\text{urine phosphate} \times \text{plasma creatinine}}{\text{plasma phosphate} \times \text{urine creatinine}}$$

A straight line through the appropriate values of plasma phosphate and TRP or phosphate/creatinine clearance passes through the corresponding value of TmP/GFR. TmP/GFR and phosphate are expressed in the same units. The scale in units of the figure is arbitrary. (From Walton, R.J. and Bijvoet, O.L.M. (1975).)

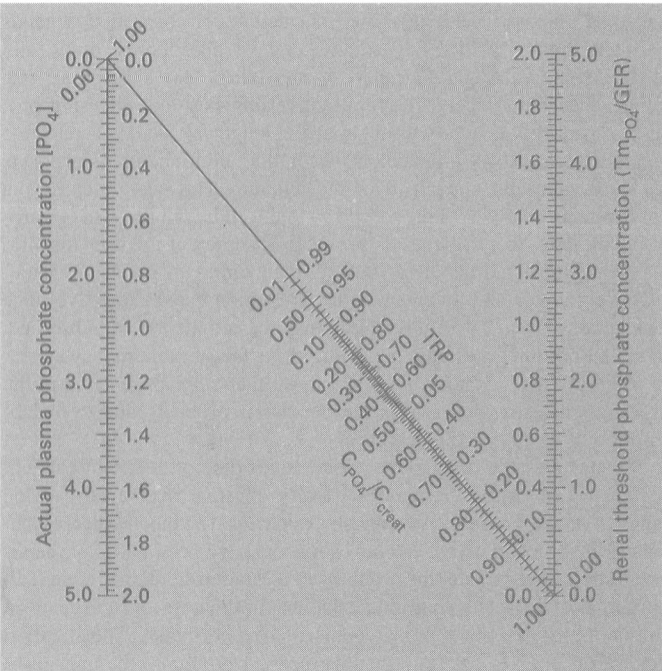

same time. These processes are governed by bone cells, including osteoblasts, which form bone matrix and are rich in alkaline phosphatase, and osteoclasts, which are multinucleate giant cells responsible for bone destruction. Alkaline phosphatase may function in calcification as a component of a membrane pump for calcium and phosphate, or it may be involved in the metabolism of potential inhibitors of calcification, such as inorganic pyrophosphate. The possible importance of alkaline phosphatase in mineralization is illustrated in hypophosphatasia (a rare and recessively inherited disorder of mineralization). This is characterized by low or absent serum activity of alkaline phosphatase. Serum activity of alkaline phosphatase provides a useful and readily measured index of osteoblast activity. It is important to note that serum activity is also partly derived from the liver and gut (and the placenta), and that diseases of these organs may also result in hyperphosphatasia. This can be resolved by the concurrent measurement of liver enzymes (for example 5′-nucleotidase) or isoenzyme studies.

Bone resorption is accompanied by a release of enzymes such as collagenase and lysosomal enzymes capable of degrading bone matrix beneath the ruffled border of the osteoclast. Proline is a major constituent of the bone collagen molecule which is hydroxylated to hydroxyproline in the post-translational stage of collagen formation. The liberation of hydroxyproline by osteoclasts into the extracellular fluid is therefore an index of collagen degradation and bone resorption which can be measured in the urine in the assessment of metabolic bone disease. Other sources of urinary hydroxyproline include the diet (meats and gelatin), non-skeletal collagen, the first component of complement, and propeptides of collagen liberated during its formation. When urine is collected under fasting conditions or on a low gel diet there is a surprisingly good correlation between hydroxyproline excretion and other indices of bone resorption. The use of the fasting urinary calcium excretion as an index of net calcium release from bone has been discussed previously.

The factors affecting bone formation and mineralization are ill-understood, and more is known of the agents that affect bone resorption, possibly because this is easier to study *in vitro*. Calcitriol and PTH are potent bone-resorbing agents, but probably act by different mechanisms. A number of agents are known to inhibit the rate of bone resorption. Administration of calcitonin inhibits bone resorption and decreases the activity and numbers of osteoclasts. Oestrogens also inhibit the rate of bone resorption, although receptors for oestrogen have not been demonstrated in bone cells. Other inhibitors of bone resorption include mithramycin corticosteroids, and the bisphosphonates which have become useful therapeutic agents in the treatment of disorders of bone turnover and of hypercalcaemia associated with increased bone resorption.

In adults the vast majority of skeletal calcium turnover is due to the remodelling of cortical and trabecular bone. The first phase of bone remodelling is the excavation of an erosion cavity. Once resorption by osteoclasts is complete, osteoblasts are attracted to the resorption surface and synthesize skeletal matrix. The mineralization of the organic matrix lags several days behind its synthesis. In a variety of both physiological and pathological states, it is clear that there is a remarkably close correlation between the rates of mineral deposition in bone and mineral resorption (Fig. 5). Even though these individual rates may be altered many fold (for example in Paget's disease) the net gains or losses of the skeletal mass are minimized by the tight balance between these rates. A component of this regulatory system, termed coupling, is due to the attraction of osteoblasts predominantly to sites of previous bone resorption. The distinction between skeletal balance and coupling is illustrated in Fig. 6. Uncoupling occurs in neoplasia affecting the skeleton. In osteoporosis, where there is a gradual diminution of bone mass, there is an imbalance in the rate of bone formation and that of bone resorption in favour of net mineral losses. However, there still appears to be a coupling mechanism in the sense that attempts to alter bone resorption, for example by calcitonin, result not only in the inhibition of bone resorption but also the later inhibition of bone formation. Thus, changes in bone turnover alone have only transient effects on plasma calcium.

A variety of techniques exist for the assessment of skeletal turnover other than the measurement of alkaline phosphatase and the urinary excretion of hydroxyproline. These include metabolic balance studies with concurrent tracer kinetic studies and other biochemical markers of bone turnover. Techniques are also available for measuring bone mass. These include density and cortical width measurements on radiography, photon absorption to measure bone density, *in vivo* neutron activation analysis, and computed tomography. The quality of bone itself can be

Fig. 5 The relationship between the rate of mineral accretion (A) and resorption (R) in patients with a variety of metabolic bone disorders. Note the logarithmic scales for accretion and resorption and the close relationship of these to measurements. The dotted line represents the state in which resorption of bone matches its accretion. (From Harris, W.H. and Heaney, R.P. (1969).)

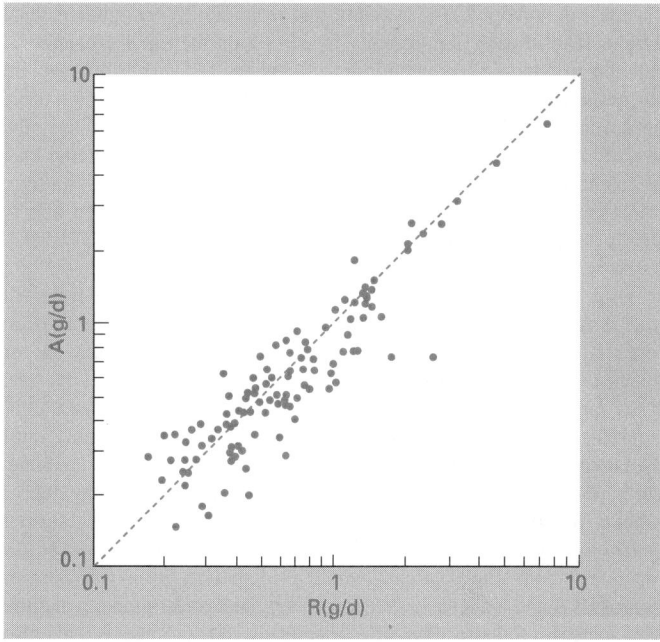

Fig. 6 Schematic diagram to illustrate the difference between skeletal balance and the coupling of bone formation with resorption. Coupling implies the recruitment of osteoblasts to sites of previous resorption irrespective of the amount of bone resorbed or formed within each resorption site.

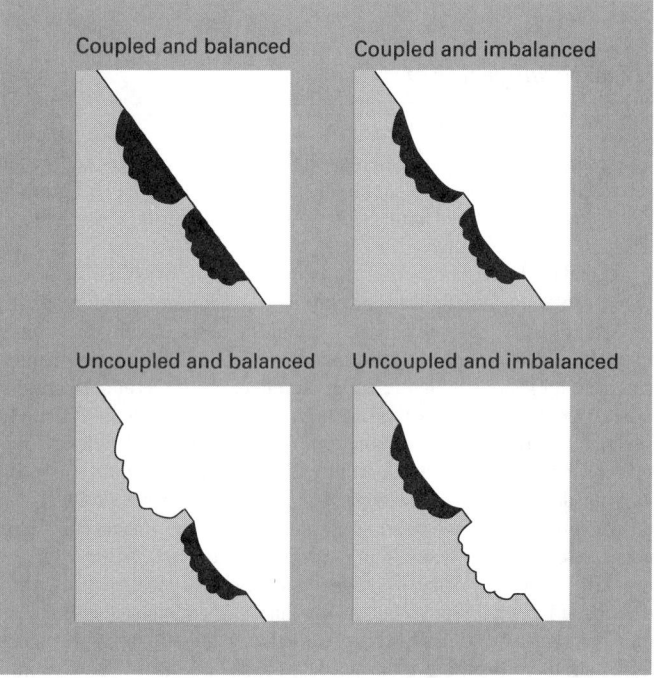

more directly estimated by the use of bone biopsy. Some of these techniques are discussed in greater detail in Section 19.

INTEGRATED RESPONSES

In considering plasma calcium homeostasis, it is useful to separate acute changes from chronic changes. When the system is disturbed a steady state no longer exists. A response occurs which adjusts the system to produce a new steady state. Deviations of plasma calcium away from its normal value are rapidly corrected by alterations in the secretion and synthesis of the regulating hormones. PTH can be considered the fast-acting component of the regulatory system, whereas vitamin D is responsible for adaptation over a longer time. The rapid control of plasma calcium by PTH is mainly due to its ability to regulate renal tubular reabsorption and possibly by effects on the rapid exchange of calcium in bone. After parathyroidectomy, the fall in plasma calcium can be largely accounted for by the continued loss of calcium into urine until a new steady state is achieved in which calcium excretion is the same as its starting value but takes place at a much reduced filtered load of calcium. During the transient state when plasma calcium is falling, urinary excretion of calcium will increase. In contrast, when a new steady state is established, urinary calcium excretion will fall to normal despite a lower level of plasma calcium.

A further example of the difference between the steady and transient state is seen during the infusion of calcium. During a calcium infusion (or, for example, increased absorption of calcium from the gut or increases in bone resorption not mediated by PTH) plasma calcium rises. If the rate of calcium entry into the extracellular fluid is constant, concentrations of plasma calcium will not rise indefinitely but only until the rate of efflux of calcium from the extracellular fluid pool (from bone, gut, and other tissues, but mainly from the kidney) matches the rate of influx. At this point, extracellular calcium levels will rise no further despite continuing the infusion, and a new steady state will prevail. In practice, the infusion of calcium would result in the suppression of secretion of PTH and a decrease in the renal tubular reabsorption of calcium. This increases the rate at which a new steady state is achieved, and also decreases the final concentration of plasma calcium obtained. It is notable that the rate of rise of plasma calcium during a calcium infusion is to some extent buffered by the exchange of calcium in bone. Thus, rises or falls in plasma calcium are partially compensated by increased net movements of calcium into or out of bone.

Hyperparathyroidism

DEFINITIONS

The term hyperparathyroidism is applied to those clinical disorders characterized by an increase in circulating concentrations of PTH. These can be arbitrarily classified into primary, secondary, tertiary, and ectopic (pseudo-) hyperparathyroidism.

Secondary hyperparathyroidism is due to hypocalcaemia, such as is seen in vitamin D deficiency or chronic renal failure, which results in the secretion of PTH and leads to hyperplasia of the parathyroid glands. In general, all four parathyroid glands are enlarged. The biochemical and skeletal lesions which result are a reflection of the underlying disorder, hypocalcaemia, as well as high circulating levels of PTH. The skeletal abnormalities seen, for example, in vitamin D deficiency, represent a combination of hyperparathyroidism, phosphate deficiency, and varying degrees of osteomalacia. Secondary hyperparathyroidism can be cured by appropriate treatment which restores the plasma calcium to normal (for example, vitamin D in simple nutritional deficiency of vitamin D). This removes the stimulus to parathyroid overactivity. Concentrations of PTH fall rapidly but the involution of parathyroid hyperplasia may take many months. More detailed considerations of secondary hyperparathyroidism are found in the sections on disorders of vitamin

Table 3 *Causes of primary hyperparathyroidism; chief-cell hyperplasia is associated with multiple endocrine abnormalities*

Single adenoma	83.0%
Multiple adenoma	4.3%
Carcinoma	1.7%
Hyperplasia	
clear cell	7.6%
chief cell	3.6%

D metabolism (see below), on renal bone disease (see Chapter 20.18), and on osteomalacia (see Section 18).

Tertiary hyperparathyroidism is a term used to denote those patients with long-standing secondary hyperparathyroidism who develop autonomous gland function and hypercalcaemia. Nowadays this is most commonly seen after renal transplantation, but may also be observed in patients with long-standing malabsorption or chronic renal failure. As in the case of many endocrine disorders, the term 'autonomous secretion' is a misnomer since PTH can be suppressed by calcium infusion, or further augmented by lowering plasma calcium. Tertiary hyperparathyroidism therefore implies a change in the set point with respect to the calcium control of PTH secretion. In this disorder, plasma calcium and PTH are both raised and treatment includes parathyroidectomy and the management of the cause.

Primary hyperparathyroidism implies hyperfunction of one or more parathyroid glands which results in a change in the set point for the control of plasma calcium such that plasma calcium values are higher than normal. Pseudohyperparathyroidism is the elaboration of PTH-like material in association with certain malignancies, particularly of the lung. This gives rise to biochemical abnormalities not unlike those of primary hyperparathyroidism.

PRIMARY HYPERPARATHYROIDISM

Primary hyperparathyroidism is usually due to a single parathyroid adenoma of the chief cells of the parathyroid gland. More rarely it is due to diffuse hyperplasia or multiple adenomata (Table 3). Hyperplasia and adenoma may be difficult to differentiate histologically. Carcinoma is very rare. Since the widespread use of multiple channel autoanalysers in clinical practice, the most common presentation (50–70 per cent of cases) is hypercalcaemia, which is asymptomatic. This has resulted in revised estimates of its prevalence, which is now estimated as between 2 and 10 per 10 000 of the population. It occurs with greatest frequency between the fourth and sixth decades of life, when it is twice as common in females as in males. At other age groups the sex incidence is roughly equal. The cause of primary hyperparathyroidism is unknown, but in women it appears to be unmasked by the menopause. An increased risk occurs some years following irradiation of the head and neck.

Since the major effect of PTH is to raise plasma calcium, the main biochemical abnormality is an increase in the circulating concentration of both PTH and calcium. There are, however, instances where patients with proven adenoma have normal total serum calcium levels or intermittent hypercalcaemia. Conversely, patients may have values of PTH within the laboratory reference range which in the presence of hypercalcaemia are inappropriately high. Thus, primary hyperparathyroidism can be defined as a circulating level of PTH that is inappropriately high for the prevailing level of plasma calcium (Fig. 7). In some instances, the patient with primary hyperparathyroidism may be normocalcaemic because of coexistent vitamin D deficiency.

As expected, the renal tubular reabsorption for calcium is enhanced at any given filtered load in primary hyperparathyroidism (see Fig. 3). There is often also increased bone resorption, reflected by increased hydroxyprolinuria and increased intestinal absorption of calcium due to the stimulation of calcitriol production. These factors will tend to increase the 24-h urinary excretion for calcium. Although resorption of bone is commonly enhanced in primary hyperparathyroidism, so too is bone formation, reflected as an increase in alkaline phosphatase. Thus the skeletal balance for calcium is usually normal, but at the expense of an increased bone turnover. Bone loss may occur, however, particularly in patients with severe bone disease and in female patients with coexisting postmenopausal osteoporosis. Calcium-containing renal stones are also a feature of primary hyperparathyroidism. The aetiology of renal stones in hyperparathyroidism is discussed elsewhere but is related in part to an increase in the filtered load of calcium and the passage of an alkaline urine.

CLINICAL AND LABORATORY FEATURES

The manifestations of primary hyperparathyroidism largely reflect the result of PTH actions and hypercalcaemia itself. Up to 50 per cent of patients present with renal stone disease, and primary hyperparathyroidism accounts for approximately 5 per cent of patients with renal stone disease.

Bone disease is usually apparent on histology of bone but it is rarely overt. Biochemical indices of increased bone turnover (raised alkaline phosphatase and increased urinary hydroxyproline excretion) are found in up to 50 per cent of patients. Radiographic manifestations of primary hyperparathyroidism occur in less than 2 per cent of patients; in these patients hyperparathyroidism is severe, and sometimes due to parathyroid carcinoma; renal calculi are uncommon in this group. The characteristic radiographic feature of hyperparathyroidism is subperiosteal erosion of bone (Fig. 8). The skeleton may also be diffusely osteoporotic or osteosclerotic, although the latter findings are usually confined to patients with severe and long-standing secondary hyperparathyroidism.

Hyperparathyroidism in growing children causes appearances which radiographically resemble rickets, but which are quite different histologically. This is due to resorption of metaphyseal bone which may give rise to crippling skeletal deformities. Cystic lesions may also be found in primary hyperparathyroidism, 'brown tumours' which may result in pathological fracture. In the skull, extensive bone resorption may give a mottled 'salt and pepper' appearance on radiographs. Subperiosteal

erosion is most frequently noted in the hands, with resorption of the phalangeal tufts, and on the radial borders of the middle phalanges. The distal ends of the clavicles are also commonly involved by resorption but are more difficult sites to examine radiographically. The loss of the lamina dura and the appearance of brown tumours in the mandible are late complications of primary hyperparathyroidism, but the radiographic appearances are not specific.

There are many other features of primary hyperparathyroidism, many of which are due to hypercalcaemia. However, it is important to realize that in one-third of patients hypercalcaemia will have been an incidental finding, and many of these patients are asymptomatic. However, the symptoms of hypercalcaemia are often very vague and include nausea, vomiting, fatigue, constipation, and hypotonicity of the muscles and ligaments. Bone pain and tenderness are seen in primary hyperparathyroidism but are more common in secondary hyperparathyroidism. Hypercalcaemia induces polyuria, and this may lead to dehydration or polydipsia. Paradoxically, hypertension may arise despite the intravascular volume depletion. The raised plasma calcium and dehydration may also lead to renal abnormalities in addition to renal stone disease such as nephrocalcinosis and progressive chronic renal failure (see Chapter 20.9.3). Calcification may also occur in other sites, such as cartilage (pseudo-gout) and blood vessels. Periarticular soft tissue calcification is more commonly seen in hyperparathyroidism due to renal failure. Calcification in the eye is reflected as a band keratopathy of the cornea or as conjunctival deposits which are as seen with the use of a slit-lamp. Proximal myopathy is an unusual feature and may be due to concurrent phosphate depletion. Gastrointestinal symptoms may be an early clue to the diagnosis of hyperparathyroidism since peptic ulceration is seen in 5 to 10 per cent of patients, possibly related to hypercalcaemia-induced secretion of gastrin. Acute or chronic pancreatitis is also associated with hyperparathyroidism and calcification of the pancreas may be evident on radiography or on radionuclide scanning. Pancreatic symptoms often precede the diagnosis of hyperparathyroidism and the failure of serum calcium values to fall during acute pancreatitis raises the suspicion of coexisting primary hyperparathyroidism.

Neurological disturbances attributable to hypercalcaemia are very

Fig. 7 Plasma values of parathyroid hormone in normal subjects (group 1) and patients with hypercalcaemia (2–6). Patients with surgically proven hyperparathyroidism (groups 2 and 3) have higher levels of PTH, but there is an overlap with the normal range. However, these patients were hypercalcaemic, indicating that values of PTH were inappropriately high for the plasma calcium. Thus, patients with vitamin D intoxication (group 4), idiopathic hypercalcaemia of infancy (group 5), and patients with skeletal metastases and hypercalcaemia (group 6) have very low or undetectable levels of PTH. (From Woodhead, J.S. and Walker, D.A. (1976).)

Fig. 8 Radiographic features of hyperparathyroid bone disease. Note the marked subperiosteal bone resorption involving the terminal phalanges. Note also the cortical porosity.

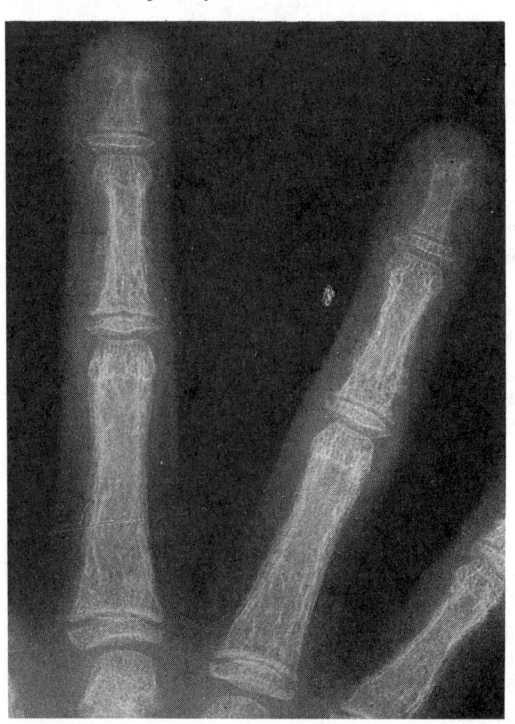

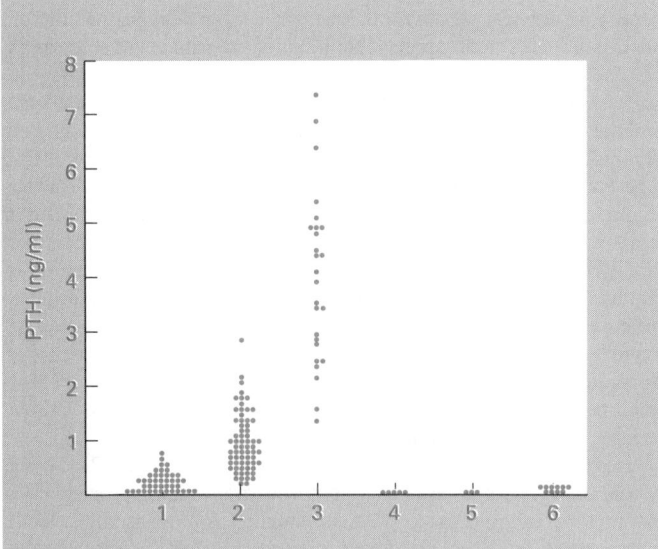

varied and often subtle. They range from behavioural disorders and mood variation to organic psychosis, dementia, and focal neurological lesions. They are associated with abnormalities in the electroencephalogram which usually disappear with treatment, unless there has been structural damage to the brain.

Less common laboratory findings in hyperparathyroidism include aminoaciduria, hypomagnesaemia, elevated erythrocyte sedimentation rate, and a shortening of the QT interval on the electrocardiogram. A monoclonal increase in immunoglobulins has been described in primary hyperparathyroidism and does not, therefore, necessarily indicate myelomatosis.

A number of other disorders have been associated with primary hyperparathyroidism, including gout, hypothyroidism, Paget's disease, and diabetes mellitus. These are relatively common disorders and it is not clear whether or not the associations are causal. Hypercalcaemia is occasionally seen in Paget's disease, particularly during immobilization, and is commonly associated with primary hyperparathyroidism. There is a familial form of hyperparathyroidism and suspicion should be alerted when hyperparathyroidism is found in young adults or children. It has an autosomal dominant mode of transmission. It may occur without other abnormalities but is frequently part of the pluriglandular syndrome. It may be associated with pituitary or pancreatic tumours, with peptic ulceration and gastric hypersecretion, or with tumours of the adrenal cortex (multiple endocrine neoplasia type 1). Combinations of hyperparathyroidism, medullary carcinoma of the thyroid, phaeochromocytoma, carcinoid tumours, and mucosal and cutaneous neurofibromata also occur (multiple endocrine neoplasia type 2). Familial benign hypercalcaemia is also an autosomal dominantly inherited form of hypercalcaemia. The aetiology of the disorder is unknown, but is associated with increased renal tubular reabsorption of calcium and normal, rather than low, circulating PTH. It is important to recognize the disorder since parathyroidectomy is rarely of benefit or required.

DIAGNOSIS

The characteristic feature of primary hyperparathyroidism is the raised plasma calcium in the presence of high or normal circulating values of PTH. Both plasma calcium and PTH should be interpreted with caution. Account should be taken of possible abnormalities in the protein concentration or in protein binding of calcium. The kidney is an important site for degradation of PTH and a degree of renal impairment is found in approximately 10 to 15 per cent of patients with primary hyperparathyroidism. Depending on the characteristics of the immunoassay, the increased values of PTH in the presence of renal failure may not reflect an increase in the biologically active fraction of PTH. The majority of patients with primary hyperparathyroidism also have low values of serum phosphate due to decreased renal tubular reabsorption of phosphate. The estimation of TmP/GFR (see Fig. 4), however, does not always discriminate various groups of patients with hypercalcaemia.

In the majority of patients, the diagnosis is quite straightforward and rests on the finding of an increase in plasma calcium, increase (or lack of suppression) in plasma PTH, reduction in tubular reabsorption of phosphate, and an increase in renal tubular reabsorption of calcium. The finding of augmented calcium absorption and high values of calcitriol, hyperphosphatasia, or increased urinary excretion of hydroxyproline support the diagnosis. It is important to recognize that renal failure makes the interpretation of these tests difficult.

Most patients with primary hyperparathyroidism present with hypercalcaemia alone or with renal stone disease. The greatest diagnostic difficulties among patients with renal calculi are encountered in distinguishing between hyperparathyroidism and idiopathic hypercalciuria. In the case of idiopathic hypercalciuria, plasma calcium is always normal but there are well-documented cases of patients with parathyroid adenoma in whom plasma calcium lies within the normal range. The administration of a thiazide diuretic such as bendrofluazide which increases renal tubular reabsorption of calcium, will induce persistent hypercalcaemia in patients with primary hyperparathyroidism and may aid in the identification of such patients.

Hypercalcaemia is commonly seen in patients with malignant disease. This is usually due to increased calcium release from bone, but in some instances may be due to the production of PTH-related protein and other factors by the tumour itself. This latter syndrome has been variously described as pseudohyperparathyroidism or humoral hypercalcaemia of malignancy, and may occur in the absence of skeletal metastases. The majority of patients with carcinoma and hypercalcaemia have overt radiographic or scintigraphic evidence for bone metastases. Patients with myelomatosis and other haematological tumours associated with hypercalcaemia may show diffuse osteoporosis rather than the more characteristic punched-out lesions. Other causes for hypercalcaemia are discussed below. A variety of tests have been advocated to distinguish these disorders, including the hydrocortisone suppression test, but are now obsolete with the development of better immunoassays for PTH. In the absence of renal impairment, a plasma bicarbonate may be useful. In hyperparathyroidism, a metabolic acidosis is commonly found which is reflected by a low plasma bicarbonate and a high plasma chloride, whereas in disorders where PTH secretion is depressed a metabolic alkalosis is to be expected. Moreover, in hypercalcaemia due to rapid bone destruction, alkalosis may be accentuated by the release of bicarbonate from bone. Patients with carcinoma frequently have low serum values of albumin and phosphate due to cachexia.

TREATMENT

A moderate increase in plasma calcium may lead to progressive renal impairment and severe hypercalcaemia may cause an immediate threat to life. At the other extreme, many patients with primary hyperparathyroidism have mild hypercalcaemia (plasma calcium < 3.0 mmol/l) without symptoms, and it is probable that many patients with adenomas of the parathyroid glands die of unrelated causes. Opinion varies whether such patients should undergo parathyroidectomy, but it is probably wise to err in the favour of surgery since many of the signs of hypercalcaemia are subtle and not always appreciated until after removal of excess parathyroid tissue. The aims of surgery are to remove the adenoma or to resect sufficient hyperplastic parathyroid tissue to render the patient euparathyroid. The best results are seen with surgeons having extensive experience.

The surgical management of patients with primary and tertiary hyperparathyroidism is often difficult because of the variable anatomy of the parathyroids, problems with the differentiation between multiple gland hyperplasia and single gland adenoma, and the incidence of postsurgical hyper- and hypoparathyroidism. The approach of many centres is to identify all cervical parathyroid tissue, since more than one parathyroid gland is affected in an appreciable minority of patients (Table 3). On the other hand, the majority of patients with primary hyperparathyroidism have a single adenoma and some surgeons, on finding an adenoma, undertake no further exploration, particularly if other glands already identified have been shown to be normal or atrophic. In cases of diffuse hyperplasia the tendency is to remove three and a half glands. This has become a standard treatment for the secondary hyperparathyroidism of renal disease requiring resection. It has recently been suggested that total parathyroidectomy may be undertaken, followed by transplantation of parathyroid tissue into the forearm muscles. This is not without technical difficulties and is, at present, experimental. Whatever the strategy employed, the operative implantation of radiopaque markers at sites of remaining parathyroid tissue is helpful if re-exploration is required. Multiple operations carry greater risk and cause difficulty for the surgeon because of distorted anatomy and local fibrosis.

Arteriography or venography with radio-immunoassay for PTH in the thyroid effluent can be used as a preoperative localizing procedure for abnormal parathyroid tissue. Venous sampling is most useful in localizing parathyroid tissue after failed surgery, although there may be difficulties with the interpretation of PTH data due to variations in venous drainage from the parathyroids, particularly after previous surgery. The technique is particularly useful for detecting mediastinal tumours and avoiding the need for mediastinal exploration. Other techniques which have proved useful include thallium pertechnetate scanning, computed tomography, ultrasonography, and selective injection of a contrast dye, such as methylene blue, to discolour the parathyroids. Unfortunately, the yield of all these techniques is better in patients not previously explored than at re-exploration.

After operation, plasma calcium should be monitored at least daily for the first few days. Postoperative tetany is common in patients who have significant bone disease. They should be treated peroperatively with intravenous calcium (10 per cent calcium gluconate, 10–30 ml in 1 litre of saline), and at the same time vitamin D should be begun. The 1α-hydroxylated derivatives of vitamin D, calcitriol and alfacalcidol, and dihydrotachysterol act quickly and are preferable in acute management. Hypocalcaemia usually persists for several days but occasionally it may take weeks or even months to reverse. Permanent hyperparathyroidism is rare where surgery is undertaken by experienced surgeons.

Medical treatment can be considered in some asymptomatic or high-risk individuals with borderline or mild hypercalcaemia. Oestrogens and progestogens have both been shown to lower plasma calcium in postmenopausal women with mild hypercalcaemia. Specific inhibitors of bone resorption, such as calcitonin and the bisphosphonates, may have effects for several months on hypercalcaemia but more lasting effects on bone loss. The bisphosphonate clodronate can be used by mouth and given for long periods to lower serum calcium. The long-term effects are disappointing but any improvement in symptoms can be used to argue a case for surgical treatment. Oral cellulose phosphate and calcium restriction may transiently lower plasma calcium in other patients, but other features of the disease may progress. The use of neutral phosphate has been advocated in doses between 1 and 2.5 g daily but may cause diarrhoea and extraskeletal calcification. Significant decreases in plasma calcium have been shown, but these have been associated with increases in serum creatinine. There is no ideal long-term medical treatment for primary hyperparathyroidism and surgery should be undertaken whenever this is feasible.

Hypoparathyroidism

DEFINITIONS

Decreased secretion of PTH may arise in hypercalcaemic disorders which suppress the secretion of PTH. The term hyperparathyroidism is, however, usually applied to hypocalcaemia arising from the defective secretion or action of PTH (the latter is termed pseudohypoparathyroidism). These disorders, irrespective of their aetiology, are characterized by hypocalcaemia, hyperphosphataemia, and the clinical manifestations of hypocalcaemia.

Many of the biochemical and metabolic abnormalities seen in hypoparathyroidism can be understood by an appreciation of the physiological effects of PTH. Serum phosphate is raised due to an increase in the TmP/GFR. Hypocalcaemia is due, in part, to a decrease in tubular reabsorption of calcium (see Fig. 3). PTH directly or indirectly stimulates the synthesis of calcitriol from its precursor calcifidiol, and hypoparathyroidism is associated with decreased synthesis of calcitriol and intestinal malabsorption of calcium. Hyperphosphataemia may be another reason for low values of calcitriol. Hypocalcaemia in hypoparathyroidism is also due to an inhibition of osteocytic calcium transfer from bone due to a deficiency of PTH or calcitriol, or both.

Hypoparathyroidism is characterized by absent or low values of plasma PTH, but it is important to interpret PTH values according to the plasma calcium, and the presence of low but detectable values of PTH with hypocalcaemia is abnormal. Indeed plasma PTH commonly falls to undetectable levels in such cases when plasma calcium is raised

Table 4 *Major causes of hypoparathyroidism*

Inadequate secretion of PTH
Surgical—thyroid, parathyroid, and radical neck surgery
Familial
Sporadic
DiGeorge syndrome
Suppression of PTH secretion from normal parathyroid glands
Neonatal—from maternal hypercalcaemia
Severe magnesium depletion
Defective end-organ response to PTH
Pseudohypoparathyroidism types I and II

during treatment. A further characteristic is that hypoparathyroid patients have normal target tissue responses to parathyroid hormone. This can be examined by the administration of exogenous PTH in the Chase–Aurbach test. The infusion of PTH normally elicits phosphaturia and an increase in plasma and urinary cyclic AMP. This contrasts with pseudohypoparathyroidism (sometimes termed PTH-resistant hypoparathyroidism) characterized by resistance of one or more target tissues to the action of PTH.

GENERAL CLINICAL FEATURES

The symptoms and signs of most forms of hypoparathyroidism are attributable to hypocalcaemia and hyperphosphataemia. Hypocalcaemia is responsible for neuromuscular irritability which may cause carpopedal spasm, paraesthaesiae of the face, fingers, and toes, and occasionally abdominal cramps. Latent tetany may be detectable by tapping of the fifth facial nerve, resulting in contraction of the facial muscles (Chvostek's sign) or by inducing carpal spasm following occlusion of the arterial circulation of the forearm (Trousseau's sign). Chvostek's sign has limited clinical usefulness since approximately 5 per cent of the normal population have a positive response. The neurological changes which accompany profound hypocalcaemia include irritability, emotional lability, impairment of memory and generalized lethargy, and convulsions which are usually of the grand mal type. Occasionally petit mal is a presenting feature. Abnormal electroencephalogram patterns are observed which disappear with effective treatment. Papilloedema occasionally associated with increased intracranial pressure may also accompany the hypocalcaemia of hypoparathyroidism, but again returns to normal with adequate treatment. A prolonged QT interval may be found in hypocalcaemia and a partial insensitivity to digoxin has been reported.

Hypocalcaemia in early life causes mental retardation which is not reversible. Cataracts are common consequences of chronic hypocalcaemia. Soft tissue calcification is not infrequent and has a curious predilection for the basal ganglia or subcutaneous tissue. If hypocalcaemia occurs in early life and is sustained, then dental abnormalities such as blunting of the roots of the teeth and enamel dysplasia occur. Nails may be malformed, brittle, and have transverse grooves. Other ectodermal changes which may be found include a dry rough skin. Certain clinical features are associated with particular forms of hypoparathyroidism, these are discussed subsequently since they aid with the differential diagnosis.

CAUSES (TABLE 4)

Simple (PTH-deficient) hypoparathyroidism most commonly results from surgery, accidental or otherwise, on parathyroid glands during thyroid, parathyroid, or laryngeal surgery. The incidence of hypoparathyroidism after thyroidectomy varies enormously, depending on the surgeon, the length of the follow-up, and the criteria used for diagnosis. Surgical hypoparathyroidism may be latent for many years, sometimes becoming manifest in association with increased calcium demands such as pregnancy and lactation.

Idiopathic hypoparathyroidism is a relatively rare condition associated with absence, fatty replacement, or atrophy of parathyroid glands. In the familial form it may be inherited as a sex-linked recessive, autosomal recessive, or autosomal dominant with variable penetrance. The sporadic form, occurring at any age, may be associated with pernicious anaemia, Addison's disease, or candidiasis. Addison's disease and candidiasis may also occur, but less commonly, in the familial form. These observations, together with the presence of antibodies to parathyroid tissue, suggest that these are autoimmune endocrine disorders. There is no evidence, however, that the antibodies to endocrine tissue are cytotoxic and they are not proven to be important in its pathogenesis.

Children with idiopathic hypoparathyroidism have impaired growth and malformations of the nails and teeth. Radiography is usually normal, although bone density may be increased and calvarial width increased. Idiopathic hypoparathyroidism is also associated with intestinal malabsorption, steatorrhoea, and osteomalacia. Candidiasis, a recognized feature of this form of hypoparathyroidism, does not complicate the surgically-induced disorder.

Rarely hypoparathyroidism may result from infiltration of the parathyroid glands by iron in haemochromatosis, copper in Wilson's disease, or from the invasion of parathyroid tissue by malignant metastases. In DiGeorge's syndrome there is a congenital absence of parathyroid glands. It is associated with immunological deficiencies (thymic aplasia) and is a consequence of failure of development of the third and fourth branchial pouches from which the parathyroids and thymus arise. Thymic agenesis leads to a severe immunodeficiency state of the cellular type. Delayed hypersensitivity and allograft rejection may be suppressed or absent, and chronic mucocutaneous candidiasis is common. Patients with this syndrome usually die in early childhood from hypocalcaemia, severe infections, or both.

Neonatal tetany may arise because of maternal hypercalcaemia which causes the fetal parathyroid glands to become suppressed. Hypocalcaemia may become overt when patients are stressed with a high phosphate diet (cow's milk). The presence of neonatal tetany should alert one to investigate the mother for primary hyperparathyroidism. Hypoparathyroidism has also been reported following ^{131}I treatment for hyperthyroidism, but radiation of the neck with X-rays appears to be one of the factors predisposing to hyperparathyroidism. Severe magnesium depletion impairs the release of PTH.

PSEUDOHYPOPARATHYROIDISM

Pseudohypoparathyroidism results from the resistance of one or more target tissues to the actions of PTH. The physiological control of PTH secretion is partially intact, in the sense that PTH levels are appropriate for the degree of hypocalcaemia. However, the administration of PTH does not produce the normal response of an increase in the renal excretion of phosphate and cyclic AMP. This is somewhat analogous to the failure of patients with nephrogenic diabetes insipidus to respond to antidiuretic hormone. There is an association between pseudohypoparathyroidism and somatic abnormalities. These include short stature, round face, short neck, and shortening of the metacarpals and metatarsals. Characteristic radiographic findings include shortening of the fourth, fifth, or all metacarpals and metatarsal bones (Fig. 9). These features are not invariably found in pseudohypoparathyroidism and may be rarely present in idiopathic hypoparathyroidism. An X-linked dominant inheritance has been postulated for pseudohypoparathyroidism, but reports of male to male transmission suggest that a recessive inheritance pattern may also occur. In contrast to idiopathic hypoparathyroidism, pseudohypoparathyroidism is associated with hypothyroidism. The defect appears to be a selective deficiency of thyroid stimulating hormone. Other associated disorders include diabetes mellitus, amenorrhoea, and gonadal dysgenesis, so there appears to be a striking overlap in the disorders associated with Turner's syndrome and pseudohypoparathyroidism.

The resistance to PTH may be partial or complete. In many patients neither phosphaturia nor increased urinary cyclic AMP production is stimulated during the infusion of PTH (type I). This type is further subdivided into those with somatic and other endocrine disorders (type Ia) and those without (type Ib). In others, a marked rise in urinary cyclic AMP occurs without a phosphaturic response (pseudohypoparathyroidism type II). In yet other patients, the responsiveness to PTH may be restored by calcium infusion. Not all target tissues need be affected, and occasionally pseudohypoparathyroidism may be associated with radiographically obvious osteitis fibrosa, indicating skeletal sensitivity to PTH.

PSEUDOPSEUDOHYPOPARATHYROIDISM

Rarely the somatic features of pseudohypoparathyroidism may be found in patients with normal plasma concentrations of calcium and phosphate. This condition is termed pseudopseudohypoparathyroidism. PTH values are usually normal but may be raised. There are patients with pseudopseudohypoparathyroidism who are relatives of patients with pseudohypoparathyroidism and who indeed may undergo transitions from hypocalcaemia to normocalcaemia or vice versa. It is notable that cataracts may develop in patients with pseudopseudohypoparathyroidism who have a consistently normal plasma calcium, suggesting that mechanisms other than hypocalcaemia are responsible for this feature.

DIAGNOSIS

The diagnosis of hypoparathyroidism rarely presents any difficulty and is based on the finding of hypocalcaemia and hyperphosphataemia in

Fig. 9 Brachydactyly in a patient with pseudopseudohypoparathyroidism. The photograph and radiograph on the left-hand side show a normal hand for comparison.

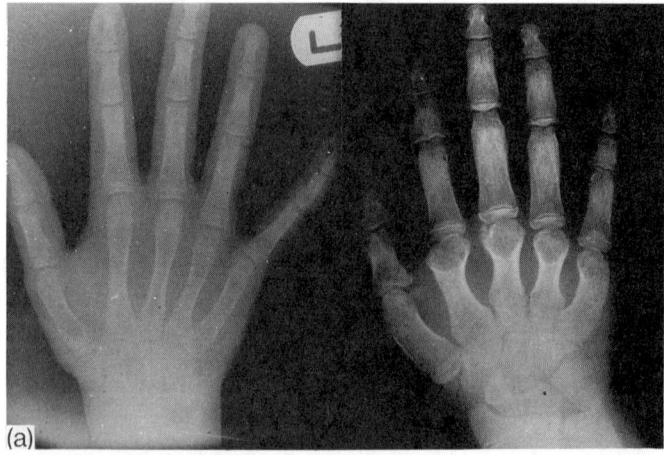

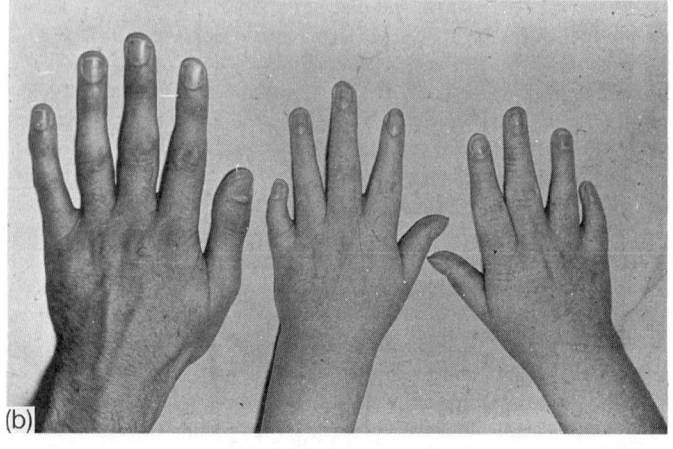

the absence of renal failure, osteomalacia, or malabsorption. The clinician should be aware of the association of hypocalcaemia secondary to magnesium deficiency. A careful history, including one of previous neck surgery and physical examination usually indicates the underlying cause. The finding of Addison's disease, pernicious anaemia, candidiasis, atypical epilepsy, or bizarre mental symptoms should alert one to the possibility of hypoparathyroidism. Apart from rare forms of vitamin D deficiency, the only other disorder commonly associated with hyperphosphataemia and hypocalcaemia is chronic renal failure. Measurement of plasma creatinine easily resolves this possibility. Since many patients with the more unusual forms of hypoparathyroidism are children, it is important to be aware that both plasma values of alkaline phosphatase and phosphate are commonly higher in children than in adults. The differential diagnosis and investigation of hypocalcaemia is discussed below. The 24-h excretion secretion of urinary calcium is commonly low but the fasting urinary calcium excretion is usually normal. In order to distinguish the various forms of idiopathic and pseudohypoparathyroidism, more detailed investigation, including the measurement of PTH and the responses to exogenous PTH, are required. The principles of treatment, however, are similar for all forms of hypoparathyroidism although the doses required of the vitamin D-like agents used may vary.

TREATMENT

The priorities of treatment are to restore normal circulating values of calcium and phosphate. This is not often attainable with the use of calcium supplements alone but they are commonly used (1–1.5 g daily) in conjunction with vitamin D or its metabolites. The use of intravenous calcium (10–30 ml of 10 per cent calcium gluconate in 500 ml or 1 litre of saline) may be required in patients with tetany. In the past, the most commonly prescribed vitamin D preparation has been calciferol (vitamin D_2) doses from 0.25 to 20 mg daily (10 000–800 000 units). One of the disadvantages of vitamin D or calcifidiol is that the onset and reversal of action of these preparations are very slow (Fig. 10). Thus it is very difficult to titrate the dose quickly according to requirements, and inadvertent hypercalcaemia may take weeks or months to resolve. The 1α-hydroxylated derivatives of vitamin D, including calcitriol, alfacalcidol,

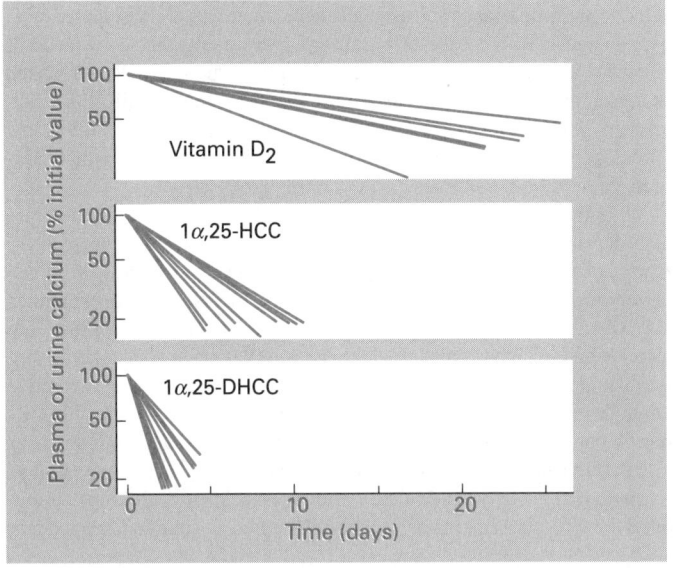

Fig. 10 The rate of reversal of biological effects after stopping treatment with vitamin D compounds. The fall in plasma or urine calcium is shown on a logarithmic scale. Note that the reversal of vitamin D toxicity is more rapid in the case of 1,25-dihydroxyvitamin D (1,25-DHC; calcitriol) and its synthetic analogue 1-hydroxyvitamin D (1-HCC; alfacalcidol) than seen with vitamin D_2. (From Kanis, J.A. and Russell, R.G.G. (1977).)

and dihydrotachysterol all have a more rapid onset and offset of action. The daily maintenance dose required of these agents is 1 to 2 μg in the case of alfacalcidol and calcitriol, and 0.25 to 2 μg of dihydrotachysterol. Occasionally higher doses are required. High doses may also be used at the start of treatment, since the rise in plasma calcium is then more rapid. It is mandatory to follow plasma calcium closely to avoid toxicity in the first 2 to 3 weeks of treatment and at least once every 6 months in patients on stable doses. The requirements for vitamin D and its derivatives may vary, particularly when the defect in PTH secretion is incomplete. Treatment may be required for concurrent hypomagnesaemia and other endocrinopathies when present.

Intercurrent illness, pregnancy, and the use of antacids, thiazide diuretics, ammonium chloride, anticonvulsants, and acetazolamide may alter the requirements for vitamin D.

The prognosis of adequately treated hypoparathyroidism is excellent. It is, however, unclear whether or not cataracts can be prevented. Major difficulties with long-term vitamin D treatment include prolonged hypercalcaemia, which may lead to renal stone formation and progressive renal failure. Further details of treatment with vitamin D and its metabolites are discussed in Chapter 20.18 and Section 19.

Disorders of vitamin D metabolism

The unravelling of the metabolism and actions of vitamin D has been one of the most rapid developments in endocrinology. An ever-increasing number of disorders has been associated with disturbances in the metabolism of vitamin D. In some instances, changes in plasma values of vitamin D metabolites reflect adaptive responses to the disorder rather than its cause.

Hypervitaminosis D

VITAMIN D TOXICITY

Vitamin D toxicity is a common finding in clinical practice and is usually iatrogenic. Since vitamin D increases intestinal absorption of calcium, and in high doses augments bone resorption, these patients develop hypercalcaemia. Plasma phosphate is commonly also elevated due to similar effects on phosphate transport. If overdosage is prolonged, increased bone resorption causes progressive loss of bone. The effects of prolonged hypercalcaemia are discussed in the sections on hypercalcaemia (see below) and hyperparathyroidism (see above), but the effects on renal function and structure are clinically the most important. Vitamin D toxicity is still an important cause of morbidity, and it should be a responsibility of the physician initiating treatment of patients with these compounds to ensure that adequate monitoring is undertaken. Vitamin D preparations should be stopped when hypercalcaemia is confirmed or suspected. The rate of fall of plasma calcium depends upon the agent used. The biological half-life of vitamins D_2 and D_3 may be months or even years, particularly when pharmacological amounts have been used over prolonged periods, resulting in high body stores. A long half-life of several weeks is also seen with calcifidiol.

The principles of treatment include the general management of hypercalcaemia (see below). In addition, protracted hypercalcaemia can be treated with corticosteroids or a specific inhibitor of bone resorption such as calcitonin or a bisphosphonate. In life-threatening situations, particularly in the face of renal impairment, patients may require haemodialysis or peritoneal dialysis.

INCREASED PRODUCTION OF CALCITRIOL

The production of calcitriol is under metabolic control. Factors augmenting the synthesis of calcitriol include hypophosphataemia, hypocalcaemia, and excessive secretion of PTH. Abnormally high values of calcitriol have been reported in patients with primary hyperparathyroidism and account for the increased calcium absorption in this disorder. Increased calcium absorption is also seen in acromegaly, which may be due to increased production of calcitriol. Many patients with calcium-containing stones are classified as having idiopathic hypercalciuria because of a normal plasma calcium, a low plasma phosphate, and increased gastrointestinal absorption of calcium. Approximately one-third of these patients have increased serum values of calcitriol, perhaps related to the hypophosphataemia. Sarcoidosis is occasionally associated with hypercalcaemia and more commonly with hypercalciuria and increased bone turnover: increased intestinal absorption of calcium is associated with high circulating values of calcitriol. Hypercalcaemia in sarcoidosis may be aggravated by relatively low doses of vitamin D_3 and also has a seasonal incidence, being more common in the summer months. Plasma levels of calcifidiol are normal, suggesting that the vitamin D sensitivity seen in this disorder is due to abnormal metabolism of calcifidiol to calcitriol. A similar syndrome of ectopic calcitriol production occurs in other granulomatous disorders (such as berylliosis, candidiasis, tuberculosis, leprosy, and silicon-induced disease) and occasionally in human T-cell leukaemia virus (HTLV)-associated adult T-cell lymphoma.

Defective production of vitamin D metabolites

The hallmarks of vitamin D deficiency include defective mineralization of bone and retardation of growth. Simple vitamin D deficiency is associated with hypocalcaemia, hypophosphataemia, and high plasma activity of bone-derived alkaline phosphatase; but in the early stages of vitamin D deficiency, plasma calcium may be normal. The hypocalcaemia is caused by malabsorption of calcium from the gut and a decrease in the calcium efflux from bone. Hypocalcaemia stimulates PTH secretion and the hypophosphataemia is due to secondary hyperparathyroidism (decreased TmP/GFR) as well as malabsorption of phosphate. Indeed, it is possible that defective mineralization of bone is due, in part, to phosphate depletion.

Not all cases of osteomalacia or rickets results from deficiency of vitamin D or its metabolites. For instance, in X-linked or sporadic hypophosphataemia (vitamin D-resistant rickets) defective mineralization of bone is probably due to abnormalities in phosphate transport rather than to impaired metabolism of vitamin D. Conversely, deficiency of calcitriol does not invariably lead to osteomalacia. Thus, osteomalacia is an unusual finding in hypoparathyroidism and is not invariably seen in end-stage chronic renal failure, even though plasma values of calcitriol are reduced in both these disorders.

The clinical manifestations of osteomalacia, its investigation and differential diagnosis are discussed in Section 19. The purpose of this section is to review the manner by which disorders associated with defective production of vitamin D metabolites arise, rather than to discuss in detail the disorders themselves.

PRIVATIONAL VITAMIN D DEFICIENCY

Simple vitamin D deficiency may be due to dietary deficiency or inadequate exposure of the skin to sunlight. In northern Europe it commonly occurs in young children, particularly at the time of adolescence, in the immigrant Asian population, and in the very old.

MALABSORPTION SYNDROMES

(See also Sections 14.9 and 19.)

Patients with long-standing malabsorption due to diseases such as cystic fibrosis or gluten-sensitive enteropathy (coeliac disease) are likely to develop osteomalacia. Not all such patients have symptomatic steatorrhoea and further investigation, such as intestinal biopsy or the determination of faecal fat excretion, may be necessary. The pathophysiology

of the disorder is related in part to malabsorption of vitamin D which is fat soluble, but in patients with active disease, the intestinal cells themselves have been destroyed and hence the vitamin D deficiency is partly related to the destruction of one of the target organs for vitamin D. The absorption of calcifidiol is also decreased in patients with intestinal disease, including those with small bowel resection, and it has been suggested that there is a defect in the enterohepatic circulation of calcifidiol. An increased prevalence of osteomalacia is also seen in patients with liver disease and those with partial gastrectomy. Malabsorption of vitamin D may contribute to the former but the cause of osteomalacia after partial gastrectomy remains somewhat of a mystery and may be more related to malabsorption of calcium.

REDUCED AVAILABILITY OF CALCIFIDIOL

Vitamin D is hydroxylated in the liver to form 25-hydroxyvitamin D. It might be expected that severe liver disease could impair this hydroxylation, and there is some evidence that the prevalence of osteomalacia is higher in patients with liver disease than in normal subjects. However, osteoporosis is more common though osteomalacia may be erroneously suspected because of hyperphosphatasia and reduced serum phosphate due to the liver disease. There is little direct evidence for defective 25-hydroxylation in liver disease. Low values of calcifidiol, when found, may be due to malabsorption or a poor dietary intake of vitamin D.

Osteomalacia has been associated with the administration of anticonvulsant drugs such as phenobarbitone and phenytoin, which are potent inducers of hepatic microsomal enzymes. Increased metabolic degradation of vitamin D to inactive metabolites is unlikely to be the sole mechanism and drug-induced target organ resistance is a major feature.

A convincing role for abnormal metabolism of calcifidiol is seen in the nephrotic syndrome. Certain features of vitamin D deficiency are common, such as reduced plasma calcium, hypocalciuria, and decreased intestinal absorption of calcium, even when the glomerular filtration rate is normal or increased. The hypocalcaemia is partly related to the low plasma concentrations of albumin which occur as a consequence of protein losses in the urine, but ionized calcium is also low, as are values of calcifidiol due to losses of the vitamin D-binding protein in the urine.

REDUCED AVAILABILITY OF CALCITRIOL

Chronic renal failure, pseudohypoparathyroidism, and hypoparathyroidism are disorders in which the conversion of calcifidiol vitamin D to calcitriol is impaired. Serum values of calcitriol are low, and physiological quantities of calcitriol reverse some of the biochemical abnormalities, whereas pharmacological amounts of vitamin D_3 are required to achieve the same response. Not all these disorders are associated with osteomalacia. In the case of parathyroid disorders, the low values of calcitriol are probably due to hyperphosphataemia as well as reduced secretion of PTH, or, in the case of pseudohypoparathyroidism, a resistance of renal tissue to respond to PTH. In chronic renal failure, low values of calcitriol reflect the destruction of the renal tissue which converts calcifidiol to calcitriol.

Vitamin D-dependency rickets (pseudo-deficiency rickets) is a rare disorder inherited as an autosomal dominant. These patients have all the features of vitamin D deficiency except that vitamin D must be given in very large doses to correct the biochemical and skeletal abnormalities (10 000–50 000 units daily). Pharmacological doses of calcifidiol are also needed, whereas physiological doses of calcitriol (1 μg daily) cure the disorder. It is thought that some of these patients have a defective 1α-hydroxylase enzyme system. However, there are patients with similar biochemical characteristics who have normal or even high levels of circulating calcitriol—the vitamin D equivalent of pseudohypoparathyroidism. This rare condition, sometimes associated with alopecia and other somatic abnormalities, has been described as vitamin D-dependent rickets type II. It reflects an inherited defect of the vitamin D receptor associated with target tissue resistance to calcitriol. An even rarer form of calcitriol deficiency is seen in patients with benign mesenchymal tumours. This is commonly associated with hypophosphataemia. It is important to identify such patients since resection of the tumour, if feasible, reverses the osteomalacia.

OTHER DISORDERS

Aside from vitamin D-dependency rickets type II, it is probable that target tissue resistance to the action of vitamin D metabolites is an important component of the osteomalacia associated with anticonvulsant treatment and with intestinal disorders.

It is thought that the osteomalacia associated with phosphate deficiency, due for example to antacid abuse or to the genetically determined disorder of hypophosphataemic rickets, is unrelated to defects in the metabolism of vitamin D. Some of the renal tubular disorders such as the Fanconi syndrome are associated with a profound metabolic acidosis which might impair the activity of the renal 1α-hydroxylase (see Chapter 20.19.1). In some cases, correction of the acidosis alone without phosphate supplements may lead to healing. Sporadic cases of acquired hypophosphataemic rickets or osteomalacia have been found in association with various mesenchymal tumours.

Low serum values of calcitriol have also been described in postmenopausal and corticosteroid-induced osteoporosis. It is unclear whether this contributes to the pathophysiology of osteoporosis, or whether the low values of calcitriol are due to the chronic efflux of calcium into the extracellular fluid by the osteoporotic process, which in turn suppresses its production. It is important to note for therapeutic reasons that osteoporosis and osteomalacia may commonly coexist in the elderly.

Disorders of calcitonin secretion

Medullary carcinoma of the thyroid

(See also Chapters 12.10 and 12.5.)

Increased secretion of calcitonin occurs in medullary carcinoma of the thyroid, a malignant disorder of the C-cells. It may be inherited in a number of distinct syndromes. Where direct evidence of inheritance is found, it is termed familial, and the term sporadic medullary carcinoma is otherwise used. Medullary carcinoma accounts for between 3 and 10 per cent of thyroid carcinomas but there is a considerable geographic variation in the incidence. The majority of patients present with a thyroid mass, often with palpable cervical lymph nodes. The tumour may spread to the mediastinum but spread beyond the neck and mediastinum usually occurs late, with the lungs, liver, adrenal glands, and bones being the most common sites. Metastases to bones are sometimes osteoblastic. The tumour may be associated with other endocrine abnormalities such as phaeochromocytoma and hyperparathyroidism—the so-called multiple endocrine adenoma syndrome (MEA Type II). Medullary carcinoma may become clinically evident by the expression of these other endocrinopathies. Severe diarrhoea may occur which is probably related to the synthesis of prostaglandins or serotonin. Hypocalcaemia is very rare.

Calcitonin is consistently produced by medullary carcinomata of the thyroid, and the measurement of serum calcitonin or its flanking peptide katacalcin is of value in establishing the diagnosis, the presence of metastases, and in following the effects of treatment. These assays are also of value in family studies for tracing asymptomatic cases. A number of other humoral agents may be synthesized by the tumour, including prostaglandins, 5-hydroxytryptamine, and adrenocorticotrophic hormone (ACTH). The last may give rise to Cushing's syndrome. Other genetically related disorders include multiple mucosal neuromata, gan-

glion neuromatosis of the gastrointestinal tract, marphanoid features, muscular weakness, and a high arched palate. A feature of associated phaeochromocytoma is the large amount of adrenaline secreted, which usually forms more than 70 per cent of the total catecholamine excretion.

Treatment is surgical, but it is advisable to screen for phaeochromocytoma pre-operatively and, if present, this should be dealt with first (see Chapter 15.28.2). Because of the high proportion of adrenaline produced by these tumours, β-adrenergic blockade should be used in addition to α-adrenergic blockade during surgery. The extent of surgery depends, in part, on the spread of disease and the associated symptoms. In the presence of distant spread it may still be worth resecting a large tumour mass to control severe diarrhoea or Cushing's syndrome.

It is important to screen members of the family, who may be submitted to partial or total thyroidectomy if raised basal plasma levels of calcitonin or katacalcin are demonstrated, or if exaggerated responses to provocative tests of calcitonin secretion (with whisky, pentagastrin, or calcium infusion) are shown. The majority of patients with medullary carcinoma have basal calcitonin levels which are clearly distinguishable from normal. In those in whom there is doubt, provocative tests of calcitonin secretion are used.

Other disorders

Until recently an elevated plasma calcitonin was considered diagnostic of medullary carcinoma of the thyroid, but high values have also been demonstrated in patients with hypercalcaemia and a variety of non-thyroidal tumours such as oat-cell carcinoma of the lung and carcinoma of the breast. There is, however, a wide variability in the reported prevalence of high calcitonin values in these disorders, probably because of the difficulties of radio-immunoassay. High values have also been described in chronic renal failure, in part, related to delayed metabolism of some of the circulating fragments. Defective secretion of calcitonin has been implicated in the pathophysiology of hyperparathyroid bone disease in chronic renal failure.

Hypercalcaemia

(See also Chapter 20.9.3.)

DIFFERENTIAL DIAGNOSIS

Many of the causes of hypercalcaemia have been reviewed previously and are summarized in Table 5. The most common cause in hospitalized patients is malignant disease. Demonstrable bone involvement with metastases occurs in approximately 20 per cent of all patients with advanced cancer. Bone lesions and hypercalcaemia are most frequently seen in patients with tumour of the breast, lung, head, neck and kidney. Skeletal metastases are rare in tumours of the gastrointestinal and the female genital tract. Carcinoma of the prostate commonly involves bone but induces osteoblastic lesions in 90 per cent of patients, and hypercalcaemia is rare. In patients with carcinoma of the breast, hypercalcaemia may be precipitated by factors which influence the tumour growth, such as the administration of oestrogen or oestrogen antagonists such as tamoxifen. Hypercalcaemia can develop rapidly in patients with malignancy and initiate a vicious cycle of increasing nausea, vomiting, dehydration, and impaired renal function, all of which accelerate the rise in serum calcium. These patients often have a hypochloraemic metabolic alkalosis, whereas hyperchloraemic acidosis is more common in primary hyperparathyroidism. Serum phosphate concentrations are variable, depending on the presence or absence of malnutrition, disturbed renal function, and increased bone resorption.

The causes of hypercalcaemia in malignancy are complex and arise by several mechanisms. Most commonly it is due to the widespread destruction of bone by metastases. In such cases the secretion of PTH

Table 5 *Causes of hypercalcaemia*

Common
  Artefactual: hyperproteinaemia due to venous stasis,
    hyperalbuminaemia (dehydration, intravenous nutrition),
    hypergammaglobulinaemia (myeloma, sarcoidosis)
  Neoplasia: carcinoma with skeletal metastases (e.g. breast,
    lung), carcinoma without skeletal metastases (humoral
    hypercalcaemia of malignancy), haematological disorders
    (myeloma, HTLV-associated lymphoma)
  Primary hyperparathyroidism

Rare
  'Tertiary' hyperparathyroidism—transplantation, chronic
    renal failure, malabsorption
  Vitamin D toxicity
  Vitamin D 'sensitivity'—sarcoidosis, other granulomatous
    disorders, ?hypercalcaemia of infancy
  Immobility—Paget's disease, adolescence
  Milk-alkali syndrome
  Thyrotoxicosis
  Thiazide diuretics
  Adrenal failure
  Phaeochromocytoma
  Familial hypocalciuric hypercalcaemia
  Haemodialysis: high dialysate calcium, aluminium toxicity
  Some other drugs, e.g. vitamin A
  Acute renal failure
  VIPoma
  Familial hypocalciuric hypercalcaemia

is suppressed. In addition, hypercalcaemia may cause intrinsic renal damage due to the deposition of calcium phosphate, which aggravates hypercalcaemia by decreasing the capacity of the kidneys to handle calcium challenges. Hypercalcaemia also decreases the renal sensitivity to antidiuretic hormone, resulting in extracellular volume depletion. Decreased renal tubular delivery of sodium increases tubular reabsorption of calcium and aggravates hypercalcaemia. In addition, tumours secrete peptides such as PTH-related protein and tumour growth factor which cause a generalized increase in bone resorption or increase renal tubular reabsorption of calcium. PTH-related protein is a 141 amino acid hormone (molecular weight 16 000), sharing sequence homology with PTH at its amino terminus. Like PTH, it increases bone resorption and renal tubular reabsorption of calcium. It is secreted by many solid tumours, including squamous carcinomas of the lung, oesophagus, head and neck, and breast. It may cause hypercalcaemia in the absence of skeletal metastases (humoral hypercalcaemia of malignancy) but may also contribute to hypercalcaemia in patients with focal lytic lesions.

The investigation and diagnosis of primary hyperparathyroidism has been discussed previously (see above). The majority of other causes may be accurately detected by a good history (including a full drug history) and the measurement of plasma calcium, phosphate, proteins, erythrocyte sedimentation rate, and creatinine, and an estimate of tubular reabsorption for phosphate. Radiography and bone scans are helpful in detecting malignant disease not otherwise clinically apparent. The investigation of the rarer forms of hypercalcaemia (Table 5) is commonly straightforward, and they are easily excluded by the appropriate investigations or history.

The major difficulties arise in those patients without overt skeletal disease and hypercalcaemia. PTH assays, together with a search for sarcoidosis or myeloma, usually resolve further diagnostic difficulties.

TREATMENT

The aims of treatment should be to reduce the high serum calcium values and to remove the underlying cause. Severe hypercalcaemia should be treated as an emergency but chronic management of hypercalcaemia is required in some patients because of difficulties in identifying or controlling the underlying disorder. Therapeutic strategy should also be based on the mechanism of the hypercalcaemia, particularly the contributions of dehydration, increased renal tubular reabsorption of calcium, and decreased renal function.

Hypercalcaemia that is neither symptomatic nor progressive requires treatment only of the underlying disorder. Mild hypercalcaemia associated with myeloma commonly responds to adequate chemotherapy alone. On the other hand, progressive and severe hypercalcaemia may be life-threatening. Patients with serum calcium concentrations greater than 3 mmol/l are commonly dehydrated and it is important to restore the extracellular fluid volume by the use of intravenous saline. Care should be taken in patients with very low plasma proteins, or impaired cardiac or renal function. Frusemide and other loop diuretics increase urinary calcium excretion and can accelerate the effects of rehydration, but the use of diuretics without adequate volume expansion may aggravate hypercalcaemia. Thiazide diuretics should be avoided since these increase the renal tubular reabsorption of calcium.

Additional, potentially helpful agents in the management of hypercalcaemia include specific inhibitors of bone resorption. Calcitonin (100–200 U intravenously or intramuscularly), commonly induces a decrease in serum calcium, but this may be of short duration. Its action may be prolonged with corticosteroids. The bisphosphonates induce a slower but more complete and sustained response. Intravenous regimens include pamidronate (up to 90 mg) or clodronate (up to 1500 mg). Less complete effects are achieved with etidronate (500 mg). Clodronate can be given by mouth (1600 mg daily) to prevent recurrence. The cytotoxic agents mithramycin (15 µg/kg intravenously) and gallium are effective but more toxic than bisphosphonates. Corticosteroids have been widely advocated in the acute management of hypercalcaemia but their efficacy is doubtful except in patients with myeloma, vitamin D intoxication, and sarcoidosis. If more prolonged treatment of hypercalcaemia is indicated, clodronate may be given by mouth (1600 mg daily). Many tumours secrete prostaglandins which resorb bone, the use of indomethacin or aspirin in long-term treatment has been disappointing but may be worthy of trials in appropriate patients. Oral phosphate has been widely employed but it frequently causes dose-dependent diarrhoea, and in patients with a high serum phosphate or impaired renal function it may lead to soft tissue calcification of kidneys, lungs, and blood vessels. Intravenous phosphate therapy is particularly likely to cause this and should be avoided.

There may be a reluctance to treat mild hypercalcaemia complicating malignant disease, but the symptoms of hypercalcaemia can be subtle and may include an increase in the pain threshold. This suggests that a more aggressive approach may have worthwhile clinical dividends.

Intestinal hyperabsorption of calcium (e.g. vitamin D toxicity or sarcoidosis) can be controlled with corticosteroids (5–20 mg prednisone daily). Additional approaches include a low-calcium diet and the use of cellulose phosphate, which is non-absorbable but binds calcium in the gut.

Hypocalcaemia and tetany

The more common causes of hypocalcaemia are shown in Table 6, most of which have been discussed earlier in this chapter. The measurement of serum calcium, phosphate, and creatinine, together with albumin, distinguishes patients with artefactual hypocalcaemia, vitamin D deficiency, chronic renal failure, and hypoparathyroidism.

The symptoms and signs of hypocalcaemia have been discussed under parathyroid disorders. The most important of these is tetany. Tetany may develop in the presence of alkalosis, and potassium and magnesium deficiency as well as in hypocalcaemia. Hyperventilation alters the protein binding of calcium such that the ionized fraction is decreased, and may therefore cause hypocalcaemic tetany in the face of normal plasma calcium. Hypocalcaemic tetany may also occur during the administra-

Table 6 *Causes of hypocalcaemia*

Low plasma albumin: malnutrition, liver disease, etc.
Vitamin D deficiency or resistance
Chronic renal disease
Hypoparathyroidism, pseudohypoparathyroidism
Magnesium deficiency
Acute pancreatitis
Drugs, e.g. calcitonin, phosphate, diphosphonates, some
  chemotherapeutic agents and chelators of calcium
Carcinoma, particularly of the prostate

tion of alkalis. This is particularly prone to occur during the treatment of acidotic patients with bicarbonate, particularly those with chronic renal failure in whom total plasma calcium may be low. Alkalosis may also occur in intestinal disorders where excess alkalis are ingested or there is excessive loss of gastric acid. Alkalotic tetany is diagnosed by an increase in plasma bicarbonate and an alkaline urine. Hypochloraemic alkalosis may be a feature of primary aldosteronism or the administration of corticosteroids. The principles of treatment are those of the underlying disorder.

Emergency treatment for hypocalcaemia has been described under parathyroid disorders, and the use of the 1α-hydroxylated derivatives of vitamin D has also been described above.

REFERENCES

Aurbach, G.D., Marx, S.J., and Spiegel, A.M. (1985). Parathyroid hormone, calcitonin and the calciferols. In *William Textbook of Endocrinology*, (7th ed), (ed. J.D. Wilson and D.W. Foster), pp. 1137–217. W.B. Saunders, Philadelphia.

Avioli, L.V. and Krane, S.M. (ed.) (1990). *Metabolic bone disease and clinically related disorders*, (2nd edition). W.B. Saunders, Philadelphia.
DeGroot, L.J., *et al.* (1979). Disorders of bone and bone mineral metabolism: relation to parathyroid hormone, calcitonin and vitamin D. *Endocrinology* **2**, 551. Grune & Stratton, New York.
Favus, M.J. (1990). *Primer on the metabolic bone diseases and disorder of mineral metabolism*. American Society for Bone and Mineral Research, Kelseyville, California.
Harris, W.H. and Heaney, R.P. (1969). *New England Journal of Medicine* **280**, 193.
Kanis, J.A. (ed.) (1980). Etiology and medical management of hypercalcaemia. *Metabolic Bone Disease and Related Research*. **2**, 143–215.
Kanis, J.A. (1992). Calcium metabolism and disorders of bone. In *Scientific foundations of clinical biochemistry*, (2nd edition), Vol. II, *Biochemistry in clinical practice*, Chapter 29. (ed. D.L. Williams, V. Marks, and W. Heinemann), Kanis, J.A. and Russell, R.G.G. (1977). *British Medical Journal* London. **i**, 78.
Kanis, J.A., Hamdy, N.A.T., and McCloskey, E.V. (1992). Hypercalcaemia and hypocalcaemia. In *Oxford textbook of clinical nephrology*, (ed. J.S. Cameron, A.M. Davison, J.-P. Grunfeld, D.N.S. Kerr, and E. Ritz), pp. 1753–82. Oxford University Press, Oxford.
Mundy, G.R. (1989). *Calcium homeostasis: hypercalcaemia and hypocalcaemia*. Martin Dunitz, London.
Nordin, B.E.C. (ed.) (1976). *Calcium, phosphate and magnesium metabolism. Clinical physiology and diagnostic procedures*. Churchill Livingstone, Edinburgh.
Nordin, B.E.C. and Peacock, M. (1969). *Lancet* 1280.
Peacock, M. (ed.) (1977). The clinical uses of 1-alpha-hydroxy-vitamin D$_3$. *Clinical Endocrinology* **7**, (Suppl.).
Walton, R.J. and Bjvoet, O.L.M. (1975). *Lancet* 309.
Woodhead, J.S. and Walker, D.A. (1976). *Annals of Clinical Biochemistry* **13**, 549.

12.7 The adrenal

12.7.1 Adrenocortical diseases

C. R. W. EDWARDS

INTRODUCTION

Three main types of hormone are produced by the adrenal cortex—glucocorticoids (cortisol, corticosterone), mineralocorticoids (aldosterone, deoxycorticosterone), and sex steroids (mainly androgens). The biochemical pathways involved in their synthesis are shown in Fig. 1.

Adrenocortical diseases are relatively rare but their importance lies in their morbidity and mortality if untreated, coupled with the relative ease of diagnosis and the availability of effective therapy. The diseases are most readily classified on the basis of whether there is hormone excess or deficiency (Table 1). In most instances this excess or deficiency arises from abnormal secretion of hormones. However, more uncommonly the defect may relate to a change in corticosteroid metabolism (for example effects of liquorice or carbenoxolone) or to defective receptors (for example glucocorticoid resistance syndromes, pseudohypoaldosteronism).

Rapid advances have been made in our understanding of the molecular pathogenesis of several of the inherited adrenocortical disorders. This progress has facilitated antenatal diagnosis and, principally in the case of congenital adrenal hyperplasia due to 21-hydroxylase deficiency, led to intrauterine therapy of affected females so as to prevent virilization (Section 13). In patients with dexamethasone-suppressible hyperaldosteronism, the discovery of the molecular defect has allowed the introduction of a simple genetic screening test. This in turn has demonstrated the very variable phenotype of the condition and has shown that in many hypertensive patients with this condition the diagnosis has been missed.

Glucocorticoid excess

Harvey Cushing first described a case of the 'polyglandular syndrome' which bears his name in 1912 in his monograph on the 'Pituitary body and its disorders'; but it was 20 years later that he wrote his definitive paper on basophil adenomas of the pituitary and their clinical manifestations, drawing attention to the association between pituitary basophil hyperfunction and adrenocortical hyperplasia. Cushing acknowledged that the first unequivocal description of the pituitary condition was by H.G. Turney, a St. Thomas' physician, in 1913 (Fig. 2). This patient had a markedly expanded sella turcica suggesting the presence of a pituitary tumour, but, when she died, was found to have an adrenal and not a pituitary tumour. A case of obvious Cushing's syndrome was also described by William Osler in 1899, but no autopsy was performed.

DEFINITION

Cushing's syndrome comprises the symptoms and signs associated with prolonged exposure to inappropriately elevated free plasma glucocorticoid levels. This definition thus takes into account the elevated corticosteroid levels which may be found in severely depressed patients but which appear to be appropriate to the condition (there is some evidence for glucocorticoid resistance in depression) and also the increased total (but normal free) glucocorticoid levels found when there is an increase in circulating cortisol binding globulin (for example in patients on oestrogen therapy). The use of the term glucocorticoid in the definition covers both endogenous (cortisol) and exogenous (for example prednisolone, dexamethasone) excess.

CLASSIFICATION OF CUSHING'S SYNDROME

The condition is most readily classified into those causes that are ACTH-dependent and those that are not (Table 2). The term Cushing's *syndrome* is used to describe all causes; that of Cushing's *disease* is reserved for cases of pituitary-dependent Cushing's syndrome in recognition of Cushing's original description.

More recently it has been recognized that there is an additional, rather poorly defined group of patients with ACTH-independent Cushing's syndrome but in whom there is bilateral adrenal disease. The two adrenals are usually enlarged and frequently contain multiple nodules. The cortex between the nodules may be described as normal, atrophic, or hyperplastic. It is likely that there are several different pathologies in this subgroup. In some there may be local production in the adrenal of a factor which enhances the response to ACTH. Alternatively, abnormal processing of the ACTH precursor molecule, pro-opiomelanocortin, may be important as the N-terminal part of this molecule appears to play

a role in adrenal growth. In some patients there may be stimulating immunoglobulins, whereas in others a somatic mutation in the stimulatory G-protein may result in continuous activation of adenyl cyclase, thus stimulating constant stimulation by ACTH.

A small group of patients has now been described in which food stimulates cortisol secretion. This led to the discovery that these patients' adrenal glands had enhanced sensitivity to the normal postprandial increase in gastric inhibitory polypeptide (GIP) (see below).

Another poorly understood condition is so-called alcohol-induced pseudo-Cushing's syndrome, in which the glucocorticoid excess associated with high alcohol intake resolves when the patients stop drinking (see below).

Aetiology of Cushing's syndrome
ACTH-dependent causes
CUSHING'S DISEASE

When the iatrogenic and ectopic groups are excluded, the commonest cause of Cushing's syndrome is Cushing's disease, which accounts for approximately 80 per cent of cases. The adrenal glands in these patients show bilateral adrenocortical hyperplasia with widening of the zona fasciculata and reticularis.

Cushing himself raised the question as to whether his disease was a primary pituitary condition or secondary to an abnormality in the hypothalamus. The release of ACTH from the pituitary is controlled by corticotrophin releasing factor (CRF) acting synergistically with arginine vasopressin (AVP). If there was hypothalamic dysfunction in Cushing's disease, it might be expected that one or other of these would be produced in excess. Measurement of CRF in both the circulation and cerebrospinal fluid has shown that the levels are low in Cushing's disease

Fig. 1 Pathways of adrenocortical steroid biosynthesis. The shaded area shows the affected steroids in a patient with salt–wasting 21–hydroxylase deficiency.

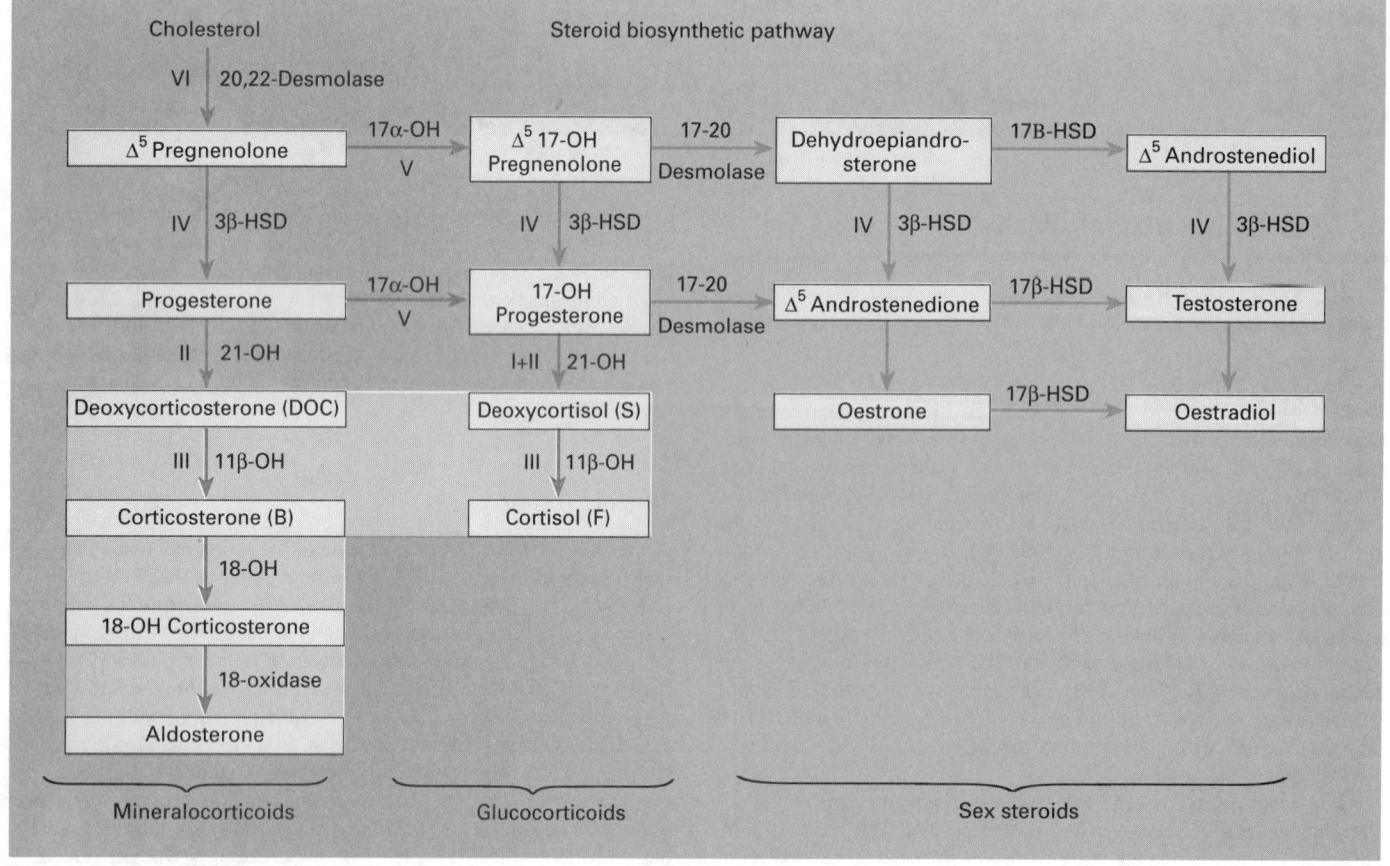

Table 1 *Adrenocortical diseases*

Glucocorticoid excess
  Cushing's syndrome
Glucocorticoid deficiency
  Primary
    Congenital àdrenal hyperplasia
      21-OHase
      Classical 3β-ol dehydrogenase
      17α-OHase
      Cholesterol desmolase
      11β-OHàse
    Addison's disease
    Hereditary adrenocortical unresponsiveness to ACTH
  Secondary
    Hypothalamic/pituitary disease
Mineralocorticoid excess
  Aldosteronism
  Other mineralocorticoids
  Glucocorticoid resistance
Mineralocorticoid deficiency
  Congenital adrenal hyperplasia
    Cholesterol desmolase
    3β-ol dehydrogenase
    21-OHase
  Congenital adrenal hypoplasia
  Disorders of terminal part of aldosterone biosynthetic
    pathway
  Pseudohypoaldosteronism
  Isolated renin deficiency
  Addison's disease
Adrenal androgen/oestrogen
  Excess
    Non-classical 3β-ol
    Non-classical 21-OHase
    PCO, tumours
  Deficiency
    17α-OHase
    17,20 lyase
    Adrenopause
    Testicular feminization

OHase = hydroxylase.

and rise to normal in the 6 months after removal of a pituitary micro-adenoma (Fig. 3). This would suggest that CRF is not involved, but patients with Cushing's disease show an exaggerated ACTH response to CRF, suggesting that there may be an enhanced sensitivity of corticotrophs to CRF. *In vitro* experiments with microadenomas from Cushing's patients, however, have not confirmed this.

There is some evidence that there may be enhanced AVP production in Cushing's disease. When bilateral blood samples were taken simultaneously from the inferior petrosal sinuses of patients with Cushing's disease the AVP levels were higher on the side of the adenoma, suggesting that increased delivery of AVP to the pituitary (possibly as a result of an aberrant blood supply) might interact with CRF to promote tumour growth and ACTH release.

Whether or not the hypothalamus has an initiating role, there is abundant evidence that at presentation the condition is pituitary- rather than hypothalamus-dependent. Thus, rare cases that have been treated by stalk section have not been cured, whereas selective removal of a microadenoma usually results in cure, gradual recovery of suppressed adjacent corticotrophs, and a very low recurrence rate.

There may be different subgroups of patients with pituitary-dependent Cushing's disease. Analyses of cortisol secretion over 24 h have shown two patterns, hypo- or hyperpulsatile, the latter perhaps hypothalamic in origin and the former pituitary-dependent.

The histopathology of pituitary adenomas from patients with Cushing's disease has been correlated with the outcome of operation and hormonal characteristics prior to surgery. In one group the adenomas contained argyrophilic nerve fibres which could not be found in the others. Nearly all those whose tumours contained the nerve fibres reverted to normal cortisol secretion rates after surgery, a rare finding in the other patients. Conversely, bromocriptine did not affect preoperative ACTH and cortisol levels in the first group, but suppressed them in the majority of patients whose tumours were free of the argyrophilic fibres. The suggestion has been made that tumours containing the characteristic fibres may arise from the anterior pituitary and those without them from the intermediate lobe.

Of particular clinical interest has been the small group of patients with cyclical Cushing's syndrome. In this condition periods of excess cortisol production (for example, 40 days) are followed by intervals of normal cortisol production (for example, 60–70 days). Some of these patients have a paradoxical rise in plasma ACTH and cortisol when treated with dexamethasone, and occasional patients show benefit with dopamine agonist (bromocriptine) or serotonin antagonist (cyproheptadine) therapy. In many of these patients basophil adenomas have been removed, some with long-term cure, but in others subsequent bilateral adrenalectomy has been required.

Two other pieces of evidence militate against Cushing's disease being a primary hypothalamic disease. Basophil hyperplasia is very uncommon. Careful application of modern histological techniques shows that in up to 90 per cent of cases there is a corticotroph microadenoma of monoclonal origin in the great majority appropriately examined.

ECTOPIC CORTICOTROPHIN RELEASING FACTOR (CRF) PRODUCTION

This is a very rare cause of pituitary-dependent Cushing's. However, a number of cases have now been described in which a tumour (for example medullary thyroid, prostate carcinoma) has been shown to contain

Fig. 2 H. G. Turney's case of Cushing's syndrome before and after developing the condition (Turney 1913).

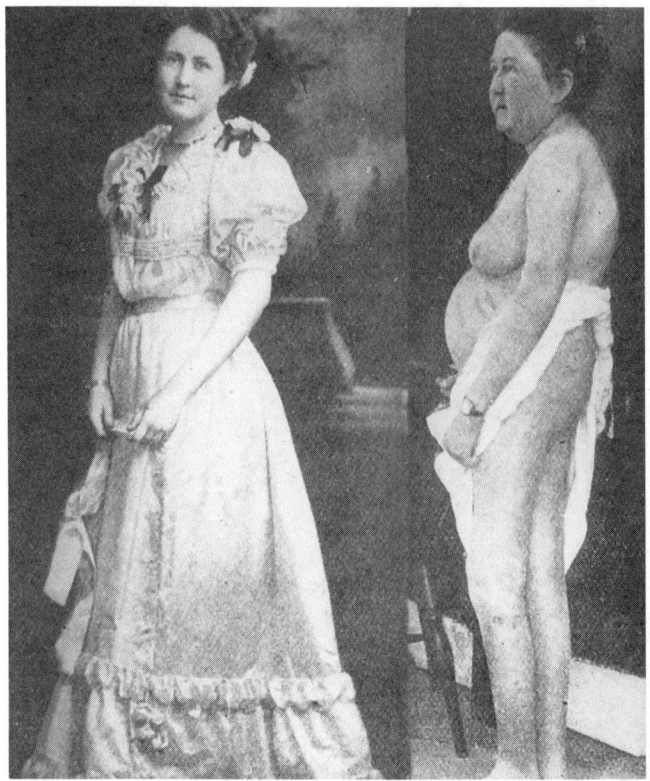

Table 2 *Classification of causes of Cushing's syndrome*

ACTH-dependent
    Iatrogenic (treatment with $ACTH_{1-39}$ or Synacthen®, $ACTH_{1-24}$)
    Cushing's disease (pituitary)
    Ectopic ACTH syndrome
    Ectopic CRF syndrome
    ?Macroscopic nodular adrenal hyperplasia
ACTH-independent
    Iatrogenic (e.g. pharmacological doses of prednisolone, dexamethasone, etc.)
    Adrenal adenoma
    Adrenal carcinoma
    Carney's syndrome
    McCune–Albright syndrome
    Gastric inhibitory polypeptide (GIP) adrenal hypersensitivity
    Alcohol

ACTH, adrenocorticotrophic hormone; CRF, corticotrophin releasing factor.

CRF but not ACTH, contrasting with the much more common situation in which a tumour contains both ACTH and CRF. It has been suggested that ectopic CRF production may explain the metyrapone responsiveness and suppression with high-dose dexamethasone found in some patients with the ectopic ACTH syndrome.

ECTOPIC ACTH SYNDROME

Cushing's syndrome may be associated with non-pituitary tumours producing ACTH, most commonly a small cell carcinoma of bronchus (Table 3). These conditions are described further in Chapter 12.11.

MACROSCOPIC NODULAR ADRENAL HYPERPLASIA

In about 20 to 40 per cent of patients with Cushing's disease there is bilateral adrenocortical hyperplasia associated with one or more nodules. These may be up to several centimetres in diameter. Such nodules are a trap for the unwary (see below) as they may be mistaken for primary

Fig. 3 Measurement of plasma immunoreactive corticotrophin releasing factor in normal subjects and patients with various adrenal diseases (data from Suda *et al*, 1987).

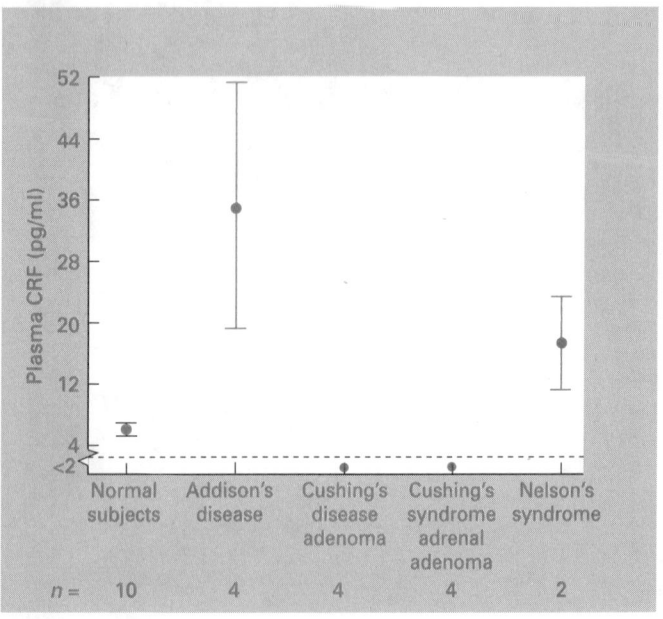

Table 3 *Tumours associated with the ectopic ACTH syndrome*

Tumour type	Approximate incidence (%)
Small cell lung carcinoma	50
Non-small cell lung carcinoma	5
Pancreatic tumours (including carcinoids)	10
Thymic tumours (including carcinoids)	5
Lung carcinoids	10
Other carcinoids	2
Medullary carcinoma of thyroid	5
Phaeochromocytoma and related tumours	3
Rare carcinomata of prostate, breast, ovary, gallbladder, colon	10

adrenal tumours. It has been suggested that this condition may be a transitional stage between a pituitary-dependent condition and an autonomous adrenal tumour. The basis for this is that the patients tend to be older; they are also more hypertensive. This situation shows remarkable parallels with that found in patients with primary aldosteronism associated with nodular hyperplasia. In these it has been suggested that the nodules might result from long-standing hypertensive vascular changes in that nodular hyperplastic glands almost invariably show arteriopathy of the capsular vessels. This is thought to produce focal ischaemia and atrophy with better perfused cells becoming hyperplastic leading to nodule formation.

An alternative explanation is that the nodules result from an autocrine or paracrine mechanism with either excess local production of growth factors or altered processing of N-terminal pro-opiomelanocortin (N-POC); this has been shown to be involved in adrenal growth. N-POC has also been found to enhance markedly the corticosteroid response to ACTH. This could then explain how it is that in macronodular adrenal hyperplasia lower circulating levels of ACTH are required to sustain hypercortisolism than in patients with diffuse bilateral adrenal hyperplasia. However, N-POC may not be the whole answer as *in vitro* studies with macronodules have shown that they show enhanced responsiveness to ACTH.

ACTH-independent causes

ADRENAL ADENOMA AND CARCINOMA

With the exclusion of iatrogenic Cushing's syndrome, adrenal adenomata are responsible for about 10 per cent of cases and carcinomata for about the same. Carcinomata are the commonest cause of Cushing's syndrome in children. The aetiology of these tumours is unknown.

CARNEY'S SYNDROME

This is an autosomal dominant condition comprising mesenchymal tumours (especially atrial myxomas), spotty skin pigmentation, peripheral nerve tumours, and various endocrine tumours, one of which may be Cushing's syndrome. The adrenals then contain multiple, small, pigmented nodules. The condition has been described as pigmented multinodular adrenocortical dysplasia. It does not appear to be ACTH-dependent and there is evidence to suggest that it results from stimulation by ACTH receptor antibodies.

McCUNE–ALBRIGHT SYNDROME

In this condition fibrous dysplasia and cutaneous pigmentation may be associated with pituitary, thyroid, adrenal, and gonadal hyperfunction. The adrenal hypersecretion may produce Cushing's syndrome. The underlying abnormality is a somatic mutation in the α-subunit of the stimulatory G protein which is linked to adenyl cyclase. The mutation results in the G protein being constitutively activated (that is, in the adrenal mimics constant ACTH stimulation). As the mutation occurs in fetal life, there is a mosaicism of cells with some containing, and others not, the mutation. In the adrenal such a mutation leads to associated local nodule formation.

GASTRIC INHIBITORY POLYPEPTIDE (GIP) HYPERSENSITIVITY

Recently two patients have been described with nodular hyperplasia, ACTH-independent Cushing's syndrome, and enhanced adrenal responsiveness to GIP. The biochemical clues were the presence of subnormal morning plasma cortisol levels and a rise in cortisol after food. This food-dependent form of Cushing's syndrome resulted from the normal increase in GIP after eating. The adrenocortical tissue of these patients responded *in vitro* to low doses of GIP, whereas there was no such effect in normal adrenal cortex, suggesting that in some unknown manner adrenal GIP receptors are linked to steroidogenesis in these patients. Not surprisingly, the clinical syndrome is related to food intake. Fasting can produce adrenal insufficiency. It remains to be seen whether abnormalities of adrenal sensitivity to GIP play a subtle role in other types of Cushing's syndrome.

ALCOHOL-ASSOCIATED PSEUDO-CUSHING'S SYNDROME

In the original description of this syndrome, urinary 17-hydroxycorticosteroid and plasma cortisol levels were elevated and failed to suppress with dexamethasone. Plasma ACTH has been found to be normal or suppressed. The frequency and pathogenesis of this condition remain unknown. With abstinence from alcohol the biochemical abnormalities rapidly revert to normal.

There appears to be little relation between the plasma cortisol levels and the degree of liver damage. Indeed, it would seem unlikely that impaired hepatic clearance of cortisol would be related as it might be expected to result in decreased ACTH secretion by negative feedback control. However, recent evidence has shown an interesting pattern of events. In both alcoholic and non-alcoholic liver disease there is impairment of 11β-hydroxysteroid dehydrogenase (11β-OHSD), the enzyme responsible for converting cortisol to inactive cortisone. Whereas in non-alcoholic liver disease this results in suppression of cortisol secretion, in alcoholic liver disease cortisol production is not suppressed. Alcohol is an inhibitor of 11β-OHSD *in vitro*; its effects could therefore be due to a direct effect on the enzyme in the liver and possibly also in the central nervous system where the enzyme appears to be involved in negative feedback control of ACTH.

Clinical features of Cushing's syndrome

The classical features of Cushing's syndrome with centripetal obesity, moon face, hirsutism, and plethora are well known following Cushing's initial description in 1912 (Figs. 2 and 4). However, this gross clinical picture is not always present. In a review of the discriminatory value of the signs and symptoms which might aid early diagnosis patients with Cushing's syndrome have been compared with those with simple obesity, using a discriminant index calculated by dividing the prevalence of a symptom or sign in Cushing's syndrome by its prevalence in simple obesity. The commonest symptoms and signs are listed in Table 4 together with the incidence of other commonly associated conditions such as diabetes and hypertension. Weight gain and obesity were the commonest symptom and sign, but the distribution of fat was not invariably centripetal; a 'buffalo hump' was present in about half the patients.

Gonadal dysfunction is very common, with menstrual irregularity in females and loss of libido in males. Hirsutism is frequently found in female patients, as is acne. All these features tend to be present more often in patients with adenoma than in those with bilateral adrenal hyperplasia.

Psychiatric abnormalities have been reported in all series of patients with Cushing's syndrome regardless of cause. Depression and lethargy are among the commonest problems, but poor concentration, paranoia and overt psychosis are also well recognized. Lowering of plasma cortisol by medical or surgical therapy usually results in a rapid improvement in the psychiatric state. In some severely affected patients it is necessary to treat the patient with metyrapone so as to improve the psychiatric condition prior to definitive investigation and treatment.

Most patients with long-standing Cushing's syndrome have lost height because of osteoporotic vertebral collapse. This can be assessed by measuring the patient's height and comparing it with their span; in normal subjects these measurements should be equal. Pathological fractures, either spontaneous or after minor trauma, are not uncommon. Rib fractures, in contrast to those of the vertebrae, are often painless. The radiograph appearances are typical, with exuberant callus formation at the site of the healing fracture.

The plethoric appearance of the patient with Cushing's syndrome is secondary to the thinning of the skin and is not due to true polycythaemia. In those with high concentration of haemoglobin, the red cell mass is usually normal and the polycythaemia due to a reduced plasma volume.

The typical red-purple livid striae of the syndrome are found most frequently on the abdomen but may also be present on the upper thighs and arms. They are very common in younger patients and less so in those over 50.

The myopathy of Cushing's involves the proximal muscles of lower limb and shoulder girdle. Complaints of weakness such as inability to climb stairs or get up from a deep chair are relatively uncommon, but observation as to whether or not as the patient can rise from a crouching position often reveals the problem.

Bruising of the skin with no known or trivial trauma is an important physical sign. Indeed the two features best discriminating Cushing's syndrome from simple obesity have been shown to be bruising and myopathy (Table 5). Hypertension is another prominent feature; even though epidemiological data show a strong association between blood pressure and obesity, hypertension is much more common in patients with Cushing's than in those with simple obesity.

Pigmentation is rare in Cushing's disease but common in the ectopic ACTH syndrome. However, in some pituitary tumours there is abnormal processing of the pro-opiomelanocortin ACTH precursor molecule, with resulting pigmentation.

Infections are more common in Cushing's patients. In many instances these are asymptomatic as the normal inflammatory response may be suppressed. In the skin, fungal infection is frequently found. Glucose intolerance may be a predisposing factor, with overt diabetes being pres-

Fig. 4 Typical facies of a Cushing's patient before and after treatment.

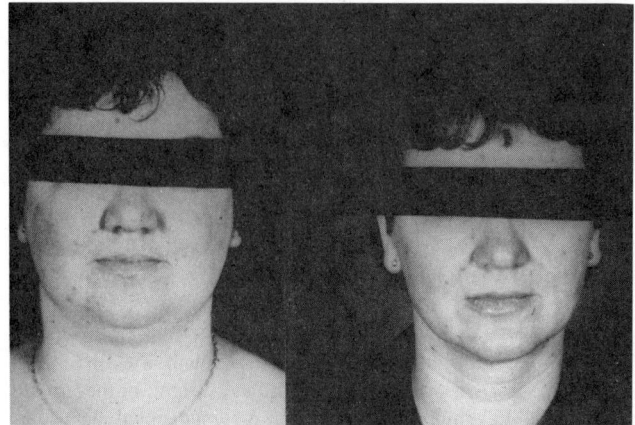

Table 4 *Prevalence of symptoms and signs in Cushing's syndrome*

	%
Symptoms	
Weight gain	91
Menstrual irregularity	84
Hirsutism	81
Psychiatric	62
Backache	43
Muscle weakness	29
Fractures	19
Loss of scalp hair	13
Signs	
Obesity	97
truncal	46
generalized	55
Plethora	94
Moonface	88
Hypertension	74
Bruising	62
Striae	56
Muscle weakness	56
Ankle oedema	50
Pigmentation	4
Other findings	
Hypertension	74
Diabetes	50
overt	13
abnormal GTT	37
Osteoporosis	50
Renal calculi	15

Data from Ross and Linch (1982).

Table 5 *Discriminant index in diagnosis of Cushing's syndrome*

	Discriminant index
Bruising	10.3
Myopathy	8.0
Hypertension	4.4
Plethora	3.0
Hirsutism	2.8
Red striae	2.5
Menstrual irregularity	1.6
Truncal obesity	1.6
Generalized obesity	0.8

Data from Ross and Linch (1982).

ent in up to one-third of patients in some series. Cataracts, a well-recognized complication of corticosteroid therapy, seem to be uncommon, except as a complication of diabetes. Cushing's report of exophthalmos in one-third of his original series was long ignored, but a recent study has confirmed exophthalmos greater than 16 mm (2 standard deviations above normal) to have been present in nearly 50 per cent of patients with Cushing's disease but was less common in other causes of Cushing's syndrome.

Special features of Cushing's syndrome

CHILDREN

In children, in addition to the above features, growth arrest is almost invariable. The dissociation between height and weight on the growth chart is obvious. It is important to try to get previous growth data so as to be able to calculate growth velocity. If the patient is growing along the same centile line, then the diagnosis of Cushing's syndrome is highly unlikely. In addition to glucocorticoid-induced growth arrest, androgen excess may result in precocious puberty.

ADRENAL CARCINOMATA

In addition to the normal features resulting from glucocorticoid excess, the patient may present with other problems relating to the tumour, for instance abdominal pain from the primary tumour or with secondary deposits; or to the secretion of other steroids, such as androgens or mineralocorticoids. Thus, in females, in addition to hirsutism, there may be other features of virilization, with clitoromegaly, breast atrophy, deepening of the voice, temporal recession, and severe acne.

ECTOPIC ACTH SYNDROME

If this is due to a small cell lung carcinoma, the clinical presentation more commonly resembles Addison's disease than Cushing's syndrome. The patients are very commonly pigmented and have lost weight, but the association of this with hypokalaemic alkalosis and glucose intolerance should alert the clinician. Patients with benign tumours, such as bronchial carcinoids which produce ACTH, present with the typical features of Cushing's syndrome.

Investigation of patients with suspected Cushing's syndrome

There are two stages in the investigation of a patient with suspected Cushing's syndrome. (1) Does the patient have Cushing's syndrome? (2) If the answer to (1) is yes, then what is the cause? Unfortunately many investigators fail to make this distinction and ill-advisedly use tests that are relevant to question (2) to try to answer question (1). The major tests are listed in Table 6.

DIAGNOSTIC TESTS
Circadian rhythm of plasma cortisol

In normal subjects plasma cortisol levels are at their highest first thing in the morning and reach a nadir at around midnight. This circadian rhythm is lost in patients with Cushing's syndrome. However, in the majority of patients the 09.00 hours plasma cortisol is normal with raised nocturnal levels. Random morning plasma cortisol levels are therefore of little value in making the diagnosis. Also various factors such as stress of venepuncture, intercurrent illness, and admission to hospital may result in normal subjects losing their circadian rhythm. It is therefore good practice to not measure plasma cortisol until the patient has been in hospital for 48 h. The morning sample is then taken at 09.00 hours together with plasma for the subsequent measurement of ACTH if other tests suggest Cushing's syndrome (see below for the importance of 08.00 hours versus 09.00 hours sampling). The midnight sample should be taken with the patient having been asleep; prior warning is not sensible as an apprehensive patient without the disease, who has not been asleep will often have an elevated plasma cortisol.

Very few laboratories have developed methods for the measurement of free levels of plasma cortisol. As more than 90 per cent of plasma cortisol is protein bound, the results of the conventional assay will be affected by drugs or conditions which alter cortisol binding globulin (CBG) levels. Thus oestrogen therapy or pregnancy may elevate CBG and hence total plasma cortisol. In normal subjects not on oestrogens midnight plasma cortisol is usually less than 180 nmol/l.

It is important to recognize two particular pitfalls in the interpretation of circadian data which may lead to a false negative test. The first of these is the pulsatile nature of cortisol secretion in some patients, espe-

Table 6 *Tests used in the diagnosis and differential diagnosis of Cushing's syndrome*

Diagnosis
Does the patient have Cushing's syndrome?
    Circadian rhythm of plasma cortisol
    Urinary free cortisol excretion*
    Low-dose dexamethasone suppression test*
    Insulin tolerance test
Differential diagnosis
What is the cause of the Cushing's syndrome?
    Plasma ACTH
    Plasma potassium
    High-dose dexamethasone suppression test
    Metyrapone test
    Corticotrophin releasing factor
    Inferior petrosal sinus ± selective venous sampling for
        ACTH
    CT/MRI scanning of pituitary/adrenals
    Scintigraphy
    Tumour markers

*Valuable outpatient screening tests (see text).

cially those with Cushing's disease. The hyperpulsatile group of Cushing's disease has the same number of spikes as the hypopulsatile group but the heights of the spikes are twice as great. There is thus a greater chance in this group of an isolated midnight sample being in the normal reference range. The second problem relates to the difficulty of investigating patients with cyclical Cushing's syndrome who may have long intervals of normal cortisol secretion.

If the 09.00 hours plasma cortisol is low then three possible diagnoses should be considered. First, the possibility that the patient is taking exogenous glucocorticoid; this is most commonly orally administered but may result from other sources such as excessive use of a potent topical steroid in a patient with severe eczema. Secondly, patients with cyclical Cushing's due to an adrenal tumour or ectopic ACTH secretion can have intermittent adrenal insufficiency. A third, but very rare example, is in patients with food-related Cushing's syndrome and enhanced adrenal responsiveness to GIP (see above).

Urinary free cortisol excretion

For many years the diagnosis of Cushing's syndrome was based on the measurement of urinary metabolites of cortisol (24-h urinary 17-hydroxycorticosteroid or 17-oxogenic steroid excretion, depending on the method used). However, the sensitivity and specificity of these methods is poor (17-hydroxycorticosteroid, 11 per cent false negative, 27 per cent false positive; 17-oxogenic steroid, 24 per cent false negative). For these reasons most investigators have abandoned these tests and use the much more sensitive measurement of urinary free cortisol excretion. The specificity of this test is very dependent on the method used for the measurement of cortisol. With radioimmunoassay it has been reported that there is a false negative rate of 5.6 per cent and false positive of 1 per cent (5 per cent in obese patients). Urinary free cortisol is an integrated measure of plasma free cortisol. As cortisol secretion increases, the binding capacity of CBG is exceeded and results in a disproportionate rise in urinary free cortisol.

Obese subjects have been shown to have an increased cortisol production rate and elevated urinary 17-oxogenic steroids. However, their urinary free cortisol is usually normal as there is an increase in metabolism of cortisol to cortisone. It is unclear whether the increase in cortisol secretion in obese subjects is related to the normal rise in ACTH and cortisol in response to food, which can be blocked by α_1-adrenoceptor antagonists.

Urinary free cortisol excretion is a useful outpatient screening test for Cushing's syndrome, but has the disadvantage of all tests requiring timed urinary collections. This can be obviated by measuring the cortisol–creatinine ratio, and can be further refined by measuring this ratio on the first urine specimen passed on waking. This should reflect the time during the 24-h cycle when there is the greatest difference between patients with Cushing's syndrome and normal subjects. Using radioimmunoassay, the upper limit of normal for cortisol → creatinine ratio in an early morning specimen of urine is about 50. Experience with this investigation in the study of cyclical Cushing's shows that urine aliquots are stable when left at room temperature for up to 7 days and can be sent by post.

Recent results have suggested that measurement of urinary 6β-hydroxycortisol may be useful in diagnosis, especially in mild cases. The enzyme 6β-hydroxylase is induced by glucocorticoid excess, resulting in a disproportionate rise in urinary 6β-hydroxycortisol in comparison to cortisol.

Dexamethasone suppression tests

In normal subjects administration of a supraphysiological dose of glucocorticoid results in suppression of ACTH and hence of cortisol secretion. In Cushing's syndrome of whatever cause there is a failure of this suppression when low doses of the synthetic glucocorticoid dexamethasone are given. Dexamethasone is used as it does not cross-react in the assays commonly used for the measurement of plasma cortisol.

Dexamethasone suppression tests are thought to have 97 to 100 per cent sensitivity in the diagnosis of Cushing's syndrome. Several types of low-dose tests have been described. In normal subjects the post-dexamethasone immunoreactive plasma cortisol is usually less than 50 nmol/l. Drugs such as phenytoin or rifampicin are a cause of false positive tests by way of their capacity to induce liver enzymes. Phenytoin, for example, increases the metabolic clearance rate of dexamethasone by about 400 per cent; as a consequence, the circulating level of dexamethasone is usually inadequate to suppress ACTH and thus cortisol secretion.

The overnight test is often used to screen outpatients. Various doses of dexamethasone have been used, usually given at midnight. The plasma cortisol is then measured at 08.00 hours or 09.00 hours. A dose of 1.5 or 2 mg gives a 30 per cent false positive rate, whereas after 1 mg this is reduced to 12.5 per cent with a false negative rate of less than 2 per cent. Thus, the outpatient overnight test has high sensitivity but low specificity, and further investigation is often required. This may not be necessary if it is possible to measure plasma dexamethasone in addition to plasma cortisol. This identifies those patients in whom inadequate plasma dexamethasone levels have been achieved. In most centres this assay is not available and the next step is to carry out the more reliable 48-h test.

In the 48-h test plasma cortisol is measured at 09.00 hours on day 0 and 48 h later. Dexamethasone is given in a dose of 0.5 mg 6 hourly for 48 h, with the last dose given 6 h before final blood sample. This test is normally carried out on inpatients. It is useful to collect 2 × 24-h urines for free cortisol prior to dexamethasone and then continue collection for the 2 × 24 h on the drug. This test is reported as having a 97 to 100 per cent true positive rate and a false positive of less than 1 per cent.

Insulin tolerance test

Patients with severe depression may show many of the biochemical features of Cushing's syndrome (loss of circadian rhythm of plasma cortisol, increased urinary free cortisol, failure of cortisol suppression with low-dose dexamethasone). Conversely, patients with Cushing's syndrome are frequently depressed. It is thus important in a depressed patient to take particular care in distinguishing the two conditions. In normal subjects and patients with severe endogenous depression insulin-induced hypoglycaemia results in a rise in ACTH and cortisol levels, a response usually not seen in Cushing's syndrome. It is important to make sure that there is adequate hypoglycaemia (i.e. blood glucose less than 2.2 mmol/l). In patients with Cushing's it may be necessary to give as much as 0.3 U soluble insulin/kg body weight, in comparison to 0.15

U/kg in normal subjects. The lack of response in Cushing's syndrome appears to be glucocorticoid-mediated as, in Cushing's disease, plasma ACTH rises in response to hypoglycaemia after adrenalectomy. The value of the insulin test is limited by the observation that there is a rise in ACTH and cortisol in some 20 per cent of Cushing's patients.

DIFFERENTIAL DIAGNOSTIC TESTS

Plasma ACTH

Having determined that the patient has Cushing's syndrome, the first key step in the differential diagnosis is to decide whether the condition is or is not dependent on ACTH. In this context it is worthwhile to take particular note of the time when plasma is taken for measurement of ACTH. In normal subjects random morning samples contain a range of concentrations from 9 to 77 ng/l; the range is much narrower (9–24 ng/l) if samples are taken only between 09.00 and 09.30 (Fig. 5). In comparison, in patients with Cushing's disease the ACTH concentrations at this time ranged from 39 to 109 ng/l. Thus the 09.00 to 09.30 hours plasma ACTH levels may help in both the diagnosis and differential diagnosis of Cushing's disease. In patients with the ectopic ACTH syndrome, plasma ACTH levels are almost invariably elevated (Fig. 6). In benign causes such as a bronchial carcinoid the levels may overlap with the levels found in Cushing's disease, but with small cell lung tumours and other malignant causes much higher levels of ACTH may be found.

In patients with adrenal tumours, plasma ACTH is usually undetectable. This can also occur with degradation of ACTH and therefore when taking blood for ACTH particular attention should be paid to taking the sample into a cold syringe and then separating the plasma in a chilled centrifuge before freezing the sample at −20°C.

The problem patients are those in whom plasma ACTH levels properly taken are low normal or intermittently detectable. This may occur in macronodular hyperplasia. The danger is that in some patients the asymmetry of the nodular hyperplasia may lead to a diagnosis of adrenal adenoma, the plasma ACTH is ignored, and a unilateral adrenalectomy performed, inappropriately, (Fig. 7). Unfortunately in some patients with this syndrome an autonomous adrenal tumour develops and, despite detectable ACTH, unilateral adrenalectomy is required (Fig. 8). These patients may be distinguished by their response to metyrapone (see below).

Fig. 6 Immunoreactive N-terminal ACTH levels in plasma samples taken between 08.00 and 10.00 hours in normal subjects (hatched area), and patients with Cushing's disease either untreated or postadrenalectomy, patients with adrenal tumours, and in the ectopic ACTH syndrome (by courtesy of Professor Lesley Rees).

Fig. 5 Plasma ACTH levels in normal controls (06.00–09.30 hours; 09.00–09.30 hours) and patients with Cushing's disease at 09.00 to 09.30 hours, (data from Horrocks and London 1982).

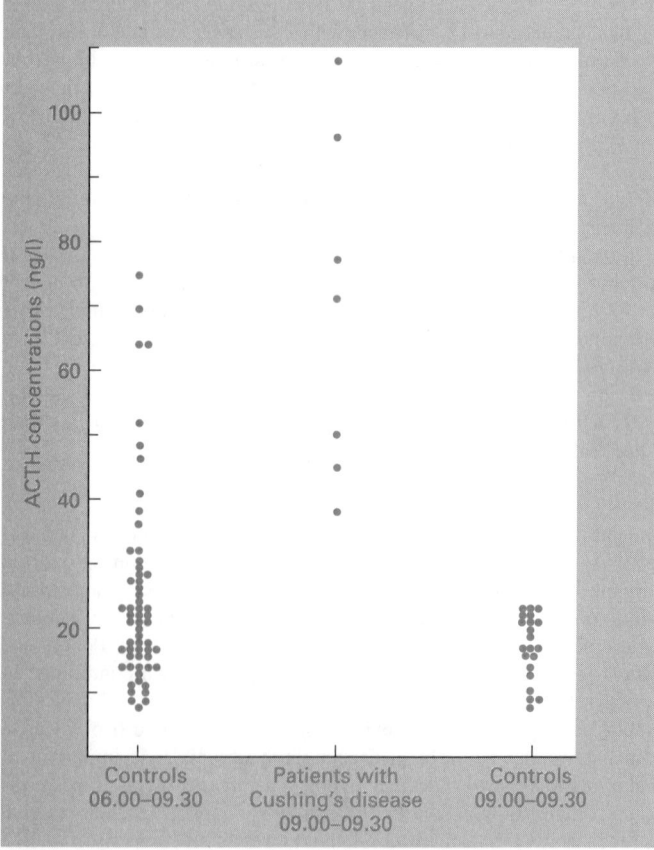

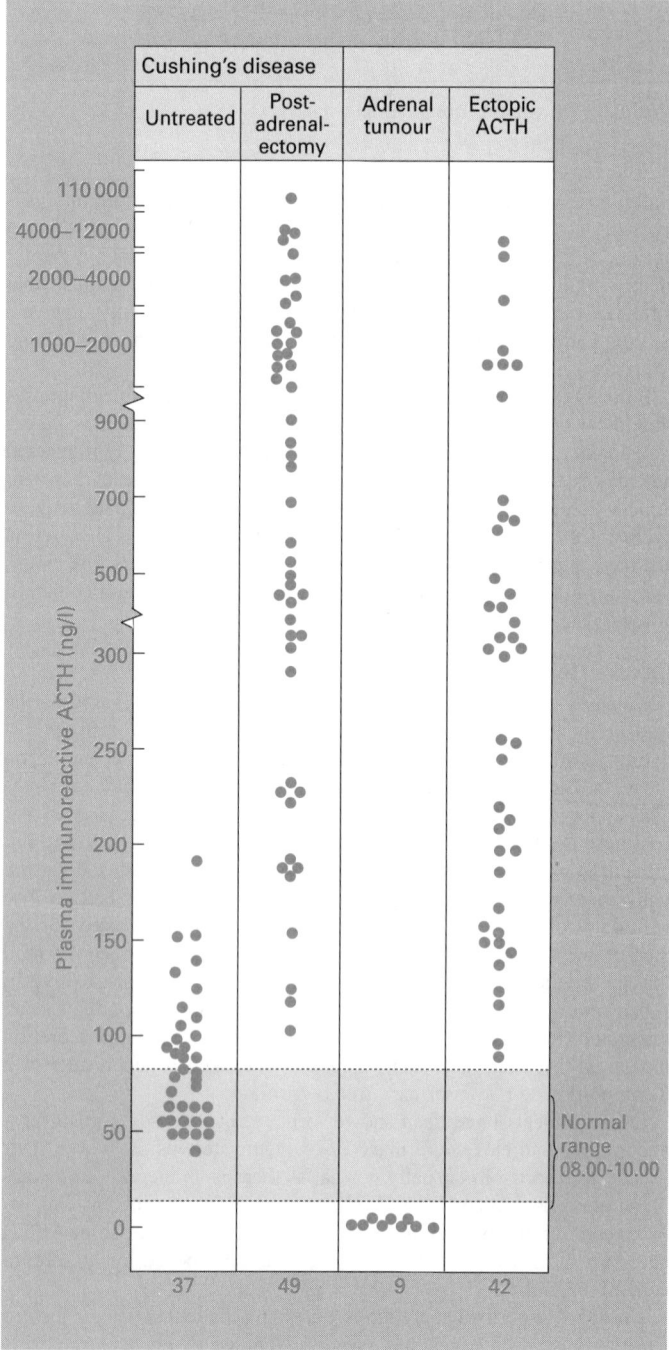

Determining the molecular species of ACTH by chromatography or by immunoradiometric assay may be helpful in making the differential diagnosis. Patients with the ectopic ACTH syndrome usually have both α_{1-39} ACTH and large molecular weight ACTH (often 22 kDa) whereas in other causes of Cushing's only α_{1-39} ACTH is found.

Plasma potassium (See also Chapter 20.2.3)

Hypokalaemic alkalosis is nearly always found in patients with the ectopic ACTH syndrome, but is present in fewer than 10 per cent of patients with Cushing's disease. The aetiology of this is now becoming clearer. Patients with the ectopic syndrome not only usually have higher plasma cortisol levels but also have impaired conversion of cortisol to cortisone. This results in a failure of the normal renal mechanism which prevents cortisol gaining access to non-specific mineralocorticoid receptors (see apparent mineralocorticoid excess syndrome, below). In addition, these patients have higher levels of the ACTH-dependent mineralocorticoid deoxycorticosterone.

High-dose dexamethasone suppression test

The rationale for this test is that in Cushing's disease there is negative feedback control of ACTH but it is set at a higher level than normal. Thus in this disease cortisol levels do not suppress with low-dose but do with high-dose dexamethasone. The original test introduced by Liddle was based on giving dexamethasone 2 mg 6 hourly for 48 h and measuring urinary 17-oxogenic steroids. Suppression was defined as a greater than 50 per cent fall in 24-h urinary 17-oxogenic steroids. In the modern test plasma cortisol is measured at 0 and +48 h or, less commonly, 8 mg dexamethasone is given orally at 23.00 hours and plasma cortisol taken at 08.00 hours on the same day (basal sample) and at 08.00 hours on the following morning. In both these tests greater than 50 per cent suppression of plasma cortisol in comparison to the basal sample has been used to define a positive response. In Cushing's disease about 90 per cent of patients have a positive 48-h test in comparison to 10 per cent with the ectopic ACTH syndrome. With overnight high-dose testing 89 per cent sensitivity and 100 per cent specificity has been reported for Cushing's disease.

The variable absorption of dexamethasone has prompted the introduction of a 5-h dexamethasone infusion test (1 mg/h). With this, plasma cortisol at 5-h shows a fall of greater than 190 nmol/l (in comparison to a mean of three basal values) in all patients with Cushing's disease but in only occasional patients with the ectopic ACTH syndrome. The latter appear to have tumours which also secrete CRF.

Metyrapone test

Metyrapone is an 11β-hydroxylase inhibitor which blocks the conversion of 11-deoxycortisol to cortisol and deoxycorticosterone to corticosterone (Fig. 1). This lowers plasma cortisol and, via negative feedback control, increases plasma ACTH (Fig. 9(a)). This in turn stimulates an increase in the secretion of adrenal steroids proximal to the block. Metyrapone is usually given orally in a dose of 750 mg 4 hourly for six doses, starting at 08.00 hours. To determine the effectiveness of cortisol blockade it is useful to measure either urinary-free cortisol (2 × 24 h samples prior to metyrapone, 1 × 24 h urine on day of metyrapone, and 1 × 24 h urine on day after metyrapone) or plasma cortisol (measured at 0, 1, 2, 3, 4, and 24 h). The measurement of urinary 17-oxogenic steroids has now been replaced by the specific radio-immunoassay of plasma 11-deoxycortisol at 0 and +24 h. This is more satisfactory than relying on the measurement of the ACTH response, as the increase in 11-deoxycortisol is much greater than that of ACTH.

In Cushing's disease metyrapone produces an exaggerated rise in plasma ACTH, and 11-deoxycortisol levels at 24 h exceed 1000 nmol/l (Figs. 9(b) and 10). In most patients with the ectopic ACTH syndrome there is little or no response, but occasional patients (possibly those producing both ACTH and CRF) have an 11-deoxycortisol response which may be similar to that in Cushing's disease (Fig. 10).

In patients with adrenal adenomas or carcinomas, ACTH is suppressed and metyrapone has little effect. Problems of interpretation arise in macronodular hyperplasia. Depending on the autonomy of the adrenal pathology there may be an ACTH and 11-deoxycortisol response typical of pituitary-dependent Cushing's (Fig. 11(a)) or of an adrenal adenoma (Fig. 11(b)).

The value of this test has been questioned. It was originally used to distinguish patients with Cushing's disease from those with a primary adrenal cause. However, these can be more reliably distinguished by measuring plasma ACTH and CT scanning of the adrenals. As indicated, the test does not reliably distinguish between Cushing's disease and the ectopic ACTH syndrome. However, when the results of ACTH assay and CT scanning are equivocal, many clinicians still perform it. Metyrapone may also be useful medical therapy prior to definitive treatment, and the test allows the clinician to determine the initial response.

Fig. 7 CT scan of adrenals in patient with asymmetrical nodular hyperplasia. The macronodule on the left was initially thought to be an adrenal tumour. The biochemistry indicating ACTH-dependent Cushing's was ignored and a unilateral adrenalectomy performed without cure of the hypercortisolism. Further investigation confirmed Cushing's disease (Figs 11 and 13) and a selective pituitary microadenomectomy resulted in cure.

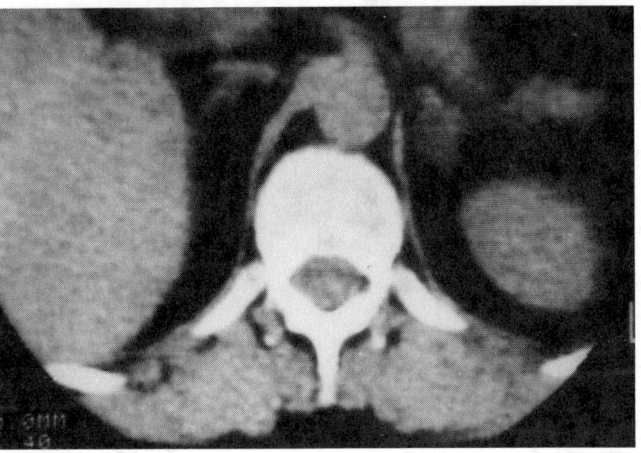

Fig. 8 CT scan of adrenals in patient with asymmetrical nodular hyperplasia. At the time of surgery the large lesion on the left was ACTH-independent and unilateral adrenalectomy resulted in cure despite the fact that adrenal scintigraphy showed that the right adrenal was not suppressed (Fig. 14).

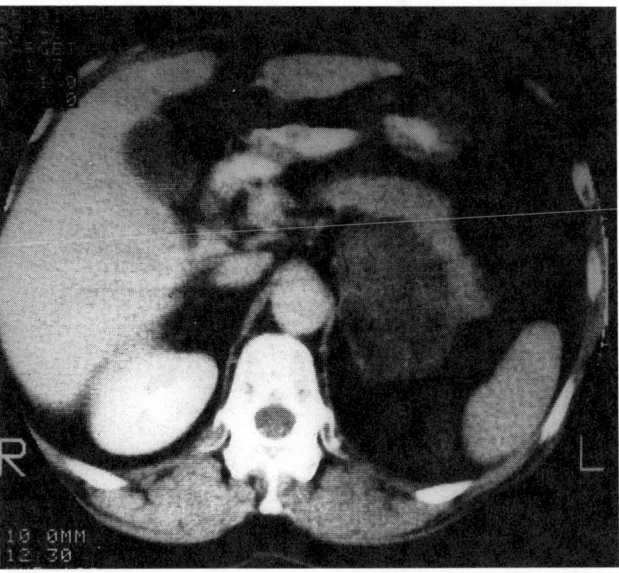

Corticotrophin releasing factor (CRF) test

CRF is a 41 amino acid peptide, identified by Vale in 1981 using ovine hypothalami. The ovine sequence differs by seven amino acid residues from that of the human, but, despite this, stimulates the release of ACTH in humans, and is used as the basis of a test usually involving the intravenous injection of 1 μg/kg body weight or a single dose of 100 μg. Human CRF has also been used and, despite producing a smaller peak cortisol response, some authors have claimed that it is more sensitive in the differential diagnosis of Cushing's syndrome; others deny this.

The test can be performed in the morning or afternoon, but for standardization many carry it out after taking a basal blood sample for ACTH and cortisol at 08.00 hours. Further blood samples for ACTH and cortisol are then taken every 15 min for 2 to 3 h after administering CRF.

In normal subjects, CRF produces a rise in ACTH and cortisol, and this response is exaggerated in Cushing's disease. It is typically absent in the ectopic ACTH syndrome and in patients with adrenal tumours. In distinguishing pituitary-dependent Cushing's from the ectopic ACTH syndrome it has been suggested that the response of ACTH to CRF has a specificity of 90 per cent, and with cortisol as the end-point, 95 per cent. Reviews of the literature suggest that, using an ACTH increase of 100 per cent over basal or a cortisol rise of 50 per cent as an end-point, this positive response eliminates a possible diagnosis of the ectopic ACTH syndrome. The slightly greater specificity of the cortisol response may relate to the release by occasional ectopic sources of large molecular weight ACTH which has lower bioactivity. However, such a response is rare, and the original case of putative ectopic ACTH syndrome which responded to CRF was subsequently found to have Cushing's disease.

As with the other tests, patients with macronodular hyperplasia may present a problem in diagnosis and show no response to CRF. The test is valuable in distinguishing patients with obesity and depression from those with Cushing's disease; in the obese and depressed the CRF response is either normal or reduced.

The administration of CRF is usually well tolerated, with a small number of patients complaining of flushing. Hypotension may occur but is rare.

Inferior petrosal sinus sampling/selective venous catheterization

In trying to distinguish Cushing's disease from the ectopic ACTH syndrome it may be necessary to identify the source of ACTH secretion. As blood from each half of the pituitary drains into the ipsilateral inferior petrosal sinus (IPS), it has been found that catheterization of both sinuses with simultaneous sampling of IPS venous blood can distinguish a pituitary from an ectopic source and aid in the lateralization of a pituitary microadenoma (Fig. 12). In patients with the ectopic ACTH syndrome, there is usually no ACTH gradient between the inferior petrosal sinus samples and simultaneously drawn peripheral venous levels. In Cushing's disease the ipsilateral : contralateral ACTH ratio is usually greater than 1.4. However, because of the problem of intermittent ACTH secretion, it is useful to make measurements before and at intervals (for example, 2, 5, and 15 min), after intravenous injection of 100 μg synthetic ovine CRF. Using this approach, patients with Cushing's disease and bilateral IPS ratios of less than 1.4 can be readily distinguished from those with the ectopic syndrome. The precise ratio that distinguishes Cushing's disease from the ectopic syndrome has been debated. Some authors use 2 rather than 1.4.

It is clear that IPS sampling is a useful technique for making the differential diagnosis in ACTH-dependent Cushing's syndrome. However, it should be reserved for those cases where the differential diagnosis is still in doubt after high-dose dexamethasone and CRF testing. IPS catheterization may also be of value to the surgeon who is planning

Fig. 10 Plasma deoxycortisol levels in response to the administration of metyrapone in patients with Cushing's syndrome of different aetiologies (data from Perry *et al.* 1980).

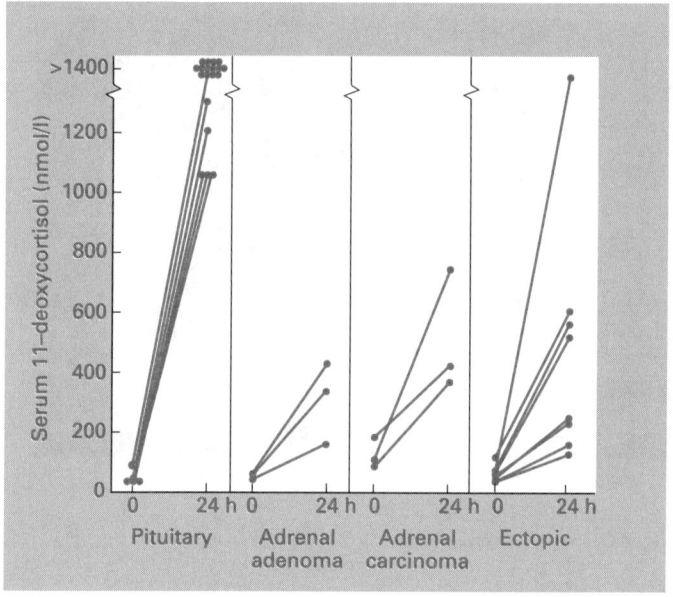

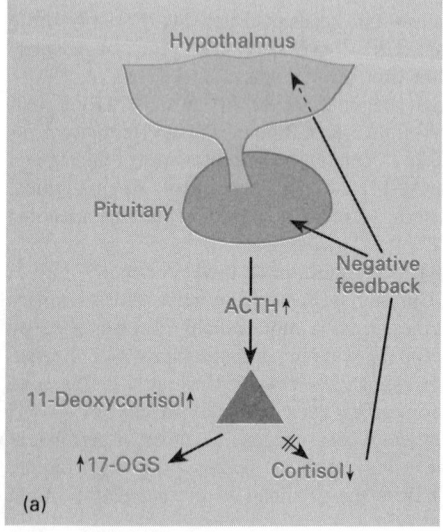

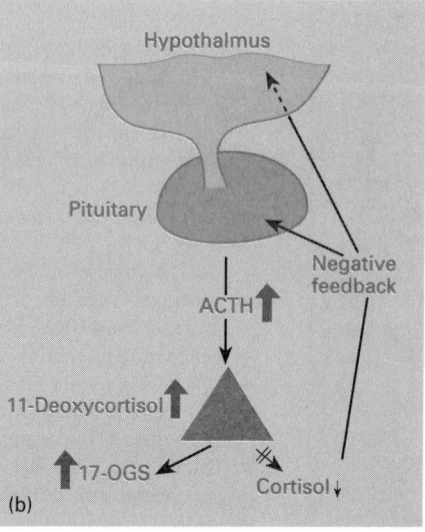

Fig. 9 Metyrapone test in (a) normal subject and (b) Cushing's disease.

to explore the pituitary in a patient with Cushing's disease and in whom other imaging techniques have not shown the localization of a microadenoma.

In some patients with the ectopic ACTH syndrome, extensive investigation may fail to reveal the source. In these, selective venous catheterization via the femoral vein with measurement of ACTH in veins draining the known possible sites of ectopic ACTH production may be required.

CT/MRI scanning of pituitary and adrenals

There is no doubt that high-resolution, thin-section contrast enhanced imaging using either CT or MRI has revolutionized the investigation of Cushing's syndrome. However, the results of the imaging must always be interpreted in the light of the biochemical results if mistakes are to be avoided. In imaging the adrenals asymmetrical nodular hyperplasia may lead to a false diagnosis of adrenal adenoma (Fig. 7). CT scanning of the pituitary may produce a very significant false positive and false negative rate for tumours less than 6 mm in diameter.

The classic CT features of a pituitary microadenoma are a hypodense lesion after contrast, associated with deviation of the pituitary stalk and a convex upper surface of the pituitary gland (Fig. 13). About 90 per cent of ACTH-secreting pituitary tumours are microadenomas (i.e. less than 10 mm in diameter); as such it is rare for the pituitary fossa to be abnormal, and hence plain radiographs of the fossa are of little value.

With such small tumours it is not surprising that the sensitivity of CT scanning is relatively low (20–60 per cent) with a similar specificity. Results with MRI suggest that this is the most satisfactory method for identifying microadenomas, with sensitivity of about 70 per cent and specificity of 87 per cent.

Not surprisingly, the results of CT scanning of the adrenals are much better than those for the pituitary. Adrenal tumours causing Cushing's syndrome are usually greater than 1.5 cm in diameter. With tumours of this size MRI has no diagnostic advantage over CT. It is important to remember that 'incidentalomas' are present in up to 8 per cent of normal subjects, and thus adrenal imaging should not be performed unless biochemical investigation suggests a primary adrenal cause.

Adrenal scintigraphy

This is of value in certain patients with primary adrenal pathology. The most commonly used agent is ^{131}I-6β-iodomethyl-19-norcholesterol. This is a marker of adrenocortical cholesterol uptake. In patients with adrenal adenomas the isotope is taken up by the adenoma but not by the contralateral suppressed adrenal. With adrenal carcinomas the tumour uptake is very low, and as the opposite adrenal is suppressed the usual result is lack of image in either adrenal area.

CT scanning in patients suspected of Cushing's and undetectable ACTH can usually accurately identify adrenal adenomas and carcinomas. Adrenal scintigraphy is useful in patients with suspected adrenocortical macronodular hyperplasia, in which CT scanning may be mis-

Fig. 11 Metyrapone tests in patients whose CT scans are shown in Figs 7 (11a) and 8. The effect of lowering cortisol secretion in a patient with macronodular hyperplasia who was successfully treated by selective removal of a pituitary microadenoma. (b) The lack of ACTH and 11-deoxycortisol response to metyrapone in a patient with macronodular hyperplasia who required unilateral adrenalectomy.

Fig. 12 Positions of bilateral catheters in inferior petrosal sinus sampling.

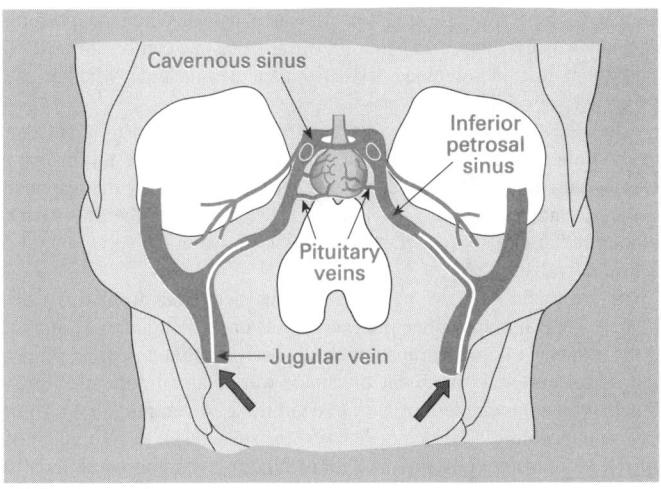

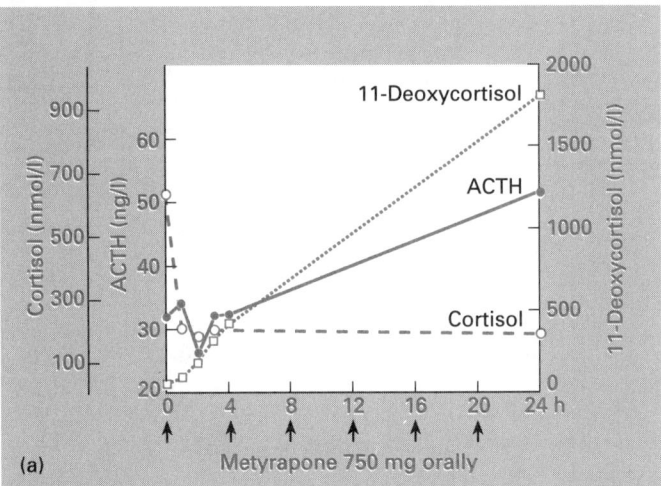

(a)

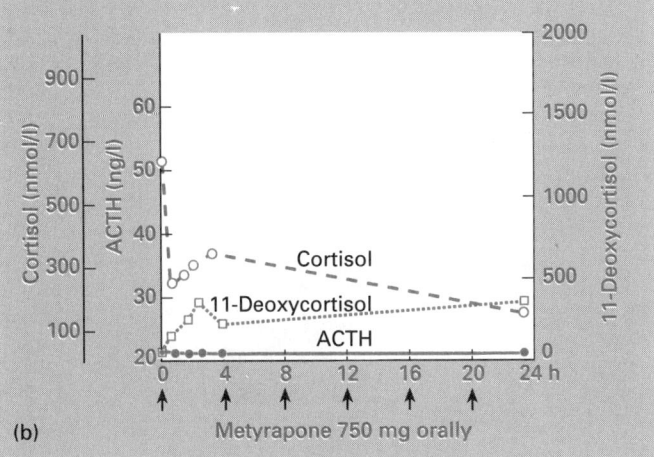

(b)

Fig. 13 Typical CT scan of pituitary in patient with Cushing's disease, showing hypodense microadenoma (A) in lateral view (top) and anteroposterior view (AP) (bottom). The pituitary stalk can be identified (B) in the AP view.

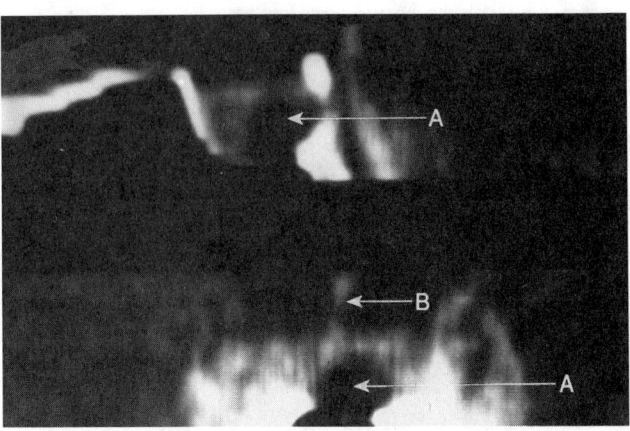

leading by suggesting unilateral pathology, whereas with isotope scanning the bilateral adrenal involvement is identified (Fig. 14).

Tumour markers

The importance of measuring tumour markers has already been stressed. Many tumours in patients with the ectopic ACTH syndrome produce other peptide hormones in addition.

Prognosis of untreated Cushing's syndrome

Studies carried out prior to the introduction of effective therapy suggested that 50 per cent of patients with untreated Cushing's syndrome died within 5 years. The relevance of this now is to the undiagnosed case.

Treatment of Cushing's syndrome

This clearly depends on the cause. Adrenal adenomas should be removed by unilateral adrenalectomy, with 100 per cent cure rate. In a clear-cut case with undetectable ACTH, unilateral tumour, and atrophic contralateral gland, a loin approach can usually be used. This has a much lower morbidity than the anterior abdominal approach required to visualize both adrenals. Following operation it may take many months or even 1 to 2 years for the suppressed adrenal to recover. It is wise therefore to give slightly suboptimal replacement therapy with dexamethasone 0.5 mg in the morning, with intermittent measurement of 08.00 hours plasma cortisol prior to taking dexamethasone. When the morning plasma cortisol is above 180 nmol/l, dexamethasone can be stopped. A subsequent insulin tolerance test may then demonstrate whether the response to stress is normal.

Adrenal carcinomas have a very poor prognosis and most patients are dead within 2 years. It is usual practice to try to remove the primary tumour even though metastases are present so as to enhance the response to the adrenolytic agent *o,p'*-DDD (see below). Radiotherapy to the tumour bed and to some metastases, such as those in the spine, may be of limited value.

The treatment of Cushing's disease has been transformed by the improvements in trans-sphenoidal surgery. Prior to the selective removal of the pituitary microadenoma which has been identified in up to 90 per cent of patients, the treatment of choice was bilateral adrenalectomy. This had an appreciable mortality even in the best centres (about 4 per cent) and morbidity. The major risk was the subsequent development of Nelson's syndrome (postadrenalectomy hyperpigmentation with locally

aggressive pituitary tumour). To try to avoid this, pituitary irradiation was often carried out following bilateral adrenalectomy. In addition, these patients required life-long replacement therapy with hydrocortisone and fludrocortisone. Nowadays bilateral adrenalectomy is reserved for the occasional patient with Cushing's disease in whom no pituitary tumour can be found, or when pituitary surgery has failed, or where the condition has recurred.

As with all types of surgery, the outcome of trans-sphenoidal microadenomectomy is crucially dependent on the skill and experience of the surgeon. This was underlined by the results of the survey carried out by Birch. In major centres the cure rate is high and the recurrence rate low (Fig. 15). However, in certain institutions where the operation is less commonly performed the converse is true.

Following selective removal of a microadenoma, the surrounding corticotrophs are normally suppressed (Fig. 16). In these cases plasma cor-

Fig. 15 Burch survey of the results of trans-sphenoidal surgery for Cushing's disease showing very variable cure rates and recurrence rates in different centres (data from Burch 1983).

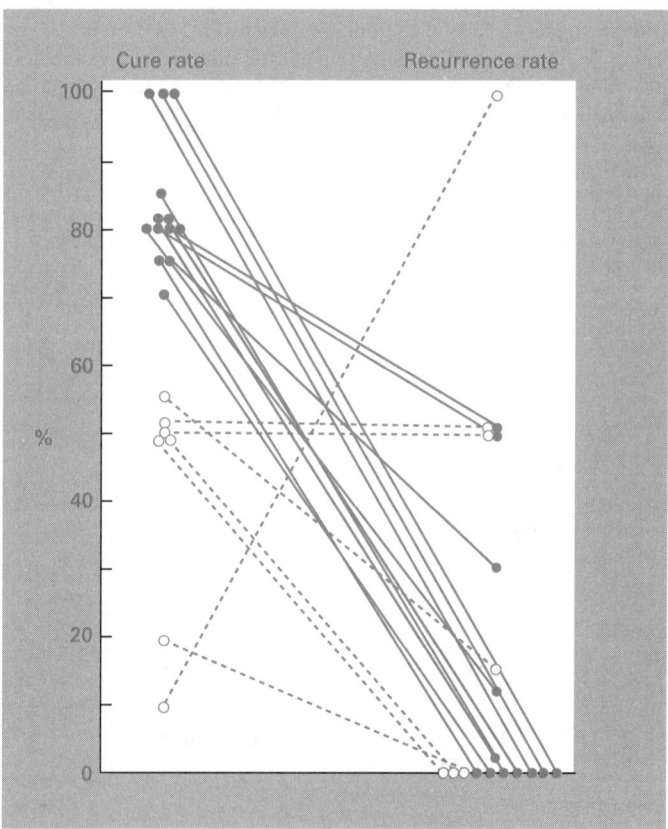

Fig. 14 Adrenal scintigraphy in patient with Cushing's syndrome and macronodular hyperplasia whose CT scan is shown in Fig. 8. Note asymmetrical uptake in the adrenals, with 1.6 per cent uptake on the left and 0.4 per cent on the right.

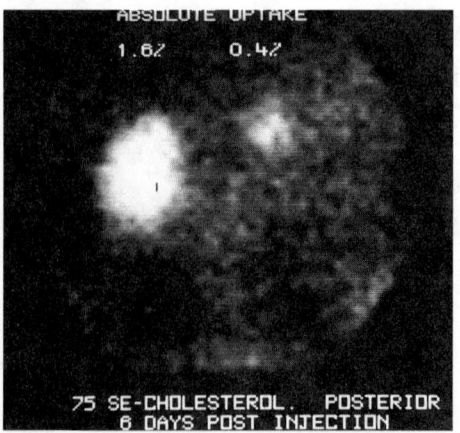

Fig. 16 Selective removal of a microadenoma and its effect on hypothalamic–pituitary–adrenal axis.

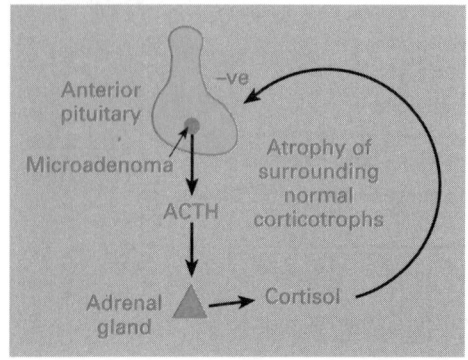

tisol levels are also suppressed postoperatively and glucocorticoid replacement therapy is required. Using the dexamethasone regime described above after removal of an adrenal adenoma, there is usually (but not invariably) gradual recovery of the hypothalamic–pituitary–adrenal axis (Fig. 17).

The incidence of hypopituitarism following pituitary microsurgery in the best centres is low (about 10 per cent). However, a much higher incidence has been reported in those patients requiring more radical pituitary surgery. Transient diabetes insipidus occurs in about 20 per cent of patients, but the permanent condition is rare.

In the past, pituitary irradiation was often used in the treatment of Cushing's disease. However, the improvements in pituitary surgery have resulted in far fewer patients being so treated. Depending on the facilities available, several types of treatment have been used, including proton beam, interstitial irradiation with implantation of radioactive seeds or rods, usually of yttrium-90, or external megavoltage X-ray therapy, most often using a linear accelerator. Even though in children pituitary irradiation appears to be effective, in adults the long-term results have not been very satisfactory, with remission rates usually lower than with trans-sphenoidal surgery, a variable time to onset of effect, and a higher incidence of hypopituitarism. For these reasons radiotherapy is not recommended as a primary treatment but is reserved for patients not responding to pituitary microsurgery or when pituitary surgery is con-

traindicated and bilateral adrenalectomy has been performed, or with established Nelson's syndrome.

Treatment of the ectopic ACTH syndrome depends on the cause. If the tumour can be found and has not spread, then its removal can lead to cure (for example bronchial carcinoid or thymoma). However, the prognosis for small cell lung cancer associated with the ectopic ACTH syndrome is poor. The cortisol excess and associated hypokalaemic alkalosis and diabetes mellitus can be ameliorated by medical therapy (see below). The treatment of the small cell tumour itself will also, at least initially, produce improvement (see Section 17.13). Sometimes, if the ectopic source of ACTH cannot be found, it may be necessary to perform bilateral adrenalectomy and then follow the patient carefully (sometimes for several years) to find the primary tumour.

Medical treatment of Cushing's syndrome

Several drugs have been used in the treatment of Cushing's syndrome. Their site of action is shown in Fig. 18. Metyrapone has been most commonly given, often to control the condition prior to definitive therapy such as pituitary or adrenal surgery, or while awaiting benefit from pituitary irradiation. It is usually easier to control cortisol secretion in patients with adrenal adenomas than with other causes. The daily dose has to be determined by measuring either plasma or urinary free cortisol. The aim should be to achieve a mean plasma cortisol of about 300 nmol/l during the day or a normal urinary free cortisol. The drug is usually given in doses ranging from 250 mg twice daily to 1.5 g every 6 h. Nausea may be produced and can be helped (if not due to adrenal insufficiency) by giving the drug with milk.

Aminoglutethimide is a more toxic drug which in high dose blocks earlier in the pathway and thus affects the secretion of steroids other than cortisol. In doses of 1.5 to 3 g daily (start with 250 mg 8 hourly) it commonly produces nausea, marked lethargy, and a high incidence of skin rash.

Trilostane, a 3β-hydroxysteroid dehydrogenase inhibitor, is ineffective in Cushing's disease, as the block in steroidogenesis is overcome by the rise in ACTH. However, it can be effective in patients with adrenal adenomas.

Ketoconazole is an imidazole which has been widely used as an antifungal agent but produces abnormal liver function tests in about 14 per cent of patients. A small number of deaths have been reported but these have usually been in patients in whom the drug was continued despite evidence of hepatic dysfunction. Ketoconazole blocks a variety of cyto-

Fig. 17 Gradual recovery of hypothalamic–pituitary–adrenal axis after removal of a pituitary ACTH-secreting microadenoma. The insulin hypoglycaemia test eventually demonstrated the return of a normal stress response.

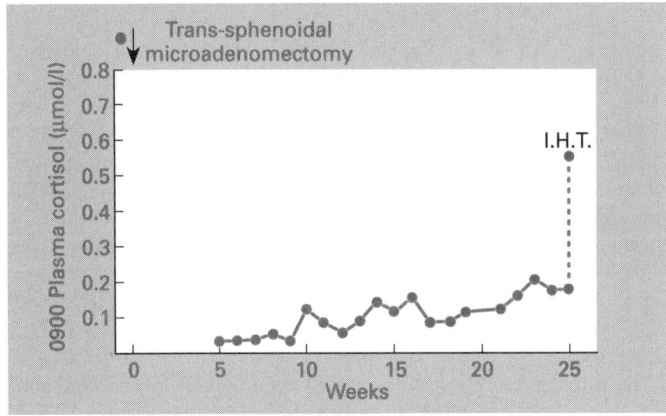

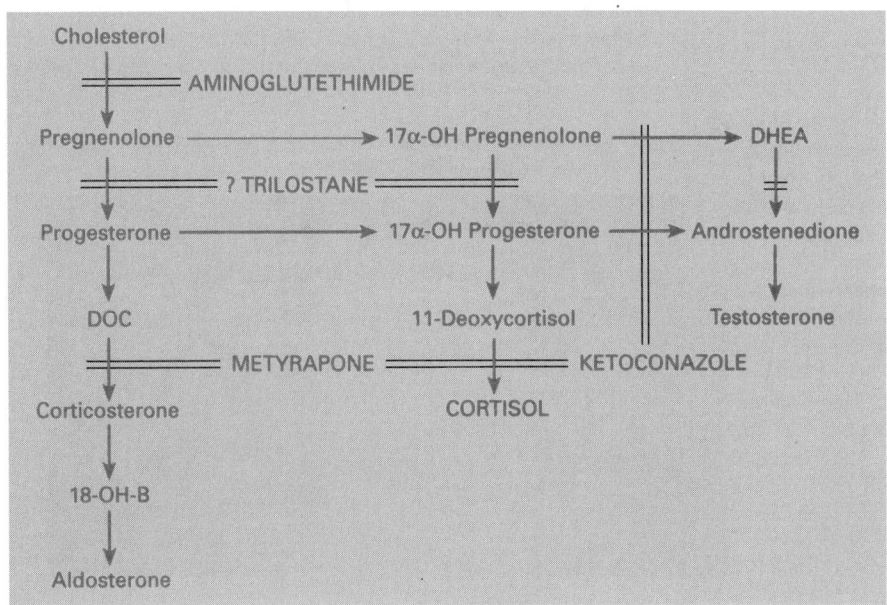

Fig. 18 Medical treatment of Cushing's syndrome: site of action of various drugs.

chrome P450-dependent enzymes and thus lowers plasma cortisol levels. For the treatment of fungal infections a dose of 200 mg daily has been used. For effective control of Cushing's cortisol hypersecretion, higher doses (for example 400–800 mg daily) have been required.

o,p'-DDD is an adrenolytic drug which is taken up by both normal and malignant adrenal tissue, thus causing adrenal atrophy and necrosis. Because of its toxicity it has been used mainly in the management of adrenal carcinoma and only rarely in Cushing's disease. In daily doses of up to 8 g it has been possible to control glucocorticoid excess and may have some beneficial effect on tumour growth. Long-term survival of patients with adrenal carcinoma is very rare. The drug will also produce mineralocorticoid deficiency. Patients may therefore require both glucocorticoid and mineralocorticoid replacement therapy. Problems such as fatigue, skin rashes, and gastrointestinal side-effects are common and limit the use of the drug.

Glucocorticoid deficiency

PRIMARY AND SECONDARY HYPOADRENALISM

Glucocorticoid deficiency can be classified on the basis of whether it is due to a deficiency of ACTH, the major trophic hormone controlling cortisol secretion (secondary hypoadrenalism) or to a defect in the adrenals which affects the synthesis of cortisol (primary hypoadrenalism). The latter condition is usually referred to as Addison's disease. By convention, congenital adrenal hyperplasia is considered separately from Addison's disease.

Primary hypoadrenalism

Congenital adrenal hyperplasia (CAH)

Various inherited enzyme defects in the synthesis of adrenocortical hormones have been identified (Table 7). This group of conditions is addressed in Chapter 12.7.2.

Addison's disease

Thomas Addison described this condition in his classic monograph published in 1855. Addison worked with Bateman, a dermatologist who produced one of the first classifications of skin disease. It seems likely that this stimulated Addison's interest in the skin pigmentation which is so characteristic of his disease.

AETIOLOGY

This is a rare condition with an estimated incidence in the developed world of 0.8 cases per 100 000 population. The causes of Addison's disease are listed in Table 8. Addison himself described tuberculous destruction of the adrenals. However, the incidence of tuberculous Addison's disease has gradually fallen, and autoimmune adrenalitis now accounts for more than 70 per cent of cases. It remains to be seen whether, with the resurgence of tuberculosis in AIDS patients, there will be a reversal of this pattern. Adrenal insufficiency is well described in AIDS and may result from a variety of causes, including tuberculosis, fungal, and other infections, such as cytomegalovirus.

In autoimmune adrenalitis the adrenal glands are atrophic with loss of most of the cortical cells. Some hypertrophied eosinophilic compact cells remain. The medulla is usually intact. By contrast, in tuberculous Addison's disease the adrenals are initially enlarged with extensive epithelioid granulomas and caseation. Calcification eventually ensues in most cases (Fig. 19). Both the cortex and the medulla are affected.

The human leucocyte antigen (HLA) associations of Addison's dis-

Table 7 *Enzyme defects and clinical syndromes in congenital adrenal hyperplasia*

Enzyme	Clinical syndrome
21-hydroxylase (21-OH)	Salt-wasting/virilization Simple virilization Non-classical

3β-hydroxysteroid
   dehydrogenase (3βHSD)
	Classical (virilization)
	       (salt-wasting)
	Non-classical (virilization)

Cholesterol desmolase	Lipoid hyperplasia Failure of all steroid production
11β-hydroxylase	Hypertension Virilization
17α-hydroxylase	Hypertension Gonadal failure (pseudohermaphroditism)
18-hydroxylase (Corticosterone methyl oxidase Type I) (CMO-I)	Salt-wasting
18-oxidase (Corticosterone methyl oxidase Type II) (CMO-II) Aldosterone synthase	Salt-wasting

ease are quite variable. Polyglandular deficiency type I is an autosomal recessive condition in which adrenocortical failure is associated with chronic mucocutaneous candidiasis, hypoparathyroidism, and a variety of other conditions (Table 8). HLA class I genes are important in determining the expression of the syndrome, with HLA-A28 being more common in affected patients. There is no association with HLA-DR genes. By way of contrast, polyglandular deficiency type II (Schmidt's syndrome) (Addison's disease, primary hypothyroidism, primary hypogonadism, insulin-dependent diabetes mellitus, and vitiligo) has an autosomal dominant mode of inheritance and is strongly associated with HLA-DR3. Sporadic autoimmune Addison's disease has the same HLA associations as the type II syndrome.

The adrenal cortex antibodies react with a 54 kDa microsomal antigen, which has been identified as the 21-hydroxylase enzyme. These antibodies are found in virtually all newly diagnosed cases of autoimmune Addison's disease, and in 70 to 80 per cent of patients the antibodies can still be found 10 years later, they are not found in other causes of the condition, but may be present in 1 to 2 per cent of patients

Fig. 19 Plain radiograph of the abdomen showing adrenal calcification in a patient with tuberculous Addison's disease.

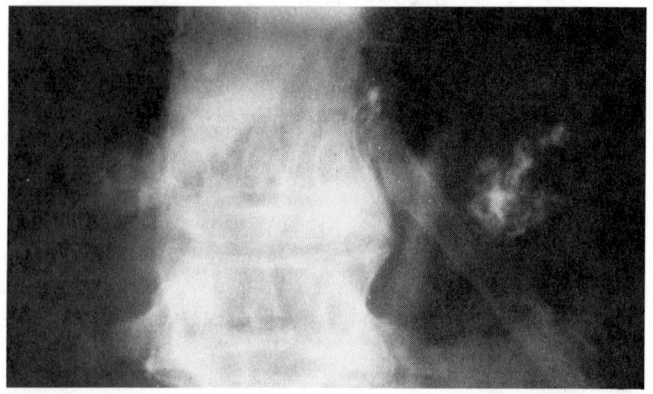

without Addison's disease but who have other organ-specific autoimmune conditions (such as hypoparathyroidism, insulin-dependent diabetes mellitus, autoimmune thyroid disease, vitiligo, and primary ovarian failure). Follow-up of these patients shows that about one-third will develop adrenal insufficiency in the next 10 years.

Patients with Addison's disease may also have antibodies which cross-react with steroid-producing cells in the ovary, testis, and placenta, and are distinct from the antibodies specific for the 21-hydroxylase enzyme. These are found in nearly all patients with both Addison's disease and primary ovarian failure, in one-third of type II polyglandular deficiency, and three-quarters of type I. The antigen recognized is a common cytoplasmic antigen (either 17α-hydroxylase or side-chain cleavage enzyme) found in the adrenals and gonads. In patients with associated pernicious anaemia the autoantigen is the gastric parietal cell $Na^+/K^+ATPase$. It is unclear why the different components of the polyglandular syndromes coexist: they do not share common determinants with the 21-hydroxylase enzyme.

In addition to the antibodies which react with steroidogenic enzymes, recent evidence suggests that many addisonian patients produce immunoglobulins which block the effect of ACTH. The binding site of these antibodies could be the ACTH receptor. The functional role that they play in producing adrenal insufficiency is unknown.

With the exception of tuberculosis and autoimmune adrenal failure, other causes of Addison's disease are rare (Table 8). Adrenal metastases are often found at postmortem examinations but adrenal insufficiency from these is uncommon. Necrosis of the adrenals with intra-adrenal haemorrhage may result from bilateral adrenal vein thrombosis. This may be due to infection, trauma, or hypercoagulability. Intra-adrenal bleeding may be found in any cause of severe septicaemia. When this is due to meningococcus the association with adrenal insufficiency is known as the Waterhouse–Friderichsen syndrome.

X-linked adrenoleucodystrophy is due to a deficiency of a peroxisomal enzyme (lignoceroyl-CoA ligase) which produces a failure of very-long-chain fatty acid oxidation. Only males have the fully expressed condition and carrier females are usually normal. Pathologically the condition is characterized by lamellar inclusions in the cells of the adrenal cortex, interstitial cells of the testis, brain macrophages, and Schwann cells. The adrenal lesions lead to a failure of steroidogenesis, with more marked effect on the zona fasciculata than zona glomerulosa. The brain lesions result in neurological symptoms from cerebral demyelination. In the childhood form of the condition (about 50 per cent of cases) the symptoms start around 5 to 10 years of age and progress eventually to a blind, mute, and severely spastic tetraplegic state. Adrenal insufficiency is usually present but does not appear to correlate with the neurological deficit. In the adult disease, which is known as adrenomyeloneuropathy, the condition develops more slowly, with spastic paresis and peripheral neuropathy in the 20s or 30s. There follows the gradual development of cerebral involvement. As both the childhood and the adult condition result from the same mutant gene, it has been suggested that there is an additional autosomal modifier gene. It had been hoped that the condition would respond to dietary restriction of very-long-chain fatty acids. One approach is to give monounsaturated fatty acids which block the synthesis of the saturated very-long-chain fatty acids. However, despite the fact that the combination of erucic acid (a monounsaturated fatty acid) and oleic acid (the combination is Lorenzo's oil) led to normal levels of very-long-chain fatty acids this does not appear to slow the rate of neurological deterioration. It remains to be seen whether early therapy before neurological dysfunction prevents it.

Another rare disease is hereditary adrenocortical unresponsiveness to ACTH. In this condition the renin–angiotensin–aldosterone axis is intact and children may present either with neonatal hypoglycaemia or later with increasing pigmentation, often with enhanced growth velocity. This condition has recently been shown to be due to a point mutation in the ACTH receptor and is inherited as an autosomal recessive.

Table 8 *Aetiology of Addison's disease*

Tuberculosis
Autoimmune
  Sporadic
  Polyglandular deficiency type I
  (Addison's disease, chronic mucocutaneous candidiasis,
    hypoparathyroidism, dental enamel hypoplasia, alopecia,
    primary gonadal failure)
  Polyglandular deficiency type II (Schmidt's syndrome)
  (Addison's disease, primary hypothyroidism, primary
    hypogonadism, insulin-dependent diabetes, pernicious
    anaemia, vitiligo)
Metastatic tumour
Lymphoma
Amyloid
Intra-adrenal haemorrhage (Waterhouse–Friederichsen
  syndrome) following meningococcal septicaemia
Haemochromatosis
Adrenal infarction or infection other than tuberculosis
  (especially AIDS)
Adrenoleucodystrophy
Adrenomyeloneuropathy
Hereditary adrenocortical unresponsiveness to ACTH
Bilateral adrenalectomy

Secondary hypoadrenalism (ACTH deficiency)

This is a not uncommon clinical problem and is most often due to a sudden cessation of exogenous glucocorticoid therapy or a failure to give glucocorticoid cover for intercurrent stress in a patient who has been on long-term glucocorticoid therapy. Such therapy suppresses the hypothalamic–pituitary–adrenal axis, with consequent adrenal atrophy. Whereas the adrenal may recover with exogenous ACTH therapy, the suppression of the hypothalamus and pituitary may last for months after stopping glucocorticoid treatment. In addition to the magnitude of the dose of glucocorticoid the circadian timing of the doses may affect the degree of adrenal suppression. Thus prednisolone in a dose of 5 mg given last thing at night and 2.5 mg in the morning may produce marked suppression of the hypothalamic–pituitary–adrenal axis, whereas 2.5 mg at night and 5 mg in the morning may produce a minimal effect. This is because the larger evening dose blocks the early morning surge of ACTH.

A list of some of the causes of secondary hypoadrenalism is given in Table 9. With the exception of glucocorticoid therapy, the other conditions are rare. In many of these, other pituitary hormones are deficient in addition to ACTH, so that the patient presents with partial or complete hypopituitarism. The clinical features of hypopituitarism make this a relatively easy diagnosis to make (see Chapter 12.4). However, if there is isolated ACTH deficiency, this diagnosis may be readily missed. In two of our recent cases of pituitary apoplexy producing isolated ACTH deficiency, one was thought to have an occult malignancy responsible for weight loss, and the other, who had been off work for 2 years, myalgic encephalomyelitis. Both responded dramatically to hydrocortisone replacement therapy.

CLINICAL FEATURES OF ADRENAL INSUFFICIENCY

The most obvious feature which differentiates primary from secondary hypoadrenalism is skin pigmentation, which is nearly always present in primary adrenal insufficiency (unless of short duration) and absent in secondary. The pigmentation is seen in sun-exposed areas, recent rather than old scars, axillae, nipples, palmar creases, pressure points, and in mucus membranes (buccal, vaginal, vulval, anal). In autoimmune Addison's disease there may be associated vitiligo (Fig. 20).

Table 9 *Aetiology of secondary hypoadrenalism (ACTH deficiency)*

Exogenous glucocorticoid therapy
Pituitary pathology
  Selective removal of ACTH-secreting pituitary adenoma
  Radical hypophysectomy for Cushing's disease
  Pituitary surgery for other pituitary tumours
  Pituitary apoplexy
  Large pituitary adenoma
  Granulomatous disease (tuberculosis, sarcoid, eosinophilic
    granuloma)
  Secondary tumour deposits (breast, bronchus)
  Postpartum pituitary infarction (Sheehan's syndrome)
  Pituitary irradiation (effect usually delayed for several years)
  Idiopathic isolated ACTH deficiency
Hypothalamic pathology
  Surgery for hypothalamic lesions (e.g. craniopharyngioma)
    or for pituitary tumours with large suprasellar extension
  Craniopharyngioma
  Head injury
  Cranial irradiation
  Third ventricular tumours or cysts
  Granulomatous disease
  Secondary tumour deposits

The cause of the pigmentation has long been debated. Three molecules derived from pro-opiomelanocortin contain melanocyte stimulating hormone (MSH) sequences, N–terminal pro-opiomelanocortin (γ-MSH), ACTH, (α-MSH), and β-lipotrophin (β-MSH). All three are elevated in Addison's disease, but the relative contribution made by each to the pigmentation is unclear.

Patients with primary adrenal failure usually have both glucocorticoid and mineralocorticoid deficiency. In contrast, those with secondary adrenal insufficiency have an intact renin–angiolensin–aldosterone system. This accounts for differences in salt balance in the two groups of patients, which in turn result in different clinical presentations.

Primary adrenal failure may present with hypotension and acute circulatory failure (addisonian crisis). Anorexia may be an early feature, which progresses to nausea, vomiting, diarrhoea, and, sometimes, abdominal pain. These crises may be precipitated by intercurrent infection or by stress, such as a surgical operation. Alternatively, the patient may present with the rather vague features of chronic adrenal insufficiency—weakness, easy fatiguability, weight loss, nausea, intermittent vomiting, abdominal pain, diarrhoea or constipation, general malaise, muscle cramps and symptoms suggestive of postural hypotension. There

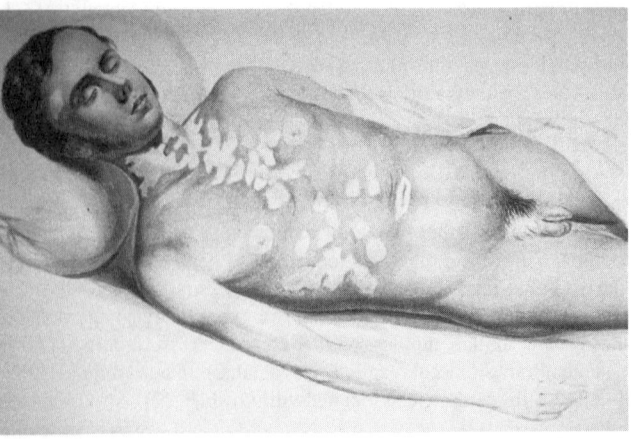

Fig. 20 Vitiligo in one of Thomas Addison's original patients. This was the only one in which he failed to get permission for a postmortem examination (Addison 1855).

may be a low-grade fever. The lying blood pressure is usually normal but almost invariably the pressure falls on standing.

In secondary adrenal insufficiency the presentation may relate to deficiency of hormones other than ACTH. In particular, gonadal failure is common, either because of hyperprolactinaemia or gonadotrophin deficiency. In Sheehan's syndrome there may be prolactin deficiency, with failure of lactation. If there is both ACTH and growth hormone deficiency, patients may present with episodes of hypoglycaemia. Secondary hypothyroidism is usually a late feature in the development of hypopituitarism. If there is isolated ACTH deficiency, the patient may present with malaise, weight loss, and other features of chronic adrenal insufficiency.

LABORATORY INVESTIGATION OF HYPOADRENALISM

Measurement of plasma electrolytes may give the first clue to the diagnosis. In established primary adrenal insufficiency hyonatraemia is present in about 90 per cent of cases and hyperkalaemia in 65 per cent. The blood urea concentration is usually elevated. In secondary adrenal failure there may be a dilutional hyponatraemia with normal or low blood urea. Eosinophilia and an elevated erythrocyte sedimentation rate may be pointers to the diagnosis. Hypoglycaemia has been found in up to 50 per cent of patients with chronic adrenal insufficiency.

Whenever there is clinical suspicion of the diagnosis it is essential to carry out definitive diagnostic tests. Basal plasma cortisol and urinary free cortisol levels are often in the low normal range and cannot be used to exclude the diagnosis. For primary adrenal insufficiency the definitive tests are either the simultaneous measurement of plasma cortisol and plasma ACTH or the measurement of the plasma cortisol response to exogenous ACTH. The typical ACTH levels found in primary and secondary adrenal insufficiency are shown in Fig. 21. The key to the diagnosis of primary adrenal failure is finding that the ACTH level is disproportionately elevated in comparison to the plasma cortisol.

The commonest ACTH stimulation test involves the intramuscular or intravenous administration of 250 μg of tetracosactrin (Synacthen ®). This comprises the first 24 amino acids of normally secreted 1–39 ACTH, the N-terminus being the biologically active end of the molecule. Plasma cortisol levels are measured at 0, 30, and 60 min. In normal

Fig. 21 Morning N-terminal immunoreactive ACTH values in patients with hypoadrenalism. The reference range is indicated by the horizontal lines. (By courtesy of Professor L. H. Rees.)

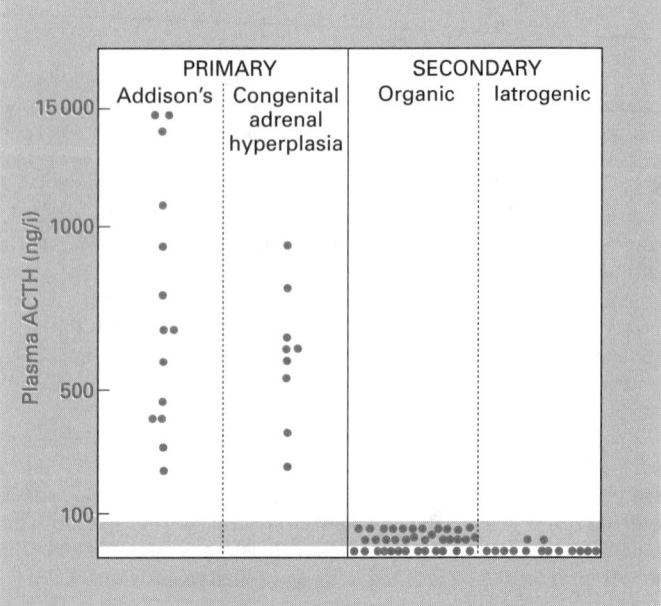

subjects the plasma cortisol at 30 min is at least 550 nmol/l. Several studies indicate that the peak level rather than the increment is the most sensitive in detecting adrenal insufficiency. Levels less than 550 nmol/l in response to the acute administration of Synacthen ® are found in both primary and secondary adrenal insufficiency. These two conditions can be distinguished either by measuring ACTH or by performing a prolonged ACTH stimulation test, usually involving administration of depot tetracosactrin in a dose of 1 mg by intramuscular injection, with measurement of plasma cortisol at 0, 4, and 24 h. In normal subjects the plasma cortisol at 4 h is greater than 1000 nmol/l and the 24-h value shows little further increase. Patients with secondary hypoadrenalism show a delayed response with usually a much higher value at 24 than at 4 h. In primary hypoadrenalism there is no response at either time. With further injections of depot tetracosactrin the difference between primary and secondary becomes even more obvious, with a progressive increase in plasma cortisol in secondary and no response in primary.

Another difference between these two conditions is in the renin–angiotensin–aldosterone axis. In primary hypoadrenalism there is normally mineralocorticoid deficiency with elevated plasma renin activity and either low or low normal plasma aldosterone. It is remarkable how frequently the investigation of zona glomerulosa activity is ignored in Addison's disease as compared to assessment of zona fasciculata function.

The insulin hypoglycaemia test remains one of the most useful in assessing ACTH and growth hormone reserve. It should not be performed in patients with ischaemic heart disease, epilepsy, or severe hypopituitarism (that is 09.00 h plasma cortisol less than 180 nmol/l). The usual test involves the intravenous administration of soluble insulin in a dose of 0.15 U/kg body weight, with measurement of plasma cortisol at 0, 30, 45, 60, 90, and 120 min. Adequate hypoglycaemia (blood glucose less than 2.2 mmol/l with signs of neuroglycopenia—sweating and tachycardia) is essential. In normal subjects the peak plasma cortisol exceeds 550 nmol/l. The use of this test has gone down markedly since the recognition that the response to hypoglycaemia can be reliably predicted (except in patients within 2 weeks of becoming ACTH deficient) by the response to acute ACTH stimulation; a safer, cheaper, and quicker test. If the ACTH test is normal, insulin hypoglycaemia testing is not necessary. Insulin is only required if, in a patient with suspected hypopituitarism, there is a subnormal response to ACTH or a need to assess growth hormone secretion. Some patients have an inadequate response to ACTH but then respond normally to hypoglycaemia. They do not require corticosteroid replacement therapy.

If the tests confirm primary hypoadrenalism, it is essential to determine its cause. Adrenal antibodies were originally detected using a complement fixation test with homogenates of human adrenals. More sensitive tests such as radio-immunoassay to detect the antibodies against the 21-hydroxylase antigen are now available. Other antibodies, such as those blocking either ACTH-induced adrenal DNA synthesis and/or cortisol secretion, are more difficult to detect. In autoimmune Addison's disease it is also important to look for evidence of other organ-specific autoimmune disease.

In long-standing tuberculous adrenal disease there may be adrenal atrophy with calcification (Fig. 19). This is most readily detected by CT scanning. At an earlier stage the adrenal glands may be enlarged and tuberculosis will then need to be distinguished from haemorrhage or neoplasm. CT and magnetic resonance imaging appear to be equally good in diagnosing adrenal haemorrhage, but CT may be better for differentiating acute inflammatory from metastatic disease. CT scanning with needle biopsy may be of particular value in some cases.

TREATMENT OF ACUTE ADRENAL INSUFFICIENCY

This is an emergency, and treatment should not be delayed while waiting for definitive proof of diagnosis. However, in addition to measurement of plasma electrolytes and blood glucose, appropriate samples for ACTH and cortisol should be taken before giving corticosteroid therapy. If the patient is not critically ill, an acute ACTH stimulation test can be performed. However, if necessary, this can be delayed and carried out with the patient on corticosteroid therapy, provided the drug used does not interfere with the plasma cortisol assay (for example, change from hydrocortisone to dexamethasone).

Intravenous hydrocortisone, 100 mg, as the hemisuccinate or sodium phosphate form should be given intravenously 6 hourly. If this is not possible, then the intramuscular route should be used. In the shocked patient 1 litre of normal saline should be given intravenously over the first hour. Because of possible hypoglycaemia, it is normal to give 5 per cent dextrose saline. The subsequent saline and dextrose therapy will depend on biochemical monitoring and the patient's condition. Clinical improvement, especially in the blood pressure, should be seen within 4 to 6 h if the diagnosis is correct. It is important to recognize and treat any associated condition, such as an infection, which may have precipitated the acute adrenal crisis.

After the first 24 h the dose of hydrocortisone can be reduced, usually to 50 mg intramuscularly 6 hourly for the second 24 h and then, if the patient can take by mouth, to oral hydrocortisone, 40 mg in the morning and 20 mg at 18.00 hours. This can then be rapidly reduced to the normal replacement dose of 20 mg on waking and 10 mg at 18.00 hours.

With high-dose hydrocortisone therapy it is not necessary to give additional mineralocorticoid replacement. However, when the hydrocortisone dose is reduced it may be necessary in primary adrenal failure to add this in the form of fludrocortisone acetate (hydrocortisone acetate which is fluorinated in the 9α position). The mineralocorticoid activity of this is about 125 times that of hydrocortisone. The usual replacement dose is 0.05 to 0.1 mg daily (see below).

REPLACEMENT CORTICOSTEROID THERAPY

Patients with primary adrenal failure may require both glucocorticoid and mineralocorticoid replacement therapy, in contrast to those with secondary adrenal insufficiency who require glucocorticoid alone.

The usual daily dose of glucocorticoid is hydrocortisone 30 mg per day, traditionally given as 20 mg on waking and 10 mg at 18.00 hours. Some patients require more than this and others less. Unfortunately, there are few good objective tests of the adequacy of glucocorticoid replacement in secondary adrenal failure. With Addison's disease which is inadequately treated pigmentation may persist and ACTH levels remain elevated. There is little point in giving cortisone acetate as this has to be converted by the liver to cortisol. If it has to be given, 25 mg of cortisone acetate is equivalent to 20 mg hydrocortisone.

Patients on glucocorticoid replacement therapy should be advised to double the dose in the event of intercurrent febrile illness, accident, or mental stress such as an important examination. If the patient is vomiting and cannot take by mouth, parenteral hydrocortisone must be given urgently, as indicated above. For minor surgery, 100 mg hydrocortisone hemisuccinate is given with the premedication. For major operations this is then followed by the same regimen as for acute adrenal insufficiency but without the saline replacement. If a patient on replacement therapy is given enzyme inducing drugs such as rifampicin or phenytoin, the replacement dose of hydrocortisone will need to be increased. The same is also true in pregnancy as the oestrogen-induced rise in cortisol-binding globulin will decrease the free cortisol.

The patient on glucocorticoid therapy should be advised to register for a MedicAlert bracelet or necklace and should carry a 'Steroid card'.

Mineralocorticoid replacement is not always necessary in Addison's disease and some patients are well on hydrocortisone alone with normal plasma electrolytes. However, in such patients plasma renin activity is usually high, indicating that they are mineralocorticoid deficient. Aldosterone cannot be given by mouth and, when deficient, is replaced with fludrocortisone, as indicated above. The adequacy of this replacement can be monitored by measuring blood pressure, plasma electrolytes, and plasma renin activity. Hypertension, hypokalaemia, and suppressed plasma renin activity indicate excess fludrocortisone. Postural hypotension, hyperkalaemia, and elevated plasma renin activity usually suggest mineralocorticoid deficiency, but occasionally may be due to inadequate salt intake. In patients with active tuberculous Addison's disease antituberculous therapy will be required. It is also important to remember that excess glucocorticoid therapy may result in the activation of latent tuberculosis.

Mineralocorticoid excess

The syndromes associated with mineralocorticoid excess can be classified on the basis of whether this is due to aldosterone (primary or secondary aldosteronism), mineralocorticoids other than aldosterone, or abnormal renal tubular function (Table 10).

Conn's syndrome—aldosterone-producing adenoma

Since Conn's original description of a patient with hypertension, neuromuscular symptoms, and hypokalaemia associated with an aldosterone-producing adrenal adenoma, it has been recognized that the same clinical and biochemical picture may be produced by other conditions in which there is aldosterone excess without adenoma. Measurement of plasma renin activity is the key to distinguishing primary aldosteronism (in which plasma renin activity is low or undetectable) from secondary, in which it is usually elevated. The exception to this is in patients with idiopathic hyperplasia of the zona glomerulosa, in which there is marked enhancement of the adrenal responsiveness to angiotensin II. Thus although this appears to be a form of primary aldosteronism with elevated aldosterone and low plasma renin activity, it is actually a type of secondary aldosteronism. The reason for the enhanced responsiveness to angiotensin II is unknown. The possibilities include ineffective dopamine inhibition of aldosterone secretion, elevated levels of a putative aldosterone-stimulating factor derived from the ACTH precursor molecule pro-opiomelanocortin or of the N-terminus of the proopiomelanocortin molecule which enhances the adrenal response to ACTH, or an abnormality of the recently described intra-adrenal renin–angiotensin system. Another aldosterone–stimulating factor has been isolated from the the urine of these patients. This is a glycoprotein with a molecular weight of 26 kDa. However, after many years of work it has yet to be further identified and nothing is known about its precise source or its control.

With the exception of glucocorticoid-suppressible hyperaldosteronism (see below), the molecular basis of the primary aldosterone excess syndromes is unknown. In about 60 per cent of patients with primary aldosteronism an adenoma is found. In most of these the tumour responds to ACTH but not to angiotensin II, and there is therefore a circadian rhythm of aldosterone similar to that of cortisol. However, an increasing number of adenomas are now being described which are responsive to angiotensin II. This is an important subgroup, as the tests may lead to an erroneous diagnosis of idiopathic hyperplasia. Aldosterone-producing adrenal carcinomas are rare (3–5 per cent of aldosterone-producing adrenal tumours).

A recently described entity is the condition of primary adrenal hyperplasia which has to be distinguished from other causes of adrenal hyperplasia. Primary adrenal hyperplasia may be either unilateral or bilateral.

Glucocorticoid-suppressible hyperaldosteronism

This syndrome has an autosomal dominant mode of inheritance and most commonly presents with the discovery of hypertension in asymptomatic young individuals. Hypokalaemia may be a clue to the diagnosis, but it is now clear that many patients with this syndrome are persistently normokalaemic despite marked aldosterone excess with suppression of the renin–angiotensin system. Gordon and colleagues have described another form of familial hyperaldosteronism which they have called familial hyperaldosteronism type II to distinguish it from

Table 10 *Mineralocorticoid excess syndromes*

Aldosterone
 Primary hyperaldosteronism
  Conn's syndrome—aldosterone-producing adrenal adenoma (APA)
  Angiotensin II-responsive APA
  Primary adrenal hyperplasia
  Aldosterone-producing adrenal carcinoma
  Glucocorticoid-suppressible hyperaldosteronism
 Secondary hyperaldosteronism

Mineralocorticoids other than aldosterone
 17α-hydroxylase deficiency
 11β-hydroxylase deficiency
 Deoxycorticosterone
 Corticosterone
 Congenital apparent mineralocorticoid excess syndromes
 Acquired apparent mineralocorticoid excess syndromes
 Ectopic ACTH syndrome
 Glucocorticoid resistance
 Exogenous mineralocorticoids

Abnormal renal tubular ionic transport (pseudoaldosteronism)
 Liddle's syndrome

the glucocorticoid-suppressible type (familial hyperaldosteronism type I). Type II familial hyperaldosteronism is not glucocorticoid suppressible and may, in some patients, be due to an adenoma.

In glucocorticoid-suppressible hyperaldosteronism (or familial hyperaldosteronism type I), as its name suggests, aldosterone secretion is under ACTH control and the condition can be treated by glucocorticoid replacement therapy. The disease results from the ectopic expression of aldosterone synthase, an enzyme normally only found in the zona glomerulosa. The genes that code for aldosterone synthase (expression limited to the zona glomerulosa) and 11β-hydroxylase (which is expressed in both the zona glomerulosa and the zona fasciculata) are 95 per cent homologous and both lie on chromosome 8. During normal meiosis homologous chromosomes pair to form bivalents, starting at the tip of the chromosome and moving towards the centromere, a process called synapsis. It is during this stage that there is a crossing-over between the chromatids of the homologous chromosomes which results in the exchange of genetic information. In glucocorticoid-suppressible hyperaldosteronism, instead of aldosterone synthase on the two homologous chromosomes aligning, aldosterone synthase on one chromatid has

Fig. 22 Chimeric gene responsible for glucocorticoid-remediable hyperaldosteronism. For details see text.

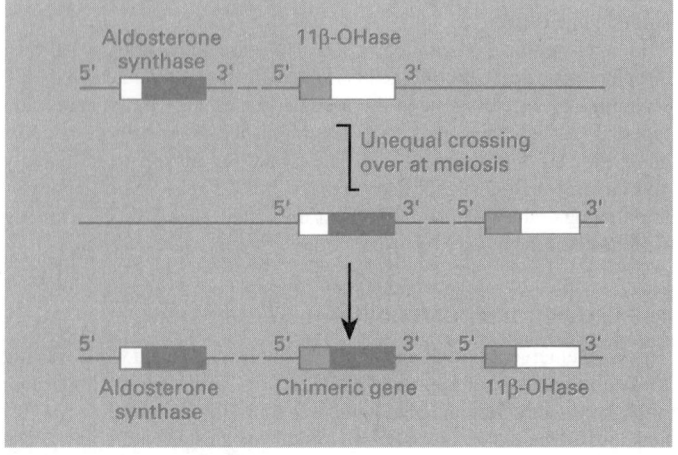

Table 11 *Drugs and the renin–angiotensin–aldosterone Axis*

Drug	Effect	Action
Spironolactone	↑ PRA especially in idiopathic hyperplasia	Stop 6 weeks before tests
Oestrogens	↑ Plasma renin substrate	Stop 6 weeks before tests
ACE inhibitors	↑ PRA ↓ aldosterone in idiopathic hyperplasia and secondary aldosteronism	Stop 2 weeks before tests
Diuretics other than spironolactone	↑ PRA	Stop 2 weeks before tests
Non-steroidal anti-inflammatory drugs	Retain sodium ↓ PRA	Stop 2 weeks before tests
β-Adrenoceptor-blocking drugs	↓ PRA	Stop 2 weeks before tests
Calcium-channel-blocking agents	↓ Aldosterone	Stop 2 weeks before tests

ACE, angiotensin-converting enzyme; PRA, plasma renin activity.

aligned with 11β-hydroxylase on the other. This has then resulted in an unequal crossing-over, with the formation of a chimeric gene which has the regulatory region of 11β-hydroxylase (therefore it is under ACTH control) with the coding sequence for aldosterone synthase (Fig. 22).

PRESENTING FEATURES

The majority of patients with primary aldosteronism are asymptomatic and the condition is only suspected when they are found to be hypokalaemic. A minority of patients will have symptoms related to hypokalaemia such as muscle weakness, polyuria and polydipsia secondary to nephrogenic diabetes insipidus, paraesthesiae, and occasionally tetany due to the decrease in ionized calcium associated with the hypokalaemic alkalosis. In Chinese patients hypokalaemic periodic paralysis is not uncommon (42 per cent in one series of Chinese patients with aldosterone-producing adenoma). The hypokalaemia may be exacerbated or precipitated by diuretic therapy, usually thiazides. However, even if the plasma potassium returns to normal after stopping such drugs, it does not mean that the diagnosis of primary aldosteronism can be excluded. In our own series of patients, identified on screening a hypertension clinic, 62 per cent of those with primary aldosteronism became normokalaemic when their thiazide diuretic therapy was stopped. Another reason for normalization of plasma potassium in a patient with Conn's syndrome can be a reduction in salt intake. This results in less sodium being available for sodium–potassium exchange in the distal nephron and hence an elevation in plasma potassium concentrations. Many hypertensive patients are on low salt diets. In the second edition of this textbook it was stated that in unselected populations normokalaemic primary aldosteronism was probably sufficiently rare to be ignored for practical purposes. This is no longer thought to be true. Recent studies in which unselected hypertensive patients have been screened using aldosterone/renin profiling have shown that 60 to 70 per cent of patients with primary aldosteronism are normokalaemic. Not surprisingly, these results have indicated that the prevalence of primary aldosteronism is much higher than previously estimated. Some centres are now suggesting that up to 10 per cent of unselected patients with hypertension may have primary aldosteronism.

DIAGNOSIS

The finding of hypokalaemic alkalosis in an hypertensive patient may first suggest the diagnosis. Confirmation then comes from the demonstration that the patient has increased aldosterone secretion (usually not measured directly but inferred from elevated plasma or urinary aldosterone) together with low or suppressed plasma renin activity. Various factors, including antihypertensive drug therapy and hypokalaemia, may affect the renin–angiotensin–aldosterone axis and make the diagnosis more difficult. If plasma potassium is less than 3 mmol/l, potassium supplementation should be given before measuring aldosterone. Some antihypertensive drugs have long-term effects on the renin–angiotensin axis and thus should be stopped several weeks before testing (Table 11).

Others have much shorter effects and some none at all. The latter group may be useful in controlling blood pressure prior to investigation (for example, bethanidine 10 mg three times daily).

If plasma aldosterone is being used as a marker of aldosterone secretion, it is normal to measure the level at a fixed time of day and with the patient in a fixed posture (for example, 08.00 hours with the patient having been lying down for 30 min). In this way the result can be compared to a known reference range. Alternatively, 24-h urinary aldosterone excretion can be measured. What is actually measured is the amount of aldosterone produced by the hydrolysis at pH 1 of the acid-labile metabolite aldosterone 18-glucuronide. The renin–angiotensin system is assessed by measuring plasma renin activity. As with aldosterone this is affected by posture and sodium intake. Thus plasma renin activity samples should be taken under the same controlled conditions as aldosterone. As it is expensive and time-consuming to control sodium intake, it is normal to infer this from measurement of 24-h urinary sodium excretion.

Because of the problems in controlling posture, sodium intake, and drug therapy several groups have now advocated the use of the aldosterone–renin ratio. Thus in patients with aldosterone-producing adenomas the ratio (plasma aldosterone pg/ml → plasma renin activity ng/ml/h) is above 400, whereas in essential hypertensive patients it is less than 200. Secondary hyperaldosteronism is characterized by elevated plasma aldosterone with a normal ratio. The only false negatives so far identified have been in patients with chronic renal failure.

Various dynamic tests have been used to further investigate aldosterone secretion in suspected primary aldosteronism. These have usually involved some form of salt loading (increased salt intake, saline infusion, exogenous mineralocorticoid administration, or a combination). The rationale behind these tests is that in normal subjects plasma volume expansion with saline will suppress plasma aldosterone concentrations, whereas in primary aldosteronism further volume expansion does not have the same suppressive effect. This is true in aldosterone-producing adenoma, but patients with idiopathic hyperplasia may show suppression. In uncomplicated patients these tests are not essential for making the diagnosis and there are better ways of making the differential diagnosis.

DIFFERENTIAL DIAGNOSIS

It is clearly important to distinguish between the various causes of primary aldosteronism (Table 10). Various tests are used to do this (Table 12). The rationale for the test involving posture and time is that in normal subjects plasma aldosterone rises with standing so that if aldosterone levels are measured lying at 08.00 hours and the patient is then up and around for the next 4 h, the 12.00 hours level will be about twice that of the 08.00 h one. In patients with aldosterone-producing adenoma or glucocorticoid-suppressible hyperaldosteronism, aldosterone is under ACTH control. Hence aldosterone levels fall during the course of the morning. In idiopathic hyperaldosteronism the enhanced adrenal responsiveness to angiotensin II results in a rise in aldosterone concentrations

Table 12 *Tests used in the differential diagnosis of primary aldosteronism*

Test	Normal subjects		Common aldosterone-producing adenoma		Rare angiotensin-responsive adenoma		Idiopathic adrenal hyperplasia		Primary adrenal hyperplasia		Dexamethasone-suppressible hyperaldosteronism	
	PRA	ALDO	PRA	ALDO	PRA	ALDO	PRA	ALDO	PRA	ALDO	PRA	ALDO
Dynamic tests of the renin–angiotensin–aldosterone axis												
Salt loading	↓	↓	↓	↑	↓	↑	↓	↑	↓	↑	↓	→
Effect of upright posture and time	↑	↑	→	↓	↓↑	↑	↓↑	↑	↓	↓	→	↑
Angiotensin-converting-enzyme inhibitor	↑	↓	↓	→	↓	↓	↓	↓	↓	→	↓	↑
Angiotensin II infusion	↓	↑	↓	↑	↓	↑	↓↑	↑	↓	↑	↓	→
Dexamethasone suppression	→	→	→	↑	→	↑	↑	↑	↑	↑	↑	↓

Plasma or urinary 18-hydroxycortisol (for details see text)

CT or MRI imaging of adrenals (for details see text)

Adrenal vein catheterization (for details see text)

Adrenal scintigraphy (for details see text)

PRA, plasma renin activity; ALDO, plasma aldosterone; ↓, decrease; →, unchanged; ↑, increase.

in response to erect posture. The levels will also rise in patients with angiotensin II responsive adenomata. It is important to measure plasma cortisol levels in addition to aldosterone. If the patient is stressed during the course of the morning and the plasma cortisol rises rather than falls, the test should be repeated.

In patients with glucocorticoid-suppressible hyperaldosteronism the administration of dexamethasone results in suppression of plasma aldosterone and a gradual return of plasma renin activity to normal. An upright plasma aldosterone level below 140 pmol/l (5 ng/dl) after overnight dexamethasone administration (1 mg at midnight and 0.5 mg at 06.00 hours) is used as a cut-off point to separate patients with glucocorticoid-suppressible hyperaldosteronism from those with aldosterone-producing adenoma and idiopathic hyperaldosteronism. Longer-term dexamethasone therapy of those with glucocorticoid-suppressible hyperaldosteronism (2 mg per day for 3 weeks) will return levels of plasma potassium and aldosterone to normal and lower blood pressure. With the discovery of the genetic defect, it is now possible to detect this specifically by Southern blotting. This is particularly valuable in studies on relatives of patients with glucocorticoid-suppressible hyperaldosteronism as the blood pressure and the plasma potassium in affected subjects may be normal.

Measurement of plasma or urinary 18-hydroxycortisol is of great value in making the differential diagnosis. This steroid is the most abundant free steroid in the urine of patients with primary aldosteronism due either to adenoma or glucocorticoid-suppressible hyperaldosteronism, in which cases the levels are significantly higher than in idiopathic hyperaldosteronism with glucocorticoid-suppressible hyperaldosteronism patients usually having higher levels than those with aldosterone-producing adenoma. (Fig. 23).

Angiotensin-converting-enzyme inhibition by blocking the production of angiotensin II will lower plasma aldosterone acutely, especially in sodium-depleted normal subjects. In aldosterone-producing adenoma and glucocorticoid-suppressible hyperaldosteronism this does not occur, but it does in the case of patients with idiopathic hyperaldosteronism. The usual test involves measuring plasma aldosterone before and 2 h after giving 25 mg captopril orally. It is important to realize that in both aldosterone-producing adenoma and glucocorticoid-suppressible hyperaldosteronism plasma aldosterone levels will fall in response to the diurnal fall in ACTH if, as is usual, the test is done in the morning; but in such patients the level usually remains above 400 pmol/l. Another problem in interpreting this test is in the case of the relatively recently recognized condition of angiotensin II responsive adenoma. These patients will respond in similar way to those with idiopathic hyperaldosteronism, despite the presence of an adenoma.

Adrenal vein catheterization is technically difficult, especially with regard to the right adrenal vein. However, it still remains the gold standard for determining whether there is unilateral or bilateral aldosterone production, and for identifying the site of it. On the side of an adenoma the adrenal venous blood contains much higher levels of aldosterone than on the contralateral side where the zona glomerulosa is suppressed (and thus the aldosterone level is the same as the periphery). Some authors suggest that this test should only be done when there is doubt about the differential diagnosis on biochemical testing, or when CT or MRI scanning is equivocal. Others suggest that it should be done in all cases, especially if surgery is being considered.

Adrenal scintigraphy with either ^{131}I-labelled ([6β-^{131}I]iodomethyl-19-norcholesterol) or ^{75}Se-6-selenomethylcholesterol can be of value in distinguishing an adenoma with mainly unilateral uptake from the var-

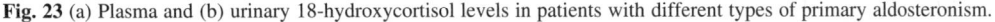

Fig. 23 (a) Plasma and (b) urinary 18-hydroxycortisol levels in patients with different types of primary aldosteronism.

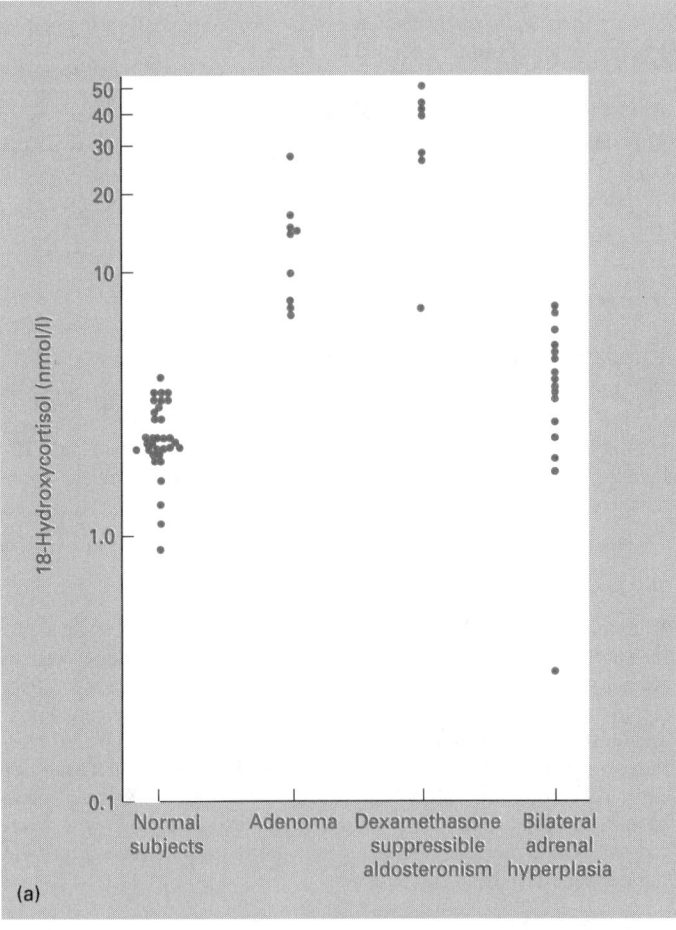

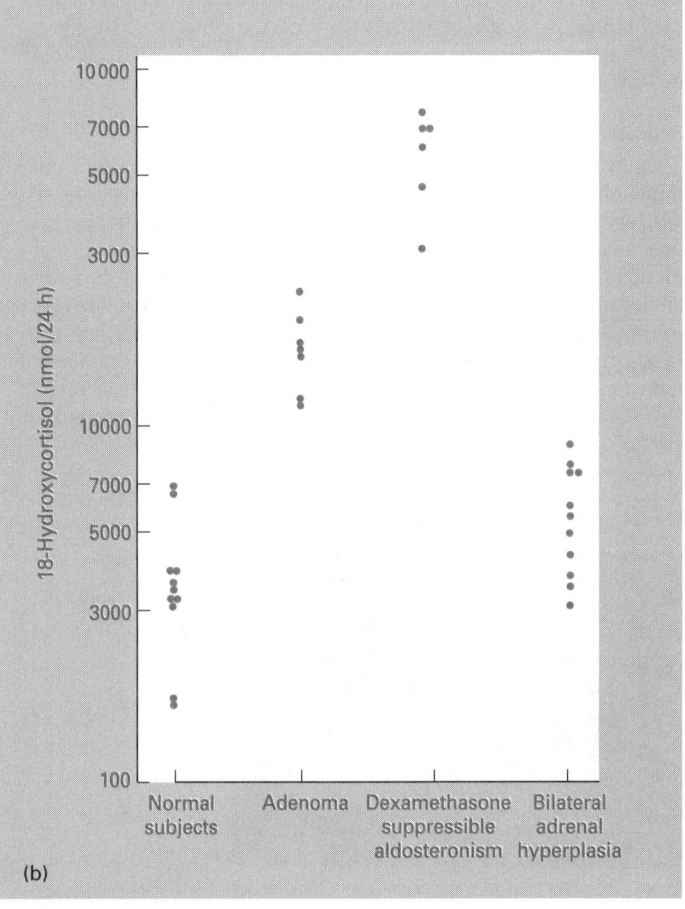

ious forms of hyperplasia with bilateral, usually symmetrical uptake. Drugs such as spironolactone must be stopped for 6 weeks before scanning. Dexamethasone treatment may improve the accuracy of diagnosis. It is important to look at the pattern of isotope uptake rather than at one single time point. In one series nearly half the patients with an adenoma had bilateral uptake and a quarter of those with hyperplasia markedly asymmetrical uptake. When dexamethasone has been given to suppress ACTH, early unilateral uptake (less than 5 days) suggests adenoma and early bilateral uptake, hyperplasia. It has been calculated that the accuracy of scintigraphy is about 72 per cent, CT scanning, 73 per cent, and adrenal vein catheterization where both veins are cannulated, 95 per cent.

CT and MRI imaging of the adrenals is of considerable value for many, but not all, tumours. Early CT scanners had relatively poor resolution and missed many small aldosterone-producing adenomata. However, even with modern CT, which can accurately diagnose tumours down to 7 mm in diameter, the sensitivity is still only about 60 per cent in some centres. There have been few comparisons of CT with MRI. In one, the sensitivity of CT for diagnosing adenomata was 82 per cent and that of MRI was 100 per cent.

Aldosterone-producing adrenal carcinoma

This may be suspected clinically as the tumours may produce cortisol or androgens in addition to aldosterone. Further clues would be a CT scan which shows either a tumour greater than 4 cm in diameter or with calcification.

TREATMENT

Glucocorticoid-suppressible hyperaldosteronism

Initial therapy is with dexamethasone in the lowest dose possible necessary to suppress ACTH (start with 0.5 or 0.75 mg on going to bed and 0.25 mg on waking). The plasma aldosterone, cortisol, plasma renin activity, electrolytes, and blood pressure can be used to assess the efficacy of therapy. It is not unusual to find that the initial effective control of blood pressure is lost, so that additional therapy with spironolactone or amiloride is required.

Aldosterone-producing adenoma

Therapy will depend on a variety of factors, such as the medical condition of the patient and drug side-effects (for example, gynaecomastia with spironolactone). In a patient fit for surgery it is usual to give preoperative treatment with spironolactone to lower blood pressure, return plasma potassium levels to normal, and to allow recovery of the renin–angiotensin system. This will stimulate the atrophic zona glomerulosa in the contralateral gland and thus avoid aldosterone deficiency with hyperkalaemia after removal of the adenoma. The dose of spironolactone required preoperatively may be up to 400 mg/day. This therapy is also useful in predicting the outcome of surgery. Thus in a group of

Fig. 24 Typical Conn's adenoma.

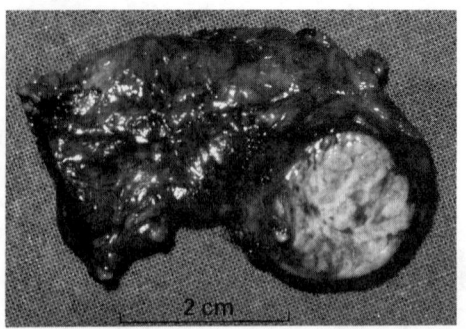

patients given spironolactone (100 mg daily for 10 days prior to operation), those who became normotensive after surgery had had a fall in mean blood pressure of greater than 15 mmHg, in contrast to those who remained hypertensive postoperatively, who had a lesser response to spironolactone. Overall, about 60 per cent of patients with adenomatous disease become normotensive within a month of surgery, and 75 per cent within a year.

Surgery for a Conn's adenoma is usually carried out via a loin incision, which has a much lower morbidity than an anterior abdominal approach. The typical Conn's adenoma is canary yellow (Fig. 24). Comparison of surgery with long term spironolactone for aldosterone-producing adenomata suggests that surgery is more effective in lowering blood pressure to normal. If medical treatment is required long term, spironolactone remains the drug of choice. After initial high-dose therapy it is often possible to reduce this to a maintenance dose of 25 to 50 mg/day. However, even with this dose patients may get unacceptable side-effects. These include impotence, gynaecomastia, and menorrhagia. Such patients should then be given amiloride in a dose of up to 40 mg daily as an alternative.

Angiotensin II responsive adenomas should be treated in the same way, but may also respond to angiotensin-converting-enzyme therapy.

Idiopathic hyperaldosteronism and primary adrenal hyperplasia

Surgery is contraindicated in patients with idiopathic hypoaldosteronism as even bilateral adrenalectomy is not curative. It would seem likely that the small minority who have responded to surgery have had primary adrenal hyperplasia. The usual therapy for idiopathic hyperaldosteronism is to start with spironolactone or amiloride. These drugs will correct the hypokalaemia but not usually the hypertension. The latter will often respond to the addition of an angiotensin-converting-enzyme inhibitor or a calcium-channel-blocking drug. Spironolactone is more often effective in lowering blood pressure in primary adrenal hyperplasia than in idiopathic hyperaldosteronism. Unilateral, subtotal, or bilateral adrenalectomy (depending on the anatomy of the disease) may be also curative in some cases of primary adrenal hyperplasia.

Aldosterone-producing adrenal carcinoma

This has a poor outlook regardless of therapy (5 year survival 25 per cent). Treatment is with unilateral adrenalectomy usually together with the adrenolytic drug *o,p'*-DDD (see above).

Mineralocorticoids other than aldosterone

Congenital adrenal hyperplasia

The two forms of congenital adrenal hyperplasia associated with hypertension and mineralocorticoid excess other than aldosterone are 17α-hydroxylase (deoxycorticosterone and corticosterone excess) and 11β-hydroxylase (elevated deoxycorticosterone secretion) deficiency (see Chapter 12.7.2).

Deoxycorticosterone and corticosterone

With the exception of congenital adrenal hyperplasia only a few patients have been described who have isolated production of deoxycorticosterone or corticosterone. Rarely, adenomas may produce deoxycorticosterone alone and aldosterone secretion is suppressed. More commonly, an aldosterone-producing adrenal adenoma will also produce deoxycorticosterone in excess. Occasional patients will have elevated levels of deoxycorticosterone with normal levels of aldosterone. Some of these have been found to have aldosterone-producing adenomata with intermittent aldosterone secretion. Most pure corticosterone-producing adrenal tumours have been carcinomata.

Congenital apparent mineralocorticoid excess syndrome

This is a rare condition in which there is hypertension, hypokalaemia, suppression of the renin–angiotensin–aldosterone axis, and deficiency of the enzyme 11β-hydroxysteroid dehydrogenase. This is the enzyme that interconverts the active steroid cortisol and inactive cortisone. The liver isoform of the enzyme converts cortisone to cortisol and the renal isoform converts cortisol to cortisone. It has now become clear that the kidney enzyme protects the non-specific mineralocorticoid receptors in the distal nephron from local effects of cortisol. This receptor has an equal affinity for cortisol and aldosterone, and given the 100-fold excess of circulating cortisol over aldosterone it would be expected that the receptor would be largely occupied by cortisol. Under normal circumstances this does not happen as 11β-hydroxysteroid dehydrogenase in the distal nephron cells prevents cortisol from reaching the receptor. If, however, the enzyme is either congenitally deficient or inhibited, cortisol reaches the receptor and produces gross mineralocorticoid excess (Fig. 25). Not surprisingly in those detected to have congenital deficiency all except one have been children and the severity of the hypertension has been associated with a high morbidity and mortality. The condition is diagnosed by the clinical and biochemical picture, with suppression of plasma renin activity and plasma aldosterone together with an elevated ratio of urinary cortisol to cortisone metabolites. In normal subjects the ratio of tetrahydrocortisol + allo-tetrahydrocortisol to tetrahydrocortisone is about 1, whereas in congenital 11β-hydroxysteroid dehydrogenase deficiency it is greater than 10. Even though spironolactone may improve the plasma electrolyte changes, it rarely controls the hypertension. Low-dose dexamethasone may be of major benefit. This drug has a much higher affinity for the glucocorticoid than for the mineralocorticoid receptor. Thus by lowering plasma cortisol it

Fig. 25 (a) The role of 11β-hydroxysteroid dehydrogenase (11β-OHSD) in protecting the non-specific type I mineralocorticoid receptor and (b) the effect of congenital or acquired deficiency of the enzyme. E = cortisone, F = cortisol.

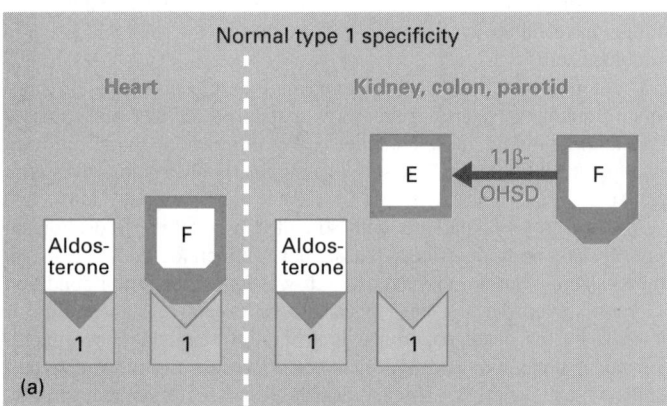

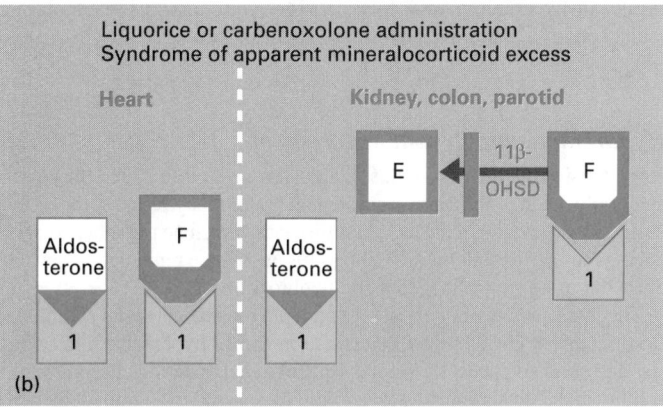

removes the major agonist for the mineralocorticoid receptor, with consequent benefit to the mineralocorticoid excess syndrome. It is usually necessary to add further drugs, such as an angiotensin-converting-enzyme inhibitor with a diuretic to achieve full control of blood pressure. The molecular basis of the syndrome is as yet unknown. Some familial cases have been described.

Acquired apparent mineralocorticoid excess syndromes

The same clinical and biochemical picture, with hypertension, hypokalaemia, and suppression of plasma renin activity and aldosterone can be found in patients who take excess liquorice or related drugs such as carbenoxolone (the hemisuccinate derivative of the active component of liquorice, glycyrrhetinic acid). These agents have now been found to be potent inhibitors of 11β-hydroxysteroid dehydrogenase and thus block the renal conversion of cortisol to cortisone. Investigation of liquorice addicts shows that the urinary ratio of cortisol to cortisone metabolites is abnormal but less so than in the congenital syndrome. With carbenoxolone there are some subtle differences. The hypokalaemia is not due to urinary loss of potassium but to a shift of potassium into cells. The drug is a potent inhibitor of the renal isoform of 11β-hydroxysteroid dehydrogenase but also blocks the hepatic conversion of cortisone to cortisol. Thus the ratio of liver metabolites of cortisol to cortisone in the urine is normal but the urinary cortisol : cortisone ratio is high. Treatment is to stop the excessive ingestion of liquorice or carbenoxolone. As with the apparent mineralocorticoid excess syndrome, dexamethasone will produce a natriuresis even if the patient continues to take the enzyme inhibitor.

Ectopic ACTH syndrome

As indicated in the section on Cushing's syndrome, patients with the ectopic ACTH syndrome are almost invariably hypokalaemic. This was once thought to be due to the excess secretion of deoxycorticosterone and/or of cortisol in this form of Cushing's as compared to others. Recent evidence has shown that there is impairment of the conversion of cortisol to cortisone, as shown either by the ratio of urinary cortisol to cortisone metabolites or of plasma cortisol to cortisone. ACTH itself does not appear to inhibit 11β-hydroxysteroid dehydrogenase and the most likely inhibitor is an ACTH-responsive steroid other than cortisol, with a high affinity for the enzyme.

Glucocorticoid resistance

A small number of patients have been described who have increased cortisol secretion but with none of the stigmata of Cushing's syndrome. These patients are resistant to suppression of cortisol with low-dose dexamethasone but respond to high doses. ACTH levels are elevated and lead to increased adrenal production of androgens and deoxycorticosterone. Thus the patients may present with the features of androgen and/or mineralocorticoid excess. Treatment with a dose of dexamethasone adequate to suppress ACTH (usually 3 mg/day) results in a fall in adrenal androgens and often return of plasma potassium and blood pressure to normal levels. Some of these patients have been found to have point mutations in the steroid-binding domain of the glucocorticoid receptor, with consequent reduction of glucocorticoid-binding affinity.

Exogenous mineralocorticoids

The administration of large doses of hydrocortisone, fludrocortisone, deoxycorticosterone (often as the acetate), or 9α-fluoroprednisolone will produce hypertension and hypokalaemia with suppression of the renin–angiotensin–aldosterone axis. With the exception of patients with asthma given prolonged high-dose hydrocortisone or patients with Addison's disease on inappropriately high mineralocorticoid replacement therapy, it is unusual to see this in clinical practice. However, several patients, especially children, have been described with severe mineralocorticoid excess resulting from 9α-fluoroprednisolone, prescribed as a spray for chronic rhinitis or as topical therapy for eczema.

Abnormal renal tubular ionic transport (Liddle's syndrome)

Liddle described a familial syndrome which simulated primary aldosteronism but in which aldosterone was suppressed. Spironolactone therapy was ineffective but an inhibitor of renal tubular ionic transport (triamterene) resulted in a natriuresis with potassium retention and return of the blood pressure to normal. An alternative drug is amiloride. Liddle suggested that there was an abnormal facility of the renal tubules to transport ions, resulting in sodium retention and potassium loss. It has recently been discovered that patients with this syndrome have a mutation of the β-subunit of the highly selective type I epithelial sodium channel. It would seem likely that some of the cases that have been thought to have been Liddle's syndrome have been due to 11β-hydroxysteroid dehydrogenase deficiency with apparent mineralocorticoid excess. This latter condition can be readily distinguished by the urinary cortisol : cortisone metabolite ratio and by its electrolyte response to high-dose spironolactone.

Mineralocorticoid deficiency

These syndromes are listed in Table 13. They can be divided into those that are congenital and others that are acquired.

Adrenal hypoplasia

This is an X-linked condition which presents in infancy with a severe salt-losing state. The external genitalia are normal and plasma and urinary steroid levels readily distinguish this from salt-losing causes of congenital adrenal hyperplasia. CT scanning confirms the hypoplastic adrenals.

Congenital adrenal hyperplasia

The various causes of congenital adrenal hyperplasia that are associated with mineralocorticoid deficiency are detailed elsewhere (see Chapter 12.7.2).

Disorders of the terminal part of the aldosterone biosynthetic pathway

Failure of conversion of corticosterone to 18-hydroxycorticosterone or of 18-hydroxycorticosterone to aldosterone results in salt-wasting (Fig.1.) The enzymes responsible for these steps have had various names (corticosterone to 18-hydroxycorticosterone catalysed by 18-hydroxylase, corticosterone methyl oxidase type I) and 18-hydroxycorticosterone to aldosterone by 18-dehydrogenase, 18-oxidase, (corticosterone methyl oxidase type II, aldosterone synthase). It was originally thought that 11β-hydroxylase and corticosterone methyl oxidase type II were the same enzyme. However, molecular studies have shown that these two enzymes have 88 per cent homology in the DNA coding region but only 52 per cent homology in the 5′ flanking region, in keeping with their very different transcriptional control mechanisms. What has become apparent from transfecting cells with cDNA sequences is that the 11β-hydroxylase gene (CYP11B1) encodes for a cytochrome P450 enzyme $P_{450}X1B1$, which only catalyses 11β-hydroxylation and converts deoxycorticosterone to corticosterone and 11-deoxycortisol to cortisol (Fig.1). In contrast, the gene CYP11B2 encodes for the isoform $P_{450}X1B2$, which converts deoxycorticosterone to aldosterone (that is, 11β-hydroxylation, 18-hydroxylation, and 18-oxidation). Depending on

Table 13 *Causes of mineralocorticoid deficiency*

Adrenal hypoplasia
Congenital adrenal hyperplasia
Pseudohypoaldosteronism types I and II
Hyporeninaemic hypoaldosteronism
Aldosterone biosynthetic defects (corticosterone methyl oxidase deficiency types I and II)
Addison's disease
Drug induced

which mutation is present in this enzyme there may be a defect of any of these steps. In corticosterone methyl oxidase II deficiency patients two mutation have been identified; one affecting 18-oxidase predominantly and the other 18-hydroxylase. The affected individuals were homozygous for both mutations.

If 11β-hydroxylase ($P_{450}X1B1$) is normal and $P_{450}X1B2$ is deficient in some way then aldosterone secretion is decreased, and patients usually present at birth with salt-wasting (hyponatraemia, hyperkalaemia, fluid depletion). The precise diagnosis can be made by finding low aldosterone and either elevated corticosterone and low 18-hydroxycorticosterone (corticosterone methyl oxidase type I deficiency) or elevated corticosterone and 18-hydroxycorticosterone (corticosterone methyl oxidase type II deficiency). The latter condition is much more common in Iranian Jews than in the Caucasian population.

Pseudohypoaldosteronism

In this condition there is a failure of the normal tissue responsiveness to mineralocorticoids. The usual presentation is with severe salt-wasting and failure to thrive in infancy. Investigation shows hyponatraemia, hyperkalaemia with very high plasma aldosterone, and plasma renin activity levels with inappropriate urinary sodium loss. The mineralocorticoid receptor appears to be defective, as judged by studies looking at the binding of aldosterone to monocytes. However, detailed molecular studies have failed to show any abnormality in the mineralocorticoid receptor itself.

The condition is heterogeneous and may be transmitted as an autosomal dominant. Heterozygotes show a reduced number of monocyte aldosterone-binding sites. Treatment is by intravenous saline followed by a high sodium intake. The salt-wasting nearly always improves with age.

Another group of patients with so-called pseudohypoaldosteronism type II has been described. These have mineralocorticoid-resistant hyperkalaemia but do not have the salt-wasting of the type I condition (Gordon's syndrome). There appears to be excessive reabsorption of chloride by the distal nephron, which then affects mineralocorticoid-dependent potassium and hydrogen ion secretion, resulting in hyperkalaemia and acidosis. The increased sodium chloride reabsorption results in hyperchloraemia, hypertension, and suppression of plasma renin activity. A similar condition has been described in obstructive uropathy.

Hyporeninaemic hypoaldosteronism

Angiotensin II is a key stimulus to aldosterone secretion, and thus damage or blockade of the renin–angiotensin system may result in mineralocorticoid deficiency. Various renal diseases have been associated with damage to the juxtaglomerular apparatus and hence renin deficiency. Of these the most common is diabetic nephropathy.

The usual picture is of an elderly patient who presents with symptoms from recurrent arrhythmias. Investigation shows hyperkalaemia, acidosis, and mild to moderate impairment of renal function. Plasma renin activity and aldosterone are low and fail to respond to sodium depletion, the erect posture, or frusemide administration. In contrast, infusion of angiotensin II usually stimulates aldosterone secretion. A similar syndrome may result from treatment with angiotensin-converting-enzyme inhibitors, but here the plasma renin activity will be high because of the lack of negative feedback ofangiotensin II on renin secretion.

Treatment of primary renin deficiency is with fludrocortisone in the first instance, to replace aldosterone, together with dietary potassium restriction. However, these patients are not salt deplete and may become hypertensive with fludrocortisone. In this case the addition of a loop-acting diuretic such as frusemide is appropriate. This will also increase the excretion of acid and thus improves the metabolic acidosis.

Other factors may also contribute to the hyperkalaemia, including the use of potassium-sparing diuretics, potassium supplementation, insulin deficiency, and β-adrenoceptor blocking drugs and prostaglandin synthetase inhibitors which inhibit renin release.

Addison's disease

This important cause of mineralocorticoid deficiency is discussed above.

REFERENCES

Cushing's syndrome

Atkinson, A.B., Kennedy, A.L., Carson, D.J., Hadden, D.R., Weaver, J.A., and Sheridan, B. (1985). Five cases of cyclical Cushing's syndrome. *British Medical Journal*, **291**, 1453–7.

Burch, W. (1983). A survey of results with transsphenoidal surgery in Cushing's disease. *New England Journal of Medicine*, **308**, 103–4.

Cauter, E. van and Refetoff, S. (1985). Evidence for two subtypes of Cushing's disease based on the analysis of episodic cortisol secretion. *New England Journal of Medicine*, **312**, 1343–9.

Cushing, H.W. (1912). *The pituitary body and its disorders*. J.B. Lippincott, Philadelphia.

Editorial. (1990). CRH test in the 1990s. *Lancet*, **ii**, 1416.

Horrocks, P.M. and London, D.R. (1982). Diagnostic value of 9 am plasma adrenocorticotrophic hormone concentrations in Cushing's disease. *British Medical Journal*, **285**, 1302–3.

Howlett, T.A., Plowman, P.N., Wass, J.A.H., Rees, L.H., Jones, A.E., and Besser, G.M. (1989). Megavoltage pituitary irradiation in the management of Cushing's disease and Nelson's syndrome: long-term follow-up. *Clinical Endocrinology*, **31**, 309–23.

Hutter, A.M. and Kayhoe, D.E. (1966). Adrenal cortical carcinoma: results of treatment with o,p'-DDD in 138 patients. *American Journal of Medicine*, **41**, 572–81.

Kaye, T.B. and Crapo, L. (1990). The Cushing syndrome: an update on diagnostic tests. *Annals of Internal Medicine*, **112**, 434–44.

Klibanski, A. and Zervas, N.T. (1991). Diagnosis and management of hormone-secreting pituitary adenomas. *New England Journal of Medicine*, **324**, 822–31.

Lacroix, A., Bolte, E., Tremblay, J. *et al.* (1992). Gastric-inhibitory polypeptide-dependent cortisol hypersecretion—a new cause of Cushing's syndrome. *New England Journal of Medicine*, **327**, 974–80.

Lamberts, S.W.J., De Lange, S.A., and Stefanko, S.Z. (1982). Adrenocorticotropin-secreting pituitary adenomas originate from the anterior or the intermediate lobe in Cushing's disease: differences in the regulation of hormone secretion. *Journal of Clinical Endocrinology and Metabolism*, **54**, 286–91.

Lamberts, S.W.J., Bons, E.G., and Bruining, H.A. (1984). Different sensitivity to adrenocorticotropin of dispersed adrenocortical cells from patients with Cushing's disease with macronodular and diffuse adrenal hyperplasia. *Journal of Clinical Endocrinology and Metabolism*, **58**, 1106–10.

Mampalam, T.J., Tyrell, B., and Wilson, C.B. (1988). Transsphenoidal microsurgery for Cushing's disease. A report of 216 cases. *Annals of Internal Medicine*, **109**, 487–93.

Meikle, W.A. (1982). Dexamethasone suppression tests: usefulness of simultaneous measurement of plasma cortisol and dexamethasone. *Clinical Endocrinology*, **16**, 401–8.

Peck, W.W., Dillon, W.P., Norman, D., *et al.* (1989). High-resolution imaging of pituitary microadenomas at 1.5T: experience with Cushing disease. *American Journal of Radiology*, **152**, 145–51.

Perry, L.A., Al-Dujaili, E.A.S., and Edwards, C.R.W. (1982). A direct radioimmunoassay for 11-deoxycortisol. *Steroids*, **39**, 115–28.

Plotz, C.M., Knowlton, A.I., and Ragan, C. (1952). The natural history of Cushing's syndrome. *American Journal of Medicine*, **13**, 597–614.

Ross, E.J. and Linch, D.C. (1982). Cushing's syndrome—killing disease: discriminatory value of signs and symptoms aiding early diagnosis. *Lancet*, **ii**, 646–9.

Suda-T, Tomori-N, Sumitomo-T, *et al.* (1987). Radioimmunoassay of corticotropin-releasing hormone: methodology and clinical application. *Hormones and Metabolism Research Supplement*, **16**, 47–51.

Tabarin, A., Greselle, J.F., San-Galli, F., *et al.* (1991). Usefulness of the corticotropin-releasing hormone test during bilateral inferior petrosal sinus sampling for the diagnosis of Cushing's disease. *Journal of Clinical Endocrinology and Metabolism*, **73**, 53–9.

Trainer, P.J. and Grossman, A. (1991). The diagnosis and differential diagnosis of Cushing's syndrome. *Clinical Endocrinology*, **34**, 317–30.

Turney, H.G. (1913). *Proceedings of the Royal Society Symposium*, **6**, lxix–lxvii.

Wittert, G.A., Crock, P.A., Donald, *et al.* (1990). Arginine vasopressin in Cushing's disease. *Lancet*, **i**, 991–4.

Zovickian, J., Oldfield, E.H., Doppman, J.L., Cutler, G.B., and Loriaux, D.L. (1988). Usefulness of inferior petrosal sinus venous endocrine markers in Cushing's disease. *Journal of Neurosurgery*, **68**, 205–10.

Mineralocorticoid excess

Conn, J.W. (1955). Primary aldosteronism: a new clinical syndrome. *Journal of Laboratory and Clinical Medicine*, **45**, 6–17.

Edwards C.R.W., Stewart, P.M., Burt, D., *et al.* (1988). Tissue localisation of 11β-hydroxysteroid dehydrogenase–tissue specific protector of the mineralocorticoid receptor. *Lancet*, **ii**, 986–9.

Gordon, R.D., Stowasser, M., Tunn T.J., *et al.* (1991). Clinical and pathological diversity of primary aldosteronism, including a new familial variety. *Clinical Experimental Pharmacology and Physiology*, **18**, 283–6.

Lifton, R.P., Dluhy, R.G., Powers, N., *et al.* (1992). A chimaeric 11β-hydroxylase/aldosterone synthase gene causes glucocorticoid remediable aldosteronism and human hypertension. *Nature*, **355**, 262–5.

Padfield, P.L., Brown, J.J., Davies, D., *et al.* (1981). The myth of idiopathic hyperaldosteronism. *Lancet*, **ii**, 83–4.

Stewart, P.M., Wallace, A.M., Valentino, R., Burt, D., Shackleton, C.H.L., and Edwards, C.R.W. (1987). Mineralocorticoid activity of liquorice: 11β-hydroxysteroid dehydrogenase deficiency comes of age. *Lancet*, **ii**, 821–4.

Stewart, P.M., Corrie, J.E.T., Shackleton, C.H.L., and Edwards, C.R.W. (1988). The syndrome of ''apparent mineralocorticoid excess'': a defect in the cortisol cortisone shuttle. *Journal of Clinical Investigation*, **82**, 340–9.

Addison's disease

Addison, T. (1855). *On the constitutional and local effects of disease of the suprarenal capsules*. S. Highley, London.

Baker, D.E., Glazer, G.M., and Francis, I.R. (1988). Adrenal magnetic resonance imaging in antibody that blocks stimulation of cortisol secretion by adrenocorticotrophic hormone in Addison's disease. *British Medical Journal*, **296**, 1489–91.

Maclaren, N.K. and Riley, W.J. (1986). Inherited susceptibility to autoimmune Addison's disease is linked to human leukocyte antigens-DR3 and/or DR4, except when associated with type I autoimmune polyglandular syndrome. *Journal of Clinical Endocrinology and Metabolism* **62**(3), 455–9.

Mugusi, F., Swai, A.B., Turner, S.J., Alberti, K.G., and McLarty, D.G. (1990). Hypoadrenalism in patients with pulmonary tuberculosis in Tanzania: an undiagnosed complication? *Transactions of the Royal Society of Tropical Medicine and Hygiene*, **84**(6), 849–51.

Stewart, P.M., Corrie, J., Seckl, J.R., Edwards, C.R.W., and Padfield, P.L. (1988). A rational approach for assessing the hypothalamo-pituitary adrenal axis. *Lancet*, **i**, 1208–10.

Wulffraat, N.M., Drexhage, H.A., Bottazzo, G.F., Wiersinga, W.M., Jeucken, P., and Van-der-Gaag, R. (1989). Immunoglobulins of patients with idiopathic Addison's disease block the *in vitro* action of adrenocorticotropin. *Journal of Clinical Endocrinology and Metabolism*, **69**(2), 231–8.

12.7.2 Congenital adrenal hyperplasia

I. A. HUGHES

Congenital adrenal hyperplasia comprises a family of inherited disorders of adrenal steroidogenesis. They have in common the net effect of an insufficient production of cortisol and/or aldosterone which, by operation of a classical endocrine negative feedback system, leads to increased trophic stimulation by adrenocorticotrophic hormone (ACTH) and hyperplastic adrenals. Genital abnormalities are not a feature of all the adrenal enzyme deficiencies so that the alternative anatomical descriptive term, adrenogenital syndrome, has now largely been abandoned.

The pathways of adrenal steroidogenesis and the required enzymes are illustrated in Fig. 1. The conversion of cholesterol to pregnenolene is a rate-limiting step controlled by ACTH-induced adenyl cyclase activation. A P_{450} mixed-function oxidase enzyme performs a side-chain cleavage reaction on cholesterol, which is the first step in the formation of steroids, whether in the adrenals, gonads, or placenta. P_{450}scc is one of two mitochondrial enzymes in the adrenal cortex, which is structurally and functionally divided into three zones. The site of expression of the genes encoding steroidogenic enzymes corresponds with functional zonation. Thus, glucocorticoids are synthesized in both the zona fasciculata and reticularis, whereas the synthesis of aldosterone is confined to the zona glomerulosa. The localization of mineralocorticoid production to this zone is the result of the absence of 17α-hydroxylase activity (the so-called 17-deoxy pathway) and the presence of corticosterone methyloxidase II required for the terminal conversion of corticosterone to aldosterone. The pathway of aldosterone biosynthesis is predominantly under the control of the renin–angiotensin system. The zona reticularis is the innermost layer of cells in the adrenal cortex and contains 17,20-lyase activity which is required to cleave the 17,20 carbon–carbon bonds in 17OH-pregnenolone and 17OH-progesterone to produce dehydroepiandrosterone and androstenedione, respectively. The last two steroids are weak adrenal androgens which mediate the growth of pubic and axillary hair (adrenarche), particularly in girls. Lyase activity predominates in the testis for the formation of testosterone. The profound virilization which is a feature of the 21-hydroxylase and 11β-hydroxylase deficiency forms of congenital adrenal hyperplasia is also associated with the action of 17,20-lyase on increased substrate concentration. Table 1 is a summary of the types of enzymes involved in adrenal steroidogenesis and the known localization of the genes that encode each enzyme. Deficiency of 21-hydroxylase activity is the cause for congenital adrenal hyperplasia in more than 90 per cent of cases. Here, the accounts of this and other forms of congenital adrenal hyperplasia deal largely with presentation and management in older children and adults; other texts should be consulted for description of these disorders in infancy.

21-Hydroxylase deficiency

CLINICAL PRESENTATION

The classical form of this enzyme deficiency presents in infancy in one of two forms. The most dramatic is with ambiguous genitalia of the newborn, whereby a female fetus becomes virilized *in utero* due to the effect of excess adrenal androgen converted peripherally to testosterone and masculinizing the external genital anlagen (see Chapter 12.9.1). Milder forms of virilization manifest either as isolated clitoromegaly or as isolated labial fusion. The latter condition should be distinguished from labial adhesions which occur quite often in normal girls. There is evidence that aldosterone biosynthesis is deficient in up to 75 per cent of cases, although frank clinical signs of salt depletion are evident in only some half of the cases.

Late-onset or non-classical forms of congenital adrenal hyperplasia are also recognized. There may be delay in the onset of virilization in the non-salt-losing male. The signs of precocious sexual development are also accompanied by tall stature, due to the growth-promoting effect of androgens. The testes remain prepubertal in size (less than 4 ml in volume), which is a useful distinguishing feature from other causes of precocious puberty associated with increased gonadotrophin secretion. The non-classical form of congenital adrenal hyperplasia in females may present with early onset of pubic hair growth or later after puberty with signs of hirsutism and symptoms of menstrual dysfunction. Evidence of 21-hydroxylase deficiency may be uncovered when a young adult female is investigated for infertility. Male infertility has also been ascribed to 21-hydroxylase deficiency, but this is usually in a known non-salt-losing patient who has long-term non-compliance with treatment. Increased testosterone production from adrenal precursor substrates inhibits pituitary luteinizing hormone secretion and hence testicular testosterone production. A high local intratesticular testosterone concentration is required for normal spermatogenesis.

TESTS TO ESTABLISH A DIAGNOSIS

Table 2 lists the investigations required when 21-hydroxylase deficiency presents in the newborn with the appearance of ambiguous genitalia.

The diagnosis of 21-hydroxylase deficiency in the later-onset forms usually requires an ACTH stimulation test to amplify marginally elevated basal values for adrenal steroid concentrations. Following a 250 μg bolus injection of tetracosactin, plasma 17OH-progesterone concentrations are inappropriately elevated. The test is also used to determine which adult females with hirsutism and menstrual disturbance have evidence of late-onset 21-hydroxylase deficiency. Ideally, the conditions should be standardized so that the test is performed during the early follicular phase of the menstrual cycle and preferably following a small dose of dexamethasone given the night before. Some of the other adrenal enzyme deficiencies, particularly 3β-hydroxysteroid dehydrogenase deficiency, have also been suggested as causes of hirsutism and menstrual disorders. Polycystic ovarian syndrome is a well recognized and more frequent cause of hirsutism and anovulation (see Chapter 12.9.1). However, to confuse matters further, congenital adrenal hyperplasia itself often results in polycystic changes to the ovaries at the time of puberty.

Fig. 1 Schematic representation of adrenal steroidogenesis. The numbers indicate the following enzymes: 1, P_{450}scc; 2, P_{450}c17 which catalyses 17α-hydroxylase and 17,20-lyase activities; 3, 3β-hydroxysteroid dehydrogenase/isomerase; 4, P_{450}c21; 5, P_{450}11β; 6, P_{450}c18 or P_{450}aldo. The dashed line denotes the extra-adrenal synthesis of testosterone, catalysed by 17β-hydroxysteroid dehydrogenase.

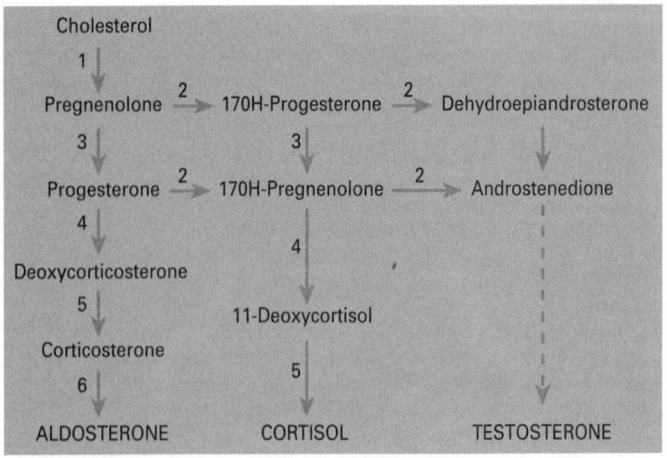

Table 1 *Genes and enzymes involved in adrenal steroidogenesis*

Enzyme activity	Site of enzyme	Gene label and chromosome
Side-chain cleavage (P_{450}scc)	Mitochondria	CYP11A;15
3β-Hydroxysteroid dehydrogenase/isomerase (3βHSD)	Endoplasmic reticulum	Type I, Type II; 1p13
17α-Hydroxylase (P_{450}17α)	Endoplasmic reticulum	CYP17; 10
21-Hydroxylase (P_{450}c21)	Endoplasmic reticulum	CYP21B, CYP21A; 6p23
11β-Hydroxylase (P_{450}11β)	Mitochondria	CYP11B1; 8q21–q22
		CYP11B2

Table 2 *Investigations for ambiguous genitalia and 21-hydroxylase deficiency*

Genetic	Peripheral karyotype
	Blood for DNA extraction
Biochemical	Urea and electrolytes
	Blood glucose
	Plasma 17OH-progesterone
	Plasma testosterone
	Plasma ACTH
	Plasma renin activity
	Urine steroid metabolites
Radiological	Pelvic ultrasound
	Sinogram

Table 3 *Parameters to monitor treatment in congenital adrenal hyperplasia*

Clinical	Linear growth velocity
	Weight gain
	Striae formation
	Blood pressure
	Skeletal age
Biochemical	Profiles of 17OH-progesterone, androstenedione
	Plasma testosterone
	Plasma renin activity
	Urinary steroid metabolites

TREATMENT IN LATE INFANCY, CHILDHOOD, AND ADOLESCENCE

Surgical reconstruction of the external genitalia is required in the virilized female infant with congenital adrenal hyperplasia. Parents are understandably anxious for the surgery to be performed as soon as possible, and some centres do so within a few weeks. However, most surgeons prefer to wait until the infant is 6 to 12 months of age. Several surgical procedures are described, but in general it is necessary to perform a reduction in the size of the clitoris and expose the opening of the vagina on to the perineum. Surgery is far more extensive when there is a high vaginal opening into the posterior urethra, and sometimes the surgeon will elect to postpone the required vaginoplasty until the child is older. Clitoral recession is performed with the intention of preserving the nerve supply to the glans.

Medical treatment for congenital adrenal hyperplasia is ongoing, with appropriate replacement doses of hydrocortisone and 9α-fludrocortisone (for salt-losers) adjusted according to body size. The hydrocortisone dose should be doubled or trebled in times of stress, such as an infection or for a surgical procedure. Other glucocorticoid preparations have been tried in congenital adrenal hyperplasia, including cortisone acetate, prednisolone, and dexamethasone. There appears to be no advantage of cortisone acetate over hydrocortisone, especially since cortisone acetate is a metabolically inactive steroid until it is converted in the liver to cortisol. Prednisolone and dexamethasone are both longer-acting glucocorticoids which appear to be useful for treatment in the postpubertal age group. Dexamethasone is often used as a single daily dose (0.5 mg) and appears to regulate menses more efficiently in the young adult female patient. Some girls, however, develop side-effects, such as excessive weight gain and striae formation on quite small doses of dexamethasone.

MONITORING TREATMENT

Several clinical and laboratory parameters can be used to monitor treatment at various ages (Table 3). The rate of linear growth is the main clinical yardstick of control before puberty. A delicate balance has to be struck between providing sufficient glucocorticoid replacement to reduce excess androgen secretion (which causes rapid growth) and to avoid the effect of excessive glucocorticoid treatment (which causes growth suppression). Growth is rapid during normal infancy, so glucocorticoid treatment must not be excessive at this time. Excessive weight gain is a sensitive sign. Linear growth in the older infant and child provides a useful yardstick of control when height is measured every 6 months. This is supplemented by periodic measurement of the bone age from a radiograph taken of the left hand and wrist. Androgens are powerful stimulators of epiphyseal maturation and changes in skeletal maturation can be detected over quite short periods of time. It is important to avoid an excessive bone age advance since this inevitably reduces the length of growing time and leads to adult short stature. The onset of the pubertal growth spurt is an important yardstick to monitor in both sexes, while delayed menarche in girls usually indicates inadequate control and increased plasma testosterone concentrations. In adult life, regular menses and ovulation in the female and normal spermatogenesis in the male are reliable clinical indicators of adequate control.

Some of the laboratory investigations listed in Table 3 are used to refine the degree of control by supplementing clinical indices. There is a marked diurnal rhythm in plasma concentrations of 17OH-progesterone so that random measurements are inadequate to monitor control. A profile of 17OH-progesterone based on measurements performed on three to four samples collected throughout the day is a useful measure of control, especially now that assays for this steroid are available in capillary blood samples spotted on to filter paper and in saliva samples. It has been possible to derive nomograms which indicate the degree of control based on profiles of 17OH-progesterone (Fig. 2). Similar analyses can be performed for androstenedione used as a marker of control. Testosterone has less of a pronounced diurnal rhythm than adrenal steroids and random plasma measurements are useful to monitor control in infants, children, and adult females. The increased production of testosterone by the testis in pubertal boys and adult males renders this steroid useless as an index of control in these two groups. It should be possible to monitor control with ACTH measurements, but this seldom seems to be used in practice. Serum electrolytes are an insensitive index of the adequacy of mineralocorticoid replacement, but the periodic measurement of plasma renin activity can be extremely useful. Elevated levels may indicate the need for 9α-fludrocortisone treatment even if the patient has had no overt evidence of salt loss. In such cases, the patient may have compensated by adjusting to a high salt intake, but this could be potentially dangerous in areas of hot climate or if a gastrointestinal upset occurs.

OUTCOME IN TREATED 21-HYDROXYLASE DEFICIENCY

The survival rate for the salt-wasting form of 21-hydroxylase deficiency seems to have improved in recent years. However, male infants in particular still die in infancy from salt-losing crisis because of unrecognized congenital adrenal hyperplasia. Achieving normal growth has long been a problem in the management of this condition. There has been an increased recognition of the importance of the type and dose of glucocorticoid to use, the need to provide adequate mineralocorticoid replacement, and the use of newer steroid assays to monitor control in more detail. A generation of patients treated in this way has yet to reach adulthood, but even so, final height is invariably lower than expected based on parental target height. Fertility is reduced in adult females. Evidence that sexual intercourse is unsatisfactory in some females because of an inadequate vaginoplasty is a contributory factor, as well as the presence of anovulatory cycles when medical treatment is insufficient. These problems can be remedied so that the reproductive potential in adequately treated females with this condition should be almost normal. Adult males who stop taking glucocorticoid replacement may develop oligospermia; this is usually reversed when treatment is re-started. Testicular tumours may also occur when treatment is stopped because of hyperstimulation of adrenal-rest cells by ACTH.

Fig. 2 Nomograms to monitor control in congenital adrenal hyperplasia using (a) blood spot and (b) saliva 17OH-progesterone profiles. Areas A, B, and C represent good, poor and extremely poor control, respectively; area D indicates overlap of B and C areas. The shaded bars denote a range of 17OH-progesterone values at 0800 h which avoids overtreatment. (Reproduced with permission of *Archives of Disease in Childhood*.)

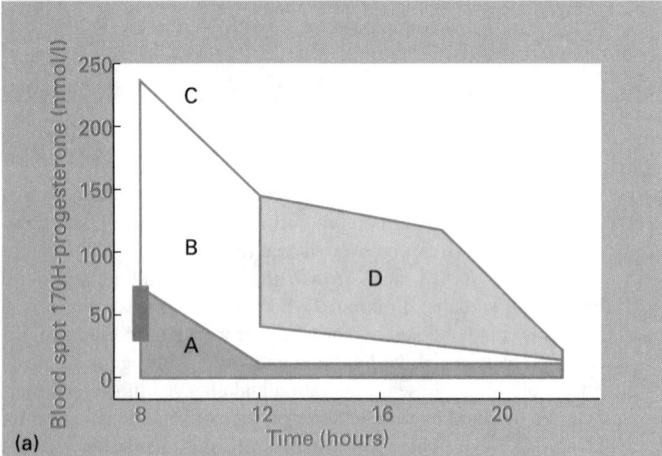

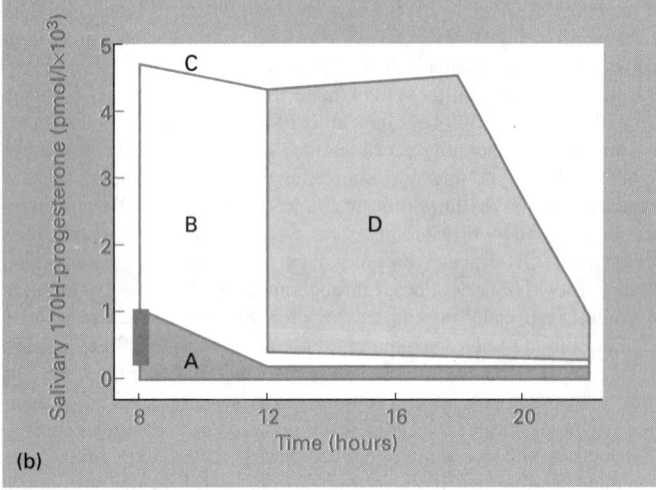

GENETICS OF 21-HYDROXYLASE DEFICIENCY

In common with other enzyme deficiency disorders, congenital adrenal hyperplasia is an autosomal recessive condition. In the case of 21-hydroxylase deficiency, linkage studies had shown the gene encoding the enzyme to be closely linked with the genes encoding the major histocompatibility complex on the short arm of chromosome 6. Studies world-wide of various HLA haplotypes in patients with congenital adrenal hyperplasia have shown an association between the uncommon A3, Bw47, DR7 haplotype in the classical condition, whereas in the non-classical variety there is a strong association with HLA-B14, DR1. With this information, it has been possible to determine carriers within affected families and also detect the condition antenatally by performing HLA haplotyping on cultured amniocytes. However, the results have not been entirely reliable because of the frequency of recombination events in this region of chromosome 6. Heterozygosity testing could be refined by also measuring the plasma 17OH-progesterone response in the individual 60 min following an injection of ACTH.

The gene for the $P_{450}c21$ enzyme was first cloned for bovine adrenals and later for the human. Two genes, labelled CYP21A and CYP21B, were identified within the class III region of the HLA complex and are approximately 30 kb apart. They are adjacent to, and in tandem repeat with C4A and C4B genes which encode for the fourth component of serum complement (Fig. 3). CYP21A is a pseudogene which is functionally inactive because of a series of deleterious mutations. The gene is 97 per cent homologous with the active gene, CYP21B. Both complement genes are functional. Early molecular genetic studies based on restriction mapping analyses suggested that approximately 25 per cent of patients had a deletion of the functional CYP21B gene. This results from unequal crossing-over during meiosis, so that a complete tandem CYP21B/C4B repeat unit is deleted. The first documented case was associated with the rare Bw47 HLA antigen, but further studies indicate that gene deletions are not just confined to patients with this HLA haplotype. A gene deletion is always associated with the severe salt-wasting form of congenital adrenal hyperplasia. The majority of patients with 21-hydroxylase deficiency can be explained on the basis of gene conversion-like exchanges between CYP21A and CYP21B. Large-scale gene conversions in which several mutations have been transferred from the pseudogene to the CYP21B gene account for up to a further 10 per cent of cases. Again, these manifest as the salt-wasting form of the

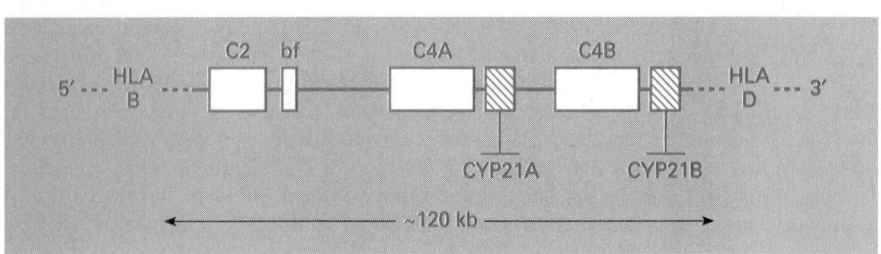

Fig. 3 A simple scheme to indicate the location of CYP21 genes on chromosome 6.

condition. Long-range restriction mapping using pulsed-field gel electrophoresis was used to resolve a vexed question regarding the interpretation of conventional restriction digest analysis in congenital adrenal hyperplasia. It appears that large gene conversions can result in one end of a CYP21B being spliced on to the beginning of a CYP21A gene, so that the resulting CYP21 gene contains no CYP21B-specific active sequences.

The majority of gene conversion events are small scale in nature and result in the transfer of a deleterious mutation from the CYP21A pseudogene to the CYP21B gene. The CYP21 gene is approximately 3.3 kb long and contains 10 exons. Several point mutations have now been identified, either by direct DNA sequencing of gene segments amplified by the polymerase chain reaction or by the use of allele-specific oligonucleotide hybridization techniques. Gene conversion events are the non-reciprocal exchange of homologous genetic information. Sequence exchanges could also occur as a result of multiple recombination events. However, a *de novo* microconversion event has recently been described which exchanges as little as 390 bp between maternal CYP21A and CYP21B genes. Although spontaneous *de novo* conversion events have been noted in mouse MHC genes, this appears to be the first occasion for the phenomenon to be characterized in humans.

Now that many groups of patients have been studied by mutational analysis, a pattern of concordance between genotype and phenotype is beginning to emerge. The most commonly found mutation in classic 21-hydroxylase deficiency affects mRNA splicing due to a nucleotide base change (A/C to G) in the second intron. A stretch of nucleotides which is normally spliced out is retained, so that the translational reading frame is altered and an inactive protein synthesized. Patients with this mutation have the salt-wasting form of congenital adrenal hyperplasia, as do others with an 8 bp deletion in exon 3. Other examples of mutations resulting in salt-wasting include a change from a conserved arginine residue to tryptophan in exon 8, and a trio of mis-sense mutations which cluster in exon 6. A specific mutation associated with the non-salt-wasting or simple virilizing form of congenital adrenal hyperplasia has been identified in exon 4, which changes an isoleucine to an asparagine. Since 21-hydroxylase activity is expressed only in adrenal cells, it has been necessary to test the activity of the altered enzyme by transfecting the mutant CYP21B gene in cultured cells such as COS monkey kidney cells. In this way it is possible to study the kinetic properties of mutant enzymes and explain the difference between salt-wasters and non-salt-wasters. Thus, the isoleucine to asparagine mutation in exon 4 produces an enzyme with about 1 per cent of normal activity, which is presumably sufficient to permit adequate aldosterone production and avoid salt-wasting. The original two gene, two enzyme hypothesis to explain the difference between salt-wasters and simple virilizers has finally been discounted for an explanation based on quantitative differences in $P_{450}c21$ activity.

The non-classical or late-onset form of 21-hydroxylase deficiency is associated with a mutant enzyme which has 50 per cent and 20 per cent of normal activity when the substrates used are 17OH-progesterone and progesterone, respectively. The gene mutation is a change from valine to leucine in exon 7 and is associated with the HLA haplotype, B14, DR1. It has been estimated that the non-classical condition occurs in about 1 per cent of the general population and in about 10 per cent of East European Jews. A further mutation described in non-classical congenital adrenal hyperplasion is a proline to leucine change in exon 1.

PRENATAL DIAGNOSIS AND TREATMENT

The deleterious mutations which cause the CYP21A to become non-functional are now well characterized but up to 10 per cent of the CYP21B alleles in patients with congenital adrenal hyperplasia do not harbour one of the known mutations. Nevertheless, prenatal diagnosis of 21-hydroxylase deficiency is now more reliable, even when the index case within an affected family is not available for study. Chorionic villus sampling at around 10 weeks' gestation is used to provide a DNA sam-

ple for mutational analysis as well as determining the sex of the fetus. Amniocentesis is now performed earlier in gestation so that the concentration of 17OH-progesterone in amniotic fluid can also be measured as an indication of 21-hydroxylase deficiency. There is the option to offer prenatal treatment with dexamethasone, given to the mother in order to prevent virilization of an affected female fetus.

Treatment needs to start as early as 6 weeks' gestation because fetal adrenal steroidogenesis is also established early. The usual daily dose of dexamethasone is 20 µg/kg maternal body weight, divided in three equally spaced doses. The diagnosis is confirmed or excluded at the time of chorionic villus sampling and treatment is continued to term only if an affected fetus is female. Male infants with congenital adrenal hyperplasia are not virilized at birth. The success of treatment has been variable with the limited number of cases reported. Partial virilization is still liable to occur when treatment is started too late, interrupted for any reason, or the dexamethasone dose is inadequate. Maternal oestriol levels should be suppressed (fetal adrenal steroids provide the substrate for formation of this oestrogen) as should the concentration of 17OH-progesterone and testosterone determined in amniotic fluid collected in mid-trimester. In ideal circumstances, one can anticipate normal external genitalia in treated females or, at least, a marked reduction in virilization compared with the previously affected female infant within the family. Treatment is not without side-effects to the mother. These can include excessive weight gain, formation of striae, hypertension, and glucose intolerance which are all reversible when treatment is stopped. No fetal malformations have been reported and early growth and development in those infants who were treated before birth has been normal.

INCIDENCE OF CONGENITAL ADRENAL HYPERPLASIA

The incidence of the classic form of 21-hydroxylase deficiency has been estimated to be about 1 in 10 000 births. When assays for 17OH-progesterone became available in filter-paper blood spot specimens, pilot screening studies were performed in several countries and the worldwide incidence was estimated to be 1 in 14 000 live births. The incidence was unusually high in the Yupik Eskimos of south-western Alaska. Only a few countries now operate a newborn screening programme for congenital adrenal hyperplasia as a matter of routine. Affected females should be recognized at birth by careful physical examination, while there is debate whether it is justifiable to screen for affected males, not all of whom would be at risk of life-threatening adrenal insufficiency. It has been decided not to add this to the list of conditions currently screened for after birth in the United Kingdom.

Other forms of congenital adrenal hyperplasia

$P_{450}scc$ deficiency

This extremely rare form of the condition has also been variously called cholesterol desmolase deficiency and lipoid adrenal hyperplasia. The latter term illustrates a feature of lipid accumulation which can lead to massive enlargement of the adrenals, visible by CT or MRI scanning. Since cholesterol cannot be converted to pregnenolone, the production of all classes of steroid hormones is deficient in gonadal as well as in adrenal tissue. Glucocorticoid and mineralocorticoid insufficiency is particularly severe and leads to infant death unless recognized and treated early. Affected males have female external genitalia or perhaps minimal virilization because of failure to synthesize testosterone. Milder cases which have survived infancy untreated are recorded. Plasma steroid and urinary metabolite levels are uniformly low and show no response to exogenous ACTH stimulation. The gene encoding $P_{450}scc$ is designated CYP11A and, in several cases studied with $P_{450}scc$ deficiency, no mutations have been found so far in the coding sequence of the gene. It is possible that the primary defect is in mobilization of cholesterol across the mitochondrial membrane.

3β-Hydroxysteroid dehydrogenase deficiency

The 3β-hydroxysteroid dehydrogenase/isomerase (3βHSD) is a non-P_{450} enzyme which is required for the conversion of Δ^5 to Δ^4 steroids in both adrenal and gonadal tissue. Recent studies have isolated two closely linked and highly homologous genes which control the expression of two isoenzymes. The type I enzyme is expressed predominantly in the placenta and peripheral tissues, whereas the type II enzyme is expressed in the adrenals, testis, and ovary. Reference to Fig. 1 illustrates that deficiency of 3βHSD activity will also result in severe glucocorticoid and mineralocorticoid deficiency. Genital abnormalities occur in affected males and females. The production of weak androgens by the testis (dehydroepiandrosterone, androstenediol) is insufficient to produce adequate virilization in the male, but their production by the adrenal does virilize the external genitalia in an affected female. The diagnosis is confirmed by demonstrating elevated concentrations of steroid precursors (particularly 17OH-pregnenolone) in plasma and their metabolites in urine.

The molecular basis of 3βHSD deficiency has been characterized in a number of affected families. Mutations such as nonsense and frame shifts have only been found in the type II 3βHSD gene while the type I gene was normal. This probably explains why some patients with 3βHSD deficiency may show normal or elevated levels of Δ^4 steroids such as 17OH-progesterone and androstenedione, particularly following ACTH stimulation. Significant amounts of type I 3βHSD enzyme activity in peripheral tissues produce sufficient amounts of active androgens to virilize some males at puberty. It has been suggested that a late-onset or non-classical form of 3βHSD deficiency is a common cause of hirsutism in adult females. This is based on an increase in the ratio of Δ^5 to Δ^4 steroids following ACTH stimulation. There are no reports yet of abnormalities in either the type I or type II 3βHSD genes in these women; however, type II 3βHSD gene mutations have recently been described in one girl with premature adrenarche and in another girl with primary amenorrhoea.

17α-Hydroxylase deficiency

A single $P_{450}17\alpha$ enzyme catalyses 17α-hydroxylase and 17,20-lyase reactions. Both are required for the synthesis of sex hormones, whereas only 17α-hydroxylase activity is required to synthesize cortisol. Mineralocorticoid biosynthesis is not dependent on the presence of the $P_{450}17\alpha$ enzyme, so that ACTH-stimulated, low renin hypertension is a typical feature of $P_{450}17\alpha$ hydroxylase deficiency. This occurs in both males and females and is accompanied by a hypokalaemic metabolic alkalosis. Lack of adequate sex hormone production leads to a variable phenotype in affected males, ranging from female genitalia to an ambiguous appearance or features of a hypospadic male. Females have lack of development of secondary sexual characteristics and primary amenorrhoea.

The biochemical pattern in this enzyme deficiency shows increased concentrations of corticosterone, deoxycorticosterone, and progesterone, with decreased levels of testosterone, oestradiol, and plasma renin. More detailed measurements of steroid metabolites by gas chromatography–mass spectrometry techniques can delineate patterns indicative of deficiencies of either 17α-hydroxylase or 17,20-lyase activities alone, or as a combination of both. Many examples of this enzyme deficiency have now been described, with the majority involving a deficiency of both activities. The human CYP17 gene is made up of eight exons, and a range of mutation types has been discovered in affected patients. One of the more frequent mutations observed is a 4 bp duplication in exon 8 which, as a result of altering the reading frame, leads to a shortened carboxy-terminal sequence. Expression studies of the mutant protein show absence of both 17α-hydroxylase and 17,20-lyase activities. This is consistent with biochemical findings and a clinical female phenotype in affected males and females.

11β-Hydroxylase deficiency

Deficiency of 11β-hydroxylase activity is a second form of congenital adrenal hyperplasia that leads to hypertension. The enzyme is required for the terminal conversion of 11-deoxycortisol to cortisol, and for the conversion of deoxycorticosterone to corticosterone. The consequences of increased ACTH stimulation are salt and water retention, low-renin hypertension, and virilization, because of the increased production of deoxycorticosterone and adrenal androgens. Virilization seems to be more profound compared with that observed in 21-hydroxylase deficiency. Prepubertal breast development is another specific and unexplained feature. Hypertension usually develops in older childhood and does not necessarily correlate with the levels of deoxycorticosterone. Hypokalaemia is not a constant finding.

The diagnosis is confirmed by elevated concentrations of 11-deoxycortisol and deoxycorticosterone in plasma and their tetrahydro metabolites in urine. In affected newborn infants, a more polar urinary metabolite called 6α-hydroxytetrahydro-11-deoxycortisol seems to be a novel marker of the enzyme defect. Plasma concentrations of androstenedione, testosterone and 17OH-progesterone are increased, although the levels of the last steroid are not as high as in 21-hydroxylase deficiency. Treatment requires glucocorticoid replacement only, although a salt-wasting state may develop transiently when plasma deoxycorticosterone levels initially fall. Hypertension should be glucocorticoid-reversible but specific antihypertensive treatment may be necessary if hypertension has been long-standing. Milder or late-onset forms of 11β-hydroxylase deficiency are also described.

The $P_{450}c11$ isoenzymes are encoded by two genes, labelled CYP11B1 and CYP11B2, respectively. They are 93 per cent identical in predicted amino acid sequences. Both genes are functional but only the CYP11B1 gene is expressed at high levels in normal adrenals. Transcripts are controlled mainly by ACTH and, to a lesser extent, by angiotensin II. The expression of CYP11B2 in the adrenal is much less and is controlled only by the presence of angiotensin II. It was originally thought that a single 11β-hydroxylase enzyme was involved in both cortisol synthesis and the production of aldosterone via 18-hydroxylase and 18-methyloxidase (or corticosterone methyloxidase II) activities. Now it is realized that the product of CYP11B2 first hydroxylates corticosterone and then oxidizes 18OH-corticosterone in order to produce aldosterone. The isoenzyme is variously termed corticosterone methyloxidase II, 18-methyloxidase, or aldosterone synthase ($P_{450}aldo$). Deficiency of 11β-hydroxylase activity accounts for about 5 per cent of congenital adrenal hyperplasia cases in general, but the incidence is higher (about 1 in 6000 births) in Moroccan Jews. A single base change mutation in exon 8 of the CYP11B1 gene has been reported. This alters the haem-binding sequence which is a unique and conserved feature of all cytochrome P_{450} enzymes. A boy of Turkish origin who was a genetic female but severely virilized and hypertensive has been reported with a frame shift mutation in exon 7 of the CYP11B1 gene, which also renders the haem domain non-functional. Similar mutations have also been reported in $P_{450}17\alpha$ deficiency.

Isolated aldosterone deficiency

Isolated defects in aldosterone biosynthesis are described, although these should strictly not be included as part of the family of congenital adrenal hyperplasia disorders. Primary hypoaldosteronism can result rarely from a deficiency in the final conversion of 18OH-corticosterone to aldosterone. Salt-wasting is the clinical feature which is indistinguishable in the male from the salt-wasting form of 21-hydroxylase deficiency. The diagnosis is established on the basis of an altered ratio of mineralocorticoid metabolites in urine in the presence of normal glucocorticoid production. Mis-sense mutations in the CYP11B2 gene have been identified in affected cases. Expression studies in cultured cells showed decreased 18-hydroxylase and 18-oxidase activities, while 11β-hydroxylase activity (a function of the CYP11B1 gene) was normal. The term pseudohypoaldosteronism has been ascribed to a condition indistinguishable in newborns from salt-wasting 21-hydroxylase and aldosterone synthase deficiencies clinically, but where aldosterone levels are elevated. There is no response to mineralocorticoid treatment, so the disorder is an example of a hormone resistance syndrome. The condition is thought to be an abnormality of the aldosterone receptor, based on binding studies in circulating mononuclear cells, but no abnormality has been described in the receptor protein. A high salt intake is required and the condition appears to improve with age. Hyporeninaemic hypoaldosteronism is probably primarily a renal disorder; diagnostic features include chronic hyperkalaemia and low plasma renin and aldosterone, which respond inappropriately to measures such as sodium restriction and diuretic administration.

REFERENCES

Azziz, R., Dewailly, D., and Owerbach, D. (1994). Nonclassic adrenal hyperplasia: current concepts. *Journal of Clinical Endocrinology and Metabolism*, **78**, 810–15.

Brook, C.G.D. (1990). The management of classical congenital adrenal hyperplasia due to 21-hydroxylase deficiency. *Clinical Endocrinology*, **33**, 559–67.

Collier, S., Tassabehju, M., Sinnott, P., and Strachan, T. (1993). A *de novo* pathological point mutation at the 21-hydroxylase locus: implications for gene conversion in the human genome. *Nature Genetics* **3**, 260–5.

Hughes, I.A. (1988). Management of congenital adrenal hyperplasia. *Archives of Disease in Childhood* **63**, 1399–404.

Hughes, I.A., Dyas, J., Riad-Fahmy, D., and Laurence, K.M. (1987). Prenatal diagnosis of congenital adrenal hyperplasia: reliability of amniotic fluid steroid analysis. *Journal of Medical Genetics* **24**, 344–7.

Miller, W. L. (1994). Genetics, diagnosis, and management of 21-hydroxylase deficiency. *Journal of Clinical Endocrinology and Metabolism*, **78**, 241–6.

Mulaikal, R.M., Migeon, C.J., and Rock, J.A. (1987). Fertility rates in female patients with congenital adrenal hyperplasia due to 21-hydroxylase deficiency. *New England Journal of Medicine* **316**, 178–82.

Pang, S., *et al.* (1988). Worldwide experience in newborn screening for classical congenital adrenal hyperplasia due to 21- hydroxylase deficiency. *Pediatrics* **81**, 866–74.

Rhéaume, E., *et al.* (1992). Congenital adrenal hyperplasia due to point mutations in the type II 3β-hydroxysteroid dehydrogenase gene. *Nature Genetics* **1**, 239–45.

Sanchez, R., Rhéaume, E., LaFlamme, N., Rosenfield, R.L., Labrie, F., and Simard, J. (1994). Detection and functional characterization of the novel missense mutation Y254D in type II 3β-hydroxysteroid dehydrogenese (3βHSD) gene of a female patient with nonsalt-losing 3βHSD deficiency. *Journal of Clinical Endocrinology and Metabolism*, **78**, 561–7.

Speiser, P.W., White, P.C., and New, M.I. (1993). Congenital adrenal hyperplasia. *Reproductive Medicine Review* **2**, 1–13.

Strachan, T. (1990). Molecular pathology of congenital adrenal hyperplasia. *Clinical Endocrinology* **32**, 373–93.

Strachan, T. and White, P.C. (1991). Molecular pathology of steroid 21-hydroxylase deficiency. *Journal of Steroid Biochemistry and Molecular Biology* **50**, 537–43.

Waterman, M.R. and Simpson, E.R. (1989). Regulation of steroid hydroxylase gene expression is multifactorial in nature. *Recent Progress in Hormone Research* **45**, 533–65.

Whitaker, R.H. (1990). Genitoplasty for virilising congenital adrenal hyperplasia. In *Operative Paediatric Urology*, (ed. J.D. Frank and J.H. Johnston), pp. 123–32. Churchill Livingstone, Edinburgh.

White, P.C., New, M.I., and Dupont, B. (1987). Congenital adrenal hyperplasia (parts 1 and 11). *New England Journal of Medicine* **316**, 1519–24 and 1580–6.

White, P.C., Dupont, J., New, M.I., Leiberman, E., Hochberg, Z., and Rösler, A. (1991). A mutation in CYP11B1 (Arg 448→His) associated with steroid 11β-hydroxylase deficiency in Jews of Moroccan origin. *Journal of Clinical Investigation* **87**, 1664–7.

Yanese, T., Simpson, E.R., and Waterman, M.R. (1991). 17α hydroxylase/ 17,20-lyase deficiency: from clinical investigation to molecular definition. *Endocrine Reviews* **12**, 91–108.

Young, M.C. and Hughes, I.A. (1990). Response to treatment of congenital adrenal hyperplasia in infancy. *Archives of Disease in Childhood* **65**, 441–4.

Young, M.C. and Hughes, I.A. (1992). Congenital adrenal hyperplasia. In *Clinical Endocrinology*, (ed. A. Grossman), pp. 421–41. Blackwell Scientific, Oxford.

Zachmann, M. (1992). Recent aspects of steroid biosynthesis in male sex differentiation. *Hormone Research* **38**, 211–16.

12.8 The reproductive system

12.8.1 The ovary

H. S. JACOBS

Approach to the patient with ovarian disorders

Synchronization of the changes in the ovary and uterus and the hypothalamic–pituitary unit is complex, and the ovulation cycle is vulnerable to disturbances at any of the levels of endocrine organization. Ovarian cylicity may also be disrupted by a deterioration in general health, a protective mechanism that prevents reproduction occurring in circumstances adverse to fetal development.

Information about the regularity of the menstrual cycle is relevant in women concerned about fertility because the chance of conception is directly related to the rate of ovulation. Oligomenorrhoea (interval between menstrual periods of more than 6 weeks but less than 6 months) is usually a consequence of the polycystic ovary syndrome (see below); amenorrhoea (no periods for more than 6 months) has a broader spectrum of causes (see Tables 1 and 2). The duration of a menstrual disturbance is relevant both to its cause and its consequences. For example, a history of delayed menarche implies the disturbance was present from the age of 12, a common finding in women with polycystic ovary syndrome. A history of weight fluctuation is important because weight loss, often in the context of mild (and denied) anorexia nervosa, is a common cause of amenorrhoea and weight increase a common precipitant of the clinical expression of polycystic ovary syndrome. Bulimia may complicate either of the above conditions and, like anorexia nervosa, requires specialist management in its own right.

The association of amenorrhoea with galactorrhoea implies hyperprolactinaemia; with symptoms of oestrogen deficiency (flushing and sweating attacks and/or vaginal dryness and discomfort during intercourse) implies an increased risk of osteoporosis. Symptoms of hyperandrogenism (seborrhoea, acne, and excessive hair growth) are, in most cases, caused by polycystic ovary syndrome. It is preferable to use the term 'unwanted hair' rather than 'hirsutism' in order to avoid debate about what is and what is not truly excessive. Whether or not treatment of unwanted hair is justified is a matter for the physician's judgement.

There is often concern that the development of unwanted hair presages a sex change. Patients with such anxieties need a clear explanation of the underlying disorder and reassurance that treatment is available.

If there has been previous use of an oral contraceptive, it is relevant to determine whether it was used for contraception or to correct a menstrual disturbance. An oral contraceptive does not cure such disturbances, which are therefore likely to recur when it is stopped; nor does oral contraception cause amenorrhoea after it has been discontinued, i.e. there is no such thing as 'post-pill amenorrhoea'. Amenorrhoea occurring after discontinuation of the pill therefore needs the same investigation as in any other case of amenorrhoea.

Most women with menstrual disturbances want reassurance about their present or future fertility. The failure to ovulate as an explanation for infertility is clearly dependent on age. Many older women need advice about the long-term effects of oestrogen deficiency and the wisdom of hormone replacement therapy.

Amenorrhoea

While the classification is usually into primary (the patient has never menstruated) or secondary amenorrhoea (interval between periods more than 6 months), most of the common causes can present as either, as seen in Tables 1 and 2. With the exception of structural abnormalities, such as an absent uterus, differences between primary and secondary amenorrhoea are outweighed by similarities, so here they are considered primarily in terms of aetiology.

In young women with primary amenorrhoea there may have been congenital abnormalities in the development of the ovaries, genital tract, or external genitalia, or a perturbation of the normal process of puberty. (Chapter 12.9.3). Investigations should be considered when menstruation has not occurred by the age of 16 in the presence of normal secondary sexual development, or by the age of 14 in its absence.

Developmental abnormalities

Developmental abnormalities of the müllerian duct, the external genitalia and the problems of intersexual abnormalities are dealt with elsewhere (Section 12.9).

GONADAL DYSGENESIS

The commonest cause of gonadal dysgenesis is Turner's syndrome, in the severest form of which a 45XO karyotype is associated with a characteristic phenotypic appearance (Chapter 12.9.3). Although spontaneous and, indeed, ovulatory cycles occasionally occur, particularly if there is chromosomal mosaicism, in the long term premature ovarian failure is inevitable. The karyotype should be determined, as the presence of a Y chromosome in an individual with gonadal dysgenesis necessitates the removal of residual gonadal tissue because of an increased risk of malignancy.

Serum gonadotrophin concentrations are elevated compared with those of normal girls of the same age, and may approach the menopausal range. Oestrogen levels are low, the uterus is small, and bone densitometry shows significant skeletal decalcification; a history of spontaneous fracture is common. In addition to a search for associated cardiovascular and renal abnormalities, autoimmune thyroiditis should be excluded.

Management includes initiation of low-dose oestrogen therapy at the time puberty would normally have occurred, starting with no more than 5 μg of ethinyl oestradiol per day in order to promote breast development without prejudicing linear growth. The dose is gradually raised over 12 to 18 months. Maintenance therapy is with a cyclical oestrogen–progestogen preparation (such as an oral contraceptive), as regular withdrawal bleeding is necessary to prevent endometrial hyperplasia and the risk of malignancy. It is now possible to provide women with Turner's syndrome with fertility through ovum donation, although the shortage of oocytes remains an important and usually critically limiting factor.

Table 1 *Causes of primary amenorrhoea in 90 consecutive cases seen in the author's clinics*

Cause	Percentage
Premature (primary) ovarian failure	36
Hypogonadotrophic hypogonadism	34
Polycystic ovary syndrome	17
Hypopituitarism	4
Congenital anomalies	4
Hyperprolactinaemia	3
Weight-related amenorrhoea	2

Table 2 *Causes of secondary amenorrhoea in 570 consecutive cases seen in the author's clinics*

Cause	Percentage
Polycystic ovary syndrome	36
Premature (primary) ovarian failure	24
Hyperprolactinaemia	17
Weight-related amenorrhoea	10
Hypogonadotrophic hypogonadism	6
Hypopituitarism	4
Exercise-related amenorrhoea	3

Hypothalamic causes of amenorrhoea

Hypothalamic hypogonadotrophic hypogonadism may be functional or organic, and occur in an isolated form or in association with more widespread endocrine defects, as in patients with infiltrating (sarcoidosis, tuberculosis), expanding (craniopharyngioma), or traumatic (head injury) lesions of the hypothalamus. Since high-definition magnetic resonance imaging has become available, lesions of the pituitary stalk, which may interfere with transport of releasing hormones from the hypothalamus to the pituitary, are increasingly recognized (Fig. 1). The clinical picture obviously depends upon the age of presentation and can therefore be with primary or secondary amenorrhoea.

KALLMANN'S SYNDROME

Isolated deficiency of secretion of gonadotrophin releasing hormone (GnRH) occurs in Kallmann's syndrome of hypogonadotrophic hypogonadism associated with hyposmia and sometimes colour blindness. Other defects, such as unilateral renal agenesis and a disorder of movement (hereditary bimanual synkinesis), may be associated.

Kallmann's syndrome occurs sporadically and as an inherited condition, of which the X-linked recessive form is the commonest. The nerve cells that synthesize GnRH originate embryologically in the epithelium of the medial olfactory placode, an ectodermally derived structure located outside the central nervous system. These neurones migrate along the cranial nerve 1 system of fibres that extends from the nasal mucosa through the cribriform plate and, by the 15th week of intrauterine life, enter the olfactory bulb, the anterior olfactory nucleus, and the arcuate nucleus of the hypothalamus. Deletions have been identified in the distal part of the short arm of the X chromosome in a gene that encodes a molecule with significant similarities to proteins involved in neural cell adhesion and axonal path-finding. X-linked Kallmann's syndrome is thus thought to arise from a genetically determined defect of the embryonic migration of olfactory and GnRH-producing neurones from the anlage of the olfactory lobes into the hypothalamus. The cause in non-X-linked Kallmann's syndrome is not yet known.

The condition presents with delayed puberty and primary amenorrhoea. Characteristically the patient cannot smell curry or the difference between tea and coffee. There are signs of marked oestrogen deficiency, usually amounting to sexual infantilism. Overall, the stature of adults with Kallmann's syndrome is normal, although the patient will not have experienced a pubertal growth spurt so skeletal proportions are abnormal.

Investigations reveal subnormal serum gonadotrophin and oestradiol concentrations. Ultrasound of the pelvis shows the small uterus and ovaries, and bone densitometry reveals marked skeletal demineralization (Fig. 2).

Management involves induction of pubertal maturation, initially with small doses of oestrogen (not more than 5 μg/day of ethinyl oestradiol) to optimize breast development. Delay in recognition and treatment impairs full development. Surgical referral for breast augmentation is appropriate if the patient considers development inadequate after a year's treatment with gradually increasing doses of oestrogen. Maintenance hormone treatment is with an oral contraceptive preparation. Bone densitometry should be repeated after a year to ensure that the dose of oestrogen is adequate (an increase of 5–6 per cent/year for 2–3 years should be obtained). Treatment with pulsatile GnRH or gonadotrophin injections allows an excellent prognosis for fertility.

FUNCTIONAL HYPOGONADOTROPHIC HYPOGONADISM

Weight-related amenorrhoea

Adequate nutrition is required for normal growth and development. Stored energy in the form of a body fat content of more than 17 per cent seems necessary for intact reproductive function. When, for any reason, body fat content falls below that figure, amenorrhoea is usual: depending on the age of onset, the patient may present with primary or secondary amenorrhoea. In clinical terms, a body mass index (normal range 20–

Fig. 1 MRI scan of sarcoid infiltration of the pituitary stalk in a patient with mild hyperprolactinaemia and hypogonadotrophic hypogonadism. (a) Sagittal view; (b) lateral view.

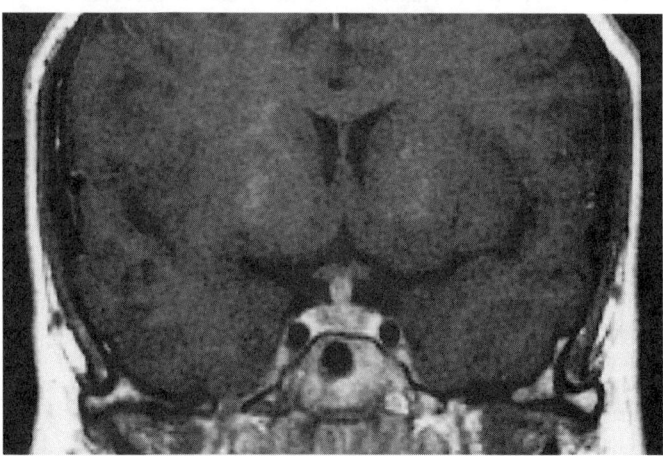

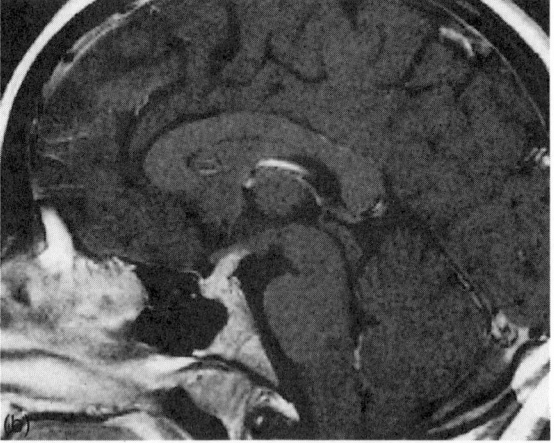

25 kg/m²) below 19 is usually associated with amenorrhoea. This figure assumes an average amount of exercise; for competitive athletes, particularly in track events, the figure would be higher.

The neuroendocrine mechanisms underlying the necessity for this critical degree of nutritional reserve are uncertain, but centre on impaired secretion of gonadotrophins, particularly luteinizing hormone, together with reduced insulin and insulin-like growth factor I levels and therefore lowered insulin drive to the ovaries and pituitary. The consequent anovulation is protective because it avoids the occurrence of reproduction in adverse circumstances. In addition to evidence of premature delivery of immature babies to women who are underweight, information is now emerging of a link between deficient fetal nutrition and the prevalence in adults of cardiovascular and pulmonary disease.

Self-imposed starvation

The cause of the weight loss is often anorexia nervosa (Chapter 10.4). Some women also lose weight as a feature of the anorexia of depression, occasioned perhaps by the break-up of a relationship; in this condition the patient does lose her appetite. The prognosis for a return of spontaneous menstrual cycles is then much better than that in women with anorexia nervosa.

Exercise related amenorrhoea

Amenorrhoea is common in ballet dancers and high-performance athletes, particularly during phases of intensive training and performance. The amenorrhoea is associated with reduced body weight and body fat content but is not common in competitive swimmers, who have a normal body fat content.

Involuntary starvation

World-wide, the most important causes of starvation are famine, war, and social disintegration. The deleterious physical effects of starvation

Fig. 2 Vertebral bone mineral density measurements in 200 young women with amenorrhoea, arranged by diagnosis. With the exception of the bone mineral density measurements in the women with polycystic ovary syndrome, the bone mineral density measurements of all other groups were significantly below those of the controls.

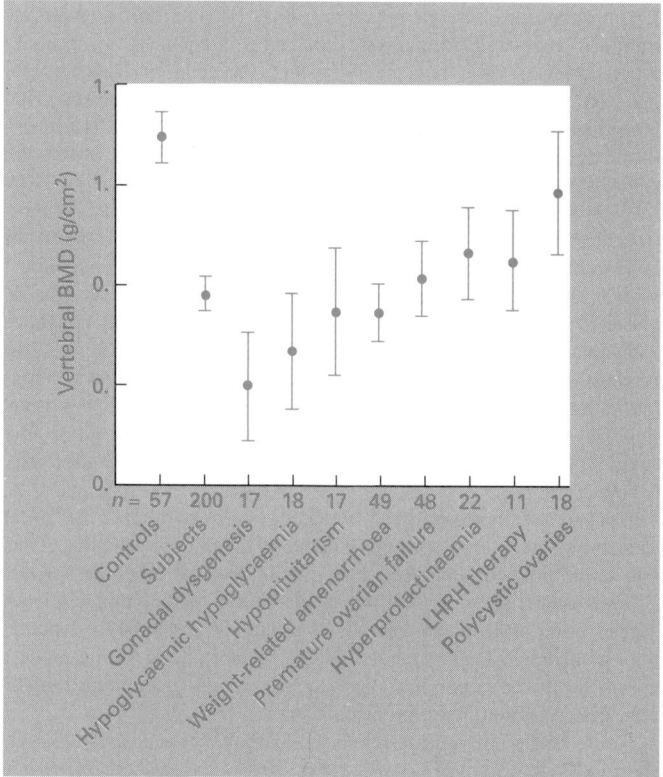

are passed on to the next generation, *inter alia*, through the adverse effects of fetal malnutrition on adult health.

Altered absorption

In patients with malabsorption, for instance in women with cystic fibrosis, amenorrhoea is associated with reduced body mass index and body fat content, and resolves when nutrition improves.

Investigation of weight-related amenorrhoea

The diagnosis is made not only by observation that the patient's weight is subnormal for her height (bearing in mind the effect of high performance training on replacing body fat with more dense muscle) but also by exclusion, because self-imposed weight loss is common in young women and may coexist with other conditions.

Women with weight-related amenorrhoea have subnormal serum gonadotrophin (particularly luteinizing hormone (LH)) and oestradiol concentrations, with small ovaries and a small uterus on ultrasound scanning. Skeletal demineralization is the rule, except in those with coexisting polycystic ovaries (see below).

Management involves explanation, identification of psychiatric conditions for which specialist advice is needed, and correction of oestrogen deficiency. Optimally the latter is achieved through weight gain alone. Oestrogen deficiency may, however, be so severe that if the patient is unable to put on weight, it may be advisable for her to take oestrogen in the form of an oral contraceptive. When the question of fertility is concerned, however, induction of ovulation using drugs should be eschewed until the patient's weight has returned to normal to avoid nutritional risks to the unborn child (and adult). In the event, when a normal body mass index is regained, induction of ovulation is rarely required.

Pituitary causes of amenorrhoea

HYPERPROLACTINAEMIA

While a non-functioning pituitary tumour sometimes causes amenorrhoea, the commonest pituitary cause is hypersecretion of prolactin. Hyperprolactinaemia may be caused by a prolactinoma, by a non-functioning pituitary tumour that compresses the pituitary stalk or hypothalamus, by dopaminergic antagonist drugs (phenothiazines, metoclopramide, and domperidone are the most frequent), by primary hypothyroidism, or it may be idiopathic. Prolactinomas account for about 60 per cent of cases of hyperprolactinaemia, the exact proportion depending on the sensitivity of the method of investigation. The mechanism by which hyperprolactinaemia causes amenorrhoea is through suppression of pulsatile gonadotrophin secretion.

Hyperprolactinaemia produces a characteristic syndrome: amenorrhoea is associated with severe oestrogen deficiency, with symptoms of vaginal atrophy (dryness and discomfort during intercourse) but almost never with the flushing and sweating attacks that occur at the menopause. Typically the patient complains of loss of libido. Galactorrhoea is uncommon, presumably because the prolactin is acting on breasts that have not been prepared for lactation by the endocrine changes of pregnancy. Serum gonadotrophin concentrations are in the low–normal range, the oestradiol level in the postmenopausal range; the ultrasound shows small ovaries and a small uterus. Skeletal demineralization may be severe (Fig. 2).

In patients with prolactinoma there is a good correlation of the serum prolactin concentration with the volume of the pituitary tumour. Thus with serum prolactin concentrations of 1000 to 4000 mU/l the MRI or CT scan usually shows a (micro)adenoma of less than 10 mm diameter. Higher serum prolactin concentrations usually imply a macroadenoma, often with suprasellar extension. A large pituitary fossa with a modest rise of the prolactin concentration suggests a non-functioning tumour with 'disconnection' hyperprolactinaemia.

The treatment of hyperprolactinaemia in the first instance is medical, using dopaminergic agonists. These agents suppress hyperprolactinaemia, permit return of pulsatile gonadotrophin secretion and thus evolution of ovulatory menstrual cycles, and, most importantly, they cause shrinkage of the prolactinoma. The drug of first choice is bromocriptine, which, if started in low doses and taken with food, is usually well tolerated. Side-effects, which usually disappear quite rapidly, include nausea and vomiting, if the drug is taken on an empty stomach, and postural hypotension. In the longer term the patient may complain of nasal stuffiness, constipation, and cold sensitivity of the extremities. Treatment is initiated with half a tablet (1.25 mg) at night with food and the dose gradually raised every few days to a usual dose of 2.5 mg three times a day. Further adjustments are titrated against the serum prolactin concentration. In patients with macroprolactinomas, particularly those with suprasellar extension, it is prudent to repeat the MRI or CT scan 12 weeks after the serum prolactin concentration has returned to normal.

Because the pituitary normally enlarges during pregnancy, in patients with macroprolactinomas conception should be delayed until there is radiological proof that any suprasellar expansion has resolved. Treatment with bromocriptine is discontinued as soon as the patient conceives; although teratogenicity has not been reported, the drug is administered during pregnancy only in the event of pituitary expansion. Such expansion has become rare in the decade since the above protocol of management was devised. In patients not wishing to conceive, bromocriptine should be administered to prevent growth of the prolactinoma and to permit re-oestrogenization and the return of normal libido. Co-treatment with an oral contraceptive to avoid pregnancy is acceptable, but requires that the serum prolactin concentration be monitored twice yearly as oestrogen treatment may elevate prolactin levels and encourage growth of a prolactinoma. In the author's experience, so long as bromocriptine is co-administered, such an adverse outcome has not occurred.

For patients intolerant of bromocriptine, alternative dopamine agonists such as pergolide, lisuride, metergoline, or carbergoline may be tried. Surgical extirpation, via the trans-sphenoidal route, is recommended for patients intolerant of medication (about 10 per cent of cases), or in the rare situation where the tumour is resistant to treatment. External radiotherapy is only recommended in the postoperative management of the patient with persistent hyperprolactinaemia that is resistant to medication and in the exceedingly rare case of malignant prolactinoma.

Ovarian causes of amenorrhoea

PRIMARY OVARIAN FAILURE

Primary ovarian failure occurs normally at the menopause ('age-appropriate primary ovarian failure') because of the process of atresia (Fig. 3) that results in almost complete depletion of oocytes and follicles by about the age of 50. If the rate of atresia is faster than normal, the causes of which are discussed below, depletion of oocytes and follicles occurs prematurely and 'age-inappropriate' or 'premature' ovarian failure develops.

Oocytes do not divide once they have been laid down in the ovary. Thus, unlike the testis, the ovary has a finite complement of germ cells. Oocytes 'used' in the process of ovulation account for a minute proportion of those that are lost, and it can be seen from Fig. 3 that most atresia occurs during intrauterine life when endocrine influences are least important. The process of atresia is controlled genetically. Loss of the second X chromosome, as in 45 XO Turner's syndrome, and destruction of genetic material by ionizing irradiation or anticancer chemotherapy are therefore predicted causes of premature ovarian failure (Table 3). Viral infections, such as mumps oophoritis, and the accumulation of compounds such as galactose and its metabolites (as in galactosaemia) can damage the ovary directly. The association of premature ovarian failure with autoimmune disorders such as thyroiditis, adrenalitis, and diabetes mellitus, has led to the hypothesis that many cases are autoimmune in origin. While reliable tests are not widely available, autoantibodies to ovarian cells, oocytes, or gonadotrophin receptors have been reported in up to 80 per cent of cases of premature ovarian failure, a result consistent with the author's finding of thyroid and adrenal auto-antibodies in almost half of the patients remaining after those with chromosomal causes had been excluded. Finally, the presence in the follicular fluid of toxic pollutants from tobacco smoke, such as cotinine, a cogener of nicotine, may account for the earlier menopause that occurs in women who smoke cigarettes.

The symptoms of primary ovarian failure are those of oestrogen deficiency, together with infertility. Investigation reveals raised serum gonadotrophin and subnormal oestradiol concentrations. While the serum LH is often elevated in patients with polycystic ovary syndrome, a rise in the follicle stimulating hormone (FSH) concentration always suggests primary ovarian failure. Autoantibodies should be sought as their presence alerts the clinician to the possible development of pluriglandular endocrine failure. Pelvic ultrasound shows undetectable or small ovaries and a small uterus. Bone densitometry usually reveals significant demineralization.

Patients with premature ovarian failure usually require hormone replacement therapy, the indications, precautions, etc. being the same as those for age-appropriate primary ovarian failure. In some women there may be a spontaneous return of ovulatory menstrual cycles, albeit usually temporary, and therefore pregnancies do sometimes occur. Treatment with glucocorticoids or immunolytic drugs for women with autoimmune ovarian failure has occasionally proven successful, but formal controlled trials are lacking and this treatment cannot be recommended. The ovaries do not respond to further stimulation with gonadotrophins and so the only chance of childbearing for most of these women is through ovum donation. The problems of supplies of donor oocytes are formidable.

RESISTANT OVARY SYNDROME

This ill-defined syndrome refers to women with amenorrhoea and elevated serum gonadotrophin concentrations in whom, paradoxically, oestrogen levels are well maintained. The persistent secretion of oestradiol

Table 3 *Causes of primary ovarian failure in 320 cases seen in the author's clinics*

Cause	Number	Percentage
Idiopathic	169	52.6
Turner's syndrome	73	22.7
Autoimmune disease*	22	6.9
Anticancer chemotherapy	21	6.5
'Resistant ovaries'	10	3.1
Surgery	7	2.2
Radiotherapy	6	1.9
Galactosaemia	6	1.9
Familial	3	0.9
Miscellaneous	4	1.2

*Sixteen had primary hypothyroidism and six had Addison's disease. Three of these patients had diabetes mellitus.

suggests persistence of ovarian follicular activity, an implication confirmed by ultrasound assessment of the ovaries or occasionally by histology and by the occasional and unpredictable occurrence of pregnancy. The ovaries do not respond to further stimulation with exogenous gonadotrophins. While both cause and prognosis remain obscure, the condition is most easily understood as a transitional phase on the way to primary ovarian failure—in effect, a premature perimenopause.

POLYCYSTIC OVARY SYNDROME

A full description of polycystic ovary syndrome is given later. Its clinical expression, typically dating from the time of puberty, involves a menstrual disorder (usually oligomenorrhoea but amenorrhoea in 26 per cent of cases), hyperandrogenization, and weight increase. Many women with polycystic ovary syndrome are hyperinsulinaemic and there is a strong correlation of the interval between menstrual periods and the fasting serum insulin concentration (see below). Since a major determinant of insulin secretion is obesity, the deterioration of menstrual cyclicity with weight increase and its improvement with weight loss is readily understood. The pubertal onset of menstrual chaos that typifies so many patients with polycystic ovary syndrome may be a consequence of the increased insulin secretion that characterizes these years.

Women with amenorrhoea caused by polycystic ovary syndrome are not oestrogen deficient (Fig. 2) because of the extraovarian conversion of (excessive) ovarian androgens to oestrogens, mainly in fat tissue but also in liver and bone marrow. Indeed, endometrial hyperplasia (which in its severe form is a precursor of endometrial carcinoma) may complicate the amenorrhoea. It may be suspected by finding a thickened endometrium at ultrasound and requires treatment by induction of menstrual shedding with cyclical progestogens. Curettage is required if the thickening persists despite hormonal treatment.

The diagnosis of polycystic ovary syndrome is described below.

The indications for treatment of amenorrhoea in women with polycystic ovary syndrome depend upon the patient's needs. For women who wish to conceive, induction of ovulation is required, combined with attempts to reduce insulin drive to the ovaries by diet and exercise. For women needing contraception, an oestrogen–progestagen pill is appropriate, the choice of preparation depending on the degree of associated unwanted hair. The oral contraceptive is also appropriate for women troubled by the lack or unpredictability of menstruation. For the remainder, it is acceptable to remain amenorrhoeic, provided annual ultrasound scans of the endometrium show that overstimulation has not occurred.

Investigation of amenorrhoea

The patient's stature, her nutritional status, the presence of unwanted hair (male pattern or the lanugo of anorexia nervosa) or acanthosis nigri-

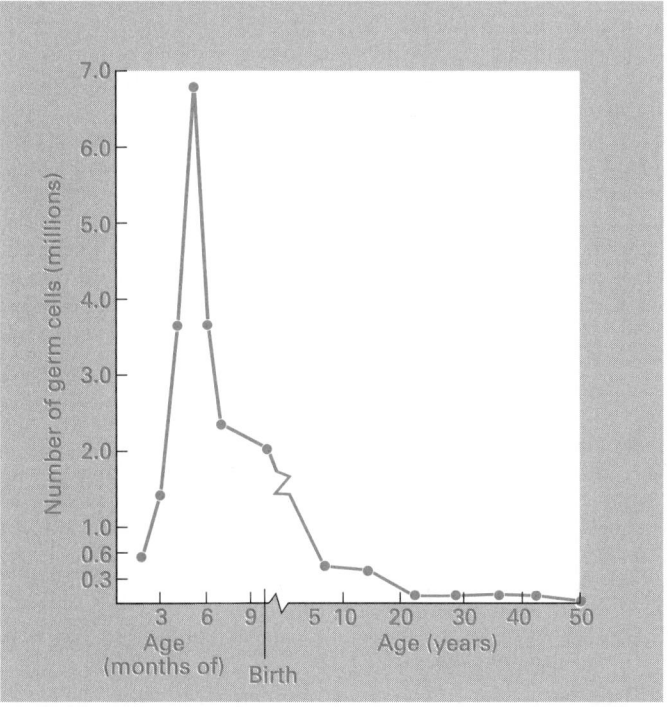

Fig. 3 The number of oocytes in the gonads in relation to age. Note that the maximum rate of atresia occurs before birth. (After Baker, T.G. (1963). *Proceedings of the Royal Society (Biology)*, **158**, 417.)

cans, and the physical stigmata of oestrogen deficiency are important parts of the physical examination. Pelvic ultrasound reveals the ovarian dimensions and whether they have the characteristic internal echoes of polycystic ovaries. Ultrasonic examination of the uterus, its size and degree of endometrial thickening provides a biological assessment of the impact of oestrogen. Hormone assays reveal subnormal serum oestradiol levels associated with elevated (primary ovarian failure) or subnormal (hypogonadotrophic hypogonadism) gonadotrophin concentrations. Assessment of white blood cell karyotype and measurement of autoantibodies is undertaken in patients with primary ovarian failure. Bone densitometry may reveal significant demineralization of spine and hips. Radiological assessment of the pituitary is undertaken in patients with hyperprolactinaemia.

Treatment of amenorrhoea

In addition to correcting the cause whenever possible, management is directed at minimizing the consequences of long-term oestrogen deficiency. When the cause cannot be corrected, oestrogen replacement therapy, usually in the form of an oral contraceptive, is appropriate. Outcome should be monitored by ensuring that sufficient oestrogen is administered to cause withdrawal bleeds and that there is an improvement in bone density if skeletal demineralization has been demonstrated.

Hyperandrogenization

Normal hair growth and androgen production in women

At birth the fetus is covered in lanugo hair which rapidly disappears and is not seen again unless anorexia nervosa develops, although very rarely such hair appears as a non-metastatic complication of malignancy. The follicles in the skin of prepubertal children grow soft, short and fair vellus hair, which, together with scalp, eyebrow, and eyelash hair, is known as non-sexual hair. In response to the secretion of adrenal androgens at puberty, both boys and girls develop terminal hair in the axillae and lower pubic triangle (ambosexual hair). Terminal hair is long, pigmented, and coarse. In boys the further increase of (testicular) androgen secretion leads to the development of terminal hair in the upper pubic triangle and on the face, chest, abdomen, and arms and legs—that is, male-pattern hair.

Perception of hairiness depends in part on its distribution and in part on its character and pigmentation. While there is racial variation in the density of hair follicles (native Americans and Orientals having few and

Fig. 4 Sources of androgens in normal women.

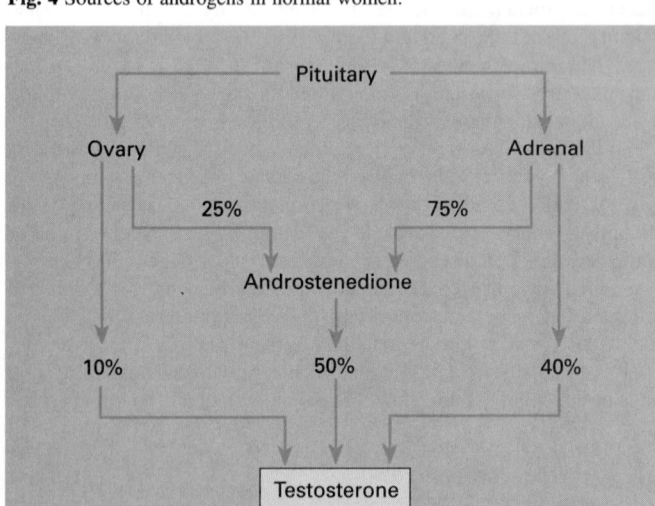

women from the Mediterranean littoral having many follicles per unit area of skin), it is the development of male-pattern hair in women which constitutes hirsutism.

The sources of androgens in normal women are shown in Fig. 4, from which it can be seen that 50 per cent of directly secreted and 75 per cent of peripherally derived testosterone normally originate from the adrenal cortex. Thus in women it is adrenal rather than gonadal failure that is associated with loss of secondary sexual hair. Testosterone circulates specifically bound to sex hormone binding globulin (SHBG), from which it disassociates and diffuses into target tissues, where it is either 5α reduced to a more powerful androgen, dihydrotestosterone or aromatized to oestradiol. The dihydrotestosterone–nuclear protein receptor complex associates with its specific DNA receptor to cause androgen-specific protein synthesis and the expression of androgen action.

Synthesis of SHBG, whose concentration largely determines the total serum testosterone concentration, takes place in the liver, stimulated by thyroxine and inhibited by insulin and to a lesser extent by androgens. The rate of clearance of SHBG is reduced by oestrogen.

Clinical hyperandrogenization

Hyperandrogenization in women is manifest as seborrhoea, persistent acne, and the development of a male pattern of distribution and quality of hair. Male-pattern scalp hair loss may also occur, particularly in women with male family members who are bald. Clitoromegaly and increased muscle bulk are signs of severe and usually long-standing overexposure to androgens.

Although defects in adrenal steroid biosynthesis (congenital and late-onset adrenal hyperplasia), Cushing's syndrome, and adrenal androgen-secreting tumours may all cause oversecretion of androgens, and therefore present with hirsutism, the commonest cause by far is polycystic ovary syndrome, in which condition there is an increase in the direct ovarian secretion of androgens.

POLYCYSTIC OVARY SYNDROME

Polycystic ovaries are readily identified by pelvic ultrasound, because they are larger than normal (average volume three times that of normal ovaries) and have a highly echo-dense central stroma in which cysts of 6 to 8 mm diameter are arranged around the circumference (Fig. 5). When ovaries with this appearance are detected in women complaining of specific symptoms, the term polycystic ovary syndrome is used (Table 4). Defined in this way, the polycystic ovary syndrome corresponds to the condition described over 50 years ago by Stein and Leventhal.

Patients with this condition commonly present in their late teens or early twenties, complaining of the consequences of hyperandrogenization or of a menstrual disturbance (Table 5). There is often a family history of similar complaints, but even when that is absent an ultrasound scan usually reveals polycystic ovaries in the patient's mother or sister. Infertility is caused by failure of ovulation, although hypersecretion of LH is also important in this regard. Obesity, often associated with an increase in the ratio of waist to hip circumference, is the third classical feature. The nature of its association with the polycystic ovary syndrome is uncertain, but it has adverse effects on most of the clinical manifestations.

Endocrine features

The classical profile is of hypersecretion of LH and androgens, with normal circulating FSH, prolactin, and thyroxine concentrations. The heterogeneity of the syndrome is reflected by a spectrum of endocrine disorders. In more than 1500 personally studied cases, 44 per cent had an elevated serum LH and 22 per cent an elevated serum total testosterone concentration. Levels of LH were raised most commonly in the women complaining of infertility, and of testosterone in those complaining of hirsutism (Fig. 6a, b).

The nature of the primary disturbance underlying these findings is uncertain. A central problem is a failure of the polycystic ovary to convert androgens, made in excessive amounts by the abundant theca and interstitial cells of the hyperplastic ovarian stroma, into oestrogens. The androgens (predominantly androstenedione and testosterone) are then released into the circulation and converted in the skin to dihydrotestosterone. In liver and fat tissue, they are converted into oestrogens at a rate which increases with the degree of obesity. The high levels of oestrogen (predominantly oestrone) inhibit secretion of FSH and may stimulate secretion of LH. The former effect contributes to persistent anovulation and the consequent lack of progesterone (which in the normal luteal phase limits the proliferative action of oestradiol) means that the action on the uterus of the normally weak oestrogen oestrone is unopposed. These patients are consequently at risk from endometrial hyperplasia and neoplasia. The raised levels of LH stimulate the excessive numbers of theca and interstitial cells to oversecrete androgens. In addition, it is thought that exposure of the ovaries to high levels of LH at inappropriate times of the cycle impairs fertility through an action on the developing oocyte.

The above model, which imputes a central role for the ovary, incorporates many of the clinical features of the polycystic ovary syndrome. It does not, however, explain its variable clinical presentation. It is likely that environmental factors, such as the development of obesity, or of a medical condition such as acromegaly or Cushing's syndrome, leads to expression of the underlying, probably inherited, condition.

Many patients with the polycystic ovary syndrome, particularly those who are anovulatory, hypersecrete insulin in association with variable degrees of insulin resistance. Three types of insulin resistance in patients with polycystic ovary syndrome are presently recognized. Type A results from one of a number of mutations in the gene that encodes the insulin receptor. The consequence is a defect in transmission of the insulin signal anywhere along the pathway from the extracellular binding of insulin to its target tissue, to phosphorylation of the intracellular receptor-associated tyrosine kinase. Type B results from circulating autoantibodies to the extracellular domain of the insulin receptor. Type C insulin resistance, probably mediated by postreceptor defects, is by

Fig. 5 Transabdominal ultrasound image of polycystic ovary. Note the enlarged ovary with the echo-dense central stroma and the necklace of cysts around the circumference.

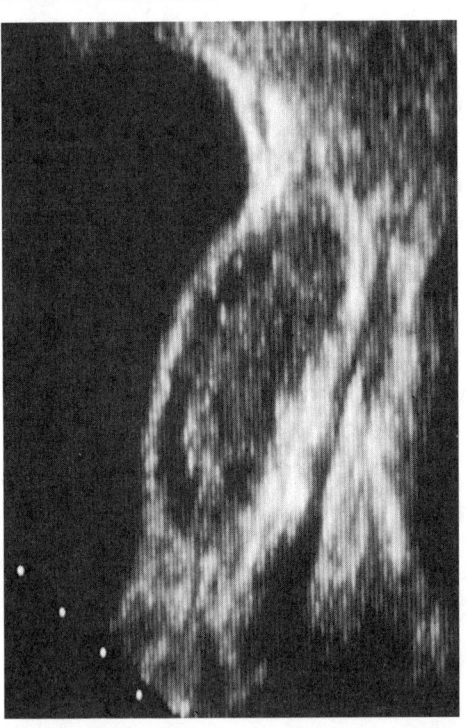

Table 4 *Diagnosis of polycystic ovary syndrome*

Ultrasound	Presence of polycystic ovaries Enlarged ovaries Ten or more cysts (6–8 mm) arranged around the periphery Echodense central stroma
Clinical	Presence of polycystic ovaries together with characteristic symptomatology Menstrual disturbance Hyperandrogenization Obesity

Table 5 *Clinical features in 1500 patients with ultrasound-diagnosed polycystic ovaries seen in the author's clinics*

	Percentage
Skin and appendages	
Hirsutism	61
Acne	24
Alopecia	8
Acanthosis nigricans	5
Menstrual cycle	
Normal cycle	25
Oligomenorrhoea	45
Amenorrhoea	26
Frequent cycles	3
Menorrhagia	1
Fertility status	
Untested	67
Primary infertility	20
Secondary infertility	9
Proven fertility	4
Body weight	
Body mass index less than 20	13
Body mass index 20–25 (normal)	52
Body mass index over 25	35

Note: Some patients had more than one symptom, so the figures do not add up to 100 per cent.

far the commonest and is the form associated with obesity. The clinical clue to the presence of severe hyperinsulinism is the presence of acanthosis nigricans (Plate 1).

Excessive insulin secretion occupies a central role in expression of the polycystic ovary syndrome. Thus receptors for insulin and insulin-like growth factor I have been identified in the ovary, and their stimulation sensitizes the ovary to stimulation by gonadotrophins, observations that may provide insight into the deleterious effects of obesity because, as body weight rises, secretion of insulin increases further. Although insulin receptors are down-regulated by exposure to persistently high levels of insulin, there is experimental evidence that receptors for the insulin-like growth factors, which can be activated by insulin, are maintained. In the polycystic ovary syndrome, when both the ovaries and the secretion of insulin are abnormal, the potential for an adverse interaction is considerable.

Hypersecretion of insulin inhibits hepatic synthesis of sex hormone binding globulin which, particularly in obese patients, results in an apparent disparity between circulating testosterone concentrations and the degree of hirsutism. In these women the concentration of unbound testosterone, and by implication the testosterone production rate, is very high despite serum total testosterone concentrations which may be within the normal range. Hypersecretion of insulin also has non-reproductive adverse effects in patients with polycystic ovary syndrome. Thus, an inverse relation of the cardioprotective HDL2 cholesterol concentration and the fasting serum insulin concentration has been demonstrated together with subnormal total high density lipoprotein concentrations (Fig. 7). These data, together with reports of high rates of coronary heart disease, hypertension, and diabetes in follow-up studies of patients with histologically verified polycystic ovaries, indicate the clinical importance of hypersecretion of insulin and its control in patients with polycystic ovary syndrome.

Other ovarian causes of hirsutism

HYPERTHECOSIS

Characterized pathologically by the presence of islands of luteinized theca cells within the ovarian stroma at a distance from follicles, the clinical features include very marked hypersecretion of androgens and of insulin. The condition is probably most easily regarded as a severe form of the polycystic ovary syndrome.

OVARIAN TUMOURS

Androgen-secreting tumours of the ovary are derived from sex cord or stromal cells and include Sertoli–Leydig cell tumours (arrhenoblastomas), hilar cell tumours, lipoid cell tumours, and adrenal rest tumours. Other non-hormone-secreting tumours (Brenner, cystadenoma, and cyst-

adenocarcinoma) have been reported to stimulate androgen secretion by the surrounding ovarian stroma. These conditions are all very rare causes of hirsutism.

Diagnosis of hyperandrogenism

Adrenal causes of hyperandrogenization include congenital and late-onset enzyme deficiencies, Cushing's syndrome, and adrenal tumours. Congenital adrenal hyperplasia is suggested by short stature and a history of surgery to the external genitalia in infancy and confirmed by measurement of steroid precursors (see Chapter 12.7.2). Cushing's syndrome is suspected clinically. Adrenal carcinoma is a rare and sinister cause of hirsutism, usually presenting with Cushing's syndrome and severe and progressive virilism. The serum testosterone is in the male range and the serum dehydroepiandrosterone sulphate concentration is very high. CT or MRI scanning confirms the diagnosis.

The vast majority of cases of hyperandrogenization are caused by direct hypersecretion of androgens by polycystic ovaries. While an ovarian tumour is suggested by a short history of rapidly advancing hirsutism, amenorrhoea, and a serum testosterone concentration in the male range, such lesions are rare; indeed, a serum testosterone concentration exceeding 10 nmol/l is more commonly associated with polycystic ovary syndrome and severe insulin resistance than with the development of an ovarian tumour.

All patients require careful assessment by pelvic ultrasound to diagnose polycystic ovaries and exclude solid or expanding lesions in the adnexae. The serum total testosterone concentration reflects in part the testosterone production rate, and in part the serum sex hormone binding globulin concentration; it should be interpreted in light of the patient's body weight, and a concentration within the normal range should not therefore be dismissed in women who are overweight. Serum LH concentrations are often raised, but the FSH level is normal. Serum prolactin concentrations are modestly elevated (up to 2500 mU/l) in 15 per cent of patients with polycystic ovary syndrome.

A small number of patients with hirsutism (fewer than 5 per cent in the author's experience) have no diagnosable cause of their cutaneous virilism. Labelled 'idiopathic hirsutism', these patients may have enhanced sensitivity of androgen-dependent tissues, perhaps caused by increased dermal activity of the 5α-reductase enzyme.

Fig. 6 (a) Serum luteinizing hormone concentrations in women with polycystic ovary syndrome complaining of infertility. Note that, using a standard radioimmunoassay with a normal range up to 10 IU/l, as the luteinizing hormone concentration rises above normal the proportion of women complaining of infertility rises from about 20 per cent to about 35 per cent. (b) The proportion of women complaining of hirsutism in relation to the serum testosterone concentration. Note that as the serum testosterone rises so the proportion complaining of hirsutism doubles.

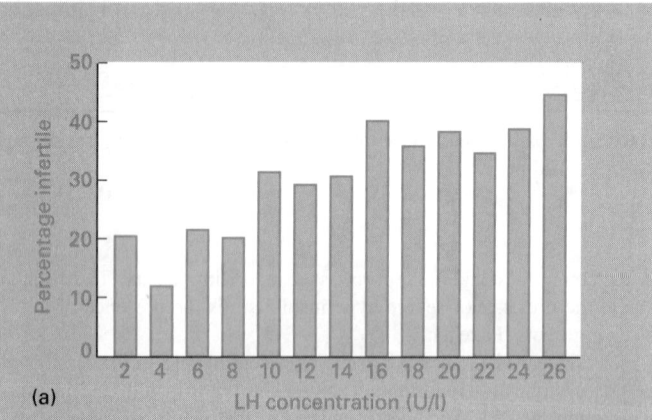

(a)

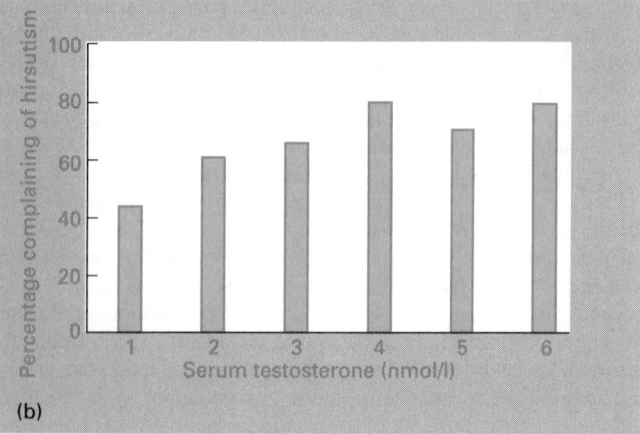

(b)

Fig. 7 Serum high density lipoprotein (HDL) concentrations in lean and obese women with polycystic ovary syndrome (PCOS). Note that despite maintaining a normal body mass index, slim women with polycystic ovary syndrome have a statistically significant depression of their fasting HDL cholesterol concentration. The HDL falls even further in women with polycystic ovary syndrome who are obese.

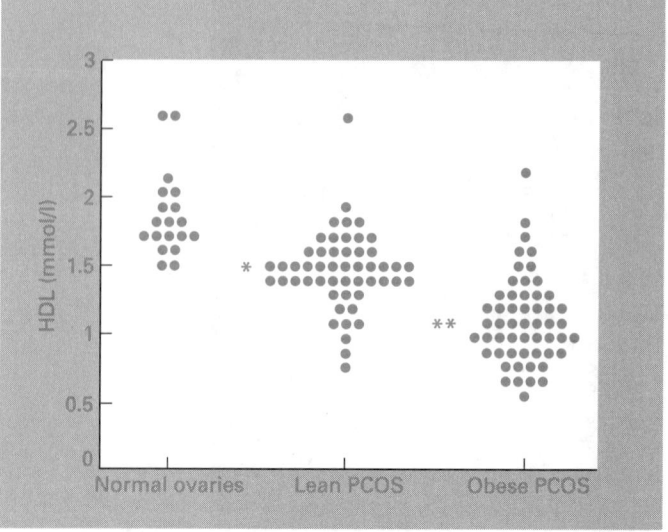

Management of hirsutism

The management of patients with the polycystic ovary syndrome is determined by the patient's priorities: thus the control of hirsutism requires suppression, and the treatment of infertility, stimulation, of the ovaries, so the patient herself has to decide which complaint to deal with first. In both cases, however, the adverse effects of hypersecretion of insulin must be recognized and so, in addition to any medication, attempts must be made to increase exercise and reduce body weight.

The preferred drug treatment of hyperandrogenization is by administration of antiandrogens. Since the Committee on Safety of Medicines of the United Kingdom has advised against long-term use of spironolactone, except for certain specific indications, the most practical regimen is with cyproterone acetate. This steroid is a peripheral antiandrogen, a progestogen, and a mild glucocorticoid. In combination with oestrogen, it suppresses gonadotrophin secretion and so reduces the secretion of ovarian androgens. The combination is also contraceptive. The glucocorticoid activity of cyproterone acetate may reduce secretion of adrenal androgens. Finally, the drug blocks uptake of the dihydrotestosterone–protein complex by the DNA acceptor protein in the nucleus of androgen-sensitive cells, and so acts as a peripheral antiandrogen.

Treatment is administered cyclically, together with oestrogen, given most conveniently in the form of Dianette® (Fig. 8). Seborrhoea and acne usually clear up in about 6 weeks but it takes 12 to 18 months to realize the maximum improvement of unwanted hair. Cosmetic treatment is continued while on the medication, the impact of therapy being assessed by a reduction in the number of episodes of electrolysis required.

Adverse reactions, contraindications, and surveillance are essentially those advised for treatment with the birth control pill. However, with high doses of cyproterone acetate, such as those used in treatment of carcinoma of the prostate (200–300 mg per day continuously), adverse effects on the liver have been reported and it seems prudent, therefore, to check liver function tests twice yearly when substantial doses of cyproterone acetate are used. Such tests are not required when the low doses that are used in medications like Dianette are given. As symptoms remit, the dose of cyproterone acetate is reduced until the patient is taking the lowest dose compatible with symptomatic relief. Eventually, treatment with Dianette® alone is usually sufficient for maintenance. In patients not responding to this regimen, newer antiandrogens, such as flutamide, may be tried. Since pure antiandrogens are not contraceptive the patient must be warned of possible feminizing effects on a male fetus if they are taken inadvertently during pregnancy. They are therefore optimally prescribed with an oral contraceptive. It is anticipated that inhibitors of testosterone 5α reductase activity will soon become available for treatment of hirsutism.

Treatment with glucocorticoids is reserved for patients with evidence of adrenal oversecretion of androgens, such as congenital or late-onset adrenal enzyme deficiencies. Since treatment with glucocorticoids may worsen insulin resistance, their use in patients with polycystic ovary syndrome should be as sparing as possible.

Infertility

Infertility is a symptom, not a diagnosis. In terms of medical intervention its definition is a matter of convention (typically no conception after a year of unprotected intercourse) but it is most logically evaluated in relation to normal fertility. Thus the maximum conception rate per ovulation is 25 to 30 per cent, so that cumulative conception rates are usually about 60 per cent after 6 months and 85 per cent after a year. Other than mechanical bars to conception (for example gynaecological problems such as occluded Fallopian tubes), the important factors that reduce a woman's fertility are her age and any condition that reduces the number of ovulations per unit time. The central strategy of medical management of female infertility is therefore the diagnosis and treatment of anovulation. An additional strategy is to ensure that ovulation, and thus conception, occurs in as favourable an environment as possible.

Ovulation is only proven by the occurrence of pregnancy, so indirect methods of detection are required. In practice, ovulation is usually inferred retrospectively by detection of a corpus luteum, indexed endocrinologically either by measurement of serum progesterone concentrations or indirectly by the effects of progesterone on basal body temperature or endometrial histology, as revealed by endometrial biopsy. Ovulation can be predicted ultrasonically be detecting the development of a preovulatory follicle of average diameter 20–22 mm, followed by its collapse and replacement by a solid structure, i.e. visualization of a corpus luteum. The preovulatory surge of LH can be detected by the patient herself using one of a number of commercially available immunological urine tests. These methods are used to determine whether anovulation can account for a couple's infertility and whether treatment has actually resulted in ovulation; prediction of ovulation is helpful for timing investigations and maximizing the chance of conception by ensuring that intercourse occurs around the time of ovulation.

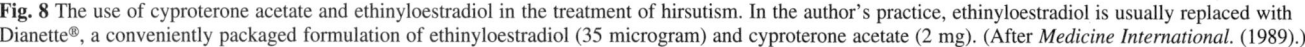

Fig. 8 The use of cyproterone acetate and ethinyloestradiol in the treatment of hirsutism. In the author's practice, ethinyloestradiol is usually replaced with Dianette®, a conveniently packaged formulation of ethinyloestradiol (35 microgram) and cyproterone acetate (2 mg). (After *Medicine International*. (1989).)

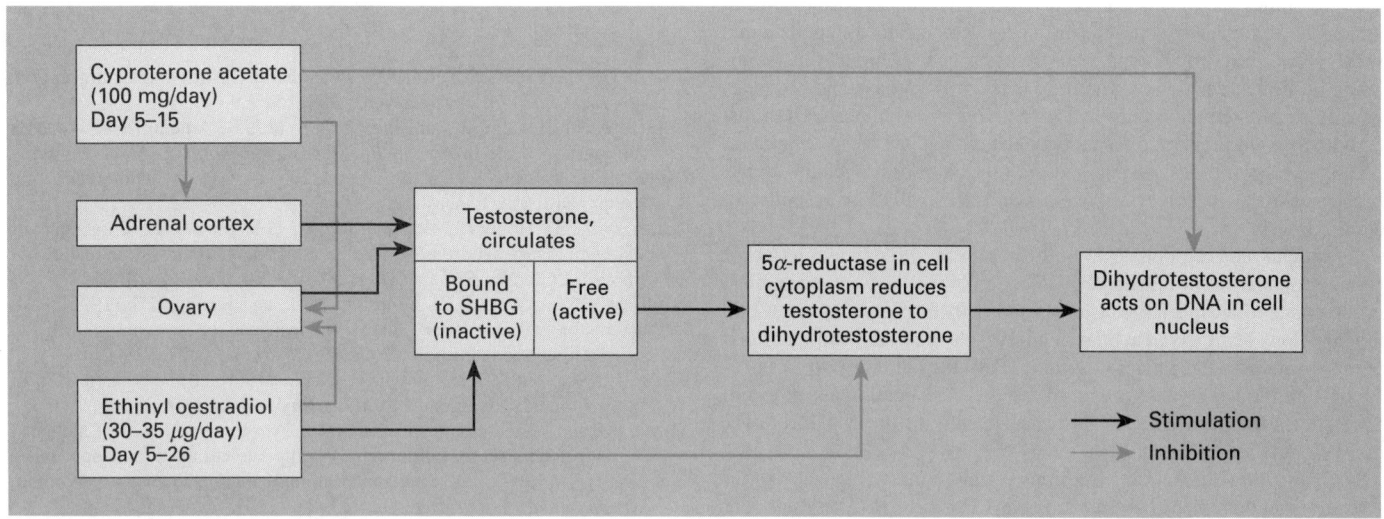

Table 6 *Induction of ovulation*

Hypothalamic level
  Enchance secretion of GnRH
    Weight increase
    Suppression of hyperprolactinaemia—bromocriptine,
      pituitary surgery
    Anti-oestrogens—clomiphene citrate, tamoxifen
  Replace secretion of GnRH
    Pulsatile GnRH therapy

Pituitary level:
  Enhance secretion of gonadotrophins
    Pulsatile GnRH therapy
  Replace gonadotrophins*
    Human menopausal gonadotrophin: 75 IU of FSH and 75
      IU of LH per ampoule
    Follitropin: 75 IU FSH, less than 0.4 IU LH per ampoule
    Human chorionic gonadotrophin: ampoule size varies

*More purified urinary extracts and recombinant versions of FSH and LH are now available.

FSH, follicle stimulating hormone; GnRH, gonadotrophin releasing hormone; LH, luteinizing hormone.

The most important factor determining normal fertility is the woman's age, conception rates after the age of 35 being half of those before the age of 25. Demographic changes in northern Europe (median maternal age at first birth in the United Kingdom is now 27 years) have resulted in a steady increase in the number of couples requesting consultations for infertility.

The causes of amenorrhoea are discussed above. All except primary ovarian failure are correctable (and that condition is treatable by oocyte donation) so the fertility prognosis for this group of patients is excellent. The commonest cause of oligomenorrhoea is polycystic ovary syndrome, and while patients with this condition usually ovulate readily in response to treatment, in about 40 per cent hypersecretion of LH impairs fertility, despite the occurrence (spontaneously or as a result of treatment) of otherwise normal ovulation. The mechanism is uncertain but may involve an adverse effect of the high levels of LH on completion of the final stages of oocyte maturation.

Failure to ovulate despite (more or less) regular menstrual cycles is an unusual but recognized cause of infertility.

Induction of ovulation

Table 6 shows the agents commonly used and the endocrine level at which they exert their actions. Anti-oestrogens enhance hypothalamic secretion of GnRH by competing with oestrogen receptors, thus simulating oestrogen deficiency. The drug is taken for 5 days and provokes gonadotrophin secretion and thence follicular development. The most commonly used preparation is clomiphene, which is a racemic mixture, one isomer having oestrogenic and the other anti-oestrogenic activity. Most patients with polycystic ovary syndrome ovulate in response to clomiphene.

In patients not responding to anti-oestrogens, pituitary secretion of gonadotrophins can be enhanced by injection of GnRH. Synthetic GnRH is administered in a pulsatile fashion, usually by the subcutaneous route, the injections being given at 90 min intervals by a portable miniaturized pump worn under the patient's clothing. Pulsatile administration is necessary to optimize gonadotrophin release because continuous exposure desensitizes the pituitary. The treatment results in the evolution of a normal ovulation cycle.

For patients with destructive lesions of the pituitary, gonadotrophin secretion can be replaced by injections of LH and FSH. At present, the preparations available are extracted from human urine and are either mixtures of equal amounts of FSH and LH bioactivity (human menopausal gonadotrophin) or compounds with varying ratios of bioactivity. Because of the substantial amounts of non-hormonal protein contained in the extracts, the injections are given by the intramuscular route. More purified preparations are available now; they, and those synthesized by recombinant technology, can be given by the subcutaneous route. Follicular development is induced by the injections of FSH and LH; ovulation is triggered and the corpus luteum is maintained by a single injection of human chorionic gonadotrophin (HCG) which has LH-like bioactivity and a very long half-life.

The objective of treatment is unifollicular ovulation with full-term delivery of a single infant. The response is monitored by ultrasound assessment of the ovaries and uterus and by measurement of plasma oestradiol concentrations. HCG is administered according to strict criteria (for example, by ultrasound not more than three follicles of diameter equal to or greater than 16 mm, or six follicles equal to or greater than 14 mm diameter). Complications include multiple birth (the perinatal mortality of twins is three times that of singletons) and the ovarian hyperstimulation syndrome. The latter condition, which occurs when treatment results in the growth of multiple large follicles followed by the development of follicular and luteal cysts, occurs almost entirely in women with polycystic ovary syndrome who have received high dose and inadequately monitored gonadotrophin therapy. It can be life-threatening.

Ovarian hyperstimulation syndrome results from massive follicular luteinization and so only occurs after ovulation has been triggered by HCG or, very rarely, by a spontaneous LH surge. Symptoms usually appear 5 to 10 days after administration of HCG. In its mildest form it consists of ovarian enlargement and discomfort but in the more severe forms abdominal distension, nausea, vomiting, and diarrhoea develop. As a result of increased vascular permeability, protein-rich fluid accumulates in the peritoneal and sometimes the thoracic cavity; hypovolaemia develops, associated with haemoconcentration, decreased central venous pressure, low blood pressure, and tachycardia. The patient develops tense ascites, respiration is embarrassed, and urine formation is suppressed. A hypercoagulable state may develop with the risk of cerebral and peripheral venous thrombosis and embolism.

In managing this syndrome, its self-limiting nature should be borne in mind. None the less hospitalization and careful observation is required if symptoms persist or worsen. Treatment is designed, first, to maintain blood volume (by monitoring the central venous pressure and infusing colloids) while correcting fluid and electrolyte balance (by infusing crystalloids, diuretics being harmful); second, to avoid thromboembolic phenomena (by full heparinization if severe hypercoagulability is detected); and, third, to relieve abdominal and pulmonary symptoms (by paracentesis under ultrasound control).

REFERENCES

Baird, D.T. and Glasier, A.F. (1993). Drug therapy: Hormonal contraception. *New England Journal of Medicine* **328**, 1543–9.

Balen, A.H., Shoham, Z., and Jacobs, H.S. (1993). Amenorrhoea – causes and consequences. In *Annual Progress in Reproductive Medicine 1993*, (ed. R.H. Asch and J.W.W. Studd), pp. 205–34. The Parthenon Publishing Group, Carnforth, Lancashire.

Conway, G.S., Honour, J.W., and Jacobs, H.S. (1989). Heterogeneity of polycystic ovary syndrome: clinical, endocrine and ultrasound features in 556 cases. *Clinical Endocrinology* **30**, 459–70.

Conway, G.S., Agrawal, R., Betteridge, D.J., and Jacobs, H.S. (1992). Risk factors for coronary artery disease in lean and obese women with the polycystic ovary syndrome. *Clinical Endocrinology* **37**, 119–26.

Davies, M.C., Hall, M.L., and Jacobs, H.S. (1990). Bone mineral loss in young women with amenorrhoea. *British Medical Journal* **301**, 790–3.

Insler, V. and Lunenfeld, B. (1993). *Infertility: male and female*, (2nd edn). Churchill Livingstone, Edinburgh. A complete and up-to-date account.

Jacobs, H.S. (1987). Polycystic ovaries and polycystic ovary syndrome. *Gynecological Endocrinology* **1**, 113–31.

Jacobs, H.S. and Homburg, R.R. (1990). The endocrinology of conception. *Ballière's Clinical Endocrinology and Metabolism* **4**, 195–205.

Regan, L., Owen, E.J., and Jacobs, H.S. (1990). Hypersecretion of LH, infertility and spontaneous abortion. *Lancet* **336**, 1141–2.

Shoham, Z., Homburg, R., and Jacobs, H.S. (1990). Induction of ovulation with pulsatile GnRH. *Ballière's Clinical Obstetrics and Gynaecology* **4**, 589–608.

Thaw, K.T. (1992). Hormone replacement therapy. *British Medical Bulletin* **48**, 240–476. A complete and authoritative account.

Wilson, J.D. and Foster, D.W. (1992). *Williams textbook of endocrinology*, (8th edn). W.B. Saunders, Philadelphia. The classic American text, exhaustive, up to date and strong on pathophysiology and basic mechanisms.

Yen, S.S.C. and Jaffe, R.B. (1991). *Reproductive endocrinology*, (3rd edn). W.B. Saunders, Philadelphia. A complete up-to-date textbook which is very strong on pathophysiology.

12.8.2 Disorders of male reproduction

F. C. W. WU

Physiology of the hypothalamic–pituitary–testicular axis

The adult testis subserves two functions—the production of androgens and of spermatozoa (Fig. 1). These functions are dependent on trophic hormones from the hypothalamus and anterior pituitary which are sensitive to the negative feedback action of testicular hormones, thus forming a closed-loop functional axis (Fig. 2).

Gonadotrophin releasing hormone (GnRH) is synthesized in neurosecretory neurones in the hypothalamus and then released episodically into the pituitary portal circulation at a frequency of 1–2 hourly. GnRH stimulates synthesis and secretion of both luteinizing hormone (LH) and follicle stimulating hormone (FSH) in the gonadotrophs of the anterior pituitary gland. Each episode of GnRH secretion elicits an immediate release of gonadotrophins. This intermittent mode of GnRH stimulation avoids desensitization of the pituitary gonadotrophs by continuous exposure to GnRH and is therefore obligatory for the maintainence of normal gonadotrophin secretion.

There is a pulsatile pattern of LH concentrations in the sytemic circulation which reflects the rapid episodic secretory bursts resulting from intermittent hypothalamic GnRH stimulation (Fig. 2). LH stimulates biosynthesis of androgenic steroids by binding to specific surface membrane receptors on the Leydig cells. This activates the cyclic-AMP/protein kinase mechanism which mobilizes cholesterol substrate and promotes the conversion of cholesterol to pregnenolone by splitting the side-chain at position C21. Figure 3 shows the major steps in the steroidogenic pathway in which the carbon skeleton of the parent compound, cholesterol, is progressively hydrolysed to form various androgenic steroids. Testosterone is the major end-product of the biosynthetic pathway in adult Leydig cells. The daily testicular production rate of testosterone is between 3 and 10 mg. As the principal circulating androgen secreted by the adult testes, testosterone exerts the major negative feedback action on gonadotrophin secretion by restricting the frequency of GnRH release from the hypothalamus and by reducing the amplitude of LH response to GnRH. Androgens are essential for the differentiation, growth, and function of the male genital ducts (epididymis) and accessory glands (seminal vesicles and prostate), male secondary sexual characteristics and sexual potency (Table 1). Testosterone circulates in plasma bound to sex hormone binding globulin (SHBG) and albumin. In man, 60 per cent of circulating testosterone is bound to SHBG, 38 per cent to albumin, and 2 per cent is free. Free and albumin-bound testosterone constitute the bioavailable fractions of the circulating hormone but recent evidence suggest that the SHBG-bound fraction may also be extractable in some tissues, namely prostate and testis. Androgen action is mediated through specific binding to intranuclear androgen receptors, which increase transcription of specific androgen-responsive genes in target cells. In target organs such as the fetal external genitalia, prostate, and facial hair follicles, full activation requires the local metabolism of testosterone by the enzyme 5α-reductase to 5α-dihydrotestosterone, an androgen which is at least tenfold more potent

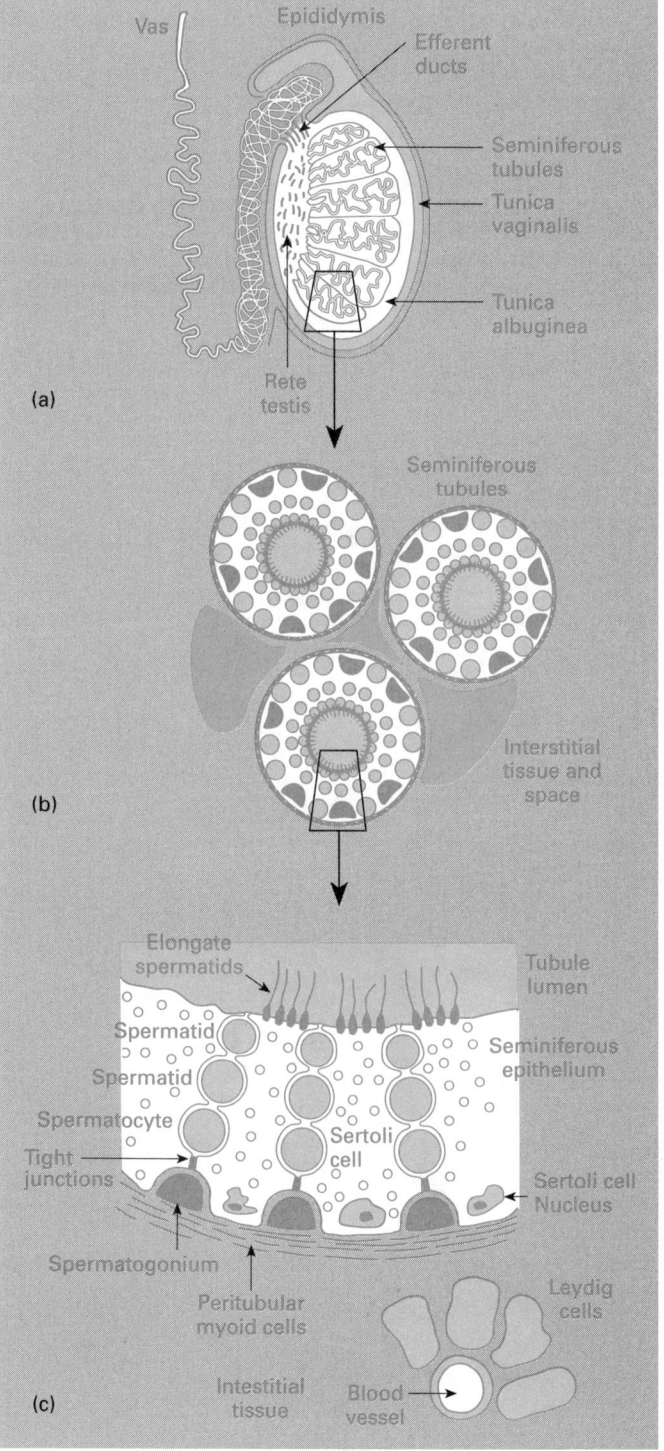

Fig. 1 (a) Human testis, epididymis, and vas deferens showing efferent ducts leading from the rete testis to the caput epididymis and the cauda epididymis continuing to become the vas deferens. (b) Cross-section through a seminiferous tubule showing central lumen, seminiferous epithelium, and interstitial space containing Leydig cells. (c) Anatomical relationships in the seminiferous epithelium between germ cells (spermatogonia, spermatocytes, and spermatids), Sertoli cells, peritubular myoid cells, and Leydig cells.

Table 1 *Physiological action of androgens and clinical features of androgen deficiency*

Physiological action	Prepubertal deficiency	Postpubertal deficiency
Penile growth	Infantile penis	Adult penis
Pubic hair growth	Scanty or absent	Decreased density and lost escutcheon
Stimulation of spermatogenesis (testes enlargement)	Spermatogenesis uninitiated (testes remain small)	Spermatogenesis regression (testes decrease in size)
Prostate growth	Prostate undeveloped	Prostate atrophy
Seminal vesicle growth	Ejaculate absent	Ejaculate volume diminished or absent
Sex drive stimulated	Sex drive not developed	Sex drive diminished or absent
Spontaneous erections increased	Spontaneous erections absent	Spontaneous erections diminished or absent
Physical stamina increased	Low physical stamina	Decreased physical stamina
Muscle mass increase	Muscle mass underdeveloped	Muscle mass atrophic
Antagonize oestrogen action on breast	Gynaecomastia may be present	Gynaecomastia may be present
Bone mass increase	Osteoporosis	Osteoporosis
Fusion of long bone epiphyses	Eunuchoid body proportion	Normal body proportion
Increase sebum secretion	Dry, smooth (low sebum), pale, fine wrinkles	Dry, smooth (low sebum), pale, fine wrinkles
Increase body hair	Scanty axillary, body, and facial hair	Decreased axillary, body hair, shaving frequency
Frontal balding	No temporal recession	No temporal recession
Laryngeal enlargement	Larynx underdeveloped, voice unbroken	Normal pitch voice
Erythropoiesis stimulated	Mild anaemia	Mild anaemia

Fig. 2 Functional relationships in the hypothalamic–pituitary–testicular axis and testicular microenvironment. Gonadotrophin releasing hormone (GnRH) is secreted into the hypophysial circulation in an episodic manner, which is reflected by an LH pulse in the systemic circulation. Open arrows represent positive stimulation and closed arrows negative feedback.

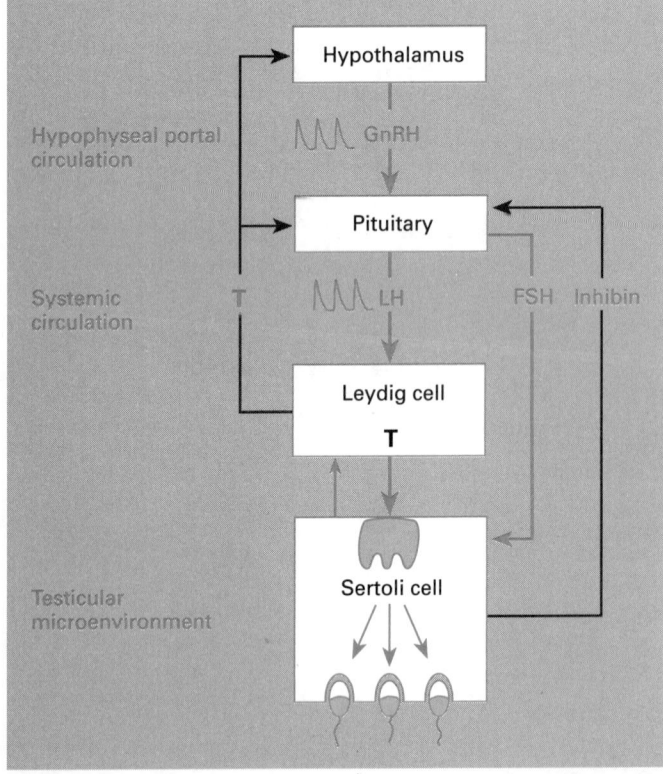

than testosterone (Fig. 3). It is not known why some but not all androgen-responsive targets require this local amplification step.

The endocrine (androgen synthetic) and gametogenic (spermatogenetic) functions in the testis are closely interlinked. Although testosterone is important as the principal circulating androgen, the local (paracrine) action of the high concentration of testosterone within the testis is crucial, together with FSH, for the initiation and maintenance of normal spermatogenesis and hence fertility (Figs 1 and 2). In response to these trophic signals, the Sertoli cells create a special microenvironment in the seminiferous tubules by providing the physical framework and chemical milieu for the developing germ cells which are embedded in their cytoplasm (Fig. 1). The Sertoli cells secrete inhibin, a group of related glycoprotein hormones, which inhibits FSH secretion by the pituitary (Fig. 2).

Spermatogenesis comprises a repetitive series of cytodifferentiation in the seminiferous epithelium whereby cohorts of undifferentiated diploid germ cells (spermatogonia) multiply and transform into haploid spermatozoa (Fig. 1). Mitotic divisions of stem cells form populations of spermatogonia which, at regular intervals of 16 days, differentiate into primary preleptotene spermatocytes to initiate meiosis. Meiotic reduction divisions of spermatocytes generate round spermatids which then transform (spermiogenesis) into compact, virtually cytoplasm-free, elongated spermatids with condensed DNA in the head and a tail capable of propelling beating movements. Mature spermatozoa are finally released from Sertoli cell cytoplasm into the tubular lumen around 74 days after their initial development from spermatogonia.

Male reproductive disorders

Male hypogonadism is a descriptive term for the clinical complex associated with androgen deficiency usually, but not invariably, due to the failure of Leydig cell function. Concomitant impairment of spermatogenesis is also likely since the seminiferous tubules will also be androgen deficient or directly involved by the same pathological process. However, infertility is usually an isolated abnormality of spermatogenesis where patients seldom show any clinical evidence of androgen deficiency.

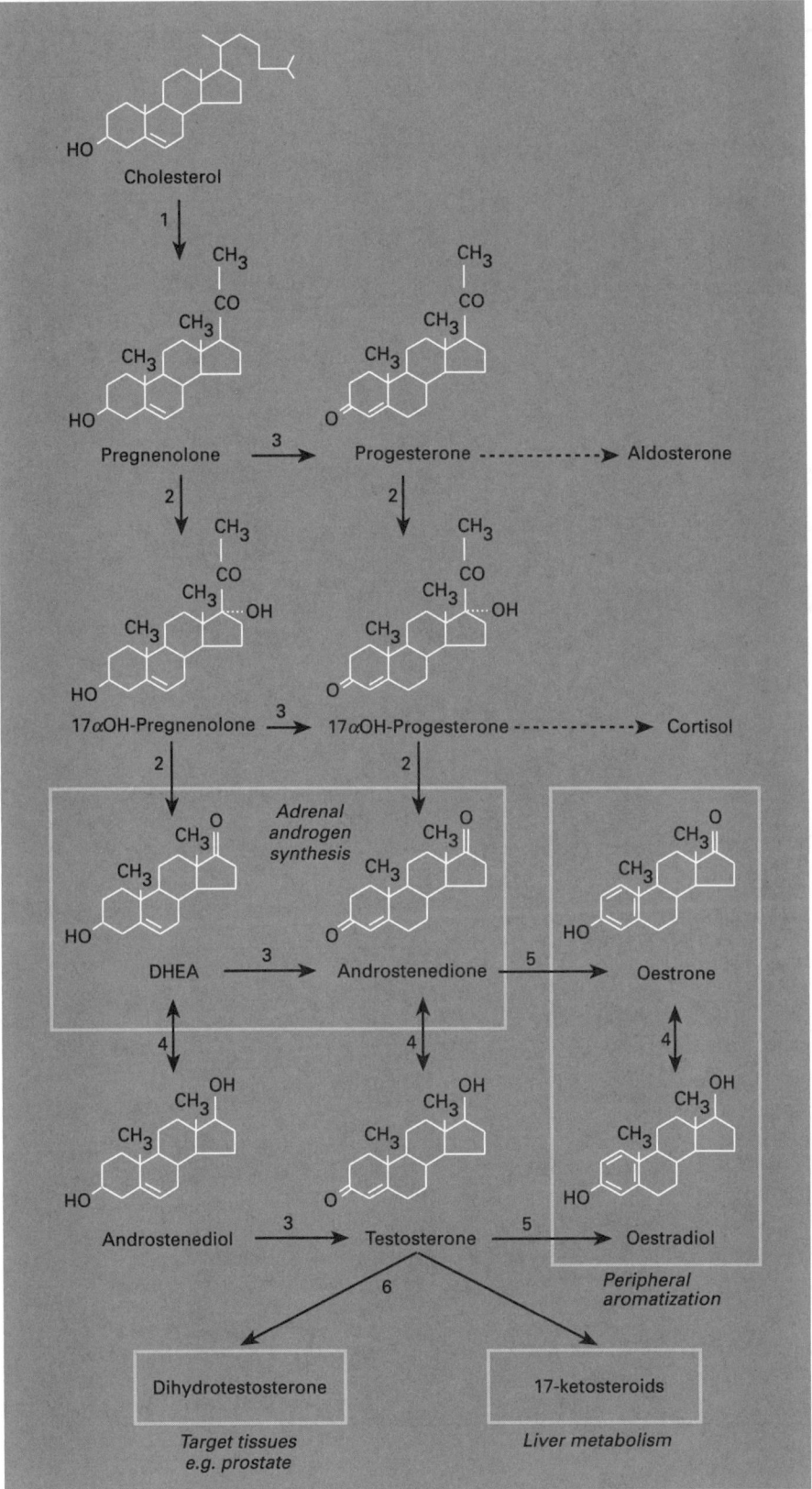

Fig. 3 Steroidogenic pathway from cholesterol to testosterone and further conversion of testosterone. 1, cholesterol side-chain cleavage; 2, 17α-hydroxylase/17,20-lyase; 3, 3β-hydroxysteroid dehydrogenase; 4, 17β-hydroxysteroid dehydrogenase; 5, aromatase; 6, 5α-reductase.

Table 2 *Aetiologies of male reproductive disorders*

Hypogonadism and infertility	Infertility
Hypothalmic 　Isolated GnRH deficiency 　Kallmann's syndrome 　Male anorexia nervosa	
Pituitary 　Craniopharyngioma 　Pituitary adenoma 　Hyperprolactinaemia 　Cranial irradiation 　Haemochromatosis 　Transfusion siderosis 　Sarcoidosis/tuberculosis/histiocytosis X 　Biologically inactive LH	
Testicular 　Congenital steroidogenic enzyme deficiencies 　Klinefelter's syndrome and variants 　Testicular agenesis (congenital anorchia) 　Testicular torsion 　Surgical orchidectomy 　Testicular trauma 　Testicular tumour 　Male Turner's syndrome	Idiopathic hypospermatogenesis Varicocele Cryptorchidism Orchitis Irradiation
Post-testicular	Sperm antibodies Immotile cilia (Kartårgener's) syndrome Young's syndrome Agenesis of epididymides and vasa Postinfection obstruction Accessory gland infection Retrograde ejaculation Coital insufficiency
Target tissues 　Androgen insensitivity syndromes (testicular feminization) 　5α-reductase deficiency 　Steroidogenic enzyme deficiencies 　Systemic diseases 　Chronic debilitating illnesses (cardiac failure, uncontrolled diabetes, neoplasia) 　Liver cirrhosis 　Chronic renal failure 　Thyrotoxicosis	
CNS diseases 　Prader–Willi syndrome 　Laurence–Moon–Biedl syndrome 　Familial cerebellar degeneration	Dystrophia myotonica Spinal cord injury
Drugs/chemicals 　Digitalis, spironolactone, 　Cyproterone acetate, flutamide 　Ketoconazole, cimetidine	Cytotoxic chemotherapy Sulphasalazine, nitrofurantoin Anticonvulsants Anabolic steroids, oestrogens Ethanol, opiates, cannabis Pesticides, fungicides, amoebicides Heavy metals

Hypogonadism

AETIOLOGY

A large number of diseases can lead to destruction or malfunction of the hypothalmic–pituitary–testicular axis (Table 2). It is important to establish the nature and site of the underlying pathology, first because the causal lesion may require specific treatment of its own, e.g. a pituitary tumour; secondly hypogonadotrophic conditions are amenable to treatment aimed at the induction or restoration of spermatogenesis, while primary testicular failure, which is usually irreversible, is not.

DIAGNOSIS

Clinical features of hypogonadism

The age of onset of androgen deficiency critically influences the manifestation of hypogonadism (Table 1).

A fetal onset of defective androgen action due to androgen receptor abnormalities or steroidogenic enzyme deficiency cause failure of masculinization of the genitalia, resulting in intersexual states (see Chapter 12.9.1).

A prepubertal onset of testosterone deficiency gives rise to sexual infantilism (Table 1) and patients will present with delayed puberty. Eunuchoidal body proportions (arm span greater than height and heel–pubis exceeding crown–pubis lengths by at least 5 cm; Fig. 2) develop due to the continued growth of long bones (growth ediated mediated) allowed by the delayed closure of their epiphyseys and failure of the testosterone-induced spinal growth in late puberty.

A postpubertal onset of testosterone deficiency leads to regression of spermatogenesis, diminished sex drive and erection, loss of ejaculation, muscle atrophy and low stamina, decreased secondary sexual hair and frequency of shaving. No change is, however, observed in body and penile proportions or voice (Table 1). The clinical diagnosis of male hypogonadism in the adult is generally not difficult since the clinical features of androgen deficiency are characteristic. However, because the symptoms and signs develop very insidiously, it is common for patients to present only after many years following the onset of hypogonadism. Furthermore, a patient who has never been adequately androgenized may not be aware that his secondary sexual function is subnormal. In contrast, young adults will often be troubled by severe and intractable hot flushes from acute withdrawal of androgens after surgical or traumatic/inflammatory castration.

Additional clinical findings

These are specific to the underlying cause and may thus be useful in identifying the aetiology of hypogonadism.

Hypothalamic–pituitary tumours are suggested by headache, impairment of visual acuity or visual field loss, polyuria and polydipsia, or evidence of pituitary hormone excess such as Cushing's disease, acromegaly, and hyperprolactinaemia. Hyperprolactinaemia is typically associated with loss of sex drive, even in the presence of normal rates of secretion of testosterone. Primary testicular failure is suggested by a past history of orchitis, testicular trauma, surgery, torsion, or irradiation and chemotherapy.

The use of recreational drugs and medications which interfere with pituitary–testicular function or androgen action should be sought (Table 2). Abuse of alcohol may be important. Ethanol causes a lowering of plasma testosterone concentrations through a direct toxic effect on Leydig cell steroidogenesis. Testicular atrophy and gynaecomastia, found in 50 per cent of men with hepatic cirrhosis, are due to altered androgen steroid metabolism, increased concentrations of sex hormone binding globulin and increased oestrogen production. These changes are usually irreversible.

Neurological diseases can be associated with hypogonadism. Postpubertal atrophy of the seminiferous tubules occurs in 80 per cent of patients with dystrophia myotonica; variable degrees of androgen deficiency also exist. Hypogonadotrophic hypogonadism is associated with familial cerebellar ataxia, Laurence–Moon–Biedl and Prader–Willi syndromes. Defective spermatogenesis is common in paraplegia or quadraplegia following spinal injury, presumably because of the inability to maintain a low scrotal temperature.

Specific condition

Klinefelter's syndrome is the commonest cause of male hypogonadism, with an incidence of 2 per 1000 live births. It is a developmental disorder of the testis resulting from the presence of an extra X chromosome. The most common karyotype is 47 XXY but rarer variants include 46 XY/ 47 XXY mosaic, multiple X + Y, and the so-called XX male syndrome. Accelerated atrophy of germ cells before puberty gives rise to sterility and small, firm testes. The degree of Leydig cell defect is very variable, ranging from the fully virilized male presenting with infertility to the eunuchoidal youth who fails to complete sexual maturation. Other features include gynaecomastia, tall stature (longer lower body segment), learning difficulties, and autoimmune endocrinopathies.

Kallmann's syndrome—with an incidence of 1 in 7500 males—is characterized by a family history (X-linked or autosomal) of hypogonadism and a number of somatic stigmata, including anosmia or hyposmia (defective smell sense), red-green colour blindness, nerve deafness, and cleft-lip or palate. This hypogonadotrophic condition is caused by a defect in embryonic migration of GnRH-secreting neurones from their site of origin in the nose. They are therefore unable to reach the hypothalamus, from where their axons normally gain access to the portal circulation in the median eminence. The same migratory defect affects the olfactory neurones in the nose, resulting in aplasia of the olfactory bulb.

INVESTIGATIONS

Confirmation of hypogonadism

Measurement of basal testosterone, LH and FSH, and prolactin, by repeated frequent sampling over 1 to 2 h if necessary, is all that is required for the diagnosis of male hypogonadism. Patients with androgen insensitivity syndromes have elevated testosterone with high LH.

Assessment of the hypothalamic–pituitary–testicular axis

The physiological basis for differentiating between hypogonadotrophic and hypergonadotrophic hypogonadism is illustrated in Fig. 2. Pathologies in the hypothalamus and pituitary will give rise to low or low–normal gonadotrophins and low testosterone, i.e. a state of hypogonadotrophic hypogonadism or secondary testicular failure. In these conditions the potential for stimulating testicular function by exogenous gonadotrophin or GnRH replacement is maintained. Conditions affecting the testes interrupt normal testicular negative feedback, resulting in elevated gonadotrophin levels with low plasma testosterone, a pattern characteristic of hypergonadotrophic hypogonadism or primary testicular failure. Failure of spermatogenesis with reduced testicular size is commonly associated with a rise in FSH alone. Inhibin cannot be measured easily for diagnostic purposes at present.

Human chorionic gonadotrophin stimulates Leydig cell steroidogenesis, and plasma testosterone increases in response. Its use can be helpful in detecting the presence of functional testicular tissue in patients with impalpable testes, assessing functional reserve of the testes prior to treatment with exogenous gonadotrophin or GnRH, and in differentiating hypergonadotrophic hypogonadism from rare patients who produce immunologically detectable but biologically inactive LH in excess.

Stimulation tests of gonadotrophin secretory reserve using clomiphene and GnRH seldom give additional information and have become largely obsolete, especially since the advent of improved sensitivity and range of modern gonadotrophin immunoassays.

Assessment of the pituitary

Patients with hypogonadotrophic hypogonadism without the stigmata of Kallmann's syndrome must undergo full pituitary functional and anatomical assessment to exclude an underlying pituitary tumour. They require pharmacological tests of growth hormone and adrenocorticotrophic hormone reserve, thyroid function tests, visual field charting, and CT scanning or MRI.

Other investigations

Suspected Klinefelter's syndrome should be confirmed by chromosome karyotyping on peripheral blood lymphocytes. Ultrasound is useful in locating ectopic or intra-abdominal testes. Androgen-receptor studies on biopsied genital skin fibroblasts or DNA analyses of the androgen receptor gene are required to confirm the diagnosis of androgen resistance in the testicular feminization syndrome.

TREATMENT

The objectives of treatment

1. To relieve the symptoms of androgen deficiency.
2. To prevent the long-term consequences of androgen deficiency, such as osteopenia.
3. To reproduce physiological levels of plasma testosterone.
4. To induce fertility, if required, in hypogonadotrophic patients.
5. To treat any specific underlying diseases.

The mainstay of treatment of the hypogonadal male is androgen replacement. Although hypogonadotrophic patients have the potential for fertility, gonadotrophin or pulsatile GnRH therapy should only be employed when there is a requirement for fertility, because of the expense and complexity of these regimens. Previous testosterone treatment does not jeopardize a subsequent response to gonadotrophin so that younger hypogonadotrophic subjects should be treated by testosterone in the same manner as hypergonadotrophic patients, to initiate and maintain virilization and sexual function.

Androgen replacement

The circulating half-life of free testosterone is short (10 min) due to rapid degradation by the liver. To achieve sustained physiological circulating concentrations, testosterone has to be administered in a modified form or by a parenteral route so that its rate of metabolism or absorption is retarded.

Parenteral testosterone administration

Testosterone esters are the most widely used androgen replacement in male hypogonadism. However, at dose regimens generally recommended, unphysiologically high levels of testosterone are invariably observed 24 to 48 h after each injection, followed by an exponential fall to subnormal levels before the next injection. Most commercially available injectable preparations of testosterone contain combinations of short- and longer-acting esters, but these inevitably produce exaggerated peak concentrations which are best avoided. Single-agent preparations containing long-acting esters (e.g. testosterone enanthate, 200 mg every 2 weeks) are therefore recommended.

Testosterone implants are cylindrical pellets containing 100 or 200 mg of crystalline testosterone which are inserted under local anaesthesia into the subcutaneous space of the lower anterior abdominal wall by means of a trocar and obturator. Peak testosterone levels are usually achieved at 2 to 4 weeks. A 600 to 800 mg dose of testosterone implants will provide relatively stable levels of plasma testosterone within the physiological range, which gradually decline towards the base-line over 4 to 6 months.

Oral testosterone administration

The long aliphatic side-chain of testosterone undecanoate makes the ester particularly lipophilic. This promotes absorption from the gut via intestinal lymphatics. The absorption of testosterone undecanoate however is variable, although this can be improved by administration with food. After a single 40 mg oral dose, peak plasma testosterone is usually observed 4 to 6 h later and levels return to base-line after 10 h. To maintain testosterone within the adult physiological range, 40 mg of testosterone undecanoate three to four times daily is required.

Mesterolone is a weak androgen which is metabolized by the liver slowly. Although commercially available, its use in hypogonadal patients as physiological replacement cannot be recommended.

Transdermal testosterone application

This new form of androgen replacement has recently become available. The testosterone is incorporated in a patch applied either to the shaved scrotal skin or on the back, and changed daily. With daily application, plasma testosterone can be maintained within the adult physiological range throughout the 24 h. The scrotal application gives elevated levels of 5α-dihydrotestosterone as a result of the abundant 5α-reductase activity in genital skin, a disadvantage not seen with non-scrotally applied systems. Early indications regarding clinical efficacy are favourable but long-term safety and acceptability are as yet unproven.

Choice of androgen preparations

The choice of preparations depends on patient preference, facilities for injections or surgical implants, and requirement for dosage adjustments. The invasive nature of the implantation procedure, the long duration of action, and the difficulties in removal make them less than ideal for the induction of puberty in adolescents and the initiation of treatment in androgen-naïve young adults, where a more gradual and flexible increase in dose is desirable. For these reasons, testosterone implant is usually reserved as maintenance treatment in young adults, replacement having been initiated with intramuscular or oral preparations. Almost all patients respond well to testosterone enanthate 200 mg every 2 weeks, 300 mg every 3 weeks, or Sustanon 250® every 2 to 3 weeks. In the absence of a satisfactory biological marker for androgen action, monitoring of treatment is best gauged by clinical response and documenting plasma testosterone in the mid-normal range 7 days after a dose of testosterone enanthate or 6 to 8 weeks after testosterone implant so that appropriate adjustments of dosing intervals can be made.

Safety and side-effects

Although systematic information from long-term treatment of hypogonadal men is not available, it is the experience of most clinicians that side-effects are very rare. These may include acne, transient priapism, gynaecomastia, fluid retention, and a clinically insignificant increase in haematocrit. The potential risks for cardiovascular disease through alteration of lipid metabolism, and exacerbation of underlying prostatic disease in hypogonadal men on androgen replacement is currently not known. Periodic digital or ultrasound examination of the prostate and measurement of circulating prostate specific antigen should be performed in patients over the age of 50 years maintained on androgens. Obstructive sleep apnoea may rarely complicate androgen therapy; those particularly at risk are older, obese men with thick necks and high upper airways resistance, identified by a raised haematocrit and a propensity to snore.

Infertility

Infertility is defined as the inability of a couple to initiate a pregnancy after 12 months of unprotected intercourse. Some 8 to 15 per cent of married couples experience involuntary infertility. Of these, male factors alone are estimated to be responsible in 30 per cent and contributory in a further 20 per cent of subfertile couples. Thus, male infertility may affect 5 per cent of men of reproductive age.

AETIOLOGIES

Male infertility implies a failure to fertilize the normal ovum arising from the deficiency of functionally competent sperm at the site of fertilization. In most instances, this is associated with defective spermatogenesis, giving rise to absent or low sperm output (azoospermia or oligozoospermia, respectively), and abnormal spermiogenesis, giving rise to spermatozoa with poor motility (asthenozoospermia) and/or abnormal morphology (teratozoospermia). The pathophysiology of hypospermatogenesis remains very poorly understood. Over three-quarters of patients with male infertility due to poor semen quality do not have any clearly identifiable cause (idiopathic hypospermatogenesis) (Table 2). Even when the underlying aetiology of hypospermatogenesis is known (e.g. Klinefelter's syndrome, cryptorchidism, orchitis, or irradiation), the pathology is rarely reversible.

Idiopathic hypospermatogensis

By far the commonest form of male infertility is idiopathic azoo/oligozoospermia, usually associated with asthenozoospermia and teratozoospermia. This probably represents the end result of a multitude of ill-defined pathologies which disrupt normal seminiferous tubular functions. Reduced velocity or vigour of sperm motility may be due to metabolic/functional defects or structural malformations in the axonemal complex of the sperm tail. Rarely, absent or extremely low sperm motility (with normal sperm density) may result from the absence of dynein arms (Na/K ATPase) of the sperm tail. This is associated with similar defects in respiratory cilia and a history of chronic respiratory infection, bronchiectasis, and sinusitis (immotile cilia syndrome). In addition, some of these patients have situs inversus (Kartagener's syndrome). Abnormal sperm morphology may indicate defective spermiogenesis. An extreme example is the failure of acrosome development leading to the formation of round-headed spermatozoa (globozoospermia).

Chromosome disorders

Abnormal chromosome karyotypes are found in 15 per cent of azoospermic patients, 90 per cent of whom have Klinefelter's syndrome (47 XXY). Other chromosomal abnormalities encountered include reciprocal X or Y autosomal translocations, XYY and XX males, reciprocal and robertsonian autosomal translocations, supernumerary autosomes, and inversion of autosomes. Recently, microdeletions of the azoospermic factor locus in chromosome Yq11.22–23 has been reported in some azoospermic patients.

Cryptorchidism

The lower temperature in the scrotum is a prerequisite for normal spermatogenesis. Undescended testes are exposed to the harmful effects of the higher temperature in the abdomen and inguinal region. Spontaneous descent of the testis rarely occurs after 1 year. A testis which is not permanently in a low scrotal position by the age of 2 years will have sustained damage to the seminiferous epithelium. Orchidopexy after 2 years of age for undescended testes does not improve fertility. For these reasons, treatment should ideally be undertaken between 1 and 2 years of age. Human chorionic gonadotrophin or intranasal GnRH are currently being used increasingly for early treatment of cryptorchidism. If hormonal treatment is unsuccessful, orchidopexy can be carried out. Undescended testes can be a feature of hypogonadotrophic hypogonadism and intersexual states. The risk of testicular tumour in a patient with a history of undescended testis, whether successfully treated by orchidopexy or not, is four- to tenfold higher than in the general population.

Varicocele

The significance of varicocele in male infertility remains controversial. Reflux of blood in the internal spermatic vein, usually involving the left side from the renal vein, gives rise to distension of the pampiniform venous plexus and reduction in ipsilateral testicular volume, associated with varying degrees of non-specific histological abnormalities in both testes. Increased scrotal temperature, hypoxia, and exposure of the testes to adrenal metabolites have been postulated as possible mechanisms by which spermatic vein reflux can induce seminiferous tubular damage. Since varicoceles can be detected clinically in 15 per cent of young fertile men, it must not be assumed that this condition is invariably or solely responsible for infertility without carefully excluding other possible aetiologies.

Sperm autoimmunity

Immunological infertility is a specific disorder caused by sperm-membrane-bound IgA antibodies found in around 5 per cent of men presenting with infertility. Conditions predisposing to sperm autoimmunity include vasectomy, testicular injury/inflammation, genital tract infection/obstruction, and family history of autoimmune disease. Male patients with significant sperm antibody usually have severely suppressed fertility potential due to sperm agglutination, poor sperm transit through cervical mucus, and blocked sperm–oocyte fusion.

Genital tract infection

Infection in the lower genital tract is a major cause of male infertility in the global context. Chlamydia, gonococci, Gram-negative enterococci, and the tubercle bacillus are the usual pathogens. If not treated by appropriate antibiotics promptly, inflammation of the accessory glands and excurrent ducts may give rise to disturbed function, formation of sperm antibody, and permanent structural damage with obstruction in the outflow tract. Asymptomatic prostatitis due to occult and usually focal infection is best diagnosed by transrectal ultrasound examination of the prostate.

Excurrent duct obstruction

Vasectomy and previous genitourinary infections are the most common causes of obstructive azoospermia. Rare congenital abnormalities include bilateral agenesis of the Wolffian duct-derived structures, corpus/cauda epididymis, vas deferens, and seminal vesicles, characterized by impalpable scrotal vasa and low volumes (< 1 ml) of acidic non-coagulating ejaculate (prostatic fluid) devoid of fructose and sperm. These patients have mutations in the cystic fibrosis (CFTR) gene and are considered to have a genital form of cystic fibrosis, while all males with typical cystic fibrosis also have the same congenital maldevelopment of Wolffian ducts. In Young's syndrome, epididymal obstruction is due to progressive inspissation of amorphous secretion in the lumen. In these patients, the high incidence of chronic sinopulmonary infection and bronchiectasis is presumably the consequence of the same abnormality in the respiratory tract.

Coital disorders

Inadequate coital technique (including the use of vaginal lubricants with spermicidal properties e.g. vaseline), low frequency, and faulty timing of intercourse may contribute to continuing infertility but are rarely the only aetiological factor in the infertile couple. Erectile and ejaculatory failure may be caused by many different conditions (see below).

DIAGNOSIS

History

Particular attention should be paid to the following aspects. Previous surgery such as herniorrhaphy in childhood, trauma, or torsion suggests possible damage to the vas or testis. History of cryptorchidism and genitourinary infections are important aetiological factors. Painful ejaculation, haematospermia, and pain in the perineum are symptoms suggestive of chronic infection in the prostate and seminal vesicles. Delayed onset of puberty may suggest the possibility of gonadotrophin deficiency. A history of recurrent chest infection, sinusitis, or bronchiectasis may be obtained in patients with epididymal obstruction (Young's syndrome), immotile cilia syndrome, and agenesis of the vasa (cystic fibrosis). Chronic disorders such as renal failure, liver disease, malignancy, diabetes, and multiple sclerosis are associated with a variety of testicular and sexual dysfunctions. Each patient should be asked about episodes of pyrexia within the past 12 weeks because of transient suppression of spermatogenesis. Careful enquiry should also be made about occupational or environmental exposure to testicular toxins and radiation, current medications, previous treatment, or the use of recreational drugs. It is important to establish that vaginal intercourse takes place with appropriate frequency and timing without the use of vaginal lubricants.

Examination

A general physical assessment of height, weight, body habitus, and secondary sexual development should be carried out in all patients. Measurement of testicular volumes by comparison with Prader's orchidometer provides a convenient clinical index of seminiferous tubular mass. Normal adult testicular volume is between 15 and 35 ml. Testicular volume is a key finding in differentiating between azoospermia due to seminiferous tubular failure (reduced volumes) and that arising from excurrent duct obstruction (normal volume). Testicular size is also a useful indicator of the degree of testicular development in hypogonadotrophic patients. If not in the scrotum, the lowest position of the testes should be defined. Irregular contour, induration or abnormal consistency of the testis suggest previous orchitis, surgery, or malignancy. Special attention should also be paid to the palpation of the epididymis and scrotal vas. An enlarged and tense caput epididymis may be palpable in cases of obstructive azoospermia. Irregularity and induration of the epididymis and vas suggest previous infection. In congenital agenesis of Wolffian duct-derived structures, the scrotal vasa are either impalpable or extremely thin. The patient should also be examined standing so that varicoceles can become visible (grade 3) or palpable (grade 2), or be detected as a venous impulse in the spermatic cord during Valsalva manoeuvre (grade 1). Rectal examination may reveal an irregular contour or abnormal consistency and tenderness in the prostate in the presence of chronic prostatitis and enlarged seminal vesicles.

Investigations

Conventional parameters of the semen analysis, such as sperm density, percentage of motile sperm, quality of sperm movements, and sperm morphology, provide a semiquantitative index of fertility potential. Although a variety of tests of sperm function, such as sperm movement analyses, mucus penetration, acrosome reaction, sperm–zona binding, and hamster oocyte penetration have been devised, none is sufficiently reliable and accurate to be used routinely in clinical practice. The continuing lack of a reliable quantitative and objective measure of male fertility is a major obstacle in patient management.

Measurement of plasma FSH is useful in distinguishing primary from secondary testicular failure and in identifying patients with obstructive azoospermia. In the presence of azoospermia or oligozoospermia, an elevated FSH, particularly with reduced testicular volume is presumptive evidence of severe and usually irreversible seminiferous tubular damage. Low or undetectable FSH (usually associated with low LH and testosterone, with clinical evidence of androgen deficiency) is suggestive of hypogonadotrophism. Conversely, azoospermia with normal FSH and normal testicular volume usually indicates the presence of bilateral genital tract obstruction. Testosterone and LH measurements are only indicated in the assessment of the infertile male when there is clinical suspicion of androgen deficiency, Klinefelter's syndrome, or sex steroid abuse. High concentrations of LH and testosterone should raise the possibility of abnormalities in androgen receptors, while the opposite suggests hypogonadotrophism. Hyperprolactinaemia is not a recognized cause of male infertility but prolactin measurement should be undertaken if there is clinical evidence of sexual dysfunction (particularly diminished libido) or pituitary disease leading to secondary testicular failure. Measurement of oestradiol is rarely indicated except in the presence of gynaecomastia.

Chromosome karyotyping should be carried out in patients with azoospermia, testicular atrophy, and elevated FSH, primarily to confirm the diagnosis of Klinefelter's syndrome. The need for testicular biopsy has largely been superseded by the use of plasma FSH in recent years to differentiate between primary testicular failure and obstructive lesions. Undetectable or very low levels of seminal fructose provides evidence to corroborate the clinical diagnosis of vasal and seminal vesicle agenesis or blocked ejaculatory ducts in the presence of obstructive azoospermia. An increase in the number of peroxidase-positive white cells in the semen is indicative of genital tract infection. Semen culture and detection of micro-organisms to identify infective pathogens are difficult because of the bactericidal properties of seminal plasma and urethral and skin commensals. Transrectal ultrasound has been advocated to diagnose asymptomatic chronic prostatitis. Sperm antibodies are detected by the mixed agglutination reaction where sheep red blood corpuscles or polyacrylamide beads are coated with rabbit antibodies to specific classes of human immunoglobulins. These will attach to motile sperm carrying specific IgA on the surface of the sperm head or tail.

TREATMENT

Since the majority of patients present no recognizable or reversible aetiological factors, the management of male infertility remains unsatisfactory.

Potentially treatable infertility

Removal or withdrawal from exposure to testicular toxins may lead to improvement in fertility. This is most commonly seen in patients with inflammatory bowel diseases changing treatment from sulphasalazine to 5-aminosalicylic acid which removes the toxic agent, sulphapyridine.

When patients with hypogonadotrophic hypogonadism desire fertility, they can discontinue androgens and start human chorionic gonadotrophin (2000 IU intramuscularly twice weekly) given alone for 6 to 12 months. If there is no sperm in the ejaculate at the end of 12 months, human menopausal gonadotrophin, which contains both FSH and LH, should be added at 75 IU intramuscularly thrice weekly. The outcome of treatment of gonadotrophin induction of spermatogenesis is variable but, in general, around 70 per cent should show some degree of spermatogenesis and 50 per cent can be expected to achieve pregnancies. In patients with hypothalamic GnRH deficiency, GnRH replacement has to be given in a pulsatile mode to avoid desensitization of the pituitary. This is accomplished by battery-driven portable infusion minipumps which can automatically deliver a desired dose of GnRH at a set time interval of 120 min; synthetic GnRH is administered subcutaneously via a needle sited in the abdominal wall or upper arm. The patient has to wear this device continuously and some have found this form of chronic therapy impractical and unsuited to their lifestyle. The outcome of treatment in terms of the induction of fertility is very similar to that obtained with exogenous gonadotrophin therapy.

Active infection in the genital tract should be treated by appropriate antibiotics (erythromycin, doxycycline, or norfloxacin) given for 4 weeks to both the patient and his partner. Bypass of epididymal obstruction with microsurgical techniques of epididymovasostomy have been reported to produce high pregnancy rates. Recently, it has become possible for sperm to be aspirated directly from the caput epididymis or efferent ducts proximal to the site of obstruction for use in assisted fertilization procedures in patients with obstructive azoospermia and agenesis of the vasa. The latter group should have genetic counselling beforehand because of the risk of cystic fibrosis in any offspring.

Infertility due to the presence of antibody to sperm can be treated by immunosuppression with high-dose prednisolone 0.75 mg/kg/day or prednisolone 20 mg twice a day on days 1 to 10 and 5 mg on days 11 and 12 of the partner's cycle for 3 to 6 cycles. Side-effects are common and may include irritability, sleeplessness, arthralgia, muscle weakness, peptic ulceration, glucose intolerance, and bilateral aseptic necrosis of femoral heads. Results of recent controlled trials have not been able to confirm the efficacy of glucocorticoid treatment. Intrauterine insemination of 'washed' sperm and in vitro fertilization have been increasingly applied to immunological male infertility.

Varicocele can be treated either by surgical ligation of the internal spermatic vein(s) above the internal inguinal ring or by transfemoral embolization of the internal spermatic vein(s). The results of treatment of varicocele are inconsistent. Until a prospective controlled therapeutic trial with sufficient numbers of patients is carried out, the significance of varicocele and its treatment in male infertility must remain an open question.

If semen of good quality can be obtained with masturbation, vibrators, or electroejaculation from patients with various coital dysfunctions, and functional spermatozoa recovered from alkalinized bladder urine of appropriate osmolality from the patient with retrograde ejaculation, artificial insemination can be reasonably successful.

Subfertility due to idiopathic hypospermatogenesis

Pregnancies can occur in some cases without treatment, albeit with a much reduced probability, depending on the duration of infertility, age, and coexisting subtle abnormalities in the female partner in addition to the defects in sperm quality. Although a wide variety of empirical treatments have been tried in attempts to improve fertility in subfertile men, none has been shown to be effective when assessed in controlled therapeutic trials. In the last few years, *in vitro* fertilization has been increasingly applied to treat male infertility, based on the premise that placing spermatozoa in close contact with multiple oocytes would increase the chance of fertilization. In patients with moderate oligozoospermia, fertilization rates of 30 per cent can be effected, with live birth rates of 8 to 10 per cent per treatment cycle. However, those with severe and multiple defects in semen fluid have significantly poorer results. Microinjection of a single spermatozoon directly into the oocyte cytoplasm has recently been shown to achieve remarkably high fertilization and live birth rates (55 and 26 per cent, respectively) even with the most severely abnormal samples. This promises to be a useful technique to overcome extreme oligozoospermia and obstructive azoospermia when sperm can be aspirated.

Untreatable sterility

Patients with azoospermia, atrophic testes, and elevated FSH have irreversible primary seminiferous tubular failure and are, to all intents and purposes, sterile. They should be informed of their prognosis and counselled regarding the options of continuing childlessness, adoption, and donor insemination.

Erectile impotence

Erectile failure may be caused by androgen deficiency, hyperprolactinaemia, neurological disorders such as autonomic neuropathy (usually complicating diabetes), multiple sclerosis and spinal injuries, vascular disease involving pelvic vessels, retroperitoneal and bladder-neck surgery, medications (commonly α- and β-adrenergic antagonists, psychotropic agents), alcohol abuse, severe systemic disease, psychological dysfunctions (including depression), and problems in personal relationships. Loss of libido characterizes androgen deficiency and hyperprolactinaemia while preservation of normal spontaneous morning erections are suggestive of psychogenic impotence. Ejaculatory abnormalities may be associated with erectile failure in neurological and drug-induced cases. Management should aim to correct any reversible underlying disease (e.g. prolactinoma) or substitute offending medications. Androgen treatment is only indicated in patients with plasma testosterone in the hypogonadal range. Vacuum devices and intracavernosal injection of vasodilator agents such as papaverine or prostaglandin E_1 have become popular in the management of neurogenic and vasculogenic impotence. Psychosexual therapy can benefit those with psychogenic impotence.

REFERENCES

Bancroft, J. (1993). Impotence in perspective. In: *Impotence: an integrated approach to clinical practice*, (ed. A. Gregoire and J.P. Pryor), pp. 3–13. Churchill Livingstone, London.

Burger, H. and de Kretser, D.M. (ed.) (1989). *The testis*, (2nd edn). Raven Press, New York.

Cantrill, J.A., Dewis, P., Large, D.M., and Anderson, D.C. (1984). Which testosterone replacement therapy? *Clinical Endocrinology* **21**, 97–107.

Carlson, E., Giwercman, A., Keiding, N., and Skakkebaek, N.E. (1992). Evidence for decreasing quality of semen during the past 50 years. *British Medical Journal* **305**, 609–13.

Griffen, J.E. (1992). Androgen resistance – the clinical and molecular spectrum. *New England Journal of Medicine* **326**, 611–18.

Hall, P.F. (1994). Testicular steroid synthesis: organization and regulation. In *The physiology of reproduction*, (ed. E. Knobil and J.D. Neill), 2nd edn. pp. 975–98. Raven Press, New York.

Handelsman, D.J., Conway, A.J., and Boyland, L.M. (1990). Pharmacoki-

netics and pharmacodynamics of testosterone pellets in man. *Journal of Clinical Endocrinology and Metabolism* **71**, 216–22.

Hargreave, T.B. (ed.) (1994). *Male infertility*, (2nd edn). Springer-Verlag, Berlin.

de Kretser, D.M. (ed.) (1992). The testes. *Ballière's Clinical Endocrinology and Metabolism* **6**, 2.

Miller, W.L. (1988). Molecular biology of steroid hormone synthesis. *Endocrine Reviews* **9**, 295–318.

Mooradian, A.D., Morley, J.E., and Korenman, S.G. (1987). Biological actions of androgens. *Endocrine Reviews* **8**, 1–27.

Nieschlag, E. (1993). Case of the infertile male. *Clinical Endocrinology*, **38**, 123–33.

Nieschlag, E. and Behre, H.M. (ed.) (1990), *Testosterone action; deficiency; substitution*, pp. 92–114. Springer-Verlag, Berlin.

Palermo, G., Joris, H., Devorey, P., and Van Steirteghem, A.O. (1992). Pregnancies after intracytoplasmic injection of single spermatozoa into an oocyte. *Lancet* **340**, 17–18.

Parvinen, M. (1982). Regulation of the seminiferous epithelium. *Endocrine Reviews* **3**, 404–17.

Russel, L.D. and Griswold, M.D. (ed.) (1993). *The Sertoli cell*. Cache River Press, Clearwater, FL.

Setchell, B.P. (1982). Spermatogenesis and spermatozoa. In: *Reproduction in mammals, Book* 2, (ed. C.R. Austin and R.V. Short) pp. 63–101. Cambridge University Press, Cambridge.

Sharpe, R.M. (1994). Regulation of spermatogenesis. In *The physiology of reproduction* (eds. E. Knobil and J.D. Neill) 2nd edn. pp. 1363–1434. Raven Press, New York.

Skinner, M.K. (1991). Cell–cell interactions in the testis. *Endocrine Reviews* **12**, 45–77.

Snyder, P.J. and Lawrence, D.A. (1980). Treatment of male hypogonadism with testosterone enanthate. *Journal of Clinical Endocrinology and Metabolism* **51**, 1335–9.

Whitcombe, R.W. and Crowley, W.F., Jr (1990). Diagnosis and treatment of isolated gonadotropin-releasing hormone deficiency in men. *Journal of Clinical Endocrinology and Metabolism* **70**, 3–7.

World Health Organization (1992). *Guidelines for the use of androgens in men*. WHO, Geneva.

12.8.3 The breast

H. S. JACOBS

Gynaecomastia

Gynaecomastia is defined as benign enlargement of the male breast caused by proliferation of the glandular components. Clinically the distinction is made from enlargement by fat tissue by examining the patient in the supine position: the breast is held between thumb and forefinger and the fingers gently moved towards the nipple. A firm or rubbery, mobile disc-like mound of tissue arising concentrically from beneath the nipple and areola indicates the presence of gynaecomastia. The most important condition that needs to be excluded is carcinoma of the male breast. Cancer usually presents as a unilateral eccentric mass that is hard and fixed to underlying tissue; it may be associated with skin tethering, nipple discharge, or axillary lymphadenopathy. Mammography and fine-needle aspiration are helpful in the differential diagnosis but if doubt remains biopsy is appropriate. While cancer of the male breast is rare, it has to be recognized that it is 16 times more common in those with Klinefelter's syndrome than in other men. Other causes of gynaecomastia are not, however, associated with an increased risk of breast cancer.

PATHOGENESIS OF GYNAECOMASTIA

Microscopically, breast tissue in both sexes appears identical at birth. It remains quiescent until puberty when, in boys, the ducts and surrounding mesenchymal tissue transiently proliferate, only to involute and ultimately to atrophy. Gynaecomastia is characterized by initial proliferation of the fibroblastic stroma and ductal system. Progressive fibrosis and hyalinization then occur in association with regression of the epithelial components. These regressive changes occur even if the stimulus (for example, oestrogen treatment) continues. When gynaecomastia has been present for more than a year, clinical regression is rarely complete, because the fibrosis persists even when the cause has been removed.

Endocrine pathophysiology

Since oestrogens stimulate and androgens inhibit development of breast tissue, gynaecomastia arises whenever there is an imbalance between these hormones. An alteration in the ratio of free androgen to free oestrogen, rather than a specific concentration of either, is thought to underlie almost all cases of gynaecomastia.

In men 98 per cent of testosterone is directly secreted by the testes, whereas the origin of oestrogen is more complex (Fig. 1): thus only about 15 per cent of oestradiol and less than 5 per cent of oestrone are directly secreted. In both cases the remainder is produced by extraglandular conversion (aromatization) of androgenic precursors in peripheral tissues, such as adipose tissue, liver, and muscle. There is also substantial interconversion of oestrone and oestradiol. Treatment of normal men with human chorionic gonadotrophin (HCG) results in an increase of directly secreted oestradiol in proportion to the increase of testosterone so that, while directly secreted oestradiol in normal men rarely amounts to more than 6 μg/day, when luteinizing hormone (LH) levels are persistently high, substantial amounts of oestradiol may be directly secreted by the testis.

CAUSES OF GYNAECOMASTIA

Gynaecomastia may be physiological or pathological. Physiologically it occurs at three times of life: the first is neonatally in response to transplacental passage of oestrogens. The second is during puberty for reasons that are not at all clear, and the third is in elderly men, probably because of the decline in Leydig cell function that occurs normally with age.

Pathological gynaecomastia is caused by a deficiency of testosterone formation or action, enhanced production of oestrogen, drugs, and unknown causes.

Testosterone deficiency

The commonest cause is Klinefelter's syndrome, about half the cases of which develop gynaecomastia at the time of puberty. The serum testosterone concentration is usually about 50 per cent of normal, the gonadotrophin concentrations are raised, and the serum oestradiol is above normal. The diagnosis is suspected clinically and confirmed by white

Fig. 1 Sources of oestrogen in men.

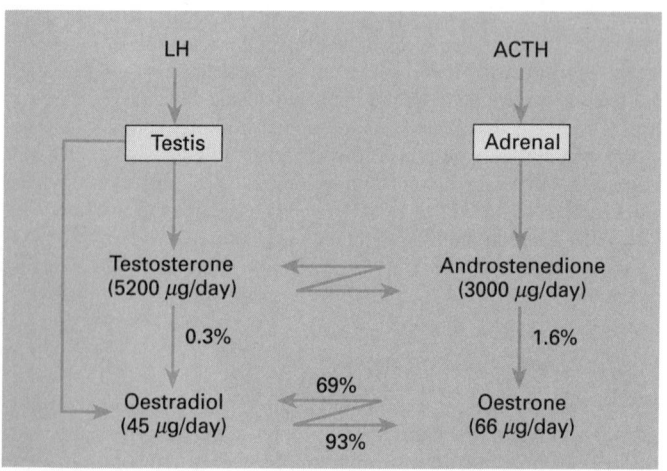

blood cell karyotype (Chapter 12.8.2). Congenital causes of testosterone deficiency include defects in testosterone biosynthesis and congenital anorchia. Acquired causes include viral orchitis (usually mumps), trauma, neurological disease (myotonia dystrophica and spinal cord lesions), and renal failure. Androgen resistance syndromes (for example, testicular feminization) are associated with high rates of secretion of testosterone and oestradiol; because of the large amounts of precursor (testosterone) there is also excessive extragonadal conversion of androgens to oestrogens.

Increased oestrogen production

An increase of oestrogen may be caused by an increase of its testicular secretion or of extraglandular production.

Increased secretion

Testicular tumours, such as Leydig and Sertoli cell tumours, may secrete androgens and oestrogens autonomously; gonadotrophin secretion is therefore suppressed and azoospermia is common. These tumours may be too small to be detected clinically but ultrasound can be very helpful. Some testicular tumours, for example choriocarcinomas, secrete HCG which then stimulates oestrogen secretion by the contralateral testis. HCG may also be secreted by non-testicular tumours such as a bronchogenic carcinoma.

True hermaphroditism may be associated with gynaecomastia because of oestrogen secretion by the ovotestis.

Increased extragonadal production of oestrogens
Adrenal disease

Congenital adrenal hyperplasia caused by 21 hydroxylase, 3β or 17β steroid dehydrogenase deficiencies results in increased availability of adrenal androgen for peripheral aromatization (Chapter 12.7.2). Adrenal carcinoma may be associated with massive oestrogen production, usually caused by extraglandular aromatization of the enormous amounts of androgen secreted by the tumour, but occasionally the oestrogen is directly secreted.

Liver disease

Cirrhosis, particularly alcoholic cirrhosis, is typically associated with gynaecomastia, testicular atrophy, and impotence. Plasma and urinary excretion of oestrogen is increased. The mechanism is in part decreased hepatic extraction of androstenedione, and consequently an increase in its extrasplanchnic aromatization, and partly reduced testosterone secretion by the testes. The gynaecomastia of starvation and refeeding may also be related to disturbed liver function.

Drugs
Oestrogens and oestrogen-like drugs

The most familiar is the use of oestrogen in the treatment of advanced carcinoma of the prostate; indeed, the development of gynaecomastia in this situation has provided the model for most of our understanding of the evolution of the histological changes in the breast in gynaecomastia. Pollution of food (via injected animals) and cosmetic products by oestrogen has been reported as a cause of gynaecomastia.

Treatment with digitalis glycosides may cause gynaecomastia, the drug acting either as an oestrogen or as an oestrogen precursor.

Drugs that enhance oestrogen secretion

Treatment with HCG and clomiphene can increase oestrogen secretion. The development of gynaecomastia in men treated with HCG usually indicates that the dose has been too high.

Drugs that inhibit testosterone secretion

Ketoconazole, an antifungal agent that is also used in the management of certain forms of Cushing's syndrome, blocks steroid synthesis in Leydig cells and, if a high dose is maintained, gynaecomastia may result.

Spironolactone causes gynaecomastia in as many as 50 per cent of men treated with 150 mg/day. The drug suppresses testosterone synthesis (by inhibiting 17,20 desmolase) but it also acts as a peripheral antiandrogen.

Drugs that block testosterone action

Cyproterone acetate and the non-steroidal flutamide are two antiandrogens, presently used in the management of advanced prostatic disease, which usually produce gynaecomastia. Cimetidine, but not ranitidine, is antiandrogenic and is associated with a significant risk of gynaecomastia.

Although, in most series, between 50 and 75 per cent of cases of gynaecomastia are labelled idiopathic because no endocrinopathy can be identified, there are increasing reasons to suspect that environmental pollution, either with oestrogens or antiandrogens, is responsible for many of the cases.

DIAGNOSIS OF GYNAECOMASTIA

The history should include enquiry about drugs as well as possible environmental exposure to oestrogens and antiandrogens. Examination should include the testes. While small, firm testes are characteristic of Klinefelter's syndrome, asymmetrical enlargement suggests a Leydig cell tumour (most readily diagnosed by ultrasound). Evaluation of alcohol intake and liver function is appropriate. Endocrine assessment should include measurement of testosterone, oestradiol, gonadotrophins, and dehydroepiandrosterone sulphate (a high level suggests adrenal disease) concentrations.

TREATMENT OF GYNAECOMASTIA

Once gynaecomastia has been present for about a year, treatment is unlikely to lead to a reduction in breast size because of the fibrosis that usually develops by this time. Consequently, surgery, usually using a circumareolar approach, is the mainstay of treatment. The psychological effects of persistent breast development in adolescent boys may be severe and surgery should be considered at an early stage; temporizing rarely produces resolution. Medical therapy with androgens or anti-oestrogens produces uncertain effects and can only be expected to have much benefit if administered early in the course of the disorder. Gynaecomastia caused by oestrogen treatment, as in the treatment of prostatic disease, can be prevented by pretreatment with low-dose irradiation of the breasts.

Galactorrhoea

Galactorrhoea is defined as a persistent discharge of milk or milk-like secretion in the absence of parturition, or beyond 6 months postpartum in a non-nursing mother. Galactorrhoea is not a sign of breast cancer and not a risk factor for it.

There are essentially two types of galactorrhoea—spontaneous galactorrhoea, or galactorrhoea present on expression only. In the latter case the menstrual cycle is usually intact and an endocrine cause is rarely found. It is spontaneous galactorrhoea that is associated with hyperprolactinaemia and amenorrhoea.

In the puerperium there is a clear correlation between the amount of prolactin released in response to suckling and the volume of milk secreted. In contrast, in inappropriate lactation, that is, in galactorrhoea, no such relation exists, presumably because the breasts have not been prepared for lactation by the oestrogen- and progesterone-rich environment of pregnancy. When this observation is considered in relation to the ease and widespread availability of prolactin measurements, one can readily appreciate that the physical sign of galactorrhoea has ceased to have much diagnostic significance. In women with amenorrhoea caused by hyperprolactinaemia, for example, only about 20 per cent have galactorrhoea. Thus the evaluation of galactorrhoea nowadays is essentially the evaluation of hyperprolactinaemia (see Chapter 12.8.1).

MANAGEMENT OF GALACTORRHOEA

The essential investigation is the measurement of serum prolactin. The management of hyperprolactinaemia is outlined in Chapter 12.8.1. For women with non-hyperprolactinaemic galactorrhoea the important advice is first to stop expressing the milk, the second is the reassurance that it is not a sign of cancer, or a risk factor for it, and the third is a trial of drug therapy with bromocriptine. In the author's experience, after they have received appropriate reassurance, patients with non-hyperprolactinaemic galactorrhoea rarely need drug therapy. Such patients are, however, very sensitive to the adverse affects of the drug, and side-effects are common, even with low doses.

12.9 Disorders of development

12.9.1 Normal and abnormal sexual differentiation

M. O. SAVAGE

Introduction

Disorders of sexual differentiation are characterized by an abnormality in the formation of the internal or external genital structures. Most are genetically determined and are associated with an ambiguous appearance of the external genitalia. During the past two decades, the study of intersex disorders has changed in orientation. The emphasis has moved away from descriptive clinical syndromes towards the biochemical and molecular nature of the defects that cause them. If such an aetiological approach is to be used, a fundamental understanding of normal sexual differentiation is required. This provides the basis for the classification, investigation, and management of patients with abnormal sexual differentiation.

Physiology of fetal sexual differentiation

In the male, it is established that the castrated embryo develops as a female, indicating that the fetal testis is essential for male development. The chromosomal sex of the embryo, established at conception, directs the development of either ovaries or testes. In the male, specific genes on the short arm of the Y chromosome, known as the sex-determining region of the Y chromosome, code for testis determination, and hence contribute to testicular differentiation. Testicular Leydig cells synthesize and secrete testosterone from 8 weeks of gestation, aided by stimulation with placental human chorionic gonadotrophin (HCG). Testosterone diffuses locally to maintain and virilize the wolffian ducts which become the vas deferens, seminal vesicles, and epididymis. Antimüllerian hormone, or müllerian-inhibitory factor, is a glycoprotein which is secreted during the same time period by testicular Sertoli cells to inhibit the formation of the uterus, fallopian tubes, and upper vagina from the müllerian structures.

In androgen-dependent tissues, testosterone is converted to dihydrotestosterone which virilizes the external genitalia. Peripheral androgen action depends on the binding of the androgen in the target tissues to a receptor controlled by an X chromosome.

In the female, ovarian development occurs in the presence of two X chromosomes and external gonadal development occurs spontaneously. Genital development in both sexes is completed by 20 weeks of fetal life. In the male, growth of the formed penis is dependent upon continued testicular testosterone secretion under stimulation by pituitary gonadotrophins.

Classification of intersex states

The classification that forms the basis of clinical assessment and management depends on gonadal morphology (Table 1). Female pseudohermaphroditism describes genital ambiguity resulting form abnormal virlization of the female with normal ovaries. The male counterpart—male pseudohermaphroditism—is the result of incomplete virilization of the male with differentiated testes. Thirdly, the true hermaphrodite possesses both ovarian and testicular tissue.

Female pseudohermaphroditism

Female pseudohermaphrodites have 46 XX karyotypes with normal ovaries and müllerian structures, but the external genitalia are virilized. The aetiology of female pseudohermaphroditism is given in Table 2. The degree of genital ambiguity can range from enlargement of the clitoris or fusion of the posterior labia to a completely male appearance, depending on the timing of androgen production and the concentration of androgens in the fetal circulation. Virilization may be caused by excessive production of either fetal or maternal androgens.

Virilization by fetal androgens

Congenital adrenal hyperplasia (see also Chapter 12.7.2)

The commonest cause of ambiguous genitalia in the newborn female is a recessively inherited enzyme defect of cortisol synthesis, with diversion of intermediates to androgen production. A reduction in steroid 21-hydroxylase or absence of 11β-hydroxylase or 3β-hydroxysteroid dehydrogenase can be the cause of this condition. These enzymes are part of the steroid biosynthetic pathways which link cholesterol with cortisol, aldosterone, and androgens. In the absence of, or lowered potential for, cortisol production, there are high adrenocorticotrophic hormone (ACTH) levels leading to adrenal hyperplasia and excess androgen production.

21-HYDROXYLASE DEFICIENCY

This form of congenital adrenal hyperplasia accounts for 90 per cent of cases of female pseudohermaphroditism, and should be excluded before proceeding to assign other causes for ambiguous genitalia. The degree of virilization can be variable (Fig. 1). In Europe, 60 per cent of all cases will develop salt depletion due to decreased production of aldosterone in the first 2 weeks of life. Usually, there is enlargement of the clitoris associated with a degree of posterior labial fusion and the formation of a hypoplastic lower vagina which may open into the urethra.

Table 1 *Classification of intersex states*

Female pseudohermaphrodite: virilization of genetic female with ovaries
Male pseudohermaphrodite: incomplete virilization of genetic male with testes
True hermaphrodite: individual with ovarian and testicular tissue

Table 2 *Aetiology of female pseudohermaphroditism*

Virilization by fetal androgens
  Congenital adrenal hyperplasia
    21-Hydroxylase deficiency
    11β-Hydroxylase deficiency
    3β-Hydroxysteroid/dehydrogenase deficiency
  Other causes of fetal androgen overproduction
    Fetal adrenal adenoma
    Nodular adrenal hyperplasia
    Persistent fetal adrenal (preterm infants)

Fetal virilization by maternal androgens
  Ovarian tumours
  Adrenal tumours

Iatrogenic fetal virilization
  Testosterone and progestins

Female pseudohermaphroditism with associated congenital malformations

17-Hydroxyprogesterone is a biosynthetic precursor of cortisol, and plasma levels are elevated in 21-hydroxylase deficiency. After the third day of life there is good discrimination between plasma levels of 17-hydroxyprogesterone in affected cases (100–800 nmol/l) and those of normal infants (< 15 nmol/l). Measurement of plasma renin activity and aldosterone help to define the extent of mineralocorticoid deficiency. Analysis of urine steroid excretion using chromatography and mass spectrometry can provide a reliable diagnostic profile from day 3 after birth.

11β-HYDROXYLASE DEFICIENCY

This defect probably accounts for about 5 per cent of all cases of congenital adrenal hyperplasia. The virilization may be severe, with affected females sometimes raised as males. The plasma concentration of 11-deoxycortisol (compound S) is elevated, and may exceed 1000 nmol/l. The urine steroid pattern will show high excretion of 6-hydroxytetrahydro-11-deoxycortisol as well as of tetrahydro-S.

Fig. 1 Variation in degree of virilization in three female infants with 21-hydroxylase deficiency.

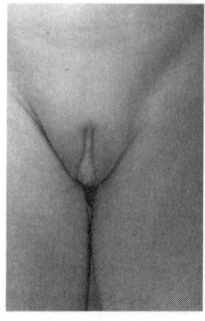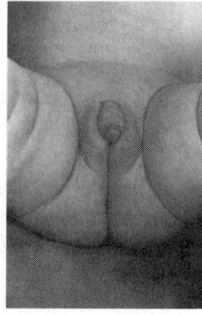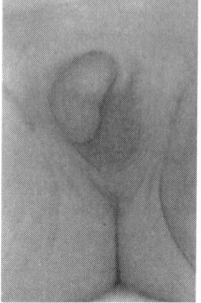

3β-HYDROXYSTEROID DEHYDROGENASE DEFICIENCY

This rare defect was originally described in male infants with incomplete virilization. However, a paradoxical androgen affect may be seen in female infants due to a very high level of dehydroepiandrosterone, the steroid precursor immediately proximal to the enzyme block. A non-classical or attenuated form of 3β-hydroxysteroid dehydrogenase deficiency has been described which presents with virilization in postadrenarchal or peripubertal females.

Virilization by maternal androgens

Virilization of the external genitalia by a maternal ovarian or adrenal androgen-secreting tumour is a rare but well-recognized cause of female pseudohermaphroditism. The degree of virilization may be striking.

Other causes of fetal virilization

Female pseudohermaphroditism due to maternal administration of progestogen preparations became recognized about 30 years ago. A number of dysmorphic childhood syndromes may also be associated with virilized female genitalia.

Male pseudohermaphroditism

Male pseudohermaphroditism arises as a result of a disturbance of male genital development in patients with testes and a 46 XY karyotype. The genital anomaly can vary from apparently female to male external genitalia with a small penis or perineal hypospadias. The three main aetiological groups (Table 3) are impaired Leydig cell activity, peripheral androgen insensitivity, and deficient testosterone and antimüllerian hormone production by incompletely differentiated testes.

Impaired testicular secretion of testosterone

Inborn errors of testosterone biosynthesis

These rare disorders (Fig. 2) lead to defective testosterone synthesis during the critical period of fetal sexual differentiation. The result is

Table 3 *Aetiology of male pseudohermaphroditism*

Impaired Leydig cell activity
  Inborn errors of testosterone biosynthesis
    Deficient formation of pregnenolone
    3β-Hydroxysteroid dehydrogenase deficiency
    17α-Hydroxylase deficiency
    17,20-Desmolase deficiency
    17β-Hydroxysteroid dehydrogenase deficiency
    Leydig cell hypoplasia

Androgen insensitivity syndromes
  Androgen receptor defects
  Complete testicular feminization
  Incomplete testicular feminization
  Reifenstein syndrome
  Infertile male syndrome
  Post-receptor resistance
  5α-Reductase deficiency

Incomplete differentiation of testes with deficient testosterone
  and antimüllerian hormone production
  Mixed gonadal dysgenesis
  Dysgenetic male pseudohermaphroditism
  XY pure gonadal dysgenesis
  Drash syndrome

Other forms
  Iatrogenic male pseudohermaphroditism
  Associated with other congenital anomalies
  Persistent müllerian structures

inadequate testosterone secretion, either locally to virilize the wolffian ducts to form the vas deferens, seminal vesicles, or epididimis, or peripherally to virilize the external genitalia. Synthesis of antimüllerian hormone, being a glycoprotein rather than a steroid, is unaffected. When the enzyme deficiency, inherited as an autosomal recessive trait, is situated early in the biosynthetic pathway, adrenal steroid synthesis may also be affected.

DEFICIENT FORMATION OF PREGNENOLONE

Three closely related microsomal enzymes (20α-hydroxylase, 20,22-desmolase, and 22α-hydroxylase) are necessary for the conversion of

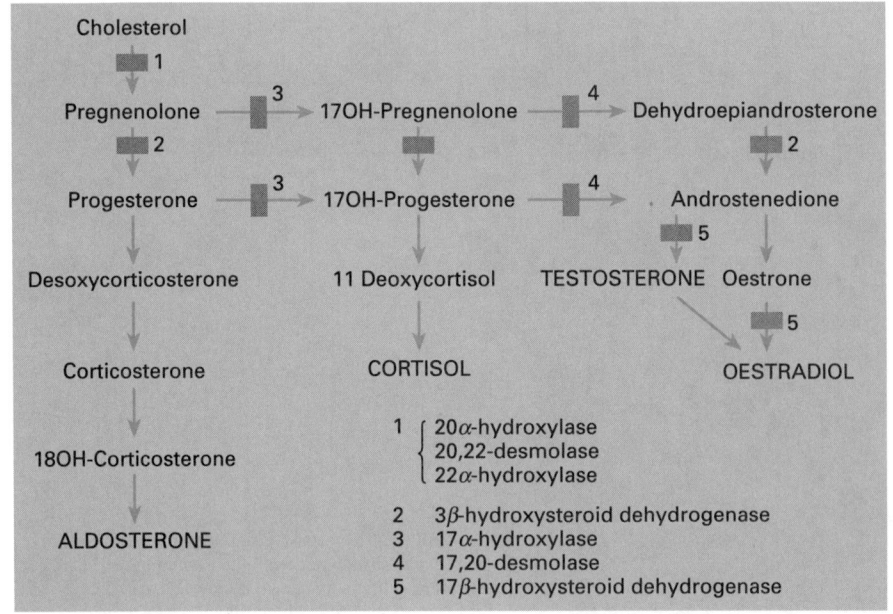

Fig. 2 Enzyme defects in testosterone biosynthesis.

cholesterol to pregnenolone. Deficiency of one of these enzymes leads to impaired synthesis of cortisol, aldosterone, and testosterone. Accumulation of cholesterol has been demonstrated in the hyperplastic adrenal.

DEFICIENCY OF 3β-HYDROXYSTEROID DEHYDROGENASE

Male patients with this enzyme deficiency are poorly virilized and usually develop salt loss and adrenal failure in infancy. Some subjects have survived puberty, which has been characterized by virilization and gynaecomastia. Urinary pregnenetriol and plasma dehydroepiandrosterone are elevated, as is plasma renin activity.

DEFICIENCY OF 17α-HYDROXYLASE

This defect results in decreased cortisol synthesis by the adrenal cortex and testosterone by the fetal testes, resulting usually in a complete lack of virilization. The disorder is identified biochemically by demonstrating high serum and urinary levels of progesterone and corticosterone. A compensatory increase in ACTH leads to excess mineralocorticoid secretion, causing hypertension, hypokalaemia, and low plasma renin activity.

DEFICIENCY OF 17,20-DESMOLASE

This rare defect is related to 17-hydroxylase deficiency as both enzyme activities are coded by the same gene. Impaired virilization may be variable in degree. Biochemically, identification of the defect relies on elevation of plasma 17-hydroxyprogesterone, 17-hydroxypregnenolone, and urinary pregnanetriolone.

DEFICIENCY OF 17-KETOSTEROID REDUCTASE (17β-HYDROXYSTEROID DEHYDROGENASE)

Patients with this defect are born with female-looking external genitalia and a phallus closely resembling a normal clitoris. There is a high prevalence within the Arab population of the Gaza Strip. The enzyme defect interferes with conversion of androstenedione to testosterone, adrenal steroid synthesis being unaffected. There is elevation of the androstenedione to testosterone ratio, particularly after HCG stimulation. Subjects are usually raised as girls; however, gender conversion to male has been described, coinciding with the marked virilization which occurs at puberty.

Androgen insensitivity syndromes

Mechanisms of androgen action

Testosterone, the principal androgen secreted by the testis, circulates bound to two proteins, sex hormone binding globulin and albumin. The protein-bound steroid is in dynamic equilibrium with the free hormone. Free testosterone enters the target cell by a passive mechanism (Fig. 3). Inside the cell, testosterone can be reduced to dihydrotestosterone by the enzyme 5α-reductase. Testosterone or dihydrotestosterone binds with high affinity to specific receptor proteins to form an androgen–receptor complex. This complex enters the cell nucleus and, after transformation into a DNA binding state, binds to specific nucleotide sequences which promote transcription of messenger RNA, resulting in clinical virilization. The gene encoding the human androgen receptor has recently been cloned.

Although testosterone and dihydrotestosterone bind to the same receptor, the two hormones perform different roles in androgen physiology (Fig. 4). Testosterone regulates secretion of luteinizing hormone, virilizes the wolffian ducts during fetal life, and may be essential for spermatogenesis. Dihydrotestosterone is responsible for formation of the external genitalia and prostate, and for most secondary sexual effects, such as hair growth and enlargement of the genitalia.

Clinical features of androgen insensitivity

Abnormalities of androgen action may have a severe effect on male sexual differentiation, resulting in incomplete virilization during fetal life and at puberty. The syndromes of androgen insensitivity probably account for the majority of cases of male pseudohermaphroditism. There are three main forms. The most important numerically is an X-linked cystolic androgen receptor defect. This may be manifested by a broad clinical spectrum from complete androgen insensitivity to a virtually

Fig. 3 Scheme of intracellular androgen action (adapted from Hughes and Pinsky 1989). T, testosterone; DHT, dihydrotestosterone; R, receptor.

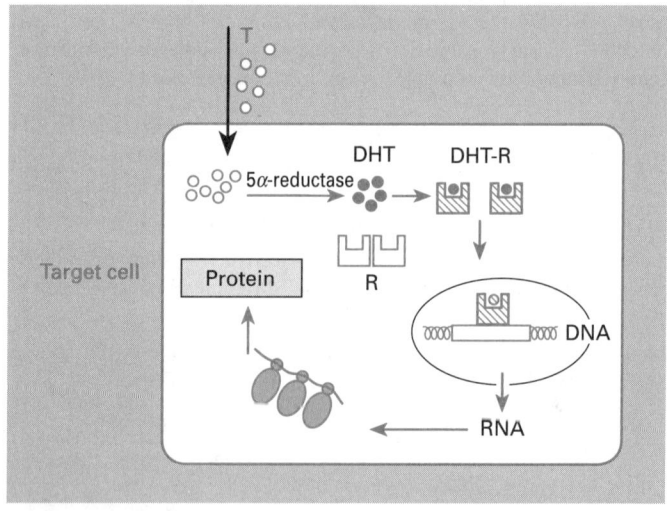

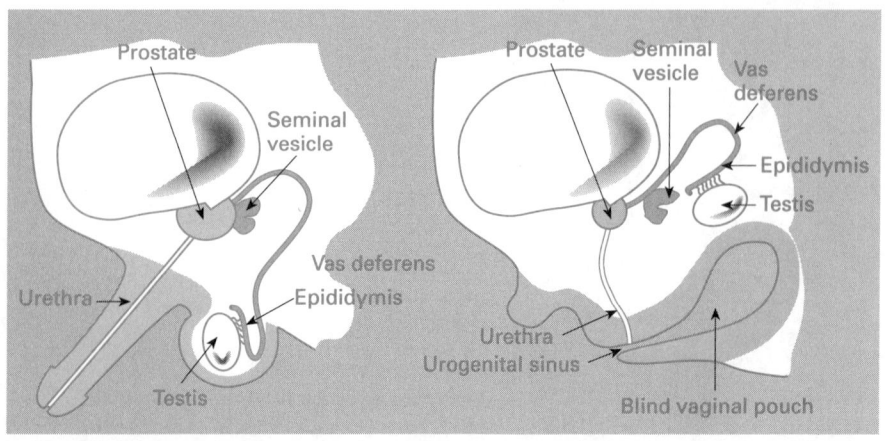

Fig. 4 Roles of testosterone and dihydrotestosterone in male sexual differentiation in the normal male (left) and the patient with 5α-reductase deficiency (right). Testosterone, heavy shading; dihydrotestosterone, light shading.

normally formed male with infertility. The second form is known as receptor-positive resistance, where a similar spectrum of clinical defects is associated with apparently normal receptor function. Thirdly, 5α-reductase deficiency is an autosomally inherited enzyme defect resulting in impaired conversion of testosterone to dihydrotestosterone in the target cell.

Androgen receptor defects

These defects may be expressed clinically as four main phenotypes, two predominantly female and two male. The female forms are complete and incomplete testicular feminization; the male forms are the Reifenstein syndrome and the 'infertile male' syndrome.

COMPLETE TESTICULAR FEMINIZATION

The typical patient with complete androgen insensitivity presents after puberty with primary amenorrhoea, or before puberty with inguinal hernias and palpable testes. The phenotype and psychosexual orientation is female. Breasts develop as in a normal woman, but pubic and axillary hair is scanty and the vagina is blind-ending due to regression of müllerian structures, which are virtually always absent. Wolffian structures are usually absent and the gonads show Leydig cell hyperplasia with no spermatogeneses. There is a significant risk of gonadal malignancy occurring after puberty, when gonadectomy is recommended.

INCOMPLETE TESTICULAR FEMINIZATION

This and the two subsequent syndromes come into the category of incomplete androgen insensitivity. Here there is more virilization than in the complete form, usually seen as clitoral enlargement and labial fusion. At puberty, feminization is dominant, with some further virilization apparent.

REIFENSTEIN SYNDROME

In this disorder the phenotype is predominantly male. Affected subjects usually have severe perineal hypospadias, most being raised as males. Virilization at puberty is more marked than in the two previous conditions, but is nevertheless incomplete and associated with gynaecomastia. Several pedigrees with family members affected according to an X-linked pattern have now been described. The degree of clinical abnormality within families may be very variable.

THE INFERTILE MALE SYNDROME

This condition represents the male end of the spectrum of androgen insensitivity. There is a normal male phenotype except for a rather small penis and small testes and possibly gynaecomastia. The main expression of the androgen receptor defect is oligospermia and infertility.

ENDOCRINE FEATURES

The endocrine features of androgen receptor defects are essentially similar in the previously described four variants. Testicular androgen secretion is normal or increased. Plasma testosterone may be elevated in infancy but is normal during the remainder of the prepubertal period. At puberty, plasma testosterone, oestradiol, and sex hormone binding globulin levels are elevated. Plasma gonadotrophins are normal in childhood but both luteinizing hormone and follicle stimulating hormone levels are consistently elevated during and after puberty, due to insensitivity of the hypothalamic androgen receptor.

5α-Reductase deficiency

This autosomal recessive disorder is characterized by impaired conversion of testosterone to dihydrotestosterone in androgen-dependent target cells. It was first described in the Dominican Republic, and occurs principally in areas of high consanguinity. The clinical features can be summarized as showing male internal genital structures and female external genitalia (Fig. 4). Fetal dihydrotestosterone-dependent development is abnormal, resulting in a rudimentary phallus and absent prostate. The wolffian structures develop normally, and the testes differentiate with spermatogenesis capable of progressing to the spermatozoa stage. Most subjects are raised as females but gender conversion to male occurs at puberty, coinciding with striking virilization of body habitus (Fig. 5) and male psychosexual orientation. Virilization during and after puberty, however, is incomplete, as the penis remains small and body and facial hair is sparse.

The endocrine features comprise low plasma dihydrotestosterone with normal testosterone and an elevated testosterone to dihydrotestosterone ratio. This abnormal ratio is the cardinal diagnostic feature. There is also elevation of the ratio of 5β : 5α androgen metabolites (i.e. aetiocholanolone to androsterone) in urine.

Male pseudohermaphroditism related to abnormal testicular differentiation

Incomplete differentiation of the fetal testes due to a defect of the Y-chromosomal genes responsible for testicular determination may cause genital ambiguity. Incompletely formed or dysgenetic testes secrete insufficient testosterone and antimüllerian hormone for normal male development. A number of clinical syndromes exist in this category.

DYSGENETIC MALE PSEUDOHERMAPHRODITISM

In this syndrome there are bilateral dysgenetic testes, persistent müllerian structures, cryptorchidism, and poorly virilized external genitalia.

MIXED GONADAL DYSGENESIS

Here there is asymmetrical gonadal differentiation with a testis present on one side and a streak gonad on the other. The internal structures are also asymmetrical, reflecting the endocrine function of the ipsilateral gonad. Many patients have a mosaic XO/XY karyotype and features of Turner's syndrome.

Fig. 5 Two Greek Cypriot brothers with 5α-reductase deficiency.

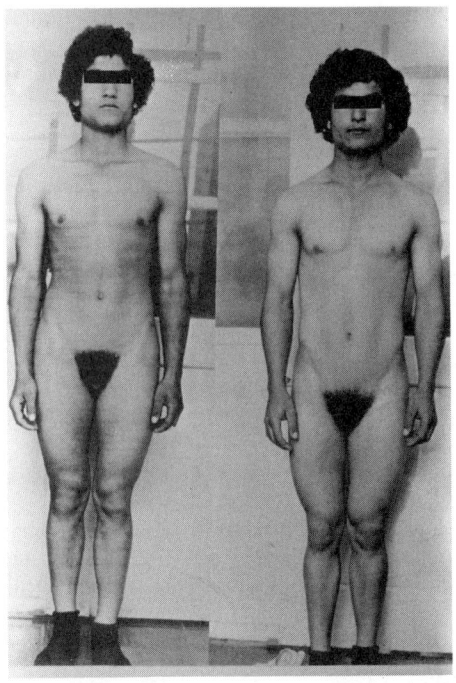

DRASH SYNDROME

This syndrome combines dysgenetic testes, genital ambiguity, glomerulonephritis, and Wilms' tumour.

True hermaphroditism

The diagnosis of true hermaphroditism is made when both ovarian as well as testicular tissue is present in the same individual. Van Niekerk has published an extensive review of the literature, including a large personal series. The most common presenting symptoms are abnormal appearance of the external genitalia. Most patients have a 46 XX karyotype: about half are pure 46 XX and about a third are mosaics or chimeras with 46 XX cell lines, i.e. 46 XX/46 XY. A few patients with a pure 46 XY karyotype have been reported. Occasional familial cases of true hermaphroditism have been described in the literature.

Other 46 XX intersex states

Pure gonadal dysgenesis

This disorder, which may be familial, is usually associated with female external genitalia. Clitoromegaly is sometimes present. The gonads are streaks and the karyotype may be 46 XX or XY. 46 XY gonadal dysgenesis, inherited as an X-linked recessive or male-limited autosomal dominant condition, has also been described.

XX male

A number of XX males have been described. These are normal-appearing males with normal intelligence and male psychosexual orientation. Gynaecomastia, sparce facial hair, small genitalia, and hypospadias may occur in this syndrome. The testes are small and resemble Klinefelter testes histologically. There is absence of spermatogenesis, leading to sterility. Families have been reported containing both an XX male and a 46 XX true hermaphrodite.

Gonadal neoplasia and intersex states

It is now established that a number of intersex disorders carry an increased risk of gonadal tumours. Two important risk factors are the presence of dysgenetic gonadal tissue and a Y chromosome. Intra-abdominal gonads are more susceptible than scrotal glands. The commonest tumour is a gonadoblastoma which is a premalignant lesion but can progress to an invasive tumour.

Clinical and laboratory assessment of patients with intersex states

The assessment of patients with intersex states may be considered from the point of view of the pediatrician assessing an infant with ambiguous genitalia. The same principles apply to the older child or adult. It must be emphasized that the general appearance of the external genitalia, while important in deciding the appropriate gender for the child, is of very little help in defining the aetiology of the disorder.

CLINICAL ASSESSMENT

The principles of clinical assessment are shown in Table 4. A history of a similar disorder in other family members may shed light on the likely diagnosis. Many of these conditions are genetically determined. Examination for other anomalies which could point to a dysmorphic syndrome known to be associated with abnormal genital development

Table 4 *Patient with intersex state: clinical assessment*

Family history, general examination for dysmorphic features
Examination of external genitalia
  No gonads palpable
    Female pseudohermaphrodite: congenital adrenal
      hyperplasia (21-hydroxylase deficiency)
    Male pseudohermaphrodite
  One gonad palpable
    Abnormal gonadal differentiation
    Mixed gonadal dysgenesis (XO/XY)
    True hermaphroditism
  Two gonads palpable
    Male pseudohermaphrodite
    Impaired testosterone biosynthesis
    Androgen receptor defect
    5α-Reductase deficiency
    True hermaphroditism

Table 5 *Patient with intersex state: laboratory assessment*

No gonads palpable
  Karyotype, plasma 17-hydroxyprogesterone, 11-
    deoxycortisol

One gonad palpable
  Karyotype, HCG test, gonadal biopsy, pelvic
    ultrasonography, laparotomy

Two gonads palpable
  Karyotype, HCG test (HCG 1000 units daily × 3), plasma
    testosterone, dihydrotestosterone, dehydroepiandrosterone,
    androstenedione on days 0 and 4

In vitro androgen binding studies

Sinogram

is also relevant. The most important aspect of the examination, however, is careful palpation of the gonads.

If no gonads are palpable, the most likely diagnosis is female pseudohermaphroditism due to congenital adrenal hyperplasia, and this is virtually certain if symptoms of salt loss develop. Other possible disorders are true hermaphroditism or male pseudohermaphroditism with intra-abdominal gonads. When both gonads are palpable in the scrotum or labial folds, the patient is likely to be a male pseudohermaphrodite, and measurement of plasma androgens will indicate whether the aetiology is a testicular or peripheral defect. A true hermaphrodite with bilateral ovotestes may also present in this way. The presence of only one palpable gonad or asymmetry of the perineum is suggestive of mixed gonadal dysgenesis; true hermaphroditism with asymmetrical gonads is the other differential diagnosis.

LABORATORY ASSESSMENT

A similar scheme may be devised as a guide to confirming the aetiology biochemically (Table 5). In all intersex patients a karyotype is indicated. If no gonads are palpable, determination of plasma 17-hydroxyprogesterone will confirm or exclude 21-hydroxylase deficiency. In 11β-hydroxylase deficiency the plasma 11-deoxycortisol concentration is elevated. The infant with two palpable gonads needs an HCG stimulation test to assess testicular androgen secretion. Numerous HCG regimens exist, of which two examples are 1000 IU daily for 3 days or a single injection of 1500 IU/m² body surface area. Basal and post-stimulatory concentrations of testosterone, dihydrotestosterone, and androstenedione should distinguish a disorder of testosterone biosynthesis from a syndrome of androgen insensitivity.

If one gonad is palpable, gonadal biopsy may be helpful, particularly if ovarian tissue is suspected. Pelvic ultrasonography or exploratory laparotomy for identification of internal genital structures may also be indicated. In any patient with incomplete virilization, urethrography should be performed to identify a vaginal cavity communicating posteriorly with the urethra.

Medical management

Choice of gender

Parents are usually shocked to learn that there is doubt as to the sex of their child; they are often under the impression that the child may grow up to be neither male nor female. Temptation to give a provisional opinion should be avoided until the nature of the disorder is known and an informed answer can be given. The decision as to the appropriate sex-of-rearing is based mainly on the appearance of the external genitalia and on the likely pattern of secondary sexual development at puberty. This decision should be taken jointly by the endocrinologist, urologist, and the parents. The gender should be assigned as soon as possible; however, in some cases of severe ambiguity, there is a case for waiting to assess the effect of early treatment with depot testosterone (25–50 mg at monthly intervals) on phallic growth as a guide to androgen responsiveness.

The concept that, once established, gender identity and role are more or less fixed has now been questioned. Although change of gender may be extremely difficult, the possibility of gender conversion should be viewed with an open mind in the individual subject who, because of spontaneous virilization or feminization at puberty, finds existence in their original gender intolerable.

Sex hormone therapy

Long-term treatment with androgens to promote phallic growth in early childhood has rightly fallen into disrepute because of the acceleration of bone maturation, which leads to loss of ultimate growth potential. While standard testosterone treatment is effective for inducing pubertal development in males with androgen-responsive syndromes, it is of limited value in patients with androgen insensitivity. Induction of full masculization in these patients is still very unsatisfactory. It has, however, been demonstrated that some further virilization in adult patients may be effectively induced using supraphysiological doses of depot testosterone (500 mg weekly). Effects, albeit slow to appear, were seen specifically in penile length and facial and body hair growth.

REFERENCES

Eckstein, B., Cohen, S., Farkas, A., and Rosler, A. (1989). The nature of the defect in familial male pseudohermaphroditism in Arabs of Gaza. *Journal of Clinical Endocrinology and Metabolism* **68**, 477–85.

Forest, M.G., (1981). Inborn errors of testosterone biosynthesis. *Pediatric and Adolescent Endocrinology* **8**, 133–55.

Hughes, I.A. and Pinsky, L. (1989). Sexual differentiation. In *Paediatric Endocrinology*, (ed. R. Collu, J.R. Ducharne, and H.S. Guyda), pp. 251–93. Raven Press, New York.

Imperato-McGinley, J., *et al.* (1982). Hormonal evaluation of a large kindred with complete androgen insensitivity: evidence for secondary 5-alpha-reductase deficiency. *Journal of Clinical Endocrinology and Metabolism* **54**, 931–41.

Kirk, J.M.W., Perry, L.A., Shand, W.S., Kirby, R.S., Besser, G.M., and Savage, M.O. (1990). Female pseudohermaphroditism due to a maternal adreno-cortical tumour. *Journal of Clinical Endocrinology and Metabolism* **70**, 1280–4.

New, M.L. and Josso, N. (1988). Disorders of gonadal differentiation and congenital adrenal hyperplasia. *Endocrinology Metabolic Clinics of North America* **17**, 399.66.

Pang, S., Lerner, A.J., and Stoner, L.S. (1985). Late onset adrenal steroid

3β-hydroxysteroid dehydrogenase deficiency: A cause of hirsutism in pubertal and post-pubertal women. *Journal of Clinical Endocrinology and Metabolism* **60**, 428–35.

Price, P., *et al.* (1984). High dose androgen therapy in male pseudohermaphroditism due to 5-alpha reductase deficiency and disorders of the androgen receptor. *Journal of Clinical Investigation* **74**, 1496–508.

Savage, M.O. (1988). Clinical aspects of intersex In *Clinical Paediatric Endocrinology*, (ed. C.G.D. Brook), pp 38–52. Blackwells, Oxford.

Savage, M.O. and Lowe, D.G. (1990). Gonadal neoplasia and abnormal sexual differentiation. *Clinical Endocrinology* **32**, 519–33.

van Niekerk, W.A. (1981). True hermaphroditism. *Pediatric and Adolescent Endocrinology* **8**, 80–99.

Williams, D.M., Patterson, M.N., and Hughes, I.A. (1993). Androgen insensitivity syndrome. *Archives of Disease in Childhood* **68**, 343–4.

Wilson, J.D., Griffin, J.E., Leshin, M., and MacDonald, P.C. (1983). The androgen resistance syndromes In *The metabolic basis of inherited disease*, (ed. J.B. Stanbury, J.B. Wyngaarden, D.S. Fredridison, J.L. Goldstein, and M.S. Brown), pp. 1001–26. McGraw-Hill, New York.

12.9.2 Normal growth and its disorders

M. A. PREECE

The normal curve of growth

The upper panel of Fig. 1 shows the height distance curve for a typical male from birth to 18 years of age. It is the most commonly used representation and the one most closely associated with height as observed

Fig. 1 The growth in height of an individual boy from birth to 18 years of age. The top panel shows the height attained or distance curve and the lower panel shows the data replotted as height gain or growth velocity. (Reproduced from Tanner 1962, with permission.)

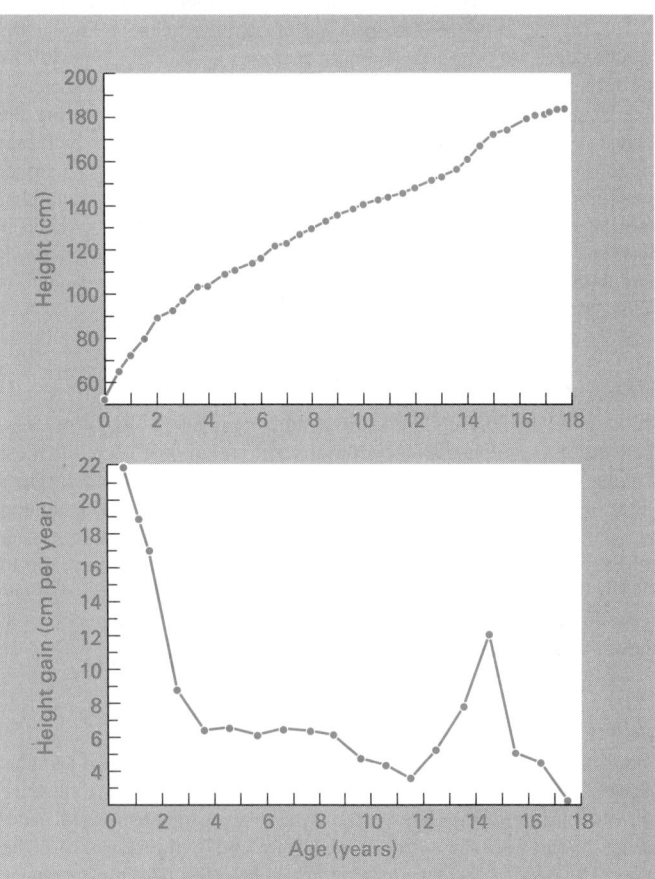

in everyday life. It contains all the relevant information about growth in height of an individual child. In the lower panel the growth data are represented in a different way, converting them to provide a record of height velocity in cm/year. This is calculated from the distance data by dividing the difference between two height measurements (as close to 1 year apart as possible) by the exact time elapsed between them. The calculated velocity is plotted at the mid-point of the time interval over which it is measured to produce the velocity curve. This representation of growth is particularly useful as it shows more detail of the growth process and is more immediate.

The growth velocity in any one year is a more sensitive measure of events that have occurred in that year than is the coincident height distance datum, which is a measurement summating all previous growth. Thus, the more sensitive measures of the velocity curve may show rather dramatic change in growth during disease or during treatment, where the simpler distance curve would be less sensitive.

There are three epochs of growth: early, rather fast growth before the age of 2 years; relatively slow steady growth during the pre-school and primary school years; and then the period around puberty when the adolescent growth spurt dominates the growth pattern.

Epochs of growth

Infancy

During the first year of life the infant has an average height velocity of about 25 cm/year. However, since this is a time when the velocity is changing dramatically, measurement over shorter time periods should be considered. The velocity during the first 3 months is equivalent to 3.3 cm/month in boys and 3.0 cm/month in girls, dropping to 1.2 cm/month and 1.3 cm/month, respectively, by the last 3 months of that year. During the next 3 years there is a further deceleration to a velocity of 0.5 cm/month, or 6 cm/year, which is the average through much of middle childhood. This continues with gentle slowing until puberty.

The first 3 years are also the time of increased channelling of the growth curve. At birth, the length of the baby is determined mostly by the fetal environment which, in turn, is much dependent on maternal size; father's height is poorly correlated with the child's. During the next 2 to 3 years, the influence of the father's genetic make-up increases progressively until there is equal influence by both parents. This phenomenon can result in some rather bizarre growth patterns where mother and father have very different heights. For example, when the child is born to a tall mother but short father, the initially rather large baby will tend to grow unusually slowly until the genetically expected channel is achieved.

Middle childhood

Although in healthy children growth is a moderately steady process, there are fluctuations that occur in the short and middle term, the most striking of which are related to seasonal changes. Most children grow faster in spring and summer, with relatively slow periods in the autumn and winter; a few children show a reversed pattern, and others no regular pattern at all. There is a rather constant, but small, growth spurt at 6 to 7 years of age in both boys and girls, with no sexual dimorphism; it has been attributed to the onset of adrenal androgen secretion that occurs at about that age.

Puberty

There is little difference in growth rates between males and females before 10 years of age. Then the typical female starts her adolescent growth spurt and, for a few years, is taller than the same-aged male. About 2 years later the male starts his spurt and by the age of 14 is the taller. The major difference in adult height between males and females (14 cm in the United Kingdom) is established at puberty. About 11 cm comes from the extra 2 years of prepubertal growth of boys and 3 cm from their more intense growth spurt.

The appearance of sexual dimorphism in height during puberty is reflected in many other body dimensions. At this time there is a generally more dramatic growth spurt in males for most body dimensions, albeit occurring about 2 years later than for females. The single major exception is the more dramatic and sustained growth spurt for bi-iliac diameter, reflecting pelvic breadth, in females. There are also associated changes in soft tissues, leading to the greater muscularity of the male.

Metabolic and endocrine factors controlling growth

Each of the epochs of growth described above is associated with particular metabolic or hormonal factors which exert their effects in an almost sequential manner. These distinctions should not be overstated however, and are only useful as a general guide to the most important factors at a given age. In essence, infant growth is dominated by nutritional considerations, the childhood period by growth hormone (GH), and puberty by the sex hormones, but nutrition has an important role throughout and GH is important in early infant growth, as shown by the reduced birth size of children with congenital GH deficiency. Thyroid hormone is also important throughout the growing period.

Disorders of growth

Growth disorders are predominantly problems of childhood, and patients seen by the adult physician are inevitably left with a legacy of events which have occurred before maturity. In many cases where the condition was successfully treated during childhood there may be no residual problem with stature in adult life. In contrast, there are many situations when this happy outcome is not achieved and there is still a persistent problem requiring attention in the adult clinic. Thus the importance of the various disorders is different and what follows reflects this.

Short stature

DEFINITION

What is considered as short (or for that matter tall) stature is essentially arbitrary. It is usually considered as a height that falls below the third centile for the relevant population; these values for adults are given in Table 1. This is easy when the discrepancy is severe but difficulties arise with patients whose height lies close to this limit. In this situation the perceptions of the patient may greatly colour the situation and its management. The most important decision is whether the apparent short stature is a symptom of a disorder that requires attention, and therefore most stress is placed upon diagnosis.

CLASSIFICATION OF SHORT STATURE

The major categories of short stature are shown in Table 2. The process of attributing such labels to an individual patient is largely one of clinical assessment, including critical appraisal of the pattern of growth, combined with appropriate confirmatory investigations.

Familial short stature

This relatively common condition is among the most difficult to manage. It is sometimes referred to as normal or idiopathic short stature. Patients usually present in childhood with heights clustered around the third centile. The parents are usually of comparable size and the child's stature is simply reflecting the genetic inheritance. This apparently straightforward situation is made difficult because of the considerable social pressures that now exist; parents and their children simply find it hard to accept the situation and want it changed.

Table 1 *Critical heights (cm) for male and female adults in the United Kingdom*

	3rd Centile	50th Centile	97th Centile
Females	152.7	163.9	175.2
Males	165.2	177.8	190.4

Table 2 *Major groups of disease processes leading to short stature*

Familial short stature
Constitutional delay of growth and/or puberty
Intrauterine growth retardation
Environmental short stature
Chronic paediatric disease
Endocrine disease
Genetic/chromosomal disorders
Dysmorphic syndromes
Bone dysplasias

Diagnosis

The clinical picture is clear: the child will be at or below the third centile for height with a normal growth velocity measured over 1 year. The height will be appropriate for the family and it is critical that parental heights are properly taken into account. The simplest way to do this is to measure both parents, if possible, and then determine their height centiles. The child's predicted adult height is calculated by an appropriate method that takes into account skeletal maturity; this predicted adult height should lie within a range of 10 cm above or below the mid-parental height centile, which represents the 3rd to 97th centiles for that family.

The general medical picture is of good health, apart from the usual childhood illnesses. Similarly, apart from short stature no abnormalities are found on general examination. In this situation no investigations are necessary other than the assessment of skeletal maturity for the prediction of adult height.

Management

The main problem is to persuade the patient and the family that there is no medical problem. Even when this is achieved, there is often a wish to change the prognosis for height. In recent years there have been many clinical trials of recombinant human growth hormone in this situation. While definitive data are still scarce, there is increasing evidence that although a short-term acceleration of height velocity is almost always achieved, this is not maintained, and adult height is unchanged. When such treatment is started after the age of 11 years this is moderately certain, but there remains some uncertainty if the recombinant human growth hormone is started at younger ages (6–8 years). Even if this is more successful, there remains a considerable debate about the ethics and cost-effectiveness of such treatment of normal healthy children.

Constitutional delay of growth and/or puberty

This problem is largely covered elsewhere (see Chapter 12.9.3). Here comment is restricted to noting that in many cases the delay in maturation is evident well before puberty when the presentation is purely of short stature associated with delayed skeletal maturation. There is often an associated element of familial short stature; the delay is highly amenable to treatment with anabolic steroids or androgens, whereas the familial element is unaffected.

Intrauterine growth retardation

This comprises a relatively large group of children who share the common feature of being born inappropriately small for gestational age; usually assessed in terms of birth weight. Many show a sustained period of accelerated or 'catch-up' growth and reach the normal centiles for height and weight. However, a significant number fail to do this and remain below the third centile although growing at a normal velocity. In some cases this clinical picture is part of a more general dysmorphic or genetic syndrome, but it may occur alone.

Diagnosis

Traditionally intrauterine growth retardation is diagnosed when a baby is born with a birth weight more than two standard deviations below the mean for gestational age, maternal height, and parity. However, this criterion is slowly changing to reflect intrauterine diagnosis by fetal ultrasound measurements.

In addition to the birth characteristics, the growth curve is characteristic and there are a number of other clinical features. The faces are small and triangular with a normal sized cranium which, compared to the small face, can give the impression of hydrocephalus. The general habitus is very lean and there may be a degree of limb asymmetry in about 50 per cent of cases. There often other minor dysmorphic features.

Many children have severe feeding problems in the first few years of life, which may compound the lean appearance and create further anxieties for the families. There may be a degree of delayed skeletal maturation, but this is very variable. General and endocrine investigations are unhelpful.

Management

In all but the most severely affected children growth velocity is normal as long as the intrauterine growth retardation is not part of a more generalized dysmorphic syndrome. However, the long-term prognosis for height is usually rather worse than appears in childhood. This is because puberty tends to be prompt and the adolescent growth spurt attenuated, so that less growth is achieved in the teenage years than might be expected.

The only active treatment that is being pursued at present is the use of recombinant human growth hormone, but it is still under clinical trial. Early results suggest short-term benefit, but in many children skeletal maturation is accelerated by the treatment and predicted mature height is probably unchanged, as in the case of familial short stature.

Environmental short stature

Over the past 30 years it has become clear that children's growth may be adversely affected by their environment other than by malnutrition or infection. This effect may be due to emotional or physical abuse or neglect and may sometimes present in the most bizarre of ways, often imitating other organic disorders such as growth hormone insufficiency. It is most common in young children but may rarely present in young teenagers and, strikingly, may present in a single child in a family where the other children thrive.

Diagnosis

This is a diagnosis which is notoriously easy to miss. In its most classical form it presents as an apparently straightforward diagnosis of growth hormone insufficiency although there will often be additional features of bizarre eating habits, behavioural abnormalities, or other evidence of abnormal family dynamics. In many where an initial diagnosis of growth hormone insufficiency is made, treatment with recombinant human growth hormone is started, often with early success. However, the accelerated growth soon falters and during the subsequent reappraisal the real diagnosis is uncovered.

As the above might suggest, endocrine investigations are often misleading. Once the suspicion is raised the only way to confirm the diagnosis is a period of time away from the family environment, either by a hospital admission or by short-term fostering. A period of accelerated growth (initially weight gain followed by height growth) makes the diagnosis. There is then the need for a detailed social and psychiatric appraisal of the family.

Management

Once the diagnosis is made the management is predominantly that of manipulation of the family circumstances, either by extensive social and psychiatric support for the family with the child *in situ*, or more commonly by removing the child from the family and placement elsewhere by fostering or adoption.

With proper management in childhood those who have suffered from environmental short stature should not present medical problems in adult life. However, it is highly likely that there may be continuing psychological problems and particularly the possibility of subsequent abuse of one or more of their own children.

Chronic paediatric disease

Any child with a long-standing chronic disease will show some degree of growth disorder if the primary disease is less than optimally managed. This may be due to the disease itself or to its treatment; the use of high doses of systemic corticosteroids is a particularly important example of the latter. However, it is very unusual for such a child to present with short stature as the primary symptom as the underlying disease is usually evident at an earlier stage. Notable exceptions to this rule are some gastrointestinal diseases, with coeliac and inflammatory bowel disease being particularly prominent. In most situations, whatever the primary disease, a degree of delayed skeletal maturation is prominent and may be the first feature of disordered growth to appear.

Management is targeted at the primary disease wherever possible. In some situations adjunct therapies, such as recombinant human growth hormone in chronic renal failure, are being studied within clinical trials. The long-term benefits of such treatments are far from clear at the present time.

Endocrine disease

The endocrine causes of short stature form the major group of readily treated growth disorders. Many of the details will have already covered in the chapters on the relevant endocrine glands and only a brief summary is given here.

Hypothyroidism

Inadequately treated congenital or acquired juvenile hypothyroidism is always associated with marked growth failure. Congenital disease ought to be diagnosed by neonatal screening programmes, such that growth is never a problem, although some delay in initiating thyroid replacement may lead to the more serious problems of intellectual impairment. On the other hand, juvenile hypothyroidism, usually due to autoimmune thyroiditis, can be far more insidious and often presents with growth failure as the sole symptom.

Diagnosis

In any undiagnosed short child there should always be a high degree of suspicion of the possibility of juvenile hypothyroidism. The classical features of adult disease such as constipation and intellectual impairment are usually absent and poor growth may be the only abnormality. Most typically the child grows with a very low velocity, rapidly crossing centiles and falling progressively further away from the third centile. General medical examination may be quite normal unless the disease is long established and severe; such symptoms and signs as may be present are no different to those in adults. A goitre may be present, depending upon the stage of the disease.

Striking delay in skeletal maturation is often seen; to the unwary this may lead to an incorrect diagnosis of constitutional delay of growth and/or puberty, as the degree of maturational delay will usually be sufficient to apparently explain the height deficit. For this reason thyroid function tests should be undertaken early and will confirm or deny the diagnosis without ambiguity. Serum T_3 or T_4 will be low, with an elevated serum thyroid stimulating hormone concentration.

Management

Thyroid replacement with L-thyroxine is relatively straightforward, with an initial dose of 100 μg/m^2/day; this is fine-tuned according to growth response, clinical examination, and maintenance of a suppressed thyroid stimulating hormone concentration with either a normal serum T_3 concentration or serum T_4 in the upper normal range. The prognosis for height is generally very good, except in those diagnosed and treated well into puberty, when the outcome is less satisfactory.

Growth hormone insufficiency

Growth hormone insufficiency may occur as an isolated disorder of uncertain aetiology, as part of more complex diseases and developmental anomalies, or as part of more extensive hypothalamopituitary disease. A list of such conditions is given in Table 3.

The principal differences arise between the congenital and acquired forms as the onset of the growth failure occurs differently. In the first case there is failure of normal growth from a very early age which can usually be detected within the first year of life. In contrast, acquired growth hormone insufficiency can lead to abnormally slow growth at any age before maturity. In the latter situation the assessment of height velocity assumes far greater importance as height may remain within the normal centiles for several years before the child becomes overtly short and below the third centile.

Particularly noteworthy is the pattern of growth in children receiving cranial or craniospinal irradiation as this may be rather different from other causes of growth hormone insufficiency. In both cases there may be associated early puberty, particularly with radiation doses below 2400 cGy, leading to a rather confusing picture as the early but rather attenuated adolescent growth spurt may mask the onset of growth hormone insufficiency. When the spine is involved in the radiation field there may be a combination of growth hormone insufficiency and direct damage to the spinal epiphyses, with subsequent failure of spinal growth which is not due to the endocrine abnormalities and not responsive to endocrine replacement.

Diagnosis

Children with growth hormone insufficiency grow with a slow height velocity and, depending on whether the insufficiency is congenital or acquired later, fall progressively further below the third centile or cross height centiles downwards. The degree of short stature can range from relatively mild to very severe, depending on the degree of insufficiency, the age of onset, and parental heights. As in many short stature disorders, the parents' heights still modify the expression of the disorder such that children with growth hormone insufficiency born to tall parents will tend to be more normal in height for longer than those with equivalent disease born to shorter parents.

Other clinical features include a rather young appearance, with immature facies and sometimes a quite striking degree of frontal bossing. There is usually an excess of subcutaneous fat, giving a rather cherubic appearance, and in boys there may be hypoplastic genitalia not necessarily due to associated gonadotrophin deficiency but secondary to intrauterine or neonatal severe growth hormone insufficiency.

The diagnosis is confirmed by a variety of endocrine measurements (see Chapter 12.2). Growth hormone (GH) is secreted in an episodic manner such that measurement in single serum samples is valueless. It is most commonly measured in several samples following pituitary stimulation by a provocative agent, of which the most important are listed in Table 4. The definition of a normal response is still rather arbitrary, but is usually set at a peak of more than 20 mIU/l at some point following the administration of the provocative agent. Arginine is probably the least satisfactory as it has the highest tendency to false positive results and its mechanism of action is unknown. The place of GH releasing hormone is uncertain; it tests the integrity of the hypothalamopituitary axis but does not detect primary hypothalamic disease, which is probably the most important cause of growth hormone insufficiency.

Table 3 *The causes of growth hormone insufficiency*

Congenital	Acquired
Genetic, usually autosomal recessive, including deletion of the hGH gene, but occasionally X-linked or dominant	Tumours of the pituitary or hypothalamus, particularly craniopharyngioma
Sporadic, usually with multiple pituitary hormone deficiencies, with hypoglycaemia and giant-cell hepatitis	Cranial irradiation, either as treatment for solid tumours or prophylaxis for childhood leukaemia
Perinatal associations, e.g. breech delivery	Head injury or surgery to the hypothalamo-pituitary region
Midline defect including septo-optic dysplasia, cleft-lip and palate, and pituitary aplasia	Langerhans cell histiocytosis
	After meningitis, particularly tuberculous
	Temporarily as part of environmental short stature

Table 4 *Provocative tests for growth hormone insufficiency*

Provocative agent	Route	Dose	Mechanism of action
Insulin	Intravenous	0.05–0.15 U/kg	Neurohypoglycaemia
Glucagon	Intramuscular	0.1 mg/kg	Neurohypoglycaemia
Clonidine	Oral	0.15 mg/m^2	β-Agonist
Arginine	Intravenous	500 mg/kg	Uncertain (basic amino acid)
GH releasing hormone	Intravenous	1 μg/kg	Physiological

Additional aids to diagnosis are the measurement of GH concentrations in serial blood samples taken frequently (every 15–20 min) over 24 h, or the measurement of basal serum concentrations of insulin-like growth factor-I (IGF-I) together with insulin-like growth factor binding protein (IGFBP-3). The former approach is laborious and labour intensive and is probably unhelpful except in some rare situations where an assessment of physiological GH secretion is required. The measurement of IGF-I and its binding protein may prove to be helpful; current experience is limited but measurement of serum IGFBP-3 concentration looks increasingly robust for identifying a disordered somatotrophic axis.

Growth hormone insufficiency may be isolated or part of a wider constellation of pituitary hormone deficiencies, and it is important to check thyroid and adrenal function at an early stage. Gonadotrophin deficiency is relatively common but difficult to confirm prior to the age of puberty, and it may not be until puberty fails to occur spontaneously that suspicion is raised (see Chapter 12.9.3).

Having confirmed the diagnosis of growth hormone insufficiency isolated or otherwise, it is important to determine the underlying aetiology and, in particular, seek an intracranial space-occupying lesion. Craniopharyngioma is the most important lesion and the use of modern imaging techniques, cranial CT or MRI, is mandatory. These lesions are most commonly associated with multiple pituitary hormone deficiencies, although these may take some years to become manifest (see Chapter 12.2).

Management

The treatment of growth hormone insufficiency is the same whatever the underlying aetiology: recombinant human growth hormone, 15 to 30 IU/m^2/week (0.6–1.2 IU/kg/week; 1 IU = 0.37 mg pure protein), by daily subcutaneous injection. The growth velocity is the best indicator of response and it should show a clear acceleration, usually to 10 cm/year or more. A poor response indicates the need to review the diagnosis. It is essential that any coexisting pituitary hormone deficiencies (such as thyroid stimulating hormone deficiency leading to secondary hypothyroidism) are adequately treated with appropriate replacement.

Treatment is continued until growth is complete and may therefore last for many years. For this reason it is particularly important to review dosage as growth occurs and ensure that injection sites are cared for adequately.

Growth hormone receptor deficiency This is a very rare disorder whose importance lies in the ability to mimic the much more common severe growth hormone insufficiency very closely. The clinical phenotypes may be indistinguishable but in the case of growth hormone receptor deficiency there is excessive secretion of GH by the pituitary gland; the fault lies in the GH receptor, which is either absent or non-functioning, leading to a deficiency of IGF-I. The abnormality is due to one of several mutations in the receptor gene, which is inherited according to an autosomal recessive pattern. Until now it has been untreatable but clinical trials of recombinant IGF-I look promising.

Adrenocortical excess (see also Chapter 12.7.1)

An excess of circulating corticosteroids is a potent cause of growth failure, whether due to endogenous overproduction or exogenous medication. In the former case, the aetiology may be hypothalamopituitary or adrenal in origin, as in adults. The diagnosis of Cushing's disease in childhood is rare and taxing to make, although, once considered, the approach does not differ from that in adults. Iatrogenic glucocorticoid excess is much more common and most often related to overuse of topical steroids for atopic disease; inhaled locally active steroids for asthma and powerful dermatological preparations for eczema are particularly important. The management of the growth failure is entirely dependent on reducing the glucocorticoid load usually by the introduction of an alternative non-steroidal treatment for the underlying condition.

Genetic/chromosomal disorders, dysmorphic syndromes, and bone dysplasias

For the purposes of this book these last three categories can be considered together. For the main part they are individually rare, but so many and varied that together they make a significant contribution to the causes of short stature. The approach to diagnosis depends heavily on clinical suspicion backed-up by chromosomal and radiological investigation.

Turner's syndrome

This is the only condition that will be discussed in any detail as it is relatively common (about 1 in 2500–3500 female births), surprisingly easy to miss, and amenable to useful treatment. Turner's syndrome tends to present in two distinct age groups: birth or infancy and mid-childhood. The young girls usually have a number of the classical features, including coarctation of the aorta leading to early clinical suspicion. However, a large number of affected girls only have subtle clinical signs, and in these patients short stature is virtually the only significant feature. Diagnosis is confirmed by chromosomal analysis, which may reveal a 45X karyotype with complete absence of one X chromosome; a more subtle structural abnormality of one X, such as an isochromosome; or a mosaic combination of cells with different chromosomal complements.

Untreated girls with Turner's syndrome reach adult heights of between 134 and 156 cm but this is dependent on their parents' heights; girls from tall families will be relatively tall for the diagnosis, even reaching into the lower part of the normal range. Puberty is usually, but not always, absent.

Treatment for both the short stature and the lack of puberty is possible. The latter requires the use of oestrogen and progestogens. A typical regimen would be the slow introduction of ethinyl oestradiol at about 12 to 13 years of age in a dose of 1 μg/day increasing to doses of 20 to 30 μg/day over 2 years. It should be given continuously at first, but when adult doses are reached it should be omitted for 1 week in every 4, when a withdrawal bleed will occur, mimicking menstruation. At the same time it is important that a progestogen, such as norethisterone 5 mg/day, is introduced for the last week of the cycle. More recently, clinical trials have shown that quite significant growth benefit can be achieved by the combined use of recombinant human growth hormone (20–30 IU/m²) and the mild anabolic steroid, oxandrolone (1.25–2.5 mg/day).

Tall stature

The causes of excessive growth are far fewer than those of short stature. Most common are variants of normal, usually with tall parents; pathological causes of tall stature are very rare.

DEFINITION

This can be defined in a complementary way to short stature (see above); it is equally arbitrary. In practical terms, boys find difficulty in accepting heights above 200 cm, whereas most girls find 185 cm the limit.

CLASSIFICATION

The major causes of tall stature are listed in Table 5; only the first will be discussed in any detail.

Familial tall stature

This is more or less the mirror image of familial short stature which is discussed above. There is often an element of advanced maturation with a skeletal age that exceeds chronological age by several years and early pubertal development. The diagnosis is made by clinical appraisal, including knowledge of parental heights and the demonstration that predicted adult height is appropriate for the family. Exclusion of other potential causes is often possible on clinical grounds, but the exclusion of excessive GH secretion may be necessary.

Management

The calculation of a predicted adult height, which because of the advanced skeletal maturation is often less than the family fears, may be

Table 5 *Principal causes of tall stature*

Familial tall stature
Pituitary gigantism
Sotos syndrome
Marfan syndrome
Homocystinuria

all that is necessary as the expected height is then acceptable. If this is not the case, then other pharmacological treatments may need discussion. At present these are unsatisfactory, although high-dose ethinyl oestradiol (100–300 μg/day) has been advocated in girls, in an attempt to accelerate skeletal maturation. However, the benefits are far from certain and there may be quite unpleasant side-effects, such as water retention. The long-term safety of this treatment is also unproven.

The use of testosterone in boys, in an analogous manner to oestrogen use in girls, is of even less value and is probably contraindicated.

Other causes of tall stature

Pituitary gigantism with excessive GH secretion is extremely rare but does occasionally require specific exclusion, usually by demonstration of normal suppression of GH secretion to undetectable levels by oral glucose (1.75 g/kg). Serum IGF-I concentrations will usually be high, but may overlap the normal range.

The Marfan syndrome is characterized by the disproportionately long limbs and digits (arachnodactyly), and is usually associated with a high-arched palate and pectus excavatum. It is an important diagnosis to make because of the risk of eye problems and dissection of the aortic root and arch. Ultrasound examination of the heart and aorta may be helpful.

Sotos syndrome and the other dysmorphic causes of tall stature are even rarer, and can usually be diagnosed on other criteria. They are not considered further here.

REFERENCES

Darendeliler, F., Hindmarsh, P.C., and Brook, C.G.D. (1990). Dose-response curves for treatment with biosynthetic human growth hormone. *Journal of Endocrinology* **125**, 311–16.

Davies, P.S.W., Valley, R., and Preece, M.A. (1988). Adolescent growth and pubertal progression in the Silver–Russell syndrome. *Archives of Disease in Childhood* **63**, 130–5.

Hindmarsh, P.C. and Brook, C.G.D. (1992) Disorders of stature. In *Clinical Endocrinology*, (ed. A. Grossman), pp. 810–36. Blackwell Scientific Publications, Oxford.

Preece, M.A. (1988). Prediction of adult height: methods and problems. *Acta Paediatrica Scandinavica (Suppl.)* **347**, 4–10.

Preece, M.A. (1992). Principles of normal growth: auxology and endocrinology. In *Clinical endocrinology*, (ed. A. Grossman), pp. 801–9. Blackwell Scientific Publications, Oxford.

Preece, M.A. (1994). Evaluation of growth and development. In *Pediatric Nephrology*, pp. 378–96. Williams and Wilkins, Baltimore.

Savage, M.O., *et al.* (1993). Clinical features and endocrine status in patients with growth hormone insensitivity (Laron syndrome). *Journal of Clinical Endocrinology and Metabolism*, **77**, 1465–71.

Tanner, J.M. (1962). *Growth at adolescence*, Blackwell, Oxford.

12.9.3 Puberty

R. J. M. Ross and M. O. Savage

Introduction

Puberty, as defined by the *Concise Oxford Dictionary*, is becoming functionally capable of procreation through the natural development of reproductive organs. The word is derived from 'puber' meaning adult, and not 'pubic', which refers to the lower part of the abdomen, the pubes. There is a popular misconception that the onset of puberty is heralded by the development of pubic hair, but in girls breast budding is usually the first sign of puberty and in boys an enlargement in testicular size. A clear understanding of normal pubertal development is essential for the management of patients with disordered puberty as in many cases counselling and reassurance is all that is required.

Sexual differentiation takes place at two stages of life; the first *in utero* extending to the perinatal period and the second occurring at puberty. Between these two stages is the 'quiescent period'. The physiological changes that accompany sexual differentiation and the hormonal factors that control these changes are well defined but what determines the duration of the 'quiescent period' and the onset of puberty remains to be established. What is known is that puberty is centrally driven and this is well illustrated by the failure of pubertal development in children with Kallmann's syndrome and the changes that occur in anorexia nervosa. In Kallmann's syndrome there is a failure in the migration of gonadotrophin releasing hormone (GnRH) neurones to the hypothalamus during fetal life. Affected patients present with hypogonadotrophic hypogonadism associated with ansomia. When puberty is delayed or arrested by anorexia nervosa it may be induced by the pulsatile administration of GnRH. The GnRH pulse generator is therefore essential for normal puberty, and the cues that switch it to pubertal mode include most importantly age and maturation of the central nervous system, environmental factors such as stress, social factors (probably the reason for an earlier onset of puberty in Western countries), and metabolic factors such as nutrition.

The onset of puberty is characterized by an increase in basal luteinising hormone (LH) levels and in the amplitude and frequency of LH pulses independent of gonadal changes. Gonadal activation stimulated by the rise in gonadotrophin (LH and follicle stimulating hormone (FSH)) secretion results in rising levels of sex steroids. Apart from their action on sexual maturation, gonadal steroids have a direct effect in stimulating skeletal growth and also a central action in stimulating increased growth hormone (GH) production. A consistent pattern of hormonal changes results in a relatively constant pattern of growth and pubertal development, characterized in girls by the development of breasts, pubic hair, and the onset of menstruation, and in boys by an increase in testicular volume, genitalia size, and the appearance of pubic hair. This is best appreciated by plotting a child's development on the Tanner–Whitehouse growth and development records. On these charts are illustrated not only the percentiles of height and weight, but also those for pubertal stages. A loss of the normal pattern of development suggests pathology. For instance, a boy who at 8 years has a height above the 97th centile, stage 3 genitalia and pubic hair, but testes less than 4 ml is likely to have an abnormal source of androgens, such as an androgen-secreting tumour or congenital adrenal hyperplasia.

Timing of puberty

Disorders of puberty can be classified by the timing of onset of sexual characteristics into either precocious or delayed puberty. Precocious puberty is characterized by signs of sexual maturation appearing less than 2.5 standard deviations (SD) from the mean; before 8 years in a girl and before 9 years in a boy. In Western society puberty is considered delayed when there are no signs of pubertal maturation in a girl aged 13.4 years (2SD) or boy aged 13.8 years. As a simple working rule, if there are no signs of puberty at 14 years of age investigation should be considered.

Precocious puberty

Precocious puberty can be classified into true (pituitary gonadotrophin dependent) or pseudo (pituitary gonadotrophin independent) precocious

Table 1 *Causes of precocious puberty*

Isolated thelarche and isolated pubarche
True precocious puberty (pituitary gonadotrophin dependent)
  Idiopathic
    sporadic
    familial
  CNS abnormalities
    congenital (e.g. hydrocephalus)
    acquired (e.g. irradiation, surgery, and infection)
    tumours, including hypothalamic hamartomas, gliomas,
      and pineal tumours
  Hypothyroidism
Pseudo precocious puberty (pituitary gonadotrophin
  independent)
  McCune–Albright syndrome (polyostotic fibrous dysplasia)
  Adrenal disorders
    adenomas and carcinomas
    congenital adrenal hyperplasia
  Gonadal disorders
    ovarian cyst
    ovarian tumours
    testotoxicosis
    Leydig cell tumour
  Ectopic gonadotrophin producing tumours
    dysgerminoma, hepatoblastoma, teratoma,
      chorionepithelioma
  Exogenous sex steroids

puberty (Table 1). In true precocious puberty, as in normal puberty, there is activation of the hypothalamopituitary axis and thus the normal pattern of puberty is preserved (complete precocious puberty). In pseudo precocious puberty as, for example that caused by an adrenal adenoma, the normal pattern of puberty is lost (incomplete precocious puberty). Pseudo precocious puberty may be isosexual, with appropriate male or female puberty, or heterosexual, when there is virilization of a girl, as in congenital adrenal hyperplasia, or feminization of a boy, as in an oestrogen-producing Leydig cell tumour. Two conditions do not fit clearly into this classification: isolated thelarche and isolated pubarche.

Isolated thelarche and isolated pubarche

Breast enlargement in the absence of other signs of puberty is called premature thelarche. It is most common under the age of 2 years and may persist from neonatal breast enlargement. There is usually spontaneous regression and later a normally timed puberty. Isolated pubarche is the early appearance of pubic hair with or without axillary hair. It is more commonly seen in girls than boys and characteristically between 4 and 6 years of age. It is associated with adrenarche, an increase in adrenal androgen secretion seen in middle childhood. There can be a slight growth spurt and advance in bone age, but this is part of normal development. It can be differentiated from abnormal forms of virilization, including adrenal tumours and congenital adrenal hyperplasia, by measuring the sex steroid hormone profile and demonstrating normal suppression of adrenal androgens by dexamethasone.

Precocious puberty

Precocious puberty presents much more commonly in girls than boys, and in the majority of girls no organic cause is found and it is idiopathic and sporadic. In contrast, in boys idiopathic precocious puberty is rare and, although there are families with familial true precocious puberty, most commonly it is due to CNS tumours, either hypothalamic hamartomas or gliomas, or dysgerminomas (Table 1).

The clinical investigation of precocious puberty is first directed towards distinguishing between a true, pseudo, isosexual, or heterosexual condition. History and examination will help establish whether there is a normal pattern of pubertal development, as in true precocious puberty, or an abnormal pattern as seen in pseudo precocious puberty. In girls, ultrasound of the pelvis will demonstrate the effect of oestrogens on uterine size and define the appearance of the ovaries. Measurement of the gonadotrophin response to GnRH should be made, as should basal measurements of β-human chorionic gonadotrophin, adrenocorticotrophic hormone, adrenal steroids (including cortisol, 17-hydroxyprogesterone, DHEA-S, and androstenedione), testosterone, oestrogen, and thyroid hormones. Steroid profiles may also be made on urine collections. Skeletal maturation should be determined by measuring the bone age.

True precocious puberty

In true precocious puberty the gonadotrophins will show a pubertal response to GnRH with a greater rise of LH than FSH. In the normal prepubertal child there is only a small rise in the gonadotrophins and the response of FSH is greater than that of LH. In pseudo precocious puberty the gonadotrophins are usually suppressed unless true puberty has also been initiated, which may occur due to excessive sex steroid secretion from any cause. Acquired hypothyroidism is associated with increased levels of FSH and may result in breast development and menstruation in girls and testicular enlargement in boys. These patients usually have stunted growth and the diagnosis is easily made by the measurement of thyroid stimulating hormone. Once a diagnosis of true precocious puberty is made, appropriate scanning of the hypothalamo-pituitary axis should be performed using either CT scanning or magnetic resonance imaging (MR).

Pseudo precocious puberty

The further investigation of pseudo precocious puberty depends on the findings of the original screening tests. Adrenal tumours will be associated with increased production of adrenal steroids which is not suppressed by a low-dose dexamethasone suppression test. CT scanning will pick up adrenal carcinomas (usually greater than 6 cm in diameter) and most adenomas, although on occasion venous catheter sampling is required. Congenital adrenal hyperplasia in girls usually presents early with virilization and ambiguous genitalia, but may present later in boys with virilization and tall stature, but prepubertal testes. There is a typical urinary steroid profile, and in the commonest form there is 21-hydroxylase deficiency, with levels of ACTH and 17-hydroxyprogesterone raised, and low levels of cortisol. Ovarian tumours are best detected by ultrasound scanning, as are testicular tumours. The McCune–Albright syndrome (polyostotic fibrous dysplasia) is an unusual cause of precocious puberty in girls which may manifest initially as autonomous ovarian activity, but this may be succeeded by true precocious puberty. Patients have patches of *café au lait* pigmentation with a ragged border and fibrous dysplasia of the bones. Testotoxicosis is an unusual inherited disorder, characterized by pubertal levels of testosterone, pubertal-sized testes, and a suppressed hypothalamogonadal axis. It is thought to be due to a circulating testicular stimulating factor. Tumours producing human chorionic gonadotrophin (HCG) can be detected by the measurement of HCG and scanning of appropriate sites, including the gonads, liver, and pineal gland.

Treatment

There are four aims in the treatment of precocious puberty:

(1) to remove the primary cause;
(2) to treat the psychosocial consequences;
(3) to allow a normal puberty; and
(4) to promote normal growth.

Table 2 *Causes of pubertal delay*

Hypogonadotrophic hypogonadism (low LH and FSH)
Constitutional delay in growth and adolescence (CDGA)
sporadic
familial
Chronic diseases
Crohn's, renal failure, thalassaemia
Malnutrition
Coeliac disease, cystic fibrosis, anorexia nervosa
Hypothalamo-pituitary
Hypopituitarism (idiopathic, tumours, craniopharyngiomas)
Isolated LH and FSH deficiency (Kallmann's, Prader–Willi, and fertile eunuch syndromes)
Isolated GH deficiency
Hyperprolactinaemia
Polycystic ovarian disease
Exercise (gymnasts)
Hormonal
Hypothyroidism, Cushing's syndrome
Hypergonatrophic hypogonadism (high LH and FSH)
Congenital
Chromosome abnormalities (Turner's and Klinefelter's syndromes)
Gonadal dysgenesis/agenesis
Steroid hormone or receptor deficiency (5α-reductase deficiency and testicular feminization)
Acquired
Radiotherapy, surgery, chemotherapy, trauma, torsion, autoimmunity

Children with precocious puberty appear much older than they are and this can result in considerable psychological difficulties and behavioral problems. Growth is stimulated both by a direct action of sex steroids on skeletal maturation and by the induction of GH secretion. This early maturation of the skeleton results in early fusion of the epiphysis, and although the child is initially tall his or her ultimate height may be very short.

Girls with only slightly advanced pubertal development often require no treatment because puberty only advances slowly, and they do not have a significant loss in height potential. GnRH analogues are now the treatment of choice in true precocious puberty. They act by down-regulating the GnRH receptor and switching off the secretion of LH and FSH. GnRH analogues have been produced as nasal sprays, daily injections, and monthly depot injections. In our experience, depot injections have proved the most effective (goserelin 3.6 mg/month). GnRH may produce an initial period of stimulation, which can be prevented by giving concomitant treatment with cyproterone acetate (100 mg/m^2/24 h for the first 6 weeks). Occasionally the acute suppression of oestrogen production at the start of treatment will precipitate an oestrogen-withdrawal bleed.

Cyproterone acetate, a peripherally acting antiandrogen, is the drug of choice for the treatment of pseudo precocious puberty. A dose of 50–100 mg daily is effective in halting the progress of the physical features of puberty, and is useful in suppressing menstruation. It is a weak glucocorticoid and may suppress ACTH and the adrenal glands.

Any effective treatment of precocious puberty will slow the growth rate by the consequent reduced secretion of sex steroids and GH. Patients treated to arrest puberty have longer to grow, but their reduced growth rate and already reduced growth potential mean that, despite the use of GnRH analogues, they will not achieve the height of which they were originally capable. Studies are currently under way to see if GH treatment can promote better growth during the treatment of precocious puberty.

Delayed puberty

The causes are summarized in Table 2. The individual conditions which may cause it are discussed in other parts of this book. Here, discussion is limited to the management of constitutional delay of growth and adolescence.

Constitutional delay of growth and adolescence (CDGA)

CDGA occurs in otherwise normal adolescents who have relatively short stature, delayed puberty and bone age, and a height prognosis appropriate in relation to their parents. It presents far more commonly in boys than girls and is the commonest cause of delayed puberty in boys with Turner's syndrome being the commonest in girls. CDGA needs to be distinguished from isolated gonadotrophin deficiency, but this is rarely easy as gonadotrophins are low with a low or prepubertal response to GnRH in both conditions. A positive family history may indicate CDGA, and associated anosmia suggests Kallmann's syndrome. If in doubt and treatment is indicated, then the patient should be reassessed after therapy (see below) to see if puberty then progresses without treatment.

Psychological problems are common in children with delayed puberty and short stature. Recent studies have suggested that delayed puberty may be associated with a reduced spinal bone density, putting adults at risk of bone fracture later in life. Thus, there are good reasons for treating this condition, which may be considered as a variant of normal growth.

Intervention with sex steroids or anabolic steroids is a safe treatment which brings forward the timing of the growth spurt without reducing height potential. The object of treatment is to stimulate normal puberty and maximize linear growth. In boys a reasonable starting dose of testosterone esters is 25 to 50 mg monthly, increasing gradually to 250 mg every 4 weeks, although puberty may be induced more rapidly over a 6 month period and the course of treatment may be as short as 3 months. Oral Oxandralone (unlicensed but available on a name patient basis from Searle, UK), 2.5 mg daily, will similarly increase growth velocity.

In girls, ethinyloestradiol at an initial dose of 2 to 10 μg daily can later be increased to 10 to 20 microgram daily, with the addition of progesterone when the oestrogen dose has reached 20 μg (for example, medroxyprogesterone acetate 5 mg on days 1–14 of the calender month).

REFERENCES

Bridges, N.A., and Brook, C.D.G. (1992). Premature sexual development. In *Clinical endocrinology*, (ed. A. Grossman), p. 837. Blackwell Scientific Publications, Oxford.

Kulin, H.E. (1989). Disorders of sexual maturation: delayed adolescence and precocious puberty. In *Endocrinology*, Vol. 3, (ed. L.J. DeGroot), Saunders p. 1873.

Stanhope, R., Albanese, A., and Shalet, S. (1992). Delayed puberty. *British Medical Journal* **305**, 790.

12.10 Non-diabetic pancreatic endocrine disorders and multiple endocrine neoplasia

P. J. HAMMOND and S. R. BLOOM

Pancreatic endocrine tumours

Pancreatic endocrine tumours (islet cell tumours, gastroenteropancreatic tumours) are rare, the commonest, insulinomata and gastrinomata, occurring with an annual incidence of one per million, with others having an incidence of less than 1 per 10 million. Functioning tumours usually present with the symptoms of hormone excess. They may secrete the pancreatic hormones insulin (see Chapter 11.12), glucagon, and somatostatin, or ectopic hormones such as gastrin, vasoactive intestinal polypeptide (VIP), or parathyroid hormone related peptide (PTHrP). (see Chapter 12.6). Non-functioning tumours can reach a large size in an apparently well patient, as characteristically these tumours cause little non-endocrine systemic upset. They were once often mistakenly identified as adenocarcinomata, but are now increasingly diagnosed as a result of detection of their secretion of functionally inactive peptides, such as pancreatic polypeptide and neurotensin, or immunohistochemical staining for neuroendocrine markers, such as chromogranin and neurone-specific enolase. They probably account for 50 per cent of all pancreatic endocrine tumours. This section will initially consider aspects of tumour biology, diagnosis, and management common to all tumours, before describing each syndrome.

NATURAL HISTORY

These tumours were originally described as APUDomata because it was thought that they had a common origin from neural crest cells with the ability to perform amine precursor uptake and decarboxylation (APUD). However, this theory has since been disproved, and it has been proposed that the neuroendocrine and mucosal endocrine cells of the gastroenteropancreatic axis are derived from a common bipotential endoplacal stem cell.

The genetic basis for the development of sporadic pancreatic endocrine tumours is largely unknown. However, about 25 per cent of them, particularly gastrinomata and insulinomata, occur as part of the familial autosomal dominant multiple endocrine neoplasia type 1 (MEN 1) syndrome (see below), in which allelic deletion in the q13 region of chromosome 11 is found, and loss of heterozygosity for this region has been demonstrated in some patients with sporadic gastrinoma and insulinoma.

Islet cells are pluripotential with respect to peptide production. Thus 70 per cent of tumours are associated with elevated pancreatic polypeptide levels, and in a small proportion of cases other hormones, particularly gastrin, may become elevated and cause secondary syndromes during the course of the disease. Altered processing of peptide precursor molecules may result in a variety of molecular weight forms of the same peptide being secreted, and not all the immunoreactive peptide is bioactive. This can have clinical implications: for example large molecular forms of glucagon (enteroglucagon) can cause villous hypertrophy and slowed intestinal transit, and large forms of somatostatin have been reported to cause hypoglycaemia, rather than the hyperglycaemia usually associated with the somatostatinoma syndrome.

The majority of pancreatic endocrine tumours are slow-growing and prolonged survival is often possible, even in the presence of metastatic spread, the median survival being about 5 years. However, some patients have aggressive, rapidly spreading disease, particularly those with non-functioning tumours, whose median survival is little over 2 years. Early in the disease, morbidity and mortality result from the effects of peptide hypersecretion rather than tumour bulk. The unpredictable nature of these tumours makes it difficult to give an accurate prognosis, occasional patients surviving for decades, and, combined with their rarity, this has made it difficult to assess the efficacy of different therapeutic strategies.

DIAGNOSIS

Pancreatic endocrine tumours can usually be diagnosed by hormonal radio-immunoassay of a single fasting plasma sample, and for certain syndromes a small number of confirmatory tests. Several conditions other than tumour are associated with increased circulating gut hormone levels (Table 1), particularly renal failure, but the elevations are usually more modest than those associated with tumour syndromes. Gut hormone radio-immunoassays are not well standardized, and the use of different antibodies and assay techniques in different laboratories can give different values on the same sample. However, concentrations are usually of the same order of magnitude in all assays and show a similar percentage increase above normal.

Most glucagonomata, non-functioning tumours, and pancreatic VIPomata and somatostatinomata are large (greater than 2 cm) tumours, which may be calcified and have metastasized to the liver in the majority of cases. Such tumours are easily localized by abdominal computed tomography (CT) scanning and ultrasonography. However, localization of tumours producing more active hormones, which are therefore detected earlier in their lifecycle, may be very difficult: for example, 40 per cent of gastrinomata and insulinomata are microadenomata, less than 1 cm in diameter. Insulinomata often occur in the distal two-thirds of the pancreas, and over 90 per cent of gastrinomata are found in the gastrinoma triangle, bounded by the third part of the duodenum, the neck of the pancreas, and the porta hepatis, about 20 per cent of these being in the duodenum. CT scanning and meticulous highly selective angiography (Fig. 1) will localize 70 per cent of these microadenomata. Magnetic resonance imaging (MRI) may be more sensitive at detecting small pancreatic lesions than CT scanning, but requires further evaluation. Transhepatic percutaneous portal venous sampling is a sensitive method of detecting hormone gradients, but cannot give accurate enough resolution to assist the surgeon in most cases, and is an expensive procedure not without risk. Recent reports suggest that, in experienced hands, endoscopic ultrasonography may be more sensitive than conventional imaging, with a resolution of 2 mm and a detection rate of over 75 per cent for tumours in the pancreatic head (Fig. 2), but visualization is poorer for lesions of the pancreatic tail and duodenum. Intraoperative ultrasonography has a sensitivity of over 90 per cent for pancreatic tumours, and endoscopic transillumination of the duodenum may allow the surgeon to detect an occult gastrinoma. Functional radiological localization has been described for both insulinomata and gastrinomata. Injection of calcium or secretin into the artery supplying the tumour causes a marked rise in insulin or gastrin levels, respectively, in the hepatic vein, and allows equivocal lesions to be verified, or the site of unlocalized lesions to be more accurately predicted. Radiolabelled somatostatin analogues have proved useful in demonstrating the extent of metastatic disease (Fig. 3), and may assist in the localization of extra-pancreatic VIPomas, but are ineffective in detecting microadenomata.

Confirmation of the diagnosis can be made by immunocytochemical analysis of resection specimens or liver biopsies, in addition to conventional histology. Antisera against non-specific markers, such as chromogranins, provide evidence for a neuroendocrine origin, while antisera to different peptides identify the specific tumour type.

TREATMENT

Surgery offers the only hope of cure for pancreatic endocrine tumours, and all sporadic tumours without evidence of metastatic spread should

Table 1 *Causes of elevated gut hormones other than pancreatic endocrine tumours*

All hormones
    Non-fasting sample
    Chronic renal failure
Gastrin
    Hypercalcaemia
    Achlorhydria
    G-cell hyperplasia
Vasoactive intestinal polypeptide
    Hepatic cirrhosis
    Bowel ischaemia
Glucagon
    Hepatic failure
    Oral contraceptives and danazol
    Stress
    Prolonged fast
    Familial hyperglucagonaemia
Pancreatic polypeptide
    Elderly
    Pernicious anaemia
    Hypercalcaemia
Neurotensin
    Fibrolamellar hepatoma

be resected if possible. Surgical cures have been reported for a few patients with hepatic metastases amenable to enucleation, and, recently, liver transplantation has been successfully performed in patients with metastatic disease confined to the liver.

In the majority of patients, surgical cure is not possible and the aim of treatment in these cases is symptomatic palliation. Until the terminal stages of the disease this is directed at reducing the symptoms of hormone excess in those with functional tumours. This can be achieved by reducing tumour bulk or inhibiting hormone secretion or action. Reduction of tumour bulk surgically is usually precluded by the operative morbidity. A variety of chemotherapy regimens have been reported as effective, although it is difficult to demonstrate that a particular regimen prolongs survival due to the small numbers of patients for analysis and the unpredictable nature of the tumours. The standard regimen consists of streptozotocin and 5-fluorouracil, with response rates of 80 per cent for functioning tumours, VIPomata responding particularly well, and about 50 per cent for non-functioning tumours. The combination of doxorubicin and streptozotocin has recently been reported to be more effective, preventing progression of disease for long periods and probably prolonging survival. Other agents advocated are dacarbazine for glucagonomata, and cisplatin and etoposide for anaplastic tumours. Another effective means of reducing tumour load in patients with exten-

Fig. 1 Venous phase of coeliac axis angiogram demonstrating gastrinoma blush in duodenal wall (arrowed).

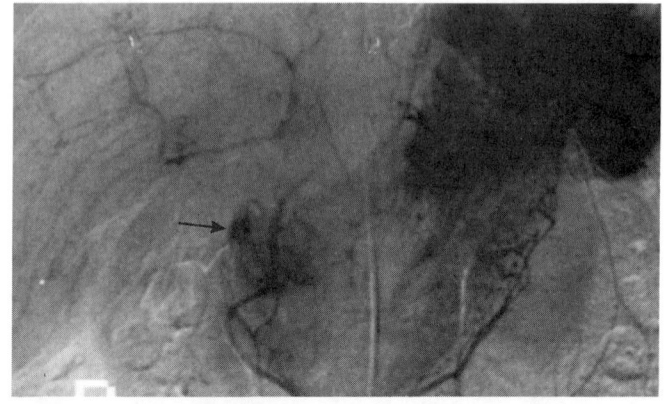

sive hepatic disease is embolization of the hepatic arterial supply to the metastases, a patent portal vein being needed to support the normal liver parenchyma. Response rates with this procedure are between 60 and 80 per cent.

Inhibition of hormone release and action is achieved by using the subcutaneous somatostatin analogue, octreotide. Native somatostatin inhibits multiple endocrine functions, acting particularly by blocking hormone effects on the target tissue, but has a half-life in circulation of only 3 minutes. Octreotide has a half-life of 2 h in the circulation and can be given in three doses daily. The clinical sequelae of peptide hypersecretion are often greatly diminished 24 h after the first injection, although patients become progressively resistant to its effects over many months or years, in part due to continued tumour growth.

Tumour syndromes

Gastrinoma

Gastrinomata are the commonest pancreatic endocrine tumour. Sixty per cent are malignant, 50 per cent of patients having metastases at the time of diagnosis, and up to 30 per cent of patients have the multiple endocrine neoplasia type 1 (MEN 1) syndrome. The majority of tumours are pancreatic, but between 20 and 40 per cent are duodenal, and these are usually microadenomata, as little as 1 mm in diameter. Sporadic duo-

Fig. 2 Endoscopic ultrasound showing a 0.7 cm insulinoma in the head of the pancreas (arrowed).

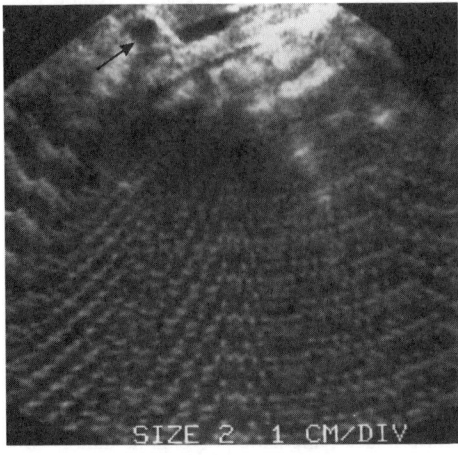

Fig. 3 [111]Indium-labelled somatostatin analogue scan showing the large primary tumour and diffuse hepatic metastases in a patient with a pancreatic glucagonoma.

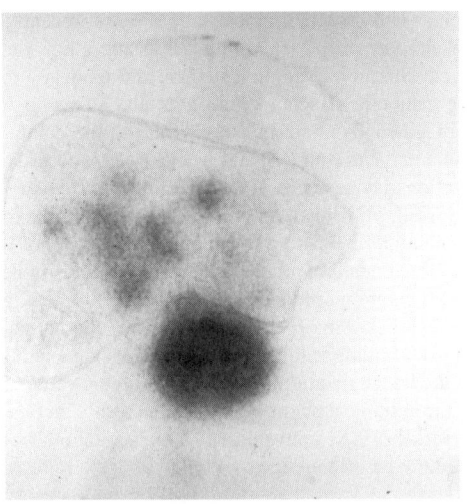

denal microgastrinomata are solitary, but in those patients with MEN 1 they are usually multiple and associated with pancreatic microadenomata. Primary lymph node gastrinomata have been described but may represent metastases from duodenal microgastrinomata.

The gastrinoma syndrome was first described in 1955 by Zollinger and Ellison, who reported the triad of fulminating ulcer diathesis, recurrent ulceration with a poor response to therapy, and pancreatic non-β cell islet tumours. The syndrome is the result of excess gastrin-stimulated gastric acid secretion. This causes severe, multiple peptic ulcers, which are usually duodenal, but may occur in the oesophagus and jejunum, and are often associated with complications such as haemorrhage, perforation, and stricture formation. Diarrhoea and steatorrhoea, due to acid inactivation of small bowel enzymes and mucosal damage, may be prominent features, frequently preceding ulcer disease by 12 months or more.

The diagnosis of the gastrinoma syndrome requires the demonstration of a raised fasting gastrin concentration, while off H_2-blockers or omeprazole, associated with increased basal gastric acid secretion. Hypergastrinaemia and raised acid output may also arise from retained antrum following partial gastrectomy or the rare condition of G-cell hyperplasia. The intravenous secretin test distinguishes these conditions from gastrinoma and can aid diagnosis when other investigations are equivocal. In the presence of a gastrinoma, gastrin levels are elevated by at least 50 per cent following secretin, while there is no such increase in association with G-cell hyperplasia or retained antrum. Furthermore, gastrin levels are increased in response to a test meal in the latter conditions but not in association with a gastrinoma. Endoscopy may be valuable in demonstrating oesophageal and duodenal ulceration and hypertrophy of the gastric mucosa, while immunocytochemical analysis of antral biopsies may demonstrate G-cell hyperplasia. Localization of microgastrinomata may be aided preoperatively by endoscopic ultrasound or selective arterial secretin injection, or intraoperatively by ultrasonography or duodenotomy with transillumination and careful palpation. Small tumours often secrete gastrin rapidly and store little peptide so that histological diagnosis may only be possible by *in situ* hybridization demonstrating synthesis of gastrin messenger RNA.

Since all gastrinomata may have the potential to metastasize, localized non-metastatic tumours should be resected, and regular attempts at localization should be made for occult tumours. In the past the morbidity and mortality of the gastrinoma syndrome resulted from the severe peptic ulceration and associated complications. The best treatment for this was total gastrectomy to remove the source of acid hypersecretion. The H_2-blockers provided relief of symptoms for many patients but often failed to suppress acid secretion adequately. The introduction of the proton-pump inhibitor, omeprazole, which almost completely inhibits gastric acid production in all cases, has transformed the management of these patients, and offers the best palliation for those with metastatic disease. Omeprazole is acid-labile and so initially should be administered with an H_2-blocker. Morbidity and mortality now occur much later and result from tumour bulk. Chemotherapy is effective in less than 50 per cent of cases, but hepatic embolization may be beneficial in the remainder.

VIPoma

VIPomata arise in the pancreas in 90 per cent of cases. The remaining tumours are mainly gangliomata or ganglioneuroblastomata originating in the sympathetic chain or adrenal medulla, and these tumours are especially common in children. Most extrapancreatic tumours are benign, but 50 per cent of pancreatic VIPomata have metastasized at the time of diagnosis, usually to local lymph nodes and the liver.

The features of the VIPoma (Verner–Morrison, pancreatic cholera) syndrome (Table 2) reflect the known biological actions of VIP. Large-volume diarrhoea without steatorrhoea is the cardinal symptom, most patients excreting more than 3 litres daily, with volumes of over 20 litres described. It is often intermittent at first, but in severe crises the volume loss coupled with the vasodilatory effects of VIP and the associated hypokalaemia may precipitate cardiovascular collapse.

Table 2 *Features of the VIPoma syndrome*

Clinical features	Biochemical features
Secretory diarrhoea	Raised plasma VIP
Severe dehydration and weakness	Hypokalaemic acidosis
Hypotension and cardiac standstill	Hypochlorhydria
Abdominal colic	Hypercalcaemia—probably due to PTHrP
Flushing	Hypomagnesaemia
Weight loss	Glucose intolerance

PTHrP, parathyroid hormone related peptide.

Hypokalaemia results from stool loss and activation of the renin–angiotensin system, and may be profound. The loss of bicarbonate in the stool leads to acidosis which may mask the true potassium deficit. Achlorhydria or hypochlorhydria occurs in over 50 per cent of patients and distinguishes this diarrhoeal syndrome from that associated with gastrinoma, but its absence in a proportion of patients makes the eponym WDHA (watery diarrhoea, hypokalaemia, and achlorhydria) syndrome inappropriate. In up to 50 per cent of cases there is glucose intolerance as a result of the glucagon-like actions of VIP. Other features include hypercalcaemia, probably due to PTHrP secretion and exacerbated by the dehydration; hypomagnesaemia due to stool loss; and flushing of the head and neck, which can occur on tumour palpation and may be associated with a marked fall in systemic blood pressure. In advanced cases extreme weight loss may occur.

VIPomata are usually associated with markedly raised plasma VIP concentrations, but because the half-life of VIP in circulation is only 2 min, the diagnosis is best confirmed by the finding of elevated circulating peptide histidine methionine, which is produced from the prepro-VIP molecule, is more stable in plasma, and is co-secreted by VIPomata. Pancreatic polypeptide levels are elevated in 75 per cent of cases and neurotensin in 10 per cent. Ganglioneuroblastomata may secrete noradrenaline and adrenaline and so be associated with elevated urinary catecholamines and catecholamine metabolites.

VIPomata are usually large and so localization is rarely a problem. Occasionally angiography may be necessary to detect small pancreatic lesions or radiolabelled somatostatin, or MIBG scanning to identify extrapancreatic tumours.

Resection specimens from pancreatic tumours show the structural and secretory patterns of epithelial endocrine tumours, while those from ganglioneuroblastomata show neurones and nerve fibres, together with Schwann cells. Immunocytochemistry detects VIP and peptide histidine methionine, and electron microscopy shows poorly granulated tumours, with characteristic small secretory granules.

Patients with non-metastatic disease should have surgical resections, and this is feasible in the majority of ganglioneuroblastomata. Chemotherapy provides very effective palliation for those with metastatic disease, and the excellent response to the comparatively non-toxic regimen of streptozotocin and 5-fluorouracil makes the use of other advocated agents, particularly α-interferon, unnecessary. Similarly, hepatic embolization is not usually indicated for metastatic VIPomas. Acute VIPoma crises should be managed with fluid and electrolyte support, and central venous pressure monitoring is usually required. A number of drugs, including prednisolone, indomethacin, metoclopramide, lithium carbonate, and opiates, have been used with varying degrees of success to treat the diarrhoea. These have now been superseded by the somatostatin analogue, octreotide. Ninety per cent of patients respond to octreotide with reduction of diarrhoea almost to normal and resolution of the electrolyte imbalance within 48 h, and it may be life-saving in an acute crisis. Unfortunately, the median duration of response to octreotide alone is less than 1 year, and so its use is probably best combined with chemotherapy.

Glucagonoma

Glucagonomata are α-cell tumours of the pancreas which secrete various forms of glucagon and other peptides derived from the preproglucagon molecule. They have an estimated annual incidence of 1 in 20 million, with a marginal female preponderance, and invariably present in adulthood. Over 70 per cent of patients have metastases at the time of diagnosis.

The characteristic feature of the glucagonoma syndrome is the rash of necrolytic migratory erythema, which occurs in almost all patients, although it often remains undiagnosed for many years. It usually starts in the groins and perineum, migrating to the distal extremities. The initial lesions are erythematous patches, which become raised and may be associated with bullae. These lesions break down and gradually heal, often leaving an area of hyperpigmentation, only to recur in another site (Plate 1). All mucous membranes may be involved, commonly leading to angular stomatitis, cheilitis, and glossitis. The cause of the rash is unknown. A direct effect of glucagon on the skin, glucagon-induced prostaglandin release, amino acid or free fatty acid deficiency, or zinc deficiency, due to the similarity with acrodermatitis enteropathica, have all been proposed as the underlying mechanism. The rash has been reported in a few patients without glucagonomata, who either had coeliac disease or cirrhosis, both of which may have led to elevation in glucagon and glucagon-like peptides. Other common features of glucagonomata include impaired glucose tolerance, and occasionally mild diabetes requiring insulin therapy; progressive weight loss, which is occasionally severe enough to be fatal; venous thrombosis, which may be life-threatening; normochromic normocytic anaemia, probably as a result of direct bone marrow suppression by glucagon; bowel disturbance and nail dystrophy. Mental slowness, depression, and paraneoplastic neurological syndromes have also been described.

The diagnosis of glucagonoma is confirmed by demonstrating raised fasting plasma glucagon concentrations by radio-immunoassay, and the elevation is usually ten- to twentyfold. Localization is almost never a problem, since tumours are invariably large and pancreatic, with metastases in the majority of cases. Barium studies often show a thickened jejunal and ileal mucosa due to the trophic effects of large forms of glucagon on the small bowel. The tumour tissue contains large quantities of extractable glucagon which is localized to α cells. Electron microscopy shows dense-core secretory granules and the core is often eccentric. Fifty per cent of tumours produce pancreatic polypeptide and co-production of gastrin and insulin has been described. Skin biopsies show necrolysis of the stratum Malpighi of the epidermis in early lesions, but only a non-specific dermatitis at later stages.

Surgical cure of glucagonomata is rarely possible, although it has been claimed for patients with resectable metastatic disease; recently, successful liver transplantation for patients with metastatic glucagonomata has been reported. Surgery is complicated by the tendency to venous thrombosis, the catabolic effects of glucagon, and anaemia. A significant proportion of glucagonomata fail to respond to the combination of streptozotocin and 5-fluorouracil, and in these cases dacarbazine or hepatic embolization may be necessary. Octreotide is particularly effective in treating the rash, with resolution usually occurring within the first month of treatment and persisting for at least 6 months, but it has little impact on the other features of the syndrome. Other simple treatments for the rash which are worth using in all cases are topical or oral zinc and a high-protein diet. Amino acid infusions and blood transfusion may also be effective, but the tendency of the rash to spontaneous remission, often following hospitalization, throws doubt on the value of such procedures. The thrombotic tendency, which can result in fatal pulmonary emboli, is refractory to conventional anticoagulation, but aspirin or dipyridamole may be of benefit.

Somatostatinoma

Somatostatinomata are extremely rare, with an estimated annual incidence of about 1 in 40 million. Fifty per cent of these tumours are pancreatic, the remainder arising in the duodenum. Approximately 50 per cent of duodenal somatostatinomata occur in association with neurofibromatosis type I (von Recklinghausen's disease; see Chapters 15.28.2, 24.17) and these tumours are usually periampullary. Pancreatic tumours usually present late with hepatic metastases, but duodenal tumours are frequently identified earlier as a result of local effects.

The somatostatinoma syndrome is characterized by the triad of cholelithiasis, diabetes mellitus and steatorrhoea, the latter occurring in almost all patients with pancreatic tumours. These features result from the inhibitory actions of somatostatin on gallbladder contraction and secretion, insulin secretion, and pancreatic exocrine secretions. Hypoglycaemia has occasionally been described, possibly due to larger molecular forms of somatostatin having a greater inhibitory effect on counterregulatory hormones than on insulin. Other features of the syndrome include hypochlorhydria, anaemia, postprandial fullness, and weight loss. The full syndrome is rarely seen in association with duodenal somatostatinomata, gallbladder disease being the only common manifestation. These tumours usually present as a result of effects on local structures, such as obstruction of the ampulla of Vater causing jaundice or pancreatitis, or intestinal obstruction or haemorrhage.

Circulating levels of somatostatin are usually elevated greater than tenfold in association with pancreatic tumours, but duodenal tumours are associated with much lower levels, probably because they are usually about one-tenth the size of the pancreatic lesions. Multiple molecular weight forms of somatostatin may be demonstrated by columning of plasma or tumour extracts, and these may explain unusual clinical features. Localization is rarely a problem, barium examinations or endoscopy identifying duodenal lesions. Duodenal somatostatinomata are classified histologically as duodenal carcinoids. Duodenal carcinoids have the usual features of neuroendocrine tumours but often contain psammoma bodies. Those associated with neurofibromatosis type I are more likely to be pure somatostatinomata and to contain psammoma bodies.

Surgical resection of duodenal somatostatinomata is usually curative, although a Whipple's procedure may be needed to ensure clearance of periampullary tumours. Pancreatic tumours have almost always metastasized by the time of diagnosis and so palliation with chemotherapy or hepatic embolization are the only therapeutic options.

Pancreatic polypeptide, neurotensin, and other hormones

Pancreatic polypeptide can be extracted from almost all pancreatic endocrine tumours and is secreted by up to 75 per cent of them. The finding of elevated circulating PP in association with other tumour syndromes indicates a pancreatic tumour source. However, PP itself has no recognized physiological role and no associated tumour syndrome, and pure PPomas can be regarded effectively as non-functioning tumours. Similarly neurotensin, which is elevated in 10 per cent of VIPomata, does not cause a characteristic syndrome. Interestingly, neurotensin is produced by fibrolamellar hepatomata.

Hypercalcaemia is a feature of the VIPoma syndrome and may also occur in association with pancreatic endocrine tumours without other hormone syndromes. Secretion of parathyroid hormone related peptide (PTHrP) by pancreatic endocrine tumours has now been reported in a number of cases, and synthesis of PTHrP messenger RNA in normal and tumorous islets has been described. It is highly probable, therefore, that almost all cases of hypercalcaemia in association with pancreatic endocrine tumours are mediated by PTHrP. In these patients the hypercalcaemia responds to both octreotide and bisphosphonates.

The hypothalamic hormone, growth hormone releasing hormone (GHRH), was originally isolated from a pancreatic endocrine tumour, and there have been subsequent reports of patients with acromegaly and gigantism as a result of GHRH secretion by pancreatic endocrine tumours. Treatment options for these patients have included surgical resection, octreotide therapy, and liver transplantation.

Another hypothalamic releasing factor, corticotrophin releasing hormone may be produced by pancreatic endocrine tumours, but only causes Cushing's syndrome when the tumour also secretes corticotrophin (ACTH). One patient with an enteroglucagon-secreting tumour of the right kidney, causing villous hypertrophy and slowed intestinal transit, steatorrhoea, and mild diabetes, has been reported, and there has been one case of acromegaly due to a growth hormone secreting pancreatic endocrine tumour. Other peptides produced by islet-cell tumours include neuropeptide Y, neuromedin B, calcitonin gene-related peptide, bombesin, and motilin, but these are not associated with recognized clinical syndromes.

Non-functioning tumours

Tumours not associated with a recognized hormonal syndrome may account for half of all pancreatic endocrine tumours. They usually present late with symptoms attributable to tumour bulk, such as anorexia and weight loss, or to effects on local structures, such as obstructive jaundice or intestinal obstruction or haemorrhage. They are often mistakenly diagnosed as adenocarcinomata, but the presence of elevated circulating gut hormones, such as pancreatic polypeptide or neurotensin, and the use of immunocytochemical analysis can point to the correct diagnosis. Non-functioning tumours usually respond poorly to chemotherapy, but hepatic embolization may be beneficial. They have a poor prognosis as a result of their late presentation and lack of response to therapy.

Multiple endocrine neoplasia

The multiple endocrine neoplasia syndromes (MEN 1 and MEN 2) are familial conditions with an autosomal dominant pattern of inheritance and a high degree of penetrance. The genetic defect in MEN 2, previously localized to chromosome region 10q11.2, has recently been identified. This will allow detection of mutations in individual families and characterization of the molecular pathophysiology of the tumour syndromes. The genetic abnormality underlying MEN 1 has been mapped only to a specific chromosomal region, so that at present only biochemical screening and linkage analysis can be offered to affected families. Identification of specific gene defects in these syndromes may provide novel therapeutic options for tumour prevention in affected individuals.

Multiple endocrine neoplasia type 1 (MEN 1)

MEN 1 is characterized by the association of parathyroid hyperplasia, pancreatic endocrine tumours, and pituitary adenomas. This association was first described by Underdahl in 1953, and the autosomal dominant inheritance was first proposed in 1954 by Wermer, whose name provided the eponym for the syndrome. The prevalence of the condition has been estimated at about 1 in 10 000. The genetic abnormality has been localized to the 11q13 region of the long arm of chromosome 11. The development of tumours fits the 'two-hit' model proposed by Knudson and demonstrated by familial retinoblastoma, whereby there is a germline mutation of the MEN 1 gene on one chromosome 11, followed by a somatic deletion of the same region on the other chromosome, leading to loss of heterozygosity for that allele and subsequent tumour formation. Loss of heterozygosity for the long arm of chromosome 11 has also been found in some sporadic parathyroid adenomas and pancreatic endocrine tumours, implying that the MEN 1 gene is a proto-oncogene. A substantial proportion of MEN 1 cases arise through sporadic mutations, and these patients present between the third and fifth decades, while familial cases can be identified earlier through screening.

Parathyroid hyperplasia and adenomata

Hyperparathyroidism is the presenting feature of MEN 1 in the majority of patients, and occurs in almost all cases. Patients present either with asymptomatic hypercalcaemia on biochemical screening or with the features of sporadic hyperparathyroidism. All four glands are diffusely hyperplastic and there may be nodule formation. Whether true adenomata develop remains controversial, but it is assumed that the presence of a capsule indicates adenomatous change. All patients should be operated on to prevent later morbidity from hypercalcaemia and there are two surgical approaches. Subtotal parathyroidectomy may be performed, but hyperparathyroidism will almost always recur, necessitating excision of the remaining parathyroid tissue. However, most surgeons would perform total parathyroidectomy, either with autotransplantation of one gland to the forearm, which can later be removed if hyperparathyroidism recurs, or with immediate replacement therapy with 1α-hydroxycholecalciferol.

Pancreatic endocrine tumours

Pancreatic endocrine tumours occur in about 70 per cent of patients with MEN 1, and usually present between the ages of 15 and 50 if not identified by screening. They account for most of the morbidity and mortality of the MEN 1 syndrome. Over 60 per cent of tumours are gastrinomata and about 30 per cent are insulinomata, the two coexisting in about 10 per cent of cases. VIPomata have rarely been described and there are only isolated reports of glucagonomata, but non-functioning tumours may occur frequently. Diffuse hyperplasia of the pancreas is usually seen, similar to the parathyroid, and in the majority of cases there are multiple adenomata, most of which are less than 1 cm in diameter. Duodenal microgastrinomata are very common, probably accounting for almost half of all MEN 1 associated gastrinomata, and are usually multiple, with up to 15 separate tumours described.

The surgical approach to pancreatic endocrine tumours in MEN 1 is controversial. Surgical cure is best achieved by removing the pancreas and duodenum with adjacent lymph nodes, but such an aggressive approach is only justified in families in which the pancreatic disease has been extremely malignant, and in these kindreds should be performed only when pancreatic disease is biochemically apparent. An alternative, potentially curative, approach is to perform a subtotal pancreatectomy with enucleation of palpable tumours in the head and careful exploration for duodenal lesions, which should also be resected. A more conservative strategy is to enucleate gross lesions to reduce the risk of developing metastatic disease and then control hormonal syndromes with appropriate medical therapy. The latter approach is probably appropriate for gastrinomata because omeprazole is such an effective treatment, but for insulinomata, where medical therapy is often unsuccessful and symptoms usually recur after enucleation alone, more aggressive surgical management may be the best option. The treatment of metastatic disease is the same as in sporadic cases.

Pancreatic endocrine tumours associated with MEN 1 are less malignant than sporadic tumours and carry a better prognosis, with a median survival of 15 years compared to 5 years for patients with sporadic tumours. This may reflect more indolent disease or earlier diagnosis.

Pituitary adenomata

The true incidence of pituitary adenomata in MEN 1 is disputed. They are detected by screening in 30 per cent of patients, but are found at autopsy in 50 per cent of patients. Unlike the pancreas and parathyroid, there does not appear to be diffuse pituitary hyperplasia, and loss of heterozygosity for the MEN 1 locus is much less common in pituitary tumours than in parathyroid and pancreatic lesions.

Prolactinomata are the commonest tumours, occurring in about two-thirds of cases, with acromegaly accounting for about 30 per cent, and other functioning tumours being rare. Treatment is the same as for sporadic pituitary tumours (see Chapter 12.6).

Other lesions

Lesions in other tissues have been reported in association with MEN 1, but their relationship to the syndrome remains controversial. Carcinoid tumours of the foregut, midgut, and thymuta occur in about 10 per cent of cases, and are often found in the pancreas, but are rarely symptomatic. Lipomata occur in a significant proportion of patients and act as a marker for affected individuals. Adrenal lesions are common autopsy findings in normal individuals, but do appear to occur more frequently in MEN 1, with an incidence of up to 40 per cent. Histology usually demonstrates nodular hyperplasia and there is no associated excess hormone secretion. Loss of heterozygosity of the MEN 1 locus is not found in these lesions and it has been proposed that there may be a circulating adrenal growth factor, possibly secreted by the pancreas, since there is a strong correlation with pancreatic tumours, particularly insulinomata. MEN 1-associated adrenal tumours showing loss of heterozygosity for 11q13 have been reported but are very rare. Thyroid disease has been reported in association with MEN 1, but does not appear to occur more frequently than in the normal population.

Screening

The screening of first- and second-degree relatives of patients with MEN 1 is aimed at early detection of parathyroid, pancreatic, or pituitary lesions in gene carriers, to reduce the associated morbidity. There is no evidence that screening reduces mortality, although the identification of affected individuals in 'malignant' kindreds with aggressive pancreatic disease may allow curative surgery which would be expected to prolong survival. Screening lowers the age of detection of the syndrome by about 20 years.

The most useful screening investigations are a serum calcium, fasting gastrin, and prolactin, although in practice a full gut hormone screen is usually performed. It has been suggested that the most sensitive markers of pancreatic disease are basal and test-meal stimulated pancreatic polypeptide and gastrin, and basal insulin and proinsulin, identifying lesions at least 3 years before there are any radiological abnormalities. Since pancreatic tumours are the only life-threatening manifestation of the syndrome, such a screening protocol may be warranted. The MEN 1 syndrome rarely develops before the age of 5 or after the age of 70, and so screening should be performed annually from 5 to 65, and at longer intervals thereafter. Eighty per cent of affected individuals will have been identified by the fifth decade. Screening of patients with apparently sporadic pancreatic endocrine tumours for evidence of MEN 1 is probably justified, especially in those with gastrinomata or insulinomata. There is little evidence to support screening in those with sporadic pituitary tumours. MEN 1 is present in 15 per cent of all patients with hyperparathyroidism, but hypercalcaemia may be associated with elevated fasting gastrin and pancreatic polypeptide, and, whereas in those at risk of MEN 1 this finding would be highly significant, in those with sporadic hyperparathyroidism this very rarely indicates pancreatic disease, so screening of all patients is not warranted.

Genetic linkage analysis has greater than 95 per cent predictive accuracy, and in most families a haplotype associated with the mutant allele can be found. If three markers can be identified, the accuracy improves to greater than 99 per cent. However, at present the use of this technique alone for detection of gene carriers cannot be advocated, and biochemical screening is still needed, although it could be performed less frequently in those whose risk of developing the syndrome is low on the basis of linkage analysis data.

Multiple endocrine neoplasia type 2 (MEN 2)

Multiple endocrine neoplasia 2 is the association of medullary cell carcinoma of the thyroid (MTC) and phaeochromocytoma. The association was first recognized in 1932, but it was not until 1961 that it was noted that the risk of phaeochromocytoma in patients with MTC was increased fourteenfold. MEN 2 has since been subdivided: in MEN 2, or Sipple's syndrome, parathyroid hyperplasia may occur; MEN 2B is associated with mucosal neuromata and marfanoid habitus. In addition, there is a familial form of MTC without other features. Germ line mutations of the *ret* proto-oncogene, a receptor tyrosine kinase, have been identified in all three syndromes. In MEN 2A and familial MTC mutations occur in the extracellular domain, and in MEN 2B a single mutation in the tyrosine kinase domain has been demonstrated. The MEN 2 phenotypes reflect the tissue expression of *ret*. Tumours in affected individuals are heterozygous for the *ret* mutation, and so it is the only known dominantly inherited proto-oncogene. It is likely that activation of *ret* leads to hyperplasia in affected tissues and that a somatic mutation in another oncogene is required for carcinogenesis. Thus loss of heterozygosity for the short arm of chromosome 1 has been described in phaeochromocytomas and MTC associated with MEN 2. New mutations are uncommon in MEN 2A, probably accounting for less than 10 per cent of cases, but account for about 50 per cent of cases with MEN 2B. Those patients with MEN 2A not identified by screening usually present in the fourth and fifth decades, while those with MEN 2B present much earlier due to their characteristic phenotype.

Medullary cell carcinoma of the thyroid (MTC)

MTC is a tumour of the C cells of the thyroid (see Chapters 12.4, 12.5), which secrete calcitonin, and this acts as a tumour marker. Twenty-five per cent of cases are familial. The incidence of MTC in MEN 2 is probably 100 per cent. Familial MTC alone is the most benign form of MTC, while MTC in association with MEN 2B is the most malignant form of the disease. In MEN 2 the initial thyroid lesion is C-cell hyperplasia, which has been found as early as the age of 3 years in MEN 2A and may be present at birth in MEN 2B. Over the subsequent 5 to 10 years microscopic MTC develops and finally gross tumours become apparent. Metastases are invariably present when tumours are already palpable, but there is speculation that they may occur with clinically occult disease. All forms of hereditary MTC are bilateral, with multifocal tumours, usually occurring at the junction of the upper third and lower two-thirds of the thyroid.

In MEN 2A, screening, using pentagastrin-stimulated calcitonin, probably identifies all cases before MTC has developed. This allows total thyroidectomy to be performed at the C-cell hyperplasia or microscopic MTC stage, which is curative in all patients. In MEN 2B, thyroidectomy with lymph node clearance should be performed at the earliest possible age in individuals with the phenotypic features, since MTC is biologically aggressive in these patients and has been reported as early as 15 months of age, with metastases by the age of 3 years. In those patients not identified by screening, thyroidectomy should still be performed, unless distant metastases, usually to lung or liver, are present. It is probable that in all patients with palpable disease metastases to local lymph nodes will be present, so a central lymph node dissection should also be performed, probably with lateral node sampling to look for further spread. The prognosis is poor in this group, with recurrent disease in about 20 per cent of patients with clinically occult but macroscopic MTC and in over 60 per cent of those with palpable MTC. It is particularly poor in individuals with MEN 2B who present with clinically apparent MTC. Their 10 year survival is about 50 per cent, and death from metastatic disease in the mid-twenties is common.

Phaeochromocytoma

Phaeochromocytoma is familial in 5 per cent of cases, 20 per cent of whom have MEN 2. Fifty per cent of individuals with MEN 2 develop phaeochromocytoma. About 70 per cent are bilateral, almost all are benign, and they are rarely extra-adrenal. The initial lesion, similar to the thyroid, is adrenal medullary hyperplasia, followed by nodule formation and, subsequently, development of multiple, multifocal phaeochromocytomata (see Chapter 15.28.2).

Symptoms and biochemical abnormalities are rare during the stage of medullary hyperplasia. MEN 2-associated phaeochromocytomata are characterized by excessive adrenaline secretion, so that palpitation and other β-adrenergic symptoms predominate initially, with hypertension a late feature, although often present by the time of diagnosis. A urine adrenaline : noradrenaline ration of greater than 0.15 in a patient with MEN 2 indicates medullary hyperplasia or phaeochromocytoma. The treatment for adrenal medullary hyperplasia or phaeochromocytoma is bilateral adrenalectomy, since the incidence of bilateral disease is high, and the mortality from phaeochromocytoma in MEN 2 about 15 per cent, usually due to sudden death. If an adrenal lesion is identified at the same time as MTC, the adrenalectomy should be performed first.

Other features of MEN 2A

Parathyroid hyperplasia occurs in up to 80 per cent of patients with MEN 2A, but less than 20 per cent have hypercalcaemia, the remainder being identified at the time of thyroidectomy. Parathyroidectomy should be performed in those with hypercalcaemia and in the remaining patients grossly enlarged glands should be removed at the time of thyroidectomy.

Cutaneous lichen amyloidosis, often preceded by intense pruritus, has been described in two kindreds with MEN 2A and provides a phenotypic marker for the syndrome.

Other features of MEN 2B

The characteristic phenotype of marfanoid habitus and mucosal neuromata (Fig. 4) identifies affected individuals with MEN 2B and allows early intervention, since these features usually predate MTC and phaeochromocytoma. Neuromata are commonly ocular and oral, causing whitish-yellow or pink nodules on the anterior aspect of the tongue, lips, and eyelids, with thickening of the mucosa and often eversion of the lower

Fig. 4 Characteristic phenotype of MEN 2B showing (a) facial appearance and (b) mucosal neuromas on tongue.

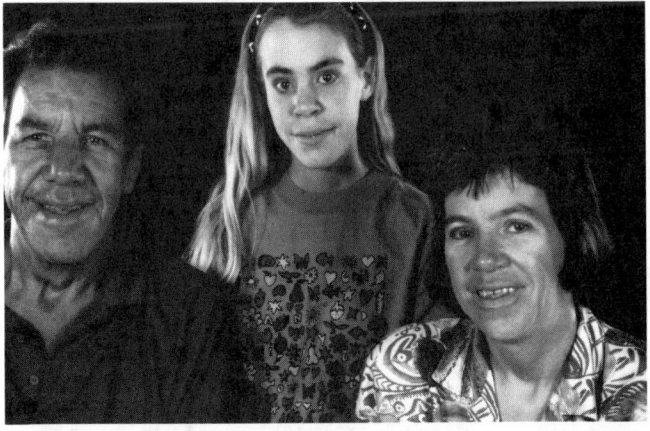

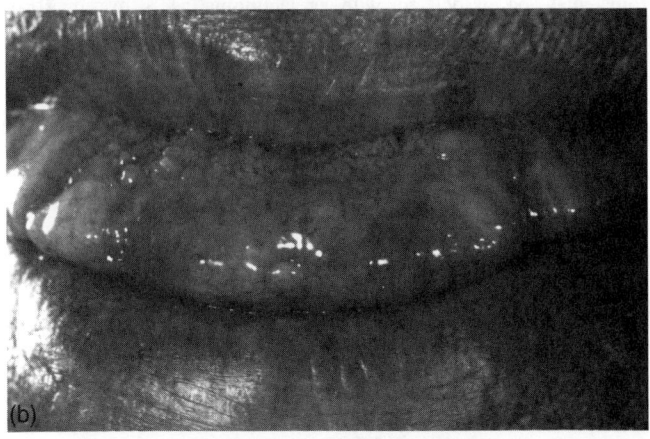
(b)

lids. The nasal bridge may be broadened, pedunculated neuromata are found on cheek mucosa, and the corneal nerves are thickened and medullated. Involvement of peripheral motor and sensory nerves can cause a peroneal muscular atrophy type picture. Intestinal ganglioneuromatosis affects about 75 per cent of cases. Neuromata involve the autonomic nerves of both the myenteric and submucosal plexi and can cause poor suckling with failure to thrive, altered bowel habit, recurrent pseudo-obstruction, toxic megacolon, and occasionally dysphagia and vomiting, possibly due to achalasia. Almost all patients have a marfanoid habitus, usually associated with skeletal abnormalities, particularly slipped femoral epiphyses. Delayed puberty is the other common feature of the syndrome.

Screening

Screening to identify affected individuals and for early detection of thyroid and adrenal disease reduces both morbidity and mortality in MEN 2. The screening investigations are a pentagastrin stimulation test, which may be combined with calcium infusion to improve the sensitivity, and measurement of 24 h urinary metanephrines and catecholamines. The pentagastrin test identifies individuals with C-cell hyperplasia or microscopic MTC, 70 per cent being detected before the age of 20, and, if a second test is positive, total thyroidectomy should be performed. Screening should commence at the age of 3 years and continue annually. The risk of developing MTC falls below 5 per cent after the age of 35, and so screening can be performed less frequently thereafter. In MEN 2B, screening for MTC is not necessary, since all affected individuals should have thyroidectomies. Urinary metanephrines and catecholamines identify at least 95 per cent of phaeochromocytomas. Urinary vanillylmandelic acid levels are less useful, being associated with a high number of false positives and negatives. MIBG and/or CT scanning or measurement of plasma catecholamines may identify phaeochromocytomas missed by urinary assays. Serum calcium should be measured at annual screening to identify overt hyperparathyroidism. Genetic linkage analysis has 98 to 99 per cent predictive accuracy, and in individuals identified as at low risk of developing MEN 2 less frequent screening would be reasonable. In families in whom a mutation has been characterized affected individuals can be identified by mutation screening.

Other syndromes associated with endocrine neoplasia

There are other syndromes which overlap with the multiple endocrine neoplasia syndromes. Phaeochromocytomata may be associated with pancreatic islet-cell tumours alone, or in combination with other syndromes: von Hippel–Lindau syndrome is associated with a high incidence of phaeochromocytomata, islet-cell tumours, cerebellar haemangioblastomata, retinal angiomata, and renal cell carcinoma; Neurofibromatosis type I (von Recklinghausen's syndrome) is often associated with phaeochromocytoma and, rarely, with duodenal somatostatinoma and medullary thyroid carcinoma; and phaeochromocytoma may be associated with prolactinoma as a mixed MEN syndrome.

FURTHER READING

Ajani, J.A., Carrasco, C.H., Charnsangavej, C., Samaan, N.A., Levin, B., and Wallace, S. (1988). Islet cell tumors metastatic to the liver: effective palliation by sequential hepatic artery embolization. *Annals of Internal Medicine* 108, 340–4.

Arnold, J., O'Grady, J., Bird, G., Calne, R., and Williams, R. (1989). Liver transplantation for primary and secondary hepatic apudomas. *British Journal of Surgery* 76, 248–9.

Gorden, P., Comi, R.J., Maton, P.N., and Go, V.L. (1989). NIH conference. Somatostatin and somatostatin analogue (SMS 201-995) in treatment of hormone-secreting tumors of the pituitary and gastrointestinal tract and non-neoplastic diseases of the gut. *Annals of Internal Medicine* 110, 35–50.

Grauer, A., Raue, F., and Gagel, R.F. (1990). Changing concepts in the management of hereditary and sporadic medullary thyroid carcinoma. *Endocrinology and Metabolism Clinics of America* 19, 613–35.

Hofstra, R.M., *et al.* (1994). A mutation in the RET proto-oncogene associated with multiple endocrine neoplasia type 2B and sporadic medullary thyroid carcinoma. *Nature*, 367, 375–6.

Jensen, R.T. (ed.) (1989). Gastrointestinal endocrinology. *Gastroenterology Clinics of North America* 18, 671–931.

Krejs, G. (ed.) (1987). Gastrointestinal endocrine tumours. *American Journal of Medicine* 82, (suppl. 5B).

Moertel, C.G., Lefkopoulo, M., Lipsitz, S., Hahn, R.G., and Klaassen, D. (1992). Streptozocin-doxorubicin, streptozocin-fluorouracil or chlorozotocin in the treatment of advanced islet-cell carcinoma. *New England Journal of Medicine* 326, 519–23.

Mulligan, L.M., *et al.* (1993). Germ-line mutations of the RET proto-oncogene in multiple endocrine neoplasia type 2A. *Nature*, 363, 458–60.

Oberg, K. (ed.) (1991). Recent advances in diagnosis and treatment of neuroendocrine gut and pancreatic tumours. *Acta Oncologica* 28, 301–449.

Rosch, T., *et al.* (1992). Localization of pancreatic endocrine tumors by endoscopic ultrasonography. *New England Journal of Medicine* 326, 1721–6.

Rossi, P., *et al.* (1989). Endocrine tumors of the pancreas. *Radiologic Clinics of North America* 27, 129–61.

Sheppard, B.C., Norton, J.A., Doppman, J.L., Maton, P.N., Gardner, J.D., and Jensen, R.T. (1989). Management of islet cell tumors in patients with multiple endocrine neoplasia: a prospective study. *Surgery* 106, 1108–17.

Skogseid B., *et al.* (1991). Multiple endocrine neoplasia type 1: a 10-year prospective screening study in four kindreds. *Journal of Clinical Endocrinology and Metabolism* 73, 281–7.

Thakker, R.V. and Ponder, B.A. (1988). Multiple endocrine neoplasia. *Baillières Clinical Endocrinology and Metabolism* 2, 1031–67.

Vasen, H.F., *et al.* (1992). The natural course of multiple endocrine neoplasia type IIb. A study of 18 cases. *Archives of Internal Medicine* 152, 1250–2.

Vinayek, R., Frucht, H., Chiang, H.C., Maton, P.N., Gardner, J.D., and Jensen, R.T. (1990). Zollinger–Ellison syndrome. Recent advances in the management of the gastrinoma. *Gastroenterology Clinics of North America* 19, 197–217.

Wynick, D. and Bloom, S.R. (1991). The use of the long-acting somatostatin analog octreotide in the treatment of gut neuroendocrine tumors. *Journal of Clinical Endocrinology and Metabolism* 73, 1–3.

12.11 Endocrine manifestations of non-endocrine disease

J. A. H. WASS

INTRODUCTION

A number of different endocrine syndromes may develop in association with diseases that are not primarily disorders of an endocrine gland. In most instances the cause is a tumour, usually but not invariably malignant, that develops in tissue not normally looked upon as the site of the particular hormone synthesized. Hence its secretion is termed 'ectopic' or 'inappropriate'.

In 1941 Albright suggested that the hypercalcaemia sometimes associated with malignant disease without osteolytic metastases might be due to the secretion by the tumour of a parathyroid hormone-like peptide; now we know that this is true (parathyroid hormone related protein, PTHrP). Later it was shown that hypersecretion of adrenocorticotrophin (ACTH), not from the pituitary but from an ectopic site, was in some 20 per cent of cases the cause of Cushing's syndrome.

Many different hormones have now been identified as being ectopically secreted by neoplasms arising in a wide variety of organs, notably the bronchus, breast, pancreas, kidney, thyroid, thymus, ovary, trachea, uterus, as well as in mesenchymal tissue. Although a particular endocrinopathy may be associated with a specific type of tumour in a particular organ, such a relationship is not invariable. Indeed, many neoplasms elaborate more than one hormonal substance at the same or at different times, and thus may produce a mixed endocrine picture (for example, pancreatic endocrine tumours). Furthermore, the amount of ectopic hormone(s) produced may fluctuate from time to time (for example, cyclical Cushing's syndrome in ectopic ACTH secretion). In some instances the changes induced by the ectopic hormone may mimic very closely, and be clinically indistinguishable, from those found in the true endocrinopathy. In others the picture is less clinically characteristic and is dominated more by abnormalities of biochemistry or hormone levels. Thus, in many cases of ectopic ACTH production by small cell lung cancer, the downhill course of the illness may be too rapid for the classical features of florid Cushing's syndrome to develop, and hypokalaemic alkalosis with diabetes predominates.

CRITERIA FOR DIAGNOSIS

The diagnosis of ectopic hormone production depends on a number of criteria, although it is seldom practicable or possible to confirm them all.

1. There is an association of the tumour with an endocrine syndrome.
2. Even though the endocrine syndrome may not be clinically florid, there is an elevated or inappropriately raised plasma level of the putative hormone.
3. Removal or suppression of the tumour induces a regression of the endocrinopathy and a fall in the hormone level.
4. The clinical picture and hormone levels are uninfluenced by removal of the gland that normally secretes the hormone.
5. The hormone level is higher in venous blood draining the tumour than in the arterial blood supplying it.
6. Extraction or immunohistochemical staining shows a higher concentration of the hormone in the tumour than in adjacent non-involved tissue.
7. *In vitro*, the tumour cells synthesize specifically identifiable hormone.
8. On Northern blot analysis of tumoural mRNA, there is evidence that the tumour tissue is producing the putative hormone.

CHEMICAL STRUCTURE

The precise amino acid sequences of hormones of ectopic origin are being increasingly defined. In general they appear to resemble closely those of their normally occurring counterparts (except parathyroid hormone (PTH) and PTHrP). There is a tendency for a greater proportion of higher molecular weight precursors, or subunits and fragments to be associated with an ectopic origin than with 'true' endocrinopathies, but it is not always clear whether this is due to differences in biosynthesis or in intracellular or extracellular processing. Minor differences in molecular structure are sometimes suggested by a disparity between bioassay and immunoassay.

PREVALENCE

Clinically evident syndromes are less common than biochemical or hormonal abnormalities. The prevalence of ectopic production of ACTH, corticotrophin-releasing hormone (CRH), parathyroid hormone related protein (PTHrP), calcitonin, chorionic gonadotrophin (HCG), prolactin or growth hormone, without clinical manifestations, is high when extensive biochemical and hormonal assays are applied to patients with cancer. Such findings bring closer the prospect of finding a diagnostic 'marker' for tumours in general and in particular, as is already the case with the monitoring of HCG or its subunits to determine the response of choriocarcinoma to treatment.

Hypercalcaemia in the absence of detectable bony metastases is the most common abnormality. It occurs in about 15 per cent of patients with squamous cell carcinoma, usually of the bronchus, and carcinoma of the kidney, ovary, or breast. Next most common in neoplastic diseases is the syndrome of inappropriate antidiuresis (SIAD), usually associated with a small cell lung cancer and reported in 40 per cent of such cases. This syndrome is also familiar in non-neoplastic pulmonary diseases and in association with intracranial disorders. Cushing's syndrome due to ectopic ACTH or CRH secretion occurs in about 5 per cent of patients with small cell lung cancer, and in association with other neoplasms. Biochemical accompaniments of Cushing's syndrome in the absence of the clinical features are much more common, occurring in 50 per cent of patients with small cell lung cancer.

PATHOGENESIS

As molecular biological technologies have evolved, it has become clear that every somatic cell contains the genes capable of synthesizing every polypeptide hormone. However, only under pathological circumstances is that capability likely to be expressed by some cells. A variety of hypotheses for ectopic hormone synthesis and secretion have been made. None explains all of the observed facts. Fundamentally all cells inherit an identical complement of DNA. They are therefore totipotential and have all the coded information required for the synthesis of all proteins and peptides, including protein hormones or part of their constituent amino acid sequences. The normal inability of non-endocrine tissue to synthesize hormones is ascribed to 'repressors' that mask specific segments of the DNA molecule. It seems possible that when a cell becomes malignant this normal repression becomes ineffective, allowing the unmasked DNA to synthesize proteins or peptides 'foreign' to the cell concerned. Such a 'de-repression' hypothesis does not explain why certain tumours are more prone to secrete certain ectopic hormones. Another hypothesis suggests that there are a small number of special proliferative cells in normal mature tissues that have fetal characteristics with the ability to produce peptide hormones—a process of 'dysdifferentiation' rather than 'de-repression'. The role of oncogenes in modulating this expression remains to be clarified.

TREATMENT

The treatment of the clinical or biochemical abnormalities associated with endocrinopathies of non-endocrine origin is best directed at the primary disorder. In neoplastic disease, this may involve surgical excision, radiotherapy, or chemotherapy. Sometimes the tumour secreting the ectopic hormone is extremely difficult to locate even with computed tomography (CT), ultrasound scanning, or selective venous catheterization.

More specific therapy may be necessary to contain the metabolic abnormality until such time as the fundamental disorder can be controlled. For example, immediate measures may be required to reduce hypercalcaemia with fluids and diphosphonates or mithramycin, or steps taken (administration of metyrapone) to diminish corticosteroid secretion from adrenal glands stimulated by ectopic ACTH secretion.

Hypercalcaemia

Hypercalcaemia may be associated with malignant solid tumours or haematological cancer. It is usually due to bone involvement. In a proportion of patients with solid tumours, however, there is no evidence using radionucleotide scanning, or indeed at autopsy, of osseous metastases. Thus in some a humoral factor, or factors, is the cause of the hypercalcaemia. Often a number of different mechanisms are involved in the same patient.

Following its discovery in 1987, it is now known that PTHrP is responsible for hypercalcaemia in a large number of patients with this tumour-associated phenomenon. PTHrP shares with PTH amino acid homology between positions 2 and 13 of the 84 residues of PTH. Infusion of synthetic 1–141 PTHrP causes hypercalcaemia in animals and it acts on PTH receptors to increase bone resorption and decrease renal excretion of calcium. The gene is located on the short arm of chromosome 12; that of PTH is on chromosome 11. PTHrP is made by squamous carcinomata as well as renal, bladder, ovary, skin, pancreas, and breast carcinomata and lymphomata.

Other factors can be involved in hypercalcaemia unassociated with osseous metastases. 1,25-Dihydroxy vitamin D_3 is not uncommonly made by lymphoproliferative tumours, which are either high grade or widely disseminated. Transforming growth factor α (TGFα) which stimulates osteoclastic bone resorption, is also made by squamous carcinoma, renal and breast carcinomata. Some tumours co-secrete both TGFα and PTHrP. Interleukin-1, which is a very powerful stimulator of osteoclastic bone resorption, is also made by squamous carcinomata as well as some haematological malignancies. Tumour necrosis factor (TNF) and lymphotoxin also stimulate osteoclastic bone resorption. These related cytokines cause hypercalcaemia *in vivo*, and lymphotoxin is produced by cultured myeloma cells *in vitro* and accounts for the hypercalcaemia seen in this condition. Prostaglandins of the E series have also been implicated in the process of hypercalcaemia, particularly in breast cancer, but they are an uncommon cause of it. It is also important to remember that primary hyperparathyroidism itself is common, particularly in the elderly; two diseases may coexist. For this reason, primary hyperparathyroidism should always be considered when hypercalcaemia occurs, even if it is in a patient within the setting of malignant disease. It is possible to differentiate between these two conditions by

using the PTH radio-immunoassay. Two-site immunoradiometric assays of PTH which detect the whole molecule show high levels in primary hyperparathyroidism and low ones in patients with excessive PTHrP secretion. Previous radio-immunoassays of PTH which picked up molecular fragments did not differentiate between the two with such confidence.

Paraneoplastic hypercalcaemia may be either asymptomatic or dominate the clinical picture and be life-threatening as a consequence of dehydration and renal failure. The features of hypercalcaemia and its general management are discussed elsewhere (see Chapters 12.6, 20.2.1, 20.9.3).

Syndrome of inappropriate antidiuresis (SIAD)

This syndrome, is usually, but not invariably, associated with high levels of circulating arginine vasopressin. Other, as yet unidentified, antidiuretic substances are sometimes involved. There is hyponatraemia and impaired water excretion in the absence of hypovolaemia, hypotension, or deficiency of cardiac, renal, thyroid, or adrenal function. In addition to the impaired urinary dilution there must also be an excess fluid intake; the mechanism of the latter is unexplained. Associated with hyponatraemia, there is a reduction in plasma osmolality and a urine concentration inappropriate to it.

Four patterns or clinical forms are thought to exist. These, the many disorders associated with SIAD diagnosis (Table 1), and management are discussed elsewhere (Chapter 20.2.1).

Ectopic ACTH secretion

Pro-opiomelanocortin (POMC) is a 31 kDa precursor for both ACTH and β-lipotrophin as well as for other polypeptides derived from it, including γ-lipotrophin and β-endorphin. A variety of non-pituitary tumours are capable of secreting POMC-derived peptides. These account for between 15 and 20 per cent of patients with Cushing's syndrome. Approximately 50 per cent of these ectopic ACTH-producing tumours are in the lung and the rest are present in a variety of other tissues (Table 2). Some tumours, particularly pancreatic islet cell tumours which are seldom (< 5 per cent) associated with Cushing's syndrome, can, in addition to ACTH, also secrete a number of other hormones, including insulin, gastrin, and glucagon (see Chapter 12.10). This accounts for the usefulness, when screening for ectopic ACTH, of measuring tumour markers, other hormones or compounds which may be co-secreted, the presence of which raises the suspicion of an ectopic hormone-secreting tumour. Very rarely, corticotrophin releasing hormone (CRH) is secreted ectopically in association with ACTH.

While small cell lung cancer is the most common source, carcinoids anywhere, but particularly bronchial carcinoids, may secrete ACTH ectopically. Thymic carcinoids, islet cell pancreatic tumours, phaeochromocytoma, and medullary carcinoma of the thyroid are other encountered sites. Others are less common (Table 2). The exact mechanism of synthesis of ectopic POMC-derived peptides is still debated. It is becoming apparent that these tumours represent undifferentiated neuroendocrine cells expressing the activity of a POMC gene outside the pituitary gland.

PRESENTATION

The clinical picture is variable. In patients with small cell lung cancer who have a rapidly progressive tumour, the physical features of Cushing's syndrome may not have time to develop. The major features are weight loss, proximal muscular weakness, polyuria, thirst, oedema, carbohydrate intolerance with glycosuria and sometimes pigmentation due to ACTH. Hypokalaemic alkalosis is a characteristic finding; the plasma potassium is less than 3.2 mmol/l and the bicarbonate greater than 30 mmol/l, the urine potassium loss being the direct cause of most of the symptoms. This hypokalaemia is in part due to the very high cortisol

Table 1 *Conditions associated with the syndrome of inappropriate antidiuresis (SIAD)*

Malignancies
  Carcinoma
    Small cell lung
    Pancreas—islet cell
    Duodenum
    Colon
    Bladder
    Prostate
    Thymus
    Cervix
    Lymphoma
Lung diseases
  Pneumonia
    viral
    bacterial
    fungal
  Tuberculosis
  Lung abscess
  Asthma
  Pneumothorax
  Chest wall injury
  Mechanical ventilation
CNS diseases
  Cerebral trauma
  Cerebrovascular accident
  Meningitis
  Encephalitis
  Brain tumours—primary or secondary (e.g. cerebellar
    haemangioblastoma)
  Cerebral abscess
  Hydrocephalus
  Guillain–Barré syndrome
  Delirium tremens
  Acute intermittent porphyria
General surgery
Drugs
  Vasopressin
  Desmopressin (DDAVP)
  Oxytocin
  Thiazides
  Vincristine, vinblastine
  Cyclophosphamide
  Phenothiazines
  Tricyclic antidepressants
  Carbamazepine
  Chlorpropamide
  Clofibrate
Metabolic causes
  Porphyria

Table 2 *Types of neoplasm causing ectopic POMC (ACTH) secretion*

Small cell carcinoma of the bronchus
Bronchial carcinoid
Thymic carcinoid
Islet cell pancreatic tumour
Phaeochromocytoma
Medullary carcinoma of the thyroid
Breast carcinoma ⎤
Tracheal carcinoma
Oesophageal carcinoma
Gastric carcinoma
Ileal carcinoma
Appendicular carcinoma ⎬ Less common
Colonic carcinoma
Ovarian carcinoma
Prostatic carcinoma
Squamous carcinoma of the cervix
Adrenal medullary paraganglioma
Melanoma ⎦

Table 3 *Response to tests used to differentiate ectopic ACTH secretion from Cushing's disease (from Howlett* et al. *1986)*

	Ectopic ACTH (% of cases)	Cushing's disease (% of cases)
Hypokalaemia		
< 3.2 mmol/l	100	10
Diabetes mellitus	78	38
Dexamethasone 8 mg/day		
(no suppression)	89	22
No response to		
metyrapone	50	36
CRH test excessive		
response	0	>90

levels which have a mineralocorticoid action, and corticosterone and 11-deoxycorticosterone may also be produced in excess. The 11β-hydroxysteroid dehydrogenase enzyme may also function abnormally, causing decreased inactivation of cortisol and corticosterone. The serum cortisol level is usually greatly elevated (>1000 nmol/l). The plasma ACTH level is also raised (>200 µg/l), and these high levels do not occur in pituitary-dependent Cushing's disease.

When the ectopic sources are other than a small cell lung cancer, the clinical picture may be quite indistinguishable from Cushing's disease and cushingoid features may antedate by months or years any evidence of a tumour causing ectopic ACTH secretion. The degree of elevation of ACTH is less marked than with small cell lung cancer and is proportional to tumour size. Some carcinoid tumours may be small and difficult to locate. The real problem is to differentiate ectopic ACTH

secretion from pituitary-dependent disease (Table 3). Hypokalaemic alkalosis (< 3.2 mmol/l) remains the most useful test in the differential diagnosis. High-dose dexamethasone (8 mg/day, 2 mg 6 hourly for 2 days) is useful, but the metyrapone test is not. CRH, the hypothalamic hormone controlling pituitary ACTH release, may be used as a stimulation test. The response is flat in ectopic ACTH secretion and exaggerated in most patients with pituitary-dependent ACTH secretion. Because most of the tumours secreting POMC are in either the chest or abdomen, computed tomography (CT) will often reveal the source of ectopic hormone secretion. In patients in whom the lesion is not readily visible by imaging techniques, selective venous catheterization and sampling may help determine a source of ACTH by comparing levels at various sites within the venous system. Such sampling should include inferior petrosal sinuses in case of pituitary-dependent disease. The presence of other tumour markers, for example HCG, calcitonin, and alpha-fetoprotein, may also suggest an ectopic source of ACTH. Chronic ethanol abuse and depression can also cause the biochemical features of Cushing's syndrome.

TREATMENT

Removal of the primary growth or its control with radiotherapy or chemotherapy will relieve the endocrine manifestations. A relapse may occur if metastases develop because these, too, usually secrete ACTH. When it proves impossible to control a primary tumour, adrenocortical hypersecretion may be reduced by 'medical adrenalectomy', giving the 11β-hydroxylase inhibitor of conversion of 11-deoxycortisol to cortisol, metyrapone (500–4000 mg daily). Aminoglutethimide (1000–1500 mg/

day) may also be used, but frequently causes a skin rash. Ketoconazole (400–800 mg/day), which can cause fatal liver damage, and the adrenolytic drug op-DDD are also useful. RU-486, a glucocorticoid antagonist at the receptor level, has been used as palliative therapy for some patients (10–30 mg/kg/day). Lastly, the long-acting somatostatin analogue, octreotide (0.3 mg subcutaneously/day), has also been used in the treatment of ectopic ACTH syndrome associated with metastatic gastrin-secreting pancreatic islet cell carcinoma.

Bilateral adrenalectomy is an alternative approach, but frequently it is not practical for patients with rapidly progressive metastatic disease. It may be possible to embolize the arterial supply of the adrenal gland if patients are not suitable surgical candidates for adrenalectomy. Medical treatment needs to be monitored carefully so that adrenal insufficiency is avoided.

Hypoglycaemia

(See also Chapter 11.12)

Malignant tumours not derived from pancreatic islet cells may be associated with hypoglycaemia. Usually the tumour is large and of mesenchymal origin, arising in the abdomen or thorax. Histology shows a mesothelioma, a fibrosarcoma, or other sarcoma such as a leiomyosarcoma. Other neoplasms associated with hypoglycaemia are haemangiopericytoma, hepatoma, adrenal carcinoma, lung carcinoma, Wilms' tumour, and colonic carcinoma. Symptoms are those of neuroglycopenia—sweating, tachycardia, disorientation, drowsiness, fits, and coma. The cause of hypoglycaemia is insulin-like growth factor II (IGF-II). IGFs I and II are simple peptides of 70 and 67 amino acids which have a considerable amino acid sequence homology with proinsulin and share some of insulin's actions. The secretion of IGF-I by the liver is much more growth hormone dependent than that of IGF-II. Fetal growth is dependent on IGF-II. The IGFs act as endocrine factors and there is now abundant evidence that they are produced in many tissues and can act locally in an autocrine–paracrine manner. The relative importance of IGFs acting as endocrine factors, or as autocrine–paracrine factors, differs from tissue to tissue and at different stages of development. IGFs circulate bound to one of six binding proteins (IGFBPs). Of these, the most important is IGFBP 3 which itself is growth hormone dependent and which binds 75 per cent of IGF-I and IGF-II. In practice, in patients harbouring the tumours mentioned above radio-immunoassay of circulating IGF-II levels are usually normal. However, there is an increase in the large molecular weight (10–15 kDa) molecules rather than the expected 7.5 kDa IGF-II. Furthermore, IGFBP 3 levels in these patients are low, possibly related to decreased growth hormone secretion. This means that there are increased amounts of 'big' IGF-II not detected on radio-immunoassay which cause hypoglycaemia. Growth hormone deficiency, decreased gluconeogenesis, and increased glucose metabolism by the tumour, which is usually large, may also contribute to the hypoglycaemia present. The blood glucose is less than 2.8 mmol/l. Treatment of these tumours is difficult. The hypoglycaemia is not responsive to diazoxide, glucagon, or corticosteroids. The underlying tumour may be resistant to radiotherapy, and surgery, although effective if possible, is not always feasible.

Hyperglycaemia

The non-endocrine causes of impaired glucose tolerance and diabetes mellitus are shown in Table 4. A number of different mechanisms of impaired glucose tolerance are involved, and these are also shown on the table. In cystic fibrosis, the incidence of diabetes mellitus rises with age, such that approximately 17 per cent of patients over the age of 35 are affected. This figure will increase as survival improves. Histologically there is fibrosis of the pancreas and hypoinsulism as well as increased insulin resistance. Patients should be treated with hypoglycaemic agents or insulin but not diet. They are already frequently undernourished.

Ectopic chorionic gonadotrophin secretion

Human chorionic gonadotrophin is a glycoprotein consisting of an α- and a β-subunit. The α-subunit is species specific and is the same for all glycoprotein hormones (luteinizing hormone (LH), follicle stimulating hormone (FSH), and thyroid stimulating hormone (TSH)). The β-subunit determines receptor interaction and specific hormone activity. The β-subunit of HCG is very similar to that of LH. In normal circumstances HCG circulates only during pregnancy, arising from the syncytiotrophoblast. Many assays do not differentiate between LH and HCG. This may lead to misinterpretation when so-called LH is measured; high levels may be due to cross-reacting HCG. A specific and sensitive HCG-β assay exists. Clinically silent ectopic secretion of HCG, with or without its free α- and β-subunits, occurs in many patients.

In the first decade of life, ectopic HCG production may cause isosexual precocious puberty in boys with hepatoblastoma. HCG, through its LH-like action, causes Leydig cell stimulation in the testes. In turn, testosterone levels reach those of a normal adult, and secondary sexual characteristics develop together with premature skeletal maturity. The testes remain small because there is no seminiferous tubule growth as this is dependent on FSH, not LH. Precocious puberty is rare in girls. This and other causes of ectopic HCG are shown in Table 5.

Intracranial teratoma, choriocarcinoma, and pinealoma are associated with ectopic HCG secretion. In men this may be associated with gynaecomastia. In some this is due to co-secretion of oestrogen which may, in women, be associated with dysfunctional uterine bleeding. These manifestations are reversible on treatment of the primary tumour. Other tumours associated with HCG secretion are testicular tumours, stomach, pancreatic, and liver tumours. In most the HCG is too low to be measured in conventional testing. Also, in most it is clinically silent. Ectopic HCG may be produced in adenocarcinoma of the ovaries.

HCG is a useful tumour marker in gestational trophoblastic disease (choriocarcinoma) and in some men with testicular tumours, giving an early warning of recurrent disease. However, it is important to measure other tumour markers, for example alpha-fetoprotein, which may also be secreted by non-seminotamous germ-cell tumours. Discordance of marker levels and tumour progress may be seen. In central nervous system disease, cerebrospinal fluid levels of HCG may be measured, and as HCG does not cross the blood–brain barrier and levels in cerebrospinal fluid remain undetectable in pregnancy, cerebrospinal fluid/plasma ratios may help in the correct localization of tumours. Thus cerebrospinal fluid levels higher than plasma suggest primary CNS disease.

In some patients, most commonly with choriocarcinoma and massive elevation of HCG, the latter, through its weak TSH activity, occasioned by its biochemical similarity to TSH, may cause goitre and hyperthyroidism. This most frequently occurs in women, is not associated with eye signs, and is mild chemically. Treatment of the tumour results in a resumption of a euthyroid state but, if this is not possible, carbimazole or propylthiouracil may be used.

Ectopic human placental lactogen

Human placental lactogen (hPL), also called human chorionic somatomammotropin (hCS), is a trophoblastic hormone not normally produced. It may be secreted ectopically and most commonly this occurs in association with lung tumours. It is usually associated with gynaecomastia in men, and these tumours may also be associated with increased levels of oestradiol and HCG.

Extrapituitary acromegaly and diseases associated with abnormal growth hormone secretion

Most patients with acromegaly (98 per cent) have benign growth hormone producing pituitary adenomas. Less than 2 per cent of patients

Table 4 *Impaired glucose tolerance/diabetes mellitus in non-endocrine diseases*

Disease	Postulated mechanism
Chronic liver disease	Impaired insulin degradation
Chronic pancreatitis (chronic calcifying and tropical calcific)	Impaired insulin release
Cystic fibrosis	Hypoinsulinaemia + insulin resistance
Haemachromatosis	Pancreatic cell toxicity (Fe) + insulin resistance
Genetic disorders	
Werner's syndrome	
Ataxia telangiectasia	Considerable insulin resistance
Mendelhall syndrome	Abnormal insulin receptor function
Acute intermittent porphyria	?
	Insulinopenia
Glycogen storage disease	
Drugs	
Streptozotocin	Beta-cell destruction
Alloxan	
Diazoxide	
Thiazide diuretics	
Loop diuretics (low incidence)	Inhibit insulin secretion by direct beta-cell effect
Verapamil (overdosage)	
Phenytoin (overdosage)	
L-Asparaginase	
Somatostatin/octreotide	
Adrenaline (α and β angonists)	Sympathetic stimulation or blockade
Clonidine (α_2 agonist)	α agonist $\rightarrow \downarrow$ insulin
Salbutamol (β_2 agonist)	β_2 agonists $\rightarrow \uparrow$ insulin
Theophylline (β_2 agonist [overdosage])	
β-Blockers	
Glucocorticoids	
Oral contraceptives	Impaired insulin action
Anabolic steroids	
Aspirin (overdosage)	
Isoniazid (overdosage)	
Rifampicin	Unknown mechanism

Table 5 *HCG in sera of patients with malignant tumours (from Vaitukaitis 1991)*

Tissue	Percentage of cases with ectopic secretion of HCG
Breast	21
Lung	10
Gastrointestinal tract	18
Pancreas (more commonly HCG-α)	33
Stomach	22
Liver	21
Small intestine	13
Large intestine	12
Biliary tract	11
Oesophagus	0
Ovary (adenocarcinoma)	40
Testis	62
Seminoma	38
Embryonal cell carcinoma	58
Choriocarcinoma	100
Mixed	73

with acromegaly have ectopic growth hormone releasing hormone (GHRH) production. Indeed, such a patient with a carcinoid tumour of the pancreas producing GHRH was responsible for the final elucidation of the structure of this important hypothalamic peptide which stimulates anterior pituitary growth hormone secretion. Besides the pancreas, lung carcinoid tumours, small cell lung cancer and phaeochromocytoma may produce GHRH ectopically and cause acromegaly by stimulation of the pituitary somatotrophs. Histologically, in the pituitary there is not an adenoma but somatotroph hyperplasia and the two can be differentiated histologically. These tumours are usually clinically apparent and GHRH levels in the circulation are elevated. GHRH can also be secreted by hypothalamic hamartomas, which also result in anterior pituitary somatotroph hyperplasia.

In McCune–Albright syndrome, polyostotic fibrous dysplasia of bone occurs in association with gonadotrophin independent sexual precocity and growth hormone and prolactin secreting pituitary adenomas, autonomous adrenal hypercortisolism, and primary hyperthyroidism. An activating mutation in the α-subunit of the Gs protein (Gsα) has been found to account for these abnormalities. Upon hormone–receptor interaction, Gsα binds guanosine triphosphate (GTP) and activates adenyl cyclase. GTPase activity inherent in Gsα then hydrolyses GTP to guanosine diphosphate, thus terminating the adenylate cyclase interaction. A mutation of Gsα (arginine 201) to either histidine or cysteine, which severely attenuates the Gsα GTPase activity, has been found in virtually all affected tissues of patients with this syndrome.

Ectopic growth hormone secretion has been reported in patients with bronchial, pancreatic, and gastrointestinal carcinoma, and *in vitro* cells cultured from an undifferentiated lung cancer have been shown to synthesize growth hormone. Breast carcinoma and ovarian tumours may also occasionally secrete growth hormone, but no clinical syndrome has been clearly identified as caused by ectopic growth hormone.

Ectopic prolactin secretion

Prolactin may be secreted by bronchial carcinoma and renal cell carcinoma; the usual endocrine manifestation is galactorrhoea and there may be marked hyperprolactinaemia. These abnormalities are reversed if the tumour is controlled or removed. Difficulties in differential diagnosis may arise unless the underlying abnormality is clinically obvious or suspected, because in most instances the hyperprolactinaemia will be attributed to a prolactin-secreting adenoma. Suspicion of an ectopic source may only arise when the prolactin level is not lowered by bromocriptine treatment.

Ectopic calcitonin secretion

Increased serum calcitonin levels are encountered in a variety of cancers apart from medullary carcinoma of the thyroid. The most common of these are small cell lung cancer, leukaemia, and neoplasms of the breast and pancreas. Ectopic calcitonin may differ from the normal hormone in having more high molecular weight components; it does not cause any apparent symptoms and does not produce hypocalcaemia.

Ectopic renin secretion

Although hypertension associated with hyper-reninism and increased aldosterone production is usually due to a renal lesion, ectopic secretion of renin has also been described in association with cancer of the lung, pancreas, and ovary. The clinical picture is usually dominated by the underlying neoplasm, but the patient has hypertension and the cause of this may be suspected from the associated hypokalaemia and its accompanying muscle weakness. Effective treatment of the primary lesion will reduce the increased renin and aldosterone levels and hence the raised blood pressure. When the underlying cause cannot be eradicated, the use of an angiotensin enzyme inhibitor will control the hypertension.

Ectopic aldosterone secretion

Hypertension and hypokalaemia related to ectopic secretion of aldosterone from a non-adrenal neoplasm have been described in patients with ovarian tumours. In its pathogenesis the situation is different from the others described above. The aberrant production of a steroid, aldosterone, rather than a peptide, is presumably due to biochemical change in the ovarian steroidogenic cells. Attention is likely to be focused on a suspected lesion of the adrenal zona glomerulosa because the hyperaldosteronism is associated with low plasma renin activity. The ovarian lesion may initially be clinically silent and only revealed by pelvic ultrasonography.

Endocrine complications of important non-endocrine diseases

ENDOCRINE COMPLICATIONS OF SARCOIDOSIS

In sarcoidosis, hypercalcaemia may result from an increase in circulating 1,25-dihydroxy-vitamin D_3. This is produced by alveolar macrophages in a dose-dependent fashion stimulated by γ-interferon, which is one factor responsible for the maintenance of the inflammatory process in sarcoidosis. However, it is possible that the increased 1,25-dihydroxy-vitamin D_3 production is a compensatory mechanism mounted by the immune system to inhibit the inflammatory process. It is the probable

mechanism of hypercalcaemia also occasionally seen in association with tuberculosis, coccidiomycosis, histoplasmosis, leprosy, and ruptured silicone implants. Vitamin D excess increases intestinal absorption and urinary excretion of calcium. Indeed, hypercalciuria is more common than hypercalcaemia. Hypercalcaemia in patients with sarcoidosis who live in the northern hemisphere is usually more pronounced in the summer months because of longer exposure to sunlight which increases the dermal production of vitamin D. Hypercalcaemia can lead to impaired renal function, nephrolithiasis, nephrocalcinosis, and chronic renal failure. Both abnormal vitamin D and abnormal calcium metabolism in sarcoidosis can be treated with glucocorticoids. The treatment lowers both 1,25-dihydroxy-vitamin D_3 and serum calcium.

Although involvement of the central nervous system occurs in 16 per cent of patients with sarcoidosis, that of the pituitary and hypothalamus is less common. The prime site of involvement is the hypothalamus. The most common manifestations of hypothalamic involvement are polyuria and polydipsia, due either to diabetes insipidus or a disordered control of thirst. Other hypothalamic symptoms may occur, including somnolence, variations in body temperature, progressive obesity, and personality changes. Hypopituitarism may also occur as a result of hypothalamic involvement resulting in decreased secretion of anterior pituitary hormones, and hypothyroidism, hypoadrenalism, hypogonadism, and, less often, impaired growth occur. Hyperprolactinaemia may be found due to impaired dopaminergic inhibition of the pituitary lactotrophs.

Treatment of hypothalamic/pituitary sarcoidosis may be difficult. Supraphysiological doses of steroids may decrease the size of the hypothalamic mass but side-effects frequently occur. Irradiation may be helpful in some cases.

The thyroid is involved in about 4 per cent of patients with sarcoidosis. Very rarely, hypothyroidism can be caused by granulomatous involvement of the gland. In the adrenal gland involvement by sarcoidosis is very rare. Although adrenal crisis and death have been reported, these, too, are very rare. Involvement of the pancreas and male and female reproductive systems have also been reported. Diabetes mellitus has not been reported.

Endocrine manifestations of acquired immunodeficiency syndrome (AIDS)

Already a considerable literature exists but confusion arises because of the difficulty of assessing whether the abnormalities are caused by the virus itself, infection, or pharmacological agents used in treatment.

For the most part, hypothalamic pituitary function is normal irrespective of the stage of human immunodeficiency virus (HIV) progression. More work is needed in assessing the pulsatility of hormones involved in the hypothalamopituitary axis. Hypogonadism is the most prevalent endocrine related disorder seen in AIDS. This may be related to infection, for example cytomegalovirus, toxoplasmosis, or tuberculosis. Testosterone levels appear to fall with progression of the disease and this may, in part, be due to non-specific ill-health and, in part, due to a functional hypothalamic disorder.

The adrenal may be affected by a number of pathological mechanisms. Cytomegalovirus, as well as cryptococcal and mycobacterial infections, may affect the adrenal, and therapy, for example with ketoconazole, may decrease the reserve of the gland and even cause insufficiency, because of its effect of decreasing cortisol production.

In the thyroid there appears to be a rise in total plasma thyroxine as the disease progresses. This may be due to a progressive rise in thyroid-binding globulin. Reverse T_3 levels fall, as seen in the sick euthyroid syndrome (see below). Infiltration of the thyroid gland is uncommon but may be the presentation of a treatable AIDS-associated opportunistic infection. Histological examination of the thyroid has revealed involvement by cytomegalovirus, Cryptococcus, *Pneumocystis carinii*, and

Kaposi's sarcoma. Further, medications that alter thyroid function tests include rifampicin, which increases thyroxine clearance by inducing hepatic microsomal enzymes.

Drug-induced and other non-endocrine causes of endocrine manifestations

A number of pharmaceutical drugs may induce manifestations of endocrine disease. More commonly they may influence the results of hormonal assays and lead to mistaken diagnosis. It may not be a major problem when it is known that the patient is taking a particular compound and from its molecular structure it is appreciated that such a substance could influence the endocrine system or the results of hormonal assays. The problem is greater, however, when the drug in question has no clear relationship to a hormone and the mechanism by which it induces an endocrine manifestation, or interferes with an assay procedure, is not readily apparent.

Thyroid

HIGH THYROID FUNCTION TESTS

A number of drugs can interfere with thyroid function tests. Some act by inhibiting the conversion of thyroxine (T_4) to triiodothyronine (T_3), others by increasing thyroid-binding globulin. β-Blockers with membrane stabilizing properties, such as propranolol, inhibit peripheral conversion of T_4 to T_3. Oral cholecystographic agents and amiodarone, a heavily iodinated antiarrhythmic agent, are also potent inhibitors of T_4 to T_3 conversion and produce decreased serum T_3 concentrations and an increase in reverse T_3. Oestrogen increases thyroid-binding globulin, the most important thyroid-binding protein, due to an increase in the sialic acid content of thyroxine-binding globulin which prolongs its half-life in the circulation with no change in the rate of its synthesis. Thus women on oestrogens, for example the contraceptive pill, have high total T_4 concentrations but are euthyroid. Such results may also be seen on tamoxifen. Heroin and methadone addicts have raised levels of thyroxine-binding globulin, as do patients on the lipid-lowering agent, clofibrate.

Pregnancy, through a similar mechanism, causes abnormal thyroid function tests—a high thyroid-binding globulin and elevated total T_4, and sometimes T_3, both of these effects being due to oestrogen stimulation of thyroid-binding globulin.

DRUG-INDUCED HYPERTHYROIDISM

In a proportion of patients on amiodarone, particularly those who are deplete of iodine, amiodarone may cause thyrotoxicosis with a marked elevation of total thyroxine, a relatively normal level of T_3, and a suppressed TSH. Often thyrotoxicosis is masked by the β-blocking effect of the drug. Because of the large iodine load, it may be very difficult to treat with antithyroid drugs, and steroids may also be necessary to suppress thyroid hormone levels into the normal range. Even if amiodarone is stopped, its effects continue for many weeks because it is predominantly stored in adipose tissue. Contrast media and iodine-containing cough medicines may similarly induce hyperthyroidism.

Hyperthyroidism is also seen in a number of other non-endocrine conditions. Struma ovarii, a rare ovarian tumour which may contain thyroid tissue, may also cause thyrotoxicosis.

Thyrotoxicosis factitia may be seen in people taking exogenous T_3 or T_4. If the subject is taking T_3, the total thyroxine level is suppressed below normal and the T_3 is raised. If T_4 is being taken in excess, the total T_4 level is more elevated than that of T_3. By contrast, in Graves' disease the T_3 is disproportionately more raised and the T_4 to T_3 ratio is lower. The diagnosis may be confirmed in these patients by performing a thyroid scan which, in the presence of high thyroid hormones, shows suppressed thyroid uptake.

LOW THYROID FUNCTION TESTS

A decreased serum T_4 does not necessarily indicate the presence of hypothyroidism. Many pharmacological agents lower the total T_4 concentration by interfering with the binding of T_4 to one or more of the thyroid-binding proteins. Therapeutic levels of phenytoin lower the level of serum T_4 and high concentrations are capable of inhibiting the binding of T_4 and T_3 to thyroid-binding globulin. Salicylates, when prescribed in high dose, have the same effect for the same reason. Diclofenac, a non-steroidal anti-inflammatory drug structurally similar to thyroxine, also interferes with thyroid hormone binding. Phenylbutazone, anabolic steroids, and glucocorticoids may also be associated with a low total T_4 and normal thyroid function. In hypoproteinaemic states, for example in the nephrotic syndrome or liver disease, total T_4 may also be low in the presence of normal thyroid function.

SICK EUTHYROID SYNDROME

A combination of reduced T_3 and T_4 is found in some patients with severe illness, including liver disease, chronic renal failure, after major surgery and burns. In general these patients are considered euthyroid, with normal basal or depressed TSH. Besides a low T_3 due to decreased conversion from T_4 there are elevated concentrations of reverse T_3, mainly due to its reduced clearance. Treatment with thyroid hormones does not affect the outcome.

The major importance of this syndrome is to exclude important thyroid disease. Primary thyroid disease is excluded by a normal TSH. Secondary (pituitary or hypothalamic) thyroid disease only occurs in advanced pituitary failure.

DRUG-INDUCED HYPOTHYROIDISM

Increased iodide intake leads to decreased iodide trapping and a decrease in synthesis of thyroid hormones, hypothyroidism, and goitre. Iodine is contained in a number of 'tonics' and cough medicines. It is also a large component of the drug amiodarone. Amiodarone, besides producing thyrotoxicosis, may be a cause in patients replete with iodine, of iodine-induced hypothyroidism. Lithium, used in manic depressive disorders, is a goitrogenic agent which acutely blocks iodine uptake and the release of thyroid hormones. Only 2 per cent of patients on lithium actually develop clinical features of hypothyroidism.

Adrenal cortex

Drugs may interfere with tests of adrenal function. Thus, for example, phenytoin accelerates metabolism of dexamethasone, and patients on phenytoin may not suppress cortisol normally during dexamethasone suppression tests. Furthermore, during the assessment of adrenal reserve, chronic topical application of steroids, as well as inhalation of steroids for asthma, may suppress adrenal function. Oestrogens, by enhancing hepatic production of cortisol-binding globulin, which binds between 90 and 97 per cent of circulating cortisol in the circulation, increases cortisol-binding globulin two- to threefold. Thus assessment of glucocorticoid replacement in patients on oestrogens is interfered with by this effect.

Chronic excessive intake of alcohol causes the syndrome of alcoholic pseudo-Cushing's. These patients behave biochemically as if they have Cushing's syndrome with absent dexamethasone suppression. This occurs through a centrally mediated mechanism with hypersection of pituitary ACTH and secondary secretion of cortisol by the adrenals.

Primary aldosteronism can be mimicked by the mineralocorticoid effect of glycyrrhizic acid contained in both carbenoxolone and liquorice. Cortisol is normally inactivated by conversion to the inactive metabolite, cortisone, by the enzyme 11β-hydroxysteroid dehydrogenase, but these compounds inhibit the enzyme, which is important in the kidney because it protects renal mineralocorticoid receptors from cortisol.

ADRENOCORTICAL INSUFFICIENCY

Aminoglutethimide, used in the treatment of Cushing's syndrome, inhibits the cholesterol side-chain cleavage enzymes and 11β-hydroxylase. It may cause adrenal insufficiency by inhibiting cortisol biosynthesis. Similarly, the antifungal agent, ketoconazole, and the short-acting anaesthetic, etomidate, are imidazole derivatives with significant inhibitory effects on 11β-hydroxylase. While they do not usually produce clinical insufficiency, they may do so in subjects with limited pituitary or adrenal reserve. Rifampicin and phenytoin, which both accelerate the metabolism of cortisol by inducing hepatic mixed function oxygenase enzymes, can also provoke adrenal insufficiency in similar patients with limited pituitary or adrenal reserve. In such patients, increased doses of replacement therapy are necessary.

THE ADRENAL MEDULLA

A number of drugs interfere with the measurement of urinary catecholamines, including labetalol.

Gonads

MALE

A number of drugs can affect testicular function, leading to hypogonadism and infertility. Mechanisms include the direct inhibition of testosterone synthesis or competitive inhibition of androgen action at receptor level. Spironolactone acts as an androgen antagonist. Alcohol reduces testosterone levels acutely and chronically by both a central and a gonadal effect. Cimetidine has been shown to block testosterone synthesis and causes an increase in serum oestradiol concentration by inhibiting its 2-hydroxylation. Anticonvulsants, for example phenytoin, increase sex hormone-binding globulin and therefore decrease free testosterone levels. They also enhance testosterone to oestradiol conversion.

Infertility with normal virilization may occur as a result of cytotoxic therapy, caused in particular by the alkylating agents such as cyclophosphamide. These produce depletion of the germinal epithelium and lead to a raised FSH level, oligo- or azoospermia, but normal LH and testosterone levels. Sulphasalazine may also cause infertility associated with oligospermia.

FEMALE

Hirsutism can be caused by a number of drugs, including danazol, phenytoin, diazoxide, and minoxidil. Hypogonadism is seen in a number of non-endocrinological conditions, including acute or chronic physical disease, usually associated with a decrease in gonadotrophin secretion ('sick eugonadal syndrome'). It is also seen in weight loss and anorexia nervosa. Excessive exercise may induce oligo- or amenorrhoea by affecting peripheral aromatization of oestrogen in decreased quantities of adipose tissue. Cirrhosis, renal failure, and β-thalassaemia are also associated with a hypogonadal state.

Prolactin

Because prolactin is controlled through dopamine, predominantly by a hypothalamic inhibitory mechanism, a number of drugs can cause hyperprolactinaemia and galactorrhoea. Most of these drugs act through a

Table 6 *Non-endocrine conditions associated with gynaecomastia*

Neoplasms
    Ectopic production of human chorionic gonadotrophin or
        human placental lactogen
Liver disease (18%)
Starvation during recovery phase (refeeding)
Renal disease and dialysis (1%)
Drugs (10–20%)
    Antiandrogens/inhibitors of androgen synthesis
        Cyproterone
        Flutamide
        Spironolactone
    Antibiotics
        Ketoconazole
    Antiulcer medication
        Cimetidine
        Omeprazole
        Ranitidine
    Cancer chemotherapeutic agents
        Alkylating agents
    Cardiovascular drugs
        Captopril
        Digoxin
        Methyldopa
        Nifedipine
    Psychoactive drugs
        Haloperidol
        Phenothiazines
    Drugs of abuse
        Cannabis

dopaminergic mechanism. They may elevate prolactin to a sufficient extent to cause a clinical suspicion of prolactinoma, and in such patients a careful drug history is particularly important. Metoclopramide, pimozide, and sulpiride all act as dopamine antagonists and may considerably elevate prolactin, with all the attendant effects thereof.

Phenothiazines, chlorpromazine, perphenazine, and trifluoperazine also act as dopamine antagonists, as do haloperidol and butyrophenone. Reserpine and methyldopa both decrease catecholamine stores and may cause hyperprolactinaemia. Oestrogens, in high dose, may slightly elevate prolactin but normal contraceptive pills do not. Verapamil, by decreasing dopaminergic tone, may also increase prolactin levels.

Because of this hypothalamic inhibition, granulomas, tumours, and other pathological processes involving the hypothalamus may cause hyperprolactinaemia, including craniopharyngioma, sarcoidosis, histiocytosis, and stalk section after head injury. Galactorrhoea may also occur in chronic renal failure.

Gynaecomastia

Palpable breast glandular tissue is prevalent in population studies of men and boys. Subareolar glandular tissue more than 2 cm diameter is found in 35 to 60 per cent of men. Alterations in the ratio of oestrogen : androgen have been found in patients with gynaecomastia on various drugs, as well as in association with testicular and adrenal neoplasms, Klinefelter's syndrome, thyrotoxicosis, cirrhosis, primary hypogonadism, malnutrition, and ageing (Table 6). An increase in free oestrogen, a decrease in free endogenous androgens, androgen-receptor defects, and partially enhanced secretions of breast tissue may underlie these changes. Increased aromatization of oestrogen precursors occurs in patients with obesity, as a result of ageing, liver disease, and hyperthyroidism, as well as in men on spironolactone. Drugs such as spironolactone and ketoconazole, which can displace steroids from sex-hormone binding globulin, displace oestrogens more easily than androgens. Activation of the oestrogen receptors in breast tissue may take place with drugs that have structural homology with oestrogen, such as digoxin; griseofulvin and cannabis may have the same effect. A decrease in androgen occurs in older men and with drugs such as spironolactone and ketoconazole that inhibit the biosynthesis of testosterone.

The mechanism for the induction of gynaecomastia by captopril and calcium-channel blockers (nifedipine) is unclear. With cimetidine and omeprazole, this effect may be due to the inhibition of liver cytochrome P450.

Posterior pituitary

The syndrome of inappropriate antidiuresis is characterized by normo-volaemic hyponatraemia with persistent secretion of vasopressin, despite a reduced plasma osmolality. A number of drugs can cause this syndrome, including thiazide diuretics, vincristine, vinblastine, cyclophosphamide, chlorpropamide, phenothiazines, carbamazepine, clofibrate, and tricyclic antidepressants (Table 1).

Nephrogenic diabetes insipidus can be induced by lithium in the therapeutic range, and up to 20 per cent of patients receiving long-term therapy may develop this complication. Demethylchlortetracycline produces dose-dependent nephrogenic diabetes insipidus, and both the concentrating defect and the unresponsiveness to vasopressin are reversible on cessation of the drug.

Parathyroid

Lithium therapy can cause an increase in parathyroid gland size, either with hyperplasia or adenoma. This hyperparathyroidism leads to mild hypercalcaemia and sometimes osteoporosis. Thiazide diuretics, by causing haemoconcentration and hypocalciuria, may also result in mild hypercalcaemia but this is usually transient (4–6 weeks); after this time, other causes of hypercalcaemia should be sought.

Vinblastine and colchicine inhibit parathyroid hormone secretion which may result in hypocalcaemia.

REFERENCES

Alberti, K.G.M.M. and Johnston, D.G. (1992). Secondary diabetes. *Clinical Endocrinology and Metabolism* **6**, 719–914.

Bell, N.H. (1991). Endocrine complications of sarcoidosis. *Endocrinology and Metabolism Clinics of North America* **20**, 645–54.

Borysiewicz, L.K. (1994). Endocrine Complications of AIDS. *Clinical Endocrinology*, in press.

Braunstein, G.D. (1993). Current concepts: gynecomastia. *New England Journal of Medicine* **328**, 490–5.

Daughaday, W.H. and Deuel, T.F. (1991). Tumour secretion of growth factors. *Endocrinology and Metabolism Clinics of North America* **20**, 539–63.

Docter, R., Krenning, E.P., DeJong, M., and Hennemann, G. (1993). The sick euthyroid syndrome: changes in thyroid hormone serum parameters and hormone metabolism. *Clinical Endocrinology*, **39**, 499–510.

Howlett, T.A., Drury, P.L., Perry, L., Doniach, I., Rees, L.H., and Besser, G.M. (1986). Diagnosis and management of ACTH-dependent Cushing's syndrome: comparison of the features in ectopic and pituitary ACTH production. *Clinical Endocrinology* **24**, 699–713.

Hung, W., Blizzard, R.M., Migeon, C.J., Camacho, A.M., and Nyhan, W.L. (1963). Precocious puberty in a boy with hepatoma and circulating gonadotropin. *Journal of Pediatrics* **63**, 895–903.

Kovacs, L. and Robertson, G.L. (1992). Syndrome of inappropriate antidiuresis. *Endocrinology and Metabolism Clinics of North America* **21**, 859–76.

Melmed, S. (1991). Extrapituitary acromegaly. *Endocrinology and Metabolism Clinics of North America* **20**, 507–18.

Penny, E., *et al.* (1984). Circulating growth hormone releasing factor concentrations in normal subjects and patients with acromegaly. *British Medical Journal* **289**, 453–5.

Vaitukaitis, J.L. (1991). Ectopic hormonal secretion and reproductive dysfunction. In *Reproductive endocrinology*, (3rd edn), (ed. S.S.C. Yen and R.B. Jaffe), pp. 795–806. W.B. Saunders, Philadelphia.

Vanderpump, M.P.J. and Tunbridge, W.M.G. (1993). The effects of drugs on endocrine function. *Clinical Endocrinology*, **39**, 389–97.

Wass, J.A.H., Jones, A.E., Rees, L.H., and Besser, G.M. (1982). HCGB producing pineal choriocarcinoma. *Clinical Endocrinology* **17**, 423–31.

White, A. and Clark, A.J.L. (1993). The cellular and molecular basis of the ectopic ACTH syndrome. *Clinical Endocrinology*, **39**, 131–41.

Section 13 *Medical disorders in pregnancy*

13.1   Benefits and risks of oral contraceptives   1723

13.2   Hypertension in pregnancy   1726

13.3   Renal disease in pregnancy   1733

13.4   Heart disease in pregnancy   1735

13.5   Thromboembolism in pregnancy   1741

13.6   Chest diseases in pregnancy   1744

13.7   Endocrine disease in pregnancy   1747

13.8   Diabetes in pregnancy   1752

13.9   Blood disorders in pregnancy   1758

13.10   Neurological disease in pregnancy   1766

13.11   Nutrition in pregnancy   1769

13.12   Infection in pregnancy   1775

     13.12.1   Viral infections in pregnancy   1775
     13.12.2   Bacterial, fungal, and protozoal infections
             in pregnancy and the newborn   1784

13.13   Liver and gastrointestinal disease in
        pregnancy   1796

13.14   The skin in pregnancy   1804

13.15   Malignant disease in pregnancy   1806

13.16   Prescribing in pregnancy   1809

13.17   Benefits and risks of hormone therapy   1813

13.1 Benefits and risks of oral contraceptives

M. P. VESSEY

Introduction

The basic physiological principles underlying a hormonal approach to contraception had already been elaborated by the mid-1930s, but the development of practical methods of hormonal birth control had to await the synthesis of potent orally active steroids some 20 years later. Much of the physiological and clinical development of 'the pill' was done by Pincus and Rock in the United States in the 1950s; great credit must be given to these two for their contribution to one of the great medical breakthroughs of the twentieth century. Indeed, in 1988 it was estimated that about 60 million women around the world were taking oral contraceptives, 38 million of them in the Third World.

There are several different types of oral contraceptive regimen, but the most important preparations include both an oestrogen and a progestogen. In the United Kingdom, only two oestrogens have been used, ethinyloestradiol and mestranol, but seven progestogens are currently available (northisterone, norethisterone acetate, ethynodiol diacetate, levonorgestrel, desogestrel, norgestimate, gestodene) while many others have been used in the past (e.g. norethynodrel, chlormadinone acetate, megestrol acetate). Since the dosage of the constituent steroids may be varied (the trend has generally been downwards over the years both for the oestrogen and for the progestogen component), it is not surprising that the number of different oestrogen–progestogen formulations marketed currently or in the past is very large—approaching 100 in the United Kingdom. This adds greatly to the difficulties confronting those trying to assess safety.

Oral contraceptives have many metabolic effects, although these are fewer with modern preparations containing norgestimate, gestodene, or desogestrel. None the less, it has been said that 'almost every metabolic parameter that is capable of laboratory investigation has been reported to be altered in one way or another by some contraceptive steroid'. This implies that the results of many routine laboratory tests may be altered by oral contraceptives, a point of considerable practical importance. In this chapter, however, attention will be largely concentrated on effects of the pill on morbidity and mortality, as revealed by epidemiological studies.

Until the mid-1970s, most of the available data about the benefits and risks of the pill had been derived from uncontrolled clinical trials and from case-control studies. One large-scale randomized study was started in Puerto Rico but it proved to have serious shortcomings. Since then, an enormous amount of epidemiological information has been obtained from two large British cohort studies, the Royal College of General Practitioners Oral Contraceptive Study and the Oxford–Family Planning Association (Oxford–FPA) Contraceptive Study. Between them, these investigations recruited 63 000 women of childbearing age who have now been carefully followed up for an average of around 20 years. Many of the findings described in this chapter are derived from these two cohort studies.

Information about the benefits and risks of oral contraception in the Third World is extremely sparse. The reader is cautioned not to extrapolate the data summarized here to parts of the world to which they clearly do not apply.

Benefits of combined oral contraceptives
HIGH EFFICACY

By far the most important beneficial effect of these preparations is their remarkable efficacy which, coupled with a high degree of acceptability (at least among the young), has given many women a new freedom from anxiety about pregnancy. If taken conscientiously, no more than about two to four women in every thousand using a combined preparation should become accidentally pregnant each year. In practice, pills are often missed and much less satisfactory results are then obtained.

SUPPRESSION OF MENSTRUAL DISORDERS

It has long been known that oral contraceptives suppress some menstrual disorders, notably menorrhagia and dysmenorrhoea, leading to a reduction in hospital admissions for dilatation and curettage and for hysterectomy, and to a lessened risk of iron-deficiency anaemia.

SUPPRESSION OF BENIGN BREAST DISEASE

Epidemiological studies have consistently shown that use of the pill is negatively associated with the occurrence of benign lumps in the breast, thus reducing the need for surgical biopsies by up to 50 per cent. The effect is most pronounced in long-term users, appears to wear off after discontinuation of use, and is probably attributable to the progestogen component of the pill. Some studies considering modern, very-low-dose pills have found less impressive effects on benign breast disease than did the earlier studies.

PELVIC INFLAMMATORY DISEASE

Oestrogen–progestogen oral contraceptives reduce the risk of pelvic inflammatory disease and possibly the severity of the disease as well. There is, however, continuing controversy about the effect of the pill on chlamydial infection.

SUPPRESSION OF FUNCTIONAL OVARIAN CYSTS

Since oral contraceptives act principally by inhibiting ovulation, it is not surprising that follicular cysts and corpus luteum cysts are relatively uncommon in pill users, although this may apply less to modern, very-low-dose pills than to older, higher-dose ones.

SUPPRESSION OF OVARIAN CANCER AND ENDOMETRIAL CANCER

Epidemiological studies reported during the past 10 years have demonstrated that the risk of both epithelial ovarian cancer and endometrial cancer is reduced by about 50 per cent in women who have used combined oral contraceptives for 2 or 3 years. Longer durations of use offer additional protection. Furthermore, the protective effect appears to persist for many years after cessation of pill use; this is important from the public health point of view since ovarian and endometrial cancer are rare in young women amongst whom oral contraceptive use is most prevalent.

OTHER POSSIBLE BENEFICIAL EFFECTS

While the beneficial effects already described may be considered established, a number of others which have been reported in some studies also deserve mention. These include a lessened risk of thyroid disease, rheumatoid arthritis, fibroids, endometriosis, and peptic ulceration. An increased peak bone mass has also been reported. Further work is necessary before the significance of these observations can be assessed.

Risks of combined oral contraceptives

Oral contraceptives are well known to cause minor side-effects such as nausea, headache, and breast tenderness. Although such symptoms are common enough and unpleasant enough to lead to the discontinuation of the pill by up to 25 per cent of women, they disappear immediately medication is stopped and so do not represent a serious problem.

CARDIOVASCULAR EFFECTS

The best known adverse effects of oral contraceptive use are the cardiovascular ones; these comprise venous thrombosis and embolism, thrombotic stroke, and acute myocardial infarction. The evidence concerning haemorrhagic stroke is rather less convincing. The risks, in most studies, are confined to current pill users and do not depend on duration of pill use. The risk of acute myocardial infarction in pill users seems to be concentrated in women with other risk factors for cardiovascular disease, notably cigarette smoking. The results of a new British case-control study have recently become available and suggest strongly that the risk with modern, low-dose oral contraceptives is greatly reduced in comparison with the risk with older, higher-dose preparations.

The mechanisms underlying adverse cardiovascular reactions to the pill are uncertain. However, oral contraceptives have effects on the coagulation system, on serum lipids, on carbohydrate metabolism, on blood pressure, and on the structure of vessels. Any or all of these effects might be of significance. However, it is important to note that modern, low-dose oral contraceptives have much less effect on each of the above possible mechanisms than did the older higher-dose oral contraceptives.

HEPATOCELLULAR ADENOMA AND CARCINOMA

Hepatocellular adenoma and carcinoma are extremely rare (but serious) conditions in women of childbearing age. In those without exposure to the pill, the incidence might be around one per million per annum. Oral contraceptive users suffer a much higher incidence than this, but there is reason to believe that the increase in risk is greatly reduced in those taking modern, low-dose pills.

IMPAIRMENT OF FERTILITY

Despite a vast literature, prior use of oral contraceptives has not been incriminated either as a cause of prolonged secondary amenorrhoea (say absence of periods for more than 6 months) or of prolactinoma of the pituitary which is sometimes associated with this condition. Many women do, however, experience some temporary impairment of fertility after stopping the pill, especially those over the age of 30 trying to have a first baby. In the majority this lasts only a month or so, but in some recovery may be much slower. It seems unlikely that oral contraceptives are ever a cause of permanent infertility.

OTHER POSSIBLE ADVERSE EFFECTS

Large epidemiological studies conducted during the 1970s and 1980s have shown that there is no general association between oral contraceptive use and breast cancer. However, a number of studies (including the particularly well-conducted United Kingdom National Case-Control Study) have suggested that prolonged early use of the pill may have an adverse effect on breast cancer risk, particularly on breast cancer manifesting itself at a young age. This matter is unresolved and may remain so until large numbers of women with prolonged early pill exposure have reached cancer age.

Likewise, a number of studies have indicated an association between long-term oral contraceptive use and cervical cancer. However, this

Table 1 *Morbidity (in terms of hospital admissions) experienced by women aged 25–39 years using either combined oral contraceptives or relying on the condom to try to prevent pregnancy for 1 year; based on data from the Oxford–FPA study*

Reason for hospital admission	Number of hospital admissions in one year among 100 000 women relying on	
	Combined oral contraceptives	Condom
Beneficial effects of oral contraceptives		
Menstrual problems	375	500
Anaemia	22	30
Benign breast disease	115	230
Pelvic inflammatory disease[a]	60	60
Functional ovarian cysts	15	60
Ovarian cancer	5	10
Endometrial cancer	2	4
Harmful effects of oral contraceptives		
Acute myocardial infarction	10	5
Thrombotic stroke	50	10
Haemorrhagic stroke	7	5
Venous thromboembolism	100	20
Hepatocellular adenoma	2	0
Hepatocellular carcinoma	0	0
Accidental pregnancy[b]		
Term birth	300	3040
Spontaneous abortion	63	640
Extrauterine pregnancy	3	20
Induced abortion	134	1300

[a]These rates are equal because both oral contraceptives and a condom offer protection against pelvic inflammatory disease.

[b]The failure rate for oral contraceptives has been taken to be 5 per 1000 per year and for the condom to be 50 per 1000 per year.

association cannot be regarded as established. Indeed, cancer of the cervix is so strongly associated with sexual activity, that it is extremely difficult to isolate any independent effect of the method of contraception used.

Several studies have examined the possible relationship between oral contraceptive use and malignant melanoma; they have not given consistent results.

In the past, there was considerable anxiety about an increase in the risk of cholelithiasis in pill users. Further work has shown the effect, at present, to be minimal. The evidence concerning chronic inflammatory bowel disease is more convincing. Many other possible adverse effects of oral contraceptives have been suggested, including depression, urinary-tract infection, and fetal malformation if taken inadvertently during pregnancy. In every case, the balance of evidence is not compelling. The most recent concern centres round human immunodeficiency virus (HIV) infection being commoner in pill users, with worrying findings in prostitutes in Nairobi. These results have not, however, been replicated elsewhere.

Progestogen-only oral contraceptives

Low doses of progestogens taken every day by mouth have been extensively investigated as contraceptives. Such preparations do not consistently inhibit ovulation and their mode of action is uncertain. Their efficacy is lower than that of the oestrogen–progestogen pill, but they can

Table 2 *Mortality in the Oxford–FPA study*

Cause of death	Oral contraceptive at entry	Diaphragm/IUD at entry
Malignant melanoma	0.7 (1)[a]	0.7 (1)
Breast cancer	23.1 (31)	27.1 (37)
Cervix cancer	4.4 (7)	0.9 (1)
Corpus cancer	0.0 (0)	1.4 (2)
Ovarian cancer	3.6 (5)	9.1 (12)
Other tumours	17.7 (26)	21.6 (27)
Ischaemic heart disease	9.2 (15)	2.8 (3)
Cerebrovascular disease	4.2 (7)	2.9 (3)
Other circulatory disease	2.4 (3)	4.1 (6)
Suicide and probable suicide	6.1 (10)	5.6 (6)
Other accidents, etc.	2.3 (4)	2.0 (2)
All other causes	9.9 (15)	11.7 (14)
All causes	84.3 (124)	90.9 (114)

[a]Rates per 100 000 woman-years with numbers of deaths in parentheses. None of the above differences reaches statistical significance.

give entirely adequate protection in older women who may prefer not to use conventional pills. A major disadvantage of progestogen-only oral contraceptives is their tendency to disrupt the menstrual cycle in many women, producing irregular bleeding, while women who become accidentally pregnant while using them have about a 5 per cent chance of having an ectopic gestation. These drawbacks probably account for the fact that progestogen-only pills represent below 10 per cent of all oral contraceptives consumed. The main advantage of progestogen-only pills is that they appear to be free from the undesirable metabolic effects of combined preparations.

Balance of benefits and risks

A number of authors have provided analyses of varying degrees of complexity in which they have attempted to weigh up the benefits and risks of taking the pill. Three approaches are described here. In the first, which uses hospital inpatient morbidity data from the Oxford–FPA study, supplemented where necessary by other epidemiological data, a comparison is made over a 1-year period of women using either oral contraceptives or a condom for contraception. The approach is fully described elsewhere, but Table 1 summarizes the main findings. Despite the sizeable cardiovascular risks (older 50 μg pills were used in the Oxford–FPA study) the overall results are quite favourable as far as oestrogen–progestogen oral contraceptives are concerned.

The second approach involves constructing models which consider what is known about the effects of oral contraceptives and other birth control methods on mortality, and estimate the balance of benefit and risk over a period of many years. This approach is too complex to describe here because of space limitations, but details are available elsewhere. It has been concluded that, in the absence of adverse effects on the breast or the cervix, women taking the pill do best whatever assumptions are made about cardiovascular disease. It was also shown that even if there is an effect on breast cancer up to age 35 and an effect on cervix cancer, there would be little to choose between oral contraceptive use and condom use. Persistence of a breast cancer effect beyond age 35 would, however, demand a reassessment.

The final approach is a more direct one. It involves examination of the mortality rates observed in the Oxford–FPA study. Table 2 shows that the available data reflect what is known about the effect of oral contraceptives in other studies. The results are reassuring thus far.

The pill has been studied extremely intensively over the past three decades. On the whole, it has stood up well to close scrutiny. It remains an excellent method of contraception for younger women. There remains some doubt, however, about its suitability for those over 40, especially if they smoke or have other cardiovascular risk factors. Women in this age group are, however, usually well served by progestogen-only pills.

REFERENCES

Brinton, L.A., Vessey, M.P., Flavel, R., and Yeates, D. (1981). Risk factors for benign breast disease. *American Journal of Epidemiology* **113**, 203–14.

Brown, S., Vessey, M., and Stratton, I. (1988). The influence of method of contraception and cigarette smoking on menstrual patterns. *British Journal of Obstetrics and Gynaecology* **95**, 905–10.

Neuberger, J., Forman, D., Doll, R., and Williams, R. (1986). Oral contraceptives and hepatocellular carcinoma. *British Medical Journal* **292**, 1355–7.

Rooks, J.B., *et al.* and the Cooperative Liver Tumor Study Group (1979). Epidemiology of hepatocellular adenoma. The role of oral contraceptive use. *Journal of the American Medical Association* **242**, 644–8.

Rubin, G.L., Ory, H.W., and Layde, P.E. (1982). Oral contraceptives and pelvic inflammatory disease. *American Journal of Obstetrics and Gynecology* **144**, 630–5.

Stadel, B.V. (1981). Oral contraceptives and cardiovascular disease. *New England Journal of Medicine*. **305**, 612–18, 672–7.

Thorogood, M., Mann, J., Murphy, M., and Vessey, M. (1991). Is oral contraceptive use still associated with an increased risk of myocardial infarction? Report of a case-control study. *British Journal of Obstetrics and Gynaecology*, **98**, 1245–53.

UK National Case-Control Study Group (1989). Oral contraceptive use and breast cancer risk in young women. *Lancet* **1**, 973–82.

Vessey, M.P. (1989). Oral contraception and cancer. In *Contraception: science and practice*, (ed. M. Filshie and J. Guillebaud), pp. 52–68. Butterworths, London.

Vessey, M.P. (1990). The Jephcott Lecture 1989. An overview of the benefits and risks of combined oral contraceptives. In *Oral contraceptives and breast cancer*, (ed. R.D. Mann), pp. 121–32. Parthenon, Carnforth.

Vessey, M.P., Smith, M.A., and Yeates, D. (1986). Return of fertility after discontinuation of oral contraceptives: influence of age and parity. *British Journal of Family Planning* **11**, 120–4.

Vessey, M., Metcalfe, A., Wells, C., McPherson, K., Westhoff, C., and Yeates, D. (1987). Ovarian neoplasms, functional ovarian cysts and oral contraceptives. *British Medical Journal* **294**, 1518–20.

WHO Collaborative Group (1985). Invasive cervical cancer and combined oral contraceptives. *British Medical Journal* **290**, 961–5.

WHO Scientific Group (1992). Oral contraceptives and neoplasia. *WHO Technical Report Series No. 817*. WHO, Geneva.

13.2 Hypertension in pregnancy

C. W. G. REDMAN

The cardiovascular system in pregnancy

Cardiac output increases during the first trimester to about 1.5 1/min above the levels of non-pregnant women. No further increase occurs in the second and third trimesters. Towards full term it declines in the supine but not lateral recumbent position, owing to the pressure of the gravid uterus on the inferior vena cava, which reduces venous return to the heart. In the third trimester about two-thirds of the additional cardiac output is distributed to the placental circulation and to augment renal plasma flow. The increased output is the result of both a greater stroke volume and a higher pulse rate. Plasma volume increases progressively during the second and third trimesters and is significantly correlated with the birthweight of the conceptus, being higher in multiple pregnancies.

Arterial pressure falls in the second half of the first trimester at about the same time as the cardiac output is increasing. This means that peripheral resistance decreases relatively more than the cardiac output increases. The uteroplacental circulation is too small at this time to cause these changes, which must therefore result from a generalized arteriolar dilatation. During the second and third trimesters the relaxation of arterial tone is associated with a marked insensitivity to the pressor action of angiotensin II.

In the later weeks of pregnancy there is a tendency for the diastolic pressure to rise slowly towards what it was before pregnancy began, the systolic pressure remaining more or less unchanged. However, in the supine position, with vena-caval compression and reduced venous return, the arterial pressure may be atypically low with a narrowed pulse pressure and reflex vasoconstriction. The fall in systolic pressure may exceed 30 per cent in 10 per cent of cases and cause 'the supine hypotension syndrome', evident as restlessness, faintness, tachypnoea, and pallor.

DEFINITION OF HYPERTENSION IN PREGNANT WOMEN

Pregnant women are young, healthy, and have lower blood pressures than those who are not pregnant. The average blood pressure during the first half of the second trimester is about 120/70; 140/85 and 160/95 correspond to two and three standard deviations above the mean, respectively. Hypertension in obstetric practice is conventionally recognized above an arbitrary threshold of 140/90. This is appropriate for the first half of pregnancy. But in the second half, about one-quarter of all women will be hypertensive by this criterion, meaning that the limits are too low to define an unusual group, who merit extra clinical attention. About 2.5 per cent have a maximum arterial pressure of 160/105 or more, and about 1 per cent of 170/110 or more; these are more relevant limits for identifying third-trimester hypertension. However, the maximum blood pressure is a biased statistic; women whose highest readings peak to 170/110 will have lower base-line blood pressures.

CONDITIONS IDENTIFIED BY HYPERTENSION IN PREGNANCY

Hypertension in pregnancy has three possible aetiologies. First, and most important, it may be caused by the pregnancy, as part of the syndrome of pre-eclampsia, a specific disorder of pregnancy that is common, dangerous, and poorly understood. Secondly, it may represent chronic hypertension which may be revealed for the first time during pregnancy, typically towards the end; but the condition is of the woman not of her pregnancy. Thirdly, and much more rarely, it may be a new medical condition by chance coinciding with pregnancy.

Pre-eclampsia (sometimes called pre-eclamptic toxaemia) is a common syndrome which becomes evident in the second half of pregnancy (although its origins may lie in the first half) and which is defined in terms of the transient development of new hypertension and proteinuria, which may be severe, but which regress after delivery. Toxaemia is an obsolete expression, previously used to describe any hypertension or proteinuria in pregnancy, whether pregnancy-induced or not; the term pre-eclampsia is to be preferred.

TERMINOLOGY

Pre-eclampsia is so called because it may precede eclampsia, which is one of a number of possible crises of the condition. Eclampsia is characterized by grand-mal convulsions. Other crises (described below) are just as dangerous and occur as commonly, or even more so. Not all cases of eclampsia are preceded by a prodromal illness of pre-eclampsia, so the terminology is not always appropriate as a description of the course of events.

Pregnancy-induced hypertension, transient hypertension of pregnancy, or gestational hypertension are terms used to describe new hypertension which appears after mid-term (20 weeks) and resolves after delivery. They denote only one of the components of the pre-eclampsia syndrome. For reasons that are historical rather than logical and, to some extent arbitrary, pregnancy-induced hypertension is deemed to be a mandatory part of pre-eclampsia; but a syndrome requires at least two specific features before it can be recognized. Thus pregnancy-induced hypertension on its own (a common clinical presentation) is not pre-eclampsia; at least one more sign is required.

The cluster of clinical features that comprise any syndrome are chosen for convenience. They describe outward appearances and embody no special truth about the underlying disease of diseases. When a syndrome such as pre-eclampsia is 'defined', rules are set that bring consistency to what is being discussed. Such rules may be sensible or not but their validity cannot be tested because there is no standard to which to refer. All the definitions of pre-eclampsia suffer from these limitations and none can be said to be the best. The conventional components of the cluster are pregnancy-induced hypertension combined with proteinuria that regresses after delivery.

Almost all hypertension presenting before mid-term (gestational age of 20 weeks) indicates pre-existing or chronic hypertension; the rare exceptions are women with atypical very early onset pre-eclampsia. However, normotension in the first half of pregnancy does not necessarily mean long-term normotension, because the fall in blood pressure induced in early pregnancy may be exaggerated in some women; many with relatively severe hypertension may have normal blood pressures by 12 weeks, without treatment. In other words, some women enjoy the benefits of pregnancy-induced normotension just as others suffer the disadvantages of pregnancy-induced hypertension. Pregnancy-induced normotension tends to be lost in the third trimester. If the pre-pregnancy blood pressures are unknown then this may be misinterpreted as pregnancy-induced hypertension rather than recognized for what it is, namely re-establishment of the hypertensive state that preceded the pregnancy.

Pregnancy-induced hypertension thus represents at least two clinical situations: early pre-eclampsia or occult chronic hypertension. In many cases the signs of pre-eclampsia are not confirmed, but nevertheless the blood pressure reverts to normal after delivery. It is possible that these represent the very early unconfirmed stages of pre-eclampsia; an alternative is that an innate tendency to hypertension has been revealed in pregnancy but will become overt only many years later. The studies have not been done to confirm or refute this suggestion.

Pre-eclampsia

Pre-eclampsia becomes evident in the second half of pregnancy, during labour, or even, for the first time, in the immediate puerperium—without apparent preceding problems. But it always resolves more remotely after delivery. It is common, can be dangerous to both mother and baby, and is of unknown cause.

Current definitions require that hypertension and proteinuria, both pregnancy-induced, should be present before the syndrome is recognized. Although part of the accepted definition of pre-eclampsia is the new occurrence of hypertension, hypertension is probably neither a necessary and certainly not a sufficient feature for diagnosis. It is one of a number of useful signs, but not a central part of the pathology, which is more extensive and can involve the maternal liver, clotting abnormalities, and nervous system disorders as well. The placenta is almost certainly the primary cause of the problem. The corollary is that pre-eclampsia is a form of secondary hypertension, probably the most common in clinical practice.

The incidence of pre-eclampsia depends on how it is defined and now assiduously the signs are sought. Thus it is possible only to estimate the size of the problem. In the United Kingdom the incidence is of the order of one in 20 to 30 maternities.

Some of the factors that affect susceptibility are listed in Table 1 and include fetal-specific as well as maternal-specific components. Primigravidae are several times more prone to the condition. In parous women pre-eclampsia particularly affects those who have had the problem before. The predisposition to pre-eclampsia is, in part, familial, probably genetic, but the pattern of inheritance is not clear. Other factors must also be relevant because pre-eclampsia does not affect identical twin sisters concordantly.

Certain medical problems including some (chronic hypertension, renal disease) that can mimic the disorder also predispose to it. Superimposed pre-eclampsia refers to the mixed syndrome comprising pre-eclampsia in an individual with pre-existing hypertension or renal disease. In the absence of a specific diagnostic test for pre-eclampsia it is sometimes difficult or impossible to disentangle what elements of proteinuric hypertension are caused by a chronic medical problem from those arising from superimposed pre-eclampsia. The conventional definitions of pre-eclampsia cease to apply. If a woman is permanently proteinuric, there are, for example, no accepted criteria for diagnosing 'proteinuric pre-eclampsia'. Nevertheless it seems that chronically hypertensive women are three to seven times more likely to develop higher blood pressures and proteinuria ('superimposed pre-eclampsia') than normotensive women. Women with hypertension associated with chronic renal disease are particularly susceptible. A history of migraine also predisposes to pre-eclampsia and eclampsia.

THE THREE LEVELS OF THE PATHOLOGY OF PRE-ECLAMPSIA

There are primary, secondary, and tertiary problems in pre-eclampsia. The primary pathology is not known for certain but is localized within the gravid uterus, for the condition always resolves after delivery. Although the presence of trophoblast is necessary, the fetus is not, because pre-eclampsia can develop with hydatidiform mole. The primary involvement of the placenta explains why pre-eclampsia is asso-ciated with two syndromes, not one. The fetal syndrome can be as, or more, important a part of the illness as the maternal syndrome.

The placental problem appears to be a relative ischaemia secondary to deficiencies in the uteroplacental circulation or to excessively large placentas (with multiple pregnancies, for example).

The uteroplacental circulation is compromised by two lesions involving the spiral arteries which are the end-arteries supplying the intervillous space. The first is a relative lack of the structural modifications of the spiral arteries that occur during placentation (between weeks 8 and 18), when the arteries become dilated in preparation for the hugely expanded uteroplacental blood flow of the second half of the pregnancy. The second is 'acute atherosis'—aggregates of fibrin, platelets, and lipid-loaded macrophages (lipophages) which partially or completely block the ends of the arteries. Neither change is specific to pre-eclampsia but can also occur with intrauterine growth retardation without a maternal syndrome. Hence the spiral artery changes may be only an associated, but not primary, feature of pre-eclampsia; an alternative concept is that 'pre-eclampsia' is a broader disorder than has been previously considered, not necessarily including hypertension. The relationship with processes that depend on placentation could mean that pre-eclampsia originates much earlier than when the maternal syndrome becomes overt.

Once pre-eclampsia is established, uteroplacental blood flow is reduced. There is no direct evidence that placental ischaemia can cause pre-eclampsia, but in various animal models a pre-eclamptic-like illness can be induced by impeding the placental blood supply. As far as is known, a comparable illness does not occur spontaneously in pregnant animals.

The secondary pathology of pre-eclampsia includes all the features of the maternal syndrome, short of decompensation. The maternal syndrome is typically variable, in the time of onset, speed of progression, and the extent to which it involves different systems including arterial, coagulation, renal, central nervous, and hepatic.

Until recently it was impossible to explain how a single pathological process might cause not only hypertension but also convulsions, disseminated intravascular coagulation, jaundice, abdominal pain, or normotensive proteinuria (among others). But the concept that the maternal endothelium is the target organ for the pre-eclampsia process has resolved this difficulty. In short, the maternal syndrome can be explained if it is seen, not as an hypertensive problem, but as the sum of the consequences of diffuse endothelial dysfunction, causing widespread circulatory disturbances in different organ systems as well as generalized arterial and coagulation abnormalities.

Under certain circumstances the secondary disturbances of pre-eclampsia can become so severe that they cause decompensation. The tertiary pathology is what makes it so dangerous for the mother or baby. It leads to a number of crises that are listed in Table 2.

CLINICAL CHARACTERISTICS OF PRE-ECLAMPSIA

Hypertension is usually the first sign of pre-eclampsia but the exact time course of the maternal syndrome is largely undefined. In most instances what is detected is what is sought, that is, changes confined to arterial pressure and urine protein content; other features of the disorder are not noted because their detection involves laboratory investigation. Usually hypertension precedes proteinuria, although the converse can happen.

However, pre-eclampsia is more variable than is generally appreciated—in the time of onset, for example. Thus although pre-eclampsia is defined as presenting after 20 weeks, it may occur earlier or, at the other extreme, become evident only after delivery. The speed with which it progresses and how it involves different maternal systems are also variable.

The hypertension of pre-eclampsia appears to be caused by an increased peripheral resistance, although the alternative that peripheral resistance is normal but cardiac output is excessive can not be discounted. The arterial constriction is probably secondary to generalized

Table 1 *Risk factors for pre-eclampsia*

| **Maternal** |
| First pregnancy |
| Previous severe pre-eclampsia |
| Age: under 20, or over 35 |
| Family history of pre-eclampsia/eclampsia |
| U nderweight and short |
| Migraines |
| Chronic hypertension |
| Chronic renal disease |
| **Fetal** |
| Multiple pregnancy |
| Hydatidiform mole |
| Placental hydrops |

Table 2 *Tertiary pathology of pre-eclampsia*

Maternal	Convulsions
	Cerebral haemorrhage
	Cerebral oedema
	Retinal detachment
	Cortical blindness
	Pulmonary oedema
	Laryngeal oedema
	Adult respiratory distress syndrome
	Disseminated intravascular coagulation
	HELLP syndrome
	Hepatic rupture
	Hepatic infarction
	Renal cortical necrosis
	Renal tubular necrosis
Fetal	Asphyxial brain damage
	Death from asphyxia

maternal endothelial dysfunction, given the evidence for increases in circulating endothelin 1 (a potent vasoconstrictor derived from endothelium), for reduced endothelial-dependent relaxation, and reduced circulating prostycyclin metabolites (presumed to be of endothelial origin). The hypertension of pre-eclampsia is not associated with a single haemodynamic pattern. Some investigators find increased cardiac output, others the converse. Some of the differences between studies may reflect the use of drugs; for example, treatment with vasodilators stimulates cardiac output by reducing afterload. Arterial pressure in pre-eclampsia is typically unstable at rest, possibly owing to reduced baroceptor sensitivity. Circadian variation is altered; first, with a loss of the normal fall in blood pressure at night, then, in the worst cases, a reversed pattern, with the highest readings during sleep.

Pre-eclampsia may cause arterial pressures which are well above the level at which arterial and arteriolar damage would be expected (i.e. a mean pressure of about 140 mmHg). It is not surprising that an important cause of maternal death from pre-eclampsia and eclampsia is cerebral

haemorrhage, the pathology of which is similar to that seen in other hypertensive states (Table 3). As far as it is known, cerebral haemorrhage is the only consequence of pre-eclampsia likely to be affected by antihypertensive treatment.

The involvement of the kidneys in pre-eclampsia has long been recognized and is one of its more consistent features. The development of proteinuria reflects advanced disease, associated with a poorer prognosis than if it is absent. The proteinuria is moderately selective, increases until delivery, and not uncommonly exceeds 10 g/24 h—pre-eclampsia being the commonest cause of heavy proteinuria in pregnancy. It is associated with impaired glomerular perfusion and filtration, both reflected in a reduced creatinine clearance and increased plasma creatinine and urea concentrations.

The typical renal glomerular lesion of pre-eclampsia is glomerular endotheliosis; the endothelial cells of the glomeruli swell and block the capillary lumina so that the glomeruli appear enlarged and bloodless. The lesion has been defined in research investigations. It represents direct histological confirmation of endothelial damage in pre-eclampsia. It should be noted that renal biopsy is never indicated for clinical management.

Hyperuricaemia is a characteristic and often early feature, preceding proteinuria and useful for diagnosis at that stage. It results from a reduced renal urate clearance, also observed in pre-eclampsia superimposed on chronic hypertension. It tends to be associated with hypocalciuria, another early change in renal function. The reduction in the renal clearance of urate is proportionally more than that of inulin. As the plasma urate rises, the plasma concentrations of urea and creatinine at first remain steady, tending to increase slowly after proteinuria has become established. The mechanisms underlying these changes are not understood. The tertiary pathology of renal involvement in pre-eclampsia is acute renal failure arising from either tubular or cortical necrosis.

The clotting system is often, but not invariably, disturbed in pre-eclampsia, with accelerated intravascular generation of thrombin and parallel changes in the platelets ascribed to increased consumption. The time course is variable, but a fall in the platelet count may be a relatively early sign—antedating proteinuria for example. However, even when eclampsia supervenes, the majority of women have normal platelet counts at the time of presentation, that is, more than $150\,000 \times 10^9/l$. The coagulation disturbances may progress to give overt disseminated intravascular coagulation, a rare endstage for which the original evidence was obtained postmortem. A further complication is microangiopathic haemolysis, which may cause a sudden drop in haemoglobin concentration associated with haemoglobinuria, fragmented or distorted red cells (schistocytes) on the peripheral blood film, and reduced serum haptoglobin concentrations.

The severe clotting abnormalities of pre-eclampsia, particularly disseminated intravascular coagulation, are often associated with liver pathology, long recognized as an important and dangerous component of the disorder. When there is also the associated complication of microangiopathic haemolysis the acronym HELLP syndrome has been used to label the concurrence of **h**aemolysis, **e**levated **l**iver enzymes, and **l**ow **p**latelet counts (see Chapter 13.13). This is merely a convenient way of

Table 3 *Maternal deaths from hypertensive disease England and Wales 1973–84; United Kingdom 1985–90**

	1973–75	1976–78	1979–81	1982–84	1985–87*	1988–90*
Number (rate/million)	34(17.7)	29(16.6)	36(18.7)	25(12.6)	27(12.1)*	27(11.0)*
Cause of death						
Cerebral haemorrhage	17(44%)	17(59%)	9(25%)	13(52%)	11(41%)	12(44%)
Other CNS pathology	6(15%)	4(14%)	8(22%)	8(32%)	0	2
Hepatic pathology	4	1	8	1	1	1
Pulmonary pathology	1	1	2	3	2(44%)	10(37%)

Figures derived from: Reports on confidential enquiries into maternal deaths in England and Wales (1973–75; 1976–78; 1979–81; 1982–84); or in the United Kingdom (1985–87; 1988–90).

bringing this aspect of pre-eclampsia, which has been documented, albeit incompletely, for many years, into focus. It is a dangerous presentation that is often not associated with marked hypertension or other conventional indices of sever pre-eclampsia. Indeed, liver damage and low platelet counts have been observed in primigravidae, without hypertension or proteinuria, but with the typical hepatic histology of pre-eclampsia, including fibrin deposition in the sinusoids. In other words, this is further evidence that pre-eclampsia is not merely an hypertensive disorder but has other features that are just as important, if not more so, which are not caused by the hypertension but by the underlying placental problem.

Epigastric pain and vomiting are the typical symptoms of the HELLP syndrome, which may present so suddenly as to be misinterpreted as renal colic, or other surgical emergency. Hepatic tenderness and raised serum liver enzymes are the signs. Serum bilirubin is usually normal but jaundice is possible and may be a presenting feature. The liver disturbances may be out of proportion to the severity of the pre-eclampsia as judged by the conventional signs of hypertension and proteinuria. In certain sever cases, typically of multiparae rather than primiparae, there may be bleeding under the liver capsule. Subsequently this may rupture to cause massive haemoperitoneum, shock, and (usually) maternal death.

Eclampsia is the most dramatic evidence of involvement of the nervous system. It resembles other forms of hypertensive encephalopathy with similar symptoms and cerebral pathology. Neither condition is associated with gross papilloedema or retinopathy. One of the complications of hypertensive encephalopathy is cortical blindness, a feature of severe pre-eclampsia and eclampsia as well. Average blood pressures in eclampsia are high (170–195/110–120), but cases with much lower blood pressures are not rare, as with non-obstetric forms of hypertensive encephalopathy.

Although the name—hypertensive encephalopathy—suggests that the syndrome is caused by hypertension this is misleading. The hypertension must be considered no more than an associated feature; there is no good evidence that hypertension causes eclampsia or other forms of hypertensive encephalopathy, and none that adequate medical control of the blood pressure prevents eclampsia.

DIAGNOSIS OF PRE-ECLAMPSIA

Pre-eclampsia is usually symptomless. Therefore its detection depends on signs or investigations. However, one symptom is crucially important, because it is so often misinterpreted. The epigastric pain, which reflects hepatic involvement and is the typical presentation of the HELLP syndrome, may easily be confused with heartburn, a very common problem of pregnancy. However, it is not burning in quality, does not spread upwards towards the throat, is associated with hepatic tenderness, may radiate through to the back, and is not relieved by antacid. It is often very severe, described by sufferers as the worst pain that they have ever experienced. Affected women are not uncommonly referred to general surgeons as suffering from an acute abdomen, for example, acute cholecystitis.

In general, none of the signs of pre-eclampsia is specific; even convulsions in pregnancy are, in modern practice, more likely to have causes other than eclampsia. Diagnosis therefore depends on finding a coincidence of several pre-eclamptic features. The final proof is their regression after delivery.

By convention the pre-eclampsia syndrome comprises pregnancy-induced hypertension and pregnancy-induced proteinuria. In practice, clinicians need to take a broader view and accept a wider range of combinations of the possible features of the syndrome, some of which are listed in Table 4. As with all syndromes, the more of the features that are clustered together, the more certain is the diagnosis. But the absence of any one feature does not exclude the diagnosis. For example, eclampsia can occur without proteinuria. Even hypertension seems not to be an essential component.

Table 4 *The pre-eclampsia syndrome, possible features*

Maternal syndrome
   Pregnancy-induced hypertension
   Excessive weight gain (>1.0 kg/week)
   Generalized oedema
   Ascites
   Hyperuricaemia
   Proteinuria
   Hypocalciuria
   Raised plasma concentration of von Willebrand factor
   Raised plasma concentration of cellular fibronectin
   Reduced plasma concentration of antithrombin III
   Thrombocytopenia
   Increased haematocrit
   Increased blood concentrations of liver enzymes
Fetal syndrome
   Intrauterine growth retardation
   Intrauterine hypoxaemia

Until the specific causes are defined we cannot diagnose the disease or diseases that underlie pre-eclampsia, but merely recognize potentially sinister clusters of signs. There is no logical reason why one or other feature must be present before there is the need for concern. Nor should the clinician limit the range of his search for signs of pre-eclampsia simply because they do not feature in one of other of the 'definitions'.

In practical terms, hypertension, proteinuria, and excessive weight gain have to be the signs of interest for screening in routine antenatal clinics. Different definitions have been proposed as to what constitutes hypertension. The details are less important than the principle of an increment from a recording taken in the first half of pregnancy; this establishes the existence of pregnancy-induced hypertension. Between weeks 20 and 30 the blood pressure is normally steady, so that even a small consistent rise is clinically important. Between week 30 and term, the diastolic pressure will rise by about 10 mmHg on average. A sustained rise of at least 25 mmHg to a threshold of 90 mmHg or more is typical of pre-eclampsia. However, it needs to be remembered that these are guidelines; there is no clinical situation in which rigid interpretation of the blood pressure is helpful.

The same applies to other measurements, such as changes in the plasma urate. As a rough guide: abnormal levels are in excess of 0.30, 0.35, 0.40, and 0.45 mmol/l at 28, 32, 36, and 40 weeks, respectively; or, if a base-line taken before 20 weeks is available, then increases of 0.10, 0.15, 0.20, and 0.25 mmol/l at 28, 32, 36, and 40 weeks, respectively.

Proteinuria and evidence of a reduced glomerular filtration rate are later signs. The changes in the measurements of renal function are usually within the normal range for non-pregnant individuals. In general, abnormal concentrations of plasma creatinine and urea are above 100 μmol/l and 6.0 mmol/l respectively. The proteinuria of pre-eclampsia ranges from 0.5 to 15 g/24 h, depending on the individual and the stage of evolution of the disorder. In terms of stick testing, 0.5 g/24 h corresponds to at least + in every specimen of urine tested. When this point is reached, the disease can be said to have entered its proteinuric phase.

Thrombocytopenia ($< 100 \times 10^9$/l) and increased plasma fibrin/fibrinogen degradation products (or specific fragments thereof, such as the D-dimer) tend to be late developments. The same is true for raised liver enzymes. In regard to the latter it should be noted that plasma alkaline phosphatase is always elevated in late pregnancy because of the contribution from the placental isoenzyme, so that its measurement is not a useful guide to hepatic function. Serum bilirubin is rarely abnormal. γ-Glutamyl transferase is increased only late in the evolution of the HELLP syndrome. Therefore the best simple tests are plasma aspartate amino-transferase or lactate dehydrogenase.

New hypertension and the *de novo* occurrence of one other sign allows the diagnosis to be made with reasonable certainty. But pregnancy-induced hypertension on its own is not pre-eclampsia, although the term is commonly, but wrongly, used to mean mild or early pre-eclampsia. It is true that pregnancy-induced hypertension may be the first indication of the onset of pre-eclampsia, but until other signs appear this remains unconfirmed. Often, spontaneous or induced delivery prevents further developments, so that a final certain diagnosis cannot be made.

COMPLICATIONS OF PRE-ECLAMPSIA

These are listed in Table 2. Eclampsia complicates 1 in 2000 maternities in the United Kingdom and carries a high maternal mortality of 2 per cent. The HELLP syndrome is more common (probably about 1 in 500 maternities) but is as dangerous as eclampsia itself. These two major maternal crises can present unheralded by prodromal signs of pre-eclampsia.

Antepartum eclampsia is likely to occur earlier in gestation and is more dangerous than that presenting in labour or after delivery. Most post-partum crises develop in the first 12 h after delivery but later is possible. Eclampsia has been documented as late as 22 days after delivery.

Cerebral haemorrhage kills women with pre-eclampsia or eclampsia (Table 3). It must be assumed, although unproven, that hypertension is a major predisposing factor in this situation. Adult respiratory distress syndrome appears to have become more common (Table 3). Whether this is more a consequence of modern methods of respiratory support than of the disease itself is not known.

PREVENTION OF PRE-ECLAMPSIA

All the evidence is that, once it becomes overt, pre-eclampsia cannot be reversed except by delivery. Reliable methods of prevention are therefore needed, although none that is completely effective is known.

It used to be believed that dietary prevention of weight gain prevented pre-eclampsia, although there was neither a rationale nor any direct evidence that this approach was effective. The concept has been supplanted by another view, that specific dietary factors may confer modest benefit. The largest randomized controlled trial of dietary supplements demonstrated a modest but significant reduction in the incidence of pre-eclampsia in a pre-war London population (People's League of Health 1946). The supplements comprised minerals and vitamins only, the latter including halibut liver oil to provide vitamins A and D. It is possible that the benefit was derived, not from the extra vitamins and minerals, but from the fatty acid content of the fish oil, which is a source of eicosapentaenoic acid that generates thromboxane A_3 and prostacyclin I_3 (PG13) instead of thromboxane A_2 and prostacyclin I_2, which are derived from arachidonic acid. These eicosanoids shift the balance of platelet reactivity away from aggregation, in effect an alternative to antiplatelet drugs (see below). Hence fish oil supplements are being investigated for their prophylactic efficacy.

The mineral supplement of interest is calcium, dietary supplements of which may reduce arterial pressure in hypertensive subjects and lessen the incidence of pregnancy-induced hypertension. Another dietary component being assessed is vitamin E, which, as an antioxidant, may help prevent the formation of free radicals which could initiate endothelial damage.

The use of drugs or other regimens to suppress one or other of the secondary features of pre-eclampsia has not proved to be useful. For example, prophylactic salt restriction or diuretics have both been advocated in the belief that excessive fluid retention is an essential part of the pathogenesis; but salt restriction increases the incidence of pre-eclampsia, and diuretics confer no benefit.

With respect to the use of antihypertensive drugs, there are two issues. First, can they attenuate the progression of early pre-eclampsia? Second, can they prevent superimposition of pre-eclampsia in chronically hypertensive women, who otherwise are more susceptible to the disorder? There is no obvious reason why uteroplacental circulatory insufficiency should be prevented by antihypertensive treatment; indeed by reducing perfusing pressure it might aggravate the problem. Nor is there any clear reason why this treatment should reduce the endothelial dysfunction that is thought to underlie the maternal syndrome.

The effect of antihypertensive treatment on the progression of pre-eclampsia is still debated. The only clear benefit is when the hypertension is so severe that delivery is essential to preserve maternal safety. Antihypertensive treatment can allow prolongation of pregnancy in this context, but the benefit is not from prevention but palliation. The extent of the presumed benefit has not been measured because severe hypertension is a reason for exclusion from randomized trials of treatment.

There is, however, clear evidence that antihypertensive treatment does not prevent superimposed pre-eclampsia in women with chronic hypertension. In essence, then, antihypertensive treatment helps to protect the mother from the consequences of raised arterial pressure *per se*, but not from the problem of pre-eclampsia itself.

The only drug-based intervention that appears to be promising is the use of antiplatelet agents; in particular, low doses of aspirin. Given that the maternal syndrome of pre-eclampsia appears to originate from diffuse systemic endothelial dysfunction, and given that it may be associated, from an early stage, with disturbances of platelet function, it could be supposed that platelet activation might either amplify, or even cause, the endothelial problems. In either case, antiplatelet therapy might have a beneficial action. This concept underpins the rationale for fish oil supplements as well as low-dose aspirin.

The results of several large trials suggest that low-dose aspirin has a modest effect in preventing or delaying the maternal syndrome, if started before the onset of signs. The benefits are greatest in preventing early onset pre-eclampsia (which is relatively rare) and least in preventing the disorder presenting at term (which is common). Antiplatelet therapy does not benefit women if it is started after signs of pre-eclampsia have appeared. As yet there has been no clear demonstration that perinatal survival is improved. Low-dose aspirin in pregnancy seems to be safe: there may be a slight increase in maternal bleeding problems around the time of delivery. No adverse effect on the fetus has yet been identified.

MANAGEMENT OF PRE-ECLAMPTIC HYPERTENSION

Pre-eclampsia is not merely a hypertensive disease but reflects a profound disturbance of pregnancy involving many maternal systems and the fetus as well, so that control of the blood pressure is only a part of management. The definitive treatment is always delivery, which removes the placenta in which lies the cause of the problem. If the affected woman can be delivered before irreversible damage has occurred (for example cerebral haemorrhage) a complete and rapid recovery is assured. Hence, the purpose of medical management is to protect the mother from the dangers of her illness, during the relatively brief interval after the disease is diagnosed and before elective delivery.

The main objective is to prevent extreme hypertension. The threshold at which antihypertensive treatment should be started is a matter of opinion. The risk of acute arteriolar damage begins at a mean arterial pressure of about 140 mmHg. For this reason, we begin treatment if maximum readings (systolic or diastolic) repeatedly reach or exceed 170 or 110 mmHg, respectively.

Hydralazine has been the preferred antihypertensive agent for the treatment of acute severe pre-eclampsia. It may be given intravenously by either continuous infusion (5–10 mg/h) or intermittent boluses (of 5 mg), or by intramuscular or subcutaneous injections (of 5–10 mg). After intravenous administration there is a significant delay in the onset of action of about 20 min. Its effect is relatively short-lived, lasting 2 to 3 h. Side-effects are common and include reflex tachycardia, anxiety, restlessness, hyperreflexia, and severe headaches. These symptoms and signs may affect 50 per cent of women and simulate the features of impending eclampsia. Then the symptoms of the disease cannot be disentangled from those caused by the treatment.

Labetalol, a combined α- and β-adrenergic blocking agent which can be given intravenously, lowers the blood pressure smoothly but rapidly without the tachycardia characteristic of treatment with hydralazine. A typical regimen starts with 20 mg/h, which is doubled every 30 min until control has been gained. There are no adequate trials of its parenteral use in pregnancy to show how it might affect perinatal outcome.

Diazoxide, sodium nitroprusside, and nitroglycerine are rapidly acting vasodilators that have been used to manage hypertensive emergencies in pregnancy. All should be reserved for use by specialists, usually in the context of intensive cardiovascular monitoring. The danger is of overdose, with problems associated with extreme and sudden hypotension. For example, an intravenous bolus dose of diazoxide may cause severe hypotension, cerebral ischaemia, or death from cerebral infarction, and a maternal death in this setting has been reported.

The calcium-channel-blocking agent, nifedipine, is an effective vasodilator which acts rapidly when given by mouth. Nifedipine capsules act within 10 to 15 min; nifedipine in slow-release tablets has a slower onset of action (about 60 min) but a more prolonged effect, whereas a long-acting preparation, formulated for once-a-day administration is less convenient for acute control of pre-eclamptic hypertension. The experience of nifedipine in pregnancy is limited, but, so far, it appears to be at least as safe as hydralazine and, in some aspects of neonatal complications of prematurity with severe pre-eclampsia, possibly superior. Tachycardia occurs but is less of a problem than with hydralazine.

As with some other drugs, the half-life is shorter than that in nonpregnant individuals, so regimens need to be adjusted accordingly. In theory, nifedipine could interact with parenteral magnesium sulphate given to prevent or treat eclampsia, because the magnesium ion inhibits calcium channels; in practice there has been a report of two cases of profound hypotension in this context. The advantage of nifedipine over hydralazine is its ease of administration; like hydralazine it can cause severe headaches. Nimodipine, another calcium-channel blocker, with a selective effect on the cerebral circulation, may have particular advantages for treating cerebral ischaemia in eclamptic women.

Diuretics are avoided because they exacerbate the hypovolaemia of pre-eclampsia, which may often be severe. However, they may be needed if complications such as pulmonary or laryngeal oedema occur.

Good blood pressure control in pre-eclampsia does not ameliorate its other features. The disease persists and remains relentlessly progressive until delivery. Therefore escape from control is common. Nor does adequate treatment prevent other complications such as eclampsia, the HELLP syndrome, abruption, or progressive fetal respiratory impairment. A persisting inability to control maternal arterial pressure is one of several indications for immediate delivery.

LONGER-TERM CONTROL OF PRE-ECLAMPTIC HYPERTENSION

The control of pre-eclamptic hypertension must always be extended for a few days at the least, and frequently for longer. Therefore, once the blood pressure has been controlled acutely, the effects need to be prolonged. The requirements are for a drug that is safe in pregnancy, has an onset of action in 6 to 12 h, allows some titration of effect, and can be safely combined with a second drug if needed. The choice lies between methyldopa and various β-adrenergic blocking agents.

Methyldopa, in adequate doses, can control the blood pressure within 6 to 12 h. A loading dose of 500 to 1000 mg is followed by 250 to 750 mg four times a day. Sedation is the rule for the first 48 h and tiredness thereafter is common. Postural hypotension is rarely a problem in the antenatal patient.

Although β-blockers cause fewer subjective side-effects, their safety in pregnancy has not been so exhaustively investigated. A preparation such as atenolol, with its slow onset of action and flat dose–response curve, is not ideal for the day-to-day titration of blood pressure control. However, its short-term safety for the fetus and neonate has been adequately demonstrated. Oxprenolol and labetalol are faster-acting alternatives. Which agent is preferred probably matters less than the clinician's familiarity with its use in achieving good blood pressure control.

PREVENTION OF ECLAMPTIC CONVULSIONS

Eclampsia is probably caused by focal cerebral vasoconstriction and ischaemia secondary to endothelial damage, and therefore is neither the result of hypertension nor prevented by antihypertensive treatment. The best mode of prevention is well-timed delivery. It is debated whether any prophylactic anticonvulsant medication needs to be offered routinely in all cases of advanced pre-eclampsia and, if so, what it should be. Intravenous diazepam is preferred to stop eclamptic convulsions, although most are self-limiting anyway. Thereafter it is reasonable to use medication to prevent recurrent convulsions. It is likely that agents that improve cerebral perfusion will be more effective than those that suppress neuronal excitability. In the former category is parenteral magnesium sulphate, widely used in the United States of America to prevent or treat eclampsia. In the latter is phenytoin. At the time of writing there is a dearth of properly controlled trials of the treatment of eclampsia that yield clear evidence about which regimen is superior.

Chronic hypertension complicating pregnancy

Pregnant women with chronic hypertension tend to be older, fatter, and slightly taller. Frequently they have clear family histories of hypertension. Their hypertension may be ameliorated or masked by the beginning of the second trimester so that the diagnosis is missed unless prepregnancy blood pressure readings are available. The blood pressure tends to climb back to the levels that characterize the non-pregnant state towards the end of the third trimester. If these are high, this normal change can be misinterpreted as pre-eclampsia. The distinction is that the blood pressure fails to settle after delivery.

Pre-eclampsia superimposed on chronic hypertension tends to be more severe, to occur at earlier stages of pregnancy, to cause more fetal growth retardation, and to be recurrent in later pregnancies. Pre-eclampsia occurring in normotensive women tends not to recur. If a blood pressure of 140/90 in the first half pregnancy is taken as evidence of chronic hypertension, then the affected individual has an approximately fivefold increased risk of later pre-eclampsia compared to normotensive women. This close link between the two conditions led earlier clinicians to conclude that chronic hypertension is extremely dangerous when combined with pregnancy. It is now clear that the particular risks of chronic hypertension are entirely attributable to the increased chance of developing superimposed pre-eclampsia; and that the majority of chronically hypertensive women, who do not get pre-eclampsia, can expect a normal and uncomplicated perinatal outcome. In other words, the dangers of chronic hypertension in pregnancy have been overemphasized.

Chronic hypertension can only be diagnosed with certainty during pregnancy on the basis of readings taken in the first half, preferably before 16 weeks of gestation. Without the benefit of such readings, hypertension in the second half of pregnancy cannot be interpreted because the possibility that it may represent pre-eclampsia can never be excluded with certainty. The signs of pre-eclampsia in chronically hypertensive women are the same as in other women except that the blood pressure increases from a higher base-line. There may be progressive hyperuricaemia, abnormal activation of the clotting system, or new proteinuria.

TREATMENT OF CHRONIC HYPERTENSION IN PREGNANCY

If antihypertensive treatment has been started before conception, the patient may seek advice about the possible effects of her medication on the growth and development of her fetus. None of the commonly used

Table 5 *Antihypertensive drug use in pregnancy*

Trimester	Drugs to avoid		Possible agents
	Relative contraindications	Absolute contraindications	
First	None known	None known	Avoid all if possible
Second	β-blockers	ACE inhibitors	Methyldopa
	Diuretics		Clonidine
			Prazosin, doxazosin
			Nifedipine
Third	Diuretics	ACE inhibitors	Methyldopa
			Clonidine
			Prazosin, doxazosin
			Nifedipine
			β-Blockers

ACE, angiotensin-converting enzyme.

antihypertensive drugs is known to be teratogenic. This does not preclude the possibility of subtle problems which are, as yet, unknown. For this reason, it is appropriate that women with no more than moderate hypertension stop treatment before conception. By the 12th week of pregnancy the normal fall in blood pressure is such that treatment may no longer be needed, at least until the beginning of the third trimester.

If chronic hypertension is diagnosed for the first time in pregnancy, it is then necessary to treat those in whom it presents an immediate (as opposed to a long-term) hazard. The precise levels at which this is necessary is a matter of opinion, not fact; a reasonable cut-off point is at 170/110 mmHg.

The problem of less severe chronic hypertension (that is 140–169/90–109 mmHg) needs to be considered. In general medical practice the purpose of treating this degree of hypertension is to prevent long-term complications such as coronary and cerebral vascular disease, heart failure, and aortic dissection. Although these problems can present in pregnant women, and are associated with hypertension, they are so rare that in themselves they cannot justify treatment for the brief period of pregnancy. Thus moderate hypertension *per se* carries no intrinsic maternal risk except in so far as it may be the precursor of more severe hypertension. However, the higher the arterial pressure the greater the eventual perinatal mortality. If the mild hypertension indicates early pre-eclampsia, the risks evolve through simple progression; if it indicates a pre-existing problem, then the risk is of later superimposition of pre-eclampsia which is several times more likely in chronically hypertensive women. Antihypertensive treatment can only be useful in this context if either it halts the progression of mild pre-eclampsia or prevents the superimposition of pre-eclampsia in women with long-term hypertension, but there is no evidence for either possibility. Indeed, there is good evidence that control of moderate long-term hypertension does not prevent superimposed pre-eclampsia. There is therefore no clear indication for the treating mild to moderate hypertension for either mother or fetus.

ORAL ANTIHYPERTENSIVE AGENTS THAT ARE USED IN PREGNANCY

The choice of drugs (Table 5) is dictated by considerations of fetal safety. Methyldopa is the preferred agent because its fetal effects have been defined much more clearly than those of any other agent. Its antihypertensive action and side-effects are the same as in non-pregnant individuals. The usual treatment schedule is 1.0 to 3.0 g/day in divided doses. It can be supplemented by nifedipine. The safety of methyldopa in pregnancy has been established by case-control studies. No serious adverse fetal effects have yet been documented. The infants in one case-control study were assessed at the age of 7 years. The group exposed to methyldopa *in utero* were as well as their controls, thus establishing the longer-term safety of methyldopa in pregnancy.

Labetalol is a popular alternative. However, long-term β-adrenergic blockade, extending throughout the second and third trimesters, has been associated with significant fetal growth retardation, and for this reason should be avoided. Angiotensin-converting-enzyme inhibitors are contraindicated in the second and third trimesters. Many reports show that they cause fetal and neonatal renal impairment or renal failure with significant perinatal mortality.

In the unlikely event that diuretics are essential for good blood pressure control, they can be continued throughout pregnancy but their use carries certain disadvantages if pre-eclampsia supervenes, as already discussed.

LONG-TERM SEQUELAE OF HYPERTENSION IN PREGNANCY

Severe pre-eclampsia and eclampsia can cause irreversible maternal complications, particularly acute renal cortical necrosis or cerebral haemorrhage. In the absence of these problems there is no evidence that long-term health is impaired. However, in terms of life expectancy, pre-eclamptic women fall into two groups. Those who become normotensive soon after delivery have a normal life expectancy. Those who remain hypertensive not only tend to suffer recurrent pregnancy-induced hypertension, but have a higher incidence of later cardiovascular disorders and reduced life expectancy, compatible with the diagnosis of an underlying disorder.

REFERENCES

Collins, R., Yusuf, S., and Peto, R. (1985). Overview of randomised trials of diuretics in pregnancy. *British Medical Journal* **290**, 17–23.

Davey, D.A. and MacGillivray,**. (1988). The classification and definition of the hypertensive disorders of pregnancy. *American Journal of Obstetrics and Gynecology* **158**, 892–8.

Department of Health (1994). Hypertensive disorders of pregnancy. In *Report of confidential enquiries into maternal deaths in the United Kingdom 1988–1990*, pp. 22–33. HMSO, London.

National High Blood Pressure Education Program (1990). National High Blood Pressure Education Program working group report on high blood pressure in pregnancy. *American Journal of Obstetrics and Gynecology*, **163**, 1691–712.

People's League of Health (1946). The nutrition of expectant and nursing mothers in relation to maternal and infant mortality and morbidity. *Journal of Obstetrics and Gynaecology of the British Empire* **53**, 498–509.

Redman, C.W.G. (1980). Treatment of hypertension in pregnancy. *Kidney International* **18**, 267–78.

Redman, C.W.G. (1991). Current topic: pre-eclampsia and the placenta. *Placenta*, **12**, 301–8.

Redman, C.W.G. and Roberts, J.M. (1993). Management of pre-eclampsia. *Lancet* **341**, 1451–4.

Roberts, J.M. and Redman, C.W.G. (1993). Pre-eclampsia: more than pregnancy-induced hypertension. *Lancet* **341,** 1447–51.

Robinson, M. (1958). Salt in pregnancy. *Lancet* **1,** 178–81.

Sibai, B.M., Mabie, W.C., Shamsa, F., Villar, M.A., and Anderson, G.D. (1990). A comparison of no medication versus methyldopa or labetalol in chronic hypertension during pregnancy. *American Journal of Obstetrics and Gynecology,* **162,** 960–6.

Sibai, B.M., Ramadan, M.K., Usta, I., Salama, M., Mercer, B.M., and Friedman, S.A. (1993). Maternal morbidity and mortality in 442 pregnancies with hemolysis, elevated liver enzymes, and low platelets (HELLP syndrome). *American Journal of Obstetrics and Gynecology* **169,** 1000–6.

13.3 Renal disease in pregnancy

C. W. G. REDMAN and J. G. G. LEDINGHAM

INTRODUCTION

Substantial changes occur in renal function and in the anatomy of the lower urinary tract in normal pregnancy. The likely effects of coincident renal disease on the progress and outcome of pregnancy and the influence of pregnancy on the progress of the underlying renal disorder are discussed here.

Urinary tract infection

Bacteriuria

Asymptomatic (covert) bacteriuria has been reported in some 2 to 7 per cent of pregnant women, the higher figure coming from surveys of those of poorer socioeconomic status. Repeated examination suggests a further 1 per cent or so will develop bacteriuria later in pregnancy, an acquisition rate similar to that of non-pregnant women. If left untreated, 25 to 30 per cent will go on to develop an attack of acute pyelonephritis, which can be prevented in more than half by adequate treatment at the asymptomatic stage. The organism most commonly found is *Escherichia coli* (in some 80 per cent) with Klebsiella, Proteus and Enterobacter comprising most of the rest. Most of the drugs commonly used in the treatment of urinary and renal infections in non-pregnant patients (see Section 20) can be used safely in pregnancy; these include ampicillin, cephalosporin derivatives, and aminoglycocides such as gentamicin and amikacin. Although there have been advocates of antimicrobial treatment for as long as 3 to 6 weeks in pregnancy, recent evidence suggests that a single dose or treatment for 3 to 5 days is equally efficacious.

Bacteriuria is recurrent in as many as 30 per cent of women, indicating the need for surveillance throughout pregnancy. In those with persistent bacteriuria, phrophylactic treatment with trimethoprim 200 mg or nitrofurantoin 100 mg at bedtime appear safe and effective in preventing pyelitis.

Bacteriuria is more common in pregnant women with pre-existing structural abnormalities of the lower urinary tract (particularly reflux nephropathy, in diabetes mellitus, and in women with the sickle-cell trait). The more persistent the bacteriuria, the higher the likelihood of finding an underlying cause. More than half the women in whom bacilluria persists despite treatment will have radiographic evidence postpartum of abnormalities of the lower urinary tract or kidneys.

Suggestions that untreated asymptomatic bacteriuria is associated with as much as a fourfold increase in premature delivery of infants of low birth rate are now disputed; even so, it is well known that an attack of acute pyelonephritis can precipitate premature labour and that an endotoxin of *E. coli* can be toxic to the fetus.

Acute pyelonephritis

Acute pyelonephritis is the most common serious medical complication of pregnancy, affecting 1 to 3 per cent of all gravid women. It may cause septicaemic shock, and blood cultures are positive in some 15 to 20 per cent of cases. It usually presents in the second or third trimesters with typical symptoms and signs of loin pain, fever, headache, nausea, and vomiting; frequency and dysuria may not be present. The right kidney is more commonly affected. Transient renal dysfunction is not uncommon and occurs more commonly than in similar infections in non-pregnant women. It is contributed to by volume depletion as well as the ill-effects of bacterial products such as lipopolysaccharide endotoxin. There is usually a good response to prompt treatment with intravenous fluids and appropriate antimicrobial therapy. Nearly one-quarter of the affected women will have recurrent attacks during pregnancy and the prevalence of persistent bacteriuria in these patients is high. The tendency of infections to recur distinguishes acute pyelonephritis in pregnancy from its natural history in non-pregnant subjects. The effect of the acute illness on the pregnancy is hard to assess, but most investigators report an increased incidence of preterm labour, fetal growth retardation, and perinatal death.

Acute renal failure

In the 1960s and the early 1970s acute renal failure complicated between 1 in 1500 and 1 in 5000 pregnancies, and obstetric disorders were the cause of renal failure in some 25 to 40 per cent of cases in renal units in Western countries. There was a bimodal pattern of occurrence, with two peaks of incidence occurring early or late in pregnancy. The most common cause was septic abortion at 12 to 18 weeks' gestation, patients presenting with fever, vomiting, diarrhoea, myalgia, and shock, complicated by haemolysis and disseminated intravascular coagulation. Renal failure in such cases is due to acute tubular necrosis, but in pregnancy, susceptibility to bilateral partial or total cortical necrosis is much increased, observed in some 5 to 30 per cent of all cases of obstetric renal failure. The reasons for this are not known, but may relate to increased sensitivity of the renal vasculature to bacterial endotoxins or abnormal activation of the coagulation system.

The incidence of acute renal failure, particularly in the first trimester, has fallen substantially with the introduction of liberal abortion laws and improved obstetric practice. It now amounts to less than 1 case in 10 000 pregnancies in Western societies. In some less-developed areas, however, the incidence remains high in both the first and last trimester.

Acute renal failure late in pregnancy is most commonly associated with severe pre-eclampsia, eclampsia, or abruptio placentae, but is also seen after prolonged intrauterine fetal death, amniotic fluid embolism, and acute fatty liver of pregnancy (see Chapter 13.13), all conditions associated with disseminated intravascular coagulation. Affected women tend to be older than average and parous.

Full recovery of renal function within 2 to 4 weeks is expected in the presence of acute tubular necrosis. Recovery is slower (extending often over several months) and less complete after partial cortical necrosis, and it does not occur in complete bilateral cortical necrosis which characteristically presents with anuria. Peritoneal dialysis, haemodialysis, or haemodiafiltration can all be used in treatment, but despite improvements in management, maternal mortality remains high at 10 to 15 per cent. The perinatal mortality is also extremely high, but this reflects the conditions that have precipitated renal failure as much as the renal failure itself.

Idiopathic postpartum renal failure

This is a syndrome of acute and rapidly progressive renal failure occurring in the first weeks after an uncomplicated pregnancy in previously healthy women. Blood pressure may be normal initially but rises rapidly and may reach the malignant phase. There is associated microangiopathic haemolytic anaemia in 75 per cent of cases, so that an alternative term is 'postpartum haemolytic uraemic syndrome' (see Chapter 20.6). Complete recovery of renal function is rarely achieved, some 10 per cent of patients requiring long-term renal replacement therapy. There may be quick improvement in function in some, but in others there is little recovery for months. Renal biopsy may show thickening of glomerular capillary walls with thrombosis and fibrinoid necrosis with intraluminal thrombosis in afferent arterioles. Another pattern is indistinguishable from that of systemic sclerosis, with major changes in intralobular arteries and ischaemic-looking glomerular tufts. This condition, and its management are further discussed in Chapter 18.11.4. In some cases a circulating 'lupus anticoagulant' or antiphospholipid antibody may be a causative association with the syndrome.

Chronic renal disorders

Women in advanced renal failure approaching the need for replacement therapy are often amenorrhoeic and infertile so that pregnancy is an unlikely event. There are, however, some reported cases of successful pregnancy even in patients on maintenance haemodialysis. Nearly all the infants have survived, but most have weighed less than 2000 g, indicating a high incidence of prematurity and fetal growth retardation. The situation is transformed by successful renal transplantation. Ovulation and menstruation are restored in about 6 months. Most of the ensuing pregnancies end successfully with the delivery of a normal infant. Whether or not pregnancy alters the natural history of the transplanted kidney is not known. A decline in graft function is relatively common during pregnancy, affecting some 10 to 20 per cent of pregnant women with renal allografts. About one-third of the episodes of deterioration occur in the puerperium. In the majority of incidents, the loss of function has been small but in some it has been total. Permanent impairment affects between 7 and 15 per cent of patients at risk. The incidence of pre-eclampsia is high (25 per cent) and this may contribute to reversible impairment of renal function. Urinary-tract infections are common (20 per cent) despite the careful supervision that these patients receive. The transplanted kidney is not at risk of damage by vaginal delivery.

The use of immunosuppressive therapy in pregnancy is discussed more fully in Chapter 20.17.3. One-quarter of mothers with renal transplants also need antihypertensive drugs.

The incidence of congenital abnormalities in the infants of mothers with renal transplants is not obviously increased but immunosuppressive therapy may result in lymphopenia, adrenal insufficiency, and infections by such organisms as cytomegalovirus or bacteria. Nearly half the infants are born prematurely which further complicates the neonatal period.

Fertility is less of a problem in women with chronic renal disease

with more modest impairment of glomerular filtration rate. It is probable that the factors chiefly determining outcome are the filtration rate itself, the degree of proteinuria, and the arterial pressure at the time of conception. There are suggestions in the literature of different prognoses according to the underlying nature of the renal disorder, but these are difficult to substantiate.

Reflux nephropathy

Reflux nephropathy is one of the more common renal disorders affecting women of child-bearing age; indeed, a complication of pregnancy such as hypertension or recurrent pyelonephritis may first draw attention to a disorder which, in the absence of gross renal failure, is often rather silent clinically. The presence of reflux scarring and modest impairment of glomerular filtration rate is, however, now compatible with a successful pregnancy, provided that hypertension and heavy proteinuria (in excess of 1 g/24 h) are not evident at conception. If, however, either creatinine clearance is less than 40 ml/min (plasma creatinine 180–220µg/l), or the patient is hypertensive at conception, there is not only a much increased risk of severe fetal growth retardation and/or intrauterine death, but also of deterioration of renal function in the course of pregnancy not reversible postpartum.

Glomerulonephritis

It is probable that, as in the case of reflux nephropathy, the factors chiefly determining the outcome of pregnancy in relation to fetal health and survival are the presence or absence of significant hypertension and the degree of loss of glomerular filtration rate; also, both probably indicate broadly the risks of further loss of maternal renal function as a consequence of pregnancy. In addition, nephrotic rates of proteinuria are likely to be aggravated and, given the now well-recognized adverse effects on prognosis of heavy proteinuria in relation to the rate of loss of renal function, this may cause more than worrisome hypoproteinaemia and fluid retention in the last trimester. There have been suggestions that particular forms of glomerulonephritis may be more liable to adverse outcome in pregnancy. Most would agree that when the kidney is involved in systemic sclerosis or polyarteritis, the risk both to mother and fetus in pregnancy is such as to advise against it. There is some evidence for a poorer prognosis in mesangiocapillary disease and perhaps also in IgA disease and focal segmental glomerulosclerosis.

Overall, proteinuria increases in more than half the women with glomerulonephritis in the course of pregnancy, with worsening or developing hypertension in some 30 to 70 per cent. Some 75 per cent of pregnancies nevertheless result in successful delivery of a viable infant, despite the presence of chronic renal impairment. Suggestions that focal and segmental glomerulonephritis may be a manifestation of pre-eclampsia as well as a contributor to its development are controversial.

Patients with previously undiagnosed chronic glomerular disease may present with proteinuric hypertension in pregnancy, and the differential diagnosis from pre-eclampsia is often difficult. The only certain discriminant is provided by renal biopsy. This presents no additional hazards to the gravid patient, provided that her blood pressure is controlled and that her coagulation status is known to be normal. However, it should only very rarely be an antipartum procedure, because the best test for pre-eclampsia is to observe what happens after delivery. Only if the proteinuria persists, for example at 6 weeks after delivery, should renal biopsy be considered.

Nephrotic syndrome

The most common cause of heavy proteinuria in late pregnancy is pre-eclampsia. More rarely it will result from a glomerulonephritis, lupus nephropathy, or diabetic renal disease. Causes such as renal vein thrombosis or amyloidosis are extremely rare. Certain women may present with heavy proteinuria which remits at the end of pregnancy only to recur cyclically with further pregnancies. The nature of this disorder has not been elucidated. In the absence of hypertension the pregnancy is not likely to be complicated.

Other renal problems

In general, the pregnancy is likely to be complicated by superimposed pre-eclampsia if there is pre-existing hypertension. Otherwise, few problems need to be anticipated. As discussed above, patients with reflux nephropathy and renal scarring are particularly prone to acute urinary-tract infection. Women with polycystic renal disease need genetic counselling so that they understand the chances of their children inheriting this autosomal dominant disorder. First trimester diagnosis of adult polycystic kidney disease should now be feasible since the gene for the disorder has been identified. Women with single kidneys tolerate pregnancy well, providing the remaining kidney is not scarred or has poor function for other reasons. Congenital abnormalities of the renal tract are associated with uterine abnormalities which can affect fertility and the success of pregnancy. Urolithiasis, being more a disease of men, is not commonly a complication of pregnancy. However, both renal colic and acute obstruction due to stones can occur in gravid women and must be managed as they are in other circumstances. At parturition the mucosa of the renal pelvis may develop small tears which can present as hae-maturia in the early puerperium. This should resolve with conservative management.

REFERENCES

Andriole, V.T. and Patterson, T.F. (1991). Epidemiology, natural history and management of urinary tract infections in pregnancy. *Medical Clinics of North America* **75**, 359–73.
Cunningham, F.G. (1987). Urinary tract infections complicating pregnancy. *Baillières Clinical Obstetrics and Gynaecology* **I**, 891–907.
European Polycystic Kidney Disease Consortium. (1994). The polycystic kidney disease-1 gene encodes on a 14 kb transcript and lies within a duplicated region on chromosome 16. *Cell*, **77**, 1–20.
Jungers, P., Houillier, P., and Forget, D. (1987). Reflux nephropathy and pregnancy. *Baillières Clinical Obstetrics and Gynaecology* **I**, 955–69.
Lancet (1989). Leading article. Pregnancy and glomerulonephritis. *Lancet* **2**, 253–4.
Lindheimer, M.D. and Katz, A.I. (1987). Gestation in women with kidney disease. *Baillières Clinical Obstetrics and Gynaecology* **I**, 922–37.
Packham, D.K., North, R.A., Fairley, K.F., Whitworth, J.A., and Kincaid-Smith, P. (1989). Primary glomerulonephritis in pregnancy. *Quarterly Journal of Medicine.* **266**, 537–53.
Pertuiset, N. and Grunfeld, J.-P. (1987). Acute renal failure in pregnancy. *Baillières Clinical Obstetrics and Gynaecology* **I**, 874–89.
Shiiki, H., *et al.* (1990). Focal and segmental glomerulosclerosis in pre-eclamptic patients with nephrotic syndrome. *American Journal of Nephrology* **10**, 205–12.

13.4 Heart disease in pregnancy

J. C. FORFAR

INTRODUCTION

Between 5 and 10 per cent of maternal deaths in the United Kingdom are a consequence of heart disease, with a significantly higher proportion in developing countries. Although the prevalence of rheumatic heart disease has declined worldwide, it remains an important and treatable condition in pregnancy. Congenital heart disease and the better survival of patients with treated complex lesions to adulthood presents new challenges and more complex decisions for planning and managing pregnancy. Information on maternal and fetal risks in such complex situations remains inadequate and optimum treatment may be unclear.

Physiological changes in pregnancy

Substantial haemodynamic and circulatory changes occur during pregnancy and the peripartum period (Table 1).

Cardiac output rises significantly (up to 50 per cent) in the first trimester and peaks between the second and third trimesters. Pressure of the gravid uterus on the cava in the supine position produces substantial falls in cardiac output and blood pressure in a minority of pregnancies, and can result in symptoms of weakness, light-headedness, dizziness, and even syncope. This supine hypotensive syndrome of pregnancy is usually relieved immediately by turning to one side. The increase in cardiac output during pregnancy arises from increases in heart rate and/or stroke volume, secondary mainly to a fall in systemic vascular resistance and increase in blood volume. The reduction in blood pressure results from vasodilatation, likely mediated by gestational hormones, increased heat production, and the low resistance uteroplacental circulation.

Table 1 *Haemodynamic changes during normal pregnancy*

	Trimester		
	1st	2nd	3rd
Cardiac output	++	+++	+++
Heart rate	+	++	+++
Stroke volume	+	++	+
Systemic vascular resistance	−	−−	−
Blood volume	++	+++	+++
Systolic blood pressure	+−	−	+−
Diastolic blood pressure	−	−	−

+− = no change; +,++,+++ = small, moderate, large increase; −, −− = small, moderate decrease.

Blood volume increases early in pregnancy and more slowly from mid-pregnancy onwards. These changes have been attributed to activation of the renin–angiotensin–aldosterone mechanism by oestrogens and secondary retention of salt and water. The rise in plasma volume (average 50 per cent) is faster and greater than the rise in red cell mass (average 25 per cent), thus accounting for the so-called 'physiological anaemia of pregnancy', when haemoglobin averages 11 g/dl.

Both blood pressure and cardiac output increase significantly with the pain and anxiety of labour and from increases in blood volume following uterine contraction. These haemodynamic changes greatly increase oxygen consumption, although appropriate analgesia or anaesthesia may limit them to some extent. Despite blood loss on delivery, blood volume is effectively (although not actually) increased by the contracting empty uterus postpartum, and augmented preload acutely increases cardiac output. These changes return to normal over 24 h.

Cardiovascular evaluation

Assessment of heart disease in pregnancy is complicated by the functional changes described above, which may simulate or mask underlying heart disease. Furthermore, the application of routine investigative methods may be limited because of potential risks to the fetus.

Fatigue, reduced exercise capacity, breathlessness, and light-headedness are common symptoms of normal pregnancy. The increase in respiratory rate and reduced tidal volume may be perceived as breathlessness and this, combined with some peripheral oedema from increased blood volume and caval compression, may lead to an erroneous diagnosis of heart failure. The increased volume, and occasionally collapsing peripheral pulses, during later pregnancy mimic aortic regurgitation or hyperthyroidism. The apical impulse is prominent and occasionally displaced laterally, simulating chronic volume loading. Heart sounds are commonly loud and may be palpable with exaggerated splitting. An apical S3 is relatively common in pregnancy but S4 is less common and its presence should promote investigation of possible underlying heart disease.

A soft systolic murmur at the base and lower left sternal edge occurs in most pregnancies and can radiate to the suprasternal notch and the neck. A continuous venous flow murmur may be audible in the neck along with a systolic or continuous murmur from increased flow to the breasts. Both of these murmurs decrease with stethoscope pressure and are less audible in the upright position.

A diastolic murmur is rare in normal pregnancy and should prompt further investigation. Murmurs associated with organic heart disease increase in intensity in pregnancy (from increased flow) and conclusions based on murmur intensity should therefore be made with caution.

ELECTROCARDIOGRAPHY (ECG)

Minor flattening of the T-waves and minor left or right QRS axis shift are common in normal pregnancy. Sinus tachycardia and atrial or ventricular premature beats are likewise frequent findings, particularly during labour and delivery.

CHEST RADIOGRAPHY

Although the radiation dose is minimal, this test is best avoided unless there are clear clinical indications. The uterus should be appropriately shielded. Straightening of the left heart border and prominence of pulmonary conus are common radiographic findings in pregnancy, along with prominent pulmonary vascular markings. A small pleural effusion may be seen early postpartum and usually resolves quickly.

DOPPLER ECHOCARDIOGRAPHY

Fetal ultrasound may be considered safe and provides valuable anatomical and functional information throughout pregnancy. A small pericardial effusion is seen late in a minority of normal pregnancies. Trivial tricuspid and pulmonary regurgitation demonstrated on colour-flow Doppler may be considered a variant of normal at this stage.

CARDIAC CATHETERIZATION

This should only be undertaken if an intervention is required for patient management. Balloon mitral valvuloplasty is an alternative to closed valvotomy for symptomatic severe mitral stenosis in pregnancy. Aortic and pulmonary balloon valvuloplasty have also been performed, as has coronary angioplasty. The brachial approach is preferable to keep radiation exposure to a minimum, and full shielding is appropriate. Radio-

nuclide imaging techniques during pregnancy are best avoided because of uncertainty of the level of radiation exposure to the fetus.

Heart diseases in pregnancy

Cardiac reserve (assessed by history and functional classification) is an important determinant of risk in pregnancy. Patients with heart disease and with no symptoms, or minimal symptoms, prior to pregnancy run a relatively small risk of complications during pregnancy and the peripartum period. Patients with moderate or severe limitation prior to pregnancy are at much higher risk, and careful monitoring, and if necessary intervention, are required. Patients who are symptomatic at rest prior to pregnancy have a high maternal and even higher fetal mortality and pregnancy is contraindicated until their functional class can be improved.

It is therefore important that accurate diagnostic and functional evaluation is undertaken in all patients prior to embarking on a pregnancy, with prediction of maternal and fetal risk as far as possible and discussion of maternal morbidity, long-term survival, and the risks of fetal heart disease. It is preferable, in patients with complex congenital heart disease, that such discussions take place as early as possible before pregnancy is contemplated so that appropriate action may be taken. For most patients where the predicted maternal mortality is above 30 per cent, sterilization or pregnancy termination may be the most appropriate course. The management of anticoagulant therapy before and during pregnancy requires special consideration (see below).

Congenital heart disease

This accounts for up to one-third of heart disease in pregnancy. Maternal and hence fetal outcome is determined by the nature of the disease, previous surgical repair, functional capacity, cyanosis, and the presence of pulmonary hypertension. Heart failure, arrhythmias, and systemic hypertension are more common with cyanotic congenital heart disease and when functional status is compromised. Infective endocarditis is a risk in the peripartum period.

Fetal mortality averages 40 per cent in maternal cyanotic congenital heart disease, over twice that for the acyanotic mother. Similarly, low birth weight for gestational age and prematurity are more common with cyanotic mothers. The risk of important congenital defects in the fetus of mothers with congenital heart disease varies greatly between 3 and 15 per cent.

Caesarean section is usually performed for obstetric reasons rather than changing maternal status. Careful haemodynamic monitoring and maintenance of ventricular filling pressures may be helpful in keeping maternal risk to a minimum. Antibiotic chemoprophylaxis is indicated during uncomplicated vaginal delivery when there is a valve prosthesis, a right to left shunt, or a surgically constructed left to right shunt. In many centres, however, prophylactic antibiotics are more widely prescribed.

Maternal risk can be classified according to structural diagnosis (Table 2).

ACYANOTIC SHUNT LESIONS

Atrial septal defect

This common lesion is usually well tolerated in pregnancy even with a substantial left to right shunt. Antibiotic prophylaxis is not indicated for an isolated secundum atrial septal defect and, in general, elective closure should be undertaken following delivery.

Ventricular septal defect

This lesion is well tolerated in pregnancy unless there is pre-existing pulmonary hypertension or impaired cardiac reserve.

Table 2 *Congenital heart disease (CHD) and maternal risks during pregnancy*

Low	Medium	High
Atrial septal defect	Cyanotic CHD without pulmonary hypertension	Eisenmenger syndrome
Small ventricular septal defect	Palliated complex CHD	Primary pulmonary hypertension
Small persistent ductus arteriosus	Hypertrophic obstructive cardiomyopathy	Symptomatic severe aortic stenosis
Mild coarctation of aorta	Symptomatic mitral stenosis	
Corrected tetralogy of Fallot	Ebstein's anomaly	

Persistent ductus arteriosus

Percutaneous transcatheter closure of a persistent ductus arteriosus has occasionally been required during pregnancy because of the development of heart failure resistant to medical therapy, but the great majority have a low risk during pregnancy provided pulmonary hypertension is absent or modest.

ACYANOTIC OBSTRUCTIVE LESIONS

Aortic valve disease

Mild aortic stenosis can be missed in pregnancy because of the prevalence of a flow-related systolic murmur and confusion between a split first-heart sound and an aortic ejection click from a bicuspid valve. Asymptomatic patients with moderate or severe aortic stenosis may require careful haemodynamic monitoring during labour and delivery. Patients with symptomatic severe aortic stenosis should be advised against pregnancy, or should consider a termination. Valvotomy and percutaneous balloon valvuloplasty have been performed successfully in the second and third trimesters for severe symptoms.

Coarctation of the aorta

Pregnancy is usually uneventful with the uncomplicated lesion, although impaired fetal development, hypertension, heart failure, and aortic dissection have all been described. If possible, aortic coarctation should be corrected prior to pregnancy.

Pulmonary stenosis

It appears that the risks associated with pregnancy in this condition are low, although heart failure has been described. Surgical valvotomy or balloon valvuloplasty are intervention options, although clinical experience of these in pregnancy is minimal.

CYANOTIC LESIONS

Tetralogy of Fallot

This is the most prevalent cyanotic congenital heart disease in adults. Pregnancy may cause major clinical deterioration because of augmented right ventricular pressure from increases in blood volume and increased left to right shunting from reduced systemic vascular resistance. Reduced arterial oxygen saturation and a high haematocrit are worrying signs, and careful monitoring of labour and deliver is essential. Maternal and fetal risk appear to be greatly reduced where the defect has been surgically repaired, and this should be performed if at all possible prior to pregnancy. Palliative aortopulmonary shunting in the tetralogy of Fallot leaves a significant risk during pregnancy.

Eisenmenger's syndrome

The high maternal mortality with this condition has been confirmed by several studies, although there are some isolated reports of success. Approximately 1 in 4 pregnancies reach term with a very high prevalence of growth retardation, prematurity, and perinatal death. Because of this, pregnancy is contraindicated and early termination should be considered for all patients. Thomboembolism is more common and anti-coagulation should be considered in late pregnancy and postpartum. Intensive haemodynamic monitoring to avoid blood loss and blood pressure swings and to maintain filling pressures is appropriate.

Complex cyanotic congenital heart disease

The increasing success of palliative and corrective surgical procedures for complex cyanotic congenital heart disease has allowed pregnancy to be contemplated through survival to child-bearing age. Successful pregnancies have been identified with a single ventricle, corrected and uncorrected transposition of the great vessels, tricuspid and pulmonary atresia, but the risks are substantial and are often inappropriate. It is likely that the literature presents an underestimate of the risk because of a tendency to report success.

Rheumatic heart disease

Although very rare in the United Kingdom, acute rheumatic fever may develop or recur during pregnancy and the associated carditis carries a substantial maternal risk. Antibiotic chemoprophylaxis has been advised throughout pregnancy in patients with a history of recurrent rheumatic fever.

Patients with valvular heart disease of rheumatic origin should be managed according to the site and severity of their valvular disease. Careful haemodynamic monitoring may be necessary in late pregnancy, labour, and postpartum.

MITRAL STENOSIS

This is the commonest lesion in pregnancy, with complications including heart failure, atrial arrhythmias (particularly fibrillation), and thromboembolism. Digoxin and β-blockade may be effective in controlling the ventricular rate and maintaining cardiac output when atrial arrhythmias ensue. Diuretics can reduce pulmonary congestion but hypovolaemia should be avoided. Asymptomatic patients, or those with mild symptoms, during early pregnancy usually progress uneventfully. Severe symptomatic mitral stenosis can be successfully relieved by closed or open valvotomy, or percutaneous balloon valvuloplasty. Both fetal and maternal risks appear to be modest with these procedures, although experience of balloon valvuloplasty is minimal. Systemic and pulmonary thromboembolism is a special complication in pregnancy and chronic anticoagulant therapy should be considered in those at higher risk based on standard criteria (see Chapter 13.5).

MITRAL REGURGITATION

This lesion is usually well tolerated in pregnancy, presumably because of reduced systemic vascular resistance. Vasodilator therapy and digoxin may be indicated.

AORTIC VALVE DISEASE

Severe rheumatic aortic valve disease is uncommon in pregnancy. Aortic regurgitation is more frequent, but like mitral regurgitation is fairly well tolerated, partly because of the fall in systemic vascular resistance and tachycardia.

Mitral valve prolapse

This has been recognized in up to 15 per cent of women of child-bearing age and, provided mitral regurgitation is not severe, there appears to be little risk for the mother or fetus.

Cardiomyopathy in pregnancy

HYPERTROPHIC CARDIOMYOPATHY

Pregnancy appears to be well tolerated in this condition, although symptoms of heart failure can develop or worsen at any stage during pregnancy. It is uncertain whether the risk of sudden death in this condition is increased by pregnancy. Careful haemodynamic monitoring may be indicated during labour and delivery, and avoidance of systemic vasodilatation, blood loss, and hypotension is essential. The role of β-blockade is uncertain, but these drugs can be useful in managing symptoms related to elevated left ventricular filling pressure and where there is an obstructive element to the condition.

PERIPARTUM CARDIOMYOPATHY

This form of dilated cardiomyopathy is associated with the development of heart failure and left ventricular systolic dysfunction in the last trimester of pregnancy or within the first 6 months postpartum. Other causes of dilated cardiomyopathy should be excluded. The disease is rare in the United Kingdom and in Europe but has a much higher incidence in certain parts of Africa, with a prevalence of up to 1 per cent. Although the causation of peripartum cardiomyopathy is unknown, age at onset, geographical frequency variation, and substantial recovery of ventricular function in the majority of individuals suggest a unique and specific syndrome. Myocarditis, nutritional deficiency, small vessel coronary disease, maternal and immunological responses to a fetal antigen have all been proposed mechanisms. Endomyocardial biopsy reveals a high prevalence of myocarditis compared to idiopathic dilated cardiomyopathy. The role of genetic factors is poorly defined.

Clinical examination reveals cardiomegaly, a third or fourth heart sound, and, commonly, functional mitral and tricuspid regurgitation. ECG abnormalities are widespread and usually non-specific, and a variety of arrhythmias have been described. The haemodynamic changes do not differ from those of other forms of dilated cardiomyopathy.

Most patients respond to conventional management with digoxin, diuretics, and vasodilators. Angiotensin converting enzyme (ACE) inhibitors may affect fetal renal function and are not recommended antepartum. The role of immunosuppressive therapy is controversial but may be indicated in patients with progressive clinical deterioration unresponsive to conventional therapy.

Fifty per cent of patients show substantial or complete recovery of ventricular function and clinical state within 6 months postpartum. In the remainder there is persistent left ventricular dysfunction and chronic heart failure. Progressive clinical deterioration and early death occur in a minority. There is a significant risk of thromboembolism and anticoagulant therapy is often appropriate.

The risk of relapse in a subsequent pregnancy is substantial (up to 40 per cent) and is greater in patients with persistently abnormal ventricular function after the initial episode.

Ischaemic heart disease

Coronary artery disease is a rare but increasingly recognized complication of pregnancy with a prevalence of around 1 in 10 000. Conventional risk factors for coronary artery disease in women apply, the combination of heavy smoking and use of oral contraceptives being powerful predictors. Peripartum myocardial infarction may be associated with normal coronary arteries on subsequent investigation, and coronary spasm or *in situ* thrombosis has been proposed as a mechanism. Coronary artery dissection has also been described.

Myocardial infarction is associated with a high maternal mortality (up to 25 per cent) and thrombolytic drugs are contraindicated. Delayed diagnosis may contribute to management difficulties. Haemodynamic monitoring is often appropriate peripartum and epidural anaesthesia and elective Caesarean section may be indicated.

The Marfan syndrome

Pregnancy in patients with the Marfan syndrome is associated with an increased incidence of aortic dissection and death, particularly if pre-existing cardiovascular disease is identified. An aortic root diameter of less than 4.5 cm and absence of progressive aortic dilatation and aortic regurgitation suggest a better outcome. However, selective literature reporting probably overestimates the true risk. In patients with established aortic root dilatation pregnancy is undesirable, and if root enlargement is progressive during the first trimester, termination must be considered. β-Blockade may reduce the rate of aortic dilatation and complications in pregnant patients with the Marfan syndrome although clinical experience is limited.

Aortic dissection in the absence of the Marfan syndrome is recognized but rare, and occurs most frequently during the third trimester of pregnancy and the peripartum period. Precordial and transoesophageal echocardiography is the diagnostic technique of choice. Emergency measures to reduce blood pressure are required, although maternal and fetal mortality is high.

Primary pulmonary hypertension

A high maternal mortality rate (up to 40 per cent) has been reported and pregnancy is contraindicated. Haemodynamic deterioration during pregnancy is not clearly predictable on the basis of preconception haemodynamics. Anticoagulation is recommended during pregnancy and early postpartum.

Cardiac arrhythmias

Atrial and ventricular premature beats occur commonly in pregnancy and appear to have no adverse maternal or fetal consequences. Patients with a substrate for supraventricular tachycardia such as atrioventricular nodal re-entry tachycardia or an artrioventricular bypass tract may experience symptomatic deterioration in pregnancy, or may develop symptoms for the first time. Bradycardia and heart block are rare during pregnancy and are usually of congenital origin. Specific causes and triggers should be sought and, if appropriate, removed in all patients. Antiarrhythmic drug therapy should be initiated only for persistent arrhythmias threatening the mother or fetus (see below). The role of radiofrequency ablation of slow atrioventricular nodal pathways or nodal bypass tracts in pregnancy has yet to be established.

Cardiac surgery in pregnancy

Closed and, less commonly, open mitral valvotomy has been frequently reported during pregnancy with a very low maternal and low fetal risk. Although many cardiac operations, including those on cardiopulmonary bypass, have been described in pregnancy, detailed information on risk is scanty. Surgery essential for maternal health should, in general, be performed during the middle trimester or towards the end of the third trimester when elective or emergency delivery can be planned. Sustained uterine contraction postpartum is essential to minimize the risk of bleeding from systemic heparinization during cardiopulmonary bypass. In appropriate circumstances balloon valvuloplasty or coronary artery angioplasty seems an attractive alternative.

Pregnancy and valve prosthesis

Increased cardiac output, a hypercoagulable state, and fetal risks from anticoagulant and other drugs potentially complicate pregnancy with a valve prosthesis. Ideally, risks should be carefully discussed prior to conception. Patients with no, or minimal, limitation prior to pregnancy usually have a favourable outcome with one or more heterograft or homograft prosthesis. The risk of thromboembolic events with mechanical valves appears increased, especially with the mitral prosthesis, although this increase in risk may, in part, result from less satisfactory anticoagulant control and the use of fixed-dose heparin regimes in the first trimester. Tissue valves are often recommended for women of childbearing age, but the long-term durability of these valves, particularly in young patients, deserves serious consideration, and there is a small but definite risk of progressive calcification in young patients.

Cardiovascular drugs in pregnancy

All drugs should be avoided where possible during pregnancy and the risk/benefit balance carefully evaluated in terms of maternal health and fetal risk. With some exceptions, the importance of maternal drugs excreted in breast milk and effects on infants are inadequately defined.

ANTICOAGULANTS

There is no ideal anticoagulant in pregnancy. Use must depend on individual assessment of risks and benefits.

Warfarin has been most widely used during pregnancy but presents significant maternal and fetal side-effects. Haemorrhage is particularly associated with delivery and this drug should be discontinued approaching term. Fetal risks are derived from the transplacental passage of warfarin. A relatively high incidence of spontaneous abortion and stillbirth has been reported. Use of this drug during the first trimester has been associated with a 'coumarin embryopathy' in 5 to 30 per cent of new-

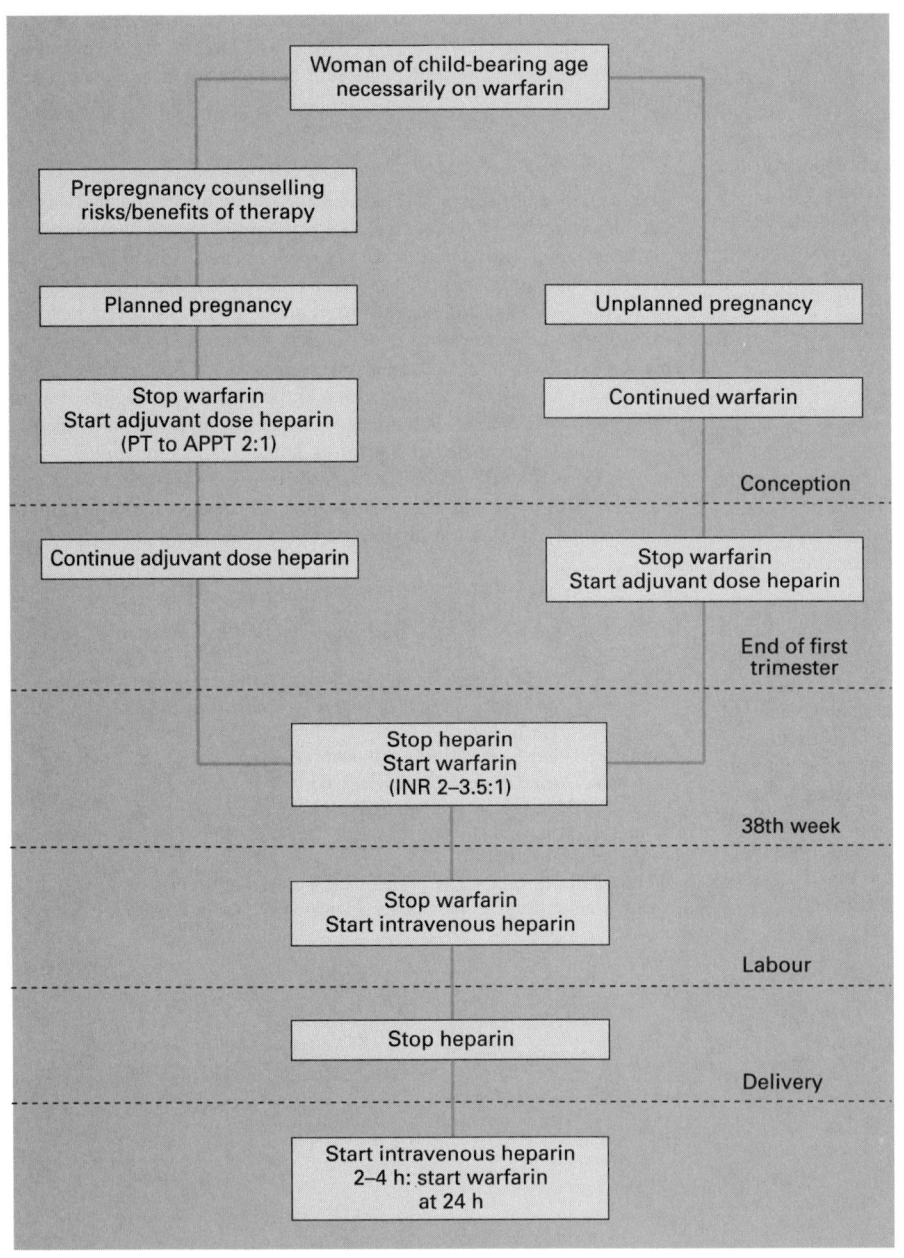

Fig. 1 Suggested strategy for anticoagulation during pregnancy.

borns. This syndrome includes hypoplasia of the nasal bone and epiphyseal stipling (chondrodysplasia punctata). Central nervous system disease, including optic atrophy and blindness, mental retardation, cerebral palsy, and intracranial bleeding have all been described and linked to warfarin.

Heparin, because of its molecular weight, does not cross the placenta. Its use in pregnancy appears to be associated with a variable incidence of maternal and fetal complications, although more recent studies have shown a favourable outcome with this treatment.

Self-injection of an adjusted dose of heparin subcutaneously every 12 h is a satisfactory approach in pregnancy. Avoidance of fixed-dose regimes is preferable. There is a consensus that intravenous heparin should be substituted close to term and discontinued at the onset of labour. Complications of long-term subcutaneous therapy include haematoma and abscess formation in the abdominal wall, thrombocytopenia, and osteoporosis.

A suggested strategy for the management of anticoagulation in pregnancy is shown in Fig. 1. This involves early substitution of heparin for warfarin (preferably prior to conception) and return to warfarin from the end of the first trimester until 2 weeks before term. Continued heparin therapy throughout the pregnancy is an alternative. With the exception of premature infants, warfarin excretion in breast milk does not cause significant anticoagulation for the infant.

DIGOXIN

Few adverse effects on the fetus have been reported for mothers treated with digoxin during pregnancy. Teratogenicity is not a problem. Digoxin crosses the placenta and maternal and fetal blood concentrations are similar. The plasma digoxin concentration tends to fall during pregnancy because of an increased volume of distribution. Although low birthweight has been reported with maternal use of this drug, it is quite likely a consequence of the underlying maternal disease rather than a drug effect.

DIURETICS

Diuretics have been used frequently in pregnancy for the management of cardiac failure and pre-eclampsia, although they should be avoided for treatment of dependent oedema because of potential effects on uterine blood flow and placental perfusion. No teratogenic effects have been reported with thiazide diuretics or with frusemide.

β-BLOCKING DRUGS

Propranolol has been used widely in pregnancy for the management of hyperthyroidism, hypertrophic cardiomyopathy, cardiac arrhythmias, and hypertension. There is controversy as to the extent of intrauterine growth retardation as a class effect of all β-blocking agents but, because of this possibility, their use should be considered carefully on an individual basis. Metoprolol and atenolol have also been used for the treatment of hypertension in pregnancy. All three drugs are secreted in breast milk, but no adverse effects have been noted in the infant.

OTHER ANTIARRHYTHMICS

Quinidine has been used successfully for the treatment of maternal and, rarely, for the treatment of fetal arrhythmias. Toxicity is described but rare. Information on the use of procainamide, disopyramide, and flecainide is limited and these drugs should be used with extreme caution for resistant arrhythmias threatening maternal health. Amiodarone has been associated with a number of fetal side-effects and should be avoided if at all possible. It is secreted in breast milk. The effects of amiodarone in infants are unknown.

Verapamil

Verapamil has been used for maternal and fetal supraventricular arrhythmias but clinical experience is limited.

Nifedipine

There is uncertainty over the possible toxic effects of nifedipine and its use in pregnancy should be avoided.

Angiotensin-converting inhibitors

Both captopril and enalapril have been used as antihypertensive drugs in pregnancy. Prolonged fetal hypotension and death has been reported in animals and there may be a risk of low birth weight, oligohydramnios, and neonatal renal failure. On present evidence these drugs should be avoided.

PROPHYLACTIC ANTIBIOTICS

The incidence of bacteraemia associated with an uncomplicated vaginal delivery is low and therefore thresholds for antibiotic chemoprophylaxis are uncertain. Routine prophylaxis is recommended for prosthetic heart valves, congenital heart disease with a right to left shunt, and where an aortopulmonary anastomosis has been created with prosthetic material. Many physicians, however, also routinely administer prophylactic antibiotics to those at conventional risk from endocarditis, including valvular heart disease, ventricular septal defect, and hypertrophic obstructive cardiomyopathy. Treatment with intravenous ampicillin and gentamicin approximately 1 h prior to delivery is recommended, with a second dose 8 h later. Slow intravenous infusion of vancomycin may be used with penicillin allergy. For patients at low risk, conventional chemoprophylaxis with oral amoxycillin is practised widely.

REFERENCES

Costanzo-Nordin, M.R. and O'Connell, J.B. (1990). *Progress in Cardiology* **2**, (2), 225–39.

Elkayam, U. and Gleicher, N. (ed.) (1990). *Cardiac problems in pregnancy; diagnosis and management of maternal and foetal disease*, (2nd edn). John Wiley, Chicester.

Hamkins, G.D., *et al.* (1985). Myocardial infarction during pregnancy: a review. *Obstetrics and Gynecology* **65**, 139–46.

Sullivan, J.M. and Ramanathan, K.B. (1985). Management of medical problems in pregnancy – severe cardiac disease. *New England Journal of Medicine* **313**, 304–9.

Weiderhorn, J., Rubin, J.M., Frishman, W.H. and Elkayam, U. (1987). Cardiovascular drugs in pregnancy. *Cardiology Clinics* **5**, (4), 651–74.

13.5 Thromboembolism in pregnancy

M. DE SWIET

This section is concerned with thromboembolism in pregnancy, specifically deep vein thrombosis and pulmonary embolism. Arterial thromboembolism, which in pregnancy usually arises because of mitral valve disease and/or arterial fibrillation, cardiomyopathy, and the presence of artificial heart valves, is considered elsewhere (see Chapter 15.26). Cerebral vein thrombosis is considered in Section 22.6..

SIGNIFICANCE AND INCIDENCE

Pulmonary embolus together with hypertension is currently the leading cause of maternal mortality in the United Kingdom, and was responsible for 33 deaths between 1988 and 1990 (eight deaths per million maternities). In addition, deep vein thrombosis is a major cause of morbidity: about 80 per cent of women who have deep vein thrombosis in pregnancy have symptoms in the same leg at follow up 11 years later. Because of the difficulties of diagnosis of non-fatal cases (see below) it is difficult to obtain precise data for the incidence of non-fatal pulmonary embolus or deep vein thrombosis, but in Western societies the incidence of both is between 2 and 12 per thousand deliveries. About two-thirds of the cases occur postnatally. In Africa and the Far East the condition is almost unknown.

RISK FACTORS

It is generally believed that pregnancy itself is a risk factor for venous thromboembolism, presumably because of the activation of the clotting system. Stasis in the lower limbs caused by obstruction of the venous return by the enlarging uterus may be another factor. Analysis of fatal cases of pulmonary embolus shows that increasing age and parity are important risk factors; the risk of dying from pulmonary embolus in a woman aged over 40 years in her fifth pregnancy is nearly 100 times greater than in a primigravid woman aged 20 to 30 years. Caesarean section (and probably other forms of complicated instrumental delivery) increase the risk about threefold. Oestrogen therapy to suppress lactation also increases the risk of thromboembolism and should no longer be used. Women who have had thromboembolism in the past have a 1 in 10 to 1 in 20 risk of thromboembolism in pregnancy. The risk is the same whether the previous episode of thromboembolism occurred while taking oestrogen-containing oral contraceptives, or whether it occurred when not taking the pill. It is not known whether previous thromboembolism in pregnancy increases the risk in subsequent pregnancies above the figures given. It is likely that prolonged periods of bed rest and obesity predispose to thromboembolism. Patients with any of the sickling conditions (Hb SS, Hb SC, Hb S thalassaemia) are particularly at risk of developing the sickle lung syndrome in pregnancy, one component of which is probably thrombosis *in situ*. Management of haemoglobinopathies in pregnancy is considered in Chapter 13.9. Patients who have the lupus anticoagulant are also at risk of pulmonary embolus; this is considered in Chapter 18.11.3. Antithrombin III and the protein C deficiencies are inherited conditions, in which the risk of venous thromboembolism is also increased (see below and Section 22).

DIAGNOSIS

In pregnancy deep vein thrombosis is much more common in the left leg than the right, presumably because the uterus obstructs the left iliac vessels more than those on the right. The clinical features of pulmonary embolus and deep vein thrombosis are considered in Chapter 15.26. These do not differ in pregnancy, although the common occurrence of leg oedema, breathlessness, minor degrees of pleural effusion in the puerperium, and abnormalities of the electrocardiograph in a normal pregnancy make the clinical diagnosis even more difficult in pregnancy than in the non-pregnant state. Furthermore, the problems of anticoagulant therapy with its associated risks to the fetus are such that every effort must be made to obtain the diagnosis by objective criteria. The implications of this policy are as follows.

Deep vein thrombosis

All patients who have a history compatible with deep vein thrombosis and supporting physical signs in the legs should now have a real-time ultrasound examination of the leg veins with additional Doppler blood flow studies if possible. This technique has been compared with venography in the non-pregnant state and shown to have high sensitivity and specificity for symptomatic femoral vein thrombosis. The direct comparison has not been made in pregnancy. Ultrasound is not yet accurate for calf vein thrombi, but these do not cause pulmonary emboli and the ultrasound test, being non-invasive, can be repeated to ensure that a calf vein thrombosis is not extending into the thigh. Ultrasound cannot be used above inguinal ligament but iliofemoral thrombosis is usually clinically obvious.

Pulmonary embolus

If a patient has a major pulmonary embolus, there is usually little doubt about the diagnosis. However, pulmonary embolus is often considered as a cause of collapse in pregnant women, particularly at the time of delivery, and the differential diagnosis of occult causes of collapse without obvious bleeding or inverted uterus is considered in Table 1. Perhaps the most important cause of confusion is intra-abdominal bleeding, with irritation of the diaphragm causing chest and shoulder-tip pain. Treatment of such a patient with anticoagulants would probably end fatally. The most important differential factors are the presence of abdominal signs and lower jugular venous pressure in abdominal bleeding, and the raised jugular venous pressure and cardiac signs of pulmonary artery obstruction in pulmonary embolus. However, the problem of diagnosis usually arises in the patient who has pleuritic chest pain with, or without, physical signs, and either absent or non-specific signs on the chest radiography. Arterial blood gas estimation may be helpful: blood samples should be taken with the patient sitting and, in cases of major pulmonary embolus, will show respiratory alkalosis with hypoxaemia. However, the definitive investigation is a lung scan, preferably a ventilation perfusion scan if there are any radiological signs in the lung parenchyma. The radiation exposure from the short-lived isotopes that are used ($^{81}Kr^m$ for ventilation and $^{99}Tc^m$ for perfusion) is trivial, and less than that of a chest radiograph. If the patient has normal blood gases and a negative lung scan, it is reasonable to exclude pulmonary embolus.

TREATMENT

Surgery

If the facilities and an expert team are available, the occasional patient who does not die from a massive pulmonary embolus, and remains shocked and hypotensive (blood pressure less than 90 mmHg systolic,

Table 1 *Features of some 'occult' causes of collapse in pregnancy**

	Predisposing circumstances	Common presenting features	Helpful diagnostic features in acute stage	
			Clinical	Investigations
Amniotic fluid embolism	Labour, not necessarily precipitate	Respiratory distress, cyanosis		Squames in SVC or sputum
Pulmonary embolus	Increasing age, multiparity, thromboembolism, operative delivery, bedrest, oestrogens haemoglobinopathy	Respiratory distress, cyanosis, chest pain	Jugular venous pressure+; 3rd heart sound, parasternal heave	ECG, chest radiograph, lung scan, blood gas, pulmonary angiography
Myocardial infarction	Increasing age	Chest pain, respiratory distress, cyanosis	Pain character, jugular venous pressure+; crepitations	ECG
Dysrhythmia	Pre-existing	Tachycardia/bradycardia	Pulse	ECG
Aspiration of gastric contents	Anaesthesia, not necessarily with vomiting	Respiratory distress, cyanosis	Bronchospasm	
Pneumothorax and pneumomediastinum	Previous history, labour	Chest pain	Chest signs	Chest radiograph
Intra-abdominal bleeding	Labour, though may occur spontaneously	Abdominal pain	Jugular venous pressure not+; signs in abdomen, laparotomy, paracentesis, culdocentesis	

Reproduced from de Swiet (1989), with permission.

Pa_{O_2} less than 60 mmHg, urine output less than 20 ml/h) 1 h after the onset of symptoms, should be considered for pulmonary embolectomy under cardiopulmonary bypass. If the patient reaches the operating theatre alive, the results are excellent. Alternatively, it may be possible to fragment the clot and improve pulmonary blood flow with a catheter introduced into the pulmonary artery. This requires only the most simple image-intensifying equipment, such as is available in most intensive care units (see Chapter 15.26).

The place of surgery (embolectomy) in massive iliofemoral thrombosis, where it might decrease the incidence of subsequent postphlebitic leg symptoms, is unclear.

Thrombolytic therapy

Streptokinase and/or urokinase treatment is probably underused for non-pregnant patients with pulmonary embolus. However, there are specific problems in pregnancy, such as bleeding, the initiation of premature labour, and the subsequent incoordinate uterine action associated with the release of fibrin degradation products. Therefore, in pregnancy, thrombolytic therapy should only be used in shocked patients with pulmonary embolus threatening life and as an alternative to embolectomy.

Anticoagulant therapy

For the reasons given above, the majority of patients will be treated with anticoagulants, the objective being to prevent further thromboembolism. As in the non-pregnant state, intravenous heparin should be used initially. Because of its highly polar nature and large molecular weight, heparin does not cross the placenta. It is not excreted in breast milk and, even if it were, it would not be absorbed from the infant's gastrointestinal tract, being denatured in the stomach. The only acute problem with heparin therapy is bleeding. Possible long-term problems are discussed below. Heparin is given by continuous intravenous infusion, starting at a dose of 40 000 units/24 h and adjusting the infusion rate to achieve a heparin level of 0.6 to 1.0 units/ml, as assayed by the protamine sulphate

neutralization test. In pregnancy, the protamine sulphate neutralization test seems to give more consistent and clinically relevant results than the more commonly used activated partial thromboplastin time. Intravenous heparin is given for 5 to 7 days. Large clots should be treated for a longer period and usually require higher infusion rates of heparin to maintain therapeutic blood levels.

After the acute phase, the therapeutic options are oral anticoagulants, of which there is far more experience with warfarin than phenindione, and subcutaneous heparin. The problems with warfarin therapy in pregnancy are maternal bleeding, particularly in the puerperium, teratogenesis (chondrodysplasia punctata), fetal microcephaly, and optic atrophy and fetal bleeding, both retroplacental and intracerebral. The latter complications can occur with warfarin therapy at any gestational age. For these reasons warfarin should not be used in venous thromboembolism in pregnancy although its use is necessary in patients with artificial heart valves. It has been said that heparin is also associated with a high fetal loss rate. However, the study on which this was based was a literature search dating back to 1948 in which heparin was used for the treatment of hypertension as well as thromboembolism. Furthermore, some of the fetal losses may have been due to the presence of lupus anticoagulant, causing the original episode of thromboembolism and also having an independent association with poor fetal outcome. A recent controlled study of heparin therapy has not demonstrated any excess fetal mortality.

Once intravenous heparin has been discontinued, the patient should be given subcutaneous heparin, 10 000 units twice daily. The majority of patients soon learn to inject themselves and can then be discharged from hospital. They should use the concentrated heparin solution, 50 000 units/ml. Bruising appears to be more related to the injection technique than the type of heparin. Subcutaneous heparin therapy is best controlled by the heparin assay, since low-dose heparin therapy does not affect any of the conventional clotting tests. This assay measures the anti-Xa activity of heparin. The heparin dose should be adjusted down in the rare event that the heparin level exceeds 0.3 units/ml. No upward adjustment of the dose in excess of 20 000 units/day is necessary. A simpler alternative to the anti-Xa heparin assay is to measure the thrombin time. This test should always be available since it is part of the normal clotting screen. The thrombin time is very sensitive to heparin. If it is not prolonged by more than a few seconds in a patient taking heparin, she will not bleed excessively because of heparin therapy. The heparin assay should be repeated whenever the patient attends the antenatal clinic; this will usually ensure that the heparin level has been checked shortly before labour. Assuming that the heparin level is less than 0.3 units/ml, there is no risk from bleeding in labour, and subcutaneous heparin therapy should be continued through labour. Although there has been concern about the possibility of epidural haematoma formation in women taking subcutaneous heparin given epidural anaesthesia, this concern is not justified. If the thrombin time is not prolonged, epidural block should not be withheld.

After delivery the dose of subcutaneous heparin is empirically reduced to 7 500 units twice daily and this treatment should be continued for the first week of the puerperium. After that time, the risk of secondary postpartum haemorrhage is small and patients may switch to oral warfarin therapy if that appears more desirable. Breast feeding is safe in patients taking warfarin, since insignificant quantities of warfarin (though not phenindione) are secreted in breast milk. Since blood-clotting parameters do not return to normal immediately after delivery, anticoagulation should be continued for some time after delivery in a patient who had thromboembolism in the antenatal period. Six weeks is often the time chosen, but the length of time is quite arbitrary.

Prophylaxis

Should any form of prophylactic therapy be given in pregnancy to women who have had an episode of thromboembolism in the past, granted the 5 to 10 per cent risk of recurrence? At present trial data are not adequate to answer the question. Warfarin therapy is contraindicated because of the complications noted above. Some clinicians would use subcutaneous heparin, as described above, throughout pregnancy. However, the incidence of maternal side-effects does not appear to warrant this form of therapy for prophylaxis in the patient who has had a single episode of thromboembolism in the past, although such treatment is reasonable in the patient who has thromboembolism in the index pregnancy. The maternal side-effects are thrombocytopenia, alopecia, and bone demineralization. Clinical bone demineralization has only been reported in patients taking more than 10 000 units of heparin/day for at least 6 months. However, there is evidence of subclinical bone demineralization in patients taking heparin 20 000 units per day for more than 3 months. The alternatives are therefore to use smaller quantities of heparin or low molecular weight heparin for shorter periods of time, or to use no prophylaxis in the antenatal period and start heparin in labour, continuing in the puerperium for at least 1 week with the option of switching to warfarin for a further 5 weeks. None of these strategies has been fully evaluated yet. Most clinicians would suggest that the patient accept the risk of prolonged subcutaneous heparin therapy if she has had more than one well-documented episode of thromboembolism, if she has the lupus anticardiolipin syndrome and previous thromboembolism, or if she has other causes of thrombophilia (see below).

Antithrombin III, protein C, and protein S deficiencies
(see also Section 22)

In these uncommon conditions there is an inherited absence of proteases which inhibit the clotting cascade. There is usually a strong family history and patients frequently develop thromboembolism in pregnancy or on the oral contraceptive pill. The risk of thromboembolism in a patient with antithrombin III deficiency in pregnancy is about 70 per cent.

Treatment of this condition in pregnancy should initially be with subcutaneous heparin, 20 000 to 45 000 units/day to achieve a 10-s prolongation of the activated partial thromboplastin time. This is equivalent to 0.1 to 0.2 units of heparin/ml of plasma measured by chromogenic sub-strate immediately prior to injection. If this level of anticoagulation cannot be achieved with subcutaneous heparin, prolonged intravenous therapy or warfarin should be considered. Before labour, warfarin should be stopped and the dose of heparin should be decreased to permit delivery without excessive bleeding. Delivery should be covered with antithrombin III concentrate or fresh, frozen plasma.

Although protein C and protein S deficiencies are probably more common than antithrombin III deficiency, there is less experience with these conditions regarding prophylaxis of thromboembolism in pregnancy. Heparin is effective in the acute phase, and therefore subcutaneous heparin may provide adequate prophylaxis. A protein C concentrate is now available for cover during labour. Care should be taken with warfarin therapy since this has caused skin necrosis, presumably due to thrombosis of the skin microcirculation. Protein S exists in both free (the physiologically active) and bound forms. Both free and bound protein S levels fall in pregnancy in a rather variable manner, and therefore the diagnosis of protein S deficiency cannot be made reliably until after pregnancy.

REFERENCES

Badaracco, M.A. and Vessey, M. (1974). Recurrence of venous thromboembolism disease and use of oral contraceptives. *British Medical Journal* **1**, 215.

Bergqvist, A., Bergqvist, D., Lindhagen, A., *British Medical Journal* and Matzsch, T. (1990). Late symptoms after pregnancy-related deep vein thrombosis. *British Journal of Obstetrics and Gynaecology* **97**, 338.

Dalhman, T., Lindvall, N., and Hellgren, M. (1990). Osteopenia in pregnancy during long-term heparin treatment: A radiological study post partum. *British Journal of Obstetrics and Gynaecology* **97**, 221.

Denson, K.W.E. and Bonnar, J. (1973). The measurement of heparin: a method based on the potentiation of anti-factor Xa. *Thrombosis and Haemostasis* **30**, 471.

Department of Health (1994). *Report on Confidential Enquiries into Maternal Deaths in United Kingdom*, 1988–1990, HMSO, London.

de Swiet, M. (ed.) (1989). Thromboembolism. In *Medical disorders in obstetric practice*, (2nd edn), p.166. Blackwell Scientific Publications, Oxford.

de Swiet, M. *et al.* (1983). Prolonged heparin therapy in pregnancy causes bone demineralisation (heparin induced-osteopenia). *British Journal of Obstetrics and Gynaecology* **90**, 1129.

Greer, I.A., Barry, J., Mackon, N. and Allan, P.L. (1990). Diagnosis of deep venous thrombosis in pregnancy: a new role for diagnostic ultrasound. *British Journal of Obstetrics and Gynaecology* **97**, 53.

Hall, J.G., Pauli, R.M., and Wilson, K.M. (1980). Maternal and fetal sequelae of anticoagulation during pregnancy. *American Journal of Medicine* **68**, 122.

Heijboer, H., Brandjes, D.P.M., Buller, H.R., Sturk, A. and ten Cate, J.W. (1990). Deficiencies of coagulation-inhibiting and fibrinolytic proteins in outpatients with deep-vein thrombosis. *New England Journal of Medicine* **323**, 1512.

Horellou, M.H., Conard, J., Bertina, R.M., and Samana, M. (1984). Congenital protein C deficiency and thrombotic disease in nine French families. *British Medical Journal* **289**, 1285.

Howell, R., Fidler, J., Letsky, E., and de Swiet, M. (1983). The risks of antenatal subcutaneous heparin prophylaxis: a controlled trial. *British Journal of Obstetrics and Gynaecology* **90**, 1124.

Hughson, W.G., Friedman, P.J., Feigin, D.S., Resnik, R., and Moser, K.M., (1982). Post partum pulmonary effusion: a common radiologic finding. *Annals of Internal Medicine* **97**, 856.

Lao, T.T., de Swiet, M., Letsky, E., and Walters, B.N.J. (1985). Prophylaxis of thromboembolism in pregnancy: an alternative. *British Journal of Obstetrics and Gynaecology* **92**, 202.

Megha, A., Finzi, G., Poli, T., Manotti, C., and Dettori, A.G. (1990). Bilateral deep vein thrombosis in a pregnant woman with antithrombin III deficiency: treatment of acute episodes and preparation for delivery with replacement treatment. *Journal of Obstetrics and Gynaecology* **10**, 220.

Orme, M.L.'E. *et al.* (1977). May mothers given warfarin breast-feed their infants? *British Medical Journal* **1**, 1564.

Villasanta, U. (1965). Thromboembolic disease in pregnancy. *American Journal of Obstetrics and Gynecology* **93**, 142.

Warwick, R., Hutton, R.A., Goff, L., Letsky, E., and Heard, M. (1989).

Changes in protein C and free protein S during pregnancy and following hysterectomy. *Journal of the Royal Society of Medicine* **82**, 591.

Winter, J.H., *et al.* (1982). Familial antithrombin III deficiency. *Quarterly Journal of Medicine* **204**, 373.

13.6 Chest diseases in pregnancy

M. DE SWIET

Physiology

The pregnant woman at rest increases her minute volume by about 40 per cent within the first trimester of pregnancy. This is achieved by an increase in tidal volume rather than in respiratory rate. The increased ventilation is more than adequate to account for the increased metabolic rate of the mother and fetus even in the later stages of pregnancy when maternal oxygen consumption increases by about 45 ml/min. The stimulus to increased ventilation is said to be increased progesterone secretion, but it is likely that this is not the only factor.

The majority view is that vital capacity and airways resistance do not change in pregnancy, although, surprisingly, transfer factor is reduced. The uterus enlarging within the abdomen partly accounts for a 20 per cent reduction in residual volume, although the reduction in residual volume occurs early in pregnancy and the chest wall changes shape early in pregnancy before there can be any mechanical effect due to the uterus. The reduction in residual volume is more marked in patients supine than in those who are sitting. PaO_2 in the sitting or erect posture is unchanged in pregnancy; $PaCO_2$ falls to about 4.0 kPa (30 mmHg). Plasma bicarbonate also falls proportionally to about 20 mmol/l, so that there is no change in the arterial pH. The PaO_2 does fall by up to 2.0 kPa (15 mmHg) in patients who are supine in late pregnancy. This fall is probably due to unequal ventilation/perfusion ratios subsequent to airways closure during tidal breathing. Therefore, where possible, blood gases for diagnostic estimation should always be taken in pregnant patients when they are sitting.

Breathlessness is a common symptom in pregnancy, presumably associated with the 40 per cent increase in ventilation that occurs in normal women. However, this cannot be the entire explanation because ventilation increases from before 4 weeks, whereas the maximum incidence of onset of breathlessness is at 28 to 31 weeks' gestation. Breathlessness is worrying for the doctor (and for the patient) because it may also be associated with cardiopulmonary disease, particularly pulmonary embolism. In the absence of other features of cardiopulmonary disease, and with normal findings on examination, useful investigations are chest radiography, arterial blood gas estimation, oximetry to determine oxygen saturation at rest and on exercise, and full lung function testing including measurement of transfer factor (see Chapter 13.5).

Lung disease in pregnancy—general considerations

Although ventilation does increase by 40 per cent in pregnancy, this increase is trivial in comparison to the marked increase (perhaps tenfold) that is possible during exercise. Women have a considerable reserve of ventilatory capacity and pregnancy does not challenge this much. Respiratory failure due to chronic respiratory disease is therefore uncommon in pregnancy. Also, the most frequent forms of respiratory disease leading to respiratory failure, chronic bronchitis and emphysema, are relatively uncommon in women, and particularly uncommon during their child-bearing years. The major problem in women with chronic conditions such as asthma or tuberculosis, is therefore a consideration of the effect of therapy on pregnancy.

Table 1 *Obstetric causes of adult respiratory distress syndrome (ARDS)*

Shock	Antepartum haemorrhage
	Postpartum haemorrhage
Aspiration of stomach contents	
Disseminated intravascular coagulopathy	Accidental haemorrhage
	Amniotic fluid embolus
	Severe pre-eclampsia/eclampsia
	Dead fetus syndrome
	Gram-negative septicaemia
Infection	Puerperal sepsis
Anaphylaxis	Acute pyelonephritis
Hydatidiform mole	

Acute respiratory failure is, however, a major cause of maternal mortality, since adult respiratory distress syndrome (ARDS) is the final common pathway for many obstetric disasters and carries a mortality of about 70 per cent. Indeed, much of the practice of modern obstetrics is directed towards the avoidance of ARDS. For example, the trend towards epidural rather than general anaesthesia reduces the risk of inhalation of stomach contents, and therefore of ARDS. Epidural, rather than general anaesthesia, is specifically indicated in all patients with significant chest disease.

Adult respiratory distress syndrome

The management of this condition is described in Section 17. Specific obstetric causes are indicated in Table 1: of these, aspiration of stomach contents is probably the most common, followed by shock with or without disseminated intravascular coagulation. Some of these obstetric causes of ARDS warrant further consideration.

Inhalation of stomach contents

This only occurs in the absence of an effective gag reflex which, in obstetric practice, is almost invariably associated with general anaesthesia. Most obstetric units starve their patients once labour is established, and it is common practice to give regular antacid therapy, since it is believed that the low pH of gastric contents makes them particularly harmful to the lungs. However, ARDS has also developed in patients given aluminium hydroxide in labour after inhalation of stomach contents at pH 6.4. The particulate nature of stomach contents (and aluminium and magnesium compounds) may therefore be important. An alternative treatment would be to use non-particulate sodium citrate. Although the results of trials of H_2-receptor antagonists, to decrease gastric acidity, and metoclopramide, to increase stomach emptying, are awaited with interest, avoidance of inhalation is the single most important preventive measure. Since the maternal mortality from inhalation has fallen from 6 per cent of all maternal deaths in England and Wales in 1976 to 1978 to 0.4 per cent of deaths in the United Kingdom in 1985 to 1987, these measures are probably having some effect.

Amniotic fluid embolism

This catastrophe occurs because amniotic fluid and other material of fetal origin enters the maternal circulation. Usually, though not invariably, it occurs at the end of a vigorous labour with intact membranes. Major elements in the pathogenesis are widespread deposition of platelet and fibrin thrombi and DIC caused by the very high thromboplastin activity of amniotic fluid. The initial presentation is with profound hypotension and cyanosis. If the patient survives this, she is at risk of dying from haemorrhage due to DIC, and if she survives the DIC she is at risk from ARDS. In the anaesthetized patient, differentiation from inhalation is important. Bronchospasm is common in inhalation, but very rare in amniotic fluid embolus. DIC is an early presenting feature in amniotic fluid embolus, but it occurs late after inhalation. The differential diagnosis of other occult causes of collapse in pregnancy is considered in Table 1 of Chapter 13.5. The diagnosis of amniotic fluid embolus can only be confirmed by finding fetal material, i.e. squames or hairs, in the maternal blood (from central venous pressure line), in the sputum or in the lungs at autopsy. Even the finding of fetal material in maternal blood is not specific since this has been reported in some normal women having Swann Ganz catheterization in labour. There is no specific treatment for amniotic fluid embolism. In the acute stage, patients will require oxygen, massive fluid therapy, and treatment for DIC. If they survive this, they may require treatment for ARDS.

Asthma

Bronchial asthma is the commonest chest disease in pregnancy (prevalence about 3 per cent). In keeping with the lack of change in airways resistance in normal pregnancy, there is no evidence that pregnancy consistently affects the clinical course of asthma. There is also little evidence that bronchial asthma affects the outcome of pregnancy, apart from an increased risk of fetal growth retardation in those patients who are severely compromised. In practice, these patients are usually taking regular steroids in excess of the equivalent of 12 mg of prednisone per day; however, it is likely that the cause of the growth retardation is intermittent hypoxaemia rather than steroid therapy. It is unusual for patients to have acute attacks of asthma in labour. Perhaps the high circulating levels of endogenous catecholamines, corticosteroids, and prostaglandins are protective.

The treatment of patients with asthma requires little modification in pregnancy. β-Sympathomimetic drugs such as salbutamol are used widely in pregnancy for the treatment and prophylaxis of premature labour. Their safety for the fetus has therefore been well documented. When given intravenously, they may cause maternal pulmonary oedema, but the dose given in this way is far greater than that given by inhalation, which is the preferred route for the treatment of asthma. Patients with asthma treated by β-sympathomimetic drugs, whether inhaled or taken orally, do not have any delay in the onset of labour, nor do they have prolonged labours. The new, long-acting β₂-agonist salmeterol is likely to be popular in patients who are not pregnant. Since very little of the inhaled drug enters the systemic circulation, it is unlikely to affect the fetus, but at present there is insufficient information to recommend its use in pregnancy. However, patients who require prophylactic therapy for asthma in pregnancy should, as in the non-pregnant state, rely on inhaled glucocorticoids (see below) with β-sympathomimetics reserved for rescue therapy.

It may be necessary or desirable to use glucocorticoids in pregnancy There is no evidence of teratogenicity in humans, and no evidence for suppression of the fetal hypothalamo-pituitary–adrenal axis when the mother is given prednisone. Prednisolone, which does not require further metabolism for activity, and other glucocorticoids, such as betamethasone, which cross the placenta more freely, may affect the fetus. The indications for the use of oral steroids in pregnancy complicated by asthma are therefore the same as in the non-pregnant state, although prednisone is preferred to any of the other glucocorticoids. Mothers who are taking prednisone may have suppression of their hypothalamo-pituitary–adrenal axis and should be given parenteral hydrocortisone during labour or at other times of stress. Inhaled corticosteroids such as beclomethasone achieve very low blood levels and are therefore safe for the fetus; the same is true for inhaled disodium cromoglycate, atropine, and ipratropium bromide.

Aminophylline is the theophylline preparation most widely used in asthma, and it, too, has been assessed in pregnancy in women at risk of premature delivery with no evidence of adverse fetal effects.

Of the commonly used antibiotics, aminoglycosides should only be given for more than 24 h in pregnancy if there is no alternative, and then with continuous monitoring of blood levels. This is because of the risk of damage to the fetal eighth nerve and kidney. Tetracycline should not be used because it causes permanent discoloration of the fetal teeth. Iodine-containing expectorants should not be used in pregnancy or in lactating women, since the iodine freely crosses the placenta, is excreted in breast milk, and may cause hypothyroidism in the infant.

It has been suggested that ergometrine can cause severe bronchospasm in patients with asthma. Syntocinon® should therefore be used for the management of the third stage of labour.

In summary, the management of patients with asthma requires little modification because of pregnancy. In the unlikely event of such a severe attack of asthma as to require ventilation, maternal hypoxaemia should be avoided because of the associated severe fetal hypoxaemia; so also should hypocapnia ($P_{CO_2} < 17$ mmHg, 2.3 kPa) and alkalosis (pH > 7.6) since these have been associated with fetal hypoxaemia, probably due to impaired placental transport.

Chronic bronchitis, bronchiectasis, and emphysema

These conditions are now very uncommon in pregnancy. Single-case reports document the relative safety of obstructive airways disease associated with α_1-antitrypsin deficiency. Since pulmonary hypertension is poorly tolerated in pregnancy, cor pulmonale is likely to be the factor limiting maternal safety. The presence of arterial hypoxaemia puts the fetus at risk from intrauterine growth retardation.

Cystic fibrosis

(See Sections 14 and 17.)

Because of better management in childhood, more patients with cystic fibrosis are surviving and therefore may want to have children. Because of the large number of cystic fibrosis mutations that have been discovered (more than 150) only 80 per cent of all heterozygotes can be identified. First-trimester prenatal diagnosis is possible on genetic material prepared from chorionic villi using linked DNA probes in at least two-thirds of couples presenting with one affected child. The prevalence of the gene in the community is said to be 1 in 20, although the overall prevalence of the disease is 1 in 2500. Therefore, patients with cystic fibrosis should be counselled that there is a 1 in 20 to 1 in 44 chance that their child will have the condition if the father's status is unknown. If the father is a heterozygote, the risk is 1 in 2. All the children of affected mothers will be carriers.

From a postal survey of 125 patients from 119 centres in the United States by Cohen, it would appear that the maternal mortality in the first 6 months following pregnancy (12 per cent) was equal to that in 1 year at other times; the perinatal mortality was considerably elevated at 11 per cent. However, these figures relate to experience before 1975, and are likely to be pessimistic. Also, it is by no means clear which are the particular factors that put a patient in a high-risk group. Many scoring schemes have been used, some based on rather subjective criteria, such as breathlessness or clinical evidence of right ventricular hypertrophy. Since the patients die from recurrent chest infection and cor pulmonale, the risk of which is related to the degree of hypoxaemia, it is suggested that these are the criteria by which the advisability of pregnancy should be judged. If there is any doubt, arterial Po_2 and pulmonary artery pressure should be measured, using a Swan Ganz catheter for the latter. Reasonable cutoff points at which the maternal and fetal outcome of pregnancy are likely to be in jeopardy, would be a Pao_2 less than 60 mmHg (8 kPa) when the patient is free from infection and breathing air, or a pulmonary artery pressure greater than 35 mmHg.

Apart from high quality and intensity of obstetric and medical care, no specific measures are necessary in pregnant patients with cystic fibrosis. Most of the drugs used have been considered above. Inhaled aminoglycosides are probably safe in pregnancy. In Cohen's series, 26 patients received intravenous and intramuscular aminoglycosides with no evidence of teratogenesis. The risk of fetal eighth nerve and renal damage from this form of therapy still remains.

Patients may have malabsorption due to pancreatic involvement in cystic fibrosis, and an increase in pancreatic supplements may be necessary. Diabetes mellitus could also become manifest for the first time in pregnancy. All patients with cystic fibrosis should be screened for diabetes early in pregnancy, and at about 28 weeks' gestation. There is also an increased risk of pneumothorax in labour (see below).

There has been concern that women with cystic fibrosis should not breast feed their infants because of the possible very high sodium content of their milk (up to 280 mmol/l). This risk has probably been exaggerated, since the samples of breast milk initially analysed were taken from women who were not lactating freely, a situation in which all breast milk has a high sodium content. More recent isolated studies have indicated that once lactation has been established, the breast milk has a normal sodium content. Nevertheless, until more data are available, the sodium content of each patient's breast milk should be checked if the mother proposes to breast feed.

Kyphoscoliosis

Mild degrees of kyphoscoliosis have no effect on pregnancy. Successful pregnancy is possible in patients with severe disease who may have a vital capacity of as little as 1000 ml. As in the other chest diseases, hypoxaemia and pulmonary hypertension will be the limiting factors. Some patients with severe kyphoscoliosis become exhausted and then hypoxaemic in the last trimester. Any suggestion of excessive fatigue should be an indication for hospital admission for rest. Progressive hypoxaemia with or without evidence of fetal compromise is an indication for delivery. Labour and/or Caesarean section are best managed with the assistance of epidural anaesthesia, since this reduces the risk of atelectasis. Epidural anaesthesia can be given to most patients, even those with very severe spinal abnormalities.

Pneumothorax and pneumomediastinum

There are rare complications of pregnancy (incidence less than 1 in 10 000) but they probably occur more commonly in pregnancy and particularly in labour, than in the non-pregnant state. Presumably the raised intrathoracic pressure due to straining in labour is a contributing factor, but there is usually some predisposing condition such as asthma, cystic fibrosis, or emphysema. Both conditions present with chest pain, and if there is a major leak of air, the patient may be hypotensive and cyanosed (tension pneumothorax, malignant pneumomediastinum). The differential diagnosis of these and other occult causes of collapse in pregnancy are considered in Chapter 13.5. The physical signs and management of the pneumothorax are no different in pregnancy from those in the non-pregnant state, and are described in Section 17.

The occurrence of pneumomediastinum is almost unique to pregnancy, apart from cases involving trauma to the chest wall. It is postulated that, as in pneumothorax, air leaks from an emphysematous bulla but instead of entering the pleural space it tracks to the mediastinum. It may also leave the mediastinum and enter subcutaneous tissue around the neck (subcutaneous emphysema). This produces a characteristic crackling sound and feel when the skin is palpated, and in pneumomediastinum the same sound may be heard, synchronous with the heart beat on auscultation (Hamman's sign). The radiological signs of air in the mediastinum and pericardium are diagnostic. Small leaks resolve spontaneously; major leaks causing haemodynamic embarrassment need to be treated with a chest drain and underwater seal as for pneumothorax. Cardiorespiratory embarrassment caused by pneumomediastinum usually requires thoracotomy. If a patient has a past history of pneumothorax or pneumomediastinum, she should have an elective forceps delivery to prevent recurrence during straining in labour.

Tuberculosis

Before the advent of antituberculous therapy, tuberculosis was the cause of many maternal deaths, particularly in the puerperium. This is no longer so, and there should be no excess mortality from tuberculosis in pregnancy. The placenta is a very efficient filter, and intrauterine infection of the fetus almost never occurs.

Rifampicin is the most effective, widely used antituberculous drug; it is safe in the second and third trimesters, and some would say throughout pregnancy. However, because of a cluster of nine variously but severely malformed children from patients taking rifampicin in the first trimester, it is sensible not to use rifampicin early in pregnancy, unless the clinical indications are overwhelming. Isoniazid and ethambutol have been used extensively in pregnancy and are safe for the fetus. Pregnant patients in particular should receive supplementary pyridoxine when taking isoniazid. A dose of 50 mg/day has been shown to give adequate blood levels in pregnancy, but the conventional dose of 10 mg/day may also be effective.

Pyrazinamide has not been used so extensively, but there is no evidence of toxicity in the fetus. Streptomycin should be avoided for the reasons given above. Ethionamide should not be used because of reports of multiple congenital abnormalities. Within these limitations, the pregnant patient with tuberculosis should be treated in the same way as she would be in the non-pregnant state.

Patients who have been adequately treated in the past for tuberculosis do not require prophylactic therapy in pregnancy. After birth, babies should only be isolated from their mothers if the mothers are still smear positive. Since modern antituberculosis regimes render the sputum sterile within 2 weeks and markedly reduce the number of organisms within 24 h, this should not occur frequently. The neonate should be treated with prophylactic isoniazid for 3 months. After this period BCG vaccination is given in the United Kingdom but not in the United States. It is not clear whether neonatal BCG vaccination adds any further protection to isoniazid prophylaxis. It is not without risks; skin ulceration and osteitis may occur, and occasionally disseminated disease, particularly if the mother has an immunodeficiency state. As isoniazid therapy does not affect the immunogenicity of BCG vaccine, there is no longer any rationale for the use of isoniazid-resistant BCG neonatal vaccination.

Sarcoid

This condition is rarely a problem in pregnancy. Patients who have had sarcoid in the past have no extra risk of relapse in pregnancy. Those who have active sarcoid during pregnancy tend to improve, possibly because of the increase in free as well as protein-bound cortisol levels. There is a tendency to deteriorate in the puerperium, but this should not be overemphasized. Since patients take many vitamins in pregnancy, those with sarcoid should be warned not to take vitamin D to which they may be very sensitive.

Pneumonia

Pneumonia is an uncommon complication of pregnancy and, unless the diagnosis is clear-cut, other conditions which produce chest symptoms and signs, such as pulmonary embolus should always be considered.

Bacterial pneumonia should be treated with antibiotics. In addition, aggressive antipyretic therapy with tepid sponging, fans, and regular paracetamol should be used, because of the association between pyrexia and premature labour. During epidemics such as the influenza epidemic in 1930 viral pneumonia has caused a high mortality in pregnancy, and clinicians should be aware that this condition should not be dismissed lightly.

Ten per cent of maternal varicella infections may be complicated by pneumonia, which has an appreciable mortality. Therefore all pregnant women who have close exposure to varicella-zoster virus and who have no demonstrable antibody should receive zoster immune globulin. Those who develop varicella should receive acyclovir 10 to 30 mg/kg daily in three divided doses for 5 days.

REFERENCES

Apter, A.J., Greenberger, P.A., and Patterson, R. (1989). Outcomes of pregnancy in adolescents with severe asthma. *Archives of Internal Medicine*, **149**, 2571–5.

Boyd, K., Walker, E. (1988). Use of acyclovir to treat chickenpox in pregnancy. *British Medical Journal*, **296**, 393–4.

Cohen, L.F., Di Sant'Agnese, P.A., and Friedlander, J. (1980). Cystic fibrosis and pregnancy. A national survey. *Lancet* **ii**, 842–4.

Department of Health and Social Security (1991) *Report on confidential enquiries into maternal deaths in United Kingdom 1985–87*. HMSO, London.

de Swiet, M. The respiratory system. In *Clinical physiology and obstetrics* (1990), (2nd edn), (ed. F. Hytten and G.V.P. Chamberlain). Blackwell Scientific Publications, Oxford.

de Swiet, M. (ed.) 1989. Diseases of the respiratory system. In *Medical disorders of obstetric practice*, pp. 1–47. Blackwell Scientific Publications, Oxford.

Grossman, III, J.H. and Littner, M.D. (1976). Severe sarcoidosis in pregnancy. *Obstetrics and Gynecology*, **50**, (Suppl.), 81s–84s.

Hague, W.M. (1980). Mediastinal and subcutaneous emphysema in a pregnant asthmatic. *British Journal of Obstetrics and Gynaecology* **87**, 440–3.

Johnson, S.R., Varner, M.W., Yates, S.J. and Hanson, R. (1983). Diagnosis of maternal cystic fibrosis during pregnancy. *Obstetrics and Gynecology* **61**, 2s–7s.

Lancet Editorial (1990). Perinatal prophylaxis of tuberculosis. *Lancet* **336**, 1479–80.

Juniper, E.F., Daniel, E.E., Roberts, R.S., Kline, P.A., Hargreave, F.E., and Newhouse, M.T. (1989). Improvement of airway responsiveness and asthma severity during pregnancy. *American Review of Respiratory Disease* **140**, 924–31.

Milne, J.A., Pack, A.I., and Coutts, J.R.T. (1977). Maternal gas exchange and acid base status during normal pregnancy. *Scottish Medical Journal* **22**, 108.

Milne, J.A., Howie, A.D., and Pack, A.I. (1978). Dyspnoea during normal pregnancy. *British Journal of Obstetrics and Gynaecology* **85**, 260–3.

Morgan, M. (1979). Amniotic fluid embolism. *Anaesthesia* **34**, 20–32.

Russell, I.F. and Chambers, W.A. (1981). Closing volume in normal pregnancy. *British Journal of Anaesthesia* **53**, 1043–7.

Siegler, D. and Zorab, P.A. (1981). Pregnancy in thoracic scoliosis. *British Journal of Diseases of the Chest*, **75**, 367–70.

Sims, C.D., Chamberlain, G.V.P., and de Swiet, M. (1976). Lung function tests in bronchial asthma during and after pregnancy. *British Journal of Obstetrics and Gynaecology* **88**, 434–7.

Snider, D.E., Layde, P.M., Johnson, M.W., and Lyle, H.A. (1980). Treatment of tuberculosis during pregnancy. *American Review of Respiratory Disease* **122**, 67–78.

Steen, J.S.M. and Stainton-Ellis, D.M. (1977). Rifampicin in pregnancy. *Lancet* **ii**, 601–5.

Turner, E.S., Greenberger, P.A., and Patterson, R. (1980). Management of the pregnant asthmatic patient. *Annals of Internal Medicine* **6**, 905–18.

Wald, N. (1991). Couple screening for cystic fibrosis. *Lancet*, **338**, 1318–19.

Weinberger, S.E., Weiss, S.T., Cohen, W.R., Weiss, J.W., and Johnson, T.S. (1980). Pregnancy and the lung. *American Review of Respiratory Disease* **121**, 559–81.

White, R.J., Coutts, I.I., Gibbs, C.J., and MacIntyre, C. (1989). A prospective study of asthma during pregnancy and the puerperium. *Respiratory Medicine* **83**, 103–6.

13.7 Endocrine disease in pregnancy

A. M. McGregor

INTRODUCTION

The intimate relationship between normal function of the endocrine system and reproduction means that in many situations pre-existing endocrine disease is likely to be associated with infertility. When fertility is not impaired, despite pre-existing endocrine disease in the mother or, more importantly, when endocrine diseases arise or are unmasked for the first time during pregnancy, the recognition of the problem, although often difficult, is exceedingly important. The considerable structural and functional changes that occur in the endocrine system as part of normal pregnancy, the alterations in circulating levels of hormone either because of altered patterns of secretion or changes in circulating binding proteins, and the clinical manifestations of these endocrine changes in the pregnant woman make the discrimination of normal from abnormal more difficult. Diseases of the endocrine system occur only rarely during pregnancy but if unrecognized, their impact on the pregnancy itself and on maternal well-being during pregnancy and in the postpartum period is considerable; failure to recognize many of these diseases may have catastrophic consequences.

Pituitary disease

INTRODUCTION

As a result of hyperplasia, predominantly of the prolactin-secreting lactotroph cells, the normal pituitary gland enlarges during pregnancy. This normal response to pregnancy may have important implications for women known to have prolactin-secreting pituitary adenomata who become pregnant. Physiological enlargement may be a contributor to the infarction of pituitary tumours, which may occur during pregnancy or immediately after delivery (see below). It may also contribute to postpartum infarction of the previously normal pituitary (Sheehan's syndrome).

Prolactin-secreting pituitary adenomas

Characteristically, women with hyperprolactinaemia due to a prolactin-secreting pituitary adenoma (prolactinoma) present with amenorrhoea and infertility (see Chapters 12.2 and 12.8.1). The tumours may be macroadenomata (> 10 mm in size) or microadenomata (< 10 mm in

Table 1 *Influence of pregnancy on the enlargement of prolactinomas*

Tumour size	Previous treatment	Symptomatic enlargement in pregnancy	Asymptomatic enlargement detected postpartum
Microadenoma	—	< 2%	< 5%
Macroadenoma	—	16–20%	9%
Macroadenoma	+[a]	< 5%	0%

[a]Pituitary surgery and/or irradiation.

Table 2 *Alterations in thyroid function in normal pregnancy*

Oestrogen-induced TBG synthesis
Free thyroid hormones
  ↑ first trimester (HCG-induced)
  ↓ second and third trimester (but always within the normal
    adult non-pregnant range)
↑ TSH
second and third trimester
within normal range
↑ Thyroid size
↑ Renal and placental iodide clearance

HCG, human chorionic gonadotrophin; TBG, thyroxine binding globulin; TSH, thyroid stimulating hormone.

size). In women keen to become pregnant treatment is influenced by the size of the lesion but also by the potential impact of therapy on surrounding normal pituitary tissue and the influence which damage to this will have on subsequent fertility. On these grounds many will prefer to use bromocriptine in all patients with macroadenomata, and provided there is a good response with evidence of reduction in both tumour size and prolactin secretion, will consider using this agent in preference to surgery and irradiation to the pituitary until the woman has completed her family. In women with prolactinomata who become pregnant on bromocriptine, less than 5 per cent of those with macroadenomata develop significant enlargement of their tumour during pregnancy. In contrast, in patients with macroadenoma who have not been treated prior to pregnancy with surgery and irradiation up to 20 per cent may develop symptomatic enlargement of the pituitary (Table 1). There is therefore a need for careful monitoring throughout the pregnancy with monthly visits to check the visual fields and to determine whether symptoms such as headache and visual disturbance, particularly field defects, are developing. Whenever evidence of tumour enlargement is suggested, a CT or MRI scan of the pituitary is required. Although a large body of evidence has accumulated over a number of years on the safety of bromocriptine medication during pregnancy, the sensible and safe approach is to withhold it once pregnancy is confirmed and, if possible, to avoid its use during the first trimester. Thereafter, particularly when evidence of tumour enlargement is obtained it can be reintroduced for the remainder of the pregnancy. It has, however, been used successfully throughout pregnancy, when evidence of tumour expansion during the first trimester has been detected.

A further important, although uncommon, consequence of an enlarging prolactinoma during pregnancy is subsequent infarction or haemorrhage into the tumour, leading to pituitary apoplexy. This diagnosis is suggested when the patient presents with sudden onset of headache, neck stiffness, nausea, vomiting, loss of consciousness, and collapse. Visual field defects and impaired eye movements resulting from extension of the haemorrhagic lesion towards the chiasma or intracavernous sinus, respectively, may also result. Prompt diagnosis and treatment with adequate replacement of glucocorticoids and circulatory support are essential in this life-threatening situation.

Growth hormone secreting pituitary adenomata

In up to a third of women presenting with acromegaly due to a growth hormone secreting pituitary adenoma, hyperprolactinaemia coexists. This may either represent co-secretion of prolactin by a mixed growth hormone and prolactin secreting adenoma or pituitary stalk compression from the tumour itself. In women with acromegaly who are hyperprolactinaemic, bromocriptine is successful in restoring fertility.

Diabetes insipidus

In normal pregnancy the placenta produces large amounts of vasopressinase which inactivates vasopressin. Pregnant women, however, experience thirst and release vasopressin at lower levels of plasma osmolality than do non-pregnant individuals, so that plasma osmolality is normally reduced in pregnancy (see Chapters 20.1 and 20.2.1). Although the development of frank diabetes insipidus is exceedingly rare in pregnancy, should significant polyuria and polydipsia develop then it is important to evaluate both anterior and posterior pituitary function to exclude the possibility of a tumour of, or infarction or haemorrhage into, the pituitary. More commonly, these symptoms are a manifestation of the enhanced degradation of vasopressin by vasopressinase. If any treatment is required DDAVP (desmopressin, which is not affected by vasopressinase) will control symptoms and can then be withdrawn with the fall of vasopressinase levels following delivery.

Diabetes insipidus that develops for the first time during the postpartum period may be a manifestation of Sheehan's syndrome and in this situation may only become a problem following the introduction of glucocorticoid replacement because in its absence the ability of the distal tubule to generate free water is impaired.

Lymphocytic hypophysitis

Women with this rare condition characteristically present in the postpartum period with symptoms either due to the effects of an enlarged pituitary (due to lymphocytic infiltration) and therefore with headaches and visual field defects, or because of hypopituitarism. Without access to pituitary tissue discrimination between lymphocytic infiltration, which is the hallmark of this disease, and a pituitary adenoma is difficult. Unlike the situation in Sheehan's syndrome, there is no evidence of haemorrhage at the time of delivery. CT scanning or MRI and assessment of pituitary function will define the extent of the lesion anatomically and functionally. Unless evidence of progression is evident, a process of careful conservative management is worth considering, since in a number of cases spontaneous remission with return of normal pituitary function has been observed. Evidence of progression of the lesion requires consideration of surgical intervention.

Sheehan's syndrome

Sheehan's syndrome describes the situation in which, following hypotension and shock due to obstetric haemorrhage, there is subsequent development of pituitary necrosis during the postpartum period. The extent of the necrosis will determine the time of presentation and also the degree of hypopituitarism. Acute pituitary infarction may present with the symptoms and signs of adrenal insufficiency and be life-threatening if unrecognized. More characteristically, however, patients present a considerable time after the obstetric event leading to the infarction with histories which may include symptoms such as failure to lactate postpartum, failure to menstruate subsequently, loss of axillary and genital hair, fatigue, and cold intolerance (see Chapter 20.1).

Thyroid disease

In the normal pregnant woman a number of alterations occur in thyroid function during pregnancy (Table 2). The oestrogen-induced increase in serum thyroxine binding globulin (TBG) levels, largely due to its altered glycosylation and the reduced metabolic clearance of TBG, has a major impact on the assessment of thyroid function using assays which measure total tri-iodothyronine (T_3) or total thyroxine (T_4). Assays which measure free T_4 and free T_3 levels suggest a small increase in both during the first trimester, which is probably accounted for by the increased levels of circulating human chorionic gonadotropin (HCG). This is then followed through the succeeding trimesters of pregnancy by a small but significant decline in thyroid function, which at all times remains within the normal adult range. This is accompanied by a small but significant rise, again within the normal range, of thyroid stimulating hormone (TSH) levels through the second and third trimesters of pregnancy. Associated with these changes in function are a significant increase in size of the thyroid gland through pregnancy and an increased iodide clearance by the kidney and later by the placenta. The increased renal iodide loss due to increased glomerular filtration rates in pregnant women is associated with a decline in the plasma inorganic iodine concentration, which in areas where iodine intake is marginal or low can be associated with absolute or relative iodine deficiency.

Fetal thyroid hormone production cannot be detected before 12 weeks of gestation but thereafter there is a gradual maturation of the hypothalamic–pituitary–thyroid axis until term. Neuronal development in the first trimester is known to be crucially dependent on maternal thyroid hormones, which at this stage of gestation cross the placenta freely. Iodide, too, will cross the placenta, and excess maternal ingestion of iodide for prolonged periods will suppress fetal thyroid function and lead to the development of a fetal goitre.

Maternal hyperthyroidism

The hypermetabolic, hyperdynamic state of normal pregnancy makes the diagnosis of hyperthyroidism during pregnancy a difficult one. Thyroid enlargement, heat intolerance, palpitations, fatigue, and emotional upset are common to both pregnancy and hyperthyroidism. A past history of thyroid disease or, on clinical assessment, evidence of Graves' disease with ophthalmopathy should raise suspicion. These signs in conjunction with a marked tachycardia, weight loss, and a bruit over the thyroid strongly suggest hyperthyroidism.

Hyperthyroidism occurs in approximately 2 of every 1000 pregnancies, which is considerably lower than the expected prevalence of the disease amongst non-pregnant women. This probably reflects (1) the effect exerted by hyperthyroidism on ovarian function, resulting in reduced fertility; and (2) the well-recognized amelioration during pregnancy of the autoimmune process inducing Graves' disease. Therefore, the majority of women presenting in pregnancy with hyperthyroidism are those in whom hyperthyroidism has been controlled by antithyroid drugs, and who may well have been on such treatment at the time of conception. The previously high fetal mortality rate in pregnancy associated with hyperthyroidism has fallen dramatically with effective antithyroid medication. Biochemical confirmation of the clinical suspicion of hyperthyroidism is essential and the combined use of assays of free T_3 and free T_4 in conjunction with measurement of TSH (undetectable in a sensitive assay in hyperthyroidism) are all that is required. Radioisotope studies of any kind are contraindicated during pregnancy because of the risk to the fetus.

The aim of management of hyperthyroidism in pregnancy is to control the maternal disease but at the same time to ensure that the treatment does not in any way interfere with the normal development and function of the fetal thyroid gland. The treatment of choice is with antithyroid drugs, although always with the recognition that should these fail to control the disease partial thyroidectomy later in pregnancy may be required. Carbimazole or propylthiouracil, which inhibit synthesis of thyroid hormones and may also suppress the autoimmune response in patients with Graves' disease, are the drugs of choice. Doses should be as low as is possible to maintain thyroid hormone levels in the upper normal range in the mother, to ensure that with the placental passage of

these drugs fetal hypothyroidism is not induced. In this context it is crucial that the regimen of high doses of antithyroid drugs in combination with thyroxine (blocking and replacement regimen) often used in the non-pregnant woman is not applied in pregnancy because of the resultant induction of hypothyroidism and a large goitre in the fetus, the latter making delivery difficult. The patient needs to be made aware of the rare but severe side-effect of agranulocytosis which may result from the use of these antithyroid drugs and should be informed of the possible consequences and therefore of the need to remain vigilant while taking them. There are no convincing reports of teratogenesis being attributable to this group of drugs. The antithyroid drugs are excreted in breast milk but at such low levels as to be insufficient to interfere with neonatal thyroid function, and therefore breast feeding is not contraindicated while mothers take this medication. When carbimazole fails to control maternal hyperthyroidism, or if compliance is a problem, surgical intervention must be considered. Preparation for surgery may require admission to hospital and in the short term the use of higher doses of antithyroid drugs may be required to establish euthyroidism, with the operation best performed late in the second or early in the third trimester.

Maternal hypothyroidism

Severe hypothyroidism is rarely seen in pregnancy because such women are commonly infertile. The prevalence of hypothyroidism in pregnant Caucasian women is estimated to be about 9 in every 1000 pregnancies. In women who become pregnant while hypothyroid there is a higher incidence of abortion, stillbirth, prematurity, pre-eclampsia, placental abruption, anaemia, postpartum haemorrhage, cardiac dysfunction, and congenital anomalies. Although the clinical features of severe hypothyroidism are easily recognized, the reduction of activity and concomitant weight gain in normal pregnancy may mask lesser degrees of hypothyroidism. The recognition of hypothyroidism in pregnant women in iodine-deficient areas of the world is of crucial importance, not only for the reasons listed above but because of the impact in such women during the first trimester of pregnancy of their iodine deficiency and hypothyroidism on the developing fetal brain. The most common cause of hypothyroidism in regions of adequate iodine intake is autoimmune thyroid disease. The detection of circulating thyroid autoantibodies will contribute to the diagnosis. A previous history of thyroid disease is of importance since women may present having been treated in the past for hyperthyroidism by partial thyroidectomy or radio-iodine, both of which can lead with time to hypothyroidism. The diagnosis of primary hypothyroidism is established by the finding of an elevated serum TSH level in the presence of a low level of free T_4. Once diagnosed, patients should be treated with T_4 replacement and the dosage increased until the TSH and free T_4 levels return to normal. This will be achieved with doses of T_4 ranging between 125 and 200 microgram daily. There is no contraindication to breast feeding while on thyroxine.

Trophoblastic disease

Hyperthyroidism may be associated with hydatidiform moles or choriocarcinomata, when it is not usually evident clinically, but is reflected only by abnormalities in biochemical indices of thyroid function. The hyperthyroidism is presumed to be due to high levels of HCG produced by the trophoblastic tumours which, at these levels, act as thyroid stimulators because of the similarity in structure of HCG and TSH. With treatment of the trophoblastic lesion the hyperthyroidism is controlled.

Hyperemesis gravidarum

(See also Chapters 13.2 and 13.13.)

A number of reports have associated hyperemesis gravidarum with abnormalities of thyroid function and in this situation treatment of the hyperthyroidism with antithyroid drugs usually allows resolution of the hyperemesis. A satisfactory explanation for the association between hyperemesis and altered thyroid function is not available, except for the recognition that the problem occurs particularly during the first trimester when HCG levels are highest and capable of thyroid stimulation.

Transient neonatal thyroid dysfunction

A number of factors (Table 3) may predispose to abnormalities of thyroid function in the new-born. The recognition that a variety of substances cross the placenta from the maternal circulation and affect the fetus is crucial. Of particular interest in women with autoimmune thyroid disease are the transient syndromes of neonatal thyroid dysfunction, which are associated with the passage across the placenta of maternal antithyroid autoantibodies, particularly of the IgG_1 subclass of immunoglobulins. Infants born to mothers with high levels of these antibodies may present with either transient neonatal hyperthyroidism or hypothyroidism, depending on whether the maternal autoantibodies to the TSH receptor on thyroid follicular cells bind to the receptor and stimulate thyroid function or bind and block thyroid cell function. Measurement of maternal TSH receptor antibody activity late in the third trimester may help to predict the likelihood of development of subsequent neonatal thyroid dysfunction. Infants are at particular risk when levels of maternal antibody are high prior to delivery. In the neonate thyroid dysfunction lasts for as long as sufficient amounts of maternal antibody remain in the baby's circulation. The baby may or may not require treatment, but the parents can at least be reassured that the condition is transient, usually resolving within 2 or 3 months of birth, and is unlikely to have any deleterious effects on the future development of the infant. With increasing use of neonatal screening programmes for congenital hypothyroidism it is important to be able to discriminate between infants with true congenital hypothyroidism and infants presenting with these transient syndromes of altered thyroid function because of transplacental passage of autoantibodies. Consideration of the criteria listed in Table 4 should help to define the subgroup of babies at risk from transient thyroid dysfunction.

Maternal postpartum thyroid dysfunction

The well-recognized improvement in clinically overt and biochemically proven autoimmune thyroid disease in pregnancy correlates with the fall in antithyroid autoantibody activity over this period. In this group of women with known autoimmune thyroid disease a characteristic rebound in antibody activity with the rise in antibody titres in the postpartum period is frequently associated with clinical and biochemical evidence of recurrence of thyroid dysfunction.

This group of women with known autoimmune thyroid disease contrasts with a group of women without a previous history of autoimmune thyroid disease who may, however, have a history of autoimmune thyroid disease in their families and the presence of detectable levels of antithyroid peroxidase autoantibodies in their circulation during pregnancy. In this group of women it is important to recognize the development of transient syndromes of thyroid dysfunction in the postpartum period. Characteristically clinically overt hyper- or hypothyroidism is not evident, but biochemically these women usually go through a phase of initial transient hyperthyroidism followed subsequently by a period of transient hypothyroidism. The disease is not associated with the characteristic TSH receptor antibodies of Graves' disease and when thyroid uptake studies have been performed in women in the postpartum period during the hyperthyroid phase the uptake of radio-isotope into their thyroids is suppressed, and therefore characteristic of a destructive thyroiditis rather than of the stimulating hyperthyroidism seen in Graves' disease. Biopsy of the thyroid at this time reveals massive lymphocytic infiltration, and as the disease proceeds into the hypothyroid phase histological evidence demonstrates thyroid follicular destruction. In the Caucasian population, about 6 per cent of women develop these transient postpartum syndromes, which are associated particularly with the HLA haplotype HLA-A1 B8 DR3, a combination of antigens well recognized

Table 3 *Maternal factors that predispose to abnormal thyroid function in the newborn*

Iodine-deficient diet
Non-thyroidal illness treated with
lithium
iodine-containing medication
Familial defect in thyroid hormone biosynthesis
Exposure to radiation while pregnant
History of autoimmune thyroid disease
Current antithyroid drug treatment
Previous surgery or radio-iodine for Graves' disease

Table 4 *Criteria for antibody-mediated transient neonatal thyroid dysfunction*

Antibody	To TSH receptor
	Blocks or stimulates receptor
	of IgG_1 sub-class which cross placenta
	Detectable in mother and newborn
Mother	Has autoimmune thyroid disease
	Has high-enough levels of the antibody
Newborn	Has abnormal thyroid function
Duration	Short (depends on rate of clearance of maternal
	IgG from infant's circulation)

to be associated with organ-specific autoimmune diseases. The importance of the recognition of this syndrome is twofold: first, a clear association has been established between the development of this syndrome and alterations in mood and behaviour that occur during the postpartum period in women. The importance of recognizing the cause and being able to offer an explanation provides reassurance to the mother and, in rare cases, because of the onset of severe depression, may indicate the need for treatment either by thyroxine for hypothyroidism or of the depression itself. The second, and important, reason for recognizing this syndrome is the clear evidence that in a significant number of women the transient syndrome may go on to permanent hypothyroidism, if not during the present postpartum period then with time and particularly with further pregnancies.

Therefore, the recognition of transient postpartum thyroid dysfunction in women as a marker of future thyroid failure, particularly after further pregnancies, provides a means for ensuring that permanent hypothyroidism is recognized early and treated appropriately, with a reduction in the likely morbidity associated with its development being prevented.

Adrenal disease

INTRODUCTION

As with the pituitary and thyroid, normal physiological changes in the hypothalamic–pituitary–adrenal axis during pregnancy need to be taken into account in trying to dissect out these changes from possible pathological changes in the system. With the marked increase in levels of cortisol binding globulin (CBG), plasma cortisol levels rise threefold by the third trimester of pregnancy. Adrenocorticotrophic hormone (ACTH) levels also rise during pregnancy, and it is possible that the placenta may make a further contribution to this increase, so that the resulting rise in ACTH levels may actually contribute to a real increase in cortisol levels, in addition to the spuriously elevated cortisol levels which result from increased levels of CBG. Diurnal variation and suppressibility to dexamethasone are, however, maintained during pregnancy. Renin and renin substrate levels are increased during pregnancy, with renin stimulating aldosterone excess via angiotensin II. However, normal pregnant women do not exhibit salt retention or potassium loss, presumably due to the antimineralocorticoid effects of the high levels of circulating progesterone. Although there is an increase in adrenal androgen production during pregnancy, the marked increase in sex hormone binding globulin (SHBG) levels results in a lowered free testosterone level.

Cushing's syndrome

Conception is rare in untreated Cushing's syndrome. In women who do become pregnant with Cushing's syndrome there is an increase in fetal loss with a fetal mortality rate of 25 per cent due to spontaneous abortion, still births, and early neonatal death due to extreme prematurity. On these grounds early and effective diagnosis and treatment are essential. Of the small number of cases of Cushing's syndrome occurring in pregnancy (fewer than 100 have been reported in the literature), the distribution of causes differs from the non-pregnant patient population, with less than half the cases being due to pituitary adenomata, a similar number having adrenal adenomata, and about 10 per cent having adrenal carcinomata. The clinical presentation of Cushing's syndrome may prove difficult to discriminate from symptoms and signs not uncharacteristically seen during pregnancy, such as weight gain of a central distribution, fatigue, oedema, emotional lability, glucose intolerance, and hypertension. Pigmentation of striae in patients with Cushing's syndrome may help in discriminating the two situations. The biochemical diagnosis of hypercortisolism is made difficult by the changes in cortisol secretion occurring during normal pregnancy. An overnight dexamethasone suppression test is usually abnormal with inadequate suppression during pregnancy itself, and therefore standard low- and high-dose dexamethasone suppression testing is required. ACTH levels should be measured but little data are available on ACTH measurement of patients with Cushing's syndrome in pregnancy and interpretation of such data is again complicated by the normal changes that occur in ACTH secretion during pregnancy itself. Discrimination of the likely aetiology of the hypercortisolism on the basis of dexamethasone suppression should be followed by radiological investigation, with assessment of the pituitary gland being carried out using MRI and that of the adrenal glands either by ultrasound or MRI. If the diagnosis is made during the first trimester, serious consideration may need to be given to termination. Although the therapeutic use of metyrapone has been reported in only a few patients, it may have a role in controlling hypercortisolism if it is felt that the stage of pregnancy is so advanced as to allow a delay in definitive treatment of the cause until after delivery. In the small number of cases in which such management has been used, the metyrapone has not had any adverse effect on the fetus. When the investigatory process suggests that an adrenal carcinoma may be the cause of the syndrome, the relatively poor prognosis makes the priority to treat the mother by surgery when feasible. When a pituitary or adrenal adenoma is the likely cause surgery should be performed as early as possible in the pregnancy and not delayed until the postpartum period, because of the impact of the disease on both maternal and fetal well-being. Although cortisol crosses the placenta, it rarely causes suppression of fetal adrenal function and this may reflect the protective effect of the placenta in converting cortisol to cortisone.

Adrenal insufficiency

Prior to the availability of glucocorticoid replacement therapy, pregnancy in patients with Addison's disease was associated with a maternal mortality rate as high as 50 per cent. Adrenal insufficiency is most commonly due to autoimmune destruction of the adrenals, and therefore a history of other organ-specific autoimmune diseases such as thyroiditis, insulin-dependent diabetes, pernicious anaemia, and vitiligo may suggest the diagnosis. In patients in whom the diagnosis pre-dates a pregnancy, those on regular glucocorticoid and mineralocorticoid replacement therapy go through pregnancy, labour, and delivery without difficulty, provided that periods of stress during the process are appro-

priately covered. In this context, during labour adequate saline hydration and an increase in glucocorticoid replacement are required, with doses of 25 to 100 mg of hydrocortisone hemisuccinate being given intravenously every 6 h, with the dose depending on the duration of labour. These doses can be reduced rapidly following delivery, with a return to normal maintenance doses within 3 days.

In the exceedingly rare situation where adrenal insufficiency presents for the first time during pregnancy, again the non-specific symptoms may prove difficult to discriminate from similar symptoms described as a result of the pregnancy. Increased skin pigmentation and evidence of other autoimmune diseases may be helpful, and hyperkalaemia may provide a clue. When suspicion is high, a low basal cortisol in the presence of an elevated ACTH level, with an absent cortisol response 60 min after an injection of synthetic ACTH, is diagnostic, and replacement therapy should be instituted immediately. Normal replacement therapy would be with hydrocortisone at a dose of 20 mg in the morning and 10 mg in the evening and fludrocortisone 0.1 mg once daily. At the time of initial diagnosis higher doses of hydrocortisone may be necessary, and at doses above 100 mg daily all the mineralocorticoid activity required is provided by this level of glucocorticoid and there is then no need to add in fludrocortisone. In addition, saline replacement in the acute phase may be essential.

Congenital adrenal hyperplasia

In women with inherited disorders of adrenal steroidogenesis due to various enzyme deficiencies, treatment of the condition will depend on the site of the enzyme deficiency in the steroidogenic pathway (see Chapter 12.7.2). In some, both fludrocortisone and a glucocorticoid will be required, whereas in others glucocorticoids alone will suffice. In such women who become pregnant steroid replacement clearly needs to be maintained throughout pregnancy, with the additional precautions described above for patients with adrenal insufficiency being observed during periods of stress, such as delivery, when additional glucocorticoid and adequate hydration will be essential. In this group of women, adequate suppression of adrenal androgens during pregnancy is essential if virilization of a female fetus is not to result from the high levels of maternal androgens crossing the placenta. Early treatment is necessary in order to deal with this situation since the virilizing effects of androgens on genital tract development may begin as early as 6 weeks of gestation; treatment should therefore be initiated before the onset of phenotypic sexual development. Beyond that time intervention may be too late and therefore unwarranted.

Primary hyperaldosteronism

(See also Chapter 12.7.1)

Primary hyperaldosteronism has been reported extremely rarely in pregnant women. Its recognition is clearly important as a possible contributor to hypertension during pregnancy. Since medical treatment with spironolactone is commonly prescribed for bilateral adrenal hyperplasia, it is important to recognize that this crosses the placenta and its antiandrogenic effects may then contribute to abnormal development of the fetal genitalia. On these grounds, once pregnancy is diagnosed the drug should be stopped; if the hypertension cannot be controlled by other means then surgical correction of disease due to an adenoma may be appropriate.

Phaeochromocytoma

(See also Chapter 15.28.2)

Although an uncommon condition, the failure to diagnose phaeochromocytomas prior to the onset of labour may have disastrous consequences, with resulting maternal and fetal mortality rates of up to 50 per cent. A high degree of suspicion is necessary in making the diagnosis. The characteristic paroxysmal or sustained presentation of the condition with hypertension, palpitation, severe anxiety, headache, and vomiting are common presenting features. These symptoms may also be accompanied during pregnancy by convulsions and an increase in the frequency of attacks particularly in the supine position, presumably due to the pressure of the gravid uterus on the tumour. Differentiation of the condition from pre-eclampsia reveals characteristically an absence of proteinuria, oedema, or elevated levels of uric acid in women with a tumour. Once biochemical evaluation suggests the diagnosis, tumour localization by MRI scanning, with or without venous sampling, is necessary (see Chapter 15.28.2), although invasive procedures carry an increased risk to the pregnancy. Radioactive scanning by MIBG (^{131}I-m-iodobenzylguanidine) is contraindicated in pregnancy.

Initial management is medical, with phenoxybenzamine which is not teratogenic and is well tolerated by the fetus. In situations where α-blockade does not control the blood pressure or a hypertensive crisis ensues, intravenous sodium nitroprusside may need to be used in addition. A normal and stable blood pressure should be achieved for at least 2 weeks before any surgery is contemplated so that re-expansion of the contracted vasculature has occurred and the risk of postoperative hypotension is thereby reduced. β-Adrenergic blockade should be added after stabilization of arterial pressure to prevent tachycardia or arrhythmias at the time of surgery. If there is a need for surgery early in pregnancy then clearly the risks to the pregnancy itself need to be taken into consideration and discussed with the mother. Surgery during the third trimester can be carried out as part of a combined operation, with caesarean section to deliver the baby at the same time as removal of the tumour. Expert anaesthetic supervision is crucial.

Parathyroid disease

INTRODUCTION

There is a significant fall in maternal plasma concentrations of calcium, total protein, and albumin during normal pregnancy. These changes are manifestations of the normal physiological haemodilution that occurs during pregnancy. In addition, considerable demands are placed on the maternal calcium stores and there is an increased maternal gastrointestinal absorption of calcium and transplacental passage of calcium to

meet the fetal calcium requirements. These requirements and the demands placed on the mother during lactation require an adequate calcium intake by the pregnant woman (see Chapter 12.6). Maternal levels of 1,25-dihydroxycholecalciferol are increased during pregnancy and contribute to the increased maternal intestinal calcium absorption.

Primary hyperparathyroidism

Hyperparathyroidism has rarely been reported during pregnancy. Whether this reflects an impact of the disease on fertility or difficulty in diagnosing the condition during pregnancy because of the changes in calcium metabolism that occur during normal pregnancy remains uncertain. In the latter context it is important to recognize that an apparent amelioration of hypercalcaemia in a patient with primary hyperparathyroidism because of the changes in maternal calcium metabolism during pregnancy may lead to the diagnosis of hyperparathyroidism being overlooked, with severe hypercalcaemia only becoming manifest in the postpartum period. The diagnosis of hyperparathyroidism in a woman found to be hypercalcaemic can be made by measurement of serum parathyroid hormone levels. Primary hyperparathyroidism in pregnancy results in increased rates of abortion, interuterine death, and premature labour, together with possible problems with neonatal tetany. A conservative approach to treatment, with adequate hydration and oral phosphate, has been used successfully. If this fails to control the disease, parathyroidectomy has been carried out successfully during pregnancy with little risk to the mother or fetus if surgery is performed after the first trimester.

REFERENCES

Burgess, G.E. (1978). Alpha blockade and surgical intervention of pheochromocytoma of pregnancy. *Obstetrics and Gynecology* **53**, 266–70.

Fudge, T.L., McKinnon, W.M.P., and Geary, W.L. (1980). Current surgical management of pheochromocytoma during pregnancy. *Archives of Surgery*, **115**, 1224–5.

Hamburger, J.I., Kaplan, M.M., and McGregor, A.M. (1992). Thyroid disease in pregnancy. *Thyroid* **2**, (1–3), 57–84, 147–70, 207–28.

Johnson, M.R. and McGregor, A.M. (1990). Endocrine disease and pregnancy. *Baillière's Clinical Endocrinology and Metabolism* **4**, 313–32.

Molitch, M.E. (1992). Endocrine emergencies in pregnancy. *Baillière's Clinical Endocrinology and Metabolism* **6**, 167–91.

13.8 Diabetes in pregnancy

M. D. G. GILLMER

Prior to the introduction of insulin treatment in 1921 diabetes was a rare complication of pregnancy due to the high incidence of amenorrhoea, infertility, and miscarriage in women with this disease. There was, in addition, a near 50 per cent maternal and fetal mortality when diabetes complicated pregnancy. Within a decade of the introduction of insulin therapy, the maternal mortality had fallen to between two and three per cent. The fetal mortality, however, remained above 40 per cent until the 1950s despite early recognition that 'rigid control' of the diabetes was vital to achieve an optimal pregnancy outcome. Although this concept has remained central to the management of the disease in pregnancy, it appears, with hindsight, that the early poor fetal outcome was due to incomplete understanding of the pathophysiology of the condition and to a lack of suitable technology for assessing adequate diabetic control.

It is now recognized that diabetes complicating pregnancy represents a unique short-term 'tissue culture', from which a great deal can and

has been learned about the long-term complications of diabetes in the non-pregnant patient and the ways in which these can be avoided.

Metabolic changes in pregnancy

Pregnancy induces major alterations in carbohydrate, lipid, and amino acid metabolism, which have been described as a combination of 'facilitated anabolism' and 'accelerated starvation'. From a teleological standpoint these changes appear to ensure the optimal availability of nutrients for both the fetus and mother.

CARBOHYDRATE METABOLISM

Fasting plasma glucose concentrations decline during pregnancy by approximately 0.5 mmol/l, reaching a nadir in the third trimester. Postprandial glucose concentrations, however, increase, despite a rise in both basal and stimulated insulin secretion. This appears to be due, in part, to peripheral insulin resistance induced by placental hormones and in part to the effects of oestrogen and progesterone on the maternal pancreas. The reduction in fasting plasma glucose is gradual. In early pregnancy it appears to result from plasma volume expansion, which causes dilution of the circulating glucose pool. In late pregnancy there is a further decline which is thought to arise from the increasing fetal and placental demand for glucose. Studies on the glucose disappearance rate in late pregnancy are, however, controversial and some suggest that the reduced plasma glucose concentrations of late pregnancy are not caused by an excessive glucose drain.

Although insulin sensitivity appears to increase transiently during the first trimester of pregnancy there is thereafter a progressive decline which is reflected by an increased insulin:glucose ratio. Human placental lactogen (hPL), a polypeptide hormone with structural and immunological similarities to human growth hormone, is one of the major causes of the insulin resistance that characterizes pregnancy. Other possible factors include increased fat stores, raised prolactin and free cortisol concentrations, sequestration of insulin by the placenta, and changes in insulin receptor affinity and number, although the evidence for these last two causes is contradictory.

Serial glucose tolerance tests indicate a progressive decline in tolerance with advancing gestation. After an oral glucose load in later pregnancy there are higher peak plasma glucose concentrations, a delay in the rise to the peak concentration, and an increase in the total area under the glucose tolerance curve compared with the non-pregnant state. Despite these changes, pregnant women maintain efficient glucose homeostasis, but with slightly lower preprandial and higher postprandial plasma glucose concentrations following mixed meals than in non-pregnant women.

Although insulin does not cross the placental barrier, glucose does so freely by a process of facilitated diffusion. This ensures that fetal glucose concentrations follow maternal fluctuations closely, but at a slightly lower level. Fetal exposure to maternal hyperglycaemia causes premature stimulation of the fetal β-cells of the pancreatic islets of Langerhans and results in fetal hyperinsulinaemia. This in turn stimulates excessive fetal growth, leading to the macrosomia which characterizes the infant of the diabetic mother.

LIPID METABOLISM

Plasma concentrations of triglycerides, cholesterol, phospholipids, and free fatty acids all increase during pregnancy. During early pregnancy increased food intake coupled with moderate postprandial hyperinsulinism create ideal conditions for lipogenesis, so-called 'facilitated anabolism'. During late pregnancy food intake declines, insulin resistance is established, and, in the presence of high circulating levels of hPL, lipolysis is enhanced during the fasting state.

Plasma triglycerides increase approximately fourfold during pregnancy, probably due to increased hepatic synthesis and possibly reduced removal, induced by placental oestrogens. This hypertriglyceridaemia reflects an increase in plasma very low density lipoprotein (VLDL), low density lipoprotein (LDL) and both fractions of high density lipoprotein (HDL), namely HDL_2 and HDL_3.

Plasma free fatty acid and glycerol concentrations decrease slightly until the early third trimester when they rise to a peak at approximately 37 to 38 weeks' gestation and thereafter decline until delivery. The late pregnancy increase in these substrates, especially in the fasting state when there is also a significant increase in ketones, is believed to indicate increased mobilization of lipid from adipose tissue under the influence of hPL and cortisol, so-called 'accelerated starvation'. This increase in circulating free fatty acid concentrations is thought to have an important influence on maternal metabolism as it provides alternate sources of maternal fuel at a time in pregnancy when fetal and maternal glucose needs are maximal.

Plasma cholesterol increases by approximately 25 per cent during pregnancy, a change that probably reflects increased synthesis and decreased catabolism.

Lipoprotein triglyceride and cholesterol do not cross the placenta but free fatty acids cross freely by simple diffusion.

PROTEIN AND AMINO ACID METABOLISM

Amino acids are crucial for fetal development, and fetal protein accumulation occurs rapidly in late pregnancy. Despite this there is an increase in maternal amino acid excretion in the third trimester which consists mainly of the non-essential amino acids glycine, histidine, serine, and alanine. In addition, most amino acid concentrations fall in pregnancy, in particular ornithine, glycine, taurine, and proline, while the postprandial peak concentrations of leucine, isoleucine, serine, and alanine following a mixed meal in late pregnancy are lower than those observed in non-pregnant subjects. These findings suggest the possibility that there may be greater retention of these amino acids by the maternal liver. Alternative explanations include the increased volume of distribution of amino acids during pregnancy or changes in their absorption and utilization. Starvation in pregnancy causes a two- to threefold rise in valine, leucine, and isoleucine but a fall in alanine concentrations.

The concentration of most free amino acids is higher in fetal than in maternal plasma, indicating placental amino acid transfer against a concentration gradient.

Gestational diabetes

In the late 1940s it was recognized that the fetal mortality in women who later developed maturity onset diabetes was much higher than normal in the years immediately preceding the diagnosis of diabetes. This led to the concept of 'prediabetes', subsequently recognized as a period of transient diabetes induced by pregnancy, now known as 'gestational diabetes'. The aetiology of gestational diabetes is, however, incompletely understood, as glucose tolerance deteriorates in all pregnant women but only a small proportion develop gestational diabetes.

Fasting and postprandial plasma insulin concentrations increase twofold on average during normal pregnancy but the peak insulin response occurs later in gestational diabetics. In addition, although the absolute insulin response to a glycaemic stimulus is similar in normal and gestational diabetic women, the relative insulin response per unit of glycaemic stimulus is lower in gestational diabetics. The insulin response to a protein-rich meal also increases to a greater extent in normal women when compared to gestational diabetics. These findings indicate an enhanced pancreatic β-cell sensitivity to glucose and amino acids in both normal and gestational diabetic women, but with some impairment of the relative response to these stimuli in women who develop gestational diabetes.

Morphological studies have shown significant maternal β-cell hypertrophy and hyperplasia in pregnancy which causes an increase in total circulating immunoreactive insulin, but without any change in relative proinsulin concentrations in either normal or gestational diabetics. In addition, although the placenta provides an alternative site for insulin degradation during pregnancy, this does not appear to have a significant effect on maternal insulin extraction which occurs mainly in the liver, as in the non-pregnant state.

The current widely accepted definition of gestational diabetes, is 'carbohydrate intolerance of variable severity with onset or first recognition during the present pregnancy'. This extends the definition to include not only those women in whom the diabetes occurs transiently during pregnancy and regresses after delivery but also those in whom type 1 diabetes arises de novo during pregnancy and persists in the long term.

Screening for gestational diabetes has traditionally involved performing glucose tolerance tests on all women with 'risk factors' or 'potential diabetic features' (see Table 1). These are, however, present in 30 per

Table 1 *Risk factors for gestational diabetes*

Family history of diabetes in a first-degree relative
Recurrent glycosuria (especially in the fasting state)
Previous macrosomic infant (> 4.5 kg) or large-for-dates baby in the current pregnancy
Polyhydramnios in the current pregnancy
Obesity
Previous stillbirth (with pancreatic β-cell hyperplasia)

cent or more women in most communities and are not present in all those who develop significant glucose intolerance during pregnancy. This means that many women are subjected to unnecessary tests while others who develop gestational diabetes are missed. 'Risk factors' are therefore of limited value for screening purposes.

Universal screening programmes based on blood glucose measurement, although controversial, have therefore become popular in recent years. The American Diabetes Association and American College of Obstetricians and Gynecologists have both endorsed the use of a 50 g oral glucose load at 24 to 28 weeks' gestation. This is given without regard to the time of the last meal or the time of day. Venous plasma glucose is measured an hour later and a value equal to or greater than 7.8 mmol/l (140 mg/dl) is recommended as the threshold for a full diagnostic oral glucose tolerance test. This screening procedure has been shown to be the most sensitive (79 per cent) and specific (87 per cent) of the screening tests available but is probably only appropriate in populations with a high prevalence of diabetes or for those at increased risk, such as older women and those who are grossly obese. A number of simpler procedures have also been introduced in recent years. These include routine random blood glucose measurement at 28 to 32 weeks' gestation, random blood glucose measurements in women who display glycosuria, and meal tolerance tests in which a single blood sample is taken after a standard 'meal'. Although these techniques generally have a high degree of specificity they display much lower sensitivities than the 50 g oral glucose load. Screening by means of glycosylated haemoglobin or plasma protein measurements, including fructosamine, have proved to be too insensitive for use in pregnancy.

The role of universal screening for gestational diabetes has been challenged in recent years, on the grounds that although there is evidence that gestational glucose intolerance is associated with an excess of heavy infants and some evidence that this can be reduced by treatment with insulin, there is little proof that there is excess fetal mortality or significant maternal or fetal morbidity in women who do not have overt diabetes. There is, however, common agreement that women identified as gestational diabetics are at increased risk of developing maturity onset diabetes in later life, and that avoidance of obesity in middle age appears to prevent development of diabetes in these women. Some authors have, however, concluded that since available data do not indicate that universal screening programmes do more good than harm, a more restrained approach should be adopted until better evidence is available.

The glucose tolerance criteria for the diagnosis of gestational diabetes are also controversial and this, together with the poor reproducibility of the test, may explain some of the inconsistent results of screening programmes. Although the American College of Obstetricians and Gynecologists has retained the 100 g oral glucose tolerance test, in Europe the World Health Organization's recommendation that a 75 g oral glucose load should be used has been accepted in preference to the 50 g, 100 g, or 1 g/kg loads. Although it has also been suggested that the criteria for 'impaired glucose tolerance' after a 75 g glucose tolerance test should be used for the diagnosis of 'gestational diabetes', this remains extremely controversial. These WHO criteria are shown in Table 2 together with the American College of Obstetricians and Gynecologist's standards for a 100 g oral glucose tolerance test; Oxford data from a study of the 75 g oral glucose tolerance test in 491 women at 28 to 34 weeks' gestation; and those from a multicentre study of the Dia-

betic Pregnancy Study Group of the European Association for the Study of Diabetes, involving 354 women in the third trimester of pregnancy.

It is apparent from these data that if gestational diabetes is diagnosed using the WHO criteria for impaired glucose tolerance this will lead to overdiagnosis of the condition, as a significant number of healthy women will have a 2 h venous plasma glucose in excess of the WHO limit of 8.0 mmol/l. Widespread acceptance of the WHO criteria for impaired glucose tolerance as diagnostic of gestational diabetes could therefore explain the continued uncertainty about potential adverse effects of gestational diabetes on the outcome of pregnancy, since many women will thereby erroneously be categorized as gestational diabetics, thus artificially improving the fetal and maternal outcome in this condition. If, on the other hand, the WHO criteria for diagnosing diabetes are adopted, women with significant hyperglycaemia may be missed. It is therefore suggested that the modified WHO criteria shown in Table 3 are used in clinical practice, and that in future a clear distinction is made between women with impaired glucose tolerance and true diabetes during pregnancy.

Medical management

In the early 1970s it was recognized that the perinatal mortality in diabetic women is positively correlated with the mean maternal blood glucose concentration during pregnancy. This finding, together with the observation that blood glucose concentrations in normal pregnant women rarely exceed 6 mmol/l, except during the hour after a meal, focused attention on the need for 'rigid control' of maternal diabetes. Glycosuria occurs in up to 90 per cent of pregnant women and it has long been recognized that the glucose content of urine cannot be used to monitor diabetic control in pregnancy. It therefore became routine practice to admit pregnant women to hospital for laboratory measurements of blood glucose from approximately 32 weeks' gestation. The development of glucose test strips and meters for objective home monitoring of blood glucose has, however, rendered this practice obsolete and it is now only necessary to consider hospital admission for complications of pregnancy or diabetes. Ideally, blood glucose concentrations should be measured preprandially, as shown in Table 4, on at least 2 days each week, or more frequently if indicated, and maintained between 4 and 6 mmol/l. Measurements of glycosylated haemoglobin or fructosamine are used in many units to provide an indication of medium- to long-term glycaemic control. Although non-essential, these measurements may prove helpful, especially in non-compliant patients.

CONGENITAL MALFORMATIONS

It has, for many years, been recognized that type 1 insulin-dependent diabetes preceding pregnancy is associated with a significant increase in the risk of major congenital anomalies of between 7 and 14 per cent. The precise aetiology remains obscure in most cases, but the frequency is undoubtedly increased in women with poor diabetic control preceding pregnancy and during the early first trimester. The incidence also varies, according to the definitions applied in diagnosing major malformations (Table 5).

There is in particular a three- to fivefold increase in the incidence of neural tube, cardiac, and renal anomalies and, although these were a relatively unimportant cause of perinatal mortality in the early postinsulin era, the gradual reduction in deaths associated with ketoacidosis, trauma, prematurity, and late intrauterine deaths means that more than half of current perinatal deaths are now caused by lethal congenital anomalies. They are also an important cause of avoidable long-term morbidity in the offspring of diabetic women. As the organ systems commonly affected in diabetes are all fully formed by 9 weeks' gestation (7 weeks after the first missed menstrual period) it is vital that all women in the reproductive age group are advised that they must make serious efforts to achieve optimal diabetic control before planning a pregnancy

Table 2 *Upper limits for normal glucose tolerance criteria in pregnancy (venous plasma glucose, mmol/l)*

	DPSG/EASD[a] (75 g)	Oxford[b] (75 g)	ADA/ACOG[b] (100 g)	WHO (75 g) IGT	WHO (75 g) Diabetes
Fasting	5.2	6.0	5.8	< 8	> 8
1 h	10.5	12.5	10.5	–	
2 h	9.0	9.5	9.2	8–11	> 11
3 h	–	7.5	8.1		–

[a]Based on 95th centile limits.

[b]Based on mean ± 2 standard deviations.

ACOG, American College of Obstetricians and Gynecologists; ADA, American Diabetes Association; DPSG, Diabetic Pregnancy Study Group; EASD, European Association for the Study of Diabetes; WHO, World Health Organization.

IGT, impaired glucose tolerance.

Table 3 *Recommended modified WHO diagnostic criteria for the diagnosis of gestational impaired glucose tolerance (IGT) and diabetes*

	Normal	IGT	Diabetes
Fasting	< 6.0	> 6.0–< 8.0	≥ 8.0
2 h	< 9.0	> 9.0–< 11.0	≥ 11.0

Table 4 *Timing of blood tests in pregnant diabetic women*

Pre-breakfast	Pre-meal
Pre-coffee	Pre-snack
Pre-lunch	Pre-meal
Pre-tea	Pre-snack
Pre-supper	Pre-meal
Bedtime	Pre-snack

Table 5 *Congenital anomalies seen in infants of diabetic mothers*

Central nervous system: anencephaly, encephalocele, meningomyelocele, spina bifida, holoprosencephaly
Cardiac: transposition of great vessels, ventricular septal defect, situs inversus, single ventricle, hypoplastic left ventricle
Renal: agenesis, multicystic dysplasia
Skeletal: caudal regression
Gastrointestinal: anal/rectal atresia, small left colon
Pulmonary: hypoplasia

and that this should be maintained throughout the period of embryogenesis. In addition, all diabetic women should be advised to take folate supplements for at least 4 weeks prior to conception to reduce the risk of delivering a child with a neural tube defect.

TEAM CARE

The concept of 'team care' for pregnant diabetic women originated in the 1930s and remains an essential part of modern management. The most important member of the team is the woman herself as she has day to day responsibility for her diabetes and usually has the clearest understanding of how optimal glycaemic control can be achieved. She should ideally attend a joint diabetic antenatal clinic where she can be seen by specialist diabetic nurses, midwives, dietitians, and medical staff, including an obstetrician, a physician, and a neonatal paediatrician with a special interest in this condition.

It is important to see these patients as early as possible in pregnancy in order to maintain good diabetic control. The frequency of clinic visits will, however, depend on several factors, including the blood glucose concentrations achieved and the occurrence of diabetic or obstetric complications. As in non-diabetic women, an average two- or threefold increase in insulin requirements occurs during pregnancy. It is therefore preferable to see all diabetic women at least every 2 weeks until 34 weeks' gestation and then weekly until delivery as this facilitates the frequent alterations of insulin dose that need to be made as the pregnancy progresses and also ensures adequate dietary advice. If control is poor and more frequent advice is required, this can usually be achieved by

telephone. This avoids the need to admit the patient, which is disruptive to both her pattern of activity and her diet, which are important components of her overall diabetic control.

DIET AND INSULIN THERAPY

The management of women who are diagnosed as gestational diabetics depends on their preprandial and postprandial blood glucose concentrations (see Table 4). If these are between 6 to 8 mmol/l, a high-fibre isocaloric diet is advised initially, and the woman retested. If the preprandial plasma glucose concentrations remain above 6 mmol/l, or if they initially exceed 8 mmol/l, then insulin therapy is begun, using a long-acting preparation in the first instance. Preprandial short-acting insulin is added before meals if the postprandial (pre-snack) values remain above 6 mmol/l. Oral hypoglycaemics are not used because they cross the placenta and stimulate the fetal pancreatic β-cells, causing fetal hyperinsulinaemia, the pathological process that insulin treatment aims to avoid.

Human insulin is preferred, as this produces least antibodies and reduces the theoretical risks of fetal β-cell damage or macrosomia due to the transplacental passage of injected insulin bound to antibody. Despite considerable controversy, there appears to be little evidence to support current concerns that human insulins lessen awareness of hypoglycaemia.

While the traditional twice-daily use of short- and intermediate-acting insulins remains widespread, a variety of new insulin regimes has become popular in pregnant and non-pregnant patients. The continuous subcutaneous insulin infusion (CSII) pump, introduced in the early 1980s, was initially hailed as the ideal means of achieving euglycaemia in pregnant diabetics. This relied on a constant basal infusion, with premeal boluses as required. However, careful studies, both in pregnant and non-pregnant subjects, have failed to identify any advantage over conventional intermittent injection regimes. In addition, the pregnant diabetic is particularly prone to overnight ketoacidosis and the absence of any insulin depot in women using this system means that disruption of the infusion through pump failure, catheter blockage, or disconnection can rapidly lead to ketoacidotic coma, with the risk of fetal or even maternal death. Much of the flexibility of CSII has, however, been retained by combining a single daily injection of long- or intermediate-acting insulin, usually administered at bedtime, with up to three intermittent preprandial injections of short-acting insulin, administered with an insulin 'pen'. In practice, the patient's prepregnancy insulin regime is only changed if it proves impossible to achieve the desired standard of control without doing so.

Pregnancy is characterized by a decline in fasting plasma glucose concentrations and a plentiful supply of alternate substrates for energy requirements, including ketones derived from the β-oxidation of free fatty acids. Hypoglycaemia is therefore rare and, unlike hyperglycaemia, does not appear to have any demonstrable adverse effect on the fetus. Despite this, pregnant diabetics are at increased risk of hypoglycaemia because of the very tight diabetic control that they must maintain throughout pregnancy. They should therefore be provided with glucagon that can be administered by a third party in the event of severe hypoglycaemia.

MANAGEMENT OF DIABETES DURING AND AFTER LABOUR

It is important to maintain normoglycaemia during labour in order to reduce the risk of neonatal hypoglycaemia. This is most easily achieved using combined insulin and dextrose infusions. Dextrose 10 per cent solution is infused at 100 ml/h and blood glucose measurements are made every hour using blood obtained from the patient's other arm. Insulin (6 units in 60 ml normal saline) is administered simultaneously, at an initial rate of one unit (10 ml) per hour using an infusion pump. The insulin infusion rate is doubled or halved as necessary to maintain the blood glucose concentration between 4 and 6 mmol/l. During labour the insulin requirement may fall dramatically, presumably because of the increased glucose demand due to uterine work, and it is frequently necessary to switch the insulin infusion off towards the end of the first stage.

After delivery the insulin infusion rate must be halved to prevent hypoglycaemia as there is a rapid decline in insulin sensitivity following the delivery of the placenta. It is also essential to return to the prepregnancy insulin dose, immediately the patient resumes her normal diet, as profound hypoglycaemia may occur if the dose required prior to delivery is administered at this time.

RETINOPATHY

Rapid reduction of blood glucose concentrations has been shown to accelerate diabetic retinopathy in both pregnant and non-pregnant subjects. There is also evidence that pregnancy and hypertension, complicating pregnancy, may act as independent risk factors for the progression of diabetic retinopathy. In addition, the duration of diabetes and the severity of the pre-existing retinopathy may accelerate this disease process. Formal retinal assessment, with dilated pupils, should therefore be performed prior to pregnancy so that improved diabetic control can be achieved over 3 to 9 months before a planned conception. This should avoid the need for acute improvement of the blood glucose concentrations in early pregnancy and thus minimize the risk of exacerbating proliferative retinopathy. All women should also have a full ophthalmic assessment in early pregnancy to assess their retinal state and determine the possible need for laser therapy.

NEPHROPATHY

Overt nephropathy is associated with various complications of pregnancy, including pre-eclampsia, growth retardation, and fetal distress, but there is little evidence to suggest that pregnancy will hasten the progression of overt nephropathy to endstage renal failure.

Patients seeking advice about pregnancy should therefore be warned that although their renal disease may have an adverse effect on pregnancy which could necessitate prolonged hospitalization, and premature delivery, possibly by caesarean section, there is usually no need to avoid or terminate pregnancy as has been advised in the past.

Obstetric management

ANTENATAL ASSESSMENT OF THE FETUS

Accurate information about the duration of pregnancy, fetal growth, and fetal well-being are vital in the management of the pregnant diabetic. Technological developments, particularly in the use of diagnostic ultrasound, have revolutionized fetal assessment and have become central to the modern obstetric management of diabetes in pregnancy.

The fetal crown–rump length (CRL) should be measured during the first trimester to confirm the duration of pregnancy. In some women this technique has identified possible 'early growth delay' in which the fetal CRL measurement is smaller than expected from the gestational age. This disputed condition is associated with an increased rate of congenital malformations and poor fetal growth, and is thought to be due to 'less-than-optimal' metabolic compensation in early pregnancy. If confirmed, this will serve to emphasize the importance of normoglycaemia before conception and during the first trimester of pregnancy.

A biparietal diameter measurement is also performed in the mid-trimester, ideally at 16 weeks' gestation, to provide additional information about gestational age. Blood for serum alpha-fetoprotein should also be taken at this time both to screen for neural tube defects and as part of the 'triple test' used to screen for Down's syndrome. In assessing the result of these investigations it must, however, be borne in mind that the serum alpha-fetoprotein and unconjugated oestriol concentrations observed in diabetic pregnancy are lower than those in non-diabetic women and this can lead to erroneous interpretation of these screening tests.

A detailed fetal examination to exclude congenital anomalies, especially of the neural, cardiac, and renal systems, is performed between 18 and 20 weeks, so that termination of the pregnancy can be considered if appropriate.

Serial studies of growth based on measurements of the fetal head and abdominal circumferences provide the best means of identifying those pregnancies in which the fetus is becoming macrosomic. It has been reported that if the fetal abdominal circumference is 1 cm or more above the mean value at this stage of pregnancy then there is a 77 per cent likelihood of fetal macrosomia at term. This observation emphasizes two points. First, it is as important to maintain optimal metabolic control during mid-pregnancy as during the first and third trimesters, because the fetal pancreatic β-cells appear to become sensitized to hyperglycaemia during the second trimester and not in the third as had been assumed in the past. Secondly, it may be possible to predict macrosomia at a time in pregnancy when it is still possible to institute optimal metabolic control and thus reduce the likelihood of this complication. In addition, although an association between birthweight and maternal blood glucose concentrations has been demonstrated during the third trimester of pregnancy, the cause of fetal macrosomia in diabetic women is still uncertain, and there are many examples of women who deliver infants with birthweights above the 97th centile despite excellent metabolic control in late pregnancy. On the other hand, a twofold increase in large-for-gestational-age infants (defined as a birthweight above the 90th centile) has been reported in women with a mean blood glucose exceeding 5.8 mmol/l, with a twofold increase in small-for-dates infants (defined as a birthweight below the 10th centile) in those diabetics with very tight control and a mean blood glucose concentration of less than 4.8 mmol/l. These data are important as they indicate that excessively tight blood glucose control may have a deleterious effect on the growth of the diabetic fetus and possibly also on its development.

OBSTETRIC COMPLICATIONS OF DIABETES IN PREGNANCY

Proteinuric hypertension

This occurs approximately twice as often in diabetics as in normal women. Serum urate and creatinine concentrations should therefore be measured at every antenatal visit and 24 h urine protein concentrations from 24 weeks' gestation, as these provide not only the earliest biochemical evidence of proteinuric pre-eclampsia but also serve to clarify those blood pressure changes in late pregnancy which are due to pre-existing essential hypertension (see Chapter 13.2).

Although the precise reason for the increased incidence of pre-eclampsia in diabetics is unknown, a link with glycaemic control has been established and the incidence of this complication is reduced with optimal metabolic control of the diabetes.

Polyhydramnios

This is one of the hallmarks of diabetic pregnancy, and is occasionally the presenting feature in gestational diabetes. The cause of this complication, which has an overall incidence of approximately 15 per cent, remains uncertain but is probably due to an osmotic diuresis induced in the fetus by fetomaternal hyperglycaemia. This would be in keeping with the fact that the degree of polyhydramnios generally reduces as the diabetic control improves. Treatment with indomethacin, which reduces fetal urine production, has been advocated when this fails to occur, although this therapy may induce premature closure of the ductus arteriosus.

Premature labour

This is more frequent in diabetic pregnancy and may, in some instances, be due to underlying polyhydramnios. Conventional management with intravenous β-sympathomimetic agents causes hepatic glycogenolysis and insulin resistance and predisposes to hyperglycaemic ketoacidosis. This treatment is therefore potentially hazardous in diabetic women and should be avoided whenever possible or used with extreme caution, even in non-insulin-dependent patients. Glucocorticoids have an additive effect and their concurrent use in diabetic pregnant women may necessitate the administration of very high doses (up to 30 units/h) of intravenous insulin to maintain normoglycaemia.

FETAL WELL-BEING AND MATURITY

Unexplained intrauterine death of the fetus during the last 3 to 4 weeks of pregnancy has been recognized as a major problem in the management of diabetic pregnancy since the pre-insulin era. The so-called 'fetal biophysical profile' a modern real-time ultrasound technique has, however, revolutionized the late pregnancy management of this condition and made it unnecessary to admit diabetic women routinely for daily monitoring in late pregnancy. These assessments, which should be performed at least weekly from 36 weeks' gestation, have also made it possible to prolong diabetic pregnancies to near term or beyond.

Antenatal Doppler ultrasound assessments have also been used widely in diabetic pregnancy in recent years. Results obtained using this technique have also provided the reassurance necessary to prolong uncomplicated diabetic pregnancies beyond term, but unlike the biophysical profile have not proved helpful in predicting fetal demise in diabetic women.

FETAL MATURITY AND TIMING OF DELIVERY

Poorly controlled diabetes is associated with fetal pulmonary and hepatic immaturity which predispose to the neonatal respiratory distress syndrome and jaundice. Some authors have therefore suggested that if delivery is planned before 38 weeks' gestation then fetal lung maturity should be assessed by measuring the lecithin:sphingomyelin ratio or phosphatidyl glycerol concentrations in amniotic fluid obtained by amniocentesis. This invasive and potentially hazardous procedure is, however, rarely if ever indicated, for if there is a pressing clinical need to deliver prematurely, then the indication alone should justify intervention, whereas if there is no urgent reason to terminate the pregnancy then no action should be taken.

The optimal time for delivery in uncomplicated diabetic pregnancy appears to be in the 39th week (273 days). Despite this, some authors have advocated deferring delivery until 40 weeks or later as this allows a larger number of women to enter labour spontaneously. This policy is, however, associated with a higher incidence of macrosomic and still-born babies and has not to date been shown to have any significant benefit.

MANAGEMENT OF LABOUR

One of the main aims in the modern management of the pregnant diabetic woman is to achieve a spontaneous vaginal delivery. Elective caesarean section may, however, be indicated with fetal malpresentations, an estimated fetal weight in excess of 4.5 kg, or a history of a previous caesarean section. The need for intravenous therapy during labour inevitably limits the mobility of the diabetic woman, but this inconvenience can be minimized by using battery-powered infusion equipment. Continuous fetal heart rate and contraction monitoring is advised because of the increased incidence of fetal distress in labour which may be due to an impaired maternal oxygen release in the uteroplacental circulation. Pain relief in labour is particularly important because painful uterine contractions cause catecholamine release, causing glycogenolysis and hyperglycaemia. Epidural anaesthesia is ideal, but not vital especially in the multiparous patient who may have a rapid and uncomplicated labour. If intravenous fluids are required for 'preloading' prior to insertion of an epidural or for the administration of oxytocin, it is essential that normal saline or Hartmann's solutions and not dextrose are used in order to avoid fetal hyperglycaemia, as this predisposes to neonatal hypoglycaemia.

Efforts to predict fetal macrosomia and, in particular the risk of shoulder dystocia, have been conspicuously unsuccessful to date. Measurement of the biacromial diameter of the shoulders using CT or MRI appear promising for this purpose but remain to be refined.

THE NEONATE

Insulin is present in the human pancreas from 11 weeks' gestation and although the pancreatic response to insulin secretogogues is sluggish in normal infants, fetal exposure to high concentrations and large fluctuations of glucose and amino acids, such as arginine, during poorly controlled diabetic pregnancy appear to produce premature maturation of the β-cells of the fetal pancreatic islets. This causes hyperinsulinaemia which predisposes to excessive fetal growth and macrosomia. It is also responsible for the neonatal hypoglycaemia that may occur during the first 24 h after delivery, when high circulating insulin concentrations inhibit both glycogenolysis and lipolysis, thus depriving the infant of alternative energy sources.

Other neonatal problems include the respiratory distress syndrome, polycythaemia, jaundice, renal vein thrombosis, hypocalcaemia, hypomagnesaemia and cardiomyopathy, all of which appear to be related directly or indirectly to fetal hyperinsulinaemia.

The respiratory distress syndrome appears to be due to suppression of surfactant production by the type 2 alveolar cells in the fetal lung caused by excessive circulating insulin. Polycythaemia, which is probably due to insulin-stimulated hepatic erythropoiesis, causes jaundice and increased blood viscosity. This, in turn, predisposes to multiple organ thrombosis, of which renal vein thrombosis is the most important. Relative hepatic immaturity, due to insulin-induced suppression of microsomal enzymes, is associated with an impaired ability to conjugate bilirubin, which results in an increased risk of kernicterus.

These infants therefore require early feeding and close supervision after delivery. The incidence and severity of neonatal complications is, however, closely related to diabetic control during pregnancy and the infant of the well-controlled diabetic mother does not usually require admission to a special care nursery, unless a problem arises after delivery.

THE PUERPERIUM AND CONTRACEPTION

Diabetics are at increased risk of wound infection following surgery, and prophylactic antibiotics are therefore advised following both elective and emergency caesarean section or operative vaginal delivery.

Breast feeding is encouraged but as this reduces the insulin requirement by approximately 25 per cent an appropriate reduction must be made once lactation is established. Women who choose not to breast feed, or in whom breast feeding is unsuccessful, should resume their prepregnancy insulin dose after delivery.

All diabetic women should be seen for a postnatal examination 6 weeks after delivery, and should be offered contraceptive advice at this time. The nature of the advice will, of course, depend on the age, parity, and future reproductive plans of each woman. The progesterone only (mini) pill has virtually no effect on carbohydrate or lipid metabolism and is therefore suitable for the breast-feeding diabetic woman. Provided she is prepared to accept the slightly higher failure rate of this method when ovulation resumes, then it may also be used long term. The potentially adverse effects on carbohydrate and lipoprotein metabolism of the older, high-dose combined oral contraceptive pills have long been a source of concern in diabetics. Recent data, however, suggest that modern low-dose preparations containing 'third-generation' progestogens have little effect on high- or low-density lipoprotein concentrations or carbohydrate metabolism, and can be used safely, especially in younger insulin-dependent and gestational diabetics. Early concerns about the apparently high failure rates of copper-containing intrauterine devices in diabetics have also been refuted in recent studies. Finally, the woman who has completed her family should be encouraged to consider a laparoscopic sterilization.

REFERENCES

Coustan, D.R. (1991). Diabetes in pregnancy. *Clinical Obstetrics and Gynaecology*, **34**, 479–580. Another up-to-date review of this subject.

Gillmer, M.D.G. and Bickerton, N.J. (1994). Advances in the management of diabetes in pregnancy: success through simplicity. In *Advances in obstetrics and gynaecology*, Vol. **18**, (ed. J. Bonnar). Churchill Livingstone, Edinburgh, in press. A review article with many up-to-date references by the author.

Oats, J.N. (ed.) (1991). Diabetes in pregnancy. *Clinical Obstetrics and Gynaecology*, **5**, 257–503. An up-to-date review of this subject.

Sutherland, H.W., Stowers, J.M., and Pearson, D.W.M. (1989). *Carbohydrate metabolism in pregnancy and the newborn IV*. Springer-Verlag, Berlin. Proceedings of a recent International Symposium on diabetes in pregnancy and its effect on the neonate.

13.9 Blood disorders in pregnancy

E. A. LETSKY

The physiological changes of pregnancy result in profound changes in the maternal haematological system. Plasma volume increases progressively, reaching a peak during the third trimester, which is about 45 per cent or 1250 ml above non-pregnant values. The change is greater in multiple pregnancy. The total red cell mass increases proportionately less, that is by about 20 to 30 per cent. The net result is haemodilution and hence a decline in haemoglobin concentration, packed cell volume, and red cell count. In the absence of iron deficiency, the mean cell haemoglobin concentration remains at non-pregnant values and there is a slight increase (approximately 4 fl) in mean cell volume. As a result of these changes, anaemia cannot be diagnosed in pregnancy using criteria applied to non-pregnant individuals.

Iron-deficiency anaemia

The expansion of red cell mass represents the largest single demand for iron in pregnancy, amounting to a net gain of about 500 to 600 mg. In addition, 250 to 350 mg is needed for transfer to the fetus by active transport across the placenta, mainly in the last 4 weeks of pregnancy. Daily requirements for iron increase three- to fourfold and are met by an increased rate of absorption from the gut, together with mobilization of maternal iron stores, The mean serum iron concentration of healthy pregnant women is about two-thirds of the levels for non-pregnant individuals. Total iron-binding capacity is increased because transferrin levels more than double as pregnancy advances. In consequence, the saturation of iron-binding capacity is, in healthy pregnancy, lower (at about 25 per cent) than is normal for other situations. Serum ferritin (reflecting iron stores) declines during the first half of pregnancy to a nadir of about 15 to 20 µg/l where it remains until delivery. Many women enter pregnancy with low or depleted iron stores even if the haemoglobin concentration is normal, and the majority of those who do not receive iron supplements have no stores at all at the end of pregnancy.

The changes in blood volume and haemodilution are so variable that the normal range of haemoglobin concentration can lie between 10.0 and 14.5 g/dl in healthy pregnancy at 30 weeks' gestation in women who have received parenteral iron. However, haemoglobin values of less than 10.5 g/dl in the second and third trimesters are probably abnormal and require further investigation. The World Health Organization (WHO) recommends that the haemoglobin concentration should not fall below 11.0 g/dl at any time during pregnancy.

The earliest effect of iron deficiency on the erythrocyte is a reduction in cell size, which appears to be the most sensitive index of underlying iron deficiency. A fall in red cell haemoglobin concentration (mean corpuscular haemoglobin, mean corpuscular haemoglobin concentration) only appear with more severe degrees of iron deficiency, or if the woman enters pregnancy with established iron-deficiency anaemia.

A fall in concentration of circulating haemoglobin is a relatively late development in iron deficiency and is preceded by depletion of iron stores followed by a reduction in serum iron levels. A state of iron deficiency can be diagnosed before anaemia has developed by finding a serum ferritin of less than 15 µg/l and a serum iron of less than 10 µmol/l, with less than 15 per cent saturation of the total iron-binding capacity. In recent years, serum ferritin, uninfluenced by recently ingested iron, has largely replaced serum iron and total iron-binding capacity as a non-invasive indicator of iron. A bone marrow examination may be necessary to assess iron stores directly and rapidly in the third trimester when there is limited time to investigate and carry out a trial of response to therapy in order to achieve a safe haemoglobin for delivery.

The anaemia of iron deficiency is the most common haematological problem in pregnancy. Because it is a late sign of iron deficiency, pregnant women are frequently given iron supplements prophylactically. The justification for doing this is still debated, although there is no question that iron deficiency is prevented. This is likely to be more important in poor than in developed countries where controlled trials demonstrate little effect of routine oral iron supplements on maternal well-being or perinatal outcome. The main point to consider is that if iron deficiency is detected in the third trimester there may not be time to correct it by either oral or parenteral supplements. Iron can be given as iron dextran, intramuscularly or intravenously, in the latter case as a total dose infusion. Intravenous administration may cause rare anaphylactic reactions and therefore should be given with caution, particularly in the first few minutes. There is no haematological benefit in giving parenteral as opposed to oral iron. The maximal response to be expected in pregnancy with oral or parenteral treatment is a rise in haemoglobin of approximately 0.8 g/dl weekly. The main advantage is that a total dose infusion ensures adequate iron for response and will avoid any undesirable side-effects associated with oral preparations. Otherwise, blood transfusions may be needed, with their associated hazards. On balance, a small daily supplement of oral iron given routinely, from the sixteenth week of pregnancy, seems the more sensible approach; it need not be considered as mandatory, but side-effects, which are most commonly bowel upsets, particularly constipation, are usually overcome by simple nutritional measures. In iron-deficient women it may take more than a year for the haemoglobin to return to pre-pregnancy levels. If iron supplements are given, the haemoglobin is in the normal pre-pregnancy range 5 to 7 days after delivery.

Non-haematological effects of iron deficiency

Tissue enzyme malfunction undoubtedly occurs even in the very first stages of iron deficiency (see Chapter 13.11). The prevention of nutritional iron deficiency is a desirable object in this period of maximal stress on the haemopoietic system during pregnancy. Overt maternal symptoms of iron deficiency are generally not prominent. However, treatment with oral or parenteral iron results in improved well-being long before the haemoglobin starts to rise significantly. Effects of iron deficiency on neuromuscular transmission may be responsible for the anecdotal reports of increased blood loss at delivery in anaemic women. The various effects of iron deficiency on cellular function may be responsible for the reported association between anaemia during pregnancy and preterm birth.

Iron deficiency—effect on fetus and newborn

The fetus derives its iron from maternal serum by active transport across the placenta in last four weeks of pregnancy. The concentrations of ferritin in the cord blood are substantially higher than those in the mother's circulation at term whether she is iron deficient or not, and all fall within normal adult range. However, babies born to iron-deficient mothers have significantly decreased cord ferritin levels compared to the others. This has an important bearing on iron stores and development of anaemia in the first year of life when iron intake is very poor.

There have also been studies to suggest that behavioural abnormalities in children with iron deficiency relate to changes in the concentration of chemical indicators in the brain. Iron deficiency in the absence of anaemia is also associated with poor performance in the Bayley Mental Developmental Index. Moreover, poor performance of 12- to 18-month-old iron-deficient, anaemic infants in mental and motor development can be improved to the level of iron-sufficient infants by treatment with

ferrous sulphate. Even more far-reaching effects of maternal iron deficiency during pregnancy have been suggested.

A correlation has recently been shown between maternal iron-deficiency anaemia, high placental weight, and an increased ratio of placental weight to birthweight. This suggests that maternal iron deficiency results in poor fetal growth compared to that of the placenta. High blood pressure in adult life has been linked to lower birthweight and with those whose birthweight was lower than would be expected from the weight of the placenta. Prophylaxis of iron deficiency may therefore have important implications for the prevention of adult hypertension.

Folic acid deficiency

When the diet is inadequate, pregnancy can lead to a state of negative folate balance. The pregnant woman needs approximately twice as much folic acid, 200 to 250 μg daily, as do non-pregnant individuals. The increase meets the needs of the growing uterus and conceptus and the expanded red cell mass. As pregnancy advances, serum folate falls to about half the non-pregnant value at term. The red cell folate content shows a slight decline over the same period.

Megaloblastic anaemia in pregnancy is usually the result of dietary folate deficiency (see Chapter 13.11). Its incidence is therefore variable, dependent on the socioeconomic status of the parturient population and whether or not folic acid supplements are given routinely as part of antenatal care. It occurs more frequently in multiple pregnancies. About half the cases present in the third trimester and the remainder after delivery. Commonly, deficiencies of iron and folate are combined; folate deficiency may then be revealed by the failure of a patient to respond to iron supplements. The peripheral blood film is unhelpful because the expected macrocytosis is often masked by microcytosis if there is also iron deficiency. Hypersegmentation of the neutrophils is also seen in pure iron deficiency. The diagnosis can only be confirmed by examination of a bone marrow aspirate. Other tests may be difficult to interpret because the results need to be related to the normal range that is expected for healthy pregnant women and not those derived from non-pregnant subjects. This applies to measurements of serum and red cell folate concentrations, as well as the excretion of formiminoglutamic acid after a histidine load (which is increased in normal pregnancy).

There is a strong case for prophylaxis during pregnancy, particularly in countries where overt megaloblastic anaemia is frequent. Women with a poor diet should be given 300 μg of folate daily. The risk of adverse effects is very small because vitamin B_{12} deficiency in pregnancy is rare (see below): subacute combined degeneration of the cord has never been reported in these circumstances. Folic acid should be given with supplemental iron. If gastrointestinal megaloblastic changes are established, oral supplements will have no effect and absorption in general will be impaired. This situation can only be reversed by administration of intramuscular folic acid. It is still argued to what extent folate deficiency may alter the outcome of pregnancy. Claims of an association between folate deficiency and placental abruption, abortion, and pre-eclampsia have not been substantiated. It has been shown that the incidence of prematurity and low birthweight can be reduced by giving supplements in poorly nourished populations, but has no effect in well-nourished women.

The fetus and folate deficiency

There is an increased risk of megaloblastic anaemia occurring in the neonate of a folate-deficient mother, especially if delivery is preterm. There are also data suggesting an association between periconceptional folic acid deficiency, harelip, cleft palate, and, most important of all, neural tube defects. The association between periconceptional folate deficiency and occurrence of neural tube defects has now been confirmed in a mass multicentre controlled trial of prepregnancy folate supplementation by the Medical Research Council.

In the United Kingdom it is recommended that women contemplating pregnancy should take folate supplements of 400 μg daily. This amount is contained in currently marketed Vitamin B complex, and such vitamin preparations should be used pending availability of specific tablets for this purpose. More recently it has also been shown in Hungary, in a large, randomized controlled trial, that periconceptional supplement of 800 μg of folic acid prevented the first occurrence of neural tube defects. The prevalence of harelip with or without cleft palate was not reduced by this supplementation.

Vitamin B$_{12}$ and pregnancy

Maternal vitamin B$_{12}$ stores, which are of the order of 3000 μg, are largely unaffected by pregnancy. The stores in the newborn infant are about 50 μg. The concentration of serum B$_{12}$ falls during pregnancy from non-pregnant levels of 205 to 1025 μg/l to 20 to 512 μg/l at term, associated with preferential transfer of absorbed B$_{12}$ to the fetus. The recommended intake of vitamin B$_{12}$ is 2.0 μg daily in the non-pregnant and 3.0 μg/day during pregnancy. This will be met by almost any diet that contains animal products, however deficient in other essential substances. Strict vegans, who will eat no animal produce whatsoever, can have a deficient B$_{12}$ intake and should be given oral supplements during pregnancy.

Vitamin B$_{12}$ deficiency in pregnancy is very rare. Addisonian pernicious anaemia does not usually occur during the reproductive years, associated as it is with infertility. Pregnancy is only likely to occur after the deficiency has been corrected.

Haemoglobinopathies

It is important to recognize the genetic defects of haemoglobin structure and synthesis early in pregnancy, or preferably before conception, because:

(1) the clinical effects may complicate obstetric management and appropriate precautions can be taken; and
(2) it is now possible to offer prenatal diagnosis to those women carrying a fetus at risk of a serious defect of haemoglobin synthesis or structure at a time when termination of pregnancy is feasible (Fig. 1).

The two clinically significant groups of haemoglobinopathies, the sickle-cell syndromes and the thalassaemias, are described in detail in Section 22. Only special problems related to pregnancy will be referred to here.

Fig. 1 Screening for haemoglobinopathies.

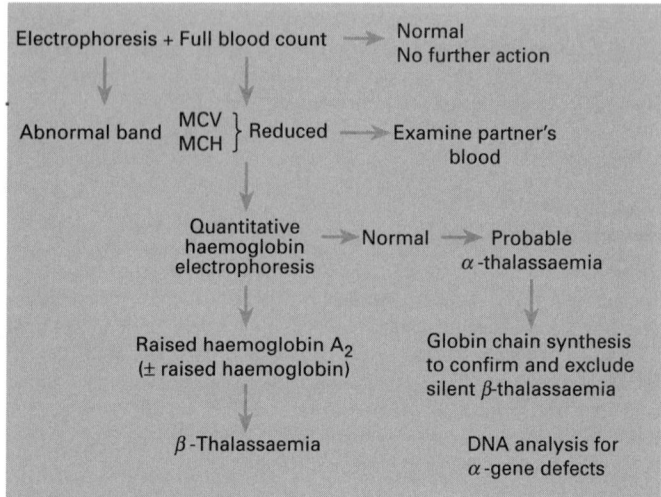

Screening procedures vary from location to location and often only involve 'high-risk' populations. The most difficult situations in the United Kingdom occur in those antenatal obstetric units which care for a small but significant proportion of immigrant mothers from varying racial backgrounds.

Figure 1 is a scheme which has been used with success in an obstetric unit serving a cosmopolitan population. This involves examination of red cell indices, haemoglobin electrophoresis, and, where indicated, quantitation of HbA$_2$ and HbF on every sample of blood taken at booking. If a haemoglobin variant or thalassaemic indices are found, the partner is requested to attend so that his blood can also be examined. By this means the chances of a serious haemoglobin defect will be assessed early in pregnancy, allowing counselling of the parents and the possibility of offering them prenatal diagnosis by fetal blood sampling or transabdominal chorion villus sampling, even though it will result in a late termination of pregnancy if indicated and desired (see Section 22).

Sickle-cell syndrome and pregnancy

It is essential to identify sickle-cell haemoglobin and the particular syndrome involved in the affected pregnant woman. The preferred procedure is to identify an abnormal band on electrophoresis at booking (see above) and to perform a sickling test only on those cases where there is such a band, to confirm that this is sickle haemoglobin. The distinction between sickle-cell trait (HbA/S), sickle-cell anaemia (HbS/S), and HbS/C disease is then immediately made and 9 out of 10 unnecessary sickling tests are avoided in women of relevant racial groups.

Women with sickle-cell trait have no difficulties in pregnancy, but care is needed if a general anaesthetic is required during labour. Tissue infarction can occur, even in the sickle-cell trait, if an adequate oxygen level is not maintained or if there is severe dehydration or shock. Most centres have developed programmes for antenatal diagnosis of sickle-cell anaemia using DNA analysis of amniotic or chorionic cells, or of fetal blood. If this is not available, it is important to identify homozygous infants by agar gel electrophoresis or isoelectric focusing immediately after birth. The first 2 years of life are particularly hazardous for an infant with sickle-cell anaemia because of the high incidence of death due to infection and splenic sequestration. Hence the mothers must be advised to present the infants early with any unusual symptoms.

Women with sickle-cell disease present special problems in pregnancy. Fetal loss is high, thought to be due to both impaired oxygen supply and sickling infarcts in the placental circulation. Abortion, preterm labour, and other complications are more common than in women with normal haemoglobin.

Although many women with sickle-cell disease have no complications, the outcome in any individual case is always in doubt. The only consistently successful way of reducing the incidence of complications due to sickling is by regular blood transfusion regimens designed to maintain the proportion of HbA at 60 to 70 per cent of the total. The management of sickle-cell syndromes in pregnancy in the United Kingdom is a relatively recent problem and longitudinal data are lacking. It is clear on review of the extensive American literature that although risks remain higher for pregnancy complicated by sickle-cell disease, modern obstetric care alone without blood transfusion has reduced the maternal morbidity and mortality dramatically, and has also improved fetal outcome.

Increasing numbers of obstetric units have adopted prophylactic transfusion regimes, but the real benefit of such prophylaxis remains to be proven by a large multicentre trial with contemporary controls. A small controlled trial in the United States suggests that the outcome is similar in women transfused prophylactically compared to those transfused only when indications arise. These prophylactic regimens are expensive and time consuming and may not be applicable in developing countries where the problem is widespread. In addition, there are problems of alloimmunization to minor blood group red cell antigens which has resulted in haemolytic disease of the new-born in some cases, not to mention the usual and apparently increasing hazards of blood transfusion, including hepatitis and human immunodeficiency virus (HIV) transmission.

Against this background of uncertainty, a reasonable compromise, particularly where blood transfusion facilities are limited, is to supervise pregnant women with sickle-cell anaemia with care throughout the pregnancy and to administer regular folate supplements. If they become severely anaemic, or have crises during the second half of pregnancy, an exchange transfusion is appropriate. Alternatively, if they present with haemoglobin values of less than 7 g/dl it is also acceptable to transfuse them up to a level of 12 to 14 g/dl, since this will reduce the level of HbS to a safe value without the need for exchange transfusion. During labour, management is directed towards preventing dehydration and acidosis. There is some controversy concerning the safest form of anaesthetic during labour or to cover delivery, but if regional, rather than general, anaesthesia is used, precautions must be taken to prevent venous pooling in the lower limbs.

Special mention should be made of the problem of HbSC disease (see Section 22) in pregnancy. Many women with this disorder go through pregnancy with no complications. However, occasionally there may be severe sickling episodes either late in pregnancy or early in the puerperium, which may lead to maternal death due to massive infarctive crises particularly in the lungs. Any women with this disorder who develop a painful crisis late in pregnancy, or who develop symptoms and signs suggestive of a chest infection or small pulmonary embolus, require urgent exchange transfusion. Examination of the stained blood film in the so-called chest syndrome will show large numbers of nucleated red cells. Cerebral sickling infarcts which, if not fatal, may result in long-term morbidity, are not unusual. The dangerous complications of this disorder are nearly always heralded by symptoms or signs of a sickling crisis; the lungs seem particularly vulnerable.

Thalassaemia syndromes

The clinical and haematological manifestations of the α- and β-thalassaemias are described in Section 22. Only certain points relevant to pregnancy will be discussed here.

α-THALASSAEMIA

The homozygous state for α°-thalassaemia produces Bart's haemoglobin hydrops syndrome. Pregnancy with an α-thalassaemia hydrops is associated with severe, sometimes life-threatening, hypertension and proteinuria, a pre-eclampsia-like syndrome (of severe rhesus haemolytic disease). Vaginal deliveries are associated with obstetric complications resulting from the large fetus and bulky placenta and the small stature of the mother (usually of Far-Eastern origin).

If routine screening of the parents shows that the mother is at risk of carrying such a child, then she should be referred as early as possible for prenatal diagnosis so that termination of an affected fetus can be carried out before these severe obstetric problems occur. Although this is not yet a common problem in the United Kingdom, it may well become more frequent if there is an influx of immigrants from Hong Kong and the Far East, as has already occurred in the United States and Australia.

β-THALASSAEMIA

Pregnancy is extremely rare in transfusion-dependent homozygous β-thalassaemics but is now being seen with increasing frequency in women with β-thalassaemia intermedia. These patients may become profoundly anaemic and require regular transfusion during pregnancy.

Perhaps the most common problem associated with haemoglobinopathies and pregnancy is the anaemia developing in the antenatal period in women who have thalassaemia minor, heterozygous β-thalassaemia. They can be identified in the usual way on examination of the blood sample taken at booking (see Fig. 1).

The level of haemoglobin in early pregnancy may be normal or slightly below the normal range. Women with β-thalassaemia minor require the usual oral iron supplements in the antenatal period. Oral iron for a limited period will not result in significant iron loading even in the presence of replete iron stores, but parenteral iron should never be given. Many women with thalassaemia minor enter pregnancy with depleted iron stores (as do many women with normal haemoglobin synthesis). A serum ferritin estimation can be carried out early in pregnancy, and if iron stores are found to be high then iron supplements can be withheld.

Folic acid, 5.0 mg daily, is recommended, to cover the requirements of ineffective erythropoiesis. If the anaemia does not respond to oral iron and folate, the latter given parenterally as well as orally, blood transfusion may be indicated. All women who are delivered in units with mixed racial background should be screened for β-thalassaemia early in pregnancy. The partners of those who are found to be carriers should also be screened so that prenatal diagnosis can be offered where there is a risk of conceiving a homozygous child.

Miscellaneous anaemias

Many systemic medical conditions may further complicate the physiological haemodilution of pregnancy, but it is impossible to cover them all here. Some of the more important are discussed below.

Haemolytic anaemias

Haemolysis is a feature of haemoglobinopathies and also of the disseminated intravascular coagulation encountered in severe pre-eclampsia (see Chapter 13.2) or postpartum renal failure (see Chapter 13.3). Autoimmune haemolysis is rarely encountered in pregnancy, although it may be a feature of active systemic lupus (see Chapter 20.5.6). The few reported cases suggest that it tends to worsen during gestation but should abate with appropriate corticosteroid therapy. As with all autoimmune conditions, the infant can be affected if the autoantibody is in the IgG class.

A rare form of haemolytic anaemia appears to be specific to pregnancy. It remits after delivery but tends to recur in about half of affected women in later pregnancies. Although no autoantibody has been identified this syndrome responds to corticosteroids or to infusion of human immunoglobulins (see below). The infant may be affected in about 20 per cent of cases.

Paroxysmal nocturnal haemoglobinuria (see Chapter 22.3.12) carries a high maternal mortality of about 10 per cent. This is largely because of the associated thrombotic tendencies that can affect the cerebral, hepatic, or intestinal circulations. The uteroplacental circulation is probably also involved because fetal wastage is so high (40–45 per cent).

Aplastic anaemia in pregnancy

Women with aplastic anaemia associated with recurrent infection or bleeding should not be allowed to become pregnant. If they do, treatment should follow the lines described in Section 22. There is a rare but interesting form of aplastic anaemia which occurs for the first time in pregnancy, remits after delivery, and then recurs again in subsequent pregnancies. The mechanism of this condition has not been worked out. It does not respond to any form of bone marrow stimulant or corticosteroid therapy and the management is symptomatic.

Leukaemia and lymphoma

These neoplastic conditions occasionally coincide with pregnancy. There is no evidence that their course is adversely affected by pregnancy, but the pregnancy becomes complicated because of the need for treatment with either radiotherapy or cytotoxic agents. Termination of pregnancy is necessary if radiotherapy needs to be started without delay, but successful pregnancies have been reported when cytotoxic therapy

Table 1 *Spectrum of severity of disseminated intravascular coagulation (DIC): its relationship to specific complications in obstetrics*

	Severity of DIC	*In vitro* findings	Obstetric condition commonly associated
Stage 1	Low-grade compensated	FDPs ↑ Increased soluble fibrin complexes Increased ratio VWF:factor VIIIC	Pre-eclampsia Retained dead fetus
Stage 2	Uncompensated but no haemostatic failure	As above, plus fibrinogen ↓ platelets ↓ factors V and VIII ↓	Small abruptio Severe pre-eclampsia
Stage 3	Rampant with haemostatic failure	Platelets ↓ ↓ Gross depletion of coagulation factors, particularly fibrinogen FDPs ↑	Abruptio placentae Amniotic fluid embolism Eclampsia

Rapid progression from stage 1 to stage 3 is possible unless appropriate action is taken.

FDP, fibrin degradation products; VWF, von Willebrand factor.

has been administered for the treatment of leukaemia. Teratogenic effects may occur with the use of folate antagonists, chlorambucil, cyclophosphamide, and vincristine. Prematurity and growth retardation seem to be the main problems in later gestation.

Disorders of haemostasis

Normal pregnancy is accompanied by major changes in the coagulation and fibrinolytic systems. There are significant increases in the procoagulant factors V, VII, and X, and a very marked increase in plasma fibrinogen. In uncomplicated pregnancy, there is no change in antithrombin III (ATIII) concentrations during the antenatal period, a fall during delivery, and then an increase 1 week postpartum. However, ATIII synthesis must be increased to maintain normal concentrations in the face of increasing plasma volume. Protein C levels appear to remain constant or increase slightly, but protein S activity falls significantly during normal pregnancy.

The result of these physiological changes is to alter the usual balance between the procoagulants and anticoagulants in favour of the factors promoting blood clotting. In addition, fibrinolytic activity appears to be reduced during healthy pregnancy but returns to normal rapidly after separation of the placenta and completion of the third stage of delivery. This effect is mediated by placentally derived plasminogen activator inhibitor type II. As pregnancy advances, the elastic lamina and smooth muscle of the spiral arteries supplying the placenta are replaced by a matrix containing fibrin. This allows an expansion of the lumen and reduces resistance to accommodate an increasing blood flow. At placental separation during normal childbirth a blood flow of 500 to 800 ml/mm has to be staunched within seconds or serious haemorrhage will occur. Myometrial contraction plays a vital role in securing haemostasis by reducing blood flow to the placental site. Rapid closure of the terminal parts of the spiral arteries will be facilitated by the structural changes described.

These changes in the haemostatic systems, together with the increase in blood volume, help to reduce the chances of abnormal haemorrhage at delivery, but convert pregnancy into a hypercoagulable state which may carry special hazards for both the mother and fetus. These hazards include a spectrum of haemostatic disorders, from thromboembolism (see Section 22) through to the many conditions associated with disseminated intravascular coagulation.

Disseminated intravascular coagulation

This is associated with a wide variety of complications of pregnancy. It may be well compensated, with little change in tests of haemostatic function and no bleeding, as seen in prolonged retention of a dead fetus and mild pre-eclampsia, or it may result in intractable haemorrhage with gross consumption of coagulation factors and platelets and raised levels of fibrin degradation products, as seen classically in abruptio placentae (see Table 1).

Other complications of pregnancy in which disseminated intravascular coagulation may take a part include amniotic fluid embolism; septic abortion and intrauterine infection; hydatidiform mole; placenta accreta; pre-eclampsia and eclampsia, and prolonged shock from any cause (see Fig. 2).

Disseminated intravascular coagulation is always a secondary process and treatment should involve removal of the triggering mechanism where this is known. In the obstetric patient it may present with haemorrhage. The principles of management are to achieve an empty and contracted uterus, and to maintain the circulating blood volume. Blood should be taken for screening tests in order to confirm or refute a diagnosis of disseminated intravascular coagulation. Useful and rapid screening tests include the platelet count, partial thromboplastin time (intrinsic coagulation), prothrombin time (extrinsic coagulation), thrombin time, fibrinogen concentration, and levels of fibrin degradation products. However, the management is the same whether bleeding is complicated or triggered by disseminated intravascular coagulation, or whether it is due to poor myometrial function or trauma to the genital tract alone. Prolonged shock from any cause will lead to endothelial damage and trigger this condition. It is very important to maintain the circulation with whatever plasma replacement therapy is to hand, until fresh frozen plasma and later cross-matched packed red cells are available. This aids the clearance of fibrin degradation products, which are potent anticoagulants in themselves and also interfere with myometrial function. The use of whole fresh blood is no longer feasible as it has to be properly processed and checked for the presence of hepatitis antigens and for HIV antibodies. To release it earlier than the usual 18 to 24 h would increase the risk of transmitting viral infection or of administering incompatible transfusions. Fresh, frozen plasma and stored red cells provide all the components apart from platelets present in whole fresh blood.

Although cryoprecipitate is richer in fibrinogen than fresh, frozen plasma, it lacks ATIII which is rapidly consumed in obstetric bleeding associated with disseminated intravascular coagulation. The use of cryoprecipitate will also expose the recipient to more donors and the associated potential hazards.

Platelets are not present in fresh, frozen plasma, and their activity rapidly deteriorates in stored blood. The maternal platelet count reflects both the degree of intravascular coagulation and the amount of bank blood transfused. A patient with persistent bleeding and low platelet count (less than 50×10^9/l) may be given concentrated platelets, although they are very rarely required in addition to fresh, frozen plasma to achieve haemostasis.

Heparin is theoretically useful but hazardous unless the circulation is intact and the uterus contracted and empty. Antifibrinolytic agents are extremely dangerous in a bleeding obstetric patient and their use is almost never indicated.

Pre-eclampsia and haemostatic changes

Pre-eclampsia may be associated with quite marked changes in the normal physiological response of the haemostatic mechanisms during pregnancy. Differential diagnosis is confused by overlapping clinical signs and symptoms and nomenclature (see Chapter 13.2). Some women who present with a raised serum bilirubin, bleeding diathesis, and renal failure may not be suffering from acute fatty liver of pregnancy but may have severe pre-eclampsia, haemolytic uraemia syndrome, thrombotic thrombocytopenia or hypertension with elevated liver enzymes and low platelets, the so-called HELLP syndrome (see Chapter 20.6).

The combination of a reduced platelet lifespan and a fall in the platelet count without platelet-associated antibodies indicates a low-grade coagulopathy. Rarely, in very severe pre-eclampsia the patient develops microangiopathic haemolysis. These patients suffer profound thrombocytopenia and this leads to confusion in differential diagnosis between pre-eclampsia, HELLP syndrome, and thrombotic thrombocytopenia.

Overall, the data concerning dysfunction of platelets in pre-eclampsia indicate that activation with increased turnover and shortening of lifespan occurs, the degree increasing with disease severity. The effect on coagulation appears to represent an augmentation of the hypercoagulable state which accompanies normal pregnancy. There appear to be some significant changes in both the factor VIII complex and antithrombin III, related to severity of the disease process. An increased ratio between von Willebrand factor and factor VIII coagulation activity has been shown to be characteristic of pre-eclampsia, which may also be associated with reduction in antithrombin III concentrations, the fall correlating broadly with the severity of the pre-eclamptic syndrome.

In relation to fibrinolysis in pre-eclampsia, most studies have shown

Table 2 *Haemostatic changes in pre-eclampsia*

Prostacyclin generation	Decreased
Platelets	Decreased numbers[a]
	Decreased lifespan
	Decreased 5HT (serotonin)
	Increased plasma β-thromboglobulin and platelet factor IV
Factor VIII complex	Increased ratio VWF[a]/factor VIIIC
Antithrombin III	Decreased
Soluble fibrinogen products	Increased, particularly fibrinopeptide-A
Fibrin degradation products	Increased in serum[a] and urine

[a]The most useful markers of severity and outcome.

VWF, von Willebrand factor.

increased levels of fibrinogen/fibrin degradation products in serum and urine. Once the disease process is established the most relevant haemostatic abnormalities appear to be the platelet count, factor VIII coagulation activity, and serum fibrin degradation products (Table 2). Those women with the most marked abnormalities in these parameters suffer the greatest perinatal loss.

Thrombotic thrombocytopenic purpura and haemolytic uraemia syndrome

These rare conditions share so many features they should probably be considered as one disease with pathological effects confined to the kidney in haemolytic uraemia syndrome and being more generalized in thrombotic thrombocytopenic purpura. In relation to pregnancy, haemolytic uraemia syndrome usually presents in the postpartum period with renal failure. These disorders are discussed more fully in Chapter 20.6.

Platelet disorders

Thrombocytopenia is a common haematological abnormality in pregnancy which has important implications for both mother and fetus. It may occur as part of the pathophysiology of pregnancy itself, or pregnancy may be superimposed on a background of haematological disease.

INCIDENTAL THROMBOCYTOPENIA

As pregnancy advances there is a progressive small but significant fall in the platelet count in individual patients, probably due to haemodilution. With the advent of automated cell counters in haematological laboratories it has become apparent that incidental thrombocytopenia during pregnancy is relatively common. Approximately 5 per cent of healthy pregnant women have been shown to have thrombocytopenia at term, with platelet counts between 90 and $150 \times 10^9/l$. These women have no history of pre-eclampsia or immune thrombocytopenia. There is no increased incidence of thrombocytopenia in their offspring.

THROMBOCYTOPENIA AND DISSEMINATED INTRAVASCULAR COAGULATION

Low-grade disseminated intravascular coagulation, as observed in pre-eclampsia, may be associated with further decrements but the platelet count rarely falls below $50 \times 10^9/l$, even in acute defibrination syndromes. Clearly thrombocytopenia and platelet consumption represent only one aspect of this condition (see above) and will be corrected quickly when haemostatic mechanisms return to normal, usually without the use of, or need for, platelet transfusion.

Fig. 2 Trigger mechanisms of disseminated intravascular coagulation during pregnancy. Interactions occur in many of these obstetric complications.

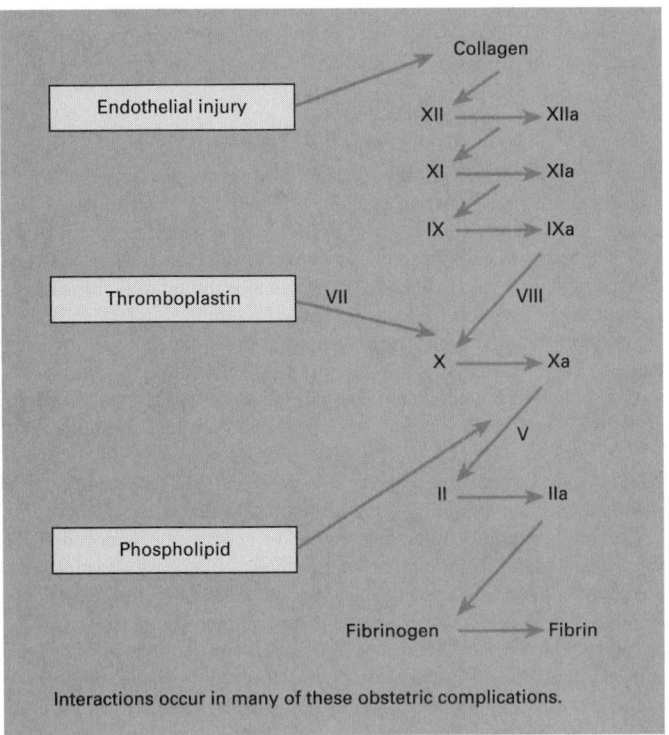

Interactions occur in many of these obstetric complications.

IDIOPATHIC THROMBOCYTOPENIC PURPURA

Idiopathic thrombocytopenic purpura is a rare condition, but relatively common in young women of reproductive years. Acute idiopathic thrombocytopenic purpura typically occurs in children, while the chronic form is more often seen in adults. Patients in remission may still have elevated levels of platelet-associated IgG (PAIgG), especially following splenectomy. This is important in pregnancy because of the possibility of placental transfer of IgG antibody resulting in fetal thrombocytopenia. In this context; measurement of maternal platelet count, serum platelet antibody, and PAIgG are useful diagnostic tools but they are not predictive of neonatal thrombocytopenia.

Although retrospective analysis of the literature in the past gave an overall incidence of neonatal thrombocytopenia of 52 per cent with significant morbidity of 12 per cent, we know now that this incidence was distorted because only symptomatic women were likely to have been investigated and reported. More recent analyses show an incidence of fetal thrombocytopenia of around 10 per cent, with severe thrombocytopenia (platelets fewer than $50 \times 10^9/l$) in less than 5 per cent overall. Fetal and neonatal morbidity and mortality is negligible even in the face of severe thrombocytopenia. Thrombocytopenia in the neonate tends to become more severe in the first few days of life and measures can be taken to correct this at birth before the nadir is reached, if indicated.

The dilemma in the pregnant woman with idiopathic thrombocytopenic purpura is that nearly all patients have the chronic form of the disease. The effects of treatment have to be considered in relation to the progress of pregnancy in both mother and fetus. The mild condition may require no treatment, but if the platelet count falls below $50 \times 10^9/l$, or there is clinical evidence of bleeding, she should be given prednisone (60 mg daily, reducing rapidly to the lowest possible dose that maintains the platelet count above $50 \times 10^9/l$). The prevalence of pre-eclampsia, gestational diabetes, postpartum psychosis, and osteoporosis are all increased by corticosteroids. The dose and duration of treatment should therefore be the minimum needed to reduce the risk of bleeding or to raise the platelet count of an asymptomatic woman at term, allowing her to have epidural or spinal analgesia if desired or indicated.

The introduction of treatment by intravenous monomeric polyvalent human IgG has altered the management options in pregnancy dramatically. Used in the original recommended dose of 0.4 g/kg for 5 days by intravenous infusion, a persistent and predictable response is obtained in approximately 80 per cent of reported cases. Recently, alternative, equally effective dosage regimens of this expensive treatment have been suggested. One g/kg is given over 8 h on 1 day. This dose will raise the platelet count to safe levels in approximately half the patients. In those in whom the platelet count does not rise a similar dose can be repeated 2 days later. Analysis of recent reports indicates that the postulated beneficial transplacental effect on fetal platelets is unreliable and that exogenous IgG may not cross the placenta.

Although there is no doubt about the value of intravenous IgG in selected cases of severe symptomatic thrombocytopenia, it would be necessary to show that its indiscriminate use in all cases dramatically improves both maternal and fetal outcome in order to justify the high cost.

Splenectomy is hardly ever indicated in the pregnant patient with idiopathic thrombocytopenic purpura and should be avoided given the success of medical management. Removal of the spleen remains an option if all other attempts to increase the platelet count to safe levels fail. Splenectomy is best carried out in the second trimester because surgery is best tolerated then and the size of the uterus will not make the operation technically difficult.

Very occasionally, immunosuppressives such as azathioprine and cyclophosphamide have to be used in severe intractable thrombocytopenia. Cyclophosphamide should be avoided in pregnancy, but azathioprine does not appear to be associated with increased fetal or maternal morbidity.

The most contentious problem in pregnancy associated with maternal idiopathic thrombocytopenic purpura is the mode of delivery of the fetus. Even if the mother has to deliver in the face of a low platelet count, she is unlikely to bleed from the placental site once the uterus is empty but she is at risk of bleeding from surgical incisions, soft-tissue injuries, or tears. Platelets should be available for transfusion but not given prophylactically. The major risk at delivery is to the fetus with thrombocytopenia who, as a result of birth trauma, may suffer intracranial haemorrhage. Maternal platelet count, maternal platelet-associated IgG, splenectomy status, and history may give a crude indication of the likelihood of fetal thrombocytopenia but can never be used in an individual case to predict the fetal platelet count. It is, however, unlikely for the fetus to have severe thrombocytopenia if the mother has no history of idiopathic thrombocytopenic purpura before the index pregnancy and if she has no detectable IgG platelet antibody. Platelet counts in blood obtained by transcervical fetal scalp sampling prior to, or early in, labour have been used to make a decision about the mode of delivery. This mode of sampling is not without risk of significant haemorrhage in the truly thrombocytopenic fetus, often gives false positive results, and demands urgent action to be taken on the results obtained. In addition, the fetus may have already descended so far in the birth canal that caesarean section is technically difficult and traumatic for the fetus.

The only way a reliable platelet count can be obtained is by a percutaneous transabdominal fetal cord blood sample. The procedure carries a risk of approximately 1 per cent for the fetus. It should be performed at 37 to 38 weeks' gestation under ultrasound guidance. The transfer of IgG increases in the last weeks of pregnancy and an earlier sample may give a higher fetal platelet count than at one taken near term. There is no point in serial fetal platelet counts because the fetus is not at risk of spontaneous intracranial haemorrhage, unlike the situation when the thrombocytopenia is alloimmune in origin (see below). For many centres the availability of planned or emergency transabdominal fetal blood sampling is severely limited, so decisions concerning the mode of delivery will have to be taken without knowledge of the fetal platelet count.

There is no good evidence that caesarean section is less traumatic than uncomplicated vaginal delivery, although this mode of delivery allows more overall control and there are usually no unpredictable complications. At the time of writing the emphasis of management is to return to a non-interventional policy of sensible monitoring, supportive therapy, and a mode of delivery determined mainly by obstetric indications and not primarily by either the maternal or fetal platelet count.

ALLOIMMUNE THROMBOCYTOPENIA

Fetal and neonatal allo-immune thrombocytopenia develop as a result of maternal sensitization to paternally derived fetal platelet antigens. The pathogenesis is analogous to that of Rh haemolytic disease of the newborn. The mother is not thrombocytopenic but the fetus may have a very low platelet count, and is at risk of spontaneous intrauterine intracranial haemorrhage. This results from the specific antibody interfering with glycoprotein-binding sites and profoundly altering platelet function, particularly aggregation. The most common platelet antigen involved is HPA-1. Ninety-eight per cent of the population in the United Kingdom are HPA-1 positive. Two allelic variants are present, HPA-1 and HPA-2. Sixty-nine per cent of the population are homozygous for HPA-1. Rarely, in the United Kingdom other platelet antigens may be involved.

A platelet incompatibility does not invariably result in alloimmunization. The maternal immune response is genetically determined by genes of the major histocompatibility complex. Response appears to be restricted to those women with HLA-B8 and HLA-DR3 antigens. Thus, although 1 in 50 pregnancies may be incompatible with respect to HPA-1 antigens, only 1 in 5000 births are affected. The children of first pregnancies (unlike rhesus disease) are often affected and the disease process can begin in early fetal life. Current management is aimed at identifying the fetus at risk and correcting the thrombocytopenia *in utero*. The approaches to this problem are all controversial. One protocol involves fetal blood sampling at 20 to 22 weeks' gestation and treating the mothers with thrombocytopenic fetuses with intravenous IgG 1 g/kg/week, with or without steroids, until delivery. This has been reported as successful in some units but not others. The overall results of multicentre trials of the efficacy of maternal intravenous IgG administration is awaited. Another approach is to administer weekly compatible platelet transfusions to the fetus. This has been successful in a number of cases but involves frequent hazardous procedures. Whatever approach is used, immediate predelivery administration of compatible platelets to the fetus is recommended. When the diagnosis is established shortly after birth, the accepted management is to transfuse specially prepared HPA-1 negative platelets from pre-selected blood-bank donors or if facilities are available, washed platelets from the mother.

Inherited defects of haemostasis

VON WILLEBRAND'S DISEASE

Von Willebrand's disease is the most frequent of all inherited haemostatic abnormalities. It has an autosomal dominant inheritance and is therefore the most likely coagulopathy to affect women in pregnancy.

There are various types of von Willebrand's disease (see Section 22), but the common type I affects platelet function and the factor VIII complex, resulting in reduced levels of both the large multimer von Willebrand factor and the smaller coagulation factor (VIIIC). In normal pregnancy a rise in both VIIIC and von Willebrand factor is observed. Patients with all but the severest forms of von Willebrand's disease show a similar but variable rise in both these factors during pregnancy, although there may not be a reduction in the bleeding time. After delivery normal women maintain an elevated level of VIIIC for at least 5 days. In women with von Willebrand's disease the duration of this elevation seems to be related to the severity of the disorder. The general consensus is that the most important determinant for abnormal haemorrhage at delivery is a low factor VIIIC level. The newly developed factor VIII concentrates do contain von Willebrand factor activity as well as factor VIIIC. Cryoprecipitate, with all the hazards of a fresh plasma product, is no longer recommended, since the concentrates, being heat treated, have the advantage of reducing the hazard of transfusion-transmittable infection dramatically. Appropriate factor VIII concentrates should be standing by to cover delivery but are rarely required to achieve haemostasis. There is virtually no place for desmopressin in obstetric practice, except perhaps in the puerperium. Any rise in factor VIII attributable to vasopressin will have been achieved under the influence of pregnancy itself. In contrast, desmopressin has a valuable place in women undergoing gynaecological or other surgery.

HAEMOPHILIA

The risks in pregnancy for the female carrier of haemophilia are twofold.

1. She may, due to lyonization (random deletion of the X chromosome), have very low VIII or IX levels and be at risk of excessive bleeding, particularly following a surgical or traumatic delivery.
2. Fifty per cent of her male offspring will inherit haemophilia. This has important implications now that prenatal diagnosis of these conditions is possible.

It is important to identify carriers prior to pregnancy, not only to provide appropriate management for the rare case with pathologically low coagulation activity but to provide genetic counselling. The changes in factor VIII complex may make the identification of carriers more difficult during pregnancy. Clinical problems occur more often in carriers for Christmas disease, since factor IX does not rise in response to healthy pregnancy in the same way as does factor VIII. Appropriate heat-treated concentrates are available to treat abnormal haemorrhage. Cryoprecip-

itate and fresh, frozen plasma should never be used unless the concentrates are not available.

Obstetric and laboratory techniques developed during the past decade have been applied successfully to the accurate prenatal diagnosis of haemostatic disorders. It is possible to obtain fetal blood suitable for coagulation factor assays from 18 weeks' gestation onwards, and to diagnose or exclude deficiencies of factors VIII and IX in male fetuses, albeit late. It is now possible to make rapid early diagnosis of these conditions by DNA analysis of chorion villus samples or amniotic fluid cells obtained earlier in pregnancy. Cloning of the genes for factors VIII and IX has facilitated prenatal diagnosis in many, but not all, cases at risk of haemophilia. Some few families remain where the recombinant DNA technology is not informative, so that fetal blood sample coagulation factor assays will continue to be of value.

REFERENCES

Anaemias and related disorders

Chanarin, I. (1985). Folate and cobalamin. In *Haematological disorders in pregnancy. Clinics in haematology*, Vol. 14, (ed. E.A. Letsky), pp. 629–41. Saunders, Eastbourne.

Czeizel, A.E. and Dudás, I. (1992). Prevention of the first occurrence of neural-tube defects by periconceptional vitamin supplementation. *New England Journal of Medicine* **327**, 1832–5.

Godfrey, K.M., Redman, C.W.G., Barker, D.J.P., and Osmond, C. (1991). The effect of maternal anaemia and iron deficiency on the ratio of fetal weight to placental weight. *British Journal of Obstetrics and Gynaecology* **98**, 886–91.

Goodall, H.B., *et al.* (1979). Haemolytic anaemia of pregnancy. *Scandinavian Journal of Haematology* **22**, 185–91.

Idjradinata, P. and Pollitt, E. (1993). Reversal of developmental delays in iron-deficient anaemic infants treated with iron. *Lancet* **341**, 1–4.

Koshy, M. and Burd, L. (1991). Management of pregnancy in sickle cell syndromes. *Hematological Oncology Clinics of North America* **5**, (3), 585–96.

Letsky, E.A. (1987). Anaemia in obstetrics. *Progress in Obstetrics and Gynaecology* **7**, 23–58.

Letsky, E.A. (1991). The haematological system. In *Clinical physiology in obstetrics*, (2nd edn), (ed. F.E. Hytten and G.V.P. Chamberlain), pp. 39–82. Blackwell Scientific Publications, Oxford.

Lewis, B.J. and Laros, R.K. (1986). Leukemia and lymphoma. In *Blood disorders in pregnancy*, (ed. R.K. Laros), pp. 85–101. Lea and Febiger, Philadelphia.

MRC Vitamin Study Research Group (1991). Prevention of neural tube defects: results of the Medical Research Council vitamin study. *Lancet* **338**, 131–7.

Perry, K.G., Jr and Morrison, J.C. (1990). The diagnosis and management of hemoglobinopathies during pregnancy. *Seminars in Perinatology* **14**, (2), 90–102.

Snyder, T.E., Lee, L.P., and Lynch, S. (1991). Pregnancy-associated hypoplastic anemia: a review. *Obstetrical and Gynecological Survey* **46**, (5), 264–9.

Tuck, S.M., James, C.E., Brewster, E.M., Pearson, T.C., and Studd, J.W.W. (1987). Prophylactic blood transfusion in maternal sickle cell syndromes. *British Journal of Obstetrics and Gynaecology* **94**, 121–5.

Haemostasis

Burrows, R.F. and Kelton, J.G. (1992). Thrombocytopenia during pregnancy. In *Haemostasis and thrombosis in obstetrics and gynaecology*, (ed. I.A. Greer, A.G.G. Turpie, and C.D. Forbes), pp. 407–29. Chapman & Hall, London.

Forbes, C.D. and Greer, I.A. (1992). Physiology of haemostasis and the effect of pregnancy. In *Haemostasis and thrombosis in obstetrics and gynaecology*, (ed. I.A. Greer, A.G.G. Turpie, and C.D. Forbes), pp. 1–25. Chapman & Hall, London.

Leduc, L., Wheeler, J.M., Kirshon, B., Mitchell, P., and Cotton, D.B. (1992). Coagulation profile in severe preeclampsia. *Obstetrics and Gynecology* **79**, (1), 14–18.

Letsky, E.A. (1995). Coagulation defects. In *Medical disorders in obstetric practice*, (ed. M. de Swiet), pp. 104–65, 3rd edn, in press.

Letsky, E.A. (1991). Mechanisms of coagulation and the changes induced by pregnancy. *Current Obstetrics and Gynaecology* **1**, 203–9.

Pillai, M. (1993). Platelets and pregnancy. *British Journal of Obstetrics and Gynaecology* **100**, 201–4.

Rock, G.A., *et al.* and the Canadian Apheresis Study Group (1991). Comparison of plasma exchange with plasma infusion in the treatment of thrombotic thrombocytopenic purpura. *New England Journal of Medicine* **325**, 393–7.

Weatherall, D.J. (1991). Prenatal diagnosis of haematological disorders. In *Fetal and neonatal haematology*, (ed. E.A. Letsky, I.M. Hann, and B.E.S. Gibson), pp. 285–314. Baillière Tindall, London.

13.10 Neurological disease in pregnancy

G. G. LENNOX

INTRODUCTION

A range of neurological problems occasionally complicate pregnancy and the puerperium. Pre-existing neurological diseases, such as epilepsy and myasthenia gravis, sometimes become more troublesome. New neurological disorders occur, from diseases of the peripheral nerves and muscles, which are relatively common but generally benign, to diseases of the central nervous system, which are rare but potentially life-threatening. In all these situations the presence of the fetus influences management.

Disorders of muscle and neuromuscular transmission

Muscle disorders

Muscle cramps, particularly on waking, are extremely common in the third trimester. They often respond to calcium supplements. Restless legs syndrome, in which there is an ill-defined sensory disturbance in the legs relieved by movement, is also common, especially on retiring to bed. It may respond to correction of any associated anaemia but otherwise management in pregnancy is aimed at promoting the rapid onset of sleep, for example by reducing caffeine intake. Drugs such as codeine, clonazepam, and levodopa are best avoided. Polymyositis, although rare in young women, can deteriorate during pregnancy; steroid treatment is thought to be safe but cyclosporin and cyclophosphamide are potentially harmful to the fetus. Most other muscle diseases are not influenced by pregnancy; the major exception is myotonic dystrophy.

Myotonic dystrophy

(See also Section 25.)

Myotonic dystrophy is an autosomal dominant disorder with a tendency to become more severe with each generation (the phenomenon of anticipation, reflecting an increasingly large CTG repeat insert within the myotonin protein kinase gene) particularly when transmitted maternally. Polyhydramnios and perinatal death are more common and surviving babies may be severely affected from birth. Myotonia affects the uterine smooth muscle, prolonging labour and increasing the risk of postpartum haemorrhage because of uterine inertia.

Myasthenia gravis

(See also Section 24.)

Myasthenia gravis deteriorates, improves, and remains stable during pregnancy in roughly equal proportions of patients, but the response is neither predictable nor reproducible in subsequent pregnancies. Approximately half of all patients worsen during the puerperium and deterioration may also occur after abortion. The mechanism of these effects is not clear. Corticosteroids, oral anticholinesterases, and plasmapheresis can all be employed in the usual ways during pregnancy. It is reasonable to continue azathioprine where it has been prescribed before pregnancy for severe myasthenia, bearing in mind the risk of inducing neonatal leucopenia. Thymectomy can be performed during pregnancy but has no immediate therapeutic effect; ideally it should be performed at least a year before pregnancy is attempted. Myasthenia does not usually influence labour, although the second stage may be prolonged by fatigue and obstetric anaesthesia is complicated by the need to avoid drugs with adverse effects on neuromuscular transmission: where possible, regional anaesthesia is preferable. Acetylcholine receptor antibodies can cross the placenta into the fetal circulation to cause neonatal myasthenia; expert paediatric support must therefore be available at delivery.

Disorders of nerves and nerve roots

Facial palsy

The incidence of Bell's palsy is substantially increased during pregnancy and the puerperium (as Bell himself described.) The reason for this is not known. There have been no studies of treatment in this specific context but it is reasonable to treat promptly with prednisolone, beginning at 40 mg daily and reducing over a 2 week course.

Mononeuropathies

Carpal tunnel due to entrapment of the median nerve at the wrist is common in pregnancy, presumably because of increasing peripheral oedema. It characteristically causes pain and paraesthesiae in the hands at night. Most cases can be managed with nocturnal wrists splints, although steroid injections into the carpal tunnel may tide the patient over until the puerperium when the symptoms almost always remit. Diuretics are of little value. Surgical decompression during pregnancy should be reserved for cases with severe pain, weakness, or wasting; occasionally delayed surgery is indicated to prevent recurrence in further pregnancies (which is common).

The lateral cutaneous nerve of the thigh can also be compressed as it crosses the inguinal ligament; this is particularly common in the third trimester in women who have put on a great deal of weight. This causes paraesthesiae and sometimes hypersensitivity in the mid lateral thigh, which may be bilateral. Usually no treatment is required but troublesome cases may respond to transcutaneous nerve stimulation or infiltration of steroid and local anaesthetic around the nerve. Remission after delivery is the rule.

Lumbar root and plexus lesions

Backache is very common in pregnancy. It is traditionally attributed to changes in posture, with an accentuation of lumbar lordosis, and the hormonally mediated relaxation of spinal and sacroiliac joints. The pain typically worsens with prolonged standing and may radiate into the buttock or thigh. Sometimes there is tenderness over one or other sacroiliac joint. Radiological investigations are not needed if there are no abnormal neurological signs, and management is conservative. Abrupt onset of pain that radiates below the knee with focal weakness or reflex loss is most likely to be due to a prolapsed intervertebral disc. Providing the signs are unilateral and there is no sphincter impairment, initial treatment should be with analgesia, muscle relaxants, and bed rest (bearing in mind the risk of deep vein thrombosis). Failing this, magnetic resonance imaging (MRI) is the best way of investigating prior to lumbar disc surgery.

The lumbosacral plexus may be compressed by the baby's head during labour, particularly if there is dystocia. Any resulting footdrop usually resolves spontaneously within a matter of weeks. The differential diagnosis includes damage to the femoral nerve, which may occur during caesarean section; again the prognosis is generally good. Long or complicated deliveries may also lead to damage to the obturator or pudendal nerves; the latter, although initially asymptomatic, probably contributes to the subsequent development of perineal descent and incontinence.

Generalized neuropathies

The combination of the increased nutritional demands of pregnancy and hyperemesis gravidarum can lead to thiamine deficiency. This most commonly causes a subacute sensory neuropathy but cases of Wernicke's encephalopathy (with any combination of altered consciousness, ataxia, and ophthalmoplegia, leading if untreated to death) have been described. Both conditions respond promptly to parenteral thiamine replacement (in doses of at least 100 mg daily). Pregnancy can precipitate relapse in women with acute intermittent porphyria; typically abdominal pain precedes the development of autonomic and sensory neuropathy, sometimes with seizures and psychiatric disturbance.

Disorders of the central nervous system

Tension headache and migraine

The most common form of headache during pregnancy is tension or muscle contraction headache. This is often the result of identifiable worry, lack of sleep, or depression, and responds to treatment of these underlying problems. In other cases the cause is less clear. None the less, the headaches usually respond to explanation, reassurance, relaxation exercises, and massage, supplemented if necessary by occasional doses of paracetamol. Aspirin should be avoided and more potent analgesics are generally no more effective than paracetamol. If frequent headaches persist, small prophylactic doses of amitriptyline may be helpful (even in patients who are not depressed).

Migraine usually improves during pregnancy. Approximately 20 per cent of patients get worse, and occasionally migraine actually begins in pregnancy. No single hormonal change has been convincingly linked to these divergent responses. Acute attacks should be treated promptly with rest and paracetamol; metoclopramide can be used for nausea or vomiting. Sumatriptan has not yet been shown to be safe in pregnancy. Ergot preparations are contraindicated in pregnancy (and lactation.) If attacks are frequent, then attention should be paid to relevant lifestyle factors, including lack of sleep and irregular meals. Prophylactic drug treatment may be necessary. The greatest experience lies with propranolol which, in doses of 20 to 80 mg three times a day, appears to be both effective and safe, despite its effect on placental blood flow (Chapter 24.11) Amitriptyline is a safe second choice. Pizotifen should be avoided because of lack of safety information; for this reason it should also be discontinued in women who are taking it prophylactically prior to pregnancy. Women with migraine are very prone to mild non-specific headaches in the first few days after delivery. These rarely require treatment, particularly if the patient is forewarned.

Table 1 *Disorders that may present with headache and focal neurological deficit during pregnancy*

Migraine	
Subarachnoid haemorrhage	Aneurysm
	Angioma
Cerebral infarction	
Cerebral venous thrombosis	
Intracranial tumour	Pituitary adenoma
	Meningioma
	Glioma
	Choriocarcinoma
Intracranial infection	Cerebral abscess
	Listeria encephalitis
Eclampsia	
Phaeochromocytoma	
Thrombotic microangiopathy	

Migraine can usually be accurately identified on clinical grounds, particularly when it precedes the pregnancy. Diagnosis is more difficult when migraine presents for the first time during pregnancy, especially when it is accompanied by transient focal deficit such as hemiplegia. Here consideration must be given to a range of other diseases that present with headache and focal deficit (Table 1).

Tumours

Although the incidence of cerebral and spinal tumours is probably no greater than at other times, some tumours expand during pregnancy and may present unusually rapidly. This probably reflects a mixture of hormonal and vascular factors; many meningiomas and some neurofibromas and gliomas contain oestrogen and progesterone receptors. Meningiomas are particularly liable to expand during the third trimester, causing local mass effects such as headache, cranial nerve palsies, hemiparesis, or paraparesis which may remit after delivery. Dexamethasone can be given to reduce surrounding oedema, and often surgery can be delayed until after delivery. Gliomas tend to present earlier in pregnancy and have a reputation for following an aggressive course. They may require early surgical intervention, and it is sometimes also appropriate to consider termination of the pregnancy. Women who come to term with intracranial mass lesions require special obstetric care. Raised intracranial pressure is worsened by Valsalva manoeuvres during labour, increasing the risk of brain-stem herniation; this can be avoided by caesarean section.

Choriocarcinoma usually presents after a molar pregnancy or an abortion, but 15 per cent occur during or after a normal pregnancy. Metastases may invade the cerebral vessels, causing strokes through infarction or haemorrhage. Spinal metastases cause cord or cauda equina compression, which again may be rapid in onset. Chest radiographs usually show multiple metastases and the serum chorionic gonadotrophin level is greatly raised.

Both the normal pituitary gland and pituitary tumours such as prolactinomas enlarge during pregnancy. Their management, the possibility of pituitary apoplexy and the differential diagnosis of lymphocytic hypophysitis are discussed elsewhere (Section 12).

Cerebrovascular disease

Although epidemiological data are limited and somewhat conflicting, there seems to be a substantially increased incidence of stroke during pregnancy and the puerperium. This is due to a mixture of cerebral infarcts (mainly from occlusion of internal carotid and middle cerebral arteries), cerebral venous thrombosis, and subarachnoid haemorrhage from aneurysms and arteriovenous malformations.

CEREBRAL INFARCTION

Ischaemic stroke is rare in young women but probably slightly more common during pregnancy and the puerperium than at other times. This is thought to reflect the mild hypercoagulable state that develops during the later stages of pregnancy and persists for a few weeks afterwards, with increased clotting factors, reduced levels of antithrombin III, and decreased fibrinolysis. In half the cases no other identifiable cause is found but a wide range of other conditions are occasionally involved. The most frequent is premature carotid atheromatous disease, with the familiar risk factors of hypertension, diabetes, smoking, and hyperlipidaemia. Cerebral vasculitis, due for example to systemic lupus erythematosus, may present or relapse during pregnancy and thereafter; it tends affect the smaller arteries, to cause a diffuse or multifocal pattern of neurological deficit, with headaches, cognitive impairment, personality change, and seizures, in addition to focal weakness, sensory loss, or chorea. A similar picture is seen in patients with antiphospholipid antibodies, whether associated with systemic lupus erythematosus or not (see Chapter 18.11.3). These women often give a history of previous spontaneous abortions or thromboses elsewhere. A personal or family history of the latter also raises the possibility of other thrombophilias, including antithrombin III, protein C, and protein S deficiencies. These can all cause major strokes due to either larger artery or venous sinus occlusion. Sickle-cell disease can lead to a similar range of major strokes, but is usually diagnosed by screening early in pregnancy. Syphilis, an infective cause of cerebral vasculitis, is also usually detected by screening tests. Finally, cardiac causes of stroke must be considered, including mitral valve disease, infective endocarditis, peripartum cardiomyopathy, and paradoxical embolus through a patent foramen semiovale.

The investigation and treatment of stroke in pregnancy follows the same lines as in any young patient. Aspirin may be given as secondary prophylaxis where there is demonstrable carotid atheroma. Anticoagulation (for thrombophilia or cardiac embolic diseases) poses particular problems. The risk of recurrent stroke in subsequent pregnancies is very remote if investigations do not reveal any specific underlying cause.

CEREBRAL VENOUS THROMBOSIS

Cerebral venous thrombosis has a predilection for the puerperium. Classically there is prominent headache and neurological deficit which evolves over several hours and may become bilateral, with seizures and papilloedema; smaller thromboses may present with the syndrome known as benign intracranial hypertension. Coexistent crural deep vein thrombosis is common. The investigation of choice is MRI which will sensitively show the characteristic distribution of venous infarction and can detect lack of flow in the major dural sinuses. If MRI is not available, then computed tomographic brain scanning may have to be supplemented with cerebral angiography. There is little information on treatment in pregnancy. Although venous infarcts frequently undergo haemorrhagic transformation, recent small studies have suggested that anticoagulation with heparin reduces overall mortality. Dexamethasone helps to relieve symptoms of raised intracranial pressure and anticonvulsants are often also required. If the patient survives then subsequent recovery may be surprisingly complete, although epilepsy tends to persist.

SUBARACHNOID HAEMORRHAGE

The incidence of aneurysmal subarachnoid haemorrhage is not increased during pregnancy, but its management is difficult. Surgical clipping of the aneurysm should be performed if technically possible; if not then most authorities recommend that the baby should be delivered by elective caesarean section (although there is in fact little evidence to suggest that there is an increased risk of rebleeding during vaginal delivery). Intracranial and subarachnoid haemorrhage from an arteriovenous mal-

formation is much less common but the principles of management are the same. Women with inoperable angiomas should be warned that there is an increased risk of bleeding (due to a mixture of haemodynamic and hormonal factors) throughout pregnancy.

Epilepsy

Most women with pre-existing epilepsy show no change in frequency of seizures during pregnancy, but some 30 per cent have more. Unsurprisingly, the patients with bad epilepsy (for example, frequent focal seizures with secondary generalization) tend to be the ones who get worse. Anticonvulsant plasma levels tend to fall during pregnancy through increased volumes of distribution and rates of elimination. Pregnancy is one of the very few situations where it may be sensible to adjust anticonvulsant dosage in the light of a change in plasma level rather than a change in the patient's condition, particularly if the patient's epilepsy has previously been difficult to control.

An equally important reason for deteriorating seizure control is reduced drug compliance because of fear of teratogenic effects. This is ideally avoided by careful preconceptual counselling, which should include an explanation of the risks of uncontrolled epilepsy to both mother and fetus. As always, the aim of treatment is to control the epilepsy using a single anticonvulsant in the lowest effective dose, and it is reasonable to try to reduce or withdraw anticonvulsants prior to pregnancy if this has not been tried before. It is unwise to attempt this during pregnancy itself, and futile to do so after the period of organogenesis (that is after 8 weeks of gestation).

All the currently used anticonvulsants are potential teratogens and the relative risk of congenital malformations in the children of women with epilepsy (compared with those of the non-epileptic population) has been reported as between 1.25 and 2.2; most of this increased risk seems to be due to the treatment rather than the epilepsy. This translates into an absolute risk in the region of 5 to 10 per cent, although many of these malformations are minor; the risk is highest in patients taking combinations of two or more anticonvulsants. Amongst the more serious abnormalities, phenytoin, barbiturates, carbamazepine, and sodium valproate all appear to be associated with facial clefts, cardiac septal defects and a pattern of craniofacial and digital dysmorphism referred to as the fetal hydantoin syndrome; sodium valproate, and to a lesser extent carbamazepine, appear to have an association with neural tube defects. Some of these defects may be secondary to drug-induced folate deficiency and it is the author's practice to recommend folate supplements to all fertile and sexually active women who are taking anticonvulsants. Carbamazepine is traditionally regarded as the safest anticonvulsant but the superior efficacy of sodium valproate in generalized epilepsy syndromes almost certainly offsets any increased teratogenic risk, particularly if screening for neural tube defects is employed (with serum alphafetoprotein levels and detailed ultrasound examination early in the second trimester).

Epilepsy presenting for the first time in pregnancy requires investigation in the same way as adult-onset epilepsy in general. Idiopathic epilepsy which only occurs in pregnancy (so-called gestational epilepsy) is rare. Women presenting with serial seizures or status epilepticus are particularly likely to have an underlying secondary cause, such as eclampsia, cerebrovascular disease, intracranial tumour, or infection. Epilepsy beginning around the time of delivery is usually either iatrogenic (for example, hyponatraemia due to inappropriate administration of intravenous fluids) or again symptomatic of serious intracranial pathology. Eclampsia (see Chapter 13.2) is clearly the first consideration. Other possibilities include phaeochromocytoma, thrombotic microangiopathy, amniotic fluid embolus, and cerebral venous thrombosis.

Pre-existing epilepsy rarely causes specific problems during labour providing the usual drug treatment is continued, but the baby may show a bleeding tendency because of hepatic enzyme induction by anticonvulsant drugs; this can be reversed with vitamin K. All the anticonvulsant drugs pass into the breast milk to some extent but this need not prevent breast feeding. Only the barbiturates occasionally cause problems, with excessive sedation. However, the risk of this must be balanced against the problems of effectively withdrawing barbiturates by not breast feeding. This can lead to the baby becoming irritable and tremulous; impaired suckling and withdrawal seizures have also been reported.

Multiple sclerosis

Pregnancy raises complex issues for women with multiple sclerosis. Preconceptual considerations include the small risk (approximately 3 per cent) of their child inheriting the disease and the practical burdens that child care imposes upon a mother with existing and potentially progressive disability. Several epidemiological studies have shown that the incidence of clinically identifiable relapses of multiple sclerosis falls during pregnancy itself but rises above the base-line rate in the puerperium (with between 20 and 40 per cent of women reporting an exacerbation of symptoms). It has been suggested this reflects the production of pregnancy-associated proteins with immunosuppressive properties, such as alpha-fetoprotein, and changes in T-lymphocyte subsets. Retrospective studies show little effect on long-term outcome. Relapses are treated in the usual way, with rest supplemented by a short course of oral or intravenous corticosteroids if there is significant new disability. High-dose steroids given late in pregnancy can cause neonatal adrenal suppression.

Many women with multiple sclerosis have impaired bladder emptying, which predisposes to urinary tract infection. Severe spinal cord disease is a particular risk factor because it may mask the usual symptoms of urinary infection; regular urine culture is a sensible precaution. Paraplegia (from any cause) otherwise has little effect on pregnancy, but can lead to premature and unheralded labour, so regular monitoring is needed during the third trimester. High spinal cord lesions can cause autonomic instability during labour; this can be blocked by careful regional anaesthesia

Listeriosis

Pregnancy predisposes to infection by the ubiquitous *Listeria monocytogenes*. This usually causes an unremarkable febrile illness in the mother followed by fetal infection and loss. Occasionally the mother may develop a subacute lymphocytic meningitis or brain-stem encephalitis. The diagnosis is made by blood and cerebrospinal fluid culture and treatment is with intravenous ampicillin.

Chorea gravidarum

Chorea gravidarum (chorea presenting during pregnancy) is becoming increasingly rare with the decline in Syndenham's chorea. In developed countries it is now more likely to be due to an incidental cause of chorea (such as systemic lupus erythematosus, thyrotoxicosis, or even Huntington's disease) than a recrudescence of previous rheumatic chorea, and should be investigated appropriately. It can be florid and exhausting; here treatment with a small dose of a neuroleptic such as haloperidol is indicated. Recurrence in subsequent pregnancies (or on taking the oral contraceptive) is common, perhaps because of the effects of oestrogens on dopamine receptor sensitivity.

REFERENCES

Birk, K., Ford, C., Smeltzer, S., Ryan, D., Miller, R., and Rudick, R.A. (1990). The clinical course of multiple sclerosis during pregnancy and the puerperium. *Archives of Neurology* **47**, 738–42.

Devinsky, O., Feldmann, E., and Hainline, B. (eds.) (1994). Neurological complications of pregnancy. *Advances in neurology*, vol. 64. Raven Press, New York. A comprehensive collection of reviews.

Donaldson, J.O. (1989). *Neurology of pregnancy*, (2nd edn). Saunders, London. This excellent monograph is the standard reference on this subject and includes an extensive bibliography.

Donaldson, J.O. (1991). Neurologic emergencies in pregnancy. *Obstetrics and Gynaecology Clinics of North America* **18**, (2), 199–212.

Fennell, D.F. and Ringel, S.P. (1987). Myasthenia gravis and pregnancy. *Obstetric and Gynecologic Surveys* **41**, 414–21.

Holcomb, W.L. and Petrie, R.H. (1990). Cerebrovascular emergencies in pregnancy. *Clinical Obstetrics and Gynaecology* **33**, 467–72.

Hopkins, A. (1989). Neurological disorders. In *Medical disorders in obstetric practice*, (2nd edn), (ed. M. De Swiet), pp. 731–74. Blackwell Scientific Publications, Oxford. An excellent pragmatic review.

O'Brien, M.D. and Gilmour-White, S. (1993). Epilepsy and pregnancy. *British Medical Journal* **307**, 492–5.

Roelvink, N.C.A. *et al.* (1987). Pregnancy-related primary brain and spinal tumours. *Archives of Neurology* **44**, 209–15.

13.11 Nutrition in pregnancy

D. M. CAMPBELL

INTRODUCTION

The importance of nutrition during pregnancy for a satisfactory outcome has been the subject of debate over many years. Reports on the effect of nutrition on perinatal mortality, birthweight, and subsequent development of the infant have been conflicting. Pregnant women have received advice ranging from needing to eat for two, to decreasing food intake to restrict weight gain. Traditionally, the nutritional needs of pregnancy have been computed as no more than the components of the products of conception and their maintenance. Thus the extra requirements for pregnancy should rise as pregnancy progresses *pari passu* with fetal growth. However, this takes no account of the large changes occurring in the maternal body. Pregnancy involves a complex interaction between maternal and fetal physiological systems which are still not fully understood, but which presumably ensure that both mother and baby have the best chance of survival even under conditions of hardship and deprivation. Impaired reproductive performance, as reflected by a high perinatal mortality, occurs in many deprived populations, both in the developing world and in the slums of better-off countries and has often been seen as an effect of poor nutrition, but it is remarkable how efficiently the fetus is protected when the mother is malnourished, and the relationship is not simply that poor nutrition leads to poor fetal growth. Women who eat badly in pregnancy have probably always eaten badly, are poorly grown, and, in general, suffer much disadvantage from poor education, poor housing, general ill-health with less medical care, an excess of cigarette smoking, and the need to do hard physical work, the latter particularly in the developing world.

Table 1 *Components of weight gain during pregnancy for women without generalized oedema (from Hytten and Leitch 1971)*

	Increase in weight up to			
	10 weeks (g)	20 weeks (g)	30 weeks (g)	40 weeks (g)
Fetus	5	300	1500	3400
Placenta	20	170	430	650
Amniotic fluid	30	350	750	800
Uterus	140	320	600	970
Mammary gland	45	180	360	405
Blood	100	600	1300	1250
Extracellular extravascular fluid	0	30	80	1680
Total weight gained	650	4000	8500	12 500
∴ Weight not accounted for	310	2050	3480	3345

Nutritional physiology in pregnancy

Normal healthy pregnant women eating to appetite gain 12.5 kg on average. The components of that increase can be calculated: the fetus, placenta, amniotic fluid, increased maternal tissue in the uterus, breasts, and blood, and an increase in extracellular fluid (Table 1). There remains approximately 3.5 kg of weight unaccounted for by this calculation at the end of pregnancy, that is about 25 per cent of the overall weight increase. Examination of the components of weight gained in normal pregnancy shows that most of the measured increase in total body water during pregnancy, at least until late pregnancy, can be accounted for by that added in specific sites (Table 2) so that the unaccounted-for weight contains no water.

As the body's capacity for storage of carbohydrate is minute, carbohydrate cannot make a significant contribution to the extra weight gain. Similarly, the body can only store protein by lean tissue containing about 80 per cent water and a recent study of nitrogen balance in late pregnancy has confirmed that nitrogen retention occurring in the late pregnancy is very close to that calculated for the growth of specific organs as detailed in Table 1. Therefore, the large amount of water-free weight can only be fat. Maternal deposition of fat increases considerably during the second trimester of pregnancy, as shown by detailed body composition studies and measurement of skinfold thickness. Fat so stored forms an energy bank during the early part of pregnancy when fetal growth is relatively slow, which can be seen as a buffer to support later fetal growth and lactation. Excess fat tends to be lost after pregnancy even in the absence of lactation.

It can be estimated that total additional energy requirement for the whole of pregnancy is approximately 70 000 kcal (293 MJ). This is needed for the accumulation of protein and fat, along with the additional energy required for the maintenance of the fetus and extra added maternal tissue (Table 3). Up to about 30 weeks of pregnancy the increase of energy requirement is dominated by the accumulation of maternal fat, but during the last 10 weeks fat deposition virtually stops and most of the energy involved is for formation of new fetal tissue, with a considerable rise in oxygen consumption for the maintenance of the new tissues. The overall effect is to spread the additions to total energy needs evenly over the entire pregnancy, at a rate of about 400 kcal/day (1.67 MJ/day). The total energy required for pregnancy will be met from two sources: increased dietary intake and a diminished energy expenditure. Both occur in human pregnancy. The specific energy requirement of pregnancy (approximately 400 kcal/day) is probably met on average by an increase in dietary intake of about 200 kcal/day (0.84 MJ/day) and a similar reduction of energy output. Reduced energy expenditure is achieved by voluntary reduction in exercise and the taking of more rest, by a general reduction in muscle tone and a slight general fall in maternal tissue metabolism due to the reduced level of thyroid hormones characteristic of pregnancy.

The specific energy requirements of pregnancy have recently been disputed by studies of energy balance undertaken in five countries. However, in all five centres the average weight and fat gain during pregnancy were less than estimated (see Table 1). Methods of assessing total body fat are inaccurate and those applicable in the absence of pregnancy have not been validated in its presence when fat is not deposited equally at all sites. The amount of fat gain in pregnancy is clearly important when determining the energy cost of pregnancy, but such marked variability as in the five centres studied makes this difficult to assess.

Dietary intake in pregnancy

Dietary intakes in pregnancy are clearly affected by factors specific to the pregnancy itself. There is an increase in appetite by the end of the first trimester which cannot possibly be related to the demands of a fetus weighing less than 50 g. The increased energy intake at this stage is used for the storage of body fat. In early pregnancy nausea, with or without vomiting, may modify the appetite response; later in pregnancy there may be heartburn, constipation, craving for specific foods and perhaps pica, that is the desire for a substance not normally considered edible.

Studies during pregnancy have shown no marked increase in the energy intake over the whole of its course. No data are available for individuals prior to pregnancy and studied longitudinally throughout pregnancy. There are many cross-sectional studies in dietary intake at different stages of pregnancy from different parts of the world. The energy and protein contents of such diets are summarized in Table 4. The most recent recommendation for energy intake for the United Kingdom still suggests an additional 200 kcal (0.84 MJ) per day over the non-pregnant allowance. Such an increase in energy intake will lead to a small increase in protein and other specific nutrients and will be met readily by the increased food intake that does occur.

Metabolic adaptations

Gastric secretions are reduced during pregnancy, as is motility of the gut. This leads to delay in gastric emptying and increased absorption times. Nevertheless, absorption of at least some nutrients may be increased. This has been shown for iron and calcium in particular, but seems to be no more than a normal adaptive response to increased needs. The reduced motility of the small intestine allows better absorption of nutrients where this has been impaired, for example, by extensive surgical resection.

Alteration in renal function, with an increase in blood flow and glomerular filtration rate together with some impairment of tubular absorption, leads to an increased urinary excretion of many nutrients during

Table 2 *The water component of weight gain in normal pregnancy compared to the measured increase in total body water (Hytten et al. 1966)*

	Estimated water content (g)		
	20 weeks	30 weeks	40 weeks
Fetus	264	1185	2343
Placenta	153	366	540
Amniotic fluid	247	594	792
Added uterine muscle	483	668	743
Added mammary gland	135	270	304
Plasma	506	1058	920
Red cells	32	98	163
Total	1820	4239	5805
	Measured increase of total body water (g)		
	20 weeks	30 weeks	40 weeks
No oedema	1740	4300	7500
Leg oedema	1810	4290	7880
Generalized oedema	2230	5740	10 880

Table 3 *Mean daily increments of protein and fat and total increments in the fetus and maternal body; and cumulative energy cost of added protein and fat, together with the energy cost of maintaining the fetus and added maternal tissues. The last line shows the metabolized (dietary) energy required to meet these costs (from Hytten and Leitch 1971)*

	Weeks of pregnancy				Cumulative total
	0–10[a]	10–20	20–30	30–40	
Protein and fat increments					
Protein (g)	0.64	1.84	4.76	6.1	925
Fat (g)	5.85	24.80	21.85	3.3	3825
kJ equivalents/day[b]					
Protein	15.0	43.1	111.6	143.0	21 652
Fat	232.4	984.8	867.8	130.8	151 889
Oxygen consumption	83.2	259.2	463.6	777.9	109 700
Total net energy (kJ)	330.0	1287.0	1442.9	1051.7	283 241
Metabolizable energy[c] (kJ)	363.7	1417.0	1588.4	1157.9	311 565

[a]For the first 10 week period total increment is divided by 56 since pregnancy is dated from the last menstrual period.

[b]Taken as 23.4 kJ/g for protein and 39.7 kJ/g for fat.

[c]Total net energy plus 10 per cent.

normal pregnancy. Glucose, amino acids, several vitamins and their metabolites are lost in the urine during pregnancy and the amount may be substantial: amounts as much as 2 g of amino acids and 10 g of glucose are not abnormal.

The concentrations of most nutrients in the circulation are reduced. This applies particularly to water-soluble nutrients, with conspicuously reduced levels in plasma of albumin, glucose, many amino acids, minerals, and water-soluble vitamins. On the other hand, lipids and fat-soluble vitamins and certain specific carrier proteins are increased in concentration. Like many of the other physiological changes that occur during pregnancy, changes in nutrient content of the blood occur so early that they cannot possibly be due to fetal demands; they are clearly the result of a changed pattern of homeostasis.

Glucose is the main fuel for fetal growth, and metabolism and maternal glucose handling is markedly altered from very early pregnancy. No one factor is thought to be responsible for the changes, but it seems likely that there is an alteration in the balance of controlling hormones such as human placental lactogen, placental steroids and their effect on insulin, glucagon, and corticoid secretion.

In the assessment of nutrition in pregnancy, failure to recognize the effect of the normal adaptation can result in errors of diagnosis. It is important that diagnostic indices specific to pregnancy, such as those summarized by the United States' National Research Council, are used.

Nutrition and outcome of pregnancy

In this context there are two aspects to be considered: first, the importance of long-term nutrition and reproductive performance and, secondly, the impact of acute changes during the course of pregnancy.

Although it was believed originally that the unexpected fall in still birth rate in England and Wales during the Second World War was due

Table 4 *Daily dietary intake, published surveys*

Study	Energy	kcal	(MJ)	Protein (g)	Survey method
Toronto, Canada 1941	Poor	1750	(4.3)	59	7 day record partial weighing
	Good	2350	(9.8)	86	
Holland 1953		2770	(11.6)	78	Dietary history
Scotland 1958	Upper Soc. Cl.	2633	(11.0)	80	Weighed 7 day record
	Middle Soc. Cl.	2521	(10.5)	78	
	Lower Soc. Cl.	2354	(9.8)	72	
DDR 1961		2753	(11.5)	77	7 day record
Holland	1st Trim.	2620	(11.0)	70	3 day recall
	2nd Trim.	2720	(11.4)	80	
	3rd Trim.	2620	(11.0)	76	
Sweden 1969	1st Trim.	2035	(8.5)	65	24 h recall
	2nd Trim.	2185	(9.1)	70	
	3rd Trim.	2137	(8.9)	73	
Sweden 1987	2nd Trim.	2200	(9.2)	54	
	3rd Trim.	2700	(9.5)	54	
Hyderabad, India 1972		1800	(7.5)	42	Questionnaire
Guatemala 1975		1500	(6.3)	40	24 and 72 h recall
United Kingdom 1977		2010	(8.4)	70	Weighed 7 day record
San Francisco, USA 1978		2000	(8.4)	86	7 day weighed record
Bogota, Columbia, 1979		1611	(6.7)	35	24 h recall
Aberdeen, Scotland, 1979		2090	(8.7)	71	7 day weighed survey
		2010	(8.4)	73	7 day weighed survey
Aberdeen, Scotland, 1989		1960	(8.2)	70	7 day weighed survey
Harlem, New York, USA 1980		2065	(8.6)	79	24 h recall
Addis Ababa, Ethiopia 1980		1600	(6.7)	47	Food weighed for 2 days
United Kingdom 1980		2152	(9.0)	70	Weighed 7 day record
France 1981	1st Trim.	2307	(9.7)	82	Recall
	3rd Trim.	2121	(8.9)	79	
Taiwan 1981		1200	(5.0)	40	Diet survey of meals only (underestimated)
Birmingham, England 1982		1740	(7.3)	54	7 day weighed record
London, England 1982		1969	(7.1)	67	7 day weighed survey
Holland 1983	2nd Trim.	2405	(10.1)	83	Dietary history
	3rd Trim.	2245	(9.4)	76	
Cambridge, England 1985	3rd Trim.	2065	(8.6)	73	4 day weighed record
Gambia 1980	Dry season	1700	(7.1)	–	24 h weighed survey
	Wet season (July–Oct.)	1350	(5.6)	–	
Glasgow 1987		2246	(9.4)		5 day weighed survey
East Java 1988		1500	(6.3)		3 day weighed record

Soc. Cl., social class; Trim., trimester.

to improved nutrition on account of the rationing system, which favoured pregnant women and children, this seems unlikely as perinatal mortality rates continued fall as rapidly in the following period, when there was no particular focus on nutrition. Adverse socioeconomic conditions prevailing in Britain during the earlier part of the twentieth century, as in other countries today, led to inability to achieve optimum reproductive efficiency. In Britain today, mothers are taller, healthier, better educated, and better nourished, and reproductive performance, an indicator of nutritional status throughout life, in particular during periods of childhood and adolescence, has improved. Taller women are known to have better outcome in pregnancy than shorter women.

The most favourable outcome of pregnancy with respect to the development of pre-eclampsia, intrauterine growth retardation, and perinatal death is associated with a gain of approximately 450 g/week, and obstetricians have aimed to keep weight gain as close to that average as possible, manipulating the diet with nutrition advice. This is clearly illogical; poor weight gain and poor fetal growth are both parts of a poor general response to pregnancy. Poor weight gain, particularly in the second trimester of pregnancy, may be used as a predictor of poor fetal growth in antenatal care.

Acute changes in nutrition, such as occur during famine, lead mainly to a massive fall in conception rates due to amenorrhoea in women and azoospermia in men. In those women who do become pregnant, the fetuses grow reasonably well, although there is a deficit in fetal weight mainly due to loss of subcutaneous fat. This was exemplified by the Dutch famine in 1940 to 1945, when there was acute deprivation in a previously well-nourished community, with dietary intake dropping to a mean level of less than 1000 kcal/day. There was a significant decrease in birth weight of about 350 g, or 9 per cent of pre-famine average birthweight, and a smaller change in birth length and head circumference, to 5 and 7 per cent, respectively, of pre-famine levels. These effects were seen when the famine coincided with the third trimester of pregnancy. Babies conceived during this period of famine and babies whose mothers were exposed to famine conditions only in the early part of pregnancy with adequate nutrition later showed no deficit in fetal growth. The impact of the famine on perinatal mortality was slight, and subsequent follow-up of the offspring to adulthood has failed to show any adverse effect on physical or mental development. This is in contrast to findings in communities that are chronically malnourished. Much of the work from the National Institute of Nutrition in Hyderabad, India, suggests that women belonging to low socioeconomic groups have very poor dietary intake throughout their lives and during pregnancy. In these situations the outcome of pregnancy is frequently unfavourable and birthweights are low. This has also been reported for other countries, such as Thailand and Central America. Clearly, the impact of famine or acute starvation in such populations is likely to have a devastating effect on reproductive performance.

As a result of epidemiological studies it has been suggested by Barker *et al.* (1992) that uterine environmental factors, in particular poor nutrition, not only influence the relationship between placental weight and birthweight but continue to exert influence into adult life, making individuals more susceptible to the development of cardiovascular disease. Alternatively, there could be a common genetic mechanism. The role of maternal nutrition during pregnancy in this interesting hypothesis remains to be elucidated.

Dietary supplementation in pregnancy

On account of the association between poor nutrition and low birthweight, many attempts have been made to increase the pregnant woman's diet by supplementation with a view to improving outcome. Most of these trials have been plagued with problems of design, selection of control groups, and appropriate assessment of total nutritional intake. In particular, in many trials no attempt was made to monitor whether nutritional supplements did not merely replace nutrients in the pregnant woman's regular diet. Table 5 summarizes the most important of the supplement studies, comments, and outcome. In general these have not had the desired effect of increasing in birthweight. Indeed, high protein supplements are associated with depression of birthweight and early delivery. There is a small increment, approximately 50 g, in mean birthweight in studies in some of the less developed countries. However, it is difficult to disentangle the effect of additional antenatal care and improved health from the part played by improved nutrition. The only demonstrable effect on mortality and morbidity has been an increase in neonatal mortality associated with high protein supplements. Targeting women at risk, such as those in the Gambia in the wet season, or by the use of skinfold thickness to identify undernutrition with subsequent supplementation, has so far been unsuccessful in improving outcome. In many such communities, women are expected to perform heavy physical work whether or not they are pregnant, and the increased energy requirement of pregnancy may not be met by increased energy intake; for example, in the Gambia in the wet season energy intakes drop to approximately 1400 kcal/day.

It has been suggested recently that a high dietary intake of fat from fish, rich in long-chain fatty acids, might prolong gestation and thereby increase birthweight. Further trials are needed to confirm or refute this hypothesis.

Fetal growth seems to be diminished only at the extremes of maternal malnutrition and many of the major adaptations in human pregnancy are such that fuel is available for fetal growth constantly, if necessary at the expense of the mother. It is not the overall supply of nutrients that is critical for fetal growth, but the delivery to the fetus, so that mechanisms likely to limit the transfer of nutrients to the fetus are crucial. These are uteroplacental blood flow, transfer across the placenta, and uptake by the fetus itself.

When uteroplacental blood flow is diminished, as it can be by factors such as obstetric disease, in particular maternal hypertensive disease (pre-eclampsia), the vasoconstrictive effect of cigarette smoking and heavy exercise when blood flow is diverted away from the uteroplacental bed to exercising muscles, fetal growth is reduced. The very heavy workload that occurs in parts of Africa is likely to be more important than low dietary intake in the aetiology of low birthweight, since hard physical work, particularly in a hot climate, diverts blood from the splanchnic vascular bed, which includes the uterus.

Nutrition and pre-eclampsia

Pre-eclampsia is associated with an above-average weight increase in pregnancy and a relatively high energy intake. Excess weight gain may be a useful antenatal indicator of developing disease. Diet restriction was therefore advocated, particularly in America, in the belief that the limitation in the amount of weight gain in pregnancy by decreasing energy intake would be beneficial. There is no good evidence that dietary restriction aimed at producing a very low weight gain during pregnancy has any beneficial effect on the incidence of pre-eclampsia. However, there is evidence from Aberdeen and Motherwell, Scotland, that iatrogenic dietary energy limitation leads to a depression in mean birthweight. Further studies from Aberdeen have indicated that dietary restriction cannot be advocated even in obese primigravidae, as it is possibly detrimental to the baby and of no benefit to the mother. It is probably best to try to reduce the weight of the obese woman mainly before or after the pregnancy.

While body weight normally fluctuates from day to day, sudden increases in body weight with a rapid increase in the rate of weight gain may be due to the acute retention of body water. However, this may be part of the normal physiological response to pregnancy and should be ignored unless there is associated hypertension. Oedema is a normal phenomenon in pregnancy and is associated with improved fetal growth and reduced perinatal mortality.

Nutrition and pregnancy anaemia

This topic is addressed in Chapter 13.9.

Nutrition and congenital abnormality

An adequate vitamin supply is necessary for normal fetal growth and development. Any association between nutrition and developmental abnormalities should be sought in the periconceptual period and very early in pregnancy when organogenesis occurs. Changing dietary practice, with the consumption of less meat and more refined foodstuffs, may mean that suboptimal trace element and vitamin nutrition is present in Western communities are well as in areas where there is known poor dietary intake.

Vitamin D deficiency may occur during pregnancy to the extent that it results in maternal osteomalacia, and may upset fetal calcium metabolism. This may be particularly so in Asian women who spend most of their time indoors with little exposure to sunlight and whose calcium absorption may be impaired by an excess of wholemeal cereals in the diet.

At present there is no evidence that most pregnant women in Britain are deficient in either vitamins or trace elements, in particular zinc.

The large Medical Research Council randomized controlled trial of periconceptional supplements of multivitamins or folic acid compared with placebo in the prevention of the recurrence of neural tube defects has shown that folic acid (4 mg/day) around the time of conception reduced the risk of recurrence by about 75 per cent. This was in women who had previously had an affected pregnancy with a neural tube defect. It remains to be shown whether such supplementation will prevent the primary occurrence of neural tube defects. The other major question posed by the results of this study is whether a small amount of folic acid would be equally effective. An intake of 4 mg/day could never be achieved by dietary measures alone (the daily dietary intake is approximately 400 μg/day). Further studies are required before there is either widespread periconception supplementation with folic acid or nutritional intervention such as fortification of foods. Other than this, vitamin and mineral supplementations in pregnancy have been reviewed by Oxford Database of Perinatal Trials, and suggest only minor benefits. The possibility that harm could be done by large supplements (of vitamin A for example around the time of conception) is real and women

Table 5 *Studies on nutritional supplementation in pregnancy*

Study	Study population	Number entering	Effect on birth weight	Comment
Taiwan	14 villages	294	+55 g for males +32 g for females	Birthweight analysis only on 213; rejected subjects because they were taking 50% supplement given
Guatemala	4 villages	671	117 g if supplement 20 000 kcal per pregnancy	38% rejected because birthweight not immediately recorded; analytical bias in favour of subjects complying
Montreal, Canada	All pregnant women at risk of low birthweight	–	+40 g	Retrospective analysis of 1213 matched pairs; programme included education and care also
Bogota, Columbia	Pregnant women with previously malnourished child	456	+89 g for males +6 g for females	Analysis only on 407–? rejects
New York, USA	Afro-American mothers at risk of low birthweight	1051	1. –3.2 g 2. +41 g	Analysis on 768 only; High protein supplement group 1 had excess preterm births with increased neonatal deaths
Birmingham	1. All Asian mothers 2. Asian mothers (selected malnourished)	1. 153 2. 128	1.(a) –60 g; (b) +40 g 2. +330 g in at risk; –180 g in rest	(a) Protein supplementation; (b) energy supplementation; analysis excludes non-compliers and those with complications; only 45 women in at-risk group
Aberdeen, Scotland	Primigravidae at risk of low birthweight	180 (90 pairs)	+37 g	Increase in energy 189 kcal/day; i.e. less than provided, indicating some replacement of diet
Keneba, Gambia	All mothers Controls over 4 years Study popl. over 2 years	181 93	+120 g	Changes in diet and birthweight varied with wet and dry season
Hyderabad, India	Inpatients—hospitalized Outpatients—admitted in labour	25 in-pat. 26 out-pat.	1. +324 g 2. +324 g	Biased because of case selection; no benefit of extra protein
San Francisco, USA	Women at risk of low birthweight	227	1. –45 g 2. +92 g	Increase in daily energy; (1) with high protein supplement 139 kcal; (2) with low protein supplement –155 kcal, suggesting replacement of normal diet; only 45% (102) of original number included in analysis
East Java	Randomized to high- or low-energy supplement Retrospective controls	687	+100 g	No difference between high- and low-energy supplements
Thailand	Women at risk	43	+236 g	Small numbers make it difficult to interpret; selection of cases not clear; low SD of birthweight

should be advised only to take such supplements as are advised by a medical practitioner.

GENERAL CONCLUSIONS

Both empirical and physiological evidence lead to the conclusion that there are powerful safeguards to the fetus and its mother even under conditions of nutritional adversity. It is thus hardly surprising that nutritional advice or intervention during pregnancy confer negligible benefit, even when there are specific indications to suggest that supplementation to the diet may be effective. Moreover, there is the danger that pharmaceutically prepared supplements may divert attention from the need to improve the circumstances which led to malnutrition in the first place. Nevertheless, the importance of good nutrition remains unquestioned: well-grown, well-nourished, and healthy mothers have the best reproductive performance, and general nutritional education during pregnancy seems likely to be the best approach to improving the nutrition of children who will be parents of future generations.

REFERENCES

Baird, D. (1980). Environment and Reproduction. *British Journal of Obstetrics and Gynaecology* **87,** 1057–67.

Barker (1992). *Fetal and adult origins of adult disease.* British Medical Journal, London.

Campbell, D.M. (1983). Dietary restriction in obesity and its effect on neonatal outcome. In *Nutrition in pregnancy*, (ed. D.M. Campbell and M.D.G. Gillmer), pp. 243–50. Royal College of Obstetricians and Gynaecologists, London.

Durnin, J. (1987). Energy requirements of pregnancy: an integration of the longitudinal data from the five-country study. *Lancet* **ii,** 1131–3.

Hemminke, E. and Starfield, B. (1978). Routine administration of iron and vitamins during pregnancy: review of controlled clinical trials. *British Journal of Obstetrics and Gynaecology* **85,** 404–10.

Hytten, F.E. and Leitch, I. (1971). *The physiology of human pregnancy*, (2nd edn), pp. 333–69. Blackwell Scientific, Oxford.

Hytten, F.E., Thomson A.M., and Taggart, N. (1966). Total body water in normal pregnancy. *Journal of Obstetrics and Gynecology,* **73,** 553–61.

Kramer, M.S. (1992). High protein supplementation in pregnancy. Record 7142. Balanced protein/energy supplementation in pregnancy Record 7141. Isocatonic balanced protein supplementation in pregnancy Record 7140. In *Oxford database of perinatal trials*, (ed. I. Chalmers), Version 1,3, Disk Issue 8, Autumn.

Mohamed, K. and Hytten, F.E. (1992). Routine iron supplementation in pregnancy. Record 3151. In *Oxford database of perinatal trials*, (ed. I. Chalmers), Version 1,3 Disk Issue 8, Autumn.

Mohamed, K. and Hytten, F.E. (1989). Iron and folate supplementation in pregnancy. In *Effective care in pregnancy and childhood*, Vol. 1, *Pregnancy*, (ed. I. Chalmers, M. Enkin, and M. Keirse), Ch. 19, pp. 301–15. University Press, Oxford.

13.12 Infection in pregnancy

13.12.1 Viral infections in pregnancy

J. E. BANATVALA

INTRODUCTION

The prevalence, severity, and outcome of viral infections in pregnancy may depend on the patient's nutritional state, and the quality of care of pregnant patients. Poor pulmonary ventilation associated with a large gravid uterus may contribute to severe pulmonary complications occurring in some viral infections in pregnancy, for example varicella and influenza.

Immunological factors may also be involved. Thus, cell-mediated immune responses are suppressed during pregnancy, reverting to normal during the immediate postpartum period. An increased concentration of placental hormones, immunosuppressive fetal products, or the presence of an identified but as yet uncharacterized serum factor which depresses lymphocyte-activated responses to mitogens may be responsible.

Severe or fatal maternal virus infections are more likely to occur during the last trimester, often being associated with premature delivery and fetal death.

Viral infections which may be unusually severe in pregnancy (Fig. 1, Table 1)

Influenza (Fig. 1(a))

The major epidemics of influenza A, which occurred in 1918 (H1N1) and 1957 (H2N2), were associated with an increased mortality among pregnant women with chronic cardiac disease, particularly rheumatic heart disease. During this epidemic, an analysis of 200 deaths from influenza in New York City showed that 10 per cent were in pregnant women; 25 per cent of 93 deaths in those aged less than 50 were pregnant. Deaths occurred most frequently during the last trimester.

Herpes virus infections (Fig. 1(b)) (see Section 7)

VARICELLA-ZOSTER

Although high mortality rates have been reported in the literature, it has not been conclusively shown that pregnant women have a higher mortality rate from varicella-zoster infection; high rates may reflect selective reporting of cases associated with an adverse outcome. Nevertheless, in view of the potential severity of varicella in adults, and because a large gravid uterus may compromise pulmonary ventilation, perhaps enhancing the development of varicella pneumonia, pregnant women without a history of chickenpox should be given varicella-zoster immune globulin. This is more likely to attenuate than prevent varicella, even if given within 72 h of exposure, and this preparation may be effective if given up to 10 days after exposure. Rapid tests of considerable sensitivity and specificity are now available for determining immune status to varicella; pregnant women without a clear history of varicella should be tested prior to the administration of varicella-zoster immune globulin. About two-thirds of adults without a history of varicella have antibodies and will therefore not require protection.

In view of the potential severity of varicella in pregnancy, particularly during its latter stages, it may be preferable to admit patients to hospital since breathlessness which may herald the onset of pneumonia may develop suddenly and disease may progress rapidly. Varicella-zoster immune globulin is not effective once varicella has developed, but since varicella pneumonia is a life-threatening complication, patients should be treated with systemically administered acyclovir. Prospective studies involving 312 acyclovir-treated pregnant patients are reassuring, showing that treatment did not appear to result in birth defects when compared with the incidence expected in the general population.

HERPES SIMPLEX (SEE SECTION 7)

Studies in London have shown that among women of child-bearing age, only about 5 per cent of Asians from the Indian subcontinent or from Africa had evidence of past herpes simplex virus type 2 (HSV-2) infection; among British Caucasians the proportion was about 10 per cent; but among those of Caribbean or African descent the proportion was about 50 per cent, antibody prevalence increasing in the late teens.

Most primary infections are inapparent but, if clinical features are present, they are usually confined to the oropharyngeal or genital tracts. However, there have been a few reports of infection in pregnancy being associated with hepatic involvement, which may sometimes be associated with thrombocytopenia, leucopenia, coagulopathy, and encephalitis. Although there have been only a few case reports, maternal mortality approaches about 50 per cent, with a similar proportion of fetal deaths, which were not necessarily associated with a fatal outcome in the mother.

Localized severe primary genital infections, usually caused by HSV-2, may occur in pregnancy. Such infections are associated with severe pain and oedema; urinary retention may occur. Studies in Britain suggest that about 80 to 90 per cent of genital lesions are caused by HSV-2.

As acyclovir does not apparently have any adverse effects on the outcome of pregnancy, severe life-threatening infections should be

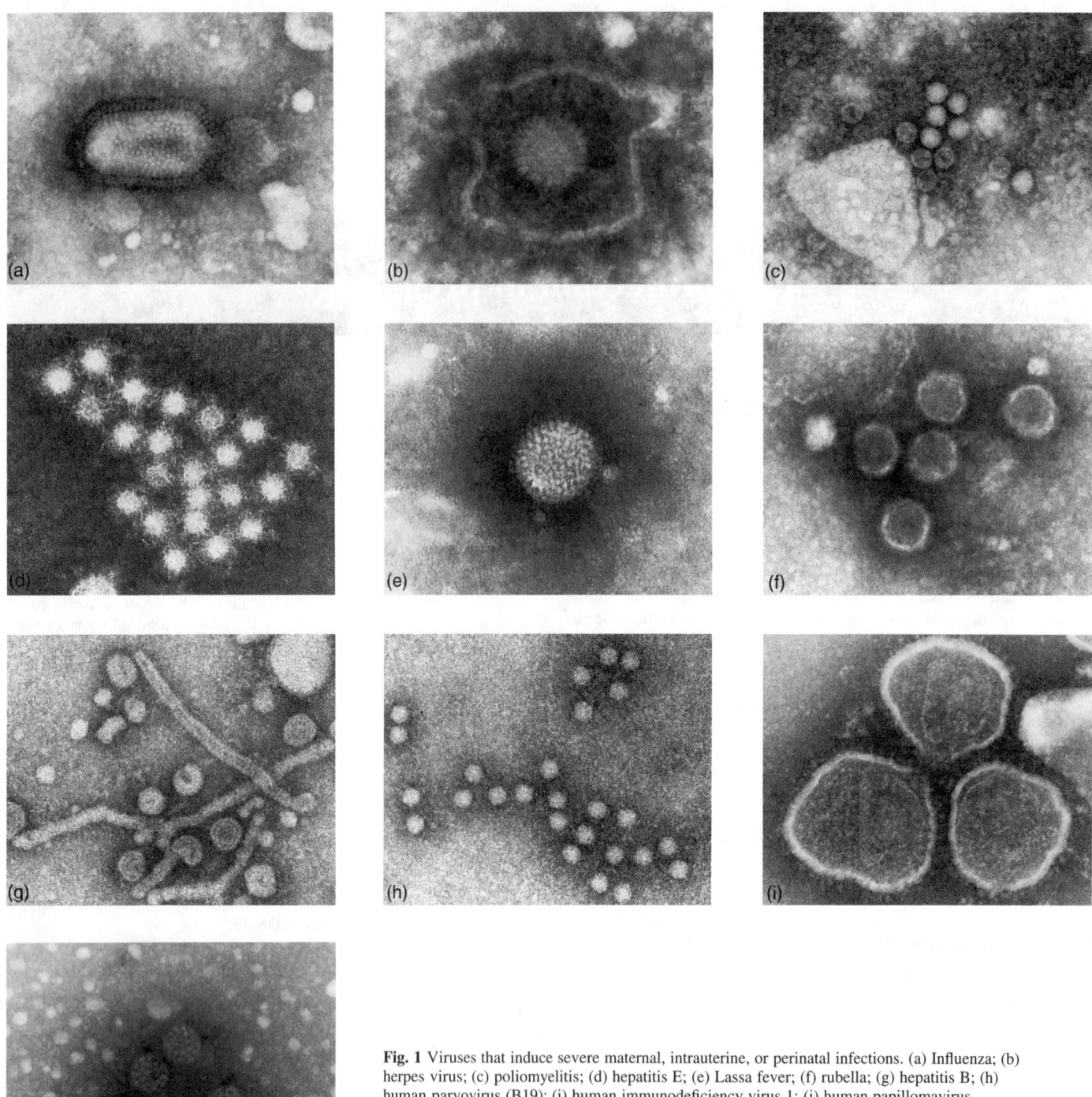

Fig. 1 Viruses that induce severe maternal, intrauterine, or perinatal infections. (a) Influenza; (b) herpes virus; (c) poliomyelitis; (d) hepatitis E; (e) Lassa fever; (f) rubella; (g) hepatitis B; (h) human parvovirus (B19); (i) human immunodeficiency virus 1; (j) human papillomavirus. Magnification of each micrograph: a 1 cm bar = 50 nm. (Electron micrographs (a)–(c) and (f)–(j) by kind permission of Dr I. L. Chrystie, Department of Virology, United Medical and Dental Schools of Guy's and St. Thomas' Hospitals, London, UK. Electron micrograph (d) by kind permission of Dr D. W. Bradley and Dr E. H. Cook Jnr, Centers for Disease Control, Atlanta, USA. Electron micrograph (e) (by kind permission of Dr D. S. Ellis, London School of Hygiene and Tropical Medicine, London, UK.)

Table 1 *Virus infections that may be severe or fatal in pregnancy*

Virus infection	Comments	Prevention
Influenza A (B)	Increased mortality in 1918 and 1957 associated with chronic heart disease	Influenza vaccine (inactivated)
Varicella	Mortality associated with pneumonia among adults Possibly more severe in pregnancy	Varicella-zoster immune globulin preferably within 72 h of contact (Treat established infections if severe with acyclovir systemically)
Poliomyelitis	Spinal paralysis increases with gestational age	Polio vaccine (attenuated or inactivated) for travellers to endemic areas
Measles	Increased mortality and complications in pregnancy	In the absence of previous vaccination or history of measles give normal human immunoglobulin
Hepatitis E	20% mortality with fetal death in last trimester Endemic in many developing countries	Locally produced immunoglobulin may be effective
Lassa fever	70–90% mortality with fetal death in last trimester Endemic in West Africa	? Prophylactic ribivarin to pregnant household contacts (Treat patient with ribivarin systemically)
Japanese B encephalitis	20–40% mortality; higher in pregnancy with fetal death Widely distributed in South-East Asia and the Far East	Vaccine available for travellers to endemic areas

treated with this drug. Consideration should also be given to its use for the more severe forms of primary genital infection, particularly if this occurs near term since, if membranes rupture early and caesarean section is delayed, the risk of an ascending infection being transmitted to the fetus is about 50 per cent.

POLIOMYELITIS (FIG. 1(c)) (SEE SECTION 7)

Studies conducted during the extensive outbreaks of poliomyelitis in the United States in the late 1940s and early 1950s showed that clinical features were related to gestational age, non-paralytic infection decreasing and spinal paralytic disease increasing with gestational age.

Most women of childbearing age in developed countries will have had a full course of polio vaccine. However, although there have been no reports of adverse effects on the fetus, it is recommended that attenuated vaccines should be avoided during the first 16 weeks of pregnancy. However, this hypothetical contraindication should be waived if pregnant women have not had a full course, or are uncertain about their immunization history, and are to be subject to the very real risks associated with travel to a polio-endemic area. Alternatively, if time permits, consideration may be given to immunization with an inactivated vaccine.

ACUTE VIRAL HEPATITIS (SEE SECTION 7)

Only hepatitis E virus (Fig. 1(d)) is known to cause severe and often fatal infections in pregnancy, with maternal mortality rates being of the order of 20 to 40 per cent. Mortality rates among pregnant women infected with hepatitis A or B viruses are 0.5 to 3.0 per cent.

Pregnant women usually die of hepatitis E infection in the immediate postpartum period, this being heralded by a sudden deterioration, coma, and massive intrauterine haemorrhage.

Locally produced immunoglobulin preparations may be of value in preventing infection. However, the high prevalence of hepatitis E virus infection in developing countries, together with its severe consequences

in pregnancy, are resulting in considerable interest in the development of vaccines.

LASSA FEVER (FIG. 1(e)) (SEE SECTION 7)

A recent prospective study in Sierra Leone showed that Lassa fever carried a high risk to the fetus throughout pregnancy, and to the mother during the last trimester. During this time, Lassa fever was the most common cause of maternal mortality (25 per cent). This study also showed that patients who abort spontaneously or in whom the uterus is evacuated had a fourfold decrease in fatality rate.

Little is known about the effect of pregnancy on other viruses causing haemorrhagic disease, such as Marburg and Ebola diseases or Congo Crimean haemorrhagic fever, and haemorrhagic fever with renal syndrome (Hantaan virus). Patients with Lassa fever treated with intravenous ribavirin have increased survival rates, and close contacts may be protected by an oral preparation.

JAPANESE B ENCEPHALITIS (SEE SECTION 7)

Case fatality rates range from 20 to 70 per cent, which may, in part, reflect poor medical care. However, particularly high mortality rates with fetal death have been reported in pregnancy. This virus has been shown to cause transplacental infection.

An unlicensed, inactivated vaccine is available on a named patient basis. Although generally well-tolerated, local and very occasionally severe allergic reactions have been reported, and this vaccine must therefore be used with caution. Although pregnancy is a listed contraindication, practitioners must evaluate the very real risks and dangers of acquiring infection, particularly during pregnancy, against the rare hazard of reactogenicity which might upset an unstable pregnancy, and the fact that there is probably insufficient information relating to the teratogenic potential of this vaccine. However, much can be done to prevent infection by such measures as ensuring that appropriate clothing is worn and insect repellents are used.

Viral vaccines in pregnancy

Although live attenuated vaccines are contraindicated in pregnancy, there is no evidence, as yet, that they induce fetal damage.

Rubella vaccine has been given, usually inadvertently, to about 500 rubella-susceptible pregnant women and follow-up studies have shown that this is not associated with an increased risk of fetal death or rubella-induced congenital malformations. In about 2 per cent of cases, a rubella specific IgM response may be detected or rubella antibodies may persist beyond 6 months of age, which suggests that rubella vaccination may have resulted in a intrauterine infection. There is therefore no need to offer termination of pregnancy to rubella-susceptible women given rubella vaccine in early pregnancy; they should be counselled and their pregnancy should be allowed to continue if this is their wish.

The theoretical risks of vaccination against such live attenuated vaccines as polio and yellow fever during pregnancy must be balanced against the risks of acquiring these infections in countries where they are endemic. Risks associated with the administration of live attenuated measles and mumps virus vaccines have not been established.

Inactivated vaccines should not provide a hazard, although those which may be reactogenic might unsettle an unstable pregnancy. Nevertheless, manufacturers and licensing authorities are reluctant to advise the use of an inactivated vaccine in pregnancy unless extensive studies have been carried out to demonstrate non-teratogenicity in animals.

Approach to the diagnosis of intrauterine and perinatal infections

Close collaboration between clinicians and the laboratory is essential so that the correct specimens, and if necessary follow-up samples, are transported to the laboratory under optimal conditions.

A prenatal diagnosis may be established by detecting the presence of specific IgM in fetal blood, isolating the organism, or by detecting its nucleic acid in fetal blood or chorionic villus samples. Since specific IgM does not cross the placenta, its presence is indicative of an intrauterine infection.

In general, specific IgM responses are unlikely to be detected until about 22 weeks' gestation but, even after this period, a negative response does not preclude intrauterine infection. Cytomegalovirus and rubella may be present in the amniotic fluid but it may take days or weeks to identify the virus by cell culture.

Molecular techniques have considerable potential. A gene amplifi-

Fig. 2 Electron micrograph of cytomegalovirus in the urine of a congenitally infected infant. Note the high concentration of virus particles. Magnification: 4.3 mm bar = 100 nm. (Electron micrograph by kind permission of Dr I. L. Chrystie, Department of Virology, United Medical and Dental Schools of Guy's and St Thomas' Hospitals, London, UK.)

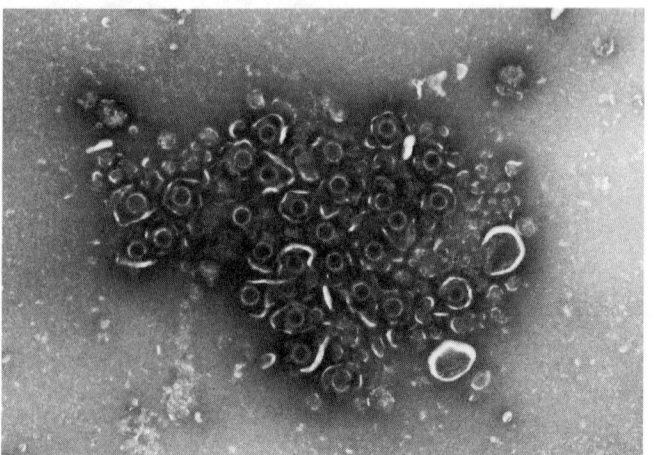

cation technique, polymerase chain reaction, can amplify a specific region of DNA up to a million fold or more, thereby greatly enhancing detection in fetal blood or a chorionic villus sample. However, the extreme sensitivity of this technique is a limiting factor since even a minimal amount of contamination from maternal cells could result in maternal infection being ascribed to the fetus.

With the possible exception of rubella, a serological diagnosis on cord blood or early neonatal serum samples is unreliable; repeat tests on further samples are often necessary. Unfortunately, many clinicians still request a TORCH screen (toxoplasma, rubella, cytomegalovirus, and herpes simplex). A Public Health Laboratory Service working party recently recommended that the use of the acronym TORCH should be discouraged and that sera collected in early pregnancy for screening for syphilis, rubella, and hepatitis B virus should be stored for at least a year so that appropriate investigations could be carried out on paired maternal and neonatal samples in cases of suspected congenitally acquired infections.

TORCH screening fails to include many other organisms which are now known to cause intrauterine or perinatal infections. However, it is usually necessary to test further serum samples to detect persistence of antibody or specific IgM responses. Second serum samples should be tested to confirm a positive specific IgM response but, if an intrauterine infection is suspected and a negative response is obtained, further samples may reveal a positive response 2 to 4 weeks later.

It is also important to collect excretions or secretions to identify the aetiological agent. Electron microscopy or cell culture techniques may be used to identify neonatal herpes simplex, cytomegalovirus, and varicella-zoster infections (Figs. 1 and 2). Molecular biological techniques for the diagnosis of congenitally or perinatally acquired infections may provide alternative and rapid methods of establishing diagnoses and are currently being evaluated.

The identification of the aetiological agent is not only of importance in the treatment of infants (for example, congenitally acquired toxoplasmosis or perinatally acquired herpes simplex) but is also of importance in preventing transmission of infection to susceptible infants in nurseries (for example, enteroviruses and herpes simplex). In the absence of strict infection-control measures, infections that carry high mortality rates have resulted in the closure of nurseries for the newborn.

Viruses that may cause intrauterine infections are listed in Table 2.

Rubella (Fig. 1(f)) (see also Section 7)

As a result of the success of the rubella vaccination programme in the United Kingdom, only 2 to 3 per cent of women of childbearing age are now susceptible to rubella. The recent augmentation of the programme whereby preschool children of both sexes are vaccinated has reduced the circulation of wild virus and notifications of rubella, including laboratory confirmed cases of rubella in pregnancy and congenitally acquired infection, are at an all-time low. In countries with poor vaccination uptake rates, outbreaks of rubella continue to occur, which result in a high incidence of therapeutic abortions or delivery of congenitally infected infants. Lack of diagnostic facilities make it difficult to assess the contribution of congenitally acquired rubella to birth defects in developing countries. However, rubella susceptibility among women of child-bearing age is often not dissimilar from that in developed countries prior to vaccination programmes (15–20 per cent); some island populations may have susceptibility rates approaching 50 per cent. Such studies as have been carried out suggest that congenitally acquired rubella may be responsible for such birth defects as blindness and deafness.

The fetus is at risk during maternal viraemia which occurs prior to the onset of the clinical features of infection. Confirmation of diagnosis serologically in pregnancy is essential since rubelliform rashes may be caused by such infections as parvovirus B19, enteroviruses, and such arbovirus infections as Ross River and Chikungunya.

Table 2 *Intrauterine viral infections*

Virus	Classification	Birth defects	Persistent infection	Fetal death
Rubella	Rubivirus	Yes	Yes	Yes
Cytomegalovirus (CMV)	Herpes CMV	Yes	Yes	Yes
Varicella	Herpes varicella/zoster	Yes	Possible	Yes
Parvovirus B19	Parvovirus	No	Yes	Yes
HIV-1 and HIV-2	Retrovirus	No	Yes	Yes
Hepatitis C	Flavivirus-like	No	Yes	Unknown
Poliomyelitis	Enterovirus	No	No	Yes
Coxsackie B	Enterovirus	No	No	Yes
Japanese encephalitis	Flavivirus	Unknown	Unknown	Yes
Lassa fever	Arenavirus	No	No	Yes

Rubella virus induces an antimitotic protein, resulting in fetal organs containing fewer cells than in an uninfected conceptus. Thus if infection occurs during the critical phase of organogenesis, in the first 8 weeks of pregnancy, multiple development defects may result.

If infection occurs during the first trimester, the fetus is almost invariably infected, developing a persistent and generalized infection, which may result in spontaneous abortion, the delivery of a still-born infant, or the birth of an infant with severe multisystem disease. Congenitally infected infants may excrete virus for up to a year despite having persistent neutralizing antibody responses.

Cardiac anomalies, cataract, and sensorineural defects occur commonly, although they may not be present at birth. Anomalies may be divided into those which are transient (for example, low birth weight, cloudy corneas, thrombocytopenic purpura), developmental (for example, sensorineural deafness, mental retardation, endocrine disturbances), and those that persist for life unless corrected. These include developmental defects, which then persist, as well as cardiac and a variety of ocular anomalies, including cataract, glaucoma, and retinopathy.

Sensorineural deafness and retinopathy are the most common defects, which may affect about 17 per cent of infants whose mothers acquire rubella between 13 and 16 weeks, but defects occur only rarely after this period. Rubella infection after the first trimester is not persistent and generalized, and infants do not excrete virus at birth.

Recent studies suggest that the fetus is not infected if rubella is acquired prior to conception. Reinfection only presents a hazard to the fetus if maternal viraemia occurs, but this is extremely rare in persons known to be immune; it may be associated with a rubella-specific defect in the host's immune mechanisms. Although the risk has not been quantified, pregnant women with naturally acquired or vaccine-induced immunity who have been exposed to rubella may be reassured that their conceptus is most unlikely to be infected.

Although congenitally acquired rubella is now rare in Britain and the United States, the legacy of previous outbreaks remains. Late-onset disease, including a subacute panencephalitis and endocrine disorders, may occur but are often delayed until adolescence or even adult life. Insulin-dependent (juvenile onset, type 1) diabetes mellitus is the commonest form of late-onset disease and has been reported in 12 to 20 per cent of patients with congenitally acquired rubella. More detailed information may be found in recent reviews.

Herpes viruses

CYTOMEGALOVIRUS

In Britain about 40 per cent of Caucasian women of childbearing age have serological evidence of previous infection, but, among the Asian population, the prevalence approaches 90 per cent. Afro-Caribbeans have an intermediate seroprevalence.

About 1 per cent of pregnant women experience a primary infection and cytomegalovirus viraemia may result in the fetus developing a gen-

eralized and persistent infection, which induces damage. However, cytomegalovirus is transmitted to the fetus in only about 40 per cent of primary maternal infections. The risks of transmission are similar throughout pregnancy. There is some evidence to suggest that those mothers whose fetuses are infected have a specific defect in cytomegalovirus-related cell-mediated immune responses. About 5 per cent of infants infected *in utero* are born with evidence of severe intrauterine infection, including such features as low birthweight, thrombocytopenic purpura, hepatosplenomegaly, and choroidoretinitis. If not present at birth, CNS anomalies, including microcephaly, periventricular cerebral calcification, and mental retardation, are likely to develop. Most congenitally infected infants are apparently healthy at birth and develop normally. However, follow-up studies show that about 10 per cent may subsequently develop sensorineural deafness, which may be unilateral or bilateral, or some degree of psychomotor retardation. Reactivation of cytomegalovirus or reinfection only very rarely results in congenitally acquired disease.

Provided specimens are collected from infants within 3 weeks of delivery, the presence of cytomegalovirus excretion is indicative of congenitally acquired infection. In developed countries, about 0.3 to 1 per cent of infants excrete cytomegalovirus at birth and this is usually the result of a primary maternal infection. However, in populations with a high seroprevalence, cytomegalovirus excretion is usually the result of maternal reactivation or reinfection.

About 10 per cent of women excrete cytomegalovirus via the cervix in the last trimester and infection may be acquired during delivery or postpartum, since cytomegalovirus is excreted in breast milk, but such infections 'immunize' and do not constitute a hazard to the infant.

Table 3 compares the impact of congenitally acquired cytomegalovirus in infants born in the United States and the United Kingdom, from which it will be seen that this infection results in a considerable number of infants being delivered with, or subsequently developing, congenitally acquired anomalies, particularly CNS defects.

Cytomegalovirus screening programmes in pregnancy have little or no part to play in preventing infection. As most patients are asymptomatic, the only way of determining whether a primary infection has occurred is by determining a cytomegalovirus-specific IgM response. However, since this response may persist for some months, primary infection may have occurred some time before conception. Furthermore, since only 40 per cent of infections are transmitted to the fetus, and as most congenitally infected infants develop normally, it would be difficult to justify pregnancy termination. Current research is being directed towards the development of suitable recombinant derived vaccines for administration to seronegative females. More detailed information may be obtained from recent reviews.

VARICELLA ZOSTER (SEE ALSO SECTION 7)

If acquired during the first 20 weeks of pregnancy, chicken pox (varicella) may cause a constellation of abnormalities (congenital varicella

Table 3 *Annual public health impact of congenital cytomegalovirus*

	United States of America	United Kingdom
Number of live births	4 000 000	700 000
Proportion congenitally infected	1%	0.3%
Number congenitally infected	40 000	2100
Number with cytomegalic inclusion disease (7%)	2800	147
Number fatal (12%)	336	18
Number with sequelae (90%)	2218	132
Number asymptomatic (95%)	37 200	1953
Number with sequelae (15%)	5580	293
Total number damaged	8134	443

Reproduced from Griffiths (1995), with permission.

syndrome) but, if acquired near term or soon after delivery, a severe and sometimes fatal infection may occur.

The congenitally acquired syndrome is rare. A prospective study including more than 1300 women with varicella and 364 with herpes zoster showed that fetal damage occurred only during the first 20 weeks of gestation, the overall risk being 1 per cent. The highest risk (2 per cent) occurred between 13 and 20 weeks' gestation. Although the proportion of abnormalities is little different from that following uninfected pregnancies, clinical features reported from this and other studies represent a distinctive constellation, and include limb hypoplasia, atrophic digits, microcephaly, cataracts, cicatricial skin scarring, and eye defects (Fig. 3). Healthy infants, whose mothers developed varicella at any stage of pregnancy, may develop shingles (zoster) in infancy. Some of the features of the varicella syndrome, particularly skin scarring, may be the result of intrauterine reactivation of fetal varicella.

Although there have been occasional reports of maternal zoster being associated with subsequent developmental defects, these observations were probably coincidental and patients with maternal zoster should therefore be reassured that infection will not affect the fetus. Varicella-

Fig. 3 (a) Child with features of congenitally acquired varicella. Note the hypoplastic limbs and some scarring of the upper limbs. (b) Upper limbs from the same child. Note the atrophic digits and pronounced cicatricial scarring. (Reproduced by kind permission of Dr P. N. Goldwater, Adelaide Children's Hospital, Adelaide, Australia.)

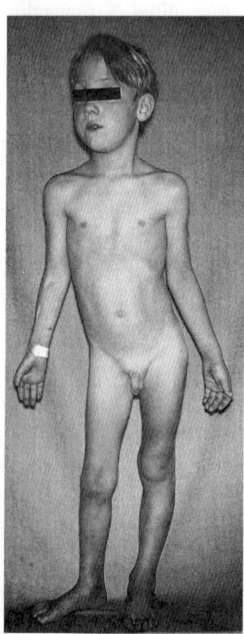

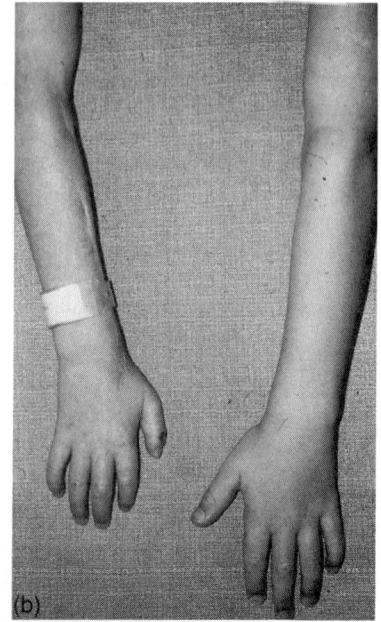

zoster-specific IgM antibody was detected at birth in 25 per cent of infants with clinical evidence of intrauterine infection, and persistent virus-specific IgG occurred in many of these infants.

Although varicella-specific IgM responses have occasionally been detected in fetal blood and varicella-zoster DNA has been found in chorionic villus samples and amniotic fluid, such findings may not be indicative of fetal damage. In any case, the rarity of the varicella syndrome makes the value of such investigations difficult to assess. Ultrasonography may be helpful in determining whether growth retardation, limb abnormalities, or gross scarring are present, but repeat examination may be necessary; some of the more subtle defects will escape detection.

Twenty-five to thirty per cent of infections among infants whose mothers acquire varicella near term are fatal, particularly if maternal rash occurs during the last 4 days of pregnancy, since there is insufficient time for maternal antibodies to cross the placenta. Such infants are likely to develop haemorrhagic varicella.

Varicella-zoster immune globulin should be given to infants whose mothers develop varicella (but not zoster) 7 days before to a month after delivery, since maternal varicella-zoster IgG antibodies are present in the infant's circulation if rash occurred 7 or more days before delivery. Between 7 and 3 days, progressively fewer infants have maternal antibody; it is absent in those delivered less than 3 days after rash. Varicella-zoster immune globulin should also be given to infants in contact with chicken pox or zoster whose mothers have no history of chicken pox or have no varicella-zoster antibody, and to those born before 30 weeks of gestation or with a birthweight of < 1 kg. Despite a history of maternal varicella, such infants may not have acquired maternal antibody. Prophylactic varicella-zoster immune globulin should also be given to susceptible infants at risk of acquiring infection from household contacts with varicella.

Varicella-zoster immune globulin may not always prevent infection, although it usually reduces its severity. However, as occasionally fatal infections have been reported despite the administration of varicella-zoster immune globulin, infants with neonatal varicella should be admitted to hospital and consideration should be given to treatment with systematically administered acyclovir.

HERPES SIMPLEX (SEE ALSO SECTION 7)

Primary maternal infection occurring during the first 20 weeks of gestation may result in fetal death with spontaneous abortion, still birth, and, much more rarely, such congenital malformations as hydrocephaly and chorioretinitis. If acquired at a later gestational age, infants may be delivered with intrauterine growth retardation.

Herpes simplex infection is more frequently acquired from contact with genital lesions during passage through the birth canal or via an ascending infection if membranes rupture early, or via fetal scalp monitoring. Infection may be acquired postpartum, infection being transmitted via maternal non-genital lesions or nosocomially via infected health-care workers.

In the United States, it has been estimated that the incidence of neonatal herpes simplex infection is about 1 in every 3500 deliveries. However, in the United Kingdom—for reasons which are not understood—the incidence is much lower; between 1986 and 1991 only 37 cases were notified, infection being equally divided between HSV-1 and HSV-2.

Newborn infants are much more likely to be infected from primary maternal lesions since, in contrast with recurrences or asymptomatic infection, high concentrations of virus are present which may persist for 2 to 3 weeks. The risk of a neonate being infected from a primary lesion is about 50 per cent but, from a recurrent lesion, less than 5 per cent.

It was previously recommended that, if pregnant women or their partners had a history of recurrent herpes, attempts should be made to culture herpes simplex prior to delivery. However, it has now been established that antepartum cultures do not predict risk at delivery and this practice has now largely been discontinued.

Caesarean section should be carried out if active genital lesions are present, provided membranes are intact or have been ruptured for less than 6 h. This reduces neonatal herpes simplex remarkably, but may not necessarily prevent it. Although consideration should be given to administering prophylactic systemically administered acyclovir to infants delivered vaginally from mothers with active lesions, this regime has not been evaluated.

The onset of neonatal herpes simplex infection usually occurs between 5 and 17 days after delivery. Although infants may present with vesicular lesions of the skin and mucous membranes, in 60 per cent of cases without treatment, herpes simplex disseminates to cause a severe and a frequently fatal infection. Some infants present with encephalitis, and others with a severe systemic disease. Treatment with acyclovir improves prognosis, although the mortality from disseminated infection recorded 1 year after treatment is 60 per cent and for encephalitis 15 per cent. Infants with infection confined to the skin and mucous membranes survive and experience no long-term defects but CNS impairment has been reported in 41 per cent and 64 per cent of infants who presented with disseminated lesions or encephalitis, respectively. In general, treated infants infected with HSV-1 experience fewer long-term sequelae than those with HSV-2 infections.

HUMAN HERPES TYPE 6 (SEE ALSO SECTION 7)

Sixty to seventy per cent of British children have antibodies to human herpes type 6 (HHV-6). Although infection may be acquired in childhood, since HHV-6 persists, intrauterine or perinatal infection is possible. A recent study showed that HHV-6-specific IgM was present in 0.25 per cent of 800 cord bloods. No abnormalities were present.

Hepatitis viruses (see also Chapter 7.10.26)

HEPATITIS B (FIG. 1(g))

It has been estimated that there are some 200 to 300 million carriers of hepatitis B virus in the world. High carrier rates with a prevalence ranging from 10 to 20 per cent occur in many developing countries, particularly in sub-Saharan Africa, the Far East, and many Pacific islands. Most of these carriers are infected perinatally or in early childhood and many develop chronic liver disease, including cirrhosis and hepatocellular carcinoma.

Maternal hepatitis B virus is likely to be transmitted during birth, regardless of gestational age, infants becoming HBsAg positive when aged 2 to 3 months. About 90 to 95 per cent of infants delivered of mothers who have markers of infectivity (HBeAg and/or hepatitis B viral DNA) will be infected and develop long-term hepatitis B virus carriage. About 30 to 40 per cent of infants delivered of mothers without either HBeAg or anti-HBe become carriers, but this only occurs in about 5 per cent of infants whose mothers have anti-HBe responses.

In about 5 per cent of cases, hepatitis B virus is transmitted transplacentally. It has been suggested that maternal antibody to the core antigen (anti-HBc) may suppress viral replication in the fetus, immune responses to hepatitis B virus associated antigens being delayed until after delivery when maternal antibodies decline.

Most infants who acquire hepatitis B virus infection via their mothers are asymptomatic, although, rarely, an acute and even a fulminating hepatitis have been reported in infants whose mothers are anti-HBe positive.

Since infants are usually exposed at birth, postdelivery immunization markedly reduces the risk of infants acquiring infection. In countries of high endemicity where perinatal transmission results in persistent hepatitis B virus infection in infancy and childhood, universal immunization of newborn infants with hepatitis B virus vaccine without prior screening of pregnant women is recommended. Although optimum protection (> 95 per cent) will be achieved if infants are given passive/active immunization with hepatitis B virus immunoglobulin (HBIG) and vaccine, many developing countries cannot afford to use HBIG; active immunization alone will protect about 75 per cent. HBIG should be given within 12 h of birth and the first dose of vaccine should be administered then or shortly after in the opposite arm. Second and third doses of vaccine should be given when the infant is aged 1 month and 6 months, respectively, although an alternative schedule in which the second and third doses of vaccine are given at 1 or 2 months of age may also be used. A booster dose may be given at 12 months.

In Britain, hepatitis B virus carrier rates among pregnant women vary from about 0.1 to 0.5 per cent, although, in some inner city areas, a 1 per cent carrier rate has been reported.

In order to prevent the long-term hepatitis B carrier state, with its attendant risk of developing chronic liver disease, the World Health Organization (WHO) has recommended that countries with an hepatitis B carrier rate of more than 8 per cent should introduce hepatitis B vaccination into the Expanded Programme of Immunization by 1995. Countries with lower carrier rates should develop programmes for the universal immunization of children by 1997.

Recently, the emergence of hepatitis B virus escape mutants is causing concern. Thus, infants vaccinated at birth, despite having adequate levels of anti-hepatitis B contracted hepatitis B virus infection. This phenomenon has now been observed in developed and developing countries, although its frequency has yet to be established. Molecular biological studies demonstrated that the virus infecting these children was a mutant having an amino acid substitution (glycine to arginine) in the *a* antigen loop of the surface antigen, this being the major protective epitope. This change resulted in the vaccine-induced anti hepatitis B response failing to neutralize the mutant virus. Mutants may be transmitted and cause disease in contacts.

HEPATITIS C

There is some evidence to suggest that hepatitis C virus may be transmitted from mothers to infants; a small study showed that the hepatitis C virus genome was detected at birth in 8 of 10 infants whose mothers had evidence of current hepatitis C infection, infants remaining positive for periods extending to 10 months. Three infants had abnormal liver function. This contrasts with a report of another study involving 116 pregnant women which showed that hepatitis C virus was not transmitted to infants unless they were also infected by HIV. In such cases, co-infected mothers transmitted hepatitis C virus in 36 per cent of cases.

Human parvovirus (B19) (Fig. 1(h)) (see also Section 7)

Seroepidemiological studies show that infection by B19 occurs throughout the world. In temperate climates outbreaks occur more commonly in late winter, spring, and early summer. Infection occurs most commonly between the ages of 4 and 10; among adults about 60 per cent are seropositive. In developing countries, acquisition of antibody occurs at an even earlier age. Women of childbearing age may be infected via the respiratory route, commonly from children who may be experiencing a non-specific respiratory-tract infection or an exanthematous disease, erythema infectiosum.

Women of child-bearing age may experience a rubelliform rash. In 80 per cent of cases, this is associated with arthralgia or arthritis. The rash may be indistinguishable from rubella, although a faint and transient, or much more florid, rash has been observed.

Maternal viraemia may result in placental and fetal infection. The B19 virus replicates in rapidly dividing cells, particularly the erythroid progenitor cells, and this may result in severe fetal anaemia. Most pregnancies proceed to term and, during the first trimester, fetal loss is no greater than expected. However, during the second trimester, fetal loss is of the order of 12 to 14 per cent, which is considerably greater than that recorded in uninfected pregnancies (0.5–0.6 per cent). Fetal loss usually occurs 4 to 6 weeks after maternal infection. Congenital malformations have not been reported. If infection occurs during the second and third trimesters, fetal hydrops may occasionally occur; in the absence of haemolytic disease, the presence of a low fetal haemoglobin is strongly suggestive of B19 infection. This may result in miscarriage or still birth (Fig. 4). It has been estimated that in Britain maternal B19 infections result in 135 to 180 miscarriages annually, although during epidemics, which occur at 3- to 4-yearly intervals, this figure may show a two-to threefold increase.

Pregnancies that reach term usually result in the delivery of a healthy infant, and follow-up studies at a year reveal no abnormalities in such infants. However, pregnant women with B19 infections should be monitored by ultrasonography for evidence of fetal hydrops; such patients may also develop rising levels of alpha-fetoprotein. Fetal infection can be established by testing blood for evidence of B19 viraemia and anaemia, although fetal virus-specific IgM is not usually present. At autopsy, B19 has been detected in the placenta and fetal liver by *in situ* hybridization or polymerase chain reaction.

Intrauterine blood transfusion has been used successfully to treat a few infants with fetal hydrops, but the procedure in itself is not without

Fig. 4 Infant delivered with parvovirus B19-induced hydrops fetalis. (Reproduced by kind permission of Professor J. R. Pattison, University College and Middlesex School of Medicine, London, UK.)

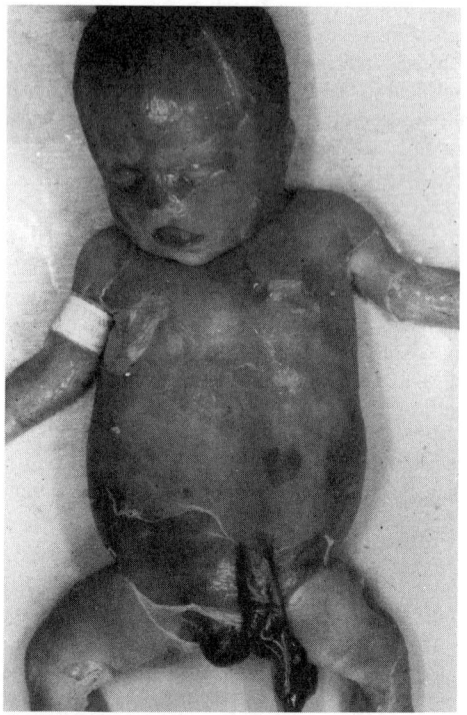

risk. It has also been shown that some infants with fetal hydrops recover spontaneously.

Retroviruses (see also Section 7)

HUMAN IMMUNODEFICIENCY VIRUSES (HIV-1, HIV-2) (FIG. 1(i))

Pregnancy does not usually result in progression of HIV-related infection, and pregnant women do not have an enhanced risk of miscarriage. Prematurity and low birthweight have been reported, but these may reflect adverse social factors rather than HIV infection.

The risk of transmission of HIV-1 from mother to infant has been estimated to vary from 10 to 40 per cent, high rates being reported in sub-Saharan Africa. However, these varying rates of transmission may reflect differences in the design of studies rather than true differences in transmission rates. The European Collaborative Study, involving 19 European centres, estimated that transmission occurs in about 15 per cent of pregnancies. In contrast, HIV-2, which is endemic in parts of West Africa but has now been imported into parts of Europe, particularly Portugal, the United States, and more recently India, is only very rarely transmitted from mother to infant (about 0 to 1 per cent). This probably reflects that, in contrast with HIV-1 infections, HIV-2 infections are associated with a much lower level of maternal viraemia.

Infection may be transmitted transplacentally, during birth, or postnatally via breast-feeding or transfusion of HIV-contaminated blood. Women transmitting HIV-1 during one pregnancy may not necessarily transmit infection in a subsequent one. Furthermore, there have been reports of monozygotic twins in which only one has been infected. The finding that some HIV-1 infected infants have histological evidence of cerebral atrophy and calcification of basal ganglia, as well as immunological abnormalities at birth, including reduced CD4 levels, diminished lymphoblastoid transformation, and low thymic hormone levels, provides evidence supporting intrauterine transmission. Further evidence is provided by the detection of HIV-1 by molecular biological techniques in the brain and thymus. However, reports of infection occurring more commonly in the first- rather than the second-born twin suggest that infection may also be acquired during birth. It is probable that the first twin is exposed to more virus from contact with maternal cervical and vaginal secretions.

There have been recent reports that various intervention procedures reduce transmission of HIV. Treatment of HIV-infected mothers and their babies with zidovudine reduced HIV transmission from mother to baby by two-thirds. Although treatment was well tolerated by mothers and babies, the potential long-term effects need to be carefully evaluated. It has also been shown that delivery by caesarean section may halve the rate of viral transmission and this adds additional weight to the theory that a high proportion of HIV infections are transmitted from mother to baby perinatally. Therapeutic vaccination, now undergoing Phase I trials, may reduce maternal viral load and, if effective, may be considerably cheaper and perhaps safer than the above methods.

The role of breast-feeding was highlighted by a recent analysis of five studies, which showed that, if mothers were infected prenatally, the additional risk of transmission through breast-feeding over and above intrauterine or intrapartum infection is of the order of 14 per cent. Although HIV-infected mothers should be discouraged from breast-feeding in developed countries, in developing countries where formula feeding is associated with high morbidity and mortality rates in infancy, mothers should be encouraged to breast feed.

Infants may present with a variety of clinical features, including failure to thrive, oral candidiasis, pneumonia, protracted diarrhoea, parotitis, and hepatosplenomegaly. Failure to thrive and *Pneumocystis carinii* pneumonia are the most frequent presenting features; HIV infection should be considered in any child presenting with an unexplained and severe illness in areas having moderate to high HIV endemicity.

Symptoms usually present at about 3 to 6 months of age; by 1 year of age about 50 per cent of HIV-infected infants will be symptomatic,

Table 4 *Laboratory diagnosis of HIV infection in infancy*

Specific IgG	Maternal IgG may persist for a year
	Test every 3 months for 18 months
Virus isolation from peripheral blood mononuclear cells	Not widely available
Polymerase chain reaction	Specificity good, may not be positive early in life
Specific IgA	Very useful (90% positive by 6 months)
In vitro HIV specific antibody production	Useful, not widely available
p24 antigen	Prognostic marker, must be confirmed by 'blocking assay'
	? transfer of maternal antigen

None of the assays can assure absolute sensitivity and specificity. A combination of tests or repeated testing is required to confirm infection.

the proportion increasing to about 80 per cent by about 3 years. Although 75 per cent die within 2 years of diagnosis, some children may remain asymptomatic for many years. However, improved management, including specific antiretroviral therapy, prophylaxis of opportunistic infections, and psychosocial support for the family, may prolong the quality and duration of life.

Current drugs under evaluation for HIV-1-infected infants include oral and continuous infusion of zidovudine, dideoxyinosine, dideoxycytosine, and soluble CD4 non-nucleoside reverse transcriptase inhibitors. Some of these drugs may be tried in combination, either simultaneously or in an alternating regime.

Unlike other viral infections acquired *in utero* or perinatally, serological investigations are of little value in establishing whether or not infants have acquired infection in early infancy, since maternal antibody may persist for up to 18 months and virus-specific IgM responses lack reliability. Table 4 lists some of the laboratory techniques that may be used to confirm the diagnosis of HIV infection in infancy.

HUMAN T-CELL LEUKAEMIA VIRUS TYPE 1 (HTLV-1) (SEE ALSO CHAPTER 7.10.31)

Studies among women attending antenatal clinics in London have shown a seroprevalence rate of 0.2 per cent. There is a higher percentage (about 2 per cent) among black women born in the Caribbean but no evidence of infection among those of Afro-Caribbean descent born in Britain. HTLV-1 does not have an adverse effect on pregnancy.

Studies in Japan have shown that HTLV-1 infection was transmitted in 28 per cent of infants whose mothers were seropositive but in none whose mothers were seronegative but whose fathers were seropositive. This suggests strongly that infection is transmitted from mother to child. Follow-up studies indicate that infection is not acquired *in utero* or during birth but postnatally via breast-feeding. The finding that HTLV-1 antigen is present in breast milk and that 21 of 31 (77 per cent) of breast-fed, but only 1 of 30 (5 per cent) of formula-fed, babies delivered of seropositive mothers is in support of the role of breast-feeding in transmitting HTLV-1.

A diagnosis of infection in the mother or baby may be established by detecting virus by co-cultivation techniques, although this is labour-intensive and expensive. Alternatively, viral genes may be identified by use of the polymerase chain reaction. However, it is more usual and convenient to employ serological tests diagnostically, relying on a reference centre for confirmation of the diagnosis and distinguishing between HTLV-1 and -2 infections.

The cumulative lifetime risk of developing acute T-cell leukaemia/lymphoma is only about 3 to 5 per cent; tropical spastic paraparesis is the result of infection acquired by older patients, often via blood transfusion. In such countries as Japan, avoidance of breast-feeding in seropositive mothers is advisable. However, in developing countries, the advantages of breast-feeding outweigh its disadvantages.

Enteroviruses (see also Section 7)

Enteroviruses are ubiquitous and, although infection occurs commonly in childhood, all age groups may be infected. Enteroviruses may be transmitted *in utero*, often via an asymptomatic maternal infection, although occasionally mothers may present with Bornholm's disease, aseptic meningitis, myocarditis, or other less specific febrile illnesses, which may be associated with abdominal pain or respiratory symptoms. Poliomyelitis is associated with an increased risk of miscarriage and, if acquired near term, may result in stillbirth or delivery of a child with paralytic disease. The most frequently reported enterovirus infections in pregnancy are coxsackie B2–5 and various echovirus infections, particularly echo II. Such infections may be transmitted transplacentally or during delivery via vaginal secretions, blood, faeces, or saliva. There have been reports of neonatal infection in infants delivered by caesarean section. Infants may be delivered with, or develop shortly after birth, clinical features of enterovirus infections, which usually present 3 to 7 days postdelivery. Outbreaks of infection have occurred as a result of nosocomial infection in nurseries for the new-born.

The early features of infection may be mild or non-specific; listlessness or transient respiratory distress may follow, with or without fever. Some infants develop a fulminating and frequently fatal disease in which encephalitis and myocarditis are dominant features. Others may develop circulatory collapse with haemorrhages and hepatic necrosis; there may be a combination of both types of presentation.

Mothers and infants who have clinical features consistent with an enterovirus infection should have appropriate specimens taken for virus isolation, which should include nasopharyngeal aspirates, stools, cerebrospinal fluid, and blood. It may be possible to isolate an enterovirus within 3 to 4 days, although it will take longer to confirm its serotype. Mothers and infants may develop a virus-specific IgM response within 3 to 4 days of the onset of symptoms.

Strict attention to infection control measures is essential in preventing spread of infection in nurseries for the newborn. It has been suggested that the administration of human normal immunoglobulin may be beneficial if given prophylactically to protect uninfected infants, as this preparation is likely to contain some neutralizing antibody to the more commonly encountered enteroviruses.

Human papillomaviruses (Fig. 1(j))

Human papillomaviruses 6 and 11 may be transmitted intrapartum or perinatally, and infected infants may subsequently develop recurrent juvenile papillomatosis. Despite infection with these viruses being common, this disease is rare.

Although epidemiological evidence suggests that the major route of infection by those human papillomaviruses implicated in the aetiology of cervical cancer (16 and 18) is sexual, infection by these viruses may also be acquired in childhood as a result of intrapartum infection. Further studies have shown that viruses may persist for at least 6 months.

REFERENCES

Ades, A.E., Peckham, C.S., Dale, G.E., Best, J.M., and Jeansson, S. (1989). Prevalence of antibodies to herpes simplex virus types 1 and 2 in pregnant women, and estimated rates of infection. *Journal of Epidemiology and Community Health* **43**, 53–60.

Ando, Y., *et al.* (1989). Bottle-feeding can prevent transmission of HLTV-1 from mothers to their babies. *Journal of Infection* **19**, 25–9.

Andrews, E.B., Yankasbas, B.C., Cordero, J.F., Schoeffler, K., Hampp, S. and the Acyclovir in Pregnancy Registry Advisory Committee. (1992).

Acyclovir in pregnancy registry: six years' experience. *Obstetrics and Gynecology* **79**, 7–13.

Best, J.M. (1992). Rubella. In *Congenital, perinatal and neonatal infections*, (ed. A. Greenough, J. Osborne, and S. Sutherland), pp. 171–84. Churchill Livingstone, Edinburgh.

Centers for Disease Control and Prevention. (1994). Zidovudine for the prevention of HIV transmission from mother to baby. *Morbidity and Mortality Weekly Report*, **43** (No. 16), 285–7.

Chaturvedi, U.C., Mathur, A., Chandra, A., Das, S.K., Tandon, H.O., and Singh, U.K. (1980). Transplacental infection with Japanese encephalitis virus. *Journal of Infectious Diseases* **141**, 712–15.

Daunter, B. (1992). Immunology of pregnancy: towards a unifying hypothesis. *European Journal of Obstetrics, Gynecology and Reproductive Biology* **43**, 81–95.

Department of Health, Welsh Office, Scottish Home Office and Health Departments, DHSS (Northern Ireland) (1982). *Immunisation against infectious diseases*. HMSO, London.

Dune, W.M. and Demmler, G.J. (1992). Serological evidence for congenital transmission of human herpesvirus 6. *Lancet* **340**, 121–2.

Eberhart-Phillips, J.E., Frederick, P.D., Baron, R.C., and Mascola, L. (1993). Measles in pregnancy: a descriptive study of 58 cases. *Obstetrics and Gynecology,* **82,** 797–801.

Enders, G., Miller, E., Cradock-Watson, J., Bolley, I., and Ridehalgh, M. (1994). Consequences of varicella and herpes zoster at successive stages of pregnancy, *Lancet*, **343**, 1548–51.

Griffiths, P. (1995). *Principles and practice of clinical virology*, (3rd edn). John Wiley and Sons, Chichester.

Levine, M.M., Edsall, G., and Bruce-Chwatt, L.J. (1974). Live-virus vaccines in pregnancy risks and recommendations. *Lancet* **ii**, 34–8.

Miller, E., Cradock-Watson, J.E., and Ridehalgh, M.K.S. (1989). Outcome in newborn babies given anti-varicella-zoster immunoglobulin after perinatal maternal infection with varicella-zoster virus. *Lancet* **2**, 371–3.

Newell, M.-L. and Peckham, C. (1993). Risk factors of vertical transmission of HIV-1 and early markers of HIV-1 infection in children. *AIDS*, **7,** (Suppl. 1), 891–7.

Pakarian, F.B., Kaye, J., Cason, J., *et al.* (1994). Cancer associated human papillomaviruses: perinatal transmission and persistence. *British Journal of Obstetrics and Gynaecology*, **101**, 514–17.

Price, M.E., Fisher-Hoch, S.P., Craven, R.B., and McCormick, J.B. (1988). A prospective study of maternal and fetal outcome in acute Lassa fever infection during pregnancy. *British Medical Journal* **297**, 584–7.

Public Health Laboratory Service (1990). *TORCH screening reassessed.* Report of a working party on diagnostic tests for congenital infections. Public Health Laboratory Service, Colindale.

Siegel, M., and Greenberg, M. (1955). Incidence of poliomyelitis in pregnancy. Its relation to maternal age, parity and gestational period. *New England Journal of Medicine* **253**, 841–7.

Thaler, M.M., *et al.* (1991). Vertical transmission of hepatitis C virus. *Lancet* **2**, 17–18.

The European Collaborative Study, (1994). Caesarean section and risk of vertical tranmission of HIV-1 infection. *Lancet*, **343**, 1464–7.

Whitley, R.J. (1991). Perinatal herpes simplex virus infections. *Reviews of Virology*, **1**, 101–10.

Zanetti, A.R., *et al.* (1995). Mother–to–infant transmission of hepatitis C virus. *Lancet*, **345**, 289–91.

13.12.2 Bacterial, fungal, and protozoal infections in pregnancy and the newborn

H. R. GAMSU

Pregnancy and susceptibility to infection

Pregnant women are more susceptible to infection and its effects. A number of factors increase this susceptibility. These include poverty, promiscuity, poor personal hygiene, alcohol and drug abuse, smoking, poor nutrition, as well as some more specific factors, such as diabetes mellitus and corticosteroid therapy.

In any pregnancy, increased oestrogen and progesterone production

cause ureteric dilatation which, when combined with the pressure of the uterus on the bladder, results in stasis and a predisposition to urinary infection. Elevation of the diaphragm in later pregnancy is likely to increase the risk and severity of respiratory infection.

Certain factors protect the woman and her fetus from infection. There is an increase in the amount and viscosity of cervical mucus, which forms a plug in the endocervical canal. The membranes form a physical barrier to ascending infection and the placenta protects against blood-borne infection, but neither is impermeable. Synthesis of vaginal mucosal glycogen is increased in response to increased hormone secretion, lactobacilli produce more lactic acid from this substrate and the acidic milieu favours their continued survival and propagation. As a result, pathogenic vaginal bacteria are less likely to colonize the vagina. Amniotic fluid has bactericidal and bacteristatic properties attributable to immunoglobulins, polymorphonuclear leucocytes, lysozyme, transferrin, and zinc polypeptides. Lectins, which inhibit bacterial binding to the membranes, are present in the amniotic fluid. The ability to inhibit the growth of organisms increases with advancing pregnancy.

However, corticosteroids, as well as placental progesterone and oestrogen production, have the effect of reducing phagocytic activity, and macrophage cytokine activity and the inflammatory response is suppressed. Alpha-fetoprotein also inhibits lymphocyte transformation and reduces macrophage activation and intracellular killing. Although the polymorphonuclear count is increased in early pregnancy and there is greater phagocytic and bactericidal activity in mid-gestation, phagocytosis, chemotaxis, and bacterial killing by these cells are all reduced. There is a fall in the population of T helper cells and a decrease in natural killer cell activity. B lymphocytes do not seem to be affected. There is a fall in total IgG concentration as pregnancy advances.

IN THE FETUS AND NEONATE

When compared to the findings in later infancy, in the fetus and newborn the stem cell proliferative pool is low, though the rate of proliferation is rapid. The polymorphonuclear neutrophil leucocyte storage pool is also low, and when infection occurs, the pool becomes exhausted and neutropenia develops. Polymorphonuclear function is poor, adherence, chemotaxis, phagocytosis, and intracellular killing are all reduced, especially in the sick or preterm neonate. Macrophage chemotaxis and T lymphocyte activation are also reduced, and complement levels remain low until the third trimester. B lymphocytes are present from 10 weeks, and by term, IgG levels are higher than in the mother. In early pregnancy, although some IgG crosses the placenta, the levels in the fetus are low.

Bacterial flora in pregnancy

In pregnancy, vaginal pH remains low. The prevalence of colonization with lactobacilli increases as pregnancy advances and there is a concomitant increase in the prevalence of *candida*. Acidic conditions favour both organisms, and there may be synergism between them.

Antimicrobials in pregnancy

As with all drugs that are used in pregnancy, antibiotics and antimicrobial drugs should be chosen with the best interests not only of the mother, but also of the baby, in mind. Certain of these drugs are either inadvisable or should be used with particular caution:

Sulphonamides, because of competitive albumin binding, predispose to bilirubin toxicity in the newborn.

Tetracycline transferred to the fetus can lead to enamel hypoplasia, retarded growth and cataracts.

Gentamicin may predispose to sensorineural deafness. Of the other aminoglycosides, streptomycin exerts an even more toxic effect on VIIIth nerve function and is normally reserved for the treatment of multiple-drug-resistant tuberculosis only.

Chloramphenicol, when given to the mother in excessive doses, can lead to 'the grey baby syndrome' if residual blood levels remain high in the new-born.

Metronidazole in high doses has been associated with carcinogenesis and teratogenesis in experimental animals.

Nitrafurantoin, nalidixic acid, and sulphonamides might precipitate haemolysis in babies with glucose 6-phosphate dehydrogenase deficiency.

Erythromycin estolate is more likely to cause cholestasis in the mother in pregnancy, especially if the course is prolonged. The stearate may also cause jaundice, but not the erythromycin base. Placental transfer of erythromycin is restricted and fetal treatment may therefore be less than adequate, particularly in conditions such as maternal syphilis.

Quinolones can cause articular damage in young experimental animals, but this effect has not as yet been demonstrated in humans.

The indications for antimicrobial therapy should be strict. They should be used for the shortest time possible. As is the case with other drugs, pregnancy exerts effects on antimicrobial pharmacokinetics. There is an increased intravascular and extravascular volume, a decreased plasma protein concentration, increased renal clearance, and an increased rate of hepatic metabolism. Vomiting is more common in early pregnancy and tends to lead to less certain absorption of drugs. The net effect is that standard antimicrobial doses result in lower serum levels towards the end of pregnancy and blood levels of some antimicrobials should be monitored and the dose increased in severe infection. Placental transfer of antimicrobials increases as pregnancy advances.

Antimicrobial dosage in the newborn also has special problems, with decreased protein binding, increased body water, and reduced renal clearance. Dosage cannot reliably be extrapolated using adult dosage formulae based on weight or surface area, and therefore in most cases although dosage schedules exist, blood levels need to be measured. Some drugs have a low therapeutic index, e.g. gentamicin and chloramphenicol. In preterm infants and in the first few days of life, smaller doses and longer dosage intervals are generally required. Intramuscular administration results in variable absorption. The small muscle mass makes this route technically difficult to use. Enteral absorption likewise is unpredictable, although with prolonged treatment it may become a more appropriate route as the baby grows older.

Prophylactic antimicrobial therapy

CAESAREAN SECTION DELIVERY

Risk factors for postoperative infection include prolonged rupture of membranes, obesity, prolonged surgery, anaemia, haematoma formation, and internal fetal monitoring. In these situations especially, a short course of antibiotics is warranted and usually adequate. There is a risk of partial suppression of neonatal infection and of alteration of the reliability of bacterial culture, and for this reason some would withhold antibiotic administration to the mother until the baby has been delivered and the cord has been clamped. It is now a recommendation of the Royal College of Obstetrics and Gynaecology that all women on whom a caesarian section delivery is carried out should have co-amoxiclav 1 to 2 g intravenously as prophylaxis.

CERVICAL CERCLAGE

As both infection and cervical weakness are causes of second trimester miscarriage and premature labour, a careful analysis of the history and the examination is important. If a previous miscarriage or premature delivery has been due to infection rather than cervical incompetence, and a cervical suture is used in error, then the situation may be further compromised rather than improved by the presence of the foreign tissue.

After cervical cerclage the vaginal flora can change dramatically and a number of pathogenic bacteria have been identified, including *Escherichia coli, Clostridium perfringens*, group B streptococci, and *Staphylococcus aureus*. It is probably best to identify the prevailing organism and its sensitivity pattern before starting antibiotic treatment.

Bacterial infections

Vaginosis

This condition results in a copious malodorous vaginal discharge and is found in about 15 to 20 per cent of pregnant women and imposes a fivefold risk of late miscarriage, preterm premature rupture of membranes, and preterm onset of labour with intact membranes. Postpartum infection and pelvic inflammatory disease may occur as a sequel in a small percentage of cases. The presence of large numbers of *Gardnerella vaginalis* in a Gram stain of material from the endocervix or posterior fornix should prompt appropriate antimicrobial treatment. Conventionally, treatment of vaginosis is with metronidazole, although there is some concern about the risk of teratogenesis and mutagenesis when it is given in high doses or in early pregnancy. Alternatives are amoxycillin/ampicillin, ciprofloxacin, cephalexin, or clindamycin in resistant cases.

Trichomonas vaginalis

This organism is present in low numbers in as many as 20 per cent of normal women antenatally. Even though most are asymptomatic, there is a reported association between *trichomonas* colonization and preterm delivery, premature rupture of the membranes, and low birthweight. A small number of female neonates will develop urinary or vaginal trichomoniasis if born to a mother who is colonized or infected. Metronidazole is effective for trichomoniasis but is usually reserved for the symptomatic woman after the first trimester. The partner should be traced and treated.

Chorioamnionitis, preterm labour, and premature rupture of membranes

Chorioamnionitis (the amniotic infection syndrome)

Various terms are used interchangeably when referring to this condition. These include amnionitis, chorioamnionitis, intrapartum infection, and intra-amniotic infection. The term can be used precisely to describe inflammation of the fetal membranes and placenta, or may be reserved for those cases in which bacteria are recovered from the amniotic fluid. Less precisely, chorioamnionitis has come to be used to describe the symptoms of amniotic infection in the pregnant woman. These include maternal fever, maternal tachycardia, fetal tachycardia, uterine tenderness, malodorous vaginal discharge, and peripheral leucocytosis with a left shift. None of these definitions is entirely satisfactory, since inflammatory change may be found in fetal membranes where there is no coexistent infection; in addition, organisms may be found in amniotic fluid in 10 per cent of otherwise normal women at term, leucocytosis may result from pregnancy itself, from labour, and after administration of steroids to the mother. The symptoms associated with chorioamnionitis, although highly suggestive of infection, are not specific and only occur in a minority of cases.

It is, however, an important entity and is a major factor predisposing to preterm labour.

PATHOGENESIS AND PATHOLOGY

Ascending infection via ruptured membranes is an established cause of chorioamnionitis, although infection is known to occur via intact membranes. Circumstances which predispose to chorioamnionitis are prolonged prelabour (premature) rupture of membranes (PPROM), prolonged labour, vaginal examinations, retained intrauterine contraceptive device, amniocentesis, fetal blood sampling, cervical incompetence, and cervical cerclage, especially if the cervix is already dilated before the stitch is inserted. Bacterial vaginosis is another predisposing factor. Coitus in pregnancy in high-risk populations with heavy vaginal colonization of pathogens is also said to predispose to infection. A number of organisms are often present in an individual case and infected amniotic fluid may contain group B streptococci, *E. coli*, *Bacteroides* spp. and other organisms frequently present in the vagina. Anaerobes predominate, especially in amniotic infection associated with preterm delivery.

The placenta and membranes are often macroscopically normal, or there may be a loss of translucency of the latter. More obvious changes include purulent exudate on the surface of the membranes and oedema and friability of the placenta. Funisitis (inflammation of the cord) may be present. Mild leucocytic infiltration is common in the membranes even in uninfected pregnancy but definite histological changes include leucocytes in the intervillus space and in the chorionic plate. Amnionitis is less frequent. Histological changes of chorioamnionitis have been found in 10 per cent of placentas at term but in 33 per cent of preterm placentas.

DIAGNOSIS

Amniotic fluid culture is a reliable test if the sample is not contaminated by vaginal organisms. Even in the presence of confirmed amniotic infection, a Gram stain of the amniotic fluid will only detect about two-thirds of infected patients. The Gram stain has a high specificity but a low sensitivity for the diagnosis of infection. White cells (more than five/high-power field) or bacteria are seen in more than 70 per cent of those with clinical infection on culture. A bacterial count of greater than $10^5/1$ is likely to be significant.

Fetal breathing movements noted on ultrasound examination imply that chorioamnionitis is unlikely.

Other tests

Leucocyte esterase in the amniotic fluid correlates only with clinically obvious infection. A raised amniotic fluid C reactive protein concentration has been found in a number of cases but it has insufficient specificity for the reliable diagnosis of infection.

The Limulus lysate assay is positive in a number of cases. Interleukin 6 is raised in the amniotic fluid, and other cytokines may also be raised, including interleukin 1, platelet activating factor, and tissue necrosis factor.

Preterm prelabour rupture of membranes (PPROM)

Rupture of the membranes (ROM) before the onset of labour occurs in 6 to 12 per cent of all pregnancies. PPROM occurs before 37 weeks of gestation in 2 to 3 per cent of all pregnancies, that is, one-third of all preterm deliveries and is more likely to occur with polyhydramnios, multiple pregnancy, cervical incompetence, and after cone biopsy of the cervix. It is also independently related to ascending infection, which may lead to rupture of the membranes as a result of dissolution of the membranes. Once the membranes have ruptured, further infection may occur as a consequence. A short interval between premature membrane rupture and the onset of labour is more likely to be associated with infection, whereas in prolonged membrane rupture, although the risk of intrauterine infection is increased, the more likely consequences are those of pulmonary hypoplasia, limb deformation, facial compression, intrauterine growth retardation, and anaemia of the fetus.

The role of infection in preterm labour

Five to 10 per cent of births in the United Kingdom are preterm, and these account for about 80 per cent of perinatal deaths. Predisposing factors are found in about 50 to 60 per cent of cases. Most of these factors are non-specific and include small maternal stature and low maternal weight, antepartum haemorrhage, a history of previous miscarriage and previous preterm delivery, multiple pregnancy, and fetal and uterine abnormality. There is increasing evidence implicating infection as a major predisposing factor, and at least 30 per cent of cases of preterm labour are associated with infection.

INITIATION OF LABOUR

In infection, micro-organisms produce proteases which digest mucin and affect the integrity of the cervical mucus plug. Intra-amniotic infection may then ensue. Bacteria can activate the peroxidase H_2O_2 halide system, leading to oxygen free-radical induced membrane damage. Some bacteria may set up low-grade inflammation, which facilitates ingress by more virulent bacteria. Infection can damage the membranes and activate phopholipases, thus leading to arachidonic acid release and prostaglandin synthesis and release. Phospholipases may also be produced by certain bacteria. In addition, inflammatory mediators, including the interleukins, tumour necrosis factor, and interferons, stimulate activation of phospholipases and lead to prostaglandin production. Macrophages are activated and in turn also release arachidonic acid. Bacterial endotoxin even resulting from distant infection, such as that of the urinary tract, may also lead to prostaglandin production and the initiation of labour.

MANAGEMENT

Clinically apparent chorioamnionitis

Even though the administration of antimicrobials could theoretically mask the signs of infection or interfere with bacterial cultures, their use remains a cornerstone of treatment. If the responsible organism has not been identified, it is usual to administer ampicillin/amoxycillin intravenously to the mother. These drugs cross the placenta readily and will be effective against a number of organisms, including group B streptococci. Alternatives are co-amoxiclav, or a second- or third-generation cephalosporin. Gentamicin may be added to ampicillin/amoxycillin particularly in severe cases, and if infection with group B streptococci or coliforms is confirmed. If anaerobic infection is suspected, metronidazole might be considered, either alone or in combination with one of the above agents. If infection is apparent in a woman with ruptured membranes, then in her own interests as well as in the interests of the fetus and newborn, delivery should be expedited. After appropriate tests, such as blood culture, culture of the external ear, or examination of a gastric aspirate, have been done, the newborn should be treated as well.

Threatened preterm labour

Evidence of chorioamnionitis is sought. Tocolytics can be employed to suppress labour long enough to administer an effective course of corticosteroids to the mother to prevent respiratory distress syndrome in the baby. Unfortunately tocolysis is less likely to be effective when underlying subclinical chorioamnionitis is present. Tocolytic therapy also imposes risks on the mother, including tachycardia, anxiety, hyperglycaemia and, most seriously, the risk of pulmonary oedema and acute cardiac failure. The treatment should therefore only be used as an adjunct to gain sufficient time to administer an effective course of steroid prophylaxis, and the tocolytic drugs should be given in the smallest possible fluid volume, employing an intravenous pump.

If infection is clearly present, then delivery should be expedited in spite of the risks associated with prematurity.

There is conflicting evidence about the effectiveness of antimicrobial treatment of mothers in preterm labour, with intact membranes and no definite evidence of infection. An international multicentre trial has just been initiated to compare the effects of various antimicrobials in the prevention of preterm delivery (Overview of the Role of Antibiotics in Curtailing Labour and Early Delivery—ORACLE).

If caesarian section is needed, antimicrobials should be administered promptly. If adequate treatment is given, mortality of the term infant should be low, but the death rate in preterm infants with preceding chorioamnionitis is still appreciable. Any infant born to a mother who had signs of chorioamnionitis should receive antimicrobial treatment promptly after birth once specimens have been taken for microbiological examination. It should be noted that in multiple pregnancy, chorioamnionitis will not lead to isolated infection of the hindmost infant but will only do so if the baby presenting first is infected.

Management of PPROM

If PPROM occurs at or near term, delivery should be expedited. If delivery has not occurred within 24 h of the membranes having ruptured, induction or stimulation with prostaglandins or oxytocin should be started. Antimicrobials should be given if there is any indication of infection. If there is evidence of infection before term, amniotic fluid should be collected at the vulva, digital vaginal examination should be avoided, and delivery expedited. Antimicrobials should be started immediately, as described earlier. If evidence of infection has not been found and the gestation is less than 34 weeks, steroids should be administered to the mother to prevent respiratory distress syndrome in the newborn, to which it is predisposed if delivery occurs prematurely. Repeated vaginal cultures should be performed at intervals if the pregnancy continues. Some would advocate direct amniotic fluid sampling as the most reliable test, though the value of this examination is still being established. It should be remembered that delivery by caesarian section in these women is associated with greater risk of puerperal infection, and antibiotics should be used.

Urinary tract infection (see Chapter 20.8.1)

Asymptomatic bacteruria occurs in 2 to 10 per cent of both pregnant and non-pregnant women. In pregnancy, it usually occurs early and persists if no treatment is given. Between 20 and 30 per cent of women with asymptomatic bacteruria will develop symptomatic urinary tract infection. Treatment of asymptomatic bacteruria will reduce this risk and also the risk of acute pyelonephritis from 40 to 5 per cent, or less than 0.5 per cent overall. In women with a past history of urinary tract infection and subsequent asymptomatic bacteruria the risk of pyelonephritis is increased tenfold.

Urinary infection even when asymptomatic will predispose to preterm labour and to early fetal loss. Preterm premature rupture of membranes and also chorioamnionitis are consequences of urinary infection.

Although dysuria and frequency occur in 20 to 30 per cent of pregnant women, acute cystitis or pyelonephritis occurs in 1 to 3 per cent. In pregnancy, factors that predispose the woman to acute cystitis or pyelonephritis include the ureteric dilatation and renal pelvic dilatation often seen after the first trimester, related in part to the effect of hormones on ureteric smooth muscle, causing diminished tone. In addition, compression of the ureters at the pelvic rim and pressure on the base of the bladder increase the angle at which the ureters enter the bladder, thus predisposing to reflux.

DIAGNOSIS

The widely held belief that urinary infection can be diagnosed by relying on urinary protein determination is spurious. All pregnant women should have at least one urine examined microscopically and cultured, and several urine tests if there is a history of previous urinary infection. Microscopic examination of a midstream sample should be carried out and the urine inoculated on to blood agar and MacConkey agar. If a delay in processing the urine is likely, then it should be stored at 4°C; alternatively, dip-slides coated with culture medium can be used and a

quantitive colony count performed. Nitrite tests or leucocyte esterase dipstick tests have a high specificity (92–95 per cent) but low sensitivity (43–77 per cent).

TREATMENT

For asymptomatic bacteruria, single dose treatment may be adequate but there is a risk of recurrence. Asymptomatic bacteruria and cystitis should be treated for 7 to 14 days, and there should be regular urine examinations thereafter to detect any relapse or recurrence. Drugs of choice include ampicillin, amoxycillin, co-amoxiclav, trimethoprim, or oral cephalosporins.

Specific infections

Group B β-haemolytic Streptococcus (see Section 7)

Group B Streptococcus (*Streptococcus agalactiae*), some strains of which cause bovine mastitis, was reported to cause postpartum sepsis in mothers more than 50 years ago, and neonatal infection at least 30 years ago. Six serotypes are usually described, although more recently two additional serotypes have been added to the list. These eight types are Ia, Ib, Ic, II, III, IV, V, and VI. In women and newborn infants the first five of these predominate, and in the newborn, group III occurs most frequently. Colonization in the newborn baby is commonly found, and though active infection is far less common, when it does occur its effects are severe. The organism is the leading pathogen, giving rise to serious perinatal bacterial infection in most developed countries. Rectal and vaginal carriage of this organism is found in up to 40 per cent of women.

Vertical transmission to the new-born results in a colonization rate of 50 to 70 per cent of babies born to colonized mothers. This is more likely in association with heavy maternal colonization, after premature rupture of membranes or if there is clinically apparent chorioamnionitis. In the United States about 1 per cent of babies of colonized women are found to develop infection, although the rate is very much lower in the United Kingdom: 1 to 2 per 1000 colonized women or 0.3 to 0.5 per 1000 live births. In the presence of recognized risk factors the infection rate rises to nearly 8 per 1000 and the rate in babies born preterm is 1 in 50. Infection is more common in multiple births.

Although the colonization rate of mothers and their babies is so high, only a small minority of newborns are infected. It is likely that the integrity of the membranes and the competence of the cervix confers some local protection to ascending infection, although the transplacental passage of type-specific antibody from the mother to the fetus, which occurs in the majority of mothers who are asymptomatic carriers, is of major importance in the prevention of infection. Mothers of infants who develop group B Streptococcus sepsis have low titres of type-specific antibody, which may be undetectable in some. Some produce IgM antibody only and since transplacental passage does not occur, the fetus would be unprotected. It should also be remembered that preterm infants are especially vulnerable since maternal antibody transmission is poor at less than 30 weeks of gestation.

MATERNAL ILLNESS

The great majority of mothers harbouring group B Streptococcus have no demonstrable illness. Infection occurs in 2 to 5 per cent of those who are colonized, and group B Streptococcus is an important cause of bacteriuria in pregnancy, although only some cases are symptomatic. There is an increased risk of mid-trimester miscarriage, premature rupture of membranes, and of preterm delivery. Symptomatic chorioamnionitis with fever, tachycardia, and abdominal tenderness may occur in the peripartum period. Postpartum endometritis, bacteraemia, infection after caesarian section, and pelvic thrombophlebitis may be caused by group B Streptococcus. Meningitis, and endocarditis in the presence of pre-existing valve disease, may also result, albeit very rarely.

NEONATAL INFECTION

Although some cases have a later onset, after the first 5 days, most manifest the disease in the first 48 h and often in the first few hours after birth. The baby is more likely to be preterm, but the disease may occur without warning in a mature baby. Similar early onset illness may result from other congenital bacterial infections, such as those caused by *Listeria monocytogenes*, *E. coli*, and, more rarely, *Haemophilus influenzae* and *Streptococcus pneumoniae*.

Septicaemia

Group B Streptococcus infection may present as septic shock with unexpected collapse of an infant who was previously well and who suddenly develops pallor, hypotension, a temperature gap between the peripheral and core readings, neutropenia, thrombocytopenia, and bleeding due to consumptive coagulopathy. Persistent pulmonary vasoconstriction refractory to ventilation may make oxygenation difficult. Persisting hypotension may lead to ischaemic cerebral lesions. The initial collapse needs to be differentiated from that caused by acute heart failure, metabolic disease, or severe haemorrhage. Purpura fulminans may complicate the septicaemia.

Pneumonia

Respiratory distress appearing within hours of birth may be difficult to distinguish from surfactant-deficient respiratory distress syndrome, especially in a preterm baby, and may even be suggested by the chest radiograph, which shows remarkably diffuse shadowing. Reticulogranularity, patchy consolidation, and pleural fluid would indicate infection to be the likely cause, as would the occurrence of respiratory distress in a mature newborn. Lower pressures are usually required to inflate the lung in the ventilated infected baby than would be needed in the treatment of surfactant deficient lung disease.

Meningitis

Meningitis occurs in 20 to 30 per cent of early onset cases, and group B Streptococcus is more common than coliform organisms as a cause of neonatal meningitis. Most cases are due to serotype III. Neurological sequelae occur in about 30 per cent of cases, sometimes as a result of ventriculitis progressing to hydrocephalus, which may be a consequence of this problem even after treatment has been given promptly.

Other manifestations

Osteomyelitis and septic arthritis occur infrequently, as do cellulitis, peritonitis, endocarditis, otitis media, conjunctivitis, ethmoiditis, and fasciitis.

Late-onset disease

There is a late-onset variant of group B Streptococcus infection which occurs after the first week; it is usually of nosocomial origin or may be acquired by maternal contact after birth. Meningitis occurs more frequently in late-onset disease than in early disease.

TREATMENT OF THE NEWBORN BABY

Symptoms compatible with infection in the newborn merit immediate treatment with suitable antimicrobials once appropriate samples have been taken to confirm the presence of group B Streptococcus. This is especially true of babies with respiratory distress. If the mother has received antibiotics prior to delivery, these might interfere with bacterial culture results. The neonate would then have to be fully treated putatively without positive proof of the presence of group B Streptococcus, though a positive latex antigen test may give further confirmation. The usual treatment given is penicillin, 60 to 90 mg/kg 12 hourly intravenously for the first 7 days followed by 30 to 60 mg/kg 12 hourly for a further 7 days. Ampicillin or amoxycillin may be used instead. An aminoglycoside such as gentamicin should be administered as well, since this combination is highly synergistic against streptococci. Other organisms causing similar signs would be susceptible to these combinations. Third-generation cephalosporins such as ceftazidime, ceftriaxone, or cefotaxime have good activity against group B Streptococcus but if the organism has been identified, penicillin is the drug of choice. Chloramphenicol is infrequently used but is an active agent against group B Streptococcus. Intrathecal or intraventricular antibiotics are not generally recommended.

PROGNOSIS OF NEONATAL INFECTION

The mortality has fallen to 5 per cent in term infants, but in the preterm baby it remains high, with an expected mortality of 25 to 30 per cent. The mortality has fallen from 35 to 50 per cent in the 1970s to 15 to 25 per cent at present. Neurological sequelae of meningitis remain an important complication.

PROPHYLAXIS

Possible strategies include:

Passive immunization

This involves the administration of intravenous immunoglobulin to the mother. This would require a high titre of type-specific antibody. However, maternal antibody does not cross the placenta in adequate concentrations until after 30 weeks of gestation, and even at 32 weeks levels are only 50 per cent of those of full-term infants.

Active maternal immunization

The mother is vaccinated with type III group B Streptococcus polysaccharide. This produces a rise in titre in at least half of the recipients. Improved vaccines are being developed. Adequate protection of the preterm infant is unlikely.

Antimicrobial treatment of the newborn

Indiscriminate penicillin administration to all newborns has resulted in a considerable reduction in group B Streptococcus infection but a rise in other infections. Treating all susceptible babies at birth is unlikely to be effective since early onset disease may be established already. It is therefore necessary to treat the mother before she gives birth.

Treatment early in pregnancy

Studies with oral antimicrobials in the second or early third trimester demonstrated that although the organism appeared to be eliminated, relapse was common. This was attributed to reinfection from the partner, but the majority still relapsed even after the partner was treated.

Chemoprophylaxis in labour

Intrapartum intravenous ampicillin markedly reduces both maternal and neonatal colonization, and in some series eliminates neonatal early onset disease. It is therefore suggested that the following scheme of prevention be followed.

1. All pregnant women should be screened at 26 to 28 weeks using a swab from the lower vagina and anorectum and using a transport medium, inoculating a selective broth culture medium. The result can be retrieved when mother is in labour. However, a negative swab in pregnancy does not necessarily predict the status at delivery. The positive predictive value is still only 67 per cent.
2. In labour all colonized mothers who have risk factors for invasive neonatal group B Streptococcus infection should receive

intravenous penicillin or ampicillin. These risk factors are shown in Table 1.

3. Rapid antigen detection tests on a vaginal swab may be used in those women who are in labour and have not been previously screened. This test can be used to identify 65 to 88 per cent of heavily colonized mothers.

4. Neonates of mothers who have received antimicrobials should be screened for infection if of less than 34 weeks' gestation and given antimicrobials; whereas those of more than 34 weeks' gestation should have surface swabs sent for cultural examination but should be treated promptly in the presence of any suggestive symptoms.

5. Mothers, and their infants, with risk factors 7 and 8 in Table 1 should be screened for group B Streptococcus and treated.

6. Consideration should be given to the use of aqueous chlorhexidine solution for vaginal disinfection during labour at term. This has been shown to be an effective means of reducing neonatal morbidity.

Listeria monocytogenes *infection (see Chapter 7.11.35)*

In 1990 in the United Kingdom there were 24 confirmed cases of listerosis associated with pregnancy, that is 1 per 30 000 births. In France, however, the number of cases in 1992 had risen to 105 in a 4 month period, whereas the expected number per year was 15. Twenty-nine per cent of these cases were associated with pregnancy.

Although the mother who has become infected with Listeria may be asymptomatic, transmission to the fetus and the newborn baby causes them to develop severe disease. Suppression of cell-mediated immunity in pregnancy probably increases the mother's susceptibility to this infection. The immunocompromised adult is more likely to have severe disease.

INFECTION OF THE MOTHER

The illness in the mother may consist of nothing more than flu-like symptoms of fever, rigors, myalgia, headache, sore throat, and cough. In some cases the illness may be severe and the mother may have meningitis or septicaemia with or without disseminated intravascular coagulation. This is especially likely if the mother has an underlying systemic disease which interferes with T-cell immunity. Infection of the fetus may result in miscarriage or still birth, although this is probably very rare. In the second and third trimesters, chorioamnionitis may occur and fetal distress may be present with decelerations, absent accelerations, and fetal tachycardia, and the liquor may become meconium-stained. Listeria is usually a blood-borne infection of the fetus and is accompanied by placentitis, funisitis, and microabscesses of the placenta.

NEONATE

Early onset infection, usually occurring within hours after birth, is the most likely result of transplacental infection, the usual route. Infection occurring as a result of exposure during delivery is of later onset. Rarely, babies may present with the appearance of non-immune hydrops at delivery but respiratory distress is usually the most prominent symptom. Signs of generalized septic shock or meningoencephalitis may predominate in some, with hepatosplenomegaly, a pustular rash, widespread petechiae, and convulsions. In others the signs of sepsis may be non-specific and include lethargy, poor feeding, apathy, apnoea, and hypotonia, although these features are more likely with late- rather than early onset infection. The early passage of meconium, especially when seen in a preterm baby, should raise the suspicion of Listeria infection.

The mortality of generalized neonatal listeriosis is high and neurological sequelae are common. Autopsy will be likely to demonstrate widespread miliary granulomata in many organs, including the placenta, usually with a mononuclear infiltrate. Late-onset infection, most commonly due to type 4b, occurs after the first week, sometimes as a result of cross-infection from another infant with listeriosis or from a mother after birth. Meningitis is more common in these cases and fever occurs in most of them. Suspected cross-infection may be confirmed by phage-typing of the isolates, although one-third of the strains are non-typeable.

TREATMENT

In the presence of suggestive symptoms in a baby in whom Gram-positive rods are seen in a sample, such as a gastric aspirate or meconium passed immediately after birth, it would be advisable to treat with ampicillin or amoxycillin plus an aminoglycoside, usually gentamicin or netilmicin.

PREVENTION

Mothers should be advised to cook food carefully during pregnancy and to avoid high-risk foods such as those poorly stored or improperly prepared, especially paté, cheeses, or cooked–chilled food. Any febrile illness in the mother should be fully investigated, especially if her symptoms are severe; these investigations should include a blood sample for culture. In the neonatal unit the possible risk of cross-infection from an infected baby must be prevented by meticulous attention to hygiene, and would certainly include hand disinfection and cleaning and disinfection of suction apparatus and common equipment.

Gonococcal infection (see Chapter 7.11.6)

In the United States antenatal gonococcal isolation rates of less than 1 per cent are reported, compared with less than 0.2 per cent in the United Kingdom, whereas in some developing countries, the percentage may be as high as 7 per cent of pregnancies, and may result in ophthalmia in 3.6 per cent of infants.

INFECTION OF THE MOTHER

Although some cases of gonococcal infection are asymptomatic or the symptoms may be trivial, they may be severe with erythema of the vulva, oedema, pain, purulent exudate, and vaginal discharge accompanied by dysuria with increased frequency of micturition. Bartholinitis may occur. Salpingitis is rare during pregnancy, although it may precede it. It may lead to subsequent sterility or to ectopic pregnancy. Conjunctival, pharyngeal, or rectal involvement may be present. In a few cases disseminated infection may occur with fever, rash, arthralgia, tenosynovitis, cardiac involvement, and hepatitis. The risk of disseminated infection is higher in pregnancy, but transplacental infection of the fetus has not been reported.

Although pelvic infection is less common in pregnancy, the disease can lead to miscarriage, chorioamnionitis, premature rupture of membranes, and preterm labour.

Table 1 *Risk factors for invasive neonatal infection*

1. Preterm labour < 37 weeks
2. Premature rupture of membranes < 37 weeks
3. Intrapartum fever or other signs of infection
4. Multiple birth
5. Prolonged rupture of membranes > 18 h
6. Maternal diabetes
7. Previous baby with invasive group B streptoccocal disease
8. Maternal group B streptococcus bacteriuria

There is a substantial risk of development of postpartum pelvic infection. *Chlamydia trachomatis* infection is reported to coexist with gonococcal infection in up to 60 per cent of cases. Other sexually transmitted diseases may also be present, including syphilis.

NEONATAL

Some babies are infected by ascending infection established via ruptured or intact amniotic membranes, others are infected during delivery. The most common manifestation is ophthalmia neonatorum occurring 1 to 12 days after birth. The most severe cases have a short incubation. Usually bilateral, there is oedema of the eyelids with profuse purulent exudate which can cause corneal ulceration if severe. The disease was an important cause of blindness when effective treatment was not available. The ulcers may perforate and lead to the development of endophthalmitis. The onset is usually earlier than the ophthalmia occurring with Chlamydia infection. Other causes of conjunctivitis in the new-born are a reaction to prophylactic eye drops and infection with other organisms, such as *Chlamydia trachomatis*, *Staphylococcus aureus*, *Haemophilus influenzae*, *Streptococcus pneumoniae*, *Enterococcus* species, and herpes simplex virus. Skin trauma, from a scalp clip for example, may become infected with gonococci, leading to abscess formation. Disseminated infection may occur leading to septic arthritis; more than one joint may be involved.

Sometimes, the baby may be infected by the mother after birth. Outbreaks of nosocomial infection have occurred and underline the need for measures to prevent cross-infection, especially in overcrowded nurseries.

PREVENTION

Women are routinely screened in pregnancy if the infection rate in that community is high. Otherwise, this screening should be reserved for those at particular risk, and certainly for those with a vaginal discharge or dysuria, for women with intrapartum fever, and premature rupture of membranes. If the mother is known to be infected prior to delivery, then the baby should be given intravenous penicillin soon after birth unless there is a high expectation of penicillin resistance, when another antibiotic such as cefotaxime should be chosen. Routine neonatal prophylaxis is advisable for populations with a high prevalence of gonococcal infection. Crede's method uses 1 per cent $AgNO_3$, 1 to 2 drops in each eye. The risk of chemical conjunctivitis in these populations is outweighed by the high risk of gonococcal ophthalmia. This method reduces subsequent ophthalmia by about 80 per cent, although it is rarely used in the United Kingdom. Tetracycline ophthalmic ointment or drops (1 per cent) or erythromycin 0.5 per cent have the advantage of efficacy against Chlamydia as well.

TREATMENT

Treatment of uncomplicated gonorrhoea in the mother when penicillin resistance is unlikely (< 5 per cent of strains are resistant) is procaine penicillin 4.8 megaunits (2.8 g) intramuscularly with 1 g of probenecid, or alternatively amoxycillin 3 g orally with probenecid.

If penicillin sensitivity is in doubt or unknown, ceftriaxone 125 to 250 mg intramuscularly, or spectinomycin 2 g intramuscularly can be used. In disseminated infection one could use ceftriaxone 1 g/day, or spectinomycin or benzylpenicillin 1.2 g intravenously 6 hourly until improvement occurs, after which amoxycillin or co-amoxiclav can be given 250–500 mg 6 hourly for 7 days.

Neonatal infection should be treated with cefotaxime 25 mg/kg intravenously or intramuscularly every 12 h for 7 days, or ceftriaxone 25 to 50 mg/kg intravenously or intramuscularly in a single dose. If the organism is penicillin sensitive, then benzylpenicillin, 30 mg/kg intramuscularly or intravenously 12 hourly for 7 days, should be used instead. The eyes should be cleaned and antibiotic eye ointment or drops applied.

Syphilis (see Chapter 7.11.34)

Although untreated yaws has been incriminated as a rare cause of congenital infection, syphilis, even in the post-penicillin era, remains the treponemal disease that gives rise to major concern. Adult, and hence congenital, syphilis is more common among the poor, in urban populations, especially in association with promiscuity and illegal drug use associated with prostitution. The number of cases decreased after the Second World War, but there has lately been a dramatic resurgence in the United States, with an increase from 158 cases of congenital syphilis in 1983 to over 7000 in 1990. This is especially to be seen in major cities such as New York where the rise is most striking in babies of mothers who are drug abusers—especially those addicted to the cocaine-based drug, 'crack'. There is a higher incidence in Afro-American and Hispanic women and hence in their babies. A rise in the number of cases is also anticipated in the United Kingdom.

PREGNANCY

Although infection may rarely result because of the administration of infected blood, the disease is usually acquired via direct sexual contact with an infected person. The infection might have been acquired prior to or during the pregnancy. The primary lesion at the site of infection may be clinically inapparent but in most cases will manifest as a relatively painless ulcer surrounded by induration, and with accompanying regional lymphadenopathy appearing after an incubation period lasting from 2 to 14 weeks. The ulcer (chancre) is teeming with spirochaetes. Spontaneous healing usually follows and, after 6 to 12 weeks or longer, the signs of secondary syphilis may become evident, with generalized skin rash, condylomata, and superficial mucosal ulceration. Fever, sore throat, headache, lymphadenopathy, and weight loss are often present. A number of organs, including the liver, kidneys, and meninges, may be involved. Subsequently, untreated cases evolve into an early latent stage lasting about 2 years, during which intermittent recurrence of systemic illness might occur. The disorder is transmissable to sexual partners during pregnancy, and to the fetus. Fetal transmission is more likely during the early course of infection, that is during the incubation period, the primary and secondary stages, and in the early latent stage.

FETAL AND NEONATAL INFECTION

Fetal infection may occur at any stage of pregnancy, and transplacental spread occurs even before 18 to 20 weeks and is not impeded by the placental Langhan's layer (which physiologically involutes at this time) as was formerly thought. Villitis occurs, associated with vascular obliteration following endo- and perivascular proliferation. Necrotizing funisitis may occur in the cord. Motile spirochaetes have been seen in the amniotic fluid, and a Venereal Disease Reference Laboratory (VDRL) or rapid plasma reagin (RPR) test of the amniotic fluid may be positive.

Early syphilis in pregnancy will almost invariably be transmitted to the fetus if untreated, and as many as 30 per cent of fetuses will die *in utero*, leading to miscarriage or still birth. In cases of unexplained stillbirth, syphilis serology must always be performed on the mother. After birth, serious or even fatal congenital syphilis may be seen early in the neonatal period, with a worse prognosis in those born prematurely. Most cases are asymptomatic. About 40 per cent of untreated survivors will develop late-onset disease.

The placenta is often pale, large, and oedematous even though the infant is likely to be growth retarded and may be preterm. The prognosis is worse in those who develop the signs of the disease early. The cerebrospinal fluid is abnormal in 40 to 60 per cent of infants with congenital syphilis, and a lumbar puncture should always be performed in cases of congenital syphilis, even in the absence of clinical signs of meningitis. The infant with missed congenital syphilis may fail to thrive, perhaps associated with pancreatitis and gastrointestinal inflammation, or may go on to develop features of late congenital infection. If syphilis is diagnosed, one should always be on the lookout for other sexually transmitted diseases, including chlamydial and gonococcal infection and human immunodeficiency virus (HIV).

DIAGNOSIS

The mother and pregnancy

All mothers are screened when they make their first antenatal visit with a VDRL test and a simultaneous *Treponema pallidum* haemagglutination antibody (TPHA) test. If a primary infection is suspected then a fluorescent treponemal antibody-absorbed (FTA-Abs) test is performed as well.

Subsequent tests are needed if there is a history of possible syphilis contact in pregnancy or to determine the effect of treatment by noting a fall in the VDRL or RPR antibody titre.

The infant

Dark-ground microscopy may give confusing results with oral lesions but is essential in the investigation of material from other suspicious lesions. Serological tests may be difficult to interpret because they may reflect passively transferred antibody. A titre higher than the mother's, or a rising titre, or antibody persisting at the same level for months are indicators that the infant is infected. Positive FTA-Abs IgM-specific tests indicate neonatal infection, but these may be falsely negative and the test should be repeated later.

A cerebrospinal fluid VDRL, long-bone radiographs, and examination of material from lymph node biopsies are useful tests in specific instances.

TREATMENT (SEE TABLE 2)

Penicillin is the preferable treatment for the mother unless there is a history of penicillin allergy, when erythromycin (not the estolate, which is potentially toxic) or cefotaxime can be used.

The infant should be given aqueous penicillin intravenously or procaine penicillin intramuscularly. One should avoid confusion between these two forms of penicillin as a fatality has occurred because the intramuscular preparation was given intravenously. Serological tests in the infant should be repeated in the first year until the VDRL is negative.

Chlamydial infection (see Chapter 7.11.41)

Of the three chlamydial species, *Chlamydia trachomatis* gives most cause for concern in pregnancy, while *C. psittaci*, which is primarily an infection of birds and mammals, has been transmitted to pregnant women after exposure to infected sheep in the lambing season, especially contact with aborting ewes. Placentitis in the sheep has been described and organisms have been seen in the placenta using electron microscopy. Pregnant women should therefore avoid contact with sheep (there is also a risk of toxoplasmosis) especially in the lambing season.

EPIDEMIOLOGY

Chlamydia trachomatis genital-tract infection is detected in about 5 per cent of women investigated during pregnancy in the United States. Prevalence rates in the United States and the United Kingdom, range from 2 to 18 per cent. Recovery rates are greater in urban women, especially those who are single, poor, and who have many sexual partners. Higher rates are also found in women with a bacterial pyuria, those who book in late during pregnancy, and those who do not habitually use barrier contraceptives. The rate is increased by one-third to one-half in women with gonococcal disease, but chlamydial infection alone is probably the most common cause of pelvic inflammatory disease in the developed world, and the associated salpingitis means that it is a common cause of infertility.

Table 2 *Treatment of syphilis*

Mother	
Early disease	Aqueous procaine penicillin, 1 g daily intramuscularly for 10–15 days
	If allergic: erythromycin (not estolate), 500 g 6 hourly for 10–15 days
	or
	Cefotaxime 500 mg daily intramuscularly for 10–15 days
Infant	
If mother adequately treated in pregnancy	
Examine the baby	
DRL, repeat every 3 months until negative	
If mother untreated or inadequately treated	
VDRL test, examine CSF, radiograph long bones	
Benzylpenicillin, 30 mg/kg intravenously 12 hourly for 10 days	
or	
Procaine penicillin, 30 mg/kg intramuscularly for 10 days	

The infection is asymptomatic in the majority of women, although some will be found to have cervicitis and even cervical erosions.

PREGNANCY

Recovery of *C. trachomatis* from the vagina is more likely in the second and third trimesters than in the first. In women with chlamydial cervicitis, salpingitis is more likely to occur after termination of pregnancy, and attempts should be made to screen for the infection and to treat it prior to the procedure. *Chlamydia trachomatis* attaches to amniotic cells and multiplies on these. There is some evidence of an association of chlamydial infection with premature rupture of membranes, miscarriage, still birth, and preterm labour. In one study treatment of half a large cohort infected with Chlamydia demonstrated decreased frequency of the above problems. Chlamydial infection can occur concurrently with bacterial vaginosis, which is an established cause of preterm labour.

Tubal damage caused by Chlamydia salpingitis increases the risk of subsequent ectopic pregnancy. More immediately, asymptomatic postpartum endometritis may occur. In some cases, symptoms of lower abdominal pain, fever, and vaginal discharge of later onset may occur. *Chlamydia trachomatis* has been isolated in up to 37 per cent of these late cases of postpartum endometritis after vaginal delivery.

FETUS AND NEWBORN

Although the organism has been shown to traverse intact membranes, fetal infection appears to be extremely rare, and the main risk to the new-born occurs during vaginal delivery, when up to 60 per cent of those exposed to *C. trachomatis* will have been infected—up to 50 per cent of them symptomatic, usually with conjunctivitis.

Purulent discharge from conjunctivitis may occur up to a month after birth. Usually this is bilateral. Sometimes pseudomembranes occur, and uncommonly may be severe enough to cause corneal ulceration. About 10 to 20 per cent of those infants exposed develop respiratory symptoms, which may be delayed for up to 3 months after birth, sometimes without conjunctivitis but often with preceding nasal congestion, otitis media, and glue ear. The baby is usually afebrile, tachypnoeic, and has a staccato paroxysmal cough which may be accompanied by weight loss and vomiting. In some cases it presents as bronchiolitis and can be accompanied by wheezing. Sometimes there is a biphasic course, with early respiratory distress and later apnoea. The chest radiograph appears hyperinflated with nodular infiltrates and bilateral diffuse symmetrical interstitial shadows with patchy atelectasis. There is often an eosinophilia in the acute stage. Chlamydia may be detected in a nasopharyngeal aspirate. The interstitial pneumonia may have a protracted course, and in some cases it may be complicated by respiratory syncytial virus infection. The disorder may predispose to asthma, with permanent lung damage and abnormal respiratory function tests in later life. In the preterm infant it has been shown to be a cause of the Mikity–Wilson syndrome.

DIAGNOSIS

Isolation of Chlamydia in cell culture is a reliable, but technically demanding test, and is no longer widely available. For conjunctivitis, a Giemsa stain of a sample of conjunctival cells provides a quick and reliable answer, but cannot be used when making a diagnosis from other sites. In sampling the conjunctiva, pus should be wiped away, and a cotton or Dacron-tipped swab then firmly stroked on the palpebral conjunctiva of the everted lower lid.

In investigating cervicitis in the pregnant mother, exudate should be removed and the area of the squamocolumnar junction then firmly swabbed to obtain cells. The swab should not be inserted too deeply into the cervical canal for fear of introducing infection. The swab should be placed in appropriate Chlamydia transport medium and/or inoculated on to a slide, depending on the technique used by the local laboratory.

TREATMENT

Drugs such as tetracycline, ciprofloxacin, co-trimoxazole, doxycycline, or azithromycin, although useful for the treatment of *C. trachomatis* infection in the non-pregnant state, cannot be used in pregnancy. One of these drugs could be used if treatment of the mother is required after birth and she is not breast-feeding. For treatment during pregnancy, the drug of choice is erythromycin (not the estolate), 250 mg 6 hourly for 14 days. The partner should be investigated for Chlamydia infection and treated if necessary.

The infant should be treated with erythromycin, 50 mg/kg/day orally in 3 to 4 doses, for up to 14 days, in those with conjunctivitis and for at least 3 weeks in those with pneumonia. Topical tetracycline ointment is used in cases of conjunctivitis.

Mycoplasma infection (see Chapter 7.11.43)

EPIDEMIOLOGY

About 30 per cent of exposed infants are colonized by *Ureaplasma urealyticum*, and the organisms can be isolated from amniotic fluid in the presence of intact membranes, but are more commonly isolated after the membranes have ruptured.

Mycoplasma hominis

IN PREGNANCY

In preterm labour and delivery, genital mycoplasmas are isolated more frequently from the amniotic fluid, placenta, fetus, and infant than after term delivery. The role of these organisms as a cause of preterm delivery has not been substantiated in large prospective studies, although in some cases there are preceding signs of chorioamnionitis. In this situation both *Mycoplasma hominis* and *U. urealyticum* may be found. Mycoplasmas have been isolated in 35 per cent of women with symptoms of chorioamnionitis and in whom there is premature rupture of membranes, compared with 8 per cent of normal controls. Seroconversion has been shown to occur during this time in some patients. Mycoplasmas are known to be associated with postpartum fever, and *M. hominis* may be isolated from the blood more commonly in women who have no detectable antibody to this organism.

THE NEONATE

The neonate may be colonized without illness, or the organism may be recovered from the blood during transient bacteraemia. Focal infection may occur causing submandibular lymphadenopathy, conjunctivitis, and scalp abscess. Pneumonia has been documented in a stillborn infant. Meningitis has been noted, especially in preterm infants with intraventricular haemorrhage. Although colonization is common, infection is not, unless the baby is premature or if there is another predisposing cause.

Ureaplasma urealyticum

IN PREGNANCY

The organism is found in the urine of pregnant women more commonly than in the non-pregnant, and in 20 per cent of those with pregnancy-induced hypertension, especially in younger women. It is often present in large numbers in the vagina of women with vaginosis. Although *U. urealyticum* has been found in the tissues of miscarried fetuses, the role of the organism as a cause of recurrent pregnancy loss is inconclusive. The organism has been cultured from the amniotic fluid in cases of chorioamnionitis but from an equal percentage (± 50 per cent) of matched control women. It has been identified in blood cultures of women with ruptured membranes and from the placenta in babies found to be colonized.

THE FETUS AND NEONATE

Colonization is more frequent in the preterm and low birthweight infant, although the role of the organism as a cause of premature rupture of the membranes and preterm labour has not been established in prospective studies. This may partly be due to the confusing effect resulting from associated organisms. There is, however, a lower rate of preterm labour in women found to be colonized with Ureaplasma and who were treated with erythromycin. Ureaplasma is a cause of congenital pneumonia and has been isolated from the lower respiratory tract in these cases. It has also been shown to be associated with babies who develop persistent pulmonary hypertension. Ureaplasma antibody is found with increased frequency in babies with respiratory distress syndrome and has been isolated from the tracheal aspirate of these babies, and in cases of chronic lung disease. Less commonly, it has been present in blood cultures and in cases of meningitis, especially those associated with intraventricular haemorrhage.

TREATMENT

Mycoplasma pneumoniae in the mother after delivery can be treated with tetracycline, unless she is lactating; although erythromycin or clindamycin is usually recommended for postpartum infection. Neonatal meningitis may be treated with chloramphenicol, although resistance may be present. If the infection is severe, one might have to use tetracycline in spite of the complication that it is deposited in bones and teeth. Resistance to this antibiotic has also been reported.

Ureaplasma urealyticum is treated with erythromycin for 10 to 14 days in the baby and in the mother, or with chloramphenicol if there are clear indications for the use of this antibiotic.

Tuberculosis (see Chapter 7.11.22)

Radiographic diagnosis of pulmonary tuberculosis in late pregnancy is made more difficult by the elevation of the diaphragm, and if performed, the abdomen should be well shielded. The radiograph should be repeated after delivery to get a certain diagnosis. Genital tuberculosis is unlikely since it usually gives rise to infertility. If, however, genital tuberculosis is suspected, three consecutive early morning (not midstream) samples of urine should be collected. Endometrial curettings or biopsy should be cultured after delivery, the diagnosis being more rapid with histology. Other material that can be sent for histological examination will depend on the site of infection and the symptoms produced, but might include cerebrospinal fluid, bone marrow, tissue biopsy, or pus.

TUBERCULOSIS DURING PREGNANCY

Pregnancy is known to predispose to the progression of tuberculosis, reactivation of existing quiescent lesions, and to miliary spread. Cell-mediated immunity is depressed and, specifically, there is a significant depression of lymphocyte responsiveness to purified protein derivative of tuberculin, probably due to a serum inhibitor which is present after 36 weeks of gestation. Reactivation usually occurs after the third trimester or in the puerperium, although in the healthy pregnant woman reactivation is unusual. In developing countries, tuberculous meningitis and miliary spread are both more likely to occur in pregnancy. In developed countries the disease most often occurs in immigrants. Clinically, the manifestations of pulmonary tuberculosis are no different to those occurring in the non-pregnant individual. The woman may be feverish in the third trimester or puerperium. The tuberculin test may initially be negative and the bacilli may be scanty and cultured only after prolonged incubation. The disease may be mild and/or asymptomatic and manifest only in the baby. With tuberculous endometritis there is a risk of pelvic infection, abortion, or fetal infection. Management of the mother is to give isoniazid (with pyridoxine) and ethambutol, neither of which are known to cause teratogenesis. Rifampicin is also though to be acceptable for the treatment of tuberculosis in pregnancy, but as with isoniazid may cause hepatotoxicity. Streptomycin should be avoided because of a possible effect on the fetal eighth nerve.

CONGENITAL AND NEONATAL TUBERCULOSIS

The placenta is usually an effective barrier but if the mother is very ill, transplacental spread may occur, usually between 7 and 9 months of pregnancy. There may be tubercles on the fetal surface and in the intervillous spaces. Organisms may then be released into the fetal bloodstream as the placenta separates. In addition there can be miscarriage, stillbirth, or inhaled or ingested amniotic fluid, leading to infection. Clinically the newborn presents with fever, poor weight gain, respiratory distress, cyanosis, vomiting, poor feeding, and cough. The primary complex is very often in the liver and there is obstructive jaundice and hepatosplenomegaly, especially in the preterm and low birthweight baby. Lymphadenopathy may occur and also ascites, oedema, skin tubercules, and, in some, a pustular rash. Hilar lymphadenopathy may be present. There may be otorrhoea, mastoiditis, and preauricular lymphadenitis. Meningitis may occur, especially with spread via the circulation through the foramen ovale. The disease has a high mortality. If the baby survives, diffuse changes in the liver can lead to subsequent cirrhosis. Diagnosis is made with gastric fluid culture, blood culture, lymph node biopsy, examination of fluid after endotracheal suction, urine, bone marrow, and the histological examination of skin nodules. The Mantoux test is usually negative initially. Treatment is with isoniazid and rifampicin for 6 to 12 months, and if meningitis is present, pyrazinamide must be given.

Fungal infections

Candida *infection (see Chapter 7.12.1)*

INFECTION OF THE MOTHER

In pregnancy, the maximum attack rate is found in the third trimester, possibly because oestrogens enhance vaginal overgrowth. Nearly all cases are due to *Candida albicans* and only a small minority to other species such as *C. glabrata*.

THE NEWBORN AND FETUS

Candida acquired from the mother during vaginal delivery commonly results in mucocutaneous infection after the first week of age. The infant presents with the familiar white plaques involving the tongue, gums, palate, buccal surfaces, and oropharynx, associated with pain during feeding. A rash involving the groins, perineum, thighs, and abdomen is often present. This consists of intense erythema, scaling with satellite papules and pustules along its leading edge.

Congenital candidiasis due to ascending intrauterine infection, although uncommon, is likely to be a severe disease associated with miscarriage or premature rupture of membranes and preterm labour. In these cases discrete yellow plaques may be seen at the base of the cord and are pathognomonic of intrauterine candidiasis. Diffuse dermatitis, comprised of papules and pustules surrounded by erythema is seen. Desquamation is frequent. Pneumonia may be present and only distinguished from other causes of respiratory infection by finding Candida in the tracheal aspirate. Haematological spread from funisitis may lead to infection of other sites including the kidneys, gastrointestinal tract, and central nervous system.

DIAGNOSIS

Congenital severe disseminated candidiasis is associated with a high peripheral leucocyte count and thrombocytopenia. Disordered coagulation tests may also be present. Yeasts may be seen in smears of tracheal and gastric aspirate and in skin scrapings from the rash. Growth of Candida from peripheral blood should not be ignored and merely ascribed to contamination in the presence of any signs suggestive of generalized infection. The same is true of Candida in the urine, although certainly this can be a transient phenomenon, especially in babies receiving antibiotics for any other reason. In the sick infant this finding should lead to a search for fungal masses in the ureters, renal pelves, or bladder using ultrasound imaging. In disseminated disease lesions may be seen in the retinae.

TREATMENT

Maternal

A topical polyene such as nystatin cream or vaginal tablets will achieve a cure rate of 75 to 80 per cent, although a topically applied azole derivative such as clotrimazole, miconazole, or terconazole results in a superior cure rate.

Neonatal

Oral candidiasis usually responds satisfactorily to oral nystatin suspension. Miconazole or clotrimazole can be used locally to the skin, as can nystatin cream to treat cutaneous candidiasis. One per cent aqueous gentian violet solution applied topically is effective treatment but the discoloration it produces is less acceptable to parents.

Intravenous amphotericin B is used to treat systemic Candida infection, usually at a starting dose of 0.5 mg/kg daily, gradually increasing to a maximum of 1.0 mg/kg in severe cases. This treatment is continued for 2 to 4 weeks. Thrombophlebitis, renal impairment, and hypokalaemia are among the possible complications that might follow, and renal function therefore needs to be carefully monitored. Liposomal amphotericin, a new formulation, is associated with fewer side-effects and the drug seems to be effective, although it is expensive. Flucytosine is used in conjunction with amphotericin, especially when meningitis is present, and has the advantage of being able to be administered orally and to be absorbed readily, but the organism rapidly acquires resistance to this drug. Bone marrow suppression and hepatotoxicity are complications. There are limited data on the safety and efficacy of fluconazole in neonates.

Protozoal infections

Toxoplasmosis

Serological studies have shown that about 25 per cent of women of childbearing age in London are immune; in Paris, Padua, and Stuttgart the proportions are higher, being 75 per cent, 56 per cent, and 36 per cent, respectively. Annual seroconversion rates are of the order of 0.5 to 1 per cent in Britain but higher in countries with a high prevalence of *Toxoplasma gondii*.

Studies in France have shown that acquisition of infection is associated with such risk factors as owning a cat, eating undercooked meat which may contain viable cysts, and eating in restaurants frequently. In adults, including pregnant women, infection is usually mild or asymptomatic. Occasionally malaise, fever, fatigue, and lymphadenopathy may occur and patients may experience a remitting or prolonged course. The peripheral blood may contain a small number of atypical lymphocytes (< 10 per cent).

The fetus is at risk during maternal parasitaemia which follows ingestion of the infectious sporocysts, and usually persists for about a month, sometimes longer. Transmission to the fetus occurs in about 25 per cent of cases during the first trimester, increasing to 60 to 70 per cent in the third trimester. However, severe fetal infection and damage occurs in about 75 per cent of first-trimester infections, declining to a negligible risk in late pregnancy.

Although only about 15 infants with congenitally acquired disease are reported annually in Britain, it is probable that this is a considerable underestimate since recent studies have shown that 2 per 1000 pregnant women experience primary toxoplasmosis. However, most infants, although asymptomatic at birth, are likely to develop chorioretinitis in later life. Unless they are treated, they are likely to develop a relapsing course which may result in considerable visual impairment. However, the effect of treating infected fetuses or newborn infants remains to be fully assessed, although treatment should be offered in all cases of congenitally acquired infection confirmed before the age of 1 year.

Infants with severe congenitally acquired disease are small for dates and may have a petechial rash at birth. In addition, such clinical features as hydrocephalus, chorioretinitis, cerebral calcification, hepatosplenomegaly, pneumonia, myocarditis, and myositis may be present. Such clinical features are usually associated with a severe degree of psychomotor retardation.

Routine antenatal screening for Toxoplasma antibodies is not usually practised in Britain but some countries screen routinely, recommending that pregnant women who have no detectable antibody should be given appropriate health education to minimize the risk of exposure to *T. gondii* during the remainder of their pregnancy. Further testing at 8 to 10 weekly intervals is arranged to ensure that seroconversion does not occur. Many patients will have antibodies to toxoplasma IgG but no specific IgM. They may be reassured that they have been infected previously and that their fetus is not at risk. Patients with Toxoplasma-specific IgG and IgM have evidence of current or recently acquired infection and may transmit *T. gondii* transplacentally. However, if highly sensitive tests are used, specific IgM responses may persist for some months and primary infection may therefore have occurred well before conception. However, there are a number of well-documented reports of maternal toxoplasmosis being acquired well before conception which have resulted in congenitally acquired infection. Although this is a rare event, persons with acute toxoplasmosis are advised not to become pregnant while a *T. gondii*-specific IgM response persists. Should the specific IgM response persist for longer than 6 months, obstetricians should take the advice of a microbiologist prior to counselling patients.

Patients acquiring infection in early pregnancy may wish to consider therapeutic abortion, although fewer than 50 per cent of infants would be infected. In such cases, ultrasonic examination may be of value since evidence of fetal involvement may be obtained by detecting such features as intracranial calcification, increased size of lateral ventricles, ascites, hepatosplenomegaly, and placental thickening. A diagnosis of fetal infection may also be established by detecting Toxoplasma-specific IgM in fetal blood or by detecting *T. gondii* DNA using the polymerase chain reaction, but such investigations can only be carried out in specialized laboratories.

Following delivery, attempts should be made to confirm the diagnosis serologically by detecting Toxoplasma-specific IgM in sequentially obtained sera. However, such responses may be absent in 30 to 50 per cent of congenitally infected infants. Persistence of IgG beyond 6 months of age is indicative of congenitally acquired disease. A diagnosis may also be established by detecting Toxoplasma DNA in neonatal blood.

Treatment is directed towards preventing fetal infection following the diagnosis of acute maternal infection, and in limiting fetal damage if infection has occurred.

Until more information has been obtained about the true incidence of congenitally acquired toxoplasmosis and cost–benefit analyses carried out, it seems unlikely that a routine screening programme in pregnancy will be recommended in Britain. Attention should be directed to preventive measures which, by health education measures carried out by health care workers responsible for the care of pregnant women, will reduce the risk of exposure to infection.

American trypanosomiasis (Chagas' disease) (see Chapter 7.13.11)

Infection may be transmitted from an infected blood transfusion or via the placenta to the fetus. An insect bite, usually on the mother's face, is followed by the development of oedema. After 2 to 3 weeks the mother becomes feverish with the development of parasitaemia. Myocarditis followed by cardiac failure is more likely in pregnancy. Encephalitis may occur. There is an appreciable mortality at this stage but most infections will enter a chronic phase. Many patients are asymptomatic but a number will develop cardiopathy, and late death occurs. In the pregnant patient the placenta is likely to be large and pale; miscarriage is more likely to occur if the placenta is severely involved.

Congenital infection leads to intrauterine growth retardation or preterm delivery, or both. Jaundice, anaemia, thrombocytopenia, hepatosplenomegaly, cardiomegaly, congestive heart failure, and hydrops may all be seen in the baby. The infection also causes congenital pneumonitis and encephalitis, and the cerebrospinal fluid will show pleocytosis. The diagnosis is made by examination of the placenta for *Trypanosoma cruzi* and by microscopic examination of stained films from the peripheral blood. There is no safe and reliable treatment for this disease in pregnancy.

Malaria (see Chapter 7.13.2)

THE MOTHER

Malaria is more severe in pregnancy, and cerebral malaria is more likely even in women living in an endemic area. The convulsions produced by this may be mistaken for eclampsia but the absence of severe hypertension and the presence of fever should suggest the possibility of cerebral malaria, especially in someone who has left a malarial area or someone who has recently arrived there. Anaemia may be severe in chronic cases, and is often exacerbated by other infections such as hookworm. Folate deficiency is more likely to occur in these instances. The effect of anaemia on the myocardium, together with the associated greatly increased blood volume which occurs, both in anaemia and in pregnancy, puts the woman at increased risk of pulmonary oedema. Fever and fetal hypoxia may both precipitate miscarriage, stillbirth, and preterm labour. Preterm labour may also be precipitated by TNF release from macrophages.

FETUS AND NEONATE

The placenta is usually enlarged and contains many parasitized red cells and macrophages. The trophoblast shows focal necrosis and there is basement-membrane thickening with deposition of fibrin. The parasites in intervillous spaces probably compete for nutrients with the fetus. Oxygen and nutrient transfer are reduced. Placental malaria is known to reduce the transfer of tetanus antibody to the fetus and the same mechanism is likely to lead to an overall reduction of antibody transfer.

CONGENITAL MALARIA (SEE CHAPTER 7.13.2)

In endemic areas congenital malaria is uncommon in the immune resident population, in spite of transient parasitaemia which often occurs during labour. Congenital malaria is said to occur in up to 4 per cent of the non-immune. In the immune mother, the fetus is more likely to be infected if the mother migrates to a non-endemic area and her immunity begins to wane. Typically at 3 to 8 weeks of age the infected baby develops fever, anaemia, splenomegaly, diarrhoea, and jaundice. Reticulocytosis is often present. Thrombocytopenia is likely. The illness may be misdiagnosed as bacterial infection unless a thick blood smear is promptly examined for parasites.

PROPHYLAXIS

1. Pregnant women should, whenever possible, avoid areas with endemic malaria.
2. Use mosquito nets and insect repellant.

REFERENCES

Microflora of the genital tract

Martins, J., and Eschenbach, D.A. (1990). The role of bacterial vaginosis as a cause of amniotic fluid infection, chorioamnionitis and prematurity – a review. *Archives of Obstetrics and Gynaecology* **247**, 1–13.

Menkoff, H. *et al.* (1984). Risk factors for prematurity and premature rupture of membranes. A prospective study of the vaginal flora in pregnancy. *American Journal of Obstetrics and Gynecology* **150**, 965–72.

Antibiotics in pregnancy

Duff, P. (ed.) (1992). Antibiotic use in obstetrics and gynaecology. *Obstetrics and Gynaecology Clinics of North America* **19**,(3).

Duff, P. (1993). Antibiotic selection for infections in obstetric patients. *Seminars in Perinatology* **17**, 367–78.

Chorioamnionitis, preterm labour, and premature rupture of membranes

Amer, T.L., and Duff, P. (1991). Intra-amniotic infection in patients with intact membranes and preterm labour. *Obstetrics and Gynaecology Survey* **46**, 589–93.

Divers, M.J., and Lilford, R.J. (1993). Infection in preterm labour. A meta-analysis. In *Contemporary Reviews in Obstetrics and Gynaecology* **5**, 71–83.

Gibbs, R.S., Romero, R., Hillier, S.L., Eschenbach, D.A., and Sweet, R.A. (1992). A review of premature birth and subclinical infection. *American Journal of Obstetrics and Gynecology* **166**, 1515–28.

Keirse, M.J.N.C., Ohlsson, A., Treffers, P.E., and Kanhai, H.H.H. (1990). Prelabour rupture of the membranes preterm. In *Effective care in pregnancy and childbirth*, Vol. 1, (ed. I. Chalmers, M. Enkin, and M.J.N.C. Keirse), pp. 666–93. Oxford University Press, Oxford.

Lamont, R.F., and Fisk, N. (1993). The role of infection in the pathogenesis of preterm labour. In *Progress in obstetrics and gynaecology*, Vol. 10, (ed. J. Studd), pp. 135–58. Churchill Livingstone, Edinburgh.

Urinary-tract infection

Gilbert, G.C. (1991). *Infectious disease in pregnancy and the newborn infant*, Harwood Academic Publishers, Switzerland. pp. 412–35.

Wang, E., and Smaill, F. (1990). Infection in pregnancy. In *Effective care in pregnancy and childbirth*. Vol. 1, *Pregnancy*, (ed. I. Chalmers, M. Enkin, and M.J.N.C. Keirse) pp. 534–8. Oxford University Press, Oxford.

Group B β-haemolytic *Streptococcus*

Burman, L.G., *et al.* (1992). Prevention of excess neonatal morbidity associated with group B streptococci by vaginal disinfection during labour. *Lancet* **340**, 65–9.

Steele, R.W. (1993). Control of neonatal group B streptococcal infection. *Journal of Royal Society of Medicine* **86**, 712–15.

Van Oppen, C., and Feldman, R. (1993). Antibiotic prophylaxis of neonatal group B streptococcal infections (editorial). *British Medical Journal* **306**, 411.

***Listeria monocytogenes* infection**

Buchdahl, R., Hird, M., Gamsu, H., Tapp, A., Gibb, D., and Tzannatos, C. (1990). Listeriosis revisited: the role of the obstetrician. *British Journal of Obstetrics and Gynaecology* **97**, 186–9.

Working Group of the Standing Medical Advisory Committee (1992). *Diagnosis and treatment of suspected listeriosis in pregnancy*. Department of Health, England.

Gonococcal infection

Cavanee, M.R., Farris, J.R., Spalding, T.R., Barnes, D.L., Castaneda, Y.S., and Wendal, G.D. (1993). Treatment of gonorrhoea in pregnancy. *Obstetrics and Gynaecology* **81**, 33–8.

Gilbert, G.L. (1991). *Infectious diseases in pregnancy and the newborn infant*, pp. 241–71. Harwood Academic Publishers, Switzerland.

Laga, M., *et al.* (1986). Epidemiology of ophthalmia neonatorum in Kenya. *Lancet* **2**, 1145–9.

Schultz, K.F., Cates, W., and O'Mara, P.R. (1987). Pregnancy loss, infant death and suffering: legacy of syphilis and gonorrhoea in Africa. *Genitourinary Medicine* **63**, 320–5.

Syphilis

BPSU quarterly bulletin (1993), Vol. 2, No. 3. The British Paediatric Surveillance Unit.

Centres for Disease Control (1988). *Guidelines for the prevention and control of congenital syphilis. Morbidity and mortality – Weekly Report.* **37**, (Suppl. 1), 15–135.

Rawstrom, S.A., Jenkins, S., Blanchard, S., Ping-Wu Li, M.A., and Bromberg, K. (1993). Maternal v. congenital syphilis in Brooklyn New York. Epidemiology, transmission and diagnosis. *American Journal of Diseases of Children* **147**, 727–31.

Candida infection

Loke, H.L., Verber, I., Szymonowicz, W., and Yu, V.Y.H. (1988). Systemic candidiasis and pneumonia in preterm infants. *Australian Paediatric Journal* **24**, 138–42.

Sobel, J.D. (1992). Candidal vulvovaginitis. *Clinics in Obstetrics and Gynaecology*, **36**, 153–65.

Chlamydial infection

Barry, W.C., *et al.* (1986). *Chlamydia trachomatis* as a cause of neonatal conjunctivitis. *Archives of Disease in Childhood* **61**, 797–9.

Ryan, G.M., Abdella, T.N., McNeeley, G., Baselski, V.S., and Drummond, D.E. (1990). *Chlamydia trachomatis* infection, pregnancy and effect of treatment on outcome. *American Journal of Obstetrics and Gynaecology* **162**, 34–9.

Smith, J.R., and Taylor-Robinson, D. (1993). Infection due to *Chlamydia trachomatis* in pregnancy and the newborn. *Ballière Clinical Obstetrics and Gynaecology*, **7**,(1), 237–55.

Mycoplasma infection

Cassell, G.H., *et al.* (1988). Association of ureaplasma urealyticum infection of the lower respiratory tract with chronic lung disease and death in very low birthweight infants. *Lancet*, **ii**, 240–5.

Dyke, M.P., Grauaug, A., Kohan, R., Off, K., and Andrews, R. (1993). Ureaplasma urealyticum in a neonatal intensive care population. *Journal of Pediatrics and Child Health* **29**, 295–7.

Tuberculosis

Gilbert, G.L. (1991). *Infectious diseases in pregnancy and the newborn infant*. Harwood Academic Publishers, Switzerland.

Gilstrap, L.C. and Faro, S. (ed.) (1990). *Infections in pregnancy*. Wiley-Liss, New York.

Malaria

Brair, M.E., Brabin, B.J., Milligan, P., Maxwell, S., and Hart, C.A. (1994). Reduced transfer of tetanus antibodies with placental malaria. *Lancet* **343**, 208–9.

Wijesundere, A. and Wijesundere, A. (1992). Malaria in pregnancy. *Contemporary Reviews in Obstetrics and Gynaecology* **4**, 137–40.

13.13 Liver and gastrointestinal disease in pregnancy

E. A. Fagan

Diseases of the liver

INTRODUCTION

These are encountered rarely, leading to delays in diagnosis and treatment. Early recognition improves outcome. In the United Kingdom between 1985 and 1987 the frequency of maternal death due to liver disease equalled that due to abortion, anaesthesia, genital sepsis, and ruptured uterus.

ANATOMY, PHYSIOLOGY, AND BIOCHEMISTRY

A palpable liver in pregnancy suggests disease. In the third trimester the liver is displaced posteriorly, superiorly, and to the right. Dullness to percussion is reduced. Percutaneous liver biopsy is safe in expert hands with normal coagulation and ultrasonographic imaging. Histology of the liver in normal pregnancy may show mild steatosis.

Palmar erythema and spider naevi occur in healthy patients during pregnancy as well as in those with chronic liver disease and acute liver failure.

In pregnancy, absolute hepatic blood flow is not increased significantly. A smaller proportion of the overall increase in cardiac output (approximately 25 per cent) passes through the liver. The increased blood volume is redistributed into the splanchnic circulation and great veins. Portal vein pressure rises in late pregnancy. The gravid uterus presses on the vena cava, diverting some of the venous return through the azygous system. Oesophageal varices are seen on endoscopy in around 50 per cent of healthy pregnant women.

Abnormalities in liver function tests suggest liver disease (Table 1). In a healthy, well-nourished pregnant woman, liver metabolism and function and handling of drugs and toxins are not altered significantly. Clearance may be reduced for drugs which rely on blood flow and volume of distribution.

Liver diseases can be divided into those peculiar, and those incidental, to pregnancy.

Liver diseases peculiar to pregnancy

Intrahepatic cholestasis of pregnancy

This is the most common condition peculiar to pregnancy, being second to viral hepatitis as a cause of jaundice in pregnancy. The incidence of severe intrahepatic cholestasis of pregnancy may be falling. The original descriptions of generalized pruritus, mild jaundice, and intrahepatic cholestasis in the third trimester were made in 1883 by Ahlfeld and later by Thorling in 1955. Svanborg in 1954 included fatigue, mild abdominal pain, and subsidence after delivery, with future recurrences.

Pruritus develops after week 30 and becomes progressively severe— 'pruritus gravidarum'. Jaundice develops 2 to 4 weeks later. Symptoms resolve rapidly post-partum. Nocturnal itching can cause insomnia and fatigue. Anorexia, malaise, mild epigastric discomfort, steatorrhoea, and dark urine are common. The predominantly conjugated hyperbilirubinaemia (total serum bilirubin < 100 μmol/l; $N < 17$) is mild, and serum levels of aspartate aminotransferase, alanine aminotransferase, and alka-

line phosphatase rarely exceed twice the upper normal limits. Vitamin K_1 replacement corrects any abnormal prothrombin ratio. Marked pain, hepatomegaly, and splenomegaly suggest other diseases. Gallstones are common. During pregnancy the gallbladder volume is increased, the ejection fraction of bile is reduced, and the metabolism of bile acids is altered.

Aetiology

A genetic predisposition alters the membrane composition of bile ducts and hepatocytes and increases sensitivity to sex steroids. The pruritus has been linked to increased availability of brain (endogenous) opioid receptors for binding their agonist ligands (endorphins, enkephalins, dynorphins) in cholestasis. Sex steroids also are implicated. Intrahepatic cholestasis is severe with multiple pregnancies and can recur with menstruation, oral contraceptive therapy, and the menopause. In some cases, reversal of the cholestasis and abolition of pruritus after high-dose S-adenosyl-L-methionine points to a metabolic defect.

A positive family history is common and associated with haplotypes HLA-B8 and HLA-BW16. Transmission is autosomal dominant. Fathers transmit the susceptibility to daughters. Intrahepatic cholestasis of pregnancy occurs in around 2 per cent of deliveries in Scandinavian and Mediterranean countries, Poland, Chile, Canada, Australia, and China. Seasonal variation suggests the involvement of environmental factors.

Management

Other causes of pruritus and jaundice, especially biliary diseases, drug hepatotoxicity, and viral hepatitis must be considered. Histological confirmation of acinar cholestasis and bile plugs may be useful when symptoms begin before the 20th week and when jaundice occurs without pruritus and persists after delivery. Ultrasonography is an important precaution for liver biopsy, helping to avoid puncturing the exceptionally large gallbladder and to exclude gallstones.

Fetal outcome

Fetal distress, premature labour, and intrauterine death occur even in mild cases, and risks increase near term. Elevated serum levels of maternal bile acids correlate with severity of pruritus and risk of fetal distress. The timing of delivery after the 37th week should follow serial estimations of fetal lung maturity and maternal levels of total bile acids. Neonatal vitamin K_1 therapy given immediately postpartum helps to prevent intracranial bleeding.

Maternal outcome

This is good. Itching and jaundice resolve rapidly but may recur with subsequent pregnancies and oral contraceptive therapy. Treatment of itching with cholestyramine, phenobarbitone, or intravenous S-adenosyl-methionine is disappointing and cholestyramine binds bile acids, anionic drugs, and fat-soluble vitamins. Vitamin K_1 corrects an abnormal prothrombin ratio and reduces postpartum haemorrhage.

Liver disorders and hypertension

Most liver diseases in late pregnancy are associated with hypertension. Acute fatty liver, HELLP syndrome (see below), hepatic rupture, and

Table 1 *Liver function tests in normal pregnancy*

No change	
Prothrombin time	Alkaline phosphatase (liver)
Total bilirubin	gamma-GT
AST/SGOT	5-nucleotidase
ALT/SGPT	Gammaglobulin
Rises	
Total alkaline phosphatase[a]	Transferrin
Alpha- and beta-globulins	Cholesterol
Fibrinogen	Triglycerides
Caeruloplasmin	Bile acids
Falls	
Albumin: 20% first trimester	

AST, aspartate aminotransferase; ALT, alanine aminotransferase; gamma-GT, gamma-glutamyl transpeptidase.

[a]Placental and skeletal isoenzymes only.

infarction form a spectrum of obscure aetiologies. Overlapping clinical features make diagnosis difficult.

PRE-ECLAMPSIA

(See also Chapter 13.2)

Hepatic tenderness, nausea, and vomiting and elevated levels of aspartate aminotransferase are common. Jaundice is infrequent. The liver is not involved primarily but becomes the target organ in advanced cases with marked hypertension (diastolic blood pressure > 110 mmHg), proteinuria with renal impairment, cerebral and visual disturbances, and intrauterine growth retardation. Hepatic petechial haemorrhages, necrosis, fibrin deposits, and thrombi are attributed to disseminated intravascular coagulation. They are secondary events because typically the prothrombin ratio and fibrinogen levels are normal. Serum levels of lactate dehydrogenase and fibrin degradation products may be elevated and antithrombin III reduced. Hormonal factors interact with vascular injury to endothelial cells, exposure of subendothelial collagen, platelet adherence, and deposition of fibrin.

THE HELLP SYNDROME

Definition

Patients with hypertension in the third trimester may present principally with hepatic dysfunction; Haemolytic anaemia, Elevated Liver transaminases (aspartate aminotransferase > 50 IU/l) and a Low Platelet count (platelet count below 100×10^9/l (100 000/mm³)). Other abnormalities include elevated levels of unconjugated bilirubin, creatinine, lactate dehydrogenase (> 180 IU/l), fibrin degradation products, fibrin D-dimer, plasminogen activator inhibitor, protein C, and anaphylatoxins (C3a, C5a). A microangiopathic haemolytic anaemia accompanies disseminated intravascular coagulation and low levels of antithrombin III. The prothrombin ratio, partial thromboplastin time, and fibrinogen levels are normal. The abnormal serum aspartate aminotransferase and unconjugated bilirubin reflect the haematological disturbances, rather than severity of liver dysfunction. The aspartate aminotransferase level recovers before the thrombocytopenia. The syndrome can also occur in postpartum eclampsia.

SPONTANEOUS HEPATIC RUPTURE

This was reported by Abercrombie in 1844. Rupture occurs once in approximately every 45 000 live births (in 250 000 pregnancies) and is most common in the third trimester, complicated by severe hypertension.

Pathogenetic mechanisms remain obscure. Subcapsular haemorrhages are common in severe hypertension with disseminated intravascular coagulation. A raised serum aspartate aminotransferase and lactate dehydrogenase usually reflect red cell destruction, but an aspartate aminotransferase level greater than 1000 IU/l and an elevated prothrombin ratio indicate extensive hepatic necrosis.

Diagnosis

Hepatic rupture should be suspected with the triad of pre-eclampsia, right upper quadrant pain, and shock. Other features include hypotension, hepatic encephalopathy, profound hypoglycaemia, fever, vomiting, absent fetal heart sounds, and bleeding *per vaginam* with a haemorrhagic diathesis. At laparotomy undertaken for suspected perforated viscus, abruptio placenta, or ruptured uterus there may be haemoperitoneum and a subcapsular tear and haematoma in the right lobe.

Serial imaging with ultrasonography, computed axial tomography (CT) scanning or magnetic resonance imaging (MRI) is essential. Diagnostic percutaneous peritoneal lavage should be carried out for suspected liver rupture. Selective transcatheter embolotherapy may arrest bleeding temporarily in haemodynamically unstable and high-risk surgical patients and those without intraperitoneal bleeding.

Prognosis

In the literature between 1976 and 1991 of around 35 cases, maternal survival exceeded 80 per cent following early surgery with evacuation of liver haematoma, packing, and drainage. Maternal mortality was around 25 per cent following lobectomy. Several authors favour immediate caesarean section. Still birth and perinatal death remain high. Uneventful pregnancies have been recorded in survivors.

ACUTE FATTY LIVER OF PREGNANCY (AFLP)

Features were described by Rokitansky in 1843 and Tarnier in 1856 before Stander and Cadden in 1934. Sheehan in 1940 differentiated AFLP from fulminant viral hepatitis.

Incidence

AFLP occurs once in every 9000 to 13 300 deliveries. Reports of mild cases and survivors do not reflect general obstetric practice. Maternal deaths seem to be increasing. In the United Kingdom between 1985 and 1987 the six deaths from AFLP were as many as for sepsis, ruptured uterus, abortion, and anaesthesia. Diagnosis is difficult without jaundice, with concurrent disease, and outside the third trimester.

AFLP occurs typically in obese women in the third trimester. Distributions in age, parity, and race do not differ from those in normal obstetric practice but there are independent associations with hypertension, twin pregnancy, and a male fetus (ratio 3 male to 1 female).

Aetiology

This remains obscure. Abnormalities in neutral triglycerides and fatty acid oxidation have been implicated. Infections of the urinary tract and chest are common accompaniments.

Diagnosis

AFLP should be suspected when epigastric pain, reflux oesophagitis, nausea, and vomiting and combined with jaundice and a bleeding diathesis. Hypertension, pedal oedema, and proteinuria are also common. Occasionally there is pruritus, fever, ascites, necrotizing enterocolitis, and backache from pancreatitis. Deterioration may be rapid with impaired consciousness, profound hypoglycaemia, and acute liver failure, renal failure, bleeding diatheses, and death. The differential diagnosis of jaundice, encephalopathy, and acute liver failure (see viral hepatitis and acute liver failure, below) is wide. The manifestations of AFLP overlap with those of the HELLP syndrome, haemolytic-uraemic syndrome, thrombocytopenic purpura, disseminated intravascular coagulation, and sepsis, but liver dysfunction is minor in the predominantly haematological conditions. Obstetrical differential diagnoses include abruptio placentae, intrauterine death, amniotic fluid embolism, toxaemia, and sepsis.

There is a marked neutrophil leucocytosis, disseminated intravascular coagulation, and microangiopathic haemolytic anaemia with thrombocytopenia, elevated levels of fibrin degradation products, and reduced antithrombin III. Renal impairment and metabolic acidosis are common. The triad of a modestly elevated serum aspartate aminotransferase with high serum alkaline phosphatase and uric acid are not discriminative. Serum levels of bilirubin may be normal. High levels of aspartate aminotransferase (> 1000 IU/l) accompany shock and hepatic ischaemia.

Profound hypoglycaemia is common and contributes significantly to fetal and maternal mortality. Increased reflectivity on ultrasonography of the liver is consistent with fatty infiltration. CT scanning and MRI show low attenuation. These tests are safe but may be falsely negative.

Histopathology

Fatty infiltration and haemorrhages are widespread. The liver is small and yellow. The microvesicular fat is characteristically panlobular with sparing of periportal areas. Microvesicular steatosis is also found in alcoholic hepatitis, in toxicity from tetracycline, sodium valproate or salicylates, vomiting disease of Jamaica, yellow fever, Reye's syndrome in children, Wolman's disease, and deficiencies of congenital urea cycle enzymes with fatty acid oxidation.

Management principles for HELLP and AFLP

Liver function tests and platelet counts should be performed in all pregnancies. Maternal and fetal outcome improve with specialized intensive care. Treatment of hypertension, severe hypoglycaemia, and caesarean section should follow severe cases presenting after week 36. Spontaneous vaginal delivery is possible for mild cases. Close monitoring is essential. Corticosteroids and low-dose salicylates occasionally improve the level of aspartate aminotransferase and platelets in HELLP. Typically, the nadir in platelet count occurs 24 to 72 h postpartum and may precipitate haemorrhage.

The benefits of early delivery remain unproven in trials, but, individually, improvement can be striking. Spontaneous recovery in severe cases is exceptional, arguing strongly for early delivery. Postpartum complications include infection, liver rupture and infarction, hypoglycaemia, pancreatitis and pseudocyst formation, and neurological dysfunction. Subsequent normal pregnancies have been successful, including after liver grafting (see liver transplantation below). Recurrences have been reported, with overlap between HELLP and AFLP. Neonatal abnormalities, especially haematological, are more common with HELLP than AFLP.

HYPEREMESIS GRAVIDARUM

Elevated levels of aspartate aminotransferase have been reported in 15 to 25 per cent of patients but return to normal with cessation of vomiting and rehydration (see gastrointestinal disorders, below).

Liver diseases coincidental to pregnancy

VIRAL HEPATITIS A TO E

Viral hepatitis remains the most common cause of jaundice in pregnancy. Presentation peaks in the third trimester. Hepatitis may be detected on screening for hepatitis B status or to detect reactivation (of the herpes viruses for example). Diagnosis relies on detection of specific serological markers of acute and chronic infection. Clinical presentation is usually delayed until cholestasis occurs. Differential diagnosis includes alcoholic hepatitis, biliary obstruction, intrahepatic cholestasis

of pregnancy, reaction to drugs, and autoimmune liver diseases. Oral contraceptive therapy has no adverse effect on acute viral hepatitis and chronic liver disease.

Maternal outcome

Reports are conflicting. In the West, overall, the outcome of pregnancy is normal, with no adverse effect of age or parity. Malnutrition and limited medical facilities affect outcome adversely in developing countries. Acute viral hepatitis in a country with high prevalence is most commonly due to hepatitis E or B; immunity to hepatitis A from childhood is almost universal. Whether the severe outcome of hepatitis E in pregnancy reported for developing countries reflects virus virulence, host factors, or suboptimal facilities, is unclear. In the United Kingdom and United States, hepatitis E seems to be confined to travellers returning from the Indian subcontinent, the former Soviet Union, Nepal, Burma, Africa and Mexico, and South America.

Management

This should be similar to that in the non-pregnant woman (see Chapter 7.10.6.

Fetal outcome

Most studies show some excess in intrauterine death, still births, and prematurity. Congenital abnormalities are not increased.

SEXUAL TRANSMISSION

Faeco-oral contamination can transmit hepatitis A and probably hepatitis E. In the West, transmission of hepatitis B is mostly horizontal from person to person (intravenous drug use in young males and heterosexual contact in young females). Sexual transmission is frequent for hepatitis B and less frequent for hepatitis C and D viruses.

VERTICAL AND PERINATAL TRANSMISSION

The risk of transmission to the neonate is maximal for acute viral hepatitis presenting in the third trimester.

Faecal contamination during delivery can transmit hepatitis A and E but the risk is limited by the short interval of viral excretion. Neonatal immunoprophylaxis for hepatitis A is rarely necessary; most neonatal infections are mild and herald life-long immunity. Vertical and perinatal transmission are infrequent for hepatitis C in the absence of HIV infection.

HEPATITIS B

Babies born of HBsAg positive mothers with virus replication (HBeAg and HBV DNA) have a 20 to 95 per cent risk of becoming infected. Infectivity depends on the HBV DNA level which relates to ethnic origin.

Chronic hepatitis B is uncommon in babies born to HBsAg positive mothers with anti-HBe and mothers also seronegative for HBeAg. These babies are at risk of severe acute neonatal hepatitis and acute liver failure. Survivors show serological evidence of clearance of virus and immunity (anti-HBs). Caesarean section does not prevent vertical transmission. Isolation is unnecessary, provided neonatal immunization has commenced. Breast feeding is not contraindicated with fetal and maternal immunization.

MATERNAL SCREENING

Hepatitis B

All pregnant women should be screened for HBsAg and IgM anti-HBc. Neonatal immunoprophylaxis against hepatitis B is optimal at birth. Universal prenatal screening in the United States is estimated to identify

22 000 HBsAg-seropositive women. This strategy should prevent 3000 chronic infections annually and is cost-saving.

Hepatitis C

Screening is recommended for high-risk patients. There are no specific recommendations in pregnancy.

PREVENTION

Isolation and barrier nursing are unnecessary for viral hepatitis with good nursing practice. Secondary spread to health-care personnel is uncommon.

Hepatitis A and E

There are no specific recommendations for passive immunoprophylaxis for hepatitis A during pregnancy. Immune globulin should be offered to symptomless contacts with an index case during the third trimester and prior to travel. Prescreening for IgG anti-HAV antibodies avoids unnecessary immunization. The hepatitis A vaccine is not licensed for pregnancy.

Pregnant medical and nursing personnel should avoid hepatitis E. Handling of faeces and bile containing A and E should be minimized by washing hands thoroughly and disposing of contaminated clothes and fomites by autoclaving and incineration.

Hepatitis B, C, and D

Direct contact with blood-soaked dressings and pads must be avoided; all attendants should wear protective clothing, cover exposed cuts and abrasions and handle body fluids with care. Goggles and masks can prevent splashes on to the eye and mouth. The few reports of transmission of hepatitis B from attendants to patients have included incidents following obstetrical and gynaecological surgery.

COMBINED ACTIVE AND PASSIVE IMMUNOPROPHYLAXIS

(See also Chapter 7.10.6)

This is the prophylaxis of choice for hepatitis B and D. Results with recombinant and plasma-derived vaccines are similar. Manufacturers do not recommend immunization during pregnancy. In specific contraindication or adverse consequence following hepatitis B immune globulin and a licensed hepatitis B vaccine.

Herpes viruses

(See also Chapters 7.10.2, 7.10.3)

Herpes simplex is the only virus in the West with a predilection to cause severe hepatitis in pregnancy. Presenting features are non-specific. Mucocutaneous lesions and jaundice may be absent. Diagnosis depends on serological markers and finding inclusion bodies and viral DNA in liver tissue. Early treatment with acyclovir in pregnancy can be successful. Caesarean section should be considered for maternal primary infection.

ACUTE LIVER FAILURE

The most common causes in pregnancy are viral hepatitis, disorders associated with hypertension (acute fatty liver of pregnancy and HELLP) and paracetamol (acetaminophen) hepatotoxicity. Paracetamol levels should be sought in all patients presenting with obscure abdominal pain and encephalopathy. Fetal hepatotoxicity from metabolites of paracetamol can impair coagulation, leading to intraventricular haemorrhage. N-acetyl-cysteine probably is safe and can be given up to 36 h following the overdose (see Section 8.2).

Management is similar to that in non-pregnant patients. Except in cases of acute fatty liver of pregnancy and HELLP (see above), delivery does not necessarily improve maternal outcome but controlled studies are lacking. Whatever the cause, survival of the fetus is exceptional in the presence of liver failure. Fetal heart sounds commonly are absent and profound fetal and maternal hypoglycaemia are likely.

LIVER TRANSPLANTATION

Successful maternal and fetal outcomes have been reported following grafting during pregnancy and in survivors of acute liver failure due to hepatitis B, acute fatty liver, and the HELLP and Budd–Chiari syndromes. Graft reinfection may be lessened when hepatitis B immune globulin is given for hepatitis B and D. Data on the efficacy of immunoprophylaxis and antiviral therapies are sparse.

The menstrual cycle returns soon after successful grafting. Continuing amenorrhoea may signify pregnancy. Early advice on contraception is necessary. Oral contraceptive drugs can enhance cyclosporin hepatotoxicity and are contraindicated in thrombogenic disorders such as the Budd–Chiari syndrome. Graft rejection and function are not altered by pregnancy. Deferral of pregnancy beyond the first year post-transplant seems sensible because of high morbidity and mortality. Successful pregnancies have been reported in grafted women maintained on cyclosporin, azathioprine, and corticosteroids. There is an increased risk of pre-eclampsia, worsening hypertension associated with cyclosporin, drug nephrotoxicity, anaemia, and preterm delivery. Cyclosporin crosses the placenta and can impair fetal growth but long-term survivors seem to be unaffected. Blood levels of cyclosporin should be monitored frequently. Shared management is essential between hepatologist, obstetrician, and perinatologist.

FETAL ALCOHOL SYNDROME

There is no safe level of alcohol intake which is certain to prevent adverse effects on the fetus. Complete abstinence throughout pregnancy is recommended, beginning before conception. Critical exposure is probably before the eighth week but the minimum dose of alcohol and its metabolites to avoid ill effects on the fetus is unknown. Cessation at any time through gestation may improve outcome.

Fetal alcohol syndrome is the third most common birth defect to cause mental retardation, after Down's syndrome and open neural tube defects. The incidence of the complete syndrome is around 1:300 and 1:2000 live births. Cardinal features are growth and mental deficiency, a characteristic facial dysmorphism (small palpebral fissures, up-turned nose, hypoplasia of maxilla, and micrognathia and prognathia in adolescence), and major malformations of organs, such as ventricular septal defect, tetrad of Fallot, small rotated kidneys and polydactyly, Klippel–Feil syndrome, scoliosis, and hernias.

Babies may present with tremor, irritability, and seizures from alcohol withdrawal. Alcohol passes into breast milk and causes sedation.

Spontaneous abortion and low birthweight are well-recognized, especially in those who smoke as well as drink. A high index of suspicion is necessary but avoid enquiry that provokes guilt. Many drinkers have normal serum liver biochemistry. Most show concern for their babies. Motivation to alter drinking habits during pregnancy is high. Intensive counselling should be continued.

CONGENITAL DISORDERS OF METABOLISM OF BILIRUBIN

Aggrevation of jaundice in pregnancy and with oral contraceptive therapy can occur with Gilbert's disease, Dubin–Johnson, and Rotor syndromes. Fetal outcome is good without especial risk of kernicterus. Differentiation is from other causes of cholestasis and jaundice which may affect maternal and fetal outcome, especially intrahepatic cholestasis of pregnancy (IHCP), biliary disease, and gallstones, viral hepatitis, and Wilson's disease. In Dubin–Johnson syndrome, unlike IHCP and many causes of cholestasis, pruritus is absent and the serum alkaline phosphatase is within the normal range for pregnancy.

Chronic hepatitis and cirrhosis

Untreated autoimmune chronic active hepatitis and Wilson's disease are associated with amenorrhoea and infertility.

AUTOIMMUNE CHRONIC ACTIVE HEPATITIS

Liver function is preserved with well-controlled disease but fetal prematurity and loss and low birthweight occur. Urinary infections and pre-eclampsia are common. Prednisolone and azathioprine have improved fertility and prognosis and should be continued in conventional doses. No specific adverse effects on the fetus have been reported. Uncontrolled disease and relapses should prompt exclusion of Wilson's disease and viral hepatitis.

WILSON'S DISEASE

(See also Chapter 11.7).

Pregnancy is uncommon with untreated disease. Subfertility and amenorrhoea are common, spontaneous abortions frequent, and maternal morbidity and mortality high.

Chelating agents

Maternal and fetal outcome are good with well-controlled disease using D-penicillamine or triethylene tetraamine dihydrochloride. Chelating agents generally are considered safe and non-toxic in pregnancy. They can reduce serum levels of iron and zinc and should not be co-administered with oral iron. Pyridoxine (vitamin B_6) counteracts the antipyridine effects of D-penicillamine. D-Penicillamine crosses the placenta. The few congenital abnormalities described probably result from copper deficiency. The normal handling of copper by the fetus may account for some improvements in neurological status and liver function in the pregnant mother.

Cirrhosis

Pregnancy is uncommon in advanced cirrhosis but the once gloomy prognosis for mother and child has improved. Infertility reflects the degree of hepatic dysfunction. Irregular menses result from disturbances of the hypothalamic–pituitary axis, malnutrition, and altered hepatic metabolism of sex steroids.

Suspected cirrhosis and portal hypertension requires full investigation. Upper endoscopy in pregnancy is safe in expert hands.

Maternal and fetal outcomes are variable, but are good for well-compensated disease. Drug therapy is non-specific and aimed at relieving symptoms such as pruritus. Cholestyramine resin binds fat-soluble vitamins. Vitamin K_1 supplements should be given throughout pregnancy and before delivery.

Maternal outcome

Prognosis depends on hepatic dysfunction rather than aetiology, although well-compensated biliary and postnecrotic cirrhosis carry the best prognoses.

Bleeding oesophageal varices

This remains the most frequent complication. Mortality is not increased with pregnancy. The progressive increase in circulating blood volume, elevations in portal pressure, and pressure from the gravid uterus on the inferior vena cava coincide to divert a greater proportion of the venous return through the azygous system. The risk of bleeding continues into the postpartum period and challenges explanations of haemodynamic alterations during pregnancy. Portal pressure can be reduced with β-blockers and vasodilators but trials in pregnancy are lacking. Upper oesophago-gastro-duodenoscopy and emergency sclerotherapy for bleeding varices are safe in expert hands and should be repeated for each episode of bleeding. Surgical portal decompression can be successful. Survivors of a variceal bleed usually have endstage irreversible disease.

Additional medical therapy may induce a remission even for large varices, such as corticosteroids for autoimmune chronic active hepatitis, D-penicillamine for Wilson's disease, and abstinence from alcohol in alcoholic cirrhosis.

General management

Pregnant patients with cirrhosis and portal hypertension should rest and avoid straining, stooping, and alcohol. Rebleeding from varices and death are likely in alcoholics who continue to drink. No specific measures are proven to protect the oesophagus in the absence of reflux.

A pregnancy should be allowed to proceed to term for well-compensated cirrhosis without jaundice and impaired liver function. In advanced cirrhosis and following surgical portal decompression, the diet should be high in carbohydrate, low in protein, and supplemented with vitamins. A high-fibre diet and lactulose lessen constipation. Management and delivery should occur in a centre experienced in oesophageal varices. Usually vaginal delivery is safe. A protracted second stage should be avoided and excess blood loss anticipated. Vitamin K_1, fresh frozen plasma, and additional coagulation factors and platelets may be required. Postpartum uterine haemorrhage is also common.

Sedatives, anaesthetics, and diuretics should be used cautiously. These and excess blood loss, hypotension, occult infection, hypoglycaemia, and constipation can precipitate hepatic encephalopathy. Dietary sodium and fluids should be restricted for ascites. Spironolactone, triamterene and thiazide diuretics cross the placenta. Their safety in pregnancy is unproven. The thiazide diuretics can precipitate hepatic coma in cirrhosis. Frusemide and a metabolite of spironolactone cross into breast milk and breast feeding is not recommended. Untreated spontaneous bacterial peritonitis and sepsis worsen the prognosis. Tetracyclines are contraindicated in pregnancy and liver disease.

Fetal outcome

Spontaneous abortion and still birth are common in advanced cirrhosis. The prognosis improves with previous portosystemic decompression.

Elective termination of pregnancy should be considered only for decompensated cirrhosis in the first trimester. Caesarean section should be reserved for saving the baby when maternal liver function is deteriorating rapidly. Abdominal surgery is difficult with the large collateral circulation and adhesions from any previous shunt surgery. Local anaesthesia with an epidural or pudendal block can be carried out safely but bleeding may occur from the raised venous pressure and abnormal coagulation.

PRIMARY BILIARY CIRRHOSIS

This may be symptomless and come to light only when a disproportionately elevated level of serum alkaline phosphatase and elevated γ-glutamyl transpeptidase are discovered. Differential diagnosis includes intrahepatic cholestasis of pregnancy which resolves in the puerperium, gallstones, and sclerosing cholangitis.

BUDD–CHIARI SYNDROME

The first description by Chiari in 1899 followed childbirth but presentation can be in any trimester. No specific abnormality in clotting factors has been found in Budd–Chiari syndrome complicating pregnancy. Hormonal factors may play a role, given the excess prevalence in females overall, in pregnancy, and in users of oral contraceptive steroids.

The prognosis is poor in pregnancy. Fetal outcome depends on maternal well-being. There is often resistance of ascites to diuretics and salt restriction. The safety of many diuretics has not been established in pregnancy. Maternal mortality with surgical intervention is high. Successful pregnancies have been reported following grafting, but risks of recurrent veno-occlusion are high despite anticoagulant therapy. Oral contraceptive drugs are contraindicated in survivors.

The gallbladder and biliary tract

Gallbladder disease in pregnancy is, after acute appendicitis, the most common non-obstetric condition requiring surgery.

PHYSIOLOGY

Gallbladder residual and fasting volumes and mean diameter of the common bile duct increase through pregnancy. Results of dynamic studies and effects of the sex steroids remain controversial. Ultrasonographic detection of symptomless stones and echogenic bile are common. Cholesterol gallstones are found in women more often than in men and particularly in users of oral contraceptive steroids. The sex difference begins at the menarche and remains throughout reproductive life. A subpopulation of women seem susceptible to early development of gallstones after oral contraceptive steroids and pregnancy. The risk of gallstones is increased in liver diseases, especially IHCP, and rises with parity in young women and declines with rising age at first pregnancy. Elevated levels of urinary oestrone are found in women with gallstones. A statistical correlation exists between gestational vomiting, gallbladder disease, and a known intolerance to oral contraceptive steroids.

BIOCHEMISTRY

Prerequisites for stone formation include the hepatic secretion of lithogenic bile. In users of oral contraceptive steroids the ratio of cholic to chenodeoxycholic acids falls, rendering the bile more saturated. In the second and third trimesters there is a progressive decrease in the size of the chenodeoxycholic acid pool but not that of cholic acid. As the overall rate of cholesterol secretion is unchanged, its concentration relative to the diminishing size of the bile acid pool is increased, rendering the bile more lithogenic. Oestrogens and progestagens have marked, different effects on metabolism of bile salts, cholesterol, and biliary lipids. Ethinyl oestradiol causes an increase in cholesterol content within the liver, but decreases the secretion of bile salts. Progesterone increases the rate of esterification, but not synthesis, of cholesterol and an increase in bile salt-independent bile secretion. The net effect is to increase saturation of the bile with cholesterol.

PRESENTATION AND MANAGEMENT

The presenting features are the same as in non-pregnant individuals. Ultrasonographic techniques are safe in pregnancy and are preferred to radiological imaging. Thickening of the gallbladder wall in severe pre-eclampsia with marked hypoalbuminaemia should not be mistaken for cholecystitis. The biliary tree outlined in a $^{99}Tc^M$-IDA (technetium-99-iododiethyl-iminoacetic acid) scan gives minimal irradiation to the fetus. Endoscopic retrograde cholecystpancreatography and percutaneous, transhepatic cholecystography are not justified without shielding from the significant doses of irradiation and monitoring radiation exposure. Laparoscopic cholecystectomy is contraindicated since the risk of bleeding is increased and the enlarged uterus obscures view. Delaying cholecystectomy until after delivery must be balanced against the risk of recurrent attack and increase in postoperative complications. Fetal outcome is optimal when surgery is carried out in the second trimester. Maternal and fetal mortalities rise with accompanying pancreatitis and pseudocyst.

In pregnancy, common bile duct stones may be painless and jaundice absent. Cholangitis is common. Surgical intervention is obligatory for large duct obstruction to avoid recurrent attacks of cholangitis, pancreatitis, and empyema of the gallbladder. Rarely, biliary obstruction may be due to cholangiocarcinoma or *Clonorchis sinensis* (see Chapter 14.24). HIV infection is associated with acalculous cholangitis and large duct dilatation. Bile acid therapy is contraindicated in pregnancy. Bile acids cross the placenta. Chenodeoxycholic acid is hepatotoxic and teratogenic in animals. Lithotrypsy is contraindicated during pregnancy.

Gastrointestinal disorders

The physiological changes in the gastrointestinal tract during pregnancy remain controversial. Most recent studies show no significant delay in gastric emptying and intestinal transit when compared with non-pregnant women. Alterations in the neuroendocrinological axis and gut motility may help explain symptoms such as nausea, vomiting, and constipation. Most are self-limiting and do not affect maternal and fetal outcome. These gestational problems must be differentiated from the many diseases with similar presentations requiring specific diagnosis and management. Self-medication with proprietary drugs is prevalent. Antacids, antiemetics, laxatives, and antidiarrhoeal agents often are taken before awareness of pregnancy and without regard for their potential teratogenicity.

Patients with known diseases require close monitoring for relapse during pregnancy. The decision to modify a therapy must be balanced against subsequent risks to mother and fetus.

Gastro-oesophageal reflux

Dyspepsia is almost invariable, especially in the third trimester. Under the influence of progestagens, oestrogens, and other hormones there is a reduction in barrier pressure in the lower oesophagus—the difference between gastric and lower oesophageal sphincter pressures. In addition, in late pregnancy the lower oesophagus fails to adapt to any rise in intragastric pressure. Severity of symptoms does not correlate with the degree of reflux, subsequent oesophagitis, and presence of a hiatus hernia. Reflux symptoms can be caused by alkaline bile as well as by gastric acid. Dyspepsia can herald many disorders, ranging from infections and infestations, liver and biliary diseases, pancreatitis, and myocardial infarction. Reflux can present as bronchospasm.

MANAGEMENT

Symptoms improve with ingestion of small, frequent meals rich in carbohydrate and low in fat. Reflux can improve by avoiding factors that reduce further the barrier pressure, such as many drugs, especially the tricyclic antidepressants, atropine, halothane, enflurane, opiates, and thiopentone; alcohol and cigarette smoking; bending; stooping; and lying supine.

In early pregnancy, first-line medication is with the simple mixtures of magnesium trisilicate, magnesium hydroxide, and non-absorbable alginates. These probably are safe and preferred to the many proprietary mixtures containing additional drugs. Anticholinergic compounds reduce further the lower oesophageal sphincter pressure and pass into breast milk. Metoclopramide and domperidone raise the barrier pressure and the H_2 antagonists have been used after the first trimester. The safety of omeprazole has not been established. Misoprostol, an analogue of prostaglandin E_1, increases uterine tone and contractions and is contraindicated in pregnancy. In late pregnancy, during labour and anaesthesia there is a risk of Mendelson's syndrome—tracheal aspiration of gastric contents leading to chemical pneumonitis, hypoxia, and pulmonary oedema. Gastric emptying can be delayed following extradural lumbar anaesthesia and fentanyl. The volume of gastric contents can be assessed using ultrasonography. Prior to anaesthesia, the pH of gastric contents should be raised with a non-particulate antacid such as sodium citrate. The H_2 antagonists take longer to act, cross the placenta, and pass into breast milk, but seem to be safe. Parenteral antiemetics commonly used are promethazine and promazine.

Nausea and vomiting

These occur most often between the sixth and sixteenth week but may continue in 20 per cent throughout pregnancy. Whether oestrogens act centrally, remains unproven. Neuroregulatory hormones such as the β-lipotrophins (endorphins) bind to opioid receptors in the vomiting centre in the hypothalamus which have been sensitized to β-human choriogonadotropin. The roles of progesterone, cortisol, and thyroxine are controversial. Gastric dysrhythmias have been demonstrated in some manometric and neuroelectrical studies. Risk factors implicated in some studies are smoking, intolerance to oral contraceptive therapy, gallbladder disease, and twin pregnancy. Statistical meta-analyses confirm a small reduction in risk of spontaneous abortion before 20 weeks with gestational vomiting. No statistical association has been found between gestational nausea and vomiting, perinatal mortality, and fetal anomalies.

MANAGEMENT

Persistent vomiting requires full investigation to exclude causes recognized in the non-pregnant population. In the third trimester, vomiting may herald acute liver failure due to fatty liver, HELLP syndrome, and other causes, such as cholecystitis and pancreatitis.

Morning sickness usually improves with reassurance, recourse to small, dry, carbohydrate-rich meals, and avoiding large-volume drinks. Concern over the teratogenic potential of many anti-emetics and sedatives follows the experience of thalidomide. No antiemetic drug is approved specifically for use in early pregnancy. Prescription should be reserved for the exceptional case and only after exclusion of intercurrent disease. Pyridoxine hydrochloride (vitamin B_6) is safe and reduces gestational nausea and vomiting in randomized, controlled trials. Metoclopramide and phenothiazines seem safe but should be used with caution. Extrapyramidal side-effects can occur with these.

HYPEREMESIS GRAVIDARUM

Definition

This diagnosis is made when persistent and severe vomiting occurs before the twentieth week, sufficient to require admission to hospital.

Pathogenesis

Mechanisms are multifactorial. Starvation and dehydration add to the central effects of high levels of oestrogens and a genetic predisposition. Associations are with multiple pregnancy, hydramnios, and hydatidiform mole. Elevated serum levels of aspartate aminotransferase up to four times the upper normal limits occur in 15 to 25 per cent of pregnant women with hyperemesis gravidarum independently of ketonuria. Elevated levels of serum cholesterol, triglycerides, and phospholipids, and alterations in low-density and high-density lipoproteins may reflect the effects of excess oestrogen on the liver. The biochemical abnormalities reverse rapidly with restoration of fluid balance, improved nutrition, and cessation of vomiting. An elevated prothrombin ratio indicates marked cholestasis and vitamin K deficiency.

Management

Symptoms improve following removal from a stressful environment, withdrawal of oral fluids and nutrition, parenteral replacement of fluids, electrolytes, vitamins and nutrition, and parenteral antiemetics with sedative properties, such as promethazine hydrochloride (25–50 mg) given by deep intramuscular injection or intravenously as a 2.5 per cent w/v solution given slowly in a tenfold dilution with sterile water (maximum parenteral dose 100 mg). Correction of weight loss improves fetal outcome. Psychiatric counselling may be beneficial.

Gluten-sensitive enteropathy

Coeliac disease should suspected with a history of delayed menarche, oligomenorrhoea, involuntary infertility, spontaneous abortion, and suspected folate and B_{12} deficiency before indiscriminate supplementation of vitamins. Outcome improves with restoration of normal gut histology following gluten withdrawal.

DIFFERENTIAL DIAGNOSIS

This is wide and includes other small bowel disorders, especially Crohn's disease, infestations and infections such as campylobacteriosis and giardiasis, and AIDS. Duodenal biopsy via fibreoptic gastroduodenoscopy is safe in expert hands. Jejunal biopsy with a capsule and radiological imaging is not recommended in pregnancy.

MANAGEMENT

Strict adherence to a gluten-free diet is essential throughout pregnancy and lactation. Supplementation with vitamin D, folic acid, vitamin B_{12}, iron, and trace metals may be necessary. Failure to respond to gluten withdrawal and clinical relapse should prompt full investigation (see Chapter 14.9.4), especially for inadvertent intake of gluten including as 'fillers' in drugs, and intercurrent infections and infestations such as giardiasis. Dyspepsia and dysphagia may rarely require fibreoptic endoscopy to exclude oesophageal malignancy.

Inflammatory bowel diseases

(See also Section 14.)

These present commonly during the reproductive years. As with coeliac disease, features are protean and the differential diagnosis is wide, especially for Crohn's disease of the small bowel. The differential diagnosis of colitis includes many infections and infestations, vascular disorders, and cocaine abuse.

FERTILITY AND FETAL OUTCOME

Recent large studies reveal a good outcome for pregnancy in all but severe inflammatory bowel disease. Voluntary infertility and male subfertility may prevent pregnancy and amenorrhoea, involuntary infertility, and spontaneous abortion may occur with uncontrolled inflammatory bowel disease, especially Crohn's disease. The risks of spontaneous abortion intrauterine growth retardation, preterm delivery, small-for-dates babies, and fetal distress are increased when Crohn's disease has been active at conception, and following previous surgical resections.

Vaginal discharge and dyspareunia are common and the chance of becoming pregnant seems to be reduced after protocolectomy. Counselling on sexual function can be beneficial.

MATERNAL OUTCOME

A normal outcome is expected in most, including when presentation occurs during pregnancy. Clinical remission is likely following conception during inactive disease. Management is not altered by pregnancy; sulphasalazine or 5-aminosalacylic acid and vitamin supplements, particularly folic acid, should be maintained throughout and during lactation. The risk of kernicterus is minimal. Topical and systemic corticosteroids are used in conventional doses after rigorous exclusion of parasitic infections. Azathioprine and 6-mercaptopurine are not recommended in pregnancy. Metronidazole seems to be non-teratogenic in humans but is best avoided in the first trimester. These drugs should be reserved for severe cases and minimum doses used. Normal fetal outcomes have followed prolonged total parenteral nutrition and elemental diets for extensive inflammatory bowel disease. Full-term vaginal delivery can follow proctocolectomy in pregnancy.

Appendicitis

This is the most common non-obstetric condition requiring surgery in pregnancy. Appendicitis can be mistaken for gestational nausea and vomiting, ectopic pregnancy, abruptio placentae, and ruptured uterus. Perforation may be silent, but maternal and fetal mortalities are increased probably through delay in diagnosis, which can be improved by the use of high-resolution ultrasonography. Appendicectomy can be safe under epidural anaesthesia, but in doubtful cases general anaesthesia and laparotomy may be necessary. Surgery can precipitate pre-term labour.

Infestations

(See also Section 7).

Up to 40 per cent of pregnant women from developing countries carry worms and other infestations. These are prevalent with congenital and acquired immunodeficiency syndromes. Common species are hookworm (*Ankylostoma duodenale, Necator americanus*), whipworm (*Trichuris trichiura*), dwarf tapeworm (*Hymenolepis nana*), roundworm (*Ascaris lumbricoides*), threadworm (*Enterobius vermicularis*), and tapeworm (*Taenia saginata* and *T. solium*). Pregnancy adversely affects parasite burden and clearance in many animal models. Data are lacking in humans. Intrauterine growth retardation is associated with multiple infestations and maternal malnutrition. Purgation should be avoided. Treatment for most parasites can be delayed until after delivery. Maternal malnutrition should be corrected and the diet supplemented with iron, folic acid, and other vitamins.

Colon and rectal disorders

Studies on intestinal transit and motility give conflicting results. Constipation and haemorrhoids are common. A diet high in fibre and fluids and hydrophilic stool bulking agents should improve most cases. Lactulose is almost unabsorbed and seems safe. Haemorrhoidectomy during pregnancy is reserved for severe cases.

The colon can become involved in endometriosis and, following caesarean section, with pseudo-obstruction (Ogilvie's syndrome) and caecal volvulus. Third- and fourth-degree tears and extensive episiotomy repair may injure the anal sphincter and result in subsequent faecal incontinence.

REFERENCES

Diseases of the liver

Burroughs, A.K., Seong, N.H., Dojcinou, D., Scheuer, P.J., and Sherlock, S. (1982). Idiopathic acute fatty liver of pregnancy in 12 patients. *Quarterly Journal of Medicine* **204**, 481–97.

Cheng, Y.-S. (1977). Pregnancy in liver cirrhosis and/or portal hypertension. *American Journal of Obstetrics and Gynecology* **128**, 812–22.

Department of Health and Social Security. (1991). *Report on confidential enquiries into maternal deaths in the United Kingdom 1985–87, pp. 1–161*.

Fagan, E.A. (1994). Disorders of the liver, biliary system and pancreas. In *Medical disorders in obstetric practice*, (ed. M. De Swiet), pp. 000–000. Blackwell Scientific Publications, Oxford.

Jones, E.A. and Bergasa, N.U. (1992). The pruritus of cholestasis and the opioid system. *Journal of the American Medical Association* **268**, 3359–62.

Kirk, E.P. (1991). Organ transplantation and pregnancy. A case report and review. *American Journal of Obstetrics and Gynecology* **164**, 1629–34.

Minakami, H., Oka, N., Sato, T., Tamuda, T., Yasuda, Y., and Hirota, N. (1988). Preeclampsia: a microvesicular fat disease of the liver. *American Journal of Obstetrics and Gynecology* **159**, 1043–7.

Morbidity Mortality Weekly Report (1990). Centers for disease control: Protection against viral hepatitis. Recommendations of the Immunization Practices Advisory Committee. *Morbidity Mortality Weekly Report* **39**, 5–22.

Morbidity Mortality Weekly Report (1991). Update on adult immunization. Recommendations of the Immunization Practices Advisory Committee. *Morbidity Mortality Weekly Report* **RR 12 40**, 33–89.

Reyes, H. (1982). The enigma of intrahepatic cholestasis in pregnancy; lessons from Chile. *Hepatology* **2**, 87–96.

Riely, C.A. (1988). Case studies in jaundice in pregnancy. *Seminars in Liver Disease* **8**, 191–9.

Rolfes, D.B. and Ishak, K.G. (1985). Acute fatty liver of pregnancy: a clinicopathologic study of 35 cases. *Hepatology* **5**, 1149–58.

Rolfes, D.B. and Ishak, K.G. (1986). Liver disease in pregnancy. *Histopathology* **10**, 555–70.

Schorr-Lesnick, B., Lebovics, E., Dworkin, B., and Rosenthal, W.S. (1991). Liver diseases unique to pregnancy. *American Journal of Gastroenterology* **86**, 659–70.

Sibai, B.M. (1990). The HELLP syndrome (hemolysis, elevated liver enzymes, and low platelets): much ado about nothing? *American Journal of Obstetrics and Gynecology* **162**, 311–16.

Stander, H.J. and Cadden, J.F. (1934). Acute yellow atrophy of the liver in pregnancy. *American Journal of Obstetrics and Gynecology* **28**, 61–9.

Svanborg, A. (1954). A study of recurrent jaundice in pregnancy. *Acta Obstetrica et Gynecologica Scandinavica* **33**, 434–44.

Tarnier, M. (1856). Note sur l'état graisseux du foie dans la fièvre puerpérale. *Comptes Réndus Séances et Mémoires Société De Biologie*, Série **III**, 209–14.

Thorling, L. (1955). Jaundice in pregnancy: clinical study. *Acta Medica Scandinavica (Suppl.)* **302**, 1–123.

Weinstein, L. (1982). Syndrome of hemolysis, elevated liver enzymes, and low platelet count; a consequence of hypertension in pregnancy. *American Journal of Obstetrics and Gynecology* **142**, 159–67.

Gastrointenstinal disorders

Brostrom, O. (1990). Prognosis in ulcerative colitis. *Medical Clinics of North America* **74**, 201–18.

Fagan, E.A. (1994). Disorders of the gastrointestinal tract. In *Medical disorders in obstetric practice*, (ed. M. De Swiet), pp. 000–000. Blackwell Scientific Publications, Oxford.

Godsey, R.K. and Newman, R.B. (1991). Hyperemesis gravidarum. A comparison of single and multiple admissions. *Journal of Reproductive Medicine* **36**, 287–90.

Grandien, M., Sterner, G., Kalin, M., and Engardt, L. (1990). Management of pregnant women with diarrhoea at term and of healthy carriers of infectious agents in stools at delivery. *Scandinavian Journal of Infectious Diseases (Suppl.)* **71**, 9–18.

Hudson, M., Flett, G., Sinclair, T.S., Brunt, P.W., Templeton, A., and Mowat, N.A.G. (1993). Fertility and pregnancy in inflammatory bowel disease – a community study of 409 patients in north east Scotland. *Quarterly Journal of Medicine*, in press.

Molteni, N., Bardella, M.T., and Bianchi, P.A. (1990). Obstetric and gynecological problems in women with untreated celiac sprue. *Journal of Clinical Gastroenterology* **12**, 37–9.

Ogorek, C.P. and Cohen, S. (1989). Gastroesophageal reflux disease: new concepts in pathophysiology. *Gastroenterology Clinics of North America* **18**, 275–92.

Singer, A.J. and Brandt, L.J. (1991). Pathophysiology of the gastrointestinal tract during pregnancy. *American Journal of Gastroenterology* **86**, 1695–712.

Villar, J., Klebanoff, M., and Kestler, E. (1989). The effect on fetal growth of protozoan and helminthic infection during pregnancy. *Obstetrics and Gynecology* **74**, 915–20.

13.14 The skin in pregnancy

F. WOJNAROWSKA

The skin undergoes profound changes during pregnancy as a result of the associated endocrine, metabolic, and physiological changes. Some of these are trivial and chiefly cosmetic, producing no or minor symptoms, but others can be distressing and/or of major medical importance. Pregnancy will profoundly modify the expression of pre-existing skin diseases and there are dermatoses which are specific to pregnancy, and which are described in detail below.

Common skin changes in pregnancy

VASCULAR CHANGES AND LESIONS

There is increased skin blood flow during pregnancy and this makes the skin more prone to itch and to oedema, manifest as tightening of rings and shoes. Spider naevi and palmar erythema are common, as are haemangiomas. Pyogenic granuloma, a benign tumour with a tendency to ulcerate and bleed may also develop during pregnancy and often recurs after local destruction.

PIGMENTARY CHANGES AND PIGMENTED LESIONS

There is darkening of the nipples, genitalia, and linea alba. The unsightly and sometimes psychologically distressing facial pigmentation of melasma (chloasma) affects 70 per cent of women; it is worse with intense sunlight and can be reduced by the use of high protection factor (SPF5) sun screens.

Pigmented naevi can increase in number, size, and pigmentation. Melanoma may occur and is associated with a poor prognosis in pregnant women (see Section 23). Any rapidly changing, irregularly shaped, or pigmented moles should be biopsied to exclude a dysplastic naevus or melanoma.

HAIR CHANGES

There is diminished shedding of scalp hair, due to prolongation of anagen, and this is perceived as thicker hair. There is often increased sebum secretion, making the hair more lustrous. The synchronized shedding of hair after parturition gives rise to the distressing postpartum telogen effluvium.

Hirsutism may begin or worsen in pregnancy as there is an associated increase in androgens.

PILOSEBACEOUS CHANGES

The increased oestrogens of pregnancy usually improve acne, but it may worsen in some unfortunate patients and the skin overall is usually greasier.

STRIAE

Striae on the breasts and abdomen are very common in pregnancy, but do not necessarily relate to either the total weight gain or the rate of weight gain. There is much individual variation.

Cutaneous Infections

Candidiasis of the vulva as well as the vagina may occur. Cutaneous and genital warts thrive in pregnancy. Treatment of genital warts is by physical destruction as discussed elsewhere, but podophyllin must not be used in pregnancy (see Chapter 21.7). Active genital herpes simplex infections can pose particular problems at the time of delivery (see Chapter 21.3.

The pregnancy dermatoses

Four major dermatoses occur specifically in pregnancy, and some can be precipitated by it.

PRURITUS OF PREGNANCY

Itching occurs in about 20 per cent of pregnancies. Sometimes this is in association with an inflammatory dermatosis. Often there are no physical signs other than scratch marks but iron deficiency must always be excluded. In about 2 per cent of women itching is related to recurrent cholestasis of pregnancy, when it is termed pruritus gravidarum. The itching of this condition begins in the third trimester and affects the abdomen. There may be a raised plasma alkaline phosphatase. It resolves postpartum, but will recur in subsequent pregnancies.

Management consists of the use of emollients and sometimes antihistamines, of which chlorpheniramine is the one usually recommended for pregnancy. The non-sedating agents are probably ineffective, but if one is to be tried, terfenadine has the best track record in pregnancy.

POLYMORPHIC ERUPTION OF PREGNANCY (PRURITIC URTICATED PAPULES AND PLAQUES OF PREGNANCY)

This dermatosis affects 1 in 240 singleton pregnancies but is more common in multiple births, and is thus seen more often nowadays in the context of in vitro fertilization. It usually begins in the third trimester and occasionally postpartum. It is most common in first pregnancies or the first multiple pregnancy.

The lesions usually begin in the striae on the abdomen and thighs, and then spread to the whole trunk and limbs, including the hands and feet. They consist of raised red papules (Plate 1) and plaques, occasionally polycyclic, and rarely may blister on the lower legs. The itching can be very severe, preventing sleep.

There are minimal changes in the histopathology of affected areas, which usually reveals no more than a few perivascular lymphocytes. Immunofluorescence does not demonstrate any circulating or bound immunoreactants. The aetiology is unknown but the increased frequency in multiple births may relate to the mechanical effect of the abdominal stretching or perhaps to an increase in circulating immune complexes.

Initial treatment is with reassurance and emollients, but this not always sufficient and antihistamines and moderate to very potent topical steroids (see Table 1) or even systemic steroids may be required. There will be significant absorption of potent topical steroids. The condition resolves over days to weeks after delivery and does not usually recur. The outcome of the pregnancy is not adversely affected by the condition.

Table 1 *Examples of topical steroids*

Group	Generic name	Trade names
Mild	Hydrocortisone 1%	Numerous
Potent		
Moderately potent	Hydrocortisone 1% with urea	Alphaderm®, Calmurid HC®
	Clobetasone butyrate	Eumovate®
	Flurandrolone	Haelan®
Potent	Betamethasone valerate	Betnovate-RD®, Betnovate®
	Betamethasone dipropionate	Propaderm®, Diprosalic®, Diprosone®
	Hydrocortisone 17-butyrate	Locoid®
Very potent	Clobetasol propionate	Dermovate®

PRURIGO OF PREGNANCY

This may affect 1 in 300 pregnancies. It begins at the end of the second or beginning of the third trimester. The eruption is scattered over the abdomen and limbs, and comprises excoriated papules. There is intense pruritus. It is essential to make sure that iron deficiency is not a contributing factor. Histopathological examination of biopsied lesions shows a perivascular infiltrate with thickened epidermis. Direct immunofluorescence of the skin and indirect immunofluorescence of the serum are both negative.

Again, treatment is with reassurance and emollients and, if this not sufficient, with antihistamines and moderate to very potent topical steroids or occlusive coal tar or icthopaste bandages, which can be applied to the limbs over topical steroids. The condition resolves in days to weeks after delivery, and does not usually recur.

PEMPHIGOID GESTATIONIS (HERPES GESTATIONIS)

Pemphigoid gestationis is the rarest but most severe of the pregnancy dermatoses. It occurs in 1 in 50 000 pregnancies. The name herpes gestationis is best abandoned as the term herpes refers to the herpetiform grouping of the blisters rather than implying herpes infection. Pemphigoid gestationis commences from the second trimester onwards and quite often as late as in the first week postpartum. It usually occurs in the first and subsequent pregnancies, although there may be skipped pregnancies. A change of partner may initiate pemphigoid gestationis for the first time or, vice versa, lead to the cessation of affected pregnancies.

The eruption begins around the umbilicus and spreads to the whole trunk, limbs, hands, and feet, including the palms and soles, and rarely the face. The mouth and vulva may be involved. The eruption usually begins as an annular red raised plaque around the umbilicus. Later lesions are annular with papules and plaques, and vesicles and blisters are seen (Plate 2). The mucosal lesions may be blisters or erosions. Pruritus is severe and often sleep impossible. Transplacental transmission to the fetus occurs in about 2 per cent of affected pregnancies, when the neonate develops transient self-limiting blisters (Plate 3).

Histopathology demonstrates eosinophilia, subepidermal blisters, and tear-drop vesicles within the epidermis, continuous with the subepidermal blisters. Direct immunofluorescence demonstrates that the C3 component of complement and IgG_1 are bound at the basement membrane zone of the dermoepidermal junction. The patient's serum has circulating IgG_1 basement membrane zone antibodies that bind C3. These immunoreactants are also found at the basement membrane zone of the amnion (Plate 4).

The aetiology is only partially understood. There is an association with tissue type HLA-DR3, HLA-DR4 and with thyroid disease and, less commonly, with other autoimmune disease. The pathogenicity of the circulating basement membrane zone antibodies is demonstrated by the transplacental transmission of the disease. Their target antigens are associated with the hemidesmosome, a structure with a crucial role in adhesion of the epidermis to the dermis. The most common target antigen is a transmembrane molecule of molecular weight 180 kDa and a less common one is intracellular of molecular weight 220 kDa. These antigens are not unique to pemphigoid gestationis but are shared with the other autoimmune blistering diseases in the pemphigoid group. The disease arises only when the mother and fetus are HLA-DR incompatible, explaining the phenomenon of skipped pregnancies and the effect of changing partner. The placentae do show increased expression of antigen-presenting cells, and it is as yet unclear why this breakdown of tolerance occurs, and why a normal component of amnion and stratified squamous epithelium becomes antigenic.

Treatment with potent or very potent topical steroids and chlorpheniramine is sometimes successful, but usually systemic steroids (for example prednisone, 30–60 mg daily) are required. The dose is varied according to disease activity. There is usually a postpartum flare, necessitating an increase in steroid dosage. The disease slowly resolves later postpartum, but often persists for several months. There is an increased incidence of premature births and small-for-dates babies. The classical teaching is that it recurs earlier and is more severe in subsequent pregnancies, but this is certainly not always the case.

Dermatoses in response to pregnancy

Urticaria (hives) and dermographism (wealing in response to pressure, for example scratching) may be precipitated by pregnancy. Erythema multiforme due to pregnancy has been described.

Dermatoses and the effect of pregnancy

ATOPIC ECZEMA

This manifestation of atopy can be severe and not only life ruining but also, if secondary infection with herpes simplex (eczema herpeticum) or Streptococcus occurs, life-threatening. The effect of pregnancy on pre-existing atopic eczema is unpredictable. The immunosuppression of pregnancy can lead to amelioration of the disease. Conversely, the tendency to pruritus may exacerbate atopic eczema, and the pruritus may make life intolerable. The eczema then becomes more widespread and may result in erythroderma in the most severe cases. Secondary infection with *Staphylococcus aureus* and Streptococcus is a frequent complication. The skin is red, dry, and scaly with areas of excoriation and thickening or lichenification (see Section 23).

Treatment is a major problem in pregnancy, as there is a dilemma between balancing the need for treatment with the wish to minimize the use of potent topical steroids which will be absorbed and may affect the fetus. The use of emollients may lessen the requirements for topical steroids, the steroids should be used in the minimum quantities and strengths necessary to control the disease, see Table 1. Many topical steroids contain antiseptics and antibiotics which will be absorbed and several of which are contraindicated in pregnancy (see Chapter 13.16). The sedating antihistamine, chlorpheniramine, may help with sleep. Secondary infection often requires systemic antibiotics, such as erythromycin or flucloxacillin.

PSORIASIS

Psoriasis may improve or deteriorate during pregnancy. Therapy poses special problems. All the systemic treatments are contraindicated; methotrexate is a folic acid antagonist, acitretin is teratogenic, cyclosporin results in intrauterine growth retardation, and psoralens with ultraviolet radiation A are still not proven to be safe. Topical therapy with steroids should be avoided if possible. Coal tars and dithranol have been widely used in pregnancy but are not proven to be safe and the new vitamin D analogue, calcipotriol (Dovonex®) is not licensed for use in pregnancy. The ideal is therefore to use the minimum treatment to render the disease tolerable, ideally with emollients alone and/or UVB and only very reluctantly with topical agents.

A severe form of pustular psoriasis, impetigo herpetiformis, may occur in pregnancy and is again best managed with bed rest and emollients.

AUTOIMMUNE DERMATOSES IN PREGNANCY

Cutaneous lupus erythematosus

Cutaneous lupus erythematosus does not seem either adversely affected or improved by pregnancy. The importance of the diagnosis in relation to pregnancy is that all such patients should be screened for anti-Ro and antiphospholipid antibodies (see Chapter 18.11.3), preferably prior to conception, to identify at-risk pregnancies.

Autoimmune bullous diseases

Linear IgA disease, an autoimmune blistering disease with IgA basement membrane zone antibodies, usually improves with pregnancy, and some patients can discontinue their dapsone therapy. Despite the deposition of immunoreactants in the amnion basement membrane zone, the fetus is not adversely affected. There is usually an exacerbation 3 months postpartum.

Pemphigus vulgaris, an autoimmune blistering disease with widespread mucosal and cutaneous erosions caused by antibodies to desmosomal components, can be transmitted across the placenta, with devastating results to the fetus, but this does not occur in the related pemphigus foliaceus, which is endemic in Brazil.

REFERENCES

Charles-Holmes, R. and Black, M.M. (1990). Herpes gestationis. In *Management of blistering disease*, (ed. F. Wojnarowska and R.A. Briggaman), pp. 93–104. Chapman and Hall, London.

Collier, P., Kelly, S.E., and Wojnarowska, F. (1994). Linear IgA disease and pregnancy. *Journal of the American Academy of Dermatology,* **30,** 407–12.

Graham-Brown, R.A.C. and Ebling, F.G.J. (1992). The ages of man and their dermatoses. In *Textbook of dermatology*, (5th edn), (ed. R.A., Champion, J.L., Burton, and F.G.J. Ebling). pp. 2886–94. Blackwell, Oxford.

Holmes, R.C., *et al.* (1982). A comparative study of toxic erythema of pregnancy and herpes gestationis. *British Journal of Dermatology* **106,** 499–510.

Kelly, S.E. and Wojnarowska, F. (1994). Pemphigoid gestationis. *European Journal of Dermatology,* **4,** 16–20.

Muller, S. and Stanley, J.R. (1990). Pemphigus: pemphigus vulgaris and pemphigus foliaceus. In *Management of blistering disease*, (ed. F. Wojnarowska and R.A. Briggaman), pp. 43–62. Chapman and Hall, London.

13.15 Malignant disease in pregnancy

P. A. PHILIP and A. L. HARRIS

Approximately 13 per cent of cancers in women develop during the child-bearing years and the incidence of cancer in pregnancy is estimated to be 0.07 to 0.1 per cent. The predominant malignancies in pregnant women are those of breast and gynaecological cancer, leukaemia, lymphoma, melanoma, thyroid carcinoma, and colon carcinoma. Although a state of immunological tolerance occurs in pregnancy, accompanied by increased production of female sex hormones and growth factors, there is no evidence of increased frequency of malignant disease in pregnant women. The improvements in the treatment of cancer raise a number of ethical issues in the management of pregnant women with cancer because of the potential serious adverse effects resulting from anticancer therapy.

Interaction between cancer and pregnancy

NATURAL HISTORY OF MALIGNANT DISEASE

The current contention is that the prognosis of malignant tumours, when corrected for stage, is largely unaffected by pregnancy. There is also no evidence of any direct effect of malignant tumours on the developing fetus or placenta.

INFLUENCE OF ANTICANCER THERAPY ON PREGNANCY

Such untoward effects include congenital malformations, intrauterine growth retardation, abortion, premature labour, and carcinogenesis. Major congenital malformations appear to occur in no more than 3 per cent of all births in the general population, yet such deformities have been reported in infants of 17 to 23 per cent of patients who received combination chemotherapy. Essentially, all such abnormalities were in the offspring of patients treated with antifolates during the first trimester. Malformations have been reported to occur in approximately 1.5 per cent after chemotherapy during the second and/or third trimester of pregnancy. Alkylating agents (such as cyclophosphamide) have also been linked to fetal malformations in approximately 14 per cent of the cases when treatment was administered in the first trimester of pregnancy. Anthracyclines and vinca alkaloids appear to be devoid of any significant teratogenic effect. Of the immunomodulators, interferons have been shown not to be associated with any fetal malformations. Existing evidence does not indicate that intrauterine exposure to chemotherapy has any late detrimental effects on children after their birth.

Radiation therapy undoubtedly causes damage to embryo and fetus. The severity is dependent on the dose received by the fetus and the stage of pregnancy. The period of organogenesis is most sensitive to radiation and small doses given then may result in severe defects. The fetus may be exposed to radiation through scatter and the amount received depends on its distance from the centre of the irradiated field, the size of the irradiated field, and the energy of radiation. The risk of irreversible harm increases significantly at doses of radiation to fetus exceeding 10 Gy. The combination of irradiation and cytotoxic therapy is considered to be particularly teratogenic.

Management of cancer patients in pregnancy

GENERAL PRINCIPLES

Assessment of the extent of disease (staging) should be undertaken after diagnosis without any delay. A multidisciplinary approach should be adopted in order to try to provide comprehensive anticancer therapy and the delivery of a healthy infant. The team will best include a medical oncologist, a radiation therapist, an oncological surgeon or gynaecologist, an obstetrician, and a neonatologist. The clinical stage of breast cancer at the time of diagnosis is known to be important in prognosis. Proper staging of disease involves the judicious use of imaging investigations to avoid harming the fetus. Sonography and magnetic resonance imaging (MRI) can be used to assess the abdomen and pelvis in pregnant patients with relatively low risk to the fetus, although the safety of MRI has not been firmly established. Computed tomographic (CT) scans and isotope studies are relatively contraindicated in pregnant women because of the teratogenic effect of ionizing radiation on fetal tissues.

The primary treatment of the majority of tumours remains surgical. Additional therapy in the form of either radiation or systemic drug therapy may be necessary to improve local tumour control and/or long-term survival. Cytotoxic therapy is indicated for patients with haematological or lymphoid malignancies and those with metastatic solid tumours. The mother and family should be informed of the possible early and delayed effects of antineoplastic drugs. The treatment strategy adopted in a given patient will depend on the type of the tumour, stage and tumour growth rate, and the trimester of pregnancy. Chemotherapy should be given in full dose, trying to avoid drugs which cause teratogenesis at an increased frequency. Diagnosis of malignancy during the pregnancy may necessitate a therapeutic abortion or elective delivery before term which should be considered in every case, according to individual circumstances and the wishes of the patient. Early termination of pregnancy allows the best management of rapidly progressing tumours which require treatment conveying high risk to the fetus, while treatment of those with slowly growing tumours may be reasonably delayed until it is possible to deliver a mature fetus.

Labour should proceed normally but may be complicated by abnormal bleeding or sepsis because of myelosuppression due to cytotoxic therapy. Babies should be examined carefully for any congenital malformations and other effects of cytotoxic therapy. It should be emphasized that exposure to irradiation or chemotherapy during the first trimester is not inevitably associated with an adverse outcome for the fetus. Breast feeding is contraindicated in patients receiving cytotoxic therapy because these drugs may reach significantly high levels in breast milk and cause neonatal myelosuppression.

CERVICAL CARCINOMA

Cervical carcinoma is the most common malignancy complicating pregnancy. Approximately 1 in every 30 newly diagnosed cases of invasive cervical cancer will occur while the patient is pregnant. There is evidence that pregnant women are more likely to present with early disease because of regular, pregnancy-related obstetric examinations. Pregnancy does not adversely affect the survival of women with invasive cervical cancer. Unfortunately, the treatment modalities used for this disease directly interfere with the maintenance of pregnancy. Although it has been customary to treat pregnant women with cervical cancer with radiotherapy recent evidence suggests that radical hysterectomy with bilateral pelvic lymph node resection for early disease is associated with acceptable morbidity and survival with preservation of ovarian function. Treatment in some patients may be delayed to achieve fetal maturity, if the diagnosis of cervical cancer is made in the late second or third trimester.

BREAST CANCER

Only 1 to 2 per cent of breast cancers are diagnosed during pregnancy or lactation. In women under 40 years of age, 8 to 11 per cent of breast cancers are diagnosed during pregnancy. There is too little evidence to suggest that hormone changes are solely responsible for the relatively poor prognosis of pregnant women with breast carcinoma. Such tumours tend to be oestrogen-receptor negative and it is not clear whether this represents a real absence of steroid receptors or an artefact arising from increased binding of the existing receptors because of the high circulating levels of oestrogens. Delays in the diagnosis of breast carcinoma in pregnant women are to be expected because the engorged breast obscures an otherwise palpable mass, and it has been demonstrated that pregnant women have a 2.5-fold higher risk of being diagnosed with advanced breast cancer and a decreased chance of diagnosis of stage I disease. A recent study of 407 women showed that there was a 3.3-fold increase in risk of dying from breast cancer, for those whose tumours were diagnosed in pregnancy compared to those who were never pregnant. This risk decreased as the interval from previous pregnancy to diagnosis increased, being evident at 1 year after pregnancy (1.9-fold risk) and 2 to 5 years later (1.1-fold risk), but not after 5 years.

Mammography is of limited value in diagnosing breast carcinoma in pregnant women because the increased radiographic density of the breasts during pregnancy and lactation. Although biopsy of breast lump is the mainstay of diagnosis of carcinoma, fine-needle aspiration is increasingly becoming a very useful mode of diagnosis in expert hands with negligible morbidity to the patients.

Many authorities would advocate treatment by modified radical mastectomy which obviates the need for adjuvant breast irradiation. Breast preservation techniques, which always require adjuvant radiotherapy, are not advisable in gestational breast cancer, unless treatment is undertaken late in pregnancy when radiation can be delayed until after delivery. Therapeutic abortion is no longer considered to be an essential component of the treatment of breast cancer during pregnancy unless the mother chooses it. Adjuvant chemotherapy significantly improves the survival of premenopausal women with axillary nodal metastases; patients with breast cancer in early pregnancy who would benefit from adjuvant chemotherapy should therefore be given the following options: to terminate pregnancy and proceed with chemotherapy; to delay treatment until the second trimester; or to proceed with chemotherapy but without antimetabolites. Some patients presenting with locally advanced breast carcinoma may require chemotherapy prior to surgery (neoadjuvant) to reduce the tumour bulk. In such instances termination of pregnancy is advisable to allow maximum therapeutic benefit. Babies delivered to women treated for breast cancer during pregnancy are more likely to be preterm and small for gestational age.

In advanced disease, decisions about treatment must be given according to individual circumstances as with early-stage disease. Strategy depends particularly on the trimester of pregnancy, as well as the patient's wishes. Little is known so far about the long-term use of hormonal treatment (such as tamoxifen) during pregnancy.

OVARIAN CARCINOMA

Carcinoma of ovary is relatively rare in pregnancy. Laparotomy for staging, subsequent surgical excision of tumours, and combination chemotherapy is the recommended therapy for ovarian cancer.

LEUKAEMIA

Leukaemia is rare during pregnancy, but when it occurs it is often detected in the course of routine antenatal care. Acute lymphoblastic leukaemia, acute myeloid leukaemia, and chronic myelogenous leukaemia are the varieties encountered during pregnancy and a significant proportion of those patients are potentially curable. Pregnancy itself does not appear to have an adverse effect on the prospects for cure either in patients with acute leukaemia or those with chronic myelogenous leukaemia. Antifolates, such as methotrexate, should be avoided during the first trimester of pregnancy because of their teratogenic potential. However, the use of cytarabine and anthracyclines, the important components in the treatment of patients with acute myeloid leukaemia, has not been associated with any increased incidence of birth defects. Other common complications of intensive therapy of acute leukaemias, such as bleeding or infection, undoubtedly increase the risk of spontaneous abortion or premature birth and may complicate delivery.

LYMPHOMAS

Lymphomas are the fourth most frequent malignant neoplasms in pregnant women. Hodgkin's disease is commoner during pregnancy than non-Hodgkin's lymphoma, since the median age at diagnosis of the latter is 42 years. Pregnancy does not influence the course of either Hodgkin's disease or non-Hodgkin's lymphoma. The stage of the disease determines the appropriate approach to treatment, radiotherapy and/or chemotherapy. Staging of the disease during pregnancy is mainly dependent on clinical findings, supplemented by bone marrow examination and a limited radiological study. Laparotomy to assess abdominal involvement should be avoided during pregnancy. Localized disease may be treated with radiotherapy. In patients with Hodgkin's disease, if systemic therapy is indicated during the first trimester, vinblastine may be given as a single agent with minimal risk to the fetus, whereas in patients with non-Hodgkin's lymphoma combination therapy offers the only chance of long-term cure. Beyond the first trimester, appropriate therapy may be given as for non-pregnant woman except for localized subdiaphragmatic disease.

MALIGNANT MELANOMA

The thickness of the lesion is a major determinant of prognosis in malignant melanoma and has been shown to be greater in tumours diagnosed during pregnancy. Delays in diagnosis and increased levels of circulating hormones and growth factors have been postulated as reasons for the greater thickness of melanoma in pregnancy. There is, however, no evidence for a direct growth stimulatory effect on melanoma cells by oestrogens. Current evidence therefore does not support termination of pregnancy as part of the treatment of patients with malignant melanoma. Recent studies have concluded that the disease-free interval is shorter in pregnant women with melanoma, due to early lymphatic spread, but is not reflected by reduced survival. Chemotherapy plays little role in the management of advanced disease. Therapy with interleukin-2 results in durable objective responses in a small proportion of patients but no data are available yet on its safety in pregnancy.

PREGNANCY AFTER TREATMENT OF MALIGNANCY

A proportion of women who have received chemotherapy will be infertile. In those who are not, it is generally recommended that pregnancy should be delayed until 2 to 3 years after the treatment of the primary tumour, especially in those patients who are at a high risk of tumour relapse, who should be advised to defer childbearing until after the period of greatest risk of recurrence. There is, however, no evidence that a new pregnancy in patients with a history of any malignancy is likely to increase the risk of tumour relapse, nor is there any evidence of significant increase in the risk of malignant neoplasms in the offspring of such women. The major facts to consider therefore when such a women contemplates pregnancy must be her individual prognosis and the perceived wish of her ultimately leaving a young family without a mother. This is a decision for the patient herself to make, albeit with expert advice.

REFERENCES

Baer, M.R., *et al.* (1992). Interferon-alpha therapy during pregnancy in chronic myelogenous leukaemia and hairy cell leukaemia. *British Journal of Haematology* **81,** 167–9.

Beeley, L. (1986). Adverse effects of drugs in the first trimester of pregnancy. *Clinical Obstetrics* and *Gynecology* **13,** 177–95.

Bottles, K. and Taylor, R.N. (1985). Diagnosis of breast masses in pregnant and lactating women by aspiration cytology. *Obstetrics* and *Gynecology* **66,** (Suppl. 3), 76S–78S.

Brent, R.L. (1989). The effect of embryonic and fetal exposure to x-ray, microwaves, and ultrasound: counselling the pregnant and nonpregnant patient about these risks. *Seminars in Oncology* **16,** 347–68.

Caligiuri, M.A. and Mayer, R.J. (1989). Pregnancy and leukemia. *Seminars in Oncology* **16,** 388–96.

Creasman, W.T., *et al.* (1971). Carcinoma of the cervix associated with pregnancy. *Obstetrics* and *Gynecology* **36,** 495–501.

Danforth, D.N. (1991). How subsequent pregnancy affects outcome in women with a prior breast cancer. *Oncology* **5,** 23–30.

Doll, D.C., *et al.* (1989). Antineoplastic agents and pregnancy. *Seminars in Oncology* **16,** 337–46.

Early Breast Cancer Trialists' Collaborative Group (1992). Systemic treatment of early breast cancer by hormonal, cytotoxic, or immune therapy. *Lancet* **339,** 1–15, 71–85.

Greene, F.L. (1988). Gestational breast cancer: a ten-year experience. *Southern Medical Journal* **81,** 1509–11.

Guinee, V.F., *et al.* (1994). Effect of pregnancy on prognosis for young women with breast cancer. *Lancet,* **343,** 1587–9.

Hass, J.F. (1984). Pregnancy in association with a newly diagnosed cancer. A population based epidemiologic assessment. *Cancer* **34,** 229–35.

Hopkins, M.P. and Morley, G.W. (1992). The prognosis and management of cervical cancer associated with pregnancy. *Obstetrics* and *Gynecology* **80,** 9–13.

Hornstein, E., *et al.* (1982). The management of breast carcinoma in pregnancy and lactation. *Journal of Surgical Oncology* **21,** 179–82.

MacKie, R.M., *et al.* (1991). Lack of effect of pregnancy on outcome of melanoma. *Lancet* **337,** 653–5.

Monk, B.J. and Montz, F.J. (1992). Invasive cervical cancer complicating intrauterine pregnancy: Treatment with radical hysterectomy. *Obstetrics* and *Gynecology* **80,** 199–203.

Nantel, S., *et al.* (1990). Treatment of an aggressive non-Hodgkin's lymphoma during pregnancy with MACOP-B chemotherapy. *Medical and Pediatric Oncology* **18,** 143–5.

Nisce, L.Z., *et al.* (1986). Management of coexisting Hodgkin's disease and pregnancy. *American Journal of Clinical Oncology* **9,** 146–51.

Slingluff, C.L. and Seigler, H.F. (1992). Malignant melanoma and pregnancy. *Annals of Plastic Surgery* **28,** 95–9.

Woo, S.Y., *et al.* (1992). Radiotherapy during pregnancy for clinical stages IA-IIA Hodgkin's disease. *International Journal of Radiation Oncology–Biology–Physics* **23,** 407–12.

Zemlickis, D., *et al.* (1992). Fetal outcome after *in utero* exposure to cancer chemotherapy. *Archives of Internal Medicine* **152,** 573–6.

Zemlickis, D., *et al.* (1992). Maternal and fetal outcome after breast cancer in pregnancy. *American Journal of Obstetrics and Gynecology* **166,** 781–7.

13.16 Prescribing in pregnancy

P. C. RUBIN

INTRODUCTION

Safe and effective prescribing during pregnancy requires an awareness of what drugs can do to the fetus and of what pregnancy can do to drugs. Concern naturally centres on the possible harm which drugs may cause to the developing fetus, but it is sometimes overlooked that pregnancy can produce clinically important changes in drug disposition. While knowledge in most therapeutic areas has grown rapidly in recent decades, information on the use of drugs in pregnancy has developed sporadically, with case reports being more usual than large, prospective clinical trials. The reasons are not surprising and largely relate to concern about causing harm to the developing fetus.

Thalidomide is a name inescapably associated with prescribing in pregnancy. Drug-induced fetal abnormality did not begin with thalidomide: Hippocrates appeared to recognize that drugs were best avoided in the first trimester. However, the scale of the thalidomide tragedy brought to the general public for the first time the realization that drugs could harm the developing baby. Thalidomide was marketed in Germany in 1956 and subsequently in other countries as a sedative and hypnotic which had the particular attraction of being safe in overdose. Indeed, the drug was considered so safe that in some countries it was available without prescription. Then in 1960 to 1961 Germany experienced what amounted to an epidemic of phocomelia: a birth defect involving absence of the long bones with hands and feet being attached directly to the trunk. What had previously been an extremely rare condition (no cases had been reported in the 10 years to 1959) was being seen almost commonly. Various causes—viral, radioactivity, food preservatives—were considered as culprits until one doctor retrospectively questioned his patients and found that 20 per cent had taken thalidomide in early pregnancy. On repeat questioning, asking specifically about the drug, 50 per cent admitted taking thalidomide, many having not mentioned it before since the drug was so obviously innocent. In fact, around 80 per cent of women who took thalidomide in the first trimester had a deformed baby. More than 10 000 such babies had been born before the drug was removed from the market.

The thalidomide experience had far-reaching ramifications. Drug regulation as we know it stems largely from the disaster. Doctors and their patients recognized that there is no such thing as a safe drug. In addition, the pharmaceutical industry has largely avoided obtaining systematic information on drug use in pregnancy. The reasons are obvious and understandable, but for the prescribing doctor the statement that 'the safety of this drug in pregnancy has not been established' is not helpful when faced with a woman who is, or may become, pregnant. A drug is unlikely to be studied comprehensively during pregnancy unless it is known to be safe, and its safety cannot be definitely established unless large studies have been performed. Thus information tends to accumulate through inadvertent use when pregnancy is not suspected, or intentional use in a few cases here and there when the risks of the disease being treated are considered to outweigh any possible harm from the drug. Therapeutic management decisions must frequently be made with the help of limited information.

The effect of drugs on the fetus

A drug can harm the fetus only if it crosses the placenta, but most drugs do. The placenta offers a lipid barrier to the transfer of drugs. The rate at which a drug crosses from mother to baby will depend on its lipophilicity and polarity. However, with the exception of drugs administered acutely around the time of delivery, the rate of transfer is of little importance, and for any course of drug treatment it should be assumed that transfer will occur. The only notable exception is heparin, a molecule of such size and polarity that it does not cross to the fetus.

Drugs can adversely affect the developing fetus in different ways depending on the gestation at which exposure occurs. For this reason it is appropriate to consider organogenesis, fetal growth and development, the breast-fed infant, and childhood growth and development separately.

Prescribing in the first trimester

Organogenesis occurs between 18 and 55 days of gestation and it is during this time that drugs can cause anatomical defects. Some drugs that are definitely teratogenic in the human are listed in Table 1. A drug can cause a teratogenic effect only if it is present in the embryo during organogenesis. Even a definite teratogen will not cause a structural defect if it is given following this period. These seemingly obvious statements become relevant in pre-pregnancy counselling and in providing advice when exposure to a possible teratogen has occurred during pregnancy. Being present in the embryo during organogenesis is not necessarily synonymous with being prescribed during this period. The retinoids are stored in adipose tissue and released slowly, so a teratogenic effect can occur many weeks after the course of treatment has been completed.

It is important to recognize that these drugs will not be teratogenic in all cases: on the contrary, most first trimester exposures will not harm the baby. The risk of fetal malformation following anticonvulsant use in the first trimester is between 5 and 10 per cent. Figures vary widely with regard to warfarin, abnormality rates from 2 to 25 per cent being quoted in different studies. Lithium is teratogenic in very few exposures, while the retinoids carry a very substantial risk. Figures are not available for danazol. Clearly there is more to drug-induced fetal abnormality than simply the drug. Some reports have claimed a direct relationship between dose and fetal abnormality. While some studies have shown a trend in this direction, the dose does not seem to be a prominent factor in human therapeutics, since epileptic women receiving anticonvulsants have been reported to 'run true' in successive pregnancies. If the first pregnancy ended with a normal baby, subsequent ones often (but not always) do so as well and vice versa.

Many of the abnormalities caused by these drugs can be detected by detailed ultrasound scanning at 18 weeks' gestation. However, the defects caused by warfarin involve mainly soft tissue and do not fall into this category.

Table 1 is not comprehensive and includes only those drugs encountered in general medical practice. Some drugs used in specialist areas are teratogenic, for example several drugs used in cancer chemotherapy (see Section 6). Many more drugs may be teratogenic in a small percentage of exposures, but definitive information is not available because both prediction and detection of human teratogens is difficult. Predicting the effect of a drug in the human usually depends on studying its pharmacology in experimental animals. This is not fruitful in the area of teratogenesis because species variation is so great. For example, thalidomide is a teratogen only in primates, while lithium causes cardiac abnormalities in humans at doses that produce no effect in the rat. Detecting teratogenic effects is complicated by the normal occurrence

Table 1 *Some commonly used drugs that are known to be teratogenic*

Drug	Abnormality
Phenytoin	Craniofacial
Carbamazepine	Limb/fingernail
	Cardiac
Sodium valproate	Neural tube
Warfarin	Chondrodysplasia punctata
	Facial anomalies
	CNS anomalies
Lithium	Cardiac (Ebstein complex)
Danazol	Virilization of female fetus
Retinoids	Multiple

of fetal abnormalities in around 2 per cent of babies. If a drug is teratogenic very occasionally, it can be very difficult to distinguish its effects from naturally occurring defects without a very sophisticated surveillance system. Information on drug-induced fetal abnormality comes from case reports, case studies, and epidemiological studies.

Case reports are a two-edged sword. Describing a single association between a drug and a fetal abnormality can be very useful in first identifying a real problem: warfarin was first linked to teratogenesis in this way. However, the problem with case reports is that they may be showing nothing more than a chance association, and caution must be exercised in their interpretation. Case studies are more secure in that they describe several patients where the same drug and malformation were linked: phenytoin and the retinoids were found to be teratogenic in this way. Epidemiological studies are of two major types: cohort studies which prospectively study exposed and unexposed groups, and case-control studies which retrospectively compare the pregnancies of abnormal and normal offspring. So far as teratogenesis is concerned, case-control studies are the norm because of the size and expense of cohort studies. The relationship between diethylstilboestrol use in the first trimester and vaginal adenocarcinoma in teenage offspring was found in a case-control study.

Among drugs that might be prescribed in the first trimester, those used in the treatment of nausea and vomiting and those used to prevent malaria deserve special mention because they illustrate important principles.

Antiemetic drugs in the first trimester

Most cases of morning sickness do not require treatment. However, some do and the drug about which most information is available was withdrawn from the market in 1983 in view of mounting public concern about its safety. This drug was a mixture of doxylamine succinate and pyridoxine hydrochloride and was marketed as Debendox® or Bendectin®. Despite having been used by over 30 million pregnant women over a quarter of a century, and notwithstanding carefully designed clinical trials suggesting that the drug was not teratogenic, individual case reports linking the use of the drug to fetal abnormality were given considerable publicity and led to its withdrawal. In view of the extremely high number of exposures, many chance associations between drug use and fetal abnormality were inevitable. Among possible alternatives, promethazine, cyclizine, or metoclopramide appear not to be teratogenic in the human.

The Debendox® saga illustrated that in an emotional area such as the use of drugs during pregnancy, well-chosen and carefully presented anecdotes can be more powerful than a substantial body of scientific data carefully accumulated over many years.

Malarial prophylaxis

Proguanil has a long record of safe use in pregnancy. However, in some areas use of chloroquine or a pyrimethamine/sulphonamide combination is necessary because of proguanil resistance. Currently available evidence suggests that chloroquine may cause a very small increase in birth defects: in one study 169 infants whose mothers took chloroquine base 300 mg once weekly were compared with 454 children whose mothers took no drug. The treated group gave rise to 1.2 per cent abnormal babies compared to 0.9 per cent in the controls: not a significant difference, but the study was too small to detect anything less than a five-fold increase in abnormality rate. Pyrimethamine/sulphonamide has not been associated with abnormality in the human but, being a folate antagonist, the possibility exists. In contrast to these minimal or theoretical risks, malaria presents a major risk to the health and life of both mother and baby, particularly when an expatriate woman is travelling in an endemic area.

While no one wishes to cause harm to the baby by prescribing a drug during pregnancy, equally it is important that harm does not befall mother or baby because treatment has been withheld.

Prescribing later in pregnancy

Beyond organogenesis, the fetus undergoes growth and development. The scope for producing anatomical defects has largely gone, exceptions being premature closure of the ductus arteriosus caused by indomethacin and bleeding into the fetal brain produced by warfarin. Growth and function tend to be the targets of drug adverse effects for the remainder of the pregnancy.

Angiotensin converting enzyme (ACE) inhibitors

The use of ACE inhibitors during the second and third trimesters has repeatedly been associated with oligohydramnios and neonatal anuria. Some series have put the perinatal mortality as high as 10 per cent, although over-reporting of poor outcomes has probably inflated this figure. None the less, a clear trend towards fetal or neonatal renal impairment when ACE inhibitors are used during pregnancy has been demonstrated. The mechanism is not known, but it seems probable that angiotensin II is necessary for fetal renal function. These drugs should not ordinarily be used in pregnancy. However, since ACE inhibitors are often used in the younger hypertensive, it is not uncommon to find a woman who has taken one through the first few weeks of pregnancy. This is not a reason for termination of pregnancy, but a detailed scan should be performed to exclude a rare skull ossification defect which may be associated with ACE inhibitors, and the woman should then be transferred to another drug, such as methyldopa.

Aspirin

Low-dose aspirin may prevent or delay pre-eclampsia in some women but may also lead to a small increase in the incidence of placental abruption. It is likely that low-dose aspirin exerts its platelet inhibiting effect entirely within the maternal portal circulation and is then metabolized in the liver with little active drug reaching the systemic circulation. Analgesic doses of aspirin have been shown to produce haemostatic problems in both mother and baby when given near the end of pregnancy. The problem seems to occur mainly when aspirin in a total dose of between 5 and 10 mg is given within 5 days before delivery. Under these circumstances a majority of mothers and almost all babies show some evidence of a bleeding tendency: in the newborn this can manifest as haematuria, cephalhaematoma, or subconjunctival haemorrhage. Since it is never quite clear when pregnancy will end, paracetamol is preferred as a mild analgesic in the third trimester.

Anticoagulants

The clinical use of anticoagulants during pregnancy is fully described in Chapter 13.5. In addition to its teratogenic effects, warfarin has been associated with central nervous system abnormalities, such as microcephaly, when used later in the pregnancy. Bleeding into the fetal brain appears to be at least one mechanism and the problem occurs more commonly in women taking higher doses of warfarin.

Heparin does not harm the fetus, but is potentially damaging to the mother because of increased bone resorption. Osteoporosis has been recognized as a complication of heparin therapy for many years. The problem is not confined to pregnancy, but many of the reports have involved obstetric cases. The osteoporosis is dose related and typically occurs in a woman who has received more than 15 000 units/day of heparin for more than 6 months. The condition can be severe and lead to vertebral collapse.

Anticonvulsants

A neonatal coagulation defect has been associated with the use of phenytoin and barbiturates. The disorder occurs earlier than haemorrhagic disease of the newborn, usually within 24 h of birth, and can be serious. The condition has similarities to vitamin K deficiency and is accompanied by low concentrations of clotting factors II, VII, IX and X together with an increased concentration of a protein induced by the absence of vitamin K (PIVKA). Administration of vitamin K to the mother for 2 weeks prior to delivery has been reported to prevent the neonatal coagulation defect.

Indomethacin

Prostaglandins are involved in maintaining patency of the ductus arteriosus, and indomethacin has been shown to produce premature closure of the ductus. When indomethacin is given during pregnancy it is usually either for the suppression of preterm labour or in the management of rheumatoid arthritis. Echocardiographic studies of the fetal vasculature when indomethacin is being given for preterm labour have shown that ductal constriction can occur in 50 per cent of cases and appears within 12 h of drug administration. The constriction reverses within 24 h of indomethacin being discontinued. These findings suggest that when it is being used in the third trimester in the management of arthritis indomethacin should be discontinued at least 24 h before delivery. However, since it is never entirely clear when labour will begin, it is preferable to avoid indomethacin in the last weeks of pregnancy if possible.

β-Adrenoceptor antagonists and agonists

β-Blockers are used in pregnancy in the management of hypertensive diseases (see Chapter 13.2), tachyarrhythmias, hypertrophic obstructive cardiomyopathy, and migraine. When given for relatively short periods of a few weeks these drugs have been found to lower maternal blood pressure with no adverse consequences for fetus or neonate. However, longer administration from early in pregnancy is associated in around 25 per cent of cases with intrauterine growth retardation, which can sometimes be severe. Methyldopa, which has a good safety record in pregnancy, is therefore the preferred drug in the management of essential hypertension during pregnancy.

β-Receptor agonists are used in the management of asthma and also in the suppression of preterm labour. A rare but potentially fatal association with the use of parenteral salbutamol or ritodrine in the management of preterm labour is maternal pulmonary oedema. Among various possible predisposing factors, fluid overload and the concomitant use of corticosteroids to accelerate fetal lung maturity are the most important. When β-receptor agonists are being used in preterm labour, the volume of fluid administered should be kept to a minimum and dextrose rather than saline should be used. Patients should be carefully monitored for the development of pulmonary oedema.

Corticosteroids

There are both maternal and fetal indications for the use of steroids during pregnancy. Women with conditions such as asthma, inflammatory bowel disease, or systemic lupus erythematosus, for instance, some-

times require therapy with prednisolone, as do those who have received a renal transplant. Betamethasone is used to accelerate fetal lung maturity in cases of spontaneous preterm labour or when early delivery is being performed because of worsening maternal disease, such as pre-eclampsia. There is no evidence that steroids are teratogenic in the human or that they significantly disturb the fetal hypothalamo-pituitary–adrenal axis. Suggestions that steroids can cause cleft palate are based on studies in rabbits and have never been confirmed in many human exposures. So far as the fetal adrenal is concerned, steroids vary in the extent to which they reach the fetal circulation. However, even those, such as betamethasone, which cross the placenta in sufficient amount to achieve a pharmacological effect on the fetal lung have been shown to have only a very transient effect on neonatal glucocorticoid levels, which become normal by 2 h following delivery.

Drugs and breast feeding

Most women now elect to breast feed their babies, and the majority will take a drug during this time. Iron, mild analgesics, antibiotics, laxatives, and hypnotics are the most commonly used. Much work has been performed on the pharmacokinetic aspects of breast feeding, but systematic studies on the effect of drug ingestion by the mother on her breast-fed baby are lacking.

Milk consists of fat globules suspended in an aqueous solution of protein and nutrients. Drugs move from plasma to milk by passive diffusion of the unionized and non-protein-bound fraction. Since breast milk has a slightly lower pH than plasma, drugs which cross most extensively into breast milk are lipid-soluble, poorly protein-bound, weak bases. However, even for drugs that do cross readily into breast milk, considerable dilution has already occurred in the mother. Thus when the concentration of a drug in breast milk and the volume of the milk consumed by the baby are translated into a dose it is often the case that the baby receives too little drug to have any detectable pharmacological effect. Some of the more commonly used drugs that, on the basis of experience, have a good safety record in breast-feeding mothers are listed in Table 2.

It will be seen from this that many of the drugs that would be indicated for common medical problems in a breast-feeding mother are safe to use. Some qualification is needed about two of the drugs listed in the table. Oestrogen-containing oral contraceptives may suppress lactation if they are taken before the milk supply is well established and in some women may do so even after this time. Progestogen-only contraceptives do not influence lactation at any stage. Metronidazole is not harmful to the baby but is said to make the milk taste bitter and may therefore interfere with feeding.

Some drugs have been shown to affect the baby when ingested in breast milk; they are listed in Table 3. There are several drugs for which theoretical risks exist, or for which isolated reports of serious adverse consequences have appeared. For example, aspirin is contraindicated in young children because of the possible association with Reye's syndrome and some authorities consider that the drug should therefore be avoided in women who are breast feeding. No evidence is available to support this view, but unless the use of aspirin is considered essential in a breast-feeding woman (and such an eventuality must be rare) then it is probably best avoided. Similarly, indomethacin has been associated with a neonatal convulsion in one case when used during lactation: a decision with regard to its appropriateness in any given patient would depend on the likelihood of real benefit accruing from its use.

Behavioural teratology

The most obvious consequences of a drug-induced fetal abnormality occur at or shortly after birth in the form of anatomical defects, and studies in teratology have largely concentrated on immediate pregnancy outcome. None the less, drugs can on occasion cause problems that

Table 2 *Some drugs that have been used in breast-feeding women without evidence of harm to the baby*

β-Blockers
Bronchodilators (inhaled)
Carbamazepine
Carbimazole (high doses may suppress neonatal thyroid)
Codeine
Corticosteroids
Digoxin
Heparin
H_2 antagonists
Methyldopa
Metronidazole
Opioids (therapeutic administration)
Oral contraceptives
Paracetamol
Penicillins
Phenytoin
Propylthiouracil (high dose may suppress neonatal thyroid)
Sodium valproate
Tricyclic antidepressants
Warfarin

Table 3 *Some drugs that may be harmful to the baby when used in breast-feeding women*

Amiodarone: risk from release of iodine
Barbiturates: drowsiness
Benzodiazepines: lethargy and weight loss
Iodine: risk of neonatal hypothyroidism
Laxatives: diarrhoea
Lithium: hypotonia, lethargy, cyanosis
Phenobarbitone: drowsiness

become manifest only after several years. The most striking example is diethylstilboestrol which, when given during early pregnancy, can lead to adenocarcinoma of the vagina in the teenage offspring. In addition to late morphological effects, concern has been expressed that drugs given during pregnancy can influence behavioural development, although the available evidence is to the contrary.

Anticonvulsants

Several studies have claimed that the use of anticonvulsants during pregnancy is associated with impaired intellectual development of the children, but it is difficult to carry out studies in this area and the choice of control group is crucially important. When all children of treated epileptic mothers in a single hospital in Finland were studied prospectively, using the offspring of untreated epileptic mothers of the same social class as controls, no difference was found in intellectual development at the age of 5.5 years. At present it appears likely that, in the absence of any obvious morphological abnormality at birth, anticonvulsant use during pregnancy is not associated with impairment of intellectual development.

Antihypertensive drugs

One of the earliest trials into the treatment of hypertension during pregnancy involved a comparison of methyldopa with no treatment. The children underwent physical and psychomotor assessment at 4 and 7.5 years. The 4-year-old children from the treatment group had slightly smaller head circumference than their untreated controls, but there was no other physical or psychomotor difference. The evaluation at 7.5 years revealed no differences between the two groups. It is largely on this very

well-conducted study that the reputation of methyldopa as a safe drug in pregnancy is based.

The effects on childhood development of atenolol and placebo have similarly shown no detrimental effects, a wide range of physical and psychomotor tests being performed on the children at the ages of 1 and 6 years.

Influence of pregnancy on dose requirements

While the emphasis on what drugs can do to the pregnancy is both understandable and appropriate, the physiological changes of pregnancy can have a clinically important influence on drug disposition and effect. The plasma concentrations of some drugs fall to a clinically important extent during pregnancy.

Among the many physiological changes in pregnancy, the most important from the standpoint of drugs are those that influence clearance. By the third trimester renal blood flow has nearly doubled and the activity of some, but not all, liver metabolic pathways is increased during pregnancy. A further factor tending to reduce drug concentrations is an increase in body water, with around an additional 7 litres being retained by the end of pregnancy.

The importance of these changes is well illustrated by the influence of pregnancy on anticonvulsant dose requirements. The concentrations of phenytoin, carbamazepine, phenobarbitone, and sodium valproate all decrease as pregnancy progresses. An increase in systemic clearance is the main reason—for example the clearance of phenytoin increases by over 100 per cent by the third trimester—with an increased volume of distribution making a further contribution. An example of the influence of pregnancy on the concentration of phenytoin is shown in Fig. 1. The reduction in anticonvulsant concentration can be substantial and if the dose is not increased then seizure control may be lost. Long before the advent of therapeutic drug monitoring it was recognized that seizure frequency in epileptics on treatment increased during pregnancy: subtherapeutic plasma drug concentrations will have been largely responsible. Drug levels should be monitored monthly during pregnancy and a falling level should initiate an increase in dose.

The physiological changes of pregnancy resolve in the 6 weeks following delivery, and there is a progressive return to pre-pregnancy dose requirements during this time.

Not all drugs metabolized in the liver show reductions in plasma concentration during pregnancy. For example, the clearance of propranolol is unchanged. This is presumably because the rate of propranolol

Fig. 1 Plasma phenytoin concentration during and following pregnancy in a woman who remained on a constant dose of 300 mg/day throughout. She had a seizure at 38 weeks gestation and delivered at 40 weeks. The dose should have been increased when the concentration began to fall.

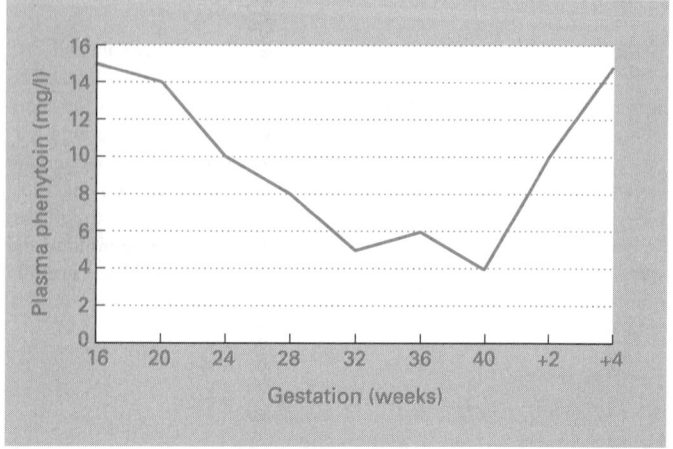

clearance is determined by liver blood flow which is not altered by pregnancy.

Since renal blood flow increases during pregnancy, the clearance of drugs eliminated by this route would also be expected to increase. Lithium clearance doubles during pregnancy and dose increases, guided by drug-level monitoring, are likely to be needed. Dose requirements fall rapidly following delivery and care must be taken to avoid the development of toxicity. The clearance of ampicillin nearly doubles during pregnancy. Formal pharmacokinetic studies have not been performed with cephalosporins, but plasma levels of around 50 per cent of those found in non-pregnant subjects have been reported. In contrast to drugs with a reasonably well-defined therapeutic range, the falling plasma levels of penicillin or cephalosporin antibiotics are of less obvious significance. However, it seems prudent to give doses at the higher end of the recommended range when using these agents to treat systemic infections during pregnancy.

Drug protein binding in pregnancy

The protein binding of drugs is also altered by pregnancy. The mechanism is not fully understood, since although the concentration of albumin falls substantially in a normal pregnancy there is not, for all drugs, a correlation between the concentration of albumin and the free fraction of the drug. The free and pharmacologically active concentration of anticonvulsants is increased in pregnancy by 30 to 50 per cent, which has consequences for the interpretation of plasma drug levels.

Therapeutic drug monitoring during pregnancy

In general, whenever therapeutic drug monitoring would ordinarily be used in the non-pregnant woman, drug levels should be monitored monthly during pregnancy. While therapeutic ranges are imprecise, they do provide a useful guide to management. In the case of anticonvulsants, a useful clinical guideline is to assume that if control has been good before pregnancy at a particular level, and if the plasma concentration is falling substantially below that level as the result of pregnancy, then the dose should be increased. Waiting for a seizure to occur is unacceptable: women die from poorly controlled epilepsy in pregnancy.

Since the free fraction of anticonvulsants increases during pregnancy, the interpretation of drug levels needs careful consideration. Most laboratories report the total (bound plus unbound) drug concentration and this may be misleading since the proportion of unbound drug increases. Given that interpretation of drug levels is an imprecise science, a pragmatic approach to the problem is not to allow drug levels to fall below the lower third of the non-pregnant therapeutic range. Alternatively, saliva samples can be used to guide treatment, since these have been shown to correlate well with the plasma concentration of unbound drug.

REFERENCES

Briggs, G.G., Freeman, R.K., and Yaffe, S.J. (1994). *Drugs in pregnancy and lactation*. 4th edn. Williams and Wilkins, Baltimore.
Rubin, P.C. (1995). *Prescribing in pregnancy*. 2nd edn. British Medical Journal, London.

13.17 Benefits and risks of hormone replacement therapy

J. C. STEVENSON

Introduction

The acute effects of female sex hormone deficiency, such as vasomotor symptoms, are well known, but the importance of the longer-term effects of ovarian failure have only recently been recognized. The menopause, the time of a woman's last menstrual period, is a useful marker for ovarian failure. The average age of natural menopause is around 51 years, although it may occur at any time after puberty. Thus with the mean female life expectancy increasing beyond 80 years, the average woman may expect to spend at least one-third of her life in a gonadal hormone-deficient state. Menopausal status can usually be confirmed by demonstration of elevated gonadotrophin levels, although transient episodes of spontaneous ovarian activity are not uncommon in the early postmenopausal years.

Clinical features of menopause

A number of symptoms may arise soon after loss of ovarian function at the menopause. These include hot flushes and night sweats, and psychological symptoms such as mood swings, depression, anxiety and irritability, and difficulties with memory and concentration. Later there may be musculoskeletal problems such as arthralgia and morning stiffness, and genitourinary problems such as vaginal dryness and dyspareunia, increased urinary frequency, and urge incontinence. Palpitation is another symptom that may perhaps be related to hormone deficiency. However, the long-term consequences of hormone deficiency, namely osteoporosis and cardiovascular disease, pose a major health problem for women.

Osteoporosis is recognized as a silent epidemic, and perhaps one in every two women will have this disease by the end of their lives (see Section 19). Health service costs of osteoporosis in the United Kingdom are of the order of several million pounds annually.

Increased cardiovascular disease risk is the most important consequence of ovarian failure. Coronary heart disease is the leading cause of death in women, and although it occurs at a later age than in men, overall more women than men die from the disease each year. The occurrence of coronary heart disease in women is frequently overlooked, and women are less likely than men to undergo both investigation and treatment for this disease. Yet middle-aged postmenopausal women more commonly experience anginal chest pain than men, and are more frequently afflicted by syndrome X (anginal pain, significant ST segment depression on exercise electrocardiogram, but no demonstrable abnormality on coronary angiogram).

Benefits of hormone replacement therapy

Hormone replacement therapy consists of oestrogen, which should be given continuously, with cyclical progestogen addition in women who have not had a hysterectomy. Progestogens are necessary to prevent endometrial hyperplasia and neoplasia, and to regulate any uterine bleeding that may occur. Oestrogen is given as oral oestradiol-17β, oestrone sulphate, or conjugated equine oestrogens. Alternatively, oestradiol-17β can be administered transdermally through adhesive skin patches, or implanted subcutaneously as pellets. The synthetic alkylated oestrogens, such as ethinyloestradiol, are not used in hormone replacement therapy because of their potency and unwanted side-effects. The

Table 1 *Usual daily doses of oestrogens and progestogens used in hormone replacement therapy*

Oral preparations	
Oestrogens	
micronized oestradiol-17β	1–2 mg
oestradiol valerate	1–2 mg
oestrone sulphate	1.5 mg
conjugated equine oestrogens	0.625–1.25 mg
Progestogens	
DL-norgestrel	0.15 mg
norethisterone acetate	0.7–1.0 mg
dydrogesterone	10–20 mg
medroxyprogesterone acetate	5–10 mg
Non-oral preparations	
Oestrogens	
transdermal oestradiol-17β	0.05–0.1 mg
oestradiol-17β implant	25–50 mg (6 monthly)
Progestogens	
transdermal norethisterone acetate	0.25 mg

Table 2 *Hormone replacement therapy and the cardiovascular system: possible mechanisms of action*

Decreased total cholesterol
Decreased triglycerides
Decreased LDL cholesterol
Decreased LDL cholesterol oxidation
Increased HDL and HDL$_2$ cholesterol
Decreased insulin resistance
Decreased circulating insulin concentrations
Decreased proportion of insulin propeptides
Improved glucose tolerance
Decreased proportion of android fat
Decreased NEFA flux
Decreased plasminogen activator inhibitor-1
Increased tissue plasminogen activator
Increased arterial wall compliance
Decreased blood pressure
Increased arterial blood flow

HDL, high-density lipoprotein; LDL, low-density lipoprotein; NEFA, non-esterified fatty acids.

progestogens used are either derivatives of 19-nortestosterone, such as norgestrel and norethisterone, or the less androgenic C-21 steroids such as dydrogesterone and medroxyprogesterone acetate. Natural progesterone can be used but is often not well tolerated because of drowsiness. Progestogens are usually given in the minimal dose necessary for endometrial protection for 12 or more days per month. Usual doses of hormones are shown in Table 1. Regimens giving continuous progestogen with continuous oestrogen in order to induce endometrial atrophy and hence abolish uterine bleeding are under investigation. Metabolic side-effects may preclude their long-term use in younger women, but such therapies may prove of use in the elderly. Tibolone, a synthetic compound with oestrogenic, progestogenic, and androgenic properties, appears to have similar effects to continuous combined oestrogen and progestogen and is thus an alternative approach.

The main indications for use of hormone replacement therapy are currently relief of menopausal symptoms and prevention of osteoporosis. It is most likely that prevention of cardiovascular disease will become a major indication in the future. Hormone replacement therapy will abolish vasomotor symptoms often within days of starting treatment, whereas psychological symptoms and genitourinary symptoms may take weeks or even months to respond. It is therefore worthwhile persisting with therapy for several months if an earlier symptomatic response is not obtained. Treatment should be continued for at least several months after symptomatic relief has been obtained. If there is any need to discontinue therapy, it should be withdrawn gradually to minimize the chance of recurrence of symptoms.

Hormone replacement therapy is well established for both the prevention and treatment of osteoporosis. It conserves, and to some extent increases, bone density and results in a reduction of fracture risk. Therapy should be offered to any woman considered at increased risk of osteoporosis, and particularly those with an early menopause. When risk of osteoporosis is uncertain, bone density measurement will greatly aid clinical decision. Hormone replacement needs to be given long term both for prevention and for treatment of osteoporosis. For the former, at least 5 years would seem to be necessary to have an appreciable impact on future risk, whereas for the latter, treatment is ideally monitored by occasional bone density assessment. Cessation of hormone replacement therapy leads to a loss of bone density but only at the usual postmenopausal rate, and the benefit gained by the skeleton from a suitable period of treatment persists into old age.

There are many mechanisms, both established and potential, whereby hormone replacement therapy may benefit the cardiovascular system, and these are summarized in Table 2. Population studies have shown that a reduction in cardiovascular disease incidence of at least 50 per cent can be achieved with hormone replacement. Most of these studies are of oestrogen alone, but preliminary data suggest that fears concerning a negation of this effect by progestogen addition may be unfounded.

Hormone replacement therapy has beneficial effects on metabolic risk markers for cardiovascular disease. These effects vary somewhat, depending on the type of oestrogen or progestogen used, and the route of administration. In general, hormone replacement produces a lowering of low-density lipoprotein cholesterol, a small increase or little change in high-density lipoprotein cholesterol, and a decrease in triglycerides, thus reversing the changes in lipids and lipoproteins brought about by the menopause. An improvement in glucose tolerance, due to an enhancement of insulin secretion and elimination or a reduction in insulin resistance, may be seen. There are also direct effects of oestrogen on arteries which improve blood flow, both by endothelium-dependent mechanisms and by calcium antagonist actions. Oestradiol may acutely reduce myocardial ischaemia in patients with angina.

Side-effects of hormone replacement therapy

The main drawback to current hormone replacement therapy regimens is the necessity of uterine withdrawal bleeding. This is often fairly light, particularly in older patients, and tends to diminish with time. With a satisfactory and regular bleeding pattern, there is usually no need for endometrial screening. Oestrogenic side-effects such as breast tenderness and nausea may sometimes be experienced on commencing therapy, particularly by older patients who are many years postmenopause. Such side-effects are transient and usually resolve by about 3 months of therapy. In older patients, it is advisable to start with a low, suboptimal dose of oestrogen initially, increasing this after a few months in order to limit such side-effects. More commonly, side-effects are due to the progestogen and can include breast tenderness, abdominal and pelvic pain, backache, depression and irritability, and migraine.

Risks of hormone replacement therapy

The major concern about hormone replacement therapy, particularly with prolonged treatment, is the risk of breast cancer. Epidemiological evidence is conflicting; although many studies show no overall increase in incidence of breast cancer, some show an increase with prolonged duration of use, usually in excess of 10 years. However, of the studies looking at mortality from breast cancer, women taking hormone replacement therapy who develop the disease appear to have a better survival than those who were not on treatment. This raises the possibility that any increase in breast cancer with hormone replacement therapy may be due to surveillance bias. Alternatively, there could be a subgroup at true increased risk who have not yet been identified. At present, it seems prudent to avoid hormone replacement therapy where possible in women with breast cancer, although the disease need not be considered a total contraindication in all cases.

Previous endometrial hyperplasia or neoplasia is not a contraindication, provided the disease has been eradicated. Similarly, endometriosis and uterine fibroids rarely cause a problem, although they may occasionally worsen. Despite previous beliefs, hormone replacement therapy does not cause hypertension except as a rare idiosyncratic reaction, nor does it increase the risk of venous thromboembolism. It is therefore not necessary to withdraw the treatment in women with, or at risk from, these conditions. Myocardial infarction and stroke may eventually prove to be indications for hormone replacement therapy in view of its beneficial effects on cardiovascular disease, as may hyperlipidaemia and diabetes mellitus. In the latter conditions, appropriate choice of types of steroid and route of administration is necessary.

Migraine is sometimes brought on by hormone replacement therapy, again as an idiosyncratic reaction, but more commonly migraine is related to oestrogen deficiency and may be relieved by replacement. Many women gain weight after the menopause but not as a result of taking hormone replacement. Weight gain may occasionally occur due to fluid retention, particularly associated with progestogen use, but increases in body fat are not seen due to hormone replacement therapy. Indeed, there is a redistribution of body fat, with a reduction in the metabolically harmful central obesity, as a result of treatment. It must be remembered that weight gain in postmenopausal women on hormone replacement therapy is most commonly due to excessive calorie intake. Most of the other reputed adverse effects of hormone replacement therapy are unsubstantiated, and have largely arisen from an inappropriate extrapolation from data obtained with oral contraceptive use.

Hormone replacement therapy is a treatment with major benefits for many women. The choice of therapeutic agents should be tailored to suit the individual woman. There are advantages and disadvantages of certain preparations and combinations, but overall the therapy used should be the one that the patient finds most acceptable. This will encourage compliance with long-term therapy which will result in the greatest health benefits.

REFERENCES

Bergkvist, L., Adami, H.O., Persson, I., Bergstrom, R., and Krusemo, U.B. (1989). Prognosis after breast cancer diagnosis in women exposed to estrogen and estrogen-progestogen replacement therapy. *American Journal of Epidemiology* **130**, 221–8.

Christiansen, C., and Riis, B.J. (1990). Five years with continuous combined oestrogen/progestogen therapy. Effects on calcium metabolism, lipoproteins, and bleeding pattern. *British Journal of Obstetrics and Gynaecology* **97**, 1087–92.

Collins, P., Rosano, G.M.C., Jiang, C., Lindsay, D., Sarrel, P.M., and Poole-Wilson, P.A. (1993). Cardiovascular protection by oestrogen – a calcium antagonist effect? *Lancet* **341**, 1264–5.

Crook, D., *et al.* (1992). Comparison of transdermal and oral estrogen/progestin hormone replacement therapy: effects on serum lipids and lipoproteins. *American Journal of Obstetrics and Gynecology* **166**, 950–5.

Drife, J.O. and Studd, J.W.W. (ed.) (1990). *HRT and osteoporosis* Springer-Verlag, London.

Knopp, R.H. (1988). The effects of postmenopausal estrogen therapy on the incidence of arteriosclerotic vascular disease. *Obstetrics and Gynecology* **72**, 23S–30S.

Ley, C.J., Lees, B. and Stevenson, J.C. (1992). Sex- and menopause-associated changes in body-fat distribution. *American Journal of Clinical Nutrition* **55**, 950–4.

Rosano, G.M.C., Sarrel, P.M., Poole-Wilson, P.A., and Collins, P. (1993). Beneficial effect of oestrogen on exercise-induced myocardial ischaemia in women with coronary artery disease. *Lancet* **342**, 133–6.

Stevenson, J.C. (1993). Today's contra-indications – tomorrow's indications. In *Safety aspects of hormone replacement therapy* pp. 131–8. Wells Medical, Tunbridge Wells.

Studd, J.W.W. and Whitehead, M.I. (ed.) (1989). *The menopause*. Blackwell, Oxford.

Sullivan, J.M., *et al.* (1990). Estrogen replacement and coronary artery disease. *Archives of Internal Medicine* **150**, 2557–62.

Whitcroft, S.I.J. and Stevenson, J.C. (1992). Hormone replacement therapy: risks and benefits. *Clinical Endocrinology* **36**, 15–20.

Section 14 *Gastroenterology*

14.1	*Introduction*	1819
14.2	*Symptomatology of gastrointestinal disease*	1819
	14.2.1 Dysphagia and other symptoms in oesophageal disease	1819
	14.2.2 Vomiting	1821
	14.2.3 Abdominal pain	1822
	14.2.4 Diarrhoea	1823
	14.2.5 Constipation	1825
	14.2.6 Gastrointestinal bleeding	1827
14.3	*Methods for investigation of gastrointestinal diseases*	1829
	14.3.1 Endoscopy	1829
	14.3.2 Radiology	1830
14.4	*Immune disorders of the gastrointestinal tract*	1836
14.5	*The mouth and salivary glands*	1846
14.6	*Disease of the oesophagus*	1865
14.7	*Peptic ulceration*	1877
14.8	*Hormones and the gastrointestinal tract*	1891
14.9	*Malabsorption*	1899
	14.9.1 Mechanisms of intestinal absorption	1899
	14.9.2 Investigation and differential diagnosis of malabsorption	1904
	14.9.3 Small-bowel bacterial overgrowth	1911
	14.9.4 Coeliac disease	1916
	14.9.5 Disaccharidase deficiency	1920
	14.9.6 Whipple's disease	1923
	14.9.7 Short gut syndrome	1925
	14.9.8 Enteropathy-associated T-cell lymphoma	1927
	14.9.9 Malabsorption in the tropics	1930
14.10	*Crohn's disease*	1936
14.11	*Ulcerative colitis*	1943
14.12	*Disorders of motility*	1951
14.13	*Functional bowel disease and irritable bowel syndrome*	1965
14.14	*Colonic diverticular disease*	1969
14.15	*Congenital abnormalities of the gastrointestinal tract*	1972
14.16	*Tumours of the gastrointestinal tract*	1980
14.17	*Vascular and collagen disorders*	1994
14.18	*Gastrointestinal infections*	2001
14.19	*The peritoneum, omentum, and appendix*	2007
14.20	*Computed tomography and magnetic resonance imaging of the liver and pancreas*	2012
14.21	*Congenital disorders of the biliary tract and pancreas*	2014
14.22	*Hereditary disease of the liver and pancreas*	2017
14.23	*Diseases of the pancreas*	2027
	14.23.1 Acute pancreatitis	2027
	14.23.2 Chronic pancreatitis	2034
	14.23.3 Tumours of the pancreas	2040
14.24	*Diseases of the gallbladder and biliary tree*	2045
14.25	*Jaundice*	2054
14.26	*Clinical features of viral hepatitis*	2061
14.27	*Autoimmune liver disease*	2069
	14.27.1 Autoimmune hepatitis	2069
	14.27.2 Primary biliary cirrhosis	2074
	14.27.3 Primary sclerosing cholangitis	2077
14.28	*Alcoholic liver disease*	2080
14.29	*Cirrhosis, portal hypertension, and ascites*	2085
14.30	*Hepatocellular failure*	2100
14.31	*Liver transplantation*	2111
14.32	*Liver tumours*	2115
14.33	*Hepatic granulomas*	2120
14.34	*Drugs and liver damage*	2124
14.35	*The liver in systemic disease*	2130
14.36	*Miscellaneous disorders of the gastrointestinal tract and liver*	2136

14.1 Introduction

This section describes the major disorders of the gastrointestinal tract, liver, and pancreas. Where possible these conditions are described in groups which have a common form of pathophysiology, for example disorders of motility or vascular disorders, rather than by the more conventional approach of considering the different pathologies of one particular of the gastrointestinal tract together. This approach seems particularly appropriate because of the increasing evidence regarding the functional interdependence of the various sections of the gastrointestinal tract and its related organs.

As is the case for most of the disorders described in this book, despite the increasing availability of sophisticated laboratory aids to diagnosis, the clinical history and thorough physical examination remain central to the diagnosis and management of diseases of the gastrointestinal tract. For this reason the section is introduced by a series of short chapters that cover the major symptoms of gastrointestinal disease and their significance.

14.2 Symptomatology of gastrointestinal diseases

14.2.1 Dysphagia and other symptoms of oesophageal disease

J. DENT

Symptom evaluation is highly rewarding in oesophageal diseases, because of the relative specificity of patterns for particular disease processes. Symptom evaluation is especially important in reflux disease because of its very high prevalence, its wide range of severity, and the need to restrict investigation to only a minority of patients. Analysis of symptom patterns is an essential preliminary to further investigation of most oesophageal diseases, as this will aid appropriate choice between endoscopy or barium study, and also determine whether investigation should progress to oesophageal function testing.

The severity of symptoms gives the best measure of how the oesophageal problem is affecting the patient's life and determines how energetically the problem should be investigated or treated.

The nature, location, and radiation of the sensation experienced by the patient is usually helpful diagnostically, but can be misleading as to disease process. The diagnostic value of analysis of oesophageal symptoms is greatly enhanced if associations, provocants and relieving factors, and the duration, progression, and frequency of symptoms are also taken into account. For instance, in a significant minority of patients with symptoms caused by episodes of gastro-oesophageal reflux these are non-specific or atypical, but the postprandial occurrence of the symptoms after ingestion of typically provocant food, and intermittent occurrence of the symptoms over many months, indicate that the most likely diagnosis is reflux disease.

Symptom evaluation is also important for recognition of alert or alarm symptoms that indicate a relatively high risk for serious disease and should lead to prompt investigation. Dysphagia that is progressive, haematemesis, and weight loss are the most important of these.

Indigestion-like symptoms arising from the oesophagus

In the great majority of patients these symptoms arise from oesophageal mucosal irritation by refluxed gastric juice, ingested irritants or damage to the mucosa caused by infective agents. This category of symptom can be considered as 'mucosal pain'.

REFLUX DISEASE

This is overwhelmingly the most common cause of mucosal pain (see Chapter 14.6).

Table 1 *Causes of hypersensitivity of the oesophageal mucosa to normal levels of gastro-oesophageal reflux*

Primary mucosal hypersensitivity or 'irritable oesophagus'
Hypersensitivity due to mucosal damage:
Infective oesophagitis
Irradiation oesophagitis
Medication-induced injury
Primary mucosal disease

Location and nature of sensation

Heartburn results from contact between oesophageal mucosa and refluxate; it is an episodic, lower retrosternal/epigastric burning that radiates upwards, sometimes to as high as the pharynx or jaw. Reflux may also induce lower retrosternal or epigastric burning without radiation, or a poorly localized lower chest/upper abdominal discomfort or unease.

Associations, provocants, and relieving factors

The following features strongly support the diagnosis of reflux-induced oesophageal mucosal pain: association with regurgitation, consistent occurrence of symptoms in the 2 h after food, provocation by large, fatty, or highly spiced meals, by bending or stooping, or heavy physical exertion, and relief by antacids.

Duration and frequency

Reflux-induced symptoms are characteristically intermittent, but only show an overall significant change in pattern and severity over months to years. Usually, symptoms will have been occurring over several months by the time of presentation, except in the case of reflux-induced symptoms associated with pregnancy.

OTHER CAUSES OF INDIGESTION-LIKE SYMPTOMS

Damage to the oesophageal mucosa from causes other than pathological gastro-oesophageal reflux can lead to similar symptoms. The causes of mucosal hypersensitivity to normal levels of gastro-oesophageal reflux are listed in Table 1. In many cases, the factor(s) that sensitize the mucosa are evident from the setting in which they occur—for instance, during an episode of infective oesophagitis or in association with radiation-induced oesophagitis. Odynophagia (painful swallowing) is often a more prominent symptom than in reflux disease. In some cases, though, especially of injury to the oesophageal mucosa from medications, the symptom pattern may mimic reflux disease, so that the primary defect may often be misdiagnosed as abnormally frequent gastro-oesophageal reflux (see Chapter 14.6).

Dysphagia

Malignancy is usually the primary concern of patients with this symptom, though most instances of dysphagia are benign. The diagnostic specificity of patterns of dysphagia is fair, but is not sufficiently high for diagnosis to rely solely on symptom evaluation in most patients.

LOCATION AND NATURE OF SENSATION

The term dysphagia implies a sensation of mechanical difficulty with movement of food from the mouth to the stomach. High and low dysphagia should be distinguished as separate patterns, as their investigation and causes differ. With high dysphagia, oral, pharyngeal or upper oesophageal structural abnormalities or motor dysfunction lead to impaired swallowing. The patient has difficulty with ejection of boluses from the mouth, takes many swallows to clear a normal-sized bolus, and usually coughs and splutters due to aspiration. With low dysphagia, successful swallowing is followed by a sensation of food hold-up. This symptom pattern is of oesophageal origin until proven otherwise. Bolus hold-up may be noted for just a few seconds, or initial dysphagia may be followed by a sensation of total, persistent blockage. Sometimes this sensation is misleading, but more often the lumen is obstructed by bolus impaction at a stricture, or above a region of muscle spasm. The surface location of the sensation of obstruction is an unreliable indication of the actual site of this in the oesophagus.

ASSOCIATIONS, PROVOCANTS, AND RELIEVING FACTORS

Regardless of the nature of the pathology, solid boluses are most likely to cause symptoms because they require more propulsive force than liquids. Close association of dysphagia with swallowing of firm/hard boluses above a particular size is strongly suggestive of a fixed narrowing, either due to extrinsic compression or oesophageal stricture. Oesophageal obstruction is confirmed by regurgitation of saliva and other oesophageal contents, and inability to swallow further boluses. Crushing chest pain with dysphagia is not always due to diffuse oesophageal spasm (see Chapter 14.6), as bolus impaction at an oesophageal stenosis can lead to secondary painful oesophageal spasm, especially in patients with a Schatski ring (see Chapter 14.6). Association of clear-cut symptoms of reflux disease with recent development of dysphagia suggests peptic stricture, but the high prevalence of reflux disease means that coincidence of this with oesophageal cancer is not uncommon.

DURATION, PROGRESSION, AND FREQUENCY

With dysphagia, these variables are especially helpful in determining the likely diagnosis and appropriate action. Typically, the dysphagia of motor disorders will have been present for many months or years at presentation. Any progression of severity is very slow. Non-specific motor disorders of the oesophageal body (see Chapter 14.6) usually cause mild, intermittent dysphagia with solids. Steady progression of severity of dysphagia over a period of weeks is especially ominous, as it is usually due to malignant obstruction and demands prompt investigation. The dysphagia of achalasia normally occurs with almost every meal and is frequently associated with regurgitation (see below). Typically, the dysphagia of diffuse oesophageal spasm is associated with crushing retrosternal pain and occurs very episodically, often only every few weeks or months. Between symptom episodes there is total freedom from dysphagia, even with challenging boluses.

Regurgitation

Regurgitation is the effortless appearance of material in the pharynx without prior nausea. Despite this distinctive pattern, it is often misdiagnosed as vomiting by both patient and doctor. Regurgitation is usually of relatively small volume, but it can be a very disabling problem when it is so voluminous that regurgitated material cannot be retained in the mouth and reswallowed.

LOCATION AND NATURE OF SENSATION

The pattern of 'vomiting' should be evaluated critically to differentiate true vomiting from regurgitation. Regurgitation of food and liquid unchanged in flavour is indicative of oesophageal retention; regurgitation of vomit-flavoured material is due to gastro-oesophageal reflux.

ASSOCIATIONS, PROVOCANTS, AND RELIEVING FACTORS

Regurgitation is provoked by any physical activity or posture that stresses the antireflux function of the upper and lower oesophageal sphincters. When there is associated dysphagia it is most probably secondary to oesophageal retention. Voluminous regurgitation of gastric content is most likely to occur after especially large meals.

DURATION, PROGRESSION, AND FREQUENCY

The regurgitation of reflux disease is typically episodic, but in particularly severe cases it can occur after every meal. It changes little in pattern over months to years. With the oesophageal retention of achalasia, regurgitation is usually a prominent symptom, occurring several times a week with gradual worsening over months to years.

Chest pain and odynophagia

These two related symptom patterns arise from a variety of conditions. The pain arising from the mucosa may be indistinguishable from the pain caused by abnormally vigorous or sustained oesophageal contraction. Furthermore, chest pain not clearly ascribable to either oesophageal or cardiac disease may also have a similar pattern. The problem of non-cardiac chest pain is discussed in Chapter 14.6.

LOCATION AND NATURE OF SENSATION

Oesophageal pain from both mucosa and muscle typically occurs retrosternally and may radiate into the arms or jaw. The sensation is often perceived as crushing, and can be very intense. Not infrequently, the pain pattern is indistinguishable from cardiac pain if it is not clearly linked in time to swallowing. When swallowing is a consistent provocant the pain may have a more burning quality if it is of mucosal origin.

ASSOCIATIONS, PROVOCANTS, AND RELIEVING FACTORS

These tend to be relatively unhelpful in patients with chronic, cardiac-like chest pain, hence the heavy reliance on oesophageal function testing in this setting. Association of severe retrosternal pain with dysphagia points strongly towards diffuse oesophageal spasm or achalasia, but absence of this association does not rule out these diagnoses. Resolution of pain during high-level acid suppression suggests that the pain is reflux induced. Consistent lack of tight association of chronic chest pain with exertion makes an oesophageal origin more likely than a cardiac source.

DURATION AND FREQUENCY

Abrupt onset of odynophagia for the first time suggests acute mucosal disease as the cause, especially if it is associated with immunodeficiency, chemotherapy, mediastinal irradiation, or infective stomatitis or pharyngitis.

REFERENCES

Arens, MJ. and Dent, J. (1993). Acid pump blockers: what are their current therapeutic roles? *Baillière's Clinical Gastroenterology*. Inhibition of gastric acid secretion, **7**, 95–128.

Dent, J. (1991). Practical issues in gastrointestinal motor disorders. *Baillière's Clinical Gastroenterology*. Vol. 5, no. 2. Bailliere Tindall, London. The first five chapters provide comprehensive reviews on swallowing disorders, non-cardiac chest pain and oesophageal motor disorders, including reflux disease.

Jamieson, GG. (1988). *Surgery of the oesophagus*. Churchill Livingstone, Edinburgh. This textbook is a valuable resource of information relevant to oesophageal surgery.

Sleisenger, M.H. and Fordtran, J.S. (1993). *Gastrointestinal disease*. (5th edn). Saunders, Philadelphia. The section on oesophageal disease is a comprehensive review which gives considerable detail.

14.2.2 Vomiting

D. P. JEWELL

Vomiting is a common symptom associated with many gastrointestinal disorders—functional, inflammatory, and obstructive. In addition it may be a symptom of many other non-gastroenterological conditions, which include: infections, metabolic disturbances, migraine, travel sickness, pregnancy, myocardial infarction, drug toxicity, raised intracranial pressure, and psychogenic syndromes.

Mechanism

The act of vomiting consists of three stages. The first stage is nausea during which there is reduced motor activity of the stomach but an increase in the activity of the duodenum and jejunum. This allows reflux of duodenal contents into the stomach. Retching is the next stage, during which there is a series of contractions of the chest muscles and diaphragm associated with the simultaneous contraction of the abdominal muscles, the glottis remaining firmly closed. During these spasms, gastric contents reflux freely into the lower oesophagus. Finally, there is a powerful and sustained contraction of the abdominal muscles with descent of the diaphragm causing a large rise in intra-abdominal pressure and emesis.

The neurophysiology of vomiting has been worked out mainly in the cat. The pathways are probably similar to those in man but obviously this has not been proven completely. Afferent stimuli from the stomach and intestine are largely carried in the vagus nerve but there are also sympathetic afferents, especially those involved in the vomiting associated with intestinal obstruction. Afferent fibres from the gallbladder, biliary tract, and peritoneum relay vomiting signals via the vagus and sympathetic nerves. Vomiting associated with cardiac pain is mainly mediated by the vagus. There are many other afferent nerves relaying emetic signs from other organs, notably the vestibular nerve and afferents from other parts of the brain. All these afferents appear to relay into the chemoreceptor trigger zone (**CTZ**), and the vomiting centre. The chemoreceptor trigger zone is located in the floor of the fourth ventricle within the area postrema. The area postrema is a vascular appendage, rather than brain substance, and lacks a blood–cerebrospinal fluid barrier. Its vascular supply is from the posterior inferior cerebellar artery, but the nature of the chemoreceptors and their exact location within the area postrema are unknown. Motion sickness and radiation sickness may be highly dependent upon the area postrema but abalation has produced conflicting results in experimental animals. Many drugs that cause vomiting, such as morphine, digoxin, ipecacuanha, L-dopa, and many cytotoxic drugs, act at this level. Signals from the stimulated chemoreceptor trigger zone are received by the vomiting centre situated in the lateral reticular formation of the medulla, although recent work has cast a doubt on whether there is a specific centre coordinating the act of vomiting. A variety of neurotransmitters is involved in these central pathways: within the vestibular system and the vomiting centre,

acetylcholine (muscarinic receptors) and histamine (H_1-receptors) are important but dopamine (D_2-receptors) and 5-hydroxytryptamine (5-HT_3-receptors) are released in the chemoreceptor trigger zone and area postrema. The efferent impulses travel in the somatic nerves supplying the pharynx, respiratory, and abdominal muscles, diaphragm, and the gastrointestinal tract. In addition, there are autonomic pathways which mediate the hypersalivation, pallor, and sweating that so frequently accompany vomiting. The neurotransmitter substances of the efferent pathways in the periphery are unknown. They are non-adrenergic and non-cholinergic. Possible candidates are substance P, vasoactive intestinal polypeptide, dopamine, and nitric oxide.

CLINICAL FEATURES

Vomiting in the morning soon after waking is characteristic of pregnancy, alcoholism, and metabolic disturbances such as uraemia. It may

Table 1 *Antiemetics and their role in clinical situations associated with vomiting*

Antiemetic	Role
Gastrokinetic	
Metoclopramide	Central and peripheral actions.
Domperidone	Domperidone lacks extrapyramidal effects
	Useful for gastrointestinal stasis, migraine, and chemotherapy-induced vomiting
Antihistamines	
Cyclizine	Effective for travel sickness and vestibular disorders
Diphenhydramine	
Promethazine	Cyclizine is often used to counteract opiate-induced vomiting, e.g. following myocardial infarction
	Useful for pregnancy.
Anticholinergics	
Hyoscine	Effective for travel sickness and causes less drowsiness than antihistamines
5-HT_3-antagonists	
Ondansetron	Especially indicated for vomiting caused by chemotherapy or by radiotherapy
Granisetron	May also be helpful for postoperative vomiting
Phenothiazines	
Prochlorperazine	D_2-receptor antagonists.
Chlorpromazine	Associated with marked sedative activity.
	Useful postoperatively or to counteract opiate-induced vomiting
Benzodiazepines	
Diazepam	Restrict to nausea and vomiting induced by anxiety states
Lorazepam	Beware addictive properties
Cannabinoids	
Nabilone	May be effective for vomiting induced by chemotherapy or radiotherapy.

Adapted from: Allan, S.G.(1992). *Gastroenterology Clinics of North America*, **21**, 597–611.

also occur after gastric surgery. Vomiting associated with psychological disorders usually occurs during or soon after a meal. Pyloric canal ulcers may also cause vomiting immediately after a meal. Delayed vomiting (more than 1 h after a meal) is the usual pattern associated with peptic ulcer, gastric carcinoma, gallbladder disease, and intestinal obstruction. Projectile vomiting, which is the forceful ejection of vomitus without retching, is often seen in pyloric stenosis and is said to occur in patients with raised intracranial pressure.

The content of the vomitus may provide some diagnostic clues. Vomiting of undigested food suggests that it is regurgitation secondary to achalasia, an oesphageal stricture, or a pharyngeal diverticulum. Intestinal contents in the vomitus suggest intestinal obstruction or ileus and the vomit usually has a faecal odour. Bilious vomiting characteristically occurs after gastric surgery. Altered blood ('coffee grounds') is of obvious significance.

Patients who are vomiting because of delayed gastric emptying (whether due to outlet obstruction or to gastric atony) may show gastric distension of physical examination and a succession splash may be present. Visible peristalsis may be seen in patients with gastric-outlet or intestinal obstruction.

METABOLIC CONSEQUENCES

Prolonged vomiting causes a metabolic alkalosis and hypokalaemia. Potassium deficiency results from a reduced intake, potassium loss in the vomit, and renal loss. The renal loss is due to hyperaldosteronism secondary to salt and water deficiency with contraction of the plasma volume. Alkalosis occurs because of the loss of H^+ in the vomit and also because there is a shift of H^+ into cells in response to potassium depletion.

TREATMENT

The treatment of nausea and vomiting partly depends on the cause. Table 1 lists the types of drug in common use and their role in clinical situations.

Drug therapy for the vomiting associated with pregnancy should be avoided wherever possible. However, if symptoms are severe, antihistamines should be used (e.g. promethazine).

SPECIFIC SYNDROMES

Psychogenic vomiting

Chronic and recurrent vomiting due to psychological causes is not uncommon and mainly affects women. There is often a long history of vomiting (e.g. vomiting associated with school examinations) and there may be a family history. Vomiting normally occurs after a meal but can usually be suppressed until the patient reaches a bathroom or lavatory. Vomiting is frequently a feature of patients with anorexia nervosa (see Chapter 10.4) and then it is often initiated by inserting a finger into the pharynx. Although organic disease must be excluded, the diagnosis should be recognized quickly and extensive investigation should be avoided. Treatment is difficult because antiemetics are not usually beneficial. Psychiatric assessment and psychotherapy may be helpful (see also Chapter 27.2.7).

Cyclical vomiting

This is a syndrome that occurs in children and is characterized by recurrent attacks of severe vomiting, which may last for several days. The onset is sudden and may be associated with headache, abdominal pain, and, occasionally, fever. Vomiting may be severe enough to cause profound dehydration and alkalosis. The syndrome usually starts before the age of 6 years and the frequency of the attacks varies from more than one a month to one or two each year. The cause is unknown but the many hypotheses that have been put forward include: epilepsy,

migraine, psychogenic, peri- or postnatal brain damage. Organic disease, especially intracranial pathology, must be excluded. Most children gradually improve with increasing age and the attacks usually stop by the end of puberty.

REFERENCE

Davis, C.J., Lake-Bakaar, G.V., and Grahame-Smith, D.G. (ed.) (1986). *Nausea and vomiting: mechanisms and treatment*. Springer-Verlag, Berlin.

14.2.3 Abdominal pain

D. P. JEWELL

Table 1 summarizes the main causes of abdominal pain.

The abdominal viscera are insensitive to cutting, tearing, and crushing, but they are sensitive to distension or tension. The nerve endings of the hollow organs are found in the muscle layers of the wall, whereas for solid organs (liver, kidneys, spleen), they are found in the capsule. The sensory nerves may also be stimulated by inflammation, ischaemia, or direct involvement by neoplasms.

As the viscera mostly receive afferents from both sides of the spinal cord, the pain is usually midline, dull, and poorly localized to the epigastrium, periumbilical area, or hypogastrium. It may be described as colicky, burning, or the gnawing sensation of hunger pains.

Parietal pain arises from the parietal peritoneum as a result of inflammation. The pain is usually sharp and can be precisely located. It is usually exacerbated by movement or coughing.

Referred pain is felt in skin or muscles remote from the affected organ and is due to the sharing of central pathways by the peripheral neurones. Examples of referred pain are the back and leg pain associated with intestinal distension.

NERVE PATHWAYS

Although 90 per cent of the nerve fibres in the vagus are sensory, none of them transmits pain. The ability to feel abdominal pain is therefore unaltered by vagotomy. The main pathways by which painful stimuli are relayed to the spinal cord are shown in Table 2. Following relay in the dorsal-root ganglion, fibres are transmitted in the posterior horn and the tract of Lissauer to synapse in the reticular formation and thalamus. From there, pain impulses are relayed to the postcentral gyrus at which point pain is experienced.

PAIN FROM SPECIFIC VISCERA

Pain from the oesophagus is felt retrosternally and is usually felt at the site of disease. It may occasionally radiate and can mimic cardiac pain. The Bernstein acid-infusion test may be useful clinically in reproducing the pain of oesophagitis. Severe oesophageal pain is referred into the back. Pain from the stomach and duodenum is usually midline in the epigastrium or in the right upper quadrant. Again, it may be felt in the back. Small-intestinal pain is central and midline, usually colicky, and radiating into the back. Colonic pain can be felt centrally, along the line of the colon, or in the hypogastrium. It is often poorly localized but frequently radiates into the back or into the thighs. Pain from the gallbladder and bile duct is colicky and is felt in the right upper quadrant. Characteristically it is also felt in the back, between the scapulae or in the right shoulder tip. Pancreatic pain is epigastric and midline, and radiates into the back. As with retroperitoneal pain, pancreatic pain is often made better by curling up and is aggravated by lying flat.

Table 1 *Causes of abdominal pain*

Intra-abdominal
  Generalized peritonitis:
    Perforated viscus; primary infective peritonitis; rupture of
    cyst
  Localized peritonitis:
    Appendicitis; cholecystitis; pancreatitis; abscesses;
    salpingitis
  Motility disorders:
    Intestinal obstruction; biliary obstruction; ureteric
    obstruction; irritable colon; diverticulosis; uterine
    contraction
  Ischaemia:
    Mesenteric angina/infarction; splenic infarction; torsion—
    ovarian cyst, testicle, omentum; tumour necrosis—
    hepatoma, fibroid
  Other:
    Peptic ulcer; inflammatory diseases; retroperitoneal
    tumours

Extra-abdominal
  Thoracic:
    Lung disease; ischaemic heart disease; oesophageal
    disease
  Neurological:
    Herpes zoster; spinal arthritis; radiculopathy from
    tumours; tabes dorsalis; abdominal epilepsy
  Metabolic:
    Diabetes mellitus; chronic renal failure; porphyria; acute
    adrenal insufficiency
  Toxins:
    Snake and insect bites; lead poisoning; strychnine

Table 2 *Nerve pathways from the abdominal viscera to the spinal cord*

Oesophagus	Unnamed sympathetic nerves
Liver, spleen	Phrenic nerve (C3-C5)
Gallbladder	
Pancreas, stomach	Coeliac plexus, greater
Small intestine	splanchnic nerves (T6-T9)
Appendix, colon	Mesenteric plexus, lesser
Pelvic viscera	splanchnic nerves (T11-L1)
Kidneys, bladder	
Rectum	Pelvic nerve (S2-S4)

DIAGNOSIS

The major features of the pain to be determined are site, intensity, character, timing, and aggravating and relieving factors. Associated symptoms, such as bowel disturbance, vomiting, heartburn, and urinary and gynaecological symptoms must be elicited. Physical examination will reveal areas of abdominal tenderness, rebound tenderness, and rigidity. Abdominal distension or visible peristalsis must be looked for. Organ enlargement and the presence of masses must be excluded. A rectal examination is essential. The hernial orifices should be carefully examined and the abdomen should be auscultated for bruits. General examination may reveal the presence of fever, tachycardia, jaundice, weight loss, or anaemia.

Investigation of abdominal pain will be directed by the clinical findings. However, in cases of chronic pain it is not usually possible to make a firm clinical diagnosis as the symptom complexes of many diseases overlap, for example gastric ulcer, gastric carcinoma, duodenal ulcer, gallstones, or irritable bowel syndrome. Radiological and endoscopic

investigations will therefore be necessary. The diagnosis of specific disorders is dealt with in the appropriate sections.

THE ACUTE ABDOMEN

Acute inflammation of any of the abdominal viscera, perforation of a hollow organ, rupture of a cyst, intestinal or ureteric obstruction, strangulation of an intestinal loop, or an aortic dissection can all present as an acute abdomen. Diagnosis rests on the history, the exact site and nature of the pain, the findings on physical examination, and the results of emergency investigations: white blood-cell count, plain abdominal radiographs and, if necessary, an intravenous pyelogram.

REFERENCES

Way L.W. (1978). Abdominal pain and the acute abdomen. In *Gastrointestinal disease*, (ed. M.H. Sleisenger and J.S. Fordtran). Saunders, Philadelphia.

14.2.4 Diarrhoea

L.A. TURNBERG

Introduction

In most cases it is easy to recognize when a patient has diarrhoea but difficulties may arise when attempts are made to define the borderline between what constitutes a normal stool output and what can be taken as diarrhoea. The passage of stools weighing more than 200 g per day is a useful definition for scientific purposes but is unhelpful in clinical practice. Usually diarrhoea is thought of in terms of frequency of evacuation and consistency of stool, but it is not easy to set the limits beyond which diarrhoea may be said to occur. A common sense attitude is indicated. For example, a patient who is habitually constipated might complain of diarrhoea when his bowel frequency reaches twice per day and he would be right to do so since it might indicate serious bowel disease even though some arbitrarily defined frequency of bowel evacuation has not been reached. The consistency of stools passed by populations consuming diets high in unrefined carbohydrate might be considered as diarrhoea in others taking highly refined diets. A clinical decision as to whether a given patient has diarrhoea or not usually depends, then, on that patient's normal bowel habit. A change to an increased frequency or looser consistency becomes suspicious without the need to define whether the patient has diarrhoea or not.

Another source of difficulty arises in the distinction between what patients and what doctors perceive as diarrhoea. Patients with carcinoma of the rectum, for example, may complain of diarrhoea when they pass blood and mucus, but may still pass normal formed stools. Faecal incontinence may also give rise to diagnostic difficulties. Many patients are reluctant to complain of incontinence, to which some social stigma is attached, and would rather complain of diarrhoea. In one study of patients complaining of diarrhoea some passed normal stools once per day but their incontinence provoked them into a complaint of diarrhoea.

These observations only re-emphasize that definitions of diarrhoea should not be slavishly adhered to and that, as experienced clinicians know well, a careful history is essential for accurate diagnosis.

Pathophysiology

To understand the underlying mechanisms of diarrhoea it is useful to think of it in terms of malabsorption of water.

Malabsorbed water-soluble nutrients such as carbohydrate and peptides in a variety of malabsorption states will add an osmotic element to the diarrhoea. In many diseases, in which there is structural damage to the intestinal mucosa, it is likely that the permeability of the intestine to salt and water will become distorted and this mechanism, too, may underlie diarrhoea. Such is the case in coeliac disease where the mucosal architecture is distorted and the, normally freely permeable, jejunum becomes less permeable to salt and water. In inflammatory bowel disease, on the other hand, an increased permeability to large molecules may play a role in the pathogenesis of the diarrhoea. Specific processes for the active absorption of sodium chloride play an important role in dehydrating luminal contents in the ileum and colon. Defects in the enzymes concerned with active transport occur in a variety of diseases. In invasive bacterial and viral gastroenteritis epithelial cell damage is associated with impaired active absorption and this plays a role in the pathogenesis of the diarrhoea. Although it seems likely that disturbances of intestinal motility can lead to diarrhoea it has proved difficult to ascribe diarrhoea to any specific abnormality of motility. Nevertheless a role for motility disturbances must be allowed.

In many diseases, of course, it is likely that a combination of these pathogenetic mechanisms is involved in contributing to the diarrhoea.

ROLE OF THE COLON

Although most of the 7 or 8 litres of fluid which enters the upper intestine each day is absorbed in the jejunum and ileum, the colon has a critical role in determining whether a patient has diarrhoea or not. The human colon normally absorbs some 1.5 to 2 litres of fluid per day and leaves less than 150 to 200 ml to escape in normal Western people's rather puny stool. Colonic diseases which result in even moderate reductions in the amount of fluid absorbed, say from 2 to 1.6 litres per day will treble the volume of stool. On the other hand, a normal colon can compensate for defective small intestinal absorption provided that the total volume reaching it does not exceed its absorptive capacity. Experimentally, the normal colon can probably cope with volumes of 4 to 5 litres of fluid per day if it is delivered at a steady rate throughout the 24 hours.

Colonic function clearly determines the presence or absence of diarrhoea in most instances and a good example of this is lactose intolerance, a condition in which it is presumed that the defect is small intestinal in origin. Malabsorbed lactose passes into the colon where it is split by bacteria into an increased number of solutes including short-chain fatty acids. The expected result of this would be an osmotic diarrhoea but most populations with this 'defect' do not usually have diarrhoea unless they take considerable quantities of milk. The colon absorbs short-chain fatty acids well and in most instances is able to compensate for the malabsorption of lactose in the small bowel. Only if colonic transit is altered, as, for example, in a colonic motility disorder, does diarrhoea occur. Indeed a careful history often suggests an 'irritable bowel syndrome' which responds better to treatment for that disorder than to milk withdrawal even though patients may be lactase deficient.

SECRETORY DIARRHOEA

In recent years much attention has been paid to the mechanisms underlying intestinal secretion provoked by a variety of exogenous and endogenous secretagogues. The classical example of this is in the diarrhoea of Asiatic cholera, in which condition the morphologically normal jejunal mucosa secretes vast quantities of salt and water. It is now known that a specific secretory process is switched on by the cholera toxin and the cellular mechanisms for this secretion have been elucidated. A central role is played by the cyclic nucleotide, cyclic adenosine monophosphate, which appears to be the 'second messenger' generated in intestinal mucosa in response to the toxin and which mediates the secretory response. Of particular importance is the recognition that a similar series of biochemical events is switched on by a variety of other secretory stimuli including a number of bacterial toxins, such as *Escherichia coli* heat labile toxin, and the toxins of *Staphylococcus aureus* and *Clostridium perfringens* (see Section 7). A similar mechanism appears to be involved in mediating the secretory diarrhoea of the Verner Morrison syndrome, in which a tumour in the islets of Langerhans secretes the peptide VIP which in turn activates mucosal cyclic AMP production. Other secretory stimuli act through different intracellular messengers, the most significant of which involves a transient rise in intracellular free calcium concentration. Acetylcholine, 5-hydroxytryptamine (carcinoid syndrome), and *Clostridium difficile* toxin appear to provoke intestinal secretion in this way. The importance of these observations lies in the clues they provide for potential therapeutic openings in which use is made of blockers of some of the biochemical steps involved in the secretory response.

Diagnosis
HISTORY

Considerable progress towards a diagnosis can be made simply by taking a careful history. Diagnosis of acute infective diarrhoeal illnesses is usually straightforward and rests on a history of recent onset, perhaps with nausea, fever, and systemic upset. Amongst the causes staphylococcal 'food poisoning' will develop soon after ingestion of the offending food and may be severe but short lived. Viral gastroenteritis is usually milder, often without systemic upset and lasts 2 to 3 days. Salmonella, Shigella, and Campylobacter can cause more severe disease with fever and prostration. Abdominal pain is a more prominent feature of Campylobacter while the presence of blood and mucus in the stool suggests shigellosis or, occasionally, salmonellosis.

That group of diseases is usually self-limiting but more difficulty is found with chronic, persistent or intermittent diarrhoeal disease. In these cases an effort should be made to distinguish diarrhoea of large bowel and small bowel origin. Large bowel diarrhoea will tend to occur maximally on waking in the morning, be associated with pain relieved by defaecation and perhaps accompanied by the passage of mucus. The presence of red blood in the stools of a patient with diarrhoea is a clear pointer towards a large bowel origin. Diarrhoea of small bowel origin does not occur at any particular time and any pain felt is not usually relieved by defaecation. A pale fatty stool, without fresh blood or mucus clearly indicates small bowel disease.

The presence of associated symptoms such as anorexia and weight loss will suggest significant organic disease while long continued diarrhoea, perhaps for many years, without weight loss or systemic upset might indicate an irritable bowel syndrome. Intermittency of diarrhoea, precipitated by stress, would point towards a functional bowel disturbance while weight loss despite a good appetite should suggest thyrotoxicosis particularly in the elderly where systemic signs of this disease may not be obvious. A complaint of persistent diarrhoea in middle-aged or elderly patients should of course be treated with more caution than the same complaint in a younger patient even if there is a clear relationship to stress and a diagnosis of functional bowel disease is suspected. More intensive investigation is indicated in such patients. A high proportion of patients with diarrhoea referred to a gastroenterologist are being treated for another disease and many of the drugs used are found to be responsible for the diarrhoea. Particular culprits are antihypertensive agents including β-blockers, diuretics, antacids, and antibiotics. Patients who drink large volumes of beer should not be surprised if they have loose stools but some come to the doctor complaining of diarrhoea. The presence of skin rashes, mouth ulcers, 'conjunctivitis', or perianal disease, which the patient may call 'haemorrhoids', should alert one to the possibility of an underlying inflammatory bowel disease particularly Crohn's disease.

EXAMINATION

In addition to a full clinical examination of a patient with diarrhoea a point should be made of inspecting the stool and performing a rectal examination. It is useful to perform a rigid sigmoidoscopy in the outpatient clinic at the patient's first visit to hospital and a positive diagnosis of inflammatory bowel disease, colonic neoplasms and polyps, and chronic amoebic dysentery may all be made. The reproduction of the patient's pain by the presence of the sigmoidoscope in a normal looking sigmoid colon lends credence to a diagnosis of the irritable bowel syndrome.

INVESTIGATION

The direction of investigation of a patient with persistent diarrhoea will be indicated by the history which may point towards a large or small bowel origin. Stool culture and sigmoidoscopy should be performed early, particularly in patients suspected of large bowel disease. Nowadays sigmoidoscopy with fibreoptic instruments is becoming increasingly used and it is often possible to examine the whole of the left side of the colon with little bowel preparation. The barium enema is less valuable in diagnosing the cause of diarrhoeal disease.

Where clinical features suggest small bowel disease evidence for deficiency of nutrients, produced by malabsorption, should be sought. Tests of absorptive capacity such as a faecal fat or xylose tolerance test may then be indicated. A radiological examination of the small bowel and a jejunal biopsy will provide anatomical and pathological indicators of underlying disease.

DIFFICULT, PERSISTENT DIARRHOEA

There remains a difficult group of patients in whom diarrhoea persists but in whom all investigation has proved unhelpful. It is useful in such patients to admit them to hospital and make some simple measurements of stool output. In practice patients with stool outputs of less than about 400 g per day, and who complain of diarrhoea for which no obvious cause has emerged on routine investigation, should be suspected of having an irritable bowel syndrome or anal incontinence. In many patients with the irritable bowel syndrome the diarrhoea frustratingly disappears on admission to hospital but that in itself is a clue. In others the complaint of diarrhoea is made because of frequency of defaecation although the amount of stool may be normal. The problem is then analogous to the frequency of micturition associated with cystitis and is due to 'irritability' of the rectosigmoid or a defect in the reservoir function of the lower bowel.

In patients who have 'large volume' diarrhoea, of say a litre or more per day, the major differential diagnosis lies between an osmotic and a secretory cause. The two simple manoeuvres which are useful in distinguishing these possibilities are the measurement of stool osmolality, and sodium and potassium concentrations. In a secretory diarrhoea the measured stool osmolality is close to the calculated total stool ionic concentration. This can be derived simply from the sum of the major cations, sodium and potassium, and multiplying that figure by two to account for the accompanying anions. Thus, in secretory diarrhoea osmolality $\simeq ([Na^+] + [K^+]) \times 2$. On the other hand, in osmotic diarrhoeas, in which some other non-absorbed solute is causing the diarrhoea, the measured stool osmolality is considerably higher than the total ionic concentration calculated from the sodium and potassium concentrations. The osmolar gap is made up by the unabsorbed solute. A further test which helps differentiate these causes is to observe the effect on the diarrhoea of a 24 to 48-h fast. Osmotic diarrhoeas are markedly reduced by fasting but secretory diarrhoeas continue unabated.

If an osmotic diarrhoea is indicated by these tests a search can be made for the non-absorbed solute. This is most commonly a disaccharide and due to disaccharidase deficiency, or occasionally an osmotic purgative such as magnesium sulphate, in a surreptitious purgative abuser. If, on the other hand, a secretory diarrhoeal disease is suspected a search may be made for very rare peptide-secreting tumours, such as the pancreatic islet adenoma of the Verner-Morrison syndrome which can be revealed by detecting raised plasma peptide concentrations. More common, but more difficult to detect, is the patient who is surreptitiously taking laxatives. The condition may be suspected where diarrhoea is severe and repeated investigation, often in several hospitals, has not revealed a cause. The patient who may work in a medical environment, and who is almost always female, will have befriended the physician so that he cannot begin to suspect her duplicity as she sits smiling sym-

pathetically before him. A previous psychiatric history, the presence of hypokalaemia, and the detection of melanosis coli are clues which should alert the most trusting of doctors. Once suspected it is a simple matter to search for the offending purgative in the patient's locker and perform a screening test of urine and/or faeces for laxatives. These should be undertaken early in the course of investigation when they may save the patient and the doctor many unnecessary, expansive, uncomfortable, and potentially dangerous investigations.

The management of diarrhoea is considered in later chapters.

REFERENCES

Cummunings, J.H. (1974). Laxative abuse. *Gut,* **15,** 758 6.

Fine, K.D., Krejs, G.J., and Fordtran, J.S. (1993). Diarrhoea. In *Gastrointestinal disease* (ed. M.H. Sleisenger and J.S. Fordtran) 5th edn. Ch. 49, pp. 1043–72. W.B. Saunders & Co., Philadelphia.

Leigh, R.J. and Turnberg, L.A. (1982). Faecal incontinence: the unvoiced symptom. *Lancet,* **i,** 1349–51.

Read, N.W. (1982). Diarrhoea: the failure of colonic salvage. *Lancet,* **i,** 481–3.

Turnberg, L.A. (1979). The pathophysiology of diarrhoea. *Clinical Gastroenterology,* **8,** 551–68.

14.2.5 Constipation

D. G. THOMPSON

INTRODUCTION

Constipation is commonly defined in clinical practice as the infrequent and/or difficult passage of hard stool. Definitions of what constitutes the normal consistency and frequency of passage of stool vary between societies, however, and depend largely upon dietary habits for most individuals. In Western Europe, passage of stool by normal individuals ranges between two to three stools per day to two to three per week. Three-quarters of the population pass approximately one stool per day, with a faecal weight of approximately 200 g. The daily stool weight is of actually little practical clinical use because it is largely dependent upon diet. Constipation ranges in its mode of presentation from an acute onset, which is usually taken to suggest organic obstruction, to a chronic lifelong disability, which usually indicates an intrinsic colonic neuromuscular disorder. Because the colon has a limited repertoire for expressing dysfunction, it is not surprising that constipation is the final event in a large number of problems. The most common causes of constipation are shown in Table 1.

When presented with a patient complaining of constipation, the main task for the clinician is to distinguish those in whom constipation is a manifestation of dietary deficiency from those in whom it is a component of a more generalized organic disease and those in whom it is the manifestation of a functional bowel disorder. In achieving this distinction, a carefully taken history and examination are generally adequate and specific investigations of the lower gastrointestinal tract and pelvic floor are usually reserved only for patients in whom organic disease is suspected, or those with particularly severe symptoms in whom simple measures fail and in whom surgery may be contemplated.

HISTORY

It is most important to establish clearly the nature of the defaecatory symptoms of which the patient is complaining, and to obtain a measure of the frequency, consistency, and volume of the stools. It is also important to determine whether the patient is describing an infrequent desire to defaecate or an inability to expel faeces, as the former suggests slow transit through the colon, while the latter suggests obstructed defaecation.

The duration of the constipation is one of the most helpful diagnostic indicators. On the one hand, the sudden onset of constipation in a previously fit individual is a serious symptom and suggests intestinal

Table 1 *Causes of constipation*

Inadequate dietary fibre and fermentable carbohydrate
Immobility, disinclination to defaecate
Organic obstruction:
  Neoplasm
  Diverticular disease
  Crohn's disease
Metabolic diseases:
  Hypothyroidism
  Hypercalcaemia
Extrinsic neurological diseases:
  Spinal-cord and sacral-nerve disease
  Pudendal-nerve damage
  Parkinson's disease
Chronic intrinsic neuromuscular disease of the colon:
  Hirschprung's disease
  Chronic pseudo-obstruction
  Systemic sclerosis
  Diabetic neuropathy
Drug therapy:
  Opiates
  Anticholinergic agents including antidepressants
  Iron therapy
Functional constipation

obstruction, particularly if accompanied by increasing abdominal pain. Such patients usually require immediate surgical attention. Alternatively, constipation since childhood, with slow deterioration in function with time, almost certainly indicates a progressive neuromuscular degenerative disorder of the colon. Between these two extremes lie the most common modes of presentation. A carefully taken dietary history is mandatory because the quantity of dietary fibre and fermentable carbohydrate ingested in a normal individual is the strongest determinant of faecal weight and defaecatory frequency. Patients who are bed-bound or find themselves in a situation where defaecation is socially inconvenient will inevitably reduce the frequency of defaecation and increase the consistency of their stool, which increases the risk of constipation. The development of progressive obstruction to the colon lumen must always be considered in adults, particularly those in whom the risk of colon cancer is high. A change in stool diameter together with the presence of blood in the stool can be indicators of malignant rectal obstruction. Metabolic diseases, in particular hypothyroidism, hypercalcaemia, and diabetes with autonomic neuropathy, should always be considered, as should the possibility of a more widespread neurological disease, particularly in elderly people. Chronic constipation in young women who are otherwise well is characteristically worse during the latter phases of the menstrual cycle and also exacerbated by pregnancy.

In women, an obstetric and gynaecological history should be obtained to determine the relation between the onset of any defaecatory difficulty and possible pelvic-floor dysfunction.

A careful drug history must be sought from all patients and consumption of constipation-inducing medication such as opiates and anticholinergic agents, including antidepressants, must be excluded.

A family history of constipation suggests a chronic neuromuscular disease of the colon, while the social and psychiatric history will help determine whether disinclination to defaecate or the social impossibility of defaecation is a factor.

CLINICAL EXAMINATION

A careful clinical examination should also be conducted. A general examination should be made to exclude disorders such as Parkinson's disease and hypothyroidism.

Examination of the abdomen should be thorough. The presence of hard faeces palpable in the colon is a useful confirmatory sign, particularly when present in the right side of the abdomen. Gross abdominal

distension is an unusual accompaniment of chronic constipation, except in individuals with severe megacolon due to colonic muscle disease or in those with psychiatric disorders and a severe disinclination to defaecate.

Examination of the perineum and anus is mandatory. A rough guide to pelvic-floor dysfunction is obtained by examination of the perineum in the left lateral position whilst the patient either strains or coughs. Absence of normal pelvic descent suggests an abnormality of pelvic-floor relaxation. The visible descent of the perineum to the level of the ischial tuberosities after straining or coughing indicates damage to neuromuscular control of the pelvic floor, which is often accompanied by rectal mucosal prolapse. Inspection of the anus for local disease, such as fissures or fistulae, is also important, as local anal pain on attempted defaecation is a powerful inhibitor of stool expulsion. A digital rectal examination and proctosigmoidoscopy should also be used to exclude organic disease of the rectum, to inspect the mucosa for melanosis coli, which is often an indicator of chronic laxative abuse, and to confirm the presence of solid faeces.

LABORATORY EXAMINATION

In most patients, an extensive battery of laboratory examinations is not warranted unless the clinical history and examination indicate a specific abnormality. A plain radiographic examination of the abdomen following air insufflation at proctoscopy is often useful in determining the diameter of the colon and excluding megacolon. Barium enema and/or colonoscopy are required in those in whom organic obstruction is suspected. Anorectal manometry and electrophysiological studies should be conducted if Hirschprung's disease is considered; a failure of the normal rectoanal inhibitory response is found in this disease.

Measurement of whole-gut and colonic transit by marker techniques is useful only if there is suspicion about the severity of the symptoms, and in those patients in whom surgery is contemplated.

MANAGEMENT

Management of a patient with constipation is dependent upon the individual concerned and whether an underlying disorder is identifiable. In the absence of a treatable underlying cause for the constipation, symptomatic relief can usually be obtained by either dietary modification, laxatives, enemata or, occasionally, by surgery.

In the vast majority of patients with simple constipation, the addition of poorly absorbed dietary carbohydrate is usually successful. Whilst this is traditionally given in the form of wheat bran, it is possible to improve symptoms using other vegetable polysaccharides such as lentils and beans, which have the advantage of being more palatable. Laxatives can be additionally prescribed if dietary modification fails. Therapy should begin with the simplest agents such as lactulose, which passes through the upper gastrointestinal tract and is fermented by colonic bacteria to produce organic acids that act both as osmotic and stimulant agents.

Specific stimulant laxatives can be tried in those individuals in whom defaecation remains a problem despite bulking agents. These drugs act directly on the neuromuscular apparatus of the colon and stimulate faecal expulsion. The prolonged unsupervised use of stimulant laxatives is to be cautioned against in view of the strong clinical suspicion that they themselves may have a deleterious effect on colonic function. In some patients, however, they are the only practical solution to an otherwise debilitating problem. Enemata may be useful in obtaining colonic clearance of impacted faeces and as a prelude to longer-term laxative use. In intractable cases, regular, intermittent enemata may be the only practical way of managing the problem.

In young persons with severe symptoms and slow transit, where the lifestyle is severely impaired, subtotal colectomy can be of great benefit. Such procedures need to be carefully planned because results depend much on the type of colonic disorder, the presence or absence of pelvic-floor dysfunction, and the integrity of the anal sphincter.

REFERENCES

McCready, R.A. and Beart, R. (1979). The surgical treatment of incapacitating constipation associated with ideopathic mega-colon. *Mayo Clinic Proceedings*, **54**, 779.

Pezim, M.E., Pemberton, J.H., Levin, K.E., Litchy, W.J., and Phillips, S.F. (1993). Parameters of anorectal and colonic motility in health and in severe constipation. *Diseases of the Colon and Rectum*, **36**, 484–91.

Reynolds, J.C. (1989). Chronic constipation. In *Pathogenesis of functional bowel disease*, pp. 199–225. Plenum, New York.

Shetty, P. and Kurpad, A. (1987). Increased starch intake in human diet increases faecal bulking. *American Journal of Clinical Nutrition*, **43**, 210–12.

14.2.6 Gastrointestinal bleeding

D. P. JEWELL

The major causes of acute bleeding from the gastrointestinal tract are listed in Table 1. In terms of diagnosis and management, they are best considered as acute bleeding from either the upper or lower gastrointestinal tract and as chronic bleeding. Chronic bleeding is discussed in Chapter 22.7.

Acute upper gastrointestinal bleeding

This presents as haematemesis and/or melaena. It is very rare for lesions distal to the ligament of Treitz to cause a haematemesis. However, brisk bleeding may occur from a proximal lesion, for example oesophageal varices, without haematemesis and present as melaena. Upper gastrointestinal bleeding can be severe enough to cause the passage of dark-red blood per rectum, which may cause diagnostic confusion. Table 2 shows the approximate frequency of lesions causing upper gastrointestinal bleeding and has been compiled from a number of recent British series. Bleeding from oesophageal varices is a common cause in those countries where the incidence of alcoholic cirrhosis is high and is being seen more frequently in Britain. It should be noted that acute bleeding from a gastric carcinoma is relatively uncommon. Bleeding from Mallory–Weiss tears usually follows an episode of violent retching. This is particularly common after large doses of alcohol. The degree of bleeding ranges from a cupful of blood to a torrent. The majority of patients stop bleeding spontaneously and, indeed, the tears may heal within 24 h. However, blood loss occasionally can be sufficiently prolonged and severe to require emergency surgery. Rare causes of acute bleeding include vascular abnormalities (telangiectasia, angiomata), leiomyoma, haemophilia, thrombocytopenia, Ehlers–Danlos syndrome, pseudoxanthoma elasticum, and rupture of the aorta into the duodenum.

The role of aspirin in initiating bleeding from whatever cause is still controversial. Certainly up to one-third of patients presenting with acute bleeding may have ingested aspirin within the previous 24 to 48 h. However, some series have shown a similar proportion of aspirin-takers amongst patients presenting with other acute medical emergencies. All the anti-inflammatory drugs may be associated with bleeding.

ASSESSMENT

A rapid clinical assessment must be made before resuscitation is begun. Except in severely shocked patients, the patient should be questioned about dyspepsia, vomiting, alcohol, drugs, previous episodes of bleeding, and jaundice. Pulse, respiratory rate, blood pressure, and the state of the peripheral circulation must be noted and recorded. Specific signs to look for are those of chronic liver disease, iron deficiency, telangiectasia (these may only be present on the undersurface of the tongue), and malignancy.

Blood should be taken for cross-matching and for determination of haemoglobin, haematocrit, platelet count, and prothrombin time. A plain radiograph of the abdomen is rarely useful.

Table 1 *Causes of gastrointestinal bleeding*

Inflammatory
Oesophagitis; gastritis; peptic ulcer; Crohn's disease; ulcerative colitis; enterocolitis—infective, ischaemic, radiation

Mechanical
Hiatus hernia; Mallory–Weiss tears; Meckel's diverticulum; diverticulosis coli

Neoplasms
Carcinoma; polyps—single, multiple; leiomyoma; carcinoid

Vascular
Varices; hereditary telangiectasia; angioma; aortointestinal fistula; mesenteric thrombosis or embolus; arteritis

Systemic
Chronic renal failure; thrombocytopenia; coagulation defects; connective tissue disorders; dysproteinaemia

Table 2 *Causes of upper gastrointestinal bleeding and their frequency*

Cause	Frequency (%)
Duodenal ulcer	35
Gastric ulcer	20
Acute gastric erosions/haemorrhagic gastritis	18
Mallory–Weiss tear	10
Gastric carcinoma	6
Oesophageal varices	5
Other	6

Assessment must be made by the physician and surgeon working as a team so that joint decisions on management can be made.

MANAGEMENT

An intravenous line is set up immediately. Saline should be given initially but, occasionally, uncross-matched blood (blood group O, rhesus negative), albumin or plasma expanders may be required if bleeding is severe. Central venous-pressure lines should be inserted into all patients over 65 years of age and into younger patients who show signs of a compromised blood volume (tachycardia in excess of 100/min; postural fall in systolic blood pressure of more than 20 mmHg). Once cross-matched blood is available, transfusion should begin with whole blood in order to raise the haemoglobin to at least 10 g/dl; this ensures the patient is in good condition should rebleeding occur. In general, one unit of blood raises the haemoglobin by 1 g/dl in an adult. In those patient in whom the central venous pressure is raised, packed cells should be used and a diuretic, such as frusemide, may also be necessary. Half-hourly observations of pulse, respiratory rate, and blood pressure are instituted, although these can be reduced in frequency once bleeding has stopped. The use of a nasogastric tube is controversial but it adds to the discomfort of the patient, it may cause fresh bleeding, and can cause erosions that may be confusing at subsequent endoscopy. Repeated nasogastric aspiration as a means of detecting a recurrent bleed is less sensitive than observing the pulse rate. The use of intravenous H_2-antagonists in the acute stage is common practice but there is little evidence to support this. Small trials have variously reported some benefit in patients bleeding from oesophageal varices, in elderly women bleeding from gastric ulcers, and in patients with upper gastrointestinal bleeding following renal transplantation. However, most studies have shown disappointing results for H_2-antagonists.

Indeed a recent trial of intravenous famotidine versus placebo in nearly 1000 patients presenting with a bleeding ulcer, and who had the endoscopic signs predicting a high risk of rebleeding, showed no benefit for the H_2-antagonist. Likewise, a similarly sized trial of oral omeprazole against placebo was also negative. Thus, it is unnecessary to lower gastric acid secretion initially; it is preferable to make a diagnosis and then start treatment. There may be some role for H$_2$-antagonists in patients in intensive care to prevent acute bleeding from stress ulcers or from gastric erosions but intragastric instillation of antacids may be a more effective measure.

For patients bleeding from oesophageal varices, further procedures may be necessary. Intravenous pitressin may be helpful, given as a continuous infusion (0.4 u/min). The arterial route confers no greater advantage. A Sengstaken–Blakemore tube is indicated if bleeding is severe and prolonged, and the decision has been made to obliterate the varices subsequently. Endoscopic sclerosis of the varices or a surgical operation may be considered. Many patients with chronic liver disease will become encephalopathic during a gastrointestinal bleed and will require the appropriate treatment.

DIAGNOSTIC PROCEDURES

Initially, the management of acute upper gastrointestinal bleeding must consist of restoring the circulation. Once bleeding has stopped, and the patient is in a good haemodynamic state, the diagnosis of the cause of the bleeding can begin. Emergency endoscopy or barium meals while the patient is still bleeding and in a state of shock are usually hazardous and often reveal little more than the fact that the stomach is full of blood. However, diagnostic procedures must be done within 24 h of bleeding because erosions and tears can heal rapidly.

The diagnostic procedure of choice is upper gastrointestinal endoscopy as this will reveal tears and acute erosions of the stomach or duodenum that may frequently be missed radiologically, even when air-contrast studies are made. Furthermore, endoscopy allows biopsies to be taken of a gastric ulcer or a tumour if found. If varices are found at endoscopy, it is safe to pass the endoscope through into the stomach (especially if a small-diameter endoscope is used) and, indeed, it is essential to make a full examination of the stomach and duodenum in order to exclude other causes of bleeding. Even if endoscopy, or radiography are delayed until bleeding has stopped, the stomach may still be full of clots. If they are troublesome, they can be washed out with a large stomach tube. However, as this procedure can damage the gastric mucosa and can cause diagnostic confusion, gastric wash-outs are best avoided. Intravenous metoclopramide can be useful in emptying the stomach of clots.

If a gastric or duodenal ulcer is found, the endoscopist should record whether there is active bleeding at the time of endoscopy, whether a visible vessel can be seen in the base of the ulcer, or whether the ulcer crater is covered by clot. These endoscopic signs of recent bleeding have a very high predictive value for rebleeding.

Angiography should be reserved for patients with continuing bleeding in whom no cause of bleeding has been found at upper gastrointestinal endoscopy. It is especially useful in detecting angiomas, the presence of duodenal or ileal varices, bleeding from Meckel's diverticulum or non-specific ulcers of the ileum, and small-bowel tumours. Small lesions, however, can only be visualized when there is active bleeding: this usually means a bleeding rate of at least 0.5 ml/min.

If patients are bleeding profusely and emergency surgery is being considered, endoscopy may be indicated immediately. In this situation, it is often best to perform the examination under anaesthetic before surgery. The presence of the endotracheal tube protects against inhalation of blood. The other possible indication for emergency endoscopy is when oesophageal varices are suspected to be the cause of bleeding, as the patients may be bleeding from mucosal lesions such as erosions or peptic ulcers. The subsequent management will obviously differ according to the endoscopic findings. Unfortunately, precise endoscopic diagnosis is often difficult under these circumstances.

INDICATIONS FOR SURGERY

As previously stated, all patients presenting with acute upper gastrointestinal bleeding must be assessed by a physician and surgeon working as a team. The precise indications for surgery will depend on the cause of bleeding. If bleeding is from a haemorrhagic erosive gastritis, surgery should be avoided if possible as the surgeon may have to do a total gastrectomy. Bleeding from a carcinoma is rarely severe and continuous enough to require emergency surgery. The management of bleeding varices is considered elsewhere (see Chapter 14.6).

For peptic ulcers, early surgery can be recommended once initial resuscitation has been achieved. This is particularly so for elderly patients if there is continuous bleeding resulting in transfusion in excess of 6 pints. Bleeding to the point at which the central venous pressure cannot be maintained is a clear indication. Patients with recurrent bleeds should also be recommended for early surgery.

ENDOSCOPIC MANAGEMENT

Increasingly, endoscopic methods are being used to control bleeding from gastric or duodenal ulcers. The methods used range from the injection of sclerosants, coagulation by diathermy or heater probes to Nd-YAG laser therapy and experimental methods of placing sutures or staples over the bleeding vessel. The most readily available technique is the injection method, the choice of sclerosant being 1 in 10 000 adrenaline, 5 per cent ethanolamine, 1 per cent polidocanol, absolute alcohol, or a combination. The most recent study suggests that absolute alcohol may be more effective than the other agents. However, the major problem with the use of these endoscopic techniques is that there have been few controlled trials comparing these various methods and they have been mostly too small for statistical validity.

COURSE AND PROGRESS

This again depends on the cause of bleeding. Patients bleeding from varices and malignant tumours are discussed in Chapters 14.6 and 14.16. The majority of patients with ulcers and erosions will stop bleeding within a few hours and, if rebleeding does not occur within 48 h, they can be considered for early discharge from hospital.

The overall mortality of upper gastrointestinal bleeding is about 8 to 12 per cent and has remained constant since the 1960s. Undoubtedly, one of the major factors contributing to this lack of progress is the increasing age of the population. So far, there is no evidence that early diagnosis by endoscopy or recourse to early surgery have greatly altered the overall prognosis. Nevertheless, the major cause of mortality is rebleeding and it is now possible to predict which patients with gastric or duodenal ulcers are at particular risk from this complication. The presence of a clot or a visible vessel at the base of the ulcer, seen at endoscopy, has been shown to predict a high risk of rebleeding. Therefore, it is possible that in this subgroup of patients with bleeding ulcers, mortality may be reduced by an aggressive interventional approach.

Hopefully, endoscopic techniques such as injection with adrenaline will prove effective so that the mortality and morbidity of surgery, especially in the case of the elderly, can be avoided.

So far, the only course of management that has reduced mortality from upper gastrointestinal bleeding has been the introduction of defined protocols of management, especially in a specialist unit. It should be possible to reduce the mortality to less than 4 per cent when patient management involves physicians, surgeons, and endoscopists with special interests in gastrointestinal bleeding.

Chronic gastrointestinal blood loss

This subject is considered in Chapter 22.7.

REFERENCES

Bernuau, J. and Rueff, B. (1985). Treatment of acute variceal bleeding. *Clinical Gastroenterology*, **14**, 185–207.

Garden, O.J. and Carter, D.C. (1992). Balloon tamponade and vasoactive drugs in the control of acute variceal haemorrhage. *Clinical Gastroenterology*, **6**, 451–63.

Langman, M.J.S. (1985). Upper gastrointestinal bleeding: the trials of trials. *Gut*, **26**, 217–20.

Rutgeerts, P., Gevers, A.M., Hiele, M., Broekaert, L., and Vantrappen, G. (1993). Endoscopic injection therapy to prevent rebleeding from peptic ulcers with a protruding vessel: a controlled comparative trial. *Gut*, **34**, 348–50.

Swain, P. (1991). Gastrointestinal bleeding: endoscopic treatment of peptic ulcer haemorrhage. *Clinical Gastroenterology*, **5**, 537–61.

14.3 Methods for investigation of gastrointestinal diseases

14.3.1 Endoscopy

D. P. JEWELL

Endoscopy not only provides the ability to visualize the oesophagus, stomach, duodenum, and colon directly but also allows biopsy specimens and cytological samples to be taken. Furthermore, therapeutic endoscopy has proved cost-effective, has improved patient comfort, and has become widely available. The introduction of electronic endoscopes over the last few years has been a major advance. These instruments avoid the need for a fibreoptic bundle; instead, they have a chip mounted at the tip of the instrument (usually three chips, one each for blue, green, and red light), which sends an electronic signal to a processor and hence an image on a television monitor. The reduction in maintenance costs, primarily due to the absence of fibreoptic bundles, and their considerable benefit for teaching and education, as everyone in the endoscopy room can see the image, has made electronic endoscopes the instruments of choice. As with fibreoptic instruments, the electronic endoscopes have four-way tip deflection, a field of view of 120° to 140°, and finger-tip controls for air insufflation, suction, and for water injection to clean the lens or mucosa.

Indications

OESOPHAGEAL DISEASE

Endoscopy with a forward-viewing instrument is essential for the diagnosis of oesophagitis and for obtaining biopsy specimens and cytological samples from strictures, Barrett's mucosa, and neoplasms. Barium studies are still required, however, because motor disorders of the oesophagus are difficult to appreciate by the endoscopist, and oesophageal reflux is much better assessed by the radiologist. Unless the endoscopist is highly experienced, patients presenting with dysphagia should have a barium swallow to determine the cause and site of the symptom before endoscopy. Benign strictures can be dilated endoscopically and malignant strictures may be treated either by inserting a tube (e.g. the Celestin tube) or by laser therapy. Although both of these procedures are associated with morbidity, mostly due to perforation, they are preferable to palliative surgery, especially as the patients are usually elderly.

GASTRODUODENAL DISEASE

Endoscopy is the investigation of choice for gastroduodenal disease. Gastritis (acute, chronic, superficial, atrophic), the presence of erosions and Mallory–Weiss tears are readily recognized and biopsy specimens can be obtained for histological diagnosis. This has become particularly important since the association between *Helicobacter pylori* and gastritis and ulcer disease has been recognized. All gastric ulcers, even if they appear benign, require biopsy and cytological brushing to exclude malignancy. Endoscopy is also essential for symptomatic patients who have had previous gastric surgery, as the postoperative stomach is notoriously difficult to examine radiologically. However, double-contrast radiography is very useful for assessing motor disorders, infiltrative tumours (e.g. linitis plastica, lymphoma), which may not be obvious endoscopically, smooth muscle tumours (leiomyoma), and for determining the degree of pyloric stenosis. Duodenal disease is always better assessed by endoscopy rather than by radiography, although the endoscopist can miss duodenal ulcers if they are just behind the rim of the pylorus.

SMALL-INTESTINAL DISEASE

Distal duodenal biopsy specimens are being increasingly used for the diagnosis of coeliac disease and appear to be as good as a jejunal biopsy taken from the ligament of Treitz. The diagnosis of coeliac disease may be obvious to the endoscopist at the time of the examination because there is often flattening and effacement of the valves of Kerckring. Distal duodenal biopsy specimens can also be useful for detecting other small-intestinal disorders such as amyloid, lymphoma, immunoproliferative disorders (α-chain disease), lymphangiectasi, and Whipple's disease. Furthermore, duodenal aspirates can be obtained to exclude giardiasis and to culture for excess bacterial populations. Recently, enteroscopes have been developed to examine the whole of the small intestine. To obtain a full examination the Sonde-type is required in which there is a balloon surrounding the tip of the instrument. The instrument is passed through the patient's nose, placed into the duodenum with the help of an ordinary endoscope passed through the mouth, and then the balloon is inflated. Peristalsis then carries the instrument forward with frequent 'feeding' of the instrument through the nose. It usually takes 6 to 8 h for the tip to travel into the ileum, and the examination of the mucosa is done on withdrawal. Clearly, it is not suitable for routine use but may have a role in the diagnosis of obscure intestinal bleeding, the diagnosis of small-bowel tumours, and the recognition of ileal ulcers. Biopsy specimens cannot easily be obtained because of the length and floppiness of the instrument.

COLONIC DISEASE

Colonoscopy is being increasingly used for the diagnosis of colonic disease in preference to a double-contrast barium enema. The major indications are: (i) either as the first-line investigation of suspected colonic disease or for patients with colonic symptoms and a negative barium enema; (ii) to perform polypectomy and to obtain biopsy specimens from tumours; (iii) to assess strictures; (iv) to investigate patients with colonic bleeding, especially for the diagnosis and treatment of angiodysplasia; (v) to assess patients with Crohn's disease or ulcerative colitis.

PANCREATIC DISEASE

Visualization of the pancreatic duct by direct endoscopic cannulation should be done when pancreatic tumours or chronic pancreatitis are suspected. This procedure, together with ultrasound or a computerized tomographic scan and possibly a pancreatic function test, will give maximal diagnostic information.

BILIARY DISEASE

Endoscopic visualization of the biliary tree is now the best diagnostic procedure for stones, tumours, and strictures of the bile duct and is the only reliable means of diagnosing primary sclerosing cholangitis. Furthermore, it offers the therapeutic procedures of sphincterotomy, stone withdrawal, and the insertion of stents across strictures. Percutaneous transhepatic cholangiography may occasionally be required for adequate assessment of high bile-duct strictures and insertion of stents at this level may require combined percutaneous and endoscopic procedures.

Premedication

In many parts of the world, upper gastrointestinal endoscopy is done with local anaesthesia to the oropharynx only and without intravenous sedation. However, the majority of units in the United Kingdom use sedation, although some patients will request local anaesthesia only and endoscopists should be sufficiently skilled to make the examination in this way. The benzodiazepines (midazolam, diazepam) are most commonly used and the dose given should be sufficient to relax the patient but maintain the ability to obey a command. Very small doses (2–3 mg) may be sufficient for the elderly. The use of diazepam can be associated with thrombophlebitis and pain at the site of injection but these problems can be overcome by using diazepam in a lipid emulsion (Diazemuls). Midazolam is not associated with these complications but it is the more potent drug and therefore it is easier to oversedate patients. At the end of the examination, the sedative and amnesic properties of these drugs can be reversed by flumazenil, a specific benzodiazepine antagonist. This should always be done for elderly patients (over 75 years of age) but its cost has prevented routine use in most units. If it is not used, it must be remembered that patients rarely remember much that has been explained about the findings of the examination, even though they appear to be comprehending well at the time.

During endoscopic examination in a sedated patient, there is frequently a fall in blood pressure and a drop in oxygen saturation. This has led to the increasing use of oxygen given nasally or by face mask at a rate of 4 l/min. Oxygen is mandatory for the following groups: elderly patients, those with ischaemic heart disease or cerebrovascular disease; patients actively bleeding or who are anaemic; the morbidly obese patient. Monitoring oxygen saturation by pulse oximetry has been recommended as it allows desaturation to be detected quickly.

There are many medicolegal implications for sedation in endoscopy units, which have led to a number of guidelines to ensure safety. The recent working party set up by the British Society of Gastroenterology made the following recommendations:

- Resuscitation equipment and drugs must be available and all staff should be familiar with their use. Specific antagonists to benzodiazepines and opiates must also be available.
- A nurse trained in endoscopic and resuscitation techniques should monitor the patient during procedures.
- Prior to endoscopy, details of the patient's medical history, blood pressure, cardiac status, and medications must be identified.
- Sedation must be kept to the minimum necessary.
- An intravenous cannula should remain in place throughout the procedure.
- Oxygen-enriched air should be given to high-risk patients and pulse oximetry is recommended.
- Monitoring must continue in the recovery area by a qualified member of the staff, usually a nurse.
- Records of management and outcome should be kept.

Disinfection of instruments

Cross-infection by contaminated endoscopes is rare but has been well documented to occur in three ways: (i) transmission of pathogenic organisms from one patient to another—the most frequent organisms being salmonellae; (ii) the transmission of infection to staff by needle-stick injury such as hepatitis B; and (iii) the introduction of opportunistic organisms that colonize the instruments on storage. These may cause serious infection in immunocompromised patients and can cause severe biliary or pancreatic sepsis if introduced during endoscopic retrograde cholangiopancreatography (ERCP). The increasing prevalence of human immunodeficiency viral (**HIV**) infection has highlighted the need for adequate disinfection.

As soon as the endoscope is removed from the patient, it should be immersed in water and detergent. Valves must be removed and all parts and the distal tip cleaned with cotton buds and a soft toothbrush. Channels are cleaned with an appropriate-sized cleaning bush and are then flushed. This mechanical cleaning reduces bacterial contamination to very low levels but disinfection is necessary to eradicate vegetative bacteria and viruses. Immersion in 2 per cent glutaraldehyde or 10 per cent succine dealdehyde for 10 min is recommended. However, a proportion of staff will become sensitized to glutaraldehyde despite wearing gloves and the installation of ventilation systems. Closed-system endoscopic washing machines with a disinfection cycle overcome these problems but they are expensive and microbiological monitoring of the machine is necessary.

Ancillary endoscopic equipment (biopsy forceps, injection needles, brushes) should be cleaned mechanically or by ultrasound, disinfected with glutaraldehyde, and then dried. Any equipment for cannulating the biliary or pancreatic ducts requires sterilization by autoclave or ethylene oxide.

Staff members should wear gloves and many wear masks and protective eyewear for patients known to be positive for hepatitis B or HIV or for patients in whom there is active bleeding. All endoscopy personnel should be immunized against hepatitis B.

Antibiotics

There is no agreed policy on the need for prophylactic antibiotics in patients with valvular disease, prosthetic valves, or a history of endocarditis. Colonoscopy and invasive procedures in the upper gastrointestinal tract (e.g. ERCP, variceal sclerotherapy) are best covered with antibiotics given intravenously just before the procedure. However, antibiotics are probably not necessary for a straightforward diagnostic oesophagogastroduodenoscopy.

14.3.2 Radiology

D. J. NOLAN and E. W. L. FLETCHER

Radiological and imaging techniques play an important part in the diagnosis and management of disorders of the digestive system. Plain radiographs may provide some help, but to obtain the required information in the majority of cases it is necessary to outline the upper gastrointestinal tract, small intestine, colon, or biliary tract with positive contrast medium. Angiography continues to have a role in the investigation of gastrointestinal bleeding and in the preoperative evaluation of the liver and pancreas. The newer imaging techniques of ultrasound, radionuclide scanning, computerized tomography, and magnetic resonance imaging are valuable for investigating the hepatobiliary system and pancreas.

The gastrointestinal tract

PLAIN ABDOMINAL RADIOGRAPHS

Plain radiographs of the chest and abdomen are the initial investigation in patients who present with symptoms or signs of an 'acute abdomen'.

Perforation or obstruction of the gastrointestinal tract may be evident on plain radiographs.

BARIUM STUDIES OF THE UPPER GASTROINTESTINAL TRACT

Barium continues to be widely used for the routine examination of the upper gastrointestinal tract, which from the radiological viewpoint consists of the oesophagus, stomach, and duodenum as far as the ligament of Treitz. The double-contrast barium meal is now used routinely in most centres as it gives much better results than the conventional single-contrast examination. The technique allows the stomach to be distended with gas while a thin coating of barium suspension enables its inner surface to be visualized (Fig. 1). The gas, introduced as an effervescent agent, puts the gastric mucosa under slight tension and lesions causing lack of distensibility result in a clearly visible series of converging folds. Carcinomas, ulcers, and ulcer scars that have a converging fold pattern

are easily detected. Small lesions and slight irregularity of the mucosa can be identified. It is possible with this examination to detect small carcinomas that have not spread beyond the mucosa and the prognosis for such patients has improved as a result. The lesions are shown *en face* and the mucosal relief pattern closely resembles the endoscopic and macroscopic appearances. Lesions most frequently seen in the upper gastrointestinal tract include carcinomas and benign strictures of the oesophagus, oesophageal varices (Fig. 2), hiatal hernias, gastric ulceration (Fig. 3), gastric carcinomas, and duodenal ulceration (Fig. 4).

Special barium studies are sometimes indicated, such as cineradiography or videoradiography, which demonstrate functional abnormalities of the pharynx and upper oesophagus. Patients who have had a previous Billroth I or Polya-type partial gastrectomy are examined by a modified double-contrast examination. If the prime interest is the duodenal loop, hypotonic duodenography should be performed as a separate study. When perforation is suspected in the upper gastrointestinal tract and plain films are inconclusive, water-soluble contrast agents are used instead of barium.

Fibreoptic endoscopy is widely used to visualize lesions and to obtain aimed biopsy and cytological specimens. It has been claimed that endos-

Fig. 1 Normal double-contrast view of the lower body and antrum of the stomach as well as the duodenal cap.

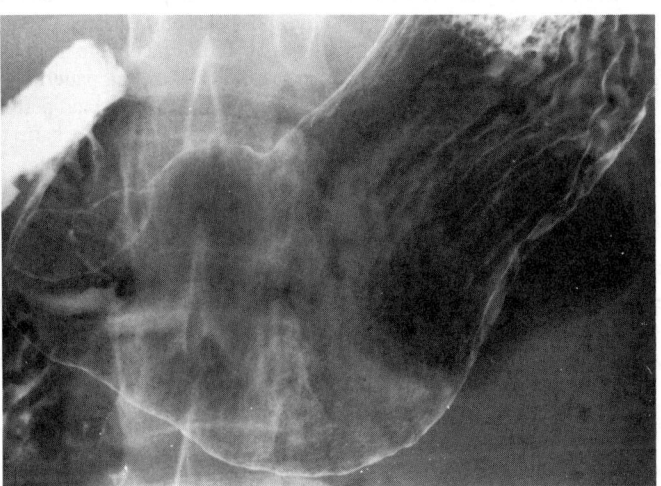

Fig. 2 Oesophageal varices shown on a barium swallow.

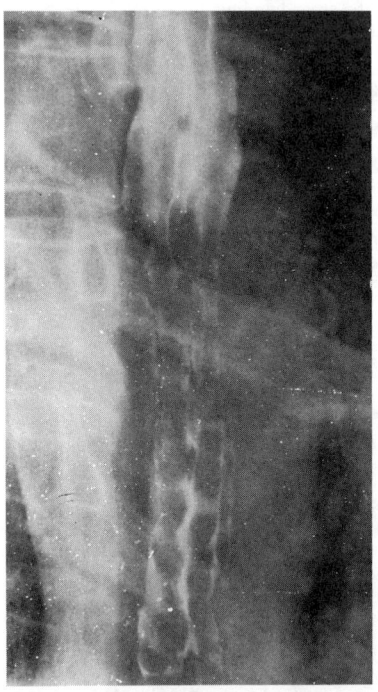

Fig. 3 Gastric ulcer. A shallow ulcer crater is seen on the posterior wall of the upper body of the stomach with distortion of the adjacent mucosal pattern. The patient presented with acute gastrointestinal bleeding.

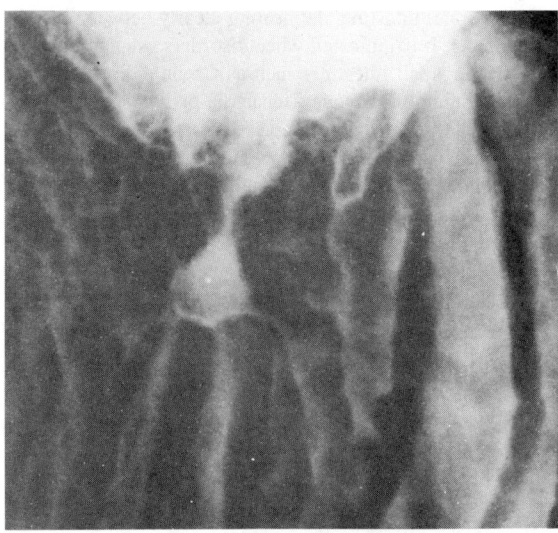

Fig. 4 Duodenal ulcer. A moderate-sized ulcer crater is seen in the base of the duodenal cap.

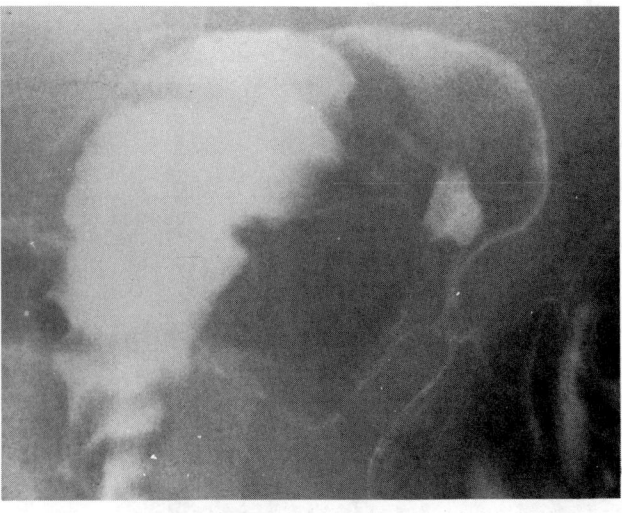

copy is more accurate in detecting lesions of the upper gastrointestinal tract than the barium meal. This was true with the single-contrast barium examination, but the argument no longer holds when proper double-contrast barium studies are done. The accuracy of both double-contrast barium studies and endoscopy depends on the experience and skill of the person performing the examination. The main advantages of the double-contrast barium examination are that it is safer and more comfortable for the patient and can be done quickly. Each radiograph obtained provides an image of a large area of the oesophagus, stomach, or duodenum that can be retained as a permanent record and is available at any time for detailed review.

BARIUM EXAMINATION OF THE SMALL INTESTINE

The follow-through is the most widely used procedure for examining the small intestine with barium. The examination is normally made following a barium-meal examination of the oesophagus, stomach, and duodenum. Large films of the abdomen are taken at half-hourly intervals as the barium progresses through the small intestine.

Many investigators are dissatisfied with the accuracy of the barium follow-through and an increasing number of centres are now adopting the enteroclysis technique (small-bowel enema) instead. A large volume of dilute barium suspension is infused directly into the small intestine through a duodenal tube (Fig. 5). The examination, including duodenal intubation, normally takes 20 to 30 min. Enteroclysis gives excellent visualization of the small intestine, delineating clearly between healthy and diseased segments. It is indicated when disorders causing morphological changes in the small intestine, such as Crohn's disease, tuberculosis, neoplasms, radiation damage, ischaemia or Meckel's diverticulum, are suspected. If coeliac disease is suspected, jejunal biopsy should be the initial diagnostic procedure and the barium studies should be reserved for patients in whom the jejunal biopsy is normal or for detecting suspected complications of coeliac disease such as lymphoma.

Reflux of barium through the ileocaecal valve may occur during barium enema examinations and this barium can be used to visualize the terminal ileum. Diseases affecting the small intestine often involve the distal ileum and the diagnostic value of refluxed barium should not be overlooked.

Fig. 5 A normal barium infusion examination of the small intestine.

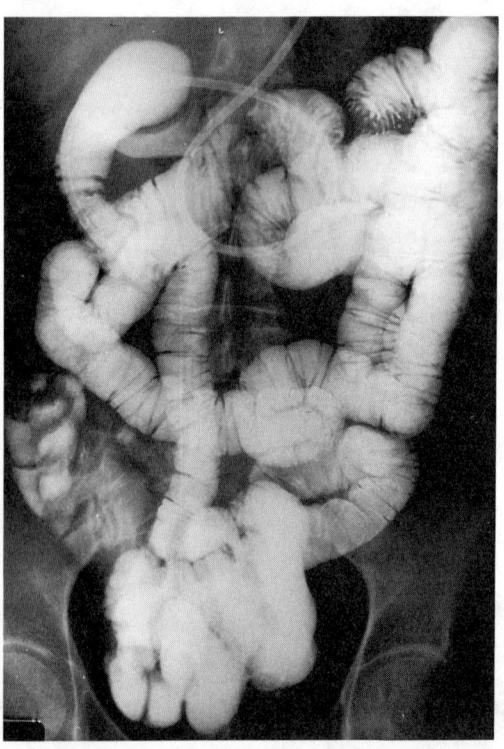

BARIUM ENEMA

Digital examination of the rectum and sigmoidoscopy should have been done before the barium enema is requested. Indications for a barium enema are to detect colorectal cancer and polyps, and in the diagnosis and management of inflammatory bowel disease. There is evidence to show that cancers of the colon develop from previously benign adenomas. If cancer of the colon is diagnosed at an early stage, the survival rate of patients is much higher than if lesions are extensive at the time of diagnosis. The barium examination of the colon is therefore a most important diagnostic procedure; it should be sensitive enough to detect small polyps of the colon as well as cancers. The double-contrast barium enema fulfils this requirement and it should be used routinely.

A clean colon, a suitable barium suspension, air insufflation, and the routine use of smooth-muscle relaxant drugs, together with a good radiographic, technique are essential for consistently good results. Barium is introduced into the rectum and it is allowed to flow in a column as far as the hepatic flexure before being drained off. A smooth-muscle relaxant such as 20 mg of hyoscine butylbromide (Buscopan) is injected intravenously and air is introduced into the rectum. Radiographs are obtained following air insufflation. Cancers and polyps of the colon are shown either as infiltrating (Fig. 6) or polypoid lesions. The changes of inflammatory bowel disease are shown as mucosal ulceration seen *en face* and in profile and as alterations in the normal mucosal pattern.

Barium enemas should not be used in patients with suspected perforation of the colon or with toxic megacolon. A single-contrast barium enema is indicated in patients with obstruction.

GASTROINTESTINAL ANGIOGRAPHY

Selective visceral angiography is indicated in certain patients who present with bleeding from the gastrointestinal tract. Angiography is done for two reasons in patients with acute bleeding—to locate the source of bleeding when it is unknown (Fig. 7), and to stop the bleeding by selective infusion of drugs or embolic material into the bleeding territory. Angiography can also yield valuable diagnostic information in patients with obscure gastrointestinal bleeding when barium studies and fibreoptic endoscopy are negative. Lesions that are likely to cause obscure bleeding include angiomatous malformations, small neoplasms, Meckel's diverticulum, and small ulcers. Selective catheterization of the coe-

Fig. 6 An infiltrating carcinoma of the ascending limb of the splenic flexure shown on a double-contrast barium enema examination.

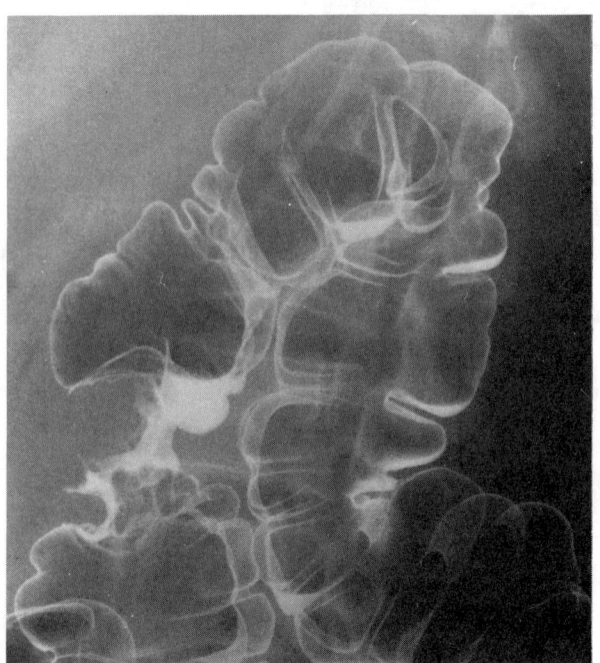

liac axis, superior mesenteric artery and inferior mesenteric artery, and superselective catherization may be required. Barium studies should be not be employed if there is evidence of gastrointestinal bleeding until the question of angiography has been considered, as the presence of barium in the gastrointestinal tract makes it impossible to carry out adequate studies.

RADIONUCLIDE STUDIES

In children, Meckel's diverticulum can be detected using $^{99}Tc^m$ pertechnetate and this should be the initial radiological procedure if this condition is suspected in neonates and children. Meckel's diverticulum is identified as an area of increased radionuclide activity in the lower abdomen, usually on the right side. In adults, ectopic gastric mucosa is an uncommon finding in Meckel's diverticulum and as a result pertechnetate scanning is often unhelpful.

Radionuclide studies can also be used to locate the site of obscured bleeding from the gastrointestinal tract. The general anatomical location of bleeding can be identified in many patients and further investigations such as angiography or barium studies can then be made to define the site and cause of bleeding more precisely.

The liver

Enlargement of the liver may be identified on plain radiographs, but adds little to clinical examination. Inflammatory masses such as subphrenic abscess under the right diaphragm may cause elevation and impairment of movement of the diaphragm, together with a pleural effusion. Calcification is occasionally seen in the liver and the most common causes are old granulomatous disease and hydatid cyst.

ULTRASONOGRAPHY

Ultrasound examination of the liver is safe, cheap, and accurate in experienced hands. Abscesses appear as black transonic areas surrounded by high-intensity echoes, whilst cysts have black transonic areas surrounded by a thin echogenic rim. Neoplasia produces areas of discontinuity in the homogeneous pattern of the liver. Most commonly, the echo amplitude is less than that of the surrounding liver, but some metas-

Fig. 7 Subtraction radiograph of a superior mesenteric arteriogram showing contrast leaking into a diverticulum of the caecum (arrow). This was successfully treated by colonoscopic diathermy.

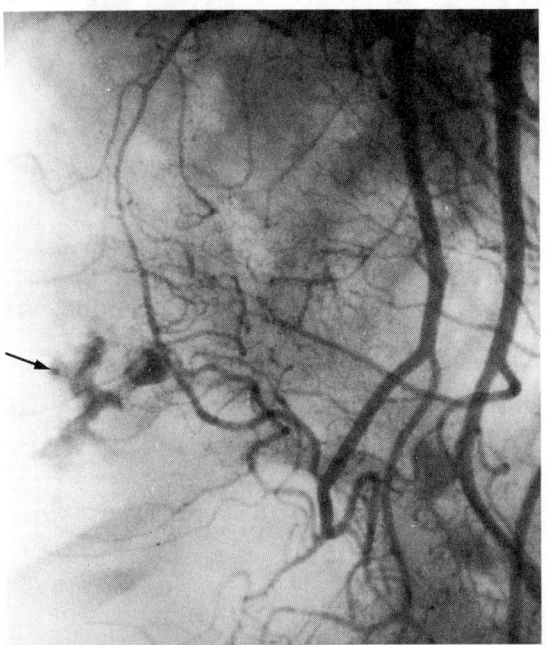

tases, particularly from the colon, produce high-intensity echoes. Direct ultrasonography of the liver exposed at surgery may show lesions not visible by the normal transcutaneous technique. Cirrhosis produces a higher amplitude of echoes than does the normal liver and a large portal vein may be demonstrated. Colour-flow Doppler can help to differentiate haemangiomas from other neoplasms and is invaluable in the assessment of the portal and hepatic veins. Diagnostic biopsy of liver tumours is greatly facilitated by ultrasound control.

RADIONUCLIDE STUDIES

Radioisotope imaging is a relatively inexpensive and accurate method of identifying metastases in the liver as they produce defects in the uptake of isotope by the Kupffer cells of the normal liver. Ultrasonography and computerized tomography have largely replaced radionuclide studies of the liver.

COMPUTERIZED TOMOGRAPHY (CT)

CT is of use in demonstrating metastatic disease and primary neoplasia of the liver. Cysts and abscesses also show well on CT, but cirrhosis may be difficult to identify with certainty.

MAGNETIC RESONANCE IMAGING (MRI)

This technique is excellent for differentiating malignant neoplasms from benign cysts, and for providing useful information in patients with cirrhosis and with metastatic deposits. The improved sensitivity produced by the use of contrast agents, the elimination of artefacts, and the characterization of tissue both by MRI and magnetic resonance spectroscopy provide a useful, radiation-free adjunct to ultrasonography and CT.

ANGIOGRAPHY

Coeliac-axis angiography is useful in identifying haemangiomas, as they have feeding vessels of normal size but with a slow flow of contrast through the lesion. Angiography will help to differentiate hepatic tumours and may be done during CT (CT arterioportography) to maximize the detection of metastases, but is more commonly used to identify the exact site and blood supply of neoplasms before partial hepatectomy. If a neoplasm is inoperable, the hepatic artery can be embolized to alleviate symptoms, which is particularly effective in secondary carcinoid.

The late films of a coeliac angiogram usually give a good picture of the portal vein, which is invaluable if portocaval shunting or transjugular intrahepatic portasystemic shunting is contemplated.

The biliary system

Plain radiographs are normally the initial diagnostic procedure in patients with acute symptoms of disease of the biliary tract. The plain film may show pathological calcification of the gallbladder, opaque calculi, gas in the biliary tree, or radio-opaque bile in the gallbladder.

ULTRASONOGRAPHY

High-definition sector scanners provide an excellent real-time image of the gallbladder, and the intrahepatic and extrahepatic bile ducts. The small probe can be used between the ribs and allows scanning with the patient erect. The accuracy in detecting gallstones (Fig. 8) is similar to that of oral cholecystography with the added advantage that the bile ducts may be examined at the same time. Ultrasonography has replaced oral cholecystography as the method of choice for detecting biliary-tract calculi and as the initial investigation for suspected gallbladder disease. A thickened gallbladder wall is sometimes seen in acute cholecystitis. Dilated hepatic and common bile ducts may be identified and, if the bowel is relatively free from gas, intraductal calculi or an enlarged head of pancreas may be identified.

ORAL CHOLECYSTOGRAPHY

About 80 to 85 per cent of gallstones are not radio-opaque and oral cholecystography remains the method of choice for examining the gall-bladder with contrast medium to detect calculi when ultrasound is not available or is inconclusive. Abnormalities causing a change in the outline of the gallbladder such as adenomyomatosis are well demonstrated at oral cholecystography.

INTRAVENOUS CHOLANGIOGRAPHY

Intravenous cholangiography is now seldom indicated and is used infrequently. It has recently been suggested that intravenous cholangiography should be routinely done preoperatively in all patients being considered for laparoscopic cholecystectomy. This suggestion is unlikely to be widely adopted.

The contrast agents used in intravenous cholangiography are water soluble and are preferentially excreted in the bile. Combined severe liver and renal disease and monoclonal IgM paraproteinaemia (Waldenström's macroglobulinaemia) must be regarded as absolute contraindications to the use of intravenous biliary contrast media. Relative contraindications include a history of asthma or allergy to contrast media or drugs. Normal or near-normal liver function is essential for satisfactory examination. Intravenous cholangiography should not be done within 1 week of oral cholecystography. When the examination is properly carried out, it is an accurate method for detecting calculi in the bile ducts, and demonstrating choledochal cysts.

RADIONUCLIDE STUDIES

^{99}Tc^{m}HIDA cholescintigraphy was once the procedure of choice but has now been mostly replaced by ultrasound for investigating suspected cholecystitis. It can accurately detect functional obstruction or patency of the cystic duct.

PERCUTANEOUS TRANSHEPATIC CHOLANGIOGRAPHY (PTC)

PTC is widely used for demonstrating the bile ducts in obstructive jaundice. The examination is carried out in the X-ray department on a fluoroscopic table with an image intensifier and television monitor. The lateral approach is used as this allows the fine needle to pass through the wide right lobe of the liver before encountering a bile duct and as a result the risk of bile and blood leakage is lessened. With adequate premedication and under local anaesthesia, the needle and stylet are passed through the liver. The stylet is removed and the needle is connected to a syringe containing contrast medium. The needle is slowly withdrawn under fluoroscopic control while contrast medium is gently injected. When contrast medium enters an intrahepatic bile duct, withdrawal is halted and the contrast medium is injected to outline the biliary tract. It may be

Fig. 8 Ultrasound of the gallbladder showing a gallstone reflecting the sound and casting a black shadow.

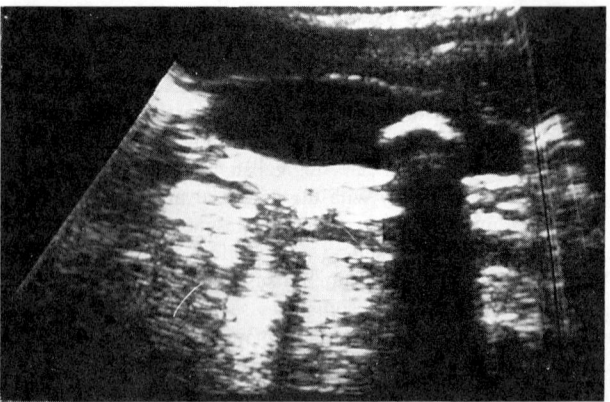

necessary to repeat the procedure a number of times before an intrahepatic bile duct is entered.

Common bile-duct calculi (Fig. 9), carcinoma of the head of the pancreas, cholangiocarcinoma, and benign bile-duct strictures are the most common causes of extrahepatic bile-duct obstruction. Contraindications to PTC include a bleeding tendency, ascites, and a history of allergy to contrast media. In the past, ascending cholangitis was a contraindication but PTC is now used to outline the bile ducts immediately before percutaneous transhepatic drainage and decompression in patients with cholangitis.

Patients with normal bile ducts should be carefully watched for evidence of bleeding or other complications following the procedure. Biliary peritonitis, cholangitis, and septicaemia are most likely to occur in patients with extrahepatic bile obstruction and the obstruction should be relieved by surgery, endoscopic sphincterotomy, percutaneous drainage, or endoprosthesis insertion without delay.

External–internal bile-duct drainage and endoprosthesis insertion by the percutaneous route are well-established alternatives to surgery in patients with benign or malignant biliary strictures. Both techniques are employed after PTC whilst the bile ducts are still outlined with contrast medium. External–internal drainage is done by passing a percutaneous catheter via the liver through the stricture. The side-holes in the catheter are positioned above and below the obstructive lesion, allowing the bile to pass from the proximal ducts to the duodenum. The technique of percutaneous transhepatic endoprosthesis insertion is similar. The indwelling endoprosthesis is inserted so that its upper end is firmly lodged above the stricture and its lower end is located in the distal common bile duct or duodenum below the stricture, allowing bile to flow freely from the proximal biliary tree to the duodenum.

ENDOSCOPIC RETROGRADE CHOLANGIOPANCREATOGRAPHY (ERCP)

Cannulation of the papilla of Vater under direct vision through a duodenoscope combined with injection of contrast medium to outline the bile and pancreatic ducts is a very useful diagnostic procedure. It is frequently used to demonstrate the ducts in patients with obstructive jaundice. Endoscopic sphincterotomy can be done during the procedure,

Fig. 9 A calculus is shown in the common bile duct at percutaneous transhepatic cholangiography. The patient presented with obstructive jaundice.

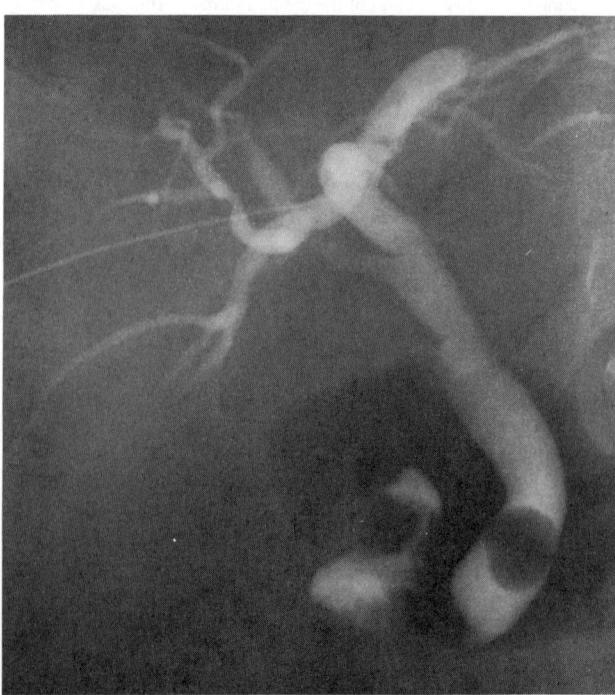

thus allowing bile-duct calculi to pass freely into the duodenum, and frequently relieving bile-duct obstruction due to calculi. Endoscopic endoprosthesis insertion through bile-duct strictures is now a well-established alternative to percutaneous biliary endoprosthesis.

The pancreas (see also Chapter 14.20)

The plain radiograph of the upper abdomen is an important investigation in patients presenting with symptoms of acute or chronic disease of the pancreas. In acute pancreatitis it may show the colon 'cut-off' sign, a sentinel loop, evidence of displacement of the stomach, or of a pancreatic abscess. Pancreatic calcification may be seen in patients with chronic pancreatitis.

ULTRASONOGRAPHY

Ultrasonography allows the measurement of size and the visualization of parenchyma of the pancreas. Acute pancreatitis, neoplasms, and pseudocysts may be identified and, if a neoplasm is diagnosed, it may be

Fig. 10 Carcinoma of the body of the pancreas is shown at endoscopic pancreatography. A tapered occlusion of the main duct has produced a 'rat-tail' appearance. (Reproduced from Baddeley, *et al.* 1978, by permission.)

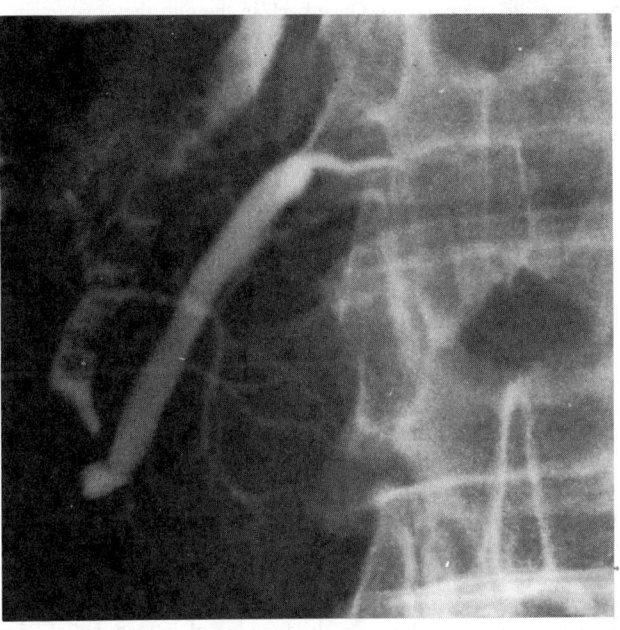

Fig. 11 Subtraction radiograph of a coeliac angiogram of a 10-year-old girl with an insulinoma of the pancreas (arrow).

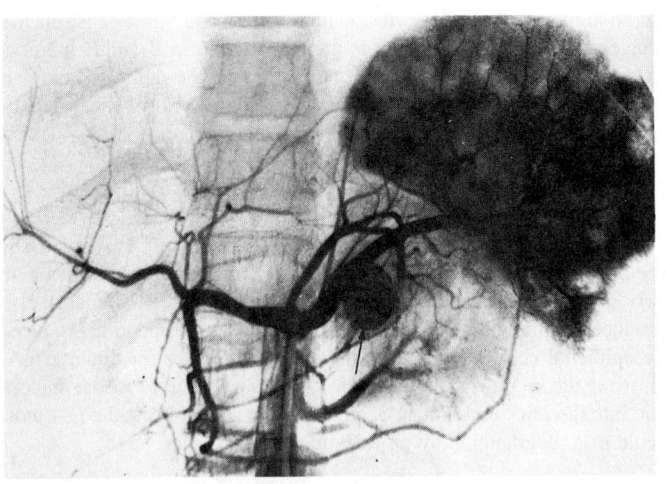

biopsied using a Chiba needle guided by ultrasound. Ultrasound is often used to investigate epigastric masses with the advantage that other organs in the region of the pancreas including the aorta, para-aortic lymph nodes, and adrenal glands may be seen. Peroperative ultrasonography may identify insulinomas not identified by other techniques.

COMPUTERIZED TOMOGRAPHY

The ability of high-resolution CT to detect small intrapancreatic pseudocysts, pseudocysts containing gas or solid contents, pancreatic calcification, and peripancreatic fascial thickening make it the most accurate method for evaluating pancreatitis. Accurate assessment of carcinoma of the pancreas is also possible with CT.

RETROGRADE PANCREATOGRAPHY

ERCP is an extremely useful procedure in the diagnosis of carcinoma of the pancreas and chronic pancreatitis. It is an accurate technique for detecting carcinoma of the pancreas; tapered strictures or occlusions of the main pancreatic duct are seen (Fig. 10). The signs of chronic pancreatitis include stricturing and irregular dilatation of the pancreatic duct, retention-cyst formation and duct concrements.

ANGIOGRAPHY

Coeliac angiography will usually show insulinomas of the pancreas (Fig. 11), but transhepatic portal catheterization will allow samples of blood to be taken from the splenic vein to localize insulinomas if CT or angiography are unsuccessful.

The spleen

The plain radiograph will usually show an enlarged spleen as is found in blood disorders of the reticuloendothelial system, infection, hepatic cirrhosis, and trauma. A single area of calcification may be seen in atherosclerosis or aneurysm of the splenic artery. Multiple calcifications occur in healed tuberculosis, phleboliths, haemangiomas, and histoplasmosis.

The spleen can be examined by radioisotopes and this may be particularly useful in trauma or where a small splenunculus is suspected. Ultrasound may be used to measure splenic size and in identifying splenic cysts, whilst CT and MRI show the spleen well and are useful following trauma.

Transhepatic portal phlebography is done by inserting a catheter through the liver into the portal vein. This technique allows obliteration of oesophageal varices to be undertaken.

REFERENCES

Allison, D.J. (1980). Gastrointestinal bleeding—radiological diagnosis. *British Journal of Hospital Medicine*, **23**, 358–65.

Baddeley, H., Nolan, D.J., and Salmon, P.R. (1978). *Radiological atlas of biliary and pancreatic disease*. HM & M, Aylesbury.

Dooley, J.S., Dick, R., Irving, D., Olney, J., and Sherlock, S. (1981). Relief of bile duct obstruction by the percutaneous transhepatic insertion of an endoprosthesis. *Clinical Radiology*, **32**, 163–72.

Foley, W.D. *et al.* (1980). Computed tomography, ultrasonography and endoscopic retrograde cholangiopancreatography in the diagnosis of pancreatic disease: a comparative study. *Gastrointestinal Radiology*, **5**, 29–35.

Joyce, W.P. *et al.* (1991). Identification of bile duct stones in patients undergoing laparoscopic cholecystectomy. *British Journal of Surgery*, **78**, 1174–6.

Kressel, H.Y. (1988). Strategies for magnetic resonance imaging of focal liver disease. *Radiological Clinics of North America*, **26**, 607–15.

Muto, T., Bussey, H.J.R., and Morson, B.C. (1975). The evolution of cancer of the colon and rectum. *Cancer*, **36**, 2251–70.

Nolan, D.J. (1980). *The double-contrast barium meal. A radiological atlas*. HM & M, Aylesbury.

Nolan, D.J. (1981). Barium examination of the small intestine. Progress report. *Gut*, **22**, 682–94.

Weissmann, H.S., Frank, M.S., Bernstein, L.H., and Freeman, L.M. (1979). Rapid and accurate diagnosis of acute cholecystitis with ⁹⁹TcᵐHIDA cholescintigraphy. *American Journal of Roentgenology*, **132**, 523–8.

14.4 Immune disorders of the gastrointestinal tract

M. R. HAENEY

Introduction

The gut is protected by several mechanisms. The acid pH of the stomach and the proteolytic enzyme content of the intestine are formidable barriers to many organisms. A change in the normal microflora of the intestine or impaired gut motility also allow pathogenic bacteria to flourish. Microbial antigens that resist these defences and penetrate the epithelial surface encounter the mucosal immune system.

FUNCTIONAL MORPHOLOGY OF THE GUT-ASSOCIATED LYMPHOID TISSUE (GALT)

Lymphocytes are found at three sites within the mucosa (Fig. 1):(i) organized lymphoid aggregates (Peyer's patches) beneath the epithelium of the terminal small intestine; (ii) lymphocytes within the epithelial cell layer (intraepithelial lymphocytes); and (iii) lymphocytes scattered among other immunocompetent cells within the lamina propria. The epithelium and Peyer's patches are the main sites of interaction between lymphocytes and antigen in the lumen of the gut.

Peyer's patches

These are covered by specialized epithelium (follicle-associated epithelium) that has no microvilli but whose surface seems wrinkled or folded under the scanning electron microscope (Fig. 1). These microfold, or **M**, cells sample and transport particulate antigens from the lumen into the 'dome' area, where T and B cells mix freely with the microfolds of the M cells and priming of both types of lymphocyte occurs. Within Peyer's patches are specialized T cells that induce immature IgM-bearing B lymphocytes to switch isotype to IgA.

Lymphocytes are mobile: an array of cell-surface receptors permits adhesion to endothelial cells and to components of the extracellular matrix. Primed B lymphoblasts, committed mainly to producing IgA antibody, migrate from Peyer's patches, via the lymphatics and mesenteric lymph nodes, to the thoracic duct and hence into the circulation. These cells return preferentially to the lamina propria, but the stimulus for this 'homing' is unknown. Once back in the gut, they mature into IgA plasma cells and are responsible for local and secretory antibody defences. The number of IgA-containing cells in the lamina propria far exceeds the numbers containing IgM, IgG, or IgE.

Intraepithelial lymphocytes

There is a similar migration pathway for T lymphocytes whereby T blasts from mesenteric nodes 'home' both to the epithelium and to the lamina propria. Intraepithelial lymphocytes (**IEL**) are phenotypically and functionally distinct from peripheral blood lymphocytes. Peripheral T cells rarely express the human mucosal lymphocyte antigen HML-1 but nearly all intraepithelial lymphocytes do. Intraepithelial lymphocytes are not a homogeneous population: about 10 per cent do not express the CD3 antigen and therefore are not T cells. These non-T cell intraepithelial lymphocytes are concentrated in the tips of the villi. Unlike the peripheral T cells, which have a CD4⁺:CD8⁺ ratio of about 2:1 most intraepithelial lymphocytes T cells express CD8 and only a few express CD4. A small proportion (8 per cent) of intraepithelial lymphocytes are CD4⁻ and CD8⁻ and express the γ/δ form of the T-cell receptor rather than the more common α/β form (see Chapter 5.1). In experimental animals, some intraepithelial lymphocytes are cytotoxic and some have natural killer activity, functions important in the control of enterovirus infection. However, the function of intraepithelial lymphocytes in man is unclear.

Lamina propria lymphocytes

Large numbers of lymphocytes, natural killer cells, mast cells, macrophages, and plasma cells occur in the lamina propria. T and B lymphocytes are both found, but T cells predominate in the ratio of about 4:1. In contrast to intraepithelial lymphocytes, 80 per cent of these T cells are CD4⁺ and only 20 per cent express CD8.

SECRETORY IMMUNOGLOBULINS

The plasma cells of the lamina propria secrete mainly IgA, which is specially adapted for its function. IgA is synthesized as a dimer with two IgA molecules linked by a smaller 'joining' peptide (J chain), also produced by the plasma cells. Secretory piece, a glycopeptide produced by epithelial cells, functions as the cellular receptor for dimeric IgA, allowing the secretory IgA molecule to be transported across the mucosa and into the intestinal lumen. Secretory piece also protects the IgA molecule from degradation by proteolytic enzymes.

Fig. 1 Organization and structure of gut-associated lymphoid tissue. On the left, T and B lymphocytes and plasma cells (Pc) can be seen in the lamina propria, with intraepithelial lymphocytes (IEL) between the columnar epithelial cells. On the right, there is a Peyer's patch covered by cuboidal epithelium with occasional M cells. The Peyer's patch comprises three areas: (i) the dome (D) of T and B lymphocytes; (ii) the thymus-dependent area (TDA); and (iii) the germinal centre (GC) containing macrophages (ma) and B lymphoblasts.

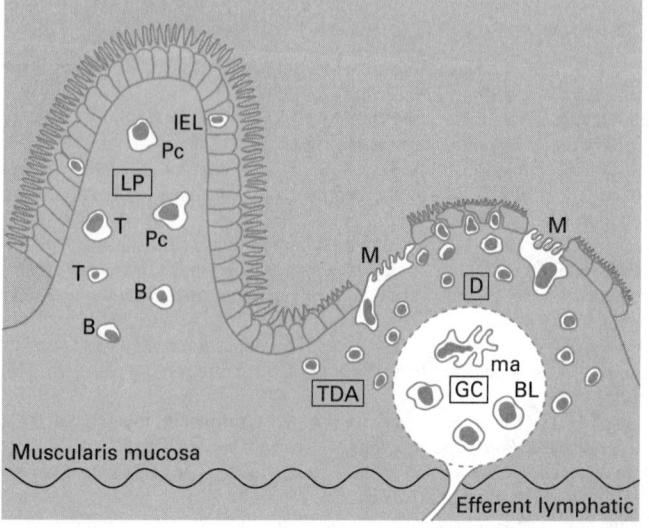

Secretory IgA predominates in the saliva and in gastric and intestinal secretions, where it tends to be concentrated in the mucous layer overlying epithelial cells. Secretory IgA neutralizes viruses, bacteria, and toxins, prevents the adherence of pathogenic micro-organisms to gut epithelium and so blocks the uptake of antigen into the systemic immune system.

SPECTRUM OF INTESTINAL IMMUNE RESPONSES

Ingestion of antigens can lead to local immunity, a systemic immune response, or a state of specific immune unresponsiveness (tolerance).

Local immune responses
These can occur independently of a systemic response. For example, immunization against poliomyelitis with oral Sabin vaccine gives better protection than the injected Salk vaccine, even though both induce serum antibodies. Local IgA antibody, produced in response to the oral vaccine, partly blocks uptake of pathogenic virus into the circulation.

Systemic immune responses
Macromolecules are absorbed by the intestine into the portal or systemic circulations, via either the glandular epithelium covering the villus or the M cells. Up to 2 per cent of a dietary protein load appears antigenically intact in the circulation. Sinusoidal phagocytes (Kupffer cells) of the liver destroy much of the antigen but enough passes through the liver to stimulate systemic antibody production, particularly in the spleen. Antibody formed in the spleen enters the portal circulation to complex with incoming antigen. Circulating immune complexes of IgA and dietary antigens are regularly found in normal people after meals.

Systemic tolerance
American Indians knew that eating the leaves of poison ivy prevented contact dermatitis on subsequent exposure to the plant. This observation can be reproduced in animals by feeding them antigen; they become immunologically unresponsive (tolerant) to subsequent parenteral injections of that antigen. Oral tolerance can affect all aspects of the systemic immune response: a single feed of protein antigen suppresses systemic IgM, IgG, and IgE responses, as well as T cell-mediated immunity. The exact mechanism is unclear.

IMMUNOLOGICAL DISORDERS OF THE GASTROINTESTINAL TRACT

Normally, the intestinal immune system steers a delicate course between the undesirable extremes of immunological incompetence, with resulting vulnerability to ingested pathogens (for instance, the gastrointestinal consequences of primary and secondary immunodeficiencies) and hypersensitivity to dietary antigens, with immunologically mediated reactions each time that antigen is eaten.

Primary immunodeficiency diseases

Immunocompromised patients are at risk from two sources of infection: common pathogens, which invade even the immunologically healthy; and 'opportunistic' agents that utilize the opportunity of weakened defences to inflict damage on the host. In the compromised host, most infections are due to common pathogens that are readily identified and controlled. The difficult problems arise from opportunistic infections because these often elude isolation, may not respond to available drugs, and carry a high fatality. Indeed, the demonstration of certain opportunistic infections implies an underlying immunodeficiency that demands further investigation.

It is beyond the scope of this section to deal with all the gastrointestinal complications of every known form of primary and secondary

Table 1 *Gastrointestinal disorders associated with common variable immunodeficiency and other forms of primary antibody deficiency*

Infective	Other
Giardiasis	Pernicious anaemia-like syndrome
Campylobacter enteritis	Hypogammaglobulinaemic sprue
Cryptosporidiosis	Coeliac disease
Strongyloides stercoralis	Carcinoma of the stomach
Salmonella/shigella infection	Nodular lymphoid hyperplasia
Viral enteritis	Inflammatory bowel disease
Bacterial overgrowth	Non-granulomatous jejunoileitis

immunodeficiency. Instead, attention will be focused on representative disorders.

Common variable immunodeficiency (CVI)

Common variable immunodeficiency is an example of one of the primary antibody deficiency syndromes described in Section 5.

DEFINITION

Common variable immunodeficiency (CVI) is a heterogeneous group of disorders characterized by low serum immunoglobulin levels, a normal or low proportion of circulating B lymphocytes and, in about one-third of patients, impaired cell-mediated immunity. It can present at any age and, in the United States and United Kingdom, the prevalence is about 20 per million of the population. Most cases are sporadic, although inherited forms have been described.

CLINICAL FEATURES

Patients typically present with recurrent sinopulmonary infections, most frequently caused by pneumococci, streptoccoci, and *Haemophilus influenzae*. Less commonly, they present with skin sepsis, meningitis, osteomyelitis, arthropathy, or other severe systemic bacterial infections (see Section 7).

With certain exceptions, these patients are not unduly susceptible to viral or fungal infections, because cell-mediated immunity is usually preserved. There are rarely any diagnostic physical signs of antibody deficiency, although examination often shows evidence of the consequences of previous infections, such as bronchiectasis, and in children, a failure to thrive.

Between 30 and 50 per cent of patients with CVI have gastrointestinal problems at some time. Virtually any part of the gastrointestinal tract may be affected (Table 1) but the most common complaints are diarrhoea (intermittent or chronic) and weight loss. An approach to the diagnosis of these complications is shown in Fig. 2.

Stomach
Achlorhydria and pernicious anaemia
Achlorhydria is found in about 30 per cent of patients and the associated atrophic gastritis occasionally leads to a syndrome resembling pernicious anaemia. It differs from classical pernicious anaemia in several respects: the atrophic gastritis involves the whole stomach without antral sparing; the serum gastrin concentrations remain normal; and autoantibodies to gastric parietal cells and intrinsic factor are absent.

Gastric cancer
Patients with CVI have an increased incidence of carcinoma of the stomach. It is sufficiently common to warrant yearly gastroscopic examination in hypogammaglobulinaemic patients who have atrophic gastritis.

The high concentrations of microbial enzymes and nitrites found in the gastric juices may lead to local production of carcinogenic *N*-nitroso compounds.

Small intestine

Infective complications

Although infestation with *Giardia lamblia* is the most common identifiable cause of malabsorption, in many patients the cause is never found. Giardiasis is virtually confined to adults and is rarely seen in boys with X-linked hypogammaglobulinaemia. Giardiasis may also cause diarrhoea, villous abnormalities, vitamin B_{12} and folate malabsorption, steatorrhoea, disaccharidase deficiency, and protein-losing enteropathy but the pathogenetic mechanisms are poorly understood.

Examination of at least three consecutive fresh stool specimens is essential to detect the cysts of *G. lamblia* (Fig. 2). If this fails, duodenal aspiration and jejunal biopsy are needed to establish the diagnosis. In particularly difficult cases, it can be useful to give a therapeutic trial of metronidazole, although infestation frequently recurs. Nevertheless, most patients show symptomatic improvement after treatment with either a 7-day course of metronidazole (2 g daily as a single dose) or mepacrin (100 mg, three times daily for 10 days). Other parasitic infestations occur. *Cryptosporidium* infection occasionally causes self-limiting diarrhoea but has a much more sinister outcome in patients with human immunodeficiency virus (**HIV**) infection.

Bacterial infections also cause diarrhoea in patients with CVI and *Campylobacter jejuni* is frequently responsible. Rarely, campylobacter

Fig. 2 A scheme for the investigation of gastrointestinal complications in patients with common variable immunodeficiency. (Reproduced from Haeney (1989) by permission of Blackwell Scientific Publications, Oxford.)

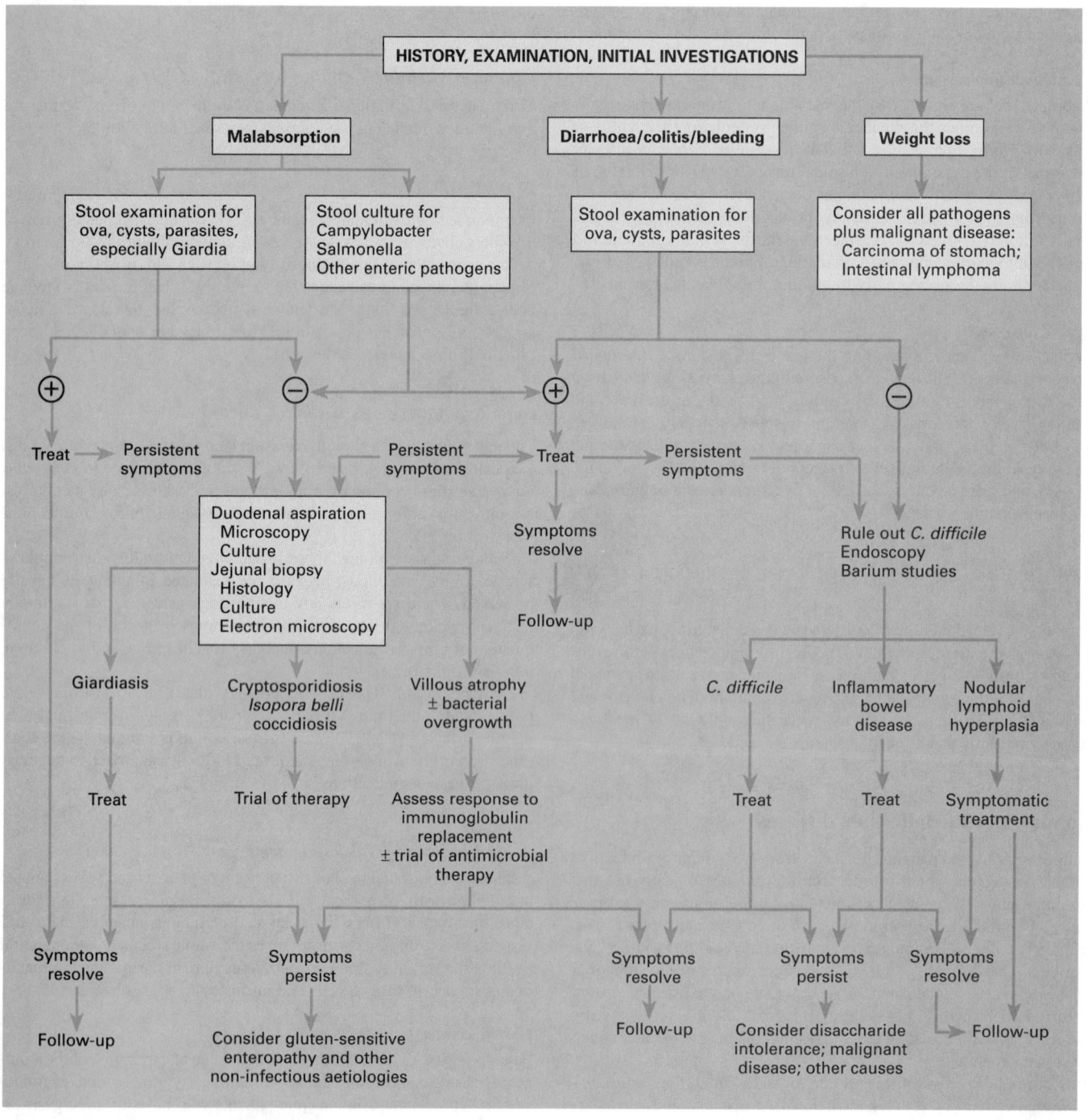

causes an ascending cholangitis and hepatitis. Treatment is a 2-week course of erythromycin (500 mg, four times daily) after which the stools should again be cultured to check that treatment has been effective.

Shigella or salmonella diarrhoea does not occur more commonly than normal. Similarly, while overgrowth of commensal bacteria is common, bacterial counts rarely exceed 10^5 organisms/ml, compared with counts of more than 10^6/ml in the blind-loop syndrome. Nevertheless, it is common practice to treat these patients empirically with tetracycline and metronidazole, often with symptomatic improvement.

Nodular lymphoid hyperplasia (NLH)

Nodular lymphoid hyperplasia describes the presence of lymphoid nodules in the lamina propria of the gut. Although described in many disorders and occasionally in healthy individuals with normal concentrations of serum immunoglobulins, nodular lymphoid hyperplasia should make the clinician suspect common variable immunodeficiency. It occurs in 20 to 50 per cent of patients but is not necessarily symptomatic. The nodules, which are 1 to 3 mm in diameter, appear as protrusions on fibreoptic endoscopy and as multiple filling defects on barium studies (Fig. 3). Nodular lymphoid hyperplasia restricted to the rectum or colon can present with rectal bleeding, abdominal pain, and features of intestinal obstruction, but rarely with diarrhoea.

The ultrastructure of these nodules is similar to that of Peyer's patches, and lymphoblasts containing IgM are found in the centres of the follicles. The condition probably represents hypertrophy of the gut associated lymphoid tissue in response to antigens in the gut lumen. In one series of nodular lymphoid hyperplasia in individuals with normal serum immunoglobulins, every patient had intestinal giardiasis, suggesting of an aetiological link with persistent infestation. Although nodular lymphoid hyperplasia is not premalignant in patients with hypogammaglobulinaemia, intestinal lymphoma has been reported in apparently immunocompetent subjects with extensive small-bowel nodular lymphoid hyperplasia.

Hypogammaglobulinaemic sprue

In a few patients with unexplained diarrhoea, the mucosal lesion resembles coeliac disease or tropical sprue but with reduced or undetectable plasma cells within the lamina propria. Indeed, in tropical regions, about 1 per cent of patients with 'sprue' may be suffering from a primary humoral immunodeficiency syndrome. Malabsorption in patients with hypogammaglobulinaemic sprue can improve rapidly after replacement immunoglobulin therapy. Although extremely rare, patients with common variable immunodeficiency may have a concomitant gluten-sensitive coeliac disease.

Fig. 3 A double-contrast barium enema showing nodular lymphoid hyperplasia in the terminal ileum (arrowed).

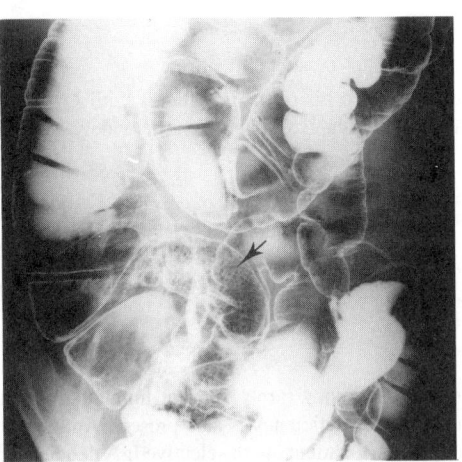

Table 2 *Gastrointestinal disorders sometimes associated with selective IgA deficiency*

Infections	Giardiasis; bacterial overgrowth
Autoimmune disease	Pernicious anaemia; antiepithelial-cell antibody
Hypersensitivity disorders	Coeliac disease; cows' milk protein intolerance; food antibodies and circulating immune complexes; inflammatory bowel disease
Neoplasia	Carcinoma of oesophagus, stomach, colon
Other	Nodular lymphoid hyperplasia; disaccharidase deficiency.

Jejunoileitis

This is a rare feature of common variable immunodeficiency and has a poor prognosis.

MANAGEMENT

The cornerstone of treatment of antibody deficiency is immunoglobulin replacement; enough must be given to prevent further infections and reduce the incidence of complications. Intravenous immunoglobulin therapy is the treatment of choice and is discussed more fully in Section 5.

Antibody-deficient patients respond as promptly as others to appropriate antibiotics but prolonged courses of treatment are usually needed to ensure complete eradication of the micro-organism.

Selective IgA deficiency (see also Section 5)

DEFINITION

Selective IgA deficiency refers to a serum IgA concentration below the limit of detection (< 0.01 g/l). By definition, the serum IgG and IgM concentrations are normal.

AETIOLOGY

Selective IgA deficiency is common and occurs in about 1 in 700 of healthy adults. Most cases are sporadic, but there is an association with inheritance of the HLA-B8, DW3 haplotype, and with deficiencies of IgG_2 and IgG_4. It is sometimes linked with defects in chromosome 18, particularly in the autosomal recessive syndrome of ataxia telangiectasia. Selective IgA deficiency may also be due to drugs such as phenytoin or penicillamine.

CLINICAL FEATURES

Although selective IgA deficiency is associated with a range of disorders, most IgA-deficient individuals are asymptomatic, possibly because IgM-producing cells provide high local concentrations of IgM antibody or because symptomatic individuals are those who also have deficiency of IgG_2.

Gastrointestinal complications (Table 2)

Pernicious anaemia

Selective IgA deficiency is associated with pernicious anaemia. Unlike CVI, the anaemia conforms to the classical Addisonian type in that atrophic gastritis and raised serum gastrin concentrations occur.

Malabsorption and steatorrhoea

IgA deficiency occurs in about 1 in 40 of patients with coeliac disease, over 15 times more frequently than in the general population. Patients

Table 3 *Gastrointestinal disease in selected types of primary immunodeficiency*

Condition	Functional defect	Typical age at presentation	Major clinical features	Gastrointestinal complications
X-linked lymphoproliferative syndrome	Inherited vulnerability to infection with Epstein–Barr virus	Childhood	Fatal or chronic infectious mononucleosis Aplastic anaemia Hypogammaglobulinaemia Malignant B-cell lymphoma	As for antibody deficiency Malignant lymphoma of the terminal ileum
Severe combined immunodeficiency	Impairment of cell-mediated immunity and antibody production—sometimes associated with inherited deficiency of enzyme adenosine deaminase	Infancy	Wide spectrum of infection Non-immunological features in subtypes	Chronic oral and intestinal candidiasis Persistent diarrhoea due to: rotavirus, cytomegalovirus, other viruses, cryptosporidium, Campylobacter; Salmonella
Malformation of the fetal 3rd and 4th pharyngeal pouches (Di George syndrome	Impairment of cell-mediated immunity and antibody production (non-familial)	From birth	Hypoparathyroidism—tetany and convulsions Cardiovascular defects Immunodeficiency Abnormal facies	Oesophageal atresia Chronic intestinal candidiasis Diarrhoea of uncertain aetiology
Wiskott–Aldrich syndrome	Progressive impairment of antibody production and cell-mediated immunity	Infancy or early childhood	Thrombocytopenia—bleeding Eczema Immunodeficiency Malignant disease	Bloody diarrhoea Food allergic disease Intestinal lymphoma
Chronic granulomatous disease	Defective neutrophil killing of catalase-producing organisms (usually X-linked)	Infancy	Severe skin sepsis due to: *Staphylococcus aureus*, fungi, Gram-negative bacilli Lymphadenopathy Hepatosplenomegaly Deep abscesses	Diarrhoea and steatorrhoea with PAS-positive histiocytes in the lamina propria
Chronic mucocutaneous candidiasis	Impaired cell-mediated immunity to *Candida albicans*	Childhood	Chronic Candida infection of: mucous membranes, nails, skin Associated endocrinopathy: Addison's disease, hypoparathyroidism, diabetes mellitus, thyroiditis	Chronic oral and intestinal candidiasis
Defective yeast opsonization	Impaired complement function	Infancy	None	Protracted diarrhoea of uncertain cause

Reproduced from Haeney (1989) by permission of Blackwell Scientific Publications, Oxford.

with selective IgA deficiency and a flat jejunal mucosa respond to dietary gluten withdrawal in a way typical of classical coeliac disease.

Antibodies to dietary antigens

Secretory IgA helps prevent absorption of food antigens through the intestinal mucosa and there is a high prevalence of serum antibodies to food proteins in patients with selective IgA deficiency. For instance, about a third of IgA-deficient blood donors have serum antibodies to milk compared with 0.3 per cent of healthy controls. IgA-deficient subjects also tend to have autoantibodies to antigens such as collagen and IgA itself (see below).

Gastrointestinal infection

With the exception of *G. lamblia* infestation, other infections rarely persist. Even giardiasis is far less frequent than in CVI. However, in the past, IgA-deficient patients were prone to develop chronic diarrhoea and malabsorption after truncal vagotomy and gastroenterostomy for duodenal ulceration. This was due to overgrowth of commensal bacteria in the upper intestinal tract, presumably because of the combined effects

of deficiency of local antibody production, achlorhydria, and impaired gastrointestinal motility.

Inflammatory bowel disease

Crohn's disease and ulcerative colitis occur in patients with IgA deficiency but their frequency is difficult to judge from the widely varying published reports.

Malignant disease

Oesophageal, gastric, and colonic neoplasms have been reported but it is not certain whether the risk of malignancy is truly increased.

MANAGEMENT

Patients with selective IgA deficiency rarely warrant immunoglobulin replacement therapy, unless IgG$_2$ deficiency is also present. Antibodies to IgA develop in about a third of patients with selective IgA deficiency: high titres of antibodies may cause severe reactions to plasma or blood transfusions or even the trace amounts of IgA present in intravenous immunoglobulin preparations.

Other types of primary immunodeficiency

Gastrointestinal problems occur in other types of immunodeficiency (Table 3) (see Section 5). These conditions are much rarer than primary antibody deficiency. Most defects involving cell-mediated immunity present within the first 6 months of life. Infants with severe combined immunodeficiency, for example, grow and develop normally for a few months but then fail to thrive, frequently with a clinical triad of pneumonia, mucocutaneous candidiasis, and intractable diarrhoea caused by one or more of a range of micro-organisms. Some disorders are associated with unusual gastrointestinal features (Table 3).

Secondary immunodeficiency

Secondary immunodeficiency describes conditions in which the immune defect results from underlying disease and is far more common than primary immunodeficiency. In many cases, the secondary immunodeficiency is of minor relevance to the clinical picture but occasionally its severity may mask the underlying condition. AIDS is a florid example of the gastrointestinal complications seen in patients with secondary defects involving cell-mediated immunity predominantly.

HIV and the gastrointestinal tract

The gastrointestinal tract is a major target organ in HIV infection and AIDS, irrespective of the route of acquisition of the infection. About half of patients with HIV infection will have gastrointestinal involvement at some time and any level of the tract, from mouth to anus, can be involved (see also Section 7).

There are three main mechanisms in the pathogenesis of gastrointestinal disease: (i) direct infection of enterocytes by HIV; (ii) opportunistic infections; and (iii) opportunistic tumours (Fig. 4). The principal change in the small intestine is a partial villous atrophy, detectable early in the natural history of HIV infection. Breast-feeding can transmit HIV in man, implying that the intestine is an important portal of entry for the virus. Enteropathogens causing intestinal infections are of the same types as in immunocompetent subjects but the infections are much more aggressive and invasive, and elicit little host immune response, so familiar symptoms and signs may be absent. A systematic and thorough search for likely pathogens is essential. Multiple infections and tumours may coexist, so the organism isolated is not necessarily the cause of the symptoms.

The clinical features of HIV infection and AIDS are discussed in detail in Section 7.

Immunodeficiency secondary to gastrointestinal disease

Hypogammaglobulinaemia, particularly involving IgG, may be due to increased intestinal loss of immunoglobulin. A useful clue to this possibility is a low serum albumin, because there are no known conditions where immunoglobulin is selectively lost from the gut. The major causes of protein losing enteropathy are discussed in Chapter 14.36.

Intestinal lymphangiectasia (see also Chapter 14.15)

This is an example of immunodeficiency resulting from increased loss of immunoglobulins and lymphocytes through the intestine. The basic defect is an abnormal dilatation of the lymphatic vessels in the intestine. There is a primary familial form in children, who present with diarrhoea,

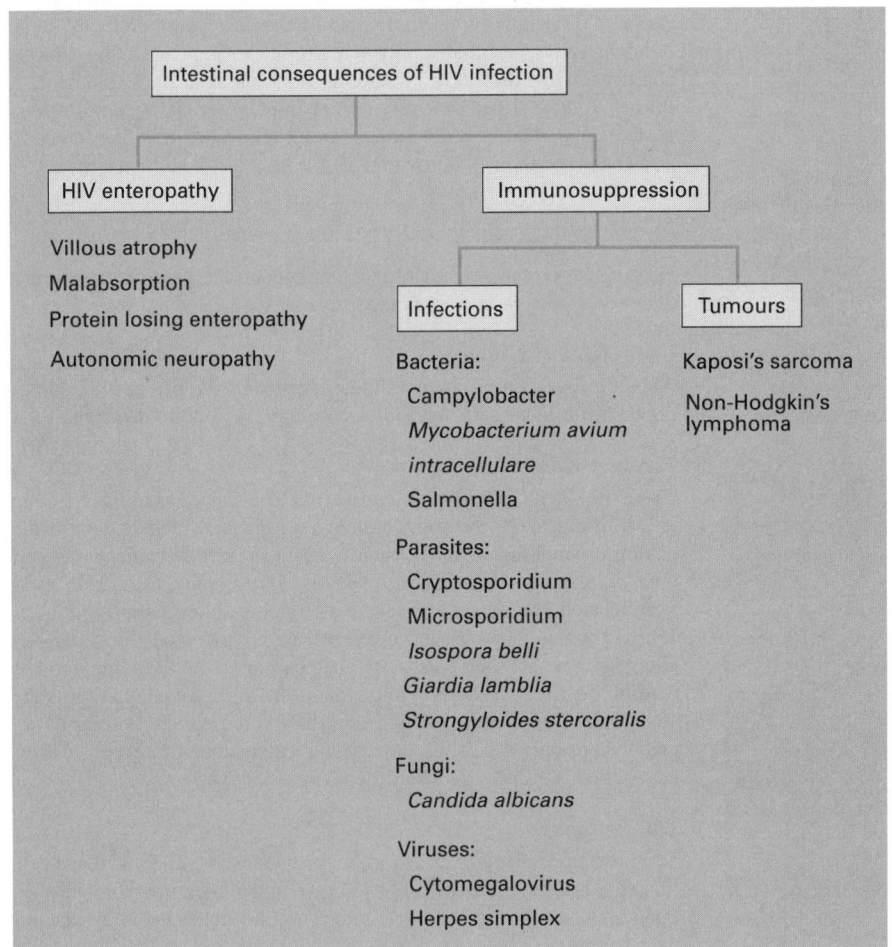

Fig. 4 Gastrointestinal consequences of HIV infection. (Redrawn from Chapel, H.M. and Haeney, M.R. (1993). *Essentials of clinical immunology*, (3rd edn) by permission of the authors and Blackwell Scientific Publications, Oxford.)

malabsorption, and growth retardation. Such children may have abnormal lymphatics elsewhere in the body causing chylous ascites, pleural effusions, and localized areas of oedema. The condition may also occur secondarily to lymphatic obstruction, for example due to lymphomas in the intestine or constrictive pericarditis (see Sections 15 and 22). The diagnosis should be suspected when there is T-cell lymphopenia, hypoalbuminaemia, and hypogammaglobulinaemia. The diagnosis is confirmed by finding dilated lymphatics in a jejunal biopsy (Fig. 5). The primary form of the disease responds well to a low-fat diet with additional medium-chain triglycerides. In secondary forms, correction of the underlying disease process is needed.

Food allergy and intolerance

INTRODUCTION

Food allergy is one of the most controversial topics in medicine. It undoubtedly exists but extravagant claims that a staggering array of symptoms are due to food 'allergy' have confused the subject. Such claims are too rarely supported by objective, scientific observations and have provoked a sceptical response from many doctors. The major cause of confusion lies in the lack of agreement on definitions and diagnostic criteria.

DEFINITION

Food allergy refers to a form of exaggerated reactivity (hypersensitivity) of the immune system to an ingested antigen. The term should be used only when the abnormal reaction is proved to be immunologically mediated, either by IgE or some other immune mechanism (Table 4). The term food intolerance should be used to describe all abnormal, reproducible reactions to food when the causative mechanism is unknown or is non-immunological. Food allergy and intolerance must be distinguished from food fads and psychological aversion to foods.

AETIOLOGY

Food allergy

Although the gut provides a physical barrier to the antigen load in the lumen, up to 2 per cent of a protein meal can appear antigenically intact in the circulation. This was shown by injecting serum from a patient with known sensitivity to fish into the skin of a normal subject. A flare at the skin test site (positive Prausnitz–Kustner reaction) was observed shortly after the normal subject ate the appropriate antigen, showing that

Fig. 5 A jejunal biopsy from a patient with intestinal lymphangiectasia showing dilated central lacteals.

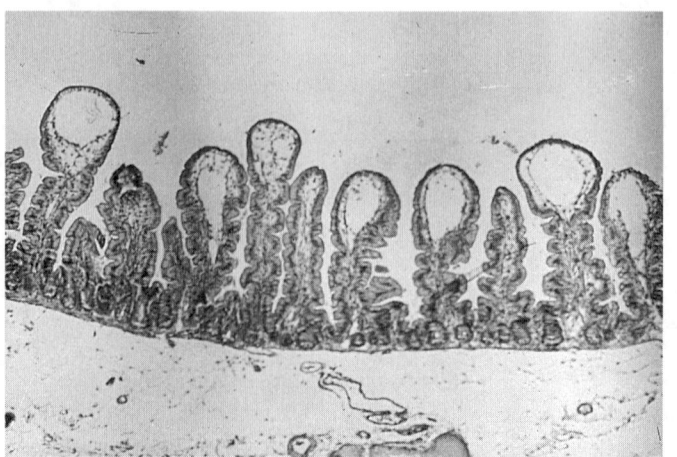

this must have crossed the gut and triggered IgE-sensitized mast cells at the skin test site.

Non-IgE antibodies to proteins in cows' milk and eggs do occur in infants, but only if a large amount of the relevant protein is ingested. However, these antibodies gradually decline in the first few years of childhood. In contrast, relatively small amounts of protein are sufficient to induce relatively high antibody concentrations, including those of IgE type, in allergic children. Such infants tend to retain high concentrations of serum antibody during childhood.

In some forms of food allergy, damage involves immune mechanisms other than IgE. For instance, in coeliac disease, there is strong evidence of exaggerated immunological reactivity to dietary gluten, but it is unclear whether local T cell-mediated hypersensitivity, immune-complex formation, or other mechanisms cause the villous atrophy.

Food intolerance

Non-immunological mechanisms of reproducible, adverse reactions to food are much more common and include irritant, toxic, pharmacological, or metabolic effects of foods, enzyme deficiencies, or even the release of substances produced by fermentation of food residues in the bowel. Some foods contain pharmacologically active substances (such as tyramine or phenylethylamine) that act directly on blood vessels in sensitive subjects to produce migraine. Traces of drugs, food additives (e.g. monosodium glutamate), colouring agents (e.g. tartrazine), or preservatives (e.g. benzoic acid) can also cause symptoms in susceptible people by mechanisms that are ill understood, but are probably due to direct effects on mast cells.

PREVALENCE

There are no reliable data. Widely varying estimates of prevalence are reported: between 0.3 per cent and 20 per cent of children suffer from, or have suffered from, symptoms caused by some form of dietary intolerance. Cows' milk protein enteropathy, the most common food allergy in infants, has an estimated prevalence of 0.5 per cent. Reactions to food additives, while they exist, are not as common as most people believe. In one study, 7.4 per cent of a survey population had symptoms suggestive of food additive tolerance; further clinical assessment and additive challenge showed a true prevalence of 0.01 to 0.23 per cent.

CLINICAL FEATURES

Food reactions can be early or late, confined to the gastrointestinal tract or occur at sites remote from the gut (Fig. 6).

Gut-related symptoms

About 75 per cent of young children, but only 10 per cent of adults, present with local gastrointestinal symptoms of food intolerance.

Early reactions

These are often 'immediate' in onset, that is occur within minutes or up to 2 h of ingestion, recur on challenge testing, and include, apart from gastrointestinal disturbances, such features as perioral rash, swelling of the lips, tingling of the throat, urticaria, angioedema, asthma, or even anaphylaxis. Such acute and severe allergic reactions are mostly due to IgE antibodies to foods and are the least controversial form of food allergy. They are fairly easy to diagnose and the offending food is readily identified, usually by the parent: the most common culprits are cows' milk (in infants), peanuts, eggs, fish, and shellfish. In some cases, anaphylaxis only occurs when the food is eaten immediately before exercise—food-induced, exercise-dependent anaphylaxis.

Late reactions

Symptoms occurring over 2 h after food ingestion, such as diarrhoea, bloating, or a fatty stool are suggestive of food intolerance, if not allergy. Features of the irritable bowel syndrome (see below) may be accom-

Table 4 *Classification of adverse reactions to foods.*

	Reproducible adverse reaction on food challenge		Immune mechanism		Non-immune mechanism	Examples
	Open	Blind	IgE	Other		
Food allergy	+	+	+	–	–	Immediate reactions to nuts, eggs, milk shellfish, fish
	+	+	–	+	–	Coeliac disease; cows' milk protein intolerance
Food intolerance	+	+	–	?	+	Irritable bowel syndrome (some); food-induced migraine; reactions to sulphites, nitrites, food additives
Food aversion	+	–	–	–	–	

panied by allergic symptoms elsewhere but usually occur in isolation, without any evidence of an immunological reaction.

Remote symptoms

Some patients with acute, IgE-mediated reactions to foods also experience rhinitis, asthma, urticaria, angioedema, or eczema. However, eating the implicated foods does not always cause these remote systems. Sneezing bouts, blocked nose, or asthma can also occur after taking wine or other alcoholic drinks because of the irritant effect of sulphite preservatives or other components. This is not an immunological reaction. Many patients with atopic eczema find that certain foods provoke a transient red and blotchy rash but it is mainly in children that food makes eczema worse. Elimination diets rarely improve atopic eczema in adults.

What is more debatable is whether food intolerance plays any part in remote symptoms such as migraine, hyperactivity, enuresis, or arthritis.

SPECIFIC SYNDROMES OF FOOD ALLERGY

Food allergy contributes to a number of common intestinal disorders. The immunological mechanisms are obscure but are not IgE-mediated.

Coeliac disease

The characteristic histological lesion in untreated cases of coeliac disease (see Chapter 14.9.4) is loss of normal villi and a marked increase in the numbers of intraepithelial lymphocytes; the infiltrate resolves on treatment with a gluten-free diet, suggesting that the intestinal damage is due to a local T cell-mediated reaction to gluten. While the evidence supports the contention that coeliac disease is a delayed and prolonged form of food allergy, the mechanism of damage is speculative.

Cows' milk protein enteropathy

Milk proteins can cause a malabsorption syndrome similar to coeliac disease. Cows' milk protein enteropathy often occurs in babies, who fail to thrive because they have diarrhoea and malabsorption and may even have intestinal bleeding and colitis. Jejunal biopsies show villous atrophy and lymphocytic infiltration.

Symptoms disappear when cows' milk is removed from the diet. Reintroduction of cows' milk causes a recurrence of symptoms and failure to thrive. After a viral gastrointestinal infection, cows' milk may also be poorly tolerated for a while because of a temporary inability to digest lactose. Thus, in babies and small children with chronic gastrointestinal symptoms and failure to gain weight, trials (under medical supervision) of milk exclusion are justified and the diagnosis can usually be confirmed by food challenge. Recovery often occurs within a few months.

RECOGNIZED SYNDROMES OF FOOD INTOLERANCE

In some conditions, a relation to specific foods can be convincingly demonstrated in a minority of patients. Sometimes, symptoms are pro-

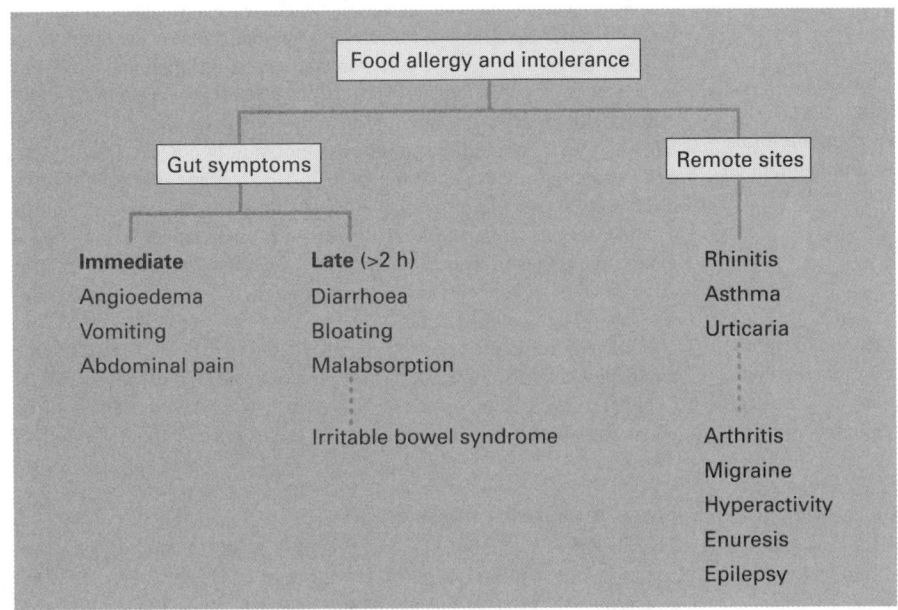

Fig. 6 Clinical spectrum of food allergy and intolerance. (Redrawn from Chapel, H.M. and Haeney, M.R. (1993). *Essentials of clinical immunology*, (3rd edn) by permission of the authors and Blackwell Scientific Publications, Oxford.)

voked by the known irritant, pharmacological, or metabolic effects of food.

Irritable bowel syndrome

The irritable bowel syndrome (**IBS**) is a descriptive term for many different conditions that produce a similar range of abdominal symptoms (see Chapter 14.13). IBS is sometimes characterized as a condition in which there is alternating constipation and diarrhoea, abdominal bloating, and pain. In a variant of this disorder, however, constipation predominates ('spastic colon') and gastrointestinal transit times are greatly increased. Most cases are unrelated to food intolerance but in a minority of others—usually those with predominant diarrhoea, with some bloating and pain—a relation to specific foods can be demonstrated. Some patients who improve on a restricted diet are able to identify foods, such as cereals and dairy products, that provoke symptoms when reintroduced. However, not all gastroenterologists are convinced that there is a causal relation between food and IBS.

Lactose intolerance

Many adults, especially non-whites, cannot digest lactose because of a deficiency of the enzyme lactase. In these subjects, undigested sugar is fermented in the lower bowel, causing diarrhoea and wind. Lactose intolerance is not common in Europeans but affects up to 90 per cent of adult Africans and Orientals. It can occur as a transient result of gastroenteritis and even as a secondary effect of cows' milk protein intolerance. This can cause confusion in diagnosis unless a lactose challenge is performed separately from a cows' milk protein challenge.

Miscellaneous syndromes

Migraine and headache

Coffee and coffee withdrawal can provoke migraine in susceptible people. Certain cheeses cause headaches in many people, probably due to the tyramine content in mature cheese. Red wines, especially port, cause headaches in susceptible people because of their content of congeners.

Asthma

Foods preserved by sulphites, particularly white wine, dried fruit, and fruit salads in supermarkets and restaurants sometimes provoke asthma by the release of sulphur dioxide.

Urticaria

Tartrazine and other coloured food dyes can sometimes trigger urticaria in sensitive subjects.

Chinese restaurant syndrome

Monosodium glutamate, used to enhance flavour in Chinese food, has been reported to cause a syndrome of chest pain, sweating, nausea, dizziness, and fainting in susceptible individuals. However, double-blind studies have not convincingly demonstrated that monosodium glutamate is the culprit.

CONTROVERSIAL ISSUES

Behavioural problems in children

The belief that foods and food additives can induce behavioural problems, particularly hyperactivity (or hyperkinesis), is a controversial one. A diet free of preservatives, salicylates, and artificial flavours has been claimed to benefit up to 70 per cent of hyperactive children but most well-designed, double-blind, placebo-controlled challenges have failed to support a causal link. Children with behaviour disorders may improve temporarily for a few weeks when given a diet avoiding food additives but this appears to be a placebo effect. Parents who suspect food additive intolerance in their child may insist of maintaining the child on a restrictive diets, even when dietary challenges prove negative.

Psychological distress in adults

Some patients with a multiplicity of vague and variable symptoms, such as unexplained fatigue and malaise, and disturbances of sleep, appetite, or libido turn to the diagnosis of food allergy as an explanation. Only a few have clear-cut psychiatric illness: others inadvertently cause symptoms by over-breathing or by somatizing their psychological distress. Having made their own diagnosis of food allergy, they have difficulty in accepting they are not allergic to foods, even though their food aversions may have resulted in a dangerously inadequate diet. They will frequently seek out practitioners who are prepared to endorse their views, whether valid or not. Early diagnosis and sympathetic management is essential if unnecessary consultations and inappropriate allergy tests are to be avoided.

DIAGNOSIS

Food allergy should not be diagnosed without clear indications, as needless dietary restrictions can seriously disrupt not only the patient's life but also the whole family and may occasionally cause malnutrition. No test can replace a careful clinical history and thorough examination to exclude other, sometimes more likely, causes of the patient's symptoms.

Skin tests and radioallergosorbent tests

Despite the enthusiasm for radioallergosorbent tests (**RAST**) to identify serum IgE antibodies to a variety of allergens, such tests have no advantage over properly done skin-prick tests (see Section 5).

Skin tests and RAST are positive in about 75 per cent of patients who have IgE-mediated, acute, early reactions to foods such as nuts, egg, or fish. Usually, the offending antigen is obvious from the clinical history and confirmatory tests are needed only if there is clinical doubt. In patients with late symptoms at sites remote from the gut (Fig. 6), skin and blood tests are notoriously unreliable for many reasons: (i) foods, as antigen sources, are poorly standardized and contain multiple, ill-defined antigens; (ii) the antigen content of the food will depend on whether it is raw or cooked; (iii) some foods cause non-specific ('irritant'), positive skin reactions; (iv) patients may have IgE antibodies but no symptoms; and (v) food reactions can be mediated by mechanisms other than IgE antibodies. For most patients with suspected food intolerance, laboratory tests are of no diagnostic value.

Elimination diets and challenge tests

In the absence of reliable tests, elimination diets and food challenge form the basis of diagnosis. In order to minimize bias and suggestion, the relation between food and symptoms should be established by a placebo-controlled, double-blind challenge under medical supervision. In some cases, for example in chronic urticaria, or when the symptoms are mild and largely subjective, it may be necessary to repeat the double-blind challenge several times before being convinced that the association between the food and the symptoms is not simply coincidental. In several series, only about a quarter of reported 'adverse reactions' can be confirmed by double-blind challenge. Although these rules are simple to state, they are often difficult to carry out in practice. However, the alternative is that of prolonged, unsupervised, dietary manipulation, usually self-imposed or inflicted by parents on their children, with the considerable risk of malnutrition.

Food challenges are not without risk: there is a danger of precipitating an anaphylactic reaction. This is well recognized in children with relatively mild symptoms of food intolerance, who develop anaphylaxis when the food, often cows' milk, is reintroduced after a period of avoidance.

Bogus or unproven laboratory tests

The absence of reliable laboratory tests has led to the promotion of controversial 'alternative' tests: these are at best misleading, at worst dangerous. New diagnostic procedures, like new drugs, require scientific validation: they must be reliable and reproducible, even when carried out by independent operators. When presented with coded, duplicate samples, some 'alternative' laboratories in the United Kingdom were unable reliably to identify food allergies in patients known to have them; they gave inconsistent results for paired samples from the same patient; they reported many allergies in non-allergic subjects; and they often gave dubious and risky dietary advice.

Provocation–neutralization testing

This has been critically evaluated by the Royal College of Physicians of London, the American College of Physicians, and the California Medical Association: these bodies concluded that reported studies on this technique were seriously flawed and that the method lacked scientific validity. Under double-blind conditions, the response of patients to active and control injections appeared to be due to suggestion and chance.

Leucocytotoxic testing

This involves incubating a patient's leucocytes with various food extracts and inspecting the cells for damage. The high number of false-positive and -negative results led the American Academy of Allergy to conclude that there was no evidence that the test was effective for diagnosis of food allergy.

Other tests

Hair analysis, Vega testing, applied kinesiology, radionics, radiaesthesia, psionic medicine, and auriculocardiac reflex testing have never been objectively evaluated and are more a matter of gullibility and faith than science.

TREATMENT

Dietary management

Recognition of the offending food and its elimination from the diet is the cornerstone of treatment. In patients with acute, IgE-mediated reactions to a single food, such as shellfish, this is usually quite straightforward. Patients with violent anaphylactic reactions to foods need to be especially careful to avoid accidental exposure. A problem for such patients is the use of a food, most notably peanut, as an undeclared ingredient in manufactured foods or restaurant meals. Where there remains a risk of accidental ingestion it may be appropriate for some patients to carry a preloaded syringe of adrenaline for self-injection, after first being instructed in its use.

In less clear-cut situations, certain foods or food additives are eliminated empirically because they are frequently implicated in that form of food intolerance: for example, a diet free of cereal grains and dairy products is beneficial in certain patients with the irritable bowel syndrome, while a diet free of azodyes, preservatives, and salicylates helps a proportion of patients with chronic intractable urticaria.

Patients who seem intolerant of a wide range of foods may need a very restricted diet—sometimes called a 'few-food' diet. If symptoms are improved, then foods can be reintroduced one at a time. This is both diagnostic and therapeutic, but care is essential, as anaphylaxis can occur on reintroduction, especially in children. Clearly, expert advice from specially trained dietitians is essential to avoid nutritional deficiency.

Sodium cromoglycate

Oral sodium cromoglycate has been used as an adjunct to diet in selected patients with food allergy, especially those with accompanying allergic reactions in the eyes, nose, and skin. Its effectiveness is still unproven.

Immunotherapy

Although immunotherapy (hyposensitization) is effective in wasp or bee venom anaphylaxis and in some forms of allergy to inhaled allergens, it is of no value in food intolerance.

'Alternative' therapies

Provocation–neutralization therapy and enzyme-potentiated desensitization are two treatments used by 'alternative' practitioners: neither is of proven value, although both induce significant placebo responses.

Food allergy seems particularly vulnerable to promoting unorthodox treatments that have not been scientifically validated by double-blind, placebo-controlled trials or confirmed by independent investigators. The hazard of the unconventional approach to therapy is that potentially serious problems can be misdiagnosed and mistreated.

REFERENCES

Ament, M.E., Ochs, H.D., and Davis, S.D. (1973). Structure and function of the gastrointestinal tract in primary immunodeficiency syndromes. A study of 39 patients. *Medicine (Baltimore)*, **52**, 227–48.

American College of Physicians. (1989). Position paper. Clinical ecology. *Annals of Internal Medicine*, **111**, 168–78.

David, T.J. (1993). *Food and food additive intolerance in childhood*. Blackwell Scientific, Oxford.

Ferguson, A. (1990). Food sensitivity or self deception. *New England Journal of Medicine*, **323**, 476–8.

Gazzard, B.G. (ed.) (1990). Gastroenterological aspects of AIDS. *Baillière's Clinical Gastroenterology*, **4**(2).

Haeney, M.R. (1989) Gastrointestinal disease in the immunocompromised host. In *Clinical gastroenterology* (ed. L.A. Turnberg), pp. 317–55. Blackwell Scientific, Oxford.

Hermaszewski, R.A. and Webster, I.N. (1993). Primary hypogammaglobulinaemia: a survey of clinical manifestations and complications. *Quarterly Journal of Medicine*, **86**, 31–42.

Hill, D.J. and Hosking, C.S. (1991). Cow's milk allergy. In *Recent advances in paediatrics 9* (ed. T.J. David), pp. 187–206. Churchill Livingstone, Edinburgh.

Jewett, D.L., Fein, G., and Greenberg, M.H. (1990). A double-blind study of symptom provocation to determine food sensitivity. *New England Journal of Medicine*, **323**, 429–33.

Metcalfe, D.D., Sampson, H.A., and Simon, R.A. (ed.) (1991). *Food allergy: adverse reactions to food and food additives*. Blackwell Scientific, Boston.

Pollock, I. and Warner, J.O. (1990). Effect of artificial food colours on childhood behaviour. *Archives of Disease in Children*, **65**, 74–7.

Ross, I.N. (1987). Primary immunodeficiency and the small intestine. In *Immunopathology of the small intestine* (ed. M.N. Marsh), pp. 283–332. Wiley, Chichester.

Royal College of Physicians and The British Nutrition Foundation (1984). Food intolerance and food aversion. *Journal of the Royal College of Physicians*, **18**, 83–123.

Royal College of Physicians (1992). *Allergy. Conventional and alternative concepts*. Royal College of Physicians, London.

Sethi, T.J., Lessof, M.H., Kemeny, D.M., Lambourne, E., Tobin, S., and Bradley, A. (1987). How reliable are commercial allergy tests? *Lancet*, **i**, 92–4.

Spickett, G.P., Misbah, S.A., and Chapel, H.M. (1991). Primary antibody deficiency in adults. *Lancet*, **337**, 281–4.

Weller, I.V.D. (1987). ABC of AIDS. Gastrointestinal and hepatic manifestations. *British Medical Journal*, **294**, 1474–6.

Young, E., Patel, S., Stoneham, M., Rona, R., and Wilkinson, J.D. (1987). The prevalence of reaction to food additives in a survey population. *Journal of the Royal College of Physicians*, **21**, 5–14.

14.5 The mouth and salivary glands

T. LEHNER

Stomatology is a branch of medicine that deals with oral diseases. For historical reasons and due to the rather technical aspects of treatment of teeth, dentistry has been separated from the main body of teaching of medicine. This has created a curious anomaly in the training of doctors, in that oral diseases receive the lowest priority in the medical curriculum. The aims of this chapter are to present briefly some aspects of stomatology of particular concern to the physician, with special reference to the differential diagnosis of the soft tissue lesions of the mouth.

Dental caries and sequelae

AETIOLOGY

Dental decay or caries is probably the most common chronic disease in man and is responsible for a great deal of pain and discomfort. The prevalence of caries is greatest in children and young adults. It affects the pits and fissures of the occlusal surfaces, and the enamel of the approximal surfaces of teeth. However, an increasing prevalence of root caries (at the neck of the tooth) occurs later in life, especially as teeth are now increasingly retained to old age. Intensive investigations during the past two decades have shown that caries is an infection caused by aggregation of bacteria on the tooth surface, usually referred to as dental plaque.

The development of dental caries requires: (a) the presence of cariogenic bacteria that are capable of rapidly producing acid below the critical pH required for dissolving enamel; and (b) sugar in the diet that favours colonization of these bacteria and that can be metabolized by the bacteria to form acid. There are a number of cariogenic organisms, which can be defined by their ability to colonize teeth, to reduce the pH to about 4.1 in the presence of a suitable sugar substrate, and to induce caries in germ-free animals. *Streptococcus mutans*, *Streptococcus sanguis*, *Lactobacillus acidophilus* and *casei*, and *Actinomyces viscosus* fulfil most of these criteria. However, *S. mutans* appears to be the most efficient cariogenic organism. Germ-free studies have clearly shown that *S. mutans* can induce caries rapidly in the absence of other organisms. *S. mutans* is a facultative anaerobic, non-haemolytic, acidogenic organism, producing extracellular and intracellular polysaccharides. The organism fulfils Koch's postulates as a cause of dental caries.

In addition to micro-organisms a sugar substrate is essential for caries formation. The most common carbohydrates in our diet are starch and sucrose, with smaller amounts of glucose, fructose, and lactose. Quantitatively and functionally the most important substrate in man is sucrose. Addition of glucose to this diet makes little difference but sucrose gives rise to heavy plaque formation, with considerable amounts of extracellular polysaccharide. The most important polysaccharide is dextran (glucan), which is synthesized in large amounts by the constitutive enzyme glucosyltransferase (dextran-sucrase). Dextran may give plaque the necessary quality of stickiness to the enamel surface.

Streptococci do not possess a cytochrome system but contain the Embden–Meyerhof glycolytic enzymes, which will convert glucose to lactic and other organic acids. The pH inside the plaque may fall within 2 to 3 min of rinsing the mouth with glucose or sucrose from a level of about 6.5 to 5; the critical pH below which decalcification of enamel occurs is thought to be about 5.5. Caries is the end-result of a complex sequence of microbial and biochemical processes terminating in acid formation.

PATHOLOGY

Caries develops as a result of acid formed by the bacterial plaque acting on sucrose. The enamel becomes demineralized and plaque bacteria penetrate along the enamel prisms. This process progresses slowly through the enamel layer, but once the dentine is reached, destruction by decalcification and proteolysis of the dentine is rapid. The pulp reacts by an acute inflammatory response that results in necrosis, as the pulp is enclosed within the rigid walls of the tooth and the exudate cannot expand to adjacent tissues. Eventually, infection and toxic materials spread from the root-canal opening to the tissues around the apex of the tooth and induce periapical inflammatory changes, which may terminate in an acute or chronic abscess, or a chronic granuloma. If epithelial proliferation takes place within the granuloma or abscess, then a cyst may develop, which will increase in size over many years before it may be revealed clinically. A dental abscess shows a mixed bacterial infection with a variety of streptococci, staphylococci, and other organisms.

The immunological changes are complex, but serum IgG, IgA and IgM antibodies, as well as cell-mediated immunity to *S. mutans*, can be correlated with the DMF (decayed, missing, and filled teeth) index of caries. Salivary IgA antibodies are also found. Although man has the potential to mount humoral and cellular immune responses to *S. mutans* under natural conditions, the immunity achieved is commonly ineffective. This might be associated with the immune responsiveness linked with the HLA class 2 gene products. Immunization experiments with *S. mutans* have been successfully carried out in rats and monkeys, with a significant reduction in caries. There are two principal immunological mechanisms of protection against caries. One involves salivary IgA antibodies, which can be induced by direct immunization of the minor salivary glands or by immunization of the gut-associated lymphoid tissue, from where sensitized B cells may home to the salivary glands. Salivary antibodies may prevent *S. mutans* from adhering to the tooth surface and thereby prevent caries. The alternative mechanism involves all the humoral and cellular components elicited by systemic immunization. Antibodies, complement, polymorphonuclear leucocytes, lymphocytes, and macrophages pass from the gingival blood vessels to the gingival domain of the tooth. Bacterial colonization of the tooth can therefore be influenced by the systemic immunity and an important mechanism is probably that of IgG-induced opsonization, binding, phagocytosis, and killing of *S. mutans* by phagocytes.

CLINICAL FEATURES

The patient complains of toothache that is made worse by any hot or cold drinks or food. The throbbing pain becomes progressively worse, affects the patient especially at night-time, and may radiate to the face and ear. If relief is not sought the pain becomes excruciating in intensity, and the tooth becomes tender to bite on. This will be followed by death of the dental pulp and the development of an acute swelling due to an abscess or cellulitis. With an acute abscess the inflammatory exudate may penetrate through the bone to the soft tissues. Whilst the pain is reduced the oedematous swelling of the face increases, and if the upper canine is involved the swelling spreads to the eyelid and may present an alarming appearance. The regional lymph nodes are tender and enlarged, there may be fever and some malaise.

Much less commonly a cellulitis or infection by β-haemolytic streptococci may give rise to a spreading infection along the fascial planes, especially of the submaxillary and sublingual spaces. The inflammatory exudate may occasionally spread along the parapharyngeal spaces into the loose connective tissue of the glottis causing oedema of the glottis and respiratory obstruction. The attendant brawny swelling of the neck and floor and the mouth, difficulty in swallowing, trismus, fever, and malaise is referred to as Ludwig's angina. An alternative chronic course is the development of a chronic pulpitis, granuloma, abscess, and eventually cyst around the apex of the offending tooth, and these may proceed without symptoms or only slight discomfort.

Although the patient may point out the painful tooth, this can be misleading, because the pain often radiates to adjacent teeth. The offending tooth is located by finding the caries, most commonly in the pits and fissures of the occlusal surfaces or the approximal surfaces of adjacent teeth. The tooth responds with pain on application of a hot or cold stimulus, and later is tender to percussion and may be discoloured. Dental radiographs may confirm or localize the carious tooth and, at a later stage, any periapical pathological changes.

TREATMENT

The principles of treatment are to remove the caries, apply a non-irritant material, such as zinc oxide and eugenol dressing, to protect the pulp, and then restore the tooth with a filling. If the pulp is damaged irreversibly it will have to be extirpated and root-canal therapy instituted. The alternative to conservative treatment is extraction of the offending tooth. A dental abscess is effectively dealt with by extraction of the diseased tooth, for this removes the source of infection and drains the pus.

If the tooth is to be saved, the pus is drained by an intraoral incision and/or establishing drainage through the root canal. Antibiotics are usually given in acute abscesses and oral penicillin, such as phenoxymethylpenicillin, 250 mg four times a day for about 7 days, is adequate. Cellulitis should first be treated by intramuscular penicillin, in the form of benzylpenicillin, 1 mega unit (MU) four times a day. The swelling should then be incised, to relieve the pressure and provide drainage; extraction of the tooth under general anaesthesia should take place as soon as the patient's condition permits it.

Prevention of dental caries is best practised by careful plaque removal by the individual, and by limiting the intake of sugar, especially the frequent consumption of sweets and sweetened drinks. The type of toothpaste used matters less than the method of tooth brushing, though fluoride in toothpaste decreases the incidence of caries in children by up to 40 per cent. Water fluoridation, however, is the most effective public-health preventive measure. One part per million of fluoride in the drinking water will decrease the incidence of caries in children by up to 60 per cent. There is no evidence of toxicity from water fluoridation. The ethical and scientific issues of water fluoridation are complex and have been the subject of a report by the Royal College of Physicians.

DIFFERENTIAL DIAGNOSIS

Toothache has a characteristic quality but occasionally needs to be carefully differentiated from sinusitis and neuralgia. The throbbing pain that is exacerbated by thermal stimuli and is more severe at night is an important diagnostic feature. An abscess or cellulitis caused by dental caries has been, on a few occasions, confused with mumps, although mumps is confined predominantly to the parotid fascia, earache may be a prominent feature, and pain is elicited by pulling on the ear lobe. A chronic granuloma or a dental cyst are usually diagnosed radiologically, unless the cyst becomes large and a swelling becomes clinically evident.

COURSE AND PROGNOSIS

The acute sequence of events from dental caries is acute pulpitis, periodontitis, resulting in an abscess or cellulitis. If treated promptly the sequelae can be prevented, but if not treated the patient will lose the

tooth and may also develop some facial scarring due to a discharging sinus. With slow progression of caries or incomplete removal of decay, a chronic pulpitis may supervene, followed by chronic periadenitis, which may result in a periapical granuloma, abscess, or cyst. Dental caries is in most instances a progressive condition and can be halted only by the dental surgeon.

Gingival and periodontal disease

AETIOLOGY

A mild inflammation of the gingiva (gum) and slight destruction of the collagen fibres of the periodontal membrane are found in most adults. Advanced destruction of the periodontal membrane, including the supporting bone, is found in about half of the middle-aged or older population. A close association has been found between accumulation of bacterial plaque and gingivitis. During this process a change occurs from a predominantly Gram-positive coccal form of plaque to a complex population of filamentous organisms, spirochaetes, vibrios, and Gram-negative cocci. Of the Gram-positive organisms, *Actinomyces viscosus* appears to be involved in the development of gingivitis. Gram-negative organisms are thought to be essential in the development of periodontal disease. *Porphyromonas gingivalis*, *Actinobacillus actinomycetemcomitans*, *Capnocytophaga* spp., and spirochaetes have been implicated in this disease. The cell walls of the Gram-negative organisms contain lipopolysaccharides and those of the Gram-positive organisms have lipoteichoic acids, dextrans or levans, which may be responsible for a variety of immunological functions.

The causative factors responsible for periodontal disease are not known, but deposits of bacterial plaque are thought to be involved in the pathogenesis of this disease. There are two views concerning the microbial aetiology: (i) that the non-specific mixed organisms in dental plaque or (ii) that specific organisms are responsible for the development of periodontal disease. The specific microbial aetiology hypothesis has recently received support from the observations that *P. gingivalis* is the predominant organism isolated from periodontal disease. Furthermore, a specific but rare type of juvenile and rapidly progressing adult periodontitis is associated with *Actinobacillus actinomycetemcomitans*. Invasiveness of these micro-organisms probably plays an important part in their virulence, and some of the periodontopathic bacteria can be found in the gingiva of adult as well as in juvenile periodontitis.

Dental plaque may calcify, especially in adults and the elderly, to produce calculus. This is often found on the lingual surface of the lower incisors and the buccal surface of the upper molars, i.e. opposite the orifices of the major salivary glands. Chronic gingival inflammation may persist for many years and breakdown of the periodontal membrane, with loss of the supporting bone, may follow and increase in severity over the years. This is referred to as periodontitis, or 'pyorrhoea', as it used to be called, and is the most important cause of loss of teeth after the age of 40, when the incidence of dental caries has greatly diminished. An important feature of periodontitis is that it affects many teeth, resulting in a complete loss of the dentition. As mentioned above, a very rare type of rapid destruction of the supporting dental tissues is found in children or young adults and is referred to as juvenile periodontitis; one or more teeth may become mobile and may be lost before 21 years of age.

PATHOLOGY

There are four immunopathological stages. (1) The initial lesion is found in the normal clinical state, with a localized inflammatory response of polymorphonuclear leucocytes; complement activation and chemotaxis generated by plaque antigens and possibly immune complexes may account for this stage. (2) The early lesion shows a localized infiltration of predominantly T with a few B lymphocytes. In the circulation, lymphocytes are sensitized at this stage to plaque antigens. (3) The established lesion is characterized by a localized plasma-cell infiltration and peripheral blood lymphocytes can be stimulated to proliferate by plaque antigens. This stage can persist for years, with early pocket formation. (4) The advanced lesion marks the transition to a destructive immuno-pathological mechanism, with ulceration of the pocket epithelium and localized destruction of collagen and bone.

Periodontitis is a progressively destructive process leading to loss of teeth. The immunological processes are complex, and may involve type I, II, III and IV reactions, with the protective–destructive mechanisms of lymphocyte and macrophage functions, antibodies, and complement activation. Repair, with collagen formation and destruction of the tissues, eventually leads to loss of support of the teeth.

CLINICAL FEATURES (FIGS. 1 AND 2)

The symptoms of chronic gingivitis or periodontitis are usually so mild that they go unnoticed by the patient. They may, however, complain of discomfort from their teeth, bleeding of gums and associated halitosis, difficulty on eating, looseness of teeth, and occasionally abscess formation. A lack of severe symptoms permits the disease to progress to an irreversible stage before help is sought, so that the loss of teeth from 'pyorrhoea' was often considered in the past as a process of ageing.

DIFFERENTIAL DIAGNOSIS

Chronic gingivitis can be differentiated from acute ulcerative gingivitis by the sudden onset, malaise, characteristic halitosis, pain, and ulceration of the gingiva in the latter. Herpetic gingivostomatitis occurs predominantly in children and again the onset is acute, with fever, malaise, pain, and ulceration of the gingiva and oral mucosa (see below). Desquamative gingivitis may cause difficulties in differential diagnosis and the points to bear in mind are that the attached gingiva shows diffuse erosive areas and evidence of bullous lesions may be found in the oral mucosa.

TREATMENT

The aims in the management of gingivitis and mild periodontitis are to remove dental plaque and calculus by scaling the teeth, and this can be done only by the dentist, or where available, by a dental hygienist. Prevention is, however, much more effective by plaque control, which involves careful tooth brushing, with the aid of plaque-disclosing solutions and regular use of dental floss and wood points. However, once

deep periodontal pockets have been formed, these can be treated by root planing, gingival curettage or surgically. It should be appreciated that the management of periodontal disease is in the hands of the patient, for any type of treatment is dependent on meticulous plaque control.

COURSE AND PROGNOSIS

If the bacterial plaque is not removed, the gingivitis may progress to periodontitis and after many years will result in increased mobility and loss of teeth. This process, however, is reversible by plaque control and, if necessary, eradication of pockets, as long as there is sufficient bone to support the teeth.

Herpes simplex and other viral infections

Herpes simplex virus type 1 is responsible for certain orofacial infections (see also Section 7).

Primary herpetic gingivostomatitis

AETIOLOGY

Clinical or subclinical primary infections by herpes simplex virus type 1 are acquired in early childhood, probably in the second and third years of life. Primary herpetic infection in the first year is rare, because most mothers have neutralizing IgG antibodies to the virus that are transferred through the placenta to the fetus. Serum virus complement-fixing and neutralizing antibodies are found in about 50 per cent of children at 5 years of age. The disease is common in children, but is also seen, less frequently, in adults.

PATHOLOGY

Herpes simplex virus is a DNA virus and there are two types: type 1 is found predominantly in the orofacial region and type 2 in the genital region. There are three genes (α, β, γ) and the β-gene codes for viral glycoproteins gB, gC, gD, and gE. These viral glycoproteins have been well characterized; gB is involved in viral penetration of the cell membrane, gC constitutes the C3b receptor (binding activated C3b), and gE is the Fc receptor for IgG. Antibodies against gD neutralize herpes simplex virus and block its penetration. Hence, this viral infection generates a number of significant immunological molecules in the host cell, in addition to expressing a viral antigen on the cell surface.

Infection starts with the herpesvirus gaining entry into epithelial cells. Virus replication takes place inside the nucleus, and this is associated with formation of intranuclear inclusion bodies and giant cells. As more

Fig. 1 Chronic gingivitis, with erythema and oedema of the gingival margin of the lower teeth and especially the upper right lateral incisor.

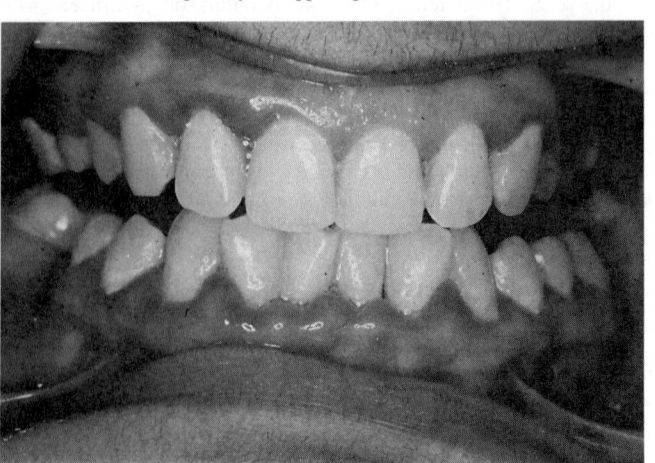

Fig. 2 Radiograph of teeth showing advanced periodontitis with loss of supporting bone of the teeth.

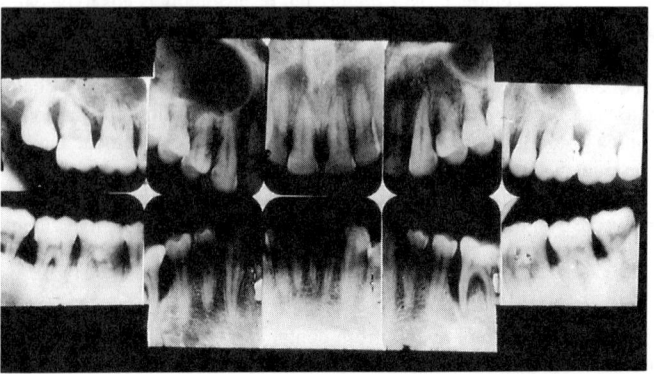

epithelial cells become infected, degenerative and oedematous changes give rise to vesicle formation. The intraepithelial vesicles contain oedematous fluid, with giant cells and degenerating cells with intranuclear inclusion bodies. The vesicles rupture early, resulting in ulcers that heal rapidly.

CLINICAL FEATURES

The disease is recognized by an acute onset of a sore mouth and often sore throat, fever, and extensive inflammation of the gum, followed by formation of vesicles and ulcers of the oral mucosa, and regional lymphadenitis. Infants display considerable fretfulness, sleeplessness, and refusal to eat. Initially there are crops of small ulcers but these coalesce to produce large, shallow, irregular ulcers with surrounding inflammation. Herpetic keratitis is not often associated with herpetic stomatitis, and herpetic encephalitis is extremely rare but may occasionally complicate herpetic stomatitis.

DIAGNOSIS

The early phase of infection can be confused with a cold but the development of vesicles and ulcers makes that diagnosis unlikely. Recurrent aphthous ulcers may occasionally be misdiagnosed in the adult, though the important differentiating points are the acute onset, sore throat, fever, and lymphadenitis in herpetic infection. Laboratory tests can be useful in confirming the diagnosis. Direct examination of a smear from the lesion can be helpful if intranuclear inclusion bodies or giant cells are found. Culture of the virus may assist in the diagnosis, but the herpesvirus is also found in carriers. A rise in antibody titre to the virus during an infection is a useful aid to diagnosis.

TREATMENT

Patients are advised to rest for 2 to 4 days; a soft diet is indicated and an adequate fluid intake is emphasized. The mouth is cleansed by thorough rinsing with hot salt water six times daily and the teeth are cleaned with a wet flannel. In infants, special attention must be paid to the fluid intake and sleep. A useful sedative to use is promethazine elixir, given in doses of 1 teaspoonful (5 mg/5 ml) at night-time.

Acyclovir tablets (200 mg), two to four times daily, can be helpful if started at an early stage of infection. However, in late onset of primary herpetic infection, tetracycline mouthwash can speed up recovery.

COURSE AND PROGNOSIS

The natural course of this infection is 7 to 14 days, during the initial days of which eating is usually difficult, but healing of the ulcers occurs spontaneously. Recurrence of herpetic lesions intraorally is rather rare in otherwise healthy subjects, but is found commonly in patients with cellular immunodeficiencies.

Recurrent herpetic infection

Synonyms

This is also called recurrent herpes labialis; cold sores.

AETIOLOGY

The lesion is caused by herpes simplex virus type 1; it is commonly found from childhood to past middle age and affects both sexes. A variety of factors may precipitate the lesions: fever, exposure to sunlight, local trauma, emotional stress, menstruation, and section of the sensory root of the trigeminal ganglion are among the best-known ones. Severe herpetic infections, affecting the lips, perioral skin, and mouth, are seen in patients receiving immunosuppressive drugs.

PATHOLOGY

Primary herpes simplex infection is followed by the virus becoming latent in the trigeminal ganglion. The relation between primary infection, latency, and recurrent infection by herpes simplex virus has not been completely elucidated but the following immunological hypothesis is supported by current evidence.

Primary infection induces immune responses to the virus, and antibody and cell-mediated cytotoxic mechanisms kill most of the virus and virus-infected cells that are accessible to killer cells. Herpes simplex virus will be sequestered to the nerves and will migrate centripetally along the axons to the trigeminal ganglia. Indeed, the entire herpes simplex virus genome can be found in the trigeminal ganglion, though the DNA is qualitatively different. Some alteration in the surface charge of neurones, triggered off by the various clinical precipitating factors, may induce derepression of the viral genome and virus replication, which will then migrate centrifugally along the axon, to be shed at the nerve endings. In the presence of some defect in cell-mediated immunity, acting at the neuroepithelial junction, a recurrent herpetic lesion will be precipitated. Cytokine production, especially interferon-γ, may be impaired, and a decrease in cytotoxic CD8 T cells is involved in recurrent herpetic infection. However, antibodies to herpes simplex virus are not impaired.

CLINICAL FEATURES (FIG. 3)

The lesions are usually limited to the vermilion border of the lips and adjacent skin. A single blister or a crop of blisters may develop a day after the prodromal phase of a burning sensation. The duration of the lesion varies usually between 3 and 10 days, but secondary infection by *Staphylococcus pyogenes* occurs commonly. The lesion recurs at various intervals often at the same site for many years, and the rate of recurrence may be related to the type of precipitating factor involved. The significance of cellular immunity is highlighted by herpes simplex virus infections found in cell-mediated immunodeficiency states, such as AIDS, and in patients receiving immunosuppressive therapy.

DIAGNOSIS

Localization to the vermilion border of the lips and the history of recurrences make this a readily recognizable condition. Laboratory assistance is rarely required but the findings are similar to those described for primary herpetic infection, except that there is an elevated initial antibody titre, which does not usually increase during recurrent infection. Staphylococcal infection from the anterior nares should be excluded.

Fig. 3 Recurrent herpes labialis vesicle on the vermilion border of the lower lip.

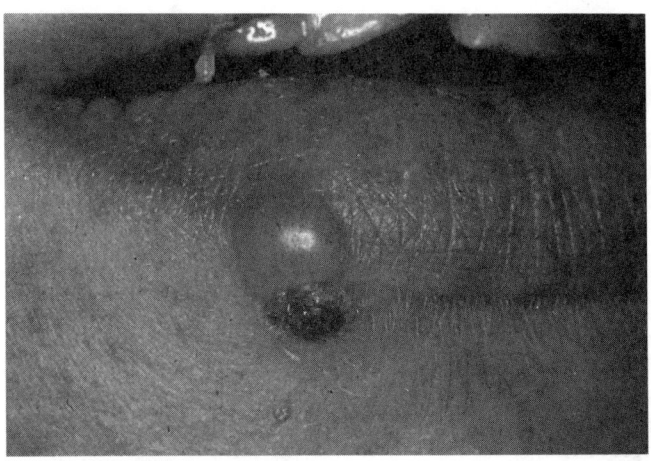

TREATMENT

Acyclovir (acycloguanosine) cream (5 per cent) can be effective if applied during the prodromal phase. Staphylococcal infection responds readily to mupirocin or fucidin ointment, applied three times daily. In the severe type of mucocutaneous herpetic infection in immunosuppressed patients, acyclovir tablets (200 mg) are administered two to four times daily.

COURSE AND PROGNOSIS

The lesions heal usually within about 7 days but recurrences are difficult to prevent. If the precipitating factors are known, some preventive measures can be taken, as by applying a barrier cream to the lips before exposure to the sun.

Herpes zoster infection

Herpes zoster infection of the skin of the face, innervated by the second or third branches of the trigeminal nerve, may be associated with unilateral oral vesicles. These break down early to produce ulcers along the oral distribution of the maxillary or mandibular branches.

Herpangina

This is a rare infection by the Coxsackie group A viruses, usually affecting the soft palate and the oropharyngeal region. Children tend to be affected more often than adults and the mode of presentation of the disease is similar to that in primary herpetic stomatitis. The diagnosis can be firmly established only by isolating the virus from a lesion or by showing an increase in antibody titre. The disease appears to be self-limiting and specific treatment is not necessary.

Hand, foot, and mouth disease

This is another virus infection caused by Coxsackie A5, 10 and 16 (see Section 7). The mouth is sore due to multiple small vesicles or ulcers, which affect most commonly the hard palate, tongue, and buccal mucosa. There are associated vesicular lesions on the hands and feet. The diagnosis is confirmed by isolating the virus from the lesion. The disease is self-limiting within about 2 weeks and no specific treatment is necessary.

Measles

This is an acute exanthematous virus infection of children (see Section 7). Whitish macules on the buccal mucosa, known as Koplik's spots, may precede the development of the red macular rash by 2 to 3 days.

AIDS (See Section 7)

AETIOLOGY

This is an infection by the human immunodeficiency virus (**HIV**) affecting primarily CD4+ cells. However, cofactors may play an important part, of which drug abuse and mycoplasma infection have been emphasized.

PATHOLOGY

Entry of HIV into the host is by the interaction between gp120 and the CD4 glycoprotein on the cell membrane, which acts as a receptor and enables the viral particle to enter the cell by fusion between viral and cell membranes or receptor-mediated endocytosis. Hence, the primary target of HIV is the CD4 subset of T cells (helper–inducer cells), but macrophages, dendritic, and Langerhans cells may also express CD4

and become infected. CD4 cells decrease in number as the cells become infected and killed, but the CD8 subset is not affected, resulting in a decrease in the CD4 : CD8 cell ratio. It is not clear how the virus kills CD4 cells; it might be mediated by interaction between CD4 protein and the HIV envelope protein that results in lethal cell-to-cell fusion (syncytium formation).

CLINICAL FEATURES

The disease affects five populations at risk. (1) Homosexual men, especially those with multiple sex partners, and the anal-receptive partner of anogenital intercourse, are at greatest risk. (2) HIV transmission during vaginal intercourse is common in parts of Africa and Asia; female prostitutes may carry the virus in their genital secretions. (3) Intravenous drug abusers spread the virus by infected needles from one person to another, directly by the vascular route. (4) Blood transfusion with HIV-infected blood, especially in haemophiliacs, treated with factor VIII. (5) Perinatal HIV infection of babies from infected mothers.

Oral transmission of HIV by orogenital intercourse, with ejaculation of infected semen into the mouth, has not been established. There is some epidemiological evidence that oral sex might enable HIV transmission, but doubt remains, as anal sex is practised more frequently than the individual is prepared to admit. The potential of salivary transmission of HIV is of immense significance to the public, as saliva is encountered during daily social interchanges of talking, coughing, sneezing, and kissing. We must recognize that oral fluid consists of saliva and gingival fluid. Most if not all the cellular components in oral fluid (whole saliva) originate from blood, passing into gingival fluid and then mixing with saliva, to result in oral fluid. Although about 90 per cent of the gingival fluid cells are neutrophils, the rest consists of T and B cells and macrophages. Oral fluid may then contain CD4+ cells, thereby creating the essential conditions for HIV transmission. Nevertheless, there is little or no evidence that salivary transmission of HIV can occur. Comparative isolation studies of HIV from body fluids have been made and their results suggest that whilst HIV can be cultured from oral fluid (whole saliva), the frequency of isolation is low (1.2–9 per cent), as compared with semen (21 per cent) or plasma (55 per cent). The quantity of HIV isolated from saliva is also low. The available evidence suggests that it is the cellular fraction of oral fluid, presumably CD4 cells and macrophages, and not the fluid fraction originating mostly from the salivary glands, in which HIV resides.

The special significance to dentists of oral transmission of HIV is self-evident, as they work in a pool of saliva and often gingival bleeding. Yet, no known seropositive conversions were found among about 1000 dental staff in the United States and the same number tested in Germany. Only 1 out of 1309 dentists in another study in the United States was seropositive and he did not wear protective gloves. This was almost a negligible prevalence of HIV seropositivity in a population of dentists among whom more than 90 per cent admitted to needlestick injuries. The possibility of HIV transmission during dental procedures remains a possibility, especially as documented by the case of the Californian dentist passing HIV to his patients. However, the details of this case are most perplexing and the route of transmission has not been established.

This section will be confined to the oral manifestations of AIDS. A variety of opportunistic infection may develop in the mouth. Fungal infections with candida, especially *Candida albicans*, is common. All varieties of oral candidiasis have been recorded in AIDS, but it appears that the chronic hyperplastic and atrophic varieties are more frequent than the pseudomembranous variety. Other fungal lesions may occur but are rare (e.g. histoplasmosis and cryptococcosis).

Viral infections with herpes simplex virus give rise to recurrent oral herpetic lesions affecting the palate or gum and present as painful vesicles that ulcerate. It should be remembered that recurrent intraoral herpetic lesions are extremely uncommon in the rest of the population (unlike recurrent herpes labialis). Orofacial lesions due to herpes zoster have also been recorded but are rather rare. Epstein–Barr virus appears to cause hairy leukoplakia, which is a raised white plaque, commonly affecting the tongue, and is clinically similar to chronic hyperplastic candidiasis. Similar lesions have not been recorded in the general population. Papillomavirus may induce single or multiple warts in the mouth of AIDS patients.

Kaposi's sarcoma is a neoplasm of the vascular endothelial cells. Oral lesions present as red or purple macules or papules, often affecting the palate and tongue. Other neoplasias are less common but non-Hodgkin's lymphomas and carcinomas have been recorded.

Gingivitis and periodontitis may show changes similar to those of acute necrotizing ulcerative gingivitis (see below), except that these may be superimposed on rapidly progressing periodontitis. The condition can be painful and can be associated with rapid loss of soft tissue and bone support, leading to loss of teeth.

Recurrent oral ulcers are probably more common in patients with AIDS than in the general population. Salivary gland enlargement, especially of the parotid glands, might be caused by a viral infection.

DIFFERENTIAL DIAGNOSIS

As oral manifestations of AIDS may occur early in the disease, oral candidiasis, herpetic infections, leukoplakia, oral or gingival ulcers, salivary gland swellings, and oral tumours should be suspected, especially in young men (and women) falling into the HIV risk populations.

TREATMENT

In addition to the general management of AIDS, the teeth and gums should receive a great deal of attention, so as to maintain a high standard of oral hygiene. Otherwise, the oral lesions should be treated topically as for any other oral condition. Routine dental treatment can be difficult to arrange in a dental practice, but most hospitals have made special arrangements for AIDS patients.

Fungal infections (see Section 7)

Candidiasis

Synonyms

This is also called moniliasis; thrush.

AETIOLOGY

Candida is a commensal organism in the mouth found in 20 to 40 per cent of the normal population. Most normal subjects show serum-agglutinating antibodies and cutaneous delayed hypersensitivity reaction to candida. It is not clear whether candida infection of the oral mucosa is endogenous or exogenous, but as the organism is ubiquitous, a suitable environment and impaired immune responses are the most important conditions conducive to infection by candida. Oral candidiasis can be an early manifestation of AIDS (see above). Although most species of candida can become pathogenic, *C. albicans* is most frequently found in oral infections.

PATHOLOGY

The different varieties of candidiasis have in common a superficial invasion of epithelium by hyphae of candida and it is unusual for the hyphae to penetrate the basement membrane. However, occasionally candida may spread by the vascular route to the heart, kidneys, and brain. Raised titres of antibodies to candida are found in serum and secretory IgA antibodies in saliva of patients with oral candidiasis. Antibodies and complement are necessary for optimal phagocytosis of candida by polymorphonuclear leucocytes or macrophages. Recent evidence suggests that serum antibodies of 44- to 60-kDa candida antigen prevent systemic candidiasis. In contrast, cell-mediated immunity is involved in chronic mucocutaneous candidiasis, with a spectrum of cellular immunodeficiencies.

CLINICAL FEATURES

Oral candidiasis develops in a variety of conditions predisposing to candidal proliferation: diabetes mellitus, anaemias, cell-mediated immunodeficiencies (such as AIDS or thymic defects), broad-spectrum antibiotics, immunosuppressive drugs, and leukaemias. Local factors commonly predisposing to oral candidiasis are dry mouth due to Sjögren's or sicca syndrome, irradiation, dentures, or steroid sprays used for asthma.

There are four varieties of oral candidiasis.

Acute pseudomembranous candidiasis (thrush)

This disease is commonly seen in infants as well as in debilitated adults, particularly in diabetes mellitus and malignant diseases, especially leukaemia and lymphoma. Iatrogenic agents are also important predisposing factors; systemic antibiotics, corticosteroids, and immunosuppressive drugs seem to enhance candida infection. Local antibiotic and corticosteroid treatment can enhance oral candidiasis. Clinical manifestations of thrush are usually symptomless white papules or cotton-wool-like exudates that can be rubbed off leaving an erythematous mucosa.

Acute atrophic candidiasis (Fig. 4)

This may follow acute pseudomembranous candidiasis and is usually associated with broad-spectrum antibiotic therapy, hence referred to as 'antibiotic sore tongue'. It is the only type of oral candidiasis that is consistently painful, showing a smooth erythematous tongue, with angular cheilitis and (less often) inflamed lips and cheeks.

Chronic atrophic candidiasis

This type of candida infection is better known as 'denture stomatitis', for it presents as a diffuse erythema of the palate, limited to the denture-bearing mucosa. The denture covering the palatal mucosa predisposes to proliferation of candida. The lesion is usually symptomless but is often associated with angular cheilitis (Fig. 5).

Chronic hyperplastic candidiasis

This lesion presents as a firm, diffuse, white patch, or as numerous white papules with intervening erythema on the tongue, cheeks, or lips. The lesion may persist for many years or for life and should be distinguished from leucoplakia. This variety of candidiasis can be associated with skin lesions and there are three clinical types of mucocutaneous candidiasis.

Fig. 4 Oropharyngeal thrush, following the application of a steroid spray in a patient with asthma.

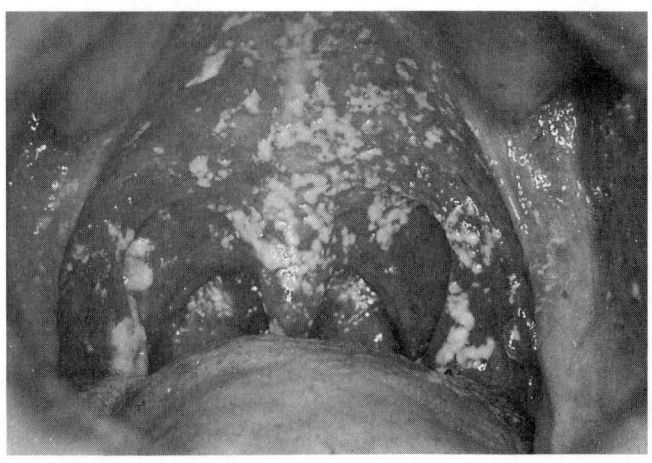

Chronic localized mucocutaneous candidiasis

This starts in childhood as an intractable oral candida infection, with involvement of nails and sometimes the adjacent skin of hands and feet. A number of other skin sites may show persistent candida infection.

Chronic localized mucocutaneous candidiasis with granuloma

The onset of this condition is in infancy and the clinical manifestations are similar to those in the previous type of candidiasis, with the important additional feature of granulomatous masses affecting the face and scalp. Recurrent respiratory tract infection has been recorded in a quarter of these children.

Chronic localized mucocutaneous candidiasis with endocrine disorder

This used to be found in children only, as the mortality was particularly high in the presence of Addison's disease, but nowadays the disease is also seen in young adults. A strong familial incidence is often found and candidiasis commonly precedes the endocrine abnormalities. The clinical features of candida infection are similar to those seen in the localized mucocutaneous variety. The association with hypoparathyroidism and Addison's disease, and less often pernicious anaemia and hypothyroidism, illustrates the relationship between cell-mediated immunodeficiencies and autoimmune endocrine disorders.

DIFFERENTIAL DIAGNOSIS

Chronic hyperplastic candidiasis can cause some difficulties in differential diagnosis from leucoplakia and the laboratory tests are useful in this, as well as in the other types of candidiasis, in establishing the diagnosis. AIDS must be considered, particularly in homosexual males. A culture from the lesion yields candida, usually *C. albicans*, and direct examination of scrapings shows Gram-positive hyphae and yeast cells of candida. Biopsy of the lesion in chronic mucocutaneous candidiasis is helpful, as in addition to the superficial invasion of epithelium by candida hyphae, there is usually extensive epithelial hyperplasia. The dermis shows an intense mononuclear cell infiltration with a large proportion of plasma cells.

A rise in convalescent serum antibody titre to candida may assist in the diagnosis of the acute types of candidiasis, but there may be an impaired antibody titre in the chronic type of candidiasis. Chronic mucocutaneous candidiasis, usually shows some defects in cell-mediated immunity and this should be determined by investigating delayed hypersensitivity, lymphocyte transformation, and macrophage migration inhibition tests to candida. It is essential that the endocrine function should be tested in children with chronic candidiasis of the mouth and nails.

Fig. 5 Angular cheilitis caused by candidal infection.

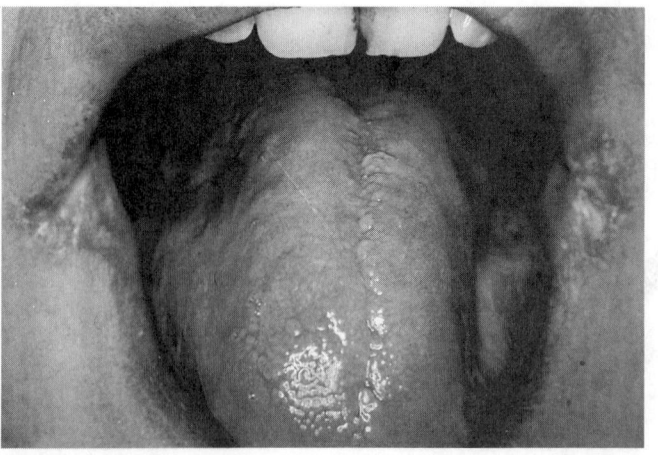

TREATMENT

Oral candidiasis responds readily to topical oral treatment with antifungal drugs; sucking tablets of nystatin 500 000 u four times a day or amphotericin B 100 mg four times a day, for 1 to 2 weeks is very effective. Alternative antifungal agents, such as miconazole, are equally effective. Chronic mucocutaneous candidiasis, however, usually does not respond to topical oral treatment and necessitates intravenous administration of amphotericin B. Although almost complete eradication of the lesions can be accomplished, amphotericin B is nephrotoxic and the disease tends to return after the drug is discontinued. This is comprehensible on the basis of an underlying immunological defect, which, if it is not rectified, will lead to reinfection with candida.

Bacterial infections

Acute (necrotizing) ulcerative gingivitis

Synonyms

This is also called Vincent's gingivitis; acute fusospirochaetal gingivitis.

AETIOLOGY

An infective cause of acute ulcerative gingivitis has been widely accepted, though the organisms thought to be responsible are disputed. *Fusobacterium fusiformis* and *Borrelia vincenti* have been favoured on account of their presence in large numbers in direct examination of smears from the lesions. *Bacteroides melaninogenicus* has been later implicated as the causative organism, but evidence is accumulating in favour of a mixed, bacterial pathogenesis of Gram-negative organisms (fusobacteria, veillonella, bacteroides, leptotrichia), which may be responsible for the lesions by their endotoxin activity.

Whatever role micro-organisms may play, a number of predisposing factors are recognized. Of the local factors, poor oral hygiene, with accumulation of dental bacterial plaque, defective restorations, and pericoronitis are most important. The prevalence of acute ulcerative gingivitis is rather high and it is seen more commonly in young adults and smokers. A lowered general resistance may also predispose to the disease, as was commonly seen in trench warfare during the First World War.

PATHOLOGY

The gum undergoes an acute inflammatory reaction, with an intense polymorphonuclear response and fibrinous exudate. This leads soon to necrosis of the epithelium and thrombosis of the small blood vessels.

CLINICAL FEATURES

Acute ulcerative gingivitis is readily recognized by the sudden onset of painful, bleeding gums and a characteristic foul breath. Except for primary herpetic stomatitis, this is the only other oral mucosal infection in which there is a rise in temperature, which may reach 39°C, regional lymphadenitis, anorexia, and significant malaise. Oral examination reveals necrotic, punched-out ulcers, affecting predominantly the interdental gingiva. At times there are shallow necrotic ulcers affecting the oropharyngeal mucosa, which shows diffuse erythema; this has been referred to as Vincent's angina. In the presence of erupting wisdom teeth, the overlying gum can show ulceration and oedema causing partial trismus of the jaws.

DIAGNOSIS

This disease is often confused with primary herpetic stomatitis, because of the acute onset. However, these patients are usually younger, their breath is stale but lacks the distinct foul quality of that found in ulcerative gingivitis. First vesicles, and then numerous well-defined ulcers are scattered over the oral mucosa unlike the tendency to localization of necrotic sites to the gingiva in ulcerative gingivitis. Direct examination of a smear from the lesion reveals a large number of spirochaetal and fusiform organisms, with a decrease in the mixed bacterial flora.

TREATMENT

Metronidazole is very effective and should be taken 200 mg by mouth three times daily for 3 to 4 days. Phenoxymethyl penicillin, 250 mg taken four times daily for a week is equally effective in clearing the symptoms. Oxidizing agents, hydrogen peroxide mouthwash, and a variety of peroxyborate preparations are also useful. During the acute phase, patients are advised to use a soft toothbrush or a soft cloth to clean their teeth, and they are encouraged to rinse their mouths forcibly with warm saline every 3 h.

Although treatment by drugs is effective in clearing the acute phase, recurrences can be prevented only by careful attention to oral hygiene. The teeth have to be scaled and polished, and the patient is instructed as to the best method of tooth brushing and dental plaque control. Frequent examinations by the dental surgeon are advisable.

COURSE AND PROGNOSIS

In the absence of treatment the acute phase may gradually disappear leaving behind a partially necrosed gingiva and chronic inflammation. Inadequate treatment commonly leads to recurrent ulcerative gingivitis over many years, with halitosis, gingival bleeding, and recession.

Cancrum oris (noma)

This is a rapidly spreading gangrene of the lips and cheeks, mostly confined to children in parts of tropical Africa. It is thought to be an extension of acute ulcerative gingivitis when associated with other diseases, especially measles. Cancrum oris is very rare in the United Kingdom, but can be seen during the terminal stages in patients with leukaemia, especially when treated by a variety of cytotoxic, anti-inflammatory, and immunosuppressive drugs.

Tuberculosis

Oral tuberculosis is rare and usually secondary to pulmonary tuberculosis. Commonly the presenting feature is a painful ulcer or a firm small swelling. Ulcers may be single or multiple, but they are usually large, with a depressed and granulomatous floor and some induration of the base. The tongue, lips, and cheeks may be affected. Diagnosis is based on microscopical and cultural demonstration of *Mycobacterium tuberculosis* and a biopsy of the lesion, which will show a tuberculous granuloma. Oral tuberculosis responds readily to specific chemotherapy.

Syphilis

Treponema pallidum may effect the mouth in all stages of syphilis (see also Section 7).

Primary stage

A chancre appears within 2 to 4 weeks of infection. The lesion that presents on the lip or tongue as a painless, small, firm nodule that breaks down and forms an ulcer with raised indurated edges. The regional lymph nodes show discrete, rubbery enlargement. The diagnosis depends on direct observation of *T. pallidum* by dark-ground illumination. This stage is highly infective, but serological tests are usually negative during the initial 3 to 4 weeks.

Secondary stage

This develops 1 to 4 months after infection and presents as a generalized maculopapular rash and lymphadenitis. Shallow, snail-track ulcers affect the tonsils, tongue, or lips, and the saliva is highly infective. The serological tests for syphilis are positive.

Tertiary stage

This is delayed by 3 to 15 years after infection. Gumma and leucoplakia are the typical oral manifestations at this stage. A gumma starts as a swelling of the palate, tongue, or tonsils; it undergoes necrosis and results in a painless, punched-out, deep ulcer, with a 'wash-leather' floor. The lesion may heal by scarring, or give rise to perforation. Leucoplakia usually affects the dorsum of the tongue as an irregular, diffuse white patch that cannot be rubbed off.

The treatment of oral syphilis is the same as that used in other sites, but the response in the tertiary stage is rather poor.

Oral ulceration

In view of the great variety of oral ulcers a classification will be given first (Table 1). Only recurrent oral ulcers will be dealt with fully and the other types of ulcers will be considered predominantly under differential diagnosis.

Recurrent oral ulcers

Synonyms

Three types of ulcers will be described: minor aphthous ulcers, also known as aphthae; major aphthous ulcers, often referred to in the literature as periadenitis mucosa necrotica recurrens; and herpetiform ulcers.

AETIOLOGY

These are the most common lesions affecting the oral mucosa and the prevalence varies between 10 and 34 per cent. Although a large variety of causes has been suggested, the aetiology of recurrent aphthous ulcers has not been fully established. Trauma is unlikely to play an essential role, though it might precipitate ulceration. There is no evidence that vitamin deficiency or food allergy are involved. Infection by the herpes simplex virus has been excluded as a cause of this type of ulceration. Whilst emotional stress may often influence the pattern of the disease, it is unlikely to be the direct cause. A family history of recurrent aphthous ulcers is often present and the highest incidence of ulcers is recorded in siblings in whom both parents have recurrent aphthous ulcers. A hormonal disturbance may play a part, as in some female patients there is a relationship between the ulcers and menstrual period; the onset of ulceration may coincide with puberty, or the ulcers may develop only after the menopause and the ulcers often disappear during pregnancy. The part that autoimmunity may play in the pathogenesis of this disease has not been fully elucidated, but the *in vitro* response of lymphocytes to epithelial antigens has been related to the clinical features, and lymphocytes are cytotoxic to oral epithelium. Oral mucosa shares common antigens with the 65-kDa heat-shock protein that is found in Gram-positive organisms and human cells. A specific peptide of 15 amino acid residues (91–105), derived from the sequence of the 65-kDa heat-shock protein has recently been found to stimulate lymphocytes from patients with recurrent oral ulcers. The role of this peptide in the pathogenesis of oral ulceration is under investigation.

PATHOLOGY

An early intense lymphomonocytic infiltration, especially with a perivascular distribution, is a constant histological finding suggesting a delayed hypersensitivity reaction. This is followed by a polymorpho-

Table 1 *Classification of oral ulcers*

Recurrent oral ulcers
Minor, major aphthous, and herpetiform
Behçet's syndrome

Microbial infection
Primary and recurrent herpes simplex infection
Herpes zoster infection
Acute ulcerative gingivostomatitis
Tuberculosis
Syphilis

Neoplastic ulcers
Carcinoma
Leukaemia

Haematological disorders
Anaemia
Neutropenia, agranulocytosis

Dermatological disorders
Erosive lichen planus
Pemphigus
Benign mucous membrane pemphigoid
Erythema multiforme and Stevens–Johnson syndrome
Reiter's syndrome

Granulomatous disorders
Histiocytosis X
Wegener's granulomatosis

Iatrogenic agents
Drug allergy
Drug-induced agranulocytosis
Cytotoxic drugs
Radiotherapy

Trauma
Denture, teeth, or foreign body
Chemical

nuclear infiltration. Immunohistological investigations suggest an enhanced immune response, with a significant increase in the number of CD4 and CD8 subsets of T cells, Langerhans cells, and macrophages and the expression of HLA-DR in the epithelial cells.

CLINICAL FEATURES (FIG. 6)

Minor aphthous ulcers

About 80 per cent of recurrent oral ulcers are of this type; they are very common, especially in the 10 to 40 year group, and they are found more frequently in females than males.

A prodromal phase is recognized by most patients, 1 to 2 days before the onset of ulceration, as a soreness or burning sensation. With the breakdown of epithelium and associated inflammatory reaction the pain increases in severity, particularly on eating. The ulcers are round or oval, up to five in number, and enlarge in size, although they remain well under 1 cm. They have a yellow floor with a slightly raised margin and often marked surrounding erythema and oedema. The most common sites of involvement are the mucosa of the lips and cheeks and margin of the tongue, and the ulcers last 4 to 14 days. The rate of recurrences varies from 1 to 4 months and is usually irregular, though in some females ulcers may precede the menstrual period. Enlargement of lymph nodes is uncommon and the patients do not have a raised temperature.

Major aphthous ulcers

These are severe variants of minor aphthous ulcers and less than 10 per cent of patients with recurrent oral ulcers have this type of ulcers. The pain that develops after the prodromal symptoms can be severe and persistent, so that patients find it difficult to eat and swallow food and often lose weight. Examination may reveal 1 to 10 ulcers at a time and some of these may enlarge to about 3 cm. The ulcers are necrotic with a raised margin and inflammation of the adjacent tissue, so they occasionally mimic a carcinomatous ulcer. In addition to the lips, cheeks and tongue, the soft palate and tonsillar region are commonly involved. Healing of an ulcer may take 10 to 40 days and recurrences are so frequent that the patient suffers from continuous ulceration. Multiple, small scars may result from the large ulcers and these may assist in the diagnosis of major aphthous ulcers. The prevalence of major aphthous ulcers is raised in ulcerative colitis. A striking association has been found in smokers who give up the habit and develop recurrent aphthous ulcers.

Fig. 6 The three types of recurrent oral ulcers: (a) minor aphthous ulcer, (b) major aphthous ulcer, (c) herpetiform ulcers.

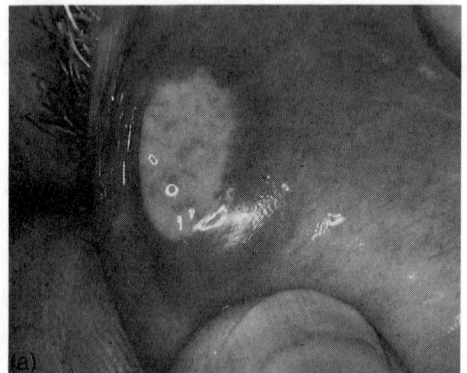
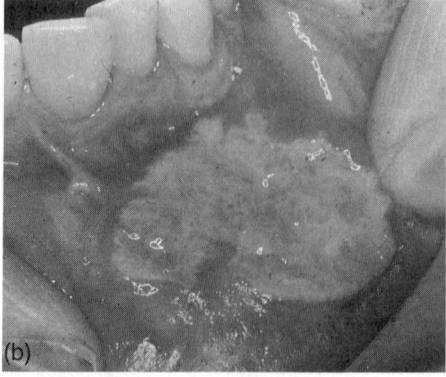
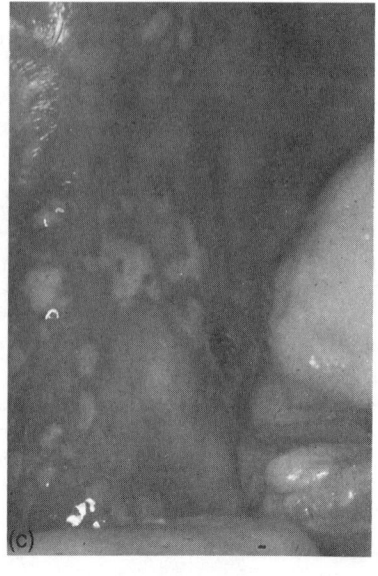

Table 2 *Differentiating features of the three varieties of recurrent oral ulcers*

	Minor aphthous ulcers	Major aphthous ulcers	Herpetiform ulcers
Sex ratio F : M	1.3 : 1	0.8 : 1	2.6 : 1
Age of onset (peak incidence)	10–19 years	10–19 years	20–29 years
Number of ulcers	1–5	1–10	10–100
Size	< 10 mm	> 10 mm	1–2 mm
Duration	4–14 days	10–30 days	7–10 days
Healing with scars	8 per cent	64 per cent	32 per cent
Recurrence	1–4 months	< monthly	< monthly
Sites	Lips, cheeks, tongue	Lips, cheeks, tongue, pharynx, palate	Lips, cheeks, tongue, pharynx, palate, floor, gum
Total duration	< 5 days	> 15 years	> 5 years
Associated oral lesions	—	Erythema migrans	—
Treatment (local)	Corticosteroids	Corticosteroids with or without tetracycline	Tetracycline

Herpetiform ulcers

These are recurrent crops of small ulcers, up to 100 in number, affecting any part of the mouth including the gum, palate, and dorsum of the tongue. They account for less than 10 per cent of recurrent oral ulcers and are much more common in females than males. Patients present with pain on eating and talking, and often with dysphagia; malaise and loss of weight can be prominent features. The lesions persist for 7 to 14 days and commonly new ulcers appear before the previous crop has healed, so that ulceration becomes continuous.

DIAGNOSIS

The differential diagnosis of the three types of recurrent oral ulcers is given in Table 2. It is important to differentiate these ulcers from those found in patients with iron, folate or vitamin B$_{12}$ deficiency, which constitutes less than 5 per cent of patients with recurrent oral ulcers. About 2 per cent may suffer from coeliac disease, due to gluten enteropathy, and these ulcers respond readily to a gluten-free diet.

Agranulocytosis or neutropenia may manifest themselves as shallow necrotic ulcers, affecting predominantly the oropharyngeal region. The ulcers tend to persist, unlike major aphthous ulcers, which recur at different sites. However, cyclical neutropenia can mimic minor aphthous ulcers and the diagnosis depends on serial weekly white blood-cell counts.

One of the most common diagnostic errors is to confuse the effects of denture trauma with aphthous ulcers, although the former are usually localized to the mucosa covering the mandibular and maxillary alveolus and the buccal and lingual sulci. The relation between denture trauma and ulceration is usually simple to find and requires the attention of a dentist.

The differential diagnosis from pemphigus, benign mucous membrane pemphigoid, and erythema multiforme will be described below.

Not infrequently, patients with major aphthous ulcers are suspected of having a carcinoma, though a careful history will make it evident that these ulcers have been recurring at different sites in the mouth. Although major aphthous ulcers may have a raised margin, this is due to inflammation and not invasion, so that palpation fails to elicit the induration usually detected in carcinomatous ulcers.

TREATMENT

Topical corticosteroids are at present the most helpful agents in alleviating aphthous ulcers. They are most effective if application is started during the prodromal phase, when the mucosa has not yet ulcerated, and the intensity of lymphocyte transformation has not reached peak values. If steroids are applied early, ulceration may be prevented, but application

at a later stage may reduce the severity and duration of ulceration. The most useful preparations are triamcinolone in orabase, containing 0.1 mg triamcinolone per 100 g of an adhesive base; hydrocortisone sodium succinate, having 2.5 mg of the steroid per tablet; and betamethasone, containing 0.5 mg steroid per tablet. The tablets are kept in the mouth, or the ointment is applied to the ulcers, three to four times daily until the ulcer disappears. Systemic prednisolone has to be resorted to occasionally in patients with major aphthous ulcers, when topical corticosteroids fail to control the ulcers.

Topical tetracycline is the drug of choice in suppressing herpetiform ulcers, but is also useful in controlling some major aphthous ulcers, particularly when there is excessive amount of inflammation. Its mode of action is not clear and an effective preparation is to use capsules containing 250 mg tetracycline; the powder from a capsule is dissolved in 10 ml of water and kept in the mouth four times daily. Chlorhexidine solution (0.2 per cent) can be used as a mouthwash, which keeps the teeth free of dental plaque, and may facilitate remission of ulceration.

COURSE AND PROGNOSIS

Minor aphthous ulcers may recur from early childhood for many years, and often these ulcers may cause only transient discomfort to which the patient becomes accustomed. However, major aphthous and herpetiform ulcers usually cause a great deal of discomfort, difficulty in eating, and loss of weight. In children, major aphthous ulcers are particularly troublesome and need careful management. In the majority of patients with recurrent oral ulceration the disease burns itself out but this may take many years. In a very small proportion of patients, extraoral sites may become involved, of which the vulvovaginal region is most common, to form part of Behçet's syndrome. There is no way of predicting the development of Behçet's syndrome in patients with recurrent oral ulcers (see Chapter 18.11.8).

Bullous lesions

These are diseases that often affect the skin and oral mucosa, but sometimes involve only one type of epithelium. Three conditions will be discussed in this section: pemphigus vulgaris, benign mucous membrane pemphigoid, and erythema multiforme (see Section 23).

Pemphigus vulgaris

AETIOLOGY

It is a rare disease, which in many instances presents in the mouth, but the mouth is involved at some stage of the disease in all patients. There is considerable evidence in favour of autoimmunity playing a part in this disease. IgG antibodies targeted to normal epithelial membrane glycoproteins (66, 150, and 210 kDa) are involved in the pathogenesis of the disease. It has been suggested that these autoantibodies bind to keratinocytes to cause a loss of interepithelial adhesion. A significant association has been established with HLA-DR4 and -DRW6 in patients with pemphigus and either of these gene products may confer disease susceptibility.

PATHOLOGY

This shows loss of interepithelial adhesion, intraepithelial bullae, and acantholytic cells, with a diffuse leucocytic infiltration of the lamina propria.

CLINICAL FEATURES (FIG. 7)

The disease affects males and females, usually over the age of 30 years. Painful, fluid-filled blisters or bullae may appear in the mouth and burst within a few hours, resulting in shallow ulcers. These persist for weeks or months, but new lesions recur throughout the disease process. Oral manifestations of the disease may persist for many months, without overt ill-health but skin lesions, malaise, and loss of weight may occur at a later stage.

DIFFERENTIAL DIAGNOSIS

Clinically the lesions can be differentiated from recurrent aphthous ulcers by the presence of bullae and when these ulcerate the edges lack the well-defined character of aphthous ulcers. Only occasionally is the Nikolsky sign helpful, by rubbing the mucosa to induce a bulla. The most important diagnostic test is the presence of acantholytic cells on microscopic examination of direct scrapings from the lesion and a biopsy must always be taken. Antibodies to interepithelial antigens also assist in the diagnosis. Pemphigus must be differentiated from pemphigoid and dermatitis herpetiformis (see below).

A less severe and rather rare variant of pemphigus vulgaris is pemphigus vegetans. Vegetation may be found on the oral mucosa and lips, and histological examination shows intraepithelial abscesses containing numerous eosinophils.

TREATMENT

Systemic corticosteroids such as prednisolone are given initially in doses of 40 to 60 mg/day and this is gradually reduced to the minimal dose that will prevent formation of new lesions. In order to keep the steroid dose to a minimum, azathioprine can also be used, with a dose of 200 mg/day.

COURSE AND PROGNOSIS

Treatment with corticosteroids must be maintained for life and has completely changed the prognosis of the disease. Patients rarely die now from the disease but they may develop the side-effects of steroid therapy.

Benign mucous membrane pemphigoid
AETIOLOGY

This is a rare disease, affecting women twice as often as men, usually over the age of 40 years. The aetiology is ill understood but there is some evidence that autoantibodies to the basement membrane of epithelium may play a part in this disease.

PATHOLOGY

This shows subepithelial bullae, and the epithelium tends to detach itself from the underlying lamina propria. IgG IgA or IgM, with or without complement, are found to the basement membrane.

CLINICAL FEATURES

Bullous lesions involve the oral mucosa, conjunctiva, and skin around the genitals and orifices, but in some patients only the mouth is involved. The bullae rupture within a day or two leaving erosions and ulcers. The gingiva is commonly involved, giving rise to persistent pain, bleeding, and a diffuse, raw, fiery red lesion. Other mucous membranes can be involved, such as the nose, larynx, pharynx, oesophagus, vulva, vagina, penis, and anus. The oral lesions usually heal without scaring unlike those of the conjunctiva.

DIFFERENTIAL DIAGNOSIS

Benign mucous membrane pemphigoid can be differentiated from pemphigus vulgaris on clinical grounds but only a biopsy examination will establish the diagnosis. There are no acantholytic cells and the bullae are subepithelial and not suprabasilar. Furthermore, autoantibodies can be detected, probably in less than half the patients, binding to the basement membrane of epithelium and not to the interepithelial substance. The disease should be differentiated from linear IgA disease, which shows linear deposition of IgA in the basement membrane, and dermatitis herpetiforms, in which IgA deposits are found in the papillae.

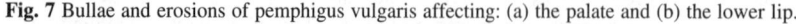

Fig. 7 Bullae and erosions of pemphigus vulgaris affecting: (a) the palate and (b) the lower lip.

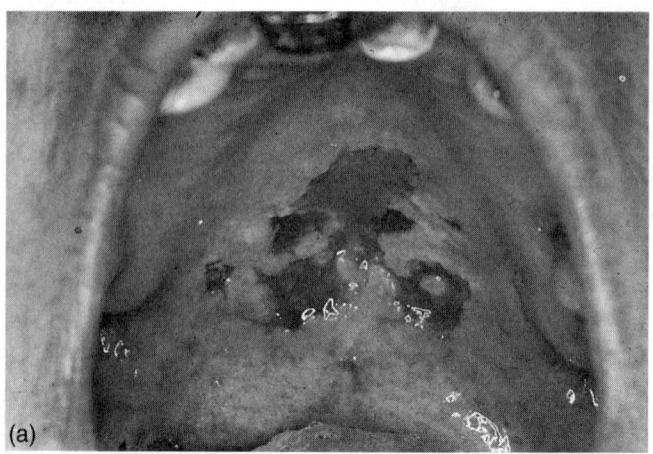

(a)

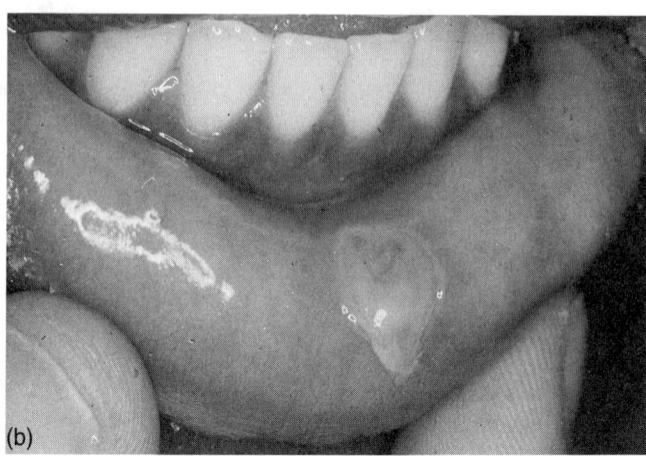

(b)

TREATMENT

If the disease is confined to the mouth, topical corticosteroids are often adequate to control the lesions. However, with involvement of other sites, systemic corticosteroids are indicated, as in pemphigus.

COURSE AND PROGNOSIS

This is a chronic disease, which persists, often with exacerbations and remissions, over many years. The conjunctivitis may result in adhesions, corneal opacity and blindness.

Erythema multiforme

AETIOLOGY

Erythema multiforme may develop at any age but often occurs in young males. Many agents have been associated with this disease: drugs, such as sulphonamides and barbiturates, microbial infections, especially with herpes simplex virus, but a large proportion appear to be idiopathic.

PATHOLOGY

There is intracellular oedema with a zone of liquefaction degeneration of the upper layers of epithelium. Often subepithelial bullae are present and the lamina propria is infiltrated with leucocytes, especially lympho-monocytic cells, neutrophils, and eosinophils.

CLINICAL FEATURES (FIG. 8)

The disease involves most commonly the skin, and oral manifestations may not be a significant feature. However, the mouth can be affected without skin involvement and the diagnosis then is more difficult. The patient develops painful, extensive erosions and ulcers with a predilection for the palate, tongue, and cheeks. The gum may show extensive erosions, which tend to bleed. Haemorrhagic crusting of the lips is often seen. A severe variant of erythema multiforme, which affects the eyes and genitalia, in addition to the skin and mouth, is referred to as Stevens-Johnson syndrome.

DIFFERENTIAL DIAGNOSIS

The diagnosis of oral lesions without the typical skin manifestation can be very difficult. The clinical features to note are the very extensive erosions affecting the palate, tongue, cheeks, and gingiva and the haemorrhagic crusting of the lips. These features should avoid confusion with aphthous ulcers. An association with drugs or microbial infection

is helpful. The age and sex prevalence differs from those in benign mucous membrane pemphigoid. A biopsy examination can definitely exclude pemphigus and erosive lichen planus. The differential diagnosis of Stevens–Johnson from Behçet's syndrome has been discussed and the points noted about Reiter's syndrome also apply here.

TREATMENT

Whenever possible the offending drug or infection should be eliminated. The oral lesions often respond to topical tetracycline. With extraoral manifestations, treatment with systemic corticosteroids may be indicated.

COURSE AND PROGNOSIS

If the offending agent is not found, the lesions may recur over many years and cause a great deal of discomfort. In Stevens–Johnson syndrome, blindness may result from intercurrent bacterial infection.

Lichen planus

This is a disease that may affect the skin, or the mouth or both muco-cutaneous surfaces (see Section 23).

AETIOLOGY

Although the prevalence of oral lichen planus is not known, it is surprisingly common in adults. Very little is known about its aetiology, but the condition can develop in graft-versus-host reaction after bone marrow transplantation. A variety of drugs is capable of inducing lichenoid changes in the mouth (e.g. penicillinase, colloidal gold). It seems to be associated with emotional or psychiatric stress. However, in most patients no cause can be determined.

PATHOLOGY

The pathological changes are hyperkeratosis, hyperplasia, and a characteristic liquefaction degeneration of the basal cell layers of epithelium. The lamina propria shows a well-defined lympho-monocytic infiltration.

CLINICAL FEATURES (FIG. 9)

In the mouth the lesions may remain symptomless for years and not infrequently they are first noticed by the dentist during routine examination. Some patients complain of a furry thickening of the mucosa and others of pain or bleeding from the gums on eating. There are three types of oral lichen planus: hypertrophic, erosive, and bullous. The

Fig. 8 Erythema multiforme: (a) haemorrhagic crusted upper lip, (b) diffuse erosion of the palate.

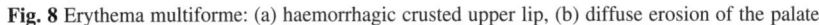

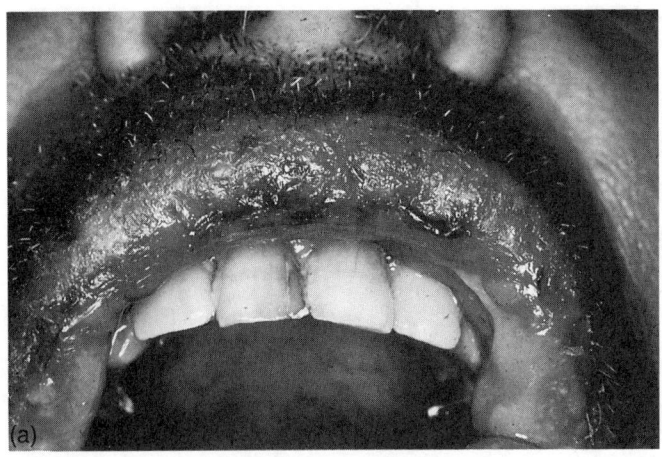

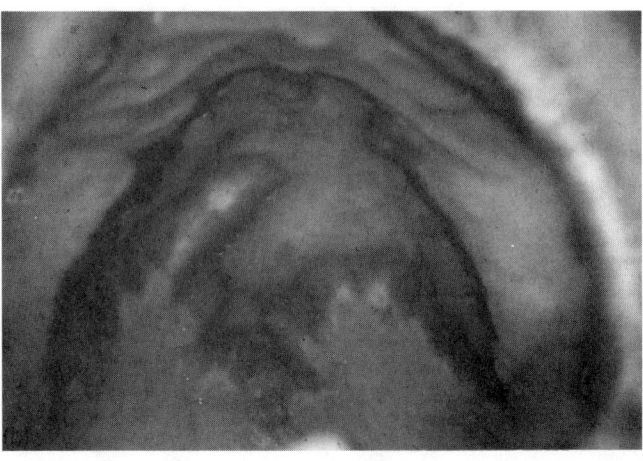

(a)

hypertrophic variety is most common and is usually seen in all three types. There are white striae and minute papules, most commonly affecting the posterior part of the buccal mucosa, lips, and dorsum of tongue, though the palate, gum, and floor of the mouth are also involved. The striae criss-cross giving rise to a fine lacy or fern-like pattern, and less commonly a honeycomb or annular patter. At times the striae may fuse together and result in a diffuse, somewhat smooth, shiny white plaque which may be difficult to differentiate from leucoplakia. Indeed, the dorsum of the tongue usually manifests diffuse white patches instead of the striated pattern.

In bullous lichen planus a bulla is rarely seen, presumably because it bursts to produce ulcers. Erosive lichen planus, however, is common, and patients complain of pain and discomfort on eating. There may be large shallow ulcers up to 3 cm in size surrounded by white striae and papules. The sites of predilection are the same as in the hypertrophic variety, and whilst the latter may break down to result in erosive lichen planus, it is remarkable how often the hypertrophic variety remains unchanged. Except for discomfort, difficulties with eating, and occasionally loss of weight, there are no general manifestations and the regional lymph nodes are not enlarged, except with secondary infection. Not infrequently lichen planus may affect only the gum, inducing a diffuse, fiery-red gingivitis and scattered erosions. This is a particularly troublesome type of lichen planus, with pain and bleeding, and tends to be resistant to treatment. It should be stressed that many patients with oral lichen planus do not have skin lesions.

DIFFERENTIAL DIAGNOSIS

The striae and papules of lichen planus are sufficiently distinctive features in the mouth to differentiate lichen planus from other lesions, without the necessity of a biopsy examination. However, the diffuse hypertrophic variety can be confused with leucoplakia and then a biopsy is helpful. Erosive lichen planus may very occasionally lack the distinctive striae, and then erythema multiforme and benign mucous membrane pemphigoid should be excluded. Both systemic and discoid lupus erythematosus can present in the mouth as central erosions, surrounded by a keratinized margin.

TREATMENT

In the absence of symptoms, hypertrophic lichen planus does not require any treatment. The patient, however, needs to be appraised as to the nature of the disease. Topical corticosteroids are usually effective in the treatment of erosive lichen planus but also suppress the striae and papules of the hypertrophic variety. Triamcinolone in orabase ointment applied four times a day is useful in localized lesions, but betamethasone

(as sodium phosphate) is more effective and is usually used in the form of 0.5 mg tablets, kept in the mouth three times daily. For these drugs to be helpful, they must be applied for one to several months. The lesions recur almost invariably, though the length of remissions vary greatly and corticosteroids may have to be applied with every remission.

Cleaning the teeth tends to be painful and the accumulation of a large amount of dental plaque aggravates the gingivitis. The patient should use a very soft toothbrush and needs to have the teeth scaled every 3 to 6 months. Chlorhexidine mouthwash can be helpful in controlling dental plaque.

COURSE AND PROGNOSIS

The disease is chronic and tends to persist for years, with natural remissions and exacerbations. Topical corticosteroids prolong the remissions, and the erosions and discomfort are kept under control. In a very small number of patients, carcinomatous transformation, especially of the erosive type of lichen planus, can take place. In view of this possibility patients should be followed up regularly at a stomatological clinic.

Leucoplakia

White patches of the oral mucosa that cannot be removed by scraping are referred to as leucoplakia. By convention, lichen planus and lupus erythematosus are excluded from this group.

AETIOLOGY

The prevalence of leucoplakia is not known, but it seems that during the past two decades it has become less frequent. There are many causes of leucoplakia and as these may have distinctive features they will be classified below. It should be noted, however, that in about half the leucoplakias a cause cannot be found. Syphilitic, candidal and AIDS leucoplakias have been discussed, elsewhere. Causes include:

(1) physical and chemical agents: frictional keratosis, smoker's keratosis;
(2) microbial infection: chronic hyperplastic candidiasis, tertiary syphilis and AIDS;
(3) congenital and hereditary leucokeratosis;
(4) idiopathic.

PATHOLOGY

The microscopical features of leucoplakia show a spectrum of changes; at the benign end is epithelial keratosis alone, followed by hyperplasia

Fig. 9 Striae of lichen planus affecting the buccal mucosa and tongue.

Fig. 10 Smoker's keratosis of the palate.

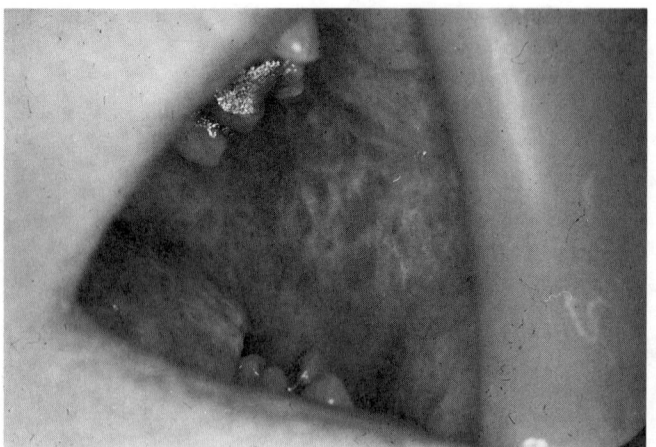

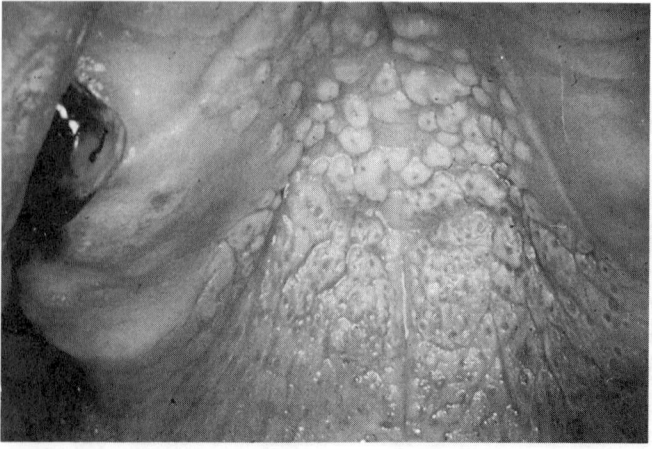

and then epithelial atypia at the premalignant end. The lamina propria shows in parallel an increase in mononuclear cells, especially plasma cells. Carcinoma *in situ* is the least common histological finding.

CLINICAL FEATURES

The white patches vary from a soft, slightly thickened mucosa, involving a small or very large mucosal surface, to hard, irregular white plaques with intervening normal, erosive, or ulcerated sites. The latter is often referred to as speckled leucoplakia and must be recognized clinically because of its greater propensity to carcinomatous transformation. Any part of the oral mucosa or gum may be involved but the cheeks and tongue are most often affected.

Frictional keratosis is usually found along the occlusal line of buccal mucosa and presents as a linear white patch of even consistency.

Smoker's keratosis (Fig. 10) shows a characteristic distribution of the soft and adjacent hard palate, as keratinized papules with central red dots. The distribution is due to involvement of the palatal mucous glands and the red dots are the openings of the ducts. It is usually caused by pipe smoking, but cigarette smoking may also lead to keratosis of a diffuse type, affecting most commonly the cheeks.

Congenital and hereditary leucokeratosis can be distinguished by the presence of diffuse, soft, white plaques, often with a folded surface. The lesions tend to be symmetrical; they affect the floor of the mouth. Members of the family may have similar lesions.

DIFFERENTIAL DIAGNOSIS

All leucoplakias should be biopsied, except smoker's keratosis of the palate, as even small white patches have at times proved to be early carcinomas (Fig. 11). It is, furthermore, essential to find out the degree, if any, of epithelial atypia as this affects the prognosis of leucoplakia. Direct examination of scrapings can be helpful in the presence of hyphae of candida; cultures should also be set up for candida. Serological tests can further aid in the diagnosis of candidiasis but are essential in the diagnosis of syphilitic leucoplakia.

TREATMENT

Smoker's keratosis is reversible in many instances, if the patient gives up smoking. Frictional keratosis can also be cleared, if some local cause of irritation is removed. Candidal leucoplakia should be treated with topical antifungal drugs, though this rarely results in permanent clearance of the lesion. Syphilis should be managed by a course of penicillin and stringent follow-up, so as to detect early any carcinomatous transformation. Leucoplakia showing evidence of epithelial atypia should be excised and if the lesion is large a skin graft may be required. However, in many cases the lesion recurs, even after repeated excision. There is no satisfactory treatment of leucoplakia and the most important point is long-term follow-up, so as to detect in time the development of an incipient carcinoma.

COURSE AND PROGNOSIS

Leucoplakia may persist for life, without any discomfort or change. However, about 5 per cent of all leucoplakias undergo malignant changes and this figure increases to about 30 per cent in leucoplakias showing histological evidence of epithelial atypia. It seems that epithelial atypia is more commonly associated with speckled leucoplakia and the latter as well as syphilitic leucoplakia have a worse prognosis. In contrast, smoker's keratosis and frictional keratosis have a very good prognosis if the offending cause is removed. Congenital or hereditary leucokeratosis were thought to be free of malignant changes, though recently a few cases with carcinomatous transformation have been reported.

Benign neoplasms, cysts, and developmental and inflammatory lesions of the soft tissues

There are numerous benign neoplasms and soft tissue lesions of the mouth. The section will be restricted to some essential features of the following lesions: papilloma, fibroma, lipoma, neurofibroma, hamartoma, pigmented naevus, lymphangioma, denture granuloma, giant-cell reparative granuloma, fibrous polyp, pregnancy tumour, mucous retention, and extravasation cysts.

AETIOLOGY

The cause of benign neoplasms is unknown and the parts that physical or chemical irritation and microbial infection may play are ill understood. Mucous retention or extravasation cysts are caused by trauma or obstruction of the duct orifice of the minor salivary glands. Whereas true benign neoplasms are rare, inflammatory lesions and cysts are commonly found in the mouth.

CLINICAL FEATURES

The soft-tissue tumours present as painless, slow-growing swellings affecting any part of the mouth, but if they originate from the gum they are referred to as epulides. Fibrous polyps are the most common inflammatory lesions of the oral mucosa and result from trauma or irritation from rough edges of carious teeth. Most of the tumours are sessile, some are pedunculated as with some fibromas, and others are flat and pigmented as with the naevi. They are usually symptomless except for bleeding from hamartomas and giant-cell reparative granulomas.

DIFFERENTIAL DIAGNOSIS

There are some distinguishing clinical features but the definitive diagnosis will depend on the histological examination of the excised specimen. A papilloma can be recognized by its firm, small, keratinized, finger-like processes. Lymphangiomas are soft swellings, which may cause considerable enlargement of the lip or tongue. Hamartomas are flat or nodular red lesions that may blanch when compressed; they are occasionally confused with pregnancy tumours, which are rather vascular granulomatous swellings of the gingiva found during pregnancy. Giant-cell reparative granulomas are also very vascular, maroon-coloured lesions originating from the gingiva. Denture granulomas can be readily recognized from their relation to the flange of a denture; the lesion is often elongated, can be indented or ulcerated by the denture.

Fig. 11 Leucoplakia of the tongue, which on biopsy examination showed a well differentiated squamous-cell carcinoma.

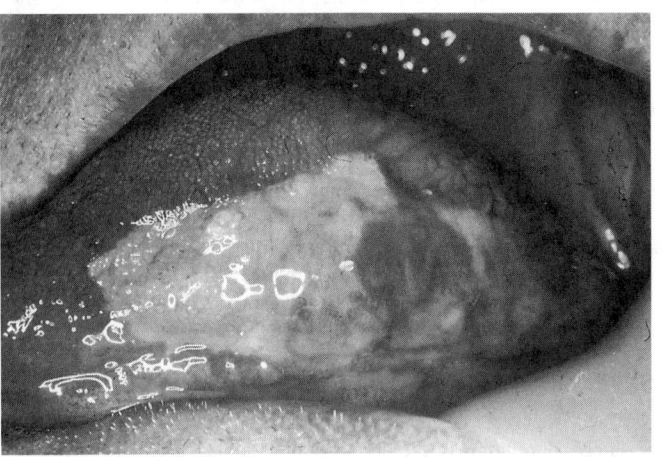

Mucous retention or extravasation cysts are small, often bluish swellings affecting the lips or cheeks.

TREATMENT

Surgical excision, with a margin of normal tissue at the base of the lesion, is usually indicated. Pregnancy tumours, however, commonly regress spontaneously.

COURSE AND PROGNOSIS

The soft-tissue neoplasms will enlarge over the years and interfere with the normal functions of the mouth. Bleeding from any of the lesions is rarely profuse. Only the giant-cell reparative granuloma has a tendency to recur after excision.

Oral carcinoma

AETIOLOGY

Carcinoma of the mouth accounts for about 2 per cent of all cancers in Britain. The prevalence increases significantly after the age of 45 years and more than twice as many men as women are affected. The incidence of oral cancer has been decreasing over the last four decades, unlike that of lung cancer. As in other carcinomas the cause is unknown, but smoking and alcohol have been implicated. There is some epidemiological evidence to support this, but unlike lung cancer it is pipe or cigar, rather than cigarette smoking that have been associated with oral cancer. The association with chronic oral sepsis and irritation has not been critically examined. There is some evidence that microbial agents, particularly *Treponema pallidum, Candida albicans*, human papillomia virus, and human immunodeficiency virus (**HIV**), may directly or indirectly influence the development of carcinoma.

Among the predisposing lesions, leucoplakia is the best-known one; in 5 per cent of all patients and in about 30 per cent of those showing evidence of epithelial atypia the leucoplakia may undergo carcinomatous transformation (Fig. 12). Submucous fibrosis is another precancerous condition and is found predominantly in India and Sri Lanka. It seems to be related to eating chillis and possibly betel-nut chewing, and affects the palate, buccal mucosa, and tongue.

PATHOLOGY

Squamous-cell carcinoma in the mouth is usually a well-differentiated keratinizing neoplasm invading the surrounding tissue. Poorly differ-

Fig. 12 Leucoplakia of the buccal mucosa, the lower edge of which is raised and on biopsy proved to be a well-differentiated squamous-cell carcinoma.

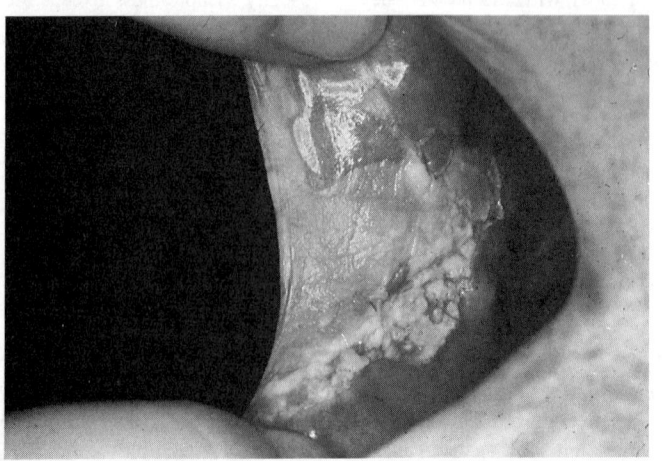

entiated and anaplastic oral carcinomas are much less frequent and especially rare with carcinoma of the lip. Spread occurs by local invasion and lymph node metastasis is less common than is generally thought, and occurs at a late stage.

CLINICAL FEATURES

The presenting features of carcinoma vary with the site of involvement but there are two types, a lump or an ulcer. The patient complains of a swelling or ulcer that is resistant to healing and gradually enlarging in size. There may be little pain initially, but at a later stage discomfort and occasional bleeding may occur. Cancer of the tongue may give rise to local pain and earache. Whereas some patients complain of excess of saliva, especially with the larger tumours, a dry mouth may be found during the early stages of malignant change and should be noted as another feature favouring malignancy. A small lump may enlarge to a hard swelling before the covering mucosa breaks down. A malignant ulcer shows a raised and often everted edge, and the most important feature is induration at the base of the lesion. Any part of the mouth can be involved but the lips (usually the lower lip) and tongue are most common, each accounting for about 25 per cent of oral carcinomas. The floor of the mouth, gingiva, cheek, hard and soft palate, and oropharynx may account for about 10 per cent of the carcinomas. In most patients there is only one lesion but some patients may have two or even multiple carcinomas. Metastasis may occur at a late stage to the submandibular or upper cervical lymph nodes, and occasionally to the submental nodes.

DIFFERENTIAL DIAGNOSIS

Any long-standing or indurated lesion in the mouth, especially of elderly or middle-aged patients, should be queried for malignancy and biopsy examination is essential. A traumatic ulcer caused by a denture can be confused with a malignant ulcer, but it may lack induration, the offending part of the denture may fit into the ulcer, and removing the denture for about a week may bring about healing of the lesion. Major aphthous ulcers have been mentioned elsewhere (see above), but the salient differentiating features are a history of recurrent ulcers at different sites of the mouth, over many years.

Adenocarcinoma of the small salivary glands may present as a lump of the soft palate, lips, or cheeks and only a biopsy will establish the diagnosis firmly. Carcinoma *in situ* is rare in the mouth, but it may present as a diffuse, erythematous, somewhat velvety lesion, affecting the mucosa of one half of the soft palate or cheek. Again a biopsy examination must be carried out for diagnosis.

TREATMENT

The principles of treatment of oral carcinomas are those applied to other carcinomas of the body. Surgical excision of the lesion and a margin of adjacent tissue is the most common practice, and this may be extended if necessary to block dissection of the regional lymph nodes. Radiotherapy is an alternative approach and is commonly used in primary treatment of cancer of the lip, in inoperable cases, or with recurrent carcinoma following surgery. Cytotoxic drugs have also been used in the management of cancer of the mouth with variable results. Management of oral cancer is a complex subject outside the scope of this section. It should be emphasized that oral hygiene is particularly important with any treatment so as to avoid ascending parotitis. A dry mouth usually follows radiotherapy and again meticulous oral hygiene should be advised, so as to prevent rampant caries and candida infection.

COURSE AND PROGNOSIS

The 5-year survival rates differ considerably with the anatomical site of the cancer. Carcinoma of the lip has by far the best prognosis, irrespective of whether treatment is by surgery or radiotherapy, and the 5-year survival rate is about 80 per cent. In contrast the figures for carcinoma of the tongue range from 25 to 35 per cent, floor of the mouth 20 to 40 per cent, cheek 30 to 50 per cent, and oropharynx, palate, and gingiva at about 25 per cent. The prognosis is significantly better in the absence of lymph node involvement.

Salivary gland diseases

Xerostomia

Xerostomia is a term describing dryness of the mouth and can be due to a variety of conditions.

AETIOLOGY

Dry mouth is a common manifestation, especially in middle-aged women, and can be caused by anxiety, emotional, and mental stress. Iatrogenic xerostomia is secondary to a number of drugs, the most common of which are antihistamines, tranquilizers (phenothiazine) hypotensive agents, diuretics, and preparations containing atropine. Another common cause is secondary to radiotherapy, but the salivary flow tends to recover, though it may take many months. Some diseases affect the salivary glands directly and cause dryness of the mouth, e.g. Sjögren's syndrome and sialadenitis. Another large group of agents cause xerostomia by inducing changes in fluid balance; diabetes, anaemia, dehydration, and oedema are common examples.

PATHOLOGY

Diseases affecting the salivary glands cause a destruction of the secretory components by a mononuclear cell infiltration and fibrosis of the salivary acini.

CLINICAL FEATURES

The patient complains of dryness of the mouth and sometimes the eyes, soreness of the mouth, especially the tongue and throat, and discomfort on swallowing of solids and at times difficulty in speaking. The best clinical evidence of xerostomia is an atrophic, dry oral mucosa, often fiery red, due to infection by candida. Inspection of the duct orifices of the major salivary glands will fail to reveal salivary flow and in severe cases stimulation by lemon juice applied to the tongue may not induce a flow of saliva. The patient may develop rampant caries, or if he/or she wears dentures these may cause difficulties with retention.

DIFFERENTIAL DIAGNOSIS

A thorough history may establish psychogenic or iatrogenic causes, and diseases affecting fluid balance. Sialography and labial gland biopsy may be necessary in the diagnosis of Sjögren's syndrome, though a raised erythrocyte sedimentation rate, rheumatoid factor, antinuclear factor, autoantibodies, and HLA-typing may assist in the diagnosis. Nevertheless there will be a large proportion of patients in whom a specific cause cannot be found.

TREATMENT

Management of the patient is clearly directed to eliminate the cause of xerostomia but this may be difficult or at times impossible to achieve. In such cases, palliative measures are helpful and these include frequent sips of water, meticulous oral hygiene, early treatment or preferably prevention of candidiasis by topical nystatin or amphotericin B. Each patient responds differently; some prefer glycerin, others carboxymethylcellulose as a lubricant, and the latter can be taken as a solution or aerosol (Glandosane). A mucin preparation can also be helpful as a spray or as a lozenge (Saliva Orthana).

Sialadenitis

Bacterial or viral infections and rarely allergic reactions may cause inflammation of the salivary glands. These agents may give rise to acute, chronic, and allergic sialadenitis, and recurrent parotitis.

AETIOLOGY

Ascending infection of the parotid gland used to be a common complication in elderly, postoperative patients who were predisposed by dehydration, reduced salivary flow, and lack of oral hygiene. Acute parotitis may also follow the use of drugs causing xerostomia. The most common micro-organisms involved are *Staphylococcus aureus*, *Streptococcus viridans*, and pneumococcus. The most common acute parotitis is mumps (see Section 7). Salivary glands are sometimes affected by HIV infection, with an enlargement of the parotid glands. Chronic sialadenitis is usually associated with duct obstruction and therefore affects usually the submandibular gland. Recurrent sialadenitis is a disease of unknown aetiology and may be associated with a decreased salivary flow causing retrograde infection. The disease may affect both adults and children.

PATHOLOGY

Acute sialadenitis shows an acute inflammatory reaction of the salivary tissue, with a predominantly neutrophil infiltration, except in mumps, which shows an infiltration by mononuclear cells. In both chronic and recurrent sialadenitis there is a marked periductal and acinar infiltration by mononuclear cells, with some duct epithelial hyperplasia, accompanied by acinar atrophy and fibrosis.

CLINICAL FEATURES

The presenting symptoms of acute sialadenitis are a painful swelling in one of the parotid glands of an elderly patient. Commonly the patient has a low-grade fever, oedema of the cheek, some trismus, and a purulent discharge may be expressed from the duct opening. In contrast, mumps affects healthy children and young adults.

In chronic sialadenitis there are usually clinical features of duct obstruction of one of the submandibular glands. There is pain and swelling in the submandibular or retromandibular region, with a reddened duct orifice discharging pus. Recurrent parotitis presents as an acute pain and swelling of one or both parotid glands, with erythema of the duct orifices and pus discharging from them. There may be an associated fever and malaise. Recurrences vary from weeks to months and after repeated attacks the affected gland may remain enlarged.

DIFFERENTIAL DIAGNOSIS

There is little clinical difficulty in the differential diagnosis between acute sialadenitis of the parotid gland in the elderly patient due to ascending infection and mumps in the healthy young subject. Any discharging pus should be cultured for organisms and its antibiotic sensitivity should be determined. Recurrent parotitis however, can cause difficulties; in addition to a history of recurrent painful swelling and discharging pus, sialography may help and show sialectasis and duct dilatation. In chronic sialadenitis there is usually clinical or radiological evidence of calculus and sialography may show duct dilatation.

A variety of granulomatous diseases may very occasionally affect the salivary glands, such as sarcoidosis, tuberculosis, syphilis, and actinomycosis. When there is bilateral salivary and lacrimal enlargement this is often referred to as Mikulicz's syndrome. Allergic sialadenitis is also rare and to determine the allergic agent can be difficult as drugs, foods, pollen, and other agents have been implicated.

TREATMENT

In acute, chronic, or recurrent sialadenitis the relevant antibiotics should be used to control the infection, but occasionally surgical drainage may also be necessary. Careful oral hygiene measures are important in all types of sialadenitis. There is no special treatment for mumps, but rest and isolation for about a week are indicated. In chronic sialadenitis the cause of obstruction, such as a calculus, should be removed. The treatment of recurrent parotitis is more difficult and if antibiotics do not control the disease, surgical intervention should be considered.

COURSE AND PROGNOSIS

Acute sialadenitis will resolve with the aid of antibiotics and general management of the patient. Mumps will resolve spontaneously and second attacks are very rare. Chronic sialadenitis may persist for many years and may lead to destruction of the gland, unless the cause of duct obstruction is removed early. Recurrent parotitis in childhood may show spontaneous recovery after puberty.

Salivary duct obstruction due to calculus

AETIOLOGY

The submandibular salivary ducts and, to a less extent, glands are the most common sites for the development of stones. Calcium phosphates and carbonates are deposited from the saliva round a nidus of desquamated cells or micro-organisms.

CLINICAL FEATURES

Salivary calculus is usually found in adults and the presenting symptoms are a sudden unilateral swelling and pain of the gland related to eating. The swelling may take minutes to appear and hours to subside. Examination reveals a soft swelling of the affected gland and careful digital palpation along the course of the salivary duct will localize the calculus. This may vary in size from a small grain to a concretion 10 to 20 mm in length. The presence and localization of a stone in a duct should be confirmed by radiographs and the presence of calculi in the gland can be diagnosed only by radiography.

DIFFERENTIAL DIAGNOSIS

Recurrent unilateral swelling associated with eating is characteristic of salivary gland obstruction but occasionally this may be caused by external agents. Trauma from a denture or sharp tooth may cause obstruction of the orifice of the parotid duct.

TREATMENT

If the calculus is near the orifice of the duct it can occasionally be teased out, otherwise surgical removal is indicated.

COURSE AND PROGNOSIS

Single calculi do not tend to recur, but if treatment has been delayed numerous calculi may have formed inside the gland, which may occasionally have to be excised.

Salivary gland tumours

A variety of epithelial tumours affects the major and minor salivary glands of which the most common is the pleomorphic adenoma, or mixed salivary tumour (74 per cent), followed by adenocarcinoma (12 per cent), adenoma (8 per cent), mucoepidermoid tumour (3 per cent), and acinic-cell tumour (2 per cent); the percentages give the prevalence in the parotid glands. Only pleomorphic adenoma will be considered in any detail and the references should be consulted for other tumours.

Pleomorphic adenoma

AETIOLOGY

The cause of this tumour is unknown, though salivary gland tumours can be produced in animals by carcinogenic hydrocarbons, polyomavirus, and other agents. The tumour originates from epithelial cells of the ducts, acini, or myoepithelial cells; the last are thought to be capable of producing the stromal mucins of this tumour.

PATHOLOGY

The epithelial cells proliferate in duct-like structures, sheets, and cords, within a connective tissue stroma, which may show mucous, cartilaginous, or hyaline appearance. The tumour is encapsulated, though satellite tumours are often found outside the capsule.

CLINICAL FEATURES

The tumour is usually found in adults and the parotid salivary gland is most commonly affected, followed by the submandibular gland and rarely the sublingual gland. The minor salivary glands, however, are also affected, and the most frequent sites are the glands of the palate, lips, and cheeks. The tumour presents as a small, painless swelling, which may take years to enlarge and is not attached to the overlying skin or mucosa.

DIFFERENTIAL DIAGNOSIS

As the tumour is slow growing it needs to be differentiated only from other tumours. Adenocarcinoma, mucoepidermoid carcinoma, and adenoid cystic carcinoma may mimic pleomorphic adenoma in its slow growth, but some may grow more rapidly, invade the adjacent skin or mucosa, and metastasize. These tumours can often be differentiated only on histopathological examination, and wherever possible an excision biopsy should be done.

TREATMENT

Surgical excision with a margin of normal tissue is always practised, as the tumour is radioresistant.

COURSE AND PROGNOSIS

If left untreated the tumour may enlarge to a grotesque size. A small proportion of pleomorphic adenomas may undergo carcinomatous transformation. The tumour has a bad record for recurrences after excision and this is thought to be due to leaving behind satellite tumours outside the capsule.

Neoplasms, cysts, developmental lesions, and dystrophies of the bones and teeth

This section covers a very large number of lesions found in the jaws. Only essential features, especially of differential diagnosis, will be covered in the following disorders: (a) benign neoplasms: osteoma, chondroma, fibroma, ossifying fibroma, and giant-cell tumour; (b) malignant neoplasms: osteosarcoma, and chondrosarcoma; (c) cysts and tumours of dental origin: periodontal and dentigenous cysts, keratocysts, and ameloblastoma; (d) dental malformations or odontomes; (e) osteodystrophies: giant-cell reparative granuloma, brown tumour of hyperparathyroidism, fibrous dysplasia, and Paget's disease.

AETIOLOGY

The cause of the neoplasms and osteodystrophies is not known. Periodontal cysts, which are the most common lesions in this group, develop as a consequence of chronic periapical infection.

CLINICAL FEATURES

The bony tumours and cysts are commonly symptomless, unless they have reached a large size and the patient notices a swelling, or a denture ceases to fit. Often pathological changes are noticed by the dentist through movement of teeth or on routine radiographic examination of the teeth. Hyperparathyroidism should be excluded, in cases when a giant-cell granuloma is suspected. Cysts can be found at any age, but giant-cell reparative granulomas, ossifying fibroma, and fibrous dysplasia are often seen in young people, unlike Paget's disease of bone, which is seen only in old people. There is a predilection for the mandible to be involved more commonly with ossifying fibroma and giant-cell reparative granuloma. Odontomes are developmental malformations of dental tissue that become calcified. This is a diverse group of disorders and varies from a simple enamel pearl, consisting of a nodule of ectopic enamel attached to a tooth, to a complex composite odontome, which is an irregular mass of calcified dental tissues. Ameloblastoma is a rare but important epithelial neoplasm of the jaws. Young adults are most often affected, the tumour is slow-growing and affects the mandible more often than the maxilla. The neoplasm is locally invasive but does not metastasize. Osteosarcoma and chondrosarcoma are found in children or young adults but may develop in the elderly with Paget's disease. They present as fast-growing, painful, and firm swellings and they may metastasize to the lungs early.

DIFFERENTIAL DIAGNOSIS

The diagnosis of bony lesions of the jaws is made on the basis of a characteristic radiological picture, coupled with the histological features of the biopsy. Periodontal cysts are very frequent and show a radiolucent rounded area with a sharply defined outline. If the crown of a tooth is enclosed within the cyst, it is referred to as a dentigerous cyst. The latter and keratocysts are usually found in the young, but with some keratocysts a tooth may be missing. Dental cysts must be differentiated from ameloblastomas, which tend to show multilocular and sometimes a honeycomb pattern on radiographs. These radiolucent lesions should also be differentiated from secondary carcinoma and myelomatosis. Giant-cell reparative granuloma and tumour (osteoclastoma) show a radiolucent area, sometimes loculated, and the outline is not as well defined as a dental cyst. Hyperparathyroidism can be excluded by radiographic appearance of other bones and by the calcium and phosphate levels in the blood. Ossifying fibromas are more common than fibromas and the radiographs show a well-defined radiolucent area with speckled calcification. This can usually be distinguished from the 'ground-glass' appearance, without a distinct border, found in fibrous dysplasia. In Paget's disease there is a distinctive 'cotton-wool' appearance on radiographic examination and the alkaline phosphatase levels are high. Odontomes can be readily recognized on clinical examination, but those that are unerupted, particularly the compound and complex composite odontomes show on radiographs a mass of overlapping denticles and an irregular radio-opaque mass, respectively. Osteosarcoma and chrondrosarcoma show patchy areas of bone resorption and deposition.

TREATMENT

The treatment of dental cysts is by enucleation of the cyst lining and usually extracting the involved tooth. The tumours and malformations are usually excised but some, such as giant-cell reparative granuloma, can be curettaged. Brown tumours will recur unless the underlying hyperparathyroidism has been dealt with. Fibrous dysplasia may require removal of excessive tissue for cosmetic or functional reasons, but this should be delayed until normal bone growth has ceased. Bony changes in Paget's disease are best not interfered with, except if there are functional reasons, such as inability to fit a denture. Composite odontomes should be removed surgically. The treatment of ameloblastoma is by local excision, with a generous margin of normal bone, or by hemimandibulectomy. Sarcoma of the jaw must be dealt with by early radical excision.

COURSE AND PROGNOSIS

If the cysts and benign tumours are removed surgically, they do not recur, except with keratocysts and the reparative granulomas. Ameloblastomas may recur after several excisions, without metastases, and this is why some surgeons prefer to do a hemimandibulectomy. The prognosis of the jaw sarcomas is very poor and the 5-year survival rate is between 25 and 40 per cent. Fibrous dysplasia tends to be self-limiting, but in Paget's disease there may be progressive enlargement, especially of the maxilla.

Miscellaneous disorders

In this section a brief discussion will be given on the following three topics: (a) oral manifestations of blood disorders, (b) halitosis, and (c) disorders of the temporomandibular joint.

Oral manifestations of blood disorders

Mild anaemias or deficiencies of iron, folate, or vitamin B$_{12}$ may manifest themselves as glossitis (Fig. 13) with a sore tongue or mouth, angular cheilitis, or recurrent ulceration (see Section 22). The tongue is commonly depapillated, the corners of the mouth may be inflamed and fissured, and occasionally there may be small shallow ulcers affecting the lips, tongue, and cheeks. The cause of any haematological deficiency should be investigated and, especially with folate deficiency, coeliac disease should be excluded. Replacement therapy usually deals with the

Fig. 13 Smooth, depapillated, erythematous tongue in a patient with iron-deficiency anaemia.

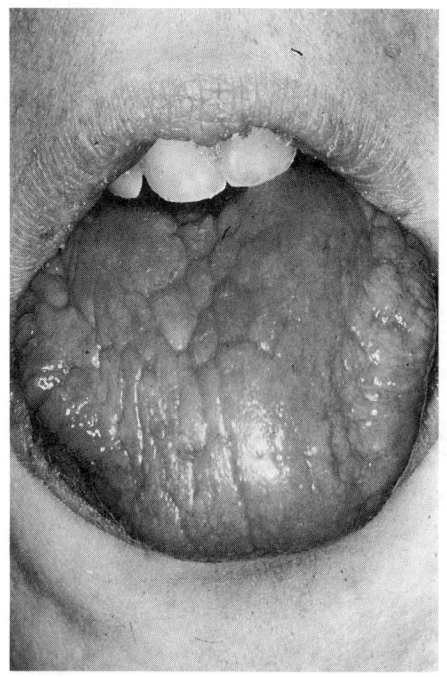

clinical features effectively. It should, however, be emphasized that the complaint of a sore tongue can be associated with many other causes, such as erythema migrans, candidiasis, lichen planus, recurrent aphthous ulceration, and black hairy tongue. Erythema migrans (geographical tongue) is particularly common and is characterized by oval, depapillated areas with a well-defined edge affecting the dorsum of the tongue (Fig. 14). The lesions move from one site to another. The aetiology of erythema migrans is unknown and treatment is rather unsatisfactory. A sore tongue is a frequent complaint in middle-aged women, often without any demonstrable aetiological factor.

Acute leukaemia, particularly the myelomonocytic form, may occasionally present in the young in the form of sore, bleeding gums. This may vary from slight inflammation to that showing bulbous enlargement of the gingiva. There are usually inadequate local causes for such a gingivitis and anaemia may be evident; blood tests should be requested to exclude leukaemia.

Leucopenia and agranulocytosis, especially those due to drugs, may become clinically evident by ulceration of the throat or the mouth. Purpura may be associated with a deficiency of platelets, so that bleeding from the gum may also be a feature.

Many haemorrhagic disorders may become evident after extraction of a tooth, because bleeding does not stop. Less commonly, gingival bleeding may attract attention to the blood disorder.

Halitosis

Bad breath is usually a trivial complaint, though it seems to be heightened by the attention drawn to it by advertising. There are four possible sources of halitosis: the mouth, nasopharynx, lungs, and the gastrointestinal tract. Altered blood round the gum may be the most important oral cause, and this may be associated with debris or pus from gingivitis and periodontal pockets. A characteristic halitosis is found in acute ulcerative gingivitis. It should be noted that bad taste and bad breath are subjective sensations which are often confused. Excessive bacterial plaque on the teeth is not a principal cause of halitosis; nevertheless, meticulous oral care should be advised.

Chronic tonsillitis may be responsible for halitosis but atrophic rhinitis causing ozena is probably the most important cause to be excluded. Occasionally, respiratory-tract infections may cause halitosis and a variety of gastrointestinal disorders have been associated with bad breath but there is little evidence to substantiate this. Frequently all these sources of halitosis may be excluded without finding a cause and these patients may have a fixation about bad breath related to emotional or sexual problems.

Fig. 14 Round or oval, depapillated lesions with a raised margin in a patient with erythema migrans of the tongue.

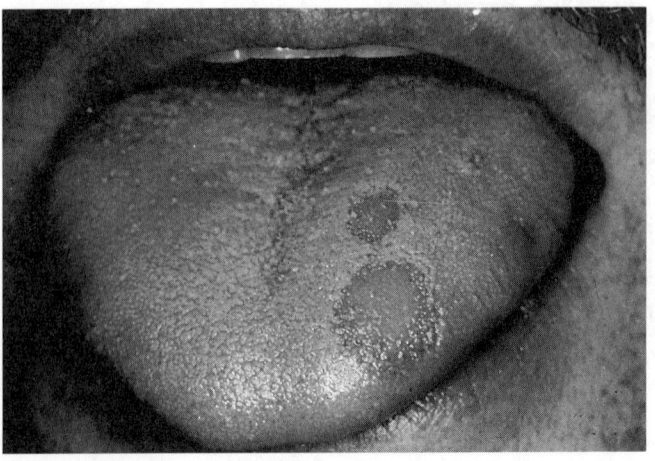

Temporomandibular-joint disorders

Temporomandibular arthrosis is the most common disorder of this joint and the patient complains of pain, clicking, or limitation of movement. It is found in young women more often than men. Examination may reveal limitations in jaw movement, tenderness of the joint, and crepitus on movement, discovered by palpating the head of the condyle through the overlying skin. The cause is difficult to establish but malocclusion might be one of several factors. The condition may clear spontaneously, but in some patients the occlusion should be checked and a bite-raising appliance is often helpful. Rheumatoid arthritis and osteoarthritis of this joint are occasionally seen clinically. Dislocation of the joint, which becomes fixed in the open position, may be caused by a blow on the jaw or during dental extractions under general anaesthesia. Ankylosis of the joint is nowadays extremely rare and used to be secondary to osteomyelitis.

REFERENCES

Atkinson, J.C., Travis, W.D., Pillemer, S.R., Bermudez, D., Wolff, A., and Fox, P.C. (1990). Major salivary gland function in primary Sjögren's syndrome and its relationship to clinical features. *Journal of Rheumatology*, **17**, 318–22.

Bouquot, J.E., Weiland, L.H., and Kurland, L.T. (1988). Leukoplakia and carcinoma *in situ* synchronously associated with invasive oral/oropharyngeal carcinoma in Rochester Minn., 1935–1984. *Oral Surgery, Oral Medicine, Oral Pathology*, **65**, 199–207.

Carlos, J.P., Wolfe, M.D., Zambon, J.J., and Kingman, A. (1988). Periodontal disease in adolescents: some clinical and microbiological correlates of attachment loss. *Journal of Dental Research*, **67**, 1510–14.

Carlsson, J. (1989). Microbial aspects of frequent intake of products with high sugar concentrations. *Scandinavian Journal of Dental Research*, **97**, 110–14.

Chau, M.N. and Radden, B.G. (1989). A clinical-pathological study of 53 intra-oral pleomorphic adenomas. *International Journal of Oral and Maxillofacial Surgery*, **18**, 158–62.

Dummer, P.M.H. *et al.* (1990). Factors influencing the caries experience of a group of children at the ages of 11–12 and 15–16 years: results from an ongoing study. *Journal of Dentistry*, **18**, 37–48.

Dzink, J.L., Socransky, S.S., and Haffajee, A.D. (1988). The predominant cultivable flora of active and inactive lesions of destructive periodontal diseases. *Journal of Clinical Periodontology*, **15**, 316–23.

Fox, P.C., Busch, K.A., and Baum, B.J. (1987). Subjective reports of xerostomia and objective measures of salivary gland performance. *Journal of the American Dental Association*, **115**, 581–4.

Genco, R.J., Christersson, L.A., and Zambon, J.J. (1986). Juvenile periodontitis. *International Dental Journal*, **36**, 168–76.

Gibbons, R.J. (1989). Bacterial adhesion to oral tissues: a model for infectious diseases. *Journal of Dental Research*, **68**, 750–60.

Greenspan, J.S., Greenspan, D., and Winkler, J.R. (1988). Diagnosis and management of the oral manifestations of HIV infection and AIDS. *Infectious Disease Clinics of North America*, **2**, 373–85.

Herrod, H.G. (1990). Chronic mucocutaneous candidiasis in childhood and complications of non-Candida infection. *Journal of Pediatrics*, **116**, 377–82.

Hogewind, W.F., van der Waall, I., van der Kwast, and Snow, G.B. (1989). The association of white lesions with oral squamous cell carcinoma: A retrospective study of 212 patients. *International Journal of Oral and Maxillofacial Surgery*, **18**, 163–4.

Holmstrup, P., Thorn, J.J., Rindum, J., and Pindborg, J.J. (1988). Malignant development of lichen planus-affected oral mucosa. *Journal of Oral Pathology*, **17**, 219–25.

Kashima, H.K., Kutcher, M., Kessis, T., Levin, L.S., de Villiers, E.M., and Shah, K. (1990). Human papilloma virus in squamous cell carcinoma, leukoplakia, lichen planus, and clinically normal epithelium of the oral cavity. *Annals of Ontology, Rhinology and Laryngology*, **99**, 55–61.

Lehner, T. (1992). *Immunology of oral diseases*. Blackwell, Oxford.

Lindhe, J., Okamoto, H., Yoneyama, T., Haffajee, A., and Socransky, S.S. (1989). Longitudinal changes in periodontal disease in untreated subjects. *Journal of Clinical Periodontal Research*, **16**, 662–70.

Lloyd, R.E. and Ho, K.H. (1988). Combined CT scanning and sialography in the management of parotid tumors. *Oral Surgery, Oral Medicine, Oral Pathology*, **65**, 142–4.

Lozada-Nur, F., Gorsky, M., and Silverman, S. (1989). Oral erythema multiforme: clinical observations and treatment of 95 patients. *Oral Surgery, Oral Medicine, Oral Surgery*, **67**, 36–40.

Moller, H. (1989). Changing incidence of cancer of the tongue, oral cavity and pharynx in Denmark. *Journal of Oral Pathology and Medicine*, **18**, 224–9.

Newbrun, E. (1989). Frequent sugar intake—then and now: interpretation of main results. *Scandinavian Journal of Dental Research*, **97**, 103–9.

Seaman, S., Thomas, F.D., and Walker, W.A. (1989). Differences between caries levels in 5 year old children from fluoridated Anglesey and non-fluoridated mainland Gwynedd in 1987. *Community Dental Health*, **6**, 215–21.

Slots, J. (1986). Bacterial specificity in adult periodontitis. *Journal of Clinical Periodontology*, **13**, 912–17.

Williams, D.M. (1989). Vesiculobullous mucocutaneous disease: pemphigus vulgaris. *Journal of Oral Pathology and Medicine*, **18**, 544–53.

Williams, R.C. (1990). Periodontal disease. *New England Journal of Medicine*, **322**, 373–82.

14.6 Diseases of the oesophagus

J. DENT

Oesophageal function testing (see also Chapter 14.2.1)

Recent advances in measurement techniques have enhanced the evaluation of oesophageal function. When oesophageal function testing is the only means for the accurate diagnosis of a treatable disorder, the benefits are clear. It is also valuable for recognition of disorders for which there is no definitive therapy, as an explanation of the cause of their symptoms is important to many patients. An oesophageal function-testing service has the added benefit of assessment of patients by an individual with more than the usual level of experience with motor and sensory oesophageal disorders. Oesophageal function testing is relatively expensive and so should not be requested for assessment of trivial symptoms, or when the information gained does not aid management.

24-h ambulatory oesophageal pH monitoring

The principal role of this procedure is to determine the association between symptoms and episodes of acid gastro-oesophageal reflux in the minority of patients in whom the mechanism of production of troublesome symptoms is unclear (Fig. 1).

Oesophageal manometry

Oesophageal manometry gives the most direct indication of patterns of functioning of oesophageal muscle. It is most helpful in the diagnosis of mechanisms of dysphagia, after exclusion of fixed, structural defects. Manometry plays only a secondary part in the management of reflux disease, usually being helpful if there is no oesophagitis and mild dysphagia is present, or when surgery is being planned. There is increasing emphasis on performance of ambulatory 24-h manometry with sophisticated, miniaturized equipment. Correlation of motor events with spontaneous symptoms has proved of little value in the diagnosis of non-cardiac chest pain.

Contrast radiology

This tends only to be used effectively as a means of screening for structural abnormalities. With specialized approaches, and analysis of repeated testings of standardized stimuli with recording of images on video tape, barium studies can give very helpful information on pharyngeal and oesophageal motor function. The technique can only be exploited successfully by the partnership of a radiologist and clinician who have a special interest in oesophageal motor disorders.

Radioisotopic transit testing

Swallowing of radiolabelled boluses can give quantitative information on patterns of movement of material down the oesophagus. This overcomes the limitation of barium contrast studies to semiquantitative information on transit. However, if good barium-contrast radiology is available, radioisotopic testing of oesophageal transit is redundant.

General management of oesophageal dysphagia

Symptomatic treatment of dysphagia is frequently necessary, because of the limited efficacy of treatment of oesophageal disorders. Though measures appear obvious, this aspect of management is commonly neglected by both patient and physician.

OPTIMIZATION OF BOLUS CONSISTENCY

Large particles of solid food may impact in strictures and require considerable propulsive forces even in the absence of stricture. Large boluses may trigger oesophageal spasm. Boluses should therefore be small and reduced to semiliquid or liquid. This can be achieved by optimization of dentition, use of fluids in bolus preparation, and avoidance of hard, fibrous foods. In some patients, defects may be so severe that the diet should be made into a purée. A dietitian will assist patients in identifying and preparing suitable foods, and in maintaining their nutrition.

ASSISTANCE WITH OESOPHAGEAL TRANSIT

Liquids assist with transit by reducing the viscosity of food and providing a pressure head in the oesophagus. Gas generated within the oesophageal body from effervescent drinks can act as a piston that displaces oesophageal contents into the stomach in the erect position, provided it is not belched prematurely into the pharynx. Forces generated by this

Fig. 1 Section of a 24-h oesophageal pH monitoring study showing the association of heartburn with episodes of acid reflux after a meal.

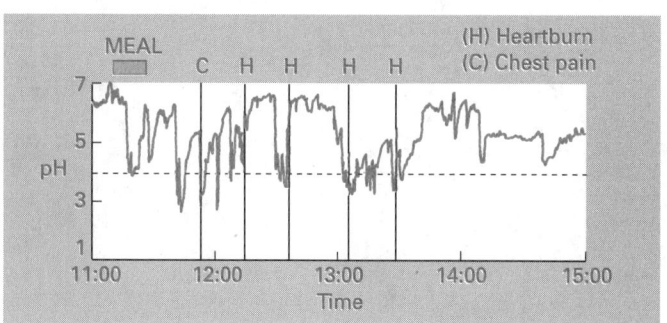

can be sufficient to overcome an achalasic sphincter. In agile patients, jumping up from crouching can accelerate the oesophagus around retained oesophageal contents. The value of gravity in assisting oesophageal transit should never be forgotten.

ALTERNATIVE/SUPPLEMENTARY FEEDING PATHS

Rarely, the above measures fail to maintain nutrition. Percutaneous endoscopic gastrostomy should then be used.

Oesophageal motor and sensory disorders (see also Chapters 14.2.1 and 14.12)

Gastro-oesophageal reflux disease

This is by far the most common oesophageal disorder, reflux-induced heartburn occurring at least once in 6 months in around one-third of people. Management should be tailored to the wide range of severity.

DEFINITION

Gastro-oesophageal reflux occurs to some degree in everybody and should only be considered a disease when it gives rise to significant symptoms or complications. The terms reflux or peptic oesophagitis should be reserved for when oesophageal mucosal injury due to reflux is clearly visible endoscopically.

AETIOLOGY

An abnormally high level of episodic exposure of the distal oesophagus to gastric contents is the most important functional defect. In most patients this is due to abnormal neural control of the sphincter and oesophageal body. Contrary to entrenched theory, in the majority of patients most reflux occurs during the day, predominantly after food. In patients with severe oesophagitis, however, nocturnal reflux and its resultant acid exposure are very important.

Slow recovery or clearance of oesophageal pH after reflux-induced acidification contributes significantly to prolonged acid exposure in about 50 per cent of patients. Hiatus hernia is probably an important amplifier of defects of sphincter function and oesophageal clearance, though the mechanisms of these effects are poorly understood.

In a small and ill-defined minority of patients, apparently normal levels of reflux induce typical symptoms, presumably because of oesophageal sensitization by a primary oesophageal mucosal sensory defect.

CONSEQUENCES OF ABNORMAL REFLUX

Oesophagitis

The chemical insult from excessive mucosal exposure to acid and pepsin leads to distal oesophageal ulceration in between one-third to one-half of patients with symptomatically troublesome reflux disease. The extent of ulceration varies greatly from tiny patches of erosion to circumferential, extensive ulceration in a small minority.

The risks of oesophagitis are not well defined, but peptic stricture and/or oesophageal columnar metaplasia (Barrett's oesophagus) are typically only associated with severe oesophagitis. Stricturing may cause debilitating dysphagia and malnutrition; its treatment by repeated bougienage is a burden and associated with significant risk of oesophageal perforation. Oesophageal adenocarcinoma is the main significance of columnar metaplasia and is dealt with in a later section. Oesophageal columnar metaplasia also carries with it the risk of deep, benign oesophageal ulceration in the metaplastic segment. Occasionally such ulcers erode into mediastinal structures or the pleural space often with a fatal outcome. Bleeding from oesophagitis is relatively common, but rarely life threatening, except when it occurs from a deep ulcer associated with columnar metaplasia.

SYMPTOMS

These are an important source of disability. Heartburn is most important, but presentation may be with less-specific patterns of dyspepsia or with regurgitation, haematemesis, and dysphagia due either to stricture or oesophageal-body motor dysfunction. Reflux-induced respiratory

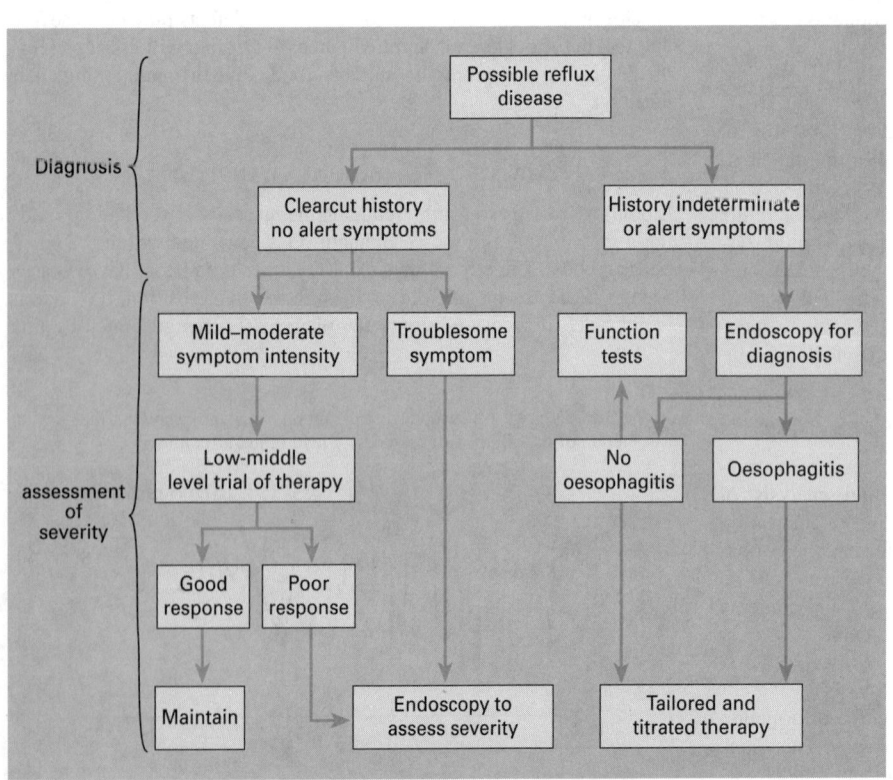

Fig. 2 Principal decision paths for management of reflux disease.

symptoms of hoarseness, persistent cough, and bronchospasm may predominate.

DIAGNOSIS AND ASSESSMENT OF SEVERITY

The history is pivotal for diagnosis because of the extremely high prevalence of reflux-induced symptoms and the lack of a definitive, inexpensive, diagnostic test for reflux disease. Fortunately, the specificity of symptom patterns of reflux disease is arguably the highest of any of the more common gastrointestinal diseases. The strategic use of the history, and initially empirical therapy, as a means to assess diagnosis and severity is summarized in Fig. 2, and discussed in detail in the section on treatment below.

Endoscopy

When investigation is needed, endoscopy is the first choice as it is the only test that can give sensitive recognition and grading of oesophagitis, and reliable diagnosis of oesophageal columnar metaplasia. Mechanically significant peptic stricture, gastric cancer, and chronic duodenal and gastric ulcer are also diagnosed with high sensitivity. The value of endoscopy as the primary initial investigation is greatly enhanced by the accurate histological diagnosis of lesions by endoscopic biopsy and cytology brushings.

Barium swallow and meal

Barium swallow and meal is an inappropriate primary diagnostic test as it is insensitive for diagnosis of oesophagitis and cannot grade it, making management less incisive. Other pathology such as gastric ulcer and oesophageal stricture is demonstrated with reasonable sensitivity, but adequate evaluation of these findings often requires endoscopic biopsy. By contrast, barium swallow has an important secondary role in the investigation of mechanisms of troublesome dysphagia, in recognizing extrinsic oesophageal compression, which may be producing symptoms that could be interpreted as due to reflux, and in assessment of anatomically complex hiatus hernia.

Oesophageal function tests

The place of these is summarized in Fig. 2 and has been outlined above.

MANAGEMENT PRINCIPLES

New treatments have transformed management in recent years, but they are often used ineffectively because the underlying principles have not been adequately distilled or communicated. The chief aims are to provide adequate relief and control of oesophagitis. Reduction of oesophagitis to minor patchy erosions is probably sufficient to prevent the complications of oesophagitis. Usually though, adequate symptom relief is achieved only when oesophagitis is completely healed. Management steps are easily confused, as endoscopy, symptom assessment, and treatment are used not only for diagnosis but also assessment of severity and grading of therapy.

Cost-efficient, secure diagnosis

Steps needed for diagnosis are shown in Fig. 2. When the history is typical endoscopy is redundant. Given the very high proportion of patients who have no endoscopic abnormality, a negative endoscopy should not detract from a diagnosis based on critical symptom evaluation. When symptoms are indeterminate, or dysphagia, haematemesis, or weight loss are a feature, endoscopy is the primary diagnostic approach.

Assessment of severity

Morbidity arising from symptoms, and the presence and severity of oesophagitis are the two most important measures; they show poor correlation. The response of symptoms to low and medium levels of therapy (see Table 1 and below) gives an indirect approximation of the severity

Table 1 *Levels of antireflux therapy*

Low: antacids, non-drug measures
Middle: normal-dose H$_2$-receptor antagonists, cisapride and sucralfate, ?bethanechol
Upper: 2–4 × normal ranitidine dose, × 2 normal famotidine dose, omeprazole 10 mg, lanzoprazole 15 mg
Combination of cisapride and standard-dose H$_2$-receptor antagonists
Highest: antireflux surgery, omeprazole 20 mg, lanzoprazole 30 mg

of oesophagitis and helps to determine further action according to the algorithm (Fig. 1). When classical symptoms are of long standing and troublesome, early endoscopy is indicated, as it will identify the most appropriate long-term treatment plan (see below).

Tailoring and grading therapy

The traditional classification of therapies by mechanism of action is impractical because it is uninformative about efficacy. Classification of therapies by level of efficacy, regardless of mechanism of action (Table 1), provides a framework for long-term management. The lowest effective dose of any agent should be used in long-term therapy. Figure 2 and Table 2 summarize the logic for using endoscopic findings to choose an appropriate type of initial therapy. As the responsiveness of patients varies, therapy needs to be graded upwards or downwards through levels of efficacy in order to find the lowest that is effective.

Most patients with reflux disease will have an initial trial of empirical therapy. There are two main options for this. Initial high-level medical therapy has become available only recently. This is most likely to confirm the diagnosis, but is relatively expensive and uninformative about the best long-term approach. Initial low–medium-level therapy is the traditional model outlined in Fig. 2. This has the disadvantage of giving less useful diagnostic information, and often, slow relief of symptoms, but it is relatively inexpensive and will usually identify patients with severe oesophagitis by their lack of response.

OPTIONS FOR TREATMENT OF OESOPHAGITIS AND SYMPTOMS ARISING DIRECTLY FROM REFLUX

Non-drug measures and antacids

The efficacy of these traditional approaches is often overrated. Most useful are avoidance of large meals and provocant foods, drinks, and physical activities. The benefits to reflux disease of stopping smoking, losing weight, and raising the bedhead are more debatable. Antacid will usually not prevent symptoms, but may be effective in controlling heartburn. These highly cost-effective measures are worth a trial within the context of their efficacy (Tables 1 and 2), and should be used as maintenance therapy if they prove effective, provided their impact on lifestyle is acceptable to the patient.

Acid suppression

Inhibition of gastric acid secretion makes gastric juice less injurious, but does not stop reflux. This has deservedly become the most widely used treatment because it is highly efficacious and adjustable. The more severe the oesophagitis, the greater the acid suppression required (Table 2). Proton-pump inhibitors have a special place, because of their effectiveness in reduction of food-stimulated acid secretion and their greater overall efficacy in control of acid secretion compared to the H$_2$-receptor antagonists.

Long-term acid suppression maintains patients free of symptoms and oesophagitis indefinitely, but withdrawal is usually associated with prompt relapse. The maintenance dose appears to be the same as the lowest effective healing dose. There have been concerns about the safety

Table 2 *Efficacy of levels of antireflux therapy*

Level of therapy	Oesophagitis grade			
	None	Mild	Moderate	Severe
Low	XX	X	0	0
Middle	XXX	XXX	X	0
Upper	XXXX	XXXX	XXX	XX
Highest	XXXX	XXXX	XXXX	XXX

Estimated proportions of patients with adequate symptom control and healing of oesophagitis where applicable.

0, 0–20%; X, 20–40%; XX, 40–60%; XXX, 60–80%; XXXX, 80–100%.

Mild, moderate, severe oesophagitis—Savary–Miller grades I, II, and II, respectively.

of long-term acid suppression ever since the introduction of H_2-receptor antagonists. To date, follow-up of patients treated continuously for 5 or more years has shown no evidence of any important effects, but more extensive follow-up is still needed and long-term treatment of reflux disease with these agents should use the lowest effective dose.

Motility stimulants

Only cisapride has been adequately researched. It has a medium level of efficacy for both short- and long-term management. It is unlikely that much is gained from an increase of dosage. The principal effect of cisapride appears to be on oesophageal acid clearance.

Other agents

Sucralfate (a complex of aluminium hydroxide and sulphated sucrose), which is of medium-level efficacy, is believed to act by protecting the oesophageal mucosa from chemical injury. Bethanechol, a parasympathomimetic, stimulates salivation and oesophageal contraction; at best it has only medium efficacy. Various formulations that include some mucosa-coating or protective agent combined with antacid are probably no better than antacid alone.

Combination medical therapy

Use of cisapride, a motility-stimulating agent, and H_2-receptor antagonists in combination gives moderately improved results, but is a relatively unattractive option given the high efficacy of monotherapy with proton-pump inhibitors.

Antireflux surgery

In skilled hands, antireflux surgery is a very effective long-term therapy. Negative factors include variation in outcome between surgeons, and the small (c. 0.5 per cent) mortality associated with the operation. Laparoscopic antireflux surgery is an important advance, as it achieves good control of reflux with marked reduction of the morbidity of the more traditional approach. More information is needed about long-term results.

Choice among therapies

Selection of medical or surgical therapy should take account of the severity of disease, the risks of antireflux surgery in individual patients, the patient's age, both from the point of view of operative risk, and the time over which they will need treatment for reflux disease, the cost of effective medical therapy, and especially importantly, the preferences of the patient. In the United States, good, conventional surgery becomes cost-effective compared to medical therapy after about 10 years, though this assessment does not take into account the cost of mortality. The choice among medical therapies should be largely governed by the local cost of the alternatives that give the necessary level of treatment, as all of the principal options are safe and well tolerated.

MANAGEMENT OF COMPLICATIONS OF REFLUX DISEASE

Peptic stricture

Dysphagia secondary to stricturing (Fig. 3) needs to be distinguished from the more common dysphagia seen in reflux disease, which is due to defective triggering and control of oesophageal-body peristalsis (see Non-specific oesophageal motor disorders below). Peptic stricturing is managed by a combination of peroral dilatation and healing of oesophagitis by either medical or surgical means. Provided oesophagitis is healed, stricture is usually not a persistent problem.

Oesophageal columnar metaplasia (Barrett's oesophagus)

This increasingly recognized consequence of oesophagitis is dealt with in the Section on oesophageal neoplasia below. The association of columnar metaplasia with oesophageal adenocarcinoma contributes to the logic of vigorous treatment of severe oesophagitis.

Respiratory complications

Respiratory disease may occur as a result of either direct aspiration of refluxed gastric contents, or from the reflex effects of gastro-oesophageal reflux. Proof of an association between coexistent reflux and respiratory disease is extremely difficult so that management of respiratory disease by antireflux surgery is a gamble supported primarily by clinical evaluation.

Regurgitation

Voluminous regurgitation is the main problem in a small subgroup of patients with reflux disease. They usually present complaining of vomiting, but a detailed history reveals that there is no prior nausea, and no effort involved in the appearance of the gastric content in the mouth. The determinants of high-volume reflux and regurgitation have not been defined. Vigorous medical therapy sometimes controls the problem, but more often antireflux surgery is the only effective management.

Non-cardiac chest pain

Reflux is an important cause, which is dealt with below.

Fig. 3 Peptic stricture: circumferential narrowing; asymmetrical; associated intramural diverticulosis suggests benign aetiology; site suggests Barrett's mucosa below proven (by courtesy of Dr. H. Harley).

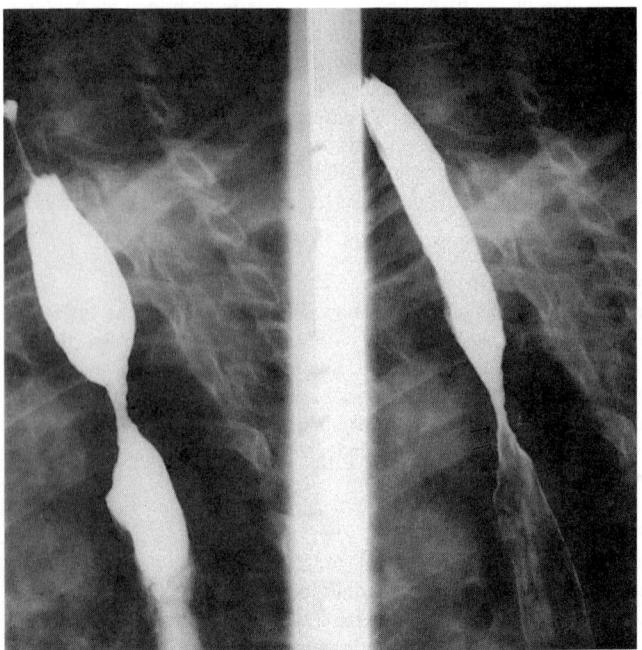

Idiopathic achalasia and achalasia-like states

DEFINITION

These disorders are characterized by absent or incomplete relaxation of the lower oesophageal sphincter and impairment of oesophageal-body peristalsis. Idiopathic achalasia, which was first described over 300 years ago, accounts for most cases and has an annual incidence of approximately 1 to 2 /200 000; it affects all ages, but is diagnosed most often in early to mid-adult life. The syndrome is also seen in Chagas' disease, sometimes as an accompaniment to the intestinal pseudo-obstructive syndrome, as a manifestation of paraneoplastic neural dysfunction, and secondary to oesophageal amyloidosis.

AETIOLOGY

Impairment of inhibitory neural control of the distal oesophagus is the universal abnormality. The syndrome can probably be produced by neural damage at several sites; evidence of myenteric inhibitory-neurone degeneration is probably most important.

Symptoms

Dysphagia with solids is the most common symptom. Regurgitation is also prominent. The regurgitated material tastes bland because it never enters the stomach (Fig. 4). Cramping chest pain occurs in some patients during the early, hypercontracting phase of the disorder. Weight loss is seen in patients with disabling dysphagia. The course of symptoms over time is variable. In some, symptoms remain static for many years, but in others there is a progression with increasing problems with regurgitation over several years, as a result of development and increase of oesophageal dilatation (Fig. 4). When this occurs, respiratory problems secondary to aspiration can become a major feature.

It takes 2 years on average for idiopathic achalasia to be diagnosed after its first presentation; delay is especially likely if oesophageal dilatation is absent. Dilatation varies in degree from a minor increase in the calibre of the oesophageal lumen to a grossly enlarged, colon-like oesophagus. Barium swallow shows oesophageal retention with a gastro-oesophageal junction that tapers smoothly to a closed sphincter, with occasional spurts of flow into the stomach (Fig. 4). In the absence of dilatation, a barium swallow is usually reported as normal. Oesophageal manometry is the only sensitive method for demonstration of the characteristic motor dysfunction, and is especially important in patients with no radiological abnormality. Idiopathic achalasia and achalasia-like states should be distinguished from constriction of the gastro-oesophageal junction by an infiltrating or encasing malignancy at the cardia. This diagnosis is often difficult to make. As a minimum, upper gastro-intestinal endoscopy should be done and mucosal biopsies should be taken. Computerized tomographic scanning is also of value.

TREATMENT

The results of reduction of lower oesophageal-sphincter pressure with drugs such as calcium antagonists and β-adrenergic agonists compare poorly with mechanical disruption of the sphincter. Oesophagomyotomy, which is now being done increasingly as a laparoscopic or thoracoscopic procedure, is highly effective but associated with a 5 to 10 per cent risk of troublesome gastro-oesophageal reflux. Balloon dilatation is an attractive approach because of its simplicity and low cost, but often needs to be repeated, and in some hands fails in up to 40 per cent of patients, especially those who are young. It also carries a risk of perforation of about 5 per cent. With the development of minimally invasive surgery for oesophagomyotomy, balloon dilatation will probably be used most in older patients who have other medical problems that increase the risks of surgery.

When oesophageal dilatation is present, prompt treatment is indicated to prevent its worsening, because of the morbidity and poor therapeutic outcome associated with a gross oesophageal dilatation. Oesophageal emptying can be assisted by effervescent drinks (see General management of oesophageal dysphagia above).

PROGNOSIS

If effective treatment is applied before the development of major dilatation, results are excellent, despite persistence of significant physiological abnormalities. Achalasia carries a very significantly increased risk for oesophageal carcinoma up to many years later; this risk ranges from 2 to 7 per cent in authoritative reports. There is no apparent reduction of this risk after treatment. The average interval from diagnosis of achalasia to development of carcinoma has been estimated as 28 years. It is not usual practice to undertake surveillance for this risk, but some clinicians recommend periodic screening endoscopy.

Diffuse oesophageal spasm

DEFINITION

Episodic chest pain and/or dysphagia result from spastic contractions of the distal half of the oesophageal body in the absence of any precipitating structural stenosis. There are no generally agreed criteria for diagnosis.

Fig. 4 Achalasia. (a) lateral chest film shows air–fluid level in mid-oesophagus just behind air column of trachea. (b) On postanterior view it was almost invisible. Barium-filled dilated oesophagus; intact mucosa in distal achalasic segment.

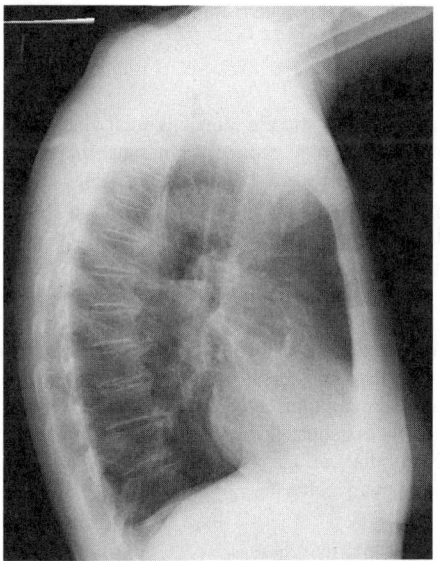

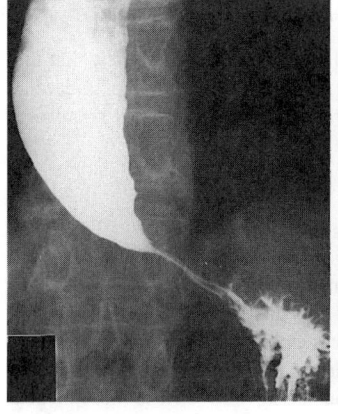
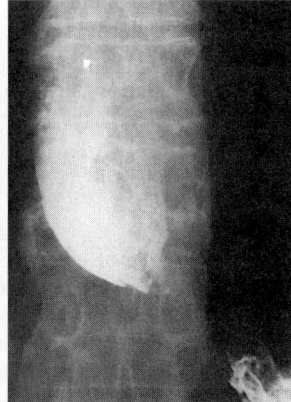

AETIOLOGY

It is widely assumed that this is a disorder of neural control, but there is no evidence that this is the case. What is known of the epidemiology is unhelpful with regard to aetiology. Stress is an unlikely primary precipitant but may exacerbate the problem. Good prevalence data are lacking. Diffuse spasm affects all ages and is much less common than achalasia.

SYMPTOMS

Virtually all patients have episodic, crushing, central retrosternal pain, which can be excruciating; cardiac ischaemia is often the first diagnosis. Intermittent dysphagia occurs in about two-thirds of patients and leads to temporary abandonment of eating until symptoms abate—usually over about 30 min, but episodes of oesophageal obstruction can last for several hours. In the majority of patients, symptom episodes occur less than once a month, but in severe cases these may occur several times a week, or each time food intake is attempted. As with any intermittent fault, full-blown dysfunction is usually absent during investigation, but in a minority of patients, there is asymptomatic motor dysfunction. Barium swallow then shows trapping of beads of contrast in the distal oesophagus—'the corkscrew oesophagus'—or sustained obliteration of the distal oesophageal lumen. Oesophageal manometry may show intermittent, simultaneous, prolonged, and vigorous oesophageal contractions interspersed with normal swallow-induced peristalsis. Relaxation of the lower oesophageal sphincter is normal.

Most frequently, the diagnosis is made from the history and the exclusion of other problems that may mimic diffuse oesophageal spasm. Most important amongst these is Schatski ring (see below). Achalasia is readily excluded by manometry, and when appropriate, myocardial ischaemia should be excluded.

Treatment

There is no specific therapy. Smooth-muscle relaxants such as nitrites, nitrates, and calcium antagonists may reduce symptoms. In many patients, reassurance is the most important management because the intensity and nature of symptoms gives rise to great concern. In the rare case of frequent, disabling spasm, long oesophagomyotomy can give good relief.

Prognosis

Of major significance are impairment of quality of life and concern about life-threatening cardiac disease. There is no consistent progression of dysfunctions and associated symptoms over time. There are several reports of progression of diffuse oesophageal spasm to achalasia, but in most of these, it seems likely that early, spastic achalasia was initially misdiagnosed as diffuse oesophageal spasm.

Non-cardiac chest pain

DEFINITION

Implicit in this rather circuitous and negative label is the view that this pain has a cardiac-like quality, but there is no evidence of a cardiac origin. The oesophagus is the next most likely origin, but it is unlikely that this is always the case.

AETIOLOGY

Long-term monitoring of oesophageal pH and motility has produced mixed results. Evidence for triggering of pain by reflux or oesophageal motor dysfunction has been found in between a fifth and a half of patients evaluated. Oesophageal mucosal pain due to gastro-oesophageal reflux is the most common and rewarding positive diagnosis. Frank oesophageal spasm associated with achalasia, and diffuse oesophageal spasm are unusual but convincing causes of non-cardiac chest pain. In the majority of patients, most episodes of pain occur independently of reflux and any motor abnormality, although many of these patients have non-specific oesophageal motor disorders or hypertensive peristalsis (Fig. 5) (see below). Opinion is shifting to the view that in many patients, non-cardiac chest pain is due to a primary oesophageal pain disorder and that any motor disorder is an epiphenomenon.

SYMPTOMS

By definition, the pain resembles cardiac pain in its sensation and distribution. It can be very intense and distressing, disturb sleep, and be worse during emotional stress. Postprandial occurrence in association with heartburn suggests triggering by reflux. When dysphagia is associated, vigorous achalasia or oesophageal spasm are very possible. Investigation is demanding and relatively low yield. Firstly, myocardial ischaemia should be assumed to be the cause until proven otherwise. Endoscopy should then follow. In patients who are having recurrent problems, oesophageal pH monitoring and oesophageal motility studies are both indicated.

TREATMENT

If the pain is triggered by gastro-oesophageal reflux, high-level therapy should be tried (see Gastro-oesophageal reflux disease). Achalasia and diffuse oesophageal spasm should be treated on their own merits. Half or more of patients will still have no clear-cut diagnosis. In these, treatment with anxiolytics and antidepressants has been found to be moderately effective. Agents that reduce oesophageal contraction strength, such as calcium antagonists, appear ineffective in hypertensive peristalsis.

PROGNOSIS

When the pain is clearly due to reflux disease, diffuse oesophageal spasm, and achalasia, the prognosis is as for these conditions. When it is not, the patient's continuing anxiety about the origin of the symptoms and the fear that this might be cardiac tends to persist, with repeated admissions to hospital because of attacks of pain.

Fig. 5 Oesophageal manometric tracing made from points along the oesophagus in a patient with hypertensive peristalsis. The time of onset of the pressure wave shows a normal peristaltic gradient, but the contraction of the distal half of the oesophagus is very vigorous so that the peak pressures are abnormally high. The high-amplitude pressure waves are also somewhat prolonged and multipeaked.

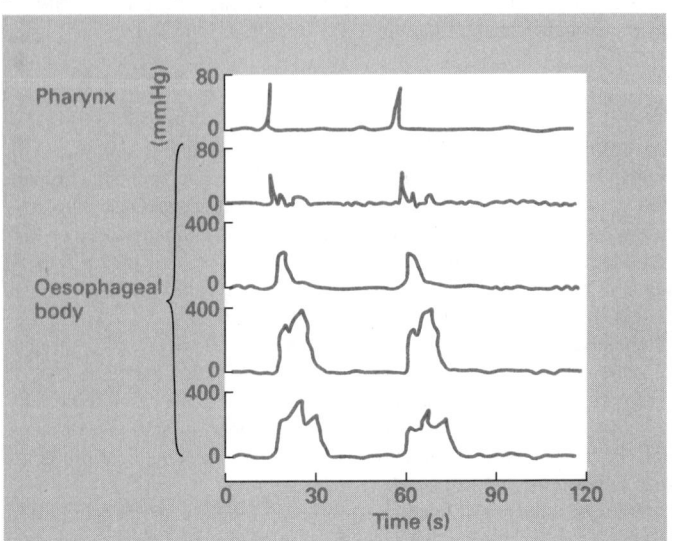

Hypertensive peristalsis or nutcracker oesophagus

DEFINITION

This is defined purely by the manometric criterion of oesophageal-body primary peristaltic pressure waves that have peaks in excess of 250 mmHg. There is preservation of the normal peristaltic pattern of aborad progression of the time of onset of the oesophageal-body contraction wave.

AETIOLOGY

This is not understood. There are indications that psychological factors can influence peristaltic amplitude. As a minority of patients with hypertensive peristalsis also experiences episodes of diffuse oesophageal spasm, the underlying dysfunction is probably closely related to diffuse oesophageal spasm and is likely to involve neural control mechanisms.

SYMPTOMS

The only clinical significance of hypertensive peristalsis is its relation to non-cardiac chest pain, a vexed question that is dealt with in the section on this problem above. Hypertensive peristalsis alone does not produce dysphagia or derangement of oesophageal transit, because, by definition, peristalsis is preserved.

TREATMENT AND PROGNOSIS

These are discussed in the section on non-cardiac chest pain.

Non-specific oesophageal motor disorders

DEFINITION

This is a ragbag of manometrically defined oesophageal motor abnormalities that occur in isolation from other more clearly defined syndromes of oesophageal dysfunction, or in association with diseases such as gastro-oesophageal reflux, diffuse oesophageal spasm, and diabetic and other autonomic neuropathies. The pragmatic definition of these dysfunctions is that they are departures from normal patterns of oesophageal motor function which do not define specific diseases, but which are of clinical significance. Non-specific oesophageal motor disorder is the most common, single functional diagnosis made in most oesophageal manometric laboratories.

AETIOLOGY

This is unknown, and it should not be assumed that only one mechanism is involved. Intermittent occurrence of dysfunctions suggests they are due to defective neural control.

SYMPTOMS

Multipeaked, swallow-induced contraction waves of the distal oesophageal body stand out from the other patterns not only functionally, but also symptomatically. This pattern is loosely associated with the hypercontraction disorders, diffuse oesophageal spasm, and hypertensive peristalsis, but sometimes does not appear to have any clinical significance.

Hypocontraction dysfunctions cause deranged oesophageal transit because of defective triggering and progression of peristalsis. This probably explains their association with mild, intermittent dysphagia, which occurs, characteristically, with solids. The non-obstructive dysphagia and slow oesophageal acid clearance seen in gastro-oesophageal reflux disease are due to such dysfunction. Secondary oesophageal-body peristalsis is not yet widely evaluated, but defects of this are probably an important cause of intermittent dysphagia as, at least in patients with non-obstructive dysphagia and reflux disease, dysfunction of secondary peristalsis is substantially more common than primary peristaltic dysfunction. Oesophageal manometry with an adequate number of oesophageal-body recording points is the only sensitive means of diagnosis.

TREATMENT

Prokinetic drugs may improve triggering and amplitude of peristaltic contractions, and so transit, but usually the symptoms arising from primary peristaltic dysfunction are not sufficiently severe to warrant continuous therapy. In most cases, patients with symptoms found to be due to non-specific oesophageal motor disorders are more in search of explanation of the origin of their symptoms, and reassurance, than symptom relief. Secondary peristaltic dysfunction may be more troublesome, but there is no good information on the effect of prokinetic or other drugs on this.

PROGNOSIS

These dysfunctions do not remit spontaneously. Patients are often helped by the measures, outlined above for dysphagia, that minimize the demands on oesophageal transport mechanisms and provide propulsive forces that substitute for oesophageal contractions.

Diseases of oesophageal muscle

The division of the oesophageal musculature into striated and smooth components is revealed clearly by these uncommon diseases. In patients with myopathy, weak or absent oesophageal contraction in the affected segment has the expected adverse impact on oesophageal transit, with a pattern of symptoms similar to the hypocontraction states of the non-specific oesophageal motor disorders described earlier. The management follows the same lines.

Oesophageal smooth-muscle diseases

Scleroderma

DEFINITION AND AETIOLOGY

This disease eventually involves the smooth muscle of the oesophagus in at least three-quarters of patients. The time of onset of symptoms from oesophageal involvement is very variable in relation to other manifestations but is sometimes the presenting symptom. Muscle atrophy and fibrosis are the cardinal features, but neuropathic abnormalities may also contribute to dysfunction. Smooth-muscle peristalsis is feeble or totally absent and the tone of the lower oesophageal sphincter subnormal or absent.

SYMPTOMS

Troublesome reflux symptoms are the most common consequence of loss of function. The pattern of dysphagia resembles that seen in non-specific oesophageal motor disorder. If dysphagia is severe, peptic stricture should be excluded; complete loss of oesophageal smooth-muscle peristalsis rarely leads to disabling dysphagia.

TREATMENT

Reflux disease is frequently severe, but can usually be managed effectively by high-level medical therapy as described earlier. Antireflux surgery is usually contraindicated because of the poor propulsive function of the oesophageal body.

Other disorders

A scleroderma-like picture of oesophageal dysfunction is sometimes seen in other connective tissue disorders such as the CREST (calcinosis, Reynaud's, (o)esophageal dysphagia, sclerodactyly, telangiectasia) syndrome, polymyositis, dermatomyositis, and mixed connective-tissue disorders, as well as in the pseudo-obstructive syndrome and with amyloidosis.

Primary striated-muscle disorders

The inflammatory myopathies, dermatomyositis, polymyositis and inclusion-body myositis, the muscular dystrophies, myotonia dystrophica and oculopharyngeal dystrophy, and myasthenia gravis are more frequent causes of this rare problem, which presents with high dysphagia often is association with oropharyngeal dysfunction (see Sections 24 and 25).

Abnormalities of oesophageal anatomy

Non-neoplastic abnormalities that distort oesophageal anatomy may interfere with normal function or merely pose difficulties of interpretation of findings.

Sliding hiatus hernia

DEFINITION

Around 90 per cent of hiatus hernias are of this type in which the gastro-oesophageal junction is displaced upwards into the thorax, giving a simple pouch of intrathoracic stomach.

AETIOLOGY

The phreno-oesophageal ligament is effaced, but it is not clear whether this is a primary defect of gastric anchorage.

SYMPTOMS

As many patients with hiatus hernia are asymptomatic, its demonstration should not be taken as diagnostic of reflux disease. Despite this, physiological studies indicate that herniation of the gastro-oesophageal junction impairs the antireflux barrier by removing normal diaphragmatic crural compression from this region.

TREATMENT

Symptoms of gastro-oesophageal reflux are the only ones of significance. These should be treated along conventional lines (see under Gastro-oesophageal reflux disease above).

PROGNOSIS

This is similar to reflux disease.

Rolling hiatus hernia

DEFINITION

In this disorder, part of the stomach herniates through the hiatus alongside a normally situated gastro-oesophageal junction. This pattern of herniation may produce a gross disturbance of gastric anatomy, usually with a narrow exit from the herniated pouch into the main stomach cavity. Some rolling hernias are also associated with displacement of the gastro-oesophageal junction above the hiatus, in which case they are known as mixed hernias.

SYMPTOMS

Obstruction and distension of the pouch causes upper abdominal discomfort and can progress to strangulation. Gastric volvulus can occur because of the laxity of the gastric anchorage and may obstruct the gastro-oesophageal junction. Both of these complications have a very high mortality and demand urgent surgery. Elective surgery is normally recommended to reduce and anchor rolling hiatus hernias in order to reduce these risks.

Prognosis

Unfortunately, there are no adequate data on the degree of risk associated with rolling hiatus hernia, or on any anatomical factors that are especially hazardous.

Schatski ring (B ring)

DEFINITION

This is a short luminal stenosis at the gastro-oesophageal junction. It may narrow the lumen to a few millimetres or cause a clinically insignificant minor indentation (Fig. 6). It is made up only of mucosa and submucosa.

AETIOLOGY

This is unknown. There is no evidence of oesophagitis to support the claim that it is reflux induced.

SYMPTOMS

With mechanically significant rings, intermittent dysphagia occurs on eating solids. Episodes of bolus obstruction are not unusual, with associated chest pain caused by powerful oesophageal contractions. Failure to recognize a Schatski ring frequently leads to the incorrect diagnosis of primary, diffuse oesophageal spasm. The diagnosis requires an expert radiologist who has been asked to look for this abnormality. Adequate distal oesophageal distension is essential for detection (Fig. 6). A less

Fig. 6 Schatzki ring: thin, 2 to 4 mm in height, annular constriction at gastro-oesophageal junction; best shown on prone-oblique views.

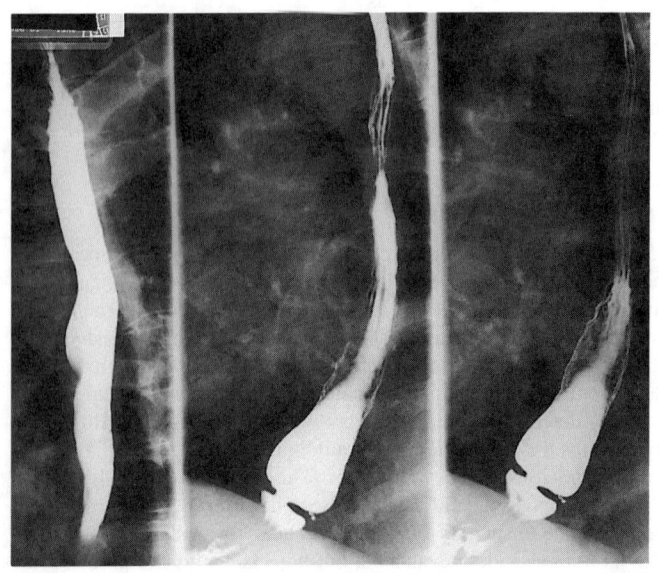

well-tailored barium examination and endoscopy frequently fail to show a symptomatic ring.

TREATMENT

Disruption of the ring by simple peroral dilatation or endoscopic diathermy or laser is very rewarding, as the dysphagia and chest pain are cured, sometimes after many years of symptoms.

Other rings and webs

Other short oesophageal stenoses are due to peptic stricture, muscular rings, and cervical webs, with (Plummer–Vinson syndrome) or without iron-deficiency anaemia.

Oesophageal diverticula and pseudodiverticula

Wide-mouthed, multiple diverticula are characteristic of scleroderma oesophagus. In the non-sclerodermatous oesophagus, diverticula occur in the mid and distal parts, both types probably caused by 'blow-outs' secondary to hypercontraction motor disorders. Though they can become very large, it is rare for them to cause symptoms. They are best left undisturbed because leakage is common after surgical removal.

Multiple intramural out-pouchings of barium are characteristic of intramural pseudodiverticulosis, which appears to be due to dilatation of submucosal gland ducts by an unknown process.

Extrinsic oesophageal compression

This is a relatively common cause of dysphagia, mainly from malignant mediastinal lymphadenopathy. Barium swallow or endoscopy usually show a relatively long, variable-calibre constriction of the oesophageal lumen, associated with a normal mucosal appearance. Dilatation of such compression is usually unrewarding because of its elastic recoil.

Mechanically significant extrinsic compression may also result from an enlarged heart, a dilated or unfolded aorta, or an aortic aneurysm. Kyphosis may accentuate the mechanical impact of these abnormalities. Congenital vascular abnormalities can also compress the oesophagus in adults, an aberrant right subclavian artery being by far the most common.

Mechanical, chemical, and radiation trauma

Mallory–weiss tear

These mucosal tears extend across the gastro-oesophageal junction and are normally induced by vigorous straining associated with vomiting. Bleeding is the only consequence of significance. In 10 per cent of cases, bleeding is severe enough to cause hypovolaemia. The history is usually characteristic, but a definitive diagnosis requires endoscopy. Continued bleeding usually responds to endoscopic injection or electrocoagulation, vascular embolization, or vasopressin infusion. Very rarely, surgery is needed to underrun a persistently bleeding artery in the base of the tear.

Boerhaave's syndrome

In this uncommon condition, straining and vomiting cause oesophageal rupture, most often in the left lower third. High-volume spillage of the gastric contents into the pleural space causes shock and chest and upper abdominal pain with radiation to the back, left chest or shoulder. The chest radiograph becomes abnormal only some hours after rupture. Surgical repair and drainage are usually necessary, and if this is delayed beyond 24 h, mortality is very high. Unfortunately, diagnostic delay is common.

Traumatic perforation

This condition usually results from trauma during dilatation of oesophageal strictures, pneumatic-bag dilatation for achalasia, or compression of oesophageal varices by balloon tamponade. Even with meticulous technique and appropriate equipment, oesophageal perforation can occur. Perforation is suggested by the development of chest or epigastric pain directly after instrumentation, sometimes with dyspnoea. Pneumothorax and surgical emphysema are diagnostic. Any suspicion of perforation should be followed by chest radiography, which, if normal, should be repeated in several hours. Broad-spectrum antimicrobials should be given on suspicion, as they are most effective in minimizing the risks of mediastinitis when used from the outset. Surgical consultation should be sought promptly; the choice between conservative and surgical management should be based on the individual circumstances. Increasingly, instrumental perforation is being managed non-surgically with nasogastric suction, antimicrobials, and intravenous nutrition, with good results primarily because the injury usually happens when the stomach is empty.

Caustic ingestion

DEFINITION AND AETIOLOGY

Strong acids and alkalis are very damaging to the oesophagus and are found in high concentrations in many agents used commonly for cleaning and maintenance. Laryngeal and gastric injuries may overshadow oesophageal injury. Because of their relative lack of taste, alkaline solutions are more likely to be swallowed accidentally in large amounts. Alkaline injury is especially deep; acid tends to form a superficial coagulant, which limits penetration.

SYMPTOMS

The severity and extent of injury are variable and cannot be predicted accurately from estimates of the volume ingested. Around half of patients with a history of caustic ingestion have no significant injury. Oropharyngeal and laryngeal injury confirm caustic ingestion and can be a major threat to the airway, but do not predict the existence and severity of oesophageal injury, which causes odynophagia, dysphagia or haematemesis. Prompt fibreoptic panendoscopy appears safe. This may be normal or show only patchy mucosal oedema, erythema, and small haemorrhagic ulcers, indicative of superficial damage with a good prognosis. Extensive and circumferential ulceration, or grey or brown/black ulceration, suggest transmural injury.

TREATMENT

Patients with severe injury must be observed closely for signs of perforation. Nasogastric suction should be used, with the administration of broad-spectrum antimicrobials, as these appear to reduce the severity of infective complications. The role of corticosteroids is controversial, the balance of evidence tending to oppose their use. Oesophageal stricture is to be expected with severe injury and appears not to be prevented by routine dilatation in the first 2 weeks after injury. A barium study should be done at 2 to 3 weeks to screen for stricturing, and then at about 3-monthly intervals thereafter for a year, so that the development of stricturing is recognized at a stage when dilatation may have some impact.

PROGNOSIS

Caustic strictures are difficult and hazardous to treat by peroral dilatation so that about half of patients require oesophageal resection. In the long term (average onset 40 years after injury), carcinoma of the oesophagus is an important hazard, the risk being 1000 to 3000 times the expected.

Medication-induced oesophagitis

DEFINITION AND AETIOLOGY

This entity was first recognized in 1970. The chemical properties of medications pose hazards to the oesophageal mucosa because of the relative susceptibility of this to injury through pH-dependent and other mechanisms. This susceptibility reflects in part the high local concentration of medications that occur in the oesophageal lumen when a tablet gets 'hung up'. Pills move surprisingly slowly through the normal oesophagus. Defective oesophageal transport, poor pill design, increased mucosal susceptibility to injury, and poor pill-taking technique contribute to the problem. Medications known to have an especially high risk for oesophageal damage are listed in Table 3.

SYMPTOMS

Symptoms are similar to any form of oesophagitis with stricturing and can be very difficult to manage. Probably, much pill-induced injury goes unrecognized. Such injury is by far the most likely cause of oesophagitis and/or benign stricture at the level of the aortic arch, where pills can lodge for prolonged periods. Injury at the distal oesophagus, the other common site of hold-up, is often misdiagnosed as due to reflux disease.

TREATMENT AND PROGNOSIS

Medications and formulations with a high risk of injury should be identified and avoided if possible, especially in elderly patients with reflux disease or abnormal oesophageal transit. Pill transit is facilitated if they are taken in the erect position with plenty of water. Pharmaceutical companies need to pay more attention to the development of pills with shapes, sizes and coatings that assist transit through the oesophagus. Stricturing may require surgery.

Chemotherapy-induced oesophageal disease

Chemotherapy causes oesophageal disease in several ways. Therapy may impair mucosal defences by affecting cell turnover. This in turn may reduce its resistance to damage from other agents, and increase susceptibility to infective oesophagitis from immune suppression. Oesophageal transit and acid clearance may be impaired through neurotoxic effects of some agents. Fistulation or perforation may occur through cytotoxic effects on malignancy in the oesophageal wall. The recent observation that combination chemotherapy is associated with development of oesophageal columnar metaplasia in women being treated for breast cancer demands further investigation.

Oesophageal neoplasms (see also Chapter 14.16)

Squamous-cell carcinoma

DEFINITION

This is defined as a squamous carcinoma arising from the squamous oesophageal mucosa. It is by far the most common oesophageal neoplasm. In some parts of the world it is the most common of all cancers, but in the Western world it accounts for approximately 4 per cent of cancer deaths and has an annual incidence in the United States of 5/100 000 in whites and 17/100 000 in blacks.

AETIOLOGY

The striking geographical variation in incidence suggests a large contribution from environmental factors. There are many proven or putative risk factors, which include heavy alcohol use and intake of carcinogens

Table 3 *Common causes of medication-induced oesophageal injury*

Severe injury—high risk
Slow-release potassium chloride
Non-steroidal anti-inflammatory agents
Tetracycline
Quinidine
Less severe injury—high risk
Many antibiotics
Iron supplements
Occasional injury
Ascorbic acid
Mexiletine
Slow-release theophylline
Captopril
Phenytoin
Zidovudin

from smoking, from soil and water, and from high levels of nitrosamines and aflatoxins. Other putative factors include vitamin A deficiency, chronic candidal infection, oesophageal mucosal injury from corrosive ingestion years previously, and chronic irritation from oesophageal retention in achalasia. Invasive carcinoma is preceded by mucosal dysplasia and carcinoma *in situ* (see also Chapter 14.15).

SYMPTOMS

Dysplasia and carcinoma *in situ* are asymptomatic, and only recognized by screening programmes set up in very high risk areas, usually using 'blind' cytological sampling methods. Inexorable progression of dysphagia over a few weeks is the almost universal presentation (see Chapter 14.2.1). Dysphagia usually occurs when the tumour has become circumferential. Rarely, malignant mucosal ulceration presents with oesophageal mucosal pain due to malignant oesophageal ulceration. Substantial weight loss has often occurred by the time of presentation.

Barium swallow typically reveals a stricture with an irregular, lobulated, mucosal outline (Fig. 7), but occasionally the appearances mimic benign peptic stricture. The diagnosis is best proven by fibreoptic endoscopy, with mucosal biopsy and brush cytology. Occasionally, an asymptomatic oesophageal carcinoma is diagnosed when endoscopy is done for some other reason. Early lesions are often unimpressive, so that any minor mucosal irregularity should be sampled thoroughly by biopsy and cytology.

TREATMENT

In very early, usually asymptomatic carcinoma, resective surgery is the management of choice as it achieves high rates of cure. Curative resective surgery should only be attempted after careful staging of the tumour by clinical examination, chest radiographs, thoracic and abdominal computerized tomographic scanning, bronchoscopy, and 'liver function tests'. Endoscopic oesophageal ultrasonography is a much needed advance in the sensitivity of definition of local extent of tumour, but is not yet widely available.

Palliation poses many challenges. There is a serious lack of critical comparison of options. Resective surgery is ineffective, especially in elderly patients, because of its morbidity and mortality. Radiotherapy, with or without chemotherapy is usually the best option for management of malignant obstruction. Repeated peroral dilatation, peroral placement of stenting tubes, laser photocoagulation, and sclerosant injection are all options for management of recurrent malignant stricture that have potential for improvement of quality of life. Oesophagopulmonary fistula is a distressing development that usually causes pneumonia and persistent cough, which is sometimes controlled by stenting.

PROGNOSIS

This remains dismal except for regions where screening programmes identify early, asymptomatic cases. Only about one-quarter of patients are deemed to be potentially curable by surgery, and of these, about one-quarter will be alive and free of disease after 5 years. Thus, the overall 5-year survival rate is approximately 6 per cent. Such figures must be interpreted cautiously, because of differences amongst studies in the scope of presurgical staging, definitions of resectability, and criteria for exclusion of patients from consideration for surgery on grounds of debility, old age, and other medical problems.

Adenocarcinoma and oesophageal columnar metaplasia

DEFINITION

Between 80 and 90 per cent of adenocarcinomas arising in the oesophagus occur in association with oesophageal columnar metaplasia, or Barrett's oesophagus. In the minority of adenocarcinomas occurring in a squamous-lined oesophagus, the oesophageal mucous glands appear to be the source of malignant change.

AETIOLOGY

Oesophageal columnar metaplasia (Barrett's oesophagus) develops as a result of healing of severe reflux oesophagitis with metaplastic epithelium. This occurs upwards from the gastro-oesophageal junction over a distance that varies from 2 or 3 cm to the full length of the oesophagus. Oesophageal columnar metaplasia carries a 40-fold risk for development of oesophageal adenocarcinoma. Surveillance programmes in patients with oesophageal columnar metaplasia have shown a rate of development of adenocarcinoma that varies from 1 in 50 to 1 in 175 patient years. Occurrence of adenocarcinoma is very strongly associated with prior development of high-grade dysplasia in the metaplastic segment. The reasons for an apparently real, marked increase in oesophageal adenocarcinoma are unclear.

Fig. 7 Squamous carcinoma: circumferential luminal narrowing; asymmetrical, irregularly shouldered, mucosal aspect ulcerated.

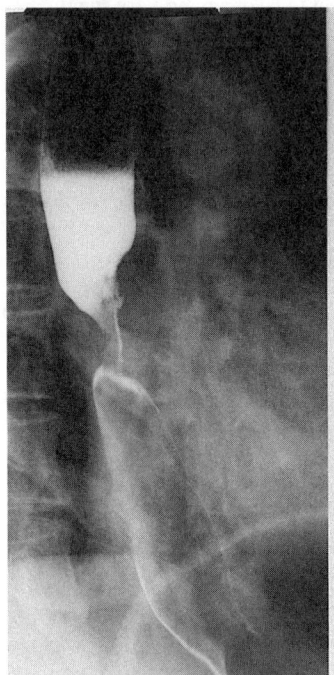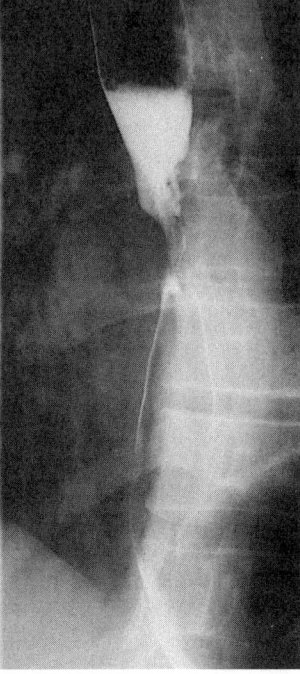

SYMPTOMS

The presentation of adenocarcinoma resembles that of squamous carcinoma (see above). Adenocarcinoma tends to be more fleshy and intraluminal, but still presents at a very late stage. Metastatic disease is more common on presentation of adenocarcinoma than squamous carcinoma.

Initial diagnosis and staging are along the same lines as for oesophageal squamous carcinoma.

TREATMENT OF ESTABLISHED ADENOCARCINOMA

Careful staging is the cornerstone of appropriate management. Because of the distal site of occurrence of oesophageal adenocarcinoma, resection with oesophagogastrostomy is usually the best approach. Adenocarcinoma appears to respond less frequently to radiotherapy and chemotherapy than squamous carcinoma.

MANAGEMENT OF THE RISK FOR ADENOCARCINOMA IN OESOPHAGEAL COLUMNAR METAPLASIA

This is a very active field of research. It is now well established that development of high-grade dysplasia in the columnar metaplastic segment precedes development of adenocarcinoma, and that this dysplasia can be recognized with sensitivity if at least four, radially spaced biopsies are taken at every 2 cm of columnar-lined oesophagus. It is controversial whether such expensive surveillance methods are justified by the relatively low rate of recognition of early adenocarcinoma. There is also controversy about how a diagnosis of high-grade dysplasia should be acted upon. Some authorities recommend oesophageal resection on confirmation of this diagnosis, whilst others favour close surveillance with endoscopic ultrasound and repeated biopsies, with oesophageal resection being reserved for when there is clear evidence of disruption of the normal structure of the oesophageal wall, indicative of early invasive carcinoma. Others advocate perendoscopic laser ablation without resection in the case of true intramucosal carcinoma. In large part, the approach to management of high-grade dysplasia is substantially moulded by the morbidity and risks of resective surgery, and the availability of endoscopic ultrasound. In younger, fit patients, the balance is more strongly in favour of early resection than it is in older, less fit patients. Lack of detailed knowledge about the natural history of high-grade dysplasia makes this decision making especially difficult.

Failure to discuss the risk for adenocarcinoma in oesophageal columnar metaplasia, and the option of endoscopic surveillance, could well be viewed as an indefensible lapse of practice, despite the uncertainties about cost-effectiveness.

PROGNOSIS

For established, symptomatic adenocarcinoma, this is every bit as dismal as for squamous carcinoma. Autopsy studies have shown that only a small proportion of patients with oesophageal columnar metaplasia are diagnosed as having this during life. Consequently, the impact of endoscopic surveillance can, at the best, only be limited. For those patients in whom screening is undertaken, it is clearly established that high-quality screening leads to diagnosis of oesophageal adenocarcinoma at a stage when it can usually be cured by resection.

Other oesophageal tumours

Malignant primary tumours

Primary malignant tumours other than squamous carcinoma and adenocarcinoma are rare and all have a poor prognosis. These include malignant melanoma, lymphoma, carcinoid, leiomyosarcoma, neuroendocrine carcinoma (small-cell carcinoma), adenoid cystic carcinoma,

Table 4 *Major causes of infective oesophagitis*

Pathogen	Management	Remarks
Immunocompetent patients		
Candida albicans	Topical/oral antifungals	By far most common
Herpes simplex	Acyclovir if severe	Unusual; may denude mucosa
Varicella zoster	Acyclovir if severe	In association with chickenpox/herpes zoster
Bacteria		Rare in well individuals
Immunocompromised patients		
Candida albicans	Systemic antifungals	Most common; oral disease almost diagnostic
Cytomegalovirus	Prophylaxis and treatment with ganciclovir or foscarnet	Part of systemic infection
		Sepiginous → giant ulcers distal half
Herpes simplex	Prophylaxis and treatment with acyclovir or foscarnet	Circumscribed ulcers, raised edges → coalescence
		Oral lesions.
Tuberculosis	Conventional	From miliary and local spread
Gram -positive cocci, -negative bacilli	IV antibiotics	Often with systemic infection
Syphilis	Conventional	Associated with tertiary syphilis elsewhere → inflammatory stricture

and pseudosarcoma. These tumours show a mixture of polypoid and infiltrating features, and are usually only clearly distinguished from the more common malignancies by histology.

Benign tumours

Leiomyoma is a relatively common oesophageal tumour, which rarely causes symptoms. It is usually intramural, but can become pedunculated. Around two-thirds of benign oesophageal tumours are leiomyomas. They usually only cause symptoms if they are very large, or on a long pedicle. Other benign intramural tumours of the oesophagus include lipoma and granular-cell tumour. The chief risk of these is that they are mistaken for malignant tumours and operated on inappropriately.

Squamous-cell papillomas of the mucosa can mimic a polypoid squamous carcinoma and so should be removed endoscopically for histological diagnosis.

Infective oesophagitis and other non-neoplastic mucosal diseases

Most of these diseases cause symptoms because of mucosal hypersensitivity. When the course is prolonged, interference with food intake may become a dominant problem in patient management. Viral oesophagitis can sometimes cause major haemorrhage. Some disorders damage the full thickness of oesophageal wall and lead to stricturing. Infective oesophagitis is by far the most important, and has become more so with the increased number of people who are immunosuppressed through HIV infection or chemotherapy.

Diagnosis is often aided by the setting in which the oesophageal problem occurs. Cutaneous or oral disease can suggest what is happening in the oesophagus, but barium swallow adds relatively little to assessment of mucosal hypersensitivity. Endoscopy is the diagnostic method of choice. Mucosal appearances and the distribution of oesophageal lesions can be virtually diagnostic. In addition, biopsies and brushings allow for histological diagnosis and identification of infectious agents. Endoscopy has most to offer in patients with chronic symptoms, or those who are immunosuppressed.

Infective oesophagitis

The more important causes are summarized in Table 4. Immune status is a major determinant of the pattern of infection. Though infective oesophagitis may be severe in immunocompetent patients, it is characteristically self-limiting and topical therapy is normally all that is needed (Table 4).

Immunocompromised patients usually need aggressive, systemic therapy, otherwise the infection does not resolve. The infection can be difficult to eradicate, tends to recur, and cause extensive disability. Two or more infections are not unusual.

Helicobacter pylori does not appear to be of any primary significance in pathogenesis of oesophageal mucosal disease.

Other non-neoplastic mucosal diseases

Rarely, Crohn's disease can cause indolent, craggy ulceration and/or stricturing. Oesophageal sarcoidosis can mimic Crohn's disease.

Skin and systemic diseases associated with lesions of the oropharynx may also involve the oesophagus. These include epidermolysis bullosa, Behçet's disease, lichen planus, pemphigus vulgaris, bullous pemphigoid, benign mucous membrane (cicatrial) pemphigoid, and drug-induced disease (Stevens–Johnson syndrome and toxic epidermal necrolysis).

Chronic, and less frequently, acute graft-versus-host disease may cause severe oesophageal problems through mucosal desquamation or mural damage. Resultant stricturing shows considerable variation in appearances.

14.7 Peptic ulceration

J. J. MISIEWICZ and R. E. POUNDER

INTRODUCTION

Chronic duodenal ulcer and chronic benign gastric ulcer are often grouped together as peptic ulcers. Although the two diseases have many similarities, they differ in some important aspects such as epidemiology, natural history, outcome, and management. These differences are important clinically, and it is therefore mandatory always to establish a precise diagnosis of either duodenal or chronic benign gastric ulcer, and to manage them clinically as separate, although related, diseases.

Duodenal ulcer

DEFINITION

Duodenal ulcer is a distinct break in the mucosa of the duodenum, almost invariably in the duodenal bulb, but occasionally more distal. The ulcer may be superficial, or may penetrate to the serosa.

AETIOLOGY

It is not known why certain patients develop duodenal ulceration, nor why the clinical course is characterized by episodes of intermittent relapses. Many aetiological factors may affect the incidence of duodenal ulcer; the relative importance of each of them in particular geographical areas or particular individuals is impossible to judge with certainty. Epidemiological evidence suggests that duodenal ulcer first became common in Western Europe around the turn of the twentieth century: similar observations cannot be made in other areas because of lack of reliable records. The clinical characteristics of duodenal ulcer appear to be changing quite rapidly with time towards a less severe clinical form: why this should be so is not known. It is now apparent that the strongest aetiological association of duodenal ulcer is with infection of the gastroduodenal mucosa by *Helicobacter pylori*. Virtually all patients with duodenal ulcer are colonized by this bacterium. *H. pylori* has important effects on gastric function. Eradication of the bacterium leads to the healing of duodenal ulcer and dramatic decrease in the incidence of ulcer relapse. *H. pylori* is an important aetiological factor in several other diseases of the foregut, including chronic gastritis, gastric ulceration, gastric cancer, mucosal associated lymphoid tissue (MALT) lymphoma, and Ménètrier's disease.

Acid and pepsin

Although the presence of acid and pepsin is essential for the appearance of a duodenal ulcer it is probably only one of several aetiological factors operating in most patients. Ulceration is generally thought to be caused by an imbalance between the damaging effects of acid and pepsin attack and the body's mucosal defences. This simplistic hypothesis does fit the extremes of acid secretion: duodenal ulcers do not occur in anacidic patients, but are almost inevitable in the presence of gross hypersecretion of acid in the Zollinger–Ellison syndrome.

As a group, patients with duodenal ulcer secrete more acid than healthy people. The previously reported overlap in maximal acid secretion values between controls and duodenal ulcer patients disappears if *H. pylori*-negative normal subjects and gastric releasing peptide (GRP) are used as controls and acid stimulant, respectively (Fig. 1). Five factors may account for the tendency to hypersecrete acid and pepsin: (i) increased parietal cell mass; (ii) increased stimulation of acid secretion;

(iii) increased parietal cell sensitivity to stimulants; (iv) decreased inhibitory control of acid secretion; and (v) *Helicobacter pylori* induced hypergastrinaemia. The evidence for these five factors is incomplete but, on average, patients with duodenal ulcer have more parietal cells than normal; their peak acid output increases as the years of disease continue (perhaps due to pyloric obstruction, antacid consumption, bile/alkaline reflux into the antrum, or continuing hypergastrinaemia); they have high basal and nocturnal unstimulated gastric-acid outputs; they also have an exaggerated gastrin response to food and continue to secrete gastrin despite increasing acidification of the antrum. Finally, increased sensitivity to exogenous pentagastrin has been reported in such patients, when compared with controls. Several of these abnormalities (hypergastrinaemia, raised basal and GRP-stimulated acid output, decreased inhibitory drive mediated by somatostatin, hyperpepsinogenaemia) disappear after eradiction of *H. pylori*.

A great deal is known about the physiology of acid secretion, but the abnormalities of acid output and gastrin release described above are subtle, difficult to investigate, and based on evidence collected from intensive study of few subjects: it is uncertain whether they apply to all patients with duodenal ulcer. Much less is known about the importance of pepsin secretion, while knowledge of factors affecting mucosal defence and integrity is fragmentary, especially in relation to the mucosa of the duodenal bulb. It is tempting to speculate that duodenal ulcer is a disease of multifactorial origin and that the importance of various factors differs. For example, excess acid output may be of greater importance in some cases with frank hypersecretion of acid [(Fig. 1)], while

Fig. 1 Peak gastric-acid secretion rates and possibility of development of duodenal (DU) or gastric ulcer (GU) (reproduced from Baron, H. (1972). *Chronic duodenal ulcer*, (ed. C. Wastell). Butterworth, London, with permission).

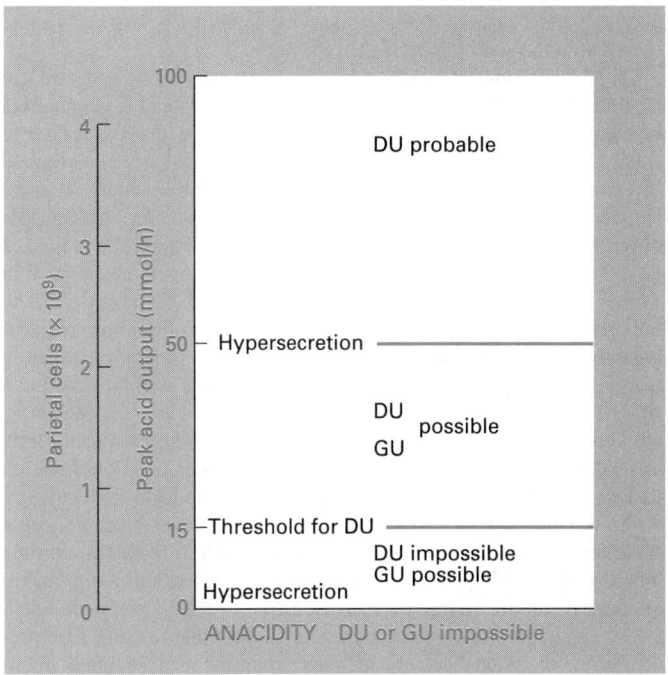

another reason, such as faulty mucosal defence, may predominate in others.

Gastric emptying

The pH in the duodenal lumen is lower (more acid) more frequently and for longer periods in patients with duodenal ulceration than in controls. These patients empty food from their stomachs faster so that after a meal there is less food available to buffer secreted acid as it passes into the duodenum. Acid is neutralized in the duodenum by bicarbonate secreted partly by the duodenal mucosa and partly by the exocrine pancreas. Patients with duodenal ulcer do not have a gross defect of pancreatic alkaline secretion, but the alkaline secretions of the duodenal mucosa are suboptimal.

Ulcerogenic drugs

Much has been written about the ulcerogenic potential of drugs, such as corticosteroids, aspirin, and other non-steroidal, anti-inflammatory agents, but the evidence that they cause chronic duodenal (or gastric ulcer) is not convincing. Anti-inflammatory agents can damage the gastric mucosa and are frequently used to produce ulcer models in experimental animals for the testing of drugs. Extrapolation from these models to man, however, should be viewed with a certain amount of scepticism. However, the incidence of consumption of non-steroidal anti-inflammatory drugs is high amongst patients with gastrointestinal bleeding, or perforation.

Psychological factors

Stress of modern life is often invoked as an important cause of duodenal ulcer, but life has always appeared modern and stressful to people living in a given period of history. Chronic (as opposed to acute) stress is difficult to measure and reproduce experimentally. Case-control studies suggest that patients with duodenal ulcer are not excessively exposed to life events, but they may be more stressed than controls exposed to similar events. Rapid urbanization in emergent countries is said to coincide with increased incidence of duodenal ulcer, but other diseases also change their pattern and the effects of stress, environment, dietary changes, and better diagnostic facilities are difficult to disentangle.

Epidemiological factors

Duodenal ulceration is very common and may effect 10 to 15 per cent of many populations. The prevalence of duodenal ulcer is subject to marked geographic variation; for example, it is much more common in Scotland and Northern England than in Southern England; it is more common in the south of India than the north.

Clinical attributes of duodenal ulcer are also affected by geographical location; for example, the rate of perforation is Scotland is greater than in metropolitan London. The characteristics of the disease appear to change with time, as evidenced by the decreasing incidence of perforated ulcers in males and the increasing rate of ulceration in elderly women. Duodenal ulceration is more common in men than women, although this difference is becoming less exaggerated, mainly because the incidence in women appears to be increasing. Duodenal ulcer is more frequent in women after the menopause, suggesting that sex hormones may be important in the aetiology of the disease; the impact of hormone replacement therapy on peptic ulceration is not known. The condition probably reached its European peak in the 1950s, but is now declining. In India and Africa the prevalence of duodenal ulcer is higher in populations who eat a low-residue diet; an American study suggested that coffee and soft drinks provoke ulceration. There are weak associations between duodenal ulceration and smoking, alcohol intake, and anti-inflammatory drugs. Although duodenal ulceration has been reported to have positive associations with other medical conditions (such as cirrhosis, chronic lung disease, and hyperparathyroidism), these correlations are probably artefactual and due to intensive investigation of patients who are liable to a second common disease. It is possible that there is a genetic predisposition to duodenal ulcers: it is more common in close family members, patients with blood group O and non-secretors of blood-group substances in the saliva.

The strongest epidemiological association is with *H. pylori* infection. Thus virtually all patients with duodenal ulcer are infected with the organism, but there are many more persons in a given community who are colonized by it but who do not develop an ulcer. The prevalence of this organism seems to be determined by socioeconomic factors and the infection is usually acquired in childhood. Thus poor housing and water supply increase the chances of infection and people living in poor conditions seem to acquire *H. pylori* earlier in life.

CLINICAL PICTURE AND NATURAL HISTORY

The main symptom of duodenal ulceration is pain. Although the pain is classically epigastric, related to food, and occurs during the night, it is clear that there can be great individual variation. Indeed, severe ulceration to the point of perforation or haemorrhage can be virtually symptomless. Thus approximately 50 per cent of patients who die from a peptic ulcer are unaware of their ulcer at the time of their final, fatal admission. The exact cause of ulcer pain is not clear: it is not always directly related to intraduodenal acidity, but is rapidly relieved by antacids.

Nausea and vomiting are relatively unusual, unless there is severe pain or pyloric stenosis; vomiting quite often brings relief from pain. Posterior penetration of a duodenal ulcer into the pancreas may cause mid-back pain, or pancreatitis. Complication rates are difficult to assess, but major complications are rare; perhaps 1 per cent per year of patients under follow-up. Haemorrhage may cause haematemesis and/or melaena, with consequent iron-deficiency anaemia. Perforation can cause acute, severe pain, collapse, and peritonitis. Of the patients recruited for long-term trials of maintenance medical treatment, 15 per cent had a history of haemorrhage but only 1 per cent had perforated.

Duodenal ulceration is a condition of spontaneous relapses and remissions. The change in the clinical picture from relapse to remission is remarkable. The patient, made miserable by severe epigastric pain and loss of sleep due to night-time symptoms, may return a few days later, feeling perfectly well. It is therefore unwise to make decisions about surgery during a relapse of duodenal ulcer as the patient's reaction may be unbalanced by the symptoms. Clinical trials suggest that within a

Fig. 2 Maintenance treatment of duodenal ulcer with cimetidine: results of double-blind trials from 22 centres (from the data of Burland, W., Hawkins, B., and Beresford, J. (1980) *Postgraduate Medical Journal*, **56**, 173).

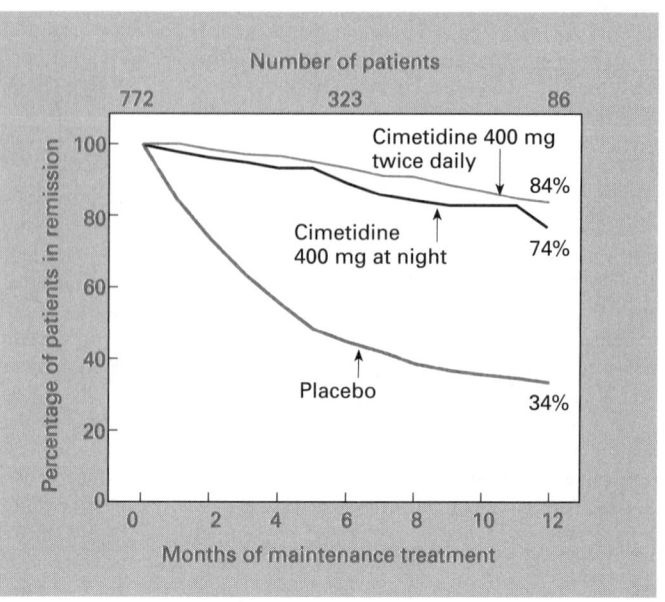

year of ulcer healing using a gastric acid antisecretory drug, 66 per cent of patients receiving a placebo will have had a symptomatic relapse (Fig. 2), but in addition approximately one-third of asymptomatic patients have recurrent ulcers when examined by endoscopy. The course of the illness is variable. Some patients suffer only a single episode of ulceration, while in others the illness is progressive, with rare remissions and severe complications. Spontaneous healing of duodenal ulcer may be delayed, and relapses are earlier and more frequent in patients who either continue to smoke cigarettes or take non-steroidal anti-inflammatory drugs.

The natural history of untreated duodenal ulceration is unclear. Although it was originally reported that the disease may go into prolonged remission after 10 to 15 years of intermittent illness, this was probably an artefact due to surgical treatment of patients with more aggressive ulcers.

DIAGNOSIS

Duodenal ulcer cannot be diagnosed by clinical history, because similar symptoms occur in other diseases, such as gastric ulcer, gastric cancer, or the irritable bowel syndrome. The patient often points to the epigastrium as site of the pain, but this is not reliable. Physical examination may show epigastric tenderness, but is otherwise unhelpful. In rare cases of severe pyloric stenosis, visible gastric peristalsis and a succussion splash are present.

The diagnosis of duodenal ulcer must be established by radiology or endoscopy. A barium meal, preferably air-contrast, will show deformity of the duodenal cap, but the differentiation between scarring, mucosal folds, and an active ulcer crater is less certain. Where available, fibre-optic endoscopy is the best method of diagnosis. Even then, pyloric stenosis with retention of gastric contents, mucosal oedema, haemorrhage, or incomplete inspection of the base of duodenal cap can all cause the ulcer crater to be missed. Diagnostic endoscopy in suspected duodenal ulcer should preferably be done at the time of a relapse. Previous therapy with ulcer-healing drugs may make the diagnosis more difficult or impossible. Duodenal ulcers are usually single, circular areas of discrete ulceration resembling oral aphthous ulcers, usually with a creamy yellow base. The surrounding duodenal mucosa may be normal, or may be erythematous, with punctate haemorrhages due to duodenitis.

Gastric secretory tests have no place in the routine diagnosis or management of duodenal ulceration. The fasting plasma gastrin concentration should always be measured in patients with severe or ectopic ulceration, or in those with continuing ulceration after adequate medical treatment or surgery, to exclude the Zollinger–Ellison syndrome.

Serological and salivary tests for specific antibodies to *H. pylori* are now becoming available. Any patient with dyspepsia who is not taking an NSAID and who is serologically negative for *H. pylori* is highly unlikely to have a duodenal ulcer. This observation has been used as a method of screening for young (aged <45 years) dyspeptic patients before endoscopy–negative serology being equated with functional dyspepsia. At the time of writing this approach needs further validation in large-scale clinical studies. In addition, commercial serology kits need careful validation in relation to the local population.

Chronic benign gastric ulcer

DEFINITION

A benign gastric ulcer is usually a single, circular or semicircular, discrete break in the gastric mucosa. Ulcers can occur anywhere in the stomach, but most develop on the lesser curvature at the junction between the acid-secreting mucosa and the mucosa of the antrum. Gastric ulcers may occur in the antrum: special care must be taken to exclude malignancy in antral ulcers. Prepyloric ulcers resemble duodenal ulcers endoscopically and are probably best managed clinically on the lines indicated for duodenal ulcers. A benign gastric ulcer can vary in size from a few millimetres to several centimetres in diameter; it often penetrates deeply into the muscularis mucosa.

AETIOLOGY

Acid secretion and duodenogastric reflux

The cause of benign gastric ulcer is uncertain but approximately 80 per cent are associated with *H. pylori* infection. Gastric ulcers are also associated with non-steroidal anti-inflammatory medication. The gastric mucosa is probably injured by the combination of acid secreted by the stomach, the reflux of duodenal contents, and by *H. pylori* colonizing the antral epithelial cells—it is noteworthy that gastric ulcer always occurs in the non-acid-secreting antral mucosa. The duodenal juice contains bile, lysolecithin, and pancreatic enzymes, all of which may damage the gastric mucosa. A number of studies have demonstrated that patients with gastric ulcer tend to reflux their duodenal contents, a tendency that is aggravated by smoking cigarettes. Gastric-emptying time in patients with gastric ulcer tends to be prolonged and retention of contents predisposes to gastric ulceration.

Gastric ulcers do not develop unless there is a degree of intragastric acidity. Patients with severe gastritis due to free biliary reflux after antrectomy rarely develop benign gastric ulceration, presumably because they secrete a negligible amount of acid. It was considered that patients with gastric ulcer secrete only a small amount of acid; this is not true—they have normal profiles of 24-h intragastric acidity. One of the defences of the gastric mucosa is a small amount of bicarbonate secreted by the mucosa into the gastric mucus. This alkaline gradient (which is only about 700 μm deep) may be an important factor for mucosal integrity and could be defective in patients with gastric ulceration.

Epidemiology

In the nineteenth century, gastric ulceration was a disease of young women but it is now common in both genders, in older age groups, and in patients of low socioeconomic class. It is less common than duodenal ulcer. Associations with other medical conditions are doubtful, but non-steroidal, anti-inflammatory drugs may cause gastric ulceration.

CLINICAL PICTURE AND NATURAL HISTORY

Benign gastric ulceration typically presents with epigastric pain that cannot be distinguished from pain due to other causes. Although exacerbations of discomfort after meals, remitting pain, weight loss, and a very long history are relatively common in this group of patients, a confident diagnosis cannot and must not be made on clinical evidence alone. Many patients with gastric ulcer are asymptomatic until they present with a complication such as acute or occult gastrointestinal haemorrhage, or perforation.

Gastric ulceration is a recurrent chronic condition; up to a half of the patients develop recurrence.

DIAGNOSIS

As in duodenal ulceration, neither clinical history nor physical examination provides evidence for a positive diagnosis. A barium-meal examination, especially if double contrast, may detect even superficial ulceration (Fig. 3). However, the important advantage of upper gastrointestinal endoscopy is that it allows a tissue diagnosis to be made using both biopsy and brush cytology. As the important differential diagnosis is between early gastric cancer and a benign gastric ulcer, all patients with gastric ulcer should be endoscoped, with multiple, targeted biopsies taken from the ulcer rim and base, followed by exfoliative brush cytology. The greater the number of biopsies, the greater the likelihood of picking up early intramucosal gastric carcinoma: the minimum number of biopsies is four, one from each quadrant of the crater margin. The importance of diagnosing early gastric cancer lies in its good prognosis after total gastrectomy.

Acute erosive ulceration

Multiple superficial ulcers may develop in the oesophagus, stomach or duodenum of acutely stressed patients, particularly after major trauma, extensive burns, or during shock or hypoxia. In only one situation (Cushing's ulceration following head injury) is there a positive relation between mucosal damage and high gastric-acid secretion. Some acid secretion is apparently necessary for stress ulceration to develop, but the main damage appears to be due to mucosal ischaemia and hypoxia. Stress ulceration is now relatively uncommon, due to the improved resuscitation and general management of severely ill patients.

This type of ulceration, which must not be confused with chronic duodenal ulcer or gastric ulcer, usually presents with haemorrhage some days after the initial insult. The patient is best investigated by endoscopy because the superficial ulceration is often not visible on conventional barium-meal radiographs. The gastrointestinal haemorrhage may be aggravated by coagulopathies associated with the primary stressful event. H_2-receptor blockers can prevent this type of ulceration and haemorrhage. They should be given orally four times per 24 h whenever feasible: the intravenous route should only be used when oral administration is definitely contraindicated by other considerations. Treatment should begin at once, because it is the preventative effect of suppressing acid secretion that is important. The recommended maximum doses are cimetidine (400 mg) or ranitidine (50 mg) intravenously 6-hourly, preferably as a continuous infusion. In the presence of renal insufficiency the dose of an H_2-antagonist should be decreased, as the drugs are mainly excreted by the kidney. Watch must be kept on the patient's mental state, because cimetidine very occasionally causes coma in severely ill people. Omeprazole is not generally available for intravenous use.

Erosive ulcers can also develop in patients whose upper gastrointestinal mucosa is damaged by either non-steroidal anti-inflammatory drugs or alcohol. Indeed, these forms of ulceration often are used in animal models and are usually prevented by pretreatment with either an antisecretory drug or a prostaglandin analogue such as misoprostol.

The management of patients with established stress ulceration involves blood transfusion, correction of clotting defects, and the use of an H_2-antagonist. Unfortunately the benefit from these drugs is smaller when used for established erosive gastritis than when used for prophylactic treatment. Surgery is to be avoided if at all possible, because the diffuse nature of mucosal damage means that radical surgery would be needed to stop the bleeding.

Oesophagitis

Oesophagitis is dealt with fully in Chapter 14.6 but is mentioned here because patients with peptic ulcer, and particularly those with duodenal ulcer, often complain of heartburn and regurgitation of acid. Inflammation of distal oesophageal mucosa is seen at endoscopy. The presence of oesophagitis in a patient with duodenal ulcers does not generally call for any modification of the adopted plan of therapy. The oesophagitis may improve as the duodenal ulcer goes into remission, but advice on weight reduction, elevation of the head of the bed, and avoidance of large meals before going to bed may be needed, if oesophageal symptoms persist.

The fall in gastric acid secretion following eradication of H. pylori should benefit oesophagitis, but so far this aspect of ulcer disease has not been studied in detail.

Non-ulcer dyspepsia

Dyspepsia is a very common presenting symptom in gastroenterological practice, but only a small proportion of patients with dyspepsia have organic disease at endoscopy or radiographically. It has been suggested that the term functional dyspepsia encompasses patients with symptoms apparently originating from the proximal gut, and that these can be further subdivided into ulcer-like, dysmotility, and reflux dyspepsias. In ulcer-like dyspepsia the symptoms suggest the presence of an ulcer, but this is absent at endoscopy. Dysmotility dyspepsia is associated with bloating and early satiety; some patients have delayed gastric emptying and symptoms may respond to motility-stimulating agents, such as cisapride. Reflux dyspepsia merges into gastro-oesophageal reflux disease. Medical treatment of ulcer-like dyspepsia is unsatisfactory in that response to gastric acid suppressants, or to eradication of H. pylori, is unpredictable; controlled trials have so far failed to show any advantage for eradication of this organism over placebo, perhaps because there is a marked placebo response. The prevalence of H. pylori in patients with functional dyspepsia is similar to that of the general population.

History of typical ulcer symptoms—epigastric pain, related to food and relieved by antacids—is not sufficient to make the diagnosis of gastric ulcer or duodenal ulcer. Many patients have the typical symptoms, but no ulcer can be demonstrated radiologically or endoscopically, even if the investigations are done in the symptomatic phase. The duodenal cap may be completely normal to endoscopic inspection, or may show minor changes of duodenitis: biopsies will likewise be normal, or display mild inflammation.

The mechanism of pain in these patients is not clear. It is possible that the duodenal mucosa may be sensitive to acid or pepsin without frank ulceration, but this is speculative. Alternatively, the patient may have very mild gastro-oesophageal reflux of acid. Another explanation is that the pain originates not in the duodenum but elsewhere in the intestinal tract, so that the condition is really a variant of the irritable bowel syndrome.

Duodenitis

Duodenitis is an ill-defined condition, characterized at endoscopy by inflamed, haemorrhagic, and friable duodenal-cap mucosa; duodenal biopsies show acute inflammatory changes. If erosions are present, the

Fig. 3 Benign gastric ulcer demonstrated by air-contrast barium meal; mucosal folds reach the rim of the ulcer crater.

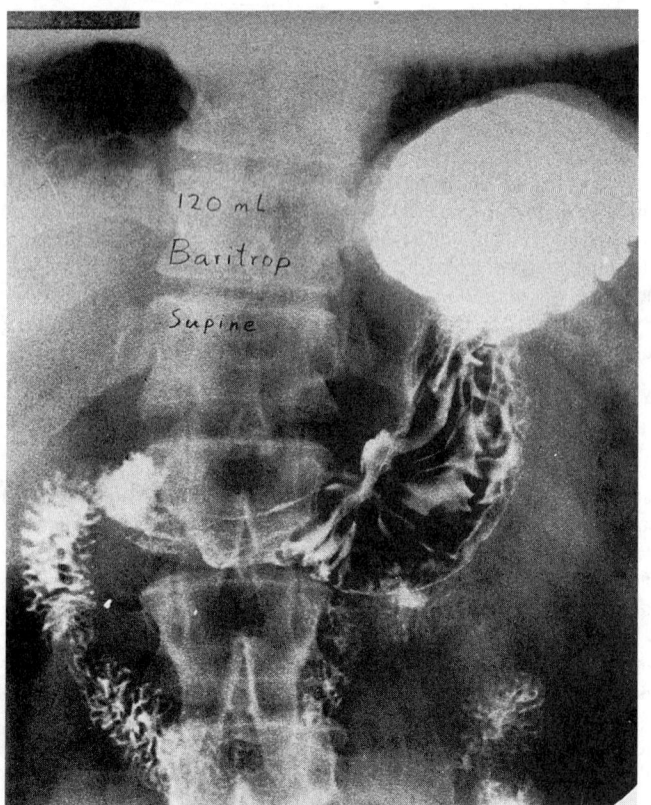

condition is called erosive duodenitis, although where erosions end and duodenal ulcers proper begin is somewhat difficult to define precisely. Erosive duodenitis may give rise to symptoms indistinguishable from those of duodenal ulcer and may be complicated by haemorrhage leading to haematemesis and/or melaena. Duodenitis is best regarded as forming one end of the spectrum of duodenal ulcerative disease. Frank duodenal ulcers are often surrounded by areas of duodenitis and the latter may persist after the ulcer has healed.

There are few trials of treatment of duodenitis. Most patients are treated as if they have a duodenal ulcer. In some patients environmental factors, such as heavy drinking, can be identified and their elimination may lead to improvement of the duodenal inflammation. Many patients with duodenitis will be colonized by *H. pylori*. At present, the effect of eradicating this organism on duodenitis has not been fully studied.

The Zollinger–Ellison syndrome

DEFINITION

In 1955 Zollinger and Ellison described a syndrome encompassing severe peptic ulceration, hypersecretion of gastric acid, and an islet-cell tumour of the pancreas.

PATHOPHYSIOLOGY

The islet-cell tumours in these patients have been shown to secrete gastrin. Gastrinomas are usually found in the body or tail of the pancreas; the tumours may be multiple and they can be histologically and clinically malignant. The gastrin secreted by the tumours is usually the G17 form (little gastrin), but smaller and larger molecular species have also been reported. Prolonged high plasma gastrin concentrations cause an increase of the parietal-cell mass with consequent high basal and maximal acid secretion. Occasionally a pancreatic gastrinoma is associated with hyperparathyroidism in Werner's syndrome (multiple endocrine adenomatosis I).

Most patients (95 per cent) have aggressive peptic ulceration. The second major symptom is diarrhoea, present in 40 per cent of the patients; it can be the only symptom. Peptic ulcers occur in the duodenum, stomach or oesophagus, but they tend to be larger, to penetrate deeper, and to be multiple. Ulceration often extends beyond the first part of the duodenum. Haemorrhage or perforation occurring soon after gastric surgery, or failure of ulcers to heal during full-dose H_2-blockade, is characteristic of the Zollinger–Ellison syndrome.

The diarrhoea is not due to hypergastrinaemia itself, for it does not occur commonly in patients with pernicious anaemia who often have higher plasma gastrin concentrations. The diarrhoea is probably due to low intestinal pH produced by sustained acid hypersecretion. The acidity denatures pancreatic enzymes, causing steatorrhoea, and precipitates bile salts, causing malabsorption of bile salts which in turn provokes water secretion by the colon.

DIAGNOSIS

The diagnosis of the Zollinger–Ellison syndrome initially depends on the detection of an elevated fasting plasma gastrin concentration, in the presence of acid in the stomach. As gastrin is measured by radioimmunoassay using antibodies with varying affinity to the different molecular species of gastrin, there is variation between the normal ranges of different laboratories. Most laboratories would be suspicious of a fasting plasma gastrin concentration of more than 50 to 100 pmol/l.

Three conditions can cause marked hypergastrinaemia (hypergastrinaemia associated with *H. pylori* is mild) with increased acid output and aggressive peptic ulceration, but without the presence of a gastrinoma. Firstly, hyperplasia of the gastrin-secreting cells of the antrum, called confusingly the Zollinger–Ellison syndrome type I (the classical condition is type II), which may represent the upper part of the normal range of gastrin and acid secretion. Secondly, a cuff of antral mucosa inadvertently retained at the end of the oversewn blind loop of a Polya partial gastrectomy results in the excluded antrum being bathed in alkaline duodenal and pancreatic secretion, thereby causing profound gastrin release. Thirdly, for a short time after massive small-intestinal resection, plasma gastrin concentrations rise markedly with consequent gastric hypersecretion: this is possibly due to transient deficiency of an inhibitory gastrointestinal polypeptide.

Treatment with gastric-acid antisecreting drugs results in a rise of plasma gastric concentration, inversely proportioned to the suppression of acid secretion. Omeprazole usually causes a fourfold rise in plasma gastric concentration, but perhaps 10 per cent of patients develop very high levels of gastrin similar to those in pernicious anaemia.

Excessive histamine release is found in rare patients with either systemic mastocytosis, or mast-cell leukaemia (see Section 22). This continuous histamine stimulation of the stomach may cause profound gastric hypersecretion, with normal or low plasma gastrin concentration. High plasma gastrin concentrations are usually found in patients with pernicious anaemia, but they are anacidic.

A number of criteria can be used to define the hypersecretion of acid in the Zollinger–Ellison syndrome: (*a*) basal acid output of more than 15 mmol/h or basal acidity greater than 100 mmol/l (pH less than 1.0): (*b*) basal acid secretion at the level of 60 per cent or more of maximal or peak acid output. Measurements of acid output and pH of gastric juice are simple and within the capabilities of most hospitals, but unfortunately they cannot be relied on to establish the diagnosis of the syndrome.

The most reliable confirmatory investigation is the secretin test. Two units GIH secretin per kg are given by slow intravenous injection with the patient fasting. In normal individuals the plasma gastrin concentration drops, but in patients with the Zollinger–Ellison syndrome there is an immediate rise (within 1 or 2 min of the injection) to more than 50 per cent above the basal values. Patients with type I Zollinger–Ellison syndrome have a normal response to secretin, but those with an excluded antrum may still be confused with type II Zollinger–Ellison syndrome. As the retained cuff of antrum will concentrate technetium in its gastric mucosa, it can sometimes be identified using a gamma-camera, particularly if the patient has not received oral perchlorate before the scan.

The pancreatic tumour may be small and difficult to identify even at laparotomy. Selective arteriography, ultrasound, or an abdominal computerized tomographic scan may help to localize the tumour before surgery, but none of these techniques is completely reliable. Percutaneous transhepatic sampling of portal-vein gastrin concentration may also aid preoperative tumour localization.

TREATMENT

The management of the classical Zollinger–Ellison syndrome is becoming less controversial. Until the mid-1970s the only possible treatment was total gastrectomy, thus removing the target organ for gastrin. This some surgeons combined with exploration and perhaps resection of the pancreas. As many patients already had previous failed gastric operations, were malnourished and catabolic, the mortality and morbidity of surgery were high.

Two advances have altered the outlook for these patients: the availability of gastrin radioimmunoassay and the proton-pump blockers. The former has made early diagnosis possible, and the latter have allowed pharmacological control of the acid-secreting parietal cell.

Most patients with the Zollinger–Ellison syndrome will respond to omeprazole, 40 mg twice daily. Failure of medical treatment is usually due to inadequate dosage. The optimal dose can be determined by measuring intragastric pH during the day after breakfast and lunch: successful treatment should keep the gastric contents between pH 2.0 and 7.0. With continued treatment, the dose of omeprazole may often be decreased, but the average total daily dose is usually 60 mg. The H_2-antagonists now have no role in the management of the Zollinger–

Ellison syndrome, except as emergency intravenous treatment, using up to six times the normal dose.

The role of surgery is now controversial. Some recommend a laparotomy to determine whether the tumour is resectable; a highly selective vagotomy done at the same time may moderate acid secretion without extra hazard to the patient and make pharmacological control of acid secretion much easier. Postsurgery plasma gastrin concentrations provide a convenient marker for tumour activity. Others argue that pancreatic surgery is hazardous, that the outlook is good with maintenance omeprazole, and that surgery should be reserved for those in whom medical treatment fails. Inoperable and progressive malignancy may respond to streptozotocin.

Complications of peptic ulcer

Perforation

Perforation is a serious complication of peptic ulcer: it is more common in men and more frequent in duodenal ulcers than in gastric ulcers. A proportion of patients, estimated at approximately 50 per cent in various studies, perforate without any preceding history of dyspepsia. The most common site of perforation is the anterior wall of the duodenal cap in duodenal ulcer or the lesser curve of the stomach in gastric ulcer. Rarely, ulcers may perforate into the biliary tract, filling it with air.

The diagnosis is not difficult in most patients. The history is of a sudden onset of abdominal pain. The abdomen is rigid, there is rebound tenderness, the abdominal respiratory movements and bowel sounds are absent, and liver dullness to percussion is diminished. A plain abdominal radiograph may show free air between the upper border of the liver and the diaphragm, but absence of this sign does not exclude perforation. Leucocytosis usually appears promptly. The symptoms are so stereotyped that the condition is eminently suitable for accurate computer diagnosis. Difficulties in diagnosis arise in the elderly, or in the mentally ill, in patients in hospital for chronic illness, or in those on high doses of corticosteroids. In this group of patients, 'silent' or painless perforations may occur; unexplained shock is the most common clinical finding, with loss of dullness on percussion of the liver.

Treatment of perforation is usually surgical, medical management being reserved only for moribund patients, or for those who are rendered inoperable by severe coexisting disease. Medical management consists of continuous nasogastric suction, treatment of shock, electrolyte and fluid replacement, and antibiotic therapy with ampicillin, gentamicin, and metronidazole. Failure of the perforated ulcer to heal leads to surgery.

Oversewing a perforated ulcer provides first-aid treatment, but no long-term cure. To avoid recurrent ulceration the patient may need either maintenance treatment with an H_2-antagonist, eradication of *H. pylori* if this organism is present, or an elective, definitive reoperation.

Haemorrhage

Haemorrhage from the stomach and duodenum is the most common life-threatening gastrointestinal emergency. The main causes of upper gastro-intestinal haemorrhage are peptic ulceration or variceal bleeding secondary to chronic liver disease; both are conditions with a highly variable prevalence throughout the world. Thus variceal haemorrhage is a relatively rare cause of upper gastrointestinal haemorrhage in the United Kingdom, although the incidence is increasing. Duodenal ulcer, gastric ulcer, erosive ulceration, and the Mallory–Weiss syndrome are all more common, in descending order of frequency (see Chapter 14.2.6).

SYMPTOMS AND SIGNS

Most patients will have a history of dyspepsia, although haemorrhage may be the first evidence of peptic ulceration, particularly if the patient is physically stressed by trauma or illness, or is taking non-steroidal anti-inflammatory drugs.

The first symptom of upper gastrointestinal haemorrhage is often sudden collapse, with weakness, sweating, and palpitations. The patient may vomit blood or may notice active bowel sounds due to stimulation of gastrointestinal motility by blood. This is often followed by lower abdominal colic, as in acute gastroenteritis, finally relieved by defaecation of normal stools and later melaena. The melaena is usually dark red or black, due to partial digestion of the blood, but fresh blood may be passed per rectum even if the haemorrhage is from the stomach or duodenum. The bleeding usually stops spontaneously and the patient gradually recovers to be left with symptoms of anaemia.

MANAGEMENT

Any patient with melaena or haematemesis within the preceding 48 h should be admitted to hospital because of the risk of further haemorrhage. Repeated bleeding rarely occurs more than 48 h after the first episode. There are three phases in the management of a patient with an acute upper gastrointestinal haemorrhage: resuscitation, exact diagnosis, and treatment.

Endoscopy is an essential step in the diagnosis and treatment of acute upper gastrointestinal haemorrhage and should be performed within 12 h of admission in all patients. The endoscopist can usually define the source of bleeding and in the case of haemorrhage from a chronic duodenal ulcer or gastric ulcer can also determine the risk of recurrence. A spurting artery in the base of an ulcer crater, a visible blood vessel or the presence of a blood clot in the crater are all indications for immediate endoscopic sclerotherapy, using 1 : 10 000 adrenaline up to 10 ml in four quadrants, and/or a sclerosant, such as polydocanol (1–2 ml) for example, injected through a variceal sclerotherapy needle in divided doses. Other techniques utilize a heater probe or a laser beam delivered by a fibreoptic bundle, which is introduced through the biopsy channel of the instrument; the injection technique is as effective, cheaper, and widely available. Recent studies indicate a significantly decreased incidence of rebleeding in patients treated with sclerotherapy, but some ulcers are technically difficult, or impossible to inject.

PROGNOSIS

The main objective in the management of upper gastrointestinal haemorrhage is to ensure the patient's survival. Most studies still show that approximately 10 per cent of patients die. However, the average age of patients presenting with haemorrhage has gradually increased, so that in Europe approximately half are 60 years old or more.

Analysis of causes of death suggests that, although occasional patients do die from exsanguination, most die from medical postoperative complications, or else the gastrointestinal haemorrhage has been a final insult in an inevitable decline of health.

The death rate from exsanguination should be minimized by appropriate resuscitation, but postoperative deaths pose more of a problem. Do the complications arise because the patients are in poor condition when presented for surgery, and would earlier surgery decrease these complications? Or would early surgery result in unnecessary operations, thereby exposing more patients to the hazards of postoperative recovery? Available data do not provide a clear answer to this problem.

The exact criteria for recommending emergency surgery are difficult to define. They include (*a*) a suitably experienced surgeon; (*b*) continuing severe haemorrhage (but the use of modern infusion techniques should mean that the most patients are fully resuscitated prior to surgery); (*c*) a combination of high-risk factors that makes major rebleeding likely and (*d*) the failure of endoscopic sclerotherapy to control the haemorrhage. Elderly patients, those with gastric ulceration, and those who have suffered a brisk initial bleed, are all more liable to recurrent haemorrhage.

High-risk patients need urgent and careful resuscitation with early medical and surgical co-operation. This co-operation might usefully be carried through to the postoperative period, allowing physicians rather than surgeons to manage the medical problems.

There are no medical treatments that decisively decrease the incidence or severity of rebleeding. Neither high-dose H_2-antagonists nor omeprazole decrease the incidence of rebleeding in duodenal ulcer and, although they may do so in gastric ulcer, their use may encourage complacency. The patient should receive standard medical treatment, aiming to speed ulcer healing. After 8 weeks of full-dose antisecretory treatment, these patients should be given not only maintenance treatment, but also a regimen to eradicate *H. pylori*. Most patients will require iron supplements, but should be warned that they will notice a grey discoloration of their stools. Ferrous sulphate, 200 mg daily, is convenient and inexpensive (see Section 22).

Pyloric stenosis

Pyloric stenosis due to long-standing peptic ulcer disease must be differentiated from infantile and adult hypertrophic pyloric stenosis. More than 80 per cent of cases are due to duodenal ulcer. The diagnosis is suggested by a long history of peptic ulcer pain, with a more recent onset of vomiting. The vomitus contains food and articles of diet consumed the previous day may sometimes be identified. Weight loss is present in most patients. Visible gastric peristalsis and succussion splash are the physical signs, but they may be absent, especially if the patient is examined soon after vomiting. Dehydration, prerenal uraemia, or metabolic alkalosis may complicate the picture.

The diagnosis can be made on the history and clinical examination. A barium-meal examination will show a dilated, often atonic stomach: food debris may be present in the lumen. Gastric emptying of barium will be grossly prolonged. Endoscopy is helpful, but the stomach must first be emptied and washed out.

Gastric-outlet obstruction due to pyloric stenosis caused by chronic duodenal ulcer must be differentiated from malignant tumours, the most common being antral carcinoma. Cancer of the head of the pancreas or lymphoma can also interfere with gastric emptying. Other causes are benign tumours (adenomatous polyp or annular pancreas), adult hypertrophic pyloric stenosis, and rarely, a pyloric or duodenal diaphragm. The treatment is surgical, after correction of water, electrolyte, and metabolic abnormalities.

Gastric-outlet obstruction can occur during exacerbations of duodenal ulcer and is probably due to oedema surrounding the duodenal or pyloric-channel ulcers. The oedema and the obstruction are relieved by medical treatment and pyloric stenosis should not be diagnosed in these patients. Pyloric stenosis requiring surgery is now very rare in the United Kingdom, although it occurs fairly frequently in other countries—for example, in India. Milder degrees of stenosis may be relieved by endoscopic balloon dilatation.

Congenital hypertrophic pyloric stenosis is considered in Chapter 14.15.

Medical treatment of duodenal and gastric ulcer

GENERAL STRATEGY

All ulcer patients should be treated medically in the first instance but, in common with many other alimentary disorders, some patients with duodenal or gastric ulcer are ideally best managed jointly by a physician and a surgeon. Surgery is reserved for emergencies such as haemorrhage or perforation, complications such as pyloric stenosis or suspicion of malignancy, unusual circumstances such as a patient residing in a remote area presenting for definitive treatment with established chronic ulcer disease, or failure of medical treatment to control the symptoms of the disease or to eradicate *H. pylori*.

EVALUATION OF THE RESULTS OF ULCER THERAPY

The aims of treatment in duodenal and gastric ulcer are the relief of symptoms, the healing of the ulcer crater, the prevention of recurrence, and the prevention of complications. The first two of these aims can be achieved with a substantial measure of success by medical therapy; prevention of recurrence or complications depends on continuous treatment with a gastric-acid antisecretory drug. Evidence is now accumulating to show that successful eradication of *H. pylori* heals ulcers and very significantly lowers the relapse rate of duodenal ulcer and probably also of gastric ulcer.

Symptomatic relief, although of paramount importance to the patient, is very difficult to measure accurately because of the subjective nature of the symptoms. Indeed, the exact cause of ulcer pain is uncertain. It is now generally accepted that evaluation of ulcer-healing drugs must be monitored by fibreoptic endoscopy and that the end-point of treatment must be the complete healing of the ulcer crater. This is because changes of ulcer size are difficult or impossible to measure accurately endoscopically and also because a partly healed ulcer is a doubtful therapeutic benefit. Relapses must also be endoscopically confirmed in drug evaluation trials. The difficulties of accurately evaluating effects of treatment on ulcers are compounded by the poor correlation between remissions and relapses of symptoms, and the healing or recurrence of the ulcer crater, especially in gastric ulcer. In both duodenal and gastric ulceration, typical symptoms may be present in the absence of the ulcer crater. On the other hand, close surveillance of patients with duodenal ulcer studied in maintenance trials has shown that approximately one-third of recurrences are asymptomatic.

Additionally, the clinical attributes of both gastric and duodenal ulcer are subject to considerable variation by ill-defined factors such as race, geographical location, diet, and the tendency of the disease to alter, quite rapidly, with passage of time. It is therefore unwise to accept uncritically results from clinical trials, important as these results are for the scientific basis of ulcer therapy. Not only may data collected in one country not be applicable to another, but it must also be remembered that clinical trials are conducted on relatively small, highly selected populations of patients and the results may not apply to everyone. The results of trials are essential if effects of treatment are to be measured scientifically, but circumstances will often modify the management of individual patients.

DIET

Diet looms very large in the consciousness of most patients with peptic ulcer. Avoidance of fatty, fried, spicy, and rich meals is almost universal, and it is sometimes difficult to be certain how much of this is due to powerful folklore, and how much to some undefined pathophysiological mechanism. The factor that has been convincingly shown to relate directly to peptic ulcer pain is low intragastric or intraduodenal pH: neutralization of acid, or its removal by vomiting or nasogastric aspiration, usually brings rapid relief of ulcer dyspepsia. Studies exploring the possibility of other factors being involved in the production of peptic ulcer pain, for example gastroduodenal motility, have not been convincing. It is therefore not clear how certain foods trigger ulcer dyspepsia, and it is quite possible that in a proportion of patients the discomfort may originate from areas other than the ulcer crater, such as the colon.

Be this as it may, the patient with a peptic ulcer will almost invariably have excluded from the diet those foods that produce pain and distension. Although many elaborate dietary regimens have been advocated in the management of peptic ulcer disease in the past, there is no evidence that any of them affects the natural history of the disease. Detailed dietary advice is therefore unnecessary and can be summed up as 'avoid what upsets you, eat little and often, and go to bed with an empty stomach. There is some scientific backing for advising frequent, small meals, because food is a powerful buffer and intragastric pH rises after meals. Only highly obsessive individuals need detailed dietary guidance, and that for their own peace of mind, rather than for any good it does to their ulcers.

SMOKING AND ALCOHOL

There is now such ample evidence of the deleterious effects of smoking on various body systems, that advice to give up should be given to everyone who smokes, regardless of the diagnosis. Having said that, there is little evidence to show that giving up smoking has an effect on the healing rate of duodenal ulcer, although faster healing rates of gastric ulcer have been reported in those patients who gave up smoking, compared with those who continued to smoke. Relapse rates of duodenal ulcer have been shown to be significantly higher in smokers than in non-smokers, indeed in one study non-smoking had the same effect on relapse frequency as prophylactic treatment of duodenal ulcer with cimetidine. Whether giving up smoking (as opposed to non-smoking) affects the outcome of peptic ulcer is not known.

Similar considerations apply to alcohol consumption. Excessive drinking must be discouraged to avoid alcoholic liver disease, but total abstinence is not a condition required for ulcer healing.

REST, SEDATION, AND PSYCHOTROPHIC DRUGS

Rest and removal from stressful circumstances at home or in the workplace will act as a non-specific adjuvant to the treatment of peptic ulcer. Admission to hospital, however, is indicated only in extreme cases and is hardly ever necessary: indeed, it is contraindicated for most patients. Sedation has no part to play in the management of either gastric or duodenal ulcer. Indiscriminate prescribing of anxiolytics, such as diazepam, to patients with duodenal ulcer is not good practice. Discussion of the particular life circumstances and lifestyle with the patient can often be more helpful and more productive of introducing changes— often quite small adjustment is all that is needed—to achieve better symptom control. There is evidence from a small number of controlled trials that tricyclic antidepressants accelerate the healing of duodenal ulcers in the short-term, when compared with a placebo. There is insufficient evidence to recommend this class of drugs as an established therapy for duodenal ulcer: depression coexisting with peptic ulcer disease should be treated on its own merits. How tricyclic anti-depressants act in peptic ulcer disease is unknown.

ANTICHOLINERGICS

Gastric-acid secretion is stimulated, at least in part, through a cholinergic pathway, mainly mediated by the efferent vagal fibres. Interruption of the vagal pathway by surgical vagotomy leads to healing of duodenal ulcer. In theory, anticholinergic drugs also block the cholinergic pathway and should have beneficial effects on the ulcer: in practice this class of compounds has been disappointing. The size of the dose is severely limited by the occurrence of unwanted effects involving other cholinergically mediated functions such as visual accommodation, salivary secretion, and bladder emptying in men. Blurred vision, dry mouth, and difficulty in micturition generally prevent the administration of effective doses of anticholinergic therapy.

There is no good evidence that conventional anticholinergics are useful in the short- or long-term healing of either gastric or duodenal ulcer. Various workers have advocated administration of anticholinergics together with other drugs, such as antacids, where slowing of gastric emptying might increase the length of time during which the antacid is available for neutralization of acid. Similarly, administration of anticholinergics together with histamine H_2-receptor antagonists has been advocated by some workers, whilst others could not demonstrate the existence of any synergistic effect between them. Anticholinergics are contraindicated in patients with glaucoma. They also probably should not be used in patients with heartburn because, by lowering oesophageal sphincter pressure, they might make this condition worse.

This picture has been modified by the introduction of an anticholinergic drug (pirenzepine), which, by virtue of its selective antimuscarinic activity, is said to be more selective in blocking cholinergic receptors on or near gastric parietal cells. Pirenzepine, 50 mg twice or three times a day, has a mild antisecretory activity, yet data from controlled trials show that the drug does speed healing of duodenal ulcer.

BISMUTH PREPARATIONS

Bismuth probably has several modes of action on ulcer healing, which include chelation with protein in the base of the ulcer, stimulation of local release of prostaglandins, and inhibition of secretion and activity of pepsin. However, probably the most important effect is the rapid and profound suppression of *H. pylori* on bismuth treatment, which probably accounted for the decreased rates of relapse of duodenal ulcer after healing with tripotassium dicitrato bismuthate, reported before *H. pylori* was discovered. Unfortunately, monotherapy with bismuth alone produces negligible eradication rates, so that the infection recurs in most patients. The main usefulness of bismuth salts at present is in their use in triple-therapy regimens for eradication of *H. pylori*, which are discussed in the next sub-section.

Helicobacter pylori

The discovery of *H. pylori* by a multidisciplinary team in Western Australia has led to the realization that this organism is one of the most common chronic infection in man, responsible for almost all cases of chronic, non-immune gastritis, which heals when the infection is eradicated. *H. pylori* is very strongly associated with duodenal ulcer, and also has associations with gastric ulcer and with gastric cancer. The bacterium affects gastric secretory function and its discovery has revolutionized the concepts pertaining to gastric physiology, aetiology of foregut disease, and its treatment, especially in relation to duodenal ulcer.

The antrum of virtually all patients with duodenal ulcer not associated with non-steroidal anti-inflammatory drugs, or with gross hypersecretion of acid, is colonized by *H. pylori*. However, the number of infected individuals in a community grossly exceeds those developing a duodenal ulcer. The factors that determine the occurrence of duodenal ulcer in a colonized individual are not fully understood at present. However, evidence is accumulating to show that some strains of *H. pylori* may be more pathogenic, and hence associated with foregut diseases other than chronic gastritis. These strains express a high molecular weight protein (about 120 kDa), associated with a cytotoxin (a product of the *CagA* gene), which has been shown to be cytopathic *in vitro*. In Western countries the prevalence of *H. pylori* increases with age, from some 20 per cent at 20 years to over 50 per cent at 50 years. This may be a cohort effect, an aftermath of poorer sanitation to which the older individuals were exposed in their youth. By contrast, the prevalence of *H. pylori* in developing countries is much higher, and may reach 80 per cent by the age of 5 years. The prevalence of *H. pylori* is inversely related to socio-economic status and to the sophistication of public health facilities; it is directly related to overcrowding. It is remarkable that some of these factors also correlate with the incidence of gastric cancer. There is no evidence to show that *H. pylori* is itself carcinogenic; the link is probably through *H. pylori*-associated chronic gastritis proceeding to gastric atrophy.

H. pylori probably spreads through the oral/faecal route and the infection is acquired in early childhood. Although the human host (there is no animal reservoir) mounts an antigenic response to *H. pylori*, this does not clear the bacterium, and once acquired the infection is very chronic.

H. pylori grows only on the surface of gastric epithelial cells and below the protecting layer of adherent mucus. It also colonizes islands of gastric metaplasia in the duodenal cap; the damage to epithelial cells and the inflammatory reaction mounted by the host (i.e. gastritis and duodenitis) presumably set the scene for the development of ulceration by other aggressive factors, such as acid, pepsin, bile, or drugs. In addition to the inflammatory and immunological responses, *H. pylori* affects gastric secretory function by increasing the release of gastrin from the antral G cells, with consequent hypergastrinaemia and hypersecretion of gastric acid. The hypergastrinaemia is probably triggered by suppression of somatostatin release from antral D cells by *H. pylori*. Gastric acid output in response to GRF is about six times greater in *H. pylori*-positive duodenal ulcer patients, when compared with *Helicobacter pylori*-negative controls; *Helicobacter pylori*-positive controls secrete about three times the normal amount of acid when stimulated by GRP. The reason for the excessive acid output in patients with duodenal ulcer is not clear, but these changes revert to normal after eradication of *H. pylori* infection. Hyperpepsinaemia is also present and all these changes are reversed by eradication of *H. pylori*. Thus colonization by *H. pylori* may result in hyperacidity, which favours gastric metaplasia in the duodenum, opening the way for epithelial damage and ulcer formation.

Diagnosis

Care is needed in the interpretation of all diagnostic tests for *Helicobacter pylori*, as they may be affected by previous medication with antibiotics, omeprazole, or bismuth-containing compounds. The most widely available diagnostic method for *H. pylori* is either one of the variants of the CLOtest (see below), or the demonstration of *H. pylori* in an endoscopic biopsy: the Giemsa technique gives satisfactory results. The guidelines laid down by the Working Party on Gastritis should be followed, viz. at least two biopsies need to be taken from the antrum, in order to avoid sampling error and false-negative results. Biopsies from the gastric corpus are indicated, if the patient has been on proton-pump inhibitors, when the antral biopsies may be negative due to changes in the distribution of the organism within the stomach.

H. pylori is rich in urease, which hydrolyses urea to NH_4 and CO_2; this is utilized in two diagnostic tests, the CLOtest (done on an endoscopic antral biopsy) and the urea breath test. In the CLOtest the NH_4 produces a colour change in a pH-sensitive indicator in a medium in which the biopsy is placed. In the urea breath test, expired air is collected after ingestion of ^{13}C- or ^{14}C-labelled urea and the excreted, labelled CO_2 is measured by mass spectrometry, or scintillation counter, respectively. Both tests are highly specific and sensitive. [^{13}C] urea breath tests are not yet widely available, but are non-invasive, can be used serially, and there are no contraindications to their use. The dose of [^{14}C] urea used in this variant of the breath test has been recently decreased with, it is claimed no loss of specificity or sensitivity; if this is confirmed, this test will be very useful.

Serological tests (based on enzyme-linked immunosorbent assay) are available, but attention must be paid to the type of antigen used. The fall in anti-*H. pylori* titre can be used to assess the results of treatment, but it takes several months for the antigen levels to decrease. Serology is valuable in epidemiological studies and it has been proposed for screening dyspeptic subjects referred for endoscopy, the hypothesis being that young (under 45 years), seronegative patients are most unlikely to have a duodenal ulcer, or a malignancy.

Culture of *H. pylori* provides the diagnostic 'gold standard' and is needed to determine the sensitivity of the bacterium to antibiotics—at present this has meant mainly its sensitivity to metronidazole, although the sensitivity to macrolides may become important in the future. Specialized techniques are necessary to grow this fastidious organism and there is a proportion of failed cultures, even in experienced hands.

Effect of **H. pylori** *on duodenal ulcer*

As duodenal ulcer is almost unknown in *H. pylori*-negative individuals, the organism must make a major contribution to the aetiology of this disease and in the maintenance of chronicity of the ulcer. Duodenal ulcer is a multifactorial disease, as evidenced by ulcer healing produced by gastric acid-suppressing drugs, such as H_2-blockers, that do not affect *H. pylori*.

This contention is further borne out by reports documenting the healing of duodenal ulcer after eradication of *H. pylori* in the absence of any other therapy. Perhaps even more exciting is the accumulating evidence suggesting that the incidence of relapse decreases very significantly after eradication of *H. pylori*. It is reasonable to state, that in the absence of other risk factors, the duodenal ulcer should remain healed as long as the patient remains free of *H. pylori* infection. As the incidence of reinfection seems to be very low amongst adults in the West, eradication of *H. pylori* appears to change the natural history of duodenal ulcer. Reinfection rates have not yet been studied in emergent countries, where they are likely to be higher than in the West.

Gastric ulcer and **H. pylori**

The association between gastric ulcer and *H. pylori* is less strong than with duodenal ulcer, with about 80 per cent of patients being *H. pylori* positive. Few trials of eradication of *H. pylori* in gastric ulcer are so far available, but they suggest that in the patients originally harbouring the organism, eradication is followed by a decreased incidence of relapse.

Treatment

The aim of treatment is eradication of *H. pylori*, defined as negative tests for the bacterium done 1 month, or longer, after the end of antimicrobial therapy. Negative tests obtained at shorter intervals from the end of treatment show suppression, not eradication, of *H. pylori* and should not be taken as indicating successful therapy.

H. pylori is difficult to eradicate because of its ecological niche on the surface of the gastric epithelium, beneath the adherent layer of mucus. This habitat is poorly penetrated by antimicrobial agents. Moreover, *H. pylori* can survive deep in the gastric pits, emerging later from these sanctuary sites. Another factor that interferes with successful treatment is the very ready development of resistant strains, principally to metronidazole, but also to other antimicrobials. Metronidazole-resistant strains of *H. pylori* exist in the community, due to previous medication with this agent, for example for pelvic infections, or tropical diarrhoeas; these resistant strains are thus more prevalent in women (20 per cent) and in developing countries (80 per cent). The use of only one agent against *H. pylori* infection (monotherapy) is thus to be discouraged. Although resistance to tripotassium dicitrato bismuthate does not develop, and although the incidence of early relapse after a healing dose of bismuth is lower than after cimetidine, eradication rates on bismuth alone are negligible at less than 10 per cent.

At the time of writing, a definitive treatment regimen for *H. pylori* infection has not yet been established. The literature is replete with numerous small therapeutic trials reporting results of a wide variety of treatment schedules, using the different combinations of antimicrobial agents, given in different doses and for different periods of time. Large blinded trials, and in particular direct comparisons of different therapies are generally lacking. Thus it is impossible to come to firm conclusions concerning efficacy, safety and cost.

The main reasons for failure of *H. pylori* treatment are resistance to the drugs, poor compliance triggered by side-effects (affecting 10 to 35 per cent of patients), or by complicated drug schedule. Triple therapies usually comprise bismuth with two antimicrobials, but there have been encouraging results with the use of non-bismuth triple regimens—for example, an antisecretory drug (ranitidine or omeprazole) together with an imidazole (tinidazole or metronidazole), and an antimicrobial (amoxycillin or clarithromycin) given for 7 to 10 days. Eradication rates are very variable, but usually range between 70 and 80 per cent.

Failure of eradication therapy

Microbial resistance, or non-compliance are the commonest causes of failure. Repeat endoscopy with bacterial culture of biopsies may help select an appropriate antibiotic regimen.

Indications for eradication

Guide-lines for eradication therapy and peptic ulceration have been the subject of much debate. Surveys of gastroenterologists in various countries disclose a general lack of agreement, with some advocating eradication treatment for all *Helicobacter pylori*-positive ulcer patients, whilst other reserve this for relapses after conventional therapy, or for patients with complications of ulcer disease. Most workers in the *Helicobacter pylori* area advise eradication therapy at the time of diagnosis. This is in line with a consensus statement of the National Institutes of Health in the United States. Thus, eradication treatment for *H. pylori* should be offered to all *H. pylori*-positive, non-NSAID associated, duodenal and gastric ulcer patients. Eradication treatment should not be offered to patients with functional dyspepsia. However, it has to be borne in mind that the treatment will not work in all ulcer patients. Thus there is a considerable need for counselling on the possible outcomes of therapy, and especially those in whom the treatment has changed. Many people are now aware of the association between *Helicobacter pylori* and gastric cancer, and they need careful and reassuring information from the doctor.

It is ideally desirable for the result of eradication treatment to be documented. This can be done using non-invasive techniques such as the ^{13}C- or ^{14}C-urea breath test, or by a repeat endoscopy and biopsy. Complete healing of gastric ulceration still needs to be confirmed by endoscopy, even if eradication has been successful to ensure that the possibility of mucosal malignancy has been eliminated.

SUCRALFATE

Sucralfate is a basic aluminium salt of sucrose octasulphate. It is said to increase in viscosity on contact with gastric acid, forming a protective coating for damaged mucosa. It is also said to absorb pepsin and bile salts. Sucralfate does not affect acid secretion. Controlled comparisons of sucralfate against placebo in the short-term treatment of duodenal ulcer show the drug to accelerate ulcer healing significantly. The drug is safe, the dose being 1 g four times daily before meals, but there is some systemic absorption of aluminium. Constipation is the only common side-effect.

CARBENOXOLONE SODIUM

Carbenoxolone sodium is a synthetic derivative of glycyrrhizinic acid, which is a naturally occurring constituent of liquorice. Liquorice root has been traditionally used for the treatment of dyspepsia. The mechanism of action of carbenoxolone sodium is unclear.

The main limitation of carbenoxolone therapy is the drug's unwanted aldosterone-like activity. Sodium and water retention, hypertension, and hypokalaemia have all been reported, and are potentially dangerous, especially in the elderly or in those with cardiorespiratory or renal insufficiency. Carbenoxolone is used rarely if at all, because a range of safer medications is now available.

HISTAMINE H₂-RECEPTOR ANTAGONISTS

Histamine, together with an enzyme system that controls its synthesis and degradation, is abundantly present in the human gastric mucosa and is a powerful stimulant of gastric acid and pepsin secretion. Histamine (released by gastric mucosal enterochromaffin-like cells), acetylcholine (released by the efferent vagal nerve endings), and gastrin (released by the antral G cells) are all involved in the stimulation of the gastric parietal cell. Experimental observations indicate that there is a close interrelation between the three secretory stimulants, and that the inhibition of one will markedly decrease the effects of the others. Antagonism of the secretory effects of histamine powerfully inhibits gastric secretion produced by hormonal or neurogenic stimulation.

Histamine H₂-receptor antagonists are a class of antihistaminic drugs, whose main pharmacological action in the body is the inhibition of gastric-acid secretion. The effects of histamine on various body systems are mediated through two populations of receptors, termed H₁- and H₂-histamine receptors. The effects of histamine on smooth muscle of the gut, the bronchial tree, and the arterial vasculature are mediated via the H₁-receptors and are blocked by the classical antihistaminic drugs such as chlorpheniramine maleate. H₁-receptor antagonists do not inhibit the powerful stimulatory effects of histamine on gastric acid and pepsin output. This observation was well known for many years, when histamine was used as a stimulant for gastric secretory tests, the patient being protected from the systemic effects of histamine by pretreatment with a conventional antihistaminic drug. It was only in 1972, however, that the concept of H₁- and H₂-histamine receptors was clearly formulated, and this then paved the way for development of specific drugs to block the action of histamine at H₂-receptor sites.

The pharmacology of histamine H₂-receptor antagonists has been studied very extensively in laboratory animals and in man. The first drug to find widespread clinical application was cimetidine, followed some 6 years later by ranitidine. In humans, histamine H₂-receptor blockade with either drug results in inhibition of acid secretion evoked by all known antagonists. Thus, either cimetidine or ranitidine administered orally or intravenously will markedly decrease acid and pepsin output stimulated by histamine, gastrin, or its analogues, cholinergic drugs, the vagus and, most importantly, food. Basal and nocturnal acid secretion can be inhibited completely, whilst doses of cimetidine (400 mg, twice daily), or ranitidine (150 mg, twice daily) will inhibit acid output and significantly decrease 24-h intragastric acidity (Fig. 4). The only other major acute pharmacological action of H₂-receptor blockade in man is the abolition of that part of histamine-induced vasodilation (histamine flush) that is not blocked by conventional antihistamines. This is because peripheral blood vessels probably have both H₂- and H₁-receptors on or near their smooth muscle. This effect is of no clinical importance.

Histamine H₂-receptor antagonists are rapidly absorbed from the upper small intestine and excreted largely unchanged by the kidneys. The metabolites, which include sulphoxide derivatives, have not been shown to have any important pharmacological effects. H₂-antagonists do not accumulate in the body.

Early histamine H₂-receptor antagonists were not evaluated clinically in large numbers of patients either because absorption was erratic (burimamide) or because of reversible granulocytopenia occasionally produced by the drug (metiamide). Cimetidine was the drug first generally available for clinical use. Other H₂-antagonists with improved specificity—notably ranitidine, famotidine, and nizatidine—have been developed and tested clinically. Although all these drugs bind at H₂-receptors, cimetidine also binds at other sites in the body and some of these interactions may rarely give rise to unwanted effects in some patients.

Fig. 4 Mean hourly H⁺ activity (i.e. intragastric acidity) over 24 h in 10 patients with duodenal ulcer receiving placebo, cimetidine 1 g daily (four divided doses), or ranitidine 150 mg twice daily. (Reproduced from Walt, R.P. *et al.* (1981). *Gut*, **22**, 49.)

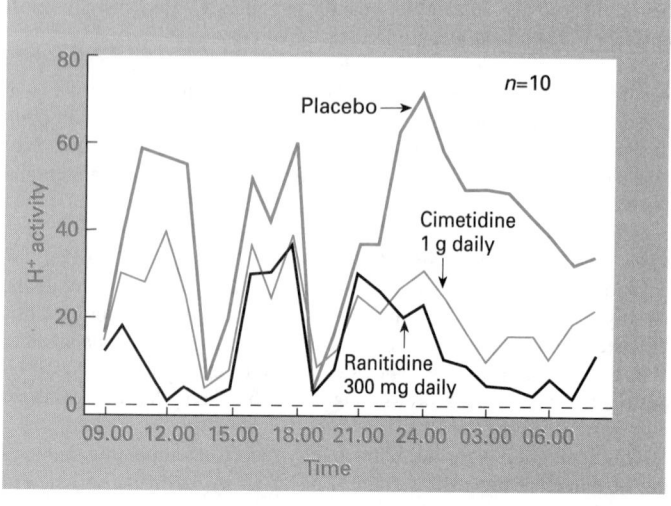

Cimetidine binds at cytochrome P450, which forms part of the mixed oxygenase metabolizing system in the liver. Inhibition of this enzyme by cimetidine can potentiate the action of drugs such as warfarin, phenytoin, or diazepam. Cimetidine also binds at androgen receptors. In terms of antisecretory activity the following oral doses are equipotent: cimetidine 800 mg, ranitidine 300 mg, famotidine 40 mg, nizatidine 300 mg. The drugs have a similar half-life in the peripheral circulation (approximately 120 min) and the duration of action is also similar.

Short-term treatment of duodenal and gastric ulcer with H$_2$-receptor antagonists

Short-term treatment usually means outpatient therapy for a period of 4 to 8 weeks. Approximately 80 to 95 per cent of gastric or duodenal ulcers will heal under this regimen, the proportion of ulcers healed being significantly higher in patients receiving the drug compared with those receiving a placebo, both groups having unlimited access to antacids.

The original dose of cimetidine in the United Kingdom and Europe was 1 g daily (200 mg three times a day and 400 mg at night), in the United States a 300 mg tablet was used and the daily dose was usually 1.2 g daily. Cimetidine 400 mg twice daily, or 800 mg at bedtime, are now the standard dose regimens. The customary dose of ranitidine throughout the world was 150 mg twice daily, but ranitidine 300 mg at bedtime is equally effective. Famotidine and nizatidine were introduced with bedtime doses at 40 and 300 mg, respectively.

Controlled comparisons between the four bedtime dosing regimens suggest that these H$_2$-receptor blockers are equipotent in terms of percentage of duodenal ulcers healed. Administration of an H$_2$-antagonist is usually accompanied by rapid relief of dyspepsia, the symptoms usually subsiding completely within a week of starting treatment.

Should H$_2$-receptor blockade be continued as monotherapy for longer than 8 or 12 weeks at full dose, if the duodenal ulcer fails to heal? Probably not as, in general, it is unlikely that H$_2$-receptor blockers will be effective if they have failed to work at the end of this time. Such a patient should be offered a repeat endoscopy to determine whether ulceration actually persists. The ulcer should be biopsied and, if the Zollinger–Ellison syndrome has been excluded, the patient should receive additional treatment in an attempt to eradicate H. pylori. The patient should be switched to omeprazole if, after a further 8 weeks, the ulcer has still not healed.

The benefit of H$_2$-blockade has been measured by the increase in the number of duodenal ulcers healed in the treated group compared with placebo, but this benefit varies considerably in different trials. The reasons for this variation are not clear, but must depend, at least in part, on dissimilarities in environment, selection of patients, and antacid consumption. It has been shown, for example, that patients in the United States with gastric ulcer consume 10 or 20 times the amount of antacid taken by patients in England or France.

Long-term (maintenance) treatment with an H$_2$-blocker is used to prevent ulcer relapse or complications. The usual dose is half that used for acute ulcer healing—for example, cimetidine 400 mg or ranitidine 150 mg at bedtime.

Unwanted effects of H$_2$-receptor blockade

Mild hypergastrinaemia does occur during H$_2$-receptor blockade. The release of gastrin from the antral G cells is partly controlled by a negative feedback mechanism dependent on the pH in the antral lumen. Drug-induced, decreased intragastric acidity slightly increases plasma gastrin concentration. As gastrin is a trophic hormone for the parietal cells, it is possible that prolonged hypergastrinaemia could lead to parietal-cell hyperplasia, with consequent hypersecretion of acid once treatment is stopped leading to severe re-ulceration. Parietal-cell hyperplasia has never been detected in man, although modest nocturnal hyperacidity persists for 3 to 6 days after withdrawal of H$_2$-blockade. The recurrence rate of duodenal ulcer is much the same in patients who have had 12 months' maintenance treatment as in those who have not.

In experimental animals and in in vitro models cimetidine has been

shown to have a weak antiandrogenic action. Sporadic instances of male erectile impotence have been reported, but this is not a serious problem in practice: the other H$_2$-blockers have no antiandrogen properties. Prolactin concentrations increase after bolus intravenous cimetidine (but not after ranitidine), but oral cimetidine does not affect prolactin metabolism. Gynaecomastia in men and galactorrhoea in women has been occasionally reported: this rare unwanted effect is most common in patients treated with cimetidine for the Zollinger–Ellison syndrome. Cimetidine (but not the other H$_2$-blockers) affects the blood concentrations of drugs metabolized by the hepatic microsmal enzymes. Blood concentrations of warfarin, labetolol, diazepam, and phenytoin are significantly higher in patients receiving cimetidine, so that smaller doses of these drugs may be necessary. Both cimetidine and ranitidine cross the blood–brain barrier in healthy subjects and are present in low concentrations in cerebrospinal fluid obtained at lumbar puncture. This is probably of little significance in healthy people. However, instances of reversible mental confusion and coma have been reported in elderly or severely ill patients in intensive care units receiving cimetidine.

Probably the most common side-effect of cimetidine is mild sedation and tiredness, which disappears when the drug is withdrawn. It is rarely severe enough to interfere with treatment. Cimetidine may cause a minor, and unimportant rise, in creatinine or hepatic transaminases. Marrow toxic effects are not a problem, although H$_2$-antagonists should be avoided in patients with a compromised bone marrow (for example, during chemotherapy for leukaemia).

Concern has been expressed about possible carcinogenic effects of long-term treatment with gastric-acid antisecretory drugs. Inhibition of acid secretion favours bacterial colonization of the stomach. Bacterial enzymes can catalyse the conversion of dietary nitrates to nitrites, with consequent formation of carcinogenic nitrosamines. Gastric anacidity in pernicious anaemia and gastric hypoacidity after partial gastrectomy are associated with an increased incidence of gastric cancer. In both these conditions, however, additional factors, such as gastritis and severe bile reflux, are also present. There are no grounds for withholding long-term H$_2$-blockade because of possible carcinogenesis, but obviously this area needs continuing careful clinical research.

H$^+$, K$^+$-ATPase INHIBITORS

Omeprazole was the first of a series of drugs that inhibit gastric-acid secretion by irreversible inhibition of the proton pump in the gastric parietal cells. This is achieved by blocking the H$^+$, K$^+$-ATPase enzyme system that provides energy for the secretion of protons into the gastric lumen. Newer, similar drugs include lansoprazole and pantoprazole.

Omeprazole is absorbed in the intestine and reaches the gastric parietal cells through the bloodstream. Omeprazole is a weak base and it can pass through cell membranes but, on exposure to a pH of less than 2, it becomes protonated. Thus the drug is trapped and concentrated in the parietal cell (an acid compartment), where it is converted into the active form, a sulphenamide. It is this active form of omeprazole that inhibits H$^+$, K$^+$-ATPase. Resumption of acid secretion by the parietal cell requires synthesis of new H$^+$, K$^+$-ATPase.

Gastric acid degrades omeprazole; hence the drug is formulated in an enteric coating that releases omeprazole when the pH is above 6. Although peak plasma concentrations of the drug occur 2 to 4 h after oral administration, bioavailability increases during the first few days of treatment, probably because increasing inhibition of acid secretion results in less intragastric degradation of omeprazole. Although omeprazole is present in the plasma for only a few hours after oral dosing, the covalent binding with H$^+$, K$^+$-ATPase results in a sustained inhibition of gastric acid secretion and 24-h control of intragastric acidity. Individuals vary in their response to an oral dose of omeprazole, with approximately one-third of patients with duodenal ulcer demonstrating a profound decrease of intragastric acidity whilst receiving omeprazole, 20 mg every morning, and almost all patients responding to omeprazole, 40 mg every morning. There is a period of sustained hypoacidity when treatment with omeprazole is stopped abruptly, with normal intragastric acidity returning 3 to 7 days later.

Safety

Treatment with omeprazole generally is extremely well tolerated by patients, with clinical trials reporting a low incidence of non-specific symptoms. The major concern is the drug's ability to cause a profound decrease of intragastric acidity—with the theoretical possibility of increased susceptibility to enteric infection or infestation, the proven development of bacterial overgrowth of the stomach and duodenum, and an unremitting rise of 24-h plasma gastrin concentration during treatment.

Gastrin is a trophic hormone for the enterochromaffin-like cell of the gastric mucosa, and rats dosed with omeprazole for up to 2 years developed dose-dependent gastric carcinoids. This phenomenon has been demonstrated with high-dose regimens of a range of other gastric-acid antisecretory drugs in the rat; similar gastric carcinoids develop in a minority of patients with pernicious anaemia. Gastric carcinoids have not developed after prolonged treatment in man using omeprazole, but proliferation of enterochromaffin-like cells may occur in such patients, superimposed on a background of accelerated gastric mucosal atrophy. Many conditions associated with aggressive peptic ulceration will require long-term treatment, and omeprazole behaves as an 'all or nothing' drug. There is no predictable, modest dose of omeprazole—for example, some patients respond to dosing with omeprazole, 10 mg daily, by marked inhibition of 24-h intragastric acidity, while others are not responsive at all. Long-term treatment with omeprazole must be inevitably associated with a long-term change of intragastric acidity.

PROSTAGLANDINS

Misoprostol is the only generally available synthetic prostaglandin analogue available for the management of peptic ulceration. Theoretical benefits of treatment with such a compound involve not only a mild gastric antisecretory activity, but also a range of potential benefits associated with enhancement of gastric mucosal defence. However, the development of these drugs has been extremely problematical—not least that the doses are in microgram quantities, and the clinical benefits are largely restricted to doses that are sufficient to control gastric-acid secretion.

Misoprostol is generally well tolerated, although a substantial minority of patients may notice either abdominal pain, or diarrhoea, particularly during the first few days of dosing. In addition, the drug has a uterotonic activity, which can induce abortion, and must therefore not be given to pregnant women, or to women of childbearing age who may conceive during the treatment period.

In general, misoprostol has not found a place in routine treatment of duodenal or gastric ulcer, because of unimpressive healing rates and fairly troublesome unwanted effects. It has been advocated as preventive therapy in patients receiving non-steroidal anti-inflammatory drugs, where clinical trials indicate a lower incidence of duodenal ulcer, or gastric ulcer, in those patients given the active treatment, on comparison with placebo.

ULCERS AND NON-STEROIDAL ANTI-INFLAMMATORY DRUGS (NSAIDS)

As the average age of the population increases, so does the incidence of arthropathies and thus the consumption of NSAIDs by the elderly. This has led to an emergence of NSAID-associated duodenal ulcers and gastric ulcers in the older patients, who are at risk to the potentially life-threatening complications of perforation or haemorrhage. A significantly increased proportion of these complications in those aged 65 or over is linked to the usage of NSAIDs. Clinical trials have shown that medication with H_2-receptor antagonists can prevent the development of duodenal ulcer, and medication with misoprostol prevents the formation of duodenal and gastric ulcer in patients receiving NSAIDs; both types of

ulcer heal on H_2-antagonists despite continued treatment with NSAIDs. However, no trial has so far shown that the incidence of ulcer complications is lowered by these therapies. At present there is no indication for treating every patient on NSAIDs with either H_2-blockers or prostaglandin analogues; patients deemed at risk—those with a history of peptic ulcer, the very elderly or frail individuals—should be selected for prophylactic treatment, which should be continued concomitantly with the NSAID. Existing peptic ulcers should be healed on H_2-antagonists, with long-term maintenance treatment thereafter, as at present the role of H. pylori in NSAID-associated ulcer is not clear. Clinically, the problems can be demanding, because symptoms of indigestion are common in patients on NSAIDs, but are not a reliable guide to the presence or absence of ulcer; doubts should be resolved by endoscopy. Even so, as pointed out above, occurrence of a major complication may be unheralded by preceding dyspepsia.

ANTACIDS

Antacids are chemicals that neutralize gastric hydrochloric acid, and are now mainly used for the symptomatic management of dyspepsia. Most antacid regimens involve the use of a mixture of several alkalis—for example, sodium bicarbonate, aluminium hydroxide, calcium carbonate, and magnesium hydroxide. To this combination there is often added a silicone (probably for the benefit of the advertising copywriter rather than medical benefit) and a carminative, usually a natural oil such as peppermint. Aluminium–magnesium antacids are usually preferred to those containing sodium bicarbonate, because of the latter's high sodium content, short duration of action, and tendency to produce alkalosis. Calcium-containing antacids are no longer popular because they tend to stimulate gastric-acid secretion and may produce hypercalcaemia with impaired renal function.

Short-term management

The management begins with the diagnosis and, as outlined above, this has to be established either radiologically or, preferably, endoscopically. The patient is given common-sense advice regarding frequent small meals and is started on ulcer-healing drugs. Strict dietary schedules are unnecessary, except for the obsessive. Smoking should be discouraged on general medical grounds; the same applies for excessive consumption of alcohol. Admission to hospital is virtually never necessary.

The main difference between the short-term management of duodenal and gastric ulcer lies in the need to exclude the presence of gastric carcinoma in patients with a gastric ulcer. It is therefore mandatory to endoscope every patient with gastric ulcer at the start of treatment, excluding only those patients who are unfit for elective endoscopy. Multiple targeted biopsies and exfoliative cytology brushings must be taken. It is then ideal to repeat the endoscopy after 8 to 12 weeks of medical therapy to check that the ulcer has healed: if still present, then histopathological evaluation must be repeated. This is because the diagnosis of early intramucosal carcinoma can be difficult to establish, while results of resection of early gastric cancer are good and quite different from the gloomy prognosis of advanced neoplasm of the stomach. The failure of an even apparently benign gastric ulcer to heal also influences the management (see below).

By contrast, once the diagnosis of duodenal ulcer is established, repeated endoscopy or radiology is unnecessary and the management is based on symptomatic assessment of the patient. Reinvestigation is only needed if the pattern of symptoms changes suggesting the need to revise the diagnosis, if complications occur, or before operation to provide the surgeon with up-to-date anatomical information.

CHOICE OF SHORT-TERM DRUGS

There is now available a range of drugs, all apparently active in accelerating the healing of peptic ulcers. Results of clinical trials indicate that there is apparently little difference between results of any of these agents in the short-term treatment of peptic ulcer. This is highly surprising, because the drugs have such dissimilar pharmacological properties. Neither carbenoxolone sodium, nor tripotassium dicitrato bismuthate, nor sucralfate, affect acid secretion. Antacids neutralize acid in the gastric lumen, while H_2-receptor antagonists and omeprazole suppress acid output to a variable extent. Despite these differences, all the drugs produce a 80 to 95 per cent healing rate after 4 to 12 weeks of outpatient treatment. Why the remaining ulcers fail to heal promptly is not clear, and analysis of variables such as age, sex, length of history, acid secretion, or consumption of tobacco and alcohol has failed to provide an answer: failure to take the tablets must play a part in some cases.

Taking the results of therapeutic trials available at their face value, therefore, the efficacy of treatment is not apparently of prime importance in deciding which drugs to use in the short-term management of peptic ulcer, and the choice of therapeutic agent must depend on other factors, such as safety, convenience, and cost.

Omeprazole produces the fastest ulcer healing and probably the best relief of daytime ulcer pain in the first days of treatment—but freedom from ulcer pain occurs before ulcer healing, and the shortest acceptable length of treatment with omeprazole is probably 4 weeks. Similar considerations apply to lansoprazole. Treatment to eradicate H. pylori could be offered to patients following remission of symptoms, but the present complicated drug regimens limit this strategy.

Pirenzepine, misoprostol, or sucralfate may be useful in some patients and can be used if H_2-receptor antagonists or omeprazole are badly tolerated or unavailable. There is no need for routine prescription of psychotropic or anxiolytic drugs, unless there is a specific clinical reason.

Long-term management

The H_2-receptor antagonists were the first drugs to be unequivocally shown to affect the incidence of peptic ulcer relapse.

The evidence was provided by data collected in maintenance trials, in which patients with ulcer healing confirmed at endoscopy were followed for 6 or 12 months, whilst receiving an H_2-antagonist or a placebo. Endoscopic examinations were done at predetermined intervals, or when symptoms recurred, and showed that long-term administration of these drugs results in a highly significant decrease in the incidence of relapse in duodenal ulcer. Maintenance therapy of gastric ulcer gives similar results, but the evidence is less strong than for duodenal ulcer, as the number of patients studied in controlled trials is smaller. Continuing benefit from H_2-blockade has been shown even after an average of 7.5 years of maintenance treatment: a switch to placebo resulted in rapid symptomatic relapse in half of a group of patients with duodenal ulcer. However, there is a definite, if slow, tendency of duodenal ulcers to recur despite maintenance treatment. The reasons for this are not clear, but failure to take the tablets probably plays a part: it is notoriously difficult to persuade symptom-free people to take any treatment regularly—with the possible exception of the contraceptive pill. Any consideration of very prolonged maintenance therapy with an H_2-antagonist, or any other agent, must take into account the fact that a number of subjects will relapse despite medical treatment. Most of these subjects will respond to a short course of full-dose H_2-blockade.

The dosage regimens commonly used in maintenance treatment are either cimetidine, 400 mg, or rantidine, 150 mg at bedtime. Two large multicentre trials comparing these regimens have shown ranitidine, 150 mg at bedtime, to be significantly better than cimetidine, 400 mg at bedtime, in prevention of relapse in duodenal ulcer.

A choice of therapeutic strategies is available for the long-term management of a patient with duodenal ulcer: either intermittent therapy (giving full-dose H_2-blockade only at time of ulcer relapse) or continuous therapy (giving low-dose bedtime H_2-blockade, with full-dose treatment only when there is rare symptomatic relapse). The best general guide to decide which regimen is suitable for the individual patient is the previous history of ulcer symptoms. The patient who has one or two well-defined relapses of duodenal ulcer each year, but who remains well

otherwise, clearly does not need continuous maintenance medication. On the other hand, the individual with continuous symptoms, or whose symptom-free periods are short, will tend to do better on continuous therapy. Preliminary attempts have been made to compare the clinical efficacy of the two regimens, but at present it is not possible to come to a definite conclusion, nor is it easy to lay down firm rules as to how long to continue H_2-receptor antagonist maintenance therapy in patients with duodenal ulcer. Patients who cannot risk an ulcer complication (the elderly or those with another serious medical problem) should receive long-term maintenance H_2-blockade. There is little or no evidence to suggest that long-term treatment affects the natural history of duodenal ulcer, so that once treatment is discontinued the ulcer recurrence rate reverts to pretreatment levels. Despite reports to the contrary, there is no convincing evidence to show that 'rebound' ulceration is a serious problem in the post-treatment period. Some physicians prefer to tail off maintenance treatment rather than stopping the drug abruptly. There are no experimental data to support this, but it is probably good practice.

The safety of prolonged medication with H_2-antagonists has been studied intensively in a small number of patients, an additional general clinical experience involving very large numbers of patients suggests that these drugs are safe for long term, or lifetime, use. Omeprazole is used rarely for the long-term treatment of uncomplicated peptic ulceration, because there is no predictable 'mild' antisecretory dose of the drug (see above).

The general view was that recurrent gastric ulcers should be treated surgically and that failure of maintenance treatment should lead to a partial gastrectomy. Exceptions to the rule were either patients for whom the risk for operation was unacceptable, or younger patients were the long-term metabolic consequences and the slightly increased risk of carcinoma in the gastric remnant would make one persevere longer with medical treatment. Although there is now a tendency to persevere with medical treatment, a non-healing gastric ulcer is unusual unless the patient is receiving an NSAID, or is covertly taking aspirin, or the ulcer is malignant.

Surgical treatment

INDICATIONS FOR SURGERY

Elective surgery for duodenal ulcer is now almost extinct. In duodenal ulcer, absolute indications for surgical intervention are continuing or life-threatening haemorrhage, perforation, or organic pyloric stenosis. In the uncomplicated patient, frequent and severe recurrences that interfere with social or professional life, poor response to, or poor compliance with, medication, residence in remote areas with limited access to medical facilities, and occupations where a sudden haematemesis or perforation may endanger the life of others all indicate the need for surgical intervention.

The general answer to the question of 'When is surgery indicated in the uncomplicated case of duodenal ulcer?' is 'When medical treatment has failed to control the symptoms adequately'. As almost every patient with duodenal ulcer does respond to H_2-blockade, or H. pylori eradication, or omeprazole, only rare patients need to be considered for surgery. Before an elective operation, the duodenal ulcer should be biopsied at endoscopy to exclude rare lymphoma, tuberculosis, Crohn's disease or carcinoma. The patients' fasting plasma gastrin concentration should also be measured to exclude the Zollinger–Ellison syndrome. Eradication of H. pylori should also be attempted before elective surgery is considered.

In gastric ulcer, absolute indications for surgery are similar to those for duodenal ulcer, except that pyloric stenosis does not occur and that suspicion of carcinoma should lead to thorough re-evaluation: if neoplasm cannot be confidently excluded, it is safer to proceed to operation. As already stated, most gastroenterologists have advocated early, rather than late surgery for benign, uncomplicated gastric ulcers, although there are a few studies suggesting that the outcome of unoperated gastric ulcer may not be as bad as generally believed.

CHOICE OF OPERATION

Uncomplicated duodenal ulcer is now almost invariably treated by some variant of vagotomy: either a truncal vagotomy with a drainage procedure (pyloroplasty or gastroenterostomy), or by selective, or highly selective vagotomy. This latter operation denervates only the parietal-cell mass, leaving the innervation of the antral pump, and thus control of gastric emptying, undisturbed. Aggressive duodenal ulceration often recurs after this type of minimal surgery, and a vagotomy plus antrectomy may be the best procedure—a good reason to persevere with medical treatment. Gastric ulcers are usually dealt with by a Billroth-type partial gastrectomy: surgical texts can be consulted for details.

OUTCOME OF OPERATIONS

Surgical treatment works well for properly selected patients with either type of ulcer. Highly selective vagotomy for duodenal ulcer is attractive, because it is a physiologically logical and least mutilating operation. The incidence of unwanted effects is very low: the main disadvantage is a relatively high recurrence rate, reported from various centres as 5 to 15 per cent. Other types of vagotomy have a lower recurrence rate, but the incidence of unwanted effects such as postvagotomy diarrhoea, or dumping, is higher at about 5 per cent. Vagotomy and antrectomy carries the lowest recurrence rate, but mortality is slightly higher than after vagotomy and drainage, where it is less than 1 per cent in good centres.

Recurrence is rare after elective partial gastrectomy for chronic gastric ulcer, but the mortality is at around 3 per cent, mainly because gastric ulcer tends to be the disease of elderly patients from low socioeconomic groups. Late or early dumping is an unwanted sequel of partial gastrectomy. Early dumping is due to hypovolaemia caused by copious secretion of fluid into the intestinal lumen provoked by the rapid emptying of a hyperosmolar load into a small gut. Late dumping is associated with hypoglycaemia: rapid absorption of a large carbohydrate load causes hypersecretion of insulin with consequent overswing of blood glucose concentration to below normal. Symptoms of dumping can be controlled in most patients by decreasing the carbohydrate intake in the diet and by advising them not to take fluids with, or immediately after, meals.

Later sequelae of partial gastrectomy include weight loss, iron-deficiency anaemia, mild steatorrhoea, and occasional osteomalacia. Death from smoking-related diseases (especially carcinoma of the lung and ischaemic vascular disease) is common in these patients. There is also a slightly increased incidence of carcinoma in the gastric remnant. For these reasons it is important that all patients with partial gastrectomy should be seen yearly at a follow-up clinic. At each visit the haemoglobin and the serum calcium, phosphate, and alkaline phosphatase should be measured and the patient's weight recorded. The anaemia usually responds to oral iron supplements. Abnormalities in calcium, phosphate, and an elevated alkaline phosphatase level should lead to bone biopsy to confirm or refute the presence of osteomalacia which, if present, can be treated by oral calcium and vitamin D supplements. Recurrence of symptoms, anorexia, further sudden weight loss, or loss of well-being should alert to the possibility of a neoplasm and lead to a gastroscopy.

POSTSURGICAL RECURRENT ULCERS

Duodenal ulcer may recur after any type of vagotomy, but recurrence is most common after the highly selective (parietal-cell) type. Reulceration becomes apparent by return of the previous ulcer symptoms, usually within 12 or 18 months after the original operation. Haemorrhage from the recurrent ulcer may be the presenting symptom. Duodenal ulcers may recur at or near their original site in the duodenal cap. If a gastroenterostomy had been fashioned, ulcers may form just distal to the stoma in the jejunal mucosa. Most recurrences after vagotomy are due to the incomplete division of the vagal fibres by the surgeon: a few are previously undiagnosed cases of the Zollinger–Ellison syndrome.

A great deal of time and effort has been devoted to the development of a reliable test for completeness of vagotomy. Most of the work is based on measurements of gastric-acid secretion produced by vagal stimulation through insulin-induced hypoglycaemia. Various criteria, based on the original work of Hollander, have been proposed, but none has proved very satisfactory in practice and the predictive value of such tests is poor. There is no point in performing routine insulin stimulation tests following vagotomy, as after several months a proportion of negative tests will become positive without recurrent ulceration.

The diagnosis of recurrent duodenal ulcer after vagotomy is best established by endoscopy. Treatment of recurrent duodenal ulcer is either by re-operation, at which undivided vagal trunks are identified and cut, or a highly selective vagotomy is converted to another type, or a partial gastrectomy is performed. Results of re-operation are good, but repeated surgical procedures carry a higher morbidity and mortality than the original operations. The alternative is aggressive medical treatment with an H_2-receptor antagonist or a proton pump inhibitor, and a further attempt to eradicate *H. pylori*. The few controlled therapeutic trials available in this area have dealt with small numbers of patients, but in general results are favourable, a significant number of recurrent ulcers healing after a few weeks of therapy. It would be illogical, however, to expect the recurrent ulcer to heal permanently after a short period of medical treatment and one is therefore committed to long-term administration of an antisecretory drug. The usefulness of *H. pylori* eradication in these circumstances remains to be investigated.

REFERENCES

Baron, J.H. (1978). Diagnostic value. In *Clinical tests of gastric secretion*, p. 79. Macmillan, London.

Blaser, M.J. (1992). Hypotheses on the pathogenesis and natural history of *Helicobacter pylori*—induced inflammation. *Gastroenterology*, **102**, 720–7.

Burget, D.W., Chiverton, S.G., and Hunt, R.H. (1990). Is there an optimal degree of acid suppression for healing of duodenal ulcers? A model of the relationship between ulcer healing and acid suppression. *Gastroenterology*, **99**, 345–51.

Burland, W.L., Hawkins, B.W., and Beresford, J. (1980). Cimetidine treatment for the prevention of recurrence of duodenal ulcer: an international collaborative study. *Postgraduate Medical Journal*, **56**, 173–6.

El-Omar, E., Penman, I., Dorrian, C.A., Ardill, J.E.S., and McColl, K.E.L. (1993). Eradicating *Helicobacter pylori* infection lowers gastrin mediated acid secretion by two-thirds in patients with duodenal ulcer. *Gut*, **34**, 1060–5.

Eurogast Study Group. (1993). An international association between *H. pylori* infection and gastric cancer. *Lancet*, **341**, 1359–62.

Feldman, M. and Burton, M.E. (1991). Histamine₂-receptors antagonists: standard therapy for acid-peptic diseases. *New England Journal of Medicine*, **323**, 1672–8; 1749–55.

Gorbach, S.L. (1990). Bismuth therapy in gastrointestinal disease. *Gastroenterology*, **99**, 863–75.

Graham, D.Y. (1993). Treatment of peptic ulcers caused by *Helicobacter pylori*. *New England Journal of Medicine*, **328**, 349–50.

Halter, F. (1992). Antacids overview. *European Journal of Gastroenterology and Hepatology*, **4**, 947–83.

Laine, L. and Peterson, W.L. (1994). Medical progress: bleeding peptic ulcer. *New England Journal of Medicine*, **331**, 717–27.

Langman, M.J.S., Weil, J., Wainwright, P. *et al.* (1994). Risks of bleeding peptic ulcer associated with individual non-steroidal anti-inflammatory drugs. *Lancet*, **343**, 1075–8.

McCarthy, D.M. Sucralfate. *New England Journal of Medicine*, **325**, 1017–25.

McIntosh, H.H., Nasery, R.W., McNeil, D., Coates, C., Mitchell, J., and Piper, D.W. (1985). Perception of life event stresses in patients with chronic duodenal ulcer: a comparison of the rating of life events by duodenal ulcer patients and community controls. *Scandinavian Journal of Gastroenterology*, **20**, 563–8.

Maton, P.N. (1991). Omeprazole. *New England Journal of Medicine*, **324**, 965–75.

Maton, P.N. (1993). The management of Zollinger-Ellison syndrome. *Alimentary Pharmacology and Therapeutics*, **7**, 467–75.

NIH Consensus Development Panel on *Helicobacter pylori* in peptic ulcer disease. (1994). *Helicobacter pylori* in peptic ulcer disease. *Journal of the American Medical Association*, **272**, 65–9.

Penston, J.G. and Wormsley, K.G. (1992). Maintenance treatment with H₂-receptor antagonists for peptic ulcer disease. *Alimentary Pharmacology and Therapeutics*, **6**, 3–29.

Peterson, W.L. (1991). *Helicobacter pylori* and peptic ulcer disease. *New England Journal of Medicine*, **324**, 1043–8.

Pounder, R. (1988). Duodenal ulcers that are difficult to heal. *British Medical Journal*, **297**, 1560–1.

Pounder, R.E. and Smith, J.T.L. (1990). Drug-induced changes of plasma gastrin concentration. *Gastroenterology Clinics of North America*, **19**, 141–53.

Soll, H. (1990). Pathogenesis of peptic ulcer and implications for therapy. *New England Journal of Medicine*, **322**, 909–16.

Sonnenberg, A. (1989). Costs of medical and surgical treatment of duodenal ulcer. *Gastroenterology*, **96**, 1445–52.

Swain, C.P. (1992). Upper gastrointestinal haemorrhage. In *Recent advances in gastroenterology—9*, (ed. R.E. Pounder), pp. 135–50. Churchill Livingstone, Edinburgh.

Talley, N.J., McNeil, D., and Piper, D.W. (1987). Discriminant value of dyspeptic symptoms: a study of the clinical presentation of 221 patients with dyspepsia of unknown cause, peptic ulcereration, and cholelithiasis. *Gut*, **28**, 40–6.

Tytgat, G.N.J. (1994). Treatments that impact favourably upon the eradication of *Helicobacter pylori* and ulcer recurrence. *Alimentary Pharmacology and Therapeutics*, **8**, 359–69.

Van Deventer, G.M., Elashoff, J.D., Reedy, T.J., Schneidman, D., and Walsh, J.H. (1989). A randomised study of maintenance therapy with ranitidine to prevent the recurrence of duodenal ulcer. *New England Journal of Medicine*, **320**, 1113–19.

Walt, R.P. (1992). Misoprostol for the treatment of peptic ulcer and anti-inflammatory drug-induced gastroduodenal ulceration. *New England Journal of Medicine*, **327**, 1575–80.

Wotherspoon, A.C., Doglioni, C., Diss, T.C., Pan, L., Moschini, A., and de Boni, M. (1993). Regression of primary low-grade B-cell gastric lymphoma of mucosa-associated lymphoid tissue after eradication of *Helicobacter pylori*. *Lancet*, **342**, 575–7.

14.8 Hormones and the gastrointestinal tract

P. J. HAMMOND, S. R. BLOOM, AND J. M. POLAK

Introduction

The discovery of secretin, the first recognized hormone, by Bayliss and Starling in 1902 marked the birth, not only of gastrointestinal endocrinology, but of endocrinology itself. This was followed in 1905 by the identification of gastrin, but the technique of identifying hormones was, thereafter, more successfully applied to the study of secretions from the ductless glands, and gastrointestinal endocrinology languished for the next six decades. The determination of the amino acid structure of gastrin following its extraction from a solid tumour in 1964 marked a renewed interest in the field, and the introduction of techniques for large-scale chemical extraction and purification of gut peptides resulted in the discovery of further gut peptides. Most of the gut peptides, such as cholecystokinin and substance P, have been identified within the central and peripheral nervous systems, playing a neuromodulatory role in many organs. These neurocrine peptides are synthesized in nerve cells rather than endocrine cells in the gut and act locally as peptide neurotransmitters or neuromodulators. The endocrine cells of the gastrointestinal tract are not grouped into anatomically distinct glands, like most endocrine cells, but are scattered through the length of the gastrointestinal tract. The principal role of gut peptides is in the integration of gastrointestinal function, and they regulate the actions of the epithelium, muscles, and nerves throughout the gastrointestinal tract. This local effect of peptides may be either autocrine, regulating the function of the cell secreting them, or paracrine, influencing the behaviour of neighbouring cells of different type. Thus somatostatin, originally identified as a hypothalamic inhibitor of growth hormone release, has been shown to have inhibitory effects in many different organ systems. It is locally released and its main mechanism of action is a direct one on neighbouring cells, for example to inhibit gastric acid and insulin secretion. In addition to altering gastrointestinal function many peptides, such as gastrin, secretin and enteroglucagon, probably play an important paracrine role in controlling the growth and development of the gastrointestinal tract. In contrast, for most gut peptides there is little evidence that they act as true hormones in an endocrine fashion.

Two techniques have made a major contribution to the increased understanding of gastrointestinal endocrinology. Molecular biology has helped identify members of peptide families by molecular cloning techniques, and has provided information about peptide processing, which has shown that a number of peptides may originate from a single common precursor. Sensitive peptide radioimmunoassay has allowed detection of gut peptides, which have very low concentrations in plasma and tissues. Furthermore, the specific peptide antibodies can be used for immunocytochemistry to demonstrate the cellular and neuronal localization of gut peptides (Fig. 1), and for immunoneutralization studies to elucidate the pathophysiological functions of gut peptides. Peptide localization is further defined by electron microscopy, which demonstrates specific peptide storage granules (Fig. 2), and *in-situ* hybridization, which allows the sites of peptide synthesis to be identified. The most recent advance in gastrointestinal endocrinology has been the molecular characterization of hormone receptors by cloning techniques. This has demonstrated different receptors for the same ligand and provides an explanation for the diverse biological actions of many gut peptides in the same tissues. The development of agonists and antagonists to specific receptors will allow the physiological roles of the gut peptides to be fully characterized, and may be of therapeutic benefit in restoring normal gastrointestinal function in a number of diverse disease states.

This section describes the gut peptide hormones and neurotransmitters, classifying them by common structure or precursor peptides, and then outlines abnormalities in gastrointestinal disease. The role of gut peptides in the syndromes associated with gastroenteropancreatic tumours are considered in detail in Chapter 14.23.3, while the carcinoid syndrome is described at the end of this section.

Hormones and paracrine peptides

GASTRIN-CHOLECYSTOKININ FAMILY

Gastrin

Gastrin occurs in a variety of molecular forms but all the biological activity resides in the four carboxy-terminal amino acids. The major molecular forms contain 17 (G17; 2098 Da), 14 (G14; pentagastrin), and 34 (G34; big gastrin) amino acids. Larger molecular forms have been described but may be artefacts. In man, gastrin is particularly localized to the gastric antrum, where G17 is the predominant form, but is also found in the upper small intestine, mainly as G34. These two are the predominant circulating forms. Gastrin is synthesized in G cells and electron microscopy shows gastrin granules to be large and electron-lucent.

Gastrin release is particularly stimulated by protein ingestion and gastric distension. Its main physiological action is the stimulation of gastric acid secretion. Gastrin's other important physiological role appears to be its trophic effect on the gastric mucosa. Infusion of gastrin stimulates gastric motor activity and contraction of the lower oesophageal sphincter, but the physiological significance of this action is unclear.

Cholecystokinin

Cholecystokinin (**CCK**) has an identical, five amino-acid, carboxy-terminal sequence to gastrin, but its specificity is conferred by the adjacent three amino acids, and this octapeptide confers its biological activity. It is found in the gut in 33, 39, or 58 amino-acid molecular forms predominantly, and is produced by the I cells of the duodenal and jejunal mucosa. The octapeptide CCK is a neurotransmitter in the central nervous system and a small amount is found in specific enteric neurones of the upper gastrointestinal tract.

CCK secretion is stimulated by long-chain fatty acids and certain amino acids. The development of CCK antagonists specific for the two CCK receptor subtypes (CCK-A, which is CCK specific, and CCK-B, which appears to be also the only gastrin receptor) has allowed the important physiological roles of CCK to be characterized. The CCK-A receptor appears to be involved in stimulation of gallbladder contraction and trophic effects on the duodenum and pancreas. The ability of CCK-A receptor antagonists potently to inhibit meal-stimulated gallbladder contraction may be of therapeutic value in biliary colic.

Fig. 1 Somatostatin cells, immunostained using the technique of indirect immunofluorescence, in the mucosa of human colon (×300).

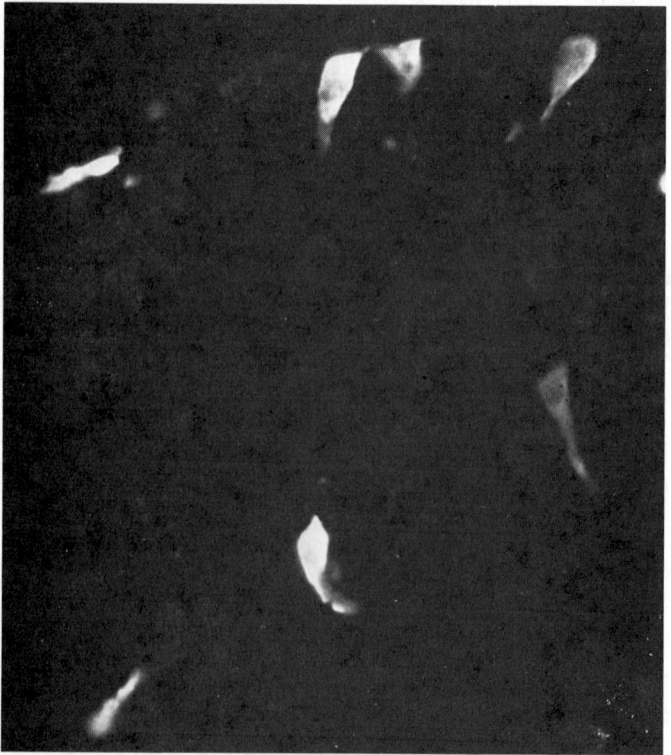

THE SECRETIN FAMILY

The secretin family comprises a number of peptides with significant sequence homology. These include, in addition to secretin, glucose-dependent insulinotropic peptide, glucagon, enteroglucagon (see below), vasoactive intestinal peptide, peptide histidine methionine, and growth hormone-releasing factor (**GRF**). GRF is released from the hypothalamus, mainly as a 44 amino-acid peptide, to stimulate release of growth hormone, but is also found in significant concentrations, mainly in a 40 amino-acid form, in the small intestinal mucosa, where its function is unknown.

Secretin

Secretin is a 27 amino-acid peptide (3056 Da), which appears to occur in only one molecular form, the whole molecule being needed for full biological activity. Circulating concentrations of secretin are lower than those of most other gut hormones. It is produced by S cells sparsely scattered throughout the duodenal and jejunal mucosa and is stored in characteristic secretory granules.

The main stimulus to secretin secretion is a duodenal pH of less than 4.5, although this occurs rarely. It is probably also secreted late after a meal but the timing and quantities of this secretion are uncertain. The main physiological role of secretin is stimulating production of watery, alkaline pancreatic juices in response to acid in the duodenum. It may play an important part in the developing gastrointestinal tract, concentrations of secretin being particularly high in the early postnatal period.

Glucose-dependent insulinotropic peptide

Glucose-dependent insulinotropic peptide (**GIP**) is a 42 amino-acid peptide (5105 Da) with considerable sequence homology at the *N*-terminal to secretin, glucagon and vasoactive intestinal peptide. It is produced by K cells, predominantly in the upper small intestinal mucosa but also in the gastric antrum and ileum, and is stored in large granules.

At pharmacological doses, GIP inhibits gastric secretions, and was originally named gastric inhibitory peptide. However, its physiological role appears to be as a component of the enteroinsular axis, being released in response to a mixed meal, particularly carbohydrates and long-chain fatty acids, and stimulating insulin release. This potentiation of insulin release in response to oral as opposed to intravenous glucose

Fig. 2 Electron micrograph of mucosal endocrine cell showing well-developed microvilli and secretory granules grouped at the basal membrane (×5500).

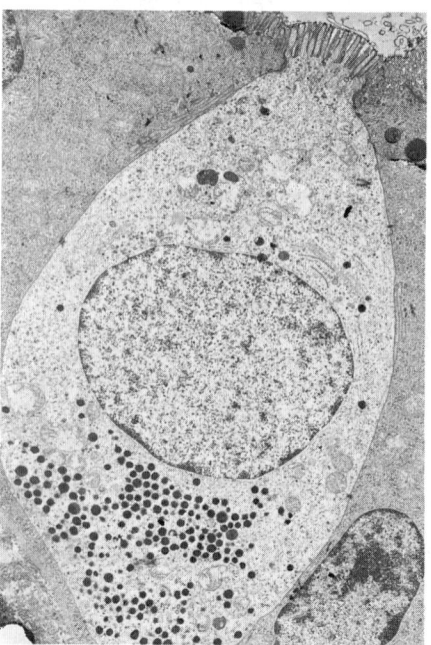

is the incretin effect. GIP has recently been implicated in the stimulation of cortisol release in two patients with ACTH-independent Cushing's syndrome whose serum cortisol rose postprandially.

Vasoactive intestinal peptide

Vasoactive intestinal peptide (**VIP**) is a 28 amino-acid peptide neurotransmitter (3326 Da) widely distributed through the central and peripheral nervous systems. The highest concentrations of VIP occur in the submucosa of the intestinal tract, where it is found in postganglionic intrinsic nerves (Fig. 3). VIP is a potent stimulator of small intestinal and colonic enterocyte secretion of water and electrolytes, acting via an elevation in cAMP. Other important actions include smooth-muscle relaxation, both in the alimentary tract and in the systemic vasculature, stimulation of insulin release, counteracted by a direct glucagon-like effect of VIP in stimulating hepatic gluconeogenesis and glycogenolysis, stimulation of pancreatic bicarbonate secretion, and relaxation of the gallbladder, pyloric sphincter, and circular muscle of the small intestine with contraction of the longitudinal muscle. VIP inhibits release of gastric acid but not at physiological concentrations in man.

Peptide histidine methionine is a 27 amino-acid neuropeptide with considerable sequence homology to VIP and derived from the adjacent exon of the preproVIP gene. It mimics the actions of VIP, probably acting via the same receptor, but is less potent.

Pituitary adenylate cyclase-activating peptide is a recently identified peptide occurring in 27 and 38 amino-acid forms and with considerable sequence homology to VIP. It has a similar tissue distribution to VIP and shares the same receptor outside the central nervous system and pituitary gland. It has similar actions to VIP on intestinal secretion and motility.

PEPTIDE PRODUCTS OF PREPROGLUCAGON

In the pancreas the major product of the preproglucagon molecule is pancreatic glucagon, but in the intestinal L cells preproglucagon is

Fig. 3 Vasoactive intestinal polypeptide fibres, immunostained using the unlabelled antibody enzyme (PAP) method, in the submucosa of human colon (×500).

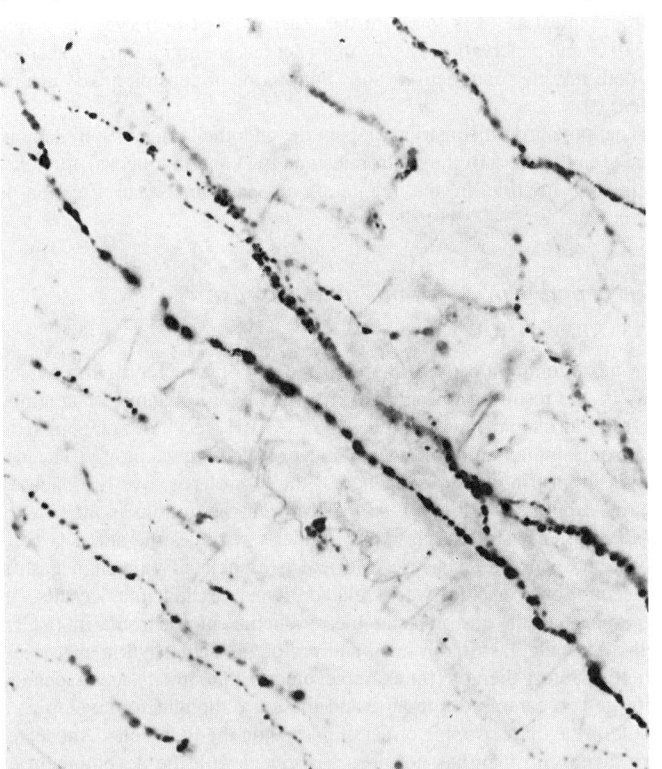

cleaved into enteroglucagon, a 69 amino-acid peptide containing the entire sequence of pancreatic glucagon, and the two glucagon-like peptides (GLP-1$_{7-36}$ NH$_2$ and GLP-2; see below).

Enteroglucagon

Enteroglucagon (also termed glicentin) is found in high concentrations in the mucosa of the ileum, colon, and rectum. It is released after a mixed meal, particularly of carbohydrate and long-chain fatty acids. Pure enteroglucagon has not become available for infusion studies and so evidence for its physiological role remains circumstantial. The amount of enteroglucagon secreted is proportional to the amount of unabsorbed food entering the colon, and high enteroglucagon concentrations are found in conditions associated with loss of the small intestinal absorptive capacity. Thus it has been postulated that enteroglucagon has a trophic effect on the small intestinal mucosa and may be important in gut adaptation. Enteroglucagon is further cleaved by the L cells to produce oxyntomodulin, a 37 amino-acid peptide released into the circulation, which is a potent inhibitor of pentagastrin-stimulated gastric acid secretion.

Glucagon-like peptide 1

Glucagon-like peptide 1 (**GLP-1**) is a 36 amino-acid peptide, which is secreted in a cleaved form containing the 30 carboxy-terminal amino acids (GLP-1$_{7-36}$ NH$_2$). It is a more potent stimulus to insulin secretion than GIP, and appears to be the most important incretin in man. It also inhibits secretion of glucagon and potentiates release of somatostatin. Infusion of GLP-1$_{7-36}$ NH$_2$ greatly reduces insulin requirements following a meal in type 1 and type 2 diabetics, and this effect may have therapeutic potential.

PANCREATIC POLYPEPTIDE, NEUROPEPTIDE Y, AND PEPTIDE TYROSINE TYROSINE

Pancreatic polypeptide, neuropeptide Y, and peptide tyrosine tyrosine are peptides with structurally similar genes and propeptide molecules probably derived from a common ancestral gene.

Pancreatic polypeptide

Pancreatic polypeptide is a 36 amino-acid peptide (4226 Da) first isolated as a contaminant during the purification of insulin. It is produced by specific cells found at the periphery of the pancreatic islets, particularly those in the head of the pancreas, and scattered through the exocrine pancreas. Pancreatic polypeptide granules are small and electron dense.

Concentrations of pancreatic polypeptide rise dramatically after a meal, particularly one high in protein, and this is at least in part due to activation of cholinergic fibres from the vagus. At physiological plasma concentrations, this polypeptide inhibits pancreatic exocrine and biliary secretion, and these may represent its biological actions, although there are no obvious consequences of its deficiency or excess.

Neuropeptide Y

Neuropeptide Y is a 36 amino-acid peptide neurotransmitter, which is often colocalized with noradrenaline. It is found in both extrinsic adrenergic nerves to the myenteric plexus and in intrinsic nerves in the myenteric and submucosal plexi, and highest concentrations occur in the upper intestine and distal colon. It is a potent vasoconstrictor, inhibits intestinal secretion, and depresses colonic motility.

Peptide tyrosine tyrosine

Peptide tyrosine tyrosine (**PYY**) is a 36 amino-acid peptide found in endocrine cells of the ileum, colon, and rectum. It has a similar distribution to enteroglucagon, with which it is often colocalized. It is released after a meal, particularly one containing carbohydrates or long-chain fatty acids, and its main function appears to be to slow intestinal transit, allowing more time for absorption. Other actions include delaying gastric emptying, decreasing intestinal motility, and inhibiting gastric acid secretion.

BOMBESIN AND THE GASTRIN-RELEASING PEPTIDES

Bombesin is a 14 amino-acid peptide (1620 Da) initially isolated from amphibian skin. It was found to be a potent stimulator of gastrin, and hence of gastric acid secretion. Its mammalian counterparts have similar properties and so were named gastrin-releasing peptides (**GRP**). In man, GRP is a 27 amino-acid peptide found in the gut in the intrinsic neurones of the myenteric and submucosal plexi, particularly in the stomach and pancreas. In addition to its effect on gastrin, it stimulates release of motilin and cholecystokinin, and pancreatic enzyme secretion. GRP has been shown to be an autocrine growth factor for small-cell lung carcinomas, and probably has trophic effects on the developing gut.

OPIOIDS

The opioid peptides leu-and met-enkephalin and dynorphin are widespread through the nerves of the myenteric and submucosal plexi of the gastrointestinal tract. Their principal actions appear to be inhibition of gastrointestinal secretion and increased smooth muscle contractility.

TACHYKININS

Substance P is an 11 amino-acid peptide (1345 Da) whose existence was demonstrated in 1931 through its ability to cause smooth muscle contraction and vasodilatation. A number of homologous peptides have now been characterized, and are collectively known as tachykinins, because of their rapid action. In man there are two tachykinin genes, preprotachykinin A encoding substance P and neurokinin-α and preprotachykinin B encoding neurokinin-β. These three tachykinins are localized to neurones in the myenteric and submucosal plexi throughout the gastrointestinal tract, with high concentrations in the duodenum and jejunum. Their principal effects are smooth muscle contraction, vasodilatation, and inhibition of intestinal absorption.

OTHER GUT PEPTIDES

Motilin

Motilin is a 22 amino-acid peptide (2700 Da) secreted by small intestinal M cells, whose density decreases from duodenum to ileum. The biological activity resides in the 9 amino-terminal amino acids. Peaks in motilin secretion coincide with initiation of the duodenal myoelectric complex, and so motilin appears to control the reflex motor activity of the small intestine, which occurs at approximately 2-hourly intervals in the fasted state, keeping the small intestine free of debris. Circulating amounts of motilin rise after a meal or drinking water and it may have a physiological role in accelerating gastric emptying and colonic transit. The macrolide antibiotics, such as erythromycin, are motilin-receptor agonists, hence their side-effects of diarrhoea and abdominal cramps.

Neurotensin

Neurotensin is a 13 amino-acid peptide (1673 Da) present throughout the central nervous system, and in enteric neurones and N cells of the ileal mucosa. It was originally isolated from bovine hypothalamus.

Plasma neurotensin concentrations rise after a meal, particularly those with a high fat content, and the rise is proportional to the size of the meal. At physiological doses, neurotensin inhibits gastric acid secretion and gastric emptying, and stimulates pancreatic exocrine and intestinal secretion. However, as with pancreatic polypeptide, there are no obvious consequences of neurotensin excess.

Somatostatin

Somatostatin was initially isolated from the hypothalamus as a 14 amino-acid peptide (1640 Da) that inhibited the release of growth hor-

Table 1 *Inhibitory actions of somatostatin*

Hormone release	Physiological function
Growth hormone	Lower oesophageal sphincter
Thyroid-stimulating hormone	contraction
Insulin	Gastric acid secretion
Glucagon	Gastric emptying and
Pancreatic polypeptide	secretions
Gastrin	Absorption of nutriments
Secretin	Splanchnic blood flow
Gastric inhibitory polypeptide	Gallbladder contraction and
Motilin	secretions
Enteroglucagon	Pancreatic enzyme and
	bicarbonate secretion

mone. It is widely distributed throughout the central and peripheral nervous system, and is found in a variety of endocrine tissues. In the gastrointestinal tract it occurs in 14 and 28 amino-acid forms. It is secreted by specific endocrine cells in the gastric and intestinal mucosa, and by the D cells on the inner rim of the pancreatic islets, and is found in the enteric neural system. Five human somatostatin receptors have now been identified and cloned, the type 1 receptor predominating in the gastrointestinal tract.

Somatostatin inhibits hormone release and blocks the response of the effector tissue, and inhibits a wide range of gastrointestinal functions (Table 1). Its acts principally as a paracrine factor or neurotransmitter, although small amounts of somatostatin are released into the plasma in response to physiological stimuli, including food ingestion, and so it may have an endocrine role.

Other peptide neurotransmitters

Calcitonin gene-related peptide is a 37 amino-acid peptide produced by alternative splicing of the calcitonin gene transcript. It is a widespread neurotransmitter, and in the gut occurs in both extrinsic sensory nerves and intrinsic neurones. It inhibits gastric acid and pancreatic secretion, and causes relaxation of vascular smooth muscle.

Galanin is a 29 amino-acid peptide neurotransmitter isolated from porcine intestine. It is found in the gut plexi and in nerves supplying the liver and pancreatic islets. Its main actions are inhibition of intestinal smooth-muscle contraction and inhibition of postprandial insulin release.

The potent vasoconstricting peptide endothelin has been demonstrated in the plexi of the gastrointestinal tract and in mucosal epithelial cells, but its role in the regulation of gastrointestinal function is unknown.

Gut peptides in gastrointestinal disease

GASTRIC PATHOLOGY

The most common cause of an elevated gastrin is achlorhydria, which may be the result of atrophic gastritis, pernicious anaemia or uraemia, or from iatrogenic causes such as the use of H_2-receptor antagonists or the proton-pump inhibitor omeprazole, or following vagotomy. The elevation in gastrin is a consequence of the loss of negative feedback on gastrin secretion by the low stomach pH. If the antrum is mistakenly retained after gastric surgery, this similarly removes the antral G cells from the exposure to gastric acid and is associated with high gastrin concentrations. Achlorhydria-related hypergastrinaemia results in hyperplasia of the gastric histamine-producing enterochromaffin (**ECL**) cells. Atrophic gastritis in man, and prolonged achlorhydria as a result of antisecretory therapy (for example, omeprazole) in rats, are associated with gastric carcinoid tumours, and these are thought to develop as a result of the direct trophic effect of gastrin on the ECL cells. Antisecretory therapy in man has not been associated with the development of these tumours, but recommended therapeutic doses should not be exceeded and in patients on long-term therapy, hypergastrinaemia should be avoided.

Peptic ulcer disease is not usually associated with abnormalities in gut peptide secretion, although a decrease in somatostatin release in patients infected with *Helicobacter pylori* may influence the paracrine regulation of gastric function.

After gastrectomy or truncal vagotomy, patients may develop the dumping syndrome due to accelerated gastric emptying. In these individuals there is a marked increase in the postprandial rise of VIP, neurotensin, PYY, and enteroglucagon, and a decrease in the release of motilin. VIP and neurotensin may both contribute to the postprandial hypotension associated with dumping, but neurotensin may have a beneficial effect in slowing gastric transit. The long-acting somatostatin analogue octreotide, which inhibits release of these peptides and inhibits gastric emptying, is often a very effective treatment for this condition.

MALABSORPTION

Malabsorptive conditions are associated with a decrease in the amount of peptides produced in the affected region, and a compensatory elevation of other peptides, particularly those trophic peptides implicated in the bowel's adaptation to loss of absorptive surface, such as enteroglucagon.

Coeliac disease is an autoimmune disease resulting from dietary gluten sensitivity and it is associated with villous atrophy of the upper small intestine (see Chapter 14.9.4). The postprandial peptide response in patients with untreated coeliac disease shows greatly reduced secretion of GIP and secretin, which originate from the affected region of bowel. In contrast, there is marked elevation of enteroglucagon, neurotensin, and PYY (Fig. 4). The decrease in secretin and increase in PYY may be responsible for the reduced pancreatic exocrine and biliary secretion found in this condition. Enteroglucagon stimulates enterocyte turnover in the affected segment, despite the villous atrophy. It may have a trophic effect on the remaining small intestinal mucosa and delay gut transit time, and neurotensin may help to improve absorption by delaying gastric emptying. In tropical sprue, a postinfective malabsorptive state usually seen in travellers to Asia and Central and South America, a different profile of postprandial peptide release is seen (Fig. 5). There is marked elevation in enteroglucagon and PYY, as in coeliac disease, but also in motilin secretion, whilst other peptides behave normally. After successful treatment of coeliac disease or tropical sprue, peptide responses return to normal.

Chronic pancreatitis (see Chapter 14.23.2) results in varying degrees of pancreatic endocrine dysfunction in addition to the exocrine insufficiency. Thus patients often have insulin-dependent diabetes, and basal and arginine-stimulated glucagon concentrations may be reduced, although they are elevated in some individuals. Basal, and meal and secretin-stimulated concentrations of pancreatic polypeptide are reduced if steatorrhoea is associated with chronic pancreatitis (Fig. 6). The early loss of pancreatic polypeptide secretion in most individuals probably reflects the location of its secretory cells throughout the exocrine pancreas and on the periphery of the islets. However, secretion of pancreatic polypeptide is occasionally preserved and its concentration is not of diagnostic value in chronic pancreatitis.

Cystic fibrosis is often associated with diabetes mellitus and pancreatic exocrine insufficiency. Fasting and milk-stimulated concentrations of pancreatic polypeptide are usually suppressed. GIP concentrations fail to rise after a milk stimulus, implying a failure of the enteroinsular axis, and this may contribute to the associated glucose intolerance.

The malabsorption associated with pancreatic exocrine insufficiency of any cause leads to an excess of nutriments in the colon, and as a result the concentrations of enteroglucagon, PYY, and neurotensin are raised. The gut adaptation resulting from the effects of these peptides may contribute to the improvement in absorptive function with age in patients with cystic fibrosis.

INTESTINAL RESECTION

Intestinal resection has profound effects on gut peptide concentrations. Jejunoileal bypass used to be constructed in patients with gross obesity. Peptide concentrations were normal preoperatively, but patients were

Fig. 4 The percentage incremental rise following a standard test breakfast in gut hormones compared to normal controls in patients with coeliac disease.

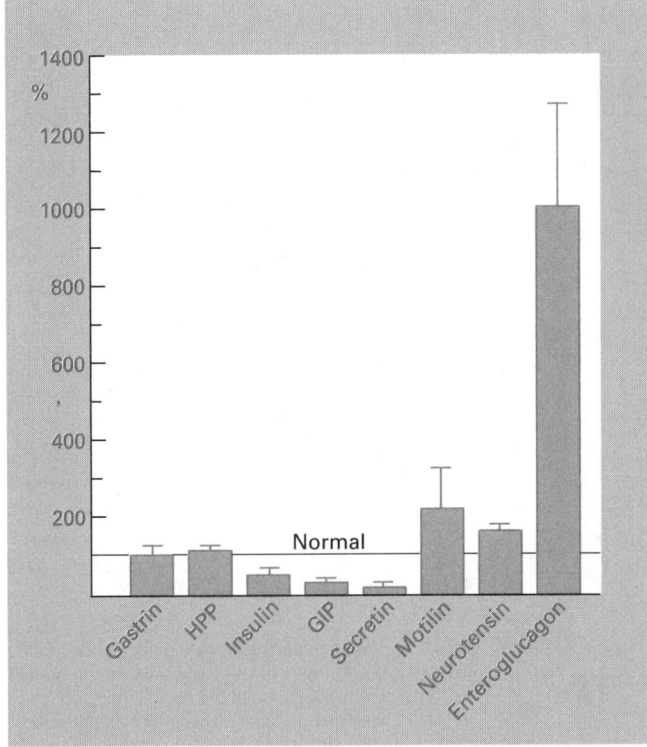

Fig. 5 The percentage incremental rise following a standard test breakfast in gut hormones compared to normal controls in patients with tropical sprue.

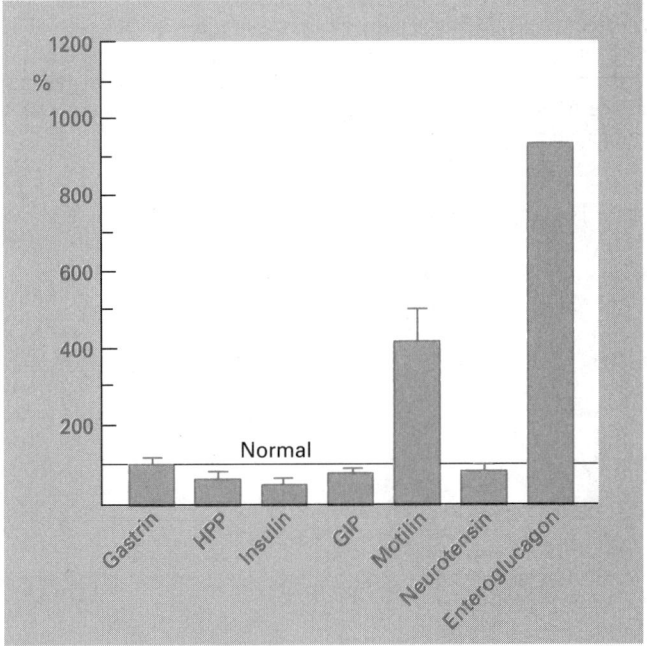

hyperinsulinaemic and glucose intolerant. After the procedure there was an almost complete absence of the prandial GIP response and consequently a much reduced first-phase insulin response. The initial beneficial effects of the operation were ultimately negated by massive hypertrophy of the remaining bowel. The appearance of large volumes of undigested nutrients in the distal ileum is associated with a 16-fold increase in enteroglucagon responses and an eightfold increase in neurotensin secretion, and this may provide an explanation for the hypertrophy. After partial ileal resection, the concentrations of gastrin, enteroglucagon, pancreatic polypeptide, motilin, and PYY are elevated, but after colonic resection only gastrin and PP are raised, as there is a decrease in production of the other predominantly colonic peptides.

DIARRHOEA

In acute infective diarrhoea, the concentrations of enteroglucagon, PYY, and motilin are increased, probably contributing to the altered gut motility and aiding mucosal repair. Patients with Crohn's disease have an elevated pancreatic polypeptide, GIP, motilin, and enteroglucagon, while in ulcerative colitis there is a modest elevation in PP, GIP, motilin, and gastrin, the last in response to the hypochlorhydria associated with the disease. No demonstrable abnormalities in gut peptides account for disordered motility in the irritable bowel syndrome.

INTESTINAL TUMOURS

The trophic effects of gut peptides may contribute to proliferation of malignant gut tumours. In particular, colon carcinoma cells have receptors for a number of potentially mitogenic peptides, including gastrin, GRP, and VIP.

NEUROPATHIC DISEASE

In conditions associated with destruction of intrinsic enteric nerves there is loss of the neurocrine peptides found in the affected region. Chagas' disease (see Section 7) results from chronic infection with *Trypanosoma cruzi* and in the gastrointestinal tract can result in mega-oesophagus and megacolon. Concentrations of VIP and substance P and of nerve fibres are greatly reduced in biopsies from affected segments. Similar changes are seen in the affected bowel from children with Hirschsprung's disease, which results from an aganglionic colonic segment. In contrast patients with the Shy–Drager syndrome, who have chronic autonomic failure with loss of preganglionic extrinsic nerves, have no abnormalities in neurocrine peptides or peptidergic nerve fibres on rectal biopsies (Fig. 7). Acquired immune deficiency disease is frequently accompanied by diarrhoea without evidence of secondary infection, and reduced immunostaining for substance P, VIP, and somatostatin in biopsies suggests a neuropathic process may be responsible.

Carcinoid syndrome

INTRODUCTION

The term *Karzinoide* was originally used by Obendorfer in 1907 to describe a carcinoma-like lesion without malignant qualities. It has now come to refer to tumours capable of producing serotonin (5-hydroxy-tryptamine; **5-HT**). However, several different cell types either synthesize or take up 5-HT and so the term carcinoid is applied to a variety of malignant tumours with different biological behaviour grouped by their similar histological appearances. This section will focus primarily on those tumours associated with the classical carcinoid syndrome.

Primary gastrointestinal carcinoid tumours are derived from the embryonic foregut (thyroid, bronchus, stomach, common bile duct, and pancreas), midgut, or hindgut. The most common sites for carcinoid tumours are the appendix and rectum, but these tumours are often found incidentally on histological examinations of appendicectomy and rectal biopsy specimens. These tumours are almost always benign. Rectal tumours are often multicentric and even when they metastasize are rarely associated with the carcinoid syndrome. The carcinoid syndrome occurs in about 10 per cent of patients with carcinoid tumours. It does not

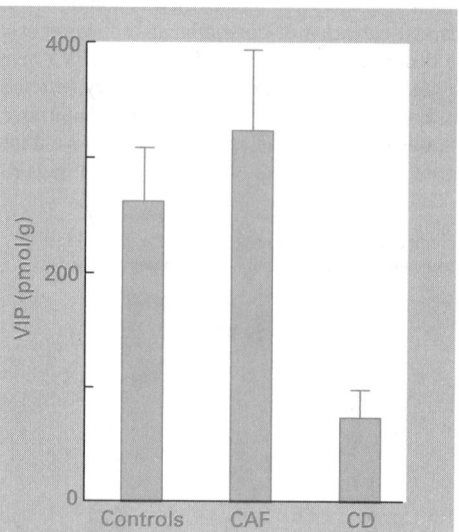

Fig. 7 Rectal vasoactive intestinal polypeptide concentrations (pmol/g wet tissue) in controls and patients with chronic autonomic failure (CAF) and Chagas' disease (CD) with gastrointestinal involvement. Reduced concentrations were seen in Chagas' specimens (reproduced from *Lancet* (1980, **i,** 559, by permission).

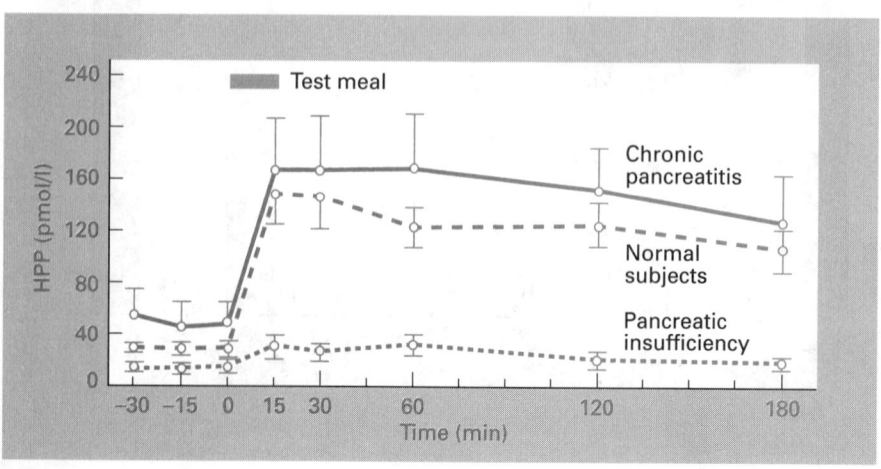

Fig. 6 The plasma human pancreatic polypeptide (HPP) response (pmol/l) following a mixed breakfast in normal controls and patients with chronic pancreatitis with and without steatorrhoea. A markedly reduced response was seen in patients with steatorrhoea.

develop when the tumour drains through a normal liver, and so midgut tumours have almost always metastasized, usually to the liver, before symptoms develop. The carcinoid syndrome is most commonly due to a metastatic midgut tumour, about 50 per cent of which metastasize to the liver. Primary carcinoid tumours are bronchial in origin in about 10 per cent of cases, and rarely occur in the ovary and testis. Tumours in these sites may be associated with the syndrome in the absence of metastases. The annual incidence of the carcinoid syndrome is about 1 in 500 000.

CLINICAL MANIFESTATIONS

The cardinal feature of the classical carcinoid syndrome is the flush. The carcinoid flush predominantly involves the head and upper thorax, and is usually associated with a tachycardia, hypotension, and increased skin temperature. Patients may have a sensation of intense heat and wheezing may occur. Rarely, flushing extends to the trunk and limbs, and may be associated with lacrimation, facial oedema, and great distress. Attacks are paroxysmal, and usually unprovoked, although precipitating factors include alcohol or food ingestion, stress, emotion, or exertion. Flushing initially lasts for only a few minutes but as the disease progresses may become almost continuous, and such patients often develop a chronically reddened and cyanotic facial hue, with widespread telangiectasia, the leonine facies. This fixed flush is more commonly seen with bronchial carcinoids, which are often metabolically inactive, but when associated with flushing can cause severe attacks lasting for hours or days, occasionally with profound hypotension and even anuria. Gastric carcinoids are often associated with raised, localized, wheal-like areas of flushing, which are usually pruritic and may migrate.

The other characteristic feature of the syndrome is secretory diarrhoea, which may be profuse, with passage of several litres a day occasionally accompanied by electrolyte disturbance. It may be associated with cramping abdominal pain, nausea, and vomiting. Rarely these symptoms may result from small bowel obstruction from a large ileal carcinoid tumour, but the majority of primary tumours are small, usually being less than 1 per cent of total body tumour weight. Hepatic metastases may cause right hypochondrial pain, particularly if the liver capsule is involved or stretched, and acute exacerbations may occur if metastases become ischaemic and undergo autonecrosis. Weight loss and, in the later stages, cachexia are common as a result of poor dietary intake, malabsorption, and increased catabolism. Pellagra with dermatitis of sun-exposed areas may occur, the increased conversion of 5-hydroxytryptophan into 5-HT causing nicotinamide deficiency.

Cardiac valve abnormalities affect about 50 per cent of patients. They occur as a result of endocardial fibrosis, with plaques of smooth muscle in a collagenous stroma deposited on the valves. Lesions are almost always on the right-hand side, left-sided valve damage only occurring in association with bronchial carcinoids, which drain into the left atrium, or atrioseptal defects with right to left shunting. The most common lesions are tricuspid incompetence and pulmonary stenosis, and the usual clinical outcome is oedema and breathlessness due to right ventricular failure, which can be fatal. The other causes of breathlessness in association with the carcinoid syndrome are bronchospasm, which affects a small number of patients, often occurring with flushing attacks, and metastatic involvement of the lung and pleura. Arthritis occurs in a small number of patients, and sclerotic bone metastases may be seen usually in association with foregut tumours.

Carcinoid tumours, in common with other gastroenteropancreatic

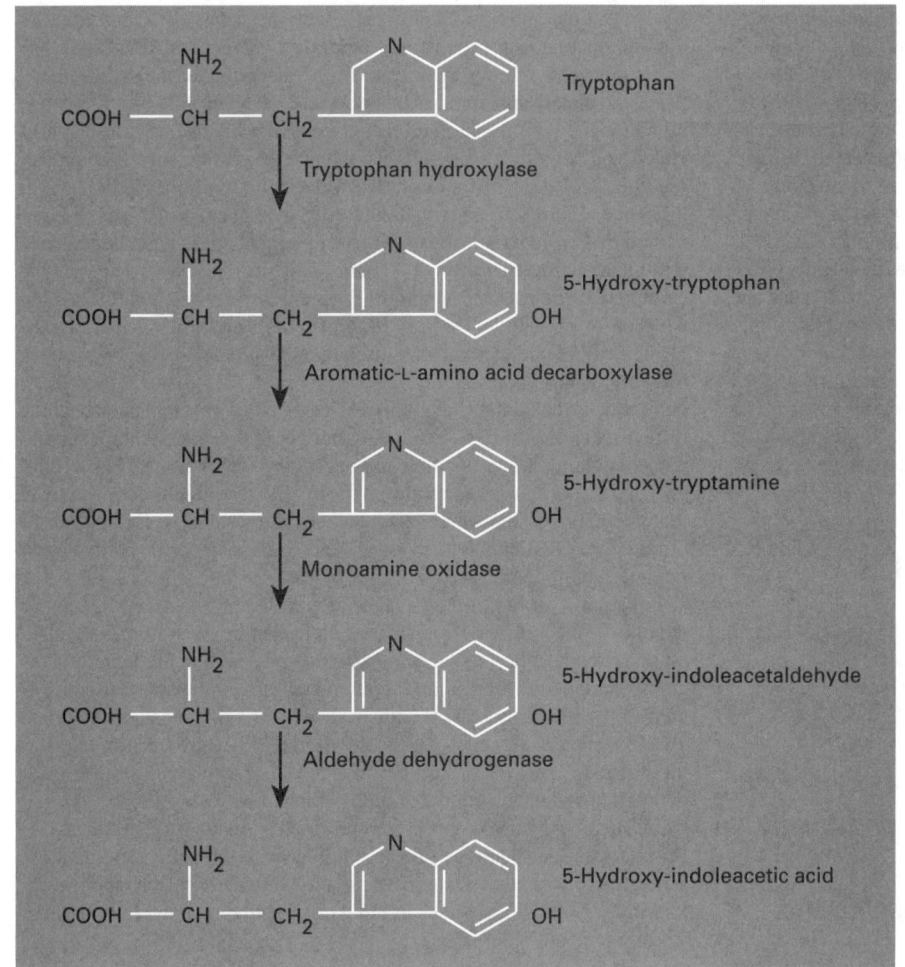

Fig. 8 Biochemical pathway for the synthesis and degradation of 5-hydroxytryptamine.

tumours, have the potential to produce a variety of peptide products and may be associated with other syndromes, with or without the carcinoid syndrome. The most common of these associated syndromes is Cushing's, due to an ectopic ACTH-secreting, bronchial or pancreatic carcinoid. Carcinoid tumours may also be a feature of multiple endocrine neoplasia type 1 (see Section 12).

BIOCHEMISTRY

The biologically active metabolite characteristically produced by metastatic carcinoid tumours is 5-HT, synthesized from the amino acid tryptophan (Fig. 8). 5-HT probably plays a part in the pathogenesis of some of the symptoms of the carcinoid syndrome, particularly the diarrhoea and bronchoconstriction. It is metabolized to 5-hydroxyindole acetic acid (5-HIAA), which accounts for 95 per cent of the urinary excretion of 5-HT.

A variety of vasoactive substances may be secreted by carcinoid tumours and have been implicated in the pathogenesis of the flush. Flushing can be provoked by intravenous noradrenaline, which has been shown to activate kallikrein in the tumour, leading to synthesis and release of bradykinin. Other possible mediators of the flush include histamine, substance P, and prostaglandins, although the flush is rarely affected by inhibitors of prostaglandin synthesis, such as indomethacin. Gastric carcinoids are derived from histamine-producing enterochromaffin cells and histamine is probably the cause of the characteristic wheal-like flush seen with gastric tumours.

INVESTIGATIONS

The diagnosis of carcinoid syndrome is made on the basis of elevated concentrations of 5-HIAA in a 24-h urine collection, and urinary 5-HIAA acts as a marker of disease progression. Various foods, including avocados, bananas, aubergines, pineapples, plums, and walnuts, should be avoided while collecting specimens to prevent false-positive results. A number of drugs and other substances interfere with the spectrophotometric assay; paracetamol, fluorouracil, methysergide, and caffeine give false-positive results, and ACTH, phenothiazines, methyldopa, monoamine oxidase inhibitors and tricyclic antidepressants false-negatives. The other products of carcinoid tumours are not routinely assayed. Circulating markers of neuroendocrine tumours, such as pancreatic polypeptide and chromogranin, may corroborate the diagnosis, and other gut hormones are occasionally elevated in association with carcinoid tumours, most frequently gastrin.

Localization of carcinoid tumours is rarely a problem, as most have gross hepatic metastases, visible on computerized tomographic (**CT**) scanning or abdominal ultrasonography, at the time of diagnosis. In those rare cases where the syndrome occurs in the absence of metastases,

tumour localization may offer the prospect of cure. These tumours are unlikely to be in the gastrointestinal tract and so chest radiographs and CT scans of the chest and pelvis should be taken. The recently developed, indium-labelled, somatostatin analogue pentetreotide may prove valuable in localizing these tumours, although the resolution is only about 1 cm and bronchial carcinoids are frequently atypical and do not bear somatostatin receptors. An alternative method of isotopic localization is using 123-*m*-iodobenzylguanidine (MIBG) scanning, which may be equally effective. These scanning techniques can be useful in patients with metastatic disease to demonstrate the extent of spread (Fig. 9), particularly in those who are being considered for liver transplantation, which would be precluded by the presence of extrahepatic metastases. Angiography may be of value in assessing suitability for hepatic embolization. Carcinoid tumours have characteristic histological features: cells showing positive staining for serotonin reduce silver salts and so are termed argentaffin positive.

TREATMENT

The principal aim of therapy in patients with the carcinoid syndrome is to provide palliation of symptoms. Simple treatments such as codeine phosphate, diphenoxylate, and loperamide may help to control the diarrhoea. Many of the symptoms can be controlled with the peripheral 5-HT antagonists: cyproheptadine, a 5-HT type 2 receptor blocker, often helps the diarrhoea, ketanserin may be effective in reducing flushing, and the 5-HT type 3 receptor antagonist ondansetron can alleviate nausea and anorexia. Parachlorphenylalanine, an inhibitor of tryptophan hydroxylase, and chlorpromazine block synthesis of 5-HT, but are rarely used. Histamine may mediate some of the features of the syndrome, especially in patients with gastric carcinoids, and in these cases H_1- and H_2-receptor blockade may be useful. These treatments, with the exception of simple antidiarrhoeal agents, have been largely superseded by the long-acting, subcutaneously administered, somatostatin analogue octreotide. This inhibits the release of the mediators of the syndrome by the tumour and antagonizes their peripheral effects. It is effective in alleviating symptoms in over 90 per cent of patients. It is rarely associated with significant side-effects: the acidic solution can cause pain at the injection site, gallstones often develop but are rarely of clinical significance, and a few patients develop steatorrhoea, which can be prevented by giving pancreatic enzyme supplements. It is now the first-line treatment in the majority of patients and may be life saving in the carcinoid crisis, when symptoms become severe and continuous. In addition to octreotide, during crises patients usually need close monitoring of fluid and electrolytes, often by measurement of central venous pressure, and appropriate replacement therapy. The major drawback to octreotide is that patients develop resistance with time, and most become refractory to any form of treatment after about 4 years. Vitamin supplements containing nicotinamide are necessary when patients have pellagra, and these can be given prophylactically. The treatment of cardiac manifestations is the same as for valve disease and cardiac failure of other causes. Patients with painful bony metastases may benefit from palliative radiotherapy.

In patients who fail to respond or are intolerant to octreotide, tumour debulking may provide palliative relief. Surgery is rarely indicated, although enucleation of large metastases may give some benefit. Carcinoid tumours rarely respond to chemotherapy, either with streptozotocin and 5-fluorouracil, or with a variety of other agents, including cyclophosphamide, and doxorubicin although recent evidence suggests interferon-α may be of more benefit. The most effective means of debulking is hepatic embolization, which devascularizes the tumour while the blood supply to the normal liver is maintained by the portal vein. Octreotide should be given in high dose to cover this intervention, as the necrotic metastases release large quantities of vasoactive mediators that can cause a severe carcinoid crisis with profound hypotension, leading to acute renal failure.

Fig. 9 Indium-111-labelled somatostatin analogue scan (left) in a patient with carcinoid syndrome showing metastases to liver, bone, and intrathoracic lymph nodes compared to a conventional base scan (right).

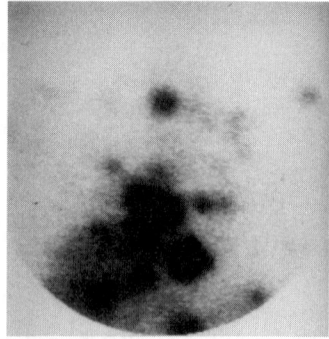
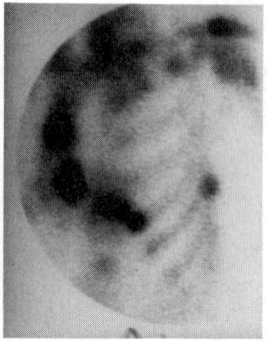

Prognosis

Carcinoid tumours behave like other gastroenteropancreatic tumours, with the majority following an indolent course. The median survival from the time of diagnosis is about 5 years, with a range of up to 20 years. Thus palliation is very worthwhile in these patients, allowing them to lead a normal life until the terminal stages of the disease.

Multiple endocrine neoplasia and non-diabetic pancreatic endocrine disorders are described in Section 12.

REFERENCES

Bloom, S.R. and Long, R.G. (ed.) (1982). *Radioimmunoassay of gut regulatory peptides*. Saunders, London.

Besterman, H.S. *et al.* (1978). Gut hormone profile in coeliac disease. *Lancet*, **i**, 785–8.

Cook, G.C., Sarson, D.L., Christofides, N.D., Bryant, M.G., Gregor, M., and Bloom, S.R. (1979). Gut hormones responses in tropical malabsorption. *British Medical Journal*, **1**, 1252–5.

Gorden, P., Comi, R.J., Maton, P.N., and Go, V.L. (1989) NIH conference. Somatostatin and somatostatin analogue (SMS 201–995) in treatment of hormone-secreting tumors of the pituitary and gastrointestinal tract and non-neoplastic diseases of the gut. *Annals of Internal Medicine*, **110**, 35–50.

Gronbech, J.E., Soreide, O., and Bergan, A.T.I. (1992). The role of resective surgery in the treatment of the carcinoid syndrome. *Scandinavian Journal of Gastroenterology*, **27**, 433–7.

Gutniak, M., Orskov, C., Holst, J.J., Ahren, B., and Efendic, S. (1992). Antidiabetogenic effect of glucagon-like peptide-1 (7–36)amide in normal subjects and patients with diabetes mellitus. *New England Journal of Medicine*, **326**, 1316–22.

Hodgson, H.J. and Maton, P.N. (1987). Carcinoid and neuroendocrine tumours of the liver. *Baillière's Clinical Gastroenterology*, **1**, 35–61.

Jensen, R.T. (ed.) (1989). Gastrointestinal endocrinology. *Gastroenterology Clinics of North America*, **18**, 671–931.

Kvols, L.K. (1989). Therapy of the malignant carcinoid syndrome. *Endocrinology and Metabolism Clinics of North America*, **18**, 557–68.

Lacroix, A. *et al.* (1992). Gastric inhibitory polypeptide-dependent cortisol hypersecretion—a new cause of Cushing's syndrome. *New England Journal of Medicine*, **327**, 974–80.

Long, R.G., Adrian, T.E., and Bloom, S.R. (1981). Gastrointestinal hormones in pancreatic disease. In *Pancreatic diseases in clinical medicine*, (ed. C.J. Mitchell and J. Kelleher), pp. 223–39. Pitman Medical, Tunbridge Wells.

Long, R.G. *et al.* (1980). Neural and hormonal peptides in rectal biopsy specimens from patients with Chagas' disease and chronic autonomic failure. *Lancet*, **ii**, 559–62.

Maton, P.N. and Jensen, R.T. (1992). Use of gut peptide receptor agonists and antagonists in gastrointestinal diseases. *Gastroenterology Clinics of North America*, **21**, 551–664.

Moss, S.F., Legon, S., Bishop, A.E., Polak, J.M., and Calam, J. (1992). Effect of *Helicobacter pylori* on gastric somatostatin in duodenal ulcer disease. *Lancet*, **ii**, 930–2.

Oberg, K. (ed.) (1989). Neuroendocrine gut and pancreatic tumours. *Acta Oncologica*, **28**, 301–449.

Oberg, K. (ed.) (1991). Recent advances in diagnosis and treatment of neuroendocrine gut and pancreatic tumours. *Acta Oncologica*, **28**, 301–449.

Reznik, Y. *et al.* (1992). Food-dependent Cushing's syndrome mediated by aberrant adrenal sensitivity to gastric inhibitory polypeptide. *New England Journal of Medicine*, **327**, 981–6.

Thompson, J.C. (1991). Humoral control of gut function. *American Journal of Surgery*, **161**, 6–18.

Wynick, D. and Bloom, S.R. (1991). The use of the long-acting somatostatin analog octreotide in the treatment of gut neuroendocrine tumors. *Journal of Clinical Endocrinology and Metabolism*, **73**, 1–3.

14.9 Malabsorption

14.9.1 Mechanisms of intestinal absorption

J. R. F. WALTERS

The principal function of the intestine is the absorption of nutrients. Before this can occur, physical solubilization and chemical breakdown of the many components of food are needed to digest them to molecular forms that can be transported across the intestinal epithelial barrier. Different mechanisms have evolved for digesting and absorbing each of the nutrients but many general principles can be described.

General principles

METHODS OF STUDYING ABSORPTION

Our knowledge about the mechanisms of absorption in man came first from clinical observations, including metabolic balance studies in patients following gastrointestinal resections or with fistulae. Experiments perfusing specific segments of the intestine with multilumen tubes added to the knowledge gained from animals. Studies with isolated tissue enabled absorptive and secretory fluxes to be separated and mechanisms could then be defined in terms of active transport, facilitated diffusion, or passive absorption. Nutrient uptake experiments with membrane vesicles and enzymatic studies led to descriptions of transporters, and these proteins were defined at the molecular level by purification, cloning, and sequencing. Increasingly, site-directed mutagenesis, expression and transfection studies are describing the critical domains in the transporter molecules and the regulation of their expression.

ABSORPTIVE CAPACITY

The overall efficiency of intestinal absorption varies for each of the classes of nutrients. Some compounds, such as components of dietary fibre, are not absorbed even in health. Others are normally almost completely absorbed, but in disease, absorption is insufficient to cope with the load, giving symptoms of diarrhoea from excess faecal water, or steatorrhoea from excess faecal fat. The principal determinants of the maximum absorptive capacity are the area of the intestinal mucosa, increased by surface folding, villi, and microvilli to about 200 m², and the function of the individual cellular transporting mechanisms. As part of the total absorptive process, the intestine also has to reabsorb endogenous secretions produced to aid digestion. Approximately 7 l of digestive fluids from salivary, gastric, biliary, pancreatic, and intestinal sources add significantly to the absorptive requirements for water, electrolytes, protein, and fat. Secretory diarrhoea and protein-losing enteropathy are conditions where endogenous output exceeds the absorptive capacity of the bowel.

SITES OF ABSORPTION

Gastrointestinal motility mixes food with digestive secretions and propels them from the mouth to the anus. During this passage, nutrients are exposed to specialized areas of the gut with specific digestive or absorptive functions. The duodenum and proximal jejunum are mostly involved with digestion and fluid secretion. However, the more acidic pH in this area means the solubility and hence the absorption of polyvalent cations such as iron and calcium are high. The bulk of nutrient absorption takes place in the more distal jejunum and ileum. The terminal ileum is specialized for cobalamin (vitamin B_{12}) and bile salt absorption. The colon salvages fluid and electrolytes not absorbed by the small intestine and absorbs short-chain fatty acids produced by colonic bacteria from poorly digested carbohydrates. Loss of specialized areas by surgical resection or disease activity produces specific patterns of malabsorption but generally the ability of the intestine to adapt is great.

The intestinal epithelial cells differentiate as they move from crypt to villus tip. The older villus-tip enterocytes perform most of the absorptive functions, though some digestive enzymes are found in less mature cells. Fluid secretion probably occurs from the crypts. Some epithelial cells are goblet cells secreting mucus. This traps an unstirred water layer, which is a relative barrier to the diffusion of large molecules but allows the smaller products of digestion to reach the surface of the epithelium. The concentration of compounds and acidity can be different in this microclimate than in the mixed contents of the lumen. Other epithelial cells secrete various hormones or have immunological functions.

CELLULAR MECHANISMS OF ABSORPTION

Absorption occurs by transcellular and paracellular pathways. The paracellular pathway is through the tight junctions that link the epithelial cells. By this pathway, passive absorption of small molecules occurs by diffusion down electrical and concentration gradients. Solvent drag is the term used to describe movement down concentration gradients, which are themselves created by the movement of water. Active transport takes place through the epithelial cell against these gradients and necessitates the expenditure of energy generated within the cell.

Three steps are involved in transcellular absorption; entry to the cell at the apical (brush-border) membrane, passage through the cytoplasm, and exit from the cell at the basolateral membrane. Polarization of the enterocyte produces differences in structure and function of the apical and basolateral membranes. Specific carrier molecules are present in one of these membranes but not the other; this asymmetry generates vectorial flow in a single direction through the cell. Several classes of carrier have been defined (Table 1). Channels allow passive movement down gradients, but can be gated to control the rate of flow. Many carriers function as exchangers enabling facilitated diffusion, and can be driven in either direction by reversing the concentration gradients of the molecules transported.

Pumps directly couple ATP to drive transport against concentration gradients in only a few instances. The Na^+/K^+-ATPase (Na^+ pump) extrudes Na^+ in exchange for K^+ at the basolateral membrane and indirectly provides the energy source needed for the absorption of many nutrients in what is called secondary active transport. The ATPase maintains a difference in intracellular and extracellular Na^+ concentrations; this Na^+ gradient is then used at the apical membrane to provide the energy for Na^+-coupled uptake of nutrients by cotransporters. Other intestinal ATPases include the basolateral Ca^{2+}-ATPase working analogously to reduce intracellular Ca^{2+} concentrations, and the colonic apical K^+-ATPase needed for active K^+ uptake.

Intracellular metabolism is important for some nutrients, particularly fats, where re-esterification forms triglycerides and chylomicron particles in the endoplasmic reticulum. These cross the basolateral membrane by a vesicular exocytotic pathway. An endocytotic pathway absorbs

Table 1 *Types of carriers across membranes*

Class	Gastrointestinal examples
Channels	Colonic apical Na^+ channel
	Basolateral K^+ channel
	Apical secretory Cl^- channel
	Apical Na^+/H^+ exchanger
Exchangers (antiports)	Anion (Cl^-/HCO_3^-) exchangers
Cotransporters (symports)	Apical Na^+/glucose cotransporter
	Apical Na^+/amino acid cotransporter
	Basolateral secretory $Na^+/K^+/2Cl^-$ cotransporter
Pumps (ATPases)	Basolateral Na^+/K^+-ATPase
	Basolateral Ca^{2+}-ATPase
	Gastric apical secretory H^+-ATPase

intact immunoglobulins and other proteins in neonatal mammals and may account for absorption of some antigens in adults.

Absorption of specific nutrients

In Table 2, the molecules involved in the absorption of each of the different classes of nutrients are described. These include digestive enzymes and other factors in the lumen of the gastrointestinal tract, enzymes and transporters at the apical brush-border membrane, intracellular enzymes that modify or interact with nutrients during absorption, and transporters at the basolateral membrane. Some important proteins in the blood that transport nutrients away from the intestine are also shown. The nucleotide and amino acid sequences of an ever-increasing number of these proteins are known.

WATER AND ELECTROLYTES

Water absorption is entirely passive and is driven by the osmotic gradients created by the transport of other nutrients, largely the principal electrolytes sodium and chloride. The mechanisms of transport of these electrolytes in the small and large intestine of various species are now well understood, which helps provide a rational basis for therapy in diarrhoeal diseases. The control of mechanisms of secretion and absorption has received much recent study following the realization that secretory diarrhoea (such as that produced by bacterial toxins, hormones, or inflammatory mediators) results from abnormal stimulation of physiological regulatory processes. Similar transport mechanisms are found in the kidney and many other tissues.

The transporters vary in different regions of the gut, partly depending on whether secretion or absorption is the predominant process. In the upper small intestine, chloride secretion (Fig. 1(a)) first involves uptake of $Na^+/K^+/2Cl^-$ by a coupled carrier at the basolateral membrane, the energy being derived from the Na^+ gradient provided by the Na^+/K^+-ATPase. Chloride leaves the enterocyte at the apical membrane down a chemical gradient and is regulated by control of the Cl^- channel. The cystic fibrosis gene product (CFTR) is one mechanism involved with this regulation in intestine and other tissues. The transcellular chloride secretion is electrogenic (no balancing ion is transported) and sodium ions follow chloride by moving passively down this electrical gradient by a paracellular route. Water secretion, also through the tight junctions, is driven by the osmotic difference created by ion movement.

Absorption of electrolytes and water in the distal small intestine and proximal large intestine is by processes that result in electroneutral NaCl absorption (Fig. 1(b)). At the apical membrane, the combined effect of Na^+/H^+ and Cl^-/HCO_3^- exchangers is to absorb Na^+ and Cl^- using the products of carbonic anhydrase activity. Carbon dioxide reforms in

Table 2 *The molecules of intestinal absorption*

Nutrient	Luminal	Brush-border membrane: digestion and uptake	Intracellular metabolism	Basolateral membrane exit from cell	Systemic carriers
Water and electrolytes		Na^+/H^+ exchanges* Cl^-/HCO_3^- exchanger Na^+ channel* K^+/H^+-ATPase*		Na^+/K^+-ATPases* Na^+/H^+ exchangers* Cl^-/HCO_3^- exchanger K^+ channels	
Carbohydrates	Salivary amylase* P. amylase*	Glucoamylase* Sucrase-isomaltase* Lactase* Trehalase* Na^+-coupled glucose/galactose transporter* Fructose transporter* (GLUT5)		Glucose transporter* (GLUT2)	
Proteins and amino acids	G. pepsin* P. trypsin* P. chymotrypsin* P. elastase* P. carboxypeptidases*	Enteropeptidase Endopeptidases (24.11 and neutral*) Ectopeptidases (aminopeptidases N* and A, dipeptidyl peptidase IV*, Gly-Leu and Asp-Lys peptidase) Di- and tripeptide transporters Na^+-coupled amino acid cotransporters (neutral*, hydrophobic, imino, acidic*, basic) Na^+-independent transporters (basic and neutral*)	Amino di- and tripeptidases Prodipeptidase	Leucine (neutral) transporter	
Lipids	P. lipase* P. colipase* P. phospholipase A_2* ? lingual lipase G. lipase* P. cholesterol esterase Breast-milk lipase	Microvillus membrane fatty-acid binding protein	Cytoplasmic fatty-acid binding proteins (intestinal* and liver*) Triglyceride synthetase (acylCoA-synthetase and mono-/di-glyceride acyltransferases) Microsomal TG transfer protein* Lysophosphatidylcholine acyltransferase	Apolipoproteins: ApoA-1* ApoA-IV* ApoB48* (also apoA-II*, C-I*, C-II*, C-III*, D*, E*)	Chylomicrons Very low-density lipoproteins High-density lipoproteins
	Biliary phospholipids Bile acids	Ileal Na^+/bile-acid cotransporter*	Sterol carrier protein-2* AcylCoA acyltransferase Bile-acid binding protein*	Bile-acid exchangers	
Calcium	Various chelators	Calmodulin*	Calbindin-D9k*	Ca^{2+}-pumping ATPase*	
Phosphate		Alkaline phosphatase* Na^+-coupled carrier			
Magnesium		? carrier			
Iron	Various chelators	Carrier	Ferritin* ?Fe-binding protein(s)		Transferrin*
Zinc	Various chelators	Carrier	Metallothionein* Cysteine-rich intestinal protein*	Carrier	
Retinoids (vitamin A)	Bile acids, phospholipids P. esterases	Esterases	Retinol-binding proteins (CRBP-II)* AcylCoA retinol acyltransferase		Chylomicrons

Table 2 (*cont.*)

Nutrient	Luminal	Brush-border membrane: digestion and uptake	Intracellular metabolism	Basolateral membrane exit from cell	Systemic carriers
Calciferol (vitamin D)	Bile acids, phospholipids				Chylomicrons Binding protein*
Vitamin K	Bile acids, phospholipids				Chylomicrons
Vitamin E	Bile acids, phospholipids				Chylomicrons
Folic acid		Pteroylpolyglutamate hydrolase Folate/OH⁻ exchanger		Carrier	Binding proteins
Vitamin C		Na⁺-coupled carrier			
Biotin		Na⁺-coupled carrier			
Riboflavin		Na⁺-coupled carrier			
Pantothenic acid		Na⁺-coupled carrier			
Thiamin		Carrier			
Cobalamin	Salivary R-proteins G. intrinsic factor* P. proteases	Ileal B₁₂ transporter			Transcobalamins*

G., gastric digestive enzymes; P., pancreatic.
*Indicates proteins where the amino acid sequence is known.

the intestinal lumen and diffuses back into the cell. At the basolateral membrane, Na⁺ is extruded by the Na⁺/K⁺-ATPase and there are likely to be roles for both a different Na⁺/H⁺ exchanger and an anion exchanger. Water follows passively. In the distal colon, electrogenic Na⁺ absorption takes place through an aldosterone- and amiloride-sensitive Na⁺ channel with paracellular water and anion movement.

Na⁺-coupled cotransport systems in the small intestine are major pathways for Na⁺ absorption (Fig. 1(c)). A large number of nutrients cross the apical membrane by this mechanism, each being accompanied by an equimolar amount of Na⁺. This is the principle justifying the use of glucose-containing oral rehydration solutions in infectious diarrhoea. Bacterial toxins (cholera or *Escherichia coli* heat-labile toxin for example) increase Cl⁻ secretion and decrease electroneutral NaCl absorption but do not affect the Na⁺-coupled processes. Glucose can thus be used to drive Na⁺, and secondarily, water absorption. Conversely, oral solutions used to prepare patients for colonoscopy contain large amounts of

water and Na⁺, but do not contain any absorbable anion or solute for Na⁺-coupled absorption and so produce copious watery diarrhoea.

K⁺ absorption has been less well studied. It now appears that there is a ATPase at the apical membrane of the colonocyte which takes up K⁺ in exchange for H⁺. K⁺ can leave the cell passively through basolateral membrane channels. Anion exchangers are involved in the colonic absorption of bicarbonate and short-chain fatty acids (acetate, propionate, and butyrate) but the mechanisms are still being clarified.

CARBOHYDRATES

The salivary, pancreatic, and brush-border enzymes that digest the various forms of carbohydrate into monosaccharides are well characterized at the functional and molecular levels (Table 2). The developmental and dietary regulation of these enzymes is currently being investigated; differences in the control of lactase expression result in the common con-

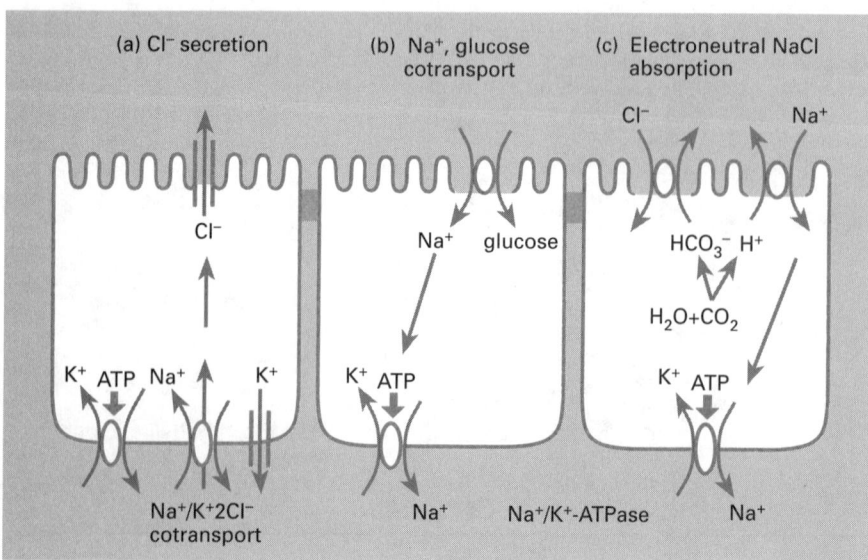

Fig. 1 Examples of ion-transport processes in jejunal enterocytes. (a) Chloride ion secretion showing the Na⁺/K⁺/2Cl⁻ cotransporter, Na⁺/K⁺-ATPase, and K⁺ channel in the basolateral membrane, and the apical chloride channel. (b) Sodium/glucose cotransport at the apical membrane with basolateral membrane Na⁺ extrusion by the Na⁺/K⁺-ATPase. (c) Electroneutral absorption of sodium and chloride with coupled Na⁺/H⁺ exchange and Cl⁻/HCO₃⁻ exchange in the apical membrane. Many other transport processes are found in these cells.

dition of lactose intolerance (see Section 11.2). Monosaccharide transport across the brush border is by the Na^+-coupled glucose/galactose cotransporter, although fructose is absorbed by a separate Na^+-independent carrier. A glucose transporter in the basolateral membrane similar to that which takes up glucose in other cells appears to be responsible for facilitated diffusion of monosaccharides out of the enterocyte. The role of colonic bacteria in digesting certain carbohydrates in fibre to short-chain fatty acids and gases should not be overlooked.

PROTEIN

The endogenous secretion of 25 g/day of digestive enzymes and another 30 g/day of desquamated gastrointestinal cells adds significantly to the average dietary intake of about 70 g/day of protein. Protein digestion takes place initially in the lumen by the gastric and pancreatic proteases (Table 2). These are activated by a complex series of reactions, which is necessary to prevent autodigestion, and is initiated by brush-border enteropeptidase. The next step in digestion is performed by the many oligopeptidases in the brush border. The products of these reactions are absorbed as di- or tripeptides as well as amino acids; specific transporters recognize different families of amino acids and are often Na^+-coupled. Further hydrolysis of the absorbed peptides occurs in the cytoplasm of the enterocyte. Amino acids leave the cell by carriers in the basolateral membrane, moving down concentration gradients. Glutamine is used as a major energy source by the intestinal cell and absorbed amino acids are also used for protein synthesis. Basolateral membrane uptake provides the amino acids needed for protein synthesis during fasting.

Fig. 2 Steps in the absorption of triglycerides. Triglycerides (TG) are digested in micelles to monoglycerides (MG) and fatty acids (FA), which after crossing the apical membrane bind to fatty acid-binding proteins (FABP). Re-esterification to triglycerides occurs in the smooth endoplasmic reticulum and chylomicrons are assembled in the Golgi by the addition of apolipoproteins (ApoA-I, ApoA-IV, and ApoB48). Secretory vesicles extrude the chylomicrons at the basolateral membrane.

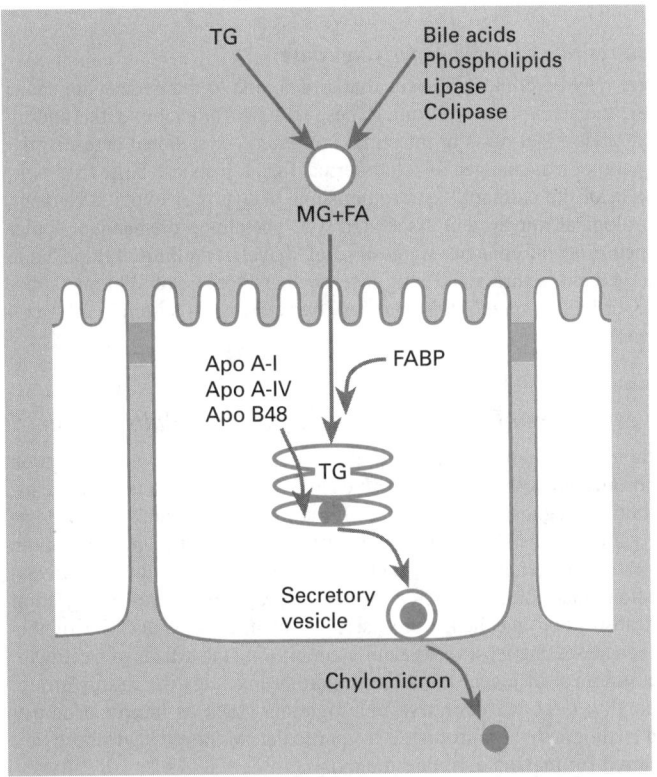

LIPIDS

The absorption of fats is affected by a different set of constraints from those for water-soluble nutrients. Solubilization in the gut lumen, cytoplasm, and blood is difficult for hydrophobic molecules; crossing the lipid bilayers of the cell membranes is less problematical. In the gut lumen, dietary fats are emulsified and then further solubilized into micelles formed by bile acids and phospholipids secreted by the liver. Pancreatic lipase is the principal enzyme needed to digest triglycerides and is aided by colipase, which anchors it to the lipid emulsion. Other enzymes break down phospholipids and cholesterol esters, and in infants, breast milk contains another lipase.

Triglyceride digestion (Fig. 2) produces fatty acids and monoglycerides, which are taken up from micelles at the brush-border membrane. It is likely that a specific protein is involved in the uptake, though this carrier is not well characterized. The cytoplasmic fatty acid-binding proteins maintain the solubility of fatty acids in the enterocyte, enabling delivery to the endoplasmic reticulum where re-esterification to triglycerides occurs. Phospholipids and cholesterol esters are also reassembled. After lipid feeding, particles that become chylomicrons in blood collect in the Golgi apparatus. The various apolipoproteins, principally apoB48, A-I, and A-IV, are synthesized in the intestinal cell and their expression is important for lipid metabolism throughout the body. ApoB48 is of particular interest as its mRNA undergoes editing in the intestine but not the liver. Apolipoproteins constitute up to 25 per cent of the chylomicron, two-thirds of the lipid being triglyceride and the rest phospholipid. Very low-density and high-density lipoproteins are also formed.

The lipoproteins move to secretory vesicles in the enterocyte and are then extruded across the basolateral membrane of the cell to enter the villous lacteals and the mesenteric lymphatics. Some lipid enters the circulation via the portal vein bound to albumin; this route is important for fatty acids derived from medium-chain triglycerides. The fat-soluble vitamins follow similar absorptive pathways to the major dietary lipids, though there are certain specialized proteins such as the cytoplasmic retinol-binding proteins and the serum calciferol-binding protein. Bile salts, which play such crucial roles in forming micelles to solublize lipids through the small intestine, are absorbed in the terminal ileum, crossing the apical membrane by a Na^+-coupled cotransporter. They are conserved by undergoing an enterohepatic circulation.

MINERALS

Calcium, phosphate, magnesium, iron, zinc, and the various trace elements all have specialized absorptive pathways, which are described in greater detail in Table 2. For iron, calcium, and the other polyvalent metals, maintaining intraluminal solubility is a problem; thus absorption is greatest in the more acidic proximal small intestine and can be increased by various chelators, or reduced by binding to form insoluble compounds such as fatty acid soaps. The bioavailability of the minerals in various dietary sources differs; on average only about one-third of dietary calcium is absorbed and the figure is much lower for iron. To avoid toxicity, intracellular concentrations are kept low by binding to proteins such as ferritin for iron, brush-border calmodulin and cytoplasmic calbindin-D9k for calcium, and metallothionein for zinc. Various transmembrane carriers have been suggested; the basolateral membrane calcium-pumping ATPase is one of the best described.

VITAMINS

The fat-soluble vitamins (A,D,E, and K) are discussed above. For many of the water-soluble vitamins, specific pathways appear to be present and in most cases involve either Na^+-coupled cotransport, or anion countertransport at the brush border. Folates require hydrolysis at the brush border before transport and have an enterohepatic circulation. Absorption of cobalamins (vitamin B_{12}) is well understood. Salivary R-proteins bind cobalamin in the stomach but are digested in the small intestine, where the vitamin is bound by intrinsic factor synthesized in the stomach. This ordinarily stabilizes cobalamin, allowing it to pass through the small intestine to the terminal ileum where the complex is recognized by a specific apical protein and absorption takes place. Transcobalamins bind the absorbed vitamin in the blood.

REFERENCES

Ahnen, D.J. (1991). Protein digestion and assimilation. In *Textbook of gastroenterology* (ed. T. Yamada, D.H. Alpers, C. Owyang, D.W. Powell, and F.E. Silverstein), pp. 381–92. Lippincott, Philadelphia.

Barrett, K.E. and Dharmsathaphorn, K. (1991). Secretion and absorption: small intestine and colon. In *Textbook of gastroenterology* (ed. T. Yamada, D.H. Alpers, C. Owyang, D.W. Powell, and F.E. Silverstein), pp. 265–94. Lippincott, Philadelphia.

Carruthers, A. (1990). Facilitated diffusion of glucose. *Physiological Reviews*, **70**, 1135–76.

Christensen, H.N. (1990). Role of amino acid transport and countertransport in nutrition and metabolism. *Physiological Reviews*, **70**, 43–77.

Davidson, N.O. and Magun, A.M. (1991). Intestinal lipid absorption. In *Textbook of gastroenterology* (ed. T. Yamada, D.H. Alpers, C. Owyang, D.W. Powell, and F.E. Silverstein), pp. 353–92. Lippincott, Philadelphia.

Ferraris, R.P. and Diamond, J.M. (1989). Specific regulation of intestinal nutrient transporters by their dietary substrates. *Annual Reviews in Physiology*, **51**, 125–41.

Field, M., Rao, M.C., and Chang, E.B. (1989). Intestinal electrolyte transport and diarrheal disease. *New England Journal of Medicine*, **321**, 800–6; 879–83.

Hopfer, U. (1987). Membrane transport mechanisms for hexoses and amino acids in the small intestine. In *Physiology of the gastrointestinal tract*, (2nd edn) (ed. L.R. Johnson), pp. 1499–526. Raven Press, New York.

Olsen, W.A. and Lloyd, M.L. (1991). Carbohydrate assimilation. In *Textbook of gastroenterology* (ed. T. Yamada, D.H. Alpers, C. Owyang, D.W. Powell, and F.E. Silverstein), pp. 334–53. Lippincott, Philadelphia.

Powell, D.W. (1987) Intestinal water and electrolyte transport. In *Physiology of the gastrointestinal tract*, (2nd edn) (ed. L.R. Johnson), pp. 1267–305. Raven Press, New York.

14.9.2 Investigation and differential diagnosis of malabsorption

M. S. LOSOWSKY

INTRODUCTION

Malabsorption is a relatively common clinical problem with divers causes. As will be apparent from the outline of the mechanisms of absorption in Chapter 14.9.1, malabsorption can arise from defective digestion of foodstuffs within the lumen of the bowel, structural changes in the bowel wall, or anatomical abnormalities in the lymphatic drainage of the bowel. In this chapter the clinical and diagnostic features of malabsorption and some of its common causes are examined. Other conditions in which malabsorption is a major feature are described in other chapters in this section; those in which malabsorption is particularly important are listed at the end of this chapter. Although some degree of malabsorption has been demonstrated in a wide variety of systemic disorders, in many cases the gastrointestinal dysfunction plays a relatively minor part in the illness.

Causes of malabsorption

The main causes of malabsorption are summarized in Table 1, in which an attempt is made to relate defective absorption to the underlying disorder of structure or function of the small bowel.

Clinical presentation of malabsorption

There are symptoms and signs that occur in the malabsorption syndrome, whatever the cause, as follows.

Diarrhoea with features to suggest steatorrhoea

In the severe case the stools are typically loose, bulky, offensive, greasy, light coloured, and difficult to flush away. Although there may be only one bulky stool per day, stool frequency is usually increased, but not to the extent seen in colonic disease. The stools may, however, appear normal and even constipated, even though steatorrhoea is shown by faecal fat measurement. Steatorrhoea may be absent in any of the diseases of the small intestine.

Abdominal symptoms

These include discomfort, borborygmi, and distension. The discomfort may follow food and thus mimic peptic ulcer, or it may be to some extent relieved by bowel action, thus mimicking the irritable bowel syndrome.

Nutritional deficiency

A patient with malabsorption may present with an apparently isolated nutritional deficiency, for example anaemia due to iron, folate or vitamin B_{12} deficiency, bleeding due to increased prothrombin time secondary to vitamin K deficiency, or bone disease secondary to vitamin D deficiency. Such deficiencies may be reflected by a variety of symptoms and signs including glossitis, pallor, pigmentation of the skin, petechiae or bruising, muscle pain, neurological abnormalities, a positive Chvostek or Trousseau sign, and skeletal abnormalities.

Features of general ill health

These include anorexia, weight loss, lethargy, tiredness on little effort, dyspnoea, and general irritability. In contrast to the usual anorexia, some patients have hyperphagia and a very high food intake. Finger clubbing occurs in some cases. In the patient with severe or prolonged disease, hypoalbuminaemia, oedema, electrolyte deficiencies, and dehydration may occur, as may amenorrhoea, infertility, and impotence.

Features related to the underlying cause

There may be clinical features that give a clue to the underlying cause of the malabsorption syndrome. These include, for example, the finding of an abdominal mass in intestinal lymphoma or regional enteritis, the dermatological changes of scleroderma, facial flush and large liver suggestive of the carcinoid syndrome, signs of hypo- or hyperthyroidism, neurological impairment associated with abetalipoproteinaemia, ocular or neurological changes suggestive of diabetes mellitus, lymph node enlargement, arthritis and lung disease characteristic of Whipple's disease, or the dermatological changes characteristic of systemic mast-cell disease.

Investigation of the patient suspected of malabsorption

Although the features described above may suggest the malabsorption syndrome, and other clinical features may suggest the correct diagnosis, definitive diagnosis requires special investigations. There is a bewildering variety of tests available for the patient suspected of malabsorption. These can, in general, be divided into two groups. First, there are investigations that point to a defect in the integrated processes of digestion and absorption and hence are useful in confirming a disorder of this type, in assessing its severity, and in monitoring the effects of treatment. Measurement of faecal fat is the important investigation in this group. Secondly, there are definitive investigations, such as intestinal biopsy and radiography, appropriate to particular diseases, and these are required for making a precise diagnosis.

Table 1 *Classification of causes of malabsorption*

Mucosal—definitive investigation: intestinal biopsy
Structure
    Food sensitivities:
      ● gluten-sensitive enteropathy*
      ● dermatitis herpetiformis
      ● cows' milk sensitivity in infants
      ● soya protein sensitivity
    Tropical sprue*
    Whipple's disease
    Intestinal lymphangiectasia
    Mast-cell disease
Function
    Alactasia
    Abetalipoproteinaemia

Structural—definitive investigation: usually small-bowel
    radiology
Crohn's disease*
Intestinal resection
Gastric surgery (see below)*
Radiation enteritis
Mesenteric arterial insufficiency
Small-intestine lymphoma or other malignancy
Blind loops, fistulae, diverticula, strictures
Idiopathic chronic ulcerative enteritis
Amyloidosis
Eosinophilic gastroenteropathy
Mechanisms of malabsorption after gastric surgery

    Poor mixing
    Decreased gastric digestion   } not important

    Lack of stimulus to bile and pancreatic secretion
    Rapid gastric emptying
    Intestinal hurry
    Afferent loop pooling of bile and pancreatic secretions
    Afferent loop bacterial overgrowth
    Pancreatic atrophy
    Unmasking of other disease: gluten sensitivity, alactasia,
      jejunal diverticula

    Inadvertent gastroileostomy
    Gastrocolic fistula   } rare

Infective—definitive investigation: usually microbiology
Acute enteritis
Travellers' diarrhoea*
Intestinal tuberculosis
Parasitic disease of the intestine, especially giardiasis
Whipple's disease
Contaminated small bowel
    Anatomical: blind loops, fistulae, diverticula, strictures
    Motility disturbance: systemic sclerosis, intestinal pseudo-
      obstruction, diabetes mellitus, abdominal radiotherapy
    Achlorhydria
    Hypogammaglobulinaemia

Defective luminal digestion
Pancreatic
    Chronic pancreatitis*
    Carcinoma of the pancreas*
    Cystic fibrosis*
    Pancreatectomy
    Zollinger–Ellison syndrome
    Defective stimulation: intestinal disease, gastric surgery
    Malnutrition
Bile-salt mediated
    Parenchymal liver disease*
    Biliary obstruction*
    Bacterial degradation (in contaminated small bowel)
    Terminal-ileum disease*
    Terminal-ileum resection*
    Cholestyramine

Drugs
Neomycin
Cholestyramine
Colchicine
p-Aminosalicylic acid
Irritant purgative abuse
Phenindione
Metformin
Methyldopa
Methotrexate
Liquid paraffin
Ethyl alcohol
Antacids

Lymphatic obstruction
Congenital lymphangiectasia
Acquired lymphangiectasia: lymphoma, tuberculosis, cardiac
    disease

Disease outside the upper gastrointestinal tract
Endocrine disorders: hyperthyroidism, hypothyroidism,
    Addison's disease, hyperparathyroidism,
    hypoparathyroidism, diabetes mellitus, carcinoid syndrome
Collagen diseases
Ulcerative colitis
Widespread skin disease
Malnutrition

Specific biochemical defects
Pancreatic enzyme deficiencies, with normal structure
Enterokinase deficiency
Disaccharidase deficiency
Cystinuria
Hartnup disease
Congenital chloridorrhoea
Vitamin B_{12} malabsorption
Folate malabsorption
Acrodermatitis enteropathica

*Relatively common.
Some disorders cause malabsorption by more than one mechanism and are thus classified under more than one heading. This has the advantage of allowing consideration of different forms of treatment in the same patient.

DEMONSTRATION OF DEFECTIVE ABSORPTION

For most substances, defective absorption cannot be demonstrated simply by comparing intake in the diet with output in the stool because of the intervention of other processes such as endogenous secretion and bacterial breakdown. Direct demonstration of defective absorption by intestinal intubation and perfusion is not of practical clinical importance.

Thus, with the exception of fat, the demonstration of defective absorption is indirect. The mechanisms in defective fat absorption are shown in Fig. 1.

In the estimation of faecal fat an abnormal result does not distinguish between inadequate digestion and inadequate absorption. Indirect assessments of the malabsorption of other substances, by estimation of their plasma concentrations or by demonstration of deficiencies, can clearly be affected by factors other than problems of digestion and absorption, and the results need to be interpreted with due caution.

FAECAL FAT

Simple measurement of the quantity of fat put out in the stools in 1 day is unsatisfactory for a number of reasons. The reservoir function of the colon is variable from day to day so that the output of fat varies greatly. Thus faeces need to be collected for several days, preferably at least five, and the result expressed as average daily excretion. Even this may not be reliable in patients with irregular bowel habits. Faecal markers, intermittent or continuous, improve the accuracy. The use of continuous markers allows reduction in the period of collection of faeces.

The quantity of fat in the stool depends on the intake of fat in the diet. Although there is a small quantity of endogenous fat in the stool, of the order of 1 to 2 g/day, this does not increase to any significant extent in patients with steatorrhoea: in such patients the excess faecal fat is unabsorbed dietary fat. In ambulant patients being investigated for malabsorption, dietary fat intake may differ by a factor of four to five. Thus, for interpretation of the faecal fat the dietary intake of fat must be known. Expressing the faecal fat as a percentage of dietary fat gives a meaningful basis of comparison between patients on different fat intakes and from time to time in the same patient if the fat intake varies with the clinical state. Ninety-three per cent absorption is the approximate lower limit of normal. Diarrhoea of any cause can lead to a modest increase in faecal fat.

Faecal fat determined in this way is useful in diseases associated with maldigestion or malabsorption because it gives an overall assessment of major physiological functions (Fig. 1). Repeated estimations are of proven value in assessing the progress of certain diseases and the effects of treatment. However, most functions concerned in digestion and absorption have considerable reserve capacity and, in the case of the small intestine, adaptation may occur with the compensatory increased function in non-diseased areas. Thus fat absorption may be normal with established disease in organs involved in digestion and absorption, for example the small intestine, the pancreas, and the liver.

To minimize collection and handling of faeces, many indirect methods of estimation of fat absorption have been devised. These include the use of radioactive fats, macroscopic or microscopic examination of faeces, and fat tolerance tests. Most correlate moderately well with faecal fat measurements.

CARBOHYDRATE ABSORPTION

The absorption of glucose cannot be directly assessed but the glucose tolerance test, which measures blood levels after a standard oral dose of glucose, tends to give a lower rise than normal with most causes of malabsorption but a higher rise than normal in patients with pancreatic disease. There are, however, so many other factors that affect the result of this test that it is of little value in the context of malabsorption.

Xylose absorption test

The test that is usually used to assess carbohydrate absorption is the xylose absorption test. An oral dose of xylose is given and the excretion in the urine measured for the ensuing 5 h. Excretion of greater than 22 per cent of a 5-g dose and greater than 17 per cent of a 25-g dose may be regarded as normal, although the limits of normal show some variation from one laboratory to another. This test rarely gives normal results in untreated coeliac disease or tropical sprue, and abnormal results rarely occur in patients with pancreatic disease. Abnormal results occur, however, for reasons other than malabsorption. These include delayed gastric emptying, low urine flow, or poor renal function.

Lactose tolerance test

This test may be performed in a similar way to the glucose tolerance test. In patients with absent or low levels of lactase in the intestinal mucosa (alactasia or hypolactasia), either primary or secondary to intestinal mucosal disease, oral lactose is followed by little rise in the blood glucose. Diminished lactose digestion may also be due to resection of a major portion of the small intestine.

The unabsorbed lactose reaching the colon is converted by bacteria to gas and lactic acid, which may cause inhibition of the absorption of

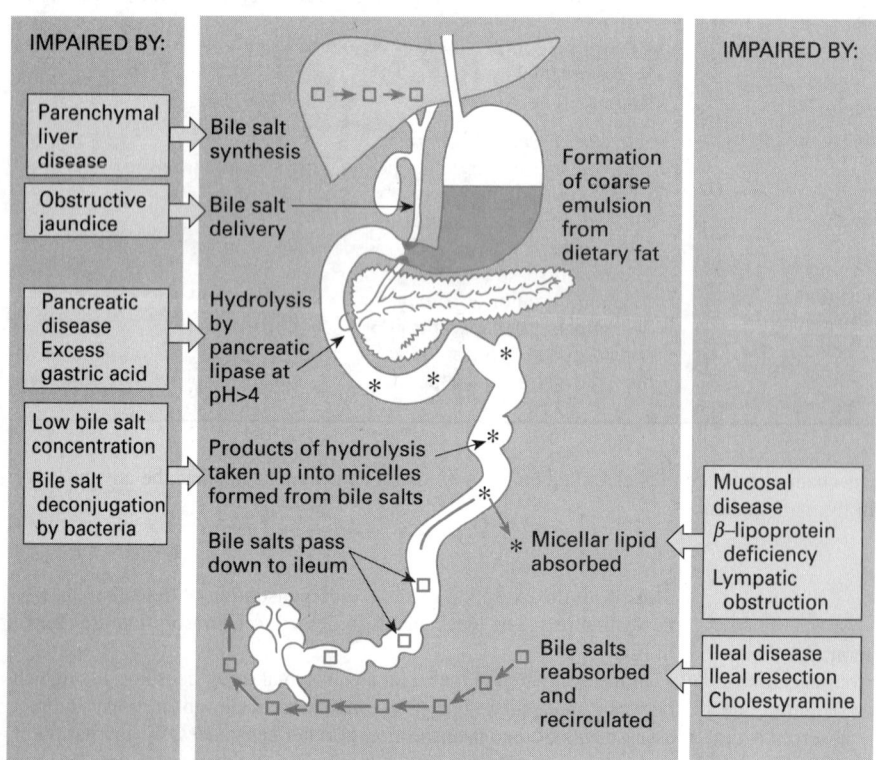

Fig. 1 Digestion and absorption of fat. Steatorrhoea may be caused by disease processes that impair different stages in the sequence of events.

salt and water by the colon and consequent abdominal discomfort and diarrhoea. These symptoms, if following oral lactose, are presumptive evidence of alactasia. Direct measurement of lactase in mucosal biopsy specimens is, in most circumstances, a better test for alactasia or hypolactasia than is the lactose tolerance test.

PROTEIN ABSORPTION

Faecal nitrogen is a measure of protein malabsorption, especially when there is gross maldigestion as in severe pancreatic disease, and parallels faecal fat in some conditions. It is, however, rarely used in diagnosis because much of the faecal nitrogen derives from sources other than dietary protein, for example bacteria and mucus.

Excessive loss of protein (protein-losing enteropathy) is a feature of many disorders of the gastrointestinal tract and is commonly responsible for hypoproteinaemia. Faecal nitrogen does not reflect this process, as most of the protein in the lumen is digested and reabsorbed. Protein-losing enteropathy is assessed by measuring faecal radioactivity after intravenous injection of radioactive protein or other substance of similar molecular weight.

VITAMIN B$_{12}$ ABSORPTION (SEE ALSO SECTION 22)

In the absence of other reasons for it to be malabsorbed, the absorption of vitamin B$_{12}$ may be used as a test of function of the terminal ileum. The Schilling test consists of an oral dose of radioactive vitamin B$_{12}$ followed by an intramuscular, large, 'flushing' dose of non-radioactive vitamin B$_{12}$ and measurement of urinary radioactivity, which reflects the amount absorbed.

Confirmation that a low value is not due to pernicious anaemia or other gastric pathology can be obtained by repeating the test and giving intrinsic factor with the oral dose of vitamin B$_{12}$. If malabsorption is due to ileal disease, the result will remain abnormal. Vitamin B$_{12}$ absorption can also be determined using a whole-body counter.

SMALL-BOWEL BIOPSY

Biopsy of the small intestine is now widely available, extremely safe, and is an invaluable aid to the diagnosis of small-bowel disease.

With the exception of endoscopic biopsy, probably most widely used is the Crosby–Kugler capsule in which a spring-loaded blade is activated by suction through a fine tube. This has the disadvantages of producing only a single specimen and of requiring the capsule to be removed before recovery of the specimen. If, for any reason, a satisfactory specimen is not obtained, the patient must swallow the capsule again. An alternative is a hydraulic capsule in which the specimen is flushed to the surface with the capsule still in position in the small intestine. The blade is automatically reset so that multiple specimens can be obtained before removal.

There are remarkably few complications to these procedures. Bleeding may occur but this is exceedingly rare provided that neither pro-thrombin time nor platelet count are grossly abnormal. In our experience on the rare occasions when bleeding has occurred it stopped spontaneously and rarely needed transfusion. Perforation of the intestine is a theoretical possibility and has occasionally been described in severely malnourished subjects. The procedure is sufficiently free of complications for us to use it routinely with adult outpatients, provided they can be observed for a few hours after completion.

Processing

The specimen can be examined and orientated on a plastic mesh, using the dissecting microscope. This enables an immediate rough assessment of the likelihood of pathology, certain recognition of severe villous loss, and an indication for sections at multiple levels if a patchy lesion is seen. The mounting and orientation of the specimen are important to obtain the best information, even though severe lesions can be diagnosed with imperfect orientation.

Histological interpretation

The biopsy of the normal upper small bowel in temperate zones shows a mixture of finger- and leaf-shaped villi (Fig. 2(a)). Histologically the epithelial cells are tall and columnar with basal, palisaded nuclei. There are a few lymphocytes between the epithelial cells. There is a scanty infiltrate of inflammatory cells in the lamina propria. The villi are several times as long as the depth of the crypts (Fig. 2(b)).

Duodenal samples with underlying Brunner's glands may show villi that are rather flattened and this may apply in areas of jejunal samples that overlie lymphoid nodules. In tropical areas a wider range of appearances may be found in subjects with no evidence of disease.

The small intestine responds in a similar way to many different diseases. Milder lesions, consisting of (i) broadening of the villi, which may be branched or fused, (ii) oedema and excess of inflammatory cells beneath the surface epithelium, and (iii) sometimes reduction in the height of the epithelial cells and loss of their regular nuclear arrangement, are very non-specific. Causes include malignancy anywhere in the body, malnutrition, small-bowel ischaemia, severe skin disease, bacterial overgrowth in the small intestine, various parasitic infestations of the small intestine, excess secretion of gastric acid as in the Zollinger–Ellison syndrome, and numerous other conditions. A severe lesion with total loss of villi and crypt hypertrophy is highly suggestive of coeliac disease but total or subtotal villous atrophy may be seen occasionally

Fig. 2 (a) Dissecting-microscopic appearance of normal jejunal mucosa showing finger-shaped and leaf-shaped villi. (b) Histological appearance of normal jejunal mucosa showing tall villi, several times as long as the crypts are deep. The epithelial cells are columnar with basal nuclei. There is a scattering of inflammatory cells deep into the mucosa.

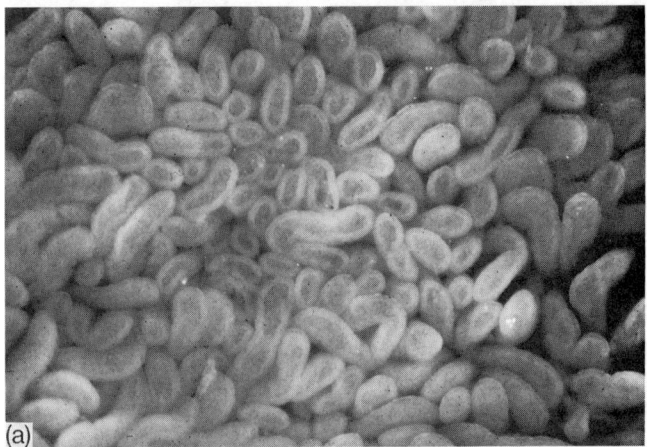

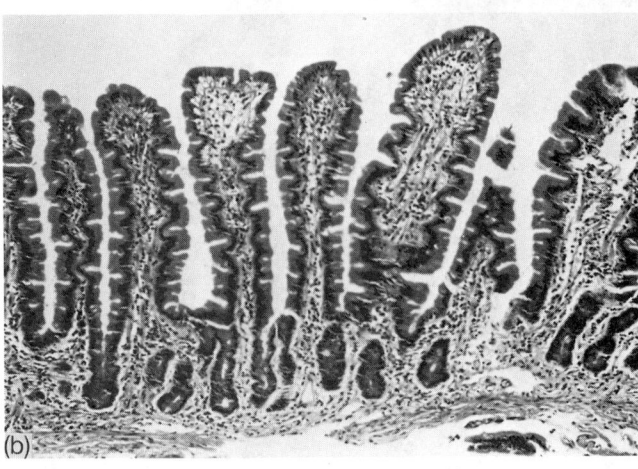

in other conditions, notably severe tropical sprue, cows' milk sensitivity in young children, and gastroenteritis in young children. Rarer causes of a severe villous lesion include soy protein intolerance, eosinophilic gastroenteropathy, immune deficiency syndromes, severe malnutrition, ischaemia of the small intestine, and damage due to drugs or irradiation.

Diseases with specific features (Fig. 3) by which a confident diagnosis may be made from the intestinal biopsy include Whipple's disease (in which the villi are seen to be stuffed with macrophages containing periodic acid–Schiff-positive material) (see Chapter 14.9.6), abetalipoproteinaemia (in which the epithelial cells are distended with lipid), diffuse lymphoma (Chapter 14.9.8), giardiasis and other infestations in which the parasites may be found (Section 7), lymphangiectasia (in which distended lymphatics can be identified in some of the villi), and humoral immune deficiencies (in which all grades of villous abnormality may be seen together with a deficiency of plasma cells in the lamina propria; Section 5). *Mycobacterium avium intracellulare*, showing up acid-fast in the lamina propria and in inflammatory cells, may be found in immunocompromised patients, especially those with AIDS.

There are certain other conditions in which a presumptive diagnosis may be made from the biopsy. In many of these the lesions are patchy and may be missed on single, or even on multiple, biopsies. Crohn's disease may show granulomas with giant cells (Fig. 3(b)). The small-bowel lesion that follows abdominal radiotherapy may show villous loss without crypt hyperplasia (a similar lesion is sometimes seen in severe coeliac disease or tropical sprue). Specific stains may reveal amyloid infiltration. Eosinophilic gastroenteropathy may be associated with eosinophilia in the blood.

ENDOSCOPIC BIOPSY

With the ready availability of upper gastrointestinal endoscopy, biopsy samples from the duodenum are frequently available. Coeliac disease may be strongly suspected from the endoscopic appearances of loss of folds in the duodenum. Endoscopic biopsy may reliably refute coeliac disease, if normal villi are shown, or suggest coeliac disease if the characteristic lesion is seen. There are, however, a number of pitfalls in

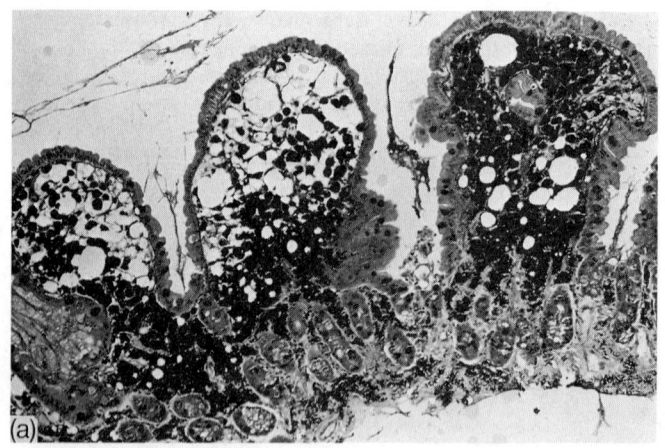

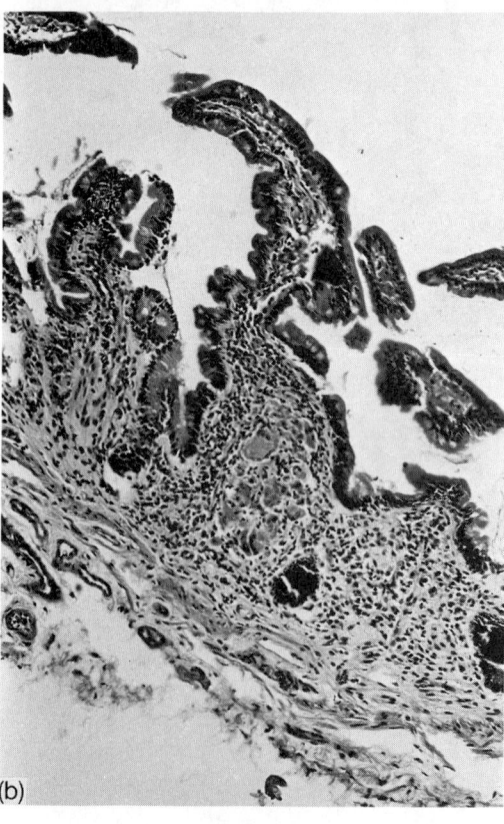

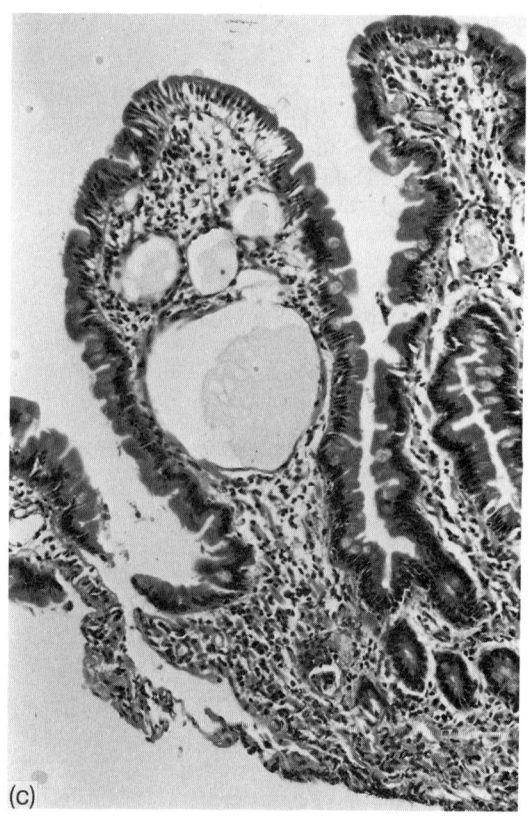

Fig. 3 Examples of conditions that may be diagnosed or suspected from jejunal biopsy material. (a) Whipple's disease: the villi are distended but the overlying epithelium is relatively normal. This periodic acid–Schiff stain demonstrates macrophages stuffed with deposits of glycoprotein, and distended lymphatic spaces within the villi. (b) Crohn's disease. At the base of a villus is a granuloma containing giant cells. (c) Intestinal lymphangiectasia. A villus is shown with grossly distended lymphatics in its core.

interpreting duodenal biopsies. Villous flattening over Brunner's glands is mentioned above. The proportion of leaf-shaped villi is higher in the duodenum and histologically this may appear as broadening of the villi. Duodenal mucosa from the vicinity of a peptic ulcer may show inflammatory changes. The relatively common condition of duodenitis must be appreciated to avoid misinterpretation. In occasional patients with coeliac disease the duodenal mucosa is much less severely affected than the jejunal mucosa.

ENZYME MEASUREMENTS

Determination of enzyme activity in biopsy tissue will reveal multiple deficiencies if there are, for any reason, gross histological abnormalities. Isolated deficiency of lactase is diagnostic of primary alactasia.

SMALL-BOWEL RADIOLOGY (SEE CHAPTER 14.3.2)

The purpose of radiological investigation of the small bowel is to reveal anatomical lesions as the cause of malabsorption and as complications of other disorders, and to indicate gross defects of motility. A small-bowel follow-through can be done as a sequel to a barium meal when metoclopramide can be used to speed the progress of the contrast medium, but we prefer the technique of small-bowel enema (enteroclysis) in which a fine tube is passed into the duodenum, and barium sulphate is followed by a propellant such as methylcellulose suspension (Fig. 4).

Non-specific findings

Non-specific findings such as dilatation, thickened folds (suggesting oedema), and poor motility occur in many disorders of the small bowel that are accompanied by malabsorption. Flocculation of the contrast medium is minimized by the technique of small-bowel enema and by the newer, relatively non-flocculating media, but when it does occur it is a non-specific indication of excessive secretion.

Specific findings

A definitive diagnosis of a cause for malabsorption may be obtained with diverticula, blind loops, strictures, or fistulae (Fig. 5).

Fig. 4 Normal small intestine shown by the technique of small-bowel enema. The loops of the small intestine and their transverse folds are well shown. The large intestine is also partially filled on this film.

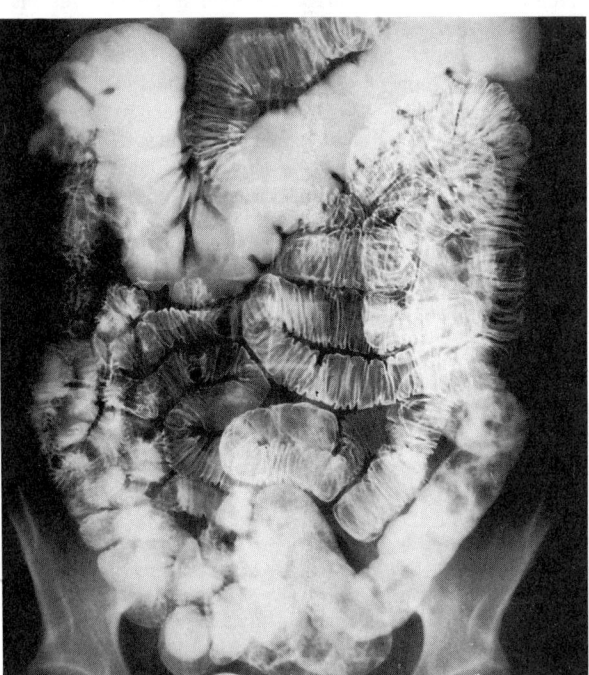

In systemic sclerosis a severe motility disturbance may be accompanied by the diagnostic feature of dilatation of the small bowel, particularly affecting the duodenum, but with the folds remaining close together (the 'hidebound' bowel) in contrast to spreading of the folds seen in other causes of dilatation (Fig. 6).

A diagnosis of Crohn's disease may be made with considerable confidence if irregular, thickened folds, ulceration, narrowing of the lumen, and thickening of the wall are seen, particularly if present in the terminal ileum and more particularly if multiple, short segments of small bowel are affected ('skip lesions'). Differential diagnosis of such appearances includes tuberculosis of the small intestine, lymphoma, Henoch–Schönlein lesions, Behçet's disease, and mesenteric venous thrombosis which sometimes occurs in young females taking the contraceptive pill.

Fig. 5 Multiple diverticula of the small intestine shown by the technique of small-bowel enema.

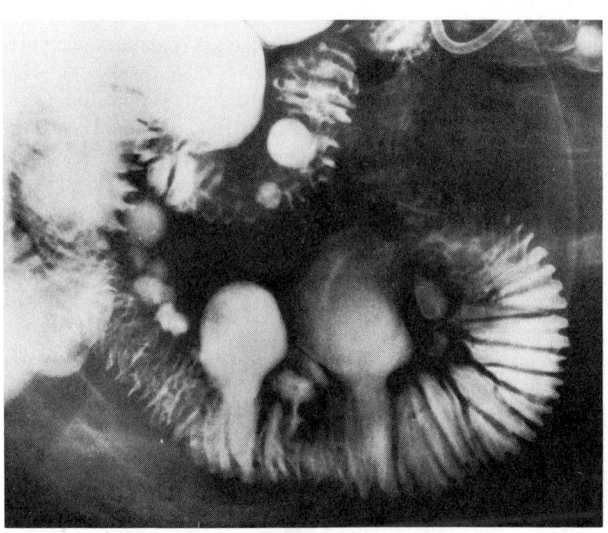

Fig. 6 Dilated small intestine with the transverse folds remaining very close together (the 'hidebound' bowel) diagnostic of systemic sclerosis of the small intestine.

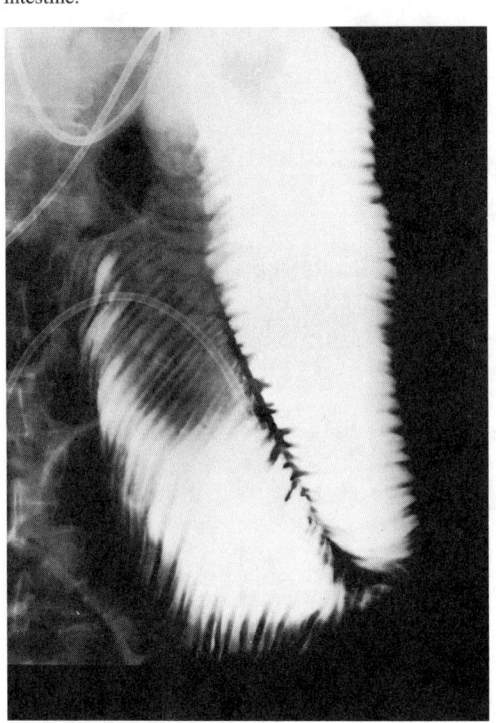

Tumours of the small intestine, usually lymphomas, may appear as mass lesions or merely as rigidity or thickening of the wall. Lymphoma of the small intestine may, however, be present with entirely normal appearances by this technique.

Complications of other disorders

In coeliac disease, strictures and ulcers may occur. A similar condition, which has been termed idiopathic chronic ulcerative enteritis, may occur in the absence of coeliac disease.

In conditions of defective humoral immunity, multiple small lymphoid nodules may be found in the small intestine (nodular lymphoid hyperplasia) and should not be mistaken for lymphoma.

After abdominal or pelvic radiation there may be defective motility of a region of small intestine and this may be accompanied by scarring, shown by tethering or rigidity of the wall, or by strictures.

NUTRITIONAL STATUS

Deficiencies of the major nutrients are reflected in a general way by loss of body weight and low serum albumin.

Investigation for deficiencies of haematinic factors (iron, folic acid, and vitamin B_{12}) and fat-soluble vitamins (A, D, and K) should be undertaken. Deficiencies of water-soluble vitamins are uncommon.

If diarrhoea is severe, water and electrolyte deficiencies need to be confirmed and managed in the usual way.

Fig. 7 The radioactive bile-acid breath test for detection of bacterial overgrowth in the small intestine. A false-positive result may be caused by ileal disease or resection, in which case there is also excess radioactivity in the faeces (see text).

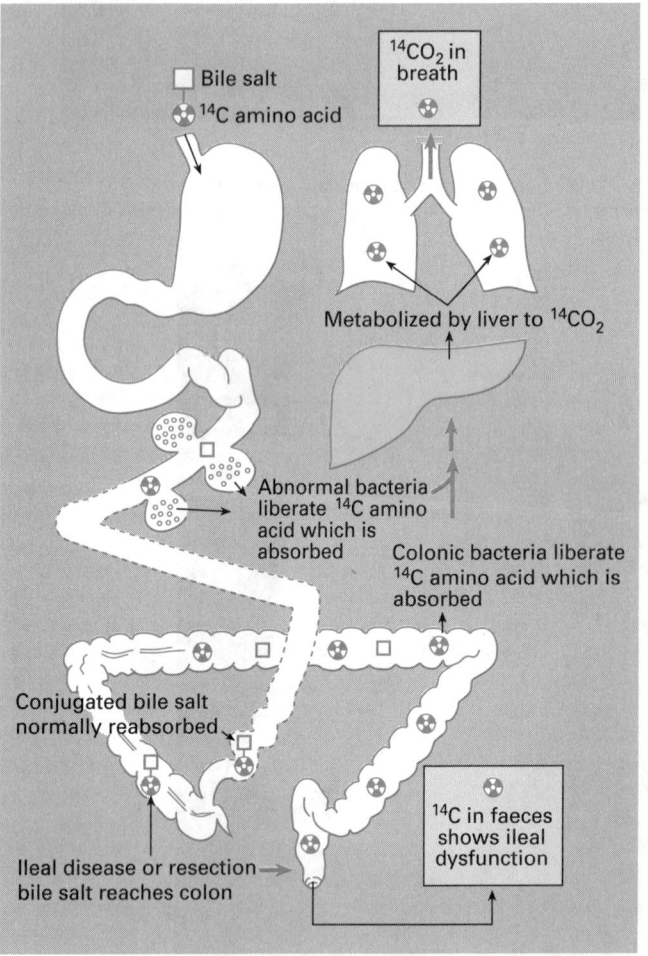

Magnesium deficiency may be suspected from low plasma and urine concentrations of magnesium.

Hypocalcaemia may need emergency treatment by intravenous calcium if tetany or other acute problems occur.

SMALL-BOWEL BACTERIOLOGY

The upper part of the small intestine has a transient and variable flora, which is received from the stomach and is derived from the resident mouth organisms and from organisms ingested in the food. Gastric acid helps to minimize the load of bacteria transmitted to the small intestine. In residents of temperate zones in the fasting state the upper part of the small intestine is remarkably free of organisms and those few present are aerobes. The further down the small intestine, the more abundant the bacterial flora becomes and the greater the concentration of anaerobes. As the terminal ileum is approached, the range of organisms comes to resemble that in the proximal colon but in much lower concentrations. The microflora in the lumen of the small intestine has beneficial nutritional effects, synthesizing vitamin K and sometimes folic acid, and also deleterious nutritional effects, consuming or binding vitamin B_{12} and deconjugating bile salts.

Diagnosis of the presence of bacterial overgrowth in the small intestine requires quantitative bacteriological investigations on jejunal aspirates, with particular attention to anaerobes. Normally fewer than about 10^5 organisms/ml are found, predominantly Gram-positive aerobes, with an absence of 'faecal' type organisms such as *Escherichia coli*, Clostridia, and Bacteroides. False-negative results occur when the overgrowth is confined to areas further down the small intestine.

Presumptive evidence of bacterial overgrowth in the small bowel may be obtained by the bile-acid breath test (Fig. 7). A conjugated bile acid, with the amino acid portion labelled with ^{14}C, is given by mouth. If there are abnormal bacteria in the upper small intestine, the bile salt is deconjugated and the radioactively labelled amino acid is absorbed, transported to the liver, and rapidly metabolized to carbon dioxide. The radioactive carbon dioxide excreted in the breath is collected and the amount of radioactivity indicates the amount of deconjugation of the bile salt that occurred in the upper small intestine. In the normal subject, very little deconjugation occurs and the conjugated bile salt passes down the small intestine, to be reabsorbed intact in the terminal ileum. In disease of the terminal ileum the conjugated bile salt is not absorbed and enters the colon, where deconjugation is produced by colonic bacteria and radioactive carbon dioxide is excreted in the breath. This false-positive result in ileal disease can be recognized by measuring the faecal excretion of radioactivity, which is high in ileal disease but not in bacterial overgrowth in the upper small intestine. The bile-acid breath test may give false-negative results, which presumably depend on the particular type of bacteria inhabiting the upper small intestine.

Breath tests that do not require the use of radioisotopes depend on the measurement of hydrogen. Bacterial fermentation of an oral dose of carbohydrate (glucose or lactulose) releases hydrogen, and if there is an increase in bacteria in the upper small bowel an early hydrogen peak occurs in the expired air. It seems likely that the sensitivity of the hydrogen breath test is similar to that of the ^{14}C bile-acid breath tests and hydrogen analysers are available that make the method easy to apply.

REFERENCES

Cook, G.C. (1984). Hypolactasia. Geographical distribution, diagnosis, and practical significance. In *Critical Reviews in tropical medicine*, Vol. 2, (ed. R.K. Chandra), pp. 117–39. Plenum, New York.

Herlinger H. and Maglinte D. (ed.) (1989). *Clinical radiology of the small intestine*. Saunders, Philadelphia.

King, C.E. and Toskes, P.P. (1983). The use of breath tests in the study of malabsorption. *Clinical Gastroenterology*, **12**, 591–610.

Losowsky, M.S. (1984). The consequences of malabsorption. In *Textbook of Gastroenterology* (ed. I.A.D. Bouchier, R.N. Allan, H.J.F. Hodgson, and M.R.B. Keighley), pp. 441–7. Baillière Tindall, London.

Losowsky, M.S. (1989). Peroral biopsy of the small intestine. In *Clinical radiology of the small intestine* (ed. H. Herlinger and D. Maglinte), pp. 237–42. Saunders, Philadelphia.

Simon, G.L. and Gorbach, S.L. (1984). Intestinal flora in health and disease. *Gastroenterology*, **86**, 174–93.

14.9.3 Small-bowel bacterial overgrowth

S. P. PEREIRA and R. H. DOWLING

DEFINITION

Small-bowel bacterial overgrowth is a syndrome characterized, in its florid form, by weight loss, diarrhoea, malabsorption of nutrients and some vitamins, and altered bile-acid metabolism. It is due to proliferation of an abnormal bacterial flora in the small intestine, and is also known as the blind loop syndrome, the contaminated bowel syndrome and, in one specific example, the afferent loop syndrome.

THE NORMAL INTESTINAL BACTERIAL FLORA

In terms of luminal bacteria, the small intestine constitutes a transitional zone between the sparsely populated stomach and the luxuriant flora of the colon. The lumen of the proximal small intestine normally contains fewer than 10^4 organisms (or, more correctly, colony-forming units) per ml of fluid. Most of these are swallowed with food, or originate in the oropharynx, and they are mainly Gram-positive aerobes and facultative anaerobes. Obligate anaerobes, such as Bacteroides, are not found in the proximal small bowel of the healthy host.

Two normal processes limit bacterial proliferation in the upper small intestine. These are: (i) the presence of secreted acid in the stomach, which largely sterilizes ingested food and decreases the load of bacteria entering the small intestine—the so-called acid trap; and (ii) normal, segmental, propulsive contractions of the intestine, which sweep bacteria that have escaped the acid trap to the distal small bowel. Intestinal immunoglobulin (mainly dimeric IgA) secretion, and the presence of a mucus barrier that inhibits bacterial adherence, may also influence the small-intestinal flora but the quantitative importance of these latter two factors is unknown.

In the ileum, the total bacterial count (aerobes and anaerobes) normally reaches 10^5 to 10^9 per ml of aspirate, and here Gram-negative bacteria begin to outnumber Gram-positive strains. Although the ileo-caecal valve is relatively weak and almost certainly not bacteriologically competent, the terminal ileum–ileocaecal valve-caecal motor unit maintains a steep bacterial concentration gradient between the distal ileum and the proximal colon. In the large bowel, bacterial concentrations increase to 10^{11} to 10^{12} organisms per ml, and anaerobic bacteria outnumber aerobes by a factor of 10^2 to 10^4. Nearly one-third of the faecal dry weight is comprised of viable bacteria.

AETIOLOGY OF SMALL-BOWEL BACTERIAL OVERGROWTH

Any situation in which gastric acid secretion is reduced, or intestinal motility is impaired, may lead to bacterial overgrowth. Anatomical disorders that result in stagnation of intestinal contents, or seeding of the proximal small intestine with colonic-type bacteria, also predispose to abnormal bacterial proliferation (Table 1). In these situations, a small-intestinal flora develops which is predominantly anaerobic and closely resembles that of the colon, with bacterial counts in the upper intestine reaching 10^5 per ml or more.

Decreased gastric acid secretion

At the normal acidic gastric pH, the stomach is essentially sterile with fewer than 10^3 organisms per ml. Hypo- or achlorhydria, secondary to chronic atrophic gastritis or pernicious anaemia (see Section 22), permits

Table 1 *Conditions associated with small-bowel bacterial overgrowth*

Gastric hypochlorhydria
Chronic atrophic gastritis/pernicious anaemia
Vagotomy and/or gastric resection
Treatment with H_2 antagonists or proton-pump inhibitors

Anatomical abnormalities of the gut
Postsurgical:
    Afferent loop of a Billroth II/Poly A partial gastrectomy
    Blind loop (side-to-end anastomosis)
    Recirculating loop (side-to-side anastomosis)
    Continent ileostomy
Diverticula:
    Duodenal
    Jejunal
Fistulae:
    Cologastric
    Ileogastric
    Colojejunal
    Ileojejunal
Obstruction:
    Strictures
    Adhesions

Disordered intestinal motility
Systemic sclerosis
Diabetic autonomic neuropathy
Intestinal pseudo-obstruction
Amyloidosis

Miscellaneous
Malabsorption in the elderly
Hypo-or agammaglobulinaemia
Cirrhosis
Bacterial cholangitis

a larger than normal fraction of the bacteria ingested with food, or present in oropharyngeal secretions, to traverse the stomach and enter the small bowel. Bacterial overgrowth in association with treatments that reduce gastric acid secretion, such as H_2 receptor antagonists or proton-pump inhibitors, has been reported recently. Gastric acid secretion is also diminished after a variety of stomach operations (vagotomy and pyloroplasty, Billroth I gastrectomy, vagotomy plus antrectomy, and Billroth II or Polya gastrectomy), and bacterial overgrowth occurs in 10 (vagotomy and pyloroplasty) to 50 per cent (Billroth II gastrectomy) of these patients. The results of studies in experimental animals suggest that bacterial overgrowth does not develop if gastric acid secretion, and antral and duodenal innervation, are preserved, and continuous gastrointestinal anatomy, without a blind loop, is maintained.

Disorders of intestinal motility

Normal intestinal motility (propulsive segmental contractions after food and migrating motor complexes in the interdigestive phase) prevents stasis of intestinal contents. Together with gastric acid secretion, the 'housekeeping' effect of motility sweeping intestinal contents distally is the other major host defence against bacterial overgrowth. Conditions associated with impaired peristalsis include systemic sclerosis intestinal pseudo-obstruction, diabetic autonomic neuropathy, and, rarely, amyloidosis.

There is also evidence that intestinal dysmotility may be a consequence, as well as a cause, of bacterial overgrowth. In experimental blind loops (rats with surgically fashioned, self-filling segments of intestine), disordered migrating motor complexes that improve after antibiotic therapy have been described. Absent or disordered interdigestive motor complexes have also been found in some 25 per cent of patients with small-bowel bacterial overgrowth. The mechanism for this disturbance in motility, or the reversibility of the motor defect with antibiotic therapy, has not been established.

Anatomical disorders

Stagnation of intestinal contents, with resultant proliferation of bacteria, may occur in the afferent limb of a Billroth II gastrectomy, within duodenal or jejunal diverticula (Fig. 1), or as a result of chronic obstruction secondary to intestinal strictures or adhesions. Contamination of the proximal intestine with bacteria from the distal small bowel and/or colon—as a result of cologastric, colojejunal, ileogastric, or ileojejunal fistulae—also predisposes to bacterial overgrowth. Underlying causes of enteric fistulae include Crohn's disease, (Fig. 2), tuberculosis, lymphoma, radiation enteritis, and colonic diverticulosis.

Resection of the distal small bowel and ileocaecal valve may result in backwash of bacteria-rich colonic contents through the anastomosis into the ileum or jejunum. Therefore, small-bowel intubation studies in these patients may show high counts of total and anaerobic bacteria in the proximal small bowel, but the clinical picture of small-bowel bacterial overgrowth is seldom seen. Even if it were present, it would be difficult to distinguish between the effects of bile acid and vitamin B_{12} malabsorption secondary to ileal resection and those of bacterial overgrowth.

Ileal bacterial proliferation and pouch inflammation have also been reported in patients with a continent ileostomy, or following proctocolectomy and ileoanal anastomoses, particularly after fashioning of a J or W pouch reservoir, or reversed (antiperistaltic) ileal segments.

Miscellaneous causes

High duodenal bacterial counts are found in 30 to 60 per cent of elderly patients presenting with clinical or biochemical evidence of malnutrition. On investigation, an explanation can be found in the majority—hypochlorhydria, duodenojejunal diverticula, or slower mouth-to-caecum transit times than those in age-matched controls. One study concluded that approximately one-third of elderly patients with high duodenal bacterial counts had 'clinically significant' bacterial overgrowth. This conclusion was based on the overall clinical picture, together with haematological and/or biochemical abnormalities consistent with malabsorption, and the fact that the abnormalities improved following treatment with broad-spectrum antibiotics.

Secretory IgA, by binding to gut bacteria, can prevent them from attaching to, and penetrating, intestinal epithelial cells. However, intestinal IgA is probably only of minor importance in maintaining the normal small-bowel flora. A few studies have suggested that patients with immunoglobulin deficiency have an abundant jejunal flora. However, gastric hypochlorhydria is common in hypogammaglobulinaemic patients with common-variable immunodeficiency, and bacterial counts in the small-bowel lumen of these patients are no higher than in those with pernicious anaemia alone. Bacterial overgrowth has only rarely been associated with selective IgA deficiency.

High counts of Gram-negative bacteria have been cultured in duodenal and jejunal juice from 20 to 75 per cent of patients with hepatic cirrhosis. Delayed small-intestinal transit, and prolonged phase-2 migrating motor complexes, have been described in cirrhosis, but whether the high counts of bacteria in the small bowel contribute to the clinical picture of cirrhosis is unknown. Paradoxically, recent experimental evidence suggests that small-bowel bacterial overgrowth itself can induce hepatobiliary injury. This is characterized by portal-tract inflammation, bile-duct proliferation, and destruction of the bile-duct epithelium. The mechanism for this induced hepatic injury is unclear. However, in rats with self-filling, blind jejunal loops, bacterial proliferation of anaerobes, such as Bacteroides results in accumulation of peptidoglycan polysaccharide (a bacterial cell-wall polymer with potent inflammatory properties), which, after absorption from the injured intestinal mucosa, may activate Kupffer cells and lead to hepatic injury.

There have been isolated reports of small-bowel overgrowth in patients with bacterial cholangitis secondary, for example, to common bile-duct stones or biliary strictures, where the infected biliary tree acts as a reservoir from which bacteria, and/or deamidated bile acids, spill into the small bowel.

PATHOGENESIS

In bacterial overgrowth, the mechanism for the malabsorption of fats, carbohydrates, proteins, bile acids, vitamins, and trace metals is due to: (i) disturbed intraluminal metabolism by the abnormal small-bowel bac-

Fig. 1 Barium follow-through in a patient with small bowel bacterial overgrowth secondary to extensive jejunal diverticulosis: supine film. (By courtesy of Dr D. MacIver.)

Fig. 2 Barium follow-through in a patient with bacterial overgrowth associated with extensive ileal Crohn's disease and a coloileal fistula. Note not only the abnormal loops of ileum showing typical features of Crohn's disease, but also the premature opacification of the rectum at a time when no barium had reached the other parts of the large bowel. (By courtesy of Dr. C. Kennedy.)

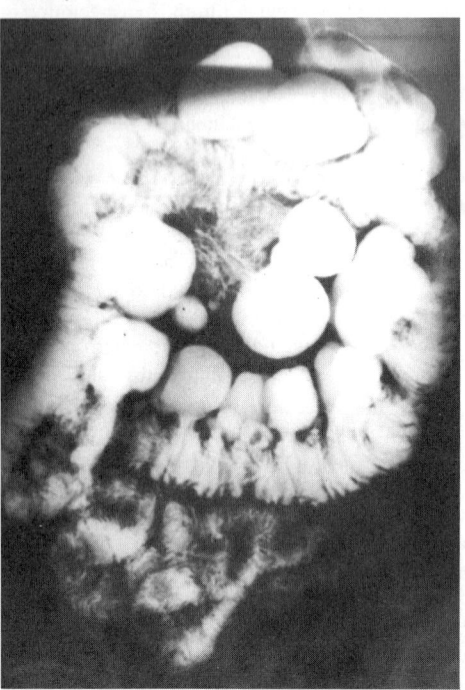

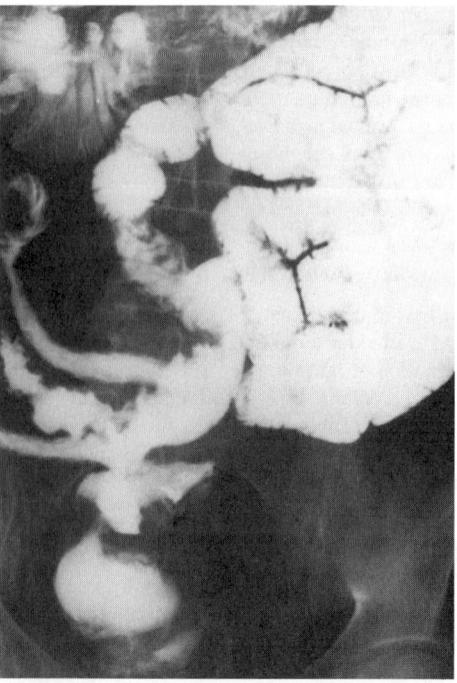

teria, and (ii) patchy damage to small-intestinal enterocytes. However, the relative importance of these two factors remains undefined. Bacterial adhesion to the small-intestinal mucosa has been demonstrated by scanning electron microscopy of peroral intestinal mucosal biopsies in 10 to 30 per cent of patients with bacterial overgrowth, but there is little evidence of direct bacterial invasion of the intestinal mucosa.

Fat malabsorption

Clinically apparent steatorrhoea has been reported in about one-third of patients who have bacterial overgrowth that is severe enough to cause vitamin B_{12} deficiency.

Under normal conditions, the digestion and absorption of long-chain triglycerides (the principal dietary form of fat) involves (i) emulsification, (ii) hydrolysis of the fatty acid ester linkages in the emulsified droplets by pancreatic lipase and colipase, (iii) solubilization and aqueous dispersion of lipolytic products (monoglycerides and fatty acids) first into vesicles and then into mixed (bile acid–phospholipid–cholesterol) micelles, and (iv) absorption of the hydrolysed lipids from the micelles, by diffusion into upper small-intestinal enterocytes.

In bacterial overgrowth, anaerobic species such as Bacteroides, bifidobacteria, enterococci, and clostridia deamidate the intraluminal bile acids, removing the glycine or taurine conjugates to a variable degree. At the pH of the proximal small bowel (5.0–6.5), the deconjugated bile acids are protonated and therefore liable to premature absorption by passive non-ionic diffusion. In turn, this leads to a premature jejunohepatic (rather than the normal ileohepatic) circulation. Given their high pK_a, deconjugated bile acids are also vulnerable to precipitation in the slightly acidic environment of the upper small-bowel lumen, as inert crystals. These two factors result in intraluminal bile-acid deficiency and, as a consequence, impaired micelle formation, fat malabsorption, and steatorrhoea. However, the fat malabsorption may not be due exclusively to the altered bile acid metabolism—mucosal injury may also play a part. Decreased mucosal uptake, reduced intracellular re-esterification of fatty acids, and impaired transfer of chylomicrons from the enterocytes into the lymphatics, have all been described in intestinal biopsies from patients with bacterial overgrowth, and in animals with self-filling blind loops.

Carbohydrates

Intraluminal fermentation of carbohydrates also occurs in bacterial overgrowth, with production of hydrogen, carbon dioxide, volatile short-chain fatty acids (acetic, butyric, and propionic acids), and small amounts of alcohol. Indeed, the generation of H_2, its rapid absorption from the intestine, diffusion into the bloodstream, and excretion by the lungs is the basis for both the glucose and lactulose breath H_2 tests for small-bowel bacterial overgrowth.

In the small intestine, high concentrations of short-chain fatty acids may damage the mucosa, and contribute to the diminished absorption of carbohydrates secondary to enterocyte brush-border injury. Certainly, decreased activity of disaccharidases has been reported in peroral jejunal mucosal biopsies from patients with bacterial overgrowth, but whether this is due to the short-chain fatty acids or to some other bacterial 'toxin' is unknown. However, in the colon, which is the predominant site of short-chain fatty acid production, the volatile fatty acids provide a 'fuel' for the mucosa, and butyrate, in particular, stimulates colonocyte growth and function. Moreover, an estimated 15 to 60 g of carbohydrate that is not absorbed in the small intestine can be 'salvaged' each day from the colon. Thus, unabsorbed carbohydrate spills into the colon and is fermented by anaerobic bacterial polysaccharidases to form short-chain fatty acids. In turn, these are avidly absorbed by both ionic and non-ionic diffusion, thereby enhancing net water and electrolyte absorption in the colon, and providing energy for the host.

Protein

Hypoalbuminaemia has been reported in patients with bacterial overgrowth. Although the mechanism for this protein deficiency is not completely understood, evidence from rats with experimental blind loops suggests that several factors play a part. Intraluminal deamidation of protein and amino acids by bacterial proteases certainly occurs. This is the basis for measuring urinary indican (indoxyl sulphate) excretion as a diagnostic test for small-bowel bacterial overgrowth. Decreased hepatic synthesis of protein (secondary to essential amino acid deficiency), reduced intestinal mucosal uptake of amino acids and peptides, and protein-losing enteropathy have all been reported in patients with small-bowel bacterial overgrowth.

Vitamins and minerals

Vitamin B_{12} malabsorption is a common feature of small-bowel bacterial overgrowth. The malabsorption is partial rather than complete, and low serum vitamin B_{12} levels are seen only in long-standing bacterial contamination of the small bowel, when hepatic stores of transcobalamin II have become depleted over several years.

The vitamin B_{12} malabsorption is usually attributed to bacterial uptake of the B_{12}–intrinsic factor complex, even though the uptake of the bound form by Gram-negative aerobes is some 20 to 95 per cent lower than their ability to take up free cobalamin. However, anaerobic bacteria avidly bind the cobalamin–intrinsic factor complex, making it unavailable to the host. This is the basis for the abnormal Schilling test, which is not corrected by intrinsic factor, in patients with small-bowel bacterial overgrowth (see Section 22). Anaerobes also metabolize the B_{12}–intrinsic factor complex to inactive analogues (cobamides), which act as competitive inhibitors of active B_{12} transport in the terminal ileum. In addition, the cobamides occupy vitamin B_{12} storage sites in the liver at the expense of the normal storage form (B_{12} bound to transcobalamin II). However, the quantitative importance of cobamide production on vitamin B_{12} stores is unknown.

Serum and red blood-cell folate levels are usually normal in bacterial overgrowth. In fact, they may even be high, due to bacterial synthesis of 5-methyl tetrahydrofolate, which is then absorbed.

While the digestion and absorption of dietary fat are facilitated by adequate luminal concentrations of bile acids, the absorption of sterols and fat-soluble vitamins is totally dependent on intraluminal bile acids. In theory, therefore, luminal deficiency of conjugated bile acids should cause more profound effects on the absorption of vitamins A, D, E, and K than on the absorption of fat. In practice, however, clinical or subclinical fat-soluble vitamin deficiency has been described only rarely in patients with small-bowel bacterial overgrowth.

Iron deficiency is also unusual, although some gut bacteria do have a high binding affinity for iron. In the experimental blind-loop syndrome, increased intestinal losses of iron and blood have been documented, but in patients with bacterial overgrowth, frank or occult bleeding in the presence of strictures or stercoral ulceration has only occasionally been reported.

Water and electrolytes

Although the mechanism for the diarrhoea in small-bowel bacterial overgrowth has not been well studied in both the small- and large-bowel lumen, secretory and osmotic processes both contribute. Bacterial metabolites, such as hydroxylated fatty acids and deconjugated bile acids, stimulate secretion of water and electrolytes although this effect is non-specific. Injury to the brush border of the enterocytes, resulting in decreased absorption of fat, carbohydrate, and protein, may also contribute to diarrhoea by increasing the osmolarity of small- and large-bowel contents.

Enterocyte damage

Although often patchy and variable in severity, a small-bowel lesion can be readily identified in experimental animals with self-filling blind loops and, less consistently, in patients with bacterial overgrowth. The lesion consists of non-specific blunting and broadening of small-intestinal villi, with or without associated crypt hyperplasia and an increase in the number of mononuclear cells within the lamina propria. In patients whose small-intestinal mucosa is normal by light microscopy, subtle degenerative changes in the enterocyte can be seen on electron microscopy. Brush-border enzyme activity (especially that of disaccharidases), and active transport of monosaccharides, fatty acids and amino acids, are also diminished. The causes of mucosal damage are unclear but have been attributed to the deleterious effects of unconjugated di-α-hydroxy-bile acids, hydroxylated fatty acids, bacterial proteases, and to mucus degradation by bacterial glycosidases.

Although morphological changes in the small-bowel mucosa have been described, there is still controversy about the overall importance of these generally minor structural changes. Thus, even if there are subtle changes in the light- and electron-microscopic appearance of mucosal biopsies from patients with small-bowel bacterial overgrowth, given the length of the small intestine and its enormous 'functional reserve' it is questionable whether the reduction in villus height, or the changes in the ultrastructure of the enterocytes described above, could cause clinically significant malabsorption in many patients.

CLINICAL FEATURES

Symptoms vary greatly, and many individuals with high duodenal/jejunal bacterial counts, with or without haematological or biochemical evidence of malabsorption, may be asymptomatic. In general, the clinical picture depends on: (i) the metabolic activity of the abnormal flora, (ii) the resultant small-bowel malabsorption, and (iii) the predisposing condition. For example, patients may have duodenal or jejunal diverticulosis for years before the classical symptoms and signs of bacterial overgrowth—weight loss, diarrhoea, steatorrhoea, and vitamin B_{12} malabsorption—develop. Other symptoms, such as recurrent abdominal pain, early satiety, and bloating, which have been reported in up to 40 per cent of patients with bacterial overgrowth secondary to jejunal diverticulosis, are non-specific. In conditions such as Crohn's disease, systemic sclerosis, or intestinal pseudo-obstruction, the clinical features of the primary disease may be difficult to distinguish from those due to intraluminal bacterial proliferation. Less commonly, patients with occult bacterial overgrowth may present with isolated vitamin B_{12} deficiency, or clinical evidence of fat-soluble vitamin malabsorption, such as night blindness (vitamin A deficiency), osteomalacia, rickets or proximal myopathy (vitamin D deficiency), or bleeding secondary to vitamin K deficiency.

DIAGNOSIS (FIG. 3)

Relevant investigations may be divided into direct and indirect tests. Direct tests for bacterial overgrowth involve small-intestinal intubation and aspiration of duodenal or jejunal contents for quantitative culture of the small-intestinal flora. Cultured bacteria are often a mixture of anaerobes (Bacteroides, clostridia, bifidobacteria, lactobacilli, enterococci) and aerobes such as coliforms (*Escherichia coli*, Klebsiella). Duodenal contents can be aspirated during upper gastrointestinal endoscopy, or after intestinal intubation under fluoroscopic control. A proximal small-intestinal aspirate, however, will not always detect distal bacterial overgrowth, so that jejunal and even ileal intubation may be required in some patients. Aspirated juice can also be examined for the proportion of deconjugated bile acids or the presence of short-chain fatty acids. These tests are highly specific for bacterial overgrowth but in most series their sensitivity is less than 60 per cent, and they are not widely used.

Indirect tests for bacterial overgrowth are based on the measurement of end-products of intraluminal bacterial metabolism of fat, carbohydrate, protein, vitamins or bile acids in the breath, urine, faeces, or serum. Although they have the advantage of being non-invasive, many do not adequately distinguish between bacterial overgrowth and other causes of malabsorption. These include measuring the urinary excretion of indican or phenols (indices of bacterial breakdown of tryptophan and tyrosine, respectively), or of xylose following either a 5 g or 25 g oral test load (the D-xylose absorption test).

In contrast, increased fasting or postprandial serum unconjugated bile acids, or an increased ratio of serum unconjugated cholic acid to total cholic acid, have a reported sensitivity for bacterial overgrowth of 70 to 80 per cent. However, serum unconjugated bile acids may also be elevated in patients with ileal resection. In small-bowel bacterial overgrowth, bile acids undergo deconjugation by anaerobic bacteria within the lumen, and are then absorbed passively across the small-bowel mucosa to enter the portal circulation. The first-pass hepatic extraction of unconjugated bile acids from the sinusoidal blood is less effective (50–70 per cent) than that of conjugated bile acids (70–95 per cent). This may be due in part to differences in protein binding (albumin binds unconjugated bile acids more avidly than the unconjugated species) and in part to differences in the kinetics of the active transport of bile acids across the sinusoidal membrane. As a consequence, there is a preferential spill-over of unconjugated bile acids from the portal, into the systemic, circulation.

Breath tests (see Chapter 14.9.2)

Breath tests rely on the pulmonary excretion of either labelled CO_2 following the administration of ^{14}C- or ^{13}C-labelled substrates, or of H_2 following the administration of glucose, lactulose, or a carbohydrate-containing test meal. The principle of the bile acid ($[^{14}C]$ glycine-labelled glycocholate) breath test, is that anaerobic bacteria in the intestinal lumen deconjugate the labelled bile acid, liberating $[^{14}C]$ glycine. After absorption, the $[^{14}C]$ glycine is transported to the liver and metabolized there to release $^{14}CO_2$, which is then excreted in the breath. However, the bile-acid breath test has a false negative rate of up to 30 per cent. Moreover, it does not easily distinguish between small-bowel bacterial overgrowth and other causes of bile-acid malabsorption, such as ileal dysfunction, unless faecal bile-acid excretion is also measured. When patients with ileal dysfunction are given $[^{14}C]$ cholylglycine, it is malabsorbed and spills into the colon where it is metabolized by colonic bacteria. This results in a delayed breath $^{14}CO_2$ peak and high faecal output of the label. Conversely, in patients with small-bowel bacterial overgrowth, the bile-acid breath test is characterized by increased breath excretion of $^{14}CO_2$ and a normal or low excretion of the label in the faeces (less than 5 per cent of the administered ^{14}C label).

The rationale for breath H_2 testing is that, in mammals, bacterial fermentation of carbohydrate within the intestinal lumen is the only known source of H_2. About 20 per cent of H_2 produced in this way is absorbed across the intestinal mucosa and excreted in the expired air. In small-bowel bacterial overgrowth, H_2 production by anaerobic bacteria occurs not only in the colon but also in the small intestine. The bacterial metabolism of ingested test carbohydrates, such as 50 to 80 g glucose or 10 to 15 g lactulose, leads to an early peak in breath H_2 excretion. Although the specificity of breath H_2 tests for bacterial overgrowth is 80 per cent or more, in recent reports their sensitivity has ranged from less than 60 to over 90 per cent.

The 1-g $[^{14}C]$ D-xylose breath test is based on the observation that xylose is absorbed in the proximal small bowel, and is minimally metabolized by the host. In patients with terminal ileal disease or resection, following the ingestion of a ^{14}C-labelled xylose load, virtually none of the sugar reaches the colon and breath $^{14}CO_2$ excretion is not increased. However, in bacterial overgrowth, Gram-negative aerobic bacteria in the small bowel metabolize the labelled xylose to $^{14}CO_2$ which, after absorption, is exhaled. Within 1 h of ingesting $[^{14}C]$ xylose, 65 to 85 per cent of patients with bacterial overgrowth will have increased quantities of $^{14}CO_2$ in the breath. The results of one study suggest that the test is reproducible in over 90 per cent of patients—compared with a reproducibility for bacterial culture of jejunal aspirates of less than 50 per cent.

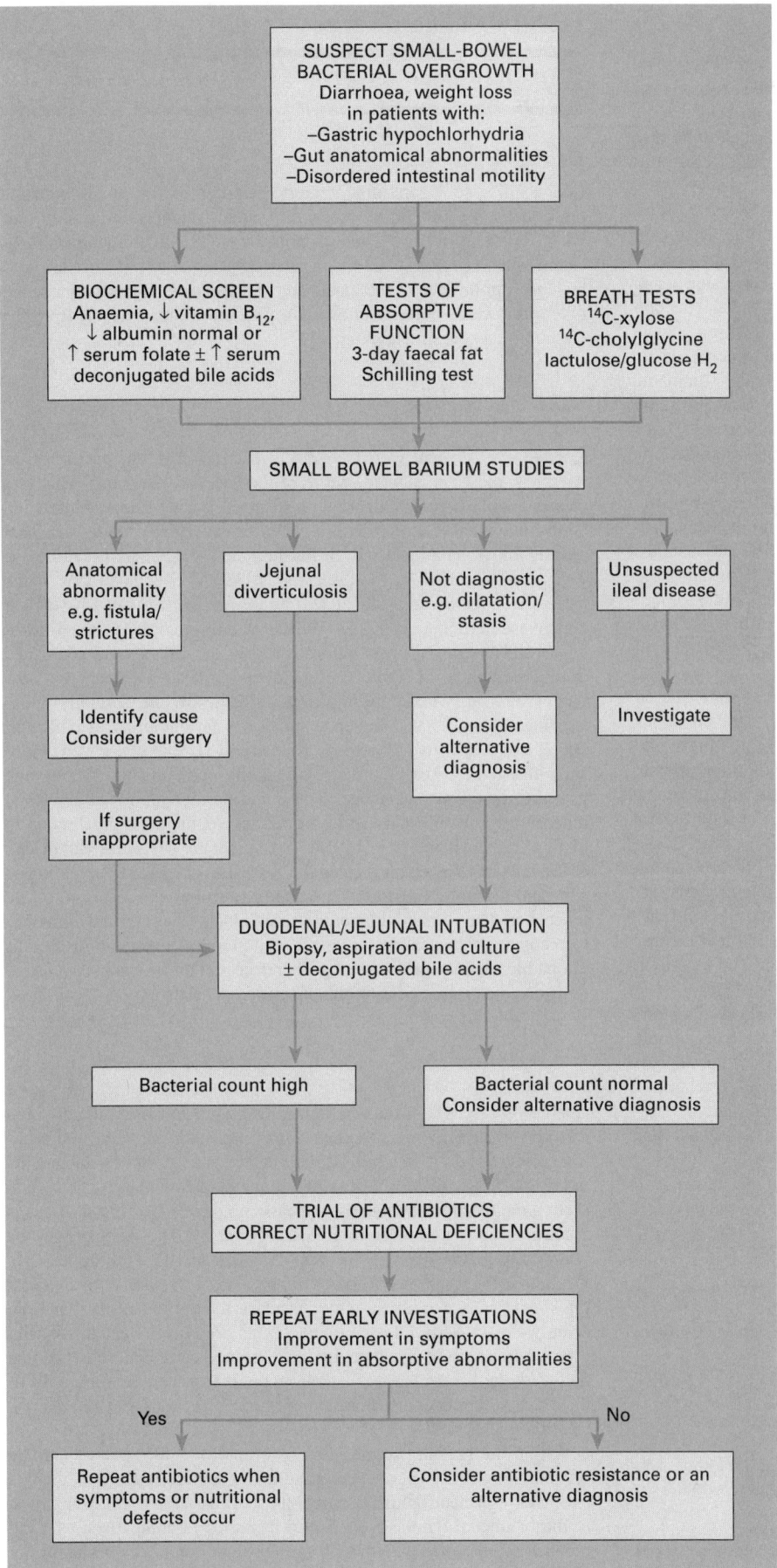

Fig. 3 Suggested scheme for the investigation of small-bowel bacterial overgrowth.

TREATMENT

Treatment is indicated in patients with small-bowel bacterial overgrowth who present with symptoms and signs such as diarrhoea and/or steatorrhoea, anaemia, and weight loss. However, there is no evidence that antimicrobial therapy is of value in asymptomatic patients who have high duodenal bacterial counts but no demonstrable absorptive abnormality.

Management of patients with small-bowel bacterial overgrowth can be divided into (i) antimicrobial treatment, (ii) nutritional support, together with correction of vitamin B_{12}, fat-soluble vitamin and possibly trace-metal, deficiencies, (iii) consideration of surgical correction of anatomical abnormalities, and (iv) medical therapy of any underlying condition, such as diabetes mellitus or small-bowel Crohn's disease.

Despite the fact that, *in vitro*, broad-spectrum antimicrobials are active primarily against aerobes, many are effective in eliminating small-bowel anaerobes. Indeed, by suppressing aerobes, broad-spectrum antimicrobials may act by creating an oxygen-rich environment that is unfavourable to the anaerobic flora, thereby reducing total bacterial counts to normal. Antimicrobials that have been shown to be effective in bacterial overgrowth include erythromycin, tetracycline, amoxycillin-clavulanic acid, trimethoprim-sulphamethoxazole, and the cephalosporins. Metronidazole is also effective, although other antianaerobic agents, such as clindamycin and chloramphenicol, are now rarely prescribed because of the risks of pseudomembranous colitis and bone marrow depression, respectively. Non-absorbable antimicrobials such as neomycin are not usually successful in eliminating the abnormal small-bowel flora.

There have been few adequately controlled studies to guide the clinician about the choice of antimicrobials, the duration of treatment, and the appropriate management of recurrent bacterial overgrowth. In general, after a 7- to 10-day course of antimicrobials chosen empirically, symptoms and absorptive abnormalities resolve and most patients remain well for months—despite the fact that small-bowel bacterial counts may return to pretreatment values within a few weeks. Consequently, the decision to prescribe repeat antimicrobial therapy should be based on symptoms and the results of absorptive function tests, and not solely on duodenal or jejunal cultures. However, if symptoms and/or absorptive abnormalities do not resolve after antimicrobial therapy, duodenal aspiration and culture, together with antimicrobial sensitivity assays, are indicated. The results of uncontrolled trials suggest that, in patients who respond initially to antimicrobials but in whom symptoms recur within several weeks, cyclical antimicrobial therapy (for example, 1 week in 6), may be effective. A minority of patients does not improve clinically after antimicrobial treatment, despite apparent correction of the abnormal small-bowel flora. Failure to respond to antimicrobial therapy may be due to antimicrobial resistance, antibiotic-associated diarrhoea, or an incorrect diagnosis.

REFERENCES

Isaacs, P.E.T., and Kim, Y.S. (1979). The contaminated small bowel syndrome. *American Journal of Medicine*, **67**, 1049–57.

King, C.E., and Toskes, P.P. (1979). Small intestine bacterial overgrowth. *Gastroenterology*, **76**, 1035–55.

Kirsh, M. (1990). Bacterial overgrowth. *American Journal of Gastroenterology*, **85**, 231–7.

Simon, G.L., and Gorbach, S.L. (1986). The human intestinal microflora. *Digestive Diseases and Sciences*, **31**, (suppl.) 147–62S.

Tabaqchali, S. (1970). The pathophysiological role of small intestinal bacterial flora. *Scandinavian Journal of Gastroenterology*, **6**, (suppl.) 139–63.

Toskes, P.P., and Donaldson, R.M. (1993). Enteric bacterial flora and bacterial overgrowth syndrome. In *Gastrointestinal disease*, (5th edn), (ed. M.H. Sleisenger and J.S. Fordtran), pp. 1106–18. Saunders, Philadelphia.

14.9.4 Coeliac disease

D. P. JEWELL

Definition

Coeliac disease is an inflammatory disorder of the small intestine induced by the prolamins of certain cereals, namely the gliadins of wheat, hordeins of barley, and secalins of rye. The inflammation is associated with loss of villous height and crypt hypertrophy that leads to malabsorption. The functional and histological abnormalities are reversed towards normal following exclusion of those cereals from the diet, but reappear on challenge.

History

Coeliac disease may well have been recognized in ancient times, as Aretaeus, the Cappadocian, wrote of the 'coeliac affection'. This was clearly a malabsorptive illness with steatorrhoea, affecting children and adults, but whether it represents a gluten-sensitive enteropathy is impossible to know. Samuel Gee of St Bartholomew's Hospital, London gave an excellent account of the disease in 1888 and concluded that 'if the patient is to be cured at all, it will be by means of a diet'. It was the Dutch paediatrician, W.K. Dicke, that finally recognized the role of wheat and his initial observations made in the 1930s were confirmed during the 'winter of starvation' in Holland in 1944. He noted that coeliac children paradoxically improved as bread became virtually unobtainable. Using dietary challenge and faecal fat output as an indicator, Dicke together with J.H. van de Kamer and H.A. Weijers went on to show that it was gliadin, the alcohol-soluble component of gluten, that was the damaging substance. The demonstration of a flat intestinal mucosa by J. Paulley in 1954 and the development of a technique to biopsy the small intestine by Margot Shiner in 1956 and Rubin and colleagues in 1960 characterized the disease histologically and allowed easy and accurate diagnosis. The ability to follow the response of the mucosa to dietary manipulation by serial biopsy also allowed clinicians to recognize that coeliac disease in children was the same disease as idiopathic steatorrhoea in adults. Therefore, the disease is now referred to as coeliac disease or as a gluten-sensitive enteropathy.

Pathology

Coeliac disease affects the small intestine but the mucosal inflammation can vary in severity and in extent. Many patients have very mild proximal disease and the mucosal damage can be patchy. The characteristic, but not specific, feature is loss of villous height so that, under a dissecting microscope, the mucosa appears completely flat (Fig. 1). This is confirmed on histological examination (Fig. 2). The mucosa may be completely flat or there may be very short, broad villi—this appearance is often called subtotal villous atrophy. However, the total mucosal thickness (surface epithelium to muscularis mucosae) is usually normal or only slightly reduced because the crypts become elongated—usually referred to as crypt hypertrophy. The surface epithelial cells become flattened, the basal polarity of their nuclei is lost, and the microvilli of the brush border become short and irregular. This last change is seen on electron micrographs.

Within the lamina propria, there is a marked infiltration of chronic inflammatory cells—plasma cells and lymphocytes. In addition, there is an increase in neutrophils, eosinophils, and mast cells. The proportion of intraepithelial lymphocytes is also increased in comparison with the number of enterocytes, although the absolute number is probably not increased.

Within the plasma-cell population, there is an increase in the cells producing IgA, G, and M isotypes, although IgA cells still predominate. There is a marked increase in the crypt cell-proliferation rate, which, in a histological section, is shown by numerous mitoses at the base of the crypts. This increase in crypt-cell proliferation is thought to be mediated by cytokines released by the underlying lymphocytes and macrophages and leads to the elongation of the crypts and the loss of villous height.

It has been proposed that three stages in the development of coeliac disease are defined—infiltrative, hyperplastic, and destructive. These stages have been identified on the basis of challenge studies as well as biopsies of asymptomatic members of coeliac families. In the infiltrative stage, the epithelium becomes infiltrated with increased numbers of lymphocytes and this is the lesion frequently seen in patients with dermatitis herpetiformis. This stage leads on to the point where there is some inflammation of the lamina propria, with elongation of crypts. Both these stages are asymptomatic and can be regarded as latent coeliac disease. The destructive stage is the full lesion with loss of villi and a marked inflammatory infiltrate. Whether this classification is helpful or, indeed representative of what actually happens, is not yet clear.

As well as these characteristic changes in the small intestine, there may be a diffuse infiltration of other mucosal surfaces with lymphocytes and plasma cells. In particular, a proctitis has been recently recognized but this is only detected if a rectal biopsy is taken and is virtually never severe enough to cause symptoms. This generalized mucosal infiltration presumably represents homing patterns of lymphocytes sensitized within the small-intestinal lamina propria.

Following a gluten-free diet, these histological changes return towards normal. For the majority of patients, a repeat biopsy after 3 months will show much less inflammation, the villous height will have increased, and the crypt elongation will have diminished. The mucosa usually returns to normal in children but, in adults, minor changes may persist with a crypt : villous ratio of 1 : 2 rather than the normal ratio of 1 : 4.

When patients in remission on a gluten-free diet are challenged with gluten, histological changes may be seen within a few days. In fact, electron-microscopic changes may occur within a few hours of challenge and a fall in brush-border disaccharidase activity occurs in 24 h. However, some patients may take much longer to relapse and there have been some individuals who have virtually no histological change for up to a year.

Epidemiology

Coeliac disease is primarily a disease of Caucasians and, as it is closely associated with the extended haplotype HLA-B8, DR3, DQ2, it is rare in those parts of the world where this haplotype is uncommon. The highest prevalence is seen in the west of Ireland, where it may be as high as 1 in 300. Throughout Europe, the prevalence ranges up to 1 in 6000, with the value in England being 1 in 1500.

There is little sex difference, although some studies have shown a preponderance of women. There is a familial incidence, with about 10 per cent of first-degree relatives being affected, and studies of monozygotic twins have shown a concordance of 70 per cent. These data indicate a strong genetic susceptibility.

Fig. 1 Dissecting microscopic appearances of a normal jejunal biopsy (a) and of coeliac disease (b).

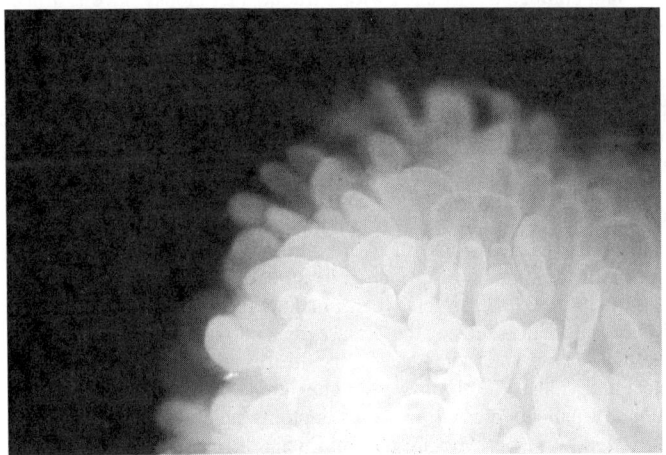

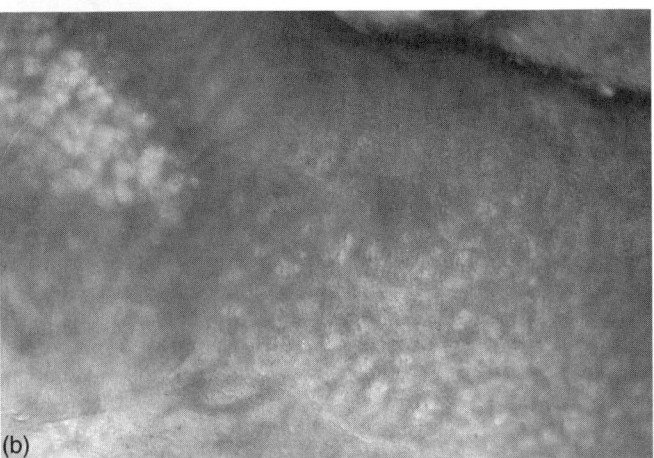

(b)

Fig. 2 Histological appearances of a distal duodenal biopsy in a patient with coeliac disease before (a) and after (b) a 3-month period on a gluten-free diet. Following treatment, there is much less inflammation and the villous pattern has begun to reappear.

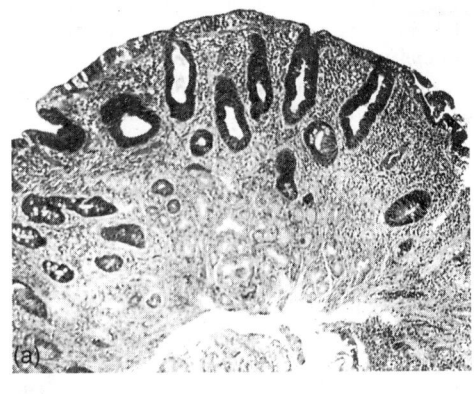

(a)

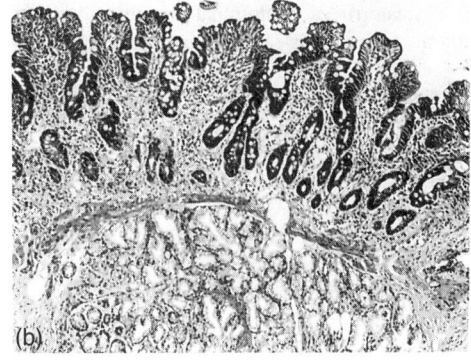

(b)

Pathogenesis

There are two clear facts about the aetiopathogenesis of coeliac disease. The first is that fractions of gliadin, the alcohol-soluble component of gluten, are the toxic dietary constituent, together with similar fractions of rye and barley prolamins. The second is that there is a genetic susceptibility to gluten intolerance because of the close association with the HLA haplotype B8, DR3, DQ2 in Northern Europeans and with B8, DR5/7, DQ2 in Southern Europeans. This difference is due to the fact that the same DRQ α-β heterodimer can be encoded on the same chromosome (*cis* position) in DR3 individuals or on opposite chromosomes (*trans* position) in DR5/DR7 individuals (see Section 5). This suggests that DRQ molecules confer most of the susceptibility. What is not clear is how this particular haplotype interacts with gluten to produce mucosal inflammation in one person whereas the majority of people with this haplotype are able to ingest gluten with impunity. The other unsolved question is the exact nature of the toxic peptide.

An attractive hypothesis to explain why certain individuals lose oral tolerance to gluten is that it occurs as a result of an infection with adenovirus 12. This hypothesis was suggested by the observation that there was a dodecapeptide on the surface of A-gliadin which was similar to a peptide contained within an E1b protein of the virus. Many coeliac patients demonstrate cellular and humoral immune responses to the virus, and so it is conceivable that the immune response to the virus cross-reacts with the gliadin peptide and thus induces intestinal inflammation. Whether either peptide binds preferentially to a particular HLA class 2 molecule, which might explain the genetic susceptibility, is not known.

Some progress has been made in determining the toxic peptide but in most studies toxicity has been assessed by *in vitro* methods rather than by direct feeding studies in patients. The amino acid sequences that seem to be shared by these toxic peptides are pro-ser-glu-glu or ser-pro-glu-glu. Thus, coeliac disease probably represents a reaction to a number of similar peptides rather than to a single epitope.

The inflammatory lesion in the small intestine seems to result from an immunological reaction to the gluten peptides, with both cellular and humoral responses being involved. The mucosal abnormality is usually a proximal one and is presumably a reflection of luminal concentration of the relevant peptides. The release of cytokines and inflammatory mediators is thought to amplify the immune response and to influence epithelial stem-cell kinetics, with subsequent crypt elongation and loss of villous height. Malabsorption occurs because of loss of absorptive area and the presence of a population of immature surface epithelial cells whose absorptive and secretory function may be additionally impaired by cytokines and inflammatory mediators.

Clinical features

Coeliac disease in infants classically presents soon after weaning at the point that cereals are introduced. The babies usually fail to thrive, are miserable, refuse to eat, and lose weight. The abdomen becomes distended, there is muscle wasting, and they may have diarrhoea, which usually has the features of steatorrhoea. Abdominal pain and vomiting may be prominent symptoms and can mislead the clinician. Rectal prolapse may occur.

In older children, growth retardation is a common presentation and if the gastrointestinal symptoms are minimal, the diagnosis can be overlooked. Nutritional deficiencies can occur and may again be the reason for presentation, anaemia being the most common deficiency. Delayed puberty is another mode of presentation.

In adults, the most common presentations are anaemia and variable abdominal symptoms of discomfort, bloating, excess wind, and an altered bowel habit. Mouth ulcers are also frequent and can be the presenting symptom. The anaemia is most commonly due to iron deficiency and frequently occurs in the absence of intestinal symptoms; the macrocytic anaemias that sometimes occur in coeliac disease are described in Section 22. Many patients presenting with diarrhoea, wind, and abdominal pain are wrongly diagnosed as having an irritable bowel syndrome and there may then be a considerable delay before the true diagnosis is made. Patients suspected of having an irritable bowel syndrome should be specifically questioned about mouth ulcers and weight loss, either of which can be a pointer of organic disease. They should also be asked about feeding difficulties as a child, about growth milestones, and the age of achieving puberty. Less commonly, patients will present with a more typical history, with features of steatorrhoea, weight loss, bruising, and other symptoms of nutritional deficiencies resulting from malabsorption.

The classical findings in infants are those of an irritable child with stunted growth, muscle wasting, and a 'pot belly'. The infant usually has feeding difficulties and may show evidence of colic, and has a marked diarrhoea. However, in toddlers and older children who present with growth failure or anaemia, there may be few signs. Similarly, in adults, there may be no physical signs in those presenting with symptoms suggestive of an irritable bowel syndrome. Signs of iron deficiency may be present and there may be aphthous ulcers in the mouth, mild finger clubbing, and evidence of recent weight loss. It is very unusual, nowadays, for patients to show evidence of bleeding and osteomalacia (or rickets in children). Even less common are patients who are so malnourished that they have signs of ascites and hypoproteinaemic oedema.

Diagnosis

The crucial test to establish the diagnosis is a small-intestinal biopsy. This has traditionally been taken from the duodenal–jejunal junction (the ligament of Treitz) using a Crosby capsule. However, a distal duodenal biopsy taken at endoscopy is being used increasingly to make the diagnosis and comparative studies with a true jejunal biopsy have justified its use.

Serological tests have been developed with the aim of screening for coeliac disease, although none of them has yet proved sufficiently reliable to replace the need for a small-intestinal biopsy. Serum antibodies to gliadin (IgA isotype), IgA antibodies to reticulin, and IgA endomysial antibodies have high specificity and sensitivity for the disease. Endomysial antibodies are proving the most useful but how they arise is unknown. They are detected by immunohistochemical methods using monkey oesophageal muscle and are found in over 90 per cent of coeliacs of all ages, in contrast to reticulin antibodies, which are more common in children (90 per cent) than in adults (60 per cent). The titre of all three antibodies falls as the disease goes into remission on a gluten-free diet. These antibodies can be useful for screening populations to select individuals for biopsy (e.g. the family members of a coeliac patient or patients presenting with symptoms suggestive of an irritable bowel syndrome but who are not improving of treatment).

ASSESSMENT OF MALABSORPTION

Careful documentation of nutritional deficiency as a result of malabsorption must be made and should include:

Full blood count

The haemoglobin level may be low, but the mean corpuscle volume may be low (iron deficiency), high (vitamin B_{12} or folate deficiency), or within the normal range. This can occur either because there is no significant deficiency of a haematinic or because there is a mixed deficiency, usually a combination of iron and folate. The red-cell folate is a more reliable indicator of folate deficiency than the serum concentration and if it is low, there may be a pancytopenia. Vitamin B_{12} concentrations are only low in patients with extensive involvement of the small intestine and so are usually normal. Serum iron, total binding capacity, and ferritin concentrations should be measured to record the patient's iron status.

Biochemistry

Quantitative estimations of faecal fat excretion are becoming progressively more difficult to obtain despite their obvious value in assessing small-intestinal function. Qualitative assessment of excess fat by staining faecal smears with Sudan black or oil red O can be a reasonable alternative but merely records the presence or absence of a steatorrhoea. Fat malabsorption is inevitably accompanied by malabsorption of the fat-soluble vitamins A, D, E, and K. Serum concentrations of β-carotene, calcium, alkaline phosphtase, vitamin D, and the prothrombin time (INR) should therefore be assayed. Patients with diarrhoea may become hypokalaemic. Serum magnesium concentrations may also be low in severe coeliac disease and, with hypocalcaemia, can lead to tetany. Serum albumin is often low, as is the concentration of zinc.

Immunological tests

In addition to the titres of diagnostic antibodies discussed above, serum immunoglobulin concentrations should be measured. The most common pattern of abnormality is a raised IgA with a low IgM but virtually any pattern may be seen. However, 10 per cent of patients with coeliac disease have an associated IgA deficiency and loss of villous height and crypt hypertrophy frequently accompany common-variable acquired immunodeficiency.

RADIOLOGY

Barium radiology cannot give a positive diagnosis of coeliac disease and is not usually necessary unless it is required to exclude other small-intestinal diseases. In mild coeliacs, the appearances may be normal but if abnormalities are present the appearances vary according to the radiological technique used. If a barium meal and follow-through is done, the small intestine may appear dilated and the barium often segments and flocculates. The proximal loops may appear smooth with a corresponding accentuation of the valvulae conniventes in the ileum—the so-called jejunization of the ileum. If a small-bowel enema is used (enteroclysis), the features are those of dilation and oedema of the valvulae conniventes.

Differential diagnosis

Few patients present with overt malabsorption, so the diagnosis of coeliac disease requires a high index of suspicion. However, once a biopsy is obtained that shows appearances compatible with coeliac disease, the differential diagnosis is limited.

For infants, the most common differential diagnosis is cow's milk allergy. An eosinophilia in the lamina propria as well as in peripheral blood is common, but this can also occur in coeliac disease. A soya milk allergy can also cause a flat small-intestinal mucosa. The precise diagnosis is usually dependent on a dietary history and the results of dietary exclusion.

In adults, infection with giardia, common-variable hypogammaglobulinaemia, lymphoma, Crohn's disease, and other small-intestinal diseases such as radiation enteritis, amyloid and Whipple's disease may all show villous flattening and mucosal inflammation. Tropical sprue is usually associated with less marked changes—so-called partial villous atrophy—but has to be considered in patients who have spent time in endemic areas. Rarely, patients may be seen with a flat biopsy but with crypt hypoplasia—these do not respond to a gluten-free diet. Some patients with crypt hypoplasia also have a thickened band of subepithelial collagen, so-called collagenous sprue. Systemic diseases such as the vasculitides and systemic sclerosis may also be associated with an abnormal mucosal biopsy. Bacterial overgrowth of the small intestine may be associated with some mucosal inflammation and minor villous changes but they are rarely sufficiently severe to be confused with coeliac disease.

Dermatitis herpetiformis is commonly associated with an abnormal mucosal biopsy. The mucosal inflammation can be as severe as coeliac disease and responds to gluten withdrawal. The skin lesions also respond to a gluten-free diet, albeit slowly.

Non-specific infections of the small intestine may lead to a degree of malabsorption and mucosal inflammation. In only a small proportion can giardia be detected, and the precise aetiology of the majority is never determined. The illness is usually sudden in onset and gets better spontaneously over several weeks. It has been named 'temperate sprue'. Although this entity is uncommon, it can mislead clinicians. Most patients presenting in this way get started on a gluten-free diet as soon as the result of the biopsy is known and their improvement is regarded as a dietary response. Thus a patient presenting with a very short history of symptoms and whose mucosal biopsy suggests coeliac disease must be considered carefully. HLA typing and the presence of serum endomysial antibodies may be very helpful in making the correct diagnosis. If there is still doubt, the patient should be given a gluten-free diet but when the mucosa has recovered, a gluten challenge with subsequent biopsy should be undertaken.

ASSOCIATED DISEASES

There is an increased prevalence of autoimmune diseases in patients with coeliac disease, especially those that are associated with HLA-B8 DR3 phenotype. These include diabetes, thyroid disease, and Addison's disease. Fibrosing alveolitis, systemic lupus erythematosus, and polyarteritis have also been reported. There may be an increase in epilepsy, especially temporal-lobe epilepsy, in coeliac patients.

About 10 per cent of coeliacs have an isolated IgA deficiency but the reason for and significance of this are not clear.

Treatment

Once the diagnosis is confirmed by a small-intestinal biopsy, patients should be started on a gluten-free diet. This diet should also exclude barley and rye but with oats the need is less clear. As the evidence for oat toxicity is confused, many clinicians allow oats and only exclude them if the repeat biopsy does not show a good histological response. However, others exclude oats as the diet is begun and then consider reintroducing them once the disease has gone into histological remission.

All patients should be advised of the diet by a dietitian and should be told to keep to it strictly. For children, the parents must be well briefed, including being told of the dangers of many sweets and 'fast foods'. For all patients, the diet is a lifelong necessity. Many children inevitably ingest small amounts of gluten during adolescence and many of them remain asymptomatic and develop normally. This has given rise to the highly erroneous view that children can 'grow out' of the disease. If the diagnosis was correct in the first place, then the patient remains a coeliac for life and if the diet is not strict, it may predispose them to complications in the future.

Patients should also be given details of the national Coeliac Society, if there is one. Most countries in which coeliac disease occurs have such a society. They provide a considerable amount of information about the disease and update patients about the gluten contents of new products appearing in the supermarkets. They also give invaluable advice about diet and foreign travel, as well as providing a social forum for patients and opportunities for fund raising to support research.

Nutritional supplements may be necessary at the start of treatment. If there are low serum concentrations of iron and folate, or biochemical evidence of osteomalacia, appropriate supplements are clearly required. However, once a gluten-free diet has begun, mucosal recovery occurs rapidly so that long-term supplementation is rarely necessary.

Patients with extensive mucosal damage are unable to digest lactose because of lactase deficiency. These patients may need a lactose-free as well as a gluten-free diet until there is histological recovery.

Once patients have been on the diet for 3 to 4 months, a further small-intestinal biopsy must be obtained to check for histological recovery. If the mucosa is still inflamed and villous height has not returned towards normal, a thorough review of the patient's diet is needed. Hidden sources of gluten (Communion wafers being a classical example) can often be found by a skilled dietitian. If oats have not been excluded, then this is worth doing. In children, additional exclusion of soya products is occasionally needed.

Long-term follow-up, preferably in specialized clinics, is desirable but need only be on an annual basis once patients are stabilized on their diet. This allows patients to be seen by a dietitian as well as their physician and reinforces the need to comply with a strict diet.

Complications

The two major complications of coeliac disease are an ulcerative jejunoileitis and a T-cell lymphoma, and some investigators consider the jejunoileitis to be a manifestation of a lymphoma. They usually occur in middle age and usually present with weight loss, anaemia, abdominal pain, and diarrhoea. Thus any coeliac presenting with these symptoms having been previously well on a gluten-free diet must be carefully screened for these complications. Biopsies should be snap-frozen in liquid nitrogen to allow immunohistochemical analysis of T-cell markers and the detection of T-cell receptor rearrangements. The prognosis of a lymphoma complicating coeliac disease is poor.

In addition, there is a slight increase in the frequency of small-bowel carcinoma, although this is still very rare. There is also an increased incidence of other gastrointestinal cancers, especially oesophageal tumours, although the reasons for this increase are obscure.

There is some evidence suggesting that the patients who develop malignant disease, especially lymphoma, are those who have been poor compliers with the diet. Although, this association is not absolutely proven, it provides the basis for continuing to advise a strict diet and to monitor compliance on a regular outpatient review.

Prognosis

Provided that patients adhere to a strict diet, the prognosis is excellent and there are no data which suggest that there is an excess mortality in this group. Children develop normally and proceed into adolescence without delay. However, as mentioned above, compliance with the diet is often poor in adolescents and some clinicians still believe that many of them can have a more liberal diet if they are asymptomatic. It is this group that often present some years later with anaemia, mouth ulcers or more serious evidence of malabsorption.

Unresponsive disease

A rare group of patients who are found to have a flat small-intestinal biopsy fail to respond to a gluten-free diet despite meticulous attention to avoid even minute amounts of gluten over many months. By definition these patients do not have coeliac disease, although they are often referred to as non-responsive coeliacs, a phrase that is misleading and should be avoided. Treatment of this group is difficult. Corticosteroids with or without azathioprine may help some, and more recent case reports suggest oral cyclosporin may also be of benefit. Excluding other dietary items such as soya can be tried, or an elemental diet that removes all dietary antigens. Some of these patients have a variety of central and peripheral neurological signs that do not fit classical vitamin-deficiency syndromes. The aetiology and pathology of these neurological lesions is unknown and the initial suggestions that they represented vitamin E deficiency have not been substantiated. The prognosis for these patients is poor because the neurological damage is slowly progressive and patients gradually lose weight despite full nutritional support.

It is always worth reviewing the intestinal biopsies in patients who do not respond to gluten withdrawal. Small-intestinal lymphoma, loss of villous height with crypt hypoplasia, and collagenous sprue are alternative diagnoses that may not have been recognized during the initial assessment.

REFERENCES

Ferreira, M., Lloyd-Davies, S., Bulter, M., Scott, D., Clark, M., and Kumar, P. (1992). Endomysial antibody: is it the best screening test for coeliac disease. *Gut*, **33**, 1633–7.

Marsh, M.N. (1992). Gluten, major histocompatibility complex, and the small intestine. *Gastroenterology*, **102**, 330–54.

Sategna-Guidetti, C., and Grosso, S. (1994). Changing pattern in adult coeliac disease: a 24-year survey. *European Journal of Gastroenterology and Hepatology*, **6**, 15–19.

van Berge-Henegouwen, G.P. and Mulder, C.J.J. (1993). Pioneer in the gluten-free diet: Willem-Karel Dicke 1905–1962, over 50 years of gluten free diet. *Gut*, **34**, 1473–5.

Weir, D.G. (1991). Pathogenesis of the coeliac syndromes. *European Journal of Gastroenterology and Hepatology*, **3**, 99–135.

14.9.5 Disaccharidase deficiency

T. M. Cox

Disaccharidases are specific glycosidases that are required for the complete assimilation of all dietary carbohydrate with the exception of free glucose and fructose. The enzymes are found on the luminal surface of the small gut; their activity may be reduced by genetically determined deficiencies of single disaccharidases or acquired by generalized disease of the intestinal mucosa. Disaccharidase deficiency causes a characteristic syndrome of carbohydrate intolerance.

Physiology of carbohydrate digestion (Fig. 1)

Free disaccharides occur in the diet or are derived from the luminal hydrolysis of starch and glycogen by salivary and pancreatic α-amylase. Because amylase cannot hydrolyse the α-1,6 branching linkages and has little specificity for α-1,4 bonds adjacent to these points, the initial products of starch digestion are branched oligosaccharides containing at least one α-1,6 bond. Maltase–glucoamylase is a mucosal α-glucosidase that removes glucose moieties sequentially from the non-reducing terminus of linear oligosaccharides. α-Dextrinase (isomaltase) continues the hydrolysis of branched carbohydrate polymers by cleaving the α-1,6 glycosidic bonds of the limit dextrins that remain. α-Dextrinase is a component of the bifunctional enzyme complex, sucrase–isomaltase, the sucrase moiety of which hydrolyses sucrose into fructose and glucose. The disaccharides sucrose, lactose, and trehalose, like the α-dextrins, are poorly absorbed: to be assimilated, they are also split into monosaccharides by glycosidases located on the brush-border membrane (sucrase, lactase, and trehalase). Mucosal disaccharidases are optimally active at pH 6.0 and are present principally in the jejunum—but are also found in the ileum.

Specific carriers in the microvilli for the transport of glucose and galactose, as well as fructose, mediate the uptake of monosaccharides released by the mucosal glycosidases—and absorption occurs rapidly. Active transport by the sodium-dependent glucose–galactose carrier is accompanied by passive flux of water from the lumen. Maldigestion of osmotically active sugars thus leads to marked retention of fluid in the gut. For most carbohydrates, hydrolysis in the lumen and at the mucosal surface is sufficiently rapid to saturate the pathways for glucose and fructose transport. For lactose, however, the rate of hydrolysis, rather than glucose and galactose uptake by the mucosa, may become limiting. Hence the functional reserve of lactase in the human intestine is restricted and assimilation of lactose is especially vulnerable to disorders of the mucosa.

Biosynthesis of surface disaccharidases continues throughout the life of the epithelium but the enzymes are only active in mature cells on the upper reaches of small-intestinal villi. Complete turnover of the enzyme molecules occurs several times during the life span of the mature enterocyte. Brush-border disaccharidases are complex glycoproteins that undergo proteolytic processing; extensive glycan modification in the Golgi apparatus occurs before insertion into the membrane. The mature enzymes are derived from large, single-chain polypeptides. At the time of writing the genetically determined mechanism by which lactase expression is normally reduced after infancy is not understood but in most individuals it appears to regulate cotranslational processing during synthesis of the enzyme molecule. Colonic epithelial cells do not express appreciable disaccharidase activity and unabsorbed carbohydrate resulting from maldigestion of disaccharides proximally is fermented by bacteria in the colon to short-chain organic acids, hydrogen, and methane. In these circumstances, ingestion of carbohydrate may cause pain by distension of the bowel with fluid and gas, accompanied by irritant and watery diarrhoea.

Carbohydrate intolerance syndrome (Table 1)

Abdominal symptoms may be noticed within an hour of ingestion of foods containing the offending sugars. There is nausea, bloating, and distension of the abdomen accompanied by borborygmi and flatulence. Colicky pain precedes watery diarrhoea that is usually associated with flatus—and may be explosive. Diarrhoea due to maldigestion of carbohydrate can occur several hours after ingestion of the noxious food or drink. These symptoms may result from consumption of only a few grams of the offending sugar. Intestinal hurry aggravates fat malabsorption in disaccharidase deficiency and may obscure the underlying cause of the diarrhoea. Deficiency of particular disaccharidases is responsible for the dietary intolerance of specific foods and drinks: milk-containing products in the case of lactase deficiency; table sugar and starch in asucrasia; mushrooms (and probably shellfish) in the rare trehalase deficiency. Identification of a cause-and-effect relation between particular items and the intolerance syndrome is often impossible, given the ubiquity of sucrose and lactose in commercial foods.

Lactose intolerance

Most patients suffering from intolerance of lactose in the diet suffer either from lactase deficiency acquired as a result of intestinal disease, especially postinfective gastroenteritis in children, or as a result of genetically determined restriction of lactase expression.

CONGENITAL LACTASE DEFICIENCY

A few infants have been reported in whom diarrhoea occurred after the first feed with breast milk and who responded completely to a lactose-free formula feed. This disorder is distinct from congenital glucose–

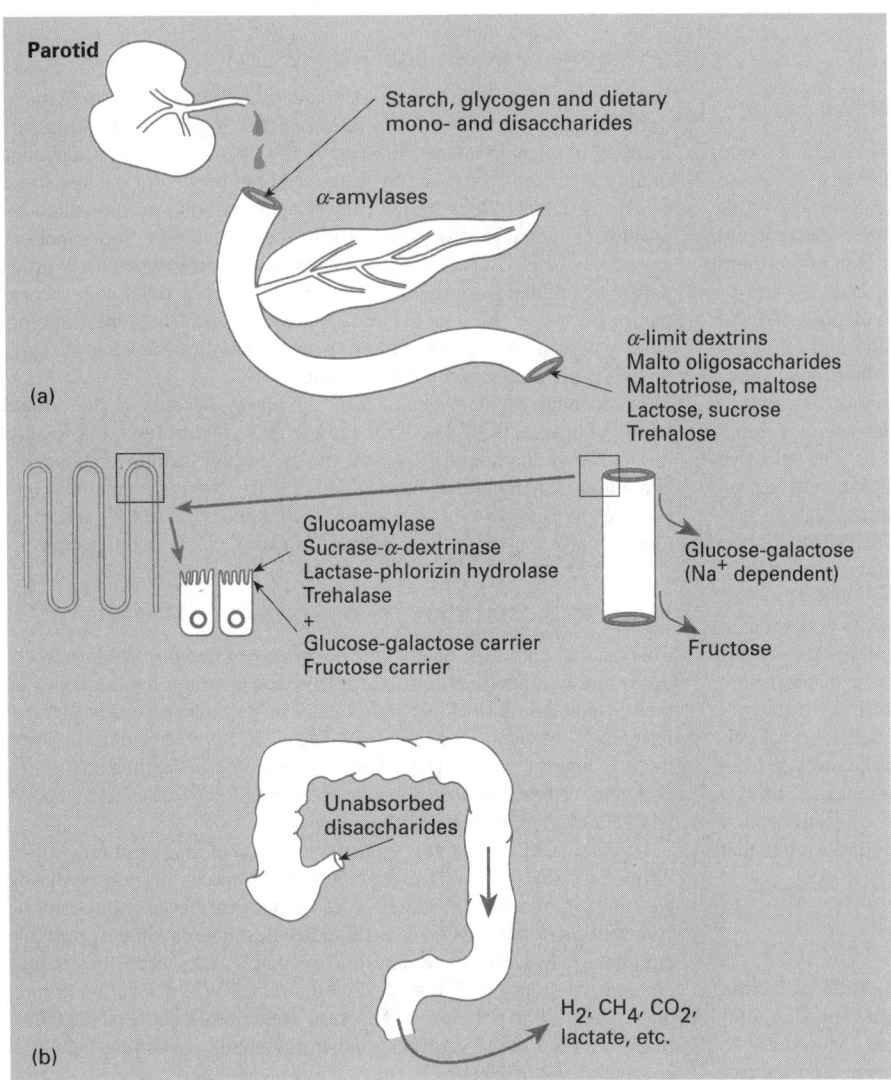

Fig. 1 Carbohydrate digestion and absorption.

Table 1 *Carbohydrate intolerance syndromes due to deficiency of disaccharidases*

Lactose intolerance
Congenital (inherited) lactase deficiency
Lactase restriction (genetically determined)
Lactase deficiency secondary to intestinal disease
Sucrose intolerance
Congenital asucrasia (inherited)
Sucrase deficiency secondary to intestinal disease
Trehalose intolerance
Congenital atrehalasia

*Accompanied by reduced tolerance of starch.

Table 2 *Foods containing lactose*

Fresh, dried, skimmed, non-fat, and condensed milks
Cream
Yoghurt
Cheese
Processed meats and sausages
Sauces, stuffings, salad dressings
Custard powder
Canned and dried soups
Biscuits, cakes, cookies, pancakes, waffles, dried cereals
Confectionery
Frozen and canned fruits
Instant coffee
Lactose is also frequently used as a filler in powdered medicines and tablets

galactose malabsorption, in which lactose exclusion alone is ineffective. Congenital lactose intolerance is associated with a severe inherited deficiency of mucosal lactase activity and, unlike intolerance of lactose associated with prematurity or secondary to diffuse intestinal disease, remains life-long.

LACTASE DEFICIENCY OF PREMATURITY

Unlike the other mucosal glycosidases, which appear early during fetal development, intestinal lactase activity is not fully expressed until after the 28th week of gestation and transient intolerance of milk feeds is common before this age. Abdominal distress due to gaseous distension and diarrhoea requires careful attention to the diet and fluid balance in premature infants.

LACTASE RESTRICTION IN CHILDREN AND ADULTS

The capacity of the infant's intestine to digest lactose is retained into adult life by only a minority of individuals. Thus, tolerance of lactose in milk, dairy products, and many processed and ready-to-eat foods (Table 2) is found mainly in peoples of Northern European descent and those with a tradition of dairy farming. In about 5 per cent of Northern European adults as compared with more than 90 per cent in parts of Africa and Asia, there is a genetically determined and physiological decline in mucosal lactase activity after weaning. Although only low levels of lactase activity remain, this is normally without any consequence because consumption of dairy products is insignificant. Symptoms develop on exposure to excessive milk-and lactose-containing foods or medicines in late childhood or early adult life. The selective pressures that maintain this physiological reduction in mucosal lactase deficiency in childhood are unknown, but the concept of 'lactase deficiency' in adults is difficult to justify, since lactase persistence is the least frequent variant. None the less, with increasing migration of peoples and the adoption of Western-style diets, this physiological loss of lactase activity is a prevalent cause of abdominal distress. A significant proportion of patients considered to have spastic colon, irritable bowel disease, or other 'functional' disturbances may prove to have lactase deficiency. The speculative possibility arises that lactase-deficient subjects are at risk from osteoporosis because of dietary deficiency of calcium. No conclusive evidence to support this theory has, however, been presented. The relative lack of functional reserve of mucosal lactase activity also explains the frequency with which lactose malabsorption becomes manifest after partial gastrectomy and related procedures that enhance delivery of carbohydrate to the jejunum.

DIAGNOSIS OF LACTOSE MALABSORPTION

Intolerance of dietary carbohydrate caused by maldigestion of lactose may be suspected from the dietary history in a patient typically complaining of abdominal pain, flatulence, and diarrhoea. Symptoms are often related to changes in social circumstances; they are reported frequently by Oriental immigrants to Western countries. The stool has an acidic pH (< 6) and the osmolality of stool water is generally greater than 350 mosmol/kg due to the presence of lactate and other organic anions. Breath hydrogen analysis is a useful confirmatory test. Hydrogen excretion determined by rebreathing 2 h after ingestion of 50 g of lactose identifies patients with lactase deficiency diagnosed by enzymatic assay of jejunal mucosa. Other investigations, such as the lactose barium-meal examination and determination of blood glucose profile after oral challenge with lactose, are cumbersome and, because they give falsely positive results, are now obsolete.

SECONDARY LACTASE DEFICIENCY

Lactase activity may be depressed by mucosal disease of the small intestine. This may occur transiently after infective gastroenteritis. It is particularly frequent in infants suffering from viral gastroenteritis, and continuing symptoms provoked by milk feeds can persist for days or some weeks. In infants, dehydration may develop rapidly, accompanied by prominent bloating; disacchariduria is found and acid, sour-smelling stools may be obvious. The symptoms resolve rapidly when dairy products are excluded from the diet. Decreased lactase activity also accompanies extensive and long-standing mucosal disease—the milk intolerance syndrome due to maldigestion may complicate coeliac disease, intestinal giardiasis, and Crohn's disease.

In secondary deficiencies of disaccharidases, because of the critical relation between lactase activity and the rate of hydrolysis, intolerance of lactose predominates. However, the use of high-calorie supplements containing disaccharides other than lactose (especially maltose and sucrose) in patients with nutritional disturbances caused by intestinal disease may also cause the syndrome of carbohydrate maldigestion.

SUCRASE–ISOMALTASE (α-DEXTRINASE) DEFICIENCY

This recessively inherited enzyme deficiency of the mucosal brush border is rare in all populations except Eskimos in whom the frequency of homozygotes is up to 10 per cent. Cetacean mammals also lack sucrase-isomaltase. Several genetic defects appear to be responsible; in some there is aberrant glycosylation and the enzyme is inefficiently transported to the brush border. Substantial degradation of the abnormal polypeptide occurs within the epithelial cell.

Intolerance of sucrose is responsible for most of the symptoms, which develop as table sugar and sugar-containing foods are introduced during weaning. Intolerance of starch is less prominent because the osmotic contribution of the larger α-dextrin molecules that remain unsplit in the gut lumen is less. However, ingestion of large, starchy meals may induce cramping discomfort, flatulence, and diarrhoea. Whilst taking a normal diet, patients with deficiency of sucrase–isomaltase have persistent diarrhoea with the passage of acid and frothy stools containing increased concentrations of lactate.

The diagnosis may be suspected on the basis of the history of diarrhoea at weaning and on the character of the stools. Differentiation from coeliac disease, cow's milk allergy, infective or postinfective gastroenteritis, pancreatic failure, and disaccharide intolerance syndromes in relation to other inflammatory disease of the bowel is important, and biopsy of the jejunal mucosa for enzymatic assay and histological examination should be considered. In inherited sucrase-isomaltase deficiency, these activities are reduced selectively to less than 10 per cent of control values in histologically normal mucosa. Hydrogen breath tests after ingestion of sucrose and isomaltose may also prove to be useful in diagnosis but experience is limited.

TREHALASE DEFICIENCY

A few patients have been reported with mushroom intolerance due to the absence of mucosal trehalase. Trehalase is a brush-border α-glycosidase that cleaves the unusual 1α-1α bond of trehalase into its component glucose moieties. Trehalose is found in the haemolymph of arthropods and in fungi, so that intolerance of crustacean shellfish as well as mushrooms in the diet might be expected. Given that intolerance of edible fungi is not uncommon, trehalase deficiency may prove to be more frequent than previously supposed.

Treatment

Dietary exclusion of the offending sugar is the best method of preventing symptoms in individuals with primary or acquired disaccharidase deficiency. Symptoms recur as soon as excessive lactose or sucrose is reintroduced and advice from a professional dietitian may be needed to avoid indiscretions. In hypolactasia, complete elimination is not usually required, as lactase deficiency is rarely absolute; nevertheless, if symptoms persist there are many potential sources of lactose that warrant investigation (see Table 2).

An early, alternative method for preventing symptoms in lactose malabsorbers was the use of β-galactosidases obtained from yeast or other microorganisms. These enzymes were added to dairy products before consumption and often changed the taste. In the United States, β-galactosidase has been produced commercially from yeast 'LactAid' and has been shown to reduce symptoms as well as breath hydrogen excretion in subjects with maldigestion of lactose. Similar studies have demonstrated the efficacy of β-galactosidase derived from *Aspergillus oryzae*, 'Lactrase', in children with late-onset intolerance of lactose. The enzymes are taken in tablet form immediately before challenge with lactose but their cost, compared with dietary exclusion, may not be justified. In the future, microbial β-galactosidases might be used for food supplementation programmes in countries where lactose intolerance and nutritional deprivation in the adult population are widespread.

Complete absence of sucrase-isomaltase activity in most patients with sucrose intolerance and the ubiquity of sucrose in modern diets complicates symptom management. Modest reduction of amylopectin-rich foods usually suffices to improve symptoms of starch intolerance but complete avoidance of sucrose-containing foods can be difficult. Recently it has been found that ingestion of dried brewer's yeast (containing invertase or sucrase but little lactase activity) after food is effective in sucrase–isomaltase deficiency.

REFERENCES

Anonymous (1992). Lactose intolerance. *Lancet*, **338**, 663–4.

Flatz, G. (1987) Genetics of lactose digestion in humans. *Advances in Human Genetics*, **16**, 1–77.

Gray, G.M. (1975). Carbohydrate digestion and absorption. Rôle of the small intestine. *New England Journal of Medicine*, **292**, 1225–30. An informative and accessible review.

King, C.E. and Toskes, P.P. (1983). The use of breath tests in the study of malabsorption. *Clinics in Gastroenterology*, **12**, 591–610.

Medow, M.S., Thek, K.D., Newman, L.J., Berezin, S., Glassman, M.S., and Schwarz, S.M. (1990) β-Galactosidase tablets in the treatment of lactose intolerance in pediatrics. *American Journal of Diseases of Children*, **144**, 1261–4. Promising results with enzyme replacement therapy.

Simoons, F.J. (1970). Primary adult lactose intolerance and the milking habit: a problem in biological and cultural interrelations. *American Journal of Digestive Diseases*, **15**, 695–700. Global review of lactase restriction in man.

Sebastio, G. *et al.* (1989). Control of lactase in human adult-type hypolactasia and in weaning rabbits and rats. *American Journal of Human Genetics*, **45**, 489–97.

14.9.6 Whipple's disease

H. J. F. HODGSON

Whipple's disease is a rare condition that may affect virtually any organ, but the clinical picture at diagnosis is usually dominated by small-intestinal involvement leading to malabsorption. Overt intestinal involvement may be preceded or accompanied by systemic symptoms such as arthralgia and fever. Affected tissues contain Gram-positive, rod-shaped bacteria, and are histologically characterized by the presence of foamy macrophages with a characteristic staining reaction. The bacterium has recently been assigned to a previously undescribed genus amongst actinomycetes. There is usually a good response to antibiotic therapy, which may have to be prolonged.

Pathology and aetiology

Whipple's initial description of a fatal case emphasized fatty deposits in the small intestine and mesenteric lymph nodes, leading to the alternative name for the disorder, intestinal lipodystrophy. In general these areas show the most severe involvement. The small intestine is thick and oedematous, with stubby or absent villi and dilated lacteals (secondary lymphangiectasia reflecting obstructed lymph flow). The intestinal lamina propria is stuffed with macrophages, which stain brilliant magenta with periodic acid–Schiff (**PAS**) reagent (diastase-resistant). PAS-positive material is also found extracellularly (Fig. 1). Apart from the macrophages, there is little inflammatory infiltrate, and the enterocytes are virtually normal. The mesenteric nodes contain fatty masses,

Fig. 1 Jejunal biopsy specimen from a 50-year-old male with Whipple's disease showing stunted villi and infiltration of lamina propria with densely staining macrophages (PAS×150).

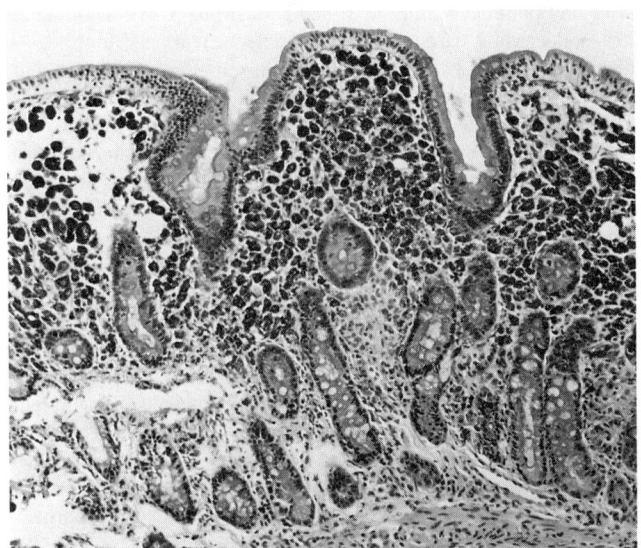

occasional granulomas, and foamy macrophages. In autopsy series most cases also show extraintestinal involvement, with foamy macrophages in spleen, lymph nodes, central nervous system, liver, lung, and heart. Cardiac involvement often leads to endocarditis with vegetations.

Both within and between the abnormal macrophages, abundant rod-shaped bacteria are usually identified in untreated cases. They are 1 to 2 μm in length, occasionally in division, and are the source of the PAS-positive material. They have been found in affected gut, lymph node, joints, liver, brain, and other tissues. They have not been convincingly cultured, although a considerable number of candidate bacterial isolates have been reported, and staining cross-reactivity of Whipple's tissue with a variety of antisera to different bacteria has been documented. Recently, two groups amplified bacterial 16s ribosomal RNA from Whipple's tissues, and phylogenetic analysis of the products suggests that the bacterium is a Gram-positive actinomycete not closely related to any known genus. The name *Tropheryma whippelii* has been proposed to describe the bacillus.

The attribution of Whipple's disease to a specific organism—which molecular analysis identified in tissues from each of five patients with Whipple's disease—appears to resolve the controversy that has surrounded the condition. The description of a number of immunological defects, in macrophage and T-cell function for example, had been taken as evidence that an underlying immunodeficiency led to colonization of the host by a variety of bacteria of low virulence. Some host factors may well be involved; a weak association with the HLA-B27 haplotype has been claimed.

The fact that the small intestine is virtually always involved at the time of initial diagnosis suggests that the organism is likely to have entered by that route. It may then spread by lymphatics and haematogenously to virtually any part of the body.

Clinical features and diagnosis

The condition is most frequently diagnosed in middle-aged men, but women and infants may be affected. The patient with advanced disease presents with malaise, weight loss, diarrhoea, and arthralgias, and on examination may show marked pigmentation, lymphadenopathy, anaemia, finger clubbing, hypotension, and oedema. Rarely, gastrointestinal bleeding may also occur. In such cases, investigation of an obvious gastrointestinal problem should quickly establish the diagnosis. Recognition is far more difficult if symptoms are limited to fever, arthritis, or another systemic manifestation. These may be transient or intermittent. The arthritis is migratory, non-deforming, and seronegative, predominantly affecting peripheral joints, and in some series has affected up to 90 per cent of patients; arthritis may precede overt gut involvement by many years. Other early features include respiratory complaints with pleurisy and pulmonary infiltrates, and pericarditis. Chylous or serous ascites, endocarditis, cardiac conduction defects, coronary arteritis, and myopathy may occur with progression of the condition. There is a wide variety of central nervous manifestations, though only 5 to 10 per cent of patients are so affected. These include depression, apathy, fits, and myoclonus, and a variety of ocular manifestations including ophthalmoplegia, papilloedema, scotomata, pseudotumour, and uveitis. Meningitis and a hypothalamic syndrome with insomnia, hyperphagia, and polydypsia also occur. An association with sarcoidosis has been suggested.

Diagnosis is by recognition of the classic histological picture. Whether or not clinical intestinal involvement is present, peroral duodenal or jejunal biopsy is a convenient, safe, and effective means of making the diagnosis in virtually all untreated cases. The endoscopic appearances may be characteristic, reflecting flattened mucosa with lymphatic dilatation. Occasionally, multiple biopsies may be required if intestinal involvement is patchy, and there are rare reports of affected tissues outside the gut (such as lymph nodes) despite normal intestinal appearances histologically. Rectal biopsy is a poor diagnostic approach, as normal colonic tissue may contain PAS-positive macrophages. In acquired immunodeficiency syndrome, intestinal involvement reminiscent of Whipple's disease has been reported when the gut is infected with *Mycobacterium avium intracellulare*.

Other investigations are of value in confirming the presence of intestinal disease or involvement of other organs, but not diagnostically. Radiographs of the small bowel characteristically show oedema and dilatation. Ultrasonography and computerized tomographic (**CT**) scanning of the abdomen may show lymphatic masses, and brain CT may demonstrate multiple ring-enhancing lesions. The sedimentation rate is elevated, and anaemia due to folate or iron deficiency may be present. Eosinophilia and thrombocytosis may be apparent on blood films. Steatorrhoea, hypocalcaemia, vitamin deficiencies, and an elevated serum alkaline phosphatase occur with advanced gut disease, as do hypoproteinaemia and a protein-losing enteropathy, although the serum IgA may be high.

Treatment and prognosis

Whipple's disease progresses slowly, but unrecognized and untreated it is eventually fatal. Antibiotic therapy is effective, although in severely ill and malnourished individuals correction of the metabolic and nutritional state, and occasionally short-term corticosteroid therapy, may be required. Many different oral and parenteral antibiotic regimens are reportedly successful, including penicillin alone, penicillin and streptomycin, tetracycline and co-trimoxazole. Without cultures to determine sensitivity, all regimens have been empirical and, for example, failure to respond to tetracycline has been reported. Clinical improvement occurs within a few days or weeks, but most recommend long-term treatment, and in particular it appears that a risk of a relapse with central nervous manifestations is reduced if the initial regimen includes agents that pass the blood–brain barrier. Parenteral penicillin and streptomycin for 2 weeks followed by doxycycline for a year is one recommended regimen. A Herxheimer-like syndrome with fever and worsening ocular manifestations have been reported after beginning treatment.

The gut mucosa returns to normal within a few months, although a few PAS-positive macrophages may persist. Even after prolonged treatment, relapse may occur, and there may be progressive central nervous involvement in the absence of other systemic involvement; more usually, however, return of the bacteria in intestinal tissues precedes clinical relapse, and offers a means of early recognition of recurrent disease.

REFERENCES

Bruggemann, A., Burchardt, H., and Lepsien, G. (1992). Sonographical findings in Whipple's disease. *Surgical Endoscopy*, **6**, 138–40.

Dobbins, W.O. (1987). *Whipple's disease*. Thomas, Springfield, IL.

Feldman, M. and Price, G. (1989). Intestinal bleeding in patients with Whipple's disease. *Gastroenterology*, **96**, 1207–9.

Fleming, J.L., Wiesner, R.H., and Shorter, R.G. (1988). Whipple's disease: clinical, biochemical and histopathological features and assessment of treatment in 29 patients. *Mayo Clinic Proceedings*, **63**, 539–51.

Geboes, K., Ectors, N., Heidbuchel, H., Rutgeerts, O., Desmet, V., and Vantrappen G. (1990). Whipple's disease: endoscopic aspects before and after therapy. *Gastrointestinal Endoscopy*, **36**, 247–52.

Gillin, J.S., Urmacher, C., West, R., and Shike, M. (1983). Disseminated *Mycobacterium avium intracellulare* infection in acquired immunodeficiency syndrome mimicking Whipple's disease. *Gastroenterology*, **85**, 1187–91.

Maizel, H., Ruffin, J.M., and Dobbins, W.O. (1970). Whipple's disease: a review of 19 patients from one hospital and a review of the literature. *Medicine (Baltimore)*, **49**, 175–295.

Pallis, C.A. and Lewis, P.D. (1980). Neurology of gastrointestinal disease. In *Handbook of clinical neurology* (ed. P. Vinken and G. Bruyn), Part II **Vol. 39**, *Neurological Manifestations of Systemic Disease*, pp. 449–68. North Holland, Amsterdam.

Playford, R.J., Schulenberg, E., Herrington, C.S., and Hodgson, H.J.F. (1992). Whipple's disease complicated by a retinal Jarisch–Herxheimer reaction. *Gut*, **33**, 132–4.

Relman, D.A., Schmidt, T.M., MacDermott, R.P., and Falkow, S. (1992). Identification of the uncultured Whipple's bacillus. *New England Journal of Medicine*, **327**, 293–300.

Silva, M.T., Macedo, P.M., and Moura-Nunes, J.F. (1985). Ultrastructure of bacilli and the bacillary-origin of the macrophagic inclusions in Whipple's disease. *Journal of General Microbiology*, **131**, 1001–13.

Wilson, K.H., Blitchington, R., Frothingham, R., and Wilson, J.A.P. (1991). Phylogeny of Whipple's disease associated bacterium. *Lancet*, **338**, 474–5.

14.9.7 Short gut syndrome

H. J. F. HODGSON

Short gut syndrome describes the clinical consequences of substantial resections of the small intestine. These include the immediate consequences of loss of absorptive capacity—diarrhoea and malabsorption—and a number of longer-term metabolic sequelae. The severity of the syndrome, and the particular range of metabolic consequences in an individual, depend upon the site and extent of resection and the state of the remaining bowel. Management of the short gut syndrome may be considered an exercise in applied gastrointestinal physiology.

Causes

Crohn's disease and bowel infarction due to vascular occlusion are the most common causes in adults. Volvulus and atresia are common precipitants in childhood. Other causes include extensive resection to achieve tumour clearance, neglected small-bowel obstruction leading to bowel infarction, and in infancy, necrotizing enterocolitis.

Factors determining severity

The normal small intestine is about 5 to 6 m in length when stretched, but is shorter *in vivo* due to muscle tone. Resections of more than half the intestine usually herald problems, and if less than 1 m remains, significant problems are inevitable. The outlook is worse if:

1. The remaining intestine is jejunum; the jejunum is usually passed through rapidly by food, and is already maximally adapted in normal life. When the remnant intestine is ileum, the organ can adapt to increase its absorptive capacity, food is slower in transit, and the specific transport mechanisms for vitamin B_{12} and bile salts are maintained. Furthermore, humoral influences from the ileum, in response to intestinal fat, slow gastric emptying (the 'ileal brake' mechanism).
2. The remaining bowel is functionally abnormal, often the case in Crohn's disease or radiation enteritis.
3. The ileocaecal 'valve' is removed: the valve both slows emptying of ileal contents into the colon, and prevents reflux of colonic contents into the ileum; its absence is associated with a tendency to bacterial overgrowth of the small intestine.
4. There is, in addition, substantial loss of colon.

Mechanisms of diarrhoea

Diarrhoea occurs in the short gut syndrome in response to eating. The mechanisms are complex and will vary between individuals. The main components are:

Failure to absorb salt and water In addition to the volume of fluid ingested, gastric, biliary, and pancreatic secretions may add a further 6 to 7 l of volume per day to the jejunal contents. Normally the distal small intestine, by active transport of sodium, with associated passive water transport, reduces this to leave about 1.5 l per day to enter the colon. Greater volumes may overwhelm the absorptive capacity of the colon.

Failure to absorb nutrients and bile acids In extensive small-intestinal resection the remaining absorptive area may be critically reduced, so that unabsorbed nutrients remain in the lumen; this retains luminal fluid by osmotic action. The reduction in total mucosal disaccharidases associated with gut resection may produce functional lactase deficiency in addition, even if surviving enterocytes individually have normal lactase activity. If the colon is still present, unabsorbed carbohydrate entering from the small intestine becomes subject to bacterial breakdown to organic acids, which both enhances the osmotic load and induces colonic secretion. Both watery diarrhoea and steatorrhoea may be particularly prominent after distal ileal resection, reflecting the loss of the bile salt-reabsorbing function of the ileum. Minor (less than 1 m) resections of the ileum are associated with watery diarrhoea, as unabsorbed bile acids enter the colon, inducing secretion. This is usually readily treated by cholestyramine. In more substantial ileal resections, the loss of bile salts is sufficient to deplete the bile-salt pool, reducing fat absorption in the upper intestine and leading to steatorrhoea. Unabsorbed fat in the colon is subject to bacterial breakdown, both increasing the osmotic load and inducing colonic secretion. Unabsorbed fat in the small intestine can also sequester cations, and even inhibit absorption of water-soluble molecules such as folate.

Small bowel overgrowth This may further inhibit fat absorption by inducing bile-acid deconjugation.

Gastric hypersecretion The mechanism is unclear, although a high concentration of circulating gastrin may contribute. A greater volume of fluid will enter the small intestine, and the low pH may destroy pancreatic enzymes and precipitate bile salts.

Nutrient malabsorption and metabolic problems

Loss of surface area, interference with fat absorption, sequestration of solutes, and loss of specific binding sites all contribute to nutrient malabsorption. More complex metabolic problems include the following three conditions.

Renal stones Hyperoxaluria occurs, particularly if the colon remains intact. The mechanism involves hyperabsorption of dietary oxalate consequent on failure to render dietary oxalate insoluble. This process normally occurs by formation of calcium oxalate in the lumen, but in the presence of unabsorbed fat, calcium is sequestered in calcium soaps and unavailable, permitting absorption of oxalate particularly in the colon. Urate stones may form with combined small- and large-intestinal resections, as the concentrated acid urine produced due to loss of bicarbonate-rich, small-intestinal fluid encourages urate precipitation.

Gallstones These are prevalent, reflecting the lithogenicity of bile associated with a depleted bile-salt pool.

D-Lactic acidosis This syndrome is best recognized in the context of jejunal–ileal bypass but occurs in short gut syndrome, usually in association with obstructive episodes. A typical episode is of 2 to 3 days extreme lethargy, with ataxia, double vision, and nausea. The biochemical basis appears to be bacterial metabolism of unabsorbed carbohydrate to D-lactate; particular forms of bacterial overgrowth (lactobacillus and torulopsis) and excess carbohydrate intake have been implicated. Both antibiotic therapy and carbohydrate restriction may be necessary.

Diagnosis and management

Diagnosis is rarely a problem, as the surgical history is usually clear. Relatively accurate assessment of the length of remaining small intestine can be made from barium radiography. Management changes over time after massive small-intestinal resection, and two important principles emerge. Generally, the absorptive capacity increases over many months, reflecting adaptive changes such as the change in the size of small intestinal villi, increasing size of enterocytes, and dilatation of the remaining bowel. However, enteral nutrition is required both for this to occur, and to prevent atrophy of the intestine, and should be therefore provided as soon as possible, even though parenteral nutrition is usually mandatory in the early stages. Whether the effect of enteral feeding is direct, or indirect via stimulation of secretion of trophic hormones such as gastrin, cholecystokinin, and enteroglucagon, is unclear. Enteral feeding also helps maintain pancreatic function.

Management after resection has been divided into three stages: early postoperative fluid and electrolyte management, including parenteral supplementation; the use of enteral (as far as possible) and parenteral nutrition to ensure adequate caloric intake for longer-term maintenance; and the management of late complications.

Early postoperative management

Following massive resection, parenteral fluid and electrolyte replacement is likely to be mandatory, at least for the period of postoperative ileus. As adequate nutrient intake orally may only become feasible after a period of weeks and months of adaptation, if at all, total parenteral nutrition is likely to be necessary and should be instituted early to prevent excessive weight loss and catabolism. Oral feeding should avoid the use of hyperosmolar high formulations, which tend to cause diarrhoea.

Subsequent dietary management

This must be tailored for individual patients. Some, usually those with between 1.25 and 1.5 m of small intestine or more remaining, can maintain a stable weight without a highly tailored diet, often by taking a greater than normal oral calorie intake, and tolerating diarrhoea. With more extensive resections, oral feeding is unlikely to provide adequate nutritional intake, and parenteral supplements are required. In patients whose ability to maintain nutritional status is marginal, enteral feeding tailored to surmount the physiological disturbances already described should be used. Meals should be small but frequent, based on solids, which are slowly released from the stomach. Lactose-containing preparations should be avoided unless it can be demonstrated that they can be tolerated. A low-fat diet, notably low in long-chain fats, should be prescribed. Restriction may need to be to less than 30 g of long-chain fats per day, with caloric requirements made up by medium-chain triglycerides, which are directly absorbed into the portal vein. Antimotility preparations such as loperamide should be prescribed. The combination of fat restriction and adequate hydration should be adequate to prevent the metabolic factors predisposing to nephrolithiasis.

These recommendations should be tested empirically to see whether they allow adequate calorie intake. It is often easier initially to introduce the entire regimen, and then relax it. In particular, some patients can tolerate a high-fat diet surprisingly well, and sufficient energy can thus be absorbed despite the potential worsening of diarrhoea. Fat in the colon can paradoxically induce constipation and this may be one mechanism.

Supplementation

Parenteral vitamin B_{12} is mandatory if the ileum has been resected. Patients should be surveyed regularly for nutritional deficiencies, and oral vitamin supplements, and a metabolic mineral mixture prescribed. Oral calcium and magnesium supplements are advisable, although poorly absorbed; parenteral magnesium may be required.

Salt and water balance

With combined small-and large-intestinal resections, loss of the reabsorptive capacity of the colon may result in oral feeding causing net loss of salt and water from the intestine on a given diet. In particular, patients with less than 1 m of jejunum remaining always need parenteral salt and water supplements. The enteral feeding principles outlined above may prevent or reduce the need for parenteral supplements by reducing diarrhoea.

'Oral rehydration' mixtures, as used for acute, diarrhoeal disease, which provide water, salt, and a fuel for active sodium transport, may be necessary. They are best taken both at an interval before breakfast and in the evening, to maximize absorption. If glucose–electrolyte mixtures are ineffective, glucose polymers, which are split at the mucosal surface, provide increased amounts of glucose to aid salt absorption whilst maintaining isotonicity. The consumption of large volumes of water without salt may be counterproductive, causing an increased small-intestinal effluent containing effectively the same water volume now rendered isotonic with body salt. Some improvement in fluid losses may be obtained by decreasing gastric secretion by H_2-receptor antagonists or proton-pump inhibitors. Long-acting somatostatin, subcutaneously, has reduced intestinal fluid loss in patients with jejunostomies on oral feeding. Potassium balance is usually less disturbed then sodium balance, but prolonged hypokalaemia in the early postoperative stage may initiate a potassium-losing nephropathy.

Other approaches

Bacterial overgrowth should be suspected if diarrhoea worsens without other cause. Screening breath tests are not always definitive. Empirically prescribed antibiotics such as tetracycline, erythromycin, and metronidazole may often be helpful.

Long-term prospects

Adaptation of the remaining gut permits progressive dietary liberalization during the first years after gut resection, eventually allowing discontinuation of parenteral supplementation. Many patients will, however, require home total parenteral nutrition, which requires meticulous education, catheter care, and supervision. Surgical procedures such as the reversal of a distal segment of the remaining small intestine, to provide an antiperistaltic break and increase absorption, have been advocated; these have obvious risks of further imperilling already limited small intestine and are of limited value. Small-intestinal transplantation has been done in a very small number of individuals, recently as part of a multiorgan transplant including liver. The procedure is formidable, but results are improving.

REFERENCES

Cooper, J.C., Williams, N.S., King, R.F.G.C., and Barker, M.C.J. (1986). Effects of a long-acting somatostatin analogue in patients with severe ileostomy diarrhoea. *British Journal of Surgery*, **73**, 128–31.

Devine, R.M. and Kelly, K.A. (1989). Surgical therapy of the short bowel syndrome. *Gastroenterology Clinics of North America*, **18**, 603–18.

Hudson, M., Pocknee, R., and Mowat, N.A.G., (1990). D-Lactic acidosis in short bowel syndrome—an examination of possible mechanisms. *Quarterly Journal of Medicine*, **74**, 157–64.

Jacobsen, O., Ladefoged, K., Stage, J.G., and Jarnum, S. (1986). Effect of cimetidine on jejunostomy effluents in patients with severe short bowel syndrome. *Scandinavian Journal of Gastroenterology*, **21**, 824–8.

Jeejeebhoy, K.N., Langer, B., Tsallas, G., Chu, R.C., Kuksis, A., and Anderson, G.H. (1976). Total parenteral nutrition at home. *Gastroenterology*, **71**, 953–63.

Ladefoged, K. and Olgaard, K., (1985). Sodium homeostasis after small bowel resection. *Scandinavian Journal of Gastroenterology*, **20**, 361–9.

Lennard-Jones, J.E. (1990). Oral rehydration solution in short bowel syndrome. *Clinical Therapeutics*, **12**, (suppl. A), 129–37.

Levine, G.M., Deren, J.D., and Yezdimir, E. (1976). Small bowel resection: oral intake is the stimulus for hyperplasia. *Digestive Diseases and Science*, **21**, 524–46.

Nightingale, M., Lennard-Jones, J.E., Walker, E.R., and Farthing, M.J. (1990). Jejunal efflux in short bowel syndrome. *Lancet*, **336**, 765–8.

Read, N.W., McFarlane, A., and Kinsman, R.I. (1983). Effect of infusion of nutrients into the ileum on gastrointestinal transport and plasma levels of neurotensin and enteroglucagon. *Gastroenterology*, **86,** 274–80.

Shenkin, A. (1988). Clinical aspects of vitamin and trace element metabolism. *Baillière's Clinical Gastroenterology*, **2,** 765–98.

Silk, D.B.A. (1987). Towards the optimisation of enteral nutrition. *Clinical Nutrition*, **6,** 61–74.

Watson, A.J.M. and Lear, P.A. (1989). Current status of intestinal transplantation. *Gut*, **30,** 1771–82.

Windsor, C.W.O., Fejfar, J., and Woodward, D.A.K. (1969). Gastric secretion after massive small bowel resection. *Gut*, **10,** 779–86.

14.9.8 Enteropathy-associated T-cell lymphoma

P. G. Isaacson

An association between malabsorption and intestinal lymphoma was first reported in 1937 by Fairley and Mackie, when it was thought that the lymphoma was in some way responsible for malabsorption. It subsequently became clear that the reverse is true and that intestinal lymphoma, in common with a variety of other tumours, was a complication of malabsorption, which in turn was most likely due to coeliac disease or gluten-sensitive enteropathy. In 1978, Isaacson and Wright characterized the lymphoma associated with malabsorption as a single entity, namely a variant of malignant histiocytosis. Later, Isaacson and colleagues showed that both the phenotype and genotype of this lymphoma were those of T cells rather than histiocytes. It had been widely assumed that the malabsorption associated with this form of T-cell lymphoma was almost certainly due to coeliac disease, but doubts about whether this was indeed the case led to the coining of the term enteropathy-associated T-cell lymphoma (**EATL**) to describe the disease. There is, however, good evidence that the malabsorption associated with enteropathy-associated T-cell lymphoma is a consequence of coeliac disease and this will be discussed in greater detail below.

Clinical features

Enteropathy associated T-cell lymphoma is characteristically a disease with an equal sex incidence that occurs in the sixth and seventh decades, although sporadic cases have been described in younger patients. The most common presentation is the sudden onset of abdominal symptoms, usually with reappearance of steatorrhoea, after a short (months to years) history of successfully treated adult coeliac disease. Some of these patients may have presented first with dermatitis herpetiformis. In a minority of cases there is a well-documented history of childhood coeliac disease. In others, the onset of lymphoma is heralded by the appearance, in a previously well patient, of severe malabsorption that is usually unresponsive to gluten withdrawal. The lymphoma may also present as an abdominal emergency without any history of malabsorption but the features of coeliac disease are found in the uninvolved portion of the resected small intestine. There is sometimes a long latent interval during which inflammation with stricture formation is seen in the small intestine, overt lymphoma manifesting only later. Finally, there is a small group of patients in whom the lymphoma presents in secondary sites such as peripheral lymph nodes, skin, lungs, or elsewhere in the gastrointestinal tract, with only a minor focus in the small intestine that may be difficult to identify. Abdominal pain, weight loss, fever, finger clubbing, and an ichthyotic rash are all common. The lymphoma usually results in intestinal perforation or haemorrhage rather than obstruction.

The jejunal biopsy in a patients with enteropathy-associated T-cell lymphoma usually shows villous atrophy with crypt hyperplasia but may only show minor changes that, in some cases, may be limited to an increase in intraepithelial lymphocytes. The biopsy may even be normal, particularly if the patient is already on a gluten-free diet. It is unusual to obtain lymphoma tissue in the biopsy but evidence of active or healed ulcers is sometimes present.

Barium studies usually show ulcers or strictures of the small intestine superimposed on a malabsorption pattern. Staging procedures may reveal evidence of disseminated lymphoma, especially in smears of bone marrow aspirate or the liver biopsy (see Chapter 22.5.3).

Most patients with enteropathy-associated T-cell lymphoma are subjected to a laparotomy, either electively, which is preferable, or as an emergency. The lymphoma may involve any segment of the small intes-

Fig. 1 Histological appearances of three different cases of enteropathy-associated T-cell lymphoma showing the cytological variability. In (a) the tumour is composed of small to medium-sized lymphocytes; in (b) the tumour is composed of monomorphic, large immunoblasts; in (c) the tumour shows striking pleomorphism.

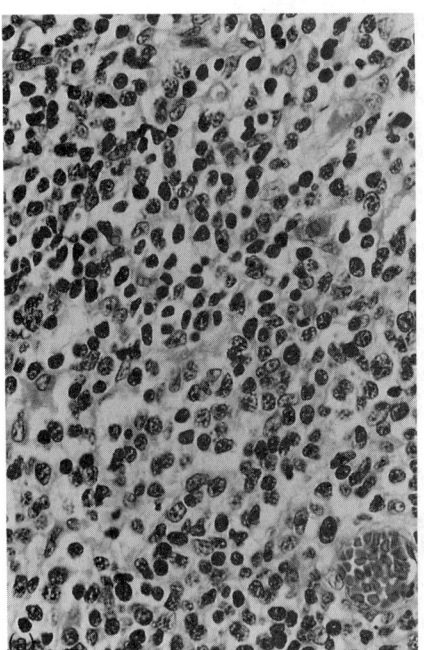
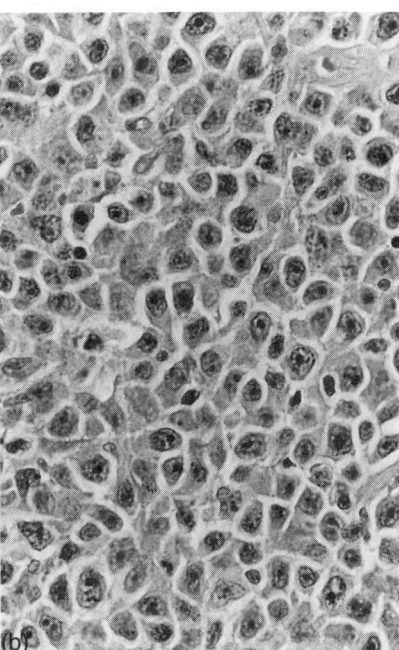
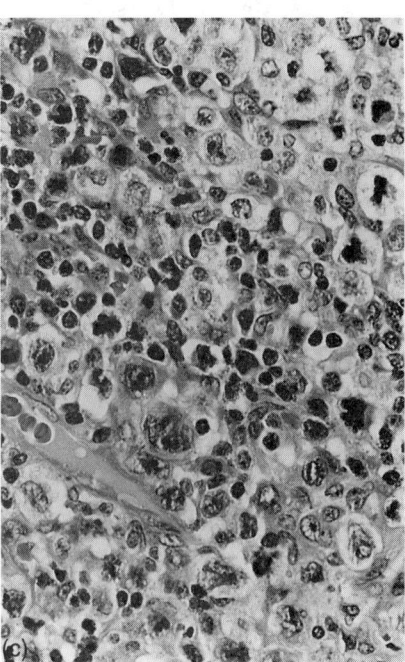

tine but is more common in the jejunum where it occurs as multiple nodules, ulcers, and strictures or, less frequently, as a single large mass. The small intestine may appear normal, although there is usually considerable enlargement of mesenteric lymph nodes. In these circumstances, multiple lymph nodes, as well as the liver, should be biopsied in the interests of making a firm diagnosis. Hepatomegaly is a common feature but the spleen may be smaller than usual as a result of splenic atrophy that occurs in coeliac disease.

The clinical course of enteropathy-associated T-cell lymphoma is very unfavourable except in a minority of patients in whom resection of a localized tumour has been followed by long remission. In most cases the lymphoma involves multiple segments of intestine, rendering resection impossible, or has already disseminated beyond the mesenteric lymph nodes and out of the abdomen.

Pathology

Enteropathy-associated T-cell lymphoma may involve any part of the small intestine and rarely other parts of the gastrointestinal tract including the colon and stomach, but most cases arise in the jejunum. The tumour is usually, but not always, multifocal and forms ulcerating nodules or large masses, which may be accompanied by benign-appearing ulcers and strictures. The mesentery is often infiltrated and mesenteric lymph nodes are commonly involved. There is sometimes remarkably little macroscopic evidence of disease in the intestine, in contrast to mesenteric lymphadenopathy.

The histological features of enteropathy-associated T-cell lymphoma show great variation both between cases and within any single case. The tumour cells may be only slightly larger than normal small lymphocytes or resemble immunoblasts but, more usually, are strikingly pleomorphic (Fig. 1). Intraepithelial tumour cells may be prominent (Fig. 2). Interpretation is further complicated by the heavy inflammatory component, often containing many eosinophils, and extensive necrosis, which, together, may mask the neoplastic infiltrate. Granulomas may be present and cause confusion with Crohn's disease.

The histological appearance of the small intestine remote from the site of the tumour is an important consideration in the diagnosis of enteropathy-associated T-cell lymphoma. In most cases the changes are identical with those of coeliac disease. Thus there is villous atrophy with crypt hyperplasia, plasmacytosis of the lamina propria, and an increase in intraepithelial lymphocytes. The degree of intraepithelial lymphocytosis may be spectacular and so extreme as virtually to obscure the epithelial cells (Fig. 3). The lymphocytes are small, without neoplastic features, and, in these extreme cases spill into the laminal propria where they may merge with the lymphomatous infiltrate. Despite their innocuous appearance these cells have, in at least two cases, been shown to be a part of the neoplastic clone. As in coeliac disease, the mucosal changes are maximal proximally and improve distally so that the lower jejunum and ileum may be normal. This must be borne in mind when the lymphoma arises in the more distal small intestine.

Episodes of ulceration followed by remission with healing may occur before the manifestation of enteropathy-associated T-cell lymphoma (so-called ulcerative jejunitis; see below) and this can lead to a confusing appearance of the mucosa, with scarring and distortion of mucosal architecture, destruction of the muscularis mucosae, and the development of florid, pseudopyloric metaplasia.

In a minority of cases the mucosal alterations are minimal, or even absent.

The mesenteric lymph nodes are commonly involved and almost always show accompanying hyperplasia that may mask the malignant cells, which may be present in remarkably small numbers. Selective necrosis of lymph nodes, often involving entire nodes, remote from the main lesion is a feature of some cases. The cause of this necrosis is obscure.

The most commonly reported phenotype of enteropathy-associated T-cell lymphoma is CD3+/−, CD7+, CD4−, CD8−. Although the cells are CD4 and CD8 negative, they do not express the γ/δ T-cell receptor. The tumour cells react with monoclonal antibody HML-1 and related reagents that recognize the normal intraepithelial T-cell population and approximately 25 per cent of T cells of the lamina propria, in contrast to only a few T cells outside the mucosae. These properties suggest that enteropathy-associated T-cell lymphoma arises from intraepithelial T cells.

Fig. 2 Mucosal infiltrate in enteropathy-associated T-cell lymphoma showing prominence of intraepithelial tumour cells (arrows).

Fig. 3 Uninvolved mucosa from a case of enteropathy-associated T-cell lymphoma showing an extreme degree of intraepithelial lymphocytosis with spilling of lymphocytes into the lamina propria.

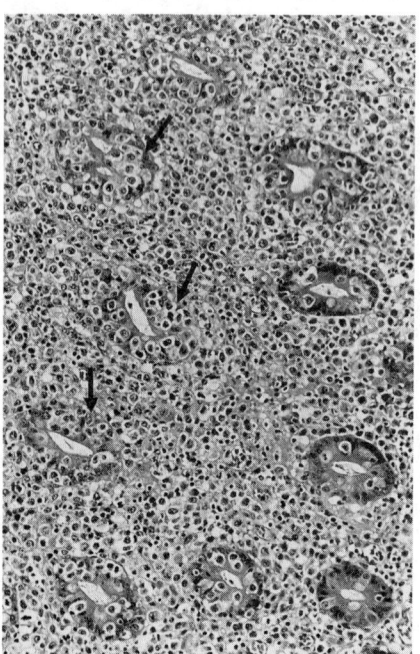

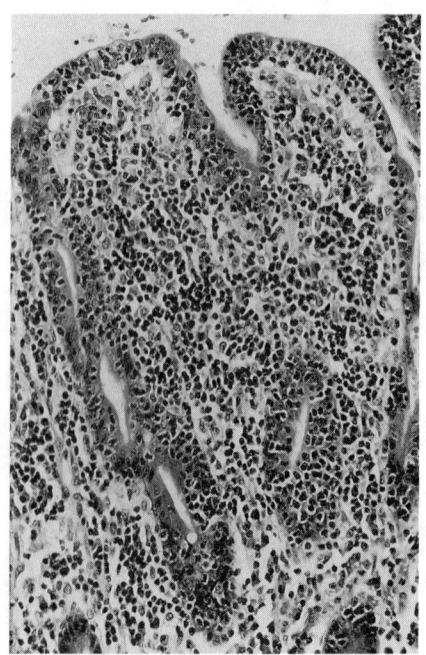

Enteropathy-associated T-cell lymphoma and coeliac disease

The original suggestion that intestinal lymphoma caused an enteropathy was subsequently countered by careful studies showing that the enteropathy was due to gluten sensitivity (i.e. coeliac disease) and preceded the lymphoma. Failure to demonstrate antibodies to α-gliadin in lymphoma cases, a common finding in coeliac disease, led to suggestions that the enteropathy was not a form of coeliac disease. Recent observations of enteropathy-associated T-cell lymphoma cases with an unusually dense and monoclonal intraepithelial lymphocyte population have turned the argument full circle, back to the proposal that some cases of adult coeliac disease may be caused by T-cell lymphoma. There is, however, strong evidence that the enteropathy in enteropathy-associated T-cell lymphoma is a consequence of coeliac disease. Its histological appearances and distribution are those of coeliac disease and the HLA type of patients with enteropathy-associated T-cell lymphoma and coeliac disease is identical. Moreover, gluten sensitivity has been demonstrated in numerous patients with enteropathy-associated T-cell lymphoma and a gluten-free diet has been shown to protect against the development of lymphoma. A significant number of patients with enteropathy-associated T-cell lymphoma have dermatitis herpetiformis, which is closely associated with coeliac disease. Given that enteropathy-associated T-cell lymphoma appears to be a malignancy of intraepithelial T cells, a dense population of these cells in some cases would not be surprising. There remains the dilemma posed by those cases with minimal or even absent enteropathy. These can be explained by observations of only mildly abnormal biopsies in patients with dermatitis herpetiformis and the demonstration of gluten sensitivity in patients with completely normal biopsies, so-called latent coeliac disease.

Chronic ulcerative jejunitis and enteropathy-associated T-cell lymphoma

Multiple, apparently benign, inflammatory ulcers may accompany enteropathy-associated T-cell lymphoma and this ulcerative component of the disease is occasionally the dominant feature. There is, thus, an overlap between enteropathy-associated T-cell lymphoma and another recognized complication of coeliac disease, namely chronic ulcerative jejunitis. The relation between the two conditions is so close that some regard ulcerative jejunitis as a manifestation of enteropathy-associated T-cell lymphoma. In support of this view are the frequent presence of ulcers in enteropathy-associated T-cell lymphoma, the finding, which is helped by using immunohistochemistry, of isolated malignant T cells in the base of one or more ulcers in some cases of ulcerative jejunitis (Fig. 4), and cases in which enteropathy-associated T-cell lymphoma has evolved following a firm diagnosis of the jejunitis. The opposite view, that the jejunitis is a disorder in its own right, is supported by those cases in which no evidence of lymphoma can be detected despite thorough investigation. Prolonged follow-up is necessary to exclude malignancy in these cases.

Management

The treatment of enteropathy-associated T-cell lymphoma is most satisfactory in those cases with a localized tumour, when surgical excision may be followed by long remission or even cure. Most cases, however, are multifocal or have already disseminated at diagnosis and require treatment appropriate for a high-grade non-Hodgkin's lymphoma, which may include bone marrow autografting (see Chapter 22.8.2). This form of therapy is particularly hazardous in enteropathy-associated T-cell lymphoma because of the danger of intestinal perforation. Some cases of ulcerative jejunitis, even when small foci of lymphoma are present, may respond to steroids.

Fig. 4 (a) 'Benign' ulcer from a case of enteropathy-associated T-cell lymphoma; (b) shows a higher magnification of the ulcer base in which isolated malignant cells are evident (arrows).

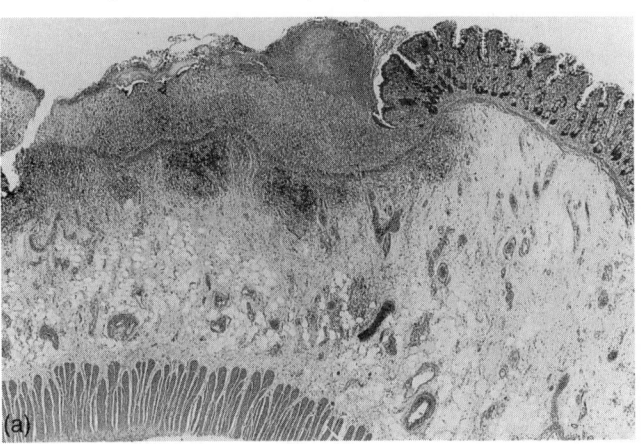

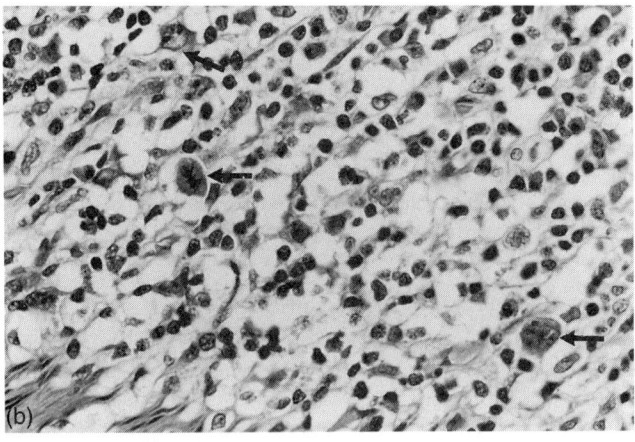

REFERENCES

Bayless, T.M., Kapelowitz, R.F., Shelley, W.M., Ballinger, W.F., and Hendrix, T.D. (1967). Intestinal ulceration—a complication of coeliac disease. *New England Journal of Medicine*, **276**, 996–1002.

Freeman, H.J., Weinstein, W.M., Shnitka, T.K., Piercy, J.R.A., and Wensel, R.H. (1977). Primary abdominal lymphoma: presenting manifestation of celiac sprue or complicating dermatitis herpetiformis. *American Journal of Medicine*, **63**, 585–94.

Holmes, G.K.T., Prior, P., Lane, M.R., Pope, D., and Allan, R.N. (1989). Malignancy in coeliac disease—effect of a gluten free diet. *Gut*, **30**, 333–8.

Isaacson, P.G. and Wright, D.H. (1978). Intestinal lymphoma associated with malabsorption. *Lancet*, **i**, 67–70.

Isaacson, P.G. and Wright, D.H. (1978). Malignant histiocytosis of the intestine: its relationship to malabsorption and ulcerative jejunitis. *Human Pathology*, **9**, 661–77.

Isaacson, P.G. *et al.* (1985). Malignant histiocytosis of the intestine: a T cell lymphoma. *Lancet*, **ii**, 688–91.

O'Mahony, S., Vestey, J.P., and Ferguson, A. (1990). Similarities in intestinal humoral immunity in dermatitis herpetiformis without enteropathy and in coeliac disease. *Lancet*, **335**, 1487–90.

Spencer, J., *et al.* (1988). Enteropathy-associated T cell lymphoma (malignant histiocytosis of the intestine) is recognised by a monoclonal antibody (HML1) that defines a membrane molecule on human mucosal lymphocytes. *American Journal of Pathology*, **132**, 1–5.

Swinson, C.M., Slavin, G., Coles, E.C., and Booth, C.C. (1983). Coeliac disease and malignancy. *Lancet*, **i**, 111–15.

14.9.9 Malabsorption in the tropics

M. J. G. FARTHING

Introduction

Malabsorption of nutrients by the small intestine has a particular relevance for the tropics, where the most common causes often differ from those in the industrialized world and its impact may be substantially greater, particularly in parts of the world where there is a background of borderline undernutrition. Tropical malabsorption is not limited to the indigenous population but also affects travellers to these regions, who are susceptible to the clearly defined infective causes of malabsorption and also to the less well-defined conditions of unknown aetiology such as tropical enteropathy and tropical sprue.

Small-intestinal absorption in the tropics can be considered to be due either to specific causes such as infections of known aetiology, inflammatory, and neoplastic disorders, or to the non-specific conditions such as tropical enteropathy and tropical sprue in which the aetiology has not been determined (Table 1).

Specific causes of tropical malabsorption

INTESTINAL INFECTION

The majority of infections that produce intestinal malabsorption in the tropics produce an enteropathy in the small intestine with varying degrees of villous atrophy, crypt hyperplasia, and inflammatory infiltrates in the lamina propria and in some cases in the epithelium. Giardiasis is the most common human protozoal infection of the small intestine worldwide and is now recognized to cause chronic diarrhoea, intestinal malabsorption and sometimes growth retardation in infants and young children. In immunocompetent individuals *Cryptosporidium parvum* usually produces an acute, self-limiting, diarrhoeal illness, often associated with mild histopathological abnormalities in the small intestine. However, in the immunocompromised, chronic diarrhoea is common and an important cause of morbidity in patients with AIDS in the tropics. *Enterocytozoon bieneusi* (microsporidium) and *Isospora belli* are also important infections causing malabsorption in AIDS patients. Helminths are not a major cause of intestinal malabsorption, although heavy infection with *Strongyloides stercoralis*, including the hyperinfection syndrome, should be included in the differential diagnosis. *Capillaria philippinensis* is an important cause of intestinal malabsorption but in a highly restricted geographic area in south-east Asia. Rotavirus, enteric adenoviruses, and the Norwalk family of viruses all produce small-bowel enteropathy, but the illness is usually self-limiting and a chronic malabsorptive state virtually never occurs. The relation between human immunodeficiency virus and small-intestinal enteropathy is controversial, although there is some evidence to suggest that the virus itself may be responsible for small-intestinal damage, even in the absence of other defined enteropathogens. Most bacterial infections of the small intestine produce acute diarrhoea and a self-limiting illness, although some enteropathogenic *Escherichia coli* strains produce chronic diarrhoea and malabsorption in infants and young children, as can diffuse small-intestinal involvement with *Mycobacterium tuberculosis*.

COELIAC DISEASE

Coeliac disease (gluten-sensitive enteropathy) is rare in the tropics but has been described in India, particularly Northern India where wheat-containing foods form an important part of the diet, and also in Africa. Coeliac disease may present for the first time in the tropics in European and North American expatriates and thus should always be considered in such individuals. Confirmation of a diagnosis of coeliac disease can be difficult in the tropical setting, particularly in distinguishing it from

Table 1 *Tropical malabsorption*

Specific	
Infection:	
Protozoa	*G. lamblia*
	C. parvum
	E. bieneusi
	I. belli
Helminths	*C. philippinensis*
	S. sterocoralis
Bacteria	Enteropathogenic *E. coli*
	M. tuberculosis
Viruses	Rotavirus
	Enteric adenoviruses
	(types 40,41)
	Norwalk viruses
	Measles virus
	HIV
Coeliac disease	
Lymphoma	
Severe undernutrition (kwashiorkor and marasmus)	
Primary hypolactasia	
Non-specific	
Tropical enteropathy	
Tropical sprue	

tropical sprue, but the morphological changes in the jejunum are usually more profound than those found in tropical sprue and will almost inevitably respond to gluten withdrawal but not to broad-spectrum antibiotics. Diagnosis should always be confirmed by gluten challenge and a further jejunal biopsy to confirm morphological relapse following reintroduction of gluten.

LYMPHOMA

Immunoproliferative small-intestinal disease (**IPSID**) and primary upper small-intestinal lymphoma (**PUSIL**) are found predominantly in those parts of the world where socioeconomic conditions are poor. Although commonly known as Mediterranean lymphoma, the condition has been found in other parts of the world including the Middle East, South Africa, and South America. There is some evidence to suggest that these conditions are related, with immunoproliferative small-intestinal disease progressing to primary, upper small-intestinal lymphoma and the implication that the former is a premalignant condition. These disorders usually occur in a younger age group, which distinguishes them from the primary intestinal lymphoma that occurs worldwide, most commonly in the elderly.

SEVERE UNDERNUTRITION

The role of undernutrition in the pathogenesis of intestinal malabsorption and small-intestinal enteropathy remains controversial. Steatorrhoea and villous atrophy have been described in children with severe kwashiorkor and marasmus, and these abnormalities can be reversed, following correction of the nutritional deficit. However, it seems unlikely that less severe degrees of undernutrition have a major impact on small-intestinal structure or function.

PRIMARY HYPOLACTASIA

Lactase activity in the small intestine is high in neonates in all ethnic groups but in many, particularly those indigenous to the tropics, activity rapidly declines within 3 to 4 months of weaning. Adult hypolactasia is found throughout most countries in south-east Asia but it is less common in the Middle East and uncommon in Northern Europe. The practical importance of hypolactasia, however, is small because African and Asian adults avoid milk unless they wish to use it as a purgative. It does mean, however, that milk-based products cannot be used reliably in these regions as a nutritional supplement. Secondary hypolactasia occurs after small-intestinal infections that produce enteropathy but this is usually short-lived and self-limiting.

Non-specific tropical malabsorption

Malabsorption in the tropics is also associated with two conditions of unknown aetiology, tropical enteropathy and tropical sprue. Despite intensive investigation during the last three to four decades, the aetio-pathogenesis of these conditions remains elusive and the relation between the two a matter for conjecture. The widespread nature of tropical enteropathy and the geographic restriction of tropical sprue continue to challenge epidemiologists and clinical investigators.

TROPICAL ENTEROPATHY

The term 'enteropathy' implies that there is a pathological process in the small intestine. The jejunal morphology of people in many tropical regions is indeed different from those living in temperate, industrialized areas. The finger-like villi characteristic of healthy people in the developed world are rare in the tropics, where broad leaf- and/or tongue-shaped villi are the usual pattern. Indeed, it has been argued that this is the 'normal' state for individuals living in this environment. The reduction in villus height is usually accompanied by increased crypt depth and an inflammatory infiltrate in the lamina propria and the epithelium. Tropical enteropathy has been detected in most tropical regions of Asia, Africa, the Middle East, the Caribbean, and Central and South America (Fig. 1). This is an acquired defect, as newborn infants in the developing world have the typical finger-like villi but by 4 to 6 months the villous architectural abnormalities and inflammatory infiltrate begin to appear. Tropical enteropathy is not limited to the indigenous population and can be acquired by travellers from the developed world who reside and work in a tropical environment for a period of several months.

Studies of migrants travelling from the developed to the industrialized world suggest that the enteropathy is reversible. However, a recent survey of small-bowel morphology in British-Indian and British Afro-Caribbean subjects who had lived in the United Kingdom for many years, some more than 30 years, has raised the question of genetic predisposition to the development of enteropathy. In both groups villous height was less than in white subjects, although there was no correlation between the reduction in villous height and the duration of stay in the United Kingdom (Fig 2). However, in Indian subjects there was a correlation between the reduction in villous height and the time since the last visit to the Indian subcontinent, suggesting that re-exposure to the tropical environment was involved in maintaining the enteropathy. No such relation was found in the Afro-Caribbean subjects, suggesting that the persisting mild abnormality of villous architecture was not related to re-exposure to a tropical environment but possibly indicated a genetic factor in enteropathy.

Small-intestinal dysfunction

Small-intestinal absorption tests in apparently healthy individuals in India, Africa, and Central and South America have demonstrated reduced absorption of D-xylose, glucose, vitamin B_{12}, and fat compared to that in Western controls. Intestinal perfusion studies using glucose, amino acids, and small peptides have confirmed reduced absorption rates compared to those in Europeans. In southern India, 50 per cent of apparently healthy adults had reduced D-xylose absorption, 10 per cent had mild steatorrhoea, and approximately 3 per cent had reduced vitamin B_{12} absorption. However, it should be stressed that these functional abnormalities are mild and represent only a subclinical malabsorptive state. These minor abnormalities appear, however, to be more common in lower socioeconomic groups living in rural environments than in more affluent city dwellers.

Aetiology of tropical enteropathy

The majority of epidemiological evidence indicates that tropical enteropathy results from environmental factors. Climate alone does not appear to be a major factor, as in locations like Singapore where water quality, sanitation, and nutritional status are similar to industrialized countries, tropical enteropathy has not been found. The major contributors to the production of the enteropathy appear to be (i) intestinal infection and (ii) nutritional insufficiency. In the developing world it is often difficult to separate these two factors and to explore, in a controlled way, their independent and combined effects on intestinal structure and function. However, evidence in human and animal studies suggests that the intestine is relatively resistant to nutritional insufficiency except when severe, and thus attention has focused on the microbiological milieu of the intestine. Studies in southern India have identified two 'infective' factors that may be important. Apparently healthy asymptomatic individuals (i) have a small intestine that is heavily colonized by aerobic and anaerobic organisms and (ii) excrete a range of established bacterial enteropathogens in their faeces. Studies in germ-free animals have clearly shown the importance of luminal and mucosal bacterial flora in modulating villous architecture and inflammatory infiltration, and thus there is compelling circumstantial evidence that it is the increased bacterial load of commensal and pathogenic micro-organisms which leads to the mucosal abnormalities in many parts of the developing world. These abnormalities are not limited to the small intestine

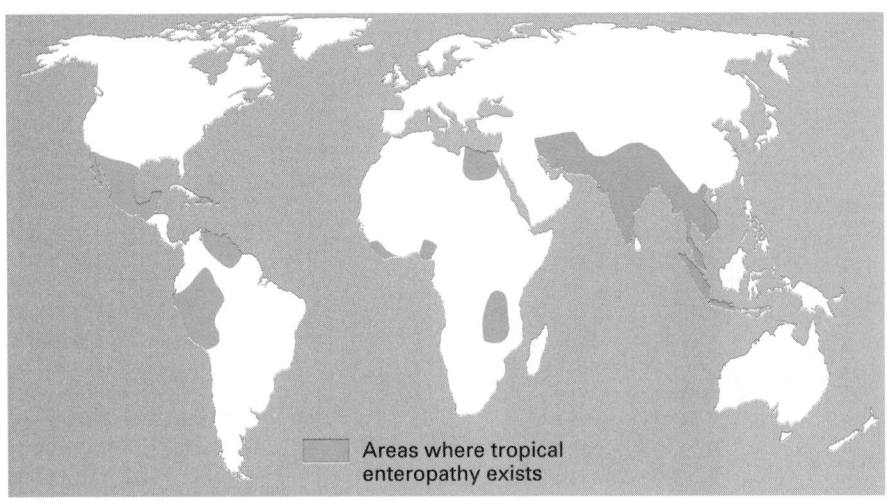

Areas where tropical enteropathy exists

Fig. 1 Geographic distribution of tropical enteropathy.

as there is also a subclinical abnormality of colonocyte structure and function, which might be called tropical colonopathy.

The broad geographical distribution of tropical enteropathy has always suggested that environmental factors are most important in the aetiology and that there is little to support a genetic basis for this condition. However, the recent description of persisting mild enteropathy in British Afro-Caribbean subjects who have not returned to their country of origin for many years suggests that there may be a genetic component.

TROPICAL SPRUE

Many controversies continue to surround the clinical entity, tropical sprue. It is epidemiologically perplexing because of its restricted geographical distribution within the tropics and, unlike most other diarrhoeal diseases, its relatively low prevalence in children. Its aetiology is unknown, though there is no lack of hypotheses. However, the varied clinical presentations make it difficult to put together a unifying theory. One of the problems has been the failure to establish a universally agreed definition of the syndrome.

Fig. 2 Villous height and crypt depth in British Indian and Afro-Caribbean subjects (adapted from Wood *et al.* (1991). *Gut*, **32**, 256–9). *$p < 0.01$ compared to white subjects.

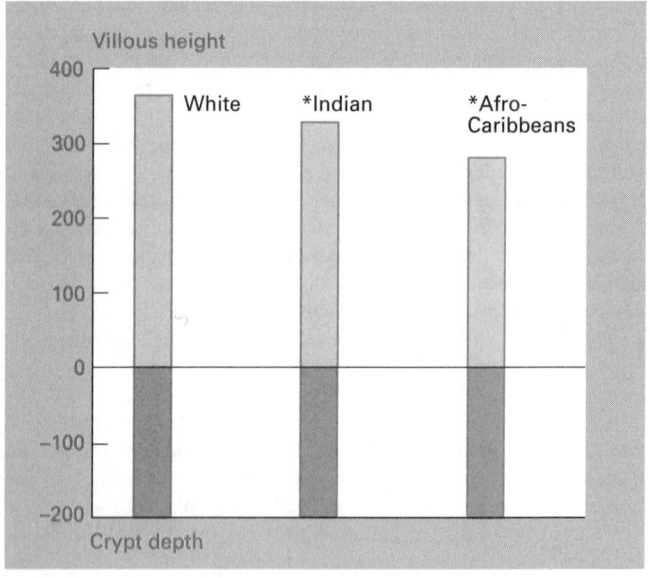

Definition

The Wellcome Trust collaborative study 'Tropical sprue and megaloblastic anaemia' published in 1971 concluded that 'tropical sprue is a syndrome of intestinal malabsorption which occurs among residents in or visitors to certain regions of the tropics'. Baker and Mathan working in Vellore added to the definition by including 'malabsorption of two or more substances in people in the tropics when other known causes have been excluded'. Cook, however, impressed by the clinical presentation that tropical sprue often followed an acute diarrhoeal illness, and the accumulating evidence that the small intestine in sprue is colonized by aerobic and anaerobic bacteria, considered that the term 'post-infective tropical malabsorption' should be used in preference to tropical sprue. Booth opposed this move on the basis that not all episodes of tropical sprue follow an acute diarrhoeal illness and that the syndrome may remain latent for many years, even after expatriates have returned to their homeland. He proposed the definition 'malabsorption in defined areas of the tropics in which no bacterial viral or parasitic infection can be detected', which carefully excludes any assumptions on cause. While the cause of sprue remains unknown, it would seem wise to resist including speculation on its aetiology in the definition.

Historical aspects

A description of a malabsorption state in the tropics appears in an ancient Indian treatise on medicine, the Charakasamhida, which was written before 600 BC. William Hillary in 1759 gave the first clear clinical description of the disease in the European literature, in which he described chronic diarrhoea and malabsorption in Barbados in the Caribbean. In the following 200 years, numerous reports came from physicians who had observed the disease, many of whom had accompanied the military to India, south-east Asia and the Far East. Manson in 1880 introduced the word 'sprue', derived from the Dutch word *sprouw*, which describes the oral aphthous ulceration in children occurring with chronic diarrhoea. By the beginning of the twentieth century it had become evident that tropical sprue was associated with morphological abnormalities in the small intestine, although all of the early observations were in autopsies and thus the significance remained controversial. Sir Phillip Manson-Bahr in 1924 was convinced that the primary lesion in sprue was in the small-intestinal mucosa and this was confirmed when peroral jejunal biopsy was introduced in the 1950s.

Epidemiology

One of the extraordinary features of tropical sprue is that it is predominantly a disease of southern and south-east Asia, the Caribbean islands and to a much lesser extent, of Central and South America. It virtually never occurs in expatriates in Africa, although there have been sporadic reports from South Africa, Zimbabwe, and Nigeria (Fig. 3). Thus,

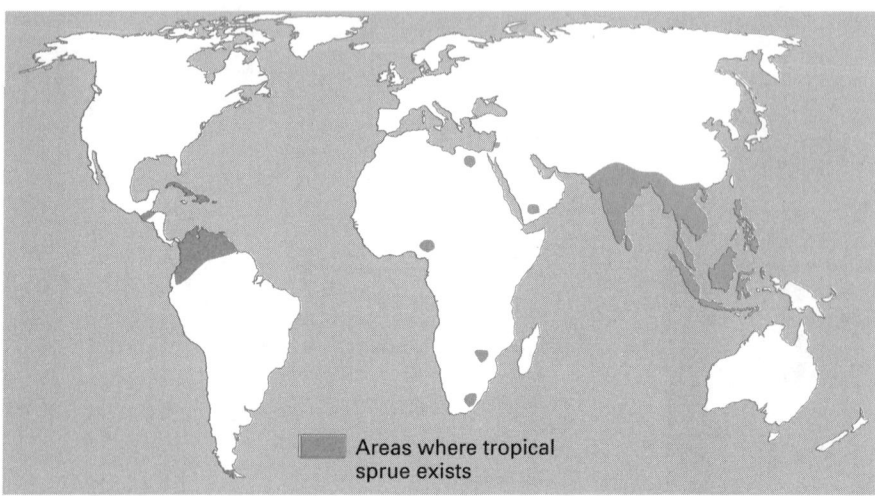

Areas where tropical sprue exists

Fig. 3 Geographic distribution of tropical sprue.

endemic tropical sprue is not found universally in tropical and subtropical regions, strongly suggesting that the aetiological factor or factors are geographically restricted. The prevalence of endemic tropical sprue has not been clearly defined, although in Europeans living in Ceylon prevalence was estimated to be 0.5 per cent, and in North Americans living in Puerto Rico, 6 per cent.

Epidemic tropical sprue has been most clearly documented in villages around Vellore in Southern India. Epidemics differ from other acute diarrhoeas in that they evolve over many months, with new cases continuing to appear after a year or more. In addition, the attack rates are higher in adults than children, although exposure during the first wave of an epidemic appears to offer protection during subsequent waves. Epidemics have also been described in Northern India and Burma. During the major epidemics in Southern India in 1960 to 1962 it was estimated that 100 000 people were affected and that tropical sprue was directly related to the death of at least 30 000 people. In southern India epidemics do not exhibit seasonality, although in Puerto Rico cases commonly present during the first trimester of the year. Clinical impressions suggest that the incidence of tropical sprue, both in the indigenous population and in visitors to endemic areas, is declining.

Clinical features

The cardinal features of tropical sprue are chronic diarrhoea, anorexia, abdominal bloating, and prominent bowel sounds. The illness in expatriates and in epidemics in the indigenous population often begins with an acute attack of diarrhoea associated with fever and malaise. The diarrhoea may then take on the features of steatorrhoea and be accompanied by weight loss. This particular form of the illness was the usual form in individuals travelling overland from Europe to India. Lactose intolerance may develop as part of this illness and may be associated with deficiencies of folic acid, vitamin B_{12}, and occasionally hypocalcaemia and hypomagnesaemia. Generally the illness remits on returning home and after treatment with broad-spectrum antibiotics and folic acid.

In some individuals the diarrhoea continues and the acute phase of tropical sprue becomes chronic. Once diarrhoea has persisted for months or even years the clinical picture becomes dominated by nutritional deficiencies producing anaemia, stomatitis, and glossitis, hyperpigmentation of the skin, and oedema as a result of hypoproteinaemia. In southern India, 1 per cent of patients with endemic tropical sprue present with nutritional deficiencies in the absence of diarrhoea. Occasionally, vitamin B_{12} deficiency can be severe enough to produce neurological signs of subacute combined degeneration of the cord.

A small number of patients has been described in whom the initial presentation of sprue involves only a mild or a subclinical illness and in whom the chronic diarrhoea and nutritional deficiencies develop months or even years after leaving a tropical environment. This form of the illness has been called 'latent sprue'. It has been described in Puerto Ricans living in New York and in Anglo-Indians in London, who typically present with steatorrhoea and megaloblastic anaemia.

Pathology

The histopathological and ultrastructural changes in the gastrointestinal tract associated with tropical sprue are highly variable but generally relate to the duration and the severity of the clinical presentation.

Chronic atrophic gastritis

Many patients with tropical sprue in southern India have reduced secretion of gastric acid and intrinsic factor as a result of chronic gastritis. This can result in vitamin B_{12} malabsorption, which is only corrected by administration of intrinsic factor. The gastritis may persist after the enteropathy has recovered.

Enteropathy

The jejunal mucosal biopsy may be normal in the early stages of sprue, although with persistent symptoms there is usually a reduction in villous height, increase in crypt depth, and an inflammatory cell infiltrate in both the lamina propria and the epithelium (Fig. 4). The changes are similar to those seen in tropical enteropathy, but more pronounced. There is a close relation between the severity of the villus architectural abnormalities and the extent of nutrient malabsorption. Electron-microscopic studies have suggested that the primary lesion in tropical sprue is in the stem cells in the crypts. It has been suggested that although crypt cell proliferation and enterocyte migration up the villus are increased in tropical sprue, the progeny of cells produced are damaged and are thus more rapidly extruded from the villus tip.

Colonopathy

Colonic epithelial cells show structural abnormalities similar to those in the small intestine. Sodium and water absorption by the colon is impaired in tropical sprue, which is thought to be related at least in part to the increased concentrations of unsaturated free fatty acids in the stool. These have a variety of effects on colonocyte structure and function, including inhibition of the enzyme sodium–potassium adenosine triphosphatase. This enzyme has a vital part to play in the absorption of sodium and water by the colonic epithelium.

Pathophysiology

Physiological disturbances in the gastrointestinal tract in tropical sprue involve the stomach, small intestine, and colon. Reference has already been made to the reduced gastric acid secretion and impaired colonic epithelial absorptive function in tropical sprue. The major pathophysiological disturbances, however, occur in the small intestine.

Fig. 4 Jejunal morphology in a traveller from the United Kingdom with tropical sprue before and after treatment with tetracycline and folic acid.

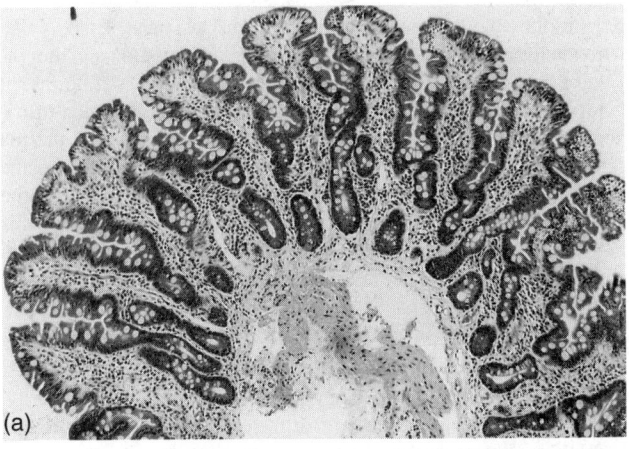

(a)

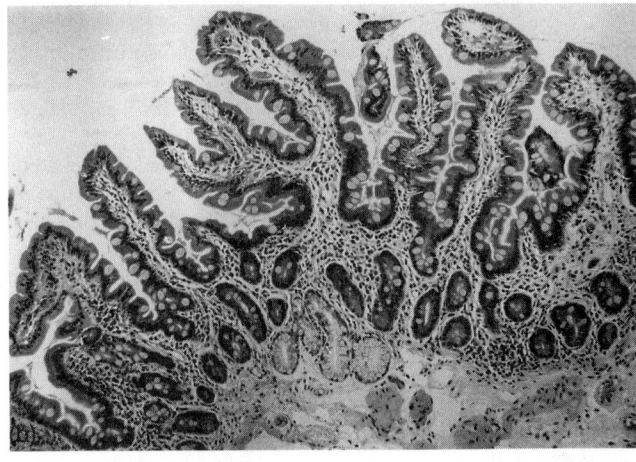

Intestinal absorption and secretion

Perfusion studies of the small intestine have indicated that some patients with tropical sprue have a net secretory state for water in the small intestine which can be dramatically improved by treatment with antibiotics. However, sprue patients in southern India did not have a secretory state and indeed absorb water and electrolytes similarly to healthy control subjects. Intestinal perfusion studies have been used to demonstrate impaired amino-acid and dipeptide absorption. Carbohydrate absorption is also impaired. D-Xylose absorption is commonly reduced in all geographical locations, as is disaccharidase activity and lactose absorption. One of the most consistent findings in patients both from Asia and the Caribbean is impaired fat absorption, with more than 90 per cent of subjects in southern India having a raised faecal fat concentration.

Absorption of micronutrients is also commonly impaired, particularly of folic acid, and as the enteropathy progresses to involve the ileum, vitamin B_{12}.

Intestinal motility

Using the lactulose hydrogen breath test, mouth-to-caecum transit time has been shown to be increased in patients with tropical sprue compared to healthy controls. In a small number of patients, the transit time was reduced after treatment with tetracycline and folic acid. It is unclear whether the increase in small-intestinal transit time is part of the primary pathophysiology of tropical sprue or whether it is secondary to bacterial colonization of the proximal small intestine. The presence of fat in the distal ileum and colon is known to increase mouth-to-caecum transit time and thus fat malabsorption in tropical sprue may be an important factor modulating small-intestinal transit.

Gut hormones

Fasting serum concentrations of motilin and enteroglucagon are increased in patients with acute tropical sprue, with a further marked increment following administration of a standard test meal. There is also a relation between the plasma enteroglucagon concentration and mouth-to-caecum transit time, suggesting that enteroglucagon is a hormonal mediator of the increase in small-intestinal transit time. Infusion of triglyceride or oleic acid into the distal small intestine increases plasma concentrations of enteroglucagon, neurotensin, and peptide tyrosine (**PYY**). However, only PYY concentrations correlate closely with the changes in small-intestinal transit and it is now considered that this peptide does have a mediator role in the so-called ileal brake mechanism induced by fat. PYY has not been measured in patients with tropical sprue.

Aetiopathogenesis of tropical sprue

The aetiology of tropical sprue is unknown. Like tropical enteropathy, epidemiological evidence indicates that the cause or causes of tropical sprue relate to factors in the tropical environment. Nutritional insufficiency, intestinal infection, and possibly toxins have all been implicated as causative agents. Tropical sprue can occur in well-nourished as well as undernourished individuals and although the disease can have a major effect on macro- and micronutrient status, there is little evidence to suggest that undernutrition has any primary role in initiating the disease process. Although bacterial enterotoxins have been identified in some patients with sprue in the Caribbean, this has not been a universal finding and thus tropical sprue cannot be attributed to a single toxic substance yet identified. The bulk of the epidemiological evidence suggests that tropical sprue does have an infective aetiology. Many people antedate their chronic diarrhoea to an episode of acute diarrhoea that fails to improve. The studies of epidemics in the Vellore area in southern India are entirely consistent with an infective aetiology, and one in which during the later phases of the epidemic, protection is confirmed consistent with the development of protective immunity.

A variety of bacteria has been isolated from the jejunum in patients with tropical sprue. In northern India, Puerto Rico, Haiti, and in Europeans travelling to India, coliforms are present in increased numbers in the jejunum. In the Europeans, *Alcaligenes faecalis*, *Enterobacter aerogenes*, and *Hafnia* spp. were found. In patients from India and the Caribbean, *Klebsiella pneumoniae*, *E. coli*, and *Enterobacter cloacae* were common. In southern India, however, the prevalence of coliforms in patients with tropical sprue was the same as in healthy controls. Thus, in some geographic areas there is bacterial colonization of the proximal small intestine with coliforms, but no single species has emerged that could explain tropical sprue in all geographic locations. However, colonization of the small intestine with coliforms can change villus architecture in animal models and similar histopathological lesions have been described in patients with bacterial overgrowth of other causes.

Viruses have been searched for as a cause of tropical sprue; viral particles resembling orthomyxo- and coronaviruses have been found in the faeces but were also found in similar numbers in local asymptomatic control subjects.

It seems possible that the syndrome of tropical sprue may have more than one cause. Tropical sprue in the Caribbean is always associated with vitamin B_{12} malabsorption, is strongly linked to the presence of enterotoxin-producing coliforms, and responds well to broad-spectrum antibiotics. Disease patterns and the bacterial profile in the small intestine differ in patients from southern India and in overland travellers, and their response to treatment is less predictable than in Caribbean sprue.

A model for pathogenesis

While the aetiology of sprue is unknown, it is presumptuous to attempt to explain confidently the pathogenetic mechanisms involved. Cook has suggested that the primary event in the pathogenesis of tropical sprue is an acute intestinal infection involving the small and possibly the large intestine. This causes non-specific mucosal injury that is responsible for the elevated plasma enteroglucagon concentration, which then slows intestinal transit and predisposes to bacterial overgrowth in the small intestine. This will then perpetuate the mucosal injury–slow transit cycle (Fig. 5). There are a number of problems with this hypothesis. It does not explain the cases of tropical sprue that do not obviously begin with an acute diarrhoeal illness and there is some question as to whether the raised concentrations of enteroglucagon are responsible for the slowing of intestinal transit. In addition, the effect of bacterial overgrowth on the small intestine is by no means clear cut, some studies demonstrating that motility is actually increased.

Whatever the initial injury or predisposing factor is, increased numbers of coliforms in the small intestine do seem to be a fairly consistent observation in many patients studied. The response to broad-spectrum

Fig. 5 Cook's hypothesis to explain the pathogenesis of tropical sprue (from *Lancet*. (1984). **i**, 721–3).

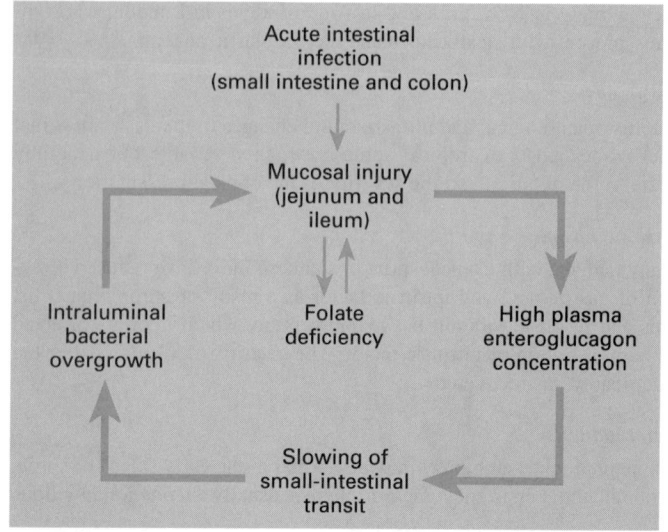

antibiotics, at least in some patients, would support the clinical importance of this finding. The importance of fat malabsorption, both with respect to the 'ileal brake' and slowing of intestinal transit, and to the effect of fatty acids on colonocyte function, would appear to be plausible mechanisms in the pathogenetic cascade. Possible routes by which these factors might interact to perpetuate the chronic diarrhoea–malabsorption cycle are shown in Fig. 6.

Diagnosis

When investigating a patient with malabsorption in the tropics or in someone who has recently returned from the tropics, the first step is to exclude the specific causes of malabsorption, specifically intestinal infections. At least three stool specimens on separate days should be examined by microscopy, using appropriate stains to search for the parasites *Giardia lamblia* and *C. parvum*, and in the immunocompromised *Isospora belli* and *Enterocytozoon bieneusi*. If faecal microscopy is negative, and any of these infections strongly suspected, then it is often worthwhile to perform jejunal aspiration and jejunal biopsy to search for the parasites in intestinal fluid or on the small-intestinal mucosa. The jejunal biopsy will also be useful in assessing whether coeliac disease is a diagnostic possibility, as are the antiendomysial and antireticulin antibodies. A barium follow-through examination and small-bowel biopsies will be necessary to exclude small-intestinal lymphoma or immunoproliferative small-intestinal disease. Once the specific aetiologies have been excluded, then with the presence of fat, vitamin B$_{12}$, and possibly D-xylose malabsorption, and a jejunal biopsy showing partial villous atrophy, the diagnosis can be assumed to be tropical sprue.

Barium follow-through in tropical sprue usually shows an increase in calibre of the small intestine and thickening of the folds (Fig. 7). The changes are present throughout the small intestine and there is usually slow transit of the barium column through the small intestine.

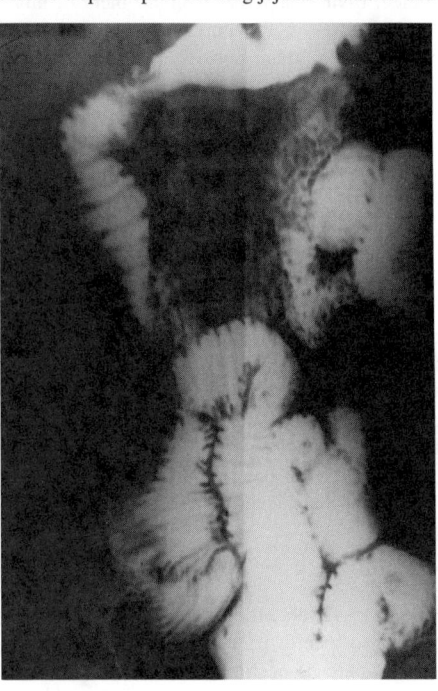

Fig. 7 Barium follow-through examination in a southern Indian patient with chronic tropical sprue showing jejunal dilatation and fold thickening.

Fig. 6 A modified model which relates the many factors that have been proposed to explain the pathogenesis of tropical sprue.

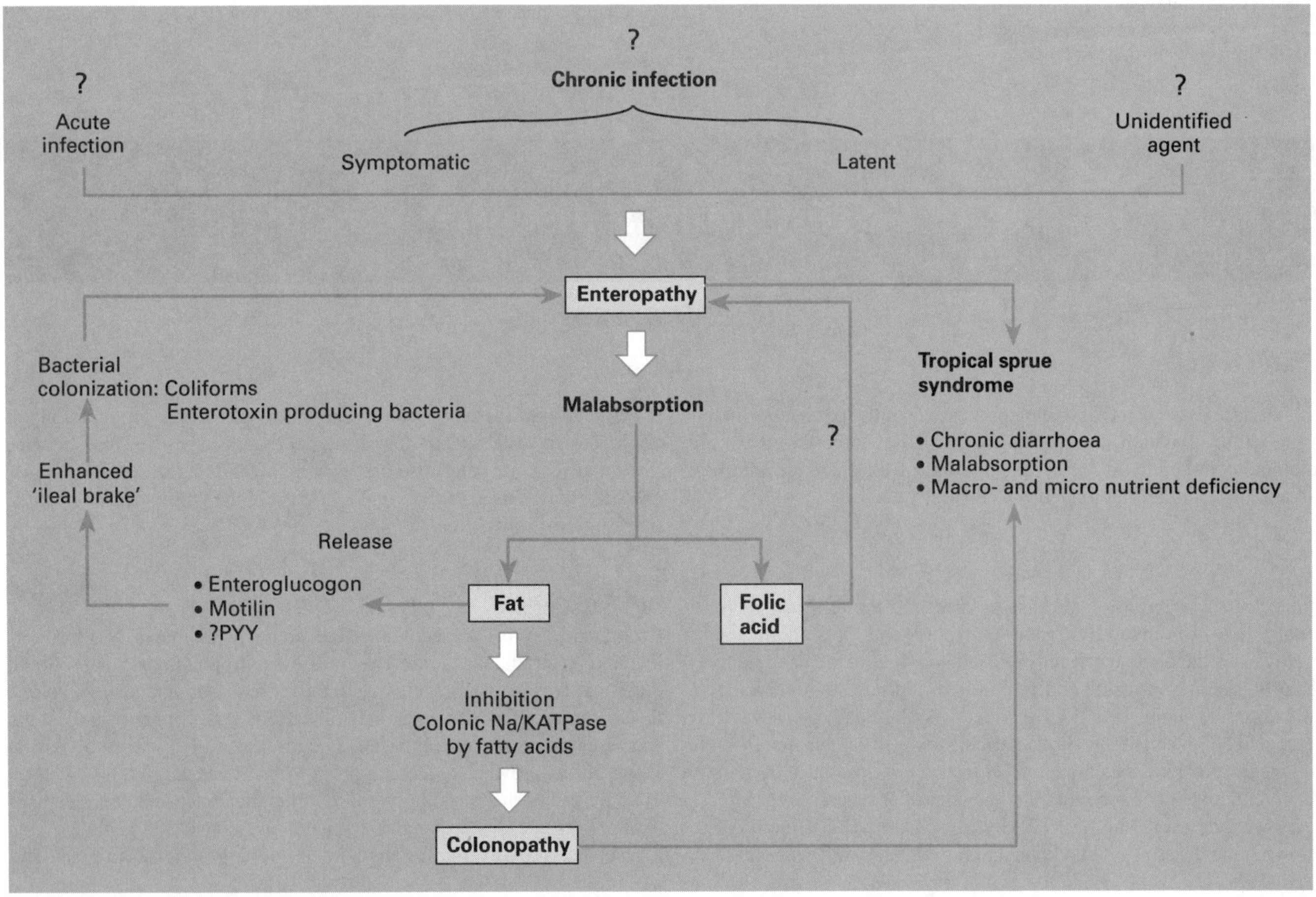

Treatment

Restoration of water and electrolyte balance and replacement of nutritional deficiencies are the priorities in the initial case management. These interventions are thought to be responsible for the dramatic decrease in mortality in epidemic sprue in southern India. It is usually recommended that vitamin B_{12} be given parenterally, although iron and folic acid may be given orally. Patients should be encouraged to take a balanced, nutritious diet to replace macronutrient deficiencies.

The question of broad-spectrum antibiotics and folic acid remains controversial. Overland travellers studied in the United Kingdom and patients in Puerto Rico are reported to make good progress on tetracyline, 250 mg four times daily, usually given over a period of several months. In a controlled trial in southern India, the addition of antibiotics to the vitamin B_{12} and folic acid regimen did not appear to improve the rate of recovery. Spontaneous recovery does occur, possibly related to a change in environment and the oral bacterial load. Symptomatic treatment with an antidiarrhoeal preparation such as loperamide is often advised. If intestinal stasis and bacterial colonization are important in the pathogenesis of this syndrome, then one might argue that slowing small-bowel transit with an antidiarrhoeal preparation could delay recovery.

Prevention

Other than the usual advice to travellers on the avoidance of contaminated food and water, there are no specific preventive measures for tropical sprue. The incidence appears to be declining in overland travellers and expatriates. This may be related to the more liberal use of antibiotics for travellers' diarrhoea. The epidemics of tropical sprue in southern India also appear to be on the decline and this again may relate to improving water quality and sanitary conditions and to the widespread availability of antibiotics.

FURTHER READING

Baker, S.J. (1982). Idiopathic small-intestinal disease in the tropics. In *Critical reviews in tropical medicine*, Vol. 1, (ed. R.K. Chandra) pp. 197–245. Plenum, New York.

Banwell, J.G. and Gorbach, S.L. (1969). Tropical sprue. *Gut*, **10**, 328–33.

Besterman, H.S. *et al.* (1979). Gut hormones in tropical malabsorption. *British Medical Journal*, **ii**, 1252–5.

Bhat, P. *et al.* (1972). Bacterial flora of the gastrointestinal tract in Southern Indian control subjects and patients with tropical sprue. *Gastroenterology*, **62**, 11–21.

Booth, C.C. (1964). The first description of tropical sprue. *Gut*, **5**, 45–50.

Cook, G.C. (1978). Delayed small intestinal transit in tropical malabsorption. *British Medical Journal*, **ii**, 238–40.

Cook, G.C. (1980). *Tropical gastroenterology*, pp. 271–324. Oxford University Press.

Cook, G.C. (1984). Aetiology and pathogenesis of post-infective tropical malabsorption (tropical sprue). *Lancet*, **i**, 721–3.

Glynn, J. (1986) Tropical sprue—its aetiology and pathogenesis. *Journal of the Royal Society of Medicine*, **79**, 599–606.

Klipstein, F.A. (1981). *Tropical sprue in travellers and expatriates living abroad.* **Gastroenterology**, **80**, 590–600.

Klipstein, F.A. and Falaiye, J.M. (1969). Tropical sprue in expatriates from the tropics living in the continental United States. *Medicine*, **48**, 475–91.

Klipstein, F.A., Engert, R.F., and Short, A.B. (1978). Enterotoxigenicity of colonising coliform bacteria in tropical sprue and blind loop syndrome. *Lancet*, **ii**, 342–4.

Manson-Bahr, P. and Willoughby, H. (1930). Studies on sprue with special reference to treatment: based upon an analysis of 200 cases. *Quarterly Journal of Medicine*, **23**, 411–42.

Mathan, V.I. (1988). Tropical sprue in Southern India. *Transactions of the Royal Society for Tropical Medicine*, **82**, 10–14.

Mathan, V.I. and Baker, S.J. (1968). Epidemic tropical sprue and other epidemics of diarrhea in South Indian villages. *American Journal of Clinical Nutrition*, **21**, 1077–87.

Tomkins, A. (1981). Tropical malabsorption: recent concepts in pathogenesis and nutritional significance. *Clinical Science*, **60**, 131–7.

Tomkins, A. and Booth, C.C. (1985). Tropical Sprue. In *Disorders of the small intestine* (ed. C.C. Booth and G. Neale), pp. 311–32. Blackwell Scientific, Oxford.

Tomkins, A., Drasar, B.S., and James, W.P.T. (1975). Bacterial colonization of jejunal mucosa in acute tropical sprue. *Lancet*, **i**, 59–62.

14.10 Crohn's disease

D. P. JEWELL

Crohn's disease is a chronic inflammatory disease of the gastrointestinal tract, the cause of which remains unknown. It is characterized by a granulomatous inflammation affecting any part of the tract, frequently in discontinuity, and by the tendency to form fistulae.

History

The first clear description of the disease affecting the terminal ileum (regional ileitis) was given by Crohn, Ginzburg, and Oppenheimer in 1932. However, the disease certainly existed long before then and many of the early descriptions of ulcerative colitis would now be regarded as Crohn's disease. Dalziel, in 1913, described an inflammatory process of the ileum and colon consisting of ulceration, submucosal oedema, fibrosis, and mesenteric lymphadenopathy. He reported the presence of granulomata on microscopy but could find no evidence of tuberculosis. Similar cases were described in the 1920s by Moschowitz and Willensky.

Following the description by Crohn and his colleagues, it was clearly recognized that the colon could also be involved and, on occasions, it could be the sole site of the disease. The disease therefore became known as regional enteritis or, preferably, Crohn's disease. Colonic disease is often referred to as Crohn's disease of the colon, Crohn's colitis, or granulomatous colitis.

Epidemiology

Crohn's disease is well recognized in Europe, Scandinavia, North America, and Australia but is rarely seen in India, tropical Africa, and South America. This may be largely due to the difficulty of diagnosing Crohn's disease in areas where intestinal tuberculosis is common and to the problems of long-term follow-up. The disease is also said to be rare in Japan but its prevalence there appears to be increasing.

There has been a striking increase in the incidence and prevalence of Crohn's disease in Europe and Scandinavia since 1950 (Table 1). This is also shown by examining the annual discharge rates in England and

Table 1 *Incidence of Crohn's disease per 100 000 population*

Aberdeen	1955–61	1.7
	1964–66	3.3
	1967–69	4.5
	1970–72	4.3
	1973–75	2.6
Cardiff	1934–70	1.1
	1971–77	4.6
Malmö	1958–65	3.5
	1966–73	6.0
Uppsala	1956–61	1.7
	1962–67	3.1
	1968–73	5.0
Stockholm	1955–59	1.5
	1960–64	2.2
	1965–69	3.6
	1970–74	4.5
	1975–79	4.1

Wales. For Crohn's disease, the rate rose from 2.8 per 100 000 in 1958 to 7.2 per 100 000 of the population in 1971, whereas the rate for ulcerative colitis during the same period was unchanged at 10 to 12 per 100 000. Recent studies in Scotland and in Stockholm have suggested that the incidence has begun to decline.

The reasons for the changing patterns of incidence are not clear. Much of the increased incidence is due to an increased frequency of colonic disease and it might be argued that this represents diagnostic transfer from ulcerative colitis to Crohn's disease. The annual discharge rates for England and Wales, quoted above, make this explanation unlikely. Whether similar changes in frequency have occurred in North America is uncertain, although the data available suggest that the incidence has probably not altered. It is possible that the changing incidence may result from an infective or environmental factor.

Crohn's disease occurs in all age groups but it is rare in early childhood and most commonly affects young adults. There is no marked sex difference, and no association with social class or occupation. There may be an increased incidence amongst Ashkenazi Jews, especially in the United States.

Genetics

There is a definite familial incidence of the disease, reports varying from 6 to 15 per cent, and the affected members of a given family may have Crohn's disease or ulcerative colitis. There is no clear mode of inheritance and, until recently, there was no established association with HLA types, apart from those patients who also have ankylosing spondylitis, who usually have the HLA-B27 phenotype. However, recent studies reanalysing the HLA association using gene typing have suggested a weak link with the HLA-DR1–HLA-DQw5 haplotype. In monozygotic twins there is a concordance rate of about 65 per cent. Discordance for the disease pairs of identical twins suggests that environmental factors may also be operating but the extreme rarity of ulcerative colitis or Crohn's disease in both husband and wife makes it unlikely that environmental factors alone are responsible for the disease.

Aetiology

The cause of Crohn's disease is unknown but clearly involves an interplay between genetic and environmental factors. The latter include smoking and intestinal luminal factors. There is a relative risk of 4 to 6 for Crohn's disease in smokers compared with non-smokers, which is in striking contrast to the reverse association seen in ulcerative colitis. Whether smoking predisposes to Crohn's disease by altering mucosal blood flow, synthesis of mucus, or by an effect on endothelial cells is

unknown. The role of luminal factors is suggested by the tendency of Crohn's colitis to heal if the colon is rendered non-functional by an ileostomy and by the effectiveness of an elemental diet for the treatment of active disease. Other mechanisms may contribute to the pathogenesis and include diet, infective agents, ischaemia, and immune mechanisms.

DIET

Several investigators have reported that patients with Crohn's disease have a higher intake of refined sugar than a control population or a matched group of patients with ulcerative colitis. In addition, patients with Crohn's disease may also have a reduced intake of fibre, especially that derived from fruit and vegetables. However, the significance of these changes is unclear, especially as a controlled trial was unable to show that a low-sugar, high-fibre diet had any effect on the cause of the disease over a 2-year period. Claims have been made that many patients will benefit from dietary exclusion determined by a period on an elimination diet followed by challenge with individual foods. This might suggest a role for dietary factors but the long-term benefit of dietary exclusion is by no means proven. Elemental diets consisting of glucose and amino acids have been shown to have equal efficacy to prednisolone for treating active Crohn's disease but whether this effect is mediated by influencing bacterial populations, by removing dietary antigens, or by some other mechanism is unknown.

INFECTIVE AGENTS

Viruses, cell-wall deficient bacteria, and atypical mycobacteria have been claimed to be the cause of Crohn's disease. Most of these claims have been discredited but there is current interest in the role of *Mycobacterium paratuberculosis* and measles virus.

Mycobacterium paratuberculosis is the organism that causes Johne's disease in cattle and other farm animals. This resembles Crohn's disease in so far as it is a granulomatous inflammatory disorder of the intestine. Over the last 10 years, an atypical mycobacterium has been isolated from intestinal tissue of a few patients with Crohn's disease and most of the isolated organisms have been shown to be identical to *M. paratuberculosis* using DNA analysis. The organism is very slow growing and it has taken 1 to 2 years of culture in order to demonstrate it. The possibility that such an organism might be involved in the aetiology of the disease was strengthened by the detection of *M. paratuberculosis* DNA in intestinal tissue in about two-thirds of patients using a specific probe and amplification by the polymerase chain reaction. However, specific DNA for the organism was also detected in 10 per cent of control tissue and other investigators have been unable to detect specific DNA in any patient with Crohn's disease. Antituberculous therapy has not proved effective so far. Thus, it is still very uncertain whether *M. paratuberculosis* is an aetiological agent, whether it is responsible for causing disease in all or just a subgroup of patients, whether some of the findings are laboratory artefacts, or whether it is a secondary invader of inflamed tissue.

Similar doubts are expressed for the role of measles virus which, using *in situ* hybridization, has been detected in Crohn's disease tissue but not in control tissues.

ISCHAEMIA

Marked abnormalities of mucosal arterioles have been detected in resected specimens of intestine affected by Crohn's disease by making resin casts of the arterial tree. Many of the small vessels have been shown to be thrombosed, but in a rather patchy distribution, suggesting that much of the inflammation may rise from multifocal infarction. However, as many cytokines and inflammatory mediators released during an immunological or inflammatory response damage endothelium, it is not possible to be sure whether these vascular changes represent a primary abnormality or are merely secondary to the inflammation. It seems more likely that they occur as a consequence of the inflammation but, nevertheless, they may still contribute to the pathogenesis of chronic inflammation.

IMMUNE MECHANISMS

Patients with Crohn's disease usually have normal serum concentrations of immunoglobulins and complement components, although raised concentration may occur in association with active disease. Neutrophil and monocyte functions, *in vitro*, show no defect although inhibitors of cell motility are often present in the serum of patients with active disease. The absolute number of peripheral blood T lymphocytes may be reduced but the proportion of phenotypic subsets (CD4, CD8) remains unchanged.

Within the inflamed tissue, there is a marked increase of plasma cells, lymphocytes, macrophages, and neutrophils. As with ulcerative colitis, the increased immunoglobulin production is predominantly of the IgG isotype but, in Crohn's disease, there is a greater proportional increase in the IgG2 subclass as compared with the IgG1 or IgG3 subclasses. However, antibodies to bacterial antigens and autoantibodies to epithelial and neutrophil antigens are much less common than they are in patients with ulcerative colitis.

T cells and macrophages in the lamina propria are activated, as shown by the increased expression of activation markers but also, in the case of macrophages, by functional assays. The possibility that chronic inflammation results because of a defect in immunoregulation has been explored in a variety of assays but no consistent defect has been described. However, recent evidence suggests that there may be an impaired facility to induce antigen-specific suppressor cells; if this is confirmed, it might explain some of the immunological overactivity that is characteristic of the disease. Cellular activation results in the release of cytokines and inflammatory mediators, which will influence the nature of the inflammatory response. The possibility that the course of the disease, whether fibrosing or fistulating, may be determined by the cytokine profile is an attractive but unproven hypothesis.

Pathology

Crohn's disease may occur anywhere in the gastrointestinal tract, although the most common pattern is an ileocolitis. The disease is often discontinuous, giving rise to the so-called skip lesions. Isolated involvement of the mouth, oesophagus, stomach, and anus is recognized but such cases are extremely rare. Macroscopically the bowel is thickened and frequently stenosed. The serosal surface may be inflamed and the mesentery becomes oedematous. The regional mesenteric nodes are usually enlarged. The earliest macroscopic lesion on the mucosal surface is an aphthoid ulcer—a small, superficial lesion often surrounded by hyperaemia. In areas of more severe disease, deep, fissuring ulcers occur in the oedematous and inflamed mucosa, giving rise to a cobblestone pattern. Long, serpiginous ulcers are a further characteristic feature. Strictures occur as a result of submucosal fibrosis and, because of serosal inflammation, the affected intestine may become adherent to adjacent loops of intestine or other structures (e.g. bladder or vaginal vault) with the subsequent formation of fistulae.

Histologically, the inflammation is transmural and consists principally of lymphocytes, histiocytes (tissue macrophages), and plasma cells. Granulomas are found in only 65 per cent of patients and they occur more commonly the more distal the disease; that is, they are present in most cases with rectal disease but are much less common in ileal disease. The granulomas appear to be in the walls of either blood vessels or lymphatics. The mucosal architecture is well preserved despite heavy inflammation and, in the colon, goblet cells are usually present even though the glands are being infiltrated with inflammatory cells. Fissures, penetrating into the submucosa and lined with histiocytic cells, are frequently present.

Quantitative histological and enzyme studies have suggested that the whole of the gastrointestinal tract is abnormal in patients with Crohn's disease even though only one segment may be overtly involved at any one time.

Immunofluorescent and immunoperoxidase studies have shown a large increase in IgG- and IgM-containing cells with a smaller rise in IgA-containing cells. Even in quiescent disease, the IgG- and IgM-containing cells appear to be increased compared with the normal intestine.

Clinical features

The manifestations of Crohn's disease are protean and are partly determined by the anatomical location of the disease. The majority of patients complain of diarrhoea (70 to 90 per cent), abdominal pain (45 to 66 per cent) and weight loss (65 to 75 per cent). Fever is also common (30 to 49 per cent). Obstructive symptoms (colic, vomiting) are much more commonly associated with ileal disease than colonic Crohn's disease. Colonic disease causes rectal bleeding more commonly than ileal disease but even so it is present in only about 50 per cent of patients with Crohn's colitis. Colonic disease is also associated with perianal disease (in about one-third of patients) and with extraintestinal manifestations, which are uncommonly seen when the disease is confined to the ileum. Symptoms of anaemia are common and usually occur as a result of iron deficiency from intestinal blood loss or, less frequently, from vitamin B_{12} or folate deficiency. Other features of malabsorption are infrequent but in patients with extensive small-bowel disease, symptoms and signs of osteomalacia may occur and there may be a bleeding tendency secondary to vitamin K malabsorption. Nutritional deficiencies may also be present, for example deficiencies of magnesium, zinc, ascorbic acid, and the B vitamins, but these are uncommon and are usually due to inadequate intake.

A few patients present with the clinical features of acute appendicitis but at operation they are found to have an acute terminal ileitis. Only a minority of these prove to be due to Crohn's disease. Diagnostic difficulties may also occur when the disease presents without gastrointestinal symptoms. These include patients presenting with fever, weight loss, and anaemia without diarrhoea or abdominal pain, and those with ileocaecal disease presenting with urinary frequency and dysuria due to ureteric involvement.

Physical examination may be normal but many patients will show evidence of anaemia. Glossitis and aphthous ulcers in the mouth, beaking or frank clubbing of the nails, evidence of weight loss, and a tachycardia are common features. Abdominal examination usually reveals tenderness over the affected bowel, which can often be felt to be thickened. An abdominal mass is frequently palpable when small-intestinal disease is present. Anal examination often shows the presence of fleshy skin tags, which have a characteristic violaceous hue. Anal fissures, perianal fistulae, and abscesses are particularly associated with colonic disease.

The extraintestinal manifestations of Crohn's disease are similar to those of ulcerative colitis. Table 2 lists those that are most frequently seen.

Complications

Patients with Crohn's disease can develop an acute dilatation of the bowel (defined as a colonic diameter of 5.5 cm or more on a plain radiograph), perforation, or massive haemorrhage especially when the disease involves the colon. These complications, however, occur less frequently than they do in ulcerative colitis. The more usual complications are intestinal obstruction due to strictures in the small or large intestine and fistulae. The latter may occur between other parts of the gastrointestinal tract (e.g. gastrocolic, enterocolic) or between the affected loop of intestine and the bladder or vagina. Pneumaturia, the passage of faeces in the urine or a faecal vaginal discharge are cardinal features of the latter forms of fistula formation. The gross malabsorption that occurs with a gastrocolic or ileocolic fistulae is largely due to bac-

Table 2 *Extraintestinal manifestations of Crohn's disease*

	Frequency (%)	Comment
Related to disease activity		
Aphthous ulceration	20	
Erythema nodosum	5–10	
Pyoderma gangrenosum	0.5	
Acute arthropathy	6–12	Large joints affected; transient, non-destructive
Eye complications:	3–10	
Conjunctivitis		
Episcleritis		
Uveitis		
Unrelated to disease activity		
Sacroiliitis	15–18	Usually asymptomatic; may be present in up to 50 per cent using isotope scanning; unrelated to HLA-B27.
Ankylosing spondylitis	2–6	75 per cent of patients have the HLA-B27 phenotype
Liver disease:	5–6	
Primary sclerosing cholangitis		Rare and poorly documented in Crohn's disease
Gallstones	Very common	Due to malabsorption of bile salts from ileum
Chronic active hepatitis	2–3	
Cirrhosis	2–3	
Fatty change	6	Very common in ill patients requiring surgery
Amyloid, granulomas	Rare	

terial overgrowth of the small intestine. External fistulae to the skin also occur, but this is usually secondary to surgical intervention. Crohn's disease affecting the terminal ileum or the right side of the colon may involve the right ureter, giving rise to frequency with a sterile pyuria, a frank urinary tract infection, or a ureteric stricture with subsequent hydronephrosis. Left-sided disease may occasionally involve the left ureter but this is very uncommon. Hyperoxaluria and oxalate stones may be complications of ileal disease associated with steatorrhoea. The mechanism is currently thought to be due to binding of calcium to unabsorbed fat, leaving the oxalate free to be absorbed from the colon.

Carcinoma of the colon may complicate Crohn's colitis. The incidence is about 3 to 5 per cent, a frequency similar to that of colonic carcinoma associated with ulcerative colitis. The risk factors are not yet established, however, although histological dysplasia has been noted in some cases of Crohn's disease. Small-bowel carcinomas have been reported in association with ileal Crohn's disease.

Amyloid is another complication of Crohn's disease; it may occur within the bowel or systemically, for example in liver, spleen, and kidney. If renal function is deteriorating, the affected bowel should be resected as the amyloid may then regress with concomitant improvement in renal function.

Radiological appearances

A plain radiograph of the abdomen should always be obtained in patients with severe disease, together with decubitus films. These are often normal but may show evidence of intestinal obstruction or suggest an inflammatory mass in the right iliac fossa. In acute Crohn's colitis, evidence of mucosal oedema and ulceration may be clearly seen on the plain films. This appearance could obviate the need for barium studies, which should, if possible, be avoided in the presence of severe, active disease. The plain film can also provide evidence of sacroiliitis or ankylosing spondylitis.

Examination of the oesophagus, stomach, and duodenum is best done endoscopically because the radiological appearances are often non-specific and biopsies are required for histological confirmation. The small intestine may be examined with a standard barium meal and follow through, but more more information is obtained with the barium infusion technique (small-bowel enema, enteroclysis). After colonic preparation, a tube is passed until the tip lies just beyond the ligament of Treitz and a dilute barium suspension is infused (800–1200 ml). The earliest lesions are thickening of valvulae coniventes and small, discrete aphthoid ulcers. In more severe disease, cobblestoning, fissure ulcers, and thickening of the wall occur (Fig. 1). Longitudinal ulcers may also occur but these are uncommon. Areas of stenosis and dilatation may be present, and sinus tracts and fistulae may be demonstrated. Asymmetry of the bowel is often present, although this may be an unreliable sign. The abnormal segment of the intestine is usually well demarcated from the normal bowel.

Radiological examination of the colon is made with a double-contrast barium enema after a thorough but gentle preparation. Characteristically there is rectal sparing but the appearances of Crohn's colitis are otherwise similar to those described for the small intestine (Fig. 2). Table 3 lists the main features that differentiate the radiological appearances of Crohn's colitis from ulcerative colitis. The barium enema is a good means of showing internal fistulae and fistulae to other organs.

If fistulae to the surface are present, sinograms should be taken to delineate the anatomy.

Endoscopy

Sigmoidoscopy and rectal biopsy should be done in all patients. The rectal mucosa is frequently normal but may show a granular proctitis and occasionally the typical appearances of Crohn's disease. Nevertheless, histological examination of a rectal biopsy specimen from a macroscopically normal rectum often shows an inflammatory infiltrate, which is often focal and may contain granulomas. The indications for colonoscopy are: (i) to examine the colon and obtain biopsies in suspected cases in whom the barium enema is normal or equivocal; (ii) to obtain biopsies from strictures; (iii) to obtain biopsies when the differential diagnosis is in doubt; and (iv) to assess activity and extent of disease in symptomatic patients when there is little clinical evidence of activity. A further advantage of colonoscopy is that biopsies can often be obtained from the terminal ileum.

Fig. 1 Small bowel enema demonstrating Crohn's disease of the terminal ileum with fissure ulcers, ileocaecal fistulae, and partial obstruction. (By courtesy of Dr D.J. Nolan.)

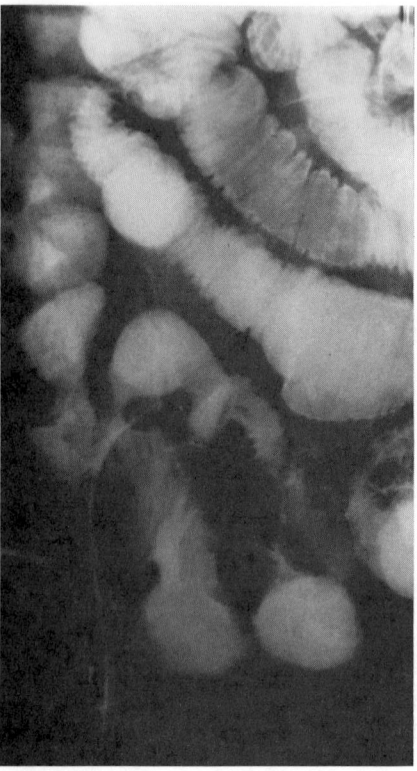

Fig. 2 Barium enema showing Crohn's disease of the colon and terminal ileum. Distal sigmoid, rectum, and a segment of ascending colon are normal. The diseased segments show loss of haustration, shortening, and fissure ulcers. (By courtesy of Dr D.J. Nolan.)

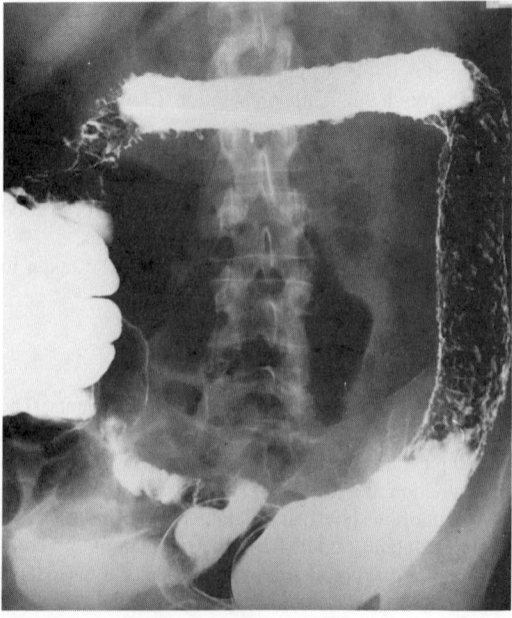

Endoscopically the earliest lesion of Crohn's disease is a small aphthoid ulcer surrounded by normal mucosa with a normal vascular pattern. This contrasts with the erythema and loss of vascular pattern seen in ulcerative colitis. In more severe disease the mucosa becomes oedematous and is penetrated by fissuring ulcers to give a cobblestone appearance. The ulcers are often linear and may eventually become confluent. A diffusely inflamed, granular, friable, and dark-red mucosa is more typical of ulcerative colitis, although discrete ulceration may occur in severe cases. Pseudopolyps and mucosal bridges occur in both diseases.

Multiple biopsies should be taken, even from apparently normal areas of mucosa, because granulomas may be present, which allows a precise diagnosis to be made.

Upper gastrointestinal endoscopy is not routinely required in these patients and is only indicated in the presence of appropriate symptoms or if abnormalities are noted on a barium meal. Although Crohn's disease of the stomach or duodenum may occur as an isolated phenomenon, most cases are associated with disease elsewhere in the gastrointestinal tract. Deep, longitudinal ulcers may occur in the stomach together with rugal hypertrophy and a cobblestone appearance. In the duodenum the major differential diagnosis is duodenal ulcer but there is usually a 'cobblestone' mucosa surrounding the frank ulceration. Biopsies are usually helpful, although granulomas are found infrequently.

Examination of the small intestine is now possible using a sonde-type enteroscope (see Chapter 14.3.1). This is an expensive procedure that takes many hours and, for these reasons, it is unlikely to become widely available. Nevertheless, it may be helpful for patients in whom the diagnosis is suspected but in whom the small-bowel enema is not diagnostic.

Laboratory data

Anaemia is common and is often due to mixed deficiencies. Iron deficiency from intestinal blood loss is the most common cause but serum folate and vitamin B_{12} concentrations may also be low. The blood film and mean corpuscular volume may therefore show microcytosis or macrocytosis. Serum ferritin is the best indicator of iron stores in those patients with chronic disease. A neutrophil leucocytosis is usually, but not invariably, associated with active disease and there may also be a thrombocytosis. The total lymphocyte count and the absolute number of circulating T lymphocytes may be reduced.

Hypokalaemia is associated with severe diarrhoea and the plasma urea concentration is often low, reflecting a poor dietary intake of nitrogen. Serum albumin is reduced in the presence of active disease, largely due to down-regulation of albumin synthesis by cytokines such as interleukin (IL)-1, tumour necrosis factor, and IL-6 but studies with ^{51}Cr-labelled albumin often demonstrate a protein-losing enteropathy. Serum immunoglobulins are normal or mildly elevated and there may be a rise in the α_2-globulins. A low serum calcium, when corrected for albumin, is unusual unless there is extensive small-bowel disease, and a low urinary calcium is more likely to reflect a poor diet rather than osteomalacia. Liver function tests are frequently abnormal, usually consisting of mild elevations of the aspartate transaminase and alkaline phosphatase. Persistence of abnormal liver tests suggests associated liver disease and should be investigated by liver biopsy and visualization of the biliary tree. Patients with extensive ileal disease or with ileal stricture may have increased faecal fat excretion. This is usually secondary to bacterial overgrowth rather than loss of absorptive surface, and is compounded by the low circulating pool and increased excretion of bile salts, which is often present in patients with long-standing ileal disease. It is important not to miss magnesium, zinc, and selenium deficiencies, which are occasionally present.

Diagnosis

This may be delayed for several years. Intermittent abdominal symptoms and diarrhoea without systemic symptoms are often labelled as an irri-

Table 3 *Differential diagnosis of Crohn's disease and ulcerative colitis*

	Crohn's disease	Ulcerative colitis
Clinical features		
Bloody diarrhoea	Less common	Common
Abdominal mass	Common	Rare
Perianal disease	Common	Less common
Malabsorption	Frequent (ileal disease)	Never
Radiological features		
Rectal involvement	Frequently spared	Invariable
Distribution	Segmental, discontinuous	Continuous
Mucosa	Cobblestones, fissure ulcers	Fine ulceration 'Double contour'
Strictures	Common	Rare
Fistulae	Frequent	Rare
Histological features		
Distribution	Transmural	Mucosal
Cellular infiltrate	Lymphocytes, plasma cells, macrophages	Polymorphs, plasma cells, eosinophils
Glands	Gland preservation	Mucus depletion, gland destruction, crypt abscesses
Special features	Aphthoid ulcers, granulomata, histiocyte-lined fissures	None

table bowel syndrome. Weight loss, fever, and anaemia without gastrointestinal symptoms are another source of misdiagnosis. The diagnosis of Crohn's disease in children may be considerably delayed when it presents as failure to thrive or delayed puberty but without gastrointestinal symptoms.

Even when the clinical diagnosis seems sound, all patients must have: (i) stool examination to exclude pathogens; (ii) sigmoidoscopy and rectal biopsy—characteristic features (e.g. granuloma) may often be present in the biopsy specimen even when the mucosa is macroscopically normal; (iii) radiographs of the small and large intestine to confirm the diagnosis and establish the extent of the disease; and (iv) colonoscopy with multiple biopsies is indicated where the above investigations are equivocal or normal and there are strong clinical reasons for suspecting Crohn's disease. Colonoscopy should also be done if the differential diagnosis is in doubt or if strictures are present.

Differential diagnosis

Few patients with an acute ileitis and a clinical picture of acute appendicitis subsequently develop Crohn's disease. Serological examination helps to diagnose those cases caused by Yersinia; the aetiology of the remainder is unknown. The main differential diagnosis of ileal Crohn's disease is tuberculosis, especially when the disease occurs in patients from areas where intestinal tuberculosis is common. Laparoscopy may be helpful if serosal tubercles are present, as they can be biopsied and cultured. Stool culture and circulating antibodies to mycobacteria are unhelpful. Colonoscopy with multiple biopsy specimens may be helpful. If genuine doubt exists, corticosteroid therapy for Crohn's disease must be covered with antituberculous therapy. Other differential diagnoses include abdominal lymphoma, α-chain disease, actinomycosis, amyloid, Behçet's disease, and carcinoma of the small bowel.

The major differential diagnosis of Crohn's colitis is ulcerative colitis (Table 3). Crohn's disease should also be considered in patients presenting with proctitis, as 30 per cent of patients with ileal Crohn's disease may have a proctitis and may present in this way. When a segmental colitis occurs, ischaemia, tuberculosis, and lymphoma have to be excluded. Young adults may present with an acute segmental colitis, which is self-limiting. The cause is unknown, although, in women, oral contraceptives have been implicated. Crohn's disease can be overlooked on the barium enema when it occurs in association with severe diverticular disease.

As indicated above, Crohn's disease may have to be considered in the differential diagnosis of a fever with weight loss, malabsorption, and delayed development.

Assessment of activity

There is no satisfactory method of assessing activity of the disease and this poses a major clinical problem. Symptoms such as fever or continuing weight loss are obvious indicators but severe disease can be present in the absence of any major symptom. Laboratory evidence of activity includes a reduced serum albumin, a rise in acute-phase reactants (C-reactive protein, orosomucoid) and in the ESR. Recently, a number of activity indices have been developed in order to standardize assessment for the purpose of multicentre studies, two examples being the American Crohn's disease activity index and the Dutch activity index. However, they are mostly too complex for normal clinical use. Furthermore, they tend to measure different aspects of disease activity. At present it is worth remembering that disease activity can be assessed by the clinical picture (symptoms and signs), morphologically (e.g. by radiography or endoscopy), and by laboratory indices. Another technique for the assessment of activity is the use of indium-labelled neutrophils. The labelled cells preferentially migrate to inflamed mucosa and the increased uptake of isotope can be detected using a gamma-camera (Fig. 3). Faecal excretion of the labelled cells can also be quantified and this has shown good correlation with the Crohn's disease activity index and albumin loss.

Labelling neutrophils with technetium-99 using hexamethyl propylene amine oxime (HMPAO) as a chelator is gradually replacing indium because it is easier, quicker, and less expensive. It appears to provide similar sensitivity and specificity but it cannot be used to assess faecal excretion of neutrophils.

Management

The management of Crohn's disease involves a team approach between physician and surgeon and includes nutritional support, medical therapy, and surgical treatment.

NUTRITIONAL SUPPORT

For the majority of patients, a well-balanced diet should be advised. A low-residue diet should be used for patients with strictures and a low-fat diet may be helpful for those with a steatorrhoea. Some centres claim good long-term results with elimination diets but the value of this approach for the generality of patients is far from proven. A lactose-free diet is obviously indicated for those with hypolactasia.

Iron and vitamin B_{12} deficiencies are common and need to be excluded. In patients with chronic active disease, the serum iron, binding capacity, and ferritin may all be low, making it difficult to know whether the anaemia is due to iron deficiency or to chronic inflammation. However, if the serum iron is less than 10 per cent of the iron-binding capacity it is reasonable to diagnose iron deficiency and treat accordingly. Many patients are intolerant of oral iron and for these a total-dose intravenous infusion is the best form of treatment. Patients with extensive small-intestinal disease may develop deficiencies of the fat-soluble vitamins (A, D, E, K). Deficiencies of folic acid and B vitamins may also occur because of poor dietary intake. Parenteral nutrition is often indicated for seriously ill patients who are being prepared for surgery or who have a short bowel syndrome.

DRUG THERAPY

In general, Crohn's disease is only treated if it is causing symptoms; there is no indication for treatment in asymptomatic patients. Active disease can usually be controlled with corticosteroids, the dose and route depending on the severity of the disease. Severe disease requires admission to hospital and treatment with intravenous prednisolone (60–80 mg daily) or hydrocortisone (400 mg daily), together with fluids and electrolytes. Most patients settle within 5 to 7 days and can then be changed to oral prednisolone (e.g. 40 mg daily). Patients with less severe disease can be treated with 20 to 40 mg prednisolone daily. There is no defined duration of corticosteroid therapy but most patients will have made a good symptomatic response by 4 to 6 weeks; the dose can then be reduced over the next 3 to 6 weeks and finally stopped.

The role of 5-aminosalicylic acid-containing drugs is not nearly so well defined for Crohn's disease as it is for ulcerative colitis. Sulpha-

Fig. 3 An Indium-111 labelled neutrophil scan in a patient with active Crohn's disease. Active inflammation in distal ileal loops is well shown (arrow).

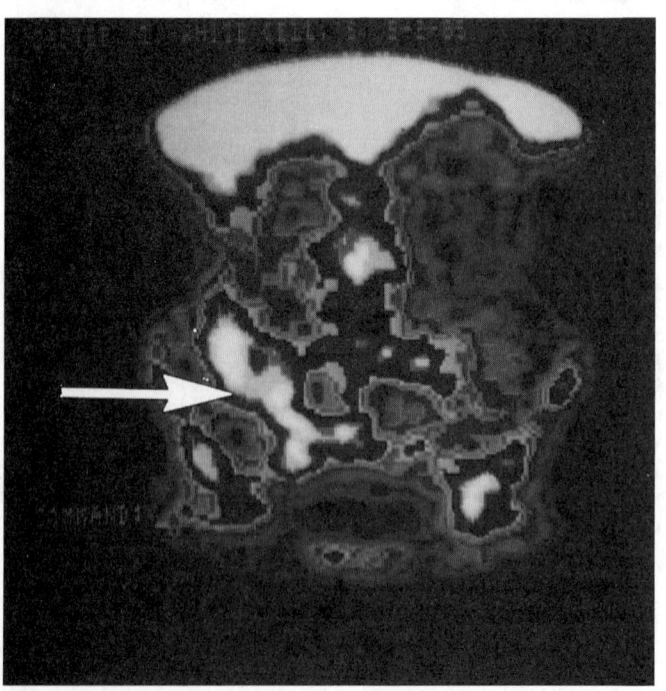

salazine has never been shown to be of value as maintenance therapy but it may have some beneficial effect on mildly active disease, especially if the disease affects the colon. Of the newer salicylate drugs, high-dose Pentasa (4 g daily) may be effective for active disease, and Claversal and Pentasa may have some benefits as maintenance treatment in order to prolong remission. However, these findings require confirmation from other trials before the efficacy of these new mesalazine formulations can be accepted. Furthermore, not all the formulations are universally available. Details of the new salicylate drugs are given in Chapter 14.11.

For patients who continually relapse when steroids are withdrawn or when the prednisolone dose falls below 10 to 15 mg daily, immunosuppressive therapy should be considered. Azathioprine or 6-mercaptopurine will benefit a proportion of such patients at a dose of 2.0 to 2.5 mg/kg but there is no way of predicting which patients will respond. These drugs usually take several weeks to exert their effects and, if a patient does respond, it is worthwhile continuing therapy for 1 to 2 years. The blood count should be checked at regular intervals (every 4 to 8 weeks) but bone marrow suppression is uncommon at those dosages. Some patients complain of nausea or myalgic symptoms, which usually necessitate stopping the drug. Pancreatitis is a rare complication and although there is a theoretical risk of malignancy, especially lymphoma, this has not been a problem with the regimen of treatment as described. Oral cyclosporin (5 mg/kg) has also been used in these patients with chronic active disease. Anecdotal experience was promising but the controlled trials have given very conflicting results. At present, cyclosporin should not be used until a full evaluation is available.

Antibiotics such as metronidazole, ciprofloxacin and Augmentin (ampicillin with clavulanic acid) are required for patients with small-intestinal bacterial overgrowth, perianal sepsis, and abscesses associated with fistulae. Whether they also have a direct effect on the inflammatory response is less certain. Certainly metronidazole has been shown to be more effective than placebo but of similar efficacy to sulphasalazine for the treatment of active disease but whether this effect is mediated by an effect on the bacterial population or by some other means is unknown.

Elemental diets have been repeatedly shown to be as effective as prednisolone in controlling active Crohn's disease but the major problem is one of compliance. Some patients intubate themselves at night with a fine-bore nasogastric tube and feed themselves during sleep. Polymeric diets may be as effective as elemental diets and are certainly more palatable. If an individual patient responds well and is willing to carry on with the diet, it should be continued until symptoms have settled and the laboratory indicators of inflammation have returned to normal. Experience then differs as to the course of the disease once normal food is introduced. Some data suggest that relapse occurs more rapidly than if remission has been achieved by the use of corticosteroids.

SURGERY

The majority of patients (70 to 80 per cent) will require at least one operation during the course of their disease. Indications for surgery include failure to respond to medical therapy, strictures causing mechanical obstruction, fistulae, and other complications such as abscess and perforation.

If surgery is required, the following principles apply. Resection should be limited to removing the most severely affected segment and an end-to-end anastomosis should be made, even if there is some inflammation in the tissue being anastomosed. Wide resections have not been shown to diminish the subsequent recurrence rate. Bypass procedures (e.g. ileotransverse colostomy) should not be done. If surgery is for fistulae, nutrition must be corrected, infection controlled, and active disease controlled with steroids before the operation. The anatomy of the fistulae must also be determined by sinograms or by computerized tomographic scans or magnetic resonance imaging. The fistula is excised together with the segment of affected intestine and the subsequent anastomosis is usually best protected with a temporary ileostomy. For colonic disease, the choice is a conservative operation of a split ileostomy or a proctocolectomy with terminal ileostomy. Colectomy with ileorectal anastomosis is associated with a high recurrence rate. Defunctioning the colonic disease with an ileostomy often allows the disease to settle and the patient's nutritional state to be restored. In Oxford, our practice is to reconnect after 12 to 18 months and the majority of patients then remain well. However, other clinicians claim a rapid relapse following restoration of continuity and will only use a split ileostomy as a means of getting patients fit for more radical surgery.

Some patients with small-intestinal disease present with multiple short strictures. Once active disease is controlled with corticosteroids, the strictures should be dealt with by stricturoplasty rather than by multiple resections. This gives good symptomatic relief and it is unusual for further stricturing to occur at sites of previous stricturoplasties. This conservative approach has greatly reduced the need for repeated resections and has therefore minimized the chances of a short bowel syndrome.

MANAGEMENT DURING PREGNANCY

Crohn's disease should be treated in the pregnant woman along the lines outlined above. Overall, the outcome of the pregnancy is not influenced by the disease except in very severe cases where there may be an increased risk of abortion. Corticosteroids and sulphasalazine are safe to use and have not been associated with fetal abnormalities. Likewise, azathioprine has not been clearly demonstrated to be teratogenic and can be used if there is sufficient clinical indication.

MANAGEMENT IN CHILDREN

There is no essential difference in the principles of management from those described for adults, although dosages may need to be reduced. Alternate-day steroids should be employed, especially if long-term treatment seems likely. Excellent but uncontrolled results have been reported in adolescents using maintenance corticosteroids, as an alternate-day regimen, which allowed puberty and growth to develop normally. One of the major effects of the disease in children is growth retardation. Corticosteroid therapy often promotes a growth spurt but great emphasis should be paid to the child's nutrition. Dietary intake should be assessed and supplemented to provide a high-calorie, high-nitrogen intake.

Course and prognosis

Patients are never cured of Crohn's disease and they are subject to relapses of their disease and to recurrence following surgical resection.

The majority of patients (70 to 80 per cent) will receive surgical treatment at some point during the course of their illness. After a resection, the disease recurs in about 30 per cent of patients during the subsequent 5 years and in 50 per cent of patients during the subsequent 10 years; of these, half will require further surgery. Although there is still some controversy, the balance of evidence suggests that the risk of requiring second or third operations is no greater than the risk of requiring the initial operation. Patients with Crohn's colitis who have proctocolectomy appear to have a lower risk of recurrence than those who have an ileal or ileocolic resection.

Recent endoscopic visualization of the neoterminal ileum has shown that the recurrence rates, when assessed by endoscopic appearance, are even higher than the rates quoted above, which are based on symptoms. For patients who have had an ileal or ileocolic resection, 70 to 80 per cent of them will show endoscopic lesions just proximal to the anastomosis within the first postoperative year. The more severe lesions, such as aphthoid ulcers, predict a high chance of symptomatic recurrence. Mesalazine has been shown to have no influence on the endoscopic recurrence rate and it remains to be seen whether steroid compounds with low systemic bioavailability (e.g. budesonide) will be effective in this context without inducing systemic side-effects.

The overall mortality of Crohn's disease varies from 10 to 15 per cent in different studies. Some of these reports have suggested a worse prognosis for women than for men, and for patients over the age of 50 years, although this was mainly associated with higher operative mortality. Overall, age, and sex probably have little influence on the outcome of the disease. The Oxford experience has suggested that mortality is not appreciably increased during the first 5 years of the disease but then becomes progressively greater during subsequent follow-up. In contrast, however, data from Birmingham suggest that the highest mortality occurs in young people during the early stages of the disease.

In general, the majority of patients with Crohn's disease will have a good prognosis with a mortality of only about twice that expected. Considerable morbidity can be expected but this will be intermittent and the overall quality of life should be good.

REFERENCES

Allan, R.N., Keighley, M.R.B., Alexander-Williams, J., and Hawkins, C. (1990). *Inflammatory bowel disease*, (2nd edn). Churchill Livingstone, Edinburgh.
Kirsner, J.B. and Shorter, R.G. (1988) *Inflammatory bowel disease*, (3rd edn). Lea and Febiger, New York.
Ginsberg, A. (ed.) (1989). *Management of inflammatory bowel disease, Gastroenterology Clinics of North America*, **Vol. 18, No 1.** Saunders, Philadelphia.

14.11 Ulcerative colitis

D. P. JEWELL

Ulcerative colitis is a chronic inflammatory disease of the colon of unknown cause. It always affects the rectum and extends proximally to involve a variable extent of the colon. It is characterized by a relapsing and remitting course.

The disease was first described in 1859 by Samual Wilks, a physician at Guy's Hospital, who recognized that 'simple, idiopathic colitis' could be distinguished from other forms of colitis, mainly bacterial dysentery. It took many years for the concept to be accepted but, finally, in 1931, Sir Arthur Hurst was able to give a complete description of the disease

including the sigmoidoscopic appearances. Nevertheless, he still considered the disease to be primarily infective, even though its chronic nature might be induced secondarily by other factors.

Epidemiology

Ulcerative colitis is a worldwide disease, although it may be difficult to diagnose in areas where infective colitis is prevalent. Accurate figures for incidence and prevalence are not universally available but the disease

Table 1 *Incidence of ulcerative colitis*

	Period of study	Incidence (per 10^5)
USA		
Minnesota	1935–64	7.2
Baltimore	1960–63	4.6
UK		
Oxford	1951–60	6.5
Wales	1968–77	7.2
Aberdeen	1967–76	11.3
Denmark		
Copenhagen	1962–78	8.1
	1981–88	9.5
Holland		
Leiden	1979–83	6.8
Sweden		
Stockholm County	1975–79	4.3
Israel		
Tel-Aviv	1961–70	3.6

is now recognized in most countries. Table 1 lists data for the high-incidence areas and also shows that there have been no trends to suggest the disease is becoming more common, which is in contrast to Crohn's disease. The low-incidence areas include Eastern Europe, Asia, Japan, and South America where the incidence rates are at least 10-fold less.

The age of onset peaks between 20 and 40 years but the disease may present at all ages from the first few months of life to the 80s. Some series show a secondary peak of onset in the 60 to 70-year-olds but this has not been a universal finding. Earlier series suggested a predominance of the disease in women but, more recently, there has been little difference between the sexes.

Both in the United States and Cape Town, Jews are more prone to ulcerative colitis than non-Jews by a factor of three to four. Within Israel, Ashkenazi Jews have a higher incidence than Sephardim but it is still less than the incidence in Jews in the United States or, indeed, than the European incidence. This suggests that environmental factors may be involved in addition to genetic factors. However, the differences in incidence between urban as opposed to rural communities or between different socio-economic groups have been slight and inconstant.

Genetics

The familial incidence of ulcerative colitis has long been recognized, with 10 to 20 per cent of patients likely to have at least one other family member affected either with ulcerative colitis or with Crohn's disease. Most of the familial association is within first-degree relatives, but there is controversy about the precise relation, with a preponderance of parent–sibling combinations being found in the United States, whereas in the United Kingdom the disease is more commonly shared by siblings.

A study of twin pairs in Sweden showed that of 16 pairs of monozygotic twins in whom one member had ulcerative colitis, only one pair was concordant for the disease whereas all 20 dizygotic twins were discordant. This gave a proband concordance rate of 6.3 per cent, which is very much lower than 58.3 per cent for Crohn's disease.

This low concordance rate might suggest that familial clustering reflects environmental influence rather than inherited genetic susceptibility. However, the incidence of ulcerative colitis in spouses of probands is extremely low, although, of course, that does not exclude environmental factors operating early in life.

Certainly it has been difficult to describe the genetic nature of the disease in terms of association with candidate genes. No consistent association with immunoglobulin (G_m) or Class III genes has been found. Furthermore, no association has been found with HLA class I or class II genes except for a weak association with *HLA-DR5* in Japan. However, recent gene-typing studies reported from California suggest that

40 per cent or so of patients with ulcerative colitis carry the *HLA-DR2* gene compared with only 20 per cent of non-colitics. It is also possible that the presence of an antineutrophil cytoplasmic antibody (**ANCA**) in serum might be a genetic marker, as the majority of patients with this antibody were HLA-DR2 positive and there was a high prevalence of the antibody in first-degree relatives. However, the association between ANCA and HLA type of family members has been disputed by other investigators.

Aetiology

The cause of the disease remains unknown. The main hypotheses that have been proposed include infection, allergy to dietary components, immune responses to bacterial or self-antigens, an abnormality in epithelial cell integrity, and the psychosomatic theory. There are virtually no data to support a primary role for psychosomatic factors in the aetiology of the disease, although they may play a secondary role in determining the pattern of symptoms and must always be considered when managing individual patients.

INFECTION

No specific infective organism has been consistently isolated from patients with ulcerative colitis. However, the recognition that the strains of *Escherichia coli* in the normal colon are continually changing has led to the concept that patients may carry strains which, by releasing enzymes or other toxic products, might damage the mucosa. The recent demonstration that, even in remission, patients with ulcerative colitis are more likely to harbour *E. coli* expressing adhesins than control subjects is a particularly interesting observation, as these may allow the bacteria to adhere readily to the epithelium.

FOOD ALLERGY

The early suggestions of allergic responses to milk proteins, eggs, and other dietary proteins have not been substantiated as an aetiological factor. Milk-free diets may be beneficial in a minority of patients but it is not clear whether this results from an associated hypolactasia, an immunological response, or some other mechanism. The failure of ulcerative colitis to respond either to intravenous nutrition with nil by mouth or to colonic isolation by means of a split ileostomy are further pointers that dietary factors play little part.

ENVIRONMENTAL FACTORS

As well as infection and diet, smoking and the use of oral contraceptives may influence disease. Many studies have now shown that ulcerative colitis is more common in non-smokers than smokers, with a relative risk of 2 to 6. Ex-smokers have a particularly high incidence and this is highest for ex-heavy compared to ex-light smokers. Women taking oral contraceptives may have a slight increased risk of the disease but this association is weak and loses significance when the data are corrected for smoking habits and social class.

Immunopathogenesis

The intense infiltration of the inflamed mucosa with plasma cells, B and T lymphocytes, and macrophages suggests immunological activity. Whether activation of both humoral and cellular immune mechanisms merely reflects increased antigenic absorption through an abnormal epithelium, a response to a specific aetiological agent, or an underlying defect in mucosal immunoregulation is unknown.

There is an increase in plasma cells synthesizing all three of the major immunoglobulin isotypes—IgA, IgG, and IgM. However, the largest proportional increase is in IgG-producing cells and this is predominantly of the IgG1 and IgG3 subclass, which is in contrast to Crohn's disease where an IgG2 response is predominant. IgG1 and IgG3 are synthesized in response to protein antigen and are effective in fixing complement. Complement activation is known to occur in active colitis, probably as a result of the formation of antigen–antibody complexes, and is likely to be one of the major effector mechanisms in establishing the inflammatory lesion. Some of the increased mucosal IgG synthesized is known to have antibody specificity for bacterial and epithelial antigens. As antibody to epithelial antigens, especially an 40-kDa protein, is a feature of ulcerative colitis, rather than Crohn's disease, it is possible that autoimmunity plays a part in ulcerative colitis. This concept is strengthened by the association with other autoimmune disorders and with circulating antibodies to neutrophils (pANCA), neither of which is associated with Crohn's disease. Nevertheless, whether anticolon antibodies or pANCA have a pathogenetic role is still very uncertain.

The major subsets of T cells (CD4$^+$, CD8$^+$) are present in increased numbers in the inflamed mucosa but their proportions do not change significantly. Several lines of evidence suggest that the T cells are activated and release a variety of cytokines. Whether there is a failure of T cells to either up-regulate or down-regulate the mucosal immune response has not been clearly shown. However, data suggest that there may indeed be a failure to induce suppression to specific antigens, which could lead to some of the immunological overactivity that is observed in this disease. Intraepithelial T lymphocytes (**IEL**) isolated from colons resected for severe ulcerative colitis also fail to suppress T-cell proliferative responses to specific antigens, a property that is not due to the increased numbers of IEL using γδ T-cell receptors.

As well as T-cell activation, there is also a marked increase in the population of activated macrophages, which not only release inflammatory mediators (reactive oxygen metabolites, leukotrienes, platelet-activating factor) but serine proteases, metalloproteinases and cytokines. The release of interleukin(**IL**)-1, IL-6, and tumour necrosis factor will not only lead to tissue damage but will initiate an acute-phase response, down-regulate albumin synthesis, and induce fever. Release of interferon-γ from activated T cells induces HLA class II molecules on colonic epithelial cells, which, in turn, are then able to present antigen to the adjacent CD4$^+$ lymphocytes and to activate the CD8$^+$ IEL. Changes in epithelial permeability induced by interferon-γ and inflammatory mediators, endothelial damage by a wide variety of cytokines and mediators leading to local ischaemia, and stimulation of collagen synthesis by transforming growth factor-β, IL-1, and IL-6 may all contribute to the inflammatory process.

Pathology

MACROSCOPIC

Ulcerative colitis always involves the rectum but in about 40 per cent of patients the disease is limited to rectum and sigmoid. In adults, only about 20 per cent will have the whole colon involved, although this proportion rises to about 50 per cent in children. In mild disease, the mucosa is hyperaemic and granular but, as the disease becomes more severe, small punctate ulcers appear, which may then enlarge and extend deeply into the lamina propria. The ulceration may be linear along the line of the taeniae coli. The mucosa can become intensely haemorrhagic. In patients with long-standing disease, inflammatory polyps (pseudopolyps) may develop. They are usually found in the colon and rarely in the rectum. Inflammatory polyps are of no significance and have no malignant potential. In occasional patients, they may regress.

When the disease goes into remission, the colonic appearances may return to normal, but, especially in patients who have had recurrent attacks, the mucosa becomes atrophic and featureless. There is often narrowing and shortening of the bowel. Fibrous strictures complicating long-standing chronic disease are extremely rare.

If an acute dilatation occurs in a patient with severe disease, the bowel becomes thin and congested. There is usually severe ulceration, with only small islands of mucosa remaining. An acute dilatation may be accompanied by a perforation.

MICROSCOPIC

The inflammation of ulcerative colitis is largely confined to the mucosa. The lamina propria becomes oedematous, with dilated and congested capillaries, and extravasation of red blood cells. There is a cellular infiltrate of acute and chronic inflammatory cells: neutrophils, lymphocytes, plasma cells, macrophages, mast cells, and eosinophils.

The neutrophils invade the epithelium, usually in the crypts, giving rise to a cryptitis and eventually to a crypt abscess. The triggers for this migration of neutrophils are unknown but chemotactic peptides of colonic bacteria (e.g. formyl methionyl leucyl phenylalanine) as well as IL-8, leukotriene B4, platelet-activating factor, and activated complement are potential candidates. Damage to the crypts leads to increased epithelial cell turnover and a discharge of mucus from goblet cells. With increasing inflammation, the surface epithelial cells become flattened, irregular, and eventually ulcerate. Deep ulcers may extend into the lamina propria, leading to inflammatory changes in the submucosa—this may be accompanied by an acute dilatation or perforation.

Many of the acute changes of ulcerative colitis are non-specific and may also be seen in infective colitides. However, the diagnosis of ulcerative colitis can be made with some accuracy (more than 80 per cent probability) if features of a chronic inflammatory process are present. These include distorted crypt architecture, crypt atrophy, basal lymphoid aggregates, and a chronic inflammatory infiltrate.

Once the disease has gone into remission, the histological appearances may return to normal. However, there is frequent evidence of bifid or shortened crypts, hyperplasia of the muscularis mucosae, neuronal hypertrophy, and Paneth-cell metaplasia at the base of the crypts.

Clinical features

Patients usually present with a gradual onset of symptoms, often intermittent, but which become progressively more severe. Occasionally, ulcerative colitis can present much more rapidly and may mimic an infective colitis. Indeed, some patients begin with a documented infection (e.g., a campylobacter or salmonella colitis) but continue to have symptoms that ultimately lead to the correct diagnosis.

The major symptoms include diarrhoea, rectal bleeding, the passage of mucus, and, less frequently, abdominal pain. When the inflammation is confined to the rectum (proctitis), patients often pass fresh blood, which is usually mixed with the stool but can be streaked on the surface. These patients often complain of constipation rather than diarrhoea and, on clinical symptoms alone, may be mistakenly diagnosed as suffering from haemorrhoids. When the inflammation extends beyond the rectum, there is usually diarrhoea with the passage of partly altered blood. The diarrhoea is often accompanied by urgency and tenesmus, and patients can be incontinent. Nocturnal diarrhoea is a common symptom in the presence of severe inflammation. With a severe ulcerative colitis affecting most or all of the colon, patients are usually anorectic, nauseated, and have lost weight. They usually have severe diarrhoea (in excess of six motions daily) that becomes a slurry of faecal material, pus, and blood—it may resemble anchovy sauce and, indeed, some patients may fail to recognize that they are passing blood.

Patients may also complain of a malaise, lassitude, and symptoms referable to chronic iron deficiency or to some of the extraintestinal manifestations, especially recurrent aphthous ulcers of the mouth.

On examination, patients with mild or moderate attacks usually look well and exhibit few abnormal physical signs. Weight should always be recorded and, for children and adolescents, both height and weight should be recorded on growth charts. Abdominal examination may reveal a tender colon but is often normal. Bowel sounds are normal and rectal examination is also normal apart from blood.

Patients with a severe attack may also look deceptively well and a tachycardia or a tender colon may be the only abnormal signs. However, many of these patients are obviously ill, with fever, salt and water depletion, anaemia, and evidence of weight loss. There may be oral candidiasis, aphthous ulceration, signs of iron deficiency, and finger clubbing. There may be the skin changes of hypoalbuminaemia and dependent oedema. The abdomen is often distended and tympanitic, with reduced bowel sounds and marked colonic tenderness.

Minor perianal disease, e.g. a fissure, may occur in patients with an active ulcerative colitis but it is never as severe as is seen in patients with Crohn's disease.

Assessment of disease severity

This can be done clinically, by grading the degree of inflammation seen endoscopically or histologically, and by using laboratory tests of inflammatory activity.

CLINICAL GRADING

Mild

Less than four stools daily, with or without blood, with no systemic disturbance and a normal erythrocyte sedimentation rate (**ESR**).

Moderate

Between mild and severe.

Severe

At least six stools daily, with bleeding, and evidence of systemic illness as shown by fever, tachycardia, a falling haemoglobin, hypoalbuminaemia, and raised ESR and C-reactive protein.

LABORATORY MARKERS OF INFLAMMATION

Active disease is often accompanied by a neutrophil leucocytosis, thrombocytosis, a rise in acute-phase proteins (C-reactive protein, orosomucoid) and in ESR. There may also be a fall in haemoglobin and albumin. These inflammatory markers are useful when measured serially during the course of treatment as an indicator of disease activity. However, if corticosteroids are used, the white-cell count can no longer be used as a marker of disease activity because it will often rise in response to the steroids. Patients with a proctitis rarely have a rise in C-reactive protein unless the inflammation is particularly severe.

Diagnosis

The diagnosis is made on the basis of the history, the absence of faecal pathogens, and the endoscopic and histological appearances of the colon.

Stool cultures should be set up for all patients presenting for the first time and, ideally, for all those presenting with a relapse of established disease. Special culture conditions are required for *Campylobacter* spp., yersinia, gonococci and *Clostridium difficile*. The possibility of an infection with *E. coli* 0157 must also be considered, especially in patients in whom bleeding and abdominal pain are predominant symptoms. An infective colitis with opportunistic organisms in patients with immunodeficiency syndromes has become much more common and has to be remembered in differential diagnosis.

Sigmoidoscopy is safe, even in patients with a severe attack, and not only confirms rectal inflammation but also allows a biopsy specimen to be taken and an assessment of severity to be obtained. Although some centres use colonoscopy in severe attacks, this is rarely necessary for diagnosis, for assessment of severity, or for determining management. It is best avoided in the acute stage. The earliest signs of colitis on sigmoidoscopy are blurring of the vascular pattern associated with hyperaemia and oedema, leading to blunting of the valves of Houston. With increasing severity, the mucosa becomes granular and then friable. With severe inflammation, the mucosa shows spontaneous bleeding and ulceration. These changes begin in the rectum, they are diffuse, and extend proximally to affect a variable length of the colon. Pseudopolyps

(inflammatory polyps) often occur in patients with long-standing disease but tend to be in the colon rather than the rectum.

Colonoscopy with multiple biopsies is useful for assessing the extent of disease and is mandatory for patients with a colonic stricture. It is also required for cancer surveillance (see later). Preparation of the colon should follow the normal methods and osmotic purgation is the most satisfactory. However, a more gentle approach is needed if colonoscopy is done in the presence of severe inflammation but this is rarely indicated.

All patients with a severe attack must have a plain abdominal radiograph. Not only does this exclude a dilated colon but it may provide prognostic information (mucosal islands, distended small bowel loops) and demonstrate the extent of the disease. An abnormal haustral pattern, thickening of the bowel wall, and mucosal oedema can be detected on a plain film (Fig. 1). As an inflamed colon does not hold faecal material, the presence of faecal matter in the ascending or transverse colon will indicate that the inflammation is distal. In a severe attack, barium radiography is virtually never indicated but, if it is done, a single-contrast study in an unprepared colon with barium entering the colon at low pressure should be used. In less severe disease, a double-contrast barium enema can be safely given (Fig. 2) but the colon must not be overdistended and the procedure must be stopped if the patient complains of pain.

Biopsy specimens must be taken at sigmoidoscopy or colonoscopy, preferably with small, cupped forceps. Histological assessment contributes to grading severity as well as the differential diagnosis.

Laboratory data

These are required for assessing severity, as discussed above, and to document haematological or biochemical complications.

Iron deficiency is common as a result of chronic iron loss; this can be exacerbated by a severe attack because 0.5 g of elemental iron can be lost thereby. Thus, a hypochromic, microcytic anaemia is frequently present. A neutrophil leucocytosis, thrombocytosis, eosinophilia, or monocytosis may also be present and are indicators of active inflammation.

Biochemical abnormalities are rare in mild or moderate attacks but

Fig. 1 Plain abdominal radiograph of a 24-year-old man with severe ulcerative colitis. The ascending and transverse colon are grossly oedematous and diseased with loss of the normal haustral pattern. In addition, there are multiple loops of distended small intestine.

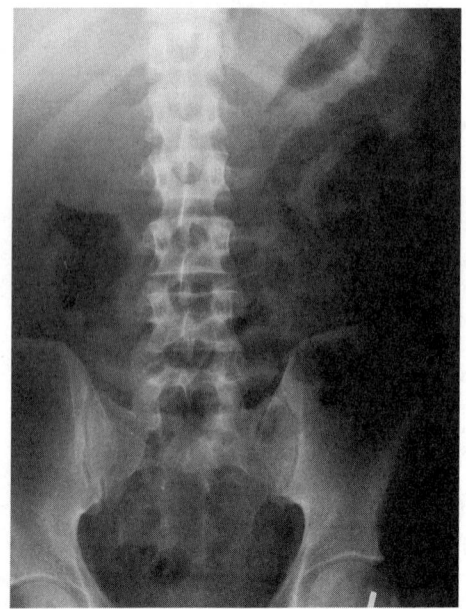

hypokalaemia, hypoalbuminaemia, and a rise in α_2-globulin frequently accompany a severe attack. Minor elevations of the aspartate transaminase or alkaline phosphatase are also frequently seen in patients with a severe attack but they return to normal when the disease goes into remission. They probably reflect a fatty liver, together with the effects of toxaemia or poor nutrition. Persistent elevation, especially of alkaline phosphatase, may indicate underlying chronic liver disease and needs further investigation (see below).

Serum immunoglobulins rarely exceed the upper limit of normal during a relapse but usually fall as remission occurs.

Differential diagnosis

If the patient has a history of slow onset of symptoms, including blood and mucus, and has diffuse inflammation on sigmoidoscopy, the diagnosis of ulcerative colitis is highly probable. The major differential diagnosis is Crohn's disease (see Chapter 14.10). If clinical, radiological, endoscopic, and histological information is considered together, less than 10 per cent of patients fall into the category of indeterminate colitis. The recently recognized collagenous colitis usually has only a mild inflammation on colonoscopy and is diagnosed on the basis of a thickened subepithelial collagen band (wider than 15 μm) seen in a rectal biopsy specimen. Microscopic or lymphocytic colitis has a normal endoscopic appearance but shows a diffuse infiltration of the lamina propria with lymphocytes and eosinophils on histological examination. Although ischaemic colitis classically occurs around the splenic flexure, it may occur in the rectum, especially in the elderly, and can be diagnosed histologically. Radiation damage to the rectum may occur, especially in men who have had radiotherapy to the prostate.

Rarely, a drug-induced colitis may occur. The drugs that have been implicated include non-steroidal anti-inflammatory drugs, gold, penicillamine, and 5-aminosalicylic acid. The last drug may cause considerable diagnostic confusion in patients who already have ulcerative colitis. An antibiotic history must be taken but a pseudomembranous colitis secondary to Cl. difficile can occur in the absence of antibiotic usage, especially in the elderly.

For those patients presenting with a much more acute history, infective forms of colitis must be excluded by stool culture. A sudden onset of symptoms, the predominance of abdominal pain, the ingestion of potentially infected food (chicken, shellfish), and evidence of diarrhoeal disease in contacts are obvious pointers to an infection. Sigmoidoscopic appearances are usually very similar to ulcerative colitis but a rectal biopsy can be very useful in distinguishing an infective from a more chronic ulcerative colitis. The presence of a chronic inflammatory infiltrate, architectural disturbances of the glands, and basal lymphoid aggregates favour ulcerative colitis. The common organisms causing an infective colitis are salmonellae, shigellae, and campylobacter. Yersinial infections may also cause a colitis and can pursue a chronic course over many months before resolving. Special culture conditions may isolate the organism from stool but a rising titre of serum antibody is often the more reliable method of identifying the infection. Escherichia coli 0157 is a recognized cause of an acute colitis, especially in institutions, and massive bleeding is often a characteristic feature. Children may develop a haemolytic–uraemic syndrome. Diagnosis is difficult because most laboratories are not equipped either to detect this strain of E. coli or to measure specific antibody. For patients who have travelled in endemic areas, amoebic and schistosomal colitis must be considered—stool examination and histological demonstration of amoebae or schistosomal ova in rectal biopsy specimens make the diagnosis.

Other causes of infective colitis can occur in immunosuppressed patients and include cytomegalovirus, herpes simplex, and Mycobacterium avium intracellulare. Although these organisms are usually associated with fairly characteristic sigmoidoscopic appearances, they can be associated with a more diffuse pattern of inflammation. Other sexually transmitted causes of proctitis (gonorrhoea, chlamydia, lymphogranuloma) do not usually cause diarrhoea and, especially with gonorrhoea, are associated with the passage of watery pus.

Ulcerative colitis also has to be differentiated from irritable bowel syndrome, colonic polyps or carcinoma, diverticular disease, solitary rectal ulcer syndrome, and factitious diarrhoea. Sigmoidoscopy usually clarifies the diagnosis but if the ulceration of the solitary rectal ulcer syndrome becomes circumferential, this can be mistaken for ulcerative colitis. A biopsy specimen showing strands of smooth muscle radiating up into the lamina propria between the glands is characteristic of the solitary ulcer syndrome.

Extraintestinal manifestations

Table 2 lists the extraintestinal manifestations.

SKIN

The most common skin rash seen in patients with ulcerative colitis is a hypersensitivity rash to sulphasalazine (related to the sulphapyridine moiety), which may be photosensitive. Erythema nodosum occurs in about 2 per cent of patients and is mostly associated with active disease. The lesions occur most commonly on the anterior aspect of the lower legs. Pyoderma gangrenosum is rare (1–2 per cent) and is usually seen in patients with active disease but occasionally persists despite inactive colitis. The lesions usually begin as sterile pustules, usually on the limbs, which break down as they enlarge and finally coalesce. Ulceration leads to necrosis and the lesions become surrounded by black, necrotic tissue. Treatment of the colitis is usually followed by regression of the skin lesions.

MOUTH

Crops of aphthous ulcers are common in patients with active disease. A sore tongue and angular stomatitis often accompany chronic iron deficiency.

EYES

Episcleritis or an anterior uveitis occur in 5 to 8 per cent of patients. Local corticosteroids and treatment of active colitis usually lead to resolution.

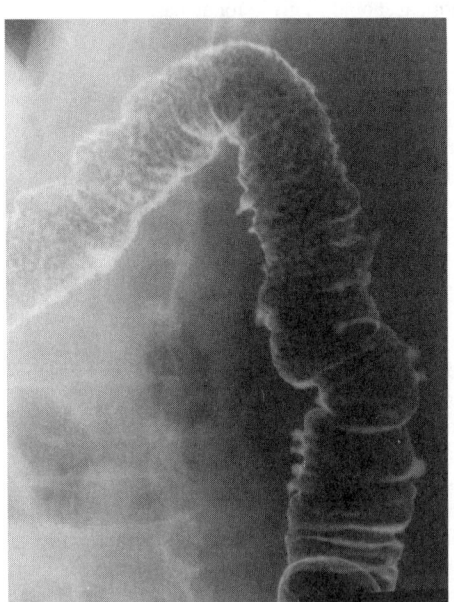

Fig. 2 A double-contrast barium enema in a patient with active ulcerative colitis. The figure is a close-up view of the splenic flexure to show extensive mucosal ulceration, loss of haustration, and narrowing of the colon. The patient also has diverticula in the descending colon.

Table 2 *Extraintestinal manifestations of ulcerative colitis*

Related to activity of colitis
Aphthous ulceration of the mouth
Fatty liver
Erythema nodosum
Peripheral arthropathy
Episcleritis
Usually related to activity of colitis
Pyoderma gangrenosum
Anterior uveitis
Unrelated to colitis
Sacroiliitis
Ankylosing spondylitis
Primary sclerosing cholangitis
Cholangiocarcinoma

JOINTS

An acute arthropathy occurs in 10 to 15 per cent of patients with active disease. It affects the larger joints (knees, hips, ankles, wrists, elbows) and is usually asymmetrical. It is a non-erosive condition and settles as the colitis goes into remission.

Low back pain is a common symptom and is usually due to a sacroiliitis, which can be seen radiologically in 12 to 15 per cent of patients. It is unrelated to disease activity, is not strongly associated with HLA-B27, and rarely progresses to ankylosing spondylitis. The last disease occurs in only 1 to 2 per cent of patients and over 80 per cent of these have the HLA-B27 phenotype. There is a 2:1 ratio in favour of males with this complication. The spondylitis may present before the colitis becomes apparent or may follow the intestinal symptoms. Its natural history is independent to that of the colitis and should be treated with physiotherapy, hydrotherapy, and, if necessary, non-steroidal inflammatory drugs. However, these drugs can occasionally worsen the colitis and should therefore be used cautiously.

LIVER DISEASE

Patients with severe attacks of ulcerative colitis often have minor elevations of alkaline phosphatase or transaminases. The cause of these enzyme rises is probably multifactorial, including malnutrition, sepsis, and a fatty liver, which occurs in up to 60 per cent of patients coming to urgent colectomy. The liver enzymes return to normal activities when remission is achieved.

However, there may be persistent abnormalities in liver enzymes in about 3 per cent of patients, usually a rise in alkaline phosphatase. The overwhelming majority of these patients will have primary sclerosing cholangitis when the bile duct is visualized by endoscopic cholangiography. Histologically, liver biopsy specimens show evidence of chronic liver disease but the spectrum of appearances ranges from those of a chronic active hepatitis to the classical picture of concentric periductular fibrosis with obliteration of bile ducts.

Many patients with ulcerative colitis and sclerosing cholangitis remain well for many years. The colitis is often very mild, though frequently affecting the whole colon, but the liver disease is progressive and ultimately leads to portal hypertension and liver failure. Sclerosing cholangitis is a premalignant condition and explains the well-recognized association between ulcerative colitis and cholangiocarcinoma. Pathogenesis and treatment of the liver disease are discussed in Chapter 14.27.3.

RARE ASSOCIATIONS

Pericarditis with or without an effusion has been described in association with an acute attack of colitis but a true association is not yet proven.

Amyloid rarely occurs in ulcerative colitis—it is much more likely to be associated with Crohn's disease.

A rapidly progressing bronchiectasis has also been described in some patients with ulcerative colitis.

Medical management

The main principles of therapy for the treatment of ulcerative colitis are: to control active disease rapidly, to maintain remission, to select patients for whom surgery is appropriate, and to ensure as good a quality of life as possible.

TREATMENT OF ACTIVE DISEASE

The most effective drugs for controlling active disease are the corticosteroids, which may be given systemically, topically, or in combination. Drugs containing 5-aminosalicylic acid (sulphasalazine, olsalazine, mesalazine) are often used to treat a mild colitis but prednisolone has been shown to be more effective and to control symptoms more rapidly, which make it the drug of choice. The dosage and route of administration are largely governed by disease severity. Once active inflammation has been controlled and remission obtained, the corticosteroids should be tailed off because they are ineffective as maintenance therapy and prolonged use puts the patient at risk of long-term side-effects such as osteoporosis.

Proctitis

Proctitis refers to disease limited to the rectum—in practice, it refers to inflammation that does not extend beyond the limits of a rigid sigmoidoscope. It can be remarkably difficult to treat. Initial therapy is usually a 5-aminosalicylic acid (**5-ASA**) drug by mouth in combination with topical therapy. The latter can be a corticosteroid or 5-ASA in the form of retention enemas, a foam preparation or a suppository. For patients who do not respond, oral prednisolone may be given. Some have sufficiently severe proctitis to warrant intravenous steroids, and occasionally colectomy may be necessary. Many patients with a refractory proctitis develop a severe proximal constipation, which can cause considerable abdominal discomfort, bloating, and nausea. Relief of the constipation, usually by gentle osmotic purgation, will often give considerable symptomatic benefit but may also be associated with a marked improvement in the inflammation.

Mildly active disease

Patients who have no more than four motions daily on average, with inflammation extending beyond the limits of the rigid sigmoidoscope, should be given oral prednisolone, 20 mg daily, together with topical steroids or 5-ASA. Treatment should be given for at least 4 weeks before being tailed off over the subsequent 3 to 4 weeks.

Moderately active disease

Patients who have, on average, more than four bowel actions daily but who are not systemically ill should be given 40 mg of prednisolone by mouth daily. Giving larger doses (e.g. 60 mg daily) provides only a marginally better effect but increases the frequency of side-effects quite considerably. The dose is reduced to 20 mg daily over 2 to 3 weeks and the regimen then follows that described for mild disease.

Severe disease

This is defined as an attack in which the patient has more than six bowel actions daily, with blood, and who is systemically ill as shown by tachycardia, fever, and anaemia. The colon is usually tender on palpation. These patients should be admitted to hospital and assessed by both physician and surgeon. Fluid and electrolyte losses are replaced intravenously; a blood transfusion should be given if the haemoglobin is less than 10 g/dl. Patients are given intravenous corticosteroids (e.g. hydrocortisone 100 mg, 6-hourly) together with a twice daily rectal drip of hydrocortisone (100 mg in 100 ml water). Parenteral nutrition is indicated for patients who are malnourished but for the majority, intravenous saline and dextrose–saline are sufficient, together with potassium supplements. Most patients with a severe attack prefer to stay on clear fluids only by mouth during the first 24 h. Thereafter, there is no evidence that continuing a light diet has any adverse effect on the disease but many clinicians will leave the patient on clear fluids only for the first few days.

Provided the patient is improving, treatment is continued for 5 to 7 days. At this time, a good response is one in which the patient feels well, there is no fever or tachycardia, the colon is not tender on abdominal palpation, and the diarrhoea has largely settled, usually to less than four motions daily. At this stage, the stools are rarely formed but macroscopic bleeding has stopped. These patients can then go on to oral prednisolone (e.g. 40 mg daily), a retention enema, an oral 5-ASA drug, and a light diet. Patients who deteriorate during the first few days of intravenous treatment or those who have not made a substantial improvement by the end of the first week should be advised to have urgent surgery. The more difficult decision is when patients have made some improvement but are still not well—they may still be anorectic, have an intermittent low-grade fever, a tachycardia, and continuing diarrhoea. Continuing intravenous therapy for more than 7 to 10 days is rarely beneficial and surgery is usually required. It is in this group of patients that the introduction of a light diet towards the end of the first week of treatment often provides a guide to future management. If the pulse rises or a niggling fever develops in response to feeding, urgent colectomy is required. Very recently, intravenous cyclosporin given as a slow infusion (4 mg/kg) has shown promise in this group of patients but its precise role is still undergoing evaluation.

Approximately 25 per cent of patients with a severe attack will require an urgent colectomy. These patients can often be identified early on using clinical and radiological features, which have been shown to have prognostic significance. These are the passage of more than nine stools, a pulse rate greater than 100/min, or a temperature greater than 38°C during the first 24 h of treatment. A serum albumin of less than 30 g/l during the first few days or the failure of acute-phase proteins such as the C-reactive protein to fall are also poor prognostic signs. Seventy-five per cent of patients showing mucosal islands in the colon or having more than three loops of distended small bowel on a plain abdominal radiograph will come to urgent surgery.

Chronic active disease

Some patients repeatedly relapse when they come off corticosteroids or get below a daily dose of 10 to 15 mg of prednisolone. Immunosuppression therapy with azathioprine or 6-mercaptopurine is often beneficial in this group. In the United Kingdom, azathioprine is the drug that is most used, in doses of 2.0 or 2.5 mg/kg, and may allow the prednisolone to be withdrawn. It usually needs 4 to 6 weeks before an effect is seen and the drug is then continued for several months. Although few long-term sequelae have been encountered, most clinicians do not usually continue therapy for more than 18 to 24 months. Oral cyclosporin (5 mg/kg) has also been used for chronic active disease but no formal clinical trials have been made. High-dose prednisolone (40 mg) given on alternate days is another approach that may be useful. However, if the patient's lifestyle is impaired by chronic disabling symptoms or by the side-effects of treatment, surgical management should be considered.

MAINTENANCE OF REMISSION

Sulphasalazine and its active moiety, 5-ASA, are able to maintain the disease in remission when given over many years and reduce the relapse rate by about four-fold. Thus, provided they are well tolerated, they should be given indefinitely.

For sulphasalazine, the optimal dose to obtain good therapeutic efficacy with the least side-effects is 2 g daily. Common side-effects are nausea, anorexia, and headache, which are dose related and are caused by the sulphapyridine component. Other side-effects, which are also usually due to the sulphonamide but are not dose related, include hypersensitivity skin rashes, male infertility, agranulocytosis, and Heinz-body

Table 3 *New salicylate drugs*

	Characteristics
Mesalazine preparations	
Enteric coated:	
Asacol	Coated with Eudragit, S 5-ASA released at pH 7.0
Claversal, Salofalk	Coated with Eudragit, L 5-ASA released at pH 6.5
Controlled release:	
Pentasa	Tablets comprise 5-ASA granules coated with ethyl cellulose; released with time at pH greater than 6.5
Prodrugs	
Olsalazine (Dipentum®)	Two molecules of 5-ASA linked with an azo bond, which is split by colonic bacteria

5-ASA, 5-aminosalicylic acid.

haemolytic anaemia. Overall, 10 to 15 per cent of patients are unable to take the drug, although the nausea and headache can often be overcome by starting at a low dose and gradually increasing it.

Sulphasalazine is an unusual drug insofar as it is poorly absorbed in the stomach and small intestine. When it reaches the colon, the azo bond linking the 5-ASA and sulphapyridine moieties is split by bacterial azoreductases. The sulphapyridine is absorbed, metabolized in the liver, and excreted in the urine. The majority of the 5-ASA (about 70 per cent) is poorly absorbed and excreted in the faeces. As it is the 5-ASA that is the active compound, several new drugs are now available that present 5-ASA to the colon without the sulphapyridine which causes the majority of the side-effects of sulphasalazine. 5-ASA cannot simply be given by mouth as it is rapidly absorbed. Thus, it is either given as a delayed release formulation (the mesalazine group) or as a prodrug (olsalazine). Table 3 lists these and details their characteristics.

Which 5-ASA-containing drug should be prescribed as maintenance therapy for ulcerative colitis? Sulphasalazine is well tolerated by 85 per cent or so of patients, it is cheap, and serious side-effects (e.g. Stevens–Johnson syndrome, agranulocytosis, pancreatitis) are very rare. The newer drugs are much more expensive than sulphasalazine but they have equal therapeutic efficacy. In general they are associated with fewer side-effects. However, occasional patients develop typical salicylate reactions (rhinitis, urticaria, and a colitis). About 10 to 12 per cent of patients will develop loose stools when given olsalazine. This gradually settles if treatment is continued, but about 5 per cent will develop a severe watery diarrhoea, which usually necessitates stopping the drug. The risk of diarrhoea can be minimized by taking the drug with food. For the resin-coated mesalazines (Asacol, Salofalk), there have been reports of renal failure, mainly due to an intestinal nephritis. It is a rare complication and the mechanism is unknown although 5-ASA has structural similarity to phenacetin. Both Asacol and, especially, Salofalk give higher plasma concentrations of 5-ASA than either Pentasa or the prodrugs (olsalazine, sulphasalazine).

Thus, it seems reasonable to use sulphasalazine as first-line maintenance treatment except in patients with known sulphonamide sensitivity and in young males who have not completed their families. The newer drugs can be used for these and for those who are intolerant of sulphasalazine.

DIET

Patients with recurrent, severe disease have a slightly higher prevalence of hypolactasia and a lactose-free diet may be beneficial. Individual patients may be intolerant of dairy products, wheat, eggs, and other dietary constituents but the majority of patients should have a normal, well-balanced diet.

Local complications

PERIANAL LESIONS

Minor lesions such a fissures, perianal abscesses, or haemorrhoids may occur in patients with ulcerative colitis but extensive lesions such as fistulae are exceptional and, if they occur, suggest Crohn's disease. Treatment of fissures involves treatment of active inflammation. Surgical treatment should be avoided wherever possible and, if necessary, should be conservative.

MASSIVE HAEMORRHAGE

This occurs in association with severe attacks but is rarely seen. Intravenous corticosteroids and transfusion usually allow the bleeding to stop. However, if patients have already received six or more units of blood and are still bleeding, urgent colectomy must be considered.

PERFORATION

This is the most dangerous of the local complications and carries appreciable mortality. In patients receiving corticosteroids, the physical signs of peritonitis may not be obvious, and malaise, tachycardia, and reduced or absent bowel sounds may be the only clinical features. Plain abdominal films usually show free intra-abdominal gas. It may complicate an acute dilatation but can occur in its absence. Management consists of immediate intravenous fluid, electrolytes, antibiotics, and hydrocortisone. As soon as the patient's condition improves, urgent colectomy is done immediately. The mortality of a perforation is as high as 16 per cent, even in specialist centres.

ACUTE DILATATION

This is defined as a transverse colon with a diameter of greater than 5.0 to 6.0 cm with loss of haustration seen on a plain radiograph in a patient with a severe attack of ulcerative colitis. It occurs in about 5 per cent of patients with a severe attack and can be precipitated by hypokalaemia or the administration of opiates. Physical signs are often minimal but the patient is usually obtunded, the bowel sounds are reduced, and the abdomen may become distended. If the colon is already dilated on presentation of the severe attack, medical therapy with intravenous steroids should be given. Approximately 50 per cent of patients will settle on medical therapy alone but urgent surgery is required for those who continue to deteriorate or do not improve within 24 h. If the colon dilates during the course of treating a severe attack, colectomy should be done.

STRICTURES

These occur very rarely in patients with long-standing ulcerative colitis with a shortened, narrow colon. Colonoscopy with multiple biopsies must be done as there must be a high index of suspicion for carcinoma.

PSEUDOPOLYPS

These are common and may be filiform, sessile, or may form bridges. They can occur throughout the colon but often spare the colon. They are not premalignant and may occasionally regress.

COLONIC CARCINOMA

The risk of cancer is mainly in patients who have had extensive disease for more than 10 years, especially if they have had recurrent attacks. The most recent series studying primary cohorts suggest that the cumulative risk for patients with extensive disease is about 7 to 15 per cent at 20 years, with very little risk up to 15 years of disease.

Carcinoma is usually, but not always, preceded by dysplasia. This can be detected histologically and has led to the use of colonoscopic surveillance programmes for patients with long-standing ulcerative colitis affecting most or all of the colon. Provided no dysplasia is found, the examination is repeated every 1 to 3 years. If high-grade dysplasia is present, prophylactic colectomy is usually considered. For low-grade dysplasia, repeat colonoscopy within a few months is usually advised. As large numbers of colonoscopies are involved in a surveillance programme the question of cost–benefit has been raised. However, two recent studies have shown that patients have a worse outcome with respect to cancer if they are not in a surveillance programme. The possibility of using flow cytometry to detect DNA aneuploidy in biopsy specimens as a means of increasing the sensitivity of surveillance is currently being explored.

Surgery

The indications for surgery have already been mentioned and are:

(1) severe inflammation unresponsive to medical therapy;
(2) for chronic active disease;
(3) to prevent cancer.

The choice of operation is partly determined by the expertise available and the activity of disease. When surgery is done for a severe attack, a one-stage proctocolectomy with a Brooke ileostomy has been shown to be a safe and effective procedure. The major problems with the operation are poor healing of the perineal wound, adhesion obstruction, and ileostomy dysfunction. Sexual dysfunction in males rarely occurs if a perimuscular excision of the rectum is made. However, with the advent of restorative proctocolectomy with the formation of an ileo-anal reservoir or pouch, many surgeons will do only a colectomy in the acute stage. The rectal stump is either oversewn (which is not recommended as it often leaks with abscess formation), or brought out as a mucous fistula either in the lower end of the wound or in the left iliac fossa. This allows histological examination of the whole colon to exclude Crohn's disease. The rectum is excised and the pouch formed some months later when nutrition has been restored and patients are not taking corticosteroids or immunosuppressive drugs.

Restorative proctocolectomy has become the procedure of choice for specialist centres provided the anal sphincter is intact. For this reason, this operation is not advised over the age of 65 years. Either the two-limb (J) or four-limb (W) pouch is now the favoured design and most surgeons preserve the anal transitional zone by anastomosing the pouch 1 to 2 cm above the dentate line. This provides much better continence but is still a matter of controversy if the operation is being done for high-grade dysplasia or cancer.

The majority of patients having a pouch operation have excellent function, with less than 10 per cent having any leakage and that usually limited to night-time soiling. Nevertheless, all patients should be advised to wear a pad at first after a pouch procedure. The pouch usually requires emptying 6 to 12 times daily within the first few weeks of functioning and loperamide is usually needed. Adaptation occurs during the first few months, and by the end of a year the emptying frequency is around four times daily but without urgency. Complications of the pouch, once the immediate surgery is over, include anal stenosis, adhesion obstruction, and pouchitis. Pouchitis occurs in 10 to 20 per cent of patients and consists of diarrhoea with blood and evidence of inflammation on endoscopy. It usually responds to antibiotics such as metronidazole or ciprofloxacin but occasionally requires topical treatment with corticosteroids or 5-ASA.

The causes of pouchitis are heterogeneous and include ischaemia, infection with a recognized pathogen (e.g. campylobacter), and poor emptying but the majority of pouchitis attacks are unexplained.

Poor emptying can be recognized by isotopic scanning using a radio-labelled artificial stool and usually responds to regular catheterization of the pouch. The idiopathic pouchitis is particularly interesting in so far as it is only seen in patients who have previously had ulcerative colitis and is rarely, if ever, seen in patients who have a pouch for other reasons. After the formation of a pouch, for whatever indication, the ileal mucosa undergoes colonic metaplasia. The triggers for this are unknown but almost certainly involve luminal stasis. Thus, whatever factors first render an individual susceptible to developing ulcerative colitis also seem to render him susceptible to developing acute inflammation in ileal mucosa that has undergone colonic metaplasia.

Course and prognosis

The majority of patients with ulcerative colitis have intermittent attacks of their disease, but the duration of remission between attacks can vary from a few weeks to many years. About 10 to 15 per cent of patients will have a chronic continuous course and rarely achieve a full remission for any appreciable time. A few (5 per cent) will have a severe first attack requiring urgent surgery but fewer, if any, have one attack only and never relapse.

Patients with extensive or total disease are much more likely to have a severe attack within 1 year of diagnosis than patients with distal disease and are therefore at greater risk of colectomy. However, a year from diagnosis the risk of colectomy is similar in all groups with a cumulative rate of about 1 per cent per year. Patients with disease limited to the rectum are a special group in so far as most of them continue to have very limited involvement. Only about 30 per cent will develop more extensive disease in the 20 years after diagnosis.

Despite having a chronic relapsing disease, 90 per cent or so of patients are able to work with very few days of sick leave each year. Nevertheless, quality of life can be impaired in many patients. During active inflammation, lassitude, discomfort, and urgency of defaecation are the major symptoms that limit everyday activities. Sexual and marital problems are not uncommon but may be no more frequent than that seen in other populations of patients with acute-on-chronic illnesses. Most of these problems disappear during remission, although fear of relapse and the need for continuing treatment and medical supervision can cause considerable anxiety. Many patients will alter their lifestyle with respect to daily activity, travel, and diet but, with prompt treatment of active disease and supportive medical care, most are able to have a normal life for most of the time. The development of patient self-help groups (e.g. The National Association for Colitis and Crohn's Disease in the United Kingdom) has been of tremendous value in providing education and an environment in which patients can regain their confidence and overcome the problem of isolation, an important and common factor in patients with an uncommon and socially unpleasant disease.

There has been a dramatic fall in the mortality rates for ulcerative colitis since the introduction of corticosteroids in the 1950s and the improvement in the management of severe attacks. The mortality rate for a severe attack, including urgent surgery, should now be less than 2 per cent. In the longer term, mortality differs hardly at all from that expected in a matched healthy population, a fact which the majority of life assurance companies fail to recognize.

Ulcerative colitis in pregnancy

Women with ulcerative colitis have normal fertility, are not at increased risk of having a spontaneous abortion, and there is no evidence that pregnancy is a risk factor for relapse. If they do become pregnant, the chance of having a normal baby is the same as for healthy women. Furthermore, there is no good evidence that corticosteroids, 5-ASA-containing drugs, or even azathioprine are harmful. Therefore, maintenance treatment should be continued throughout the pregnancy and, if a relapse does occur, it should be treated aggressively with corticosteroids to obtain a rapid remission.

Ulcerative colitis in childhood

Ulcerative colitis is less common in children than in adults and, for the United Kingdom, the prevalence is about 6 to 7 per 100 000. Nevertheless it can present within the first few weeks of life, although the mean age of presentation is about 10 years. The symptoms are those of diarrhoea, rectal bleeding, abdominal pain, and failure to thrive. There may be evidence of delayed growth but this is more commonly a feature of childhood Crohn's disease. The proportion of children with a total colitis is about 50 per cent, which is higher than in adults, and probably accounts for the higher rate of colectomy reported in most series.

Treatment follows the same principles as for adults, although dosages are adjusted for the child's weight. In addition, great attention must be made to nutrition to allow for adequate growth. For children requiring repeated courses of corticosteroids, an alternate-day regimen usually controls the disease activity but prevents growth retardation. If colectomy becomes necessary, a restorative proctocolectomy should be done.

REFERENCES

Allan, R.N., Keighley, M.R.B., Alexander-Williams, J., and Hawkins, C. (1990). *Inflammatory bowel disease*, (2nd edn). Churchill Livingstone, Edinburgh.

Kirsner, J.B. and Shorter, R.G. (1988). *Inflammatory bowel disease*, (3rd edn). Lea and Febiger, New York.

Ginsberg, A. (ed.) (1989). Management of inflammatory bowel disease. *Gastroenterology Clinics of North America*, **Vol. 18, No. 1**. Saunders, Philadelphia.

14.12 Disorders of motility

D. L. WINGATE

INTRODUCTION

The main function of the gastrointestinal tract is the assimilation of water and nutrients. Of the major processes contributing to this, two—digestion and absorption—have been relatively well understood for much of the twentieth century. The third, motility, describes the propulsive activity of the digestive tract which allows that the transit of material through the gut is so governed as to ensure that the residence of material in the sites where mechanical and chemical breakdown and absorption take place is optimal for efficient assimilation; motility also ensures that unwanted material is ejected from the gut. In contrast to the other important physiological functions of the gut, motor activity has been, until recently, a topic shrouded in ignorance and exciting little interest among gastroenterologists. Perhaps clinicians tended to share the convenient lay view of the gut, which is that of a system akin to a slot machine; something inserted in an upper orifice proceeds by gravity while being transformed into something else that is ejected at a lower level. As the gut is a hollow tube with an upper and lower opening, in which the progress of material—in an upright biped—is in the direction dictated by gravity, such a view is understandable, but it is wrong. Material is propelled along the gut by active patterns of propulsive motor activity, and without these motor programmes, there are, despite gravity, only stasis and obstruction, constituting intestinal motor failure.

There is a changing perception of the nature of gastrointestinal motility and its relevance to clinical gastroenterology, stemming from three decades of research in this field. Two themes dominate this altered view. For the clinician, it is now increasingly appreciated that motility disorders are not rare and exotic syndromes but, on the contrary, include two of the most common problems presenting in gastroenterology clinics, gastro-oesophageal reflux and constipation. For the scientist, it has become clear that the control of motility is not limited to the operation of the peristaltic reflex, but is dominated by complex neurochemical controls involving both the peripheral and central nervous systems.

In the future, what are now seen as recent advances will become incorporated into standard undergraduate teaching materials, but for many of the readers of this book who have already entered practice, this will be too late. It is particularly for the latter group that an overview of normal anatomy and physiology is included, because some familiarity with the current state of knowledge is essential to appreciate not only the present view of motility disorders, but also further progress in this field.

The motor system

Smooth muscle

MORPHOLOGY

The digestive tube is composed of three muscle layers: the muscularis mucosa adjacent the mucosal layer, the circular muscle, with muscle fibres arranged in a circumferential syncytium, and the longitudinal muscle whose fibres run parallel to the lumen of the bowel. The function of the muscularis is unknown; it is only a thin layer incapable of generating

forces sufficiently powerful to perturb the contents of the bowel lumen. The propulsive nature of smooth muscle is explicable in terms of the circular and longitudinal layers, which, when contracted, respectively constrict and shorten the bowel. These layers are present throughout the bowel, but the gross morphology of the tube is specialized in different regions according to function. The fundamental unit of gastrointestinal motility is peristalsis, the propulsive movement that comprises a repetitive, broad sequence of relaxation distal (caudad) and contraction proximal (orad) to material within the lumen. In the oesophagus, where transit is rapid, the muscular tube is straight and featureless, so that the forces of peristalsis are directed along a single, caudad vector. In contrast, the complex contours of the stomach, and of the antropyloroduodenal segment, allow the simple sequence of peristalsis to be utilized as a pressure head to feed a pumping segment that is more retropulsive than propulsive. In the colon, where the speed of transit is slow, the longitudinal layer is not continuous around the circumference of the gut, but condensed into bands as the taenia coli.

Segments of the muscular tube are interrupted by sphincteric regions; these serve as potential barriers to transit, but also demarcate the boundary between regions with different intrinsic electrical characteristics (Fig. 1). In the absence of pathological change, sphincters—with the exception of the internal anal sphincter—do not obstruct, or even regulate forward flow; they serve to prevent retrograde flow (reflux).

ELECTRICAL AND CONTRACTILE ACTIVITY

The smooth muscle of the gut has two distinct characteristics: it is, for the most part, intrinsically rhythmic with a regular wave of depolarization, and it functions as a syncytium, with electrical contact between adjacent cells that allows synchronous depolarization. In this respect it resembles myocardial smooth muscle, and the electrical frequency is similarly driven by pacemaker zones. The degree and frequency of rhythmicity varies between regions of the gut (Fig. 1); it is dominant in

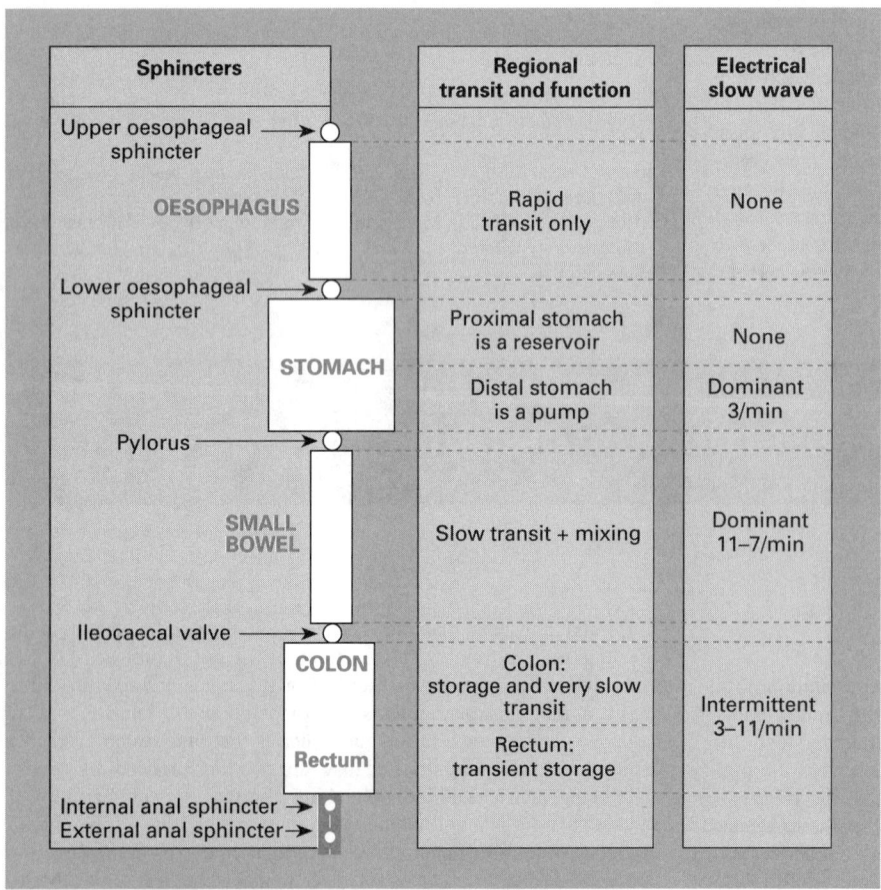

Fig. 1 Sphincters, transit, and electrical characteristics of the different regions of the digestive tract.

the distal stomach and small intestine, but less so in the colon and rectum, while the proximal stomach and oesophagus do not appear to possess intrinsic rhythmicity. It was previously believed that the property of rhythmicity resided within the smooth-muscle cells, but recent studies have revealed that the pacemaking activity appears to be generated by the interstitial cells of Cajal, which are closely applied to the smooth-muscle layers. It has been shown that the interstitial-cell population in the gut closely parallels the dominance of pacemakers; such cells are numerous in the antroduodenal region but not in the colon or oesophagus.

There is, however, one important difference between cardiac and gut smooth muscle. In the heart, the relation between electrical depolarization and contraction is obligate; each depolarization results in contraction, and there is normally complete correlation between the QRS complex of the electrocardiogram and the myocardial contraction. In the gut, however, depolarization is a permissive event (Fig. 2); the plateau of depolarization provides the opportunity for the generation of action potentials and, hence, contraction, but whether this occurs is determined by neurochemical regulatory mechanisms. It is this permissive property that allows the simple reflex of peristalsis to be built up into complex, spatiotemporal patterns of movement.

The completely denervated small-bowel smooth muscle exhibits continuous contractile activity, as can be demonstrated on isolated smooth muscle in an organ bath. When the intrinsic nerves are blocked by the application of tetrodotoxin, the previously inert muscle exhibits regular contractions. This implies that the neural input into the smooth muscle is predominantly inhibitory.

Innervation

OVERVIEW

The innervation of the gut is extrinsic and intrinsic. The extrinsic innervation comprises part of two divisions of the autonomic nervous system, parasympathetic and sympathetic. The parasympathetic innervation is mainly provided by the vagus nerves, whose territory extends from the oesophagus to the proximal colon, with the pelvic nerves supplying the distal gut. The sympathetic innervation consist of the splanchnic nerves from the dorsal-root ganglia of the spinal cord. For most of the twentieth century, since Langley first described the autonomic nervous system, the control of gastrointestinal motility was attributed to the extrinsic innervation (Fig. 3).

The intrinsic innervation consists of the intramural nerve plexuses of the gut. There are two major plexuses, the myenteric (Auerbach's)

plexus between the two major layers of smooth muscle, and the submucosal (Meissner's) plexus between the smooth muscle and the mucosa. First clearly described more than a century ago, no functional role was ascribed to the plexuses beyond providing the circuitry for the peristaltic reflex. In the last two decades it has become clear that the intrinsic innervation, formerly described as the enteric division of the autonomic nervous system, and now known collectively as the enteric nervous system, is the major regulatory system controlling gut function in general, and motility in particular. The enteric nervous system is the only part of the peripheral nervous system possessing not only afferent and efferent neurones, but also interneurones; its structure, consisting of a network of neurones connecting ganglia, has homology with the cerebral cortex, and in common with the central nervous system, it contains large families of neuropeptides.

The changing perception of neural control of the gut is not only a product of systematic research into gut function; it follows from two important observations: that (i) the vagus nerve is predominantly a sensory nerve; only about 20 per cent of vagal fibres are efferent motor fibres, equivalent to about 10 000 neurones—similar considerations apply to other extrinsic nerves; and (ii) that the enteric nervous system is a very large nervous system, comprising, in man, about 100 million neurones. The ration of vagal motor fibres to enteric nervous-system neurones is thus about 10 000 : 1. Given this disproportion, it is clearly impossible for individual effector cells to be directly innervated by extrinsic motor neurones.

It is now clear that the function of the enteric nervous system is not only the operation and regulation of peristalsis through intrinsic afferent and efferent neurones, but also the operation of specific and complex programmes of motor activity according to the material that is present within the lumen of the gut. The function of the extrinsic innervation is

Fig. 3 The classical concept of dual control of gastrointestinal motility by opposing excitatory (cholinergic) and inhibitory (adrenergic) innervation. This concept, which ignored the contribution of the enteric nervous system, is outmoded and incorrect.

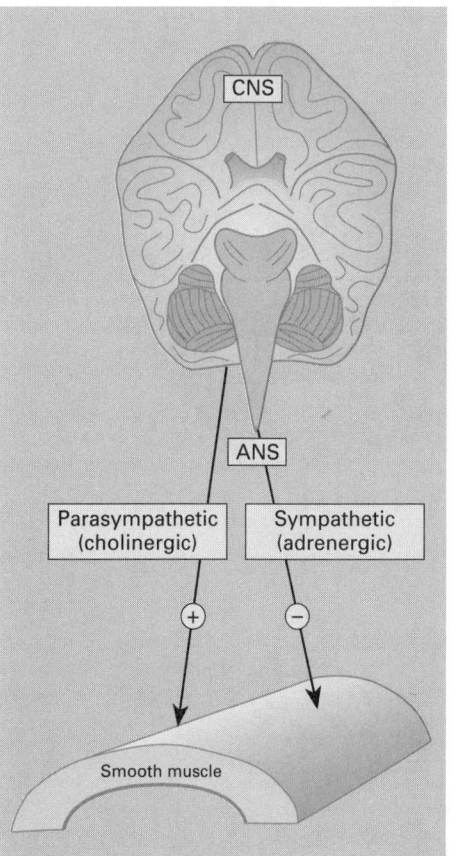

Fig. 2 Schematic comparison of intracellular activity of smooth muscle (upper trace), electrical activity as recorded by serosal electromyography (middle trace), and tension change in the muscle (lower trace). Intracellular depolarization is represented extracellularly as a QRS-type complex, the slow wave. Tension change does not occur with the slow wave, but with the associated action potentials, if present; summated action potentials are detected extracellularly as spike bursts.

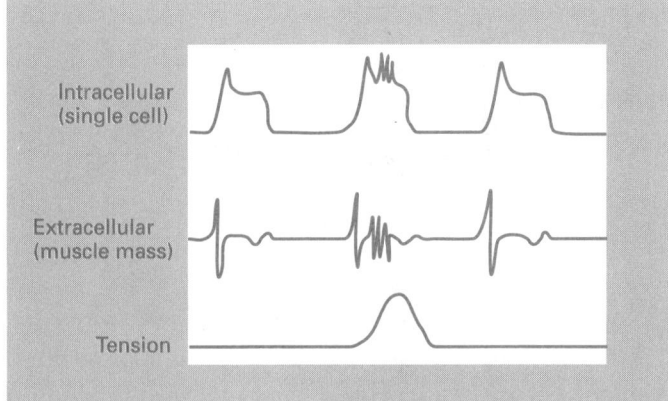

mainly sensory; the afferent nerves provide the central nervous system with continuous information about conditions within the lumen of the bowel, and the function of the effector systems in the gut. The motor function of the extrinsic innervation is to modulate the programming activity of the enteric nervous system according to the overriding needs of the organism: for example, during stress, the motor activity of the gut is profoundly modified; this is not due to direct neuronal input into smooth muscle, rather it is the motor programmes of the enteric nervous system that are thus modulated.

This concept of neural control is illustrated in Fig. 4.

MOTOR PROGRAMMES

The classical view of integrative motor activity in the digestive tract was derived from the conclusions, published in 1833, of William Beaumont, who maintained that motor activity was stimulated by food, and that when food was absent, so was motor activity. This view was challenged at the beginning of the twentieth century by Boldyreff, a Russian sur-

Fig. 4 The current concept of neural control of the gut; the enteric nervous system (ENS), represented by a hatched plane, has its own afferent and efferent communication with the muscle and mucosa. The extrinsic efferent and afferent innervation terminates in the ENS; some extrinsic afferents (not illustrated here; see Fig. 6) serve the gut mucosa and bypass the enteric nervous system.

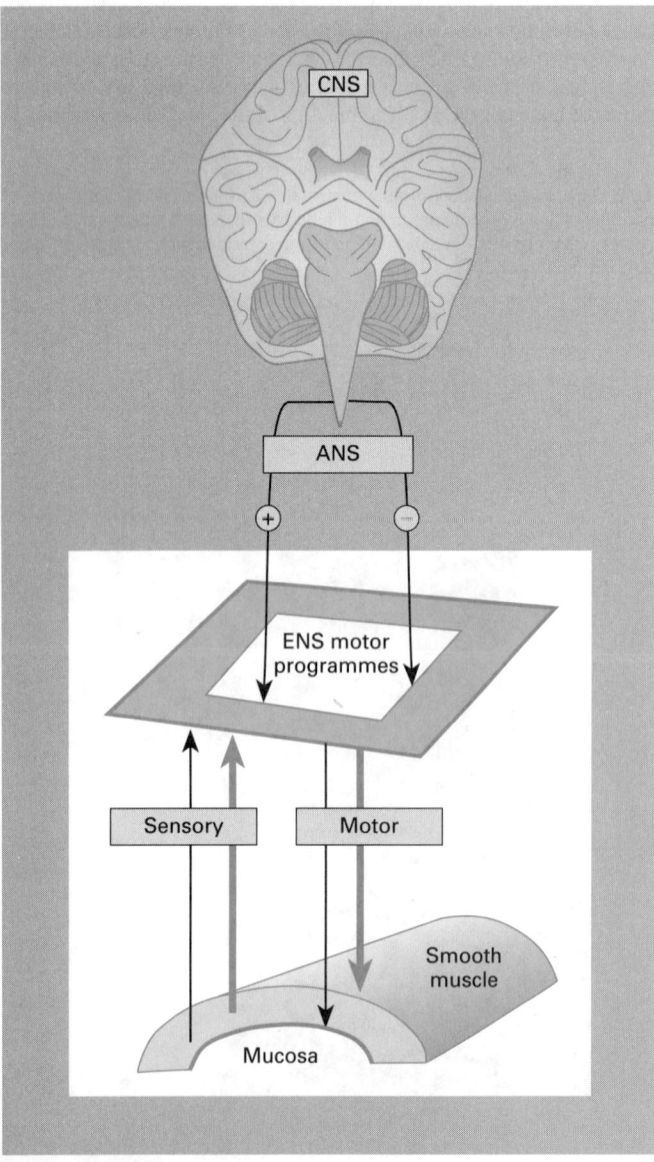

geon, who documented intermittent but recurring—or periodic—motor and secretory activity in the stomach and duodenum of fasting, conscious dogs. These observations were soon forgotten and remained so until 1969, when Szurszewski elegantly demonstrated the migrating myoelectric (or motor) complex (**MMC**) in fasting dogs. In 1975, Marlett and Code showed that, on feeding, the periodic MMC activity of the stomach and duodenum is replaced by a different pattern of apparently irregular contractions that persist until gastric emptying of nutrient is complete (Fig. 5). Within the next few years, several investigators confirmed the presence of a similar phenomenon in man.

At any point in the distal stomach and small bowel, the periodic sequence of the MMC has three phases. Phase I is motor quiescence, followed by the irregular contractions of phase II. This is succeeded by a brief phase of regular contractions at the frequency of the slow wave—3/min in the human stomach and 11/min in the duodenum—that lasts for about 5 min, to be replaced once more by the quiescence of phase I. This stereotypical pattern appears to migrate down the bowel at a speed that is an order of magnitude slower than the rate of propagation of peristalsis. The same pattern is found in virtually all mammalian and avian species studied so far, but the disruption on feeding is confined to carnivores who eat discrete meals that are high in nutrient density.

In dog and man under laboratory conditions the period of the MMC is remarkably constant, but this is not so in humans who are normally mobile and active. Sleep and stress are important modulating factors of the biorhythm. It is now clear that the MMC biorhythm is generated within the enteric nervous system; the contribution of the extrinsic innervation is to modulate the period of the MMC and its constituent phases.

Extrinsic innervation has one other important function. The arrival of food in the gut is signalled by stimulation of duodenal chemoreceptors. These chemoreceptors are, however, vagal, and therefore the signal that food has arrived is conveyed by a vagovagal reflex pathway through the dorsal motor complex in the brain-stem. In this scheme, both ipsilateral and contralateral vagi are effectively acting as sensory neurones for the programming function of the enteric nervous system (Fig. 6). It is, therefore, scarcely surprising that the major functional impairment resulting from truncal vagotomy in man is an inappropriate motor response to food, but during the era when this was a common procedure for the treatment of chronic duodenal ulcer, the sensory contribution of the vagus was not known.

One important consequence of emerging importance on the enteric rather than central control of the motor function of the gut is that the transplanted gut contains a functioning control system, which rapidly adapts to a new host.

Fig. 5 Schematic illustration of periodic fasting motor activity in the proximal gut (above) and its interruption on feeding (below). For explanation of the phases of the MMC, see text.

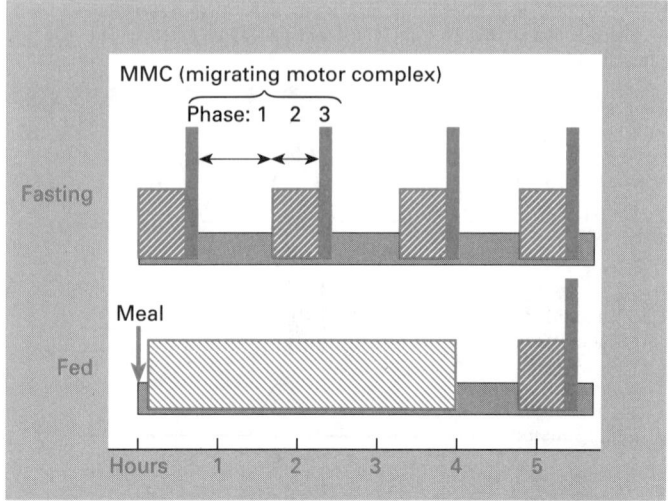

REGIONAL INTEGRATED ACTIVITY

Oesophagus

The swallowing reflex is initiated and controlled by the central nervous system. When the swallowed bolus has passed the striated muscle structure of the oropharynx, upper sphincter, and proximal oesophagus, the peristaltic activity is propagated onwards through the smooth muscle of the lower two-thirds of the oesophagus; as it arrives at the cardia, the lower sphincter relaxes.

Stomach

With the arrival of food, the stomach relaxes (receptive relaxation), and its tone gradually decreases to accommodate the ingesta, which are stored in the proximal stomach. The process of gastric emptying is not completely understood, but appears to depend upon the proximal stomach acting both as a reservoir and a pressure head that fill the antrum. Regular contractions, starting in the mid stomach, sweep through the distal stomach to the pylorus; some of the antral contents escape through

the pylorus, but the remainder, including all solid particles of more than 5 mm in diameter are retropelled back into the proximal stomach. This mechanical retropulsion in a chemical medium that contains acids and pepsin gradually breaks down (trituration) all digestible solids. Any remaining indigestible solid that is not broken down is emptied from the stomach by the first fasting MMC. In diabetic gastroparesis, when trituration is inadequate and fasting MMCs are absent, retained solids accumulate to form bezoars.

Small intestine

The average transit time through the small bowel is approximately 3 h and is similar during fasting and postprandial states. Following food, however, activity is not periodic and flow is therefore continuous and gradual; contractions are more frequent and vigorous than during phase II of the MMC and serve to mix the contents with pancreatobiliary secretions. The intensity and frequency of contractile activity is neurally modulated, with vagal receptors responding to the chemical content and receptors of the enteric nervous system responding to the physical qualities such as viscosity and the particle content.

Colon

The colon is a large elongated cavity where the content, being semisolid, moves slowly. The normal motor patterns of the colon are not clearly defined; there is general agreement on only two phenomena. First, during sleep, the colon appears to enter a state of almost total motor quiescence, unlike the stomach and small bowel, which exhibit marked periodicity. Secondly, while most colonic motor events do little to move the contents, infrequent (two to four per day) high-pressure contractions traverse the entire colon; these correspond to the mass movements seen by radiologists, and result in a considerable redistribution of the contents, sometimes including rectal filling. Feeding may serve as a stimulus to the large, propagated contractions, and it also induces an increase in local segmenting motor activity (the gastrocolonic response). The arrival of stool in the rectum stimulates the defaecatory reflex, with relaxation of the internal sphincter; in social animals and man, continence is maintained for a time by the external sphincter alone; if a suitable opportunity for defaecation presents, the rectum will be voided.

Abnormal motility

The classification of motility disorders is, in the present state of knowledge, a problem. Disorders of motility become apparent because of the abnormal propulsion, or lack of propulsion, of ingesta and/or secretions rather than from symptoms arising from focal lesions of the neuromuscular apparatus of the digestive tract. The pathological basis of some motility disorders remains to be clarified; further, it is even uncertain to what extent some syndromes, currently labelled as 'functional', are primarily disorders of motility.

As there is no agreed taxonomy for these disorders, it seems reasonable to divide them into primary disorders caused by specific nerve or muscle dysfunction, and secondary disorders where derangements of motility are incidental to systemic disease. According to this scheme, primary disorders have been classified according to the disturbance of transit—delayed, retrograde, or accelerated—that they present, while secondary disorders have been classified in terms of the underlying systemic pathology.

Investigation

At the present time, the methods available for the investigation of motility disorders are largely directed at documenting disorders of transit. Techniques for the direct evaluation of the neuromuscular system of the digestive tract are, for the greater part, not yet developed to the point where they yield reliable and reproducible information, and they remain in the domain of the research worker. With the exception of oesophageal disorders, standard protocols of investigation have not been established,

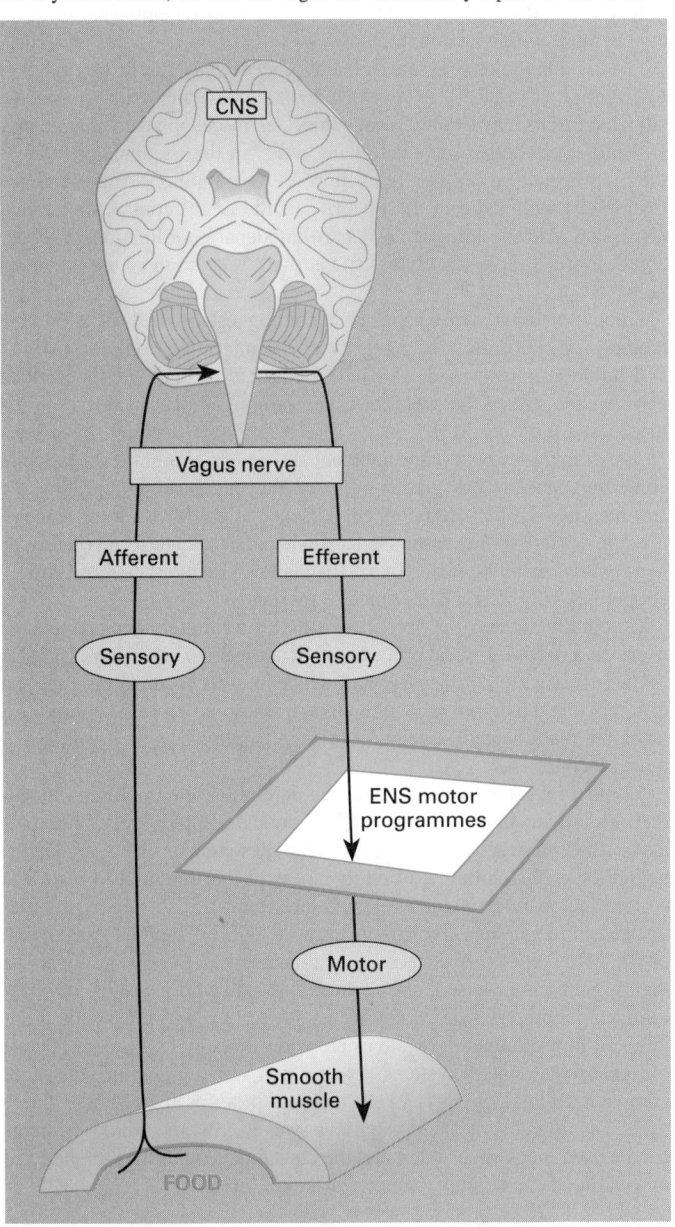

Fig. 6 The enteric response to feeding is mediated by sensory information received by vagal afferents and conveyed to the programming network of the enteric nervous system (ENS) by the vagovagal route. In transmitting this sensory information, the efferent vagus acts as a sensory input into the ENS.

and some of the methods that are likely to become established—such as proximal small-bowel manometry—are not yet widely available. The application of the techniques that are described will therefore depend not only on the clinical judgement of the physician, but all the resources that are available.

RADIOLOGY

Except in the oesophagus, where a barium swallow is often diagnostic of a motility disorder, conventional gastrointestinal radiology is often unhelpful, and a 'normal barium meal' or 'normal barium enema' by no means excludes a motility disorder. As has been pointed out, the motor activity of the digestive tract is markedly altered in the presence of food. Barium sulphate is not a nutrient, and the transit of barium through the digestive tract is dissimilar from the transit of food, except in the oesophagus. Barium radiology is effective in the observation of oesophageal motility because there is no difference in the oesophageal transit of barium bolus from the transit of a nutrient bolus; the swallowing reflex activated in each case is identical. Distally, conventional barium radiology may yield some clues: a stomach that still contains significant residue after the normal period of fasting usually indicates delayed gastric emptying, and it is sometimes possible to suggest from the rate of transit of barium that the transit of food and secretions may be abnormal. Gastro-oesophageal reflux may be demonstrated radiologically, but failure to demonstrate reflux may reflect technical failure on the part of the radiologist rather than the absence of reflux in the patient.

The admixture of contrast media with food, originally used by Cannon to study gastric emptying, is disliked by radiologists because the mucosal pattern is impaired, but this is the simplest relevant technique for the study of motility disorders. Barium sulphate can be incorporated into food during preparation, as a 'bariumburger', or more simply, the patient can be asked to take sips of barium sulphate between mouthfuls of food. Given close collaboration between physician and radiologist, the 'nutrient barium meal' can be a useful diagnostic procedure.

The investigation of the progress of the solid phase of a meal without conventional fluid radiographic contrast media has been done by using solid radiopaque markers, usually small pieces of plastic into which barium sulphate has been incorporated. These are most valuable for studying colonic transit. In the presence of normal gastric emptying and small-intestinal transit, it is reasonable to assume that all the opaque markers eaten with a meal will have passed into the colon after 6 to 8 h. Subsequent radiological study of their distribution may give useful information about colonic stasis or accelerated transit. Essentially similar information but which avoids exposing the patient to ionizing radiation can be obtained by making radiographs of all stool samples subsequent to marker ingestion until all the markers have been recovered.

The importance of radiology in the investigation of motility disorders resides more in the fact that the services are widely available than on its intrinsic value. While conventional examinations with contrast media may be unhelpful, particularly if the radiologist has not been clearly informed of the clinical problem, the intelligent use of radiology and the application of some ingenuity may yield a diagnosis as precise as that which can be obtained by more refined techniques.

MANOMETRY

Manometric techniques, until recently largely within the domain of the research worker, are of increasing importance in clinical practice. In general, clinical manometric techniques depend upon transducers that can transform applied pressure into an electrical signal. Originally, the size of transducers dictated their use external to the body, with pressure being transmitted to them from through a tube perfused with fluid with an open tip in the cavity of the digestive tract. Multiple perfused-tube assemblies allow pressure changes to be recorded simultaneously from several sites, but such systems have two disadvantages. Perfused-tube

systems introduced through the nose or mouth are uncomfortable, and the mobility of the patient is restricted because of the need to stay tethered to the infusion system. Miniaturization of strain-gauge transducers allows them to be incorporated in fine-bore flexible catheters, similar in size and pliability to enteric feeding tubes, and these are readily tolerated for hours or days. The use of digital electronics allows pressure data to be captured, if required, on miniature portable dataloggers for subsequent downloading to desktop computers, and such systems can be used either in the controlled conditions of the clinical laboratory or on ambulant subjects pursuing their normal activities.

Discrete sensors, such as the open tips of perfused tubes, or miniature strain gauges, are only accurate when the wall pressure results in occlusion of the lumen; they are thus useful in the oesophagus, small intestine, and—theoretically—within sphincter zones. They give little or no indication of pressure change in large, hollow cavities such as the stomach or colon, where fluid-filled balloons connected to external transducers must be used. Within the sphincter zones of the oesophagus and pylorus, discrete sensors attached to catheters are easily dislodged; this problem has been overcome by locating the sensors within elongated, fluid-filled sleeves, such the Dent sleeve.

Oesophageal manometry using multiple sensors is the 'gold standard' for the diagnosis of disordered oesophageal motility but is, in practice, rarely required because radiology has usually provided a diagnosis, and is readily available. This situation is changing as oesophageal manometry is more widely available.

Gastric manometry as an isolated procedure is rarely helpful, but observation of motility in a selected region together with that in the adjacent viscus may be of clinical value. Gastro-oesophageal manometry will indicate whether the swallowing reflex in the oesophagus induces the appropriate receptive relaxation in the fundus. Antroduodenal manometry will indicate the integrity of the antral contractile mechanism, and also the integrity of gastro-duodenal coordination, whereby antral contraction is closely associated with relaxation of the duodenal bulb.

Duodenojejunal manometry is becoming established as a reliable method for confirming the integrity of the migrating complex (MMC) and its abolition by food. The new electronic technologies, described above, have solved the problem of the prolonged observation required to observe multiple MMC cycles, preferably over a period of at least 18 h that includes both a normal meal and a normal night's sleep, while computer analysis has greatly reduced the labour of interpreting the complex records that are obtained. Absence of the MMC, or absence of the appropriate motor response to food, indicate enteric myopathy or neuropathy; again, it seems likely that as this procedure is more widely adopted, it will increase in clinical importance.

Colonic manometry is not, at the time of writing, either practical or useful as a routine clinical procedure, but anorectal manometry is helpful in the investigation of faecal incontinence in order to study the function of internal and external anal sphincters; it is also an essential component of biofeedback systems, which have been employed in the treatment of faecal incontinence.

Clinical investigators should not be deterred from employing manometry by the technical refinements and arcane complexities of interpretation that preoccupy research workers. Research projects demand a degree of precision that is often in excess of that required to resolve a simple diagnostic point; absolute pressure values are not needed in order to determine whether a normal pattern of motility such as swallowing or the MMC exists. A decade ago, clinicians had to rely on apparatus that might be improvised, or borrowed from the cardiovascular or physiological laboratory, which may well serve to resolve a diagnostic problem, but now commercial systems are widely available. The capital cost of modern manometry systems remains high, although in line with other computer technology, it is likely to fall rapidly as it becomes widely used. The unit cost of manometry is, however, low; the sensing systems can be used many times over, and the consumable materials, in the form of alkaline batteries and computer diskettes, are cheap.

RADIONUCLIDES

The problems of observing the transit of ingesta with radiology include the fact that contrast media do not resemble food, and also the radiation hazards of observation over long periods of time. Radionuclides, which can be incorporated in tracer quantities into palatable meals, offer an answer to the first problem, while imaging techniques using a γ-camera scan allow detailed observation over prolonged periods of time. The current disadvantage of these techniques is the poor resolution of the image in comparison with radiology, and the difficulty of reconstructing continuous movements from serial scans.

Radionuclides offer the best available method of studying gastric emptying at the present time. Considerable ingenuity has been employed in developing methods of incorporating isotopes into food to ensure that the isotope remains with the solid phase of the meal. The technique now widely employed for assessing the emptying of solids is a meal consisting of scrambled eggs to which technetium sulphur colloid has been added before cooking. Liquid emptying relies on an isotope such as indium or labelled DPTA added to a drink, and with appropriate scintiscanning equipment, double isotope studies can assess solid and liquid emptying at the same time. Scintiscanning is the current method of choice for the evaluation of gastric emptying, and is now most often used for the detection of diabetic gastroparesis and for the study of postsurgical problems.

Radionuclides have been used to study all levels of the digestive tract. The isotopic measurement of oesophageal clearance has become possible with the refinement of scanning and computer analysis techniques, although it remains to be seen whether the diagnostic yield is improved in comparison with contrast radiology and manometry. Small-bowel transit can also be studied using isotopes, but the length and convolution of the small bowel do not allow for anything less than major disturbances of transit to be studied; the same is true of the colon. One problem is common to all radionuclide investigations, which is the biohazard of ionizing radiations.

BREATH TESTS

Breath tests have the attraction of providing a non-invasive method of studying intestinal transit. All of them are based upon the principle that transformation of ingested nutrients by colonic flora will release gases that can be detected in expired air, either as hydrogen from non-absorbed carbohydrates or labelled carbon dioxide from lipids or bile acids labelled with ^{13}C or ^{14}C. These tests are used to measure orocaecal transit; alternatively, the labelled substrate can be introduced by gavage at a selected level of the gut. Clinical equipment for the measurement of breath hydrogen down to a level of 1 part/10^6 in end-expiratory breath samples is now commercially available. Care is required to eliminate sources of error such as exercise, smoking, and hydrogen production by oral bacterial flora. These techniques have proved to be useful in the physiological assessment of small-bowel transit time, but their value in clinical practice is limited, because when motility is disordered, invasion of the small bowel by colonic flora is common, and will result in spurious assumptions of rapid transit from the results of a breath test.

ENDOSCOPY

The introduction of fibreoptic endoscopy, which has proved so fruitful in the accurate diagnosis of mucosal lesions in the digestive tract, has little to offer in the study of motility. This is hardly surprising, as the muscle and nerve of the digestive tract are out of sight, and beyond the reach of the biopsy forceps; moreover, the premedication required for endoscopy, and the need for a void viscus, mean that the movements observed through an endoscope do not correspond to normal physiology. Endoscopy has a limited place in determining the degree of damage due to refluxed secretions; endoscopic biopsy is a useful diagnostic adjunct in confirming the presence of oesophagitis due to refluxed gastric acid, and gastritis due to refluxed bile. Endoscopic visualization of bile reflux is not diagnostic, as a degree of bile reflux is physiological, but its appearance should prompt the endoscopist to biopsy the antral mucosa. Endoscopic diagnosis of hiatus hernia and pyloric stenosis is possible, but dynamic tests of function are required in order to determine whether the lesion that has been seen is of functional importance.

Published studies have shown that it is dangerous to rely on endoscopy in the diagnosis of oesophageal dysmotility; in particular, achalasia of the cardia is easily missed, as in less advanced cases, the oesophageal body is not dilated or filled with fluid residue, nor is the lower sphincter markedly spastic. The author is not alone in having experience of patients referred following unsuccessful fundoplication for 'reflux' who have proved to be suffering from achalasia.

ELECTROMYOGRAPHY

Gastrointestinal electromyography is widely used in motility research in animals and should, in theory, offer a definitive means of investigation of motility disorders. This is not the case, because of the difficulty of placing sensors in relation to the smooth muscle, and because of the complexity of the recorded signal. In clinical practice, manometry offers a much simpler method of obtaining analogous information about muscle contraction. There are rare cases of gastrointestinal myopathy and neuropathy in which electromyography might be regarded as definitive, and it is possible that the range of such disorders will increase with advancing knowledge. Electromyography of the sigmoid colon has been alleged to be of value in the diagnosis of the irritable bowel syndrome, but the electromyographic abnormalities that have been reported are not always present in all cases with characteristic symptoms, and the putative abnormalities can only be detected by the application of sophisticated methods of computer analysis. For the present, electromyography rests firmly in the domain of the specialist research worker.

NON-INVASIVE ASSESSMENT OF GASTRIC FUNCTION

As indicated above, dynamic assessment of gastric motor function presents problems; manometry is not helpful, and scintigraphy assesses only the rate of emptying. Three techniques are of current interest, and may well make a significant impact on clinical diagnosis in the near future.

Ultrasonographic scanning

Ultrasound imaging has rapidly improved in quality, and it is now possible to obtain clear rapid sequential images of the antrum and pylorus under physiological conditions.

Electrical impedance

The impedance to a high-frequency current passed through the abdomen from surface electrodes will depend upon the fluid content of the stomach, and the change in impedance following a standard fluid load with an ionic content that differs from extracellular fluid can be continuously monitored from a pair (impedance epigastrography, IE) or an array (applied potential tomography, APT) of surface electrodes to give an estimate of gastric emptying. Equipment for these techniques is available, but their utility is hampered by the difficulty of obtaining a clear signal, particularly in obese patients. However, they can be valuable in the investigation of neonates, where more invasive methods are not acceptable.

Electrogastrography (EGG)

Because gastrointestinal smooth muscle has, like cardiac muscle, the properties of a rhythmic syncytium, the detection of the electrical signal by remote electrodes on the body surface has been the target of research for many years. In general, this is not possible because the convolutions of the different regions of the gut lack a strong vector that would allow remote detection. This is less true of the stomach, and, in recent years there has been some success with the technique of electrogastrography; active skin electrodes and Fourier transforms of the signal enable the fundamental frequencies to be detected. There is a clear link between gastric dysrhythmias (tachygastria and bradygastria) and nausea from any cause (including motion sickness and pregnancy). The technology for clinical measurement is now available; its value in diagnosis remains to be established.

Primary disorders of motility

Retrograde transit (reflux)

GASTRO-OESOPHAGEAL REFLUX DISEASE (GORD)

Reflux of gastric juice, containing hydrochloric acid and pepsin, into the oesophagus causes pain and damage to the mucosal squamous epithelium. This is the most common primary disorder of motility in Europe and North America. GORD is common in the presence of a hiatus hernia (the protrusion of the proximal stomach through the diagphragmatic hiatus into the chest (Fig. 7)), but may also occur without any apparent anatomical displacement. The association of a hiatus hernia with reflux is evidence that the sphincteric mechanism which normally prevents reflux is not only due to the action of the intrinsic lower oesophageal sphincter, but also to the normal anatomical relation of oesophagus, cardia, and proximal stomach.

Symptomatic reflux usually involves the association of two factors, hiatus hernia and obesity. It may occur in the absence of hiatus hernia, especially in the obese; conversely, a non-obese subject with a radiologically demonstrable hiatus hernia is often free of symptomatic reflux. Both duodenal ulcer and cholelithiasis are said to be associated with an increased degree of reflux, as is smoking.

The clinical features and management of GORD are discussed in Chapter 14.6

Delayed transit

OESOPHAGEAL SPASM (SEE ALSO CHAPTER 14.6)

Oesophageal spasm is caused by spontaneous, non-propagated contraction of the oesophageal smooth muscle. Asymptomatic abnormal con-

tractions are sometimes found by chance in elderly patients undergoing a barium meal; but, in other patients, oesophageal spasm presents with dysphagia or pain, or both. The diagnosis can usually be made with a barium swallow, when the bolus of barium is seen to travel normally only as far as the smooth-muscle segment of the oesophagus; thereafter, it may be delayed, occluded or compressed by a number of ring contractions ('corkscrew oesophagus') (Fig. 8). Abnormal contractions may sometimes be seen during fibreoptic endoscopy. If the abnormality is not severe and is intermittent, oesophageal manometry is the investigation of choice. Ambulant monitoring of oesophageal pressure over 24 h may be required to detect the abnormality. As with GORD (see above), angina pectoris is an important differential diagnosis.

The condition is largely unresponsive to treatment, and prognosis is variable. Some patients benefit from glyceryl trinitrate sublingually for the relief of pain arising from the spasm; others may benefit from calcium-channel antagonists such as nifedipine. In some patients, progression to the characteristic syndrome of achalasia has been reported, but this is probably due an incorrect initial diagnosis.

ACHALASIA (SEE ALSO CHAPTER 14.6)

Achalasia is chronic and progressive obstruction to the passage of contents through the lower oesophageal sphincter. The cause is degeneration of the ganglion cells of the myenteric plexus, or vagal nuclei, and the major pathophysiological consequence is failure of relaxation of the sphincter; although the resting pressure of the lower oesophageal sphincter may be mildly elevated, the previous term 'cardiospasm' is somewhat misleading. The pathology also effects the rest of the smooth-muscle portion of the oesophagus; as a consequence, peristalsis is usually weak and uncoordinated. The condition usually presents in adults but it can occur in childhood. The aetiology is unknown except in Latin America, where achalasia may be one manifestation of Chagas' disease (see Section 7). Rarely, achalasia may be the presenting manifestation of a diffuse enteric neuropathy that will progress to chronic intestinal pseudo-obstruction.

The condition presents as dysphagia, sometimes associated with pain, occurring both with fluids and with solids. A barium swallow will reveal

Fig. 8 Oesophageal spasm, shown here with the classic radiological appearance of 'corkscrew oesophagus'. Instead of proceeding as a smooth bolus, the barium column in indented by a series of ring contractions. (Reproduced by courtesy of Dr Kreel.)

Fig. 7 Hiatus hernia, shown in this case by the presence of the gastric air bubble within the thoracic cavity. The anatomical distortion of the gastro-oesophageal junction impairs the resistance to reflux, which cannot be maintained by the intrinsic lower gastro-oesophageal sphincter.

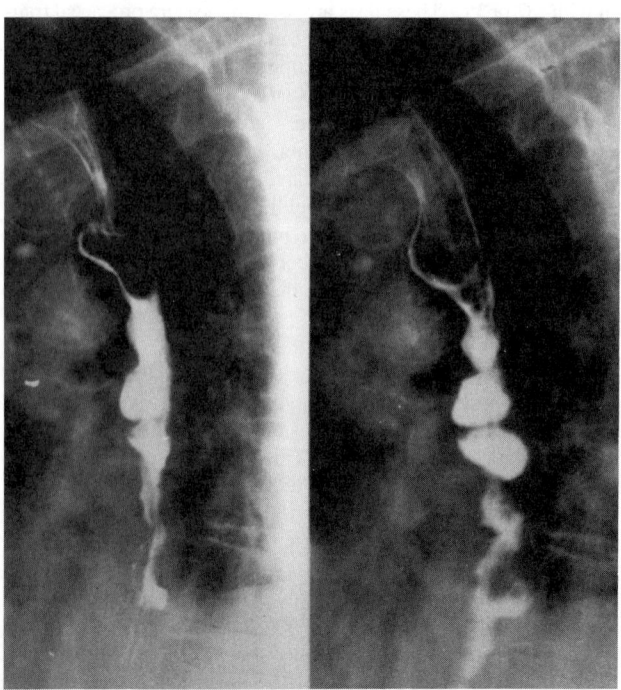

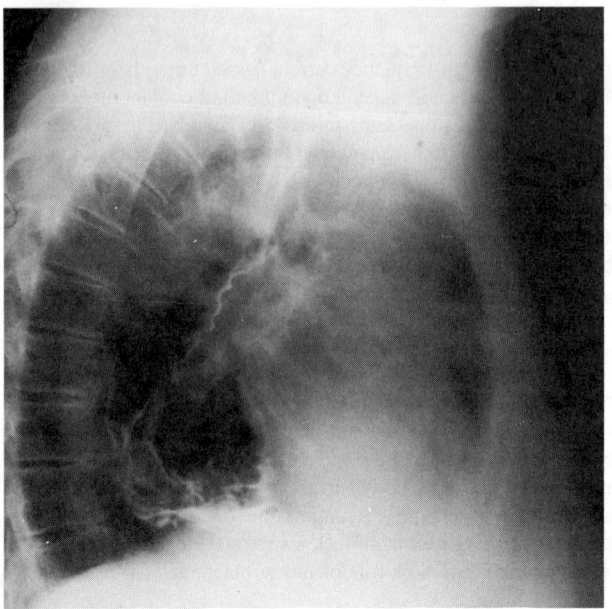

failure of the sphincter to relax and, additionally, disordered peristalsis on swallowing in the distal oesophagus. The oesophagus becomes dilated and elongated, and acts as a reservoir of unassimilated nutrient (Fig. 9). Spillage from this reservoir into the airway may result in aspiration pneumonia, which is one (uncommon) presentation of achalasia. In the early stages of the disease, impaired peristalsis reduces the oesophageal clearance of physiological acid reflux, so that what would otherwise be transient episodes of reflux are prolonged, leading to symptoms of GORD.

Oesophagoscopy may reveal a dilated oesophagus, usually containing retained food, but the endoscope will traverse the lower oesophageal sphincter, showing that the obstruction is not a true organic stenosis. Manometry is diagnostic and will demonstrate the failure of relaxation. Because a tissue deprived of its autonomic nerve supply is unduly sensitive to the missing neurotransmitter, the diagnosis may be confirmed by the administration of small doses of methacholine (5–10 mg subcutaneously) during manometry, which will, in the achalasic patient, induce powerful, prolonged, and sometimes painful contractions of the oesophageal body, but with improved manometric techniques, such tests are now largely of historical interest only.

The condition is progressive and the degenerative process is unresponsive to treatment. Therefore, therapy must be directed to mechanical relief of the functional obstruction. The majority of patients will obtain lasting relief from forcible dilation of the lower oesophageal sphincter by bouginage or, more commonly, pneumatic dilation, presumably because the procedure ruptures significant numbers of muscle fibres. The success rate of dilatation is such that only a minority of patients will require surgery. Heller's operation, a longitudinal myotomy with preservation of the mucosa, is the most successful procedure; radical destruction of the sphincter is to be avoided because of the subsequent postoperative reflux and oesophagitis. One problem which follows surgery is that it greatly increases the risk of oesophageal rupture during subsequent dilatation. With failure of the lower oesophageal sphincter, any procedure designed to ease the antegrade passage of food will also increase the retrograde passage of gastric acid, and therefore the long-term management of achalasic patients is similar to the management of GORD, with appropriate advice on posture and maintenance administration of acid-suppressing medication.

Apart from the pulmonary complications of achalasia, carcinoma of the distal oesophagus is a late, and rare, complication.

Fig. 9 Achalasia of the cardia, showing gross dilation of the oesophagus, which is filled with food debris. (Reproduced by courtesy of Dr Kreel.)

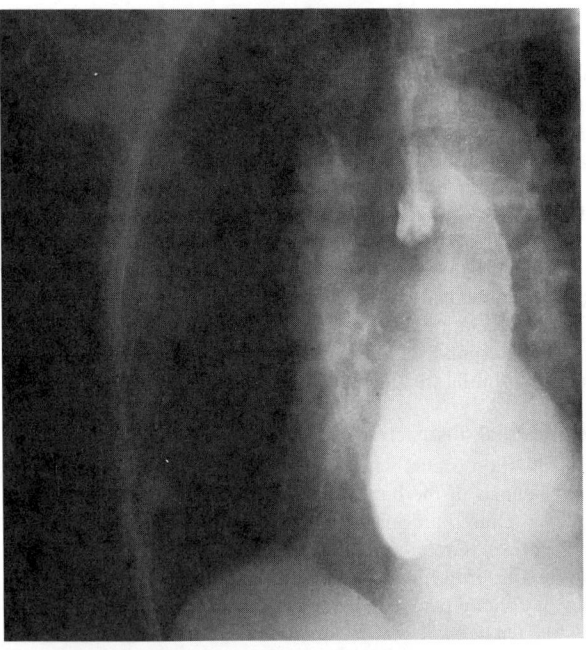

GASTRIC STASIS (IDIOPATHIC GASTROPARESIS)

Gastric stasis may be caused by mechanical obstruction, or more commonly it may be a sequel of abdominal surgery; it can also be caused by autonomic neuropathy. These secondary disorders of motility are discussed below. Gastric stasis can, however, also occur as a primary motility disorder, when it is known as idiopathic gastroparesis. The cause, incidence, and nature of this disorder remain matters of controversy. Idiopathic gastroparesis presents with symptoms of gastric stasis, mainly postprandial epigastric discomfort and distension, nausea, and vomiting. If, in such patients, investigation reveals: (a) delayed emptying of solids and liquids with scintigraphy; (b) hypomotility of the gastric antrum with manometry; (c) normal motor function in the rest of the digestive tract; or (c) absence of any associated systemic disease; then most physicians would concur with a diagnosis of idiopathic gastroparesis.

Unfortunately, the diagnosis is often made without all of these conditions being fulfilled and, moreover, values for the normal range of function with scintigraphy and manometry have not been agreed; this accounts for the disparity between the reported incidence of this condition from different centres. Some investigators maintain that the condition can be diagnosed by the detection of gastric dysrhythmias in the presence of appropriate symptoms; others would suggest that the gastric dysrhythmias are no more than the physical correlate of nausea, and have little do with the function of emptying.

In the relatively few patients in whom the diagnosis can be made with confidence, the cause remains unknown, and therapy is often ineffective. 'Prokinetic' drugs such as metoclopramide and cisapride may produce some symptomatic improvement, and erythromycin (a motilin agonist as well as an antibacterial drug) is sometimes helpful. There are no reliable data on the natural history of this condition.

ADYNAMIC ILEUS

Acute and reversible motor failure of the whole bowel is a normal occurrence after major abdominal surgery, and is considered in more detail under the heading of postoperative ileus below. It also occurs, but much less frequently, after major traumatic injury, and in some states of metabolic imbalance; the principles of diagnosis and management are as for the postsurgical state.

CHRONIC IDIOPATHIC INTESTINAL PSEUDO-OBSTRUCTION (CIIP)

The label of chronic pseudo-obstruction includes a variety of rare disorders in which the patient presents, usually in childhood or early adult life, with the clinical features of subacute or acute intestinal obstruction, but in whom no actual obstruction can be found. The cause of pseudo-obstruction is an intrinsic disorder of function of the bowel, which is usually due to myopathy of the smooth muscle or neuropathy of the enteric nerves, or a combination of both. The disorder may be familial, and some varieties of pseudo-obstruction are associated with disorders of other smooth muscle, usually in the urinary tract. One of the more common presentations of this uncommon clinical problem is that of megaduodenum, which appears to be due to a localized neuropathy of the duodenum; duodenojejunostomy is indicated.

The rarity of pseudo-obstruction is such that the physician will always be relatively unfamiliar with the condition, and the lack of consistent pathology means that there is no established routine of investigation. Ingenuity and perseverance is required from the physician, as well as understanding from a patient who is resentful of having been dismissed previously as a malingerer or neurotic and who faces a lifetime of likely disability.

In severely affected patients, treatment is difficult and demanding, and usually requires close collaboration between physician and surgeon. In such patients, drugs intended to stimulate motility are rarely effective, because the pathophysiology is, in neuropathy, disordered rather than absent motility, while in myopathy the problem is a failure of the contractile apparatus of the smooth-muscle cells. Surgery should be avoided unless life is threatened or the bypass of a segment of bowel is clearly indicated. Bacterial overgrowth secondary to stasis leads to chronic malnutrition; antibacterial therapy with metronidazole or tetracycline may lead to temporary improvement. When stasis is severe, the patient may be unable to eat enough to avoid malnutrition. Nutritional support, either enterally—via an orojejunal feeding tube, gastrostomy, or enterostomy—or parenterally, may be required. When CIIP is less severe, and the sufferer can develop eating strategies that maintain nutrition and body weight, cisapride has been shown to produce short-term benefits in some of these patients.

Patients suffering from CIIP with evidence of significant obstruction are rare, but they may (or may not) be the tip of an iceberg. There are many more patients with symptoms of 'functional' disorders, often resembling the irritable bowel syndrome, who probably have neuropathy or myopathy of the bowel. In these patients, unlike those suffering from irritable bowel syndrome, manometry of the upper small bowel can reveal significant abnormalities suggesting malfunction or damage to the enteric nervous system or to the smooth muscle. To date, such patients have been little investigated, and are usually classified as having irritable bowel syndrome, albeit atypical. The increased use of manometry and the availability of laparoscopy to obtain full-thickness bowel biopsies that allow histopathological study of nerve and muscle will help to clarify the size of this problem.

SIMPLE CONSTIPATION (SEE CHAPTER 14.2.5.)

By definition, constipation implies delayed transit of faeces. In the absence of neuropathy (as in Chagas' disease and Hirschsprung's disease), or systemic disorders, such as myxoedema, there is no evidence that it is due to any local lesion in the colon, and it has, therefore, been considered as a functional or psychomotor disorder.

HIRSCHSPRUNG'S DISEASE

This is a localized neuropathy of the colorectum, in which there is an aganglionic segment that acts as an obstruction to the transit of faeces; proximal to the segment, the bowel is dilated. Surgery is indicated.

DIVERTICULAR DISEASE (CHAPTER 14.4)

This is not a motility disorder, but hypersegmentation of the colon has been implicated in the pathogenesis of this condition, and various histological abnormalities of smooth muscle have been reported.

Accelerated transit

INTESTINAL HURRY

Intestinal hurry is another ill-defined disorder of motility, in which the transit of ingesta through the small intestine is excessively rapid, too rapid to permit the normal assimilation of water and solute. The result is the delivery to the colon of an excess fluid and nutrient load, the latter being then subject to bacterial fermentation, which causes osmotic dilution; the outcome is diarrhoea.

The circumstances in which intestinal hurry occur are far from clear. Damage to the intrinsic innervation of the bowel as in diabetes, or to the extrinsic innervation as a sequel of vagotomy, are known factors. Another possibility is the persistence of powerful peristaltic activity, resembling the interdigestive migrating complex, in the postprandial phase.

The truth is that too little is yet known about this condition; at the present time, the physician will continue to encounter occasional cases of chronic 'motor diarrhoea', in which the only abnormality is excessively rapid transit of the intestine, or intestinal hurry. Until further light

is shed on this condition, specific therapy does not exist, and the only form of management is conventional antidiarrhoeal medication. This condition is sometimes labelled as one form of the 'irritable colon syndrome', but even though there may be a psychogenic component, the label is probably a misnomer.

RECTAL INCONTINENCE

Chronic faecal incontinence is a distressing disability, which may occur in the absence of anorectal disease. The primary disorder appears to be defective tonic contraction of the internal anal sphincter with defective compensation by the external sphincter, as shown by anorectal manometry. Various surgical procedures have been attempted in this condition, and the results have been variable.

A new approach to this procedure, pioneered in the United States, is treatment by biofeedback using 'operant conditioning'. With this technique, the pressure changes recorded on manometry are displayed to the patient on a visual display that also shows a normal manometric trace. The patient is encouraged to attempt to achieve a normal manometric pattern, and is able to compare his or her performance with the normal pattern. Where there is no associated organic disease or anatomical defect, a high rate of success is claimed for this technique by some.

Secondary disorders of motility

Associated with surgery

Many motility disorders are associated with surgery, either as presenting symptoms of structural disorders that require surgical relief, or as the sequelae of surgery of the digestive tract.

MECHANICAL OBSTRUCTION

Obstructed gastric outflow

Congenital hypertrophic pyloric stenosis is a congenital thickening of the pyloric smooth muscle, and usually presents as projectile vomiting, with constipation and weight loss, 10 days to 3 months after birth. The condition occurs in about 2/1000 live births and is four times as frequent in male infants. Physical signs may include visible gastric peristalsis and a palpable mass; barium radiography will show an elongated and symmetrically narrowed pylorus. The treatment is a surgical pyloromyotomy (Ramstedt's operation), after correction of nutritional and electrolyte deficiency.

Rare forms of congenital outflow of obstruction, such as duodenal bands or duodenal stenosis, may occur, and may not be diagnosed until early adult life, as the obstruction is usually less severe. These conditions are considered in more detail in Chapter 14.15.

Adult pyloric stenosis occurs as a late complication of chronic duodenal ulcer disease. It is characterized by vomiting, usually of copious amounts of food some hours after a meal, in an individual with a long history of ulcer disease; occasionally a history of dyspepsia may not be volunteered, as patients may have trained themselves to disregard 'indigestion'. The stenosis may be due entirely to long-standing fibrosis of the pylorus and duodenal bulb; more commonly it presents during a period of active ulceration, in which case there is an inflammatory component that will respond to conservative treatment. Even if there is a rapid response to initial treatment, surgery is inevitable.

Subacute intestinal obstruction

Subacute obstruction occurs when there is any condition which creates a functional stenosis of the bowel that falls short of complete obstruction. The usual causes are intrinsic obstruction, due to inflammatory disease of the bowel (Crohn's disease, tuberculosis) or extrinsic obstruction due to tumour or fibrous adhesions. The condition usually presents as episodes of colicky pain, sometimes associated with abdominal distension and vomiting. Localized tenderness may indicate the site of obstruction.

The diagnosis of subacute obstruction is not always simple. Any episode of abdominal pain in a patient at risk, such as a patient with known Crohn's disease, will give rise to the suspicion of subacute obstruction, but many of these episodes are not obstructive. The diagnosis of subacute obstruction is important; in the absence of any known predisposing cause, explanatory laparotomy is indicated, but conversely, it is important to prevent unnecessary exploration of patients with known enteric disease.

It is probably true (although unproved) that subacute obstruction is always accompanied by abnormal transit proximal to the site of obstruction. Careful radiology may indicate abnormal transit of contrast medium. Some have reported that manometry will reveal a gross disturbance of the normal pattern of motility proximal to the site of obstruction, where repeated bursts of powerful contractions are seen at intervals of a few minutes; it is these bursts that are presumably projected into the sensorium as pain. This is an example of one condition in which the increasing availability of diagnostic intestinal manometry may prove to be helpful.

FOLLOWING ABDOMINAL SURGERY

Postoperative ileus

Postoperative (or paralytic ileus) is a functional motor paralysis of the digestive tract. It is a neurogenic condition in which the normal electrical slow wave is present in the smooth muscle, but either, as in the colon, does not excite any action potentials or, as in the stomach or small bowel, is not associated with normal patterns of motor activity. The motor pathophysiology shows species variations: in some species, such as dog and rat, postoperative small-bowel motor activity is characterized by total motor inertia, but in man, periodic activity starts shortly after wound closure with a rapid sequence of MMCs that slows gradually

Fig. 10 Adynamic ileus of the small bowel, shown by dilated air-filled loops of bowel in this plain film taken in the supine posture. A few liquid levels were seen in an erect film taken at the same occasion. Severe degenerative changes in the spine and a calcified fibroid are also visible. (Reproduced by courtesy of Dr Kreel.)

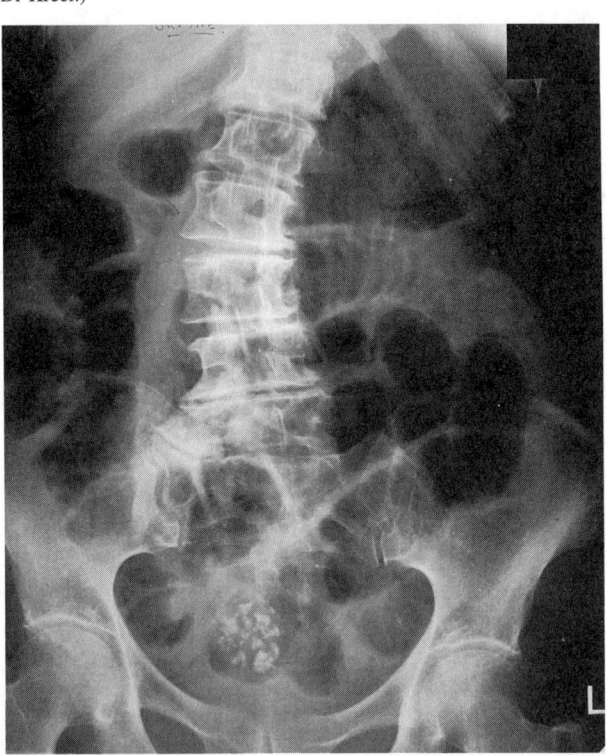

over the next 60 h. The human colon is inert after surgery, but motor activity returns to the stomach almost as rapidly as in the small bowel. But, although contractions are present, they are ineffective, and it is possible that a change in non-electrogenic tone is involved. The mechanism is thought to be adrenergic postsynaptic inhibition, possibly involving dopamine release, but adrenoceptor blockade or dopamine inhibition have not been shown to be therapeutically effective. The motor inhibition is triggered by a variety of stimuli including peritoneal inflammation, but much the most common cause is tactile stimulation of the bowel wall during surgery. It is an inevitable sequel of resection of the digestive tract, but is much diminished after abdominal procedures such as cholecystectomy in which the bowel remains intact. Minimally invasive abdominal surgery is accompanied by a marked diminution of postoperative ileus.

The signs of ileus are the apparent cessation of any motor activity: bowel sounds are absent, flatus is not passed, and there is consequent gastric stasis, which may lead to vomiting of accumulated secretions. The radiological appearances are diagnostic: a plain radiograph of the abdomen in the upright posture shows dilated loops of bowel with multiple fluid levels indicating distension with both fluid and gas (Fig. 10).

Treatment is conservative, as the condition is usually self-limiting. Recovery is hastened by the correction of any fluid or electrolyte imbalance, and by measures to 'defunction' the small bowel by aspirating gastric contents and administering fluid and nutrients by the parenteral route. Occasionally, the condition appears to be prolonged, and many drugs have been tried in an attempt to terminate prolonged ileus, but with little uniform success. Cisapride, a cholinergic agonist, has so far shown the most promising results with the fewest unwanted side-effects.

FOLLOWING SURGERY FOR PEPTIC ULCER DISEASE

The drastic reduction in the surgical treatment of peptic ulcer disease that has followed the introduction of the H_2-receptor antagonist drugs means that in the United Kingdom at least, the sequelae of ulcer surgery are now much less common, but even though few indigenous residents of the United Kingdom now develop such problems, the growth in migration from less-developed to more-developed regions of the world means that patients will present in the developed world suffering from the effects of treatment that is obsolete. The following group of disorders can result from different types of operation for peptic ulcer disease.

Gastric stasis

Non-obstructive gastric stasis is an expected sequel of section of the vagus nerve, and consequently occurs during the early postoperative period after a vagotomy. It rarely persists, as there is considerable functional adaptation after vagotomy.

Biliary gastritis

Experimentally, it has been shown that the gastric mucosa is damaged by bile acids, possibly due to their detergent action on the protective layer of mucus. It is also known that if the pylorus is a true sphincter, its major role is to prevent the reflux of duodenal contents into the antrum. Biliary gastritis may occur when the functional integrity of the pylorus as an antireflux barrier is compromised by surgery. Unfortunately, there are no histological features which, on light microscopy, distinguish the antrum damaged by bile from other forms of antral gastritis, although characteristic changes on scanning electron microscopy have been reported.

A diagnosis of biliary gastritis may reasonably be made when dyspeptic symptoms persist following vagotomy and pyloroplasty, provided that: (a) there is an antecedent history of gastric surgery; (b) active ulcer disease is excluded and biliary reflux is confirmed at endoscopy; (c) antral gastritis is confirmed on biopsy; and (d) gastric aspiration repeatedly confirms the presence of bile.

Treatment of biliary gastritis is difficult; antacids are often ineffective because the lesion is not acid induced. Medical treatment is a matter of trial and error: some cases will respond to antacids, some to carbenox-olone, and some to 'prokinetic' drugs such as metoclopramide or cisapride that are sometimes effective in improving gastric clearance and antroduodenal motor coordination. Some cases do not respond to medical treatment and, if this is the case, and the persistence of antral damage is confirmed, surgery may be indicated. A Roux-en-Y gastrojejunostomy is the operation of choice, and has shown to be an effective, if drastic treatment, if medical treatment has failed.

Gastric incontinence and the dumping syndrome

Gastric incontinence, or excessively rapid gastric emptying, is an uncommon sequel of gastric surgery that included a procedure to alter gastric drainage, usually pyloroplasty. The presence of gastric incontinence is indicated by manifestations of excessive input into the small bowel, of which the most common is the dumping syndrome. The syndrome of dumping includes postprandial weakness, sweating, flushing, and cramping abdominal pain. The mechanism is thought to be due both to the rapid delivery of hypertonic contents to the small intestine resulting in osmotic diminution of blood volume, and to disturbances of carbohydrate metabolism leading to excessive insulin activity. The problem is entirely food related and does not occur during fasting; consequently, it is best managed by the regulation of food intake. Small, frequent meals should be substituted for large, infrequent meals and carbohydrate intake should be reduced as it is the carbohydrate moiety of a meal that makes the greatest osmotic contribution. Recently, it has been shown that the addition of colloids, such as guar or pectin, to carbohydrate is also helpful in reducing the rate of effective delivery of carbohydrate to the small intestine.

The presence of a dumping syndrome is diagnostic of gastric incontinence, but if there is an associated motility disorder of the small bowel, as may occur after truncal vagotomy, gastric incontinence may lead to diarrhoea. Under these circumstances, further investigation of gastric emptying by methods outlined previously may be required; above all, the physician should remember that the rate of emptying of barium sulphate from the stomach may be a very poor, or even misleading, indicator of the rate of emptying of a meal.

Where the problem cannot be managed by the adoption of a different pattern of eating by the patient, or the use of food additives, further surgery may be indicated. Reversal of a segment of proximal intestine, in combination with a Roux-en-Y procedure, may be helpful, and it is likely that the success rate of this type of palliative surgery will increase as diagnostic techniques become more refined.

Associated with metabolic disease

DIABETES MELLITUS (SEE SECTION 11)

Disordered motility is encountered in diabetes mellitus as a consequence of autonomic neuropathy. The precise nature of the lesion has not been defined, but there are two types of disorder, which may coexist in the same patient.

Diabetic gastroparesis is delayed gastric emptying due to gastric atony. The prolonged retention of food may be diagnosed by radiology, or become apparent on endoscopy after normal fasting, and it may provoke vomiting in addition to abdominal distension and discomfort. Radiology reveals a dilated, hypotonic stomach with poor emptying. Radionuclide imaging shows delayed emptying of solids rather than liquids. Manometry shows diminished or absent postprandial antral contractions, and absence of phase III of the MMC during fasting. The reported incidence of diabetic gastroparesis depends upon whether impaired function or symptoms are used as the diagnostic criteria; it has been established that functional impairment in diabetics is common, with only a relatively small proportion of patients suffering from symptoms. In the past, metoclopramide and cisapride have been shown to be beneficial in some, but not all, symptomatic cases, but the improvement is usually temporary. More recently, erythromycin has emerged as an effective form of

therapy. There is now little doubt that poor diabetic control is contributory, leading to a vicious circle in which euglycaemia is difficult to achieve because of uncertain delivery of carbohydrate to the small bowel, thereby further aggravating the condition.

Diabetic diarrhoea is uncommon and is assumed to be due to autonomic denervation in the small bowel. It is characterized by intestinal atony, can be detected manometrically, and results in variable combinations of diarrhoea and steatorrhoea. There is no specific therapy for denervation, but as bacterial overgrowth of the small intestine may occur, antibacterial therapy sometimes affords a degree of relief.

THYROID DYSFUNCTION (SEE SECTION 12)

Diarrhoea may be one presenting feature of hyperthyroidism and, conversely, hypothyroidism is usually accompanied by constipation. It is assumed, on the basis of very little evidence, that these extremes are due to disordered motility, although altered smooth-muscle activity in thyroid disease has been demonstrated. Treatment is that of the underlying metabolic disorder. Given the incidence of these symptoms in the normal population, it must not be assumed that these symptoms are always a consequence of the disease, or that their occurrence should always provoke investigations of thyroid status.

ADRENAL INSUFFICIENCY (SEE SECTION 12)

Abdominal pain and vomiting form one presentation of adrenal insufficiency. Although it is not clear whether this is due to disordered motility, the assumption seems to be at least reasonable. The symptoms disappear with appropriate adrenocortical supplementation.

PORPHYRIA (SEE SECTION 11)

Autonomic neuropathy affecting gastrointestinal motor function may occur in porphyria, but there is no characteristic manifestation.

Associated with neurological disease (see also Section 24)

OROPHARYNGEAL DYSKINESIA

Under this heading may be grouped disorders of the voluntary muscles involved in swallowing. These include bulbar poliomyelitis and vascular disease of the brain-stem; both may lead to permanent impairment. Myasthenia gravis is an important cause of oropharyngeal dyskinesia, because of the risk of aspiration pneumonia. Disordered swallowing also characterizes the early recovery phase after cerebrovascular accidents.

PARKINSON'S DISEASE

A large proportion of patients with Parkinson's disease suffer from motor impairment of the gut, usually in the form of constipation, but sometimes affecting swallowing. These are often attributed (and sometimes justifiably) to the unwanted side-effects of therapy for the underlying disease, but as Loewy bodies have been identified in the oesophagus and the colon, it is likely that the enteric nervous system is also directly affected by the disease.

Associated with pathogens

CHAGAS' DISEASE (SEE SECTION 7)

Chagas' disease is caused by the protozoan *Trypanosoma cruzii*, the vector being a beetle. It is endemic in parts of South American, affecting poverty-stricken people in particular, as it is the barefoot and those who sleep on the ground who get bitten. Infection also occurs through transfusion with blood from an infected donor. The parasite has a predilection for smooth-muscle regions, but it is the digestive tract that is particularly affected. The result of infection is a cellular-type immune response. T lymphocytes are sensitized by antigens from the parasite and cross-react with antigens on enteric neurones. The result is destruction of the myenteric plexuses and the disease is characterized by various manifestations of denervation; achalasia of the cardia, chronic pseudo-obstruction, and colon may occur independently or in combination. Although clinical evaluation suggests that the small bowel is relatively spared in the disease, manometry of the small bowel has confirmed abnormal fasting motor activity. Once denervation has occurred, treatment consists only of palliative surgery; current therapeutic efforts are directed toward the development of an effective prophylactic vaccine.

ACUTE INFECTIOUS DIARRHOEA

Acute infectious diarrhoea is usually considered to be the consequence of impaired absorption and/or increased net secretion in the bowel, with altered motor activity as a consequence rather than a cause. One recent study of patients with acute salmonellosis has shown markedly deranged motor activity in the jejunum, suggesting that pathogen-induced, abnormal propulsive activity may be implicated. The spasms of colic experienced by patients who have managed to treat the secretory state with opiate antidiarrhoeal drugs may have a similar origin, as these drugs do not induce similar symptoms in non-infectious diarrhoeas.

Associated with connective tissue disease

SCLERODERMA (SEE SECTION 18)

The digestive tract may be affected in scleroderma (progressive systemic sclerosis). The regions most commonly affected are the oesophagus and small intestine, where replacement of smooth muscle by collagen, and destruction of autonomic nerves may occur. These lesions may result in failure of oesophageal peristalsis, leading to dysphagia, and an adynamic small intestine in which bacterial overgrowth may occur. Manometry of the small intestine has shown diminished or absent MMC activity in affected intestine.

Associated with malignancy (see Section 6)

DIFFUSE NEUROPATHY

Diffuse neuropathy, presenting as pseudo-obstruction, has been described in association with malignancies.

RADIATION ENTERITIS

Damage to the bowel from radiotherapy affects all tissues; nerve and muscle damage has been demonstrated in animal models. Radiation damage usually presents as diarrhoea, but obstructive symptoms are also common.

Functional and psychomotor disturbances of motility

Functional disorders of the digestive tract constitute the most frequent conditions confronting physicians. Their classification as motility disorders is not, for the greater part, based on scientific grounds but simply because the presenting symptoms suggest a disturbance of motility, or manifest themselves, as in vomiting, by an actual disorder of function.

The psychogenic nature of some of these complaints is also, for the most part, an unverified assumption. Yet the assumption does not appear to be without justification for, of the major functions of the digestive tract—secretion, absorption and motility—it is motility that is modulated from moment to moment in accordance with the function of the whole individual, and it is motility that is dominated by neural control. The 'brain–gut axis', although still largely unexplored, is not a scientific myth. The stressful effect of emotional and social life, as well as overt psychiatric illness, produce dysfunction in all systems of the body, as somatic pain, migraine, asthma for example. The digestive tract is no exception and it appears to be motility that is the gastrointestinal function which is most susceptible to stress, psychiatric illness and, most commonly, unhappiness.

These considerations mean that the physician who wishes to deal effectively with the majority of patients presenting with apparent dysfunction of the digestive tract must understand that many of these symptoms are manifestations of unsuccessful adaptation to the demands of life. Successful management of these patients includes some common principles.

A careful history

Gastrointestinal diagnosis depends little on physical signs of disease, but very largely on an accurate history, which should not only consist of an enumeration of symptoms, but also the chronology of the illness (periodicity, duration, association with environment, and activity) and also some consideration of the psychosocial aspects of the patient's life.

A positive diagnosis

Many patients with functional disorders fear that they are suffering from some serious disease, usually malignancy. It is important that the physician make a positive diagnosis, and not a diagnosis by exclusion. The attitude of 'well, we've done all the tests that we can think of and we can't find anything wrong' is not reassuring to the patient, who may well assume that the diagnostic routine omitted a crucial test. Once sure that the problem is indeed functional (and a long history of symptoms combined with manifest physical well-being is often a sure indicator), the physician should refrain from further investigations, and should explain to the patient that a positive diagnosis is now clear. It is important for the physician to have some understanding of the motor function of the bowel, so that a rational explanation of the pathophysiology can be given to the patient.

A full explanation

The physician who dismisses functional symptoms as of little importance is not likely to help a patient whose social and private life may be considerably impaired by discomfort. An explanation of the problem, and any possible association with provocative factors in the lifestyle of the patient, must be offered. The limitations of effective therapy must be explained, and patients must be firmly reassured that they are not suffering from the prodromal manifestations of serious organic disease. The prognosis of most functional complaints is that, by and large, there will be little change, and this should not be concealed from the patient. In fact, when the patient gains insight into the problem, symptoms often lessen or even disappear; alternatively, the provocative factors in the patient's life may be removed with the passage of time. Even so, this should be regarded as an unexpected bonus; the wisest attitude for the physician is that of 'no disease and no cure'. A sensible physician will also avoid attribution of symptoms to a specific occupational or conjugal situation, as not only are individuals rarely free to change these circumstances at will, but also the association of symptoms with such specific circumstances may be coincidental rather than causal.

Although functional symptoms may present in a bewildering variety of permutations, certain syndromes predominate, and are more easily recognized.

Globus hystericus

This curious condition presents as apparent dysphagia at the level of the upper oesophageal sphincter, which may be only related to swallowing, or also as a persistent feeling of 'a lump'. Investigation reveals no abnormality, but anxiety is a common feature of this condition. Because the syndrome is remarkably specific, it may well be that this is a sensory disorder of motility, in which abnormal tension of voluntary muscle plays a part. As the principal fear of the patient is usually of oesophageal malignancy, adequate investigation followed by strong reassurance is required.

Rumination

Rumination, or merycism, comprises the effortless regurgitation of a meal into the mouth. This condition is now well recognized, although this was not the case at the beginning of the twentieth century. Rumination is normal in infants, and is perpetuated through childhood in mentally retarded children. Children are taught not to regurgitate, and the presence of rumination in later childhood or early adult life might be regarded as a failure of early training. In rumination, boluses of food are retropelled into the mouth at intervals during the first one or two postprandial hours, when the acidity of gastric contents is still insufficient to render them unpalatable. The retropulsion is due to a complex sequence of efforts that involve a rise in intra-abdominal pressure at the moment when the lower oesophageal sphincter opens during swallowing. Patients tend to be encouraged to seek medical attention by their relatives or spouses; halitosis is one of the side-effects of the habit. It is important not to confuse this syndrome with normal gastro-oesophageal reflux. There is no known method of treatment beyond persuasion, which is rarely successful.

Psychogenic vomiting

Unlike the retropulsion of rumination, which is often intrinsically satisfying to the patient, psychogenic vomiting, which is self-induced, is a conversion symptom; that is, a symptom designed to draw attention to the patient as an invalid. Patients are commonly adolescent girls, but not invariably so. There is usually a discrepancy between the alleged volume and frequency of vomiting, and an apparently adequate state of nutrition with unaltered body weight. Treatment of this condition requires the elimination of the existence of possible organic causes of vomiting and attention to the underlying psychological disturbance. As with other functional complaints with a presumed psychogenic origin, admission to hospital for close observation often results in complete remission.

One cause of vomiting, which is not psychogenic and with which this should not be confused, is retching associated with spasms of coughing in bronchitis. This usually occurs on getting out of bed in the morning, and is usually found in heavy smokers.

Irritable bowel syndrome

This condition is discussed in Chapter 14.13.

Constipation (see also Chapter 14.2.5)

Because the bowel habit of normal individuals is so varied, constipation defies precise definition. Empirically, it may be defined as occurring when defaecation is sufficiently infrequent to cause the sufferer discomfort or alarm, and to induce recourse to self-medication or medical attention. Some individuals are content to open their bowels once every 2 or 3 days, while others are not. The aim of the physician should be to increase the regularity of defaecation by the patient to a frequency that satisfies the patient, and also to persuade the patient to discontinue excessive self-medication with potentially hazardous purgatives. Most patients who suffer from constipation never consult a physician, but resort to self-medication; it is the failure of self-medication that usually drives the patient to the doctor.

Constipation in children may be an expression of psychological disturbance, in which there is conscious, forced retention of faeces or encoparesis. This may lead to spurious diarrhoea, in which there is leakage of liquid faeces around a mass of hard, retained faeces. Expert paediatric management is required in these cases as attempts to treat only the bowel disorder may aggravate the situation. Spurious diarrhoea may also be the presentation of constipation in the elderly, where a hypnotic colon and a lax abdominal musculature and also anal problems, such as haemorrhoids, which render defaecation painful, are often additional aggravating factors. Where there is spurious diarrhoea, manual movement of a retained mass may be required before a normal bowel habit can be regained.

Apart from the special circumstances that may obtain in the very young and in the elderly, constipation in the majority of patients in the absence of any organic disease resolves around twin defects: the suppression of the defaecation reflex, and the absence of habit. In the normal individual, on sensory stimulation of the rectum when it fills as a result of the postprandial gastrocolic reflex, which initiates a mass movement, the act of defaecation becomes a reflex that is perpetuated as a postprandial habit; one act of defaecation following the first meal of the day is sufficient for the majority of individuals. Constipation develops when the habit is disturbed. This may be because a change of job requires the individual to leave the house in a hurry, whereas previously there was time for adequate defaecation. Overcrowding may mean lack of access to a lavatory at the appropriate time. Schoolchildren may dislike the lack of privacy and cleanliness that is too often the hallmark of communal school facilities. As the habit is abolished, so is rectal sensation suppressed from consciousness, and the patient becomes unaware of the call for stool. Once the reflex is disturbed, attempts at self-regulation of defaecation may be unsuccessful; with the loss of rectal sensation, the patient may be straining to void an empty rectum out of a sense of social obligation. Suppression of defaecation leads to gradual colonic distension with inspissated faeces, causing a sensation of abdominal discomfort. In addition, patients may complain of a host of generalized somatic discomforts, such as headache, fatigue, and nausea; these do not arise from constipation, but more probably from the patient's need to convert an undignified inadequacy into an illness. One curious feature of simple constipation is that sufferers in early adult life are almost invariably female. There is no satisfactory explanation for this phenomenon, but the fact that constipation is sometimes eased during menstruation and during pregnancy suggests that endocrine factors may be responsible.

When a patient presents with constipation, the history should be directed into determining under what circumstances did an acceptable bowel habit lapse into constipation, in addition to simple enquiries about the frequency of bowel habit and the nature of the patient's diet. Physical examination will usually reveal a palpable, firm, descending colon and often a rectum loaded with faeces; if the latter is the case, the patient will usually deny any sensation of rectal fullness or desire to defaecate.

Treatment should be directed towards restitution of a lost habit. Bran and hydrophilic colloids may provide faeces that give strong stimulation to the colon. Laxatives are permissible initially, but should be prescribed so as to induce a physiological bowel habit. Anthracene purgatives (such as senna) should be avoided; osmotic laxatives (such as lactulose and magnesium sulphate) are better. The patient's diet is of less consequence than is generally imagined, as myriad individuals live with a great variety of diet but an acceptable bowel habit, but emphasis on breakfast, preferably including a bran cereal, is important, as it is following breakfast that attempts to establish a normal bowel habit are most likely to be successful. Reassurance and explanation to the patient are important, and the physician should explain the logic of the regimen he or she is advocating. Adjunctive therapy may include treatment of anal and perianal discomfort that sometimes causes the individual to strain at stool with a closed external anal sphincter. Self-medication should be firmly discouraged, and the dangers of anthracene purgatives, which cause gradual autonomic denervation of the colon with prolonged use, should be emphasized to the patient.

Purgative abuse

Given the degree of cultural concern over the alleged dangers of constipation (a concern that has been assiduously cultivated by the vendors of patent medicines since the invention of advertising), self-medication with purgatives is to be expected. Less expected is the fact that some individuals may surreptitiously take purgatives to the point where troublesome chronic diarrhoea prompts recourse to the physician. The psychopathology that leads such an individual to deny the use of purgatives is varied and the causes are often obscure. Diarrhoea due to purgative abuse must be differentiated from other forms of chronic diarrhoea. Suggestive features include hypokalaemia, finger clubbing, and persistence during abstention from food. Barium enema may reveal a colon lacking in haustrations, similar to the appearance of chronic ulcerative colitis, but the mucosal pattern is normal and this may be confirmed by endoscopic examination and biopsy. If anthracene purgatives are being used, pigmentation of the colonic mucosa may be present (melanosis coli). The abnormal outline of the colon together with the absence of mucosal damage suggests that disordered motility as well as disordered absorption may contribute to the diarrhoea.

The condition is only treatable when the purgatives are found and the patient is confronted with the evidence; this usually requires hospital admission. Removal of the purgatives results in prompt remission; if the colonic innervation has been damaged by prolonged use of anthracene derivatives, such as senna, the diarrhoea may be replaced by troublesome constipation; this should be treated with osmotic purgatives. Psychiatric referral may be helpful in determining the cause of the habit.

Proctalgia fugax

Attacks of anorectal pain occur in some individuals without evidence of anorectal disease; the disease is said to be more common among physicians than among other socioeconomic groups. The cause of the attacks, which often occur at night and are sometimes associated with emotional stress, is disputed but spasm of the levator ani musculature has been implicated. In some individuals, spasm of the anal sphincter may also play a part; in such cases, rectal examination may reveal a tight sphincter. Reassurance over the absence of organic disease is sometimes helpful, but there is no generally effective treatment.

REFERENCES

Normal motility

Code, C.F. and Marlett, J.A. (1975). The interdigestive myoelectric complex of the stomach and small bowel of dogs. *Journal of Physiology*, **246**, 298–309.

Holle, G.E. and Wood, J.D. (ed.) (1992). *Advances in the innervation of the gastrointestinal tract*. Excerpta Medica, Amsterdam.

Szurszewski, J.H. (1969). A migrating complex of the canine small intestine. *American Journal of Physiology*, **217**, 1757–63.

Thompson, D.G., Wingate, D.L., Archer, L., Benson, M.J., Green, W.J., and Hardy, R.J. (1982). Normal patterns of human upper small bowel motor activity recorded by prolonged radiotelemetry. *Gut*, **23**, 517–23.

Wingate, D.L. (1981). Backwards and forwards with the migrating complex. *Digestive Diseases and Sciences*, **26**, 641–66.

Wood, J.D. (ed.) (1989). Motility and circulation. In *Handbook of Physiology*, Vol. 1, Section 6, (ed. S.G. Schultz. American Physiology Society, Bethesda, MD.)

Abnormal motility

Kumar, D. and Wingate, D.L. (ed.) (1993). *An illustrated guide to gastrointestinal motility*. Churchill Livingstone, London.

Schuster, M. (ed.) (1993). *Atlas of gastrointestinal motility in health and disease*. Williams & Wilkins, Baltimore.

Vantrappen, G., Janssens, J., Hellemans, J., and Ghoos, Y. (1977). The interdigestive motor complex of normal subjects and patients with bacterial overgrowth of the small intestine. *Journal of Clinical Investigation*, **59**, 1158–66.

14.13 Functional bowel disease and irritable bowel syndrome

D. G. THOMPSON

INTRODUCTION
Functional bowel disorders

Symptoms suggestive of disturbed lower gastrointestinal function without adequate explanation are very common in the adult population of the Western world. Surveys from the United Kingdom and United States indicate that up to 15 per cent of the adult population experience such symptoms at any one time. Most of these people do not seek medical advice and regard themselves as being perfectly normal. The chief question that is still largely unresolved, therefore, is whether the symptoms of those individuals who do see their doctors have a different pathophysiological basis from those who do not, and whether the seeking of medical advice is an indication of a worried personality rather than disturbed gut function.

Given these difficulties with a clear identification of a diagnostic group, currently used terms such as irritable bowel syndrome are best viewed as an attempt by clinicians to organize rational thought about such patients and their symptoms. Knowledge of the pathophysiology and the psychology of the problem remains incomplete and therapy is still largely empirical. Current observations about functional bowel disorders should be regarded as the latest (but not necessarily the last)

attempt at symptom rationalization. Terms such as 'mucus colitis' or 'spastic colon' are now best avoided.

Definitions

Many attempts have been made to provide a definition of functional bowel disease. It is not surprising that most have failed to stand the test of time, as the symptoms suffered, whilst being genuine and troublesome to the patient, are often difficult to define, variable in their expression, and continue to defy pathophysiological explanation. The latest and perhaps the best of the attempts to categorize functional lower-bowel diseases was made by a working group at the 13th International Congress of Gastroenterology in 1990. Their recommendations, known as the 'Rome criteria', are becoming widely accepted. Whether these criteria will stand the test of time will depend upon whether they turn out to provide a better understanding of the pathogenic mechanisms of the disease or aid therapy. The Rome working party has suggested a division of functional bowel disease into a number of categories on the basis of symptoms (Table 1). Because they seem to have some practical value in approaches to management, this chapter is based on some of the Rome categories, with emphasis on those previously encompassed by the term irritable bowel syndrome. The Rome criteria do not necessarily include all symptoms due to abnormal bowel function. Failure to allocate a patient into one or other category should therefore not be taken to mean that the patient does not have a functional bowel disorder.

The author wishes to thank members of the Rome Working Group (Dr W.G. Thompson, Professor D. Drossman, and Professor F. Creed) for permission to use the 'Rome Criteria' as the basis for this chapter.

Table 1 *Categorization of functional bowel disease according to the 'Rome criteria'*

Functional bowel disorders
Irritable bowel syndrome
Functional abdominal bloating
Functional constipation
Functional diarrhoea
Functional abdominal pain

From Thompson *et al.* (1992).

Irritable bowel syndrome

DEFINITION

This syndrome is characterized by the presence of abdominal pain associated with defaecation, or a change in bowel habit together with disordered defaecation and the sensation of abdominal distension. For clinical purposes, the diagnosis relies upon the presence of at least 3 months' abdominal pain that is relieved by defaecation and is associated with a change in frequency in defaecation and/or consistency of stool, together with two or more of the following symptoms: (a) altered stool frequency; (b) altered stool consistency; (c) altered ease of defaecation; (d) passage of mucus; (e) sensation of abdominal distension. These criteria are based on the studies of Manning and of Kruis, which identified that the above features were reported most frequently in patients with functional bowel problems, and were very unusual in patients with structural disease of the lower gut.

DIAGNOSIS

The diagnosis of the irritable bowel syndrome is clinically based, and relies on an adequately taken history and examination, there being no specific endoscopic, radiological or laboratory investigation that is yet capable of providing a positive diagnosis. Despite the absence of a specific pathological indicator, the identification of irritable bowel syndrome is usually not difficult and in most cases it is unnecessary to investigate the patient extensively in an attempt to exclude other, more serious disease.

CLINICAL FEATURES

The history

In addition to the careful elicitation of the above specific symptoms, other features may be found that serve to increase clinical confidence. For example, many patients have upper-gut symptoms suggestive of such as food-related abdominal distension. Women may also complain of menstrual and bladder symptoms, and there is also an increased prevalence of psychosexual problems.

Examination

Clinical examination is important. Whilst there is no physical abnormality that is diagnostic of irritable bowel syndrome, a number of features occur commonly. Palpation over the site of the lower colon, particularly in the left iliac fossa, commonly produces discomfort, and a sigmoid colon containing faeces is often palpable. Similar tenderness may be present in the right iliac fossa.

Rectal examination and sigmoidoscopy are commonly done as part of the initial clinical assessment in patients with symptoms of irritable bowel. Characteristic findings are the presence of pelletty stools in the rectum and a mucosa of normal appearance, evidence of mucosal inflammation being incompatible with the diagnosis. A further helpful pointer is the response to air insufflation during sigmoidoscopy; abdominal dis-

comfort is often reproduced by insufflation and relieved by its expulsion. Evidence of a pigmented rectal mucosa (melanosis coli) may sometimes be found in patients who have been taking stimulant laxatives and is a useful indicator of the chronicity of the problem.

Further laboratory investigations are at the discretion of the clinician, depending upon the confidence with which a clinical diagnosis is made. Routine haematological and biochemical screening is usually done on the assumption that they will be normal and to provide reassurance both to the patient and the doctor. Radiological and endoscopic examination of the colon is not mandatory unless a clinical suspicion of a structural colonic disorder, particularly neoplasia, remains after the history and examination.

Features indicating a need to investigate the patient further would include those symptoms that raise the suspicion of organic disease, particularly the onset of symptoms in a middle-aged or elderly patient together with weight loss or blood in the stool. The development of new colonic symptoms in a patient with a long history of irritable bowel syndrome should also be taken seriously, as there is no evidence that the syndrome protects against the development of other disease and the incidence of colonic neoplasia increases with age.

PATHOPHYSIOLOGY

Despite much interest and many painstaking clinical studies, our understanding of the pathophysiology of irritable bowel syndrome remains limited. The hypothesis that many patients have a disorder of neuromuscular function of the gastrointestinal tract seems eminently plausible but incontrovertible evidence is lacking. Manometric studies of the colon do show an increased contractile activity in patients with this syndrome, particularly after food, but the neurophysiological basis of this finding remains to be determined. Another currently popular hypothesis is that in these patients, visceral sensation from the gastrointestinal tract is somehow enhanced. This is based on the observation that distension of the rectum and colon produces greater discomfort at lower volumes of distension than in people with normal bowel function. This increased sensory awareness appears to be viscerally specific, as cutaneous responsiveness is normal. It remains to be determined whether the mechanism for this hypersensitivity is peripheral (abnormal mechanoreceptor responsiveness in the gut) or central (abnormal sensory processing by the central nervous system).

There is also powerful evidence that psychiatric disease and abnormal illness behaviour are more prevalent in patients with irritable bowel syndrome. Again, the relation between the psychological problem and any neuromuscular abnormality remains uncertain, although it is recognized that a heightened awareness of visceral sensation is a feature of affective disorders.

It has been traditional to regard diet as being a major pathogenic factor, and to attribute most symptoms to fibre deficiency, on the basis that irritable bowel syndrome is uncommon in those parts of the world where a high-fibre diet is consumed. While it is true that faecal bulk can be increased by increasing fibre ingestion and that some symptoms are improved, careful studies of fibre intake and symptom development do not show a clear causal relation. Food 'allergy' or sensitivity is occasionally confused with irritable bowel syndrome because abdominal pain and diarrhoea can accompany such problems. True food allergy with measurable immunological responses to a particular food (e.g. egg, shellfish) is readily distinguishable from irritable bowel by its extraintestinal symptoms and by a clear relation between ingestion of the food and symptom development. More subtle forms of foodstuff intolerance (e.g. lactose intolerance, fructose intolerance) that produce gut symptoms without an accompanying immune response are much more difficult to recognize because the nutrient in question is often present throughout the diet. Recognition of such problems requires a painstaking dietary history and clear relation between symptoms and food intake. In most patients such a relation cannot be found.

Functional abdominal bloating

DEFINITION

This is a disorder characterized by symptoms of abdominal fullness or distension, awareness of audible bowel sounds, and excessive flatus for at least 3 months without any evidence of either maldigestion and malabsorption or excessive consumption of poorly absorbed fermentable carbohydrate.

PATHOPHYSIOLOGY

This syndrome seems to be a variant of irritable bowel in which abdominal discomfort predominates over disordered colonic transit and defaecatory difficulty.

Distension of the colon at sigmoidoscopy characteristically produces greater discomfort than normal, suggesting increased gut sensitivity. There is no evidence that intestinal gas production is increased. As in irritable bowel syndrome, the prevalence of psychological disorders is high.

CLINICAL FEATURES

The clinical assessment of such patients is identical to that for irritable bowel syndrome.

Functional constipation

DEFINITION

Functional constipation is arbitrarily defined by the 'Rome criteria' as persistently difficult, infrequent defaecation, or the sensation of incomplete defaecation. The criteria required are two or more of the following for at least 3 months:

- straining at defaecation at least a quarter of the time;
- lumpy or hard stools at least a quarter of the time;
- the sensation of incomplete evacuation at least a quarter of the time;
- two or fewer bowel movements per week.

Unlike the irritable bowel syndrome, abdominal pain is not a prerequisite for the diagnosis.

CLINICAL EVALUATION

As with the other categories of functional bowel disease, the diagnosis is based on a carefully conducted history and examination designed to exclude the possibility of more serious colonic disease, particularly cancer. When considering the diagnosis, it is important to enquire about immobility, concomitant drug therapy (particularly opiate analgesia), and a low roughage diet, which are well recognized to contribute to constipation, particularly in the infirm elderly.

An abnormality of pelvic-floor relaxation on attempted defaecation is an unusual but important cause of constipation that should be suspected in those individuals who feel the need to defaecate but cannot expel faeces despite severe straining. Clinical evidence of diabetes, hypothyroidism, and hypercalcaemia must also be sought, as these also produce constipation.

Physical examination should include a rectal and vaginal examination. The absence of perineal descent on straining or coughing is a simple indicator of pelvic-floor dysfunction, while descent below the level of the ischial tuberosities indicates pelvic-floor weakness. Sigmoidoscopy is required to confirm the diagnosis of functional constipation, to identify the presence of formed faeces, and to exclude faecal impaction and organic obstruction of the lower colon.

LABORATORY EXAMINATION

In the absence of clinical indicators of systemic disease and in the presence of the above diagnostic criteria, extensive laboratory investigation is usually unnecessary. A plain abdominal radiograph is often helpful to confirm the presence of faecal material throughout the colon and to indicate the diameter of the small intestine and colon, which helps exclude the rare cases of intestinal pseudo-obstruction and megacolon caused by intestinal myopathies and neuropathies.

Transit studies using radio-opaque markers are commonly done as part of the research investigation of constipated patients in order to determine the severity of transit delay and to distinguish those with a pancolonic abnormality from a more localized problem of pelvic relaxation. However, measurement of whole-gut transit should not be regarded as necessary for the diagnosis; documented infrequent defaecation is usually sufficient. The electrophysiological and radiological assessment of anorectal function is indicated if there is evidence of abnormal perineal descent or rectal prolapse, as the accurate recognition of pelvic-floor dysfunction can influence the choice of therapy. Such investigations are indicated when Hirschsprung's disease (Chapter 14.15) is suspected.

PATHOPHYSIOLOGY

The cause of functional constipation is uncertain. Factors purported to be of relevance are similar to those proposed for irritable bowel syndrome, in particular, dietary-fibre insufficiency and visceral neuropathy.

In the mildest cases, dietary-fibre deficiency may be relevant; however, in the more severely affected patients, fibre supplementation does not abolish the problem and may even worsen symptoms, making a causal role for fibre untenable. In the most severe cases an abnormality of colonic enteric nerves or muscle may be found; for the great majority, no structural abnormality has been identified.

In a proportion of patients, almost invariably female, defaecatory dysfunction appears to be the major factor and colonic function is normal. A failure of relaxation in appropriate pelvic-floor muscles on attempted stool expulsion is identifiable in these patients; this appears to be a 'learned' phenomenon with a psychophysiological aetiology rather than peripheral nerve dysfunction. However, the relation between constipation and pelvic-floor dysfunction remains obscure in many instances. In other patients, low tone in the pelvic floor and rectal prolapse appear to be the result of damage to the pudendal nerve from straining at stool and thus may be a consequence of the constipation rather than its cause.

In some severely affected women, there is a relation between symptom severity and the luteal phase of the menstrual cycle, which has led to the suggestion of a sex-hormonal aetiology. In support of this hypothesis is the fact that colonic muscle tone is reduced by progesterone and that constipation is a frequent accompaniment of normal pregnancies. Against the hypothesis is the failure to demonstrate abnormal colonic sensitivity to progesterone in constipated women, so that the possibility remains that the menstrual cycle-related events are merely the expression of a normal cyclical progesterone effect on a malfunctioning colon.

Functional diarrhoea

DEFINITION

This is defined as the frequent passage of unformed stool without the presence of other features of irritable bowel syndrome.

The diagnosis of functional diarrhoea depends on the presence of two or more of the following findings for at least 3 months:

- unformed stool for more than three-quarters of the time;
- three or more bowel movements per day for more than half the time;
- increased stool weight of greater than 200 g/day.

Note that neither abdominal pain nor the frequent passage of formed stools are present in this diagnostic category.

CLINICAL FEATURES

Because of its non-specific nature and its clinical overlap with many other pathological processes in the gastrointestinal tract, the diagnosis of functional diarrhoea is usually achieved by exclusion. A careful history is required to exclude inflammatory bowel disease and to rule out secretory diarrhoeas. The possibility of surreptitious laxative use should always be borne in mind. Some patients identify the time of onset of the problem to a specific life-event, particularly a bout of severe gastroenteritis. The possibility of a chronic intestinal infection needs to be considered carefully in such patients, although in most evidence of an infective agent will be lacking.

Physical examination must be done to determine the extent of nutritional deficiency, to exclude metabolic disorders such as hyperthyroidism, and to rule out intra-abdominal structural abnormalities. Careful biochemical and microbiological examination of stool samples is mandatory.

LABORATORY INVESTIGATIONS

Unlike the other functional diseases, a careful search for a structural mucosal disease is usually made in such patients. Key diagnoses that must be excluded are chronic malabsorption diseases such as chronic pancreatic insufficiency and gluten sensitivity, together with inflammatory bowel diseases, infections, and infestations of the gastrointestinal tract.

PATHOPHYSIOLOGY

In the absence of any definable structural abnormality of exocrine function or intestinal epithelial transport, functional diarrhoea is generally assumed to be a disorder of neuroenteric function. In favour of this assertion are the findings of accelerated upper-intestinal transit following ingestion of a meal, and reduced rectal compliance, both of which would be expected to contribute to symptom development.

In some patients, there is a clear relation between psychological state and symptoms, with diarrhoea developing whenever anxiety occurs, suggesting that the diarrhoea is a secondary phenomenon.

Functional abdominal pain

DEFINITION

This symptom category is commonly included amongst the functional bowel disorders. However, the relation between the abdominal pain and a disturbance of gastrointestinal-tract function is difficult to ascertain in the majority of patients.

The term refers to the presence of frequent, recurrent, or continuous abdominal pain for at least 6 months together, without relation between pain and recognizable physiological events such as eating, defaecation or menstruation, and in the absence of evidence of organic disease in the abdomen. Most of these patients show a major loss of daily functioning capacity and exhibit chronic illness behaviour. Detailed discussion of such patients is outside the scope of this chapter.

Management of functional bowel diseases

The management of patients with functional bowel disorders remains empirical. It is not surprising that in an area of human suffering with such symptom diversity and in which the pathophysiological mechanisms remain obscure, no single pharmacological agent or group of agents have been found to be consistently effective.

A recent review of randomized, double-blind, placebo-controlled trials for the treatment of irritable bowel syndrome examined 43 trials and concluded that none offered convincing evidence that any therapy was effective. Such a conclusion is perhaps as much an indictment of the design of the trials as the efficacy of the drug therapy. In a condition in which the patient's mental state appears to play such an important part in symptom severity, it is not surprise that in most clinical trials the placebo responses have been very high, usually up to 50 per cent. Also, short-term trials of therapeutic agents in diseases where symptoms are intermittent may be unable to distinguish a true drug effect from a placebo response.

So what can the clinician do to help patients with functional bowel disease? As in all chronic problems without a clear cure, a principal task is explanation and reassurance. Therapy must be patient centred, designed to provide a solution for the patient's personal needs and expectations. The clinician should give a full explanation of the likely nature of the problem and firm reassurance that organic disease is not present. Attention to the patient's psychological state is very important, as it is clear that mood is a powerful modulator of symptom severity.

In more severe cases of irritable bowel syndrome, psychological treatment using a variety of methods, including 'dynamic psychotherapy', has been found to provide greater improvement than drug therapy alone. Good prognostic factors for improvement by psychological therapy seem to be overt psychiatric symptoms, particularly anxiety or depression, together with intermittent pain exacerbated by stress. In contrast, patients in whom the abdominal pain is constant, and who exhibit evidence of chronic illness behaviour, do not seem to be helped by a psychotherapeutic approach but may respond to antidepressants.

In less severe cases, attention to treatment of the individual and his/her symptoms is usually the approach taken. In patients with predominantly constipational symptoms, supplementary dietary fibre and additional, poorly absorbed fermentable carbohydrates (e.g. pulses) increase faecal bulk, soften the stool, and may ease defaecatory difficulties. On occasions, this approach can exacerbate symptoms of abdominal distension, probably as a result of increased quantities of colonic gas produced by the fermentation of the unabsorbed carbohydrate. Wherever possible, long-term use of stimulant laxatives is best avoided because of the concern that such drugs may themselves damage the colonic enteric–neural function and eventually make the problem worse. Osmotic laxatives and enemas are the mainstay of therapy of the severely constipated patient with slow transit.

For the patient with normal colonic function but who is unable to relax musculature of the pelvic floor on attempted defaecation, a variety of biofeedback techniques are now available that help the individual to 'relearn' the process. Success is high in those able to comply.

For patients with diarrhoea-predominant symptoms, attention to dietary intake is also often helpful, as the size of and timing of meals is likely to influence the frequency and social inconvenience of the diarrhoea. Poorly absorbed foods such as fermentable carbohydrates are best taken in moderation because they can exacerbate symptoms. In the more persistent cases of diarrhoea, symptoms can be improved by antidiarrhoeal agents, the dose provided being adjusted according to the symptoms and administered before the meal rather than after it, so that its effect is exerted on transit at the time of ingestion.

In the management of patients with pain-predominant irritable bowel syndrome, it is tempting to provide analgesic drugs, but therapy with opiate-derivative analgesics is unlikely to benefit patients in the long term and may even exacerbate symptoms because of their constipating effects. Antidepressants are often provided empirically in low doses to patients with irritable bowel syndrome, as are 'antispasmodics' (e.g. hyoscine butyl bromide). Whilst there are undoubtedly patients who are convinced of the clinical benefit of such medications, a beneficial effect has yet to be proven beyond doubt by clinical trial.

Relaxation therapy, in particular hypnosis, seems to provide benefit in those individuals who are prepared to participate. If the initial results are confirmed more widely by other groups, then a programme of symptom management involving self-delivered 'autohypnosis' may offer a satisfactory approach for many sufferers.

Surgical intervention for symptoms of functional bowel disease is usually best avoided, as benefit is unlikely and symptoms may worsen. On occasions, subtotal colectomy and ileorectal anastomosis will provide marked symptomatic benefit in severe, slow-transit constipation.

Although the management of patients with functional bowel disease remains a large therapeutic challenge, it should not be shirked by clinicians, with whom responsibility rests for providing careful, individually oriented explanation and support. Carefully conducted, double-blind controlled trials of the many therapies currently used in practice, designed to satisfy the most stringent criteria for acceptability, must now be a priority.

REFERENCES

Anuras, S. (ed.) (1992). *Motility disorders of the gastrointestinal tract.* Raven Press, New York.

Afzalpurkar, R.G., Schiller, L.R., Little, K.H., Santangelo, W.C., and Fordtran J.S. (1992). The self-limited nature of chronic idiopathic diarrhoea. *New England Journal of Medicine*, **327**, 1849–52.

Christensen, J. (1992). Pathophysiology of the irritable bowel syndrome. *Lancet*, **ii**, 1444–7.

Creed, F.H., Craig, T., and Farmer, R.G. (1988). Functional abdominal pain, psychiatric illness and life events. *Gut*, **29**, 235–42.

Guthrie, E., Creed, F., Dawson, D., and Tomenson, B. (1991). A controlled trial of psychological treatment for the irritable bowel syndrome. *Gastroenterology*, **100**, 450–7.

Klein, K.B. (1988). Controlled treatment trials in the irritable bowel syndrome: a critique. *Gastroenterology*, **95**, 232–41.

Kruis, W., Thiemo, C.H., Weinzierl, M., Schussler, P., Hall, J., and Paulus, W. (1984). A diagnostic score for the irritable bowel syndrome: its value in the exclusion of organic disease. *Gastroenterology*, **87**, 1–7.

Manning, A.P., Thompson, W.G., Heaton, K.W., and Morris, A.F. (1978). Towards a positive diagnosis of the irritable bowel. *British Medical Journal*, **2**, 653–4.

Read, N.W., Timms, J.M., and Barfield, L.J. (1986). Impairment of defaecation in young women with severe constipation. *Gastroenterology*, **90**, 53–61.

Thompson, W.G., Creed, F., Drossman, D., Heaton, K., and Mazzacca, G. (1992). Functional bowel disease and functional abdominal pain. *Gastroenterology International*, **5**, 75–91.

Wexner, S.D., Cheape, J.D., Jorge, J.M.N., Heymen, S., and Jagelman, D.G. (1992). Prospective assessment of biofeedback for the treatment of paradoxical puborectalis contraction. *Diseases of the Colon and Rectum*, **35**, 145–50.

Whorwell, P.J., Prior, A., and Faragher, E.B. (1984). Controlled trial of hypnotherapy in the treatment of severe refractory irritable bowel syndrome. *Lancet*, **ii**, 1232–4.

14.14 Colonic diverticular disease

N. J. McC. MORTENSEN and M. G. W. KETTLEWELL

Diverticula can be found throughout the gastrointestinal tract, but are seen most commonly in the sigmoid and descending colon.

EPIDEMIOLOGY

Asymptomatic diverticular disease is much more common than clinical diverticulitis. Autopsy studies in the United Kingdom and Australia have shown that the prevalence of colonic diverticula increases with age. It is rare in those under 30 years of age but occurs in more than 50 per cent of those over 70 years. On the other hand, colonic diverticulosis is very rare in African and Asian countries and right-sided disease predominates in Japan. This geographical distribution is not due to race, as West Indians and Asians living in Britain, American blacks, and Japanese who have moved to Hawaii or the mainland United States are just as prone to the disease as Caucasians. Patients presenting with complicated diverticular disease have a low dietary-fibre intake, whilst vegetarians have a low incidence of the disease.

In Edinburgh, 23 per cent of all barium enemas demonstrated diverticula. The annual incidence increased from 0.17/1000 in those under 45 years to 5.7/1000 in those over 75 years of age. Women were affected more than men. In spite of the introduction of high-fibre diets, there is no evidence that the incidence of acute diverticulitis is declining.

AETIOLOGY

Diverticular disease is said to be a disease of the twentieth century. It was rarely described in the nineteenth century literature, and in Britain there is a correlation between the rising incidence at the beginning of this century and an increased consumption of refined flour and sugar. Sugar consumption has trebled since 1860, and in the late 1870s the stone grinding of flour was replaced by roller milling, which removes more fibre. Modern white and some brown breads contain little fibre compared to the amount in wholemeal bread, which was previously a staple part of the diet.

The development of diverticula therefore can be ascribed to a lifelong diet deficient in dietary fibre. An unrefined, high-fibre diet produces swiftly passed, soft stools that subject the colon to little strain. Modern, fibre-deficient diets on the other hand give rise to stiff, viscous stools that need high intracolonic pressures to propel them. High luminal pressures cause a protrusion of the mucosa through vulnerable points in the sigmoid and descending colon. They usually occur at the site where colonic blood vessels penetrate the wall. This hypothesis is supported by the observation that, although basal intracolonic pressures are similar in health and diverticular disease, when the diseased colon is activated by emotion, eating, mechanical stimuli or drugs such as morphine or prostigmine, high pressures are generated in those segments that have diverticula. This is due to hypersegmentation by the colonic smooth muscle, and the difference has been recorded in the earliest stage of disease and may explain its progressive nature. In symptomatic patients an increase in dietary fibre causes a relief of symptoms in many cases.

Changes in the colon wall also play a part. With age, and following episodes of diverticulitis, the colonic wall becomes stiff and less distensible, aggravating the effects of raised intracolonic pressure. An increase in elastin and changes in collagen have been reported. Diabetic patients are prone to diverticular disease at an earlier stage, suggesting a defect in glycolysation of colonic collagen with advancing age. In those with connective tissue disorders such as Ehlers–Danlos syndrome or Marfan's disease, diverticula are also seen at an unusually early age.

The distinction between symptomatic and asymptomatic diverticular disease is important, for whilst something is known about the formation of diverticula it is not known why some diverticula become symptomatic.

PATHOLOGY

A diverticulum consists of a herniation of mucosa through the colonic musculature, and as it enlarges its muscle covering atrophies, so that the fully developed diverticulum consists of mucosa, connective tissue, and peritoneum. The striking abnormality is in the thickening of the circular and longitudinal muscle, which both narrows the colonic lumen and shortens the sigmoid like a concertina to give a saw-tooth appearance on barium enema. The diverticula occur as slit-like apertures between the muscle clefts.

Inflammation in diverticular disease is the result of infection around diverticula, which spreads within the pericolic fat to form a dissecting abscess. Usually a single diverticulum is the cause of a pericolic abscess, perhaps initiated by the presence of a faecolith. Involvement of the peritoneum results in local peritonitis, which may become generalized in the event of a perforation. This may also give rise to intra-abdominal abscesses or fistulae to the bladder, small bowel, vagina, or uterus. Repeated episodes of diverticulitis lead to a contracted, narrowed sigmoid colon surrounded by fibrous tissue. Bleeding in diverticular disease can often be traced to an infected diverticulum. This may cause either the erosion of a vessel in its wall or the formation of granulation tissue inside the diverticulum, which then bleeds.

CLINICAL FEATURES

As diverticulosis is so common, most diverticula are asymptomatic. They are usually discovered incidentally and only some 10 per cent produce symptoms, and around 1 per cent require surgery. The symptoms usually result from disordered motility rather than secondary complications of the disease.

Uncomplicated diverticular disease

Pain can be felt along the course of the colon, particularly over the sigmoid, and is often accompanied by a change in bowel habit with the passage of broken, pellety stools after considerable straining. These symptoms may be indistinguishable from those of the irritable bowel syndrome. The passage of blood with an unformed stool is unusual and should alert one to the possibility of other pathology.

Management

All patients should have a rigid or flexible sigmoidoscopy in addition to a barium enema to exclude a rectal or sigmoid carcinoma (Fig. 1). They should be reassured that there is no serious underlying disease and a high-fibre diet should be recommended. This must include wholemeal

Fig. 1 Barium enema showing a narrowed sigmoid colon with a few diverticula. This appearance can be confused with those of a carcinoma and colonoscopy would be indicated to clarify the diagnosis.

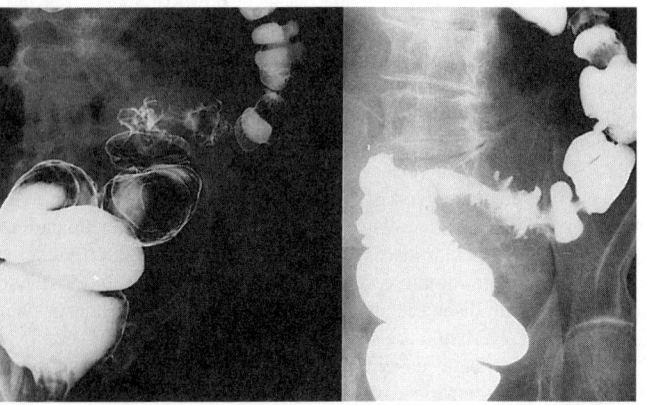

Table 1 *Indications for surgery*

Sepsis
Recurrent diverticulitis
Perforated diverticulitis
Purulent peritonitis
Faecal peritonitis
Pelvic or paracolic abscess

Colonic obstruction
Inflammatory stricture
Fibrotic stricture
Suspected malignancy

Fistulae
Colovesical
Colovaginal
Ileocolic

Major haemorrhage

bread, whole-wheat breakfast cereals, rough porridge or muesli, and fresh fruit and vegetables daily. Fibre increases stool bulk in three ways—by holding water, by proliferation of bacteria, and from the by-products of bacterial fermentation. The coarser the fibre the greater is the faecal bulk, and unpalatability, and although cooking bran improves its taste, it reduces its water-holding capacity. A good clinical response is usually achieved by including two tablespoons of bran with the morning cereal, but about half the patients will experience gaseous distension or cramps on starting the high-fibre diet. It is worth warning them that this is likely to happen and that it will resolve within a month or so if they persist with the diet.

In patients with pain, antispasmodics such as mebeverine may be useful, and in a minority with repeated severe attacks an elective resection is then indicated (Table 1). This is probably more effective than sigmoid myotomy, an operation popularized in the mid-1960s. In this procedure the circular muscle is divided with a longitudinal incision to widen the colonic lumen. The incision is made through the taenia so as to avoid opening diverticula, and is deepened until the mucosa is just seen. The operation lowers the sigmoid intraluminal pressures and improves symptoms but, after 3 years, pressures return to their former levels. The need for myotomy has declined but it may still be useful in some elderly or obese patients.

Complicated diverticular disease

It is important to distinguish the minority of patients who suffer from a febrile attack with left iliac-fossa peritonism, sometimes called left-sided appendicitis, from those with chronic pain and diarrhoea. The inflammation may settle with minimal symptoms or develop into a pericolic abscess or peritonitis.

Acute diverticulitis

Pain is felt over the left lower abdomen, and the patient may have a pyrexia, malaise, anorexia, and nausea. The white blood count is raised.

Treatment is with rest, antibiotics, usually cefuroxime 750 mg and metronidazole 500 mg 8-hourly, and analgesia. Most cases settle and the diagnosis can be confirmed after 2 to 3 weeks by barium enema. A narrow segment can sometimes be difficult to distinguish from a carcinoma and any doubtful cases can be clarified by subsequent colonoscopy (Fig. 2).

If symptoms fail to resolve, or recur, resection of the sigmoid colon may be necessary. When it is necessary to resect an acutely inflamed and unprepared colon, a Hartmann's operation may be safer than a primary anastomosis.

For recurrent diverticulitis operated electively, a primary anastomosis would be ideal.

Diverticular abscess

Acute diverticulitis can lead to a local peritonitis with abscess formation, either in the paracolic or pelvic area. There may be a palpable mass and a swinging fever. When in doubt the diagnosis can be confirmed by ultrasound or computed tomography (**CT**) with rectal contrast (Fig. 3).

It is wise to let an abscess localize whilst treating the patient with rest, antibiotics, and analgesia. Some abscesses will be amenable to drainage by direct incision, over them or via the rectum or vagina. More complicated collections are best drained by CT-guided aspiration or drain placement. There is rarely any need to do a proximal transverse colostomy. If drainage persists, an elective sigmoid colectomy with primary anastomosis can be done at a later time. Even when an abscess is localized, however, the condition remains potentially dangerous as it may rupture into the peritoneal cavity giving rise to peritonitis.

Perforated diverticulitis

Acute diverticulitis can be complicated by generalized purulent peritonitis, either by direct spread from the inflamed colon or by rupture of a peridiverticular abscess. The clinical picture is of severe intraperitoneal sepsis with toxaemia, ileus and abdominal pain, and septicaemia will often follow. Emergency laparotomy is almost always required, although time must be allowed for adequate rehydration, correction of electrolytes, and starting antibiotic therapy—again cefuroxime and metronidazole.

Other causes of the acute abdomen that may not require surgery should be excluded, including pelvic inflammatory disease, ureteric calculus, and even pulmonary embolus. In these circumstances a CT scan is invaluable.

There has been a shift away from the more conservative procedures in this situation. At one time, peritoneal toilet, pelvic drainage, and a defunctioning transverse colostomy was the favoured procedure, but this has the disadvantage that the 'septic colon' is left in place and that there is a column of faecal material below the stoma and above the perforation. There is the further problem of the unsuspected carcinoma within the inflammatory mass.

For these reasons more radical measures are favoured by experienced surgeons. A Hartmann's procedure—removing the diseased sigmoid, oversewing the distal rectum, and bringing out an end colostomy, is the most frequently used procedure (Fig. 4). In favourable cases it may be possible to do an on-table colonic lavage via the appendix stump and make an immediate anastomosis but this carries the risk of leakage.

Hartmann's procedure is safe and effective, although subsequent reconnection may involve a major operation in elderly patients. Purulent peritonitis carries a mortality of around 15 per cent.

Faecal peritonitis

This is a catastrophic complication with a mortality of around 50 per cent particularly in the elderly. A diverticulum ruptures, often with little or no inflammation, liberating quantities of faeces into the peritoneal cavity. Rapid and severe shock with septicaemia ensues. Energetic resuscitation is necessary, followed promptly by surgery and a Hartmann's operation. These patients often need to be stabilized in an intensive care unit postoperatively.

Fig. 2 The typical appearance of diverticula seen at colonoscopy. Note the muscular haustra and the mouths of diverticula—one with a faecolith. (Reproduced from the *Slide Atlas of Gastroenterology*, Gower Medical Publishing Ltd., London, with permission.)

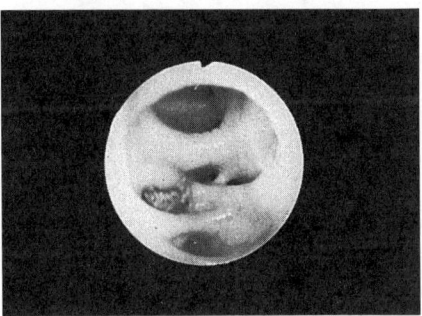

Fig. 3 Computerized tomography of the pelvis in a patient with acute diverticulitis. The sigmoid colon is grossly thickened, the lumen narrowed, and pockets of air are seen in the diverticular disease.

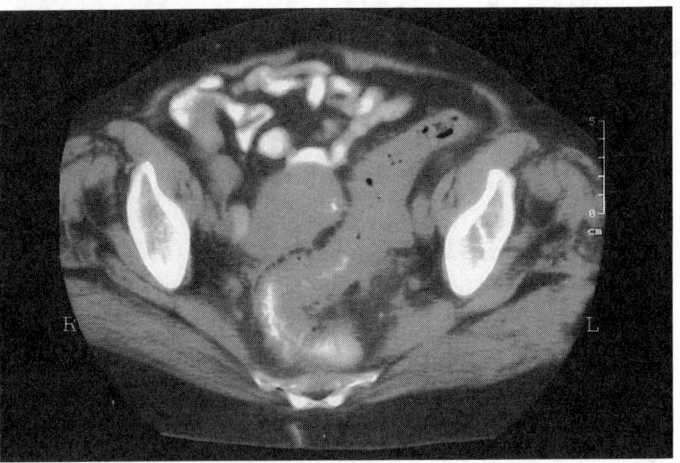

Fig. 4 (a)The area of sigmoid colon resected for perforated diverticular disease. (b) Hartmann's operation—the sigmoid colon has been resected, the rectum oversewn, and a left iliac-fossa colostomy fashioned.

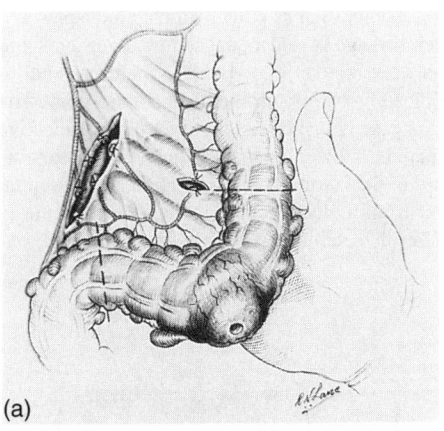

(a)

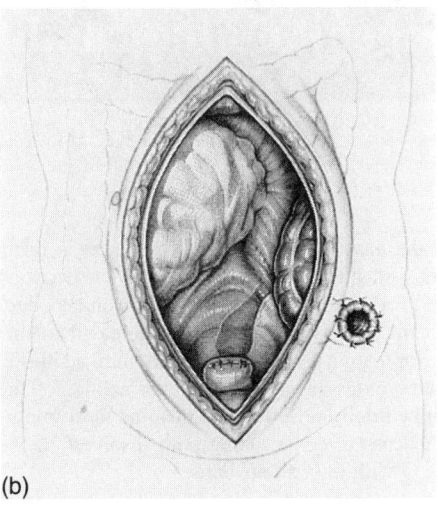

(b)

Intestinal obstruction

Recurrent inflammation with fibrosis and muscular hypertrophy can lead to progressive stenosis and colonic obstruction, which is usually chronic but may present acutely. Conservative treatment is worth trying at first, provided a carcinoma has been excluded. With the aid of a stool softener the symptoms may resolve and the stricture gradually dilate. If these measures fail, the bowel should be prepared for a resection, with care taken not to aggravate the obstruction.

Small-bowel obstruction is sometimes a complication of acute diverticulitis, as the bowel may adhere to the inflammatory mass. It usually resolves as the inflammation subsides but on occasion a laparotomy and division of adhesions or even a small-bowel resection may be necessary.

Colonic fistulae

A colovesical fistula usually presents with recurrent urinary-tract infections together with pneumaturia or faecuria. The fistula arises in the sigmoid, which has often folded over into the pouch of Douglas, and adheres to the apex of the bladder. This is the most frequent cause of colovesical fistula but carcinoma and Crohn's disease should be excluded.

Fistulae may also occur between the sigmoid and vagina, uterus, ureter, and ileum. They seldom heal spontaneously but do not always give rise to disabling symptoms and so represent a relative indication for surgery. Sigmoid colectomy as a one-stage procedure is the best option, and colostomy is rarely required. A fistula into the bladder is simply closed and urethral catheter drainage continued for a week.

Haemorrhage

Major haemorrhage is an uncommon but well-recognized complication. It is usually self-limiting, only requiring transfusion and supportive measures. The precise reason for the bleeding is not known but angiographic and colonoscopic studies suggest that many bleeds attributed to diverticula are caused by other lesions such as polyps and angiodysplasia.

Repeated or minor haemorrhage is seldom caused by diverticula and is more likely to be due to carcinoma or polyps. It is therefore vital to exclude other sources of bleeding by barium enema or colonoscopy. The source of a persistent major bleed must be sought urgently and selective angiography whilst the patient is bleeding is essential. As the haemorrhage can be from any part of the colon, good localization is an essential prelude to any operation. Blind colonic resections have a particularly poor record and if the site of bleeding has still not been located, on-table colonic lavage via the appendix stump and intraoperative colonoscopy will usually target the bleeding segment.

REFERENCES

Boulos, B.P., Karamanolis, D.G., Salmon, P., and Clark, G.C. (1984). Is colonoscopy necessary in diverticular diverticula disease? *Lancet*, **i**, 95–6.

Eastwood, M.A., Sanderson, J., Pocock, S.J., and Mitchell, W.D. (1977). Variation in the incidence of diverticular disease within the city of Edinburgh. *Gut*, **18**, 571–4.

Eastwood, M.A., Smith, A.N., Brydon, W.G., and Pritchard, J. (1978). Comparison of bran, ispaghula and lactulose on colon function in diverticular disease. *Gut*, **19**, 1144–7.

Gear, J.S.S. *et al.* (1979). Symptomless diverticular disease and intake of dietary fibre. *Lancet*, **i**, 511–14.

Gianfranco, J.A., and Abcarian, H. (1982). Pitfalls in the treatment of gastrointestinal bleeding with blind subtotal colectomy. *Diseases of the Colon and Rectum*, **25**, 441–5.

Grief, J.M., Fried, D.O., and McSherry, C.K. (1980). Surgical treatment of perforated diverticulitis of the sigmoid colon. *Diseases of the Colon and Rectum*, **23**, 483–7.

Heaton, K.W. (1985). Diet and diverticulosis—new leads. *Gut*, **26**, 541–3.

Hughes, L.E. (1969). Postmortem survey of diverticular disease of the colon. *Gut*, **10**, 336–51.

Hyland, J.M.P. and Taylor, I. (1980). Does a high fibre diet prevent the complications of diverticular disease? *British Journal of Surgery*, **67**, 77–9.

Kettlewell, M.G.W. and Moloney, G.E. (1977). Combined horizontal and longitudinal colomyotomy for diverticular disease: preliminary report. *Diseases of the Colon and Rectum*, **20**, 24–8.

Krukowski, Z.H. and Mattheson, N.A. (1985). Emergency surgery for diverticular disease complicated by generalised and faecal peritonitis: a review. *British Journal of Surgery*, **71**, 921–7.

Krukowski, Z.H., Koruth, N.M., and Mattheson, N.A. (1985). Evolving practice in acute diverticulitis. *British Journal of Surgery*, **72**, 684–6.

Painter, N.S. (1975). *Diverticular disease of the colon*. Heinemann Medical, London.

Reilly, M. (1966). Sigmoid myotomy. *British Journal of Surgery*, **53**, 859–63.

Smith, A.N., Attisha, R.P., and Balfour, T. (1969). Clinical and manometric results one year after sigmoid myotomy for diverticular disease. *British Journal of Surgery*, **56**, 895–9.

Whiteway, J. and Morson, B.C. (1985). Elastosis in diverticular disease of the sigmoid colon. *Gut*, **26**, 258–66.

14.15 Congenital abnormalities of the gastrointestinal tract

V. M. WRIGHT AND J. A. WALKER-SMITH

Congenital disorders of the gastrointestinal tract are present at birth. Although they are usually manifest shortly after birth, on occasion symptoms may be delayed for months or even years. For example, duodenal atresia presents in the first few days of life whereas duodenal stenosis may not present for many years, sometimes not until adult life.

In this chapter the embryology of congenital abnormalities of the gastrointestinal tract will be briefly reviewed and then the most important conditions will be discussed, commencing with disorders of the oesophagus and concluding with imperforate anus.

Embryology of the congenital abnormalities of the gastrointestinal tract

The primitive gut is initially a simple tube of endoderm, the muscle and connective tissue developing from the splanchnopleuric mesoderm. Cranially, the gut terminates at the buccopharyngeal membrane and caudally at the cloacal membrane. Both membranes disappear; failure of the cloacal membrane to do so results in one of the rarer forms of imperforate anus. The primitive foregut diverticulum gives rise to the respiratory system, oesophagus, stomach, duodenum to the level of the ampulla of Vater, liver, and pancreas. The primitive oesophagus lengthens rapidly, becomes narrow, and frequently the lumen is transiently obliterated. A longitudinal, ventral diverticulum of the foregut forms the trachea with ridges on either side that fuse, initially caudally with progression cranially, until the primitive respiratory system is separated from the oesophagus. Failure of this complex process results in the various forms of oesophageal atresia and tracheo-oesophageal fistula. Dilatation of the foregut distal to the oesophagus produces the stomach, initially slung from the dorsal body wall by the dorsal mesentery and from the septum transversum by the ventral mesentery. Rapid differential growth results in the stomach rotating through 90° on its long axis, the dorsal border becoming the greater curvature, and the ventral border the lesser curvature. The dorsal mesentery forms the greater omentum. The ventral mesentery, into which the liver bud grows, forms the falciform ligament and coronary ligaments attaching the liver to the diaphragm, and the lesser omentum. Congenital abnormalities of the stomach are excessively rare. The liver arises as a shallow groove on the ventral aspect of the duodenum. The groove becomes tubular and invades the septum transversum and the ventral mesentery. Bile is secreted from the fifth month, and gives meconium its characteristic dark-green appearance. The mesoderm of the septum transversum forms the fibrous tissue of the liver.

The pancreas develops as two outgrowths of the duodenum. One comes from the dorsal aspect, the other from the ventral. The dorsal bud grows into the dorsal mesentery and the ventral bud is swept around dorsally into the mesentery when the duodenum rotates to the right. These two primordia fuse, the ducts fuse, and the main pancreatic duct joins the bile duct to enter the duodenum at the ampulla of Vater. If the ducts do not fuse, an accessory pancreatic duct persists. Annular pancreas is a congenital anomaly where the pancreas surrounds the duodenum, which may be atretic or intrinsically stenosed. Annular pancreas is not the primary cause of the duodenal obstruction in these cases.

The duodenum is derived partly from foregut and partly from the midgut. The loop of primitive duodenum is fixed at the pyloric end, and by the ligament of Treitz at the duodenojejunal flexure to the left of the first lumbar vertebra. By rotating to the right, the entire duodenum comes to lie retroperitoneally in a curve around the head of the pancreas. Failure of the duodenum to fix in this position is a fundamental reason for the gut failing to rotate correctly. During rapid growth the duodenal lumen is obliterated and partial or total failure of recanalization will result in the anomalies of duodenal atresia or stenosis. The small intestine and colon, suspended on the dorsal mesentery, rapidly lengthen and outgrow the primitive peritoneal cavity, and herniation occurs into the umbilical sac during the fifth week of development. Growth in length continues, the loop of bowel rotating through 180° anticlockwise, the cranial limb lengthening more than the caudal limb. About the tenth week the loops of bowel return to the peritoneal cavity. The small intestine goes first, the large intestine subsequently. Thus the large intestine lies in front of the small. The caecum is initially subhepatic, the large liver occupying the right side of the abdomen, eventually retreating to the right upper quadrant and allowing growth in the length of the ascending colon. The caecum, ascending colon, and descending colon become fixed to the posterior abdominal wall; thus the small bowel is suspended from a mesentery that runs from the left side of the first lumbar vertebra to the right iliac fossa. Failure of the duodenum to rotate and fix, coupled with a failure of normal rotation of the bowel with consequent lack of normal fixation, gives rise to malrotation of the intestine. Abnormal bands run from the caecum, which lies to the left of the midline, to the region of the gallbladder and may compress the duodenum. The narrow mesentery of the small intestine predisposes to a volvulus of the entire midgut.

At the apex of the midgut loop, the primitive gut is in continuity with the extraembryonic yolk sac via the vitellointestinal duct, which runs in the umbilical cord. Obliteration and disappearance of this duct occurs,

allowing the bowel to return from the umbilical sac to the enlarged peritoneal cavity. Failure of the duct to disappear may result in a Meckel's diverticulum, a band connecting the ileum to the umbilicus, a communication between the lumen of the ileum and the umbilicus, or failure of the gut to return completely to the peritoneal cavity, resulting in a small umbilical hernia.

Persistence of the umbilical sac will result in an exomphalos, with the sac containing a variable amount of gut and much of the liver. The embryology of gastroschisis is disputed. It may be due to early rupture of the umbilical sac allowing the primitive gut to extrude into the extra-embryonic coelom, or failure of fusion of the lateral body folds producing a defect in the anterior abdominal wall adjacent to the umbilicus.

The midgut comprises the duodenum distal to the ampulla of Vater, jejunum, ileum, caecum, and colon as far as the left transverse colon. Atresia affecting the midgut may occur at single or multiple sites. The cause is probably intrauterine interference with the blood supply to that part of the gut which is affected, with consequent resorption of the ischaemic bowel.

The hindgut gives origin to the left third of the transverse colon, the descending colon, sigmoid, rectum, and upper part of the anal canal, and a considerable part of the urogenital system. The hindgut terminates in the primitive cloaca, which is separated from the proctodaeum (a shallow ectodermal depression) by the cloacal membrane. The primitive cloaca communicates with the hindgut and the allantois. Early in development the cloaca is joined by the pronephric ducts. A coronal septum (the urorectal septum) arises in the angle between the allantois and hindgut, grows caudally, fuses with the cloacal membrane, and divides the cloaca into a dorsal primitive rectum and a ventral primitive urogenital sinus. The cloacal membrane breaks down, establishing continuity between the endodermal hindgut and the ectodermal part of the anal canal. There are many varieties of imperforate anus. Absence of a variable length of rectum and anal canal, known as the 'high' anomaly, is frequently associated with the bowel terminating via a rectourethral or rectovaginal fistula. Ten per cent of babies with an imperforate anus will have oesophageal atresia, with or without a fistula, suggesting that the division of trachea and oesophagus and urogenital system and rectum must be occurring at a similar time in gestation, with possibly a similar mechanism producing the division. Anomalies of the urogenital system occur in a very high proportion of affected infants. Abnormalities of the ectodermal component of the anal canal result in 'low' imperforate anus.

The ganglion cells of the gut lie in the submucosa and intermyenteric plane. Ectodermal in origin, they migrate caudally along the length of the gut. Failure of migration down to the internal sphincter of the anal canal results in an aganglionic segment extending for a variable distance proximally, and is the underlying abnormality in Hirschsprung's disease.

Mucosal differentiation occurs in the early months. The inner circular muscle differentiates earlier than the outer longitudinal. Thus the fetal intestinal tract is prepared for digestion, absorption, and propulsion at a comparatively early stage in development.

Oesophageal atresia and tracheo-oesophageal fistula

The incidence of this condition is approximately 1 in 3500 live births.

The upper oesophagus ends in a blind pouch. In the majority of cases the lower oesophagus communicates at its upper end with the trachea, that is, there is a tracheo-oesophageal fistula. Although much less common, there are a number of well-recognized anatomical variations illustrated in Fig. 1.

CLINICAL FEATURES

Frequently the infant with oesophageal atresia is premature or small for gestational age. In 50 per cent there is a history of polyhydramnios. Shortly after birth, because swallowing is impossible, copious amounts of frothy saliva dribble from the mouth, associated with choking, dyspnoea, and cyanotic episodes. Frequent suction is required to keep the airway clear. The infant with a tracheo-oesophageal fistula without associated oesophageal atresia coughs, chokes, and becomes cyanosed during feeds. Because air escapes through the fistula into the oesophagus, gaseous distension of the abdomen is frequently present. Aspiration of feed into the airway results in pulmonary collapse/consolidation.

Over 50 per cent of infants with oesophageal atresia will have significant associated anomalies. Of particular importance are cardiac, anorectal, urogenital, and skeletal anomalies. The premature infant or the infant who is small for gestational age are more likely to have multiple anomalies than is the full-term infant.

Survival of infants with oesophageal atresia depends on birth weight and associated abnormalities. All infants with a birth weight greater than 1.8 kg and no associated abnormalities or pneumonia should survive; this is also true of the larger infant with a moderately severe associated abnormality or pneumonia. The mortality for the infant less than 1.5 kg, or one with multiple severe congenital abnormalities, remains in the region of 20 to 30 per cent.

DIAGNOSIS

When oesophageal atresia is suspected a size 10 or 12 FG catheter is passed through the mouth and into the oesophagus. If the oesophagus is obstructed, the catheter meets a resistance 9 to 11 cm from the gum margin. A smaller catheter may curl up in the obstructed oesophagus. Contrast studies of the oesophagus are rarely necessary. A chest and abdominal radiograph will show the position of a radio-opaque tube in the upper oesophagus, and the presence of gas in the bowel, if a tracheo-oesophageal fistula is present. Complete absence of gas in the abdomen is diagnostic of an oesophageal atresia without a distal tracheo-oesophageal fistula. The radiograph will also reveal any abnormalities of ribs or vertebrae, signs of pneumonia, and may provide evidence of an associated cardiac abnormality.

In isolated tracheo-oesophageal fistula, very careful contrast studies of the oesophagus are required to demonstrate the fistula. Endoscopic examination of trachea and oesophagus is usually diagnostic.

MANAGEMENT

Early division of the tracheo-oesophageal fistula and anastomosis of the oesophagus are possible in the majority of cases. Postoperatively, mechanical ventilation may be necessary, but usually the full-term infant with no preoperative complications only needs careful suction of the nasopharynx to maintain a clear airway. A gastrostomy or a transanastomotic nasogastric tube is usually used to enable the infant to be fed within 48 h of operation. A primary anastomosis may not be feasible in pure oesophageal atresia, extreme prematurity, or where the infant's general condition is poor. In such cases a tracheo-oesophageal fistula, if present, would be divided and a feeding gastrostomy established. Subsequently, an oesophageal anastomosis after a delay of 4 to 6 weeks,

Fig. 1 Anatomical variations of oesophageal atresia and tracheo-oesophageal fistula, indicating the relative frequency.

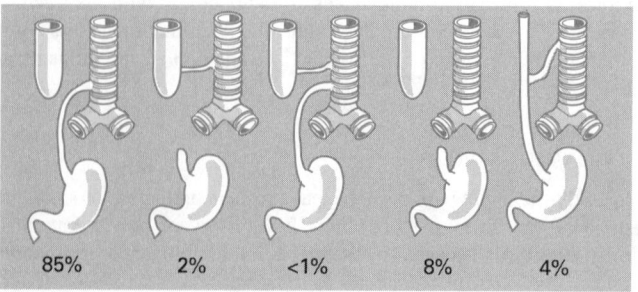

| 85% | 2% | <1% | 8% | 4% |

having left the upper oesophageal pouch intact and kept empty of saliva by continuous suction, may be feasible. Alternatively a cervical oesophagostomy is done with the intention after some months of establishing continuity between mouth and stomach, using a length of colon, a tube of stomach, or the whole stomach. The decision depends on the clinical situation and the surgeon's preference.

Anterior abdominal wall defects

The incidence of exomphalos and gastroschisis is approximately 1 in 3000 births. An exomphalos occurs because the intra-abdominal contents herniate through the umbilical ring into the base of the umbilical cord and are covered by a translucent membrane composed of peritoneum and amnion. Exomphalos major indicates that the diameter of the defect is greater than 5 cm, exomphalos minor that the defect is less than 5 cm. The contents of the exomphalos almost always include liver and a variable amount of bowel. On occasion a very small amount of bowel alone herniates into the base of the cord. The diagnosis is frequently made on a prenatal ultrasonographic scan and prompts a search for associated major abnormalities, particularly anencephaly, chromosomal trisomies, major cardiac anomalies, and the Beckwith–Wiedemann syndrome. Associated abnormalities occur in 40 per cent.

The Beckwith–Wiedemann syndrome also termed the EMG (Exomphalos Macroglossia Gigantism) syndrome, usually presents as a large-for-dates infant with a small exomphalos. The tongue is strikingly large, there are frequently ridges in the ear lobes, and a prominent naevus flammeus on the forehead. Hypoglycaemia as a result of hyperinsulinism produced by islet-cell hyperplasia is a common early problem, which may require steroids, glucagon, and rarely subtotal pancreatectomy to effect control. In the long term, children with this syndrome have an increased incidence of solid tumours, particularly nephroblastoma and hepatoblastoma.

In gastroschisis there is a full-thickness defect in the anterior abdominal wall, usually to the right of the umbilical cord. The defect is small but most of the gastrointestinal tract may be extruded through it, and appears grossly thickened, very short, and covered with a densely adherent, gelatinous membrane. In contrast to exomphalos, other intra-abdominal organs are rarely eviscerated and abnormalities outside the gastrointestinal are unusual. Again, prenatal diagnosis on ultrasonographic scan is common.

EXOMPHALOS

Clinical features

The lesion will be obvious at birth. Occasionally the membrane will rupture during, or shortly after, delivery. Careful examination for associated defects is essential.

Management

A nasogastric tube is passed to keep the bowel decompressed and prevent unnecessary enlargement of the exomphalos by air-filled bowel. The sac can be very satisfactorily covered and supported by wrapping clingfilm around the exomphalos and the baby's trunk. Plain radiographs of chest and abdomen are taken preoperatively in order to study the cardiac contour, the intestinal gas pattern, and to look for evidence of an associated diaphragmatic hernia. If the contents of the sac can be reduced into the peritoneal cavity, the abdominal wall can be closed in layers. If closure of all layers of the abdominal wall is impossible, skin closure alone may be used, with or without excision of the membrane, or a synthetic material such as silastic sheeting or Prolene mesh is used to enclose the sac after suturing it to the margins of the defect. Gradual reduction, over a number of days, of the contents into the peritoneal cavity is then possible, with delayed closure of the abdominal wall. An alternative is to paint the sac with an antiseptic solution such as 70 per cent alcohol, or one of the iodine-based preparations. This results in the formation, after a few days, of a dry eschar that separates after some weeks, leaving a granulating surface, which gradually epithelializes. Any method that does not achieve muscle closure will leave a ventral hernia, which requires surgery at a later date.

Postoperatively, ventilatory support may be necessary. Antibiotics commenced preoperatively are continued postoperatively, particularly if an artificial material is used. Parenteral nutrition will be necessary if oral feeds cannot be given. Survival is related to the size of the lesion and the presence of severe associated abnormalities.

GASTROSCHISIS

Clinical features

Babies with this abnormality are frequently small for gestational age. After delivery, heat loss from the exposed bowel rapidly causes hypothermia. Hypoproteinaemia is very common. The small size of the defect in the anterior abdominal wall and the often narrow pedicle from which the bowel is suspended may impair the blood supply and result in infarction of much of the extruded intestine. Atresia may have occurred because of intrauterine impairment of the blood supply.

Management

A nasogastric tube is passed and the bowel decompressed. The bowel can be enclosed in clingfilm wrapped around the baby's trunk, or the baby can be placed in a large polythene bag taped around the chest. This keeps the bowel moist and prevents excessive heat loss. Antibiotics are commenced preoperatively and plasma is given to counteract the existing hypoproteinaemia and hypovolaemia. At operation the anterior abdominal wall is stretched and any meconium washed out *per rectum* to reduce bulk. Reduction of the extruded bowel is attempted and abdominal wall closure achieved where possible.

In a proportion of cases a Silastic sheet or Prolene mesh are used to form an artificial sac over the intestine. The material is sutured to the margins of the defect and the size of the sac gradually reduced over some days, squeezing the bowel back into the peritoneal cavity until closure of the abdominal wall becomes feasible—usually after 10 to 14 days. Ventilatory support postoperatively is often necessary. Parenteral nutrition is essential and may need to continue for many weeks until gastrointestinal motility and absorption are adequate. Sepsis is a considerable hazard. The mortality is now 5 to 10 per cent compared with 80 per cent 10 years ago. Improved postoperative management is largely responsible for this.

Congenital pyloric stenosis

Congenital hypertrophic pyloric stenosis is a disorder characterized by hypertrophy of the circular muscle of the pylorus and so obstruction to the gastric outlet. The incidence is 2 per 1000 live births. The aetiology is unknown. Theories include primary muscle hypertrophy, abnormalities of the maturation of ganglion cells, absence of a certain type of ganglion cell, or a response to abnormally high concentrations of circulating gastrin. Genetic and environmental factors play an important part. There is an increased incidence of pyloric stenosis in siblings of an affected child and in the offspring of a woman who has had the condition. Environmental factors include social class, type of feeding, and a seasonal variation with an increase in the winter months. In any large series the male:female ratio is 3 or 4:1 and half the cases will be first-born children.

CLINICAL FEATURES

The onset of symptoms is usually between 3 and 6 weeks of age, but may present shortly after birth. Vomiting of increasing severity is the cardinal symptom, eventually occurring after most feeds and becoming projectile. The vomitus is milk and mucus, and may contain altered blood suggesting an oesophagitis or gastritis; bile is never present. The baby stops gaining weight and becomes constipated. Characteristically the baby is alert, anxious, and hungry. If diagnosis is delayed, severe malnutrition may develop.

Examination reveals evidence of weight loss and in advanced cases signs of dehydration will be evident. When the stomach is full, waves of peristalsis travelling from left to right in the epigastrium will be seen (visible peristalsis). The thickened pylorus is felt as an olive-sized tumour lying deep to the edge of the right rectus and is often most easily felt when the stomach is empty. The diagnosis of pyloric stenosis is made on clinical grounds in the majority of cases. A plain radiograph of the abdomen may be very helpful in revealing a large stomach with a paucity of distal gas. A barium meal is diagnostic when the 'string' sign of the elongated pylorus is demonstrated. The barium study may also reveal gastro-oesophageal reflux, which is commonly associated with pyloric stenosis. In experienced hands, ultrasound can accurately delineate the elongated, thickened pylorus.

MANAGEMENT

In the child presenting early, electrolyte disturbance and dehydration are minimal. In the later case, dehydration with hypochloraemic alkalosis and marked potassium depletion occurs. Preoperative correction of water and electrolyte deficits is essential. The operation of pyloromyotomy, described by Ramstedt in 1912, splits the hypertrophied muscle longitudinally allowing the mucosa to bulge through the defect, thus enlarging the pyloric canal. Postoperatively, various feeding regimens are advocated; all aim to have the baby on a normal feeds by 48 to 72 h postoperatively. The prognosis is excellent.

Atresia and stenosis of the small intestine

An intrinsic obstruction may produce either complete or partial obliteration of the bowel lumen. Complete obliteration may be due to a gap between the two ends of the small intestine, with or without a connecting band between these ends, or a complete mucosal diaphragm. Such complete obstruction is known as atresia. When obstruction is incomplete it may be due to a narrowing of the lumen—a stenosis—or a complete mucosal diaphragm with a hole. Small-intestinal atresia is a more common finding than is stenosis. The duodenum is most often affected, followed by jejunum and least often ileum.

Associated abnormalities of the gastrointestinal tract, including malrotation, oesophageal atresia, imperforate anus, biliary atresia, and annular pancreas, are a feature of duodenal atresia/stenosis. Localized volvulus and meconium ileus are associated with jejunoileal atresias.

Intrinsic obstruction of the small intestine of congenital origin presents most often in the neonatal period but when the obstruction is partial it may first present much later, in infancy and childhood.

CONGENITAL INTRINSIC DUODENAL OBSTRUCTION

When duodenal obstruction is complete, vomiting usually occurs within a few hours of birth and is bile stained unless the obstruction is proximal to the ampulla of Vater, when the vomiting is persistent and copious but not bile stained. Meconium may be passed normally and there may be obvious epigastric distension. In view of the association with other abnormalities, these should be sought carefully. In particular the infant should be examined for evidence of Down's syndrome. Duodenal lesions are an association of this syndrome and occur in 10 per cent of cases.

When obstruction is incomplete the symptoms may be intermittent and the diagnosis delayed.

Congenital intrinsic duodenal obstruction may be accompanied by an annular pancreas; this is a sign of failure of duodenal development rather than an obstructive lesion *per se*. In infants with duodenal atresia, at operation, it often looks as if there is an annular pancreas because there is interposition of the pancreas between the two ends of the duodenal atresia.

Congenital intrinsic duodenal obstruction is not in general associated with multiple atresias in the remainder of the small intestine, but there may be obstruction at two levels in the duodenum.

JEJUNOILEAL OBSTRUCTION

Symptoms, typically bile-stained vomiting and abdominal distension, usually occur within the first 2 days of life. Meconium may or may not be passed. When obstruction is incomplete the diagnosis may again be long delayed and the child may present with intermittent vomiting, abdominal distension, and even with features of malabsorption—a clinical picture that may resemble coeliac disease.

Diagnosis

Plain radiographs of the abdomen are usually diagnostic in infants who present with a complete obstruction. In duodenal atresia there is the characteristic 'double bubble' (Fig. 2). When duodenal obstruction is incomplete there may be small amounts of air in the lower bowel. A barium meal may be necessary to demonstrate the obstruction and may suggest an associated malrotation. When there is complete jejunoileal obstruction there are usually dilated loops of intestine. A barium enema may reveal an unused microcolon. When obstruction is incomplete a barium follow-through may be needed to establish the diagnosis. Rarely, laparotomy may be the final court of appeal.

Management

A nasogastric tube is passed to empty the stomach and allow accurate measurement of gastric losses. Correction of fluid and electrolyte disturbances, if present, should precede surgery, provided that gangrenous or ischaemic bowel is not suspected. At laparotomy, care should be taken to exclude any accompanying gastrointestinal abnormality. In duodenal obstruction, the operation of choice is duodenoduodenostomy. In jejunoileal lesions, resection is obviously indicated but there should be adequate resection of the proximal dilated gut. This reduces the great discrepancy in size between the two blind ends and so facilitates end-to-end anastomosis, although an oblique-to-end anastomosis is sometimes necessary. Leaving the dilated gut immediately proximal to an atresia results in ineffective peristalsis above the anastomosis.

Fig. 2 Plain radiograph of the abdomen of an infant with duodenal atresia showing characteristic 'double bubble'.

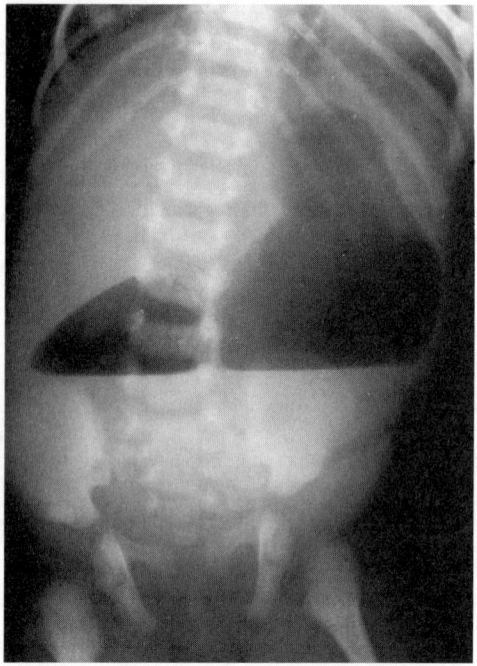

Considerable loss of intestinal length may occur as a result of the intrauterine process producing the atresia; surgical correction, particularly of multiple atresias, will result in further loss. Every effort is made to preserve some ileum and the ileocaecal valve. Loss of considerable lengths of jejunum is well tolerated. Loss of ileum, particularly if the ileocaecal valve is also lost, presents considerable management problems throughout childhood because malabsorption of a variety of important nutrients occurs. The enterohepatic circulation is disrupted. Liver damage is compounded by episodes of sepsis and the need for long-term parenteral nutrition.

Duplication of gastrointestinal tract

DEFINITION

Duplications are cystic or tubular structures whose lumen is lined by a mucous membrane, usually supported by smooth muscle. They occur most often within the dorsal mesentery of the gut. They are also sometimes described as enteric cysts, neurenteric cysts, and reduplications. Duplications may occur anywhere along the alimentary tract but they are found most often in relation to the small intestine, particularly the ileum. They may not communicate with the lumen of the gastrointestinal tract. Duplications may be found in association with intestinal atresias. Sometimes those associated with the small intestine are lined by gastric mucosa and peptic ulceration of the adjacent small-intestinal mucosa with bleeding may occur. Those associated with the colon never contain ectopic gastric mucosa.

CLINICAL FEATURES

These are congenital malformations that present most often in early infancy. Later presentation, even into adult life, is well recognized. Duplications may present in infancy as a small-bowel obstruction, or a small cystic duplication may form the lead point of an intussusception. A palpable abdominal mass in infancy, as well as rectal bleeding and volvulus, may also be modes of presentation of this disorder. The clinical diagnosis is often difficult and the diagnosis may sometimes be made only at laparotomy. A technetium scan may be helpful by demonstrating ectopic gastric mucosa. Some cases may present as a posterior thoracic space-occupying lesion and may go through the diaphragm and be related to an extensive upper small-intestinal duplication as well. The presence of an abnormal cervical or thoracic vertebra on radiographs may suggest the diagnosis of a duplication.

MANAGEMENT

Excision of a cystic duplication with or without the adjacent intestine is usually straightforward. Any associated thoracic cyst will also need excision. Short tubular duplications can be excised with the adjacent intestine; very extensive tubular duplications can be opened longitudinally and the mucosa stripped out, leaving the common muscle wall.

Small-intestinal malrotation with or without volvulus

Malrotation of the small intestine is due to disordered movement of the intestine around the superior mesenteric artery during the course of embryological development.

Two main abnormalities that produce clinical syndromes may occur. First, there is a gross narrowing of the base of the mesentery, which may allow the midgut to twist around and cause a volvulus. This may occur acutely, causing complete obstruction, or it may occur intermittently, producing bouts of partial or complete obstruction that release themselves spontaneously. Secondly, there may be partial duodenal obstruction from extrinsic compression of the small intestine by peritoneal bands (Ladd's bands) that extend from the caecum to the subhepatic region.

Malrotation may be associated with duodenal atresia or stenosis. It may also be found in association with diaphragmatic hernia, omphalocele, and gastroschisis. However, malrotation may not produce symptoms and is sometimes discovered only as an incidental finding on a barium study. The majority of children who develop symptoms related to malrotation do so within the neonatal period, presenting with features of intestinal obstruction, complete or incomplete. When there is a volvulus there may also be obstruction to the blood supply to the bowel, which if complete will lead to extensive gangrene of the small bowel. The passage of melaena stools may be an early sign of this complication.

Those children with malrotation who present later in childhood may do so with features of intermittent obstruction such as episodes of vomiting, often bile stained, and abdominal pain, but sometimes they may manifest with features of malabsorption and many clinical features suggestive of coeliac disease. This is due to intestinal stasis with bacterial overgrowth in the lumen of the small intestine. Steatorrhoea may be accompanied at times by protein-losing enteropathy from obstruction of the mesenteric lymphatics, and chylous ascites may also occur.

DIAGNOSIS

The diagnosis needs to be considered in the differential diagnosis of small-intestinal obstruction in infancy.

Plain radiographs of the abdomen may be very useful, typically revealing some distension of the stomach and duodenum, but unlike duodenal atresia this is accompanied by some gas scattered through the lower part of the abdomen. However, a malrotation may not be accompanied by any abnormality on the plain radiograph of the abdomen and a barium meal will then be necessary to reveal the presence of malrotation by outlining the duodenum. A barium enema may be useful if it demonstrates the abnormal position of the caecum, but a barium meal is more reliable.

MANAGEMENT

Surgical intervention is indicated when a firm diagnosis is established. Ladd's operation is usually the procedure of choice. This involves, in general, the placement of the colon on the left and the small intestine on the right, having divided any bands and adhesions between the duodenum and large bowel, and by dissection broadened the base of the mesentery as much as possible. After a volvulus, total bowel necrosis is untreatable, but severe bowel ischaemia can be reversible and a 'second look' laparotomy may be necessary.

Small-intestinal lymphangiectasia

Small-intestinal lymphangiectasia has been described as a primary, that is a congenital, abnormality or as a secondary manifestation of some other disease process such as constrictive pericarditis. The primary abnormality may be accompanied by generalized lymphatic abnormalities including lymphoedema, chylous ascites, and hypoplasia of the peripheral lymphatic system, but the lymphatic abnormality may be confined to the small bowel and its mesentery. It is usually, but not invariably, accompanied by hypoproteinaemic oedema. Radioisotope studies have demonstrated that the hypoproteinaemia is due to abnormal protein loss into the gut. The pathogenesis of the hypoproteinaemia has been attributed to the rupture of dilated lymphatic channels or to protein exudation from intestinal capillaries via an intact epithelium, where there is obstruction of lymphatic flow.

CLINICAL FEATURES

It is a rare condition, which may present throughout life but most often in the first 2 years with diarrhoea and failure to thrive and, later, generalized oedema with hypoproteinaemia. The clinical picture may resemble coeliac disease. There is lymphopenia in the presence of a normal bone marrow and reduction of serum albumin, serum IgG, and carrier proteins such as protein-bound iodine. The severe protein loss may be accompanied by enteric calcium loss, leading to hypocalcaemia. Steatorrhoea is often found in this disorder.

DIAGNOSIS

Diagnosis is made by showing the characteristic lymphatic abnormality on small intestinal biopsy, that is dilated lacteals, but the lesion is patchy. One negative biopsy does not exclude the diagnosis. Radioisotope demonstration of abnormal enteric protein loss using a technique such as intravenous $CrCl_3$ is helpful in diagnosis but is not specific. Barium studies in most cases show coarse mucosal folds.

PATHOLOGY

Autopsy studies reveal a considerable variation in the distribution of the lymphatic abnormality along the length of the small intestine. Dilated lacteals may occur irregularly along the small bowel and there may be gross dilatation of lymphatics projecting into the lumen. Lymphatic proliferation and dilation may also occur within the mesentery, as well as the serosal, muscular, and submucosal layers of the small-intestinal wall, and extend into the lymph nodes and occupy part of the nodal tissue.

TREATMENT

This is usually dietetic, as the lymphangiectasia is rarely localized enough to allow surgical excision to effect a permanent cure. The amount of long-chain fat in the diet, which is normally absorbed via the intestinal lymphatics, should be limited. This leads to a reduction in the volume of intestinal lymph and in the pressure in the dilated lymphatics. It is best done by placing the child on a low-fat diet (5–10 g/day) and adding medium-chain triglycerides, instead of the usual long-chain dietary fats, in unrestricted amounts. A milk containing medium-chain triglyceride such as Pregestimil^R may be used with medium-chain triglyceride oil for cooking. Some children may be resistant to this therapy when the abnormality is very extensive and, on occasion, death may result despite therapy. Albumin infusions are of little value in management as their benefit is so transitory. Steroids have been advocated but there is little evidence to justify their use. In a follow-up study of children, although there was a continuing chyle leak, as shown by persistent lymphopenia and hypoalbuminaemia, there was a rapid and sustained improvement in dependent oedema following the use of the diet recommended above, although asymmetrical oedema from peripheral lymphatic abnormalities was unaffected. Their growth rate improved on the diet. Clinical relapse occurred quickly when the diet was relaxed. Continued adherence to a strict diet, at least through puberty, is therefore recommended. Indeed it seems probable that this is a life-long disorder and that some dietetic management may usually need to be permanent.

Meckel's diverticulum

This diverticulum is the vestigial remnant of the vitellointestinal duct. Although most people who have such a diverticulum are asymptomatic, complications may arise, which may present in a variety of ways. In children these complications chiefly arise in association with the presence of ectopic gastric mucosa in the diverticulum. Other ectopic tissue, for example pancreatic tissue and colonic mucosa, may be found in some cases.

The diverticulum is located in the distal ileum within 100 cm of the ileocaecal valve. It is always antemesenteric.

CLINICAL FEATURES

Rectal bleeding is the main symptom. This is usually the passage of bright blood rather than tarry melaena stools. Typically the stool is at first dark in colour but later bright red. Bleeding may be acute, with shock requiring urgent blood transfusion, or it may be chronic. From a practical viewpoint any child who has a massive, painless, rectal bleed should be regarded as a case of Meckel's diverticulum until proved otherwise. Most often bleeding from Meckel's diverticulum is associated with ulceration of the small bowel adjacent to ectopic gastric mucosa but this is not always the case as such bleeding on occasion may occur in the absence of ectopic gastric mucosa.

Small-intestinal obstruction may also be a mode of presentation. This may be as a volvulus or an intussusception with the diverticulum as the leading part. Acute diverticulitis occurs and may produce a picture indistinguishable from acute appendicitis.

DIAGNOSIS AND MANAGEMENT

This depends upon the mode of presentation. When rectal bleeding occurs, other causes such as anal fissure, intussusception, peptic ulcer, oesophagitis, and colonic polyps must be considered. Investigation may include colonoscopy to exclude colonic causes and upper endoscopy to exclude peptic ulceration or oesophagitis.

Barium follow-through is usually an unrewarding investigation but introduction of barium via a duodenal tube, the so-called small bowel enema, may be more successful. Angiography to exclude a haemangiomatous malformation may sometimes be done but a technetium scan is usually the most important investigation. The radionuclide technetium-99m concentrates in the gastric mucosa. When it is given intravenously, ectopic gastric mucosa appears as an abnormal localization on abdominal imaging with a gamma-camera. In this way a Meckel's diverticulum with ectopic gastric mucosa or indeed a duplication with such ectopic tissue may be diagnosed. However, although the use of this technique should lead to an earlier and more accurate diagnosis of Meckel's diverticulum, a negative result in a child with severe bleeding should not deter a surgeon from proceeding with a diagnostic laparotomy, which even in the 1990s remains the final diagnostic test. Indeed, when considering the other modes of presentation of Meckel's diverticulum it is often only at laparotomy that the role of a Meckel's diverticulum in the child's intestinal obstruction is appreciated.

Meconium ileus

This is a manifestation of cystic fibrosis, the disorder sometimes known as fibrocystic disease of the pancreas. Meconium ileus is the earliest mode of presentation of this disorder during the neonatal period. A similar syndrome in older children and young adults who have cystic fibrosis may occur—the meconium ileus equivalent. The abnormally viscid consistency of the meconium produces an intraluminal obstruction. It may result from several factors including the lack of pancreatic enzymes during fetal life, which may account for its high protein content, a characteristic of the meconium from these children. There is also evidence of reduced secretion of water and electrolytes in such infants, which may further render the meconium more viscid. The meconium, because of its high viscosity and tendency to adhere to the mucosa, cannot be propelled along the bowel and so small-intestinal obstruction results. This occurs most often in the distal ileum.

CLINICAL FEATURES

The neonate with this disorder usually develops signs of intestinal obstruction within the first 24 to 48 h of life, with the classical signs of bile-stained vomiting, progressive abdominal distension, and failure to pass meconium. In simple meconium ileus the meconium is the sole source of the obstruction but meconium ileus may be complicated by perforation of the gut, and when this occurs in utero, intraperitoneal calcification may be observed on a plain radiograph of the abdomen, providing evidence of meconium peritonitis. Perforation may also occur in the neonatal period. Volvulus and atresia may also complicate meconium ileus.

In simple meconium ileus, the plain radiograph of the abdomen may show dilated bowel but unaccompanied by many fluid levels. Sometimes there is the appearance of bubbly meconium in the right lower quadrant. Bowel loops may be palpable. If a contrast enema is performed a microcolon, a consequence of disuse, will be demonstrated. The finding of this radiographic appearance in the presence of a family history of cystic fibrosis makes the diagnosis of meconium ileus highly probable, but a similar appearance occurs with jejunoileal atresia.

MANAGEMENT

When meconium ileus is complicated by atresia or perforation, gangrene, peritonitis, or associated volvulus, surgical intervention is essential. Surgical options include the formation of a double-barrelled stoma with subsequent irrigation of the meconium from the distal bowel over a week or so, or intraoperative irrigation of the bowel with an immediate end-to-end anastomosis. In both options, an associated atresia or necrotic bowel are resected. The treatment of uncomplicated meconium ileus using enemas containing pancreatic enzymes, mucolytic agents such as acetylcysteine, and the detergent Tween 80 had been advocated for some time. Noblett in Melbourne, in 1969, used a Gastrografin enema to relieve intraluminal obstruction. Gastrografin is a radioopaque, hyperosmolar solution that is effective because of its hypertonicity. This technique should not be used until a plain radiograph of the abdomen has excluded the possibility of complicated meconium ileus. An initial barium enema should exclude Hirschsprung's disease and demonstrate a microcolon extending to the proximal colon. The retrograde passage of contrast medium through the ileocaecal valve should demonstrate intraluminal meconium with passage into proximal dilated ileum, thus excluding an ileal atresia. After a successful Gastrografin enema, large amounts of meconium will be passed.

Although there may be no signs clinically or radiologically of pulmonary complications in the neonatal period, immediate physiotherapy of the chest should be started and any chest infections treated with antibiotics when they occur (as for older children with cystic fibrosis). A pancreatic enzyme preparation should also be started, at first in small dosage when milk feedings have begun. The diagnosis should be confirmed by sweat electrolyte estimations; concentrations of sweat sodium above 60 mmol/l are abnormal. In the majority of infants with cystic fibrosis the finding of the abnormal gene *deltaF508* or one of the other recognized mutations confirms the diagnosis. In a minority the abnormal gene is not identifiable.

Congenital short intestine

There is a syndrome of congenital short intestine in association with malrotation with clinical features similar to those that follow massive intestinal resection. There is also another syndrome of congenital short intestine in association with pyloric hypertrophy and malrotation. This latter syndrome is due to an absence or diminution of argyrophil ganglion cells in the small-intestinal wall. These cells normally organize peristalsis and ensure that the bolus moves forward at the correct speed. In the absence of such innervation, smooth muscle of the small-intestinal wall contracts spontaneously and rhythmically, but segmentation is not coordinated and the food bolus does not move forward, and there is work hypertrophy of smooth muscle.

Both syndromes are rare and often only diagnosed at laparotomy.

Colonic atresia

Atresia of the large intestine is rare. In any series of cases of intestinal atresias, fewer than 10 per cent will have isolated colonic atresia.

CLINICAL FEATURES

The baby presents in the first 24 to 48 h with marked abdominal distension, vomiting, and failure to pass meconium.

DIAGNOSIS

Abdominal radiographs reveal multiple dilated loops of bowel with fluid levels; the position of the loops may suggest a large bowel obstruction. Confirmation of the level of the atresia is obtained by barium enema.

MANAGEMENT

Nasogastric suction and intravenous fluids are commenced preoperatively. At laparotomy the lesion may be an isolated atresia or associated with multiple atresias of small and large bowel. If the atresia is solitary, it may be possible to make an anastomosis after resection of the atresia and a length of the grossly dilated proximal bowel. Frequently a colostomy is made to allow the dilated proximal bowel to contract before an end-to-end anastomosis some weeks later.

Hirschsprung's disease

In this condition, ganglion cells are absent in the bowel wall. The distal rectum is always aganglionic and the aganglionosis extends proximally for a variable distance. In 70 per cent the rectosigmoid is involved, in 20 per cent the aganglionosis extends proximal to the sigmoid for a variable distance up the colon, and in 10 per cent the aganglionosis extends into the small intestine. The aganglionic bowel is incapable of coordinated peristalsis and passively constricts, resulting in a mechanical obstruction. The incidence is approximately 1 in 5000 births.

CLINICAL FEATURES

Hirschsprung's disease is not associated with a high incidence of prematurity, and most of the babies have a birth weight appropriate for gestational age. This contrasts sharply with most of the other congenital obstructions of the alimentary tract. Associated abnormalities are rare. The most important association is with Down's syndrome.

Symptoms of Hirschsprung's disease are present in the first few days of life in almost all cases. Exceptionally a baby will have no symptoms during the early neonatal period. The major symptoms are failure to pass meconium within 36 h of birth, abdominal distension, vomiting, and poor feeding. These may occur singly or in combination. Frequently a rectal examination will relieve the obstruction by passively dilating the aganglionic segment. Twenty to fifty per cent of patients with Hirschsprung's disease are not diagnosed in the early weeks of life. Later presentation is with constipation that dates back to the neonatal period. It is not accompanied by soiling and is frequently associated with failure to thrive. Presentation may be delayed for months or years.

Hirschsprung's enterocolitis may be the mode of presentation in the infant of a few weeks of age. This condition, the precise cause of which is unknown, presents with abdominal distension, profuse diarrhoea, and circulatory collapse. The infant is gravely ill and the mortality is 20 per cent. The child with this complication, successfully treated initially, may have absorptive problems for some time, suffer recurrent episodes of enterocolitis despite successful surgery, and the surgery is attended by a higher rate of complications. The incidence of enterocolitis can be greatly reduced if the diagnosis of Hirschsprung's disease is made in the first week of life.

DIAGNOSIS

In the neonatal period a plain abdominal radiograph will reveal distension of small and large bowel. A barium enema may show the narrow aganglionic bowel with dilated proximal bowel (Fig. 3) but a normal barium enema does not exclude Hirschsprung's disease. A 24-h film showing retained barium in the colon is often more helpful than the actual enema in confirming the clinical suspicion of Hirschsprung's disease. The definitive diagnostic procedure is a rectal biopsy. Suction biopsy enables the pathologist to look for ganglion cells in the submucosal plexus; full-thickness biopsy provides the intermyenteric plexus as well but this is usually unnecessary. In Hirschsprung's disease, ganglion cells are absent, hypertrophic nerve trunks are present, and if a histochemical stain for acetylcholinesterase is used, this reveals excessive amounts of this enzyme in the bowel wall. Anorectal manometry in Hirschsprung's disease typically shows failure of relaxation of the internal sphincter in response to rectal distension but this reflex is frequently absent in normal-term babies until after the second week of life. This method of diagnosis is therefore unreliable in the neonatal period, requires considerable expertise to obtain reliable results, and cannot be regarded as suitable for the routine diagnosis of Hirschsprung's disease.

MANAGEMENT

Having established the diagnosis, the initial procedure in the majority of patients is a colostomy in the ganglionic bowel to relieve the obstruction and allow the dilated hypertrophied proximal bowel to return to normal. If the diagnosis is made in the neonatal period, the colostomy is usually left for 4 to 12 months to allow the child to reach a reasonable size. Definitive surgery consists of excision of aganglionic bowel with a 'pull through' procedure, enabling an anastomosis to be made between the anus and ganglionic colon. The three operations most often performed are those described by Swenson, Duhamel, and Soave. Provided that the surgery is uncomplicated, the long-term complications, which include faecal and urinary incontinence, and impotence, should be minimal. Bowel control is likely to be imperfect for a number of years, with soiling as a major problem, but good bowel control will be achieved in the majority of patients treated by experienced surgeons.

Imperforate anus

The exact incidence of this abnormality is not known but the usual incidence quoted is 1 in 5000 births. The basic classification differentiates between the high anomalies, where the bowel terminates above the pelvic floor, the bowel narrowing down to communicate with the urethra in the male—a rectourethral fistula—and the vagina in the female—a rectovaginal fistula—in the majority of cases. In the low

Fig. 3 Barium enema in Hirschsprung's disease illustrating a narrow aganglionic rectum with dilation proximally.

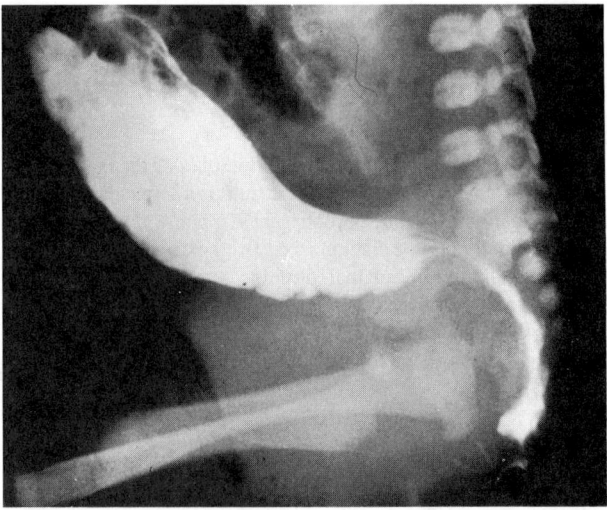

anomalies, the bowel passes through the pelvic floor and either opens on to the perineum in an ectopic position, or lies just beneath the skin-covered anus. The high anomaly is more likely to occur in boys, the low in girls. Overall, more boys than girls present with an imperforate anus. Associated anomalies of the urogenital tract, oesophagus, heart, and skeletal system are common.

CLINICAL FEATURES

Early examination of the perineum will establish the presence of an anorectal anomaly. In the male the presence of meconium on the perineum usually indicates a low anomaly. In the female, careful inspection is necessary to differentiate meconium being passed *per vaginum*, indicating a high anomaly, from meconium emerging from a perineal site, suggesting a low anomaly. Careful probing of any opening will enable the direction in which the bowel is running to be established. In the female, doubt about the precise anatomy of the anomaly may be resolved by contrast studies. In the male, differentiating a completely covered anus from a high anomaly may be difficult in the early hours after birth. Examination of the urine microscopically may reveal the presence of squamous cells or debris, suggesting a fistula between bowel and urethra. Occasionally meconium is passed *per urethra*.

A lateral film of the pelvis taken after the infant has lain 'bottom up' over a foam wedge for some minutes will often reveal the level at which the rectum terminates, but this film cannot be reliably interpreted in the first few hours after birth because air may not have reached the distal bowel. In boys a micturating cystourethrogram will demonstrate a recto urethral fistula in a high proportion of cases, but is rarely necessary as an initial diagnostic procedure. Having defined the nature of the anorectal anomaly, evidence of any associated abnormality should be sought by careful clinical examination and radiographs of chest, abdomen, and the vertebral column.

MANAGEMENT

A low anomaly usually requires a perineal procedure to enlarge the opening. Dilatation alone may suffice, but in the majority of cases a simple anoplasty produces a more satisfactory result. In the long term the functional results for the low anomalies should be very good. A high anomaly necessitates a defunctioning colostomy in the neonatal period. Definitive surgery involves division of any fistula and bringing the bowel through the puborectalis sling to the perineum. Delay in achieving bowel control is common and a number of secondary operations designed to improve control have been advocated. However, if the initial surgery is meticulous and the importance of the puborectalis sling is recognized, acceptable continence should be achieved in over 80 per cent of children within the first 10 years. A permanent colostomy should rarely be necessary. The high incidence of associated genitourinary abnormalities makes it mandatory to investigate carefully the urinary tract at an early stage. The mortality for anorectal anomalies is largely dictated by the presence of other serious abnormalities.

REFERENCES

Coppens, B. and Vos, A. (1992). Duodenal atresia. *Paediatric Surgery International*, **7**, 435–7.
Coran, A.G. (ed.) (1986). Hirschsprung's disease. *Paediatric Surgery International*, **1**, 79–104.
Hamilton, W.J., Boyd, J.D., and Mossman H.W. (1972). *Human embryology*. Williams and Wilkins, Baltimore.
Huysman, W.A., Tibboel, D., Bergmeijer, J.H., and Molenaar, J.C. (1991). Long-term survival of a patient with congenital short bowel and malrotation. *Journal of Pediatric Surgery*, **26**, 103–5.
Lister, J. and Irving, I.M. (1990). *Neonatal surgery*. Butterworth, London.
Myers, N.A. (ed.) (1992). Oesophageal atresia. *Paediatric Surgery International*, **7**, 83–100.
Patrapinyokul, S., Brereton, R.J., Spitz, L., Kiely, E., and Agrawal, M. (1989). Small-bowel atresia and stenosis. *Paediatric Surgery International*, **4**, 390–5.
Pena, A. (ed.) (1988). Anorectal malformation. *Paediatric Surgery International*, **3**, 81–119.
Reyes, H.M. and Vidyasagar, D. (ed.) (1989). Neonatal surgery. *Clinics in Perinatology*, **16**(1).
St-Vil, D., Brandt, M.L., Panic, S., Bensoussan, A.L., and Blanchard, H. (1991) Meckel's diverticulum in children: a 20-year review. *Journal of Pediatric Surgery*, **26**, 1289–92.
Stephens, F.D., Smith, E.D., and Paul N.W. (ed.) (1988). *Anorectal malformations in children: update*, pp. 1–604. Liss, New York.

14.16 Tumours of the gastrointestinal tract

M. L. CLARK, I. C. TALBOT, and C. B. WILLIAMS

Oesophageal tumours (see also Chapter 14.6)

Benign

Leiomyomas are the most common benign tumours of the oesophagus. They are often discovered incidentally or at autopsy. Typically, a barium swallow examination for vague oesophageal symptoms reveals an intramural lesion, which must be distinguished from extrinsic compression. Mucosal ulceration is rare so that bleeding is uncommon (compare below with stomach). Only tumours that are large and cause dysphagia should be removed, by enucleation rather than resection. Rarely, fibrovascular polyps, lipomas, and other benign tumours are found.

Malignant

The majority of malignant tumours of the oesophagus are squamous carcinomas. Adenocarcinomas occur in the lower third and at the cardia. The proportion of adenocarcinomas appears to be on the increase over the last decade.

Other malignant tumours—malignant melanomas, secondary tumours, plasmacytomas, and leiomyosarcomas—are rare.

Kaposi's sarcoma is a frequent manifestation of AIDS; gastrointestinal Kaposi's sarcoma is found in 50 to 60 per cent of patients dying with AIDS. The tumours are widely disseminated throughout the gastrointestinal tract but are particularly found in the mouth and hypopharynx. These tumours rarely lead to symptoms and do not require treatment, but gastrointestinal involvement with Kaposi's indicates a poorer prognosis than in patients without such involvement.

EPIDEMIOLOGICAL AND AETIOLOGICAL FACTORS

Squamous carcinoma

In the United Kingdom the overall incidence of oesophageal carcinoma ranges from 5 to 10 cases per 100 000 people or 2.5 per cent of all malignant disease. The incidence varies considerably throughout the world, being high in China, parts of Africa, and in the Caspian region of Iran, where the incidence is the highest observed for any type of cancer in general populations anywhere in the world. This global variation in incidence is greater than for any other commonly occurring cancer and is unusual in that there are sharp differences between regions only a few hundred miles apart. There is no simple explanation for this geographical variability, which is probably multifactorial.

It seems likely that possible causative agents differ between geographical areas. Alcohol (particularly spirits) and tobacco consumption have been strongly implicated as aetiological factors in many areas of the world. In Chinese populations there is an association between pickled vegetable consumption and oesophageal cancer risk. These pickled vegetables contain high concentrations of *N*-nitroso compounds, which are thought to be carcinogenic in man. A number of other exogenous factors (e.g. contaminated foods or repeated minor trauma from ingestion of hot liquids) may also result in increased individual susceptibility and it is probable that many of these factors are additive.

There is an increased incidence of malignancy in patients with oesophageal strictures due to ingestion of corrosives as well as in patients who have been treated with radiation therapy. An increased incidence also occurs in patients with achalasia, possibly due to stasis above the narrow segment, and in patients with coeliac disease.

The Patterson–Kelly (Plummer–Vinson) syndrome, consisting of hypochromic anaemia with an associated postcricoid web in young women, is becoming rare but is historically associated with carcinoma of the oesophagus.

There is no evidence of an inherited basis for oesophageal cancer except in the rare skin disease tylosis, which is characterized by hyperkeratosis of the palms and soles and in which oesophageal carcinomas affect up to 40 per cent of patients.

Adenocarcinoma (see also Chapter 14.6)

The large majority of these tumours arise in the columnar-lined epithelium of the lower oesophagus or occasionally in islands of columnar epithelium higher up (Barrett's oesophagus). This columnization arises from long-standing reflux, although up to one-third of such patients have never had symptoms of reflux. There is an estimated 30 to 40 times increased risk of developing cancer with Barrett's oesophagus. This has led to surveillance programmes being set up for known cases of Barrett's but such initiatives are unlikely to reduce the death rate overall from adenocarcinoma. Adenocarcinoma of the gastric cardia with involvement of the lower oesophagus has become an increasing cause of malignant oesophageal obstruction.

CLINICAL FEATURES

The median age for the presentation of oesophageal cancer is 68 years for both males and females, and the disease is virtually unknown in children. The dysphagia of malignancy is progressive and unrelenting; initially it causes difficulty in swallowing solids but eventually dysphagia with liquids also occurs. Benign strictures, in contrast, often produce intermittent dysphagia. Impact pain after eating occurs with malignancy but more persistent pain in the front and back of the chest suggests infiltration and is a bad prognostic feature. Loss of appetite and weight loss are often present, partly because of the difficulty in swallowing but also because the patient may have advanced disease. Metastases, most commonly to regional lymph nodes, are found at diagnosis in approximately 50 per cent of cases. The earliest spread is through the mediastinal tissues around the oesophagus but subsequently downwards to the gastric glands and to the liver. Direct spread of the tumour involves neighbouring structures, especially the bronchi, lungs and pleura, but also the aorta. Perforation and local sepsis may occur, resulting in tracheo-oesophageal or other fistulas, or mediastinitis. Involvement of the recurrent laryngeal nerve causes hoarseness. By the time that oesophageal obstruction is causing difficulty in swallowing saliva, cough and other features of aspiration are common and may result in terminal bronchopneumonia. Physical signs, apart from weight loss, are often absent. Anaemia may be present and palpable lymph nodes can be found in the neck.

DIAGNOSIS

Diagnosis relies on endoscopy and radiology. Barium swallow gives an accurate picture of the extent of any deformity, characteristically showing a narrowing with an abrupt shoulder and irregular mucosa, as opposed to the smooth narrowing of a benign stricture. A patient with dysphagia may proceed directly to endoscopy where biopsies can be taken and, if appropriate, palliative dilatation or intubation performed. Combining brush cytological samples with biopsies will produce a diagnostic accuracy rate of 95 per cent. In tumours of the distal oesophagus it is important to differentiate between a squamous carcinoma and an adenocarcinoma as the latter does not respond to radiotherapy.

The differential diagnosis is from a peptic stricture following reflux oesophagitis, which can produce similar symptomatology and radiological or endoscopic appearances.

A computerized tomographic (**CT**) scan will show the volume of the tumour and also possible spread outside of the oesophagus (Fig. 1). It has been used to attempt to stage tumours before surgery but results are disappointing. Endoscopic ultrasound (endosonography) is being used in some centres with an accuracy rate of nearly 90 per cent for assessing depth of tumour infiltration and 80 per cent for staging lymph-node involvement.

TREATMENT

The overall results of the treatment for carcinoma of the oesophagus are poor. A recent review concludes that surgery over the last 10 years has produced no improvement in long-term prognosis despite postoperative mortality having been reduced by half. Overall, of 100 patients presenting with an oesophageal cancer, approximately 50 per cent have resectable disease. Seven per cent of these will die postoperatively and of the remaining approximately 40 patients, 25 will survive 1 year, 10 will survive a second year, and 10 will survive into the fifth year.

It is important to differentiate between tumours that have not completely infiltrated the oesophageal wall and those that have spread beyond the wall; the latter are inoperable and patients should, if at all possible, be spared from surgery. Conversely, 'cure' is only achievable by surgery, with some 5-year survival rates in favourable cases approaching 25 per cent. The hope is that with better preoperative staging by endosonography, only patients with resectable lesions will have surgery, with palliative measures on the remainder done endoscopically (with or without radiotherapy) to improve the quality of life.

Fig. 1 CT scan of oesophageal carcinoma demonstrating invasion of the left main bronchas (thin arrow) and aorta (thick arrow) with extensive mediastinal lymph-node (arrow heads) involvement.

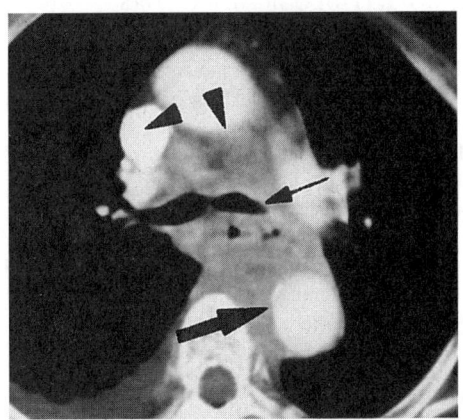

Attempts to improve survival using adjuvant chemotherapy and/or radiotherapy as well as surgical resection have been made but there has been no universally accepted regimen that has improved overall survival. Radiotherapy alone has been used in some centres, with similar results to surgery for squamous carcinoma. There are, however, no controlled studies and radiotherapy is mainly used for palliation. Adenocarcinoma of the oesophagus does not respond to radio- or chemotherapy.

Many patients with oesophageal cancer have inoperable lesions and are elderly, so that only symptom relief is possible by dilating a stricture endoscopically and placing an oesophageal tube or metal expanded stent through the tumour. The tube allows passage of saliva and soft food but the patient is unable to eat a normal diet.

Laser photocoagulation of the tumour is also done for palliation. Comparisons of the two approaches show little difference, although complication rates in those treated with intubation are higher. Laser requires more endoscopic procedures and is expensive and not universally available. Ethanol injection to induce tumour necrosis is quick, cheap and safe, and can give good results, often combined with intubation. Nutritional support and control of pain are needed, as well as good support for the patient and family affected by this distressing disease.

Stomach tumours

Benign tumours and polyps

The most common benign tumour of the stomach at autopsy is a leiomyoma, which arises from the smooth-muscle tissue but projects into the lumen. Most are asymptomatic but occasionally there can be superficial ulceration and the patient develops gastrointestinal haemorrhage. Local surgical removal is done for any symptomatic lesion and is curative. Other rare benign gastric tumours include lymphomas, angiomas, and gastric carcinoids.

Gastric polyps are relatively uncommon lesions and are found by chance in a patient being investigated for unrelated dyspepsia.

The most common is the regenerative or hyperplastic polyp, which probably develops following mucosal damage. These polyps have no malignant potential. They are often multiple and small and after biopsy to ascertain their nature, they can be safely left and not removed. Adenomatous polyps of the stomach are much less common and have a villous or tubular/villous architecture. Unlike the large bowel there is no evidence to suggest that gastric cancers commonly arise from pre-existing adenomas. Nevertheless, because of the slight risk of malignant potential, if a polyp is biopsied and shown to be adenomatous the whole of it should be removed endoscopically. In rare cases, larger pedunculated polyps may ulcerate and bleed or obstruct the pyloric outflow.

Carcinoma of the stomach

EPIDEMIOLOGICAL AND AETIOLOGICAL FACTORS

The occurrence of gastric carcinomas varies considerably both within and between different countries. There is a high incidence in Japan, parts of Chile, and the mountainous regions of Costa Rica but a low incidence in the United States. In the United Kingdom, approximately 15/100 000 males per year are affected. Gastric cancer is the sixth most common fatal malignancy in the United Kingdom and accounts for about 10 per cent of all deaths from malignant disease. There is a continued fall in incidence of gastric cancer worldwide. However, there appears to be an increase in the number of cases of carcinoma of the cardia.

Epidemiological data are accumulating that link *Helicobacter pylori* infection to an increased risk of carcinoma of the body and antrum of the stomach. *H.pylori* seropositivity in American men and women and Japanese men was associated with a 3.5- to 6-fold risk of gastric cancer in case-control studies. Emerging evidence from China and Peru has revealed an association between early (childhood) acquisition of *H.pylori* and high prevalence rates of gastric cancer. Pathological studies provide possible explanations for these observations. *H.pylori* infection results in chronic active gastritis (Fig. 2). Gastric atrophy and intestinal metaplasia are consequences of long-standing, *H.pylori*-associated gastritis, which may account for the age-related increase in gastric carcinoma prevalence. Gastric carcinoma is more frequent in those with a lower socioeconomic status, which again may reflect the increased prevalance of *H.pylori* infection in this group. It has also been suggested that *H.pylori* impairs gastric antioxidant defences, supported by the observation that vitamin C levels in gastric juice are low in infected subjects. Studies that have failed to show a relation between *H.pylori* and gastric cancer are generally those that have been based on identification of *H.pylori* at the time of diagnosis of cancer.

People from countries with a high incidence of carcinoma, such as Japan, continue at high risk when they migrate to a low-risk area, such as North America, but a decrease occurs in succeeding generations. The higher prevalence of infection with *H.pylori* amongst children in Japan than America is the suggested mechanism.

Dietary factors may still be important, as both initiators and promoters may have separate roles in carcinogenesis. Dietary factors that have been implicated include spiced or pickled foods, salt, and alcohol, as well as a diet low in fresh fish and vegetables. Levels of dietary or water nitrate ingestion are high in areas of high incidence of gastric carcinoma. Nitrates can be converted to nitrosamines by bacteria at neutral pH and nitrosamines are known to be carcinogenic in animals. Nitrosamines are present in the stomach of patients with achlorhydria, who have an increased cancer risk. Smoking is also associated with stomach cancer and may account for the age-related increase in gastric cancer. Gastric cancer is increased in blood-group A patients; further evidence on genetic susceptibility is required.

PRECANCEROUS CONDITIONS

Pernicious anaemia

Patients with pernicious anaemia have a two to three times increased incidence of stomach cancer but, even so, surveillance programmes are unwarranted as the overall incidence is still low; 1 in 80 patients with

Fig. 2 Flow chart of pathogenesis of gastric cancer.

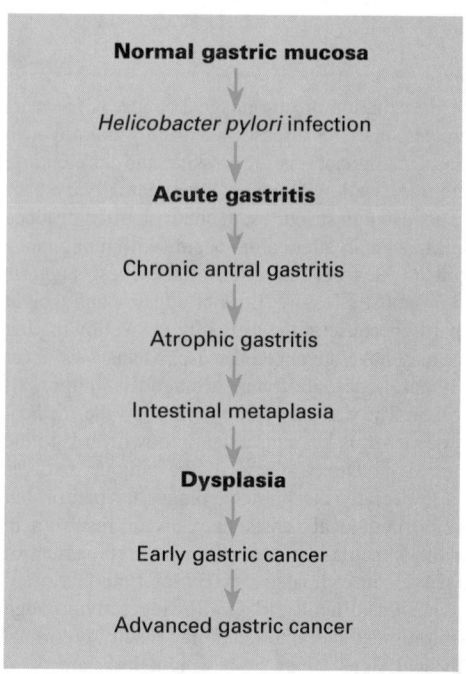

Normal gastric mucosa

↓

Helicobacter pylori infection

↓

Acute gastritis

↓

Chronic antral gastritis

↓

Atrophic gastritis

↓

Intestinal metaplasia

↓

Dysplasia

↓

Early gastric cancer

↓

Advanced gastric cancer

pernicious anaemia studied prospectively over a number of years developed cancer. The association is usually explained by the precancerous nature of gastric atrophy that is invariably present in the body and fundus of the stomach in patients with pernicious anaemia.

Peptic ulcer

There is no good evidence that cancer ever develops in a proven benign gastric ulcer, nor is there unequivocal evidence of a previous gastric ulcer having occurred at the site of a carcinoma. Thus, benign gastric ulcers are not premalignant. It can, however, be very difficult to differentiate clinically, radiologically, and endoscopically between some benign and malignant ulcers, and malignant ulcers can heal on medical treatment. For these reasons it was originally thought that gastric ulcers could become malignant.

Intestinal metaplasia

Intestinal metaplasia occurs more frequently in stomachs that contain a carcinoma, and in some early cases of carcinoma of the stomach there appears to be a transition between metaplastic mucosa and carcinoma. Most cases of intestinal metaplasia develop after chronic, active gastritis, which is now thought in most cases to be secondary to infection with *H.pylori*.

Postgastrectomy

Intestinal metaplasia and chronic active gastritis are also found in the resected stomach, which, in most series, shows an increased incidence of gastric cancer (especially after gastrojejunostomy). This is seen regardless of whether the gastric resection was for a gastric or a duodenal ulcer. Prolonged contact of bile with the stomach remnant leading to gastritis is one suggested mechanism, but again *H.pylori* may be involved.

SCREENING

Gastric cancer has an appalling prognosis. In an attempt to improve this, earlier diagnosis has been advocated. In Japan, mass screening by

Fig. 3 Barium meal showing early gastric cancer with distortion of normal fold pattern.

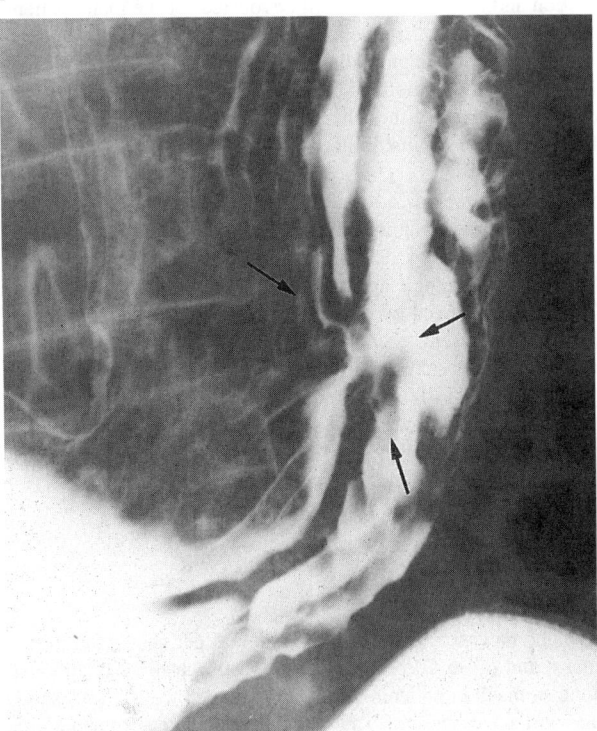

mobile radiographic units has increased the proportion of early gastric cancer; diagnosed (Fig. 3) Early gastric cancer is defined as a carcinoma that is confined to the mucosa or submucosa. As resection of early gastric cancer results in 5-year survival rates of approximately 90 per cent, it has been suggested that mass screening might be introduced more widely. In a large series of British patients with gastric cancer, only 0.7 per cent were identified as having early gastric cancer, with this small number, mass screening would not be warranted. Even in Japan, with its very high incidence of gastric cancer, it is debatable whether mass screening is cost-effective. An effective screening procedure needs to be cheap, applicable to all social groups so that they attend for examination, have a good discriminatory index from benign lesions, and, ultimately, reflect an improvement in prognosis. Gastric screening is expensive and the compliance is low, and the incidence of gastric cancer is decreasing. On present evidence, therefore, screening is unwarranted, except possibly for individuals with an increased susceptibility to the disease. Patients with the precancerous conditions discussed earlier would fall into this category. It seems doubtful, however, even in this relatively high-risk group, whether screening asymptomatic subjects could be justified.

An alternative approach to screening asymptomatic patients is to investigate symptomatic patients as quickly as possible. At present the mean interval between the onset of symptoms and attendance at hospital is approximately 6 to 9 months. Dyspepsia is, however, very common in the general population without any significant gastric lesion. It would obviously be impractical for every dyspeptic member of the population to consult a physician on each occurrence of this symptom, and most physicians would be unlikely to be prompt in arranging a complicated series of investigations.

CLINICAL FEATURES

There may be no symptoms in cases of early gastric cancer, although in some series weight loss has been a frequent feature. Symptoms of carcinoma of the stomach may be exactly the same as for benign disease. The most common is epigastric pain, which may be relieved by food and antacids. The pain can vary in intensity, but can be constant and severe. Most patients with carcinoma of the stomach have advanced disease at the time of presentation so, in addition to pain, they have anorexia and weight loss. Nausea frequently accompanies the anorexia, and vomiting occurs in approximately half of the patients. Vomiting can be severe if the tumour is near the pylorus, whereas dysphagia can occur with tumours involving the fundus. Gross haematemesis is unusual but anaemia from occult blood loss is frequent. Patients can also present with problems related to metastases, in particular abdominal swelling due to ascites or jaundice due to liver involvement. Metastases, however, can occur to bone, brain, and lungs, producing appropriate symptoms.

The presence of a palpable epigastric mass has been reported in up to 50 per cent of patients. Abdominal tenderness may be found but often the only feature will be that of weight loss. A palpable lymph node is sometimes found in the left supraclavicular fossa (Virchow sign). Signs of metastases are present in up to a third of patients. Carcinoma of the stomach is the cancer most frequently associated with dermatomyositis and acanthosis nigricans.

PATHOLOGY

Gastric cancer occurs most frequently in the antrum of the stomach. It is almost invariably an adenocarcinoma. The most widely used histological classification (of Lauren) recognizes two types of carcinoma. The more common, intestinal type occurs in high-frequency areas, in elderly patients, and is usually polypoid; it is often associated with intestinal metaplasia in the surrounding mucosa and *H.pylori* is frequently found. The diffuse type is composed of scattered or small clusters of cells, occurs in low-frequency area, and in younger people; it is associated with extensive submucosal spread, which may result in the picture of 'linitis plastica' and has a worse prognosis than the intestinal type.

Early gastric cancer is defined as carcinoma limited to the mucosa or submucosa and not invading the muscle layer. The complex Japanese classification of early gastric cancer is not used worldwide, differentiation often being made simply between those that are raised and those that are ulcerated. Early gastric cancers are not necessarily small; they can be multifocal and they may spread superficially to cover a considerable area.

DIAGNOSIS

Early gastric cancer is occasionally identified in patients outside Japan, either by double-contrast barium study (Fig. 3) or by very careful endoscopy often using dye staining of the gastric mucosa. These lesions are usually identified by chance in patients investigated for dyspepsia.

The more usual advanced gastric cancer can be identified either radiologically (Fig. 4a) or by endoscopy. Good-quality, double-contrast radiology of the stomach is very accurate (90 per cent) in diagnosing gastric cancer but, because radiographic quality varies and because of the ability to obtain biopsy, endoscopy is becoming increasingly utilized as the diagnostic procedure of choice.

Positive biopsies can be obtained in almost all cases of obvious car-

cinoma. However, one or more negative biopsies from the edge of an ulcer do not rule out malignancy, and it is recommended that eight to ten biopsies be taken around the ulcer margin and from its base. Taking superficial brushing specimens for exfoliative cytology during the same procedure in addition to the biopsies will further improve the diagnostic rate.

ADDITIONAL INVESTIGATIONS

Once the diagnosis is established an attempt should be made, in most patients, to stage the disease (unless frailty or a medical condition prevents this).

In an attempt to stage for operability, CT has been used (Fig. 4(b)) but so far results have been disappointing, particularly at revealing nodular and peritoneal deposits. Endoscopic ultrasound is becoming increasingly used and is said to be very accurate at staging the depth of the primary tumour invasion, which often decides operability.

Routine blood tests and biochemistry help to rule out metastases and most patients have an upper-abdominal ultrasonographic examination to look for liver secondaries.

TREATMENT

The 5-year survival rate of patients who have undergone surgery for early gastric cancer in Japan is over 90 per cent but outside Japan early gastric cancer is uncommon. In more advanced stomach cancer, 5-year survival rates of 30 to 40 per cent have been obtained in Japan and it is to achieve this latter figure that is the surgeon's goal. A recent analysis of 5-year survival rates published in English language journals from 1970 shows an improvement in recent years. The overall operation rate has decreased over the last 20 years, suggesting better selection, and the 5-year survival rate of all resections has increased from 20.7 to 28.4 per cent since 1970. Five-year survival rates following curative resection have also increased from 37.6 to 55.4 per cent over the same period. More depressing is the 5-year survival rate of only 5 per cent in patients with carcinoma of the cardia. These results suggest that improvements in preoperative staging and perioperative care are producing worthwhile improvments in survival.

Palliative surgery to relieve symptoms and to prevent complications of obstruction and haemorrhage is still advocated for the many patients found to be inoperable as far as a potential cure is concerned. A number of patients do benefit symptomatically from palliative procedures for local advanced disease but radical total gastrectomy should not be done.

Adjuvant therapy with either chemotherapy or radiation continues to be tried but so far the results do not show significant improvements in survival.

Chemotherapy alone for advanced disease can be used, with new combinations of drugs being introduced into treatment regimens at regular intervals. The results of these clinical trials still show little improvement over the use of a single agent such as 5-fluorouracil and, although survival may be prolonged by a few months, the toxicity of the drugs limit their use. At present, chemotherapy should normally be administered only as part of a clinical trial and its indiscriminate use is not justified. The quality of life in the remaining months is more important to the patient and family than minimal gains in survival figures.

Cimetidine has been shown in a Danish study to improve survival and further trials with this agent are being conducted.

Other malignant tumours of the stomach

PRIMARY LYMPHOMA

Gastric lymphoma accounts for approximately 5 per cent of all gastric malignancies and 50 to 60 per cent of all gastrointestinal lymphomas occur in the stomach in patients from the developed world. It is usually a non-Hodgkin's lymphoma of the B-cell type arising from mucosa-

Fig. 4 (a) Barium meal demonstrating circumferencial narrowing and irregularity of the distal body and antrum of the stomach. (b) CT scan in same patient with water used as intraluminal gastric contrast and dynamic intravenous contrast enhancement to demonstrate markedly thickened gastric wall, the fat plane between the stomach and pancreas (arrowheads) and prepancreatic lymph node involvement (arrow).

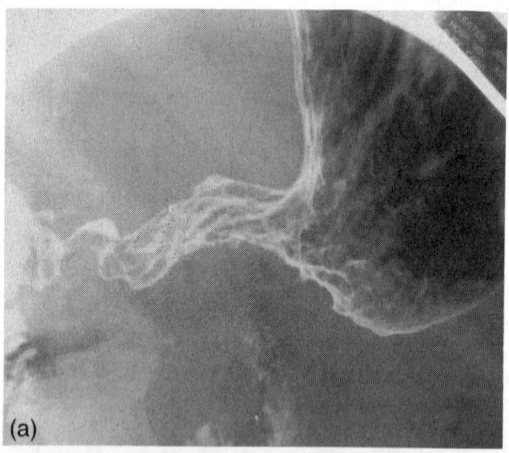

(a)

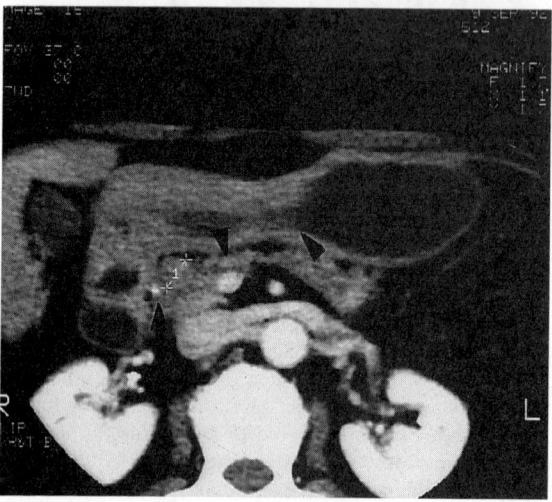

associated lymphoid tissue (MALT). MALT tumours are associated with *H. pylori* gastritis. The tumours vary in degree of blastic transformation; the more blastic, high-grade tumours are categorized as centroblastic or, rarely, immunoblastic. The clinical features are indistinguishable from those of other benign or malignant lesions of the stomach; usually the patient presents with advanced disease similar to carcinoma of the stomach. Treatment is surgical combined with radiotherapy; chemotherapy is used for widespread disease although some MALT tumours respond to *H. pylori* eradication. The prognosis for primary gastric lymphoma varies from 75 to 95 per cent 5-year survival, depending on whether a low- or high-grade B-cell lymphoma is present.

Small-bowel tumours

The small intestine is relatively resistant to the development of neoplasia; only 3 to 6 per cent of all gastrointestinal tumours and fewer than 1 per cent of all malignant lesions occur in the small bowel. This contrasts with the long length of gut involved and the complexity of the different histological structures of the gut. The reason for the rarity of the tumours is not known; explanations include the fluidity and relative sterility of the small-bowel contents and the rapid transit time, which reduces any exposure to potential carcinogens. It may also be due to the unique part that the gut plays an immunological surveillance. It can be argued that IgA, secreted mainly by the gut musoca, may have an important role in preventing malignancy—possibly by forming complexes with potentially damaging agents such as viruses or carcinogens.

Malignant tumours are more common than solitary benign lesions and 90 per cent of the malignant tumours are symptomatic.

Benign

Adenomas, leiomyomas, and lipomas are the three most common solitary benign tumours (excluding Peutz–Jeghers syndrome and other forms of polyposis discussed later). They are frequently asymptomatic and often found incidentally at operation or necropsy. If symptoms occur, pain is the most common, usually due to intussusception, but insidious loss of blood leading to anaemia is another frequent manifestation. Haemangiomas are rare, occurring as small polyps that are usually not seen on the conventional barium examination of the small bowel or small intestine but may be found on angiography or by pre- or perioperative fibreoptic endoscopy of the small intestine. The duration of history of some of these cases is extremely long, the diagnosis being unsuspected because of its rarity. When found, resection is curative.

Malignant

The jejunum and ileum account for 1 to 5 per cent of all alimentary-tract malignancies, and a carcinoma in these regions is 40 to 60 times less common than a colonic cancer. Surprisingly, despite this 'resistance' to malignancy, the small bowel is the most common site in the gastrointestinal tract for metastic melanoma.

Adenocarcinoma is the most common malignancy of the small intestine, accounting for about 50 per cent of primary tumours. Carcinoid tumours form the next major group, whilst lymphoma and smooth-muscle tumours make up the remainder. Adenocarcinomas are found most often in the duodenum, periampullary region, and jejunum (Fig. 5), with lymphomas and carcinoid tumours most often in the ileum. The small intestine may also be involved secondarily, by direct extension from other intra-abdominal or retroperitoneal tumours or by haematogenous spread from a carcinoma of the bronchus or breast.

Lymphoma

Some 20 to 30 per cent of gastrointestinal non-Hodgkin's lymphomas occur in the small bowel in patients in the developed world, whereas in the Middle East over half of the lymphomas occur in the small bowel. In developed countries the most common tumour is of the B-cell type

arising from musosa-associated lymphoid tissues. B-cell lymphomas tend to be annular or polypoid masses in the distal ileum (Fig. 6).

In coeliac disease and dermatitis herpetiformis there is an increased incidence of lymphoma, which is often T cell in origin. These T-cell lymphomas are usually ulcerated plaques or strictures in the proximal small bowel. Treatment of coeliac disease with a gluten-free diet seems to protect against the development of lymphoma.

Fig. 5 Prone compression view of mid-jejunum demonstrating annular 'apple core' lesion with prestenotic dilatation typical of an adenocarcinoma.

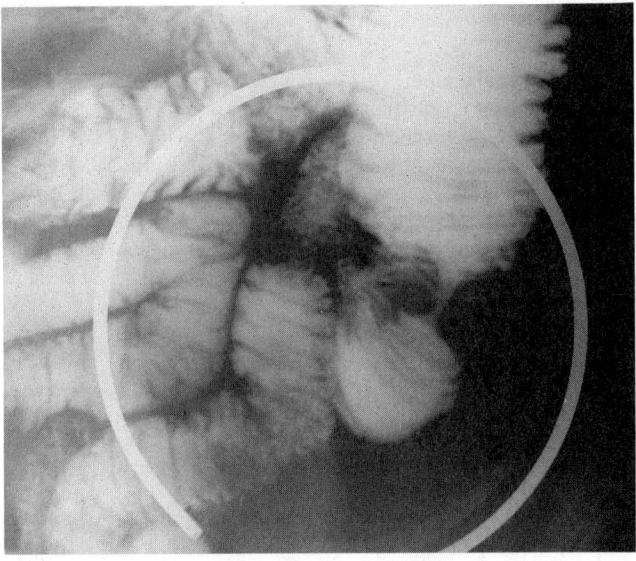

Fig. 6 Small-bowel follow-through demonstrating extensive thickening of folds in the mid and distal small bowel indicating submucosal infiltration that proved to be a lymphoma.

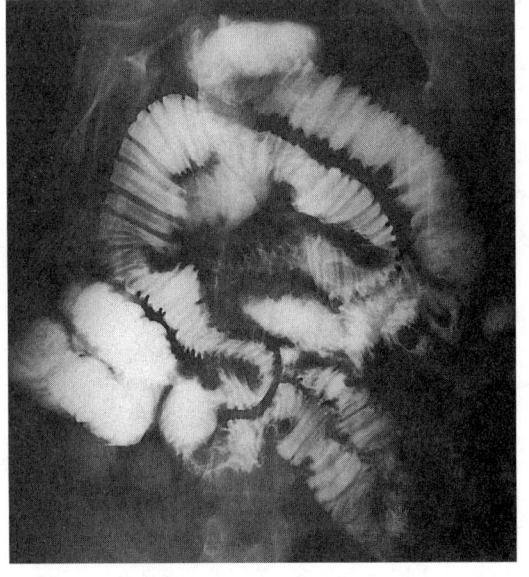

A tumour similar to Burkitt's lymphoma also occurs and commonly affects the terminal ileum of children in North Africa and the Middle East.

Small-intestinal lymphoma is a frequent manifestation in patients with AIDS.

IMMUNOPROLIFERATIVE SMALL-INTESTINAL DISEASE (IPSID)

This is a B-cell lymphocyte disorder in which there is proliferation of plasma cells in the lamina propria of the upper small bowel. These cells produce truncated monoclonal heavy chains but lack associated light chains. The α-chains are found in the gut mucosa on immunofluorescence and these can also be detected in the serum. IPSID occurs usually in countries surrounding the Mediterranean but it has also been found in other developing countries in South America and the Far East, and has recently been documented in the developed world. IPSID affects predominantly people in lower socioeconomic groups in areas with poor hygiene and a high incidence of bacterial and parasitic infection of the gut. IPSID presents as a malabsorptive syndrome, associated with diffuse lymphoid infiltration of the small bowel and neighbouring lymph nodes, which responds to tetracycline. This then progresses in some cases to an immunoblastic lymphoma.

Adenocarcinoma

Familial adenomatous polyposis

Patients with this condition are being increasingly shown to have polyps throughout their small gut, particularly in the periampullary region of the duodenum (Plate 1). These adenomas, as in the colon, have malignant potential. Approximately 12 per cent of such patients eventually develop an upper gastrointestinal malignancy, usually an adenocarcinoma of the ampulla of Vater. Screening by duodenoscopy has been suggested by some for patients with polyposis.

Coeliac disease

This is associated with an increased incidence of adenocarcinoma of the small bowel (as well as lymphoma) and, in addition, an unexplained increase in incidence of all malignancies throughout the gastrointestinal tract (e.g. oesophagus) and elsewhere in the body (e.g. testes). Again, there is some evidence that a gluten-free diet protects against the development of malignancy.

Crohn's disease

Crohn's disease of long duration results in an increased incidence of adenocarcinoma of the small bowel. This is a rare occurrence and does not influence the overall management of the Crohn's disease.

CLINICAL FEATURES

Malignant tumours commonly present with abdominal pain, anorexia, and weight loss with associated anaemia; a number of patients have diarrhoea. A palpable mass is sometinmes found. Most lesions can be detected on small-bowel follow-through (Fig. 5) but it is sometimes necessary to use an intubation technique with air insufflation as the lesion can be extremely small. Lymphomas tend to appear on the small-bowel follow-through either as a diffusely infiltrating lesion (Fig. 6) or a nodular or polypoid mass. CT and ultrasound will demonstrate the bowel-wall thickening and the involvement of the mesentery and lymph nodes, which is common with lymphoma. Biopsies are normally taken to ascertain the histological type of the lesion before treatment is decided, using a flexible enteroscope if necessary.

TREATMENT

Adenocarcinoma is treated surgically with wide excision of the lymph nodes. The 5-year survival is 10 to 20 per cent. Radiotherapy and some-times chemotherapy can be given but the evidence for their benefit is minimal. Lymphoma is also treated by surgical excision, with radiotherapy and/or chemotherapy added in most cases. No universal treatment regimen for small-gut lymphomas has yet been agreed. The 5-year survival for T-cell lymphomas is only around 25 per cent; for B-cell lymphomas it varies from 75 to 50 per cent, depending on whether the lyhmphoma is low or high grade.

Colon polyps and polyposis syndromes

A polyp is an elevation above the mucosal surface, the word deriving from the Greek *polypous* for squid, which a stalked polyp broadly resembles. The majority of colorectal polyps prove to be adenomas with malignant potential (whereas they are in the minority in the stomach) and thus their detection and removal are important.

Polyps range in appearance from tiny, translucent, and almost invisible bumps only 1 to 2mm in diameter to those having a head of 1 to 3 cm in diameter on a vascular stalk or peduncle of normal tissue (Plate 2). A small number are sessile, little raised but between 1 and 10 cm in diameter. Polyps may be single, may occur together in small numbers, or may carpet the colon in hundreds or thousands as part of the rarer polyposis syndromes. Histological examination is essential because it is usually impossible to be sure of the type of polyp by direct macroscopic or radiological inspection; the pathologist prefers to examine representative whole polyps rather than small biopsies in order to assess malignancy. Table 1 gives a general classification of large-bowel polyps, most individual types occasionally occurring as polyposis.

Non-neoplastic polyps

Metaplastic (hyperplastic) polyps

These are the most common type seen on proctosigmoidoscopy, appearing as 2 to 4 mm pale shiny nodules in the rectum. They have a characteristic histological appearance with 'saw toothing' of the elongated mucosal crypts but normal-looking nuclei; this makes microscopic distinction from the heavily staining neoplastic nuclei of adenomas easy. Hyperplastic polyps have no clinical consequence, although large ones may need removal for reassurance that they are not adenomas and 'mixed' polyps containing both adenomatous and hyperplastic tissue may occur. Multiple hyperplastic polyps proximal to the rectum (hyperplastic polyposis) may be associated with malignant potential and such patients need follow-up endoscopy.

Inflammatory polyps

These may be equally numerous and extremely variable in size and shape, although classically filiform (thread-like). Inflammatory polyps are seen in the healed phase after one or more severe attacks of colitis (ulcerative colitis, Crohn's disease, schistosomiasis, etc.). They are sometimes dramatic-looking on endoscopy or radiographs but histologically are usually only tags covered by normal or mildly distorted epithelium ('postinflammatory' polyps). Larger inflammatory polyps may be composed of granulation tissue or be sufficiently inflamed to cause bleeding or protein loss; they may require removal or biopsy for distinction from adenomas. Mucosal traumatization from straining or other causes can result in local prolapse or even, rarely, multiple inflamed-looking polyps (cap polyposis) (Plate 3).

Hamartomatous polyps

Principally juvenile or Peutz-Jeghers in type, these are developmental malformations containing a disorganized mixture of normal intestinal tissues. Hamartomatous tissues have no malignant tendency but the polyps occasionally harbour a focus of dysplastic (adenomatous) tissue, which probably explains the sporadic reports of malignancy in the stomach or colon in Peutz-Jeghers syndrome and the greater cancer risk in the colon in juvenile polyposis. Hamartomatous polyps are commonly

Table 1 *Colonic polyps and polyposis: a classification*

Pathogenesis	Polyps	Polyposis
Metaplastic	Hyperplastic	Hyperplastic polyposis
Inflammatory	Inflammatory	Inflammatory polyposis
Lymphatic	Benign lymphoid	Malignant lymphomatous polyposis
Traumatic	Mucosal prolapse syndrome	Inflammatory cap polyp polyposis
Neoplastic	Adenoma	Familial adenomatous polyposis if >100
Hamartomatous	Juvenile	Juvenile polyposis
	Peutz–Jeghers	Peutz–Jeghers syndrome
		Cronkhite–Canada syndrome
Stromal origin		
Type/neoplastic	Leiomyomatous polyp	Cowden's syndrome
	Lipomatous polyp	
Hamartomatous	Vascular hamartoma	
	Neurofibroma	
	Ganglioneuroma	

large and stalked, the histology of juvenile polyps showing mucus-retention cysts and inflammation, whereas Peutz-Jeghers polyps have characteristic fibromuscular fronds radiating between the disorganized mucosal crypts. Juvenile polyps are a cause of bleeding in childhood, which may be acute if the polyp head twists and autoamputates. They can intussuscept and present at the anus or may be an incidental finding in the middle age. Juvenile polyposis, defined as more than three to five colonic polyps (the small intestine and stomach are sometimes involved), requires careful endoscopy surveillance and polypectomy, and perhaps even colectomy and ileorectal anastomosis, as these patients have a considerably increased risk of colon cancer. There is no evidence that solitary juvenile polyps have neoplastic potential and children with one or two polyps do not normally require follow-up. Histologically similar polyps occur throughout the gastrointestinal tract in the rare Cronkhite–Canada syndrome, resulting in diarrhoea and steatorrhoea associated with ectodermal abnormalities such as alopecia, nail dystrophy, and skin hyperpigmentation.

Peutz-Jeghers syndrome of mucocutaneous pigmentation (circumoral (Fig. 7), hands and feet) and gastrointestinal polyposis is inherited as a mendelian dominant. Peutz-Jeghers polyps may occur anywhere in the intestine but associated malignancy is rarer in the colon than in the duodenal region and stomach. The lip and mouth pigmentation is a very useful clinical marker. Operation may be advised if polyps over 1 cm in diameter are found radiographically in the small intestine, because there is a risk of intussusception and infarction. Gastroduodenal and colonic polyps may also bleed and cause anaemia; they are best removed by 2-yearly endoscopy with snare polypectomy.

Fig. 7 Peutz–Jeghers patient showing characteristic lip pigmentation.

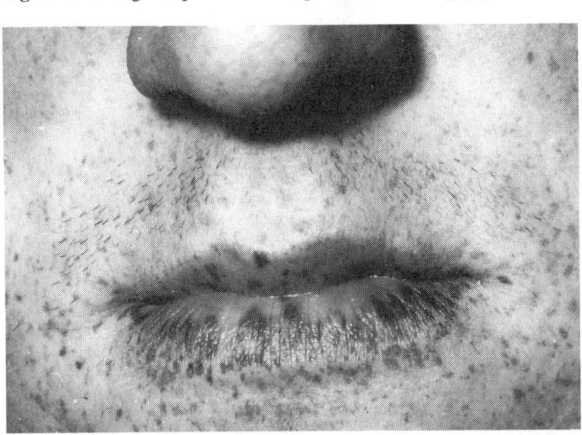

Other non-neoplastic polyps

These are less common. Lipomas are found in the right colon but do not normally require removal. Fatty enlargement of the ileocaecal value may produce an abnormal radiographic appearance but is equally unimportant. Endometriosis involving the bowel is usually on the serosal aspect or in the muscle layer of the distal colon, causing deformity but no symptoms; rarely, it may result in a submucosal polypoid mass that bleeds and needs to be distinguished from carcinoma. Benign tumours can also arise from other tissue elements of the wall of the intestine and include neurofibromas, leiomyomas, and polypoid haemangiomas. Lymphoid tissue is present in the colon as tiny lymphoid follicles dotted across the mucosa. These are normally visible only in childhood, when nodular lymphoid hyperplasia may cause radiological appearances that, in the colon, can resemble polyposis or, in the terminal ileum, mimic Crohn's disease. Pneumocystic disease (pneumatosis cystoides) causes multiple, raised, colonic mucosal blebs, sometimes haemorrhagic, which can be punctured and collapsed; treatment, if clinically indicated, is with oxygen therapy.

Neoplastic polyps

The majority of neoplastic polyps in the colon and rectum are adenomas, a generic name covering the spectrum of benign dysplastic epithelial growths having malignant potential. They range from the most frequent tubular adenomas, those with mixed or intermediate tubulovillous characteristics, to the rarer but larger and often sessile villous adenomas (villous papilloma), which have the greatest tendency to malignancy (Fig. 8). The differing use of histological terms in the literature can be confusing. The above terms are the recommended World Health Organization nomenclature.

AETIOLOGICAL FACTORS AND PATHOLOGY

Adenomas occur, usually asymptomatically, in around 30 per cent of a middle-aged Western population but more rarely in Africa, Asia, and South America. Adenomas are uncommon in Japanese unless they adopt a Western diet, whether at home or after emigration. The factors affecting adenoma development are probably the same as those relating to carcinoma. All observations suggest an influence of environmental or ecological factors, probably dietary, which may result in changed bacterial flora and the production of chemical carcinogens by bacterial action. Additionally, there is evidence of genetic influences, of which the most obvious is the dominant inheritance of familial adenomatous polyposis, which seems to occur with approximately equal incidence in all countries throughout the world.

A change in the normal processes of epithelial cell maturation results in an unstable, adenomatous epithelium (Fig. 9). Contrary to common belief this neoplastic epithelium has a normal rate of cell turnover. Available clinical evidence also suggests that adenomas are extremely slow growing, in most cases taking several years to reach 1 cm in size and significant cancer potential. They often cause no sequelae in the life-span of the patient; 30 per cent of an older Western population will have a colonic adenoma but only 3 to 5 per cent develop colon cancer, so 90 per cent of adenoma-bearing subjects die of other causes.

All forms of adenoma have similar abnormal or 'dysplastic' epithelium, analogous to precancerous changes in bronchial epithelium or the cervix uteri. The severity of the changes may be graded as mild, moderate, or severe dysplasia, which reflects the malignant potential of the polyp. Endoscopically there is a clearly visible junction between the darker red, neoplastic epithelium and pale, shiny, normal mucosa, which makes local excision easy. Histological examination will determine if dysplastic epithelium has invaded across the muscularis mucosa into the submucosa of the head of the polyp (Fig. 10); this is the only accepted proof that carcinomatous change has occurred. Although localized foci of severe dysplasia may occur on the surface of an adenoma and are sometimes described as 'carcinoma in situ', this term is best avoided, as, without invasion across the muscularis mucosa, there is no contact with lymphatics and therefore no possibility of metastasis. The frequency with which invasive carcinoma arises in adenomas increases with the size of the polyp and the degree of dysplasia. It is greater in villous adenomas because they are often large and severely dysplastic. Older data from surgical series suggest an average incidence of carcinoma in adenomas of 10 per cent, whereas figures from endoscopic series find it to be around 5 per cent (Table 2). The difference between these results is probably due to case selection, as the surgical figures were biased by the inclusion of polyps found during cancer resection.

THE ADENOMA-ADENOCARCINOMA SEQUENCE

There is considerable circumstantial evidence that most colon carcinomas originate from an adenoma. No one disputes that some adenomas progress to invasive carcinoma; the average interval for a medium-sized adenoma to develop malignancy is thought to be about 5 to 7 years but the progression can be quicker or slower. Many small carcinomas contain areas of benign adenomatous change but these are found less often in more advanced cancers, presumably because the carcinoma has outgrown and destroyed the benign tissue. Patients with adenomas have a higher risk of coexisting (synchronous) colon carcinomas or of developing one subsequently, the risk of cancer increasing with the number of adenomas found up to the 100 per cent lifetime risk in familial adenomatous polyposis. The distribution of colorectal carcinomas and adenomas is similar, with increasing incidence distally towards the rectum; there is a small increased incidence of villous adenoma and cancer formation in the caecum of elderly people.

Epidemiological patterns for colorectal cancer also mirror those for adenomas: for example, Japanese emigrating to Hawaii acquire an increased prevalence of both adenomas and cancer. Systematically

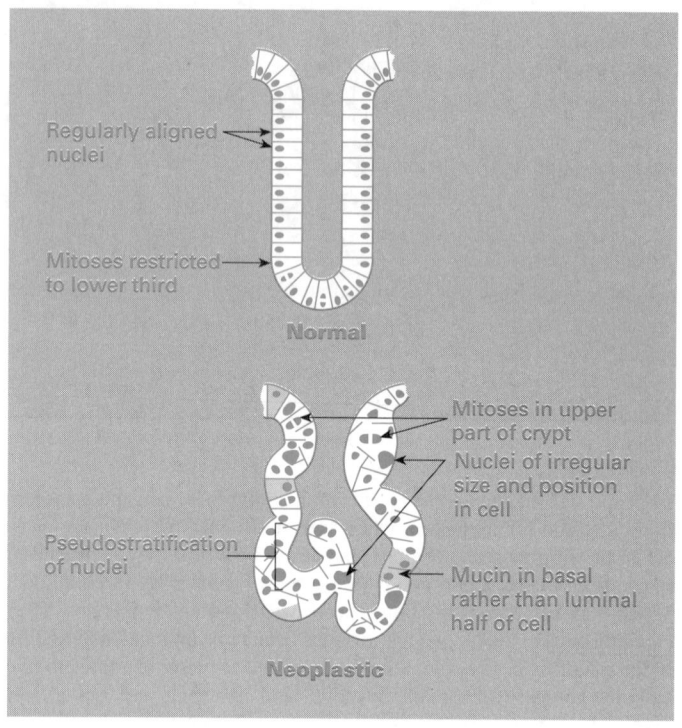

Fig. 9 Diagrammatic representation of the difference between the ordered histology of a normal colonic crypt and the disorder of a neoplastic (dysplastic) crypt.

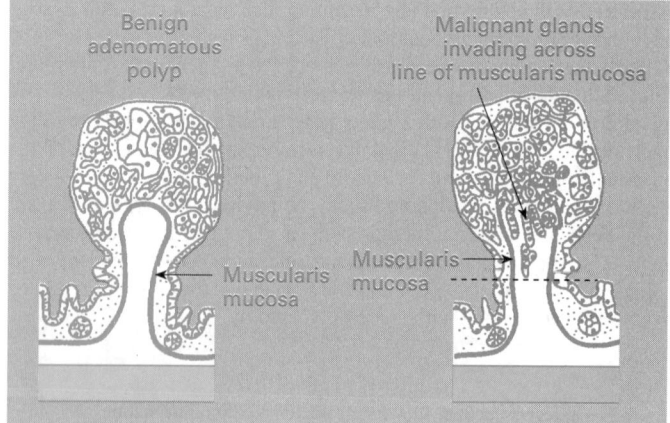

Fig. 10 Diagrammatic representation of the histology of a benign adenoma and a 'malignant polyp' showing adenoma and invasive adenocarcinoma (dotted line indicates snare transection line for complete removal).

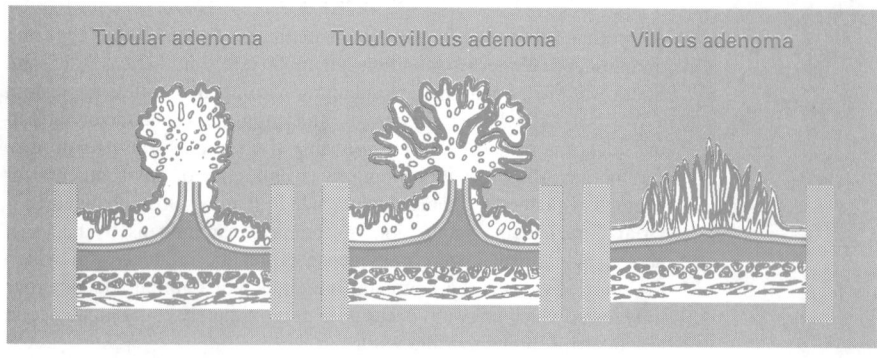

Fig. 8 Diagrammatic representation of the histology of adenomatous polyps.

Table 2 *Frequency of invasive carcinoma in different types of sizes of adenomas in an endoscopic series*

	Type as percentage of all adenomas	Percentage with malignancy			
		<1.1cm	1–2cm	>2cm	All sizes
Tubular	75	1	3.0	10	2
Tubulovillus	20		5.0	11	6
Villous	5		6.0	38	18
All adenomas		1	5.5	16	5 (overall)

From Gillespie *et al.* (1979).

destroying adenomas in the rectum of normal subjects or those with familial polyposis is found markedly to decrease the expected local incidence of carcinoma formation.

Very small or intramucosal carcinomas are rarely found except in association with the unique flat pattern of dysplasia of chronic extensive colitis (ulcerative colitis, schistosomiasis, and possibly Crohn's disease). The rare occurrence of a so-called *'de novo'* carcinoma of 1 cm or so in diameter in other patients can perhaps be explained by the known existence of 'microadenomas' where only one or more individual epithelial crypts show neoplastic abnormality; such a tiny initial focus would be undetectable after the development of carcinoma. Although small foci of adenoma cause a proportionately lower risk of malignant change than large masses, their existence means that even the most fastidious follow-up regimens are unlikely completely to remove the risk of carcinoma formation.

CLINICAL FEATURES AND MANAGEMENT

Most colonic polyps are symptomless and are diagnosed on radiographs or by endoscopy. Larger ones may bleed intermittently. Obvious mucus production, altered bowel habit, or abdominal pain are uncommon presenting features. The largest, sessile, villous adenomas of the rectum can, rarely, present with profuse mucoid diarrhoea and electrolyte depletion, especially hypokalaemia.

Once found a polyp must be completely removed for histological assessment. Over 95 per cent are removable by endoscopic snare polypectomy or local electrocoagulation. Even small colonic polyps are worth destroying (except in the most elderly patients) because they are usually adenomatous and because when the colon is known to be polyp free the patient can be spared frequent follow-up examination, which is the alternative if the polyp is left. The mucosal surface of the colon is without pain sensation, so the action of snaring and electrocoagulating the polyp stalk to prevent bleeding is not felt at all by the patient and can be done on outpatients with or without sedation. Some 90 per cent of patients with polyps have only one or two of them, and 90 per cent of polyps are under 2 cm in diameter, thick stalked, and easy to snare. Larger polyps have more extensive feeding vessels with a greater tendency to bleed after polypectomy. Very large or sessile polyps may have to be removed 'piecemeal' in multiple portions but few are so large as to need surgical resection. Within 5 cm of the anus there is a likelihood of pain sensation and general anaesthesia may sometimes be advisable. Skilled management by a colorectal surgeon is needed for large, sessile, villous adenomas in the rectum or caecum although laser photocoagulation or urological resectoscopes have been used.

When carcinoma is identified in an endoscopically removed adenomatous polyp the decision for or against further surgical resection of the bowel is a matter of balance. There is a less than 2 per cent chance of finding resectable metastatic carcinoma in the draining lymph nodes, which must be weighed against the risk of operation in the elderly. If the carcinoma is well or moderately well differentiated, and histologically completely removed, operation is not advised.

Follow-up

Once a patient has had one or more polyps removed and they are shown to be adenomas, some form of long-term surveillance is recommended because, over the ensuing years, adenomas are found in over 30 per cent of patients and carcinomas in 2 to 4 per cent. If only one or two small (under 1 cm) tubular adenomas are found no follow-up may be needed. For multiple, larger, or villous polyps the first colonoscopy check can usually be at 3 years, unless the polyps are very numerous or not certainly removed. After a normal 3-year examination it may be safe to increase the subsequent intervals to 4–5 yearly. Follow-up stops at around 75 years of age. Villous adenomas have both a high incidence of invasive carcinoma and a remarkable tendency to recur locally.

Familial adenomatous polyposis

Familial adenomatous polyposis (**FAP**) is now known to affect the whole gastrointestinal tract and, as well as the colon, the duodenal region is particularly involved. The term 'polyposis coli' is thus best avoided. At least a hundred and often thousands of polyps are present throughout the colon (Fig. 11). The qualification 'adenomatous' is included to ensure distinction from other non-neoplastic forms of polyposis. The condition is inherited as a mendelian dominant but 30 per cent of cases occur without a preceding family history, presumably due to mutation.

Fig. 11 Familial adenomatosis polyposis (FAP) colectomy specimen–close-up view showing carpeting of colon by hundreds of adenomas.

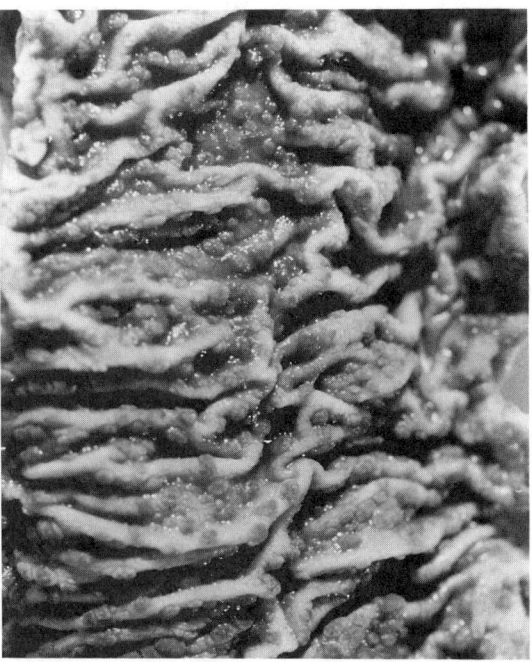

The prime reason for concern is the inevitable occurrence of colorectal carcinoma in all affected patients followed for long enough. Carcinoma of the duodenum, ampulla or bile ducts occurs in a small but significant percentage of patients secondary to the adenomatous polyps found in this region. Gardner's syndrome, in which adenomas coexist with meso-dermal tumours (desmoid tumours of the abdomen, osteomas of the mandible and skull, sebaceous cysts, and soft-tissue tumours of the skin), and the even rarer Turcot's syndrome, (in which there are brain tumours and adenomatosis), are both variants within the broad spectrum of clinical presentation of FAP.

It is unusual for the adenomas to appear before adolescence and symp-toms usually only occur when a carcinoma has developed. The mean age of symptomatic presentation in the St Mark's polyposis registry is 36 years, whereas the diagnosis can be made much earlier and before the development of cancer if all members of known 'polyposis families' are called to attend a screening clinic at 12 to 14 years of age. Screening of FAP family members is currently by a combination of methods that together establish the individual's risk. DNA analysis, looking for muta-tions of the *APC* (adenomatous polyposis coli) gene at the q21–22 region on chromosome 5, is theoretically possible *in utero* or at birth. In prac-tice, gene-probe methodology is, however, not applicable to all families and in any case many parents prefer to leave screening until adolescence for psychosocial reasons (see below). The presence of congenital hyper-trophy of the retinal pigment epithelium (**CHRPE**), visible to an expert as small, dark blobs on the periphery of the retina is, for the present, a valuable adjunctive clinical screening method, being present in two-thirds of FAP patients even before adenomas are apparent. Flexible sig-moidoscopy is a more accurate examination than rigid proctosigmoid-oscopy in looking for polyps. Any polyps seen must be biopsied to make a positive diagnosis and to differentiate from the less serious, non-neo-plastic forms of polyposis, which do not require surgery. Although neg-ative DNA testing with absence of CHRPE on ophthalmological exam-ination and lack of polyps on sigmoidoscopy by the age of 20 virtually guarantees that the individual does not have the FAP genotype, sur-veillance should continue intermittently until the age of 35.

Colectomy with ileorectal or ileoanal anastomosis is usually done in FAP subjects at the age of 17 to 18 years for social convenience, as there is no significant risk of carcinoma before this. Careful long-term follow-up is needed; if rectal mucosa is left, 10 per cent of polyposis patients with ileorectal anastomosis develop cancer of the rectal stump over a 30-year period. Total proctocolectomy with ileostomy is reserved for those with unmanageable numbers of rectal polyps wishing to avoid the greater operative risks of ileoanal anastomosis with formation of a pelvic pouch.

A screening programme is necessary (flexible sigmoidoscopy) for all blood relations, including cousins, nephews, and nieces of relevant age, in addition to constructing a careful family tree and keeping a register of affected families. As a result of such precautions, familial adeno-matous polyposis has become the classic example of practical colorectal cancer prevention, though a small risk persists when the rectal stump remains and also from intra-abdominal desmoids and duodenal or ampullary tumours in later life.

Colorectal cancer

Adenocarcinomas of the colon and rectum present a major challenge to medical practice, being common, potentially curable, and possibly pre-ventable. The other malignancies of the region—lymphoma, sarcoma and carcinoid—are very rare.

EPIDEMIOLOGY AND AETIOLOGICAL FACTORS

Colorectal carcinoma is the most common malignancy in the United Kingdom after lung cancer, and in the United States after skin cancer. In the United Kingdom, 19,000 deaths are reported annually. Exact sta-tistics are uncertain because anatomical distinction between rectum and colon is sometimes arbitrary. At least another 6000 colorectal cancers a year are successfully resected. There is evidence from the United States that the percentage of colon cancers is steadily increasing compared to rectal cancers. There are differing reports on sex incidence but men appear to be slightly more at risk for rectal cancer and women for colon cancer. The incidence of both cancers increases with age, the average age at diagnosis being around 60 to 65 years.

The epidemiology of colorectal cancer suggests that environmental (probably dietary) and genetic factors are both important. The incidence of colorectal cancer is higher in Northern Europe and North America than in Southern Europe and South America or in Africa and Asia. Japan is a low-risk area for carcinoma of the colon compared to carcinoma of the rectum, but Japanese of higher socioeconomic status who adopt a 'Westernized' diet or who emigrate to North America change to high risk for both adenoma formation and colon cancer. Sporadic examples of colorectal cancer occur even in low-risk countries, unfortunately often in young people, who develop an anaplastic carcinoma with poor prog-nosis. There is some evidence that carcinogens or cocarcinogens may be produced by bacterial metabolism of bile salts or other sterols derived from animal fat. A contributory factor in populations eating a low-fibre diet may be explained by slow colonic transit, which gives more time for carcinogen production, concentration, and contact with the mucosa. Ethanol consumption, particularly beer drinking, has also been associ-ated epidemiologically with colon carcinogenesis.

Surgical implantation of the ureters into the sigmoid colon (uretero-sigmoidostomy) results, after 10 to 20 years, in a high incidence of colonic adenoma or carcinoma adjacent to the ureteric stoma, possibly due to carcinogen formation from bacterial action on nitrates/nitrites excreted in the urine. There is long-term risk of mucosal cellular dys-plasia or atypia (precancerous charge) and subsequent cancer in patients with previous extensive or total ulcerative colitis, and probably in Crohn's colitis also.

GENETIC FACTORS

Besides the extreme example of familial polyposis, the importance of genetic factors is suggested by an increased incidence of cancer within families: 15 per cent of siblings and 10 per cent of offspring of colorectal cancer patients develop the disease. Hereditary non-polyposis colon can-cer (**HNPCC**) includes site-specific colorectal cancer families (Lynch type I) and other 'cancer families' (Lynch type II) with associated malig-nancies including breast, female genital tract, perhaps prostate, stomach, and skin cancer. In both of these there is mendelian dominant inheritance of cancer risks; the putative gene responsible is localized to chromosome 2. Although HNPCC families contribute only 5 to 10 per cent of colo-rectal cancers, there is potential for screening colonoscopy to detect and destroy precursor adenomas in family members. Genetic risk is consid-ered certain if there has been cancer in three successive generations, probable when there are three or more affected relatives, one being a first-degree relative (parent, sibling, child) of the other two with suc-cessive generations being involved and one diagnosed before age 50 (Amsterdam Criteria for HNPCC). A single first-degree relative affected at older age indicates only slightly increased risk, probably insufficient to justify screening.

The molecular genetic basis for colorectal carcinogenesis is increas-ingly understood, and involves a number of genetic events, which, in a generally stepwise manner, cumulatively result in the progression from normal epithelium to adenoma and finally to invasive adenocarcinoma (Fig. 12). The changes include activation of dominantly acting onco-genes regulating cell division and differentiation (k-*ras* and possibly c-*myc*), and inactivation of tumour-suppressor genes, including *APC* (adenomatous polyposis coli/FAP) and *MCC* (mutated in colorectal can-cer), both on chromosome 5, *DCC* (deleted in colorectal cancer) on chromosome 18, and *P53* on chromosome 17. In addition to these muta-tions on chromosomes 5, 17, and 18, some colorectal carcinomas may show deletions, insertions and mutations on chromosomes 1, 4, 6, 8, 9 or 22, suggesting that other tumour-suppressor genes may sometimes be inactivated.

The redeeming factor from the clinical point of view is that the sequence of events in the colon is slow moving, making it possible to find and remove the lesion at its precancerous stage; additionally, most colorectal cancers are well- or moderately well-differentiated and usually present without distant metastases. Furthermore, colorectal neoplasms, whether precancerous or invasive, tend to grow into the lumen of the bowel, which makes them easier to diagnose and resect. Only the carcinoma of chronic ulcerative colitis is characteristically intramucosal and even this appears usually to be preceded by a period of superficial dysplastic change, potentially allowing biopsy diagnosis and colon resection in the precancerous phase.

PATHOLOGY

The majority of bowel carcinomas occur distally in the rectosigmoid. A convenient rule, acceptably accurate considering the difficulties of definition and measurement of site, is that 30 per cent occur in the rectum, 30 per cent in the sigmoid colon, and 30 per cent proximal to that.

The typical carcinoma is a polypoid mass with central ulceration and irregular, easily bleeding edges, which may spread to become a stricture (Fig. 13). Infiltrating scirrhous colon carcinomas are rare. Colorectal carcinoma initially spreads by local invasion rather than by venous or lymphatic routes, which accounts for its good prognosis when confined to the bowel wall. It invades through the mucosa and muscle coats of the bowel to penetrate the extramural tissues and may involve adjacent organs such as the bladder, giving rise to secondary complications (e.g. fistula formation). Involvement of larger veins results in early spread to the liver and poor prognosis, although occasionally liver metastases may be single and resectable. When lymphatics are invaded the spread is to nodes nearest to the growth before those lying more centrally in the mesentery. This gradual progression through mainly free-slung and easily resected tissues improves the chances of complete surgical removal of large-bowel cancer.

In 1932, Dukes described a staging classification (Fig. 14) for resected carcinoma of the rectum, subsequently applied to colonic carcinomas as well, in which the extent of local spread and presence or absence of lymph node metastases were related to 5-year survival (Table 3). A major modification to this incorporating the degree of lymphocytic reaction (Jass) or alternatively the extent of tumour nodal or metastatic involvement (TNM classification) seem to offer little predictive advantage. Classification is also possible by histological grade (well differentiated, moderately well differentiated, poorly differentiated) but is less accurate than the Dukes' classification in predicting survival. The poorly differentiated carcinomas are usually the most extensive and have a poorer prognosis, disproportionately worse if larger veins are involved. The most frequent sites of metastases are liver (over 60 per cent), lung (50 per cent), peritoneum (15 per cent) or skeleton (15 per cent).

CLINICAL FEATURES

Once a colorectal carcinoma has reached moderate size it is likely to produce symptoms according to its site in the colon. Any large-bowel cancer will bleed intermittently but rectal and sigmoid colon cancers are more likely to bleed overtly because their friable tumour surface is buffeted by solid stool, the blood being mixed in with the stool (in contrast to the bright red and separated blood of haemorrhoids). Similarly, alteration in previously regular habit, whether bowel frequency or constipation, only occurs if tumour obstructs the passage of solid stool in the narrow left colon. The flow of liquid contents through the capacious caecum or ascending colon is unaffected even by large tumours. For this reason the caecum is known as a 'silent area' in which large but symptomless carcinomas may occur, eventually presenting with iron-deficiency anaemia consequent on long-continued minor blood loss, altered by bacterial action and therefore passing unnoticed in the stools. The problem of diagnosis in the caecum is further compounded by the difficulty of cleansing it completely and of obtaining good radiography of the area. Pain, suggesting obstruction or invasion, and weight loss are late symptoms, which are most common in advanced cancers with poor prognosis. Even at this stage, however, the slow-moving nature of colon cancer means that it may be resectable. The presence of a palpable mass equally does not invariably mean a bad prognosis, for the carcinoma may be small with considerable faecal holdup, or most of the mass may be due to surrounding inflammatory change or abscess formation.

The problem in clinical diagnosis of colorectal cancer is that the symptom patterns are very variable and non-specific. The most common causes of anorectal bleeding are trivial haemorrhoids or fissures; the patients most troubled by colonic pain, altered bowel habit, or mucus

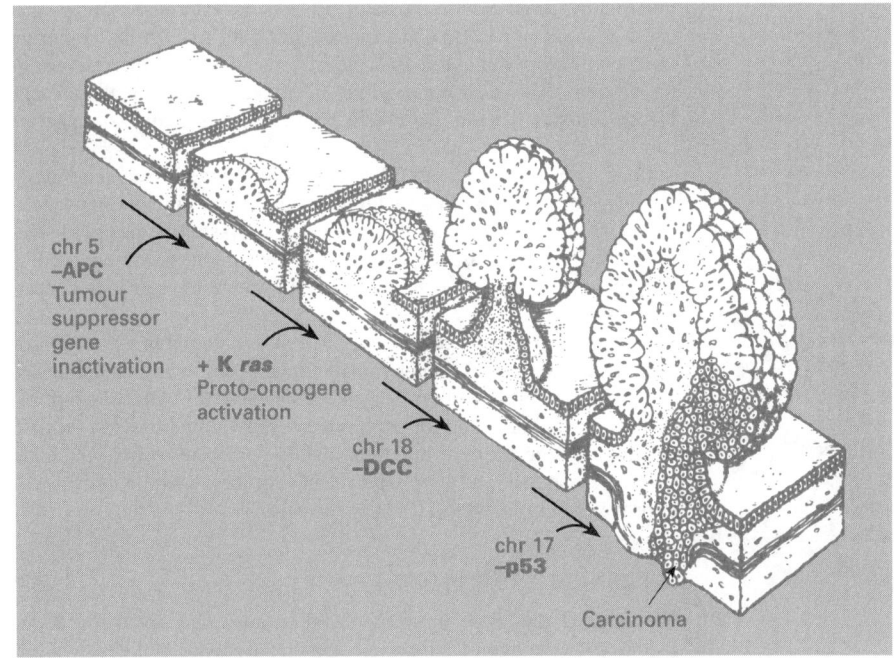

chr 5
–APC
Tumour suppressor gene inactivation

+ K ras
Proto-oncogene activation

chr 18
–DCC

chr 17
–p53

Carcinoma

Fig. 12 The 'adenoma–carcinoma sequence'–a possible genetic model. Accumulated genetic changes in the stepwise progression from normal epithelium to increasing size of polyp and eventual malignant change include inactivation of tumour suppressor genes (adenomatous polyposis coli (*APC*), deleted in colorectal cancer (*DCC*) and p53, as well as the activation of proto-oncogenes such as K-*ras*. These alterations do not occur in a rigid sequence. (Adapted from Fearon and Vogelstein (1990). *Cell*, **61**, 759.)

loss are those with irritable or spastic colon, who often also have an obsessive and cancerphobic personality. Nevertheless, the importance of early diagnosis of colon cancer is such that any new colonic symptoms should be taken seriously, particularly bleeding and especially in patients over 45 years of age. Every patient should be clinically examined with initial digital examination of the rectum and proctosigmoidoscopy, preferably with the flexible sigmoidoscope.

Flexible sigmoidoscopy requires a single enema as preparation, needs no sedation, takes only two to three minutes longer to do than rigid examination but examines three to four times the extent of colon with

Table 3 *Modified Dukes' classification and life prognosis for potentially curative colorectal cancer*

Dukes' classification	Cases resected (%)	5-year survival (corrected for other causes of mortality %)
A	15	95–100
B	40	65–75
C₁ (local nodes)	35	30–40
C₂ (apical nodes)	10	10–20

proportionately increased reassurance and pathological yield. Its range over the distal colon (sometimes to the splenic flexure) covers both the highest risk area for adenomas and carcinoma and the region where most radiological misses occur. Examination of the proximal colon is also most accurate with the colonoscope but the technique is difficult and traumatic in about 30 per cent of patients, such that some sedation is normally required. The air- or double-contrast barium enema gives reasonable accuracy for large lesions such as cancers, but is inaccurate for small precursor lesions.

Patients with unexplained and persistent rectal bleeding or severe anaemia should be preferentially referred for endoscopy. About 20 per cent of patients with rectal bleeding referred for colonoscopy are found to have polyps or cancer. Patients with strictures of the colon can have malignancy excluded more certainly by the passage of a small calibre fibrescope (Plate 4) than by diagnostic laparotomy, because of the mucosal view and biopsy capability of the endoscope although extracolonic tumours cannot be diagnosed endoscopically. Even those patients with the diagnostic 'apple-core' appearance of stricturing colon carcinoma on radiographs (Fig. 13) need high-quality examination of the rest of the colon either radiologically or by endoscopy because of the 20 per cent incidence of coexisting benign or malignant neoplasms elsewhere in the colon.

Differential diagnosis must be made from other benign lesions such as localized ischaemic areas, solitary ulcer of the rectum, granulation-tissue masses, endometriosis, or inflammatory lesions such as amoebomas, all of which can exactly mimic carcinoma on radiographs and at endoscopy. Palpable masses with radiological features simulating carcinoma can be caused in the caecal area by an appendix abscess, tuberculosis, actinomycosis, or Crohn's disease, and in the sigmoid colon by diverticular disease with pericolic abscess formation. Strictures that cause suspicious radiographic appearances but prove to be benign on endoscopic biopsy or cytology occur in Crohn's disease, ulcerative colitis, or after severe ischaemic colitis. Whenever practicable, therefore, a forceps biopsy should be taken before operating on an apparent carcinoma.

Imaging by other methods (ultrasound, CT, magnetic resonance imaging, etc.) are generally disappointing except where spread of advanced cancer requires assessment. In a few early lesions of the rectum or rectosigmoid, local ultrasonography, by probe or ultrasound endoscope, may indicate the presence or absence of local invasion and so help decision taking.

Other indirect diagnostic means such as haemoglobin estimation or sedimentation rate make an obviously limited contribution to diagnosis. The lack of specificity of serological tests such as the carcinoembryonic antigen has so far been a disappointment; they are now used routinely in only a few institutions and then mainly postoperatively in the hope that early diagnosis and aggressive management of recurrent tumour will improve prognosis, which is rarely the case.

SCREENING AND FOLLOW-UP

Screening studies have been attempted on large, asymptomatic populations over the age of 40 using commercially available, occult-blood test packs. Those cancers detected by such screening (about 1/1000 per-

Fig. 13 Air-contrast radiograph of 'apple-core' stricture caused by colonic carcinoma.

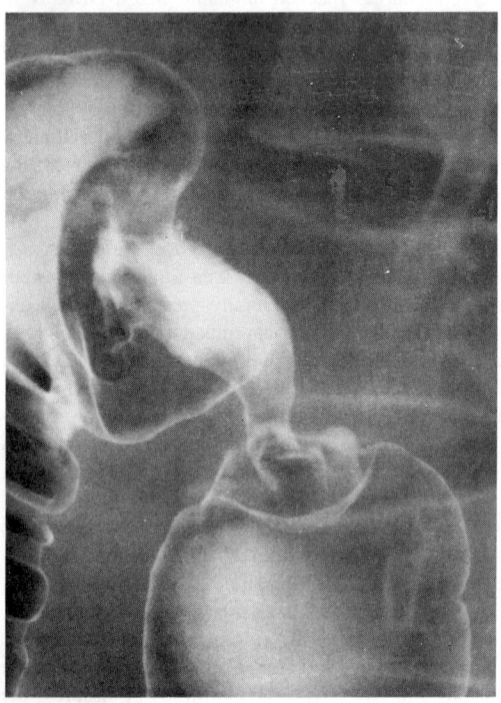

Fig. 14 Dukes' classification of colorectal carcinoma.

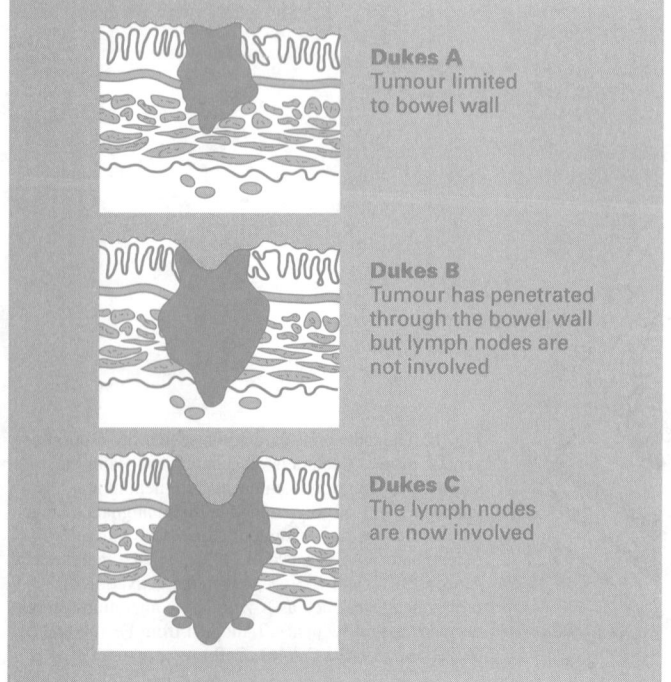

Dukes A
Tumour limited to bowel wall

Dukes B
Tumour has penetrated through the bowel wall but lymph nodes are not involved

Dukes C
The lymph nodes are now involved

sons tested) are usually at an earlier stage with improved prognosis, but occult-blood testing will miss about 40 per cent of cancers and 80 per cent of larger adenomas. The costs of screening are enormous, as futher investigation is required for the 30 to 40 subjects per 1000 tested positive, 80 per cent of whom have no significant pathology. Most unbiased observers conclude that to extend such screening programmes to the general population is unrealistic unless more effective methodology, such as DNA probes, can be applied. For high-risk subjects, such as those with previous adenomas or members of colorectal cancer families, occult-blood screening is insufficient and colonscopy is required.

After resection of colorectal cancer, follow-up is indicated mainly as a preventative measure as these patients have an increased risk of developing future polyps or carcinoma. As for polyp follow-up, colonoscopy is the preferred technique because of its accuracy and ability to destroy or remove any lesions found. A careful whole-colon examination should usually be made within months of surgery and 2- to 3-yearly thereafter depending on whether additional adenomas are found on first examination.

TREATMENT AND RESULTS

The best treatment for colorectal carcinoma is excision, usually by surgical resection, except for snared polyps with invasion limited to the head, or occasional small and circumscribed rectal cancers suitable for local excision. There have been enthusiastic reports on radiotherapy for rectal carcinoma and it may decrease the risk of local recurrence. Chemotherapy with 5-fluorouracil in combination with folinic acid agents has shown some improvement in survival time in advanced disease. Combining levamisole with 5-fluorouracil may increase the cure rate for these advanced (Dukes' C) cases or adjuvant therapy in patients undergoing curative surgery. The hope of the surgeon is to be able to perform a radical operation, removing the growth with an adequate margin of normal tissue and the entire draining lymphatic field. Even in the 20 per cent of patients in whom the presence of metastases or extensive infiltration makes radical surgery impossible, resection of the primary tumour is usually desirable as palliative treatment in order to prevent obstruction and the unpleasantness of bloody discharge. In particularly poor-risk patients, palliative tumour destruction by repeated laser photocoagulation is an alternative.

Preoperatively the surgeon attempts to assess by palpation the resectability of any tumour accessible to digital examination, but involvement of liver or pelvic organs is best assessed by ultrasonography or CT scanning. Urography is sometimes used to check for ureteric involvement. The bowel is prepared for surgery by cleansing with oral lavage or a purgative regimen with enemas and an antibiotic combination to reduce the risk of postoperative sepsis. Obstructing carcinomas clearly make effective cleansing impossible, spillage more likely, and the hazards of surgery greater; endoscopic canalization or deflation is sometimes possible.

The choice of operation is usually straightforward because the object is to remove a wide area of the supplying vasculature and the associated lymphatic field. Substantial resections are therefore made, such as right hemicolectomy for proximal lesions, transverse colectomy, left hemicolectomy or sigmoid colectomy distally, the feeding artery or arteries to the region being tied off and dissected close to their origin from the aorta. By combining laparoscopic mobilization of the relevant area with modified surgical techniques the speed of postoperative recovery can be considerably increased.

Improved surgical suturing technique or the use of the stapling gun have also made it possible to resect and reanastomose rectal carcinomas down to about 5 cm above the anus. The exact limit depends on circumstances including the apparent extent of tumour spread, as a 3- to 5-cm margin of excision is desirable. 'Low' anterior resections are now commonplace and the results of restorative surgery or local excision are so good that rectal excision is often avoidable. When the tumour involves the region of the anal sphincter there is no alternative to rectal excision and a permanent colostomy. A temporary colostomy is sometimes per-

formed when the likelihood of postoperative anastomeotic leakage of sepsis is high, for instance after low anterior resections, technically difficult operations, or when there is obstruction and imperfect perparation. The operative mortality of colorectal resections is around 5 per cent overall, although much lower when considering only elective resections by skilled colorectal surgeons and higher in old people.

The long-term results of surgery for colorectal cancer depend on the centre reporting as well as on the stage and grade of tumour. Specialist centres quote over 90 per cent of cases as being suitable for radical or curative surgery, with corrected 5-year survival of 50 to 60 per cent overall and 100 per cent for Dukes' A cases. District general hospitals find only 50 per cent to be suitable for radical surgery and, even so, have only 30 per cent corrected 5-year survival. The overall figures reflect the problems of less experienced surgeons in general hospitals, elderly patients with a more advanced stage of disease due to late referral or inadequate diagnostic methods, and emergency operations (obstruction, perforation) done under unfavourable conditions. In spite of this the results for colorectal cancer are cheerful in comparison to those for gastric or pancreatic cancer, reflecting the differences in pathology rather than medical skill. Surgical technique and advances in anaesthesia, postoperative care, and antibiotic cover have in the past improved the results considerably but they have not changed in the past 30 years. Further improvement in survival figures must rest on public attitude towards early reporting of bleeding or bowel symptoms, early referral for investigations with modern diagnostic techniques, screening of those over 55 years of age for adenomas by flexible sigmoidoscopy, and identification of those at increased genetic risk.

Carcinoma in ulcerative colitis

Patients who have had previous ulcerative colitis for more than 8 to 10 years affecting the whole colon are at increased risk of developing colon cancers. A similar tendency is thought to exist in patients with longstanding, extensive, Crohn's colitis. The risk remains even when the colitis is inactive and the patient symptom free, but is probably greater when the colitis has been persistently active or started in childhood. After 20 years from the onset of symptoms of extensive ulcerative colitis, 5 to 10 per cent of patients are likely to develop carcinoma. Unlike other colon cancers, these are more likely to be multifocal and histologically of mucinous or signet-ring type, although any variety may occur. Although this risk is a matter for concern in the individual patients, the numbers involved are small and account for less than 0.5 per cent of all colon cancers. There appears to be no significant risk in patients with a short history and lesser risk in those with proven left-sided colitis.

Some centres report relative success in screening patients with longstanding, extensive colitis by periodic rectal and colonoscopic biopsies looking for precancerous or severely dysplastic changes analogous to those in adenomas or in the cervix uteri. Others report mainly frustration due to 'breakthrough' cancers without dysplasia in spite of careful and expensive surveillance regimens. The rectum of patients with previous ileorectal anastomosis is similarly at risk and requires surveillance. Symptomless patients with dysplasia on biopsy are recommended to have prophylactic surgery. This dysplasia surveillance policy is still under evaluation but it appears to offer a reasonable alternative to the blunderbuss approach of total colectomy in all patients with chronic extensive colitis or the nihilism of doing nothing in young patients with known cancer risk.

Other colonic and anal tumours

Carcinoid tumours of the large bowel occur mainly as yellowish rectal nodules that are usually benign, do not produce the carcinoid syndrome, and can be locally resected. Violaceous nodules of Kaposi's sarcoma may be found in AIDS patients. Primary lymphoma of the colon is rare but polyposis-like involvement can occur either in primary malignant lymphomatous polyposis or as part of generalized lymphoma with multiple, umbilicated nodules present in the distribution of the lymphoid follicles in the colon and elsewhere in the gastrointestinal tract; diagnosis is made on forceps biopsy, the polyps disappearing on chemotherapy. Localized lymphoma may be treated by resection or irradiation, depending on its site.

In the anal region a number of tumours may occur relating to the different structures and embryology of the area. They include (epidermoid) carcinomas, anal-gland adenocarcinomas, condylomas, and malignant melanomas. Rarely, the anal region may be the site of precancerous skin conditions such as leucoplakia, Paget's disease, or Bowen's disease.

REFERENCES

Akoh, J.A. and MacIntyre, I.M.C. (1992). Improving survival in gastric cancer: review of 5 year survival rates in English language publications from 1970. *British Journal of Surgery,* **79,** 293–9.

Brunetaud, J.M., Maunoury, V., Cochelard, D., Cortot, A., and Paris, J.C. (1989). Laser palliation for rectosigmoid cancers. *International Journal of Colorectal Diseases,* **4,** 6–8.

Clen, K.K., Day, N.E., Duffy, S.W., Lam, T.H., Fok, M., and Wong, J. (1989). Pickled vegetable in the aetiology of oesophageal cancer in Hong Kong China. *Lancet,* **339,** 1314–17.

Correa, P. and Haenszel, W. (1978). The epidemiology of large bowel cancer. *Advances in Cancer Research,* **26,** 1–141.

Craven, J.L. (1991). Gastric cancer. *Current Opinion in Gastroenterology,* **7,** 933–8.

De Meester, T.R., Attwood, S.E.A., Smyrik, J.C., Therkildsen, D.H., and Hinder, R.A. (1990). Surgical therapy in Barrett's esophagus. *Annals of Surgery,* **212,** 528–40.

Domizio, P., Owen, R.A., Shepherd, N.A., Talbot, I.C., and Norton, A.J. (1993). Primary lymphoma of the small intestine. *American Journal of Surgical Pathology,* **17,** 429–42.

Earlham, R. and Cunha-Melo, J.R. (1980). Oesophageal squamous cell carcinoma. I Review of Surgery. II Review of radiotherapy. *British Journal of Surgery,* **67,** 381–90; 457–61.

Fitzgibbons, R.J., Lynch, H.T., Stanislav, G.V. and Watson, P.A. (1987). Recognition and treatment of patients with hereditary non-polyposis colon cancer (Lynch syndromes I and II). *Annals of Surgery,* **206,** 289–95.

Gillespie, P.E., Chambers, T.J., Chan, K.W., Doronzo, F., Morson, B.C., and Williams, C.B. (1979). Colonic adenomas—a colonoscopic survey. *Gut,* **20,** 240–45.

Haenzel, W., Kurihara, M., Segi, M., and Lee, R.K. (1972). Stomach cancer amongst Japanese in Hawaii. *Journal of the National Cancer Institute,* **49,** 969–88.

Haggitt, R.C., Glotzbach, R.E., Soffer, E.E., and Wruble, L.D. (1985). Prognostic factors in colorectal carcinomas arising in adenomas: implications for lesions removed by endoscopic polypectomy. *Gastroenterology,* **89,** 328–36.

Jass, J.R., Williams, C.B., Bussey, H.J.R., and Morson, B.C. (1988). Juvenile polyposis–a precancerous condition. *Histopathology,* **13,** 619–30.

Lynch, H.T. *et al.* (1993). Genetics, natural history, tumour spectrum and pathology of hereditary nonpolyposis colorectal cancer: an updated review. *Gastroenterology,* **104,** 1535–9.

Müller, J.M., Erasmi, H., Stelzner, M., Zieran, U., and Pichmaier, H. (1990). Surgical therapy of oesophageal carcinoma. *British Journal of Surgery,* **77,** 845–57.

Nomura, A., Stemmermann, G.N., Chyou, P-H., Kato, I., Perez-Perez, G.I., and Blaser, M.J. *Helicobacter pylori* and gastric carcinoma among Japanese American in Hawaii. *New England Journal of Medicine,* **325,** 1132–6.

Parsonett, J. *et al.* (1991). *Helicobacter pylori* infection and the risk of gastric carcinoma. *New England Journal of Medicine,* **325,** 1127–32.

Potet, F., Fléjou, J.F., Gervaz, H., and Pafaf, F. (1991). Adenocarcinoma of the lower oesophagus and the oesophagogastric junction. *Seminars in Diagnostic Pathology,* **8,** 126–36.

Spigelman, A.D., Murday, V.A., and Phillips, R.K.S. (1989). Cancer and the Peutz-Jeghers syndrome. *Gut,* **30,** 1588–90.

Thomas, W.M., Pye, G., James, P.D., Amar, S.S., and Moss, S.M. (1989). Randomised, controlled trial of faecal occult blood screening for colorectal cancer. Results for first 102,349 subjects. *Lancet,* **i,** 1160–4.

Vogelstein, B. *et al.* (1988). Genetic alterations during colorectal tumour development. *New England Journal of Medicine,* **319,** 525–32.

Vogelstein, B., Fearon, E.R., Hamilton, S.R., Kern, S.E. Preisinger, A.C., and Leppert, M., (1988). Genetic alterations during colorectal tumor development. *New England Journal of Medicine,* **319,** 525–32.

Williams, C.B. and Bedenne, L. (1990). Quadrennial review: management of colonic polyps—is all the effort worthwhile? *European Journal of Gastroenterology and Hepatology,* **5** (suppl. 1), 144–65.

Wotherspoon, A.C., Doglioni, C., Diss, T.C., *et al.* (1993). Regression of primary low-grade B-cell gastric lymphoma of mucosa-associated lymphoid tissue type after eradication of *Helicobacter pylori.* Lancet, **342,** 575–7.

14.17 Vascular and collagen disorders

G. NEALE

Clinical disorders of the gastrointestinal tract caused by vascular and collagen diseases are rare in general medical practice. They may cause ulceration, strictures, infarction, perforation, or bleeding. Although clinicians have become increasingly aware of the possibilities, progress in developing methods for assessing the adequacy of blood flow have been slow. Thus the diagnosis and medical management of many of the conditions described in this section remain unsatisfactory; all too often a potentially life-threatening acute episode is the first indication of gastrointestinal involvement.

Ischaemic disease of the gut

Aetiology

Ischaemic lesions may occur in the small or large intestine with or without evidence of gross vascular occlusion. The stomach is rarely affected. A list of causes is shown in Table 1.

OCCLUSION OF MAJOR ARTERIES

Atheromatous occlusion

This is the most common cause of mesenteric vascular insufficiency, which often remains undiagnosed in life, probably because the slowness of the pathological process allows for the development of a compensatory collateral circulation. Intestinal infarction secondary to atheromatous occlusion of one major vessel is uncommon. Indeed, all three vessels may be occluded without visceral damage.

Thrombosis

This often develops on an ulcerated atheromatous plaque but may also occur spontaneously in polycythaemia, sickle cell disease, cryoglobulinaemia, and amyloidosis. Thromboangiitis obliterans (Buerger's disease) (see Section 15) only rarely affects mesenteric vessels but in such cases the prognosis is poor.

Table 1 *Causes of ischaemic disease of the gut*

Atheromatous occlusion of arteries
Thrombosis of major vessels
Systemic emboli
Miscellaneous lesions damaging or compressing the arterial
   tree
Inflammation (usually non-infective) of blood vessels (see
   Table 2)
Diffuse microthrombosis
Non-occlusive intestinal infarction (see Table 3)
Occlusion of large veins

Systemic arterial embolism

This has accounted for up to one-third of cases of mesenteric vascular occlusion in some series. Emboli arise from the heart, especially in patients with mitral stenosis and atrial fibrillation, with myocardial infarction and endocardial thrombosis, and with bacterial endocarditis. Paradoxical embolism through a patent foramen ovale and embolism from aortic mural thrombi are uncommon causes.

INFLAMMATION OF BLOOD VESSELS

Vasculitis may affect the splanchnic circulation in several multisystem disorders including polyarteritis and the collagen disorders (Table 2). Resulting thrombosis may cause oedema, mucosal haemorrhages, focal ulceration, and focal necrosis with perforation. Occasionally the healing process leads to the development of intestinal strictures.

Primary gastrointestinal angiitis without systemic lesions has been described but in such cases one must take care to exclude conditions that may cause secondary inflammation of vessels, such as inflammatory bowel disease, potassium-induced ulceration, and eosinophilic granuloma. Granulomatous pathology as in Wegener's disease and lethal midline granuloma may also have an associated angiitis of the gastrointestinal tract. Irradiation of abdomen leads to vascular necrosis and thrombosis, which in turn may cause ischaemic ulceration that on healing leaves a fibrosed intima and a poorly perfused segment of intestine.

MISCELLANEOUS LESIONS

Many other conditions occasionally cause frank intestinal ischaemia. For example, blood vessels may be compressed by retroperitoneal haematomas from leaking aneurysms and following trauma, by neoplastic infiltration, and rarely by proliferating fibrous tissue such as occurs in retroperitoneal fibrosis and very rarely around carcinoid tumours.

The wall of mesenteric arteries may be involved in fibroelastic hyperplasia and in Takayasu's disease. In malignant hypertension, intimal hyperplasia and fibrinoid necrosis of arteriolar walls may lead to patchy ischaemia of the intestines.

Damage to the arterial wall in the splanchnic circulation may also occur a few days after surgical correction of coarctation of the aorta. There is necrotizing arteritis with fibrinoid necrosis, most marked at arterial bifurcations, and similar changes may be seen in the small vessels of the liver, kidney, and spleen. These changes, which appear to be related to the sudden sustained increase in blood pressure, usually resolve spontaneously but occasionally may lead to intestinal infarction requiring operative intervention.

Diffuse microthrombosis

This may occur as a result of disseminated intravascular coagulation (as in the Schwartzman reaction). The haemolytic–uraemic syndrome and thrombotic thrombocytopenic purpura appear to be related conditions in which platelet aggregation occurs in small vessels (see Sections 20 and 22). Renal failure often dominates the clinical picture but in most patients there is evidence of widespread involvement of the intestine and related organs. A plasma factor that stimulates the production of

Table 2 *Vasculitides that may affect the gut*

Involving vessels of all sizes
Polyartertis nodosa
(Churg–Strauss disease)
Giant-cell arteritis
Takayasu's arteritis
Transplant rejection

Involving predominantly medium and small vessels
Wegener's granulomatosis
Kawasaki disease
Buerger's disease
Vasculitis of collagen–vascular disorders*:
   Rheumatoid disease
   Systemic lupus erythematosus
   Progressive systemic sclerosis
   Dermatomyositis

Involving predominantly small vessels
Hypersensitivity angiitis (microscopic polyarteritis)
Henoch–Schönlein purpura
Serum sickness
Infective angiitis (e.g. typhoid, tuberculosis)

*The vasculitides of these disorders often involve only small vessels and the histological features may be indistinguishable from hypersensitivity angiitis. However, significant gastrointestinal pathology rarely occurs without the involvement of medium-sized vessels.

Table 3 *Intestinal infarction without vascular occlusion*

Neonatal
Necrotizing enterocolitis

Haemorrhagic enteritis or colitis
Bacterial toxins (e.g. *E.coli* 0157:H7; *Clostridium perfringens*)

Focal ulceration
Stress ulcers (especially stomach and duodenum)
Drug-induced ulcers (e.g. potassium, NSAID)
Radiation enteritis
Uraemic ulceration (especially in colon)

After prolonged period of poor perfusion
Low-output cardiac failure (? digitalis predisposed)
Hyperviscosity syndromes
Polycythaemia and haemoconcentration

NSAID, non-steroidal anti-inflammatory drug.

prostacyclin from the endothelial cells, thereby inhibiting the aggregation of platelets, appears to be reduced or absent in many patients with these rare disorders. Infusions of plasma often lead to a good therapeutic response.

Non-occlusive intestinal infarction (Table 3)

Sporadic and epidemic cases of necrotizing enteritis presumably due to ischaemia have been described from many parts of the world and in all age groups, from premature neonates to the very elderly. Neonatal necrotizing enterocolitis may occur in the first week of life of premature and low birth-weight infants. It follows an episode of splanchnic underperfusion after the establishment of oral feeding, which encourages the proliferation of normal gastrointestinal bacteria. Breast milk appears to be protective, possibly by providing passive enteric immunity; artificial hyperosmolar feeds may promote damage. Lesions occur most frequently in the stomach, the distal ileum, and the colon; as mucosal integrity disintegrates, bacterial invasion enhances the damage. The condition may also occur in normal birth-weight infants with a hyperviscosity syndrome or who have been exposed to cocaine *in utero*.

In adults, infarction of the gastrointestinal tract without vascular occlusion is seen mainly in the elderly with severe, low-output cardiac failure and occasionally in the severely shocked. In tropical and sub-tropical areas the condition occurs at any age and may be related to environmental factors including diet, infection, and infestation.

Pathogenetic mechanisms

Experimentally, morphological damage of the mucosa can be demonstrated 1 h after the complete cessation of blood flow to the colon. After 3 h the structure of the microcirculation breaks down and coagulative necrosis develops. During reperfusion, damage appears to be enhanced by the generation of reactive oxygen metabolites (including superoxide, hydrogen peroxide, and hydroxyl radicals). These alter the vascular permeability of endothelial cells and damage epithelial cells by the peroxidation of cell membranes. The reactive oxygen metabolites are strongly chemotactic for neutrophils and this leads to an acute inflammatory response. The hallmark of ischaemic bowel pathology is extensive coagulative necrosis, which commences in the mucosa and then spreads to deeper layers. The muscularis propria and the serosal surface are not involved until the process is well established. The appearences are similar in both occlusive and non-occlusive forms of ischaemia.

Although the appearances of the gut are similar in non-occlusive pathology, the mechanisms are less well defined. In most cases, micro-vascular occlusion cannot be demonstrated in the affected segments of gut. There is diffuse haemorrhage into the mucosa and submucosa with coagulative necrosis. Pseudomembranes may form in the absence of specific pathogenic organisms and may represent an acute inflammatory response mediated by reactive oxygen metabolites.

Non-occlusive focal ischaemia appears to underlie the pathogenesis of uraemic colitis, radiation enteritis, potassium-induced ulcers, and multiple stress ulcers of the upper gastrointestinal tract. The verotoxin of *Escherichia coli* 0157:H7, which causes haemorrhagic colitis, is another aetiological agent. This is a particularly potent cause of disseminated intravascular coagulation, which may occur as a result of the absorption of bacterial endotoxin and thromboplastins from damaged tissues. It is associated with the development of the haemolytic–uraemic syndrome in children and more rarely with thrombotic thrombocytopenic purpura in adults.

Clinical syndromes

The clinical effects of mesenteric vascular insufficiency are becoming more clearly recognized. Four major syndromes have emerged in medical literature (unfortunately under a variety of titles): (i) acute intestinal ischaemia (affecting much of the intestine); (ii) chronic intestinal ischaemia; (iii) focal ischaemia of the intestine; and (iv) ischaemic colitis.

ACUTE INTESTINAL ISCHAEMIA

Acute intestinal ischaemia is primarily a condition of older people with degenerative cardiovascular disease. Occasionally it may cause an acute abdomen in the newborn infant. It correlates with necrosis, threatened or complete, of that part of the gut supplied by the superior mesenteric artery.

Clinical features

The onset of the condition is usually abrupt but may be insidious. Abdominal pain is the key symptom and at the onset is generally colicky in nature and poorly localized. As the condition progresses the pain becomes constant and unremitting. Initially it is felt in the right iliac fossa and then spreads over the entire abdomen. Diarrhoea is usual and frequently the motions contain blood. Vomiting occurs in some cases but haematemesis is rare. In the early stages of illness the distress of the patient is out of all proportion to the physical signs. There may be slight tenderness in the right iliac fossa and some exaggeration of bowel sounds. As the condition develops over the course of hours (or at the

most a day or two) the abdomen becomes distended and silent with increasing tenderness and a positive rebound sign. At the same time there are usually signs of peripheral circulatory failure. The patient is pale, anxious, sweating, and tachypnoeic. Later the blood pressure falls, the patient becomes cyanosed and anuric. At this stage, intestinal necrosis has almost certainly gone beyond the point of recovery.

The diagnosis may be suspected on the basis of clinical correlations but is often difficult and delayed. Experimentally, the CK-BB isoenzyme is released into the circulation 3 to 9 h after intestinal infarction and in clinical practice may provide a useful pointer to diagnosis. Unfortunately this laboratory test is not sufficiently sensitive to exclude the condition. Duplex Doppler ultrasonography and magnetic resonance imaging may be useful in specialist units. But, for practical purposes, diagnosis still depends on the efficiency with which other causes of an apparent abdominal catastrophe can be excluded. Needling the peritoneal cavity may be a helpful procedure: with intestinal infarction it usually produces bloodstained fluid. Plain radiographs of the abdomen may show non-specific dilatation of loops of intestine with multiple fluid levels. The presence of gas bubbles in the portal vein is diagnostic of intestinal necrosis at a stage when the patient is beyond recovery. The place of aortography is not yet clearly defined.

Management

In the management of this condition the clinician has to combat the effects of (i) loss of water, electrolytes and protein leading to hypovolaemia and impaired tissue perfusion; (ii) bacterial invasion; and (iii) disseminated intravascular coagulation. The value of pharmacological agents (such as phenoxybenzamine, glucagon, or dopamine) to improve the mesenteric circulation remains uncertain. Similarly there is no clear evidence of the benefit of large doses of corticosteroids.

As soon as the patient is sufficiently fit, laparotomy must be done. If a large vessel is occluded, the surgeon may be able to undertake embolectomy or reconstruct an occluded artery. In both occlusive and non-occlusive vascular disease it is necessary to decide how much intestine to resect. If there is doubt about the viability of the residual intestine the abdomen may be closed and, 24 h later, re-explored. Infiltrating the coeliac and mesenteric plexuses with local anaesthetic may help relieve vascular spasm.

Many patients with acute intestinal ischaemia causing necrosis die. Those who do recover may present major problems in the management of their nutrition.

CHRONIC INTESTINAL ISCHAEMIA

All too often, warning symptoms of impending mesenteric vascular occlusion go unnoticed or undiagnosed. The prodromal period is usually short but the history of rather characteristic abdominal pain occurring shortly after eating may raise the possibility of chronic intestinal ischaemia. Unfortunately, in the absence of any definitive test to show functionally significant intestinal ischaemia, the diagnosis often remains uncertain. Artheroma of the visceral arteries commonly involves the coeliac axis and superior mesenteric artery. The inferior mesenteric artery is affected to a much lesser extent. Stenotic lesions occur at the aortic origins of the vessels. Diffuse, severe atheroma throughout the intestinal arterial tree is uncommon and therefore arterial reconstruction may be very rewarding.

Clinical features

Classically the patient suffers cramping abdominal pain 20 to 60 min after eating. This may be relieved by simple analgesics or by vasodilator drugs. As the condition progresses the patient becomes afraid to eat and loses weight.

The finding of a loud systolic bruit on auscultation of the abdomen is a doubtfully valid physical sign. Bruits may be detected in normal subjects, young as well as old, and may be absent in patients with severe visceral arterial disease.

In practice the diagnosis is made by excluding other conditions and correlating clinical symptoms with angiographic findings. The descriptions of methods of correcting of arterial abnormalities leave one more impressed by the degree of surgical enthusiasm and operative ingenuity than by the standard of care in evaluating the results.

Coeliac-axis compression

In occasional patients with chronic abdominal pain and an abdominal bruit (which may be exacerbated by inspiration), aortography shows apparent constriction of the coeliac axis by the median arcuate ligament. It has been claimed that the arteries in the territory of the coeliac axis 'steal' blood from that of the superior mesenteric artery, thereby causing intestinal angina that may be relieved by dividing the median arcuate ligament and possibly by reconstructing the coeliac axis.

Unfortunately, symptomless compression of the compression coeliac axis has been demonstrated frequently and some symptomatic patients are not helped by operation. Although patients claim to have been cured by surgery to the coeliac axis, the validity of the syndrome remains uncertain.

FOCAL ISCHAEMIA OF THE SMALL INTESTINE

Ischaemia of a segment of small intestine may cause local ulceration that on healing leads to stenosis. This may occur as a result of any of the vascular disorders already described as causing acute, diffuse, intestinal ischaemia, whether these be thrombotic, embolic or non-occlusive.

More specific entities include ischaemic damage by a strangulated hernia, by an episode of blunt trauma to the abdomen, by irradiation, and rarely by localized vasculitis secondary to infective disease (e.g. typhoid or leprosy) or collagen–vascular disorders (e.g. polyarteritis).

Drug-induced ulceration is an important entity, of which that associated with the ingestion of potassium salts is the most clearly defined. It has been shown that a high concentration of potassium in the lumen of the intestine causes venous spasm and subsequently local arterial thrombosis. This may lead to ulceration and fibrosis of a segment of intestine especially if there is pre-existing large-vessel disease.

Clinical features

The patient presents with features of subacute obstruction of the small intestine. Colicky abdominal pain occurs 2 to 3 h after meals, associated with nausea, abdominal distension, and occasional vomiting. The stricture is located by radiological examination of the small intestine and the obstruction needs to be relieved by operation.

ISCHAEMIC COLITIS

The colon has distinctive features that make it more prone to ischaemic damage than the small intestine. The transverse and descending segments of the colon are supplied by marginal branches of the middle colic (superior mesenteric territory) and left colic (inferior mesenteric territory) arteries. An arterial and lymphatic watershed exists close to the splenic flexure, which is supported to a variable extent by an additional vascular arcade. A deficient marginal artery or an absent anastomotic arcade may imperil the blood supply of the splenic flexure in occlusive disease of either mesenteric artery.

If the blood supply fails, damage to the large intestine may be more rapid and more severe than that occurring in the small intestine because of the effects of the high concentration of bacteria in the faecal stream.

Again, blood flow to the colon may be impaired by any of the mechanisms described previously. In addition, colonic obstruction may reduce blood flow by increasing the intraluminal pressure. Thus the pathological changes of ischaemic colitis may occur in the segment of intestine immediately proximal to an obstructing carcinoma (stercoral ulceration) or in association with prolapse or volvulus of the colon.

Venous occlusion is also a possible cause of ischaemic colitis. Inevitably the contraceptive pill has been incriminated as a cause but the condition has been described in young men as well as young women. The evidence regarding the pill remains suggestive rather than conclusive.

Clinical features

In the acute phase of ischaemic colitis the clinician has to differentiate between mild disease, which responds quickly and effectively to supportive measures and treatment with appropriate antibiotics, and severe disease in which gangrene may develop. Most patients are between the ages of 50 and 70 years and often have a background history of atheromatous arterial disease, collagen disorder, or local colonic pathology. Typically the affected person complains of pain in the left iliac fossa, nausea, and vomiting followed by the passage of a loose motion containing dark blood.

Marked tenderness in the left iliac fossa is the most constant physical sign. At colonoscopy the mucosa may be blue and swollen without contact bleeding. The rectum is invariably spared. Plain radiographs of the abdomen may show an abnormal segment of large intestine outlined with gas. Angiography is only occasionally helpful in showing occlusive arterial disease.

Contrast enema examination of the colon is a most useful way of demonstrating ischaemic damage. In the early phase, 'thumb printing' is the characteristic sign, which may persist for several days (Fig. 1). Subsequently the mucosal appearances may return to normal or progress to the next phase of mucosal ulceration, giving an appearance that may be indistinguishable from segmental ulcerative colitis or Crohn's disease, although the haustral pattern is usually not seriously disrupted and the ulcers are patchy and do not penetrate deeply.

Again, these changes may resolve spontaneously or progress to tubular narrowing of the intestine with or without sacculation on the antimesenteric border.

Ischaemic colitis may be confused with dysenteric conditions, acute diverticular disease of the colon, acute inflammatory bowel disease, perforation of a hollow viscus, or left-sided peritonitis secondary to pancreatitis. The most important distinguishing features are the characteristic age range, the association with degenerative cardiovascular disease, and the distinctive, although not pathognomonic, radiographic and colonoscopic appearances.

Fig. 1 Ischaemic colitis: barium enema showing thumb-printing at the splenic flexure. (By courtesy of Dr A. Freeman, Addenbrooke's Hospital.)

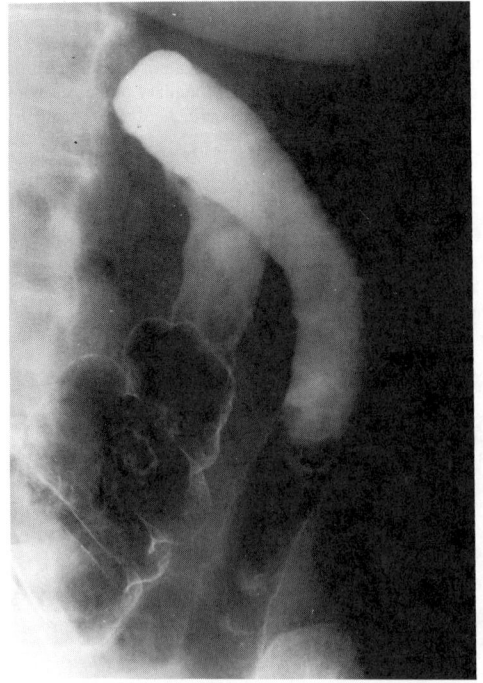

Management

On establishing the diagnosis of ischaemic colitis the treatment is initially expectant. The patient should be given intravenous fluid as necessary, together with systemic broad-spectrum antibiotics (on the basis of experimental rather than clinical evidence).

Well over 90 per cent of recognized cases resolve spontaneously. A stricture may develop in up to a third of patients but this is usually asymptomatic and only rarely needs to be resected.

Surgery is indicated if there is evidence of peritonitis, persistent bleeding, or of an underlying colonic disorder (such as carcinoma).

Non-inflammatory vascular disorders that may affect the gut

ANEURYSMS OF THE AORTA AND ITS MAJOR BRANCHES (SEE SECTION 15)

Rarely, aneurysms fistulate into the stomach or duodenum. This usually causes catastrophic bleeding and rapid death. Even more rarely there is intermittent bleeding (for example from the splenic artery into the stomach), which may be difficult to diagnose.

Fig. 2 Angiodysplastic lesion in the caecum, photographed through a colonoscope. (By courtesy of Dr R. Hunt, RN Hospital, Haslar.)

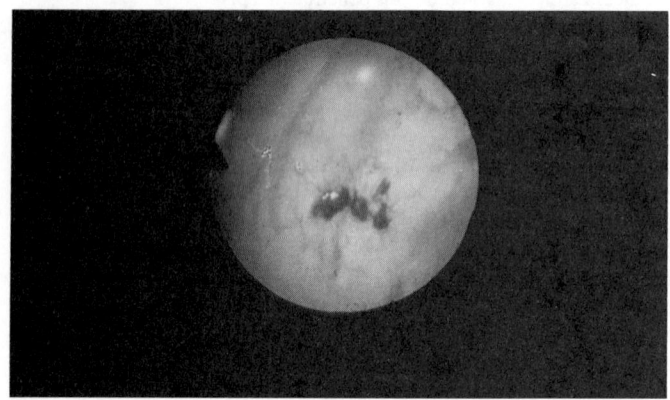

SUPERIOR MESENTERIC ARTERY SYNDROME

A syndrome of postprandial epigastric pain, distension, and vomiting may occur in asthenic young people, especially those who have lost weight or who are fixed in a position of hyperextension after spinal injury. Barium studies show a distended proximal duodenum with a sharp cut-off at the line where the superior mesenteric artery crosses the duodenum. Symptoms may be relieved if the patient adopts the prone position after meals and may disappear as the patient gains weight. Occasionally surgery is necessary. The condition must be distinguished from duodenal ileus caused by mesenteric bands, a condition that is associated with partial malrotation of the midgut.

HAEMANGIOMA

Haemangiomas are uncommon lesions of the gut that may cause painless bleeding, especially from the jejunum.

INTESTINAL TELANGIECTASIA

These lesions occur most commonly with Osler–Weber–Rendu disease (see Section 22) and may lead to microscopic bleeding with anaemia, especially in adult life.

VASCULAR DYSPLASIA

This is a more recently recognized and not uncommon disorder causing occult bleeding from the gut in older subjects. The lesions occur as small arteriovenous malformations or as foci of ectatic capillaries or veins with little supporting stroma; they are found predominantly in the caecum and ascending colon. There may be an association with aortic stenosis but none with cutaneous telangiectases and no familial aggregations are yet described.

Patients give a history of recurrent anaemia or episodes of bleeding from the gut; usually have been investigated repeatedly without getting a firm diagnosis; and sometimes have had one or more operations, including resection of a segment of the gastrointestinal tract, without relief of symptoms. The diagnosis of vascular dysplasia should be considered in all cases of obscure gastrointestinal haemorrhage and may be made by direct visualization of the intestinal mucosa (Fig. 2) or by selective mesenteric arteriography (Fig. 3). The lesions may be multiple,

Fig. 3 Angiodysplastic lesion in the caecum: superior mesenteric angiogram in a 53-year-old man with anaemia for 20 years (no lesion found at previous operations). (a) Vascular lake in caecum (arrowed). (b) Capillary phase, showing early-filling vein arising from lesion. (c) Injected specimen magnified ×30). (By courtesy of Dr D. J. Allison, Royal Postgraduate Medical School and reprinted with permission of the Editor of the *British Journal of Medicine*.)

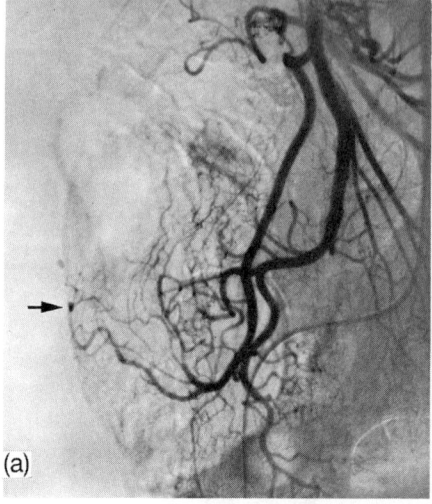
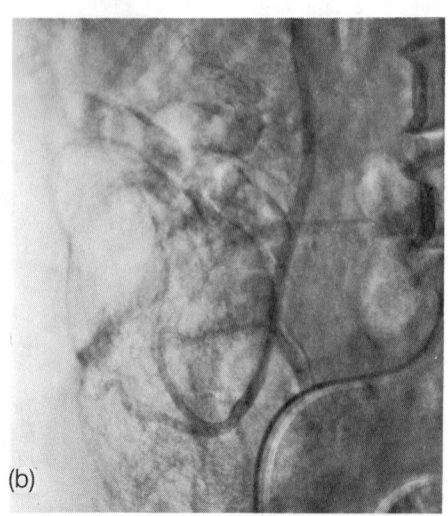
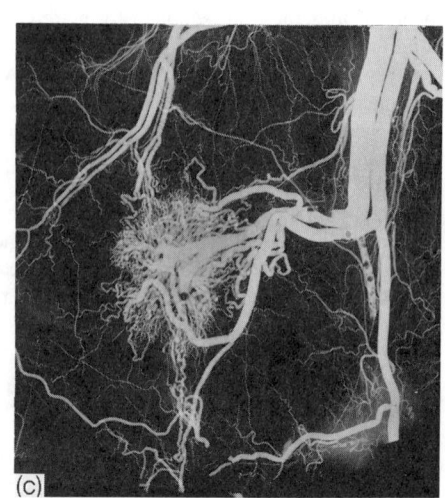

in which case resection of the affected segment of gut may be necessary. Many patients, however, can be treated successfully by fulguration of the lesion through an endoscope.

INTRAMURAL BLEEDING

Bleeding into the wall of the bowel may occur as a result of treatment with anticoagulants or from the inflammation of small vessels (as occurs classically in Henoch–Schönlein purpura). The usual presentation is with colicky abdominal pain, with bleeding into the lumen of the gut. Appropriate barium examination may show the classical sign of 'thumb printing'. The condition usually resolves spontaneously providing the underlying disorder can be treated. A blood transfusion may be needed.

Vasculitis and the collagen disorders

The gut may be involved in any of the systemic collagen and inflammatory vascular disorders. Vasculitis may cause focal ischaemic damage of the intestine and any of the syndromes described previously. In addition the visceral muscle may be damaged and the resulting dysmotility may cause dysphagia, delayed gastric emptying, small-intestinal stasis with bacterial overgrowth, or colonic inertia. Gas may infiltrate the tissues, giving rise to pneumatosis intestinalis.

The specific pathological diagnosis is usually based on the systemic features of the illness and the laboratory findings rather than on the mostly non-specific abdominal complications. But the inquisitive physician may also recognize curious associations in patients with multisystem disorders. Thus, intestinal malabsorption and protein-losing enteropathy have been described in association with systemic lupus erythematosus and rheumatoid arthritis, pancreatic insufficiency with systemic sclerosis, acute pancreatitis during the course of Behçet's disease, and apparently classical inflammatory bowel disease with systemic lupus erythematosus.

Thus, it is difficult to provide clear-cut clinical descriptions of typical disorders of the gut in this group of conditions.

SYSTEMIC SCLEROSIS

Pathology

In primary systemic sclerosis (see Chapter 18.11.4), fibrous connective tissue proliferates. In the gastrointestinal tract it may replace smooth muscle, especially in the oesophagus (involved in 80 per cent of cases), to a lesser extent in the small intestine (although duodenal involvement is quite common), and rather rarely in the colon.

Overt vasculitis is a less common feature but occasionally causes intestinal infarction. Pneumatosis cystoides intestinalis is also described, especially in association with intestinal pseudo-obstruction or pneumoperitoneum.

Symptoms

Difficulty in eating may be caused by induration of the gums, by restriction of the size of the oral cavity as a result of subcutaneous fibrosis, and in advanced cases by impaired sensation because of atrophy of the buccal mucosa and taste buds.

Progressive dysphagia is the most frequent gastrointestinal symptom in systemic sclerosis. Initially there is a decrease in the incidence and amplitude of contractions of the lower oesophagus and incomplete relaxation of the lower oesophageal sphincter. In addition, the resting tone of the sphincter is reduced, allowing reflux of gastric juices, oesophagitis, shortening of the oesophagus, and occasionally stricture formation. Associated hiatal herniation is common.

More rarely the stomach is involved, causing delayed emptying that on occasion is exacerbated by associated stenosis of the pyloric canal. Changes lower down the gastrointestinal tract are readily found when looked for. Characteristically the duodenum is dilated, the valvulae of the small intestine are thickened, and pseudodiverticula may form. These changes may give rise to abdominal discomfort, distension, and borborygmi, especially after the taking of meals. The impaired motility of the small intestine leads to stasis of its contents and bacterial overgrowth causing malabsorption, especially of fat and vitamin B_{12} (see Chapter 14.9.2). Occasionally this is sufficiently severe to cause acute or chronic pseudo-obstruction with persistent abdominal distension and vomiting (Fig. 4).

Colonic involvement is rare. Clinically, there is progressive constipation, sometimes going on to a large-bowel obstruction secondary to impaction of faeces. Radiologically there is a loss of the normal haustral pattern, the development of wide-necked pseudodiverticula on the antimesenteric border of the transverse and descending colon, and generalized dilatation of the lumen. If the internal sphincter (smooth muscle) of the rectum is involved, an already troublesome tendency to constipation will be exacerbated. A significant reduction of intestinal secretions (gastric, biliary, and pancreatic) appears to occur in perhaps one-third of patients with primary systemic sclerosis but this is rarely, if ever, severe enough to cause malabsorption.

Management

There is no specific treatment of primary systemic sclerosis. Lesions in the gastrointestinal tract need management on their merits. It is important to recognize early the patient with gastro-oesophageal reflux. A proton-pump inhibitor should be given to prevent the ravages of acid-peptic digestion of the oesophageal mucosa. Repeated oesophagoscopy is the best way of documenting the progress of pathology, and when strictures occur these should be dilated by bouginage. If a stricture becomes fixed and unyielding, surgical intervention may be necessary.

A breath test (see Chapter 14.9.2) is a useful screening test for delayed passage of contents and bacterial proliferation in the small intestine. Patients with a positive breath test should be assessed for evidence of malabsorption and if this is found, intermittent therapy with antibiotics for an indefinite period may be of clinical value.

Patients with severe colonic disease are often difficult to manage. Efforts should be made to avoid the development of severe constipation. A combination of a high-roughage diet and aperients as necessary is usually sufficient but occasionally it may be necessary to resort to the repeated use of enemas.

SYSTEMIC LUPUS ERYTHEMATOSUS

Systemic lupus erythematosus (**SLE**) (see Chapter 18.11.3) may cause abdominal symptoms arising from any part of the gastrointestinal tract,

Fig. 4 Systemic sclerosis. Typical 'sacculation' appearance of the bowel.

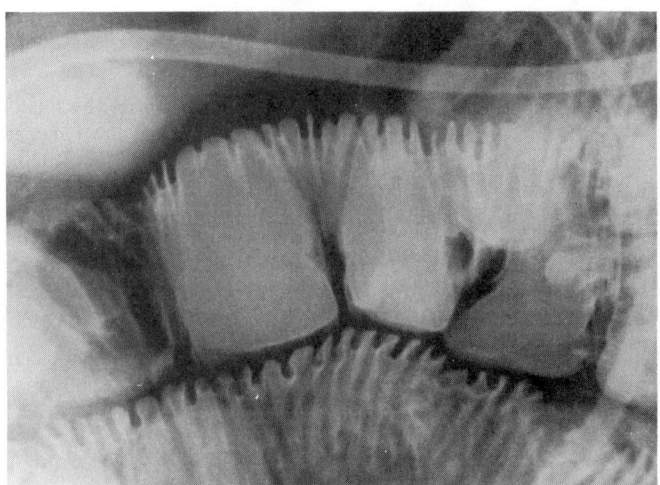

although these symptoms are rarely part of the presenting picture. Anorexia, weight loss, nausea, vomiting, and diarrhoea are relatively common. Dysphagia, abdominal pain, distension due to ascites, and gastrointestinal bleeding are less frequent symptoms. Occasionally, a patient with SLE develops an acute abdomen, which may be due to localized or widespread lupus vasculitis causing ischaemic damage to the gut or its related organs, including the gallbladder and pancreas. Arteriography may be helpful in diagnosis by revealing diffuse irregularities in the branches of mesenteric vessels.

Treatment

Treatment with oral corticosteroids usually relieves minor abdominal symptoms and will lead to rapid resolution of simple ascites. In the acute stage of the disease, however, surgery may be necessary to deal with infarcted intestine, serious bleeding, or intestinal obstruction.

RHEUMATOID ARTHRITIS

Vasculitis secondary to rheumatoid arthritis is associated with long-standing disease, seropositivity, and florid subcutaneous nodule formation (see Chapter 18.4). It may affect small arteries, arterioles, capillaries, and venules, and often causes little in the way of symptoms. Occasionally, a severe diffuse and necrotizing angiitis causes infarction in the gallbladder, pancreas, or intestine. Symptoms vary from vague abdominal pain, with or without diarrhoea, to the development of an acute abdomen. Malnutrition is present in many such patients and for the most part is due to decreased intake of nutrients rather than malabsorption, although this has been described in association with rheumatoid arthritis.

DERMATOMYOSITIS

This inflammatory disease (see Sections 18 and 23) of muscle and skin rarely causes damage to the viscera. Thrombosis of small vessels occasionally causes gastrointestinal ulceration.

BEHÇET'S SYNDROME

The triad of relapsing iritis, painful ulcers of the mouth, and genital ulceration is only part of the syndrome of this multisystem disorder (see Chapter 18.11.8). Again, vasculitis appears to be the underlying histopathological lesion. In the gastrointestinal tract this may lead to ulceration of colon, malabsorption (sometimes with lymphangiectasia), and pancreatitis.

Primary vasculitis

HENOCH–SCHÖNLEIN SYNDROME OR ANAPHYLACTOID PURPURA

This is a self-limiting disorder of unknown cause characterized by small-vessel vasculitis (see Chapter 18.11.2). Gastrointestinal involvement occurs in at least two-thirds of cases and is manifest as abdominal pain and gastrointestinal bleeding. Intramural haematomas are common and rarely may be complicated by intussusception, perforation, or an infarcted segment of gut.

POLYARTERITIS NODOSA

Abdominal pain and other gastrointestinal symptoms are common in patients with polyarteritis nodosa. The underlying cause is usually rec-

ognized by evidence of systemic disease such as skin lesions, renal involvement, hypertension, and eosinophilia. Mesenteric angiography is useful as a diagnostic tool because up to two-thirds of cases have recognizable aneurysms of mesenteric and renal vessels. A small proportion of patients with polyarteritis have acute abdominal episodes including ulceration, haemorrhage, perforation and segmental necrosis of intestine, cholecystitis, pancreatitis, and hepatic infarction. Kohlmeier–Degos syndrome is a variant of polyarteritis characterized by a papular skin eruption and occlusive lesions of small arteries.

Kawasaki disease (infantile acute febrile mucocutaneous lymph-node syndrome) (see Chapter 18.11.9) proceeds to a disorder indistinguishable histopathologically from infantile periarteritis nodosa. Cardiac involvement is most common but the gastrointestinal tract is affected in up to a third of cases.

ANCA-POSITIVE VASCULITIDES

Wegener's granulomatosis, Churg–Strauss syndrome, and microscopic polyarteritis (see Section 18.11) are conditions frequently associated with the finding of antineutrophilic cytoplasmic antibodies (ANCA). Gastrointestinal symptoms are common in these conditions, although the intra-abdominal pathology has not been well characterized except when it has led to a life-threatening condition such as visceral perforation or infarction.

Giant-cell arteritis

This characteristically affects the larger cranial arteries including the ciliary and central retinal arteries (see Chapter 18.11.7) and rarely limb arteries. Very occasionally a similar pathology affects mesenteric arteries and causes bowel infarction.

Localized arteritis

This has been described affecting appendix, gallbladder, and pancreas. Its relation to systemic polyarteritis is uncertain. Similarly, localized leucocytoclastic (hypersensitivity) vasculitis has been described in the abdominal cavities.

REFERENCES

Bisceglia, M., Germani, G., Tardu, B., Di Mattia, A., and Li Bergoli, M. (1989). Leucocytoclastic vasculitis of the colon. *Italian Journal of Surgical Science*, **19**, 269.

Hunder, G.G. (ed.) (1992). Vasculitic syndromes. *Current Opinion in Rheumatology*, **44**, 1–55.

Ito, M., Sano, K., Inaba, H., and Hotchi, M. (1991). Localised necrotising arteritis. *Archives of Pathology and Laboratory Medicine*, **115**, 780.

Jamieson, C.W. (1986). Coeliac axis compression syndrome. *British Medical Journal*, **293**, 159.

Krant, J.D. and Ross, J.M. (1992). Extracranial giant cell arteritis restricted to the small bowel. *Arthritis and Rheumatism*, **35**, 603.

Marston, A. (1986). *Vascular disease of the gut*. Arnold, London.

Miyake, T., Kawamori, J., Yoshida, T., Nakano, H., Kohno, S., and Ohba, S. (1987). Small bowel pseudo-obstruction in Kawasaki disease. *Paediatric Radiology*, **17**, 383.

Musemeche, C.A., Kosloske, A.M., Barton, S.A., and Umland, E.T. (1986). Comparative effects ischaemia, bacteria and substrate in the pathogenesis of intestinal necrosis. *Journal of Pediatric Surgery*, **21**, 536.

Norris, H.T. (1991). Re-examination of the spectrum of ischaemic bowel disease. In *Pathology of the colon, small intestine and anus. Contemporary issues in surgical pathology*, Vol. 17, (ed. L.M. Roth). Churchill Livingstone, New York.

Toskes. (1991). Hope for the treatment of intestinal scleroderma. *New England Journal of Medicine*, **325**, 1058.

14.18 Gastrointestinal infections

C. P. CONLON

Introduction

Infections of the gastrointestinal tract produce a variety of symptoms and can be due to a large number of different infective agents. The most common symptom is diarrhoea, which leads to considerable morbidity and mortality worldwide, particularly among children in developing countries. In the tropics, diarrhoea in childhood is intimately linked with malnutrition. Recurrent bouts of gastroenteritis lead to nutritional deficiencies, while malnutrition may increase susceptibility to further infections; the cycle ultimately results in significant mortality. In developed countries, acute gastroenteritis is still common and, although mortality is low compared to the tropics, there is significant morbidity and many days of work lost.

The types and severity of gastrointestinal infections are determined by a variety of epidemiological factors. Different age groups will have different risks, with the extremes of age being the most vulnerable. Underlying medical conditions, such as immunosuppressive diseases, may influence the response to infections. Overcrowding and poor sanitation predispose to epidemics of gastrointestinal infection. Certain organisms, such as *Entamoeba histolytica*, are much more common in the tropics than in temperate zones. Most enteric infections in the tropics occur in the summer months, whereas in temperate regions, winter is the time of peak prevalence.

The organisms that cause the different gastrointestinal infections are considered in detail in Section 7. Here, the spectrum of different gastrointestinal disorders due to infection is summarized.

Pathophysiology

HOST FACTORS

The response to potential enteric pathogens depends on a variety of non-specific and specific host defences.

Gastric acid

Food and drinks are rarely sterile, but the low pH in the stomach (pH < 4) kills most ingested bacteria within minutes, so that enteric infection is prevented. However, achlorhydria or drugs, such as antacids or H_2-antagonists, that inhibit gastric acid secretion may allow survival and multiplication of ingested organisms. In these circumstances, only a small inoculum may be required to cause disease.

Intestinal motility

Normal gut motility ensures a regular distribution and flow of normal gut flora, as well as optimizing the adequate absorption of fluid from the bowel contents. Bowel stasis may lead to bacterial overgrowth and a malabsorption syndrome. Antimotility drugs, such as diphenoxylate hydrochloride, may lead to prolonged carriage of pathogens and may increase the risk of bacterial invasion.

Normal bowel flora

There are about 10^{11} organisms per gram of faeces, and of the 300 to 400 difference species identified as normal commensals, more than 99 per cent are anaerobes. The bacteria in the normal flora may physically prevent potential pathogens from adhering to enterocytes—so-called colonization resistance. We know that the administration of broad-spec-

Table 1 *Inocula of organisms required to produce symptoms*

Pathogen	No. of organisms
Shigella	10^{1-2}
Salmonella	10^5
Campylobacter	10^{2-6}
V. cholerae	10^8
Giardia	10^{1-2}
Entamoeba histolytica	10^{1-2}

trum antibiotics may disrupt the usual protective effect of the bowel flora, reducing the size of inoculum of pathogens needed to cause disease.

Intestinal immunity (see Chapter 14.4)

The gut is the largest lymphoid organ in the body. Gut-associated lymphoid tissue comprises cells in the lamina propria, lymphoid nodules (particularly Peyer's patches in the distal small bowel), and intraepithelial lymphocytes. In Peyer's patches, B and T lymphocytes are present in discrete areas. These cells traffic to mesenteric nodes and the thoracic duct with some primed cells 'homing' back to the lamina propria as IgA-producing plasma cells. Plasma cells are confined to the lamina propria and are the main cells there. Of the specific antibody in the gut, IgA predominates. It is produced locally and is mainly secretory (dimeric) IgA. Secretory IgA is resistant to proteolysis and blocks bacterial adhesion to enterocytes. It may well be able to lyse bacteria in the presence of complement. Although some of the other immunoglobin classes are made in small amounts in the gut, most IgG and IgM probably comes from leakage of serum immunoglobins. In addition, neonatal immunity may be acquired from colostrum, which contains specific antibody and non-specific agents such as lactoferrin.

MICROBIAL FACTORS

There are wide variations in the numbers of organisms that need to be ingested in order to cause disease (Table 1). Smaller inocula may be sufficient in certain circumstances, such as achlorhydria or immunosuppression. The key factors in microbial pathogenesis in the gut are the elaboration of toxins, the ability to adhere to intestinal mucosa, and the ability to invade enterocytes.

Toxins

The ability of enteric organisms to elaborate pathogenic toxins was first shown by using cell-free filtrates from bacterial cultures to produce changes in gastrointestinal structure and function. There are three categories of toxins produced: neurotoxins, enterotoxins, and cytotoxins.

Neurotoxins such as botulinum toxin are usually ingested as preformed toxins and some, like those produced by *Staphylococcus aureus* or *Bacillus cereus*, cause enteric symptoms, particularly vomiting, by acting on central pathways. Enterotoxins act directly on cells in the gut, resulting in excessive secretion of fluid into the lumen. The best known example of this is cholera toxin (see Chapter 7.11.11). The B subunits of the toxin bind to monoganglioside GM_1 on the enterocyte brush-border membrane and the A subunit then enters the cells, activating adenyl cyclase. This leads to a rise in intracellular AMP, inhibition of sodium/chlorine-linked absorption, and a net flow of chlorine ions and water into the lumen. Other organisms such as *Staph. aureus* and *Escherichia coli* produce pathogenic enterotoxins. Cytotoxins lead directly to mucosal damage, often causing acute inflammatory changes in the bowel wall. Examples of these cytotoxins are produced by organisms such as *Shigella dysenteriae*, *Clostridium perfringens*, and enterohaemorrhagic *E. coli* (**EHEC**).

Adherence

Even though bacteria may produce toxins, they often cannot cause disease unless they can attach themselves to mucosal cells. Attachment takes place via various adhesins, or fimbriae. Different types of fimbriae may be encoded by plasmids, which can be transferable. Parasites may have specially adapted means of adhesion, such as the suction plates of *Giardia lamblia* or the sucker and hooklets on the scolex of *Taenia solium*.

Invasiveness

Some organisms retain the ability to invade and destroy intestinal epithelial cells. Invasiveness may be associated with certain antigens in the lipopolysaccharide cell wall (e.g. Shigella) and may be encoded in plasmids. It is likely that the production of cytotoxins aids the invasive process.

Other factors associated with virulence

Although the mechanisms outlined above are clearly important, other factors are probably also involved. The motility of some organisms, such as *Vibrio cholerae*, may aid colonization of the mucosa. *Salmonella typhi* appears to depend on the presence of a Vi antigen as well as on other specific virulence antigens associated with the lipopolysaccharide cell wall. Some viruses, for example rotavirus, can selectively destroy cells at the tip of intestinal villi, which are most concerned with absorption, while leaving relatively unscathed the secretory cells in the villus crypts. This leads to a secretory diarrhoea.

Clinical syndromes of gastrointestinal infection

Gastrointestinal infection, although caused by many different pathogens, usually results in one of three clinical syndromes:

Non-inflammatory diarrhoea Usually caused by viruses or bacterial enterotoxins affecting the proximal small bowel and leading to a secretory diarrhoea.

Inflammatory diarrhoea Predominantly affecting the colon, there may be bacterial invasion of the mucosa. Cytotoxins are often involved and the inflammation may lead to blood and pus in the diarrhoea.

Systemic infections Organisms may penetrate the distal small bowel leading to local problems and, in addition, produce systemic symptoms due to tissue invasion and bacteraemia.

NON-INFLAMMATORY DIARRHOEA

Infections in the proximal small bowel often result in a secretory, watery diarrhoea, frequently in association with nausea and vomiting. There is very little bowel inflammation and no colonic involvement so pus cells are not found in faeces. Viruses, bacteria, and protozoa may all affect the bowel in this manner (Table 2).

Viruses

Virus infections are a common cause of vomiting and diarrhoea in babies and children. Rotavirus infections are particularly common below the age of five, with most infections occurring in autumn and winter in temperate climates. This virus disrupts the normal cuboidal epithelium

Table 2 *Causes of non-inflammatory infective diarrhoea*

Viruses	Bacteria	Parasites
Rotavirus	EPEC	Giardia
Norwalk	ETEC	Cryptosporidium
SRSV	*V. cholerae*	*Isospora belli*
Calicivirus	*V. parahaemolyticus*	
Astrovirus	*Staph. aureus*	
Adenovirus	*B. cereus*	
	C. perfringens	

Abbreviations are explained in the text.

at the villus tips, leading to impaired absorption, while the secretory crypt cells are unaffected. The more severe the microvillus damage, the more severe the diarrhoea and dehydration. An incubation period of 1 to 3 days is followed by vomiting and then diarrhoea, sometimes in association with a fever. Symptoms usually resolve after about a week.

Older children and adults may be subject to attacks of severe nausea and vomiting due to viruses (sometimes called winter vomiting disease). Although this can be due to rotavirus, usually other agents are involved. A small virus (30–33 nm) was identified during an outbreak of vomiting in Norwalk, Ohio in 1968. Most patients had vomiting for less than 24 h, and less than half had diarrhoea or fever. The Norwalk virus has similar effects to rotavirus on the microvillus and villus architecture, with complete resolution of these changes by about 2 weeks after infection.

Other Norwalk-like agents subsequently have been identified as causing similar symptoms (sometimes referred to as small round structural viruses (SRSV)), as have other viruses such as astroviruses, adenoviruses, and caliciviruses.

Bacteria

The most well-known and perhaps best-studied bacterial cause of non-inflammatory diarrhoea is *V. cholerae*. The mechanism of adenyl cyclase activation in intestinal mucosal cells has already been described and can lead to a severe secretory diarrhoea. The fluid and electrolyte loss from the gut leads to the depletion of water and salts from both intravascular and extracellular spaces, producing the classical clinical picture of cholera. Although there may be some initial borborygmi, abdominal bloating, and nausea and vomiting, the disease begins with watery diarrhoea. The diarrhoea then becomes profuse with so-called rice-water stools, which are usually odourless and are isotonic with serum. When severe, the diarrhoea can lead to extreme dehydration, shock, and death. However, *V. cholerae* can produce anything from asymptomatic excretion to mild watery diarrhoea through to fulminant disease and death. Many other bacteria can produce secretory diarrhoea via the elaboration of toxins. Cholera-like syndromes may result from infection with ETEC. These *E. coli* produce two types of enterotoxins, one heat labile (**LT**) and one heat stable (**ST**). LT is very similar to cholera toxin while ST is smaller and activates guanylate cyclase with an earlier onset of action than LT. Different strains of ETEC may produce only one or the other enterotoxin or both.

Food poisoning (see Section 7)

Several bacteria associated with food poisoning elaborate toxins that lead to diarrhoea and, sometimes, vomiting. When preformed toxins are ingested (e.g. *Staph. aureus* and *Bacillus cereus*) the incubation period is short (usually less than 6 h) and vomiting is often a prominent feature. *Bacillus cereus* also produces a toxin after it is ingested, as do other organisms like *Clostridium perfringens*, so that the incubation period is longer (8–16 h). Much of the length of the small bowel may be involved, with diarrhoea and abdominal cramps being the main symptoms and little in the way of vomiting. Other bacteria, such as ETEC or *V. parahaemolyticus* produce toxins *in vivo* that take longer to act, leading to long incubation periods (16–72 h).

Travellers' diarrhoea

When tourists or business people from more affluent countries travel to less developed regions of the world, they may succumb to a bout of acute diarrhoea soon after arrival. The risk increases in hot climates where bacteria in food and water multiply more rapidly and there are increased numbers of flies to contaminate food. Symptoms usually arise within 2 weeks of arrival and normally only last for 3 to 5 days. Nausea and abdominal cramps are soon followed by the sudden onset of watery diarrhoea of mild to moderate severity. Vomiting may occur and, with some infections, there may be blood in the stool.

The organisms responsible for these infections are acquired from contaminated water or food, particularly unwashed fruit and raw vegetables. ETEC is responsible for about 50 per cent of cases of travellers' diarrhoea worldwide, with viruses, particularly rotavirus, responsible for a significant minority. Other organisms include shigellae, salmonellae, campylobacter, giardia, and sometimes *Entamoeba histolytica*.

The risk of travellers' diarrhoea can be reduced by prudent eating and drinking. Water sterilization tablets and portable water filters are now readily available and simply boiling water for about 10 min will kill many enteric pathogens. Avoiding salads, raw vegetables, and ice also helps. Although prophylactic antibiotics, such as co-trimoxazole or doxycycline, have been shown to reduce the incidence of travellers' diarrhoea, their routine use cannot be recommended because of the risk of toxicity and the increasing emergence of multiply drug-resistant enteric bacteria. Antibiotic prophylaxis should be reserved for those at highest risk, such as patients with achlorhydria or those who are immunosuppressed.

CHRONIC NON-INFLAMMATORY DIARRHOEA

Some infections may lead to a more chronic diarrhoea of small-bowel origin. Giardiasis may cause chronic symptoms and eventually even lead to a malabsorptive state. In some children and in immunosuppressed adults, the protozoal parasite cryptosporidium may cause chronic diarrhoea. Viral, bacterial, and protozoal infections may all cause sufficient damage to small intestinal microvilli to lead to a secondary disaccharidase deficiency. Most commonly, lactase deficiency develops so that if diarrhoea is prolonged, it is worth trying a lactose-free diet before embarking on more invasive investigations.

Occasionally, Europeans develop diarrhoea and sometimes malabsorption after prolonged stays in the tropics. The exact aetiology of this condition, often called tropical sprue, is not understood but is thought to be partly infective as it usually responds to prolonged courses of broad-spectrum antibiotics.

A number of conditions can give rise to bacterial overgrowth in the small bowel, leading to an increase in the faecal flora in the proximal small bowel with numbers of organisms in excess of 10^5/ml. Factors favouring bacterial overgrowth include achlorhydria, stasis due to diverticula or blind loops, and decreased motility as may occur with diabetes mellitus or scleroderma. The mechanisms by which the bacteria lead to diarrhoea are unclear but may involve deconjugation of bile salts in addition to the effects of toxic bacterial products.

INFLAMMATORY DIARRHOEA

Acute inflammatory diarrhoea is usually bacterial and occasionally parasitic in origin, and may present with several distinct syndromes. Organisms commonly responsible include salmonellae, campylobacter, and shigella. In all cases, both the distal small bowel and the colon are involved and the inflammation leads to pus cells in the stool.

Acute dysentery

Patients may present with diarrhoea of sudden onset, often associated with abdominal cramps and a mild fever, when infected by some bacteria or parasites (Table 3). The frequent bowel movements often contain blood and mucus and there may be tenesmus. Microscopy reveals red

Table 3 *Infective causes of dysentery*

Bacterial	Parasitic
Shigella spp.	*Entamoeba histolytica*
EHEC	*Balantidium coli*
Salmonella spp.	*Schistosoma mansoni*
Campylobacter jejuni	*S. japonicum*
V. parahaemolyticus	*Trichinella spiralis*
C. perfringens	
C. difficile	

EHEC = enterohaemorrhagic *E. coli*.

cells and pus cells in the stool. Sigmoidoscopic examination of the rectum may show an active proctitis, sometimes with ulceration; shallow and widespread with shigellae, deeper and more discrete with amoebiasis. Common causes of this syndrome are *Shigella* spp., non-typhoidal salmonella, and *Campylobacter jejuni*.

Bacteria

Shigella may produce symptoms after a very small inoculum ($< 10^2$ organisms) and although *S. dysenteriae* and *S. flexneri* cause the most severe disease, *S. sonnei* and *S. boydii* are more common in the United Kingdom. Intestinal inflammation is caused by a combination of cytotoxin production and local mucosal invasion. Certain strains of *E. coli* (ETEC) may produce a very similar syndrome via identical cytotoxins. *Campylobacter jejuni* is emerging as one of the most common causes of inflammatory diarrhoea in developed countries, although the dysenteric symptoms tend to be milder than is seen with shigella infections. Salmonella infections are also an increasing problem with notable outbreaks of *Salmonella enteritidis* (phage type 4) gastroenteritis in the United Kingdom in the past few years. This particular species is associated with the consumption of undercooked eggs and poultry but many other *Salmonella* spp. can lead to inflammatory diarrhoea. Rarely, the abdominal pain may be severe enough with campylobacter or salmonella infections to mimic appendicitis and both infections have been known to cause toxic megacolon. All of the above organisms may be associated with a postdysenteric reactive arthropathy (often as part of Reiter's syndrome) in patients with HLA-B27.

Both enteroinvasive *E. coli* (**EIEC**) and EHEC may cause bloody diarrhoea. The former can be indistinguishable from shigellosis, with probably identical pathogenesis. One type of EHEC, *E. coli* 0157:H7 is responsible for a haemorrhagic colitis, particularly in children, that is associated with haemolytic–uraemic syndrome and presents in a manner similar to thrombotic thrombocytopenic purpura.

Parasites

Several parasites may cause acute, bloody diarrhoea. *Entamoeba histolytica* can cause a range of problems from asymptomatic cyst excretion to fulminant, severe colitis, but most adults with symptoms have a mild to moderately severe dysentery. The onset is gradual, with abdominal discomfort and flatulence followed by the frequent passage of watery, bloody stools. Fever is uncommon. Occasionally, the parasite invades deep into the bowel mucosa resulting in an amoeboma, either in the ascending colon or in the rectosigmoid. Unlike amoebic abcesses, amoebomas are usually associated with an active dysentery. *Balantidium coli* may present in a manner indistinguishable from amoebic dysentery but mucosal invasion is limited to the rectum and there are no extraintestinal manifestations. Rarely, this parasite can cause acute appendicitis and sometimes chronic diarrhoea.

Acute schistosomiasis may cause bloody diarrhoea when the adult worms of *Schistosoma mansoni* or *S. japonicum* initially invade the gastrointestinal tract and start producing eggs. Sometimes these trematodes and their eggs are a cause of chronic, intermittent diarrhoea. Acute trichinosis may sometimes start with an inflammatory diarrhoea a week or two before the systemic features of this disease are manifest.

Antibiotic-associated colitis

Ever since the introduction of antibiotics it has been recognized that some patients develop diarrhoea as a complication of therapy. In the late 1970s it was shown that most cases of antibiotic-related diarrhoea are due to infection with a spore-forming, Gram-positive rod, *Clostridium difficile*. Although found in the normal intestinal flora of about 3 per cent of adults, growth of *C. difficile* is favoured by the suppression of other faecal flora by broad-spectrum antibiotics. This organism produces two well-characterized cytotoxins, A and B. Cytotoxin A is probably responsible for damaging colonic mucosa and causing the symptoms (*C. difficile* is not invasive) but cytotoxin B is detected diagnostically by its cytotoxic effects on tissue cultures. Patients with antibiotic-associated colitis may develop symptoms during a course of antibiotics or not until some weeks after finishing a course. Most antibiotics have been implicated at one time or another but cephalosporins are perhaps the most common culprits. There is usually a moderately severe diarrhoea, with red cells and pus in the stool but symptoms can range from mild, self-limiting watery diarrhoea to severe colitis culminating in a toxic megacolon and perforation. Often there is a characteristic sigmoidoscopic appearance of a pseudomembranous colitis with the pale nodules or plaques (the pseudomembrane) on the rectal mucosa. Histologically, the pseudomembrane consists of mucus, fibrin, and sloughed epithelial cells with no evidence of bacterial invasion of the mucosa. *Clostridium difficile* can be the cause of nosocomial outbreaks of diarrhoea and may recur after specific treatment.

Necrotizing enteritis (pig bel)

In Papua New Guinea, infection with *Clostridium perfringens* type C has been associated with a fulminant colitis, usually following feasting on undercooked pork. Probably due to a β-toxin produced by *C. perfringens*, the symptoms are usually vomiting, severe abdominal pain and bloody diarrhoea, sometimes progressing to toxaemia and shock if the bowel perforates.

CHRONIC INFLAMMATORY DIARRHOEA

Some infections lead to chronic symptoms due to more low-grade inflammation. This may occur with recurrent or relapsing bacterial infections, such as salmonellosis, or with protozoal infections, such as amoebiasis. Intestinal tuberculosis, though relatively rare, may lead to diarrhoea, although fever, abdominal pain, and weight loss are more common. Complications of intestinal tuberculosis include bowel obstruction, tuberculomas, strictures, and, occasionally, perforation. Infection may occur primarily through ingestion of bacilli (for example from unpasteurized milk) or spread during miliary infection, or secondarily from swallowing infective sputum in cases of pulmonary tuberculosis.

Rarely, fungi like South American blastomycosis (*Paracoccidiodes brasiliensis*) or histoplasmosis may affect the gut, producing ulcerating or granulomatous lesions and causing abdominal discomfort and diarrhoea.

INVASIVE INFECTIONS

Not all intestinal infections present with diarrhoea; some present with a systemic illness in which fever and non-diarrhoeal abdominal symptoms predominate. This often takes the form of an enteric fever, typhoid being the best example.

Typhoid

Enteric fever due to *Salmonella typhi* results from systemic spread of the ingested organism. The bacilli penetrate the intestinal epithelium and multiply in Peyer's patches before being disseminated by either the lymphatic or haematogenous route. Initially there is a sustained bacteraemia with further multiplication in cells of the reticuloendothelial sys-

Table 4 *Bacteria causing enteric fever syndromes*

Salmonella typhi
S. paratyphi A and B
Campylobacter fetus
Yersinia enterocolitica
Y. pseudotuberculosis

tem. Most patients present with fever that may initially be remittent but is later sustained. Many patients complain of headache and a dry cough is common. Diarrhoea does occur but in less than half of the cases. There may be abdominal tenderness and sometimes hepatosplenomegaly. Up to 50 per cent of patients will have a relative bradycardia with their fever but only about 25 per cent will develop the classic rose spots in the second week of the illness. Complications include small-bowel ulceration with haemorrhage, and sometimes perforation, and occasionally patients develop a frank meningitis.

Other causes of enteric fever

In addition to *S. typhi*, other enteric pathogens may present with typhoid-like illnesses (Table 4). Unlike *Campylobacter jejuni*, *C. fetus* causes diarrhoea relatively uncommonly and may just present with fever. Yersinia infections usually occur in patients with underlying medical disorders, particularly chronic liver disease, but unlike typhoid the illness usually starts with acute diarrhoea followed by fever. Both *Yersinia enterocolitica* and *Y. pseudotuberculosis* may be associated with a polyarthritis and sometimes a frank septic arthritis. Yersinia may also present with acute mesenteric adenitis that may mimic appendicitis. *Campylobacter fetus* also can present with a septic arthritis and is associated with thrombophlebitis, which is unusual with other forms of enteric fever.

PARASITES

Many parasites may, at some stage of their life cycle, cause abdominal symptoms and fever, often with eosinophilia. Infection with *Strongyloides stercoralis* can cause abdominal pain, diarrhoea, and abdominal distension. This important helminth can persist through autoinfection and, in patients who become immunosuppressed (e.g. by steroid therapy), can lead to a severe hyperinfection syndrome. Many other nematodes, such as *Ascaris lumbricoides* or *Trichinella spiralis*, may present with gastrointestinal problems but may also be discovered during investigation of extraintestinal symptoms.

Invasive trematode infections may also have extraintestinal presentations. Schistosomal infection may present with bowel disturbance but may first present with 'swimmer's itch' or a more serious illness, Katayama fever, characterized by fever, urticaria, lymphadenopathy, diarrhoea, and eosinophilia. Other flukes, such as *Fasciola hepatica* or *Clonorchis sinensis*, may present with hepatomegaly or cholangitis.

Cestode infections do not often cause symptoms unless tapeworm segments are noticed in the stool. However, the larval form of *Taenia solium* may cause cysticercosis in man if excreted eggs are ingested.

Trypanosoma cruzi, the protozoal cause of Chagas' disease in South and Central America may damage the myenteric plexus anywhere in the gastrointestinal tract leading to motility problems. Most commonly this affects the oesophagus, leading to mega-oesophagus and dysphagia. The colon is also involved, resulting in chronic constipation and megacolon, similar to Hirschsprung's disease.

ABDOMINAL TUBERCULOSIS

Intestinal tuberculosis may present with diarrhoea and occasionally presents as an acute abdomen because of obstruction or perforation. The terminal ileum and caecum are most commonly involved and some patients may present with a mass in the right iliac fossa. Occult gastrointestinal blood loss is quite common, sometimes presenting as an iron-deficiency anaemia, but frank rectal bleeding is rare. Malabsorption is common and will present with weight loss, with or without bulky stools. Some patients will present only with fever and/or malaise and others may be diagnosed incidentally, sometimes at autopsy.

Tuberculous peritonitis is relatively rare, usually resulting from local spread of infection from mesenteric lymph nodes infected via blood-borne spread. Ascites is a common presenting feature, although some cases present with a thickened, doughy-feeling omentum and perito-neum. Rarely, abdominal tuberculosis may present with a mass of enlarged retroperitoneal lymph nodes.

SEXUALLY TRANSMITTED INTESTINAL INFECTION

A number of organisms transmissable by sexual intercourse may cause diarrhoea or other gastrointestinal symptoms. These pathogens are usu-ally transmitted by anal intercourse but orogenital and oroanal contact may also be implicated. Gonococcal or chlamydial proctitis may cause diarrhoea or anal discomfort. Herpes simplex perianal infection may cause rectal bleeding in addition to pain, and warts due to human pap-illomavirus may involve the anal canal as well as the perineal skin. Giardia and cysts of *Entamoeba histolytica* are often found in the stools of homosexual men but they usually do not appear to cause symptoms.

In the tropics, both chancroid due to *Haemophilus ducreyii* and gran-uloma inguinale due to *Calymmatobacterium granulomatis* can cause perianal bleeding; lymphogranuloma venereum resulting from infection with *Chlamydia trachomatis* may present with proctocolitis or even a rectal stricture.

Diarrhoea is a very common symptom in human immunodeficiency virus (**HIV**) disease. This may reflect the alteration in gut permeability brought about by a direct effect of HIV or it may be caused by a wide variety of opportunist infections of the intestine, such as *Cryptosporid-ium*, cytomegalovirus, and the newly recognized pathogens, microspor-idia. Oesophagitis due to *Candida albicans* is also a common problem, usually presenting with dysphagia. Viral infections, such as HSV or cytomegalovirus may also cause oesophagitis or, sometimes, solitary ulcers. In addition, Kaposi's sarcoma and HIV-associated lymphoma may affect the gut, causing diarrhoea (see Chapter 14.4).

HELICOBACTER PYLORI

This Gram-negative, curved or spiral bacillus has recently been impli-cated in the aetiology of gastritis and peptic ulcer disease. Acute infec-tion may lead to acute gastritis with nausea and vomiting that settles after a week or two, but there may be a longer-lasting achlorhydria. Most attention has recently focused on the association between *Heli-cobacter pylori* and ulceration. The organism lives in the layer of gastric mucus, is motile, and produces a powerful urease, all factors that con-tribute to its survival in acid environment of the stomach. *Helicobacter pylori* is associated with an antral gastritis, with chronic inflammation found on biopsy. When the bacteria are found in the duodenum there is always duodenitis or ulceration. There is also an association between this organism and adenocarcinoma of the stomach.

Although it has been shown that elimination of the organism improves the histological appearance of gastric tissue and reduces the relapse rate of duodenal ulcer, the role of *H. pylori* is still not completely worked out. *Helicobacter pylori* can only reliably be cultured from mucosal biopsies and, although sensitive *in vitro* to a number of antibiotics, pro-longed antibiotic courses are needed and resistance may emerge. Stan-dard antiulcer drugs, such as H_2-antagonists and antacids, have no effect on bacterial growth, but the organism is susceptible to omeprazole. At present, a 2- to 4-week course of a combination of tetracycline and metronidazole offers a good chance of elimination, particularly if pre-ceded by a course of bismuth salts. Unfortunately, as the mode of trans-mission and the pathogenesis are still not well understood, infection and reinfection cannot be prevented.

WHIPPLE'S DISEASE (SEE CHAPTER 14.9.6)

This systemic disease that primarily affects middle-aged men causes most morbidity because of its effects on the gastrointestinal tract. An infective cause has been sought for some time because most affected tissues have macrophages stuffed full of rod-shaped organisms. The macrophages appear to be foamy and stain intensely with periodic acid–Schiff stain. Recently, molecular biological techniques have been used to identify a probable cause; a novel organism that is a Gram-positive actinomycete and has been tentatively named *Tropheryma whippelii*.

Arthralgia is a common manifestation that comes and goes before the gut involvement predominates. Diarrhoea then ensues, which if untreated progresses to malabsorption, weight loss, and eventual death. If recognized, treatment with an initial course of parenteral penicillin and streptomycin followed by at least a year of oral co-trimoxazole can effect a cure.

Although this is a rare condition, now that a putative cause has been found it should be possible to unravel the pathogenesis of Whipple's disease.

Diagnosis and management of gastrointestinal infections

DIAGNOSIS

Clues to the aetiology of gastrointestinal infections should first be sought in the history. Particular note should be taken of foreign travel, the dietary history, the possibility of associated causes, and the underlying medical problems of the patient. Vomiting in association with watery diarrhoea may indicate a non-inflammatory intestinal infection, while the presence of blood in the faeces points to an inflammatory enteritis. A history of current or recent antibiotic treatment may suggest *C. dif-ficile* colitis. The clinical signs that should be noted are the presence and degree of dehydration, fever, evidence of toxaemia, and any extraintes-tinal manifestations.

Investigations should include culture of blood and stool, with light microscopy of stool to look for pus cells and parasites. If a viral cause is suspected, stool should be examined by electron microscopy. In addi-tion, rotavirus may be detected by a commercially available enzyme-linked immunosorbent assay, and other viruses may be found by tissue culture or radioimmunoassay.

Sigmoidoscopy and rectal biopsy may sometimes be helpful, partic-ularly to identify parasites such as *Entamoeba histolytica* or *Schistosoma mansoni* and to help in the differential diagnosis of inflammatory bowel disease. Occasionally small-bowel biopsies and duodenal fluid aspirates may be needed to sort out chronic diarrhoea and in the differential diag-nosis of conditions such as gluten enteropathy. Plain abdominal radio-graphs may be required to exclude a toxic megacolon and barium studies are useful in the work-up of bloody diarrhoea that is not settling or if intestinal tuberculosis is a consideration.

DIFFERENTIAL DIAGNOSIS

Non-inflammatory diarroea

Although this syndrome is usually due to infective causes, other pos-sibilities need to be considered, particularly if the symptoms persist. A variety of toxins can produce acute diarrhoea and vomiting, including heavy metals, such as cadmium and arsenic. Mushroom poisoning, for example, with *Amanita phalloides*, may result in severe vomiting and sometimes diarrhoea along with other symptoms. Some fish contain tox-ins that may affect the gastrointestinal tract in addition to other systems. The best known of these is ciguatera poisoning, which has been asso-ciated with several hundred different species of fish in the Pacific and Caribbean. The toxin, probably produced by a fish parasite, produces neurological and gastrointestinal symptoms, the latter comprising nausea, vomiting, abdominal cramps, and diarrhoea. Scromboid poisoning results from the ingestion of poorly refrigerated fish in which bacteria have caused breakdown of histine in fish muscle to saurine, a histamine-like substance. The symptoms are like those of histamine poisoning, with diarrhoea in association with a constellation of other reactions, such as flushing, generalized urticaria, myalgia, and swelling of the tongue and throat.

There are also endocrine causes of diarrhoea that may work through activation of adenyl cyclase. These include carcinoid tumours, medullary carcinoma of the thyroid, and non-β islet-cell tumours. Tumours producing vasoactive intestinal peptide may also present with diarrhoea. Sometimes, diarrhoea is a major feature of thyrotoxicosis or hypoadrenalism. More chronic diarrhoea may result from coeliac disease or from inherited disaccharidase deficiency.

Inflammatory diarrhoea

When patients present with bloody diarrhoea, the main differential diagnosis is between infection and idiopathic inflammatory bowel disease. Although histological examination of the rectal biopsy may distinguish between Crohn's disease, ulcerative colitis, and infection, the diagnosis of inflammatory bowel disease may only be made with the passage of time in the absence of an infective cause being found. Sometimes acute diverticulitis or ischaemic colitis may present acutely with bloody diarrhoea and mimic infection. This rarely occurs with colonic cancers.

Enteric fever

In the early phases, when fever is the main symptom and sign, many infections may suggest typhoid. These include malaria, acute trypanosomiasis, bartonellosis, and intra-abdominal collections. Other non-infective conditions, such as connective tissue disease and tumours, may present with fever. Usually, other symptoms and signs or initial investigations will point to the correct diagnosis but blood cultures are an essential part of the work-up.

MANAGEMENT

Rehydration

The mainstay of managing diarrhoeal diseases is the recognition and correction of water and electrolyte depletion. This is particularly the case with acute non-inflammatory diarrhoea in the very young and the very old, when large, rapid fluid losses can quickly lead to circulatory collapse and renal failure. If vomiting is not a major feature then rehydration can usually be achieved using oral rehydration solutions (ORS) (Table 5). The World Health Organization (WHO) 'universal formula' has simplified the management of childhood gastroenteritis in the tropics. This takes the form of a powder containing 20 g glucose, 3.5 g sodium chloride, 1.5 g potassium chloride, and either 2.5 g sodium bicarbonate or 2.9 g trisodium citrate per litre of solution, usually packaged in aluminium foil in quantities appropriate to the volume of containers used for water in different tropical regions. However, in Western countries where faecal sodium losses are less and where formula feeds are more common than breast feeding, there are real fears of hypernatraemic dehydration. In these areas an ORS with a lower sodium content than the WHO one is preferable, for example Dioralyte (Rorer Pharmaceuticals). In addition, in the tropics there is evidence that fluids from cooked cereals, such as rice water, may be used as ORS. Clearly, depending on the ability of the patient to take fluid orally and the severity of the dehydration, parenteral fluids may need to be given intravenously or even subcutaneously.

Antidiarrhoeal agents

A variety of agents, such as diphenoxylate sodium and codeine phosphate, are used to inhibit intestinal motility and hence relieve the symptom of diarrhoea. There are unsubstantiated fears that these drugs may increase the risk of toxic megacolon but there is some evidence to sug-

Table 5 *Oral rehydration solutions*

Constituents (mmol/l)	WHO	Dioralyte (Rorer)
Sodium	90	60
Potassium	20	20
Chloride	80	60
Base (citrate)	10	10
Glucose	110	90
Osmolality	310	240

gest that they may slow the clearance of organisms from the intestine and slightly increase the risks of some organisms, such as shigella, becoming invasive. However, these agents may provide useful symptomatic relief in many cases of mild diarrhoea as an adjunct to rehydration. Loperamide, which has some activity as a calcium antagonist, may inhibit intestinal secretion but only in very large doses. Prostaglandin synthetase inhibitors, such as indomethacin, may inhibit the sodium pump in small-bowel epithelial cells and thus decrease secretion caused by toxins that stimulate adenylate cyclase. However, this is probably not useful clinically. Other agents like kaolin pectin have been promoted as absorbents of bacteria and their toxins but there is no evidence to suggest that they are any more effective than placebo and their use cannot be recommended. Solutions of bismuth salts may have an antiseptic role and have been shown to be useful in the prevention of travellers' diarrhoea and to have some activity against *Helicobacter pylori*.

Antibiotics

Specific antimicrobial chemotherapy is rarely indicated for diarrhoeal illnesses; rehydration and time will usually effect a cure. In some instances, antibiotics may actually prolong carriage and excretion of the pathogen while at the same time increasing the chances of multiply resistant enteric pathogens emerging. However, in some circumstances specific therapy is indicated. Cholera symptoms will settle more quickly, and transmission in epidemics will be reduced, if tetracycline is given in addition to ORS. Clearly, typhoid and other enteric fevers need to be treated with an appropriate systemic antibiotic according to the sensitivity of the causative organism. In many cases chloramphenicol, trimethoprim, or ampicillin are adequate, although quinolone antibiotics are being used increasingly. Infections with non-typhoidal salmonellae or *Campylobacter jejuni* rarely require treatment unless the patient is ill and immunocompromised or there is a documented bacteraemia. Here, again, the newer quinolones are being used but there are already quinolone-resistant campylobacter isolates reported. Many cases of antibiotic-associated colitis will settle once the offending antibiotics have been withdrawn but, if not, both oral metronidazole and oral vancomycin are equally effective against *C. difficile*. Parasitic infections such as amoebiasis or giardiasis will require specific chemotherapy.

Surgery

Surgery has little role in the management of gastrointestinal infection unless there is a bowel perforation or torrential bleeding. Some infections may present as an acute abdomen and the decision to explore the abdomen in these patients is a difficult one requiring experience and judgement. Surgery may be needed to remove strictures or to make a diagnosis in cases of intestinal tuberculosis.

Public health

Patients admitted to hospital with presumed infectious diarrhoea should be nursed in side rooms to minimize the risk of nosocomial spread of the infection. Cases of food poisoning, typhoid, tuberculosis, etc. are notifiable and the local public health physician should be informed. The public health official should also be told of any food handler who presents with gastroenteritis.

Prevention

Most diarrhoeal illnesses can be prevented through good hygiene and adequate sanitation, including a safe water supply. In neonates and infants, breast-feeding significantly reduces the incidence of gastroenteritis compared to bottle feeding, especially in the tropics. Antibiotic prophylaxis is rarely indicated, even though drugs such as co-trimoxazole and doxycycline have been show to reduce the risk of travellers' diarrhoea. These drugs may be useful for immunocompromised individuals at high risk but their routine use cannot be recommended as this is likely to increase the antibiotic resistance of enteric pathogens, might lead to unacceptable toxicity, and the cost would be high.

Immunization against enteric pathogens is an ideal aim but has, so far, been relatively unsuccessful. Vaccines against *S. typhi* are relatively effective, those against *V. cholerae* less so. There are no effective vaccines against ETEC, campylobacter, protozoa, or enteric viruses (other than polio).

REFERENCES

Avery, M.E. and Snyder, J.D. (1990). Oral therapy for acute diarrhea. The underused simple solution. *New England Journal of Medicine*, **323**, 891–4.

Baird-Parker, A.C. (1990). Foodborne salmonellosis. *Lancet*, **336**, 1231–5.

Bartlett, J.G. (1992). Antibiotic associated diarrhoea. *Clinical Infectious Disease*, **15**, 573–9.

Blacklow, N.R. and Greenberg, H.B. (1991). Viral gastroenteritis. *New England Journal of Medicine*, **325**, 252–64.

Blaser, M.J. (1992). *Helicobacter pylori*: its role in disease. *Clinical Infectious Disease*, **15**, 386–93.

Chant, H., Smith, H.R., Scotland, S.M., Rowe, B., Milford D.V., and Taylor, C.M. (1991). Serological identification of *Escherichia coli* 0157:H7 infection in haemolytic uraemic syndrome. *Lancet*, **337**, 138–40.

Chen, L.C., Rohde, J.E., and Sharpe, G.W.G. (1971). Intestinal adenylcyclase activity in human cholera. *Lancet*, **i**, 939–41.

Cover, T.C. and Aber, R.C. (1989) *Yersinia enterocolitica. New England Journal of Medicine*, **321**, 16–24.

Gianella, R.A., Broitman S.A., and Zamcheck, N. (1973). Influence of gastric acidity on bacterial and parasitic enteric infections: a perspective. *Annals of Internal Medicine*, **78**, 271–6.

Klimach, O.E. and Omerod, L.P. (1985). Gastrointestinal tuberculosis: a retrospective review of 109 cases in a district general hospital. *Quarterly Journal of Medicine*, **56**, 569–78.

Laughton, B.E. *et al.* (1988). Prevalence of enteric pathogens in homosexual men with and without acquired immunodeficiency syndrome. *Gastroenterology*, **94**, 984–93.

Leading Article (1989). HIV-associated enteropathy. *Lancet*, **ii**, 777–8.

Levine, M.M. (1986). Antimicrobial therapy for infectious diarrhea. *Review of Infectious Diseases*, **8**, S207–16.

Levine, M.M. (1987). *Escherichia coli* that cause diarrhea: enterotoxigenic, enteropathogenic, enteroinvasive, enterohemorrhagic and enteroadherent. *Journal of Infectious Diseases*, **155**, 377–89.

Lucas, S.B., Papadaki, L., Conlon, C.P., Sewankambo, N., Goodgame, R., and Serwadda, D. (1989). Diagnosis of intestinal microsporidiosis in patients with AIDS. *Journal of Clinical Pathology*, **42**, 885–7.

Morgan, M.R.A. and Fenwick, G.R. (1990). Natural foodborne toxicants. *Lancet*, **336**, 1492–5.

National Institutes of Health Consensus Conference. (1985). Travelers' diarrhea. *Journal of the American Medical Association*, **253**, 2700–4.

Pizarro, D., Posada, G., Sandi, L., and Moran, J.R. (1991). Rice-based oral electrolyte solutions for the management of infantile diarrhea. *New England Journal of Medicine*, **324**, 517–21.

Reed, S.L. (1992). Amebiasis: an update. *Clinical Infectious Disease*, **14**, 385–93.

Relman, D.A., Schmit, T.M., MacDermott, R.P., and Falkow, S. (1992). Identification of the uncultured bacillus of Whipple's disease. *New England Journal of Medicine*, **327**, 293–301.

Simon, G.L. and Gorbach, S.L. (1982). Intestinal microflora. *Medical Clinics of North America*, **66**, 557–74.

Wicks, A.C.B., Holmes, G.S., and Davidson, L. (1971). Endemic typhoid fever: a diagnostic pitfall. *Quarterly Journal of Medicine*, **40**, 341–54.

14.19 The peritoneum, omentum, and appendix

M. IRVING

INTRODUCTION

Diseases of the peritoneal cavity and its contents remain a challenge to the diagnostic skills of the clinician. Thus, despite all the imaging techniques now available, the combination of a careful history with a physical examination that pays particular attention to the facial appearances, cardiovascular responses, and abdominal physical signs is still the basis of the diagnosis of acute peritonitis. However, the development of fibreoptic peritoneoscopy, enabling minimal access, direct examination of the peritoneal cavity (laparoscopy), together with ultrasonography and computerized axial tomography, have undoubtedly brought a new degree of accuracy to clinical assessment.

The peritoneal cavity and its diseases

The peritoneum consists of a mesothelial lining containing fibroblasts and macrophages that produce an intense cellular response to inflammatory and neoplastic processes. Anatomically it is a closed sac that is invaginated from behind by the abdominal viscera, most of which are invested by the peritoneal lining on at least two or three surfaces. Between the two layers is a potential space (the peritoneal cavity), with only a small amount of fluid to lubricate movement between the layers.

It only becomes actual when distended by fluid or gas outside a viscus. The parietal peritoneum receives a somatic innervation whilst the visceral peritoneum is innervated by autonomic nerves. Secretory responses of the peritoneum vary from the fibrinous response to inflammation to the ascitic exudatory responses to neoplasia. The apron-like duplication of the peritoneum is known as the omentum, which, because of its tendency to wrap itself in a protective fashion round sites of inflammation, has been called the 'policeman' of the abdomen. The peritoneum is capable of giving rise to lesions itself, for example pseudomyxoma, and recurrent adhesions.

Peritonitis

Most cases of infective peritonitis are secondary to diseases of intra-abdominal organs. Commonly, enteric organisms gain entry into the peritoneal cavity by passing through the wall of a diseased organ or by perforation of a hollow viscus. Among the more common disorders causing peritonitis are necrosis of the bowel, resulting from ischaemia that may be due to strangulating obstruction or mesenteric vascular occlusion, perforation of a neoplasm, inflammatory diseases such as appendicitis, Crohn's disease, colitis, diverticulitis, and perforation of peptic ulcer. Gynaecological disorders such as salpingitis give rise to pelvic peritonitis. Less commonly, peritonitis may occur in the absence of an intra-abdominal lesion. For example, patients with cirrhosis or the nephrotic syndrome and ascites are prone to spontaneous bacterial peritonitis. The most common causative organism is *Escherichia coli*, but pneumococci or streptococci may be implicated. Pneumococcal peritonitis used to be encountered as an apparently primary phenomenon but is not often seen now in the United Kingdom. Peritonitis may also arise as a result of bacterial contamination of the catheter used in peritoneal dialysis. Peritonitis can be divided into acute, as typically develops in association with an inflammatory lesions such as appendicitis, or chronic, as occurs in tuberculosis. Not all peritonitis is bacterial and a 'chemical peritonitis' may arise when acid or blood are released into the peritoneal cavity. A special type of peritonitis occurs with foreign material such as talc and glove powder

CLINICAL SIGNS

Bacterial or chemical contamination of the peritoneal cavity with blood or acid leads to the production of an exudate, paralytic ileus, and reflex spasm of the abdominal muscles. It results in immediate depletion of circulatory volume and hypoperfusion. This, if untreated, progresses to circulatory shock and its associated complications such as renal and multiple organ failure. The characteristic picture of acute generalized peritonitis is one of agonizing abdominal pain in a patient who is pale and sweating, with shallow breathing, and who is lying absolutely still because every movement causes exacerbation of pain in the abdomen. Even respiration is painful, and the patient tends to breathe with the thorax whilst holding the abdomen immobile. When confronted with such a patient the temptation is to move immediately to physical examination but valuable information can be obtained just by observing the patient's responses. This is especially so in children, who may be terrified by the thought of their abdomen being palpated; they may be observed and examined more successfully whilst being held in the parent's lap.

At the beginning of the physical examination the patient should be asked to sit up. One with generalized peritonitis will be unable to do so and one with localized peritonitis will find it difficult. If asked to cough, the patient with generalized peritonitis will give an inadequate effort whilst one with localized peritonitis will wince and immediately put a hand over the inflamed area. These responses are signs of rebound tenderness. Another useful technique is for the examiner to place a hand 2 cm above the patient's abdomen and ask the patient to raise the abdomen to touch the hand. This will prove impossible for one with acute generalized peritonitis. Palpation will reveal widespread guarding, or rigidity in generalized cases, and similar signs over the inflamed organ in localized peritonitis. These classical physical signs may not be present in the very young or the very old, or may become less obvious when the disease is progressing or has been modified by treatments such as analgesia, antibiotics or corticosteroids. However, even those without the classical physical signs will usually manifest systemic changes such as tachycardia, oliguria, hypotension, ileus, and vomiting.

Simple investigations such as radiographs of the chest and abdomen may show air under the diaphragm, distended loops of bowel, and fluid between loops. Aspiration of the peritoneal cavity through a fine catheter may show leucocytes and organisms. Ultrasonography will reveal thickened bowel, and air and fluid in the peritoneal cavity and its recesses.

TREATMENT

Peritonitis is an acute surgical emergency and the cause should be dealt with as soon as possible. Resuscitation is the priority and the patient should be started on intravenous fluids to correct hypovolaemia and restore satisfactory renal perfusion as judged by urine output. Infusion should begin with normal saline and progress as soon as possible to colloids such as a gelatin preparation. A nasogastric tube and should be passed and the urinary bladder catheterized. Antibiotics should be given intravenously. Local protocols will govern the choice of regimen but a

combination of cefuroxime and metronidazole is a reasonable one to cover most gastrointestinal emergencies.

Analgesic agents should be given intravenously as absorption is unpredictable after intramuscular administration in such patients. The perceived danger of such analgesia masking physical signs is more apparent than real. Surgical treatment, either by conventional laparotomy or laparoscopy, should proceed as soon as possible to deal with the underlying cause of the peritonitis and to cleanse the peritoneal cavity. Infected fluid should be washed out of the cavity initially with copious volumes of warm normal saline solution and finally with saline containing an antibiotic such as tetracycline. There is no point in trying to excise fibrinous exudates adherent to the bowel wall but all traces of solid material such as faeces and food debris should be meticulously removed.

Intraperitoneal abscesses

Abscesses arise when infection in the peritoneal cavity is walled off. They can occur anywhere but typically are found in the peritoneal recesses, such as the subphrenic spaces and hepatorenal spaces, and the pelvis. They can be located between loops of bowel (interloop abscesses).

Subphrenic and pelvic abscesses

These are the two more common sites of intra-abdominal abscesses. They usually arise secondary to a source of infection in the abdomen such as a perforated appendix or colonic diverticulum, or following a leak from an intestinal anastomosis. Occasionally, they may arise without obvious cause. The clinical picture is characterized by malaise, fever, and pain, often referred to the shoulder tip in the case of a subphrenic abscess. A polymorphonuclear leucocytosis is an almost invariable finding. Physical signs are usually minimal, although in subphrenic abscess there may be a small, reactive pleural effusion on the affected side, and in pelvic abscess a boggy swelling may be felt on rectal examination. Plain radiographs of the abdomen may show gas and a fluid level under the diaphragm and a sympathetic pleural effusion on the same side as a subphrenic abscess. Screening may show impaired movement of the diaphragm. The diagnosis may be facilitated by ultrasound examination and computerized tomographic scanning. Treatment is by percutaneous drainage under ultrasonographic or computerized tomographic guidance. A fine catheter is inserted into the cavity and is left in place until the abscess cavity contracts. Open surgical drainage is virtually never required other than in thick, multilocular abscesses.

Peritoneal abscesses in other classical sites can also be readily detected by ultrasonography or computerized tomographic scanning and can be drained percutaneously. This is the treatment of choice for most intra-abdominal abscesses. However, it is often difficult to detect interloop abscess and therefore hard to ensure adequate drainage by this technique. In such patients, laparotomy with separation of the individual bowel loops may be the only way to ensure that the abscesses are detected and adequately drained. In very difficult cases of intraperitoneal sepsis, where infection is diagnosed late or keeps on recurring, more radical treatment, such as leaving the peritoneal cavity open, may be necessary. This technique, termed 'laparostomy', has a small and decreasing place in management.

Glove powder peritonitis

A special type of peritonitis caused by glove powder was first described in the 1950s. Initially it was thought to be confined to the use of talc, which was subsequently withdrawn from use. However, it was then appreciated that the substitute, starch powder, could also give rise to similar problems. The condition has almost been eliminated by the use of starch-free gloves. Patients who develop this type of peritonitis suffer abdominal pain and discomfort, associated with an intermittent pyrexia, about a week to 10 days after operation. The abdomen is often swollen, with signs of free fluid and subacute intestinal obstruction. The condition can be treated conservatively but often the patient requires a further laparotomy. At operation the abdomen is found to contain fluid and the loops of bowel are often stuck together. The serosal surface of the bowel and the parietal peritoneum are often covered with small nodules of white material, sometimes having the appearance of neoplastic secondaries. Biopsy of these will show the classical appearances of birefringent material diagnostic of starch peritonitis.

Tumours of the peritoneum

The vast majority of tumours in the peritoneal cavity are the result of metastases from carcinomas arising in the gastrointestinal tract, the uterus, the ovary, the lung, and the breast. The only primary tumour of any significance arising from the peritoneum is the mesothelioma. This occurs more commonly in the pleura and is associated with occupational exposure to asbestos. The diagnosis will come to mind when a patient with a history of such exposure presents with abdominal symptoms and weight loss associated with a raised erythrocyte sedimentation rate.

Pseudomyxoma

In this rare condition the peritoneal cavity becomes distended with loculated masses of semitranslucent mucinous material. Although the usual cause is associated with ovarian cystic lesions (e.g. mucinous cystadenoma), pseudomyxoma may arise from rupture of a mucocele of the appendix at appendicectomy, with peritoneal adhesions resulting from the organizing mucus. It may also arise from seeding throughout the peritoneum of a mucus-secreting neoplasm of the appendix or even *de novo*. Patients present with abdominal distension, which on investigation is shown to be the result of the characteristic fluid. Pseudomyxoma is a difficult condition to treat because of its tendency to recur and of its lack of response to chemotherapy. The cystic masses can occasionally be excised but ultimately they accumulate, causing intestinal, ureteric, and sometimes vascular obstruction, and eventually become inoperable. In my experience, debulking by surgical excision has a part to play and very vascular pseudomyxomas may occasionally be controlled by arterial embolization. Because of the slowly progressive nature of the condition, patients with chronic intestinal obstruction not amenable to operation and causing nutritional problems may be successfully treated with home parenteral nutrition.

Adhesions

Adhesions are part of the healing process that follows surgical operation or peritonitis. Their extent varies according to individual responses and they can sometimes be so extensive as to virtually obliterate the peritoneal cavity. It is generally agreed that adhesions are related to alterations in peritoneal cellular fibrinolytic activity, but their extent is associated with the amount of tissue damage caused by the operation, the extent of infection and blood loss into the peritoneal cavity, and the amount of ischaemic tissue resulting from ligation and strangulating sutures. It has been clearly demonstrated that suture reperitonealization of peritoneal defects leads to increased adhesion formation.

Do adhesions give rise to pain? This is a difficult question to answer. Most surgeons are well aware that an abdomen can be full of adhesions that do not give rise to any symptoms. Other abdomens have single bands that can give rise to obstruction. Since the advent of laparoscopic surgery there is no doubt that some patients with abdominal adhesions can be relieved of their pain by division of these adhesions. The adhesions in question tend to be small and may well give rise to pain by traction on a small area of parietal peritoneum.

Tuberculous peritonitis (see Section 7)

Tuberculous peritonitis may be generalized or localized. The source of the bacillus in generalized tuberculous peritonitis may be a caseous mesenteric lymph node or it may enter via the fallopian tube in women. The bacillus may also derive from the bloodstream. The macroscopic appearance of the peritoneum varies widely and there may or may not be a serofibrinous exudate. The omentum is often extensively involved and forms a palpable mass in the upper abdomen. The diagnosis and management of this condition is described in Section 7. Unlike acute bacterial or chemical peritonitis the symptoms are usually insidious and consist of fever, anorexia, and weight loss. On two occasions the author has seen Asian patients presenting with impotence as the first sign of their condition. In about 70 per cent of cases there is abdominal distension resulting from ascites, and when fluid is removed a mass can sometimes be palpated. The diagnosis is made by cytological and bacteriological examination and culture of the removed ascitic fluid or by biopsy of the peritoneum or the intra-abdominal mass, both of which may be seen at laparoscopy.

Fungal and parasitic peritonitis

These rare forms of peritonitis present a similar clinical picture to that of tuberculosis. Fungal peritonitis usually occurs in patients who are immunosuppressed, particularly those on corticosteroids and peritoneal dialysis. Cryptococcal infections have been reported in immunosuppressed patients. Peritoneal schistosomiasis has been recorded, simulating malignant diseases.

Drug-induced peritonitis

Obliterative peritonitis and retroperitoneal fibrosis have been described as a consequence of treatment with a number of drugs. For example, practolol may produce a sclerosing peritonitis in which the whole of the small bowel is wrapped in a cocoon. This had to be divided or excised to free the bowel.

Familial paroxysmal peritonitis

This condition occurs mainly in ethnic groups from the Mediterranean and is part of the syndrome of familial polyserositis or familial Mediterranean fever. It is described in Chapter 11.13.2.

Appendicitis and other appendiceal conditions

In 1886, Fitz described the pathological sequence of acute inflammation of the appendix, right iliac-fossa peritonitis, and abscess formation. The lifetime incidence of appendicitis, once put at 12 per cent in Western communities, is now falling, possibly as the result of the more widespread use of high-residue diets. Nevertheless, people still die from the condition. Of the 80 000 people in the United Kingdom admitted to hospital in 1990 with appendicitis, approximately 100 died as a result of their disease.

AETIOLOGY

There is still considerable discussion about why the appendix should so commonly become inflamed. The usual explanation, although still not proven, attributes the inflammation to obstruction of the mouth of the lumen with a faecalith. This obstruction is more likely to occur if the lumen becomes narrowed by lymphoid follicular hypertrophy or fibrosis. If this is the explanation, then it seems reasonable to accept that some patients may have repeated attacks of appendicular pain associated with peristaltic efforts by the appendix to expel the obstructing faecalith. The classical explanation for acute appendicitis based on luminal obstruction, venous engorgement, ischaemia, suppuration, and gangrenous perforation is challenged by some. Thus, it is suggested that physiological changes such as occur in the postoperative period may predispose to acute inflammation of the appendix, and some workers have suggested a familial association.

Although there does not seem to be a sustainable pathological basis for a clinical diagnosis of 'chronic appendicitis', the long-held belief in a 'grumbling appendix' could be explained by recurrent faecalithic obstruction. However, it is more likely that patients with such symptoms are afflicted by the irritable bowel syndrome. The association of faecalith-induced appendicitis with Western diet seems to be supported by epidemiological studies. Burkitt pointed out that acute appendicitis is rare in African communities who consume a traditional, high-residue diet but that the incidence of the disease increases when Africans change to a Western type of diet.

AGE AND SEX

Acute appendicitis can occur at any age but is rare in infants. The incidence rises rapidly in children over the age of 5 years and reaches a peak during the second and third decades of life. The disease is not uncommon in elderly people and can occur in extreme old age. Some have reported a sex difference for appendicitis in young people, with it being twice as common in males than females in the age group 15 to 25 years.

DIAGNOSIS

Appendicitis can be a particularly challenging diagnosis to make in children, elderly people, and pregnant women. The classical signs are seen most often in young and middle-aged individuals. The symptoms commence with colicky abdominal pain in the periumbilical region. This coincides with peristaltic efforts by the appendix to overcome the obstruction caused by the faecalith at its base. The patient almost invariably vomits during this stage. There is little doubt that in some patients the pathological process ends at this point if the faecalith is expelled into the caecum. Where this does not happen, venous congestion occurs and the appendix is distended and becomes turgid, at which time bacterial growth occurs in the lumen. The appendix wall becomes inflamed and the arterial blood supply is impaired. The greater omentum moves over to wrap itself around the inflamed organ. Peristaltic contractions cease and the peritoneum adjacent to the appendix becomes inflamed. This gives rise to pain in the right iliac fossa as the parietal peritoneum becomes inflamed.

In children, appendicitis may present as gastroenteritis. Frequently the history is atypical and the vomiting is more likely to be the presenting symptom. In elderly people the incidence of perforation increases, possibly because it is more difficult to make the diagnosis, or because the disease progresses more rapidly. These patients may have fewer of the classical physical signs and indeed may present with features of intestinal obstruction. They are less likely to have a leucocytosis than are younger patients. As a result they suffer longer delays before operation and consequently have a higher postoperative mortality.

In patients with retrocaecal appendicitis the ureter may be involved in the inflammatory process, leading to dysuria and inflammatory cells in the urine. An appendix in this position or one lying in the pelvis may also involve the psoas muscle, leading to the so-called psoas sign, that is, flexion contracture of the hip.

Examination usually reveals tenderness and guarding in the right iliac fossa. Rectal examination rarely provides useful signs and indeed appendicitis should not be diagnosed just on a finding of rectal tenderness. In children, if the diagnosis is apparent from the history and abdominal examination, rectal examination should be omitted. Gentle percussion of the abdomen will elicit the signs of rebound tenderness, which are usually maximal in the right iliac fossa. If the appendix perforates, which it usually does at its base (the site of the faecalith), localized peritonitis results and may be contained by the omentum and form an abscess. If not, then a spreading, generalized peritonitis ensues.

DIFFERENTIAL DIAGNOSIS

Differential diagnosis from gynaecological causes may be difficult, especially in a woman, where pelvic peritonitis may mimic the signs of appendicitis. In young adults, the presence of an element of small-bowel obstruction raises the possibility of Crohn's disease. Frank obstruction and dilated loops of bowel can be a feature of late appendicitis. Mesenteric adenitis, once a popular diagnosis, and a common explanation for the finding of a normal appendix at laparotomy, is probably only a rare cause of abdominal pain. Enlarged nodes in the ileocaecal mesentery are a frequent incidental finding at laparotomy for other conditions. Whereas it is undeniable that young patients with viral infections and generalized lymphadenitis may suffer abdominal pain that can be difficult to differentiate from appendicitis, the cause is just as likely to be constipation associated with a sore throat and pyrexia as inflammation of the mesenteric nodes. In such cases, surgical exploration depends upon the interpretation of the whole clinical picture and the investigations. The use of laparoscopic surveillance of the abdomen may avoid unnecessary laparotomy in such cases.

SPECIAL INVESTIGATIONS

The white-cell count is rarely of value in contributing to the diagnosis. Nevertheless, a low white count should always lead to a review of the diagnosis before operating. Plain radiographs of the abdomen can reveal a large faecalith lying in the right iliac fossa or a dilated loop of small or large bowel caused by an associated ileus. Barium enema can show a filling defect at the base of the appendix or incomplete filling of the appendix. Ultrasonography is increasingly capable of showing the presence of the distended appendix.

Peritoneal aspiration with a fine catheter can show a cellular response diagnostic of appendicitis. In confusing cases, a computerized tomographic scan can occasionally be of value. It has been found that computer-aided diagnosis of abdominal pain can increase the diagnostic accuracy of those making the clinical assessment and reduce the number of 'negative' laparotomies for suspected appendicitis. Overnight observation in doubtful cases may reduce the 'negative' appendicectomy rate.

TREATMENT

The standard management of the inflamed appendix is surgical removal. However, experience in the armed forces with patients distant from sophisticated medical services has demonstrated that, with antibiotic treatment and analgesia, it is possible to manage the condition conservatively. Nowadays, there is no doubt that skilfully performed open or laparoscopic appendicectomy is the treatment of choice. Laparoscopic appendicectomy, whilst more time consuming than conventional techniques, is associated with less postoperative pain and wound infection. Postoperative appendicitis presents a particular diagnostic problem and it is here that investigations such as ultrasonography are of particular value. Similarly, appendicitis in the immunosuppressed patient may be difficult to diagnose because of atypical presentation. However, it is reassuring to find that, overall, appendicitis in human immunodeficiency virus-infected patients presents in the same way as in immunocompetent patients, though the usual preoperative leucocytosis is absent and pyrexia is only low grade. A wish to avoid operation in these cases should be resisted; indeed a reported 44 per cent perforation rate indicates that operation should hastened, after confirmation by laparoscopy.

Appendix abscess

The incidence of appendix abscess is now much less than it used to be because of earlier diagnosis. When patients present with a 2- to 3-day history of appendicitis and a mass in found in the right iliac fossa, ultrasound examination should be undertaken. If an abscess is found it should be drained percutaneously. In the absence of persisting symptoms or recurrence of the abscess there is no need for interval appendicectomy. However, any residual mass should be investigated with colonoscopic examination of the caecum to ensure there is no underlying neoplasia.

Non-acute inflammation of the appendix

The days when chronic appendicitis, or so-called grumbling appendix, was an acceptable diagnosis have long since passed. Elective removal of the appendix for non-specific pain in the right iliac fossa is no longer acceptable, as most patients with these symptoms turn out to have the irritable bowel syndrome. On the other hand, chronic inflammation of the appendix resulting from obstruction of its base with consequent accumulation of mucus in the lumen and the development of a globular swelling is an undoubted entity and can present as a mucocele. Such patients complain of discomfort in the right iliac fossa and occasionally a mass may be felt. The true nature of the underlying condition can be revealed by ultrasound examination, which will show a distended appendix.

Carcinoid tumour (see Chapter 14.8)

Carcinoid tumour is often an incidental finding presenting either as a rounded nodule in the appendix or being revealed histologically after appendicectomy. Very few of them metastasize to regional lymph nodes. If they do so the treatment should be right hemicolectomy. A small proportion will go on to metastasize to the liver and develop carcinoid syndrome.

Adenocarcinoma

Adenocarcinoma of the appendix is well recognized but rare. Such tumours may present as acute appendicitis or may be an incidental finding at laparotomy. They can also present as a mass in the right iliac fossa. In my own experience the diagnosis resulted from investigation of a patient presenting with anaemia and the findings of a positive occult blood. Colonoscopy showed blood coming out of the appendicaecal lumen. The patient was treated by right hemicolectomy, which is accepted as being preferable to appendicectomy.

Other appendiceal tumours

Benign tumours of the appendix are rare. Leiomyoma, fibroma, neuroma, neurofibroma, and ganglioneuroma have all been described but are curiosities. Similarly, occasional rare malignancies have been described, such as sarcoma and a condition called malignant mucocele. The treatment of these lesions follows the general principles outlined above.

REFERENCES

Ashley, D.J.B. (1967). Observations on the epidemiology of appendicitis. *Gut*, **8**, 533–8.

Binderow, S.R. and Shakeed, A.A. (1991). Acute appendicitis in patients with AIDS/HIV infection. *American Journal of Surgery*, **162**, 9–12.

Burns, R.P., Cochran, J.C., Russell, W.L., and Bard, R.M. (1985). Appendicitis in mature patients. *Annals of Surgery*, **201**, 695–704.

Clifford, P.C., Chan, M., and Hewitt, D.J. (1986). The acute abdomen— management with microcomputer aid. *Annals of the Royal College of Surgeons of England*, **68**, 182–4.

Coder, D.M. and Olander, G.A. (1972). Granulomatous peritonitis caused by starch glove powder. *Archives of Surgery*, **105**, 83–6.

Crossley, I.R. and Williams, R. (1985). Spontaneous bacterial peritonitis. *Gut*, **26**, 325–31.

DeDombal, F.T., Leaper, D.J., Horrocks, J.C., Staniland, J.R., and McCann, A.P. (1974). Human and computer-aided diagnosis of abdominal pain: further report with emphasis on performance of clinicians. *British Medical Journal*, **1**, 376–80.

Dunning, P.G. and Goldman, M.D. (1991). The incidence and value of rectal examination in children with suspected appendicitis. *Annals of the Royal College of Surgeons of England*, **73**, 233–4.

Gazelle, G.S., Haaga, J.R., Stellato, T.A., Gauderer, M.W.L., and Plecha, D.T. (1991). Pelvic abscesses: CT-guided transrectal drainage. *Radiology*, **181**, 283–4.

Goletti, O. *et al.* (1993). Percutaneous ultrasound-guided drainage of intra-abdominal abscesses. *British Journal of Surgery*, **80**, 336–9.

Harland, R.N.L. (1991). Diagnosis of appendicitis in childhood. *Journal of the Royal College of Surgeons of Edinburgh*, **36**, 89–90.

Jones, P.F. (1976). Active observation in the management of acute abdominal pain in childhood. *British Medical Journal*, **2**, 551–3.

Lau, W.Y., Fan, S.T., Yiu, T.F., Chu, K.W., and Lee, J.M.H. (1985). Acute appendicitis in the elderly. *Surgery, gynaecology and Obstetrics*, **161**, 157–60.

McLean, A.D., Stonebridge, P.A., Bradbury, A.W., and Rainey, J.B. (1993). Time of presentation, time of operation and unnecessary appendicectomy. *British Medical Journal*, **306**, 307.

Mughal, M.M., Bancewicz, J., and Irving, M.H. (1986). 'Laparostomy': a technique for the management of intractable intraabdominal sepsis. *British Journal of Surgery*, **73**, 253–9.

Ooms, H.W.A., Kouman, R.K.J., Ho Kang You, P.J., and Puyalert, J.B.C.M. (1991). Ultrasonography in the diagnosis of acute appendicitis. *British Journal of Surgery*, **78**, 315–18.

Parsons, J., Gray, J., and Thorbarnson, B. (1970). Pseudomyxoma peritonei. *Archives of Surgery*, **101**, 545–9.

Pearson, R.H. (1988). Ultrasound for diagnosing appendicitis. *British Medical Journal*, **297**, 309–10.

Rasmussen, O.O. and Hoffman, J. (1991). Assessment of the reliability of the symptoms and signs of acute appendicitis. *Journal of the Royal College of Surgeons of Edinburgh*, **36**, 89–90.

Rubin, S.Z. and Martin, D.J. (1990). Ultrasonography in the management of possible appendicitis in childhood. *Journal of Paediatric Surgery*, **25**, 737–40.

Stewart, R.J., Gupta, R.K., Purdie, G.L., and Ibister, W.H. (1986). Fine-catheter aspiration cytology of peritoneal cavity improves decision-making about difficult cases of acute abdominal pain. *Lancet*, **ii**, 1414–15.

Tamir, I.L., Bongard, F.S., and Klein, S.R. (1990). Acute appendicitis in the pregnant patient. *American Journal of Surgery*, **160**, 571–5.

Tsuji, M., McMahon, G., Reen, D., and Puri, P. (1990). New insights into the pathogenesis of appendicitis based on immunocytochemical analysis of early immune response. *Journal of Paediatric Surgery*, **25**, 449–52.

Underwood, M.J., Thompson, M.M., Sayers, R.D., and Hall, A.W. (1992). Presentation of abdominal tuberculosis to general surgeons. *British Journal of Surgery*, **79**, 1077–9.

Williams, N. and Kapila, L. (1991). Acute appendicitis in the pre-school child. *Archives of Diseases in Childhood*, **66**, 1270–2.

14.20 Computed tomography and magnetic resonance imaging of the liver and pancreas

R. Dick

Computed tomography (**CT**) is used to image the solid organs of the abdomen (liver, pancreas) and has an increasing role in inflammatory and neoplastic disease of the oesophagus, stomach, and bowel (Fig. 1). It may also detect retroperitoneal tumours, abdominal lymphadenopathy, and intra-abdominal abscesses.

CT of the liver and biliary system

Because of its bulk and anatomical relations the liver is an organ well suited to CT diagnosis (Fig. 2). Abnormalities of size and shape are well demonstrated. In focal lesions, the attenuation number may point to the nature of the tissue (cyst, abscess, neoplasm), but it is the enhancement characteristics after contrast that may clinch the diagnosis, such as occurs with haemangiomas.

Most primary and metastatic neoplasms show diminished attenuation compared with normal tissue. Intravenous or intra-arterial contrast may highlight the difference, and in some patients lipiodol may have been given before CT, either to detect tumour or, when linked to a cytotoxic agent, to treat it (Fig. 3).

Cysts are well shown down to a diameter of 1.0 cm, their attenuation value being 0 to 20 Hounsfield units. Calcification not shown on plain films will be seen on CT, and infiltration of liver by fat or iron gives a dramatic change in liver density.

In established cirrhosis, contour irregularities and ascites are common, though the nature of the cirrhosis cannot be gauged. A dynamic enhanced scan may provide dramatic information in the presence of portal hypertension (Fig. 4).

Neither gallbladder calculi nor biliary-duct information are as reliably shown, as with ultrasound.

CT of the pancreas

Lying in the transverse axial plane, the pancreas is an organ well suited to CT, which is the best current method for showing pancreatic morphology (Fig. 5). It is particularly good for lesions in the pancreatic head, a site where ultrasound may have difficulty because of gas in adjacent hollow organs (Fig. 6).

Fig. 1 CT reveals extensive gastric carcinoma with extragastric spread into the omentum anteriorly.

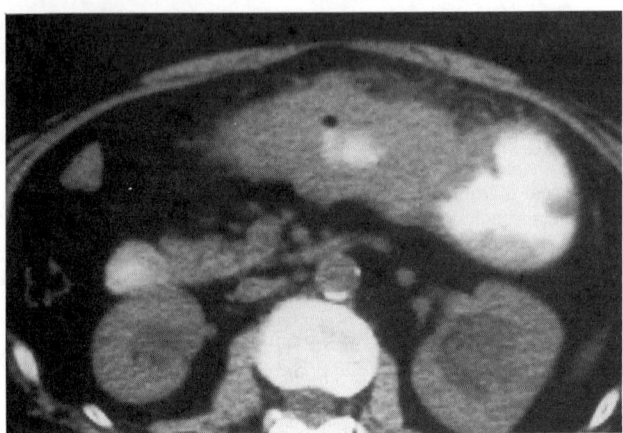

Fig. 2 CT, normal liver: the negative tubular structure at the porta hepatis in the portal vein; a contrast-enhanced scan is invariably required or disease will be missed.

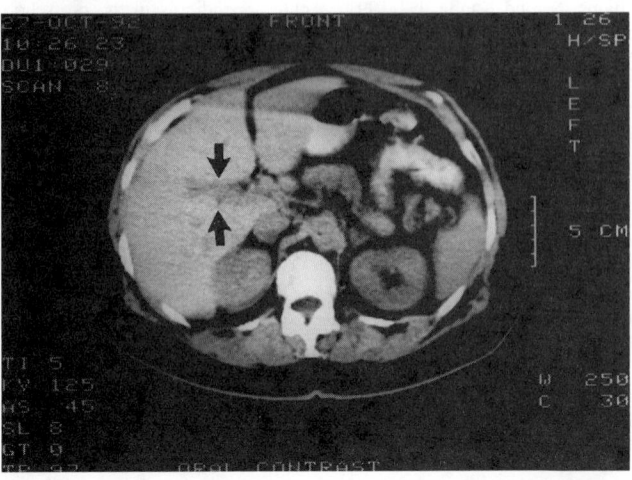

Fig. 3 CT/lipiodol outlines recurrent tumour in the left lobe of the liver (previous right hepatectomy for primary liver cancer).

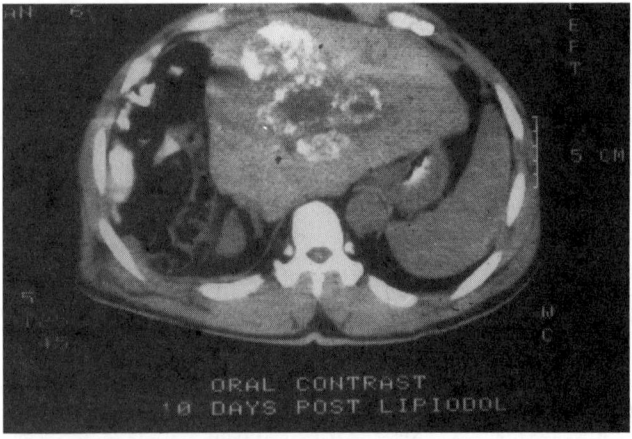

Fig. 4 Dynamic CT: portal vein thrombosis consequent to chronic pancreatitis.

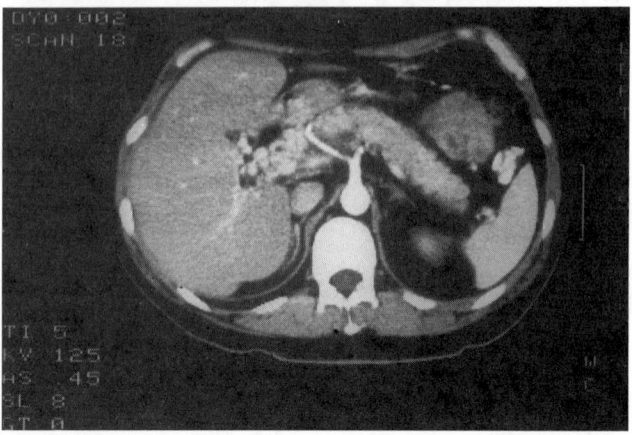

Scanning is done with the patient supine. The organ is well seen in most patients, as it is surrounded by a layer of retroperitoneal fat. One-centimetre cuts are obtained, and if the head of the pancreas is not clearly shown, CT may be repeated with the patient lying on the right side to allow the dilute oral contrast, given before scanning, to gravitate into the duodenal loop.

In acute pancreatitis there is general enlargement with loss of peripancreatic fat planes; in chronic pancreatitis (Fig. 7), calcification, cyst formation and dilatation of the main duct may be present, though the pancreas sometimes appears normal. Fine-needle aspiration or mini-Trucut biopsy of any pancreatic abnormality may safely be done with CT guidance.

Magnetic resonance imaging (MRI) of liver and pancreas

In many centres, MRI is used mainly to clarify problems not fully evaluated with CT and ultrasound, particularly if there is a conflict between their findings (Fig. 8). In the liver, the relation of tumours to vessels can be shown preoperatively, and MRI is advantageous (compared to CT) in allowing imaging in multiple planes. There are still problems of resolution where long breath-holds are required and if respiratory and cardiac 'gateing' are not employed.

Careful choice of sequences and variation of flip angles can aid in differential diagnosis, for example between haemangioma and metas-tasis; MR angiography is promising, though its spatial resolution is limited. The ultimate goal would be to obtain three-dimensional imaging of a tumour in relation to the intrahepatic vessels, biliary tree, and liver surface.

Good quality pancreatic imaging may be difficult. Oral superpara-magnetic iron oxide has been used to help pancreatic delineation by producing a negative signal from the adjacent stomach and upper small bowel.

REFERENCES

Brailsford, J., Ward, J., Chalmers, A.G., Ridgway, J. and Robinson, P.J. (1994). Dynamic MRI of the pancreas—Gadolinium enhancement in normal tissue. *Clinical Radiology*, **49**, 104–8.

Dixon, A.K. (1984). CT of the abdomen for general surgical problems. *Radiology Now*, **4**, 2–5.

Husband, J.E. and Fry, I.K. (1981). *Computer tomography of the body—a radiological and clinical approach.* Macmillan, London.

Saifuddin, A., Ward, J., Ridgway, J., and Chalmers, A.G. (1993). Comparison of MR and CT scanning in severe acute pancreatitis initial experiences. *Clinical Radiology*, **48**, 111–16.

Suramo, I., Paivansalo, M. and Pamilo, M. (1984). Unidentified liver metastases at ultrasonography or computed tomography. *Acta Radiologica et Diagnostica.* **5**, 385–9.

Ward, J., Martinez, D., Chalmers, A.G., Ridgway, J., Robinson, P.J. and Smith, M.A. (1993). Rapid dynamic contrast-enhanced magnetic resonance imaging of the liver and portal vein. *British Journal of Radiology*, **66**, 214–22.

Fig. 5 CT: normal head, body, and tail of pancreas; it is unusual to see all positions of the gland in one slice.

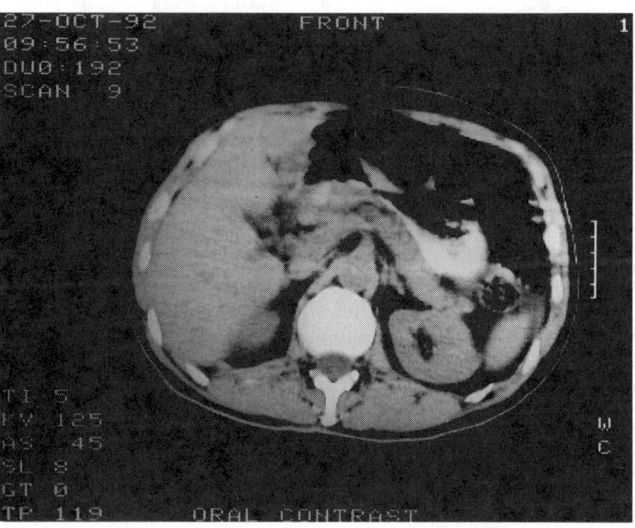

Fig. 6 CT reveals a mass in the pancreatic head; note biliary prosthesis in its centre. Percutaneous CT biopsy showed adenocarcinoma. Splenomegaly due to splenic vein encasement.

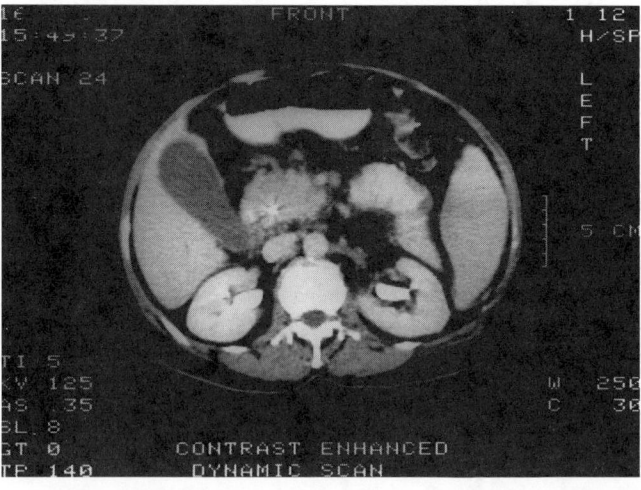

Fig. 7 CT in chronic pancreatitis; note dilated pancreatic duct and gland calcification.

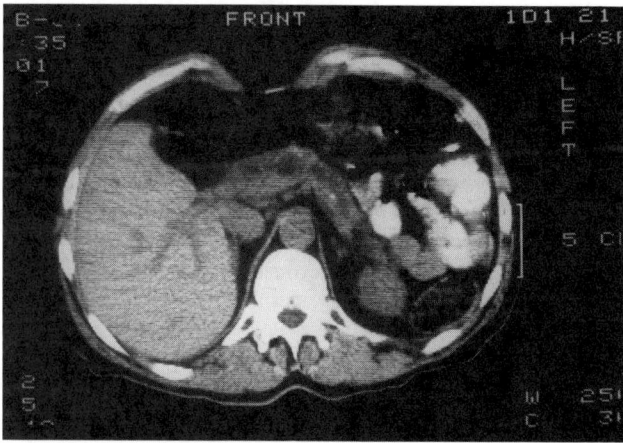

Fig. 8 MRI: recurrent fibrolamellar carcinoma of the left lobe of the liver extending through a diaphragmatic hiatus adjacent to the inferior vena cava. CT and ultrasound did not demonstrate this satisfactorily.

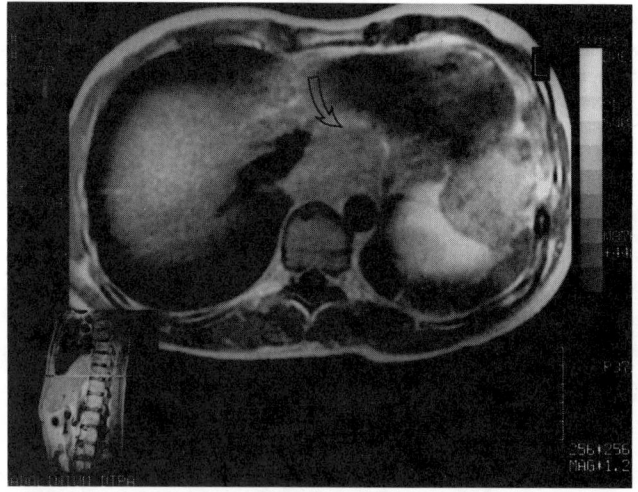

14.21 Congenital disorders of the biliary tract and pancreas

J. A. SUMMERFIELD

Congenital disorders of the biliary tract

PATHOGENESIS

During the fourth week of gestation the liver arises as a bud of cells (the hepatic diverticulum) from the ventral wall of the foregut. At about the eighth week of gestation a layer of liver precursor cells around the portal vein branches differentiate to form a sleeve, termed the ductal plate. This sleeve duplicates to form a double layer of cells, which by 12 weeks is remodelled by dilatation of segments of the double layered ductal plate to form tubules that become the intrahepatic bile ducts. Non-tubular parts of the plate disappear and the bile ducts form part of the portal tracts.

Congenital disorders of the biliary tract can be classified into two main groups: diseases characterized by inflammatory destruction of the bile ducts (the biliary atresias) and diseases marked by ectasia of the bile ducts with varying degrees of fibrosis (the fibropolycystic diseases). Both of these groups of disorders are related to the persistence or lack of remodelling of the embryonic ductal plate. They are termed 'ductal plate malformations'.

Ductal plate malformations can be seen on ultrasound or computerized tomographic (**CT**) scans as a circular lumen containing a fibrovascular cord. Figure 1 shows ductal plate malformations in a CT scan of a patient with Caroli's disease (a fibropolycystic disease).

Biliary atresia

CLASSIFICATION

Biliary atresias can be classified into extrahepatic and intrahepatic (paucity of intrahepatic bile ducts). Biliary atresia does not represent agenesis of the bile ducts but is the result of progressive bile-duct destruction from an inflammatory disease of unknown cause. In extrahepatic biliary atresia the destructive cholangitis affects not only part or all of the extra-hepatic bile duct but also intrahepatic bile ducts and leads to paucity of intrahepatic bile ducts. In intrahepatic biliary atresia the destructive cholangitis is restricted to the intrahepatic bile ducts. Intrahepatic biliary atresia can be classified further into those with a non-syndromatic and those with a syndromatic type (Alagille's syndrome or arteriohepatic dysplasia). About a quarter of patients with extrahepatic biliary atresia have evidence of ductal plate malformation, indicating that the destructive cholangitis started early in fetal life.

SYMPTOMS AND SIGNS

Biliary atresia presents as cholestatic jaundice starting after the first 2 weeks of life. The infant develops jaundice with pale stools, dark urine, and hepatomegaly. Itching is often prominent. Bile pigments may stain the growing teeth greenish. The jaundice steadily deepens and xanthomas of the palm and knees, rickets, a bleeding tendency and growth failure may develop. Biliary atresia may eventually cause biliary cirrhosis with pigmentation (due to melanin), portal hypertension, ascites, and liver failure.

The progress of biliary atresia depends on the type. Infants with extrahepatic biliary atresia (usually girls) have a steadily deepening jaundice and biliary cirrhosis soon develops. Untreated, these children usually die by 6 months. The fate of infants with intrahepatic biliary atresia depends on whether it is syndromatic or non-syndromatic. Children with non-syndromatic intrahepatic biliary atresia survive longer than those with extrahepatic biliary atresia but biliary cirrhosis eventually develops in later childhood. In contrast, patients with syndromatic intrahepatic biliary atresia (Alagille's syndrome) tend to recover normal liver function as they become adolescent. Infants with Alagille's syndrome can be recognized by the associated features, which include a characteristic facies (a flattened and triangular face), pulmonary stenosis, vertebral abnormalities, and a change in the eyes (embryotoxon). Some have growth and mental retardation.

DIFFERENTIAL DIAGNOSIS

Jaundice is common in early infancy. In the early neonatal period, jaundice is usually due to haemolysis and impaired bilirubin conjugation. After 2 weeks, jaundice is usually cholestatic. There are many causes of cholestasis in infancy and childhood. The most common are extrahepatic and intrahepatic biliary atresias, neonatal hepatitis (e.g. hepatitis A, B, and C, rubella, and cytomegalovirus infection), metabolic causes (e.g. galactosaemia, α_1-antitrypsin deficiency, and tyrosinaemia) and the 'inspissated bile syndrome' (e.g. congenital spherocytosis).

LABORATORY INVESTIGATIONS

Liver function tests show a cholestatic (biliary obstructive) pattern. The serum bilirubin and alkaline phosphatase are markedly raised, with only modest elevations of serum transaminases. Later very high concentrations of serum cholesterol may develop.

Histological examination of the liver cannot distinguish between intrahepatic and extrahepatic biliary atresia. Liver biopsy shows severe centrizonal cholestasis and a prominent giant-cell reaction. In the portal tracts, bile ducts are reduced. Later in the course of the disease the portal tracts are devoid of bile ducts and biliary cirrhosis is present.

Fig. 1 Caroli's disease: intravenous contrast-enhanced CT scan of the liver shows dilated intrahepatic bile ducts containing filling defects which are portal vein branches (arrowed); this is an example of a ductal plate malformation (reproduced from Sherlock, S. and Summerfield, J.A. (1991) with permission).

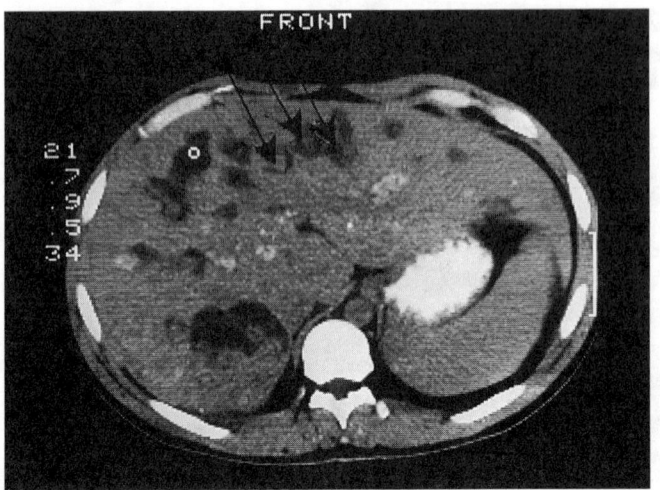

IMAGING

The initial step in the management of cholestatic infants is to differentiate between intrahepatic and extrahepatic biliary atresia. Because the clinical and laboratory findings are similar this distinction requires imaging techniques. In extrahepatic biliary atresia, scintiscanning with ^{99}Tc^{m}-labelled HIDA (dimethyl acetanilide iminodiacetic acid) (see Section 14.3) shows accumulation of the label in the liver but none enters the biliary tree. Percutaneous and endoscopic cholangiography provide more precise anatomical detail.

TREATMENT AND PROGNOSIS

General supportive measures include parenteral administration of fat-soluble vitamins A, D, K, and E. Medium-chain triglycerides, as a source of fat, cholestyramine to relieve itching, and ursodeoxycholic acid, as a choleretic, help some patients.

Extrahepatic biliary atresia

Hepatic portoenterostomy (Kasai's operation) has been the treatment of choice for extrahepatic biliary atresia and is still widely used. However, long-term follow-up of patients submitted to this bilioenteric reconstruction has shown that it does not cure most patients. About 80 per cent will require liver transplantation at a later date. At present it appears reasonable to continue to submit these infants to the Kasai operation because children under 1 year have a relatively low survival rate after liver transplantation and because appropriate organ donors for this age group are rare.

Intrahepatic biliary atresia

All infants should receive general supportive measures. Definitive treatment depends on the type of intrahepatic biliary atresia. Non-syndromatic atresia eventually progresses to biliary cirrhosis and liver failure. Liver transplantation should be done before the onset of failure. Syndromatic atresia (Alagille's syndrome) has a good prognosis in most children and few develop biliary cirrhosis. General supportive measures are usually sufficient until the cholestasis disappears.

Fibropolycystic disease

Fibropolycystic disease encompasses a family of rare congenital hepatobiliary diseases that arise from malformations of the embryonic ductal plate. These diseases include fibropolycystic disease (polycystic liver), congenital hepatic fibrosis, congenital intrahepatic biliary dilatation (Caroli's disease), choledochal cysts, and microhamartomas (von Meyenberg complexes). Many patients will have more than one disease. The combination of congenital hepatic fibrosis and Caroli's disease is characteristic, as these patients develop first variceal haemorrhage (due to congenital hepatic fibrosis) and later recurrent cholangitis (due to Caroli's disease). Associated kidney defects are common. Malignant change may complicate congenital hepatic fibrosis, Caroli's disease, choledochal cysts, and microhamartomas. These diseases are of widely differing severity and the prognosis in an individual patient is determined by the fibropolycystic diseases present.

POLYCYSTIC LIVER DISEASE

The infantile type is inherited as an autosomal recessive and is usually rapidly fatal because of the associated renal disease. Adult polycystic liver disease is more common and has a dominant inheritance. The patient is usually a woman presenting in the fourth or fifth decade. The liver contains many thin-walled cysts filled with a clear or brownish liquid (altered blood). The cysts vary in size from a pinhead to about 10 cm in diameter. The remainder of the liver is normal. Patients present with right upper quadrant pain and increasing girth. Examination reveals an enlarged liver as the cause of the upper abdominal swelling. Liver function tests are normal. Provided no other fibropolycystic diseases are present, polycystic liver disease is benign. Some patients with polycystic liver disease also have polycystic kidneys or nephrocalcinosis. (see Section 20). The associated renal disease may cause serious complications including renal failure. The diagnosis can be confirmed by ultrasonography or CT scanning, which show numerous thin-walled cysts of low density (Fig. 2). The enlarged polycystic liver causes some patients considerable discomfort. It is best treated by percutaneous aspiration of the larger cysts using ultrasound guidance in order to reduce liver size. Percutaneous aspiration can be done repeatedly.

CONGENITAL HEPATIC FIBROSIS

This is a rare autosomal recessive condition that is usually diagnosed before 10 years of age. The main complication is portal hypertension. Children present with a large very hard liver and splenomegaly or bleeding from oesophageal varices. Congenital hepatic fibrosis may be misdiagnosed as cirrhosis. Liver function tests are normal or only slightly deranged. Ultrasound scans show the liver contains many bright areas due to the dense bands of fibrous tissue. The diagnosis is made by liver biopsy, which shows a normal parenchyma surrounded by fibrous septa containing bile duct-like structures.

Patients with congenital hepatic fibrosis bleed repeatedly from oesophageal varices but because liver function is well preserved they do not develop portosystemic encephalopathy. Portocaval shunts will stop the variceal bleeding and are well tolerated. Liver transplantation has also been used successfully.

The long-term prognosis in congenital hepatic fibrosis is usually determined by the associated renal disease. Renal lesions include renal dysplasia, medullary cystic disease, and infantile-or adult-type polycystic kidneys. The kidneys are rarely normal and renal failure eventually develops in many patients. However, renal transplants have been successful.

CONGENITAL INTRAHEPATIC BILIARY DILATATION (CAROLI'S SYNDROME)

In Caroli's syndrome the common bile duct is normal but the intrahepatic ducts have bulbous dilatations with normal ducts between (Fig. 3). The mode of inheritance is unknown. While the cystic dilatations of the bile ducts remain uninfected the patient is symptom free. Eventually ascending infection leads to cholangitis, which can be intractable, with the formation of gallstones and liver abscesses. Caroli's syndrome usually presents in early adulthood as cholangitis. Most patients are male. Liver function tests are cholestatic with elevations of serum bilirubin and alkaline phosphatase and modest elevations of the transaminases. The diagnosis is made by endoscopic cholangiography. CT scans can also demonstrate the syndrome (see Fig. 1). The natural history of Caroli's disease is of recurrent cholangitis that is very resistant to antibiotics. Biliary cirrhosis eventually develops. Bile-duct cancer develops in about 10 per cent. Treatment is difficult; antibiotics are usually only

Fig. 2 Polycystic liver disease: CT scanning shows the liver contains many cysts of low density indicating that they are fluid filled (reproduced from Sherlock, S. and Summerfield, J.A. (1991) with permission).

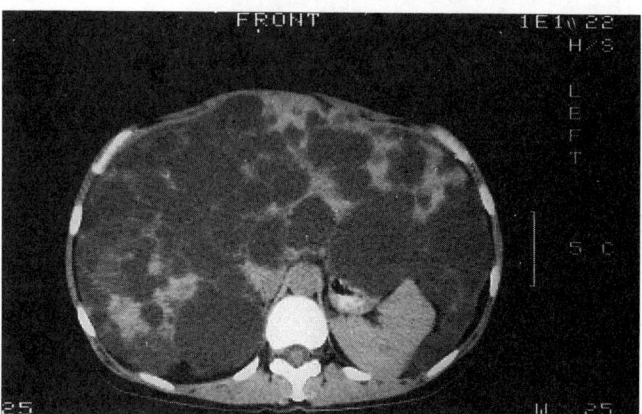

partially effective and liver transplantation is compromised by the extensive sepsis.

About half the patients with congenital hepatic fibrosis or Caroli's disease will also have the other disease. The clinical presentation in these patients is distinctive. As in Caroli's disease, males predominate. The first complication is variceal haemorrhage, followed about 10 years later by recurrent cholangitis.

CHOLEDOCHAL CYST

Choledochal cyst is a congenital dilatation of part or whole of the common bile duct (Fig. 4). It is more common in girls and usually presents in childhood but may appear in early adulthood. Choledochal cysts classically cause a triad of intermittent pain, jaundice, and a right hypochondrial mass. They are particularly common in Japanese and Chinese. Liver function tests are cholestatic, similar to Caroli's disease. Ultrasound and CT scans show cystic dilatation of the bile duct. The diagnosis is made by endoscopic or percutaneous cholangiography. Choledochal cysts should be treated by surgical excision because of the risk of bile-duct malignancy. Caroli's disease is a common associated disease.

Fig. 3 Caroli's disease: an endoscopic cholangiogram shows bulbous dilatations of the intrahepatic bile ducts; the rest of the biliary tree is normal (reproduced from Sherlock, S. and Summerfield, J.A. (1991) with permission).

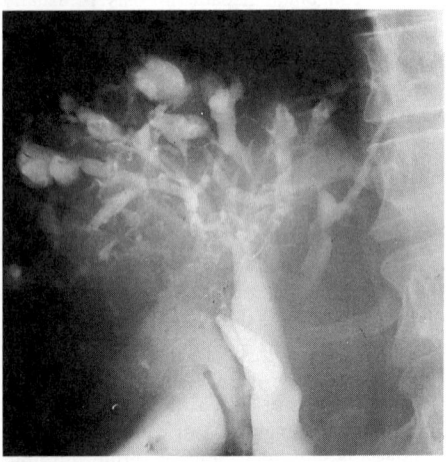

Fig. 4 Choledochal cyst in a 20-year-old woman: the endoscopic cholangiogram shows a massively dilated common bile duct; the gallbladder was normal but obscured by the dilated bile duct (reproduced from Sherlock, S. and Summerfield, J.A. (1991) with permission).

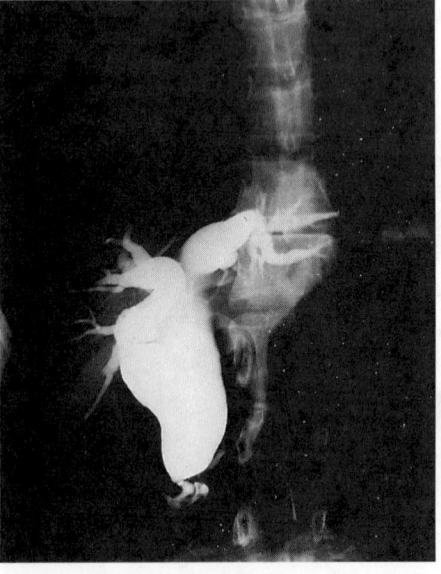

MICROHAMARTOMAS (VON MEYENBERG COMPLEXES)

Microhamartomas are groups of rounded biliary channels embedded in a collagen stroma located around portal tracts. The appearances are of localized islands of congenital hepatic fibrosis. Microhamartomas are usually asymptomatic and discovered incidentally on liver biopsy. They may be associated with other fibropolycystic diseases and are a rare cause of portal hypertension. Bile-duct and pancreatic cancers are more common in these patients.

Congenital disorders of the pancreas

AGENESIS OF THE PANCREAS

Pancreatic agenesis is rare and may occur as an isolated anomaly or be associated with other defects. These children usually die soon after birth. Agenesis of either the dorsal or ventral pancreas may also occur, although agenesis usually involves the dorsal segment.

ANNULAR PANCREAS (SEE CHAPTER 14.23.2)

This is a rare condition where pancreatic tissue encircles the descending duodenum. It results from persistence of part of the ventral pancreas during embryonic development. Annular pancreas is the most common cause of duodenal obstruction in infancy and often involves growth of pancreatic tissue into the duodenal wall. However, the clinical presentation is variable and annular pancreas may first present as an incidental finding at surgery or autopsy.

PANCREAS DIVISUM (SEE CHAPTER 14.23.2)

Pancreas divisum results from failure of fusion of the ducts of the dorsal and ventral portions of the pancreas. The body and tail of the pancreas drain through the narrow duct of Santorini into the accessory papilla. Only the head of the pancreas drains into the ampulla of Vater (Fig. 5). This is the most common congenital abnormality of the pancreas, occurring in about 5 per cent of patients. Pancreas divisum appears to be associated with an increased incidence of pancreatitis affecting the body and tail of the pancreas, which drains into the accessory papilla. Endoscopic sphincterotomy of the accessory papilla is reported to lead to clinical improvement in this type of pancreatitis.

HEREDITARY PANCREATITIS (SEE ALSO CHAPTER 14.22)

This rare form of pancreatitis is inherited as an autosomal dominant. Recurrent attacks of abdominal pain start in childhood or the second decade. Hereditary pancreatitis tends to be troublesome rather than life-threatening and attacks become less severe as the patient gets older. They often disappear by middle life.

Fig. 5 Pancreas divisum: an endoscopic pancreatogram following injection of contrast medium into the ampulla of Vater shows only the ducts of the head of the pancreas, characterized by a trefoil pattern; the body and tail of the pancreas drain via the accessory ampulla.

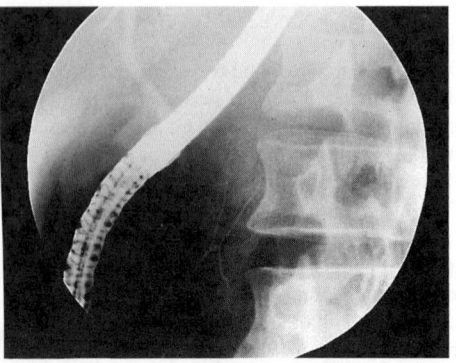

Other rare abnormalities causing pancreatic disease

Congenital abnormalities adjacent to the pancreas are rare causes of pancreatitis. These include duodenal diverticulum, duplication of the duodenum, stenosis of the sphincter of Oddi, and choledochal cyst. These abnormalities seem to cause pancreatitis by obstructing the pancreatic duct.

REFERENCES

Desmet, V.J. (1992). Congenital diseases of intrahepatic bile ducts: variations on the theme 'ductal plate malformation'. *Hepatology*, **16,** 1069–83.

Laurent J. *et al.* (1990). Long-term outcome after surgery for biliary atresia: study of 40 patients surviving more than 10 years. *Gastroenterology*, **99,** 1793–7.

Misiewicz, J.J., Pounder, R.E., and Venables, C.W. (1994). *Diseases of the gut and pancreas*. 2nd edn. Blackwell Scientific, Oxford.

Sherlock, S. (1992). *Diseases of the liver and biliary system*, (9th edn). Blackwell Scientific, Oxford.

Sherlock, S. and Summerfield, J.A. (1991). *A colour atlas of liver disease*, (2nd edn). Wolfe Medical, London.

Summerfield, J.A., Nagafuchi, Y., Sherlock, S., Cadafalch, J., and Scheuer, P.J. (1986). Hepatobiliary fibropolycystic diseases; a clinical and histological review of 51 patients. *Journal of Hepatology*, **2,** 141–56.

14.22 Hereditary disease of the liver and pancreas

C. A. SEYMOUR

INTRODUCTION

Because its blood supply comes from both arterial and portal venous circulations, the liver is well adapted to the central part it plays in many metabolic processes. It is therefore not surprising that congenital and acquired metabolic defects may affect its structure and function, regardless of whether they originate in the liver or elsewhere.

This chapter will focus on inherited metabolic disorders arising in the liver and pancreas. Although the liver is often involved in inborn errors of metabolism and may be the main site for accumulated materials, trace metals, glycogen or lipid for example, only a few of them cause permanent liver damage. They can be divided into those that damage parenchymal cells and those that affect biliary canalicular cells, which may also secondarily affect parenchymal-cell function. Emphasis will be placed on conditions presenting in adult life; the liver has such regenerative capacity that if cellular components are damaged sequentially rather than globally, some inherited disorders affecting the liver may not be diagnosed until adolescence or later, often presenting with hepatomegaly (Table 1). These disorders, some of which are described in other chapters, are summarized in Tables 1 and 2.

With any metabolic liver disease, early diagnosis is important if cirrhosis is to be prevented. Until recently, this meant diagnosis after birth and thus treatment was directed towards limiting and preventing further damage. However, with advances in understanding of the genetic basis of inherited diseases and the mechanisms of cellular damage, it is now possible to diagnose some of these conditions, glycogen storage disease and cystic fibrosis for example, *in utero* by amniocentesis, and genetic counselling of patients and their families can be expected to change our approach to the management of these diseases. For example, an affected individual (index case) acts as an effective 'biopsy' for a family at risk of inherited disease, and other members of the family can be screened to detect carriers of the gene (see Section 4).

In diagnosing and following up hepatic disorders, physicians need to work closely with other specialists such as paediatricians and clinical geneticists, as well as with obstetricians involved in prenatal diagnosis. Not every hospital will have access to these facilities, and it is therefore important to suspect these relatively uncommon conditions, regardless of the age of the patient, and, where appropriate, to link with or refer to other specialists.

General approach to metabolic disease affecting the liver

Metabolic abnormalities may originate in, or secondarily affect, hepatic function (Fig. 1). It is important in assessing a patient with suspected inherited liver disease, primary or secondary, to know what weight to place on the history and physical signs before using the 'technology' that is now increasingly available both for initial diagnosis and for monitoring progress and treatment.

EVALUATION OF HISTORY IN HEPATIC METABOLIC DISORDERS

The clinical history, including a family history, is important in diagnosis and evaluation of suspected metabolic liver disease. The identification of general pointers to liver abnormality is as important as specific diagnostic features, because otherwise secondary problems arising in other organs may be missed, portal hypertension for example (see Chapter 14.29), where shunting of blood containing toxic material normally degraded by the liver can affect the kidneys and brain; such patients could present with renal, neurological, or psychiatric symptoms. In addition, an individual with compensated liver damage and established cirrhosis may become decompensated by dehydration, intercurrent infection, or drugs.

Often important features of the patient's medical history, particularly transient jaundice at birth or during childhood, may have been missed but may be an important factor in the diagnosis of the cause of liver damage—haemolysis in Wilson's disease for example (see Section 22). It is well known that the neonatal and childhood liver has a remarkable capacity for regeneration and recovery from transient damage. Similarly, a detailed family history is essential in the diagnosis of inherited disorders and may lead to the diagnosis of unsuspected disease in presymptomatic individuals. Common symptoms and signs of increasing liver dysfunction and disease are outlined in Table 3.

INVESTIGATION OF LIVER DISEASE

Biochemical investigations play a major part in the diagnosis of liver disease, alone or in combination with other, more invasive, investigations. Specific biochemical investigations for inborn errors of metabolism are outlined in Table 4. It is important to distinguish between those that are indicators of liver-cell damage and those that reflect changes in functional liver-cell mass (Table 4). With increasing understanding of subcellular anatomy and of alterations in intracellular organelles it is now possible to recognize specific organelles or enzyme-system abnormalities in metabolic liver disease, for example lysosomes in glycogen storage diseases, mitochondria in Wilson's disease and lipid disorders; and peroxisomes in Zellweger's and Reye's syndromes.

Table 1 *Inherited metabolic disorders affecting liver (presenting in childhood and adult life)*

Disorder	Clinical features	Defect/deficiency	Genetic type	Diagnosis (tissue enzyme assay)
Iron and porphyrin metabolism				
Primary haemochromatosis	Pigmentation, multisystem disease, enlarged liver/spleen, diabetes, and arthropathy	Absorptive abnormality of intestine to iron (? ferritin, ? non-transferrin bound iron abnormality)	AR	HLA -A3, -B7, -B14 (chromosome 6) Liver biopsy—iron, serum ferritin
Porphyria cutanea tarda	Skin light sensitivity, and enlarged liver	Uroporphyrinogen decarboxylase:		
	Personality change	familial	AD	(a) RBC, urine/faecal porphyrins
		liver	AD	(b) Liver iron content
Copper metabolism				
Primary copper toxicosis:				
Wilson's disease	Haemolytic anaemia	Chromosome 13 defect	AR	Plasma caeruloplasmin
	Hepatic presentation including hepatic failure	↓ Biliary copper excretion ↓ Plasma caeruloplasmin		Serum copper, urine copper Liver biopsy—copper
	Neurological syndromes (Parkinson's disease)	Biliary duct damage		
Secondary copper toxicosis:				
Indian childhood cirrhosis	Insidious onset, Indians predisposed Anorexia, jaundice, hepatomegaly	Increased copper in diet	(AR)	Liver copper/Mallory's hyaline
Primary biliary cirrhosis	Jaundice, skin pigmentation, pruritus, enlarged liver/spleen	Immune damage to bile ducts (antibodies to M2 antigen)		Liver histology Antimitochondrial antibody (E$_2$ antigen)
Storage diseases				
α$_1$-Antitrypsin deficiency	Emphysema Liver disease—cirrhosis (neonatal hepatitis, childhood cirrhosis)	α$_1$-Antitrypsin (Pi ZZ, chromosome 4)	AD	Serum phenotypes Pi ZZ (chromosome 4) Liver accumulation of α$_1$-antitrypsin
Cholestatic syndromes				
Inherited:				
Cystic fibrosis of liver	Lung, pancreas, liver abnormality	CFTR protein abnormality	AR	Raised sweat sodium In neonates, increased immunoreactive trypsin
Hepatic cystic fibrosis Congenital biliary tract Abnormalities: Biliary atresia Congenital hepatic fibrosis Focal intrahepatic biliary dilatation (Caroli's disease)				
Acquired:				
Primary biliary cirrhosis (autoimmune)	See 'Secondary copper toxicosis'	See 'Secondary copper toxicosis'		See 'Secondary copper toxicosis'
Secondary biliary cirrhosis: Secondary to biliary tract surgery Sclerosing cholangitis Cystic fibrosis				
Reye's syndrome				
In childhood	Rare, acute, fatal encephalopathy → death	Mitochondrial abnormality		Liver E/M abnormal mitochondria
Aspirin induced	History of viral infection Aspirin ingestion			Reduction in mitochondrial enzymes

AD, autosomal dominant; AR, autosomal recessive; CFTR, cystic fibrosis transmembrane regulator protein; RBC, red blood cell.

Table 2 *Inherited metabolic disorders resulting in liver damage (presenting in childhood)*

Disorder	Clinical features	Defect/deficiency	Genetic type	Diagnosis (tissue enzyme assay)
Carbohydrate metabolism				
Diabetes mellitus	Fatty infiltration of liver, liver cirrhosis and gallstones	Insulin dependent (IDDM)		Fasting blood glucose, ultrasound, fatty change, liver biopsy
		Non-insulin dependent (NIDDM)		Postprandial glucose, glucose tolerance test, liver biopsy
Glycogen storage disease (types I–XII)	Fasting hypoglycaemia, hyperlipidaemia, Massive hepatomegaly, bleeding, gout	Enzymes in glycogen/glycolytic cycles	AR	Types I, VI–X—liver Types III–IV—leucocyte
Galactosaemia	Growth/mental retardation, liver disease Cataracts, bleeding tendency	Galactose I-P uridyl transferase	AR	RBC, galactosuria
Hereditary fructose intolerance	Benign, vomiting, diet-induced hypoglycaemia Hepatomegaly, liver disease, hyperuricaemia	Fructose I-P aldolase	AR	Small-intestine mucosal biopsy Liver biopsy
Complex carbohydrate metabolism				
Mucopolysaccharidoses	Cloudy cornea	α-+L-iduronidase	AR	Leucocytes
	Mental retardation	N-acetyl β-glucosaminidase	AR	Fibroblasts
Mucolipidoses	Corneal lesions, hepatosplenomegaly	Aryl sulphatase	AR	
Lysosomal storage diseases	Mild dementia, cardiomegaly	α-mannosidase	AR	Sweat with high [Na]
		α-fucosidase	AR	Fibroblasts
Protein metabolism				
Tyrosinaemia	Progressive hepatocellular damage Hypophosphataemia	Fumaryl acetoacetate hydrolase	AR	Plasma amino acids Excess urine succinyl acetone
Urea-cycle disorders (six different disorders)	CNS abnormalities Hepatomegaly	Partial deficiency of enzymes converting ammonia to urea. Ornithine transcarbamylase	AR X-linked	Serum ammonia Specific urine amino acid
Lipid metabolism				
Gangliosidoses:	Dementia, bone/joint abnormalities Mental/motor retardation	Hexosaminidase A + B β-galactosidase	AR	Serum, fibroblasts Leucocytes, fibroblasts
Gaucher's disease	Splenohepatomegaly Bone, skin, lung infiltration, skin pigmentation	Glucosyl ceramide β-glycosidase	AR	Serum, leucocyte enzyme
Sphingomyelin storage disease:				
Niemann–Pick disease	A—Hepatosplenomegaly, first 6 months of life Vomiting, death under 14–30 months	Sphingomyelinase	AR	A—Fibroblast
	B—Growth retardation, liver/spleen			B—Fibroblast
	C—Lung involvement			C—Fibroblast enzyme deficient Liver enzyme normal
Cholesterol ester hydrolase deficiency:				
Wolman's disease	Cirrhosis, diffuse adrenal calcification	Lysosomal acid lipase	AR	Liver tissue—cholesterol ester
Cholesterol storage disease	Liver/spleen, death by 6 months Enlarged liver, hepatic fibrosis	Lysosomal acid lipase	AR	Peripheral blood lymphocytes

Table 2 (*cont.*)

Disorder	Clinical features	Defect/deficiency	Genetic type	Diagnosis (tissue enzyme assay)
Familial hyperlipoproteinemia:				
Hypercholesterolaemia	Xanthelasma/xanthomata Coronary artery disease, atherosclerosis	II—LDL receptor defects	AD	Fibroblast
Hypertriglyceridaemia	Eruptive skin xanthomata, abdominal pain, pancreatitis, lipaemia retinalis	I—Lipoprotein lipase IV V	AR AD AD	I—Chylomicrons IV—VLDL V—VLDL and chylomicrons
Zellweger's syndrome	Mental retardation, liver fibrosis Multiple congenital abnormalities Renal cysts, retinal degeneration, deafness	Absent peroxisomes and defective peroxisomal enzymes	AR	Prenatal chorionic villus biopsy Defect in C29 bile acids

AD, autosomal dominant; AR, autosomal recessive; LDL, low-density lipoprotein; VLDL, very low-density lipoprotein.

Inherited metabolic disease affecting the liver

Tables 1 and 2 summarize some of the main clinical features of diagnostic tests for inherited metabolic diseases. In all but the cholestatic syndromes, damage is likely to involve hepatocytes, and only in the later stages of disease to affect biliary cells as the cirrhotic process progresses. Certain diseases (Table 1) are therefore singled out because they are often not detected until early adulthood. In addition, some (e.g. cystic fibrosis) are 'new' entities, arising because patients with these genetic disorders are living longer.

Inherited diseases of trace-metal toxicity are good models for the acquired trace-metal toxic disorders. Most common are haemochromatosis (iron toxicosis) and Wilson's disease (copper toxicosis), both of which occur in hereditary and secondary forms.

HAEMOCHROMATOSIS (SEE ALSO SECTION 22)

This term refers to a group of conditions in which iron in the body is increased and is deposited in and damages the parenchyma of various organs. It is therefore a multisystem disease. In the primary form, idiopathic haemochromatosis, iron overloading of liver is a major feature, determined by a gene situated on the long arm of chromosome 6 near

Fig. 1 Clinical approach to metabolic liver disease.

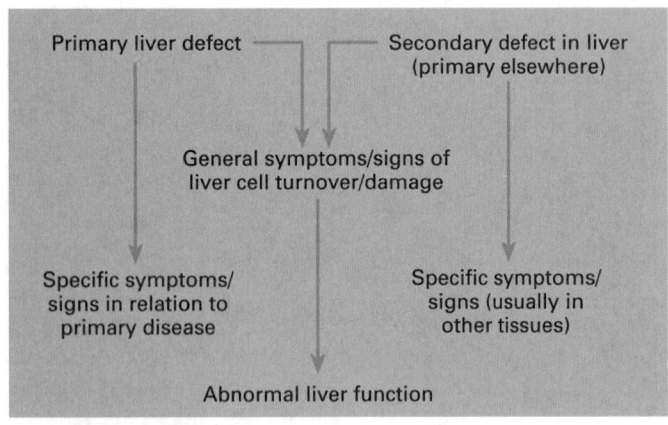

the *A* locus of the HLA system. Secondary forms of iron overload, such as occur with iron-loading anaemias, and which are described in Section 22, present with similar features as far as the liver involvement is concerned.

Clinical features

Primary haemochromatosis is described in Section 22. Hepatomegaly in association with diabetes, skin pigmentation, cardiomyopathy, and joint disease is the typical presentation. Hepatomegaly occurs in 75 to 95 per cent of patients, often predominantly with an increase in size of the left lobe of the liver, which may be palpable in the epigastrium. In the early stages, it is rarely associated with clinical symptoms or signs of hepatic dysfunction, probably because damage to parenchymal cells is insidious, and liver enzyme tests are often normal when the patient first presents. A major complication is the development of hepatocellular carcinoma in association with cirrhosis and iron overload.

Secondary haemochromatosis

In this form of hepatic iron toxicosis, hepatic fibrosis develops within the first decade. The most common cause is thalassaemia major, and, as discussed in Section 22, other systems are involved, with failure to develop secondary sexual characteristics and increasing iron damage to the heart.

Hepatic pathology

In primary haemochromatosis, the diagnosis is made on liver biopsy; parenchymal iron loading is found in conjunction with cirrhosis and is demonstrable by blue staining of iron granules with Perl's reagent (potassium ferricyanide). Any therapy that reduces or depletes the iron stores will often leave lipofuscin granules ('wear and tear' pigment), which do not stain for iron. In secondary haemochromatosis, iron granules may be more prominent in reticuloendothelial cells.

Initial investigations

Iron overload can be detected by indirect and direct methods. Indirect methods include measurement of serum iron concentrations, which are increased, in genetic haemochromatosis, to values in excess of 36 μmol/l, increased transferrin saturation, and increased serum ferritin concentrations, which correlate with iron overload in both forms of haemochromatosis. Liver enzymes and function tests may be normal or show slightly increased transaminase (alanine, aspartate) activities suggestive of increased hepatocyte turnover. Acute or chronic

Table 3 *Symptoms and signs associated with liver disease*

Symptoms		Signs		
General	Specific	General	Specific	Disease association
Anorexia	Polyuria/polydypsia (diabetes)	Skin stigmata	Palmar erythema	Cirrhosis
Weight loss	Pruritus (biliary disease)	Bruising/purpura	Spider naevi	Chronic liver disease
Nausea, vomiting	Abdominal swelling, ascites	Clubbing	Leuconychia	
Diarrhoea	(cirrhosis)	Oedema	Splenomegaly	Storage disease
Abdominal	Steatorrhoea (fat malabsorption,	Ascites		Portal hypertension
discomfort	biliary disease)	Hepatomegaly	Skin xanthelasma	Primary biliary cirrhosis
Bleeding tendency	Reversal of sleep rhythm	Splenomegaly		Familial
Epilepsy	(precoma)	Parotid gland		hypercholesterolaemia
	Asterixis	enlargement	Eye: Kayser-Fleischer	Wilson's disease
			ring	
			Pigmentation	Haemochromatosis
				Alcohol cirrhosis

Table 4 *Biochemical tests of liver function*

(a) General indicators of liver function

Blood glucose (glycogen stores)
Urea synthesis
Clotting factors (II, V, VIII, X)
Albumin, globulins
Lipoprotein — cholesterol
Vitamin B_{12} (store)

(b) Markers of liver disease

General markers			Specific markers	
	Cell type		*Serum proteins*	
			Caeruloplasmin	$\downarrow$ in Wilson's disease
Test	Hepatocyte	Biliary tract		$\uparrow$ cholestatic syndromes
			α-antitrypsin:	$\downarrow$ specific forms in α_1-antitrypsin deficiency
AST, ALT	$\uparrow - \uparrow\uparrow$	$N - \uparrow\uparrow$	Ferritin:	$\uparrow$ in primary
Alkaline phosphatase	$N - \uparrow$	$\uparrow\uparrow - \uparrow\uparrow\uparrow$		haemochromatosis
γ-Glutamyl transferase	$N - \uparrow$	$\uparrow\uparrow - \uparrow\uparrow\uparrow$		
	$\uparrow - \uparrow\uparrow$ (alcohol)		*Fetal proteins*	
Albumin	$\downarrow$	N	α-fetoprotein	$\uparrow$ in hepatocellular carcinoma
Prothrombin time	Prolonged	N		
Bilirubin	$N - \uparrow$	$\uparrow - \uparrow\uparrow$	Carcinoembryonic	$\uparrow$ in hepatocellular
Bile salts	N	$\uparrow\uparrow$	antigen:	carcinoma
Immunoglobulins				Present with secondary
IgG	$\uparrow$ (chronic liver disease)			metastases in the liver
IgA	$\uparrow$ (alcoholic liver disease)	$N - \uparrow$ (sclerosing cholangitis)	*Antibody tests*	(*Positive in*)
IgM	$\uparrow$ (acute liver disease)	$N - \uparrow$ (primary biliary	Hepatitis IgM/IgG:	hepatitis A
		cirrhosis)	Hep Bs Ag:	hepatitis B
			Hep Bc Ag:	
			Hep Bc Ab:	
			Hep C IgG:	hepatitis C
			Specific antibodies:	CMV, HIV
				Herpes simplex
				Epstein-Barr virus
			Autoantibody	
			Smooth muscle:	chronic active hepatitis
			Mitochondrial Ab	primary biliary cirrhosis
			(E_2):	

ALT, alanine transaminase; AST, aspartate transaminase; CMV, cytomegalovirus; HIV, human immunodeficiency virus; N, normal; $\uparrow$ increased, $\downarrow$ reduced.
Ag, antigen; Ab, antibody

liver dysfunction may lead to a further increase in the serum iron and ferritin.

Specialized investigations

Genetic markers such as HLA (-A3, -B14) and DNA analysis have proved important in identifying genetic haemochromatosis. Direct methods of confirming the disease and monitoring treatment involve liver biopsy, where the histological appearances of the liver are diagnostic of iron overload. Histological grading establishes the extent of overload and identifies the predominantly periportal and hepatocytic iron distribution. Genetic haemochromatosis has a more parenchymal distribution, whereas in secondary haemochromatosis, iron is localized to Kupffer cells and fibrotic areas. Measurement of the hepatic iron concentration by atomic absorption spectrophotometry correlates closely with measurement of iron stores by a desferrioxamine test (moderate iron overload, liver iron of less than 70 μmol/g dry weight; major liver iron overload, in excess of 160 μmol/g dry weight). Other investigations such as computerized tomography (**CT**) and magnetic resonance imaging (**MRI**) have proved useful for assessing liver iron loads semiquantitatively, but may be more appropriate, in association with serum ferritin estimations, for monitoring the effects of therapy.

Mechanisms of iron toxicity

These have been well established in liver tissue and are discussed in detail elsewhere (Section 22). Severity of hepatic damage relates to the degree of iron overload, and the toxic effect of iron is further demonstrated by the development of hepatic fibrosis in untreated livers and by some regression of hepatomegaly in iron-depleted livers. The basic mechanism of hepatocyte damage involves iron-induced lysosomal fragility, probably secondary to peroxidative injury; the released hydrolytic lysosomal enzymes are thought to damage the hepatocyte. Lysosomal fragility has been reversed on iron depletion by phlebotomy. Studies in iron-loaded rats have suggested that peroxidative damage also affects mitochondria and microsomes.

Management of haemochromatosis

In the genetic type (see Section 22), iron depletion can be achieved by phlebotomy, with monitoring of liver iron concentrations by ferritin measurements and CT scanning. Screening of relatives of the 'index case' by HLA typing and DNA studies is an essential prophylactic measure. In secondary forms of haemochromatosis, phlebotomy may be helpful. Iron overload in the iron-loading anaemias, thalassaemia for example, is best treated with prolonged subcutaneous desferrioxamine infusions or oral chelating agents such as hydroxypyridones (see Section 22).

OTHER CAUSES OF SECONDARY IRON LOAD CONDITIONS

Chronic alcoholic liver disease

Iron overload is found in about 30 per cent of alcoholics. The clinical pattern is very similar to primary haemochromatosis, both in skin pigmentation and damage to the endocrine system. The histological appearance of liver tissue shows signs of alcohol damage (Mallory bodies) in addition to classical iron-induced damage to hepatocytes. Differentiation between alcoholic siderosis and the genetic haemochromatosis heterozygote may be difficult in the absence of familial evidence of genetic haemochromatosis.

Porphyria cutanea tarda

This is a chronic hepatic porphyria resulting from a deficiency of uroporphyrinogen decarboxylase (Section 11). The liver form is sporadic and the enzyme abnormality is restricted to the hepatocyte (i.e. the red-cell enzyme level is normal). Clinical expression of this disease is usually exacerbated by alcohol, oestrogens, iron, and other liver disease.

The iron overload is of moderate order (less than four times the normal value) and responds, as does the porphyrin overload, to iron depletion by phlebotomy, which also resolves the skin lesions and reduces the light sensitivity of exposed areas of skin. The mechanisms involved in this form of iron overload are incompletely understood. They are discussed in more detail in Section 11.

COPPER TOXICITY

Liver damage due to copper toxicity may be inherited, Wilson's disease for example, or secondary, such as occurs in Indian childhood cirrhosis or chronic biliary obstruction (Table 1).

Wilson's disease

This is an inherited disorder of copper metabolism, transmitted in a Mendelian recessive fashion, due to mutation of a gene on the long arm of chromosome 13. It is characterized by increased body copper, predominantly in hepatocytes but also in the kidneys, cornea, and brain. A pathognomonic feature and cause of the disease is a reduction in the biliary excretion of copper, the regulatory site of body copper balance, and an invariably absent or reduced plasma caeruloplasmin, the copper-binding protein.

Clinical features

These are as outlined in Table 1 and described in detail in Section 11. There are three modes of presentation: haemolytic jaundice (usually in children), hepatic, and neuropsychiatric, accounting for all but 10 per cent of cases.

Hepatic symptoms and hepatomegaly arise at younger ages, usually 8 to 10 years, than neurological disease (usually 14 to 40 years), and may be indicative of non-specific liver involvement. Less commonly, acute fulminant hepatic failure may be the first manifestation. In many untreated patients, hepatic fibrosis and cirrhosis with portal hypertension develop, after which copper bypasses the liver to reach the central nervous system and basal ganglia, causing lenticular degeneration. Abnormalities such as behavioural disorders, truancy at school, dysarthria, tremor, and difficulty with fine movements with some parkinsonian features are common neurological problems. Cirrhosis is invariably present in adult patients with neurological disease, though basic biochemical tests of liver function may be normal. Involvement of kidneys may be reflected by renal rickets and a Fanconi syndrome. Complications of untreated disease include hepatic decompensation, portal hypertension, and increasing neurological disability (see Section 11).

Diagnosis

Wilson's disease should be considered in any patient with cirrhotic liver disease, particularly in late childhood. Kayser–Fleischer rings, copper deposition in the limbus of the cornea, are pathognomonic of Wilson's disease, and can be confirmed by slit-lamp examination.

Plasma caeruloplasmin concentrations are markedly reduced or absent (less than 20 mg/dl, normal range 20–45) and an increase in the non-caeruloplasmin serum copper (normal 80–135 μg/dl, 13–21 μmol/l) and 24-h urinary excretion of copper (normal $\leq$40 μg/24 h, $\leq$0.628 μmol/24 h; Wilson's disease 100–1000 μg/24 h, 1.57–15.7 μmol/24 h) strongly suggest the diagnosis.

Penicillamine, a copper-chelating agent, given in a single dose of 0.5 g, increases urinary copper excretion (by ninefold or more). A liver biopsy is usually diagnostic, showing classical cirrhosis, and copper may be detected by staining for copper-associated protein (orcein) or, specifically, for copper (rubeanic acid). However, these qualitative estimations do not correlate well with copper overload and quantitation of the hepatic copper load is best assessed by atomic absorption spectrophotometry. Liver copper is often increased by between 1.5 and 25 times normal in Wilson's disease (normal range, less than 50 μg/g dry weight).

Where doubt exists, increased copper uptake and reduced excretion can be demonstrated using radioactive copper.

Treatment

Use of copper-chelating agents, penicillamine (dimethylcysteine) and trientine (triethylene tetramine) can deplete the liver and central nervous system of copper, by promoting urinary copper excretion to the point of negative balance. Small doses of pyridoxine need to be given daily to compensate for depletion. Often agents such as zinc sulphate and ammonium thiomolybdate (discussed in more detail in Section 11) have also been used to reduce absorption of intestinal copper. It should be noted, however, that, unlike iron in haemochromatosis, this is not the site of copper regulation and is unlikely to deplete copper overload *per se.*

Symptomatic treatment is the same as for any patient with chronic liver disease—vitamin supplements, management of ascites and portal hypertension, and where necessary of hepatic failure.

Fulminant hepatic failure may develop, even in the early stages of chelating therapy, when orthotopic liver transplantation is the only life-saving measure available. Management of other complications and monitoring of therapy are discussed in Section 11.

Prognosis

Early diagnosis and the use of chelation therapy remain the most effective ways to ensure a good prognosis. However, a poor outcome is likely in patients with a delayed diagnosis, acute and extensive neurological damage, severe liver disease, and bleeding varices or liver failure. As treatment with chelating agents is lifelong, the compliance of patients and their families is very important and can be achieved by regular discussion of the disease, its complications and prognosis, as well as the possible complications of treatment.

Chronic cholestatic syndromes

Intra- and extrahepatic disturbances in secretion of bile, the major route of copper excretion from the body, can also lead to copper accumulation in the liver and elsewhere. These can arise with congenital abnormalities of the biliary tract (e.g. biliary atresia) or from secondary damage to the liver and biliary tract (e.g. primary biliary cirrhosis, Indian childhood cirrhosis). Unlike Wilson's disease, biliary-cell damage precedes the accumulation of copper, which increases with progressive cholestasis and exacerbates the destruction of hepatocytes and biliary cells. The major features were shown in Table 1; childhood forms are detailed elsewhere (Chapter 14.21).

The liver in cystic fibrosis

Until recently, cystic fibrosis had been regarded as a disease of infants and children. However, with better techniques for earlier diagnosis and advances in the treatment of lung and pancreatic disease, 60 per cent or more of children are now surviving to adult life and cystic fibrosis is now becoming the province of the non-paediatric physician. There is an increasing awareness of hepatic involvement in this disease, which can impair and affect the quality of life, although pulmonary manifestations are still the main determinants of survival. This has become particularly important now that lung transplantation is available for selected patients with cystic fibrosis.

INCIDENCE AND GENETICS (SEE ALSO CHAPTER 17.9.2)

Cystic fibrosis is a genetically determined disorder of exocrine glands characterized by abnormal composition of exocrine secretion with abnormalities of salt and calcium, and increased viscosity of mucus. It is these viscid secretions that damage the intestine, lungs, pancreas, and also intrahepatic bile ducts. Details of the recent advances in genetics and their use in prenatal diagnosis are covered in Sections 4 and 17. To date, there is no mutation that identifies the patient at specific risk of developing liver disease, although gene probes are available for clinical use. Liver involvement must be sought for in every patient with cystic fibrosis. The incidence varies between 20 and 50 per cent of patients studied and about 2 to 5 per cent of these patients develop significant liver damage and cirrhosis. These are likely to be minimum estimates, as with better prognosis of the lung disease and more lung transplantations, the prevalence of cirrhosis is likely to increase.

CLINICAL FEATURES

Hepatic disease may occur at any age (Table 1), with cholestasis due to bile plugs and fatty change in association with meconium ileus being common in neonates, and focal biliary cirrhosis, as well as portal hypertension and liver failure, in adolescents and young adults. Some patients have bile-duct strictures, which may also contribute to liver damage.

Apart from features of obstructive jaundice in neonates with hepatitis, few die in childhood of hepatic complications of cystic fibrosis. Cirrhosis is found in 10 to 15 per cent of adolescents, but hepatomegaly and portal hypertension is now found increasingly in patients with cystic fibrosis in their 20s. However, only 13 per cent of patients undergoing lung transplantation for severe cystic fibrosis have abnormal liver tests, and only 2 per cent of patients have had heart, lung, and liver transplants. More commonly, hepatomegaly is found by chance and its significance is made more difficult to assess by lung disease, which may, by depressing the liver, make it more palpable.

INVESTIGATIONS

Common liver enzyme abnormalities include increased biliary-tract enzymes, i.e. alkaline phosphatase and γ-glutamyl transferase. Their levels do not correlate well with the degree of portal fibrosis and it is essential to make an ultrasonographic examination of the liver and gall-bladder to exclude gallstones. Although technetium colloid and CT scans of the abdomen may be helpful in defining the size of liver and spleen, and for demonstrating varices, liver biopsy may be the most informative investigation for suspected liver involvement and cholestasis.

PATHOLOGY

The liver in cystic fibrosis may vary in appearance from fatty change at birth to different degrees of bile-duct obstruction. Mucous plugs in cholangioles, almost certainly present to some degree in all patients, are believed to be the cause of inflammation and proliferation, and predispose to chronic liver damage and cirrhosis. However, the parenchymal architecture and hepatocyte integrity are relatively well preserved, even when changes in the portal tract are extensive. Although some have noted periportal changes without excess mucous plugging or inflammation in children under 1 year of age, for most adult patients presenting to a physician, focal biliary cirrhosis due to mucous plugs is the characteristic lesion of hepatic cystic fibrosis. Initially, eosinophilic material accumulates in ducts in focal areas, and in older patients these fibrotic areas increase to involve the portal tracts and, later, the hepatic parenchyma (5 to 20 per cent in older children and adults). Established cirrhosis, with disordered hepatocytes and regenerating nodules, follows focal biliary fibrosis. Electron-microscopic studies suggest an increase in Ito cells, with hypertrophy of smooth endoplasmic reticulum and the Golgi apparatus, and large, distended lysosomes.

Bile-duct abnormalities predominate in cystic fibrotic livers and multilobular biliary cirrhosis follows focal biliary fibrosis. Recent studies have suggested that up to 25 per cent of patients have abnormal liver function due to intrahepatic bile plugs, and that extrahepatic lesions (such as strictures) of the common bile duct are present in nearly all patients suffering from liver disease. Some of these features are also found in sclerosing cholangitis.

PATHOGENESIS

At present, there is no clear indication as to which patients will develop biliary-tract and liver disease or to which particular complications within the hepatobiliary system they might be predisposed. There is some evidence that intrapancreatic strictures of the common bile duct are more common in patients with biliary cirrhosis; but these may still be explained by viscid bile plugs.

However, 60 per cent of patients with cystic fibrosis do not develop clinical hepatic manifestations. To date no increase in severity of the lung disease has been demonstrated in those who also have liver disease. It is likely that any explanation must account for the effects of altered bile-acid metabolism related to malabsorption, fatty acid deficiency, an altered cellular immune response to liver membrane antigens, and abnormal secretions from bile-duct epithelium. The most reasonable explanation, which would link with genetic studies and an altered cystic fibrosis transmembrane regulator protein (CFTR), is that biliary-tract cells and hepatocytes may have the same impaired handling of electrolytes that has been described for respiratory and secretory epithelia, (pancreas, salivary, and sweat glands) and that these cells are more susceptible to injury and progressive fibrosis.

MANAGEMENT OF HEPATIC CYSTIC FIBROSIS

There is, at present, no treatment for severe liver damage in cystic fibrosis other than orthotopic liver transplantation. However, as portal-tract changes predominate, treatment is directed prophylactically towards portal hypertension (including sclerotherapy if varices bleed) and hypersplenism/splenic infarction (including splenectomy), and to the management of gallstones, biliary obstruction, and liver failure. In order to reduce the incidence of bile plugging, it is now accepted practice to use chenodeoxycholic acid in patients who have pancreatic, biliary, or liver problems.

Management of hepatic encephalopathy is aimed at the correction of precipitating factors such as systemic infection, hypokalaemia, and constipation.

Liver transplantation may be appropriate in chronic liver failure; in selected patients it is combined with lung transplantation.

PROGNOSIS

Survival of patients with cystic fibrosis, including those with liver disease, is now markedly improved. Literature reviews suggest that liver disease during adult life may affect as many as 20 per cent, and an increase in lung transplantation programmes may well add to this number.

Less common metabolic disorders of liver in adulthood

In all diseases affecting liver, patients may present with similar basic symptoms and signs of a liver defect (see Table 3) and simple indicators of liver dysfunction (see Table 4). The more specific clinical features and investigations diagnostic of a particular metabolic liver disease were outlined in Table 2.

DISORDERS OF CARBOHYDRATE METABOLISM

Diabetes mellitus

In childhood this often presents acutely with hepatomegaly during episodes of ketosis, and histological examination of the liver confirms increased deposition of glycogen. Hepatomegaly, in juvenile diabetics, and more frequently in adults (maturity-onset), is due to fatty change and fat infiltration, which in adults often resolves with weight loss and

'control' of the diabetes. Mauriac syndrome is associated with massive hepatomegaly, growth retardation, and hypercholesterolaemia that does not respond solely to management of the diabetes.

In other disorders, such as fructose intolerance and galactosaemia, where fatty vacuole infiltration is an early feature eventually leading to necrosis and cholestasis, it is important to suspect such defects from the history, because, with appropriate dietary restrictions, hepatocyte damage can be reversed, limited, or prevented.

Glycogen storage diseases (see Section 11)

These disorders are associated with inefficient glycogen utilization due to specific enzyme defects (Table 2). They are characterized by episodes of hypoglycaemia and glycogen deposition, predominantly in the liver and spleen, leading to hepatosplenomegaly, but also in other tissues and organs. With increasing damage to hepatocytes symptoms and signs of general liver dysfunction and damage occur (Table 4) in addition to the more specific symptom of hypoglycaemia. Type I glycogen storage disease is an exception, in that cirrhosis is rare.

AMINO ACID AND UREA-CYCLE DISORDERS (SEE SECTION 11)

Hereditary tyrosinaemia (Table 2 and Section 11)

This is characterized by progressive hepatocellular damage, renal tubular dysfunction and hypophosphataemic rickets, with increased urinary excretion of succinyl acetone diagnostic of the condition, urinary tyrosine metabolites (p-hydroxyphenylacetic acid) and increased plasma concentrations of tyrosine, phenylalanine, and methionine. Parenchymal cells are damaged by succinyl acetone reacting with sulphydryl groups in both liver and kidneys. The hepatocytes show fatty change, followed by necrosis and cholestasis. Dietary restriction of tyrosine, phenylalanine, and methionine, together with symptomatic management of liver disease, and vitamin D and phosphate supplements, improve growth of affected individuals, but do not prevent liver failure. Liver transplantation is the treatment of choice at present.

Urea-cycle disorders

These conditions (Table 2) usually present in childhood with hyperammonaemia together with a normal blood urea and increased precursor substrates for the specific enzyme deficiencies. As well as the brain, the liver is also involved as indicated by hepatomegaly and increased turnover of hepatocytes, leading to an increase in blood transaminases. These conditions are often brought to the attention of a paediatrician or physician by intercurrent infection, or at surgery. Very exceptionally a chronic form persists that is associated with a slowly developing cirrhosis and an increased incidence of hepatocellular carcinoma.

STORAGE DISORDERS

As outlined in Table 2, these are associated with a specific enzyme deficiency leading to accumulation of the non-degradable substrates of the defective enzyme reaction, usually in liver lysosomes but, in the more complicated mucopolysaccharidoses, with accumulation in the brain leading to mental retardation (see Section 11).

Lipid storage disease and the liver

The liver is the main source of very low-density lipoproteins (**VLDL**) in plasma and is responsible for secretion of high-density lipoproteins (**HDL**) as nascent HDL particles containing non-esterified cholesterol. The important lipid storage diseases are shown in Table 2.

Niemann–Pick diseases

These are a heterogeneous group of disorders, characterized by abnormal sphingomyelin, that may present early in childhood (Niemann–Pick A and B), or in later adolescence (Niemann–Pick C), with increasing hepatomegaly due to sphingomyelin accumulation, associated with growth and behavioural disorders and motor/mental retardation. In some patients, asymptomatic cirrhosis develops, only to present in late adolescence or early adulthood with portal hypertension in association with the neurological and psychomotor disturbances. There is little possible treatment, and liver transplantation does not provide control, unlike the glycogen storage diseases.

Wolman's disease

This is characterized by deposition of cholesterol esters and triglycerides in hepatocytes and Kupffer cells as well as in spleen and intestinal mucosa cells. Death often occurs by 6 months of age, preceded by a failure to thrive, diarrhoea, vomiting, and hepatosplenomegaly with cirrhosis. Early diagnosis can lead to successful treatment with bone marrow transplantation (see Chapter 22.8.2).

Cholesterol ester storage disease

This is similar to, but less severe than, Wolman's disease and is a cause of asymptomatic hepatomegaly in childhood and in early adulthood. Cirrhosis occurs rarely and the spleen is palpable in only about one-third of patients. Deficiency of lysosomal acid lipase results in accumulation of cholesterol esters and triglyceride in many tissues including the liver and intestinal mucosa. The liver enzymes and function tests are normal. Hepatic histological appearances are diagnostic, with orange-coloured tissue due to parenchymal cells, Kupffer cells, and portal macrophages containing intracellular lipid in the form of cholesterol ester. Hepatic septal fibrosis rather than cirrhosis occurs progressively but slowly. Thus liver function is usually well preserved.

Zellweger's syndrome

This defect leads to accumulation of lipid in hepatocytes. It is an autosomal recessive condition in which a peroxisomal enzyme deficiency and absence of peroxisomes lead to abnormalities in bile-acid synthesis, with abnormal C29 bile acid, increased synthesis of dihydroxy and trihydroxy coprostanoic acids, increased pipecolic acid (as in Refsum's disease; see Section 11) and impaired oxidation of long-chain fatty acids, a specific function of peroxisomes.

Hepatic damage occurs during the first few weeks of life, and micronodular cirrhosis with jaundice is established by 6 months. Liver enzymes and function tests are abnormal, with reduced concentrations of albumin and prothrombin.

Although these individuals usually die in infancy, there is an increasing number of survivors into adulthood. It is disappointing that, to date, there is no specific therapy for these disorders and eradication of the disease must therefore rely on prenatal diagnosis and genetic counselling.

Gaucher's disease (see also Section 11)

Gaucher's disease exists in three forms, which all result from deficiency of the lysosomal enzyme, glucocerebrosidase, leading to the accumulation of glucosylceramide in lysosomes of reticuloendothelial cells. Although the classical presentation (see Table 2) involves the spleen, bone, and blood, an early, non-tender hepatomegaly is often present and the liver may become huge. Liver damage is caused by involvement of Kupffer cells or of portal macrophages, which may be located in scattered foci throughout the liver. These 'Gaucher's cells' are autofluorescent, periodic acid–Schiff positive (diastase resistant), and also stain for acid phosphatase. Pericellular fibrosis is common, usually with a centrizonal distribution, but some patients progress to cirrhosis. There are minor elevations of circulating transaminases, and alkaline phosphatase (which is normally of bone origin). Decompensated liver failure occurs only rarely but can be precipitated by infection and is associated with jaundice, a poor prognostic sign. Portal hypertension occurs but splenomegaly is more usually due to Gaucher-cell infiltration. Patients may bleed from gastric varices or suffer splenic infarcts. Treatment of this condition has been radically improved by splenectomy and the availability of genetically produced glucocerebrosidase (cerisidase) (see Section 11).

Hyperlipoproteinaemias

As shown in Table 2, hyperlipoproteinaemias may be associated with liver abnormalities. In the autosomal dominant hypercholesterolaemic conditions, familial and combined, the liver is rarely damaged but may be affected by interventions such as portocaval anastomosis and ileal bypass, which usually cause fatty change. In selected patients with the homozygous condition, liver transplantation may be curative.

Predominantly hypertriglyceridaemic conditions, such as hyperchylomicronaemia (type I) and pure and combined hypertriglyceridaemia (Types IV and V) with abnormalities of VLDL and triacylglycerol-rich lipoproteins, are usually associated with easily palpable hepatomegaly, and occasionally with splenomegaly due to reversible triglyceride deposition in foam cells, in association with abdominal pain and pancreatitis. Secondary forms of these conditions can occur with severe obesity, diabetes, or alcohol ingestion. These disorders are discussed in Section 11.

REYE'S SYNDROME

Definition

Reye (1963) defined the syndrome of fulminant encephalopathy and acute hepatocyte dysfunction in previously healthy children occurring in the week following a viral infection. It is a rare, acute, and often fatal encephalopathy that can arise in children of any age. It should be clearly distinguished from any inborn errors of metabolism presenting with encephalopathy (Table 2), including urea-cycle defects, carnitine deficiency, and organic acidaemias. There are now increasing reports of Reye's syndrome in adults following flu-like illness.

CLINICAL FEATURES

A typical patient is usually between 6 and 14 years of age. Frequently there is a preceding history of epidemic viral infection such as influenza but as yet the link between viral disease and liver damage is unknown. Initial features are a trivial viral illness followed by persistent vomiting with increasingly severe encephalopathy, deepening confusion, and rapid progression to coma. Clinical staging of encephalopathy, from grade I to V, aids in management decisions. In the latter stages, seizures occur in association with flaccidity, loss of deep tendon reflexes, and respiratory arrest. Typically, there are no clinical features of liver disease, and the diagnosis must be suspected if weight is to be given to the interpretation of transient increases in transaminases, an increased plasma ammonia, and hypoglycaemic episodes with prolonged prothombin times. Tests of liver enzymes and function are often normal. Abnormalities include a low plasma VLDL, and increased serum concentrations of uric acid and creatine phosphokinase (CK-MM).

Diagnosis

When Reye's syndrome is suspected, liver biopsy done under cover of infused clotting factor (fresh frozen plasma) is important as diagnostic features are present within a few days of onset of vomiting. Hepatocytes typically show a swollen, rounded contour with central nuclei, cytoplasmic fragmentation, and glycogen depletion. There is no hepatic necrosis or inflammation and the triglyceride found in hepatocytes is not the typical lipid droplets of chronic fatty liver. Ultrastructural changes include swollen, pleomorphic mitochondria; there is a reduction in mitochondrial enzyme activities with preservation of cytoplasmic enzymes. Progressive mitochondrial deformity occurs and is self-limiting over about 2 to 6 days after the onset of encephalopathy. Some recent evidence suggests a genetic predisposition to Reye's treatment, which may be helpful in making the diagnosis.

Treatment

Early diagnosis and intensive care may improve the outcome. Maintenance of cerebral circulation and oxygenation is important whilst the mitochondria recover, and mechanical ventilation is necessary to prevent hypoxia. Hypothermia should be avoided. Hypoglycaemia should be averted by dextrose infusions, and patients should be nursed and given appropriate therapy to reduce intracranial pressure; in some circumstances, decompression may be necessary. Serum and urine should be collected as early as possible and screened to exclude a range of inborn errors of metabolism.

Prognosis

Many patients are treated successfully but death rates vary from 10 to 50 per cent. Some survivors have permanent brain damage, which is probably related to the duration of the encephalopathic phase of the illness.

The most effective way of preventing complications or death is to suspect the disease, particularly after or during epidemics of influenza B and chickenpox. Incidence rates vary, but in a large American study, the incidence was higher in blacks than whites, and varied with the location of residence and social class. In addition, there is a link with the use of aspirin and an increased predisposition to a Reye-like syndrome. Limiting the use of aspirin in children under 5 years has been associated with a significant reduction in the disease. It is therefore suggested that aspirin should not be used during episodes of influenza, upper respiratory tract infections, and varicella.

INHERITED PANCREATITIS

Acute and chronic pancreatitis have several aetiological factors in common, but it is rare for acute attacks, even if recurrent, to proceed to chronic pancreatitis. Chronic pancreatitis may occur with autosomal dominant or more rarely autosomal recessive inheritance, often involving several generations of affected families. The major forms are idiopathic, and associated with cystic fibrosis, hereditary hyperlipoproteinaemia (types I and V), and hereditary hyperparathyroid disease.

Hereditary pancreatitis

This disease occurs in Caucasians as a rare autosomal dominant and presents in childhood. The mode of inheritance is unclear, although there is evidence for suppression of the gene for pancreatic structural protein (**PSP**) and its secretory form (PSP-S), which inhibit the growth of calcium carbonate crystals, and levels of these were three times lower in chronic calcific pancreatitis than in controls. There is a possible association between this pancreatitis, expression of the erb-B_2 receptor, and development of pancreatic carcinoma.

Clinical features

The condition usually presents in children, with recurrent episodes of acute abdominal pain lasting 1 to 2 days for which no other cause can be found. Rarely, there are associated features of acute pancreatitis.

After some years, secondary damage to the pancreas may ensue, with chronic inflammation and exocrine insufficiency with clinical features of steatorrhoea. Pancreatic calcification eventually occurs, which is clearly apparent on radiographs. Other complications include pancreatic pseudocysts, thrombosis of splenic and portal veins, and, in up to 25 per cent, the development of pancreatic carcinoma. Surprisingly, diabetes is rare.

Diagnosis

Increased serum amylase and lipase activities can be detected during attacks of abdominal pain, associated with positive tests of fat malabsorption and pancreatic hypofunction. Pancreatic calcification can be noted on plain abdominal radiographs. About half the patients have aminoaciduria, predominantly of cystine and lysine.

Differential diagnosis

Other causes of chronic pancreatitis associated with inherited disorders need to be excluded, such as cystic fibrosis, haemochromotsis, hereditary hyperlipoproteinaemias, and primary hyperparathyroidism.

REFERENCES

Cystic fibrosis

di Sant' Agnese, P.A. *et al.* (1953). Abnormal electrolyte composition of sweat in cystic fibrosis pancreas. *Pediatrics*, **12**, 549–63.

Riordan, J.R. *et al.* (1989). Identification of the cystic fibrosis gene: cloning and characterisation of complementary DNA. *Science*, **245**, 1066–73.

Rommens, J.M. *et al.* (1989). Identification of the cystic fibrosis gene: chromosome walking and jumping. *Science*, **245**, 1059–65.

Seymour, C.A. (1991). The liver in cystic fibrosis. In *Oxford textbook of clinical hepatology* (ed. N. McIntyre *et al.*), pp. 967–74. Oxford University Press.

Haemochromatosis

Bonkovsky, H.L. (1991). Iron and the liver. *American Journal of Medical Science*, **301**, 32–43.

Brissot, P. and Deugnier, Y. (1991). Genetic haemochromatosis. In *Oxford textbook of clinical hepatology* (ed. N. McIntyre *et al.*) pp. 948–58. Oxford University Press.

Cox, T.M. (1990). Haemochromatosis. *Blood Reviews*, **4**, 75–87.

Cox, T.M. and Lord, D.K. (1989). Hereditary Haemochromatosis. *European Journal of Haematology*, **42**, 113–25.

Simon, M. and Brissot P. (1988). The genetics of haemochromatosis. *Journal of Hepatology*, **6**, 116–24.

Simon, M., Fauchet, R., LeGall, J.Y., Brissot, P., and Bourel, M. (1988). Immunogenetics of idiopathic haemochromatosis and secondary iron overload. In *Immunogenetics of endocrine disorders* (ed. N.R. Favid), pp. 345–71. Liss, New York.

Hereditary pancreatitis

Chait, A. and Brunzell, J.D. (1992). Chylomicron syndrome. *Advances in Internal Medicine*, **37**, 249–73.

Fojo, S.S. and Brewer, H.B. (1993). Hypertriglyceridaemia due to genetic defects in lipoprotein lipase and apolipoprotein. *Journal of Internal Medicine*, **231**, 669–77.

Miller, A.R., Nagorney, D.M. and Sarr, M.G. (1992). The surgical spectrum of hereditary pancreatitis in adults. *Annals of Surgery*, **215**, 39–43.

Moir, C.R., Konzen, K.M., and Perrault, J. (1992). Surgical therapy and long term follow-up of childhood hereditary pancreatitis. *Journal of Paediatric Surgery*, **27**, 282–6.

Stafford, R.J. and Grend, K.J. (1982). Hereditary diseases of exocrine pancreas. *Clinical Gastroenterology*, **11**, 141–70.

Robechek, P.J. (1967). Hereditary chronic relating pancreatitis: a clue to pancreatitis in general. *American Journal of Surgery*, **113**, 819–824.

Reye's syndrome

Hurwitz, E.S. (1989). Reye's syndrome. *Epidemiologic Review*, **11**, 249–53.

Osterlok, J., Cunningham, W., Dixon, A., and Combest, A. (1989). Biochemical relationships between Reye's and Reye's-like metabolic and toxicological syndromes. *Medical Toxicology Adverse Drug Experience*, **4**, 272–94.

Wilson's disease

Bearn, A.G. (1960). A genetic analysis of 30 families with Wilson's disease. *Annals of Human Genetics*, **24**, 33–43.

Bull, P.C., Thomas, G.R., Rommens, J.M., Forbes, J.R., and Wilson Cox, D. (1993). The Wilson disease gene is a putative copper binding P-type ATPase similar to the Menkes gene. *Nature Genetics*, **5**, 327–38.

Chelly, J. and Monaco, A.P. (1993). Cloning the Wilson disease gene. *Nature Genetics*, **5**, 317–18.

Frydman, M. (1990). Genetic Aspects of Wilson's disease. *Journal of Gastroenterology and Hepatology*, **5**, 483–90.

Houwen, R.H. *et al.* (1991). Isolation and regional localisation of 25 anonymous DNA probes on a chromosome 13 hybrid panel. *Cytogenetics Cell Genetics*, **57**, 87–90.

Petrukhin, K., *et al.* (1993). Mapping, cloning and genetic characterization of the region containing the Wilson disease gene. *Nature Genetics*, **5**, 338–44.

Sternlieb, I. (1990). Perspectives on Wilson's disease. *Hepatology*, **12**, 1234–9.

Sternlieb, I. and Scheinberg, I.H. (1991). Wilson's disease. In *Oxford textbook of clinical hepatology* (ed. N. McIntyre *et al.*), pp. 945–8. Oxford University Press.

Tanzi, R.E., *et al.* (1993). The Wilson disease gene is a copper transporting ATPase with homology to the Menkes disease gene. *Nature Genetics*, **5**, 344–51.

Walshe, J.M. and Yealland, M. (1993). Chelation treatment of neurological Wilson's disease. *Quarterly Journal of Medicine*, **86**, 197–204.

Yarze, J.C., Martin, P., Munoz, S.J., and Friedman, L.S. (1992). Wilson's disease: current status. *American Journal of Medicine*, **92**, 643–54.

14.23 Diseases of the pancreas

14.23.1 Acute pancreatitis

C. W. Imrie

Incidence and epidemiology

There is a considerable range in incidence of acute pancreatitis, from 40 to 500 new cases per million of the population per annum. The two main aetiological factors are biliary disease and alcohol abuse, with the majority of prospective studies showing a dominance of biliary aetiology, from 40 to 60 per cent of all patients. All female and the older male patients tend to have biliary pancreatitis, while younger males are the group most commonly affected by alcohol-abuse pancreatitis. American and Scandinavian populations have shown a preponderance of alcohol-induced disease. This is typified by a study from Gothenburg, where, from the late 1950s to the mid1970s, there was a change from a 68 per cent association with biliary disease to exactly the same proportion with alcohol-abuse pancreatitis.

In the only recent large population studies (from Scotland and Finland with similar populations of around 5 million), the incidence of the disease has shown a steady rise, while from 1960 onwards, the mortality has remained fairly stable.

Aetiological factors (Table 1)

MAJOR FACTORS

The two major aetiological factors, biliary disease and alcohol abuse, together account for over 80 per cent of patients in most prospective studies. In many studies, almost a quarter of cases remain unexplained, but with recent diagnostic advances, particularly the early use endoscopic retrograde cholangiopancreatography (**ERCP**), it is clear that almost all of these patients have very small stones. Biliary sludge or bile crystals may also be indicative of a tendency to stone formation. Studies in the United Kingdom reveal an incidence of pancreatitis of between 40 to 57 per cent with small gallstones. In Ohio in the United States a similar incidence has been detected, while in Argentina over 80 per cent of patients have been shown, by faecal sieving, to have small gallstones. The way in which the transient migration of small stones causes acute pancreatitis is not understood. But it is clear that risk is much greater with small stones.

Alcohol-abuse pancreatitis occurs in over 80 per cent of patients in published series from New York, and around 70 per cent in Scandinavian studies. This association is usually found in young males who drink in excess of 80 g alcohol/day. Up to 10 per cent of patients may have both a biliary pathology and alcohol abuse. Alcohol may cause acute pancreatitis by acinar stimulation with ampullary spasm.

Table 1 *Aetiological factors in acute pancreatitis*

Major
Biliary disease
Alcohol abuse
Minor
Post-ERCP
Blunt trauma
Coxsackie B
Mumpsvirus
Hyperlipoproteinaemia
Ampullary tumour
Hyperparathyroidism
Worm infestation[1]
Scorpion bites[2]
Drugs

[1]S.E. Asia;

[2]Trinidad.

MINOR FACTORS (TABLE 1).

Iatrogenic causes

Iatrogenic acute pancreatitis may be induced by surgical or endoscopic procedures involving the ampulla of Vater. The frequency of post ERCP pancreatitis is increasing, even though the procedure only carries a risk for acute pancreatitis of about 1 per cent. Following a therapeutic endoscopic sphincterotomy the risk of acute pancreatitis is approximately 3 per cent. It is possible that failure to clear the duct of stones and inadequate sphincterotomies are the two most common predisposing features because they often allow stones to impact at the ampullary area. Manometric studies in the small group of patients with sphincter of Oddi dysfunction are associated with acute pancreatitis in around 30 per cent of cases.

Viral infection

Viral infection, particularly mumpsvirus, Cocksackie B, and hepatitis can cause acute pancreatitis, and is often missed if appropriate serological samples are not collected. One clinical feature that may prove useful is prodromal diarrhoea, which is rare in all other types of acute pancreatitis.

Drug-induced acute pancreatitis

The drugs most commonly implicated in acute pancreatitis are valproic acid, azathioprine, L-asparaginase, and corticosteroids. However, unless viral titres have been determined, together with adequate biliary investigations, it is unwise to ascribe an acute pancreatitis to a particular drug.

Hyperparathyroidism

This is now recognized to be an uncommon accompaniment of acute pancreatitis. Indeed, many of the reported patients have also had gallstones. The association is calculated at 0.1 per cent. Removal of the parathyroid adenoma usually relieves further acute pancreatitis.

Hyperlipoproteinaemia

Patients with type I and V hyperlipoproteinaemia (see Chapter 11.6) may develop acute pancreatitis. The significance of this association may be difficult to validate. It has been found that hyperlipoproteinaemia-associated acute pancreatitis is rare in patients who do not, at the same time, have a high alcohol intake. In such patients the increased level of lipoproteins may simply be an epiphenomenon rather than a cause of pancreatitis. Nevertheless, several experimental studies point to the importance of this association, and, clinically, some patients with primary hyperlipoproteinaemia are prone to attacks of acute pancreatitis.

Hypothermia

This is a particularly important association in the elderly. In younger patients, alcohol abuse may be linked, particularly if patients fall asleep out of doors or in a cold, unheated house. Histologically, the acute pancreatitis is perilobular.

Blunt trauma (Fig. 1)

This is an important cause of acute pancreatitis, particularly in young children. Sports injuries from rugby, football, ice hockey, martial arts, and similar activities may result in acute pancreatitis, usually from a crush injury to the body of the pancreas against the vertebral column. Of greater importance numerically are victims of road traffic accidents.

Periampullary adenoma or cancer

This is an important association, which is best diagnosed by ERCP; with the increase in this approach to diagnosis, tumours at or close to the ampulla have been shown to have a greater association with acute pancreatitis than hyperparathyroidism (0.4 per cent). Effective treatment of the tumour abolishes recurrent attacks. This usually involves surgical resection.

LEAST COMMON CAUSES

Unusual causes of acute pancreatitis are listed in Table 2. The link with pancreatic cancer and metastases to the pancreas is well documented.

Fig. 1 Blunt trauma causing pancreatitis by transection at arrowpoint on CT scan.

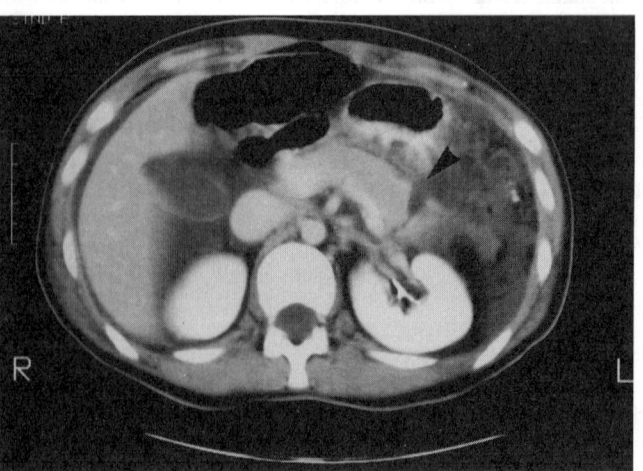

Table 2 *Conditions that may occasionally be involved in the aetiology of acute pancreatitis*

Hypothermia
Sclerosing cholangitis
α_1-Antitrypsin deficiency
Pancreatic cancer
Cancers metastatic to pancreas:
Renal
Stomach
Breast
Ovarian
Lung
Virus infection:
Hepatitis
ECHO
Duodenal reduplication
Annular pancreas

Microscopical pathology

All patients with acute pancreatitis have microscopic evidence of necrosis, while macroscopic changes, particularly black discoloration, are confined to the most severe cases. It is more frequent for this gross form of necrosis to occur in the peripancreatic fatty tissue than in the pancreas itself. When evident in the pancreas there is usually a panlobular necrosis and it is impossible to delineate where the disease initiated.

In a classical paper, Foulis claimed that the most common microscopic abnormality seen in man, periductal necrosis, is typical of biliary and alcohol causation. Less commonly a perilobular necrosis is found, usually in patients with hypothermia or gross hypotension.

In experimental acute pancreatitis the initial lesion is now considered to be intracellular, featuring coalescence of lysozymes and zymogen granules. Acinar-cell disruption is found with many of the hyperstimulation models such as caerulein-induced acute pancreatitis. It is now believed that this initial event may be associated with oxidative stress. Although this is very difficult to prove, it has formed the basis of new approaches to treatment.

Clinical presentation and laboratory abnormalities

CLINICAL FEATURES

Sudden onset of upper abdominal pain with vomiting is the most common manner of presentation.

The pain may focus in the epigastrium, right or left upper quadrant, with penetration through to the back. Occasionally it encircles the upper abdomen. Patients who have experienced both a myocardial infarct and acute pancreatitis usually describe the latter pain as being much more severe. However, it tends to lessen in severity progressively over the first 72 h, and it is unusually a significant factor beyond this time. The pain on presentation is very similar to that of a perforated duodenal ulcer, but vomiting is less common in those who perforate ulcers.

Up to 90 per cent of patients with acute pancreatitis have troublesome vomiting in the first 12 h of illness, and this contributes to hypovolaemia and hypotension.

Patients with stones in the common bile duct may well be jaundiced, and cholangitis can supervene in a minority. Much milder degrees of jaundice may occur from compression of the lower bile duct in patients with alcohol-induced disease.

Gross hypotension only occurs in the very severe cases, but loss of circulating volume due to the extravasation of albumin, coupled with vomiting, leads to dehydration; the patient is thirsty, but fears drinking because of vomiting.

Bowel sounds are rarely present in the early phase of the disease and paralytic ileus may extend beyond 4 days. Indeed the duration of ileus is a useful marker of severity of disease.

The course of mild acute pancreatitis

Those patients who fail to meet objective criteria of severe acute pancreatitis tend to have a low mortality (maximum 2 per cent) and rarely need to be in hospital beyond 7 to 10 days. Simple therapeutic measures usually suffice through the first 48 h, at which time nasogastric suction and urinary catheterization can usually be discontinued. It is safer to assume that a patient may move into the more severe group and to provide early monitoring of the volume of nasogastric aspirate and urinary output to maintain adequate fluid replacement. Even in this category of patients it may occasionally be necessary to provide 4 to 5 litres of intravenous fluid in the first 24 h of the illness.

The course of severe acute pancreatitis

Patients who meet objective criteria of severe acute pancreatitis may be pyrexial, and are hypotensive, markedly tachypnoeic, and suffer from acute ascites, pleural effusions, and prolonged paralytic ileus. Body-wall staining at the umbilical area (Cullen's sign) or in the flanks (Grey Turner's sign) can occur.

Renal and respiratory compromise are very common and must be anticipated. The urine output and arterial oxygen saturation must be monitored. Pulse oximetry is useful in monitoring, but arterial gas analysis may be needed three or four times in the first 24 h in order to make sensible decisions about humidified oxygen therapy and ventilator support. Single-organ insufficiency or failure necessitates high-dependency care and often full intensive-care management, as this may be a prelude to multiorgan failure.

The cardiovascular system

The initial hypovolaemia is of great importance in cardiac and renal function, and low-dose dopamine may be particularly helpful. Where the cardiac output is more compromised and simple fluid replacement does not restore circulating volume, support drugs such as dobutamine, catecholamines, and high-dose dopamine may well be necessary. In the most severe acute pancreatitis the cardiovascular changes are very similar to those encountered in septic shock, with a high cardiac output and low peripheral vascular resistance. Stress on the heart may cause arrhythmias and ischaemic changes necessitating amiodorone or glycosides.

Renal compromise

Not only do hypotension and hypovolaemia threaten renal function but localized intravascular coagulation in the glomerular capillaries may be an important element in patients who develop renal failure. In addition, a significant vasoconstrictor effect involving the main blood vessels to the kidneys has been demonstrated.

The single most important corrective measure is to provide adequate fluid replacement. Low-dose dopamine is the most useful drug, but diuretics such as frusemide and mannitol may still have an important place.

Additional measures are required in any patient failing to produce 30 ml of urine per hour. Most respond to increasing the rate of intravenous infusion but more vigorous measures are necessary in the most ill patients, including haemoperfusion, peritoneal dialysis, or haemodialysis.

Respiratory insufficiency or failure

Hypoxaemia is the hallmark of acute pancreatitis and reflects its severity. The basic mechanism of the hypoxaemia is unknown but high levels of cytokines, particularly leucocyte elastase may be involved, together with factors that contribute to localized intravascular coagulation. Shunting of blood in the pulmonary vascular bed may account for up to 30 per cent of cardiac output.

The initial clinical sign, which may easily be overlooked, is a fast respiratory rate, but there is no substitute for the measurement of arterial oxygen saturation. Almost all of the scales for objective monitoring of severity of disease include an arterial oxygen saturation of less than 60 mmHg (8 kPa) as an index of severity. Hypoxaemia can usually be reversed by the provision of humidified oxygen, and in severe cases, the pattern is similar to adult respiratory-distress syndrome of other causes. Pleural effusions may be large enough to warrant aspiration, and when humidified oxygen is insufficient to reverse the hypoxaemia, assisted ventilation is necessary. Hyaline membrane formation has been found in severe cases, and even in milder cases, reversal of the respiratory insufficiency takes many weeks.

BIOCHEMICAL ABNORMALITIES

A multitude of biochemical phenomena are found in acute pancreatitis, but it is the gross elevations of various pancreatic enzymes that are useful as diagnostic markers. With acinar-cell disruption, high levels of amylase, lipase, trypsin, chymotrypsin, phospholipase, elastase, as well as breakdown products such as trypsinogen activation peptide (**TAP**) and phospholipase activation peptide (PLAP), are all found. The cheapest and most durable of these measurements as a diagnostic marker has been the total level of serum amylase. Levels over four times the upper limit of normal in blood are usually taken as diagnostic of acute pancreatitis, provided the clinical course corresponds. The lipase level is a more specific measure and is now almost as cheap to measure; levels of twice the upper limit of normal are significant. Other body fluids contain elevated levels of these enzymes.

Measurements of trypsin and chymotrypsin are expensive and the antiprotease defence mechanisms are so well designed that α_2-macroglobulin and α_1-antiprotease (also known as α_1-protease inhibitor and α_1-antitrypsin) rapidly degrade free trypsin and chymotrypsin within body fluids. Thus measurement of both trypsin and chymotrypsin can be unrewarding, while measurement of TAP shows great potential. This small peptide molecule is found at very high levels in urine very early in the disease course in patients with severe acute pancreatitis. It is therefore a good measure of the degree of disruption of acinar cells and a commercial method of its assessment is being pioneered. In time this may be a valuable investigation, both for diagnosis and gauging severity of acute pancreatitis.

For many years it was believed that the antiprotease defence mechanisms required supplementation in patients with acute pancreatitis. Thus aprotinin (Trasylol), gabexate mesolate (FOY), and purified plasma derivatives have all been given intravenously in the hope of improving the clinical course. It is now clear, however, that the antiprotease defence works very effectively and that there is no need to boost them in this way, a conclusion that is supported by many clinical trials. Aprotinin was also given into the peritoneal cavity in the hope that it would improve survival and lower complications, but was unsuccessful.

In the last few years it has become appreciated that there are very high levels of circulating cytokines at an early stage in the disease. In particular, it is believed that tumour necrosis factor-α (**TNF-α**), platelet-activating factor, and interleukin 6 (**IL–6**) are present in greatest concentration in those with severe acute pancreatitis. The stimulus to the release of cytokines is thought to be endotoxin, probably from the gut, and there is great interest in the possibility of administering agents that inhibit endotoxin or the cytokines as a potential therapy.

CALCIUM–ALBUMIN

It has been known since the 1940s that low levels of calcium are a feature of a acute pancreatitis but some 30 years later it was found that a significant proportion of patients had only a drop in protein-bound calcium and that the primary pathology was the loss of albumin from the intravascular space, rather than a drop in levels of ionized calcium. However, even after correction factors are applied there is an undoubted tendency for ionized calcium levels to fall but this is usually counteracted by a marked elevation in parathyroid hormone.

HAEMATOLOGICAL ABNORMALIES

There is marked haemoconcentration associated with hypovolaemia so that initial haemoglobin levels of over 16 g/100 ml may be found. After rehydration, the haemoglobin level falls, but it is unusual for blood transfusion to be required as the degree of haemorrhage in and around the pancreas is usually not of great moment. Later in the course of the disease, bleeding from gastric erosions, peptic ulcer, or haemorrhage into a pseudocyst may require blood products and endoscopic, angiographic or surgical intervention.

Due to mobilization of leucocytes, monocytes, and macrophages, there is a marked elevation of elastase, TNF-α, and similar substances. In addition the acute-phase response results in high levels of liver derived C-reactive protein, α_1-antiprotease, factor V, factor VIII, and fibrinogen. Platelet and α_2-macroglobulin levels fall in the first week, usually returning to normal by days 8 to 10. The common finding in patients with severe acute pancreatitis is hypercoagulation, and disseminated intravascular coagulation, while it does occur, is very uncommon; its management is considered in Section 22. The rapidity of mediator response makes leucocyte elastase, TNF-α, and IL-6 potentially excellent markers of severity; C-reactive protein levels in excess of 150 mg/l, though a slower response, are another useful marker of severe disease.

PYREXIA

This is a reflection of cell damage and necrosis in a similar fashion to the initial pyrexia that can be a feature of myocardial infarction. A low-grade fever is typical of the first 3 to 4 days of illness. Especially in those who have the clinical signs of obstructive jaundice, ascending cholangitis should be suspected and appropriate antimicrobials given. In the most severely ill patients, transudation of bacteria from the transverse colon into necrotic tissue around the pancreas, and occasionally in the gland itself, has been detected within 48 to 96 h of onset, although it is more typical to find sepsis at a later stage.

Diagnosis and grading of severity

The diagnosis is usually made from the clinical presentation, particularly the rapid onset of upper abdominal pain and vomiting. Gross elevations of amylase and lipase in blood usually support the diagnosis, while urinary amylase levels of greater than five times the upper limit of normal can be helpful in less typical cases.

Peritoneal aspiration (after catheterization of the urinary bladder and nasogastric intubation) can be very helpful where diagnostic doubt still exists. The aspiration of more than 20 ml of free fluid without bacterial contamination (evident by smell and Gram film) is indicative of a severe form of the disease. The darker the colour of the fluid, the more severe the disease. This procedure is especially effective in patients with alcohol-induced acute pancreatitis. The presence of bacterial contamination indicates an alternative diagnosis and the need for an immediate laparotomy, as visceral perforation of the duodenum or small bowel is more likely.

Computerized tomography (**CT**) may reveal pancreatic swelling, fluid collection, and change in density of the gland. Angiogram-enhanced CT scanning is mandatory to obtain the most useful information.

DIFFERENTIAL DIAGNOSIS (TABLE 3)

A dissecting aortic aneursym usually presents with an initial history of chest pain in a known hypertensive; abdominal pain and loss of femoral pulses may occur later. A minor degree of pancreatitis due to ischaemia of the pancreas should not obscure the main diagnosis. Elevated amylase levels are frequently present in patients with renal failure, while a lifetime of high amylase occurs in those with macroamylasaemia; failure to filter the macromolecule of amylase results in very low urine levels.

Table 3 *Differential diagnosis of acute pancreatitis*

Perforated duodenal ulcer
Acute cholangitis
Acute cholecystitis
Mesenteric ischaemia/infarction
Small-bowel obstruction/perforation
Atypical myocardial infarction
Ectopic pregnancy
Renal failure
Macroamylasaemia
Ruptured aortic aneurysm
Dissecting aortic aneurysm
Diabetic ketoacidosis

High amylase levels in ectopic pregnancy come from the fallopian tubes, but the clinical presentation should not be mistaken for acute pancreatitis. Patients with diabetic ketoacidosis may occasionally have very high levels of amylase, but this should not distract from the major pathology requiring therapy.

Small-bowel obstruction is associated with multiple gas–fluid interfaces on erect abdominal radiographs. The differentiation of an early perforated duodenal ulcer (less than 5 h) will rest on the combination of the finding of free gas under the diaphragm on radiographs and the lack of a significant rise in blood amylase to greater than twice the upper limits at the acute stage of illness.

A more difficult diagnostic problem arises in the patient who has had a perforated duodenal ulcer for some hours; a marked elevation of amylase can occur. Similarly, mesenteric ischaemia or infarction can be associated with biochemical changes similar to those of acute pancreatitis, but in both these situations bacterial contamination of the peritoneal cavity will be detected by peritoneal aspiration. A CT scan also helps to distinguish between these conditions.

GRADING DISEASE SEVERITY

The importance of objective grading of disease severity is that less experienced clinicians can direct the more serious cases to high–dependency or intensive care facilities at an early stage of their illness, or institute CT angiogram scanning and early ERCP for patients who will derive most benefit. Grading is also useful for trials of different forms of therapy.

The original Ranson grading system of 11 prognostic factors was developed for patients with acute pancreatitis due to alcohol abuse, but later a system was introduced for those with gallstones. An alternative single system, validated for both the common causes, is the Glasgow scoring system of eight prognostic factors (Table 4). Validation came from a multicentre British study that assessed the place of peritoneal lavage in the management of severe acute pancreatitis.

CT scanning

This can be very useful in confirming the diagnosis and also to grade severity of disease (Table 5). This is not a more accurate system of grading than the Glasgow score but it is very helpful in assessing the individual patient (Fig. 2) and for guiding accurate needle aspiration.

The APACHE II system (Fig 3)

This can be used to grade severity of many diseases and has been shown to be valuable in acute pancreatitis. It takes time for an individual clinician to learn to use the system, but it has the particular advantage that it can be applied throughout the first week of illness. The higher the score the worse the prognosis; patients with the most severe acute pancreatitis have scores in excess of 10.

Table 4 *Glasgow Prognostic Score*

WBC	>	15 000/mm³
Glucose	>	10 mmol/l (no diabetic history)
Urea	>	16 mmol/l (despite IV infusion)
pO₂	<	8 kPa (60 mmHg)
Albumin	<	32 g/l
Calcium	<	2.0 mmol/l
LDH	>	600 international units/l
AST/ALT	>	200 units/l

Any 3 or more factors = severe acute pancreatitis. The greater the number of factors, the poorer the prognosis.

WBC = white blood count, LDH = lactic dehydrogenase, AST = aspartate transferase, ALT = alanine transferase.

Table 5 *CT scanning in severe acute pancreatitis*

Angiogram-enhanced CT essential for pancreatic assessment; grading systems are based on:
Degree of pancreatic swelling
Peripancreatic fluid collection
Size of the section of non-perfused (or poorly perfused) pancreas

Details of grading are described by Balthazar *et al.* (1985), London *et al.* (1989), and Lucarotti *et al.* (1993) - see References.

C-reactive protein

As an acute-phase reactant the main value of this marker is at 36 to 48 h into the illness when the baseline levels of less than 10 mg/l are far exceeded in those with severe acute pancreatitis. A cut-off at 150 mg/l is a useful guide in groups of patients being assessed, but rogue results can be obtained and cause difficulty (Fig 4). Of all the simple markers of severity, most experience has been gained with C-reactive protein.

Polymorphnuclear (PMN) elastase

Retrospective assessment of frozen serum samples from patients with acute pancreatitis have shown that this marker can accurately separate severe from milder acute pancreatitis. However, there are no published data on the clinical application of PMN elastase measurement. Preliminary clinical studies have shown that patients with mild disease may have high levels, suggesting that this may not be a valuable marker of severity.

IL-6

Findings in groups of frozen plasma samples assayed for IL-6 suggest that its level correlates with severity. It is an expensive assay and has not yet been used prospectively.

Trypsinogen activation peptide (TAP)

The activation of trypsinogen releases trypsin and a small peptide (TAP) that passes unchanged in the urine, where its level can be used as a marker of severity. It has only been employed in one clinical study thus far.

Clinical management

Pain is usually treated with pethidine or buprenorphine; intravenous benzodiazepines may be required in severe cases. The effect of the combination of intravenous midazolam and pethidine can be particularly difficult to predict and the combination must be used with great care. Morphine has a strong spastic effect on the sphincter of Oddi and is contraindicated.

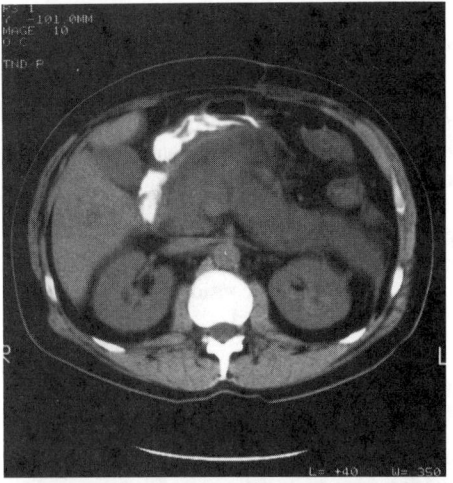

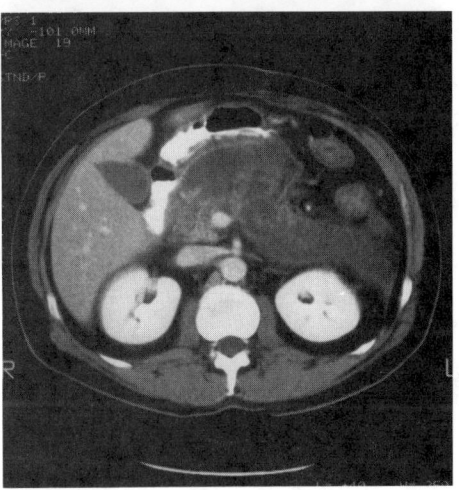

Fig 2 (a) Severe acute pancreatitis with diffuse pancreatic swelling on plain CT scan. (b) Same scale level as in (a) with angiogram enhancement, revealing hypodense areas of poor perfusion.

Fig. 3 Mean daily APACHE II scores by outcome in 119 patients with an uncomplicated course (–.–.–), 26 patients with a complicated course (– – – –), and 12 patients with a fatal outcome(——). The differences between fatal and uncomplicated and between complicated and uncomplicated were highly significant ($p < 0.001$) for each day (Mann-Whitney U test). (Published with permission from *British Journal of Surgery*.)

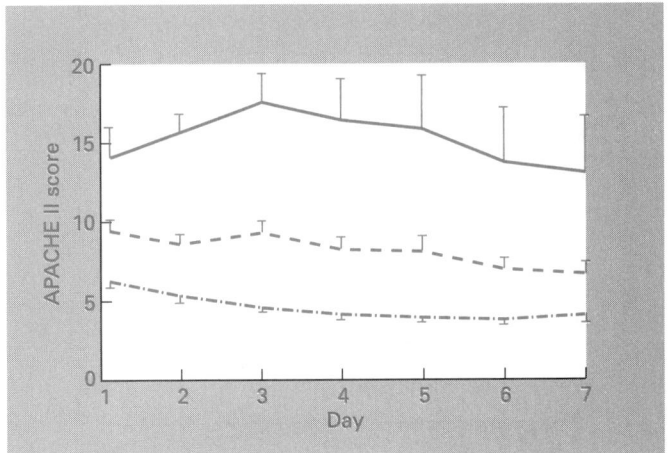

Correction of hypovolaemia requires the rapid infusion of high-volume electrolyte solutions (and albumin-rich solution). There is a tendency to underestimate fluid requirements in the initial 12 h of treatment and monitoring the central venous pressure is essential.

Catheterization of the bladder to monitor urine output should be done at an early stage and a minimum flow of 30 ml/h obtained. Nasogastric aspiration is particularly beneficial and both this and urinary catheterization can be discontinued at an early stage if the disease proves to be mild. In such patients there is little justification for the routine use of antimicrobials or H_2-receptor antagonists as nearly all of them improve within a few days. If gallstones have been identified by ultrasound scanning, laparoscopic or open cholecystectomy should be done in the same admission to minimize the risk of a recurrent attack. In older and infirm patients, ERCP sphincterotomy alone is considered a satisfactory alternative.

THE SEVERELY ILL PATIENT

Those who are graded as having severe acute pancreatitis or who are severely ill at the time of admission, warrant high-dependency or intensive care therapy. Monitoring for system failures and biochemical or haematological abnormalities is now routine. An algorithm for suggested steps in the management of severe acute pancreatitis (Fig. 5) may prove valuable.

Fig 4 (a) Sequential C-reactive protein concentrations in 47 patients with mild pancreatitis (——) and 25 with complicated attacks (– – –). Results are expressed as mean ± s.e.m.; * $p < 0.05$; ** $p < 0.01$; *** $p < 0.001$ (mild versus complicated); (—..—), upper limit of normal for C-reactive protein. (b) Scattergram showing discrimination between mild and complicated attacks of pancreatitis based on the peak C-reactive protein concentration recorded on days 2–4. —..—. The peak concentration providing the best discrimination was ⩾ 210 mg/l. (Published with permission from *British Journal of Surgery*.)

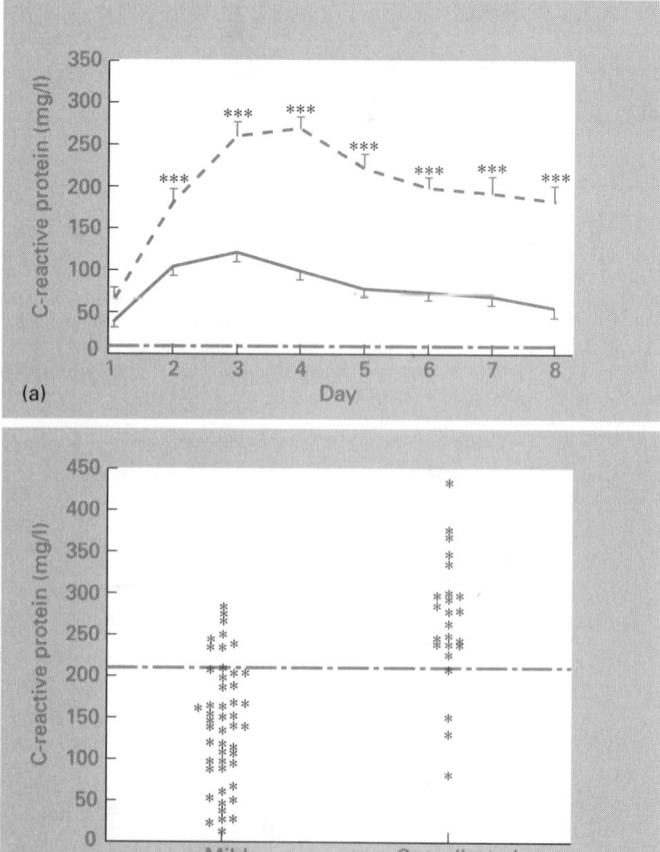

In addition to monitoring individual systems and providing support, the most revolutionary step has been the early provision of diagnostic and therapeutic ERCP. As recently as 1984 it was considered that ERCP was contraindicated in acute pancreatitis. However, two controlled studies and a large body of clinical data indicate that endoscopic sphincterotomy in those with gallstone acute pancreatitis provides a significant therapeutic advantage. It has also been my experience that rapid improvement can occur in some of the most severely ill patients with early endoscopic sphincterotomy and duct clearance.

Intravenous antimicrobial therapy is recommended as a cover for ERCP sphincterotomy and the drugs most widely used include the third-generation cephalosporins and piperacillin. The administration of imipenem to patients with objectively graded severe acute pancreatitis throughout the first 2 weeks of illness has been found to be of value in several studies, possibly because of its high tissue penetration. Some advocate a more selective use of antimicrobials depending on specific indications such as proven cholangitis, the use of ERCP, and evidence of specific culture of organisms at percutaneous needle aspiration in patients with infected necrosis. Fungal infection may be a problem in long-term management of those with severe acute pancreatitis where broad-spectrum antimicrobials are given for more than 10 days.

Another approach has been to strive to lower the concentration of intestinal organisms by methods of gut irrigation combined with antimicrobial therapy. A large study is nearing completion in The Netherlands that shows an initial trend in favour of this approach.

The reasons for this attention to the lowering of the risk for sepsis is the belief that transudation of organisms from the transverse colon into the peripancreatic necrotic tissue is one of the most serious complications of this disease. While this is usually a late complication, around the end of the first week of illness, it has been claimed that it may occur much earlier.

Fig. 5 Summary of management of acute pancreatitis.

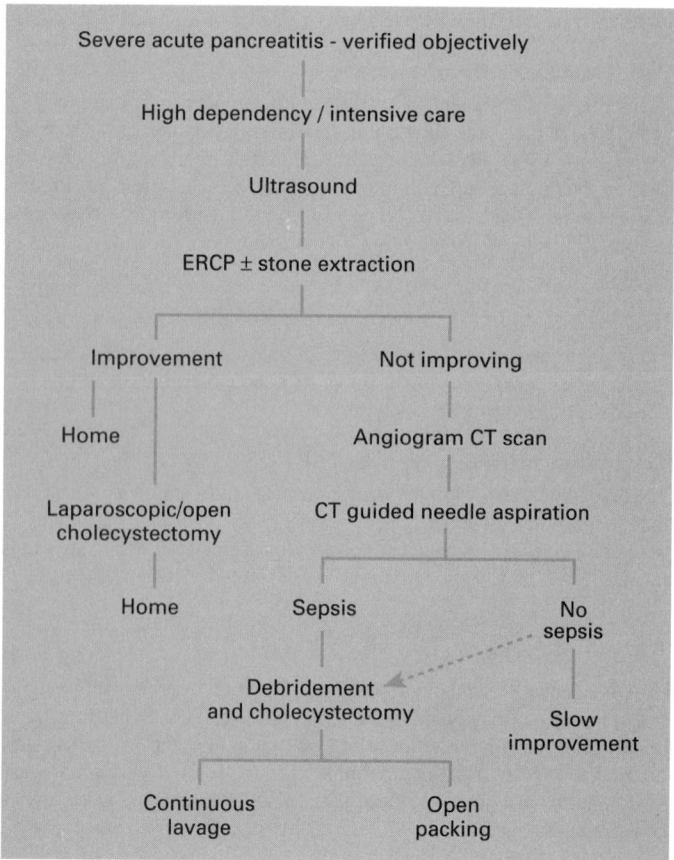

Table 6 *Role of surgery in acute pancreatitis*

To establish diagnosis without laparotomy
To remove all gallstones within same admission, if possible
To remove infected necrotic tissue in the most severe cases; and possibly to remove non-infected necrotic tissue
To drain pseudocysts

THE ROLE OF SURGERY (TABLE 6)

Patients who develop infection in the necrotic tissue around the pancreas and in the pancreas itself require open surgical debridement of the necrotic tissue by a combination of gentle finger and forceps dissection; the infected necrotic tissue will not readily drain along percutaneously introduced tubes. After the removal of the infected tissue there are two options. One is to establish a postoperative lavage system, which may necessitate up to three inflow and three outflow drains because of the retroperitoneal extension of the infected necrosis down the paracolic gutters and upwards towards the diaphragm. Alternatively, if venous ooze of blood is a particular problem, packing of the abdominal cavity with large cotton packs wrapped in non-adhesive paraffin gauze, together with limited or non-closure of the abdominal wall, has been advocated. Such patients are invariably in intensive care on ventilation. Hence the packs can be changed at 24-to 48-h intervals, with removal of any extension of infection or necrosis.

Debate continues as to whether only patients with infected necrosis warrant such surgical intervention. Proof of infection depends on either the presence of retroperitoneal gas radiologically or the results of needle aspiration guided by ultrasound or CT scanning. Some have strongly advocated that uninfected necrosis can be managed very successfully without surgical intervention, while others are concerned about the limitations of methods for detecting infection, and would therefore widen indications for surgical intervention. Irrespective of approach, the proportions of patients coming to surgery vary between 4 and 15 per cent or approximately 35 per cent of those with objectively graded, severe acute pancreatitis.

THE ROLE OF ANGIOGRAM-ENHANCED CT SCANNING. (FIG. 2)

A standard CT scan gives limited information about the pancreatic circulation, but large-bolus intravenous contrast (dynamic or angiogram-enhanced) CT scanning provides very helpful information on the perfusion of the pancreas. Areas of non-perfusion on such scans have been shown to correlate very closely with necrosis.

NUTRITION AND GALLSTONE ERADICATION

At the time of surgical debridement it is important to provide for postoperative nutrition by the insertion of a feeding jejunostomy. This is preferred to continued intravenous nutrition, which is customarily introduced at the time of intensive supportive management. It has the advantage of safety and being a more physiological route for feeding.

Cholecystectomy and common-duct clearance are indicated in patients with stones or biliary sludge.The later complication of pancreatic pseudocyst is more common and has a higher morbidity and mortality in those with biliary than alcohol-abuse pancreatitis. This is largely attributable to postoperative complications of sepsis and haemorrhage, which are much more common in the gallstone group, particularly if they have not had the gallbladder removed at the primary operation. Thus, all patients with severe acute pancreatitis coming to surgery should have a cholecystectomy, especially as it is often impossible to identify small stones.

PANCREATIC PSEUDOCYST

This condition is probably overdiagnosed. A recent international conference on nomenclature agreed that the fibrous wall around a pseudocyst took approximately 4 weeks to develop from the onset of acute pancreatitis. It is recommended that the term 'acute fluid collections' be used at an earlier stage in the disease process because these frequently disappear spontaneously. Even established pseudocysts can spontaneously resolve in around 50 per cent of patients. For those not resolving, synthetic somatostatin therapy (octreotide) given subcutaneously three times a day, can be helpful, either alone or combined with percutaneous tube drainage of the pseudocyst cavity.

Percutaneous aspiration alone invariably results in recollection of the fluid quite rapidly, while infection is potentially associated with long-term percutaneous drainage. In younger patients this later complication of acute pancreatitis is best dealt with by internal surgical drainage to the stomach or a defunctioned loop of jejunum. Cystogastrostomy has been done laparoscopically, an approach that can also be used for cholecystectomy. Pancreatic pseudocyst most commonly occurs in the lesser sac and often represents a closed pancreatic fistula; a breach in the main or a major pancreatic duct can often be demonstrated at ERCP. This investigation is potentially hazardous as it may lead to the introduction of infection and should not be done without an appropriate antimicrobial in the injection fluid.

PANCREATIC ASCITES

This condition occurs either when a pancreatic pseudocyst spontaneously decompresses into the peritoneal cavity or a major pancreatic duct disrupts after trauma or pancreatitis, with escape of pancreatic juice into the peritoneal cavity. Treatment comprises either a combination of intravenous nutrition and octreotide therapy or surgical excision of the disconnected segment of pancreas. Some success has also been obtained with intrapancreatic main-duct stents passed endoscopically.

RARE COMPLICATIONS

Rarer complications of severe acute pancreatitis include splenic vein thrombosis and subcutaneous fat necrosis. The latter condition can mimic erythema nodosum.

REFERENCES

Acosta, J.M., and Ledesma, C.L. (1974). Gallstone migration as a cause for acute pancreatitis. *New England Journal of Medicine*, **290**, 480–7.

Allam, B.F., and Imrie, C.W. (1976). Serum ionized calcium in acute pancreatitis. *British Journal of Surgery*, **64**, 655–68.

Balthazar, E.J. *et al.* (1985). Acute pancreatitis: prognostic value of CT. *Radiology* **156**, 767–72.

Bradley, E.L. (1987). Management of infected pancreatic necrosis by open drainage. *Annals of Surgery*, **206**, 542–50.

Braganza, J.M., and Rindernecht, H. (1988). Free radicals and acute pancreatitis. *Gastroenterology*, **94**, 1111–12.

Corfield, A.P. *et al.* (1985). Prediction of severity in acute pancreatitis: prospective comparison of three prognostic indices. *Lancet*, **ii**, 403–7.

Corfield, A.P., Cooper, M.J.C., and Williamson, R.C.N. (1985). Acute pancreatitis: lethal disease of increasing incidence. *GUT*, **26**, 724–9.

Croton R.S., Warren, R.A., Stott, A., and Roberts, N.B. (1981). Ionized calcium in acute pancreatitis and its relationships with total calcium and serum lipase. *British Journal of Surgery*, **68**, 241–4.

Fan, S.T. *et al.* (1993). Early treatment of acute biliary pancreatitis by endoscopic papillotomy. *New England Journal of Medicine*, **328**, 228–32.

Fenton-Lee, D. and Imrie, C.W. (1993). Pancreatic necrosis: assessment of outcome related to quality of life and cost of management. *British Journal of Surgery*, **80**, 1579–82.

Foulis, A.K. (1982). Morphological study of the relation between accidental hypothermia and acute pancreatitis. *Journal of Clinical Pathology*. **35**, 1244–8.

Gudgeon, A.M. *et al.* (1990). Trypsinogen activation peptide assay in the early prediction of severe AP. *Lancet*, **i**, 4–8.

Gupta, R.K. (1971). Immunohistological study of glomerular lesions in acute pancreatitis. *Archives of Pathology*, **92**, 267–72.

Heath, D.I. *et al.* Role of interleukin-6 in mediating the acute phase protein response and potential as an early means of severity assessment in acute pancreatitis. *Gut*, **34**, 41–5.

Imrie, C.W., Ferguson, J.C., Murphy, D., and Blumgart, L.H. (1977). Arterial hypoxia in acute pancreatitis. *British Journal of Surgery*, **64**, 185–8.

Imrie, C.W. *et al.* (1978). Parathyroid hormone and homeostasis in acute pancreatitis. *British Journal of Surgery*, **65**, 717–20.

Imrie, C.W. *et al.* (1978). A single centre double blind trial of Trasylol therapy in primary acute pancreatitis. *British Journal of Surgery*, **65**, 337–41.

Kelly, T.R. (1976). Gallstone pancreatitis: pathophysiology. *Surgery*, **80**, 488–92.

Kivisaari, L. *et al.* (1984). A new method for diagnosing of acute haemorrhagic necrotising pancreatitis using contrast enhanced CT. *Gastrointestinal Radiology*, **9**, 27–30.

Larvin, M. and McMahon, M.J. (1989). APACHE II score for assessment and monitoring of AP. *Lancet*, **ii**, 201–4.

Leese, T. *et al.* (1987). Multicentre clinical trial of low volume fresh frozen plasma therapy in acute pancreatitis. *British Journal of Surgery*, **74**, 907–11.

London, N.J.M. *et al.* (1989). Contrast enhanced abdominal computed tomography scanning and prediction of severity of acute pancreatitis: a prospective study. *British Journal of Surgery*, **76**, 268–72.

Lucarotti, M.E., Virjee, J., and Alderson, D. (1993). Patient selection and timing of dynamic computed tomography in acute pancreatitis. *British Journal of Surgery*, **80**, 1393–5.

Murphy, D., Pack, A., and Imrie, C.W. (1980). The mechanisms of arterial hypoxia occurring in AP. *Quarterly Journal of Medicine*, **49**, 151–63.

Neoptolemos, J.P., Carrlocke, D.L., Leese, T., *et al.* (1987). Acute cholangitis in association with acute pancreatitis: incidence, clinical features, outcome and the role of ERCP and endoscopic sphincterotomy. *British Journal of Surgery*, **74**, 1103–6.

Pickford, I.R., Blackett, R.L. and McMahon, M.J. (1977). Early assessment of severity of acute pancreatitis using peritoneal lavage. *British Medical Journal*, **2**, 1377–9.

Poulakkainen, P. *et al.* (1987). C-reactive protein (CRP) and serum phospholipase A2 in the assessment of severity of AP. *Gut*, **28**, 764–71.

Ranson, J.H.C. *et al.* (1974). Respiratory complications in acute pancreatitis. *Annuals of Surgery*, **179**, 559–66.

Ranson, J.H.C. *et al.* (1974). Prognostic signs and the role of operative management in acute pancreatitis. *Surgery, Gynecology and Obstetrics*, **139**, 69–81.

Rindernecht, H. (1986). Activation of pancreatic zymogens: normal activation, premature intrapancreatic activation, protective mechanisms against inappropriate activation. *Digestive Diseases and Science*, **24**, 80–6.

Viedma, J.A., Perez-Mateo, M., Dominguez, J.E., and Carballo, F. (1992). Role of interleukin-6 in acute pancreatitis. Comparison with C-reactive protein and phospholipase A. *Gut*, **33**, 1264–7.

Werner, M.H., Hayes, D.F., Lucas, C.E., and Rosenberg, I.K. (1974). Renal vasoconstriction in association with AP. *American Journal of Surgery*, **127**, 185–90.

Wilson, C., McArdle, C.S., Carter, D.C., and Imrie C.W. (1988). Surgical treatment of acute necrotising pancreatitis. *British Journal of Surgery*, **75**, 1119–23.

Wilson, C., Heads, A., Shenkin, A., and Imrie, C.W. (1989). C-reactive protein, antiproteases and complement factors as objective markers of severity of AP. *British Journal of Surgery*, **76**, 177–81.

14.23.2 Chronic pancreatitis

P. P. TOSKES

INTRODUCTION

Patients with chronic pancreatitis come to medical attention largely due to two complaints—abdominal pain or maldigestion (diarrhoea, steatorrhoea, weight loss). The true frequency of chronic pancreatitis has been underestimated because many patients with these complaints are inaccurately evaluated by physicians. The realization that significant impairment of pancreatic exocrine function can occur without obvious dilation of the main duct, that is 'small-duct disease', has had a large effect on the approach to management of these patients. The great variability in symptoms and the many causes of this disease have made its classification problematical.

In the most recent attempts at classification, three forms of chronic pancreatitis have been recognized: (i) chronic calcifying; (ii) chronic obstructive; and (iii) chronic inflammatory. Alcohol abuse and/or malnutrition are the most common causes of the calcifying type. Obstruction of the main pancreatic duct with secondary fibrosis in that part of the pancreas proximal to the obstruction leads to the obstructive type. Chronic inflammatory pancreatitis is not well characterized and many patients with idiopathic chronic pancreatitis fall into this group. Often irreversible changes occur in the gland, making a cure improbable. Nevertheless, the chief complaints of pain and/or maldigestion are frequently well managed medically or surgically.

Histologically, in advanced stages of chronic pancreatitis the gland may be fibrotic, calcified, and there may be marked dilation of the main duct. Inflammation and sclerosis with progressive damage to the acini and ducts are the histological hallmarks of chronic pancreatitis. Islet cells are usually lost more slowly than the exocrine part, thus preserving endocrine function relative to exocrine function.

AETIOLOGY

Table 1 classifies chronic pancreatitis into a number of different conditions associated with this disease. Chronic alcoholism and cystic fibrosis are the most frequent causes in adults and children, respectively. Cholelithiasis rarely, if ever, causes chronic pancreatitis because a cholecystectomy is almost always done after the first or second attack of acute pancreatitis related to gallstones and the pancreas returns to normal after removal of the gallbladder. It has not been generally appreciated that hypertriglyceridaemia may cause chronic as well as acute pancreatitis. Tropical pancreatitis (Africa and Asia) is characterized by calcific disease, glucose intolerance, and infrequent pain. Pancreatic exocrine impairment is not infrequent in patients with haemochromatosis and α-antitrypsin deficiency but the pancreatic disease is usually not symptomatic. Secondary pancreatic exocrine insufficiency may occur after gastric surgery, leading to postcibal asynchrony; usually the maldigestion is not very severe. Similarly, the acid hypersecretion associated with gastrinoma may irreversibly inactivate lipase, causing steatorrhea. Hereditary pancreatitis and developmental anomalies leading to pancreatitis will be discussed later in this chapter.

Idiopathic chronic pancreatitis remains the controversial category. It may account for up to 20 per cent of cases of chronic pancreatitis, depending on the patient population being served. Many patients with idiopathic pancreatitis present solely with unexplained abdominal pain and no evidence of maldigestion. These patients have small-duct disease, often without radiographic abnormalities. It is necessary to make a direct intubation (hormone stimulation) test to detect these cases—a test not done at many medical centres. Endoscopic retrograde cholangiopancreatography (**ERCP,**) which is often used to diagnose chronic pancreatitis, may miss up to 30 per cent of those with chronic pancreatitis who have abnormal hormone-stimulation tests. It is provocative to con-

Table 1 *Conditions associated with chronic pancreatitis*

Alcohol abuse
Cystic fibrosis
Malnutrition (tropical)
Pancreatic cancer
Gastrinoma
Trauma
Familial pancreatitis
Schwachmann's syndrome (pancreatic insufficiency and bone marrow dysfunction)
Trypsinogen deficiency
Enterokinase deficiency
Isolated deficiencies of amylase or lipase
Haemochromatosis
α_1-antitrypsin deficiency
Postsurgery:
    Pancreatic resection
    Subtotal gastrectomy with Billroth I or II anastomosis
    Truncal vagotomy and pyloroplasty
Idiopathic pancreatitis

sider how many patients with unexplained abdominal pain may fit into this category of small-duct chronic pancreatitis! No doubt some are labelled as having non-ulcer dyspepsia. Others with idiopathic pancreatitis may present at an older age with painless diarrhoea, steatorrhoea, and secondary diabetes mellitus. They often have pancreatic calcification.

PATHOPHYSIOLOGY

Although alcohol-induced chronic pancreatitis has been extensively investigated, controversy continues as to whether the biochemical and histological lesions are secondary to a primary reduced secretion of pancreatic-stone protein or a direct toxic effect of alcohol on the pancreas. The reduced secretion theory suggests that, in a predisposed individual, ingestion of large amounts of alcohol may decrease the stone protein below a critical level, allowing calcium and other components within the secretion to precipitate and form protein plugs, which ultimately lead to ductal obstruction. The toxic theory suggests that alcohol may cause abnormalities in acinar cells, leading to a deficiency of protease inhibitors with resulting inflammatory changes. In tropical pancreatitis a combination of protein deficiency and a toxin found in the diet, which is high in cassava or sorghum, may cause the disease. A primary defect in the electrolyte permeability of epithelium within the pancreatic ducts of patients with cystic fibrosis results in reduced fluid flow, producing hyperconcentrated proteinaceous secretions that precipitate and obstruct the ducts. The pathophysiology of the other causes of chronic pancreatitis is not understood.

Although it is commonly believed that at the time a patient presents with the first attack of clinically apparent acute pancreatitis, secondary to alcohol abuse, they have already sustained chronic damage to the pancreas, recent clinical experiences suggest that some individuals with no history of chronic alcohol ingestion may develop acute pancreatitis following the ingestion of large quantities of alcohol (binge drinking).

INCIDENCE

There is a lack of data on the prevalence and incidence of chronic pancreatitis. Most opinions are based on clinical experiences, which vary greatly. The prevalence in autopsy studies varies from 0.04 to 5.0 per cent. The only prospective study (Copenhagen Pancreatic Study) found a prevalence of 26.4 cases per 100 000 population and an incidence of 8.2 new cases per 100 000 per year. Yet, it must be stressed that this study is largely based on alcohol-induced pancreatitis and does not accurately reflect the prevalence and/or incidence of other kinds.

CLINICAL FEATURES

Abdominal pain is the cardinal clinical manifestation of chronic pancreatitis; its pattern, severity, and frequency vary considerably. Whereas the pain of acute pancreatitis is often located in the epigastrium and bores through to the back, the pain of chronic pancreatitis has no characteristic features: it may be constant or intermittent. Eating may often increase the severity of the pain, resulting in avoidance of food and weight loss. The pain may be mild, requiring no therapy, or severe, leading to frequent use of narcotics and addiction.

Patients with abdominal pain may develop steatorrhoea and/or diarrhoea, or the abdominal pain may remain their main symptom. Approximately 15 per cent never suffer with abdominal pain but present initially with steatorrhoea, diarrhoea, and weight loss. In those who only have abdominal pain, there is a paucity of physical findings except for abdominal tenderness and mild pyrexia. Indeed, there is a marked disparity between the severe nature of the abdominal pain and the lack of physical findings.

In patients with maldigestion and weight loss secondary to alcohol-induced pancreatitis, signs and symptoms of liver disease may be present. Clinically apparent deficiencies of fat-soluble vitamins are uncommon.

DIAGNOSIS

Computed tomographic scans may reveal diffuse enlargement of the pancreas and, occasionally, a pseudocyst (Fig. 1). Ultrasonography may reveal calcification and dilatation of the pancreatic duct (Fig. 2); calcification may also be seen on plain abdominal radiographs (Fig. 3). Blood chemistry is usually not very helpful in making a diagnosis of chronic pancreatitis. The levels of pancreatic enzymes (amylase, lipase, trypsin) are usually not elevated except in patients who have a pseudocyst of the pancreas. There may be evidence of cholestasis (elevated alkaline phosphatase, elevated bilirubin) secondary to an inflammatory reaction around the common bile duct as a result of the pancreatitis. Some patients with severe disease may have elevated fasting blood-glucose levels.

Table 2 lists selected tests of pancreatic function and structure. In general, abnormalities of function precede abnormalities in structure. The most sensitive tests are at the top of the table, the least sensitive at the bottom. Currently, the most accurate means of detecting chronic pancreatitis is a combination of a hormone stimulation test and ERCP. As many as 30 per cent of patients with chronic pancreatitis may have a normal ERCP but an abnormal hormone-stimulation test. Occasionally

Fig. 1 CT scan demonstrating a pseudocyst (PC) in the head of the pancreas, diffuse enlargement of the pancreas (P) a normal liver (L), and normal gallbladder (GB).

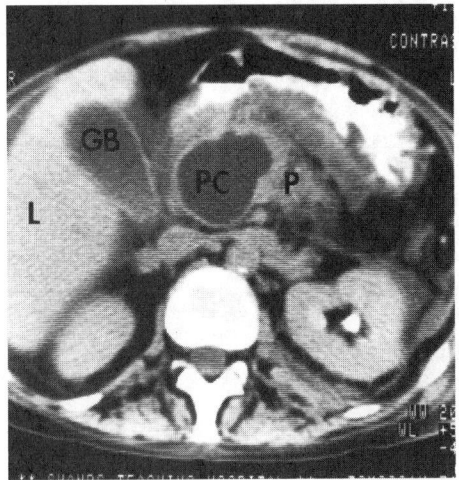

the converse will be true. Two significant causes of a false-positive (abnormal) ERCP are normal ageing and performing the investigation within several weeks of an attack of acute pancreatitis. Ageing does not appear to affect the hormone stimulation test. Simple, non-invasive tests (bentiromide, pancreolauryl, trypsin) are not sensitive and are used to confirm the clinical impression. The same can be said for radiography other than ERCP.

Almost any test listed in Table 2 will detect patients with severe disease but a hormone stimulation test is often needed to diagnose those with abdominal pain only. Although it is generally accepted that a hormone stimulation test is the most sensitive way to detect mild to moderate impairment of exocrine function, comparisons of the true 'gold standard' (histological examination of the pancreas) with any pancreatic

Fig. 2 Ultrasonogram of chronic pancreatitis. The large closed arrow points to pancreatic calcification, the small closed arrow shows a dilated pancreatic duct, and the open arrow identifies the splenic vein.

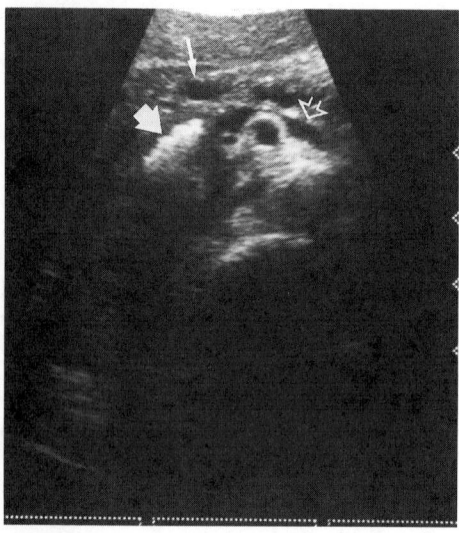

Fig. 3 Plain film of the abdomen showing diffuse pancreatic calcification; the arrow points to one of the calcified areas.

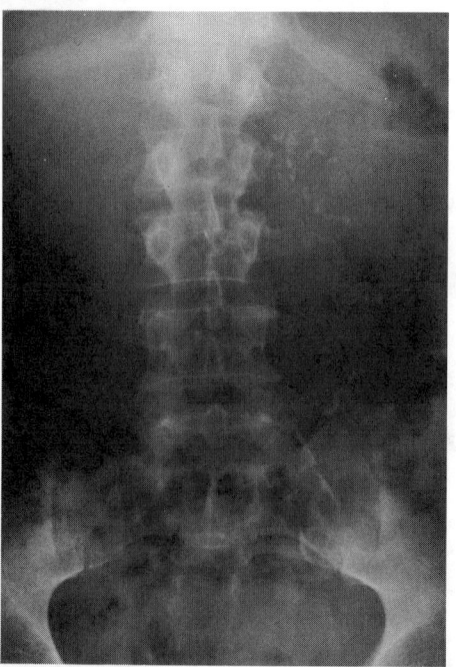

test have been lacking until recently. A recent study compared the hormone stimulation test to pancreatic histological findings obtained at surgery in 108 patients. The most discriminatory function was the maximum bicarbonate concentration, followed by volume and amylase output. A significant correlation was found between pancreatic function and histology. In 29 of these patients with histologically confirmed pancreatitis, the cholecystokinin-secretin test had a sensitivity of 79 per cent and ERCP, 66 per cent. What is sorely needed is a simple, inexpensive test that has a sensitivity and specificity approaching that of hormone stimulation. A cost-effective approach to the evaluation of patients suspected of having chronic pancreatitis would be, first, a simple, non-invasive test like serum trypsin (or bentiromide). If the result is abnormal, pancreatic enzyme therapy should be initiated. If this first-order test is normal, proceed to a hormone stimulation test and finally, if needed, an ERCP.

MANAGEMENT

The cornerstone of the medical management of chronic pancreatitis is the use of pancreatic enzyme formulations. The principles of therapy are similar for treating pain or steatorrhoea. A potent enzyme formulation must be used to ensure that the relevant enzymes (proteases for pain, lipase for steatorrhea) escape destruction by gastric acid and reach the duodenum.

Abstinence from alcohol is recommended. The diet should be moderate in fat (30 per cent), high in protein (24 per cent), and low in carbohydrate (40 per cent). Non-narcotic analgesics are the pain-relieving medications of choice.

Three controlled trials have shown that pancreatic enzymes decrease abdominal pain in some patients with chronic pancreatitis. Pain relief was obtained in 75 per cent of the patients evaluated. Those most likely to respond have small-duct disease, that is minimal to moderate impairment of exocrine function (abnormal hormone-stimulation test, minimal abnormalities on ERCP, normal fat absorption) (Fig. 4). Patients with severe (large-duct) disease (abnormal hormone-stimulation test, marked abnormalities on ERCP, steatorrhoea) (Fig. 5) do not respond well to enzyme therapy for pain. These clinical observations fit well with findings in both experimental animals and man, which demonstrate negative feedback regulation of pancreatic secretion controlled by the amount of proteases within the lumen of the proximal small intestine. Eight tablets or capsules of a potent, non-enteric-coated enzyme preparation should be given at mealtime and at bedtime, with appropriate adjuvant therapy (Table 3). Enteric-coated preparations are not the preparations of choice because they often release their proteases in the jejunum or ileum, rather than the duodenum, thus failing to deliver to the feedback-sensitive segment of the intestine.

Figure 6 outlines an approach to patients with abdominal pain thought to be secondary to chronic pancreatitis. After other causes of abdominal pain have been excluded, an ultrasonogram should be obtained. If no pseudocyst or mass is found, a hormone stimulation test should be done. In patients with abdominal pain secondary to chronic pancreatitis, the hormone stimulation test will invariably be abnormal. A 4-week trial of pancreatic enzymes (with adjuvant) is indicated, as described above. If pain is not relieved, ERCP is appropriate to characterize the pancreatitis as small- or large-duct disease, and possibly to define the surgical approach.

If there is large-duct disease (diameter of the main pancreatic duct greater than 8 cm), a lateral pancreaticojejunostomy (Peustow procedure) should be done. Immediate pain relief occurs in 80 per cent of patients, with satisfactory pain relief sustained in about 50 per cent at 1 to 3 years, follow-up. If the ducts are not significantly dilated, most patients can eventually have their pain controlled by adjusting enzyme and adjuvant therapy; for example, substitution of omeprazole for H_2-receptor antagonist, total parenteral nutrition with no food orally for several weeks, or performing a nerve block. It is now rare for a major

Table 2 *Selected pancreatic diagnostic tests*

	Principle	Comment
Test pertaining to function		
Hormone stimulation test	Secretin stimulates bicarbonate output, CCK stimulates enzyme output	Most sensitive and specific pancreatic test; requires intestinal intubation; not done at most centres
Bentiromide test	Synthetic peptide specifically cleaved by chymotrypsin freeing PABA, a metabolite of which is excreted into the urine	Not very sensitive; will detect 80% of patients with severe disease
Pancreolauryl test	Fluorescein dilaurate is hydrolysed by elastase; fluorescein measured in urine	Sensitivity and specificity similar to bentiromide
Faecal chymotrypsin	Pancreatic secretion of proteases	Not sensitive; significant number of false positives and false negatives; disadvantage of analysing stool
Serum trypsin-like immunoreactivity	Pancreatic secretion of proteases	Not sensitive; high specificity, simple, inexpensive
Quantitative faecal fat	Lipase deficiency leads to maldigestion	'Gold standard' for diagnosing maldigestion/malabsorption; does not distinguish between pancreatic steatorrhoea and other causes of steatorrhoea; not cost-effective, requires high-fat diet, low sensitivity; disadvantage of analysing stool
Test pertaining to structure		
Endoscopic retrograde cholangiopancreatography (ERCP) (Figs 4, 5)	Direct cannulation of pancreatic-biliary ducts	Sensitivity 70%, specificity 90%; differentiation of chronic pancreatitis from cancer may be problematical; may cause acute pancreatitis in 3%; expensive
CT scan (Fig. 1)	Detailed visualization of pancreas and surrounding structures	Permits early detection of calcification, masses, dilated main pancreatic duct; may not distinguish inflammatory masses from cancer; expensive
Ultrasonography (fig. 2)	Can provide information on pseudocysts, calcification, phlegmon	Simple; inexpensive; no radiation exposure
Plain films of abdomen (Fig. 3)	Diffuse calcification indicates severe damage; hallmark of alcohol-induced pancreatitis	Simple, inexpensive; focal calcification does not have same meaning; calcification also seen in trauma, islet-cell tumours, hypercalcaemia, familial pancreatitis, malnutrition, idiopathic pancreatitis

Fig. 4 Early ERCP changes of chronic pancreatitis. A non-dilated main pancreatic duct (PD) and accessory duct (AD) with mild dilation and clubbing of the side branches (arrow) are shown.

Fig. 5 ERCP showing a dilated main pancreatic duct with a communicating pseudocyst (PC).

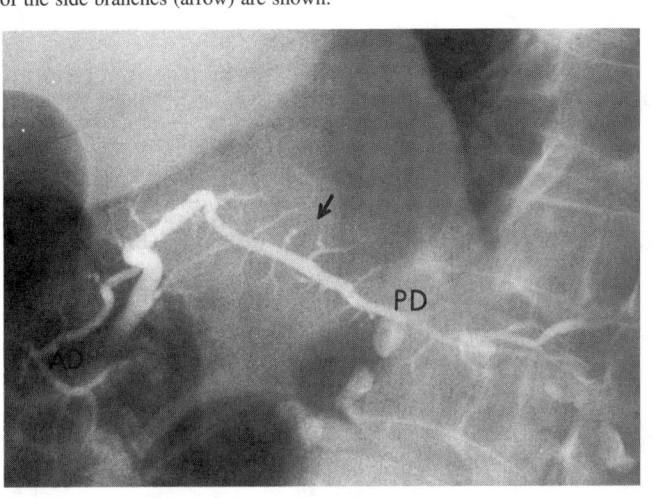

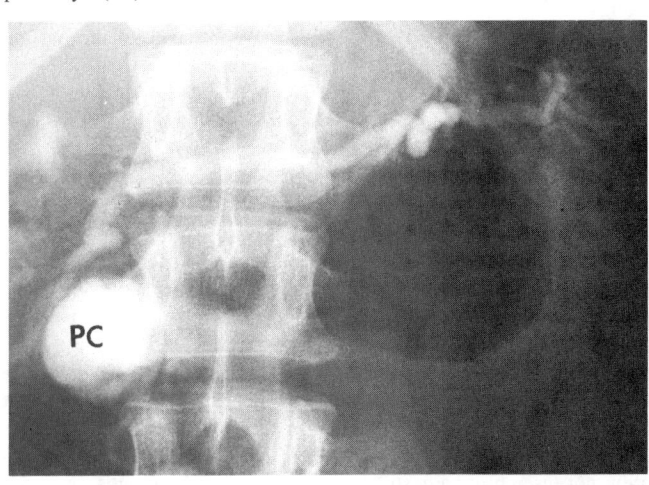

Table 3 *Frequently used pancreatic enzyme therapy*

Pancrelipase
Viokase (C), 8 tablets each time
Pancrease (E), 3 capsules each time

Pancreatin
Creon (E), 3 capsules each time

Adjuvant
Sodium bicarbonate, one 650-mg tablet before and after each
    meal and 1300 mg at bedtime for pain
H$_2$-receptor antagonists in usual acid-suppressive doses, twice a
    day
Omeprazole, 20 mg every day

The enzymes should be administered before meals; a bedtime
    dosage should be given if the enzymes are being used to
    treat pain

C, conventional preparation; E, enteric-coated preparation.

pancreatic resection to be done for pain control. In some preliminary controlled trials, octreotide in doses up to 200 µg three times daily given subcutaneously has been effective in lessening pain in severe chronic pancreatitis. Whether ductal decompression or major resection are done, enzyme therapy for enhancing digestion should be given.

Endoscopic therapy for the pain of chronic pancreatitis has been disappointing. This therapy has included dilation or stenting of duct strictures, removal of calculi, and treatment of biliary obstruction. With the exception of acute biliary decompression, none of these therapies has been shown to be effective in controlled trials. It is noteworthy that following stent placement, complications such as bleeding, sepsis, pancreatitis, and perforation have occurred. Stents can induce progressive ductal changes similar to the abnormalities seen in chronic pancreatitis.

Steatorrhoea in chronic pancreatitis is a late finding and does not occur until less than 10 per cent of lipase is secreted. With eight conventional or three enteric-coated tablets or capsules (Table 3), control of steatorrhoea and diarrhoea, and weight gain, can be readily achieved, even though steatorrhoea is not fully corrected. Enzyme formulations containing lipase in amounts of 25 000 units or higher have recently been associated with the occurrence of colonic strictures in patients with cystic fibrosis who were taking large doses of these high-potency preparations. No such problems have occurred in adult patients with chronic pancreatitis. In the United States, all pancreatic enzyme preparations with more than 20 000 units of lipase per capsule have been taken out of clinical use. The cause of the colonic strictures remains obscure.

Decreasing the amount of long-chain triglyceride in the diet and/or adding medium-chain triglycerides (which do not require pancreatic lipase for absorption) may decrease the steatorrhoea and enhance weight gain and energy.

COMPLICATIONS

Table 4 lists the structural and metabolic complications of chronic pancreatitis. Inflammatory masses are common. Ultrasonography and computerized tomography have helped immensely in sorting out phlegmon from pseudocyst from abscess. The management of pseudocysts is currently being re-evaluated. Most clinicians have followed an aggressive approach, that is drainage, if the pseudocyst persists for longer than 7 weeks. It now appears that the ability of pseudocysts to undergo late resolution may have been underestimated and the incidence of serious complications overestimated. Recent clinical experience suggests that in patients who have pseudocysts but minimal symptoms, no evidence of active alcohol abuse, and a mature pseudocyst on radiographic evaluation not resembling a cystic neoplasm, non-intervention is appropriate. There is a reasonable chance that the pseudocyst will resolve, and approximately a 10 per cent chance of complications.

Pancreatic ascites occurs when there is a rent in the pancreatic duct or a leaking pseudocyst. The amylase content in the ascitic fluid is extraordinarily high, averaging 20 000 i.u./l. True pancreatic ascites should be distinguished from 'reactive ascites' in patients with pancreatitis. In reactive ascites the ascitic amylase content, while increased, is not nearly as high as in the pancreatic ascites. Patients with pancreatic ascites should have complete pancreatic rest, including total parenteral nutrition and no food by mouth. Surgery may be needed if the ascites persists after several weeks of conservative therapy. An ERCP may be needed to determine the site of the leakage.

Although obstruction of the common bile-duct is common, it may be temporary, owing to the resolution of inflammation. Even obstruction due to fibrosis of the pancreas rarely leads to cholangitis. Conservative management is suggested unless the alkaline phosphatase remains very high or cholangitis develops. In a small percentage of patients the obstruction may have to be relieved surgically by anastomosing the dilated common bile duct to the duodenum or jejunum.

Gastrointestinal bleeding may arise from portal hypertension associated with splenic-vein thrombosis caused by inflammation of the tail of the pancreas. It may also occur if a pseudocyst erodes into the duodenum or from a pseudoaneurysm within the wall of a pseudocyst. Of course, the most common reason for bleeding in chronic pancreatitis is a related duodenal ulcer or alcohol-induced gastritis.

Up to 30 per cent of patients with chronic pancreatitis have glucose intolerance. Although the diabetes is usually manageable, hypoglycaemia is not uncommon. If the data are corrected for the duration of the

Fig. 6 Approach to management of chronic pancreatitis and abdominal pain.

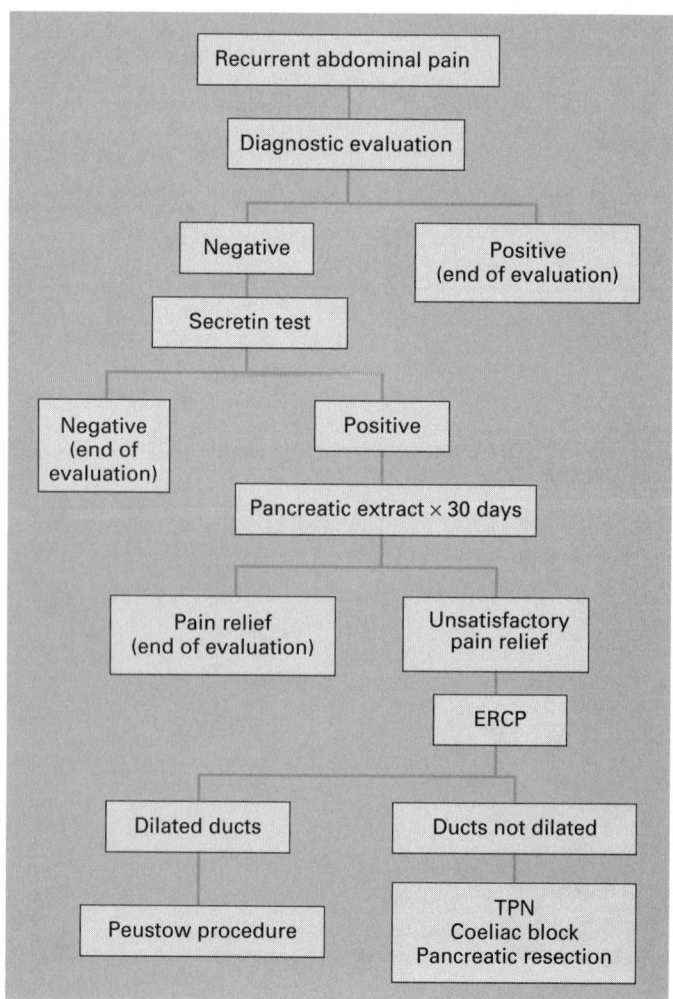

Table 4 *Complications of chronic pancreatitis*

Structural
Phlegmon
Pseudocyst
Abscess
Ascites
Common bile-duct obstruction
Duodenal obstruction
Splenic-vein thrombosis
Gastrointestinal bleeding

Metabolic
Narcotic addiction
Diabetes mellitus
Cobalamin (vitamin B$_{12}$) malabsorption
Subcutaneous fat necrosis
Bone pain
Non-diabetic retinopathy
Pancreatic cancer

diabetes, diabetic retinopathy occurs as often in this secondary form of diabetes as in idiopathic diabetes mellitus. Retinopathy due to zinc or vitamin A deficiency may occur.

Cobalamin (vitamin B$_{12}$) malabsorption is common in chronic pancreatitis but clinical vitamin B$_{12}$ deficiency is rare. It is caused by excessive binding of cobalamin by non-intrinsic factor cobalamin-binding proteins. Exogenous administration of pancreatic enzymes corrects the malabsorption.

Hereditary and familial diseases

Hereditary pancreatitis (see Chapter 14.22)

Hereditary pancreatitis (autosomal dominant with incomplete penetrance) is a rare disease with many similarities to chronic pancreatitis of other causes. Severe, acute attacks of abdominal pain with or without elevations of pancreatic enzymes in the blood occur in childhood. It is usual for these individuals to progress to chronic pancreatitis with marked dilation of the main pancreatic duct, calcification of the pancreas, and steatorrhoea. Ductal decompression is the usual therapy.

Schwachmann's syndrome (pancreatic insufficiency and bone marrow dysfunction)

This is a familial disorder involving the pancreas, bone marrow, and skeletal system. It is second to cystic fibrosis as a cause of pancreatic insufficiency in infants. Unlike cystic fibrosis the sweat chloride test is normal. Neonates with this condition present with severe steatorrhoea. The associated neutropenia leads to frequent infections. The steatorrhoea is well treated by pancreatic enzymes but severe skeletal defects result in dwarfism.

Isolated pancreatic enzyme deficiencies

Protease deficiencies may result from a deficiency of enterokinase (proximal small-intestine mucosal enzyme) or a deficiency in trypsinogen. The addition of exogenous enterokinase to duodenal secretions will distinguish these two deficiencies from each other; it will not activate duodenal secretions that have no trypsinogen. Both of these conditions will respond to pancreatic enzyme therapy. Lipase and colipase deficiency may occur, resulting in steatorrhoea. Patients with these deficiencies still manifest some fat absorption, presumably from the action of other lipases such as gastric lipase.

Developmental anomalies (see Chapter 14.21)

Annular pancreas

A failure of the ventral and dorsal anlage of the pancreas to unite produces a ring of pancreatic tissue encircling the duodenum. This may lead to intestinal obstruction in the neonate or the adult. Non-specific symptoms of postprandial fullness, nausea, abdominal pain, and vomiting may be present for years before the diagnosis is made. The radiographic findings are symmetrical dilation of the proximal duodenum with bulging of the recesses on either side of the annular band, effacement of the duodenal mucosa without obstruction of the mucosa, accentuation of the findings in the right anterior oblique position, and lack of change on repeated examinations. The differential diagnosis should include duodenal webs, tumours of the pancreas or duodenum, postbulbar peptic ulcer, Crohn's disease of the proximal intestine, and adhesions. Patients with annular pancreas have an increased incidence of pancreatitis and peptic ulcer. Because of these and other intestinal complications, surgery may be necessary, even though the condition has been present for years.

Retrocolic duodenojejunostomy is the procedure of choice, although some surgeons prefer a Billroth II gastrectomy, gastroenterostomy, and vagotomy.

Pancreas divisum (see Chapter 14.21)

Pancreas divisum is the most common, congenital, anatomical abnormality of the human pancreas. It occurs when the ventral and dorsal parts of the pancreas fail to fuse, so that pancreatic drainage is accomplished mainly through the accessory papilla. Current evidence indicates that this anomaly is not often a predisposing factor to the development of pancreatitis. The combination of pancreas divisum and a small accessory orifice could result in dorsal-duct obstruction. The challenge is to identify this subset of patients. Cannulation of the dorsal duct by ERCP is not as easy as cannulation of the ventral duct. Patients with pancreatitis and pancreas divisum demonstrated by ERCP should be treated conservatively, including pancreatic enzyme therapy. Many of them have idiopathic pancreatitis unrelated to the pancreas divisum and will respond well to pancreatic enzymes. Endoscopic or surgical intervention is indicated only when these methods fail. If marked dilation of the dorsal duct can be demonstrated, surgical ductal decompression is indicated. The appropriate therapy for those patients without dilation of the dorsal duct is not yet defined. It should be stressed that the ERCP appearance of pancreas divisum (i.e. a small-calibre ventral duct with an arborizing pattern) may be confused with an obstructed main pancreatic duct secondary to a mass lesion.

REFERENCES

Forsmark, C.F. and Grendell, J.H. (1991). Complications of pancreatitis. *Seminars in Gastrointestinal Diseases,* **3,** 165–76.
Forsmark, C. and Toskes, P. (1995). What does an abnormal pancreatogram mean? *Gastrointestinal Endoscopy Clinics of North America,* in press.
Gulliver, P.J. *et al.* (1992). Stent placement for benign pancreatic disease: correlation between ERCP findings and clinical response. *American Journal of Roentgenology,* **159,** 751–5.
Hayakawa, T. *et al.* (1992). Relationship between pancreatic exocrine function and histological charges in chronic pancreatitis. *American Journal of Gastroenterology,* **87,** 1170–4.
Huibreg, K. *et al.* (1988). Endoscopic pancreatic drainage in chronic pancreatitis. *Gastrointestinal Endoscopy,* **34,** 9–15.
Jacobson, D.G. *et al.* (1984) Trypsin-like immunoreactivity as a test for pancreatic insufficiency. *New England Journal of Medicine,* **310,** 1307–9.
Moosa, A.R. (1987). Surgical treatment of chronic pancreatitis. An overview. *British Journal of Surgery,* **74,** 661–7.
Owyang, C., Louie, D.A., and Tatum, D. (1986). Feedback regulation of pancreatic enzyme secretion. Suppression of cholecystokinin release by trypsin. *Journal of Clinical Investigation,* **77,** 2042–7.

Slaff, J. *et al.* (1984). Protease specific suppression of pancreatic exocrine secretion. *Gastroenterology*, **87**, 44–52.

Toskes, P.P. (1991). Medical therapy of chronic pancreatitis. *Seminars in Gastrointestinal Diseases*, **3**, 804–16.

Toskes, P.P. (1993). Chronic pancreatitis. *Current Opinion in Gastroenterology*, **9**, 767–973.

Vitab, G.J. and Sarr, M.G. (1992). Selected management of pancreatic pseudocysts: operative versus expectant management. *Surgery*, **III**, 124–30.

Walsh, T.N. *et al.* (1992). Minimal change chronic pancreatitis. *Gut*, **33**, 1566–71.

14.23.3 Tumours of the pancreas

R. C. G. RUSSELL

Introduction

A diagnosis of carcinoma of the pancreas carries a particularly poor outlook. Progress in our understanding of this appalling disease remains disappointingly slow despite major improvements in our ability to detect it. Current methods of adjuvant treatment offer little prospect of significantly prolonging useful life; fewer than 20 per cent of patients with a pancreatic carcinoma survive the first year and only 3 per cent are alive 5 years after the diagnosis. Of more than 60 cancer sites, pancreatic carcinoma is the one with the lowest 5-year survival rate.

Biology and epidemiology

INCIDENCE

Worldwide, there are large variations in the incidence of pancreatic carcinoma. In the United States, the incidence, which had been increasing since the 1930s, has been unchanged since 1973 and was 9/100 000 in 1988, with a male : female ratio of 1.3 : 1. The disease is rare before the age of 45 years, but its occurrence rises sharply thereafter. Afro-Caribbeans are more frequently affected than Caucasians, with an incidence of 15.2/100 000 black men. In India, Kuwait, and Singapore the rate is less than 2.2/100 000; in Sweden it is 12.5 and has remained practically unchanged for the past 20 years; however, in Japan the rate has risen sharply from 1.8 in 1960 to 5.2/100 000 in 1985. In the United Kingdom there were 6750 of deaths from pancreatic carcinoma in 1991.

RISK FACTORS

No single external factor has been unequivocally linked with the causation of pancreatic carcinoma in man. Cigarette smoking has the firmest link. Many cohort and case-controlled studies have found that the relative risk of pancreatic cancer in smokers is at least 1.5. The risk increases with the numbers of cigarettes smoked; the excess risk levels off 10 to 15 years after stopping smoking. Pancreatic tumours can be induced experimentally in animals by lifelong administration of tobacco-specific nitrosamines in drinking water as well as by parenteral administration of other *N*-nitroso compounds.

The second most important risk factor appears to be diet, notably a high intake of fat, meat, or both. A protective effect is ascribed to diet containing fresh fruits and vegetables. Lower than normal serum concentrations of leicopene, a carotenoid present in fruits, and selenium were found in persons in whom pancreatic cancer subsequently developed. A possible mechanism is the induction of premalignant pancreatic hyperplasia by cholecystokinin release. It appears that the type of fat is important, as giving linoleic acid increased the number of experimentally induced rat tumours, and giving eicosapentanoic acid reduced it. Animal studies have suggested that high levels of protease inhibitors might be carcinogenic.

Much controversy was generated by a report suggesting that coffee consumption could contribute to the development of pancreatic cancer; however, a recent comprehensive review of 30 epidemiological studies concluded that, although certain ecological and case-controlled studies suggest a possible increase in risk, only a few of the case-controlled studies and none of the prospective studies has confirmed a statistically significant association.

There is little doubt that pancreatic carcinoma and chronic pancreatitis coexist; there are families who develop hereditary pancreatitis and have a markedly increased risk of pancreatic cancer, suggesting that there may be a link between the two. Available studies of non-hereditary chronic pancreatitis do not, however, suggest an association. Nevertheless, the clinical coexistence of the two makes for clinical dilemmas, and the physician must be aware that either may mimic the other. Diabetes mellitus is associated with pancreatic cancer, although the nature and sequence of this association has not been established. It is suggested that there is a fourfold increase in the risk ratio. Experimentally, the diabetic state enhances the growth of pancreatic cancer.

Gastric resection with biliary reflux has been indicted as a precursor of pancreatic malignancy, increased levels of cholecystokinin being the proposed mechanism. Even after correction for smoking there appears to be a two-to fivefold increased risk of pancreatic cancer 15 to 20 years after partial gastrectomy. It has been proposed that increased formation of *N*-nitroso compounds by nitrate reductase-producing bacteria that proliferate in the hypoacidic stomach could be responsible for both the gastric and pancreatic cancers. Pancreatic tumours can be induced experimentally by long-term duodenogastric reflux, which is associated with increased amounts of cholecystokinin.

Other possible carcinogenic influences include industrial toxins, socioeconomic status (though probably less so than for malignancy in general), and viruses; oncogenic viruses produce pancreatic sarcomas in animals.

TUMOUR BIOLOGY

The genesis and biology of these tumours is complex. Differences between species and milieux may make the translation of experimental animal data to the human state invalid. As spontaneous pancreatic tumours are rare in laboratory animals, models of tumour production have been developed. They include: (i) *N*-nitrosobis(2-oxopropyl)amine (**BOP**) or *N*-nitroso(2-hydroxypropyl)-(2-oxopropyl)amine-treated Syrian golden hamsters, in which all forms of pancreatic ductal tumours are produced; (ii) azaserine-treated rats, which yield mostly acinar tumours; (iii) transgenic mice produced by insertion of an elastase antigen fusion gene into germinal cells. It is unclear in all three models whether the tumours arise from cells already differentiated into acinar or ductal cells or from pluripotent stem cells. The identification, by monoclonal antibodies, of cell markers that reliably relate a tumour cell to its cell of origin is awaited. Most research has been directed by the initiator–promoter concept wherein the effects of various entities are studied to determine whether they promote the already induced tumour. Promoters studied include cholecystokinin, sex steroids, bombesin, epidermal growth factors, secretin, cholecystectomy, and bile salts. Possible inhibitors include somatostatin, selenium deficiency, and inhibitors of polyamine synthesis such as cyclosporin. Studies of initiating influences in man have centred on oncogenes. Pancreatic tumours are known to express sex-steroid receptors (androgen–oestrogen), with male hamsters having two forms of oestrogen receptors. Allied to this, testosterone may promote and oestrogens inhibit azaserine-induced neoplasms. This possible promoter role of sex steroids may explain the high incidence of pancreatic carcinoma amongst human males and provide a rationale for hormone treatment. The use of tamoxifen as an antioestrogen would therefore seem illogical; its experimental and perhaps clinical value, if any, may derive from its direct pro-oestrogenic activity. Bile acids have been studied in BOP-treated hamsters. Lithocholic and deoxycholic acid enhanced the induction of ductal adenocarcinoma of the pancreas. The suggested mechanism *in vivo* is bile reflux.

Table 1 *Classification of exocrine primary pancreatic neoplasia*

Benign	Malignant
Epithelial origin	
Duct/ductile/centroductal (acinar) cell	Duct/ductule cell origin:
Polyp?	Duct-cell carcinoma
Papilloma, papillomatosis, villous papilloma	Giant-cell carcinoma (including osteoclastoid)
Adenoma:	Adenosquamous carcinoma (including spindle-cell type)
	Microadenocarcinoma (solid microglandular)
Solid	Mucinous ('colloid') carcinoma
Duct (ductule)	Mucinous-carcinoid carcinoma
Centroductular (centroacinar)	'Oat-cell' carcinoma
Cystadenoma	
Serous: Simple	
Papillary	Papillary cystic tumour
Mucinous: Simple	Mucinous (''colloid'') carcinoma
Papillary	
Carcinoid	Carcinoid
Oncocytoma	Oncocytic carcinoma/carcinoid
Ciliated cell?	Ciliated-cell carcinoma?
Acinar cell:	Acinar cell:
Adenoma	Acinar cell carcinoma
Cystadenoma	Acinar cell cystadenocarcinoma
Mixed epithelial cells:	Mixed cell:
Duct/islet; Duct/acinar	Duct/islet; duct/islet/acinar
Duct/acinar/islet;	Acinar/islet; carcinoid/islet
Acinar/islet; carcinoid/islet?	
Connective tissue origin	
Fibroma	Fibrosarcoma
Leiomyoma	Leiomyosarcoma
Neurilemmoma	Malignant neurilemmoma
Fibrous histiocytoma	Malignant fibrous histiocytoma
Vascular:	
Lymphangioma	
Haemangioma	
Miscellaneous	Osteogenic/lipo/rhabdomyosarcoma
Mixed epithelial–connective tissue origin	
Fibroadenoma?	
Uncertain histiogenesis/other	
	Pancreatoblastoma (simple and mixed types)
	Unclassified (large-, small- or clear-cell type)

Armed Forces Institute of Pathology, 1984.

The probable importance of genetic influence is illustrated by the transgenic mouse model, wherein an oncogene (SV40 early-transforming oncogene region) is placed under the control of elastase-1 promoter and enhancer, which increases gene expression by 1000-fold in acinar cells, producing diffuse hyperplasia and dysplasia. Focality of tumour development in the face of a diffuse genetic change demands that it requires a further factor. This could be environmental or genetic. Specific chromosomal deletions in malignant tissue but not adjacent non-malignant tissue have been found in man. The most widely reported oncogene from human pancreatic cancer cell lines is K-*ras* sequences, but it is still unclear whether these transforming gene sequences are truly activated or merely overexpressed.

Finally, a possible role for viruses and exocrine/endocrine interaction in human exocrine pancreatic tumorigenesis should not be totally disregarded: guinea fowl develop pancreatic ductal adenocarcinoma after injection of virus-containing plasma; endocrine tumours may also be derived from influences similar to those in exocrine tumours as single doses of streptozotocin or alloxan can produce endocrine tumours in rats. This last phenomenon is enhanced by retinoids.

Pathology

Primary malignant epithelial neoplasms of the pancreas can occur either in the exocrine parenchyma or the endocrine cells of the islets of Langerhans but they are far more frequent in the former. Non-epithelial tumours are exceedingly rare. Ductal adenocarcinoma makes up between 75 and 92 per cent of pancreatic neoplasms and is twice as frequent in the head of the pancreas as in the body or tail. At the time of diagnosis, over 85 per cent of tumours have extended beyond the pancreas. Pancreatic adenocarcinoma has a proclivity for perineural invasion within and beyond the gland, although lymphatic spread also leads to early metastasis to adjacent and distant lymph nodes. The most common sites of extralymphatic involvement are the liver and peritoneum, and the lung is the most frequently affected extra-abdominal organ. Two histological pathological classifications are used commonly; the Armed Forces Institute of Pathology (**AFIP**) classification deals primarily with exocrine neoplasia (Table 1). The other widely recognized classification is from the World Health Organization, which combines endocrine and exocrine neoplasia as well as some non-neoplastic lesions. Though simpler and more standardized, it is in many ways less clinically useful than the AFIP classification. Some of the non-ductal carcinomas are of clinical importance. The giant-cell carcinoma has no clinical distinguishing feature from ductal adenocarcinoma except for a tendency to a larger size at presentation and a shorter survival, with a median of only 2 months and few, if any, documented survivors at 1 year from diagnosis. The histopathological appearance is unmistakable, with large polypoid, often bizarre, giant mononucleated or multinucleated tumour cells that are obviously malignant. The exact origin of the giant cells is unclear but they are thought to come from non-specific metaplasia rather than an all-encompassing stem cell.

Adenosquamous carcinoma presents in an identical manner to the ductal carcinoma. The ductal component is usually well differentiated but may be very small in quantity. Squamous metaplasia rather than squamous carcinoma may occur. The prognosis is poor. Microadenocarcinoma is characterized by sheets of small oval or round cells with small or moderate amounts of cytoplasm and no neurosecretory granules. Necrosis is common but fibrosis is rare. These tumours are found more commonly in the body than the head and have a median size of 14 cm at presentation. They have a particularly poor prognosis.

Mucinous adenocarcinoma presents identically to a ductal adenocarcinoma but is associated with a much longer survival. Histologically, the mucin-filled cystic spaces are separated by internal collagen septa. Tumour cells may float in the mucus as clumps or strands. The mucin itself may produce biliary obstruction, and jaundice as a result of these tumours is not relieved by the insertion of a stent, which blocks with mucus, and thus a surgical bypass is required.

Mucinous carcinoid, as the name suggests, features both mucin-producing ductal adenocarcinoma and carcinoid tumour. It is important that the usual mucinous cystadenocarcinomas may normally have up to 10 per cent of cells positively staining for neurosecretory granules and that carcinoid tumours may normally produce some mucus.

Mucinous cystadenocarcinoma is a variant that tends to occur in younger females and rarely involves the pancreatic head. The median size at presentation is large and the survival is generally better than for ductal adenocarcinoma. These tumours may show calcification on plain radiographs. Again, at endoscopic retrograde cholangiopancreatography, thick mucin may be seen pouring from the dilated main pancreatic duct. The cysts are completely lined by columnar cells showing a wide range of histological appearance from benign to definite invasive malignancy. It is probable that the smaller tumours are truly benign but the larger invariably become malignant.

Pancreatoblastoma is a neoplasm of childhood and has a mixed cell type with ductal, acinar, epidermoid, and islet cells present. The cell predominance is variable. No neoplastic mesodermal element is present. The prognosis is poor but rare long-term survivors have been recorded.

Papillary cystic tumour presents as a gradually enlarging, painful mass in the left upper quadrant in young women. It has a relatively good prognosis. The solid areas consist of sheets of small polyhedral cells with a moderate amount of eosinophilic cytoplasm. It is important to recognize this tumour as resection can occasionally cure the patient.

Acinar-cell carcinoma is clinically associated with polyarthritis, skin lesions, and metastatic fat necrosis, possibly due to raised levels of serum pancreatic lipase. It consists of large, polyhedral acinar cells with basal, round nuclei and an abundant, dense, eosinophilic, granule-containing cytoplasm. It has a particularly poor prognosis.

Lymphoma can occasionally involve the pancreas and, on account of its response to therapy, must be differentiated from other pancreatic masses.

Clinical features

SYMPTOMS AND SIGNS

The early symptoms of non-hormone-producing pancreatic neoplasms transmitted by visceral afferent nerves are usually non-specific and compatible with numerous benign conditions; therefore the early symptoms are often ignored by patient or medical attendant. Examples include epigastric bloating and flatulence (31 per cent), general fatigue and weakness (31 per cent), diarrhoea (25 per cent), vomiting (23 per cent), and constipation (13 per cent). Even if an early diagnosis is pursued with investigations, the findings are normal on less-invasive investigations. Therefore, up to 90 per cent of patients will present with incurable advanced disease, with one or other of the classical triad of symptoms of pain, jaundice or weight loss. Symptoms depend largely on the site and extent of the tumour.

Painless jaundice as a presentation carries the best prognosis if it is due to a tumour in the pancreatic head, as it need only be small and local to produce intrapancreatic bile-duct obstruction. If the jaundice is present when the tumour is in the body or tail of the pancreas, there is invariably metastasis to the lymph nodes in the porta hepatis. Pain is, overall, the most common symptom and is diffuse in the early stages. More localized discomfort only occurs later as somatic afferent nerves are involved. The pain may be posture related, similar to musculoskeletal disease, intermittent at onset, mimicking of biliary disease, and food related, suggestive of peptic ulcer. It is usually epigastric but one-quarter of patients also have back pain; some only have back pain. Pain in the left upper quadrant may occur and is suggestive of body and tail disease. Cramping abdominal pain may be secondary to fat malabsorption with colonic fermentation and palliated by oral enzyme supplementation. Weight loss may be rapid despite normal appetite, due to steatorrhoea. There is usually loss of appetite, however. There are other uncommon presenting symptoms: acute cholecystitis or acute pancreatitis; upper gastrointestinal haemorrhage; neuropsychiatric disturbance; diabetes mellitus; polyarthritis or painful skin nodules due to metastatic fat necrosis (especially with acinar-cell adenocarcinoma); pyrexia of unknown origin; clinical steatorrhoea; and, migratory thrombophlebitis (Trousseau's sign) or thromboembolic disease.

Important signs include an upper abdominal mass, icterus and scratch marks, hepatomegaly, palpable gallbladder (Courvoisier's sign), supraclavicular lymphadenopathy (usually left-sided), splenomegaly (due to portal or splenic vein compression, thrombosis or diffuse liver involvement), periumbilical mass (due to lymphatic spread along the line of the umbilical vein), ascites and/or peripheral oedema (including inferior vena caval obstruction), and thrombophlebitis. Clinical manifestations in which the diagnosis of pancreatic cancer should be entertained early and appropriate investigations instituted are: a recent onset of unexplained upper abdominal pain and/or thoracolumbar back pain suggestive of retroperitoneal origin accompanied by negative upper gastrointestinal investigations; extrahepatic obstructive jaundice; unexplained weight loss of more than 10 per cent; unexplained acute pancreatitis after the age of 50 years; and unexplained sudden onset of diabetes after the age of 50 years (no family history, obesity or steroids).

Investigation

BLOOD TESTS

The blood count may show a normochromic normocytic anaemia; the erythrocyte sedimentation rate and concentration of C-reactive protein may be raised. The concentration of albumin is usually reduced in advanced disease and 'liver function tests' may show evidence of hepatic metastatic disease or extrahepatic biliary obstruction. Serum markers of three varieties may be elevated. The first group includes enzymes that are normally found in the blood, such as amylase (or isoenzymes thereof), lipase, pancreatic ribonuclease or galactyl transferase, pancreatic secretory trypsin inhibitor, and pancreatic elastase-1. The second consists of ectopically produced regulatory peptides and hormones. Finally, there are tumour-related antigens such as carcinoembryonic antigen, pancreatic oncofetal antigen, CA 19-9, DuPan-2, pancreatic cancer-associated antigen, and CA 50. Some of these antigens may be found in pure pancreatic juice. The tumour-related antigens offer the best chance so far of serodiagnosis of pancreatic malignancy but as yet they are only reliable in late, disseminated disease. Measurement of combinations of antigens has little advantage. These markers are usually absent in the early stages of pancreatic cancer and are thus unsuitable for screening. No tumour-related antigen, because of lack of sensitivity and specificity, can independently establish a diagnosis of pancreatic cancer. Their use is limited to acting as an adjunct to clinical diagnosis, to monitoring of established disease, as yardsticks for newly developed tests, and for research into of carcinogenesis.

An interesting marker is the ratio of testosterone to dihydrotestosterone. It is normally about 10 but has been shown to be below 5 in over 70 per cent of men with pancreatic cancer, presumably because of the increased metabolic conversion of testosterone by the pancreatic tumour. Although less sensitive than CA 19-9, a low ratio is more specific for the diagnosis of pancreatic cancer.

PANCREATIC FUNCTION TESTS

These carry 89 per cent sensitivity and 80 per cent specificity for pancreatic disease. However, they are usually negative in body and tail tumours, and in head lesions that do not obstruct the main pancreatic duct. There are false positive results arising from disease of the small-bowel mucosa; reproducibility is limited with non-tube tests; differentiation of benign from malignant disease suffers the same uncertainties as the measurement of tumour-related antigens. Samples in the tube tests sent for cytological examination at the time of the study can be of value. Overall, however, these tests of pancreatic function have no current role in the diagnosis of pancreatic malignancy.

PANCREATIC ISOTOPE SCANNING

Iodocholesterol and [75]selenomethionine scanning has a high rate of false positives and an unacceptable rate of false negatives, and thus has no role in the diagnosis of pancreatic cancer. There is, however, a possibility that isotope scanning may be used in the future for radiolabelled, monoclonal antibody-directed scintigraphy.

IMAGING

The main methods of imaging are percutaneous ultrasonography, computerized tomography, endoscopic retrograde cholangiopancreatography, percutaneous cholangiography, and endoscopic ultrasound. Magnetic resonance imaging, though available and applicable, has yet to gain a place except perhaps where an equivocal vascular imaging requires further definition. Both cytological (fine-needle aspiration) and histopathological (Tru-cut biopsy) samples should be obtained with radiological techniques in all patients not submitted to surgery. It must be remembered that all radiological procedures are operator and equipment dependent so the results or experience of one centre do not necessarily apply universally.

Ultrasonography and computerized tomography

These are the methods most frequently used to confirm a clinical suspicion of pancreatic cancer. Both can detect pancreatic masses as small as 2 cm and occasionally smaller, dilatation of the pancreatic and bile ducts, hepatic metastases, and extrapancreatic spread. Ultrasonography, because it is cheaper, is the primary investigation and should rapidly distinguish between obstructive and non-obstructive jaundice, the presenting feature in 50 per cent of patients. Modern, high-resolution, real-time ultrasound scanners with digital processors and synthetic focusing systems may give resolutions of below 5 mm. Meticulous technique is essential, with gas displacement by orally administered fluids, variations in patient posture and position, and the use of antikinetic agents as required. Modern computerized tomography of the pancreas necessitates oral bolus intravenous contrast and close collimation of scans (Fig. 1). When using intravenous contrast, careful attention must be paid to hydration to prevent renal damage in hyperbilirubinaemic patients.

Findings on computerized tomography and ultrasound scanning fre-

quently confirm that a particular pancreatic neoplasm is unresectable. Approximately 70 per cent of patients at presentation will have local extension, 40 per cent contiguous organ involvement, 40 per cent hepatic metastases, 30 per cent regional lymphadenopathy, and 85 per cent vascular involvement. Computerized tomography tends to overestimate resectability.

Endoscopic retrograde cholangiopancreatography (ERCP) and percutaneous transhepatic cholangiography (PTC)

PTC was the original method for preoperative delineation of bile-duct anatomy. It has been supplanted by ERCP in patients in whom the ultrasound scan shows dilatation of the common hepatic duct suggestive of a carcinoma of the lower end of the bile duct. With the development of stenting, PTC is still preferable for high bile-duct strictures provided that it is done by a radiologist competent in the immediate placement of a stent should this be deemed appropriate.

ERCP has the advantage of avoiding liver puncture; it allows other gastrointestinal disease to be excluded, determines duodenal patency, defines periampullary tumours with the possibility of biopsy, and enables imaging of both the bile and pancreatic ducts (Fig. 2). Cytolog-

Fig. 1 CT scan showing mass in the head of the pancreas surrounding a stent and involving the major vessels.

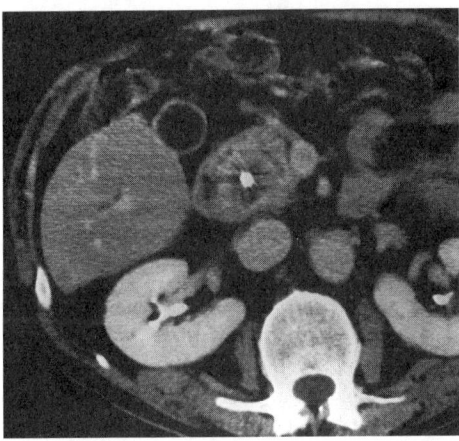

Fig. 2 Cholangiogram from a patient with primary sclerosing cholangitis showing a diverticular appearance of the common bile duct.

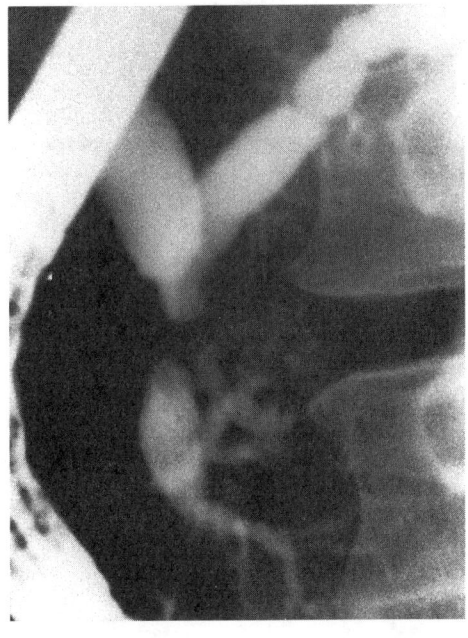

ical sampling from both ducts can be achieved and a stent can be placed at the time of the study. It must be remembered that the pancreatic ductal system is normal in up to 12 per cent of patients with pancreatic carcinoma.

Endoscopic and intraoperative ultrasonography

With these techniques higher-frequency ultrasound can be used, ensuring better definition of tumour margins and a greater chance of defining local lymphadenopathy and metastases in the liver. With improved technology, endoscopic ultrasonography enables pancreatic tumours to be clearly evaluated, with clear views of the pancreas in over 90 per cent of studies. It is possible to define contiguity with the superior mesenteric artery and portal vein, and even invasion into the inferior vena cava. Peroperative ultrasonography has limited value except as a method of imaging the liver more accurately and defining the presence of metastases.

Angiography

The role of angiography as a method of diagnosis of small pancreatic tumours and as a determinant of resectability has largely been replaced by ultrasonography, computerized tomography, and ERCP. With the Doppler facility on the ultrasound, flow characteristics within vessels can be determined and the presence or absence of tumour involvement predicted as accurately as with angiography. Even in the diagnosis of APUDomas, endoscopic or peroperative ultrasound are superior.

Percutaneous biopsy and cytology

Radiological techniques to obtain cytological specimens by aspiration of histological specimens by Tru-cut biopsy are well established either using ultrasound or computerized tomographic guidance. Histological confirmation of the diagnosis is mandatory. The main disadvantage of the percutaneous technique is the small risk of tract seeding, which occurs only in patients with disseminated disease. The incidence of major complications is small (less than 2 per cent), with acute pancreatitis and haemorrhage being the most common. Localized leakage of pancreatic juice appears to be unimportant.

Laparoscopy

There has been a resurgence of interest in this technique as a result of recent enthusiasm for laparoscopic surgery. Its only value is in the determination of seedling deposits not visible by current imaging techniques. Nevertheless, laparoscopy has a significant role as an independent predictor of operability and can be of great value when alternative methods of imaging are unavailable.

Treatment

Once preliminary investigation has suggested that the patient has obstructive jaundice or a serious illness due to a carcinoma of the pancreas, a decision has to be made on management. Previously, the decision was simple and rested between no treatment or a surgical exploration with a view to possible curative resection or a palliative bypass. With the advent of stents placed endoscopically into the bile duct to relieve the jaundice (Fig. 3), it is now no longer necessary to do a laparotomy and thus a decision has to be made early as to how best to manage the patient. It is best to proceed, after the preliminary ultrasonographic examination confirming the diagnosis, to an ERCP and immediate stent placement. This has the advantage of advancing the diagnosis, relieving the jaundice and, occasionally, providing confirmatory histological evidence. Its disadvantage is the possible risk of infection or pancreatitis, which may delay the chance of curative surgery. Such a risk is small in the hands of a competent endoscopist and is acceptable.

Biliary drainage to reverse the ill-effects of cholestasis has not been of proven benefit in prospective controlled trials. Its major advantage is the time that it gives for a full assessment by computerized tomographic scanning, endoscopic ultrasound and biopsy, so that the disease can be staged.

Once the cholestasis has resolved a dynamic computerized tomographic scan and endoscopic ultrasonography should be used to determine the size of the tumour, involvement of major vessels, lymph node metastases, or the presence of liver metastases or direct extension into major structures. Involved local lymph nodes, that is nodes adjacent to the pancreas, are not a contraindication to operation but large nodes or those within the porta hepatis suggest that inoperability is inevitable.

The ideal patient for surgical resection with a view to cure is one with a tumour of less than 3 cm in diameter that does not involve major veins or other structures, and in whom there is no evidence of lymph node or distant metastases. Such patients should be referred for a laparotomy with a view to surgical resection.

All others should be considered for palliative therapy. The elderly and unfit person is best managed by a stent placed endoscopically. The fitter patient may be better managed by a surgical bypass. In addition, the 15 per cent of patients who present with duodenal obstruction or who have significant obstruction at the initial endoscopy are preferably treated surgically. There is good evidence that the difference in palliation between treatment by stents or surgery is marginal. The major disadvantage of surgery is the perioperative mortality and morbidity, while the major disadvantage of stent placement is recurrent blockage. Approximately 60 per cent of patients die with their initial stent in place and free of jaundice, but the remainder may have several stent changes with repeated attacks of cholangitis. The more expensive Wallstent may overcome this problem (Fig. 3) and thus provide better palliation than surgery, except in the presence of duodenal obstruction.

Surgical treatment

In 1987, Gudjohnsson comprehensively reviewed the results of surgical treatment for pancreatic cancer. Of 4100 patients whose tumours were resected, only 144 (3.5 per cent) survived 5 years. He concluded that surgery had such a small effect on survival that resections for cure should be abandoned. Subsequent data suggest that a 5-year survival of 24 per cent can be achieved in selected groups of patients, that is those under 70 years with small tumours (2 cm or less in diameter) and no evidence of distant disease. Tumours of the ampulla of Vater have a very much better 5-year survival (40 per cent) and should be resected.

Fig. 3 The hepatic histological changes of early primary sclerosing cholangitis showing a concentric (onion skin) fibrosis around the bile ducts.

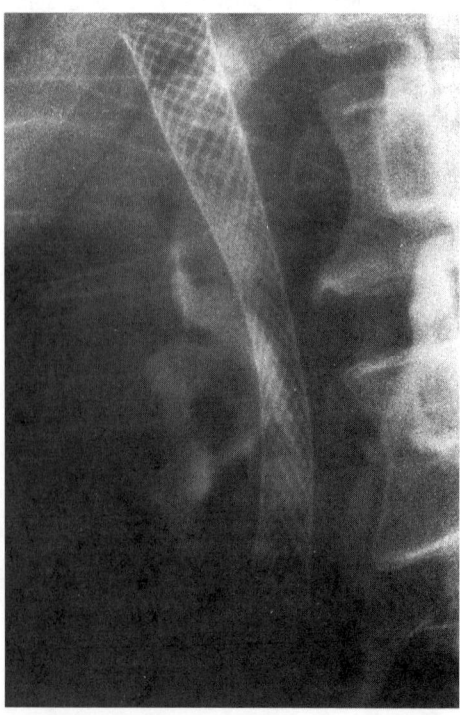

The standard resection for tumours in the head of the pancreas is a pancreatoduodenectomy. This resection should now have an operative mortality of less than 5 per cent, with a low morbidity.

Radiotherapy

Radiation therapy may be useful in the treatment of 40 per cent of pancreatic cancers that are not resectable but are localized. The use of conventional external-beam radiotherapy alone does not improve outcome but when combined with fluorouracil therapy it can significantly improve survival from a median survival of 5.5 months to 10 months. External-beam radiotherapy has a role as an adjuvant treatment after surgical resection and can be of value in the palliation of pain.

Chemotherapy

Chemotherapy for advanced cancer has been hampered by the poor state of many patients with pancreatic cancer, who are unable to tolerate radical chemotherapy. Of all chemotherapeutic agents, 5-fluorouracil has been studied most extensively and has been shown to improve median survival. Combination chemotherapy with other agents such as doxorubicin and cisplatin can relieve pain. There are likely to be developments in this area and the younger patient should have the benefit of an oncological opinion.

Endocrine therapy

On the basis of epidemiological and experimental evidence linking pancreatic carcinoma to sex hormones, antioestrogen and antiandrogen treatment has been prescribed. To date, neither is of proven benefit.

Palliative care

An important part of the management of patients with pancreatic cancer is the relief of symptoms that impair quality of life. After diagnosis, and, if necessary, the relief of jaundice, most patients will have good quality of life for a period of weeks to several months. This time can be improved by the careful management of their diabetes and steatorrhoea. The latter is often neglected and can be completely relieved by the new, high-lipase, enzyme preparations. Pain occurs in more than half the patients during the course of the disease. A coeliac plexus block is effective and should be arranged early in the course of the pain history. Because of the bad reputation of this disease, many patients are concerned about the discomfort in the preterminal phase. This can be completely controlled by good nursing and referral to a local palliative care team.

Pancreatic cancer is one of the most predictable cancers, with a 5-year survival of 0.04 per cent. Therapy either after early or late diagnosis makes little difference to the outcome and the only hope for the patient with pancreatic cancer is good palliation. Rapid diagnosis and early treatment to relieve the jaundice and pain will ease the patient's progress. Careful symptomatic treatment of all their problems will enormously enhance the quality of survival and counteract the nihilism of the therapeutic approach.

REFERENCES

Arbuck, S.G. (1990). Overview of chemotherapy for pancreatic cancer. *International Journal of Pancreatology*, **7**, 209–22.

Bakkevold, K.E., Pettersen, A., Arnesjo, B., and Espehaug, B. (1990). Tamoxifen therapy in unresectable adenocarcinoma of the pancreas and papilla of Vater. *British Journal of Surgery*, **77**, 725–30.

Brandt, K.R., Charboneau, J.W., Stephens, D.H., Welch, T.J., and Goellner, J.R. (1993). CT- and US-guided biopsy of the pancreas. *Radiology*, **187**, 99–104.

Cameron, J.L. *et al.* (1991). Factors influencing survival after pancreato-duodenectomy for pancreatic cancer. *American Journal of Surgery*, **161**, 120–5.

Cubilla, A.L. and Fitzgerald, P.J. (1984). *Tumours of the exocrine pancreas*: *Atlas of tumour pathology*, 2nd Series, Fascicle 19. Armed Forces Institute of Pathology. Washington DC.

Freeny, P.C. (1989). Radiologic diagnosis and staging of pancreatic ductal adenocarcinoma. *Radiologic Clinics of North America*, **27**, 121–8.

Friess, H. *et al.* (1993). CA 494—a new tumour marker for the diagnosis of pancreatic cancer. *International Journal of Cancer*, 759–63.

Geer, R.J. and Brennan, M.F. (1993). Prognostic indicators of survival after resection of pancreatic adenocarcinoma. *American Journal of Surgery*, **165**, 68–73.

Gudjonsson, B. (1987). Cancer of the pancreas. Fifty years of surgery. *Cancer*, **9**, 2284–303.

Merrick, H.W., III. Dobelbower, R.R., Jr. (1990). Aggressive therapy for cancer of the pancreas: does it help?. *Gastroenterologic Clinics of North America*, **19**, 935–62.

Sarr, M.G. and Cameron, J.L. (1982). Surgical management of unresectable carcinoma of the pancreas. *Surgery*, **91**, 123–33.

Warshaw, A.L. and Fernandez-del-Castillo, C. (1992). Pancreatic carcinoma. *New England Journal of Medicine*, **326**, 455–65.

14.24 Diseases of the gallbladder and biliary tree

J. A. SUMMERFIELD

Anatomy

The biliary system comprises the collection of ducts extending from the biliary canaliculus of each hepatocyte to the ampulla of Vater opening into the duodenum. The biliary canaliculi drain into interlobular and then septal bile ducts. These further ramify to form the intrahepatic bile ducts, which are visible on cholangiography (Fig. 1). They eventually form the right and left hepatic ducts draining bile from the right and left lobes of the liver, respectively. The junction of the hepatic ducts at the porta hepatis forms the common hepatic duct. The cystic duct, linking the gallbladder to the bile duct, arises from the lower end of the common hepatic duct. The gallbladder rests in a fossa under the right lobe of the liver. Anatomical variations in the size and position of the gallbladder and the insertion of the cystic duct into the bile duct are of major surgical importance. The common hepatic duct becomes the common bile duct below the insertion of the cystic duct. The common bile duct passes through the head of the pancreas and the sphincter of Oddi to drain into the duodenum via the ampulla of Vater. The bile duct usually leaves through a common channel with the pancreatic duct in the ampulla of Vater, although anatomical variations are frequent.

The investigation of biliary disease

OBJECTIVES

The clinical and laboratory features of biliary disease may also be caused by hepatic disorders. Consequently, the primary objective of the investigation is to establish that the cause is biliary and not hepatic disease. The secondary objective is to define the anatomy of the lesion to permit a rational choice of the many surgical and non-surgical therapeutic options now available. To achieve these objectives requires not only a careful history and physical examination, but also the use of various imaging techniques and sometimes aspiration liver biopsy.

SYMPTOMS AND SIGNS

Disorders of the biliary system usually give rise to the symptoms and signs of biliary obstruction (cholestasis). The repertoire is rather limited: pain, jaundice, itching, nausea and vomiting, fevers, and rigors. The pain can range between abdominal discomfort described as 'dyspepsia' to severe right hypochondrial colic caused by a sudden rise in biliary pressure. Jaundice, dark urine, and pale stools indicate obstruction of the bile duct. Itching is an important sign of biliary obstruction. Nausea and vomiting may be prominent in sudden obstruction of the bile duct, usually by a gallstone. The milder symptoms of flatulence and intolerance of fatty food are more common. Fever and rigors indicate bacterial infection of the biliary tract, which frequently accompanies partial obstruction. In jaundiced patients, weight loss is usual and results from fat malabsorption due to the lack of bile acids reaching the gut; it may also indicate a malignant tumour. Prolonged biliary obstruction leads to skin changes: increased pigmentation (due to melanin) and cholesterol deposits (xanthelasma and xanthoma). Finally, biliary cirrhosis may develop, causing the signs of portal venous hypertension and liver-cell failure.

LABORATORY INVESTIGATIONS

In general, disorders of the biliary system give rise to the biochemical picture of biliary obstruction (cholestasis). A notable exception is gallstones in the gallbladder (cholelithiasis) where the liver function tests are usually normal. In cholestasis, the serum bilirubin concentration may be normal or raised and most of the bilirubin is esterified (conjugated).

Fig. 1 The normal biliary tree. The intrahepatic bile ducts (IHD) taper smoothly and extend deep into the liver. The gallbladder (GB) drains via the cystic duct (CD) into the common bile duct (CBD). The pancreatic duct (PD) has also been opacified in this endoscopic retrograde cholangiogram (ERCP).

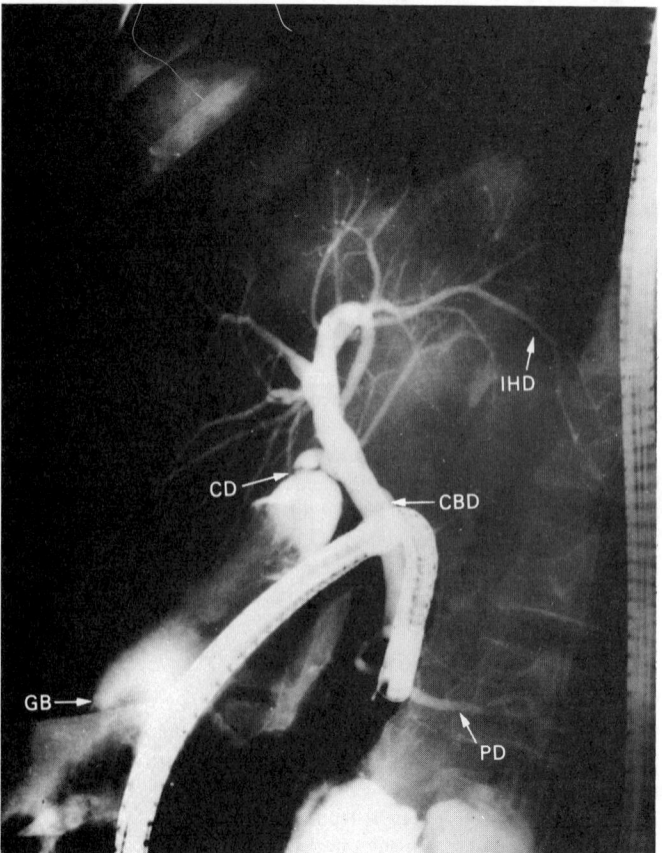

Bilirubinuria is present. The disappearance of urobilinogen from the urine indicates complete biliary obstruction. Elevation of the serum alkaline phosphatase is an important but not invariable sign of biliary obstruction; the rise is usually greater than three times normal. Other biliary canalicular enzymes accumulate in the blood, including 5'-nucleotidase and γ-glutamyl transpeptidase. These enzymes are found only in the liver and are estimated if there is doubt as to whether the alkaline phosphatase is of bony or hepatic origin. This may be required in children and patients with malignancy. Serum transaminases, such as aspartate aminotransferase, show only modest elevation in contrast to the rises that occur in hepatitis. The serum cholesterol concentration rises and may cause abnormalities of red-cell shape (target cells) (see Chapter 14.20). A raised serum bile-acid concentration is a sensitive index of biliary disease. A prolonged prothrombin time reflects intestinal malabsorption of fat-soluble vitamin K due to a lack of bile acids. Vitamin A and D deficiency may also develop. The serum albumin and gammaglobulin concentrations are normal until biliary cirrhosis develops. A polymorphonuclear leucocytosis accompanies bacterial infections of the biliary system.

IMAGING TECHNIQUES

A plain radiograph of the abdomen may reveal an enlarged liver, calcified gallstones, or air in the biliary tree. Plain radiographs of the abdomen are now rarely taken. The preferred first investigation is ultrasonography (ultrasound) (Fig. 2). Computerized tomography (**CT** scan) and magnetic resonance imaging (**MRI**) are used in complicated diagnostic problems (see Chapter 14.20). These tests reveal dilated bile ducts and may also indicate the position of the obstruction in the biliary tree and dense structures such as gallstones. Hepatic scintiscanning with 99Tc^m-labelled HIDA (dimethyl acetanilide iminodiacetic acid) is an alternative and is of value in the diagnosis of acute cholecystitis. Oral cholecystograms are taken if ultrasound is not available and to determine whether the gallbladder functions in patients with gallstones being assessed for oral bile-acid dissolution therapy (see below). Intravenous cholangiography is obsolete. However, these non-invasive investigations usually provide insufficient anatomical detail for diagnosis or planning of treatment. An invasive cholangiographic technique such as percutaneous transhepatic cholangiography (**PTC**) and endoscopic retrograde cholangiopancreatography (**ERCP**) is necessary. ERCP is the preferred investigation in the first instance. PTC is reserved for patients in whom ERCP fails. Both these techniques carry small risks, including haemorrhage, biliary peritonitis, and cholangitis (PTC) and bowel perforation and cholangitis (ERCP). Should cholangiography reveal a normal biliary system in a jaundiced patient, a liver biopsy is indicated.

Fig. 2 Ultrasound scan of the gallbladder shows gallstones (arrowed) as bright round objects which cast acoustic shadows.

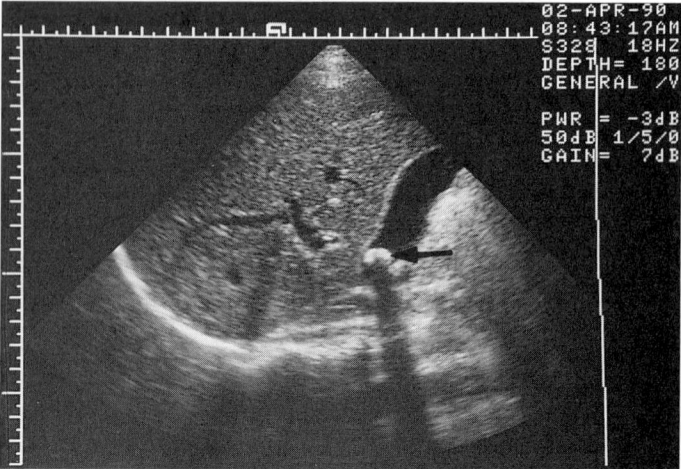

This diagnostic approach is ideal but expensive both in terms of human and material resources. The apparatus required is costly and procedures such as ERCP require considerable expertise. Local factors will determine the diagnostic pathway that is adopted. Nevertheless, these techniques have revolutionized the management of the patient with biliary disease. It is now a routine matter to achieve rapidly a precise diagnosis. In addition, a series of non-operative therapeutic options ranging from the introduction of endoprostheses for the management of benign and malignant biliary strictures to endoscopic sphincterotomy for the removal of the biliary calculi are direct consequences of these new diagnostic approaches.

Bile composition and gallstone formation

BILE COMPOSITION

Bile is secreted by the hepatocytes and its water and electrolyte composition altered during its passage down the biliary system. Between meals much of the bile is diverted to the gallbladder, where it is concentrated by the removal of sodium, chloride, bicarbonate, and water. In response to food, the gallbladder contracts, emptying bile into the duodenum. Apart from water (97 per cent) the major components of bile are bile acids, phospholipids, and cholesterol. Bile is also the major excretory route of other compounds including bilirubin and certain drugs and their metabolites. Cholesterol is insoluble in water but is held in solution by the detergent action of bile acids with the aid of phospholipids.

Cholesterol is synthesized primarily in the liver and small intestine. The rate-limiting enzyme for cholesterol production is hydroxymethyl-glutaryl-CoA reductase, which catalyses the first step, the conversion of acetate to mevalonate. Subsequently, non-esterified (free) cholesterol is secreted into bile. Dietary cholesterol also contributes to biliary cholesterol secretion. The control of cholesterol metabolism is complex. It is not yet clear what proportion of biliary cholesterol is derived from circulating lipoproteins and what proportion is newly synthesized by the liver.

The primary bile acids, cholic and chenodeoxycholic acid, are synthesized in the liver from cholesterol. The economy of the bile-acid pool is preserved by efficient reabsorption, principally in the terminal ileum. About 95 per cent of the bile acids are reabsorbed and pass back to the liver in the portal venous system (enterohepatic circulation). The remainder enters the colon where bacteria form the secondary bile acids, deoxycholic and lithocholic acid, from cholic acid and chenodeoxycholic acid, respectively. Some of the secondary bile acids are absorbed from the colon but most are excreted in the faeces. The normal bile-acid pool is about 3 to 5 g and circulates six to ten times each day. Synthesis is controlled by the negative feedback of bile acids returning in the portal venous blood, which act on the rate-limiting hepatic enzyme, cholesterol-7α-hydroxylase. The principal phospholipid in bile is lecithin. It is produced in the liver and secreted into the bile. In the intestine, lecithin is hydrolysed to lysolecithin by pancreatic phospholipase and is subsequently reabsorbed.

Above a certain level (the critical micellar concentration), bile acids coalesce to form micelles that have a hydrophilic external surface and hydrophobic internal surface. Cholesterol is incorporated into the hydrophobic interior. Phospholipids are inserted into the micellar wall so that the micelles are enlarged; these 'mixed micelles' are thus able to hold more cholesterol.

Consequently, the solubility of cholesterol in bile depends on the concentrations of bile acid and phospholipid. In the presence of a relative excess of bile acids and phospholipid (on a molar basis), the cholesterol-holding capacity of bile is increased and it is said to be unsaturated. However, if there are insufficient micelles of bile acid and phospholipid to hold the cholesterol, the solution is referred to as saturated and the excess cholesterol tends to precipitate. With a knowledge of the molar concentration of cholesterol, phospholipid and bile acids, the cholesterol saturation of bile can be predicted using triangular coordinate diagrams.

GALLSTONE FORMATION

Gallstone disease is common and afflicts between 10 and 20 per cent of the world's population. Gallstones are classified according to their composition into two main groups: cholesterol stones and bile pigment stones. Cholesterol stones are composed mainly of cholesterol (more than 70 per cent) and can be subdivided into pure cholesterol stones, usually solitary, and mixed stones which contain cholesterol in a matrix of calcium bilirubinate, calcium phosphate, and protein (Figs. 3 and 4). Mixed stones are usually multiple and faceted. Bile pigment stones can also be divided into two main groups. Brown pigment stones are soft and friable and consist of calcium bilirubinate, cholesterol, and calcium soaps. Pure pigment stones ('black stones') are black, hard, and brittle and contain an insoluble black pigment, calcium bilirubinate, calcium carbonate and phosphate, calcium salts of fatty acids and bile acids. All pigment stones contain a large amount of mucoprotein matrix (up to 70 per cent). Gallstones are rare before the age of 10 years. The incidence increases progressively with age. Cholesterol gallstones account for about 75 per cent of the gallstones in Europe and the United States.

CHOLESTEROL GALLSTONES

Cholesterol gallstones result from the secretion of cholesterol-saturated bile by the liver. The cause of the saturation is unclear. Gallstone patients usually have a smaller bile-acid pool than control subjects and it circulates more frequently. The rapid recycling of bile acids may be responsible for the smaller bile-acid pool by excessive inhibition of the enzyme that controls bile acid synthesis, cholesterol-7α-hydroxylase. However, diminished bile-acid synthesis is probably not the most important factor in the production of saturated bile. This appears to be an elevated biliary cholesterol secretion rate, due either to increased hepatic cholesterol synthesis or increased transfer of plasma lipoprotein cholesterol into bile. Nevertheless, saturated bile may be encountered in normal subjects,

Fig. 3 Calcified gallstones. Gallstones contain sufficient calcium to be visible on a plain abdominal radiograph in about 10 per cent of patients. The gallbladder stones are surrounded by a ring of calcium salts. (Reproduced from Sherlock, S., and Summerfield, J. A. (1979). *A colour atlas of liver disease*, Wolfe Medical Publications, London, with permission.)

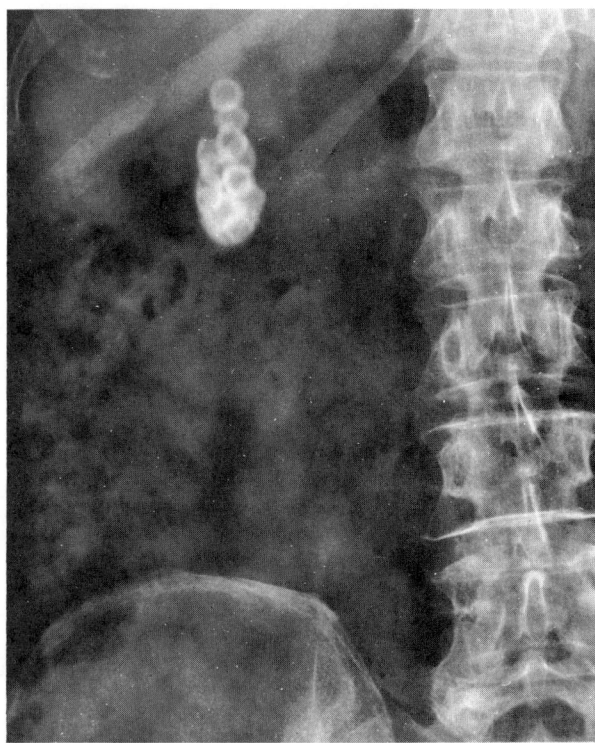

especially during fasting. It is therefore likely that other factors such as the condition of the gallbladder, the mechanism of seeding (nucleation) of gallstones and the control of gallstone growth are important. Furthermore, racial differences, advancing age, female sex, obesity, diet, drugs (such as the contraceptive pill and clofibrate), and gastrointestinal disease (such as Crohn's disease) are known to have a significant influence on the development of gallstones.

BILE PIGMENT GALLSTONES

In contrast to cholesterol stones, little is known of the aetiology of bile pigment stones. The soft, friable brown pigment stones are especially common in the Far East and are associated with *Escherichia coli*, Bacteroides, and clostridial infection of the biliary tract. It is probable that these bacteria contribute to stone formation by producing β-glucuronidase, which deconjugates bilirubin diglucuronide to form free unconjugated bilirubin. This combines with calcium to form sparingly soluble calcium bilirubinate, which precipitates.

The black, hard, and brittle, pure pigment stones are the type commonly encountered in the West. The incidence of pure pigment stones increases with age and they are found in patients with cirrhosis, chronic bile-duct obstruction (e.g. biliary strictures), and chronic haemolytic anaemias including prosthetic heart valve-induced haemolysis and malaria. Pure pigment stones affect both sexes equally. The mechanism of their production is unclear, but does not appear to be due to cholesterol saturation of hepatic or gallbladder bile. About 50 per cent of all pigment stones are radio-opaque and they account for about 70 per cent of all opaque stones.

NATURAL HISTORY OF GALLSTONES

The majority of gallstones remain in the gallbladder (cholelithiasis) and may give rise to no symptoms ('silent' gallstones), being discovered incidentally during investigation or at autopsy. Impaction of a gallstone in the neck of the gallbladder results in its inflammation and the symptoms and signs of acute or chronic cholecystitis. Acute cholecystitis will subside if the stone spontaneously disimpacts or may progress to gangrene and perforation, or empyema, of the gallbladder. Gallstones may pass through the cystic duct into the bile duct (choledocholithiasis),

Fig. 4 Cholesterol gallstones. An intravenous cholangiogram has opacified the gallbladder showing multiple faceted radiolucent gallstones. These are typical features of cholesterol stones.

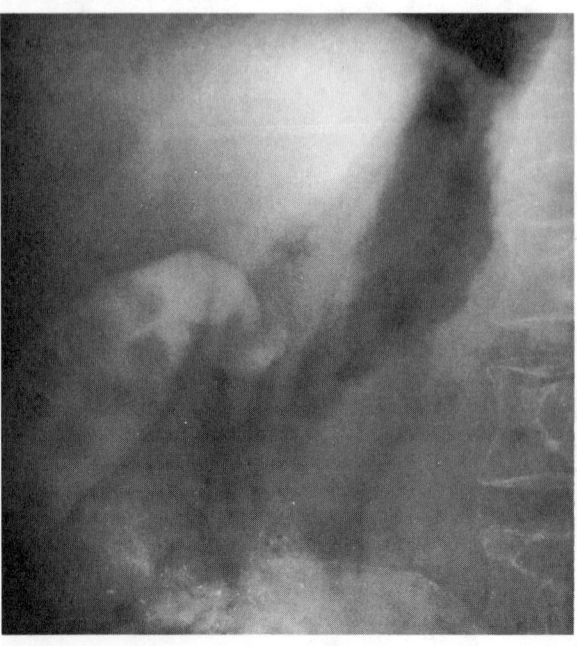

resulting in biliary obstruction and jaundice. Bacterial infection (cholangitis) commonly accompanies choledocholithiasis and can lead to a liver abscess. Gallstones may perforate through the inflamed gallbladder wall to form an internal fistula, usually to the small intestine or colon. A large gallstone passing into the small intestine may impact in the ileum, resulting in intestinal obstruction (gallstone ileus). Finally, surgical treatment for gallstones, while usually curative, may result in a postcholecystectomy syndrome or a benign stricture of the bile duct.

TREATMENT

The usual treatment for gallstones remains cholecystectomy, although medical treatments may be employed in selected patients (see below). The advent of laparoscopic cholecystectomy is swinging the balance again in favour of surgery, as this technique carries so little morbidity. Treatment is obviously indicated for symptomatic gallstones and for their complications. However, in patients in whom 'silent' gallstones are discovered incidentally and in patients with minimal symptoms it is by no means clear that treatment is always the best solution. The problem revolves around the probability of serious complications in the future. It is appropriate to offer treatment to young patients (who, with many years ahead of them, will have a greater likelihood of developing the complications of gallstones) and to advise against treatment in the elderly with other major medical problems. However, in fit, middle-aged patients with no or minimal symptoms it is reasonable to tell the patient of the finding and to withhold surgery until it is warranted by symptoms or complications.

GALLSTONE DISSOLUTION AND DISRUPTION

Cholesterol gallstones can be removed from the gallbladder and bile ducts in a proportion of patients by medical treatments. These techniques avoid the discomfort, disability, and risks of general anaesthesia and surgical exploration of the abdomen and bile ducts. There are two types of medical method: chemical agents, which dissolve gallstones, and physical methods such as endoscopic sphincterotomy and extracorporeal shock-wave lithotripsy (**ESWL**). Judicious combinations of chemical and physical methods yield the best results.

Chemical methods
Oral bile-acid therapy
Oral treatment with chenodeoxycholic acid or ursodeoxycholic acid can dissolve cholesterol gallstones. These bile acids, normal constituents of bile, reduce the cholesterol saturation of bile and result in the leaching of cholesterol from gallstones. They act by reducing the hepatic synthesis and biliary excretion of cholesterol. Ursodeoxycholic acid has advantages over chenodeoxycholic acid in that it does not cause diarrhoea or elevations of serum transaminases. These bile acids differ in the way that they remove cholesterol from gallstones and have been shown to dissolve gallstones better in combination than singly. Combination therapy is the preferred treatment.

Contact dissolution of gallstones
Cholesterol stones in the gallbladder can be dissolved by the direct instillation of methyl tert-butyl ether (**MTBE**) into the gallbladder via a percutaneous catheter. MTBE is a foul-smelling, volatile, inflammable, colourless liquid that remains liquid at body temperature. The gallbladder is catheterized by the transhepatic route, entering it through the area of attachment to the liver, and MTBE is continually infused and aspirated with vigour until the stones have disappeared (which typically takes 5 to 7 h).

Physical methods
Extracorporeal shock-wave lithotripsy
ESWL is a non-invasive and safe but expensive way of rapidly shattering gallstones into a coarse powder. The gallbladder must contain no more than three stones to allow accurate focusing of the shock waves.

Endoscopic sphincterotomy

Endoscopic sphincterotomy can remove gallstones from the bile duct. The bile duct is entered by a cannula passed via a duodenoscope and the bile duct is opened by diathermy cutting of the ampulla of Vater. Stones are removed by balloon or wire catheters.

Patient selection and results

Medical treatment with oral bile-acid therapy, ESWL, or contact dissolution are suitable for patients with cholesterol gallstones in a functioning gallbladder (as judged by an oral cholecystogram). Calcified gallstones do not dissolve. Radiolucent gallstones are usually, but not always, composed of cholesterol. CT scans are useful for detecting low levels of gallstone calcification. These treatments should be reserved for patients with mild or no symptoms in whom the risk of cholecystectomy is high, including those with pre-existing disease, the elderly, and the very obese. They are also of value in patients who refuse surgery. Drugs that increase the cholesterol saturation of bile should be avoided; these include oestrogens, the oral contraceptive pill, and clofibrate.

Oral bile-acid therapy is protracted but safe. It dissolves gallstones in about 25 per cent of patients, fulfilling the selection criteria by 6 months. It should not be taken during pregnancy. The preferred treatment is combination therapy with chenodeoxycholic acid (7 mg/kg) and ursodeoxycholic acid (7 mg/kg). Proprietary combination tablets are available. Gallstone dissolution usually requires 6 to 24 months of therapy, depending on stone size. Oral cholecystograms are performed every 6 months to assess progress. Combining oral bile-acid therapy with ESWL speeds up the process greatly: gallstones will be cleared in more than 90 per cent of patients within 18 months. Furthermore, slightly calcified gallstones can be treated this way. MTBE therapy is invasive and the ether is unpleasant to use but dissolution is rapid. Endoscopic sphincterotomy removes gallstones from the common bile duct. Any type of stone can be removed up to about 20 mm diameter.

Side-effects and toxicity

The most frequent side-effect of oral bile-acid therapy is diarrhoea. It is dose related and usually mild and transient. It can be minimized by slowly increasing the dose to the required level. Transient elevations of serum transaminase activity are also common; liver function tests should be monitored. Ursodeoxycholic acid may cause calcification of gallstones. Gallstone recurrence remains a major problem with oral bile-acid therapy. One year after gallstone dissolution about 30 per cent of patients will have had a recurrence. Unwanted effects of ESWL include biliary colic, skin petechiae, and haematuria. The principal unwanted side-effects of MTBE are sedation, burning upper abdominal pain, nausea, and vomiting. Endoscopic sphincterotomy can cause gastrointestinal haemorrhage and acute pancreatitis.

Acute cholecystitis

AETIOLOGY

Acute cholecystitis is associated with gallstones in over 90 per cent of patients. It follows the impaction of a gallstone in the cystic duct. Continued secretion by the gallbladder leads to a rise in pressure. Inflammation of the gallbladder wall results from the toxic effects of the retained bile and bacterial infection. The gallbladder bile is usually turbid but may become frank pus (empyema of the gallbladder). Intestinal organisms, especially anaerobes, are commonly cultured from the gallbladder. Ischaemia in the distended gallbladder wall may lead to infarction and perforation. Generalized peritonitis may follow but the leak is usually localized to form a chronic abscess cavity. Some patients have repeated attacks of acute cholecystitis, which are probably exacerbations of chronic cholecystitis. Acute cholecystitis in the absence of gallstones (acalculous cholecystitis) is usually very rare. However, acalculous cholecystitis is a particular problem in patients with the acquired immune deficiency syndrome (**AIDS**). Cytomegalovirus and cryptosporidium are the most commonly associated organisms in acalculous cholecystitis in AIDS.

SYMPTOMS AND SIGNS

The typical patient is an obese, middle-aged female, and the acute attack is often precipitated by a large or fatty meal. However, there are many exceptions to this pattern. The principal symptom is pain, of fairly sudden onset, which is severe, continuous, or minimally fluctuating, and localized to the epigastrium or right hypochondrium. The pain often radiates to the back. The constancy of the pain is in contrast to the repeated short bouts of biliary colic. In uncomplicated cases the pain gradually subsides over 12 to 18 h. Flatulence and nausea are common but persistent vomiting suggests the presence of a stone in the common bile duct. Examination reveals an ill, sweating patient with shallow, jerky respiration. Fever indicates a complicating bacterial cholangitis. Jaundice may accompany acute cholecystitis but is usually a sign of a stone in the bile duct. The abdomen moves poorly with respiration. Right hypochondrial tenderness is present and is exacerbated by inspiration (Murphy's sign). Muscle guarding and rebound tenderness are common. The gallbladder is usually impalpable but occasionally a tender mass of omentum and gallbladder may be felt under the liver.

LABORATORY INVESTIGATIONS

The white-cell count is usually moderately elevated ($12-15 \times 10^9$/l) due to a polymorphonuclear leucocytosis. Serum bilirubin concentrations between 17 and 68 μmol/l (1–4 mg/dl) may be seen in uncomplicated acute cholecystitis but should raise the suspicion of a stone in the bile duct. Modest rises in the serum alkaline phosphatase, aspartate transaminase, and amylase may also be seen. An abdominal radiograph will show gallstones in about 10 per cent of patients. Ultrasound scanning of the gallbladder is the preferred first investigation. Scintiscanning with ^{99}Tc^m-labelled HIDA provides similar information. It is important to establish the correct diagnosis before surgery is performed.

DIFFERENTIAL DIAGNOSIS

Acute cholecystitis maybe confused with other abdominal emergencies including perforated peptic ulcer, acute pancreatitis, retrocaecal appendicitis, perforated carcinoma or diverticulum of the hepatic flexure of the colon, and liver abscess. Cardiac infarction and pneumonia with right-sided pleurisy should also be considered.

COMPLICATIONS

Gangrene of the gallbladder

Pain, tenderness, and fever progressively increasing or persisting for longer than 24 to 48 h are indications of gangrene of the gallbladder. The prognosis is poor if necrosis and perforation occur. In the elderly and obese, perforation of the gallbladder can occur without definite signs. Perforation into an adjacent viscus may produce a cholecystenteric fistula and may lead to gallstone ileus.

Cholangitis

Intermittent high temperatures, often accompanied by rigors, indicate bacterial infection of the bile duct and usually follow the passage of a stone into the bile duct.

TREATMENT

In most patients acute cholecystitis subsides in a few days with conservative treatment. Cholecystectomy is done either a few days after the symptoms have settled or 2 to 3 months later. In the latter event, if the symptoms recur during the interval, cholecystectomy is done without delay. Immediate surgery is mandatory if signs of gangrene or perforation develop.

Conservative treatment

Oral feeding is stopped. Intravenous fluids, and analgesia with nalbuphine or pethidine (demerol) and atropine, are given. Antibiotics are given to all but the most mild cases; tetracycline, ampicillin, or a cephalosporin are satisfactory for general use. The patient should be observed frequently, with abdominal examination and sequential leucocyte counts to detect signs of gangrene of the gallbladder or cholangitis.

Surgical treatment

Cholecystectomy is the operation of choice. Laparoscopic cholecystectomy is the preferred approach. As 10 per cent of patients with acute cholecystitis will have stones in the common bile duct they should first be assessed by ERCP and have bile-duct stones removed by endoscopic sphincterotomy. If an open cholecystectomy is done, intraoperative cholangiography may be used to determine whether bile-duct stones are present. In poor-risk patients and when technical difficulties are encountered a cholecystotomy may be done.

Chronic cholecystitis

This is the most common form of gallbladder disease that results from gallstones. Pathologically it is characterized by chronic inflammation and thickening of the gallbladder wall. In addition to stones the gallbladder may contain a brown sediment ('biliary mud'). A proportion of these patients have cholesterolosis of the gallbladder ('strawberry gallbladder'). This describes the deposition of yellow specks of cholesterol in the pink gallbladder wall and is a consequence of cholesterol-saturated bile. Cholesterolosis of the gallbladder is asymptomatic but about half the patients develop gallstones. Chronic cholecystitis usually develops insidiously but may follow an attack of acute cholecystitis.

SYMPTOMS AND SIGNS

Some patients complain of bouts of constant right hypochondrial or epigastric pain. If it is intermittent, i.e. biliary colic, the height of the pain is separated by 15- to 60-min intervals. The pain may last several hours or be as brief as 15 to 20 min. It may radiate to the right shoulder or the back. More commonly the symptoms are vague and ill-defined, and include abdominal discomfort and distension, nausea, flatulence, and intolerance of fatty foods. Unfortunately, many patients who do not have chronic cholecystitis complain of these symptoms. Examination of the abdomen may reveal tenderness over the gallbladder and a positive Murphy's sign. Laboratory investigations are usually unhelpful.

IMAGING TECHNIQUES

A plain radiograph of the abdomen may reveal calcified stones or opacification of the gallbladder caused by high concentrations of calcium carbonate ('limey bile'). An ultrasound scan is used to detect gallstones. If these investigations fail to show stones but stones are still suspected on clinical grounds an ERCP should be done before surgery is undertaken.

DIFFERENTIAL DIAGNOSIS

Dyspepsia and fat intolerance are common symptoms that may be caused by many conditions including peptic ulcers, hiatus hernia, irritable bowel syndrome, chronic relapsing pancreatitis, and tumours of the stomach, pancreas, colon, or gallbladder. Other functional disorders may also mimic chronic cholecystitis.

COMPLICATIONS

The complications of chronic cholecystitis include acute exacerbations (acute cholecystitis), passage of stones into the bile duct (choledocholithiasis or Mirizzi's syndrome), pancreatitis, cholecystenteric fistula formation and gallstone ileus, and rarely carcinoma of the gallbladder. Occasionally the accumulation of mucus and gallstones produces hydrops of the gallbladder, which is characterized by a tender mass without the symptoms of acute cholecystitis.

TREATMENT

In established cases of chronic cholecystitis the treatment of choice is cholecystectomy. When the diagnosis is in doubt, especially when vague symptoms are associated with a well-functioning gallbladder containing stones, a conservative approach is worth trying. This includes weight reduction and a low-fat diet, especially if fatty food is associated with the symptoms. Oral bile-acid therapy may also be considered (see above).

PROGNOSIS

Chronic cholecystitis carries a good prognosis. Cholecystectomy is curative and should have a mortality below 1 per cent. However, if cholecystectomy is done indiscriminately on patients with 'dyspeptic' symptoms who happen to have incidental gallstones the results will be unpredictable and often unsatisfactory.

Choledocholithiasis

Most stones in the common bile duct originate in the gallbladder. About 15 per cent of patients with cholelithiasis have common-duct stones. This proportion rises with age so that in the elderly nearly 50 per cent of patients with cholelithiasis may have common-duct stones. Stones may develop in the bile duct in diseases causing chronic biliary obstruction, such as benign bile-duct strictures and sclerosing cholangitis.

CLINICAL FEATURES

The classical triad of symptoms is right upper abdominal pain, jaundice, and fever. The abdominal pain is typically colicky, severe, and persists for hours. It is often associated with vomiting. Fever and rigors indicate cholangitis, which commonly accompanies bile-duct stones. Jaundice is variable; it may be mild or deep and is often intermittent. The urine is dark due to conjugated bilirubin and the faeces are pale. Frequently, the amount of pigment in the faeces varies. Itching may be prominent. However, common bile-duct stones may also be silent, especially in the elderly. Alternatively, only one of the triad of symptoms may be present; the patient presenting with jaundice, abdominal pain, or cholangitis. The liver is moderately enlarged and there may be tenderness in the right upper quadrant. Prolonged biliary obstruction lasting months or years eventually leads to biliary cirrhosis with portal venous hypertension and liver cell failure.

LABORATORY INVESTIGATIONS

Liver function tests show a cholestatic (biliary obstructive) pattern. The prothrombin time may be prolonged due to inadequate absorption of vitamin K. A polymorphonuclear leucocytosis is common and indicates biliary infection. Blood cultures should be made repeatedly during the fevers to isolate the organism and determine sensitivities.

IMAGING TECHNIQUES

A plain radiograph of the abdomen will show calcified gallstones in 10 per cent of patients. Ultrasonography is useful for demonstrating the dilated biliary tree that results from obstruction and may reveal biliary gallstones. Unfortunately, ultrasound frequently fails to detect common-duct stones obstructing the lower end of the bile duct. Cholangiography by ERCP is required in these patients (Fig. 5). Common bile-duct stones should be removed by endoscopic sphincterotomy before the patient is submitted to cholecystectomy.

DIFFERENTIAL DIAGNOSIS

Common-duct stones are the most common cause of cholestatic (biliary obstructive) jaundice. Next in frequency are carcinomas of the head of the pancreas, bile duct, and ampulla of Vater (Table 1). Intrahepatic diseases may also cause a cholestatic jaundice; these include viral and alcoholic hepatitis, drugs, and pregnancy.

TREATMENT

Common bile-duct stones must be removed. The optimal treatment is endoscopic sphincterotomy to remove bile-duct stones, followed by laparoscopic cholecystectomy. This approach avoids the hazards of open exploration of the common bile duct. Endoscopic removal of common-duct gallstones without cholecystectomy is appropriate in patients unfit for surgery. Few patients will have further problems from the gallbladder that remains. Stones overlooked at surgery (residual calculi) are best treated by endoscopic sphincterotomy or, if a T tube is in place, removed by a steerable basket catheter manipulated down the T-tube track. Open exploration of the common bile duct is required if gallstones are too large to be removed endoscopically (> 2 cm). Preoperative preparation includes appropriate antibiotics for cholangitis, the correction of fluid and electrolyte balance, nutrition, and anaemia, and if the prothrombin time is prolonged, parenteral vitamin K.

POSTCHOLECYSTECTOMY SYNDROMES

After cholecystectomy a proportion of patients continue to complain of symptoms such as pain in the right upper quadrant, flatulence, and intolerance of fatty foods. However, the vast majority of patients with gallstones are improved by surgery. The persistence of symptoms in many is probably a consequence of the wrong diagnosis being made before surgery, and other disease such as oesophagitis, pancreatitis, or functional bowel disease should be sought. In others, technical problems during surgery may have resulted in a benign post-traumatic biliary stricture or residual calculi. However, there remains a group of patients

Fig. 5 Choledocholithiasis. An endoscopic retrograde cholangiogram shows multiple faceted radiolucent stones in a dilated bile duct. The gallbladder has not been opacified.

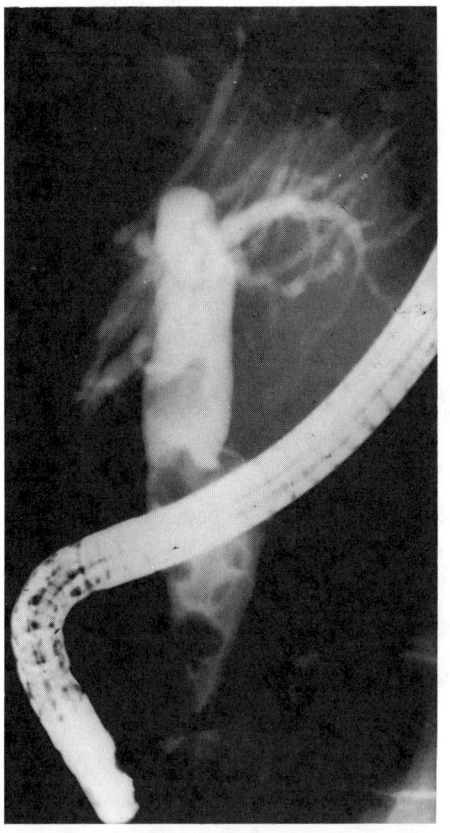

Table 1 *Causes of bile-duct obstruction*

Intrinsic causes
Common bile-duct gallstones
Cholangitis
Carcinoma of the bile duct
Carcinoma of the gallbladder
Benign post-traumatic stricture
Sclerosing cholangitis (primary and secondary)
Haemobilia

Extrinsic causes
Carcinoma of the pancreas
Carcinoma of the ampulla of Vater
Metastatic carcinoma
Lymphoma
Pancreatitis (acute and chronic)
Pancreatic cysts

Congenital causes
Biliary atresia
Choledochal cyst
Congenital intrahepatic biliary dilatation (Caroli's disease)

where the cause appears to be due to less common biliary disorders such as long, dilated cystic-duct remnants, amputation neuromas of the cystic duct, and spasm or stenosis of the sphincter of Oddi. The biliary tract must be carefully investigated in these patients, especially if colicky pain, fever, jaundice, or cholestatic liver function tests persist. Manometry of the biliary tract may be of value when spasm or stenosis of the sphincter of Oddi is suspected.

Biliary infections

BACTERIAL CHOLANGITIS (SUPPURATIVE CHOLANGITIS)

This is usually associated with common bile-duct calculi and benign biliary structures. Malignant structures produce complete obstruction and the bile remains sterile. Other conditions associated with cholangitis are biliary enteric fistulas, both spontaneous and surgical, sclerosing cholangitis, and congenital intrahepatic biliary dilation (Caroli's disease). Organisms of the gut flora are usually cultured in these infections including aerobes such as *E. coli, Streptococcus faecalis, Proteus vulgaris* and staphylococci, and anaerobes such as bacteroides, aerobacter, and anaerobic streptococci.

CLINICAL FEATURES AND TREATMENT

The onset of malaise, fever, and rigors is followed by pain, vomiting, jaundice, and itching. The urine turns dark and the faeces pale. The biliary obstructive features are probably due to oedema of the bile-duct wall. Recurrent attacks are common. Hepatic abscesses may result. Repeated blood cultures are made during the fever to isolate the organisms. Culture of a liver biopsy fragment may also yield the organism. The main element of treatment is drainage of the biliary tract, which is best achieved by emergency endoscopic sphincterotomy. Additionally, appropriate antibiotics such as cefuroxime and metronidazole are given. For recurrent attacks of cholangitis, tetracycline, amoxycillin, or cephalexin are usually effective.

INFESTATIONS (SEE ALSO SECTION 7)

Infestations with the round worm *Ascaris lumbricoides* and the liver fluke *Clonorchis sinensis* are particular problems of the Far East. Both lead to cholangitis. Infestation with *C. sinensis* predisposes to bile-duct carcinoma and primary liver cancer. The common sheep fluke *Fasciola hepatica* may be encountered as a cause of cholangitis in Europe during wet summers.

Benign biliary strictures

In about 95 per cent of patients these are a consequence of biliary-tract surgery. The remainder are caused by gallstones eroding the bile duct and, rarely, blunt injury to the abdomen. Signs of biliary stricture may be detected in the immediate postoperative period but are often delayed. Disasters such as ligation or section of the bile duct present early with jaundice and drainage of bile from the wound drains. With lesser damage to the duct the patient presents after an interval with cholangitis and jaundice. Liver function tests reveal a cholestatic pattern and blood cultures may yield an organism. The precise delineation of the stricture requires ERCP or PTC. Biliary stricture is not a benign condition; untreated it will often progress to biliary cirrhosis with portal venous hypertension and liver failure. Treatment is surgical and should be done by a surgeon skilled in this difficult repair.

Malignant biliary stricture

This is most commonly due to adenocarcinoma of the head of the pancreas but may also be caused by adenocarcinomas of the bile ducts, of the ampulla of Vater, and rarely of the gallbladder. Occasionally the cause is lymph node enlargement at the porta hepatis due to malignant metastases or lymphoma.

SYMPTOMS AND SIGNS

Cancers of the pancreas and biliary tree (Figs. 6 and 7) usually affect the middle aged and elderly. The onset is insidious with deepening jaundice, itching, and weight loss. A dull, nagging upper abdominal pain that radiates to the back is common. In contrast to choledocholithiasis and benign strictures, cholangitis is unusual. Examination reveals a deeply jaundiced patient, often excoriated from scratching. The liver is enlarged but not tender. If the malignant obstruction is below the level of the cystic duct, the gallbladder is distended and may be palpable (Courvoisier's law). The urine is dark and the stools pale. In cancer of the ampulla of Vater a film of blood on the pale stool may give it a silvery colour ('silver stools').

LABORATORY INVESTIGATION

Liver function tests reveal a cholestatic pattern. The serum bilirubin may be very high (600 μmol/l; 35 mg/dl). A microcytic hypochromic anaemia indicates blood loss from the tumour.

IMAGING TECHNIQUES

An abdominal radiograph shows an enlarged liver. An ultrasound or CT scan examination will reveal dilatation of the biliary tree and may demonstrate the level of the obstruction. Ultrasound guided percutaneous needle biopsy may be employed to provide a histological diagnosis. Bile-duct carcinoma frequently causes obstruction at the porta hepatis and consequently at laparotomy the extrahepatic biliary tract appears non-dilated. Even if operative cholangiography is performed, the contrast medium frequently fails to pass the obstruction and fill the dilated intrahepatic biliary tree. Therefore it is important to establish the diagnosis precisely, before surgery is contemplated, by ERCP or PTC. This is particularly important because most of these patients are best treated by endoscopic or percutaneous biliary stents rather than surgery (see below).

TREATMENT

Occasionally, small tumours confined to the head of the pancreas and ampulla of Vater may be treated curatively by a Whipple's operation. Unfortunately the great majority of pancreatic and bile-duct cancers can only be treated palliatively with a bypass procedure such as a chole-

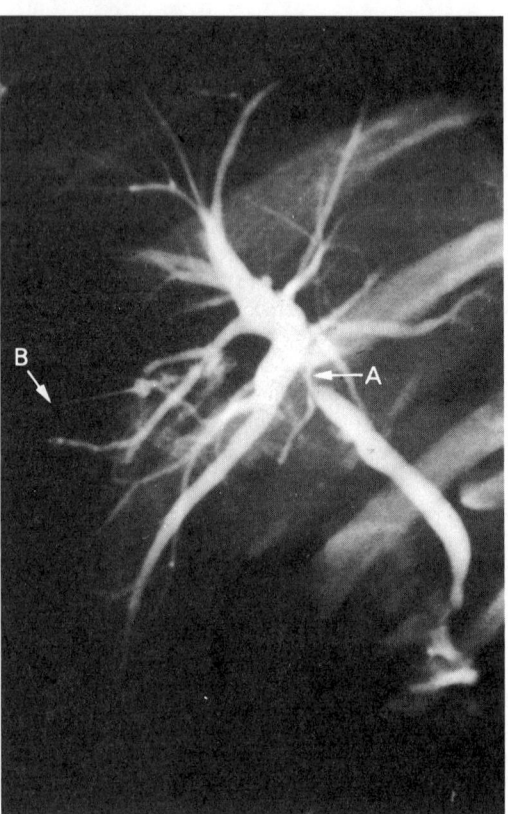

Fig. 6 Carcinoma of the bile duct. A percutaneous transhepatic cholangiogram (PTC) shows a stricture (A) high in the bile duct at the porta hepatis. The intrahepatic bile ducts are moderately dilated. The transhepatic track of the 'skinny' needle used for the PTC is also visible (B).

Fig. 7 Carcinoma of the pancreas. The percutaneous transhepatic cholangiogram (PTC) shows a very dilated biliary tree which terminates in a blunt 'nipple-like' obstruction (arrow) at the lower end of the common bile duct. This is the usual finding in the cancers of the head of the pancreas which obstruct the biliary system.

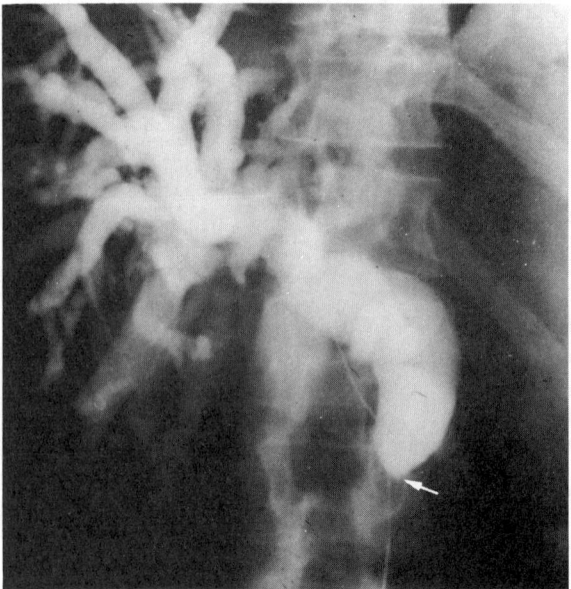

cystojejunostomy. The prognosis for these patients is poor. An alternative treatment is endoscopic or percutaneous transhepatic introduction of prostheses (stents) through the biliary stricture. Patients with endoscopic prostheses have the same median survival as those with a surgical bypass procedure but the operative mortality and morbidity is much less for endoscopic prostheses. Endoscopic prostheses are the preferred treatment for unresectable biliary and pancreatic cancers. The prostheses may block after about 3 months and need to be replaced.

Other causes of bile-duct obstruction

Pancreatitis may obstruct the common bile duct where it passes through the head of the pancreas. Transient jaundice is common in acute pancreatitis, owing to compression by pancreatic oedema. In chronic pancreatitis, especially alcoholic, persistent jaundice can develop, requiring a surgical bypass procedure such as a cholecystojejunostomy. This biliary obstruction is probably a consequence of pancreatic fibrosis. Pancreatic cysts may rarely cause extrinsic compression of the bile duct. Haemobilia or haemorrhage into the biliary tract is uncommon but may follow trauma, liver biopsy, biliary tumours, and gallstones. In addition to jaundice the blood clots cause biliary pain. Massive gastrointestinal haemorrhage may occur. The diagnosis of these conditions relies on accurate cholangiography (usually ERCP).

SCLEROSING CHOLANGITIS

Sclerosing cholangitis is the description applied to multiple strictures and bead-like dilatations of the intrahepatic and extrahepatic biliary tree. It is discussed in detail in Chapter 14.27.3.

Fig. 8 Primary sclerosing cholangitis. The intrahepatic bile ducts show alternate strictures and dilatations ('beading'). The common bile duct, cystic duct, and gallbladder appear normal in this study but may also be involved.

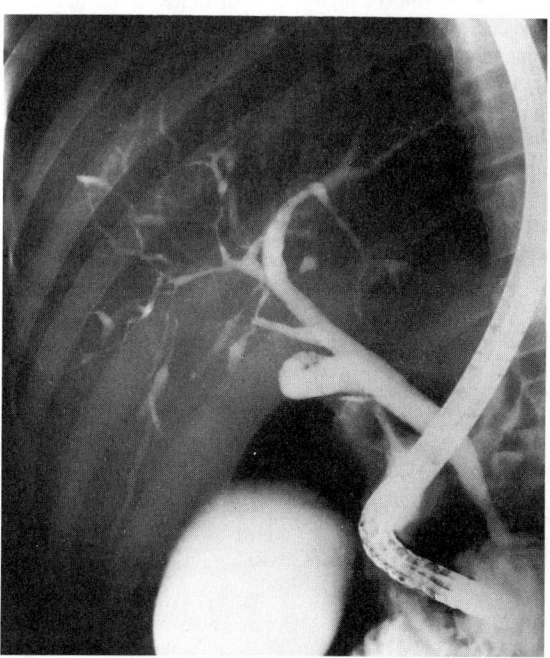

Primary sclerosing cholangitis (Fig. 8)

This should only be diagnosed if the following criteria are satisfied: (i) absence of gallstones; (ii) absence of previous biliary surgery, and (iii) sufficiently long follow-up to exclude carcinoma of the bile duct. Primary sclerosing cholangitis affects males more than females (2:1) and about 70 per cent of patients have ulcerative colitis. The usual clinical presentation is cholestatic jaundice and cholangitis. However, a significant proportion of patients are asymptomatic or present with cirrhosis and portal venous hypertension. There is associated retroperitoneal fibrosis or Riedel's thyroiditis in some cases. Serum biochemistry shows cholestatic liver function tests. A raised serum alkaline phosphatase is almost invariable. Consequently the diagnosis should be considered in cirrhotic patients whose liver function tests show cholestatic features. The IgM concentration is commonly elevated. Liver biopsy may be helpful and usually indicates large bile-duct obstruction. The diagnosis is established by cholangiography with ERCP or PTC. Laparotomy should not be done. Lone tight strictures and stones can be treated by endoscopic techniques. Primary sclerosing cholangitis is being recognized more frequently as a result of the widespread use of ERCP and PTC. It may be confused with primary biliary cirrhosis but the serum mitochondrial antibody is always negative in primary sclerosing cholangitis. Treatment is unsatisfactory; neither corticosteroids nor azathioprine are of proven value. Ursodeoxycholic acid is under clinical trial. Pruritus may be helped by cholestyramine. The prognosis is variable but most patients eventually develop cirrhosis and liver failure. Liver transplantation yields excellent results in these patients. Bile-duct adenocarcinoma is a late complication.

Secondary sclerosing cholangitis

Several causes of secondary sclerosing cholangitis are now recognized. These include recurrent bacterial cholangitis due to gallstones or benign biliary strictures. Children with primary immunodeficiency syndromes and patients with AIDS also develop sclerosing cholangitis. Cytomegalovirus and cryptosporidium are the organisms most commonly associated with AIDS-related sclerosing cholangitis. Sclerosing cholangitis may also develop in patients treated by hepatic arterial infusion of cytotoxic drugs and after the introduction of caustics into hydatid cysts.

REFERENCES

Bonacini, M. (1992). Hepatobiliary complications in patients with human immunodeficiency virus infection. *American Journal of Medicine*, **92**, 404–11.

Chapman, R.W. (1991). Aetiology and natural history of primary sclerosing cholangitis—a decade of progress? *Gut*, **32**, 1433–5.

Donovan, J.M. and Carey, M.C. (1991) Physical–chemical basis of gallstone formation. *Gastroenterology Clinics of North America*, **20**, 47–66.

Jacyna, M.R. and Summerfield, J.A. (1992). Endoscopic management of biliary tract obstruction in the 1990s. *Journal of Hepatology*, **14**, 127–32.

Jazwari, R.P., Pigozzi, M.G., Galatola, F., Lanzini, A., and Northfield, T.C. (1992). Optimum bile acid treatment for rapid gallstone dissolution. *Gut*, **33**, 381–6.

Schiff, L. (1987). *Diseases of the liver*, (6th edn). Lippincott, Philadelphia.

Sherlock, S. (1992). *Diseases of the liver and biliary system*, (9th edn). Blackwell Scientific, Oxford.

Sherlock, S. and Summerfield, J.A. (1991). *A colour atlas of liver disease*, (2nd edn). Wolfe Medical, London.

Tint, G.S. *et al.* (1992). Lithotripsy plus ursodiol is superior to ursodiol alone for cholesterol gallstones. *Gastroenterology*, **102**, 2042–9.

Trotman, B.W. (1991). Pigment gallstone disease. *Gastroenterology Clinics of North America*, **20**, 111–26.

14.25 Jaundice

E. ELIAS

Jaundice is the yellow discoloration of sclerae, mucous membranes, and skin caused by accumulation of bilirubin. Involvement of the sclerae helps distinguish jaundice from other causes of pigmentation such as melanosis, hypercarotinaemia, and mepacrine therapy. Bilirubin is the major bile pigment in man and is formed as an end-product of the catabolism of haem-containing proteins. Jaundice results from either excessive production or defective elimination. There may be detectable differences in the tint produced by haemolytic (lemon-yellow), hepatocellular (orange-yellow), and cholestatic (greenish-yellow) causes of jaundice but no diagnostic reliance should be based on such impressions alone. In medicine, icterus, from the Greek *ikteros*, is used synonymously with jaundice, though it can also refer to a disease of plants in which the leaves turn yellow, or to a certain yellowish-green bird.

Metabolism of bilirubin

PRODUCTION

Bilirubin is a tetrapyrrole compound formed when the ring structure of haem is broken open by microsomal haem oxygenase, thus liberating a bridge carbon as carbon monoxide (CO) (Fig. 1) and total production of CO has been used to estimate the rate of bilirubin formation in healthy persons. Biliverdin and carbon monoxide are formed in equimolar amounts, but because haem oxygenase and biliverdin reductase are present in man in all tissues where senescent red cells are destroyed, bilirubin is formed instantaneously so there is virtually no detectable biliverdin in plasma. Haem oxygenase exhibits maximal activity for free haem, intermediate activity for haemoproteins such as haemoglobin, cytochrome P450, and catalase, in all of which the haem and apoprotein are linked solely through the iron and therefore freely dissociable, and lesser activity for compounds such as carboxyhaemoglobin in which the haem is tightly bound to its apoprotein. The major source of bilirubin in man is from breakdown of red cells. Because all of the four nitrogen atoms are derived from glycine it is possible to investigate haem metabolism after administration of ^{15}N-glycine. As would be expected peak production of ^{15}N-bilirubin and its derivatives occurs between 90 and 120 days later and coincides with the disappearance of ^{15}N-labelled erythrocytes from the circulation. However, a significant peak of ^{15}N-bilirubin production is also seen within the first 2 weeks and does not appear to be due to destruction of circulating erythrocytes. This has been termed 'early labelled bilirubin' and is thought to result from ineffective erythropoiesis and catabolism of non-haemoglobin haemoproteins such as hepatic cytochromes, catalase or myoglobin. An increase of the early-labelled bilirubin peak occurs in pernicious anaemia, erythropoietic porphyria, the thalassaemia syndromes, shunt hyperbilirubinaemia, refractory sideroblastic anaemia, and lead poisoning. In these conditions it may be due to defective synthesis of haemoglobin, but destruction of erythrocytes in the bone marrow before they have entered the circulation will also enhance production of early labelled bilirubin (see Section 22).

Although bilirubin may be regarded as a waste product of haem catabolism, the constituent amino acids of its apoprotein (e.g. globin in haemoglobin) and iron are conserved and reutilized. Other minor degradation pathways for haemoglobin have been described in which biliverdin and bilirubin may not be intermediates, and in one such pathway the denatured haemoglobin of Heinz bodies is converted to water-soluble compounds that are not detected by the van den Bergh reaction.

TRANSPORT IN PLASMA

Bilirubin is transported from its site of production to the liver bound to albumin. The molecular configuration of bilirubin secludes potentially polar groups and renders it non-polar and lipophilic. Even physiological concentrations of plasma bilirubin vastly exceed its solubility in water (4–7 nmol at pH 7.4) and are only achieved because of protein binding. Each albumin molecule has one binding site for bilirubin which is of such high affinity (K_a 10^8/mol) that when molar ratios of bilirubin : albumin do not exceed 1 : 1 there is virtually no free bilirubin in solution. Each albumin molecule has two additional binding sites of moderately high affinity and a third group of low-affinity binding sites. However, when bilirubin : albumin ratios exceed 1 : 1, binding affinities are such that there is a disproportionate increase of the unbound freely diffusable fraction of bilirubin in plasma and in newborn infants brain damage leading to kernicterus may occur. A molar ratio of 1 : 1 exists between albumin 40 g/l and bilirubin 578 μmol/dl, but in newborn infants there is a danger of saturation with relatively less bilirubin. The situation is exacerbated by agents that compete with bilirubin and displace it from the binding sites on albumin (e.g. salicylates, sulphonamides, diazepam, vitamin K analogues, and contrast media for cholangiography). Drugs that are not protein bound may be used safely. The brain is not susceptible to kernicterus in later life though in deep jaundice all tissues other

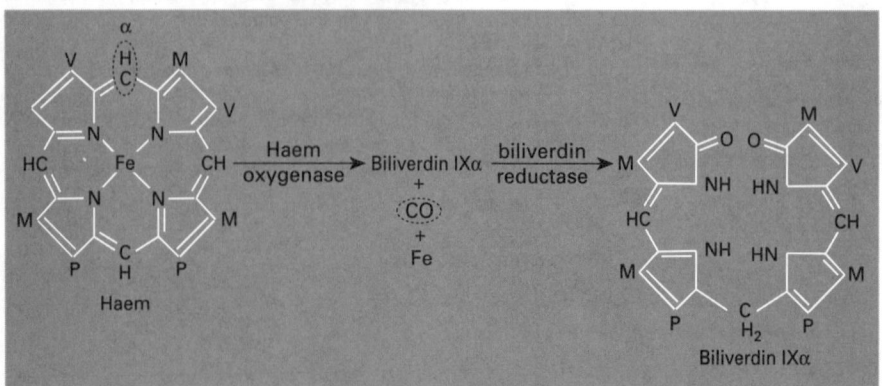

Fig. 1 Production of bilirubin from haem. M, CH$_3$; V, CH; P, CH$_2$—CCH$_2$—COOH. Of the four bridge carbon atoms (α, β, γ, δ), the ring is usually opened at α.

than the brain may become pigmented. Rarely, bilirubin in the eye will produce yellow vision (xanthopsia). In cholestatic jaundice some conjugated bilirubin becomes covalently bound to serum albumin. Resolution of obstructive jaundice is initially rapid due to clearance of dissociable bilirubin and followed by a much slower phase corresponding to disappearance of the irreversibly bound albumin–bilirubin complex. The existence of the latter accounts for persistent conjugated hyperbilirubinaemia long after resolution of bilirubinuria during recovery from cholestasis.

HEPATIC UPTAKE

Uptake of bilirubin by the liver is rapid and occurs independently of albumin uptake though involving interaction of the hepatocyte membrane with the albumin : bilirubin complex. Animal experiments show up-regulation by oestrogens and down-regulation by testosterone of the high-affinity transporter protein that mediates bilirubin uptake via the sinusoidal membrane. This may account for females generally having a lower serum bilirubin and for the tendency for Gilbert's syndrome to present in postpubertal males. Within the cell, bilirubin is bound by ligandin (glutathione S-transferase B) and Z protein (also known as fatty acid-binding protein). Other organic anions, including bromsulphthalein, indocyanine green and cholecystographic agent, compete with bilirubin for hepatocyte uptake and for binding to ligandin and Z protein. Clearance of these agents is enhanced by phenobarbital, which increases ligandin synthesis, and reduced by fasting or oestrogen therapy, which diminish hepatic levels of ligandin and Z protein.

CONJUGATION

Within the liver cell, free bilirubin is rendered water soluble by conjugation with glucuronic acid. This reaction is catalysed by the microsomal enzyme glucuronyl transferase or **UDPGT** (bilirubin uridine diphosphate glucuronate glucuronyl transferase) (Fig. 2). The major conjugate in human bile is bilirubin diglucuronide, with lesser quantities of monoglucuronide and other conjugates, for example glucosides and xylosides. The proportion of mono- and diglucuronide in bile varies, monoglucuronide formation being favoured by a high bilirubin load, low enzyme activity or microsomal injury. Enzyme induction by phenobarbitone increases diglucuronide formation.

BILIARY EXCRETION

The concentration of bilirubin in bile greatly exceeds that in the liver but the nature of the concentrative step is unknown. When bilirubin or bromsulphthalein are administered by intravenous infusion their plasma concentration and biliary excretion rise until a plateau level of biliary excretion is reached. Further infusion produces a progressive rise of plasma concentration without an increment of biliary excretion. Reflux of increasing amounts of conjugated bilirubin into plasma then occurs, suggesting that canalicular excretion rather than conjugation is the rate-limiting step. Transport of bile acids and bilirubin into the canaliculus appear to be mediated by separate transporter proteins. Thus, in the Dubin–Johnson syndrome, transport kinetics for bile acids are usually normal though there is a marked excretory defect for the organic anions bilirubin, bromsulphthalein, and indocyanine green.

Fig. 2 Sequential formation of bilirubin mono- and diglucuronide is catalysed by microsomal glucuronyltransferase and dependent on UDP-glucuronic acid.

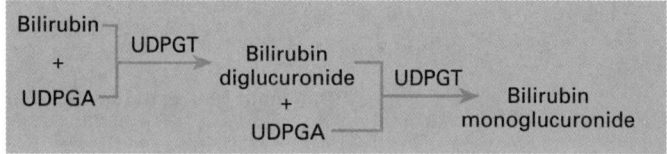

UROBILINOGEN METABOLISM

Metabolism of bilirubin by intestinal bacteria produces a number of breakdown products, which include the readily absorbable, water-soluble urobilinogen. Most of the absorbed urobilinogen is immediately extracted by the liver and excreted in bile, thus undergoing an enterohepatic circulation. The small fraction of urobilinogen that passes through the liver to enter the systemic circulation is available for urinary excretion. An increased urinary urobilinogen output may be caused by a diminished hepatic fractional extraction rate, when its detection is a very sensitive index of early liver disease. Alternatively, increased urinary urobilinogen may occur in the face of a normal hepatic fractional extraction rate when it has been produced and absorbed in proportion to excessive bilirubin production, e.g. in haemolysis (see Section 22). If there is complete biliary obstruction, absence of bile from the gut will be reflected by absence of urobilinogen from the urine.

CLINICAL CHEMISTRY

Plasma bilirubin may be measured by the van den Bergh reaction. Conjugated bilirubin forms a violet colour immediately on addition of sulfanilic acid (direct-reacting bilirubin); the colour is intensified by unconjugated bilirubin following addition of alcohol (indirect-reacting bilirubin). Urobilinogen in the urine may be detected by addition of Ehrlich's reagent (2 per cent p-dimethyl-aminobenzaldehyde in 50 per cent HCl), which produces a red colour. Both urobilinogen and porphobilinogen produce a red colour, but only that due to urobilinogen may be extracted by chloroform. Precise quantitation of free bilirubin, its monoglucuronide and diglucuronide conjugates, and the fraction bound covalently to albumin, requires high-pressure liquid chromatography.

Additional 'liver function tests'

The measured levels of various substances in blood, including bilirubin, have traditionally been described as liver function tests, though as can be seen from the preceding discussion, the concentration of serum bilirubin depends on many factors, of which liver function is only one. The term is equally inappropriate for the measurements of hepatocellular enzymes in serum, as these more precisely reflect the degree and extent of damage to hepatocytes; thus the highest levels are found in massive hepatic necrosis. Liver function is more truly reflected by levels of circulatory proteins that are exclusively synthesized by the liver (e.g. albumin and some clotting factors; II, V, VII, IX, and X), and by the liver's ability to clear certain substances (e.g. bile acids and bromsulphthalein) from the blood, though for each of these, too, there are important determinants other than the health of hepatocytes and patency of the biliary tree.

Hepatocellular damage is reflected by a rise in the activity of serum aspartate aminotransferase (**AST**, formerly glutamic oxalacetic transaminase, GOT), and alanine aminotransferase (**ALT**, formerly glutamic pyruvic transaminase, GPT). Because the enzymes are not specific for the liver, elevated serum levels of, say, AST and lactate dehydrogenase could reflect either muscle or hepatic damage. Even when the tissue of origin is known with certainty, the diagnostic significance of individual values must be interpreted with caution; nevertheless, in liver disease, when serum AST or ALT activity reaches levels that exceed normal by more than 30-fold, jaundice is almost certainly due to a hepatitis, whether of viral, drug, or toxic origin.

High levels of serum alkaline phosphatase (**SAP**) activity are characteristic of cholestasis of both intra- and extrahepatic origin. Electrophoresis permits discrimination between isoenzymes of alkaline phosphatase that are characteristic of liver, bone, kidney, placenta, and intestinal mucosa. Total SAP levels that exceed two and a half times normal because of an increase of the hepatic isoenzyme are rare in jaundice due to hepatocellular disease but common in biliary disorders. Serum 5′-nucleotidase is more specific to liver than alkaline phosphatase and its estimation or that of the more commonly available γ-glutamyltransferase can be substituted for isoenzyme analysis in order to discriminate between hepatic and bony origins of raised SAP activity. Measure of the serum bile-acid concentration has a high specificity for detection of minor degrees of hepatic dysfunction. The sensitivity is enhanced by performing estimations on blood taken 2 h after a fatty meal, when hepatic clearance has been stressed by the bile-acid load returning in the portal blood as part of the enterohepatic circulation.

Quantitative 'liver function tests'

Many have sought a test that can quantitatively express the liver's functional capacity in order to monitor serially disease progression and hepatic regeneration, provide prognostic information, and precisely measure benefit from any attempted therapy. No such single test exists, those generally proposed being able to reflect on only part of the liver's function.

The galactose elimination capacity can be derived from the rate of fall in its blood concentration following a single bolus intravenous injection of galactose (0.5 g/kg) and analysis of blood samples taken at 5-min intervals between 20 and 40 min later. Galactose elimination is a safe and accurate way of measuring hepatic cytosolic functional mass.

Bromsulphthalein and indocyanine green are organic anions that compete with bilirubin for hepatocyte uptake. Bromsulphthalein can rarely cause anaphylactoid reactions and its clinical use has been abandoned. Indocyanine green is not metabolized by the liver but its clearance can be used to measure hepatic blood flow because the liver is solely responsible for its removal from blood.

The ^{14}C-aminopyrine breath test is done by giving the patient a small amount of radioactive aminopyrine by mouth and measuring radioactive $^{14}CO_2$ released by N-demethylation in trapped breath 30 and 60 min later. Like antipyrine and caffeine clearance and the **MEG-X** (mono-ethylglycine xylidide) test, which measures N-de-ethylation of lignocaine, the result is a measure of hepatocyte P450 enzyme activity. The MEG-X test is done by injecting lignocaine (1 mg/kg IV over 2 min) and measuring the concentration of the metabolite MEG-X before and 15 min after its administration. It has been proposed as a rapid test for confirmation of hepatic integrity before the removal of donor livers for transplantation. Clearance of antipyrine and caffeine have the advantage that they can be accurately worked out from serial sputum samples.

Causes and pathophysiology of jaundice

Hyperbilirubinaemia with jaundice may result from excessive bilirubin production, reduced hepatic uptake of bilirubin, reduced hepatic conjugation of bilirubin, or reduced excretion of conjugated bilirubin (Fig. 3).

Excessive production of bilirubin

Excessive production of bilirubin occurs in the haemolytic anaemias. It also may occur in patients with a marked degree of ineffective erythropoiesis and intramedullary destruction of red-cell percursors, as occurs, for example, in thalassaemia and pernicious anaemia. These conditions are considered in detail in Section 22.

Reduced uptake of bilirubin

A defect in the transfer of bilirubin to the hepatocyte may explain the unconjugated hyperbilirubinaemia associated with Gilbert's syndrome, severe congestive heart failure, portocaval shunts, and the action of certain drugs including rifamycin.

Reduced hepatic conjugation of bilirubin

Reduced hepatic conjugation of bilirubin is probably the cause of neonatal jaundice and occurs in the Crigler–Najjar syndrome, where it results from a specific deficiency of glucuronyl transferase. Inhibition of the activity of that enzyme by steroids excreted in maternal milk is a rare cause of neonatal jaundice.

Reduced excretion of conjugated bilirubin

Very rarely this occurs because of congenital defects of hepatic excretion in the Dubin–Johnson and Rotor syndromes. Commonly, it is a consequence of hepatocellular injury as in viral hepatitis or drug jaundice; inflammatory, granulomatous or neoplastic infiltration of the liver, or extrahepatic bile duct obstruction by gallstones, pancreatic carcinoma, and other disorders (Table 1).

Clinical approach to the jaundiced patient

Urine testing differentiates between unconjugated and conjugated hyperbilirubinaemia. If bilirubin is absent from the urine, the detection of excess urinary urobilinogen, splenomegaly, anaemia, reticulocytosis, and a family history of anaemia suggest a haemolytic cause for jaundice. If there is no haemolysis or ineffective erythropoiesis, and other 'liver function tests' are normal, the patient may be fasted for 48 h to differentiate between benign hepatic hyperbilirubinaemia (see below) and liver disease such as inactive cirrhosis. In newborn babies, action may be required to prevent brain damage.

If bilirubin is present in the urine, the common causes are hepatitis and obstruction of the biliary system. Inquiry should be made regarding family history, travel, exposure to toxins, viral hepatitis, drugs, or a recent anaesthetic. In viral hepatitis, jaundice is usually preceded by a prodromal phase involving anorexia, nausea, and aversion to smoking, sometimes with an influenza-like illness: the liver is characteristically enlarged and tender at the onset, and serum transaminase levels (ALT, AST) are markedly elevated. When the typical features of hepatitis are absent, jaundice with bilirubinuria, especially if accompanied by pale stools and pruritus, prompts the question of whether cholestasis is due to an intrahepatic or extrahepatic cause. In certain cholestatic conditions (e.g. primary biliary cirrhosis or sclerosing cholangitis), jaundice may be a very late sign, preceded by raised SAP levels, pruritus, and xanthelasma for several years. Severe abdominal pain of abrupt onset preceding jaundice by a couple of days suggests gallstone obstruction. A

Fig. 3 Classification of jaundice.

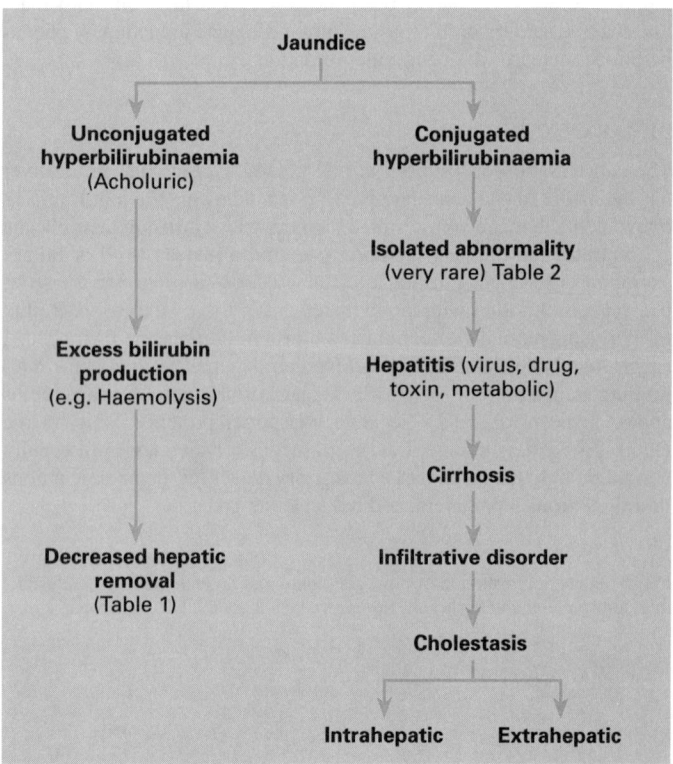

Table 1 *Hyperbilirubinaemia in the absence of overt liver or biliary-tract disease or haemolysis*

Unconjugated	Conjugated
Gilbert's syndrome	Dubin–Johnson syndrome
Crigler–Najjar type I	Rotor's syndrome
Crigler–Najjar type II	
Physiological jaundice of the newborn	
Transient familial neonatal hyperbilirubinaemia	
Breast-milk jaundice	

rigor in association with dark urine due to bilirubinuria is extremely strong evidence that mechanical biliary obstruction is causing cholangitis. Painless cholestatic jaundice when accompanied by the absence of urinary urobilinogen and a palpable gallbladder usually indicates a neoplastic cause (Courvoiser's law). Ultrasonography is used to determine the diameter of the bile ducts, and when the ducts are not dilated may be followed by liver biopsy or endoscopic retrograde cholangiography, and when the ducts are dilated, percutaneous transhepatic cholangiography may be the preferred method for clarifying the diagnosis (Fig. 4). When jaundice and bilirubinuria are accompanied by none of the features mentioned above, and 'liver function tests' are otherwise normal, one of the rare familial causes of conjugated hyperbilirubinaemia is probable.

During examination of the jaundiced patient, other features that may indicate whether liver disease is chronic or due to alcoholism should be sought, including spider naevi, bruises, parotid enlargement, gynaecomastia, testicular atrophy, and loss of body hair, leuconychia, palmar erythema, and Dupuytren's contracture. Fetor hepaticus, mental impairment, and asterixis may accompany hepatic encephalopathy. In addition, portal hypertension may be suspected because of dilated veins on the abdominal wall, splenomegaly, and ascites. In cirrhosis the liver may be enlarged or very small. Absence of any signs of chronic liver disease in a jaundiced patient with an enlarged, irregular, hard liver suggests the presence of an infiltrative disorder, possibly a secondary neoplasm.

Unconjugated hyperbilirubinaemia

The main causes of unconjugated hyperbilirubinaemia are summarized in Table 1.

Gilbert's syndrome

In 1901, Gilbert noticed a familial occurrence of hyperbilirubinaemia in the absence of apparent liver disease. He subdivided subjects according to whether or not there was any splenomegaly, the splenomegalic group later being shown to be due to haemolysis. Gilbert's syndrome now refers to mild unconjugated hyperbilirubinaemia in the absence of liver disease or overt haemolysis, although if careful red-cell survival studies are done, up to half the cases are shown to have slightly diminished survival. Estimates of its frequency vary from 0.5 to 8 per cent, giving a mean prevalence of 1 to 2 per cent of the population.

Some patients with Gilbert's syndrome complain of symptoms such as abdominal pain, weakness, and malaise, but these are non-specific and may represent a coincidental occurrence rather than true association. Plasma bilirubin levels fluctuate markedly, but are usually not sufficiently high to produce jaundice. Most patients are discovered incidentally, many as a result of scleral icterus brought on by reduced caloric intake during an illness that causes anorexia.

Though a strong familial tendency exists, the precise mode of inheritance is unclear. An autosomal dominant defect has been suggested, but it is likely that Gilbert's syndrome embraces a heterogeneous group of biochemical defects including abnormalities of hepatic uptake, intracellular binding and conjugation. In most though not all patients, hepatic UDPGT activity is diminished, suggesting a primary defect in glucuronidation. However, this is a highly inducible enzyme and decreased levels may be due to decreased hepatic uptake of substrate. Furthermore, in some, clearance of indocyanine green is defective, though this organic anion is excreted unconjugated; in one other subgroup abnormal bromsulphthalein clearance suggests a defect in hepatic uptake of organic anions. Conventional 'liver function tests' are normal. Liver histology is grossly normal, though an increase of lipofuscin may be seen especially in centrolobular hepatocytes. Electron microscopy suggests heterogeneity between patients, with evidence of mitochondrial changes and proliferation of the smooth endoplasmic reticulum in some. The diagnosis is based on clinical and laboratory findings. Demonstration of unconjugated hyperbilirubinaemia with otherwise normal 'liver function tests' and no overt haemolysis may suffice. Plasma bilirubin levels approximately double in both normal individuals and those with Gilbert's syndrome when dietary intake is reduced to 1680 J (400 cal) daily for 48 to 72 h. The percentage increase is similar in normal and Gilbert's subjects; however, the increment and final value is much higher in Gilbert's, and this may be diagnostically useful because such increases are not seen in patients with hyperbilirubinaemia due to hepatocellular disease or cirrhosis. As an alternative to fasting, 50 mg of nicotinic acid may be injected intravenously. Unconjugated serum bilirubin is increased by nicotinic acid as the result of complex mechanisms that include increased erythrocyte fragility, increased splenic haem-oxygenase activity, and increased formation of bilirubin in the spleen. An increase of unconjugated serum bilirubin of more than 17 μmol/l is highly suggestive of Gilbert's syndrome and the concentration versus time curve shows a significant delay in the clearance of unconjugated bilirubin at the end of the test compared to controls. This provocation test is especially recommended in patients with suspected Gilbert's syndrome whose serum bilirubin is normal at the time of investigation. Liver biopsy is required when there is reasonable doubt about the diagnosis, but is not essential.

The prognosis is excellent, and there is no substantive evidence for the association of Gilbert's syndrome with other more serious disorders. Patients require no more than the reassurance derived from an understanding of the commonness of their condition and its totally benign nature.

Crigler–Najjar syndrome

The Crigler–Najjar syndrome results in severe unconjugated hyperbilirubinaemia in the absence of any other evidence of hepatic dysfunction or haemolysis. Where they have been studied, hepatic clearance of bromsulphthalein and indocyanine green, red-cell survival, and 'early labelled bilirubin' peak are all normal. The underlying defect appears

Fig. 4 Investigation of jaundice: ERCP, endoscopic retrograde cholangiopancreatography; PTC, percutaneous transhepatic cholangiography.

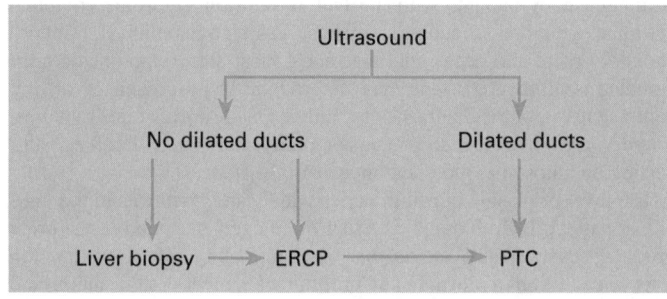

to be a deficiency of UDPGT activity. There are two genetically distinct groups, types I and II.

TYPE I

In type I Crigler–Najjar there appears to be a complete absence of UDPGT activity, and no bilirubin glucuronide is formed though other compounds may be glucuronidated by the liver. Severe unconjugated hyperbilirubinaemia occurs in the neonatal period, leading to kernicterus and early death in most infants. A minority survives the neonatal period without apparent brain damage but may also succumb in later childhood.

The diagnosis is based on clinical and laboratory findings. There is no Rhesus, ABO or other blood-group incompatibility and no haemolysis. Other 'liver function tests' are normal and there is no bilirubin in the urine. Bilirubin conjugates are not present in bile, which may be colourless. Nevertheless, the colour of faeces has been normal, and urobilin is present though quantitatively diminished in the faeces. The explanation for this is unclear, but is thought to result from diffusion of a small amount of unconjugated bilirubin into the bowel lumen across the intestinal mucosa and biliary tract. Consanguinity is common in the parents of affected offspring, suggesting an autosomal recessive mode of inheritance. Heterozygotes are usually not jaundiced.

TYPE II

Type II Crigler–Najjar is associated with only partial deficiency of UDPG activity, and is a less well-defined entity than type I embracing those unconjugated hyperbilirubinaemias of hepatic origin that are intermediate between Gilbert's syndrome and type I Crigler–Najjar. Jaundice is usually of less acute onset and less severe than seen in type I, and occasionally jaundice may not be apparent in early childhood. Kernicterus is rare. Bile contains bilirubin and therefore is deeply pigmented. Familial occurrence is common. Gilbert's syndrome is frequently found in relatives; in some families Crigler–Najjar type II syndrome appears to represent the homozygous state for a variant of Gilbert's syndrome present in both parents, but the incidence of Crigler–Najjar is much lower than it would be if this was true for all cases.

TREATMENT

In Crigler–Najjar type II syndrome the time course of the response to phenobarbitone therapy suggests than an enzyme with a relatively long half-life is being induced. The lack of any such responsiveness to phenobarbital in type I, a rare indication for replacing a histologically normal liver by transplantation, suggests a complete absence of the enzyme, and constitutes the most useful method clinically for differentiating the two types. In type II, phenobarbital treatment reduces plasma bilirubin levels, which patients may welcome for its cosmetic effect.

Phototherapy is effective in alleviating hyperbilirubinaemia in infants. Bilirubin has an intense absorption band in the visible spectrum between 425 and 475 nm, and exposure of the skin to light of this wavelength reduces the plasma bilirubin concentration. A series of highly polar, water-soluble derivatives of bilirubin result from its photodegradation, and these pass readily into urine, bile or across the intestinal wall. This treatment has become established as a means of preventing kernicterus in neonatal units. However, it is probably impractical as a lifelong measure, even in patients with Crigler–Najjar type I syndrome, and its freedom from undesirable side-effects in the long term is unproven. Photodegradation may be enhanced by riboflavin.

Physiological jaundice of the newborn

A rise in plasma bilirubin concentration occurs very commonly in the first few days of life, but infants born prematurely with low birth weights are most likely to become jaundiced. *In utero*, bilirubin is transported across the placenta and removed by the maternal liver. After birth, the fetal liver may be incapable of maintaining low plasma bilirubin levels, its immaturity being shown by low levels of ligandin, glucuronyl transferase activity, and capacity for excretion of conjugated bilirubin into bile. After birth, glucuronyl transferase activity increases exponentially to reach adult levels by 14 weeks of age, regardless of full-term or premature birth. Susceptibility to hyperbilirubinaemia in the neonate may be compounded by a shortened red-cell lifespan, reduced caloric intake or shunting past the liver through a patent ductus venosus.

Plasma bilirubin levels must be monitored in jaundiced infants because of the risk of kernicterus. Though levels in excess of 340 μmol/l have, traditionally, been thought to constitute a risk of kernicterus, recent work suggests that plasma levels half as high may be associated with some impairment of subsequent psychomotor development. This problem can be averted by reduction of plasma bilirubin concentrations with phototherapy or exchange transfusions. In addition, reabsorption of unconjugated bilirubin, formed in the intestine by the action of β-glucuronidase, may be prevented by the oral administration of a non-absorbable agar, which binds the bilirubin. Drugs that displace bilirubin from albumin should be avoided.

Transient familial neonatal hyperbilirubinaemia

Occasionally there is a familial tendency to develop neonatal hyperbilirubinaemia, and affected infants are at risk of developing kernicterus even following full-term gestation. There is no haemolysis and the onset of jaundice occurs earlier than is seen with breast-milk jaundice. The management is the same as for physiological jaundice. Jaundice is transient and the long-term prognosis is excellent. Neonatal jaundice associated with glucose 6-phosphate deficiency is considered in Section 22.

Breast-milk jaundice

A small number of infants have been reported in whom jaundice due to unconjugated hyperbilirubinaemia has occurred, apparently as a result of breast feeding. Kernicterus is not a complication. There appears to be an icterogenic factor in breast milk that is not detectable in maternal serum. Siblings of affected individuals are also liable to jaundice if breast fed. High levels of the steroid 3α, 20β- pregnanediol, an inhibitor of glucuronyl transferase, in the milk of these mothers has been implicated. However, whether this is the true identity of the icterogenic factor remains to be confirmed.

Conjugated hyperbilirubinaemia

Conjugated hyperbilirubinaemia results from reflux into plasma of bilirubin which has previously been taken up and conjugated by the liver. In most instances it is found in association with retention of other biliary constituents such as bile acids, but typical families have been described in which defective excretion of conjugated bilirubin occurs as an isolated defect.

The Dubin–Johnson syndrome

Although many patients with the Dubin–Johnson syndrome complain of vague symptoms of anorexia, malaise, easy fatiguability, right hypochondrial pain, and occasional diarrhoea, most are asymptomatic until jaundice is discovered. This may be brought on by pregnancy or oral contraceptives, or the diagnosis may only be made during family studies. There is a high incidence of consanguinity in reported families, suggesting an autosomal recessive mode of inheritance.

The level of plasma bilirubin varies widely and fluctuates in the individual patient. Bilirubin and excess urobilinogen are found in the urine in the absence of any haemolysis or abnormalities of 'liver function tests'. In addition to bilirubin and urobilinogen, other organic anions are affected, and non-visualization of the gallbladder with cholecysto-

Table 2 *Differential features of the two more common types of familial conjugated hyperbilirubinaemia*

	Dubin–Johnson syndrome	Rotor's syndrome
Cholecystography	Usually unsuccessful	Usually successful
Liver biopsy	Pigment loaded	No excess pigment
BSP clearance	Normal initial phase	Slow initial clearance
	Late rise of BSP-GSH	No late rise of BSP-GSH
Urinary coproporphyrin:		
Total excretion	Normal	Raised
Ratio I : III	Raised	Raised

BSP, bromsulphthalein; GSH, reduced glutathione.

graphic media is the rule. The pattern of bromsulphthalein clearance is also helpful diagnostically. Early plasma disappearance of bromsulphthalein appears normal and retention at 45 min may not be markedly deranged. However, plasma levels subsequently rise so that at 90 min they exceed those at 45 min, due to reflux of glutathione-conjugated-bromsulphthalein. The diagnosis may be confirmed by measurement of urinary coproporphyrin excretion. In homozygous Dubin–Johnson patients the ratio of urinary coproporphyrin I to coproporphyrin III is at least 4 : 1, compared to a ratio of approximately 1 : 3 in normal subjects. The intermediate ratios found in heterozygous carriers support an autosomal recessive mode of inheritance. Similarly increased ratios occur in erythropoietic porphyria but the markedly increased overall excretion of coproporphyrins seen in that situation are not a feature of the Dubin–Johnson syndrome.

The liver is deeply pigmented, and the diagnosis may be suspected if a liver biopsy specimen appears black to the naked eye. Histologically, liver cells contain much granular pigment that is not bilirubin and has been variously ascribed to lipofuscin and melanin. There is no recognized treatment for the condition, which is benign, and the patient can be reassured accordingly. Very rarely there has been a coexistent dyserythropoietic anaemia or a defect in blood coagulability.

Rotor's syndrome

Rotor described the familial occurrence of conjugated hyperbilirubinaemia in natives of the Philippines. Originally considered a variant of the Dubin–Johnson syndrome, it is now thought to have a different pathology with demonstrable uptake and storage defects similar to those found in Southdown sheep and Indigo snake. There is no apparent abnormality of bile acid transport and other liver function tests are normal. Plasma concentrations of bilirubin fluctuate widely as in the Dubin–Johnson syndrome but formal testing distinguishes between the two conditions (Table 2).

Intrahepatic cholestasis

Cholestasis describes a constellation of clinical, biochemical, and histological findings in which the predominant abnormality is a failure of bile secretion. The earliest detectable abnormality may be elevation of serum bile-acid levels, but accumulation of other biliary constituents including cholesterol and conjugated bilirubin often follows. Derangement of 'liver function tests' characteristically produces an elevation of alkaline phosphate and 5′-nucleotidase as the more striking features. When biliary obstruction is recent and complete, liver histology reveals oedematous portal tracts, bilirubin in hepatocytes, and plugs of inspissated bile within canaliculi, especially in centrolobular zones. Prolonged cholestasis with partial obstruction as in early primary biliary cirrhosis or primary sclerosing cholangitis is suggested histologically by accumulation of copper-associated protein within periportal hepatocytes, bile-ductular proliferation at the periphery of portal tracts, and portal fibrosis. Absence or diminution of intestinal bile acids may lead to steatorrhoea, and if cholestasis is prolonged, deficiency states affecting the fat-soluble vitamins A, D, E, and K may be anticipated. The classical triad of symptoms in cholestatic disorders is of dark urine, pale stools, and pruritus. When biliary obstruction is incomplete, pruritus is often first to appear and may be the sole feature for an extended period of time.

Cholestasis may result from obstruction of the extrahepatic biliary system, and from obstruction of intrahepatic interlobular bile ducts (e.g. with primary biliary cirrhosis) and sclerosing cholangitis or parasitic infestations. However, intrahepatic cholestasis may be due to secretory failure at the level of the hepatocellular canaliculus in the absence of any obstruction to flow within the bile ductules or ducts. This is seen with drug-induced cholestasis and occasionally when liver disease is due to alcohol or viral hepatitis.

Vanishing bile-duct syndrome

Severe progressive cholestasis may ensue in conditions that destroy bile ducts of predominantly interlobular size. Normally, portal tracts contain arterioles and bile ducts of approximately equal size and in a ratio of 1 : 1. In vanishing bile-duct syndrome, sensitive and specific stains for biliary epithelium reveal none in more than a half, and occasionally all, portal tracts. The process is always insiduous in conditions such as primary biliary cirrhosis, primary sclerosing cholangitis, sarcoidosis, and mucoviscidosis but can also occur either insidiously or abruptly in liver allograft rejection, graft-versus-host disease and extremely rarely in Hodgkin's disease and cholestatic drug reactions (e.g. reactions to flucloxacillin). When the syndrome is severe, liver failure supervenes and liver transplantation is the only curative option.

Benign recurrent intrahepatic cholestasis

This is a relatively rare condition, affecting males more than females and characterized by recurrent attacks of cholestasis in the absence of any mechanical biliary obstruction and with restoration of completely normal hepatic structure and function between attacks. The first attack usually occurs during childhood or adolescence: attacks last for several weeks or months and are separated by intervals of normality lasting many months or years. Pruritus usually precedes jaundice and may sometimes subside without occurrence of jaundice. Patients tend to recognize a precise pattern common to all of their attacks, though the features vary between individuals. There may be vague, right hypochondrial pain and malaise preceding pruritus but fever and chills are not a feature.

Serum bile acids and alkaline phosphate levels are characteristically raised during attacks. Jaundice is due to conjugated hyperbilirubinaemia; bilirubin is present in the urine and urinary urobilinogen is extremely low. Disappearance from plasma of unconjugated bilirubin is always normal, but during episodes of jaundice there is a subsequent rise of conjugated bilirubin. Cholestasis may also cause steatorrhoea and significant hypoprothrombinaemia with bruising. If the diagnosis is not established, cholangiography may be used to rule out mechanical obstruction. Histological examination of the liver reveals centrilobular cholestasis. Electron microscopy shows changes common to many forms of cholestasis: canalicular dilation with loss of canalicular microvilli, widening of the pericanalicular ectoplasm, enlargement of the Golgi, and proliferation of the smooth endoplasmic reticulum.

Benign recurrent intrahepatic cholestasis has a familial incidence but no hereditary pattern is apparent. One family has been reported in which there were several members with benign recurrent intrahepatic cholestasis, cholestasis of pregnancy or contraceptive steroid-induced cholestasis, which suggests a related mechanism in these conditions. Because of the early changes in bile-acid metabolism in each attack it has been postulated that the bile acids have a primary pathogenetic role.

Patients can be reassured of the benign, non-progressive nature of their disease. Early experience suggests that ursodeoxycholic acid is useful both for prophylaxis and in controlling attacks in some patients. Despite their wide usage there is no convincing benefit from corticosteroids or cholestyramine.

Cholestasis of pregnancy (see also Chapter 13.13)

Intrahepatic cholestasis which clinically resembles that described under benign recurrent intrahepatic cholestasis is seen in some women during pregnancy, usually in the third trimester. Pruritus is usually the first symptom and cholestasis may progress to jaundice with unconjugated hyperbilirubinaemia, bilirubinuria, and low urinary urobilinogen levels. Hypochondrial pain is uncommon and fever is not a feature. Serum bile acids are characteristically raised from the onset of pruritus. Serum ALT is the most sensitive of the conventional tests but becomes abnormal later and only in the more severely affected. Steatorrhoea may be produced, with hypoprothrombinaemia that is corrected rapidly by parenteral administration of vitamin K. Pruritus is much more common than jaundice in cholestasis of pregnancy but should probably be regarded as a mild form of the same condition. Cholestasis characteristically resolves rapidly after parturition, and normality is usually restored within 2 to 3 weeks. Incomplete resolution of the cholestasis after delivery may indicate underlying disease, such as primary biliary cirrhosis, that has been unmasked by pregnancy. The differential diagnosis includes cholelithiasis, which has increased incidence during pregnancy; even so, cholangiography can usually be avoided in cholestasis of pregnancy if the course is typical. Also, viral hepatitis is a more common cause of jaundice during pregnancy than either intrahepatic cholestasis of pregnancy or choledocholithiasis. The viral illness is usually less cholestatic and proportionately higher serum transaminase levels reflect the hepatitic nature of the illness.

There is a strong tendency for cholestasis to recur in subsequent pregnancies, and these women are also predisposed to develop cholestasis if given oral contraceptive steroids. There is a relatively strong familial tendency, though the precise mode of inheritance is unclear. Particularly high incidences of recurrent intrahepatic cholestasis of pregnancy has been observed in certain countries, notably in Scandinavia and Chile. Spontaneous labour occurs prematurely and, although outcome is usually benign, there is an increased risk of fetal distress and unexplained stillbirth. No long-term ill effects on infant or mother have been described. However, these women have two to three times the prevalence of gallstones found in their unaffected peers of similar parity.

The concurrence of cholestasis in the third trimester of pregnancy when oestrogen levels are at their highest, with a predisposition of the same subjects to develop cholestasis when given contraceptive steroids points to a pathogenetic role for oestrogens. The importance of progestogens is less certain. At present it appears that these women suffer from a high susceptibility to develop cholestasis due to normal oestrogens, rather than from formation of an abnormal compound with cholestatic properties.

Reports of benefit from treatment with S-adenosyl methionine lack confirmation. Ursodeoxycholic acid reverses liver dysfunction and pruritus in some patients, but its protective effect on the fetus remains to be determined. Cholestyramine, even in high doses, is less beneficial. Early delivery of the fetus following confirmation of lung maturity is recommended, at least in those with a prior history of fetal distress or stillbirth.

Contraceptive steroid-induced cholestasis

Pruritus progressing to jaundice occurs in some women taking oral contraceptive steroids (see Chapter 13.1). Symptoms usually appear during the first three monthly cycles, and recede spontaneously when 'the pill' is discontinued. Those who have experienced cholestasis on the 'contraceptive pill' have a high likelihood of developing cholestasis of pregnancy and vice versa. If possible, oral contraceptive steroids should be avoided in women with a prior history of cholestasis of pregnancy or benign recurrent intrahepatic cholestasis. Rarely, progressive biliary disorders such as primary biliary cirrhosis or sclerosing cholangitis may first become symptomatic due to the unmasking effect of contraceptive steroids and also constitute contraindications to their use. There is no evidence to suggest an increased risk of oral contraceptive-induced cholestasis during convalescence from viral hepatitis.

REFERENCES

Burra, P. and Elias, E. (1992). The vanishing bile duct syndrome. *British Journal of Surgery*, **79**, 604–5.

Elias, E. (1989). Clinical and biochemical diagnosis of jaundice. *Ballières Clinical Gastroenterology*, **3**, 357–85.

Merkel, C. *et al.* (1991). Prognostic value of galactose elimination capacity, aminopyrine breath test, and ICG clearance in patients with cirrhosis: comparison with the Pugh score. *Digestive Disease Science*, **36**, 1197–203.

Sherlock, S and Dooley, J. (1993). *Diseases of the liver and biliary system*, (9th edn). Blackwell. Oxford.

Tiribelli, C. and Ostrow, J.D. (1993). New concepts in bilirubin chemistry, transport and metabolism: Report of the Second International Bilirubin Workshop. *Hepatology*, **17**, 715–36.

Westwood, A. (1991). The analysis of bilirubin in serum. *Annals of Clinical Biochemistry*, **28**, 119–30.

14.26 Clinical features of viral hepatitis

H. C. Thomas

At least five viruses (A,B,C,D,E) cause hepatitis without significant damage to other organs. These agents, which are described in detail in Section 7, may result in an acute infection with hepatitis (A,B,C,D,E), or persistent infection with chronic hepatitis (B,C,D), sometimes leading to cirrhosis and hepatocellular carcinoma. Other viruses that infect and damage many tissues of the body may also cause hepatitis. These include Epstein–Barr, cytomegalo, herpes simplex, herpes zoster, coxsackie A and B, measles, Lassa fever, Marburg fever, and Ebola viruses.

Acute viral hepatitis

This is a self-limiting episode of predominantly hepatocytic damage caused by one or other of the above viruses.

CLINICAL FEATURES

Many patients present with an influenza-like syndrome associated with malaise and arthralgia. These symptoms, probably due to circulating interferon-α, last a few days and are followed by clinical and biochemical evidence of hepatocellular necrosis. The first biochemical signs of liver-cell necrosis are increased concentrations of aspartate and alanine aminotransferases; these enzymes, normally present within the cell, increase in the serum to between 3- and 50-fold the normal range. Conjugated bilirubinaemia then follows in some cases and is associated with leakage of this water-soluble pigment into the urine, causing it to darken. In patients who develop intrahepatic cholestasis, where swollen liver cells compress the biliary cannulicular system and small intrahepatic biliary ductules, the alkaline phosphatase will rise and the patient subsequently develops pruritus and pale stools (steatorrhoea). Thus, in an acute viral hepatitis, the sequence of clinical and biochemical events is first caused by the patient's interferon response due to viraemia, then liver-cell necrosis, and finally by intrahepatic cholestasis.

In many patients the hepatitis is mild and they do not develop icterus. Jaundice is most common in acute hepatitis due to hepatitis B and least frequently seen in patients with hepatitis C (Table 1). Once jaundice has appeared there is often rapid symptomatic improvement, although in the rare clinical syndrome of fulminant or subfulminant hepatic failure, deterioration continues and proceeds within either 1 week (fulminant) or 8 weeks (subfulminant) to liver failure and coma.

SPECIFIC FEATURES OF DIFFERENT FORMS OF VIRAL HEPATITIS

Hepatitis A virus infection

This virus (**HAV**) is enterically transmitted and is most common in countries where hygiene is poor. Faecal contamination of drinking water is the usual source of infection. The incubation period is between 15 and 50 days, and a febrile onset is commonly seen. In young people the disease is usually anicteric, but from middle age onwards it may cause a severe hepatitis, often with deep icterus. The concentrations of transaminases rise, sometimes to several thousand, in the first week of the illness and this is followed rapidly by jaundice. Intrahepatic cholestasis is seen commonly and is identified by a rising alkaline phosphatase associated with pruritus.

The diagnosis is made by demonstration of IgM antiHAV in the patient's blood (Fig. 1), which is present within 10 days of the onset of viraemia and therefore is positive at presentation in virtually all cases. This is followed by an IgG antibody response that is lifelong and confers protective immunity. Although the virus can be detected in faeces from the time of prodromal symptoms through many weeks, direct isolation of the virus is clinically inconvenient and rarely used. A short period (24–48 h) of viraemia does occur and transmission by blood and blood products (factor VIII concentrates) has been reported.

The icteric patient is often confined to bed because of severe lethargy. Bedrest, however, does not accelerate recovery. The patient should be allowed to undertake a level of exercise consistent with the symptoms. No antiviral compounds active against this agent are available.

Family contacts should be offered either an injection of pooled globulin, which has a protective content of antibody and confers protection for 3 months after a single injection, or active immunization with vaccine.

A heat-inactivated, whole-virus vaccine is now available and may be used to protect family members as an alternative to the use of globulins. The immune response to this vaccine is rapid and is sufficient to either prevent or reduce the infection. It should also be used to protect trav-

Table 1 *Clinical features of viral hepatitis*

	HAV	HBV	HCV	HDV	HEV
Transmission	Enteral	Parenteral	Parenteral	Parenteral	Enteral
Incubation period (days)	15–50 %	28–160%	14–160%	28–160% (coinfection of HBV + HDV)	20–40%
Severity of hepatitis	Increases with age (rarely icteric in childhood)	50% icteric	Rarely icteric	Usually icteric	Severe, with high mortality in pregnant women
Progression to chronic disease	Never	At birth: > 90% > 2 years < 5%	50%	Coinfection: < 5% Superinfection: > 95%	Never
Risk of hepatocellular carcinoma	None	High in cirrhotics	High in cirrhotics	High in cirrhotics	None

ellers to areas of the world endemic for HAV and high-risk groups in developed countries (primary schoolteachers, sewage workers, and attendants in mental health institutions).

Hepatitis B virus infection

Hepatitis B virus is transmitted by contact with infected body secretions. The virus is present in saliva, urine, and plasma. Inoculation of these fluids through the skin, mucous membranes, or conjunctival sac will result in hepatitis within 28 to 160 days. Again, prodromal symptoms of fever and arthralgia with malaise are commonly seen. These are followed by a marked increase in serum transaminases to concentrations usually between 300 and 800 u/l. In approximately half of the cases, jaundice will follow.

Persistent hepatitis B virus infection occurs with differing frequency dependent on the time of exposure (Fig. 2). Exposure at birth from an infected mother invariably results in persistent infection. These infants initially have minimal hepatitis but as the years progress, chronic persistent will change to chronic active hepatitis (see Fig. 3 for definition of these histological entities) and up to half of these children will develop cirrhosis with or without liver-cell cancer and will die of the

complications of these two conditions. Infection between birth and 2 years of age results in a persistent infection in 40 per cent of cases and these children run the same risks as the neonatally infected children. From 2 years of age onwards, infection rarely results in persistent infection, only 2 to 5 per cent developing this complication. Again, the disease may start with minimal hepatitis but as time passes, chronic active and lobular hepatitis intervene and approximately 25 to 50 per cent of patients will develop cirrhosis and run the risk of hepatocellular carcinoma.

Diagnosis of acute infection involves the identification of hepatitis B surface antigen (**HBs**) in serum (Table 2). This, however, is also present in the chronic infection, and the acute disease is differentiated from the chronic by the presence of high-titre IgM antiHBc (core antigen). During the first month of the acute infection the infected liver cell secretes the viral protein HBe; its presence in serum indicates intense viraemia and infectivity. After approximately 4 weeks, there is seroconversion from HBe antigen to anti-HBe, associated with resolution of the hepatitis, clearance of the virus from serum and, usually, recovery. Some patients remain HBs antigen positive because hepatitis B virus sequences have become integrated into cellular DNA, continuing to encode for the envelope proteins of the virus but without production of virus particles.

Management of patients with acute hepatitis is conservative. Those with severe symptoms may require admission to hospital. No specific therapy is required. They must be followed until HBs antigen is cleared and they have developed anti-HBs. Patients who remain HBe antigen

Fig. 1 Hepatitis A: clinical and virological course. Hepatitis A virus (HAV) is shed into the faeces before clinical presentation and before appearance of IgM antiHAV.

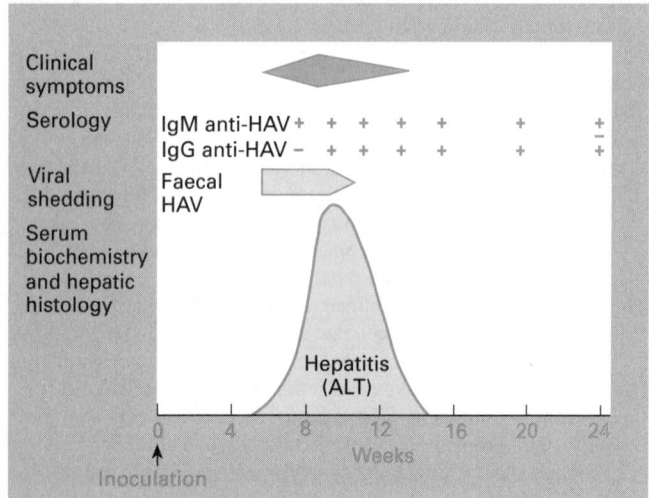

Fig. 3 Histological classification of chronic hepatitis dependent on distribution of inflammatory (mononuclear cell) infiltrate.

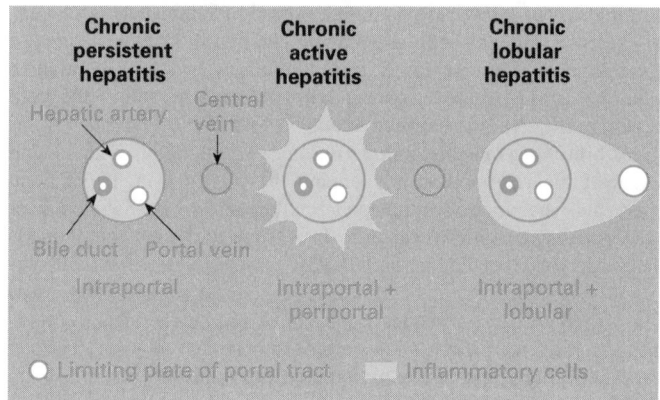

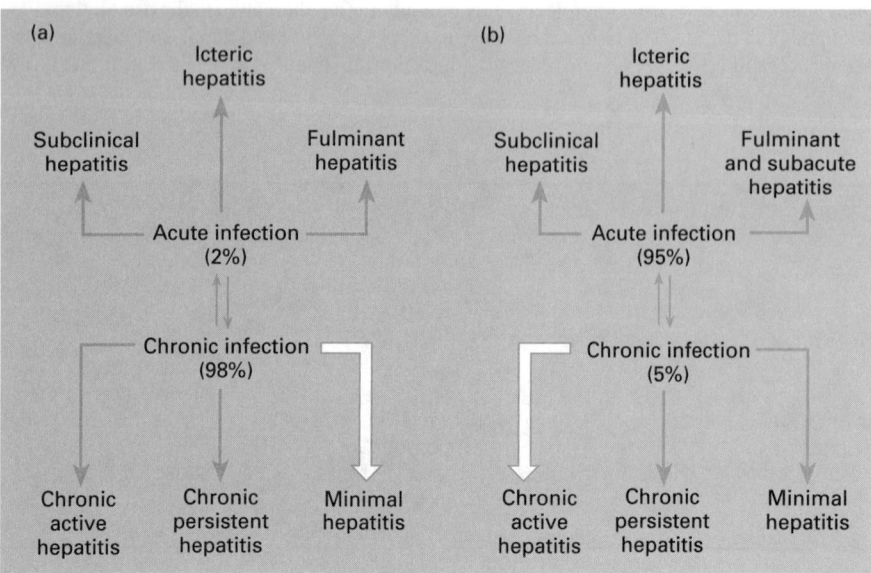

Fig. 2 Clinical syndromes occurring after hepatitis B virus infection in (a) neonates, (b) children (over 2 years old) and adults. CAH, chronic active hepatitis; CPH, chronic persistent hepatitis.

Table 2 *Diagnosis of viral hepatitis*

	Acute infection	Chronic infection	Recovered infection
HAV	IgM anti-HAV	Not seen	IgG anti-HAV
HBV	HBsAg	HBsAg	IgG anti-HBs
	IgM anti-HBc (high titre, 19S)	IgG anti-HBc; IgM anti-HBc in low titre (usually 7S)*	IgG anti-HBc
HCV	IgM anti-HCV	IgG anti-HCV	IgG anti-HCV
	IgG anti-HCV	(polymerase chain reaction is used to detect HCV-RNA to differentiate)	
HDV	Coinfection (HBV and HDV):	Superinfection (HDV on HBV):	
	IgM anti-HDV	IgM anti-HDV	IgG anti-HDV
	IgM anti-HBc	IgG anti-HBc	IgG anti-HBs
HEV	IgM anti-HEV	Not seen	IgG anti-HEV

*This low titre 7S IgM anti-HBc is not detectable by the standard IgM anti-HBc assay which utilizes dilute serum.

positive after 1 month or HBs positive for longer than 6 months will remain HBs antigen positive and will require further management. Monthly monitoring of these proteins is required to differentiate the recovering acute from the chronic infection.

Prevention of secondary spread is important. Sexual and close family contacts should be vaccinated with the recombinant subunit envelope (HBsAg) vaccine. Over 95 per cent of patients will develop protective immunity after three injections spaced over 6 months. A minority, more frequent amongst older people, will not develop antibody, and they will probably remain susceptible to infection.

Hepatitis C virus infection

This flavivirus is parenterally transmitted (Table 1). It is present in blood in low titre, approximately 10^3 to 10^5 virus particles/ml. This concentration is lower than in hepatitis B virus infection (10^7–10^9 particles/ml). The majority of patients develop hepatitis within 14 to 160 days of exposure. The disease is invariably anicteric and can be diagnosed by screening for elevated serum transaminases. Jaundice is rare. The usual prodromal symptoms of fever and malaise may occur at the beginning of the hepatitic phase.

Only 50 per cent of patients recover from this virus infection. The remainder develop persistent viraemia with hepatitis. One in five develops cirrhosis and runs the risk of hepatocellular carcinoma (Fig. 4). The rate of progression of the disease is slow. Sequential studies in Japan have shown that patients pass from acute to chronic persistent hepatitis, to chronic active hepatitis, to cirrhosis, and eventually to hepatocellular carcinoma over 20 to 40 years.

Antibodies to structural and non-structural proteins of the virus (Fig. 5) can be detected at various times after infection. Diagnosis in the acute phase is difficult; antibodies to the nucleocapsid proteins of the virus (anti-c22) are the first to appear but may be delayed for 3 to 6 months (Fig. 6). Antibodies to the non-structural proteins appear even later. Viraemia can be detected by polymerase chain reaction (**PCR**) techniques (see Section 4) as early as 2 weeks after exposure, but this technique is only just becoming available.

Management of the acute hepatitis is symptomatic. Patients with severe symptoms may require bedrest, but the majority need only outpatient follow-up with monitoring of transaminases to identify those going on to develop persistent infection. Sexual transmission may occur and therefore patients should be advised to use barrier contraceptives.

Fig. 4 Clinical course of hepatitis C virus infection.

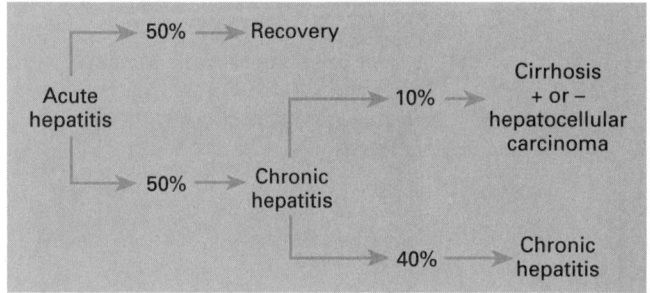

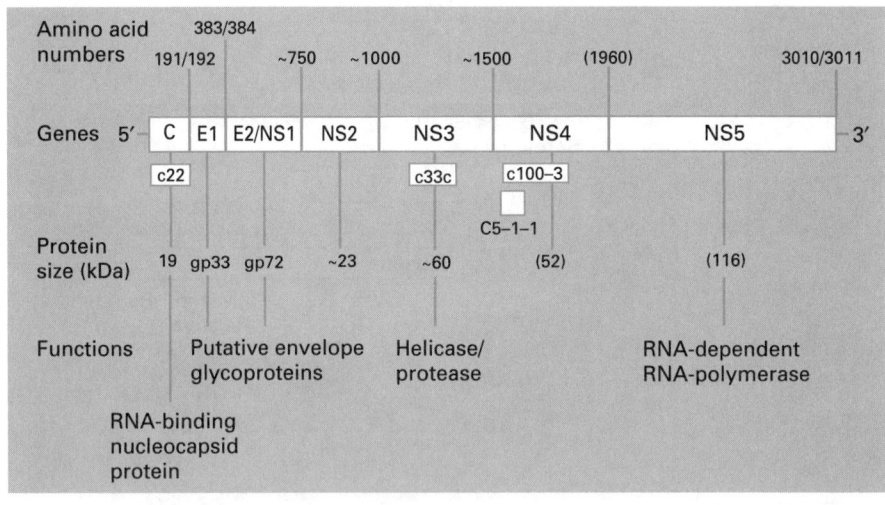

Fig. 5 Map of antigens of hepatitis C virus (HCV): c22–nucleocapsid; C33–NS3; and C100–NS4 proteins are used in the current assays to detect HCV antibodies. NS5 proteins are to be added to the third generation assays.

The frequency of sexual transmission is much lower than with hepatitis B virus infection. Transmission from mother to infant occurs infrequently.

Hepatitis D virus

This virus only replicates in patients already infected with hepatitis B virus. Infection is common amongst hepatitis B carriers in the Mediterranean area. In Northern Europe it is only seen in intravenous drug abusers and haemophiliacs.

The delta virus requires the envelope proteins of hepatitis B virus to produce infectious virions. Infection may occur at the same time as hepatitis B virus, so-called coinfection (Fig. 7(a)). Ninety-five per cent of patients under these circumstances clear both viruses; 5 per cent go on to persistent virus infection with both agents. The latter have a rapidly progressive disease. Hepatitis B virus carriers may be superinfected with hepatitis delta virus (Fig. 7(b)). The majority of them develop persistent delta virus infection and, again, a rapidly progressive course follows.

The management is similar to that of acute hepatitis B. Sexual and family contacts should be immunized with the HBsAg subunit vaccine. Immunization against hepatitis B protects against both B and delta virus coinfection. Hepatitis B carriers cannot be protected against hepatitis D virus superinfection.

Hepatitis E virus

This is an enterically transmitted virus that is common in Africa and Asia. Infection usually follows faecal contamination of drinking water. The incubation period is approximately 20 to 40 days. There is a febrile illness followed by an elevation of transaminases. Intrahepatic cholestasis is reported in approximately one-third of patients. Pregnant women suffer a particularly severe disease, many running a fulminant course. Persistent infection has not been described. The diagnosis involves screening for IgM antibodies to the virus or, if available, immunoelectronmicroscopy. The management is along the lines for hepatitis A. Although no vaccines are currently available, they are being developed.

OTHER VIRUSES

Cytomegalovirus and Epstein–Barr virus infections are commonly seen in immunocompromised individuals. The hepatitis is often anicteric. Their management is considered in Chapters 7.10.4 and 7.10.6.

Chronic viral hepatitis

Chronic hepatitis is defined as hepatic inflammation continuing without improvement for longer than 6 months. Inflammation of the intrahepatic biliary tree is usually excluded from this group of diseases but may occur to a minor degree. The diagnosis is made by liver biopsy. When there is historical evidence of an attack of acute hepatitis, the biopsy should not be undertaken earlier than 6 months after the acute episode. Premature biopsy usually gives an equivocal result: chronic persistent hepatitis cannot usually be differentiated from the changes of resolving acute hepatitis. Early biopsy may be indicated when there is no historical evidence of an acute hepatitis and the duration of the symptoms and signs and the biochemical tests of liver function are consistent with a chronic disease that has already progressed to a severe stage. A prolonged period of lethargy, jaundice, fluid retention, or gastrointestinal bleeding from oesophageal varices would suggest advanced disease. Laboratory data such as a low serum albumin, high gammaglobulin, and a markedly prolonged prothrombin time would support this diagnosis. In these cases, liver biopsy must be undertaken to establish the type and severity of the disease process. In some cases, fresh frozen plasma may be needed to correct the coagulopathy before percutaneous biopsy can be safely undertaken. If this is ineffective, transjugular hepatic biopsy may be tried. Biopsy should be delayed until ascites has been cleared.

Several aetiological factors may initiate chronic hepatitis. These

Fig. 7 Coinfection and superinfection with hepatitis D virus (HDV): (a) coinfection results in the development of IgM antiHBc and IgM antiHDV; (b) superinfection of an hepatitis B virus carrier with HDV results in IgM anti-HDV in the absence of IgM anti-HBc.

Fig. 6 (a) Acute hepatitis C. (b) acute progressing to chronic hepatitis C (50 per cent of cases).

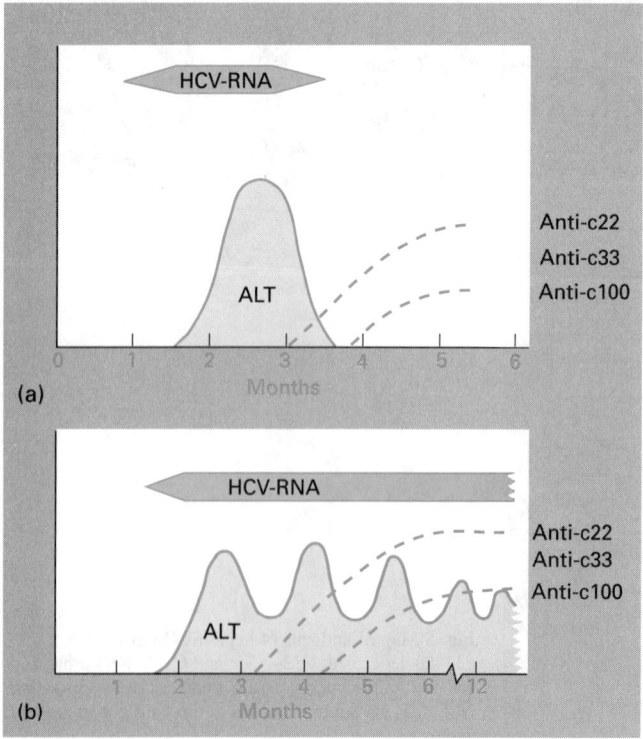

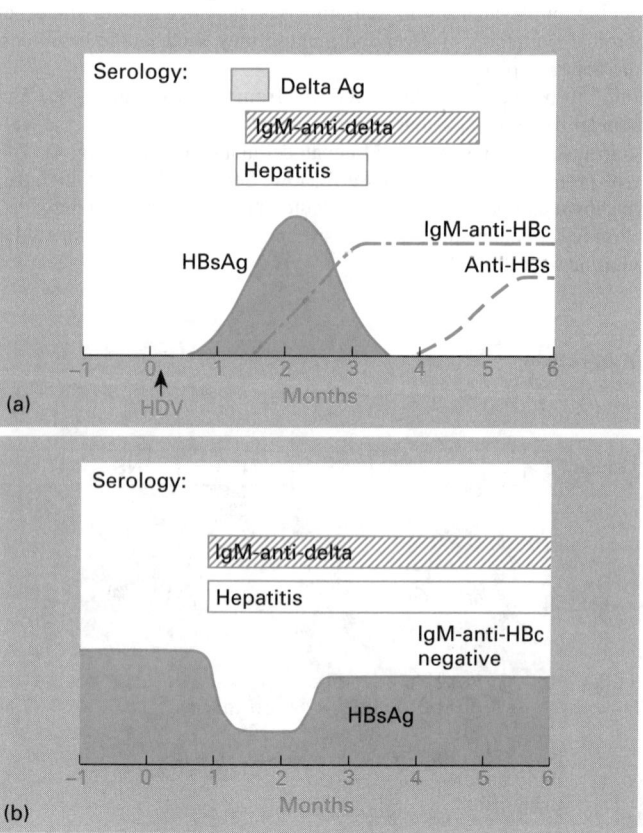

include persistent viral infection (type B and C hepatitis viruses). Other conditions, including a primary defect in the regulation of the immune response (autoimmune), drug-induced hepatitis (oxyphenisatin, methyldopa, isoniazid, and nitrofurantoin), alcohol, and Wilson's disease, should be excluded.

The distribution of the inflammatory infiltrate in the portal tracts and hepatic lobules, established by hepatic biopsy, allows a further classification (Fig. 3), which is justifiable on prognostic grounds. These lesions may be seen with any of the aetiological factors.

CHRONIC PERSISTENT HEPATITIS

Definition

This diagnosis can only be made by liver biopsy. The histological picture is of a mononuclear cell infiltrate of the portal tracts with no spillover into the periportal area (Fig. 3). There may, however, be areas of focal liver-cell necrosis in the lobule, and in these cases the histological picture should be described as chronic persistent hepatitis with a lobular component.

Clinical features

Patients with this condition are asymptomatic, with no physical signs of chronic liver disease. The liver and spleen are not enlarged. The concentrations of aspartate and alanine aminotransferases are increased by approximately two to five times above the upper limit of the normal range. The bilirubin, alkaline phosphatase, serum albumin, globulin, and prothrombin time are always normal.

Some cases present because abnormal aminotransferases are found six or more months after an episode of acute hepatitis. Others come to clinical attention on autoanalyser biochemical screening, and presumably have followed asymptomatic acute hepatitis. Only a few cases are attributable to hepatitis B virus infection and the role of hepatitis C is now being assessed; preliminary data would suggest that many cases of chronic persistent hepatitis are due to this agent.

Prognosis and treatment

The disease has a good prognosis: over the first 5 years there is no increased mortality. The majority of cases do not progress to chronic active hepatitis and cirrhosis. HBs antigen-positive patients who have evidence of active viral replication (HBe antigen positivity) may progress slowly to active hepatitis and cirrhosis over many years. In studies in Taiwan, 50 per cent of asymptomatic HBs antigen-positive patients died of the complications of cirrhosis or hepatocellular carcinoma. These patients may need antiviral therapy (see below). Twenty per cent of patients with chronic hepatitis C progress to cirrhosis and they may also require antiviral therapy.

CHRONIC LOBULAR HEPATITIS

Definition

The histological picture is virtually identical to that of acute lobular hepatitis, chronicity being recognized by careful biochemical follow-up. The hepatic lobule is infiltrated from portal to central areas with chronic inflammatory cells and there are scattered areas of necrosis of hepatocytes (focal necrosis) (Fig. 3).

Clinical features

These patients are usually asymptomatic but some may be icteric with symptoms of general malaise. The course is often fluctuating. A viral aetiology is usual (hepatitis B or C), but in some cases, high titres of smooth muscle and nuclear antibodies suggest an autoimmune aetiology. The biochemical picture is similar to that seen in acute hepatitis. The aspartate and alanine aminotransferases and bilirubin may be markedly elevated. A low serum albumin and prolonged prothrombin time indicate severe disease.

Prognosis and treatment

Hepatitis B virus-induced chronic lobular hepatitis has a variable prognosis. A benign course has been described but others progress rapidly to cirrhosis. Chronic lobular hepatitis due to hepatitis C virus infection may have a more benign course. Patients with high-titre autoantibodies also have a benign prognosis.

Antiviral therapy is a logical approach in some of these patients in whom hepatitis B or C virus infection can be established, but clinical experience with this is inconclusive. In patients with autoantibodies, immunosuppressant therapy has been tried. Its value is difficult to assess because of the fluctuating course of the disease; controlled studies have not been done.

CHRONIC ACTIVE HEPATITIS

Definition

In this disease there is mononuclear and plasma-cell infiltration of the portal and periportal areas of the liver (Fig. 4). The limiting plate, which delineates the portal zone from the periportal area of the hepatic lobule, is breached by the infiltrate and there is 'piecemeal' necrosis of the hepatocytes adjacent to this plate. Groups of hepatocytes ('rosettes') are surrounded by chronic inflammatory cells. When liver cells are destroyed, the reticulin framework may collapse. This may be followed by collagen accumulation and regeneration of hepatocytes, resulting in disorganization of the lobular architecture and the development of a coarse, macronodular cirrhosis. The picture of chronic active hepatitis may be accompanied by varying degrees of chronic lobular hepatitis and occasionally by cholangitic features. When the 'piecemeal' necrosis is severe, bands of necrotic tissue may extend from one portal tract to another or to the central vein (bridging necrosis). This histological picture is usually seen in patients with subacute hepatic necrosis, a term used to describe those who develop fluid retention and encephalopathy between 1 and 2 months after the onset of acute hepatitis.

The histological entity of chronic active hepatitis may be the result of the same pathogenetic processes that cause chronic persistent hepatitis: only the viral causes will be dealt with here.

Hepatitis-B virus-induced chronic active hepatitis

There are probably 300 million people in the world who are chronically infected with hepatitis B virus, the highest prevalence being in tropical Africa, Central and South America, China, Japan, and Indonesia. The virus may produce chronic persistent, lobular, or active hepatitis and, in some studies, up to 50 per cent of patients progress to develop cirrhosis, some developing primary hepatocellular carcinoma. In others there is no significant inflammatory or malignant liver disease (Fig. 3). In a few patients, usually those with mild inflammatory liver disease (chronic persistent hepatitis or inactive cirrhosis), extrahepatic pathology—polyarteritis nodosa or membranoproliferative glomerulonephritis—may be evident. The deposition of viral antigen/antibody complexes, particularly HBe antigen/antibody, may be involved in the pathogenesis of these diseases.

The factors that determine whether an individual suffers an acute or chronic infection are unknown. Various immune defects, genetically determined or acquired, have been described but none of these is of proven pathogenetic significance. The elimination of infected hepatocytes in acute hepatitis B is associated with a CD8, cytolytic T-cell response to peptides derived from various proteins including HBc. In chronically infected patients this cytotoxic response is much reduced or absent. At some stage the viral genome integrates into the hepatocyte DNA but the relation between this event and the duration of persistent infection and malignant transformation is unknown. The virus is not directly cytopathic and the variety of pathological changes exhibited in chronically infected people is related to variation in the ability of the host's immune system to respond to the virus.

The mechanism of liver damage in chronically infected patients is not fully established. There is a cytotoxic T-cell immune response to some viral antigens (HBc) but, as stated earlier, this is weaker than in acute hepatitis B. In addition there is a response to native liver membrane antigens such as liver-specific protein. The relative importance of these cellular responses to viral and hepatocyte membrane antigens in mediating liver-cell damage in chronic hepatitis B is unknown. Humoral responses to these and other antigens are also present and may play a part in viral neutralization or in hepatocytic necrosis. Immune complexes containing viral antigens, particularly HBe antigen, have been demonstrated in the serum and tissues of patients with polyarteritis and glomerulonephritis.

Patients with chronic hepatitis B are initially HBe antigen positive with intense viraemia—concentrations of hepatitis B viral DNA in serum are high (1–300 pg/ml)—and little inflammatory necrosis of infected hepatocytes (Fig. 8). Over months and years the inflammatory liver disease becomes more severe, reflecting destruction of hepatocytes supporting productive viral replication. As a result, the viraemia diminishes and, eventually, HBe antigen is cleared and antibody appears in the serum. During HBe antigen/antibody seroconversion there is usually an exacerbation of the hepatitis and in some cases, if this phase is prolonged, cirrhosis will develop. In many patients the appearance of antiHBe is associated with control of viraemia (the viral DNA can only be detected by PCR) and resolution of the hepatitis. The continued production of HBs antigen in such cases is dependent on the presence of viral DNA integrated into cellular DNA sequences. The HBs antigen-positive patient with antiHBe in the serum and normal transaminases is called the 'normal carrier'.

Patients with chronic hepatitis B who have developed cirrhosis run an increased risk (200-fold) of developing hepatocellular carcinoma many years (7–40) after infection. In a few cases, hepatitis B virus promoters are reportedly inserted into cellular DNA upstream of proto-oncogenes (erb-, c-myc) and cellular genes controlling cell division (cyclin gene)—insertional mutagenesis. In the majority of cases the integration site is distant from such cellular genes and alternative mechanisms such as transactivation of cellular proto-oncogenes by viral proteins, including HBx and truncated HBs, probably contribute to malignant transformation. Approximately half of hepatocellular carcinomas secrete alpha-fetoprotein: screening for elevated serum concentrations of this protein in high-risk patients, together with ultrasonographic scanning, allows the early detection of such tumours, which may then be resected.

In some 'normal carriers', after months or years, viraemia, detectable by dot-blot techniques (see Section 4), reappears but HBe antigen is not secreted by the infected liver cell. This variant of the hepatitis B virus has undergone genetic mutation to generate a novel, translational stop codon in the precore region of the viral genome (Fig. 9), preventing synthesis of the 25-kDa precore/core molecule (p25c) from which HBe antigen (p15–18e) is derived. The appearances of this mutant virus in HBs antigen-, antiHBe-positive carriers is associated with increased hepatitis and progress to cirrhosis. This HBe antigen-negative mutant virus is common in the Mediterranean, Asia, and the Far East, but is uncommon in Northern Europe and North America. This mutant has been associated with fulminant hepatitis B but a causal relation has not been established.

Fig. 8 Clinical course of chronic hepatitis B. Note that the natural history of this chronic infection may arrest at any stage: the patient may remain in the stage of HBe positive viraemia or never enter the stage of HBe negative viraemia. The HBe positive and negative stages of viraemia may run into each other.

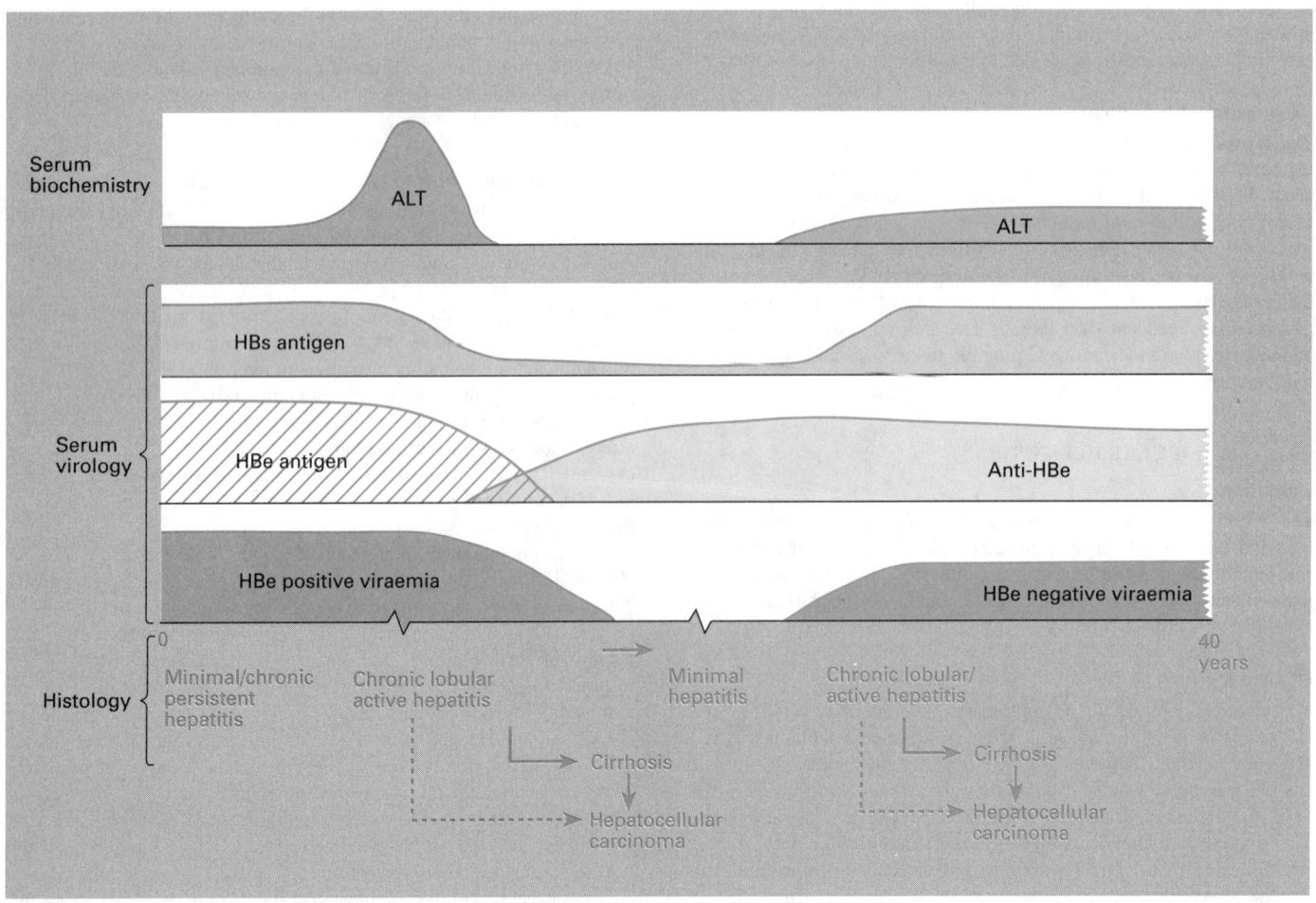

Clinical features

The majority of patients are asymptomatic, coming to medical attention as a result of testing for HBs antigenaemia during blood donation, or on routine screening during hospital admission for unrelated diseases. They usually have chronic persistent hepatitis or are carriers with a histologically normal liver, and more rarely have chronic active hepatitis or cirrhosis. They rarely give a history of acute hepatitis, and presumably have suffered either a subclinical attack or have been infected at birth. Infection during the neonatal period or in early childhood is common in the Tropics and Far East, but probably of lesser importance in Western Europe and North America, where infection probably occurs in the second and third decades of life as a result of sexual contact or drug abuse. When infection occurs at birth, 95 per cent develop chronic disease, whereas infection during childhood or adult life results in chronic carriage in less than 5 per cent.

Some cases follow acute hepatitis. Approximately 95 per cent of adult patients will have cleared the virus and its antigens (HBs) from the blood within 3 months of the clinical onset of the hepatitis (Fig. 2). Others will clear the virus up to 1 year after infection but thereafter spontaneous recovery from infection is rare. The majority of persistently infected patients will develop chronic active hepatitis. During the first years of the chronic infection the virus replicates rapidly and virus particles can be demonstrated in both the liver and blood. At this stage the patient is HBe antigen positive and is highly infectious. At a later stage the rate of replication is lower and the virus cannot be detected in the blood in spite of the continued presence of HBs antigen. These patients are HBe antibody positive and are of much lower infectivity. In some cases, many years after the onset of infection, the HBs antigen may be undetectable in the blood but can be found in the liver. These patients usually produce antibodies to HBc but not to HBs antigen.

Some patients present relatively late in the course of the infection, usually with the complications of cirrhosis, including ascites, bleeding, oesophageal varices, and hepatic failure. These symptoms may indicate the development of hepatocellular carcinoma.

The importance of hepatitis B virus infection as a cause of chronic active liver disease (chronic active hepatitis, with or without cirrhosis) varies considerably in different countries. In the United Kingdom, Western Europe, and North America it accounts for less than 5 per cent of the clinically overt cases. In tropical Africa, India, Japan, and China it is probably the most common cause. It is more common in men.

Management

The initial assessment will require the determination of: (i) the level of viral replication; (ii) the severity and type of inflammatory liver disease; (iii) the degree of fibrosis or cirrhosis.

The level of replication will determine the infectivity of the patient's blood. In general, blood from HBe antigen-positive patients is highly infectious, injection of less than 0.01 ml being sufficient to transmit the disease. These patients may infect their sexual partners by oral or genital contact. Of epidemiological importance is the fact that HBe antigen-positive mothers have a 95 per cent probability of infecting their infants and most of these children develop chronic infections. HBs antigen-positive patients who are HBe antibody positive are of much lower infectivity. Larger volumes of their blood are required to transmit the infection and therefore sexual transmission is uncommon. The infants of HBs antigen-positive, HBe antibody-positive mothers have a less than 5 per cent chance of being infected at birth.

The level of inflammatory activity will influence the prognosis. Those with severe chronic active hepatitis or active cirrhosis have progressive disease and should be offered appropriate therapy (see below). Those with chronic persistent hepatitis and inactive cirrhosis have quiescent disease and should only be treated if they have evidence of active viral replication (HBe antigen positivity) and therefore a high level of potential infectivity.

An assessment of the degree of fibrosis or cirrhosis is an indication of the amount of damage already accrued. It is of prognostic value only.

Treatment of HBe antigen-positive patients

Alpha interferons These have been shown to cause transient inhibition of viral replication and, in 40 per cent of cases, treatment for several (3–6) months has produced permanent inhibition with conversion from HBe antigen to antibody (Fig. 10), followed up to several years later by clearance of HBs antigen. Clearance of HBe antigen is followed by reduced inflammatory activity and histological resolution of the hepatitis. Patients with high concentrations of transaminases and severe chronic active hepatitis on biopsy are most likely to respond, while those with minimal hepatitis have only a 20 per cent chance of seroconversion.

Vidarabine (adenine arabinoside) This drug has been evaluated in controlled trials and shown to be effective in producing an increased rate of conversion from HBe antigen to antibody, a reduction in HBs antigen concentration, and improvement in liver function tests. More recently, adenine arabinoside 5'-monophosphate, a water-soluble derivative of the parent compound, has been shown to be effective when given twice daily by intramuscular injection for 3 to 4 weeks. Neurotoxicity has limited general acceptance of the value of this treatment.

Immunostimulation This has been proposed as an alternative approach. Synthetic (levamisole) and bacterial (BCG) adjuvants have been studied. No beneficial effect has yet been established and these should still be considered experimental procedures. Their aim is to stimulate the host's

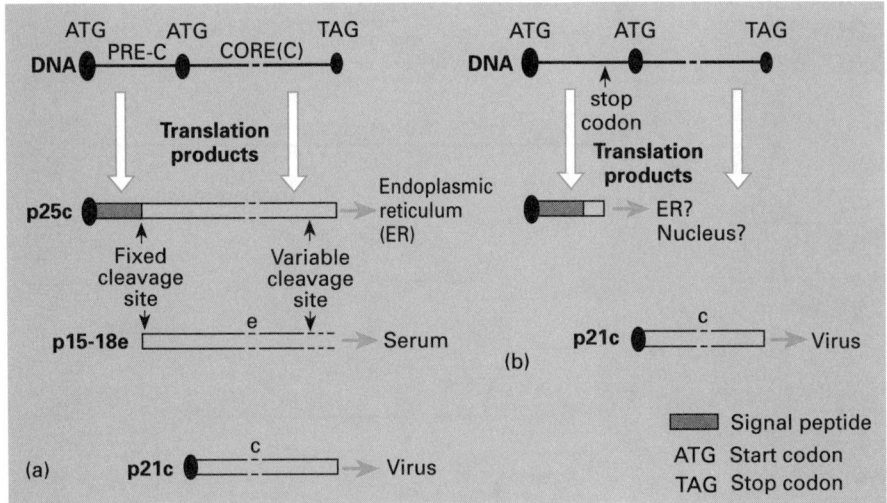

Fig. 9 Translation of nucleocapsid reading frame in (a) HBe antigen-positive (wild type), (b) HBe antigen-negative (precore mutant) viraemia. The latter virus contains an additional stop codon at position 28, preventing translation of the p25c molecule from which HBe is derived.

immune system to facilitate clearance of the virus. Ultimately their use may be in combination with the synthetic antiviral agents.

Immunosuppression This results in increased replication of the virus with no improvement in the level of inflammatory activity in the liver. It is contraindicated in patients with active viral replication. Prednisolone 'priming'—a 4-week course of prednisolone, rapidly withdrawn—followed by interferon-α for 3 months may improve results in patients with minimal hepatitis. 'Rebound hepatitis' may precipitate liver failure in cirrhotic patients near to decompensation and prednisolone priming should not be used in these individuals.

Treatment of antiHBe-positive patients

In these patients continued HBs antigenaemia is usually the result of expression of viral sequences that are integrated into the hepatocyte genome. There is usually no replication of hepatitis B virus and therefore antiviral therapy is not appropriate. In 50 per cent of patients with HBe antigen-negative viraemia and hepatitis, inteferon-α may be valuable in controlling viraemia.

Occasionally, superinfection with the delta virus may have occurred and be responsible for continued liver damage. No effective therapy has been developed, although interferons are being evaluated. Concurrent infection with hepatitis C virus should be excluded, particularly in drug abusers.

Prognosis

The natural history of hepatitis B virus-induced, chronic active hepatitis is variable. In a few cases the disease may progress rapidly to cirrhosis but in most the evolution is slow. In general, progression is fastest during the phase of conversion of HBe antigen to antibody. If this is protracted, cirrhosis may develop (Fig. 8). When the patient converts to HBe antibody, the inflammatory activity subsides. Thus, chronic active hepatitis may become chronic persistent hepatitis and active cirrhosis change to inactive cirrhosis. The rate of conversion from HBe antigenaemia to HBe antibody positivity varies from 5 to 10 per cent per annum in different populations. Antiviral therapy is designed to accelerate the HBe antigen/antibody seroconversion to minimize the degree of liver damage. Emergence of the HBe antigen-negative variant is associated with progression of the liver disease.

Hepatitis C virus-induced chronic hepatitis

Hepatitis C is parenterally transmitted causing a mild (anicteric) acute hepatitis. Fifty per cent of patients develop chronic infection and hepatitis, 20 per cent of whom develop cirrhosis. These patients are at risk of hepatocellular carcinoma.

In Britain, 0.1 to 0.5 per cent of the population are infected with this virus. It is a common cause of chronic liver disease hitherto called cryptogenic hepatitis. Most cases of post-transfusion hepatitis are caused by this virus but in the United Kingdom, sporadic, community-acquired, non-A, non-B hepatitis is not due to this agent. These patients usually recover and do not develop chronic disease. In contrast, in the United States, sporadic hepatitis is usually due to hepatitis C virus infection and chronic hepatitis is rather common. Many of these patients are abusing drugs.

Clinical features

Hepatitis C is a relatively mild, usually asymptomatic illness. The transaminases fluctuate rapidly during the early course of the illness, the peak values becoming gradually lower (Fig. 6(b)). This pattern was prominent in haemophiliac patients infected by hepatitis C virus transmitted by factor VIII concentrates. About 80 per cent of them developed chronic hepatitis, the lesions ranging from chronic persistent to active hepatitis and cirrhosis, and being characterized by the presence of an intense lobular infiltrate of mononuclear cells. These patients had a predominantly short (2- or 4-week) incubation period. Factor VIII concentrates are now rendered safe by heat inactivation.

There are other reports of chronic hepatitis developing after blood transfusion or plasma donation (plasmapheresis). In the majority of these patients the incubation period is 7 to 10 weeks and the hepatic biopsies show predominantly chronic persistent hepatitis with a low incidence of periportal 'piecemeal' necrosis and lobular hepatitis. These differences may be the result of infection with different genotypes of hepatitis C virus (five are currently known) or variation in the size of the viral inoculum.

Fig. 11 Treatment of chronic hepatitis C virus (HCV) infection (usually for 6 to 12 months). The graphs show the pattern of transaminase change. Viraemia can be determined by polymerase chain amplification of HCV-RNA from serum. Patients with a complete response clear HCV-RNA from their serum: this response is seen in 20 per cent of patients treated.

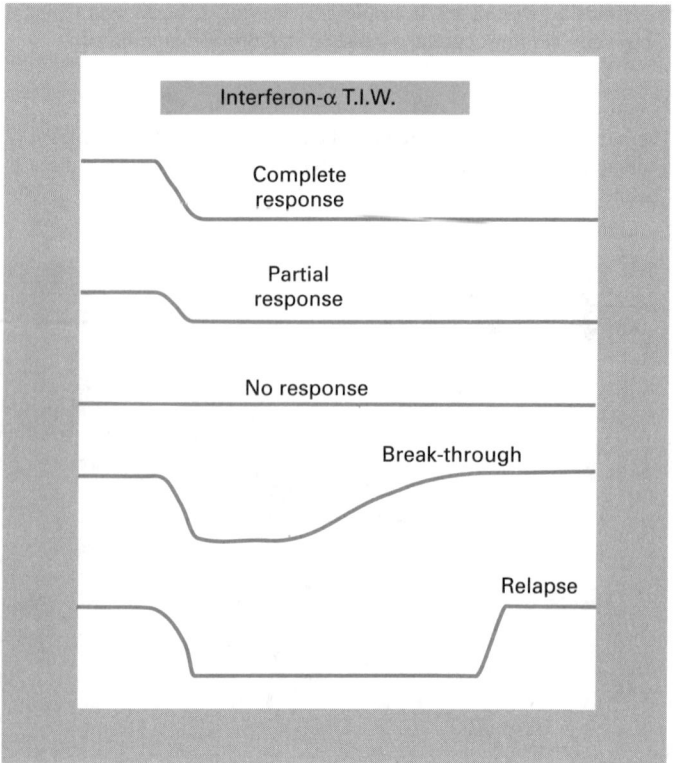

Fig. 10 Treatment of chronic HBe antigen-positive hepatitis with interferon-α. Note that HBe antigen/antibody seroconversion is preceded by exacerbation and is followed by resolution of the hepatitis. Clearance of HBs antigen is often delayed for five or more years.

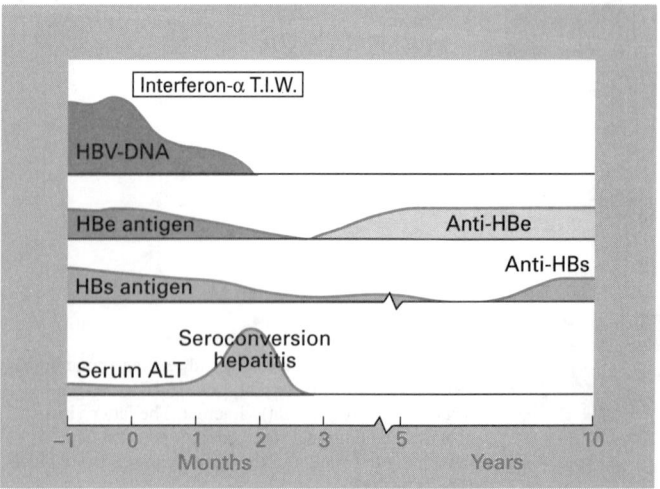

The immunological features of this form of chronic hepatitis are more similar to hepatitis B virus-induced disease than to the autoimmune type. Concentrations of serum immunoglobulins are normal until the stage of advanced cirrhosis when IgG concentrations increase. Smooth muscle and nuclear antibodies may be found in patients with chronic active hepatitis or cirrhosis, but the titres are much lower than in autoimmune chronic active hepatitis and cirrhosis.

Management and prognosis

The rate of progression of the disease is variable. In 20 per cent of cases, cirrhosis develops in 5 to 10 years but in the majority the prognosis is good. In some series there has been a tendency for the inflammatory process to subside over several years, and in others progression is very slow.

Interferon-α (3–5 megaunits thrice weekly for 6–12 months) has normalized transaminases in 50 to 85 per cent of cases but relapse is common (60 per cent) (Fig. 11). Long-term control is seen in about 10 to 20 per cent of treated patients. Longer periods of therapy are being studied.

Tribavirin (Ribavirin) has some beneficial effect but its role is not yet defined. Combination therapy is being evaluated.

REFERENCES

Carman, W.F. and Thomas, H.C. (1992). Genetic variation in hepatitis B virus. *Gastroenterology*, **102**, 711–19.

Garem, D. and Varmus, H.E. (1987). The molecular biology of the hepatitis viruses. *Annual Review of Biochemistry*, **56**, 651–93.

Houghton, M., Weiner, A., Han, J., Kuo, G., and Choo, Q.L. (1991). Molecular biology of hepatitis C viruses: implications for diagnosis, development and control of viral disease. *Hepatology*, **14**, 381–8.

Jacyna, M. and Thomas, H.C. (1990). Antiviral therapy: hepatitis B. *British Medical Bulletin*, **46**, 368–82.

Lau, J.Y.N. and Wright, T.L. (1993). Molecular virology and pathogenesis of hepatitis B. *Lancet*, **342**, 1335–1340.

Lemon, S. (1992). Hepatitis A virus; current concepts of the molecular virology, immunobiology and approaches to vaccine development. *Reviews in Medical Virology*, **2**, 73–87.

Monjardino, J. and Saldanha, J. (1990). Delta hepatitis: the disease and the virus. *British Medical Bulletin*, **46**, 309–407.

Okuda, K. (1992). Hepatocellular carcinoma; recent progress. *Hepatology*, **15**, 948–63.

Tam, A.W. *et al.* (1991). Hepatitis E virus (HEV): molecular cloning and sequencing of the full-length viral genome. *Virology*, **185**, 120–31.

Tsarev, S.A. *et al.* (1992). Characterisation of a prototype strain of hepatitis E virus. *Proceedings of the National Academy of Sciences (USA)*, **89**, 559–63.

14.27 Autoimmune liver disease

14.27.1 Autoimmune hepatitis

P. J. JOHNSON and A. L. W. F. EDDLESTON

DEFINITION

Chronic hepatitis in young women with extreme hyperglobulinaemia was first described in detail by Waldenström and Kunkel in the early 1950s. The detection of the lupus erythematosus (**LE**) cell and the presence of antinuclear antibodies in a subset of these patients led to the introduction of the term 'lupoid hepatitis'. However, the disease is clearly different from systemic lupus erythematosus, particularly in the occurrence of serious glomerulonephritis, which is rare in autoimmune liver disease. The term 'autoimmune' chronic active hepatitis has been the most widely used label, but as the disease may become inactive for long periods during treatment-induced or spontaneous remission, an international expert group meeting in 1992 recommended adopting the name autoimmune hepatitis for this subgroup of patients with chronic active hepatitis, and it is likely that this will be widely accepted.

Chronic active hepatitis is characterized histologically by piecemeal necrosis of periportal hepatocytes with prominent plasma-cell infiltration of the portal tracts (Plate 1) and persistence of symptoms or signs for more than 6 months. It is now recognized as aetiologically heterogeneous. Hepatitis viruses B, δ (D), or C are the most clearly defined causative agents but chronic active hepatitis is also a recognized feature of other primary liver diseases and may arise as an adverse reaction to certain therapeutic drugs (Table 1). A diagnosis of autoimmune hepatitis implies that all other known aetiological factors have been excluded and that immunological features, particularly high titres of certain non-organ-specific autoantibodies and polyclonal hyperglobulinaemia, are prominent. A scoring system that is of help in providing an objective assessment has been devised (Table 2).

The different types of autoimmune hepatitis

Type-1 autoimmune hepatitis

This form, previously called 'classical' autoimmune chronic active hepatitis, corresponds most closely with the early description of 'lupoid' hepatitis. The patient is typically a young woman, who presents with either an acute hepatitic or a chronic, rumbling illness characterized by lethargy, arthralgia, oligomenorrhoea, fluctuating jaundice, and a cushingoid appearance with striae, hirsutism, and acne. Particularly in those with a more protracted onset of symptoms, cutaneous manifestations of chronic liver disease and signs of cirrhosis may be prominent. Other 'autoimmune' diseases such as hyperthyroidism and Coombs' positive haemolytic anaemia may also be present. There may be cirrhosis at first presentation, or it may develop during the course of the disease.

Characteristically, corticosteroids in moderate doses lead to a prompt disappearance of symptoms and 'normalization' of liver biochemistry but the disease often relapses rapidly when treatment is stopped. This 'classical' form appears to be getting less common, or at least to form a smaller proportion of the range of autoimmune hepatitis. Only a minority of patients, perhaps 10 to 15 per cent have LE cells, and such patients have no distinctive clinical or histological features and do not fall within the range of systemic lupus erythematosus.

DIAGNOSIS AND LABORATORY INVESTIGATIONS

The diagnosis cannot be established without liver biopsy for histological examination. However, when the prothrombin time is prolonged and cannot be corrected, it may be necessary to institute immunosuppressive treatment before biopsy or to use the transjugular approach to obtain liver for histological examination. Treatment usually returns the coagulation profile towards normal quite quickly, while the histological features of chronic active hepatitis persist for some weeks, allowing confirmation of the diagnosis to be obtained by liver biopsy.

Table 1 *Causes of, and diseases associated with, chronic active hepatitis*

| Autoimmune hepatitis: |
| Type 1—with ANA/SMA antibodies |
| Type 2—with LKM antibodies |
| Chronic hepatitis virus infection: |
| Hepatitis B virus |
| Delta virus |
| Hepatitis C virus |
| Other non-A, non-B, non-C viruses |
| Wilson's disease |
| Alcoholic liver disease |
| α_1-Antitrypsin deficiency |
| Drugs:[1] |
| α-methyldopa |
| -Oxyphenisitin |
| -Nitrofurantoin |
| -Isoniazid |
| -Tienilic acid |
| Cryptogenic[2] |

[1]Reactions associated with therapeutic drugs closely resemble, and are sometimes categorized with, the autoimmune types.

[2]The distinction between autoimmune and cryptogenic types is not always made (see text).

ANA, antinuclear antibody; LKM, liver/kidney microsomal (auto-) antibody; SMA, smooth-muscle antibody.

Laboratory investigations reveal hepatitic features. In younger patients, who tend to have more active disease at presentation, serum aspartate aminotransferase levels are often more than 10 times greater than the upper limit of the reference range and the gammaglobulin concentration is grossly raised, often in the range 50 to 100 g/l. The gammaglobulin is polyclonal and largely accounted for by IgG. Antinuclear antibodies are found in the serum of about 70 per cent of patients, many of whom, together with the remaining 30 per cent, have smooth-muscle autoantibodies. Antimitochondrial antibodies are detectable in about 15 per cent.

With the widespread availability of autoanalysers for 'liver function tests', many patients are being diagnosed before they develop symptoms. In a study of 47 asymptomatic patients with chronic elevations of aspartate aminotransferase, 34 had histological features of chronic active hepatitis and 18 of these were ultimately classified as autoimmune. Ten had already reached the stage of cirrhosis, implying prolonged chronicity. This is in agreement with the common finding that symptomatic patients are often cirrhotic at presentation.

It is now recognized that there is an older age group of patients with a disease that broadly conforms to autoimmune hepatitis but which also affects males, although females still predominate (4 : 1). The most common presenting symptoms are profound lethargy, epigastric pain, and fluctuating (often mild) jaundice. Antinuclear, antismooth-muscle, and antimitochondrial antibodies are found as frequently as in the younger age group, but the hyperglobulinaemia tends to be less marked and there may be only mild to moderate elevation of serum aminotransferases.

Non-organ-specific autoantibodies
Antinuclear antibodies are a useful diagnostic marker for autoimmune hepatitis but are also found in other liver disorders. They give a 'homogeneous' pattern of immunofluorescent staining on tissue sections, similar to that seen with antinuclear antibodies in patients with systemic lupus erythematasus; in both conditions they are usually associated with serum autoantibodies against double-stranded DNA (**dsDNA**). They react with a different antigen from that recognized by anti-dsDNA in

systemic lupus. High titres (in excess of 1 : 80) of IgG class smooth-muscle autoantibodies with anti-actin specificity are particularly associated with autoimmune hepatitis.

Liver-specific autoantibodies
Antiliver-specific lipoprotein represents a population of autoantibodies, some of which react with non-organ-specific liver-cell determinants and others with liver-specific components. One of the latter is the galactose-specific hepatic asialoglycoprotein receptor (**ASGP-R**) and autoantibodies (antiASGP-R) against this hepatocyte-specific component, which is preferentially expressed on the surfaces of periportal liver cells, can be measured separately. Antiliver-specific lipoprotein is found in serum in a number of chronic liver disorders, primarily those with an underlying immunopathology and in which periportal inflammation is a feature, but is rare in chronic non-A, non-B hepatitis. AntiASGP-R is more specific for chronic active hepatitis but is found in lower titre than antiliver-specific lipoprotein.

Type-2 autoimmune hepatitis

The presence of circulating antiliver/kidney microsomal antibodies (anti-LKM-1) has been used to define a separate subgroup of autoimmune hepatitis 'type 2'. In the United Kingdom these cases appear less frequently than antinuclear/smooth-muscle antibody-positive autoimmune hepatitis and have been described most often in continental Europe. Whilst the disease conforms in many respects to type-1 autoimmune hepatitis, certain distinctive features are apparent. It tends to present predominantly in childhood and is more often associated with other 'autoimmune' disorders such as insulin-dependent diabetes, autoimmune thyroid disease, and vitiligo. The presentation is more often acute, even fulminant, with severe histological features and a marked propensity to progress rapidly to cirrhosis. The anti-LKM autoantibodies comprise a group of at least three distinct antibodies. Anti-LKM-1 reacts with cytochrome P450db_1 (now termed P450 IID6), while anti-LKM-2 (associated with tienilic acid-induced hepatitis) reacts with cytochrome P450-8, and anti-LKM-3 (found in chronic δ-virus infections) recognizes a third microsomal antigen glucuronyl transferase.

Patients without antinuclear smooth-muscle or LKM antibodies

Some patients with 'cryptogenic' chronic active hepatitis (i.e. no aetiological factors and seronegative for antinuclear smooth-muscle and LKM autoantibodies) are, in all respects other than their autoantibody status, similar to those classified as 'autoimmune'. Such patients may either never have had autoantibodies or lost them during a prolonged asymptomatic phase. Most respond well to immunosuppressive therapy.

Differential diagnosis

All the factors listed in Table 1 need to be excluded. This involves serological screening for hepatitis viruses B, C and D, and a careful drug and alcohol history. It is very important to rule out Wilson's disease in any young person presenting with features characteristic of chronic active hepatitis (see Chapter 14.22). This should include, at a minimum, estimation of serum caeruloplasmin, serum copper, and examination of the eyes for Kayser–Fleischer rings. The serum concentration of α_1-antitrypsin should also be measured together with the phenotype if available (see Chapter 11.15).

OVERLAP WITH OTHER CONDITIONS

The distinction between autoimmune hepatitis and primary biliary cirrhosis is not always clear-cut and histological, clinical, and immunological overlap has been well described. Many children with florid, anti-

Table 2 *Scoring system for diagnosis of autoimmune hepatitis*

Required measures		
Gender		
Females		+ 2
Males		0
Serum biochemistry		
Ratio of elevation of serum alkaline	> 3.0	− 2
phosphatase vs. aminotransferase	< 3.0	+ 2
Total serum globulin **or** gammaglobulin **or** IgG		
Times upper normal limit:		
> 2.0		+ 3
1.5–2.0		+ 2
1.0–1.5		+ 1
< 1.0		0
Autoantibodies (titres by IF on rodent tissues)		
Adults		
ANA, SMA, or LKM-1:		
> 1 : 80		+ 3
1 : 80		+ 2
1 : 40		+ 1
< 1 : 40		0
Children		
ANA, or LKM-1:		
> 1 : 20		+ 3
1 : 10 or 1 : 20		+ 2
< 1 : 10		0
or SMA:		
> 1 : 20		+ 3
1 : 20		+ 2
< 1 : 20		0
Antimitochondrial antibody		
Positive		− 2
Negative		0
Viral markers		
IgM anti-HAV, or HBsAg, or IgM anti-HBc positive		− 3
Anti-HCV positive by ELISA and/or RIBA		− 2
or positive by PCR for HCV-RNA		− 3
Positive test indicating active infection with any		
other virus		− 3
Seronegative for all of the above		+ 3
Other aetiological factors		
History of recent hepatotoxic drug usage	Yes	− 2
or parenteral exposure to blood products	No	+ 1

Required measures (cont.)			
Alcohol (average consumption)			
Males: < 35g/day	Females: < 25g/day		+ 2
35–50 g/day	25–40 g/day		0
50–80 g/day	40–60 g/day		− 2
> 80 g/day	> 60 g/day		− 1
Genetic factors			
Other autoimmune diseases in patient or first-degree			
relatives			+ 1

Additional measures	
Histology	
Chronic active hepatitis with piecemeal necrosis:	
(a) with lobular involvement and bridging necrosis	+ 3
(b) without lobular involvement and bridging necrosis	+ 2
Rosetting of liver cells	+ 1
Marked/predominantly plasma cell infiltrate	+ 1
Biliary changes	− 1
Any other change(s), e.g. granulomas, siderosis, copper	
deposits, etc., suggestive of a different aetiology	− 3
Autoantibodies	
In patients who are seronegative for ANA, SMA, and	
LKM-1	
Any defined 'liver autoantibody' (e.g. anti-SLA,	
-ASGP-R,	
-LSP, -LC1, -LP, -HHPM, -sulphatide, etc.):	
Positive	+ 2
Negative	0
Genetic factors	
HLA-B8,-DR3 haplotype, or -DR4 allotype	+ 1
Response to therapy	
Complete response	+ 2
Partial response	0
Treatment failure	0
No response (in terms of disease activity)	− 2
Relapse during or after treatment withdrawal	
following 'complete' initial response	+ 3

Interpretation of aggregate scores:

Before treatment	After treatment	
> 15	> 17	= 'definite' AIH
10–15	12–17	= 'probable' AIH

Abbreviations: AIH, autoimmune hepatitis; ANA, antinuclear antibody; ASGP-R, asialoglycoprotein receptor; ELISA, enzyme-linked immunosorbent assay; HAV, hepatitis A virus; HBs Ag, hepatitis B surface antigen; HBc, hepatitis B core antigen; HCV, hepatitis C virus; HHPM, human hepatocyte plasma membranes; IF, indirect fluorescence; LC1, liver cytoplasmic antibody 1; LKM, liver/kidney microsomal; LP, lipoprotein; LSP, liver-specific lipoprotein; PCR, polymerase chain reaction; RIBA, recombinant immunoblot assay; SLA, soluble liver antigen; SMA, smooth-muscle antibody.

actin positive, autoimmune hepatitis ultimately progress to primary sclerosing cholangitis and the same progression has also been noted in some young adults. Patients with well-documented Wilson's disease may develop very high titres of smooth-muscle and antinuclear antibodies. The development of autoantibodies in patients with hepatitis C treated with interferon has recently been reported, suggesting that these were people with autoantibody-negative autoimmune hepatitis whose disease was unmasked by this immunomodulatory therapy.

Aetiology

The most reasonable hypothesis is that autoimmune hepatitis arises in a genetically susceptible host who, by chance, encounters an appropriate environmental trigger. In common with a number of other autoimmune conditions, autoimmune hepatitis is strongly associated with the *HLA-A1,-B8,-DR3* haplotype and recent evidence suggests a secondary association with DR4 and a protective role for DR1. As *DR3/DR4* heterozygotes are no more common in this condition than would be expected by chance it would appear that the *HLA-A1,-B8,-DR3* haplotype and DR4 are acting independently of each other and may identify two distinct subgroups of the disease. In support of this contention, those with DR4 tend to present at an older age than those without and relapse on treatment less frequently. In Japan, where DR3 is very rare in the population, the association is almost entirely with DR4, and it is of considerable interest that the patients there belong almost exclusively to the older age group.

Although hepatotropic viruses have always been assumed to be the most likely environmental triggers, no trigger can be detected in most cases. Instances of the development of autoimmune hepatitis following infection with hepatitis A have now been described in patients with disturbed immunoregulation. In others, hepatitis C has been implicated (see below). Autoimmune hepatitis may follow the ingestion of certain therapeutic drugs, notably oxyphenisatin and methyldopa. Tienilic acid (ticrynafen) may induce a specific antiLKM antibody that is associated with chronic hepatitis in up to 10 per cent of cases.

MECHANISM OF HEPATOCYTE DAMAGE

A specific target antigen for both humoral and cellular immune reactions is the asialoglycoprotein receptor (**ASGP-R**), which, in contrast to targets of the other autoantibodies so far described, is expressed on the membrane of periportal hepatocytes and as such provides an explanation for the focus of the disease in the liver. More than 90 per cent of patients with active disease will have high titres of circulating autoantibodies reacting with ASGP-R and most will also have T cells sensitized to ASGP-R both in the peripheral blood and liver. These antigen-specific T cells are predominantly of the CD4 (helper/inducer) subset, as are the T-cell clones isolated from the liver of patients with autoimmune hepatitis.

The mechanism of tissue damage may be by T-cell-mediated immune responses to the ASGP-R either directly or through antibody-dependent cellular cytotoxicity in which ASGP-R antibodies bound to the surface of periportal hepatocytes sensitize these cells to attack by cytotoxic non-T (K) cells carrying Fc receptors. In common with other autoimmune diseases there appears to be a non-antigen-specific defect in immunoregulation, linked to the *HLA-A1,-B8,-DR3* haplotype, which can be reversed *in vivo* and *in vitro* by corticosteroid therapy.

THE ROLE OF HEPATITIS C

When a test for antibodies to the hepatitis C virus (**HCV**) became available towards the end of 1989 there were reports that nearly half of patients categorized as having type-1 autoimmune hepatitis also tested positive for anti-HCV. An even higher percentage of those with type 2 (anti-LKM positive) were anti-HCV positive. In fact, many of these proved to be 'false positive' results in patients with hypergammaglobulinemia, and the application of more specific, second-generation, anti-HCV tests revealed only very weakly positive results in less than 10 per cent of British and North American cases of autoimmune hepatitis. However, when the same specific tests were applied to patients from Italy, a high percentage remained strongly positive, particularly among those with type-2 disease. Further studies in Germany and France have shown clear-cut differences between the two groups of LKM-1-positive patients. Those with chronic HCV infection tend to be older, have less active disease, and have lower titres of LKM-1 antibodies (Table 3).

The implications of these findings for treatment remain unclear, particularly in those with type-1 autoimmune hepatitis. In general the choice of treatment for an anti-HCV-positive patient who otherwise fulfils the criteria for the diagnosis of autoimmune hepatitis is between corticosteroids and interferon-α. Interferon is an immunostimulant and can lead to exacerbations if given to patients with autoimmune hepatitis, while it is also an antiviral that can substantially reduce serum aminotransferases in more than half the patients with chronic HCV infection. On the other hand, corticosteroids are the mainstay of treatment for

Table 3 *Hetereogeneity in type-2 autoimmune hepatitis according to anti-HCV (hepatitis C virus) status in serum*

	Anti-HCV + ve	Anti-HCV− ve
Mean age (years)	50 ± 16	13 ± 11
Males (%)	34	7
Serum transaminases	Moderate	High
Histological activity	Moderate	Severe
LKM titre > 1 : 1000(%)	17	61

LKM, liver/kidney microsomal (autoantibody).

autoimmune hepatitis (see below) and will also reduce aminotransferases in patients with HCV infection, but only at high doses. In practice, most specialist units will begin treatment in truly doubtful cases with prednisolone, and if serum transaminases are not controlled by the usual low maintainance doses, then interferon-α is given cautiously. In the general hospital it would be wise to seek specialist advice before starting treatment.

Natural history of autoimmune hepatitis

Early studies emphasized the serious, invariably fatal, nature of the disease and the prognosis was also grave among patients in the untreated arm of three controlled clinical trials of immunosuppressive therapy reported in the 1970s. In the Royal Free Hospital trial, 62 per cent were dead within a mean follow-up period of 4 years and in the Mayo Clinic trial the survival figure was only 50 per cent at 2 years. As already noted, patients with very mild disease are being detected more frequently nowadays and whilst those with severe disease still have a poor outlook without treatment, the prognosis of the whole group is probably not as poor as initially reported.

In the absence of cirrhosis, piecemeal necrosis, the hallmark of the disease, appears to be a relatively benign feature that seldom progresses to cirrhosis. By contrast that group in whom both piecemeal and bridging necrosis is present frequently progresses to cirrhosis. Many workers consider that, as piecemeal necrosis on its own is a relatively benign lesion, treatment should be confined to those with bridging necrosis and/or cirrhosis. There is also a widespread feeling that those patients in trials showing efficacy of corticosteroid therapy were a highly selected group with advanced and severe disease seen at referral centres. On the other hand, in view of the fluctuating nature of the illness and the possibility that it may at any time become more severe, early intervention with corticosteroid therapy would seem sensible and may account, in part, for the improvement in survival seen since the early 1970s. The extent to which corticosteroid therapy can reduce symptoms, irrespective of any prolongation of survival, should also not be underestimated.

Treatment

If the patient is symptomatic, has histological evidence of bridging necrosis, an aminotransferase activity of greater than 10 times the upper limit of reference, or is jaundiced, then immunosuppressive therapy is clearly indicated. Under these circumstances, prompt resolution of symptoms and improvement of histological features may be anticipated and there is good evidence that survival is markedly prolonged. On the other hand, if the patient is asymptomatic, with no histological evidence of bridging necrosis and only mildly abnormal 'liver function tests', the decision whether or not to use immunosuppressive treatment is more difficult. Our current policy, on the basis of the arguments outlined above, is to treat both groups of patients similarly, whilst awaiting the results of clinical trials that address the problem of optimal management of mild disease.

The standard approach is to induce remission with prednisolone, 0.5 mg/kg body weight. Higher doses are very seldom required. When the aminotransferase level has fallen to less than twice the upper limit of the reference range (usually after 2 to 8 weeks), the dose of prednisolone is decreased to 0.25 mg/kg and azathioprine 1 mg/kg is added. Azathioprine is used as a 'steroid sparing' agent, but takes 3 to 6 months to be fully effective; it has no role in induction of remission. The aim should be to maintain the aminotransferase levels within the reference range; once this has been achieved (5 to 10 mg prednisolone and 50 to 75 mg azathioprine is a typical regimen) the dosages should be kept constant for a minimum of 2 years and not further titrated. Measurement of aminotransferase activity is not an infallible method of assessing disease activity and a liver biopsy should be done after biochemical remission has been obtained to confirm histological remission.

Even after 2 years of remission, attempts to withdraw corticosteroid therapy are often unsuccessful. The resulting relapse can be dangerous if liver function is not monitored very closely and treatment reinstituted before symptoms recur. Recently it has been demonstrated that it is usually possible to withdraw the corticosteroid component, after prolonged remission, if the dose of azathioprine is increased from 1 mg/kg to 2 mg/kg per day. This approach is particularly useful in those patients in whom corticosteroid side-effects are prominent. Frequent measurement of platelet and white-cell counts are important when the high dose of azathioprine is used, particularly over the first 6 months.

After many years the disease does enter a 'burnt-out' phase when all treatment can be withdrawn, but patients should still be checked at least at yearly intervals, as relapses can occur at any time over the next 10 years.

Fig. 1 Survival of patients with chronic active hepatitis in relation to (a) presence or absence of cirrhosis at presentation and (b) aetiology. The poor survival of those with 'cryptogenic disease' is accounted for by their high frequency of cirrhosis.

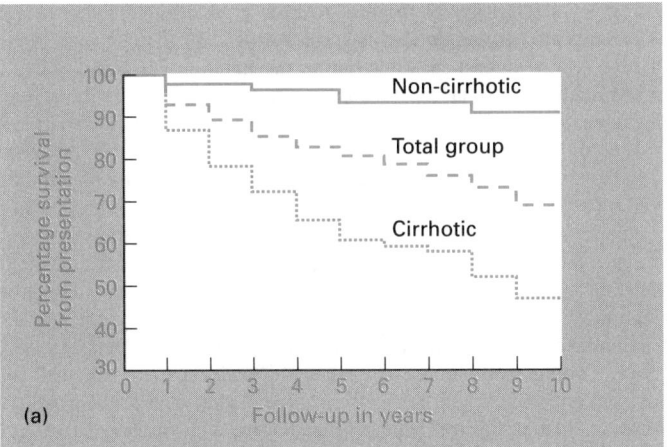

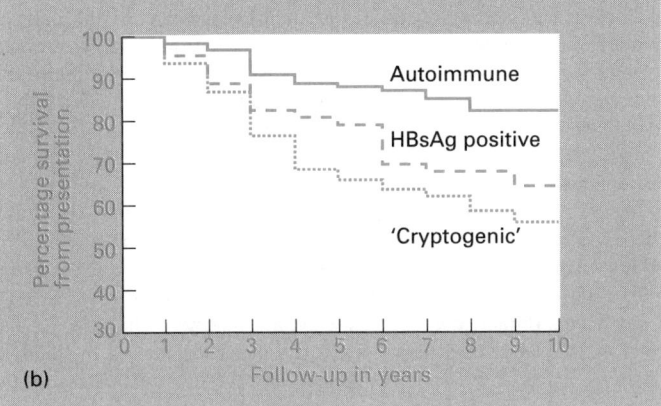

STEROID INSENSITIVITY

About 10 per cent of patients will never achieve a remission with corticosteroids and a smaller percentage will become unresponsive after an initial response. Occasionally, remission can be induced by high-dose corticosteroid therapy (prednisolone, 1 mg/kg per day) but more often there is progressive liver failure and early referral to a liver transplant unit is indicated.

SPECIAL CONSIDERATIONS

When the presentation is with liver failure (deep jaundice, ascites, variceal haemorrhage), fulminant (encephalopathy), or if the liver is very small, a trial of immunosuppressive therapy may still be indicated, but the outcome depends on the underlying liver function more than control of disease activity. The risk of fulminating septicaemia and rapid deterioration is high and such trials should only be undertaken in units with experience in managing liver failure and preferably with facilities for liver transplantation.

PROGNOSIS AND SURVIVAL

In a large retrospective analysis of our own experience, in whom all patients received immunosuppressive therapy, the 5-year survival in autoimmune hepatitis was 85 per cent and in cryptogenic chronic active hepatitis, 65 per cent. This difference is accounted for by the significantly higher frequency of cirrhosis in the cryptogenic group at presentation (Fig. 1). Patients with LKM antibody-positive disease are reported to have a worse prognosis, with a 10-year survival of about 75 per cent, but, allowing for the high frequency of cirrhosis in this group, the figure is very similar to that in autoimmune hepatitis.

CAUSES OF DEATH

Other than incidental, non-hepatic causes, death is now largely a consequence of cirrhosis. In the small group of steroid-resistant cases, and the few who present acutely with fulminating disease, death may be due to acute hepatic failure and its complications—although liver transplantation is increasingly becoming a life-saving option in these cases. In the vast majority, hepatocellular failure secondary to cirrhosis is the major cause of death, followed by variceal haemorrhage, septic complications, and hepatocellular carcinoma.

REFERENCES

Cooksley, W.G.E. *et al.* (1986). The prognosis of chronic active hepatitis without cirrhosis in relation to bridging necrosis. *Hepatology*, **6**, 345–8.

Donaldson, P.T. *et al.* (1991). Susceptibility to autoimmune chronic active hepatitis: human leucocyte antigens DR4 and A1-B8-DR3 are independent risk factors. *Hepatology*, **13**, 701–6.

Homberg, J-C. *et al.* (1987). Chronic active hepatitis associated with anti liver/kidney microsome antibody type 1: a second type of 'autoimmune' hepatitis. *Hepatology*, **7**, 1333–9.

Johnson, P.J. and McFarlane, I.G. (1993). Meeting Report. International Autoimmune Hepatitis Group. *Hepatology*, (in press).

Johnson, P.J., McFarlane, I.G., and Eddleston, A.L.W.F. (1991). Natural course and heterogeneity in autoimmune type chronic active hepatitis. *Seminars in Liver Disease*, **11**, 000–000.

McFarlane, B.M. *et al.* (1986). Serum autoantibodies reacting with the hepatic asialoglycoprotein receptor (hepatic lectin) in acute and chronic liver disorders. *Journal of Hepatology*, **3**, 196–205.

McFarlane, I.G. *et al.* (1990). Hepatitis C virus antibodies in chronic active hepatitis: pathogenetic factor or false-positive result? *Lancet*, **335**, 754–7.

Murray-Lyon, I.M., Stern, R.B., and Williams, R. (1973). Controlled trial of prednisolone and azathioprine in active chronic hepatitis. *Lancet*, **i**, 735–7.

Soloway, R.D. *et al.* (1972). Clinical biochemical and histological remission in severe chronic active liver disease: a controlled study of treatments and early prognosis. *Gastroenterology*, **63**, 820–33.

14.27.2 Primary biliary cirrhosis

M. F. BASSENDINE

Primary biliary cirrhosis is a chronic, cholestatic, inflammatory liver disease most commonly seen in middle-aged women. The cause is unknown but increasing evidence suggests that autoimmune phenomena are in some way involved, in particular the strong association with auto-antibodies reacting predominantly against mitochondria but, also in a minority of cases, against nuclear factors. The disease has an insidious onset and patients with early disease are usually only recognized following the incidental discovery of antimitochondrial antibodies or elevated levels of serum alkaline phosphatase during screening for other disease. Progression is slow but eventually many patients develop cirrhosis and, ultimately, death may occur from liver failure or complications of cirrhosis such as bleeding oesophageal varices. Primary biliary cirrhosis was previously considered to be rare and account for fewer than 5 per cent of patients dying of cirrhosis in Western communities, but recognition of cases earlier in the evolution of this chronic disease has allowed a more accurate estimate of its incidence to be made. In Britain its prevalence is between 90 and 150/1 000 000 (276/1 000 000 in women over 18 years) and in Europe it is now the most common indication for liver transplantation.

AETIOLOGY AND PATHOGENESIS

Genetic factors may be important. Familial clustering is well documented, the disease having been reported in siblings, twins, parents, and cousins. A high familial incidence of autoantibodies, including antimitochondrial antibodies, has been noted. There is no association of the disorder with major histocompatibility complex (**MHC**) class I antigens but several associations with class II antigens have been reported, in particular HLA-DR8. Earlier serological and recent DNA studies have independently shown a two- to sixfold increase in HLA-DR8 in patients compared to controls. Data on MHC class III associations are conflicting.

The presence of antibodies reacting against mitochondria in the serum of over 90 per cent of patients with primary biliary cirrhosis may provide a clue to aetiology. It is now known that the major disease-specific antigens reacting with these autoantibodies are components of the 2-oxo-acid dehydrogenase multienzyme complexes located in mammalian mitochondria (Table 1). The main immunodominant autoimmunizing B-cell epitope has been localized to the lipoyl domains of the dihydrolipoamide acyltransferase (E2) components of these complexes. Of possible relevance to pathogenesis is that cell-surface expression of this autoantigen has been found on biliary epithelial cells of patients with primary biliary cirrhosis, raising the possibility that antibody-directed cell cytotoxicity has a part to play in tissue damage.

Other autoantibodies reacting against nuclear antigens are found in a minority of patients with primary biliary cirrhosis. Disease-specific nuclear antigens reacting with these autoantibodies have also been characterized and include an integral glycoprotein of the nuclear-pore membrane and the nuclear envelope lamin-B receptor (Table 1).

Study of the autoantibody response in primary biliary cirrhosis has helped identify potential autoantigens, but as yet little is understood of the way in which the autoimmune response is induced or the effector mechanisms that cause tissue damage. Multiple abnormalities often coexist in the immune systems of patients with primary biliary cirrhosis, including raised IgM levels in serum, chronic activation of the complement system with depletion of C4 and aberrant expression of MHC class II antigens on biliary epithelial cells; it is not clear whether these are the cause or consequence of liver damage. Available evidence suggests that CD8+ cytotoxic T cells play a significant part in the destructive lesion of the bile ducts. These T cells infiltrate the portal tract and can be found adjacent to biliary epithelial cells at the time of maximal damage. The biliary epithelial cells express MHC class I antigens and the cellular adhesion molecules that are necessary for cytotoxic cell adherence. T cell clones derived from liver tissue of patients with primary biliary cirrhosis contain a high proportion of CD8+ cells, and possess cytotoxic ability. The role of the other effector systems of the immune response in the inflammatory destructive lesions of bile ducts is less clear.

PATHOLOGY

The characteristic early lesion of primary biliary cirrhosis is inflammatory duct destruction. Later there is fibrosis, often patchy, and eventually a frank cirrhotic picture. Histologically this disease appears to evolve from a florid duct lesion to cirrhosis. This has led to a morphological classification into four stages. It must be recognized, however, that overlaps between stages is common in different parts of the liver. In stage 1, the duct lesion is florid (Fig. 1) with the epithelium irregular, hyperplastic or ulcerated. There is a heavy infiltrate of lymphocytes, plasma cells and neutrophils, with occasional eosinophils. Aggregates of histocytes with granulomas ranging from foci of epithelioid cells to rounded lesions with multinucleated giant cells are present. In stage 2 there is established duct destruction and the bile ducts may be replaced by lymphoid aggregates with fibrosis. In stage 3 there is relatively little inflammation, though lymphoid aggregates may be present and fibrous septa extend from the portal tract. In stage 4 there is an established cirrhosis, paucity of bile ducts, and lymphoid infiltration (Fig. 2). Mallory bodies similar to those seen in alcoholic liver disease may be present adjacent to the areas of inflammation and there is excess stainable copper-binding protein, a reflection of the cholestasis.

CLINICAL FEATURES

Over 90 per cent of patients are women, usually between the ages of 40 and 60 years. It is a slowly progressive disorder. A substantial proportion of patients are 'asymptomatic' with respect to liver disease when their disease is first diagnosed, often due to the finding of hepatomegaly, a raised alkaline phosphatase or a positive antimitochondrial antibody during investigation of another putative autoimmune disorder. Such patients may complain only of fatigue or symptoms associated with collagen-vascular disease or thyroid disease. Classical descriptions of patients with more advanced primary biliary cirrhosis emphasize the presence of clinical cholestasis, with jaundice, pruritus, light stools, easy bruising, and weight loss. Occasionally, patients present with gastrointestinal bleeding from oesophageal varices or associated peptic ulcer. The pruritus may first be noticed during pregnancy or when the patient is on the contraceptive pill. Diarrhoea due to steatorrhoea may be a feature.

The findings on examination when the patients first seek medical advice vary widely. At one extreme, there may be no abnormality, whereas at the other the patient is jaundiced, with scratch marks and signs of long-standing cholestasis. The planus form of xanthoma occurs characteristically as xanthelasmas around the eyes and in the palmar creases. Tuberous lesions develop late on the extensor surfaces around the knees, elbows, wrists, ankle, and on pressure points such as buttocks. Occasionally they affect tendon sheaths and nerves, producing xanthomatous peripheral neuropathy.

The liver is usually enlarged and firm, and splenomegaly may be present, with or without portal hypertension. Spider naevi and palmar erythema are less frequent than in patients with alcoholic cirrhosis. Bleeding from oesophageal varices is a late complication of primary biliary cirrhosis. Liver failure with encephalopathy and fluid retention with ascites and oedema are also usually late manifestations. Steatorrhoea occurs primarily in patients who have advanced cholestasis. The chief consequence of steatorrhoea is the malabsorption of fat-soluble vitamins, especially vitamin D. Bone pain due to osteomalacia, with tenderness and fractures involving vertebrae, can occur. Osteoporosis

Table 1 *Disease-specific autoantigens in primary biliary cirrhosis*

	Molecular weight ($\times 10^3$)	Sera reacting to antigen (%)
Mitochondrial antigens		
Pyruvate dehydrogenase complex:		
E2 acetyltransferase	74	94
Protein X	52	94
E1α decarboxylase	41	40
E1β decarboxylase	36	10
2-oxoglutarate dehydrogenase complex:		
E2 succinyl transferase	50	53
Branched-chain 2-oxo-acid dehydrogenase complex:		
E2 acyltransferase	50	89
Nuclear antigens		
Glycoprotein of the nuclear-pore membrane	210	10
Lamin-B receptor (protein of inner nuclear membrane)	58	10
Protein with dot-like distribution within cell nuclei	100	27

may also complicate primary biliary cirrhosis. Deficiency of vitamin K sometimes results in easy bruising or other haemorrhagic phenomena. Clubbing of the fingers and leuconychia are rare findings. There is an increased incidence of gallstones and peptic ulceration, and features of these conditions may form part of the clinical picture. Male patients with established cirrhosis (histological stage 4) are at increased risk of developing primary hepatocellular carcinoma.

ASSOCIATED DISEASES

Primary biliary cirrhosis is associated with a number of other putative autoimmune diseases. These include scleroderma, Sjögren's syndrome, seropositive and seronegative arthropathy, thyroiditis, and renal tubular acidosis. The CRST syndrome (calcinosis, Raynaud's phenomenon, sclerodactyly, and telangiectasia), pulmonary fibrosis, and coeliac disease have also been reported (see Section 18).

DIAGNOSIS

The diagnosis is based on the clinical findings, the histology, and serological and biochemical changes. A positive antimitochondrial antibody may antedate all other abnormalities. Immunofluorescence is the technique in routine use to detect these autoantibodies but assays using expressed recombinant or purified mitochondrial polypeptides have recently been developed and shown to have greater sensitivity and specificity. 'Liver function' tests indicate cholestasis, with an elevated serum alkaline phosphatase, paralleled by increased γ-glutamyl transferase and 5′-nucleotidase. The aminotransferase activity is only moderately elevated. At presentation the level of total serum bilirubin is usually normal or only modestly increased. The serum globulins are usually raised, particularly the IgM, but the serum albumin is usually maintained until late in the disease. Other tests such as erythrocyte sedimentation rate, cholesterol, and autoantibodies other than antimitochondrial antibodies are less specific. Liver biopsy is mandatory in the evaluation of a patient suspected of having primary biliary cirrhosis.

The main differential diagnosis is from other causes of cholestasis. Scanning of the liver with ultrasonography and computerized tomography is necessary to exclude extrahepatic biliary obstruction or gallstones, and to provide information about the nature of the liver and biliary system. The biliary tract may need to be evaluated by endoscopic retrograde cholangiopancreatography (**ERCP**), particularly in the small minority of patients with a negative test for antimitochondrial antibody. Many such patients will have a positive antinuclear factor and may be diagnosed as having 'autoimmune cholangitis'. There is an overlap with

Fig. 1 Bile-duct lesion in primary biliary cirrhosis. There is granulomatous destruction of a medium-sized bile-duct radicle in which the epithelium appears hyperplastic. Epithelioid macrophages are surrounded by a chronic inflammatory cell infiltrate. Haematoxylin and eosin. (By courtesy of A.D. Burt.)

Fig. 2 Stage 4 primary biliary cirrhosis: an established micronodular cirrhosis; the halo effect seen around the nodules is a characteristic feature of biliary cirrhosis. Haematoxylin and eosin. (By courtesy of A.D. Burt.)

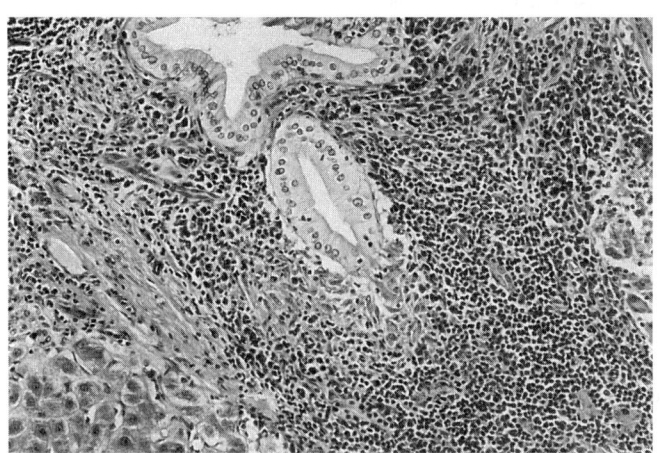

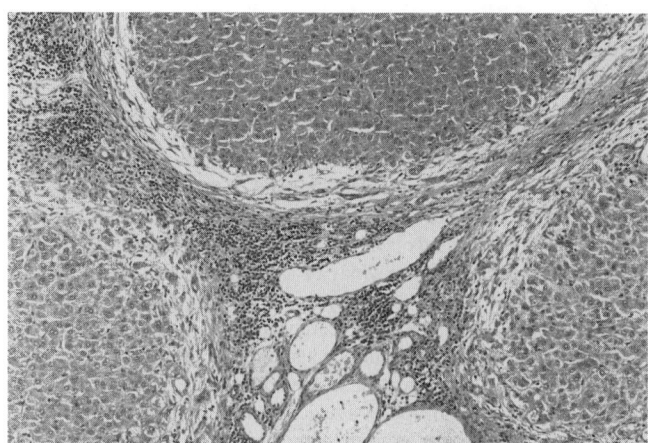

Table 2 *Therapeutic agents evaluated in primary biliary cirrhosis*

Agent	Dosage	Comment
Immunosuppressive		
Cyclosporin	3–4 mg/kg/day	Improved hepatic function but renal toxicity and hypertension
Methotrexate	15 mg/week	Under evaluation Some benefit but toxicity possible
Prednisolone	30→10 mg/day	Improved hepatic function in one small study
Azathioprine	0.5–2 mg/kg/day	Minor benefits ?Improved survival
Chlorambucil	0.5–4 mg/day	Potentially toxic Benefits unclear
Antifibrotic		
Colchicine	1–1.2 mg/day	Minor benefits
Malotilate	1.5 mg/day	Minor benefits
Cpruretic		
D-penicillamine	250–1000 mg/day	No convincing benefit Excessive toxicity
Bile acid		
Ursodeoxycholic acid	10–15 mg/kg/day	Improvement in biochemistry

autoimmune chronic active hepatitis, which can be diagnosed on liver histology, whilst primary sclerosing cholangitis will be evident on ERCP. Laparotomy is no longer necessary to establish the diagnosis but is sometimes done because of misdiagnosis and inadequate investigation.

COURSE AND PROGNOSIS

No spontaneous remissions of primary biliary cirrhosis have been documented and hence the long-term prognosis is poor. However, the course is very variable and patients without symptoms often have a good prognosis, remaining free of hepatobiliary symptoms for years following diagnosis. Once symptoms develop, several biochemical and histological features have been shown to have prognostic significance. Models have been developed to predict mortality and assist in identifying those most likely to benefit from liver transplantation. There is an inverse relation between serum bilirubin and survival, and most models also use age, albumin, and presence of cirrhosis or a marker of advanced liver disease such as increased prothrombin time. These models have been used to show, mathematically, that transplantation prolongs life in primary biliary cirrhosis.

TREATMENT

This consists of therapy aimed at modifying the disease process and progression to cirrhosis, and treatment of symptoms and late complications.

Although numerous trials of treatment have been undertaken in the last 30 years, none has produced an agent for which there is clear evidence of benefit at an equivalent level to that seen for corticosteroids in autoimmune chronic active hepatitis. The aim of therapy must be disease remission but it is unlikely that significant alteration in the outcome of the disease can be expected once irreversible liver damage (i.e. cirrhosis) has occurred, though symptoms may be ameliorated. In addition, earlier diagnosis combined with difficulty in predicting clinical course in asymptomatic patients has led to uncertainty as to which patients should be treated, when treatment should be started and what is the best treatment to administer. The agents that have been assessed fall into four main categories: immunosuppressive drugs (azathioprine, prednisolone, chlorambucil, cyclosporin, and methotrexate), antifibrotic agents (col-

chicine, malotilate), the cupruretic agent D-penicillamine, and bile acid therapy (ursodeoxycholic acid) (Table 2). At present there is no obvious treatment of choice, though it is arguable that ursodeoxycholic acid, being safe and with some benefit on cholestasis and possibly pruritus, could be used by all physicians not considering referral to centres running controlled trials.

Itching can be an intolerable symptom in primary biliary cirrhosis and the first line of treatment is usually with cholestyramine, one sachet before and after breakfast, and one before lunch and dinner. Improvement in itching has also been reported with rifampicin and opioid antagonists (nalmifene and naloxone). There is no indication for a fat-free diet unless the patient has symptoms related to steatorrhoea or xanthelasma with high serum cholesterol levels. Supplementation with medium-chain triglycerides may be necessary if adequate weight or nutrition cannot be sustained. Deficiency of fat-soluble vitamins is a logical consequence of long-term cholestasis and parenteral supplements are usually given to jaundiced patients. A prolonged prothrombin time is treated with intramuscular vitamin K, 10 mg monthly. Injections of vitamin A (100 000 i.u.) and vitamin D (100 000 i.u.) are usually given every 2 months. Vitamin E supplements may also be required. Osteomalacia is now rarely seen with the use of vitamin D supplements but prevention of osteoporosis is more problematical. Oral calcium, 1 g daily by mouth, may be helpful, possibly combined with cyclical diphosphonate treatment if there is evidence of progressive bone loss on serial bone-densitometric measurements.

The complications of portal hypertension, such as variceal bleeding and ascites, and of liver failure, such as hepatic encephalopathy, are treated appropriately. Liver transplantation is now the accepted treatment for endstage primary biliary cirrhosis. Debate continues as to whether the disease recurs post-transplant but if so, this does not appear to significantly affect the outcome of the graft. Timing of transplantation requires careful evaluation of quality of life and life expectancy. Referral to a transplant centre should be considered as the bilirubin approaches 100 μmol/l, though patients with particular problems such as intractable itching or bleeding may need to be considered individually.

REFERENCES

Balan, V., Batts, K.P., Porakyo, M.K., Krom, R.A.F., Ludwig, J., and Wiesner, R.H. (1993). Histological evidence for recurrence of primary biliary cirrhosis after liver transplantation. *Hepatology* **18**, 1392–6.

Bassendine, M.F. *et al.* (1993). Molecular basis of mitochondrial autoantigens associated with acyltransferases. In *Immunology and liver*, (ed. K.H. Meyer Zum Buschenfelde, J.H. Hoofnagle, and M. Manns), pp. 361–372. Kluwer Academic, New York.

Gershwin, M.E. and Mackay, I.R. (1991). Primary biliary cirrhosis: paradigm or paradox for autoimmunity. *Gastroenterology*, **100**, 822–33.

Heathcote, E.J., *et al.* (1994). The Canadian multicenter double-blind randomized controlled trial of ursodeoxycholic acid in primary biliary cirrhosis. *Hepatology*, **19**, 1149–56.

James, O.F.W., and Mysor, M. (1990). Epidemiology and genetics of primary biliary cirrhosis. In *Progress in liver disease*, (ed. H. Popper and F. Schaffer), pp. 523–36. Saunders, Philadelphia.

Jones, D.E.J., Gregory, W.L., and Bassendine, M.F. (1993). Primary biliary cirrhosis. In *Immunology of liver disease*, (ed. H.C. Thomas and J. Waters), pp. 121–43. Kluwer Academic, New York.

Joplin, R., Lindsay, J.G., Johnson, G.D., Strain, A., and Neuberger, J. (1992). Membrane dihydrolipoamide acetyltransferase (E2) on human biliary epithelial cells in primary biliary cirrhosis. *Lancet*, **339**, 93–4.

Leung, P.S.C. *et al.* (1992). Use of designer recombinant mitochondrial antigens in the diagnosis of primary biliary cirrhosis. *Hepatology*, **15**, 367–72.

Lindor, K.D., *et al.* (1994). Ursodeoxycholic acid in the treatment of primary biliary cirrhosis. *Gastroenterology*, **106**, 1284–90.

Lombard, M. *et al.* (1992). Cyclosporin A treatment in primary biliary cirrhosis. Results of a long-term placebo controlled trial. *Gastroenterology*, **105**, 519–26.

Markus, B.H. *et al.* (1989). Efficacy of liver transplantation in patients with primary biliary cirrhosis. *New England Journal of Medicine*, **320**, 1709–13.

Mitchison, H.C. and Bassendine, M.F. (1993). Rolling review: autoimmune liver disease. *Alimentary Pharmacology and Therapeutics*, **7**, 93–109.

Scheuer, P.J. (1989). Primary biliary cirrhosis. In *Liver biopsy interpretation*, (4th edn), pp. 53–65. Baillère Tindall, London.

Wiesner, R.H., Graubsch, P.M., Lindor, K.D., Ludwig, J., and Dickson, E.R. (1988). Clinical and statistical analysis of new and evolving therapies for primary biliary cirrhosis. *Hepatology* **8**, 668–76.

Weisner, R.H. *et al.* (1992). Selection and timing of liver transplantation in primary biliary cirrhosis and primary sclerosing cholangitis. *Hepatology*, **16**, 1290–9.

Worman, H.J., and Courvalin, J.C. (1991). Autoantibodies against nuclear envelope proteins in liver disease. *Hepatology*, **14**, 1269–79.

14.27.3 Primary sclerosing cholangitis

R. W. CHAPMAN

Primary sclerosing cholangitis is a chronic cholestatic liver disease characterized by an obliterative inflammatory fibrosis of the biliary tract. It may lead to bile-duct obstruction, biliary cirrhosis, hepatic failure and, in some patients, cholangiocarcinoma. Primary sclerosing cholangitis was initially considered to be a rare disease; however, the advent of endoscopic retrograde cholangiopancreatography in the early 1970s established the diagnosis in a progressively larger number of patients. This led to the realization that primary sclerosing cholangitis has a much wider clinical and pathological spectrum than was previously recognized. Indeed, in the United Kingdom it has become the second most common reason for orthotopic liver transplantation in patients with chronic liver disease.

The generally accepted diagnostic criteria of primary sclerosing cholangitis are: (i) generalized bleeding and stenosis of the biliary system on cholangiography (Fig. 1); (ii) absence of choledocholithiasis or a history of bile-duct surgery; (iii) exclusion of bile-duct cancer, usually by prolonged follow-up.

The term secondary sclerosing cholangitis is used to describe the typical bile-duct changes when a clear predisposing factor to duct fibrosis, such as previous bile-duct surgery, can be identified. The causes of secondary sclerosing cholangitis are:

- previous bile-duct surgery;
- bile-duct stones causing cholangitis;
- intrahepatic infusion of 5-fluorodeoxyuridine;
- formalin insertion into hepatic hydatid cysts;
- AIDS—probably infective (cytomegalovirus or cryptosporidium).

AETIOLOGY

The cause of primary sclerosing cholangitis remains unknown. There is a very close association, however, between primary sclerosing cholangitis and inflammatory bowel disease, particularly ulcerative colitis. Approximately two-thirds of patients with primary sclerosing cholangitis have coexisting ulcerative colitis, and primary sclerosing cholangitis is the most common form of chronic liver disease found in ulcerative colitis. Three to 10 per cent of patients with ulcerative colitis will develop primary sclerosing cholangitis, and the prevalence is greater in patients with substantial or total colitis than in those with distal colitis only. Any proposed factors in the aetiopathogenesis of primary sclerosing cholangitis clearly have to explain this close association with inflammatory bowel disease. It has been suggested, therefore, that the diseased colon may give rise to either abnormal, toxic bile acids or chronic, low-grade, portal bacteraemia, leading to portal inflammation. Current evidence does not support either hypothesis and recent studies have suggested that genetic and immunological factors are important in the pathogenesis of primary sclerosing cholangitis.

Immunogenetic factors

Case reports of a number of families in whom members developed ulcerative colitis and primary sclerosing cholangitis led to the search for an HLA association. A close link with the *HLA-A1, -B8, -DR3* haplotype has been found, in common with other organ-specific autoimmune diseases such as autoimmune chronic active hepatitis. *HLA-DRw52a*, which is in linkage disequilibrium with *-DR3*, is also closely linked to the development of primary sclerosing cholangitis. In patients who are -DR3 and -Drw52a negative, an increased prevalence of HLA-DR2 is found. HLA-A1,-B8,-DR3 and -DR2 are equally distributed in patients with primary sclerosing cholangitis, with or without ulcerative colitis.

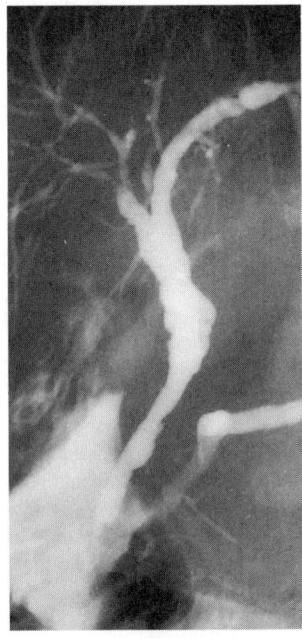

Fig. 1 Cholangiogram showing the typical features of primary sclerosing cholangitis with stricturing and dilatation of the intra- and extrahepatic biliary tree.

Moreover, these HLA antigens are not found universally in increased frequency in patients with ulcerative colitis although some studies have found an increased prevalence of -DR2. These data suggest that *HLA-DR3/DRW52a*, *-DR2*, and ulcerative colitis are separate independent risk factors for the development of primary sclerosing cholangitis. It has been suggested that both *-DRw52a* and *-DR2* encode for amino acids in the HLA β-chain that may enhance antigen presentation by the HLA molecule to the T-cell receptor. Further evidence of an autoimmune basis for this condition has been provided by many studies that have shown humoral and cellular immune abnormalities.

Humoral immune abnormalities

Like primary biliary cirrhosis, a disease with which it shares many features (see Chapter 14.27.2), symptomatic primary sclerosing cholangitis is characterized by hypergammaglobulinaemia, often with a disproportionate elevation of serum IgM concentrations in adult patients. In contrast, high concentrations of serum IgG are found in all children with primary sclerosing cholangitis. Smooth-muscle antibody and antinuclear factor are also found in approximately one-third of patients with primary sclerosing cholangitis, usually in low titres.

Recently, a cytoplasmic antineutrophil antibody was found in the serum of 80 per cent of patients with primary sclerosing cholangitis and approximately 30 per cent of patients with ulcerative colitis. It appears to be relatively specific for primary sclerosing cholangitis and is not found in other chronic liver diseases, apart from in a minority of patients with autoimmune chronic active hepatitis. Unlike the antigens in Wegener's granulomatosis, which have been shown to be proteinase 3 and myeloperoxidase, the antigen in neutrophils from primary sclerosing cholangitis has yet to be identified. The pathogenetic significance of the circulating antibody is not clear, but it may prove to be useful in a diagnostic test.

Cellular immune abnormalities

Elevated circulating immune complexes associated with activation of complement via the classic pathway have been found in the serum and bile of patients with primary sclerosing cholangitis.

In common with other autoimmune diseases, there are reduced levels of T-suppressor cells circulating in the serum of these patients, leading to an increased ratio of T-helper to T-suppressor cells. Infiltration of portal tracts by increased numbers of mononuclear cells is seen in liver biopsies from patients with primary sclerosing cholangitis. The majority of these cells are activated T lymphocytes.

Current evidence suggests that primary sclerosing cholangitis is an immunologically mediated disease, perhaps triggered in genetically susceptible subjects by acquired toxic or infectious agents, which are presented through antigen-presenting cells to activated T lymphocytes. Unlike normal biliary cells, the biliary epithelial cells in primary sclerosing cholangitis express HLA class II molecules and also intercellular adhesion molecules (**ICAM**) such as ICAM-I. It has not yet been confirmed, however, that bile-duct cells can act as antigen-presenting cells.

CLINICAL FEATURES

There is a clear male predominance, with a male : female ratio of 2 : 1. The majority of patients present between the ages of 25 and 40 years, although primary sclerosing cholangitis may be diagnosed at any age. Indeed, it has become recognized recently as an important cause of chronic liver disease in children.

The clinical presentation is variable: some patients may present with fatigue, intermittent jaundice, weight loss, right upper-quadrant pain, and pruritus. Attacks of acute cholangitis are surprisingly rare and usually follow instrumental biliary intervention, such as endoscopic retrograde cholangiopancreatography. Physical examination is abnormal in approximately half of symptomatic patients; the most common findings are jaundice and hepatosplenomegaly. Many patients with primary sclerosing cholangitis are asymptomatic at diagnosis, which is made inci-

dentally when a persistently raised serum alkaline phosphatase is discovered, usually in the setting of ulcerative colitis.

Serum biochemical tests usually indicate cholestasis but primary sclerosing cholangitis may not cause any abnormality of serum biochemistry. The serum alkaline phosphatase is often raised to greater than three times normal, and mild elevations in liver transaminases are seen in the majority of patients. Serum bilirubin is not usually elevated until later stages of the disease. Levels of bilirubin and alkaline phosphatase may fluctuate widely in an individual patient during the course of the disease. Hypoalbuminaemia is unusual until the disease becomes advanced. As mentioned above, increased serum IgM concentrations are seen in about half of the symptomatic adult patients, but high concentrations of IgG are always found in children with primary sclerosing cholangitis.

In addition to the serum antineutrophil antibodies, low levels of antinuclear antibody and smooth-muscle antibody may be found in approximately one-third of patients, but serum mitochondrial antibodies are absent.

DIAGNOSIS

Radiological features

The cholangiographic appearances after endoscopic retrograde cholangiopancreatography are usually diagnostic and consist of multiple, irregular stricturing and dilatation (beading of the intrahepatic and extrahepatic biliary ducts) (Fig. 1). Occasionally, involvement is localized to the intrahepatic system, and even more rarely, only the extrahepatic bile ducts may be involved. Small diverticula are found along the common bile duct in about 20 per cent of patients and are pathognomonic (Fig. 2).

Pathological features

The histological appearances of liver are not usually diagnostic of primary sclerosing cholangitis, although some form of biliary disease can usually be identified. The characteristic early features of primary sclerosing cholangitis are periductal 'onion skin' fibrosis and inflammation, portal oedema, and bile ductular proliferation resulting in the expansion of the portal tracts (Fig. 3). Later, fibrosis spreads into the liver paren-

Fig. 2 Cholangiogram from a patient with primary sclerosing cholangitis showing a diverticular appearance of the common bile duct.

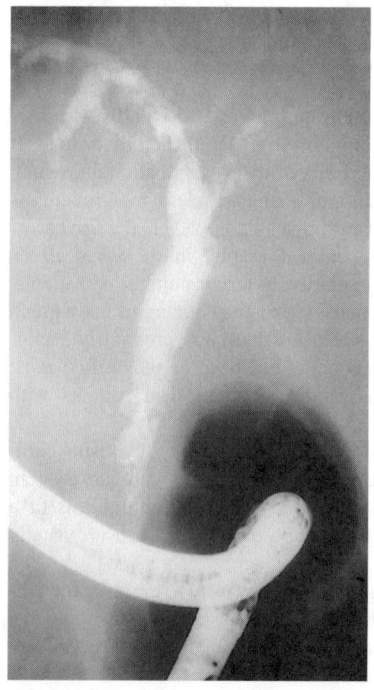

chyma to form fibrous septa, leading inevitably to biliary cirrhosis. As in primary biliary cirrhosis, with disease progression an obliterative cholangitis occurs, leading to complete replacement of the intralobular bile ducts by connective tissue—the so-called vanishing bile-duct syndrome. In addition, piecemeal necrosis, copper-binding protein, cholestasis, and occasional portal phlebitis may be present.

ASSOCIATION WITH OTHER DISEASES

A large number of diseases have been associated with primary sclerosing cholangitis (Table 1). The most important association, as discussed above, is with inflammatory bowel disease, particularly ulcerative colitis. The extent of the colitis is usually total but symptomatically and, paradoxically, mild, often with no rectal bleeding and characterized by prolonged remission. Although the symptoms of ulcerative colitis usually develop before those of primary sclerosing cholangitis in some patients, the onset of primary sclerosing cholangitis may precede the symptoms of colitis by some years. The outcome of primary sclerosing cholangitis is completely unrelated to the activity, severity, or clinical course of the colitis, and colectomy has no effect on the progression of the cholangitis. Primary sclerosing cholangitis is less common in Crohn's disease, occurring in less than 1 per cent of patients and only in those with Crohn's colitis.

NATURAL HISTORY AND PROGNOSIS

The course of primary sclerosing cholangitis is highly variable. The median survival from presentation to death or liver transplantation is approximately 10 to 12 years. The majority of patients die in hepatic failure following deepening cholestatic jaundice. However, approximately 10 to 30 per cent of patients with long-standing primary sclerosing cholangitis die from the development of bile-duct carcinoma, which often follows a very aggressive course. Unfortunately, there are no factors that will predict which patients will develop this cancer. Attempts to identify factors that will predict the risk of progression to liver failure and death have yielded conflicting data from different centres. It is clear that the majority of asymptomatic patients will progress insidiously to symptomatic liver disease, liver failure, and death.

TREATMENT

Symptomatic measures

There is no curative treatment for primary sclerosing cholangitis. This is indicated by the plethora of medical, endoscopic, and surgical approaches that has been advocated.

Fig. 3 The hepatic histological changes of early primary sclerosing cholangitis showing a concentric (onion skin) fibrosis around the bile ducts.

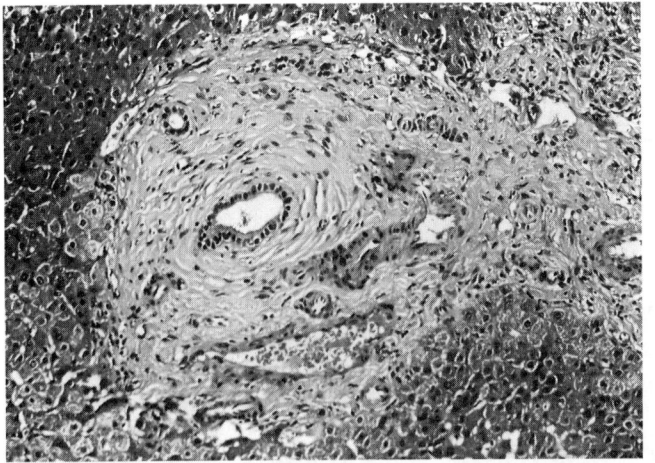

Table 1 *Diseases associated with primary sclerosing cholangitis*

Ulcerative colitis
Crohn's colitis
Chronic pancreatitis
Retroperitoneal fibrosis
Riedel's struma
Retro-orbital tumours
Immunodeficiency states
Sjögren's syndrome
Angioimmunoblastic lymphadenopathy
Histiocytosis X
Autoimmune haemolytic anaemia

Management of cholestasis

Symptomatic patients are frequently troubled by pruritus. This is best managed initially by cholestyramine and the dose should be increased until relief is obtained. In addition, replacement of fat-soluble vitamins is necessary when patients become jaundiced.

Management of complications

Broad-spectrum antibiotics should be given for acute attacks of cholangitis, but they have no proven prophylactic value and should not be used in the long term routinely. If cholangiography shows a well-defined obstruction to the main extra hepatic bile ducts, then mechanical relief must be considered. In many patients the best approach is to introduce a prosthesis (stent) through the obstruction. This may be placed nonoperatively by the percutaneous transhepatic route or at endoscopic retrograde cholangiography. Balloon dilatation of the strictures before stenting may prove useful in a minority of patients with well-defined localized strictures and can lead to a striking improvement in symptoms and serum biochemistry.

Another common complication is the development of small biliary stones (brown pigment) and biliary sludge, which can lead to a rapid clinical or biochemical deterioration. In these patients, endoscopic sphincterotomy with extraction of the biliary debris can be beneficial. Some have advocated endoscopic biliary drainage, but no long-term results are available.

Specific treatment
Medical

The medical treatment of primary sclerosing cholangitis has included trials of corticosteroids, immunosuppressive drugs, cholecystogogues, and antibiotics, either alone or in combination. The results have been universally disappointing, although assessment of treatment of this uncommon disease is difficult because the clinical course fluctuates, survival is variable, and some patients may remain asymptomatic for long periods of time. The role of corticosteroid therapy is unclear. There have been no large controlled trials, but corticosteroids have been used topically and systemically in small and generally uncontrolled studies. However, there is evidence that, even in male patients, metabolic bone disease may be accelerated by corticosteroids and in general they should not be used in this condition.

Ursodeoxycholic acid is a non-hepatotoxic hydrophilic bile acid. Small, controlled trials have confirmed that it improves clinical symptoms and reduces the levels of cholestatic enzyme markers, but larger studies are needed to show a long-term effect on morbidity and mortality. The drug, however, is free of side-effects.

A number of immunosuppressant agents have been tried, either alone or in combination, including azathioprine, methotrexate, and cyclosporin. Overall, the results have been disappointing.

Surgical

The role of hepatobiliary surgery in the treatment of primary sclerosing cholangitis remains controversial. Good results have been claimed for the resection of the extrahepatic biliary tree followed by biliary reconstruction with silastic transhepatic stents. However, controlled trials are needed to confirm the efficacy of these and other surgical techniques, as previous biliary surgery will increase perioperative mortality from hepatic transplantation.

Transplantation

Orthotopic liver transplantation is the only option available in young patients with primary sclerosing cholangitis and advanced liver disease. Primary sclerosing cholangitis is now the second most common indication for liver transplantation in the United Kingdom. Recent results have been very encouraging, with 4-year survival rates of 80 to 90 per cent being obtained in some centres. These rates compare favourably with those for other forms of chronic liver disease. Interestingly, there have only been a few case reports of primary sclerosing cholangitis recurring in the transplanted liver.

REFERENCES

Chapman, R.W. *et al.* (1980). Primary sclerosing cholangitis—a review of its clinical features, cholangiography and hepatic histology. *Gut*, **21**, 870–7.

Donaldson, P.T., Farrant, J.M., Wilkinson, M.L., Hayllar, K., Portmann, B.C., and Williams, R. (1991). Dual association of HLA DR2 and DR3 with primary sclerosing cholangitis. *Hepatology*, **13**, 129–33.

Farrant, J.M. *et al.* (1991). Natural history and prognostic variables in primary sclerosing cholangitis. *Gastroenterology*, **100**, 1710–17.

Low, S.K., Fleming, K.A., and Chapman, R.W. (1992). Prevalence of anti-neutrophil antibody in primary sclerosing cholangitis and ulcerative colitis using an alkaline phosphatase method. *Gut*, **33**, 1370–5.

Ludwig, J. *et al.* (1981). Morphological features of chronic hepatitis associated with primary sclerosing cholangitis and ulcerative colitis. *Hepatology*, **1**, 632–40.

Johnson, G.K., Geenen, J.E., Venu, R.P., Schmalz, M.J., and Hogan, W.J. (1991). Endoscopic treatment of biliary tract strictures in sclerosing cholangitis: a large series and recommendations of treatment. *Gastrointestinal Endoscopy*, **37**, 38–43.

McEntee, G., Wiesner, R.H., Rosen, C., Cooper, J., and Wahlstrom, E. (1991). A comparative study of patients undergoing liver transplantation for primary sclerosing cholangitis and primary biliary cirrhosis. *Transplant Proceedings*, **23**, 1563–4.

Wiesner, R.H. and LaRusso, N.F. (1980). Clinical pathological features of the syndrome of primary sclerosing cholangitis. *Gastroenterology*, **79**, 200–6.

14.28 Alcoholic liver disease

O. F. W. JAMES

The association between alcohol abuse and liver disease was recognized by the ancient Greeks and by Indian physicians many centuries ago. The causal connection between excess alcohol and cirrhosis was noted by Baillie in 1793, and between alcoholism and fatty liver by Addison in 1836.

Epidemiology

After the Second World War there was a general increase in alcohol consumption in most European countries, North America and, later, the Far East, until around 1975. From comparison between countries, a generally close relation between per capita ethanol consumption and both deaths from cirrhosis and the total mortality attributable to excess alcohol consumption (including accident, suicides and hypertension) may be deduced. Thus in the former West Germany, mortality from cirrhosis rose fourfold between 1950 and 1980; and threefold in England between 1959 and 1978. This causal connection is further confirmed by the dramatic fall in deaths from cirrhosis that had occurred in France between 1941 and 1945 during the years of wine rationing. After the mid-1970s, per capita ethanol consumption fell in Mediterranean, largely wine-drinking countries including Italy, France, Spain, and Portugal, and in the United States, whereas in countries where beer or spirits are predominant, no trend can be observed. In Sweden, the United States, and Canada there have been slight declines in mortality from cirrhosis between the late 1970s and the late 1980s *pari passu* with a moderate decrease in *per capita* ethanol consumption. There is no good epidemiological evidence that the type of drink consumed (beer, wine, spirits), or pattern of drinking has a marked influence on cirrhosis or its mortality.

Individual susceptibility

Only 10 to 30 per cent of heavy, persistent alcohol drinkers develop cirrhosis, although well over 50 per cent may have fatty livers. Whether an individual develops alcoholic liver damage is not only a function of how much alcohol he or she consumes and for how long; it is becoming clear that individual susceptibility also depends upon many other factors (Fig. 1). In a large group of males with alcoholic cirrhosis, average alcohol consumption was 160 g/day (equivalent to over two bottles of wine, 4.5 litres of average-strength lager, two-thirds of a bottle of spirits) for over 8 years. It was suggested that to have a 50 per cent chance of cirrhosis a man must drink 210 g of ethanol a day for 22 years. In a recent case-control study, relative risk for cirrhosis was 100 for men consuming 80 g of ethanol per day compared to those taking less than 40 g/day. Similar trends were seen for women. Another case-control study from Australia also reported that the risk of alcoholic liver disease probably began to develop in those men and women reporting consumption of over 40 g/day. It seems likely that almost no risk of significant alcohol-related liver damage exists below about 40 g/day (280

Fig. 1 Susceptibility to alcoholic liver disease.

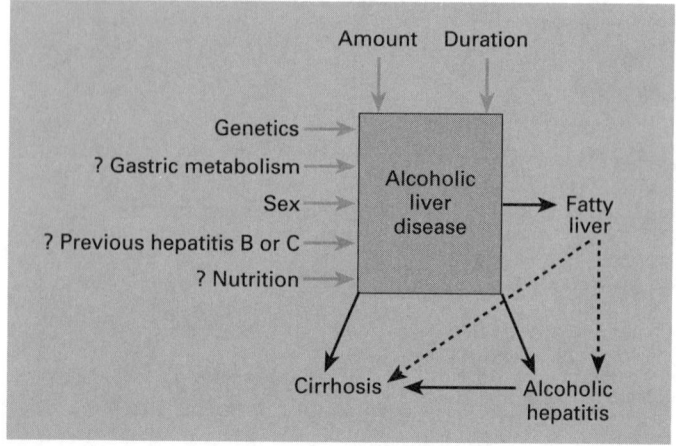

g/week, equivalent to about 30 units) for men or women. Current 'safe' limits for ethanol consumption recommended in the United Kingdom are 21 units (about 200 g) ethanol per week for men and 14 units (about 130 g) ethanol per week for women, but these figures are somewhat arbitrary.

GENETIC FACTORS

Individual susceptibility to both alcoholism and alcoholic liver damage has important genetic components. Probably one out of three alcoholics will have at least one parent who is alcoholic; analysis of twin studies suggests hereditability of alcohol-drinking behaviour in the range 0.3 to 0.6 (where 0 = no hereditability, 1.0 = complete hereditability). Recently several possible biological markers of alcoholism have been described. These include (i) the A1 allele of the D_2 dopamine receptor in the brain, present in significantly more alcoholics than controls; (ii) monoamineoxidase B activity in platelets: this enzyme, which catalyses the oxidation of monoamine neurotransmitters, is present in two iso-forms—one of these, the B form, is present in platelets and its activity is markedly decreased in alcoholics; (iii) P_{300} event-related potentials. These potentials measure brain-wave response to external sensory stimuli by computer averaging. One part of the event-related potential is a positive wave occurring about 300 ms (the P_{300}) after a sensory stimulus that has required an individual to attend to and interpret its meaning. It is thought that P_{300} measures the sensory, perceptual, and cognitive responses of an individual. Several studies have found reduced P_{300} in alcoholics, former alcoholics, and in young sons of alcoholics.

Several studies have examined variation in the genes encoding the two principal alcohol-metabolizing enzymes—alcohol and aldehyde dehydrogenase (**ADH** and **ALDH**). The ADH isoenzyme subunits are encoded by at least seven different loci and polymorphisms have been identified in two, *ADH2* and *ADH3*. The isoenzymes arising from these subunits oxidize alcohol to acetaldehyde at widely differing rates. The most important isoenzyme for acetaldehyde metabolism is encoded by the *ALDH2* locus; about 50 per cent of orientals possess a dominant null allele that encodes an inactive form of the enzyme. Individuals with the more active forms of ADH, and hence more rapid production of acet-aldehyde, or the inactive form of ALDH2 and slower metabolism of acetaldehyde, are less likely to be alcoholic, due to the aversive effects of acetaldehyde in the circulation—the alcohol flush. However, in a Japanese population, homozygotes for ALDH2 drank less for the same degree of liver disease than heterozygotes. Homozygosity for ALDH2 thus renders individual less likely to become alcoholic but if they do drink heavily, more likely to develop alcohol-related liver injury. Meta-analysis of two recent European studies suggests that possession of the active form of ADH3, and hence more rapid production of acetaldehyde, may carry an increased risk of the development of cirrhosis. A recent meta-analysis of 28 studies of HLA phenotypes in patients with alcoholic liver disease found no significant correlations.

GASTRIC FIRST-PASS METABOLISM

The majority of oral ethanol is rapidly absorbed by passive diffusion from the stomach and duodenum but it has recently been suggested that after food a significant first-pass metabolism of ethanol occurs in the stomach, mediated by gastric ADH, thus delivering less ethanol load to the liver. Furthermore, one group has suggested that there is less gastric ADH in women than men, offering a possible explanation for the increased susceptibility of women to develop alcoholic liver disease. This remains to be confirmed.

SEX

The assertion that women are more susceptible to alcoholic liver disease is supported by several studies showing lower *per capita* ethanol consumption for a given degree of histological damage in women than men,

even allowing for the lighter weight of women. This susceptibility may be attributed partly to differences in pharmacokinetics related to body composition. Furthermore, women with alcoholic hepatitis are more likely to progress to cirrhosis than men with a similar histological picture, whether they abstain or not. Social changes now mean that the proportion of women among patients with alcoholic liver disease has risen dramatically in most countries.

NUTRITION

The contribution of nutrition to the development of alcoholic liver disease remains controversial but it seems possible that under nutrition and direct alcohol toxicity synergistically increase the likelihood of liver damage. Certainly, most patients with alcoholic liver disease have evidence of protein-calory malnutrition using well-validated criteria. Furthermore, the severity of malnutrition has been shown to correlate with the severity of the liver disease. A causal relation has not been fully established, however. Experimental studies have suggested that ethanol may increase nutritional requirements—particularly the essential amino acid choline. The finding of a histological picture indistinguishable from that of alcoholic liver disease in nutritionally related disorders such as jejunoileal bypass or intestinal resection, or associated with total parenteral nutrition, adds some weight to the concept of synergy between nutritional factors and alcohol in producing liver damage.

HEPATITIS B AND C

Although in several European countries there is more serological evidence of past or present infection with hepatitis B virus (HBV) among patients with alcoholic liver disease than in controls, it now seems that this is due to such confounding factors as more blood transfusions among the alcoholics. Furthermore, there is no correlation between HBV DNA levels in serum and the histological severity of alcohol-related liver damage.

The relation between hepatitis C viral (**HCV**) infection and susceptibility to alcoholic liver disease is controversial. Studies from Spain, France, and the United States have shown that HCV antibodies detected by ELISA are more common in patients with alcoholic liver disease. Furthermore, those who were HCV positive had more severe liver disease. These findings could not be explained on the basis of the same confounding factors as for HBV. But in the American study, use of a more specific RIBA for HCV reduced the proportion of positive subjects by 80 per cent; the high rate of ELISA positivity may relate to high serum levels of IgG in the patients with the worst liver disease.

Continuing significant alcohol consumption may possibly worsen liver disease related to chronic HBV or HCV infection and patients with known chronic HBV or HCV liver disease should be advised to abstain or radically reduce their alcohol consumption.

Previous infection with HBV or HCV acts in synergy to increase substantially the risk of development of primary hepatocellular cancer in patients with long-term alcoholic cirrhosis, particularly men.

Pathogenesis

To understand the diversity of mechanisms of alcoholic liver injury, one must first review ethanol metabolism. Ethanol must be metabolized by oxidation, mainly in the liver, because it cannot be stored. In relatively low quantities in a normal individual, most is oxidized to acetaldehyde, and hence to acetate by the enzyme ADH (see Fig. 2). At higher quantities and in regular drinkers a second alcohol metabolic pathway is recruited, the microsomal ethanol oxidizing system, whose major enzyme, cytochrome P450 IIE1, has been identified. This cytochrome has a high affinity for a number of carcinogens and for paracetamol (acetaminophen). By inducing the activity of this enzyme, chronic ethanol consumption increases metabolism not only of ethanol itself but of paracetamol to unstable intermediates rather than to stable (excretable) conjugates, thus causing liver damage. Increased carcinogen metabolism by this route may contribute to the increased incidence of cancers at several sites found in chronic alcohol abusers. The many ways, direct and indirect, by which ethanol may cause liver damage are summarized in Table 1. Many interact together and the dissection of their individual contributions in man is by no means complete. Ethanol can be considered a direct, predictable hepatotoxin, but one whose toxicity to any particular individual is, as we have seen, governed by several genetic and other factors.

Pathology

Some confusion has arisen over the description of the pathology of alcoholic liver disease, first because of the considerable overlap between the three major morphological changes—fatty liver, alcoholic hepatitis and cirrhosis—and, second, because these changes are also used clinically as descriptive terms. Predominant fatty liver is the first histological lesion seen; it occurs in most heavy drinkers at one time or another. At the stage of pure fatty change the picture is completely reversible on alcohol withdrawal. At present it is unclear what proportion of individuals with fatty liver progresses to alcoholic hepatitis and cirrhosis, and what proportion develops cirrhosis without going through a phase of hepatitis, or why some individuals develop gross fatty change and others very little. The answers must lie in individual susceptibility to the different mechanisms whereby ethanol causes liver damage.

More serious than simple fatty change is alcoholic hepatitis, which may occur in up to 40 per cent chronic ethanol abusers. The most severe changes are seen in zone 3 of the liver lobule, the perivenular area. These include: (a) ballooning and necrosis of liver cells, in some of which eosinophilic perinuclear inclusions (Mallory bodies) may be seen; (b) pericellular fibrosis (chicken-wire fibrosis)—fibrosis may also been seen around hepatic venules and suggests the likelihood of subsequent progression to cirrhosis; (c) a patchy inflammatory-cell infiltrate, mainly polymorphs, often seen only around a few hepatocytes, although occasionally lymphocytes predominate. In many instances these changes may be mild, but the more widespread they are the worse the disease.

Ultimately, as with other forms of liver injury, fibrous septa link hepatic veins to portal tracts and regeneration occurs, disturbing normal liver architecture with the formation nodules, (Fig. 3 (a–c)) and indicating that cirrhosis which is irreversible has developed.

Clinical features

The clinical range of alcoholic liver disease extends from asymptomatic to very severe, life-threatening, multisystem failure. Conventionally, the clinical syndromes are considered in terms of underlying histology but it is emphasized that the full range of clinical severity can be found at each histological stage and it is impossible confidently to determine histological severity on the basis of clinical presentation or conventional 'liver function tests'.

Fig. 2 Major pathways of ethanol metabolism.

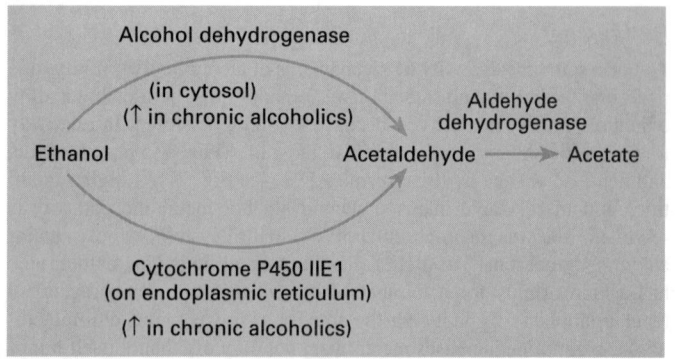

FATTY LIVER

Most patients present with such non-specific symptoms as malaise, nausea, or tiredness, or they are found to have an enlarged, possibly tender, liver or have abnormal 'liver function tests' on screening. Occasionally, very severe fatty liver can lead to cholestsis, liver failure, and portal hypertension.

ALCOHOLIC HEPATITIS

Mild alcoholic hepatitis is clinically indistinguishable from fatty liver and may be asymptomatic. In more severe cases, symptoms of anorexia, abdominal pain, nausea (often in the morning), and weight loss become prominent. Despite abdominal enlargement, many patients show signs of undernutrition and they may develop marked spider naevi remarkably quickly. Severe alcoholic hepatitis with or without underlying cirrhosis is a very serious disease, demanding urgent hospital treatment. Such patients may develop hepatic decompensation—ascites, bleeding diathesis, and encephalopathy. They are susceptible to infections—urinary tract, pneumonia, or spontaneous bacterial peritonitis—and the diagnosis is rendered more difficult because persistent, swinging fever and neutrophil leucocytosis, often over $20\,000 \times 10^9/l$, are themselves features of alcoholic hepatitis. The most severely ill patients may develop profound cholestasis and hypoglycaemia. Alcoholic hepatitis in women almost always progresses to cirrhosis, even following abstinence.

ALCOHOLIC CIRRHOSIS

Again, the clinical picture is very wide. Some patients who have cut down alcohol consumption may become asymptomatic and have normal or near normal 'liver functon tests'. More commonly, cirrhotics present either with a constellation of non-specific symptoms—weight loss, abdominal discomfort, and malaise—or with signs and symptoms of hepatic decompensation—jaundice, ascites, or haemorrhage from oesophageal or gastric varices. Rarely, patients present with marked jaundice, a combination of cholestasis and haemolysis associated with gross hyperlipidaemia (Zieve's syndrome). Patients with advanced alcoholic liver disease often show other manifestations of alcoholism (Table 2).

Investigation

It is vital to obtain an accurate drinking history, both to establish a causal relation between alcohol and the presenting liver disease, and to demonstrate this to the patient. Typically, long-term problem drinkers have a history of divorce or separation, work problems or depression. The investigation of a patient with suspected alcoholic liver disease differs little from that for other chronic liver diseases.

Conventional 'liver function tests' are often unhelpful in establishing the severity of the disease, except at the late stage. Early abnormalities may include raised serum γ-glutamyl transferase, a fairly sensitive but not specific abnormality, and macrocytosis, which, though common in alcohol abusers, is non-specific. Outpatient measurement of blood, breath or urinary ethanol is helpful if high levels are found. There may be a disproportionate elevation of serum aspartate transaminase compared to alanine transaminase. Confusingly, the serum ferritin may be very elevated in active heavy drinkers and does not indicate haemochromatosis. Alcoholism is the (often forgotten) most common cause of combined hyperlipidaemia.

There is no substitute for liver biopsy. This allows accurate confirmation of the histological severity and exclusion of other pathologies. Claims that ultrasonography or other imaging techniques of the liver can obviate the need for histological examination have been made but these methods have not been widely adopted.

Table 1 *Mechanisms of alcoholic liver damage*

Type of effect	Mechanism of effect	Mechanism of hepatocyte damage/fibrosis
1. Direct ethanol effect	'Fluidizes' membranes	Altered function of membrane proteins (enzymes/receptors)
2. Acetaldehyde mediated	Formation of protein–acetaldehyde adducts leads to: (i) appearance of 'neo-antigens' (ii) altered protein function including damage to the microtubular system of cytoskeleton (iii) reduction in levels of glutathione (GSH)	(a) Immunologically-mediated cytotoxicity (b) Impaired enzyme and receptor function, impaired protein secretion leading to hepatocyte swelling (c) contributes to oxidative damage (see 4)
3. Induction of a hypermetabolic state	Redox changes (increased [NADH]/[NAD] ratio) associated with ethanol metabolism increases hepatocyte's oxygen requirements	Hypoxic cell necrosis in zone 3 (perivenular zone)—area of sinusoid farthest from arteriole—hence most susceptible to hypoxia
4. Oxidative stress	(i) Increases production of free radicals, via: • microsomal enzyme induction • increased [NADPH]/[NADP] ratio • increased hepatic free iron (ii) Reduces [GSH] (free radical scavenger) (iii) Reduces the activity of 'protective' enzymes that metabolize free radicals	(a)(i)–(iii) combine to induce cell-membrane damage via membrane phospholipid peroxidation (b) Leads to increased susceptibility to other environmental toxins that produce oxidative damage, e.g. paracetamol (acetaminophen)
5. Immune mediated (these may be epiphenomena)	Induces appearance of several 'candidate' antigens including: acetaldehyde adducts, Mallory's hyaline, altered plasma membranes, and liver-specific proteins	(a) Humorally mediated immune attack—antibodies detected to many of these antigens in sera of alcoholic patients (b) Cell-mediated immune attack—evidence of increased lymphocyte-mediated cytotoxicity *in vitro*
6. Proinflammatory effects	(i) Increases cytokine (IL-1, IL-6, TNF) release—probably endotoxin mediated (ii) Increases expression of leucocyte adhesion molecules including: ICAM-1, E-selectin, and VCAM-1. May be secondary to (i), alcohol metabolites or cell damage	(a) TNF directly induces hepatocyte necrosis (b) Neutrophil (alcoholic hepatitis)- or direct lymphocyte (cirrhosis)-mediated cell damage (c) Kupffer-cell infiltration activates fibrogenesis by lipocytes
7. Direct stimulation of fibrosis (in addition to that occurring secondary to hepatocyte necrosis/Kupffer-cell infiltration)	Increases levels of lactate and acetaldehyde	Both shown directly to stimulate collagen-gene transcription by activated lipocytes
8. Factors associated with the development of fatty liver	(i) Increases substrate supply—fatty acids (due to inhibition of β-oxidation and increased hepatic uptake) and glycerol 3-phosphate (ii) Direct stimulation of esterification due to increased activity of phosphatidate phosphohydrolase (iii) Decreases hepatic export of triglyceride as VLDL	Increased [fatty acid] may be cytotoxic—explaining correlation between fatty liver severity and risk of progressive liver disease

ICAM, intercellular adhesion molecule; IL, interleukin; TNF, tumour necrosis factor; VCAM, vascular-cell adhesion molecule; VLDL, very low-density lipoprotein.

Prognosis

Prognosis is related to continuing consumption above all else. In patients with fatty change alone the outlook is excellent, provided patients stop or substantially cut down drinking. It is now becoming clear that fatty change is not 'protective' as was once thought, and patients whose biopsies show fatty change alone may progress to more advanced liver disease with a correspondingly poorer outlook. Clinically and histologically, mild alcoholic hepatitis has a similar prognosis to fatty change. In severe, acute alcoholic hepatitis, whether or not superimposed upon cirrhosis, there is a 12 to 50 per cent mortality within 6 months of presentation. Particularly adverse features are a raised bilirubin level and abnormal blood clotting. This has led to the use of a discriminant functon to help assess prognosis and decide upon treatment (Table 3). Many studies have suggested that among cirrhotics, overall survival at 5 years is around 50 per cent, among abstainers 70 per cent, and in those who continue to drink 35 per cent. A second important prognostic feature is age at presentation. In a recent United Kingdom study, 3-year survival was 77 per cent in patients under the age of 60, and 46 per cent in those presenting over that age. Among cirrhotics, nutrition (possibly reflecting socioeconomic status) influences survival. Thus, in one large group of patients from the United States from largely a lower socioeconomic class, median survival was 33 months, lower than in the majority of other studies from the United States, Europe, or Australia.

Treatment (see also Section 28)

The first and best form of treatment remains withdrawal of alcohol and subsequent long-term abstinence in all patients with liver disease worse than moderate fatty change alone, in whom controlled, very moderate drinking after a period of abstinence may be an option. Good prognostic features include recognition of the alcohol problem by the patient, a supportive family, steady employment, and willingness to accept treatment or help. There is no clear evidence as to which long-term model of treatment is best; certainly an interested team prepared to follow up and support patients is important. No other treatment is required for patients with fatty liver or mild alcoholic hepatitis (on biopsy).

WITHDRAWAL

The syndrome of acute alcohol withdrawal occurs in over 50 per cent of alcohol abusers; at its worst this amounts to the syndrome of delirium tremens, a severe medical emergency. Alcohol withdrawal of patients who have alcoholic liver disease should take place in hospital over 5 to 8 days; in this setting delirium tremens should be almost completely avoidable. Conventionally, the benzodiazepine chlordiazepoxide, 30 to 120 mg/day orally, together with atenolol, 50 to 100 mg/day, are used. Alternatively, chlormethiazole may be given. During the first few days, parenteral vitamin supplements, together with oral thiamine, 200 mg daily, and a high-protein, easily absorbed diet should be given. Complications of the liver disease should be treated appropriately. Patients who present with persistent alcohol-withdrawal fits should initially be treated with intravenous diazepam, up to 50 mg over 2 min; rarely they also need paralysis and ventilation. Severe hallucinations may be treated with haloperidol, 2.5 or 5 mg by mouth, repeated after 4 h if necessary.

SEVERE ALCOHOLIC HEPATITIS

Because of its poor prognosis, several treatments have been evaluated. Recent meta-analysis of more than 10 trials of high-dose corticosteroid treatment in addition to conventional therapy in severe, complicated

Table 2 *Clinical signs of alcoholism*

Undernutrition
 Thin arms and legs (reduced muscle mass), frequently with
  swollen abdomen
 Red tongue
 Dry, scaly, cracked skin (zinc and/or essential fatty-acid
  deficiency)

Endocrine
 Gynaecomastia
 Testicular atrophy
 Loss of body hair
 Signs of pseudoCushing's (red face, hump, striae)

Face/skin
 Parotid enlargement
 Spider naevi
 Paper-money skin
 Easy bruising
 Dupuytren's contracture

Neuromuscular
 Tremor
 Proximal myopathy
 Painful peripheral neuropathy
 Specific neurological syndromes
 Memory loss and cognitive impairment

Cardiovascular
 Hypertension
 Signs of heart failure (cardiomyopathy)
 Hyperdynamic circulation (in advanced liver disease)

Bone
 Unexplained rib fractures on chest radiographs
 Spinal osteoporosis (often in men)

General
 Signs of personal neglect
 Smells of drink

alcoholic hepatitis led to the following recommendation. In patients with a bad prognosis (discriminant function over 32), but who have no overt sepsis or active bleeding, 40 mg oral prednisolone for 21 days probably provides a 20 per cent improvement in mortality. Acute treatment with insulin and glucagon, anabolic steroids, colchicine, enteral or parenteral nutrition, and several 'hepatoprotectve' agents, including (+)-cyanidol-3, thioctic acid, silymarin, and malotilate over periods of up to 1 month following acute presentation of severe alcoholic hepatitis with or without cirrhosis, have all been the subject of one or more trials and have

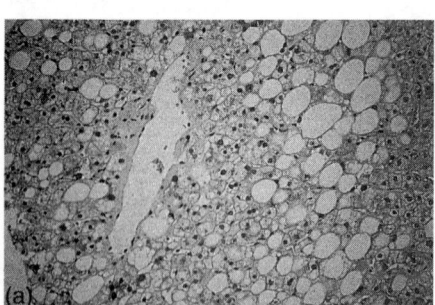
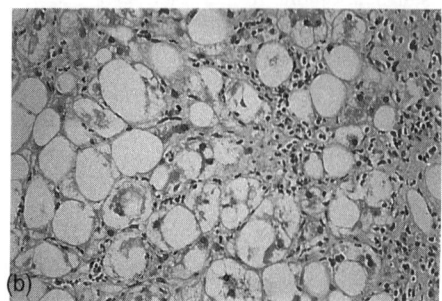
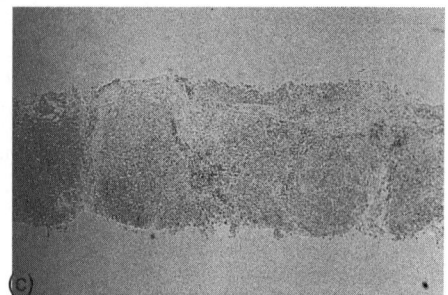

Fig. 3 Histopathology of alcoholic liver disease. (By courtesy of Dr. A. D. Burt.) (a) Macrovesicular steatosis. Perivenular hepatocytes are distended by large lipid droplets (H & E × 80). (b) Alcoholic hepatitis. The hepatocytes show ballooning degeneration and contain Mallory bodies. There is an accompanying inflammatory cell infiltrate and pericellular fibrosis (H & E × 140). (c) Alcoholic cirrhosis. This shows a micronodular pattern. Within some areas there is residual pericellular fibrosis (Van Gieson × 45).

Table 3 *Alcoholic liver disease discriminant function*

Discriminant function (number) = [4.6 × (prothrombin time − control PT) + serum bilirubin (mg%)]

Over 32 = poor prognosis.

shown no benefit with respect to mortality, even after meta-analysis of several trials, and cannot at present be recommended.

In general, attention to nutrition (replacement of vitamin and mineral deficiencies, high protein and carbohydrate) is recommended. No benefit can be discerned for parenteral delivery of nutritional supplementation.

Longer-term treatments of alcoholic liver disease have been difficult to carry out because of high rates of drop-out. One large, controlled trial examined the effect of the antithyroid drug, propylthiouracyl, 300 mg daily for 2 years. Although there were many drop-outs in this study, cumulative mortality in the 157 patients given the drug was 13 per cent versus 25 per cent in those receiving placebo ($p > 0.05$). The clinical benefit appeared to be in those patients with more severe disease. There was a similar number of individuals in both groups who abstained from, or substantially reduced, alcohol consumption. At present propylthiouracyl is not widely used and a repeat controlled trial is urgently needed. No other long-term treatment has shown benefit in a large, well-conducted, controlled trial. Attention has turned to increasing the proportion of abstinent patients and in this context, early studies suggest that fluoxetine may reduce alcohol drinking behaviour by 10 to 15 per cent. Naltrexone, the opioid antagonist, may reduce drinking days and the likelihood of relapse in abstainers. Disulfiram (Antabuse) has no place in modern therapy.

CIRRHOSIS

Treatment of cirrhosis is directed against its complications, particularly portal hypertension, ascites, spontaneous bacterial peritonitis and encephalopathy, and towards their prevention. There are few aspects of the management of alcoholic cirrhosis that are unique to this form of cirrhosis, exept that alcohol withdrawal may complicate the picture.

TRANSPLANTATION

The medical indications for transplantation in alcoholic cirrhosis are similar to those for other endstage liver diseases (see Chapter 14.31). There is one important difference, namely the question of abstention. Whereas in end-stage cirrhosis of other causes the illness is irreversible and likely to be progresssive, this may not be the case in patients with even advanced alcoholic cirrhosis, in whom abstention can dramatically and unpredictably lead to enormous clinical improvement and long-term survival. A recent controlled study in France showed that 2-year survival of patients transplanted for alcoholic liver disease was similar to that in a closely matched group of patients who simply abstained. The advent of transjugular intrahepatic portosystemic stents for long-term treatment of portal hypertension could further reduce the need for transplant. At present, many liver units consider patients for transplantation only after a 6-month period of abstention, both to detect patients in whom transplantation is no longer necessary and to exclude individuals who continue to drink heavily, as their operative risk may well be higher. In future it may be that, despite attendant ethical issues, transplantation will increasingly be used for patients with very severe liver failure accompanying alcoholic hepatitis.

REFERENCES

Day, C.P. and Bassendine, M.F. (1992). Genetic predisposition to alcoholic liver disease. *Gut*, **33**, 1444–7.

Derr, R.F., Porta, E.A., Larkin, E.C., and Ananda Rao, G. (1990). Is alcohol *per se* hepatotoxic? *Journal of Hepatology*, **10**, 381–6.

Hayes, P.C. (ed.) (1993). Alcoholic liver disease. *Clinical Gastroenterology*, **7**, No. 3.

Hislop, W.S. *et al.* (1983). Alcoholic liver disease in Scotland and North-eastern England, presenting features in 510 patients. *Quarterly Journal of Medicine*, **206**, 232–3.

International Group (1981). Alcoholic liver disease: morphological manifestations. *Lancet*, **i**, 707–10.

Lieber, C.S. (1988). Biochemical and molecular basis of alcohol induced injury to liver and other tissues. *New England Journal of Medicine*, **319**, 1639–50.

Poynard, T. *et al.* (1993). Efficacy of transplantation in patients with alcoholic cirrhosis—evaluation using a case control study and simulated controls. *Hepatology*, **18**, 57–60.

Ramond, K.J. *et al.* (1992). A randomised trial of prednisolone in patients with severe alcoholic hepatitis. *New England Journal of Medicine*, **326**, 507–12.

Salaspuro, M. (1991). Epidemiological aspects of alcohol and alcoholic liver disease, ethanol metabolism, and pathogenesis of alcoholic liver injury. In *Oxford textbook of clinical hepatology*, (ed. N. McIntyre, J.-P. Benhamou, J. Bircher, M. Rizzetto, and J. Rodes), pp. 791–810. Oxford University Press.

Zakim, D., Boyer, T.D., and Montgomery, C. (1971). Alcoholic liver disease. In *Hepatology. A textbook of liver disease*, (2nd edn), (ed. D. Zakim and T.D. Boyer), pp. 821–68. Saunders, Philadelphia.

14.29 Cirrhosis, portal hypertension, and ascites

N. McINTYRE AND A. K. BURROUGHS

Cirrhosis is a diffuse 'septal' fibrosis of the liver, associated with regenerative parenchymal nodules and a disturbed intrahepatic circulation; fibrous sheets link portal tracts (portal–portal fibrosis), central zones (central–central), and/or portal tracts and central zones (portal–central). Cirrhosis results from prolonged, widespread, but patchy hepatocellular necrosis, which may have many causes. Necrosis may be absent if the causative factor is no longer operative, or if its effects have been ameliorated.

The most important classification of cirrhosis is based on aetiology (Table 1). The most common and important causes are chronic infection with the hepatitis viruses B and C, and prolonged alcohol abuse.

Clinicians often refer to 'compensated' and 'decompensated' cirrhosis. A patient with compensated cirrhosis has no major problems resulting from the disease. Decompensated cirrhotics show evidence of impaired liver function, including jaundice, hypoalbuminaemia, prolonged prothrombin time, or of a complication of cirrhosis, such as ascites, encephalopathy, or gastrointestinal bleeding. Irreversible decompensation results from the inexorable progress of the disease;

Table 1 *Causes of cirrhosis*

Alcohol
Chronic viral infection—HBV, HBV + HDV, HCV
Drugs and toxins
Autoimmune chronic liver disease
Metabolic disorders
Haemochromatosis
Wilson disease
α_1-antitrypsin deficiency
Cystic fibrosis
Glycogen storage disease
Galactosaemia
Hereditary fructose intolerance
Hereditary tyrosinaemia
Ornithine transcarbamylase deficiency
Byler's disease
Abetalipoproteinaemia
Porphyria

Biliary tract disease (prolonged)
Extrahepatic biliary obstruction
Intrahepatic biliary obstruction:
Primary biliary cirrhosis
Primary sclerosing cholangitis

Venous outflow obstruction
Veno-occlusive disease
Budd–Chiari syndrome
Cardiac failure
Obesity/diabetes mellitus
Intestinal bypass for obesity
Sarcoidosis
Syphilis
Indian childhood cirrhosis
Hereditary haemorrhagic telangiectasia
Cryptogenic
?Schistomiasis, malnutrition, mycotoxins

decompensation may be reversible if brought on by an insult that resolves spontaneously, or one that responds to treatment, bleeding, bacterial infection, acute viral hepatitis, or drug hepatotoxicity for example.

Pathology and pathophysiology

Cirrhotic livers are firm and may be large (even very large), of normal size, or small and shrunken. Their lower edge is blunted, and there may be considerable distortion of the normal shape. The surface is nodular, but the size of the nodules is very variable.

With cirrhosis there is increased resistance to portal blood flow through the liver; the portal venous pressure rises, the portal vein and its tributaries distend, and venous collaterals may develop, allowing some blood to pass from the portal to the systemic circulation without traversing the liver. The spleen enlarges due to the high splenic-vein pressure; it may become very large, particularly in patients with small, shrunken livers.

Histology

The main histological features are diffuse 'septal' fibrosis and regenerative nodules. With 'micronodular' cirrhosis, which is usually obvious in a needle-biopsy specimen, the nodules are uniformly small (and similar in size to the liver lobules). In 'macronodular' cirrhosis the nodules are variable in size and may be more than 10 mm in diameter: it may be difficult to diagnose on needle biopsy as complete nodule formation may not be evident (Fig. 1); other histological features, such as frag-

mentation and the pattern of fibrosis, especially on a reticulin stain, may suggest the correct diagnosis.

Cell necrosis, evidence of active regeneration, and cellular infiltration indicate that the aetiological agent is still active. The nature of that agent may be evident on histological examination, if, for example, special stains are used to demonstrate infection with hepatitis B and D, excessive iron stores, or the presence of α_1-antitrypsin globules.

Clinical features

Cirrhosis can be present without symptoms or signs, and may be found unexpectedly at autopsy or during abdominal surgery. Symptoms alone are not useful pointers to cirrhosis, unless due to a major complication such as ascites, hepatic encephalopathy, or gastrointestinal bleeding (from oesophageal varices), because similar symptoms occur with other liver diseases and with diseases of other systems. Clues to the presence of cirrhosis and its cause often come from other points in the history, for example previous jaundice or 'hepatitis', blood transfusion, intravenous drug abuse, alcoholism, treatment with hepatotoxic drugs, or a strong family history of liver disease.

Symptoms

Jaundice is usually absent in cirrhosis. It suggests either that the causative agent is still active, that there is a reason for decompensation, or that a drug may have caused further impairment of bilirubin metabolism. It is also common after a blood transfusion, owing to the increased bilirubin load.

Fig. 1 (a) Clear-cut micronodular cirrhosis; (b) fibrous septa suggestive of nodule formation compatible with macronodular cirrhosis.

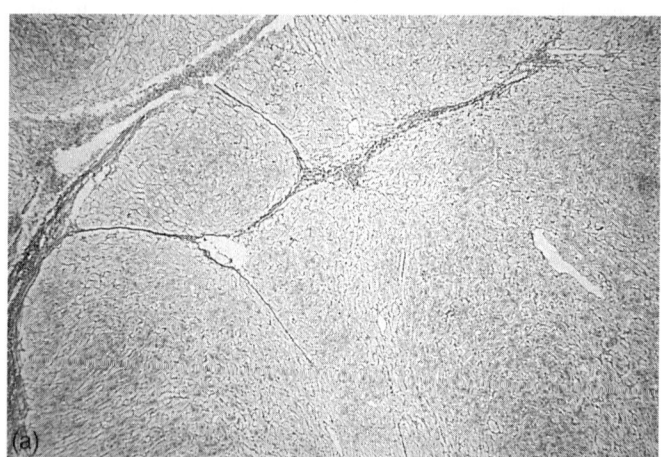

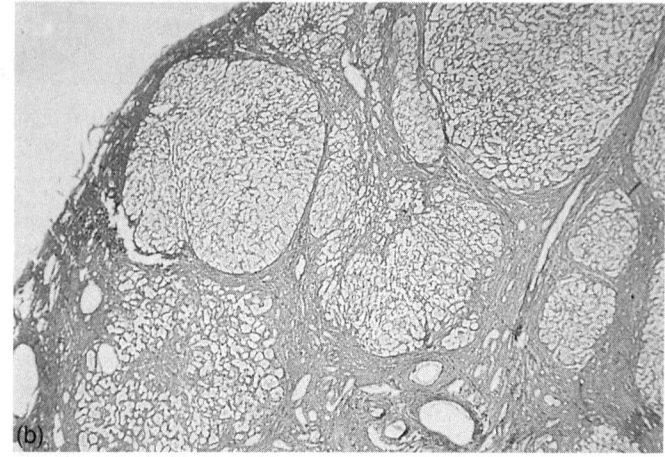

Weakness (asthenia), easy fatiguability, and tiredness are very common and contribute to the general 'malaise' of cirrhosis, though objective evidence of weakness is unusual. They are often present for months or years before diagnosis. There is no effective treatment for these symptoms, which usually improve with specific therapy for the underlying disease.

Anorexia is frequently present; when severe it is an ominous sign unless caused by a drug or another treatable condition. Loss of adipose tissue and muscle, and other features of malnutrition, often result. The cause of the anorexia is unknown. Weight loss is an unusual presenting feature, but is common in end-stage cirrhosis because of anorexia and reduced food intake; in some there is a superimposed hypercatabolic state due to infection or tumour. Weight gain is usually due to simple obesity, or to fluid retention (when the complaint is usually of ankle or abdominal swelling rather than weight gain).

Nausea is also common in cirrhosis; vomiting is unusual unless there is hepatocellular decompensation or another complication. A remediable cause for nausea and vomiting should be sought—alcohol or a drug for example. Clarifying the nature of any vomitus allows early identification and management of small haematemeses. Metoclopramide reduces nausea (and heartburn) in cirrhotics but, as it stimulates aldosterone secretion, it should be used cautiously in patients with fluid retention, for whom domperidone is preferred.

Abdominal pain or discomfort is common, usually in the right upper quadrant or over the right lower ribs (front, side or back). There is rarely an obvious cause, unless a tumour has developed, when spread to the liver surface may cause 'pleuritic' pain (with referral to the shoulder if there is a diaphragmatic involvement). Tenderness over the liver, rather than pain or discomfort, is found occasionally in cirrhosis; some tumours are extremely tender on palpation. Pain or discomfort can also occur with gross splenomegaly. Generalized discomfort may occur with abdominal distension due to ascites, and is related to the rate of fluid accumulation and the tension in the abdominal wall.

Increased stool frequency, with soft or loose stools, is common, particularly in alcoholics, but not usually a presenting symptom. Severe diarrhoea, or a marked alteration in bowel habit, should suggest another cause. Diarrhoea may be a presenting feature of hepatocellular carcinoma; the reason is unknown. Black or very dark stools, in the absence of a dietary cause (iron, bismuth, or Guinness (a dark beer)) suggests upper intestinal bleeding.

Constipation is an unusual consequence of cirrhosis, although it may persist in habitual sufferers. It may precipitate encephalopathy in patients with decompensated cirrhosis and should be treated. It may develop as a result of drug therapy.

In patients with cirrhosis, fluid retention causes swelling of the ankles and legs (or other types of dependent oedema), and/or ascites, and these findings (with no other obvious cause) should suggest the possibility of cirrhosis. The symptoms and complications of ascites are discussed later. Brief episodes of abdominal distension also occur in cirrhotics and are presumably due to intestinal gas.

Dyspnoea may be associated with gross ascites (see below). In patients with some types of cirrhosis it is associated with disorders such as fibrosing alveolitis, pulmonary arteriovenous shunting, and pulmonary hypertension.

Pruritus is an important symptom in primary biliary cirrhosis (in which it is often the presenting symptom, preceding other features of the disease by months or years); it may occur in other types of cirrhosis, but is said to be rare in alcoholic liver disease, even when cholestatic features are present.

Patients with cirrhosis may complain of spontaneous bleeding, from the nose or gums, or of easy bruising. The severity of the complaint is usually related to thrombocytopenia, or to the degree of hepatic decompensation (which affects hepatic synthesis of clotting factors and the fibrinolysis system).

Cirrhotics may develop hepatic encephalopathy (see below). The patients themselves rarely complain of the resulting mental disturbance, but it is a source of distress to relatives and friends.

Fever is common in cirrhosis and may have no obvious cause. It is often due to infection. Rigors suggest bacteraemia. Impotence, more common and more severe in alcoholic cirrhosis, is often accompanied by loss of libido. Women often complain of amenorrhoea or oligomenorrhoea and may be sterile (but many successful pregnancies have been reported). Painful muscle cramps, in the calves, hands, feet, and thighs, are more common in cirrhotics than in normal subjects and appear unrelated to diuretic therapy or to electrolyte disturbances. They may respond to quinine sulphate. Depression is common in patients with liver disease; it is important to identify it as it often responds to appropriate therapy.

Physical signs

Most patients with cirrhosis look well until the late stage of their disease, when muscle wasting and loss of adipose tissue may be prominent features. An acute worsening of appearance should suggest an infection (especially bacteraemia or spontaneous bacterial peritonitis) or gastrointestinal bleeding; a more prolonged deterioration results from hepatic decompensation or the development of hepatocellular carcinoma.

Overt jaundice suggests hepatic decompensation; it is an ominous sign unless there is a reversible precipitating factor. Conjunctival pallor may result from recent gastrointestinal bleeding from varices, or from iron deficiency anaemia due either to chronic blood loss (with portal hypertensive gastropathy, peptic ulcer, or oesophagitis) or to inadequate iron supplementation after an earlier variceal haemorrhage. Evidence of 'dehydration' may be found over the upper body (i.e. with reduced skin turgor over the sternal manubrium), even when there is ascites and/or dependent oedema; this is usually a consequence of diuretic therapy. Postural hypotension may result from dehydration or hypovolaemia.

Cyanosis is uncommon but occurs when there is marked intrapulmonary shunting. Mild clubbing is common in cirrhosis, particularly in primary biliary cirrhosis and when there is associated hypoxia and pulmonary hypertension. Hypertrophic osteoarthropathy may also be present, with periostitis (subperiosteal new bone formation) at the distal diaphyses of the long bones.

Spider naevi should suggest cirrhosis (but are often absent, and are found in other liver diseases); when they are large and numerous, alcoholic liver disease should be suspected. Related signs include white spots, 'paper money' skin, and erythema of the thenar and hypothenar eminences ('liver palms'). Excessive bruising, usually due to mild trauma (often unrecognized), may be noted when hepatocellular function is poor. Petechial haemorrhages are often found over the lower legs, but also on the arms or abdomen (at points of trauma or pressure from tight clothing). They suggest thrombocytopenia due to hypersplenism. A crop of new lesions suggests a fall in the platelet count, due to bacteraemia or disseminated intravascular coagulation (and therefore indicate a need for urgent treatment).

Many cirrhotics, particularly those with primary biliary cirrhosis or haemochromatosis, show widespread melanin pigmentation with local areas of hyperpigmentation, particularly at sites of minor trauma or irritation. Vitiligo occurs with autoimmune chronic liver diseases, and stands against a background of generalized pigmentation (as in primary biliary cirrhosis, for example). Lichen planus, commonly associated with primary biliary cirrhosis, also appears to have a higher prevalence in other types of liver disease.

Gynaecomastia (with palpable and often tender glandular tissue beneath the areola) is found in some males with cirrhosis. It may result from sex hormone imbalance, or as a troublesome side-effect of spironolactone. Testicular atrophy is common in cirrhotic males, particularly those with alcoholic liver disease or haemochromatosis, and is usually accompanied by thinning of body hair and other signs of feminization.

Dupuytren's contracture is more common in alcoholic cirrhotics than in the general population. It is related to alcoholism, not to cirrhosis.

Physical signs may be found in other systems in patients with liver disease. Two signs of particular interest in patients with liver disease are the flapping tremor of hepatic encephalopathy (see Chapter 14.30), and the Kayser–Fleischer ring (see Chapter 11.7), which is a particularly valuable sign of Wilson's disease.

Abdominal examination

The physical signs of ascites are discussed later. Ascites is often associated with peripheral oedema, which, when gross, may involve the abdominal wall and genitalia. Surface venous collaterals are a particularly important sign of cirrhosis and of other types of portal hypertension. Their significance is discussed below in the section on portal hypertension.

Enlargement of the liver or spleen may give rise to localized bulgings of the upper abdominal wall, which are often more evident when the organs move with respiration.

The firm, cirrhotic liver is usually easy to feel when it is enlarged, either across the upper abdomen, in the epigastrium alone, or below the right lower ribs. Its shape may be markedly deformed and this occasionally causes diagnostic confusion. The spleen is often palpable, and may be very large, particularly when the liver is very small; it is not usually palpable in alcoholic cirrhotics. With tense ascites it may be difficult or impossible to feel a large liver and/or spleen, but it is sometimes possible to feel them by 'dipping'.

Percussion is useful for detecting a large liver that cannot be felt, a small liver (when there is resonance above the costal margin), and for identifying the presence of ascites (see later).

Auscultation may reveal an 'arterial bruit' over the liver (suggesting a hepatocellular carcinoma), a 'venous hum' (in patients with portal hypertension and rapid, turbulent flow in collateral veins), or a 'friction rub' over the liver or spleen when the patient breathes deeply. In a cirrhotic a friction rub over the liver suggests tumour invasion of the visceral peritoneum, while a rub over a large spleen suggests splenic infarction.

Investigations (cirrhosis per se)

LIVER FUNCTION TESTS (ABBREVIATIONS FOR ENZYMES ARE EXPLAINED IN CHAPTER 14.25).

Liver 'function' tests are used to detect liver disease, to assess its severity, and to monitor its progress. They are of little value for differential diagnosis. In established cirrhosis the results may be entirely normal.

AST and ALT levels are often normal in cirrhosis if the causative agent is no longer active (e.g. with abstention from alcohol or withdrawal of drugs) or with effective therapy (e.g. immunosuppression in autoimmune cirrhosis).

In alcoholic cirrhosis (and hepatitis) the AST/ALT ratio is often 2 or greater, due in part to a relative reduction of ALT. With alcoholic cirrhosis, serum ALT levels may be normal when there is an obvious elevation of AST; for this reason ALT alone should not be used to screen for liver disease. A ratio in excess of 2 is also seen with other types of cirrhosis, as the AST/ALT ratio tends to rise with the transition from chronic hepatitis to cirrhosis; it therefore has a limited diagnostic value.

While the serum total bilirubin is often normal, there is usually a reduction in the liver's ability to excrete bilirubin. An increase in bilirubin load, with blood transfusion or an episode of haemolysis for example, or the use of drugs that impair bilirubin transport, such as oestrogens or androgenic steroids, may therefore cause an increase in serum bilirubin and obvious jaundice. An increase in bilirubin with no obvious cause suggests hepatic decompensation; it is an important prognostic feature in assessment for transplantation.

In most patients with cirrhosis the serum alkaline phosphatase is either normal or only modestly elevated. With 'biliary' cirrhosis, more marked increases are found, and this has diagnostic relevance.

A low serum albumin in cirrhosis is usually attributed to reduced hepatic albumin synthesis. However, hypoalbuminaemia may be present with ascites due to the expanded extracellular volume; the albumin pool may be increased and synthesis normal or even high. Other factors also affect plasma albumin—gastrointestinal or renal loss, increased catabolism, altered vascular permeability or overhydration for example; albumin levels must therefore be interpreted with caution in cirrhotics.

OTHER BIOCHEMICAL TESTS

Plasma electrolytes are often abnormal in cirrhosis and may change rapidly with complications such as bleeding, infections, fluid retention, and diuretic therapy, and with inappropriate use of fluid and electrolytes. Careful monitoring is necessary.

Hyponatraemia is common and usually results from excessive administration of water (because of a reduced ability to excrete a water load), or with diuretic therapy (due to a 'differential' loss of salt and water). Hypernatraemia is less common but can occur with gastrointestinal bleeding (due to an urea diuresis), use of lactulose, or with severe fluid restriction and increased insensible water loss.

Serum potassium concentrations are usually normal in cirrhosis. Low concentrations result from diuretic therapy, a poor diet, vomiting, or diarrhoea. Potassium-losing diuretics, such as frusemide, should be stopped and potassium chloride given, preferably orally. If a diuretic is needed, spironolactone should be used. Hyperkalaemia occurs with renal failure, and with the use of spironolactone or other 'potassium-retaining' diuretics such as amiloride. Such drugs should not be given together, nor should they be given with potassium supplements. Hypokalaemia and hyperkalaemia are both potentially dangerous; the serum potassium requires careful monitoring, particularly in those on diuretic therapy.

Urinary Na and K measurements are valuable in patients with fluid retention—to assess the need for, and the efficacy of, diuretic therapy; the dose of spironolactone should be increased until the urinary Na:K ratio is greater than one.

Hypomagnesaemia occurs in cirrhotics, particularly alcoholics and decompensated patients, but is not usually accompanied by clinical evidence of magnesium deficiency. The mechanism is unclear but increased urinary loss may result from secondary hyperaldosteronism, or the use of loop diuretics such as frusemide.

In well-compensated cirrhosis the serum urea is usually normal. In decompensated cirrhosis, urea production falls and the serum urea is then low. Mild renal failure can occur without the serum urea rising above the normal range; this can be identified if there is a gradual rise in urea, or if there is an increased serum creatinine. Renal failure is common in cirrhosis, due to dehydration (often associated with diuretic therapy), hypotension (with bleeding or infection), or the development of the hepatorenal syndrome.

Fasting blood glucose is usually normal in cirrhotics, but most are insulin resistant, are intolerant to an oral glucose load, and have postprandial hyperglycaemia. Overt diabetes mellitus, with a high fasting glucose, is more common in cirrhotics than in the general population.

The serum total cholesterol is normal in most cirrhotics. Lecithin cholesterol acyltransferase (**LCAT**), a plasma enzyme secreted by the liver, catalyses formation of cholesteryl ester in plasma. With end-stage disease, plasma LCAT activity falls; there is a decrease in cholesteryl ester and total cholesterol, while free cholesterol is normal or increased. In primary biliary cirrhosis the total cholesterol tends to rise, as in other forms of biliary obstruction, and may reach very high levels.

HAEMATOLOGICAL INVESTIGATIONS

Routine haematological values may be normal in cirrhosis. Mild anaemia is common, due in part to hypersplenism. More severe anaemia results from overt bleeding or from iron deficiency (see above). On blood films, target cells are usually visible, and in rare cases acanthocytes are found in association with features of haemolytic anaemia.

The anaemia of cirrhosis is characteristically macrocytic (the mean corpuscular volume (**MCV**) may be very high in alcoholics). As a result, the MCV is often normal despite marked iron deficiency. Routine measurement of serum iron and total iron-binding capacity is therefore of particular value in cirrhosis, and may also identify haemochromatosis as the cause. Serum ferritin is of less value for identifying iron deficiency as it may be normal or high due to hepatocellular damage.

The white-cell count tends to fall in patients with cirrhosis, due to hypersplenism, and may be an important factor in their susceptibility to bacterial infections. With such infections there may be an increase in the neutrophil count, but it may remain within the normal range.

The platelet count is usually low in cirrhosis, also due to hypersplenism, and may fall to very low levels. Other factors should be suspected when the platlelet count is relatively high in a patient with cirrhosis or portal hypertension without cirrhosis, for example a tumour, infection, or myeloproliferative disorder. Changes in coagulation factors are considered in Section 22.

Diagnosis and differential diagnosis

The main diagnostic tasks are (i) to establish that cirrhosis (and not another condition) accounts for the clinical findings; (ii) to identify the cause; and (iii) to search for complications, including those associated with the underlying cause.

ESTABLISHING THAT CIRRHOSIS ACCOUNTS FOR THE CLINICAL FINDINGS

When a patient presents with clinical signs of liver disease the first step is to establish whether acute or chronic liver disease is present. The mode of presentation may be of little value: acute disorders such as viral or drug-induced hepatitis may have few symptoms and signs; patients with cirrhosis may present with jaundice and malaise. However, some physical signs are strongly suggestive of cirrhosis (e.g. spider naevi, liver palms, gynaecomastia, ascites and oedema, and abdominal venous collaterals).

Diseases other than cirrhosis presenting with a palpable liver and/or spleen are listed in Table 2. Disorders associated with portal hypertension and/or ascites are considered in the relevant sections below.

A definitive diagnosis of cirrhosis requires a liver biopsy, which may also establish the cause. Routine percutaneous liver biopsy is contraindicated when the prothrombin time is prolonged or the platelet count low. The use of alternative methods of liver biopsy (transjugular, plugged, or open biopsy) in high-risk patients is rarely justified simply to establish the presence of cirrhosis. A working diagnosis of cirrhosis may still be made on clinical grounds, with strong confirmatory evidence from ultrasonography, computerized tomographic (**CT**) scanning (see Chapter 14.20), or peritoneoscopy. Oesophageal varices on endoscopy suggest cirrhosis, but there may be another cause of portal hypertension (see below).

It may be important to distinguish between chronic hepatitis and cirrhosis, particularly if the underlying cause is treatable, as it may be possible to prevent progression from chronic hepatitis to cirrhosis, and thus to prevent the complications of cirrhosis. Unfortunately, many patients who are considered to have chronic active hepatitis on histological examination are already cirrhotic.

IDENTIFYING THE CAUSE OF CIRRHOSIS

It is important to establish the cause of cirrhosis; it dictates the choice and monitoring of treatment and may lead to a search for the same disease in relatives or contacts. A rigorous diagnostic approach is needed; when it is half-hearted, less common conditions such as Wil-

Table 2 *Other conditions often presenting with a palpable liver and/or spleen*

Some other forms of congestive splenomegaly
Primary biliary cirrhosis
Sclerosing cholangitis
Biliary atresia
Chronic active hepatitis
Graft-versus-host disease
Granulomatous hepatitis
Storage disorders
Cystic fibrosis?
Schistosomiasis
Nodular regenerative hyperplasia
Gaucher's disease
Niemann–Pick disease
Hurler's syndrome
Lymphomas and leukaemias
Extramedullary haemopoiesis
Histiocytosis X
Leishmaniasis
Amyloid

*Other conditions with a palpable spleen alone**
Congestive splenomegaly
Portal venous obstruction/thrombosis
Splenic tumours and cysts
Infections (infectious mononucleosis, septicaemias, bacterial endocarditis, tuberculosis, malaria, trypanosomiasis, AIDS, congenital syphilis, splenic abscess)
Rheumatoid arthritis (Felty's syndrome)
Systemic lupus erythematosus
Immune haemolytic anaemias, thrombocytopenias, and neutropenias

*See also Chapter 22.5.4.

son's disease, haemochromatosis, and autoimmune disease may be missed, and treatment delayed. When a firm diagnosis cannot be made the patient should be referred to a specialist unit. It is also important to realize that in an individual patient more than one factor may be causing hepatic damage; for example, hepatitis B and C may coexist, either of these viral infections may occur in association with schistosomiasis or alcoholic liver disease, and cirrhosis of any cause may be complicated by the use of hepatotoxic drugs.

The cause of cirrhosis is sometimes obvious on clinical grounds (see above) or it may be identified from biochemical and serological investigations (see Table 3). Liver biopsy can establish some causes of cirrhosis with a high degree of probability if specific stains are used, or if chemical measurements are made on the tissues (Table 4).

SEARCHING FOR COMPLICATIONS OF THE CIRRHOSIS

Major complications
Portal hypertension and ascites

Two of the most important complications of cirrhosis, portal hypertension and ascites, are major problems in their own right and are caused by conditions other than cirrhosis. They are considered in detail below.

Hepatic encephalopathy

Hepatic encephalopathy, another major complication of cirrhosis, is considered in Chapter 14.30. It is not the only cause of cerebral disturbance in cirrhotics; others include drugs, to some of which cirrhotics may be unduly sensitive, alcohol, hypotension, and renal failure. Alcoholics may develop Wernicke–Korsakoff syndrome due to thiamin deficiency, alcohol withdrawal problems (see Chapter 24.19) or hypoglycaemia (rarely). It is particularly important to detect a subdural haematoma, which may result from unrecognized trauma.

Table 3 *'Routine' investigations for identifying the cause of cirrhosis*

Investigation	Cause
HBV, HDV and HCV markers	Chronic viral infection
ANA (to ds-DNA); SMA (antiactin); LKM-1 Ab; Ab to SLA	Autoimmune chronic hepatitis (see Chapter 14.27.1)
Antimitochondrial antibodies (M2, M4, M8, M9) (ELISA techniques for purified AMA)	Primary biliary cirrhosis (see Chapter 14.27.2)
Serum copper and caeruloplasmin, urinary copper, Kayser-Fleischer rings	Wilson's disease
Serum iron and iron-binding capacity, serum ferritin	Haemochromatosis
Serum α_1-antitrypsin, α_1-chymotrypsin	α_1-Antitrypsin and α_1-chymotrypsin deficiency
Detailed drug history	Drug-induced cirrhosis (see Chapter 14.34)

AMA, antimitochondrial antibody; ANA, antinuclear antibody; ELISA, enzyme-linked immunosolvent assay; SLA, soluble liver antigen; SMA, smooth muscle antibody.

Table 4 *Special tests that may be made on liver tissue in investigation of cirrhosis*

Special stains
Perl's stain for iron
DPAS (periodic acid–Schiff stain after diastase digestion) for α_1-antitrypsin globules
PAS (without diastase digestion) for glycogen

Biochemical measurements
Copper (Wilson's disease, Indian childhood cirrhosis)
Iron (haemochromatosis)
Glycogen
Fructose 1-phosphate aldolase (hereditary fructose intolerance)

Hepatocellular carcinoma

One of the most serious complications of longstanding cirrhosis is hepatocellular carcinoma (see Chapter 14.32). The prognosis is poor, and the best treatment is resection if the tumour can be detected early. For this reason, patients with cirrhosis should, ideally, be screened at regular intervals (4- to 6-monthly) with measurement of serum alpha-fetoprotein and the use of ultrasound or CT scanning. Up to 15 per cent of cirrhotics without a carcinoma have an increased concentration of serum alpha-fetoprotein, but the elevation is generally minor compared with that seen with hepatocellular carcinoma. A very high level, or a gradual increase, should lead to a search for a hepatocellular carcinoma.

Infections

An acute deterioration is usually due to bacteraemia or gastrointestinal bleeding. Both conditions may cause tachycardia, hypotension, tachypnoea, mild fever and/or confusion, and impaired renal function with oliguria. With bacterial infections the white cell count may be lower than expected, due to hypersplenism. Fresh petechiae suggest bacteraemia; there may be evidence of intravascular coagulation. Volume expansion may be necessary to maintain the blood pressure. Cultures should be taken of blood, urine, ascites, and intravenous drip lines and insertion sites. As soon as bacterial infection is suspected the patient should be started on a third-generation cephalosporin. The response to antibiotics may be the best 'diagnostic test', to be confirmed later by the cultures.

More gradual deterioration, over days or weeks, may also result from infections such as spontaneous bacterial peritonitis, or urinary or chest infections.

Other complications of cirrhosis

A number of other complications of cirrhosis have been mentioned earlier, including fluid and electrolyte disturbances, anaemia, cardiopulmonary problems, diabetes mellitus, and feminization.

The prevalence of peptic ulcer is higher in cirrhosis than in the general population. The prevalence of gallstones is also higher; the stones are pigment stones, which appear to cause fewer problems (e.g. biliary obstruction) than cholesterol stones.

Management

Many causes of cirrhosis have specific treatments, including immunosuppression for autoimmune chronic hepatitis, penicillamine for Wilson's disease, venesection for haemochromatosis, and abstention from alcohol for alcoholic cirrhosis. These are discussed in other chapters. Patients with cirrhosis, regardless of cause, require regular follow-up in order to identify complications (see above), new symptoms, or changes in physical signs or in the results of laboratory tests.

PATIENT EDUCATION

Patients, or their relatives, should be advised to seek help quickly for deepening jaundice, fever/rigors, haematemesis and/or melaena, ankle or abdominal swelling, or signs of confusion, or if other symptoms and signs cause concern. They must appreciate the value of prompt treatment for these problems.

Patients with cirrhosis are often given erroneous advice. Their daily life should be disrupted as little as possible. However, constraints are inevitable in certain circumstances. They are more likely to follow advice if the reasons are clearly explained. Written instructions about their disease are helpful.

DIET

Most cirrhotics should eat a normal mixed diet. Obese patients should lose weight; obesity causes abnormal liver function tests and, rarely, significant liver damage. Fat restriction is necessary only for troublesome steatorrhoea, which is uncommon in cirrhosis. Low-fat diets are unpalatable, compound problems with anorexia, and reduce intake of fat-soluble vitamins. Furthermore, deficiency of essential fatty acids may impair platelet aggregation and contribute to a worsening of renal function; the daily fat intake should therefore contain some corn or safflower oil.

The dietary management of ascites and oedema is considered below, and the management of hepatic encephalopathy in Chapter 14.30. Although short-term protein restriction may be needed for acute attacks of encephalopathy, long-term restriction should be avoided in order to avoid protein depletion.

Patients with alcoholic hepatitis and/or cirrhosis should abstain from alcohol. There is no evidence that abstention significantly affects outcome in non-alcoholic cirrhotics who drink in moderation.

REST AND PHYSICAL ACTIVITY

Many cirrhotics suffer from asthenia and tire easily; they may reduce physical activity. However, reduction of muscle mass with inactivity may increase the sense of fatigue with mild effort. Prolonged bedrest should be avoided. Patients with well-compensated cirrhosis should exercise, to promote general well-being and delay bone thinning, particularly common in primary biliary cirrhosis and in those on long-term steroids. They should also be encouraged to remain at work, but patients with encephalopathy, overt or latent, should not make major decisions, or do work involving risk of serious physical injury.

SEXUAL ACTIVITY

Impotence and loss of libido are symptoms of cirrhosis; impotence appears more common and more severe in alcoholic patients with cirrhosis than in non-alcoholics and may improve with abstinence. In women, fatigue and depression seem more important causes of sexual dysfunction than cirrhosis *per se*; women with cirrhosis can be reassured that they can maintain normal sexual relations if they so wish.

Although there have been many successful pregnancies in women with cirrhosis, there is a significant risk to the mother and to the fetus.

FOREIGN TRAVEL AND RESIDENCE IN UNDERDEVELOPED AREAS

Cirrhotics travelling abroad should appreciate the potential dangers and financial implications. They should avoid places where treatment facilities are poor or unavailable, or where the risks of contracting viral hepatitis or AIDS after blood transfusion are high. They should carry an adequate supply of essential drugs, and a summary of their medical history; a MedicAlert bracelet is a sensible precaution. When patients with portal hypertension must live in an underdeveloped area, portal–systemic shunt surgery should be considered, as this reduces the risk of variceal bleeding.

Cirrhotics can take standard prophylaxis for malaria, and can be actively immunized against bacterial and viral diseases, but may have a reduced immune response. Non-immune cirrhotics should probably be vaccinated against hepatitis A and B, particularly if visiting endemic areas, as an acute hepatitis will cause more severe illness in a cirrhotic.

DRIVING AND LIVER DISEASE

Patients with overt encephalopathy should be discouraged or prevented from driving. Most patients with compensated cirrhosis can drive safely. However, studies by neuropsychologists suggest that some patients, particularly alcoholic cirrhotics, with portal hypertension but without electro-encephalographic changes of encephalopathy, are unfit to drive. Further studies are needed in this area.

DRUGS AND LIVER DISEASE

Patients with cirrhosis often need to take medication. All prescriptions should be considered carefully in cirrhotics as many drugs are removed, metabolized, and/or excreted by the liver. Clearly, drugs that often cause liver disease are best avoided; they may cause diagnostic confusion and may have a greater hepatotoxic effect in cirrhotics.

Drugs with a high extraction ratio are removed in relatively large amounts during their first passage through the liver (e.g. propranolol, labetalol, pentazocine, morphine, lidocaine, verapamil, nifedipine, and ergotamine tartrate). When they are given orally to normal subjects a relatively small amount of the drug enters the systemic circulation. However, in cirrhotics (with portal–systemic shunting) the systemic availability of these drugs may be markedly increased and toxicity may result; ergot derivatives are particularly dangerous and may cause peripheral gangrene. The oral dose of these drugs needs to be reduced. Drugs that are metabolized by the liver, even if they are removed slowly, tend to accumulate when liver function is impaired; repeated doses of such drugs should be given at less frequent intervals. Narcotics, such as morphine and pethidine, and benzodiazepines have additional dangers in cirrhosis because many patients are unduly sensitive to them.

For simple analgesia, paracetamol, despite its dose-dependent hepatotoxicity, is the drug of choice but no more than 3 g a day (six tablets) should be given on a long-term basis. Codeine is also useful, as it has a smaller first-pass uptake than most other opiates, but it can accumulate and cause cerebral depression. Aspirin and other non-steroidal anti-inflammatory drugs should be avoided: they cause gastrointestinal bleeding, have an antiplatelet effect, and are toxic to the kidneys, particularly in patients with fluid retention. D-Propoxyphene is of doubtful efficacy and is hepatotoxic.

For hypertension, β-blockers are the drugs of choice, having an additional, beneficial effect on portal hypertension. Little adjustment of dosage is required for atenolol or propanolol, despite their marked first-pass hepatic uptake; however, treatment should be started with a low dose. Calcium antagonists such as diltiazem, nifedipine, nitrendipine, and verapamil can be used, but they tend to show a marked first-pass effect, and small doses should be used initially (a quarter to a half of the normal dose). Thiazide diuretics should be avoided: they enhance kaliuresis, may precipitate encephalopathy, and impair glucose tolerance. Methyldopa should not be used because of the risk of further liver damage.

Subclinical vitamin deficiencies are relatively common. Routine prescription of water-soluble vitamins is sensible as they are harmless in normal doses, but large doses of nicotinamide or nicotinic acid should be avoided. Of the fat-soluble vitamins, A is potentially hepatotoxic, and D and K can cause other problems.

Patients with cirrhosis should be discouraged from taking herbal medicines on the advice of friends or homeopathic practitioners.

It is considered that oral contraceptive pills are contraindicated in cirrhosis. Oestrogens reduce the excretory capacity for bilirubin and other anions, but jaundice does not appear until it falls below 10 per cent of normal. Long-term use of the pill is associated with an increased (though small) risk of hepatic-vein thrombosis, gallstones, hepatic adenoma, and hepatocellular carcinoma); it is best avoided in cirrhosis, particularly in jaundiced women or those with marked abnormalities of other liver function tests. If a woman insists on using it, a low-dose oestrogen or a progestogen-only preparation can be tried after the risks are explained. Serum bilirubin and aminotransferases should be monitored regularly (weekly for 1 month, monthly for the next 3 months, and every 3 months thereafter): if the test results deteriorate the drug should be stopped; the liver function tests are likely to improve on stopping treatment.

Similarly, hormone replacement therapy can be tried, with careful monitoring, if menopausal symptoms are particularly severe or if there is osteoporosis.

SURGERY IN PATIENTS WITH CIRRHOSIS

Surgical operations are potentially more dangerous in cirrhotics, the risk increasing with the degree of hepatic decompensation. Surgery should only be done in decompensated cirrhotics when there a clear and important indication. Furthermore, the good results now being achieved with liver transplantation have changed the approach to the management of end-stage liver disease. If transplantation is feasible, every effort should be made to maintain the patient in as good a condition as possible until the operation can be done. Procedures that might jeopardize transplantation should be carried out only if they are for life-threatening conditions.

Patients must be told the truth about their illness. They may need to attend to their affairs, and discussion about liver transplantation is impossible unless patients recognize the seriousness of their condition; occasionally, patients refuse transplantation because they have been given an overoptimistic view of their prognosis.

Portal hypertension

Anatomy and physiology of the portal circulation

Venous blood from the gut, spleen, and pancreas drains into the portal vein, passes through the liver, and enters the inferior vena cava via several hepatic veins. This portal circulation is represented in Fig. 2, which shows the large tributaries of the portal vein and the main sites of obstruction.

Portal vein flow is about 900 to 1200 ml/min, hepatic arterial flow about 500 to 700 ml/min. The portal venous pressure is normally about 5 to 10 mmHg, only a little higher than that in the inferior vena cava. Vascular resistance to portal flow is thus very low. Little is known about the factors controlling splanchnic and thus portal blood flow; the increase after meals is proportional to the increase in splanchnic arterial flow.

Definition and causes of portal hypertension

Portal hypertension may be arbitrarily defined as an increase in resting portal venous pressure above 12 mmHg, but it may rise as high as 50 mmHg. It results from increased resistance to portal flow and/or an increase in portal flow. There are many causes (listed in Table 5). Portal hypertension is usually classified as 'presinusoidal', 'sinusoidal', or 'postsinusoidal', on the basis of aetiology, when this is known. In difficult cases, measurements of hepatic venous pressure are useful for determining the site of resistance; the hepatic venous-pressure gradient (**HPVG**) is the difference between the wedged hepatic venous pressure (**WHVP**) and the free hepatic venous pressure. With presinusoidal portal hypertension, due to a blocked portal vein or narrowing of the smaller intrahepatic portal vein branches, the WHVP is normal. Portal hypertension in cirrhosis is considered to be 'sinusoidal' (with a high WHVP and HPVG), but the exact site of the increased resistance is not clear; it may be due to pruning of portal vein branches, narrowing of sinusoids due to hepatocyte enlargement or collagen deposition in the space of Disse, or to distortion of the intrahepatic vasculature due to fibrosis and/ or nodule formation. Varices in the oesophagus tend to develop in cirrhosis when the HPVG rises above 12 mmHg.

Consequences of portal hypertension

An elevated portal venous pressure distends the veins proximal to the block and the spleen enlarges. Capillary pressure rises in organs drained by the obstructed vein; fluid exudation and lymph flow both increase. Small anastomoses connecting the portal and systemic circulations may enlarge (often markedly) because of the increased portal pressure and allow portal blood to pass directly into the systemic circulation. The extent of collateral flow is variable, as are the routes taken by the diverted blood. Patients with cirrhosis tend to have a high cardiac output,

Fig. 2 A diagrammatic representation of the main tributaries of the portal vein, and the sites of obstruction to portal flow causing portal hypertension.

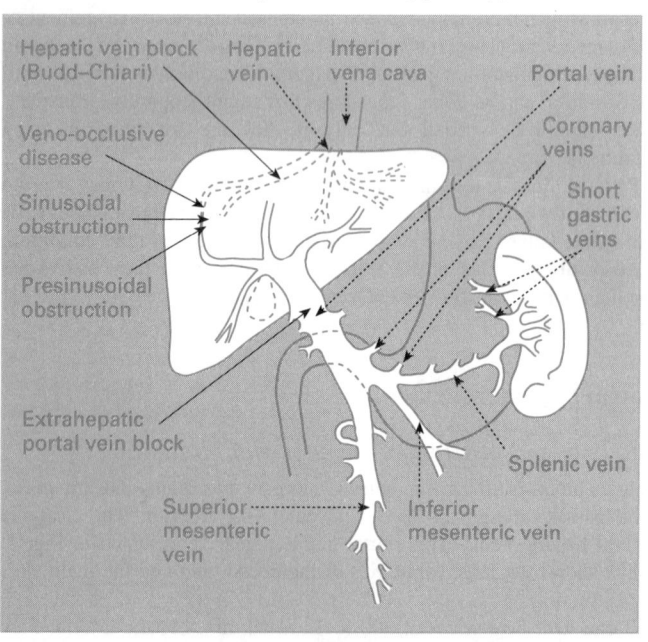

Table 5 *Causes of portal hypertension*

Extrahepatic obstruction of portal vein and its tributaries
Portal-vein thrombosis (idiopathic, umbilical and portal sepsis, malignancy, hypercoagulable states, pancreatitis)
Splenic-vein thrombosis

Hepatic venous outflow 'obstruction'
Suprahepatic
  Budd–Chiari syndrome (see Table 10)
  Constrictive pericarditis
  Right heart failure
Smaller hepatic veins and venules
  Veno-occlusive disease (due to ingestion of pyrrolizidine alkaloids; antileukaemic drugs, radiation)
  Sclerosing hyaline necrosis

Hepatic causes (in some cases there may be presinusoidal and sinusoidal resistance to flow)
Presinusoidal
  Schistosomiasis
  Idiopathic portal hypertension
  Primary biliary cirrhosis (early stage)
  Sarcoid
  Myeloproliferative diseases
  Arsenic, vinyl chloride
  Fibropolycystic disease (including congenital hepatic fibrosis)
Sinusoidal
  Cirrhosis
  Chronic active hepatitis
  Alcoholic hepatitis and fatty liver
  Partial nodular transformation

Increased hepatic blood flow (rare causes)
Tropical splenomegaly syndrome
Haematological and other conditions with massive splenomegaly
Hepatoportal arteriovenous fistula

and increased splanchnic blood flow may maintain an elevated portal pressure despite the development of large anastomoses.

There are three main types of anastomosis:

1. Veins at the oesophagogastric junction shunt blood from the left gastric and short gastric veins into the inferior oesophageal plexus and on to the superior vena cava via the azygous system. 'Varices' are dilated submucosal veins projecting into the lumen of the oesophagus and stomach; they often cause gastro-intestinal bleeding. Anastomoses at the anorectal junction rarely cause bleeding.
2. Venous channels from retroperitoneal viscera may communicate directly with systemic veins on the posterior abdominal wall.
3. The obliterated umbilical vein and paraumbilical veins may open up, allowing blood to pass from the left branch of the portal vein to the umbilicus and thence into abdominal-wall veins. Anterior abdominal-wall collaterals also occur where adhesions exist between abdominal viscera and the parietal peritoneum (e.g. at surgical incisions), or at ileostomy or colostomy sites. Localized varices, colonic for example, may be related to previous surgical operations.

Thrombosis of individual tributaries of the portal vein causes local venous hypertension; with splenic-vein block, oesophageal and gastric varices may result from short gastric collaterals. When hepatic veins are occluded (Budd–Chiari syndrome), collaterals open up within the liver; blood tends to be diverted through the caudate lobe whose short hepatic veins drain directly into the inferior vena cava.

Clinical signs of portal hypertension

Patients may show physical signs associated with the underlying disease process (e.g. hepatomegaly, jaundice, spider naevi), or with complications of portal hypertension (e.g. ascites, hepatic encephalopathy, or haemorrhage).

The spleen is usually palpable, and may be very large in young patients, in patients with extrahepatic portal block, and in those with small, shrunken livers. In alcoholics the spleen is less often palpable than in other forms of cirrhosis.

Prominent abdominal-wall veins are often found with portal hypertension, and are easier to see if the skin of the abdominal wall is stretched. Veins radiating away from the umbilicus are a valuable diagnostic sign as they indicate that the block is distal to the main portal vein branches (usually due to cirrhosis); they disappear if the main portal vein subsequently becomes thrombosed.

With simple, extrahepatic, portal-vein block there are no abdominal-wall collaterals (as the pressure in the left branch of the portal vein is not elevated). However, if abdominal surgery has been performed, adhesions between viscera and the abdominal wall may result in the development of surface collaterals. Such collaterals radiate out from the scar and can result from intrahepatic portal hypertension or from portal-vein block; unlike true umbilical collaterals they indicate only a high portal pressure, not the site of the block.

Prominent abdominal-wall veins also result on the side of an ileofemoral block, or with inferior vena caval obstruction (when they are bilateral and may be visible over the back). When hepatomegaly and ascites are present with signs of inferior vena caval obstruction they suggest coexisting obstruction of hepatic veins (the Budd–Chiari syndrome), which may also cause narrowing of the cava due to pressure from an enlarged caudate lobe. The sudden development of 'umbilical' collaterals in a patient with cirrhosis suggests an acute hepatic-vein block; 'inferior vena caval' collaterals suggest a blocked cava. Both conditions can be a consequence of hepatocellular carcinoma, which can also cause portal venous obstruction.

A venous hum, loudest during inspiration, is sometimes heard over large upper abdominal collaterals ('Cruveilhier–Baumgarten syndrome') and there may be an accompanying thrill.

Investigation of portal hypertension

When portal hypertension is suspected, endoscopy should be done to look for oesophageal and gastric varices; they confirm the diagnosis. If oesophageal varices are large (in excess of 5 mm in diameter), blue, or have red wheals or cherry-red spots on their surface, there is an increased risk of bleeding. Endoscopy may also reveal the features of portal hypertensive gastropathy; in its most severe form, which causes chronic anaemia or frank bleeding, red spots similar to petechiae are seen, particularly in the antrum and fundus.

In a patient with splenomegaly and/or prominent abdominal-wall veins, but without varices, portal hypertension can be confirmed by direct measurement of portal pressure, by splenic puncture or transhepatic cannulation of a portal vein branch. Measurement of WHVP and HVPG might also help, but the WHVP is not elevated if the portal hypertension is presinusoidal. Intravariceal pressure, which is slightly lower than portal pressure, can be measured endoscopically. All these techniques require special facilities.

Alternatively, other evidence of diseases causing portal hypertension can be sought. Liver biopsy is particularly useful as it may reveal cirrhosis (and its cause), hepatic outflow obstruction, schistosomiasis, or congenital hepatic fibrosis. An apparently normal biopsy may be found with idiopathic portal hypertension, partial nodular transformation, or with macronodular cirrhosis, but the most likely cause of portal hypertension with a normal biopsy is extrahepatic portal venous obstruction.

The site of the block to portal flow can be demonstrated by examining the venous phase of a coeliac or superior mesenteric arteriogram, by splenic portography following injection of dye into the splenic pulp (the splenic pressure can be measured at the same time), or by retrograde portography (via a hepatic vein). Both techniques give information about the extent and direction of flow through collaterals.

In skilled hands, ultrasound and CT are useful. They may show the characteristic changes of portal hypertension and give clues to its cause (Chapter 14.20). Doppler ultrasound examination gives information about the direction of flow in individual vessels, and allows quantitation of blood flow in major vessels. Magnetic resonance imaging is also valuable for investigating the hepatic vasculature.

Catheterization of the hepatic vein with venography is helpful when hepatic-vein block or idopathic portal hypertension are suspected, as characteristic venograms have been described. Special investigations allow measurement of hepatic blood flow, or the study of the collateral circulation (e.g. azygos venous flow, or the concentration in the systemic blood of substances injected into the portal veins). They are rarely required in clinical practice.

Management of portal hypertension

Patients with portal hypertension suffer complications from the high portal pressure, or the development of collaterals allowing intestinal venous blood to bypass the liver. Gastrointestinal bleeding, ascites, and hepatic encephalopathy are common and serious complications.

GASTROINTESTINAL BLEEDING

The most important source of bleeding is bleeding from oesophageal varices; a varix explodes as a result of increased pressure, an increase in size, and thinning of its wall.

Other sources of bleeding are gastric varices, portal hypertensive gastropathy, sclerotherapy ulcers which usually cause only minor bleeding, peptic ulcers (which are more frequent in cirrhotic patients) and oesophageal or gastric erosions, which are common in alcoholics and which may result from ingestion of non-steroidal anti-inflammatory drugs. Bleeding from erosions may be more severe with portal hypertension because of the high intravascular pressure.

Frank haemorrhage from any of these sources causes haematemesis and/or melaena, and other clinical features of acute blood loss, the severity depending on the amount and rapidity of blood loss. Bleeding may be relatively mild; variceal bleeding can be torrential. Bleeding from rectal varices is rare.

Diagnostic endoscopy is mandatory when portal hypertension is a possibility, as identification of the source directly influences therapy. If endoscopy is delayed for more than 24 h it may be impossible to identify the source of bleeding. Early endoscopy, within a few hours and after resuscitation, nearly always reveals the source, even if bleeding has stopped. Delirium tremens must be controlled before endoscopy, using intravenous chlormethiazole; it has a short half-life and is easily titrated.

A definitive endoscopic diagnosis of bleeding varices is made if there is: a venous (non-pulsatile) spurt, or venous ooze from a varix; a white 'fibrin–platelet' plug on the varix; or an adherent blood clot, which is rare.

If these signs are absent a presumptive diagnosis of variceal bleeding should be made if varices are present and no other lesions are seen in the stomach or duodenum. If blood obscures the view, or if more than one potential bleeding source is seen, further endoscopy should be done if rebleeding occurs. Gastric varices account for no more than 10 per cent of bleeding in cirrhotics, but the diagnosis is more difficult to establish. Non-variceal sources may account for up to 30 per cent of cases.

Treatment of acute variceal haemorrhage

Acute variceal haemorrhage is often severe and there may be repeated bleeding over days or weeks. Ideally it should be treated by an experi-

Table 6 *Pugh-Child's grading of the severity of liver disease*

Clinical and biochemical measurements	Points scored for increasing abnormality		
	1	2	3
Encephalopathy*	None	1 and 2	3 and 4
Ascites	Absent	Slight	Moderate
Bilirubin (μmol/l)	34	34–51	> 51
Albumin (g/l)	> 35	28–35	< 28
Prothrombin (s prolonged)	1–4	4–6	> 6
For primary biliary cirrhosis bilirubin (μmol/l)	< 68	68–170	> 170

*According to grading of Trey *et al.* (1966). *New England Journal of Medicine*, **274**, 473.

enced clinical team. When facilities for dealing with variceal bleeding are not available early referral is indicated.

Initially, the severity of the bleeding, and the degree of hepatic dysfunction, a major determinant of subsequent mortality, which is usually classified using Pugh-Child's grading (Table 6), should be assessed. The average mortality with variceal bleeding is less than 10 per cent in grade A patients, about 25 per cent in grade B, and 50 per cent or more in grade C patients. Renal function should also be assessed, and evidence of infection sought by chest radiography, ascitic tap, and blood and urine cultures.

The aims of therapy are to correct hypovolaemia and shock, to stop the bleeding, and to prevent complications of bleeding. At least one large-bore venous cannula must be inserted, together with a central venous line. Colloid may be needed to maintain circulating volume while waiting for cross-matched whole blood. After restoring the systolic pressure to 80–90 mmHg, packed cells should be given to maintain the haemoglobin at 10 g/dl and the urine output at 40 ml/h or more. Fresh frozen plasma is only needed to correct the effect of a large transfusion of stored blood. Platelet transfusions have only a transient effect, but are indicated when there is massive transfusion or a profound basal thrombocytopenia. Vitamin K (10 mg, intravenous) should be given.

The major complications of variceal bleeding (which may lead to multiorgan failure and cause death) are:

1. Pneumonia due to aspiration, especially during endoscopy or placement of balloon tamponade tubes; tracheal intubation should be used if the level of consciousness is poor. Standard treatment should be given if aspiration pneumonia is suspected. Pulse oximetry is useful, even in patients without obvious pneumonia, as hypoxaemia is common, particularly in cirrhotic patients, and may be aggravated by shock, sepsis, and massive transfusion.
2. Hepatic encephalopathy—which should be prevented or treated using lactulose or lactitol (orally or via a nasogastric tube), and twice-daily cleansing enemas.
3. Infection, usually due to enteric organisms causing septicaemia or spontaneous bacterial peritonitis. Prophylaxis against Gram-negative enteric organisms reduces the risk of infection. A third-generation cephalosporin, given intravenously, is the antibiotic of choice. As soon as infection is suspected it should be treated. Nephrotoxic antibiotics should be avoided.
4. Water/electrolyte imbalance—with increasing ascites and the development of renal failure. Close monitoring of fluid balance is necessary to maintenance an adequate circulating volume while minimizing fluid overload. Saline solutions should be avoided. Electrolyte abnormalities should, if possible, be

corrected as they exacerbate encephalopathy. Ascites should be treated (see below).
5. Undernutrition—oral feeding should be started as soon as possible, usually 24 h after admission. Consideration should be given to enteral or parenteral supplementation, depending on the state of nutrition and renal function.

Specific therapy

Several types of treatment may be needed to stop bleeding. Vasoactive drugs, balloon tamponade, endoscopic sclerotherapy, banding ligation, surgical transection, and shunts (surgical or radiological) have all been used. Reduction of gastric pH does not affect variceal bleeding, but is indicated for erosive gastritis or oesophagitis, and for bleeding from sclerotherapy ulcers; omeprazole, with or without topical agents, heals these ulcers and minimizes the risk of bleeding.

Vaso-active drugs

Vasoactive drugs are thought to act as splanchnic arteriolar vasoconstrictors, thus reducing portal inflow and flow through the bleeding varices. A recent meta-analysis of randomized clinical trials identified the following as regimens as effective:

1. Vasopressin (0.20–0.40 units/min for 24–48 h) with nitroglycerin (by infusion or patch). Nitroglycerin prevents some deleterious systemic vasoconstrictor effects of vasopressin. The systolic pressure should be maintained at 100 mmHg or more.
2. Glypressin (2 mg every 6 h for 24–48 h)
3. Somatostatin (250 μg/h for 2–5 days)
4. Octreotide (50 μg/h for 2–5 days)

These drugs control bleeding more effectively than placebo, but may not alter hospital mortality. Somatostatin or octreotide have fewer side-effects, and can be given for longer; they may reduce early rebleeding from varices.

Balloon tamponade

Severe variceal bleeding can be controlled by balloon tamponade. The most frequently used tube has two balloons: the oesophageal balloon compresses the oesophageal varices; the gastric balloon prevents laryngeal obstruction due to upward movement of the oesophageal balloon, and may occlude some gastric varices and control bleeding from oesophageal varices. Balloon tamponade can also be used to stabilize the patient before more definitive therapy or for transfer to another centre. Before insertion the patient should be head down in the left lateral decubitus position. There should be suction facilities to cope with a massive haemorrhage. If the patient is uncooperative or comatose, tracheal intubation is necessary. External traction is not necessary. Bleeding is controlled in at least 90 per cent of cases. Continued bleeding is often due to incorrect placement, a wrong diagnosis about the source of bleeding, or the presence of overwhelming coagulopathy. Tamponade should not be maintained for more than 12 h, and more definitive therapy should be planned as rebleeding is very common. Unfortunately, the placement of balloons by inexperienced users is accompanied by many complications, particularly aspiration pneumonia.

Endoscopic therapy

Endoscopic sclerotherapy, using one of many sclerosants (e.g. 5 per cent ethanolamine, 1 per cent polidocanol), is the mainstay of acute management of bleeding varices. The sclerosant can be injected into the varix, or alongside it to compress it. Tissue adhesive (bucrylate), which polymerizes instantly on contact with blood, may be useful for gastric varices, for which sclerotherapy is not very effective. For oesophageal variceal bleeding a single session of sclerotherapy is effective in over 65 per cent of cases; the success rate is at least 85 per cent with two sessions. No more than two sclerotherapy sessions should be used in a 5-day period; this minimizes oesophageal complications, and allows endoscopic banding ligation or a later surgical transection to be done if necessary. Severe complications of sclerotherapy, such as mediastinitis, deep oesophageal ulceration and stenosis, occur in less than 2 per cent of cases in experienced hands.

Endoscopic banding ligation of oesophageal varices is a new technique, akin to banding of haemorrhoids. It has fewer complications than sclerotherapy in the long term but has no advantage in the emergency situation.

Portal-systemic shunting

Emergency portal–systemic shunting has a high mortality and is now rarely done. Oesophageal staple transection can be used if endoscopic therapy is not available or if it fails, if bleeding continues, or if early rebleeding occurs despite vasoactive therapy. It is as effective as emergency sclerotherapy, with no difference in mortality. There should be no undue delay, as prolonged bleeding and complications increase the operative risk. Devascularization procedures should only be considered for patients with extrahepatic venous obstruction in whom shunts cannot be fashioned. If transplantation is contemplated, abdominal surgery should, if possible, be avoided because of the risk of adhesions.

The transjugular intrahepatic portosystemic stent shunt (**TIPSS**) achieves shunting without need for surgery and will probably replace emergency surgical shunting. Preliminary data suggests that it is very effective but has a high thrombosis rate within 12 months. Further experience will define its role more precisely.

Prevention of variceal rebleeding

Cirrhotic patients who survive their first variceal bleed have a 70 per cent or more chance of rebleeding, which accounts for 20 to 35 per cent of deaths during follow-up. Rebleeding is most frequent in the first 6 weeks. Meta-analysis reveals that all treatments (surgery, endoscopic therapy, and β-blockers) reduce the frequency of rebleeding but have variable effects on mortality. The choice of therapy depends on individual circumstances, particularly the severity of liver disease and the feasibility of the different methods of treatment.

Portal–systemic shunts reduce risk of rebleeding to 10 per cent or less but do not prolong survival. Non-selective shunts (end-to-side or side-to-side portacaval; mesocaval; proximal splenorenal) divert portal flow from the liver; encephalopathy is therefore a problem, particularly in cirrhotics. The distal splenorenal shunt, which is technically more difficult, selectively shunts blood from the splenic region and maintains some portal perfusion; encephalopathy is less common within the first 2 years. It also avoids surgery at the liver hilum (which affects liver transplantation) but has a higher rate of shunt thrombosis.

Repeated sclerotherapy reduces the rebleeding rate (to about 50 per cent) and reduces mortality. Complications are fewer than with emergency sclerotherapy, but depend on the experience of the operator. In four recent studies, banding ligation of varices caused fewer complications than sclerotherapy; there was less rebleeding but the effect on survival must still be determined.

Drug therapy is more convenient for patients and cheaper to administer. β-Blockers reduce variceal flow by reducing cardiac output, allowing unopposed α-vasoconstriction of splanchnic arterioles, and acting directly on collaterals feeding the varices. The reduction in portal pressure is modest (10 to 20 per cent), and intrahepatic resistance increases slightly. It appears that lowering the hepatic venous pressure gradient to less than 80 per cent of pretreatment values at 3 months reduces the risk of rebleeding. Meta-analysis shows a reduction in rebleeding with β-blockers, to about 50 per cent, and suggests a lower mortality. Complications are fewer than with sclerotherapy but their use is contraindicated in some patients. The portal hypotensive effect of β-blockers may be enhanced by adding isosorbide mononitrate, which lowers intrahepatic resistance and thus further lowers portal pressure. β-Blockers also reduce the risk of bleeding and chronic anaemia due to portal hypertensive gastropathy.

In some trials, in which patients were fit for surgery, shunt surgery (distal splenorenal) reduced the rebleeding rate compared with sclerotherapy, but did not improve survival and the risk of encephalopathy was increased. In trials comparing sclerotherapy with β-blockers, higher-risk patients were included; there were no differences in survival or rebleeding rates. No advantage accrued by combining β-blockers with sclerotherapy. No trials have been reported comparing endoscopic banding of varices, or TIPSS, with other therapies.

Primary prevention of gastrointestinal bleeding

Attempts at primary prevention of variceal bleeding, using surgical shunts or sclerotherapy, have shown no overall benefit; mortality increased in several studies. However, primary prevention studies of β-blocker therapy have shown a reduction in bleeding from varices and portal hypertensive gastropathy, and have suggested a decrease in mortality. β-Blocker therapy should therefore be offered to patients with 'at risk' varices who have no contraindications to these drugs. Preliminary evidence suggests that the HVPG should be reduced to 12 mmHg or below to eliminate the risk of bleeding.

Ascites

'Ascites' (Greek *askitos*—bladder, belly, bag) denotes excessive free fluid in the peritoneal cavity. The volume of ascites is variable; up to 70 l have been recorded. It is usually a clinical finding, which should be confirmed by routine diagnostic paracentesis. Ascites is also detectable by ultrasonography or CT, which reveal subclinical amounts of fluid (i.e. less than 1.5 l). Depending on the cause, ascites may appear gradually or accumulate rapidly. When ascites is a presenting feature in cirrhosis, particularly in young patients, Wilson's disease should be suspected.

Moderate ascites may cause no symptoms. When large amounts of fluid accumulate girth and weight increase, and there may be abdominal discomfort, particularly with tense ascites. Hernias (particularly umbilical hernias) may appear or enlarge. Some patients with gross ascites complain of numbness or paraesthesiae, with sensory loss, in the distribution of the lateral cutaneous nerve of the thigh. Gross ascites is a hindrance; mobility may be limited and diaphragmatic elevation and restriction may cause breathlessness. In some, breathlessness may be unduly severe because of an associated pleural effusion (see below).

Physical signs

Gross ascites is usually obvious, but striking abdominal distension can occur with other conditions (see below). The important physical signs of ascites are: bulging of the flanks; dullness to percussion in the flanks (while the umbilical region may be hyperresonant due to floating bowel); shifting dullness (the uppermost flank becoming resonant when the patient lies on his or her side); and a fluid thrill (palpable vibrations on one side of the abdomen when the other side is flicked). None of these signs is reliable in doubtful cases, when they would be most useful. Ascites is unlikely to be present (less than 10 per cent of cases) in the absence of flank dullness; the converse is not true.

Dependent oedema (ankle or sacral) often occurs with ascites. Scrotal or abdominal-wall oedema may be present, particularly after paracentesis or after abdominal surgery (presumably through leakage of peritoneal fluid). Ascites and dependent oedema may both be found while the upper body shows evidence of extravascular fluid depletion (best sought by pinching the skin over the upper sternum where loss of skin turgor is evident regardless of age). Sometimes, particularly with aggressive diuretic therapy, there may be generalized cutaneous evidence of 'dehydration', and postural hypotension, indicating a reduced intravascular volume. Other physical signs may give clues to the cause of the ascites (see below).

Ascites is not the only cause of marked abdominal swelling. Gross obesity, gaseous distension, abdominal masses, or large organs may cause diagnostic problems. Massive ovarian or hydatid cysts, and occasionally pregnancy with hydramnios can be confusing as they may be associated with a fluid thrill.

Causes of ascites

The causes of ascites are presented in Table 7. In Europe and North America cirrhosis, malignant neoplasms, congestive heart failure, and tuberculosis account for more than 90 per cent of cases. Portal venous hypertension is an important contributory factor in cirrhosis—and in congestive heart failure, constrictive pericarditis, and hepatic outflow obstruction. Congestive heart failure is usually obvious, but confusion can arise because ascites can elevate the jugular venous pressure through its mechanical effects. Constrictive pericarditis (with ascites, hepatosplenomegaly, and little or no peripheral oedema) is often mistaken for cirrhosis, as is the Budd–Chiari syndrome.

Acute portal-vein thrombosis may cause transient ascites; chronic portal-vein block does not usually cause ascites in the absence of liver disease, but it may appear transiently after variceal bleeding. Hepatocellular carcinoma can result in portal or hepatic venous thrombosis, both may cause or exacerbate ascites.

Most of the other diseases listed in Table 7 can be diagnosed if their presence is suspected, often by examination of the peritoneal fluid (see below) or by percutaneous peritoneal biopsy.

Leakage from the biliary tract (e.g. after surgery or blunt trauma) may cause the gradual development of ascites rather than an acute bile peritonitis. Diagnosis is difficult, particularly if there is pre-existing cirrhosis; the leak can be demonstrated by endoscopic retrograde cholangiopancreatography. Leakage from the urinary tract (again after surgery or trauma) is a rare cause of ascites.

EXAMINATION OF THE ASCITIC FLUID

Diagnostic paracentesis is done by aspirating through a needle inserted in the flank. The main reason for routine diagnostic paracentesis is to check for spontaneous bacterial peritonitis (see below).

In ascites due to portal hypertension or hypoalbuminaemia the fluid is clear and straw coloured. Turbid ascites may indicate infection; chylous or pseudochylous ascites is a milky colour. Blood-stained ascites is usually due to malignancy but may occur with tuberculosis, pancreatitis, hepatic-vein thrombosis, recent abdominal punctures, or with a 'bloody tap'.

Low-protein ascites (less than 25 g/l) is a 'transudate'; it usually occurs with portal hypertension or hypoalbuminaemia. A higher-protein ascites (an 'exudate') is usually found with malignancy, tuberculosis, pancreatitis or myxoedema, but the protein content is not a reliable method of diagnostic classification. It tends to rise during successful diuretic therapy.

A high ascitic-fluid (and serum) amylase suggests pancreatic ascites; a low glucose (relative to blood) is found in malignant ascites. Cytological examination may reveal malignant cells, and the finding of a high concentration of carcinoembryonic antigen in ascitic fluid is of diagnostic value even in the absence of malignant cells. The triglyceride content should be measured when the ascites is milky. It is low in pseudochylous ascites, when scattering of light is due to aggregates of cholesterol, phospholipid, and protein from degenerating malignant or inflammatory cells. A high triglyceride, the fat floating on standing, indicates true chylous ascites. This is usually due to malignant or inflammatory lymphatic obstruction, or to trauma, but is also common in ascites due to the nephrotic syndrome. Chylous ascites also occurs in cirrhosis, presumably due to rupture of overloaded lymphatics.

Complications of ascites

Some consequences and complications of ascites have already been mentioned. Spontaneous leakage from a large umbilical hernia requires

Table 7 *Causes of ascites*

> *Venous hypertension*
> Cirrhosis
> Congestive heart failure
> Constrictive pericarditis
> Hepatic venous outflow 'obstruction'
>   (a) Hepatic-vein block (Budd–Chiari syndrome)
>   (b) Veno-occlusive disease
> Portal-vein block (acute thrombosis)
>
> *Hypoalbuminaemia* (may be contributory in above causes, especially cirrhosis)
> Nephrotic syndrome
> Malnutrition and protein-losing enteropathy
>
> *Malignant disease*
> Secondary carcinomatosis
> Lymphomas and leukaemias
> Primary mesothelioma
>
> *Infections*
> Tuberculous peritonitis
> Fungal (candida, cryptococcus)
> Parasitic (strongyloides, entamoeba)
>
> *Miscellaneous*
> Chylous ascites
> Bile ascites
> Pancreatic ascites
> Urinary ascites
> Ovarian disease
>   Meig's syndrome
>   Struma ovarii
> Ovarian overstimulation syndrome
> Myxoedema
> Pseudomyxoma peritonei
> Eosinophilic gastroenteritis
> Whipple's disease
> Sarcoidosis
> Starch peritonitis
> Systemic lupus erythematosus

surgical repair. Some patients with ascites develop a pleural effusion; usually right-sided, it can be left-sided or bilateral. It results from passage of fluid through small holes in the diaphragm. These effusions may be very large and cause symptoms; they usually respond to salt restriction and diuretics, and may respond to TIP55, but chemical obliteration of the pleural space may be necessary. In rare cases of cirrhosis a large pleural effusion may be found in the absence of detectable ascites.

With marked ascites, liver biopsy and other procedures involving percutaneous puncture of liver or spleen are more difficult and dangerous, because the organs may separate from the parietal peritoneum and move with the impact of the needle.

SPONTANEOUS BACTERIAL INFECTION OF THE ASCITIC FLUID

This is usually due to a single enteric organism, occurs in 10 to 15 per cent of patients with ascites, and is sometimes associated with bacteraemia. Abdominal pain and tenderness may occur but spontaneous bacterial peritonitis (**SBP**) often presents with general malaise or fever, hypotension or hepatic encephalopathy. SBP should be suspected whenever sudden deterioration occurs in a patient with ascites. Certain diagnosis requires bacterial culture of ascitic fluid (10 ml should added to blood-culture bottles at the bedside) but this involves inevitable delay. Culture-negative ascites is common, but a white-cell count of ascitic fluid helps in diagnosis. If the initial white-cell count is in excess of

500/mm³, if the neutrophil count is in excess of 250/mm³, or if a lower count is present with clinical features suggesting SBP, fever, abdominal pain and tenderness, and decreased bowel sounds for example, a third-generation cephalosporin should be given immediately without waiting for the results of culture. Early antibiotic therapy is mandatory as rapid deterioration can occur, and the course of infection is the same in culture-negative and culture-positive cases. A 5-day course of treatment is sufficient.

In secondary bacterial peritonitis there are usually multiple organisms. If this is suspected, or when cultures are returned, intravenous metronidazole should be added.

Pathogenesis and therapy

PATHOGENESIS

Ascites due to liver disease results from several factors:

- avid salt (and thus water) retention;
- decreased colloid pressure of plasma due to reduced albumin synthesis in the liver;
- portal hypertension, which localizes the fluid within the peritoneal cavity;
- increased hepatic lymph production, possibly due to obstruction by cirrhotic nodules at the postsinusoidal level.

The mechanism of sodium retention is complex. There is now an unified hypothesis of 'peripheral arterial vasodilatation', which combines the older 'underfill' and 'overfill' hypotheses. Plasma volume expansion, with renal water and sodium retention, occurs before ascites formation, which goes against an 'underfill' theory. However, the 'overfill' theory cannot explain activation of the renin–angiotensin–aldosterone system, increased amounts of vasopressin, or activation of the sympathetic nervous system causing increased concentrations of plasma noradrenaline. All of these occur in cirrhotics with salt and water retention, owing to an inadequate intravascular volume relative to the intravascular space ('underfilling'), which may result from 'peripheral arterial vasodilatation'. This hypothesis also accounts for the changes seen in the systemic circulation.

In patients with ascites, renal secretion of prostaglandins (**PG**), (mainly PGE₂) may help to preserve renal function by maintaining glomerular filtration and free water clearance. When renal PGE₂ production falls, due perhaps to renal deficiency of the precursor arachidonic acid, renal function deteriorates. Deterioration also occurs with drugs which inhibit prostaglandin synthetase, non-steroidal anti-inflammatory drugs for example, which should not be given to patients with fluid retention. A list of other drugs which should be avoided in patients with ascites is given in Table 8.

MANAGEMENT

Some patients with relatively high urinary sodium output may respond simply to a modest reduction in sodium intake. Most patients with ascites have avid urinary sodium retention (under 10 mmol/day). Some have a diuresis with bedrest and/or moderate dietary sodium restriction. If renal function is good, as evidenced by a normal creatinine and ability to clear free water, there is usually a good response to diuretics.

When diuretics are effective, patients are more comfortable on a sodium intake of around 60 mmol/day. A strict low-salt diet is unpalatable and may increase the likelihood of renal failure. Medicines rich in sodium, such as standard magnesium trisilicate mixture, should be avoided. When patients have renal failure and cannot generate free water the response to dietary sodium restriction and diuretics is poor; hyponatraemia may develop, which requires water restriction to about 1 l/day. The prognosis is then poor unless there is a remediable cause of renal deterioration, such as infection or haemorrhage. A classification of renal failure in liver disease is presented in Table 9.

Table 8 *Drugs to avoid in treatment of ascites*

Direct nephrotoxins	Demeclocyline, aminoglycosides, amphotericin, cephalosporins penicillins, etc.
Prostaglandin synthetase inhibitors	NSAID; aspirin, indomethacin, phenylbutazone, etc.
Sodium-rich drugs	Antacids, i.v. metronidazole, etc.
Potassium-rich drugs (with spironolactone, tramterene, amiloride, etc.)	'Salt substitutes'
Renin–angiotensin blockers	Captopril, saralasin
Drugs increasing aldosterone secretion	Metoclopramide
Others	Lithium, radiographic contrast materials; care with lactulose

In view of the potential hazards of diuretic therapy it is sensible to begin their use in hospital. Spironolactone is the drug of choice, at an initial dose of 100 mg daily; the dose can be increased by 100 to 200 mg every third day, up to a dose of 800 mg/day, until the urinary sodium:potassium molar ratio exceeds one, when a diuresis usually results. The serum potassium should be monitored, as severe hyperkalaemia can occur with spironolactone therapy. Potassium supplements should be avoided, unless obvious potassium depletion is present (NB: 'salt substitutes' are potassium rich). Some men develop painful reversible gynaecomastia on spironolactone; other distal-tubular diuretics such as triamterene (100–500 mg/day) or amiloride (10–60 mg/day) can then be tried. These also cause hyperkalaemia and they should not be given with spironolactone or potassium supplements. In some patients, spironolactone causes marked metabolic acidosis.

If no diuresis results with spironolactone, frusemide should be added, starting with 40 mg on alternate days; the dose can be increased to 160 mg/day. With diuresis induced by frusemide, hypokalaemia may occur despite concurrent use of a potassium-sparing drug, and potassium supplements may then be necessary. Hyponatraemia may develop or worsen and metabolic alkalosis may occur. Hepatic encephalopathy is often precipitated by diuretic therapy, although spironolactone alone seems relatively safe in this regard.

One should try to limit the diuretic response to salt loss of 50 to 100 mmol/day more than intake; or to a weight loss of about 0.5 kg/day in those with only ascites, and up to 1 kg/day when there is also peripheral oedema. It is not advisable to try to remove all the excess fluid. Rapid fluid loss is better tolerated in ascitics with peripheral oedema; patients with ascites only may show deterioration in renal function due to an excessive initial loss from the systemic fluid space.

If diuresis does not result from combined diuretic therapy, other methods are needed to control severe ascites. Therapeutic paracentesis is now standard therapy for tense ascites, for refractory ascites (i.e. which does not respond to diuretics), and when electrolyte changes or hypovolaemia limit the use of diuretics. It is best done with a Kuss needle (with additional side holes) and low-grade suction. Total paracentesis can be carried out; 6 to 8 g of albumin or colloid equivalent should be infused for every litre of ascitic fluid removed to prevent depletion of intravascular volume and renal failure. The length of hospital stay is shorter and the complication rate less with therapeutic paracentesis than with diuretic therapy.

For short-term control, ascites can be concentrated before reinfusion; this conserves plasma proteins and expands the intravascular volume. For longer-term control, a shunt, such as the LeVeen shunt, can be inserted surgically between the peritoneum and a jugular vein. Both methods have dramatic effects in some patients, but there is a high

Table 9 *Renal failure in liver disease*

Type	Causes	Treatment	Prognosis
Spontaneous (functional)	Underlying liver disease		Bad
Diuretic induced	Frusemide, spironolactone, amiloride, etc.	Stop drug	Good
Induced by NSAIDS	Phenylbutazone, indomethacin, aspirin, etc.	Stop drug	Good
Acute tubular necrosis	Infections, viral hepatitis, nephrotoxic drugs (e.g. gentamycin)	Dialysis	Bad (mortality 70%)
Chronic renal failure with liver damage			Bad

morbidity and mortality due to infection, consumption coagulopathy, pulmonary oedema, and variceal bleeding. They should only be used in specialist centres, and on selected patients resistant to other forms of therapy.

Portal–systemic shunt surgery may relieve ascites but has a high operative mortality (see below under Budd–Chiari syndrome). Recently, the TIPSS has been used to treat resistant ascites, but its role is still being assessed.

Treatment of other forms of ascites

For some causes of ascites there is a specific treatment. Surgery is required for constrictive pericarditis, ovarian tumours, and biliary and urinary ascites. Appropriate chemotherapy is needed for infective causes, and thyroxine for myxoedematous ascites. The triglyceride content of chylous ascites usually falls if medium-chain triglyceride is substituted for the normal long-chain triglyceride of the diet, but this may have little effect on ascitic fluid accumulation and conventional therapy with diuretics and salt restriction should be used. Surgical relief of obstructed lymphatics is rarely possible.

The management of malignant ascites is an important clinical problem when ascites causes severe symptoms and does not respond to conventional systemic therapy (see Section 6). A complete paracentesis should be done initially as a diagnostic and therapeutic procedure; colloid replacement does not appear to be necessary. The fluid may not reaccumulate; if it does, repeated paracentesis may be needed to control discomfort and breathlessness. Although malignant ascites is often refractory to diuretics, some do well on high doses of spironolactone.

If malignant cells are present in the ascitic fluid, and there are no large intra-abdominal tumour masses, palliation may be achieved in patients with drug-sensitive malignancies by the intraperitoneal injection of the appropriate cytotoxic drug (see Section 6). This treatment should be carried out by an experienced oncologist. Good results have also been achieved in many patients with intraperitoneal administration of a colloidal suspension of radioactive phosphate (^{32}P) or gold (^{198}Au). Immunotherapy with intraperitoneal injection of OK-432 (a penicillin/heat-treated lyophilized powder of a *Streptococcus pyogenes* strain) gives good short-term results in about 60 per cent of patients. In patients without malignant cells in the ascitic fluid a peritoneovenous shunt may be of value in the control of resistant ascites.

Budd–Chiari syndrome (hepatic vein obstruction) and veno-occlusive disease

Budd–Chiari syndrome results from obstruction of the major hepatic veins, usually from thrombosis. A thrombogenic disorder, including paroxysmal nocturnal haemoglobinuria (see Chapter 22.3.12), is responsi-

ble in about 75 per cent of cases. There may be clear evidence of myeloproliferative disorders such as polycythaemia rubra vera and essential thrombocythaemia. In some patients with definite Budd–Chiari syndrome the only suggestion of a myeloproliferative disorder is a specific abnormality of bone-marrow progenitor cells; spontaneous formation of erythroid colonies occurs when progenitor cells are cultured in appropriate erythropoietin-poor medium. Other patients may suffer from antithrombin III, protein S or protein C deficiency, or may have an underlying tumour. Other causes are shown in Table 7 and are discussed in Section 22. Pregnancy and oral contraceptives are associated with Budd–Chiari syndrome, but a thrombogenic tendency should also be sought in these cases.

There is an associated thrombosis in the inferior vena cava in up to 20 per cent of cases, and in the portal vein in about 10 per cent. Thus detailed visualization of the systemic and/or splanchnic venous circulations may be necessary. The thrombus eventually organizes, with recanalization and/or fibrosis of the vein wall.

Hepatic congestion is worst around the hepatic vein radicles and causes necrosis. Acute portal hypertension may develop if the process is widespread. If congestion is unrelieved fibrosis results, leading to chronic portal hypertension and eventually cirrhosis. The thrombosis is often asynchronous, with late changes (fibrosis and atrophy of hepatocytes) in some areas, and recent changes (congestion and necrosis) in others. In many cases the caudate lobe enlarges and obstructs the inferior vena cava, making it difficult to perform a side-to-side portacaval shunt, the best shunt for relieving the ascites and portal hypertension.

The speed and extent of hepatic-vein thrombosis determine the presentation. A few patients present with fulminant liver failure, and high aminotransferase levels; without intervention death usually occurs within 2 weeks. About 25 per cent of cases evolve over a month or so, with rapid onset of ascites, abdominal pain (and jaundice in about half). The most common presentation is with progressive ascites over several months, and tender hepatomegaly in the later stages. Dependent oedema occurs, due to caval compression or thrombosis. Jaundice is unusual, and there may be little disturbance of liver function tests. 'Asymptomatic' cases, that is without ascites, are now being recognized. Variceal bleeding can occur across the spectrum of Budd–Chiari syndrome, and the emergency treatment is similar to that for cirrhotics.

Ultrasound usually confirms the diagnosis. The hepatic veins and inferior vena cava should be examined by venography, and the portal vein by superior mesenteric angiography. Hepatic venography allows identification of thrombus or webs in the hepatic veins. Sometimes the hepatic veins are completely occluded; hepatic venography is then impossible, but a wedged venogram may still show the characteristic 'spider web' pattern. Venography allows assessment of inferior vena caval compression, and measurement of caval pressures above and below the liver. These investigations help to plan surgery. A liver biopsy is mandatory to evaluate fibrosis and necrosis, and to help to estimate reversibility of liver injury. Transjugular liver biopsy may be necessary

Table 10 *Causes and associations of Budd–Chiari syndrome and veno-occlusive disease*

Budd–Chiari syndrome
Haematological disorders—polycythaemia rubra vera, other myeloproliferative disorders, paroxysmal nocturnal haemoglobinuria, sickle cell anaemia, prothrombotic disorders, antithrombin III deficiency, protein C, protein S, antiphospholipid antibody
Tumours—hepatocellular carcinoma, renal-cell carcinoma, adrenal carcinoma, leiomysarcoma of inferior vena cava or right atrium, carcinoma of stomach or pancreas
Drugs—oral contraceptives, antitumour drugs (doxorubicin, vincristine, vinblastine, etc.)
Pregnancy and post-partum period
Infections—amoebic abscess, aspergillosis, other fungal infections, hydatid cysts, schistosomiasis, syphilis
Membranous webs (common in the Far East)
Trauma
Miscellaneous—inflammatory bowel disease, protein-losing enteropathy, nephrotic syndrome, sarcoidosis, mixed connective tissue disease, nodular regenerative hyperplasia, Behçet's syndrome

Veno-occlusive disease
Pyrrolizidine alkaloids (plants of Crotalaria, Senecio, and Heliotropium families)
Irradiation
Antitumour and immunosuppressive drugs (cytarabine, carmustine, mitomycin, azathioprine).
Graft-versus host disease following bone marrow transplantation, following liver transplantation

---

if clotting is severely disturbed; if this is difficult due to the hepatic venous occlusion a plugged transhepatic liver biopsy can be done.

If there are no contraindications to their use (e.g. the presence of varices), anticoagulants should be given to prevent progression of thrombosis. A few patients have regression of the disease and can then be treated with expectant medical management; however, fibrosis and cirrhosis usually supervene. Ascites is treated in standard fashion, but is often refractory.

If a venous web is present, which is common in the Far East, balloon dilatation may relieve the obstruction of the hepatic vein and/or inferior vena cava. However, there may be involvement of veins deep in the liver; this prevents complete resolution of the syndrome and the liver disease may progress.

Patients with a patent portal vein, and without significant fibrosis or marked obstruction of the cava, should have a portacaval shunt (side-to-side portacaval, mesocaval, or TIP55) to decompress the liver, relieve ascites, and reduce the risk of variceal bleeding. In patients operated on within 16 weeks of onset of symptoms the results are good, with a long-term survival of about 85 per cent. Ascites resolves, fibrosis is often arrested, and in some a normal histological appearance of liver is restored. Patients having a shunt procedure should continue their anticoagulation irrespective of the type of shunt.

When the inferior vena cava is blocked a mesoatrial shunt can be used; its length predisposes to graft thrombosis despite anticoagulation. If the inferior vena cava is patent, but severely compressed (by the caudate lobe), a stent across its intrahepatic portion will reduce the pressure distally, allowing construction of a shunt to the cava.

Liver transplantation should be considered for all patients with severe forms of the Budd–Chiari syndrome. A major problem is assessment of viable hepatocyte mass. With the fulminant presentation, very early decompressive surgery may be life saving, but death can result from extensive necrosis before regeneration can occur. With the acute presentation the degree of necrosis may be such that shunt surgery precip-

itates acute liver failure, thus accounting for some perioperative deaths. Transplantation should be used if there is fibrosis and/or marked necrosis on biopsy, and if hepatocellular failure persists because a shunt has thrombosed (although this increases the risk of the operation). Liver transplantation should be considered in chronic cases, especially if the patient is seen some months after the onset of symptoms, and if marked fibrosis or cirrhosis is present on liver biopsy. Survival is very good, particularly in those without previous surgery. Anticoagulation should be administered for life.

Veno-occlusive disease

The term 'veno-occlusive disease' is given to a non-thrombotic obliterative process with luminal narrowing of small intrahepatic tributaries of the hepatic veins. The clinical picture mimics the Budd–Chiari syndrome, with acute, subacute, and chronic presentations. The original cases resulted from ingestion (in 'bush teas') of pyrrolidizine alkaloids found in plants of the Crotalaria, Senecio, and Heliotropium families, but there are other causes (Table 10). Cytotoxic drugs, particularly when used before bone marrow transplantation, are the most common cause in Western countries. Some acute cases improve spontaneously, but many are progressive and fatal. Some improve with antifibrinolytic therapy. Liver transplantation has been used successfully. Some non-fatal cases have been associated with nodular regenerative hyperplasia. The distinction between Budd–Chiari syndrome and veno-occlusive disease is not always clear cut, as histological changes may be found in large and small vessels. Changes of veno-occlusive disease may be seen with thrombosis of large hepatic veins, and fibrin may be found in the lumina of veins with alkaloid- or radiation-induced veno-occlusive disease.

REFERENCES

General

McIntyre, N., Benhamou, J-P., Bircher, J., Rizzetto, M., and Rodes, J. (ed.) (1991) *Oxford textbook of clinical hepatology*. Oxford University Press.

Schiff, L. and Schiff, E.R. (ed.) (1982). *Diseases of the liver*, (5th edn). Lippincott, Philadelphia.

Sherlock, S. and Dooley, J. (1992). *Diseases of the liver and biliary system*, (9th edn). Blackwell Scientific, Oxford.

Wright, R., Alberti, K.G.M.M., Karran, S., and Millward-Sadler, G. (ed.) (1992). *Liver and biliary disease*, (3rd edn). Saunders, London.

Zakim, D. and Boyer, T.D. (ed.) (1990). *Hepatology: a textbook of liver disease*, (2nd edn). Saunders, Philadelphia.

Ascites

Albillos, A. *et al.* (1990). Ascitic fluid polymorphonuclear cell count and serum to ascites albumin gradient in the diagnosis of bacterial peritonitis. *Gastroenterology*, **98**, 134–40.

Epstein, M. (ed.) (1988). *The kidney in liver disease*, (3rd edn). Williams & Wilkins, Baltimore.

Gines, P. *et al.* (1987). Comparison of paracentesis and diuretics in the treatment of cirrhotics with tense ascites: results of a randomized study. *Gastroenterology*, **93**, 234–41.

Schrier, R.W., Arroyo, V., Bernardi, M., Epstein, M., Henriksen, J.H., and Rodes, J. (1988). Peripheral arterial vasodilation hypothesis: a proposal for the initiation of renal sodium and water retention in cirrhosis. *Hepatology*, **8**, 1151–7.

Tito, L. *et al..* (1990). Total paracentesis associated with intravenous albumin management of patients with cirrhosis and ascites. *Gastroenterology*, **98**, 146–51.

Portal hypertension

Huet, P.M., Pomier-Layrargues, G., Villeneuve, J.P., Varin, F., and Viallet, A. (1986). Intrahepatic circulation in liver disease. *Seminars in Liver Disease*, **6**, 277–86.

North Italian Endoscopic Club for the Study and Treatment of Oesophageal Varices (1988). Prediction of the first variceal haemorrhage in patients with cirrhosis of the liver and oesophageal varices: a prospective multi-centre study. *New England Journal of Medicine*, **319**, 983–9.

Pagliaro, L. *et al.* (1989). Therapeutic controversies and randomised controlled trials (RCTs): prevention of bleeding and rebleeding in cirrhosis. *Gastroenterology International*, **2**, 71–84.

Pagliaro, L. *et al.* (1992). Prevention of first bleeding in cirrhosis. A meta-analysis of non-surgical randomized clinical trials. *Annals of Internal Medicine*, **117**, 59–70.

Webb, L.J. and Sherlock, S. (1979). The aetiology, presentation and natural history of extrahepatic portal venous obstruction. *Quarterly Journal of Medicine*, **48**, 627.

Zemel, G., Katzen, B.T., and Becker, G.J. (1991). Percutaneous transjugular portosystemic shunts. *Journal of the American Medical Association*, **266**, 390.

Budd–Chiari Syndrome and Veno-Occlusive Disease

Mitchell, M.C., Boitnott, J.K., Saufman, S., Cameron, J.L., and Madrey, W.C. (1982). Budd–Chiari syndrome: etiology, diagnosis, and management. *Medicine*, **61**, 199–218.

Zafrani, E.S., Pinaudeau, Y., and Dhumeaux, D. (1983). Drug induced vascular lesions of the liver. *Archives of Internal Medicine*, **143**, 495–502.

14.30 Hepatocellular failure

E. A. JONES

Introduction

Hepatocellular failure is the functional syndrome resulting from severe impairment of the function of hepatocytes. Its clinical manifestations include hepatic encephalopathy, a haemorrhagic diathesis, fluid retention, and hepatocellular jaundice. The syndrome may complicate any disease in which the pathophysiology includes hepatocellular necrosis or hypofunction of hepatocellular organelles. The duration of evidence of hepatic dysfunction before the onset of hepatocellular failure is variable, ranging from a few days to many years. The term hepatocellular failure does not necessarily imply impaired function of hepatic cells other than hepatocytes (i.e. Kupffer cells, sinusoidal endothelial cells, fat-storing cells, pit cells). Although many biochemical lesions induced by hepatotoxic agents have been defined, the precise mechanisms by which such agents induce hepatocellular necrosis or organelle failure are, in general, poorly understood, a notable exception being hypoxia. An influx of calcium ions appears to be a late event in the sequence of biochemical events culminating in hepatocellular necrosis.

Definitions

Acute liver failure

The syndrome of hepatocellular jaundice, hypertransaminasaemia, and prolongation of the prothrombin time associated with an acute liver disease.

Fulminant hepatic failure

Classically defined as the syndrome of acute liver failure complicated by hepatic encephalopathy occurring within 8 weeks of the onset of clinical evidence of liver disease. The King's College Hospital (London) group have introduced the term late-onset liver failure for the syndrome in which hepatic encephalopathy occurs 8 to 24 weeks after the onset of clinical evidence of liver disease. In addition, the Beaujon Hospital (Paris) group have proposed that the term fulminant hepatic failure be applied to acute liver failure with a plasma factor V level of less than 50 per cent of normal and hepatic encephalopathy occurring less than 2 weeks after the onset of jaundice. This group also proposed use of the term subfulminant hepatic failure for acute liver failure with a plasma factor V level of less than 50 per cent of normal and hepatic encephalopathy occurring 2 weeks to 3 months after the onset of jaundice. An advantage of the French definitions is that they permit inclusion of cases in which an acute liver failure-like syndrome is the first clinical manifestation of a previously asymptomatic chronic liver disease (e.g. Wilson's disease).

Chronic hepatocellular failure

The syndrome of decompensated chronic liver disease, that is, a chronic liver disease complicated by hepatic encephalopathy, a coagulopathy, fluid retention, and/or hepatocellular jaundice (see Chapter 14.25).

Aetiology

The most common causes of fulminant hepatic failure are acute viral hepatitis (particularly types A and B) and drug-induced hepatocellular injury. Some cases appear to be due to a non-A, non-B, non-C hepatitis of undetermined aetiology. Markers of acute infection with specific viruses (e.g. IgM anti-HAV, IgM anti-HBc, IgM anti-HDV) may be useful in suggesting a viral aetiology of acute liver failure. An acute liver failure-like syndrome and encephalopathy associated with other viruses (e.g. herpes, varicella), particularly in immunocompromised patients, do not always meet the criteria of fulminant hepatic failure. Only drugs that can cause acute hepatocellular injury (rather than cholestasis) have the potential of inducing fulminant hepatic failure. The most common are paracetamol (acetaminophen) and halothane. Fulminant hepatic failure from poisoning may be due to paracetamol overdose (suicide attempts), Amanita mushrooms or industrial solvents, particularly chlorinated hydrocarbons such as carbon tetrachloride. Hypoxic hepatocellular injury may be attributable to reduced hepatic perfusion, but rarely leads to fulminant hepatic failure (e.g. following cardiac arrest). Important vascular causes of fulminant hepatic failure include the Budd–Chiari syndrome and veno-occlusive disease. The latter may be induced by pyrrolizidine alkaloids, chemotherapy or irradiation. A rare cause of fulminant hepatic failure is heat-stroke. Fulminant hepatic failure has also been attributed to intrasinusoidal invasion by secondary neoplasia. Intravascular haemolysis in the presence of a fulminant hepatic failure-like syndrome suggests Wilson's disease. Autoimmune chronic active hepatitis may present with a syndrome similar to subfulminant hepatic failure associated with type 1 antibodies to liver and kidney microsomes. Fulminant hepatic failure may be precipitated by partial hepatectomy (removal of more than 80 per cent of normal liver or about 50 per cent of cirrhotic liver). Fulminant hepatic failure soon after liver transplantation may be due to hyperacute allograft rejection or hepatic arterial thrombosis. Viral hepatitis may be responsible for late-onset liver failure after liver transplantation. The HBsAg chronic carrier state appears to be a major predisposing factor for fulminant hepatic failure.

Fulminant hepatic failure is usually associated with massive hepatocellular necrosis, but rare cases due to acute fatty liver of pregnancy,

Table 1 *Clinical stages of hepatic encephalopathy*

Stage	Mental status	Asterixis	EEG changes
I (prodrome, often diagnosed in retrospect)	Alert; euphoria; occasional depression; decreased attention; slow mentation and affect; untidiness; irritability; inverted sleep rhythm	Usually absent	Often lacking
II (impending coma)	Increased drowsiness; agitation; lethargy; major personality changes; inappropriate behaviour; inability to perform mental tasks or maintain sphincter control; confusion; slurred speech; disorientation; palilalia	Present (with or without incoordination)	Generalized slowing
III	Stupor; somnolent but rousable; incoherent speech; marked confusion; fits of rage; amnesia; restlessness	Usually present (if patient can cooperate)	Always present
IV	Coma; with (IV-A) or without (IV-B) response to painful stimuli	Usually absent	Always present

intravenous tetracycline, valproic acid, and pirprofen are associated with microvesicular hepatocellular steatosis. Reye's syndrome includes cerebral changes not specific for acute liver failure. When Wilson's disease, alcoholic hepatitis, jejunoileal bypass syndrome, chronic active hepatitis, or the HBsAg carrier state present with hepatic encephalopathy and an acute liver failure-like syndrome, only the French definition of fulminant hepatic failure can be applied.

Chronic hepatocellular failure may complicate any progressive chronic hepatocellular disease or any lesion causing chronic hepatic central venous congestion.

Manifestations

The four cardinal manifestations of hepatocellular failure are hepatocellular jaundice, hepatic encephalopathy, ascites, and a haemorrhagic diathesis. Severe hepatocellular failure leads to an increased susceptibility to infections and is often associated with foetor hepaticus, and acid-base and electrolyte changes. Cerebral oedema and raised intracranial pressure as well as hypoglycaemia complicate fulminant and subfulminant hepatic failure. Clinically important phenomena associated with incipient or overt chronic hepatocellular failure include cardiovascular, renal, pulmonary, skin, and endocrine changes, fatigue, increased protein catabolism, fever, and anaemia.

Cardinal features

HEPATIC ENCEPHALOPATHY

This is the syndrome of impaired mental status and abnormal neuromuscular function attributable to impaired hepatocellular function. Hepatic encephalopathy is associated with increased delivery of constituents of portal blood to the systemic circulation. The spectrum of psychiatric and neurological abnormalities that can occur is broad. A subclinical phase may be detected by electrophysiological or psychometric tests. The earliest clinical signs are psychiatric and behavioural

changes that may be more apparent to the patient's family and close friends than to the physician. These changes are primarily due to subtle impairment of intellectual function that reflects predominantly bilateral forebrain dysfunction. Conventionally, four clinical stages of hepatic encephalopathy are recognized (Table 1). During the encephalopathy there is often increased muscle tone with cogwheel and neck rigidity. Asterixis ('liver flap') is often found (Fig. 1). The mouth may be difficult to open. Myoclonic twitchings may be evident and deep tendon reflexes

Fig. 1 The 'liver flap' is a slow, flapping tremor, which can be elicited by asking the patient to dorsiflex the hands with the arms outstretched and the fingers extended and parted, as if trying to stop traffic. It is due to neuromuscular incoordination between flexor and extensor muscles. The hands tend to fall forward, but this involuntary movement is rapidly corrected by readoption of the dorsiflexed position, thereby creating a 'flap'. The same phenomenon may be elicited by asking the patient to squeeze the physician's extended finger. Neuromuscular incoordination is indicated by repeated intensification and relaxation of the intensity of the squeeze ('milkmaid's grip').

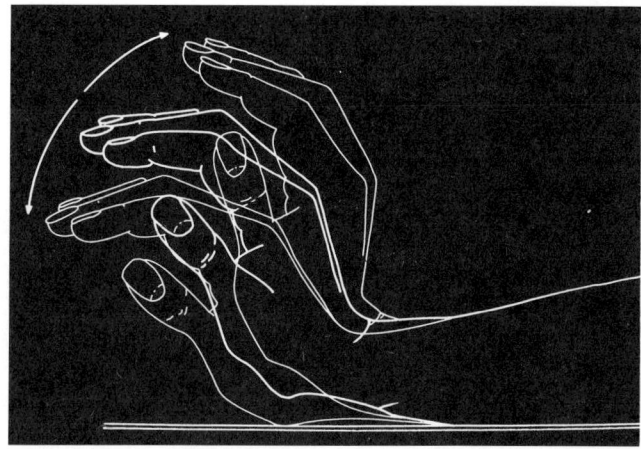

tend to be increased. One or both plantar responses may be extensor. The electroencephalogram (**EEG**) is always abnormal in stage II to IV hepatic encephalopathy. As the encephalopathy progresses the frequency of the EEG decreases and initially its amplitude increases. With further progression, the amplitude decreases. Triphasic waves may occur in severe hepatic encephalopathy. Flattening of the EEG is a preterminal event. The clinical and electrophysiological manifestations of hepatic encephalopathy are non-specific.

Hepatic encephalopathy complicating chronic liver disease may be either acute or chronic. Acute hepatic encephalopathy in a cirrhotic patient is usually associated with one or more clearly definable precipitating factors (Table 2). With the notable exception of benzodiazepines, the relationship between common precipitating factors and pathogenesis is poorly understood. The term chronic portal–systemic encephalopathy is often applied when hepatic encephalopathy is persistent or episodic (with or without complete resolution between episodes) in a patient with chronic liver disease. The encephalopathy may be precipitated by a surgically created portal–systemic shunt or a transjugular intrahepatic portal-systemic shunt.

Hepatic encephalopathy is considered to be a reversible metabolic encephalopathy primarily due to impaired hepatic extraction of substances that can modulate central neuronal function. Most of its manifestations appear to be attributable to a net increase in neuronal inhibition. The pathogenesis is probably multifactorial.

Ammonia is an established potent neurotoxin that is widely believed to play a part in the pathogenesis. The gastrointestinal tract is one of the major sites of ammonia production. Ammonia is normally converted into either urea or glutamine in the liver and accumulates in the brain in liver failure. Encephalopathy and seizures occur in children with congenital hyperammonaemia syndromes but seizures are unusual in hepatic encephalopathy. Furthermore, experimental hyperammonaemia does not reproduce the behavioural or electrophysiological manifestations of hepatic encephalopathy. A decrease in cerebral energy metabolism may be a result rather than a cause of ammonia-induced neurotoxicity. Ammonia promotes transformation of glutamate to glutamine and consequently has the potential of decreasing excitatory neurotransmission mediated by glutamate. Direct electrophysiological effects of ammonia include neuronal excitation (dysinhibition). Although ammonia has documented neurochemical and electrophysiologic effects its contribution to hepatic encephalopathy remains poorly defined. Other neurotoxins (e.g. mercaptans, short-chain fatty acids, phenols) have also been implicated. However, abnormalities of visual-evoked responses in experimental hepatic encephalopathy have not been reproduced by combinations of putative neurotoxins.

In liver failure, particularly if chronic, the ratio of serum concentrations of branched-chain amino acids to those of aromatic amino acids decreases. This abnormality may promote transfer of aromatic amino acids from plasma to brain. Changes in cerebral metabolism induced by aromatic amino acids may lead to depletion of normal catecholaminergic neurotransmitters, including dopamine, and an accumulation of 'false' neurotransmitters. However, the plasma ratio of branched chain to aromatic amino acids in patients with cirrhosis correlates poorly with hepatic encephalopathy and neither dopaminergic drugs (L-dopa, bromocriptine) nor branched-chain amino acids have been shown to improve hepatic encephalopathy in controlled clinical trials.

Increased neurotransmission mediated by γ-aminobutyric acid (**GABA**) the principal inhibitory neurotransmitter in the brain, is associated with impaired motor function and decreased consciousness. The GABA$_A$benzodiazepine receptor/chloride ionophore complex is an oligomeric glycoprotein complex that has been pharmacologically and biochemically subdivided into three components: GABA$_A$ receptors, central benzodiazepine receptors, and chloride ionophores. These units are allosterically linked to form a 'supramolecular' complex. Binding of GABA to the GABA$_A$ receptor induces opening of the Cl$^-$-ionophore, allowing Cl$^-$ to enter the neurone and hence cause membrane hyperpolarization. This phenomenon is the basis of GABAergic inhibitory

Table 2 *Factors that may precipitate hepatic encephalopathy (HE)*

	Comments
Constipation Oral protein load Upper gastrointestinal bleed	Gut factors contribute to HE
Diuretic therapy Paracentesis Diarrhoea and vomiting	Dehydration, electrolyte and acid–base imbalance
Hypoglycaemia Hypoxia Hypotension Anaemia	Factors with adverse effects on both liver and brain function
Sedative/hypnotic drugs	Benzodiazepines and barbiturates enhance the action of GABA
Azotaemia	
Infection	May cause dehydration and increased protein catabolism

GABA, γ-Aminobutyric acid.

neurotransmission. Benzodiazepine-receptor agonists (e.g. diazepam) increase the neuroinhibitory potency of GABA. Enhancement of GABAergic tone in hepatic encephalopathy could occur if the availability of GABA at GABA$_A$ receptors is increased and/or if agonist ligands (e.g. benzodiazepines) that potentiate the action of GABA are present. A functional increase in GABAergic tone has been demonstrated in experimental hepatic encephalopathy and may apply to the syndrome in general, as increased levels of benzodiazepine agonists, including diazepam, have been found in body fluids and brain of patients with hepatic encephalopathy. Thus, a rationale exists for giving a benzodiazepine-receptor antagonist in hepatic encephalopathy. However, brain levels of benzodiazepine receptor ligands in hepatic encephalopathy have not been fully characterized and appear to be insufficient to account for all of the manifestations of the syndrome.

HAEMORRHAGIC DIATHESIS (SEE ALSO SECTION 22)

The basis of the haemorrhagic diathesis is multifactorial, but the predominant factor is impaired synthesis of liver-produced blood-clotting factors, which is reflected in prolongation of the prothrombin time. A prolonged prothrombin time, which is not corrected by parenteral vitamin K, is presumptive evidence of hepatocellular failure, unless an alternative explanation is readily apparent. Thrombocytopenia is often present and may reflect the hypersplenism of portal hypertension (see Section 22). However, in fulminant hepatic failure, platelet structure and function are abnormal and the capillary bleeding time tends to be greater than that expected from the platelet count. Mild disseminated intravascular coagulation is often detectable but is rarely of clinical significance. Spontaneous haemorrhage may not occur, even when the coagulopathy is profound (as in the typical case of fulminant hepatic failure), and intracranial haemorrhage is rare. However, upper gastrointestinal haemorrhage (e.g. from gastritis, gastro-oesophageal varices, peptic ulcer) frequently occurs. A common clinical feature of the bleeding tendency is bruising around venepuncture sites.

ASCITES

Ascites due to hepatocellular failure complicates lesions that cause sinusoidal portal hypertension or impaired hepatic venous drainage. It is more common in subfulminant hepatic failure and decompensated cirrhosis than in fulminant hepatic failure. Hepatocellular failure is not invariable when ascites is associated with hepatic venous congestion, but is more likely to be present if the primary lesion is veno-occlusive disease or the Budd–Chiari syndrome that if it is of cardiac origin. Ascites due to hepatocellular failure is invariably associated with hepatic dysfunction and portal hypertension (see Chapter 14.29).

HEPATOCELLULAR JAUNDICE

The jaundice of hepatocellular failure has an orange tint and is attributable to conjugated hyperbilirubinaemia due to impaired secretion of conjugated bilirubin into the bile canaliculus. In acute hepatitis the degree of conjugated hyperbilirubinaemia reflects the extent of hepatocellular necrosis, but, even when jaundice is deep, other features of hepatocellular failure (e.g. a prolonged prothrombin time) are often absent, reflecting the large normal hepatic reserve. In contrast, in chronic liver disease, hepatocellular jaundice usually reflects severe hepatocellular failure.

Other features

INCREASED SUSCEPTIBILITY TO INFECTION

Hepatocellular failure predisposes to a high incidence of infections. Most are bacterial, but about one-third are complicated by tissue invasion by fungi (e.g. aspergillosis, candidiasis). Such complex infections are usually associated with leucocytosis and a high mortality. Fungal infection is suggested by antibiotic-resistant fever. The frequency of infections may be related to reduced amounts of complement components and opsonins, reduced phagocytic and bactericidal properties of polymorphonuclear leucocytes, and a reduced clearance function of reticuloendothelial cells, especially Kupffer cells. Spontaneous bacterial peritonitis is a common and potentially fatal complication of ascites (see Chapter 14.29). Bacteraemia may occur in the absence of fever, rigors, or a substantial leucocytosis. In about one-quarter of patients dying of fulminant hepatic failure, sepsis appears to be the immediate cause of death and sepsis is often present in patients dying of chronic hepatocellular failure.

FOETOR HEPATICUS

Foetor hepaticus is the term applied to a particular smell of the breath that may be detected in patients with cirrhosis and extensive portal–systemic shunts or acute liver failure. Descriptions vary and include a sweetish, slightly pungent or faecal smell, similar to that of a rotten apple, mice, or a freshly opened corpse. Being subjective there is considerable variation in its recognition by different physicians. It has been attributed to gut-derived, sulphur-containing products of methionine metabolism, such as mercaptans. For the individual experienced physician, foetor can be a useful sign in the clinical recognition of severe hepatocellular disease and in the differential diagnosis of coma.

ACID–BASE AND ELECTROLYTE CHANGES

A wide range of abnormalities of acid–base and electrolyte balance occurs, particularly in fulminant hepatic failure, and may contribute to altered neurological and cardiac function. Hyponatraemia may be attributable to impaired renal free-water clearance, failure of the sodium pump, or the effects of giving fluids, diuretics, or mannitol; hypernatraemia is usually iatrogenic. The most common acid–base change in fulminant hepatic failure is respiratory alkalosis secondary to hyperventilation. Also common is hypokalaemic metabolic alkalosis precipitated by loop diuretics. Metabolic acidosis may be associated with extensive tissue damage, hypoxia, and lactic acidaemia. Respiratory acidosis may be associated with hypercapnia and respiratory-tract infection.

CEREBRAL OEDEMA AND RAISED INTRACRANIAL PRESSURE

Cerebral oedema and raised intracranial pressure frequently complicate fulminant hepatic failure, occurring in 80 per cent of patients with this syndrome and grade IV encephalopathy. It is useful to classify these complications separately from hepatic encephalopathy and terminal hypoxic events. Herniation of the cingulate, uncus, or cerebellar tonsil secondary to raised intracranial pressure is a major cause of death in fulminant hepatic failure. Antemortem diagnosis of cerebral oedema and raised intracranial pressure can be difficult, but is suggested by sudden deterioration in consciousness and certain neurological signs, which include increased muscle tone, unequal pupils, abnormally reacting pupils, myoclonus, focal seizures, decerebrate posturing, fixed pupils with spontaneous respiration, and absent ciliospinal reflexes. Sudden changes in pulse and blood pressure unrelated to haemorrhage, rapid deterioration of the EEG, sweating, tachycardia, arrhythmias, intermittent systemic hypertension, sudden severe hypotension, bursts of hyperventilation, and fever may all be manifestations of raised intracranial pressure. Papilloedema is rare. Signs of raised intracranial pressure may become apparent when intracranial pressure exceeds 30 mmHg.

The metabolic basis for cerebral oedema in fulminant hepatic failure has not been established. Possibilities include increased blood to brain transfer of fluid across the blood–brain barrier (vasogenic), a failure of cellular osmoregulation (cytotoxic), or expansion of the extravascular space (interstitial or hydrocephalic).

HYPOGLYCAEMIA

Severe hypoglycaemia (blood glucose of less than 40 mg/dl) occurs in about 40 per cent of patients with fulminant hepatic failure (particularly children) and exacerbates encephalopathy. The clinical and EEG features of hepatic and hypoglycaemic encephalopathy are similar. In acute liver failure, hypoglycaemia can occur independently of hepatic encephalopathy. It may develop rapidly and recur with sepsis. It is often associated with neurological and electroencephalographic deterioration. It is due primarily to impaired hepatic glucose release secondary to glycogen depletion. In contrast to hepatic encephalopathy, hypoglycaemic coma may cause irreversible brain damage.

CARDIOVASCULAR CHANGES

Hepatocellular failure is associated with systemic vasodilation and a hyperdynamic circulation. Cardiac output is increased, peripheral vascular resistance decreased, blood pressure reduced, and splanchnic and capillary flow increased, but perfusion of the renal cortex is decreased. Features of a hyperdynamic circulation include a bounding pulse, capillary pulsation, vasodilated extremities, a praecordial heave, and an ejection systolic murmur. The increased cardiac output has been attributed to an increased vascular capacitance and hence relative hypovolaemia with low jugular venous pressure. Hypotension is present for about 16 per cent of the time a patient with fulminant hepatic failure is in stage IV encephalopathy. In only about 40 per cent of instances can hypotension be attributed to clinically identifiable complications of hepatocellular failure, such as haemorrhage. Arrhythmias and other cardiac abnormalities occur in more than 90 per cent of patients with fulminant hepatic failure in stage IV encephalopathy. Cardiac arrest (unrelated to respiratory arrest) may occur. Arrhythmias, other than sinus tachycardia, tend to occur in patients with hypoxia.

HEPATORENAL SYNDROME

Renal failure is common and may be rapidly progressive; in only a minority of cases is it attributable to hypovolaemia. It is typically functional and characterized by reduced glomerular filtration rate and oliguria. Acute tubular necrosis may supervene and be difficult to differentiate from uncomplicated, progressive, functional renal failure. Some cirrhotic patients with diuretic-resistant ascites develop a stable, moderately elevated plasma creatinine. Absorption of large quantities of nitrogenous substances from the gut after a gastrointestinal haemorrhage may contribute to azotaemia. Plasma urea and creatinine are not reliable indices of renal function in fulminant hepatic failure; hepatic synthesis of urea is decreased and tubular secretion of creatinine is increased. Renal failure in fulminant hepatic failure is often associated with cerebral oedema.

Functional renal failure is associated with intense renal arterial vasoconstriction. The kidneys in this syndrome function normally when transplanted into non-cirrhotic subjects. Several neurohumoral systems and endogenous substances have been implicated in the pathogenesis of the hepatorenal syndrome.

HEPATOPULMONARY SYNDROME

Intrapulmonary peripheral vascular dilatation with decreased pulmonary vascular resistance occurs in hepatocellular failure. Hypoxaemia ($Pa_{O_2} < 70$ mmHg) is present in about one-third of patients and may be associated with cyanosis. In the absence of gross pulmonary pathology, the hypoxaemia is usually reversed by 100 per cent oxygen and is attributable to abnormal ventilation–perfusion ratios and diffusion capacity. However, in some cirrhotic patients, pulmonary arteriovenous shunts may be responsible for hypoxaemia that is not reversible by 100 per cent oxygen. Chest radiographs may show a high diaphragm (due to ascites, ileus, delayed gastric emptying), basal pulmonary infiltrates, or (in fulminant hepatic failure) pulmonary oedema. Pulmonary oedema occurs in about one-third of cases of fulminant hepatic failure; it is not attributable to left ventricular failure, but tends to be associated with cerebral oedema. Hyperventilation of central origin with hypocapnia occurs early in fulminant hepatic failure. With progression of encephalopathy the cough reflex becomes suppressed and there is increasingly impaired protection of the airway. This problem can be compounded by ileus and delayed gastric emptying. Respiratory arrest of central origin may occur.

The mechanism of the pulmonary vasodilation is unknown. Oxygen does not diffuse readily into the centre of dilated vessels and increased cardiac output (see above) limits the time for gas exchange.

SKIN CHANGES

Recognition of certain skin changes in a patient with chronic liver disease alerts the clinician to the possibility of incipient or overt hepatocellular failure. However, there are no skin changes that are specific for hepatocellular failure.

Spider naevi are often present in cirrhotic patients; these consist of a central protuberant arteriole from which small vessels radiate in a manner that has been likened to the appearance of a spider's legs (Fig. 2). Their diameter is usually less than 0.5 cm. They occur in the area of drainage of the superior vena cava. One or two may be found occasionally in normal subjects and they may occur transiently in pregnancy and viral hepatitis. They may occur with chronic alcoholism, oestrogen therapy, thyrotoxicosis, and rheumatoid arthritis. Spider naevi should be distinguished from telangiectasia, corkscrew scleral vessels, and purpura. Development of new 'spiders' suggests progressive hepatocellular disease; conversely their disappearance may indicate improving hepatocellular function.

Palmar erythema occurs less frequently than spider naevi in advanced chronic liver disease. It is characterized by an exaggeration of the normal mottling of palmar surfaces of the hands, resulting in well-demarcated redness of the thenar and hypothenar eminences, and of the pulps of the fingers. Palmar erythema may also occur in normal subjects and as a family trait; it may occur in association with pregnancy, oestrogen therapy, rheumatoid arthritis, chronic pulmonary disease, thyrotoxicosis, chronic leukaemia, subacute bacterial endocarditis, hyperglobulinaemia, and chronic febrile disease.

Dilated, thread-like blood vessels in the skin having an apparently random distribution may occur, particularly on the upper arms, in chronic (usually alcoholic) liver disease. They may resemble a US dollar note ('paper money' skin). Patients with chronic liver disease may exhibit white nails with loss of demarcation of the lunulae (leuconychia, Terry's nails) (Fig. 3). Finger clubbing (Lovibond's angle in excess of 180 °) in the absence of hypertrophic osteoarthropathy occurs in a small minority of patients with cirrhosis (Fig. 4). Dupuytren's contracture and

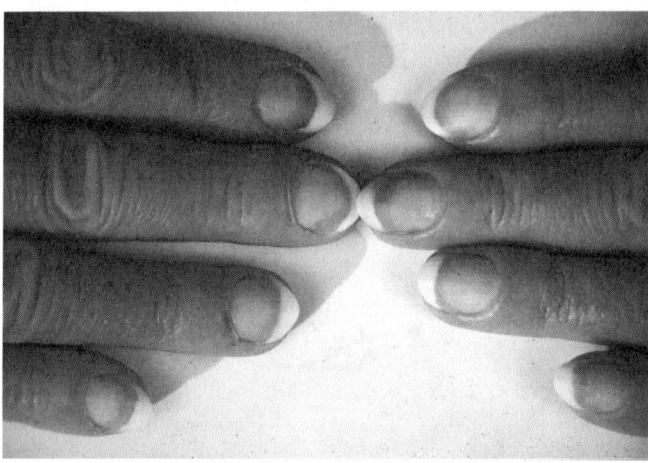

Fig. 3 White nails (leuconychia) in a cirrhotic patient.

Fig. 2 Spider naevi in a cirrhotic patient.

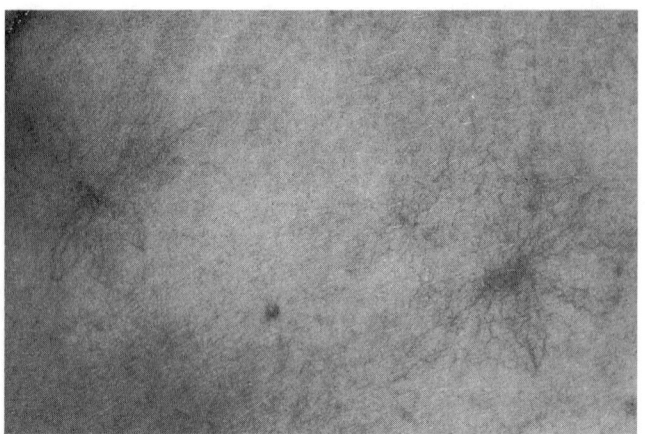

Fig. 4 Finger clubbing in a cirrhotic patient.

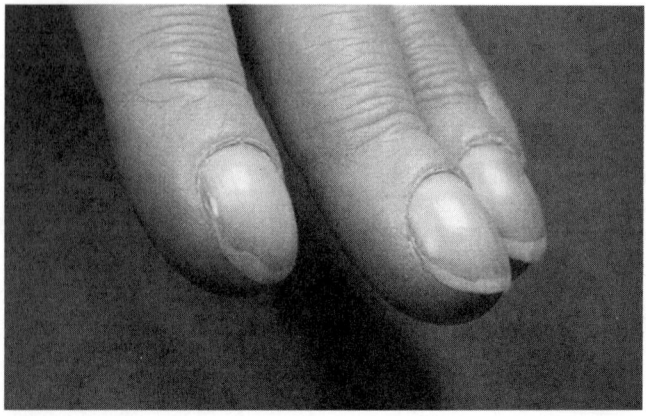

parotid-gland swelling are typically associated with chronic alcoholism and do not necessarily imply hepatocellular failure.

ENDOCRINE CHANGES

Chronic liver disease may be associated with reduced concentrations of testosterone. Some male cirrhotics develop hypogonadism and feminization. The former is characterized by testicular atrophy, decreased potency and libido, and reduced need to shave; the latter is characterized by gynaecomastia and female hair distribution and body habitus. Some female cirrhotics develop infertility, scanty, irregular menstruation, and an asexual appearance due to loss of female characteristics. It is common for these changes to be associated with alcoholism. However, the presence of chronic liver disease appears to be a requisite for feminization to occur. Accordingly, it is important to distinguish between signs of hypogonadism and signs of feminization. Gynaecomastia, which may be unilateral or bilateral, occurs in alcoholic and non-alcoholic cirrhosis (Fig. 5). In cirrhotic patients, spironolactone often precipitates (tender) gynaecomastia.

FATIGUE

Severe disabling fatigue, which seems out of proportion to the patient's general physical condition, may occur before the onset of overt hepatocellular failure in chronic liver disease.

ABNORMAL PROTEIN METABOLISM

Reduced synthesis of liver-produced plasma proteins involves not only blood-clotting factors but also albumin. In chronic liver disease the degree of hypoalbuminaemia reflects both decreased hepatic synthesis and an increase in plasma volume. Because of the long plasma half-life of albumin (about 20 days), hypoalbuminaemia may not be present early in fulminant hepatic failure. Chronic hepatic decompensation is associated with a loss of skeletal muscle mass. The mechanism of the increased protein catabolism is unknown.

FEVER

A low-grade fever may occur in severe hepatocellular disease (e.g. alcoholic hepatitis) (and with hepatocellular carcinoma) in the absence of evidence of infection.

ANAEMIA

A normochromic normocytic anemia, unassociated with deficiency of any haematinic, is a feature of chronic hepatocellular failure.

Fig. 5 Gynaecomastia in a cirrhotic patient.

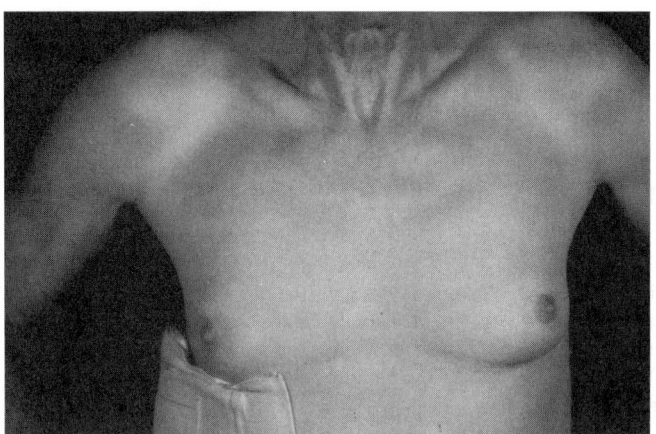

Diagnosis

The syndrome of hepatocellular failure constitutes a clinical spectrum from acute liver failure at the one extreme to decompensated chronic hepatocellular disease at the other. No single abnormality is pathognomonic of hepatocellular failure. A patient dying of hepatocellular failure usually exhibits all four of the cardinal manifestations with or without complicating sepsis.

HEPATIC ENCEPHALOPATHY

This is a clinical diagnosis that is made by excluding other forms of encephalopathy in a patient with severe hepatocellular disease. The diagnosis can usually be made with a high degree of confidence on the basis of the history, physical examination, and routine blood tests alone, but no individual clinical or laboratory abnormality is specific. By definition, the presence of hepatic encephalopathy implies hepatocellular failure. Special attention is paid to changes in personality, hypersomnia, and deterioration of performance at work or school. Stages I to III of the encephalopathy are often associated with asterixis (liver flap) (Fig. 1), although this useful sign is not pathognomonic; it occurs also in hypercapnia, uraemia, and heart failure. Signs of portal hypertension may be useful and include not only ascites, but also splenomegaly and dilated veins in the wall of the abdomen (with flow away from umbilicus). Furthermore, non-specific stigmata of liver disease, such as spider angiomata and palmar erythema, may be found. Foetor hepaticus suggests hepatocellular failure and/or increased portal–systemic shunting. It is necessary to recognize disorders with neurological manifestations that may mimic hepatic encephalopathy, such as Wernicke's encephalopathy, alcohol intoxication, or subdural haematoma.

Psychometric tests are useful in detecting and monitoring subtle mental dysfunction in patients with subclinical or prestupor stages of hepatic encephalopathy. Qualitative tests include orientation to time, person and place, recall of current events, subtraction of serial 7s, handwriting, figure drawing, and constructing a five-pointed star. The number connection test is a useful quantitative test. Allowance must be made for the effects of learning on test scores.

EEGs are helpful in the assessment of hepatic encephalopathy but must be interpreted with caution. The abnormalities seen are not specific, and occur in other metabolic encephalopathies such as uraemia, hypercapnia and hypoglycaemia, as well as drug-induced encephalopathies. EEG changes typical of those found in overt hepatic encephalopathy may develop before clinical features of the syndrome are apparent. Usually there is a good correlation between the clinical stage of the encephalopathy and the degree of abnormality of the EEG. The EEG is of value in differential diagnosis because it can reveal focal defects in the brain, seizure activity, and other findings that might suggest an alternative diagnosis. Visual event-related potentials that depend on cognitive function are promising for the detection of subclinical hepatic encephalopathy.

In uncomplicated hepatic encephalopathy, abnormal liver function tests reflect the underlying liver disease. Laboratory tests aid in the differential diagnosis of encephalopathies, such as uraemia and hypoglycaemia, and in the detection of factors that may precipitate hepatic encephalopathy, such as hypokalaemic metabolic alkalosis. Plasma ammonia concentrations are increased in the majority of patients with hepatic encephalopathy. However, they correlate poorly with the clinical stage, are not specific for this syndrome, and are not useful in management. An elevated plasma ammonia may be helpful in suggesting an hepatic origin for an undiagnosed encephalopathy.

HAEMORRHAGIC DIATHESIS

The most important readily obtainable laboratory marker of this phenomenon is a prolonged prothrombin time, uncorrected by parenteral vitamin K (see Section 22).

ASCITES

When the presence of ascites on physical examination is in doubt, the issue may be resolved by ultrasonography of the abdomen, which can detect as little as 100 to 200 ml of intraperitoneal fluid. It is usually inappropriate to obtain a needle biopsy of the liver when ascites is present, but the presence of chronic liver disease may be apparent from clinical findings or the results of a previous biopsy. Careful clinical examination of the jugular venous pressure wave is necessary in the exclusion of cardiac causes of ascites. Difficulty in visualizing major hepatic veins on ultrasonography suggests Budd–Chiari syndrome.

HEPATOCELLULAR JAUNDICE

The conjugated hyperbilirubinaemia of hepatocellular failure has to be distinguished from that due to rare congenital bilirubinopathies, such as Dubin Johnson and Rotor syndromes, in which other routine liver tests, including the prothrombin time, are normal. It has also to be distinguished from acquired intrahepatic cholestatic disease, including drug-induced cholestasis, primary biliary cirrhosis, and primary sclerosing cholangitis, and acquired large-duct biliary obstruction, which may be due to stones, biliary strictures, pancreatitis or neoplasms. Recognition that conjugated hyperbilirubinaemia is attributable to hepatocellular failure is usually possible from clinical and routine serum biochemical data alone, but, if large-duct biliary obstruction is suspected, endoscopic retrograde cholangiography is indicated. Unconjugated hyperbilirubinaemia is not a feature of hepatocellular failure.

Acute hepatocellular failure

Acute hepatocellular disease associated with a conjugated hyperbilirubinaemia may be classified as acute liver failure when prolongation of the prothrombin time occurs. Acute liver failure due to hypoxia may erroneously be attributed to viral hepatitis. If hypoxia is implicated, a cause is usually obvious, such as a hypotensive episode during surgery.

The diagnosis of fulminant hepatic failure requires routine serum biochemical and haematologic data consistent with acute hepatocellular dysfunction including a markedly elevated serum alanine aminotransferase early in the course, hepatocellular hypofunction reflected by a markedly prolonged prothrombin time, and the presence of hepatic encephalopathy. Serum alanine aminotransferase concentrations of more than 50 times the upper limit of normal are common in massive hepatocellular necrosis, but may be less than three times the upper limit of normal with minimal hyperbilirubinaemia in hepatic steatosis (see Pathology). In fulminant hepatic failure, the serum albumin may be normal, but foetor hepaticus is almost always present. Abdominal pain may occur with poisoning. Rarely, hepatic encephalopathy precedes jaundice and the patient may present with abnormal behaviour that has to be distinguished from non-hepatogenous acute psychiatric disease. However, patients with fulminant hepatic failure due to massive hepatocellular necrosis who survive more than a few days develop deep jaundice. Special tests such as lumbar puncture, are only necessary if atypical clinical findings are present, but a baseline computerized tomographic (**CT**) scan of the head may be useful. Evidence for the presence of other types of encephalopathy, including uraemic and hypoglycaemic, is routinely sought. Fulminant and subfulminant hepatic failure and late-onset liver failure are differentiated on the basis of the time of onset of liver disease (see Definitions above). The syndrome of fulminant hepatic failure may occasionally be mimicked by severe sepsis or falciparum malaria. It may be difficult to assess whether acute viral hepatitis is responsible for fulminant hepatic failure from the profile of viral markers. In approximately one-fifth of cases of fulminant type B hepatitis, HBsAg is undetectable. In subfulminant hepatic failure, ultrasonography may reveal hepatic nodules.

Chronic hepatocellular failure

The diagnosis of chronic hepatocellular failure involves the demonstration of an appropriate chronic liver disease and evidence of hepatocellular failure. Conjugated hyperbilirubinaemia and a modest prolongation of prothrombin time tend to occur before the development of overt hepatic encephalopathy or ascites. In contrast to diseases causing sinusoidal portal hypertension, those that cause presinusoidal portal hypertension (e.g. schistosomiasis) do not usually progress to hepatocellular failure and are rarely associated with ascites.

Pathology

There is no single hepatic histological change that is pathognomonic of hepatocellular failure. Most agents responsible for acute liver failure or fulminant hepatic failure induce massive or confluent hepatocellular necrosis, whereas a few induce microvesicular fatty metamorphosis of hepatocytes, without displacement of nuclei from their central location within the cell. In patients with fulminant hepatic failure who succumb to brain death, about one-third, there is typically evidence of cerebral oedema, such as increased brain weight, and raised intracranial pressure, such as tense dura, flattened cortical gyri, dilated ventricles, and cingulate, uncal, or cerebellar herniation. The histological appearances of the brain are essentially normal. In some patients with chronic hepatocellular failure, an increase in the number and size of astrocytes, particularly Alzheimer type 2, may be found at autopsy. These changes may be an epiphenomenon. Functional renal failure is associated with no gross pathological changes in the kidney, except in those patients who develop acute tubular necrosis.

Course and prognosis

Acute hepatocellular failure

In patients with acute liver failure who do not develop encephalopathy, such as the typical case of acute icteric viral hepatitis, complete recovery is the rule.

The course of fulminant hepatic failure is variable. There are no reliable criteria that enable prediction of whether an individual patient will die or regain consciousness and ultimately survive. Overall survival is about 20 to 25 per cent with standard intensive medical care alone. Mortality tends to be greater when the encephalopathy and the electroencephalographic abnormalities are more severe and prolonged and when coagulopathy is severe (prothrombin time in excess of 100 s). Mortality also tends to be greater if the age of the patient is below 5 or over 40 years. The mortality is particularly high (over 80 per cent) in cases caused by halothane, non-A, non-B hepatitis, or drugs other than paracetamol, but is about 50 per cent when paracetamol is implicated. The development of a major complication, such as severe gastrointestinal haemorrhage or renal failure, reduces the chances of survival. Small or decreasing liver size, convulsions, cardiac arrhythmias (other than sinus tachycardia) and marked foetor hepaticus are ominous signs. Concentrations of serum aminotransferases may decrease abruptly but are not of prognostic value. The course of fulminant hepatic failure can be divided into five phases, as follows.

Pre-encephalopathy

It is not possible to predict reliably whether an individual with acute liver failure will develop fulminant hepatic failure. However, a progressively increasing prothrombin time often precedes the onset of hepatic encephalopathy. After paracetamol overdosage the onset of encephalopathy may be predicted from plasma concentrations of the drug. Encephalopathy may occur at any time during the course of acute liver failure, but usually within a few days of onset.

Encephalopathy

About one-third of patients die within 2 days of the onset of stage IV encephalopathy. Variations in survival rates in different series may be related to differences in the severity and duration of encephalopathy, the intensity of critical medical care, and the aetiology of the liver disease. In patients who are in stage IV encephalopathy and are not on a ventilator, sudden respiratory arrest may occur. In about 20 per cent of cases, death appears to be due to acute liver failure with progressive encephalopathy. In other cases, death can be attributed to one or more complications of the syndrome, including upper gastrointestinal haemorrhage, cerebral oedema, sepsis, and renal failure. In general the more advanced and more prolonged the encephalopathy or the sooner stage IV encephalopathy develops, the worse the prognosis. In subfulminant hepatic failure, brain death is more uncommon and death due to sepsis more frequent than in fulminant hepatic failure. Subfulminant hepatic failure more frequently complicates drug hepatotoxicity than viral hepatitis. In patients who develop subfulminant hepatic failure, prolonged consciousness may occur with factor V levels below 20 per cent.

Hepatic regeneration

The key factor in determining the outcome of fulminant hepatic failure, in the absence of liver transplantation, is the ability of the liver to regenerate. Nodules of hyperplastic regenerating liver tissue may be found at autopsy in patients who survive more than 10 days after the onset of hepatic encephalopathy. In general, such patients have usually died of a complication of fulminant hepatic failure, such as sepsis, at a time when indices of hepatocellular function may have been improving. Increased serum concentrations of alpha-fetoprotein, regarded as an index of hepatic regeneration, do not usually occur for at least 10 days after the onset of hepatic encephalopathy. The concentrations tend to correlate fairly well with the amount of hepatic regeneration found at autopsy. Recovery is usually heralded by clinical improvement in the encephalopathy, which may be preceded by a decreasing prothrombin time. The EEG may remain abnormal for several days after consciousness is regained.

Cholestasis

A phase of profound cholestasis often develops 2 to 3 weeks after patients regain consciousness. When death has occurred during this phase, large regenerative nodules and intense cholestasis in hepatocytes have been found at autopsy. The pathogenesis of the cholestatic syndrome is poorly understood.

Long-term sequelae

Complete restoration of normal hepatic function and structure usually occurs in survivors of fulminant hepatic failure, even after cerebral oedema, decerebrate rigidity, and episodes of flattening of the EEG. Serum biochemical liver tests and hepatic histological features typically return to normal 45 to 75 days after the onset of hepatic encephalopathy. It is rare for chronic liver disease to develop as a sequel of fulminant hepatic failure. Permanent neurological sequelae have been reported when recovery has occurred after respiratory arrest.

Chronic hepatocellular failure

In patients with chronic hepatocellular disease, hepatic encephalopathy is likely to be reversible if overall hepatocellular function remains relatively well maintained or if a precipitating factor can be clearly identified. Elevated serum conjugated bilirubin in cirrhosis or acute alcoholic hepatitis is associated with a poor prognosis. A rising serum conjugated bilirubin in a patient with a chronic cholestatic disease may reflect progression of the disease and/or development of hepatocellular failure. The serum bilirubin is regarded as a good index of prognosis in primary biliary cirrhosis. When ascites first develops in a patient with cirrhosis, 1-year survival is about 50 per cent and 5-year survival about 20 per cent. Survival after the onset of the hepatorenal syndrome is usually only a few weeks or months.

Management

The first issue in management of hepatocellular failure is whether it is possible to give any effective therapy for the underlying liver disease. It is useful to consider management of the syndromes of chronic and acute hepatocellular failure separately. The chronic syndrome accounts for the great majority of cases of hepatocellular failure, whereas the acute syndrome, when severe, is one of the most challenging in clinical medicine, presenting the physician with a unique constellation of difficult problems. Whether liver transplantation is an appropriate therapeutic option must be considered in all patients with severe hepatocellular failure.

In addition to discontinuing any drugs that might have contributed to the clinical condition, especially neuroactive, hepatotoxic, and nephrotoxic drugs, it is necessary to take into account liver disease-associated abnormalities of drug metabolism and pharmacokinetics, and abnormal brain sensitivity to drugs, when prescribing for the patient in hepatocellular failure. Drugs may modify the clinical manifestations of hepatocellular failure. For example, exogenous benzodiazepines may decrease muscle tone and exacerbate encephalopathy to degrees greater than suggested by levels of clotting factors.

Liver disease

A treatment that suppresses the pathological process responsible for impairing hepatocellular function may decrease, arrest, or reverse manifestations of hepatocellular failure. For acute liver failure, corticosteroids are ineffective and may be harmful. For acute viral hepatitis, antiviral therapy does not have an established place. Acetylcysteine has been shown to improve survival in patients who have taken an overdose of paracetamol, and this may apply even when the antidote is given after hepatic encephalopathy has developed. When viral infections, other than viral hepatitis, are diagnosed, appropriate antiviral treatment is instituted. Interruption of pregnancy is advocated to improve survival in a patient with fulminant hepatic failure due to acute fatty liver of pregnancy. Infant mortality in such cases is high.

Chronic hepatocellular failure

As the patient has irreversible architectural changes in the liver there is no potential for complete recovery with medical treatment. In such cases, management consists of trying to reduce the manifestations of hepatocellular failure that are amenable to treatment, especially encephalopathy and ascites, treating complicating infections and assessing suitability for liver transplantation. Non-specific clinical deterioration raises the possibility of bacteraemia, bacterial peritonitis, or hepatocellular carcinoma. Endocrine changes in a male are not an indication for androgen therapy.

HEPATIC ENCEPHALOPATHY

The following general principles are relevant in the management of hepatic encephalopathy: (a) removal or correction of any precipitating factors (Table 2); (b) reduction of absorption of nitrogenous substances from the gut; (c) reduction of increased portal-systemic shunting; and (d) reversal of contributing neuropathophysiological events with drugs that act directly on the brain. Approaches (a) and (b) are routine, (c) is practical only in rare instances, and (d) is experimental (Table 3).

Acute hepatic encephalopathy

Treatment should begin with a search for, and appropriate management of, precipitating factors. All drugs that could be implicated, including

Table 3 *Treatment of hepatic encephalopathy*

	Comments
1. Correction or removal of precipitating factors	Mandatory
2. Institution of manoeuvres to minimize absorption of nitrogenous substances: Dietary protein restriction Evacuation of the bowel Non-hydrolysed carbohydrate (lactulose or lactitol) and/or oral broad-spectrum antibiotics	Routine
3. Reduction of portal–systemic shunting	Rarely practical
4. Direct reversal of neuropathophysiology Flumazenil.	Experimental

diuretics, are stopped and consideration is given to administering an appropriate antidote, such as naloxone or flumazenil. Meticulous attention is paid to maintaining fluid and electrolyte balance, and an adequate urine flow. Dietary protein intake is completely withheld. Enemas, such as MgSO$_4$ or phosphate, are given to encourage bowel emptying with loss of nitrogenous substances. Lactulose, or a related carbohydrate with similar properties, such as lactitol, is given routinely. There is no disaccharidase on the microvillus membrane of enterocytes that hydrolyses lactulose. Its metabolism by colonic bacteria leads to production of lactic acid and other organic acids, a fall in colonic pH, and increased ionization of nitrogenous compounds. These changes may lead to a decrease in the absorption of nitrogenous substances. Lactulose is a cathartic and is widely considered to be effective in the management of hepatic encephalopathy. It may induce hypernatraemia due to increased faecal fluid loss. Broad-spectrum, poorly absorbed antibiotics are given to reduce the enteric bacterial flora. Neomycin (up to 6 g daily) has been most extensively used, but many potent alternatives are available, such as kanamycin, paramomycin, tetracycline, and ampicillin. Metronidazole, which is effective against anaerobes, may also be given. With return of protein tolerance, dietary protein is reintroduced promptly but gradually to prevent sustained negative nitrogen balance.

Chronic portal–systemic encephalopathy

In the absence of protein intolerance a nutritious diet that includes a high protein intake (80–100 g/day) is encouraged to maintain a positive nitrogen balance and optimize liver function. Vitamins are given empirically and thiamine replacement may be indicated in malnourished alcoholics. Vegetable protein diets seem to be well tolerated and tend to be cathartic due to their fibre content. Oral branched-chain amino acids may decrease protein catabolism and facilitate maintenance of positive nitrogen balance. When protein intolerance develops, management consists of reducing dietary protein intake to as low as 40 g/day. Lactulose or lactitol is given in doses sufficient to produce two to three semiformed bowel actions daily, and precipitating factors are carefully avoided. Long-term protein intake of less than 40 g/day may induce negative nitrogen balance and consequently is contraindicated. If lactulose or lactitol intolerance develops, broad-spectrum antibiotics can be tried. However, long-term neomycin should be avoided because it may cause ototoxicity and nephrotoxicity. Metronidazole may induce a peripheral neuropathy.

If intractable portal–systemic encephalopathy occurs in a patient with a large, surgically induced or spontaneous portal–systemic shunt, the invasive technique of balloon occlusion, coupled with embolization of a collateral (e.g. coronary) vein, may reverse the portal venous blood flow from hepatofugal to hepatopedal. Restoration of portal perfusion in this way can improve hepatocellular function appreciably and achieve a dramatic and sustained amelioration of the encephalopathy.

A new therapeutic approach is to give a drug that acts on the target organ of hepatic encephalopathy, the brain, by reversing contributory neuropathophysiological events. The benzodiazepine antagonist, flumazenil, is the first promising drug of this type. It competes with high specificity with other benzodiazepine-receptor ligands for binding to the benzodiazepine receptor, and rapidly and completely reverses the sedative and other neurological effects of the benzodiazepine agonists, such as diazepam. Anecdotal reports have suggested that when given as a bolus parenterally flumazenil induces a transient and incomplete clinical and electrophysiological improvement in hepatic encephalopathy in about two-thirds of patients with acute liver failure or cirrhosis. However, in a single case study, long-term orally administered flumazenil was associated with a sustained complete reversal of manifestations of chronic, intractable, portal–systemic encephalopathy. Use of this drug is currently experimental.

ASCITES

The place of bedrest, sodium and fluid restriction, diuretics, and therapeutic paracentesis with intravenous infusion of a plasma expander in the management of ascites due to hepatocellular failure is discussed in Chapter 14.29. Diuretic therapy may precipitate hepatic encephalopathy in cirrhotic patients.

Acute hepatocellular failure

PREVENTION

The incidence of fulminant type B hepatitis should be substantially reduced by widespread vaccination against hepatitis B. Fulminant hepatic failure may be prevented by avoiding re-exposure to an agent that has induced an idiosyncratic hepatocellular reaction (e.g. halothane) or by giving *N*-acetycysteine after paracetamol overdose.

ACUTE LIVER FAILURE

Treatment for acute liver failure in the absence of hepatic encephalopathy is expectant, but frequent monitoring is necessary when the prothrombin time is prolonged and prompt admission to hospital is indicated at the first sign of hepatic encephalopathy. Referral to a specialized liver unit has been recommended before encephalopathy develops, when levels of clotting factors are reduced by less than 50 per cent.

FULMINANT AND SUBFULMINANT HEPATIC FAILURE

All patients are considered to have potentially reversible disease. Treatment is designed to buy time for hepatic regeneration to take place and to avoid iatrogenic deterioration. No factors reported to stimulate hepatic regeneration experimentally are of proven clinical benefit. Conventional intensive care for the unconscious patient is instituted. The urinary bladder is catheterized, a nasogastric tube passed, and a central venous line inserted via a jugular vein for infusing fluids and monitoring venous pressure. A Swan–Ganz catheter may be inserted. A fluid intake of 1 to 2 litres daily is usually adequate. The nasogatric tube is used to decompress the stomach and detect upper gastrointestinal haemorrhage. An arterial catheter is useful for continuous blood-pressure monitoring, frequent blood sampling and measurements of blood gases. Caloric intake is maintained by infusing hypertonic dextrose (10 to 50 per cent), usually 200 to 300 g/day. Intravenous lipids and amino acids are contraindicated, but folic acid and vitamins may be given empirically.

Blood and all secretions are considered to be infectious. Attending personnel should wear gowns, gloves, and masks. Enteric isolation procedures are enforced and all specimens from the patient are labelled as infectious. Blood is withdrawn at the outset for serological investigation (e.g. for hepatitis viruses, cytomegalovirus), screening for common drugs, and estimation of serum copper. Blood sugar is monitored as frequently as 1 to 2 hourly. The following investigations are done every 12 h: haemoglobin, total and differential leucocyte and platelet counts, urea, creatinine, potassium, sodium, chloride, and bicarbonate; daily investigations include prothrombin time, reticulocyte count, total and direct bilirubin, alkaline phosphatase, alanine and aspartate aminotransferases, cholesterol, albumin, amylase, calcium, phosphate, magnesium, fibrinogen and fibrinogen split products. Chest radiographs are obtained daily. Measurements of blood gases are necessary despite the coagulopathy. Serial ultrasonic determinations of liver size may be useful in following the course. Needle biopsy of the liver is contraindicated. This procedure is hazardous because of the coagulopathy and management decisions have to be made promptly before the results of a biopsy are available.

Frequent semiquantitative assessments of the neurological status (e.g. Glasgow coma score) and continuous monitoring of the electrocardiogram and EEG are necessary. The value of intensive care is emphasized by the appreciable proportion of patients who die of potentially treatable complications and have evidence of hepatic regeneration at necropsy. Accordingly, patients should be monitored frequently for complications, which must be treated vigorously. A major goal is prevention of brain damage. If agitation, piercing cries, delerium, or seizures occur, the patient should be restrained in a quiet room and the temptation to administer sedatives should be resisted. With the onset of stage II hepatic encephalopathy, intensive care should be instituted and transfer of the patient to a unit with the potential of undertaking orthotopic liver transplantation is recommended, by helicopter if necessary.

Specific problems

Some of the complications of hepatocellular failure present problems in the management of both the acute and chronic syndromes; for example, increased susceptibility to infection, acid–base and electrolyte disturbance, renal failure, and impaired cardiovascular and pulmonary function. The haemorrhagic diathesis tends to be more profound in acute than in chronic liver failure, and cerebral oedema, raised intracranial pressure, hypoglycaemia, agitation, delerium, and seizures are more commonly associated with fulminant and subfulminant hepatic failure.

SUSCEPTIBILITY TO INFECTIONS

Intensive microbiological monitoring is necessary. In fulminant hepatic failure, daily cultures of blood, urine, sputum, and swabs of intravenous cannulae are recommended. Prophylactic antibiotics are not advocated but antibiotics are given promptly when there is bacteriological or other evidence of infection. Nephrotoxic aminoglycosides are avoided. Antibiotics are recommended to cover invasive procedures.

Potential sources of infection, such as intrauterine devices, are removed. Antifungal therapy is given when fungal cultures are positive or there is evidence of tissue invasion by fungi.

HAEMORRHAGIC DIATHESIS (SEE ALSO SECTION 22)

The haemorrhagic diathesis requires no treatment in the absence of overt bleeding, although parenteral vitamin K is given empirically (10 mg subcutaneously daily). Fresh frozen plasma is not given routinely, so that plasma levels of clotting factors can be used as indices of prognosis. Skin puncture sites may require protracted pressure to achieve haemostasis. An H_2-antagonist, when given to maintain the gastric pH above 5.0, has been associated with decreased transfusion requirements in fulminant hepatic failure; dose reduction may be necessary with renal failure. Infusion of platelets and fresh-frozen plasma may be indicated to cover invasive procedures. Clotting factor concentrates, which exacerbate disseminated intravascular coagulation, are contraindicated. Heparin is not indicated for mild disseminated intravascular coagulation. Standard regimens of endoscopic diagnosis and therapy are instituted when haemorrhage occurs from the gastrointestinal tract. A haematocrit of 30 to 35 per cent should be maintained. A dramatic increase in intracranial pressure may be due to an intracranial haemorrhage and is an indication for a CT scan of the head.

ACID–BASE AND ELECTROLYTE DISTURBANCES

Alkalosis does not require treatment. Acidosis should be managed by specific treatment of the cause; intravenous sodium bicarbonate increases body sodium. Hypokalaemia (K < 3.5 mmol/l) is corrected promptly by adding KCl to intravenous fluids; about 120 mmol daily is usual, but up to 600 mmol may be required. The serum potassium is not increased above 4.0 mmol/l if liver transplantation is an option as graft reperfusion may precipitate marked hyperkalaemia. Addition of NaCl to intravenous fluids is not indicated in the presence of hypnonatraemia unless there is clear evidence of excessive losses of sodium. Sudden changes in sodium concentration should be avoided; they have been causally related to central pontine myelinolysis.

CEREBRAL OEDEMA AND RAISED INTRACRANIAL PRESSURE

Encephalopathy in fulminant hepatic failure, which is initially hepatic encephalopathy, may be compounded by cerebral oedema and raised intracranial pressure, hypoglycaemia, hypoxia, renal failure, acid–base/electrolyte changes, and the preterminal state. Routine management for acute hepatic encephalopathy is instituted (see above), with particular attention to correcting any possible aggravating metabolic abnormalities or precipitating factors. Cerebral oedema precedes raised intracranial pressure and is not always demonstrable on CT scan; it may be indicated by a loss of demarcation between grey and white matter. To avoid precipitating an increase in intracranial pressure, patients are nursed in a quiet room with the trunk and head elevated 40°; jugular venous compression is avoided and oculovestibular and oculocephalic reflexes are not elicited. Intracranial pressure cannot be quantitated clinically; this problem can be overcome by direct monitoring. A right parietal or temporal bur hole is required to place an extradural or subdural pressure transducer; this procedure is controversial—it is potentially hazardous due to the coagulopathy and should be undertaken by a neurosurgeon in an operating theatre. Epidural monitoring is safer but less accurate than subdural monitoring. The cerebral perfusion pressure (mean arterial pressure minus intracranial pressure) should be maintained at a minimum of 60 mmHg and the intracranial pressure at below 25 mmHg. The best time to introduce a transducer is uncertain, but may be when progression to stage III encephalopathy occurs or when the patient becomes a candidate for liver transplantation. Although monitoring intracranial pressure has not been associated with increased survival, it may facilitate optimal management before liver transplantation. When raised intracranial pressure is diagnosed an attempt is made to reduce it. Mannitol has been shown to reduce elevated pressures that are not greater than 60 mmHg. It is given as an intravenous bolus of a 20 per cent solution (1 g/kg), which can be repeated 4-hourly (0.5 g/kg) if the previous infusion induced a diuresis, plasma osmolarity does not exceed 315 mosmol/kg, and azotaemia is not present. Mannitol has variable and potentially deleterious effects on intracranial pressure when the initial pressure is over 60 mmHg and should probably not be given without prior knowledge of the intracranial pressure. The efficacy of mannitol suggests a cytotoxic component to the cerebral oedema. Thiopentone (185–500 mg intravenously over 15 min) may reduce raised intracranial pressure if mannitol is ineffective. Corticosteroids and controlled hyperventilation are not effective treatments.

HYPOGLYCAEMIA

Hypoglycaemia must be detected promptly and corrected vigorously by intravenous dextrose to maintain a plasma glucose of 60 to 200 mg/dl. Large amounts of dextrose are occasionally required (e.g. in excess of 2 kg).

CARDIOVASCULAR CHANGES

Maintenance of blood pressure may reduce the risk of cerebral oedema or lessen its severity. Ionotropes may increase tissue hypoxia and have not been shown to improve prognosis. However, if sepsis is suspected as the cause of hypotension, an ionotrope infusion may be warranted. If hypertension occurs, hypotensive or vasodilator drugs, which might adversely affect intracranial pressure, are not given. Arrhythmias may subside with correction of acid–base or electrolyte disturbances.

HEPATORENAL SYNDROME

Optimization of blood volume by infusing 20 per cent albumin may transiently improve renal function by correcting haemodynamic disturbances. Care is taken not to overload the circulation to avoid an adverse effect on intracranial pressure. Any therapeutic agents that may contribute to impaired renal function, including diuretics, are avoided. Severe acid–base/electrolyte disturbances or fluid overload, and, rarely, azotaemia, may be an indication for ultrafiltration or renal dialysis. Such therapy, which must be undertaken carefully because of cardiovascular instability and coagulopathy, may be necessary to optimize a patient's condition before liver transplantation, but should not be expected to alter the course of the hepatic or renal dysfunction. In the presence of raised intracranial pressure, ultrafiltration is preferred. Continuous venous access may be obtained using a double-lumen tube. The left femoral vein may not be used to facilitate venovenous bypass during liver transplantation. Use of vasopressin analogues is experimental.

Fig. 6 Three hypothetical courses of fulminant hepatic failure (FHF) (as envisaged by N. Tygstrup). In group I patients, although liver function deteriorates below the coma limit with conventional intensive supportive therapy, liver function does not fall below the survival limit; these patients should survive with intensive conventional medical care alone. In group II patients, liver function deteriorates below the survival limit, but, if it can be maintained above this limit for a sufficient time by providing effective temporary hepatic support (rational hepatic assist), liver function would not fall below the regeneration limit and these patients should also survive. In group III patients, liver function deteriorates below the survival and regeneration limits irrespective of whether temporary hepatic support is provided. Liver transplantation offers the only hope of survival for group III patients. To facilitate optimal selection of patients for temporary hepatic support and liver transplantation it is necessary to develop reliable criteria that indicate which course an individual patient will follow.

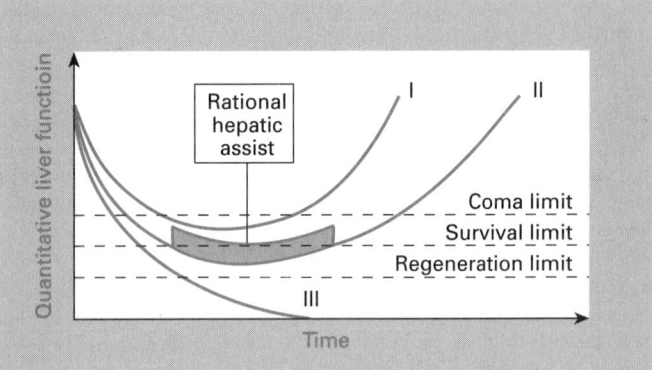

HEPATOPULMONARY SYNDROME

No attempt should be made to correct hyperventilation. Hypoxaemia is an indication for 100 per cent oxygen by face mask. Endotracheal intubation is recommended at the onset of stage III encephalopathy. A tube large enough to permit bronchoscopy should be used. Tracheal intubation may be difficult due to trismus and may be associated with mucosal haemorrhage. This procedure may be facilitated by curarization. Assisted mechanical ventilation is indicated for patients with stage IV encephalopathy, respiratory failure (increasing PCO_2) or pulmonary oedema. Positive end-expiratory pressure, which may reduce hepatic blood flow and increase intracranial pressure, should be avoided.

CONVALESCENCE

Abstinence from alcohol for a period of 6 months is recommended after recovery from an episode of acute liver failure not precipitated by alcohol. If alcohol is incriminated in either acute or chronic hepatocellular failure, life-long abstinence is advocated. Other identified precipitants must be rigorously avoided, such as halothane following halothane-induced elevations of serum aminotransferases.

Temporary hepatic support

The original rationale for providing temporary hepatic support was based on the assumption that the hepatic lesion in fulminant hepatic failure is reversible, provided that the patient can be kept alive sufficiently long for hepatic regeneration to take place. Theoretically, the patient selected for treatment with temporary hepatic support would die if treated by conventional medical management alone and would survive if the functions of the liver could be provided artificially over a finite period (Fig. 6). Temporary hepatic support should not only maintain the general condition of the patient, but also prevent life-threatening complications of fulminant hepatic failure. As there is a lack of detailed understanding of the biochemical disturbances that need to be corrected in fulminant hepatic failure, the design of artificial support systems is largely empirical. Attempts have been made to remove substances that have accumulated in the body (e.g. charcoal haemoperfusion) and/or provide deficient factors normally synthesized by the liver (e.g. haemoperfusion using devices containing hepatocyte preparations). All of the methods tried are time-consuming, expensive, demanding, and potentially dangerous. Complications include hypervolaemia, hypovolaemia, sepsis, and bioincompatibility. It is not clear that the risk:benefit ratio associated with the use of any such device favours the patient.

The provision of temporary hepatic support has no place in the management of chronic irreversible liver disease, such as cirrhosis, unless it is given in the context of preparing a patient for liver transplantation. When a patient with fulminant hepatic failure or chronic hepatocellular failure is a candidate for liver transplantation, effective temporary hepatic support may not only reduce operative mortality but may also beneficially increase waiting time for a donor liver.

REFERENCES

Agusti, A.G.N., Roca, J., Bosch, J., and Rodriguez-Roisin, R. (1990). The lung in patients with cirrhosis. *Journal of Hepatology*, **10**, 251–7.

Arroyo, V., Gines, P., Jimenez, W., and Rodes, J. (1991). Ascites, renal failure, and electrolyte disorders in cirrhosis. Pathogenesis, diagnosis and treatment. In *Oxford textbook of clinical hepatology* (ed. N. McIntyre, J-P. Benhamou, J. Bircher, M. Rizzetto, and J. Rodes), pp. 429–70. Oxford University Press.

Basile, A.S., Jones, E.A., and Skolnick, P. (1991). The pathogenesis and treatment of hepatic encephalopathy: evidence for the involvement of benzodiazepine receptor ligands. *Pharmacology Review*, **43**, 27–71.

Bernuau, J. and Benhamou, J-P. (1991). Fulminant and subfulminant liver failure. In *Oxford textbook of clinical hepatology* (ed. N. McIntyre, J-P. Benhamou, J. Bircher, M. Rizzetto, and J. Rodes), pp. 923–42. Oxford University Press.

Blei, A.T. (1991). Cerebral edema and intracranial hypertension in acute liver failure: distinct aspects of the same problem pressure. *Hepatology*, **13**, 376–9.

Butterworth, R.F. and Layrargues, G.P. (ed.) (1989). *Hepatic encephalopathy. Pathophysiology and treatment.* Humana, Clifton, NJ.

Canalese, J. *et al.* (1982). Controlled trial of dexamethasone and mannitol for the cerebral oedema of fulminant hepatic failure. *Gut*, **23**, 625–9.

Conn, H.O. and Bircher, J. (ed.) (1988). *Hepatic encephalopathy: management with lactulose and related carbohydrates.* Medi-Ed, East Lansing, MI.

Ede, R.J., Gimson, A.E.S., Bihari, D., and Williams, R. (1986). Controlled hyperventilation in the prevention of cerebral oedema in fulminant hepatic failure. *Journal of Hepatology*, **2**, 43–51.

Epstein, M. (ed.) (1988). *The kidney in liver disease*, (3rd edn). Williams & Wilkins, Baltimore.

Jones, E.A. and Schafer, D.F. (1990). Fulminant hepatic failure. In *Hepatology: a textbook of liver disease*, (2nd edn), (ed. D. Zakim and T.D. Boyer), pp. 460–92. Saunders, Philadelphia.

Kelly, D.A. and Summerfield, J.A. (1987). Hemostasis in liver disease. *Seminars in Liver Disease*, **7**, 182–91.

Kugler, C.F.A., Lotterer, E., Petter, J., Wensing, G., Taghavy, A., Hahn, E.G., and Fleig, W.E. (1992). Visual event-related P300 potentials in early portosystemic encephalopathy. *Gastroenterology*, **103**, 302–10.

Lidofsky, S.D. *et al.* (1992). Intracranial pressure monitoring and liver transplantation for fulminant hepatic failure. *Hepatology*, **16**, 1–7.

MacDougall, B.R.D. and Williams, R. (1978). H$_2$-receptor antagonist in the prevention of acute upper gastrointestinal hemorrhage in fulminant hepatic failure: a controlled trial. *Gastroenterology*, **74**, 464–5.

O'Grady, J.G., Gimson, A.E.S., O'Brien, C.J., Pucknall, A., Hughes, R.D., and Williams, R. (1988). Controlled trials of charcoal haemoperfusion and prognostic factors in fulminant hepatic failure. *Gastroenterology*, **94**, 1186–192.

O'Grady, J.G., Alexander, G.J.M., Hayllar, K.M., and Williams, R. (1989). Early indicators of prognosis in fulminant hepatic failure. *Gastroenterology*, **197**, 439–45.

Ostrow, J.D. (ed.) (1986). *Bile pigments and jaundice.* Dekker, New York.

Pappas, S.C. and Jones, E.A. (1983). Methods for assessing hepatic encephalopathy. *Seminars in Liver Disease*, **3**, 298–307.

Rolando, N. *et al.* (1990). Prospective study of bacterial infections in acute liver failure: an analysis of fifty patients. *Hepatology*, **11**, 49–53.

Trewby, P.N., Casemore, C., and Williams, R. (1978). Continuous bipolar recording of the EEG in patients with fulminant hepatic failure. *Electroencephalography and Clinical Neurophysiology*, **45**, 107–10.

Trewby, P.N. *et al.* (1978). Incidence and pathophysiology of pulmonary edema in fulminant hepatic failure. *Gastroenterology*, **74**, 859–65.

Weston, M.J. *et al.* (1976). Frequency of arrhythmias and other cardiac abnormalities in fulminant hepatic failure. *British Heart Journal*, **38**, 1179–88.

Wiesner, R.H. *et al.* (1992). Selection and timing of liver transplantation in primary biliary cirrhosis and primary sclerosing cholangitis. *Hepatology*, **16**, 1290–9.

Williams, R. (ed.) (1986). Fulminant hepatic failure. *Seminars in Liver Disease*, **6**, 97–173.

14.31 Liver transplantation

R. WILLIAMS

The concept of a vascularized liver graft in the normal anatomical position (orthotopic transplantation) resulted from pioneering experimental work on dogs carried out by Moore and Starzl independently in America during the 1950s. The grafting of an additional (accessory) liver to a heterotopic site was successfully accomplished in the experimental situation and a few long-term human survivors were reported from the early attempts with this technique. The bulk of an extra liver is not easily accommodated in the abdomen and many of the conditions that might be treated in this way, for instance cirrhosis, have a malignant potential. However, during the past few years there has been a resurgence of interest in this approach, based on a new programme of heterotopic liver transplantation developed by the Rotterdam group, with improved surgical techniques and using the right lobe only of the donor organ as the accessory graft.

The first patient to receive an orthotopic graft in the United Kingdom was in 1968 in a joint Cambridge/King's College Hospital programme, but until the early 1980s only a few patients were transplanted each year. The much improved survival reported by Starzl and his group when cyclosporin was introduced as the main immunosuppressive agent led to an important National Institutes of Health Consensus Development Conference in 1983. This decided that liver transplantation was no longer an experimental procedure and one that deserved wider application. Following this the number of transplants increased rapidly (Fig. 1) and the procedure has since become widely adopted throughout the world. In the United Kingdom during 1991, 424 transplants were made and the number is increasing about by 15 to 20 per cent per year. This remarkable increase reflects a greater awareness of the excellent survival figures currently being obtained with liver grafting (Fig. 2), together with the greater expertise of the centres using the procedure and the very considerable work of the United Kingdom Transplant Support Service Authority in donor organ provision.

Selection of patients and pretransplant evaluation

Transplantation should be considered whenever a patient with a progressive or otherwise fatal liver disorder is no longer able to enjoy a reasonable existence, although still well enough to withstand the considerable trauma of the surgery involved. Almost every type of end-stage liver disease has been treated by transplantation but in practice the decision as to which patient should have a transplant, and when, can be very difficult.

Transplantation below the age of 2 years is accompanied by a greater number of technical difficulties because of congenital anomalies. Above the age of 50, cardiopulmonary disease is increasingly frequent, although many patients in their 60s and 70s have been successfully transplanted. The risks are considerably greater if the patient has had previous upper abdominal surgery: this increases the hazard of dissection and can be the critical factor in blood loss and other complications such as damage to the bowel. The poor nutrition and wasting of patients with chronic parenchymatous liver disease is another adverse factor. Body defences against infection are known to be reduced in such patients and every effort has to be made to eradicate infections preoperatively before exposure to the added risks of immunosuppression. Common to all types of cirrhosis and portal hypertension are two specific cardiorespiratory complications—anoxia from pulmonary shunting (based on capillary vasodilatation) and right heart strain from pulmonary hypertension consequent on spasm/narrowing of the small pulmonary arterioles. Although both syndromes are reversible over a period of time by a successful liver transplant, the immediate post-transplant period, when there is major shunting or pulmonary hypertension, can be very difficult to manage.

Specific diseases

MALIGNANT TUMOURS OF THE LIVER

The realization of the high rate of tumour recurrence has led to a decrease in the frequency of liver grafting for malignancy. None the less, the younger patient with a relatively slow-growing primary hepatocellular carcinoma, often serum alpha-fetoprotein negative and without underlying cirrhosis, may be a suitable candidate. The fibrolamellar variant of hepatocellular carcinoma, which tends to metastasize late, is one of the more favourable histological types. Hepatoma development in the long-standing cirrhotic, which has been recognized at an early presymptomatic stage by serial ultrasonographic examination or screening for alpha-fetoprotein, is another favourable indication. Recent analyses show how closely the risk of tumour recurrence is related to the size of tumour at the time of transplantation (Table 1). Nevertheless, even with moderately sized tumours (4–8 cm diameter) over 40 per cent are cured and in some of the others long periods of palliation are obtained.

Extrahepatic spread must be excluded, as far as is possible, before transplantation by a lung and abdominal computerized tomographic scan together with a radioisotope bone scan. Small tumour deposits may be missed on imaging and tumour dissemination may also occur during the transplant operation. Recurrence of tumour may develop even in cases where the serum alpha-fetoprotein has fallen to normal after transplantation. Diagnostic needle biopsy should be avoided when liver transplantation is being considered, as the subsequent appearance of tumour

in the needle tract is well described. The suggestion that tumour growth is enhanced after the transplant by the immunosuppressive drugs given is not proven.

CIRRHOSIS

Most of the patients within this category have had end-stage disease from chronic active hepatitis, cirrhosis of the cryptogenic variety, or biliary cirrhosis (primary or secondary). In cirrhotic patients, the relief of pruritus and of the deep jaundice and pigmentation after transplantation is remarkable. As a rule of thumb, transplantation should be done once the serum bilirubin is greater than 150 μmol/l, for the prognosis then is likely to be less than a year. Patients may be transplanted when the serum bilirubin is lower if they are disabled by osteodystrophy, severe pruritus, or uncontrollable variceal haemorrhage. Cases of chronic encephalopathy in association with a large spontaneous or surgically induced (shunt) collateral circulation, and who are poorly controlled by dietary restriction and lactulose, can also show a dramatic response to successful transplantation. The procedure should also be considered for the cirrhotic patient with recurrent variceal haemorrhage in whom all other measures have been tried.

In those with end-stage liver decompensation for cryptogenic cirrhosis and end-stage active chronic hepatitis the proper timing of the operation is very difficult. When cases are separated into low-, intermediate- and high-risk groups for surgery on the basis of encephalopathy, ascites, nutritional status, serum bilirubin, prothrombin time, and age, considerable differences in the 1-year survival rates become apparent, ranging from 90.5 per cent after transplantation in the low-risk subgroup to 44.5 per cent in the high risk.

Patients with hepatitis B-related cirrhosis have a poorer early survival due to recurrence of the hepatitis B virus (**HBV**) infection and ensuing damage to the graft. A particular form of rapidly progressive liver failure, associated with extensive fibrosis and deep cholestasis, was iden-

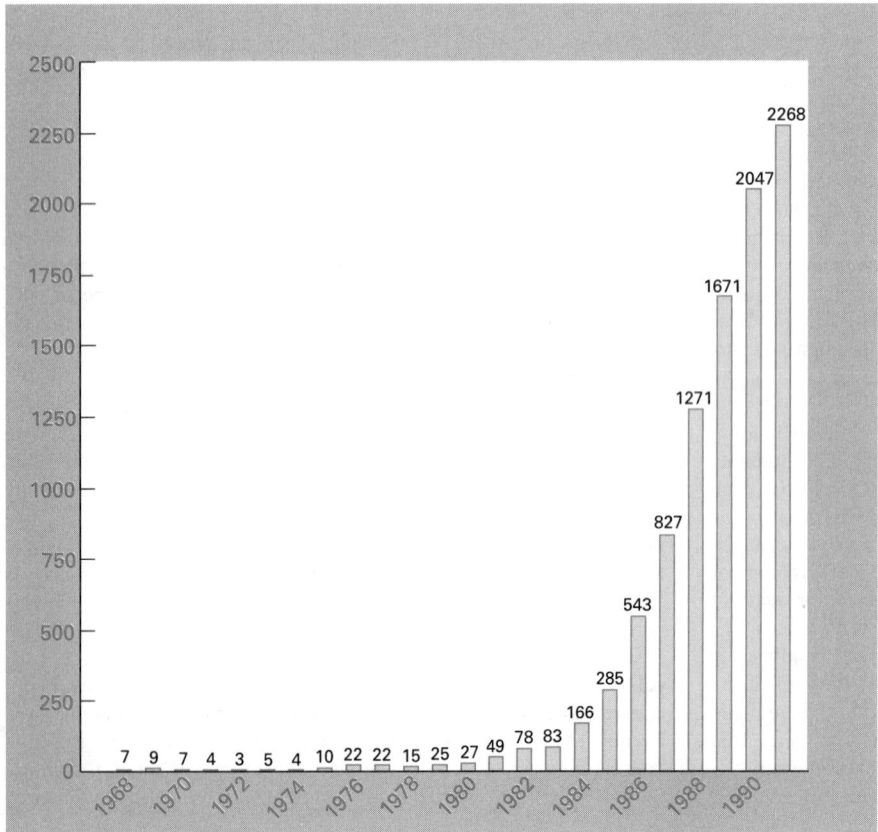

Fig. 1 The evolution of liver transplantation over the period May 1968 to December 1991 (reproduced by courtesy of Professor H. Bismuth, Director, European Transplant Registry).

tified by the King's group and termed fibrosing cholestatic hepatitis. Evidence from Europe suggests that the long-term use of immunoglobulin can decrease the frequency of recurrence and appearance of severe disease, particularly in cases at the non-replicating stage, with HBV-DNA negative in the serum.

The proportion of patients with alcoholic cirrhosis who will constitute suitable candidates for transplantation in relation to the total number of patients with this condition is small. The heavy use of alcohol is associated with cardiac and cerebral impairment, which, in addition to malnutrition, will add to the hazards of the operation. There is also a significant risk of return to harmful drinking habits. Nevertheless, excellent results can be achieved in carefully selected patients.

BUDD–CHIARI SYNDROME

In severe cases, transplantation probably carried less risk overall than a side-to-side shunt and offers the chance of greater long-term benefit. Experience has shown the importance of maintaining patients on long-term anticoagulation after the transplant, otherwise thrombosis of the portal vein and/or hepatic veins may occur.

INBORN ERRORS OF METABOLISM

Grafting may be curative in several of these congenital disorders in which the primary defect arises in the host liver and leads to its irreversible damage. These include α_1-antitrypsin deficiency (after transplantation, the α_1-antitrypsin phenotype changes to the donor type), some glycogen storage disorders, and galactosaemia. In the case of Wilson's disease, not only the chronic form, with its disabling neurological and/or hepatic disorders, but also the fulminant variety, which carries a very high mortality, can be treated in this way with correction of the disordered copper metabolism. Liver transplantation may also be done for inherited metabolic disorders in which the liver, although the site of the defect, is not damaged by it, as in the case of the patient with an irreversibly damaged heart from familial hypercholesterolaemia, who can be treated successfully by combined heart and liver grafting. Sufficient low-density lipoprotein receptors are present in the normal donor liver to restore lipid metabolism to normal. Another instance of combined grafting is in patients with renal failure from primary hyperoxaluria, where the grafting of a normal liver together with a kidney corrects abnormal oxalate pools by providing the defective hepatic enzyme, and prevents the grafted kidney from becoming damaged by oxalate deposition.

Table 1 *Liver transplantation for hepatocellular carcinoma: analysis of recurrence and survival in relation to size of original lesion*

	N	Cirrhosis	Recurrence	Duration of survival (years)
A < 4 cm	14	14*	0	0.6–4.1
B 4–8 cm	15	14	6 (40%)	0.4–16
C > 8 cm and multifocal	27	12	21 (78%)	0.3–5.2

*Includes four incidental findings.
Reproduced from McPeake *et al.* (1992). *Journal of Hepatology*, **18**, 226–34, with permission.

ACUTE LIVER FAILURE

Selection of cases is based on strict criteria derived from a multivariate analysis of prognostic indicators. It is important that such criteria are followed because survival rates with intensive liver care can reach 39 to 67 per cent for hepatitis A and B and paracetamol overdoses. Patients with presumed non-A, non-B fulminant hepatitis or drug hepatotoxicity reactions have the highest mortality. Potential cases need to be referred early to a transplant centre to allow for the likely delay in obtaining a donor organ. The 1-year survival in the first 100 patients transplanted at King's for acute liver failure was 58 per cent.

BILIARY ATRESIA

Despite the difficulties of obtaining organs in this age group, an increasing number of children in whom a Kasai operation of portal enterostomy has failed are now being treated by transplantation. With cyclosporin as the main immunosuppressive agent, retardation of growth is no longer a problem; indeed there is a growth spurt after a successful transplant. Reduction techniques allow adult organs to be used and results are as good as with the whole organ. The use of voluntary donation of a left lobe from a parent is another approach for which there is a good ethical justification.

Donor–recipient matching and organ preservation

Matching the size of the donor organ to the recipient is extremely important, as is matching for blood-group compatibility. ABO blood group-incompatible grafts should be used only in exceptional, life-threatening situations. Although studies at King's have shown a relation between tissue matching and occurrence of chronic rejection, the interrelation between mismatching of HLA class 1 antigens, HLA-DR class 2 matching, and cytomegalovirus infection of the bile ducts (which are the site of the chronic rejection process) is complicated. In any event, the urgent needs of the recipient combined with time constraints on liver preservation will preclude efforts at HLA tissue matching.

Current organ procurement policy means that several organs may be removed from the same donor, including heart, liver, kidneys, pancreas, and cornea. Removal of the liver requires between 2 and 3 h of careful dissection in a donor with brain death whose circulation is supported. The quality of the organ that is removed is of great importance to the success of the transplantation, although it is often not possible to make more than a superficial assessment of its function and viability. Donors who have been in serious accidents may have been heavy drinkers, and anoxic death, drowning for instance, can also damage the liver. A satisfactory cardiovascular state before liver removal is essential. To avoid damage from warm ischaemia, cold perfusion of the liver through the portal vein is started *in situ* using the University of Wisconsin (**UW**) solution, which contains potassium lactobionate, phosphate buffer, raffinose, and glutathione. Its introduction in 1988 was a major advance; the longer preservation obtained allows transplant operations to be

Fig. 2 Three-year survival curves for 4243 adult patients transplanted during the period January 1988 to June 1991 (reproduced by courtesy of Professor H. Bismuth, Director, European Transplant Registry).

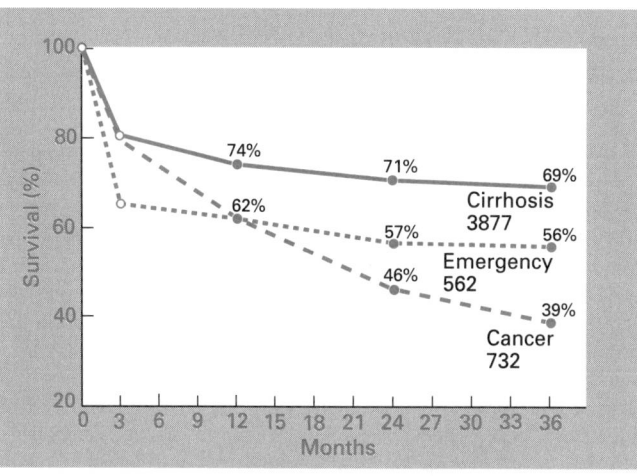

planned for the daylight hours. Once the liver is removed it is placed in a bowl of cold saline surrounded by ice, and the hepatic artery is then perfused with UW solution. The gallbladder is also washed free of bile, otherwise this will damage the mucosa during the period of preservation. A liver can be kept in this way for up to 24 h, although its function will almost certainly be better if the period of cold ischaemia is kept to less than 12 to 15 h.

Recipient hepatectomy and orthotopic transplantation

Control of haemorrhage during the dissection preceding removal of the liver can be extremely difficult in the cirrhotic patient when portal hypertension is associated with many thin-walled collateral vessels. Occlusion of both splanchnic and vena caval circulations is necessary during the final stages of removal and although patients can tolerate this for a time, the current practice in adult patients is to institute venovenous bypass with decompression of both portal and systemic circulation.

The order of anastomoses is, first, the inferior vena cava above the liver and then the portal vein, before completion of which a cannula is inserted into the portal vein and the organ perfused with plasma protein fraction at room temperature to wash out preservation fluid, which will have a high content of potassium ions and acid radicals. The portal venous anastomosis is then completed and some blood is allowed to flow through the liver and out through the inferior vena cava below. The clamp is then removed from the vena cava above the liver and the lower anastomosis of the inferior vena cava carried out. Arterial supply to the liver is re-established by joining the hepatic artery to the coeliac axis or to a Carrell patch on the aorta. The biliary tract is then reconstructed. A direct end-to-end anastomosis of donor and recipient common bile duct is the favoured technique. In patients with biliary atresia or sclerosing cholangitis, the gallbladder or donor common bile duct is anastomosed to a jejunal Roux loop. Unfortunately there is still an appreciable number of early as well as longer-term biliary tract complications, with stricture formation and recurrent cholangitis. An occlusion/thrombosis of the hepatic artery anastomosis has been shown to be the main factor affecting the viability of the extrahepatic bile ducts and the development of strictures.

POSTOPERATIVE MANAGEMENT

A high level of medical and nursing care is essential at this stage. When the donor organ is undamaged by ischaemia or by difficulties during the implantation procedure there is immediate function and the patient recovers consciousness within a few hours and may be extubated within 24 h. During the first few days, thrombosis of the hepatic artery or of the portal vein may occur and result in rapid deterioration in liver function; the prothrombin time and serum transaminases are the best markers. One of the most serious complications in the early postoperative period is continuing haemorrhage, and re-exploration to search for bleeding points may become necessary. Patients whose grafts are functioning poorly for any reason are best treated by early retransplantation.

Rejection and immunosuppression

Studies in several animal species have shown that the liver is rejected less aggressively than other organs such as skin, kidneys, or heart. Indeed, liver transplantation has been done against recipient antidonor T-warm antibodies, which would cause hyperacute rejection of kidney homografts. However, occasional instances of hyperacute liver rejection are recorded and certainly the liver can be aggressively damaged by acute and chronic rejection processes. Cyclosporin, the principal agent in immunosuppressive drug regimens, has significant nephrotoxic properties and considerable care is needed in the postoperative period when intravenous administration is necessary, particularly when renal function is already impaired. Careful monitoring of the blood concentration of

cyclosporin is essential. Most centres use azathioprine and prednisolone in combination with cyclosporin for initial immunosuppression. Cyclosporin is not adequately absorbed after oral administration until the T-tube is clamped and there is bile in the duodenum. Oral dosage with cyclosporin is 10 mg/kg per day, the dose being adjusted subsequently so as to maintain a trough blood concentration of 100 to 150 ng/ml (by monoclonal assay). Long-term maintenance regimens vary according to centre, with all three drugs being used in combination (each in somewhat lower dosage to minimize side-effects), or with cyclosporin and azathioprine together, or with cyclosporin alone in cases where the drug is well tolerated. A new immunosuppressive drug, FK506, is now under controlled clinical evaluation. The frequency of acute rejection episodes appears to be reduced and the need to give high-dose corticosteroids decreased, but nephrotoxicity and neurotoxicity similar to that experienced with cyclosporin are undoubtedly observed.

Acute rejection is common between the seventh and fourteenth postoperative day. The diagnosis may be confirmed by liver biopsy, which shows characteristic histological appearances. Liver biopsy is also essential in the diagnosis of later rejection episodes and in confirming chronic rejection, particularly the variety with deep cholestasis consequent to progressive damage of the bile ducts known as the 'vanishing bile-duct syndrome'. Acquired hepatitis virus infection of the graft, particularly cytomegalovirus, will require histological confirmation and is an important complication in relation to bile-duct damage; it responds in most instances to gancyclovir, which in some centres is also used prophylactically from the third week onwards in recipients receiving cytomegalovirus-positive grafts, who are the most likely group to develop this complication. Ultrasonographic examination, non-invasive and easily repeatable, is particularly useful in distinguishing obstructive jaundice (and other biliary-tract complications) from rejection or hepatitis infection of the graft.

The treatment of acute rejection is with a course of intravenous solumedrone, 1 g daily for 3 days. This usually results in a rapid improvement of liver function. Repeated episodes of acute rejection may be followed by chronic rejection of the vanishing bile-duct type, although this can also develop insidiously. Although usually considered as irreversible, at least 50 per cent of cases, in which the serum bilirubin is less than 200 μmol/l respond to FK506. The frequency with which chronic rejection is encountered has undoubtedly decreased and is no more than 5 to 10 per cent of cases in most series.

With the discovery of hepatitis C and the introduction of a diagnostic serological test it has become apparent that many cases of so-called cryptogenic cirrhosis are attributable to this infection; additionally, when transplantation is done the rate of reinfection in the graft is very high, a situation similar to that for hepatitis B, as described earlier in this chapter. The antiviral agents interferon and ribavirin are of some value in controlling the effects of such reinfection.

Long-term rehabilitation and overall results

Even when immunosuppression has been reduced to maintenance levels, patients remain susceptible to infection and it is important that both patients and general practitioners are alerted to this possibility. Other long-term complications include those directly related to the immunosuppressive drugs. Hypertension, renal impairment, and severe headaches are common with cyclosporin. The long-term nephrotoxic effects of FK506 are not yet established, although hypertension appears to be less frequent than with cyclosporin. One of the most troublesome complications of continued corticosteroid therapy is osteoporosis, particularly vertebral collapse. In many patients with primary biliary cirrhosis, osteoporosis is already present and is further aggravated by immobilization during the postoperative period.

In those who survive beyond 1 year, rehabilitation is usually excellent and the majority of patients in the King's College Hospital series have returned to a full-time occupation. Of immense satisfaction to many women is the ability to look after their families and homes again. In those who have died after a year, the cause of death was often unrelated to the transplant or even to the original disease. The longest current survivor in the United Kingdom is now in his sixteenth year after transplant for hepatocellular carcinoma in association with familial HBV infection. One-year survival figures are running at 75 to 80 per cent for elective operations, with 5-year survival of 65 to 70 per cent.

Recurrence of primary biliary cirrhosis in the graft was originally described in patients who survived for 3 or more years after liver grafting. Although subsequently disputed on the basis that such changes are the consequence of a continuing mild rejection process, several recent reports have confirmed the original observation. In autoimmune chronic active hepatitis where, as in primary biliary cirrhosis, immune mechanisms play a major part in pathogenesis, recurrence of the disease might also be anticipated. This was first reported in a single instance of a 21-year-old woman who underwent grafting in 1980, and the most recent report from the Pittsburgh group describes some histological evidence of recurrence in approximately 25 per cent of cases. Such patterns of disease recurrence are of little clinical significance to the patient for many years and, as with recurrence of hepatitis B and C, can often be satisfactorily managed.

REFERENCES

Calne, R.Y. (ed.) (1987). *Liver transplantation*, (2nd edn). Grune & Stratton, London.

Lowe, J., O'Grady, J.G., Calne, R.Y., McEwen, J., and Williams R. (1990). Quality of life following liver transplantation: a preliminary report. *Journal of the Royal College of Physicians*, **24**, 43–50.

O'Grady, J.G., Alexander, G.J.M., Hayllar, K.M., and Williams, R. (1989). Early indicators of prognosis in fulminant hepatic failure. *Gastroenterology*, **97**, 439–45.

Polson, R.J., Portmann, B., Neuberger, J.M., Calne, R.Y., and Williams, R. (1989). Evidence for disease recurrence after liver transplantation for PBC. *Gastroenterology*, **97**, 715–25.

Samuel, D. *et al.* (1991). Passive immunoprophylaxis after liver transplantation in HBsAg-positive patients. *Lancet*, **337**, 813–15.

Singer, P.A. *et al.* (1989). Ethics of liver transplantation with living donors. *New England Journal of Medicine*, **321**, 620.

Starzl, T.E. (1992). *The puzzle people: memoirs of a transplant surgeon.* University of Pittsburgh Press.

Starzl, T.E., Todo, S., Fung, J., Demetris, A.J., Venkataramman, R., and Jain, A. (1989). FK506 for liver, kidney and pancreas transplantation. *Lancet*, **ii**, 1000–4.

14.32 Liver tumours

I. M. MURRAY-LYON

Benign and malignant tumours may arise in the liver from the hepatocytes, bile-duct epithelium, or supporting mesenchymal tissue. With the exception of hepatocellular carcinoma all the primary malignant tumours are rare but the liver is frequently the site of secondary (metastatic) deposits of malignant tumours elsewhere in the body.

Hepatocellular carcinoma

This occurs either as a single mass or as scattered nodules of tumour and in around 80 per cent of patients there is pre-existing cirrhosis. The tumour tends to invade the portal and hepatic veins, and spreads to the abdominal lymph nodes, and bones. Histologically the tumour is typically composed of cells resembling hepatocytes, which are arranged in cords. A number of other distinct histological subtypes are now recognized, including the fibrolamellar variant in which clumps of eosinophilic carcinoma cells are surrounded by a characteristic fibrous stroma. This tumour occurs in young adults in a non-cirrhotic liver.

EPIDEMIOLOGY

Although this is a comparatively rare tumour in Western Europe and North America where the annual incidence is around 1 to 2 per 100 000 population, it seems to be becoming more common, and in Africa and South-East Asia the incidence is 20 to 30 times higher. The highest annual incidence is recorded in Mozambique (98 per 100 000 males). In patients with underlying cirrhosis, males greatly outnumber females but in non-cirrhotic cases this sex difference is less striking. In areas of high incidence the peak age is in the third and fourth decades but in Europe and North America most cases occur in the fifth and sixth decades.

AETIOLOGY

In all countries of the world, cirrhosis, particularly the macronodular form, is present in about 80 per cent of cases and in Western Europe and the United States this is due usually to chronic alcoholism or chronic active hepatitis and at least 10 to 15 per cent of such patients will develop a hepatocellular carcinoma. In Africa and Asia, chronic liver disease is usually associated with hepatitis B or C virus infection and the percentage of these patients who develop this tumour may be higher than in other types of cirrhosis. Rare cases may follow prolonged use of the oral contraceptive pill or prior investigations using the radioactive contrast agent Thorotrast. In parts of Africa and the Far East there is circumstantial evidence implicating aflatoxin. This is a potent carcinogen derived from the mould *Aspergillus flavus*, which often contaminates food, and a number of field surveys have shown a correlation between aflatoxin levels in food and the incidence of hepatocellular carcinoma.

The hepatitis B virus (**HBV**) is now recognized to have an important role in the development of hepatocellular carcinoma, especially in areas of high incidence (see also Chapter 7.10.26). Evidence comes from several lines including the similar geographic distribution of areas of high prevalence of the HBV and hepatocellular carcinoma, and viral markers of HBV infection are found in a substantially higher proportion of patients with the tumour than in matched controls. Long-term follow-up studies of large numbers of HBV carriers have confirmed that the risk of developing hepatocellular carcinoma is much higher than in matched uninfected controls. The HBV can be identified in tumour as well as the surrounding liver and integration of viral DNA in the genome of hepatocellular carcinoma has been shown. This HBV DNA integration may result in major structural rearrangements in adjacent cellular

DNA, and a range of deletions, duplications, and translocations between chromosomes has been reported. In geographical areas of high endemicity of HBV as well as exposure to aflatoxins, mutation of the *p53* gene on chromosome 17 is a frequent finding. These mechanisms add additional evidence for a close association between HBV and hepatocellular carcinoma.

The hepatitis C virus (**HCV**) is also closely linked with the development of hepatocellular carcinoma, especially in geographical areas such as Japan, Italy, and Spain, where HBV is not hyperendemic. Almost all cases are associated with cirrhosis. Prospective studies of patients with chronic post-transfusion HCV infection indicate the latent period before tumour development may be as long as 25 to 30 years.

It is to be hoped that over the next few decades extensive use of vaccines against hepatitis B in areas of high prevalence will lead to a reduction in incidence of this tumour. Until such time as a vaccine against HCV is available, introduction of all possible measures to reduce transmission of this virus is important.

CLINICAL FEATURES

In Africa and other high-incidence areas, patients usually present with a short history of right upper abdominal pain, often associated with fever and weight loss. There may be considerable abdominal swelling due to liver enlargement, with or without ascites. Sometimes catastrophic intraperitoneal bleeding occurs, owing to tumour rupture. In low-incidence areas the disease is often more insidious and presents as a general deterioration in the health of a patient already known to have cirrhosis. There is usually hepatomegaly and a bruit may be heard over the liver. A number of non-metastatic systemic manifestations may also rarely occur, such as hypoglycaemia, hypercalcaemia, and porphyria cutanea tarda.

Because of the use of screening in high-risk groups, more small (less than 3 cm diameter), asymptomatic tumours are increasingly being detected.

INVESTIGATIONS

The haematological and biochemical changes apart from alpha-fetoprotein are non-specific and reflect the space-occupying lesion as well as the underlying cirrhosis present in about 80 per cent of cases.

Alpha-fetoprotein is a glycoprotein synthesized by fetal liver and its plasma concentrations reach their maximum at the end of the first trimester (3–4 mg/ml) and then decline. After birth concentrations fall rapidly to adult levels (1–10 ng/ml). Raised levels are found in about 80 per cent of patients with hepatocellular carcinoma and tend to be higher in those in Africa and the Far East than in the low-incidence areas. Concentrations of above 500 ng/ml in a patient with liver disease are highly suggestive of hepatocellular carcinoma but in interpreting alpha-fetoprotein values it should be remembered that high plasma levels are found in some patients with germinal-cell tumours of the testis and ovary as well as occasional patients with carcinoma of the stomach or pancreas, usually with hepatic metastases. Below 500 ng/ml there is a diagnostic 'grey zone', for such levels may be found in patients with severe viral hepatitis and active cirrhosis, but in these conditions subsequent readings tend to fall towards normal whereas in patients with hepatocellular carcinoma the levels rise exponentially. Sequential readings are therefore of great diagnostic value.

Other tumour markers for hepatocellular carcinoma have been described in the serum, including an abnormal vitamin B_{12}-binding protein, which is usually present with the fibrolamellar histological variant, and tumour-specific alkaline phosphatase and ferritin.

Liver imaging
Real-time ultrasound

This is a sensitive and specific test and picks up hepatocellular carcinoma in 85 to 90 per cent of cases. False-negative results usually occur in patients with tumours of less than 2 cm diameter.

Abdominal computerized tomographic (CT) scanning

This technique is probably no more accurate in detecting hepatocellular carcinoma than ultrasound and should be reserved for cases in which doubt persists. Sensitivity can be increased by combining CT scanning with a variety of arteriographic techniques (see below)

Hepatic arteriography

Excellent visualization of the hepatic artery can usually be obtained by selective catheterization using the Seldinger technique. As the major vascular supply to hepatocellular carcinoma is usually arterial, diagnostic changes are seen in a high proportion of cases. Information gained on the anatomical distribution of the tumour and the vascular anatomy is essential if surgical resection is being contemplated, and consideration can also be given at the time of arteriography to intra-arterial chemotherapy and hepatic artery embolization. The sensitivity of arteriography can be increased considerably by combining it with simultaneous CT

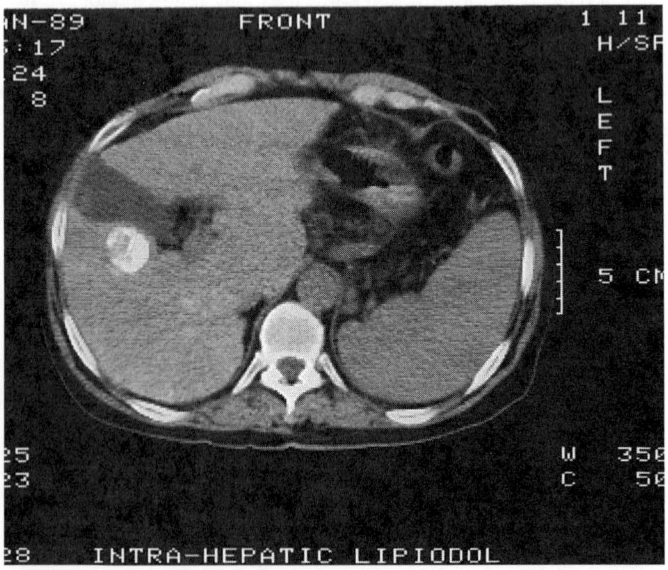

Fig. 1 CT scan of upper abdomen 10 days after Lipiodol angiography showing a cirrhotic liver with Lipiodol retained in a hepatoma (by courtesy of Dr John Karani).

scanning together with late films to show the portal venous system (arterioportography). Furthermore, the recent technique of Lipiodol angiography followed by CT scanning 10 to 14 days later can visualize tumours as small as 2 to 3 mm in diameter (Fig. 1). Lipiodol is an iodine-containing lymphographic contrast medium that is selectively retained in foci of hepatocellular carcinoma.

Magnetic resonance imaging (MRI)

The diagnostic role for this technique is still being assessed. It seems to add little to the results obtained using other techniques.

Liver biopsy

For definitive diagnosis, liver biopsy is essential, although this is not always possible because of prolongation of the prothrombin time. The diagnosis can be considered highly likely without liver biopsy proof if the alpha-fetoprotein level is greater than 500 ng/ml and the hepatic arteriogram shows a tumour circulation. Biopsy may be conveniently done at the time of laparoscopy or ultrasonography, and suspicious areas can be sampled under direct vision.

SCREENING

Patients with an increased risk of developing hepatocellular carcinoma, such as those with cirrhosis or chronic infection with HBV or HCV, should be considered for regular screening with assay of alpha-fetoprotein and abdominal ultrasonography. While such a strategy has been shown to pick up early tumours, and there is evidence of improved survival figures for these patients in the Far East, the benefits of screening have so far proved disappointing in Europe.

PROGNOSIS

This is usually a highly malignant tumour and the mean survival in most series is around 4 months. In Africa the disease tends to run a more malignant course. Patients with cirrhosis have a poorer prognosis than those without. Encapsulated tumours and the fibrolamellar histological variant have a better prognosis.

TREATMENT

Curative

Only complete resection or orthotopic transplantation hold out any chance of cure and these procedures should be considered in every case (see Chapter 14.31). Resection is possible, however, in only about 10 per cent of cases, because of underlying cirrhosis or spread to both lobes. Often a major resection is needed and the anatomical possibilities are illustrated in Fig. 2. In the presence of cirrhosis a limited resection only

Fig. 2 Diagram to illustrate the main types of hepatic resection.

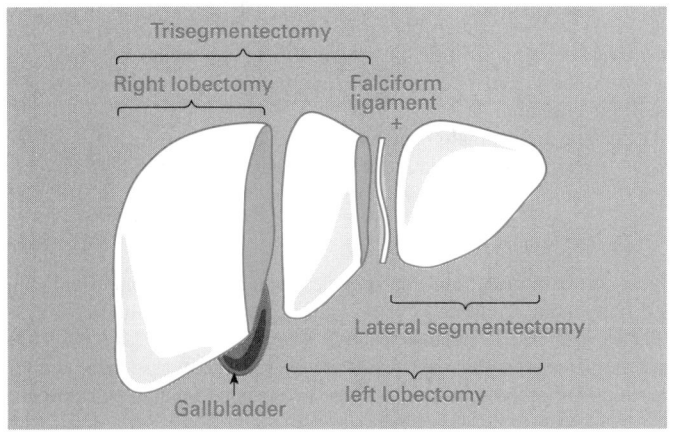

is possible as liver regeneration is defective, but this procedure may be curative if the tumour is small. In China, screening programmes to detect early hepatocellular carcinoma have led to higher rates of tumour resection in cirrhotic patients and improved long-term survival figures. There are also some long-term survivors after transplantation but all too often micrometastases are present at the time of operation and there is tumour recurrence later. The best results obtain when a hepatocellular carcinoma is discovered incidentally in the resected liver when transplantation is done for liver failure, and with the fibrolamellar histological variant. Otherwise most transplantation units now restrict the operation to patients with tumours less than 3 cm in diameter. It is unknown whether the results of transplantation are any better than limited resection for these small tumours.

Palliation

X-irradiation

External-beam irradiation alone has not produced consistent improvement and results are no better when used in combination with the cytotoxic drugs so far available.

Cytotoxic drugs

Doxorubicin (Adriamycin) is one of the few drugs tried so far which has produced worthwhile regression, but only 20 to 30 per cent of cases respond. It is given intravenously as a bolus every 3 weeks in a dose of 60 mg/m^2. The total dose is usually limited to 540 mg/m^2 because of cardiotoxicity; the only other significant side-effects are hair loss and marrow depression. In patients with a raised plasma alpha-fetoprotein the response can be gauged after one or two courses; its concentrations fall in patients with responsive tumours and there is no point in continuing Adriamycin treatment if the levels are unchanged or rise.

Mitozantrone (Novantrone), which is structurally similar to doxorubicin, gives a similar response rate. It has the advantage of fewer toxic side-effects.

Continuous intra-arterial infusion of cytotoxic drugs has now largely been abandoned.

A variety of other cytotoxic drugs, antihormones, and other agents have been assessed in trials, but none has shown convincing activity.

Targeted therapies

A wide variety of local targeted therapies have been developed and assessed in recent years. None, however, has yet been submitted to a prospective randomized controlled trial.

Percutaneous ethanol injection

Sterile alcohol is injected directly into the tumour under ultrasound guidance causing tumour necrosis. Repeated injections may be given into more than one tumour mass. The best results are obtained with tumours less than 3 cm diameter and the survival figures are comparable with those of limited surgical resection.

Lipiodol-targeted chemotherapy and radiotherapy

Cytotoxic drugs may be emulsified with Lipiodol (see above) and delivered directly into the liver at selective hepatic arteriography. There are some data to show that the duration of action of the drugs is prolonged because of the retention of Lipiodol in the tumour. There is, however, no convincing evidence of benefit from therapy.

Lipiodol has also been used in the same way to deliver radioactive ^{131}I to the tumour. Early clinical experience is encouraging.

Transcatheter arterial embolization (TAE)

Embolization with foreign material such as gel foam can be achieved at the time of hepatic arteriography and may result in substantial tumour necrosis, particularly in highly vascular tumours, which derive the bulk of their blood supply from the hepatic artery. In patients with decompensated cirrhosis and those with portal vein occlusion the procedure is contraindicated. Total occlusion of the hepatic arterial vasculature should be avoided. Broad-spectrum antibiotics are given for some days because of the risk of anaerobic infection in the ischaemic liver. As tumour necrosis is never complete, embolization of the tumour should be combined with targeted chemotherapy (chemoembolization). The gel-foam particles may be soaked in doxorubicin or the TAE may be immediately preceded by Lipiodol-targeted chemotherapy. While such treatment may result in tumour necrosis, shrinkage, and symptomatic improvement, controlled trials are needed to establish whether survival is prolonged.

Cholangiocarcinoma

Carcinoma may arise in the biliary tree in any part from the small intra-hepatic bile ducts down to the lower end of the common bile duct. Two clinical varieties occur in the liver—a peripheral form, which consists of multiple nodules often scattered throughout both lobes, and a hilar form usually situated at the confluence of the right and left hepatic ducts. This invades locally and causes obstruction of the biliary tree. Micro-scopically it is an adenocarcinoma with a simple ductular arrangement of columnar or cuboidal cells, usually with a prominent fibrous stroma, and the histological appearances are identical whatever the site of origin.

EPIDEMIOLOGY

This tumour is much less common than hepatocellular carcinoma and accounts for about 7 to 10 per cent of primary malignant tumours, except in the Far East where it makes up about 20 per cent. The peak age is in the sixth and seventh decades and is older than for hepatocellular carcinoma. The sex incidence shows only a slight male predominance.

AETIOLOGY

Thorium dioxide (Thorotrast) is a well-recognized but rare cause of the intrahepatic variety of tumour. In the Far East, infestation with one of a variety of distomes (*Clonorchis sinensis*; *Opisthorchis viverrini*) is probably commonly related.

Patients with long-standing ulcerative colitis occasionally develop carcinoma in the biliary tract and the risk is about 10 times greater than for the general population. Patients with total involvement of the colon of more than 10 years duration are the ones usually affected and the tumour may develop some years after panproctocolectomy. Either the intra- or extrahepatic biliary tree may be affected. Various types of cystic disease of the biliary tree such as congenital hepatic fibrosis, polycystic disease of the liver, and Caroli's disease may all be complicated by the development of malignant change. The role of gallstones has been emphasized in the aetiology of extrahepatic cholangiocarcinoma but the association does not necessarily indicate causation. Unlike hepatocellular carcinoma, neither long-standing HBV infection nor cirrhosis seem to predispose to cholangiocarcinoma but secondary biliary cirrhosis may develop, owing to prolonged biliary obstruction.

SYMPTOMS AND SIGNS

In the peripheral intrahepatic type, patients present with upper abdominal pain, anorexia, malaise, and weight loss. With hilar tumours, jaundice is an early feature. Hepatomegaly is usual and splenomegaly may be found if secondary biliary cirrhosis develops.

DIAGNOSIS

The liver function tests show cholestatic features with elevation of bilirubin and alkaline phosphatase. Alpha-fetoprotein concentrations are usually normal or only slightly raised and tests for HBV infection are negative.

Ultrasonography and CT scanning may demonstrate the tumour mass and with hilar tumours show dilation of the intrahepatic biliary tree. On hepatic angiography the tumour tends to be avascular but encasement and occlusion of vessels occurs. Biliary-tree obstruction in the hilum may be demonstrated by percutaneous transhepatic cholangiography using the skinny (Chiba) needle or by endoscopic retrograde cholangiography (**ERCP**).

PROGNOSIS

Most patients deteriorate progressively, with average survival from diagnosis around 4 to 6 months. If biliary drainage can be achieved in patients with hilar tumours, the prognosis is considerably better, for these tumours are often slow growing.

TREATMENT

For the peripheral tumours the principles of treatment are the same as for hepatocellular carcinoma (see above) but the response to chemotherapy is disappointing. A variety of different drug combinations, with or without radiotherapy, is being tried but none can currently be recommended.

Hilar tumours may sometimes be resectable with reanastomosis of the biliary tree or anastomosis of a Roux loop of jejunum to the biliary tree in the hilum. More usually curative excision is not possible, and the aim must be to establish biliary drainage. A stent can be placed through the growth at laparotomy, or at ERCP, or via the percutaneous transhepatic route, thus avoiding surgery. The use of self-expanding metal stents is a recent advance. Conventional radiotherapy may also produce useful symptomatic relief, and high-dose local irradiation has been given within the biliary tree by means of iridium-192 wire. Excellent palliation can be achieved by these procedures and survival for 1 to 2 years is not unusual. Because of a high risk of tumour recurrence, liver transplantation is seldom indicated.

Angiosarcoma (Kupffer-cell sarcoma; malignant haemangioendothelioma)

This is a rare tumour consisting of malignant endothelial cells supported on a reticulin framework. It is often multifocal and may arise in a cirrhotic liver.

Considerable progress has been made in identifying aetiological agents. Like hepatocellular carcinoma and cholangiocarcinoma, it occurs in patients who were exposed to Thorotrast 15 to 25 years earlier, and chronic exposure to arsenic has also been implicated. More recently the tumour has been found in workers in the vinyl chloride industry, particularly those exposed to high concentrations of vinyl chloride monomer while cleaning the autoclaves. Since this discovery, strict safety regulations have been introduced but because of the long latent period new cases continue to present. A few cases have occurred in long-term androgen takers but in the majority of patients no aetiological factor has yet been identified. As with other liver tumours, patients present with abdominal pain and hepatic enlargement and blood-stained ascites is common.

This is a highly malignant tumour and curative resection is rarely possible. No form of palliative treatment has so far proved effective.

Other primary malignant tumours

These are extremely rare and include fibrosarcoma, leiomyosarcoma, and lymphoma. Children develop both hepatoblastoma and hepatocellular carcinoma. The former usually occurs in the first 2 years of life and the latter after the age of 5. Both are frequently associated with a raised alpha-fetoprotein. Resection or transplantation may be curative.

Hepatic metastases

The liver is a favoured site for metastatic spread and about 50 per cent of malignant tumours in the portal venous drainage area eventually give rise to hepatic metastases.

DIAGNOSIS

The diagnosis is easy when physical examination reveals a large nodular liver but detection of small or solitary deposits is difficult. Liver function tests may be normal, but as the tumour mass enlarges, the alkaline phosphatase usually rises. Ultrasound scanning should pick up tumours greater than 1 cm in diameter but accuracy is greatest when the metastases are large and numerous. In one large autopsy study, metastatic deposits were all less than 2 cm in diameter in one-third of the cases. 'Blind' liver biopsy is positive in only about 50 per cent of cases but accuracy can be greatly increased by target biopsy at the time of laparoscopy or ultrasonography.

PROGNOSIS

The prognosis is obviously worse when there is extensive liver replacement by tumour with severe disturbance in liver function tests or ascites. The site of primary growth is also relevant and deposits from colorectal cancer have a better prognosis (untreated mean survival, 9 to 12 months) than most other tumours, especially if the deposits first appear some years after resection of the primary.

TREATMENT

The range of possible treatments is the same as has been discussed for hepatocellular carcinoma. Partial hepatectomy to remove a solitary deposit may occasionally lead to prolonged survival or cure and the results are best in patients with colorectal cancer. The number of cases, however, with solitary deposits suitable for resection is small. A special situation exists with respect to hepatic metastases from the carcinoid tumour. This is often a slowly growing neoplasm and the main problem is the distress caused by flushing and diarrhoea. Resection of tumour bulk without any attempt at total removal often gives symptomatic relief for some years, as does embolization. Transplantation should be considered for slowly growing tumours.

Chemotherapy

The choice of drugs will be determined by the origin of the primary tumour and this will not be discussed in detail here. The most common drug used for deposits from gastrointestinal cancer is 5-fluorouracil but responses are infrequent (10–15 per cent) and short lasting. Better results are achieved when 5-fluorouracil is combined with folinic acid.

As with hepatocellular carcinoma the poor results with systemic chemotherapy led to trials with intra-arterial perfusion. Such treatment has been simplified by the recent development of implantable pumps, but while objective tumour regression may occur, there is as yet no certain evidence that survival is prolonged and the technique cannot be recommended for general application.

Ligation of the hepatic artery at laparotomy or embolization at the time of hepatic arteriography are occasionally used for patients with severe pain due to their metastases. Like X-irradiation these treatments may produce tumour shrinkage and give pain relief for a time.

Benign tumours

HAEMANGIOMA

This is the most common benign tumour and is usually asymptomatic, being found incidentally either during ultrasonography or CT scanning. Occasionally it may cause abdominal pain or shock due to rupture. Rarely it may be associated with thrombocytopenia, hypofibrinogenaemia, or microangiopathic haemolytic anaemia. Although the appearances at ultrasonography are usually diagnostic, it may be necessary to proceed to CT scanning with contrast, angiography, or MRI.

A similar tumour also occurs in infants and usually presents before the age of 6 months with cardiac failure secondary to the arteriovenous shunt. Many of these tumours regress as the child develops but if symptoms are troublesome, involution may be speeded by corticosteroids or X-irradiation. Ligation of the hepatic artery that feeds the angioma may be needed as a life-saving measure.

HEPATIC ADENOMA

The incidence of this tumour seems to have increased markedly since the introduction of the oral contraceptive pill and most reported cases have occurred in females who have been on the pill for 5 years or more. It should be emphasized, however, that the risk for the individual woman is infinitesimal. Patients are often asymptomatic and a mass is discovered on physical examination but some complain of upper abdominal pain and others present acutely with shock due to intraperitoneal bleeding. The tumour is usually solitary but may be multiple; it consists of cords or acini of hepatocytes without bile ducts or portal tracts, and fibrous tissue septa are sparse. It may be encapsulated. There is little or no disturbance in liver function and alpha-fetoprotein concentrations are normal. A filling defect is seen on the isotope scan and hepatic arteriography demonstrates a highly vascular mass. In some cases the tumour has regressed after withdrawal of the pill but surgical resection is usually recommended because of the risk of intraperitoneal bleeding and the occasional development of malignant change.

FOCAL NODULAR HYPERPLASIA

This is a benign condition of uncertain pathogenesis that is frequently confused with the hepatic adenoma. It is much more frequent in women than men but no relation to the contraceptive pill has been established. The liver mass is usually solitary and is divided into nodules by bile duct containing fibrous tissue septa that radiate out from a central focus. It is usually asymptomatic but rupture with intraperitoneal bleeding occasionally occurs. The findings on investigation are closely similar to those for a hepatic adenoma. The prognosis is excellent and malignant change is not recorded. Surgical excision is usually recommended, however, for diagnostic certainty.

OTHER BENIGN TUMOURS

These are very much rarer and include fibroma, lipoma, leiomyoma, and cystadenoma.

REFERENCES

Blumgart, L.H. (ed.) (1988). *Surgery of the liver and biliary tract.* Churchill Livingstone, Edinburgh.
Colombo, M. (1992). Hepatocellular carcinoma. *Journal of Hepatology*, **15**, 225–36.
Dunk, A.A. *et al.* (1985). Mitozantrone as single agent therapy in hepatocellular carcinoma. *Journal of Hepatology*, **1**, 395–404.
Dusheiko, G.M., Hobbs, K.E.F., Dick, R., and Burroughs, A.K. (1992). Treatment of small hepatocellular carcinomas. *Lancet*, **340**, 285–8.
Okuda, K. (1992). Hepatocellular carcinoma: recent progress. *Hepatology*, **15**, 948–63.
Penn, I. (1991). Hepatic transplantation for primary and metastatic cancers of the liver. *Surgery*, **110**, 726–35.

14.33 Hepatic granulomas

G. M. DUSHEIKO

The term granuloma describes a cellular reaction comprising a focal accumulation of modified macrophages that transform to predominantly secretory cells in response to ingested antigens. Histopathologists may report the presence of granulomas in liver biopsies under the light microscope, sometimes confirming the clinical diagnosis. At other times the finding of granuloma is unexpected. Hepatic granulomas are not uncommon findings in patients who have liver biopsies; they are found in 3 to 10 per cent of 'blind' needle at general hospitals. Granulomas in the liver may be accompanied by other morphological signs of inflammation, including bile-duct damage, vasculitis, cholestasis, and fibrosis.

There are many different causes; frequently the disorder is part of a generalized disease process. The differential diagnosis can be difficult. Consequently, an orderly approach is required, particularly because the therapy of infectious diseases associated with granuloma may be very effective.

Pathology

The typical granuloma is a focal accumulation of modified macrophages surrounded by a rim of mononuclear cells, predominantly lymphocytes; the modified macrophages are often called epithelioid cells because of their pale-staining cytoplasm and a superficial resemblance to epithelial cells. Epithelioid cells may fuse to form multinucleated giant cells in certain conditions, and these cells may contain inclusions. Langhans' giant cells are classically found in tuberculosis, but are also found in other granulomas. Granulomas are usually found throughout the liver, but are generally clustered near portal tracts; there may be associated necrosis within the granuloma. Caseous necrosis, referring to material resembling cheese, is associated with tuberculosis, but similar necrosis may be found in sarcoidosis. Other forms of necrosis, including purulent or eosinophilic, occur, depending upon the cause.

PATHOGENESIS

Granulomas are part of a process by which antigen, activated macrophages, and activated T lymphocytes coalesce into epithelioid and giant cells. In infectious causes, micro-organisms, or their products, are the sensitizing exogenous antigens. Alternatively, sensitizing endogenous antigens, for example tumours or immune complexes, may trigger sensitized lymphocytes, monocytes, macrophages, and Kupffer cells to form aggregates, and undergo epithelioid transformation. Granulomas thus represent an immunological reaction to a local antigen, which is not always identifiable. Discrete T-cell- and lymphokine-dependent mechanisms are involved in the initial acquisition of resistance as opposed to established immunity. However, granuloma formation by itself may not be required, nor necessarily sufficient, to confer antimicrobial activity. This may explain why ingested particles including bacteria may be seen within vacuoles.

The morphological appearances of hepatic granulomas may be a functional arrangement: monoclonal antibody subtyping suggests that T cells within the granuloma are predominantly of the T4 phenotype, and that the centres of sarcoid granuloma are populated by HLA-DR-positive macrophages. T8 suppressor cells are found within the periphery. Activated T cells release monocyte chemotactic factor and macrophage migration inhibitory factor. The cells within the granuloma have secretory activity, and granulomas in sarcoidosis, for example, are accompanied by production of several cytokines, including interleukins, serum angiotensin-converting enzyme, lysozyme, glucuronidase, collagenase, elastase, calcitriol, and fibronectin.

Experimental studies

Several experimental studies have pointed to potential mechanisms of granuloma formation. Egg deposition is the major stimulus for the cytokine response in murine schistosomiasis. T-cell chemotactic factors are released, and the cytokine response in *Schistosoma mansoni*-infected mice suggests that T cells must play a major part in the formation of egg granulomas. Transforming growth factor-β (**TGF-β**) secreted by Kupffer cells after stimulation with streptococcal-wall antigen may enhance receptor expression and TGF-β_1mRNA. This produces autocrine amplification. Several fibrogenic factors are secreted by the granulomas formed around *S. mansoni* eggs and one such factor, 'fibroblast-stimulating factor', has been isolated and shown to be a novel lymphokine; CD4$^+$ cells are the source.

Interleukin 5 (**IL-5**) is important in maturation of eosinophils; vasoactive intestinal peptide (**VIP**) released from eosinophils interacts with lymphocyte VIP receptors and influences IL-5 production as part of a feedback regulatory circuit. Streptococcus-induced hepatic granulomatous lesions in mice are under genetic control. Tumour necrosis factor (**TNF**) is inductive in the development of bactericidal granulomas during bacillus Calmette–Guérin (**BCG**) infection. TNF released from macrophages in developing granulomas acts in an autocrine or paracrine way, to enhance its own synthesis and release; this favours further accumulation and differentiation of macrophages, leading to bacterial elimination. *In vivo* molecular analysis of lymphokines involved in the murine immune response during *S. mansoni* infection has shown that IL-4 mRNA is abundant in the granulomatous livers, mesenteric lymph nodes, and spleens of infected mice.

CLASSIFICATION

A clinicopathological classification is often used to facilitate diagnosis; this is because there are many causes of granulomas within the liver (Table 1). The most common specific causes are infections, particularly tuberculosis and other mycobacterial infections, histoplasmosis and other fungal infections, brucellosis and other bacterial infections, Q fever, schistosomiasis, syphilis, sarcoidosis, some hypogammaglobulinaemias, and Hodgkin's disease. Drugs and toxins, and specific liver diseases (particularly primary biliary cirrhosis), are also important causes. Sarcoidosis and tuberculosis are apparently the most common causes of granulomatous hepatitis, but the several studies showing this may be biased because the results of unselected liver biopsies and autopsy reports are included. In some series, idiopathic granulomatous hepatitis confined to the liver is relatively common.

There is geographical variation in the prevalence and aetiology of hepatic granuloma. Infectious causes may be more important in tropical regions.

CLINICAL FEATURES

Fever is the major presenting manifestation of many patients with granulomatous hepatitis, irrespective of the cause. Almost half of the patients present with fevers of unknown origin. The clinical features of other common causes of hepatic granulomas vary according to the underlying disease.

Table 1 *Causes of hepatic granulomas*

Infections
Mycobacteria:
    Tuberculosis (typical and atypical)
    Leprosy
Bacteria:
    Brucellosis
    Tularaemia
    Yersiniosis
    Proprioni/listeriosis
    Melidiosis
    Whipple's disease
Spirochaetes:
    Syphilis
Fungi:
    Blastomycosis
    Histoplasmosis
    Cryptococcosis
Protozoa:
    Leishmaniasis
    Toxoplasmosis
Metazoa:
    Schistosomiasis
    Visceral larva migrans
Rickettsia:
    Q fever
    Boutonneuse fever
Viruses:
    Epstein–Barr virus
    Cytomegalovirus
    Hepatitis A
Helminths

Chemicals
Beryllium
Copper

Drugs (see Table 2)

Immunological disorders
Sarcoidosis
AIDS
Bowel and liver disease
Crohn's disease
Ulcerative colitis
Primary biliary cirrhosis
Hypogammaglobulinaemia
Systemic lupus erythematosus
Polymyalgia rheumatica

Idiopathic
Granulomatous hepatitis

Enzyme defects
Chronic granulomatous disease of children

Neoplasia
Lymphoma
Carcinoma

Miscellaneous
BCG vaccine

Diseases associated with hepatic granulomas

Infections

Tuberculosis, and infections caused by *Mycobacterium tuberculosis, M. leprae*, and atypical mycobacteria including *M. bovis, avium intracellulare, kansasii*, or *scrofulaceum* may involve the liver. These pathogens, although of low virulence, are often resistant to most antituberculous drugs; the response to treatment is slow, and late relapse is frequent. Granulomatous hepatitis due to atypical mycobacteria is recognized with increasing frequency in immunosuppressed patients and patients with acquired immune deficiency syndrome (**AIDS**).

Granulomas are seen within the liver in leprosy, particularly in the lepromatous type; leprosy bacilli are readily demonstrated within Kupffer cells. The diagnosis is based on epidemiological factors, and a positive lepromin skin test. Brucellosis, caused by *Brucella abortus, B. suis*, and *B. melitensis*, is seen in abattoir workers exposed to pigs and after ingestion of goat cheese or unpasteurized milk; *B. abortus* infection may progress to fibrosis. The diagnosis is made by positive blood culture or antibody titre. Tularaemia, a bacterial disease caused by *Francisella tularense*, a Gram-negative bacillus, may lead to hepatic infection; true granulomas are rare, but the liver has necrotic nodules. Granulomatous hepatitis may occur in cat-scratch disease; affected patients have high fever for several weeks. Computerized tomography of the liver has shown focal hepatic defects or periportal and periaortic lymphadenopathy. The Warthin–Starry silver stain shows organisms consistent in appearance with the cat-scratch bacillus in the liver or periaortic lymph nodes.

Granulomatous hepatitis has been observed in approximately 5 per cent of patients admitted to hospital for yersinial infection. *Listeria monocytogenes* may cause bacteraemia and microabscesses in multiple organs, including the liver. Meliodosis, caused by the Gram-negative bacillus *Pseudomonas pseudomallei* is endemic in south-east Asia. Treponemal infections, notably secondary and tertiary syphilis, may cause diffuse hepatitis associated with granulomas, or localized gummas. The diagnosis is made by a positive treponemal antibody test.

Many fungi may cause granulomatous hepatitis. Histoplasmosis is the most common cause in the United States. A high proportion of patients with disseminated histoplasmosis have liver abnormalities; the diagnosis is made by chest radiography and antibody titres. Fungus can be cultured from the liver biopsies, or seen on microscopic examination; blood and bone marrow culture may be positive. Blastomycoses and coccidiodomycosis are prevalent in the western United States.

Several parasites may cause hepatic granulomas. Leishmaniasis, the disease caused by the protozoon *Leishmania donovani*, may cause intermittent fever, night sweats, weight loss, and anaemia. Progressive hepatosplenomegaly occurs. Pancytopenia is common. The patient may have elevated concentrations of IgG. The parasite is found in Giemsa-stained bone marrow smears as oval, intracellular bodies, 2 to 4 μm in diameter. Many parasites are found in liver in Kupffer cells. Hepatic fibrosis may develop.

Schistosomiasis due to *S. mansoni* (in Africa and Brazil) and *S. japonicum* (in the Orient) is associated with liver disease. Ova are found in the fine radicles of the portal vein; these provoke a granulomatous reaction within the periportal tissues, which organize into characteristic pipe-stem fibrosis, ultimately producing presinusoidal portal hypertension. The disease is seen in patients who live in endemic areas. Firm hepatomegaly may be the only abnormality. Signs of portal hypertension may appear. Eggs in stool confirm the diagnosis, or viable ova may be found in rectal biopsies, or are seen in the centre of granulomas. Granulomas are also observed in *Toxocara cani* infection, which causes visceral larval migrans.

The aetiological agent of Q fever is *Coxiella burnetti*. The disease may mimic viral hepatitis, but may cause characteristic hepatic granulomas. The granulomas contain fibrin, which produces a halo effect surrounding a central area of fat, necrosis, and inflammatory cells. However, similar granulomas are seen in Hodgkin's disease, visceral leishmaniasis, cytomegalovirus infection, and drug reactions. Epstein–Barr virus (**EBV**) and hepatitis A have been associated with granulomatous hepatitis. The diagnosis of EBV infection is made by a monospot test or testing for IgM EBV antibodies.

Chemicals and drugs

Beryllium exposure, causing berylliosis, induces an immunological reaction. The diagnosis is made by chest radiography, and from a history of industrial exposure. Copper sulphate toxicity may lead to hepatic

Table 2 *Drugs causing hepatic granulomas* (see also Chapter 14.34)

Allopurinol
Beryllium
Carbamazepine
Chlorpromazine
Chlorpropamide
Clofibrate
Contraceptive steroids
Diazepam
Diphenylhydantoin
Halothane
Hydralazine
Hydrochlorothiazide
Methyldopa
Nitrofurantoin
Oxyphenbutazine
p-Aminosalicylic acid
Perhexiline maleate
Phenylbutazone
Phenytoin
Procainamide
Quinidine
Silicon
Starch
Sulphonamides
Sulphonylureas
Talc
Tolbutamide

Adapted from James and Scheuer (1991).

granulomas. Hepatic granulomas due to hyperaluminiumaemia have been described in patients on long-term haemodialysis. Reactions to starch, talc, suture material, polyvinyl pyrrolidone, silicone, barium sulphate, and thorium dioxide may also lead to granulomas within the liver.

Drug causes are usually the result of a hypersensitivity reaction; numerous drugs have been implicated (Table 2). Patients with drug-induced or toxic granulomatous hepatitis may be asymptomatic. Usually, however, they present with an acute febrile illness, with or without a rash and eosinophilia, jaundice, and biochemical evidence of hepatic dysfunction. The diagnosis of drug-induced granulomatous hepatitis depends upon excluding other causes. Liver biopsy is important in confirming the diagnosis. The patient may develop a rise in temperature and recurrent symptoms if challenged with the offending drug. Morphologically, drug-induced granulomas may be impossible to distinguish from those due to other causes. Patients usually recover if the drug is stopped. Associated lesions suggesting a reaction to a drug include significant tissue eosinophilia, unicellular hepatocytic degeneration and necrosis, cholestasis, and acute cholangitis or vasculitis. Special stains, polarizing and phase-contrast microscopy, and transmission or scanning electron microscopy play a part in the diagnosis of some types of granulomas.

Immune disorders

Hepatic granulomas in AIDS are often due to disseminated *M. avium intracellulare*. Patients with AIDS may also have other causes of hepatic granulomas, including lymphomas, drugs (particularly sulphonamides, antibiotics, antifungals, isoniazid), cytomegalovirus infection, histoplasmosis, toxoplasmosis, or cryptococcal infection. Liver biopsy is clinically useful in patients with antihuman immunodeficiency viral antibodies and unexplained fever or abnormal serum biochemistry.

Sarcoidosis This is the most common non-infectious cause of hepatic granulomas. The disease is considered to be immunologically mediated. The sensitizing antigens are unknown. Twenty per cent of patients with sarcoidosis have hepatomegaly, and hepatic granulomas are found in

two-thirds of cases submitted to aspiration liver biopsy. Patients often have splenomegaly. The granulomas, which are all at the same stage of development, cluster in the portal tracts, embedded in dense fibrous tissue. Central necrosis is less obvious than in tuberculosis. The lesions are often up to 2 mm in diameter. Systemic disease including erythema nodosum may be present.

Laboratory tests usually indicate a high alkaline phosphatase and elevated serum aminotransferases. The Kveim–Sitzbach skin test is positive in 80 per cent; the antigen used in this test is derived from sarcoid spleen. Hypercalcaemia and hypercalcuria occur. Concentrations of serum angiontensin-converting enzyme are increased in 80 per cent of patients. Bilateral hilar lymphadenopathy is seen on chest radiography. Rare complications of hepatic sarcoidosis include cholestasis, portal hypertension, and progressive liver disease. These complications are most often seen in black males, who present with jaundice, pruritus, and hepatosplenomegaly. After many years, the disease may eventually lead to hepatic fibrosis and cirrhosis. The portal hypertension is of the presinusoidal type, owing to involvement of the smaller portal venous radicles. Patients may present with fever, malaise, weight loss, jaundice, and pruritus; the serum alkaline phosphatase is elevated and the serum aminotransferases increased two- to fivefold. Ductopenia is seen on liver biopsy. The disease associated with portal hypertension has a poor prognosis, and is not responsive to steroids. In other patients, long-term corticosteroid therapy may reduce hepatosplenomegaly, and may improve the cholestasis.

Other non-infectious causes Granulomas are found in the intestine and occasionally in the liver in Crohn's disease. Hepatic granulomas are also found in ulcerative colitis. Patients with primary biliary cirrhosis are usually women and older than 40 years. Pruritus is relatively common, and hepatomegaly is usual. Clubbing and xanthomas are seen in those with more advanced disease. In contrast to patients with sarcoidosis, those with primary biliary cirrhosis infrequently have erythema nodosum, uveitis, and respiratory involvement. Hilar adenopathy is absent. Serum antimitochondrial antibodies are positive in the majority of patients with this cirrhosis. The granulomas are relatively sparse but bile-duct damage, in contrast to sarcoidosis, is extensive. Granulomas may have prognostic implications in this disease; they are found less often in patients who subsequently die of the disease than in survivors.

Granulomas have been described in patients with hypogammaglobulinaemia, systemic lupus erythematosus, and Wegener's granulomatosis; however, hepatic granulomas are actually rare in Wegener's. Whipple's disease may present in older patients: typical changes are polyarthritis, steatorrhoea, and granulomas of the alimentary tract; the diagnosis is made by intestinal biopsy.

Enzyme defects

Chronic granulomatous disease of childhood This condition is characterized by the inability of phagocytic leucocytes to produce hydrogen peroxide and a consequent bactericidal defect following phagocytosis. Neutrophil enzymes needed for the superoxide respiratory burst are deficient. Granuloma formation in the liver is characteristic, and the lesions may undergo caseation necrosis. Persistent infection is common in this X-linked disorder. Patients present with hepatosplenomegaly, weeping skin lesions, or miliary lung infiltration. The diagnostic test is based on neutrophil failure to reduce nitroblue tetrazolium to form blue–black formazan granules.

Neoplasia

Epithelioid granulomas occur in Hodgkin's and non-Hodgkin's lymphoma, even in the absence of malignant deposits in the liver. These granulomas may be related to tumour antigens. The diagnostic work-up includes chest radiographs, computerized tomographic scans, and lymph node or bone marrow biopsy. Granulomas are also found in specific carcinomas.

Miscellaneous

BCG vaccination may produce intrahepatic granulomas; these probably represent an immunological response to antigens of the vaccine. They have been reported in patients who have had intravesical instillation of BCG for bladder cancer, and may respond to corticosteroids. Granulomas have also been reported in polymyalgia rheumatica, Still's disease, and regional enteritis. A type of granuloma may be formed in fatty liver when fat-laden cells rupture. An entity called familial granulomatous hepatitis was recently reported in two West Indian parents and three of their seven offspring who presented over a 12-year period with identical systemic illnesses. Granulomata were found in the liver, and also in muscle, lymph nodes, and pleura in some of these affected individuals.

Investigation of the cause of hepatic granulomas

Laboratory abnormalities are often not specific or diagnostic. The erythrocyte sedimentation rate is frequently elevated, as is the serum alkaline phosphatase. Patients may have mildly elevated concentrations of alanine transaminase. Hyperglobulinaemia may be present. Elevated serum bilirubin concentrations are unusual, and the prothrombin time is usually normal. A liver biopsy confirms the pathological diagnosis, and may even indicate the cause of the disease. Multiple sections should be searched if granulomas are suspected. Other morphological features may be helpful, for example damage to bile ducts in patients with other features of primary biliary cirrhosis. In some patients, the lesions are found unexpectedly, but the cause may be found histologically (for example, schistosomiasis). Associated hepatic changes, or special stains, such as Ziehl–Nielsen for mycobacteria, silver staining for fungi or immunostaining for specific organisms, may be diagnostic. There may be other useful morphological features including eosinophils, purulent lesions, or an associated vasculitis. Alternatively, the diagnosis may be obvious from other features, for example if the patient is known to have a particular disease, such as active tuberculosis, or primary biliary cirrhosis. If a diagnosis is suspected, the pathologist and clinician can pursue a rational series of investigations.

In other cases, the cause is not found and no further histological clues are present. In these patients all causes relevant to the clinical presentation and probable epidemiological background must be considered. Although a multitude of diseases may be responsible, investigations in a patient with granuloma in the liver should initially be directed to rule out sarcoid, tuberculosis, brucellosis, histoplasmosis, syphilis, leprosy, cytomegalovirus, EBV, schistosomiasis, berylliosis, lymphomas, Crohn's disease, primary biliary cirrhosis, drugs, AIDS, or drug reactions. These represent the common causes in the Western world. A undiagnosed group accounts for approximately 10 per cent of patients. It may be appropriate to institute investigation for a possible neoplasm, or rare causes.

Treatment

The underlying disease cause should be treated. It is particularly important to rule out an infectious cause requiring specific therapy. Any drugs incriminated should be stopped. In idiopathic granulomatous hepatitis, the response to corticosteroids is often prompt. Treatment is started with 40 to 60 mg of prednisone daily. This regimen improves symptoms, subdues the fever, and reduces the hepatic granulomas. The alkaline phosphatase and ESR improve. Alternate-day corticosteroids can be used after initiating treatment with daily steroids. The dose is gradually lowered over a period of months.

If there is concern over unproven tuberculosis, then a trial of anti-tuberculous therapy may be necessary. Corticosteroids can be added if there is no response in 2 months. Isoniazid prophylaxis can be added. The patient's course should be monitored with liver biopsies. Fever may recur every time steroids are stopped. Indomethacin may also alleviate fever, and cyclophosphamide therapy of idiopathic hepatic granulomatosis may be indicated in patients in whom prednisone is contraindicated.

Propranolol apparently reduced the development of portal–systemic shunting in a murine model of chronic schistosomiasis with portal hypertension. The role of this treatment in endemic areas is being assessed.

REFERENCES

Biest, S. and Schubert, T.T. (1989). Chronic Epstein–Barr virus infection: a cause of granulomatous hepatitis? *Journal of Clinical Gastroenterology*, **11**, 343–6.

Cappell, M.S., Schwartz, M.S., and Biempica, L. (1990). Clinical utility of liver biopsy in patients with serum antibodies to the human immunodeficiency virus [see comments]. *American Journal of Medicine*, **88**, 123–30.

Chen, C.Y., Cohen, S.A., Zaleski, M.B., and Albini, B. (1992). Genetic control of streptococcus-induced hepatic granulomatous lesions in mice. *Immunogenetics*, **36**, 28–32.

Fauci, A.S. and Woolf, S.M. (1976). Granulomatous hepatitis. In *Progress in Liver Diseases* (ed. H. Popper and F. Schaeffner). Volume V, pp. 609–21. Grune & Stratton, New York.

Ferrel, L.D. (1990). Hepatic granulomas: a morphologic approach to diagnosis. *Surgical Pathology*, **3**, 87–94.

Guckian, J.C. and Perry, J.E. (1969). Granulomatous hepatitis: an analysis of 63 cases and review of the literature. *Annals of Internal Medicine*, **65**, 1081–100.

Henderson, G.S., Conary, J.T., Summar, M., McCurley, T.L. and Colley, D.G. (1991). *In vivo* molecular analysis of lymphokines involved in the murine immune response during *Schistosoma mansoni* infection. I. IL-4 mRNA, not IL-2 mRNA, is abundant in the granulomatous livers, mesenteric lymph nodes, and spleens of infected mice. *Journal of Immunology*, **147**, 992–7.

Ishak, K.G. and Zimmerman, H.J. (1988). Drug-induced and toxic granulomatous hepatitis. *Baillières Clinical Gastroenterology*, **2**, 463–80.

James, D.G. and Scheuer, P.J. (1991). Hepatic Granulomas. In *Oxford textbook of clinical hepatology*, (ed. N. McIntyre, J-P. Benhamou, J. Bircher, M. Rizzetto, and J. Rodes.), pp. 750–8. Oxford University Press.

Kindler, V., Sappino, A.P., Grau, G.E., Piguet, P.F., and Vassalli, P. (1989). The inducing role of tumor necrosis factor in the development of bactericidal granulomas during BCG infection. *Cell*, **56**, 731–40.

Kurumaya, H., Kono, N., Nakanuma, Y., Tomoda, F., and Takazakura, E. (1989). Hepatic granulomata in long-term hemodialysis patients with hyperaluminumemia. *Archives of Pathology and Laboratory Medicine*, **113**, 1132–4.

Lenoir, A.A. *et al.* (1988). Granulomatous hepatitis associated with cat scratch disease. *Lancet*, **i**, 1132–6.

Light, R.W. (1990). Hepatic mycobacterial disease and AIDS. *Hepatology*, **11**, 506–7.

Longstreth, G.F. and Bender, R.A. (1989). Cyclophosphamide therapy of idiopathic hepatic granulomatosis. *Digestive Disease and Sciences*, **34**, 1615–16.

McCullough, N.B. and Eisele, C.W. (1951). Brucella hepatitis leading to cirrhosis of the liver. *Archives of Internal Medicine*, **88**, 793–802.

Mahida, Y., Palmer, K.R., Lovell, D., and Silk, D.B. (1988). Familial granulomatous hepatitis: a hitherto unrecognized entity. *American Journal of Gastroenterology*, **83**, 42–5.

Marazuela, M., Moreno, A., Yebra, M., Cerezo, E., Gomez-Gesto, C., and Vargas, J.A. (1991). Hepatic fibrin-ring granulomas: a clinicopathologic study of 23 patients. *Human Pathology*, **22**, 607–13.

Mathur, S., Dooley, J., and Scheuer, P.J. (1990). Quinine induced granulomatous hepatitis and vasculitis. *British Medical Journal*, **300**, 613.

Modesto, A. *et al.* (1991). Renal complications of intravesical bacillus Calmette–Guerin therapy. *American Journal of Nephrology*, **11**, 501–4.

Moreno, A. *et al.* (1988). Hepatic fibrin-ring granulomas in visceral leishmaniasis. *Gastroenterology*, **95**, 1123–6.

Prakash, S., Postlethwaite, A.E., and Wyler, D.J. (1991). Alterations in influence of granuloma-derived cytokines on fibrogenesis in the course of murine *Schistosoma mansoni* infection. *Hepatology*, **13**, 970–6.

Prakash, S. and Wyler, D.J. (1992). Fibroblast stimulation in schistosomi-asis. XII. Identification of CD4$^+$ lymphocytes within schistosomal egg granulomas as a source of an apparently novel fibroblast growth factor (FsF-1). *Journal of Immunology*, **148**, 3583–7.

Saebo, A. and Lassen, J. (1992). Acute and chronic liver disease associated with *Yersinia enterocolitica* infection: a Norwegian 10-year follow-up study of 458 hospitalized patients. *Journal of Internal Medicine*, **231**, 531–5.

Sarin, S.K. *et al.* (1991). Propranolol ameliorates the development of portal–systemic shunting in a chronic murine schistosomiasis model of portal hypertension. *Journal of Clinical Investigation*, **87**, 1032–6.

Sartin, J.S. and Walker, R.C. (1991). Granulomatous hepatitis: a retrospec-tive review of 88 cases at the Mayo Clinic. *Mayo Clinic Proceedings*, **66**, 914–18.

Satti, M.B. *et al.* (1990). Hepatic granuloma in Saudi Arabia: a clinicopath-ological study of 59 cases. *American Journal of Gastroenterology*, **85**, 669–74.

Simon, H.B. and Wolff, S.M. (1973). Granulomatous hepatitis and pro-longed fever of unknown origin: a study of 13 patients. *Medicine (Balti-more)*, **52**, 1–21.

Warren, K.S., Domingo, E.O., and Cowan, R.B.T. (1967). Granuloma for-mation around schistosome eggs as a manifestation of delayed hypersen-sitivity. *American Journal of Pathology*, **51**, 735–6.

14.34 Drugs and liver damage

J. NEUBERGER

Introduction

Drug-induced liver injury is relatively uncommon but unless recognized early may cause death. Adverse drug reactions are responsible for between 0.1 and 3 per cent of all hospital admissions. Reliable data are difficult to come by: a relatively recent study has shown that in 1986 to 1987 about 1600 cases per year of adverse drug reactions were reported in England. Hepatic reactions accounted for 3.5 per cent, of which 7 per cent were fatal. Most reactions are of jaundice and hepatitis; the more common are due to halothane, antibiotics such as sodium fusidate, anti-inflammatory drugs, and oral contraceptives. These figures are likely to represent only a small proportion of drug reactions. The wide regional and individual variation in reporting rates and failure to report reactions after deliberate overdose combine to underestimate their frequency. In most instances, withdrawal of the drug will lead to resolution of the liver damage. It is important therefore to consider the possible contri-bution of drugs in a patient with any type of hepatic dysfunction. Almost all patterns of liver disease can be induced by drugs (Table 1) and some drugs may be associated with more than one type of drug reaction. For example, oral contraceptives are associated not only with the develop-ment of cholestasis but also with adenoma, hepatocellular carcinoma, peliosis hepatis, and Budd–Chiari syndrome.

The diagnosis of drug-induced liver damage is largely circumstantial and by exclusion of other causes of liver disease. The increasing rec-ognition of the contribution of hepatitis viruses, as yet not all serolog-ically definable, makes it impossible to implicate a drug reaction with certainty. Thus, it must be remembered that the reporting of an associ-ated drug reaction does not prove causality. The temporal association between the onset of damage and timing of drug exposure, and the response to drug withdrawal (Table 2), and the known patterns of drug reaction all help in establishing the drug as the cause of liver damage. Rarely, the presence of specific serological markers may help confirm the association between the drug and liver damage. For example, an antibody to trifluoroaceylated proteins is found in halothane-associated hepatitis, and anti-LKM antibodies occur in tienilic-associated hepatitis. Use of a clinical challenge is rarely justified, may be misleading, and may prove fatal.

Acute hepatitis

The range of liver-cell necrosis associated with drugs varies from a mild subclinical elevation of serum transaminases to the clinical picture of fulminant hepatic failure. Many drugs have been associated with acute liver failure (Table 3). Clinically, the picture may be indistinguishable from that of viral hepatitis. Occasionally, pain may be so severe as to lead to the mistaken diagnosis of acute cholecystitis. The serological changes are those of acute hepatitis with initial elevations of serum aminotransferases. Prolongation of the prothrombin time and jaundice may occur in more severe cases. Histologically, the appearances vary from a mild focal necrosis to massive liver-cell damage. In some cases, paracetamol for example, the damage is predominantly centrilobular, whereas in others, such as α-methyldopa, the whole lobule is affected. Steatosis, granulomas, and eosinophilia are variable features. The most common causes of drug-associated fulminant hepatic failure are para-cetamol overdose and halothane hepatitis. There is a current increase in liver failure due to 'recreational' drugs such as 'Ecstasy'.

The development of abnormalities of liver function tests during pro-longed drug use poses particular problems, as for example, with anti-tuberculous therapy. Derangement of serum aminotransferases occurs in approximately 10 per cent of patients and, if the drug is continued, up to 10 per cent of these develop severe hepatic necrosis. Identification of those patients who will develop severe hepatic failure is difficult and the clinician has to decide whether the risks of continuing therapy out-weigh the potential benefits. Drugs such as heparin are commonly asso-ciated with abnormal liver enzymes but very rarely with liver disease. The reason is not known but it may be due to loss of a few sensitive hepatocytes or to adaptation.

Conventionally, hepatic drug reactions are classified into predictable and idiosyncratic (Table 4). Predictable reactions are dose dependent; that is, the greater the amount of drug ingested, the greater the proba-bility of developing liver damage. Because animal models can usually be developed, screening will detect many of these drug reactions and stop the drug reaching the market. Hence this type of drug reaction is uncommon, except in overdose. The classic example is paracetamol tox-icity, which is described in detail elsewhere. None the less, between individuals there may exist great variability in the probability of devel-oping predictable drug reactions.

With very few exceptions, drugs require metabolism before cytotox-icity develops. Variations in susceptibility may, therefore, be a conse-quence of genetic variations in drug metabolism. Well-recognized genetic polymorphisms include variations in the cytochrome P450 iso-enzymes, drug oxidation, acetylation, and hydroxylation (see Section 9). Age, too, is associated with differences in susceptibility to toxicity. In general, children metabolize drugs differently from adults. Those taking enzyme inducers such as alcohol, rifampicin, or phenobarbitone are at a greater risk of increased metabolism of the drug and hence of forming

Table 1 *Patterns of hepatic drug reactions*

Hepatitis	
Fulminant	Halothane
Acute	
Subacute	
Chronic	Methyldopa, nitrofurantoin
Cholestatic	Phenothiazine, erythromycin
Granulomatous	
Cirrhosis	
Cholestasis	
Bland	Anabolic steroids, oestrogens
Vanishing bile-duct syndrome	Chlorpromazine
Sclerosing cholangitis	Floxuridine
Granulomas	
	Sulphonamides, phenylbutazone, allopurinol
Steatosis	
Microvesicular	Valproic acid, tetracycline
Macrovesicular	Methotrexate, amiodarone
Tumours	
Adenoma	Oral contraceptive, anabolic steroids
Carcinoma	Oral contraceptive
Angiosarcoma	Thorium dioxide, arsenicals
Cholangiocarcinoma	Thorium dioxide
Vascular	
Peliosis	Oestrogens
Budd–Chiari syndrome	Oestrogens
Veno-occlusive disease	Azathioprine, urethrane
Fibrosis	
	Vitamin A, arsenicals

toxic metabolites. Those with reduced glutathione stores, due to fasting, malnutrition or associated disease for example, may be at greater risk of developing paracetamol toxicity because detoxification mechanisms are impaired. Finally, liver disease itself may alter susceptibilities to drug toxicity. However, because of potential alterations in absorption, volume of distribution, protein binding, detoxification, and excretion it is difficult to predict the effect.

In contrast, idiosyncratic drug reactions are dose independent and may be due either to metabolic idiosyncrasy or the involvement of immune mechanisms. Immune involvement rather than metabolic idiosyncracy is suggested by a rapid onset after subsequent exposure and the appearance of markers such as peripheral and intrahepatic eosinophilia, granulomas, circulating immune complexes, autoantibodies, and other autoimmune phenomena, for example, haemolytic anaemia. Two drugs in particular have been well studied with respect to immune-mediated hepatitis—halothane and tienilic acid. Halothane hepatitis occurs rarely and after multiple exposures. Risk factors include female sex, obesity, and repeated or subsequent exposure within 3 months. Immune involvement is suggested by an increased incidence of organ non-specific autoantibodies, peripheral eosinophilia and circulating immune complexes, and the presence of antibodies reacting with a variety of halothane-associated liver-cell macromolecules. In other examples, antibodies to drug-metabolizing enzymes are present in serum. Tienilic acid-associated hepatitis is associated with a circulating liver/kidney microsomal antibody that reacts with the cytochrome P450, cytochrome $2c_3$, associated with metabolism of the drug; antibodies to cytochrome $1a_w$ are associated with hydralazine hepatitis. Whether these antibodies are involved in the pathogenesis of the disease remains uncertain.

Cross-reaction between two drugs may occur. Thus, halothane sensitization may predispose to toxicity from other halogenated hydrocarbon anaesthetic agents such as isoflurane. This may be due to the two drugs inducing similar antigenic determinants, leading to cross-sensitization, or to a different mechanism of toxicity, as suggested for captopril and enalpril hepatoxicity, where a similar metabolic pathway of toxicity has been postulated.

Acute cholestatic hepatitis

Acute cholestatic hepatitis is characterized by jaundice, pruritus, pale stools, and dark urine. There are usually few clinical findings, although the liver may be enlarged. Serologically, in the early stages there is elevation of the serum alkaline phosphatase and γ-glutamyl transpeptidase; as the disease progresses, hepatocellular enzymes start to rise. Histologically, the liver shows dilated sinusoids with cholestasis often predominating in the centrilobular region. There may be an associated portal inflammation and liver-cell necrosis. In the majority of cases there is rapid resolution following withdrawal of the drug, although with chlorpromazine and other phenothiazines the cholestasis may take up to 1 to 2 years to resolve. Many drugs cause a mixed hepatitis, where there are features both of cholestasis and liver-cell damage (Table 5).

Bland cholestasis

Bland cholestasis is characterized by cholestasis in the absence of hepatitis and is due to specific interference with bile secretion. The two main groups of drugs associated with this condition are oral contraceptives and oestrogens, and anabolic steroids. Cholestasis occurs in women taking oral contraceptives and in pregnancy. Prevalence varies, being low in southern Europe and North America (1 in 10 000) to high (1 in 4000) in parts of Chile and Scandinavia. Cholestasis associated with

Table 2 *Establishing the diagnosis of drug-associated liver damage by the pattern of symptoms, their timing, and the effect of withdrawal*

	Suggestive	Compatible	Incompatible		
	From onset	From onset	From cessation	From onset	From cessation
Hepatitis					
Initial treatment	5–90 days	< 5 or > 90 days	< 15 days	Drug taken after onset	> 15 days
Subsequent	1–15 days	> 15 days	< 15 days	Drug taken after onset	> 15 days
Acute cholestasis					
Initial treatment	5–90 days	> 5 or > 90 days	< 1 month	Drug taken after onset	> 1 month
Subsequent	1–90 days	> 90 days	< 1 month	Drug taken after onset	

After Danan (1990).

Table 3 *Main drugs causing hepatocellular necrosis*

Anaesthesia		*Neuropsychiatric diseases*	
Chloroform	Halothane	Amitriptyline	Nomifensine
Cyclopropane	Isoflurane	Bromocriptine	Pemoline
Enflurane	Methoxyflurane	Carbamazepine	Peogamide
Ethyl ether	Trichloroethylene	Dantrolene	Phenacetamide
Fluroxene	Vinyl ether	Desipramine	Phenelzine
		Ferpexide	Pheniprazine
Antineoplastic		Imipramine	Phenoxyproperazine
Carmustine	Hydroxycarbamide	Iproniazid	Phenytoin
Chlorozotocin	Mithramycin	Isaxonine	Phethenylate
Cyclophosphamide	Procarbazine	Lergotrile	Tetrahydroaminoacridine
Cytarabine	Streptozotocin	Levodopa	Valproate
Dacarbazine	Vincristine	Loxapine	Viloxazine
		Methylphenidate	
Cardiovascular disease		*Nutritional and metabolic diseases*	
Captopril	Nicotinic acid	Clofibrate	Gemfibrozil
Enalopril	Papaverine	Fenofibrate	Nicotinamide
Frusemide	Quinidine	*Radiological examinations*	
Hydralazine	Tienilic acid	Iodipamide	Iopanoic acid
Methyldopa		*Rheumatic and musculoskeletal diseases*	
Gastroenterological		Allopurinol	Dantrolene
Chenodeoxycholic acid	Omeprazole	Aspirin	Glafenine
Disulfiram	Salazosulphapyridine	Baclofen	Paracetamol
		Benorilate	Piroxicates
Endocrine disease		Benoxaprofen	Salicylates
Acetohexamide	Metahexamide	Clometacin	
Carbutamide	Propylthiouracil	*Skin diseases*	
Flutamide		Etretinate	Povidone–iodine
Infectious and parasitic disease		Methoxsalen	Tannic acid
p-Aminosalicylic acid	Isoniazid	*Others*	
Amodiaquine	Ketoconazole	Cocaine	Ecstasy
Carbenicillin	Levamisole		
Ciprofloxacin	Mebendazole		
Clindamycin	Mepacrine		
Co-trimoxazole	Minocycline		
Dapsone	Oxacillin		
Dideoxyinosine	Piperazine		
Fluconazole	Sulphonamides		
Fusidic acid	Zidovudine		
Hycanthone			

Table 4 *Cholestasis of acute hepatitis associated with drugs*

Type	Onset	Reaction to re-exposure	Dose effect	Reproducible in animals	Hypersensitivity features
Predictable	Rapid	Rapid	++	+	−
Idiosyncratic	Variable	Delayed	+/−	−	−
	Variable	Rapid	−	−	+

anabolic and contraceptive steroids is well recognized and may occur in association with virtually all the anabolic steroids with a C17 group; these drugs include norethandrolone, oxymethalone, danazol, stanozalol, and methyltestosterone. Other drugs are listed in Table 6.

Steatosis

Steatosis may be micro- or macrovesicular. Differentiation is important because the clinical features and outcomes are different. (Table 7).

MICROVESICULAR STEATOSIS

In microvesicular steatosis, the fat is distributed in small lipid droplets; the hepatocellular nucleus is not displaced. There may be an associated hepatitis. Extensive microvesicular steatosis, even in the absence of liver-cell necrosis, may lead to a serious clinical syndrome with haemorrhage, syncope, hypotension, lethargy, coma, or hypoglycaemia. In some cases, renal failure and pancreatic inflammation may occur. Biochemically, serum aminotransferases and bilirubin are not greatly

Table 5 *Main drugs causing mixed or cholestatic hepatitis*

Cancer

Aminoglutethimide	Cisplatin
Arabinoside	Cyclosporin
Azathioprine	Cytosine
Chlorambucil	Mitomycin
Chlorozotocin	Streptozotocin

Cardiovascular disease

Ajmaline	Phenindion
Captopril	Prajmaline
Diltazem	Procainamide
Disopyramide	Propafenone
Flecainide	Quinine
Hydralazine	Spironolactone
Methyldopa	Verapamil
Mexiletine	Warfarin
Nifedipine	

Gastroenterological diseases

Cimetidine	Ranitidine
Penicillamine	

Endocrine diseases

Acetohexamide	Methimazole
Carbimazole	Propylthiouracil
Chlorpropamide	Tamoxifen
Glibenclamide	Thiouracil
Metahexamide	Tolbutamide

Infectious and parasitic diseases

p-Aminosalicylic acid	Nitrofurantoin
Arsphenamine	Phenazopyride
Cefalexin	Quinine
Chloramphenicol	Rifampicin
Cloxacillin	Sulphadiazine
Co-trimoxazole	Sulphonamides
Erythromycin	Tiabendazole
Griseofulvin	Troleandomycin
Nalidixic acid	Tryparsamide

Neuropsychiatric diseases

Amitriptyline	Iprindole
Bromocriptine	Isocarboxazid
Carbamazepine	Mianserin
Chlordiazepoxide	Phenobarbital
Chlorpromazine	Phenytoin
Desipramine	Prochloperazine
Diazepam	Promazine
Fluphenazine	Thioridazine
Flurazepam	Triazolam
Haloperidol	Trifluoperazine
Imipramine	Zimelidine

Rheumatic and musculoskeletal diseases

Allopurinol	Kebuzone
Baclofen	Naproxen
Colchicine	Oxyphenbutazone
Diclofenac	Penicillamine
Diflunisal	Phenopyrazone
Fenbufen	Phenylbutazone
Feprazon	Piroxicam
Flurbiprofen	Probenecid
Gold salts	Propoxyphene
Ibufenac	Proquazone
Ibuprofen	Sulcindac
Indomethacin	Zoxazolamine

Skin diseases

Isotretinoin

Table 6 *Drugs causing acute cholestasis*

Antimicrobials

Erythromycin	Co-trimoxazole
Penicillin, oxacillin, cloxacillin	Sulphones
	Nitrofurantoin
Rifampicin	Thiobendazole
Cephalosporins	Triacetyloleandromycin
Novobiocin	Amoxycillin/clavulanic acid
Ketoconazole	Flucloxacillin
Griseofulvin	Trimethoprim

Antithyroid drugs

Thiouracil	Methimazole
Carbimazole	

Hypoglycaemics

Tolbutamide	Chlorpropamide
	Glibenclamide

Anticancer drugs

Azathioprine	Busulphan
Chlorambucil	Cytarabine

Steroids

C17 anabolic sex steroids	Tamoxifen
Danazol	Aminoglutethimide
Stanozolol	

Cytokines

Tumour necrosis factor	Interleukin 2

Anti-inflammatory/analgesic drugs

Dextropropoxyphene	Piroxicam
Benoxaprofen	Diflunisal
Naproxen	D-Penicillamine
Phenylbutazone	Gold

Anticonvulsants

Phenytoin	Phenobarbitone
Carbamazepine	

Psychiatric drugs

Chlorpromazine	Amitryptyline
Haloperidol	Prochlorperazine
Imipramine	Zemeldene
Chlordiazepoxide	Nomifensine
Flurazepam	Thioridazine

Cardiovascular

Ajmaline	Captopril
Chlorthalidone	Disopyramide
Hydralazine	Nifedipine
Thiazides	Verapamil

Others

Warfarin	Cimetidine
Phenindione	Ranitidine
Allopurinol	Cyclosporin A

increased, although the prothrombin time may be greatly prolonged. Microvesicular steatosis is thought to be related to drug inhibition of mitochondrial β-oxidation of fatty acids.

MACROVESICULAR STEATOSIS

In contrast, macrovesicular steatosis is far less serious. The hepatocyte contains a large droplet of fat, which displaces the nucleus to the periphery. Liver function tests are usually only minimally deranged. Damage is thought to be related to impaired release of lipids from liver cells.

Table 7 *Drugs causing steatosis*

Microvesicular
Amineptine
Aureomycin
Pirprofen
Tetracycline
Valproate
Macrovesicular
Asparaginase
Glucocorticosteroids
Methotrexate

Table 8 *Drugs inducing hepatic granulomas*

Antineoplastic
Procarbazine
Cardiovascular
α-Methyldopa
Diltiazem
Hydralazine
Procainamide
Quinidine
Tocainide
Endocrine
Chlorpropamide
Glibenclamide
Tolbutamide
Gastroenterological disease
Ranitidine
Sulphasalazine
Infectious diseases
Amoxycillin/clavulanic acid
Cephalexin
Dapsone
Isoniazid
Nitrofurantoin
Oxacillin
Penicillin
Sulphonamides
Neuropsychiatric disease
Carbamazepine
Chlorpromazine
Diazepam
Nomifensine
Rheumatological
Allopurinol
Aspirin
Gold salts
Oxyphenbutazone
Phenylbutazone

Table 9 *Drug-related vascular diseases of the liver*

Veno-occlusive disease
Azathioprine
Mercaptopurine
Pyrrolizidine alkaloid
Thioguanine
Budd–Chiari syndrome
Actinomycin
Dacarbazine
Oral contraceptive
Perisinusoidal fibrosis
Arsenicals
Azathioprine
Mercaptopurine
Methotrexate
Vitamin A

Table 10 *Malignant hepatic tumours associated with drugs*

Hepatocellular carcinoma
Anabolic/androgenic steroids
Oral contraceptive
Thorium dioxide
Cholangiocarcinoma
Thorium dioxide
Angiosarcoma
Anabolic/androgenic steroids
Arsenicals
Thorium dioxide

Phospholipidosis

Phospholipidosis is characterized by the accumulation of phospholipids in liver-cell lysosomes. The major drugs to be associated with this form of liver damage, perhexiline and amiodarone, are cationic, amphiphilic compounds that accumulate within the liver-cell lysosomes, where they form complexes with phospholipids. Accumulation can be detected by immunohistochemistry or electron microscopy. The compounds are stored in these complexes and may be released very slowly, even after ingestion has stopped. The extent to which these complexes accumulate in patients without toxicity remains uncertain.

Non-alcohol steatotic hepatitis syndrome (NASH)

Long-term treatment with perhexiline and amiodarone may be associated with a syndrome that clinically and histologically is identical to alcoholic hepatitis. The disease develops insidiously and may be characterized by hepatomegaly, jaundice, ascites, and encephalopathy. Other drugs implicated in this syndrome include diltiazem and nifedipine.

Fibrotic and vascular disease (Table 9)

PERISINUSOIDAL FIBROSIS

Perisinusoidal fibrosis is characterized by accumulation of collagen within the space of Disse. This may be asymptomatic or lead to hepatomegaly and portal hypertension. The most common cause of perisinusoidal fibrosis due to drugs are large doses of vitamin A given for prolonged periods, or methotrexate. Liver damage may be associated with alopecia. Characteristically the liver shows hyperplasia of the Ito cell as a consequence of vitamin A accumulation. Serum concentrations

Granulomatous hepatitis (see also Chapter 14.33)

The spectrum of granulomatous hepatitis varies from an asymptomatic finding to a systemic illness characterized by generalized aches and pains, pruritus, jaundice, and hepatomegaly. Serologically, the main abnormality is that the serum alkaline phosphatase is increased. Histologically the liver is infiltrated by granulomas—small, rounded foci of epithelioid cells with multinucleated giant cells. Drugs associated with granulomatous hepatitis are listed in Table 8.

Table 11 *Main drugs causing subacute hepatitis, chronic hepatitis, or cirrhosis*

Acetohexamide
Amiodarone
Amodiaquine
Aspirin
Benzarone
Busulphan
Chlorambucil
Cimetidine
Clometacin
Dantrolene
Diclofenac
Iproniazid
Isoniazid
Methotrexate
Methyldopa
Nicotinic acid
Nitrofurantoin
Oxyphenisatin
Perhexiline
Propylthiouracil
Tienilic acid
Urethrane
Valproate
Vitamin A

Table 12 *Causes of chronic cholestasis*

Phenothiazines
Especially chlorpromazine

Tricyclic antidepressants
Amitriptyline, imipramine

Sex steroids
Methyl testosterone, norandrosterone

Sulphonylureas
Carbutamide, tolbutamide

Antimicrobials
Cloxacillin, dicloxacillin, flucloxacillin

Others
Arsenicals, cyproheptidine, haloperidol, thiobendazole
   troleandomycin, piroxicam

In contrast, hepatocellular carcinoma is also associated with the anabolic and androgenic steroids, oral contraceptives, and thorium dioxide. Although the risk of malignancy increases with the prolonged use of oral contraceptives, up to eightfold after 8 years, it must be emphasized that the overall risk of developing hepatocellular carcinoma with oral contraceptives is extremely small, and must be balanced against their protective effects. Angiosarcomas and cholangiosarcomas may also be related to drugs, although the association is less clear-cut.

of vitamin A may be normal, even in the presence of marked liver damage. Patients with a high intake of alcohol are at greater risk of fibrosis.

PELIOSIS HEPATIS

Peliosis hepatis is a histological diagnosis characterized by blood-filled cavities, bordered by hepatocytes, which may be distributed throughout the liver. Originally described in association with tuberculosis, it is now appreciated that peliosis hepatis is drug-induced and is often asymptomatic. The major drugs involved are the anabolic steroids, androgenic steroids, azathioprine, vinyl chloride, and pyrazolide derivatives.

HEPATIC VENOUS DAMAGE

Obstruction of the large hepatic veins results in the Budd–Chiari syndrome, characterized by the onset of the abdominal pain and ascites, often with diarrhoea. In the acute form the patient may develop liver failure. Most cases of Budd–Chiari syndrome are due to myeloproliferative disorders, either clinically apparent or latent, but it may be associated with the use of oral contraceptives and some antineoplastic drugs such as dacarbazine, doxorubicin, and cyclophosphamide.

Obstruction of the small veins leads to hepatic veno-occlusive disease, characterized by non-thrombotic, concentric narrowing of the small centrilobular veins. Clinical presentation is often chronic but rarely may be acute. Veno-occlusive disease was initially described in association with ingestion of the pyrrolizidine alkaloids present in Senecio plants but may be seen in patients treated with immunosuppression, especially with organ transplantation.

Hepatic tumours

Hepatic tumours may be benign or malignant (Table 10). Hepatocellular adenoma has been associated with the use of oral contraceptives and anabolic steroids. These tumours have a potential for malignant transformation. Usually withdrawal of the steroid results in a reduction in the size of the tumour.

Chronic disease

CIRRHOSIS AND CHRONIC HEPATITIS

Some drugs are associated with chronic liver disease. It may be that the initial lesions develop subclinically and that only prolonged use of the drug will result in cirrhosis. Rarely, a short-term exposure to a drug results in chronic liver disease. It has been suggested that some drugs may trigger an autoimmune response but this has yet to be proved. None the less, drugs must be considered in all cases of chronic liver disease. Some of the drugs associated with the development of cirrhosis and chronic hepatitis are listed in Table 11.

INTRAHEPATIC CHRONIC CHOLESTASIS

In some instances of drug-related cholestasis, jaundice or cholestatic liver function tests persist for 6 months or more (Table 12). In these cases it is important to exclude other causes of cholestatic disease, such as primary biliary cirrhosis or primary sclerosing cholangitis, which may have been brought to light by drug-induced disorder. However, some drugs may be associated with a chronic vanishing bile-duct syndrome, which may be indistinguishable from primary biliary cirrhosis. A syndrome virtually identical to primary sclerosing cholangitis can be induced by infusion into the hepatic artery of floxuridine for the treatment of intrahepatic malignancy. Sclerosing cholangitis may develop several months after starting chemotherapy. The outcome is variable. A vanishing bile-duct syndrome has been associated with carbamazepine, thiobendazole, flucloxacillin, haloperidol, ajmaline, cyproheptidine, and chlorpromazine. There has been a suggestion that primary biliary cirrhosis is associated with the use of benoxaprofen. The cause of the chronic cholestasis is uncertain; both immune mechanisms and the recirculation of toxic metabolites have been implicated.

REFERENCES

Bem, J.L., Msann, R., and Rawlins, M.O. (1988). Review of yellow cards. *British Medical Journal*, **296**, 1319.

Danan, G. (1990). Consensus Meeting. Criteria of drug induced liver disorders. *Journal of Hepatology*, **11**, 272–6.

Friis, H. and Andreason, P. (1991). Drug induced hepatic injury: an analysis of 1100 cases reported to the Danish Committee on Adverse Drug Reactions between 1978 and 1987. *Internal Medicine*, **232**, 133–42.

Kaplowitz, N. (ed.) (1990). Recent advances in drug metabolism and hepatotoxicity. *Seminars in Liver Disease*, **10**, 235–338.

Lewis, J. and Zimmerman, H. (1989). Drug induced liver disease. *Medical Clinics of North America*, **73**, 775–96.

Neuberger, J. (1989). Drug induced jaundice. *Clinical Gastroenterology*, **3**, 447–66.

Stricker, B.H. and Spoelstra, P. (1985). *Drug induced hepatic injury*. Elsevier, Amsterdam.

Zimmer, H.J. (1990). Update of hepatoxicity due to class of drugs in common clinical use. *Seminars in Liver Disease*, **10**, 322–33.

14.35 The liver in systemic disease

J. Neuberger

The liver may be affected in a wide variety of systemic diseases. In most instances, disturbance of liver structure and/or function is a minor component of the illness, but in some cases abnormalities of liver function may be the presenting symptom. In this section, some of the abnormalities of liver function seen in systemic diseases are discussed.

Cardiovascular disease

CONGESTIVE CARDIAC FAILURE

Most patients with congestive cardiac failure have few symptoms related to hepatic congestion, although nausea, vomiting, and pain in the right upper quadrant may occur occasionally. Hepatomegaly is found in most patients with moderately severe heart failure and, when cardiac cirrhosis develops, may be associated with splenomegaly and ascites. With progressive failure, jaundice occurs in about one-quarter of patients.

The standard liver tests may show a rise in serum bilirubin, which rarely exceeds 50 μmol/l. Unconjugated bilirubin usually exceeds conjugated bilirubin. The aminotransferases (both of aspartate and alanine) may also be elevated but rarely rise above twice the upper limit of normal. However, in severe, acute heart failure, concentrations in excess of 1000 u/l may be found. Serum alkaline phosphatase is rarely elevated. The prothrombin time is often prolonged by a few seconds.

The liver is enlarged, with a tendency to purple discoloration. A cut section shows the classical nutmeg appearance, with the pale periportal zones alternating with darker centrilobular zones. Microscopically the liver shows congestion and areas of centrilobular necrosis. With chronic heart failure there may be features of centrilobular necrosis and fibrosis. This may progress to a true cirrhosis.

CONSTRICTIVE PERICARDITIS

Hepatic complications of constrictive pericarditis occur late in the course of the illness. Cardiovascular features of constrictive pericarditis are described elsewhere (see Section 15). The liver is enlarged and there may be associated splenomegaly. As the condition progresses, jaundice and ascites develop. Treatment is related to correction of the underlying cause. It is therefore important in any patient with unexplained cirrhosis to examine the neck veins carefully, as an elevated jugular venous pressure should raise the possibility of constrictive pericarditis. In addition to the typical radiographic and ultrasonographic appearances of constrictive pericarditis, ultrasonography of the liver will show enlargement with dilated hepatic veins.

TRICUSPID INCOMPETENCE

Tricuspid incompetence most commonly occurs as a result of right heart failure but may also result from congenital or acquired disease of the tricuspid valve. The liver is enlarged and pulsatile.

TUMOURS OF THE HEART

Tumours of the right atrium, including myxoma and myosarcoma, may infiltrate the hepatic veins resulting in a Budd–Chiari syndrome. Cardiac myxoma may be associated with abnormalities of liver function tests, including increased serum bilirubin and alkaline phosphatase, and a reduction in serum albumin and total protein.

DRUG REACTIONS

As described elsewhere (see Chapter 14.34), many drugs used for the treatment of heart disease may be associated with adverse reactions that involve the liver. Thus, chronic active hepatitis may be associated with methyldopa, and granulomatous hepatitis with hydralazine. Quinidine, amiodarone, and perhexiline may cause phospholipidosis and a syndrome resembling alcoholic hepatitis.

Pulmonary disease

CIRRHOSIS

Lung disease is not uncommon in patients with cirrhosis; the hepatopulmonary syndrome, discussed elsewhere, resolves after treatment of the underlying liver disease. In contrast, abnormalities of liver function in patients with pulmonary disease may arise either as a consequence of that disease or of diseases affecting both lung and liver. In the majority of patients with chronic lung disease, abnormalities of liver function are mild and may be manifest only by abnormalities of bromsulphophthalein clearance. In more advanced disease, associated with hypoxia, there may be more widespread disturbances of liver function, with elevation of aminotransferase, bilirubin, alkaline phosphatase, and γ-glutamyltransferase. However, abnormality of liver function in patients with pulmonary disease is associated mainly with pulmonary hypertension rather than lung disease or hypoxia *per se*.

PNEUMONIA (SEE ALSO SECTION 7)

Some patients with pneumococcal pneumonia may have jaundice. It is usually manifest in the fourth or fifth day of the illness and is seen particularly in patients with consolidation of the right lower lobe. The serum bilirubin rarely exceeds 100 μmol/l, and abnormalities of other liver tests are unusual. The cause of the jaundice is not known: factors that have been implicated are glucose 6-phosphatase deficiency, associated acute haemolysis, hypoxia, fever, and direct toxicity. The increased amounts of inflammatory cytokines seen in such patients may also contribute to the jaundice.

Abnormal liver function tests are also seen in patients with legionnaire's disease and are characterized by elevation of aspartate aminotransferase and alkaline phosphatase. Jaundice is less common and tends to occur only in patients who are severely ill.

Other infections that may involve the lung and liver are considered later.

Diseases affecting both lung and liver

α_1-ANTITRYPSIN DEFICIENCY (SEE ALSO CHAPTER 11.15)

α_1-Antitrypsin deficiency was initially described in relation to pulmonary emphysema but it subsequently became clear that the liver, kidney, and pancreas can also be involved. In children, liver disease often presents as neonatal hepatitis: in one-third it resolves, one-third develop fibrosis, and the remainder develop progressive cirrhosis, often requiring transplantation. In adults the disease often presents with cirrhosis or its complications. The diagnosis is made on a basis of clinical suspicion, the demonstration of α_1-antitrypsin deficiency, and the characteristic histological features of periodic acid–Schiff-positive, diastase-resistant globules in the liver. These globules are not diagnostic of the disease, however.

The natural history is unpredictable but many patients develop progressive disease, often requiring liver transplantation. There is no proven effective treatment. The onset of cholestasis often heralds liver failure. In cases where lung and liver disease coexist, the only effective therapy is with a triple transplant (heart, lung, liver).

CYSTIC FIBROSIS

The increasing success in treating respiratory complications in children with cystic fibrosis has resulted in a greater number surviving to develop liver disease. Abnormal liver tests are found in up to half the children, and in adults up to a quarter of patients with cystic fibrosis develop a biliary cirrhosis. Clinically, these patients present with cholestasis and jaundice. The pathogenesis and aetiology of this cholestasis are poorly understood. In most cases, liver disease is characterized by the development of a focal biliary cirrhosis that increases with the age of the patient. Early involvement of the liver is characterized by the presence of eosinophilic granular material in the portal ducts. There is proliferation of bile ducts and portal fibrosis. This progresses to a focal biliary cirrhosis, which then develops into a multilobular cirrhosis with onset of symptoms of cholestasis and jaundice. However, many patients have evidence of biliary obstruction on endoscopic retrograde cholangiopancreatography (**ERCP**). There is some evidence that infusion of *N*-acetyl cysteine into the biliary tree may relieve the obstruction in the extrahepatic biliary tree. The onset of jaundice and ascites is associated with a poor prognosis.

Other causes of cholestasis in patients with cystic fibrosis include gallstones and pancreatic insufficiency associated with increased loss of faecal bile salts, a consequent decrease in the size of the bile-salt pool and the development of lithogenic bile.

Treatment is uncertain. Open studies have suggested that ursodeoxycholic acid, 10 mg/kg per day, may result in biochemical improvement, weight gain, and improved nutrition. However, whether this agent has any long-term effect remains to be established.

SARCOIDOSIS

Sarcoidosis is a systemic granulomatous disease of unknown aetiology (see Section 17). The liver is commonly involved, with evidence of granulomatous infiltration in up to 70 per cent of cases. However, symptoms and signs are relatively uncommon. Hepatomegaly and splenomegaly occur in about a quarter of patients. While jaundice is extremely rare, elevation of the serum alkaline phosphatase is not uncommon. Complications of granulomatous infiltration of the liver are unusual. There is one case report of liver failure developing. More commonly, portal hypertension may occur, with bleeding varices or ascites.

As with sarcoid elsewhere, the diagnosis is made on the basis of an elevated concentration of serum angiotensin-converting enzyme, confirmation by Kveim test, and, most importantly, by the finding of non-caseating granulomas around the portal tracts. These granulomas are usually large and consist of multinuclear giant cells with lymphocytes and areas of epitheloid cells. Most patients respond to corticosteroids, although the portal hypertension may persist, possibly due to established presinusoidal fibrosis.

Overlap with primary biliary cirrhosis is well recognized, and cases have been described with typical sarcoid involvement of both lungs and liver in the presence of bile-duct damage consistent with primary biliary cirrhosis. These patients are antimitochondrial antibody positive. Treatment should be directed against the sarcoid because, as yet, there is no treatment that improves survival in primary biliary cirrhosis. Other causes of granulomatous hepatitis are discussed in Chapter 14.33.

DRUGS (SEE CHAPTER 14.34)

As indicated elsewhere, many drugs used for the treatment of lung diseases may be associated with abnormal liver function. Inhaled disodium chromoglycate reportedly causes a syndrome that transiently resembles primary biliary cirrhosis. However, inhaled medications otherwise rarely cause significant abnormality of liver function.

Gastrointestinal-tract disorders

INFLAMMATORY BOWEL DISEASE (SEE CHAPTERS 14.10 AND 14.11)

The spectrum of liver abnormality associated with inflammatory bowel disease ranges from fatty change to pericholangitis, sclerosing cholangitis, chronic active hepatitis, cirrhosis, and amyloidosis. The reported incidence of liver abnormalities in inflammatory bowel disease varies from 3 to 10 per cent. In general, abnormalities of liver function tests correlate poorly with severity of liver disease determined histologically. Ulcerative colitis more commonly is associated with abnormality of liver function tests than is Crohn's disease.

There is no clear-cut relation between the onset of symptoms of inflammatory bowel disease and of the liver abnormalities. In general, symptoms of ulcerative colitis precede changes in liver function tests by about 8 years but liver disease may precede by many years the onset of clinically apparent inflammatory bowel disease; conversely, liver disease may become manifest several years after colectomy. Furthermore, there is no clear-cut correlation between the severity of inflammatory bowel disease and the incidence or severity of liver disease. Indeed, in many patients with liver disease the colitis tends to be a pancolitis but is often quiescent. (Table 1).

Fatty change is relatively common on histological examination of liver in patients with inflammatory bowel disease and is probably multifactorial in origin, relating to the degree of ill health, poor nutrition, and use of corticosteroids. As a patient's condition improves, the fatty infiltration resolves.

In contrast, features of sclerosing cholangitis are becoming increasingly recognized as ERCP has become a routine investigation. The presence of the perinuclear antineutrophil cytoplasmic antibody, as a further aid to the diagnosis, may increase the detection of patients with this complication. It is a premalignant condition, associated with bile-duct carcinoma.

Cirrhosis occurs in up to 10 per cent of patients dying with colitis. The cause of the cirrhosis is not known, but it may, in some cases, relate to chronic hepatitis C infection from drug transfusions or to drug toxicity, rather than primary sclerosing cholangitis.

Although chronic active hepatitis in association with inflammatory bowel disease is rare, it is important to diagnose it because many cases have features similar to autoimmune chronic active hepatitis and respond well to corticosteroids.

Other hepatic complications of inflammatory bowel disease include

Table 1 *Hepatic disorders associated with inflammatory bowel disease*

Parenchymal Granulomas Pericholangitis Chronic active hepatitis Cirrhosis Amyloid Hepatocellular carcinoma Primary biliary cirrhosis Liver abscess *Biliary* Gallstones Primary sclerosing cholangitis Cholangiocarcinoma

Table 2 *Possible contributing factors in liver disease associated with total parenteral nutrition (TPN)*

Underlying disease
Sepsis:
   Systemic
   Local
   Anaerobic colonization of small bowel
Duration of TPN
Pre-existing liver disease
Neonatal factors:
   Pre-existing liver disease
   Excess non-protein calories
   Deficiency of essential fatty acids
   Amino-acid toxicity
   Carnitine deficiency
   Bile-acid abnormalities

granulomatous hepatitis, amyloid infiltration of the liver, bile-duct carcinoma, gallbladder cancer, and gallstones.

COELIAC DISEASE (SEE CHAPTER 14.9.4)

In patients with coeliac disease there may be minor abnormalities of liver function tests, characterized by elevation of serum aminotransferases; they usually resolve with treatment. Coeliac disease may also be associated with autoimmune diseases affecting the liver, including primary biliary cirrhosis, cryptogenic cirrhosis, sclerosing cholangitis, and chronic active hepatitis.

BYPASS SURGERY

Jejunoileal bypass surgery may be associated with a significant degree of liver impairment; the changes in the liver range from simple fatty infiltration to cirrhosis. In a few cases there may be features identical to those of alcoholic hepatitis. In those in whom liver function tests are deranged there is a likelihood of progression, and although treatment with metronidazole has been advocated, restoration of normal anatomy appears to be the only effective treatment.

DRUGS

Many drugs associated with the treatment of inflammatory bowel disease are associated with a variety of patterns of liver damage (see Chapter 14.34).

TOTAL PARENTERAL NUTRITION (TPN)

The association of hepatobiliary disorders with TPN has been recognized over the last two decades. Although the pathogenesis remains obscure, most studies suggest that the incidence is falling to less than 5 per cent of patients. Clinically, TPN-associated hepatobiliary disease varies from a mild, asymptomatic disease with acalculous cholecystitis, biliary sludge, or hepatomegaly to jaundice, cirrhosis, and liver failure. Biochemically, the severity of abnormalities will reflect the severity of the disease but elevations of liver enzymes such as aspartate and alanine transferases, lactate dehydrogenase, and alkaline phosphatase, and serum bilirubin, are common. The histological features vary from a mild fatty infiltrate or cholestasis to a more severe picture resembling alcoholic fatty liver. In chronic cases, cirrhosis will develop.

The mechanism is uncertain. Suggestions include hypoxic enterocytes, nutritional depletion, sepsis, toxicity of certain unidentified amino-acids, and even carnitine deficiency (Table 2).

Once a patient develops abnormal liver function, and provided that other causes have been excluded, there is little alternative other than to reduce or stop parenteral nutrition and find other ways of providing adequate nutrition.

Liver in haematological diseases (see also Section 22)

In general, diseases of the blood do not cause significant hepatic dysfunction. However, diseases associated with abnormal blood clotting, such as protein C or S deficiency and paroxysmal nocturnal haemoglobulinuria may lead to a Budd–Chiari syndrome.

HAEMOLYSIS

Jaundice may accompany haemolysis, usually through an increase in unconjugated bilirubin. In patients with underlying liver disease there may be an elevation of both conjugated and unconjugated bilirubin, out of proportion to the degree of haemolysis. Patients with chronic haemolytic anaemia are at risk of developing haemosiderosis. Iron is deposited initially in the Kupffer cells, but spread to the parenchyma will subsequently occur. The haemolytic anaemias are associated with an increased risk of pigment gallstones, which may lead to liver and biliary-tract disease.

SICKLE-CELL DISEASE

Most of the abnormalities of liver function in sickle-cell disease are due to haemolysis or infections transmitted by blood. Kupffer cell hyperplasia, haemosiderosis, fibrosis, or cirrhosis may be due to iron overload following multiple transfusions. Sometimes, patients present with severe pain in the right upper quadrant and rapid enlargement of the liver is part of the hepatic sequestration syndrome (see Section 22).

MULTIPLE TRANSFUSIONS

Patients who are maintained on regular blood transfusion, or blood products, those with thalassaemia or haemophilia for example, are at risk of developing viral hepatitis B or C. It is now clear that there is an increased risk of hepatitis C, which may lead to cirrhosis and liver-cell cancer. Treatment for chronic hepatitis B or C is considered elsewhere (see Chapter 14.26). With more screening and improved preparation of blood and blood products, the incidence is likely to fall.

LYMPHORETICULAR DISEASE

In patients with Hodgkin's disease, liver function tests are of limited value in predicting liver involvement; although jaundice is a recognized feature, it may be due to a number of different causes. For example, haemolysis may complicate Hodgkin's disease, and occasionally there is a bland cholestasis in the absence of infiltration, which resolves when the disease is treated. The clinical manifestations of liver involvement in Hodgkin's disease relate to the degree of infiltration. In rare cases, patients present with fulminant hepatic failure: the clue to infiltration is a large liver, as most cases of viral or drug-related, fulminant hepatic failure are associated with small livers. Liver biopsy may be diagnostic. Primary lymphoma of the liver has been described but is rare. The liver may be involved in both non-Hodgkin's lymphoma and leukaemia. The diagnosis is usually made by biopsy. Some patients with non-Hodgkin's lymphoma have a chronic hepatitis preceding diagnosis or treatment. A casual effect cannot be excluded. Both Hodgkin's disease and non-Hodgkin's lymphoma may be associated with obstructive jaundice due to hilar obstruction by nodes; this is more common in the latter and resolves with treatment.

The liver and infection (full descriptions of individual infections are given in Section 7)

Abnormal liver function may occur during systemic infections but it is rare for patients with sepsis to present primarily with liver symptoms (Table 3). However, jaundice, abnormal liver function tests or even, occasionally, fulminant hepatic failure may be the major presenting feature.

BACTERIAL INFECTIONS

Pneumococcal infections were discussed earlier. Meningococcal infections are occasionally associated with features suggestive of viral hepatitis. Gonococcal infection is a well-recognized cause of liver disease. The classical Fitzhugh–Curtis syndrome, perihepatitis (see also Section 7), is characterized by sudden onset of severe pain in the right upper quadrant, occurring classically in a woman with a previous history of pelvic inflammatory disease. On examination there may be little to find, although tender hepatomegaly and an hepatic rub may be present. Where laparotomy has been done in the mistaken diagnosis of cholecystitis, perihepatitis with adhesions and pus around the liver may give the clue to the diagnosis. In chronic infection, adhesions develop between the surface of the liver and the anterior abdominal wall. The condition usually resolves without treatment, although the use of penicillin causes a more rapid resolution. Abnormalities of liver function may occur in gonococcal bacteraemia, peritonitis, and endocarditis. Perihepatitis is also reported in association with syphilis and chlamydial infections.

In childhood, some infections with *Escherichia coli* may be associated with hepatitis and jaundice. Jaundice is rare in older patients, although pregnant women seem more susceptible. Abnormalities of liver function occur in systemic streptococcal and staphylococcal infection and in enteric fevers, paratyphoid, and typhoid. In typhoid infection, hepatomegaly is common and jaundice occurs in about 10 per cent of patients, although up to a third have abnormal liver function tests, with increased levels of aminotransferases and normal values for alkaline phosphatase. The hepatomegaly rapidly responds with treatment.

Brucellosis may also be associated with jaundice and abnormal liver function tests. All three forms of brucellae have been associated with abnormal liver function. Characteristically, the liver biopsy shows a marked inflammatory infiltrate and fibrosis with multiple, large or small granulomas scattered throughout the parenchyma. Although some reports have suggested granulomatous hepatitis due to brucellae may progress to cirrhosis, the data are not convincing. (The common causes of liver granulomas, including infections, are described in Chapter 14.33.)

In gas gangrene (*Clostridium welchii*), deep jaundice may occur in occur up to a fifth of patients. The liver may be infected and a plain radiograph of the abdomen may show gas within the liver.

Actinomycosis israelii and *bovis* are commensals that rarely cause disease. Actinomycotic infection of the liver may occur, the patient presenting with abdominal pain, anorexia, and fever. In one case report the liver was found to have small, multilocular abscesses.

Tuberculosis may present with granulomatous hepatitis, biliary tuberculosis, a solitary tuberculoma, or tuberculosis of the biliary tract. The liver is involved in up to 85 per cent of patients with tuberculosis, being greatest in those with miliary disease. The presence of multiple granulomas in the liver should raise the possibility of tuberculosis, although the differential diagnosis of granulomatous hepatitis is long. With the increasing incidence of atypical mycobacterial infections, lesions similar to tuberculosis can be found. In those infected with *Mycobacterium avium intracellulare*, there are numerous acid-fast bacilli, often in the absence of granulomas.

LEPTOSPIROSIS

Leptospiral infections are described in Chapter 7.11.32. Acute leptospirosis is frequently accompanied by jaundice, although frank liver failure is uncommon. The jaundice is mainly cholestatic, although there may be liver-cell damage.

Table 3 *Systemic infections affecting the liver*

Bacteria
Actinomycosis
Brucellosis
Chlamydial
Clostridium welchii
E. coli
Gonococcal
Granuloma inguinale
Listeriosis
Melioidosis
Meningococcal
Nocardiosis
Shigellosis
Streptococcal
Staphylococcal
Paratyphoid
Typhoid
Tularaemia
Yersiniosis
Mycobacteria
Tuberculosis
Leprosy
Other mycobacteria
Protozoa
Giardiasis
Kala-azar
Malaria
Toxoplasmosis
Fungi
Aspergillosis
Blastomycosis
Candidal
Cryptococcosis
Coccidioidomycosis
Histoplasmosis
Rickettsia
Q fever
Rocky Mountain spotted fever
Spirochaetes
Leptospirosis
Lyme disease
Relapsing fever
Syphilis (congenital/acquired)

RICKETTSIAL INFECTION

Liver involvement in Q fever (*Coxiella burnetii*) is recognized, although symptoms of liver disease are uncommon. Hepatomegaly is frequent and liver function tests may show an elevation of serum alkaline phosphatase and, rarely, a picture resembling viral hepatitis. Histologically, the liver has areas of focal necrosis, Kupffer cell proliferation, lipogranuloma formation, and mononuclear cell infiltration in the portal tracts. The characteristic histological feature of Q fever is eosinophiliic fibrinoid necrosis but this is not specific. Treatment is with chloramphenicol or tetracycline. Liver involvement has a much greater incidence in Rocky Mountain spotted fever (*Rickettsia rickettsia*).

FUNGAL INFECTIONS

The liver may be involved in fungal infection, often in patients with immunodeficiency such as with AIDS, following chemotherapy, and after organ transplantation. Histoplasmosis, cryptococcosis, aspergillosis, blastomycosis, and candidiasis are all described. The liver is usually involved in disseminated fungal infections. Cryptococcal infection has also been associated with a primary biliary cirrhosis-like condition.

PROTOZOAL INFECTIONS

Protozoal infections are described in detail in Section 7.13; many of them involve the liver.

In toxoplasmosis, while most patients are asymptomatic and liver involvement is mild, hepatitis may occur and on biopsy *Toxoplasma gondii* may be found in the liver. In malaria, due to either *Plasmodium falciparum* or *vivax*, abnormality of liver function may be observed. Hepatomegaly is common and is often associated with jaundice. The jaundice is in part due to haemolysis but liver tests may provide a picture suggestive of viral hepatitis. Histological examination may show characteristic features of Kupffer-cell proliferation with black malarial pigment and mononuclear cell infiltrate. Frank hepatic failure is extremely rare.

TREMATODE INFECTIONS

Schistosomiasis is one of the most common worldwide causes of liver disease. A heavy infection of fertile schistosomes in the portal system results in deposition of eggs that induce an immune response, leading to portal fibrosis and granuloma formation, portal hypertension with consequent splenomegaly, ascites, and variceal haemorrhage. Hepatocyte function is well preserved. There is a complex interaction between schistosomal eggs and the immune system; the degree of fibrosis is directly related to the number of eggs and the duration of infection. The diagnosis is made on stool examination or finding schistosomes in the liver. At present, serological tests are unreliable. Treatment is described in Chapter 7.16.1. Successful treatment is associated with a significant but variable improvement in the degree of portal hypertension. Treatment of the portal hypertension is dependent on the medical facilities available. As parenchymal function is well preserved, these patients usually tolerate a portosystemic shunt.

Coinfection of patients with schistosomiasis and hepatitis B virus appears to be a particularly serious combination.

Pyogenic liver abscess

Pyogenic liver abscesses may occur as part of a systemic illness as a consequence of portal phlebitis, often associated with bowel sepsis, biliary-tract disease, direct trauma, septicaemia, and in association with carcinoma of the colon or bacterial endocarditis. Most commonly they

Table 4 *Sources of pyogenic liver abscess*

Obstructed biliary tree	30–40%
Intra-abdominal pain	15–25%
Systemic infections	25%
No source identified	20%

arise out of portal phlebitis, with the primary focus being the appendix, colon, diverticular disease, or in the pelvis (Table 4). Although abscesses may occur in patients with inflammatory bowel disease, this is relatively rare.

The patient presents with abdominal pain, pyrexia, nausea, and weight loss. However, fever is less common in children. Hepatomegaly may be present and the liver is sometimes tender. The serum albumin is often reduced and alkaline phosphatase elevated. There is usually marked neutrophil leucocytosis, but this is not invariable. The diagnosis is made on imaging of the liver. A chest radiograph may show elevation of the right hemidiaphragm with an associated pleural effusion or even lung consolidation. Ultrasound, computerized tomographic scanning and magnetic resonance may define an hepatic abscess. With the increasing sensitivity of these techniques, radioisotope scanning is now less important.

Treatment of a solitary abscess is by percutaneous drainage in the first instance. Under ultrasound or computerized tomographic guidance, a percutaneous drain should be established for single abscesses, and even in some cases of multiple abscesses. The abscesses should be drained to dryness, and antibiotics should be given according to the sensitivities of the organisms isolated. Pathogens are usually anaerobic or aerobic gut coliforms, especially *Streptococcus milleri*. In children, *Staphylococcus aureus* is common. The success rate of treatment with drainage and systemic antibiotics is 80 to 90 per cent. Mortality is high in children and the elderly, in those with coexisting disease such as diabetes, and those with delayed diagnosis. Once the abscess has been drained, the primary source of infection must be sought and appropriate management instituted. Surgery may be required for patients with multiple abscesses or for those with abscesses that do not respond to simple drainage and antibiotic therapy. Liver abscess due to hydatid and amoeba is discussed elsewhere.

AIDS and liver disease

Liver disease in patients with human immunodeficiency virus (**HIV**) infection may be due to pre-existing hepatitis virus, opportunistic infections, or neoplasms. In some cases the abnormality of liver function may be due to HIV virus itself. Such patients have non-tender hepatomegaly with anorexia, weight loss and low-grade fever. Liver function tests show slight derangement with cholestasis. The liver biopsy shows non-specific features including Kupffer-cell hyperplasia, fat infiltration, non-caseating granulomas, and portal-tract inflammation; occasionally, Mallory bodies may be present.

Other causes of hepatobiliary abnormality in HIV patients include primary hepatic infection due to viral hepatitis.

OTHER CAUSES OF LIVER DAMAGE IN AIDS

Many patients with AIDS are also at risk from hepatitis B, C, and D. As discussed elsewhere, HIV patients respond less well to interferon-α than those who are HIV negative. It is not yet clear whether patients with hepatitis C who are HIV positive respond similarly. Other infections that are more common in HIV patients include cytomegalovirus, herpesvirus, cryptosporidiosis, and mycobacteria including tuberculosis and *M. avium intracellulare*. Drug-induced liver damage must always be considered in HIV patients with abnormal liver tests and it has been suggested that HIV patients are more susceptible to drug hepatotoxicity. Thus, many of the anticonvulsants, analgesics, and antimicrobials are associated with hepatocellular damage, and antibiotics may also be associated with cholestatis. Other abnormalities that may be of less significance clinically include peliosis hepatis and fatty infiltration.

The biliary tree may also be affected in HIV infection inducing a syndrome superficially resembling primary sclerosing cholangitis. This is characterized by a rapid elevation of the serum alkaline phosphatase, which may be associated with pain in the right upper quadrant and, later, jaundice. Ultrasonography may be unhelpful, although dilated and thickened walls of the bile duct may be seen. Otherwise, ERCP will show the characteristic changes of sclerosing cholangitis with bleeding, dilatation, and stricture. Both cryptosporidial and cytomegaloviral infections have been associated with this form of sclerosing cholangitis.

The liver may be involved in a number of other ways. There is an association between AIDS and lymphomas, be they Burkitt's, large cell, or immunoblastic. The liver and/or spleen may be the site of these tumours and hepatic involvement may be present in up to a third of those with gastrointestinal lymphomas. Tumours may be microscopic or macroscopic. The hepatic masses are often asymptomatic but if large may cause pain in the right upper quadrant, fever, jaundice, and abnormalities of liver function tests, especially of the serum alkaline phosphatase. Kaposi's sarcoma may affect the liver and biliary tree but is often asymptomatic.

Liver and rheumatological disease (see Section 18)

Liver abnormalities are not uncommon in patients with rheumatological disorders, although rarely prove a significant problem. More significant involvement may either be a consequence of treatment or occur in association with other autoimmune diseases. For example, those diseases assumed to have an autoimmune basis, such as autoimmune chronic active hepatitis or primary biliary cirrhosis, may be associated with extrahepatic rheumatological diseases such as the sicca syndrome.

RHEUMATOID ARTHRITIS

Abnormalities of liver structure and function are uncommon in patients with rheumatoid arthritis, although minor abnormalities of liver function tests occur in 20 to 50 per cent. Nodular regenerative hyperplasia may cause complications of portal hypertension.

FELTY'S SYNDROME

Felty's syndrome is characterized by the triad of splenomegaly, hypersplenism, and seropositive rheumatoid arthritis. Liver function tests tend to be more commonly deranged than in uncomplicated rheumatoid arthritis. Anti-inflammatory therapy may contribute to the abnormal liver tests. Histological examination of the liver shows lymphocytic infiltration and, rarely, an established cirrhosis. Nodular regenerative hyperplasia has been described in patients with Felty's syndrome, as with rheumatoid arthritis. Although portal hypertension and variceal haemorrhage may occur, jaundice is unusual.

Connective tissue disease (see Section 18.11)

SYSTEMIC LUPUS ERYTHEMATOSUS (SLE)

Usually minor abnormalities of liver function occur in patients with SLE, although spontaneous rupture of the liver has been described. The pattern of liver disease in patients with SLE varies from minimal change to chronic persistent hepatitis, chronic active hepatitis, and cirrhosis. In others, a granulomatous hepatitis has been described.

POLYARTERITIS NODOSA

In contrast to rhematoid arthritis, liver involvement in polyarteritis nodosa is relatively uncommon, although an hepatic arteritis may occur, leading to aneurysm. Rupture of an aneurysm is rare and is characterized by fever, pain in the right upper quadrant, and jaundice.

POLYMYALGIA RHEUMATICA

Abnormalities of liver function are well recognized in patients with polymyalgia rheumatica. These abnormalities usually resolve with effective treatment. Histologically, the liver shows mild portal inflammation with occasional liver-cell necrosis.

SJÖGREN'S SYNDROME

Symptoms of sicca syndrome are common in patients with liver disease, particularly primary biliary cirrhosis, and abnormalities of salivary gland function have been described in all patients in some series. Sicca syndrome is also found in patients with cryptogenic cirrhosis and autoimmune chronic active hepatitis. In patients with Sjögren's syndrome there is often hepatomegaly and minor derangement of liver function tests, particularly serum alkaline phosphatase, in 25 per cent. The liver may show non-specific inflammatory infiltration.

Amyloid (see Chapter 11.13.1)

The liver is involved in both primary and secondary amyloidosis; liver involvement is found in over 80 per cent of patients with either form. In general, however, liver involvement has few significant clinical consequences, although jaundice, hepatitis, portal hypertension, and spontaneous rupture have been described. Clinically, the liver is enlarged. The serum alkaline phosphatase is usually greatly elevated; jaundice is uncommon. It is believed that liver biopsy may be particularly hazardous in patients with amyloid because there may be an increased risk of bleeding after biopsy. There is no specific treatment, which depends on the underlying cause.

Cryoglobulinaemia (see Chapter 18.11.10)

The reported incidence of liver disease in essential, mixed cryoglobulinaemia varies greatly. In 20 to 80 per cent of patients there is an association with hepatitis C viral infection. Up to half of patients have evidence of infection with hepatitis B virus, and up to 10 per cent have chronic active hepatitis or cirrhosis with jaundice.

Pregnancy

Liver disease in pregnancy is discussed in Chapter 13.13.

REFERENCES

Bjornson, H.S. (1989). *Biliary tract and hepatic infections in humans.* Academic Press, London.

Bossingham, D. and Hawkey, C.J. (1993). Gastroenterology in the rheumatic diseases. In *Oxford Textbook of Rheumatology,* (ed. P.J. Maddison, D.A. Isenberg, P. Woo, and D.N. Glass). pp. 138–45. Oxford University Press.

Civardi, G., Filice, C., Careman, M., and Giorgio, A. (1992). Hepatic abscesses in immunocompromised patients: ultrasonically guided percutaneous drainage. *Gastrointestinal Radiology,* **17,** 175–8.

Collins, P. and McIntyre, N. (1981). The liver in cardiovascular and pulmonary disease. In *Oxford Textbook of Clinical Hepatology.* (ed. N. McIntyre, J.-P. Benhamou, J. Bircher, M. Rizzetto, and J. Rodes). pp. 1159–70. Oxford University Press.

Gertz, M.A. and Kyle, R.A. (1988). Hepatic amyloidosis (primary AL): natural history in 80 patients. *American Journal of Medicine,* **85,** 73–80.

Kibbler, C.C. (1991). Bacterial infections of the liver. In *Oxford Textbook of Clinical Hepatology*. (ed. N. McIntyre, J.-P. Benhamou, J. Bircher, M. Rizzetto, and J. Rodes). pp. 656–82. Oxford University Press.

Laxer, R.M., *et al.* (1990). Liver disease in neonatal lupus. *Journal of Pediatrics,* **116**, 238–42.

LeBovies, E., Dworkin, B.M., Heier, S.K. and Rosenthal, W.S. (1988). The hepatobiliary manifestations of human immunodeficiency virus infection. *American Journal of Gastroenterology,* **83**, 1–7.

McIntyre, N., Benhamou, J.-P. Bircher, J., Rizzetto, M., and Rodes, J. (1991). *Oxford Textbook of Clinical Hepatology.* Oxford University Press.

Pottipati, A.R., Dave, P.B., Gumaste, V., and Vieux, U. (1991). Tuberculosous abscess of the liver in acquired immunodeficiency syndrome. *Journal of Clinical Gastroenterology,* **13**, 549–53.

Trevino, H., Tsianos, E.B. and Schenker, S. (1987). Gastrointestinal and hepatobiliary features in Sjögren's syndrome. In *Sjögren's syndrome: clinical and immunological aspects.* (ed. N. Talal, H.M. Moutsopoulos, and S.S. Kassan). pp. 89–95. Springer-Verlag, Berlin.

Tsianos, E.B., *et al.* (1990). Sjögren's syndrome in patients with primary biliary cirrhosis. *Hepatology,* **11**, 730–4.

14.36 Miscellaneous disorders of the gastrointestinal tract and liver

D. P. Jewell

This chapter reviews some of the conditions which do not fall naturally into any of the other major sections that deal with disorders of the gastrointestinal tract and liver.

Cystic disorders of the bowel

There is a variety of disorders of the small and large bowel associated with cyst formation. All of them are rare and present major diagnostic and therapeutic problems.

COLITIS CYSTICA

There are several varieties of benign cystic lesions involving the colonic mucosa. Colitis cystica superficialis occurs in patients with pellagra and has also been reported in adult coeliac disease. The presenting feature is usually diarrhoea and the condition is characterized by the presence of small mucus-filled cysts that lie superficially to the muscular layer of the colon. The disease seems to respond to therapy for pellagra. In colitis cystica profunda the cysts occur below the muscular layer of the colon. The pathogenesis and aetiology of this condition are unknown. It is usually characterized by cramping lower abdominal pain, tenesmus, and diarrhoea associated with blood and mucus in the stools. The diagnosis is made by sigmoidoscopy, rectal biopsy, and barium enema examinations. Treatment consists of local surgical excision.

PNEUMATOSIS CYSTOIDES INTESTINALIS

This disorder is characterized by the presence of multiple, gas-filled cysts in the wall of the colon and, less frequently, the small intestine. The stomach and mesentery may also rarely be affected. The condition is usually seen in middle-aged patients and may be associated with obstructive airways disease or pyloric obstruction. It has also been found in association with a variety of other conditions, including mesenteric vascular disease, small-bowel tumours, and Whipple's disease, and following small-bowel surgery. It can also occur after sigmoidoscopy or colonoscopy.

The pathogenesis of the condition is unknown. The composition of the gas within the cysts is similar to atmospheric air with the addition of small quantities of methane and a higher concentration of hydrogen. Thus, the gas may diffuse into the lamina propria from the intestinal lumen. Suggestions that the gas is formed by excessive bacterial fermentation of carbohydrate or that, in patients with obstructive airways disease, alveolar air tracks down through the muscle planes of the posterior abdominal wall and out into the mesentery lack firm evidence.

Pneumatosis cystoides can be an incidental finding during radiological examination of the abdomen. However, it can present with symptoms, which include lower abdominal pain, recurrent diarrhoea, rectal bleeding, and tenesmus. Obstructive symptoms can occur. The cysts can frequently be detected at sigmoidoscopy and rectal biopsy specimens may show the characteristic giant cells that frequently line the cyst walls. Double-contrast radiology is the best method to establish the diagnosis but computerized tomographic scans may detect serosal or mesenteric cysts.

If the disease is detected incidentally and the patient has no abdominal symptoms, no treatment is necessary. However, treatment is indicated for symptomatic patients, especially those with severe obstructive symptoms. The most effective therapy is oxygen in high concentration. Most patients will benefit from a concentration of 60 to 70 per cent given by a face mask or a nasal catheter. Hyperbaric oxygen may rarely be indicated for resistant pneumatosis. The aim of oxygen therapy is to wash out the nitrogen from the cysts and replace it with oxygen, which can be resorbed, with collapse of the cysts. Other treatments that have been tried are antibiotics (metronidazole), a low-carbohydrate diet, and an elemental diet. Surgical resection may be necessary for patients who do not respond and for those with severe obstructive symptoms, especially if there is a suspicion of volvulus.

Microscopic and collagenous colitis

These two disorders are primarily seen in middle-aged women presenting with a watery diarrhoea. Although claims have been made for microscopic colitis progressing to a collagenous colitis, this has not been universal experience and so the disorders will be described separately.

Collagenous colitis was first recognized by the Swedish physician Lindstrom in 1976. Patients usually present in the fifth and sixth decade, mostly in women, but the disorder can occur in young adults as well as in the elderly. A watery diarrhoea accompanied by abdominal cramps, wind, distension, and nausea are the usual symptoms. The diarrhoea can be severe and is often secretory in nature. There may be some mucus but bleeding is not a feature. Despite severe symptoms, these patients are usually well, with a good appetite, and they do not lose weight. There are no abnormal physical signs on examination and, on sigmoidoscopy, the rectal mucosa is hyperaemic with some oedema and granularity. These endoscopic changes occur throughout the colon but are usually patchy and never severe. The diagnosis is made on the appearance of colonic biopsies. There is a thickened band of subepithelial collagen exceeding 15 μm compared with the normal thickness of 2 to 6 μm. The collagen band is of maximal thickness in the right colon and tends to become thinner more distally—there may rectal sparing, which may lead to misdiagnosis if the only histological material available is from the rectum. Immunohistochemical studies have shown the band to consist predominantly of collagen type III but why the pericryptal fibroblasts synthesize abnormal collagen in this disorder but not in other inflammatory disorders is not understood. There is a patchy and variable inflammatory infiltrate in the lamina propria consisting of lymphocytes, plasma cells, and some neutrophils. The disease is confined to the colon and does not extend into the ileum. It is therefore a separate entity to collagenous sprue.

Microscopic colitis shares the same clinical features as collagenous colitis but the colonic mucosa always looks normal at colonoscopy. Nevertheless, histological examination of biopsy specimens shows a diffuse inflammatory infiltrate throughout the lamina propria with no architectural changes of the glands. The infiltrate is predominantly lymphocytic but there are also plasma cells and eosinophils. A characteristic feature is the marked increase in intraepithelial lymphocytes, which clearly separates this disease from ulcerative colitis in which the intraepithelial lymphocyte counts are normal or reduced. It is this feature that has led some clinicians to use the term 'lymphocytic colitis'. A microscopic colitis can be seen in some patients with untreated coeliac disease and in some patients receiving non-steroidal anti-inflammatory drugs. These possibilities need to be excluded before the diagnosis of microscopic colitis can be made.

Both of these disorders have a variable clinical course and the symptoms can spontaneously remit and relapse. However, in general, treatment is difficult, especially if a large-volume secretory diarrhoea occurs. Antidiarrhoeal agents, such as loperamide, should be used initially but, if no response is seen, then 5-aminosalicylic acid compounds or oral corticosteroids can be tried. If symptoms persist, dietary exclusion and even an elemental diet are sometimes helpful. Other treatments that have had some anecdotal benefit are metronidazole, cholestyramine, and mepacrine.

Patients may have intermittent symptoms over many years and, unless a rectal biopsy is obtained and correctly interpreted, the true diagnosis is not made. Many of these patients are thus labelled as having an irritable bowel syndrome. A few cases of microscopic colitis have been reported as progressing to a collagenous colitis but this seems rare. Neither disease progresses to a frank ulcerative colitis.

Miscellaneous vascular disorders of the bowel

INTRAMURAL BLEEDING

The most common cause of bleeding into the wall of the bowel is anticoagulant therapy. Occasionally, intramural haematomas form in patients with congenital coagulation defects such as haemophilia or in conditions such as vasculitis. The usual presentation is with abdominal pain and symptoms of intestinal obstruction and bleeding. The diagnosis is made by barium follow-through or enema examination and the condition can usually be treated conservatively with blood replacement and, if necessary, nasogastric suction.

AORTIC ANEURYSM

Aneurysmal dilatation of the aorta is relatively common in elderly patients, the usual site being the segment distal to the origin of the renal arteries. Aneurysms larger than 6 to 7 cm or those that show increasing

enlargement are probably best resected. Rarely, a spontaneous fistula into the duodenum may develop with catastrophic gastrointestinal haemorrhage. This condition is considered in more detail in Section 15.

In patients who have had prostheses inserted into the abdominal aorta or into other retroperitoneal arteries the complication of paraprosthetic–enteric fistula may occur. This is characterized by the abrupt onset of abdominal pain and shock. Treatment is surgical and the prognosis is extremely poor.

VASCULAR MALFORMATIONS

The vascular ectasias of the colon are described in Chapter 14.17. Haemangiomas of the small intestine are rare. They usually present as recurrent anaemia due to gastrointestinal bleeding. They are best diagnosed by angiography. Telangiectasia may also occur throughout the stomach and bowel as part of the Osler–Rendu–Weber syndrome.

Endometriosis

The term endometriosis describes the presence of extrauterine endometrial tissue and its clinical manifestations. The disorder occurs most frequently between the ages of 30 and 40 years and is rare below the age of 20. Intestinal involvement is most common in those parts of the bowel adjacent to the uterus and fallopian tubes, particularly the rectosigmoid colon. It is not certain how heterotopic endometrial tissue reaches the bowel, and spread may be direct, via the bloodstream or via the lymphatics. The mucosa of the bowel is seldom penetrated by ectopic endometrial tissue and therefore gastrointestinal bleeding is an unusual accompaniment of endometriosis of the bowel.

The usual symptoms of endometriosis include dysmenorrhoea, menorrhagia, sterility, and intermenstrual pelvic pain and backache. If the rectosigmoid region is involved, there may be cyclic pains in the rectum and, occasionally, mild diarrhoea and tenesmus. Implants in the small intestine may produce symptoms of obstruction or volvulus. However, endometriosis affecting the intestine is frequently asymptomatic and much of the pain and altered bowel habit attributed to this condition is more often caused by an irritable bowel syndrome.

The diagnosis of endometriosis requires a thorough pelvic examination to demonstrate tender nodules in the rectosigmoid region or in the rectovaginal area. The diagnosis may be suggested by radiological evidence of the presence of lesions in the rectosigmoid region, but ultimately depends on biopsy of these lesions. Laparoscopy is often helpful in making the diagnosis. The differentiation from carcinoma may be extremely difficult and when in doubt surgical exploration should be carried out.

The management of this condition requires expert gynaecological help. Mildly symptomatic cases are probably best managed by analgesics and sedation. More severe cases may require hormonal therapy with danazole, gestrinone or gonadorelin analogues. These drugs inhibit gonadotrophin release from the pituitary.

Malakoplakia

This is a rare granulomatous disease involving the urinary tract and occasionally the colon or stomach. Histologically the condition is characterized by the presence of histiocytes containing dark inclusions that are PAS positive and seem to contain both calcium and iron. There appears to be an acquired abnormality of macrophage function associated with defective digestion of phagocytosed bacteria.

Colonic malakoplakia is usually found as an incidental finding in elderly debilitated individuals, quite often in association with a malignant disease of the colon. Occasionally it presents as a systemic illness characterized by fever, diarrhoea, and other gastrointestinal symptoms. It can only be diagnosed by histological examination of the bowel. There is no effective treatment, although there has been a recent report of improvement in otherwise unresponsive cases by the use of cholinergic drugs.

Isolated ulcers of the large intestine

Caecal ulcers

These occasionally occur but their aetiology is unknown. They can present with abdominal pain, either acute or chronic, and may be a cause of an acute abdomen. Laparotomy may show perforation or local abscess formation. More commonly, they present with bleeding. Similar ulcers may occur elsewhere in the colon, especially at the flexures.

Solitary rectal ulcer syndrome

This refers to the occurrence of an ulcer in the rectum, usually 4 to 10 cm from the anal verge. It is usually found in young adults, mostly in women, but can arise at any age. The ulcers are most commonly on the anterior wall but they can be multiple and can be sufficiently extensive to encircle most of the rectum. There may be an associated anterior-mucosal prolapse. Symptoms include rectal bleeding, which is the most common mode of presentation, tenesmus, and abdominal and rectal pain. The bowel habit may be normal, but many of these patients have a history of constipation and straining. At sigmoidoscopy the ulcer is readily seen and usually has a greyish base. However, there may be just an area of inflamed mucosa or the ulcer can be a polypoid lesion simulating a carcinoma. In either case, a biopsy specimen should allow the correct diagnosis to be made. Histologically, there is often evidence of ischaemia but the characteristic feature is hypertrophy of the muscularis mucosae with smooth-muscle fibres extending between the crypts towards the epithelium. There may be considerable fibrosis. Treatment is often difficult. Correction of constipation with bulking agents (with or without lactulose) is important and patients should be warned not to strain. Topical treatment with 5-aminosalicylic acid or corticosteroids may be helpful but there are no controlled data to confirm their efficacy. As these ulcers can remit spontaneously, it is difficult to be sure whether treatment has been effective in an individual patient. For patients with continuing and disabling symptoms, anorectal physiological measurements should be made because there may be evidence of denervation of the pelvic-floor muscles. A defaecating proctogram should also be obtained to demonstrate whether the anorectal angle changes when the patient attempts to empty the rectum and to record the degree of mucosal prolapse. Surgical therapy such as an anterior and posterior rectopexy may be helpful in some patients.

Stercoral ulcers

These occur in association with faecal impaction and are most commonly found in the sigmoid–rectal area. Most patients are elderly but they can occur in any patient who is severely constipated, including patients with neurological causes of constipation (e.g. paraplegia, multiple sclerosis). The common symptoms are those associated with the constipation—nausea, abdominal distension and pain, anorexia—and there may be overflow incontinence. The ulcers are frequently asymptomatic but may be a cause of anaemia from chronic blood loss. They are normally revealed because of an acute bleed or a perforation. Treatment of these acute complications requires surgery but, otherwise, the ulcers are treated by relieving the faecal impaction.

Acute colonic pseudo-obstruction (Ogilvie's syndrome)

This syndrome describes a massive and acute dilatation of the caecum and right colon in the absence of organic obstruction or inflammatory disease of the colon. It may occur following intra-abdominal surgery, including urological or gynaecological surgery, but can also happen in any sick patient. Hence, it can occur in association with severe systemic sepsis, respiratory or cardiac disease. Most patients have a constant, rather dull pain with marked abdominal distension and they frequently vomit. There is constipation but usually patients continue to pass wind and some may actually have diarrhoea. On examination, there is a distended and tympanitic abdomen that is tender to the point of mild

rebound tenderness. Bowel sounds are variable in pitch and frequency but are rarely absent. The diagnosis is made on a plain radiograph of the abdomen. The danger is that of a colonic perforation if treatment is not instituted immediately. Intravenous fluids and electrolytes are given together with nasogastric suction. Any drugs that might be implicated (e.g. tricyclic antidepressants, anticholinergics) are stopped. Rectal tubes and enemas are often used but there value is dubious. It is usually recommended that the patient is turned from side to side at regular intervals. Theoretically this should distribute the intracolonic gas and hence reduce a continuous high pressure in the right colon—again, evidence that this is effective in reducing the incidence of perforation is not clear-cut. If the dilatation does not resolve, decompression can sometimes be achieved by colonoscopy but as it is dangerous to prepare the colon the procedure is difficult. Surgical decompression with a caecostomy may be needed, which may be accompanied by resection if there is an obviously ischaemic segment of colon.

Melanosis coli and related disorders

The term melanosis coli is used to describe black or brown discoloration of the mucosa of the colon. It results from the presence of dark pigment in large mononuclear cells or macrophages in the lamina propria of the mucosa. The coloration is usually most intense just inside the anal sphincter and is less dark higher up in the sigmoid colon. Similar pigment has been found in the appendix and mesenteric nodes. The condition is thought to result from faecal stasis and the use of anthraquinone cathartics such as cascara or senna. Chronic cathartic abuse may also cause radiological changes of the colon that go under the general heading of cathartic colon. The changes are characterized by loss of haustral markings and appearances resembling multiple strictures, although in fact these areas are capable of distension. These changes may involve all parts of the colon and the terminal ileum, and have to be distinguished from those of ulcerative colitis, Crohn's disease, and other inflammatory bowel diseases.

Miscellaneous vascular disorders of the liver

The important vascular disorders of the liver include underperfusion in conditions of shock and left ventricular failure, the wide variety of diseases that give rise to portal hypertension, and acute and chronic venous congestion due to cardiac failure, diseases of the pericardium or, rarely, primary obstruction of the hepatic veins. Portal hypertension is considered in Chapter 14.29.

ACUTE CARDIAC FAILURE AND SHOCK

Reduced hepatic blood flow primarily causes ischaemia in Rappaport zone III, which leads to centrilobular necrosis. This occurs frequently in acute congestive heart failure or in severe hypotension from any cause.

In acute congestive cardiac failure, the liver may be enlarged and tender if the central venous pressure is elevated. There may be biochemical features of liver-cell damage or intrahepatic cholestasis. Liver function may be interfered with sufficiently to cause a reduction of prothrombin synthesis and hence increased sensitivity to anticoagulant drugs.

In patients with severe hypovolaemic shock there may be marked biochemical changes of deranged liver function, and, in severe cases, jaundice. These changes are transient and revert rapidly to normal following restoration of a normal blood pressure and perfusion.

CHRONIC VENOUS CONGESTION

A persistently elevated central venous pressure due to right-sided heart failure or constrictive pericarditis results in hepatic venous congestion and hepatomegaly. The associated histological changes are characterized by centrilobular congestion with surrounding fatty change (the typical 'nutmeg liver'). If the disorder is of long standing, there may be progressive fibrosis extending peripherally from centrilobular to portal areas, although regenerative nodules are not prominent.

Apart from the underlying cardiac lesion, this disorder is characterized by hepatic enlargement and signs of congestive cardiac failure. The serum bilirubin level is usually increased and there may be a slight elevation in the serum alkaline phosphatase and in the transaminases.

It should be emphasized that, although the changes outlined above are relatively common in patients with long-standing heart failure, true cirrhosis of the liver with regenerative nodules is very rare, as is the clinical picture of portal hypertension that accompanies other forms of cirrhosis of the liver; it is very unusual to find oesophageal varices in patients with cardiac cirrhosis.

HEPATIC ARTERIAL OCCLUSION

This is a rare condition. It usually follows surgical trauma but has been found in association with arteritis and bacterial endocarditis.

The condition is characterized by an acute onset of pain in the upper abdomen, tenderness over the liver, and progressive shock and liver failure. Most cases have a fatal outcome.

HEPATIC ARTERIAL ANEURYSM

This condition is recognized by the triad of upper abdominal pain, jaundice, and haematemesis following rupture of the aneurysm into the stomach or duodenum. The diagnosis is made by hepatic angiography. Treatment is by surgical resection.

SEPTIC VENOUS THROMBOSIS OF THE PORTAL SYSTEM

This condition results from infection anywhere in the abdominal cavity leading to pylephlebitis of the portal venous system. It may occasionally result from a systemic septicaemia or from inflammatory disorders of the bowel, such as ulcerative colitis.

The acute phase of the disorder is usually characterized by features related to the underlying abdominal sepsis. This is followed by an episode of high fever, worsening abdominal pain, and rigors. There may be obvious evidence of septic embolization to the liver. This may lead to abdominal pain and hepatic tenderness with mild jaundice. All the systemic features of a severe infection develop and there is usually a polymorphonuclear leucocytosis and abnormal liver tests. Occasionally, multiple large intrahepatic abscesses may develop.

The condition should be suspected in any patient with abdominal sepsis who develops an acute systemic illness with abdominal pain and deranged liver tests. Management consists of intensive antibiotic treatment directed particularly towards Gram-negative organisms and microaerophilic streptococci. In some patients the clinical picture associated with portal venous thrombosis may develop after the acute phase has settled.

Protein-losing enteropathy

Rarely, hypoproteinaemia may result from excessive loss of plasma proteins into the gastrointestinal tract. All plasma proteins are affected; those showing the greatest reduction in concentration are the ones with the longest half-lives, including albumin. The resulting oedema is largely due to the low albumin, this being the main molecule responsible for the plasma colloid osmotic pressure. Although uncommon, this is an important condition to recognize because the resulting oedema or ascites may overshadow the intestinal symptoms and hence the underlying condition is easily missed.

This condition has been found in association with a wide variety of inflammatory or neoplastic disorders of the small bowel and abdominal lymphatic system. It is also associated with allergic disorders involving the small bowel. In most of these conditions protein loss is mild and incidental. Severe protein loss occurs mainly in lymphatic disorders and in Menetriér's disease, a curious condition characterized by the presence of giant gastric rugae.

CLINICAL FEATURES

When severe, the condition is characterized by peripheral oedema and occasionally by ascites and pleural effusions. There is marked hypoalbuminaemia in the absence of liver or renal disease. There may be associated steatorrhoea, particularly if the condition occurs in association with lymphoma of the bowel.

DIAGNOSIS

The diagnosis is made by determining the rate of loss of protein into the intestine using a radioactive label, usually, $^{51}CrCl_3$, which attaches to all plasma proteins, or as ^{51}Cr albumin which redistributes the label, to some extent, to other proteins. ^{67}Cu-labelled caeruloplasmin is theoretically a better marker but has a short half-life. The proportion of radioactivity in the stool is measured during the succeeding 4 days; 0.7 per cent is taken as the upper limit of normal. In comparison with plasma radioactivity, more sophisticated measures of plasma clearance can be derived to give quantitative data. Alternatively, measurements of α_1-antitrypsin in the stool has been shown to be a useful marker of protein-losing enteropathy, without necessitating radioactive labelling.

The further diagnosis of the condition is directed towards determining the underlying cause.

TREATMENT

Treatment is directed towards raising the plasma albumin and correction of the underlying disorder. For example, cases associated with neoplasm of the stomach or colon require surgical resection. Those secondary to coeliac disease, sprue, Whipple's disease, or allergic gastroenteropathies should be treated appropriately.

Jejunoileal bypass

The majority of patients with massive obesity have fatty infiltration of the liver. Following jejunoileal bypass, 55 per cent of them show further fatty change, although this is usually asymptomatic. The increase in fat is due entirely to an accumulation of triglyceride. There is frequently a mild elevation of liver enzymes in serum but this returns to normal once weight reduction has been achieved. The mechanism for the increased fatty change is unknown but it may be a result of protein-calorie malnutrition. An alternative possibility is that the steatosis may be secondary to bacterial overgrowth in the excluded loop of small intestine, as steatosis may diminish with metronidazole therapy.

Acute liver failure may develop in a few patients and is associated with considerable mortality. It is thought to be due to bacterial colonization of the included and excluded small intestine with the production of 'hepatotoxins', which are then absorbed. Treatment consists of intravenous amino acids and broad-spectrum antibiotics. If the condition recurs, further treatment should be given and the ileal bypass reversed.

A micronodular cirrhosis may develop 1 to 6 years after a bypass operation. Histologically, the liver often shows appearances similar to those induced by alcohol. If liver function deteriorates, small-bowel continuity should be restored. Patients may still progress to liver failure and death, but there are reports of the cirrhosis arresting or even reversing with complete recovery of the histology.

Parenteral nutrition and the liver

Abnormalities of serum liver enzymes and bilirubin are commonly seen in patients receiving total parenteral nutrition. Thirty to 60 per cent of patients will show a rise in at least one liver test of greater than 50 per cent of baseline, a rise in alkaline phosphatase being the most frequent abnormality. The changes occur towards the end of the first week and peak between 9 and 12 days. Patients receiving intravenous lipid are particularly at risk but biochemical cholestasis can occur when no fat is given. Liver histology shows steatosis, mild portal inflammation and fibrosis, bile-duct proliferation, and bile plugs. The changes in serum liver tests and in liver histology are reversible once parenteral nutrition is discontinued, although persistent histological changes have been reported. The abnormal liver-enzyme concentrations may also return to normal if the calorie–nitrogen ratio is reduced by reducing the amount of dextrose given, or may even settle spontaneously if parenteral nutrition is continued without change.

The cause of the intrahepatic cholestasis is unknown. Direct toxicity of the intravenous solutions (especially those containing tryptophan), calorie excess or a deficiency of essential fatty acids have been proposed as possible mechanisms. A more likely explanation is the possibility of an overgrowth of anaerobic bacteria in the intestine with subsequent production of endotoxin and lithocholic acid, both of which induce liver damage in animals with similar histological features to that seen in humans receiving total parenteral nutrition. Patients who develop a rise in serum transaminases and alkaline phosphatase have a high concentration of lithocholic acid in the bile compared with patients being parenterally fed who do not have abnormal liver tests. Furthermore, metronidazole has been shown to prevent cholestasis developing in these patients. Hence, the situation may be analogous to the cholestasis associated with a jejunalileal bypass (see above).

PELIOSIS HEPATITIS

This consists of venous lakes within the liver, which probably occur as a result of sinusoidal ectasia. It may be seen in association with oral contraceptive usage, terminal cachexia from carcinoma, and with androgenic steroid therapy. Clinically there are usually few symptoms, although hepatomegaly may be present. Mild to moderate increases in transaminases may occur. Diagnosis is usually made coincidentally on liver biopsy and the prognosis is that of the underlying condition.

REFERENCES

Adibi, B.A. and Stanko, R.T. (1984). Perspective on gastrointestinal surgery for the treatment of morbid obesity: the lesson learned. *Gastroenterology*, **87**, 1381.

Baddeley, R.M. (1980). Surgical management of severe obesity. In *Topics in gastroenterology* 8, (ed. S.C. Truelove and H.J. Kennedy). Blackwell Scientific, Oxford.

Bolt, R.J. (1976). Disease of the hepatic blood vessels. In *Gastroenterology*, (3rd edn), (ed. H.L. Backus), p. 471. Saunders, Philadelphia.

Chatel, A., Garnier, Th., Bigot, J.M., Toneg, C., and Hélénon, Ch. (1979). L'arteriographie dans la periartérite noueuse. *Journal of Radiology*, **60**, 113–20.

Dockerty, M.B. (1972). Primary malakoplakia of the colon. *Mayo Clinic Proceedings*, **47**, 114.

Drenick, E.J., Fisler, J., and Johnson, D. (1982). Hepatic steatosis after intestinal bypass—prevention and reversal by metronidazole, irrespective of protein-calorie malnutrition. *Gastroenterology*, **82**, 535.

Lambert, J.R. and Thomas, S.M. (1985). Metronidazole prevention of serum liver enzyme abnormalities during total parenteral nutrition. *Journal of Parenteral Nutrition*, **9**, 501.

Lazenby, A.J., Yardley, J.H., Giardello, F.M., Jessurum, J., and Bayleis, T.M. (1989). Lymphocytic ('microscopic') colitis: a comparative histopathologic study with particular reference to collagenous colitis. *Human Pathology*, **20**, 18–28.

Long, R. and James, O. (1974). Polymyalgia rheumatica and liver disease. *Lancet*, **i**, 77.

Ranney, B. (1975). The prevention, inhibition, palliation and treatment of endometriosis. *American Journal of Obstetrics and Gynecology*, **123**, 778.

Runyon, B.A., La Brecque, D.R., and Anuras, S. (1980). The spectrum of liver disease in systemic lupus erythematosus. *American Journal of Medicine*, **69**, 187.

Sheldon, G.F., Peterson, S.R., and Sanders, R. (1978). Hepatic dysfunction during hyperalimentation. *Archives of Surgery*, **113**, 504.

Sherlock, S. (1981). *Diseases of the liver and biliary system*, (6th edn). Blackwell Scientific, Oxford.

Sleisenger, M.H. and Fortram, J.S. (1993). *Gastrointestinal disease*, (4th edn). Saunders, Philadelphia.

Steer, H.D. and Colin-Jones, D.G. (1975). Melanosis coli. Studies of toxic effects of irritant purgatives. *Journal of Pathology*, **115**, 119.

Whaley, K. and Webb, J. (1977). Liver and kidney disease in rheumatoid arthritis. *Clinics in Rheumatic Diseases*, **3**, 527.

Section 15 Cardiovascular disease

15.1 Physiological considerations: biochemistry and cellular physiology of heart muscle 2143

15.2 Clinical physiology of the normal heart 2152

15.3 Symptoms of cardiac disease 2162

  15.3.1 Breathlessness 2162
  15.3.2 Chest pain 2165
  15.3.3 Oedema 2169
  15.3.4 Fatigue 2171
  15.3.5 Syncope and palpitation 2173
  15.3.6 Cardiac cachexia 2176

15.4 The clinical assessment of cardiovascular function 2177

  15.4.1 Chest radiography in heart disease 2177
  15.4.2 The electrocardiogram 2182
  15.4.3 Doppler echocardiography 2200
  15.4.4 Nuclear techniques 2204
  15.4.5 Magnetic resonance and computed X-ray tomography 2212
  15.4.6 Cardiac catheterization 2220
  15.4.7 Exercise testing 2225

15.5 The syndrome of heart failure 2228

15.6 The treatment of heart failure 2238

  15.6.1 Diuretics 2238
  15.6.2 Digitalis 2241
  15.6.3 Vasodilators 2246
  15.6.4 Catecholamines and the sympathetic nervous system 2253

15.7 Cardiac transplantation 2255

15.8 Cardiac arrhythmias 2259

  15.8.1 Cardiac arrhythmias 2259
  15.8.2 Pacemakers 2285

15.9 Atheroma, the vessel wall, and thrombosis 2289

  15.9.1 Pathogenesis of atherosclerosis 2289
  15.9.2 Vascular endothelium, its physiology and pathophysiology 2295
  15.9.3 Haemostatic variables in ischaemic heart disease 2300

15.10 Ischaemic heart disease 2305

  15.10.1 Epidemiology and prevention 2305
  15.10.2 The pathophysiology of ischaemic heart disease 2318
  15.10.3 Angina and unstable angina 2321
  15.10.4 Myocardial infarction 2331
  15.10.5 Coronary angioplasty 2349
  15.10.6 Coronary artery bypass grafting 2353
  15.10.7 Vocational aspects of coronary artery disease 2356

15.11 Peripheral arterial disease 2362

15.12 Cholesterol embolism 2375

15.13 Takayasu's disease 2377

15.14 The cardiomyopathies 2380

  15.14.1 The cardiomyopathies, myocarditis, and specific heart muscle disorders 2380
  15.14.2 HIV-related heart muscle disease 2394
  15.14.3 The hypereosinophilic syndrome and the heart 2396

15.15 Congenital heart disease in adolescents and adults 2398

15.16 The cardiac aspects of rheumatic fever 2432

15.17 Infective endocarditis 2436

15.18 Valve disease 2451

15.19 Cardiac myxoma 2472

15.20 Pericardial disease 2474

15.21 Cardiovascular syphilis 2482

15.22 The pulmonary circulation in health and disease 2484

15.23 Pulmonary oedema 2495

15.24 Pulmonary hypertension 2505

15.25 Cor pulmonale 2515

15.26 Pulmonary embolism 2522

15.27 Essential hypertension 2527

15.28 Secondary hypertension 2544

  15.28.1 Renal and renovascular hypertension 2544
  15.28.2 Phaeochromocytoma 2553
  15.28.3 Coarctation of the aorta as a cause of secondary hypertension in the adult 2557

15.29 Lymphoedema 2559

15.1 Physiological considerations: biochemistry and cellular physiology of heart muscle

P.A. POOLE-WILSON AND P.H. SUGDEN

Structure of the myocardial cell

The heart of normal man weighs 250 to 300 g, contracts at a rate of 70 to 75 beats/min at rest, and pumps blood at a rate of 5 l/min. On exercise, the heart rate may increase to 200 beats/min and the cardiac output to 20 l/min. The organ is made up of many different cell types. Cardiac myocytes constitute about 75 per cent of the heart mass but only about 25 per cent of the cell number. Contraction of these myocytes provides the force needed for the ejection of blood from the ventricles. Specialized cells, such as those in the sinoatrial node, the atrioventricular node, the bundle of His, and Purkinje fibres, are adapted for the purpose of initiating and transmitting the cardiac action potential in a regular and coordinated manner to the myocytes in the atria and ventricles. In addition, the heart contains cells (vascular smooth-muscle cells, endothelial cells, and others) that comprise its own extensive circulatory system. Fibroblasts and nerve cells provide systems for controlling the extracellular matrix of the heart and the neural control of cardiac function. The importance of non-cardiac muscle cells such as the endothelium and endocardium in controlling cardiac events is an area of increasing interest. Although the cardiac myocyte has features in common with many cell types, it is in many ways uniquely adapted for its role *in vivo*.

The cardiac myocyte is approximately 100 μm long and 15 μm wide (Figs. 1 to 3). It interdigitates in a 'stepwise' manner with up to nine adjacent myocytes and is in intimate contact with a rich microcapillary network. At the ends of its long axis, each cell is in contact with another through a specialized area of cell membrane called the intercalated disc.

This contains particular structures, the fascia adherens, desmosomes, and gap junctions. The fascia adherens links adjacent cells mechanically so that force can be transmitted between them when the heart contracts. It is linked to the contractile apparatus by a series of specialized proteins such as titin, α-actinin, filamin, and vinculin. Cadherins [in the heart these are N-cadherins, otherwise called A-CAM (cell-adhesion molecule)] connect adjacent cells at the fascia adherens. The desmosomes

Fig. 2 Electron micrograph of part of a single myocardial cell. The glycocalyx (surface coat) and the T-tubules have been stained with potassium ferrocyanide and appear black. Note that the T-tubules penetrate deep into the cells, are connected to the extracellular space, and are aligned with the Z-lines of the sarcomeres. Scale bar: 1 μm.

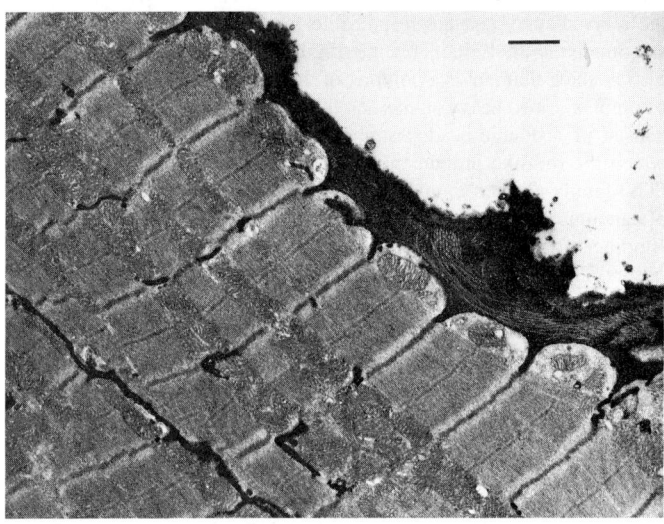

Fig. 1 A single myocardial cell (myocyte). The picture was obtained by scanning electron microscopy. The black holes in the background are part of the supporting material on which the cell has been placed. The cell is approximately 100 μm in length. (Provided by courtesy of Professor N. Woolf and Dr E. M. Steen, Middlesex Hospital.)

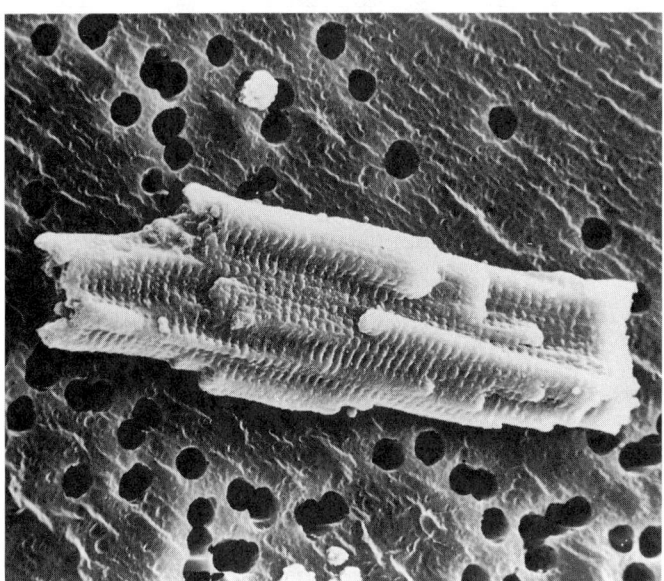

Fig. 3 Diagrammatic representation of organelles in a myocardial cell.

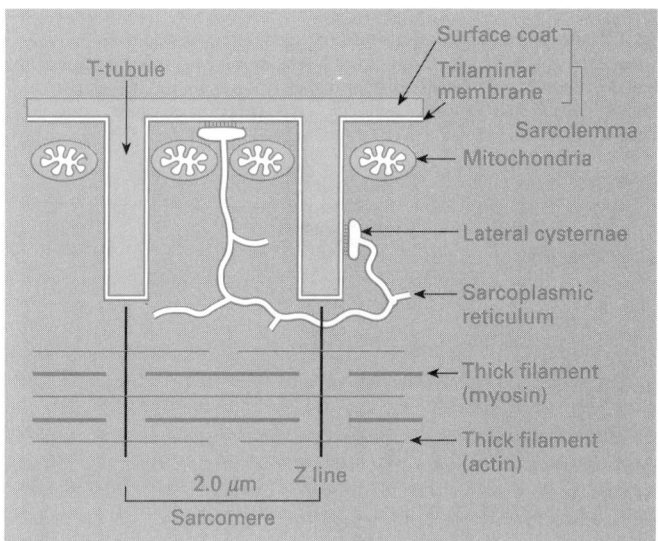

are where the intermediate filaments of the cytoskeleton, which provides an intracellular supporting lattice, attach to the cell membrane. Adjacent cells are linked at the desmosome by integrins of the cadherin super-family of proteins. The gap junctions are the areas of the intercalated disc where the membranes of adjacent cells are particularly close. Here there are specialized gap-junction proteins (the connexon, each made up of six connexins with a central pore) that allow cell-to-cell communication through micropores. The permeability of the cell membrane to ions is high in the gap-junction region so that electrical impulses can pass easily between cells. Gap junctions may also allow the passage of other small molecules between myocytes.

An organized matrix of structural proteins within the cell comprises the cytoskeletal structure or cytoskeleton. This is made up of intermediate filaments and microtubules. The intermediate filaments are so called because they are intermediate in size (10 μm) between actin and myosin. The main protein of these filaments is desmin, which forms a weave around the Z-line and anchors the proteins to the cell surface membrane at the desmosomes. Integrins at this site make connections with the extracellular matrix. Intracellular microtubules (made of the protein tubulin) provide a means for the movement within the cell of intracellular organelles.

Each myocyte has a highly ordered fibrillar structure consisting of bundles of myofibrils (approximately 1 μm in diameter and 150/cell) running the length of the cell. As in skeletal muscle, myofibrils are made up of a basic, repeating, sarcomeric unit that is about 2 μm in length in the relaxed state, and are responsible for muscle contraction. In each sarcomere the thick filaments interdigitate with thin filaments (Figs. 4, 5). The thick filament is a polymer of the rod-like protein myosin (itself a complex of two heavy chains and four light chains). The thin filaments consist of a double-beaded strand of the globular protein actin with which the rod-like protein tropomyosin and members of the troponin (**TN**) family (TN-I, -C, and -T) are associated (Fig. 6). In the absence of calcium, TN-I maintains the myofibrillar ATPase in an inactive state. Binding of Ca^{2+} ions to TN-C removes this restraint and contraction occurs. The thin filaments within adjacent sarcomeres are aligned at the Z-line. The alignment and the overlapping of thick and thin filaments give the myofibril its striated appearance in micrographs (Figs. 2, 5, and 7). The basic process of myofibrillar contraction in the heart is not greatly different overall from that in skeletal muscle. Increases in cytosolic Ca^{2+} concentrations cause the myosin heads in the thick filaments to move along the actin beads in the thin filaments to bring about a shortening of the sarcomeric length, the hydrolysis of ATP providing the energy for contraction. The genetic defect in familial hypertrophic cardiomyopathy (see Section 15.14) involves a mutation, which can be

in any one of a number of sites in the myosin heavy chain, but does not involve the site of attachment to actin or the hinge site in the myosin molecule.

The myocardial cell is surrounded by the sarcolemma, which is made up of a trilaminar membrane (10 nm thick) and an outer layer (70 nm thick) called the surface coat or glycocalyx. As with all such membranes, the structure consists of a phospholipid bilayer in which the polar heads are facing outwards and the lipid tails are within. Numerous proteins are located in the cell membrane and move freely in it. These include proteins anchored at the cytoplasmic or extracellular face of the membrane, and those that cross the membrane. The last mentioned include the proteins constituting the channels and transporters that allow passage of ions through the membrane, and receptor sites for hormones and pharmacologically active substances. Outside the trilaminar membrane, but attached to it, is the glycocalyx (surface coat, external lamina) made up of glycoproteins, glycolipids, and polysaccharides.

Although much of the myocytic volume is occupied by myofibrils, about 30 per cent is taken up by mitochondria. As in other oxidative

Fig. 5 An electron micrograph of a single sarcomere, the basic contractile unit of heart muscle. Below is a diagrammatic interpretation of how the thick and thin filaments interdigitate. The heads protruding from the thick filament are not shown.

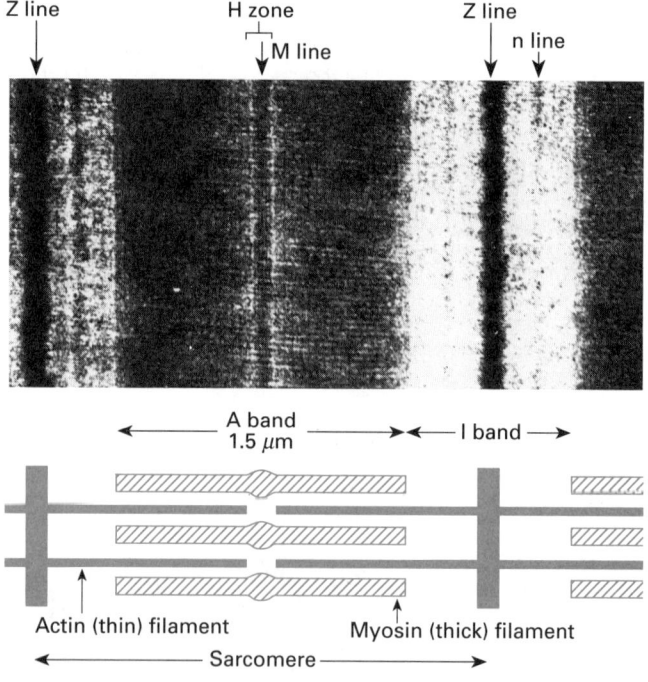

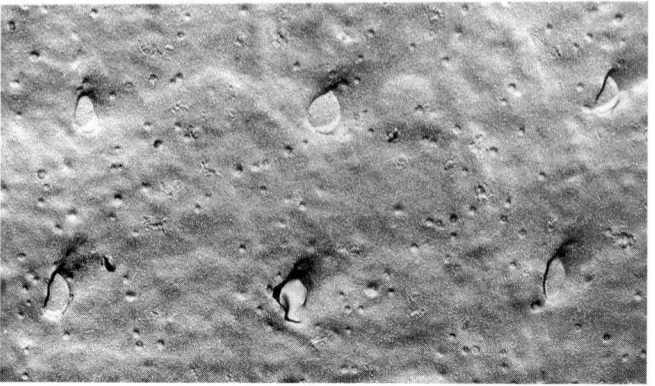

Fig. 4 Picture of the surface of a single myocardial cell viewed from the extracellular space. The openings of six T-tubules can be seen arranged in a regular pattern. The T-tubules are approximately 2 μm apart. The smaller dimples are caveolae. In the background very small particles can be seen. These are individual proteins in the trilaminar cell membrane.

Fig. 6 Diagrammatic representation of the contractile proteins. The thick filament is made from myosin, the thin filament from actin.

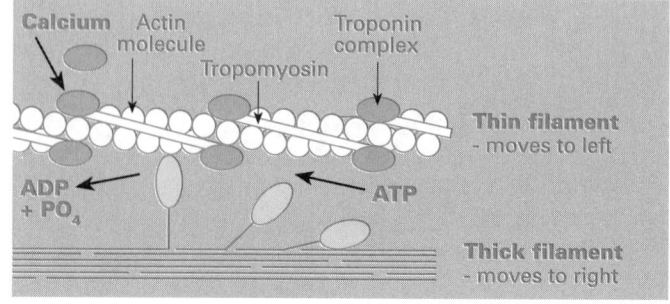

tissues, these subcellular organelles convert the energy released by oxidation of metabolic fuels to catalyse the regeneration of the energy-transducing molecule ATP from ADP and inorganic phosphate. In the cardiac myocyte, the chief pathway for hydrolysis of ATP is myofibrillar contraction but there are also other essential pathways that require energy (for instance, biosynthetic pathways and ion transport). The ATP content of the heart is only sufficient to allow contraction for a few beats and its supply of endogenous fuels (e.g. glycogen, endogenous triglyceride) is limited given the amount of work it has to perform. Thus, in order to maintain fuel oxidation, ATP regeneration and muscle contraction, a highly developed coronary circulation and a continuous coronary blood flow is necessary to ensure delivery of adequate oxygen and fuels, and to remove the products of metabolism. Increased work of the heart is accompanied by an immediate increase of coronary blood flow.

The cardiac myocyte possesses a well developed array of T-tubules and an extensive sarcoplasmic reticulum (see Figs. 2 and 3). The T-tubules are invaginations from the cell surface with openings up to 200 nm in diameter. They are regularly spaced (approximately 2 μm apart) so that one T-tubule penetrates to each Z-line of each myofibril. Unlike skeletal muscle, cardiac muscle is reliant (to varying degrees, dependent on species) on extracellular Ca^{2+} for contraction. The T-tubules allow the passage of Ca^{2+} through the L-type Ca^{2+} channels across the cell membrane to be in close proximity to the Z-line and also allow the necessary ion movements for membrane depolarization that precede the entry of Ca^{2+}. The sarcoplasmic reticulum is a lace-like, tubular structure (30 nm in diameter) spreading over the myofibrils and throughout the whole cell. Where it comes close to the surface membrane or T-tubules, swellings develop called lateral cisternae. Feet, seen as dark opacities under the electron microscope, connect the lateral cisternae to the T-tubule membrane. During diastole, when cytoplasmic Ca^{2+} concentrations are low (0.1–1 μmol/1), Ca^{2+} ions are sequestered in the sarcoplasmic reticulum as a complex with the protein calsequestrin. Entry of extracellular Ca^{2+} through the sarcolemma stimulates release of Ca^{2+} from the sarcoplasmic reticulum through a second Ca^{2+} channel (the ryanodine receptor, so called because of its sensitivity to inhibition by the plant alkaloid ryanodine) in a process known as Ca^{2+}-stimulated Ca^{2+} release. Cytoplasmic concentrations of Ca^{2+} ions are raised (maximally to about 10 μmol/l) and systolic contraction is initiated. The process is terminated by the activation of ATP-requiring Ca^{2+} pumps and ion exchangers (e.g. the Na^+/Ca^{2+} exchanger) that remove calcium from the cell.

In common with most other cells, the cardiac myocyte has one or more nuclei, many ribosomes, and a Golgi apparatus. The nucleus directs the transcription of DNA-encoding protein into mRNA. The mRNA in the cytoplasm is translated into proteins by the ribosomes. The ability of mammalian cardiac myocytes to divide is lost early in life, so that most of their maturational growth occurs through enlargement. A complicating factor is that the nuclei in the cardiac myocyte may be polyploid (i.e. possess more than two chromosome pairs) and/or the cell may contain more than one nucleus; non-mitotic division cannot therefore be excluded. The reasons for the withdrawal of the cardiac myocyte from the cell cycle are not understood. In other cells, proteins known as cyclins are synthesized at specific stages in the cycle. These interact with regulatory protein kinases (the cyclin-dependent kinases), which control *inter alia* the sequestration of transcription factors involved in the regulation of the cell cycle by 'tumour suppressor' proteins such as the retinoblastoma protein. An ability to allow the cardiac myocyte to re-enter the cell cycle in a controlled manner could have considerable clinical significance as it would be one step towards allowing the damaged heart to regenerate its contractile capacity. As it is, the cardiac myocyte can only increase its contractile capacity by enlargement, leading to the clinical entity of cardiac hypertrophy.

The extracellular structure of the heart is made up of collagen and fibronectin. The collagen forms tendons, a network that weaves around cells, and struts, which adhere to the cell membrane at the site of desmosomes and at lateral costamere junctions. The thicker strands are made of type 1 collagen (85 per cent) and the weave from type III. The normal heart contains 5 per cent collagen but in pathological conditions this can increase to 25 per cent. Fibronectin in the extracellular space is concerned with cell adhesion, migration, proliferation and growth, clotting, and is a chemoattractant for macrophages and fibroblasts. The collagen matrix is responsible for the alignment of cells, prevents overstretching, transmits force, determines the shape and architecture of the heart, and stores energy during systole.

Energy for contraction

The heart relies on aerobic metabolism for its energy supply. In normal humans at rest, it extracts 60 to 65 per cent of O_2 passing through it. This corresponds to a rate of O_2 utilization of about 4.5 μmol/min per g wet weight (0.1 ml/min per g wet wt.), increasing three- to four-fold during exercise. The comparable rates (in μmol/min per g wet wt.) are: brain 1.7; kidney 7.1; liver 1.6; skeletal muscle at rest 0.08; and skeletal muscle during exercise 6.4. Thus the maximal physiological O_2 uptake of the heart is higher than that of any other tissue.

The heart will utilize any fuel presented to it, within the constraints of metabolic regulation. Furthermore, because it is contracting continuously, an uninterrupted exogenous provision of fuels through the coronary circulation is essential. The principal substrates for oxidation in man are lipid-derived substances (long-chain fatty acids), principally palmitate, triglycerides and ketone bodies, and the carbohydrate-derived fuels (glucose, lactate, and pyruvate). Although the heart can oxidize amino acids, these probably represent a relatively minor source of energy. The relative contribution of each substrate to the supply of fuels to the heart depends principally on their individual concentrations in plasma.

CARBOHYDRATE METABOLISM

Glucose crosses the myocardial cell membrane by two carrier-mediated mechanisms (the type 1 and type 4 glucose transporters (**GLUT-1** and

Fig. 7 Diagrammatic representation of the structure of the contractile proteins in longitudinal and transverse sections.

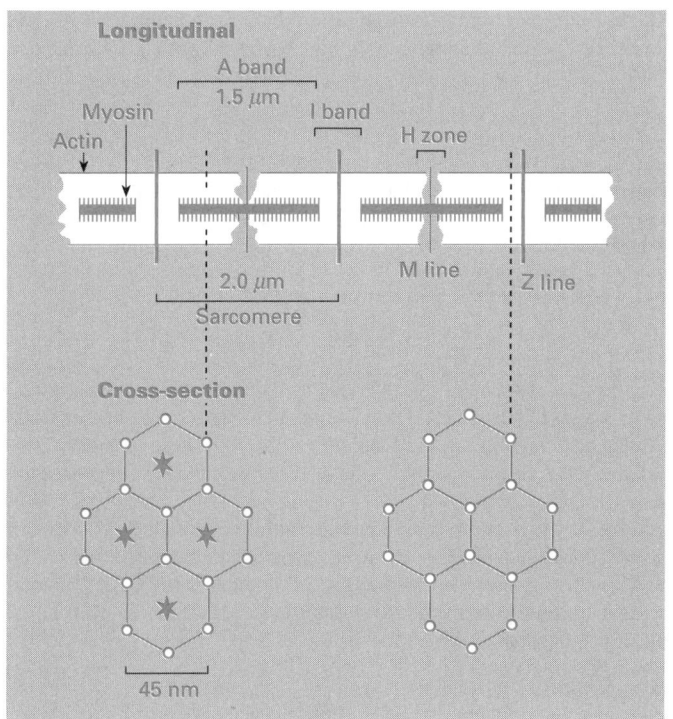

-4)). The activity of GLUT-1 is largely independent of insulin but controlled by the intra- and extracellular concentrations of glucose. Insulin can increase glucose uptake by recruiting intracellular GLUT-4 transporters to the sarcolemma. Each molecule of glucose is degraded to pyruvate through the exclusively cytoplasmic glycolytic pathway, with the concomitant production of reducing equivalents (NADH) and the regeneration of two molecules of ATP. This pathway can function anaerobically but is then inefficient in terms of the quantity of ATP regenerated. In the absence of O_2, pyruvate is reduced by NADH to lactate in a reaction catalysed by cytoplasmic lactate dehydrogenase and NAD^+ is regenerated:

$$\text{Pyruvate} + \text{NADH} + \text{H}^+ \rightleftharpoons \text{Lactate} + \text{NAD}^+.$$

Lactate is then released into the circulation. Lactate release occurs in anaerobic ('white') skeletal muscle (where the carbohydrate source is glycogen) and in the more aerobic muscles ('red' skeletal muscle and cardiac muscle) under hypoxic conditions. This anaerobic pathway of glucose metabolism to lactate is not significant in the normal heart and is utilized only under pathological conditions such as ischaemia.

Under aerobic conditions, pyruvate is transported into the mitochondria and the glycolytically derived reducing equivalents enter on a shuttle mechanism (the malate/aspartate shuttle), regenerating cytoplasmic NAD^+. The electron-transport chain transfers the reducing equivalents to molecular O_2, thereby producing water, the energy released being used to drive regeneration of ATP from ADP and inorganic phosphate. Under aerobic conditions, exogenous lactate or pyruvate can also be utilized by the heart, the former being first oxidized to pyruvate and NADH by lactate dehydrogenase. These enter oxidative metabolism in the same way as glycolytically derived pyruvate and NADH.

The remaining steps of carbohydrate metabolism take place in mitochondria. Pyruvate is oxidized to acetyl coenzyme A (**acetyl CoA**) and NADH by the pyruvate dehydrogenase multienzyme complex (**PDH-MEC**). This is a critical regulatory step in man and many other organisms because it is physiologically irreversible and commits pyruvate (hence glucose) to oxidation. Before the actions of the PDH-MEC, glucose can be resynthesized in liver from lactate or pyruvate by gluconeogenesis. The activity of the PDH-MEC is subject to stringent regulation.

Acetyl CoA enters the tricarboxylic acid cycle, which is also known as the citric acid or Krebs' cycle. By a series of decarboxylations and oxidations, the carbon in the acetyl moiety of acetyl CoA is oxidized to CO_2 and the reducing equivalents used to regenerate ATP by the electron-transport chain. The bulk of the mitochondrially generated ATP is then transported into the cytoplasm (where it is available for myofibrillar contraction) in exchange for cytoplasmic ADP. This exchange is mediated by the adenine nucleotide translocase of the inner mitochondrial membrane.

The combined metabolism of glucose through anaerobic glycolysis and the tricarboxylic acid cycle allows a much greater release of free energy than metabolism through anaerobic glycolysis alone. Whereas metabolism of glucose to lactate results in the regeneration of 2 mol ATP/mol glucose, the complete oxidation of pyruvate to CO_2 and water yields 18 mol ATP/mol pyruvate. Thus, the complete oxidation of 1 mol of glucose results in the regeneration of $2 + 18 + 18$ (i.e. 36) mol ATP. Complete oxidation of glucose is therefore far more efficient in terms of energy release than its fission to lactate but is dependent on a well-developed blood supply to provide both O_2 and glucose.

METABOLISM OF FATTY FUELS

Long-chain fatty acids (**LCFA**), triglycerides, and ketone bodies are all capable of providing energy for the heart. LCFAs (principally palmitate) are present in the plasma either non-covalently bound to albumin or covalently bound as triglycerides, which are in turn complexed with apolipoproteins. The albumin-bound LCFAs enter the cardiac myocyte by a process that is still relatively ill-defined. Triglycerides are hydrolysed by lipoprotein lipase on the capillary wall to form LCFA and glycerol. Ketone bodies are synthesized in the liver from LCFA and probably diffuse readily across cell membranes.

LCFA CoA and ketone bodies can only be metabolized aerobically and exclusively in mitochondria. Two-carbon fragments are successively removed from LCFA CoA in a series of reactions known generically as β-oxidation to form acetyl CoA. Each turn of β-oxidation generates sufficient reducing equivalents to regenerate 5 mol of ATP; acetyl CoA is then oxidized through the tricarboxylic acid cycle. The energy yield from LCFA oxidation is considerable. In the case of palmitic acid ($CH_3(CH_2)_{14} \cdot CO_2^-$), 2 mol ATP equivalents may be used in the activation of 1 mol palmitate to palmitoyl CoA. Thereafter, seven rounds of β-oxidation will produce 8 mol acetyl CoA and the regeneration of 35 mol ATP/mol palmitate, and eight turns of the tricarboxylic acid cycle will regenerate 96 mol ATP/mol palmitate, a net synthesis of 129 mol of ATP/mol palmitate.

REGULATION OF CARDIAC FUEL METABOLISM BY LIPID-DERIVED FUELS

Under normoxic conditions, presentation of lipid-derived fuels (LCFA, ketone bodies) to the heart suppresses glucose utilization, a process achieved by the regulation of the activity of three important enzymes: PDH-MEC, phosphofructokinase, and hexokinase, the latter two regulating the rate of glycolysis.

REGULATION OF CARDIAC FUEL AND ADENINE NUCLEOTIDE METABOLISM DURING HYPOXIA

Ischaemia is the most common cause of hypoxia in the heart. Ischaemia in the context of myocardial infarction is regional. Part of the myocardium is almost totally deprived of its blood supply, so that the supply of exogenous metabolic fuels as well as of O_2 and removal of the products of metabolism are prevented. Maintenance of ATP regeneration is then impossible, given that heart muscle contains relatively little glycogen relative to its workload. Anaerobic carbohydrate metabolism would have to increase about 10-fold (not possible given the activity of the glycolytic pathway) to maintain ATP. Concentrations therefore fall rapidly and contractile activity ceases. Two mechanisms to maintain ATP operate short term in ischaemia before the onset of infarction. First, the creatine phosphokinase equilibrium is driven to the right by retained lactic acid (see below):

$$\text{Phosphocreatine} + \text{ADP} + \text{H}^+ \rightleftharpoons \text{Creatine} + \text{ATP}.$$

This alone allows limited ATP regeneration, sufficient only for a few beats, but secondly, glycogenolysis is increased. A small proportional decrease in ATP concentration leads to a large proportional increase in that of AMP by the operation of the adenylate kinase equilibrium:

$$\text{ATP} + \text{ADP} \rightleftharpoons \text{2ADP}.$$

At physiological ATP concentrations, AMP is a powerful activator of phosphofructokinase, leading to an increase in glycolytic rate. Glycogen breakdown is stimulated by AMP and by catecholamine release, resulting in increased lactate formation. Failure to remove lactate causes intracellular acidification and an increase in NADH. These changes eventually produce a profound inhibition of glycolysis and ATP regeneration ceases.

Lesser degrees of ischaemia produce similar metabolic effects, with the additional deposition of droplets of endogenous triglyceride within cells. These are probably derived from accumulation of LCFA CoA and LCFA-carnitine (intermediates of fatty acid oxidation) as well as of glycerol-3-phosphate, which results in synthesis of triglycerides:

Glycerol-3-phosphate
$$+ \text{ 3 LCFA CoA} \rightarrow \text{Triglyceride} + \text{P}_i + \text{3 CoA}.$$

LCFA CoA and LCFA-carnitine are also powerful detergents. Their accumulation may therefore lead to disruption of membrane systems within the cardiac myocyte, to the detriment of the cell.

Transmembrane and intracellular signalling pathways in the heart

Myriad information in the form of signalling molecules (e.g. catecholamines, insulin) impinges on the outside of the cardiac cell. These bind to transmembrane receptors that transfer information to the inside of the cell. Intracellular signalling pathways then transmit information from one part of the cell to another. Other substances (for instance, thyroid hormone or oestrogen) interact directly with intracellular receptors, and are mainly concerned with effects at the level of transcription achieved by the formation or presence of a signal–receptor complex in the nucleus.

G PROTEIN-COUPLED RECEPTORS

These receptors are proteins with seven transmembrane-spanning regions ('serpentine' receptors). Their extracellular domains interact with individual agonists, whilst their intracellular domains interact specifically with one or more of the large family of heterotrimeric ($\alpha\beta\gamma$) GTP-binding proteins (G proteins), which in their inactive state contain GDP bound to the α-subunit. The receptor–G protein interaction that follows binding of the extraneous signal to the receptor stimulates the exchange of GDP for GTP and dissociation of $\alpha\beta\gamma$ into $\alpha\cdot$GTP and $\beta\gamma$. This dissociation is reversed by the innate GTPase activity of the α-subunit and α(GDP). $\beta\gamma$ is reformed. $\alpha\cdot$GTP (and possibly $\beta\gamma$) are effectors of membrane-bound enzymes that produce so-called second messengers. The archetypal second messenger is cyclic AMP (cAMP), which is formed from ATP by membrane adenylyl cyclase when catecholamines have bound to the β-adrenergic receptor and formed the appropriate $\alpha\cdot$GTP. cAMP then activates cAMP-dependent protein kinase A by dissociating its catalytic subunits from its regulatory (inhibitory) subunits. The catalytic subunits, freed from inhibition, phosphorylate specific serine/threonine in certain enzymes/proteins, thereby modulating their activities/properties. In the heart, β-adrenergic agonists are positively inotropic, chronotropic, and lusitropic (that is, they increase the rate of relaxation). The positive inotropism is the result of a protein kinase A-catalysed phosphorylation of the L-type Ca^{2+} channel that enhances Ca^{2+} entry into the cell, as well as the direct activation of the L-type Ca^{2+} channel by $\alpha\cdot$GTP, and increased phosphorylation of the sarcoplasmic reticulum protein phospholamban and the myofibrillar protein TN-I. Phosphorylation of phospholamban activates the ATP-requiring Ca^{2+} pump, stimulating Ca^{2+} uptake and increasing the rate of myofibrillar relaxation. Phosphorylation of TN-I stimulates dissociation of Ca^{2+} from TN-C, again increasing the rate of relaxation. The positive chronotropic effect of catecholamines is probably exerted at the level of the pacemaker and presumably also involves cAMP.

A second G protein-coupled transmembrane signalling system is the phosphoinositide-based system. Extraneous signals (such as from the α_1-adrenergic agonists or endothelin) interact with receptors and stimulate membrane phospholipase Cβ, the coupling mechanism again involving heterotrimeric G proteins. Phospholipase Cβ hydrolyses the membrane phospholipid phosphatidylinositol 4,5-bis-phosphate to the dual second messengers inositol 1,4,5-tris-phosphate and diacylglycerol. In many cell types (e.g. hepatocytes, vascular smooth-muscle cells), inositol trisphosphate regulates release of Ca^{2+} from the endoplasmic reticulum by binding to its receptor there. In the cardiac myocyte, the physiological function of the trisphosphate is still controversial. It does not seem to be able to release sufficient Ca^{2+} from the sarcoplasmic reticulum to initiate contraction. The diacylglycerol limb of the signal is concerned with the regulation of phospholipid-dependent protein serine/threonine protein kinases that comprise the protein kinase C family.

Protein kinase C is concerned with the regulation of growth in a variety of cell types. Its participation in cellular processes is inferred by the fact that the tumour-promoting phorbol esters, by acting as diacylglycerol analogues, activate it directly.

PROTEIN TYROSINE KINASE RECEPTORS

These receptors are transmembrane proteins that possess an extracellular domain to which the agonist binds, a transmembrane domain, and an intracellular domain that has a protein tyrosine kinase activity essential for signalling activity. The insulin receptor is an example. These receptors frequently mediate the effects of growth factors such as fibroblast growth factors and epidermal growth factor. The subsequent signalling pathway is complex but one limb may involve the small G protein Ras. Ras is the cellular homologue of a viral oncogene-encoded protein and shows similarities to the α-subunits of heterotrimeric G proteins. The adult heart possesses insulin receptors that probably mediate the stimulatory effects of insulin on glucose uptake and protein synthesis.

OTHER SIGNALLING PATHWAYS

The endothelium produces endothelium-derived relaxing factor, which is now thought to be nitric oxide (NO). NO is synthesized from arginine by NO synthase and is very short lived. Amongst other effects, it causes vasodilatation. There is also evidence that it is negatively inotropic in the cardiac myocyte.

Growth of the cardiac myocyte during cardiac hypertrophy

In response to an increased workload, the cardiac myocyte enlarges and, because of its increase in myofibrillar content, its capacity to perform contractile work increases. This enlargement of the myocyte contributes to the increase in ventricular mass that constitutes the clinical entity of 'cardiac hypertrophy'. Cardiac hypertrophy can be seen (although not invariably) when the heart is pressure overloaded or when it is volume overloaded. Each form of hypertrophy produces a characteristic anatomical pattern of enlargement. Pressure overload causes thickening of the chamber walls in the absence of any increase in chamber volume. Volume overload produces enlargement of the chamber with an increase in wall thickness in proportion to the increase in the radius of the cavity. These changes allow peak systolic wall stress to be held at normal values. In addition, following myocardial infarction and myocyte death, the surviving myocytes hypertrophy in order to replace the contractile capacity that has been lost ('reactive' hypertrophy). The shape of the heart may then alter, with slippage of cells ('remodelling').

As described earlier, the cardiac myocyte loses the capacity to divide at an early age in mammals so that a mitotic pathway of cardiac enlargement is not possible. The enlargement of the myocyte that occurs during normal maturational growth is a process quite distinct biochemically from cardiac hypertrophy. Cell dimensions, protein content, and myofibrillar content increase in both, but the hypertrophied myocyte displays a number of transcriptional alterations not shown by the maturing myocyte. There is an increase in the total cellular RNA and in the RNA/protein ratio in hypertrophy. Because the bulk of RNA in any cell is ribosomal RNA, the increased RNA/protein ratio indicates an increase in the number of ribosomes per cell and hence an increase in the capacity for protein synthesis. An early response is the activation of the transcription of certain immediate-early (or primary response) genes that encode DNA-binding proteins involved in the regulation of transcription (transcription factors). These include c-*fos*, c-*jun* (the cellular homologues of viral oncogenes), and *egr*-1. There is up-regulation of constitutive gene expression, for instance that for myosin light-chain 2.

Finally, the pattern of gene expression reverts to a more fetal type, with re-expression in the ventricular myocyte of genes encoding atrial natriuretic factor, skeletal muscle α-actin and, in some species, β-myosin heavy chain. The functional significance of these changes is not clear.

The initiating stimulus (or stimuli) for hypertrophy, be it neurohumoral or mechanical, has been difficult to identify. In cultured cardiac myocytes, two neurohumoral stimuli are particularly effective in stimulating hypertrophy. These are the α₁-adrenergic agonists and endothelin, suggesting that sympathoadrenal and vasomotor tone may regulate the response. Endothelin, produced by the endothelial cells lining the vasculature, stimulates vascular smooth-muscle cell contraction and is positively inotropic in the cardiac myocyte. Both α₁-adrenergic agonists and endothelin stimulate hydrolysis of phosphoinositide and activate protein kinase C in the cardiac myocyte. There is increasing evidence that activation of protein kinase C may be important in the mediation of the hypertrophic response. One current hypothesis is that such activation, by a mechanism that is not yet understood, leads to the sequential activation of a protein kinase cascade that activates mitogen-activated protein kinase, which is thought to be important in the regulation of transcriptional events, probably because, by phosphorylation, it modifies the activities of transcription factors.

Intracellular calcium ion concentration—regulator of contraction

Contraction of cardiac muscle is brought about by changes in the cytoplasmic concentration of Ca^{2+} (Fig. 8). As the Ca^{2+} concentration in the region of the myofibrils rises, it binds to TN-C, relieving the inhibition of the actomyosin ATPase by TN-I, and contraction ensues. The raised cytoplasmic Ca^{2+} concentration then activates Ca^{2+} exchangers and Ca^{2+}/ATPase pumps to return cytoplasmic Ca^{2+} concentrations to the basal state, and tension declines. There are two sources of Ca^{2+} for contraction. Some enters the cardiac myocyte through the L-type Ca^{2+} channel (the dihydropyridine receptor), which gives rise to the slow Ca^{2+} current of the action potential. This calcium triggers release of Ca^{2+} from a second source, the sarcoplasmic reticulum through a distinct sarcoplasmic reticulum Ca^{2+} channel (the ryanodine receptor), thereby amplifying the signal. During relaxation, Ca^{2+} is taken up by the sarcoplasmic reticulum by a Ca^{2+} ATPase or returned to the extracellular space through the sarcolemmal Na^+/Ca^{2+} exchanger.

The Na^+/Ca^{2+} (3 Na^+ for 1 Ca^{2+}) exchange mechanism in the cell membrane is important for the extrusion of Ca^{2+} from the cell. It is driven by the difference between the intracellular and the extracellular concentration of Na^+ (10 and 140 mmol/l, respectively). Intracellular Na^+ is subsequently exchanged for extracellular K^+ by the energy-requiring sarcolemmal Na^+/K^+ ATPase. Ca^{2+} can also be pumped out of the cell against the gradient between the extracellular Ca^{2+} concentration (1 mmol/l) and the intracellular concentration (0.1–1 μmol/l) by a sarcolemmal Ca^{2+} ATPase, a mechanism which may remove the small amount of Ca^{2+} that enters the cell passively.

Electrophysiology

Each heart beat is initiated by a spontaneous electrical discharge in the sinoatrial node. The electrical signal passes across the atrium to the atrioventricular node, through the bundle of His, and down the Purkinje fibres to the ventricular myocardium.

Within a ventricular cell the concentrations of K^+ and Na^+ ions are 140 and 10 mmol/l of cell water, respectively (Fig. 8). Negative charges are carried by intracellular proteins. In the extracellular fluid, the concentrations of K^+ and Na^+ are 4 and 140 mmol/l, respectively, and the principal negatively charged ions are Cl^- (110 mmol/l) and HCO_3^- (24 mmol/l). In the resting state, the cell membrane is more permeable to K^+ than any other ion. K^+, therefore, passes down its concentration gradient to the outside of the cell. As K^+ is positively charged and proteins remain in the cell, the inside of the cell becomes negatively charged. An equilibrium is reached where the electrical force retaining K^+ inside the cell balance its tendency to diffuse out of the cell down its concentration gradient. The transmembrane potential is then the equilibrium potential for that ion. It can be calculated from the Nernst equation:

$$E = \frac{RT}{zF}\ln\frac{(\text{Activity outside})}{(\text{Activity inside})}$$

where E is the equilibrium potential in mV, T is the absolute temperature, R is the gas constant, F is the Faraday constant, and z is the valency. For K^+:

$$E_{K^+} = 61.5 \log_{10}\frac{(4)}{(100)} = -86 \text{ mV}$$

The calculated equilibrium potential for Na^+ is +70 mV and for Ca^{2+}, +120 mV.

In resting cardiac muscle (diastole), the membrane is permeable to K^+ and the inside of the cell is at −80 mV relative to the outside. The difference between this value and the equilibrium potential for K^+ (−86 mV) is attributable to a small leakage of other ions and differences between activity and concentration of intracellular ions. The Na^+/K^+ ATPase is electrogenic (3Na^+ extruded for 2K^+ entering) and also contributes to the negative resting membrane potential. The pump maintains the intracellular ion concentrations despite small leakage currents.

When a cell is electrically excited, its membrane allows Na^+ ions to enter (Figs. 9 and 10). The membrane potential increases to approximately +20 mV (depolarization). The rate of change of the potential is related to the propagation velocity of the action potential across the heart. The increase in Na^+ conductance lasts only a few milliseconds ('fast' Na^+ channel current) and is followed by a transient outward current, probably carried by K^+ (phase 1). Phase 2 is caused largely by the 'slow' inward current, sometimes called the 'second' inward current. This current is made up predominantly of Ca^{2+} ions entering through the slow Ca^{2+} (L-type Ca^{2+}) channel with a smaller contribution from entry of Na^+ ions. At the same time, the conductance to K^+ is reduced so that despite depolarization a large outward K^+ current does not occur (anomalous rectification). Phase 2 of the cardiac action potential is referred to as the plateau and is not present in skeletal muscle, which has a much shorter action potential. Finally, the cell repolarizes (phase 3). Repolarization occurs because of an increase in K^+ conductance and termination of the Ca^{2+} current.

Fig. 8 Calcium exchange in heart muscle. Note the two intracellular stores in the mitochondria and sarcoplasmic reticulum. Three methods for influx and efflux of calcium are shown.

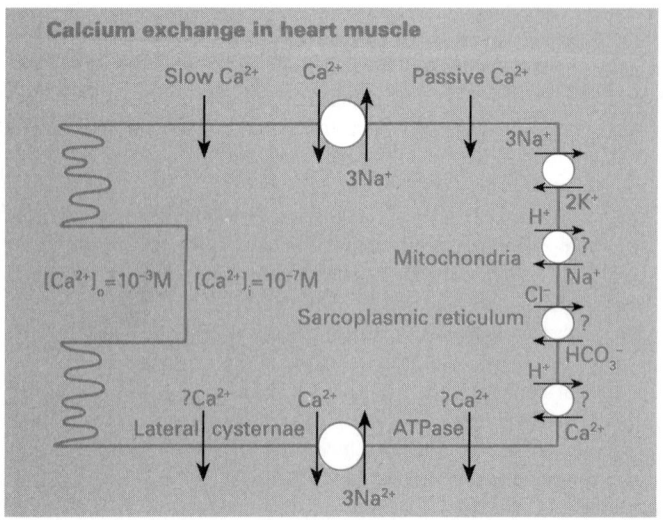

The configuration of the cardiac action potential differs regionally (Fig. 11). The longest action potential is in Purkinje fibres. They act as a gate, preventing retrograde activation by depolarization of adjacent ventricular muscle cells. The action potential is longer in the epicardium than endocardium and apex than base of the heart. The reason is not clear but the discrepancy is the probable explanation for the upright T-wave on the electrocardiogram.

In specialized cardiac tissue (sinoatrial node, atrioventricular note) and in damaged myocardial cells, the resting membrane spontaneously depolarizes (phase 4). This is mainly due to a decrease of K^+ conductance, although Na^+ and Ca^{2+} conductance may increase. When the membrane potential reaches a value of approximately -50 mV (threshold voltage), the cell spontaneously depolarizes and an action potential is initiated.

Electrical disequilibrium in the heart leads to arrhythmias. There are at least three cellular mechanisms. The first is called 'automaticity'. Injured myocardial cells or Purkinje fibres develop spontaneous phase-4 depolarization. Conditions that make the resting membrane potential less negative, the threshold voltage more negative or increase the rate of phase-4 depolarization favour automaticity. The second mechanism is 're-entry'. The requirements for this are unidirectional block of an electrical impulse and slow propagation of the action potential. Under these circumstances the electrical wavefront may pass round diseased tissue through the block retrogradely and stimulate again cells that have had sufficient time to repolarize and not be refractory. A circus movement is established. The third mechanism relates to after potentials. These can occur during the plateau phase of the action potential (called **EAD**s, early after depolarizations) or after repolarization (called **DAD**s,

delayed after depolarizations). EADs are caused by a reduction of the normal repolarizing current or abnormal prolongation of the inward current carried by calcium and sodium. DADs are due to intracellular calcium overload and are carried either by the Na^+/Ca^{2+} exchanger or a calcium non-specific cation channel. Injured cells are often partly depolarized, particularly in ischaemic tissue where the extracellular K^+ can be high (up to 18 mmol/l) because of leakage of the ion out of the cell. Under these conditions, spontaneous depolarization can occur and is often caused by Ca^{2+} currents. It can be initiated by mechanical stretching of injured myocardium. If the phenomenon occurs in a sufficient number of cells, the current density can bring about depolarization of adjacent healthy cells and initiate an ectopic heart beat.

The exact cause of an arrhythmia in an individual patient is rarely known and the classification of antiarrhythmic drugs is based on electrophysiological and pharmacological observations.

Mechanics

The basic unit of contraction in cardiac muscle is the sarcomere. In resting muscle, the sarcomere is between 1.8 and 2.0 μm long. If the pressure at the end of the diastole (the left-ventricular filling pressure) is increased as in acute heart failure, the volume of the ventricle is increased and the sarcomere lengthens to a maximum of 2.3 μm. Only when acute dilatation of the ventricle occurs, for example, by accident during cardiac surgery, is the length of the sarcomere increased beyond 2.3 μm. This is associated with tearing of the muscle and irreversible damage. The enlargement of the heart in severe chronic heart failure is due to slippage of the myofibrils and adjacent myocardial cells and is not due to excessive elongation of the sarcomere.

Laser diffraction techniques have allowed the measurement of sarcomere length, and resting and developed tension during a single heart beat in which either length is maintained constant or shortening is allowed to occur. Some results are shown in Figs. 12 and 13. Regardless of the resting length of the muscle or whether the muscle shortens against an afterload, there is a constant relation between maximum developed tension and minimum sarcomere length. This generalization is not precisely true, as shortening and stretch of myocardial cells can both bring about a small reduction in the duration of the action potential and the degree of activation of myofibrils. The relation between tension and minimum sarcomere length is analogous to the relation in the whole heart between pressure and volume. There is an almost fixed relation between end-systolic volume and end-systolic pressure (Fig. 13). The

Fig. 9 Action potential of ventricular myocardium. The action potential is the voltage measured between a microelectrode inserted into the intracellular fluid (cytosol) of a myocardial cell and a reference electrode in the extracellular fluid. The action potential is recorded after the muscle has been stimulated by an electrical impulse.

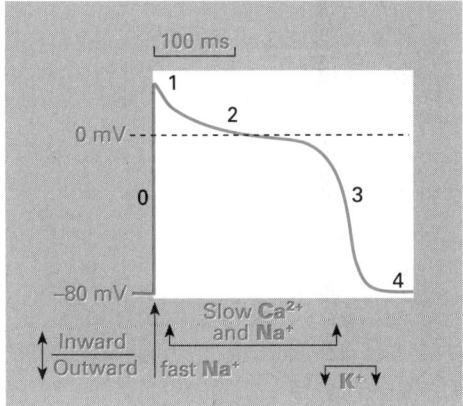

Fig. 10 The relation of the action potential to the generation of tension. The absolute refractory period is the period when a second electrical stimulus will elicit no response.

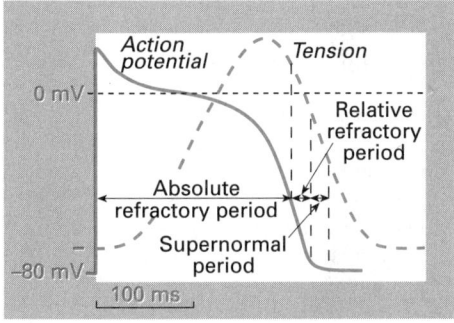

Fig. 11 The action potential has a different configuration in different parts of the heart. In the sinoatrial and atrioventricular nodes the cell spontaneously depolarizes during diastole (phase 4 depolarization). When the voltage reaches the threshold potential a complete action potential is initiated. Thus, the sinoatrial node with the fastest phase 4 depolarization acts as the primary pacemaker for the heart.

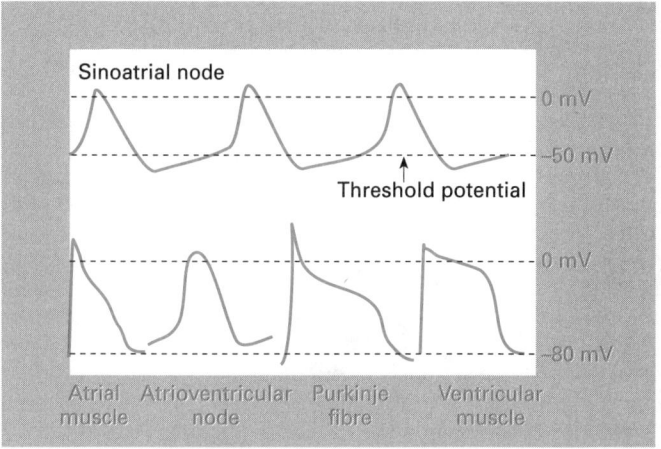

relation is altered by inotropic agents and by the extracellular Ca^{2+} concentration.

The extent to which the sarcomere can shorten determines the stroke volume. During severe exercise or in the presence of powerful inotropic drugs, the sarcomere at end-systole may be only 1.4 μm long. At this length, cardiac muscle recoils. A negative pressure is present during early diastole and filling of the ventricle is partly due to suction. With zero filling pressure, the length is about 1.6 μm. Under normal resting conditions in man the ventricle is filled by a positive pressure and the sarcomere is between 1.8 and 2.0 μm long.

From Figs. 12 and 13 it is apparent that as the initial sarcomere length is increased the greater is the degree of shortening which occurs for a given afterload (tension or blood pressure). Because the greater degree of shortening occurs in a similar time, the velocity of contraction is also increased. If no shortening is permitted (isometric contraction), then the maximum developed tension increases with increasing resting sarcomere length. These observations form a basis for understanding the well-known Frank–Starling mechanism. Frank showed that the systolic pressure in systole increased in isovolumic hearts as end-diastolic volume increased. Starling showed than an increase in atrial pressure resulted in an increase in end-diastolic volume and cardiac output. This latter effect is often referred to as 'heterometric' regulation of the cardiac output, as resting sarcomere length is altered. In cardiac muscle the slope of the Starling curve is much greater than in skeletal muscle. In skeletal muscle, the mechanism for the increased developed force on increasing resting length is believed to be related to the greater overlap of the

Fig. 12 Resting and active tension in isolated cardiac muscle at different initial sarcomere lengths. In intact tissue the sarcomere length at the end of systole (maximal contraction) is determined by the end systolic tension against which the muscle contracts and shortens. This relation at end systole is shown by the middle curve.

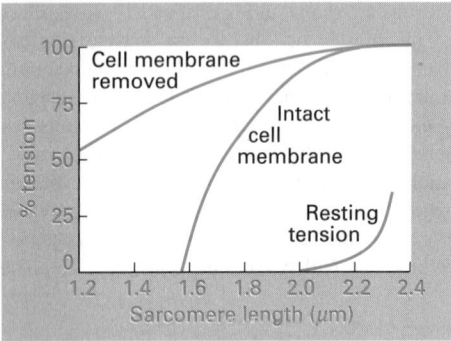

Fig. 13 The pressure-volume relation in the intact heart. A single heart beat is represented by the dotted line ABCD. EF is the line showing the end systolic relation between pressure and volume. The relation is almost constant provided myocardial contractility is unaltered.

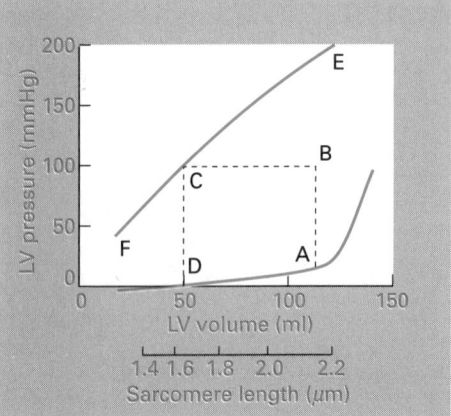

contractile proteins. In cardiac muscle the curve is too steep for this explanation to be possible. The increased tension developed is probably related to an increased Ca^{2+} sensitivity of the contractile apparatus as the muscle is stretched.

A second intrinsic mechanism by which heart muscle increases the force of contraction is referred to as 'homeometric' regulation or the Anrep effect. After a sudden increase in afterload, end-diastolic pressure and ventricular volume rise but decrease again over several minutes so that the heart finally ejects against an increased afterload from almost the initial end-diastolic volume. The mechanism of this effect is probably related to intracellular control mechanisms for Ca^{2+}. The effect is only of slight importance in man.

The third intrinsic mechanism by which the heart can increase the force of contraction is by an increase of heart rate (Bowditch effect, rate staircase, interval–strength relation). If stroke volume remains constant, an increase of heart rate will cause an increase of cardiac output. However, experiments in isolated hearts show that, in addition, the strength of contraction is increased. This phenomenon is present in man but is weak. A possible mechanism is that the increased number of depolarizations per minute increases the entry of Na^+ into the cell. The Na^+ pump reaches a new equilibrium when the intracellular Na^+ is slightly increased. The raised intracellular Na^+ concentration increases the net Ca^{2+} movement into the myocardial cell and more Ca^{2+} is available during each contraction.

Positive and negative inotropes

The action of drugs on the myocardium can be due to an effect on the calcium transient (upstream regulation) or on the sensitivity of the contractile proteins to calcium (downstream regulation). No inotrope currently used in clinical practice increases the force of contraction by a direct effect on the myofibrils. A group of drugs known as calcium sensitizers is currently under investigation. Cyclic nucleotide phosphodiesterase inhibitors (e.g. caffeine, milrinone) raise cAMP concentrations and activate protein kinase A. This increases Ca^{2+} entry through L-type Ca^{2+} channels, increases the rate of Ca^{2+} release from troponin C, and increases the ability of the sarcoplasmic reticulum to sequester Ca^{2+}. The net effects are positive inotropy and positive lusitropy (improved relaxation).

All other drugs act primarily on the cell membrane. Cardiac glycosides (e.g. digoxin) inhibit the Na^+/K^+ ATPase, preventing the extrusion of intracellular Na^+. This in turn inhibits Ca^{2+} extrusion via the Na^+/Ca^{2+} exchanger and may even stimulate Ca^{2+} entry by reversing the physiological direction of the exchanger. Cytoplasmic concentrations of Ca^{2+} increase, thereby increasing the force of contraction. Ca^{2+} may also be taken up by the sarcoplasmic reticulum, thereby increasing the cardiac Ca^{2+} pool, and it also may facilitate Ca^{2+}-stimulated Ca^{2+} release from the sarcoplasmic reticulum. The net effect is to increase the cytoplasmic concentration/availability of Ca^{2+} and increased force of contraction results.

Catecholamines (adrenaline and isoprenaline) raise cAMP and protein kinase A activity and are powerful positive inotropic drugs. The influx of Ca^{2+} is increased by phosphorylation of the L-type Ca^{2+} channel, relaxation is augmented by activation of phospholamban, which increases the uptake of Ca^{2+} by the sarcoplasmic reticulum, and the contractile proteins are rendered less sensitive to Ca^{2+} by phosphorylation of troponin I.

The 'calcium antagonists' (verapamil, nifedipine, diltiazem) have the property of inhibiting the slow Ca^{2+} current of the action potential and thus causing a fall in contractility, relaxation of muscle, and reduced conduction in the sinoatrial and atrioventricular nodes. Therapeutically, their chief effects are through their antiarrhythmic action and their vasodilator activity (which increases blood flow and oxygen delivery). The vasodilator activity is related to their ability to relax vascular smooth muscle by decreasing intracellular concentrations of Ca^{2+} ions.

Ischaemia (see also Section 15.10)

Whatever the initiating mechanism for acute myocardial ischaemia, the three important consequences are a failure of contraction, arrhythmias, and cell death. Myocardial ischaemia is traditionally regarded as that state that exists when myocardial oxygen supply is less than demand. Oxygen demand reflects the rate of consumption of ATP and oxygen supply is related to blood flow. Furthermore, blood flow not only provides a source of oxygen and substrate for heart muscle but also removes the products of metabolism. Two key products are heat and carbon dioxide. Ischaemia is better defined as an imbalance between ATP consumption and blood flow or as the state that exists when anaerobic metabolism occurs because of a low blood flow.

Total ischaemia results in cessation of contraction within 60 s. An important but not the sole mechanism is the rapid development of an intracellular acidosis. An intracellular rise in the concentration of the phosphate ion from the breakdown of ATP is another contributory factor. Total tissue ATP does not decline within 60 s but the rapid fall of tissue creatine phosphate is suggestive that ATP in some compartment within the cell does fall rapidly. A low ATP might affect contraction if insufficient ATP were available to maintain the normal functioning of ionic channels in the cell membrane or to allow shortening of the myofibrils.

The exact mechanism of cell death is at present unknown but may be related to free radical damage and Ca^{2+} overload. Under normal resting conditions, the myocardium will recover almost completely after 10 to 15 min of ischaemia. More prolonged periods of ischaemia cause the cell membrane to become permeable to cations and recovery is reduced. If limited blood flow is present from collateral coronary arteries or from 'stuttering ischaemia' due to periodic opening and closing of the native coronary artery the cell gains Na^+ and loses K^+. After 60 to 90 min of ischaemia, the cell membrane is destroyed. This may be attributable to a low tissue ATP, acidosis, activation of phospholipases, and lysosomal activity.

Reperfusion of ischaemic heart muscle results in further damage (reperfusion damage). There is an immediate swelling of the cell, release of intracellular enzymes, and a large influx of Ca^{2+}. Ca^{2+} is taken up by the mitochondria and can be seen as dark granules under the electron microscope. A large gain of Ca^{2+} is an indicator of cell death, as it prevents the normal functioning of mitochondria and the regeneration of ATP. Many theories seek to explain the sudden influx of Ca^{2+}. A popular one is that the reintroduction of oxygen causes an increased generation of oxygen radicals that damage the cell membrane and in particular render the membrane permeable to Ca^{2+}. The normal mechanisms within the cell for the removal of radicals are partly destroyed during the period of ischaemia. Recovery from a period of ischaemia is slow. This is partly because the myocardium loses nucleotides. ATP is broken down to ADP and AMP, which in turn are broken down to inosine and adenosine. These latter two are lost from the cell. Regeneration of nucleotides takes several days and is the probable reason why, even if a cell does not die, total recovery may taken days even weeks.

Drugs that are now used in an attempt to reduce the size of a myocardial infarction act either by reducing ATP consumption (cardioplegic solutions, hypothermia, afterload reduction, negative inotropic agents) or by increasing coronary flow (afterload reduction, coronary vasodilators) through collaterals or the native coronary. The introduction of thrombolytic therapy for selected patients with myocardial infarction will reduce infarct size if the occlusion is due to thrombus, if the thrombus can be dissolved, and if the occlusion has not been present for more than a few hours. No drug has been shown to benefit the ischaemic myocardial cell by a mechanism that acts directly on the cell structure or cell metabolism, with the possible exceptions of insulin, glucose and K^+ therapy, corticosteroids, and hyaluronidase. Hypothermia is effective partly because metabolic pathways are inhibited.

Four new concepts have emerged, 'hibernating myocardium', 'stunned myocardium' and 'preconditioning' and 'remodelling'. Hibernating myocardium describes a state of persistently impaired myocardial and left ventricular function at rest, due to reduced coronary blood flow, that can be partially or completely restored to normal if the myocardial oxygen supply/demand relation is favourably altered, either by improving blood flow and/or reducing demand. Stunned myocardium refers to the mechanical dysfunction that persists after reperfusion despite the absence of irreversible damage and despite restoration of normal or near-normal coronary flow. Preconditioning describes the greater tolerance to ischaemia that develops if the myocardium has previously been exposed to a transient period of ischaemia of between 2 and 10 min. Remodelling refers to changes in the size, shape, and architecture of the heart that can follow the successful treatment of heart failure, particularly after myocardial infarction. Remodelling may be a consequence of haemodynamic changes or biological processes involved with repair, inflammation, growth, and hypertrophy of the myocardium. The cellular mechanisms for these concepts are not fully understood. Indeed, their relevance to many clinical conditions is also uncertain.

Mechanism of heart failure

Acute heart failure is most commonly caused by reduced myocardial contractility secondary to acute ischaemia (e.g. acute myocardial infarction, diminution of oxygen supply). More rarely the cause is associated with a high ATP consumption and an increased requirement for force development (e.g. aortic stenosis, malignant hypertension, increased 'demand' for oxygen). Reduction of cardiac function due to structural derangement of the heart as a pump (e.g. acute mitral regurgitation due to papillary muscle rupture) is another cause.

The causes of chronic heart failure are more complex, as coronary blood flow, oxygen supply, and removal of metabolites are often normal and no initiating haemodynamic factor is present. Under these circumstances (e.g. heart failure in the presence of coronary arterial disease or cardiomyopathies), abnormalities have been reported in the cell membrane, sarcolemma, and myofibrils. The control mechanisms for calcium homeostasis are abnormal in the hypertrophied and failing heart. Loss of coordinate contractility is common. Furthermore, changes in the size, shape, fibre orientation, and architecture of the heart may be key mechanisms for the abnormal function of the heart as a pump despite normal or near-normal function of individual myocytes. Fibrosis increases in the dilated and damaged myocardium. Whether these abnormalities are primary or merely secondary to myocardial damage or reduced contractility is unclear. The primary cellular event is different in the many forms of heart failure.

REFERENCES

Chien, K.R., Knowlton, K.U., Zhu, H., and Chien, S. (1991). Regulation of gene expression during myocardial growth and hypertrophy: molecular studies of an adaptive physiologic response. *FASEB Journal*, **5**, 3037–46.

Fozzard, H.A., Haber, E., Jennings, R.B., Katz, A.M., and Morgan, H.E. (1991). *The heart and cardiovascular system. Scientific foundations.* Raven Press, New York.

Folkow, B. and Neil, E. (1971). *Circulation.* Oxford University Press.

Ganote, C. and Armstrong, S. (1993). Ischaemia and the myocyte cytoskeleton: review and speculation. *Cardiovascular Research*, **27**, 1387–403.

Katz, A.M. (1992). *Physiology of the heart.* Raven Press, New York.

Marban, E. (1991). Myocardial stunning and hibernation. The physiology behind the colloquialisms. *Circulation*, **83**, 681–8.

Milnor, W.R. (1990). *Cardiovascular physiology.* Oxford University Press.

Murry, C.E., Jennings, R.B., and Reimer, K.A. (1986). Preconditioning with ischemia: a delay of lethal cell injury in ischemic myocardium. *Circulation*, **74**, 1124–136.

Newsholme, E.A. and Leech, A.R. (1983). *Biochemistry for the medical sciences.* Wiley, Chichester.

Opie, L.H. (1991). *The Heart. Physiology and metabolism,* Raven Press, New York.

Rahimtoola, S.H. and Griffith, G.C. (1989). The hibernating myocardium. *American Heart Journal,* **117**, 211–21.

Suga, H. (1990). Ventricular energetics. *Physiology Reviews, 70*, 247–77.

Sugden, M.C. and Holness, M.J. (1994). Interactive regulation of the pyruvate dehydrogenase complex and the carnitine palmitoyltransferase system. *FASEB Journal*, **8**, 54–61.

Taegtmeyer, H. (1994). Energy metabolism of the heart: from basic concepts to clinical applications. *Current Problems in Cardiology*, **19**, 57–116.

Weber, K.T. *et al.* (1992). Remodeling and reparation of the cardiovascular system. *Journal of the American College of Cardiology*, **20**, 3–16.

15.2 Clinical physiology of the normal heart

D.E.L. WILCKEN

Introduction

The function of the heart is to pump sufficient oxygenated blood containing nutrients, metabolites, and hormones to meet moment-to-moment metabolic needs and preserve a constant internal milieu. The heart has two essential characteristics, contractility and rhythmicity. The nervous system and neurohumoral agents modulate relationships between the venous return to the heart, the outflow resistance against which it contracts, the frequency of contraction, and its inotropic state; there are also intrinsic cardiac autoregulatory mechanisms. This section describes normal cardiac function and discusses the principal mechanisms contributing to its regulation.

The cardiac cycle

Electrical events initiate the cardiac cycle with depolarization of the sinoatrial node in the upper right atrium near the orifice of the superior vena cava (Fig. 1). Cardiac muscle acts as a functional syncytium. Cell-to-cell conduction is possible because the intercalated discs offer a low electrical resistance. The action potential in an active cell causes current flow, which depolarizes the adjacent cells. The generated action potential spreads from the sinoatrial node across the functional syncytium at a speed of 1.0 to 1.2 m/s. The first mechanical response is atrial systole.

The valvular attachments and connective tissue in the atrioventricular groove normally prevent cell-to-cell conduction of the electrical impulse from atrium to ventricle. This conduction occurs only through the specialized cells of the atrioventricular node (Fig. 1). The atrioventricular node is a region of slow conductance, from 0.02 to 0.1 m/s. This delays activation of the cells of the bundle of His and allows time for completion of ventricular filling. The conduction velocity in the bundle of His is from 1.2 to 2.0 m/s. The impulse passes via the right bundle branch and the two branches of the left bundle, and spreads rapidly (2.0 to 4.0 m/s) through the Purkinje fibres and each muscle cell to produce an orderly sequence of ventricular contraction (Fig. 1). Atrial and ventricular depolarization (P wave and a QRS complex) and repolarization (T wave) can be recorded on the electrocardiogram as the summation of the spread of the electrical potentials over all the cells of the heart (Fig. 2). Electrocardiography is considered in Chapter 15.4.2.

The specialized cells of pacemaker tissue have an inherent rhythmicity which is shared by the sinoatrial node, the atrioventricular node, and Purkinje tissue. Unlike other myocardial cells these cells do not maintain a diastolic intracellular potential of about −90 mV but tend to depolarize spontaneously. Because the sinoatrial node has the fastest inherent discharge (depolarization) rate, and because there is a brief period after depolarization of the whole heart during which a further stimulus is ineffective – the absolute refractory period – the sinoatrial node is normally the pacesetter for the heart. However, if for some reason this does

Fig. 1 Diagram of the heart showing the impulse-generating and impulse conducting system. (Reproduced from Junqueira, L.C., Carneiro, J., and Kelly, R.O. (1992). *Basic histology*. 7th edn, Appleton and Lange, Norwalk, Connecticut, with permission.)

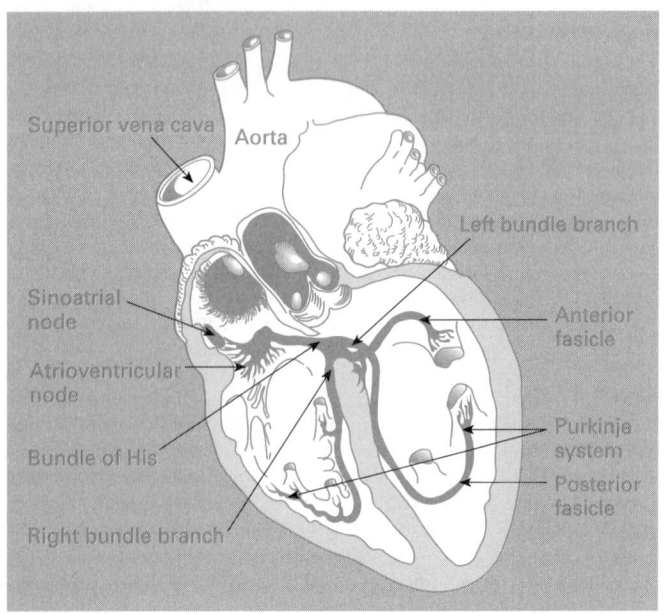

Fig. 2 Diagram of electrocardiographic complexes, intervals, and segments. VAT, ventricular activation time. (Reproduced from Goldman, M.J. (1986). *Principles of clinical electrocardiography*. 12th edn, Lange, Los Altos, California, with permission.)

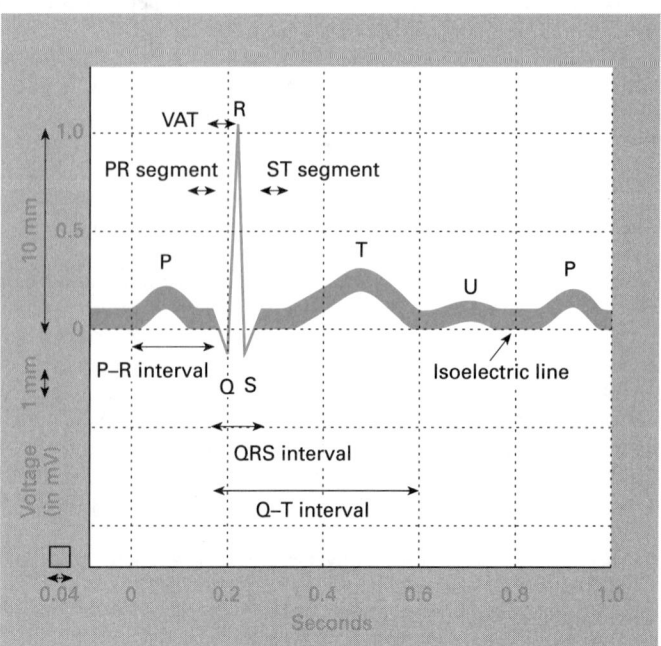

not function, pacemaker tissue in the atrioventricular node, bundle of His, or Purkinje system, will assume this role. The heart rate is then considerably slower.

MECHANICAL EVENTS

The mechanical events following depolarization of the atrial and ventricular muscle and their timing in relation to the electrocardiogram, to pressure and flow changes, and to heart sounds are shown in five phases in Fig. 3. After the P wave, and coinciding with atrial systole, 'a' waves appear in left atrial and right atrial pressure tracings due to atrial contraction, and an 'a' wave can be seen in the jugular venous pulse. Atrial contraction increases ventricular filling by about 10 per cent (phase 1).

The onset of ventricular contraction coincides with the peak of the R wave of the electrocardiogram and there is a rapid rise in intraventricular pressure, which closes the mitral and tricuspid valves. The first heart sound is heard at the time of maximum displacement of these valves as they reach their closing positions. During this short isovolumetric period (phase 2 of Fig. 3) the pressure rises rapidly in the ventricle, which changes in shape but not in volume. When ventricular pressures exceed those in the pulmonary artery and aorta, the outflow valves open and ventricular ejection follows, with the highest flow rate occurring in early systole, and pressures in the aorta and pulmonary artery rise. Normally between 50 and 70 per cent of the ventricular volume is ejected during systole, and this can be seen in the volume curve included in Fig. 3 (phase 3).

The jugular venous pulse during ventricular contraction has a positive deflection in early systole, the 'c' wave, due to right ventricular contraction and bulging of the tricuspid valve into the right atrium. Descent of the tricuspid ring caused by ventricular contraction then produces a negative 'x' descent, but as atrial inflow continues the pressure rises in the atria and great veins, producing the 'v' wave. This reaches its peak just before the opening of the tricuspid valve, declining during early ventricular filling as the negative 'y' descent. The changes in the pulmonary veins and left atrium are similar.

As the strength of ventricular contraction declines, and coinciding with the end of the T wave of the electrocardiogram, the aortic and pulmonary valves close, producing the dicrotic notch seen on both aortic and pulmonary artery pressure tracings in Fig. 3. Aortic closure slightly precedes pulmonary closure, and together these are responsible for the two components of the second heart sound. A short period of further rapid decline in ventricular pressure ensues without changing ventricular volume (the period of isovolumetric ventricular relaxation, phase 4) and at the end of this the mitral and tricuspid valves open. There is a pressure gradient from atrium to ventricle so that a period of rapid ventricular filling follows, which coincides with the timing of the third heart sound. The rapid ventricular filling is reflected in the shape of the ventricular volume curve, and is followed by a period of slower filling (phase 5) with a final sudden small increment from the next atrial contraction as diastole ends (phase 1).

Third heart sounds are audible with the stethoscope in normal children and young adults. The hearing of these sounds in patients over the age of about 40 years, however, usually indicates elevation of ventricular end-diastolic pressure (most frequently in the left ventricle). This is probably because the myocardium and valvular structures become stiffer with ageing, and large increases in ventricular end-diastolic pressure are then required to tense valvular structures and generate audible vibrations. The hearing of a fourth heart sound almost always indicates abnormal ventricular function. The end-diastolic pressure in the affected ventricle (usually the left) is increased, and the already stretched inflow valve responds to atrial systole and further filling with oscillations, producing a low pitched sound often palpable, as well as audible, at the cardiac apex. A fourth heart sound precedes the Q wave of the electrocardiogram and must be distinguished from a normal splitting of the two components of the first heart sound. The latter occurs after the Q wave (Figs. 2 and 3).

Normal volumes, pressures, and flows

The blood volume in normal adults is about 5 litres (haematocrit 45 per cent) and of this about 1.5 litres are in the heart and lungs – the central blood volume. The pulmonary arteries, capillaries, and veins contain about 0.9 litres and at any one instant only about 75 ml are in the pulmonary capillaries. The volume of blood in the heart is about 0.6 litres. Left ventricular end-diastolic volume (EDV) is about 140 ml, the stroke volume (SV) about 90 ml, so that the end-systolic volume is around 50 ml, and the ejection fraction (SV/EDV) from 50 to 70 per cent. The right ventricular ejection fraction is of the same order of magnitude.

Of the 3.5 litres in the systemic circulation most, at least 60 per cent of the total blood volume, is in the veins. The term 'mean circulatory

Fig. 3 Events of the cardiac cycle at a heart rate of 75 beats/min. The phases of the cardiac cycle identified by the numbers at the bottom are: (1) atrial systole; (2) isovolumetric ventricular contraction; (3) ventricular ejection; (4) isovolumetric ventricular relaxation; and (5) ventricular filling. Note that late in systole, aortic pressure actually exceeds left ventricular pressure. However, the momentum of the blood keeps it flowing out of the ventricle for a short time. The pressure relationships in the right ventricle and pulmonary artery are similar. The jugular venous pulse is similar in form to that seen in the right atrial pressure tracing. The 'c' wave interrupts the 'x' descent of the 'a' wave. The decline in pressure from the peak of the 'v' is the 'y' descent; the rate of decline reflects speed of ventricular filling. Atr. syst, atrial systole; ventric. syst, ventricular systole. (Modified from Ganong, W.F. (1993). *Review of medical physiology*. 16th edn, Appleton and Lange, Norwalk, Connecticut, with permission.)

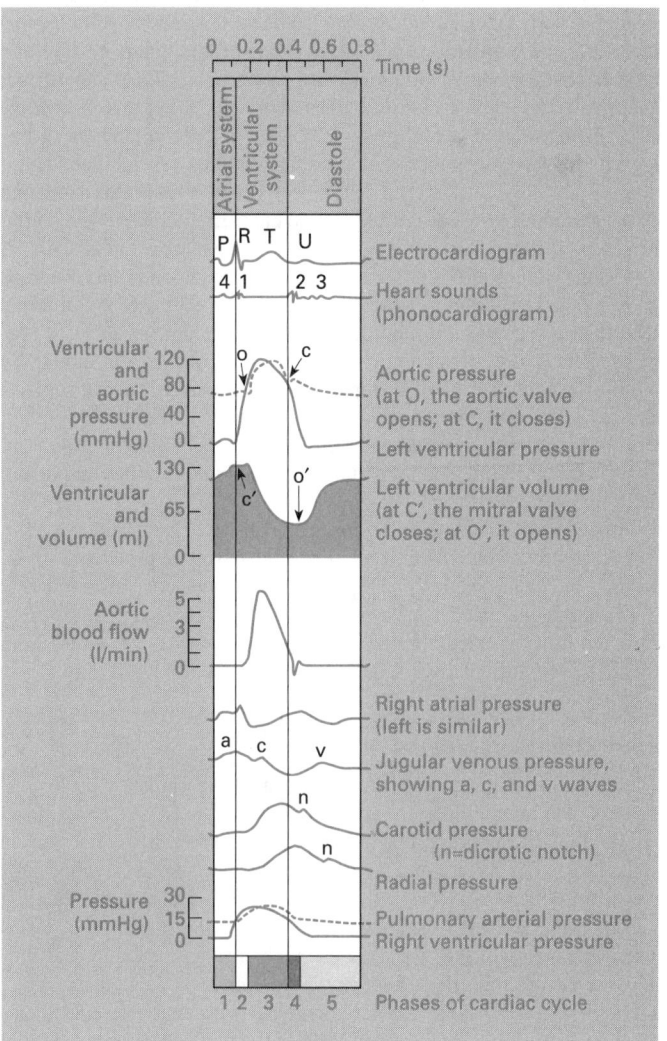

Table 1 *Normal resting values for pressures in the heart and great vessels*

Site	Systolic pressure (mmHg)	Diastolic pressure (mmHg)	Mean pressure (mmHg)
Right atrium	'a' up to 7 'v' up to 5	'x' up to 3 'y' up to 3	Less than 5
Right ventricle	Up to 25	End pressure before 'a' up to 3; End pressure on 'a' up to 7	Not applicable
Pulmonary artery	Up to 25	Up to 15	Up to 18
Left atrium (direct or indirect pulmonary capillary wedge)	'a' up to 12 'v' up to 10	'x' up to 7 'y' up to 7	Up to 10
Left ventricle	120	End pressure up to 7 End pressure on 'a' up to 12	Not applicable

pressure' introduced by Guyton is useful and refers to the equilibrium pressure measured in the entire circulation within a few seconds of stopping the heart; in dogs this is about 7 mmHg. The systemic veins containing most of the blood volume are easily distensible, and input of blood into the contracting heart is associated with only small changes in venous pressure. Ejection of blood into the much less distensible arterial tree, on the other hand, produces large pressure changes.

The normal values for pressures generated in the heart and great vessels during the cardiac cycle are shown in Table 1. Pressures are measured with reference to a zero pressure arbitrarily set at 5 cm below the sternal angle with the patient recumbent. 'Normal' arterial blood pressure is considered later (see below).

Cardiac output is the product of stroke volume and heart rate. It is related to body size and is best expressed as litres/min/m² of body surface area: the 'cardiac index'. Mean cardiac index under resting and relaxed conditions is 3.5 l/min/m², and values below 2 and above 5 are abnormal. The cardiac index declines with age. In persons of average size, resting oxygen consumption is about 240 ml/min, and the difference in oxygen content between arterial and mixed venous blood about 40 ml/l (arteriovenous oxygen difference), giving a basal cardiac output of 6 litres/min from the direct Fick equation. In normal subjects, arteriovenous difference at rest is maintained within narrow limits, from 35 to 45 ml/l; values of 55 ml/l and above are always abnormal.

Pulmonary or systemic vascular resistance is estimated by dividing the difference between mean inflow pressure (pulmonary artery or aortic) and mean outflow pressure (left atrial or right atrial) in mmHg by the flow in l/min through the respective circulations. In normal subjects and patients without intracardiac shunts this flow is the cardiac output. Normal pulmonary vascular resistance is less than 2 mmHg/l/min (160 dyne/s/cm⁵). Arterial blood pressure is the product of cardiac output and total peripheral resistance.

Stroke work is the integral of instantaneous ventricular pressure with respect to stroke volume but is usually estimated as the product of stroke volume and mean ejection pressure. The orderly sequence of contraction in the normal cardiac cycle co-ordinates changes in instantaneous pressure and flow, so maximizing the transfer of energy to the circulation. Normal left ventricular work output at rest is about 6 kg/m²/min.

Myocardial mechanics

A more rational approach to the understanding of cardiac muscle contraction and altered performance in disease states has come from renewed interest in the results of classic experiments in skeletal muscle physiology. The three-component model for muscular contraction proposed by Hill in 1938 (Fig. 4) comprises, first, a contractile element which, when activated, develops force and shortens; second, a series elastic element which is stretched passively during shortening and produces a dampening effect; and, third, a parallel elastic element which supports resting tension. The latter, together with the series elastic element, is responsible for the extensibility or compliance of relaxed mus-

cle. It is not known which precise structures are responsible for the series elastic and parallel elastic components, but there is no doubt of their functional significance.

When a muscle is activated to contract, it develops a potential for doing work. In isolated skeletal and heart muscle preparations (for example, frog sartorius or cat papillary muscle) the stretching force applied to the muscle, and therefore the length of the muscle, can be varied before contraction; this is the preload. The activated muscle will begin to shorten when it has generated a force sufficient to overcome that exerted by the attached weight or load against which it is caused to contract. When the force exerted by the load is so arranged that it is not applied to the relaxed muscle and is applied only after the muscle has begun to develop tension it is termed the afterload. If the load is so large that the activated muscle is unable to overcome it, and so cannot shorten, the contraction produces tension only, and the contraction is isometric. When shortening does occur, external work is done. If the load is constant during the shortening, the contraction is said to be isotonic; if it changes it is auxotonic.

It is known that the tension produced by both skeletal and cardiac muscle during contraction depends on initial fibre length; also, that during afterloaded isotonic contractions from a particular length, the amount and the speed of fibre shortening and the tension developed all depend upon the afterload. Over a range of loads the initial velocity of muscle shortening is most rapid when the load is smallest and slowest with the largest load. The most extensive shortening occurs with the smallest load and the least with the load just less than that which would cause the contraction to be isometric.

The inverse relationship between initial velocity of fibre shortening and load in an isotonic contraction is a fundamental one for both skeletal and cardiac muscle (Fig. 5). There is, however, a major difference

Fig. 4 A representation of the model A. V. Hill used to illustrate the three mechanical components of functioning muscle.

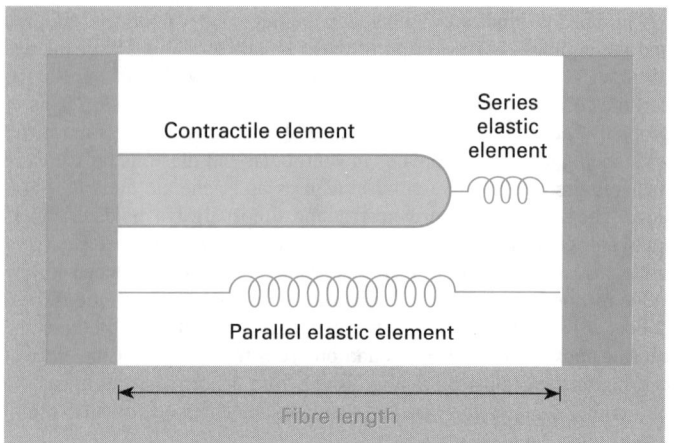

between the two types of muscle in that the relationship at any one length is constant in a skeletal muscle, whereas in cardiac muscle there are variations in inotropic state which are accompanied by considerable changes in the force–velocity relationship. A positive inotropic effect produces a more extensive contraction from the same initial length and afterload, and a faster maximum velocity of shortening (V_{max}). An increase in initial fibre length with no increase in inotropic state increases the force of contraction but does not, however, change maximum velocity of shortening. This is illustrated in Fig. 5.

The contraction of the intact heart can be visualized as being similar mechanically to the afterloaded contraction of an isolated muscle strip. For the left ventricle, the preload is the distending force which stretches the muscle fibres in end-diastole, and the initial afterload is the force the ventricle must generate in order to open the aortic valve and eject blood. At the end of ejection, the ventricular muscle is isolated from the peripheral circulation, as the afterload is then supported by the competent aortic valve, and the muscle relaxes against a comparatively small force. Relaxation of the heart is an active process due to withdrawal of calcium ions from the cytoplasm surrounding the myofibrils. The relaxation rate is faster with smaller than with larger loads. 'Active' relaxation is still proceeding in the ventricular wall when the atrioventricular valves open, and, if it is delayed, as in the hypoxic heart, it increases the stiffness of the ventricular wall and reduces filling. Wall thickness is also a determinant of relaxation rate and compliance. For this reason filling pressures are higher for the thicker and stiffer left ventricle than for the thinner and more distensible right ventricle (Table 1). When the left ventricle is hypertrophied due to chronic pressure overload, as in systemic hypertension or aortic stenosis, it becomes more stiff and filling pressures may then be abnormally high.

Regulation of cardiac function

Four essential factors determine the performance of the heart: (1) venous return; (2) outflow resistance (afterload); (3) inotropic state or contrac-

tility; and (4) heart rate. Changes in cardiac performance are accomplished by mechanisms which alter these four determinants.

VENOUS RETURN, PRELOAD, AND THE FRANK–STARLING RELATIONSHIP

The relationship described independently by Frank and Starling between end-diastolic fibre length and force of contraction is shown in Fig. 6. When the right or left ventricle ejects against a constant pressure, variations in venous return alter the degree of stretch of the muscle fibres in diastole, and this determines contraction strength and work output. The number of active force-generating sites in each fibre increases as it lengthens so that, within limits, force of contraction and stroke work are positively related to end-diastolic fibre length. The relationship is curvilinear when stroke work is plotted against end-diastolic pressure as an index of preload, but this curvilinearity reflects the exponential relationship between end-diastolic pressure and end-diastolic volume. When stroke work is plotted against end-diastolic volume the stroke work–preload relationship is linear. Fenely and coworkers have recently shown that the left ventricular stroke work/end-diastolic volume relationship in the human heart is linear, and that this is also true for the right ventricle.

The response of any particular heart at any particular time depends upon certain factors: (1) the intrinsic state of the muscle itself; i.e. the nature of its own biochemistry and contractile machinery; (2) the prevailing neurohumoral state; i.e. increased sympathetic outflow produces a more forceful contraction at any end-diastolic fibre length and shifts the curve upward and to the left; (3) extrinsic inotropic influences; digitalis preparations, for example, have a positive inotropic effect and shift the curve upward and to the left (at least in the short term), whereas myocardial depressants such as barbiturates in high blood concentration have a negative inotropic effect and shift the curve downward and to the right.

End-diastolic fibre length is determined by the force distending the ventricle at end-diastole, and end-diastolic pressure provides a reasonable indication of this force when the ventricle has normal distensibility or compliance; this is the preload. The systemic venous return and the elastic properties of the myocardium produce the end-diastolic distend-

Fig. 5 Idealized relationships between velocity of fibre shortening and afterload or force developed during contraction of a strip of cardiac muscle under three different conditions. Curves 'a' and 'b' were obtained with the muscle in the same inotropic state but with a longer initial fibre length (greater preload) for curve 'b'. Curves 'b' and 'c' were obtained with initial fibre length the same but with contractility increased in 'c' by the addition of a drug producing a positive inotropic effect. The terms V_{max} and P_o were used by Hill to describe, respectively, a hypothetical maximum shortening velocity in the absence of any load (hence the broken lines), and the force developed in an isometric contraction. An increase in initial fibre length increases P_o but not V_{max}; a positive inotropic change increases both P_o and V_{max}.

Fig. 6 The relation between left ventricular end diastolic fibre length and left ventricular stroke work showing displacement upward and to the left with an increase in contractility and downward and to the right with a reduction in contractility. Similar but not identical curves are obtained by plotting left ventricular stroke work as one measure of the force of contraction against ventricular end-diastolic pressure or volume (see text). Similar function curves may be obtained from both ventricles and both atria.

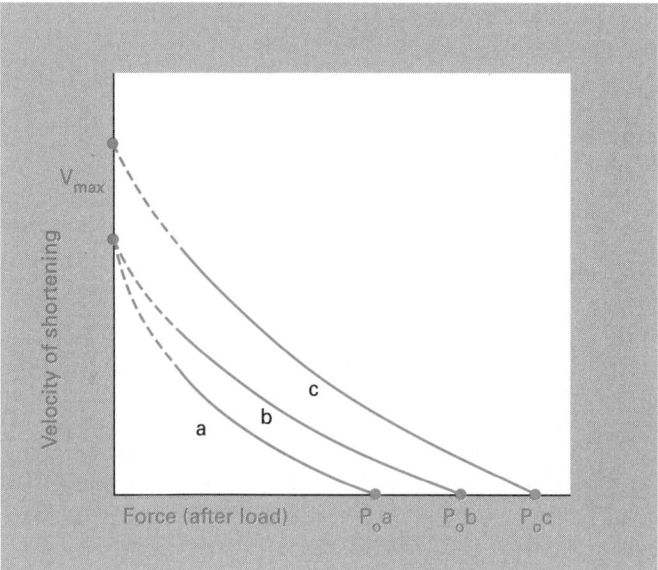

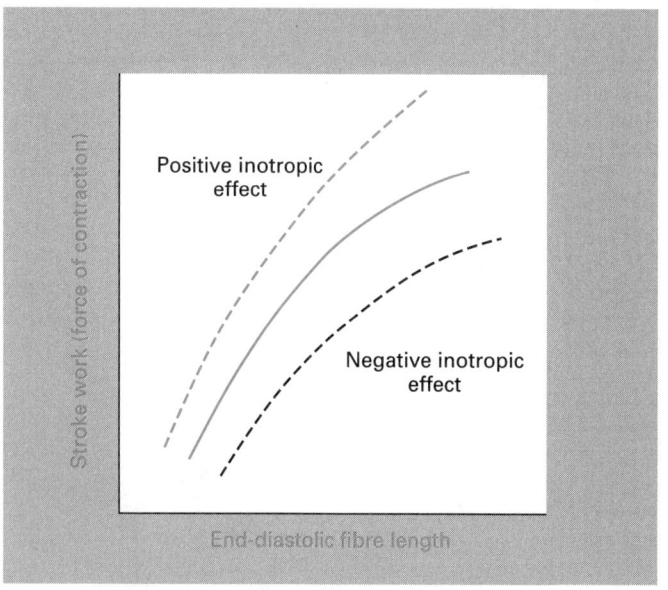

ing pressure for the right ventricle, and the pulmonary venous return and myocardial elasticity that for the left ventricle. For clinical purposes it is convenient to equate venous return with preload because, as it changes from beat to beat, it adjusts the strength of the subsequent ventricular (and atrial) contraction by varying the force stretching the relaxed cardiac muscle and changing end-diastolic fibre length.

OUTFLOW RESISTANCE OR AFTERLOAD

The pressure which the ventricle must develop to exceed that in the pulmonary artery and the aorta and open the pulmonary and aortic valves is determined largely by the pulmonary and systemic vascular resistances as shown for the latter in Fig. 7. These resistances, together with an inertial component dependent upon the mass of blood within the vessels, the compliance (stiffness) of the vessels and the physical characteristics of each vascular tree combined with the pulsatile nature of the flow, constitute the impedance to ventricular outflow. This is the load against which the ventricle must contract and shorten. As this load is not applied in diastole to the relaxed muscle, it then being supported by competent aortic and pulmonary valves, it is usefully described clinically as the afterload; it becomes applied to the muscle only after the ventricle has begun to develop tension.

REGULATION OF SYSTEMIC ARTERIAL BLOOD PRESSURE

The regulation of the systemic circulation is well adapted to the particularly vital function of maintaining constant, adequate cerebral perfusion. There is a need to maintain a relatively constant arterial blood pressure when there are changes in posture and circulating blood volume. The baroreceptors mediate rapid responses to alterations in aortic pressure whilst a variety of hormonal and physical factors regulate the circulating blood volume.

BARORECEPTORS

The baroreceptor regulatory system comprises two groups of stretch receptors: (1) one group in the carotid sinuses near the bifurcations of the common carotid arteries in the neck; and (2) a second group in the

Fig. 7 Diagram of the changes in pressure as blood flows through the systemic circulation. TA, total cross-sectional area of the vessels. This increases from 4.5 cm² to 4500 cm² in the capillaries. The major resistance to flow is at the arteriolar level. (Modified and reproduced, with permission, from Ganong, W. F. (1993). *Review of Medical Physiology.* 16th edn. Appleton & Lange, Norwalk, Connecticut)

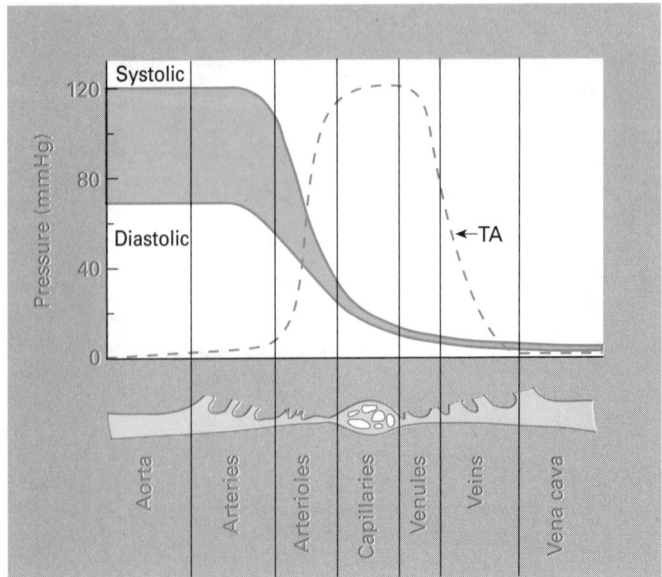

arch of the aorta. The receptors respond to an increase in central arterial pressure by the firing of impulses which pass by the glossopharyngeal and vagus nerves to the solitary tract nucleus in the medulla and inhibit sympathetic outflow. Efferent impulses from these central connections pass via the right vagus nerve mainly to the sinoatrial node, and via the left vagus mainly to the atrioventricular node. The effect is to decrease the heart rate and force of atrial contraction. There is also attenuation of sympathetic discharge via the thororacolumbar sympathetic outflow to arteriolar smooth muscle in the limbs and visceral circulation. This results in a release of peripheral arteriolar constriction and therefore peripheral vasodilatation. Thus the immediate response to a rise in arterial pressure is slowing of the heart rate, reduced force of atrial contraction, and reduced vascular resistance. The net effect of this negative feedback system is to offset the elevation in blood pressure. Conversely a lowering of blood pressure diminishes stimulation of the stretch receptors and reduces afferent traffic to the solitary tract nucleus resulting in reduced inhibition of sympathetic outflow. As a consequence there is a quickening of heart rate and peripheral vasoconstriction so that the blood pressure increases. The heart rate changes take place within 1 to 2 s and changes in vasomotor control within 5 or 6 s.

Baroreceptor mechanisms effectively modulate blood pressure responses to postural change. They also adapt to maintain the normal circadian variation in blood pressure (see below) and to prolonged arterial blood pressure increase in systemic hypertension to keep blood pressure relatively constant at an abnormally high level. Sensory input to the reflex is reduced in disorders of the autonomic nervous system, and in the prolonged weightlessness of space flight.

BLOOD VOLUME

The circulating blood volume is relatively small and a large proportion is contained in the veins (Fig. 7) so that any change in blood volume will affect venous return and therefore cardiac output and blood pressure. When blood volume is large and the veins full there is little reduction in venous return on standing and cardiac output is maintained. However, when effective blood volume is reduced and the veins are relatively empty on standing there is pooling of blood in the veins of the legs and a reduction in venous return and cardiac output so that arterial blood pressure falls. Baroreceptor responses become evident within a couple of beats, the heart rate increases and cardiac output and blood pressure are restored. One would predict that orthostatic changes would be more evident in tall people and this is indeed the case. Circulating blood volume is kept relatively constant by a combination of mechanisms which involve the actions of atrial natriuretic factor (ANF), the renin–angiotensin–aldosterone system, vasopressin, and osmolality.

Atrial natriuretic factor

The discovery of natriuretic granules which resemble secretory tissue in the atria of the heart, had important implications for the understanding of the regulation of blood volume. In 1981 it was shown that these granules produce atrial natriuretic factor, which inhibits the reabsorption of sodium in the distal tubule of the kidney. Atrial natriuretic factor also has a vasodilator action and opposes the constricting effects of noradrenaline and angiotensin II and depresses plasma aldosterone concentration, either directly or through effects on angiotensin II. The peptide nature and amino acid content of atrial natriuretic factor have been determined. Atrial naturietic factor is present in the circulation, and concentrations increase during volume expansion tending thereby to reduce blood volume and offset the effects of the blood volume increase. The right atrium contains about 2 to 4 times as much activity as the left and release of the hormone is mediated largely by atrial distension. Atrial natriuretic factor has stimulated much recent research and, whilst its overall effect is to produce a diuresis and to reduce cardiac and circulating blood volume, its precise role in cardiovascular homeostasis and therapeutic potential await further study.

The renin–angiotensin system

This system which is both local and systemic, is of major importance in the regulation of circulating blood volume and the maintenance of normal blood pressure. Enhanced activity of systemic renin and angiotensin increases aldosterone production, which promotes sodium reabsorption by the kidney and expansion of circulating blood volume. All components of the system are distributed widely throughout tissues, including the brain and the heart. The angiotensin converting enzyme inhibitors in clinical use diminish angiotension II production locally and in the circulating blood. It is not clear whether local or more general effects are more important in mediating the benefits that have followed the use of these drugs in the management of hypertension and congestive cardiac failure and in the reduction in rates of recurrence of coronary events in ischaemic heart disease associated with impaired left ventricular function. The mechanisms mediating this latter effect in particular await clarification.

A recent relevant finding is that the insertion (I)/ deletion (D) polymorphism of the angiotensin converting enzyme gene signals an independent risk of developing coronary artery disease. The D/D genotype, which is associated with higher levels of circulating angiotensin converting enzyme than the I/D or the I/I genotypes, has been found significantly more frequently in patients with myocardial infarction, and also in individuals with a parental history of ischaemic heart disease. Angiotensin II is a potent vasoconstrictor which also enhances smooth muscle cell proliferation. Attenuation of both these effects by angiotensin converting enzyme inhibitors is likely to be important for the reduction of cardiovascular risk in appropriate clinical settings.

Blood pressure, gender, and age

In all adult populations surveyed in developed countries blood pressure in normal men has been consistently slightly higher than that in normal women. The reasons are not clear but may be hormonally related. The effect of ageing in both men and women is to reduce the compliance of systemic arteries. The vessels become stiffer and as a consequence there is a more rapid transmission of pressure and velocity waves to the periphery. Reflections of these from the periphery amplify pulse pressure in the periphery and this tends to increase brachial artery systolic pressure in older people, at least those living in developed countries.

The pulmonary circulation

The pulmonary circulation is characterized by high flow at low perfusion pressure. This promotes maximal gas exchange and exposes blood to a wide expanse of endothelial surface facilitating biochemical effects, for instance, the conversion of angiotensin I to angiotensin II by converting enzyme. Hypoxia is the principal factor affecting pulmonary vascular resistance. Low alveolar oxygen tension produces pulmonary vasoconstriction. In the lung this vasoconstriction may restrict blood flow to areas of reduced ventilation and help to prevent ventilation perfusion inequality. Reflex control of the pulmonary vasculature is minimal.

The regulation of the pulmonary circulation is covered fully in Chapter 15.22.

VENTRICULAR VOLUME AND AFTERLOAD

Ventricular volume also has a major effect on afterload, as pressure comprises force per unit area. The force acting radially on the inner surface of the whole ventricle at any time during systole is the product of the intraventricular pressure and ventricular surface area at that time. If the left ventricle is assumed to be a sphere (surface area $= \pi d^2$), the force opposing ejection at any time during contraction is the product of the intracavity pressure and πd^2 at that time. Thus, a change in left ventricular diameter from a normal value of 5 cm to one of 10 cm would result in a four-fold increase in the force opposing ejection for the same intracavity systolic pressure; the ventricle would need to develop greatly increased wall tension to overcome that force. Even taking into account

the oversimplification of the spherical model, the contraction clearly will be much less efficient in the larger heart for the same stroke volume and ejection pressure (stroke work), as wall tension developed during systole is the major determinant of myocardial oxygen consumption.

During a normal heart beat the afterload is greatest at the beginning of ejection (rapid rise in pressure and maximum volume; Fig. 3), but thereafter decreases as the pressure reaches a plateau and then declines as the ventricle becomes smaller. There is therefore a matching of the afterload to the declining intensity of the contraction as it proceeds to completion, and fibres shorten at a relatively constant rate. This is less obvious in a large heart where the volume change during ejection is a smaller proportion of the total ventricular volume.

The end-diastolic volume is influenced by preload, afterload, circulating blood volume, the inotropic state of the ventricle, heart rate, and neurohumoral influences. For example, it is smaller in the erect than in the horizontal position because of reduced venous return, and it decreases with a moderate increase in heart rate because of an associated positive inotropic effect. The proportion of end-diastolic volume ejected during systole, the ratio of stroke volume to end-diastolic volume (SV/EDV), is the ejection fraction (normal 50 to 70 per cent). It is a useful index of overall left ventricular function, which is easily measured noninvasively by gated blood pool scanning and two-dimensional echocardiographic techniques. The ejection fraction increases with exercise and with positive inotropic interventions. Values for right ventricular ejection fraction are of the same order as those for the left side of the heart.

MYOCARDIAL CONTRACTILITY AND INOTROPIC STATE

Myocardial function is greatly altered by changes in inotropic state or contractility. Positive inotropic effects are thought to be mediated by activation of excitation–contraction coupling mechanisms and are associated with an increased influx of calcium ions into myocardial cells and a more powerful contraction. Changes in the intensity of excitation–contraction coupling are independent of the Frank–Starling mechanism, with increases shifting the curve upwards and to the left and decreases shifting it downwards and to the right (Fig. 6). With a positive inotropic effect, the force of contraction, however measured, is increased for a given end-diastolic fibre length and, if the afterload is the same, the initial velocity of fibre shortening is also increased (Fig. 5); in the intact heart, there is more complete emptying during systole. Increased sympathetic stimulation, digitalis, and other drugs, and an increase in heart rate itself (the staircase or Bowditch phenomenon; postectopic potentiation, see below) have positive inotropic effects. Myocardial depressants, such as hypoxia and most anaesthetic drugs, have negative inotropic effects. Increased parasympathetic stimulation produces acetylcholine-mediated negative inotropic effects which are confined almost entirely to the atria, because of the anatomical distribution of vagal endings in the myocardium.

It is difficult to measure inotropic changes accurately in the human heart because changes in the intensity of excitation–contraction coupling and changes in the Frank–Starling relationship, though separate, are nevertheless closely linked. Whilst Hill's classic model (Fig. 4) has been important conceptually, attempts to define contractility as predicted by the model – by deriving an extrapolated maximum velocity of fibre shortening which would obtain with the muscle contracting against zero load – have not been rewarding. Peak rate of change of intraventricular pressure (peak dp/dt) is a useful index of change in contractility provided that preload, afterload, and heart rate remain constant.

Little has demonstrated a linear relationship between left ventricular dp/dt_{max} and end-diastolic volume which is relatively insensitive to afterload. But an approach that is apparently relatively insensitive to changes in both preload and afterload is that of Suga and Sagawa using the ventricular pressure–volume loop diagram. There is an approximately linear relationship between end-systolic pressure (or wall stress) and end-systolic volume when measured over a narrow physiological range in the human left ventricle. Increased contractility shifts the relationship upward and to the left, as illustrated in Fig. 8, allowing the separation of enhanced from reduced contractility in the same heart, and poorly contracting from normally contracting ventricles. Stroke volume is shown on the abscissa as the difference between end-diastolic and end-systolic volumes. The efficacy of afterload reduction in assisting reduced ventricular function is also easily explained from the diagram. With a reduced afterload, the aortic valve opens at a lower pressure and a greater stroke volume is ejected; a new end-systolic pressure-volume point is reached which is shifted downwards on the same linear relationship. There has been no change in contractile state.

Recent work indicates that the end-systolic pressure/end-systolic volume relationship may exhibit significant non-linearity when measured over a sufficiently wide pressure–volume range. The degree of non-linearity varies with altered contractility, and the relationship may be sensitive to altered ventricular afterload. The concept of a relationship is nevertheless useful. It helps to identify those changes which result simply from variations in afterload from those which derive from a true change in contractility.

HEART RATE

Frequency of contraction is the fourth essential determinant of cardiac performance. Heart rate during rest and exertion may vary from 45 to 200 beats/min in the healthy young adult and as changes can occur within seconds. An increase in heart rate is the usual and most effective way of producing a rapid increase in cardiac output. It plays the major role in the response to exercise, during which Stroke volume does increase (more so in athletes and when in the erect rather than the supine position) but the changes are less marked than those of rate. In addition, an increase in contraction frequency itself produces a positive inotropic effect, whereby the force of contraction increases and reaches a new steady state within a few beats. This is termed the 'positive staircase', Treppe, or Bowditch effect. It may be a consequence of an augmented movement of calcium ions into myocardial cells with increased frequency of action potentials, combined with diminished time for outward

Fig. 8 Diagrammatic representation of intraventricular pressure and volume relationships during the cardiac cycle at two levels of myocardial contractility; three separate beats with the same end-diastolic volume are shown for each. The loops on the left of the diagram were obtained when contractility is increased and those on the right when it is reduced. There is a linear end-systolic pressure–volume relationship with different afterloads (pressures) for each level of contractility. The slope of the end-systolic pressure–volume relationship for any inotropic state is relatively insensitive (see text) to changes within physiological ranges in afterload and preload, although changes in preload are not shown in this diagram. The volume change seen on the horizontal axis for each beat is the stroke volume. This increases with reduction in pressure (afterload).

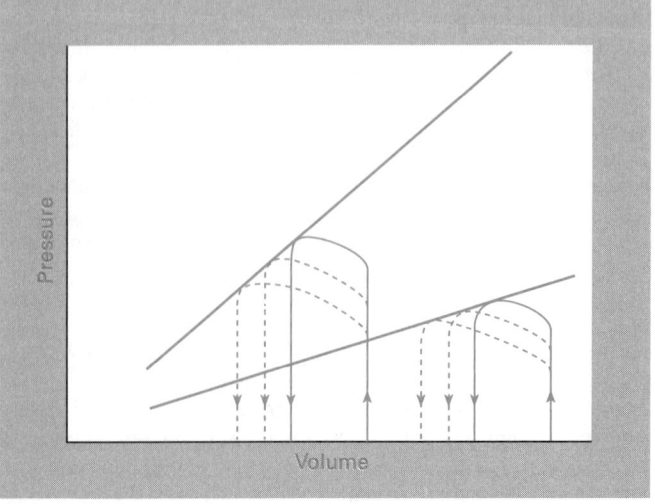

movement of calcium between beats. More forceful contractions also follow premature beats – the phenomenon of postextrasystolic potentiation – and the mechanism is probably the same. The extrasystole occurring prematurely is a weak contraction because of decreased filling time and an uncoordinated activation of the ventricle when the ectopic focus is within the ventricle. The next beat is delayed because of the refractory period of the extrasystolic beat but is a more powerful contraction because of increased filling time and ventricular volume, and increased contractility. Calcium-dependent changes similar to those of the Bowditch effect are probably responsible for the latter.

CORONARY BLOOD FLOW

Coronary blood flow accounts for about 4 per cent of the cardiac output. The heart extracts most (70 per cent) of the oxygen carried in the coronary circulation; the arteriovenous difference for oxygen across the heart is about 110 ml/l whilst that for the whole body is only about 40 ml/l under resting conditions. Therefore, large increases in myocardial oxygen requirements must be met largely by increases in coronary blood flow and this may increase five- or six-fold during strenuous exercise. The greater part of this flow is to the left ventricle, of which at least two-thirds occurs during diastole, because of the throttling effect systole has on myocardial perfusion. The main coronary arteries are on the superficial surface of the heart, and because of this, and the hindrance to coronary flow during systole, the subendocardial region of the left ventricle is more vulnerable to perfusion deficits in relation to oxygen need than the outer two-thirds of the muscle wall. Despite these mechanical problems flow is normally evenly distributed throughout the myocardium so that, when regional coronary blood flow is measured using injected radioactive microspheres (in dogs), the ratio of endocardial to epicardial flow is approximately unity. In fact the inner layers of the heart probably receive slightly more blood (up to 10 per cent) than the outer layers. This is consistent with the subendocardium developing more tension than the subepicardium, and is evidence for a greater rate of myocardial oxygen consumption in the inner layers.

REGULATION OF CORONARY BLOOD FLOW

Myocardial oxygen requirements and coronary blood flow are finely adjusted. The mechanisms are incompletely understood, but it is clear that the control resides largely in the heart itself. The major determinants are aortic pressure, myocardial extravascular compression, myocardial metabolism, and neurohumoral control.

Pressure gradients and extravascular compression

As with any vascular bed, the available pressure gradient is a determinant of blood flow. The input pressure for the coronary circulation is that of the aorta. As myocardial extravascular compression with each left ventricular contraction nearly stops coronary blood flow during systole, coronary inflow occurs mostly during diastole, probably entirely so in the subendocardial layers. Thus high diastolic intramyocardial pressure, secondary to elevated intraventricular (cavity) pressure, may restrict flow, particularly to the inner layers. This is particularly so when there is left ventricular hypertrophy due to chronic pressure overload.

The effective coronary perfusing pressure is the coronary pressure (aortic pressure) minus the outflow pressure. The outflow pressure may be the intramyocardial pressure or the coronary venous pressure or the diastolic zero flow pressure (see below) whichever is the largest. In dogs, end-diastolic flow at slow heart rates may be zero in the circumflex coronary artery when coronary pressure at the moment of zero flow may be between 20 and 40 mmHg, the lower pressures occurring with maximal coronary vasodilation. There is doubt about the reason(s) for the diastolic zero flow pressure. In conscious humans, distal coronary artery diastolic pressures at zero flow, determined during complete occlusion of the left anterior descending coronary artery at percutaneous transluminal angioplasty, are usually between 10 and 20 mmHg. The significance of these zero flow pressures is uncertain but they may reflect collateral flow. Extravascular factors are responsible for up to 50 per cent of hindrance to coronary flow however, and these are largely due to systole.

Autoregulation

A relative constancy of coronary blood flow in relation to changes in driving pressure is readily demonstrated in isolated animal heart preparations; changes in coronary perfusion pressure ranging from 40 to 200 mmHg result in a return of coronary blood flow to approximately control levels in 30 to 60 s indicating that alterations in arteriolar calibre may occur through intrinsic mechanisms. This may be brought about by adjustments to local release of vasodilator metabolites, which are increased when myocardial oxygen pressure falls. The ensuing vasodilation restores myocardial oxygenation and reduces local vasodilator metabolite release. Intrinsic coronary vascular smooth muscle stretch mechanisms may also contribute by adjusting vessel calibre in response to changes in coronary transmural pressure, although this is difficult to establish. However, similar myogenic mechanisms do operate in the peripheral circulation. The myogenic hypothesis suggests that elevation of vascular transmural pressure stretches arteriolar smooth muscle cells, inducing lengthened myofibrils to contract more forcefully, and that the ensuing vasoconstriction keeps contained a potential increase in blood flow, a mechanism which stems from the work of Bayliss in 1902. It is very likely, however, that interactions between locally acting vasoactive agents produced by the endothelium – endothelin-1 and endothelial derived relaxing factor (EDRF) – contribute to these responses (see below).

Metabolic regulation

Myocardial metabolism is the main factor in the local control of the coronary circulation. An increase in cardiac metabolism is accompanied by functional coronary vasodilation. With an increase in heart rate and ventricular pressure, there is an increase in cardiac metabolism and local release of vasodilator metabolites. Almost any cardiovascular response will alter coronary blood flow secondary to a change in myocardial metabolism. There is a linear relationship between coronary blood flow and myocardial oxygen consumption, and a hyperbolic relationship with coronary venous oxygen content (which reflects myocardial oxygen partial pressure). Sharp increases in flow occur when coronary venous oxygen content falls below 5 ml per 100 ml. The mechanism of this vasodilation is unknown. Although oxygen itself might have a direct effect, it is unlikely that a change in coronary perivascular oxygen tension alone is the principal mechanism for metabolically induced vasodilation.

A number of vasoactive substances link coronary blood flow to the metabolic requirements of the heart. A role for dissolved carbon dioxide is likely, as arterial hypercapnia results in coronary vasodilation independent of changes in myocardial oxygen consumption: a 1 mmHg increase in coronary venous carbon dioxide tension reduces coronary vascular resistance by about half that occurring with a 1 mmHg decrease in coronary venous oxygen tension. Potassium ions produce coronary vasodilation in a concentration of 1 to 10 mmol/l. Potassium release may be involved in the initial vasodilation seen with an increase in heart rate. Carbon dioxide and locally released potassium may act as vasodilator mediators under certain circumstances, without fully accounting for responses. There is also evidence favouring a vasodilator role for prostaglandins in human coronary flow regulation. Adenosine, however, has been most extensively investigated as a possible regulatory metabolite.

Berne and his associates have provided impressive evidence that adenosine is an important metabolic coupling agent linking coronary blood flow to myocardial oxygen demand. Adenosine monophosphate production reflects the degree of adenosine triphosphate utilization and hence the energy state of the cell. The enzyme which dephosphorylates adenosine monophosphate to adenosine, 5'-nucleotidase, appears to be conveniently situated at the cell membrane, in the T tubules, and in the cells surrounding capillaries – the pericytes. Adenosine moves quickly through cell membranes into the interstitial space. There it may dilate arterioles and enhance oxygen delivery, which then reduces the production of adenosine monophosphate and adenosine. Additional adenosine may re-enter the cell or be deaminated in red cells by adenosine deaminase. The evidence for the adenosine hypothesis is best for hypoxic conditions and remains to be established for normal conditions. Indeed recent direct measurement of left ventricular interstitial adenosine in relation to metabolic changes have failed to reproduce the expected correlations, suggesting that adenosine may be less of a coupling agent and more a 'fellow traveller'.

Considering the importance of metabolic vasodilation for normal cardiac function, a unitary theory of regulation of coronary blood flow with a single vasodilator would seem to lack built-in safety factors and flexibility. It is unlikely that there is any one sole mediator of every kind of physiological coronary vasodilation. Evidence is accumulating for interrelations between naturally occurring coronary vasodilators, with links provided by prostaglandins. Overall, coronary flow is very closely related to coronary perfusing pressure and myocardial oxygen consumption although the mechanisms responsible are still unclear.

Neurohumoral control

Whilst metabolic factors, however mediated, are undoubtedly the principal mechanisms operating to adjust coronary flow to oxygen needs, stimulation of α-adrenoreceptors and β-2-receptors in coronary vascular smooth muscle cells does play a subsidiary role in the regulation of the coronary circulation. These receptors mediate vasoconstriction and vasodilation, respectively. Large epicardial and small coronary arteries have a similar density of innervated vasoconstrictor α-receptors. Stimulation of these receptors limits local metabolic vasodilation by about 30 per cent in animal experiments. Adrenergic α-receptor coronary vasoconstriction may be unmasked by β-receptor blockade. There is parasympathetic coronary innervation restricted apparently to small vessels distal to the epicardial arteries, which produces vasodilation, but at present the functional significance is uncertain. In animals such nerves mediate reflex coronary vasodilation resulting from stimulation of chemoreceptors in the carotid body.

Whilst the functional significance of reflex activity in the human coronary circulation remains uncertain, changes in reflexly mediated α-adrenergic receptor activity may be responsible for periodic spontaneous increases seen in coronary blood flow (up to two-fold). This has been documented in sleeping baboons without changes in heart rate or aortic blood pressure. Alterations in sympathetic discharge may also be relevant to the pathogenesis of coronary artery spasm, which is now known to occur in a subset of patients whose coronary arteries usually also have detectable fixed atherosclerotic luminal obstructions. The functional integrity of endothelium may also be important in this regard since the endothelium itself produces vasodilators and a powerful vasoconstrictor.

Endothelium-induced vasodilation and vasoconstriction

The endothelial cells release at least two powerful vasodilator substances. Vane showed that prostacyclin is synthesized in endothelial cells by the cyclo-oxygenase pathway, and that it is both a vasodilator and also an inhibitor of platelet aggregation. It opposes the vasoconstrictor effects of thromboxane, released locally from platelets aggregating at sites of endothelial damage. In 1980, Furchgott and Zawadzki identified another locally acting vasodilator, endothelial-derived relaxing factor, or EDRF. It is released from endothelium by the vasodilators acetylcholine, substance P, bradykinin, and adenosine diphosphate and by increased shear stress and also inhibits platelet aggregation. It has a half-life of less than 1 min and is now known to be nitric oxide. Endothelium-dependent relaxations are accompanied by an accumulation of cyclic guanosine monophosphate (cGMP) in the vascular smooth muscle.

Nitric oxide is produced in vascular endothelium by nitric oxide synthase during the conversion of L-arginine to L-citrulline. Studies with inhibitors of this enzyme (L-arginine analogues) have established that endothelial cells release nitric oxide under basal conditions in the systemic and coronary circulations, and that there is an increased release during reactive hyperaemia. The latter effect is thought to be due to enhanced shear stress accompanying the initial high-flow velocity in the artery after release of a brief occlusion.

Endothelial cells also produce a 21-amino acid vasoconstrictor peptide with mitogenic properties, endothelin-1. It also has a short half-life (1 to 2 min). Its production is inhibited by endothelial-derived relaxing factor and stimulated by angiotensin II, vasopressin, and thrombin. Whilst the vasodilator action of endothelial-derived relaxing factor has a rapid on–off response time (seconds) the constrictor action of endothelin may last minutes. Recent evidence suggests that modulation of the complementary actions of endothelial-derived relaxing factor and endothelin may make important contributions to flow-dependent dilatation and reactive hyperaemia, and to autoregulation and myogenic responses in the heart. Changes in the activities of these locally acting vasoactive agents are also relevant to a variety of clinical situations in which endothelial cell dysfunction is a common factor. Non-invasive assessment of endothelial function in the systemic circulation is now possible by precise measurement of reactive hyperaemic responses using high-resolution ultrasound. Endothelial dysfunction reduces flow-dependent vasodilatation.

MYOCARDIAL OXYGEN SUPPLY AND DEMAND

At present it is difficult to measure myocardial oxygen supply and demand directly in humans. However, the product of systolic pressure and heart rate is a useful index of myocardial oxygen requirement at rest and on exercise. Also, Hoffman and his colleagues have derived an index of left ventricular oxygen supply in relation to demand, by dividing the area under the diastolic aortic pressure trace by the area enclosed by the left ventricular pressure trace (see Fig. 3). This ratio is normally about 0.9, and a value below 0.5 is associated with subendocardial ischaemia in dogs. This is almost certainly true in humans also, in the absence of coronary atherosclerosis. The rationale for using coronary perfusion pressure to estimate myocardial oxygen supply depends upon the assumption that flow is primarily pressure dependent when the coronary vasculature becomes maximally dilated, as a level of 0.5 is approached. Obviously, coronary obstructions producing local pressure gradients could result in subendocardial ischaemia with values above 0.5.

THE NERVOUS SYSTEM AND THE HEART

The heart is richly supplied with adrenergic nerves. Terminals reach atrial and ventricular muscle fibres and impinge upon all pacemaker tissue including sinoatrial and atrioventricular nodes and Purkinje fibres. Sympathetic stimulation leads to an increase in myocardial contractility and heart rate, and in the rate of spread of the activation wave through the atrioventricular node and the Purkinje system. This is mediated by local noradrenaline release, which interacts with β-adrenergic receptors. The key elements in these regulatory mechanisms are calcium ions and cyclic AMP. The activated β-receptor increases adenylcyclase activity and conversion of ATP to cyclic AMP. Peptide co-transmitters released with noradrenaline and acetylcholine have been recently isolated, and also influence autonomic function. Neuropeptide Y is a 36-amino acid peptide which is co-localized with noradrenaline in most sympathetic nerves and is released with sympathetic stimulation. It is a powerful pressor agent which has a direct arteriolar vasoconstrictor action and also potentiates the pressor action of noradrenaline.

The distribution of parasympathetic fibres is much more limited, being confined to the sinoatrial and atrioventricular nodes and the atria, with few if any fibres reaching the ventricles in humans, except perhaps in relation to coronary arteries and Purkinje tissue. The effects of para-

sympathetic nerve stimulation are mediated by local acetylcholine release which slows the heart rate and speed of conduction through the atrioventricular node and Purkinje tissue, and depresses atrial contractility. The negative inotropic effects are associated with a lowering of intracellular cyclic AMP concentration.

The effect of the nervous system on the heart at any one time is the sum of the activities of these two opposing control systems. They usually vary reciprocally. Under resting conditions, vagal inhibitory effects predominate, maintaining a slow heart rate, there being virtually no sympathetic outflow. With exercise, there is withdrawal of vagal activity and an increase in sympathetic outflow. Afferents from stretch receptors in the carotid sinus and aortic arch – the baroreceptors – also have a considerable effect on cardiac performance, this effect being mediated via the adrenergic nervous system. A fall in blood pressure reduces carotid sinus stretch and inhibitory afferent traffic so that sympathetic outflow increases. As a consequence there is a quickening of the heart rate within one or two beats, a positive inotropic effect on the heart and also a constriction of veins and arterioles which increases preload and afterload. Elevation of carotid sinus pressure has the reverse effects.

There are also mechanoreceptors in all four chambers of the heart in dogs and in the coronary vessels which give rise to depressor reflexes. Their clinical relevance is uncertain, but they may contribute, for example, to the bradycardia and hypotension occurring in some patients with acute myocardial infarction and to the syncope which patients with critical aortic stenosis may experience with the onset of exercise when there is sudden left ventricular distension. Vagal afferents from reflexogenic areas in the infarcting left ventricle may be responsible for the bradycardia, gastric distension, nausea, and vomiting which frequently occur with the onset of inferior or posterior myocardial infarction, but not usually of anterior infarction which is generally associated with a marked increase in sympathetic activity. The cardiac receptors connected to afferent fibres running in cardiac sympathetic nerves, however, are very important because they are responsible for the impulses which are perceived as cardiac pain. Receptors have also been identified (in animals) at the junction of pulmonary veins with the atrial wall. These respond to mechanical distension with increased sympathetic outflow to the sinus node and inhibition of antidiuretic hormone secretion from the posterior lobe of the pituitary gland. The result is quickening of the heart rate and a diuresis, effects which could contribute to the regulation of cardiac volume.

Autonomic efferent activity

The autonomic outflow to the heart is controlled by multiple integrative sites within the central nervous system, with complex interactions between afferent and central inputs. Autonomic responses are mediated through suprapontine and bulbospinal pathways, both those arising 'reflexly' and those arising from various types of volitional or central 'command'. Nevertheless, intrinsic mechanisms are sufficient for adequate cardiac function in the absence of autonomic control, as prolonged survival after cardiac transplantation has shown. But in the denervated heart there is blunting of the normally rapid physiological adjustments mediated by the autonomic nervous system.

DIURNAL VARIATION IN AUTONOMIC FUNCTION

Variations in vascular tone and blood pressure control and of hormone secretion and platelet function occur in a predictable way throughout the 24 hours of the day. There is a circadian rhythm of blood pressure changes in normal subjects not seen in patients after cardiac transplantation who have denervated hearts. There is a decline in blood pressure at night and an increase soon after wakening. This is due to a normal adrenergic surge in the early mornings which results in increased vascular tone and blood pressure. Increased forearm vascular resistance in the mornings with a reduction in the afternoon and evening can be clearly identified in humans by assessing responses to α-adrenergic blockade. It is presumed that this occurs in coronary vessels as well.

Measurable early morning increases in circulating catecholamines and in the propensity for platelets to aggregate can also be documented.

The circadian rhythm of autonomic function is correlated with a significant tendency for myocardial infarction and sudden cardiac death to occur more frequently in the mornings soon after wakening. There is also evidence for an increase in the occurrence of angina pectoris in the early morning, independent of the level of physical activity.

EXERCISE AND THE HEART: CARDIAC RESERVE

The heart responds to exercise with an increase in cardiac output, and values of 30 l/min may be achieved in a trained athlete. Exercising muscles extract more oxygen from the blood perfusing them, but the cardiac output response is the ultimate determinant of oxygen delivery to tissues and is the limiting factor for aerobic exercise.

The cardiac response to exercise involves all the mechanisms already discussed. Interaction within the central nervous system between higher and autonomic centres augments sympathetic discharge and there is a withdrawal of parasympathetic outflow. The heart rate increases immediately, and redistribution of peripheral flow increases venous return and preload. There is venoconstriction, particularly in the large-volume splanchnic circulation, and vasoconstriction and increased oxygen extraction in non-active parts. In active parts there is vasodilation. This is most evident in the vascular beds of the exercising skeletal muscles and of the heart. The overall effect is a marked lowering of total peripheral vascular resistance, which reduces afterload and encourages greater systolic emptying of the left ventricle. Stroke volume increases during exercise in the upright position. During light to moderate exercise, up to about 80 per cent of maximum exercise capacity, there is an almost linear relationship between work intensity and heart rate response, cardiac output, and oxygen uptake. With further exercise the heart rate and cardiac output responses level off whilst additional increases in oxygen consumption (about 500 ml) occur by increased oxygen extraction and a greater widening of the arteriovenous difference for oxygen.

The venous return increases in relation to the elevated cardiac output. Vasodilation in the working muscles which receive the bulk of the redirected blood permits high flow rates into the capacitance vessels. Because of adrenergically mediated venoconstriction the capacity of this system is reduced, so that blood moves rapidly into the right atrium. Venous return is also enhanced by an increase in intra-abdominal pressure, a decrease in intrathoracic pressure with forced inspiration, and by the pumping action of the rhythmically contracting working muscles. The augmented pulmonary blood flow results in only slight increases in pulmonary artery pressure due to the distensibility of the large pulmonary arteries, an increase in the area of the pulmonary capillary bed due to the recruitment of more capillaries, and the low resistance offered by the normal pulmonary circulation (see Table 1).

Because of the elevated cardiac output and larger stroke volume, systolic blood pressure and pulse pressure increase even though the afterload itself is reduced. Enhanced neurohumoral activity from adrenergic stimulation of the heart and the suprarenal glands (increased circulating adrenaline and noradrenaline) effect positive inotropic changes, to which tachycardia also contributes because of the Bowditch effect. There is a shift in the Frank–Starling relationship to the left accompanied by greater speed and force of cardiac contraction which tends to elevate further the ejection fraction and stroke volume. Peak dp/dt is increased and there is a rapid rise in coronary blood flow to meet myocardial oxygen requirements which increase linearly with the product of systolic blood pressure and heart rate. During moderate exercise these changes together result in a decreased or unaltered end-diastolic volume and, as mentioned, a decreased end-systolic volume. With severe exercise, end-diastolic dimensions and end-diastolic fibre length are slightly increased and the Frank–Starling mechanism then operates and augments further the force of contraction.

The haemodynamic and ventilatory responses evoked by an increase to a new steady work load take about 2 to 3 min to equilibrate and adjust

oxygen supply to the greater demand. Protocols for exercise testing are therefore usually based on work increments at 3-min intervals to allow time for a new 'steady state' to occur as, for example, in the standard Bruce Exercise Protocol. A steady state becomes progressively more difficult to maintain as maximal exercise capacity is approached. Glycogen is used by the working muscles as a source of stored energy and the anaerobic metabolism which ensues produces lactic acidosis which further increases ventilation. As all cardiopulmonary transport mechanisms reach maximum levels, shortness of breath, fatigue, and muscle pain become limiting symptoms; motivation is then the final determinant of duration of exercise. Ageing reduces the efficacy of cardiopulmonary transport mechanisms and, of course, exercise capacity. The heart rate response at peak exercise reflects this. In healthy individuals aged 20 years it is about 200 beats/min and at 65 years about 170 beats/min.

When exercise stops, the cardiopulmonary and metabolic changes return rapidly to resting levels, the rate following an exponential pattern in the first few minutes; the excretion and metabolism of lactate and other substances, and the dissipation of heat generated take longer (time constant of about 15 min or more). Reduced circulatory function slows the recovery rate. The mechanisms responsible for dyspnoea and ventilatory responses to exercise are considered in a later section.

Training effects

Regular exercise to about 60 per cent of maximal heart rate for 20 to 30 min three times a week is the minimum requirement for a training effect. The resting heart rate becomes slower whilst the cardiac output is maintained by an increased end-diastolic volume and ejection fraction, and therefore stroke volume. In a 'trained' exercising individual there is a reduced heart rate response to a standard submaximal work load, and systemic blood flow is more effectively distributed away from visceral and skin circulations to working muscles. Adaptive changes in muscle mitrochondria occur, permitting improved oxygen extraction from perfusing blood so that maximum oxygen consumption increases. There is suggestive evidence for prolonged endurance training increasing the calibre of coronary arteries and enlarging capillary surface area relative to cardiac muscle mass (in animals). Myocardial protein synthesis increases. Adrenergic mechanisms appear to be involved in mediating this response. It should be noted that rhythmic exercise (e.g. running) and isometric exercise (e.g. weight lifting) have different physiological effects. The blood pressure rises disproportionately during the latter. The mechanisms are partly reflex, and partly mechanical from the contracting muscles. Isometric exercise training is not recommended for cardiac patients because of the increased afterload it imposes on the heart.

Reports of exercise-induced mood changes are difficult to validate scientifically, although feelings of well-being seem to occur. There is evidence, however, for increased concentrations of circulating β-endorphin during exercise, and recent studies with the opiate receptor antagonist, naloxone, to block the effects of opioid peptides suggest that β-endorphin release may reduce exercise-induced adrenaline and noradrenaline responses. Regular exercise lowers blood pressure in normotensive and mildly hypertensive subjects, and modulation of catecholamine release by changes in endogenous opioid peptide secretion may be a possible contributing mechanism. There are other diverse exercise-induced hormonal changes but one of particular clinical relevance is reduced glucose-stimulated insulin secretion. This is beneficial for type II diabetics, whose basal hyperinsulinaemia is the result of both hypersecretion and hypocatabolism of insulin, and for patients with insulin resistance and hyperinsulinaemia, obesity, hypertension and dyslipidaemia – so-called syndrome X.

To summarize, changes in the four essential determinants of cardiac function – preload, afterload, heart rate, and contractility – combine to augment cardiac output and oxygen delivery during exercise. Measurement of the cardiovascular response to exercise is essential for the objective assessment of cardiac function and is the subject of a later chapter.

FURTHER READING

Braunwald, E. (1992). *Heart disease: a textbook of cardiovascular medicine* 4th ed. W.B. Saunders, Philadelphia.

Brenner, B.M., Ballerman, B.J., Gunning, M.E., and Zeidec, M.L. (1990). Diverse biological actions of atrial natriuretic peptide. *Physiological Reviews,* **70,** 665–99.

Cheitlin, M.D., Sokolow, M., and McIlroy, M.B. (1993). *Clinical cardiology.* 6th edn. Appleton and Lange, Norwalk, Connecticut.

Eckberg, D.L. and Sleight, P. (1992). *Human baroreflexes in health and disease.* Clarendon Press, Oxford.

Ganong, W.F. (1993). *Review of medical physiology.* 16th edn. Appleton and Lange, Norwalk, Connecticut.

Hill, A.V. (1970). *First and last experiments in muscle mechanics.* Cambridge University Press, Cambridge.

Hoffman, J.I.E. and Spaan, J.A.E. (1990). Pressure–Flow relations in coronary circulation. *Physiological Reviews,* **70,** 331–390.

Moncada, S. and Higgs, A. (1993). The L-arginine–nitric oxide pathway. *New England Journal of Medicine,* **329,** 2002–12.

Villarreal, D. and Freeman, R.H. (1991). ANF and the renin–angiotensin system in the regulation of sodium balance: longitudinal studies in experimental heart-failure. *Journal of Laboratory and Clinical Medicine,* **118,** 515–22.

15.3 Symptoms of cardiac disease

15.3.1 Breathlessness

S.W. DAVIES and D. LIPKIN

Introduction

The sensation of breathlessness (dyspnoea) is a common symptom of many different forms of cardiac disease. It is unpleasant and distressing, and dyspnoea on exertion may severely limit the exercise capacity of patients and impair their quality of life. Despite its prevalence, the pathophysiology of dyspnoea is complex and surprisingly poorly understood.

Dyspnoea has been defined as 'the consciousness of the necessity for increased respiratory effort' and as 'the sensation of difficult, laboured, uncomfortable breathing'. All normal subjects will have experienced dyspnoea on heavy exertion—pathological dyspnoea is the same sensation occurring at lower workloads or at rest, and includes a perception that the awareness of breathing is unpleasant and/or inappropriate to the situation. It is not known whether dyspnoea serves any useful purpose—it may deter the patients from imposing an excess strain on the cardiorespiratory system, but this is speculation.

Clinical types of cardiac dyspnoea

Dyspnoea is a cardinal symptom of left heart failure and occurs in many other cardiovascular conditions; these are listed in Table 1.

Different types of dyspnoea can be distinguished in clinical practice, although they often coexist.

1. Exertional dyspnoea: this may be graded according to the revised New York Heart Association scale (Table 2). The severity of cardiac disease may be underestimated if the patient's physical activities are restricted for any other reason—sedentary habit, intermittent claudication, or arthritis.
2. Orthopnoea: dyspnoea worse when lying flat than when sitting up or standing is common. It is a non-specific feature of any cause of severe dyspnoea and does not necessarily indicate a cardiac cause. Marked orthopnoea occurs in left heart failure, but also in asthmatic attacks and in paralysis of the diaphragm.
3. Platypnoea: dyspnoea worse when erect than when lying flat is rare. It occurs with large pulmonary arteriovenous malformations and in selective paralysis of the intercostal muscles with sparing of the diaphragm. In children, dyspnoea which is

worse when erect and is relieved by squatting suggests Fallot's tetralogy.
4. Paroxysmal nocturnal dyspnoea: acute dyspnoea wakening the patient from sleep. Characteristically the patient sits upright or stands up, and may throw open the windows for air. Paroxysmal nocturnal dyspnoea can be crudely graded by the number of pillows that the patient uses to prop himself up to allow uninterrupted sleep.
5. Acute dyspnoea at rest: this is uncommon. It may complicate myocardial infarction, severe arrhythmias, or a number of other catastrophic events.

Other respiratory symptoms may occur with dyspnoea in cardiovascular disease.

1. Acute pulmonary oedema: acute severe dyspnoea accompanied by cough producing copious white or pale pink frothy sputum. There is usually cyanosis, sweating, tachycardia, and raised systemic blood pressure. Dyspnoea with copious pale pink frothy sputum also occurs in the rare condition of alveolar cell carcinoma of the lung.
2. Dry cough: a persistent dry cough may occur in chronic left heart failure, particularly after exercise and when lying flat in bed at night. A dry cough may persist for about half an hour after an episode of paroxysmal nocturnal dyspnoea. Treatment with angiotensin-converting enzyme inhibitors sometimes causes troublesome cough.
3. Wheeze: noises during breathing can be audible to the patient. They are usually musical in character, polyphonic, and slightly worse during expiration.
4. Haemoptysis: coughing large amounts of blood is a dramatic symptom and has many causes. Small haemoptyses occur in severe mitral stenosis and occasionally in severe left ventricular failure. Massive or exsanguinating haemoptysis may occur with rupture of a thoracic aortic aneurysm, pulmonary artery aneurysm, or arteriovenous malformation.
5. Irregular respiration: Cheyne–Stokes periodic respiration is well known to occur in advanced cardiac failure, but is uncommon. Cyclical variation in ventilation without frank apnoeic phases is relatively common during sleep in moderate and severe heart failure.

Myocardial ischaemia usually produces chest pain typical of angina, but the perception of ischaemia is very variable and episodes of ischaemia and even infarction can be 'silent'. It is not surprising that some patients

Table 1 *Some common causes of dyspnoea*

	Cardiovascular	Other

Exertional dyspnoea	Left heart failure
	    Left ventricular failure, acute and chronic
	    mitral valve disease, atrial myxoma
	Congenital heart disease
	Pulmonary vascular disease
	    Pulmonary embolism, acute and chronic
	    Other causes of pulmonary hypertension
	Angina equivalent
		Lung disease
		Upper airway obstruction
		Fluid overload
		Anaemia
		Obesity
		Psychogenic
		Neuromuscular weakness

Orthopnoea	Left heart failure	Lung disease Diaphragmatic weakness
Platypnoea	Pulmonary arteriovenous malformation	Intercostal weakness
Paroxysmal nocturnal dyspnoea	Left heart failure	Nocturnal asthma Gastro-oesophageal reflux with aspiration
Acute dyspnoea at rest	Acute myocardial infarction Supraventricular or ventricular tachycardia Acute dissection of the aortic root Mitral chordal or papillary muscle rupture Large pulmonary embolism Mitral obstruction by left atrial ball thrombus or left atrial myxoma Obstruction or dehiscence of an artificial valve Infundibular spasm in Fallot's tetralogy	Asthma Pneumothorax Aspiration/inhaled foreign body Metabolic acidosis Massive haemorrhage

Table 2 *The New York Heart Association scale*

Class I
Patient with cardiac disease but without resulting limitation of physical activity; ordinary physical activity does not cause undue dyspnoea (or fatigue, palpitation, or anginal pain)

Class II
Patients with cardiac disease resulting in slight limitation of physical activity; they are comfortable at rest; ordinary physical activity results in dyspnoea (or fatigue, palpitation, or anginal pain)

Class III
Patients with cardiac disease resulting in marked limitation of physical activity; they are comfortable at rest; less than ordinary physical activity causes dyspnoea (or fatigue, palpitation, or anginal pain)

Class IV
Patients with cardiac disease resulting in inability to carry on any physical activity without discomfort; symptoms of dyspnoea (or of angina) may be present even at rest; if any physical activity is undertaken, discomfort is increased

cannot distinguish between tightness or pressure in the chest due to angina and the sensation of dyspnoea, and describe their 'angina' as 'difficulty in breathing'.

Pathophysiology of cardiac dyspnoea

There is little doubt that in acute heart failure pulmonary venous congestion causes pulmonary oedema and hypoxia which are potent stimuli to dyspnoea and are relieved by diuresis, vasodilatation, and venesection. In patients with right-to-left shunts systemic arterial desaturation contributes to dyspnoea. Orthopnoea in left heart failure is due to increased systemic venous return which increases pulmonary venous congestion and leads to a progressive decrease in pulmonary compliance, narrowing of the airways by bronchial mucosal oedema, and early pulmonary oedema.

The causes of exertional dyspnoea in chronic left heart failure are less clear. It has long been supposed that pulmonary venous congestion is responsible. In 600 BC the Yellow Emperor's Text of Internal Medicine stated 'if the breathing is noisy, then the veins of the lungs are in disorder . . . the water disturbs the rest, and causes the troubled breathing'. In 1831 James Hope proposed that when the left ventricle failed to discharge its contents, blood accumulated and caused 'backward pressure' in the atrium and the pulmonary veins, causing dyspnoea. In patients with chronic heart failure who have pulmonary venous congestion but no frank pulmonary oedema, it has been postulated that decreased lung compliance stimulates J-receptors to produce dyspnoea. Thus pulmonary venous congestion provides a simple explanation for orthopnoea and exertional dyspnoea in both acute and chronic heart failure. Why then should this convenient and simple hypothesis be questioned?

A number of studies now suggest that there is no direct relationship between dyspnoea and pulmonary venous congestion in chronic heart failure. Although the pulmonary wedge pressure is elevated, and may rise dramatically on exercise, there is little correlation between pulmonary wedge pressure and either exercise capacity or symptoms. Ambulatory monitoring of pulmonary artery diastolic pressure, which approximates to pulmonary wedge pressure, reveals little correlation with the episodes of dyspnoea during everyday life. In both long-term and short-term drug trials the changes in pulmonary wedge pressure follow a different time course from the changes in dyspnoea and in exercise capacity. If increased pulmonary venous pressure is the stimulus to dyspnoea and increased ventilation during exercise, peak ventilation might be expected to be greater at the end of a prolonged submaximal test than at the end of a brief maximal test because pulmonary venous pressure will have been elevated for longer. However, when submaximal and maximal exercise tests are compared in the same patients, both forms of exercise are limited at similar levels of ventilation.

Other mechanisms which might be responsible for the sensation of dyspnoea include blood gas and pH changes, the effects of a variety of intrapulmonary receptors including the J-receptors (chemoreceptors in the respiratory muscles), awareness of the level of ventilation, and awareness of the level of 'wasted' ventilation due to the increased physiological dead space (Fig. 1). Campbell and Howell have suggested that dyspnoea arises when the patient experiences an excessive effort needed to achieve a given level of ventilation; in sensory terms this corresponds to excessive tension in the respiratory muscles for a given length or rate of change of length of the muscle, and it is known as the 'length–tension inappropriateness' concept. This sense of inappropriateness of respiratory effort might originate from the muscle spindles in the respiratory muscles or at cortical level. The proponents of this hypothesis have demonstrated length–tension inappropriateness in a number of different situations associated with dyspnoea. However, the elegant work of Guz and colleagues in normal subjects and patients with chronic airflow limitation suggests that exertional dyspnoea has a complex and multifactorial origin without necessarily involving length–tension inappropriateness.

Similar mechanisms may apply in chronic heart failure. There is no simple relationship between dyspnoea and the level of ventilation or of dead-space ventilation. Decreased lung compliance has not been studied in relation to dyspnoea in chronic left ventricular failure, but in patients with mitral stenosis there is no correlation between the level of dyspnoea and decreased lung compliance. Dyspnoea is unaffected by inhalation of aerosols of local anaesthetic which block the pulmonary J-receptors, and dyspnoea occurs in heart–lung transplant recipients in whom the lungs are denervated. Dyspnoea may instead relate to respiratory muscle fatigue on exertion, caused by limitation of the blood supply to the respiratory muscle during exercise. Profound deoxygenation of the intercostal muscles and a slowing of inspiratory muscle relaxation rate during exercise in heart failure are compatible with respiratory muscle fatigue. While the concept of respiratory muscle fatigue is attractive, its definition is controversial and the methodology for demonstrating it is fraught with difficulties. Patients with chronic heart failure have increased small airways resistance, bronchial hyperreactivity to inhaled methacholine, and heightened cough reflex to inhaled capsaicin and other irritants. However, inhaled bronchodilators have minimal effects on exercise capacity or exertional dyspnoea.

Whether or not these other mechanisms contribute to dyspnoea in chronic heart failure, it is still likely that pulmonary venous congestion plays a role. The lack of apparent correlation between pulmonary capillary wedge pressure and dyspnoea might be due firstly to inadequacy of measurement of pulmonary capillary wedge pressure as an index of pulmonary venous pressure, particularly during exercise. Secondly, there may be individual variation in pulmonary microvascular permeability or in pulmonary lymphatic capacity, affecting the propensity to develop pulmonary oedema. Thirdly, there seems to be individual variation in the perceptual threshold for dyspnoea. Thus we cannot dismiss

pulmonary venous congestion as a factor in the genesis of exertional dyspnoea in heart failure. Indeed, the various mechanisms which have been postulated for dyspnoea need not be mutually exclusive; pulmonary venous congestion and reduced pulmonary compliance might combine with reduced cardiac output on exercise to cause respiratory muscle fatigue leading to length–tension inappropriateness.

It seems unlikely that there will prove to be a single mechanism for dyspnoea in heart failure. In a memorable phrase, Campbell and Howell warned that 'a respiratory physiologist offering a unitary explanation for dyspnoea should arouse the same suspicions as a tattooed archbishop offering a free ticket to heaven'! Even if there is no simple explanation, it is to be hoped that a better understanding will eventually lead to new symptomatic treatments for dyspnoea.

Treatment of cardiac dyspnoea

Whenever possible, the specific cause of cardiac dyspnoea should be determined and treated. Acute pulmonary oedema responds to intravenous loop diuretics such as frusemide, which also has a rapid venodilator effect. The patient should sit erect with legs dependent over the edge of the bed or chair, and be given 60 to 100 per cent oxygen by face-mask. Lower concentrations of oxygen are only necessary in patients with chronic lung disease and carbon dioxide retention; they are quite inadequate in pulmonary oedema. Intravenous or intramuscular opiates act as vasodilators as well as relieving pain and dyspnoea. Sublingual nitrates, intravenous infusion of nitrates, urgent venesection, or rotating limb tourniquets may all help, but sometimes endotracheal intubation and ventilation is required, and this is best anticipated before the patient is *in extremis*.

Exertional dyspnoea in chronic heart failure is improved by standard therapy with diuretics and angiotensin-converting enzyme inhibitors. β-Blockers should be discontinued when possible. Domiciliary or ambulatory (portable) oxygen therapy does not seem beneficial in chronic heart failure, unlike chronic lung disease. The addition of large oral doses of long-acting nitrates may help on an empirical basis. Long-term therapy with oral or nebulized opiates has small benefits but obvious risks of tolerance and dependence. Exercise training programmes increase exercise capacity in chronic heart failure and may improve dyspnoea.

Dyspnoea may be improved by cardiac surgery for particular conditions such as valvular disease, left ventricular aneurysmectomy, and correction of congenital cardiac defects. In many cases there is irre-

Fig. 1 The possible mechanisms of dyspnoea in cardiac disease.

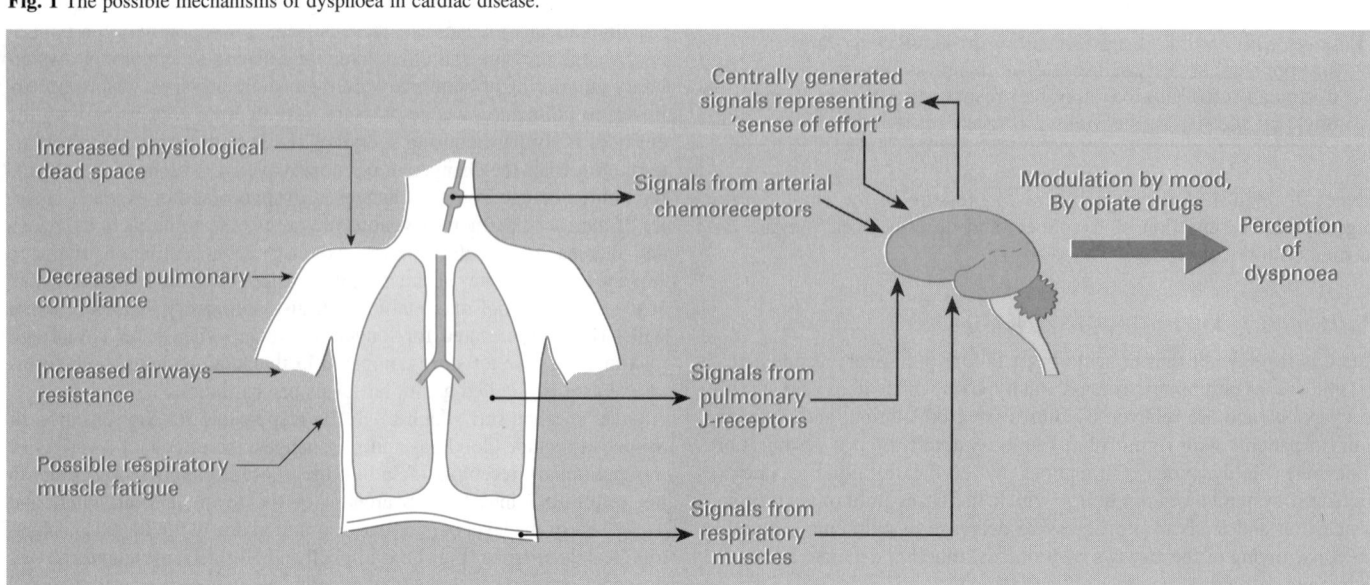

versible impairment of ventricular function or pulmonary vascular disease, and the patient should understand that surgery will prevent further deterioration but may fail to improve the present level of dyspnoea.

REFERENCES

Campbell, E.J.M. and Howell, J.B.L. (1962). The sensation of dyspnoea. *British Medical Journal*, **2**, 868–90.

Cockroft, A. and Guz, A. (1987). Breathlessness. *Postgraduate Medical Journal*, **63**, 637–41.

Davies, S.W., Emery, T.M., Watling, M.I.L., Wannamathee, G., and Lipkin, D.P. (1991). A critical threshold of exercise capacity in the ventilatory response to exercise in heart. *British Heart Journal*, **65**, 179–83.

Davies, S.W., Wilkinson, P.W., Bailey, J., Timmis, A.D., Balcon, R., Rudd, R., and Lipkin, D.P. (1992). Reduced pulmonary microvascular permeability in severe chronic left heart failure. *American Heart Journal*, **124**, 637–41.

Gibbs, J.S.R., Keegan, J., Wright, C., Fox, K.M., and Poole-Wilson, P.A. (1990). Pulmonary artery pressure changes during exercise and daily activities in chronic heart failure. *Journal of the American College of Cardiology*, **15**, 52–61.

Hayward, G.E. and Knott, J.M.S. (1955). The effect of lung distensibility and respiratory work in mitral stenosis. *British Heart Journal*, **17**, 303–11.

Lipkin, D.P., Canepa-Anson, R., Stephens, M.R., and Poole-Wilson, P.A. (1986). Factors determining symptoms in chronic heart failure: comparison of fast and slow exercise tests. *British Heart Journal*, **55**, 439–45.

Poole-Wilson, P.A. (1988). The origin of symptoms in patients with chronic heart failure. *European Heart Journal*, **9**, (Suppl. H), 49–53.

Restrick, L., Davies, S.W., Noone, L., and Wedzicha, J.A. (1992). Ambulatory oxygen in chronic heart failure: symptoms, exercise capacity, and oxygen desaturation. *Lancet*, **340**, 192–3.

Uren, N.G., Davies, S.W., Jordan, S.L., and Lipkin, D.P. (1993). Inhaled bronchodilators increase maximum oxygen consumption in patients with chronic left ventricular failure. *European Heart Journal*, **14**, 744–50.

15.3.2 Chest pain

A.H. HENDERSON

Chest pain – its diagnosis and its management – looms large in the life of the cardiologist. To the patient who experiences it, the possibility that it may be due to 'heart disease' is likely to raise its head. There are however many different causes of this very common symptom and the great majority are non-cardiac, particularly as it presents in general practice. Pain in the chest is also a common presenting symptom to general physicians and physicians specializing in a number of other disciplines, though the case-mix of causes will differ. Textbooks carry lists of causes. They may be grouped as cardiac, chest wall, other intrathoracic viscera, abdominal viscera, or psychogenic.

In practice, the clinician's approach is weighted by probabilities (there is also an aphorism that uncommon presentations of common diseases are commoner than common presentations of uncommon diseases). Patients referred with chest pain to a cardiologist are preselected as those in whom a cardiac cause is suspected, or at least merits excluding. The alternative causes which make for most diagnostic difficulty are oesophageal pain and musculoskeletal pain. In more general medical practice, the physician will see more patients with non-anginal pain, as well as patients with mild angina thought not to merit referral for specialist management or more definitive diagnosis. Diagnostic difficulty however is similarly most likely when faced with the not-quite-typical case of cardiac, oesophageal or musculoskeletal pain. Each of these main groups of causes can pose difficulties even for their respective specialists, in that uncertainties remain about some of the underlying mechanisms and simple diagnostic tests are not always available. Not only will this common problem differ in the emphasis of its presentation to the primary care doctor and to different specialists, but the investigative approach to its diagnosis and management will also differ. The gastroenterologist, for example, is more likely to see those patients where the presentation is more clearly related to the gastrointestinal tract, whereas the cardiologist (and the general in-taking physician) is more likely to see those patients presenting with severe chest pain masquerading as angina or even myocardial infarction. The clinical viewpoint thus colours the perception of chest pain as a presenting symptom, particularly when it is atypical and mild and where, inevitably, its precise cause is not definitively established. The process of diagnosis generally concerns assessment of probabilities, the need for further investigation being determined by the relative importance of establishing and further defining that diagnosis with certainty. The differential diagnosis between cardiac, oesophageal and musculoskeletal causes of chest pain is not always as easy as it may seem. It can however with care be made and indeed it must for the spectre of possible heart disease raises the diagnostic stakes for the patient with chest pain. A careful and detailed history is the essential first step.

A good history remains the first and often most important approach to diagnosis. Nowhere is this more true than in diagnosing the cause of chest pain, when the history may be the overriding contribution to establishing the diagnosis. History-taking skills graduate from straight reportage of the patient's story, to what has been called the clinician's 'art' but is in fact attention to detail against a carefully ordered personal database of accumulated experience. History taking is an active process. It involves matching the patient's symptoms to the archetype of a particular cause of chest pain. Obtaining a complete and accurate picture of the patient's symptoms requires the establishment of rapport and, contrary to conventional teaching, judicious direct questioning: specific promptings are generally necessary both to check details and to confirm common understanding of the words used to describe the pain. Archetypes are learned from textbook descriptions but they need then to be clothed and honed with experience. The patient's symptoms should be matched both positively against the archetype of the likely diagnosis, and negatively against the archetypes of differential diagnoses to be excluded. It is often helpful to ask the patient to recall the very first episode of the pain in question: this may be more typical of the archetype.

An awkward rider is that more than one cause may coexist, for chest pain is common: the patient however will often know, if asked, whether there are two fundamentally dissimilar types of chest pain which can be dissociated at least sometimes.

Angina

The word 'angina' describes a classic symptom. In common usage, however, it implies also that the symptom is due to myocardial ischaemia. Where doubt exists about whether pain is cardiac in origin, it is wiser to describe the symptom as 'angina-like', if only to avoid falsely categorizing the patient as suffering from myocardial ischaemia. The symptoms of angina vary widely from one individual to another in their characteristics. In any individual though, these generally run true to form (albeit with varying intensity) on different occasions. The principal characteristics of angina are nevertheless well-known and usefully define the archetype.

Site

Angina, being referred pain, is determined by the patient's inborn innervation and is constant and characteristic for each individual. Visceral pain is sensed in the somatic region with which it shares common nerve root innervation. Its localization, however, is less precise than that of somatic pain, probably because its sensory innervation spreads over a larger number of nerve roots. Afferent sensory fibres from free nerve endings in the endocardium and more complex free nerve endings around veno-atrial junctions, run predominantly with sympathetic fibres to thoracic roots 1 to 5. What stimulates these nerve endings, and thus what the fundamental mechanism of ischaemic pain is, remains unknown; there is some evidence that adenosine may be responsible. Angina can occur in patients some years following cardiac transplantation, implying reinnervation.

Angina is most commonly felt in the central chest (sometimes slightly to the left but not 'inframammary'), and/or spreading to or primarily to the jaw, neck, arms (most commonly the upper, inner aspect of the left arm, with paraesthesiae in the hands), back, or epigastrium.

Character

This is generally described as gripping or tight, not stabbing or sharp (though it is important to ensure that the word used by the patient means the same as for the clinician, e.g. by 'sharp' the patient sometimes means severe).

Severity

This varies from an ill-defined discomfort (nociceptive sensation) to great pain, the severity of which is unrelated to the severity of ischaemia, its duration or the amount of myocardium involved. Myocardial ischaemia and even infarction may however occur without pain in some patients; moreover, in patients with typical angina of effort, some 50 per cent of electrocardiographically monitored episodes of ischaemia are painless ('silent angina'). Why some episodes are associated with pain and others not remains unknown.

Onset

The pain is not 'abrupt' in onset, in contrast to musculoskeletal pain, though patients may say it is 'sudden', and it may be helpful to act an abrupt onset to ensure mutual understanding. The pain is either present or absent, unlike some other types of chest pain which may be described as a background ache not clearly present or absent unless the patient thinks about it.

Factors influencing pain when present
None (cf. other types of chest pain).

Duration and relief

Angina generally lasts 3 to 10 min, easing with rest/relaxation/sublingual or oral spray of glyceryl trinitrite, the pharmacological response to which occurs within 2 or 3 min (note that nitrites relax smooth muscle and may also relieve oesophageal spasm). If severe, it may be more prolonged, but infarction ensues if ischaemia lasts for more than 30 min. Prolonged chest pain without subsequent evidence of infarction thus raises doubts about its cardiac origin.

Associated features

Angina may be associated with other features of myocardial ischaemia. Ischaemic regional myocardial dysfunction, if it involves a sufficiently large region and/or occurs in the context of a pre-existing reduction of cardiac reserve, can reduce cardiac output to the extent of causing clinically overt acute heart failure, with hypotension, faintness/syncope, dyspnoea, pallor, sweating, anxiety ('angor animi'), nausea and arrhythmias – to which increased sympathetic activity induced by pain or reduced cardiac output contribute. Angina may be associated also with

fatigue and is not uncommonly followed for some hours by unaccountable fatigue.

Initiating factors

The pathogenesis of myocardial ischaemia accounts for the circumstances in which angina is experienced:

1. In stable effort angina, with fixed coronary artery stenosis, angina is predictably related to the additional myocardial energy consumption of exercise or acute stress. The threshold is often lower in the mornings, in cold (or sometimes particularly hot) weather, at times of associated general stress or after a heavy meal, and with concomitant general or cardiovascular conditions which increase cardiac workload, such as paroxysmal tachycardia, high blood pressure, aortic valve disease or anaemia.
2. Unstable angina represents a period of coronary instability, due to plaque fissure and platelet thrombus (which may be intermittently occlusive and associated with local vasoconstriction by platelet-derived products). Angina occurs at rest and/or the severity of effort-related angina becomes worse. Cardiac pains may thus become more prolonged and less predictable, and infarction ensues if ischaemia is prolonged. The unstable plaque may be at an angiographically demonstrable coronary artery stenosis, but atheroma only obtrudes into the lumen when advanced and can cause arterial (endothelial) dysfunction with undue susceptibility to local vasoconstriction (vasospasm) even in angiographically 'normal' or near normal arteries. Prinzmetal's angina, described before the days of angiography, is a condition of apparently spontaneous occlusive vasoconstriction, in the absence of stable effort angina and (it came to be accepted) of underlying coronary stenosis, causing full thickness myocardial ischaemia and thus ST segment elevation on the electrocardiogram, occurring typically in the early mornings (when clinical manifestations of coronary artery disease generally are slightly more common) for self-limiting periods of months or years. Once a 'sought after' curiosity, it is now regarded as representing one extreme end of the spectrum of unstable angina in which the vasomotor component is predominant. It is very rarely encountered as such in Britain – a reflection perhaps of changing medical fashion where definition and data deficit allow – but it is more common in Japan, where atheroma is less common, coronary artery disease less advanced, and arteries presumably more mobile.
3. In Syndrome X (or microvascular angina, as it is coming by inference to be called) the usual history is indistinguishable from that of stable effort angina though there may be atypical features, the angina tending to last slightly longer and be somewhat less predictable.
4. Angina due to haemodynamic imbalance, as in aortic valve disease, presents as stable effort angina: with aortic stenosis, exercise may induce prolonged and potentially dangerous myocardial ischaemia, and arrhythmias may complicate the picture.

Atypical features

Not every patient will present a textbook description of angina, both because of natural biological variation and because of inadequacies of recall or communication. Nevertheless the presence of atypical features should alert the clinician to the possibility that the pain may not be anginal. Angina has many mimics which can deceive the most experienced clinician more often than many appreciate unless they are routinely rigorous in seeking confirmation. Once labelled it is difficult to 'undiagnose' angina.

Confirmation of diagnosis

STABLE ANGINA

The diagnosis of stable angina is confirmed and its severity estimated by stress testing (exercise or pharmacological) with electrocardiographic monitoring. This carries a predictive accuracy of only about 70 per cent (though this figure will be influenced by its prevalence in the population, according to Bayesian theory) so that false positive and false negatives occur; nuclear perfusion scans (e.g. with thallium) increase predictive accuracy to approximately 90 per cent; ultrasound or nuclear scans for ischaemic regional contractile dysfunction are alternative means of assessing myocardial ischaemia during stress testing. Coronary angiography shows underlying coronary anatomy – stenosis and/or spasm (or their absence in Syndrome X), thus providing circumstantial evidence that myocardial ischaemia is the cause of the chest pain.

UNSTABLE ANGINA

In unstable angina, stress testing is potentially dangerous, and the history is more difficult because it lacks the feature of a predictable relationship of the pain to exercise. Unstable angina, however, carries high risk of preventable infarction. Clinical suspicion is thus sufficient to merit urgent admission to hospital, where continuous electrocardiographic monitoring can provide confirmatory evidence that the pains are due to myocardial ischaemia.

SYNDROME X

Syndrome X (microvascular angina) causes diagnostic problems, if only because the existence of the syndrome means that a normal coronary arteriogram cannot be used to exclude myocardial ischaemia as the cause of angina-like pain. Special investigations in such patients have confirmed inducible ischaemia, with reduced coronary artery perfusion reserve due, by implication, to microvascular dysfunction; its underlying cause(s) remains unknown as does its prevalence. The syndrome is defined empirically as angina, with positive stress test, but normal coronary arteriogram, in the absence of overt cardiovascular disease (e.g. valve disease, cardiomyopathy). These patients present just like any other patient with stable effort angina and it is the negative findings on coronary angiography that lead to its diagnosis following rigorous re-evaluation of the evidence for or against myocardial ischaemia. In the great majority of patients with angina-like chest pain subsequently shown to have normal (or near normal) coronary arteriograms, however, the pain turns out to be non-cardiac and the diagnosis is not microvascular angina. The normal coronary arteriogram therefore prompts critical re-evaluation of the history and reconsideration of alternative diagnoses.

The diagnosis of microvascular angina can be confirmed only by inference from convincing evidence of impaired coronary perfusion reserve, inducible myocardial ischaemia, absence of haemodynamic cause and a 'normal' coronary arteriogram – by which is meant the absence of angiographically demonstrated fixed stenosis and/or spasm of sufficient severity (reduction in luminal diameter ≥ 50 per cent) to be the cause as demonstrated at the time of induced pain, as spasm and local thrombus may be transient.

Other cardiovascular causes of chest pain

Myocarditis

Myocarditis commonly causes chest pain, reflecting associated myocardial ischaemia (angina) or pericarditis.

Pericarditis

The site of the pain is similar to that of angina but is sharper and, as it arises from inflammation of the pericardium which is adjacent to the pleura, is commonly 'pleuritic', i.e. exacerbated by inspiration. It may be relieved by sitting up and leaning forward, and exacerbated by swallowing, twisting or sternal pressure.

Aortic dissection

Dissection of the aorta can cause extremely severe pain, which is generally abrupt in onset, prolonged, and commonly felt in the back.

Mitral stenosis

Angina can occur with mitral stenosis, either because of incidental or embolic coronary artery disease or, it has been suggested, from right ventricular ischaemia attributable to excessive systolic load with severe pulmonary hypertension.

Pulmonary embolism

Angina-like pain or chest discomfort (as distinct from pleuritic pain with pulmonary infarction) can occur with major pulmonary embolism and may similarly reflect right ventricle overload and ischaemia.

Mitral valve prolapse

This is often cited as a cause of chest pain but the evidence is unconvincing.

Oesophageal pain

Oesophageal pain may be manifest as: (1) retrosternal 'heart burn' due to acid regurgitation; or (2) angina-like pain due to oesophageal dysmotility ('spasm'). The site, character, and radiation of oesophageal pain may be indistinguishable from those of cardiac pain, reflecting common root innervation. These two types of oesophageal pain may however be difficult to distinguish from each other. They may coexist. Acid regurgitation often induces oesophageal dysmotility but each can occur without the other, while either or both can be associated with chest pains or cause no symptoms. Oesophageal pains in mild form are extremely common in the community, respond readily to simple antacid therapy and do not present medically. The spectrum, however, is wide and the type of patients who present with oesophageal symptoms will vary considerably in different types of clinical practice.

Gastro-oesophageal acid reflux also is extremely common. It can be induced by lying down or bending or with exercise. It may cause no symptoms or it may cause chest pain, characterized typically as burning and often associated with acid regurgitation. It may lead to endoscopically confirmed oesophagitis and more intractable symptoms, complicated sometimes by dysphagia with or without stricture formation. Gastro-oesophageal reflux appears to occur more commonly with duodenal ulcer or gallbladder disease, thereby mediating the symptom of chest pain in association with these conditions.

Angina-like pain of oesophageal origin is typically attributable to oesophageal dysmotility. Oesophageal dysmotility may thus, like angina, be induced by exercise, but unlike angina it tends to follow rather than coincide with the exertion. For probably similar reasons, oesophageal pain characteristically wakes the patient during the early hours of the morning, without the background of critically severe effort angina that characterises nocturnal decubitus angina. Another potentially misleading feature is that the pain of oesophageal dysmotility can, like angina, be relieved by smooth muscle relaxants such as nitrites or calcium antagonists. The pain of oesophageal spasm varies widely in severity and can be very severe, with associated pallor, tachycardia, sweating, and 'dyspnoea', attributable to activation of the sympathetic nervous system. It may be indistinguishable from unstable coronary syndromes, and it frequently occasions emergency admission to coronary care units. Where a longer history is available, it becomes apparent that episodes have been occurring for longer than the relatively short duration of an unstable coronary syndrome, without infarction and without confirmatory evidence of myocardial ischaemia. There may or may not be associated evidence of oesophageal symptoms such as acid regurgitation, heartburn or dysphagia. A useful (and potentially reassuring) test to be undertaken during an episode of chest pain is to swallow a bolus of saliva which will transiently relieve the pain of oesophageal spasm but not that of angina.

Pains arising from specific oesophageal disease such as diverticulum, rupture, or carcinoma may be localized over the site of the lesion. Associated features in the history, relationship to swallowing, and time course are such that they do not pose diagnostic problems relative to cardiac pain. Dysphagia is an indication to seek a gastroenterological opinion because of its potentially serious implications, whether or not it is associated with chest pain.

Oesophageal pain under test conditions can reduce coronary flow, to the point possibly of inducing true angina when coronary perfusion reserve is already compromised by coexistent coronary artery disease. Specific reflex mechanisms have long been postulated but a simpler explanation may be the increased sympathetic activity which can cause coronary vasoconstriction in these often abnormal vascular beds. Conversely, oesophageal pain can lower the threshold for experiencing the pain of angina during exercise without altering the haemodynamic response or the electrocardiographic evidence of ischaemic exercise tolerance.

Confirmation of diagnosis

Given the uncertain correlation of symptoms to acid reflux and dysmotility in group studies and the fact that both are common, it is important to ensure that a finding of either is not simply coincidental. Confirmation that the chest pain in question is oesophageal in origin demands rigorous criteria, and temporal correlation of valid manometric criteria of dysmotility and of pH measurements with the symptom in question, both in its onset and its offset. An episode of oesophageal dysmotility can be provoked pharmacologically and the response measured by manometry, but this approach is now tending to be superseded by ambulatory monitoring for naturally occurring episodes. Because of the roles both of acid regurgitation and of smooth muscle contraction, trials of omeprazole (even in single high dose) and, during pain, of smooth muscle relaxants such as glyceryl trinitrate or nifedipine can be diagnostically as well as therapeutically useful, and have practical and economic advantages over the sophisticated investigations described.

Other gastrointestinal causes

Dyspeptic pains, as from peptic ulcer, are generally experienced in the epigastrium rather than the chest (but see above) and are generally related to eating or hunger, but they can also cause discomfort in the lower substernal or left inframammary regions.

Pancreatic and gallbladder pain are subcostal, rarely felt in the chest.

Colonic distension can be felt in any quadrant of the abdomen and does not usually include a component of chest pain. Colonic pains may be influenced by breathing and by bowel action and do not generally cause diagnostic difficulty in relation to possible cardiac pain.

Musculoskeletal and neurological causes

These comprise a *pot pourri* of very common, generally ill-understood but benign causes, and some rare specific and potentially serious causes.

Local bone pain from neoplasm, trauma, osteoporotic vertebral crush fracture or rib stress fracture (e.g. from coughing) are associated with local tenderness and with pain on rib springing, the diagnosis being confirmed radiologically. The sudden onset of pain and subsequent local tenderness following a coughing bout without radiological evidence of rib fracture has been attributed to subperiostial haematoma. Local intercostal muscle pain as from trauma will similarly be associated with local tenderness. Pain associated with local tenderness over the costochondral junctions, known as Tietze's syndrome, is a self-limiting condition which may be common in general practice but appears to be only rarely encountered by cardiologists. Band-like often unilateral thoracic root pains due to specific causes – herpes zoster, diabetic mononeuritis, tabes – can also occur. Far more common, however, are musculoskeletal pains without local tenderness and of uncertain origin. They may be acute or intermittent and chronic. Their clinical features are suggestive of non-specific root pain, analogous to the more familiar cervical or lumbar root pain associated with degenerative changes in the spine or prolapsed intervertebral discs – though thoracic disc and other spinal lesions in the thoracic region generally present with evidence of spinal cord lesions.

These common non-specific thoracic musculoskeletal pains may present acutely with the abrupt (sic) onset of chest pain, typically during some minor movement such as turning or bending. They may be very severe, causing the patient to sit stock still, because the pain is exacerbated by the slightest movement including that of breathing (so that the patient feels 'short of breath'). They may cause pallor due to the sympathetic nervous system activity evoked by the severity of the pain. The acute severe pain generally resolves or eases spontaneously, but can be followed by recurrent episodes which may not be so typical. These may be felt in an ill-defined manner in different regions of the chest but they generally retain a relationship to movement or position. To elicit this feature of the history often requires specific questioning, such as the relationship to position in bed, or to twisting or coughing, both in the initiation of an episode and to its exacerbation while present. Pain may be near constant or intermittent, and it does not occur in such discrete episodes as does angina, often being felt as a background ache of which the patient is variably conscious. Sometimes such pains can be reproduced by forced rotation of the thoracic spine, thus confirming their musculoskeletal nature (even, gratifying but rarely, curing them!)

Confirmation of the diagnosis

Radiographic and, in particular, magnetic resonance imaging may be indicated when potentially sinister bony lesions are suspected. Radiological evidence of degenerative spinal changes such as spondylosis, however, is common, correlates poorly with symptoms and is more likely to be misleading than helpful. Investigations otherwise are generally unhelpful.

Psychological

Familiarity with the range of characteristics within which the chest pain could be consistent with that of cardiac, oesophageal, or specific musculoskeletal pain leaves little room for diagnostic doubt *vis-a-vis* other more vaguely defined symptoms which reflect the somatic symptoms of anxiety and/or the consequences of general muscle tension.

Tension

A vaguely described symptom of discomfort attributable to muscle tension on a background of anxiety can usually be distinguished as such by a careful history.

Overlay

Anxiety, attention-seeking, or pending litigation provide an overlay to the presentation of pain from any cause – amplifying rather than explaining chest pain, whose cause must still be sought and managed.

Hyperventilation

Psychogenic hyperventilation – said to have Freudian origins of sub-conscious claustrophobia – can cause symptoms which patients find hard to describe. They generally include sensations of panic, shortness of breath, chest discomfort, tingling in the hands, and perhaps palpitations. True hyperventilation (as distinct from the increased ventilation associated for example with exercise) leads to increased elimination of carbon dioxide and respiratory alkalosis, accounting for peripheral paraesthesiae. Hyperventilation may also induce coronary constriction in specifically susceptible subjects, although this is not a well-documented event in clinical practice.

The combination of hyperventilation (awareness of breathing, or difficulty in getting enough air into the lungs), left submammary pain (often described as 'stabbing' or 'knife-like') and palpitation occurs sufficiently often to be considered an entity, however ill-defined and heterogeneous. This triad of symptoms has had a variety of names including circulatory neurasthenia, Da Costa's syndrome, effort syndrome, soldier's heart or, more plainly, cardiac neurosis. It appears most commonly at least, to be a manifestation of anxiety about the heart and responds well to confident diagnosis and firm reassurance without recourse to more than a minimum of investigation. Observations that in at least some of these patients there is evidence of an increased heart rate, cardiac output, and pulse pressure with reduced peripheral resistance (the 'hyperkinetic heart') are compatible with an increase in sympathetic tone associated with anxiety about the presence of heart disease.

Bronchopulmonary

Pleurisy

Pleuritic pain due to inflammation of the pleura is the main bronchopulmonary cause of chest pain and is quite unlike angina. It is a sharp, superficial pain which catches on inspiration. Parietal pleural innervation is represented across many spinal cord roots and pain may thus be felt anywhere in the chest or back or be referred from the diaphragm to the shoulder, depending on the location of the pleural inflammation. Pleurisy may be infective (e.g. bacterial or viral pneumonia involving the pleura, or primarily pleural), malignant, traumatic, or inflammatory from other causes (e.g. systemic lupus erythematosus, Dressler's syndrome following acute myocardial infarction). Pulmonary infarction is an important cause of pleuritic pain, though the absence of pleurisy by no means excludes pulmonary emboli which do not necessarily result in pulmonary infarction. Pneumothorax can cause acute pleuritic chest pain.

Other bronchopulmonary

Mesothelioma can present with chest pain which is aching rather than pleuritic.

Mediastinal lesions can cause unpleasant 'deep' chest pain. The temptation to avoid a chest radiograph on grounds of economy should be resisted when faced with unexplained chest pain.

Pneumomediastinum is a rare cause of chest pain with pleural and pericardial components, associated diagnostically with subcutaneous emphysema.

Conclusion

Chest pain is one of the most common of symptoms and one of the most testing of the clinician's diagnostic skills. The range of its causes, from the trivial, self-limiting benign to the serious and life-threatening, independent of severity, emphasises the importance of establishing the diagnosis. This in turn emphasises the importance of the history.

REFERENCES

Cannon, R.O. (1993). Chest pain with normal coronary angiograms. *New England Journal of Medicine*, **328**, 1706–8.

Editorial. (1992). The oesophagus and chest pain of uncertain cause. *Lancet*, **339**, 583–4.

Hutchison, S.J., Poole-Wilson, P.A., and Henderson, A.H. (1988). Angina with normal coronary arteries: a review. *Quarterly Journal of Medicine* **72**, 677–88.

15.3.3 Oedema

J.D. FIRTH and J.G.G. LEDINGHAM

Oedema in heart disease is associated with an expansion of extracellular fluid volume. It can only occur as a consequence of a period of positive sodium and water balance, during which renal excretion fails to keep pace with input. Once established, however, oedema will persist even if sodium output and input become equal; a period of negative sodium balance is required for its removal. A number of questions arise: what causes the kidney to retain sodium in heart failure? how does it do so? and why does sodium retention lead to oedema? Complete answers to these seemingly simple questions are not available.

What causes the kidney to retain sodium in heart failure?

In severe heart failure the kidney behaves in a manner that closely resembles its response to haemorrhage, yet at no time in clinical or experimental heart failure is blood volume reduced – indeed, it usually appears to be increased. The stark contrast between the expansion of actual (measurable) blood volume and renal behaviour was recognized by Peters in 1948, who commented, regarding the circulatory blood volume, that 'it must be so expanded that the kidneys are unaware of it ... it may be not the actual volume of circulating plasma but some function usually related to the volume of circulating plasma – such as renal blood flow – that apprises the kidney of the need to conserve water'. Subsequent authors have spoken of a reduction in 'effective blood volume' in cardiac failure to reflect this concept. When blood volume is reduced, most dramatically following haemorrhage, a large number of neural and humoral mechanisms are invoked which, amongst other functions, serve to induce vasoconstriction, maintain arterial pressure, and sustain perfusion of vital organs. In cardiac failure the same pattern of neurohumoral changes occur, and it is this which supports the contention that erroneous perception of reduced blood volume (reduced 'effective blood volume') occurs somewhere within the circulation. It is not clear from precisely where this perception arises. There are many possibilities: on the arterial side the baroreceptors in the carotid sinus and aortic arch are obvious candidates; on the low pressure side of the circulation there are atrial (type B), ventricular and juxtapulmonary capillary (J) receptors connected to vagal afferents. Observations made by Epstein on changes in renal function following the opening and closing of arteriovenous (AV) fistulae suggest that in man receptors in the arterial tree exert the dominant influence over renal sodium handling. By shunting blood directly from the arterial to the venous side of the circulation the presence of such a fistula can reasonably be said to simultaneously reduce arterial and increase venous 'filling'. If the effect of arterial afferents were to dominate, then opening an arteriovenous fistula would be predicted to induce renal sodium retention; whereas if the venous afferents were to dominate, a natriuresis would be expected. In practice, the formation of a fistula leads to sodium retention, and natriuresis results when it is closed. Impairment of the pump function of the heart is bound to lead to alteration, perhaps subtle, of perfusion of the arterial tree, disturbing the relationship between cardiac output and peripheral resistance in a manner which may be analogous to the situation of the arteriovenous fistula. Intuitively, it seems reasonable to imagine that this might stimulate arterial receptors in a similar manner and thus initiate a similar pattern of responses. Proof (or disproof) of the greater importance of arterial rather than venous receptors will only come with a more complete understanding of the basic physiological mechanisms involved in the sensing of circulatory volume and perfusion.

By contrast with the difficulties involved in determining whether the same afferent pathways are activated in cardiac failure as in blood loss, there is no doubt that the same efferent responses are turned on. Patients with cardiac failure have increased sympathetic tone and levels of plasma noradrenaline correlate both with the degree of left ventricular dysfunction and with prognosis. High levels of plasma renin and aldosterone are observed, although not invariably, and there is a potential role for local intrarenal generation of renin and angiotensin, not necessarily reflected by increases in plasma levels. In cardiac failure plasma arginine vasopressin (AVP) levels are consistently elevated and the ability to excrete a water load is reduced: abnormalities which are ameliorated by afterload reduction leading to increased cardiac output.

Each of these efferent mechanisms could plausibly be involved to explain the renal inability to excrete sodium and water normally. However, the situation is complex, and sodium retention is likely to result from the summation of many influences on the kidney. Manoeuvres designed to block the renal effect of any single sodium-retaining system rarely produce significant natriuresis. For instance, changes in electrolyte excretion induced by adrenergic blockade in patients with heart failure are generally small, and the characteristic picture of renal dysfunction in cardiac failure can be seen in transplanted and denervated kidneys. The natriuresis that can be induced by angiotensin converting enzyme (ACE) inhibitors almost certainly results from improvements in cardiac output caused by afterload reduction, rather than specifically from lowering of plasma angiotensin II and aldosterone levels, although changes may occur as a result of inhibition of local angiotensin generation. The aldosterone antagonist spironolactone rarely produces substantial sodium excretion when given alone in heart failure.

Although the renal response to heart failure is to retain sodium, it is noteworthy that mechanisms which would tend to increase sodium excretion are also activated, and the degree of activation is greatest in those whose cardiac failure is most severe. Plasma levels of atrial natriuretic peptide, released directly from atrial myocytes in response to atrial distension, are usually elevated. Plasma levels of prostaglandin I_2 and E_2 metabolites may be markedly increased, and the dramatic decreases in renal perfusion and glomerular filtration rate sometimes precipitated in heart failure by non-steroidal anti-inflammatory agents, which inhibit cyclo-oxygenase and thereby prostaglandin production, suggests that they may be important in maintaining renal function in this condition. Circulating levels of dopamine are also increased in heart failure. Aside from the possible 'renoprotective' effect of prostaglandin activation, the biological significance of activation of these humoral vasodilator / natriuretic systems is uncertain. The renal response to them is blunted, either by hypotension or by a combination of the factors tending to encourage sodium retention.

The term 'high output cardiac failure' appears in the literature and is worthy of mention. In patients with hyperthyroidism, an arteriovenous fistula, anaemia or beriberi, sodium and water retention can occur despite much increased cardiac output. A pattern of hormonal activation similar to that seen in haemorrhage and 'low output cardiac failure' is observed. The explanation is thought to be a perception of reduced 'effective blood volume' due to diminished peripheral arterial vascular resistance. As primary impairment of cardiac function is not thought to be to blame, and the heart appears to be responding normally to an abnormal situation, we view the term 'high output cardiac failure' as a misnomer.

How does the kidney retain sodium in heart failure?

In patients with clinically moderate or severe heart failure there is striking and consistent reduction in renal blood flow. Glomerular filtration

rate (GFR) is relatively preserved, necessarily implying an increase in filtration fraction at the glomerulus. In patients with less severe disease, renal blood flow and glomerular filtration rate are often within the normal range if measured at rest, but minimal exercise may precipitate a dramatic reduction in both. The effects of exercise may have bearing on two clinical observations: the efficacy of bed rest as a treatment for severe cardiac failure, and the benefit of physical training in patients with milder forms of the condition.

Intrarenal haemodynamic changes have been examined in rats with ventricular dysfunction following myocardial infarction. The observed changes in glomerular plasma flow and single nephron glomerular filtration rate mirrored those found in whole organ animal studies and in man, and were due to intense constriction of the efferent arteriole. These hemodynamic changes, very similar to those induced by infusion of angiotensin II, would be predicted to increase the reabsorption of fluid from the proximal tubule. This is because blood flow in the peritubular capillaries arises solely from the effluent of the glomerular circulation. Efferent arteriolar constriction and resultant increase in glomerular filtration fraction therefore serves to increase the oncotic pressure and reduce the hydrostatic pressure in the peritubular capillaries, both factors tending to favour uptake of fluid from the peritubular interstitium into the capillaries (as opposed to the alternative of back leak into the tubular lumen). In some, but not all, animal models of heart failure increased proximal tubular sodium reabsorption has been demonstrated. In man the increase in free water clearance induced by mannitol infusion, and the lack of effect in heart failure of diuretics acting solely on the distal nephron, have also been taken as evidence that at least part of the increased tubular reabsorption of sodium takes place in the proximal tubule. Parts of the nephron beyond the proximal tubule are much less accessible to study. The sheer magnitude of the response that sometimes occurs when loop diuretics are given to patients with heart failure suggests that enhanced sodium resorption may occur in this nephron segment, as these agents work primarily by inhibition of the sodium–potassium–chloride cotransporter in the thick ascending limb of the loop of Henle. There is, however, no direct evidence to corroborate this suspicion. In other states associated with sodium retention abnormal behaviour of the distal tubules and collecting ducts has been invoked. Indeed, it is clear that the final 'fine tuning' of sodium excretion must occur in the distal nephron, as tubular fluid flows immediately thereafter into the urine. In several animal models bearing some resemblance to heart failure increased distal sodium resorption has been reported. This possibility cannot be excluded in man, but pharmacological blockade studies would strongly suggest that abnormal handling in more proximal segments must occur concurrently.

A further possibility that has been raised is that abnormal sodium handling in heart failure might be attributable to intrarenal redistribution of blood flow. On the basis of washout studies using inert gases in man, and microsphere infusion in animals, it has been proposed that blood flow be redirected from cortical to juxtamedullary nephrons in heart failure, and that the latter might have greater avidity for sodium. The technical difficulties involved in such studies are formidable, and there remains considerable doubt as to whether redistribution of blood flow actually occurs. With current technology the hypothesis and its implications cannot be properly tested.

Why does sodium retention lead to oedema?

Before Peters focused attention on the hypothesis that a reduction in effective blood volume might be the stimulus driving sodium retention in heart failure, an alternative hypothesis concentrated on events on the venous side of the circulation (the so-called 'backward', as opposed to 'forward', failure hypothesis). This depended on the observation that in many patients with oedematous heart failure the jugular venous pressure was considerably raised. The argument suggested that impairment of cardiac function led to a primary increase in central venous pressure, that this induced a parallel increase in tissue capillary pressure, leading via Starling forces to increased filtration and decreased reabsorption of fluid, resulting in both oedema and a reduction in plasma volume, which served as a further stimulus for sodium retention. This simple analysis is untenable. In many patients sodium retention clearly precedes any rise in central venous pressure. At no stage in the development of clinical or experimental heart failure has blood volume been shown to be reduced. There are, however, situations in which an elevation of venous pressure may correlate with the generation of cardiac oedema. In one study of patients with severe valvular heart disease, the only haemodynamic parameter measured that separated the oedematous from oedema-free individuals was an elevation of right ventricular end-diastolic pressure. However, the association does not prove cause and effect, and even if a rise in central venous pressure is linked in some instances to the development of oedema, the mechanism by which this happens is not known. The vessels taking blood to and from the capillaries are not simple passive conduits. Formation of tissue fluid is critically dependent on the control of pre and post capillary resistances. Without these elements, moving from the supine to the upright position would lead to massive changes in hydrostatic pressure in the capillaries in the feet. Indeed, a complete explanation for the failure of the feet of normal individuals to accumulate oedema on standing is not yet known. It probably depends on regulation of hydrostatic pressure by the pre-capillary arteriolar sphincter, as well as on changes in the rate of removal of interstitial fluid by lymphatic vessels. Given that these processes are crucial in the normal defence against the development of dependent oedema, they must either become deranged in some way, or their capacity must be overwhelmed, in cardiac failure. A reduction in lymphatic fluid return because of an increased central venous pressure is certainly a possible factor, but once again an appreciation of pathophysiology will have to wait for a better understanding of basic physiological processes.

Summary

In heart failure neurohumoral mechanisms are activated, and the kidney behaves as if blood volume were reduced. The sensing of an apparent loss of blood volume probably arises in the arterial side of the circulation, but why and where remain unknown. The end result is renal retention of sodium and water. Oedema arises from local imbalance between the rate of formation and rate of removal of interstitial fluid. The control of these processes at the capillary level is complex, but recent work indicates the importance of the precapillary arteriolar sphinctre. Why and how imbalance arises in heart failure, such that oedema results, is not known.

REFERENCES

Cohn, J.N., Levine, T.B., Olivari, M.T., Garberg, V., Lura, D., Francis, G.S., Simon, A.B., and Rector, T. (1984). Plasma norepinephrine as a guide to prognosis in patients with chronic congestive heart failure. *New England Journal of Medicine, 311*, 819–823.

Dzau, V.J. (1987). Renal and circulatory mechanisms in congestive heart failure. *Kidney International, 31*, 1402–1415.

Epstein, F.H., Post, R.S., and McDowell, M. (1953). Effects of an arterio-venous fistula on renal hemodynamics and electrolyte excretion. *Journal of Clinical Investigation, 32*, 233–241.

Hollander, W. and Judson, W.E. (1956). The relationship of cardiovascular and renal hemodynamic function to sodium excretion in patients with severe heart disease but without edema. *Journal of Clinical Investigation, 35*, 970–979.

Laragh, J.H. (1985). Atrial natriuretic hormone, the renin aldosterone axis and blood pressure-electrolyte homeostasis. *New England Journal of Medicine, 113*, 1330–1340.

Mancia, G. (1990). Neurohumoral activation in congestive heart failure. *American Heart Journal, 120*, 1532–1537.

Michel, C.C. (1984). Fluid movements through capillary walls. In *Handbook of physiology. The cardiovascular system IV* (Eds. E.M. Renkin, and C.C. Michel), pp. 375–409. American Physiological Society, Washington DC.

Oberg, B. (1964). Effects of cardiovascular reflexes on net capillary transfer. *Acta Physiologica Scandinavica, 62* (Suppl 229), 1–98.

Peters, J.P. (1948). The role of sodium in the production of oedema. *New England Journal of Medicine, 239*, 353–362.

Schrier, R.W. (1988). Pathogenesis of sodium and water retention in high output and low output cardiac failure, nephrotic syndrome, cirrhosis and pregnancy. *New England Journal of Medicine, 319*, 1065–1072; 1127–1134.

15.3.4 Fatigue

S. W. DAVIES and D. LIPKIN

Introduction

The sensation of fatigue is a non-specific symptom of many cardiac and non-cardiac diseases. It limits the exercise capacity of patients and impairs the quality of life. As with dyspnoea, the pathophysiology of fatigue is complex and not well understood.

An explicit definition of fatigue is elusive: it may be defined as 'weariness of mind and body following exertion, associated with a desire for rest and a disinclination or inability to make further effort.' Fatigue, like dyspnoea, can be normal after heavy exertion—pathological fatigue is the same sensation occurring at lower workloads or at rest. Fatigue ranges from slight lassitude to exhaustion. Physiologists define fatigue as failure of a muscle or muscle group to maintain a given force or workrate, but this is unhelpful in clinical practice.

Clinical types of cardiac fatigue

Fatigue is a cardinal symptom of heart failure but is very non-specific. In obtaining the history two types of fatigue should be distinguished.

1. Local fatigue: tiredness of particular muscle groups during exercise, often with local muscular discomfort. The muscles may be described as feeling heavy or stiff. Local fatigue of the leg muscles, and in particular of the quadriceps, is a common symptom limiting cycle exercise in normal subjects.
2. General fatigue: tiredness of all parts of the body during exercise. General fatigue is a common symptom limiting treadmill exercise in normal subjects.

Almost any type of cardiac disease may cause fatigue, and as in normal subjects the distinction between local fatigue and general fatigue often depends upon whether the exercise involves predominantly restricted muscle groups (as in cycling) or all the limb and trunk muscles (as in treadmill exercise). However, the differential diagnosis of fatigue differs for the local and generalized forms (Table 1).

The exercise causing fatigue should be related to the patient's age and previous level of physical fitness. Fatigue includes lassitude—a sensation of weariness at rest—but should be distinguished from malaise which denotes an indefinite sensation of discomfort and uneasiness.

Fatigue is often regarded as a symptom of heart failure, but it is also common in patients with a diagnosis of any serious cardiac disease in whom cardiac function is objectively unimpaired. In such cases there is probably a large psychological component in the symptom.

Pathophysiology of cardiac fatigue

In the past, fatigue has been regarded as evidence of a low cardiac output, sometimes termed 'forward failure', and has been contrasted with dyspnoea supposedly due to pulmonary venous congestion or 'backward failure'. This accords pleasingly with Starling's law of the heart, and gives an explanation for the fact that an increased diuresis which reduces central venous pressure alters the balance from backward failure towards forward failure, lessening dyspnoea but exacerbating fatigue. It is also true that in terminal heart failure, when resting cardiac output is reduced, there is severe fatigue and lassitude.

Table 1 *Causes of fatigue*

	Cardiovascular	Other
Local fatigue	Heart failure—all causes	Localized neuromuscular disease—poliomyelitis, myopathies Local vascular disease

General fatigue	Heart failure—all causes
	Some cardiovascular drugs
	  β-Blockers
	  α-Methyldopa
		Lung disease
		Psychogenic—depression, myalgic encephalomyelitis
		Obesity
		Anaemia
		Chronic renal disease
		Chronic liver disease
		Generalized neuromuscular disease—following stroke, myopathies
		Hypokalaemia, hyponatraemia

However, there is controversy as to whether skeletal muscle blood flow is adequate or inadequate during exercise in heart failure. Many studies have found that in mild and moderate heart failure the reduction in peak cardiac output and in maximal limb blood flow during exercise is in direct proportion to the reduction in exercise capacity—at a given workrate muscle blood flow is similar in heart failure patients and in controls. However, there is no evidence of a disproportionate reduction in exercise skeletal muscle blood flow which might account for fatigue. It seems likely that reduced blood flow at peak exercise is secondary to the reduced muscle bulk and to the reduced peak workrate performed by the muscles. These inferences must be cautious as a causal relationship is difficult to test directly in patients. Vasodilators which acutely increase limb blood flow fail to improve exercise capacity or fatigue, but it can be argued that the increased flow is through the skin, other soft tissues, and intramuscular arteriovenous shunt vessels, and not to working muscle bed.

Recently it has been suggested that when large masses of muscle are exercised, blood flow to exercising skeletal muscle is disproportionately reduced. The profound desaturation of femoral venous blood during exercise suggests that the oxygen supply to exercising muscle is limited, and limb muscle deoxygenation has been measured directly using infrared spectroscopy. The reduction in the vasodilatory capacity of large muscle groups during exercise in patients with heart failure may reflect the drive to maintain central arterial pressure. Intraneural recordings from the peroneal nerve using tungsten microelectrodes reveal increased efferent sympathetic nerve traffic to skeletal muscle.

One of the principal determinants of fatigue is the reduced bulk of skeletal muscle in chronic heart failure. In severe chronic heart failure there is "cardiac cachexia", and even in mild and moderate heart failure lean body mass is reduced. Reduced skeletal muscle mass probably results more from reduced habitual exercise and deconditioning, than from chronic hypoperfusion of the muscles; resting muscle blood flow is normal until heart failure is very severe indeed. The increased circulating levels of tumour necrosis factor (cachectin) found in severe heart failure may contribute to muscle resorption, but its quantitative importance has not been proven.

Many workers have sought to explain fatigue in chronic heart failure in terms of the abnormal findings on skeletal muscle biopsies, usually taken from the quadriceps. Mitochondrial oxidative enzymes are decreased while cytosol glycolytic enzymes are normal, and there are reductions in the number of mitochondrial cristae and in capillary numbers. However, it is debatable whether there is any specific abnormality of the skeletal muscles in chronic heart failure. The many abnormalities of histology, ultrastructure, and biochemistry of the skeletal muscles in moderate and severe heart failure are similar to those seen in deconditioning. These abnormalities tend to be reversed by treatment with angiotensin-converting enzyme inhibitors and by exercise training programmes.

Nuclear magnetic resonance (NMR) spectroscopy using the phosphorus isotope ^{31}P provides information on the metabolism of working skeletal muscle *in vivo*. The ratio of phosphocreatine to inorganic phosphate, which gives an index of high energy phosphate levels in the cells, can be estimated from the areas under their peaks in the ^{31}P NMR spectrum. Changes in pH cause small shifts in the location of the peaks in the ^{31}P

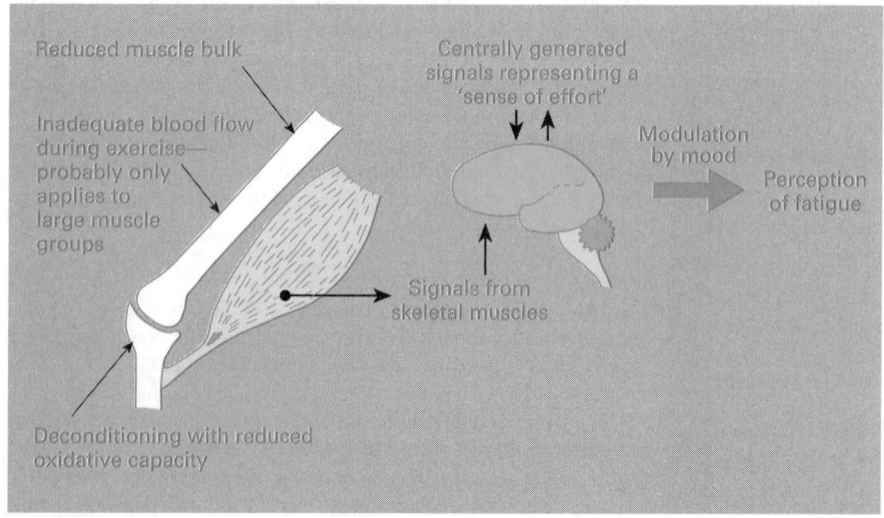

Fig. 1 The possible mechanisms of fatigue in cardiac disease.

spectrum so that intracellular pH can also be estimated. ^{31}P NMR spectroscopy reveals abnormally rapid depletion of phosphocreatine and rapid development of acidosis in exercising forearm and leg muscles in heart failure patients compared with normal subjects. Two observations suggest that this may be due to decreased oxidative capacity of the muscles in heart failure rather than to differences in blood flow during exercise. First, the difference between patients with heart failure and normal subjects persists when both perform exercises with tourniquets occluding all blood flow to the exercising limb. Second, at the same low workrate the phosphocreatine ratio is lower in patients with heart failure than in controls, although limb blood flow is similar.

The genesis of the sensation of muscular fatigue is unknown (Fig. 1). Accumulation of lactic acid has been held responsible, but this particular metabolite may not be wholly to blame. Fatigue occurs even if the production of lactic acid is inhibited by dichloroacetate, and in conditions such as inherited myophosphorylase deficiency (McArdle's syndrome) in which lactic acid levels do not rise during exercise.

Finally it should be recalled that even when there is an organic cause for fatigue, psychological factors are often important. Fatigue occurs less readily when exercise is undertaken congenially in pleasant and familiar surroundings, and more readily under conditions of boredom or stress.

Treatment of cardiac fatigue

When a specific cause such as anaemia is present it can be treated directly. Standard treatment for heart failure with diuretics and angiotensin-converting enzyme inhibitors ameliorates fatigue and improves exercise capacity. Other vasodilators such as hydralazine and nitrates are also effective. Drugs known to cause or exacerbate fatigue include β-blockers and α-methyldopa, which are still used occasionally in the treatment of hypertension.

Patients with severe fatigue attributable to acute heart failure or to an exacerbation of chronic heart failure are best treated with several days bed or chair rest until the heart failure is better controlled. However, patients with stable chronic heart failure benefit from physical exercise training, even when cardiac failure is severe, provided that the heart failure is clinically stable. Graded exercise programmes for heart failure are increasingly being used.

REFERENCES

Arnolda, L., Conway, M., Dolecki, M., Sharif, H., Rajagopolan, B., Ledingham, J.G.G., *et al.* (1990). Skeletal muscle metabolism in heart failure: a 31P nuclear magnetic resonance spectroscopy study of leg muscle. *Clinical Science*, **79**, 583–9.

Buller, N., Jones, D., and Poole-Wilson, P.A. (1991). Direct measurement of skeletal muscle fatigue in patients with chronic heart failure. *British Heart Journal*, **65**, 20–4.

Coats, A.J.S., Adamopolous, S., Meyer, T.E., Conway, J., and Sleight, P. (1990). Effects of physical training in chronic heart failure. *Lancet*, **335**, 63–6.

Davies, S.W. and Lipkin, D.P. (1991). Exercise physiology and changes in the periphery. *Current Opinion in Cardiology*, **6**, 352–7.

Lavine, B., Kalman, J., Mayer, L., Fillit, H., and Packer, M. (1990). Elevated circulating levels of tumor necrosis factor in severe chronic heart failure. *New England Journal of Medicine*, **323**, 236–41.

Massie, B., Conway, M. Yonge, R., Frostick, S., Ledingham, J., Sleight, P., *et al.* (1987). Skeletal muscle metabolism in patients with congestive heart failure: relation to severity and to blood flow. *Circulation*, **76**, 1009–19.

Sylven, C., Jansson, E., Cederholm, T., Hildbrand, I.L., and Beermann, B. (1991). Skeletal muscle depressed calcium and phosphofructokinase in chronic heart failure are upregulated by captopril—a double-blind, placebo-controlled study. *Journal of Internal Medicine*, **229**, 171–4.

Wilson, J.R., Mancini, D.M., Ferraro, N., and Egler, J. (1988). Effect of dichloroacetate on the exercise performance of patients with heart failure. *Journal of the American College of Cardiology*, **12**, 1464–9.

15.3.5 Syncope and palpitation

R. Sutton

Symptoms of syncope and palpitation where of primary cardiac origin are most usually caused by arrhythmias. Syncope is the term used to describe loss of consciousness due to a reduction in cerebral blood flow sufficient to prejudice cerebral metabolism, whilst palpitation describes an awareness of the heart beat.

Patients complain of fainting, falls, or 'blackouts' when they describe syncope. Palpitation is described in many different ways, of which a fluttering sensation in the chest or epigastrium is perhaps the most common.

Syncope

AETIOLOGY

The causes of syncope can be considered to be related to the electrical function of the heart, to structural disease of the heart and to disease of the vasculature – both systemic and pulmonary. Table 1 summarizes the various causes. Neuroendocrine disturbances of the control heart rate and vascular tone can also cause syncope; these are summarized in Table 2.

Electrical disturbances of cardiac function cause syncope either by reduction of the mechanical efficiency of the heart thereby reducing cardiac output, blood pressure, and cerebral blood flow, or by complete interruption of cardiac activity due to asystole complicating atrioventricular block or ventricular tachyarrhythmia most commonly seen in coronary heart disease. Technical faults in pacing systems can result in asystole due to sudden complete lack of pacing or, occasionally, very rapid pacing may occur. Inappropriate choice of pacing mode, mostly ventricular, may be associated with retrograde conduction to the atria causing them to contract during ventricular systole with regurgitation of blood into pulmonary veins. This has the effect of ventricular under filling and resultant low cardiac output known as pacemaker syndrome. Such retrograde conduction is most difficult for patients to tolerate when it occurs intermittently.

The neuroendocrine causes of syncope largely have two components: cardioinhibition and vasodepression. All these conditions (Table 2) can be considered together as being separate trigger points that lead to a common dual component reaction.

Vasovagal syncope is the most frequent and in many ways the best understood. Upright posture is an almost invariable feature, leading critically to the pooling of 500 to 1000 ml of blood in the lower limbs and to reduction in central blood volume. Susceptible people show higher than normal plasma concentrations of adrenaline and vasopressin prior to the attack. These cause vigorous left ventricular contraction and sensitization of left ventricular baroreceptors, respectively. Reduced cardiac filling on standing then triggers the sensitized baroreceptors to manifest a reflex that is appropriate in left ventricular dilatation – bradycardia and vasodilatation. In the context of low central blood volume this reflex is disastrous for maintenance of blood pressure. In addition to the increased sensitivity of left ventricular baroceptors, there is some evidence in sufferers of recurrent vasovagal attacks of an abnormal positive gain in the reflex at brainstem level. In the autonomic neuropathies the mechanism is different and results from a failure of the normal adaptations to the erect posture.

There are many other causes of repeated episodic events, often described by the patient as 'blackouts'. The history is all important here and, apart from epilepsy, an important diagnosis to consider is hyperventilation. This is a common condition often masquerading as a primary cardiac disorder when the symptoms include the triad of left submammary pain (often stabbing in nature), severe palpitation, and what is described as breathlessness. The last, on careful questioning, is found

Table 1 *Cardiovascular causes of recurrent syncope*

Cardiac–electrical
Tachyarrythmias
supraventricular tachycardias
ventricular tachyarrhythmias
Bradyarrhythmias
sinoatrial node disease
atrioventricular block
Pacemaker malfunction
technical faults
pacemaker syndrome
Cardiac–structural
Aortic stenosis
Hypertrophic cardiomyopathy
Pulmonary stenosis, including tetralogy of Fallot
Myocardial infarction
Obstruction of a prosthetic valve
Atrial ball thrombus
Cardiac tumour
Cardiac tamponade
Vascular
Dissection of the aorta
Takayasu's disease
Carotid stenosis
Vertebrobasilar disease
Subclavian steel
Pulmonary embolism
Pulmonary hypertension
Migraine
Transient ischaemic attack

Table 2 *Neuroendocrine causes of syncope*

Carotid sinus syndrome
Vasovagal syndrome
Glossopharyngeal syndrome
Cough
Micturition
Defaecation
Deglutition
Postural or orthostatic hypotension
Autonomic neuropathies
Diabetes mellitus
Alcohol
Idiopathic
Prolonged bed rest
Sympathectomy
Other central nervous diseases, e.g. Shy–Drager syndrome
Drug-induced
α-adrenoceptor blockade
methyldopa and levodopa
tricyclic antidepressants
thiazide diuretics
phenothiazines
benzodiazepines

to consist of an uncomfortable and worrying awareness of breathing and a compulsion to take deep, sighing breaths. Not all components of this syndrome (variously called Da Costa's syndrome, effort syndrome, neurocirculatory asthenia, cardiac neurosis, etc.) are always described in the initial history, but a clear account is valuable in preventing cardiological investigation which may, in some cases, aggravate rather than relieve anxiety about an underlying serious cardiac disorder.

PRESENTATION

True syncope is of sudden onset and brief duration, typically lasting less than 1 min. A careful history taken from both patient and observer is vital if an accurate diagnosis is to be made. When syncope has been caused by structural cardiac or vascular causes, other symptoms may emerge; for instance in obstructive cardiac disease (classically aortic stenosis) it tends to occur on exertion. When the cause is a bradyarrhythmia, and in some of the neuroendocrine disturbances, sudden loss of consciousness tends to be devoid of warning, whereas, syncope due to tachyarrhythmia is often heralded by palpitation and the vasovagal syndrome is typically is preceded by tiredness, yawning, air hunger, boredom, nausea, and occasionally palpitation, which lead to dizziness and a rather gradual greying into syncope. Only a minority of vasovagal sufferers, usually older patients, give no history of prodrome.

The observer reports striking pallor in syncope and often wonders if the patient is dead. Cyanosis supervenes in the second half of the first minute there may be epileptiform movements and after onset, incontinence of urine (but rarely faeces). Recovery from cardiac syncope is associated with a bright flush; episodes that are due to neuroendocrine causes do not end with a flush because of the longer time course of vasodepression. Estimates of the duration of syncope by an observer tend to be exaggerated because of the dramatic nature of the event. Attacks typically last less than 1 min: episodes lasting up to 2 min do occur and, when longer than this, cerebral damage may be sustained. There is a mortality of attacks of syncope but, in the whole picture of sudden cardiac death, bradyarrhythmias contribute only a small per-

centage and ventricular tachyarrhythmias dominate. An experienced observer, perhaps the patient's spouse, may be able to anticipate a vasovagal episode even before the patient by observing the characteristic initial pallor, glazed look, and deeper than normal respiration. Recovery from cardiac syncope is rapid with almost immediate orientation.

When there is a neuroendocrine cause, syncope can be prolonged, occasionally with compromised cardiac output for hours due to vasodepression which resolves slowly. Although the cardiac contraction is restored, bradycardia also tends to persist so that more time is taken to restore cerebral perfusion to normal.

RELATED SYMPTOMS

Dizziness (faintness) is the symptom which precedes syncope and represents an incomplete form in which the blood pressure and cerebral blood flow have not fallen sufficiently to cause loss of consciousness. It consists of a floating feeling or lightheadedness, darkening of vision, and sometimes a feeling of falling backwards and the sensation of an impending loss of consciousness. Those prone to recurrent attacks learn to sit, often with their head between their knees, or lie – reactions that may prevent loss of consciousness.

SEQUELAE OF SYNCOPE

Syncopal attacks may result in injury because the lack of warning prevents any self-protective measures. Some patients present to the fracture clinic because of falls and injury. The possibility that such injury resulted from syncope must always be considered and appropriate questions asked. Syncope is occasionally followed by a transient neurological defect. This may lead to diagnosis of a transient ischaemic attack but unconsciousness is rarely associated with transient ischaemic attacks. The cause of any neurological sequelae may be either systemic embolism from the left atrium in sinoatrial node disease or focal cerebrovascular disease giving a more persistent and severe perfusion defect than that experienced by the brain overall.

INCIDENCE AND MORTALITY

The incidence of syncope is difficult to ascertain but it has been estimated that as many as 30 per cent of the population experience at least one episode in a lifetime and perhaps every individual is capable of fainting given unfavourable circumstances. One per cent of all emer-

Table 3 *Differential diagnosis of syncope*

	Syncope	Epilepsy

Warning	Cardiac
	  minimal or none
	  rushing noise in head
	  falling backwards
	Vasovagal
	  definite prodrome
		Minimal typical prodrome

Colour changes	Cardiac
	  White, blue, red
	Vasovagal
	  White, blue, white
		Red, blue

Timing of convulsion and incontinence	After 30s	Before 30s
Injury	Trauma on falling	Trauma on falling plus that self-inflicted
Recovery	Usually rapid	Slow
Pre-ictal amnesia	None	Present
Physical examination	No pulse	Pulse present

gency room attendances is reported to have been for syncope. The most common cause of these is vasovagal syncope (up to 58 per cent) but in some 50 per cent of cases the cause remains undiagnosed, even after extensive and expensive inpatient investigation. Unexplained syncope carries a much better prognosis for survival than cardiac syncope; one series has given the respective mortalities as 6 versus 30 per cent. Recurrent syncope, despite investigation and treatment of a probable cause, seems to carry an appreciable mortality and justifies detailed investigation including tilt testing and cardiac electrophysiological studies with ventricular extrastimulation to reveal a tendency to ventricular tachyarrhythmias.

DIFFERENTIAL DIAGNOSIS

The challenge to the clinician in this field is separation of syncope and epilepsy (Table 3). The value of the history from patient and observer cannot be overstated. The type or lack of warning, the sequence and timing of colour changes, the timing of convulsions and incontinence, the type of injury, the speed of recovery and the existence of pre-ictal amnesia are most important. The chance of observation of an attack by a medical or paramedical person is slim but this may provide very persuasive evidence of, for example, a bradycardia.

Palpitation

This is a symptom experienced by most people at some time in their lives. Ambulatory electrocardiography has shown that some extrasystolic activity – supraventricular or ventricular – occurs in everybody. These events may or may not be perceived by the patient. When palpitation is severe or frequent enough for medical consultation, careful analysis of the patient's description can often reveal the type of arrhythmia underlying the symptoms. Extrasystoles, often reported as missed beats, typically have a compensatory pause and potentiation of the post-pause beat. This sequence can often be drawn from the patient without using leading questions. Such extrasystoles are usually of no pathological significance but cause worry, which is likely then to be self-propagating, because anxiety is the most prominent cause of awareness of perhaps long-standing and previously asymptomatic extrasystoles. The history should include questions about alcohol consumption, caffeine, nicotine, and other drugs, as all of these agents favour extrasystolic activity.

Tachyarrhythmias will be given different descriptions by the patient and it is usually possible to ascertain with accuracy whether the arrhythmia is regular or irregular and approximately how fast. A useful way of appreciating these features is to ask the patient to imitate the arrhythmia

by tapping on the desk. If this fails then a series of choices illustrated by the clinician doing the tapping may be helpful. Symptoms of impending or actual syncope are often features associated with palpitation and, in general, the most important rhythm disturbances are those associated with dizziness and syncope. The clinician will also want to know about onset and its timing, duration and mode of termination, including the effect on the attack of any spontaneous Valsalva-type manoeuvres, for example, vomiting. The other symptoms which coincide with arrhythmias are also of great importance: dyspnoea, sweating, chest pain, polyuria. Polyuria tends to occur only in arrhythmias where atrial and ventricular systole are simultaneous, resulting in great atrial wall stretch and release of large quantities of atrial natriuretic peptide. That this is not a hard and fast rule may depend on release of brain natriuretic peptide, the role of which is not yet fully understood. From this approach to history taking it is usually possible to diagnose extrasystoles, atrial fibrillation, supraventricular tachycardias, and malignant arrhythmias especially ventricular tachycardia (Table 4).

Palpitation may also accompany bradyarrhythmias, with symptoms resembling those of missed beats. Unpleasant awareness of the heart beat may also be experienced in relation to its forcefulness, for instance with impending vasovagal syncope, in the postprandial state, and in hypertrophic cardiomyopathy.

Because palpitation is such a ubiquitous symptom it does not lend itself to the detailed and exhaustive descriptions of all its associations. The management of both syncope and palpitation is discussed in other sections of the book in the context of the underlying associated conditions. Perhaps the most common cause of each symptom is vasovagal syncope and innocent extrasystoles; in both, diagnosis must be followed immediately by patient explanation and firm reassurance.

FURTHER READING

Buxton, A.E., Marchlinski, R.E., Doherty, J.H. et al. (1984). Repetitive, monomorphic ventricular tachycardia: clinical and electrophysiologic characteristics in patients with and patients without heart disease. *American Journal of Cardiology*, **54**, 997.

Dermskian, G. and Lamb, S.E. (1958). Syncope in a population of healthy adults: incidence, mechanisms and significance. *Journal of the American Medical Association*, **168**, 1200.

Doherty, J.U., Pembrook-Rogers, D., Grogan, E.W., *et al.* (1985). Electrophysiologic evaluation and follow-up characteristics of patients with recurrent unexplained cyncope and presyncope. *American Journal of Cardiology*, **55**, 703.

Hinckle, L.E. and Carrer St Stevens, M. (1969). The frequency of asymptomatic disturbances of cardiac rhythm and conduction in middle aged men. *American Journal of Cardiology*, **24**, 629.

Table 4 *Historical analysis of palpitation*

	Bradycardias	No arrhythmia	Extrasystoles	A Fib	SVT	VT
Timing						
Onset	–	–	Sudden	Sudden	Sudden	Sudden
Timing of onset	–	–	When quiet	Any time, effort, rest	Any time, effort, rest	Any time, effort
Duration	–	–	Usually short	Variable	Variable	Variable
Termination	–	Syncope evasion	Exertion	Sudden, Valsalva (slow)	Sudden, Valsalva (slow)	Sudden (slow)
Symptoms						
Dizziness	Possible	Possible	Unlikely	Possible	Possible	Likely
Syncope	Possible	Vasovagal syncope	No	Possible	Possible	Likely
Dyspnoea	Possible	–	Hyperventilation, not dyspnoea	Possible	Possible	Likely
Chest pain	Unlikely	–	Unlikely	Possible (atypical)	Possible (atypical)	Likely (typical)
Polyuria	No	No	No	Unlikely	Possible	Unlikely

A Fib, Atrial fibrillation; SVT, Supraventricular tachycardia; VT, Ventricular tachycardia.

Exceptions and variations must be expected when applying a table such as this to the clinical scene.

Jarisch, A. (1941). Vasovagal syncope. *Zeitschrift für Kreislaufforschung,* **23,** 267–79.

Kapoor, W.N., Karpf, M., Maher, Y., *et al.* (1982). Syncope of unknown origin: the need for a more cost-effective approach to its diagnostic evaluation. *Journal of the American Medical Association,* **247,** 2687.

Kenny, R.A., Bayliss, J., Ingram, A., *et al* (1986). Head-up tilt: a useful test for investigating unexplained syncope. *Lancet,* **ii,** 1352.

Lown, B., Ganong, W.F., and Levine, S.A. (1952). The syndrome of short PR interval, normal QRS complex and paroxysmal rapid heart rate. *Circulation,* **5,** 693.

Morley, C.A. and Sutton, R. (1984). Carotid sinus syndrome – editorial review. *International Journal of Cardiology,* **6,** 287.

Sander-Jensen, K., Secher, N.H., Astrup, A., *et al.* (1986). Hypotension induced by passive head-up tilt: endocrine and circulatory mechanisms. *American Journal of Physiology,* **251,** R742.

Shy, G.M. and Drager, G.A. (1960). A neurological syndrome associated with orthostatic hypotension. *Archives of Neurology,* **2,** 511.

Sloane, P.D., Linzer, M., Pontinen, M., *et al.* (1991). Clinical significance of a dizziness history in medical patients with syncope. *Archives of Internal Medicine,* **151,** 1525–628.

Takahashi, N., Seki, A., Imataka, K., and Fujii, J. (1981). Clinical features of paroxysmal atrial fibrillation: an observation of 94 patients. *Japanese Heart Journal,* **22,** 143.

Travill, C.M. and Sutton, R. (1992). Pacemaker syndrome: an iatrogenic condition. *British Heart Journal,* **68,** 163–6.

Wayne, H.H. (1961). Syncope: physiological considerations and an analysis of the clinical characteristics in 510 patients. *American Journal of Medicine,* **30,** 418.

Wellens, H.J.J. (1983). Woff–Parkinson–White syndrome Part 1. Diagnosis, arrhythmias and identification of the high risk patients. *Modern Concepts in Cardiovascular Disease,* **52,** 53.

Wood, P. (1946). DaCosta's syndrome (effort syndrome). *British Medical Journal,* **1,** 767, 805, 845.

15.3.6 Cardiac cachexia

W.L. MORRISON

Weight loss may occur as a consequence of heart disease. Long-standing severe congestive heart failure is commonly accompanied by a loss of total body fat and lean body mass, principally skeletal muscle, which in its most severe form is described by the term cardiac cachexia. This generally implies a fall in total body mass of 20 per cent below pre-dicted. The term is not generally used to include those conditions in which cachexia is due to infection involving the heart such as endocarditis.

Aetiology

Cardiac cachexia has been recognized since Withering's 1785 description: 'His countenance was pale, his pulse quick and feeble, his body greatly emaciated except for his belly which was very large ...'. Although formerly seen in patients with severe mitral valve disease and pulmonary hypertension in the early days of cardiac surgery, this is now less common, as these patients tend to undergo surgery at an earlier stage. Cardiac cachexia now more commonly occurs in patients referred for transplantation, in the main due to endstage coronary artery disease or cardiomyopathy. Right-sided cardiac dysfunction with tricuspid regurgitation is generally present. Cachexia *per se* may lead to cardiac atrophy with further deterioration in cardiac function. Patients with cardiac cachexia generally complain of effort intolerance, muscle weakness, and fatigue.

Pathogenesis

Cardiac cachexia is characterized by loss of body fat and lean body mass, the principal component of which is skeletal muscle. The mechanism of the muscle wasting is a reduction of protein synthesis, coupled with an increase in the rate of breakdown of protein in skeletal muscle. Various factors have been postulated to explain the mechanism of cardiac cachexia (Fig. 1). Reduced nutrient limb blood flow exists in severe cardiac failure as a result of diminished cardiac output, neurohumoral compensatory mechanisms, and increased vascular stiffness, and this may supply tissues inadequately with the substrates necessary for normal protein turnover and growth.

Relative immobility as a result of breathlessness and effort intolerance is common in patients with severe cardiac failure. Immobility *per se* has been shown to produce wasting and reduced protein synthesis in skeletal muscle with atrophy of the type I fibres. Disuse atrophy and deconditioning may contribute to the tissue wasting seen in cardiac failure.

Anorexia is commonly present in patients with cardiac cachexia. When central venous pressure is chronically elevated the resultant increased back pressure on splanchnic vessels and lymphatics may result in malabsorbtion of nutrients. Hepatic congestion, hypoxia, and drug toxicity may all result in delayed emptying and hypomotility of the gut, and these factors can also contribute to malassimilation of nutrients and,

Fig 1. Pathogenesis of cardiac cachexia.

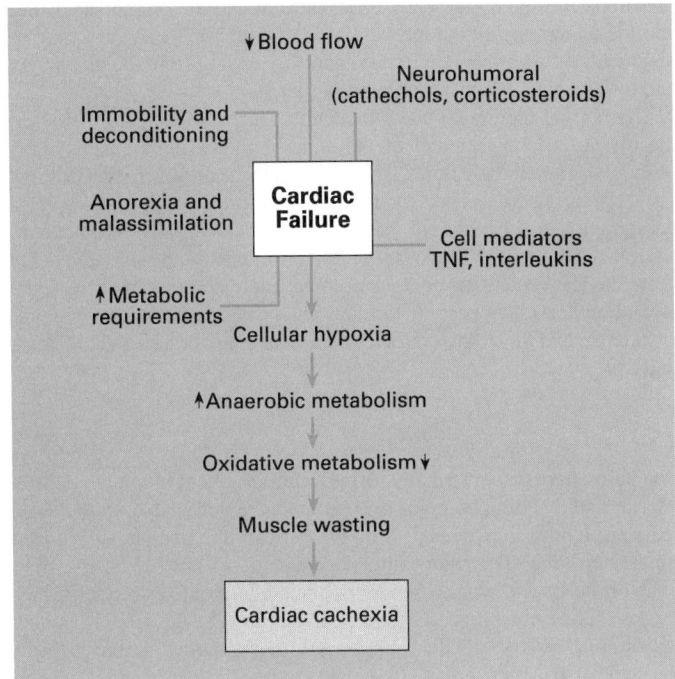

consequently, an inadequate energy supply to maintain normal tissue growth. If anorexia is severe, skeletal muscle may be utilized as an energy source. Protein losing enteropathy and steatorrhoea may also occur.

Sympathetic nervous system activity is increased in heart failure, and neurohumoral compensatory mechanisms result in elevated catecholamine and corticosteroid secretion. Both have been shown experimentally to result in increased breakdown of skeletal muscle and are associated with type IIb fibre atrophy.

Cellular hypoxia is likely to play a central role in the pathogenesis of cardiac cachexia. Phosphorus magnetic resonance spectroscopy has demonstrated a reduction in oxidative metabolism and an increase in anaerobic (glycolytic) metabolism on exercise. This suggests that there are intrinsic changes in skeletal muscle energetics that could reflect alterations in fibre composition, recruitment patterns, contractile efficiency, and metabolism. Muscle histology has demonstrated a reduced percentage of slow twitch type I oxidative fibres, and a higher percentage of type IIb glycolytic fibres (fast twitch, fast fatigue), which are smaller than normal type IIb fibres. These histological changes are accompanied by a reduction in mitochondrial oxidative enzyme capacity. Cell mediator responses are also important in cardiac cachexia. Tumour necrosis factor (cachectin; TNF) is a 17 kilodalton cytokine, originally isolated from rabbits with trypanosomiasis, and thought to be responsible for the development of fever and a wasting diathesis. High concentrations of tumour necrosis factor have been found in the blood of patients with heart failure and cardiac cachexia, appearing to correlate inversely with body weight. But high concentrations have not been found universally in all patients with cardiac cachexia. Several other cell mediators may subsequently be found to be important in cardiac cachexia.

Treatment

Treatment of cardiac cachexia is very limited. Diuretics, cardiac glycosides, angiotensin converting enzyme inhibitors and vasodilators may improve cardiac function somewhat, but patients often remain wasted. The only longer-term solution for most patients with cardiac cachexia is transplantation, after which reversal of the tissue wasting has been demonstrated. Improved diet with enteral or parenteral feeding is useful to build patients up prior to transplantation. Physical training may lead to improvement in both exercise tolerance and skeletal muscle oxidative metabolism, but it is currently unknown if this can help to reverse the muscle wasting in true cardiac cachexia.

REFERENCES

Levine, B., Kalman, J., Mayer, L., Fillit, H.M., and Packer, M. (1990). Elevated circulating levels of Tumor Necrosis Factor in Severe Chronic Heart Failure. *New England Journal of Medicine.* **323**, 236–241.

Massie, B., Conway, M., Yonge, R., Frostick, S., Ledingham, J., Sleight, P., Radda, G., and Rajagopalan, B. (1987). Skeletal muscle metabolism in patients with congestive heart failure: relation to clinical severity and blood flow. *Circulation.* **76**, 1009–1019.

Morrison, W.L. and Edwards, R.H.T. (1991). Cardiac cachexia. *British Medical Journal* **302**, 301–302.

Pittman, J.G. and Cohen, P. (1964). Pathogenesis of cardiac cachexia. *New England Journal of Medicine* **271**, 453–460.

15.4 The clinical assessment of cardiovascular function

15.4.1 Chest radiography in heart disease

M.B. RUBENS

Introduction

The chest radiograph is often abnormal in patients with congenital heart disease, but in most patients with acquired heart disease it is normal and rarely provides a precise diagnosis. None the less, a chest radiograph remains part of the routine work-up of virtually all patients with known or suspected heart disease. The chest radiograph is relatively inexpensive and non-invasive. It provides a record of cardiac size and shape, and it may suggest specific chamber enlargement. Abnormal cardiac calcification may be visible, and analysis of the pulmonary vessels may indicate precise physiological disturbances. Analysis of the skeleton may provide evidence of associated systemic disease or previous surgery, and abnormalities of situs may be apparent. Occasionally, unsuspected non-cardiac abnormalities are discovered.

A routine examination always includes a frontal view and usually a lateral view. Ideally, the frontal view is posteroanterior (PA), with the patient upright and at end-inspiration. Patients who are too ill to be taken to the X-ray department may be examined with mobile equipment and an anteroposterior (AP) film is taken. In this projection the heart appears magnified because it is further from the film.

A lateral film may give additional further information on heart size and shape, and cardiac calcification is often best demonstrated in this view. Frontal and lateral films combined with a barium swallow may provide data on left atrial size and the presence of aberrant branches of the great vessels.

The normal chest radiograph

The cardiovascular silhouette (Fig. 1)

The right border of the cardiovascular silhouette comprises, from above downwards, the superior vena cava, the body of right atrium, and the inferior vena cava. The normal superior vena cava produces a low-density vertical shadow, just lateral to the spine. The azygos vein may be visible as a convex density above the origin of the right main bronchus and superimposed on the superior vena cava. The lower part of the right cardiovascular silhouette is convex and produced by the body of the right atrium. Occasionally, the inferior vena cava is visible as a short vertical shadow in the right cardiophrenic angle (Fig. 1).

The left border of the cardiovascular silhouette comprises, from above downwards, the aortic knuckle, the pulmonary trunk, the left atrial appendage and the left ventricle. The aortic knuckle is produced by the posterior part of the aortic arch. The proximal descending aorta may be visible as a vertical shadow, continuous with the knuckle and eventually merging with the left paraspinal shadow. The pulmonary trunk is situated below the aortic knuckle, and below this is a short segment of left atrial appendage. The bulk of the left heart border is formed by the body of the left ventricle. The left cardiophrenic angle may be occupied by a low-density shadow representing an apical pericardial fat pad. Less often, a fat pad is visible in the right cardiophrenic angle.

On the lateral film (Fig. 2) the heart is seen to be situated immediately posterior to the inferior half of the sternum. The anterior border of the cardiac shadow is formed almost entirely by the right ventricle, although in atrial diastole the right atrial appendage may come in contact with the sternum. The right ventricular outflow tract is continuous with the main pulmonary artery, which arches posteriorly and continues into the left pulmonary artery. The branches of the right pulmonary artery cast an ovoid shadow anterior to the right bronchus. Part of the ascending aorta may be visible above the pulmonary trunk, and the aortic arch is seen passing posteriorly and then descending for a variable distance. The aortic arch is separated from the left pulmonary artery by the sub-

aortic fossa. The upper part of the posterior aspect of the cardiac silhouette is formed by the body of left atrium and the pulmonary veins, and the lower part by the left ventricle. The inferior vena cava may be visible as a short straight vertical shadow extending from the diaphragm and overlapping the posterior heart border.

The normal cardiovascular silhouette changes with age. In infancy, the thymus occupies much of the anterior mediastinum, and it may obscure the aorta, the pulmonary trunk, and the right ventricular outflow tract. By early adolescence, the thymus is no longer visible on the chest radiograph, and the normal pulmonary trunk is often prominent. In adulthood, the pulmonary trunk is less prominent, and with advancing years the left ventricular contour becomes more convex. In old age, the ascending aorta may become tortuous and project lateral to the superior vena cava, and the aortic knuckle and descending aorta may be increasingly prominent.

The pulmonary vasculature

The pulmonary trunk normally forms a short segment of the left cardiovascular silhouette. The pulmonary arteries are not visible on the chest radiograph until they emerge from the pericardium and are surrounded by aerated lung. The right pulmonary artery lies anterior to the right main bronchus and usually divides into upper lobe and descending arteries just before emerging from the pericardium. The descending branch is usually clearly seen lateral to the right heart border, where it forms the bulk of the right hilum. Its diameter should not exceed 15 mm in females and 16 mm in males. The left pulmonary artery arches posteriorly over the left main bronchus, and, therefore, the left hilum is higher than the right. The branching pattern of the pulmonary arteries is similar to that of the bronchi. As the pulmonary arteries pass peripherally, they taper smoothly and are not normally visible in the outer third of the lung.

Fig. 2 Lateral chest radiograph. Patient with calcific aortic stenosis. The aortic valve is heavily calcified (arrowheads). AA, aortic arch; IVC, inferior vena cava; LA, left atrium; LPA, left pulmonary artery; LV, left ventricle; RPA, right pulmonary artery; RV, right ventricle.

Fig. 1 Normal chest radiograph. The right border of the cardiovascular silhouette comprises superior vena cava (SVC), right atrium (RA), and inferior vena cava (IVC), and the left border comprises aortic knuckle (AK), pulmonary trunk (PA), left atrial appendage (LA) and left ventricle (LV). Transverse cardiac diameter = a + b. Cardiothoracic ratio = (a + b)/ T.

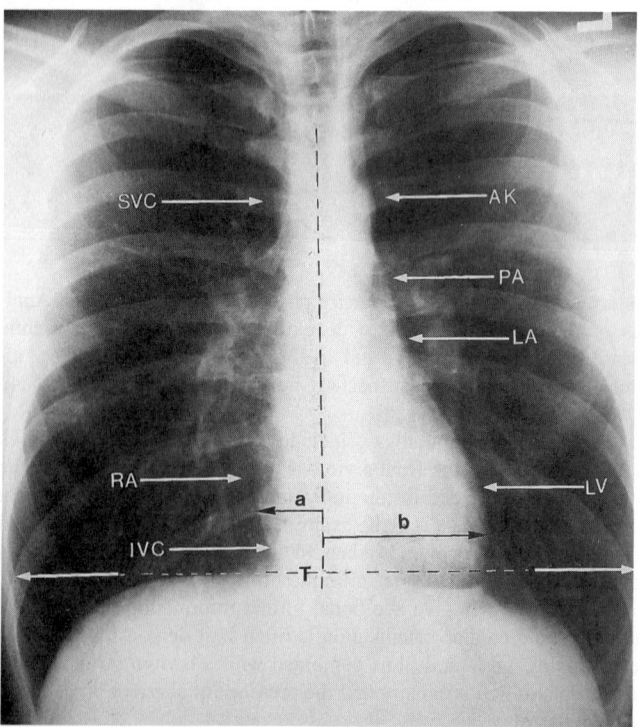

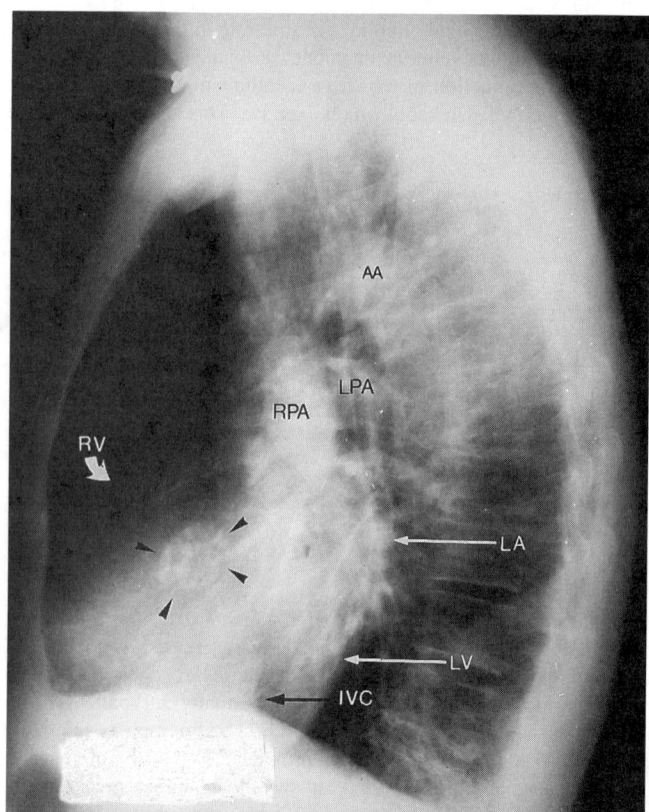

The anatomy of the pulmonary veins is somewhat variable. The upper lobe veins run lateral to the corresponding pulmonary arteries and can often be identified crossing the pulmonary arteries at the hilum prior to entering the left atrium. The lower lobe veins run more horizontally and medially than the accompanying arteries.

On the frontal chest radiograph of a normal, erect subject, the pulmonary vessels should be clearly visible and are larger in the lower zones than in the upper zones. The upper zone veins in the first anterior intercostal space should not exceed 3 mm in diameter. On a supine film, the upper zone and lower zone vessels appear similar in size.

Heart size

The most common methods of assessment of cardiac size using the chest radiograph are the measurement of the transverse cardiac diameter and the measurement of cardiothoracic ratio (see Fig. 1).

The transverse cardiac diameter is measured on a posteroanterior film by adding the maximum distance of the right heart border from the midline to the maximum distance of the left heart border from the mid-line. The upper limit of normal is 16 cm for men and 15 cm for women. A change of 1.5 cm in cardiac diameter should be regarded as significant. Apparent increase in heart size may be due to a poor inspiration; on anteroposterior films geometric magnification of the heart shadow occurs.

The cardiothoracic ratio is the ratio of transverse cardiac diameter to maximum internal diameter of the thorax. There are racial differences in the normal ratio, which should not exceed 50 per cent in white subjects or 55 per cent in black subjects.

Analysis of the chest radiograph

As in all areas of clinical examination, the chest radiograph should be analysed in a careful, systematic manner. It must be remembered that poor radiographic technique may produce spurious appearances. Moreover, the cardiovascular silhouette is such an obvious focus of attention that the bones, soft tissues and upper abdomen may be overlooked. The cardiac shadow provides information about anatomy, but the lungs provide information about haemodynamics. A recommended order of analysis is as follows: technical factors, the bones, the upper abdomen, the lungs and, finally the cardiovascular silhouette.

The abnormal chest radiograph

Technical considerations

On an overexposed chest radiograph the lungs appear blacker than usual and may mimic pulmonary oligaemia. Conversely, an underexposed film may accentuate the pulmonary vascular pattern, or even suggest diffuse lung disease. A chest radiograph taken on expiration may show increased basal shadowing and suggest pulmonary oedema or other some other interstitial pulmonary abnormality, and the heart may appear enlarged. A rotated film may make some structures appear unusually prominent and others unusually small.

The bones

Deformity of the thoracic skeleton may alter the appearance of the heart. Sternal depression (pectus excavatum) usually displaces and rotates the heart to the left producing a characteristic straight left heart border). In the 'straight back syndrome', the anteroposterior diameter of the thorax is decreased and the heart may be compressed between sternum and spine producing a spurious appearance of cardiomegaly on the frontal chest radiograph. Severe scoliosis may not only alter the shape of the mediastinum but may actually cause cardiopulmonary disease.

Congenital deformity of the thoracic skeleton may be associated with cardiac disease. Both sternal depression and 'straight back' may be associated with mitral valve prolapse. Many systemic diseases and congen-ital syndromes which involve the cardiovascular system may also have skeletal manifestations, e.g. in Down's syndrome there may be an atrioventricular septal defect and only eleven pairs of ribs.

Rib notching is usually associated with coarctation of the aorta, but it may be seen in pulmonary atresia and vena caval obstruction or following creation of a Blalock–Taussig shunt. Evidence of previous surgery, such as rib deformity, sternal sutures and prosthetic valves, may also be seen on the chest radiograph.

The upper abdomen

Rarely, patients presenting with chest pain have a hiatus hernia or gallstones, which may be visible on the chest radiograph. In patients with congenital heart disease, information about situs may be visible. In these cases, it is worth noting whether the stomach and liver are normally situated, and also whether the spleen is visible and its location. However, the best indication of atrial situs is given by the tracheobronchial anatomy.

The lungs

The normal radiographic appearance of the lung is produced by pulmonary vessels outlined by aerated lung. Any opacity that is not a vessel should be carefully considered. Since smoking is an important aetiological factor in both cardiovascular and pulmonary disease, it is not surprising that the routine chest radiograph in a cardiac patient may uncover previously unsuspected lung disease.

The pulmonary vascular pattern may be normal, increased, decreased or uneven. Normal pulmonary vascularity does not exclude significant myocardial disease, mild valvular disease or a small intracardiac shunt.

There are four distinct patterns of increased pulmonary vascularity.

1. Pulmonary venous hypertension.
2. Pulmonary arterial hypertension.
3. Pulmonary over-circulation.
4. Systemic supply to the lungs.

Any of these patterns may coexist.

PULMONARY VENOUS HYPERTENSION

Pulmonary venous hypertension is most commonly caused by left ventricular failure, mitral valve disease or aortic valve disease. Rarely, it is due to pulmonary venous obstruction. When pulmonary venous pressure rises, the upper lobe veins distend and become similar in size to the lower lobe veins, and eventually they become larger. This phenomenon may be described as 'upper lobe blood diversion' (Fig. 3). When the pulmonary venous pressure exceeds the plasma osmotic pressure, fluid accumulates in the interstitial spaces of the lung. Radiographically, this appears as interstitial pulmonary oedema. The lower zone and hilar vessels may become indistinct (perihilar haze) and interstitial lines may appear. Kerley B lines are caused by fluid-filled interlobular septa and appear as fine non-branching horizontal lines in the periphery of the lower zones (Fig. 4). Kerley A lines are less common and are longer, fine-line shadows that radiate from the hila into the mid and upper zones. They also represent distended interlobular septa. Excess interstitial fluid around bronchi may appear as peribronchial cuffing. A further rise in pulmonary venous pressure leads to accumulation of fluid in the alveolar spaces (Fig. 5). Classically, alveolar oedema is perihilar, but it may be patchy and asymmetric, or even nodular, and it may be indistinguishable from other forms of pulmonary consolidation. Pleural effusions are common in pulmonary venous hypertension.

In the untreated patient, there is a fairly close correlation between the pulmonary capillary wedge pressure and the radiographic signs of pulmonary venous hypertension. A normal vascular pattern corresponds to a wedge pressure of less than 12 mmHg, redistribution of blood flow corresponds to 12 to 18 mmHg, and interstitial oedema to 18 to 22 mmHg; above 22 mmHg, there is usually overt alveolar oedema. If a patient has received diuretic therapy, this correlation is less reliable.

In patients with long-standing pulmonary venous hypertension radiographic signs of pulmonary arterial hypertension may also be present. Chronic pulmonary venous hypertension may also be associated with pulmonary haemosiderosis or pulmonary ossicles. The former appears as a fine nodular pattern throughout both lungs, and the latter as calcified basal nodules of up to 1 cm in diameter.

Although redistribution of blood flow and septal lines are most often a manifestation of pulmonary venous hypertension, there are other causes which should be considered. Redistribution of blood flow may occur in patients who have basal emphysema and no evidence of pulmonary venous hypertension. Septal lines may be seen in non-cardiogenic pulmonary oedema, lymphangitis carcinomatosa, sarcoidosis, and silicosis.

PULMONARY ARTERIAL HYPERTENSION

Pulmonary arterial hypertension may be defined as a pulmonary artery systolic pressure exceeding 30 mmHg. The most common causes of this condition are chronic lung disease, pulmonary emboli, pulmonary venous hypertension, and intracardiac shunts. It may also be idiopathic. The typical radiographic appearances are enlargement of the central pulmonary arteries and attenuation of the peripheral arteries. In severe long-standing pulmonary arterial hypertension, calcification may be seen in the central pulmonary arteries.

An indication of the underlying cause may be present on the chest radiograph; for example, there may be signs of chronic obstructive airways disease or pulmonary embolism. Bilateral hilar lymph node enlargement may mimic enlarged central pulmonary arteries, but usually lymphadenopathy is lobulated, whereas enlarged arteries have a smooth outline.

PULMONARY OVERCIRCULATION

Pulmonary overcirculation or plethora implies increased blood-flow through the lungs. It is usually due to a left-to-right shunt, less commonly due to bidirectional shunting and rarely due to increased cardiac output. Small shunts may not be perceptible on the chest radiograph, but shunts with a pulmonary-to-systemic flow ratio of 2 : 1 or greater should be apparent unless there is coexisting heart failure. The central pulmonary arteries are larger than normal and peripheral pulmonary vessels are visible in the outer third of the lung (Fig. 6). Pulmonary plethora in a non-cyanosed patient indicates a left-to-right shunt, whereas in the presence of cyanosis it indicates bidirectional shunting.

SYSTEMIC SUPPLY TO THE LUNGS

Systemic arterial supply to the lungs, which is sometimes referred to as 'bronchial circulation', develops in patients with severe right ventricular

Fig. 3 Upper lobe blood diversion. Patient with mitral valve disease. The extra density over the right heart border (arrowheads) is due to left atrial enlargement.

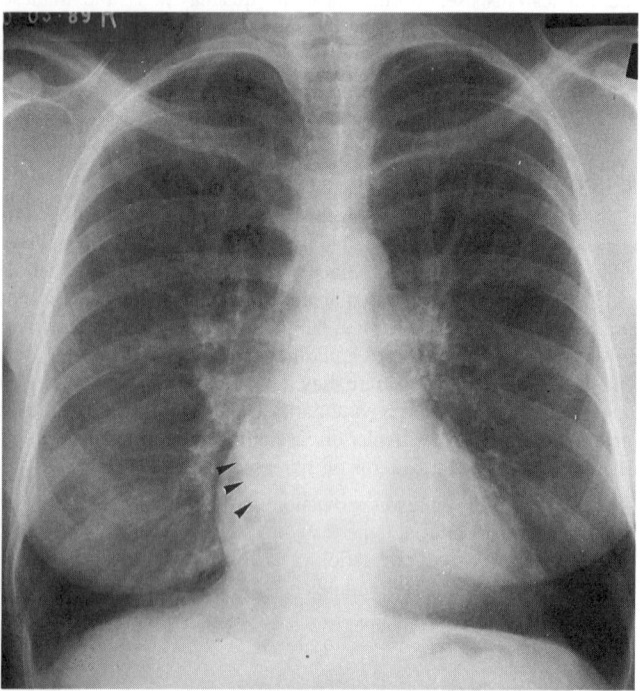

Fig. 4 Kerley B lines. Patient with interstitial pulmonary oedema due to mitral stenosis.

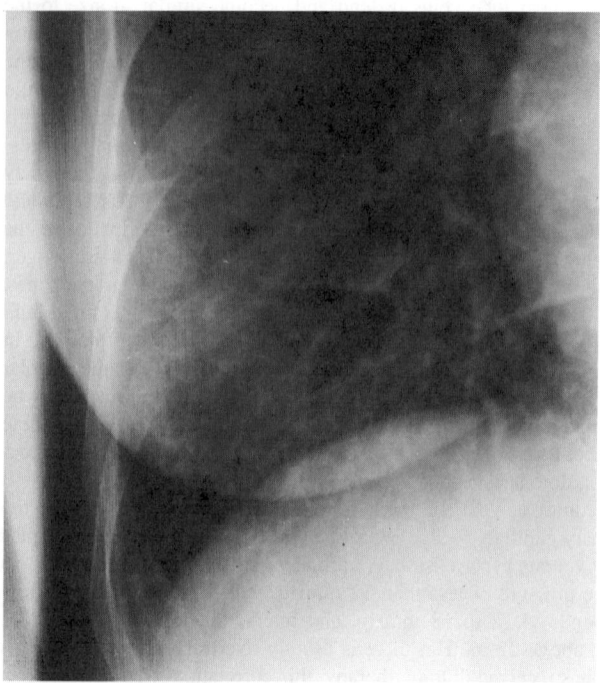

Fig. 5 Severe pulmonary venous hypertension. Patient with acute myocardial infarction. In addition to upper lobe blood diversion, perihilar haze and basal septal lines indicate interstitial oedema, and right lower zone consolidation indicates alveolar oedema.

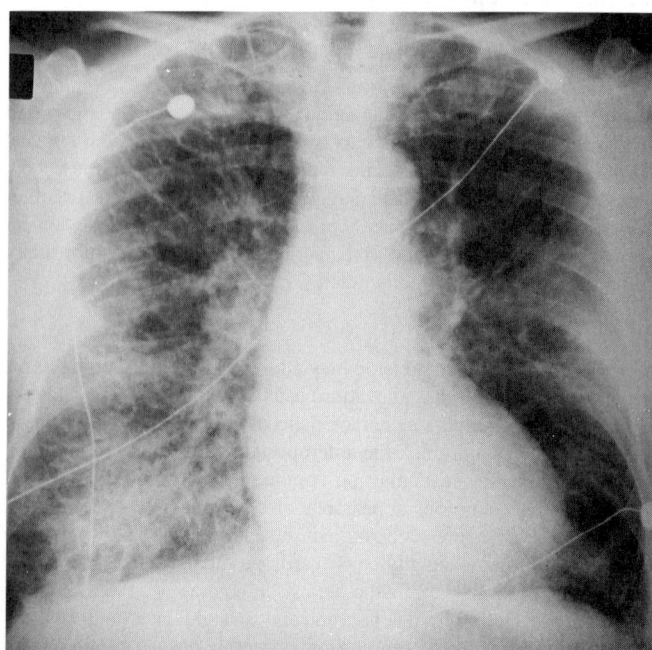

outflow obstruction. The pulmonary trunk is either small or absent, and the peripheral vessels are disorganized and may produce a reticular or nodular pattern that mimics diffuse lung disease.

PULMONARY OLIGAEMIA

Pulmonary oligaemia implies decreased blood flow through the lungs. It is usually due to right ventricular outflow obstruction in association with a right-to-left shunt, e.g. tetralogy of Fallot. The lungs appear to have fewer and smaller vessels than usual, and the pulmonary trunk may be small or inapparent. Pulmonary oligaemia due to restricted filling of the right heart, such as occurs in cardiac tamponade, is rarely perceptible on the chest radiograph.

UNEVEN VASCULARITY

Uneven pulmonary vascularity is most commonly due to pulmonary disease. A previous lung resection will obviously alter the vascular pattern. Apart from pulmonary thromboembolism, cardiovascular causes of uneven vascularity are rare but include previous shunt operations for congenital heart disease, pulmonary artery stenoses, and pulmonary arteriovenous fistulae.

Abnormalities of the heart and great vessels

THE SYSTEMIC VEINS

Enlargement of the superior vena cava may be caused by either increased flow or increased pressure. Increased flow occurs in supracardiac anomalous pulmonary venous return. Increased pressure occurs in right heart failure, tricuspid valve disease, cardiac tamponade, and constrictive pericarditis. The superior vena cava may also dilate secondary to obstruction caused by mediastinitis or mediastinal tumour. The superior vena cava may be displaced laterally by a tortuous or dilated ascending aorta or a right-sided aortic arch.

The azygos vein may enlarge for the same reasons as enlargement of the superior vena cava. An enlarged azygos vein is also seen in superior vena caval obstruction, portal vein obstruction and absence of the hepatic portion of the inferior vena cava in polysplenia.

The inferior vena cava may enlarge secondary to tricuspid valve disease and right heart failure.

Fig. 6 Pulmonary plethora. Infant with transposition of the great arteries. The pulmonary vascular pattern is accentuated; there is also cardiomegaly.

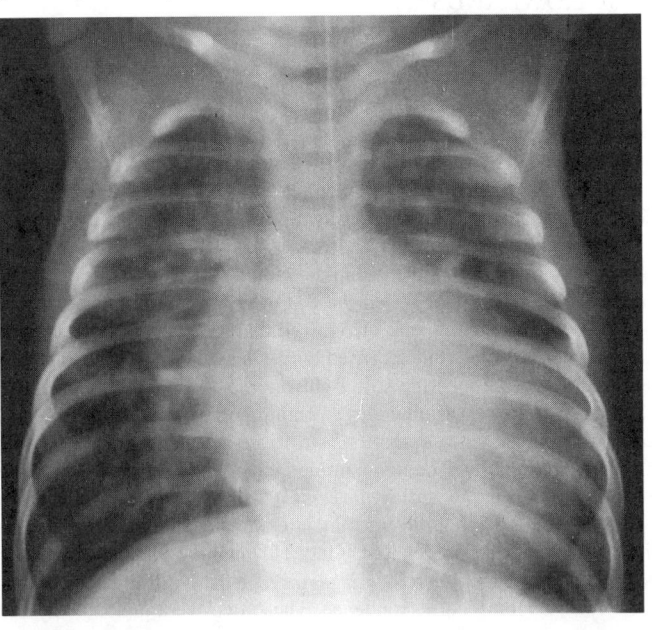

THE RIGHT ATRIUM

Right atrial enlargement rarely occurs in isolation, and is usually associated with right ventricular enlargement. Classically, right atrial enlargement produces increased prominence of the lower half of the right side of the cardiac shadow. Right atrial enlargement occurs in right heart failure, tricuspid valve disease and in atrial septal defect and other shunts that enter the right atrium.

THE RIGHT VENTRICLE

The normal right ventricle is not a border-forming structure on the frontal chest radiograph. An enlarging right ventricle tends to displace the left ventricle laterally so that the cardiac apex becomes elevated. In gross right ventricular enlargement, the right ventricle may actually form the left heart border, and dilatation of its outflow tract may produce a bump just below the pulmonary trunk. On the lateral view, right ventricular enlargement may manifest as increased contact of the heart with the sternum. Right ventricular enlargement occurs in pulmonary arterial hypertension, tricuspid valve disease, pulmonary valve disease, left-to-right shunts and tetralogy of Fallot.

THE PULMONARY TRUNK

Enlargement of the pulmonary trunk is due to increased pressure, increased flow, post-stenotic dilatation or idiopathic dilatation (Fig. 7). In pulmonary arterial hypertension it may be associated with enlargement of the central pulmonary arteries and peripheral pruning. In situations of increased flow, it is associated with pulmonary plethora. In cases of post-stenotic and idiopathic dilatation, it is usually associated with enlargement of the left pulmonary artery and normal peripheral vascularity.

In corrected transposition of the great arteries, the pulmonary trunk

Fig. 7 Patient with mitral stenosis. The transverse cardiac diameter size is normal, but the left atrial appendage is enlarged (curved arrow), and there is also prominence of the pulmonary trunk (arrowhead).

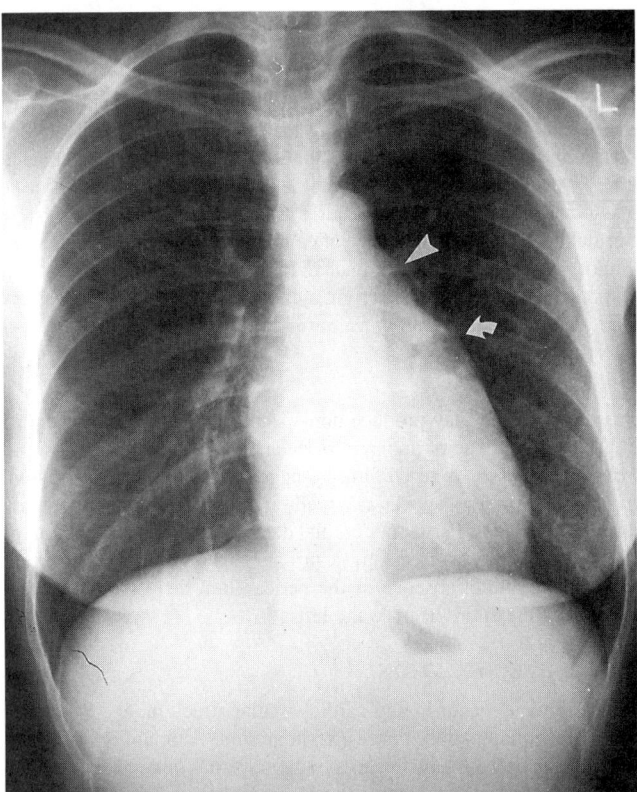

is not visible on the chest radiograph. In tetralogy of Fallot and pulmonary atresia, the pulmonary trunk is small, producing an obvious pulmonary bay.

THE LEFT ATRIUM

The body of the left atrium is situated beneath the carina and in front of the oesophagus. Enlargement superiorly may increase the angle between the left and right bronchi by elevating the left bronchus and displacing it posteriorly. Posterior enlargement may displace the oesophagus posteriorly. Enlargement to the right may produce an extra density over the right heart border (Fig. 3), and if grossly enlarged the left atrium may actually form the right heart border. Enlargement of the left atrial appendage causes straightening or convex bulging of the upper left heart border (Fig. 7). Left atrial enlargement occurs most obviously in mitral valve disease, but is seen in other forms of left heart failure, in shunts at ventricular and great vessel level, and in association with left atrial tumours.

THE LEFT VENTRICLE

Left ventricular hypertrophy produces increased convexity of the left heart border, but not cardiac enlargement unless heart failure develops. Left ventricular dilatation causes displacement of the cardiac apex downward and to the left. On the lateral view, the heart shadow extends more posteriorly than usual. Left ventricular hypertrophy results from systolic overload, and dilatation from diastolic overload. In left ventricular aneurysm, a discrete bulge may develop on the left heart border.

THE AORTA

Selective enlargement of the ascending aorta is seen in post-stenotic dilatation due to aortic valvar stenosis and in association with aneurysms. The aortic knuckle may be prominent due to aneurysm, patent ductus arteriosus, tetralogy of Fallot, and pulmonary atresia. In coarctation of the aorta, the knuckle always appears abnormal – it may be prominent, flat, high, low, or have an abnormal contour. In non-obstructing coarctation or pseudocoarctation, the arch appears elongated and kinked. Selective enlargement of the descending aorta may be due to aneurysm. Generalized prominence of the thoracic aorta may be part of the ageing process but is also seen in systemic hypertension and aortic regurgitation.

The aortic arch is usually left-sided, arching posteriorly over the left main bronchus, but may be right-sided when it arches over the right bronchus and indents the right side of the trachea; the usual shadow of the left arch is then absent, and the superior vena cava may be displaced laterally. A right arch with an aberrant left subclavian artery is not usually associated with heart disease, but if its branches are the mirror image of normal there is a high incidence of congenital heart disease. Tetralogy of Fallot, pulmonary atresia, truncus arteriosus, and ventricular septal defect may be associated with a right arch. An aberrant subclavian artery can be identified on a barium swallow.

THE PERICARDIUM

Pericardial effusion may produce non-specific globular enlargement of the heart shadow. The pulmonary vascularity is usually normal. Rapid increase in heart size on serial films is suggestive of pericardial effusion. A pericardial cyst may appear as a well-circumscribed rounded opacity adjacent to the heart. Partial pericardial defects may allow herniation of the left atrial appendage causing a prominent bulge on the left heart border. In congenital absence of the pericardium there is usually displacement of the entire heart to the left.

CARDIAC CALCIFICATION

Calcification may occur in any cardiovascular structure, and is usually the result of inflammatory disease or infarction. Although cardiac calcification may be visible on the chest radiograph it is better demonstrated by fluoroscopy when movement of an abnormally calcified structure aids its detection, in contrast to the plain film when movement causes blurring.

Myocardial and endocardial calcification most commonly occur in the left ventricle secondary to coronary artery disease. Curvilinear calcification may occur in the wall of left ventricular aneurysms, in thrombi and in infarcts. Left atrial wall calcification may be due to rheumatic myocarditis, and left atrial thrombi may calcify.

Aortic valve calcification usually lies over the spine on the frontal chest radiograph and may, therefore, be obscured. It is best seen on the lateral view (see Fig. 2), and tends to lie mostly above a line drawn from the carina to the anterior costophrenic angle. Mitral valve calcification usually lies to the left of the spine, and on a lateral view lies below the line drawn from carina to the anterior costophrenic angle. Calcification is rarely seen in the tricuspid and pulmonary valves, but commonly occurs in right ventricular outflow tract homografts.

Calcification is frequently seen in the aortic arch of older patients as part of the normal ageing process. Extensive aortic calcification is most likely to be due to atheroma, but it may be the result of an arteritis or syphilitic aortitis, which characteristically involves the ascending aorta. Calcification in a healed dissecting aneurysm may be seen in any part of the aorta. Chronic traumatic aneurysms in the region of the aortic isthmus may calcify.

Coronary artery calcification indicates atheroma, but does not necessarily correspond to significant coronary artery narrowing. A patent ductus arteriosus may calcify, and calcification may develop in the central pulmonary arteries in long-standing, severe pulmonary arterial hypertension.

Pericardial calcification may be a sequel to pericarditis and haemopericardium, and it may be associated with pericardial constriction.

Rare causes of cardiac calcification include tumours, hydatid disease, and coronary artery fistulae.

REFERENCES

Elliott, L.P. (1991). *Cardiac imaging in infants, children and adults.* Lippincott Co., Philadelphia.
Elliott, L.P. and Schiebler, G.L. (1979). *X-ray diagnosis of congenital cardiac disease* 2nd edn. Charles C. Thomas, Springfield.
Jefferson, K. and Rees, S. (1980). *Clinical cardiac radiology,* 2nd edn. Butterworth, London.

15.4.2 The electrocardiogram

D. J. ROWLANDS

Historical introduction

The first electrocardiographic recording of the human heart was made in 1887 by A. D. Waller, who expressed the view that it was unlikely that such recordings would be of much use in clinical practice. This view was not shared by Einthoven, who noted the differences between recordings taken from healthy and from sick persons and was, in consequence, convinced that the technique would prove to be of great clinical value. Einthoven suggested the P, QRS, T, U terminology, which is in universal use today, and recognized that a better recording device than the capillary electrometer (used by Waller) would be necessary. He modified and developed the string galvanometer for this purpose. The resulting instrument was unwieldy, weighing over a quarter of a ton and requiring five people to operate it, but it produced electrocardiograms of remarkable quality. The first commercially available machine for the recording of the electrocardiogram (ECG) was made in England in 1911 by the Cambridge Scientific Instrument Company and was delivered to Sir Thomas Lewis at University College Hospital in London. In the early 1900s Einthoven and Lewis had a series of most fruitful meetings and a vigorous, ongoing correspondence. These two were undoubtedly the pioneers who at that time did most to advance the clinical study of electrocardiography. In the early 1930s the most productive research worker in this field was Frank N. Wilson. Whereas Lewis had concentrated on the cardiac rhythm, Wilson's work was centred on the QRS complexes and T waves. It was Wilson who developed the unipolar recording system, by developing an 'indifferent' electrode that gave a stable reference potential, with respect to which the potential at a single exploring electrode could be measured. This reference potential was obtained from a central terminal which was connected to the left arm, the right arm, and the left leg through equal resistors.

The development of electrocardiographic recording techniques continues (witness the rapidly expanding use of electrophysiological studies of the heart) but the standard 12-lead ECG still forms an essential part of any full clinical cardiological assessment – more than 100 years after the first human ECG recording. It is estimated that in excess of 100 million 12-lead ECGs are recorded annually worldwide, a fact that would surely have astonished Waller. Electrocardiography developed empirically and its basic diagnostic criteria remain empirical. The criteria given here represent a reasonable compromise between sensitivity and specificity.

Normal electrocardiographic appearances

The basic ECG waveform

The basic ECG waveform consists of three recognizable deflections termed 'P wave', 'QRS complex', and 'T wave', by Einthoven (Fig. 1). The P wave is the surface electrocardiographic manifestation of atrial myocardial depolarization. Depolarization of the sinoatrial node is not recognizable on the surface ECG and can only be inferred – from the shape and direction of the P wave. The QRS complex is the surface electrocardiographic manifestation of ventricular myocardial depolarization. The S–T segment and T wave represent ventricular myocardial repolarisation. Atrial myocardial repolarization is indicated by the Ta wave, which is a small, asymmetrical negative wave following the P wave. The Ta wave is usually obscured by the QRS complex, which occurs at the same time. The Ta wave usually becomes easily recognizable during sinus tachycardia (especially during exercise) as it then increases in size and becomes a rounded negative wave begining before the QRS complex and extending into the S–T segment. A prominent atrial repolarization wave occurring during an exercise stress test is frequently wrongly interpreted as S–T segment depression. The key to avoiding this error is to recognize that the negativity begins before the QRS complex. The P wave and T wave have relatively simple shapes which exhibit few variations. The QRS complexes exhibit more readily recognizable differences in pattern in different leads within the same ECG.

QRS waveform nomenclature

The QRS complexes usually have the largest voltages and virtually always the highest frequency components of the various ECG deflections and usually consist of 'sharp', pointed deflections. The presence and relative size of the several possible components of the QRS complex may be indicated by a convention using combinations of the letters q, r, s, Q, R, S (Fig. 2). If a given component is considered to be large, an UPPER CASE letter is used, if it is considered to be small a lower case letter is used.

The twelve conventional ECG leads

Unipolar, bipolar, and augmented leads

Leads I, II, and III are the bipolar limb leads, introduced originally by Einthoven. The remaining three limb leads and the six precordial leads are unipolar (they involve the use of the central terminal of Wilson) and

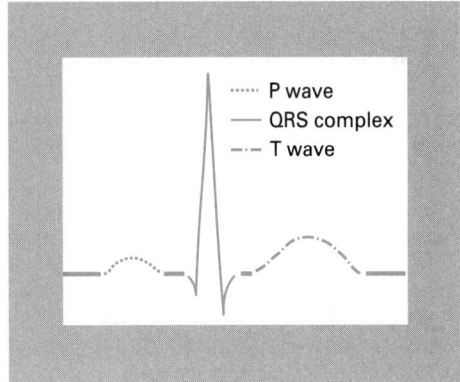

Fig. 1 The basic electrocardiogram waveform.

...... P wave
—— QRS complex
—·— T wave

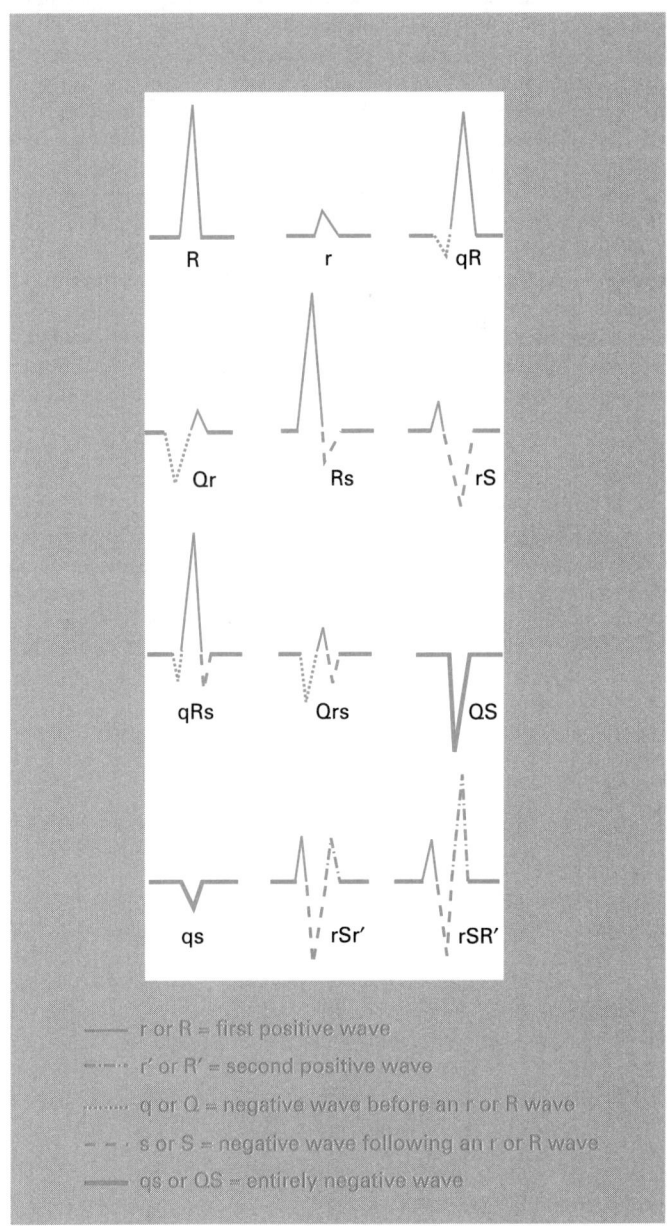

Fig. 2 QRS waveform nomenclature.

R   r   qR

Qr   Rs   rS

qRs   Qrs   QS

qs   rSr′   rSR′

—— r or R = first positive wave
—·— r′ or R′ = second positive wave
······ q or Q = negative wave before an r or R wave
— — s or S = negative wave following an r or R wave
—— qs or QS = entirely negative wave

are termed V leads (the 'V' originally stood for 'voltage', to reflect the fact that these unipolar leads effectively measure the voltage at the location of the recording electrode). All currently available ECG machines use augmented limb leads (i.e. they record aVR, aVL, and aVF as opposed to VR, VL, and VF) as a result of the use of a no-longer-necessary but now standard modification of the original Wilson central terminal. This modification was originally introduced to produce a 1.5 times amplification in the recorded voltage.

The six limb leads (frontal plane leads)

The limb leads are remote from the heart and give (spatially) general rather than localized (i.e. spatially specific) information. In this respect they differ markedly from the precordial leads. The limb leads consist of the three bipolar leads (leads I, II, and III) and the three augmented, unipolar leads aVR, aVL, and aVF. The orientation around the heart of the six limb leads is illustrated in Fig. 3. The orientation of leads aVR, aVL, and aVF with respect to the heart is intuitively obvious because the limbs act as linear conductors (like wires). The left arm connection is therefore effectively 'looking at the heart' from the left shoulder (i.e. the left arm is acting as part of the wire connecting the ECG machine to the patient's left shoulder), the right arm connection from the right shoulder, and the foot lead connection from the pelvic area. One practical consequence of the fact that the limbs act as linear conductors is that it does not matter whereabouts on any given limb the electrode is attached. The orientation of the bipolar leads with respect to the heart is not intuitively obvious (simply because they are bipolar leads) but may be worked out from the known polarities of the conventional connections used in the bipolar leads. Thus, for example, because lead I is recorded with the left arm connected to the positive and the right arm to the negative terminal of the recorder, the position of lead I is effectively that obtained by subtracting the right arm vector from the left arm vector. To subtract vector R from vector L one reverses the direction of vector R and adds it to vector L. Inspection of Fig. 3 reveals that if this is done the resulting 'direction' of lead I is effectively horizontally to the left of the heart. In a similar manner it can be shown that the effective orientations of leads II and III with respect to the heart are as shown in Fig. 3.

The six precordial leads (chest leads)

For each precordial lead, the positive (recording) terminal is connected to an electrode at an agreed site on the chest wall. As the connection to the negative terminal of the recorder is the 'indifferent' one formed by joining together leads R, L, and F, the chest leads are 'V' leads and are designated V_1, V_2, V_3, V_4, V_5, and V_6. As the torso, unlike the limbs, acts as a volume conductor, the waveform obtained depends critically on the siting of the recording electrode. A standard anatomical siting of the precordial electrodes was agreed between the British Cardiac Society and the American Heart Association and is shown in Fig. 4. The important relationships of the precordial leads to the cardiac chambers are shown in Fig. 5.

The twelve conventional ECG leads

Figure 6 shows the relationship of the 12 conventional electrocardiographic leads to one another and to the heart.

Recognizing the normal electrocardiogram

This is the most difficult and the most important aspect of understanding the electrocardiogram. The electrocardiogram is recognized as being within or beyond normal limits by the normality or otherwise of the shape and dimensions of its various substituent deflections, and the frequency of the deflections and their relationship in time to the deflections preceding and succeeding them. This introduction to the subject consid-

Fig. 4 The positions of the precordial leads. V_1, is located at the right sternal margin in the fourth intercostal space, V_2 at the left sternal margin at the fourth intercostal space, V_4 at the intersection of the left midclavicular line and left fifth intercostal space, V_3 mid-way between V_2 and V_4, V_5 at the intersection of the left anterior axillary line with a horizontal line through V_4, and V_6 at the intersection of the left midaxillary line with a horizontal line through V_4 and V_5 (reproduced, with permission, from Rowlands, 1991).

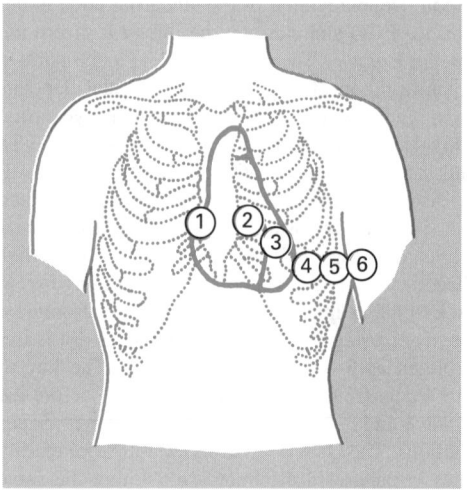

Fig. 5 The precordial leads and their important anatomical relationship to the main cardiac chambers (reproduced, with permission, from Rowlands, 1991).

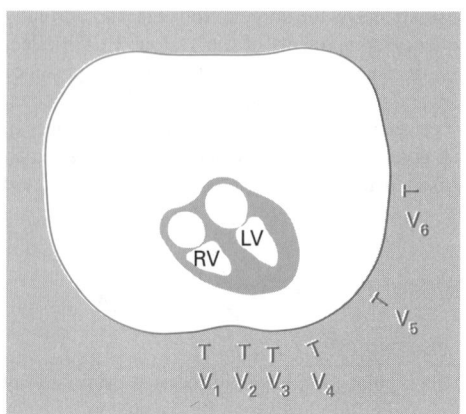

Fig. 3 The arrangement of the frontal plane leads. Note that leads Il, III, and F are inferior to the heart, I and L are anterolateral to the heart, and R looks into the cavity of the heart (reproduced, with permission, from Rowlands, 1991).

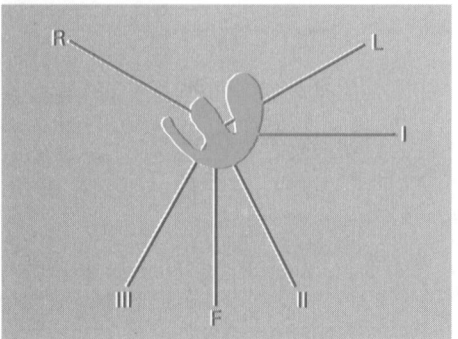

ers only morphological normality or abnormality. The presence of sinus rhythm will therefore be assumed. The criteria for normality of the P waves obtain in any rhythm where atrial depolarization is of sinus origin (sinus tachycardia, sinus bradycardia, sinus arrhythmia, first, second, or third degree heart block). Those for the QRS complexes, S–T segments, and T waves obtain in any rhythm of supraventricular origin, provided the rate is not so rapid as to induce functional bundle branch block. A supraventricular rhythm is one initiated at a site above the bifurcation of the His bundle.

Normal QRS appearances in the precordial leads

QRS morphology

The QRS complex in V_1 typically shows a small initial positive wave followed by a larger negative wave and in V_6 a small initial negative wave followed by a large positive wave. In general the size of the initial positive wave (r or R wave) increases progressively from V_1 to V_6 (Fig. 7(a)). The direction of the initial part of the QRS is generally upward (i.e. positive) in V_1–V_3, and downward (i.e. negative) in V_4–V_6. That is, V_1–V_3 show initial r waves and V_4–V_6 initial q waves. Leads showing an rS complex are being primarily influenced by right ventricular myocardium and leads showing a qR complex by left ventricular myocardium. The transition zone between right and left ventricular epicardial leads is seen (Fig. 7(b)) to be between V2 and V4. When the transition zone falls outside this region the heart is said to be rotated. If the transition zone occurs further to the left in the precordial series (for example between V_5 and V_6) then the heart is said to be clockwise rotated. Conversely if the transition zone is moved to the right in the precordial series, the heart is said to be counter-clockwise rotated. Clockwise and counter-clockwise rotation refer to a normal state of variability between one subject and another and are not in themselves indicative of abnormality. For a detailed understanding of clockwise and counter-clockwise rotation, more extensive works should be consulted. Although, as stated above, V_1 usually shows an rS complex and V_6 a qR complex, it is also possible for V_1 to show a QS complex and for V_6 to show a monophasic R wave, a QRS complex or an Rs complex (Fig. 7(c)).

QRS dimensions

The dimensions of the individual waves making up each part of the precordial QRS complexes are of crucial importance in determining normality or otherwise. Figure 8 shows how measurements within the QRS complexes are obtained. The criteria for normality of these individual waves are:

1. *Minimum voltage*: at least one R wave in the precordial leads must exceed 8 mm in height.
2. *Maximum voltage*: (a) the tallest R wave in the left precordial leads must not exceed 27 mm; (b) the deepest S wave in the right precordial leads must not exceed 30 mm; (c) the sum of the tallest R wave in the left precordial leads and the deepest S wave in the right precordial leads must not exceed 40 mm.
3. *Maximum duration*: the total QRS duration in any one precordial lead must not exceed 0.10 s (two and a half small squares).
4. *q wave criteria*: (a) no precordial q wave must equal or exceed 0.04 (one small square); (b) precordial q waves must not have a depth greater than a quarter of the height of the R wave in the same lead and
5. *The ventricular activation time*, also known as 'intrinsic deflection time', in leads facing the left ventricle (i.e. showing qR complexes) must not exceed 0.04 (one small square).

Normal precordial T waves

The criteria given below for normality of the T waves are applicable to adults only.

T waves in lead V_1

In this lead 80 per cent of normal adults have upright T waves and 20 per cent have flat or inverted T waves. Therefore, the finding of an inverted T wave in V_1 cannot be considered an abnormality (unless it was upright in a previous ECG).

T waves in lead V_2

About 95 per cent of normal adults show upright T waves and 5 per cent have flat or inverted T waves in V_2. Therefore there is a 1 in 20 possibility of inverted T waves in V_2 occurring by chance and not indicating an abnormality. However, if the T wave in V_2 is inverted when it was formerly upright, it is abnormal. Further, if there is T wave inversion in V_2 with an upright T wave in V_1 the T wave in V_2 is abnormal.

T waves in leads V_3–V_6

The T wave is normally upright in these leads. T wave inversion in V_4, V_5, or V_6 is always abnormal. T wave inversion in V_3, as well as in V_1 and V_2, may (rarely) be found in healthy young adults.

T wave size

There are no strict criteria for T wave size. In general the tallest precordial T wave is found in V_3 or V_4, and the smallest in V_1 and V_2 and, as a general rule, the T wave should not be less than 1/8 and not more than 2/3 of the height of the preceding R wave in each of the leads V_3–V_6.

Normal precordial S–T segments

There is a single rule for normality of the S–T segment. It must not deviate by more than 1 mm above or below the isoelectric line in any precordial lead. The isoelectric line is that vertical position of the ECG recording when no part of the heart is being depolarized or repolarized

Fig. 6 The conventional 12 electrocardiogram leads and their relationship to the heart.

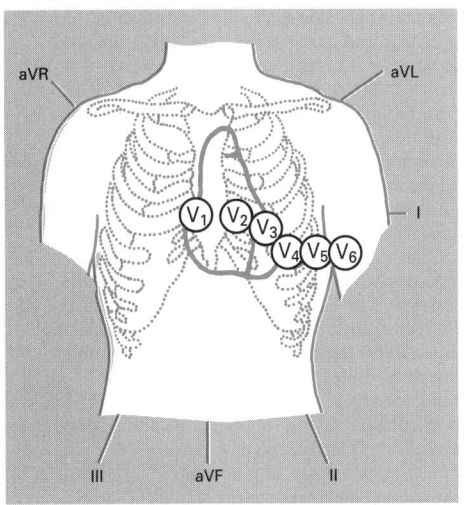

15 CARDIOVASCULAR DISEASE

(i.e. the interval between the end of one T wave and the beginning of the next P wave).

Normal precordial P waves

The P waves are usually upright from V_4–V_6. Upright or biphasic P waves may occur in V_1 and V_2. If the P waves are biphasic, the negative (terminal) component of the P wave should have an area no greater than the positive (initial) component.

Normal limb lead QRS complexes

Only three criteria need to be applied to the limb leads to determine the normality or otherwise of the QRS complexes:

(1) the size of any q waves in aVL, I, II, or aVF;
(2) the size of the R waves in aVL and aVF;
(3) the electrical axis of the heart.

Q wave size

Any q wave present in lead I, II or aVF must not exceed 1/4 the height of the ensuing R wave and must not equal or exceed 0.04 s in duration. Any q wave present in aVR or lead III should be ignored irrespective of its size. Q waves present in aVL should fulfil the same criteria as those in leads I, II, or aVF unless the frontal plane QRS axis is more positive than $+ 60°$, in which case large q waves in aVL are acceptable, as aVL is then a cavity lead (and may therefore have a QS complex as aVR, which is virtually always a cavity lead, usually has).

R wave size

The R wave in aVL must not exceed 13 mm and that in aVF must not exceed 20 mm.

The frontal plane axis

The electrical axis of the heart must not lie outside the limits of $- 30°$ to $+ 90°$ (travelling clockwise). The significance and technique of determination of the electrical axis are described in larger texts.

Normal limb lead S–T segments

Normal S–T segments do not deviate above or below the isoelectric line by more than 1 mm.

Normal limb lead T waves

In general, the T waves and QRS complexes in the limb leads are concordant, i.e. when the QRS complexes are upright, the T waves are

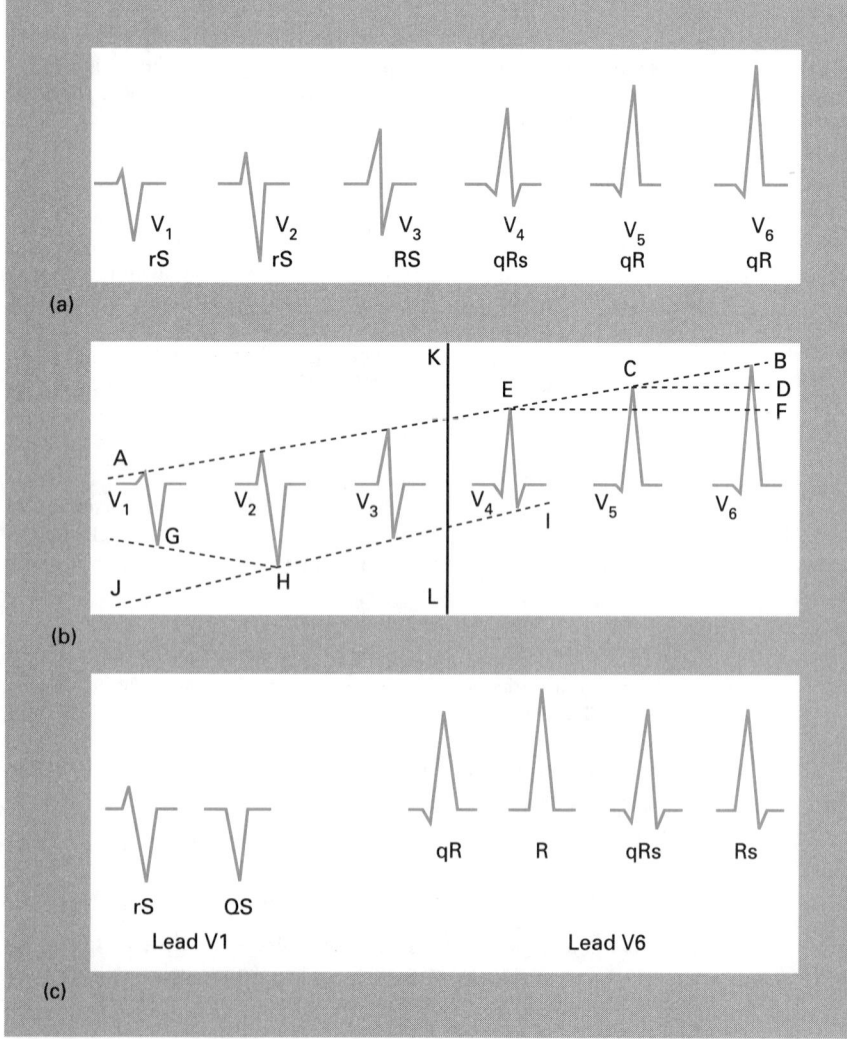

Fig. 7 Morphology of the precordial QRS complexes. (a) Typical normal QRS morphology of the precordial leads (reproduced, with permission, from Rowlands, 1991). (b) Normal variations of R wave amplitude and S wave depth in the precordial leads. The R wave in each precordial lead is usually larger than in the preceding lead in the series from V_1–V_6 (line AB). However, it is quite normal for the R wave in V_6 to be smaller than that in V_5 (line CD) or for the R wave in V_5 to be smaller than that in V_4, provided that the R wave in V_6 is also smaller than that in V_5 (line EF). The size of the S wave diminishes progressively across the precordial leads (line JI), although the S wave in V_2 is often greater than that in V_1 (line GHI). Leads before line KL have an initial deflection which is positive and those after line KL have an initial deflection which is negative. This line marks the transition zone between right and left ventricular QRS configurations (i.e. between rS and qR configurations, respectively) (reproduced, with permission, from Rowlands, 1991). (c) Possible normal QRS configurations in leads VI and V6. Typically, V_1 has an rS configuration but a QS configuration is also normal in this lead. Typically V_6 has a qR configuration but it is also normal for V_6 to show an R wave, a qRs complex or an Rs complex.

upright and when the QRS complexes are negative the T waves are negative. A normal T wave will always be negative in aVR and positive in I and II. T waves can be positive or negative in aVL, aVF, and II without necessarily indicating abnormality. A rough guide to assess normality of the T waves in the limb leads is:

(1) in any lead in which the QRS is predominantly upright, the T wave must be clearly upright;
(2) in any lead in which the QRS is predominantly negative, the T wave should be clearly negative;
(3) in any lead in which the algebraic sum of QRS deflections is close to zero, the T wave may be positive or negative (though small in either case) or isoelectric (flat);
(4) the normal T wave is always upright in leads I and II.

Normal limb lead P waves

The limb lead which normally best shows the P wave is lead II. In this lead the normal P wave duration does not exceed 0.12 s and its height does not exceed 2.5 mm

All the above criteria are dependent upon a normal (standard) calibration and a normal paper recording speed.

Myocardial hypertrophy

Appreciable hypertrophy of the right or left ventricle produces characteristic changes in the electrocardiogram. Lesser degrees of hypertrophy may be present without electrocardiographic changes or with only minor, non-specific changes. This is more often true of right than of left ventricular hypertrophy.

Left ventricular hypertrophy

The increased bulk of the left ventricle increases the voltage induced during left ventricular depolarization. This results in taller R waves in the left precordial leads and deeper S waves in the right precordial leads. The increased ventricular wall thickness also results in prolongation of the time taken to for the depolarization wave to travel from endocardium to epicardium, i.e. it increases the ventricular activation time. In addition, secondary changes in depolarization occur changing the S–T segments and T waves. The electrocardiographic criteria for left ventricular hypertrophy are:

(1) at least one R wave in the left precordial leads exceeds 27 mm;
(2) at least one S wave in the right precordial leads exceeds 30 mm;
(3) the sum of the tallest R wave and the deepest S wave in the precordial leads exceeds 40 mm;
(4) the largest positive or negative deflection in the limb leads exceeds 20 mm;
(5) the intrinsic deflection time (ventricular activation time) exceeds 0.04 s;
(6) S–T segment depression and T wave inversion may occur in the left precordial leads and in those limb leads which face the left ventricle.

The presence of one or more of the above abnormalities indicates the presence of left ventricular hypertrophy only provided that the total QRS duration does not exceed 0.10 s. Left ventricular hypertrophy is a graded, rather than an all-or none diagnosis. The greater the number of criteria fulfilled, the more confident one can be of the diagnosis. The voltage criteria have the greatest sensitivity and the intrinsic deflection time the greatest specificity. Caution should be exercised when diagnosing left

ventricular hypertrophy on the basis of voltage criteria alone, especially if the patient is slim. An example of clearcut electrocardiographic changes of left ventricular hypertrophy is shown in Fig. 9.

Right ventricular hypertrophy

Increased bulk of the right ventricle gives rise to higher voltages during right ventricular depolarization, increasing the size of the positive deflection in the right precordial leads. In addition, it shifts the electrical axis towards the right and changes the S–T segments and T waves, in leads facing the right ventricle, because of secondary changes in the repolarization process. The electrocardiographic criteria for right ventricular hypertrophy are:

(1) a positive deflection equal to or greater than the negative deflection in V_1 (RS, Rs, qR, rR′) in the presence of a normal total QRS duration;
(2) a mean frontal plane QRS axis more positive than + 90°;
(3) S–T segment depression and T wave inversion in right precordial leads.

The more features present, the more convincing is the electrocardiographic evidence for right ventricular hypertrophy but, in general, the combination of a dominant positive deflection of the QRS in V_1 and an abnormal degree of right axis deviation (axis more positive than + 90°) establishes the diagnosis. Examples are shown in Fig. 10. In both exam-

Fig. 8 The dimensions of constituent waves within QRS complexes. (a) Wave voltage measurements. (b) Wave duration measurements (reproduced, with permission, from Rowlands, 1991).

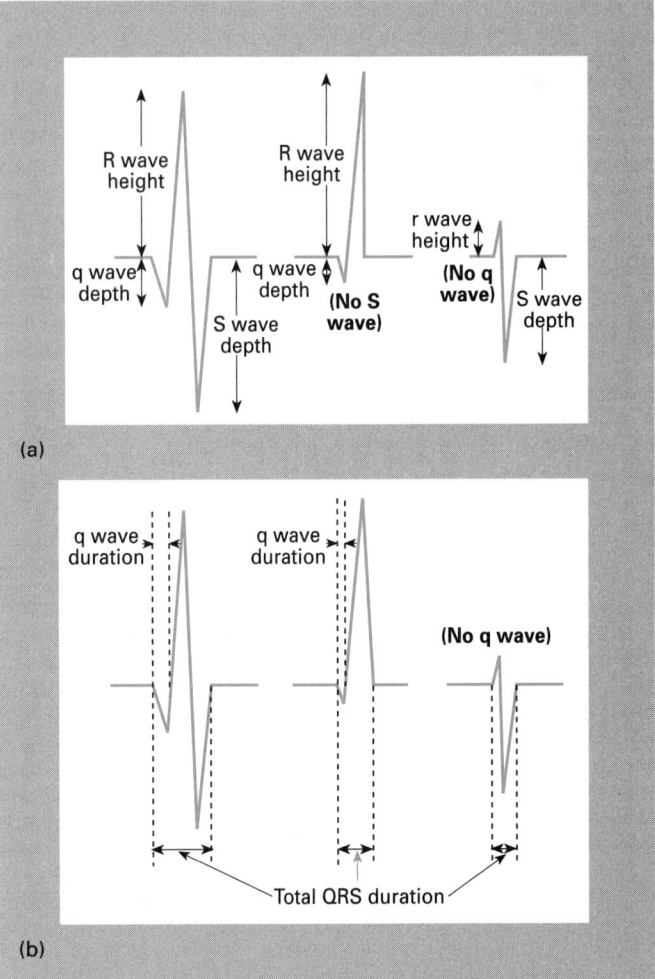

ples there is abnormal right axis deviation and a dominant R wave in V_1. Figure 10(a) shows an Rs complex in V_1 and Fig. 10(b) shows a qR complex. Figure 10(b) also shows pronounced clockwise cardiac rotation, which often accompanies right ventricular hypertrophy.

Atrial hypertrophy

The electrocardiographic changes produced by left atrial hypertrophy are those produced by an increase in the voltage and duration of the left atrial depolarization wave. As the terminal part of the normal P wave is produced by left atrial depolarization, it follows that the total P wave duration is prolonged in left atrial hypertrophy. In addition, the P wave tends to be bifid in lead II and biphasic in V_1. In V_1 the area of the (terminal) negative component exceeds the area of the (initial) positive component (see Figs 9 and 11).

The electrocardiographic change produced by right atrial hypertrophy is an increase in the peak voltage of the P wave. This is usually best seen in lead II. In lead II the P wave voltage is abnormal when it exceeds 3 mm (see Fig. 10(b)).

Bundle branch block

Total failure of conduction in the right or left branches of the bundle of His (bundle branch block) can only be diagnosed with confidence from the appearances in the precordial leads, although there are also changes in the appearances of the limb leads.

Right bundle branch block

In right bundle branch block, the primary change induced is a delay in depolarization in the right ventricular free wall. This results in the development of a second positive wave in right ventricular leads (and a second negative wave in left ventricular leads), and prolongs the total QRS duration. The essential electrocardiographic features of right bundle branch block are:

(1) a total QRS duration of 0.12 s or more;
(2) the presence of a secondary positive wave in V_1 (rsR′, rR′). In addition, secondary changes occur, but these are not in themselves essential for the definitive diagnosis. These include:
(3) deep and slurred S waves in lead I, aVL, and V_4–V_6;
(4) secondary S–T, T changes in leads V_1–V_3.

An example of the appearances in right bundle branch block is shown in Fig. 12.

Left bundle branch block

Left bundle branch block induces more extensive changes in the electrocardiographic appearance than right bundle branch block. Not only is depolarization of the free wall of the left ventricle delayed (a precise corollary of the changes in right bundle branch block), but also the direction of depolarization of the interventricular septum is from right to left instead of from left to right as in the normal electrocardiogram. This reversal of the direction of septal depolarization gives rise to widespread and major alterations in the QRS complexes in every lead of the electrocardiogram. The diagnostic criteria for left bundle branch block are:

(1) a total QRS duration equal to or in excess of 0.12 s;
(2) absence of the normal (septal) q waves in lead I, aVL, and V_4–V_6;
(3) the absence of a secondary r wave in V_1.

This last criterion is necessary to prevent confusion in cases of right bundle branch block, which gives a QRS deviation of 0.12 s or more, occurring in the presence of pronounced clockwise cardiac rotation, which gives loss of q waves in left ventricular leads. The finding of a

Fig. 9 Left ventricular hypertrophy. There is evidence also of left atrial hypertrophy (reproduced, with permission, from Rowlands, 1991).

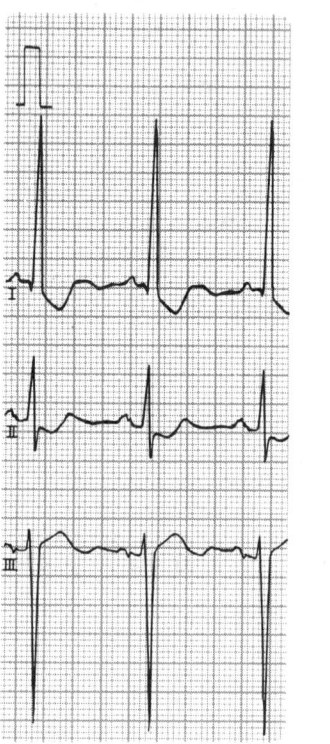
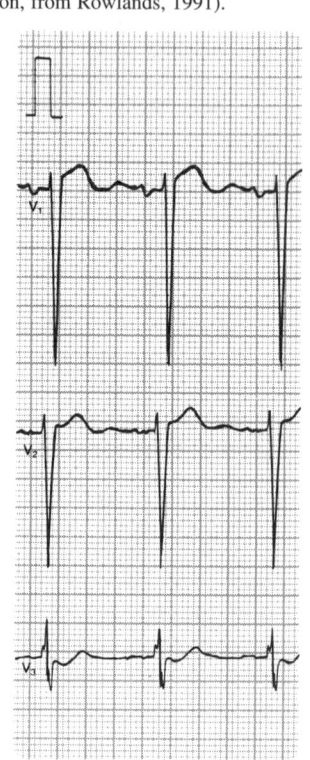
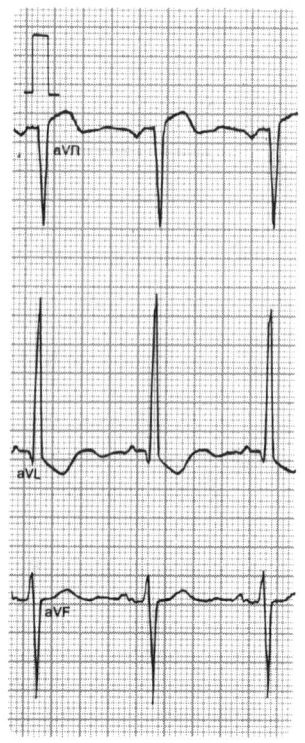
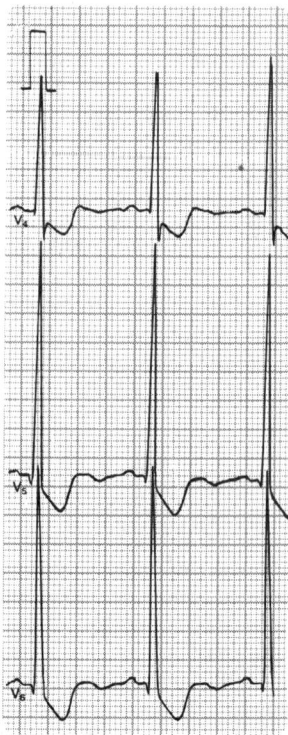

secondary r wave in V_1 in the presence of an abnormally wide QRS complex indicates the presence of right bundle branch block.

Secondary changes also inevitably occur but these are not part of the diagnostic process. These include:

(4) secondary S–T depression and T wave inversion in leads I, aVL, and V_4–V_6;

(5) broad QS waves in V_1–V_3;

(6) notching of the R waves giving rise to rsR′ or M-shaped QRS complexes;

(7) broad, R waves in leads I, aVL, and V_4–V_6.

An example of the ECG appearances in left bundle branch block is shown in Fig. 13. The changes in left bundle branch block so disturb the normal pattern of the ECG that none of the usual criteria can be applied for determining any other abnormality of

Fig. 10 Two examples of right ventricular hypertrophy. There is also right atrial hypertrophy (reproduced, with permission, from Rowlands, 1991).

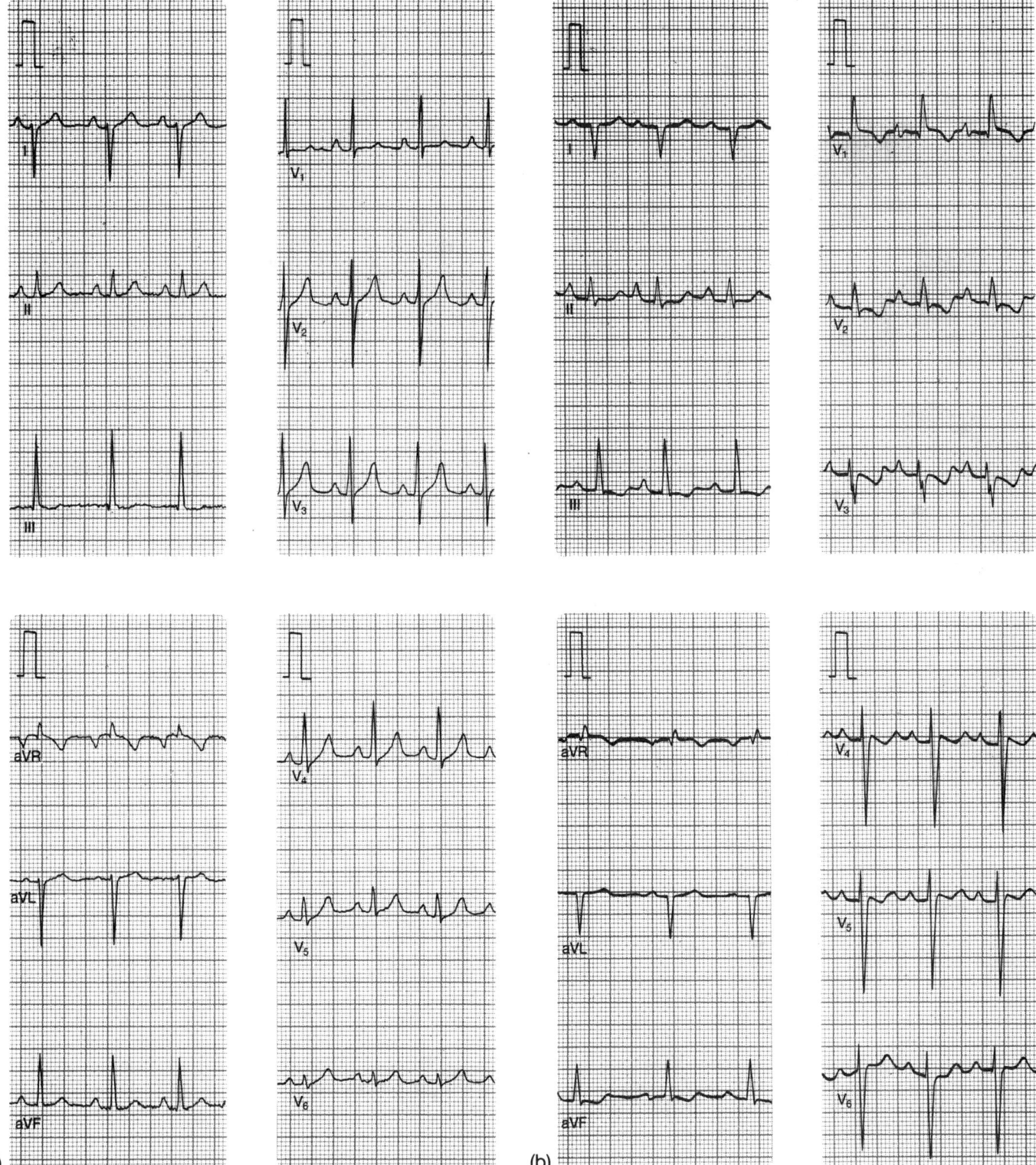

(a)

(b)

the QRS complexes, S–T segments, or P waves. When left bundle branch block is present, a diagnosis of right or left ventricular hypertrophy, myocardial ischaemia or infarction, or of non-specific changes in the S–T segments and T waves cannot easily or reliably be made.

Fig. 11 Left atrial hypertrophy. Broad, bifid P waves in lead ll. Biphasic P waves in V_1, with dominant negative component (reproduced, with permission, from Rowlands, 1991).

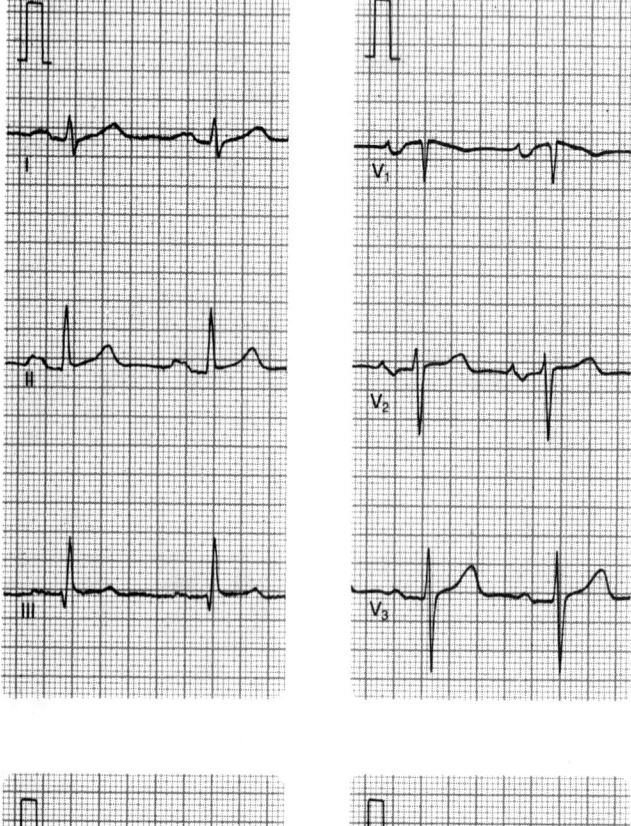

The electrocardiogram in ischaemic heart disease

ECG changes in ischaemic heart disease are very variable, depending on the site and severity of the ischaemic damage. However, certain patterns are commonly produced.

Fig. 12 Right bundle branch block (reproduced, with permission, from Rowlands, 1991).

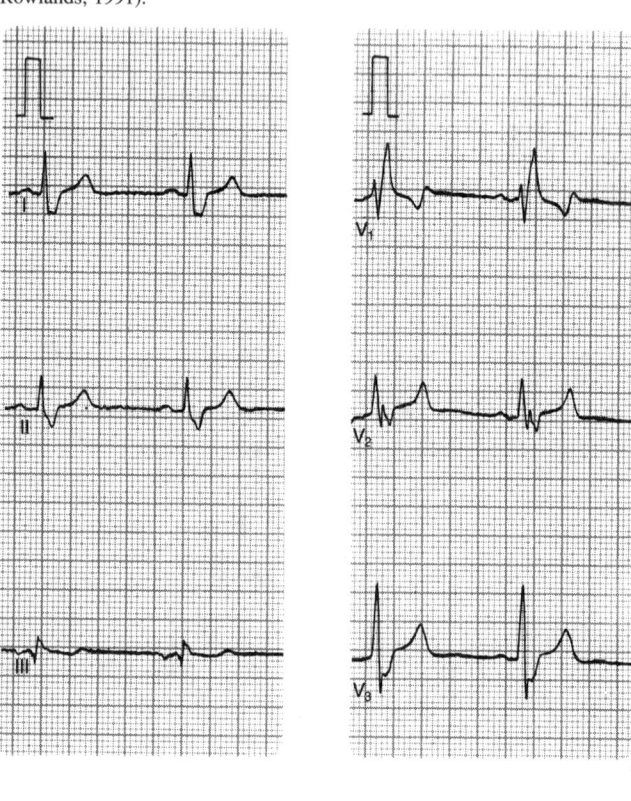

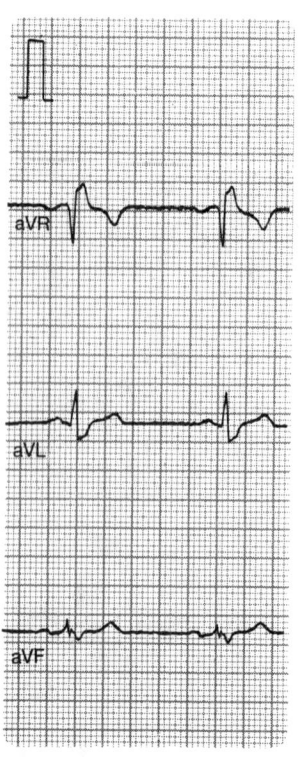

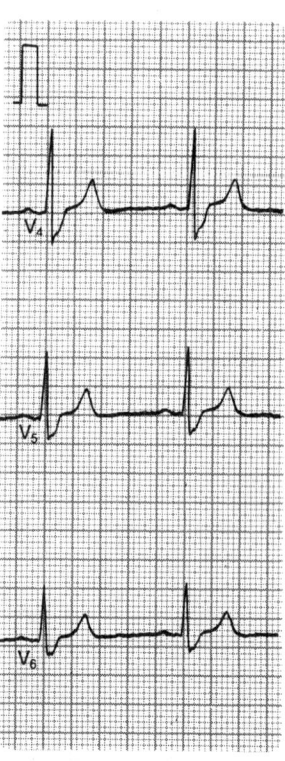

Myocardial infarction QRS changes

Two QRS changes are indicative of myocardial infarction. These are:

    (1) inappropriately low R wave voltage in a local area;
    (2) abnormal q waves.

Fig. 13 Left bundle branch block (reproduced, with permission, from Rowlands, 1991).

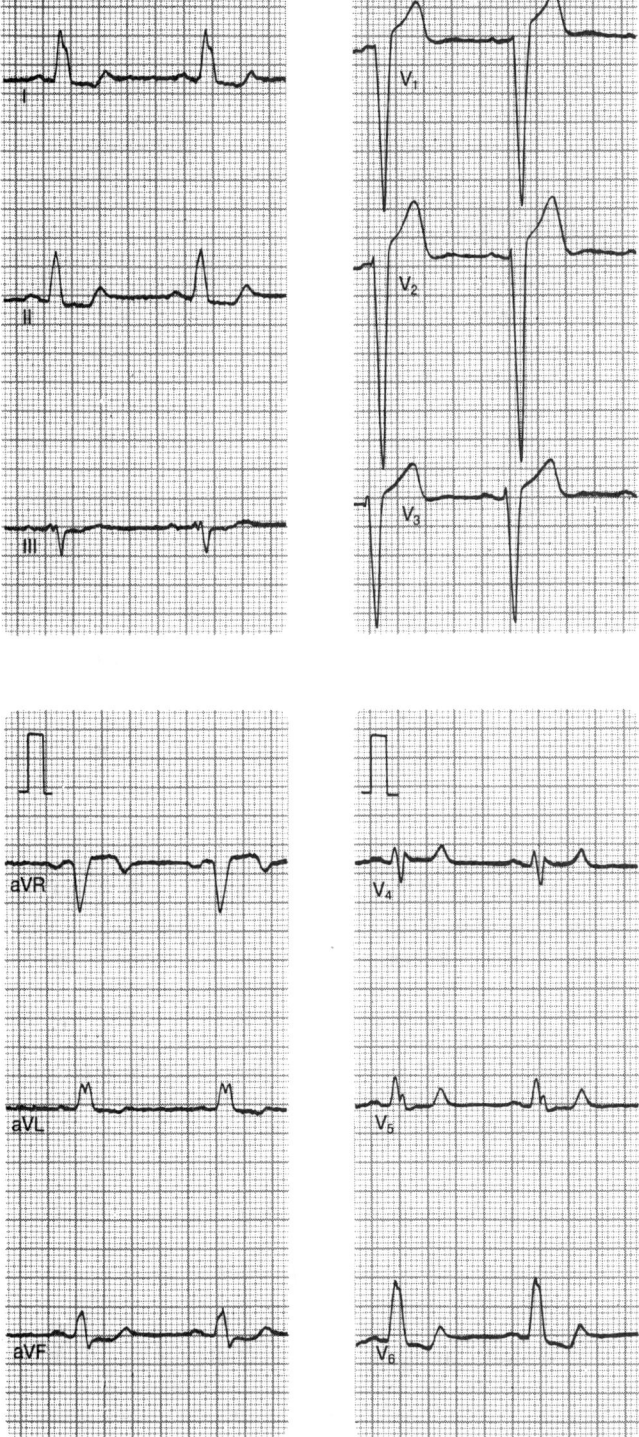

These two changes represent parts of the same process. The development of increased negativity (abnormal q waves) and the reduction in the normal positivity (loss of R wave height) of QRS complexes in the precordial leads each result from a loss of underlying viable muscle, with a consequent reduction in the normally generated positive voltage. When there is full thickness (transmural) myocardial infarction in an area of myocardium underlying the precordial leads there is total loss of the positive deflection. In this situation a totally negative wave (QS complex) occurs. This totally negative wave occurs as a result of depolarization of the posterior wall of the ventricle travelling (posteriorly) from endocardium to epicardium in the normal way and no longer swamped by the usual simultaneous and dominant depolarization towards the exploring electrode of the anterior wall of the ventricle.

The normal precordial QRS complexes show a progressive increase in the R wave height from V_1–V_6 (Fig. 14). The positive (upgoing) part of the deflection in each precordial lead is predominantly the result of depolarization from underlying endocardium to epicardium. In the presence of infarction of part of the left ventricle, the positive waves overlying the necrotic area will be reduced in size (Fig. 15). Loss in R wave height can only be used as a criterion for myocardial infarction if either: (1) larger, normal R waves are visible on both sides of the infarcted zone; or (2) previous ECGs are available demonstrating the normal R wave height for that particular lead in that particular subject. If a major part of the thickness of the myocardial wall is infarcted, the positive wave generated by any remaining viable left ventricular myocardium underlying the electrode is insufficient to overcome the negative deflection induced by the normal depolarization of the interventricular septum from left to right and of the free wall of the right ventricle (or the posterior wall of the left ventricle) from endocardium to epicardium. In this situation an abnormal q wave will develop. In the precordial leads, a q wave is abnormal if its duration is equal to or in excess of 0.04 s or if its depth is greater than 1/4 the height of the ensuing R wave in that lead. In Fig. 15, the q wave in V_4 satisfies this criterion. If the infarction involves the full thickness of the ventricular wall (transmural infarction), no R wave is generated at all and an entirely negative (QS) wave develops (Fig. 16). Figure 17 shows (in diagrammatic form) the appearances produced in the precordial leads when infarcts of varying thickness occur under each of three precordial electrodes. The QRS complex in V_3 is of QS type and indicates transmural infarction at this site. The appearances in V_4 indicate a substantial loss of myocardium underlying that electrode. The q wave is abnormal in duration and depth. The appearances in V_5 indicate a thinner zone of infarction. The q wave is not, in itself, abnormal but the R wave height is less than would be predicted from the height of the R waves present in V_2 and V_6.

The diagnosis of myocardial infarction in the limb leads depends entirely on the presence of abnormal q waves. Q waves of any size may be seen in the normal ECG in aVR and in lead III. In leads I, II, and aVF, q waves equal to or greater than 0.04 s in duration or with a depth in excess of 1/4 the height of the ensuing R wave are abnormal and, unless a defect of intraventricular conduction is known to be present, indicate myocardial infarction. The same is also true of abnormal q waves in aVL, except when the mean frontal plane QRS axis is equal to or more positive than + 60°; in this situation aVL becomes a cavity lead like aVR.

S–T segment changes of infarction

Only changes in the QRS complexes provide definitive evidence of infarction, but in the acute stages of myocardial infarction S–T segment shift occurs. Strictly speaking this shift is evidence of injury to, rather than infarction of, the myocardium. Thus, although in the vast majority of cases the development of typical S–T segment elevation is followed by the development of definitive QRS changes, occasionally the ECG with S–T segment changes of myocardial injury will revert to normal within hours or days. This does not happen if definitive QRS changes of infarction are also present. It is marginally more likely to occur following the use of thrombolytic therapy but is still relatively uncommon. The essential change of myocardial injury is deviation of the S–T segment above the isoelectric line. The S–T segment shift must be in excess of 1 mm to be significant. Minor degrees of S–T segment elevation in the right precordial leads are very common in normal ECGs and S–T segment elevation of up to 2 mm may be accepted as within normal limits in V_1 and V_2. Significant S–T segment elevation occurs in transmural and subepicardial infarction in leads facing the infarct. S–T segment depression occurs in leads facing the infarct when it is subendocardial. S–T segment depression also occurs as a reciprocal change (see below) in leads opposite to those showing the primary changes of acute infarction.

T wave changes of infarction

A variety of T wave changes occurs in association with myocardial infarction. These include flattened, diphasic, and inverted (negative) T waves. None of these changes is specific. Whilst they are always abnormal in leads V_4–V_6 and in those limb leads showing clearly upright QRS complexes, they may be caused by factors other than infarction or ischaemia, including electrolyte changes, digitalis effect, pericarditis, myocarditis, changes in body position, and changes in oesophageal temperature. T wave changes are never, in themselves, reliable indicators of infarction although characteristic T wave changes do occur in relation to the latter. The most typical T wave change associated with infarction is the development of deep, symmetrically inverted T waves (Fig. 18).

The sequence of ECG changes in infarction

Any combination of the QRS, S–T segment, and T wave changes described above may occur in relation to acute infarction of the myocardium but commonly a typical sequence of changes can be recognized (Fig. 19). Typically, S–T segment elevation (which is convex upwards) appears within hours of the onset of symptoms. At this stage no change in the QRS complex can be recognized. Within one to three days, reduction in the R wave height occurs, abnormally deep and broad q waves

Fig. 14 Normal R wave progression in the precordial series (reproduced, with permission, from Rowlands, 1991).

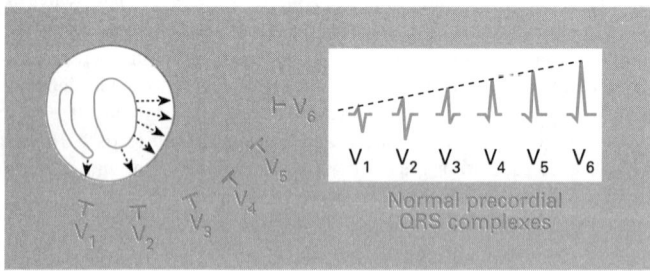

Fig. 15 Loss of R wave height in myocardial infarction. The R wave height is reduced in leads V_3 to V_5 (reproduced, with permission, from Rowlands, 1991).

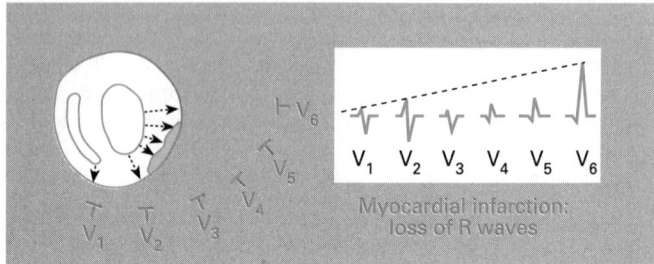

develop, some reduction in the extent of S–T segment elevation occurs, and there is development of T wave inversion. After the first few days the S–T segment elevation disappears completely. The deep, symmetrical T wave inversion typically persists for weeks before reverting to normal. The changes in the QRS complex are usually permanent. The QRS changes may occasionally disappear altogether if the infarct is small and the myocardial scar subsequently shrinks.

Location of ECG changes in myocardial infarction

Primary ECG changes of the type described above occur in leads facing the infarct. It follows that the leads in which such primary changes occur indicate the location of the infarct (Table 1).

Reciprocal changes

In addition to the primary changes, 'reciprocal' changes occur in leads opposite those facing the infarction. Reciprocal changes are the inverse of primary changes (e.g. S–T segment depression instead of S–T segment elevation and tall, pointed T waves instead of symmetrical T wave inversion). The inferior limb leads (II, III, and aVF) are reciprocal to the anterior leads (the precordial leads, lead I, and aVL) and vice versa.

Examples of ECGs showing recent and old anterior and inferior infarctions are shown in Figs 20 to 24.

Subendocardial infarction

Subendocardial infarction does not always produce recognizable changes in the ECG and such changes as do occur are usually apparent only in the S–T segments or T waves. Persistent deep symmetrical T wave inversion or persistent flat S–T segment depression may be found.

Pitfalls in the diagnosis of myocardial infarction

Left bundle branch block so distorts the normal ECG that the usual criteria for the diagnosis of myocardial infarction are no longer applicable. Although it is possible to diagnose myocardial infarction in the presence of left bundle branch block, such diagnoses should be left for experts to make. In the presence of ventricular pre-excitation neither left branch bundle block nor myocardial infarction should be diagnosed by the non-expert.

Miscellaneous abnormalities of the electrocardiogram

Abnormalities associated with the effects of drugs (including digitalis), hypokalaemia, hyperkalaemia, pericarditis, and hypothyroidism are discussed in other parts of this text. It is appropriate here, however, to mention ventricular pre-excitation, even though this is also dealt with in more detail elsewhere. The reason for this is that an incorrect diagnosis of bundle branch block (right or left), ventricular hypertrophy (right or left) or myocardial infarction may easily be made if ventricular pre-excitation is present but is not recognized.

Ventricular pre-excitation (see also Chapter 15.8.1)

The meaning and clinical significance of ventricular pre-excitation

The term 'ventricular pre-excitation' implies that some part of the ventricular myocardium is depolarized (during normal sinus rhythm or during some other supraventricular rhythm) earlier than would be anticipated. This occurs as a result of the presence of one or more accessory (anomalous) pathways linking atrial and ventricular myocardium in such a way as to permit the depolarization wave descending through the atria from the sinoatrial node to bypass the atrioventricular node, partially or completely, intermittently or consistently. A variety of pathways exist which may, for example, pass: (1) from atrial myocardium to ventricular myocardium; (2) from atrial myocardium to the distal part of the atrioventricular node; or (3) from the atrioventricular node to the ventricular myocardium. The most common are those that link atrial and ventricular myocardium directly, and such pathways can exist at any point around the atrioventricular junction, as embryologically the atrial and ventricular muscle masses were in continuity around the whole atrioventricular junction. These muscular remnants bear no resemblance to the junctional structures described by Kent, and the use of the term 'Kent bundle' to describe the anomalous atrioventricular muscular connections that form the anatomical substrate for ventricular pre-excitation, though widespread, is anatomically unjustifiable.

The presence of an accessory atrioventricular conduction pathway (in addition to the atrioventricular node) provides a substrate that facilitates the development of circus movement tachycardia and the patients with such pathways are at risk of developing paroxysmal tachycardia. Only a proportion of patients with anomalous pathways develop such tachycardias (10 per cent in the 20 to 39 age group and 36 per cent in those over 60s). In the presence of such a pathway an appropriately timed atrial or ventricular premature beat may initiate atrioventricular re-entrant tachycardia (AVNRT).

Recognition of the presence and of the location of such pathways has assumed greater practical importance with the advent of the technique of radiofrequency ablation, which makes it possible to destroy, or at least to render non-functional, the accessory conduction pathway, thereby removing the anatomical substrate upon which the occurrence of AVNRT is dependent.

Electrocardiographic appearances in the presence of anomalous atrioventricular pathways

Space constraints prevent a detailed discussion of this important topic but the fundamental principles of the electrocardiographic appearances in the presence of an (anomalous) atrioventricular accessory pathway will be described. Ventricular pre-excitation is found in approximately 0.1 per cent of the general population and failure to recognize it may lead to serious misdiagnosis. The typical electrocardiogram in this condition has the following features:

(1) an abnormally short PR interval (0.11 s or less);
(2) an abnormally wide QRS complex (0.11 s or more);
(3) slurring of the initial 0.03 s of the QRS complex (a delta wave).

An example is shown in Fig. 25(a).

Location of the accessory pathways

Accessory pathways may remain at any site around the atrioventricular junction but the sites can be broadly categorized as: (1) anteroseptal; (2) posteroseptal; (3) right free wall; and (4) lateral (left free wall). If lead V_1 has a negative delta wave and QRS the accessory pathway is situated in that part of the atrioventricular groove adjacent to the right ventricle and if the delta wave and QRS are positive it is adjacent to the left ventricle. Of the left ventricular locations, those with negative delta waves and negative QRS complexes in II, III, and aVF have pathways situated in the posteroseptal area and those with isoelectric or negative delta waves in I, aVL, V_5, and V_6 have lateral (left ventricular free wall) pathways. Of the right ventricular locations, those with negative delta waves and negative QRS complexes in II, III, and aVF have pathways situated in the posteroseptal area, those with an inferiorly directed QRS axis have an anteroseptal pathway and those with a leftward directed QRS axis have a right free wall pathway.

Figure 25(a) shows an example of ventricular pre-excitation via a left free wall ('lateral') accessory pathway. The delta wave is clearly positive in V_1, indicating a left-sided pathway and the delta waves are negative in aVL and virtually isoelectric in V_6. Figure 25(b) shows an electrocardiogram from the same patient in which only the third beat during the recording of aVR, aVL, and aVF, the first beat during the recording of leads V_1, V_2, and V_3 and the third beat during the recording of V_4, V_5, and V_6 are fully pre-excited. All other beats are conducted predom-

Fig. 16 Transmural myocardial infarction. QS complexes are seen from V_3 to V_5 (reproduced, with permission, from Rowlands, 1991).

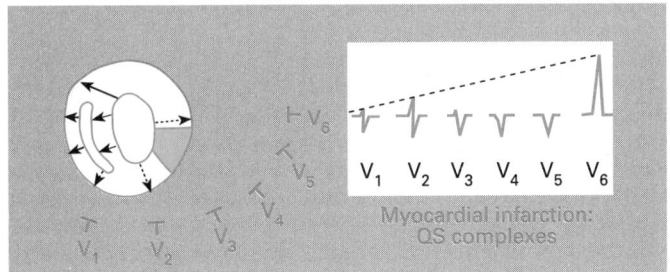

Fig. 17 Varying thickness infarction (reproduced, with permission, from Rowlands, 1991).

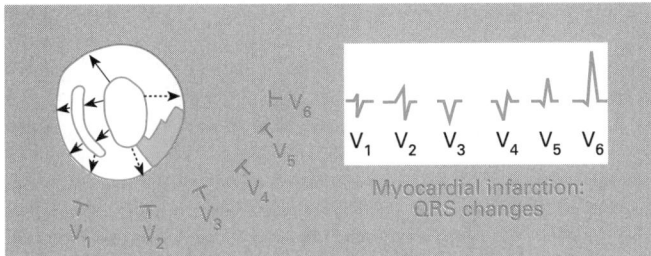

Fig. 18 Deep symmetrical T wave inversion. This is not truly specific but is typically found in association with myocardial ischaemia or infarction (reproduced, with permission, from Rowlands, 1991).

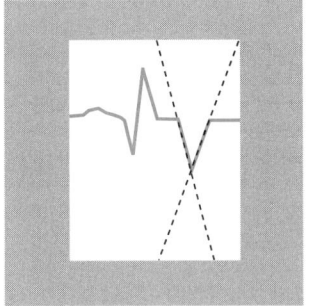

Fig. 19 Sequential changes in acute myocardial infarction (reproduced, with permission, from Rowlands, 1991).

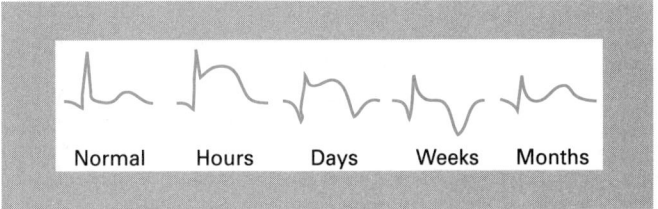

Table 1 *Location of myocardial infarction by the primary changes in the 12 lead electrocardiogram*

Location of infarction	Leads showing primary changes
	Typical changes
Anteroseptal	V_1, V_2, V_3
Anterior	V_2, V_3, V_4
Anterolateral	V_4, V_5, V_6, I, aVL
Extensive anterior	V_1, V_2, V_3, V_4, V_5, V_6, I, aVL
High lateral	aVl (plus high precordial leads)
Inferior	II, III, aVF
Inferolateral (apical)	II, III, aVF, V_5, V_6, I, aVL
Inferoseptal	II, III, aVF, V_1, V_2, V_3
	Other changes
Posterior	V_1, V_2
Subendocardial	Any lead (usually multiple leads)

inantly via the atrioventricular node. Figure 25(c) shows an electrocardiogram from the same patient following successful radiofrequency ablation of the accessory pathway. The fact that the QRS complexes are not exactly the same as in the apparently non-pre-excited beats in Fig. 25(b) suggests that there may have been partial pre-excitation in those beats with atrioventricular conduction occurring both via the atrioventricular node and also via the accessory pathway to give fusion beats in which the main contribution is from depolarization via the atrioventricular node.

Ambulatory electrocardiography

The technique of ambulatory electrocardiographic monitoring was first introduced by Holter in 1961 and is still sometimes referred to as Holter monitoring. It is a technique designed to permit long-term electrocardiographic recording in patients during their normal, everyday activity. It is useful in the detection, diagnosis, and quantification of arrhythmias, the evaluation of anti-arrhythmic therapy, and in detecting pacemaker malfunction. It may also be useful in the recognition of the intermittent myocardial ischaemia from changes in the configuration of the S–T segments and T waves.

Equipment used, recording technique, playback technique

Several manufacturers now produce a range of equipment for ambulatory monitoring, most of which will be adequate for the recording of the cardiac rhythm. However, higher specifications are needed for the recording system if reliable assessments of S–T segment and T wave changes are to be made and more complex play back equipment is needed if the assessment of the resulting record is to be automated or semi-automated. The most commonly used type of equipment is the battery operated continuous electrocardiogram recorder. The recording box is about the same size as a 'Walkman' type of recorder and is worn strapped under the patient's clothing. The electrocardiogram electrodes are connected to the patient via gel-type patch electrodes. The siting of the leads determines the size and configuration of the P waves and QRS complexes in the resulting recording. Sometimes it is worthwhile selecting a lead to give a maximum monophasic QRS amplitude (by inspecting the subject's resting 12-lead electrocardiogram). Typically, electrodes are placed in the V_1 and V_6 positions with an indifferent electrode in the suprasternal area (electrode positions should avoid large muscle masses to minimize interference from electromyographic potentials from skeletal muscle). The electrocardiogram scanner or playback unit either provides a full printout in miniaturized form of 24 h of recording

Fig. 20 Acute inferior myocardial ischaemic damage. Primary S–T elevation is visible in leads 11. 111, and aVF. S–T elevation is also visible in V_4–V_6 indicating that the damage extends to the lateral wall of the ventricle. There is reciprocal S–T segment depression in I. aVL, aVR, and from V_1–V_3 (reproduced, with permission, from Rowlands, 1991).

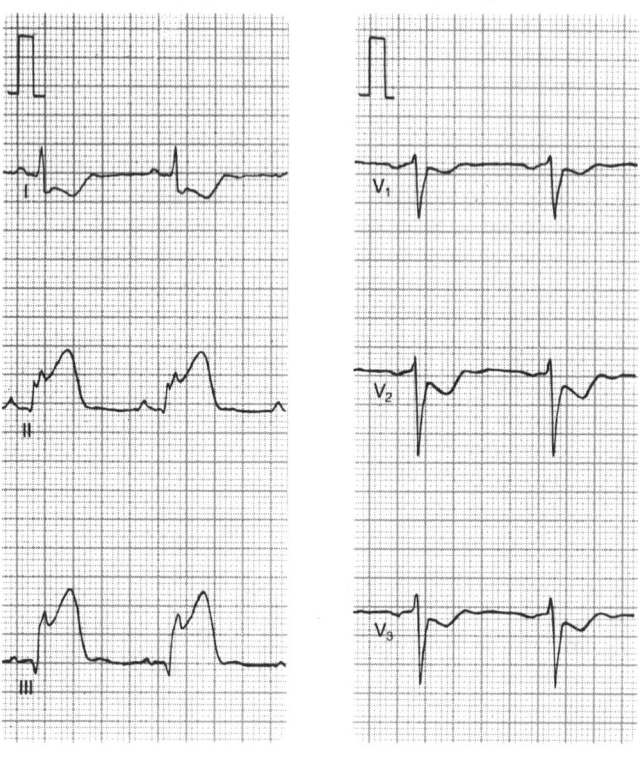

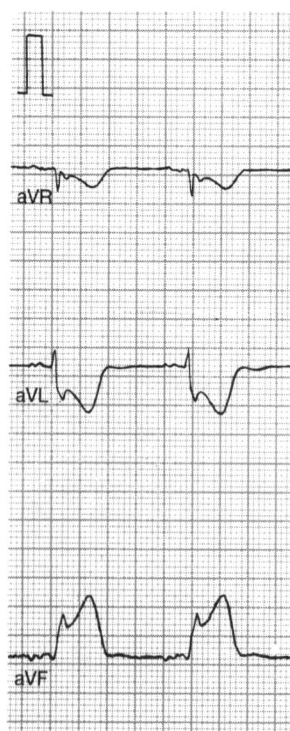

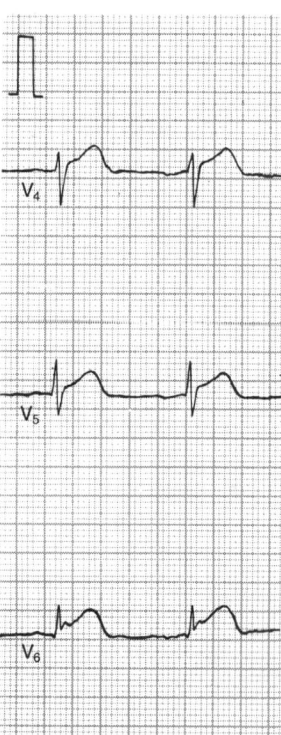

Fig. 21 Inferior myocardial infarction of intermediate age. The Q waves are abnormal in aVF (and also in III) and the q waves in II are borderline abnormal. There is T inversion in II, III, and aVF. The S–T segments are still minimally elevated in these leads. There is inversion of the terminal part of the T wave in V_5 and V_6 suggesting that the ischaemic area extends to the lateral wall of the ventricle. The T waves are strikingly tall in V_2 and V_3. This is not necessarily abnormal but could indicate true posterior ischaemia (reproduced, with permission, from Rowlands, 1991).

Fig. 22 Acute anteroseptal infarction. There is obvious S–T elevation in V_1–V_4 with minimal reciprocal S–T depression in III and aVF. There is obvious loss of initial R wave height in V_2 and V_3 (reproduced, with permission, from Rowlands, 1991).

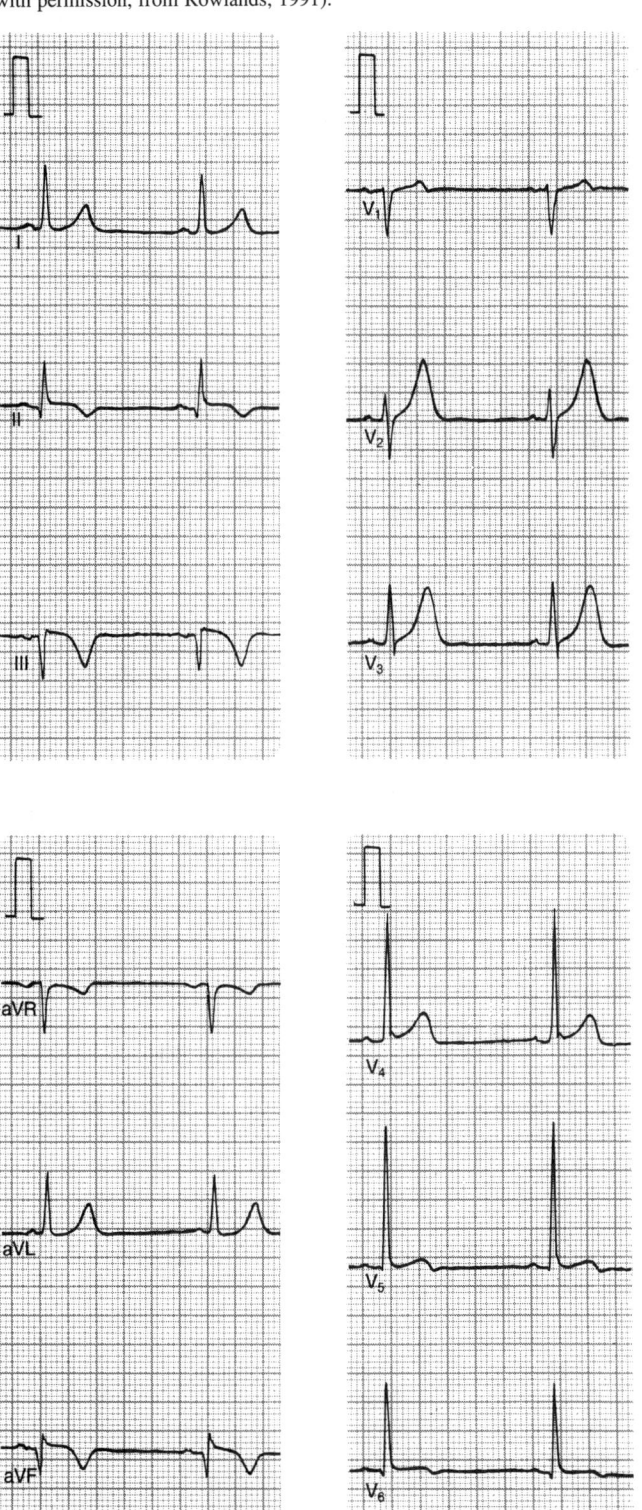

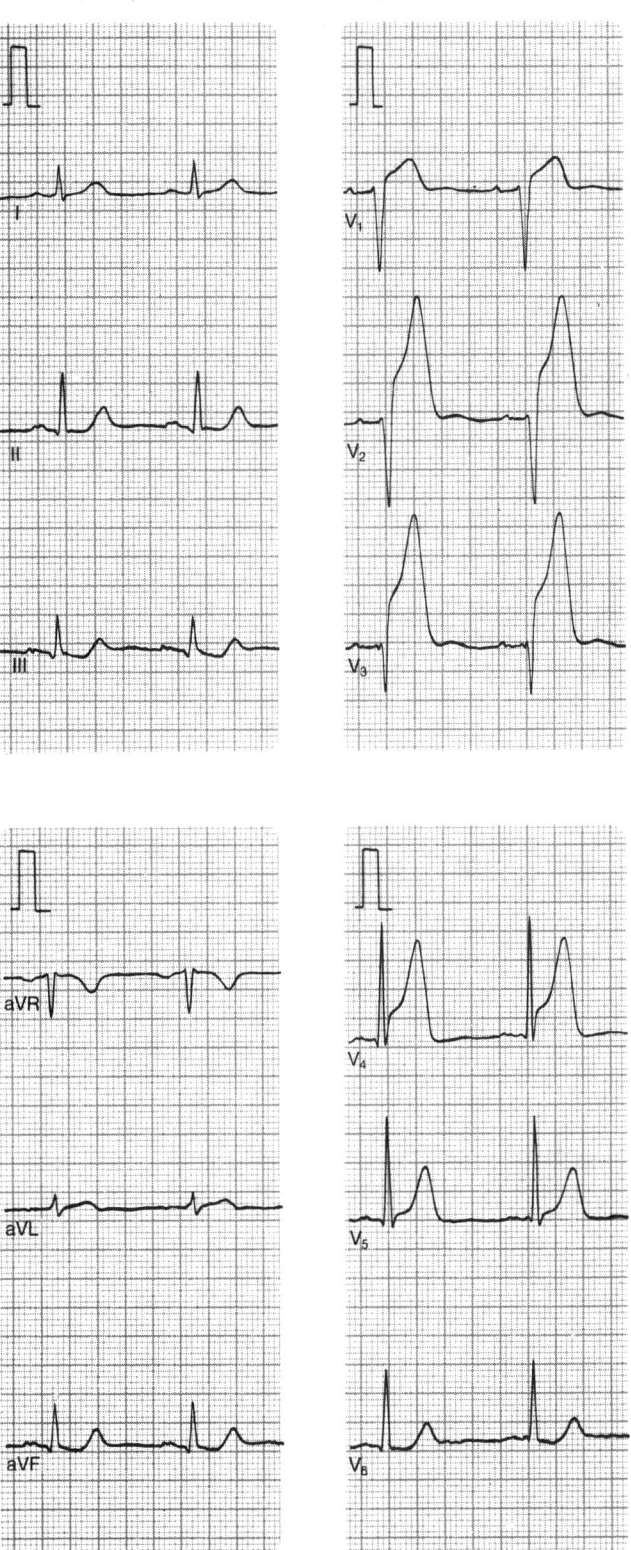

(one sheet per hour) or it permits a technician to view the electrocardiogram signal on an oscilloscope screen at 60 to 120 times natural speed. In the former system the clinician sees (albeit with difficulty) the entire recording. In the latter system the technician may, noticing a deviation from normal, obtain a 'natural' speed printout of the relevant parts of the record. Computer-assisted techniques are available to provide further help in the tedious, time-consuming, and error-fraught tech-

niques of visual analysis. In addition to the commonly used continuous recording systems there are systems available for the brief recording of the electrocardiogram following the recognition by the patient of some significant event. In one variety the patient carries a pocket-sized device that contains a solid state memory capable of recording the electrocar-

Fig. 24 Extensive anterior infarction. There are abnormally wide, abnormally deep Q waves from V_3–V_6 and in I. The T waves are of low voltage in most leads. This latter abnormality is non-specific (reproduced, with permission, from Rowlands, 1991).

Fig. 23 Old anterior myocardial infarction. There are QS complexes in V_2 and V_3 (reproduced, with permission, from Rowlands, 1991).

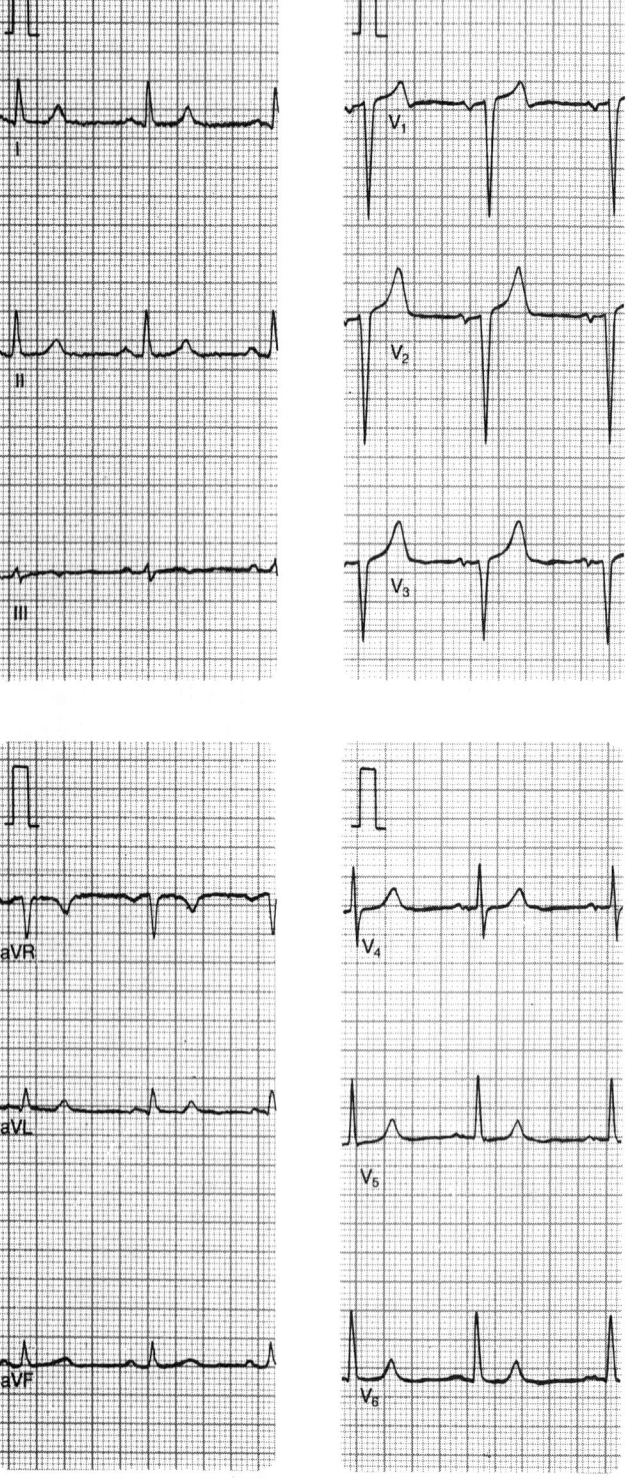

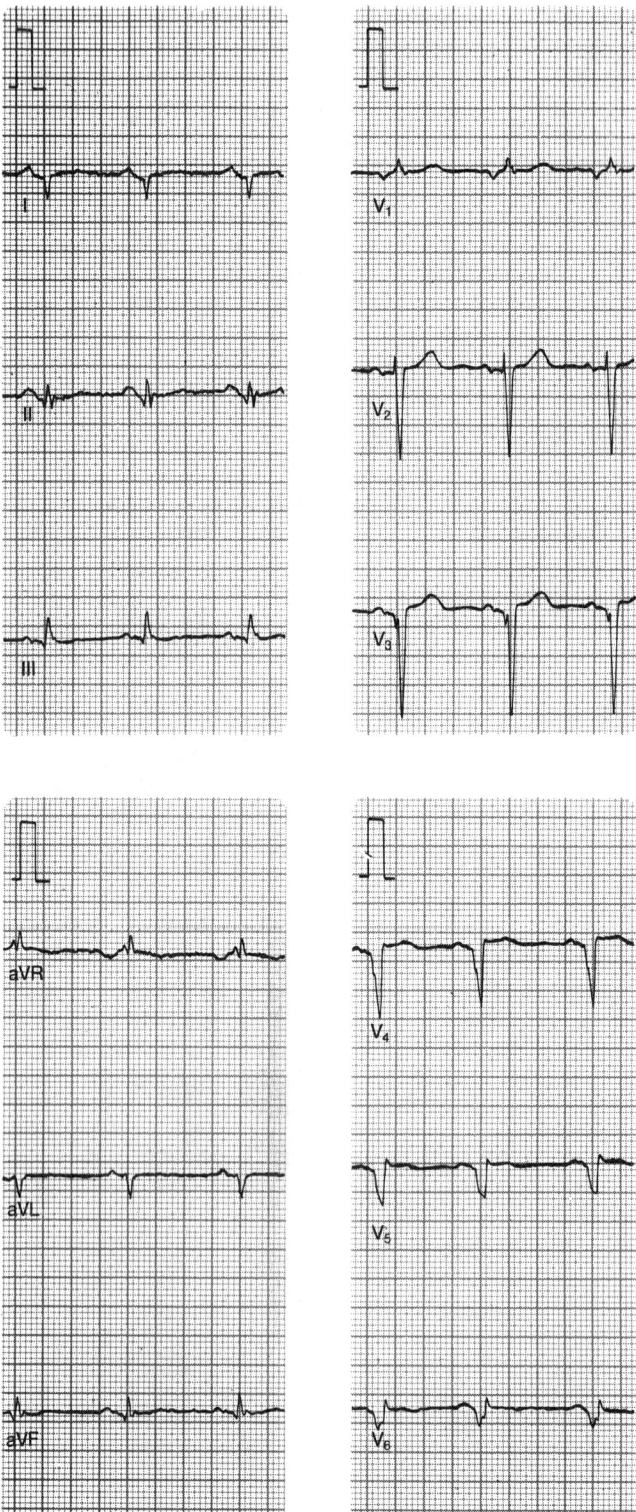

diogram for a limited period (typically 30 s). The device has metal 'feet', which are applied directly to the bare chest and also has a button to activate the recording. All the patient has to do is to open his shirt place the device on his chest with the 'feet' electrodes touching the skin, and then press the button. The recording takes place automatically. The memory is non-volatile (though it can be overwritten, if required, by a further push on the button) and the equipment is taken to the recording centre for subsequent analysis (or if the appropriate model is available the contents of the memory can be transmitted via a telephone to the recording centre). Such intermittent devices are useful when arrhythmias are associated with symptoms (especially palpitation or tachycardia, but occasionally dizziness), but this technique is not useful when the patient presents with syncope.

Fig. 25 Ventricular pre-excitation. Three 12-lead electrocardiograms from the same patient. Three channel recordings with the standard layout of (from left to right) leads I, II, III; leads aVR, aVL, aVF; leads V_1, V_2, V_3; leads V_4, V_5, V_6. (a) Sinus-initiated rhythm with ventricular pre-excitation via a left free wall accessory pathway. (b) The majority of the beats are conducted normally via the sinoatrial node. (c) After radiofrequency ablation of the accessory pathway. For details see text (reproduced, with permission, from Rowlands, 1991).

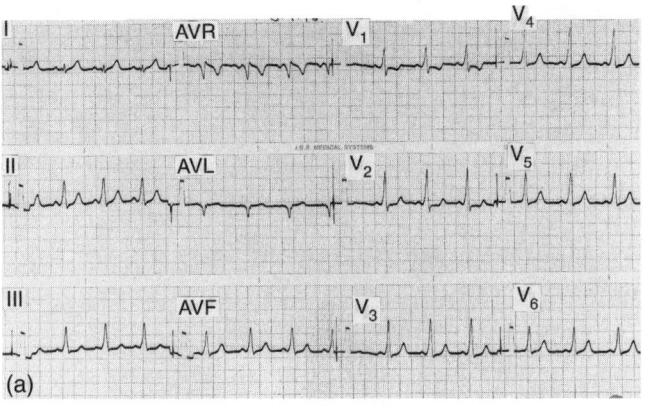

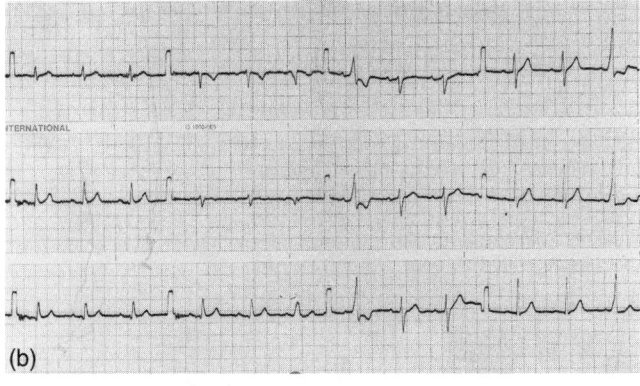

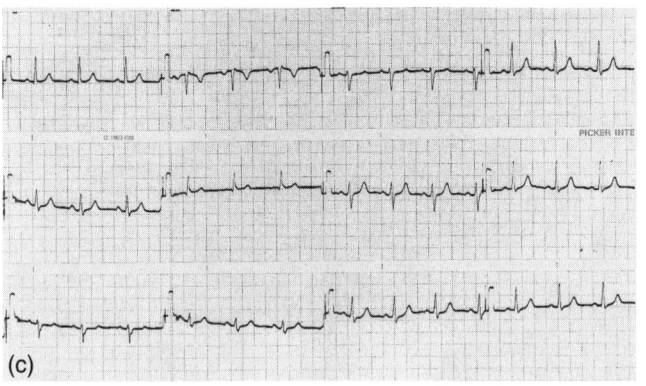

Patient diary

A very important part of ambulatory monitoring is the daily log kept by patients of all relevant activities and symptoms and the times when various medications (especially anti-arrhythmic drugs) are taken. Most recorders are equipped with an event marker which the patient is instructed to press when any relevant symptoms occur. Events coincidental with these symptoms and the timing of these symptoms should be logged in the patient diary.

Normal database

The widespread availability of ambulatory electrocardiogram recordings has revealed how much more variation occurs in the electrocardiogram of normal subjects than was formerly recognized. Normal, healthy subjects at rest (and especially during sleep) not uncommonly demonstrate profound sinus bradycardia (35 to 40 per min), sinus arrhythmia with R–R intervals of up to 2 s, the Wenckebach phenomenon (Mobitz type I second degree atrioventricular block), junctional escape beats, and occasional atrial and ventricular premature beats. However, some arrhythmias are not known to occur in normal subjects. Such arrhythmias are always significant. These include Mobitz type II second degree atrioventricular block, ventricular tachycardia, and complete heart block. Brief episodes of atrial fibrillation not uncommonly occur without any patient awareness. S–T segment shifts may be artefactual unless the low frequency response of the recording equipment is of the highest calibre, but with top class equipment primary, spontaneous (commonly 'silent', i.e. painless) ischaemic S–T segment shift can be recognized.

Artefacts

Artefactual 'arrhythmias' may occur from inadequate skin preparation, poor electrode localization or securement or from inadequate recorder or playback quality. Most systems record two electrocardiogram channels simultaneously and this minimizes the possibility that the artefactual nature of the problem could be overlooked. However, the clinician using this technique should be alert to the possibility that a transient loss of signal (as a result of electrode movement) can mimic asystole and that sinus pauses and intermittent heartblock can be mimicked by transient slowing or sticking of the tape during playback. In addition, pseudotachycardia can occur because of slowing of the tape speed during recording in cases of battery depletion. These pseudotachycardias can usually be recognized as such because the heart rate progressively increases towards the end of the recording and because the P waves, QRS complexes, and T waves all become progressively narrower at the same rate as the R–R interval appears to shorten.

Ambulatory monitoring for palpitation

Palpitation, or unusual awareness of the cardiac action, frequently disturbs patients and often constitutes an indication for ambulatory monitoring in the hope that an electrocardiographic explanation of the symptoms will become apparent and that suitable treatment will then be possible. Examples of rhythm strips obtained from 24-h ambulatory records used in this way are shown in Figs 26 to 31.

Ambulatory monitoring for dizziness or syncope

Palpitation, occurring in association with frequent premature beats or with episodic tachydysrhythmias, is often symptomatically disturbing to patients but symptoms of dizziness or syncope are potentially of much greater importance as they can be indicative of serious or even life-threatening arrhythmias. Complaints of transient lightheadedness, feelings of impending loss of consciousness or episodes of actual syncope may all be cardiac in origin. Equally, of course, they may not. A full clinical history and examination and appropriate investigations other than electrocardiography are required in addition to one or more periods of 24 h ambulatory electrocardiogram recording. The use of *ad hoc* transient recording techniques with short-term memory devices (applied by patients to their own chests) is inappropriate in the context of this symptom as it is unlikely that the patient will have sufficient time to activate the equipment before the symptoms induce diability. In the context of such symptoms the use of ambulatory electrocardiogram recordings is appropriate. It is important to appreciate that it is only when the patient experiences typical symptoms at the precise time when definitive and significant electrocardiographic changes occur in the ambulatory recording that the 24-h electrocardiogram recording contributes to management. Definitive electrocardiogram appearances can

be defined as: (1) a cardiac rhythm likely to be, or inevitably, associated with loss of consciousness; or (2) a cardiac rhythm which could not possibly cause loss of consciousness (although it might occur in association with or in response to a loss of consciousness). Examples of the former group include ventricular fibrillation, rapid ventricular tachycardia, profound bradycardia, or asystole; examples of the latter group include sinus rhythm with rates of 60 or more, sinus rhythm with occasional atrial or ventricular ectopic beats, and first degree heartblock. Unfortunately there will be many occasions when the electrocardiogram

Fig. 26 Sinus rhythm. Varying sinus rate. The first four complexes show a very rapid sinus rate (approximately 115 per min) with each P wave superimposed on the preceding T wave. The sinus rate then slows spontaneously and rapidly. This patient complained of pounding of the heart. Treatment with a β-blocker suppressed the symptoms (reproduced, with permission, from Rowlands, 1991).

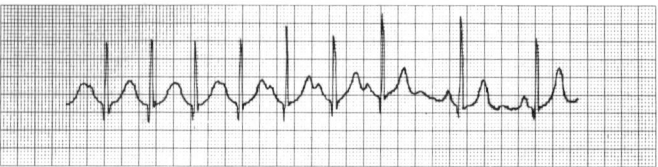

Fig. 27 Sinus rhythm with three junctional ('nodal') premature beats. The fourth, sixth, and eighth beats are junctional ('nodal') premature beats. The patient complained of occasional irregularity of the heart. No treatment was necessary (reproduced, with permission, from Rowlands, 1991).

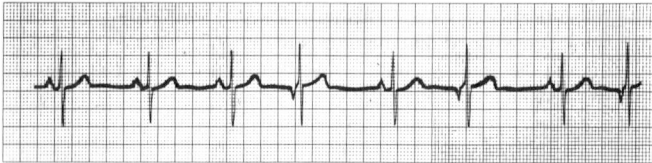

Fig. 28 Sinus rhythm with unifocal, coupled 'interpolated' ventricular premature beats. Such an arrhythmia may or may not result in symptoms Hypokalaemia and digitalis toxicity should be considered (reproduced, with permission, from Rowlands, 1991).

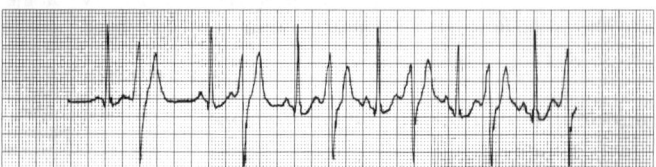

Fig. 29 Onset of atrial fibrillation. The first three beats are sinus beats. The remainder of the strip shows atrial fibrillation. The patient complained of repeated attacks of irregularity of the heart which he found disturbing. The ventricular rate during atrial fibrillation is surprisingly slow, suggesting atrioventricular nodal dysfunction (reproduced, with permission, from Rowlands, 1991).

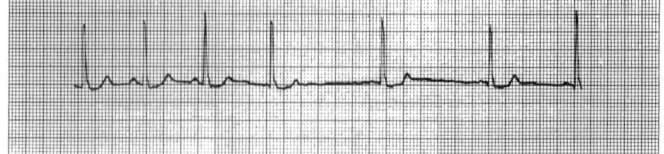

Fig. 30 Sinus rhythm with a run of wide QRS complex tachycardia, suggesting ventricular tachycardia. The P wave rhythm appears undisturbed – supporting this diagnosis – (but it is difficult to follow the P waves through the QRS complexes) and the ventricular rate is very irregular An alternative explanation of the wide QRS tachycardia explanation would be a burst of rapid atrial fibrillation with aberrant intraventricular conduction, but the long R–R interval during the wide QRS tachycardia is not followed by a more normal QRS, which is a little against aberration as an explanation of the wide QRS complexes. This record illustrates the difficulty of interpretation often experienced with ambulatory records. The correct diagnosis is probably non-sustained ventricular tachycardia (reproduced, with permission, from Rowlands, 1991).

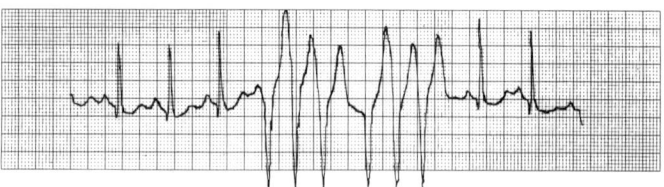

Fig. 31 Sustained wide QRS complex tachycardia (ventricular flutter). The difference between ventricular flutter and ventricular tachycardia is merely one of rate. In the case of ventricular flutter the rate is in the region of 300 per min, as here (reproduced, with permission, from Rowlands, 1991).

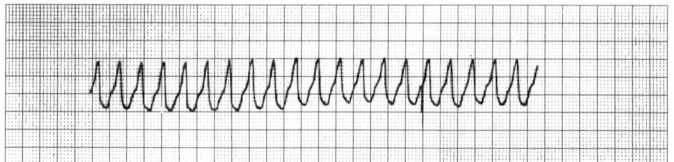

Fig. 32 Sinus arrest. The first two beats are sinus beats, followed which there is a brief period of sinus arrest. The pause is ended by a junctional escape beat. The fourth beat is an echo beat followed again by sinus arrest, a junctional escape beat and a further echo beat. The appearances leave little doubt that the sinoatrial and atrioventricular nodes are diseased (reproduced, with permission, from Rowlands, 1991).

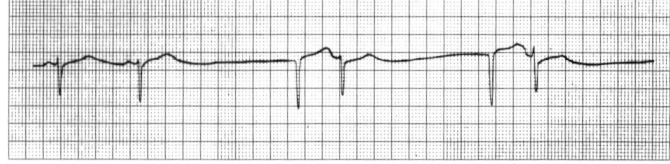

Fig. 33 Sinoatrial disease with sinus arrest. The first two beats are sinus beats. There is then a period of atrial and junctional arrest for more than 4.7 s before a junctional escape beat occurs. The tracing coincided with syncope; permanent pacing was necessary (reproduced, with permission, from Rowlands, 1991).

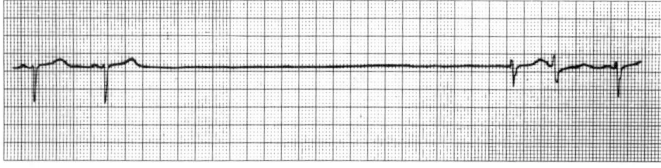

is not definitive (e.g. when it shows atrial fibrillation with a rapid ventricular rate, short bursts of supraventricular or ventricular tachycardia, pauses of 1 to 3 s, etc.). In such situations it may not be possible to reach a definitive conclusion about the possible role of the rhythm in producing the symptoms. If the symptoms of dizziness or syncope do not occur during the monitoring period and if no significant arrhythmia occurs, the investigation makes no contribution to the diagnosis.

Although a 24-h ambulatory record represents a considerable advance in the magnitude of data collection compared with a 12-lead electrocardiogram it still represents a very small time window and has, for example, only a 1 in 30 chance of catching an event which occurs monthly. Even so it has proved to be a very useful advance and examples of its value in the investigation of patients with dizzy spells are shown in Figs 32 to 36.

Innocent arrhythmias recorded by ambulatory monitoring

Ambulatory electrocardiographic recordings from subjects with no overt evidence of heart disease have demonstrated that a wide range of arrhythmias may occur in apparently normal hearts. Occasional atrial or

Fig. 34 Atrial flutter with varying atrioventricular block and a short run of ventricular tachycardia. The basic rhythm is atrial flutter. There is varying 3 : 1 and 2 : 1 atrioventricular conduction. A single ventricular premature beat is seen near the beginning of the trace and there is a run of four beats of ventricular tachycardia (reproduced, with permission, from Rowlands, 1991).

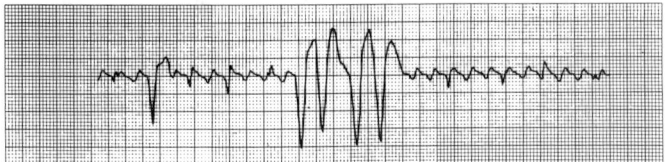

Fig. 35 Atrial fibrillation with a slow mean ventricular rate. Two pauses of 2 s each are seen in a short segment of trace. The pauses indicate atrioventricular nodal dysfunction either as a result of disease or as result of medication (especially if digitalis β-blockers, verapamil, or diltiazem) are used singly or in combination (reproduced, with permission, from Rowlands, 1991).

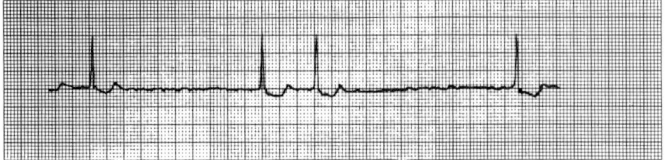

Fig. 36 Torsade de pointes. Note that the record runs continuously from top left to bottom right. There is frequent ventricular ectopic activity and there are two runs of non-sustained ventricular tachycardia of the 'torsade de pointes' variety. This arrhythmia is commonly the result of the injudicious use of anti-arrhythmic drugs.

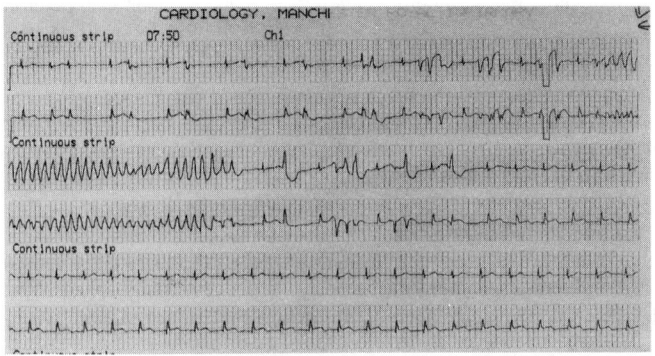

ventricular premature beats are found in 25 to 50 per cent of normal young subjects and in 60 to 70 per cent of subjects in the older age groups. Profound bradycardia (Fig. 37) is usual during sleep. Transient Wenckebach (Mobitz type I) second degree atrioventricular block is occasionally seen in normal subjects, especially those with an active vagus. When it occurs, it commonly presents against the background of a slow sinus rate as during sleep (Fig. 38).

Ambulatory monitoring in ischaemic heart disease

Subjects with ischaemic heart disease and symptoms suggestive of cardiac arrhythmias are also candidates for ambulatory monitoring, which is sometimes of value in demonstrating electrocardiographic evidence of ischaemia. In the absence of increases in heart rate or blood pressure such changes are often thought to be indicative of coronary artery spasm (Fig. 39).

Ambulatory monitoring in pacemaker patients

Pacemaker malfunction may be intermittent and in suspected cases ambulatory monitoring can demonstrate intermittent failure of capture of the pacing stimulus or intermittent failure of sensing (in the case of

Fig. 37 Sinus bradycardia. The rate is 30 per min. This record was obtained during the early hours of the morning and such slow heart rates are not abnormal during sleep (reproduced, with permission, from Rowlands, 1991).

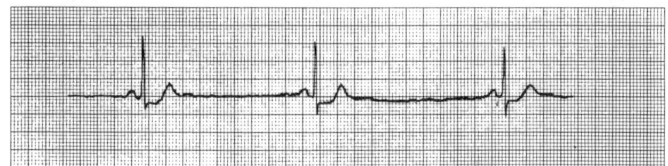

Fig. 38 Wenckebach type second degree atrioventricular block. The first two beats show atrioventricular conduction with increasing P–R interval. The third P wave is not followed by a QRS. The fourth P wave is followed by a QRS at a normal P–R interval. Subsequent cycles once more show progressive prolongation of the P–R interval. The Wenckebach phenomenon can occur in healthy hearts (reproduced, with permission, from Rowlands, 1991).

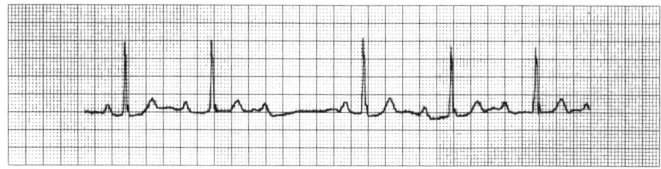

Fig. 39 Electrocardiographic appearances in during spontaneous (non-exercise induced) angina. (a) Control record in the absence of pain. (b) Record taken during an anginal episode. There is marked T wave inversion in the absence of a tachycardia (reproduced, with permission, from Rowlands, 1991).

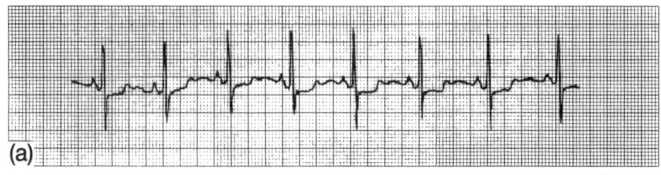

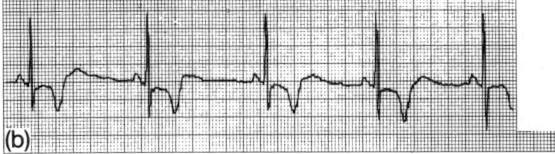

pacemakers with demand function). The ambulatory electrocardiographic recording can also be useful in showing absence of pacing malfunction at the time the patient experiences symptoms.

REFERENCES

Rowlands, D.J. (1978). The electrical axis. *British Journal of Hospital Medicine*, **19**, 472–481.
Rowlands, D.J. (1991). *Clinical electrocardiography*. Gower, London.
Schamroth, L. (1976). *An introduction to electrocardiography*. Blackwell Scientific Publications, Oxford.

15.4.3 Doppler echocardiography

I. A. Simpson

Introduction

The Doppler effect was first described by Christian Doppler 1842. He described the change in the colour of light stars caused by their rapid movement towards or away from the earth, but the Doppler effect holds true for any source of wave production, be it light, sound or, in the case of cardiac investigation, ultrasound. As the transmitted ultrasound from an echocardiographic transducer is reflected from moving blood, the red cell reflectors will interact with the ultrasound waves, altering their frequency as a function of the velocity of blood flow. This Doppler frequency shift can be detected from the reflected ultrasound waves and used to estimate blood flow velocity by the Doppler equation:

$$V = \frac{c \, \Delta F}{2F \cos\theta}$$

where V = the velocity of blood, c = the velocity of ultrasound in biological tissue, F is the frequency of the transmitted ultrasound and θ is the angle of incidence between the ultrasound beam and the direction of blood flow.

If Doppler echocardiography is to measure blood flow velocity accurately, the ultrasound beam must be directed as close as possible to the direction of blood flow within the heart and great vessels. As not all blood cells move at exactly the same velocity, even where flow within the heart is laminar, a spectrum or range of frequency shifts will be detected, rather like the different musical notes used to make up a chord. These can be separated into their individual components using a spectrum analyser, which then displays the whole range of velocities throughout the cardiac cycle. At any given time the intensity of the signal on the spectral display will be dependent on the number of red cells travelling at a given velocity. This spectral display of velocity against time is the conventional way to record cardiac spectral Doppler ultrasound information (Plate 1). Directional information is shown with velocities towards the transducer displayed above the zero velocity line and those away from it below. If blood flow is laminar and Doppler information is acquired from a single position within the heart, the range of velocities will be small and there will be a narrow band of high signal intensity on the spectral display. When blood flow is highly turbulent, there will be a wide range of velocity values at the point of Doppler interrogation and a broad band of values on the spectral display.

Doppler ultrasound can provide the following information:

1. The velocity of blood flow derived from the Doppler frequency shift, assuming a minimal angle between the ultrasound beam and blood flow.
2. The direction of blood flow in relation to the ultrasound transducer.
3. The distinction of normal laminar flow from turbulent flow,

the latter seen as a broad band of velocities on spectral Doppler or a multicoloured mosaic pattern on colour Doppler flow mapping.

Doppler ultrasound modalities

There are a number of ways in which cardiac Doppler information can be acquired (Table 1). Spectral Doppler ultrasound uses either pulsed or continuous wave Doppler interrogation along any single line of a simultaneously obtained two-dimensional echocardiographic image or with a dedicated transducer without the image. In contrast to the spectral technique, colour Doppler flow mapping provides a two-dimensional colour-coded display of information superimposed on an echocardiographic image. The different Doppler modalities listed in Table 1 each have particular strengths and limitations but they are rarely used in isolation. Rather, all three modes are used in combination to provide a more coordinated and comprehensive clinical assessment of the spatial distribution, localization, and measurement of velocities in patients with a wide range of cardiovascular abnormalities.

Pulsed wave Doppler

Pulsed wave Doppler allows information to be obtained from a single position, or sample gate, within the two-dimensional image. The velocity resolution of pulsed wave Doppler is limited because of the need to send a pulse of ultrasound and wait for its return to the transducer, but it is well within the resolution of normal intracardiac flow velocities (usually less than 1.5 m/s) and its allows the position of the Doppler signal to be directly related to the two-dimensional image.

Continuous wave Doppler

Continuous wave Doppler is achieved by continuously transmitting and receiving Doppler information. This allows velocities in excess of 6 m/s to be measured accurately. This is necessary to identify patients with critical valve stenosis, but the resultant spectral display is a compilation of all the velocities along the ultrasound beam and the exact position of highest velocity cannot be determined from the Doppler recording. However, the data provided by the two-dimensional echocardiogram is usually sufficient to indicate the origin of the high velocity flow.

Colour Doppler flow mapping

Colour Doppler flow mapping allows a dynamic real-time two-dimensional spatial display of velocities superimposed on an echocardiographic image. As Doppler information is displayed not only along a single line of ultrasound but also over a portion of a two-dimensional image, there is a vast amount of information inherent in a single image. Time constraints negate the use of the spectral format for colour flow mapping and a mean velocity value is colour encoded for each pixel in the two-dimensional image, in order to display this information in a dynamic real-time format. Conventionally, blood flow towards the ultrasound transducer is encoded as red, and flow away encoded as blue, with the colour brightness proportional to the blood flow velocity. Colour Doppler flow mapping is basically a pulsed system and it is therefore limited in the maximum velocity it can encode. The major advantage of colour flow mapping is its ability to relate spatial velocities to the surrounding structural detail. High velocity, turbulent jets often related to valve or congenital abnormalities, produce characteristic multicoloured mosaic patterns on colour flow mapping, which are ideally suited to the identification and localization of abnormalities within the heart.

Table 1 *Doppler echocardiography modalities*

Modality	Advantages	Disadvantages
Pulsed wave Doppler	Single sampling point Depth resolution Spectral velocity display	Limited velocity resolution No spatial velocity distribution
Continuous wave Doppler	Unlimited velocity resolution Spectral velocity display	No depth resolution Sampling from a single line
Colour Doppler flow mapping	Spatial velocity information Real time display	Slow frame rate Limited velocity resolution No spectral display

Doppler assessment of valve disease

Concept of estimation of pressure drop by Doppler echocardiography

The ability to estimate the pressure drop across a valve stenosis accurately is one of the most important clinical applications of modern cardiac Doppler ultrasound. As velocity of flow and pressure drop are related, it is possible to derive the pressure drop across a valve from the velocity of blood flow through it. This is based on the Bernoulli equation, which has been modified for clinical purposes to the following:

$$\Delta P = 4 \ (V_2^2 - V_1^2)$$

where ΔP = the pressure drop across the valve obstruction in mmHg, V_2 = the velocity of blood flow (in m/s) at the obstruction, and V_1 = the velocity of blood flow (in m/s) proximal to the obstruction.

The greater the difference in velocities, the more severe the pressure drop. In most circumstances, the proximal velocity is ≤ 1 m/s and the calculation of pressure drop is almost entirely determined by the velocity at the site of obstruction. The modified equation of $\Delta P = 4V^2$ can then be used in the majority of clinical conditions, but this is only valid when the proximal velocity is low. High cardiac output or severe valve regurgitation may significantly increase the proximal velocity above 1 m/s and lead to an erroneous overestimation of the true pressure drop if this increased proximal velocity is not taken into account.

Mitral valve disease

The diagnosis of mitral stenosis is usually apparent clinically, and confirmed by echocardiography. However, the precise severity of stenosis is less easy to estimate, particularly in patients with mixed valve disease or previous mitral valvotomy. Doppler ultrasound is particularly useful in the non-invasive assessment of these patients because of its ability to provide an accurate quantitative estimate of the severity of mitral stenosis. Plate 2 demonstrates the velocity pattern across a normal mitral valve compared to one from a patient with significant mitral stenosis (Fig. 1). Normal flow past the mitral valve produces a characteristic M-shaped spectral Doppler signal with an initial peak velocity, or E wave, due to early rapid filling. The velocity then falls rapidly towards zero with further rapid increase towards the end of diastole associated with atrial contraction, the so-called A wave. In mitral stenosis (Fig. 1(a)), the initial E wave velocity is increased as a consequence of the high left atrial pressure and the resultant pressure difference between the atrium and the ventricle. This E wave velocity is altered to some extent by changes in cardiac output and is not particularly useful in isolation for assessing the severity of mitral stenosis. It is possible to estimate the mean mitral valve gradient from planimetry of the mitral inflow velocity and this does correlate well with similar measurements obtained at cardiac catheterization. More valuable, is an assessment of the rate at which the initial E wave velocity decreases. Figure 1(a) demonstrates that the

Fig. 1 (a) Spectral continuous wave Doppler recordings from a patient with significant mitral stenosis. The peak velocity in early diastole is increased to over 2 m/s[1] with a much slower decrease in velocity than Plate 2. The late diastolic peak due to atrial contraction has been lost as the patient is in atrial fibrillation. Note that continuous wave Doppler has been used in order to accurately record the increased velocity, but the narrow band of velocities on the spectral trace has been lost and the spectral trace has been 'filled in' by velocities recorded along all of the ultrasound beam rather than solely at the mitral valve. (b) Spectral continuous wave Doppler recording from the same patient as Fig. 1(a). The mitral velocity curve has been traced to measure the maximum velocity and pressure drop, and estimate the mitral pressure half-time (230 ms) from which an value for mitral valve area has been calculated (0.96 cm²).

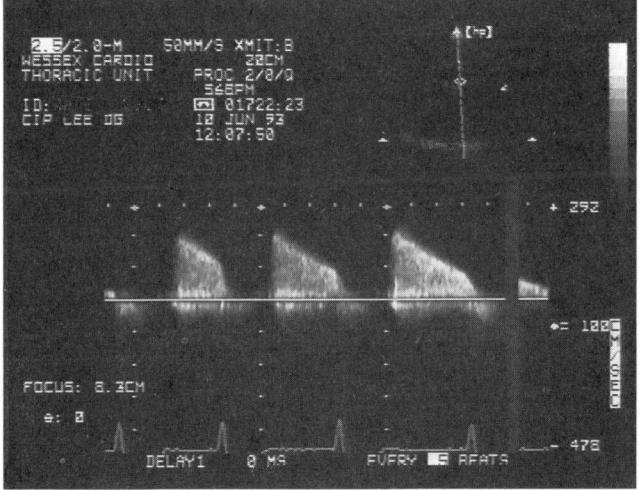

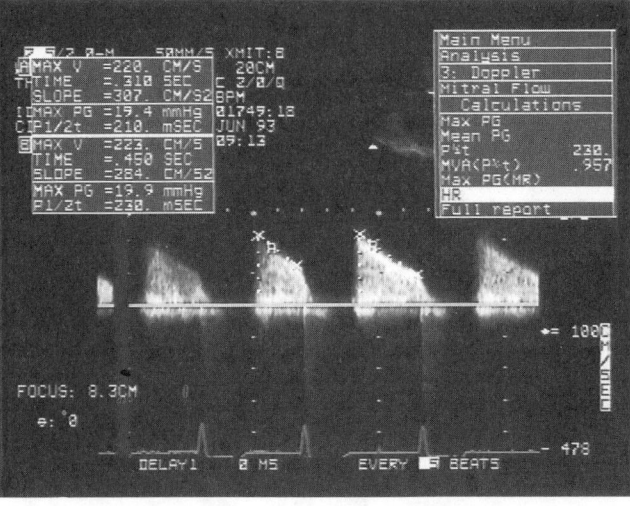

velocity falls more slowly in mitral stenosis. This can be quantified by measuring the mitral pressure half-time in milliseconds, which is the time taken for the initial peak velocity to fall to a value equivalent to half the initial peak pressure drop (Fig. 1(b)). In effect, this is a measurement of the slope of the velocity decrease from its initial peak value. The longer the mitral pressure half-time then the more severe the mitral stenosis. As the rate of velocity decrease is largely unaffected by changes in cardiac output, the pressure half-time provides an accurate quantification of the severity of mitral stenosis. Indeed, the mitral valve area can be estimated directly from the pressure half-time measurement from the equation:

$$\text{MVA (cm}^2) = 220/\text{pressure half-time (ms)}$$

When, as in most patients with mitral stenosis, there is atrial fibrillation, the A wave component of the mitral inflow velocity pattern is lost, but the pressure half-time remains unaltered and continues to provide the single most accurate non-invasive estimate of the true severity of mitral stenosis irrespective of cardiac output or the presence of significant mitral regurgitation.

Mitral regurgitation

The ability of Doppler ultrasound to display high velocities is ideally suited to the detection of valve regurgitation. Mitral regurgitation is characteristically visualized from the cardiac apex as a high velocity, systolic jet away from the transducer on spectral Doppler ultrasound (Plate 3) and on colour Doppler flow mapping, a multicoloured mosaic jet of regurgitation is seen within the left atrium (Plate 4). Colour flow mapping is also useful for identifying multiple jets and the direction of regurgitation in the left atrium which correlates with the structural abnormalities seen in mitral valve prolapse. Doppler echocardiography is so sensitive to high velocity jets that it is likely to easily detect even trivial mitral regurgitation.

The ability of Doppler echocardiography to quantify mitral regurgitation is somewhat more complex. Colour Doppler flow mapping was initially hailed as an 'ultrasonic angiogram' with the potential to quantify mitral regurgitation in a similar manner to left ventricular angiography. However, as a velocity mapping technique, the size of regurgitant jets are highly dependent on the driving pressure of regurgitation and quantification is limited to assessing mild, moderate or severe regurgitation. Some assessment of regurgitation severity can be obtained using spectral Doppler ultrasound (Table 2) but again the accuracy of this is limited by the use of a velocity encoding technique rather than one related directly to regurgitant volume.

Aortic stenosis

Doppler ultrasound is an important clinical investigation for patients with suspected aortic stenosis. The relationship of velocity to pressure drop is particularly applicable to aortic stenosis where a significant pressure drop across the valve results in a marked increase in peak aortic velocity. In severe stenosis the peak aortic velocity may be as high as 6 m/s, indicating a pressure drop in excess of 140 mmHg. It is necessary to use continuous wave Doppler in order to estimate velocities of this magnitude accurately. Distortion of the aortic valve, often in the presence of heavy calcification, may effect the direction of the high velocity jet within the aortic root. In order to ensure that the highest velocity is being recorded it is essential that ultrasound examination is performed from all possible precordial positions including the apex, suprasternal notch, right parasternal region and the subcostal approach, though the peak velocity is most often recorded from the apex or right parasternal regions. When care is taken to obtain the highest recordable velocity, continuous wave Doppler will predict the peak pressure drop across the aortic valve with great accuracy. Doppler ultrasound estimates a peak

Table 2 *Severity of mitral regurgitation*

	Mild regurgitation	Severe regurgitation
Spectral intensity	↓	↑
Peak diastolic flow velocity	Normal	↑
Systolic flow reversal in pulmonary veins	Absent	Present
Width of colour jet at origin	↓	↑

or instantaneous pressure drop, rather than the peak to peak value traditionally measured at cardiac catheterization. The peak instantaneous pressure drop may be slightly higher than the peak to peak value though this discrepancy is usually of little clinical relevance. Significant aortic regurgitation will increase the velocity proximal to the stenotic value. When such an increase is identified in the left ventricular outflow tract using pulsed wave Doppler, this should be used as part of the modified Bernoulli equation (see above) to reflect the true pressure drop across the aortic valve.

Aortic regurgitation

The large pressure difference between the aorta and left ventricle in diastole is reflected in the Doppler signal of aortic regurgitation by a high velocity throughout diastole (Fig. 2). Doppler ultrasound will identify the presence of even trivial aortic regurgitation, which is often not apparent clinically, because of the sensitivity of the technique for high velocities, but quantifying aortic regurgitation is fraught with difficulties. If the velocity of regurgitation falls rapidly during diastole, this represents a change towards equalization of aortic and left ventricular diastolic pressures. This may be due to severe aortic regurgitation but it can also result from a high left ventricular diastolic pressure secondary to severe dysfunction. The width of the regurgitant jet at its origin on colour flow mapping is related to severity of regurgitation to some extent

Fig. 2 Spectral continuous wave Doppler recording of aortic regurgitation. Note that from the transducer position at the apex of the heart, the diastolic signal of aortic regurgitation is directed towards the transducer. There is a high velocity value (5 m/s in this example) in early diastole. The velocity falls slowly during diastole but remains high even at end diastole (3 m/s in this example) reflecting the sustained pressure difference between the aortic pressure and left ventricular diastolic pressures. The rate at which velocity falls during diastole provides some indication as to the severity of aortic regurgitation.

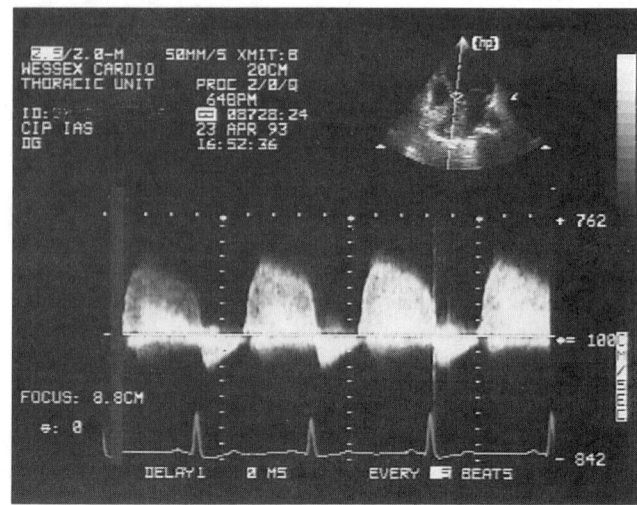

and the combination of this with spectral Doppler recordings may provide an indication of the severity of the regurgitation, though similar information is often apparent clinically, especially when combined with conventional echocardiography.

Right heart valves

As with aortic stenosis, Doppler ultrasound can predict the pressure drop in pulmonary valve and subvalve stenosis with accuracy. The obstruction of subvalvular stenosis is often a dynamic one related to muscular hypertrophy with the maximum pressure drop occurring in late systole rather than mid-systole is the case with the fixed valve obstruction. The shape of the Doppler signal can be useful in differentiating these different obstructive components (Fig. 3). The detection of pulmonary and particularly tricuspid regurgitation by Doppler techniques is important not so much to determine the function of these valves but in order to predict pulmonary artery pressure. The peak velocity of tricuspid regurgitation will reflect the systolic pressure difference between the right ventricle and right atrium. As the right atrial pressure is low, or predictable from the jugular venous pressure, the right ventricular systolic pressure, and hence pulmonary artery pressure, can be estimated. Even in the presence of pulmonary stenosis, the pulmonary artery systolic pressure can still be estimated from the predicted right ventricular systolic pressure and the Doppler derived pressure drop across the pulmonary valve.

Physiological regurgitation

The sensitivity of Doppler ultrasound for detecting high velocities has lead to some interesting insights into cardiac function, not least the presence of physiological regurgitation. Following the widespread use of cardiac Doppler echocardiography it rapidly became apparent that regurgitation through the right heart valves could be detected in the vast majority of normal individuals, up to 95 per cent in some studies. It is not possible to detect this clinically, and it is of no haemodynamic importance, yet it would appear to be true regurgitation rather than merely displacement of blood due to valve closure. It is likely that the lower pressures within the right heart predispose to physiological regurgitation by failure of complete apposition of the leaflets but physiological mitral regurgitation has also been reported, particularly in children. The presence of tricuspid regurgitation on Doppler echocardiography even in normal individuals allows the prediction of pulmonary artery systolic pressure in most patients in whom adequate echocardiographic images have been obtained.

Fig. 3 Schematic representation of the differing shape of the spectral continuous wave Doppler signal in fixed and dynamic obstruction. A fixed obstruction produces a parabolic velocity profile with a peak velocity in mid-systole as would occur with valvar pulmonary stenosis. In comparison, a dynamic obstruction produces a 'scimitar'-type signal of increasing velocity during early and mid systole with the peak velocity in late systole. This is the expected pattern in dynamic subvalve muscular obstruction such as infundibular pulmonary stenosis.

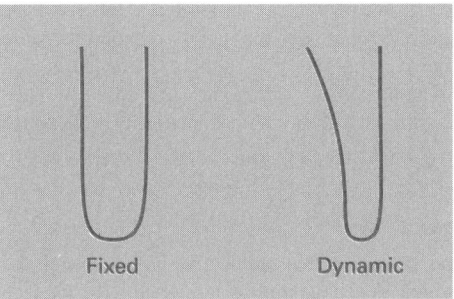

Prosthetic valves

The use of Doppler ultrasound to examine prosthetic valves has had a similar impact to its use in native valve disease. Tissue valve replacements in the aortic and mitral positions can be evaluated in the same way as in native valve disease but the mild obstructive nature of the replacement valves, particularly the smaller ones used in the aortic position, does cause a slight increase in peak velocity reflecting a small pressure drop across the valve. Mechanical valves, especially the tilting disc variety, are inherently regurgitant to a small extent and this can be detected by Doppler echocardiography. Regurgitation through a mechanical aortic valve is detectable by transthoracic Doppler echocardiography, whereas the acoustic shadowing in the left atrium of the mechanical mitral valve masks the regurgitation. This can be overcome by using transoesophageal echocardiography combined with colour Doppler flow mapping.

Other Doppler applications

Left ventricular function

Although M-mode and two-dimensional echocardiography remain the mainstay for assessment of ventricular function, Doppler echocardiography has provided additional insights into the mechanisms and evaluation of ventricular disease. The pattern of mitral inflow velocities has been used to assess 'diastolic' disease but the complex interplay of haemodynamic variables that contribute to this pattern make it of limited clinical value when used as an isolated measurement without knowledge of ventricular pressure, though this can be estimated by using a simultaneous apexcardiogram. It is also possible to evaluate left ventricular systolic function by estimating cardiac output from Doppler recordings of aortic velocity combined with the diameter of the left ventricular outflow tract measured by echocardiography. Although there are limitations of this technique for absolute estimates of cardiac output, it can detect changes in cardiac output in an individual patient with accuracy.

Congenital heart disease

The complex anatomy of congenital heart disease and the associated flow abnormalities are ideally suited to investigation by Doppler echocardiography (Table 3). Obstructive lesions such as pulmonary stenosis, aortic stenosis, and coarctation of the aorta can be localized and characterized using echocardiography whereas the severity of the obstruction can be quantified with a high degree of accuracy using spectral continuous wave Doppler. As excellent Doppler echocardiographic images are usually obtained in infants and children, cardiac catheterization in patients with pulmonary stenosis is now reserved for balloon valvotomy, the diagnosis and severity of stenosis having been made using Doppler echocardiography.

Shunt lesions are best evaluated using colour Doppler flow mapping, by which the abnormal flow velocity patterns are displayed in relation to the surrounding, often complex, structural abnormalities. The size of an atrial septal defect imaged by echocardiography can be confirmed by the distribution of low velocity shunt flow across the defect. In comparison, the sensitivity of colour Doppler flow mapping for high velocity flow will allow imaging of small and/or multiple ventricular septal defects even if these are not apparent using echocardiography alone. The presence of a high velocity jet on colour Doppler flow mapping can then be used to direct the continuous wave Doppler beam in order to measure the peak velocity. In patients with a ventricular septal defect this peak velocity will represent the pressure difference between the ventricles and allow an alternative estimation of right ventricular systolic pressure by subtracting this pressure difference from the systolic arterial pressure, usually measured by cuff sphygmomanometry.

Table 3 *Doppler echocardiography in congenital heart disease*

Spectral Doppler	Colour Doppler flow mapping

Obstructive lesions
    Estimation of pressure drop in:
        pulmonary stenosis
        aortic stenosis
        coarctation of the aorta
 	
Shunt lesions
    Ventricular septal defect:
        detection of ventricular septal
            defect
        estimation of RV systolic
            pressure
    Detection of patent ductus arteriosus
	Obstructive lesions
	    Localizing site of obstruction in congenital lesions for
	        quantification by spectral Doppler
	
	Shunt lesions
	    Site, number, and size of ventricular septal defects
	    Site and size of atrial septal defect
	    Detection of patent ductus arteriosus
	    Detecting shunt flow in complex congenital heart
	        lesions with multiple shunts, e.g. atrioventricular
	        septal defects

Tabel 4 *Common applications of Doppler echocardiography*

Valvar heart disease
  Pressure drop in valve stenosis
  Detection of valve regurgitation
  Assessment of prosthetic valve function
  Estimation of RV pressure from velocity of tricuspid
    regurgitation

Ischaemic heart disease
  Evaluation of systolic and diastolic LV function
  Detection of post-infarction mitral regurgitation
  Detection of post-infarction ventricular septal defect

Congenital heart disease
  Detection and quantification of shunt lesions
  Evaluation of valvar and subvalvar pulmonary stenosis
  Congenital aortic stenosis
  Coarctation of the aorta

Summary

Doppler echocardiography is complementary to conventional echocardiography and, as an ultrasound technique, is subject to many similar limitations, including poor quality recordings in difficult patients. The value of the true maximum velocity may be underestimated if its site is missed by the Doppler beam or if there is a significant angle between the ultrasound beam and blood flow. The strength of Doppler echocardiography lies in its ability to quantify the severity of stenotic lesions and the identification of abnormal high velocity, often turbulent jets associated with valve regurgitation and congenital heart defects (Table 4).

REFERENCES

Hatle, L. and Angelsen, B. (1985). *Doppler ultrasound in cardiology* 2nd edn. Lea & Febiger, Philadelphia.
Wilde, P. (1993). *Cardiac ultrasound: clinical ultrasound, a comprehensive text.* Churchill Livingstone, Edinburgh.

15.4.4 Nuclear techniques

D. J. ROWLANDS and H. J. TESTA

Nuclear imaging of the heart has evolved over the last 20 years and techniques are currently available to demonstrate the extent and distribution of viable myocardium, localized areas of ischaemia induced by exercise or by drugs, recent myocardial cell damage, and global and regional left ventricular function. These investigations involve very low invasiveness and little discomfort or inconvenience to the patient. However, there are limitations inherent in the resolving power of nuclear techniques in general. Tissues less than one cubic centimetre in volume are not demonstrable with reliability, infarcts involving less than 3 to 7 g of myocardium are unlikely to be shown, and edge detection is less reliably accomplished with nuclear angiography than with contrast radiography. Nuclear techniques currently provide a very useful complement to rather than a substitute for electrocardiography, plane chest radiography, echocardiography, and cardiac catheterization.

Scintigraphic determination of left ventricular function

The assessment of left ventricular function is one of the most important aspects of the evaluation of the cardiac status. Traditionally, left ventricular performance has been evaluated by the determination of cardiac output and left ventricular end-diastolic pressure, and by cine-angiography following the injection of contrast material into the left ventricular cavity. These are relatively or highly invasive investigations. Scintigraphic approaches now provide the possibility of obtaining a good deal of information on left ventricular performance by non-invasive means. This information consists of:

1. Estimates of left ventricular ejection fraction (the fraction of the ventricular end-diastolic volume ejected per beat), which is an overall measure of left ventricular performance.
2. Estimates of regional ventricular performance by observation of the movements of the margins of the ventricle.

There are two distinct approaches to the assessment of left ventricular function – the 'first pass technique' and the 'gated equilibrium' method. Both methods involve the intravenous injection of a radioactive tracer, technetium-99m is almost universally used as the tracer. For first pass studies it may be used in its ionic form as technetium-99m-pertechnetate. If multiple studies are to be carried out technetium-99m-diethylene-triaminepenta-acetic acid (DTPA) is preferable because it is cleared rapidly from the blood (as a result of which background activity will be decreased). For gated equilibrium studies the more common procedure is to label the patient's own red blood cells, although labelled human serum albumen may also be used. Both techniques (first pass and gated equilibrium) may be performed with a single injection of radioactive tracer.

The first pass technique

In this technique the first passage of the radioactive bolus through the central circulation is studied. As sequential images follow the passage of the tracer through the central circulation, the right and left ventricular images are separated in time. As a result of this separation, any desired view of the ventricles can be obtained without the problem of overlap of the two ventricular images. The single most useful view is probably the right anterior oblique which is the projection of choice in single plane contrast radiography of the left ventricle. With the gamma-camera positioned over the patient in the right anterior oblique projection, sequential images are obtained after the administration of the tracer and are stored in the computer. Figure 1 shows a sequence of 16 such images obtained at 1-s intervals.

DETERMINATION OF EJECTION FRACTION BY THE FIRST PASS TECHNIQUE

Using the computer display of stored data, a region of interest (ROI) over the left ventricle is outlined and a high frequency activity–time curve for that region of interest plotted. Each point on the curve represents accumulated counts for a period of 0.04 s. The amount of radioactivity in the heart is proportional to the volume of blood in the cardiac cavities. Thus the change in the precordial count rate reflects the cyclical volume changes in the heart. A second region of interest is taken (usually as a horse-shoe-shaped region surrounding the left ventricular region of interest) to sample the background activity variation with time. Digital smoothing processes are applied to the background curve to minimize statistical 'noise' components. The background curve is then 'normalized' to the left ventricular curve (to correct for the different areas of the two). This normalized, smoothed background curve is then subtracted point-for-point from the high frequency left ventricular activity–time curve to give the corrected high frequency left ventricular activity–time curve. (Fig. 2). The ejection fraction (*EF*) is then obtained as:

$$EF = EDc - \frac{ESc}{EDc}$$

where *EDc* is the background-corrected count of end-diastole and *ESc* the background-corrected count of end-systole. Although up to 10 or 12 cycles may be available for analysis, it is usual to take 4 to 6 cycles around the peak of the left ventricular curve and to average the calculated ejection fractions from these cycles.

DETERMINATION OF REGIONAL WALL MOTION BY THE FIRST-PASS TECHNIQUE

It is possible to assess regional wall motion by the first pass technique but this does not represent a good approach to the problem and it is rarely done in practice.

The gated equilibrium technique

This technique is also referred to as gated cardiac blood pool imaging or as multigated acquisition (MUGA) imaging. It is dependent upon complete mixing of the marker throughout the circulating volume and it therefore requires a marker which remains intravascular. The marker of choice is technetium-99m-labelled red blood cells. The cells do not have to be removed from the patient for labelling, for the 'in vivo labelling' technique may be used. This involves predisposing the patient's red cells to accept the technetium label by the administration, 30 min prior to the technetium, of non-active stannous pyrophosphate. Subsequently, 600 to 800 MBq (approximately 15 to 20 mCi) of technetium-99m-pertechnetate are injected intravenously and imaging is begun after a further 10 min or so. As there is complete mixing of the marker throughout the blood volume, all four cardiac chambers are seen simultaneously and various degrees of superimposition of the chambers is inevitable. Proper alignment of the gamma-camera is therefore crucial for the optimal separation of the cardiac chambers. In general, maximal separation of the right and left ventricles is achieved in the left anterior oblique view, to which a caudal tilt of 15° may be added.

DETERMINATION OF EJECTION FRACTION BY THE GATED EQUILIBRIUM TECHNIQUE

A region of interest over the left ventricle and a second horse-shoe-shaped region around the left ventricle (for background correction) are assigned in the same manner as for the first pass technique. A background-corrected activity–time curve of the left ventricular area is obtained (Fig. 3 (normal) and Fig. 4 (abnormal)). With the equilibrium technique this is usually displayed as a single cycle representative activity–time curve being produced as a composite of many (typically hun-

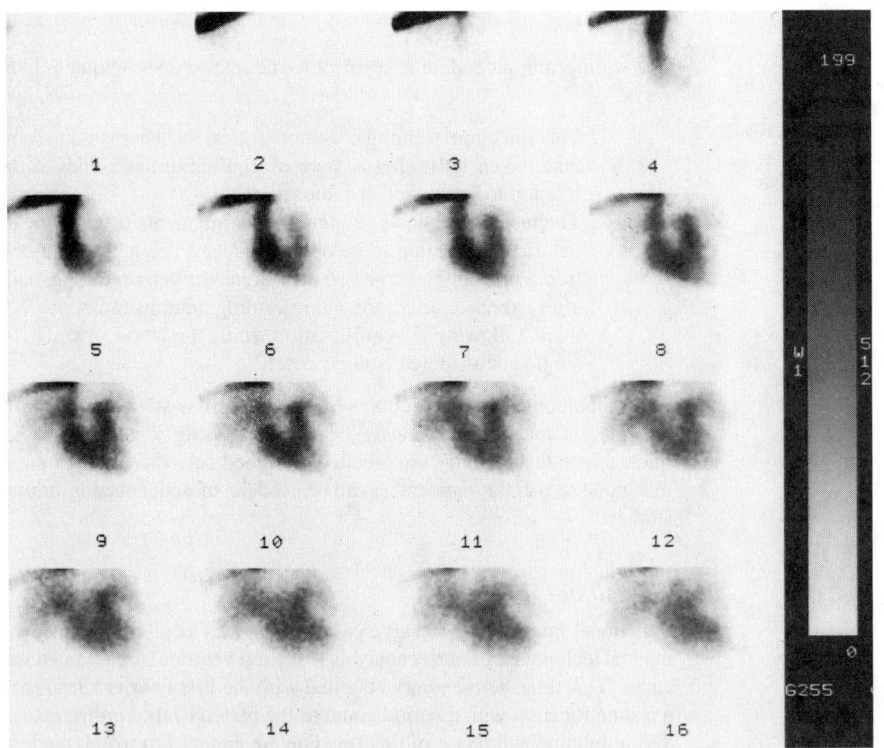

Fig. 1 The first pass technique. Anterior view of the first passage through the central circulation of radioactive tracer injected intravenously via the right arm. In the first frame no activity is seen. In frames 2 and 3 activity is seen in the right subclavian vein. In subsequent frames it is seen descending in the superior vena cava, passing through the right heart, the pulmonary circulation, the left heart, and into the aorta. The right ventricular image is well seen at 6 to 11 s and the left ventricular image at 12 to 16 s.

dreds) consecutive cycles, synchronization of the cycles being achieved by means of the R wave of the electrocardiogram. As the count rate is proportional to the ventricular volume, the ejection fraction can be determined in the same way as with the first pass procedures:

$$EF = EDc - \frac{ESc}{EDc}$$

REGIONAL WALL MOTION STUDIES BY THE GATED EQUILIBRIUM TECHNIQUE

Left ventricular images are collected for each of many short time intervals and the images from corresponding parts of numerous cardiac cycles are summed to produce a composite. Typically, the 'exposure' time for each individual image collection might be 0.03 s, so that if the heart rate were 80 per min (i.e. R–R interval = 0.75 s), there would be 28 images per cardiac cycle. The summed image would typically be collected from several hundred cardiac cycles. In this way 28 'frames' of a 'representative cine-cycle' (i.e. representative of the several hundred actual cycles which occupied the data collection period) are produced. Figure 3 shows an example of end-diastolic and end-systolic 'frames' of such a representative cine-cycle, obtained from the normal heart in the left anterior oblique view. A zone of decreased activity is seen between the two ventricles. Comparison of the end-diastolic and end-systolic ventricular boundaries permits the assessment of regional ventricular contractile performance. (In this example there is uniform contraction of those parts of the ventricular wall which are displayed in this view.) Figure 4 shows end-systolic and end-diastolic frames from a patient with congestive cardiomyopathy. There is uniformly reduced myocardial contraction.

Scintigraphic determination of right ventricular function

Techniques for the assessment of ventricular function are, in general, less satisfactory when applied to the right than to the left ventricle. The differences are less marked in respect of nuclear techniques than of most other techniques and scintigraphic procedures currently offer one of the best approaches to the assessment of right ventricular function.

The basic techniques involved are the same as for the left ventricle. First pass radionulide angiography provides adequate temporal anatomical separation of activity within right-sided and left-sided cardiac structures and provides an ideal method for the assessment of right ventricular ejection fraction. The gated equilibrium technique is, in general, less useful in the assessment of right ventricular function because of the overlap between the two ventricles, but it is possible to obtain useful information concerning right ventricular size and regional wall motion (usually just visually assessed) from this technique and the best approach is to combine the two techniques to obtain a gated first pass study.

Relative advantages and drawbacks of 'first pass' and 'gated equilibrium' scintigraphic ventriculography

The first pass procedure is superior to the equilibrium technique in the following ways.

1. Because of the temporal separation of right and left ventricular studies, it is possible to use the right anterior oblique view for the analysis of regional left ventricular function. This is the projection of choice for single plane contrast cine-angiography (where, of course, any view could be chosen).
2. The first pass technique can also provide information on mean transit times between various sections of the circulation and it permits the production of indicator–dilution curves and of shunt ratios. As absolute cardiac output (from which stroke volume is easily calculated) can be measured from the indicator dilution curves, and as the ejection fraction is determined, the venticular end-diastolic volume can easily be calculated from the equation which defines ejection fraction:

$$EDV = \frac{SV}{EF}$$

where EDV is end diastolic volume; SV is systemic volume, and EF is ejection fraction.
3. The procedure is brief, the complete data being collected from the patient within a minute of the injection. This is less exacting for the patient and it is, of course, more likely that the heart rate will remain regular for a brief period than for a long period.

The equilibrium procedure is superior to the first pass technique in two ways.

1. The injection technique is not critical because studies are undertaken only after a state of equilibrium is achieved in relation to intravascular radioactivity.
2. The technique allows sequential measurements of global and ventricular function to be obtained after a single tracer injection. For example, repeated measurements before, during, and after exercise, or before and after drug administration can be made following the equilibration within the blood stream of a single administered isotope dose.

A combination of both procedures (a gated first pass study) gives most information and this can easily be achieved using a non-diffusable marker (e.g. technetium-99m-labelled red blood cells) for the first pass technique so that the same tracer can be used for subsequent equilibrium studies.

Functional images

Functional images of the heart can be obtained by applying the mathematical technique of Fourier analysis to the left ventricular volume–time curve. This time–activity curve is fitted with the first Fourier harmonic, a cosine function with a period equal to the period of the cardiac cycle. The amplitude and phase of this function are adjusted to match the left

Fig. 2 High frequency activity–time curve recorded from the region of the left ventricle during the first passage of radioactive tracer through the central circulation. The time, in seconds, after the injection is shown on the abscissa. The ordinate displays the scintillation counting rate on a linear scale, after background correction. The early hump shows increased activity during the passage of the tracer through the right ventricle (RV). The later, larger hump shows the count rate during the passage through the left ventricle. Peaks and troughs are visible in relation to each cardiac cycle. Estimates of ejection fraction can be made for each cardiac cycle: $(ED_1 - ES_1/ES_1$, $(ED_2 - ES_2/ED_2$, etc.

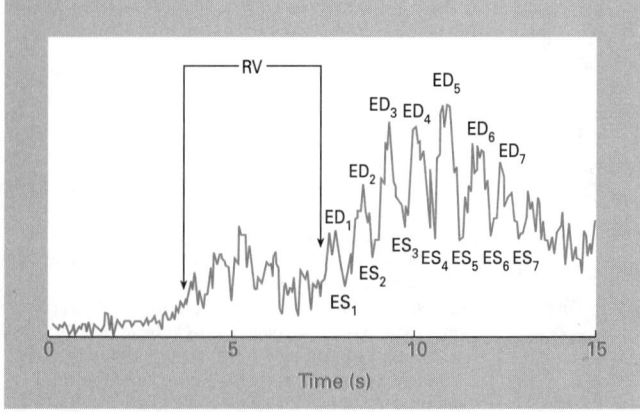

ventricular curve optimally. The amplitude image reflects the change in ventricular volume throughout the cycle. It is similar to the stroke volume but may give a more reliable index of the change in chamber volume.

The phase image represents the time at which the maximum contraction occurs, and gives information on the mechanical contractility of the heart. The atria will contract out of phase with the ventricles. Phase data are also presented as a histogram in which the number of pixels in an image with a particular phase is plotted against the phase.

Radionuclide imaging in the diagnosis of myocardial infarction

Two general approaches have been used for the detection of myocardial infarction or ischaemia.

1. *Recent myocardial damage* may be demonstrated using radiopharmaceuticals, which concentrate selectively in acutely injured cells. This is called positive imaging, infarct-avid imaging, or 'hot-spot' scanning. Clearly, this technique can only be applied within a brief time window (of the order of several days) of the onset of infarction.

2. *Non-viable myocardium* (i.e. recent or long-standing infarction) may be demonstrated by the absence of uptake of certain tracers. The greatest experience is with ionic tracers, and particularly with thallium-201. These tracers, which behave in a fashion similar to the potassium ion, accumulate in viable, perfused myocardium but are not taken up by infarcted myocardium and are taken up to a less than normal extent by ischaemic myocardium. This is called negative imaging, ionic tracer scanning, or 'cold-spot' scanning. The use of lipid-soluble complexes, which appear to diffuse passively into myocardial cells and to bind to cytosol, is being investigated as an alternative to the use of ionic agents. To date the most commonly used such alternative is technetium-99m-2-methoxyisobutyl isonitrile (MIBI). Another recently developed myocardial perfusion imaging agent is technetium-99m-labelled teboroxime. Experience with this agent is currently very limited.

Infarct-avid imaging (hot-spot scanning)

A large number of agents have been used for hot-spot scanning of myocardial infarction but the one most extensively used to date has been technetium-99m-stannous pyrophosphate. The observation that calcium is deposited in irreversibly damaged myocardial cells led to the idea of using technetium-99m-stannous pyrophosphate, a bone scanning agent, as a means of demonstrating myocardial necrosis. The cellular death of myocardial infarction is accompanied by an influx of calcium ions, which are deposited in crystalline and subcrystalline form within mitochondria. It has been suggested that calcium accumulation in this way might be used as an index of irreversible myocardial cell damage after ischaemia. However, it may be that the tracer is associated with cytoplasmic denatured macromolecules rather than with mitochondrial hydroxyapatite.

Technetium-99m-stannous pyrophosphate is not a specific marker of necrosis but is a marker both of irreversible damage (necrosis) and of severe but reversible injury. Clearly, it would be of clinical value to be able to differentiate between these two conditions and other approaches to hot spot scanning have been tried. Those in current clinical usage include: (1) the use of indium-111-labelled leucocytes; and (2) the use of labelled antimyosin monoclonal antibodies. In the first of these techniques the patient's own white blood cells are labelled *in vitro* and then reinjected. This procedure is indicated on the second or third day after the onset of symptoms suggestive of infarction. The migration of white cells into freshly infarcted myocardium can then be visualized by imaging with the indium-111. More recently some experience has been gained with the use of indium-111-labelled monoclonal antimyosin, which binds selectively to irreversably damaged myocytes. The clinical usefulness of this agent remains to be determined but preliminary work suggests that the technique is reliable. In addition to its use in the diagnosis of acute infarction this approach has found some value in the investigation of myocarditis, cardiac transplant rejection, and cardiomyopathy.

The greatest experience by far, however, is with technetium-99m-tin-pyrophosphate. The three most important determinants of the uptake of this agent by the myocardium are as follows.

1. There must be significant myocardial necrosis (it seems that at least 3 g of necrotic tissue are necessary for a positive scan).

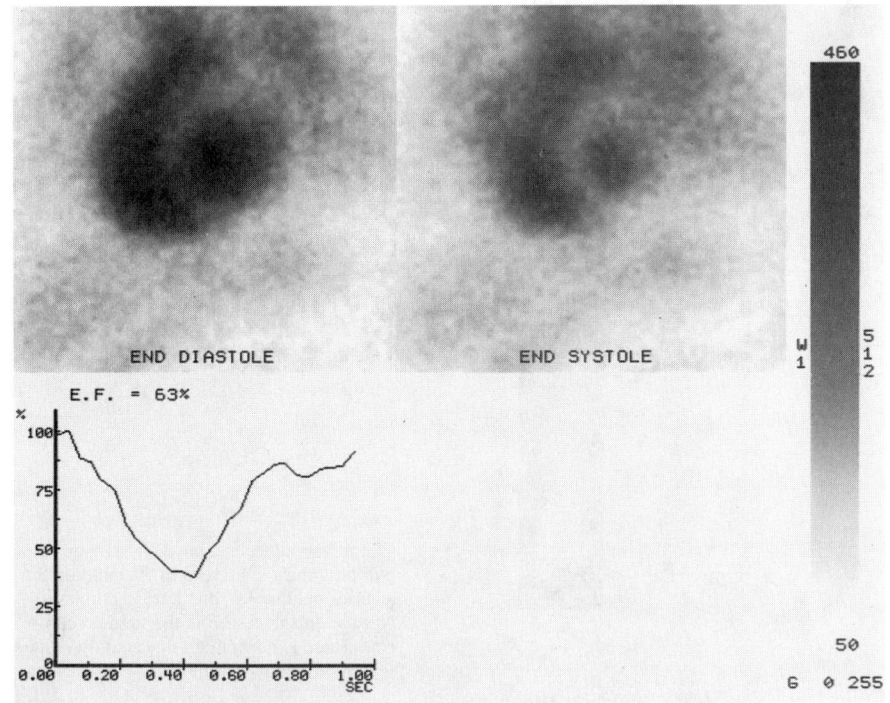

Fig. 3 Normal, resting multigated acquisition scan in the left anterior oblique 45° view. *Top left.* End-diastolic frame. The circular outline of the left ventricular cavity and the crescentic outline of the right ventricular cavity are seen. The curved zone of decreased activity between the two represents the interventricular septum. *Top right.* End-systolic frame. The left ventricular end systolic volume is clearly much smaller than in the end-diastolic frame and all regions of the left ventricle have contracted well. *Bottom left.* Background corrected activity–time curve showing the overall count rate from the region of the left ventricle with the end-diastolic count rate normalized to 100 per cent. The ejection fraction is normal at 63 per cent.

2. There must be persistent residual collateral coronary blood flow into the area of irreversible myocardial damage (something of the order of 20 to 40 per cent of the normal flow being required).

3. The time interval between the clinical onset of infarction and the scanning is critical. Scans are unlikely to be positive in the first 12 h and the optimum scanning time is 24 to 96 h. Ideally two or more scans should be undertaken within this time. Scans may occasionally be positive 2 weeks after an isolated episode of infarction.

Between 200 and 600 MBq (approximately 5 to 15 mCi) of technetium-99m-stannous pyrophosphate are given intravenously. Scanning is undertaken 60 to 90 min following the injection of radionuclide. Scans taken earlier than this are obscured by appreciable residual radioactivity in the cardiac blood pool. Scans taken much later demonstrate marked skeletal uptake. An example of a negative (normal) is shown in Fig. 5 and of a positive (abnormal) technetium-99m-stannous pyrophosphate scan is shown in Fig. 6. The ribs and sternum normally take up the isotope and are always apparent in both normal and abnormal technetium-99m-stannous pyrophosphate scans.

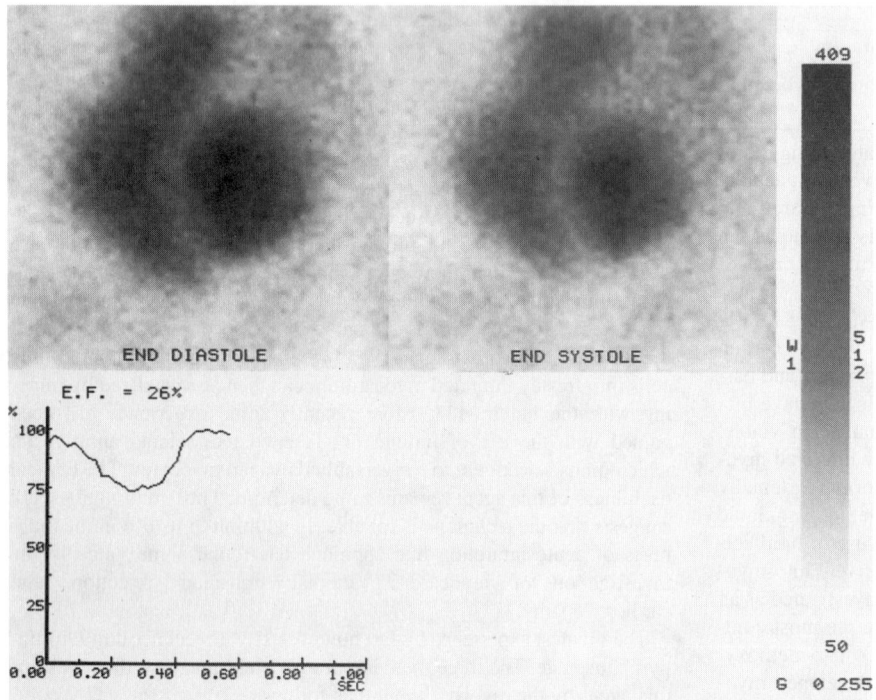

Fig. 4 Abnormal, resting multigated acquisition scan in the left anterior oblique 45° view. The format and layout are as in Fig. 3. There is very little difference between the end-diastolic and end-systolic left ventricular activities and, therefore, volumes (top left and top right respectively) and the reduction in left ventricular contractile performance is uniform. The background corrected activity–time curve shows an ejection fraction of only 26 per cent. The appearances are typical of a congestive cardiomyopathy.

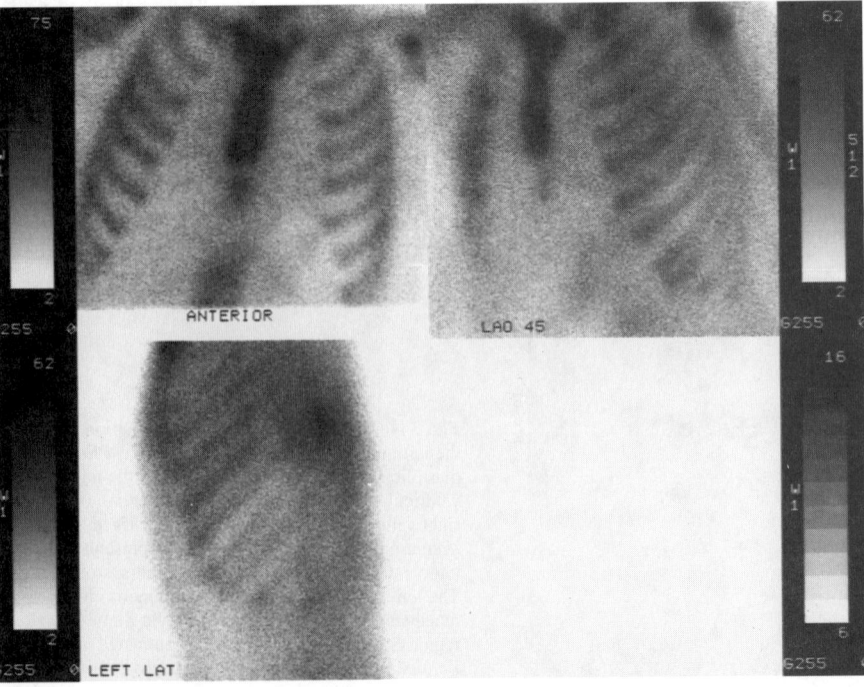

Fig. 5 Normal technetium-99m-stannous pyrophosphate scan, seen in the anterior, left anterior oblique 45°; and left lateral views. Normal uptake is seen in the sternum and ribs. There is no recognizable activity in the region of the myocardium.

DIAGNOSIS OF INFARCTION

False negative and false positive results occur. In 14 different series involving 562 patients with acute myocardial infarction diagnosed by all the usual criteria, the false negative rate was 6 per cent. A further group of 15 different series involving 1083 patients with no evidence of acute infarction showed a false positive rate of 17 per cent. The 'efficiency' of the procedure (i.e. its overall ability correctly to classify patients as to whether or not they had acute infarctions) is 86 per cent. The recorded causes of false positive technetium-99m-stannous pyrophosphate scans include unstable angina, left ventricular aneurysms, cardiomyopathy, valvular calcification, myocardial contusion, persistent blood pool activity, rib fractures, breast tumours, calcified costal cartilages, skeletal muscle damage, and recent cardioversion (giving skeletal muscle or myocardial damage).

LOCALIZATION OF INFARCTION

In general, infarct localization by hot-spot scanning agrees with electrocardiographic localization when the infarct is transmural. Subendocardial infarction cannot be accurately localized. Posterior extension of infarction is more commonly found by hot-spot scanning than would be suggested by standard electrocardiographic criteria.

SIZING OF INFARCTION

Although experimental work shows a good correlation between the scintigraphic estimate of infarct size and infarct size estimated histologically at post-mortem examination, *in vivo* scintigraphic studies in man do not permit accurate sizing because of the limited resolution of scintigraphic images and the complex geometry of infarction.

Myocardial perfusion imaging (cold-spot scanning)

For many years it has been known that radio-isotopes of potassium and of some of its homologues from Group I of the periodic table are actively taken up by myocardial cells. Extensive work has been done on isotopes of potassium, caesium, and rubidium. At present perfusion studies of the myocardium are mainly performed using thallium-201. Although thallium is not in the same group of the periodic table as potassium, its biological behaviour is analogous to that of potassium because of the similarity in size of the hydrated ions. Thallium appears a suitable isotope for myocardial scanning at present because of its physical characteristics. It has a long physical half-life (72 h), providing a longer shelf-life than potassium-43 but with a lower total body radiation dose. Thallium is cleared rapidly from the blood; 5 min after intravenous injection the plasma activity has decreased to 50 per cent of its initial maximum. The myocardial extraction efficiency is high (80 per cent) but as the coronary artery blood flow is only 5 per cent of the total cardiac output, only some 5 to 10 per cent (after several circulations) of the administered dose is concentrated in the myocardium, most of the rest being taken up by kidneys, liver, stomach, and skeletal muscle. Thallium uptake is dependent upon both perfusion and viability of myocardial cells and its concentration in the myocardium depends therefore not only upon normal blood flow distribution but also upon the integrity of the myocardial cell membrane. Defects in the normal distribution of thallium may thus indicate infarction or ischaemia. Experience has shown that defects in scans obtained with the patient at rest indicate infarction, and that defects that are seen on scanning during exercise, but that are not present on scanning at rest indicate local myocardial ischaemia. Typically the patient undergoes an exercise stress test following standard protocols. Exercise is continued until the target heart rate is achieved or until there are clinical indications to discontinue exercise (whichever is the sooner). At peak exercise, or during induced cardiac pain, 80 MBq (approximately 2 mCi) thallium-201 are injected intravenously and (when the safety of the patient permits) exercise is continued for a further 2 min. Scans are taken immediately after cessation of exercise and 3 to 4 h later (to allow time for redistribution of the tracer). An example of a normal myocardial perfusion scan is shown in Fig. 7. The scan shows a doughnut-shaped outline of the left ventricular mass with an area of lesser activity indicating the left ventricular cavity. The cavity is often best delineated in the anterior and left anterior oblique views. The myocardium of the atria and right ventricle is not normally visualized because the mass of myocardium involved per unit

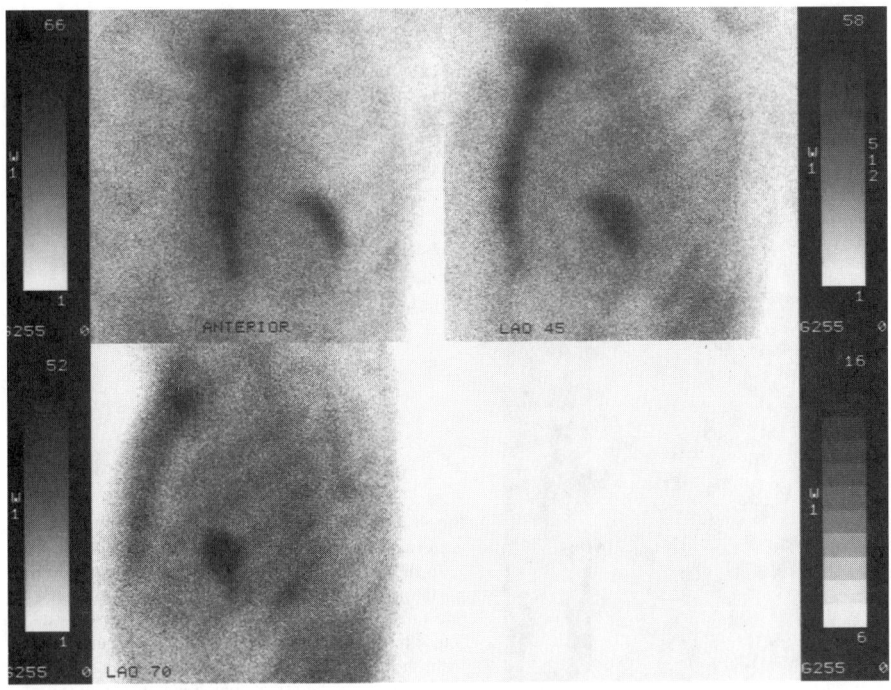

Fig. 6 Abnormal technetium-99m-stannous pyrophosphate scan, seen in the anterior, left anterior oblique 45°; and left lateral views. In addition to the normal uptake in the sternum (well seen) and ribs (less well seen), there is clearly a large area of localized uptake lateral and posterior to the sternum, in the region of the left ventricle. The patient had had an acute myocardial infarction.

area of scan is much less than is the case with the left ventricle. The use of three or more views permits separate visualization of most of the regions of the left ventricular myocardium. An example of an abnormal myocardial perfusion scan (showing infarction) is shown in Fig. 8.

DIAGNOSIS OF INFARCTION

The sensitivity of thallium scintiscanning in the diagnosis of myocardial infarction is related to the size and age of the infarct. Infarcts involving less than 7 g of myocardium may be missed. It is claimed that no false

negatives occur if the scans are undertaken within 6 h of the onset of symptoms. With increasing intervals between the time of onset of symptoms of infarction and the time of scanning there is a moderate reduction in the sensitivity for detection of transmural infarcts and appreciable reduction in the sensitivity for detecting subendocardial infarcts.

LOCALIZATION OF INFARCTION

The use of multiple views with thallium scans permits the localization of defects (whether the defect be an infarct or ischaemia). The scans

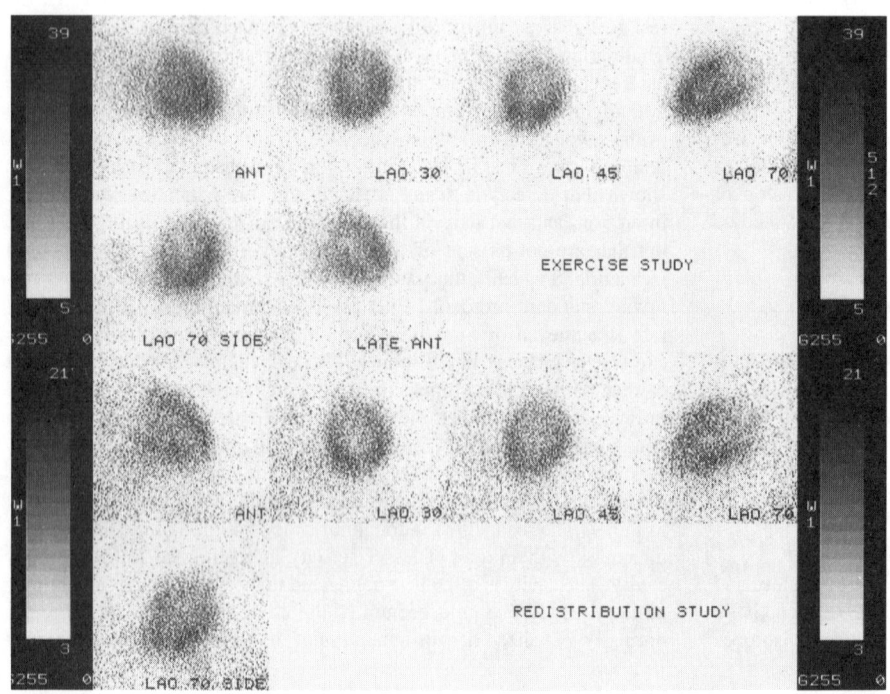

Fig. 7 Normal exercise and resting thallium-201 scan. Anterior and four anterior oblique views are seen. The 'late anterior' view helps to reduce the possibility of missing a defect in this view (which could happen because of the rapid ventricular movement which is occurring at peak exercise). The doughnut-shaped outline of the left ventricular myocardial activity is seen. Tracer concentration appears uniform throughout the left ventricular myocardium and there is no apparent difference between the appearances during exercise and after a period of 3 to 4 h rest.

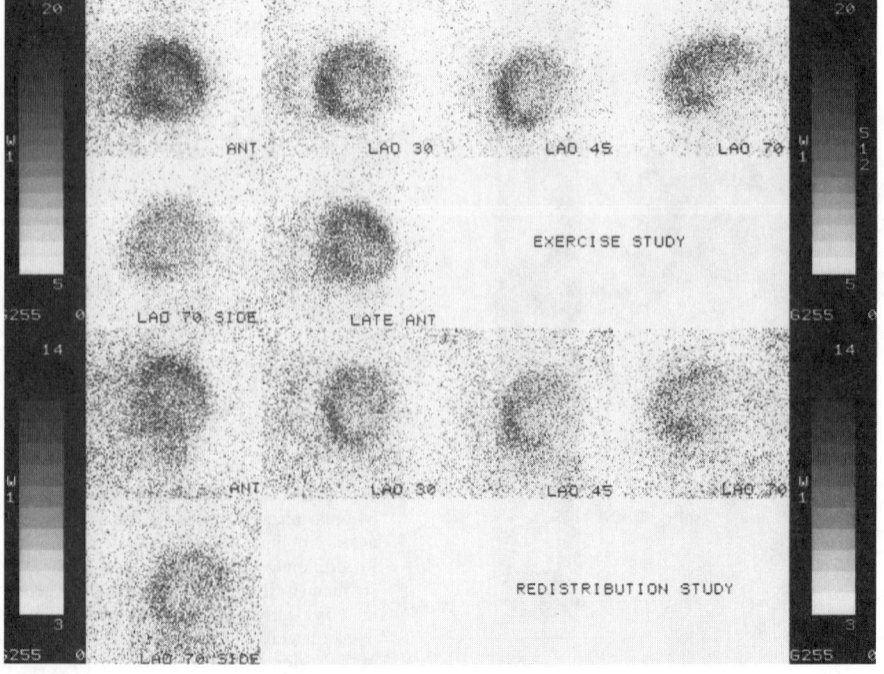

Fig. 8 Abnormal exercise and resting thallium-201 scan (infarction). The format and layout are as in Fig. 7. In the exercise study there is reduced uptake in the posteroinferior wall of the left ventricle. This could be due to ischaemia or infarction. The resting scan (taken 3 to 4 h later) shows appearances indistinguishable from those obtained during exercise, indicating that the myocardium in the affected area is non-viable (i.e. the patient has had a posteroinferior infarction).

have a tendency to underestimate the incidence of inferior infarction (compared with the electrocardiogram) but they are more likely to diagnose true posterior infarcts than the standard electrocardiogram.

SIZING OF INFARCTION

No reliable clinical method currently exists for the assessment of infarct size. Early hopes that cold-spot scanning would provide such an estimate have not been sustained. There is certainly a correlation between the size of infarction as assessed isotopically and as assessed by electrocardiography or by serial enzyme estimation, but precise sizing of infarcts by any technique is not possible.

Myocardial perfusion imaging in the recognition and assessment of myocardial ischaemia

The ionic tracers have extensively and increasingly been used in the recognition and assessment of myocardial ischaemia, irrespective of the presence or absence of established infarction. Although the technique can be used to demonstrate spontaneously occurring ischaemia, opportunities for such studies are necessarily limited and in general are fortuitous. Most perfusion scintigraphic studies are undertaken as formally conducted stress tests. Exercise is usually the chosen mechanism for the induction of stress but not infrequently stress tests are conducted using infusions of pharmacological vasodilators such as dipyridamole or adenosine as the mode of stress induction. After injection at maximal chosen or achievable exercise, thallium-201 accumulates rapidly in myocardium that is both viable and also adequately perfused. Any localized defects occurring in association with stress (exercise- or vasodilator-induced) are indicative of non-viability (infarction) or underperfusion (ischaemia). Defects of thallium uptake occurring in the absence of stress (or after redistribution during a period of rest following the stress) correlate well with areas of infarction. Scans from a patient with exercise-induced myocardial ischaemia are shown in Fig. 9. A defect in tracer uptake is seen on the immediate postexercise scan. In the course of the next few hours redistribution of thallium occurs within myocardium (as the ischaemic but viable area continues to take up thallium

from residual blood pool activity). The ultimate near normality of uptake indicates viability of the myocardium and the immediate postexercise deficit is thus seen to be indicative of ischaemia.

Use of other agents: technetium-99m-labelled isonitriles

Lipid soluble complexes such as technetium-99m 2-methoxy-isobutyl isonitrile (MIBI) have been proposed and used in humans as a possible replacement for thallium. The mechanism of uptake of these compounds is not completely understood but technetium-99m-2-methoxy-isobutyl isonitrile diffuses passively into the myocardial cell and concentrates in the cytosol of normally perfused myocardium. Technetium-99m-2-methoxy-isobutyl isonitrile does not redistribute from its initial pattern of uptake and as a consequence two injections are necessary: one at peak exercise and the second one at rest. After injection, images start at 5 to 10 min, but because of the absence of redistribution, images can also be acquired at a later time.

In clinical practice technetium-99m-labelled compounds have the advantage of continuous availability and of better energy with a higher photon yield than thallium-201. The latter feature gives the potential for better images. In addition because of the shorter half-life of technetium-99m the radiation dose to the patient is less. The disadvantages of technetium-99m-2-methoxy-isobutyl isonitrile compared with thallium-201 are the rapid liver and lung uptake, and the need to perform two injections, which, in most centres, are carried out on two consecutive days.

Single photon emission computed tomography

This technique has been applied mainly to myocardial perfusion imaging, either using thallium or technetium labelled isonitriles. It allows tomographic images of the heart to be obtained. The patient is positioned supine on the single photon emission computed tomography (SPECT) couch with the left arm placed over the head to avoid attenuation artefacts. The gamma-camera rotates around the patient through 180° from the right anterior oblique 30° to the left posterior oblique 30°, at 6° increments of 30 s duration. The orbit of rotation may be circular or non-circular; the latter is preferred. The acquired data are fed into the

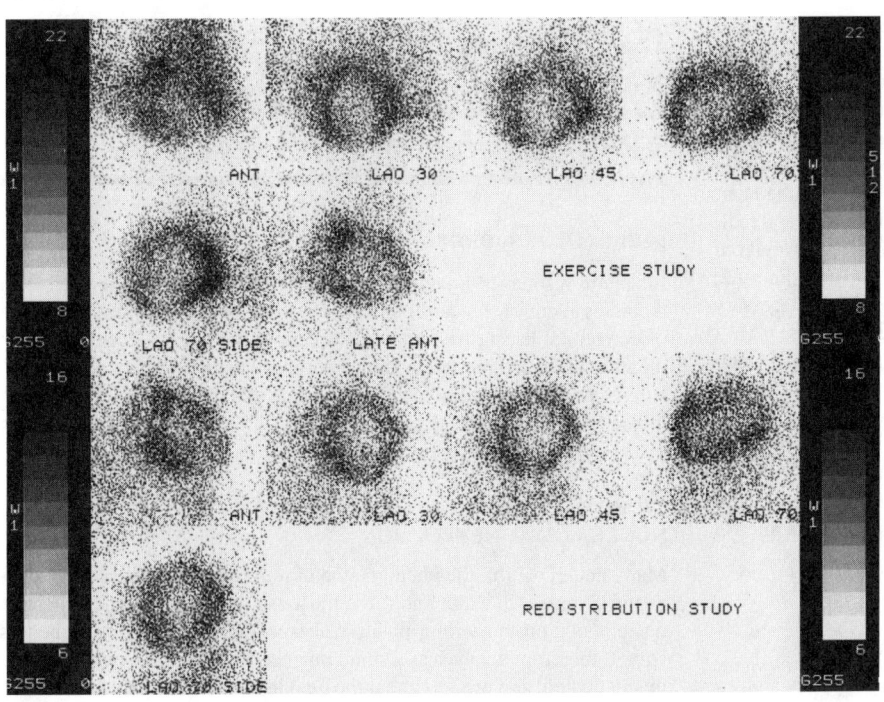

Fig. 9 Abnormal exercise and resting thallium-201 scan (ischaemia). The format and layout are as in Figs 7 and 8. In the exercise study there is reduced uptake in the inferior wall of the left ventricle. This could be due to ischaemia or infarction. The resting scan (taken 3 to 4 h later) shows improvement in the uptake in the inferior wall. The reversible defect indicates the occurrence of exercise-induced inferior wall ischaemia.

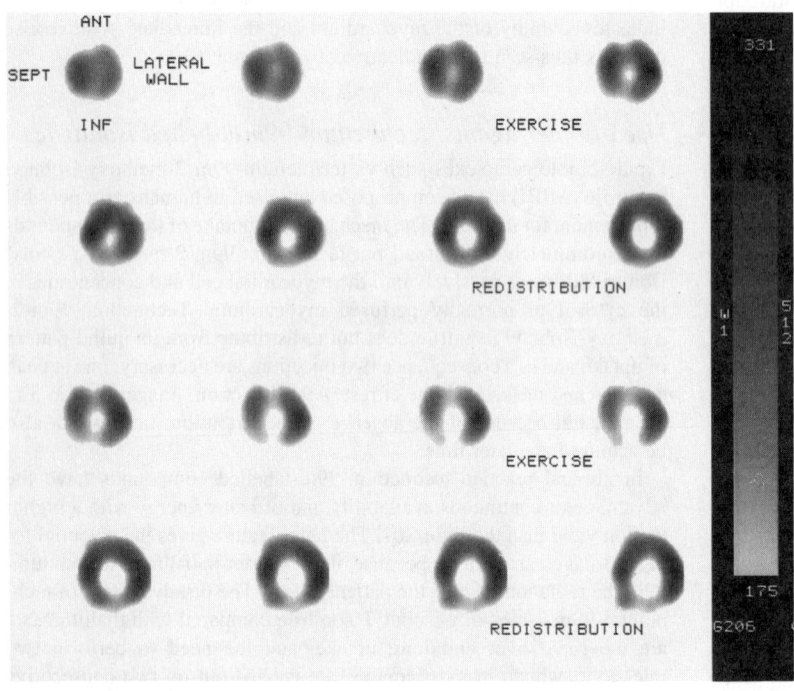

Fig. 10 Abnormal tomographic thallium scan. The appearances during exercise and following redistribution after 3 to 4 h rest are shown. The first and third rows were taken during exercise and the second and fourth rows after redistribution. The tomographic planes are at right angles to the long axis of the left ventricle. The top left hand cut is taken from the region of the left ventricular apex and cuts further to the right and in the third row are taken progressively further from the apex and nearer to the base of the heart. Eight cuts are shown for the exercise and for the subsequent resting study. In each cut the anterior, septal, free wall, and inferior zones of the left ventricular myocardium are as indicated. During exercise, there is decreased activity in the anterior and inferior walls of the left ventricle. Following redistribution (period of 3 to 4 h) there is no longer any defect in the anterior wall but the inferior wall defect is still apparent, though less striking. The findings would be interpreted as indicating exercise-induced ischaemia of the anterior left ventricular wall together with partial thickness infarction and exercise-induced ischaemia of the inferior left ventricular wall.

computer system and slice images are constructed using the techniques of filtering back projection at approximately 1 cm intervals. Sagittal, coronal, short- and long-axis slices are reconstructed for clinical evaluation. An example of images obtained in this way is shown in Fig. 10. This study was obtained in a patient with an inferolateral myocardial infarction.

It is not yet clear whether single photon emission computed tomography has real clinical advantages over multiprojection planar images. The theoretical advantages of tomography include the ability to produce a true three-dimensional image of the distribution of tracer in the myocardium with improved image contrast due to the elimination of overlying structures.

Positron emission tomography

This relatively new technique uses positron emitting radionuclides and emission computed axial tomography to produce tomographic images of coronary flow and cardiac metabolism. The instrumentation consists of detector systems working in coincidence to register the paired anihilation photons emmitted from the radiopharmaceuticals. Positron emission tomography (PET) devices record multiple slices of the heart simultaneously (usually between three and eighteen slices). Several radiopharmaceuticals have been used; perfusion studies may be carried out injecting patients with either ammonia-13, $H_2^{15}O$, or rubidium-82. Because of the very short half-life of these radionuclides, it is necessary to inject the patient twice (at rest and during maximum exercise). Metabolic studies of the heart have been carried out using carbon-11-palmitate or glucose analogues such as fluorine-18-deoxyglucose. These procedures are relatively new and still in the process of evaluation. There is the suggestion that perfusion studies are more accurate than thallium scanning in the detection of exercise induced ischaemia, and equal to thallium in the detection of infarction. The main drawback to this technique is cost. It requires expensive detectors and a cyclotron in site for the production of most of these radionuclides.

REFERENCES

Feiglin, D. (1989). The cardiovascular system. In *Practical nuclear medicine* (ed P.F. Sharpe, H.G. Gemmell, and F.W. Smith), pp. 137–159. IRL Press, Oxford.

Isakandrian, A.S. and Heo, J. (1991). Nuclear cardiac imaging. *Current Opinion in Cardiology*, **6,** 953–964.

Pennell, D.J., Underwood, R., Costa, D.C., and Ell, P.J. (1992). *Thallium myocardial perfusion tomography in clinical cardiology*. Springer-Verlag, Berlin.

Rigo, P. and De Landsheere, C. (1989). Radionuclide imaging in the assessment of cardiac disease. *Current Opinion in Cardiology*. **4,** 824–833.

Tamaki, N., Fishman, A.J., and Straus, W.H. (1991). Radionuclide imaging of the heart. In *Clinical nuclear medicine*, (2nd edn) (ed M.N. Maisey, K.E. Britton, and D. L. Gilday), pp. 1–40. Chapman and Hall, London.

Waldenström, A. and Långstrom, B. (1991). Assessment of cardiac metabolic disorders with positron emission tomography. *Current Opinion in Cardiology*, **6,** 695–971.

15.4.5 Magnetic resonance and computed X-ray tomography

S.R. Underwood and P.F. Ludman

Magnetic resonance

Magnetic resonance imaging has a small but important clinical role in the assessment of the cardiovascular system, particularly in the context of congenital heart disease and disorders of the aorta. Recent developments such as magnetic resonance coronary angiography and the measurement of myocardial perfusion mean that it is likely to have an increasing role in cardiac patients.

Physical principles

NUCLEAR MAGNETIZATION

Many nuclei exhibit the phenomenon of magnetic resonance, but hydrogen is abundant in water and is the most useful clinically. The hydrogen nucleus is a proton with a positive charge and a property described as spin. It therefore behaves as a small magnet. It will align with an applied magnetic field and precess about the field in the same way that a spinning top precesses in a gravitational field. The frequency of precession depends on the strength of the magnetic field but at a typical imaging field of 0.5 Tesla the precessional or resonant frequency is approximately 21 MHz.

It is easiest to understand magnetic resonance by considering the net effect of many protons. Quantum mechanics dictates that individual protons can take up only two orientations with respect to an applied field, parallel and antiparallel. At normal temperatures there is a small excess of nuclei in the lower energy parallel orientation and so there is a net magnetisation vector in the direction of the applied field (Fig. 1). Because precession of individual protons is uncoordinated, there is no net magnetisation in the plane perpendicular to the field. Applying radio waves at the resonant frequency, however, excites some protons to the higher energy antiparallel orientation and these protons initially precess in phase together. The net effect is to rotate the net magnetisation vector at an angle to the applied field, and this initial flip angle is determined by the amount of energy applied (Fig. 2). Flip angles of 90 degrees and 180 degrees are common. After absorption of energy, the net magnetization vector precesses and relaxes back to its equilibrium position tracing out a spiral. As long as there is a component of magnetization perpendicular to the applied magnetic field, an emitted radio signal at the precessional frequency will be detected.

The rates at which the net magnetization parallel and perpendicular to the applied field return to equilibrium after a disturbance are called the longitudinal (T_1) and transverse relaxation times (T_2) respectively. They depend upon the fluctuating magnetic fields experienced by the nuclei, and hence upon their biochemical and biophysical environment.

MAGNETIC RESONANCE IMAGING

Conventional magnetic resonance images are maps of the amplitude of the emitted radio signal at each point in the imaging plane (Fig. 3). The

Fig. 1 Individual nuclear magnetization vectors align parallel and antiparallel (but at an angle) to an applied magnetic field (B_0). The net effect is a magnetization vector (M) in the direction of the applied field.

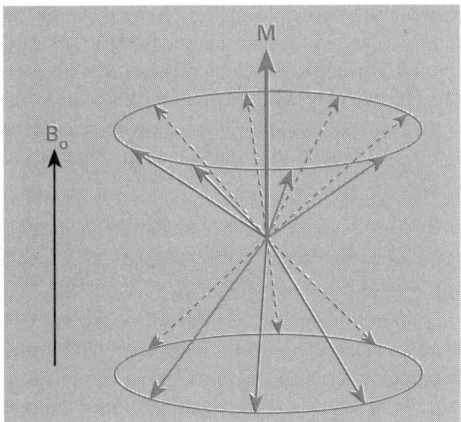

Fig. 2 The net magnetization vector (M) can be displaced from its equilibrium position parallel to the applied magnetic field (B_0). Its component in the xy plane (M_{xy}) can be detected as a radio signal.

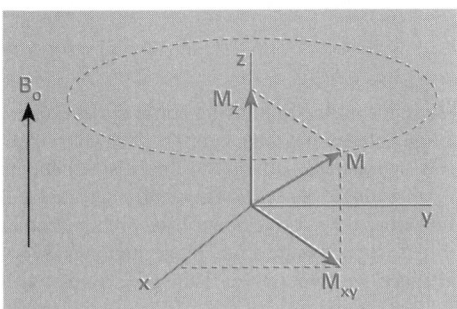

signal is stimulated and localized by pulses of radiofrequency energy and magnetic field gradients superimposed upon the main field. A common combination of pulses (or sequence) is the spin echo sequence. In spin echo images, moving blood gives no signal and appears black, in contrast to other tissues which give some signal and appear in increasing shades of grey. The strength of the signal, and hence the contrast in the images, depends partly upon proton density and upon the relaxation times of the nuclei. The timing of the sequence can be altered to weight the signal towards any of these three parameters and so limited biochemical information can be obtained. Fat, for instance, normally appears with a high signal, other soft tissues with intermediate signal, and fibrous tissue or cortical bone with a low signal. Abnormal increases in signal can be used to detect pathology, such as the oedema related to acute myocardial ischaemia.

Another common sequence is the gradient echo sequence in which blood gives high signal and appears white, except where it is turbulent when it can lose signal. Such gradient echo images can be repeated rapidly in the same plane to generate a cine image consisting of a number of frames through the cardiac cycle (typically 16 to 32). A modification of gradient echo imaging is used to measure flow by encoding velocity in the phase of the magnetic resonance signal. A map of the phase of the signal rather than the amplitude then becomes a velocity map, and the images show velocity in a chosen direction with respect to the imaging plane.

MAGNETIC RESONANCE SPECTROSCOPY

The frequency of the emitted radio signal is determined by the magnetic field experienced by the nucleus. Because nuclei in different chemical environments are screened from the external field by surrounding electrons to varying extents, the same nucleus in different chemical environments will emit signal at different frequencies. The spectrum of frequencies gives important information since the position of the peaks identifies chemical species and the size of each is proportional to the number of emitting nuclei.

Magnetic resonance imaging is almost entirely restricted to the hydro-

Fig. 3 Spin echo images showing normal anatomy. (Top left, coronal; top right, transverse; bottom left, horizontal long axis; bottom right, short axis. LV, left ventricle; RV, right ventricle; LA, left atrium; RA, right atrium; Ao, aorta; DA, descending aorta; PA, pulmonary artery.)

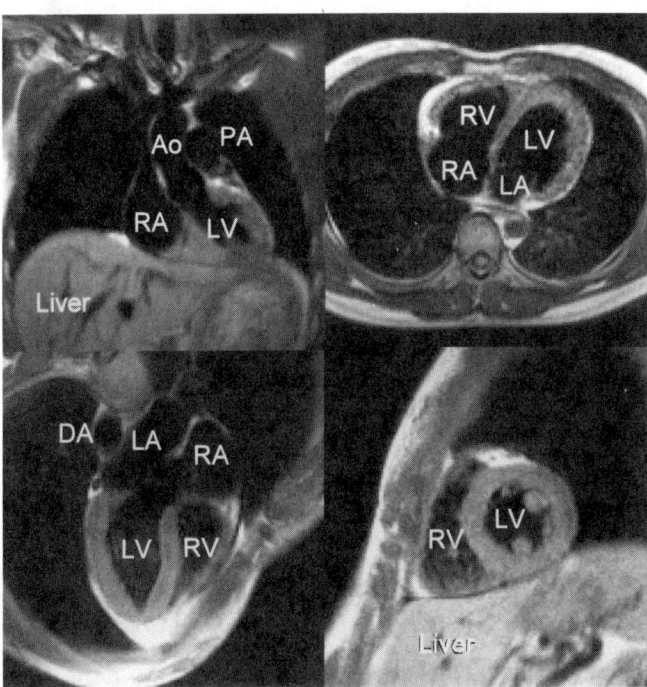

gen nucleus because of its abundance and the need for a strong signal. Although hydrogen spectroscopy is possible, the number of different chemical environments in which it is found make interpretation difficult. Phosphorus-31 spectroscopy is more useful, and its value lies in the importance of phosphorus-containing compounds in cellular metabolism. The ratio of high energy phosphates (phosphocreatine and adenosine triphosphate) to inorganic phosphate is a measure of tissue energetics, and the position of the inorganic phosphate peak reflects intracellular pH.

CONTRAST MEDIA

Magnetic resonance contrast agents are paramagnetic compounds that influence the relaxation times of tissues with which they have close contact, by virtue of unpaired electrons in the outer shell of a central atom or ion. Gadolinium (Gd) is a particularly powerful paramagnetic substance because of the seven unpaired electrons in its outer shell. Uncomplexed gadolinium ions are toxic but non-toxic organic complexes such as diethylene-triamine penta-acetic acid (DTPA) can be used as magnetic resonance contrast agents. In addition to complexes of gadolinium, manganese ethylene diamine tetraphosphonate (Mn-TP), manganese bis-pyridoxal ethylene diamine diacetate (Mn-DPDP), and dysprosium-DTPA have been studied in animal models.

SAFETY

There are no known hazards associated with occasional exposure to radiofrequency radiation or high intensity magnetic fields. The absorption of radiowaves generates heat but this does not produce significant heating in well perfused tissues. The rapidly changing magnetic field gradients induce currents in the body but these are small. Flashes of light from retinal stimulation and muscle twitching have been reported using fast imaging techniques in high magnetic fields. Patients with pacemakers should not be scanned because of the effect of the magnetic field upon the pacemaker electronics and because of the theoretical possibility of inducing currents in the pacing lead which might cause arrhythmias. The confines of the magnet cause 5 per cent of patients some anxiety, but this is reduced by careful explanation, the company of relatives, and mirrors allowing vision out of the magnet. About 1.5 per cent of patients fail to complete the examination.

Clinical applications

CONGENITAL HEART DISEASE

Spin echo images in multiple contiguous slices and in several planes provide excellent anatomical information. Magnetic resonance compares favourably with echocardiography and cardiac catheterization in providing a complete anatomical diagnosis in 90 per cent of cases although congenital anomalies of the valves and small defects of the interatrial and interventricular septum are often difficult to visualize on spin echo images alone. Cine gradient echo images provide additional information such as ventricular function, particularly on the right. They also show turbulent blood flow in a manner similar to colour coded Doppler and this improves the detection of small ventricular and atrial shunts. The combination of cine imaging with velocity mapping provides further information, improving the detection of shunts and allowing flow to be measured in conduits, great vessels, and within the heart. Shunts can therefore be measured either from the difference in stroke volumes of left and right ventricles or more flexibly by measuring flow directly in the aorta and pulmonary artery.

Pulmonary arteries

Several studies have shown the ability of magnetic resonance imaging to identify the central pulmonary arteries in patients with pulmonary atresia and this is particularly helpful to determine the feasibility of creating a shunt surgically and to monitor the growth of the pulmonary artery after shunting. In these patients, magnetic resonance is also able to assess shunt patency accurately, although complete evaluation of systemic collateral arteries, particularly their distal connections, may require selective angiography. Peripheral pulmonary artery stenoses can be missed by magnetic resonance imaging.

Pulmonary and systemic veins

Normal pulmonary veins can be identified in most patients and 95 per cent of pulmonary venous abnormalities can be diagnosed. This is superior to cardiac catheterization and to transthoracic echocardiography. Abnormalities of the systemic veins such as a left-sided superior vena cava and its drainage are clearly seen.

Transposition of the great arteries

In patients with transposition that has been surgically repaired, postoperative follow-up with magnetic resonance imaging is a valuable addition to transthoracic echocardiography for the detection of superior vena caval obstruction. Cine gradient echo imaging can improve the assessment by demonstrating abnormal flow patterns associated with residual ventricular septal defects, subpulmonary stenosis, obstruction of the pulmonary venous atrium, and baffle leaks. Because the right ventricle supports the systemic circulation in these patients, outcome is determined in part by right ventricular function and competence of the tricuspid valve. Magnetic resonance can be used to monitor both of these accurately and reproducibly. In a minority of patients, artefacts caused by sternal wires may preclude complete assessment of the right ventricle.

Surgical conduits

Obstruction of conduits between the right ventricle and the pulmonary circulation, such as in tricuspid atresia after the Fontan operation, may be difficult to detect clinically because patients may be asymptomatic despite significant obstruction. Magnetic resonance imaging can demonstrate the anatomy of the proximal and distal anastomoses and obstruction within the conduit caused by intimal proliferation or 'peel' (Fig. 4). A pressure gradient can be determined by velocity mapping and invasive investigation can be avoided in many cases. In contrast, echocardiography often fails to visualize the conduit because of its position behind the sternum. Palliative systemic to pulmonary shunts are also difficult to assess by echocardiography but magnetic resonance imaging is able to provide anatomical and functional information in most patients.

Complex disease

Another group of patients in whom magnetic resonance imaging has advantages over other techniques are those with complex congenital disease such as single or common ventricles. These anomalies are frequently associated with abnormal thoracic or abdominal situs, and abnormal venous and ventriculoarterial connections. Spin echo imaging is as effective as angiography in demonstrating ventricular morphology and size, the orientation of the septum relative to the atrioventricular valves, and the origins and relationships of the great vessels. Magnetic resonance imaging is superior to other imaging techniques for assessing thoracic and abdominal situs and systemic and pulmonary venoatrial connections.

THE AORTA

The advantages of magnetic resonance in imaging aortic dissection are its ability to image in oblique planes and the fact that it does not require contrast injection, but it is undoubtedly difficult to image sick patients in the current generation of scanners. Dissection is readily detected and its extent can be seen including the involvement of the arch and other vessels (Fig. 5). The ability to demonstrate aortic regurgitation and rupture into the pericardial space are important additional features when assessing these patients. Because the intimal flap is thin it may not be easily seen in spin echo images unless static blood in the false lumen leads to natural contrast with the true lumen. If there is any doubt, then the flap will be more easily seen using a gradient echo sequence, and velocity mapping will confirm the diagnosis by demonstrating the differential flow velocities in each lumen.

Comparisons of magnetic resonance imaging with other imaging techniques have indicated that magnetic resonance should be the primary investigation in stable patients and transoesophageal echocardiography the primary investigation in patients who are too ill to be imaged by magnetic resonance. In most cases, the investigation performed will depend upon practical problems such as local expertise and availability of equipment.

Other aortic abnormalities that can be seen by magnetic resonance are aneurysms and coarction. The combination of anatomical imaging with velocity mapping to assess the gradient across the coarction mean that surgical decisions can be taken without invasive investigation in many cases. It is an ideal method for the long-term follow-up of patients following coarction repair and patients with Marfan's syndrome. A further application is in suspected abscess in the heart or around the aortic root in postoperative patients with infection which is difficult to control. Echocardiography often gives equivocal results in such patients, whilst magnetic resonance will usually produce a definitive answer.

TUMOURS

Magnetic resonance imaging can provide additional information in many patients with masses previously identified by echocardiography. Although it is not possible to identify the nature of a mass from its signal with certainty, the high signal of lipomata and the appearance of angiomata are often characteristic. Gadolinium-diethylene-triamine penta-acetic acid (Gd-DTPA) may be helpful to demonstrate vascularity and to distinguish myxoma from thrombus. Even in the absence of typical signal, a diagnosis can often be made from the site and size of the tumour and from its involvement of neighbouring tissues.

Metastatic tumours are much more frequent than primary cardiac tumours. These can also be imaged successfully, whether they come from direct invasion of the heart such as in carcinoma of the bronchus or are distant metastases as in melanoma. Involvement of the myocardium or pericardium can be identified if present and the large field of view is a considerable advantage over echocardiography for determining the extent of tumour.

THROMBUS

Atrial and ventricular thrombus is easily identified by magnetic resonance although tranoesophageal echocardiography is also reliable in the left atrium and the transthoracic approach often provides clear images in the ventricles. It is important to combine spin echo magnetic resonance imaging with cine gradient echo imaging because it may be difficult to distinguish signal from thrombus and from slowly moving blood in spin echo images. Although contrast is not as great in cine gradient echo images it is more consistent and the presence of a fixed filling defect is characteristic of thrombus.

PERICARDIUM

Pericardial thickening is readily demonstrated by magnetic resonance and by computed X-ray tomography and both techniques are more accurate than echocardiography. The most common clinical question is to distinguish between pericardial constriction and myocardial restriction, when a thickened pericardium with the haemodynamic features of constriction makes the distinction reliably. Cine imaging shows immobility of the pericardium and additional features that indicate constriction are dilated atria and caval veins, small ventricles with retained systolic function, and a reduced diastolic caval flow peak suggesting impaired right ventricular filling. Magnetic resonance cannot detect calcification reliably and this may be a drawback if pericardectomy is planned.

Pericardial effusion is also clearly seen on spin echo images but its appearance is variable. Moving fluid gives no signal but static fluid gives a high one particularly if haemorrhagic. It can also appear with varying signal in cine gradient echo imaging because rapid through plane refreshment of fluid reduces magnetic saturation. Cine imaging is there-

Fig. 4 Transverse spin echo images from superior (top left) to inferior (bottom right) in a patient with tricuspid atresia (TA) and a Fontan conduit (F) connecting right atrial appendage (RAA) to pulmonary artery (PA). The right ventricle is hypoplastic and has a ventricular septal defect (VSD). There is also an atrial septal defect (ASD).

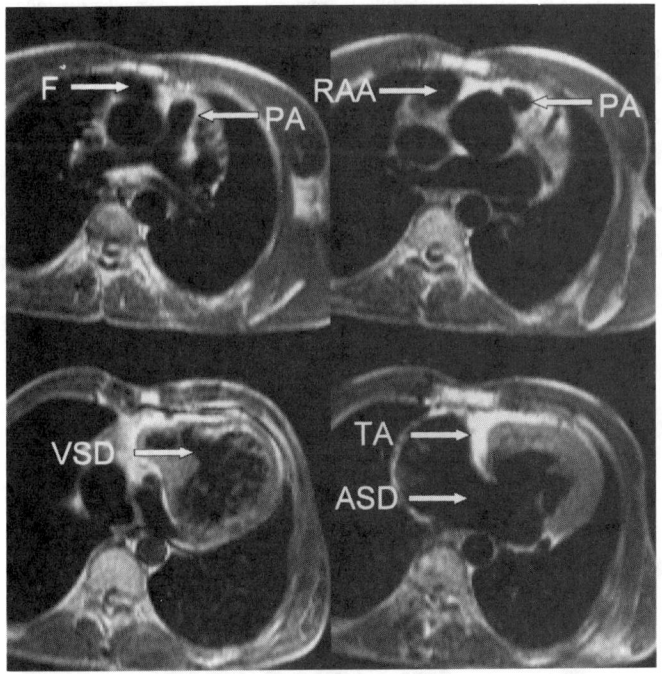

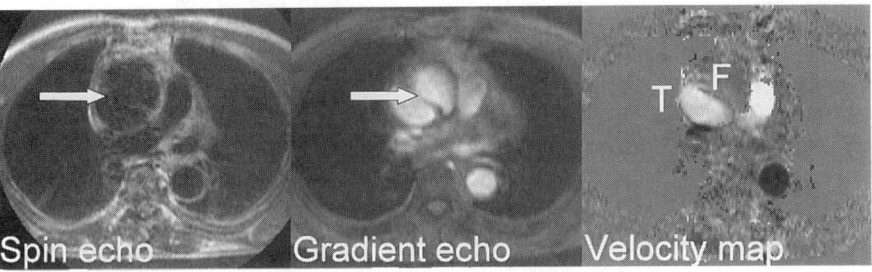

Fig. 5 Three images in the same plane in a patient with aortic dissection. The ascending aorta is dilated and there is an intimal flap (arrow), better seen in the gradient echo image. The velocity map shows rapid systolic flow in the true lumen (T-white), and absent flow in the false lumen (F-in grey).

fore particularly helpful to distinguish thickened pericardium from a pericardial effusion.

MYOCARDIUM

Hypertrophy

The measurement of myocardial volume and mass has been extensively validated in animal experiments and in humans and because of its accuracy, magnetic resonance should now be the standard against which other techniques are judged. Increased muscle volume (and hence mass) can be observed in athletes and patients with left ventricular hypertrophy, and the regression of hypertrophy following treatment of hypertension can be monitored.

Hypertrophic cardiomyopathy

The location and severity of hypertrophic cardiomyopathy is readily assessed. Many patients do not have the classic form of asymmetric septal hypertrophy, and apical hypertrophy in particular is better shown by magnetic resonance imaging than by echocardiography. Metabolic abnormalities have also been observed using phosphorus-31 spectroscopy. A reduced ratio of phosphocreatine to adenosine triphosphate has been described in hypertrophic cardiomyopathy of the right ventricle in a few patients. Similar changes have also been detected in ventricular failure in dilated cardiomyopathy and in valvular disease, and are therefore likely to reflect myocardial failure rather than hypertrophy.

Dilated cardiomyopathy

Chamber dilatation and impaired myocardial thickening are clearly demonstrated. Because of the reproducibility of magnetic resonance measurements even modest changes of systolic and diastolic function can be monitored serially.

Other myocardial disease

Non-coronary myocardial disease can manifest itself by abnormalities of global and regional left ventricular function or by abnormalities of relaxation times, which lead to differential contrast within the myocardium. Myocardial sarcoidosis is an example where magnetic resonance may have a clinical role because there is a high incidence of subclinical involvement. Conventional methods of detection include electrocardiography, echocardiography, and thallium-201 or gallium-67 scintigraphy, but the sensitivity of all of these techniques is limited. Magnetic resonance can show active involvement either as increased myocardial signal indicating active inflammation, or as abnormal regional wall motion.

Generalized thickening of the myocardium and valves is seen in advanced cardiac amyloidosis. Early involvement may not be apparent although abnormal diastolic function may be suggestive. Other myocardial diseases in which abnormalities have been demonstrated include myocarditis, systemic lupus erythematosus, Pompe's disease, and Fabry's disease.

ENDOCARDIUM

Magnetic resonance is not as good as echocardiography at demonstrating small moving structures such as thickened valves and vegetations, but it is able to detect complications of infective endocarditis such as aneurysms and abscesses. The interpretation of spin echo images is only minimally compromised by the presence of a prosthetic valve and because infection of these valves is a frequent cause of perivalvular abscess magnetic resonance imaging should be used if there is any doubt after echocardiography.

Fig. 7 Cine velocity mapping in an oblique plane through the aortic valve in a patient with aortic stenosis and regurgitation. Twelve frames are shown through the cardiac cycle (top left to bottom right). There is a systolic jet from left ventricle to aorta in systole (black, frames 1 to 8), and a smaller diastolic jet of regurgitation in diastole (white, frames 10 to 12). Peak systolic velocity in the jet was 4 m/s compatible with a pressure gradient of 64 mmHg. (With acknowledgement to Dr P.J. Kilner, Royal Brompton Hospital, London.)

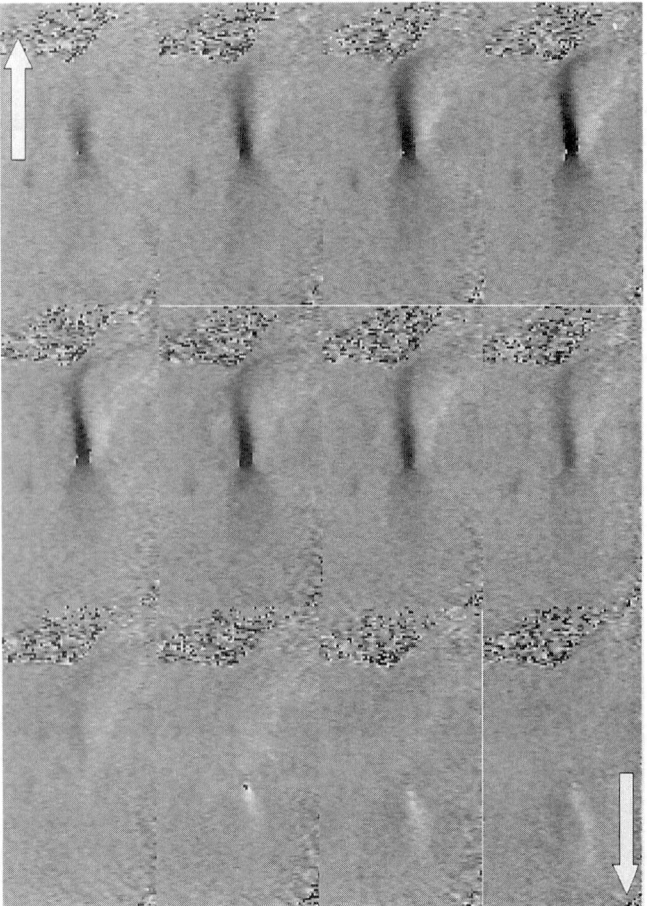

Fig. 6 Four systolic frames from a cine gradient echo acquisition in the vertical long axis plane in a patient with rheumatic mitral stenosis and regurgitation. The regurgitant jet from left ventricle (LV) to left atrium (LA) is seen by virtue of signal loss (black) from the turbulence. The size of the jet indicates that regurgitation is moderate.

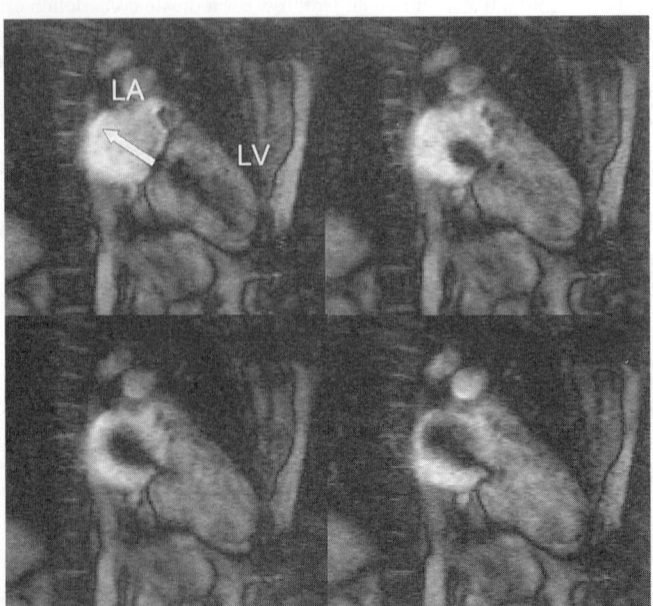

VALVULAR DISEASE

Regurgitation

If only a single valve is regurgitant, comparison of left and right ventricular stroke volumes allows the regurgitant fraction to be calculated. If single valves on both sides of the heart are regurgitant, the method can be extended by comparing ventricular stroke volumes with great vessel flow measured by magnetic resonance velocity mapping. The regurgitant fraction then compares well with the regurgitant grade assessed by Doppler echocardiography. The method still fails if both valves on one side of the heart are regurgitant, but flow studies in the proximal aorta (or pulmonary artery) can be used to measure aortic (or pulmonary) regurgitation alone from the amount of retrograde diastolic flow in the artery, and it is then possible to assess even the most complex cases.

Regurgitation can also be detected using cine gradient echo imaging when a turbulent jet of regurgitation is seen as an area of signal loss (Fig. 6). The size of the jet can be used as a semiquantitative measure of regurgitation although factors other than the size of the jet can affect the area of signal loss.

Stenosis

As with regurgitant jets proximal to a valve, a turbulent distal jet can be used to detect potential stenosis, although abnormal valves which are not stenosed can also generate turbulence. The best method of assessing stenosis is therefore to use cine velocity mapping to measure the peak velocity within the jet (Fig. 7). The modified Bernoulli equation, commonly used in Doppler echocardiography, can then be used to estimate the pressure gradient across the stenosis. A disadvantage of magnetic resonance is that it is not yet real time and so careful alignment of the imaging plane is required in order to obtain an accurate measurement.

ISCHAEMIC HEART DISEASE

Myocardial infarction

Magnetic resonance imaging can be used in a number of ways to detect and measure the size of an area of acute myocardial necrosis. The simplest methods are to use spin echo or cine gradient echo imaging to image the associated wall motion abnormality and the findings agree well with X-ray left ventriculography. Alterations in myocardial signal can also be observed and an increase of signal in T_2 weighted spin echo images occurs only a few hours after occlusion of a coronary artery. The changes are most likely related to oedema and the abnormal area may include viable as well as necrotic myocardium.

Abnormal signals can also be observed in T_1 weighted images although these changes follow a different time course to the changes of T_2 and are maximal at 6 weeks, possibly corresponding to cellular infiltration and repair rather than to oedema. Intravenous contrast agents can highlight the abnormalities and they have helped to distinguish reperfusion from continuing ischaemia in animal models. The same has not been possible in humans.

Reversible ischaemia

Dynamic exercise is impractical within a scanner, but pharmacological intervention using dipyridamole or dobutamine is a suitable alternative. Regional function is assessed using cine gradient echo imaging and global function can also be measured from cine velocity mapping of aortic flow. New wall motion abnormalities imply myocardial ischaemia and there is a close correspondence between these abnormalities and regional perfusion assessed by radionuclide perfusion imaging. The sensitivity of this approach for detecting coronary artery disease depends upon whether a vasodilator or a β-agonist is used. Because the heterogeneities of myocardial perfusion provoked by dipyridamole do not always cause myocardial ischaemia, sensitivity is not as high (60 per cent) as with with dobutamine (91 per cent). The latter is therefore the preferred agent for provoking abnormalities when using a wall motion technique.

An alternative method of assessing reversible perfusion abnormalities is to study the transit of a bolus of magnetic resonance contrast through the myocardium. This is not possible using conventional triggered images but with ultra-fast gradient echo (or echo planar) techniques, images can be acquired in 200 to 400 ms (or less). Images in each cardiac cycle show the arrival and transit of a bolus of contrast (Gd-DTPA) injected into a central vein. Territories supplied by diseased arteries have delayed arrival of contrast and reduced signal increase, and abnormalities can be provoked by dipyridamole vasodilation. Such bolus-tracking studies of perfusion cannot yet replace radionuclide techniques but they have the advantage of higher resolution and the potential to provide measurements of myocardial perfusion in absolute terms.

CORONARY VESSELS

Bypass grafts

Coronary artery bypass grafts can be imaged relatively easily using conventional spin echo or gradient echo techniques. In spin echo images, the appearance of low intraluminal signal contrasting with the high signal of the surrounding fat or other soft tissue, implies that the graft contains moving blood and is patent, particularly if it can be followed distally to its insertion. If a graft cannot be identified, or if its origin is seen but it cannot be followed distally, it is likely to be occluded. Using these criteria, sensitivity and specificity for the detection of patent grafts in the region of 90 per cent can be achieved. Internal mammary artery grafts are more difficult to visualize than saphenous vein grafts, partly because of their smaller size and partly because they can be tortuous and are therefore more difficult to follow through multiple slices.

Cine gradient echo imaging has been used with similar results and the cine technique is helpful to identify a graft if there is doubt from the spin echo images alone. Metallic clips and sternal sutures produce larger artefacts in gradient echo than in spin echo images. They are not ferromagnetic and imaging is perfectly safe but the artefacts can complicate image interpretation.

Native arteries

The coronary arteries are small, tortuous, and rapidly moving: three properties which conspire against successful imaging. Despite this, the proximal vessels can nearly always be identified in conventional spin echo images and their appearance with low intraluminal signal implies that they contain moving blood and are patent. Unfortunately, resolution is not sufficient to identify stenoses reliably. Rapid gradient echo techniques and acquisition within a single breathhold provide much better images and the resolution is adequate to detect atheromatous disease (Fig. 8). Spiral and echo planar imaging have also been used, and all of these can be combined with velocity mapping. Further development may allow magnetic resonance to provide reliable coronary artery imaging and flow measurements non-invasively.

Computed X-ray tomography

Conventional computed X-ray tomography is widely available and has an established clinical role in imaging the heart, particularly the pericardium and great vessels. Resolution, however, is reduced by cardiac and respiratory motion. Electrocardiographic gating can overcome this problem but there are limitations. A more robust method is to increase the speed of acquisition and this has been achieved in two forms of scanner by eliminating the need to rotate the X-ray source mechanically. One is the dynamic spatial reconstructor which has an arc of X-ray sources activated in turn with opposing detectors. The other uses an electron beam which is focused and deflected onto a stationary target to generate a fan of X-rays which is swept through the patient (Fig. 9). At its most rapid, this scanner can acquire two contiguous 8 mm thick tomograms in 50 ms, with a repetition rate of 17 images a second.

Although electron beam technology has significantly improved X-ray tomography of the heart, only a limited number of scanners are available at the time of writing (Table 1).

Pericardium

The normal parietal pericardium is seen in 95 per cent of patients by conventional computed tomography, particularly over the anterior surface of the heart. The posterior pericardium is most frequently seen at its caudal insertion into the central tendon of the diaphragm, where it may be 3 to 4 mm thick. It is often not so well seen laterally and posteriorly because of the absence of epicardial fat. Congenital anomalies, thickening, calcification and effusion can be readily identified. The presence of thickening can distinguish pericardial constriction from restrictive cardiomyopathy, although thickening is also seen in a variety of conditions without necessarily implying constriction (Fig. 10).

Aortic dissection

Computed tomography is sensitive (83 to 100 per cent) and highly specific (90 to 100 per cent) for the identification of thoracic aortic dissection. This is similar to magnetic resonance imaging and transoesophageal echocardiography but computed X-ray tomography is more widely available. The two lumina are commonly seen separated by an intimal flap, and other features that indicate dissection include differential opacification of true and false lumens, compression of the true lumen by a thrombosed false lumen, inward displacement of intimal calcification, and irregularity of the contrast enhanced lumen (Fig. 11). Although computed tomography is particularly successful in identifying the distal extent of dissection and the presence of a haemopericardium, it has limitations. Artefacts may create difficulties, and the intimal tear or flap may not be identified in all cases. Thus if findings are negative but there is a strong clinical suspicion of dissection, further investigation is necessary.

Intracardiac masses

The presence, location, and extent of thrombus and tumour in the cardiac chambers can be defined with conventional and electron beam computed tomography. This provides advantages over transthoracic echocardiography, particularly in the assessment of the left ventricular apex, the left atrial appendage, and the site of attachment of tumours. Electron beam is superior to conventional tomography for these patients because left ventricular wall motion and thickening can also be measured. It may be helpful when magnetic resonance images are degraded by arrhythmia or patient motion.

Congenital heart disease

Patient movement during electron beam computed tomography does not reduce image quality. Experience is limited to a few centres but anatomical assessment of congenital heart disease in infants, small children and adults is very successful. The anatomy of the heart and great vessels can be assessed, myocardial mass and ventricular volumes can be monitored after surgical correction, the patency of surgical conduits can be assessed from the appearance and washout of contrast, and shunts can be detected and quantified. In disorders such as tetralogy of Fallot where intracardiac pressures do not need to be measured pre-operatively, electron beam computed tomography may avoid invasive investigation.

Cardiac structure and function

Using electron beam computed tomography and intravenous contrast, cine images at multiple contiguous levels can be obtained in approximately eight cardiac cycles. This allows a qualitative and quantitative assessment of ventricular function and morphology. Planimetry can be used to measure cavity and muscle area and hence volume at any part of the cardiac cycle. Regional and segmental left ventricular wall motion

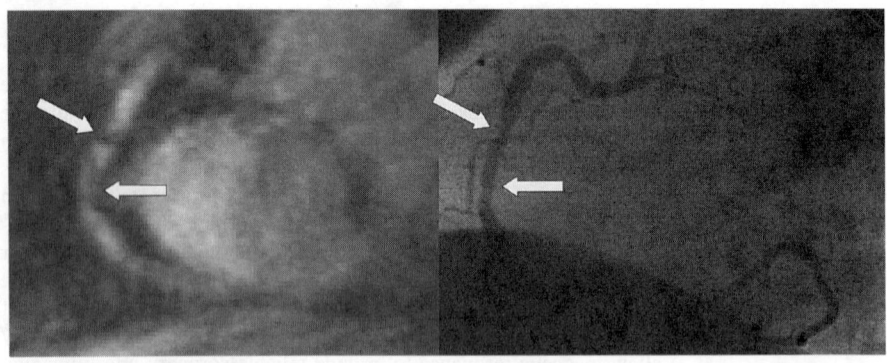

Fig. 8 Rapid gradient echo magnetic resonance image acquired in 20 s during a single breath hold (left), with corresponding radiographic contrast angiogram (right). The right coronary artery is seen with two stenoses in its mid course (arrows). (With acknowledgement to Dr D.J. Pennel, Royal Brompton Hospital, London.)

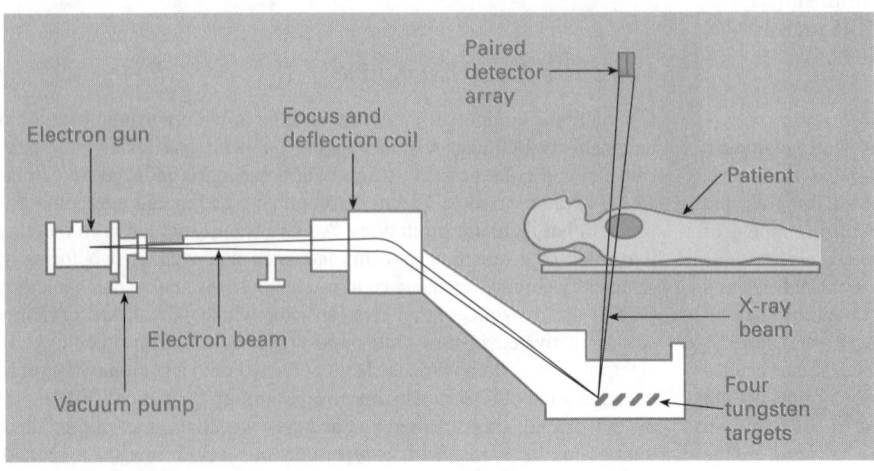

Fig. 9 Electron beam X-ray computed tomography scanner. The electron beam is swept around each of four targets in an arc around the patient. Two contiguous tomograms are generated from each target.

Table 1 *Common applications of conventional and ultrafast computed X-ray tomography*

Application	Conventional	Ultrafast
Clinical	Pericardium and pericardial fluid	Pericardium and pericardial fluid
	Aortic dissection	Aortic dissection
	Cardiac tumours	Cardiac tumours
		Coronary calcification
Specialist	Bypass graft patency	Bypass graft patency
		Intracardiac masses
		Congenital heart disease
		Cardiac structure and function
Research		Myocardial perfusion

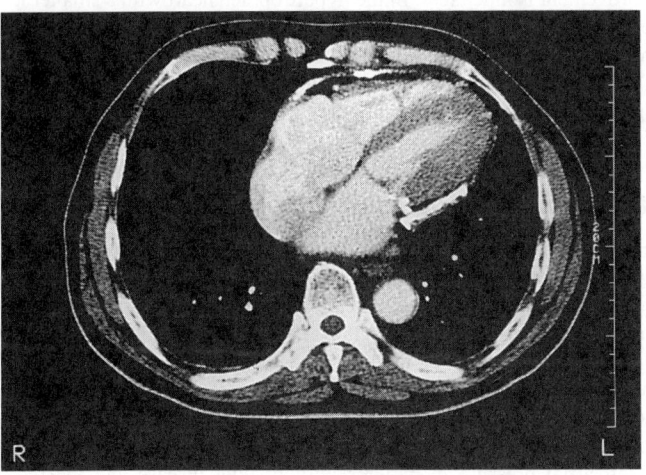

Fig. 10 Constrictive pericarditis. Electron beam CT scan with contrast showing thickened and calcified pericardium, dilated atria, and normal sized ventricles.

can be assessed at rest and during pharmacological stimulation and changes induced by exercise in patients with ischaemic heart disease can be measured.

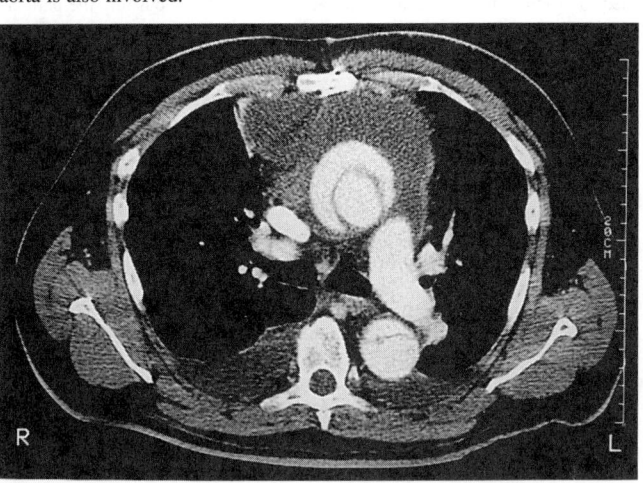

Fig. 11 Aortic dissection. Electron beam CT scan with contrast showing a dilated ascending aorta with almost circumferential dissection. The descending aorta is also involved.

Coronary calcification

Because acute coronary occlusion may occur on atheromatous plaques that do not limit flow, techniques that image the arterial wall may be better suited to the early detection of disease than those that depend upon narrowing of the lumen. Unlike the medial calcification of larger arteries, coronary calcification is normally associated with atheroma. Electron beam computed tomography is highly sensitive for the detection of coronary calcium and it is possible to score the extent and density of the deposits semiquantitatively (Fig. 12). Its prevalence is high even in asymptomatic subjects, rising from 25 per cent in the fourth decade to 75 per cent in the seventh decade. The score is related to the extent of coronary atheroma assessed angiographically, although there is only a weak relationship with the degree of luminal narrowing. The absence of calcium does not exclude histologically defined coronary atheroma, although it does imply a low likelihood of flow limiting stenoses.

Myocardial perfusion

The relatively high spatial resolution of electron beam computed tomograms and the ability to acquire images rapidly as a bolus of contrast passes through the myocardium, imply the potential to measure myocardial perfusion in absolute terms. The techniques are based on the principles of first pass distribution using contrast medium as an indicator, and successful studies have been performed with injection into the aortic root and intravenously. Myocardial perfusion measured using these techniques compares well with microspheres at low and moderate values, although there is an underestimate at high values. These techniques may be able to differentiate epicardial and endocardial perfusion but the results have yet to be validated.

REFERENCES

Agatston, A.S., Janowitz, W.R., Hildner, F.J., Zusmer, N.R., Viamonte, M.J., and Detrano, R. (1990). Quantification of coronary artery calcium using ultrafast computed tomography. *Journal of the American College of Cardiologists,* **15,** 827–832.

Gibson, D.G. (1989). Non-invasive cardiac imaging. *British Medical Bulletin,* **45.**

Higgins, C.B., Hricak, H., and Helms, C.A. (1992). *Magnetic resonance imaging of the body* 2nd edn., Raven Press, New York.

Kanal, E., Shellock, F.G., and Talagala, L. (1990). Safety considerations in MR imaging. *Radiology,* **176,** 593–606.

Ludman, P.F., Coats, A.J.S., Burger, P., *et al.* (1993). Validation of measurement of regional myocardial perfusion in man by ultrafast X-ray computed tomography. *American Journal of Cardiac Imaging* (in press).

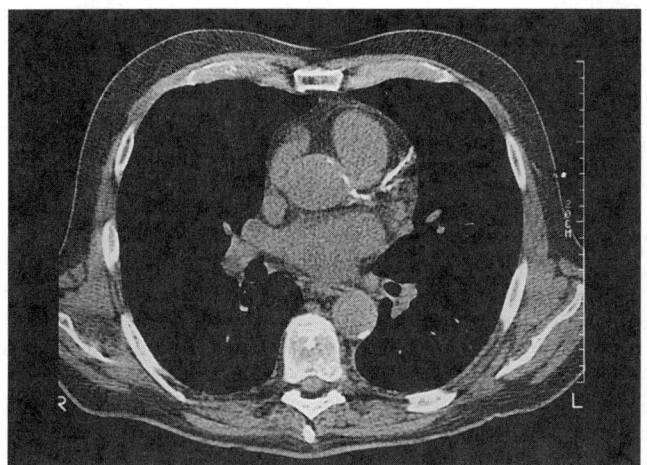

Fig. 12 Coronary calcification. Electron beam CT scan without contrast. There is high intensity calcification in the aortic root, the left main stem, left anterior descending, and diagonal coronary arteries.

Manning, W.J., Atkinson, D.J., Grossman, W., Paulin, S., and Edelman, R.R. (1991). First-pass nuclear magnetic resonance imaging studies using gadolinium-DTPA in patients with coronary artery disease. *Journal of the American College of Cardiologists*, **18**, 959–965.

Manning, W.J., Li, W., and Edelman, R.R. (1993). A preliminary report comparing magnetic resonance coronary angiography with conventional angiography. *New England Journal of Medicine*, **328**, 828–832.

Marcus, M.L., Schelbert, H.R., Skorton, D.J., and Wolf, G.L. (eds), (1991). *Cardiac imaging*: a companion to Braunwald's heart disease. W.B. Saunders Co, Philadelphia.

Nienaber, C.A., Vonkodolitsch, Y., Nicolas, V., *et al.* (1993). The diagnosis of thoracic aortic dissection by noninvasive imaging procedures. *New England Journal of Medicine*, **328**, 1–9.

Pennell, D.J., Underwood, S.R., Manzara, C.C., *et al.* (1992). Magnetic resonance imaging during dobutamine stress in coronary artery disease. *American Journal of Cardiology*, **70**, 34–40.

Rees, R.S.O., Firmin, D.N., Mohiaddin, R.H., Underwood, S.R., and Longmore, D.B. (1989). Application of flow measurements by magnetic resonance velocity mapping to congenital heart disease. *American Journal of Cardiology* **64**, 953–956.

Roig, E., Chomka, E.V., Castaner, A., *et al.* (1989). Exercise ultrafast computed tomography for the detection of coronary artery disease. *Journal of the American College of Cardiologists*, **13**, 1073–1081.

Stehling, M., Chapman, B., Glover, P., *et al.* (1987). Real-time NMR imaging of coronary vessels. *Lancet*, **ii**, 964–965.

Underwood, S.R. and Firmin, D.N. (1991). *Magnetic resonance of the cardiovascular system*. Blackwell Scientific Publications, Oxford.

15.4.6 Cardiac catheterization

R.H. SWANTON

Introduction

Cardiac catheterization provides a unique technique for the assessment of cardiovascular function and provides more information about the heart than any other currently available investigation. Although echocardiography has rendered catheterization unnecessary in some cases of valve disease prior to cardiac surgery, the latter is still necessary for the diagnosis and assessment of associated coronary artery disease, providing at the same time information on a large number of haemodynamic variables. Echocardiography can be used for non-invasive assessment of segmental wall motion abnormalities, ejection fraction, ventricular volumes, valve anatomy, and gradients, but cardiac catheterization will provide additional information on intracardiac pressures, and cardiac output, as well as quantitating intracardiac shunts. Numerous derived variables are available including the measurement of pulmonary and systemic vascular resistance, cardiac work, power, and efficiency.

Echocardiography has relieved the paediatric cardiologist of a great deal of investigative cardiac catheterization but an accurate measurement of pulmonary artery pressure and pulmonary vascular resistance together with information on pulmonary artery, pulmonary vein, and collateral anatomy is still necessary and these are best achieved by cardiac catheterization.

Cardiac haemodynamics

Cardiac output can be altered by changing one of four variables: heart rate, contractility, preload (ventricular filling pressure and volume), and afterload (represented by aortic or pulmonary pressure as impedance to ejection). A fall in contractility must be compensated by an increase in heart rate or by homeostatic autoregulation mechanisms. The best known of these is the Frank–Starling mechanism: increasing myocardial fibre length increases the velocity of contraction and hence stroke vol-

ume. However, filling pressures above about 20 mmHg do not generate much benefit in terms of stroke work (the ventricular function curve flattens out) and may well precipitate pulmonary oedema once the colloid osmotic pressure is exceeded. Representative left ventricular function curves are shown in Fig. 1.

Although the stroke volumes of the right and left ventricles will be the same (assuming no valve regurgitation), their filling pressures will be very different, especially in diseased states where one ventricle may be functioning virtually normally and the other very abnormally with very high filling pressures. It is essential not to assume the filling pressure of the left ventricle from the venous pressure on the right side. For correct management the filling pressures of both ventricles should be known. If the diastolic pressure is measured directly then two figures are quoted (beginning and end-diastolic). If the left ventricular filling pressure is measured indirectly (via a Swan–Ganz catheter) then the single figure quoted is the left ventricular end-diastolic pressure.

In the diseased heart manipulation of the filling pressure will have different effects from the normal. Increasing the filling pressure in the normal heart by a fluid challenge briskly increases stroke volume and cardiac output (Fig. 1). In the dilated heart with poor ventricular function a much larger increase in filling pressure will be needed and the improvement is much less. In the hypertrophied heart with a smaller left ventricular cavity and a stiff muscle a small increase in volume will produce a very sharp and possibly unexpected rise in filling pressure. It is vital that the filling pressure is accurately measured to avoid overfilling the patient and risking pulmonary oedema.

Measurement of filling pressure

The use of the Swan–Ganz catheter to determine the left ventricular filling pressure has revolutionized the care of the cardiac patient in intensive care units. Following subclavian vein or internal jugular vein puncture, the balloon-tipped Swan–Ganz catheter can be advanced into the right ventricle with the balloon deflated. Once in the right ventricle the balloon is inflated and by careful manipulation floated into a distal pulmonary artery without radiological screening. By gentle balloon inflation a pulmonary capillary wedge pressure is obtained. This is equivalent to left atrial pressure in patients without lung disease and the mean pulmonary capillary wedge pressure is a measure of left ventricular end-diastolic pressure in the absence of mitral stenosis. If a satisfactory wedge position cannot be obtained then the pulmonary end-diastolic pressure is used.

A triple lumen thermodilution Swan–Ganz catheter provides for mea-

Fig. 1 Left ventricular function curves. Three representative curves are shown in a normal heart, a normal heart following inotropic stimulation and in a failing heart. In the failing heart substantial increases in filling pressure are needed to produce any increase in cardiac output, and risk pushing the patient into pulmonary oedema.

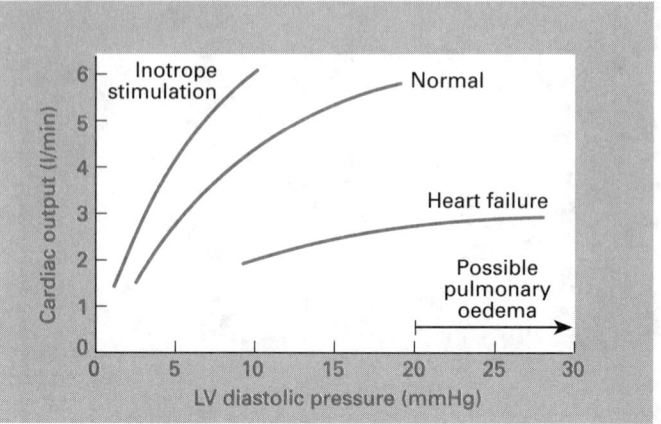

surement of the pulmonary capillary wedge pressure, the pulmonary artery pressure, the cardiac output, the mixed venous oxygen saturation (from the pulmonary artery), and the central core temperature (from the distal thermistor). Saturations can also be checked from the right atrium if there is any suspicion of a left to right shunt at ventricular level. The pulmonary and systemic vascular resistances are easily calculated once a radial artery or femoral artery pressure is known. The effects of acute or chronic drug administration on these variables can be studied. In addition a catheter is available with pacing electrodes for right atrial and/or right ventricular pacing.

A normal pulmonary vascular resistance and a transpulmonary gradient of less than 15 mmHg (mean pulmonary artery pressure − mean left atrial pressure) is needed before patients can be accepted for cardiac transplantation, and cardiac catheterization is important in this context.

The risks of Swan–Ganz catheterization are minimal in experienced hands, but subclavian vein puncture itself may, on occasion, cause pneumothorax, haemothorax, or damage to the subclavian artery and brachial plexus. Carotid artery injury can occur with internal jugular punctures. Excessively enthusiastic manoeuvring of the catheter itself may result in its knotting and damage to the tricuspid and pulmonary valves has been reported. An incorrect inflation technique may result in pulmonary infarction, if the balloon is left inflated too long, or pulmonary artery rupture – the risk of this being higher in pulmonary hypertensive patients. The greatest risk is of infection being introduced at the catheter entry site. A specially designed sheath enables the catheter position to be changed in a sterile condition, but the risk of infection increases with the time the catheter is in place. It should always be removed at the earliest opportunity and should remain for longer than 3 to 4 days only in exceptional circumstances.

Indices of ventricular function

An ideal index of ventricular function still eludes the cardiologist and no single index can be used to diagnose early myocardial damage. Compensatory mechanisms make it difficult to detect early ventricular wall damage, independent of changes in preload or afterload. The more commonly used indices listed shown on Table 1 may be obtained at cardiac catheterization by pressure measurement using a micromanometer tipped catheter (frequency response of a fluid filled catheter is inadequate) or by angiographic volume analysis or both. Many of the indices referred to below are for the left ventricle and not the right. Particular problems have arisen in attempts by angiographic and nuclear techniques to measure right ventricular volumes. Formulae that have been derived have made assumptions of right ventricular cavity shape which are even more unfounded than those made for the left ventricle; right ventricular volume analysis will not therefore be discussed here.

Cardiac output

This is one of the most commonly used indices of cardiac function in the catheter laboratory and in the coronary and intensive care units. It is not a good measurement of ventricular function dependent as it is on so many other variables, e.g. blood volume, intra- or extracardiac shunts, valve lesions, haemoglobin level and saturation, total oxygen consumption, and endocrine/hormonal status.

The most common techniques used to measure cardiac output are: the direct or indirect Fick method, indicator dilution, thermodilution, and angiography.

The Direct Fick method

This method provides a measure of cardiac output calculated as follows:

$$\text{Cardiac output} = \frac{\text{Measured oxygen consumption in ml/min}}{\text{Arteriovenous oxygen content difference}}$$

Table 1 *Indices of ventricular function*

Angiographic indices
    Left ventricular end-diastolic volume (LVEDV) (ml)
    Left ventricular end-systolic volume (LVESV) (ml)
    Angiographic stroke volume (ml)
    Ejection fraction (LVEDV−LVESV/LVEDV) (%)
    LV ejection rate (ml/s)
    LV mass (g)
    Regional wall motion studies

Pressure and haemodynamic indices
    Left ventricular peak systolic pressure (LVP)
    Left ventricular end-diastolic pressure (LVEDP)
    Cardiac index (CI) l/min/m^2
    Stroke work index (g/m/m^2)
    Minute work index (kg/m/m^2/min)
    LV power (g/m/s)
    Myocardial O$_2$ consumption (ml/min)

Response of the ventricles to exercise
    Response of LV indices to dynamic or isometric exercise on the catheter table
    Response of LV indices to atrial or ventricular pacing
    Ventricular function curves derived from atrial pacing

Pre-ejection phase/isovolumic indices
    Systolic time intervals
    Max dP/dt; min dP/dt; mmHg/s
    Derivatives of max dP/dt which correct for preload:

$$\text{e.g.} \quad \frac{\max dP/dt}{\text{LVEDP}} \quad \text{or} \quad \frac{\max dP/dt}{\text{LV DP40}} \quad \text{or} \quad \frac{\max dP/dt}{\text{LVEDV}}$$

    V_{pm}, maximum measured rate of contractile element shortening from the force–velocity loop.
    V_{max}, maximum rate of contractile element shortening at zero pressure (extrapolated from force velocity loop)

Ejection phase indices
    These are derived either from the angiogram or the echocardiogram. These may either be measured throughout the ejection phase or just in the first third of ejection, e.g. peak V_{cf}, peak circumferential fibre shortening velocity; mean V_{cf}, V_{cf} at peak stress

Diastolic indices
    Diastolic stiffness (dP/dV)
    Diastolic compliance (dV/dP)

DP = Developed pressure (LVP−LVEDP).

$$\text{Cardiac output (l/min)}$$
$$= \frac{\text{Measured oxygen consumption in ml/min}}{\text{(Aorta} - \text{PA) O}_2 \text{ content (ml/100ml)} \times 10}$$

The main difficulties with this approach are the accurate measurement of oxygen consumption and of the oxygen content of systemic and mixed venous pulmonary artery (PA) blood. Any artery can be used for arterial sampling but only the main pulmonary artery is sampled for mixed venous blood.

Oxygen consumption can be measured in the basal state by a variety of techniques. The oxygen content of blood can be measured directly using a galvanic fuel cell, or by a manometric method. Alternatively it can be calculated from:

$$\text{O}_2 \text{ content (ml/100 ml) blood} = \text{(Haemoglobin} \times 1.34$$
$$\times \text{ percentage saturation)} + \text{plasma O}_2 \text{ content}$$

When fully saturated, 1 g haemoglobin combines with 1.34 ml oxygen. Tables are available for the plasma correction factor (e.g. for blood saturation of 97 per cent the correction factor is 0.3, for 80 per cent it is 0.14, and for 70 per cent it is 0.11).

THE INDIRECT FICK METHOD

This method uses the principles above but uses an estimated oxygen consumption based on the patient's body surface area. Tables of estimated oxygen consumption in the basal state are available. Some also include estimates at a variety of heart rates, but the indirect Fick method, although a useful check of cardiac outputs measured by other techniques, should not be used as a sole guide.

The cardiac output is divided by the body surface area (obtained from table of height and weight) to yield the cardiac index in l/min/m². The normal cardiac index is 2.5 to 4.0 l/min/m².

INDICATOR DILUTION

Until the development of the thermodilution method this was the standard invasive technique for the measurement of cardiac output. Indocyanine green dye is injected into the right atrium or main pulmonary artery and systemic arterial blood (e.g. from femoral artery) is continuously sampled through a densitometer. Peak absorption of indocyanine green is at 800 nm.

The technique is cumbersome and justifiably unpopular. First, a calibration factor (K) must be calculated from known concentrations of green dye in fresh heparinized non-smokers blood. Second, two catheters are required. Third, the dye curve has a recirculation component and the true primary curve must be reconstructed to obtain the area under this primary curve. This is most accurately performed by plotting the the time–concentration curve on semilogarithmic paper with the indicator concentration on the semilog axis. The straight line on the descending limb is extrapolated assuming the decay in the primary curve is exponential. The technique cannot be repeated rapidly as time must be allowed for the green dye to equilibrate in the plasma and this increase in background dye causes a baseline shift. Finally small volumes of blood are lost with each estimate.

$$\text{The calibration factor K} = \frac{\text{Indicator concentration in mg/l}}{\text{Deflection of densitometer in mm}}$$

$$\text{The cardiac output} = \frac{I \times 60}{C \times t} = \frac{I \times 60}{A/L \times K \times t}$$

Where I = the amount of green dye injected (mg), C = the mean concentration of dye (mg/l), and t = duration of curve (s). The product $C \times t$ is the area under the reconstructed primary curve excluding the recirculation component. A = the planimetered area under the curve; L = the length of baseline in cm, and K = the calibration factor.

There are many mathematical short cuts to primary curve reconstruction but the many practical difficulties with the technique have largely resulted in its being replaced by the thermodilution method.

THERMODILUTION

This is the most common technique used to estimate cardiac output using the Swan–Ganz thermodilution catheter described above. 10 ml of cooled 5 per cent dextrose at known temperature are injected into the right atrium and the thermistor at the catheter tip in the pulmonary artery senses the transient fall in temperature as a slight rise in resistance. A variety of cardiac output computers are available which electronically integrate the area under the curve of change in resistance against time. There are many advantages of this technique over indicator dilution: the equipment needed is a great deal simpler, the recirculation component can be ignored, and only one catheter is needed. The technique can be used in the very sick patient and repeated measurements quickly performed following drug intervention or manipulations of plasma volume.

Table 2 lists normal values for cardiac haemodynamics.

ANGIOGRAPHIC VOLUME ANALYSIS

In spite of the facts that the angiographic estimation of ventricular volume involves assumptions about the shape of the left ventricular cavity, that magnification errors may arise and that single plane cine is most commonly used, the angiographic assessment of left ventricular volume correlates very closely with other methods and in particular with measurements from ventricular casts. It is particularly valuable in studies of regional wall motion in ischaemic heart disease. Ventricular volume measurements are proving useful in the timing of valve replacement for aortic or mitral regurgitation: mitral valve replacement is recommended for chronic mitral regurgitation once the left ventricular end diastolic volume reaches 110 ml/m².

Although angiographic volume analysis was originally computed from biplane cineangiography most centres use single plane cineangiography in the 30 degree right anterior oblique projection with the film taken during maximum inspiration. It is assumed that the left ventricle is an ellipsoid of revolution, thus assuming that the minor axes are identical. A representative tracing from a left ventricular cineangiogram is shown in Fig. 2. The long axis is drawn from the mid-point of the aortic valve to the apex, and the minor axis at the mid-point of the long axis and at right angles to it.

$$\text{LV volume (V)} = \frac{4\pi}{3} \times \frac{D}{2} \times \frac{D}{2} \times \frac{L}{2}$$

(uncorrected for magnification)

where D is the minor axis and L the major axis or length in centimetres. The magnification factor (f) is calculated by filming a grid or ruler of known length at mid chest level. The formula corrected for magnification and simplified becomes:

$$V = \frac{\pi D^2 \times L \times f^3}{6} = 0.524 \times D^2 \times L \times f^3$$

(Greene formula)

An alternative method, which is probably more accurate is the area-length method in which the only measurements required are the long axis (L) and the area of the ventricle (A) in cm². The area can be calculated by planimetry or, more easily, by digitized X-Y plotters or a light pen computer system.

Substituting the semi-minor axis $\frac{D}{2} = \frac{2A}{\pi L}$ in the Greene formula and applying the correction factor the area–length method formula becomes:

$$V = \frac{0.849 \times A^2 \times f^3}{L} \quad \text{(Dodge formula)}$$

Programming this formula into the computer allows rapid sequential estimations of LV volumes. Table 3 shows the normal values for angiographically derived left ventricular volumes in resting and stable patients.

Left ventricular mass can be calculated by assuming a uniform wall thickness measured at the point of intersection of the short axis (W).

Fig. 2 Angiographic volume analysis. Single plane angiography in the 30 degree right anterior oblique projection. End-diastolic and end-systolic frames are superimposed. The long axis (L) and the short axis (D) are shown drawn for the end-diastolic frame. The Greene and Dodge formulae are shown for left ventricular volume calculation.

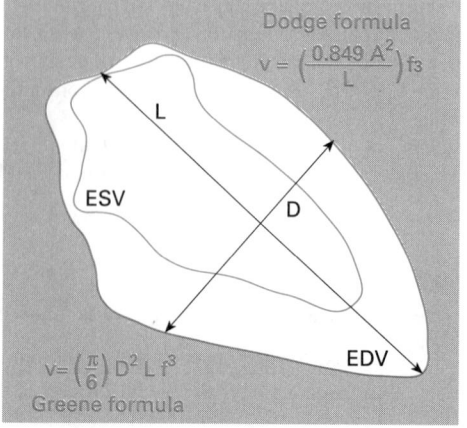

Table 2 *Normal values for cardiac haemodynamics*

Cardiac index	2.5 to 4.0 l/min/m²
Stroke volume index (SVI)	40 to 70 ml/m²
Left ventricular end-diastolic pressure	5 to 10 mmHg
Right ventricular end-diastolic pressure	2 to 5 mmHg
Systemic arterial pressure	120/80 (mean 95 mmHg)
Pulmonary artery pressure	20/10 (mean 13 mmHg)
Systemic vascular resistance (SVR)	770 to 1500 dynes s/cm⁵ or 10 to 20 units
Pulmonary vascular resistance (PVR)	< 200 dynes s/cm⁵ or < 2.5 units
Left ventricular stroke work index	40 to 80 g/m/m²
Left ventricular minute work index	4.5 to 5.5 kg/m/m²/min
Left ventricular dP/dt max	1000 to 2400 mmHg/s
V_{max} (developed pressure)	2.0 to 3.3/s

Table 3 *Normal values for left ventricular volumes derived from angiographic analysis* (Kennedy *et al.* 1966)

Left ventricular end-diastolic volume index	70 ± 20 (mean ± SD) ml/m²
Left ventricular end-systolic volume index	24 ± 10 ml/m²
Ejection fraction	0.67 ± 0.08
Left ventricular mass	92 ± 16 g
Wall thickness	10.9 ± 2.0 mm

Using the Greene formula the volume of the left ventricular cavity is subtracted from the volume of cavity plus left ventricular wall and the result multiplied by 1.05, the calculated specific gravity of heart muscle. Estimates using this method have shown a very close correlation with weighed postmortem hearts.

The angiogram film can be timed with the electrocardiograph and left ventricular pressure, and a pressure volume curve constructed. The area within the curve is a measure of systolic work. The slope of the line in diastole can be used to calculate diastolic stiffness (dV/dP) and compliance (dP/dV). If a time/volume curve is constructed the ventricular filling and ejection rates can be obtained. These time related indices need to be calculated with a fast film speeds (50 frames/s), and are best normalized to the end-diastolic volume or circumference. Thus the peak systolic ejection rate is normalized to the end-diastolic volume, and peak velocity of circumferential fibre shortening (peak V_{cf}) to the end-diastolic circumference. Circumferential wall stress can be derived from the left ventricular pressure, wall thickness and the axes measured above. At least four different equations for wall stress calculation may prove to be a valuable prognostic indicator in the volume loaded ventricle.

Angiography is rarely used to calculate the stroke volume for cardiac output measurements, but is valuable in the absolute measurement of end-diastolic or end systolic volume, ejection fraction and for studies of regional wall motion.

Regional wall motion

A major drawback in the use of the ejection fraction as a measure of left ventricular function is the fact that it is an overall measurement and may still be normal with early left ventricular disease. An area of hypokinesia occuring after a myocardial infarction may be compensated for by hyperkinesis in another area, the overall ejection fraction being maintained. The best way that this can be documented is by studies of regional wall motion.

Two of the many methods for studying regional wall motion are shown in Fig. 3. Figure 3(a) shows the volume analysis of the same patient as in Fig. 2. Seven frames have been analysed from end-diastole to end-systole. The long axis is quadrisected and the shortening of each hemiaxis calculated. A different technique is shown in Fig. 3(b). This is the computerized printout of angiographic volume analysis in a patient with a recent small anterior infarct. The technique involves the drawing of radians every 4 degrees from the computerized centre of the left ventricular end-systolic frame. The percentage shortening of each radian from the end-diastolic to the end-systolic frame is calculated starting at the mid-point of the aortic valve and working clockwise. It can be seen that the anterior wall is hypokinetic, and the inferior wall hyperkinetic. However the overall ejection fraction is 0.82, above the normal range.

Fig. 3(a) Regional wall motion analysis. Same patient (normal) and projection as in Fig. 2. Seven frames of the cine-cycle shown from end-diastole to end-systole. The long axis is quadrisected producing eight regions of interest and six hemiaxes. The percentage shortening of each hemiaxis can be calculated. (b) Regional wall motion analysis. Recent small anterior infarct. Upper panel shows superimposed end-diastolic and end-systolic frames in 30 degree right anterior oblique projection. The frames are superimposed at the mid-point of the aortic valve. 90 radians are plotted from the computerized geometric centre of gravity of the left ventricular end-systolic frame. Only 8 radians are shown for clarity. The percentage shortening of each radian is plotted starting at the mid-point of the aortic valve and working clockwise. The lower panel shows the plot with the normal range within the dotted lines. The anterolateral segment is hypokinetic, and the inferior wall shows compensatory hyperkinesis.

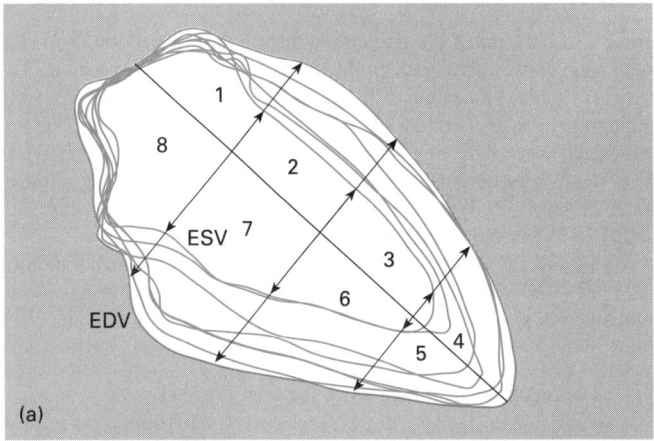

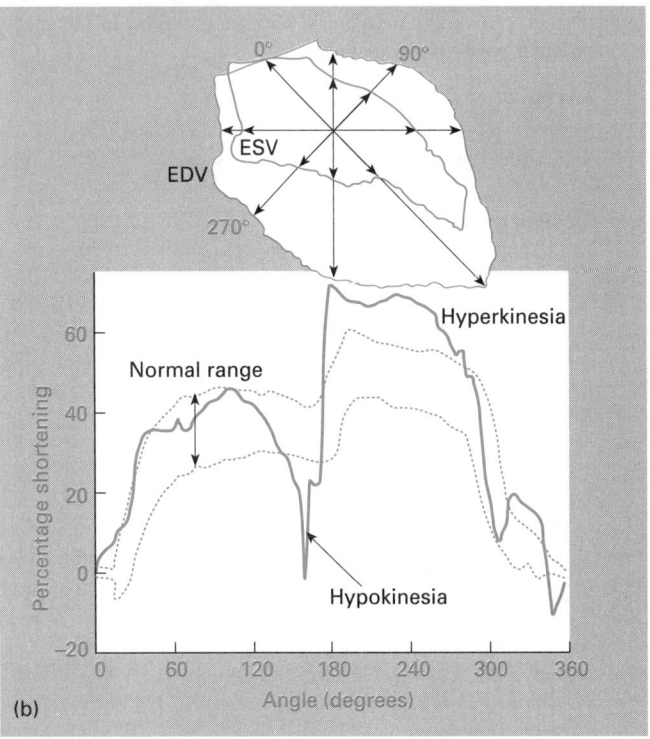

The compensatory hyperkinesis in the non-infarcted segment does not persist and is due to the effect of initially high endogenous catecholamines on normal cardiac muscle. Attempts to show an improvement in ejection fraction following thrombolysis have at best only shown very small improvements in overall ejection fraction and have been thwarted by this problem of early compensatory hyperkinesis in the non-infarct segment. Studies of regional wall motion have proved more informative.

A further abnormality of wall motion, which only may be appreciated after computerized wall motion analysis is the timing of inward movement of different segments of the left ventricle. It may be found that inward movement is delayed in ischaemic areas, and may even continue into the iso-volumic relaxation phase when other areas are relaxing and left ventricular pressure is falling. A true end-systolic frame may then be difficult to determine. The left ventricle does not necessarily have to be dilated. Paradoxical outward movement (dyskinesis) may be seen over the infarct area. This asynchronous movement of wall segments is an important cause of left ventricular dysfunction and inefficiency.

Left ventricular work

The most common measurement of left ventricular work is the left ventricular stroke work index (LVSWI) calculated as:

$$\text{Left ventricular stroke work index} = \text{LV} \times \text{SVI} \times 0.0136 \text{ g m/m}^2$$

where LV is the mean LV pressure in mmHg during ejection. Provided there is no aortic valve gradient mean aortic pressure may be used. SVI is stroke volume index ml/m²/beat. This must be calculated from the angiogram or from thermodilution cardiac output measurement. Net left ventricular work may be calculated by substituting (LV − LVED) or Ao − PAW) in the position of LV in the equation where Ao = mean aortic pressure, PAW = mean pulmonary artery wedge pressure, and LVED left ventricular end-diastolic pressure.

A modification of the stroke work index allows for consideration of heart rate (HR) in the calculation as heart rate tends to to have an inverse relation with stroke volume. This is the left ventricular minute work index.

$$\text{Left ventricular minute work index} = \text{LVSWI} \times \text{HR}/1000 \text{ kg/m/m}^2/\text{min}$$

Left ventricular power is a measure of work per unit time. Instantaneous left ventricular power is calculated as:

$$\text{LV power} = P \times \text{dV/dt} \times 0.0136 \text{ g/m/s}$$

where P is the instantaneous left ventricular pressure or aortic pressure during ejection and dV/dt change in volume in ml/s.

In man these measurements require simultaneous measurement of left ventricular pressure and volume in the catheter laboratory.

Pre-ejection phase indices of ventricular function

Numerous indices have been derived from measurement of pressure changes during the isovolumic phase in an attempt to produce an index of contractility which is easy to measure, independant of both preload and afterload and which is sensitive enough to detect early changes in left ventricular function. Some of these are shown in Table 1. Unfortunately it has become clear that there is no single ideal contractility index, and that assumptions from isolated muscle preparations do not necessarily hold for the intact human heart.

Early work using fluid filled catheters to study these isovolumic phase indices are invalidated by the poor frequency response of the system. Catheter tip micromanometers must be used. Also the index is measured during the isovolumic period and the figures are probably meaningless in patients with significant mitral regurgitation where there is no iso-volumic period. Only two pre-ejection phase indices will be briefly discussed.

Maximum dP/dt (peak dP/dt) is one of the most simple and useful indices of contractility. It is preload-dependent and will increase as the preload increases, but is relatively independent of afterload. It is affected not only by the inotropic state of the muscle but also by end-diastolic fibre length. It increases with increasing heart rate, exercise, and inotropic intervention, but there is considerable variation between patients and a normal range in man is difficult to establish. It is thus of little value in studies between patients but is useful as an index of contractility in studies within the same patient. Minimum dP/dt (peak negative dP/dt) occuring during the isovolumic relaxation phase has been less studied but is known to be dependent not only on the inotropic state of the muscle, but on afterload and end-systolic fibre length. Figure 4 shows max and min dP/dt falling after intravenous propranolol 0.1 mg/kg during atrial pacing at constant heart rate. Table 1 shows some of the many other indices that have been derived from maximum dP/dt in an attempt to correct for preload. None is in routine use.

V_{max} is the maximum velocity of contractile element shortening at zero load. The left ventricular pressure is differentiated and divided by the developed left ventricular pressure. This is plotted on the vertical axis with left ventricular pressure on the horizontal axis. Using numerous assumptions about the left ventricle it can be shown that:

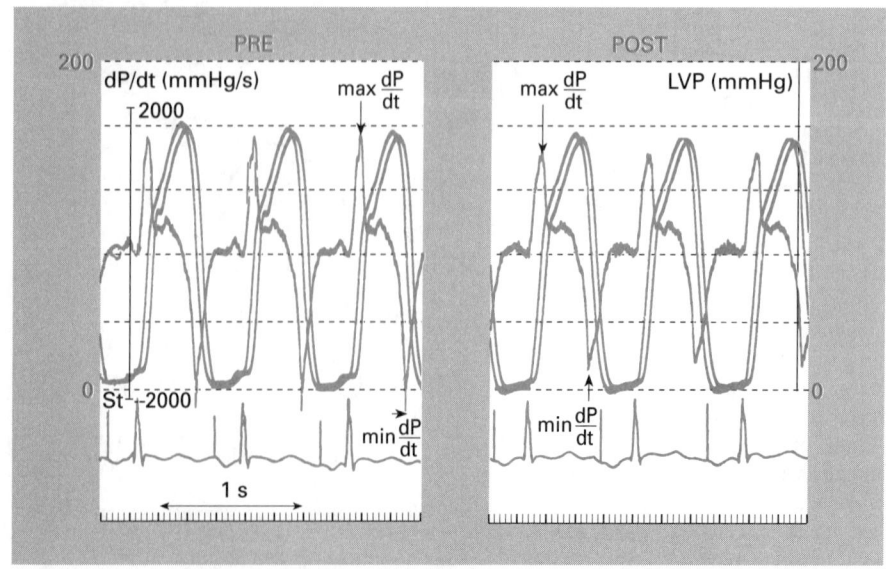

Fig. 4 Max and min dP/dt post-propranolol. Atrial pacing to hold heart rate constant. Left ventricular pressure recorded from both micromanometer tip and fluid filled lumen. Both maximum and minimum dP/dt fall after 0.1mg/kg intravenous propranolol.

Fig. 5 Force–velocity analysis. Atrial pacing 90/min. LVP, left ventricular pressure; LVEDP, left ventricular end-diastolic pressure; V_{max}, maximum velocity of contractile element shortening; K, stiffness constant; DP, developed pressure (LVP − LVEDP). The vertical axis is converted to a log scale (right-hand panel) and the straight part of the loop extrapolated to zero-developed pressure. β-Blockade results in a fall in kV_{max}.

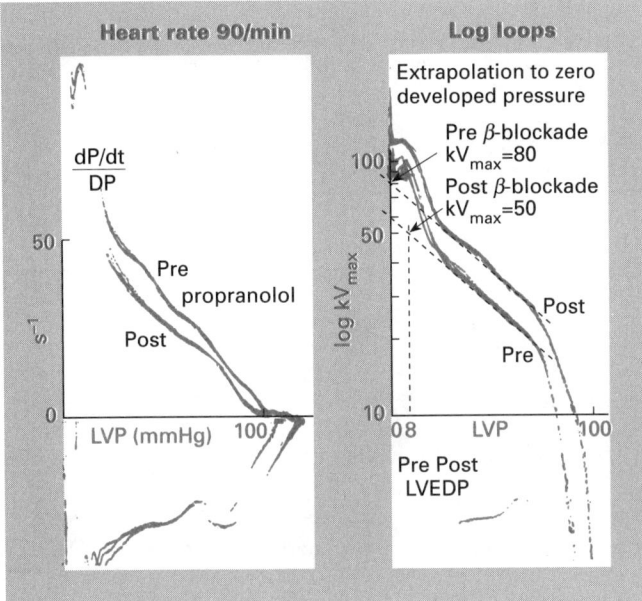

$$VCE = \frac{dP/dt}{KP} \quad or$$

$$kV_{max} = \frac{dP/dt}{DP}$$

where VCE = velocity of contractile element shortening in circ/s, P = left ventricular pressure, DP = developed pressure, and K = the coefficient of series elasticity. This constant has never been calculated in man and is assumed to be 28, a figure estimated from studies in dogs. The force–velocity loop can be extrapolated to zero or, better, to left ventricular end-diastolic pressure (i.e. zero-developed pressure). An example of force velocity loops is shown in Fig. 5, before and after propranolol with atrial pacing at 90/min. kV_{max} is the extrapolated maximum shortening velocity and falls following β-blockade.

V_{max} is relatively independent of preload and afterload, and the normal range is a great deal narrower than for dP/dt max, making it theoretically more useful in interpatient comparisons. Its measurement is more complex than max dP/dt, which remains one of its most limiting factors.

Summary

The measurement of cardiac function is complex and only briefly touched on here. The most valuable indices clinically still remain the pulmonary artery wedge pressure, the cardiac output, the ejection fraction and end-diastolic and end-systolic volumes. Although these measurements have major limitations, they are relatively easy to perform, and of great management and prognostic value.

REFERENCES

Bradley, R.D. (1977). *Studies in acute heart failure*. Edward Arnold, London.

Branthwaite, M.A. and Bradley, R.D. (1968). Measurement of cardiac output by thermal dilution in man. *Journal of Applied Physiology*, **24**, 434–8.

Forrester, J.S., Diamond, G., Chatterjee, K., and Swan, H.J.C. (1976). Medical therapy of acute myocardial infarction by application of hemody-namic subsets. *New England Journal of Medicine*, **24**, 1356–62; 1404–13.

Gibson, D., Mehmet, H., Schwarz, F., Li, K., and Kubler, W. (1986). Asynchronous left ventricular wall motion early after coronary thrombosis. *British Heart Journal*, **55**, 4–13.

Grossman, W. and Baim, D.S. (1991). *Cardiac catheterisation, angiography and intervention*, 4th edn. Lea and Febiger. Philadelphia.

Jefferson, K., and Rees, S. (1980). *Clinical cardiac radiology*. Butterworths, London.

Kennedy J.W., Baxley W.A., Figley M.M., Dodge H.T., and Brackman J.R. (1966). Quantitative angiocardiography. The normal left ventricle in man. *Circulation*, **34**, 272–8.

Miller, G. (1989). *Invasive investigation of the heart*. Blackwell Scientific Publications, Oxford.

Rickards, A.F., Seabra-Gomes, R., and Thurston, P. (1977). The assessment of regional abnormalities of the left ventricle by angiography. *European Journal of Cardiology*, **5**, 167–82.

Swan, H.J.C., Ganz, W., Forrester, J.S., Marcus, H., Diamond, G., and Chonette, D. (1970). Catheterisation of the heart in man with use of a flow-directed balloon tipped catheter. *New England Journal of Medicine*, **283**, 447–51.

Sutton, M.G.St.J., Sutton, M.St.J., *et al.* (1981). Valve replacement without preoperative cardiac catheterisation. *New England Journal of Medicine*, **305**, 1233–8.

Yang, S.S., Bentivoglio, L.G., Maranhao, V., and Goldberg, H. (1978). *From cardiac catheterisation data to haemodynamic parameters*. F.A. Davis Company, Philadelphia.

15.4.7 Exercise testing

K. DAWKINS

Introduction

Exercise testing is a pivotal investigation in the assessment of the patient with possible coronary heart disease. As the resting electrocardiogram lacks both sensitivity and specificity for the presence of myocardial ischaemia, some form of stress test is required in an attempt to provoke symptoms (e.g. angina) and record any associated changes on the electrocardiogram. Exercise protocols are safe, non-invasive, reproducible, simple to perform, and, in many patients, allow a decision to be made regarding the need for coronary arteriography. The exercise test should be regarded as an extension of the clinical history and examination; ideally, it should be supervised by the referring physician, although for practical reasons this goal is rarely achieved. The correct interpretation of the test requires a knowledge of the protocol used, the exercise duration achieved, the symptom(s) limiting exercise, the haemodynamic response observed, together with any electrocardiographic changes provoked by the test.

History

The association between symptoms of angina and repolarization changes on the electrocardiograph were first reported in 1918, and in the 1920s it was appreciated that ST segment changes were related to underlying myocardial ischaemia. The first attempt to formalize the exercise test used a two-step technique to monitor heart rate and blood pressure, and later the electrocardiograph after completion of exercise. Reproducibility was increased with the development of treadmill and then bicycle stress testing using a variety of protocols and lead systems.

Physiological changes with exercise

During upright dynamic exercise there is an increase in oxygen intake in relation to raised metabolic demands up to a maximum (V_{O_2}max),

Table 1 *Bruce protocol*

Stage	Speed (mph)	Gradient (%)	Time (min)	Cumulative time (min)
1	1.7	10	3	3
2	2.5	12	3	6
3	3.4	14	3	9
4	4.2	16	3	12
5	5.0	18	3	15
6	5.5	20	3	18

Table 2 *Indications for exercise testing*

Investigation of the patient with chest pain to determine the presence and/or severity of coronary heart disease
Stratify patients for risk after acute myocardial infarction
Evaluation of therapy in patients with known coronary heart disease (drug treatment, angioplasty, bypass grafting)
Provocation of exercise induced arrhythmias
Assessment of rate response (atrial/ventricular) prior to permanent pacing
Monitoring of blood pressure response to exercise
Screening asymptomatic individuals for the presence of occult coronary heart disease

Table 3 *Contraindications to exercise testing*

Contraindications
 Acute myocardial infarction (during the first few days)
 Unstable/progressive angina at rest
 Arrhythmias with rapid ventricular response at rest
 Congestive cardiac failure
 Cardiac infection (myocarditis, endocarditis, pericarditis)
 Systemic illness (anaemia, hyperthyroidism, pyrexia, etc.)

Relative contraindications
 Severe aortic valve stenosis
 Severe systemic or pulmonary hypertension
 Unfavourable coronary anatomy (left mainstem stenosis)
 Hypertrophic obstructive cardiomyopathy

above which oxygen uptake reaches a plateau despite the increasing metabolic requirements. V_{O_2}max for an individual depends on age, gender, weight, muscle mass, and level of fitness. The normal cardiovascular response to dynamic exercise includes an increase in heart rate, blood pressure, venous return, stroke volume, and oxygen extraction. Heart rate increases almost immediately with the onset of exercise due to a reduction in vagal tone and an increase in sympathetic activity: for a given amount of exercise heart rate is lower in fit subjects. The increase in heart rate with exertion correlates well with oxygen consumption such that oxygen uptake need not be measured in routine clinical practice. Peak heart rate correlates well with V_{O_2}max, but declines with increasing age. For a patient population the maximum predicted heart rate can be calculated from the equation, heart rate$_{max}$ = 0.65 × age (years). In untrained individuals, changes in stroke volume are of secondary importance to alterations in heart rate as a means of increasing cardiac output with exercise. Systemic blood pressure increases linearly with increasing work until V_{O_2}max is reached, at which point there may be a slight decrease in diastolic blood pressure due to a fall in systemic vascular resistance secondary to both arterial and venous dilatation. Alterations in oxygen extraction documented with increasing levels of exercise are particularly important as a method of increasing oxygen delivery in patients with a low cardiac output. Major determinants of myocardial oxygen consumption (also linearly related to V_{O_2}) are heart rate, contractility, and circumferential wall stress.

Protocols and equipment

A number of exercise testing protocols are in common use and provide satisfactory results, but it is clear that a maximum symptom-limited protocol increases the sensitivity of the test. For example, a submaximal test carried out to 85 per cent of the maximum predicted heart rate may miss 50 per cent of the ischaemic responses that could have been identified had the test been continued to maximal effort. A protocol should be chosen that can be applied to a wide variety of individuals; an aggressive protocol should not be applied to children, the elderly, or the infirm, whereas too gentle a protocol will be time-consuming and may result in failure to reach the maximum heart rate (and therefore V_{O_2}max) because of the prior onset of muscle fatigue. In using one of the standard protocols there is the advantage that data are available relating to the predicted performance of a variety of subsets of patients; one of these, the standard or modified Bruce protocol is in common use (Table 1). The major practical advantage of the treadmill over the bicycle ergometer is that the conduct of the test is under the control of the supervisor rather than the patient; therefore the level of exercise achieved is higher with the treadmill.

The choice of lead system determines in part the sensitivity of the test. Most current systems use a conventional 12-lead ECG; other lead arrangements include a bipolar (CM_5) system and the XYZ orthogonal or vector system.

Many of the current exercise testing systems consist of an integrated treadmill and electrocardiograph machine with pre-programmed protocols which can be selected by the operator. During the test the speed and gradient increase automatically and a full 12-lead electrocardiograph is recorded after each stage. Proper skin preparation and the correct application of disposable skin electrodes, together with a screened electrocardiograph cable are necessary to obtain high quality traces with minimal movement and respiratory artefact.

Indications

Table 2 lists the common indications for exercise testing in cardiology. The majority of exercise tests are undertaken to determine the presence or severity of coronary disease, to stratify patients for risk following acute myocardial infarction, or to evaluate the effect of therapy (e.g. drug treatment, coronary angioplasty, or coronary artery bypass grafting) in a patient with known coronary artery disease. Less frequent indications include the provocation of arrhythmias and the assessment of heart rate response prior to permanent pacing. Monitoring of the blood pressure response to exercise in a patient with borderline hypertension may also occasionally be useful. Exercise testing in asymptomatic individuals is more contentious (see below).

Contraindications

Exercise testing is contraindicated in patients who have suffered a very recent myocardial infarction, unstable angina, or who are known to have high risk coronary anatomy (e.g. left mainstem stenosis) (Table 3). Patients with infections including myocarditis, pericarditis, infective endocarditis should not undergo exercise testing. Exercise testing is unlikely to be of value and may be dangerous in patients with arrhythmias with a rapid ventricular response at rest (e.g. atrial fibrillation, supraventicular or ventricular tachycardia). Patients with certain conditions, for example aortic stenosis, or dilated or hypertrophic cardiomyopathy, can undergo exercise testing with care, but it is wise to use a submaximal protocol.

General medical conditions that should preclude exercise testing include septicaemia, severe anaemia, and thyrotoxicosis.

Risks of exercise testing

Exercise testing in the patient with coronary artery disease is associated with a small but finite risk. Procedure related mortality varies from 0.2

to 1.0 per 10 000, with an incidence of ventricular tachycardia or ventricular fibrillation requiring DC cardioversion of 1 in 5000. Exercise testing in inappropriate subsets of patients, for example, those with unstable angina, congestive cardiac failure, or uncontrolled hypertension is associated with a significant increase in morbidity/mortality. An exercise testing laboratory should be equipped with all the equipment needed for full resuscitation, although it is usual for ventricular arrhythmias to be managed with cardioversion alone without the need for intubation or additional drug therapy. Other documented complications of exercise testing include acute myocardial infarction, stroke, and retinal detachment.

In the United Kingdom written informed consent is not normally required for exercise testing, but it may be a prerequisite in some hospitals and in the United States. All exercise tests should be undertaken with a physician and technician present. A lack of medical supervision cannot be recommended and is unlikely to be defensible in a court of law.

PROBABILITY THEORY

The sensitivity of exercise testing reflects the ability of the test to detect the presence of significant (usually 50 to 75 per cent obstruction) of a major epicardial coronary artery. The more sensitive a test the higher the probability that an individual with coronary disease will have an abnormal result when tested. The specificity of exercise testing reflects the ability to detect normality; the higher the specificity the more likely a patient with normal coronary arteries will have a normal test. A highly sensitive test gives rise to few false negatives, and a highly specific test results in few false positives. There is therefore a trade-off between sensitivity and specificity, and an increase in sensitivity is only achieved at a cost of reducing specificity. For example, if the magnitude of the exercise induced ST segment depression used to define positivity is increased from 1.0 to 1.5 mm, the specificity increases from 89 to 100 per cent but the sensitivity decreases from 62 to 48 per cent.

The clinical usefulness of a test is dependent on the prevalence of the disease in the study population, i.e. the pretest likelihood of the disease. The predictive accuracy of a positive exercise test is defined as the probability that a patient with an abnormal test does truly have significant coronary artery disease. Similarly, the predictive accuracy of a negative test is defined as the probability that a patient with a normal test is free of coronary artery disease. The pretest likelihood of the disease is incorporated in Bayes' theorem. Other terms used in probability analysis are outlined in Table 4. In a population with a low prevalence of coronary artery disease, for example asymptomatic young men, there may be more false-positive responders than true-positive responders, thereby rendering the test clinically useless in this subset of patients.

FALSE-POSITIVE AND FALSE-NEGATIVE RESPONDERS

Numerous causes of false-positive response have been reported (Table 5). Many protocols specify a resting electrocardiograph in both the lying and standing position before beginning exercise to exclude patients with repolarization changes provoked by changes in posture, which significantly reduces the false-positive rate. False-negative tests occur in subjects taking β-blocking drugs, which should therefore be withdrawn 24 h before testing. Most commonly a false-negative result occurs because the test is discontinued prematurely and is therefore not truly 'maximal'.

Exercise test interpretation

The provocation of symptoms constitutes an important part of the exercise test. Both their nature and severity should be ascertained, in particular whether the symptoms provoked on the treadmill reflect those experienced during day-to-day activities. In the patient with significant coronary artery disease, typical angina occurs with or without associated breathlessness; less commonly the patient may experience a non-cardiac symptom (e.g. claudication). Angina occurring at a low workload, either

Table 4 *Definitions used in probability analysis*

Sensitivity
True positives
True positives + false positives
Specificity
True negatives
True negatives + false positives
Positive predictive accuracy
True positives
True positives + false positives
Negative predictive accuracy
True negatives
True negatives + false positives
Risk ratio
Percentage of subjects with an abnormal test result who develop CHD
Percentage of subjects with a normal test who develop CHD

Table 5 *Causes of a false-positive exercise test response*

Changes in posture
Hyperventilation
Left or right ventricular hypertrophy (e.g. systemic hypertension, aortic stenosis)
Pre-excitation (e.g. Wolff–Parkinson–White syndrome)
Left or right bundle branch block
Mitral valve prolapse syndrome
Dilated cardiomyopathy
Elevated right ventricular end-diastolic pressure (e.g., pulmonary embolism, pulmonary stenosis)
Vasoregulatory asthenia
Drug therapy (e.g. digoxin, lithium, phenothiazines)
Hypokalaemia
Food or glucose ingestion

de novo or following a myocardial infarct is associated with a poor prognosis.

Changes in the ST segment remain the primary variable in exercise testing. The timing, distribution, magnitude, and severity of ST segment depression, together with the speed of normalization during recovery are all important factors in identifying the presence, severity and prognosis of coronary artery disease. ST segment depression is recognized in three basic patterns (upsloping, horizontal, and downsloping) measured in millimetres of depression 80 ms after the J point. Other features of myocardial ischaemia include the inability to increase the heart rate (chronotropic incompetence), a fall in blood pressure, an increase in R-wave amplitude (indicative of ventricular cavity dilatation), exercise-induced ventricular arrhythmias, and a flat blood pressure response to exercise. Isolated T wave changes are unreliable as a manifestation of myocardial ischaemia.

There is a tendency to over-report ST segment changes on the exercise trace. Therefore a convention of two mm (or more) depression 80 ms after the J point should be regarded as a 'positive' response offering an acceptable compromise between sensitivity and specificity (see Probablity theory above).

Reasons for terminating an exercise test

An experienced supervisor will insure that the patient undertakes a maximal symptom limited effort; too often a test is terminated prematurely with the associated reduction in sensitivity such that no useful clinical data are obtained. Similarly, an arbitrary cutoff at some heart rate below maximum (e.g. 150 beats/min or 75 per cent maximum) limits the usefulness of the test. The onset of angina is reproducible on repeat testing at a similar rate-pressure product. Reasons for terminating an exercise test are shown in Table 6.

Invasive exercise testing

Exercise testing maybe combined with cardiac catheterization when there is a need to assess the haemodynamic response to an increase in cardiac output. Specific indications include the measurement of transvalve gradients (e.g. mitral stenosis), the evaluation of cardiac function in patients with valve regurgitation (e.g. aortic regurgitation), and the assessment of the patient with unexplained breathlessness. Valve lesions of borderline significance at rest may become important on exercise due to the increase in transvalve flow secondary to the change in cardiac output. Stress testing in the catheterization laboratory takes various forms and is constrained by the need for the patient to lie flat; these include dynamic exercise (e.g. straight leg raising), isometric exercise (e.g. handgrip), and atrial pacing.

EXERCISE ECHOCARDIOGRAPHY

M-mode and cross-sectional echocardiography have been used as methods of assessing changes in left ventricular dimensions and regional wall motion abnormalities provoked by exercise. The echocardiogram is usually recorded immediately after completion of a maximal treadmill exercise test, or occasionally during upright bicycle ergometry or during isometric exercise using static handgrip. Movement artefact seriously limits the application of theses techniques which are likely to remain in the research domain. The more recent utilization of dobutamine stress echocardiography may supersede exercise echocardiography in the majority of patients.

RADIONUCLIDE EXERCISE TESTING

The sensitivity and specificity of treadmill exercise testing for the detection of coronary artery disease can be enhanced by the addition of myocardial imaging using a number of agents including thallium-201 and, more recently, technetium-99m-sestamibi. Stress and rest images are compared thereby identifying 'fixed' defects indicative of myocardial infarction and 'reversible' defects as a consequence of myocardial ischaemia. The addition of single photon emission tomography (SPECT) allows the identification of abnormalities of regional myocardial perfusion. Exercise perfusion scintigraphy is indicated in four groups of patients:

Table 6 *Reasons to terminate an exercise test*

Symptoms (severe/progressive chest pain, breathlessness, dizziness/syncope)
Profound ST segment depression (> 5 mm)
Change of rhythm (e.g. ventricular tachycardia)
Progressive fall in blood pressure or heart rate
Patient appears unwell (pale, vasoconstricted, etc.)
Elevated blood pressure (> 200 mmHg systolic)
Patient unable to continue

1. Patients performing an inadequate amount of exercise (due to fatigue, arrhythmias, β-blocking drugs, etc.).
2. Patients with a resting electrocardiographic abnormality (e.g. left bundle branch block).
3. When exercise precipitates chest pain without associated electrocardiographic abnormalities.
4. If an 'ischaemic' electrocardiographic response occurs in the absence of symptoms.

FURTHER READING

Bayes, T. (1763). An essay toward solving a problem in the doctrine of chance. *Philosophical Transactions of the Royal Society of London,* **53,** 270.

Bousfield, G. (1918). Angina pectoris: changes in electrocardiogram during paroxysm. *Lancet,* **ii,** 457–8.

Bruce, R.A. (1971). Exercise testing of patients with coronary heart disease. *Annals of Clinical Research,* **3,** 323–30.

Cumming, G.R. (1972). Yield of ischaemic exercise electrocardiograms in relation to exercise intensity in a normal population. *British Heart Journal,* **34,** 919–23.

Ellestad, M.H. (1986). *Stress testing: principles and practice.* F.A. Davis Co., Philadelphia.

Fletcher, G.F. (1993). *Cardiology clinics: exercise testing and cardiac rehabilitation.* W.B. Saunders Co., Philadelphia.

Master, A.M. (1935). The two step test of myocardial function. *American Heart Journal,* **10,** 495.

Martin, C.M. and McConahay, D.R. (1972). Maximal treadmill exercise electrocardiography; correlations with coronary angiography and cardiac hemodynamics. *Circulation,* **46,** 95–162.

Pardee, H.E.B. (1920). An electrocardiographic sign of coronary artery obstruction. *Archives of Internal Medicine,* **26,** 247.

Schlant, R.C., Friesinger, G.C., and Leonard, J.J. (1990). Clinical competence in exercise testing. *Circulation,* **82,** 1884–8.

15.5 The syndrome of heart failure

A.J.S. COATS AND P. A. POOLE-WILSON

Definitions

'Heart failure' is an unfortunate term. It has negative connotations for the patient and describes imprecisely several different clinical situations. Left and right heart failure are quite distinct clinical syndromes, although they frequently coexist (biventricular failure). Historically, heart failure has been further subdivided on the basis of presumed pathophysiological mechanisms into: (1) 'forward' or 'backward' heart failure, depending on whether congestion or organ underperfusion was the predominant clinical feature; (2) 'congestive' or 'non-congestive',

depending on the presence or absence of oedema; and (3) 'high-output' or 'low-output'. These subdivisions have not proved to be particularly useful. A more recent and more useful classification is dependent on the predominant pattern of left ventricular dysfunction, be it systolic, diastolic, or mixed. Whatever the complexities of the ventricular pathophysiology that initiates events, a well-recognized clinical pattern is identifiable as 'heart failure', one which has proved a useful description of a complex clinical syndrome for many years.

The pertinent features of any definition of heart failure (of which there have been several) are that the clinical picture is: (1) initiated by a reduction in effective cardiovascular (usually left ventricular) functional reserve; (2) associated with symptoms either at rest or at an unexpectedly low level of exertion; and (3) associated with characteristic pathophysiological changes in many disparate organ systems. The last can include biochemical, hormonal, metabolic, or functional alterations. In simple terms heart failure is a syndrome in which a reduction in left ventricular function causes pathophysiology which produces symptoms and exercise limitation.

A clinical picture similar to that of heart failure can develop when ventricular function itself is normal, but where there is an extreme volume or pressure overload on the ventricle. These include volume overload conditions such as endotoxic high-output shock, severe anaemia, arteriovenous fistulae or shunts, and pressure overload conditions such as acute hypertensive crisis or prosthetic heart valve occlusion. It is probably more useful clinically and for research purposes to separate these from cases where the initiating cause is a reduction in ventricular function.

Acute and chronic heart failure

It is conventional, because of differences in assessment and management, to separate acute and chronic heart failure. Both are, of course, different stages of a single disease process, and in the clinical course of a patient with chronic heart failure acute exacerbations may be common, often described as 'acute decompensation' or 'acute on chronic' heart failure. Acute heart failure usually has a dramatic clinical presentation, with an acutely dyspnoeic patient demonstrating visible signs of cardiovascular insufficiency such as tachycardia, pulmonary or peripheral oedema, and underperfusion of systemic organs. Chronic heart failure, by contrast, can be a subtle disorder, which, if gradual in onset, can be missed by both patient and physician. The salient features are the initiating and persisting left ventricular dysfunction, and the pathophysiological changes in other organs which produce symptoms and which limit exercise. In severe chronic heart failure a chronic persistent state of circulatory insufficiency can exist with pulmonary and peripheral oedema and symptoms and signs of distress even at rest.

Epidemiology

Heart failure is a common condition with an estimated incidence of 20 to 30 per thousand per year and a prevalence overall of about 1 per cent. The prevalence increases in frequency with increasing age, reaching 30 per cent in the over-80 year olds. The ageing of the population in industrialized societies is leading to more elderly people and as a result heart failure is increasing as a major health care cost. Paradoxically, improvements in the management of acute myocardial infarction and chronic coronary heart disease has lead to more heart failure, as more people survive to develop heart failure later in life.

Because of its multiple debilitating symptoms, heart failure is a frequent cause of both acute hospital admission and long-stay residential care. It is the most common diagnosis on discharge from hospital in the United States in people over the age of 65, and the second most common overall. It is also the one with the greatest rate of re-admission to hospital and the most expensive single diagnosis of the US diagnosis-related groupings. Heart failure is a feature of the clinical condition of approximately 5 per cent of patients in hospital at any one time. It is therefore of major importance in the health economics of developed countries.

Aetiologies

Heart failure is a clinical syndrome, not a single diagnosis; it can have a number of separate causes. In Western industrialized societies the most common are ischaemic heart disease, hypertension, and idiopathic dilated cardiomyopathy. The Framingham study suggested that hypertension, especially when complicated by left ventricular hypertrophy, was by far the most common antecedent of heart failure; but most recent intervention trials have included a preponderance of patients whose heart failure was secondary to ischaemic heart disease and, in cross-sectional studies in the community, hypertension is cited as a relatively minor cause of heart failure. This change has been attributed to better detection and treatment of hypertension, but may also reflect re-labelling when, for example, in a hypertensive patent who later develops coronary disease and then heart failure, the initial hypertension may either never have been detected or superseded in the clinical picture by coronary artery disease. Some cases of hypertension may develop a dilated poorly functioning heart with an eventual normalization in arterial pressure; such cases may be diagnosed as idiopathic dilated cardiomyopathy, the only clue to the true underlying cause being greater than expected left ventricular hypertrophy.

In industrialized societies, previously common causes such as nutritional deficiency disorders or chronic complications of rheumatic valvular disease are now rare. In less developed societies infective causes still underlie the majority of cases. Particular disorders may be common in individual societies and these should always be borne in mind in assessing a patient from these regions. These include Chagas' disease in Central and Southern America, iron overload in certain tribes in southern Africa, and nutritional deficiency states in the world's poorest countries.

Classification of cause

More than one underlying cause of heart failure can coexist, such as hypertension and ischaemic heart disease. Table 1 lists the major causes of heart failure subdivided by the mechanisms by which ventricular disease leads to the clinical syndrome. Such a differentiation is important because of specific strategies available for certain diagnoses, such as nutritional support, cardiac valve or bypass surgery, endocrine therapy and avoidance of a toxic agent.

Pathophysiology

Cardiac

STRUCTURAL CHANGES

Structural changes in the heart are common, both at macroscopic and microscopic levels. The clinical picture usually includes enlargement of the left ventricular cavity (with the exception of diastolic dysfunction and restrictive or constrictive cardiomyopathies). The shape of the ventricle also changes becoming more spherical. This can occur quickly after an initial myocardial infarction via a passive process of stretching of the infarcted territory (infarct expansion) or more slowly over a period of weeks to months in a process termed 'remodelling'. A similar change in shape is seen in dilated cardiomyopathies but not in the restrictive cardiomyopathies. The more spherical shape of the 'remodelled' and enlarged ventricle increases the stress of the myocardial wall and may thereby worsen myocardial ischaemia. Change in shape may also disrupt the complex conformational changes which normally occur during the isovolumic contraction phase in which the apex of the ventricle constricts in a twisting motion and pushes the blood into the base of the ventricle. Where the ventricle is already spherical at rest this intraventricular redistribution of blood during isovolumic contraction is not possible and the net effect is a reduction in the efficiency with which the blood is ejected.

Cardiac enlargement has long been known to be an adverse prognostic sign, even when estimated crudely as cardiothoracic diameter on chest radiograph. More precise measurements of the internal dimensions of the left ventricle by echocardiography have confirmed the prognostic value of cardiac enlargement in patients recovering from a myocardial

Table 1 *Causes of heart failure*

Loss of myocytes
  Ischaemic heart disease
  Idiopathic dilated cardiomyopathy
  Familial cardiomyopathies
  Infective cardiomyopathies, e.g. Chagas' disease
  Toxic cardiomyopathies including alcoholic cardiomyopathy
  Infiltrative conditions: sarcoid, amyloid, iron overload
  Cardiac neoplasms

Myocyte dysfunction
  Nutritional deficiencies
  ? Chronic ischaemia ('hibernating myocardium')
  Hypertrophic cardiomyopathy
  Restrictive cardiomyopathy
  Secondary to chronic tachyarrhythmia
  Endocrine disorders, e.g. thyrotoxic, hypocalcaemic,
    acromegalic

Alterations in myocardial interstitium
  Senile myocardial fibrosis
  Endomyocardial fibrosis

Valvular disorders
  Rheumatic heart disease
  Congenital valve disease
  Senile valve calcification
  Mitral valve prolapse
  Paravalvar dysfunction, e.g. paraprosthetic leak, dissection of
    aortic valve
  Infective endocarditis
  Non-infective endocarditis, e.g. secondary to connective
    tissue diseases

Pericardial disorders
  Constrictive pericarditis
  Cardiac tamponade

Extracardiac causes
  Volume overload, e.g. anaemia, arteriovenous shunt
  Pressure overload, e.g. coarctation, severe hypertenion

infarction, even when accounting for the size of the myocardial infarct. Prevention of the late remodelling process was the theory behind the use of angiotensin-converting-enzyme inhibitors given early after myocardial infarction. These agents have been shown to reduce ventricular size and to reduce late mortality if given between 2 and 14 days after the infarction, but not if given intravenously within the first few hours. Whether this beneficial effect is directly related to any reduction in ventricular remodelling is not, however, known.

Changes at the microscopic level

The failing heart also shows alterations in cardiac structure at microscopic and ultrastructural levels. There is an increase in the collagen content of the extracellular matrix, a process thought to be in part related to increased wall stress and in part due to neurohormonal activation, particularly of aldosterone. This change reduces ventricular wall distensibility and may affect the efficiency with which active restorative forces can assist the diastolic filling process. As a result this microscopic structural change may help explain the frequent coexistence of systolic and diastolic functional deterioration in an enlarging ventricle in chronic heart failure.

The enlargement of the ventricle is associated with a thinning of the ventricular wall and, as there is believed to be no increase in the total myocyte population there must be a realignment of the intercellular attachments between individual myocytes. This process whereby there is a continual breaking and reforming of cell-to-cell junctions to allow

remodelling has been called 'cell slippage', although exactly how this occurs has not been established. There are changes in the microscopic structure of the failing ventricle with a reduced number of tight junctions between myocytes.

FUNCTIONAL ABNORMALITIES

Overall circulatory function

The description of an objective measurement of systolic function in intact humans has proved difficult. In simplest terms the left ventricle is a pump which generates both pressure and flow. It has a theoretical operating range from a pure pressure generator to a pure flow generator, although it always functions as a mixed pump. The function of this pump can be described in terms of the kinetic and potential energy it imparts to the blood ejected each beat, or in terms of the average power output of the circulation (flow times mean pressure drop) assuming the left ventricle is the only significant power source in the circulation. Thus overall ventricular function can be described as cardiac output times the pressure drop across the systemic circulation, a quantity described as cardiac power output. Cardiac power output is well-preserved at rest, even in severe heart failure. The maximal reserve of cardiac power output is reduced progressively as heart failure progresses, and a significant reduction in maximal power output during inotropic stimulation is a poor prognostic sign. However, the measurement of cardiac power output tells us little of the mechanisms underlying any reduction in ventricular performance. This may be due reduced ventricular filling, or emptying, or to wasted myocardial power such as in aortic stenosis. Attempts have been made, therefore, to define the components of ventricular function in attempt to explain the nature of a reduced overall circulatory function and to assist in monitoring a patient's clinical course and the response to treatments.

Systolic dysfunction

Systole can be defined either clinically as the ejection phase between mitral valve closure and aortic valve closure, or in terms of ventricular dynamics as the phase of contraction of the myocytes within the ventricle. These two definitions do not coincide, for there is a period of isovolumic contraction at the onset of ventricular systole in which myocyte contraction generates a pressure increase within the ventricle and a conformational change in its shape but during which no blood is ejected. Similarly, during the latter phase of ventricular ejection the blood is flowing passively from the left ventricle and the myocardial elements may already be relaxing.

In clinical practice, systolic dysfunction is most easily recognized by direct haemodynamic measurements showing a reduced peak rate of pressure rise within the ventricle (positive dP/dt maximum), an increased filling pressure (left ventricular end-diastolic pressure, LVEDP) or by indirect measurement of ventricular volumes. If there is a reduction in myocardial contractile function an enlargement of the ventricle will develop in which a greater preload will enhance ventricular emptying via the Frank–Starling mechanism. As a result the ventricle will operate at an increased end-diastolic and end-systolic volume. This can be measured by pressure and volume estimations for instance by ventriculography (either radiographic or radionuclear) or echocardiography. Although not a direct measure of ventricular performance, ejection fraction, being the fractional emptying of the ventricle with each beat, carries information about ventricular volumes and global ventricular function. It has been shown to be an important predictor of longevity in heart failure, independent of other measures of severity, and it has the advantage of simplicity. However, it is a poor predictor of the severity of symptomatic limitation in these patients. At the most simple level, systolic heart failure can be recognized by signs of cardiac insufficiency in the presence of an enlarged ventricle. Clinically it is most conveniently estimated as left ventricular ejection fraction.

Diastolic dysfunction

Diastole is the opposite to systole, the period of filling of the ventricle or the period of relaxation of the myocyte. Objective measurements of diastolic function are, however, more problematic than of systolic function. Whereas systole occurs rapidly and in one action, diastole is complex, with an initial rapid and active ventricular recoil producing rapid filling of the ventricle, then a period of relative stasis as atrial and ventricular pressures equilibrate, followed by a second period of ventricular filling produced by the effects of atrial contraction. These processes are affected by many factors including heart rate, atrioventricular delay, atrial contractility, active myocardial recoil, passive ventricular wall stiffness, and the efficacy of ventricular systole and the residual end-diastolic volume and pressure within the ventricle. As a result of all these interacting factors, it is not surprising that no simple measure of 'diastolic function' has been developed, and those measures that have been used clinically are affected profoundly by systolic function and heart rate. Diastolic functional disturbance is, however, important, as there are cases of definite clinical heart failure, in which the patient has a small heart with normal or even increased left ventricular ejection fraction, and in whom the only demonstrable abnormalities of ventricular mechanics are those related to diastolic filling. These may include increased filling pressures, delayed pressure fall within the ventricle and a greater than normal dependence on the effects of atrial contraction for ventricular filling. Such cases form the minority of cases of heart failure (estimates vary from a few percent to about one-fifth of cases) but are seen with increasing frequency in older patients in whom senile myocardial fibrosis occurs more frequently as the major pathology underlying the heart failure. Other, rarer, causes include hypertrophic cardiomyopathy, infiltrative conditions such as amyloid heart disease, and the acute effects of ischaemia or the chronic effects of advanced hypertrophy in response to hypertension.

Diastolic dysfunction can be quantified by a variety of measurements: haemodynamic, echocardiographic, radionuclear, or ventriculographic. The most commonly employed are the rate constant of isovolumic relaxation of the ventricle during early diastole (tau), the early to late peak filling velocity ratio (E/A) across the mitral valve on Doppler echocardiography, and the peak rate of ventricular filling on radionuclear gated acquisition (MUGA) scans in end-diastolic volumes per second. None of these parameters is independent of the loading conditions of the ventricle, nor of atrioventricular delay and heart rate, nor of the effect of systolic dysfunction. Pure diastolic dysfunction is rare, as indeed is pure systolic dysfunction, as the two are almost inseparably interdependent. One can speak, however, of cases where the heart failure is predominantly due to systolic or diastolic impairment of the ventricle, and the simplest separation is via the size of the end-diastolic volume; if large, systolic dysfunction is likely to be the major abnormality; if small, diastolic. As will be discussed in later chapters, this differentiation is important because of differing effects of treatment, in particular vasodilators which may be less useful in diastolic dysfunction because of the requirement for high ventricular filling pressures in this condition.

Pericardial

Pericardial dysfunction is not a common cause of heart failure. In pericardial constriction such as after tuberculous pericarditis (or in pericardial tamponade such as in connective tissue diseases, infections or after heart surgery) the effects on net cardiac function can be catastrophic and a clinical picture of acute or more rarely chronic heart failure can develop. Detailed clinical investigation will identify tell-tale signs, and the reader is referred to Section 15.4 for further details. Pericardial dysfunction in cases of heart failure due to myocardial disease is not common. It is perhaps surprising that a considerable degree of cardiac enlargement can be accommodated without signs of pericardial restriction if the enlargement occurs slowly. The key to detection of important pericardial dysfunction is a high index of suspicion, careful clinical examination and access to echocardiography where such clinical suspicion exists.

Non-cardiac

GENERAL SYNDROME

Although initiated by ventricular dysfunction, in its chronic form heart failure is a multisystem disorder: the syndrome of chronic heart failure. The causes of many of the disparate organ pathologies which develop are poorly understood, as are the mechanisms by which these are (slowly) corrected by effective therapy including transplantation of the heart. Much remains uncertain about this non-cardiac pathology and pathophysiology, including its genesis, symptomatic effects, and correct management. A variety of evidence has suggested, however, that non-cardiac factors become the major factors which generate both the symptoms and the objective limitation to exercise in chronic heart failure.

SPECIFIC ORGAN SYSTEMS

Peripheral vascular

The microvasculature

Changes occur in the microvasculature in many organ systems and these may contribute to the organ underperfusion seen in this syndrome. There have been few reports of definite structural changes in the microvasculature but functionally the endothelial-dependent vasomotor control systems are disordered. The endothelial-dependent vasodilator system is impaired both in the myocardial vessels and in the periphery. Tumour necrosis factor, which is elevated in some cases of chronic heart failure, has been implicated in impaired endothelial vasodilator function, and there have been reports of enhanced activity of the endothelin vasoconstrictor system. This generalized endothelial dysfunction may contribute to some of the organ dysfunction described below, including renal, hepatic, and pulmonary vascular impairment. Specific treatments for endothelial abnormalities have not been described for heart failure.

Large arterial function

In heart failure, there is a reduction in large arterial compliance and this in turns leads to an increase in the impedance to ventricular outflow. Thus the efficiency of ventriculo-aortic coupling is reduced, the impaired ventricular reserve is further stressed and there is an increase in myocardial wall stress. The cause of the large arterial changes probably relate to sympathetic and possibly local renin–angiotensin activation. Specific treatments have not been developed for these changes.

Respiratory

The lungs

Despite the frequency of dyspnoea as a central complaint of a patient with heart failure, relatively little is known of the role of the lung in chronic heart failure. In acute heart failure, changes within the lung are profound and easily explain much of the acute respiratory distress of the syndrome. With an acute reduction in left ventricular performance a rapid increase in left ventricular filling pressures and hence pulmonary venous pressures will lead to fluid accumulation in the lung parenchyma. Initially this will decrease the compliance of the lung, thereby reducing vital capacity and increasing the work of breathing. It may also, via oedematous swelling of the bronchial mucosa, cause a non-asthmatic bronchial constriction which can mimic asthma and further increase respiratory muscle work.

With more severe pulmonary venous hypertension the alveolar membrane becomes thickened and oedematous and this may impair gas exchange leading to an increase in the alveolar–arterial oxygen gradient and eventually arterial hypoxaemia. Eventually frank pulmonary oedema can form, further exacerbating the above processes and leading to the clinical picture of gross dyspnoea, hypoxaemia, lung crepitations, and the production of copious quantities of pink frothy sputum (the alveolar oedema fluid itself). The management of this medical emergency is dealt with elsewhere in this section.

In chronic heart failure, the patent remains dyspnoeic but the changes in the lungs are far less marked. With well-diuresed and non-oedematous patients very few changes can be detected in lung histology. The changes of pulmonary siderosis seen with chronic untreated mitral stenosis are not seen in well treated chronic heart failure. Even pulmonary venous pressures may be normal if diuretic treatment is effective. There have been reports of subtle changes in lung function in chronic heart failure including a reduction in gas diffusing capacity, intermittent non-asthmatic bronchial constriction and a purported increase in dead space ventilation, but these are largely functional changes which have not an established anatomical cause. One pathophysiological change which can lead to respiratory distress is an alteration in the volume, structure, strength and fatiguability of the respiratory musculature. Such changes have been described in chronic heart failure, but other features of these changes such as their cause, effect on the sensation of dyspnoea, or most appropriate therapy are unknown. Similar changes are seen in skeletal muscle (see below).

Respiratory control

The mechanisms of normal respiratory control during exercise are not fully understood. It is not surprising, therefore, that the mechanisms underlying the abnormal respiratory response seen in chronic heart failure are also unclear. Patients with heart failure, even in the absence of pulmonary oedema, have an increased ventilatory response to exercise, whilst maintaining normal arterial blood gas tensions. They show a reduced maximal oxygen consumption, an early dependence on anaerobic metabolism and an increased ventilatory equivalent for carbon dioxide even at low work levels. This latter feature can be best appreciated by the plot of ventilation against the rate of carbon dioxide production (the $V/V\text{co}_2$ slope) during progressive exercise. This slope is significantly steeper (up to three-fold) throughout both aerobic and anaerobic levels of exercise, and its steepness correlates closely with the reduction of maximal oxygen consumption. Although it is clear that this increased ventilation relative to the external work rate must indicate wasted ventilation, exactly why it occurs in non-oedematous patients is not certain. It has been assumed that there is a primary increase in dead-space ventilation due to a reduction in the ability of the right ventricle to perfuse adequately all lung regions, or the development of significant ventilation/perfusion mismatching within the lung. These hypotheses have not, however, been proven, and an alternative is that something other than the rate of carbon dioxide production causes the increased exertional ventilation in heart failure patients. In support of this second hypothesis is the finding that, rather than being abnormal, arterial carbon dioxide during exercise is often lower than in normal subjects suggesting the presence of a degree of relative hyperventilation or the action of a non-carbon dioxide ventilatory stimulus. There are several candidate stimuli including an increased release of, or sensitivity to known ventilatory stimuli such as lactate, arterial potassium or adenosine. Skeletal muscle in heart failure is abnormal (see below) and releases metabolites earlier in exercise than age-matched normal subjects. In addition there is a neural pathway (the ergoreflex) in the control of ventilation utilizing group III and IV afferents from skeletal muscle. These are sensitive to the metabolic state of exercising muscle and transmit signals via the lateral spinothalamic tract to mediate reflex increases in ventilation as well as peripheral vasoconstriction and sympatho-excitation. This mechanism may also be activated in chronic heart failure given the abnormalities of metabolism of the exercising skeletal muscle.

Airflow

Expiratory airflow can be restricted in patients with heart failure, even when all smokers and patients with a history of intermittent bronchospasm have been excluded. These patients can exhibit considerable dips in their peak expiratory flow rate on occasion especially at night. This may lead to episodes of respiratory distress as well as adding to the work of breathing, and through that to the perception of dyspnoea. The mechanisms of this 'bronchoconstriction' are not known but they may involve oedema of the bronchial mucosa. Thus a variety of lung factors can add together to contribute to dyspnoea in chronic heart failure, even in the absence of frank pulmonary oedema. Recently methoxamine has been reported to improve peak flow rates and lead to an increase in exercise tolerance in these patients.

Gas exchange

Although arterial oxygen desaturation and carbon dioxide retention are rare in well-diuresed patients with heart failure, more mild alterations in the gas exchange function of the lung can occur in heart failure. These could reduce the rate of delivery of oxygen to the metabolizing tissues and act as a stimulus to increased ventilation. They may also explain the compensatory increase in arterial oxygen content seen in chronic heart failure, if mild but intermittent hypoxia develops in this condition. This could also explain the beneficial effects of oxygen supplementation, even acutely, on exercise tolerance in patients with chronic heart failure.

It is not certain, however, that a reduction in diffusing capacity is either quantitatively important nor that oxygen supplementation works via increasing net oxygen delivery to the tissues. Alternative explanations are that the effect of high inspired oxygen is non-specific in reducing peripheral chemoreflex drive and thereby relieving the sensation of dyspnoea, in a way akin to that produced by narcotic analgesics. Similarly reduced gas exchange especially for oxygen may have more to do with inadequate expansion of the pulmonary capillary network and an inadequate time for gas transfer rather than to any alteration in the alveolar blood–gas barrier itself. The very low mixed venous oxygen saturations seen in chronic heart failure may mean that even a normal capillary transit time is inadequate for full oxygen exchange.

The sleep–apnoea syndrome

Nocturnal oxygen saturation monitoring of patients with chronic heart failure has demonstrated the presence of episodes of desaturation often to below 80 to 85 per cent. These episodes coincide with, and are caused by episodes of apnoea; they are also followed by semi-arousal from sleep and hyperventilation which may awaken and frighten the sleeping partner. The pattern is reminiscent with Cheyne–Stokes respiratory patterns which are well recognized in severe heart failure. The mechanisms of both abnormalities of respiratory rhythms are incompletely understood. In some cases of nocturnal desaturations there is an obstructive element with obesity and pharyngeal occlusion by the tongue flopping back. In others there appears to be an alteration in the central sensitivity to carbon dioxide so that oscillating levels of respiratory drive and hence arterial oxygen saturations develop. This second mechanism may be partly the cause for Cheyne–Stokes breathing as well. A possibly related finding is that patients with chronic heart failure exhibit reduced total and high frequency heart rate variability but relatively enhanced variability of heart rate at very low frequencies (less than 0.01 Hz, or 1 cycle every 100 s). Although rhythmic variations in heart rate at higher frequencies are related to homeostatic mechanisms controlling blood pressure, in particular the vagal and sympathetic limbs of the arterial baroreflex, the genesis of this very low frequency rhythm is not known. It does, however, have several features which suggest that chemoreflex activity may play a role in its genesis. First, this rhythm is particularly prominent in heart failure, where circulation time is long. Second, it is of similar frequency to the more obvious rhythm of Cheyne–Stokes breathing, and third, the chemoreflex loop has sufficient delay characteristics and possesses sufficient interactions with the baroreflexes and control of heart rate for an harmonic of oscillatory arterial gas concentrations to set up a similar harmonic oscillation in respiration which would then entrain heart rate via an effect of the baroreflex. Last, similar rhythms are particularly prominent in heart failure in pulmonary arterial pressure tracings. Thus it may be that periodic sleep–apnoea (at least that which is not obviously obstructive), very low frequency rhythms of heart rate variability and Cheyne–Stokes respiration may all be reflections of harmonic oscillation of chemoreflex–baroreflex interactions. If this is the case then they may respond to therapies which alter chemoreflex gain or drive, and in this regard the promising reports of nocturnal oxygen supplementation and of nasal positive pressure ventilation may be supportive for this theory. It is in any case surprising, and perhaps chastening, to note that in a condition so associated with dyspnoea that the state of chemoreflex drive at rest, during sleep or exercise is not known.

Musculoskeletal

Structure

Skeletal muscle biopsies in patients with moderate to severe chronic heart failure have shown a variety of pathological changes ranging from individual fibre atrophy and a shift in the distribution frequency of types IIa and IIb fibres, to changes at an ultrastructural level including a reduction in mitochondrial density, volume, and the number of cristae. It has proved impossible to define a specific pathological change characteristic of heart failure, partly because of the enormous variation in a control population, but also because muscle becomes abnormal in a limited number of ways in a variety of diseases associated with skeletal myopathy. It is also important to be sure that it is a specific heart failure-related change that is being observed and not a subclinical skeletal myopathy as part of an inherited cardioskeletal myopathy. That such changes are seen with equal frequency and severity in ischaemic heart failure makes this unlikely to be the only explanation, however.

One of the most marked structural changes in peripheral muscle which has frequently been ignored is the substantial reduction in total skeletal muscle bulk. Although it has long been recognized that in some cases of endstage heart failure a catabolic wasting syndrome can develop (cardiac cachexia), it has only recently been stressed that more subtle evidence of muscle wasting may be both common and functionally important in chronic heart failure. If less muscle is available to do the work of a limb, then each fibre will be more easily fatigued, be able to accept a lower total blood flow, will appear metabolically more stressed, and require anaerobic metabolism at an earlier point in exercise. These have all been taken as indicators of a deficiency in blood and oxygen delivery, rather than the alternative explanation that there simply is too little muscle for the exercise to be performed efficiently.

Function

In chronic heart failure there is a reduction in the peak strength of both small and large muscle groups. In the case of the small muscles of the hand this clearly cannot be due solely to a reduced cardiac pumping capacity because of its tiny blood flow requirement. This suggests that there may be inherent defects in the quality of the muscle itself. Given the difficulty of exactly matching for active muscle bulk the difference may, however, be partly a reflection of muscle wasting.

In addition to reduced peak strength, there is early fatiguability of muscle in heart failure. As a result patients frequently complain that muscle fatigue is the major limitation to the performance of their daily tasks. Weakness and fatigue may both contribute to reduced physical activity which may induce physical deconditioning and further muscle wasting and dysfunction.

Metabolism

Skeletal muscle metabolism during exercise has been investigated by magnetic resonance spectroscopy. This technique allows an exploration of the rate of utilisation of high energy phosphate bonds associated with phosphocreatine and of intracellular pH, and through these the efficiency of aerobic and anaerobic metabolism within the muscle during exercise. These experiments have shown that there is an early depletion of phosphocreatine, an early acidification and accumulation of inorganic phosphate, a reduction in the rate of resynthesis of phosphocreatine and in the removal of adenosine diphosphate (ADP). These changes cannot be explained by the acute effects of impaired blood flow because the difference between normal controls and heart failure patients is seen even when both groups perform exercise in ischaemic conditions produced by regional circulatory occlusion. The metabolic abnormalities described by magnetic resonance spectroscopy probably reflect alterations in oxidative enzymic content of skeletal muscle described in biopsy studies. The cause of these metabolic changes is not understood, but it has been estimated that muscle wasting alone cannot explain the changes because the half-time of adenosine diphosphate removal is independent of both the work-load per unit muscle mass or the blood flow.

The only treatment which has been definitely shown to correct these metabolic abnormalities is physical exercise conditioning of the muscle, either localised or general. The time course of the possible correction of the muscle changes after cardiac transplantation has not been determined nor has any definite effect of angiotensin converting enzyme inhibitor treatment been described.

Autonomic and neuroendocrine systems

Much has been written about the importance of neuroendocrine activation in chronic heart failure, partly because of the established benefits of blocking one aspect of this with the angiotensin converting enzyme inhibitors. There is an undoubted activation of neuroendocrine systems involved in the 'fight or flight' reaction. These probably evolved, in a teleological sense, as a way of compensating for blood or fluid loss or sodium depletion, but in heart failure, although initially helping to support the circulation, continuous activation may be harmful. These include the renin–angiotensin–aldosterone system, the sympathetic nervous system, and the vasopressin system, as well as the counteracting atrial natriuretic peptides. Simultaneously with neuroendocrine activation there is a reduction in vasodilator influences and in vagal tone which, when maintained chronically, may be harmful. Adverse consequences have been described such as organ hypoperfusion, myocardial toxicity, an increased susceptibility to ventricular arrhythmias, and a possible progression of the underlying disease process whether it be myocardial ischaemia or cardiomyopathy.

The renin–angiotensin–aldosterone system

In untreated heart failure there is a mild activation of the renin system. This is dramatically augmented by the first use of diuretics in the treatment of the heart failure. After that there is a reasonable relationship between the severity of the heart failure and further increases in circulating renin and angiotensin II levels. In addition, all the components of the circulating renin–angiotensin system also exist in tissue sites and there is probably activation of these local tissue systems in the heart, kidney, brain, and blood vessel walls. The role and effects of these in health and in the progression of heart failure are unknown, but some of the beneficial effects of angiotensin-converting enzyme inhibition described in other sections stress how important these systems may be in the syndrome of chronic heart failure.

At an organ level, the effects of elevated local and circulating angiotensin II can be very profound. In the kidney it can cause either a preservation of glomerular filtration rate (GFR) in the presence of low arterial pressure or a reduced renal blood flow and glomerular filtration rate if the kidney is already dependent on angiotensin II-mediated efferent arteriolar constriction to maintain an adequate filtration pressure in the Bowman's capsule. Such a dependence can be seen in renal artery stenosis. In the heart local increases in angiotensin II can cause coronary vasoconstriction and toxic effects on the myocytes, and in the periphery local angiotensin activation can elevate systemic vascular resistance and thereby increase the afterload to the failing heart.

The clinical effects of inhibition of the renin–angiotensin–aldosterone system are dealt with more fully in other sections, but it is important to note that we still do not know how they mediate their beneficial effects, whether by reduced circulating or tissue-based angiotensin II or by augmentation of bradykinin or other kinin systems.

The autonomic nervous system

Early in the progression of heart failure from mild asymptomatic left ventricular dysfunction to the full clinical picture of chronic heart failure there is an activation of the sympathetic nervous system and a concomitant reduction in resting vagal tone. These changes are further enhanced by the administration of diuretics. There is no clear mechanism for either the activation of the sympathetic system in mild heart failure, or why the activation should persist and progress in the chronic syndrome. In severe heart failure there may be a reduction in blood pressure but this is often the result of aggressive therapy. In asymptomatic left ventricular dysfunction or mild heart failure, in contrast, no perceptible change in blood pressure occurs at a stage when sympathetic activation commences. It has been said that the activation is secondary to the withdrawal of the chronic sympathoinhibitory effects of the arterial baroreflexes but there are flaws in this explanation. Even complete denervation of the baroreceptors does not lead to such persistent sympatho-excitation as seen in chronic heart failure, and in heart failure it also begs the question as to what caused the baroreceptor inhibition in the first place. If it is thought to be sympathetic activation, as seems likely, then we are left with a circular argument. No significant sympatho-excitatory influence, active in heart failure, has been demonstrated to underlie the very high levels of sympathetic tone in the established syndrome. Two candidate mechanisms which have received little attention are the skeletal muscle ergoreceptor system and an interaction between the arterial chemoreflex and the baroreflex and cardiovascular autonomic centres. Both the ergoreflex and the chemoreflex cause sympathetic activation and may be abnormal throughout the progression of chronic heart failure.

The investigation of sympathovagal balance is limited by the lack of precise and quantifiable methods. Apart from a measurement of plasma noradrenaline levels there is no easily available clinical test for the activity of the sympathetic limb and for the vagal limb the problem is even more difficult. Recently analysis of variations of heart rate variability has identified characteristic frequency harmonic oscillations in cardiovascular parameters, the relative oscillatory power of which show promise in the estimation of sympathovagal balance. The pattern in heart failure is very abnormal with a dramatic reduction in total heart rate variability and a selective loss of the higher frequency (predominantly vagally mediated) rhythm characteristic of respiratory sinus arrhythmia, and a relative preservation of low and very low frequency rhythms which have their genesis more in the action of the sympathetic (low frequency) and renin–angiotensin or chemoreflex systems (very low frequency). Analysis of total heart rate variability and, in particular individual frequency components, has shown that the pattern seen in heart failure is one associated with high risk for the development of unstable ventricular arrhythmias and cardiac sudden death, although why this should be the case is not certain.

β-Receptor function

With chronic sympathetic activation there is a depletion in myocardial catecholamine stores and a down-regulation of β-1 receptors on the myocardium. There is also a decoupling of receptors from the post-receptor response, all of which lead to a loss of myocardial response to increased sympathetic drive. Clinically this manifests as chronotropic incompetence, loss of response to sympathomimetic stimulation and a further impaired exercise tolerance. Specific treatments are few but there has been some improvement after β-blockade, angiotensin-converting-enzyme inhibition, and even very short duration intermittent sympathomimetic stimulation.

The natriuretic peptide systems

The atria and ventricles contain granulated cells which release peptides, atrial natriuretic peptide (ANP or ANF), brain natriuretic peptide (BNP), and C-type natriuretic peptide (CNP) in response to stretch. These peptides are natriuretic agents which also relax peripheral vasculature and thereby mildly oppose the actions of the sympathetic and renin–angiotensin systems. There is an increased release of these peptides in chronic heart failure associated with cardiac enlargement, but the significance of the increased plasma levels is uncertain. Certainly the use of exogenous atrial natriuretic peptide or increasing endogenous levels by inhibiting their breakdown by neutral endopeptidase inhibitors have produced only minor natriuretic and haemodynamic effects in heart failure. It appears that the natriuretic effects are blunted in heart failure. At the present time there is some interest in the measurement of brain natriuretic peptide as a marker for early ventricular enlargement in asymptomatic left ventricular dysfunction and mild heart failure.

The vasopressin system

Vasopressin, also known as antidiuretic hormone (ADH), is a hormone released from the posterior pituitary gland. It is found in elevated plasma concentrations in chronic heart failure, but its importance in the pathophysiology of chronic heart failure is not certain. Its actions are a combination of haemodynamic, with a profound arteriolar vasoconstriction increasing peripheral resistance and renal, with an action on the collecting duct to increase reduce free water reabsorption and thereby antidiuresis.

Other hormonal systems

Abnormalities have been described in several other hormonal systems in chronic heart failure, but the significance of these changes is uncertain. Thyroid hormone handling in the cells is deranged with an increase in reverse T3 similar to that seen in the so-called 'sick cell syndrome'. Plasma insulin levels are increased in heart failure, whether of ischaemic, valvular or idiopathic aetiology, and this is associated with a decreased sensitivity to the glucose transport effects of insulin. In advanced cardiac cachexia alterations in sex hormones and growth factors are likely but to what extent these are specific to the syndrome of chronic heart failure is uncertain.

The kidney

Disturbed function of the kidney is of major importance in heart failure. Control of fluid and electrolyte balance is impaired in heart failure. This is due to the reduced renal perfusion pressure in advanced heart failure, to the effects on intrarenal haemodynamics of the neuroendocrine activation described above, and to the effects and side-effects of commonly prescribed medication for heart failure.

Fluid overload and hence oedema is common in heart failure, and electrolyte disturbances are both common and important. In mild heart failure fluid retention is due to the effects of aldosterone, vasopressin, and catecholaminergic renal vasoconstriction. The kidney itself is a partly a passive organ responding to neuroendocrine activation outside its control, but it is also an active endocrine and autocrine organ responding to reduced renal perfusion pressure in heart failure.

The renin–angiotensin–aldosterone system

The juxtaglomerular apparatus adjacent to the distal convoluted tubule senses the reduction in the rate of delivery of sodium to the distal tubule and releases renin in response. This plays an important part in the activation of the circulating renin–angiotensin system described above. The homeostatic role of this system is to divert blood flow to the kidney and to increase the glomerular filtration rate and active reabsorption of sodium. An additional effect of angiotensin on thirst and possibly salt hunger completes the response ensuring an increased retention of salt and water.

All the components of the renin–angiotensin system also exist within the kidney and there can be a local autocrine activation which can have important effects on intrarenal haemodynamics. These may either increase or decrease glomerular filtration rate depending on the level of renal perfusion pressure and other factors operating on the kidney such as the renal sympathetic nerves and circulating vasoactive factors.

The kallikrein–kinin system

This second autocrine system of the kidney is less well studied because of the short-half life of some of its active components and the difficulty in isolating how and where they are operative. In simplest terms the kinin system appears complementary to the renin–angiotensin system causing vasodilatation where the latter causes vasoconstriction. It is also thought to be involved in the control of renal tubular function, but its precise role in heart failure and the effects of angiotensin converting enzyme inhibitors (which also block the enzyme which breaks down bradykinin) are unknown.

The cardiorenal syndrome

Some of the causes of heart failure, most notably atherosclerotic arterial disease and hypertension can have direct effects on the kidney which can cause a increased coexistence of cardiac and renal failure. Other less common conditions which can cause both organs to fail include amyloid, sarcoid, and certain vasculitides. A more common finding is that an apparently reasonably well-functioning kidney can fail progressively in the presence of severe heart failure. This is partly due to the effects of hypovolaemia and low blood pressure (prerenal azotaemia) but also to the circulating and intrarenal neurohormonal systems described above, and the renal effects of drugs used for the condition. The net effect is that renal failure is an extremely common and clinically important complication of severe heart failure. Aggressive diuretic therapy can precipitate a significant worsening of renal function which then blunts their effectiveness. The angiotensin-converting-enzyme inhibitors usually lead to a small increase in serum creatinine concentrations and in a few patients can precipitate clinically important renal failure.

Electrolyte disturbances

In untreated heart failure these are not common except in severe heart failure. There is initially a retention of sodium and a loss of potassium due to the effects of increased levels of aldosterone. Later, and especially after diuretics have been administered, there is a further depletion of potassium and also magnesium. Both of these disturbances may be important in generating cardiac arrhythmias, especially in digoxin toxicity. In severe heart failure a dilutional hyponatraemia can develop which can be both difficult to manage and a poor prognostic sign.

The careful management of fluid and electrolyte balance in heart failure can lessen renal complications and improve both symptoms and prognosis. There is no simple therapeutic regime which will ensure this, just careful clinical examination and measurement, judicious use of drugs and knowledge of their potential side-effects.

Haematological system

Haemoglobin

An increased arterial haemoglobin content has been described as an adaptive response in heart failure. This may be secondary to chronic tissue hypoxia, perhaps most importantly in the kidney in which it may stimulate an increase in erythropoietin production. It is doubtful if the increase in haemoglobin is very effective in increasing oxygen delivery to the tissues for if the haematocrit increases too much increased whole blood viscosity will reduce net tissue perfusion by increasing the resistance to blood flow.

Other haematological changes

Impaired clotting factor production can result from hepatic dysfunction (see below) and abnormalities in haemostatic function as a result are not uncommon. White blood cell counts may be mildly elevated in heart failure as part of a more generalized but poorly understood immune activation in this syndrome.

Other organ systems

The liver

In heart failure the liver can be affected by increased venous back-pressure, by an impaired arterial supply, and by the metabolic compli- cations of the syndrome. It can also be affected by the underlying process which lead to heart failure, for example alcohol excess or haemachromatosis.

The most common hepatic abnormality in chronic heart failure is congestion due to the effects of right heart failure on venous pressures. This leads to increased venous engorgement of the liver and can result in a noticeable increase in hepatic size, local tenderness and minor derangements in liver function. In its mildest form this causes modest increases in transaminase levels. In more severe cases nausea and right hypochondrial discomfort develop, and in severe cases jaundice, impaired albumin and clotting factor production, and malabsorption of fats may result. These changes can have clinically important effects on clotting, especially as warfarin is commonly prescribed, and also of hepatic metabolism of certain drugs. The nausea and malabsorption can worsen the catabolic state of the patient and can contribute to the wasting seen in cardiac cachexia. There is no specific treatment for this complication of chronic heart failure other than the correct dosage of diuretics and maximizing cardiac function with vasodilators.

Gastrointestinal tract

This is mainly affected by the increased venous pressure of right heart failure. Intestinal mucosal oedema can contribute to malabsorption and possibly nausea. Cardiac conditions are also associated with a higher rate of intestinal angiodysplasia and this can lead to recurrent blood loss which can be a considerable management problem for a patient who requires anticoagulation.

Central nervous system

Certain conditions which cause heart failure can also produce neurological effects, these include alcoholism, amyloid, and heavy metal poisoning. Apart from the abnormalities of autonomic and neuroendocrine function described earlier, specific neural complications of heart failure are not common.

Immune function

Release of cytokines involved in the inflammatory and immune responses have been described in advanced heart failure. These include increased levels of tumour necrosis factor. The cause and significance of these changes in heart failure remain speculative.

Cause of non-cardiac pathophysiology in heart failure

The changes described in different organ systems as part of the syndrome of chronic heart failure remain largely unexplained. We have proposed a 'muscle hypothesis' in which we explain the generation of many of these abnormalities via the combined effect of physical deconditioning effects and metabolic dysfunction combining a release of catabolic factors with a loss of normal anabolic function. Figure 1 describes the general pathway by which we believe these changes could lead to skeletal and respiratory muscle abnormalities and via these to fatigue, dyspnoea, exercise limitation and sympatho-excitation.

Clinical assessment

The assessment of a patient with heart failure requires a careful history and examination both at initial presentation and when assessing progress and response to treatment. Confirmation of heart failure can be aided by chest radiograph, echocardiography, and, in selected cases, cardiac catheterization, radionuclide ventriculography and other imaging modalities. Invasive haemodynamic monitoring has a role in the assessment of acute severe heart failure.

Cardiopulmonary exercise testing with respiratory gas analysis can help establish the cause of symptoms in patients with coexisting heart and lung disease and can establish whether the heart failure is causing the symptoms limiting the patient. When the respiratory exchange ratio (carbon dioxide produced per unit oxygen consumed) exceeds 1.0 muscle metabolism has become anaerobic indicating that a point of limiting cardiac reserve has been approached. If it does not exceed 1.0 at peak exercise then the true cardiac limitation cannot be assessed. Significant hypoxaemia and/or hypercapnia on exercise is rare in non-oedematous chronic heart failure, and when present suggests the limiting pulmonary or a right to left shunt.

Regular assessment of the severity of heart failure is usually by taking a history of symptomatic limitation and clinical examination. The occasional use of chest radiography, echocardiography, and cardiopulmonary exercise testing can also help. Repeated haemodynamic monitoring has little role in the management of chronic heart failure. Whether monitoring levels of plasma noradrenaline or atrial natriuretic peptides would materially assist in clinical management is uncertain. Certainly regular assessment of clinical biochemistry is essential.

Treatment

The major elements of treatment of heart failure are shown in Table 2. Specific therapies are described in detail in the chapters on diuretics, digitalis, vasodilators, and cardiac transplantation. Other treatments, which play a more limited role in chronic heart failure, include anticoagulants and non-digitalis antiarrhythmics. The former are definitely indicated in heart failure with atrial fibrillation but whether they have a role in heart failure with sinus rhythm is disputed. The latter have not been shown to improve prognosis, in fact many may worsen prognosis by their proarrhythmic effects. They should be reserved for troubling arrhythmias which are symptomatically limiting the patient in their own right. Treatment options for the management of severe or endstage heart failure are shown in Table 3.

There are many other aspects of the management of this syndrome which do not involve the use of the drugs and these are briefly discussed below.

Non-pharmacological treatments

Patient education

Patients and their families are often confused and bewildered by the term heart failure. Alternatives such as 'weak heart', 'congestion', or 'large heart' may be better at giving the correct impression as to the nature of the condition. It can be extremely useful for long-term adher-

ence to treatment recommendations to spend some time explaining to the patient and spouse some simple physiology of left ventricular dysfunction, the body's compensatory mechanisms and, why these lead to symptoms and signs which the patient may have already noted. The patient will then be much more aware of the need for diuretics and vasodilators, and the effects of alterations in fluid and salt intake, or intercurrent illness, for instance. This could improve control of oedema and lessen the frequency with which a patient needs to attend outpatient clinics or be admitted for stabilization. Simple measures such as information on low salt diets, fluid restrictions, and the monitoring of daily weight at home can significantly improve long-term management of heart failure.

Rest and exercise

There is very good evidence in acute heart failure, or in an acute decompensation in chronic heart failure, that bed rest can improve renal blood flow and the response to diuretics. This is presumably via a reduction in the level of stimulation of the sympathetic and renin–angiotensin systems. Thus admission to hospital for a few days rest is a common treatment for heart failure, and one with a very long history. Initial enthusiasm for the benefits of longer periods of bed rest (weeks to months) as a management strategy for chronic heart failure and cardiomyopathy have not been borne out; in fact this practice is accompanied by the considerable and well-known complications of prolonged bed rest. On the contrary benefits have been shown from exercise training in carefully selected patients with chronic heart failure. Improvements are seen in exercise tolerance, skeletal muscle, and respiratory function and in autonomic balance. This raises the possibility that profound physical deconditioning may be contributing to some of the pathophysiological changes described in the sections above. In a patient with stable chronic heart failure, with no evidence of exercise-induced ventricular arrhythmias regular exercise should be encouraged rather than prohibited.

Prognosis

In severe heart failure where patients are symptomatic at rest (NYHA class IV) the prognosis is very poor, with a survival rate of 1 year or less. The prognosis remains considerably reduced even in mild heart failure (class II to III), with a mortality rate of 20 to 30 per cent per

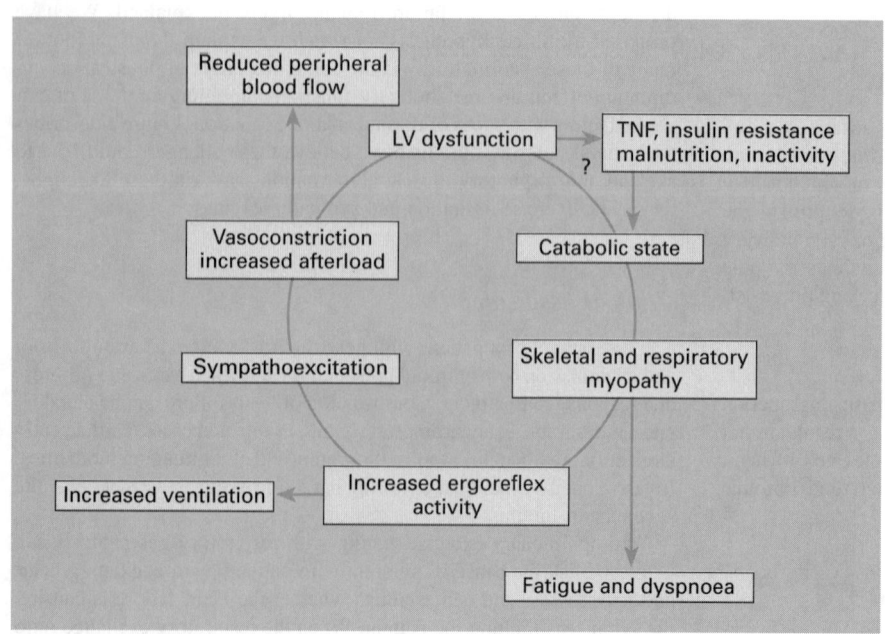

Fig. 1 The muscle hypothesis in chronic heart failure. A proposal to explain the genesis and effects of several components of the non-cardiac pathophysiology of heart failure. TNF, tumour necrosis factor (proposed by Coats 1994).

Table 2 *Treatment of chronic heart failure*

General	
No added salt	Treat hypertention
Maintain optimal weight	Detect alcohol abuse
Stop smoking	Prevent coronary disease
Encourage exercise	
Mild	
Thiazide/loop diuretic	?? potassium therapy
ACE inhibitor	
Digoxin if atrial fibrillation	
Moderate	
Loop diuretic	?? potassium therapy
ACE inhibitor	
Combine diuretics	
Severe	
Increase loop diuretic	Transplant
Combine diuretics	? cardiomyoplasty
Metolazone	? inotropic drug
ACE inhibitor	? digoxin
Nitrates	? spironolactone

Table 3 *Options in the treatment of severe chronic heart failure*

Drugs
  Diuretics (loop, thiazide, and potassium sparing
    combination)
  ACE inhibitors
  Vasodilators (nitrates, hydralazine)
  Postive inotropes (digoxin, IV intermittent inotrope)
  Anticoagulants
  β-Blockers, calcium antagonists or anti-arrhythmics

Implantable cardiac defibrillator (ICD)

Haemofiltration

Peritoneal dialysis of haemodialysis

Aortic balloon pump or ventricular assist device

Transplantation or cardiomyoplasty

Table 4 *Adverse prognostic markers in heart failure*

Left ventricular dysfunction
  Low ejection fraction
  Increased cardiothoracic ratio
  Increased left ventricular end-diastolic diameter
  Reduced peak cardiac power output

The degree of functional limitation
  Reduced exercise time
  Reduced peak oxygen consumption
  Advanced New York Functional Class

Electrolyte disturbances
  Hyponatraemia
  Hypomagnesaemia

Neurohormonal or autonomic dysfunction
  Increased plasma noradrenaline
  Increased cardiac natriuretic peptide levels
  Reduced heart rate variability
  Impaired baroreflex sensitivity

Markers of ventricular arrhythmogenesis
  Non-sustained ventricular tachycardia on Holter monitoring
  Late potentials

year. Although major treatment advances have been achieved in mild, moderate, and even severe heart failure, these have lead to only a very partial correction of the excess mortality associated with this condition.

Prognostic factors and markers

Many separate parameters have been described as having prognostic value in patients with heart failure. It is important to differentiate between those that have a direct functional link to increased mortality, and those that merely reflect a worse prognosis, without themselves being involved in the mechanism. It can be dangerous to base treatments on the supposition that improving an adverse prognostic feature will improve outlook. The treatment can improve the marker but have either a neutral or even a detrimental effect on survival.

The presence of non-sustained ventricular tachycardia on Holter monitoring is a sign of an increased probability of mortality from sudden death. Class I antiarrhythmic agents can reduce the frequency of ventricular tachycardia, and as a result they have been suggested for this purpose in heart failure. The Cardiac Arrhythmia Suppression Trial (CAST), a randomized controlled trial of three such agents in left ventricular dysfunction, showed that, despite reducing the frequency of ventricular arrhythmias, there was an increased rate of sudden death, presumably due to some proarrhythmic effects. Similarly a low ejection fraction is an adverse prognostic sign in heart failure, and it was expected that agents which improve ejection fraction should increase survival. Positively inotropic oral agents, such as milrinone (a phosphodiesterase inhibitor), in controlled studies increase ejection fraction but with a reduced survival. Thus we should never use the justification for treatment of improving a risk marker unless we have proof that in so doing we improve survival. The only justifications for treatment are to slow the progression of the underlying disease, to relieve symptoms which trouble the patient, or to use agents proven to improve survival.

Specific prognostic indicators

These can be grouped into several relatively independent features (Table 4). The most important factors are: (1) the extent of the left ventricular dysfunction; (2) the degree of functional limitation; (3) the electrolyte disturbance; (4) the degree of neurohormonal or autonomic dysfunction; and (5) certain electrophysiological or electrocardiographic indicators of ventricular arrhythmogenesis. There are also general factors such as age or the presence of second diseases. It has not been established whether estimation of these predictive variables materially improves patient management.

REFERENCES

Bristow, M.R., Ginsburg, R., Minobe, W., *et al.* (1982). Decreased catecholamine sensitivity and b-adrenergic receptor density in failing human hearts. *New England Journal of Medicine,* **307**, 205–11.

Clark, A., and Coats, A. (1992). The mechanisms underlying the increased ventilatory response to exercise in chronic stable heart failure. *European Heart Journal,* **13**, 1698–1708.

Coats, A.J.S., Adamopoulos, S., Radaelli, A, *et al.* (1992). Controlled trial of physical training in chronic heart failure: exercise performance, hemodynamics, ventilation and autonomic function. *Circulation* **85**, 2119–2131.

Coats, A.J.S., Clark, A.L., Piepoli, M., Volterrani, M. and Poole-Wilson, P.A. (1994). Symptoms and quality of life in heart failure; the muscle hypothesis. *British Heart Journal,* 72 (suppl), S36–S39.

Drexler, H., Banhardt, U., Meinertz, T., Wollschläger, H., Lehmann, M., and Just, H. (1989). Contrasting peripheral short-term and long-term effects of converting enzyme inhibition in patients with congestive heart failure. A double-blind, placebo-controlled trial. *Circulation,* **79**, 491–502.

Firth, B.G. and Dunnmon, P.M. (1990). Left ventricular dilatation and failure post-myocardial infarction: pathophysiology and possible pharmacological interventions. *Cardiovascular Drug Therapy,* **4**, 1363–74.

Francis, G.S. (1985). Neurohumeral mechanisms involved in congestive heart failure. *American Journal of Cardiology*, **55**, 15A–21A.

Kannel, W.B. and Belanger, A.J. (1991). Epidemiology of heart failure. *American Heart Journal*, **121**, 951–7.

Lipkin, D.P., Perrins, J., and Poole-Wilson, P.A. (1985). Respiratory gas exchange in the assessment of patients with impaired ventricular function. *British Heart Journal*, **54**, 321–8.

Massie, B., Conway, M., Yonge, R., *et al.* (1987). Skeletal muscle metabolism in patients with congestive heart failure: relation to clinical severity and blood flow. *Circulation*, **76**, 1009–19.

Moore, D.P., Weston, A.R., Hughes, J.M.B., Oakley, C.M., and Cleland, J.G.F. (1992). Effects of increased inspired oxygen concentrations on exercise performance in chronic heart failure. *Lancet*, **339**, 850–3.

O'Rourke, M. (1990). Arterial stiffness, systolic blood pressure, and logical treatment of arterial hypertension. *Hypertension*, **15**, 339–47.

Poole-Wilson, P.A. (1989). Chronic heart failure: causes, pathophysiology, prognosis, clinical manifestations, investigations. In *Diseases of the Heart*. (ed P.A. Poole-Wilson), pp. 48–57. Balliere Tindall, London.

Rahimtoola, S.H. (1989). The pharmacological treatment of chronic congestive heart failure. *Circulation*, **80**, 693–9.

Smith, T.W., Braunwald, E., and Kelly, R.A. (1988). The management of heart failure. In *Heart Disease*. (ed E. Braunwald), pp. 485–543. W.B. Saunders Co., Philadelphia.

Sullivan, M.J., Green, H.J., and Cobb, F.R. (1990). Skeletal muscle biochemistry and histology in ambulatory patients with long-term heart failure. *Circulation*, **81**, 518–27.

Sullivan, M.J., Higginbotham, M.B., and Cobb, F.R. (1988) Increased exercise ventilation in patients with chronic heart failure: intact ventilatory control despite hemodynamic and pulmonary abnormalities. *Circulation*, **77**, 552–559.

Wasserman, K. and Casaburi, R. (1988). Dyspnea: physiological and pathological mechanisms. *Annual Reviews of Medicine*, **39**, 503–15.

15.6 The treatment of heart failure

15.6.1 Diuretics

J. G. G. LEDINGHAM AND A. E. G. RAINE

Why treat cardiac oedema?

The need to treat pulmonary oedema urgently needs no discussion, but there is a place for circumspection in deciding how hard to press treatment in patients retaining fluid other than in the lungs. Massive oedema is unsightly and can be physically inconvenient and sometimes incapacitating. But on occasions physicians substitute a low cardiac output, a feeling of physical exhaustion, and an electrolyte disturbance with renal failure for a relatively mild degree of oedema by overenthusiastic treatment with potent diuretic drugs. There are, too, cardiac conditions in which removal of fluid from the circulation is quite inappropriate, despite clear evidence of an elevation in central venous pressure. These include constrictive pericarditis, pericardial tamponade, right ventricular infarction, pulmonary embolism or mitral valve disease when cardiac output is severely compromised.

Conservative measures

The value of bed rest and moderate sodium restriction in the treatment of all forms of fluid retention has been known for years, but these simple approaches have been neglected more than they should have been since the advent of potent diuretics, effective given by mouth. An early consequence of cardiac failure is of renal vasoconstriction, aggravated by exercise and the erect posture. Supine bed rest enhances venous return, increases cardiac output and the secretion of atrial natriuretic peptide and increases the proportion of the output reaching the kidneys, thus facilitating natriuresis and diuresis and enhancing the efficacy of diuretic therapy. Strict sodium restriction to an intake of 20 to 30 mmol/day is an unpleasant treatment, found impractical or unacceptable by most patients, but more modest restriction may reduce the need for drugs and thus reduce risks of toxicity. It is surprising how often house staff report a patient's oedema to be uncontrolled by diuretics when the 24-h urinary sodium excretion exceeds 100 mmol, implying an intake well in excess of that quite generous figure.

Fluid restriction (intake confined to 500 to 1000 ml per 24 h) was once commonly prescribed for heart failure and there are still good reasons for this approach in advanced failure, as a number of factors combine to reduce the ability of the kidneys to excrete free water.

Diuretics

By increasing urinary excretion of salt and with it water, diuretics reduce cardiac preload and thereby the symptoms and signs of congestion. Most diuretic agents, with the exception of spironolactone, influence renal tubular reabsorptive mechanisms in relation to their concentration in the tubular fluid which they reach largely by the organic ion transport mechanisms in the proximal convoluted tubule. Because of strong protein binding, loop agents and thiazides do not enter tubular fluid by glomerular filtration in significant amounts. The efficacy of a diuretic in individual cases depends therefore not only on the inherent potency and site of action of the drug, but also critically on renal perfusion and tubular function as well as the antinatriuretic neurohumoral factors associated with heart failure, these latter commonly enhanced by previous drug therapy (see Chapter 15.3.3). In the presence of heavy proteinuria, protein binding of diuretics in tubular fluid may also limit their efficacy.

When fluid retention is mild but requires relief, one of the benzothiadiazine agents should be the first choice. There has been a tendency since the more potent 'loop' agents became available to prescribe these potentially dangerous drugs unnecessarily. The hazards of extreme hypovolaemia, of aggravating any tendency to urinary retention, and of serious electrolyte disturbance are less with thiazides, agents which inhibit sodium transport in an area just proximal to the distal convoluted tubule. Inhibition at this site, where sodium is reabsorbed without water, impairs maximal urinary dilution, but the excretion of free water is not completely inhibited since the diluting site in the ascending limb of the loop of Henle is not affected. In maximal effective doses, the thiazide diuretics are capable of inhibiting reabsorption of some 5 per cent of the filtered load of sodium, quite enough for many patients with cardiac oedema. The dose–response curve of thiazides is flat, with little difference between small and large doses. Most thiazides affect urinary salt excretion for some 8 to 10 h but some, like chlorthalidone, last for as long as 24 to 36 h.

The response to thiazides and other diuretics is characterized by an initial increase in sodium and water excretion, resulting in net negative sodium balance, provided dietary sodium intake remains constant. Within several days, activation of neurohumoral and intrarenal compensatory mechanisms results in re-establishment of equal sodium intake and excretion but with the desired diminution in body water, extracellular volume, and right atrial pressure.

Potassium supplements

Because the site of action lies proximal to the area in the distal nephron where potassium is secreted, all thiazide drugs tend to increase urinary potassium losses to a degree dependent on tubular flow rate, the delivery of sodium to the distal nephron, and the extent of secondary aldosteronism present. Chloruresis and potassium loss both tend to produce alkalosis of the extracellular fluid, which, when present, further inhibits renal potassium conservation (see Chapter 20.2.3). The rate at which potassium may be lost during treatment by thiazide diuretics is, therefore, variable and the need to provide supplements or not, is equally variable. Arguments as to whether they are required in general are somewhat futile as so much depends on the response of the individual patient and the features of the underlying disease. There is no doubt that severe potassium depletion can be provoked by thiazide treatment, especially perhaps by chlorthalidone, and that such depletion can potentiate cardiotoxic effects of digitalis analogues. When in doubt the wisest course is to prescribe supplements, or to combine treatment with one of the distally acting agents which promote potassium retention. Enteric coated potassium preparations can cause jejunal ulceration and stricture formation. Potassium given as bicarbonate aggravates alkalosis, inhibits renal potassium conservation, and is much less effective than the chloride preparations in correcting deficits. Slow-K (Ciba) or Kay-Cee-L (Geistlich) or equivalents are probably the preparations of choice, but much can be achieved by advising a high intake of foods naturally rich in potassium content.

Preparations providing thiazide diuretics and potassium in the same tablet are widely available and advertised. They are often prescribed, but the amounts of potassium incorporated may not suffice to prevent hypokalaemia; separate preparations of the diuretic and of potassium supplements are preferable as they allow precision and flexibility of dosage.

Potassium-sparing diuretics

Spironolactone, amiloride, and triamterene all act on the distal nephron at the site of potassium secretion, promoting modest increases in sodium excretion but a very significant inhibition of potassium secretion. Spironolactone is a true antagonist of aldosterone, competing for its cytosolic receptor and has no effect after bilateral adrenalectomy. Effective doses range from 25 to 400 mg daily and depend on the degree of aldosteronism present. Treatment with spironolactone stimulates increased formation of renin, angiotensin, and aldosterone so that dose requirements may increase. Gastrointestinal side-effects of nausea and abdominal discomfort complicate higher dosage and prolonged use of the drug is remarkably commonly complicated by the development of gynaecomastia which may be unilateral or bilateral. The onset of action of spironolactone is delayed for a full 24 to 72 h.

Triamterene and amiloride also act on the distal nephron to inhibit sodium reabsorption and potassium secretion. They are not antagonists of aldosterone, but block luminal sodium channels directly. Triamterene is rather less potent and less well tolerated by patients than is amiloride, which is perhaps the best of the three distally acting agents for general use. Just as effective in conserving potassium and excreting sodium as spironolactone, it is free of the unpleasant side-effects of gynaecomastia. Effective doses range between 5 and 20 mg daily.

The addition of spironolactone, triamterene, or amiloride to thiazides or 'loop' agents augments sodium excretion and reduces potassium loss, but to a variable degree between patients depending on haemodynamic factors and the activity of the renin-aldosterone system. It is *not* safe to assume potassium homeostasis without regular checks of plasma levels, particularly in the first 1 to 2 weeks after their introduction.

Given alone, triamterene, spironolactone, or amiloride are of little value, except perhaps in the oedema of liver cirrhosis in which natriuresis needs to be more than usually slowly induced, and hyperaldosteronism probably plays a much larger part in aetiology than it does in cardiac or nephrotic oedema.

More resistant oedema

When patients have been shown to be unresponsive to thiazide diuretics combined with amiloride, spironolactone or triamterene, one of the 'loop' agents should be introduced. Frusemide (furosemide), ethacrynic acid, bumetanide, and piretanide all act principally by inhibiting sodium chloride cotransport in the ascending limb of the loop of Henle. This is the site in the nephron at which the capacity for sodium reabsorption is difficult to saturate and which is critical to the mechanisms of urinary concentration and dilution. Dilution is achieved here and more distally by the reabsorption of sodium without water. Hypertonicity of the medulla, on which urinary concentration depends, is greatly reduced by inhibition of electrolyte transport at this site. Although they differ structurally, and there is some evidence of additional sites of action in the proximal nephron and perhaps in the second diluting site for frusemide, there is little to choose between these agents clinically. All are extremely potent, capable of blocking reabsorption of 25 to 40 per cent of the sodium filtered at the glomerulus in experimental conditions. All are chloruretic agents and promote a considerably greater excretion of chloride than of sodium. Because they act at a point proximal to the site of potassium secretion, which is itself dependent on tubular flow rates and the rate of delivery of sodium, all tend to increase urinary potassium losses in an amount dependent on the extent of secondary hyperaldosteronism present and the degree of alkalosis induced by chloride deficiency or any pre-existing potassium depletion.

These 'loop' diuretic agents are potentially dangerous drugs particularly in the elderly. Their remarkable potency results in a very real risk of extreme hypovolaemia, postural hypotension, circulatory failure, and uraemia when they are given without proper supervision, particularly to patients whose disease could well be controlled by less drastic agents. Weight loss from diuretic therapy should be achieved ideally at a rate not exceeding 1 to 2 kg/day. Unlike the thiazides, which rarely reduce plasma potassium levels below 3 mmol/l, the 'loop' agents can reduce concentrations to dangerously low levels and a remarkable degree of hypochloraemic hypolalaemic alkalosis can arise over a period of treatment as short as 48 h.

These caveats apart, the value of 'loop' diuretics properly prescribed and supervised has constituted a major advance in the care of patients whose oedema cannot be controlled by less powerful drugs. Given by mouth, all begin to induce natriuresis and diuresis within 1 to 2 h and have a peak effect at about 4 h, which is complete at about 6 h. The dose response range for oral frusemide extends from 20 to 400 mg per day or more, of ethacrynic acid from 50 to 200 mg, for bumetanide from 1 to 8 mg, and piretanide from 6 to 24 mg. The relatively short period of action can be used to tailor treatment for individual patients. When the diuretic response is good, patients can take a single dose at a time of day which suits their domestic and work commitments, although in a few who continue to take an unrecognized high salt diet, the relatively short duration of action of frusemide (6 h), followed by 18 h of antinatriuresis may result in no net change in salt and water balance. This phenomenon, best treated by a reduction in sodium intake or by twice daily doses of frusemide, should be distinguished from true 'resistance'. However, the threshold dose required to produce a natriuresis in any given case may be increased for a number of reasons, including slow gastrointestinal absorption, reduced renal perfusion, impaired secretory function of the proximal tubule, as well as the sodium-retaining consequences of increased activity of the renin–angiotensin system and other neurohumoral mechanisms. In this situation, larger individual doses are required as a first step, with increased frequency of administration as the second.

As in the case of thiazides, the natriuretic effect of loop agents can be considerably augmented by the addition of spironolactone, amiloride or triamterene. Potassium losses are reduced, but severe hypokalaemia can still complicate combined therapy of this sort. Potassium concentrations must be checked regularly and supplements given according to need. Again, chloride preparations are mandatory since alkalosis is almost invariable when hypokalaemia complicates treatment by potent loop diuretics.

Resistant oedema

A small minority of patients exists in whom sodium restriction, bed rest, and combinations of loop agents, thiazides, and potassium-conserving distal acting drugs fail to control fluid retention. This problem arises particularly when cardiac failure or oedema co-exists with impaired renal function. In this setting thiazides are of limited use as sole agents, their efficacy being greatly reduced as glomerular filtration rate declines to 30 ml/min or lower, and distally acting potassium sparing diuretics should be avoided because of the risk of serious hyperkalaemia. In such cases, metolazone in place of standard thiazides has been shown to be remarkably effective when combined with a loop agent, even in the presence of renal failure. Indeed its addition may produce an excessive natriuresis and it is often wise to begin with a small dose, e.g. 2.5 to 5 mg on alternate days, increasing if necessary to a maximum dose of 20 mg per day.

The use of drugs which reduce cardiac afterload, of which the angiotensin converting enzyme (ACE) inhibitors are most effective, may increase cardiac output, renal perfusion, and thus initiate diuresis which once begun tends to continue. Some patients are resistant even to these measures, and in extreme cases angiotensin converting enzyme inhibition may result in an acute fall in glomerular filtration rate, oliguria, and uraemia secondary to inhibition of angiotensin-mediated efferent arteriolar tone. Withdrawal of the angiotensin converting enzyme inhibitor in such cases usually restores renal function, although in occasional cases when severe intrarenal microvascular disease is present, renal impairment caused by angiotensin converting enzyme inhibition may be irreversible.

When fluid retention persists despite therapy, there is a need to decide whether to increase the dose of angiotensin converting enzyme inhibitor or of a diuretic first. Cold extremities and a rise in blood urea concentration above 20 mmol/l (blood urea nitrogen (BUN) over 60 mg/100 ml) indicates predominance of poor cardiac output, probably best treated by the introduction of or an increase in angiotensin converting enzyme inhibition or other methods of decreasing afterload, together with a reduction in diuretic dose. When blood urea concentrations are below some 12 to 18 mmol/l (BUN 36 to 54 mg/100 ml) and the extremities are warm, it may be more effective to increase the dose of diuretic first.

The diuretic resistance which may occur in heart failure is in part explained by the activation of neurohumoral systems, most of which – the renin–angiotensin system, arginine vasopressin, the sympathetic nervous system – act to increase renal sodium reabsorption. It appears that these effects override those of cardiac secretion of atrial natriuretic peptide, which is also greatly enhanced in heart failure. Although trials of infusion of atrial natriuretic peptide itself in heart failure have been relatively disappointing, initial results with inhibitors of neutral endopeptidase (E-24.11) which increase atrial natriuretic peptide concentrations by inhibiting its degradation, are encouraging. The natriuresis achieved with this approach is most pronounced in states of hypervolaemia, when endogenous atrial natriuretic peptide concentration is elevated, and it has the theoretical advantage of not causing hypokalaemia or renin–angiotensin system activation, in contrast to conventional diuretics.

In some cases of advanced heart failure there may be delayed, or inadequate absorption of loop agents due in part to intestinal oedema

and therefore a failure to achieve the concentrations in plasma necessary to provide critical amounts of diuretic in the tubular fluid for natriuresis to occur. Higher blood levels can then be achieved by the use of bolus doses of diuretics given intramuscularly or intravenously. More effective and more comfortable for the patient is a slow infusion of the drug given intravenously by a low volume pump delivering the total 24-h dose in 100 ml or less of 5 per cent dextrose. Remarkably low total doses may be effective given this way; for instance 40 to 80 mg of frusemide may induce diuresis when 500 mg given by mouth is ineffective. Patients resistant even to this manoeuvre are rare indeed, and it is doubtful whether the underlying cardiac disorder is then worthy of more drastic measures of support, but there are advocates for the use of 'low dose' dopamine, peritoneal dialysis, or haemofiltration. Good indications for such approaches must be vanishingly rare.

Complications

Prolonged treatment with loop agents or thiazides induce hyperuricaemia and may cause gout. Hyperglycaemia and overt diabetic ketoacidosis can be provoked by thiazides particularly, and the risk appears greatest in the elderly. The modest hyperlipidaemia associated with thiazides may not be sustained during prolonged treatment, and is of doubtful significance. Hypercalcaemia is increasingly recognized as a consequence of thiazide treatment, which should be considered as a possibility before full investigation is begun to seek other causes. Thiazides are also associated with hypersensitivity reactions including photosensitive skin rashes, thrombocytopenia, and acute interstitial nephritis. Hypokalaemia and alkalosis are easily recognized and treated, but hyponatraemia represents more of a problem and, until recently, hypomagnesaemia has not been sufficiently recognized.

DIURETIC-INDUCED HYPONATRAEMIA

Advanced degrees of chronic heart failure are often accompanied by hyponatraemia of greater or lesser degree. This complication is never, or almost never, due to sodium depletion, but almost always due to a relative water overload.

Mechanism

A number of factors contribute. Increased tubular reabsorption of sodium occurs in the proximal tubule in response to raised oncotic pressure in the post glomerular circulation and to activation of neurohumoral factors in severe cardiac insufficiency. As a result, less sodium and chloride are delivered to the diluting sites where chloride and sodium are reabsorbed without water in the ascending limb of the loop of Henle and in the early distal nephron. The capacity of the kidney to excrete free water is thereby decreased. It is decreased further by the use of diuretics, which inhibit electrolyte transport at these diluting sites. These include all thiazides, frusemide, ethacrynic acid, bumetanide, xipamide, and piretanide; indeed all agents except acetazolamide and the relatively weak distal tubular agents. There is very good reason, therefore, why the kidney's ability to excrete a water load is gravely reduced in heart failure. In addition, patients with cardiac insufficiency are often thirsty. Whether thirst is induced by volume–receptor-mediated neurological mechanisms or by an increase in the plasma concentrations of angiotensin II induced by diuretics or poor renal perfusion is not known. Thirst in the presence of hyponatraemia due to water retention is clearly inappropriate to both volume and osmotic status. Finally, plasma levels of antidiuretic hormone are increased in severe heart failure and this may add to the reduced ability of the kidney to excrete free water.

Management

Mild hyponatraemia probably needs no treatment, although it may be taken as a sign of a guarded prognosis. More severe hyponatraemia accompanied by constitutional symptoms may require treatment. If diuretics cannot be reduced, the addition of an angiotensin converting enzyme inhibitor may, by improving cardiac performance and renal perfusion, restore normal levels of plasma sodium, but on occasion hyponatraemia follows angiotensin converting enzyme inhibition, probably because in that situation renal perfusion is reduced rather than increased, perhaps because of adverse changes in systemic arterial pressure. Water restriction (see above) is then only moderately effective and is rarely tolerated by patients. Demethylchlortetracycline, a drug which in doses of 600 to 1200 mg daily induces a degree of nephrogenic diabetes insipidus, has been tried in this situation but usually without great benefit.

Reports that diuretic-associated hyponatraemia may reflect a shift of sodium into cells by inhibition of membrane sodium–potassium adenosine triphosphatase by magnesium depletion draw attention to the importance of magnesium homeostasis in patients treated chronically with diuretics.

MAGNESIUM DEPLETION

Some 15 to 30 per cent of filtered magnesium is normally reabsorbed in the proximal renal tubules, 50 to 60 per cent in the ascending limb of Henle's loop, and a further 5 per cent or so in the distal nephron. Both 'loop' diuretics and thiazides (particularly the former) may on occasion provoke magnesium depletion, especially in subjects whose dietary intake is low, in soft water areas, among alcoholics, and in malabsorptive states. Symptoms and signs are rare but can include depression, muscle weakness, refractory hypokalaemia, hypertension, and ventricular or atrial dysrhythmias resistant to treatment. The classic features of magnesium depletion – paraesthesiae, cramp, and tetany associated with accompanying hypocalcaemia – are probably never the result of diuretic treatment alone.

In the context of cardiac disease, the risks of hypomagnesaemia include supraventricular and ventricular arrhythmias, including ventricular tachycardia and fibrillation. Magnesium therapy after acute myocardial infarction was originally introduced with these considerations in mind, but the evidence now suggests that any benefit that they bring in this situation may be related rather to limitation of infarct size.

Treatment with magnesium glycerophosphate is quite well accepted in doses of 3 to 6 g daily providing 12 to 24 mmol of magnesium per 24 h. Other possible preparations include magnesium hydroxide which gives approximately 20 mmol in 15 ml but at the risk of diarrhoea and less efficient absorption.

Distal tubular agents (amiloride, spironolactone, or triamterene) do not increase urinary magnesium.

Acute pulmonary oedema (see Chapter 15.6.3)

Apart from morphine, the most effective agent in the immediate relief of dyspnoea in pulmonary oedema are intravenous injections of 'loop' diuretics. There is probably little to choose between them, but there is most experience with frusemide. Given in a dose of 20 to 40 mg there is an increase in urinary salt and water excretion within 2 min, which reaches a peak at 5 to 10 min and is complete within 25 or 35 min unless there is renal retention of the drug secondary to gross impairment of renal function. There is some evidence that the beneficial effects can be contributed to not only by natriuresis and diuresis but also by falls in left atrial pressure which precede the renal effects and may be attributable to dilatation of venous capacitance vessels. If ethacrynic acid is the loop agent chosen and is given intravenously (50 to 100 mg), particular care must be taken to avoid extravasation of the drug into the tissues where it is highly irritant and painful.

REFERENCES

Dzau, V.J. and Hollenberg, N.K. (1984). Renal response to captopril in severe heart failure: role of furosomide in natriuresis and reversal of hyponatraemia. *Annals of Internal Medicine,* **100**, 777–82.

Ellison, D.H. (1991). The physiologic basis of diuretic synergism: its role in treating diuretic resistance. *Annals of Internal Medicine,* **114**, 886–94.

Fliser, D., Schröter, M., Neubeck, M., and Ritz, E. (1994). Co-administration of thiazides increases the efficacy of loop diuretics, even in patients with advanced renal failure. *Kidney International,* **46**, 482–8.

Kau, S.T. (1992). Basic pharmacology and pharmacological classification of diuretics. *Progress in Pharmacology and Clinical Pharmacology,* **9**, 33–113.

Mujais, S.K., Nora, N.A., and Levin, M.L. (1992). Principles and clinical uses of diuretic therapy. *Progress in Cardiovascular Diseases,* **35**, 221–45.

Nicholls, M.G. (1990). Diuretics and electrolytes in congestive heart failure. *American Journal of Cardiology,* **65**, 17E–23E.

Rose, B.D. (1991). Diuretics. *Kidney International,* **39**, 336–52.

Wilkins, M.R., Unwin, R.J., and Kenny, A.J. (1993). Endopeptidase-24.11 and its inhibitors: potential therapeutic agents for edematous disorders and hypertension. *Kidney International,* **43**, 273–85.

15.6.2 Digitalis

D. A. CHAMBERLAIN

Digitalis and related glycosides have been used sporadically as a medicine for more than two millennia and became established after Withering's famous treatise of 1785. Most haemodynamic benefits of the drug follow from two basic actions on the heart: modification of electrical events in the pacemaker and conducting system, which may slow heart rate and stabilize some rhythm disorders, and modification of the mechanical properties of the muscle, which thereby augments the force of myocardial contraction. Manifestations of failure may regress as a result—excess filling pressure may be relieved, diuresis promoted, and heart size reduced. The effect on cardiac output is inconsistent, reflecting the complexity of the mechanisms that control it.

Mechanisms of action

At a cellular level the mechanical (inotropic) effect is mediated principally by the inhibition of membrane Na^+/K^+-ATPase. The concentration of sodium within the cell tends to increase, leading in turn to an augmented exchange, through another dedicated pathway, of intracellular sodium for extracellular calcium. The result is an increase in intracellular calcium that augments contractile power. Not all the inotropic effects of digitalis are readily explained by this mechanism alone. Depression of this one enzyme system can be amplified by actions that involve other membrane channels. For example, the increases in calcium mediated by Na^+/K^+-ATPase inhibition may be amplified by a positive feedback signal acting through slow calcium channels. Sodium–hydrogen exchange may also have an indirect role in augmenting the calcium available to the contractile proteins of the myocardium for conversion into mechanical force. Thus several ion pumps, exchangers, and channels of the cell membrane may be involved in the modification of function induced by digitalis.

The electrical effects of the drug (which account for all the important arrhythmias of digitalis toxicity as well as much of the clinical benefit) are also complex. The influence of glycosides on action potential and refractory period within the Purkinje system, on automaticity and conductivity in the sinoatrial and atrioventricular nodes, and on conduction velocity and refractory period within atrial and ventricular muscle is detailed in standard pharmacology texts. At therapeutic plasma concentrations, the most important electrical effects are those on the sinoatrial and atrioventricular nodes. Slowing of sinus rate is slight in normal subjects but may be prominent when heart failure responds to treatment. Slowing of ventricular response in atrial fibrillation and control of the reciprocating mechanism of junctional tachycardias account for much of the clinical benefit of the cardiac glycosides. These actions depend only slightly upon direct cardiac effects. Indirect effects on the level of autonomic activity, and on the sensitivity to it of both nodes, are of much greater importance. Details of mechanisms are not well understood, but actions that have been described include central nervous effects, changes in baroreceptor sensitivity, and the modulation of release and uptake of noradrenaline from adrenergic nerve endings. Sympathetic influences are reduced and vagal influences enhanced at therapeutic doses. Conversely, sympathetic activity may be increased at toxic concentrations of cardiac glycosides.

Therapeutic effects of digitalis in patients with heart failure are likely to depend upon additional mechanisms. Renin release is suppressed by the inhibition of $Na^+/K^+ - ATPase$, so that the activity of the renin–angiotensin system will be reduced. The growing appreciation of the neurohormonal disturbances in heart failure underline the likely importance of this effect. Changes also occur in peripheral arterial and venous tone mediated directly and through the autonomic system.

Preparations of digitalis

1. Digitalis leaf (digitalis folium) is now of mainly historical interest. Until recently it was available in tablet form as prepared digitalis (BP), consisting of the powdered leaves of *Digitalis purpurea,* and contains a number of glycosides, of which digitoxin is probably the most important.
2. Digitoxin (Digitaline Nativelle) is a purified glycoside, available as tablets usually of 100 μg. The solution for injection is no longer available in the United Kingdom.
3. Digoxin (Lanoxin; Diganox) is a glycoside obtained from *Digitalis lanata,* available as tablets usually of 62.5, 125, or 250 μg, as an elixir containing 50 μg/ml, and as a solution for injection containing 250 μg/ml.
4. Medigoxin (Lanitop) is β-methyl digoxin, available in some countries as tablets of 100 μg and as a solution for injection containing 100 μg/ml.
5. Ouabain (Strophanthin-G) is another naturally occurring glycoside—usually from the seeds of *Strophanthus gratus*—that should be used only by intravenous injection as absorption from the gut is unpredictable. Solutions contain 250 μg/ml. Haemodynamic effects occur somewhat more rapidly than with digoxin. Elimination is also faster (plasma half-life of approx. 18 h) and mostly renal. It is no longer available in Europe.

The most popular oral agents are digoxin and digitoxin, but with marked regional preferences for one or the other. For parenteral use most physicians use digoxin. Though choice of glycoside depends primarily upon the prescriber's familiarity with them, clinical considerations may also influence the balance between the relative advantages and disadvantages of the various agents.

Pharmacokinetics—influences on dose requirements

Four principal factors influence dose requirements: first, the absorption, metabolism, and excretion of the glycosides, which determine plasma concentrations obtained during therapy; secondly, other metabolic variables that affect potency at cellular level; thirdly, the sensitivity or vulnerability of the myocardium and conducting system to digitalis; finally, drug interactions that can modify digitalis requirements through any of the preceding three dose determinants. The difficulties imposed by these complex variables are compounded because therapeutic and toxic doses are close or even overlap, and toxicity is always important and may be lethal. Decisions on dosage are therefore more critical for digitalis than for most other drugs.

ABSORPTION, METABOLISM, AND EXCRETION

Digitoxin is rapidly and fully absorbed after oral administration. Digoxin, however, is incompletely absorbed: on average, about 70 per

cent enters the circulation but some variation can occur. In the past, tablet brands and even batches differed widely in the bioavailability of their digoxin content, but the introduction of a standard for dissolution rate led to acceptable uniformity. Differences in capacity for absorption between individuals are usually slight and timing of administration relative to meals makes little difference. But concomitant administration of some drugs has an appreciable effect (see below). Another unusual factor can markedly affect absorption in some individuals, leading to a dose requirement even several times larger than usual: digoxin can be metabolized within the gut by *Eubacterium lentum,* an otherwise harmless, anaerobic saprophyte. Agents that alter the gut flora may have a profound and even dangerous effect on drug half-life in such instances. Metabolism is important only for digitoxin: at least 50 per cent undergoes transformation in the liver, though some of the resulting compounds may retain cardioactivity. Digitoxin and its metabolites are excreted in the bile but the parent compound is absorbed again in an enterohepatic cycle, which accounts in part for the relatively long plasma half-life of nearly 5 days (slightly longer in the presence of hepatic dysfunction). Ultimately, most digitoxin is lost by metabolism, in the urine, and in the faeces. Digoxin is removed from the body almost entirely by renal excretion, and in an unchanged form except in those individuals—about 10 per cent of patients—who have extensive bacterial metabolism of the glycoside within the gut. Glomerular filtration is most important, but digoxin clearance exceeds inulin clearance so that another mechanism must be involved. Tubular secretion is now thought to be responsible for at least part of the digoxin eliminated by the kidney. The half-life of digoxin depends almost entirely upon renal function, which is therefore a prime determinant of maintenance dose requirements. The half-life is about 32 h in healthy young adults and up to 48 h in elderly patients with normal serum creatinine concentrations, but it can reach more than 2 weeks in the presence of renal failure. The half-life of digitoxin, on the other hand, is influenced much less by renal failure. In summary, the relation of blood level to dosage of digoxin depends principally on renal function and to a lesser degree on absorption. For digitoxin, the relation tends to be more consistent: it depends principally on hepatic metabolism, but this is usually well maintained even with hepatic failure.

OTHER METABOLIC VARIABLES

The activity of cardiac glycosides is influenced by protein binding of the moiety in plasma. Only about 20 per cent of the digoxin in plasma is bound to albumin, compared with over 90 per cent of digitoxin. Since only the free fraction exchanges readily with tissue sites, the ratio of tissue to plasma levels is smaller for digitoxin than digoxin (myocardium to plasma ratios are less than 10: 1 for digitoxin but about 100:1 for digoxin, though for both glycosides the correlation is poor). The avid protein binding of digitoxin is responsible for its limited renal excretion. This, together with the enterohepatic cycle, are the factors that help retain digitoxin in the body so that maintenance doses are usually smaller than those for digoxin.

The activity of cardiac glycosides is influenced by electrolyte concentration. Hypokalaemia is particularly important in this respect because potassium affects binding of digitalis to its specific receptor sites (membrane Na^+-K^+-ATPase). Binding of glycosides at these sites is enhanced either by a high plasma concentration of the drug or by a reduced concentration of potassium. Magnesium depletion, high concentrations of serum calcium, and hypothyroidism are other metabolic factors thought to increase sensitivity to digitalis. Conversely, thyrotoxicosis seems to decrease sensitivity to at least some actions of digitalis.

SENSITIVITY AND VULNERABILITY OF THE MYOCARDIUM AND CONDUCTING SYSTEM

Some of the therapeutic effects of digitalis, and also the susceptibility to cardiac manifestations of toxicity, depend not only on the concentration of glycosides at receptors but also upon the state of the myocardium and the conducting system. This is most readily appreciated by considering the use of the drug to slow ventricular rate in atrial fibrillation. Whilst in any one patient increasing the plasma levels causes progressive cardiac slowing, the correlation of plasma levels with ventricular rate between patients is very poor. Not only does the responsiveness of the atrioventricular node vary but the heart rate in the untreated state determines how much effect is needed for an adequate therapeutic action. Thus a relatively low plasma level of the drug many cause bradycardia in one patient whilst a high level bordering on toxicity may be insufficient to prevent undue tachycardia in another. Similarly, a sinus node may be vulnerable to the effects of digitalis because of degenerative changes that were latent before treatment had been given. Sinoatrial block may then be an unwanted effect of digitalis provoked by only a low plasma level of digitalis. Whether or not this should be called toxicity is a matter of semantics, but the principle of interaction between drug and end-organ is important and often ill understood by clinicians. This explains much of the confusion that arises over the value of plasma levels in the diagnosis and assessment of digitalis toxicity.

Not only does the presence or absence of disease within the conducting system influence the effects of digitalis but the state of the myocardium is also important. For example, vulnerability to ventricular arrhythmias is very variable among patients, depending upon the presence and extent of underlying disease (especially ischaemic heart disease). Thus, the threshold at which digitalis will provoke arrhythmias depends upon an interaction of drug and end-organ: the tendency to arrhythmias does not correlate closely with any critical plasma concentration of drug, but rather develops steadily with increasing plasma concentrations, especially above about 2.0 ng/ml.

DRUG INTERACTIONS INFLUENCING DIGITALIS REQUIREMENTS

The interactions of digoxin and digitoxin with other agents have been described in over 500 papers listed in *Index Medicus* since 1980, and the wise physician will pause before prescribing a glycoside with any other drug. Such caution is important because the drug has a relatively narrow therapeutic ratio. The mechanisms of drug interaction influencing digitalis therapy are manifold and influence most of the factors relating to the pharmacokinetics of the glycosides.

Influence on absorption

Antacids and cholestyramine readily combine with both digoxin and digitoxin and can thereby reduce absorption if they are administered concurrently. Other drugs can influence digoxin absorption more readily than that of digitoxin, which is complete under most circumstances. Transit time through the jejunum is probably the most important factor. For example, metoclopramide reduces plasma levels of digoxin whilst propantheline increases them. Antibiotics may increase absorption in individuals who have previously required a large ingested dose to compensate for the metabolism of digoxin within the gut lumen by *Eu. lentum*.

Influence on metabolism

Microsomal enzymes that are responsible in part for hepatic metabolism of digitoxin are inducible by other drugs. Phenytoin and phenobarbitone can substantially reduce digitoxin concentrations by this mechanism.

Influence on excretion

The enterohepatic cycle of digitoxin is subject to interference. The drug can be bound in the gut by cholestyramine, which thereby breaks the cycle and reduces the plasma half-life. As excretion of digoxin depends principally upon renal function, its elimination is less susceptible to drug interaction. Spironolactone and triamterene, however, seem to reduce the fraction actively secreted by renal tubules and thereby cause a slight increase in plasma levels. This is unlikely to be important clinically.

Amiodarone, verapamil, and quinidine also reduce digoxin excretion, and possibly the renal component of digitoxin excretion. Toxicity can occur from the increased plasma concentrations, and dosage of the glycosides should be reduced to avoid adverse effects associated with high plasma concentrations. Captopril also causes a small increase in plasma digoxin concentrations, probably by a combination of a decrease in glomerular filtration and an effect on tubular secretion. Severe hypokalaemia may reduce tubular secretion of digoxin, and thereby add to the risk of an augmented digitalis effect induced by low potassium concentrations mentioned below.

Influence on binding to plasma proteins

Most digoxin in plasma is free, so the decrease in protein binding found experimentally with some drugs such as prazosin is unlikely to be important clinically. The greater protein binding of digitoxin may be thought a potential hazard when other drugs that are also albumin bound are administered. In practice, these interactions also seem to be of little clinical significance.

Influence on tissue binding

Quinidine administration has been shown to increase plasma concentrations of digoxin, and part of this effect is probably due to displacement of the glycoside from tissue sites. Amiodarone may have a similar effect, though the mechanism has not been investigated fully.

Influence on metabolic factors

A well-known and important interaction concerns the propensity of some diuretics to enhance digitalis effect by causing hypokalaemia, which enhances digitalis binding to Na^+/K^+-ATPase. Spironolactone and potassium-retaining diuretics may be more effective than potassium supplements at countering drug-induced hypokalaemia. Treatment of hyper- or hypothyroidism also changes digitalis requirements.

Modification of digitalis-induced augmentation of intracellular calcium

As mentioned earlier, some of the increase in the availability of calcium for the contractile proteins depends indirectly on the slow calcium channels. Calcium channel-blocking agents may therefore decrease the availability of intracellular calcium and thereby impair the inotropic effect of digitalis. This mechanism has been suggested only for diltiazem. Verapamil has complex interactions with digoxin that increase plasma concentrations, and these may obscure small membrane effects.

Summation or competition of drug effects on the heart

Drugs that have similar effects to digitalis may change dose requirements. For example, β-adrenoceptor-blocking agents or verapamil may reduce the need for digitalis in atrial fibrillation and are often useful in the control of ventricular rate in this setting. Catecholamines and parasympatholytic drugs, on the other hand, may increase heart rate and suggest a need for increased dosage. Caution is necessary because toxicity may be precipitated under these circumstances.

Measurement of digoxin and digitoxin concentrations

Until 1961, the clinical pharmacology of the cardiac glycosides was poorly understood because no adequate assay system was available to measure therapeutic plasma or tissue concentration. Since then, the introduction of isotopically labelled glycosides and later the sensitive radioimmunoassays have contributed much to our knowledge of these drugs. Assays are of value in the management of patients, provided clinicians understand the complex relation between plasma levels and therapeutic and toxic effects. Blood samples should be drawn when the plasma concentrations after oral dosage have passed the absorption peak and fallen to a plateau, which then decays slowly at a rate corresponding to the elimination half-life of the drug. In practice this requires venesection after an interval of about 8 h from the last oral dose. Another variable has been recognized over the past decade. Exercise increases the binding of digoxin (and presumably of digitoxin) to exercising skeletal muscle. The plasma concentrations after a period of rest can be increased by as much as 75 per cent compared with concentrations during exercise. Even everyday activities can have a pronounced effect, and a steady state may not be reached for 2 h. Pregnancy and renal impairment have been reported to produce false-positive (or elevated) plasma glycoside concentrations in some assay systems.

Most therapeutic plasma concentrations of digoxin are in the range of 1 to 2 μg/l. The usual therapeutic concentrations for digitoxin are approximately 10 to 15 times higher than for digoxin, due chiefly to the greater protein binding of the drug: free levels of the glycosides will be similar. Measurements of plasma concentrations of glycosides are not required as a routine, but they can be useful when the therapeutic response is greater or less than expected, when digoxin is used in patients with renal impairment, when unusually large maintenance doses seem to be required, and when digitalis toxicity is suspected. Creatinine concentration or other measures of renal function should be known before the dose of digoxin is prescribed for maintenance therapy.

Therapy with cardiac glycosides

RAPID DIGITALIZATION: INDICATIONS AND REGIMENS

Urgent digitalization may be required for the control of some tachyarrhythmias. A rapid ventricular response in atrial fibrillation is the most common indication. Some cases of recurrent supraventricular tachycardia or atrial flutter may be treated by digitalization, particularly if agents with negative inotropic properties are contraindicated. Early experimental observations indicating a positive inotropic effect with acute administration were confirmed by clinical measurements of increased contractility using force–velocity curves obtained with radiopaque markers sewn on to the myocardium. Some observations were associated with slight falls in cardiac output that were incorrectly interpreted as denying the possibility of clinical benefit. They are now known to depend on reflex adjustments of venous return in a complex system replete with possibilities for autoregulation. The role of digitalis for acute heart failure due to coronary disease is, however, limited because of the risk of inducing ventricular arrhythmias and because failure of diastolic relaxation may be more important than loss of contractile power. But prompt digitalization can still be recommended for acute left-ventricular failure if appropriate doses of opioids, diuretics, and vasodilators fail to bring rapid relief—particularly if tachycardia limits the use of other inotropes. Glycosides are best given intravenously in all urgent situations. An infusion of digoxin in 5 per cent dextrose may be used to avoid the very high plasma levels that cause nausea and other central nervous effects: 500 μg over 30 min may be followed by 500 μg over 1 h, and if necessary a third dose may be given over 2 h (doses for children, small adults, patients with hypokalaemia or hypothyroidism, or those already receiving glycosides should be less). The intramuscular route is much less satisfactory; indeed plasma concentrations are attained more reliably after oral administration if this is feasible.

MAINTENANCE THERAPY: INDICATIONS AND REGIMENS

Maintenance therapy is indicated for the long-term control of most cases of atrial fibrillation or flutter, for suppression of some supraventricular tachycardias, and for the management of symptomatic heart failure due to systolic ventricular dysfunction. Much debate has centred around the value of digitalis as an inotropic agent for long-term use in patients with sinus rhythm, and until recently the matter has been contentious. A review of evidence published up to 1982 provided no clear guidance on the value of long-term treatment for patients with congestive heart failure and sinus rhythm, but the situation has been clarified by 14 studies using digoxin, reported in the 6 years from 1988 to 1993. These have included one large-scale, randomized comparison against captopril and placebo, and another against xamoterol and placebo. Another large-scale

trial involving milrinone tested the effects of digoxin withdrawal in patients with severe heart failure. Methodologies in other trials have involved withdrawal studies with or without concomitant converting-enzyme inhibitor therapy, comparisons with enalapril, and detailed cross-over studies in relatively small numbers of patients. The type of observation varied widely among trials. While findings have not been entirely consistent, in most studies significant benefits that could be ascribed to digoxin included one or more of the following: subjective measures, heart failure scores, haemodynamic measures, exercise capacity, time to treatment failure, and frequency of hospital admission. One of the trials showed that the benefits of digoxin in heart failure were additive to those of converting-enzyme inhibitors. A subsequent randomized study showed that withdrawal of digoxin in patients treated with diuretics and converting-enzyme inhibitors led to worsening heart failure and deterioration of functional capacity as compared with those who continued to receive digoxin. The differences between the two groups continued to widen over 12 weeks. Thus the symptomatic benefits of digitalis for patients in sinus rhythm who have chronic heart failure due to systolic dysfunction is additional to the benefits of other current conventional treatments.

Against the evidence of benefit from digitalis in chronic heart failure must be set the possibility of harm. Toxicity in routine clinical practice has been relatively common in the past, and the potential risk may remain greater than any observed in recent trials—which have generally been reassuring in this respect. Some authorities consider that cardiac glycosides should be used with particular caution in patients with severe coronary heart disease because the threshold to ventricular fibrillation may be lowered. Patients treated with digitalis have sometimes been shown to have a higher mortality than those not so treated, but they also tend to have worse failure and thus to be a higher-risk group. Evidence is inconclusive that digitalis is an independent risk factor for death, but it cannot be pronounced innocent in this regard. The case at present is 'not proven', and the danger of inducing ventricular fibrillation in vulnerable patients should be taken into account when decisions are made on long-term treatment, especially for those with coronary disease whose failure is often predominantly due to diastolic dysfunction that does not respond well to cardiac glycosides. Important new information will become available, probably in 1995, from the report of the Digitalis Investigations Trial (DIG). This is a large randomized placebo-controlled mortality study that has enrolled approximately 8000 patients. Decisions on the most appropriate dose of digitalis for patients in sinus rhythm are sometimes guided by plasma concentrations, although usually they are empirical. Evidence on dose response in patients with heart failure is not available. Without it, the risk benefit ratio for digoxin and digitoxin may be less than optimal for many patients.

Some assessment of ventricular rate during exercise should preferably be made before deciding dose requirements for control of atrial fibrillation, but in the presence of normal or near-normal renal function up to twice daily administration of 250 μg digoxin may be needed. Very rarely, higher doses may be used but only with careful observation and preferably with confirmation that plasma concentrations remain within the therapeutic range. More commonly, the need for smaller doses is dictated by impaired renal function, by unwanted effects even with usually acceptable plasma concentrations, or by a ventricular rate that is not unduly fast at rest or that rises only modestly on exercise. Extra caution is needed when atrial fibrillation is not present, for this provides a useful yardstick of dose requirement. For most patients with sinus rhythm and blood urea concentrations within the normal range, a dose of digoxin of 250 μg daily is usually appropriate, though with caution larger doses may be used. These larger doses, appropriate for some patients with normal renal function, should be divided (usually twice-daily administration) because plasma half-life is relatively short and because of unwanted effects that can occur with plasma concentrations that may be transiently high after absorption. With impaired renal function, relatively small doses should be prescribed, and daily administration is then always appropriate because half-life is prolonged. Digitoxin may be a better glycoside to use in this situation because cumulation is less likely to occur with a drug that is predominantly metabolized. The usual dose of digitoxin is 100 µg daily, but 200 µg daily may be necessary in some patients with sustained atrial fibrillation or with other troublesome supraventricular arrhythmias. Impaired hepatic function dictates the need for smaller-than-average doses of digitoxin.

Although many patients on maintenance cardiac glycosides do not require them, the strong evidence for continuing benefit in individuals with heart failure and sinus rhythm should not be disregarded. The potential risk for some of continued treatment with glycosides must be weighed carefully against the risks—now clearly demonstrated—of inappropriate withdrawal, even for those also receiving converting-enzyme inhibitors.

Digitalis toxicity

Digitalis has both cardiac and extracardiac toxic effects. There is considerable variation in the plasma and tissue concentrations at which these occur because of differences among patients in sensitivity and vulnerability of the myocardium, the conducting system, the central nervous system, and other tissues. Serious manifestations of toxicity are unusual with plasma concentrations below 2 µg/l, and are likely to be present with concentrations more than 3 µg/l. Between these figures some patients have a satisfactory therapeutic response whilst others have troublesome adverse effects.

The extracardiac effects of high plasma concentrations were studied systematically by two Dutch physicians (Lely and van Enter) in an epidemic of toxicity that occurred when digitoxin was inadvertently substituted (weight for weight) for digoxin in prepared tablet form. Nearly all patients had fatigue with profound muscular weakness and also severe visual disturbances. Nausea and anorexia also occurred in the majority, whilst abdominal pain, vomiting, and diarrhoea were experienced by about half of them. Headache, restlessness, and agitation were also prominent.

In the absence of myocardial disease or massive overdose (as may occur with suicidal intent), the cardiac manifestations of high plasma concentrations are usually relatively benign. First, second, and third degree atrioventricular block may occur, but severe bradycardia or long pauses are unlikely to be seen because the rate of subsidiary junctional pacemakers tends to be accelerated by the glycosides. In patients with heart disease the manifestations are more complex and usually more serious. Whilst almost any rhythm disturbance can occur, the following may be regarded as characteristic: frequent ventricular extrasystoles, junctional and ventricular rhythms or tachycardias, the association of atrial tachycardias with varying degrees of atrioventricular block, bradycardia due to sinoatrial block, an unduly slow ventricular response with atrial fibrillation, progressive regularization of ventricular response in atrial fibrillation due to the emergence of accelerated junctional beats, and ventricular fibrillation. Some digitalis-induced arrhythmias are very complex and difficult to analyse. The disturbances of heart rhythm that occur in toxicity are the result of both direct effects on the heart and on autonomic effects, mostly mediated though the vagus. In addition to the well-understood effects on conduction and automaticity that occur as a result of transmembrane ionic shifts, some tachyarrhythmias occur because of the increased magnitude of delayed after-depolarizations and because of enhanced triggered activity. With very high plasma levels, asystole may occur. This may be associated with refractory hyperkalaemia and is difficult to manage.

Many of the adverse effects are related to the central nervous system. As with the therapeutic actions, the vagus also plays an important part in the emergence of some cardiac arrhythmias, notably those associated with sinoatrial and atrioventricular block. Vagal effects, and perhaps some other central nervous manifestations of toxicity, seem to be related more closely to plasma concentrations than to tissue concentrations of the drug. These may therefore occur within an hour of oral administra-tion or rapidly following intravenous administration, before equilibra-tion with tissue sites has occurred.

Other extracardiac effects such as weakness, and the cardiac manifestations of toxicity involving the emergence of ectopic pacemakers, are almost certainly more dependent on tissue concentrations, but the different mechanisms interrelate and are not readily separable.

Digitalis toxicity or troublesome unwanted actions were very common in the past during maintenance therapy with glycosides; up to 20 per cent of patients on digoxin had some adverse effects. Toxicity should occur in a smaller proportion of patients now that the pharmacokinetics are well understood. Toxicity is less likely to occur with digitoxin than with digoxin because levels do not depend upon renal function and are therefore more predictable; but toxicity is more persistent if it does occur because of the longer half-life. The importance of digitalis toxicity as a clinical problem has also receded as its use in heart failure has been partially superseded by other drugs.

TREATMENT OF DIGITALIS TOXICITY

In most patients it is sufficient to withhold the drug, and, especially in the presence of hypokalaemia, to give potassium. Some believe potassium to be contraindicated when atrioventricular block is present because the conduction defect may be exacerbated. Atropine and per-venous pacing have an occasional role in the management of bradyarrhythmias.

A specific antidote—digoxin-specific antibody fragments (Fab) prepared from IgG produced in sheep—has been available commercially since 1986 (Digibind, Ovine). Antibody therapy is particularly valuable because of the risk to life with severe toxicity and the limited clinical benefit from conventional treatment. The antibody fragments rapidly bind intravascular and interstitial digoxin. The small molecular size permits rapid diffusion into the interstitial space where the binding of free digoxin sets up a concentration gradient leading to the egress of tissue stores of the glycoside. An initial clinical response can usually be expected within 60 min, and complete reversal of toxicity within about 4 h. If renal function is normal, the digoxin bound to Fab is excreted with a half-life of approximately 16 h. Although the affinity of the Fab is less for digitoxin than for digoxin, limited experience suggests it is high enough to achieve a satisfactory clinical response for toxicity caused by this glycoside too. The dose of Fab is based on body weight and plasma digoxin concentration for patients toxic from excessive maintenance therapy or on the amount ingested after a single dose. Failure to respond may occur if the patient is already moribund, but otherwise an incorrect diagnosis or an inadequate dose of Fab should be suspected. Allergic reactions have occurred in less than 1 per cent of patients treated with Fab. Recrudescence of toxicity occurs rarely, but caution is needed if renal failure is severe enough to prolong greatly the elimination of the digoxin–antibody complex, which may eventually release free digoxin.

Lignocaine or phenytoin may be effective for established serious arrhythmias, even if they are of supraventricular origin. β-Adrenoceptor-blocking agents are useful for ectopic ventricular arrhythmias but may precipitate heart failure or bradyarrhythmias in susceptible patients. Electrical cardioversion may precipitate ventricular fibrillation and should be considered only for the most pressing indications. The lowest effective energy should be used. Toxicity with digitoxin can be made less persistent by the oral administration of cholestyramine, which binds the glycoside and interrupts the enterohepatic cycle. Dialysis and haemoperfusion are ineffective for both digoxin and digitoxin toxicity (except to control hyperkalaemia) because the large tissue stores equilibrate relatively slowly with the much lower concentrations in the plasma.

REFERENCES

Editorial (1989). Digoxin: new answers; new questions. *Lancet*, **ii**, 79.
Jaeschke, R., Oxman, A.D., and Guyatt, G.H. (1990). To what extent do

congestive heart failure patients in sinus rhythm benefit from digoxin therapy? A systematic overview and meta-analysis. *American Journal of Medicine,* **88,** 279.

Gheorghiade, M. and Zarowitz, B.J. (1992). Review of randomized trials of digoxin therapy in patients with chronic heart failure. *American Journal of Cardiology,* **69,** 48G.

Hickey, A.R. *et al.* (1991). Digoxin immune Fab therapy in the management of digitalis intoxication: safety and efficacy results of an observational surveillance study. *Journal of the American College of Cardiology,* **17,** 590.

Kelly, R.A. and Smith, T.W. (1993). Digoxin in heart failure: implications of recent trials. *Journal of the American College of Cardiology,* **22,** 107A.

Lely, A.H. and van Enter, C.H.J. (1970). Large-scale digitoxin intoxication. *British Medical Journal,* **iii,** 737.

Marcus, F.I. (1985). Pharmacokinetic interactions between digoxin and other drugs. *Journal of the American College of Cardiology,* **5,** 82A.

Packer, M. *et al.* for the RADIANCE Study (1993). Withdrawal of digoxin from patients with chronic heart failure treated with angiotensin-converting-enzyme inhibitors. *New England Journal of Medicine,* **329,** 1.

Smith, T.W. (1988). Digitalis. Mechanisms of action and clinical use. *New England Journal of Medicine,* **318,** 358.

Smith, T.W. and Haber, E. (1973). Digitalis. (Review in four parts.) *New England Journal of Medicine,* **289,** 945, 1010, 1063, and 1125.

Uretsky, B.F. *et al.* for the PROVED Investigative Group. (1993). Randomized study assessing the effect of digoxin withdrawal in patients with mild to moderate chronic congestive heart failure: results of the PROVED trial. *Journal of the American College of Cardiology,* **22,** 955.

Withering, W. (1785). *An account of the foxglove and some of its medicinal uses: with practical remarks on dropsy and other diseases.* C.G.J. and J. Robinson. London. (Reprinted in *Medical Classics* (1937), **2,** 305.)

Several of the selected references above are very recent. They can provide a gateway to the many important papers of the last decade that have modified perceptions on the mode of action of digitalis and on its potential for the treatment of patients with heart disease.

15.6.3 Vasodilators

J. H. DARGIE

Introduction

When vasodilator therapy for heart failure was first introduced in the early 1970s it was greeted with enthusiasm and optimism. The then recent availability, simplicity, and safety of invasive haemodynamic measurements in the clinical setting had allowed a greater appreciation of the importance of factors other than contractility, especially loading conditions, in the determination of cardiac output. It also made possible the measurement of the acute effects of vasodilators in counteracting the marked vasoconstriction found to be present in many patients with heart failure.

The ensuing two decades have witnessed some tempering of that early zeal; indeed it is mainly due to the introduction and subsequent extensive clinical experience with angiotensin converting enzyme inhibitors that a more balanced view of what can and what cannot be achieved by vasodilators now prevails.

Haemodynamic considerations relevant to vasodilatation

Cardiac output is dependent on several factors, principally preload, afterload, myocardial contractility, compliance, and heart rate. Preload is represented by the end-diastolic volume which is determined by venous tone, the intravascular volume, ventricular compliance, and the extent of ventricular emptying. In clinical practice, the left ventricular end-diastolic pressure or filling pressure provides a useful indicator of pre-

Table 1 *Vasodilators in common clinical use*

Drug	Mechanism	Arterial	Venous
Nitrates	Cyclic GMP	+	++
Hydralazine	Unknown	++	−
ACE inhibition	Angiotensin II	++	+
Calcium antagonists	Calcium entry	++	−
Angiotensin receptor antagonist	AT$_1$ receptor	++	+
Renin inhibitor	Renin	++	+
Neutral endopeptidase inhibitors	ANP breakdown	+	+

load. In the absence of any physical obstruction to blood flow, left ventricular end-diastolic pressure correlates well with the pulmonary capillary wedge pressure and usually with the pulmonary artery end diastolic pressure.

Afterload, the left ventricular wall stress that must be overcome for ejection of the stroke volume, is mainly determined by the radius of the ventricle, its thickness and its pressure and by the peripheral vascular resistance. Since preload affects the volume and therefore the radius of the ventricle, it also influences the afterload. Systemic vascular resistance is the main contributor to and is used as a clinical approximation for the afterload.

In the treatment of heart failure, preload and afterload are often considered separately, but as they are, to a significant extent, interdependent this distinction is artificial. It can be shown that, in most cases, balanced vasodilatation with agents that reduce both preload and afterload leads to the greatest haemodynamic improvement and, ultimately, clinical benefit.

Both preload and afterload contribute to the mitral regurgitation found in many patients with left ventricular systolic dysfunction. Therefore an additional factor responsible for the increase in cardiac output following vasodilator treatment is redistribution in a forward direction of the mitral regurgitant volume.

Other important consequences of reduced loading conditions include a decrease in myocardial oxygen consumption and improved right as well as left ventricular function.

Classification of vasodilators

In a complex and intricately regulated system like the human circulation, there are many vasodilatory and vasoconstrictor mechanisms or mediators. Increased vascular tone typifies the state of heart failure and indicates that vasoconstrictor predominate over vasodilatory influences. Vasodilators which are used in clinical practice in heart failure are relatively few; classification of them, for instance as directly/indirectly acting are clinically unhelpful, though of pharmacological interest. The likely haemodynamic effects of such a drug and its mechanism of action are important considerations, allowing anticipation of and safe-guarding against excessive effects and giving some guidance on how these may be reversed if necessary. For example, a fall in preload and arterial pressure might be expected with venous dilators and reflex tachycardia with arterial vasodilators.

Additional effects may be of considerable importance as exemplified by the angiotensin converting enzyme inhibitors, which are the first vasodilators to antagonize a specific abnormality of known pathophysiological importance in heart failure.

The best classification of vasodilators for clinical purposes would be one based on mechanisms and site of action. Incomplete information on mechanisms, however, together with clinical convenience has led to the adoption of a simpler descriptive classification based on relative actions on arteries or veins or various combinations of these effects.

Table 1 lists those agents that are: (1) in common clinical use; and (2) under investigation.

The way in which reduction in preload or afterload or both affect the cardiac output is illustrated schematically in Fig. 1. This simple scheme has served well as the basis for the management of acute heart failure with intravenous therapy, usually with the aid of bedside haemodynamic monitoring. It also reveals the reason for the poor efficacy of the earlier vasodilators during chronic ambulatory treatment; long-term reduction in breathlessness and tiredness did not reliably occur despite acute haemodynamic effects that were often both salutory and striking.

NITROPRUSSIDE

In dilating both arterioles and veins equally, nitroprusside is a balanced vasodilator which can only be given intravenously and whose rapid onset and offset of action renders it only suitable, but eminently so, for the acute situation; close haemodynamic monitoring both of systemic arterial and right heart pressures are essential during its use. As light degrades the parent compound, the delivery system must be shielded. The dose ranges from 10 μg/kg/min up to 30 μg/kg/min depending on response. A typical indication for its use would be a patient with acute or chronic low cardiac output and high filling pressures due to poor systolic left ventricular function resulting from dilated cardiomyopathy, acute myocardial infarction (AMI), chronic coronary heart disease, acute or chronic aortic or mitral incompetence, or acute ventricular septal defect following acute myocardial infarction. Two main problems complicate the use of nitroprusside infusion. The first is hypotension, which is best avoided by starting at a very low dose and by close continuous monitoring of systemic arterial and pulmonary capillary wedge pressures. Second, toxic metabolites of cyanide or cyanate accumulate in patients with liver or renal dysfunction. Intravenous nitroprusside remains a very useful treatment option; but the problems associated with its use lead many physicians to opt for intravenous nitrate on the insecure assumption that it is safer and as effective.

NITRATES

All the various preparations of nitrates available for angina pectoris may also be used in the treatment of patients with heart failure. Glyceryl trinitrate is prepared in intravenous, sublingual, and transcutaneous formulations, while the mainstays of oral therapy are isosorbide mono- or dinitrate. It is impossible to say whether the subtle differences in hae-modynamic effects sometimes claimed with different nitrate preparations are of any clinical relevance.

They all cause vascular smooth muscle relaxation particularly in veins by increasing intracellular cyclic guanine monophosphate (cGMP). Though some decrease in arteriolar tone also occurs, this effect is seen predominantly in the capacitance and pulmonary vessels resulting, acutely, in a reduction in preload. Frequently repeated doses of nitrate lead to the rapid development of tolerance in heart failure, as in other conditions. Recent experimental data suggest that the use of hydralazine may prevent the development of tolerance to nitrates.

HYDRALAZINE

The mechanism of action of this drug still eludes discovery. It is an arteriolar smooth muscle relaxant formerly used in the treatment of hypertension. Its haemodynamic profile is illustrated in Fig. 1 but these impressive effects did not translate into long-term clinical benefit in controlled trials when this drug was used as a single agent. Subsequent partial popularization of its use in combination with nitrate suggests that preload reduction is an essential component of any vasodilator regimen in chronic heart failure. The combination of hydralazine with isosorbide dinitrate is now the only way in which hydralazine is used in chronic heart failure. The value of this combination has received much publicity as a result of two major large trials by the Veterans Administration in the United States – the so-called Veterans' Heart Failure or V-HeFT I and II trials (Fig. 2).

Fig. 2 (a) Cumulative mortality rates with time (months) in V-HeFT I. Hydralazine/isosorbide dinitrate (Hyd-iso) group has a lower mortality trend than prazosin and placebo. (b) Cumulative mortality rate with time in V-HeFT II. Enalapril group has a significantly lower mortality (*P* = 0.08) than hydralazine/isosorbide dinitrate.

Fig. 1(a) Schematic diagram of normal and depressed left ventricular function curves relating filling pressure and cardiac output. (b) Effects of vasodilatation. (i) arteriolar vasodilatation with hydralazine (H); cardiac output rises more than filling pressure falls. Tiredness expected to improve; (ii) venous dilatation with nitrates (N); filling pressure falls more than cardiac output rises. Dyspnoea expected to improve; (iii) 'balanced' vasodilation with nitroprusside (NP); both cardiac output and filling pressure improve. Dyspnoea and tiredness expected to improve.

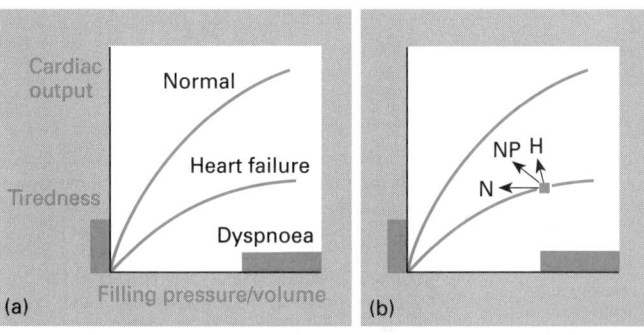

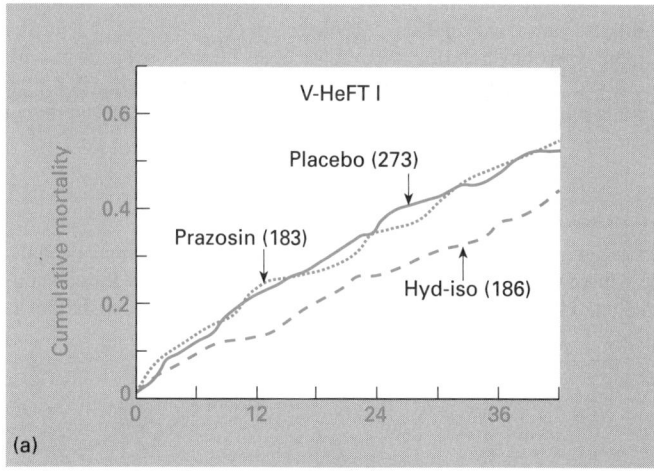

(a)

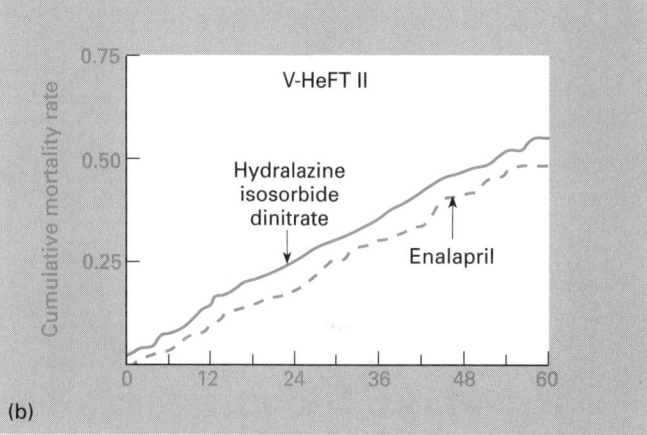

(b)

Effect on symptoms and exercise tolerance and mortality

There is no consistent evidence of symptomatic benefit from nitrates or hydralazine when given separately in heart failure. Furthermore, captopril has been shown to be superior to hydralazine in terms of symptom control and exercise capacity. There is also surprisingly little hard evidence that the combination of hydralazine and isosorbide dinitrate (H-ISDN) is of symptomatic benefit. In V-HeFT I, for instance, there was no consistent benefit in functional capacity over placebo. The combination of hydralazine and isosorbide dinitrate is also less efficacious than angiotensin converting enzyme inhibitors, both in terms of symptom control/functional capacity and reduction in mortality; and about one-third of patients will be unable to tolerate it, usually on account of headache, palpitation, or nasal congestion. These observations clearly relegate hydralazine and isosorbide dinitrate to second line therapy for patients who have failed to tolerate an angiotensin converting enzyme inhibitor. The beneficial effect of adding hydralazine and isosorbide dinitrate to diuretic/angiotensin converting enzyme inhibitor in heart failure was evident in the trial comparing the effects of hydralazine and captopril in severe heart failure, underpinning an increasingly common clinical practice.

Use of hydralazine and isosorbide dinitrate to treat heart failure

Treatment should be started with hydralazine 37.5 mg four times daily and hydralazine and isosorbide dinitrate 20 mg four times daily and increased until the maximum tolerated doses are found. These average 400 mg and 150 mg/day respectively.

Joint symptoms and the development of positive antinuclear antibody tests are uncommon complications of this treatment. Angiotensin converting enzyme inhibitors may result in an increase in urea, creatinine, and potassium concentrations, problems which do not occur with the combination of hydralazine and nitrates. Many heart failure patients with exertional symptoms may also benefit from the prophylactic use of nitrates prior to exercise in a manner analogous to their use to prevent chest pain in patients with chronic stable angina.

Calcium channel blockers

These agents are specific arteriolar vasodilators acting by decreasing the slow inward calcium current that promotes arterial smooth muscle contraction. The main concern in considering their use in heart failure is that they also decrease calcium availability within cardiac myocytes, which decreases contractility. Most interest in heart failure is therefore centred on those agents with relatively greater effects on the peripheral vascular calcium channels, such as nifedipine, felodipine, and amlodipine. There are few long-term studies on the value of these agents in heart failure but several reports have shown that the use of nifedipine may lead to clinical deterioration in patients with heart failure, probably reflecting its negative inotropic effects and, in some cases, the ill effects of secondary reflex neuroendocrine activation.

More recently, amlodipine, a dihydropyridine without an abrupt onset of action and with a prolonged effect, has been found to be of benefit in patients with heart failure. Its use in one study was associated with suppression of reflex neuroendocrine response to vasodilatation. A survival study of amlodipine in heart failure is now underway.

Angiotensin converting enzyme inhibitors

Angiotensin converting enzyme inhibitors have been the most significant advance in the treatment of heart failure since diuretics, superior to other vasodilators despite the observation that their acute haemodynamic effects (at least in terms of increasing cardiac output) seem less impressive than, say, the combination of isosorbide dinitrate (Fig. 3). But angiotensin converting enzyme inhibitors have many other actions depending primarily on local and systemic alternation of the production of angiotensin II.

NEUROENDOCRINE ACTIONS

As angiotensin II stimulates aldosterone, and vasopressin (AVP) secretion, facilitates sympathetic neural transmission and inhibits vagal activity, angiotensin converting enzyme inhibition leads to reduced plasma concentrations of aldosterone and vasopression; decreased sympathetic activity is reflected in lower plasma catecholamine levels. Angiotensin converting enzyme inhibitors also facilitate parasympathetic activity. It is also possible that increased bradykinin (and resultant vasodilator prostaglandins) are important in mediating the actions of angiotensin converting enzyme inhibitors. However, when the effects of angiotensin converting enzyme inhibitors are compared with those of renin inhibitors and angiotensin II receptor antagonists, the results argue against a major role for kinins and prostaglandins as a result of inhibition of kininase II.

Angiotensin converting enzyme inhibitors decrease the concentration of atrial natriuretic and brain natriuretic peptides in heart failure, reflect-

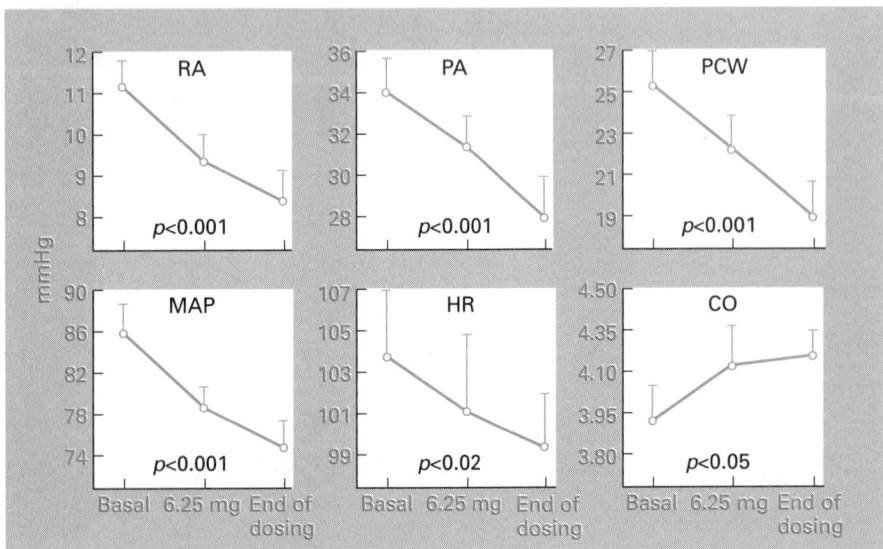

Fig. 3 Acute haemodynamic effects of captopril in heart failure following acute myocardial infarction. Haemodynamic effects of a cumulative dose of captopril (6.25 mg or 12.5 mg orally) in 18 patients with left ventricular failure following acute myocardial infarction. CO, cardiac output; HR, heart rate; MAP, mean arterial pressure; RA, right atrial pressure; PA, pulmonary arterial pressure; PCW, pulmonary capillary wedge pressure.

ing a reduction in ventricular filling pressures. This effect may underlie the transient reduction in sodium excretion that often occurs on initiation of an angiotensin converting enzyme inhibitor.

Angiotensin converting enzyme inhibitors also reduce plasma erythropoietin concentrations, presumably by their effects on renal blood flow. The resultant fall in haemoglobin concentration may contribute to improve peripheral blood flow. Recently it has also been reported that angiotensin converting enzyme inhibitors can increase the plasma concentration of opioid peptides.

VASCULAR ACTIONS

A major effect of angiotensin converting enzyme inhibitors is arterial and venous vasodilatation, one important consequence of which is an increase in resting and exercise skeletal muscle blood flow. Angiotensin converting enzyme inhibitors have also been shown to increase coronary blood flow in a number of clinical situations.

As angiotensin II and other neuroendocrine mediators may also act as growth factors, it is possible that angiotensin converting enzyme inhibitors also alter vascular structure in a way that improves peripheral blood flow.

MYOCARDIAL ACTIONS

Angiotensin converting enzyme inhibitors reduce cardiac filling pressures, wall stress, chamber size, and myocardial hypertrophy. As angiotensin II has a mild inotropic effect, intracoronary infusion of an angiotensin converting enzyme inhibitor can reduce myocardial contractility; however left ventricular ejection fraction increases after systemic angiotensin converting enzyme inhibition as a result of vasodilatation. The improvement in cardiac output in these circumstances may be less than seen with conventional vasodilators as there is usually a slight fall in heart rate (see Fig. 3).

In experimental models, high circulating concentrations of angiotensin II can cause myocyte necrosis. This direct cardiotoxic effect of angiotensin II is inhibited by angiotensin converting enzyme inhibition. The renin–angiotensin system has also been shown to be important in the development of the interstitial fibrosis associated with experimental myocardial hypertrophy. This fibrosis can be reduced by angiotensin converting enzyme inhibitor treatment.

RENAL ACTIONS

In patients with advanced heart failure, glomerular filtration may become dependent on angiotensin II. In the face of reduced renal perfusion pressure, angiotensin II, by constricting the efferent arteriole, increases intraglomerular hydrostatic pressure and filtration fraction. Loss of this action of angiotensin II then reduces glomerular filtration despite an increase in renal blood flow. This accounts for the usually small increase in plasma urea and creatinine concentrations that often occur following the introduction of an angiotensin converting enzyme inhibitor. It may also contribute to the less well recognized early antidiuretic and antinatriuretic effects of starting an angiotensin converting enzyme inhibitor. The longer-term effects of angiotensin converting enzyme inhibitors on filtration rate and sodium excretion have not been studied so thoroughly. Should renal perfusion pressure fall below the autoregulatory threshold, glomerular filtration may decline precipitously in the absence of angiotensin II leading to acute renal failure, which is reversible on withdrawing angiotensin converting enzyme inhibition.

EFFECTS ON ELECTROLYTES

Although there were early reports of angiotensin converting enzyme inhibition correcting hyponatraemia in patients with severe heart failure, more recent studies have demonstrated that a small fall in serum sodium concentration is more commonly seen, at least in patients with less severe congestive heart failure. This may reflect an early reduction in free water clearance that occurs on starting an angiotensin converting enzyme inhibitor in some patients, perhaps the result of a temporary increase in vasopressin release in response to an initial fall in blood pressure.

By suppressing aldosterone secretion, angiotensin converting enzyme inhibitors can attenuate the potassium losing effects of loop and thiazide diuretics and indeed cause hyperkalaemia in patients with coincident renal failure.

As magnesium excretion is also partially controlled by aldosterone, angiotensin converting enzyme inhibitors should reduce renal magnesium loss and replenish plasma and tissue stores, but this has not been a consistent finding.

ELECTROPHYSIOLOGICAL ACTIONS

In view of the effects of angiotensin converting enzyme inhibitors on coronary perfusion, myocardial function, neurohumoral activity, and electrolyte status, a beneficial effect on ventricular arrhythmias is to be expected, confirmed, however, only in the V-HeFT II and SAVE trials. Very little is known about the effect of angiotensin converting enzyme inhibitors on supraventricular arrhythmias, especially atrial fibrillation.

Effect on symptoms and exercise capacity

The vast majority of studies have shown that angiotensin converting enzyme inhibitors lead to an improvement in reported symptoms, clinical signs, exercise capacity, and NYHA class. 'Quality of life' assessments, however, have not demonstrated such clear improvements.

Effect on disease progression

Heart failure is a progressive disorder. Most patients pass through a phase of asymptomatic cardiac dysfunction (e.g. 'asymptomatic left ventricular dysfunction'), ultimately becoming symptomatic. We are much less clear as to the cause of progression (Fig. 4). The concept of a

Fig. 4 Schematic diagram of 'progression' of ventricular dysfunction following acute myocardial infarction. Following initial injury, a variable period of asymptomatic or symptomatic ventricular dysfunction is followed by the features of clinically obvious heart failure and its complications.

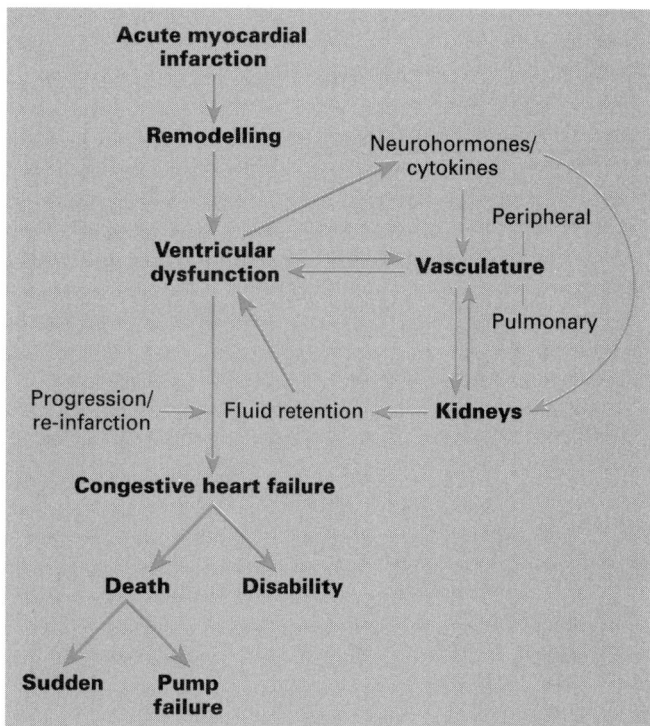

'vicious cycle' of increasing neurohumoral activation, vascular resistance, and renal dysfunction, leading to escalating myocardial dysfunction has gained much credence. It is easy to see, theoretically, how angiotensin converting enzyme inhibitors might break this cycle. More abrupt deterioration might be precipitated by further myocardial infarction; here too angiotensin converting enzyme inhibitors appear to be of benefit.

A number of studies have now shown that angiotensin converting enzyme inhibitors do indeed reduce the rate of progression of the heart failure syndrome. Others have shown that they also delay the development of symptomatic heart failure in patients with asymptomatic left ventricular dysfunction. Angiotensin converting enzyme inhibitors have also been shown to reduce mortality in all grades of symptomatic heart failure, including that occurring soon after acute myocardial infarction (Fig. 5).

MECHANISM OF REDUCTION IN MORTALITY?

At least half of all cases of heart failure die suddenly and unexpectedly, usually, it is presumed, due to a lethal ventricular arrhythmia. Brady-arrhythmias may also account for sudden unexpected death. Alternatively patients may die from progressive pump failure, whilst in some, sudden death may be precipitated by myocardial ischaemia/infarction.

In the CONSENSUS I and SOLVD studies enalapril reduced death due to pump failure but did not reduce presumed arrhythmic death. In the V-HeFT II trial however, enalapril reduced sudden unexpected death, while in the SAVE study captopril reduced both modes of death. Other trials have confirmed that captopril results in a reduction in sudden

death in heart failure. There is now also evidence from SOLVD and SAVE that angiotensin converting enzyme inhibitors also reduce myocardial ischaemia/infarction.

SIZE OF REDUCTION IN MORTALITY

The percentage reduction in mortality seen with angiotensin converting enzyme inhibition, especially in mild congestive heart failure, is small (e.g. approximately 4 per cent in the treatment arm of SOLVD), but because of the overall high mortality the absolute reduction is substantial. Nevertheless, even with angiotensin converting enzyme inhibitor treatment, mortality remains high and the benefit falls far short of that obtained with transplantation (Fig. 6).

Effect on myocardial ischaemia and infarction

Several studies have investigated the potential anti-ischaemic effect of angiotensin converting enzyme inhibitors in patients with coronary artery disease, hypertension, and heart failure. Conflicting results have been obtained, with some studies showing a reduction, some no effect, and, in one study, an increase in angina. These disparities may reflect a variable decrease in blood pressure and, therefore of coronary perfusion that may occur after starting the angiotensin converting enzyme inhibitor.

The effect of angiotensin converting enzyme inhibitors on myocardial infarction seems more consistent; in both the SOLVD and SAVE studies there was a reduction of about 25 per cent in the risk of myocardial infarction. A 20 per cent reduction in admissions for unstable angina was also reported in SOLVD, although this did not become apparent until after 6 to 12 months treatment.

These findings require explanation. An association between the renin–angiotensin system activation and myocardial infarction has been described in hypertension. More recently angiotensin converting enzyme genotype has been related to the risk of myocardial infarction, the DD deletion increasing the risk. Experimentally, angiotensin converting enzyme inhibitors reduce the development of atherosclerosis, but other possible explanations exist. Whatever the explanation, SOLVD and SAVE do not support the 'J-shaped curve' hypothesis for the failure of blood pressure-lowering therapy to reduce the rate of myocardial infarction in hypertensives.

Place in management

The unique effects of angiotensin converting enzyme inhibitors on survival, disease progression and the development of myocardial infarction make them mandatory treatment in all grades of symptomatic heart failure. In most studies angiotensin converting enzyme inhibitors have been combined with diuretics and, when used alone they have proved inadequate.

Fig. 5 (a) Cumulative mortality in CONSENSUS I. Clear survival advantage of enalapril is obvious as is the overall poor prognosis of severe heart failure. (b) Cumulative mortality in SOLVD Treatment trial (T). Significant survival advantage of enalapril is noted.

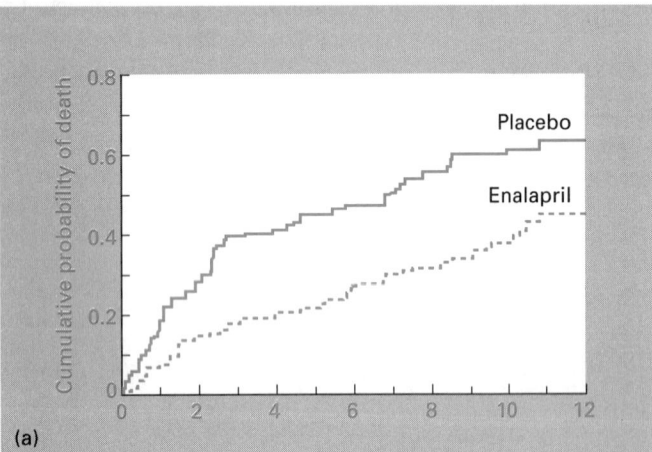

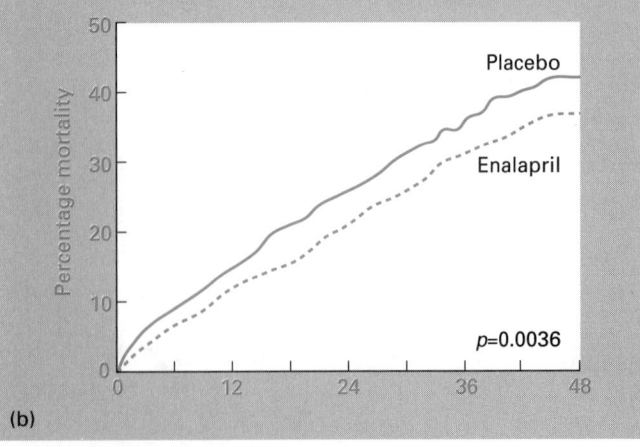

Fig. 6 Comparison of effects on survival of enalapril in CONSENSUS I and of transplantation.

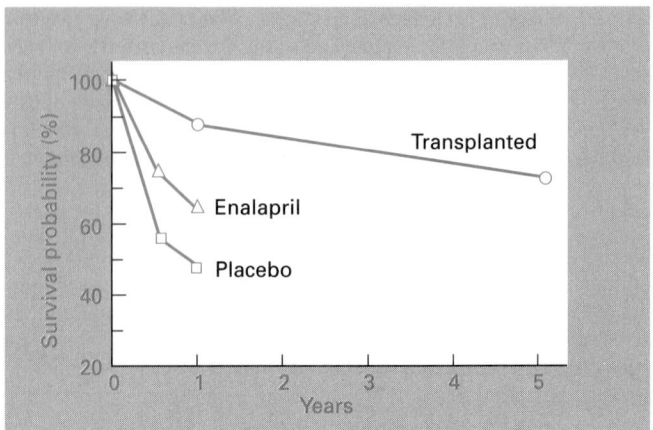

Use of angiotensin converting enzyme inhibitors to treat heart failure

An angiotensin converting enzyme inhibitor is indicated primarily in heart failure due to left ventricular systolic dysfunction. Patients with mitral or aortic valvular regurgitation should also be considered. Only a minority show intolerance of an angiotensin converting enzyme inhibitor, though certain precautions should be taken before treatment is started (Table 2).

It should be possible to begin angiotensin converting enzyme inhibition in most patients with mild or moderate heart failure without admission to hospital, but in those with severe heart failure on high doses of diuretics admission is essential.

A low dose should be given initially (e.g. 2 to 6.25 mg captopril, 2.5 mg enalapril). The patient should remain seated or supine until the peak haemodynamic effect of the drug has been observed (1 to 2 h with captopril, 2 to 6 h with other angiotensin converting enzyme inhibitors). Head-down tilt of the bed and intravenous saline will usually correct symptomatic hypotension. Once treatment has been successfully introduced, the dose can be increased to achieve maximum symptomatic benefit, though this may be delayed for weeks or months.

WHAT DOSE SHOULD BE USED?

Most published studies showing efficacy have used large doses, e.g. captopril 50 mg thrice daily and enalapril 10 mg twice daily. More recently, in a retrospective study of patients awaiting cardiac transplantation, those receiving higher dose captopril fared significantly better and neuroendocrine suppression was greater than did the low dose group. The available evidence, therefore, favours using the highest tolerated dose.

Adverse effects

First dose hypotension

The term 'first dose' hypotension refers to the uncommon occurrence of a sometimes precipitous fall in blood pressure, occasionally accompanied by a bradycardia in response to the first dose of an angiotensin converting enzyme inhibitor. Severe reductions in blood pressure of this type are usually only seen in volume depleted patients, and the incidence of first dose hypotension is greater in more ill patients on larger doses of diuretic. In patients at risk a small test dose of a short-acting angiotensin converting enzyme inhibitor is advisable, e.g. captopril 2 mg or perhaps 6.25 mg, with close observation of the blood pressure response over the subsequent 1 to 2 h. Correction of fluid–volume status may permit subsequent uncomplicated reintroduction of an angiotensin converting enzyme inhibitor in patients who have shown this phenomenon. It is also important to ensure that significant pulmonary or obstructive valve disease has not been missed and that the patient does not have an unusual type of heart muscle disease causing poor compliance (diastolic dysfunction), for example, amyloid.

SUBSEQUENT HYPOTENSION

Hypotension is often a feature of advanced heart failure, but angiotensin converting enzyme inhibitors rarely exacerbate this significantly. Symptomatic hypotension, when it occurs, is often due to volume depletion in response to overuse of diuretics. In such a case the first move should be to reduce the dose of diuretic rather than of the angiotensin converting enzyme inhibitor; arrhythmias as a cause of 'dizziness' must not be forgotten.

RENAL DYSFUNCTION

Long-term small increases in creatinine (i.e. > 175 μmol/l) are common when angiotensin converting enzyme inhibitions are used to treat advanced heart failure, but serious renal dysfunction is rare. As with hypotension, renal dysfunction can be aggravated by volume depletion. Therefore, if a significant increase in creatinine (> 200 μmol/l or > 25 per cent rise) occurs, and the patient has no overt evidence of fluid retention, the diuretic dose should be reduced. Conversely, if the patient is volume overloaded, the dose of angiotensin converting enzyme inhibitor should be reduced. In both circumstances, great care must be taken and frequent monitoring of blood chemistry is essential.

Coprescribing of a non-steroidal anti-inflammatory drug may lead to renal impairment and must be avoided or only employed with caution.

HYPERKALAEMIA

Modest hyperkalaemia (plasma potassium 4.6 to 5.8 mmol/l) is to be expected when angiotensin converting enzyme inhibitors are given to patients whose glomerular filtration rate is less than 20 to 30 ml/min. Hyperkalaemia was also detected in 6.3 per cent of placebo-treated and 18.9 per cent of enalapril-treated patients in the CONSENSUS I study, but no patients in either group were withdrawn for that reason; approximately half of patients randomized in this trial were taking spironolactone. Volume depletion and extrarenal uraemia increase the likelihood of hyperkalaemia with angiotensin converting enzyme inhibitors and coprescription of a non-steroidal anti-inflammatory or potassium-conserving diuretic also much increases the risk.

COUGH

Cough is commonly reported by patients with heart failure. There is a small but significant increase in its incidence during angiotensin converting enzyme inhibitor therapy but, in the trials, this has not led to more withdrawals in the actively treated patients. Cough should therefore not be attributed immediately to angiotensin converting enzyme inhibitor, and pulmonary congestion or airways obstruction must be excluded; even if it is due to the angiotensin converting enzyme inhibitor, the patient may be able to tolerate it and in some it may, on occasion, resolve spontaneously.

OTHER ADVERSE EFFECTS

Taste disturbance, skin rash, proteinuria, and leucopenia have been rare in the recent trials. Angio-oedema certainly occurs but was no more common after enalapril than placebo in the SOLVD study.

Drug interactions

The most important is between an angiotensin converting enzyme inhibitor and a non-steroidal anti-inflammatory when serious renal dysfunction may ensue. Careful serial checking of blood chemistry is mandatory when a non-steroidal anti-inflammatory is given to a patient with heart failure being treated with an angiotensin converting enzyme inhibitor.

Table 2 *Guidelines for starting ACE inhibitors*

Confirm left ventricular systolic dysfunction (e.g. by echocardiography)
Check routine blood chemistry
Temporarily omit diuretic for 24 to 36 h
Stop potassium supplements or potassium-sparing diuretics
Initiate therapy under supervision
Consider admission if:
  > 80 mg frusemide/equivalent
  systolic blood pressure < 100 mmHg
  serum creatinine > 200 μmol/l
  serum potassium > 5.0 mmol/l
  History of CVA or TIA
  Peripheral vascular disease

Other inhibitors of the renin–angiotensin system

The renin inhibitors and angiotensin II receptor antagonists are as yet agents used in research rather than clinical practice. It may be that the sometimes troublesome side-effect of angiotensin converting enzyme inhibition of cough, will be eliminated, but on the other hand, any contribution to peripheral vasodilatation afforded by the presumed increase in bradykinin as a result of angiotensin converting enzyme inhibition will be lacking.

NEUTRAL ENDOPEPTIDASE INHIBITORS

In patients with heart failure, circulating levels of atrial and brain natriuretic peptide are elevated. Indeed it has been suggested that plasma concentrations of these agents are directly and closely related to the extent of left ventricular dysfunction and might provide for the future a marker for the presence of underlying left ventricular systolic dysfunction.

A number of inhibitors of the breakdown of atrial natriuretic peptide are under investigation in clinical trials. In theory such agents by causing peripheral vasodilatation and an increase in sodium and water excretion without stimulation of the renin angiotensin system would have an ideal haemodynamic and neuroendocrine profile. Preliminary haemodynamic studies confirm a reduction in preload and afterload but with little effect on cardiac output and heart rate. In short-term studies of oral candoxatril, one such neutral endopeptidase inhibitor, persistent elevations of atrial natriuretic peptide have been found in association with natriuresis and diuresis which over 24 h is similar to 40 mg of frusemide. It remains to be seen whether these agents will find a place in clinical practice.

EPOPROSTENOL (PROSTACYCLIN)

Epoprostenol is an unstable prostaglandin with pulmonary and, to a lesser degree, systemic vasodilator activity. One small study suggested beneficial effects on symptoms, signs and functional capacity. However a large multicentre controlled trial has just been terminated prematurely because of adverse effects on well-being and survival in the epoprostenol group.

PRAZOSIN

Prazosin is an α-adrenoceptor antagonist with acute venous and arterial vasodilator effects. Rapid tachyphylaxis, with neuroendocrine activation, is seen. Prazosin has no sustained beneficial effect on symptoms or functional capacity. In V-HeFT I prazosin did not reduce mortality in men with mainly NYHA Class II/III heart failure. At the present time, neither prazosin nor other of the adrenoceptor antagonists play a major role in the routine treatment of patients with heart failure.

Conclusion

Despite side-effects, tailored vasodilator therapy can have impressive effects on some individuals with severe heart failure. In selected patients, results comparable to those of cardiac transplantation can be achieved in terms of effort capacity and quality of life.

Vasodilators having been the most important advance in the therapy of heart failure for many years, and there is considerable interest in the development of new compounds. As research into vascular function in heart failure becomes more sophisticated, so a larger number agents targeted to specific mechanisms are likely to emerge.

REFERENCES

Ambrosioni, E., Borghi, C., Degli Esposti, D., Bacchelli, S., Magnani, B. on behalf of the SMILE investigators (1992). Effects of early ACE-inhibition on short-term mortality and congestive heart failure in patients with acute anterior myocardial infarction. The SMILE experience. *European Heart Journal,* **13** (Suppl.), 154.

Binkley, P.F., Haas, G.J., Starling, R.C., *et al.* (1993). Sustained augmentation of parasympathetic tone with angiotensin-converting enzyme inhibition in patients with congestive heart failure. *Journal of the American College of Cardiologists,* **21,** 655–61.

Cambien, F., Poirer, O., Lecerf, L., *et al.* (1992). Deletion polymorphism in the gene for angiotensin-converting enzyme is a potent risk factor for myocardial infarction. *Nature* **359,** 641–644.

Captopril–Digoxin Multicenter Research Group (1988). Comparative effects of therapy with captopril and digoxin in patients with mild to moderate heart failure. *Journal of the American Medical Association,* **359,** 539–44.

Cleland, J.G.F., Dargie, H.J., Hodsman, G.P., *et al.* (1984). Captopril in heart failure: a double blind controlled trial. *British Heart Journal,* **52,** 530.

Cleland, J.G.F., Henderson, E., McLenachan, J., Findlay, I.N., and Dargie, H.J. (1991). Effect of captopril, an angiotensin-converting enzyme inhibitor, in patients with angina pectoris and heart failure. *Journal of the American College of Cardiologists,* **17,** 733–9.

Cohn, J.N., Johnson, G., Ziesche, S., *et al.* (1991). A comparison of enalapril with hydralazine-isosorbide dinitrate in the treatment of chronic congestive heart failure. *New England Journal of Medicine,* **325,** 303–10.

CONSENSUS Trial Study Group (1987). Effects of enalapril on mortality in severe congestive heart failure. *New England Journal of Medicine,* **316,** 1429–35.

Firth, B.G. (1988). The multifacetted role of angiotensin converting enzyme inhibitors in congestive heart failure. *American Journal of Medical Science,* **296,** 275–88.

Flapan, A.D., Davies, E., Waugh, C., Williams, B.C., Shaw, T.R.D., and Edwards, C.R.W. (1991). Acute administration of captopril lowers the natriuretic and diuretic response to a loop diuretic in patients with chronic cardiac failure. *European Heart Journal,* **12,** 924–7.

Gottlieb, S.S., Robinson, S., Weir, M.R., Fisher, M.L., and Krichten, C.M. (1992). Determinants of the renal response to ACE inhibition in patients with congestive heart failure. *American Heart Journal,* **124,** 131.

Handa, K., Sasaki, J., Tanaka, H., *et al.* (1991). Effects of captopril on opioid peptides during exercise and quality of life in normal subjects. *American Heart Journal,* **122,** 1389.

Heber, F.X., Niemolier, L., and Doering, W. (1992). Impact of converting enzyme inhibition on progression of chronic heart failure: results of the Munich Mild Heart Failure Trial. *British Heart Journal,* **67,** 289–296.

Ljungman, S., Kjekshus, J., Swedberg, K. for the CONSENSUS Trial Group (1992). Renal function in severe congestive heart failure during treatment with enalapril (the Cooperative North Scandinavian Enalapril Survival Study [CONSENSUS] Trial). *American Journal of Cardiology,* **70,** 479–87.

McLay, J., McMurray, J., Bridges, A.B., and Struthers, A.D. (1993). Captopril attenuates the natriuretic and diuretic responses to frusemide in chronic heart failure. *American Heart Journal,* (in press)

McMurray, J. and Dargie, H.J. (1992). ACE inhibitors for myocardial infarction and unstable angina. *Lancet* **340,** 1547–48.

McMurray, J. and McInnes, G. (1992). The J-curve hypothesis. *Lancet* **i,** 561–562.

Nishimura, H., Kubo, S., Ueyama, M., Kubota, J., and Kawamura, K. (1989). Peripheral hemodynamic effects of captopril in patients with congestive heart failure. *American Heart Journal,* **117,** 100–5.

Oster, J.R. and Materson, B.J. (1992). Renal and electrolyte complications of congestive heart failure and effects of therapy with angiotensin-converting enzyme inhibitors. *Archives of Internal Medicine,* **152,** 704–10.

Pfeffer, M.A., Braunwald, E., Moye, L.A., *et al.* (1992). Effect of captopril on mortality and morbidity in patients with left ventricular dysfunction after myocardial infarction: results of the Survival and Ventricular Enlargement Trial. *New England Journal of Medicine,* **327,** 669–77.

SOLVD Investigators (1991). Effect of enalapril on survival in patients with reduced left ventricular ejection fractions and congestive heart failure. *New England Journal of Medicine,* **325,** 293–302.

SOLVD Investigators (1992). Effect of enalapril on mortality and the development of heart failure in asymptomatic patients with reduced left ventricular ejection fractions. *New England Journal of Medicine,* **327,** 685–91.

Suki, W.N. (1989). Renal hemodynamic consequences of angiotensin-converting enzyme inhibition in congestive heart failure. *Archives of Internal Medicine,* **149,** 669–73.

Tan, L.-B., Jalil, J.E., Pick, R., Janicki, S., and Weber, K.T. (1991). Cardiac myocyte necrosis induced by angiotensin II. *Circulation Research,* **69,** 1185–1195.

15.6.4 Catecholamines and the sympathetic nervous system

J.C. FORFAR

Introduction

Many of the minute-to-minute adjustments in performance of the circulation depend on changes in sympathetic nervous activity through regulation of systemic vascular resistance, the inotropic state of the myocardium and venous capacitance. Understanding of the nature and consequences of activation of this control system has been progressive over this century and has led to the development of natural and synthetic agents of value in circulatory support.

Adrenergic neurotransmission

Sympathetic preganglionic efferent nerves represent the final common pathway for neural impulses to the cardiovascular system. They connect cardiovascular centres in the medulla to the heart and vasculature, receiving both excitatory and inhibitory impulses from many levels within the central nervous system, especially from mechanoreceptors in the carotid sinus, aorta, and the heart. Higher centre influences from the cerebral cortex, hypothalamus and pons regulate the medullary vasomotor centre.

The cell bodies of the preganglionic neurons lie within the spinal cord and exit via the thoracic and upper lumber nerves to synapse in the peripheral sympathetic ganglia running in a paraspinal chain. The adrenal medulla is innervated directly by preganglionic fibres passing through the splanchnic nerves to synapse directly with the secretory cells that predominantly release adrenaline. Sympathetic nerves from the right stellate ganglion are distributed mainly to the sinus node and right atrium and ventricle while on the left, the ventrolateral cardiac nerve provides a major sympathetic supply to the left atrium and posterior and lateral surfaces of the left ventricle.

Noradrenaline, the natural transmitter for sympathetic nerves is synthesized and stored in sympathetic nerve terminals in neurosecretory granules. Neuronal depolarization releases intraneuronal calcium causing the granules to migrate to the neuronal membrane and release noradrenaline into the synaptic cleft. The effects of released neurotransmitter are terminated principally by neuronal uptake, an energy dependent process. Intraneuronal noradrenaline may be taken back up into the neurosecretory granule or oxidized (monoamine oxidase, MAO) to the principal intraneuronal metabolite, dihydroxyphenylethylene glycol (DHPG). Smaller quantities of released noradrenaline escape to the circulation or are taken up into the effector cell for methylation by catechol-O-methyl transferase (COMT) to normetranephine. Both oxidation and methylation of noradrenaline can occur in many organs including the liver, kidney and gut.

Adrenergic pharmacology

The descriptive classification of adrenergic receptors into alpha and beta subtypes has been considerably refined since their discovery 45 years ago (Table 1) and now includes α-1, α-2, β-1, β-2, and dopamine receptor subtypes. Further subtypes have been described although their clinical importance is less certain. Activity of the sympathetic nervous system has been defined in terms of efferent neural discharge, noradrenaline release at nerve terminals, target receptor availability and occupancy and effector cell response. From a clinical perspective each element of activity may be important. In chronic heart failure, for example, cardiac efferent sympathetic activity is increased coupled with impairment of neuronal reuptake further increasing intrasynaptic noradrenaline con-

Table 1 Adrenergic receptor subtypes

Receptor	Action on circulation
α-1	Vasoconstriction (increase in contractility)
α-2	Vasoconstriction. Presynaptic sympathetic inhibition.
β-1	Increase in heart rate (sinus node)
	Increase in contractility (atrium, and ventricle)
	Increase in conduction (atrioventricular node)
β-2	Vasodilatation (bronchodilatation).
Dopaminergic-1	Renal and mesenteric vasodilatation.
Dopaminergic-2	Vasodilatation

centration. However, tolerance to the action of both endogenous and exogenous catecholamines arises through β-adrenoceptor down regulation.

The physiologically occurring catecholamines – noradrenaline, adrenaline, and dopamine and their synthetic derivatives, isoprenaline, dobutamine, salbutamol, and dopexamine – interact with the six adrenoceptor subtypes shown in Table 1 according to the specificity and affinity of the various agonists for these receptors (Table 2). Stimulation of the β-adrenoceptor increases the intracellular concentration of cyclic adenosine monophosphate (cAMP) through a transcription process involving activation of membrane adenylate cyclase. The molecular mechanisms involve the β-adrenoceptor, the catalytic unit (adenylate cyclase) and a guanyl nucleotide-binding regulatory protein. The latter exchanges guanine triphosphate (GTP) for guanine diphosphate and modulates the affinity of agonist for its receptor (leading to dissociation) while activating the adenylate cyclase complex. An opposite change in cyclic adenosine monophosphate follows stimulation of α-2-adrenoceptors, the process requiring guanine triphosphate. The main intracellular signal following α-1-adrenoceptor stimulation appears to be a rise in cytoplasmic calcium. Membrane phosphatidylinositol turnover is increased and cytoplasmic cyclic guanine monophosphate levels rise.

Phosphodiesterase (PDE) is the intracellular enzyme responsible for degradation of the cyclic adenosine monophosphate 'second messenger' system. Phosphodiesterase exists in several distinct forms characterized by affinity for cyclic adenosine monophosphate, membrane binding, and response to calmodulin. Drugs such as theophylline act through a nonselective inhibition of phosphodiesterase. Milrinone is a bipyridine derivative that selectively inhibits the third isoform of phosphodiesterase and shows inotropic activity through augmentation of the intracellular cyclic adenosine monophosphate messenger system. Enoximone is an imidazolone inhibiting the fourth isoform of phosphodiesterase.

The concept of adrenoceptor classification suggests that different receptor subtypes are coupled to different cellular signals. However, differentiated signal transformation by receptor subtypes has not been clearly demonstrated throughout the heart and circulation. A further mechanism of differential response can be achieved by receptor prevalence and availability in different organs. Human ventricular muscle contains predominantly β-1-adrenoceptor subtypes in close proximity to the adrenergic synapse, mediating an inotropic response. The sinoatrial node, however, may respond preferentially to β-2-adrenoceptors distributed throughout the specialized tissue and responsive to circulating catecholamines (adrenaline/noradrenaline) as well as neuronally released noradrenaline.

Haemodynamic profiles and usage of catecholamines

Catecholamines are mainly used intravenously to enhance the inotropic state of the heart, although both salbutamol and low-dose dopamine have

Table 2 *Adrenergic receptor activity of endogenous and synthetic catecholamines*

Catecholamine	Receptor subtypes					
	α-1	α-2	β-1	β-2	DA-1	DA-2
Dopamine	++	+	++	0	+++	++
Noradrenaline	+++	++	+++	+−	0	0
Adrenaline	++	++	+++	++	0	0
Isoprenaline	0	0	+++	+++	0	0
Dobutamine	+	+−	+++	++	0	0
Salbutamol	0	0	+	+++	0	0
Dopexamine	0	0	+	++	++	+

the useful actions of peripheral, splanchnic or renal vasodilatation and noradrenaline may cause vasoconstriction. Catecholamines are used principally to provide short-term circulatory support, for example during ventilation with positive end-expiratory pressure, following cardiac surgery and in various shock states. Adrenaline also has a role in the emergency management of anaphylactic shock and during cardiopulmonary resuscitation.

An increase in inotropic state of the heart, while increasing stroke volume for a given filling pressure, also increases myocardial oxygen consumption to a greater or lesser extent. An increase in heart rate will further augment oxygen demand as will the development of tachyarrhythmias. Catecholamine usage in an individual patient requires careful consideration of the balance between augmented short-term cardiac performance and longer-term adverse effects of myocardial oxygen demands.

DOPAMINE

This endogenous catecholamine is the biosynthetic precursor of noradrenaline and a central nervous system transmitter. Effects on the circulation are dose-dependent. Vasodilatation is mediated by specific dopaminergic receptors distributed widely in the peripheral circulation as well as the nervous system. The renal and mesenteric circulation, and to a lesser extent the coronary and cerebrovascular circulation dilate at low-dose infusion (Table 3). The most important clinical effect is on the kidney with increased renal blood flow, glomerular filtration, and natriuresis. This action is especially useful in the management of persistent heart failure associated with reversible reduction in myocardial contractility or with impaired diuretic responsiveness as a result of renal artery vasoconstriction. Dopaminergic vasodilatation is antagonized by phenothiazines such as chlorpromazine and by butyrophenones such as haloperidol.

Higher doses of dopamine activate β-1-adrenoceptors leading to an increase in myocardial contractility and heart rate. Tachycardia is restrained through a baroreceptor reflex mechanism after activation of α-1-adrenoceptors and increase in blood pressure and through some effect on presynaptic α-2-adrenoceptors decreasing noradrenaline release. These actions increase myocardial oxygen demand yet may augment coronary perfusion pressure. High-dose dopamine infusion leads to dominant α-1-adrenoceptor actions and peripheral vasoconstriction.

Infusion of dopamine has greatest clinical use at low and medium dose when the renal vasodilator action and some inotropic effect are of greatest value.

NORADRENALINE

The main clinical actions of noradrenaline are α-receptor mediated vasoconstriction and β-1-adrenoceptor mediated enhancement of contractility. Arteriolar vasoconstriction significantly increases blood pressure and cardiac output usually decreases. Heart rate usually falls because of dominance of baroreceptor mediated vagal stimulation and sympathetic

Table 3 *Catecholamine dosage*

Drug	Infusion rate (μg/kg/min)
Dopamine dopaminergic	1–5
β-1	5–10
β-1/α	10–40
Noradrenaline	0.01–0.07
Adrenaline	0.06–0.18
Isoprenaline	0.01–0.15
Dobutamine	2.5–10

withdrawal (as a result of elevated blood pressure) over β-1-adrenoceptor stimulation. Vasoconstriction is most intense in peripheral vascular beds with substantial reductions in muscle, skin, hepatic, and renal blood flow. Noradrenaline actions on the myocardium result from increased after-load (arteriolar vasoconstriction), increased preload (venoconstriction) and increased contractility. Myocardial oxygen demand will increase along with coronary perfusion pressure.

Noradrenaline has clinical usefulness in short term improvement in the cerebral and coronary circulations in some shock states and during resuscitation and may be used to counteract hypotension as a result of vasodilator therapy. It has little role in the longer term especially with primary cardiac disease when adverse effects on oxygen demand are likely to be hazardous. As with other catecholamines used over a prolonged period, there is a risk of peripheral gangrene.

ADRENALINE

The endogenous adrenal medullary hormone is widely used as an exogenous catecholamine and acts on α- and β-adrenoceptors most notably the β-1-adrenoceptors in the heart. Augmented cardiac contractility and increases in heart rate, automaticity and conduction are progressive and dose-dependent. Vasoconstriction and increase in blood pressure are less pronounced than with noradrenaline. At low dose, systemic vascular resistance may fall while at higher doses vasoconstriction is evident. Myocardial oxygen demand is substantially and progressively increased by this drug and tachycardia and cardiac arrhythmias may limit clinical usefulness particularly with acute circulatory failure. The main use of adrenaline is for short-term acute inotropic support, for example during cardiopulmonary resuscitation.

ISOPRENALINE

Isoprenaline is a synthetic catecholamine with powerful β-adrenoceptor stimulatory actions. Direct effects include increases in heart rate, inotropic state and atrioventricular conduction and automaticity. Peripheral vascular and pulmonary vascular resistance fall from β-2-adrenoceptor stimulation. Systolic blood pressure may rise from the cardiac effects of this drug although diastolic pressure normally falls. Myocardial oxygen consumption increases greatly as a result of these actions and arrhythmias and provocation of myocardial ischaemia frequently limit dose.

Isoprenaline is most frequently used for its chronotropic action as a short-term intravenous infusion in patients with symptomatic bradycardia, for example heart block. The infusion rate may be adjusted to achieve a heart rate alleviating acute symptoms and pending longer term management such as cardiac pacing. Rarely, oral medication (30 to 60 mg 6-hourly) is necessary if other chronotrophic measures are not available.

DOBUTAMINE

Substitution of the isoprenaline molecule has allowed a drug with some β-1-adrenoceptor selectivity and hence less effect on the sinus node and on heart rate. Enhancement of left ventricular contractile activity provides a useful short-term role for this drug in shock states with primary or secondary ventricular disease. Effects on heart rate and arrhythmogenesis, however, are not infrequently limiting.

SALBUTAMOL

This β-2-adrenoceptor agonist is of greatest value in the management of bronchial asthma but causes peripheral vasodilatation and hence afterload reduction. Increases in heart rate, however, limit clinical usefulness and alternative vasodilator agents are usually to be preferred.

DOPEXAMINE

Dopexamine is a dopamine analogue acting on β-2-adrenoceptors and some dopamine receptors. The combined effects of renal, hepatic, and splanchnic vasodilatation with peripheral vasodilatation offer a hae-modynamic profile that may be of value although increases in heart rate, as with dobutamine, can restrict its use.

PHOSPHODIESTERASE INHIBITORS

Emoximone and milrinone are selective phosphodiasterase inhibitors with primary myocardial effects. These drugs increase cardiac contractility, promote ventricular relaxation and cause modest peripheral vasodilatation. As with catecholamines, improvements in myocardial performance are short lived, although it has been claimed that increases in myocardial oxygen consumption are modest. Both atrial and ventricular arrhythmias may be increased.

The search for effective orally active inotropic agents effective in the long term has been elusive. Catecholamine derivitives, partial β-adrenoceptor agonists and phosphodiesterase inhibitors have all been evaluated but, while short-term haemodynamic benefit has been confirmed, long-term adverse effects on survival have led to withdrawal of the product or limitations of its use. Intermittent pulsed therapy of certain catecholamines are under current investigation to determine whether β-adrenoceptor down regulation is reversed and functional capacity improved in chronic heart failure.

REFERENCES

Curfman, G.D. (1991). Inotropic therapy for heart failure: an unfulfilled promise. *New England Journal of Medicine,* **325,** 1509–10.

Hoffman, B.B. and Lefkowitz, R.J. (1990). Catecholamines and sympatho-mimetic drugs. In *The pharmacological basis of therapeutics* (eds L.S. Goodman, and A.G. Gilman), pp. 187–220. Pergamon Press, New York.

Smith, T.W., Braunuald, E., and Kelly, R.A. (1992). The management of heart failure. In *Heart disease: a textbook of cardiovascular medicine.* (ed E Braunuald), (pp. 500–509). WB Saunders, Philadelphia.

Stiles, G.L. and Lefkowitz, R.J. (1984). Cardiac adrenergic receptors. *Annual Reviews of Medicine,* **35,** 149–64.

15.7 Cardiac transplantation

J.H. DARK

The surgical technique of cardiac replacement had been described in 1960 by Lower and Shumway, but only with effective immunosuppression, and particularly the introduction of cyclosporin in 1981, was widespread clinical success achieved. After rapid expansion in the past decade, numbers of patients transplanted have reached a plateau, with approximately 300 annually in the United Kingdom and 3000 to 4000 throughout the world.

Patient selection

INDICATIONS FOR TRANSPLANTATION

The aetiology of heart failure will be either idiopathic dilated cardiomyopathy or ischaemic heart disease in more than 90 per cent of all recipients. Of those aged over 55 years, 75 per cent will have ischaemic disease, with a striking male predominance. Other presenting diagnoses are shown in Table 1. Patients with congenital heart disease are often excluded because of a high pulmonary vascular resistance secondary to uncorrected shunts. However, an increasing number of those who had palliative procedures as children are now presenting with irreversible ventricular failure in early adulthood.

Transplantation for an active myocarditis is associated with a poor outcome, in some instances because the inflammatory process goes on

Table 1 *Indications for transplantation*

Ischaemic cardiomyopathy
Idiopathic dilated cardiomyopathy
Congenital heart disease
Valvular heart disease
Restrictive/obstructive cardiomyopathy
Anthracycline toxicity

to affect the new heart. When the heart is involved in a systemic disease, such as sarcoid or amyloidosis, compromise of other organs, such as the lungs or kidneys will often determine survival, and thus the long-term results may be poor.

Almost regardless of aetiology, referral for transplantation should only be made when conventional treatment, both medical and surgical, has failed to control the symptoms and signs of cardiac failure, and the anticipated prognosis is clearly worse than that offered by transplantation. Most patients will have had a thorough trial of angiotensin-converting enzyme inhibitors and high-dose diuretics, together with digoxin and antiarrythmic drugs when indicated. If there is any suggestion of reversible ischaemic damage, for instance in the patient with angina in addition to dyspnoea, coronary artery surgery should be seriously considered before transplantation.

Although the prognosis of even optimally treated patients with heart failure is poor in the long term, selection of those to be given an early transplant may be difficult. Up to 40 per cent of recipients will have been unable to leave hospital prior to transplantation often because they were receiving intravenous inotropes. Other markers of poor prognosis such as low left ventricular ejection fraction, cardiac index, or serum sodium (and the list is almost endless) do not consistently predict the patients at risk of early death, which should be the criterion for selection for urgent transplantation. Although complex, exercise testing with measurement of maximum oxygen uptake (MVo_2) may be the best available means of predicting confidently those with the worst prognosis. In one study, only 30 per cent of patients with an MVo_2 below 14 ml/kg/min survived for 12 months.

CONTRAINDICATIONS TO TRANSPLANTATION

Not every patient with endstage cardiac failure is suitable for a cardiac transplant. Careful screening of individuals with irreversible failure of other organs is essential to success. A list of standard exclusions is shown in Table 2. The 'absolute' contraindications are universally accepted and imply a low chance of survival if they are ignored. Thus if there is a high, fixed pulmonary vascular resistance there will be fatal, acute right ventricular failure of the previously normal donor heart after transplantation. In practice, all patients with any degree of left ventricular failure will have at least some pulmonary vasoconstriction and the risk of early death is related to the pulmonary vascular resistance as well as to many other factors.

All the 'relative' contraindications are associated with a higher postoperative risk, and, in general, the sickest patients are both those with the greatest need of transplantation, and also those with the least chance of surviving after the operation. An individual assessment has to be made in each case, considering not only his or her need, but also the best use of a limited number of donor organs.

THE NUMERICAL DISCREPANCY BETWEEN RECIPIENTS AND DONORS

The number of patients who could benefit from cardiac transplantation is estimated to be 20 to 60 per million of population. Against this figure must be set the number of cardiac donors, approximately 6 per million in the United Kingdom, although a little higher in the United States, and up to 10 per million in some countries, for instance France. It is clearly important to avoid transplanting those who are too sick to have any worthwhile chance of survival.

Perioperative management

THE CARDIAC DONOR

After brain-stem death occurs, the heart continues to beat but there is a progressive loss of homeostatic control. This includes hypotension with loss of vascular tone, compounded by a polyuria and hypothermia. Appropriate corrections include administration of antidiuretic hormone analogues (usually intranasal DDAVP), intravenous fluids, and often peripheral vasocontrictors.

The initial damage to the brain is usually intracerebral or subarachnoid haemorrhage, or head trauma. Positive serology for HIV and hepatitis B, previous cardiac surgery, or a known history of ischaemic heart disease are contraindications to cardiac donation, as are prolonged periods of hypotension. Older donors, into their fifties or even sixties are acceptable if they have normal coronary arteries. Intravenous drug abuse (because of its association with HIV infection) is a contraindication, as is more than occasional use of cocaine. Brain-steam death following

Table 2 *Contraindications to transplantation*

Absolute
Coexistent systemic illness with poor prognosis
Active infection
Malignancy
Elevated PVR > 8 Wood units
Severe peripheral or cerebrovascular disease
Relative
Insulin dependent diabetes
Obesity
Recent pulmonary embolism
Peptic ulcer disease
Elevated PVR > 4 Wood units
Psychosocial instability

PVR, pulmonary vascular resistance.

tricyclic antidepressant overdose or carbon monoxide poisoning may be associated with specific damage to the heart.

The heart to be transplanted will often come from a 'multiorgan donor' comprising lungs, liver, kidneys, and occasionally pancreas. After removal, the heart is cooled rapidly to 4 °C and will remain viable for up to 4 to 5 h, allowing transport across hundreds or even thousands of miles.

MATCHING OF RECIPIENT AND DONOR

The donor should be blood-group compatible (but not necessarily identical) with the recipient, and size discrepancies of more than 20 to 30 per cent should be avoided. Although HLA matching, particularly of the DR antigens, would probably reduce rejection of the transplanted heart, time constraints and the clinical state of many recipients often makes this impossible.

Some 5 to 10 per cent of recipients are presensitized to HLA antigens by blood transfusion, pregnancy, or a previous transplant, and preformed antibodies can cause immediate or hyperacute rejection, usually fatal. Before a transplant is performed from a particular donor, recipient serum is tested against donor cells to exclude a positive or cytotoxic crossmatch in this group of patients.

IMPLANTATION

The native heart is removed, leaving most of the atria and length of aorta and pulmonary artery, after the recipient has been placed on cardiopulmonary bypass. Implantation is technically straightforward but small doses of inotrope (usually isoprenaline) are used for the first 24 to 48 h and temporary pacing may be required for up to 3 weeks. A permanent pacing system will be required by 3 to 5 per cent of patients.

Postoperative management is as for any cardiac surgical procedure, with transfer to an intensive care unit and thence to the recovery ward within a few days. Reverse barrier nursing is no longer used unless the patient is undergoing augmented immunosuppression (see below) and discharge from hospital within 12 to 15 days is to be expected.

Immunosuppression and rejection

From shortly after it is re-perfused, the allografted heart evokes an immune response in the recipient, mediated principally by T lymphocytes (cellular rejection) although antibodies play a supplementary role. The immune response is most vigorous early after the transplant, and gradually diminishes towards (but does not reach) a state of acquired immune tolerance. The response is greatly modified by immunosuppressant drugs, required in high doses early after the transplant, reducing to a maintenance level after a few months. Control of the immune process is variable, because drug activity may fluctuate (due to changes in absorption, rate of metabolism, or because doses have to be reduced) as may the strength of the immune response. Temporary loss of control is seen as an episode of rejection, with a histological appearance of necrosis of myocytes and infiltration of lymphocytes into the myocardium.

IMMUNOSUPPRESSION

Immunosuppression is achieved with three principal drugs: corticosteroids (usually prednisolone), cyclosporin A, and azathioprine. In some centres, particularly in the United States, induction therapy with specific antilymphocyte antibodies, such as the murine monoclonal OKT3, is also given. This reduces early rejection but at a cost of increased risk of infection and has little long-term advantage.

All the components of this triple drug regime are given in maximum tolerable doses for the first 4 to 6 weeks. Cyclosporin A is monitored by measuring trough levels: doses of 5 to 10 mg/kg/day are required for levels of around 400 ng/l, but deteriorating renal function often dictates a reduction in dose. For azathioprine a target leucocyte count of below 5000/mm^3 usually requires a dose of 1.5 to 3 mg/kg/day.

Prednisolone is typically given in a dose of 1 mg/kg/day, reducing to 0.2 mg/kg/day after a few weeks. Steroids may be successfully stopped after 3 months in a proportion of patients, and this is of particular advantage in the elderly who are less tolerant of steroid-induced morbidity. All of these drugs have short- and long-term side-effects, as shown in Table 3.

MONITORING FOR REJECTION EPISODES

Acute rejection, with infiltration of inflammatory cells and myocardial oedema causes diastolic dysfunction of the ventricle with preservation of systolic function. Clinical clues are often sparse, with perhaps a third sound, elevated filling pressures, and occasionally atrial flutter. Non-invasive tests are not generally helpful, although echocardiography has a role in children. Monitoring of the adequacy of immunosuppression is achieved by regular transvenous endomyocardial biopsy. Early after the transplant this is performed weekly, with lengthening intervals as time passes. If the biopsy shows a dense infiltrate of lymphocytes, and in particular, myocyte necrosis, augmented immunosuppression with intravenous methylprednisolone is given in a dose of 10 mg/kg/day for 3 days.

Infection after transplantation

The need for high levels of immunosuppression creates a substantial risk for infection, which is at its greatest in the early months. In the first few weeks typical postoperative bacterial infections predominate. These include pneumonias, wound and urinary tract infections, and sepsis related to indwelling arterial or venous catheters. Common organisms are *Haemophilus influenzae* and pneumococcus in the chest, coliforms in the urine, and staphylococcus in wounds or grown from line tips. Avoidance of broad-spectrum antibiotics helps to prevent overgrowth with Gram-negative organisms and emergence of fungal infections. The latter are usually associated with repeated augmented immunosuppression and can be life-threatening. Oral nystatin is used routinely to prevent oral pharyngeal candidiasis. Aspergillosis is the most significant fungal infection, usually as a pneumonia but sometimes in a disseminated form which is often fatal. Amphotericin B remains the drug of choice, although the orally administered itraconazole may have a role in prophylaxis of those who, for instance, are known to have their airways already colonized with Aspergillus.

Cytomegalovirus, the most common single agent to infect the post-transplant population occurs later, at 1 to 2 months. About 50 per cent of adults in the United Kingdom will have had previous exposure to this herpes virus, with seropositivity. A seronegative recipient of a heart

Table 3 *Side-effects of immunosuppressant drugs*

Cyclosporin
   Nephrotoxicity
   Hypertension
   Hirsutism
   Gingival hypertrophy
   Tremor, fits
Azathioprine
   Neutropenia
   Cholestatic jaundice
Steroids
   Cushingoid appearance
   Osteoporosis
   Myopathy
   Peptic ulceration
   Hyperglycaemia, hypercholesterolaemia

from a seropositive donor will almost certainly suffer a donor-acquired primary cytomegalovirus infection. This may be mild, with flu-like symptoms, or life-threatening, particularly if there is pneumonitis or gastrointestinal involvement. Prophylactic administration of pooled immunoglobulin, although expensive, will largely prevent serious complications after seropositive to seronegative cardiac transplants. Cytomegalovirus-seropositive patients may have a similar illness, either a reactivation of their previous infection after immunosuppression or a primary infection as a result of transmission of a different strain of cytomegalovirus from the donor. The illness tends to be less severe in this group.

The diagnosis of a serious cytomegalovirus infection is best made by biopsy of the appropriate organ (lung, stomach, colon), when the characteristic inclusion bodies may be seen. Ganciclovir is an effective drug, although side-effects, particularly neutropenia, can be troublesome.

INVESTIGATION OF PYREXIAL TRANSPLANT PATIENTS

Except for what appear to be life-threatening septic states, empirical antibiotics must be avoided. Cardiac rejection occasionally presents with a pyrexia and, certainly within the first year, this should be excluded by biopsy. Blood, urine, and sputum cultures should be obtained and, unless an obvious pathogen is easily identified, chest radiograph changes must be investigated by bronchoscopy and broncho-alveolar lavage. *Pneumocystis carinii* pneumonia may present with a relatively normal chest radiograph and inappropriate hypoxia; it is then best detected by bronchoalveolar lavage (see Section 7).

Treatment must be guided by specific diagnosis; some antibiotics, particularly erythromycin and rifampicin have serious interactions with cyclosporin.

Long-term complications

Despite excellent survival and functional rehabilitation, the transplant patient remains exposed to three areas of morbidity—drug side-effects, risks of continuous immunosuppression, and chronic rejection, usually manifested as accelerated coronary artery disease in the transplanted heart.

SIDE-EFFECTS OF IMMUNOSUPPRESSANTS

Almost all cardiac transplant recipients develop significant hypertension that in the past has been simply related to the use of cyclosporin. However, recipients of other solid organs, such as liver or lungs also given cyclosporin have a lower incidence of hypertension and there seems little doubt that a combination of preoperative disease, denervation of the heart, and inappropriate fluid retention puts these patients at particular risk. The antihypertensive drug of first choice is nifedipine, which ameliorates nephrotoxicity and does not interact with cyclosporin. Other calcium antagonists, particularly diltiazem, can lead to very high blood levels of cyclosporin.

Impaired glucose tolerance is common in patients receiving steroids and may require insulin treatment. Elevation of plasma lipids, including cholesterol, is similarly common and may be related to both the steroids and cyclosporin. Management is complicated by further drug interactions, particularly between 3-hydroxy-3-methylglutaryl-CoA reductase inhibitors and cyclosporin.

Many long-term recipients have considerably impaired renal function, and dialysis and/or renal transplantation is occasionally required. They may also have gout, but treatment with allopurinol must be cautious, because it potentiates the effects of azathioprine, and the latter may even have to be stopped.

THE EFFECTS OF CHRONIC IMMUNOSUPPRESSION

The transplant patient remains exposed to the risks of infections, particularly with opportunistic organisms, and in addition there is an increased risk of malignancy. The most common cancers after transplantation are of the skin, particularly those associated with exposure to the sunlight, and appropriate precautions must be taken.

POST-TRANSPLANT LYMPHOPROLIFERATIVE DISEASE

An increased incidence of non-Hodgkin's lymphoma has long been associated with chronic immunosuppression. It is now evident that these 'tumours' are nearly always of B-cell type and are an uncontrolled response to latent Epstein–Barr virus infection. Cyclosporin, and probably the other immunosuppressants as well, inhibit the suppressor T cells which usually exert an immunological control on Epstein–Barr virus-infected lymphocytes. With loss of control these lymphocytes proliferate, usually at extranodal sites and often in association with the transplanted organ. Reduction of the immunosuppression together with high-dose intravenous acyclovir will usually result in shrinkage and disappearance of these so-called 'lymphomas', which clearly are not truly malignant.

CORONARY DISEASE IN THE TRANSPLANTED HEART

Even in the absence of overt acute rejection there is probably continued immunological damage to the endothelium of the coronary arteries of the transplanted heart, which is the zone of contact with the recipient. This damaged endothelium leads to subintimal hyperplasia and thickening of the wall of the artery, which can be detected as early as 6 weeks after transplantation and is progressive. By 5 years after transplantation, 40 to 50 per cent of recipients will have developed qualitative angiographic evidence of this disease, and it will go on to be the most common late cause of death after transplantation.

Pathologically, this accelerated coronary disease differs substantially from typical atherosclerosis. It comprises a diffuse, symmetrical, and proliferating process resulting in cylindrical narrowing and involving intramuscular as well as epicardial vessels. It is not associated with pretransplant diagnosis, age of donor, blood pressure, lipids, or smoking. It does seem to be more severe in patients with a history of frequent early rejection episodes, lending credence to the immunological hypothesis of its origin. Because the transplanted heart undergoes complete denervation, angina seldom occurs and the usual presentation is either with sudden death or a silent myocardial infarction. Surveillance angiography remains the only effective means of diagnosis. Angioplasty for focal lesions has been described, but restenosis is frequent and the long-term benefit is questionable. The only effective treatment is retransplantation.

Results of transplantation

If conventional selection criteria are followed, most centres will report a 1-year survival of 85 to 90 per cent and a 5-year survival of 75 per cent. Long-term experience is scanty but extrapolation of survival curves suggests that 50 per cent of patients will live 10 or 12 years after their transplant. The great majority of late deaths will be due to accelerated coronary disease.

Functional rehabilitation is excellent. Patients may return to work and resume the full range of sporting and leisure pastimes.

REFERENCES

Billingham, M.E. (1987). Cardiac transplant atherosclerosis. *Transplantation Proceedings* **19**, 19–25.

Billingham, M.E., *et al.* (1990). A working formulation for standardisation of a nomenclature in the diagnosis of heart and lung rejection: heart rejection study group. *Journal of Heart and Lung Transplantation,* **9**, 587–93.

Dummer, J.S. (1990). Infectious complications of transplantation. *Cardiovascular Clinics* **20**, 163–78.

Freeman, R., Gould, F.K., and McMaster, A. (1990). Management of cytomegalovirus antibody negative patients undergoing heart transplantation. *Journal of Clinical Pathology* **43**, 373–6.

Frist, W.H., Oyer, P.E., Baldwin, J.C., Stinson, E.B., and Shumway, N.E. (1987). HLA compatibility and cardiac transplant recipient survival. *Annals of Thoracic Surgery* **44**, 242–6.

Kahan, B.D. (1989). Cyclosporin. *New England Journal of Medicine* **321**, 725–38.

Keogh, A.M., Barren, D.W. and Hickie, J.V. (1990). Prognostic guides in patients with idiopathic or ischaemic dilated cardiomyopathy assessed for cardiac transplantation. *American Journal of Cardiology* **65**, 903–8.

Mancini, D.M., Eisen, H., Kussmaul, W., Mull, R., Edmunds, L.H., and Wilson, J.R. (1991). Value of peak exercise oxygen consumption for optimal timing of cardiac transplantation in ambulatory patients with heart failure. *Circulation* **83**, 778–86.

Mark, A.L. (1990). Cyclosporine, sympathetic activity and hypertension. *New England Journal of Medicine* **323**, 748–50.

Miller, L.W. (1991). Long-term complications of cardiac transplantation. *Progress in Cardiovascular Disease* **33**, 229–82.

Opelz, G., and Henderson, R. (1993). Incidence of non-Hodgkin lymphoma in kidney and heart transplant recipients. *Lancet* **342**, 1514–16.

Rodeheffer, R.J. and McGregor, C.G.A. (1992). The development of cardiac transplantation. *Mayo Clinic Proceedings* **67**, 480–4.

Schroeder, J.S., *et al.* (1993). A preliminary study of Dilitazem in the prevention of coronary artery disease in heart transplantation recipients. *New England Journal of Medicine* **328**, 164–70.

Tazelaar, H.D. (1990). Spectrum and diagnosis of myocardial rejection. *Cardiology Clinics* **8**, 119–39.

15.8 Cardiac arrhythmias

15.8.1 Cardiac arrhythmias

S.M. COBBE AND A.C. RANKIN

General principles

Definition

The term cardiac arrhythmia (or dysrhythmia) is used to describe an abnormality of cardiac rhythm of any type. Normal sinus rhythm is arbitrarily defined as a rate between 60 and 100 per minute, and any disturbance from this is by definition an arrhythmia. The spectrum of cardiac arrhythmias ranges from innocent extrasystoles to immediately life-threatening conditions such as asystole or ventricular fibrillation. Arrhythmias may be present in the absence of cardiac disease, but are more commonly associated with structural heart disease or external provocative factors.

Fig. 1 The electrophysiology of the heart. The sinus node, atrioventricular node, and conducting system (His bundle, bundle branches, and Purkinje fibres) are illustrated. Examples of actions potentials are shown.

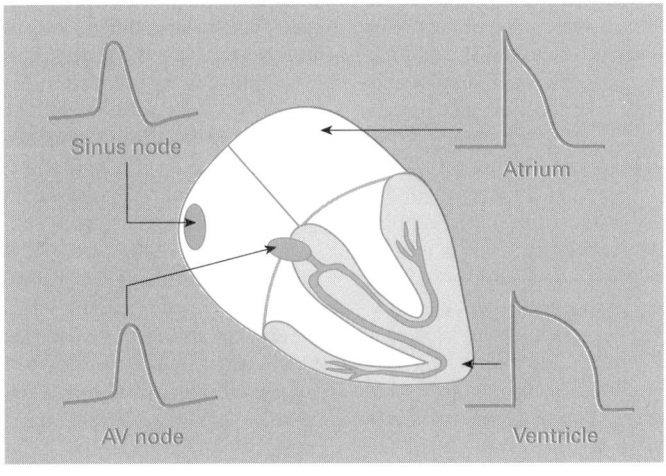

Aetiology and mechanisms

NORMAL ELECTROPHYSIOLOGY

The normal cardiac impulse originates from the pacemaker cells in the sinus node. These cells have an unstable membrane potential which tends towards spontaneous depolarization during diastole (Fig. 1). The rate of diastolic depolarization is accelerated by sympathetic stimulation and slowed by vagal stimulation. Conduction proceeds from the sinus node through the atrial myocardium to the atrioventricular (AV) node, through which it is conducted slowly resulting in the normal atrioventricular delay. Conduction distal to the atrioventricular node is via the bundle of His, the bundle branches, and the ramifications of the Purkinje system, which results in rapid activation of both ventricles. The atrioventricular node and the His–Purkinje system are also capable of spontaneous pacemaker activity, but at slower rates than the sinus node.

The electrophysiology of cardiac muscle differs from that of nerve in that the action potential is much longer (200 to 300 ms). During the plateau phase of the action potential, the heart is refractory to further stimulation. Excitability is regained during phase 3 of the action potential, which corresponds to the T wave of the surface electrocardiogram. The effective refractory period of the atrium or ventricle may be determined by timed extra stimuli, and is defined as the longest interval between two successive stimuli which fails to elicit a second cardiac depolarization (Fig. 2).

The upstroke of the action potential in sinoatrial and atrioventricular nodal cells is generated by the slow inward calcium current (i_{Ca}). Repolarization arises as a result of decay of the inward current with an increase in the outward potassium current (i_K). In contrast, the action potential upstroke in atrial and ventricular myocardium and in the His–Purkinje system is determined by the rapid inward sodium current (i_{Na}). This results in a much more rapid depolarization than in sinoatrial or atrioventricular nodal tissue, and a much faster conduction velocity of the depolarization wavefront. These differences are of particular importance in understanding the differential effects of antiarrhythmic drugs (see below).

DISORDERS OF IMPULSE FORMATION AND CONDUCTION

Bradyarrhythmias may result from impairment of impulse formation or conduction in the sinoatrial node or of conduction in the atrioventricular

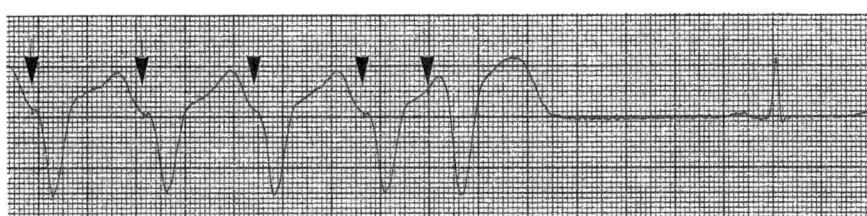

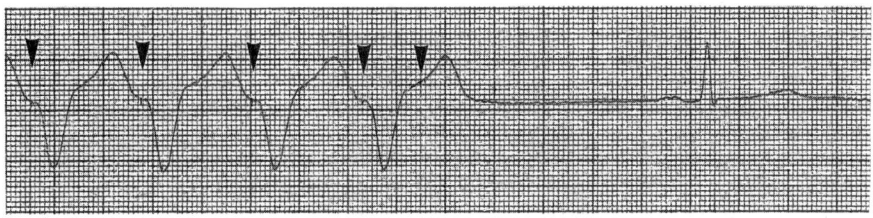

Fig. 2 Ventricular effective refractory period. The top tracing shows the end of a train of ventricular paced beats which are followed by an extra stimulus, which captures the ventricle. In the lower tracing the extra stimulus has been delivered 10 ms earlier, and it fails to capture.

node due to extraneous factors such as sympathetic withdrawal, vagal stimulation or drugs. In addition, intrinsic degenerative disease of the sinus node may result in failure of normal sinus rhythm. Idiopathic conducting system disease may result in impairment of atrioventricular conduction, which may also be affected by myocardial ischaemia, infarction, infiltration, or surgical trauma.

MECHANISMS OF ARRHYTHMOGENESIS

The exact electrophysiological mechanism responsible for cardiac tachyarrhythmias is not known in all cases. There is commonly a complex interaction between an underlying substrate such as previous myocardial infarction, a triggering event such as an extrasystole and modulating influences of which sympathetic stimulation and myocardial ischaemia are the most important. The principal mechanisms responsible for tachyarrhythmias are those of abnormal automaticity, triggered activity and re-entry (Fig. 3).

Automaticity

Abnormal automaticity is defined as an inappropriate increase in the rate of discharge of a tissue having physiological pacemaker properties (i.e. sinus node, atrioventricular node or Purkinje fibres) (Fig. 3(a)). Such abnormalities are most commonly seen in the presence of ischaemia, sympathetic stimulation, or drug toxicity, especially digoxin. Automatic

Fig. 3 Mechanisms of arrhythmias. (a) Increased automaticity; (b) triggered activity due to delayed after-depolarizations; (c) triggered activity due to early after-depolarizations; (d) re-entry circuit. See text for details.

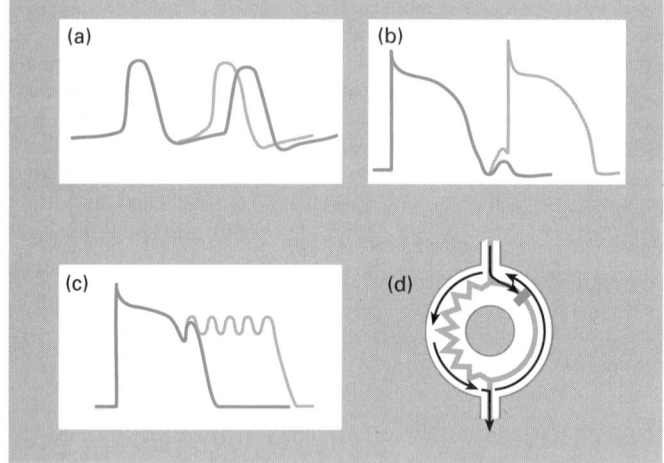

tachycardias are characterized by an absence of initiation by extrasystoles either spontaneously or during electrophysiological testing.

Triggered Activity

The term 'triggered activity' is used to define the appearance of automaticity as a result of external stimulation, and may arise in tissues which do not demonstrate physiological automaticity. Their relevance to clinical arrhythmias is difficult to establish with certainty, but certain arrhythmias behave in a manner consistent with triggered activity. Two characteristic forms of depolarization have been demonstrated to cause triggered activity *in vitro*. Delayed after-depolarizations are seen as small, subthreshold depolarizations after full repolarization of the action potential (Fig. 3(b)). Their amplitude is increased by tachycardia or intracellular calcium overload, and may reach a level at which a spontaneous action potential is generated, potentially initiating a sustained tachycardia. Delayed after-depolarizations can be induced experimentally by digitalis overload, and are the likely mechanism of digitoxic arrhythmias. Early after-depolarizations, in contrast, are seen during the plateau phase of the action potential, prior to repolarization (Fig. 3(c)), and are more evident at slow heart rates, particularly in the presence of hypokalaemia and hypomagnesaemia. Drugs that prolong myocardial repolarization (class IA and class III antiarrhythmics, tricyclic antidepressants, organophosphorus insecticides, and many others) predispose to the appearance of early after-depolarizations *in vitro*. These agents are associated with the acquired long QT syndrome and the arrhythmia of torsades de pointes (see below). It seems likely that this particular arrhythmia arises as a result of triggered activity due to early after-depolarizations.

Re-entry

The majority of the clinically important sustained tachycardias, whether of atrial, junctional or ventricular origin, appear to arise on the basis of re-entry. The establishment of a re-entry tachycardia requires the presence of a potential circuit comprising two limbs with different refractoriness and conduction properties (Fig. 3(d)). A premature beat may result in the development of block in one limb of the circuit, while the activity is conducted by the other. If this conduction is sufficiently slow, the tissue distal to the site of block in the other limb is no longer refractory on the arrival of the depolarizing wavefront and conducts the activity retrogradely. This, in turn, results in reactivation of the slowly conducting pathway and thus a circus movement tachycardia is established. Macro re-entry is defined as the occurrence of a re-entry circuit over a large area of the heart such as in the presence of an accessory pathway (Fig. 4(a)). In contrast, micro re-entry may occur in a relatively small area of the heart (possibly as little as 1 cm²), for example, when normal myocardium is adjacent to the border zone of an old myocardial infarc-

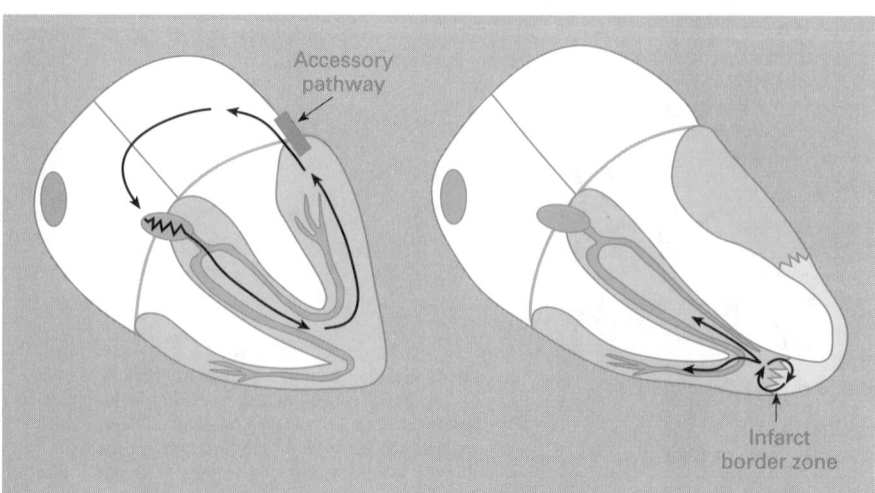

Fig. 4 Clinical examples of re-entry tachycardias. (a) Macro re-entry circuit involving an accessory pathway, which results in atrioventricular re-entry tachycardia; (b) micro re-entry circuit at the border zone of a myocardial infarction.

tion in which conduction velocity is slowed (Fig. 4(b)). The characteristic feature of re-entry tachycardias is their initiation by appropriately timed extrastimuli, which induce unidirectional block and thus initiate the arrhythmia. The tachycardia may be terminated by extrastimuli which depolarize the tissue ahead of the circulating wave front and thus interrupt the circus movement.

Symptoms of arrhythmias

The extent to which tachyarrhythmias are symptomatic depends on a variety of factors including the absolute rate, the difference between the rate during the arrhythmia and the patient's own sinus rate, the degree of irregularity of the rhythm, and the presence or absence of underlying cardiac disease. Tachycardias sufficient to cause low cardiac output and profound falls in cerebral blood flow may cause syncope. Other symptoms of tachycardia include a feeling of rapid palpitation, angina or dyspnoea. Episodes of paroxysmal supraventricular tachycardia may be associated with polyuria due to release of atrial natriuretic peptide. Ectopic beats are commonly asymptomatic, but may produce a sensation of the heart 'missing a beat' often followed by a bump in the chest due to the more powerful post-ectopic beat.

The symptoms produced by bradyarrhythmias will depend on the extent of cardiac slowing or ventricular standstill. They may include sudden death, syncope (Stokes–Adams attacks) or dizziness (presyncope). Continuous bradycardia without asystolic pauses may produce symptoms of fatigue, lethargy, dyspnoea, or mental impairment.

Investigation of arrhythmias

A detailed description of the symptoms associated with the arrhythmia is essential. Evidence should be sought for factors which may precipitate the arrhythmia (e.g. exercise, alcohol) and for the presence of underlying cardiac disease, in particular a history of valvular heart disease, myocardial ischaemia/infarction or of congestive heart failure. Examination of the pulse may be unremarkable if the arrhythmia is intermittent. Careful physical examination for evidence of structural heart disease is essential. Further investigations to establish the presence of structural heart disease and to determine ventricular function may include 12 lead electrocardiography, chest radiography, echocardiography, or exercise stress testing.

ELECTROCARDIOGRAPHY

The key to successful diagnosis of cardiac arrhythmias is the systematic analysis of the electrocardiogram during the arrhythmia in question (Table 1). The electrocardiogram should be of the optimal quality, ideally comprising all 12 leads recorded on a multi-channel recorder. This may allow the identification of P waves in one lead while they may be absent or equivocal in another. Where arrhythmias are intermittent, continuous monitoring may be necessary for identification. This may include inpatient monitoring in the cardiac care unit, particularly in the acute stages of myocardial infarction, or outpatient ambulatory (Holter) monitoring for periods of 24 to 48 h using a portable recorder. High speed or automatic replay facilities for ambulatory electrocardiographic recordings enable identification of intermittent arrhythmias, as well as the quantification of extrasystoles. Patients who have infrequent, sustained palpitations may be taught to use a patient activated recorder which has the advantage of identifying those arrhythmias which are symptomatic, and avoiding unnecessary and time consuming analysis of continuous ambulatory recordings.

Recently, attempts have been made to identify patients at high risk of ventricular tachyarrhythmias by demonstrating evidence of areas of slow conduction in the myocardium which may provide a component of the substrate necessary for re-entrant arrhythmias. This is undertaken by high resolution electrocardiography using the technique of signal averaging to reduce background noise (Fig. 5). Low amplitude signals

Table 1 *Principles of ECG diagnosis of arrhythmias*

Obtain 12-lead or multichannel recordings if possible	
Atrial activity	P waves visible?
	Normal P wave morphology and axis?
	Flutter/fibrillation waves?
	Atrial rate?
Ventricular activity	Ventricular rate?
	Regular or irregular?
	Normal QRS morphology and duration?
	Bundle branch block or bizarre QRS morphology?
	Variation in QRS morphology/axis?
Atrioventricular relationship	PR interval–fixed or varied?
	Retrograde P waves?
	Atrial versus ventricular rate?

in the terminal QRS complex and ST segment have been associated with an increased risk of the development of sustained ventricular tachycardias or arrhythmic sudden death. Another abnormality which appears to be predictive of sudden cardiac death is reduction in heart rate variability on Holter recording, which is thought to reflect abnormalities in autonomic control of the heart.

CARDIAC ELECTROPHYSIOLOGICAL STUDY

More detailed investigation of cardiac arrhythmias may be undertaken by invasive cardiac electrophysiological testing. Multipolar electrodes are inserted to record electrograms from the atrium, ventricle, His bundle and commonly from the coronary sinus if accessory pathways are suspected (Fig. 6). The site of conduction delays within the heart may be identified, but the principal indication for electrophysiological study is in the evaluation of tachyarrhythmias. Sustained arrhythmias may be initiated and terminated by extrastimuli (Fig. 7), and their pattern of activation in the heart can be studied in detail. This may allow, for instance, the localization of an accessory pathway prior to ablation. The technique of programmed stimulation to induce tachycardia can be used to assess whether antiarrhythmic drugs have been effective in preventing the initiation of an arrhythmia, and thus to predict the likely efficacy of long-term antiarrhythmic drug therapy.

Management of arrhythmias

Many cardiac arrhythmias are benign and require no active intervention. The major indications for treatment are relief of symptoms, prevention of complications such as myocardial ischaemia, cardiac failure or embolism, or an attempt to improve survival. The presence of structural heart disease is an important factor in the decision to institute active therapy. The same arrhythmia may be treated in a patient with underlying heart disease but left untreated in a patient with a structurally normal heart. Precipitating factors such as infection, thyrotoxicosis, alcohol, electrolyte disorders, or drug toxicity must be sought. Avoidance of these may be sufficient to prevent recurrence of the arrhythmia without further specific intervention. The type of therapy used will commonly be influenced by the presence of underlying ischaemic heart disease or left ventricular impairment.

OBJECTIVES OF THERAPY

The objectives of therapy, and the choice of treatment will depend upon the clinical context. Patients presenting with a sustained tachyarrhythmia will normally require therapy to restore sinus rhythm. However, in the case of chronic atrial fibrillation it may be unrealistic to expect that sinus rhythm will be maintained even if it can be restored briefly. Under these circumstances, the objective of therapy will be to control the ventricular rate by slowing conduction through the atrioventricular node. If sinus rhythm can be restored, a decision must be made regarding the requirement for long-term prophylaxis. This will be indicated in the presence of a life-threatening tachyarrhythmia or if the patient has a history of recurrent, symptomatic attacks of palpitation.

In the case of bradyarrhythmias, the initial treatment will be to increase the ventricular rate either by pharmacological means or by pacing. Permanent pacing may be necessary unless the cause of bradycardia was transient.

ANTIARRHYTHMIC DRUG THERAPY

As indicated above, antiarrhythmic drugs may be used for the termination of tachyarrhythmias, for rate control or for prophylaxis. All antiarrhythmic drugs have potentially serious side-effects and must be used with caution. The ability of antiarrhythmic drugs to worsen cardiac

arrhythmias or to produce new, possibly life-threatening, arrhythmias (proarrhythmia) is recognized increasingly. The possibility of a proarrhythmic response should be borne in mind as part of the risk/benefit assessment whenever antiarrhythmic drugs are prescribed. No classification exists which provides accurate predication of the efficacy of a given drug for a given arrhythmia; thus therapy is initiated on the basis of trial and error, supported if necessary by more detailed investigation such as Holter monitoring and cardiac electrophysiological testing.

The most commonly used classification of antiarrhythmic drug action was proposed by Vaughan Williams (1970) and is based on the effects on the cardiac action potential. It should be emphasized that this is a classification of antiarrhythmic drug effects and that many antiarrhythmic drugs may have multiple actions, the net result of which cannot be predicted easily. Furthermore, the classification is based on drug effects in isolated tissue, and does not predict effects mediated indirectly via the autonomic nervous system such as the vagotonic action of digoxin or the vagolytic action of disopyramide. The electrocardiographic features of the major Classes of antiarrhythmic drug activity and the prin-

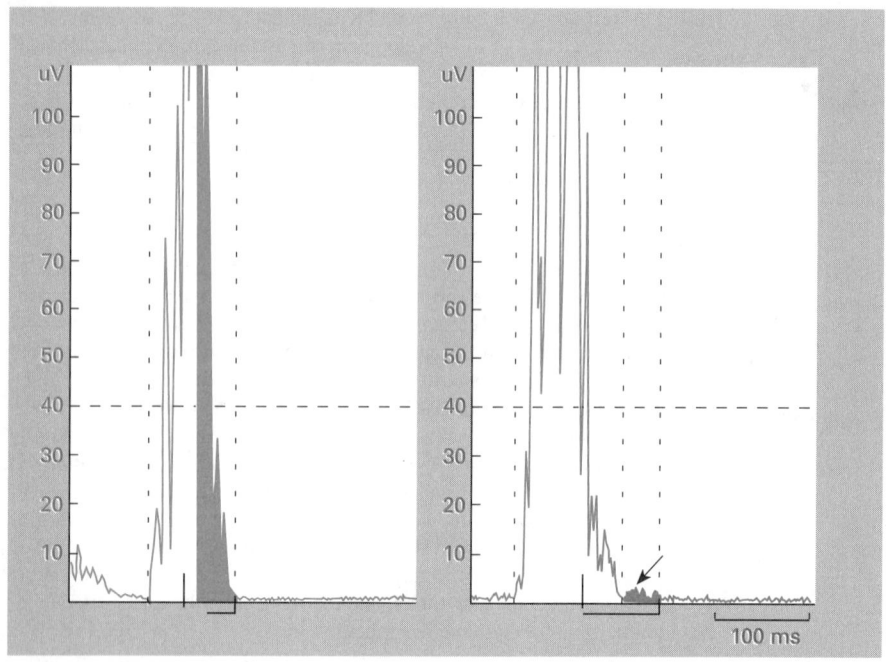

Fig. 5 Signal averaged electrocardiograms. The high amplitude deflection corresponds to the QRS complex, with the last 40 ms shaded in black. The normal tracing (left) shows no evidence of slow activity. The abnormal record (right) has a low amplitude 'late potential' (arrow). Criteria for late potentials include (1) a total filtered QRS duration of > 114 ms (2) duration of low amplitude signal (less than 40 μV) of > 38 ms; (3) terminal (last 40 ms) voltages of < 25 μV.

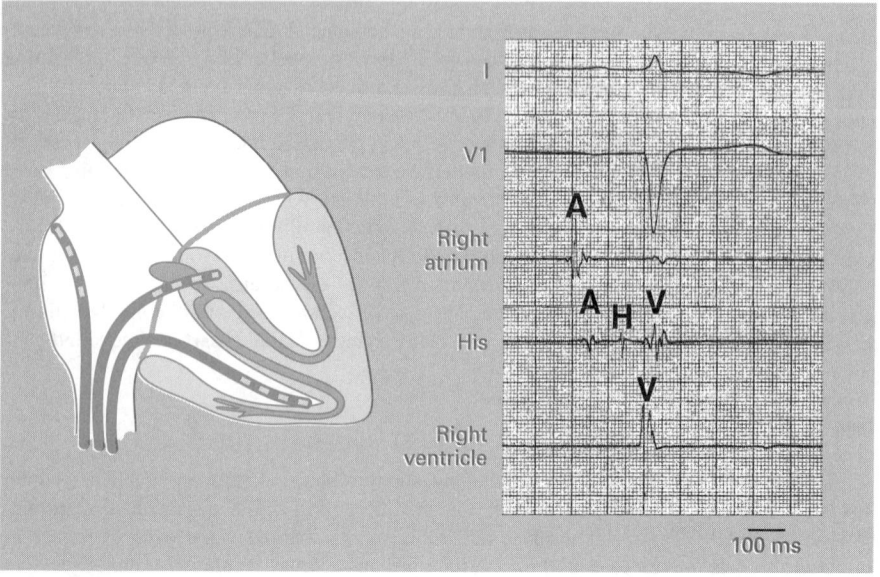

Fig. 6 Electrophysiology study. Illustration of lead placement (left). Quadripolar leads have been inserted from the femoral vein and the tips are shown positioned to allow recording and pacing from the high right atrium, the His bundle and the right ventricular apex. Intracardiac electrograms (right) show recordings from atrium (A), His bundle (H) and right ventricle (V).

cipal sites of action are listed in Table 2. Individual drugs are described in Table 3.

Class I activity

Class I antiarrhythmic drugs act by inhibition of the rapid inward sodium current and have local anaesthetic activity. Three subdivisions of class I activity have been proposed. Class Ia agents cause lengthening of action potential duration, and have intermediate effects on the onset and recovery kinetics of the sodium channel and hence on intracardiac conduction. Examples of this class in clinical use are quinidine, procainamide and disopyramide. Class Ib agents shorten the cardiac action potential duration, and have very rapid offset kinetics which result in minimal slowing of normal intracardiac conduction. Examples in clinical use include lignocaine, mexiletine and tocainide. Class Ic drugs have no major effect on action potential duration, but produce the most long-lasting effect on cardiac sodium channel kinetics, and the most marked slowing of intracardiac conduction. Examples in clinical use include flecainide, encainide, and propafenone.

Class II activity

Vaughan Williams originally defined class II activity as antagonism of the arrhythmogenic effects of catecholamines. The most common agents in this class are the competitive β-adrenoceptor blockers. Other agents such as propafenone have a weak β-receptor blocking activity, while amiodarone (see below) exhibits a non-competitive sympatholytic effect.

Class III activity

The class III mode of antiarrhythmic activity comprises lengthening of the cardiac action potential duration and hence of effective refractory period. Drugs of this class possess a broad spectrum of activity against atrial, supraventricular and ventricular arrhythmias. No 'pure' class III antiarrhythmic drug is currently available, although a number are undergoing clinical evaluation. Amiodarone is a complex drug which has class I, II, III, and IV antiarrhythmic actions. Sotalol is a non-selective β-adrenoceptor antagonist which also possesses class III activity. Bretylium is a sympathetic neuronal blocker which acts by initial release of noradrenaline from the sympathetic nerve terminal. In addition it possesses moderate class III activity.

Class IV activity

Class IV antiarrhythmic activity is manifest by a reduction of the inward calcium current in sinoatrial and atrioventricular nodal tissues. In clinical practice, the effects of these drugs is almost exclusively on atrioventricular nodal conduction, where slowing of conduction may interrupt a re-entry tachycardia involving the atrioventricular node (e.g. atrioventricular nodal re-entry tachycardia), or slow the ventricular response in atrial fibrillation. Verapamil and diltiazem are examples of this class of action. The dihydropyridine calcium antagonists such as nifedipine have no antiarrhythmic action.

Fig. 7 Induction of ventricular tachycardia by programmed stimulation. Ventricular pacing at a cycle length of 400 ms is followed by two extrastimuli (290 and 270 coupling intervals). Sustained monomorphic ventricular tachycardia is induced by these double extrastimuli. Leads II (above) and V$_1$ (below) are shown.

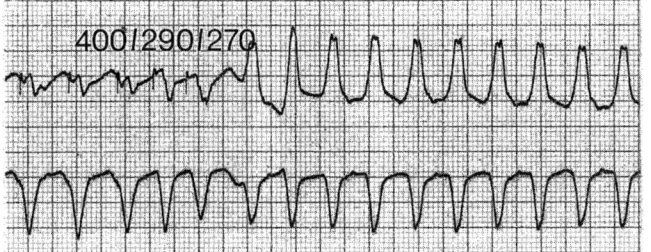

Digoxin

The antiarrhythmic activity of digoxin is not explained within the Vaughan Williams classification. Although its inotropic actions are based on inhibition of cardiac sodium/potassium adenosine triphosphatase (Na$^+$K$^+$ATPase), the antiarrhythmic activity appears to be mediated predominantly via vagal stimulation. Digoxin exerts its effects by slowing of atrioventricular nodal conduction which may terminate or prevent the initiation of tachycardias involving the atrioventricular node, or slow the ventricular rate in atrial fibrillation. As vagal tone is withdrawn during exercise, the effect of digoxin in slowing the ventricular rate in atrial fibrillation is less evident on effort than at rest.

Adenosine

Adenosine is a naturally occurring purine nucleoside which may be used pharmacologically to produce transient slowing of the sinus node or atrioventricular node, and is thus effective for the termination of arrhythmias involving the atrioventricular node. Adenosine is of particular value in view of its extremely short plasma half-life (approximately 2 s), which confers safety. Unlike other drugs, it must be administered by rapid intravenous injection, using incremental bolus doses from 3 to 12 mg, to achieve the desired therapeutic effect.

NON-PHARMACOLOGICAL THERAPY

Physical manoeuvres

Tachycardias involving the atrioventricular node may be terminated by manoeuvres which produce transient vagal stimulation. Although carotid sinus massage is the time-honoured technique, comparative studies indicate that the Valsalva manoeuvre, particularly if performed in the supine position, is more effective. Patients with recurrent supraventricular tachycardias should be taught these manoeuvres, which may abort attacks and avoid the need for hospital treatment.

Pacing

Re-entry tachycardias may be terminated by the delivery of appropriately timed extrastimuli which depolarize part of the re-entry circuit prior to the arrival of the wave front, and interrupt the arrhythmia. In the absence of sophisticated equipment for programmed stimulation, simple overdrive pacing may be effective in the termination of atrial flutter, atrioventricular nodal re-entry, atrioventricular (orthodromic) re-entry tachycardia, or sustained ventricular tachycardia (Fig. 8). The cardiac chamber in question is paced at a rate just above that of the tachycardia for periods of 10 to 15 beats. Repeated attempts may be necessary at gradually increasing rates. Overdrive atrial or ventricular pacing may result in degeneration into atrial and ventricular fibrillation, respectively, and facilities for cardioversion must be available. Implantable antitachycardia pacemakers have been used in patients with recurrent, drug refractory tachycardias. Although many modalities of pacing have been tried, the most successful are based on a train of overdrive stimuli in a manner analogous to that described above. Antitachycardia pacing in the ventricle must be combined with facilities for defibrillation.

Occasionally, continuous pacing may be effective in suppressing frequently recurring attacks of tachyarrhythmia. The basis of this effect is that an increase in the underlying cardiac rate will tend to suppress the occurrence of the extrasystoles which initiate the tachyarrhythmia. The rate in question has to be determined by trial and error, but it is common to start continuous pacing at a rate of 90/min and increase stepwise up to a maximum of 120/min according to efficacy and haemodynamic tolerance.

External cardioversion/defibrillation

Direct current cardioversion remains the most effective and immediate means of terminating sustained tachycardias. R-wave synchronized cardioversion using low energies may be effective in terminating atrial flutter or atrial fibrillation, although in the latter case, higher energies

Table 2 *Classification of antiarrhythmic drug activity*

	ECG effect				Tissue effect			
	HR	PR	QRS	QT	SA node	Atrium	AV node	Ventricle
Class Ia	0	0/−	+	++	0	++	−	++/−−
Ib	0	0	0	0/−	0	0	0	++/−
Ic	0	+	++	+	0	++	0/+	++/−−
Class II	−	+	0	0	++	++	++	+/0
Class III	0/−	0/+	0	++	0/+	++	0/+	++/−−
Class IV	0/−	+	0	0	0/+	0/−	++	0/+
Digoxin	0/−	+	0	0	0/+	0/−	++	0/−
Adenosine	−	+	0	0	++	0/−	++	0/+

ECG effect: + increases; − decreases; 0 no effect; HR heart rate.

Tissue effect: + antiarrhythmic activity; − potential adverse or proarrhythmic effect; 0 no effect.

Table 3 *Commonly used antiarrhythmic drugs*

	Principal indication	Dose		Adverse effects
		IV	Oral	
Class Ia				
Quinidine	AF cardioversion VT prophylaxis	–	1–2 g/day	Hypersensitivity, gastrointestinal symptoms, QT prolongation, hypotension
Disopyramide	VT prophylaxis VT termination	2 mg/kg	300–600 mg/day	Negative inotropy, QT prolongation, Parasympathetic blockade, (urinary retention, dry mouth, blurred vision)
Procaineamide	AF cardioversion VT termination VT prophylaxis	100 mg/5 min up to 1000 mg 1–6 mg/min	2–6 g/day	Hypotension, QT prolongation, gastrointestinal upset, lupus syndrome
Class Ib				
Lignocaine	VT termination VT/VF prophylaxis	100 mg bolus 1–4 mg/min	Ineffective	CNS–confusion, dysarthria, fits
Mexiletine	VT prophylaxis	–	600–1000 mg/day	CNS–dizziness, ataxia, gastrointestinal symptoms
Class Ic				
Flecainide	AF cardioversion AF prophylaxis WPW prophylaxis VT prophylaxis	2 mg/kg	100–300 mg/day	Proarrhythmia, negative inotropy, CNS disturbance
Class II				
Atenolol	AF prophylaxis AF rate control SVT prophylaxis	–	50–100 mg/day	Bradycardia, negative inotropy, Cold extremities, bronchoconstriction, lethargy
Class III				
Sotalol	AF termination AF prophylaxis WPW prophylaxis VT prophylaxis	2 mg/kg	160–480 mg/day	Bradycardia, negative inotropy, cold extremities, bronchoconstriction, lethargy, QT prolongation
Amiodarone	AF termination AF prophylaxis WPW prophylaxis VT prophylaxis	300 mg in 30 min then 1200 mg/24h	600–1200 mg/d loading first 2 weeks then 100–400 mg/day	Photosensitivity, skin pigmentation, hypo- or hyperthyroidism, alveolitis, hepatitis, peripheral neuropathy, epididymitis
Class IV				
Verapamil	SVT termination SVT prophylaxis AF rate control	5–10 mg	240–480 mg/day	Negative inotropy, AV block flushing, constipation
Other				
Digoxin	AF rate control	0.5–1 mg	0.0625–0.5 mg/day	Anorexia, nausea, vomiting, AV block, atrial and ventricular arrhythmias, toxicity
Adenosine	SVT termination	3–12 mg by incremental bolus	ineffective	Flushing, chest pain, bronchospasm, transient AV block

AF, atrial fibrillation; SVT, supraventricular tachycardia (atrioventricular nodal and atrioventricular re-entrant tachycardia); VT, ventricular tachycardia; WPW, Wolff–Parkinson–White syndrome.

may be necessary. Sustained ventricular tachycardia may be terminated by synchronized direct current shock, normally requiring energies of 100 to 360 J. The most important use of direct current counter-shock is in the termination of ventricular fibrillation (Fig. 9). A non-synchronized shock is used, initially at 200 J, with further shocks at 360 J as necessary. Recent technological developments have led to the widespread use of advisory external defibrillators, which analyse the cardiac rhythm automatically and advise as to whether a shock should be delivered. These devices have allowed individuals such as ambulance crew to defibrillate successfully without extensive training in electrocardiographic recognition.

Implantable cardiovertor defibrillators

Patients at high risk of sudden cardiac death as a result of previous sustained ventricular arrhythmias or out-of-hospital cardiac arrest may be treated with an implantable cardiovertor defibrillator if no alternative pharmacological or surgical option exists (Fig. 10). Earlier devices

required thoracotomy for the insertion of patch electrodes on to the epicardium. Newer devices utilize transvenous electrodes, and avoid the need for thoracotomy. The latest implantable cardiovertor defibrillators have the facility for antitachycardia pacing to minimize the number of shocks which need to be delivered. However, the devices remain complex and expensive with a limited battery life.

Ablation

Selective ablation of part of a re-entry circuit or of the bundle of His is increasingly used in the management of troublesome arrhythmias. Energy is delivered between the tip of an intracardiac electrode positioned at the appropriate site, and an indifferent electrode placed over the scapula. His bundle ablation is indicated in cases of intractable paroxysmal atrial fibrillation or flutter (Fig. 11), or in sustained atrial fibrillation or flutter where the ventricular rate cannot be controlled adequately by pharmacological means. The energy source is provided by a conventional defibrillator discharge, a modified low energy direct cur-

Fig. 8 Termination of ventricular tachycardia by overdrive ventricular pacing.

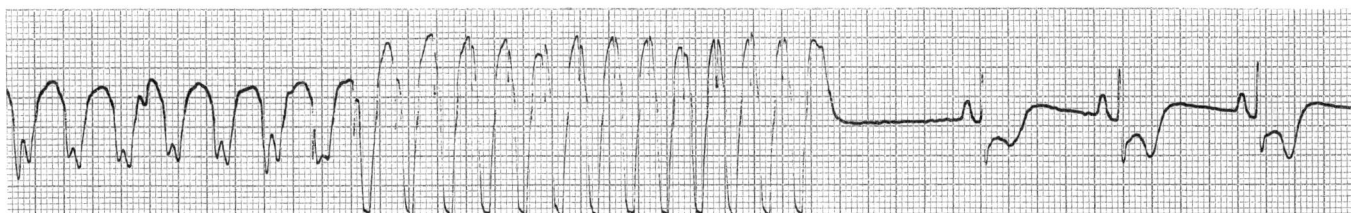

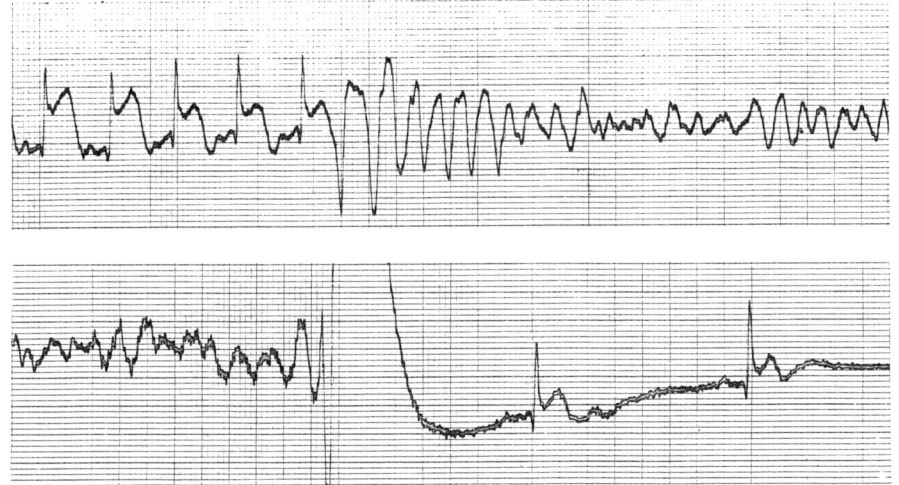

Fig. 9 Ventricular fibrillation is initiated by an 'R-on-T' ventricular extrasystole (above). Defibrillation (200 J direct current shock) terminated the ventricular fibrillation and restored sinus rhythm.

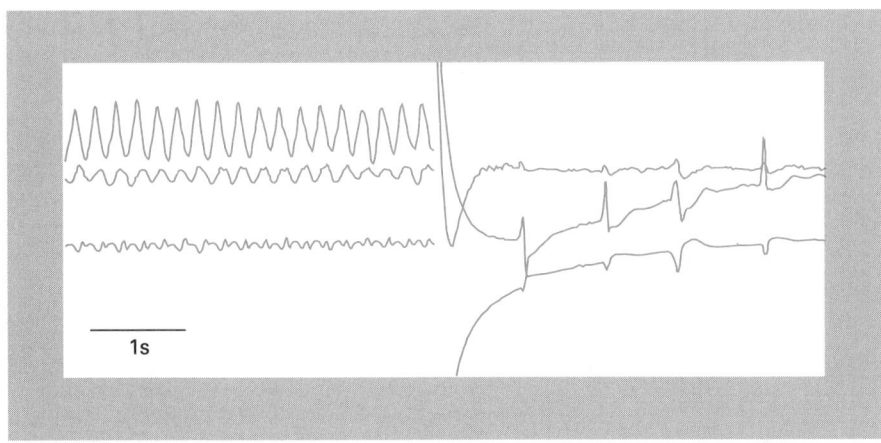

Fig. 10 Discharge from an Implantable Cardioverter Defibrillator. A rapid polymorphic ventricular tachycardia is terminated by a 20 J shock from the device.

rent shock, or by radiofrequency energy. Following His bundle ablation, patients require lifelong permanent pacing.

Radiofrequency ablation provides definitive treatment of the Wolff–Parkinson–White syndrome and atrioventricular nodal re-entry tachycardia. Careful mapping of the accessory pathway will identify a site at which radiofrequency current can be passed, with the disappearance of accessory pathway conduction within a few seconds (Fig. 12). Applications of radiofrequency energy for up to a minute are sufficient to achieve permanent interruption of the accessory pathway and a complete cure.

Surgery

The role of cardiac surgery in the management of intractable arrhythmias is diminishing with the development of techniques for ablation. Surgical ablation of the bundle of His or of accessory pathways is now largely superseded by catheter ablative techniques. Surgical management of recurrent ventricular tachycardia is suitable for a selected group of patients with adequate left ventricular function in whom the site of origin of the tachycardia can be mapped preoperatively and at surgery. This micro re-entry circuit in sustained ventricular tachycardia commonly arises from the subendocardial area at the border zone between normal and aneurysmal tissue (see Fig. 4(b)), and subendocardial resection of this area will result in permanent suppression of the tachycardia. However, most of these patients have extensively damaged ventricles and the operative mortality is over 10 per cent in most series.

Individual arrhythmias

Bradycardias

A bradycardia is defined as a ventricular rate less than 60 per minute, and results from a reduction in the rate of normal sinus pacemaker activity, or from disturbances of atrioventricular conduction. A reduction in sinus rate may occur as a result of extrinsic influences, largely modulated through the autonomic nervous system, or as a result of an intrinsic abnormality of the sinus node (Table 4).

SINOATRIAL DISEASE

The presence of inappropriate sinus bradycardia, sinus pauses or junctional rhythm (Fig. 13) in the absence of extrinsic factors is indicative of sinoatrial disease, often referred to as 'sick sinus syndrome'. This condition is most commonly caused by idiopathic degeneration of the sinus nodal cells particularly in the elderly, and is associated in about 20 per cent of cases with idiopathic bundle branch fibrosis (see below). Conduction block may occur between the sinus node and the atrium (sinoatrial block), resulting in 'dropped' P waves (Fig. 14). More prolonged suppression of sinus node activity results in periods of sinus arrest (Fig. 15). A period of sinus arrest may be terminated by an escape beat from the sinus node, atrioventricular junction or ventricle. Where the sinus rate is permanently slower than the junctional rate, continuous atrioventricular junctional rhythm will be present (Fig. 16). These patients may also have an increased predisposition to atrial tachyarrhythmias (bradycardia/tachycardia syndrome) (Fig. 17). Sinoatrial disease may be associated with coronary artery disease, particularly involving the right coronary artery. However, many patients with sinus nodal disease have normal coronary arteries.

Patients with sinus node disease may be asymptomatic, or may present with symptomatic bradycardia, dizziness, or syncope. The diagnosis is made is most cases from 12 lead or ambulatory electrocardiographic recording. Investigation should focus on exclusion of extrinsic causes of bradycardia, and on demonstration of the correlation between bradycardia or sinus pauses and the patient's symptoms. If such a correlation can be demonstrated, permanent pacemaker implantation is indicated for relief of symptoms. Prognosis is not improved by pacemaker implantation in sinus nodal disease and thus pacemaker implantation in asymptomatic patients is not indicated.

CAROTID SINUS HYPERSENSITIVITY

A hypersensitive carotid sinus reflex may lead to reflex bradycardia or cardiac standstill resulting in symptomatic dizziness or syncope. The condition is diagnosed by the demonstration of a sinus pause greater than 3 s (Fig. 18) or the appearance of atrioventricular block in response

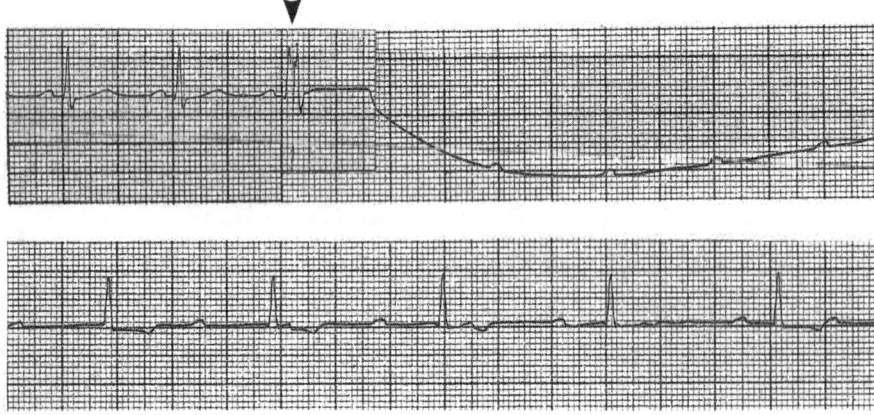

Fig. 11 His bundle ablation. Delivery of a 50 J DC shock (arrow) via an intracardiac lead to a patient with paroxysmal atrial fibrillation resulted in complete heart block. Ventricular pacing was switched on following the brief period of ventricular standstill (above). The patient subsequently developed a junctional rhythm at 50 b.p.m. (below).

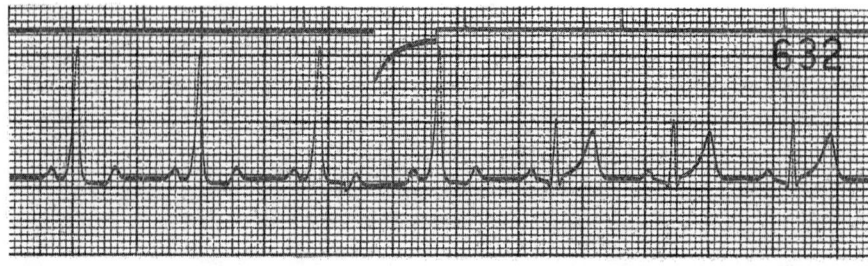

Fig. 12 Radiofrequency ablation of an accessory pathway. The patient had Wolff–Parkinson–White syndrome with evidence of ventricular pre-excitation on the surface electrocardiogram during sinus rhythm (short PR interval, delta wave). One beat after switching on the current (indicated by deflection in marker channel, above) the QRS becomes normal, indicating successful ablation of the accessory pathway.

Table 4 *Causes of sinus bradycardia*

Physiological–sleep, young people, athletes.
Sinoatrial disease
Drugs–β-blockers, amiodarone, Ca^{2+} channel blockers
Vagotonia–vasovagal syndrome, inferior myocardial infarction
Hypothyroidism
Hypothermia
Other medical conditions–jaundice, raised intracranial pressure

to 5 s right carotid sinus massage. The carotid sinus reflex comprises both bradycardia and hypotension due to vasodilation. Where a clear association between bradycardia and symptoms can be documented, implantation of a permanent pacemaker is indicated.

VASOVAGAL SYNDROME

Vasovagal syncope is a common occurrence, particularly among young people. The malignant vasovagal syndrome is recognized in older patients who are subject to episodes of dizziness and syncope, particularly when in the upright position, which are not provoked by identifiable noxious stimuli. There is no evidence of conventional sinoatrial disease, but provocation by tilt table testing, for example head upright tilting at an angle of 70 ° for up to 45 min, will provoke bradycardia and hypotension. The basis of effective treatment in this condition is as yet uncertain, but vagally mediated bradycardia may be prevented by pacemaker implantation.

ATRIOVENTRICULAR CONDUCTION DISTURBANCES

The normal function of the atrioventricular node is to delay ventricular activation and thus allow optimum haemodynamic benefit from atrial filling of the ventricle. In addition, physiological atrioventricular block will occur in the face of rapid atrial rates to avoid excessive tachycardia. Pathological atrioventricular conduction disturbance is defined as an abnormality of atrioventricular conduction despite a normal sinus rate. Impairment of atrioventricular conduction may occur either within the atrioventricular node (intranodal) or within the His–Purkinje system (infranodal). The site of conduction block cannot be identified from the surface electrocardiogram. Intracardiac recording can identify intranodal conduction block by prolongation or block between the atrial and His

bundle electrograms, while infranodal block is identified by slowing of His bundle conduction or prolongation of the interval between the His bundle and ventricular electrograms. Intranodal block is not associated with QRS abnormalities, while distal (infranodal) block is commonly associated with bundle branch block.

Electrocardiographic features

The normal upper limit of PR interval is 0.20 s and, if the value exceeds this, first degree atrioventricular block is present (Fig. 19). In second degree atrioventricular block, there is intermittent failure of conduction from atrium to ventricle. In type I (Wenckebach) second degree block, a characteristic pattern of increasing PR interval duration followed by a non-conducted P wave is seen (Fig. 20). The QRS morphology is commonly normal. In type II second degree atrioventricular block there is sudden failure of conduction, without preceding increase in PR interval (Fig. 21). This condition is commonly associated with distal conducting system disease resulting in the presence of bundle branch block. Regular non-conducted P waves may result in high degree block, with 2 : 1 or 3 : 1 conduction. In third degree (complete) atrioventricular block, there is complete dissociation between atrial and ventricular activity (Fig. 22). The ventricular rate is slower than the atrial rate, regular and with a QRS morphology dependent on the site of the escape rhythm. An escape rhythm arising above the bifurcation of the bundle of His will produce a narrow QRS morphology, commonly with a relatively rapid escape rhythm (50 to 60 per minute). A more distal escape rhythm arising from Purkinje fibre automaticity results in widened bundle branch block morphology complexes with a slower escape rate (20 to 30 per minute). Atrial fibrillation may coexist with complete atrioventricular block, and is recognized by the presence of a slow, regular ventricular response.

Patients may present with symptomatic bradycardia and have evidence of atrioventricular conduction disturbance on the resting electrocardiogram. However, the resting electrocardiogram may be normal or may only show evidence of mild conducting system disturbance such as first degree atrioventricular block or bundle branch block. Ambulatory electrocardiographic recording, for prolonged periods if necessary, may be required to obtain evidence of higher degrees of atrioventricular block.

Atrioventricular conduction disturbances may be preceded by or associated with evidence of distal conducting system disease resulting in bundle branch block. The left bundle branch has a fan-like radiation without obvious distinction into anterior and posterior divisions, but electrocardiographic patterns of marked left and right axis deviation are

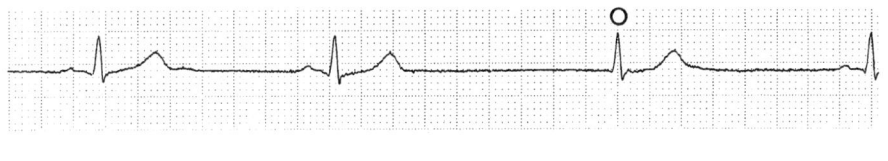

Fig. 13 Sinus bradycardia. The heart rate is less than 40 b.p.m., and the sinus rate is so slow that an escape junctional beat is seen (open circle), preceding the P wave.

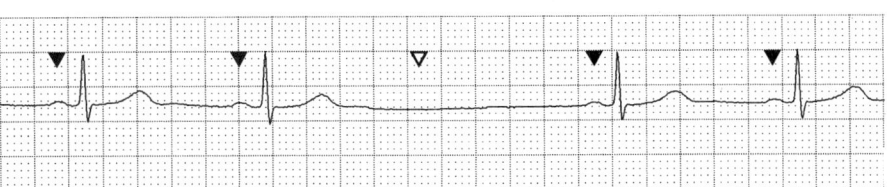

Fig. 14 Sinoatrial exit block. A pause occurred because of the absence of a P wave (open arrow). The timing of the sinus beats, however, is not interrupted, indicating that the sinus node discharged but the impulse failed to excite the atria.

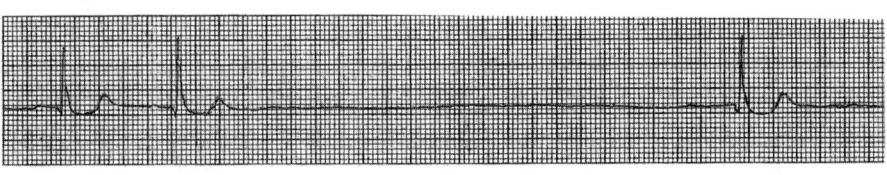

Fig. 15 Sinus arrest. A pause of 4.5 s results from failure of the sinus node to discharge.

commonly described as left anterior and posterior fascicular (hemi-) block. The term bifascicular block is used to describe the combination of (1) right bundle branch block with left anterior or posterior fascicular block (Fig. 23) or (2) complete left bundle branch block. Trifascicular block is defined as the coexistence of bifascicular block with a prolonged PR interval, normally implying slowed conduction through the remaining fascicle.

Aetiology

The causes of atrioventricular block are listed in Table 5. The most common is idiopathic fibrosis of the conducting system, which affects the His–Purkinje system and occurs with increasing frequency from the seventh decade of life onwards. This condition results in progressive impairment of atrioventricular conduction, and is associated in up to 25 per cent of cases with sinoatrial disease. There is no specific association with coronary arterial disease, although the two may coexist in elderly patients. Atrioventricular block may occur acutely in myocardial infarction (Fig. 24). Inferior myocardial infarction predominantly affects atrioventricular nodal conduction by vagal overactivity, and possibly adenosine release from ischaemic myocardium. First degree, Wenckebach second degree atrioventricular block, or third degree atrioventricular block may occur, but these are usually transient. In contrast, atrioventricular conduction disturbance secondary to anterior myocardial infarction is normally due to extensive infarction of the interventricular septum involving the left and right bundle branches after the division of the bundle of His. This may result in type II second degree block or complete atrioventricular block, with a lower probability of recovery of normal conduction. Atrioventricular nodal blocking drugs may potentially produce significant conduction disturbance, particularly when used in combination. The combination of intravenous verapamil in patients already receiving β-adrenoceptor blockers is particularly hazardous. Vagally mediated conduction disturbances may occur as a physiological

finding in highly trained athletes, or in conjunction with carotid sinus syndrome or vasovagal syndrome. Atrioventricular conduction disturbances may arise in structural congenital heart disease such as endocardial cushion defects, but may also arise as an isolated congenital abnormality, commonly in association with maternal systemic lupus erythematosus in the presence of the Ro/La antibody.

Management

First degree atrioventricular block produces no symptoms and does not require active treatment. Wenckebach-type second degree atrioventricular block is normally associated with a reliable subsidiary pacemaker and a low risk of progression to complete heart block. In the majority of instances, active treatment is not necessary. However, the finding of Wenckebach block on ambulatory monitoring in a patient presenting with recurrent syncope may indicate the occurence of higher degree block at other times and may require consideration of pacemaker implantation. Type II second degree atrioventricular block is generally indicative of extensive infranodal conduction abnormality, with a high risk of progression to complete atrioventricular block. Most authorities therefore recommend permanent pacemaker implantation even in the absence of symptoms. The presence of complete atrioventricular block except in the context of an acutely reversible condition should be regarded as an indication for permanent pacemaker implantation. This is particularly urgent in cases where Stokes–Adams attacks are occurring, but even in asymptomatic patients the prognosis appears to be improved by permanent pacemaker implantation. One exception to this general rule is congenital complete heart block, where the escape rhythm is often relatively fast (50 to 60 per minute) with a narrow QRS morphology. Many patients remain asymptomatic well into adult life, although there is a small risk of syncope or sudden death. Pacemaker implantation should be considered if there are symptoms, or if the ventricular rate on ambulatory recording remains persistently below 50 beats per minute.

Temporary pacemaker implantation is indicated where frequent Stokes–Adams attacks are occurring, or where the conduction disturbance is likely to be transient such as in cases of drug intoxication or inferior myocardial infarction. In the latter case, even the presence of complete heart block may be associated with an adequate ventricular rate and pacing need only be undertaken if there is haemodynamic compromise. Spontaneous recovery of normal conduction generally occurs within the first 7 to 10 days.

The risk of progression from chronic bifascicular block to complete heart block is low, and patients with asymptomatic bifascicular block do not require prophylactic pacemaker implantation. The presence of trifascicular block implies advanced conducting system disease, and permanent pacing is usually advised.

Fig. 16 Junctional rhythm. No P wave precedes the QRS complexes, but P waves are seen following them (arrows).

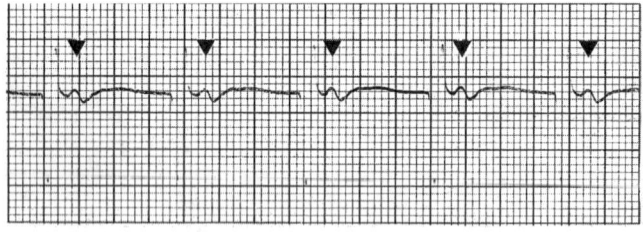

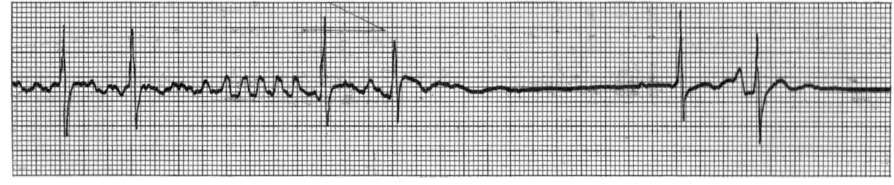

Fig. 17 Bradycardia/tachycardia syndrome. Termination of atrial fibrillation is followed by a pause and bradycardia.

Fig. 18 Carotid sinus hypersensitivity. Pressure applied to the carotid sinus (arrow) causes sinus arrest and a pause of 5.5 s.

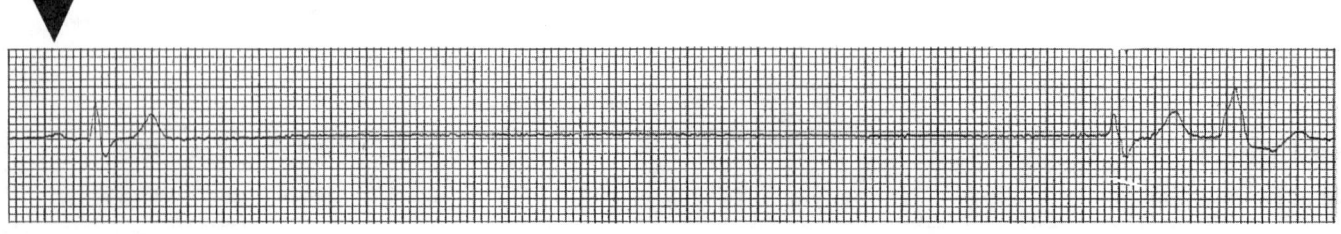

Prognosis

The prognosis of patients with complete atrioventricular block having Stokes-Adams attacks is poor without pacemaker implantation, and has been shown to improve markedly following permanent pacing. In contrast to sinoatrial disease, therefore, most cardiologists regard the presence of established type II second degree or third degree atrioventricular block as an indication for permanent pacemaker implantation regardless of symptoms. Following pacing, the prognosis will depend on the underlying cardiac disease. In patients with idiopathic bundle branch fibrosis and no other cardiac abnormality, the prognosis is restored to that of a comparably aged population.

Fig. 19 First degree heart block. The PR interval is prolonged (0.32s).

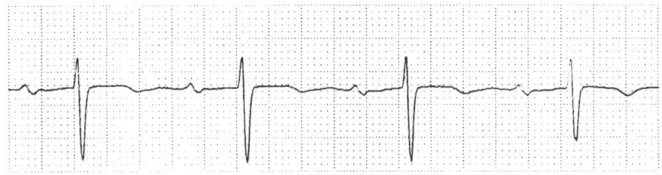

ASYSTOLE

The term asystole is used when the electrocardiogram shows a complete cessation of both atrial and ventricular activity. The electrocardiographic appearances of asystole may be mimicked by disconnected electrocardiograph cables or other artifact, but since asystole causes cardiac arrest, the distinction is usually obvious. Asystole is usually the end point of all arrhythmias resulting in cardiac arrest, and will occur following ventricular fibrillation if defibrillation is not instituted within 10 to 15 min. In addition, asystole may occur as the initiating rhythm of cardiac arrest. This has been reported as a result of profound vagal discharge, and is the likely cause of cardiac arrest in strangulation or hypoxia. The occurrence of persisting P waves without ventricular activity due to complete atrioventricular block is normally termed ventricular standstill rather than asystole (Fig. 25). The management of asystole is discussed below in the section on cardiac arrest.

Fig. 20 Second degree heart block, type I (Wenckebach). The PR interval progressively prolongs until there is failure of conduction following a P wave (arrow).

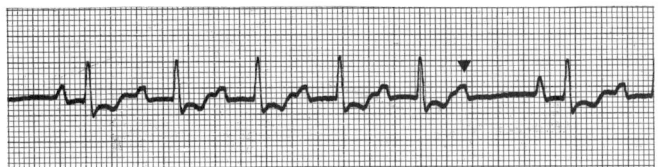

Estrasystoles

The term extrasystole is used to describe premature beats arising from a focus other than the sinus node. They are also described as premature beats, premature contractions, premature depolarizations or ectopics. Extrasystoles may arise in the atrium, atrioventricular junction or ventricle. The underlying mechanism is unknown in most instances, although abnormal automaticity, triggered activity and re-entry are all capable of initiating extrasystoles.

Fig. 21 Second degree heart block, type II. A non-conducted P wave occurs without preceding prolongation of the PR interval (above). Higher grade block developed with 2:1 atrioventricular conduction (below).

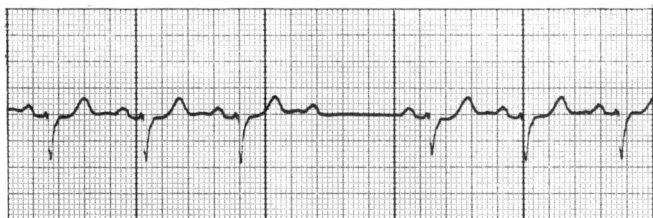

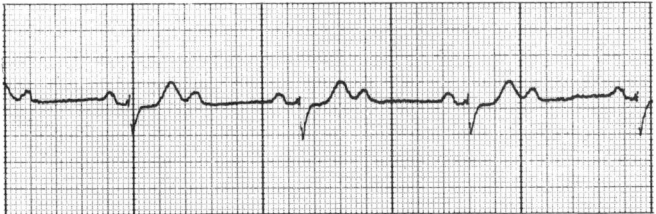

ATRIAL EXTRASYSTOLES

Atrial extrasystoles are recognized by a premature P wave of different morphology from the sinus P wave (Fig. 26). It may be necessary to inspect several leads on the electrocardiogram to identify the P wave, which may be hidden within the ST segment or T wave of the preceding sinus beat. If atrioventricular and bundle branch conduction has recovered fully following the previous sinus beat, the atrial extrasystole will be followed by a normal QRS complex (Fig. 26). Premature atrial extrasystoles may occur before full recovery of the atrioventricular node, in which case there may be prolongation of the PR interval, or if sufficiently premature the extrasystole may encounter complete atrioventricular nodal refractoriness and not be conducted (Fig. 27). It is important to distinguish non-conducted atrial extrasystoles from second degree atrioventricular block or sinus arrest. Sometimes, atrial extrasystoles are conducted through the atrioventricular node but encounter bundle branch refractoriness in which case a bundle branch block pattern of the QRS complex will be identified (Fig. 28).

Atrial extrasystoles are a common finding in healthy people, particularly with increasing age. Their frequency is increased by toxins such as alcohol or caffeine and by increased atrial pressure or stretch, as in cardiac failure or chronic mitral valve disease. In these situations they may be harbingers of the development of atrial fibrillation. Atrial extrasystoles may occasionally be symptomatic.

Management should involve exclusion of underlying organic heart disease and avoidance of any external precipitating factors. Drug treatment is rarely necessary, and patients should be reassured that the arrhythmia is benign. If treatment is required on symptomatic grounds, β-adrenergic blockers may be used; class I antiarrhythmic drugs should be avoided in view of their proarrhythmic risk.

Fig. 22 Third degree (complete) heart block. The escape rhythm may have narrow (above) or broad (below) QRS complexes.

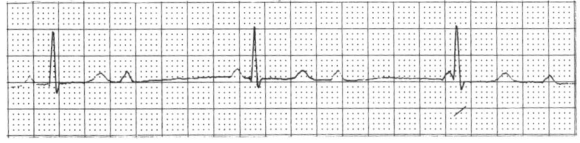

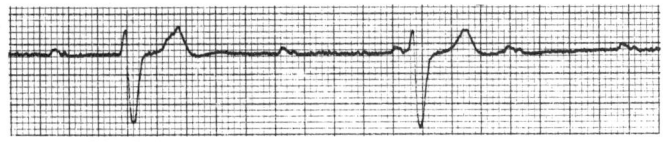

ATRIOVENTRICULAR JUNCTIONAL EXTRASYSTOLES

Junctional extrasystoles are identified on the electrocardiograph by the appearance of a premature, normal QRS complex in the absence of a preceding atrial extrasystole. The atria as well as the ventricles may be activated, resulting an inverted P wave which may be simultaneous with the QRS complex, or inscribed within the ST segment. The significance and management of junctional extrasystoles are similar to those of atrial extrasystoles.

VENTRICULAR EXTRASYSTOLES

Ventricular extrasystoles are identified by the appearance of a bizarre wide QRS complex not preceded by a P wave. There is commonly ST segment depression and T wave inversion. Ventricular extrasystoles commonly bear a constant coupling interval to the previous QRS complex. Retrograde activation through the atrioventricular node may occasionally produce an inverted P wave. If retrograde atrial activation does not occur, the interval after the extrasystole will be fully compensatory, i.e., the interval between the pre- and post-extrasystolic beats will be twice the normal sinus cycle length (Fig. 29). Retrograde depolarization of the atria may reset the sinus node and result in a less than compensatory pause. Ventricular extra systoles may be intermittent, or occur with a fixed association to the preceding normal beats, i.e. 1 : 2, 1 : 3 (bigeminy or trigeminy) (Fig. 30). Where extrasystoles are of differing morphologies the terms multi-focal or multi-form are used (Fig. 31). Two extrasystoles in a row are described as a couplet, while three or more in succession is defined as a salvo. Occasionally, a focus may arise which discharges at its own intrinsic rate, independent of the preceding QRS complex, with variable myocardial capture. This arrhythmia, termed parasystole, results in extrasystolic beats which bear no consistent relationship to the preceding QRS complex, but have an interectopic interval which is normally a multiple of the intrinsic cycle length of the parasystolic focus.

Ventricular extrasystoles occur in otherwise normal hearts, but are found particularly in the presence of structural heart disease. They occur commonly in the acute phase of myocardial infarction, but are also seen in the post infarction phase, in the presence of severe left ventricular hypertrophy, hypertrophic cardiomyopathy or congestive heart failure. Extrasystoles may produce symptoms which require treatment in a minority of cases. The major controversy regarding the management of extrasystoles has centred on their prognostic significance. Natural history studies have demonstrated that the presence of frequent ventricular extrasystoles (>10/h) is an independent risk factor for mortality, particularly sudden death, in convalescent patients after myocardial infarction. Frequent extrasystoles also appear to confer an adverse prognosis in patients with congestive cardiac failure. Numerous clinical trials have attempted to demonstrate an improvement in prognosis in patients after myocardial infarction by suppression of extrasystoles with class I anti-arrhythmic agents. None of these has demonstrated a statistically significant reduction in mortality, and a meta-analysis of all available trials suggests that class I agents are associated with a tendency towards an increased mortality. This was particularly clearly demonstrated in the best designed of the trials, the Cardiac Arrhythmia Suppression Trial (CAST), which was terminated prematurely following the demonstration of a statistically significant increase in sudden death and all-cause mortality in patients treated with flecainide or encainide, compared to placebo. These results are to be contrasted with the evidence that β-blockade will reduce sudden death and all-cause mortality in post infarction patients, although β-blocker trials have not been performed specifically in patients with frequent extrasystoles. There is at present no convincing evidence from randomized trials that the suppression of asymptomatic extrasystoles in any clinical context is associated with an improvement in prognosis, with the possible exception of the use of amiodarone in dilated cardiomyopathy. The use of class I agents for suppression of extrasystoles is to be avoided in view of the accumulating evidence that they may increase the risk of death. If extrasystoles require suppression on symptomatic grounds, the safest option is β-blockade.

Supraventricular tachycardias

Tachycardias arising from the atria or atrioventricular junction are commonly labelled supraventricular in order to distinguish them from ventricular tachycardia. However, the term encompasses tachycardias of different origins and mechanisms, which should be clearly distinguished from each other because their mechanism, significance, and management differ widely.

DIFFERENTIAL DIAGNOSIS OF NARROW QRS COMPLEX TACHYCARDIAS

The majority of supraventricular tachycardias have normal atrioventricular conduction and therefore demonstrate normal QRS morphology. In certain instances, rate-related (functional) bundle branch block may produce widening of the QRS complex and result in difficulty in distinguishing supraventricular from ventricular tachyarrhythmias. The differential diagnosis of wide complex tachycardias is discussed below. The characteristic electrocardiographic features of the principal supraventricular arrhythmias are listed in Table 6. Careful study of all leads of the electrocardiogram is necessary to identify the presence of retrograde P waves. Flutter waves are most commonly evident in the inferior limb leads or in lead V1. Transient interruption of atrioventricular nodal conduction by vagal stimulation or intravenous adenosine is of particular value in revealing the mechanism of tachycardia (see Figs. 34 and 35). Atrial tachycardias will not be terminated, but an increase in atrioventricular block will reveal the underlying atrial tachycardia. In contrast, tachycardias utilizing the atrioventricular junction as part of the re-entry circuit will be terminated by transient atrioventricular block.

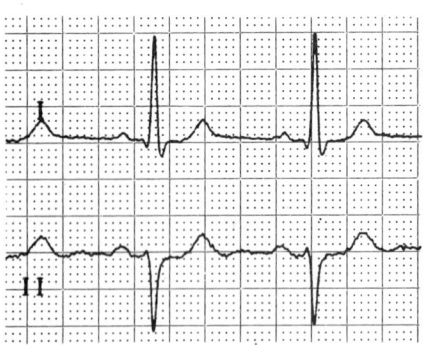
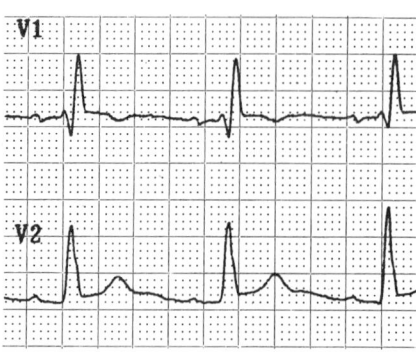

Fig. 23 Left anterior hemiblock (left axis deviation) and right bundle branch block (bifasicular block). This is the electrocardiogram of the patient who had intermittent second degree heart block, type II (Fig. 21).

Table 5 *Causes of AV block*

Drugs–digoxin, verapamil, β-blockers, class I antiarrhythmics
Idiopathic conducting system fibrosis
Acute myocardial ischaemia/infarction
Infiltration–calcific aortic stenosis, sarcoid, scleroderma,
   syphilis, tumor
Infection–diphtheria, rheumatic fever, endocarditis, Lyme
   disease
Vagal–athletic heart, carotid sinus, and vasovagal syndrome
Dystrophia myotonica

Fig. 24 Complete heart block in a patient with acute myocardial infarction. There is a narrow QRS complex escape rhythm, with ST segment elevation.

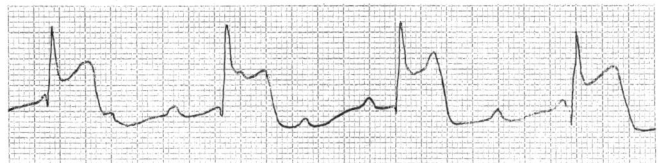

Fig. 25 Complete heart block with ventricular standstill.

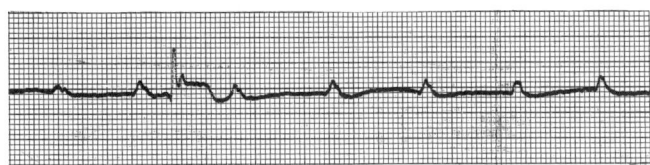

Fig. 26 Atrial extrasystole (arrow).

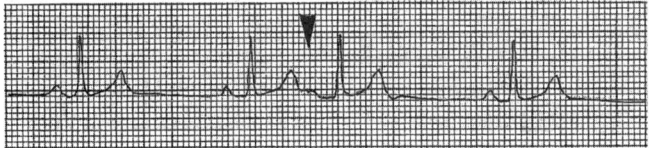

Fig. 27 Blocked atrial extrasystoles. Inverted P waves (arrowed) occur following each sinus beat. The atrioventricular node is refractory because of the proximity of the atrial extrasystole to the preceding beat, and conduction is blocked.

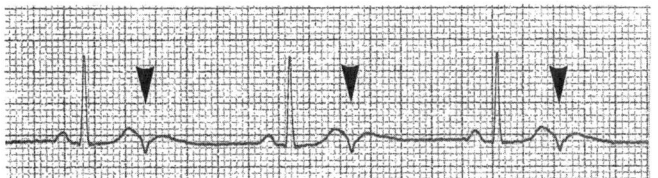

Fig. 28 Atrial extrasystoles with aberrant conduction. The second QRS complex has left bundle branch block morphology, while the fourth and sixth show a right bundle branch block pattern. Lead V₁ is shown.

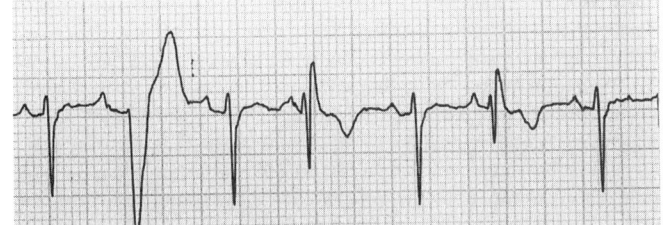

Atrial arrhythmias

ATRIAL FIBRILLATION

Atrial fibrillation is the most common sustained tachycardia. Its prevalence increases with advancing age and may be as high as 5 per cent in the very elderly. The underlying mechanism is thought to be macro reentry in most instances. The characteristic electrocardiographic findings in atrial fibrillation of recent onset are of rapid, irregular 'f' waves at a rate of 350 to 600/min. These are associated with an irregular ventricular response because of variable conduction through the atrioventricular node (Fig. 32). With increasing duration of chronic atrial fibrillation, the amplitude of the 'f' waves diminishes until they are no longer visible. Under these circumstances, atrial fibrillation is diagnosed solely by the absence of P waves and the irregular ventricular response.

Clinical features

Atrial fibrillation may present in a paroxysmal or sustained form. Characteristically, the earliest manifestation is of paroxysmal attacks of fibrillation which may last anything from a few seconds to a few days. At this stage, the ventricular rate is often rapid and the patient may be

Fig. 29 Ventricular extrasystole. No retrograde atrial activation occurs, and the P wave sequence is undisturbed (arrowed).

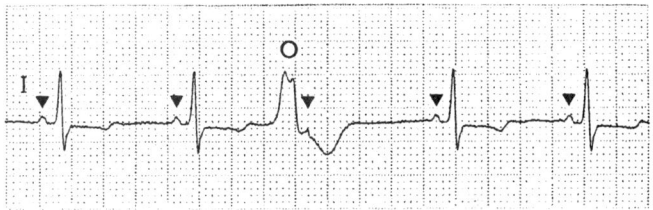

Fig. 30 An interpolated ventricular extrasystole (above) occurs in mid diastole and does not interfere with the following sinus cycle. Ventricular bigeminy (below), with ventricular extrasystoles following each sinus beat. The extrasystoles occur earlier and are followed by a compensatory pause.

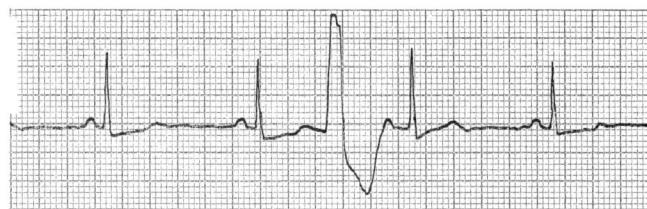

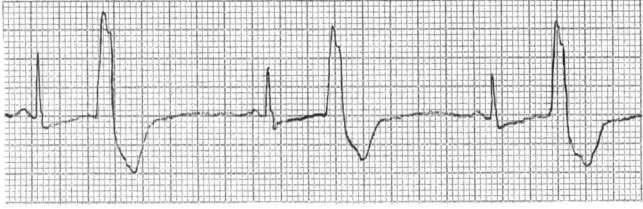

Fig. 31 Multiform ventricular extrasystoles.

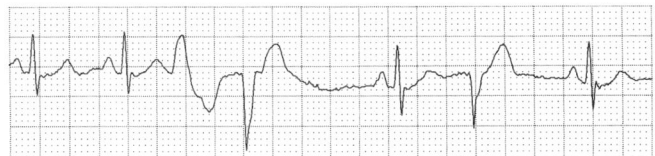

Table 6 *Diagnosis of narrow QRS tachycardias*

| Arrhythmia | P waves | | P–R relationship | Other |
	Rate/min	Morphology/axis		
Sinus tachycardia	100–150	Normal	1:1 normal PR	Rarely >150 except exercise
Sinus re-entry	100–140	Normal	1:1 normal PR	Abrupt ↑ HR
Atrial tachycardia	150–200	Abnormal	1:1 with prolonged PR or 2:1	
Atrial flutter	300	Flutter waves Negative II, III and a VF	Variable 1:1 to 4:1 or Wenckebach	Ventricular response regular or irregular
Atrial fibrillation	450–600	'f' waves or isolectric	–	Irregular ventricular response
AVNRT	140–220	Retrograde	Usually synchronous	Normal resting ECG
AVNRT fast/slow	120–150	Retrograde	R–P' > P'R	Frequent/incessant
AVRT	150–220	Retrograde	RP' < P'R Inverted P' in ST segment	WPW or concealed accessory pathway

P', retrograde P wave; AVNRT, atrioventricular nodal re-entry tachycardia; AVRT, atrioventricular (orthodromic) re-entry tachycardia; WPW, Wolff–Parkinson–White syndrome.

severely symptomatic. After a variable period which may be as much as several years, atrial fibrillation typically becomes chronic. At this stage, the ventricular rate is often slower and the patient is commonly unaware of the irregular pulse or of palpitations. There are numerous causes of atrial fibrillation (Table 7), but in some instances no obvious aetiological factor can be identified, and the individual is described as having 'lone' atrial fibrillation. Many studies have demonstrated the adverse prognostic significance of atrial fibrillation. This is due in part to its association with organic heart disease. In addition, atrial fibrillation is a clearly recognized risk factor for the development of stroke. The risk is small in patients with paroxysmal atrial fibrillation in the absence of organic heart disease, but is significantly greater in the presence of chronic atrial fibrillation. The risk of stroke is increased 5-fold in such patients, and as much as 17-fold in patients with mitral stenosis and chronic atrial fibrillation where stasis and thrombus formation in the left atrium are particularly common.

Atrial fibrillation results in loss of the atrial contribution to left ventricular filling, which may result in a modest reduction in cardiac output. This may be important in the presence of impaired ventricular function, and result in a worsening of heart failure. More commonly, symptoms arise as a result of a rapid uncontrolled ventricular rate. This may result in impairment of ventricular filling such as in mitral stenosis, or in the development of angina in patients with coexisting coronary artery disease. A sustained high rate may precipitate cardiac failure.

Fig. 32 Atrial fibrillation, with rapid (above) and controlled (below) ventricular response.

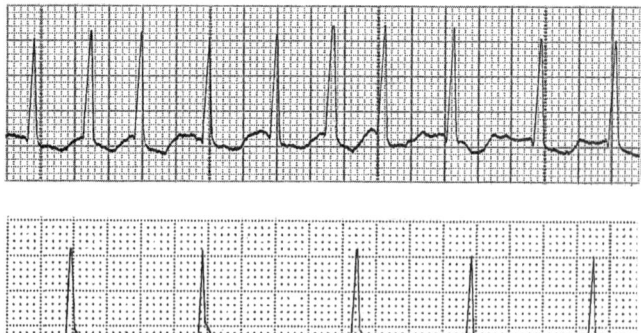

Table 7 *Aetiology of atrial fibrillation*

Increased atrial pressure/wall tension–mitral valve disease, congestive heart failure, left ventricular hypertrophy, restrictive cardiomyopathy, hypertrophic cardiomyopathy, pulmonary embolism, atrial septal defect
Myocardia ischaemia/infarction
Thyrotoxicosis
Alcohol
Sinoatrial disease
Infiltration–constrictive pericarditis, tumour
Infection–myo/pericarditis, pneumonia
Retrograde activation–WPW syndrome, ventricular pacing
Cardiac or thoracic surgery
Idiopathic–'lone' atrial fibrillation

WPW, Wolff–Parkinson–White.

Management

The management of a patient presenting in atrial fibrillation will depend upon the duration of the episode, the presence of organic heart disease and any precipitating factors. An attempt to restore sinus rhythm should be made unless atrial fibrillation is obviously of long standing or associated with advanced organic heart disease. Underlying precipitating factors such as thyrotoxicosis should be corrected before attempting cardioversion. Chemical cardioversion may be achieved with class Ia, Ic or III agents. Class Ia agents may accelerate the ventricular rate by virtue of their anticholinergic action on the atrioventricular node, and must be used in combination with digoxin. The most common agent used is quinidine (1 to 2 g/day), but more recently satisfactory results have been reported with flecainide given intravenously (2 mg/kg over 30 min), sotalol (1.5 mg/kg intravenously over 30 min) or amiodarone (300 mg intravenously over 30 min followed by 1200 mg per 24 h until cardioversion). Normally, only one drug should be tried in any individual patient. If drug therapy fails, direct current cardioversion under general anaesthesia is commonly effective.

Following successful cardioversion, or in the presence of paroxysmal atrial fibrillation, prophylactic therapy may be necessary, particularly if multiple episodes have occurred. No drug is entirely satisfactory. Quinidine, the traditional mainstay of prophylaxis, appears to increase mortality and is best avoided. Sotalol 80 to 160 mg twice a day is well tolerated and appears to be the drug of choice. Amiodarone is effective in controlling paroxysmal atrial fibrillation, but its side-effect profile is such that it is rarely indicated for this use unless the arrhythmia is extremely troublesome and fails to respond to other drugs. If drug therapy fails completely, His bundle ablation may be indicated. However, it is wiser to defer ablative therapy where at all possible, since the natural history of paroxysmal atrial fibrillation is to revert into chronic atrial fibrillation with a marked improvement in symptoms.

If restoration of sinus rhythm is not practical or is unsuccessful, chronic management of atrial fibrillation involves control of ventricular rate. The mainstay of treatment is digoxin, at a dose titrated to achieve adequate slowing in ventricular rate at rest, with therapeutic plasma concentrations. Despite adequate rate control at rest, patients with atrial fibrillation commonly have an uncontrolled heart rate on exercise. This is normally well tolerated, and attempts to slow the rate response with additional atrioventricular nodal blocking drugs such as verapamil or beta blockers do not improve exercise tolerance, except if the duration of diastole is critical as in mitral stenosis or ischaemic heart disease.

Prophylaxis against thromboembolism should be considered in all patients in atrial fibrillation. Cardioversion may be associated with embolism, and patients who are scheduled to have elective chemical or electrical cardioversion should ideally be treated with warfarin for up to four weeks before admission. Where the arrhythmia is of only a few days origin, intravenous heparin for 24 to 48 h is acceptable. Chronic prophylaxis with warfarin anticoagulation is indicated in patients in atrial fibrillation with mitral stenosis or regurgitation. Recent studies have shown that even patients with non-rheumatic atrial fibrillation will benefit from prophylaxis against thromboembolism. The risk of thromboembolism is low in paroxysmal atrial fibrillation, but increases with chronic atrial fibrillation. Warfarin anticoagulation has been shown to reduce the risk of thromboembolic events. There is some evidence that low dose aspirin may also be effective, but studies are still underway to determine this with certainty.

ATRIAL FLUTTER

Atrial flutter is a characteristic arrhythmia producing a typical electrocardiographic 'saw tooth' pattern of atrial activity with a rate close to 300/min (Fig. 33). Flutter waves are commonly negative in the inferior limb leads and positive in lead V1. Atrial flutter may be associated with either a regular or irregular ventricular response.

Two to one atrioventricular conduction producing a regular tachycardia of 150/min is common, and atrial flutter should always be considered in the differential diagnosis of a regular, narrow QRS tachycardia of this rate. Occasionally, flutter occurs with 1 : 1 atrioventricular conduction producing a ventricular rate approaching 300/min. The flutter waves may not be seen easily with faster ventricular rates, and transient slowing of atrioventricular conduction may be necessary to make the diagnosis (Fig. 34).

The underlying causes of atrial flutter are the same as those of atrial fibrillation. Although atrial flutter may last for many months or occasionally years, it usually degenerates into chronic atrial fibrillation unless cardioversion is undertaken. Atrial flutter carries a lower risk of thromboembolism, presumably because there is some organized contractile activity in the atria and the duration of the arrhythmia is shorter.

Termination of atrial flutter may be achieved by chemical or electrical

Fig. 33 Atrial flutter, with variable ventricular response.

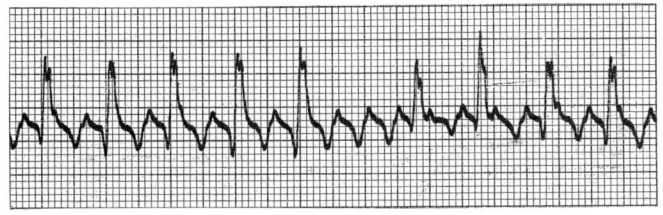

cardioversion as described above for atrial fibrillation. Atrial flutter is due to a re-entry mechanism and an additional mode of termination is by rapid atrial pacing at a rate approximately 10 per cent above the atrial flutter rate. Bursts of atrial pacing may restore sinus rhythm, or precipitate atrial fibrillation. It is important to attempt to terminate atrial flutter, since the ventricular rate is often poorly controlled by digoxin and the patient may remain symptomatic. Prophylaxis against atrial flutter is undertaken using the same agents as in paroxysmal atrial fibrillation. Indeed, the conditions often coexist and patients may manifest either flutter or fibrillation at different times.

ATRIAL TACHYCARDIA

The term atrial tachycardia is used when the atrial rate is slower than in atrial flutter, usually between 120 and 250/min. As in atrial flutter, there may be a degree of atrioventricular block although 1 : 1 atrioventricular conduction may occur. The electrocardiogram shows regular P waves which do not show the same 'saw tooth' appearance as in atrial flutter (Fig. 35).

Atrial tachycardia may occur as a result of sinus node re-entry, in which sudden paroxysms of tachycardia with a normal P wave morphology will arise. Automatic atrial tachycardia manifests a different P wave morphology, commonly with a longer PR interval. The rate characteristically accelerates or 'warms up' before reaching a rate of 125 to 200/min. This arrhythmia is not started or terminated by atrial extrasystoles. Atrial tachycardia with block is a manifestation of digitalis tox-

Fig. 34 Atrial flutter with 1 : 1 atrioventricular conduction (above), 2 : 1 conduction (middle) and following adenosine administration (below) (6 mg intravenous injection 10 s previously).

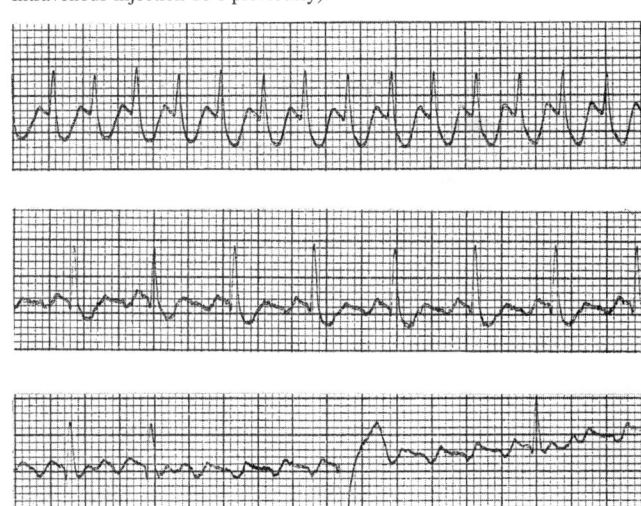

Fig. 35 Atrial tachycardia with 1 : 1 atrioventricular conduction (above). The underlying atrial tachycardia is revealed following intravenous administration of 6 mg adenosine (below).

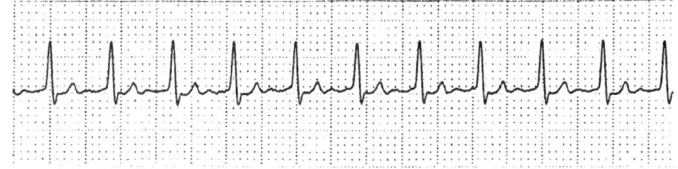

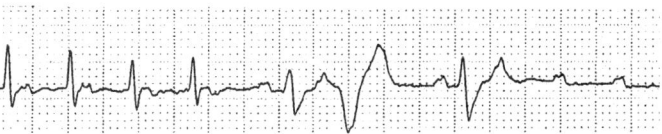

icity. The ventricular rate may be relatively slow in view of the atrio-ventricular block and careful evaluation of the electrocardiogram is necessary to identify this arrhythmia. Multifocal atrial tachycardia, in which rapid irregular, discrete P-waves of three or four different morphologies are seen, may occur in severely ill, elderly patients or may be associated with acute exacerbation of pulmonary disease. It is rarely responsive to digoxin, but success with intravenous verapamil, or magnesium, has suggested triggered activity as the underlying mechanism.

The clinical context of atrial tachycardia is commonly the same as for atrial fibrillation and flutter, except for the association with digitalis toxicity. The approach to management is identical to that of atrial fibrillation.

Junctional re-entry tachycardias

All regular, paroxysmal tachycardias with narrow QRS complexes were previously grouped together as 'supraventricular tachycardias', or even more loosely as 'paroxysmal atrial tachycardias'. Greater understanding of the underlying mechanisms responsible for these arrhythmias has rendered these terms obsolete, and it is now possible to identify the exact mechanism underlying regular narrow complex tachycardias with confidence in most instances. When atrial arrhythmias are excluded, the vast majority are junctional re-entry tachycardias, either atrioventricular nodal re-entry or atrioventricular re-entry (see below), which involve the atrioventricular node in the re-entry circuit. Correct recognition of these arrhythmias has achieved additional importance with the development of effective curative measures, such as ablative techniques.

ATRIOVENTRICULAR NODAL RE-ENTRY TACHYCARDIA

This is the most common cause of paroxysmal re-entry tachycardia manifesting regular, normal QRS complexes. The basis of the arrhythmia is the presence of two functionally distinct atrioventricular nodal pathways (Fig. 36). The fast pathway conducts more rapidly, but has a longer refractory period. The slow pathway has slow conduction properties but a shorter refractory period. During sinus rhythm, atrioventricular nodal conduction occurs via the fast pathway with a normal PR interval. If a sufficiently premature atrial extrasystole arises, conduction in the fast pathway is blocked. Slow pathway conduction may continue, resulting

in an abrupt increase in the AH interval as recorded in the His bundle electrogram corresponding to an increased PR interval on the surface electrocardiogram. Conduction may be sufficiently slow as to allow the fast pathway to recover excitability prior to activation reaching the distal end of the pathways, allowing retrograde activation to occur via the fast pathway. The stage is then set for a re-entry circuit with antegrade conduction via the slow pathway and retrograde conduction via the fast pathway. The arrhythmia circuit is functionally distinct from the atria and ventricles, which may be perturbed by extrastimuli without interruption of the tachycardia. Characteristically, antegrade activation of the ventricles and retrograde activation of the atria occur virtually simultaneously, resulting in the P wave being 'buried' within the QRS complex, or producing a very small distortion of the terminal QRS, which cannot be recognized easily without careful comparison with the electrocardiogram during sinus rhythm (Fig. 37). The tachycardia is readily initiated by atrial premature stimulation, and terminated by appropriately timed extrastimuli or by overdrive pacing. A less common variant of atrioventricular nodal tachycardia may arise where antegrade conduction during tachycardia is via the fast pathway with retrograde conduction via the slow pathway. Under these circumstances, the atrium is activated well after the QRS complex, characteristically producing an inverted P' wave with the R–P' interval greater than the P'R interval during tachycardia (Fig. 38). Occasionally, slow/fast and fast/slow tachycardias may coexist in the same patient.

Atrioventricular nodal re-entry tachycardia commonly presents for the first time in childhood or adolescence, although it may appear at any age. The natural history is of episodic paroxysmal tachycardia. Attacks occur at random intervals, although clustering of attacks may occur with periods of relative freedom from symptoms in between. Atrioventricular nodal re-entry tachycardia has no specific association with other organic heart disease. Palpitations are normally well tolerated unless the tachycardia is particularly rapid, prolonged or if the patient has other heart disease.

Termination of an attack of atrioventricular nodal re-entry tachycardia is achieved by producing transient atrioventricular nodal block. This may be achieved by vagotonic manoeuvres, by intravenous verapamil (5 to 10 mg) or by intravenous adenosine (3 to 12 mg) (Fig. 39). Intravenous β-blockade is occasionally used, but is less effective. Drug prophylaxis of atrioventricular nodal re-entry tachycardia is undertaken

Fig. 36 Atrioventricular nodal re-entry tachycardia. Mechanism of initiation by atrial extrasystole. See text for details.

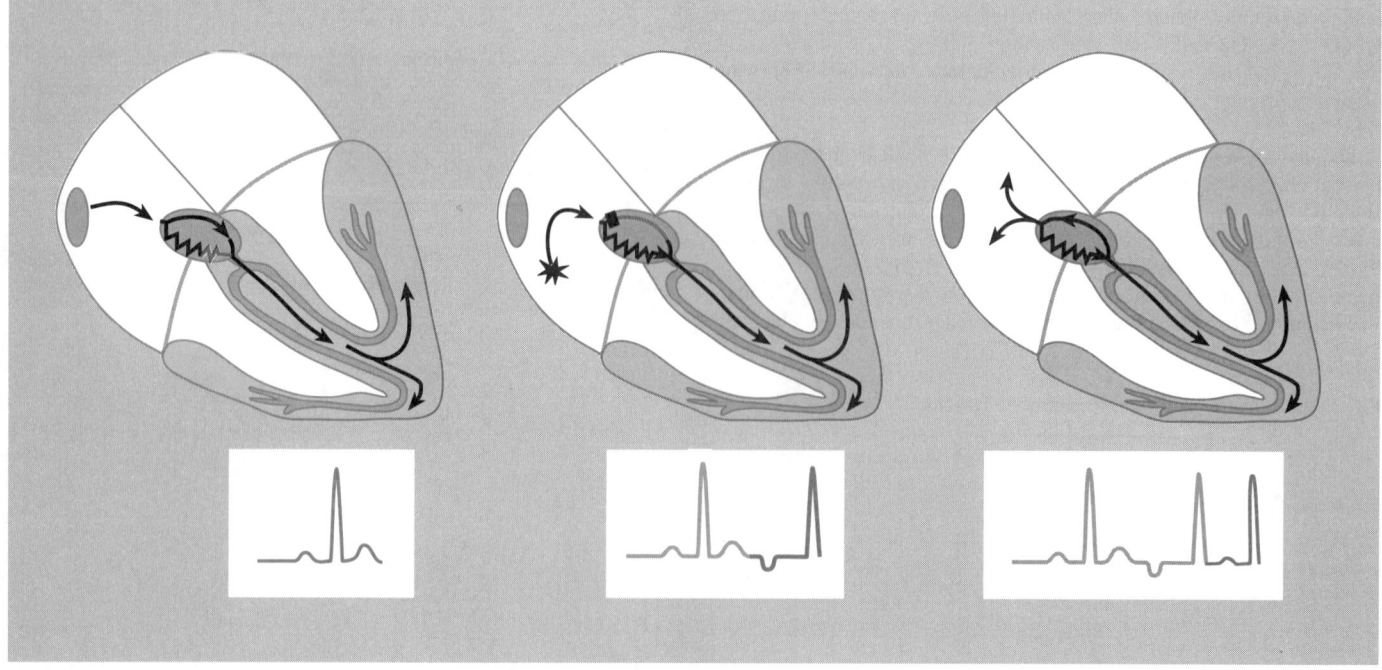

with β-blockers, a combined β-blocker class III agent such as sotalol, or with atrioventricular nodal blocking drugs such as verapamil or digoxin. Atrial anti-tachycardia pacemakers have been used successfully in patients refractory to drugs or intolerant of side-effects. These pacemakers do not prevent attacks of tachycardia, but can usually terminate them by overdrive pacing salvoes within a minute or so. Recently, attempts at curative treatment of atrioventricular nodal re-entry tachycardia have been reported, initially by surgical means and more recently by radiofrequency ablation. Most authors have attempted to ablate the slow pathway, which appears anatomically distinct from the site of the atrioventricular node despite its electrophysiological properties. Ablation of the slow pathway carries a low risk of induction of complete atrioventricular block, and produces excellent results.

ATRIOVENTRICULAR RE-ENTRY TACHYCARDIA

The re-entry circuit in atrioventricular re-entry tachycardia also involves the atrioventricular node but, in addition, uses an anomalous atrioventricular connection, or accessory pathway. The mechanism of the common form of atrioventricular re-entry tachycardia, orthodromic tachycardia, is illustrated in Fig. 40. The refractory period of the accessory pathway is commonly shorter than that of the atrioventricular node; hence a premature atrial extrasystole may find the accessory pathway refractory, but be conducted through the atrioventricular node. If sufficient delay has occurred, the accessory pathway will have recovered excitability sufficiently to allow retrograde activation from the ventricle to atrium, with the establishment of a re-entry circuit. Since the circuit involves activation of the ventricles via the His–Purkinje system, the QRS morphology during re-entry tachycardia will be normal, unless rate related bundle branch block develops. Retrograde atrial activation may be identified by the presence of an inverted P′ wave inscribed early in the ST segment. The presence of a P′ wave in this position during a

regular narrow complex tachycardia is suggestive of an atrioventricular tachycardia utilizing an accessory pathway rather than of atrioventricular nodal re-entry tachycardia. In sinus rhythm, the presence of an accessory pathway may be revealed by the characteristic features on the electrocardiogram of 'pre-excitation' (Fig. 41).

PRE-EXCITATION SYNDROMES (WOLFF-PARKINSON-WHITE SYNDROME)

The term pre-excitation refers to the premature activation of the ventricle via an accessory pathway which bypasses the normal atrioventricular node and His–Purkinje system. The most common of the pre-excitation syndromes is the Wolff–Parkinson–White syndrome in which one or more accessory pathways with electrophysiological properties of normal myocardium are present. The accessory pathways may lie at any point in the atrioventricular ring, although the commonest sites are in the left free wall and the posteroseptal region.

The electrocardiographic appearances of the Wolff–Parkinson–White syndrome arise from early activation of the myocardium adjacent to the ventricular insertion of the accessory pathway (Fig. 40). There is no atrioventricular delay, hence the PR interval is shortened but slow intraventricular conduction results in a slurred initiation of the QRS complex (the δ wave) (Fig. 42). The remainder of the ventricle is excited via the normal His–Purkinje system. The degree of pre-excitation during sinus rhythm is variable. Pre-excitation may be intermittent, if the refractory period of the accessory pathway is close to the sinus cycle length, or latent, if the δ wave is obscured due to rapid atrioventricular nodal conduction. Agents which enhance atrioventricular nodal conduction will increase the proportion of ventricular tissue activated via the His–Purkinje system and will lessen the appearances of pre-excitation. In contrast, transient slowing of atrioventricular nodal conduction will enhance the proportion of the ventricle excited by the accessory pathway. This feature may be used to diagnose latent pre-excitation by the administration of adenosine or verapamil.

The characteristic tachycardia of the Wolff–Parkinson–White syndrome is atrioventricular (orthodromic) re-entry tachycardia. Rarely, the refractory period of the atrioventricular node may exceed that of the accessory pathway, and a tachycardia may arise which has antegrade conduction via the accessory pathway and retrograde conduction via the atrioventricular node (antidromic tachycardia). The QRS morphology of this tachycardia will be grossly abnormal with appearances dependent upon the site of insertion of the accessory pathway (Fig. 43).

Not all accessory pathways conduct antegradely to cause pre-excitation. The term 'concealed accessory pathway' is used to denote a pathway which can only conduct in the retrograde direction. Patients with concealed accessory pathways will have a normal resting electrocardiogram. They are not at risk of pre-excited atrial fibrillation (see below) but may be prone to attacks of atrioventricular re-entry (orthodromic) tachycardia.

Other forms of pre-excitation include the Mahaim pathway, previously thought to be a connection between the atrioventricular node and the ventricle or bundle branches, but recent evidence based on catheter ablation suggests that many, if not all, Mahaim pathways are direct atrioventricular or atriofasicular connections with slow conduction properties typical of atrioventricular nodal tissue. Evidence for direct atrionodal pathways associated with a short PR interval but no delta wave (Lown–Ganong–Levine syndrome) remains controversial and has not been established histologically.

Pre-excited atrial fibrillation

Patients with Wolff–Parkinson–White syndrome are at increased risk of the development of atrial fibrillation, possibly as a result of rapid atrial stimulation during prolonged orthodromic tachycardia. Although orthodromic tachycardia is an important cause of symptoms, the major prognostic concern in Wolff–Parkinson–White syndrome is pre-excited atrial

Fig. 37 Atrioventricular nodal re-entry tachycardia.

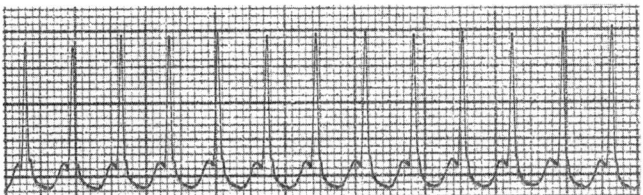

Fig. 38 Atypical atrioventricular nodal re-entry tachycardia ('long RP'). Inverted P′ waves precede the QRS complex during tachycardia (compare with preceding sinus beats).

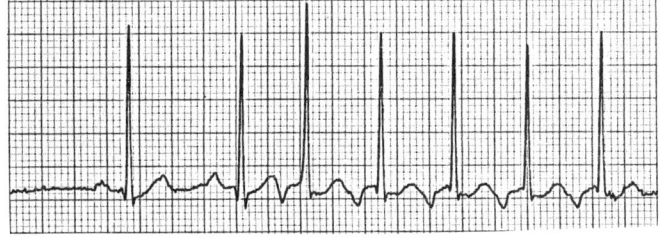

Fig. 39 Termination of atrioventricular nodal re-entry tachycardia 20 s after intravenous injection of adenosine (6 mg).

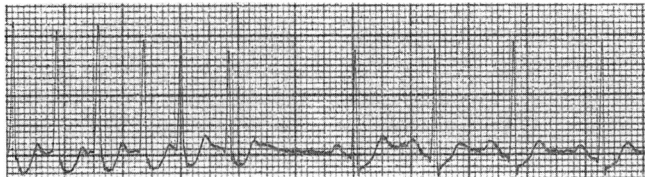

fibrillation because conduction via a fast accessory pathway, bypassing the normal atrioventricular nodal slowing, may result in atrial fibrillation being conducted at a rapid rate to the ventricles (Fig. 44). If the refractory period of the accessory pathway is sufficiently short, atrial fibrillation may result in very rapid ventricular conduction which may degenerate into ventricular fibrillation. The degree of pre-excitation during atrial fibrillation may vary, giving a characteristic pattern of an irregular ventricular response with QRS morphology varying from normal to fully pre-excited. The exact QRS morphology will depend on the site of insertion of the accessory pathway.

Clinical features

Accessory pathways are a common anomaly, with the electrocardiographic appearances of a delta wave occurring in approximately 1.5 per 1000 of the population. Many of these patients never experience paroxysmal tachycardias. The major concern in Wolff–Parkinson–White syndrome is the risk of sudden death due to rapid pre-excited atrial fibrillation. This risk appears to be very low among patients who have not had any symptomatic tachycardias, and increases in symptomatic patients, particularly if episodes of pre-excited atrial fibrillation have been documented. Analysis of spontaneous or induced episodes of pre-excited atrial fibrillation is important in assessing risk. The identification of consecutive pre-excited RR intervals of less than 250 ms identifies a higher risk group, although even in this group the absolute risk remains low. The general tendency is for accessory pathway conduction to become slower with increasing age. Patients who have experienced atrial fibrillation with relatively slow ventricular rates are unlikely to develop faster ventricular responses subsequently. Spontaneous disappearance of antegrade accessory pathway conduction is well documented in

patients with low risk pathways. Wolff–Parkinson–White syndrome may be associated with Ebstein's anomaly but has no other clinical associations.

Careful analysis of the electrocardiogram is helpful in predicting the likely site of the accessory pathway, and may avoid erroneous diagnoses. For instance, a positive delta wave and QRS complex in lead V1 may be mistaken for right bundle branch block, while negative delta waves in the inferior leads may be mistaken for previous inferior myocardial infarction (see Fig. 42).

Management

Management of the Wolff–Parkinson–White syndrome includes termination of individual attacks of tachycardia, risk assessment, drug prophylaxis and ablative therapy. Orthodromic re-entry tachycardia may be terminated by atrioventricular nodal blocking manoeuvres such as vagal stimulation, verapamil or adenosine. The management of pre-excited atrial fibrillation requires particular care, since digoxin or verapamil may paradoxically accelerate ventricular rate and are contraindicated. In the presence of severe haemodynamic disturbance, direct current cardioversion is the treatment of choice. Where patients are more stable, the use of an agent which slows antegrade conduction through the accessory pathway and ideally restores sinus rhythm is advised. Intravenous flecainide, sotalol, or amiodarone are all effective for this indication.

Patients with symptomatic Wolff–Parkinson–White syndrome should be evaluated carefully for the risk of pre-excited atrial fibrillation. If pre-excitation is intermittent, this is commonly associated with a long accessory pathway refractory period and a low risk of life-threatening tachycardias. Disappearance of the δ wave in response to administration of a class Ia or Ic antiarrhythmic drug also suggests a low risk. Ideally, all

Fig. 40 Atrioventricular re-entry tachycardia. Mechanism of initiation by atrial extrasystole. See text for details.

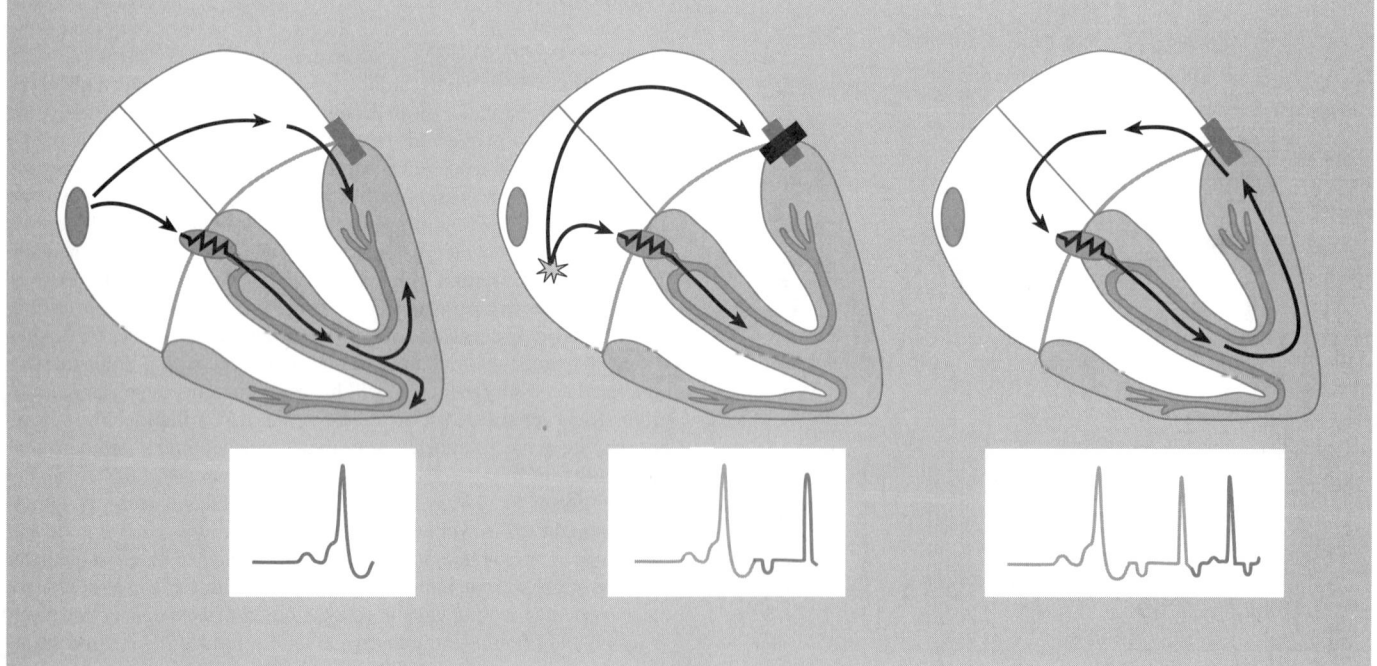

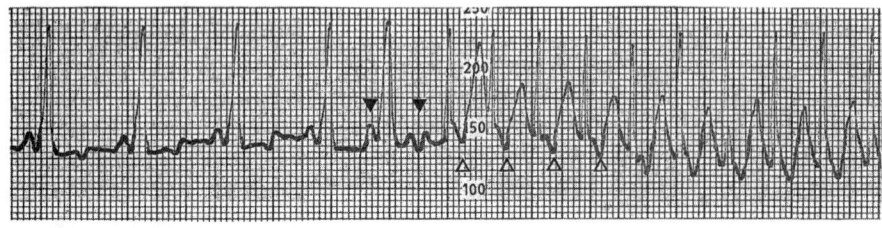

Fig. 41 Initiation of atrioventricular re-entrant tachycardia by atrial extrasystoles (arrows). Note the presence of short PR interval and delta wave during sinus rhythm, with normalization of QRS complex and appearance of retrograde P′ waves (open arrows) during tachycardia.

patients with symptomatic Wolff–Parkinson–White syndrome should undergo electrophysiological assessment. The principal objective is to assess the accessory pathway refractory period by premature stimulation, and to determine the ventricular rate during induced atrial fibrillation. The site of the accessory pathway is mapped at electrophysiological study, and, in many centres, ablation of the pathway will be attempted at the same session.

Fig. 42 Electrocardiographic features of Wolff–Parkinson–White syndrome, from a patient with a posteroseptal accessory pathway.

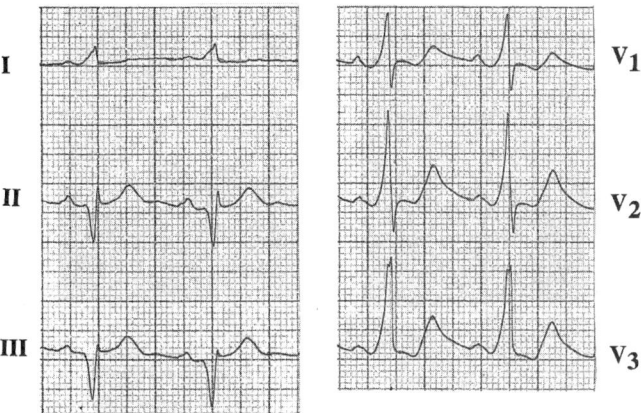

Fig. 43 Antidromic tachycardia.

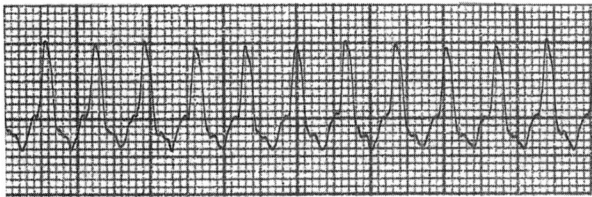

Fig. 44 Pre-excited atrial fibrillarion.

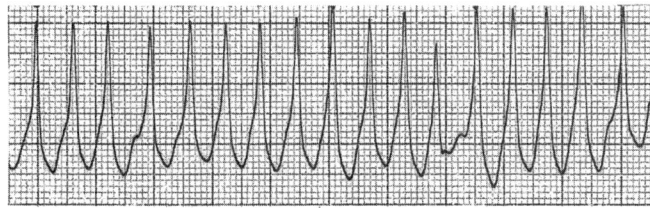

Fig. 45 Broad complex tachycardia is revealed as supraventricular tachycardia with bundle branch block following spontaneous loss of aberrant conduction.

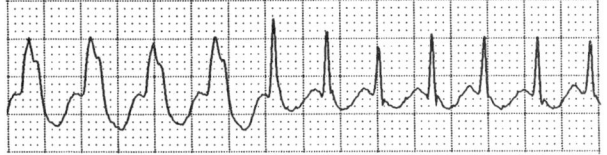

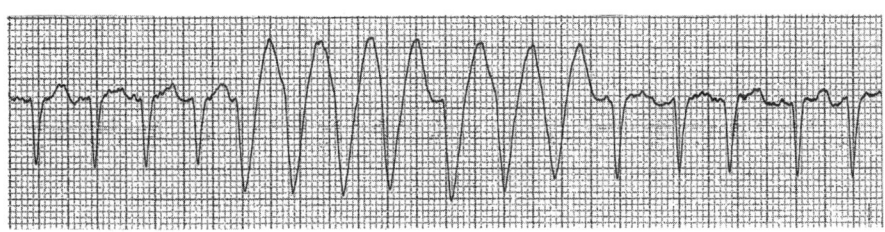

Fig. 46 Atrial fibrillation with intermittent bundle branch block.

Drug prophylaxis of Wolff–Parkinson–White syndrome should attempt to minimize the frequency of orthodromic re-entry tachycardia and of atrial fibrillation. For this reason, drugs acting only on the atrioventricular node such as verapamil are less effective than agents having an action on the accessory pathway in addition such as flecainide and sotalol. Although amiodarone is effective in the prophylaxis of Wolff–Parkinson–White syndrome, its use is not desirable in otherwise fit young people who may require long-term drug therapy, because of its potential for adverse effects.

In patients who are shown to be at high risk of pre-excited atrial fibrillation, those with troublesome symptomatic arrhythmias or those who do not wish to consider long-term drug therapy, radiofrequency ablation of the accessory pathway is an attractive option. Careful electrode positioning on the atrioventricular annulus is necessary to identify the site at which the atrioventricular interval is at a minimum, ideally with a discrete accessory pathway potential between the atrial and ventricular signals. Application of radiofrequency current at this site will produce rapid interuption of accessory pathway conduction, and more prolonged energy application results in a permanent ablation of the pathway (see Fig. 12). The procedure may be undertaken under local anaesthesia, and multiple pathways may be ablated. The success rate of this procedure in experienced centres is over 90 per cent, with a very low incidence of complications. Although surgical techniques for ablation of accessory pathways were comparably effective, their use has fallen dramatically since the introduction of radiofrequency ablation.

LOWN–GANONG–LEVINE SYNDROME

The Lown–Ganong–Levine syndrome consists of a short PR interval and a normal QRS complex in association with supraventricular tachycardias. The basis of the short PR interval has not been established with certainty, but may reflect a small atrioventricular node, the presence of excess adrenergic tone, or partial bypass of the normal atrioventricular nodal tissue. Paroxysmal tachycardias may be of the atrioventricular nodal re-entry tachycardia or atrioventricular re-entry tachycardia type. Treatment of this condition is along the lines indicated for atrioventricular nodal re-entry tachycardia.

Diagnosis of wide QRS complex tachycardias

Few areas in cardiology cause more difficulty, or result in more mismanagement, than the diagnosis of wide complex tachycardias. While it is safe to assume that virtually all narrow complex tachycardias have a supraventricular origin, wide complex tachycardias may arise either from the ventricle, or from supraventricular mechanisms (Figs 43, 44, 45 and 46) when associated with pre-excitation or bundle branch block (Table 8). Misdiagnosis and mismanagement most commonly arise when ventricular tachycardia is not recognized and is misdiagnosed as 'SVT with aberration'. This can arise as a result of a number of failings or misconceptions:

1. The clinical context is not considered. Middle-aged or elderly patients presenting with a recent history of wide complex tachycardia and who give a history of myocardial infarction or congestive heart failure are more likely to have ventricular than supraventricular tachycardia. Supraventricular tachycar-

Table 8 *ECG features of wide complex tachycardia*

	Atrial rhythm	Atrioventricular relationship	ECG morphology	
			Tachycardia	Sinus rhythm
Irregular ventricular response				
AF/AF1 with previous BBB	'f' or flutter waves	Irregular	Typical BBB	BBB
AF/AF1 with functional BBB	'f' or flutter waves	Irregular	Typical BBB	Normal
Pre-excited AF	'f' waves	Irregular	Varying normal/pre-excited	WPW
Torsades de pointes	Obscured	–	Varying QRS axis	Long QT
Regular ventricular response				
Ventricular tachycardia	Sinus or retrograde VA conduction	AV dissociation or 1:1/2:1 VA conduction	Abnormal wide complexes QRS > 0.14 s Extreme axis deviation Fusion/capture beats Concordance RBBB tachycardia with Rsr' in V1 or qS in V6	?Old MI
AF1 with BBB	Flutter waves	2:1	Typical BBB	WPW or normal
AVRT with functional BBB	Retrograde atrial activation	1:1		
AVNRT with functional BBB	Synchronous with QRS	1:1	Typical BBB	Normal
Antidromic tachycardia	Obscured in QRS	1:1	Pre-excited	WPW

AF, atrial fibrillation; AF1, atrial flutter; AV, atrioventricular; AVNRT, atrioventricular nodal re-entry tachycardia; AVRT, atrioventricular (orthodromic) re-entry tachycardia; BBB, bundle branch block; MI, myocardial infarction; RBBB, right bundle branch block; VA, ventriculoatrial; WPW, Wolff–Parkinson–White syndrome.

Table 9 *Diagnostic use of intravenous adenosine*

Arrhythmia	Response
Atrial tachycardia Atrial flutter Atrial fibrillation	Transient AV block reveals atrial arrhythmia. Rarely terminated
AVNRT AVRT	Terminates tachycardia by antegrade (AV) block)
Ventricular tachycardia	Not terminated 1:1 VA conduction may be blocked, revealing AV dissociation

AV, atrioventricular; AVNRT, atrioventricular nodal re-entry tachycardia; AVRT, atrioventricular (orthodromic) re-entry tachycardia; VA, ventriculoatrial.

dias due to accessory pathways or atrioventricular nodal re-entry normally present in adolescence or early adult life. However, ventricular tachycardia may arise even in young patients.

2. Ventricular tachycardia is invariably assumed to cause haemodynamic collapse. Patients in ventricular tachycardia may be haemodynamically stable if the rate is not excessively fast or if underlying cardiac function is good. Conversely, supraventricular tachycardias may cause syncope, hypotension or shock if sufficiently rapid.

3. History of tachycardias. Ventricular tachycardia may present with a typical history of paroxysmal self-terminating tachycardia, just as in the case of supraventricular tachycardia.

4. Electrocardiographic analysis. Lack of detailed analysis of the electrocardiogram during tachycardia may lead to misdiagnosis. A 12-lead electrocardiogram should be obtained wherever possible. Characteristic electrocardiographic features of wide complex tachycardias are presented in Table 8.

In addition to careful analysis of the history and electrocardiogram, the response to transient atrioventricular nodal blockade will assist consid-erably in diagnosis. Vagal stimulation may be inadequate to achieve sufficient atrioventricular block, but the response to adenosine (Table 9) will permit distinction between atrial, junctional and ventricular tachycardia in many patients (Fig. 47).

The importance of making a correct diagnosis in wide complex tachycardia is two-fold. First, inappropriate acute therapy of the tachyarrhythmia can be avoided. In particular, the use of verapamil in ventricular tachycardia misdiagnosed as supraventricular tachycardia is associated with a high risk of haemodynamic deterioration as a result of the negative inotropic effect of verapamil coupled with its lack of efficacy in terminating ventricular tachycardia. Cardiac arrest may be precipitated. Verapamil should not be used in a wide complex tachycardia unless the

Fig. 47 Responses of broad complex tachycardias to intravenous adenosine. Supraventricular tachycardia is terminated (above), atrial flutter is revealed (middle) and ventricular tachycardia is not terminated (below), although retrograde ventriculoatrial block results in atrioventricular dissociation (P waves are arrowed) and a fusion beat (open circle).

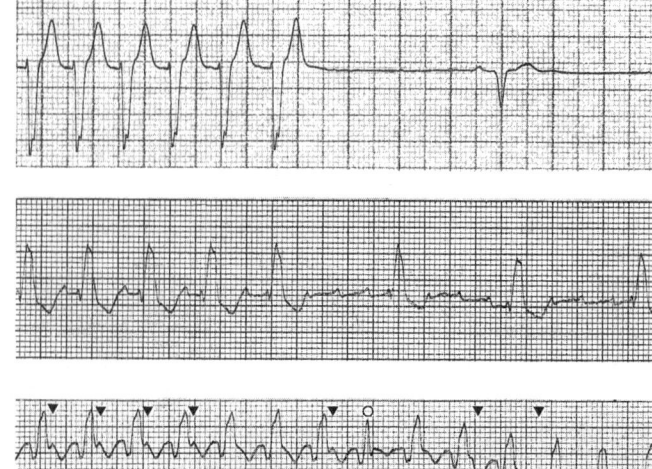

diagnosis of supraventricular tachycardia is made beyond doubt. Adenosine is a safer diagnostic aid. Second, the correct diagnosis has prognostic implications. It may be argued that any wide complex tachycardia can be terminated effectively by cardioversion. However, if the original tachycardia has been misdiagnosed, the prognostic significance of ventricular tachycardia may be overlooked and appropriate investigation and long term management may not be instituted.

Ventricular tachyarrhythmias

DEFINITIONS

Ventricular tachycardia is defined as the presence of five or more consecutive ventricular beats at a rate of 120 per min or greater. Ventricular tachycardia is defined as sustained if an individual salvo lasts for 30 s or more, and non-sustained if the duration is between five beats and 30 s. Monomorphic ventricular tachycardia demonstrates a consistent QRS morphology during each paroxysm, although patients may have paroxysms of monomorphic ventricular tachycardia of different morphologies at different times. Polymorphic ventricular tachycardia demonstrates a constantly changing QRS morphology, often without discrete QRS complexes. Polymorphic ventricular tachycardia may degenerate into ventricular fibrillation and the electrocardiographic distinction between the two is difficult. Torsades de pointes is a characteristic type of polymorphic ventricular tachycardia with a typical undulating variation in QRS morphology as a result of variation in axis. The term is best reserved for the arrhythmias arising in association with QT interval prolongation.

SUSTAINED MONOMORPHIC VENTRICULAR TACHYCARDIA

This arrhythmia occurs most commonly in the presence of structural heart disease, particularly recent or remote myocardial infarction. Operative mapping studies suggest that the usual mechanism is one of micro re-entry with slow conduction occurring at the border of the infarcted area where surviving muscle fibres are interdigitated with fibrous tissue (see Fig. 4). Less common mechanisms of sustained monomorphic ventricular tachycardia include macro re-entry involving the bundle branches, or triggered activity.

Electrocardiographic characteristics

The electrocardiographic characteristics of ventricular tachycardia have been listed in Table 8. The presence of atrioventricular dissociation is a particularly important feature to seek in a wide complex tachycardia as it makes the diagnosis of ventricular tachycardia virtually certain (Fig. 48). Careful search for P waves perturbing the QRS complex or T waves is necessary, ideally using multichannel recordings. A fusion beat may be present, where activation of the ventricle occurs partly via the normal His–Purkinje system and partly from the tachycardia focus (Fig. 49).

Occasionally, a fortuitously timed P wave may allow the development of a capture beat of normal QRS morphology without interupting the tachycardia. Fusion and capture beats are diagnostic of ventricular tachycardia and should be carefully sought, but are commonly present only if the ventricular rate is relatively slow. Where dissociated P wave activity cannot be recognized with certainty on the surface electrocardiogram, direct recording of atrial activity by an oesophageal or right atrial electrogram may aid the diagnosis. Echocardiography and Doppler cardiography may also permit identification of dissociated atrial activity. Although atrioventricular dissociation is diagnostic of ventricular tachycardia, it is not invariable. Retrograde ventriculoatrial conduction may occur, giving either 1 : 1 ventriculoatrial conduction or higher degrees of ventriculoatrial block (Fig. 48). If 1 : 1 ventriculoatrial conduction can be interupted temporarily by adenosine, this may allow the identification of atrioventricular dissociation or the appearance of a fusion or capture beat (see Fig. 47). The QRS duration in ventricular tachycardia is commonly greater than 0.12 s, and values greater than 0.14 s are particularly suggestive of ventricular tachycardia. Although the QRS morphology may superficially resemble left or right bundle branch block, the morphology is commonly atypical. Specific morphological patterns may be identified (Table 8). The presence of concordant positive or negative QRS complexes across the chest leads is suggestive of ventricular tachycardia, as is the existence of extreme axis deviation (Fig. 50). The occurrence of different abnormal QRS morphologies during tachycardia on different occasions is highly suggestive of ventricular tachycardia.

Aetiology

Although sustained ventricular tachycardia may occur in acute myocardial infarction, it is more commonly of an unstable, polymorphic type, which either terminates spontaneously or degenerates into ventricular fibrillation. Sustained monomorphic ventricular tachycardia may be seen in the subacute phase, or at any time after myocardial infarction. Episodes may arise many years after the index infarction, particularly in association with left ventricular dilatation and aneurysm formation. Sustained ventricular tachycardia may occur in other conditions associated with ventricular dilatation or fibrosis such as dilated cardiomyopathy, hypertrophic cardiomyopathy or previous ventriculotomy (e.g. following repair of Fallot's tetralogy). Ventricular tachycardia in younger patients may arise in association with right ventricular dysplasia, an idiopathic condition associated with replacement of the right ventricular free wall with fibrous tissue and fat. These patients may have no other symptoms or signs of cardiac disease, but dilatation of the right ventricle may be demonstrated on echocardiography or angiography. Ventricular tachycardia has been associated with mitral valve prolapse. Sustained monomorphic tachycardia may occur as a proarrhythmic response to antiarrhythmic drugs, particularly class Ic agents, which may produce a characteristic slow, incessant tachycardia at a rate of 120 to 150 per

Fig. 48 Sustained monomorphic ventricular tachycardia. Atrioventricular dissociation (above) and 2 : 1 ventriculoatrial conduction (below). P waves are shown by arrows.

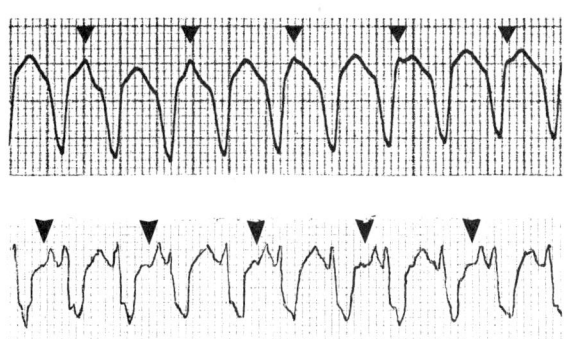

Fig. 49 Ventricular tachycardia with fusion beat (arrow).

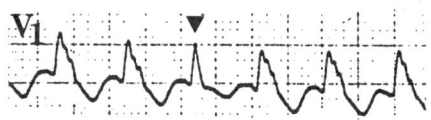

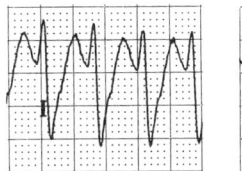 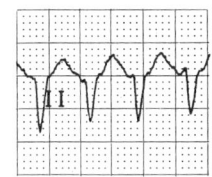 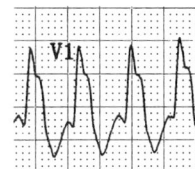

minute, especially after intravenous administration. There remains a minority of patients with documented ventricular tachycardia in whom no structural heart disease is evident on clinical, electrocardiographic or echocardiographic examination. Some of these patients have biopsy evidence of subclinical right ventricular dysplasia, and in others the tachycardia appears to arise from the posterior fascicle of the left bundle branch.

Clinical features

Clinical findings of a patient in ventricular tachycardia will depend on the rate, the duration of the arrhythmia and the underlying cardiac reserve. Rapid ventricular tachycardia may present as cardiac arrest, syncope, shock or left ventricular failure. Slower tachycardias in patients with good cardiac function may present only as palpitations, or may be asymptomatic. Physical examination will reveal a rapid, regular pulse rate and possible signs of shock or left ventricular failure. If atrioventricular dissociation is present, intermittent cannon waves may be seen in the jugular venous pulsation and variation of the intensity of the first heart sound may be heard. In the presence of ventriculoatrial conduction, there will be regular cannon waves with a 1 : 1 or 1 : 2 relationship with the arterial pulse.

Management

Ventricular tachycardia is a medical emergency and normally requires admission to the cardiac care unit. If cardiac arrest is present, or the patient is unconscious, immediate synchronized direct current cardioversion is necessary. If the patient is conscious but hypotensive, urgent elective direct current cardioversion under general anaesthesia or diazepam sedation is used. Tachycardias which are better tolerated may be terminated by drug therapy. The most common agent used is intravenous lignocaine 100 mg, repeated if necessary after 5 min. Second-line drugs for the termination of ventricular tachycardia include procainamide, disopyramide, and amiodarone. Amiodarone normally has a slow onset of action but may be effective if the tachycardia is well tolerated. Flecainide is not advised in view of the risk of developing incessant tachycardia. All antiarrhythmic drugs have significant negative inotropic actions which may further impair the haemodynamic status of the patient if sinus rhythm is not restored. For this reason, no more than two antiarrhythmic drugs should be given before recourse to alternative therapy. Pacemaker termination of ventricular tachycardia following insertion of a temporary pacing lead may be very effective (see Fig. 8), particularly if the tachycardia is relatively slow, or has been slowed by drug therapy. Overdrive pacing is instituted as described previously. Facilities for cardioversion must be available in view of the risk of acceleration of the tachycardia or degeneration into ventricular fibrillation.

Having terminated an episode of ventricular tachycardia, it is essential that the patient be assessed carefully and appropriate prophylactic therapy instituted before discharge from hospital. The risk of recurrent ventricular tachycardia or sudden cardiac death is up to 40 per cent in the first year after the initial event. Evaluation of the patient after restoration of sinus rhythm includes detailed history and physical examination for evidence for organic heart disease, plus electrocardiography to identify evidence of previous myocardial infarction. Further investigation should be undertaken to assess ventricular structure and function by echocardiography and/or radionuclide ventriculography. Particular attention should be paid to the possibility of right ventricular dysplasia in young patients. In patients with a previous history of ischaemic heart disease, exercise testing will be undertaken to identify the presence of reversible ischaemia which may act as a trigger to ventricular tachycardia. Demonstration of exercise induction of ventricular tachycardia is also important, although unusual. Patients with ischaemic-related ventricular tachycardia should undergo coronary arteriography to determine the extent of arterial disease, and to obtain detailed assessment of left ventricular function and of the possibility of left ventricular aneurysm. The underlying mechanism of ventricular tachycardia may be assessed by signal averaged electrocardiography. The presence of ventricular late

potentials indicates an area of delayed conduction which may contribute to a re-entrant substrate for further ventricular tachycardia.

Unless there is a clear precipitating factor such as drug toxicity, electrolyte abnormality, or acute ischaemia, patients who have had documented ventricular tachycardia require antiarrhythmic drug prophylaxis. Unfortunately, the efficacy of any given antiarrhythmic drug cannot be predicted; thus it is necessary to demonstrate antiarrhythmic drug efficacy and to exclude proarrhythmic responses. If episodes of ventricular tachycardia, sustained or non-sustained, are occurring frequently, it is sufficient to administer antiarrhythmic drugs under continuous electrocardiographic monitoring, and to demonstrate that salvoes of tachycardia have been suppressed completely. Unfortunately, many episodes of sustained ventricular tachycardia are infrequent, and suppression of brief salvoes of non-sustained ventricular tachycardia may not correlate with protection from recurrence of sustained tachycardia. Under these circumstances, cardiac electrophysiological testing is indicated. The initial objective of electrophysiological testing is to initiate a tachycardia of similar rate and QRS morphology to the spontaneous arrhythmia. This is attempted by introducing ventricular extrastimuli following trains of ventricular pacing to the right ventricular apex or outflow tract (see Fig. 7). Most protocols start with single extrastimuli at a slow rate, and proceed with increasingly premature stimuli with subsequent increase of the underlying pacing rate and introduction of multiple extrastimuli. Ventricular tachycardia induced at programed stimulation can commonly be terminated by overdrive pacing (see Fig. 8), although cardioversion may be necessary.

If a sustained monomorphic tachycardia can be induced, drug therapy is then administered and a repeat study is undertaken once stable plasma levels of the drug have been achieved. Suppression of inducibility of the tachycardia is associated with a substantially reduced risk of arrhythmia recurrence and an improved prognosis in comparison with patients whose arrhythmia is not suppressed. The choice of antiarrhythmic drug is dictated principally by the underlying left ventricular function and by the adverse effect profile of the drug. Class Ia antiarrhythmic drugs (procainamide, quinidine, or disopyramide) have been the traditional agents of first choice, although recently the class III agent sotalol has been shown to be more effective. Orally active class Ib agents tend to be relatively ineffective in the suppression of ventricular tachycardia, while class Ic agents may be moderately effective but are associated with a high risk of proarrhythmic responses. Amiodarone is generally reserved as the second line agent if no other antiarrhythmic drug is shown to be effective. Because of the slow onset of action of amiodarone, programmed stimulation should not be performed until 10 to 14 days of loading. If arrhythmia is totally suppressed, the prognosis is good. Even if ventricular tachycardia is still inducible, the presence of marked slowing (increase in cycle length greater than 100 ms) associated with good haemodynamic tolerance appears to indicate a good long-term prognosis.

There remains a subgroup of patients in whom no effective antiarrhythmic drug can be found, or in whom antiarrhythmic therapy is not tolerated due to poor ventricular function. These patients are at particularly high risk if treated empirically, and may be candidates for non-pharmacological therapy. Direct surgical management of recurrent ventricular tachycardia involves aneurysmectomy, endocardial mapping, and resection of the subendocardial area containing the micro re-entry circuit. Endocardial resection is often combined with coronary artery bypass grafting. Surgery is most commonly undertaken in patients with a localized anterior aneurysm who have stable monomorphic ventricular tachycardia without multiple morphologies. Patients with diffuse left ventricular dilatation and multifocal origin of ventricular tachycardia are poor risks for antiarrhythmic surgery. The overall surgical mortality is 10 to 15 per cent according to patient selection.

Patients who are unsuitable for surgery may be considered for an implantable cardioverter defibrillator. The device is most appropriately used in those who have had one or more life threatening episodes of ventricular tachycardia or ventricular fibrillation, in whom drug therapy has been shown to be ineffective and surgery is contraindicated. In view of the cost and complexity of the therapy, it is not appropriate in patients with advanced congestive heart failure and, hence, limited prognosis. Earlier devices which provide only defibrillation shocks cannot be used in patients having frequent episodes of tachycardia. However, more recent devices combine antitachycardia pacing with 'backup' defibrillation, which widens the indications for implantation and reduces the frequency of painful defibrillation shocks. To date, no randomized prospective trial has compared the survival of patients treated with the implantable cardioverter defibrillator in comparison with drug therapy. Retrospective studies using historical controls suggest that the incidence of sudden cardiac death is markedly reduced by the implantable cardiovertor defibrillator, although death due to progression of left ventricular dysfunction and congestive cardiac failure still occurs. Nevertheless, these comparisons may be confounded by inappropriate selection of control groups, and the results should be viewed with caution. Where medically intractable ventricular tachyarrhythmias are associated with very poor left ventricular function, the only possible therapeutic option is cardiac transplantation.

Prognosis

It is essential to recognize that sustained ventricular tachycardia is a potential life-threatening condition. Unless the acute episode was clearly precipitated by some transient or reversible factor, there is a high probability of recurrent attacks, which may result in sudden death rather than a sustained tachycardia. The 3-year cardiac survival varies from 80 per cent in patients in whom arrhythmia induction is suppressed by antiarrhythmic drug therapy to 40 per cent in those in whom no effective suppression is achieved and empirical therapy is used.

ACCELERATED IDIOVENTRICULAR RHYTHM

The term accelerated idioventricular rhythm is used to describe a continuous ventricular rhythm with a rate less than 120/min. Idioventricular rhythm commonly occurs in the setting of acute myocardial infarction, and appears to be a marker of successful thrombolytic therapy (Fig. 51). No active treatment is necessary.

NON-SUSTAINED VENTRICULAR TACHYCARDIA

The mechanism and causes of non-sustained ventricular tachycardia are similar to those of sustained ventricular tachycardia. As episodes are, by definition, short-lived, the electrocardiographic appearances are more commonly obtained on single channel monitor or ambulatory electro-

cardiographic recordings rather that on a full 12-lead electrocardiogram (Fig. 52). There is often slight variation in the RR interval, particularly if the salvo involves only a few beats. Salvoes of non-sustained ventricular tachycardia have been reported in association with severe left ventricular hypertrophy due to hypertension, aortic stenosis, or hypertrophic cardiomyopathy. The arrhythmia may also present as an incidental finding in patients with no evidence of organic heart disease.

Clinical features

If salvoes of non-sustained ventricular tachycardia are short and not particularly rapid, they may be entirely asymptomatic. More prolonged episodes may result in dizziness or presyncope, and occasionally in syncope. Apart from the instances where non-sustained ventricular tachycardia produces troublesome symptoms, the major clinical significance of the arrhythmia is as a risk marker for sustained ventricular tachycardia or sudden cardiac death. Long-term follow-up of patients with non-sustained ventricular tachycardia in the absence of structural heart disease has indicated a good prognosis with no excess risk. However, non-sustained ventricular tachycardia recorded by ambulatory electrocardiographic monitoring in the convalescent phase of myocardial infarction is an independent risk factor for subsequent sudden cardiac death, particularly if it is associated with impaired left ventricular function. Non-sustained ventricular tachycardia is also an adverse prognostic feature in patients with hypertrophic cardiomyopathy, but its prognostic significance in hypertensive left ventricular hypertrophy remains to be established. Asymptomatic non-sustained ventricular tachycardia is commonly recorded in patients with advanced congestive heart failure. It is associated with an increased risk of cardiac death, but not selectively of sudden death. It may therefore represent a marker for advanced cardiac disease rather than a specific mechanism for sudden death.

Management

The management of non-sustained ventricular tachycardia involves identification of underlying organic heart disease as described in the section on sustained ventricular tachycardia. If no significant organic heart disease is present, and the patient is asymptomatic, no treatment is indicated. Symptomatic treatment in the absence of significant heart disease should be with antiarrhythmic drugs least likely to be complicated by proarrhythmic reactions such as β-blockers. Calcium channel blockers are effective occasionally and may be tried. Failing these, sotalol or a class I agent may be necessary. The management of asymptomatic non-sustained ventricular tachycardia in patients with organic heart disease is controversial. There is no evidence that antiarrhythmic drug

Fig. 51 Accelerated idioventricular rhythm.

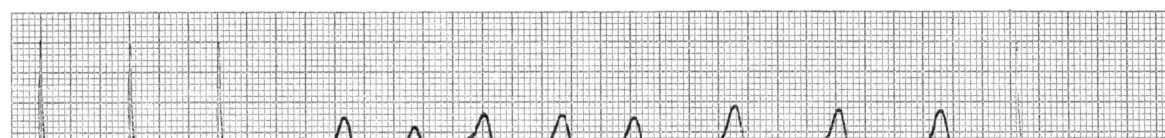
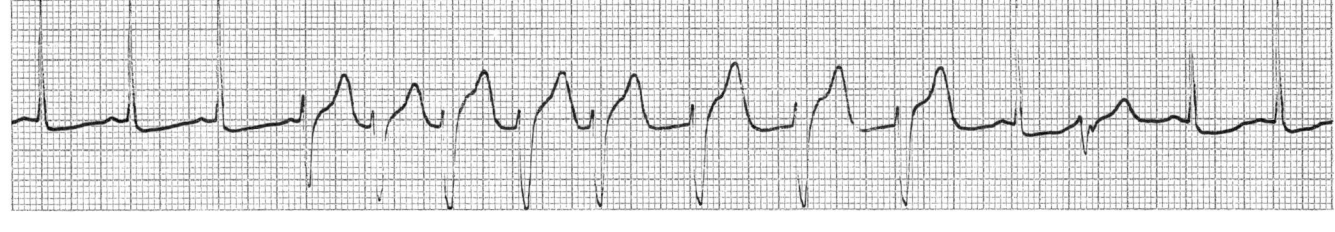

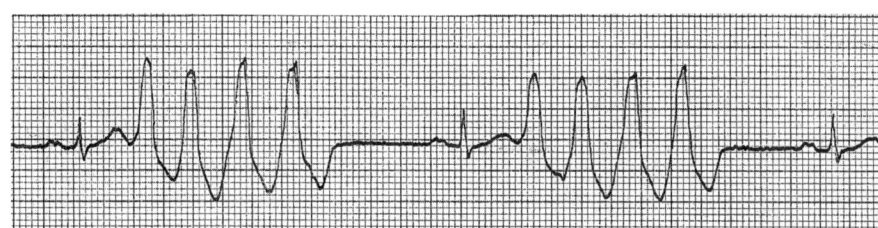

Fig. 52 Non-sustained ventricular tachycardia.

therapy improves survival in post infarction patients. Low dose amiodarone therapy has been recommended in the management of patients with hypertrophic cardiomyopathy and non-sustained ventricular tachycardia, although the evidence for its efficacy is based on comparison with historical controls rather than on a randomized prospective study. Amiodarone has been shown to improve survival in one study of patients with congestive heart failure, but this result is yet to be confirmed.

If non-sustained ventricular tachycardia is sufficiently troublesome to produce symptoms in the presence of organic heart disease, it may be a precursor of sustained ventricular tachycardia. Patients should be evaluated non-invasively by echocardiography or radionuclide ventriculography and signal averaged electrocardiography. Patients with well preserved ventricular function and a normal signal averaged electrocardiogram are at low risk of sustained ventricular tachycardia, and may be treated empirically with β-blockers. Patients with impaired ventricular function and an abnormal signal averaged electrocardiogram are likely to have the substrate for sustained ventricular tachycardia. It is appropriate to undertake programmed ventricular stimulation in this group and management of any induced sustained ventricular tachycardia should be along the lines indicated above.

POLYMORPHIC VENTRICULAR TACHYCARDIA

Polymorphic ventricular tachycardia is an unstable rhythm with varying QRS morphology. It is most commonly seen in the acute phase of myocardial infarction and is due to unstable re-entry circuits. As such, it commonly undergoes spontaneous termination, although it may degenerate into ventricular fibrillation. If episodes of polymorphic ventricular tachycardia are frequent in the early hours of myocardial infarction, they can be suppressed by intravenous lignocaine. However, short, infrequent episodes are commonly left untreated.

TORSADES DE POINTES AND THE LONG QT SYNDROMES

Torsades de pointes is an atypical ventricular tachycardia characterized by a continuously varying QRS axis ('twisting of points') (Fig. 53). Paroxysms of torsades de pointes are commonly repetitive and normally self terminating, although they may degenerate into ventricular fibrillation. Paroxysms of torsades de pointes are associated in the preceding beats with evidence of marked QT prolongation, and frequently with morphological abnormalities of the T waves such as T-U fusion, gross increases in T wave amplitude or T wave alternans. Paroxysms of torsades de pointes in the congenital syndromes are often associated with increases in sinus rate, while in the acquired syndromes a slowing of the heart rate, and in particular a post extrasystolic pause is often associated with initiation of the arrhythmia. This produces a characteristic 'short–long–short' sequence of initiation. The combination of QT interval prolongation during sinus rhythm with intermittent torsades de pointes is described as the long QT syndrome.

The long QT syndromes may be congenital or acquired. The underlying arrhythmic mechanism is not established with certainty. The arrhythmias have some characteristics consistent with triggered activity. The congenital syndrome appears to be associated with an imbalance of

Table 10 *Acquired (pause dependent) long QT syndromes*

Drug-induced
Antiarrhythmic drugs–classes Ia, III
Vasodilators–prenylamine, ketanserin, lidoflazine
Psychotropics

Electrolyte disturbances
Hypokalaemia, hypomagnesaemia, hypocalcaemia

Metabolic
Hypothyroidism, starvation, anorexia nervosa, liquid protein
    diet

Bradycardia
Sinoatrial disease, atrioventricular block

Toxins
Organophosphorus insecticides, heavy metal poisoning

right and left sympathetic innervation to the heart resulting in left-sided sympathetic overactivity and right sided underactivity. The right-sided sympathetic innervation affects principally the sinus and atrioventricular nodes, and accounts for the sinus bradycardia commonly seen in the congenital long QT syndrome. Left-sided overactivity may account for the increased risk of ventricular arrhythmias. In the acquired long QT syndrome the predisposing factors to arrhythmogenesis are QT prolongation, bradycardia, hypokalaemia and hypomagnesaemia. All of these predispose to early after depolarizations *in vitro* and this mechanism appears the likely cause of torsades de pointes in the acquired syndromes.

A variety of congenital long QT syndromes have been identified. The Jervell–Lange–Nielsen syndrome is an autosomal recessive condition associated with neural deafness. The Romano–Ward syndrome is an autosomal dominant condition without deafness. Sporadic cases of idiopathic, presumed congenital long QT syndrome have been reported. Attacks of torsades de pointes in the congenital syndromes are commonly associated with sympathetic stimulation such as exercise, wakening, or fright. Paroxysms may produce syncope which if prolonged may be complicated by convulsion. For this reason, the syndrome may often may be misdiagnosed as epilepsy. A family history of recurrent syncope or sudden death may be obtained.

Many factors may predispose to the development of the acquired long QT syndrome (Table 10). Episodes of torsades de pointes are most likely to occur as a result of a combination of factors including prolongation of the QT interval in association with bradycardia or pauses, hypokalaemia and hypomagnesaemia. The clinical presentation is of recurrent dizziness and syncope, and the condition may easily be misdiagnosed as self-terminating polymorphic ventricular tachycardia or ventricular fibrillation unless the characteristic morphology of torsades de pointes and the associated QT interval prolongation is recognised.

Management

Individual paroxysms of torsades de pointes are normally self-limiting but, if they are persistent, cardiac arrest will occur and emergency defi-

Fig. 53 Torsades de pointes. Note the marked QT interval prolongation in the sinus beats.

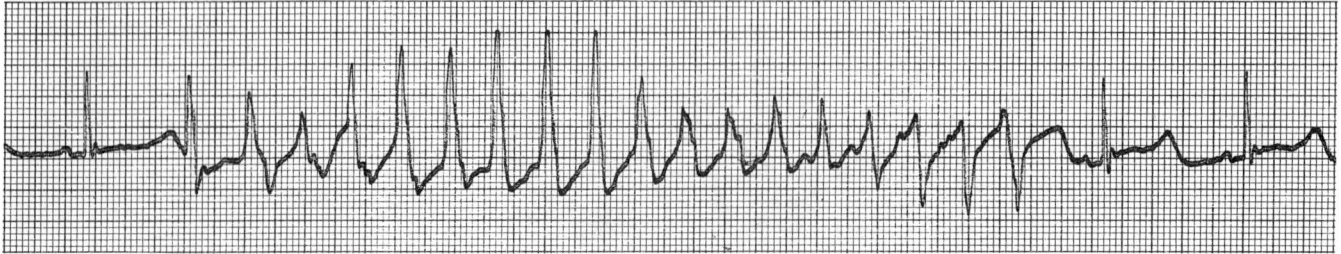

brillation is necessary. The essential feature in management of both the congenital and acquired forms of long QT syndrome is the diagnosis, and the avoidance of empirical antiarrhythmic drug therapy which may worsen the arrhythmia. Indeed, antiarrhythmic drug therapy is one of the commonest causes of torsades de pointes. Attacks of syncope in the congenital long QT syndrome are effectively treated with high dose β-blockade, e.g. propranolol. If this is unsuccessful, selective high left stellate ganglionectomy has been employed successfully. Occasionally, pacemaker or defibrillator implantation is necessary for resistant cases.

Prevention of recurrent attacks of torsades de pointes in the acquired long QT syndrome involves discontinuation of predisposing drugs or other agents. Intravenous magnesium sulphate (1 to 4 g) appears to be a safe and effective emergency measure. In view of the association of paroxysms of tachycardia with bradycardia and pauses, an attempt to increase heart rate should be made. If facilities for temporary pacing are available, atrial or ventricular overdrive pacing at a rate of 90 to 100/min is successful. Alternatively, isoprenaline infusion may be utilized to raise the sinus rate comparably. Caution must be exerted in cases of acute ischaemia. Hypokalaemia should be sought and corrected if necessary.

The prognosis of untreated congenital long QT syndrome is poor, with a high incidence of sudden death in childhood. Retrospective data from the International Registry has indicated that the 15-year survival in patients following their first episode of torsades de pointes has been improved from 50 per cent in untreated cases to 90 per cent following treatment with β-blockade and/or left stellate ganglionectomy. The prognoses of acquired long QT syndrome is excellent provided the underlying predisposing factors are identified and avoided.

VENTRICULAR FIBRILLATION

Ventricular fibrillation is defined as a chaotic, disorganized arrhythmia with no identifiable QRS complexes (see Fig. 9). The mechanism is of multiple, unstable re-entry circuits. The electrocardiographic pattern depends on the duration of fibrillation. Recent onset fibrillation is described as 'coarse', with a peak-to-peak amplitude of around 1 mv (1 cm). With increasing duration of cardiac arrest, the amplitude of ventricular fibrillation diminishes and 'fine' ventricular fibrillation is less likely to be amenable to successful electrical defibrillation.

Ventricular fibrillation may represent the end point of cardiac disease of many aetiologies. Fibrillation may occur during acute myocardial ischaemia, and is the principal cause of death in the first 2 h following acute myocardial infarction. Ventricular fibrillation during myocardial infarction is subdivided into primary, occurring without warning in an otherwise stable patient, and secondary, where fibrillation occurs in the context of left ventricular failure and cardiogenic shock. In acute myocardial infarction, ventricular fibrillation is often initiated by an R on T extrasystole. Ventricular fibrillation occurring in chronic heart disease is most commonly a result of degeneration of rapid ventricular tachycardia, whose causes have been described above. Rarer causes of fibrillation are listed in Table 11.

Ventricular fibrillation is rarely self terminating, and normally causes cardiac arrest with the rapid onset of pulselessness, unconsciousness and apnoea. The management of cardiac arrest due to ventricular fibrillation is discussed below.

Cardiac arrest

Cardiac arrest is defined as the sudden cessation of a circulation adequate to maintain consciousness and, ultimately, life. Cardiac arrest may arise as a result of a ventricular tachyarrhythmia, asystole or ventricular standstill, or to electromechanical dissociation, where cardiac output is absent despite continuing electrocardiographic evidence of cardiac electrical activity (Table 12).

The initial clinical signs of cardiac arrest are pulselessness and rapid

Table 11 *Causes of ventricular fibrillation*

Acute myocardial ischaemia
Acute myocardial infarction–primary or secondary
Advanced organic heart disease with poor LV or RV function
Severe LV hypertrophy
Ventricular tachycardia/torsades de pointes
Electrical–electrocution, lightning, unsynchronized direct current shock, competitive ventricular pacing
Pre-excited atrial fibrillation
Profound bradycardia
Hypoxia, acidosis

LV, left ventricular; RV, right ventricular.

Table 12 *Causes of cardiac arrest*

Electrical
Ventricular fibrillation
Rapid ventricular tachycardia
Pre-excited atrial fibrillation
Asystole
Complete atrioventricular block with ventricular standstill
Hypoxia/acidosis
Respiratory arrest
Metabolic
Hyperkalaemia
Electromechanical dissociation
Massive haemorrhage/hypovolaemia
Circulatory obstruction–massive pulmonary embolism, myxoma, prosthetic valve obstruction, air embolism
Cardiac tamponade
Tension pneumothorax
Massive infarction–'dying heart'
Drug overdose/intoxication
Hypothermia

loss of consciousness, usually associated with pallor or a grey appearance. The diagnosis of pulselessness should be based on an attempt to feel a large pulse such as the carotid. Respiratory activity may persist for some time after cessation of circulation, and the presence of agonal respiratory efforts in no way excludes the diagnosis of cardiac arrest. Pupillary dilatation is a relatively late occurrence. From the onset of cardiac arrest, the likelihood of successful resuscitation with recovery of cardiac and cerebral function declines rapidly with increasing delay. The majority of successful resuscitations occur within the first five minute of the collapse, and long-term success is rare if resuscitation is delayed more than 15 min.

Management of cardiac arrest

BASIC LIFE SUPPORT

All medical and paramedical staff should be capable of performing basic life support in the presence of cardiac arrest. The first rescuer should shout or telephone for assistance to ensure that definitive treatment is on its way as quickly as possible. The vital steps are as simple as ABC. A is for *airway,* indicating that airway obstruction should always be excluded by passing a finger to the back of the tongue. The airway should be cleared by extending the cervical spine and pulling the jaw forwards. B is for *breathing,* using expired air by a mouth-to-mouth or mouth-to-mask approach, pinching the nose to avoid leakage. C is for *circulation.* External cardiac massage should be initiated by chest compression of the lower sternum at a rate of 60 per min. The ratio of chest compressions to lung inflations should be 5 : 1 if two rescuers are present or 15 : 2 if the rescuer is single-handed.

ADVANCED CARDIAC LIFE SUPPORT

Effective cardiopulmonary resuscitation will maintain some circulation to the brain and myocardium and will buy time for the institution of definitive therapy. Advanced cardiac life support involves application of a defibrillator or electrocardiographic monitor to identify the cardiac rhythm, with appropriate therapy as determined by the findings. Protection of the airway and avoidance of aspiration requires endotracheal intubation. A large vein should be cannulated for drug administration, although endotracheal administration is an alternative. The guidelines recommended by the European Resuscitation Council are shown in Fig. 54. Of all causes of cardiac arrest, the probability of survival is greatest in ventricular fibrillation, and it is vital that defibrillation should be initiated without unnecessary delay. Provision of advisory external defibrillators has allowed more rapid provision of defibrillation by individuals without detailed training in electrocardiographic recognition.

MANAGEMENT OF INITIALLY SUCCESSFUL RESUSCITATION

If a spontaneous circulation has been restored by means of advanced cardiac life support, the patient requires skilled management to obtain the best possibility of survival. Continued attention to airway, breathing, and circulation are necessary. If the patient remains unconscious, the airway will be at risk and should be protected by endotracheal intubation if this has not already been performed. Artificial ventilation will need to be continued until adequate spontaneous respiration is restored. Early analysis of arterial blood gases and serum potassium are necessary to correct any abnormalities arising during the resuscitation. The cardiac rhythm may remain unstable and, if multiple episodes of ventricular fibrillation have occurred, lignocaine prophylaxis by bolus and continuous infusion is indicated, although care should be taken to avoid lignocaine overdosage. Persisting bradycardia may require treatment with atropine or temporary pacing. If the patient remains severely hypotensive, inotropic support with dobutamine (2.5 to 10 µg/kg/min) may be necessary, with the use of low dose dopamine (2.5 to 5 µg/kg/min) to minimize renal vasoconstriction. An unconscious patient should have a urinary catheter inserted and urine output measured hourly. If adequate circulatory stability has been achieved, the short-term outlook is principally determined by the extent of neurological damage. Patients who are defibrillated rapidly may recover consciousness almost immediately, although there may be a period of cerebral irritability if hypoxia is more prolonged. Patients in whom a more prolonged period of cardiac arrest was present may remain unconscious for longer periods. Severe anoxic cerebral damage may result in convulsions, which may require treatment with anticonvulsant agents. The persistence of coma after initial resuscitation indicates a poor prognosis. The majority of patients in whom a successful outcome will occur have regained consciousness within 24 to 48 h, although they may remain confused and suffer memory loss for more prolonged periods. There is no evidence that elective hyperventilation or the use of dexamethasone or mannitol will improve cerebral recovery after cardiac arrest.

PROGNOSIS

The short-term outcome after cardiac arrest depends on the mode of arrest, the speed of resuscitation and the nature of the underlying heart disease. For example, the survival of ventricular fibrillation which

Fig. 54 Guidelines for advanced life support from the European Resuscitation Council. DC, direct current.

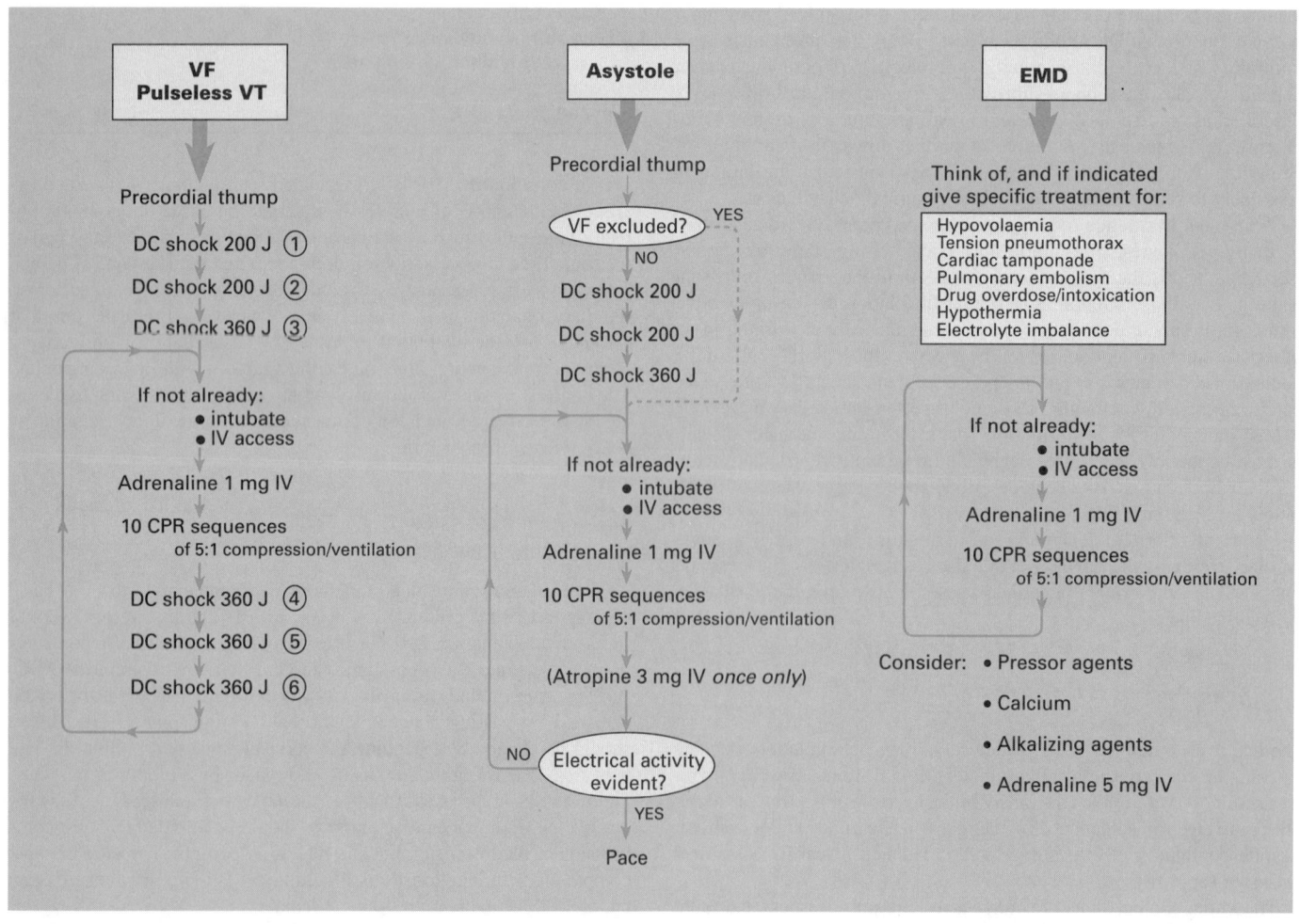

occurs as a complication of cardiac electrophysiological study is almost 100 per cent, and that occurring during exercise stress testing is 90 per cent in view of the immediate availability of defibrillation. The survival rate of primary ventricular fibrillation occurring in the cardiac care unit after acute myocardial infarction is good, whereas that of secondary ventricular fibrillation in patients with left ventricular failure or cardiogenic shock is very poor. The outcome of cardiac arrest occurring in general medical wards is generally lower than that in cardiac care units, as a result of slower response times, greater average age, and differing underlying pathology. The survival rate of witnessed ventricular fibrillation occurring out of hospital varies between 15 to 25 per cent, but is markedly lower if cardiac arrest is unwitnessed, or in the presence of asystole. The low survival following asystolic cardiac arrest is a feature of both in hospital and out of hospital series and reflects the nature of cardiac pathology and the fact that asystole is commonly an agonal event following prolonged ventricular fibrillation. Similarly, electromechanical dissociation is normally caused by a catastrophic cardiovascular event which is rarely amenable to immediate correction, thus survival is unusual.

Patients who survive an episode of ventricular fibrillation should be assessed carefully to determine the risk of recurrence. If ventricular fibrillation has occurred in the first few hours of a typical Q wave myocardial infarction, the risk of recurrent cardiac arrest is low, and no specific prophylactic therapy other than conventional post infarction beta blockade is indicated. In many instances, ventricular fibrillation arises as a result of acute ischaemia in patients with known, extensive heart disease who have not sustained an acute infarction. These patients remain at high risk of recurrent ventricular fibrillation, and should be evaluated fully by exercise testing and coronary arteriography with a view to revascularization. Finally, patients may sustain a cardiac arrest without any preceeding chest pain, but in the presence of a known risk factor for ventricular tachycardia such as previous myocardial infarction. In these individuals, it is likely that ventricular fibrillation arose as a result of degeneration of rapid ventricular tachycardia. These patients are at risk of further cardiac arrest, and require full electrophysiological evaluation along the lines outlined for ventricular tachycardia. Antiarrhythmic prophylaxis or implantation of an implantable cardioverter defibrillator is normally required in such patients. The long-term survival after discharge from hospital following a cardiac arrest will depend upon the nature of the underlying pathology. Overall survival is of the order of 50 to 60 per cent at 5 years.

REFERENCES

Advanced Life Support Working Party of the European Resuscitation Council (1992). Guidelines for advanced life support. *Resuscitation*, **24**, 111–121.

Akhtar, M., Garan, H., Lehman M.H., and Troup, P.J. (1991). Sudden cardiac death: management of high-risk patients. *Annals of Internal Medicine*, **114**, 499–512.

Camm, A.J. (1989). The recognition and management of tachyarrhythmias. In *Diseases of the Heart* (eds D.G. Julian, A.J. Camm, K.M. Fox, R.J.C. Hall, and P.A. Poole-Wilson), pp. 509–583. Bailliere Tindall, London.

Echt, D.S., Liebson, P.R., Mitchell, L.B., *et al.* (1991). Mortality and morbidity in patients receiving encainide, flecainide or placebo. The Cardiac Arrhythmia Suppression Trial. *New England Journal of Medicine*, **324**, 781–788.

Jackman, W.M., Friday, K.J., Anderson, J.L., Aliot, E.M., Clark, M. and Lazzara, R. (1988). The long QT syndromes: a critical review, new clinical observations and a unifying hypothesis. *Progress in Cardiovascular Diseases*, **31**, 115–172.

Jackman, W.M., Wang, X., Friday, K.J., *et al.* (1991). Catheter ablation of accessory atrioventricular pathways (Wolff–Parkinson–White syndrome) by radiofrequency current. *New England Journal of Medicine*, **324**, 1605–1611.

Mehta, D., Wafa, S., Ward, D.E., and Camm, A.J. (1988). Relative efficacy of various physical manoeuvres in the termination of junctional tachycardia. *Lancet*, **i**, 1181–1185.

Pritchett, E.L.C. (1992) Management of atrial fibrillation. *New England Journal of Medicine*, **326**, 1264–1271.

Rankin, A.C., Rae, A.P., and Cobbe, S.M. (1987). Misuse of intravenous verapamil in patients with ventricular tachycardia. *Lancet*, **ii**, 472–474.

Rankin, A.C., Oldroyd, K.G., Chong, E., Rae, A.P., and Cobbe, S.M. (1989). Value and limitations of adenosine in the diagnosis and treatment of narrow and broad complex tachycardias. *British Heart Journal*, **62**, 195–203.

Task Force of the Working Group on Arrhythmias of the European Society of Cardiology (1991). The Sicilian Gambit. A new approach to the classification of antiarrhythmic drugs based on their actions on arrhythmogenic mechanisms. *Circulation*, **84**, 1831–1851.

Turrito, G., Fontaine, J.M., Ursell, S.N., Caref, E.B., Henkin, R., and El-Sherif, N (1988). Value of the signal-averaged electrocardiogram as a predictor of the results of programmed stimulation in nonsustained ventricular tachycardia. *American Journal of Cardiology*, **61**, 1272–1278.

Tzivoni, D., Banai, S., Schuger, C., *et al.* (1988). Treatment of torsade de pointes with magnesium sulfate. *Circulation*, **77**, 392–397.

Ward, D.E. and Camm, A.J. (1987). *Clinical Electrophysiology of the Heart*. Edward Arnold, London.

Wellens, H.J.J., Smeets, J.P., Vos, M., and Gorgels, A.P. (1991). Antiarrhythmic drug treatment: need for continuous vigilance. *British Heart Journal*, **67**, 25–33.

Wilson, J.S. and Podrid, P.J. (1991). Side effects from amiodarone. *American Heart Journal*, **121**, 158–171.

15.8.2 Pacemakers

R. SUTTON

Pacemakers are employed in the management of arrhythmias, in the majority of case for control of bradycardia but there are now increasing indications for their use in tachycardias. The first pacemaker implant was reported in 1959 and now more than 250 000 devices are inserted worldwide per year.

Aetiology of conditions requiring pacing

Bradycardias requiring pacing can be considered in three categories: (1) diseases of the ventricular conduction system and of the atrioventricular node; (2) pathology of the sinoatrial node and atria; and (3) disturbances of the neuroendocrine heart rate control mechanisms. The most common pathological process found in the His–Purkinje conduction system in Western countries is patchy fibrosis that is considered to be autoimmune in origin. Similar fibrotic damage is found in sinoatrial node disease, whereas the aetiology of the neuroendocrine disturbances is entirely unknown. In South America the most common conduction system lesion is that caused by Chagas' disease. Other conditions and therapies affecting ventricular conduction include coronary artery disease, cardiomyopathy, calcific aortic valve disease, surgical correction of some congenital defects, congenital atrioventricular block and the effects of drugs such as digitalis.

Tachycardias arising from the ventricles when implantation of a pacemaker may be considered are mostly related to coronary artery disease or cardiomyopathy, whereas atrial tachyarrhythmias share their aetiology with that of sinoatrial node disease.

Presentation

Cardiac arrhythmias may present simply with palpitation, but, in cases requiring pacemakers, more often with more severe symptoms.

Bradycardias present most frequently with dizziness or syncope. These are disturbances of consciousness due to an associated profound fall in blood pressure, which can also be the result of tachycardia. Cardiac syncope occurs typically without warning and often with resultant self-injury. These attacks, known as Stokes–Adams syncope, are usually of short duration and self-limiting but they have mortal potential. During the attack the unconscious patient is pale but, if the episode is prolonged, cyanosis ensues with epileptiform seizures. On recovery the patient flushes and full consciousness is restored rapidly, usually without amnesia or neurological sequelae, but on occasion neurological damage may result from systemic embolism, particularly in sinoatrial node disease, or may be the consequence of coexisting local cerebral arterial disease.

In the neuroendocrine disturbances of heart-rate control, inappropriate vasodilation in some arteriolar and venous beds also invariably occurs but the time frame of the event is longer than in attacks caused by bradycardia. The effect of this is to make unconsciousness longer and recovery unassociated with such marked skin hyperaemia. As a result, these patients may be misdiagnosed as epileptic.

Another presentation of arrhythmias requiring treatment by pacemakers is with congestive heart failure. In this context presentation is more often a bradycardia than sustained tachycardia. Severe bradycardia, particularly in the elderly may result in mental confusion, dementia, or renal dysfunction due to low cardiac output. It is important to recognize that recurrent falls may be due to transient disturbances of consciousness when cases may be referred to orthopaedic geriatric or neurological departments. There is no difference in incidence of bradycardia due to sinoatrial node disease or atrioventricular block between the sexes and the average age of presentation is 70 years. The disturbances of neuroendocrine heart rate control are more common in males with a similar age of presentation.

Investigation and diagnosis

When the history suggests syncope, information from an observer is of paramount importance. The underlying arrhythmia or other evidence of heart disease may be evident on physical examination, but in many cases the diagnosis emerges only as the result of investigation which begins with electrocardiography. Evidence of complete or second degree atrioventricular block (of Mobitz types I and II) will provide an immediate diagnosis. Sinus rhythm is more common, but clues may be available from evidence of abnormalities of ventricular conduction. Prolongation of the PR interval combined with bundle branch block raises the strongest likelihood of intermittent episodes of complete heart block and asystole.

If the electrocardiogram is normal, a series of investigations is prompted, beginning with carotid sinus massage on each side separately during rhythm monitoring for 5 to 10 s, unless the patient has had a transient cerebral ischaemic episode or has a carotid bruit. If more than 3 s asystole results, with reproduction of symptoms, the diagnosis is carotid sinus syndrome. Proof of symptomatic bradycardia or tachycardia may also be gained by ambulatory electrocardiography, often needed for more than 24 h and most valuable in sinoatrial node disease.

The next investigation to be considered is 60° head-up tilt-testing, which employs passive postural stress for up to 45 min and may reproduce the patient's symptoms yielding a diagnosis of vasovagal syncope. Attempts have been made to shorten and improve the sensitivity of this test by using an intravenous drug challenge such as isoprenaline but an accompanying loss of specificity appears inevitable. If the patient's condition still remains undiagnosed, measures to provoke any underlying arrhythmia, such as exercise stress testing and an electrophysiological study, may be employed. Electrode catheters introduced percutaneously under local anaesthesia into the femoral vein are positioned in the right heart to obtain atrial, His bundle and ventricular signals. In patients with intermittent atrioventricular block the His bundle to ventricular conduction time may be prolonged (normal 35 to 55 ms; clearly pathological > 100 ms). Rapid atrial pacing is used to stress the integrity of the atrioventricular node and ventricular conduction, and to assess the ability of the sinoatrial node to recover after a period of pacing, which is abnormally delayed in sick sinus syndrome. None of these electrophysiological tests is performed routinely.

Indications for pacing

Symptoms provide the major indications for permanent cardiac pacing: syncope, dizziness, and heart failure. When complete or second degree atrioventricular block exist, a pacemaker is advisable, even in the absence of symptoms, as asystole is common and mortality is significantly reduced by pacing. In sinoatrial node disease it has been conventional, hitherto, to pace only to obviate symptoms without any expected benefit in mortality, but in more recent studies using atrial and dual chamber pacing as opposed to ventricular only, survival is improved and systemic embolism may be avoided. The weight of this evidence is now sufficient to consider these types of pacing in patients with asymptomatic sinoatrial node disease.

In carotid sinus syndrome, pacing has been shown to have symptomatic benefit but the place for pacing in vasovagal syndrome is not yet defined. In other conditions prophylactic pacing is controversial; these include evidence of conduction tissue disease without symptoms following myocardial infarction or cardiac surgery. Temporary cardiac pacing may be employed in cardiac or intensive care units to control many transient arrhythmias but these do not usually require such treatment for longer than 72 h.

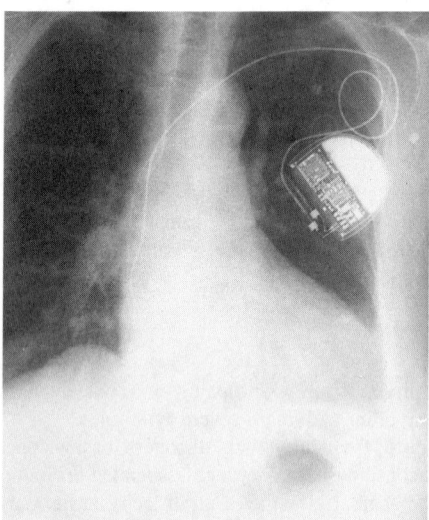
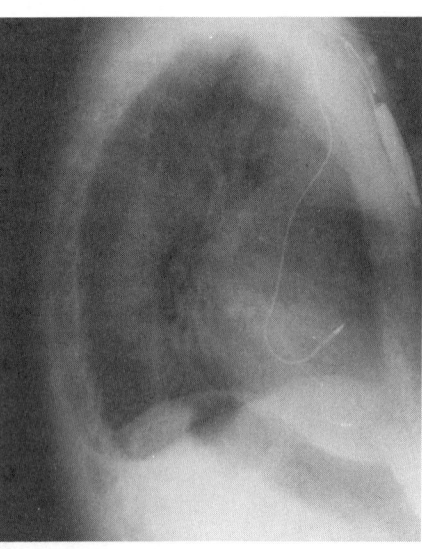

Fig. 1 A posteroanterior and a lateral chest radiograph of a patient with a dual chamber unipolar pacemaker system.

Techniques

The implantation of a pacemaker is a surgical procedure requiring full sterile precautions performed by surgeons or cardiologists usually under local anaesthesia. The central cephalic approach by incision or the subclavian percutaneously are the veins of choice for the lead, which consists of a multistrand conductor wire insulated by silicone rubber or polyurethane with an electrode tip usually of platinum alloy and a connector plug at the distal end. The lead is passed with the aid of fluoroscopy and a stiffening stylet in the core of the lead to the right atrium through the tricuspid valve, and positioned in the apex (anterior) of the right ventricle. Lateral fluoroscopy is useful to confirm the position. Close to the electrode an anchoring device is fitted to the lead which engages the right ventricular trabeculae. The most effective of these is a group of tines which project outwards and backwards from the tip at an angle of 60°.

If an atrial lead is to be used it is guided through the same vein to the right atrium. Most atrial leads are designed with a curved (or J) tip, which can be straightened temporarily by the stylet. When the stylet is withdrawn the lead takes up its J shape, which can be manipulated to position its electrode tip in the right atrial appendage. This is also a trabeculated area, which provides the means for stability of the electrode against the endocardium. Lateral fluoroscopy is used to be sure that the electrode is pointing upwards just behind the sternum. Once the lead is in position tests are made of the signal that the heart will convey to the pacemaker via the lead (electrograms) and the ability of an external pacemaker attached to the lead to pace the heart (threshold testing). If the lead is found satisfactory, it is sutured in the vein and subcutaneous tissues and a subcutaneous pocket over pectoralis major is constructed for the pacemaker which is attached to the lead and implanted (Fig. 1). Prophylactic antibiotics are recommended for a few days after surgery. The patient is mobilized on the same day and discharged the next. These procedures can often be performed as day cases providing home support is adequate.

This has been a description of transvenous or endocardial pacing; epicardial pacing with placing of the lead on the surface of the heart or in the myocardium is a much more extensive procedure requiring general anaesthesia, and, as a result, it has almost disappeared. Even children are now usually paced by the endocardial route. Growth can be accommodated by good electrode fixation combined with redundant loops of lead both within and outside the venous system.

Technology

Pacemakers are manufactured under rigorous conditions of cleanliness and quality assurance. The unit, now weighing 25 to 40 g, contains a battery, which is commonly a lithium–iodine cell developed especially for pacemakers. This cell has the advantage of high power to weight and size ratios, predictable discharge behaviour, and long life. Present-day cells offer up to 10 years life with low current drain from circuit and electrode. The other major component is the pulse forming circuitry, which is now of hybrid type using a silicon chip with the addition of a few discrete components. All pacemakers have a 'sensing' capability where an amplifier picks up spontaneous cardiac activity and uses this to recycle the pacemaker's output. Thus, if the patient returns to normal sinus rhythm, the pacemaker output is inhibited; as soon as the rate of the spontaneous rhythm falls below the set rate of the pacemaker, stimulation of the heart recommences. This is known as demand function. It can be excluded by placing a magnet over the pacemaker, excluding the sensing amplifier from the circuit, rendering the unit asynchronous or fixed rate. The hybrid circuit is usually sealed hermetically, as is the battery, and the outer coat of the pacemaker offers another hermetic seal, usually being constructed of titanium. There is a feed-through connection to the lead plug, which permits electrical connection without loss of hermetic seal. The sealing is necessary to prevent access of body fluids. Part or all of the metal shield may be used as the indifferent pole of the pacemaker system, which has implications for local stimulation and sensing: due to the low current density the pectoralis major is not stimulated. The problem of skeletal muscle activity (electromyogram) being 'sensed' as spontaneous cardiac activity is minimized by filtering at the amplifier. An alternative is to use a lead with a second ring electrode close to the tip (bipolar system) and the pacemaker's metal casing then plays no part in the circuit. The bipolar lead has, in the past, been more vulnerable to fracture.

Recent developments include trifilar conductor wires and improved insulation materials and are encouraging a trend towards dominant use of bipolar leads. Pacemakers now are programmable and telemetric by means of an external programmer which can communicate bidirectionally by radiofrequency. It can receive the present settings of rate, output, sensitivity and refractory periods as well as information on lead and battery impedance and current drains allowing assessment of remaining battery life and alter settings to adjust the pacemaker to suit the patient's need or prolong pacemaker life. Similar tests of sensitivity and stimulation thresholds to those made at implant may reveal problems which, with the pacemaker's flexibility, settings can be altered to solve.

PHYSIOLOGICAL PACEMAKERS

Pacing the heart at a single rate is clearly not physiological. In the last decade technology has successfully overcome many of the difficulties that previously prevented the patient's physiological state from determining the pacing rate. Two approaches have been followed. First, use of the atria which often function normally in atrioventricular block. Atrial activity is detected via an atrial lead and ventricular pacing via a ventricular lead follows after a suitable 'PR' interval (Figs. 1 and 2). The second approach has been to determine the body's needs for heart rate by means of a sensor. The most common of these used is a piezo-electric crystal, which acts as a vibration sensor or accelerometer, but many other more physiological systems are in use or development. These devices were first combined with ventricular pacemakers, but more recently have been combined with dual chamber systems, thus moving the pacemaker system closer to a true imitator of sinus rhythm in all conditions.

Pacemaker clinic

Prior to discharge from hospital the pacemaker is checked by electrocardiography (12-lead) for proper capture of the heart with a magnet over the pacemaker if necessary. Chest radiography for lead position is performed, as well as use of the programmer to check that there has been no significant change in sensitivity and stimulation thresholds and to adjust the pacemaker to the patient's needs. Battery saving adjustments are not made at this stage as a rise in stimulation threshold is expected in the first 3 months of pacing except where electrodes are used which contain 1 mg dexamethasone. This permeates the surrounding endocardium and inhibits the fibrotic process, which causes stimulation threshold rise. The patient should attend the pacemaker clinic after 1 month for checking and again at 6 months when battery saving settings can be employed. Thereafter attendance is annual until changes in basic rate and pulse duration signal battery depletion when closer monitoring is required. The objectives of the consultation are not only to diagnose and solve clinical problems but also to prolong the life of the pacemaker. When physiological pacing systems have been introduced, more sophisticated techniques are required, including exercise testing, echocardiography and ambulatory electrocardiography to achieve the best settings for the patient.

Results

Permanent pacing results in abolition of dizziness and syncope and a marked prolongation in life expectancy in atrioventricular block. It is now emerging that dual chamber pacing gives improved life expectancy over ventricular pacing when heart failure is a presenting feature and atrial or dual chamber pacing also offers benefits in life expectancy in sick sinus syndrome. No such benefits have yet been demonstrated in the case of neuroendocrine disturbances of heart rate.

With modern pacing systems reoperation is rarely necessary until battery exhaustion is imminent.

Complications

SURGICAL

With proper techniques the incidence of infection should be less than 1 per cent. Erosion of the pacemaker through the skin, probably due to pressure necrosis has now been almost eliminated with modern lightweight units. Thromboembolism is extremely rare. Local problems such as pain and haematoma are very rarely severe.

LEAD

Perforation of heart or venous system is usually benign: proper techniques and modern leads have rendered this rare. If a lead becomes displaced from the endocardium, loss of capture results. This tends to occur in the first few weeks after implant and may be fatal because of sudden cessation of pacing. Modern tined leads have reduced this incidence to less than 2 per cent. Fracture of the wire, insulation, or both may also result in loss of pacing. This occurs rarely and may be anticipated by alterations in the electronic analysis of the pacemaker pulse. Infection may result in endocarditis at the lead tip and, because of the presence of a foreign body, may necessitate the removal of the whole pacemaker system, and the use of temporary endocardial pacing until eradication of the infection when a new permanent endocardial system can be placed or an epicardial system may be preferred. The power required to capture the heart may rise progressively, instead of the normal early rise followed by stabilization or fall, known as exit block. Its treatment may require a higher pacemaker output or a new lead.

PACEMAKER

Premature failure presents either by excessive slowing, loss of output or by acceleration (runaway). International bodies now collect data on all pacemaker types in order to provide early warnings of pacemaker batch failures, allowing explantation of many before they fail. Runaway protection is now built into all pacemakers. Human error may occur with pacemaker programming; record keeping and appropriate check lists are essential. Most pacemaker circuit faults occur either as a result of ingress of body fluids or failure of connections between the discrete components and the silicon chip. Hermetic sealing and manufacturer's quality assurance must prevent this as far as is possible. The environment provides most hazards to the pacemaker patient. Electromagnetic interference may arise from many sources, including weapon and theft detectors. Most pacemakers revert to asynchronous mode under these conditions without risk to the patient. Some new software-based highly complex pacemakers may dump their programmes in the face of surgical diathermy. Special care is required in these cases. Halothane and related anaesthetic gases raise the energy required for capture of the heart and should be avoided. Close contact with leaky microwave ovens and working with special apparatus, such as arc-welders, are contraindicated for pacemaker patients because of possible inappropriate inhibition or acceleration.

Ventricular extrasystoles are not uncommon immediately following lead implant. Competition by the pacemaker with spontaneous rhythm is almost always excluded by the demand function and is further minimized by rate hysteresis where there is a longer interval before the pacemaker takes over than the set pacing interval. Occasionally ventricular pacing may be associated with retrograde atrioventricular conduction. This may be asymptomatic or may cause syncope or dizziness, by fall in blood pressure, or heart failure. Treatment is by use of an atrioventricular sequential pacemaker with careful programming to avoid an endless loop pacemaker mediated tachycardia.

DEFIBRILLATORS

Implantable cardioverter defibrillators (ICD) are now being used much more widely for control of ventricular tachyarrhythmias that have either failed medical therapy or where failure is anticipated. New systems are transvenous which permits implantation by a cardiologist using almost identical techniques to those for pacemakers. Most devices now offer some form of antibradycardia pacing. Implantation requires testing of efficacy against ventricular tachycardia and fibrillation at moderate output (in the region of 18 J). Follow-up should be more frequent than for pacemakers and patients require more support. Results compare favourably with medical therapy but exhaustive controlled trials have not yet

Fig. 2 An electrocardiograph (12-lead) of the same patient as illustrated in Fig. 1. The pattern is of sensing of spontaneous P waves followed by ventricular pacing. There is one atrial premature complex, which is also sensed and is followed by ventricular pacing. This is an example of physiological pacing.

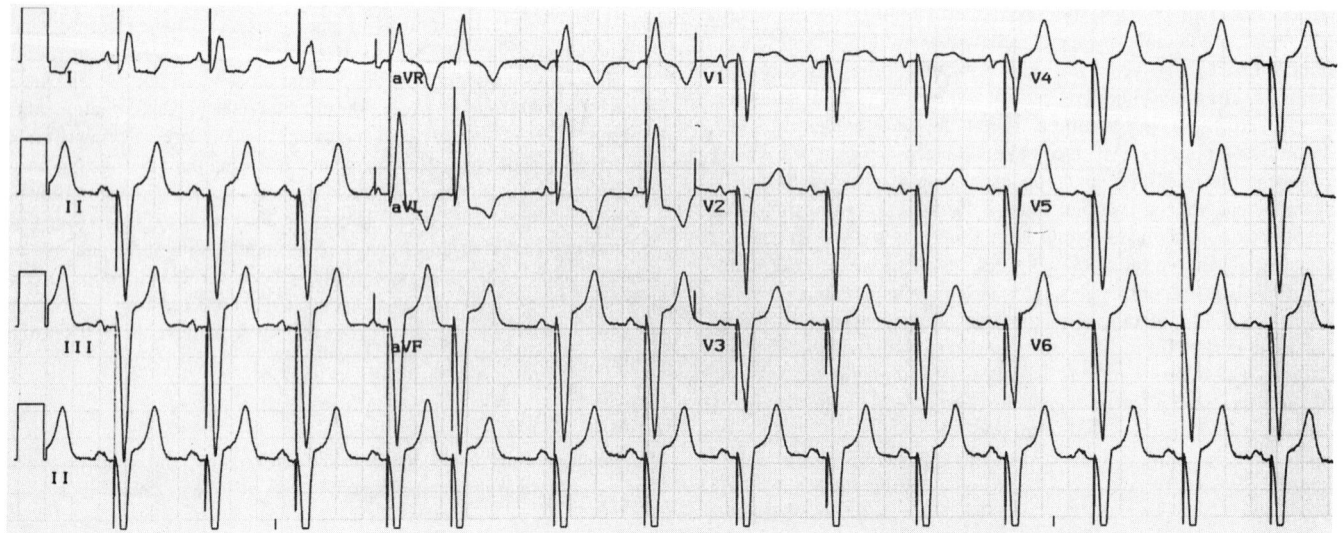

been completed. Complications are similar to those experienced with pacemakers.

Developments

Pacing is being considered in more and more patients. Recent reports suggest a role for dual chamber pacing in both hypertrophic and dilated cardiomyopathy. Pacing may find clear indications in vasovagal syndrome and more sinoatrial node disease patients can be expected to benefit in terms of symptoms of fatigue and palpitation and possibly a reduction in thromboembolism with dual chamber rate response systems. Use of physiological pacing is increasing and has exceeded 35 per cent of implants in some countries.

One field in which pacing is now almost unused is that of supraventricular tachycardias, because of the introduction of the techniques of precise ablation of small areas of cardiac tissue by radiofrequency. Thus, antitachycardia pacing for these conditions is now obsolete.

REFERENCES

Andersen, H.R., Thuesen, L., Bagger, J.P., Vesterlund, T., and Bloch Thomsen, P.E. (1994). Prospective randomised trial of atrial versus ventricular pacing in sick sinus syndrome. *Lancet,* **344,** 1523–8.

Davies, M.J. (1971). *The pathology of the conducting tissue of the heart.* Butterworth, London.

Hochleitner, M., Hortnagl, H., Ng C-K. et al. (1990). Usefulness of physiologic dual-chamber pacing in drug-resistant idiopathic dilated cardiomyopathy. *American Journal of Cardiology,* **66,** 198–202.

Jeanrenaud, X., Goy, J.J., Kappenberger, L. et al. (1992). Effects of dual-chamber in pacing in hypertrophic obstructive cardiomyopathy. *Lancet* **339,** 1318–1323.

Kenny, R.A., Ingram, A., Bayliss, J., and Sutton R. (1986). Head-up tilt: a useful test for investigating unexplained syncope. *Lancet* **i,** 1352–1355.

Morley, C. and Sutton, R. (1984). Carotid sinus syndrome. *International Journal of Cardiology,* **6,** 287–293.

Rosenqvist, M., Brandt, J., and Schüller, H. (1988). Long-term pacing in sinus node disease: Effects of stimulation mode on cardiovascular morbidity and mortality. *American Heart Journal,* **116,** 16–22.

Santini, M., Alexidou, G., Ansalone, G. *et al.* (1990). Relation of prognosis in sick sinus syndrome to age, conduction defects and modes of permanent cardiac pacing. *American Journal of Cardiology,* **65,** 729–735.

Sutton, R. and Bourgeois, I. (1991). *An illustrated practical guide to basic pacing. Foundations of cardiac pacing, Vol. 1.* Futura Publishing Co. Inc., Mount Kisco, New York.

Sutton, R., Citron, P., and Perrins, J. (1980). Physiological cardiac pacing. *Pace* **3,** 201–219.

Sutton, R., Rydén, L., and Bourgeois I. (1995). *An illustrated practical guide to rate variable pacing. Foundations of cardiac pacing, Vol. 2.* Futura Publishing Co. Inc., Armonk, New York.

Travill, C.M. and Sutton, R. (1992). Pacemaker syndrome: an iatrogenic condition. *British Heart Journal,* **68,** 163–166.

15.9 Atheroma, the vessel wall, and thrombosis

15.9.1 The pathogenesis of atherosclerosis

J. SCOTT

Introduction

Atherosclerosis, the underlying cause of heart attacks, strokes, and peripheral vascular disease, is one of the major killers in the world. The disease develops slowly over many years in the innermost layer of large and medium-sized arteries. It does not usually become manifest before the fourth or fifth decade, but then often strikes with devastating suddenness. Fifty per cent of individuals still die (25 per cent immediately) from their first heart attack; and morbidity from coronary heart disease is significant. The disease has a profound impact on health-care services and on industrial economies.

Progress has been made in identifying the risk factors that predispose to atherosclerosis, its medical and surgical treatment, and the consequences of the disease once it has developed. Cellular and molecular biology have allowed an understanding of how risk factors contribute to the process of atherogenesis and are providing the rationale for development of new and effective treatments; as a consequence the prevalence of and mortality from atherosclerosis are decreasing.

Epidemiology

The demonstration of coronary heart disease in an individual is taken as a reliable index of the presence of more general atherosclerosis. The highest death rates from coronary heart disease are found in Britain, northern Europe, the United States, Australia, and New Zealand. Death from coronary disease in industrialized countries rose dramatically after the end of the First World War. Rates peaked in the late 1960s in the United States and have since declined rapidly, with a reduction of 45 per cent for all persons. In Britain and the rest of Europe this peak and decline lagged behind the United States by some 10 years, but is now evident. Changes in diet, exercise, smoking, and affluence account for much of this decline. Better medical and surgical intervention has also been important. By contrast, the countries of eastern Europe and the former Soviet Union are showing a marked increase in the prevalence of coronary heart disease and are now equal to our own (Table 1). This can be attributed to the influence of the risk factors that have, until recently, operated in the industrialized West (see Table 2).

Substantially lower death rates are found in southern Europe, Latin America, and Japan, but the largest differences exist between the industrialized nations and less-developed countries such as China. The most obvious difference between these groups of individuals is in lifestyle—diet and physical activity—and this must account for much of the differences in risk. This is best exemplified by migrants from Japan to Hawaii and in turn to the United States, who adopt the North American lifestyle and then have the same risk of coronary heart disease as those of their host nation.

The Natural History of Atherosclerosis

THE NORMAL ARTERY

Anatomy

An artery consists of three histologically discrete concentric layers. The innermost, luminal part of the artery, the intima, contains a densely adherent monolayer of endothelial cells, bound together by tight junctions, which provide a barrier that strictly controls the entrance of substances to the arterial wall. The endothelial cell layer is adherent to the internal, or basal, elastic lamina, a network of areolar and elastic tissue. This layer is more marked in medium-sized and larger arteries. The

Table 1 *Deaths by cause in the United Kingdom and in Poland, 1990*

| | Standardized death rates, age 35–69[a] | | | |
| | United Kingdom | | Poland | |
Causes of death	Male	Female	Male	Female
All causes	1072	626	1814	751
All vascular diseases	494	206	812	327
All cancer	358	282	496	246
Accidents	50	20	174	35
Other	170	118	332	143

[a] Defined as the means of seven 5-yearly rates.

media contains vascular smooth muscle cells arranged in a closely adherent monolayer or multiple layers, depending on the size of the artery. Smooth muscle cells secrete a mixture of collagen, elastic tissue, and glycosaminoglycans, which form a dense matrix around them. The adventitia forms the external layer and is separated from the media by an external elastic lamina. It contains a meshwork of collagen and elastic fibrils, smooth muscle cells, and fibroblasts. The adventitia receives its blood supply from a series of externally derived small arteries, the *vasa vasora,* which also supply the outermost layers of the media. The intima and innermost layer of the media receive their nutritional support from luminal blood.

The media and adventitia together provide a strong, elastic, contractile wall, which provides the physical strength to deal with the hydrodynamic and sheer stress of the pressurized vascular system. It serves to propagate the flow of blood towards the periphery, and to smooth out the pulse as blood reaches small peripheral arteries and capillary beds.

Physiology and biochemistry

Endothelial cells serve several important metabolic functions. They deter thrombosis and regulate the access of luminal substances and white blood cells to the arterial wall, synthesize compounds that control vascular tone and cell division, and secrete matrix substances from their abluminal surface.

The unbroken endothelial layer protects against thrombosis and maintains normal blood fluidity by a number of constitutive mechanisms. Mucopolysaccharides such as heparin are synthesized and secreted on to the luminal surface by endothelial cells. Heparin binds and activates antithrombin III, thereby providing the endothelial cell surface with a potent anticoagulant. The other endothelial cell anticoagulant is thrombomodulin, which binds thrombin and activated protein C. Activated protein C and protein S serve as potent anticoagulants by innactivating clotting factors Va and VIIIa.

Additional endothelial cell activities inhibit thrombosis. Prostacyclin is the endothelial cell product of arachidonic acid. It blocks platelet activation and aggregation, and promotes vasodilatation through the suppression of platelet cyclic AMP. Nitric oxide (NO) synthesized in endothelial cells stimulates relaxation of smooth muscle cells, thereby supporting reduced platelet activity. Endothelial cell membrane ADPases reduce local ADP levels and decrease platelet activation at the lumenal surface.

The endothelial cell is freely permeable to water and small hydrophilic molecules. The tight junctions between endothelial cells are impervious to macromolecules. To gain access to the subendothelium, macromolecules, and macromolecular complexes must traverse the cell in vesicles. This rapid, unidirectional process is called transcytosis. It is mediated by specific proteins such as caveolin and *N*-ethylmaleamide-sensitive factor. Insulin, transferrin, albumin, and low-density lipoprotein (LDL) traverse the endothelial cell by this route, and provide nutrition for arterial wall cells.

White blood cells and platelets do not adhere to normal vascular endothelium. The activation of endothelial cells, platelets, or white blood cells leads to the production of specific sets of adhesion molecules, which promote this. Adhesion molecules are only expressed at very low levels on the normal endothelial cells.

Endothelial cells elaborate the matrix proteins that form the basement membrane on which they lie. They also synthesize a variety of substances that control vascular tone and blood volume, including NO, the endothelins, and angiotensin-converting enzyme, which activates the renin–angiotensin system.

Smooth muscle cells and a few fibroblasts are the only cells in the normal artery wall. Smooth muscle cells provide the tone of the artery wall and elaborate the matrix proteins, which give it its tensile strength and elasticity. These include collagen, elastin, and glycosaminoglycans. With increasing age, arteries become more rigid, dilated, and tortuous. This is due to a symmetrical increase in the smooth muscle cells and matrix components of the intima. Such arteries are more prone to aneurysmal dilatation and rupture, particularly when affected by atherosclerosis.

THE LESIONS OF ATHEROSCLEROSIS

Autopsy studies show that in humans atherosclerosis develops slowly over many years. A similar disease can be produced in experimental animals, where diet and genetics can be manipulated to produce accelerated lesions. The earliest lesions are fatty streaks. These consist of an accumulation of lipid-engorged macrophages (foam cells), and T lymphocytes in the arterial intima. The fatty streaks progress to intermediate lesions, composed mainly of foam cells and smooth muscle cells. With time these develop into the advanced plaques which are characterized by a dense fibrous cap of connective tissue and smooth muscle cells overlying a core containing necrotic material and lipid, mainly cholesteryl esters, which may form cholesterol crystals on histological section. Advanced plaques also contain foam cells and T cells, and undergo vascularization. This promotes plaque growth, but may also provide a channel for the access of inflammatory cells and thus weaken the plaque.

Plaques may impede the flow of blood to an organ, giving rise to ischaemia and the symptoms of angina and intermittent caudication; or undergo denuding injury with limited thrombosis and unstable angina, or deep fissuring with sudden complete occlusion of coronary arteries and myocardial infarction. In the cerebral circulation the same process causes transient ischaemic attacks and completed stroke. In arteries weakened by the ageing process and complicated by atherosclerosis, aneurysmal dilatation and rupture may occur. Unsupported cerebral arteries are particularly prone to rupture.

THE PATHOGENESIS OF ATHEROSCLEROSIS

It is now generally accepted that atherosclerosis develops as a healing response to repeated vascular-wall injury, and that risk factors (Table 2)

Table 2 *Risk factors for atherosclerosis*

Male gender
Race (East Indian)
Diet high in saturated fat and cholesterol, low in fruit, grain, and vegetables
Family history of coronary heart disease before 55 years in first-degree relative
Hypercholesterolaemia (greater than 5.2 mmol/l (210 mg/dl))
Cigarette smoking
Hypertension
Low high-density lipoprotein–cholesterol (less than 0.9 mmol/l (35 mg/dl))
Diabetes mellitus
Personal history of cerebrovascular disease or peripheral vascular disease
Severe obesity (>30% overwieght)
High lipoprotein(a)
High fibrinogen
Homocysteinaemia

operate by promoting chronic cycles of damage and repair. Oxidatively damaged low-density lipoprotein, the toxins in tobacco smoke, the sheer stress of hypertension, homocysteine, and viruses can all cause endothelial cell dysfunction. The dysfunctional endothelium undergoes a protective response, with the expression of adhesion molecules, growth-promoting substances, and activation of the blood coagulation cascade. Monocytes and T lymphocytes adhere to the activated endothelium and themselves become activated and produce growth factors, cytokines, and chemoattractants. The adherent white blood cells migrate into the arterial intima and smooth muscle cells are recruited from the intima and media. With the repeated rounds of injury and repair, palisades of smooth muscle cells, matrix proteins, lipid-laden macrophages, and T lymphocytes accumulate to form the atherosclerotic plaque (Fig. 1).

LDL has a central place in the pathogenesis of atherosclerosis. It may enter the intima either through the damaged endothelium or, more usually, by transcytosis. In the intima LDL undergoes low grade modification by oxidative free-radicals to form minimally modified LDL (mmLDL) (Fig. 2). This adheres to the matrix proteins of the arterial wall, where it undergoes more extensive oxidation. Free radicals are produced from macrophages and from NO derived from endothelial cells. This is compounded by the products of tobacco smoke and by homocysteine. Oxidized LDL in the intima is the major ligand for the scavenger receptor, which is expressed in the macrophages that accumulate at the site of vessel wall injury. The accumulation of cholesteryl esters in these cells gives the cytoplasm its characteristic foamy appearance.

Hypertension accelerates atherogenesis by activating genes that respond to hydrodynamic stress, the products of which perturb vascular tone, worsen oxidative damage, and promote smooth muscle cell accumulation.

Advanced atherosclerotic lesions, particularly those with a necrotic fatty core, are susceptible to rupture, with sloughing of their endothelial cap or deep fissuring into the plaque. This leads to platelet adherence and activation of the coagulation cascade. Mural thrombus may progress to vascular occlusion or become incorporated into the atherosclerotic plaque.

THE CELLS OF THE ATHEROSCLEROTIC PLAQUE

Endothelial cells

In the earliest stages of atherogenesis, damaged endothelial cells become dysfunctional (non-denuding injury). Sloughing of the endothelium occurs at a later stage in the disease, when plaques become complicated and split or fissure (denuding injury). The dysfunctional endothelial cell produces growth factors, cytokines, chemoattractants, clotting factors, and adhesion molecules. The result is the recruitment and transformation of monocytes into macrophages, and the recruitment and proliferation of smooth muscle cells. Thrombotic processes are activated. There is chronic alteration of vascular tone as a result of disordered NO production and signalling.

Monocyte/macrophages

The lipid-laden macrophage is the hallmark of atherosclerosis and the instrument of its development. The process of the monocyte conversion from a quiescent cell to the phagocytically active macrophage is associated with the expression of the scavenger receptor. The uptake of oxidatively modified LDL thus accompanies macrophage activation. The macrophage scavenger receptor is expressed in two differentially spliced forms. Both forms contain a collagen-like domain that binds polyanionic ligands, such as modified LDL. In modified LDL apolipoprotein B loses its overall basic charge due to oxidation of lysine residues, such as those that mediate binding to acidic residues on the LDL receptor, and becomes covalently associated with lipid peroxidation products including short-chain aldehydes and ketones. This material is no longer taken up by the LDL receptor, but is avidly taken up by the macrophage scavenger receptor. The cholesteryl ester released from LDL is broken down in lysosomes and re-esterified in the cytoplasm.

The activated macrophage secretes a wide variety of growth-modulating substances and chemoattractants. Phagocytic macrophages produce free radicals and are induced to produce NO; this itself generates free radicals and promotes further oxidative damage to LDL. Macrophages also secrete proteolytic enzymes (collagenase, elastase, stromolysin, and gelatinases). Proteases contribute to the necrosis and liquefaction of the core of advanced fatty plaques and render the plaque prone to rupture, either into the arterial lumen or through the external wall.

Vascular smooth muscle cells

In the normal artery wall smooth muscle cells contain mainly contractile proteins, such as actin and myosin. These cells are said to display a contractile phenotype. They respond to vasoregulatory substances such as catecholamines, angiotensin II, prostaglandins, leukotrienes, endothelin, NO, and other regulatory compounds. Under the influence of proinflammatory cytokines and growth factors, smooth muscle cells in the atherosclerotic plaque switch from a contractile to a secretory phenotype. These secretory cells have large amounts of endoplasmic reticulum and Golgi apparatus. They produce extracellular matrix. The local release of growth factors, cytokines, and chemoattractants leads to autocrine and paracrine effects on growth and cell recruitment. Smooth muscle cells also express a scavenger receptor and they, too, become lipid-loaded.

T lymphocytes

These accompany macrophages into the atherosclerotic plaque. T cells also produce proinflammatory cytokines, which compound the atherosclerotic process by attracting further macrophages and T lymphocytes and perpetuating endothelial cell activation. T cells in the plaque become sensitized to new antigens in the lesion, such as modified LDL.

Platelets

Platelets undergo activation in response to agonists such as thrombin, ADP, adrenaline, and platelet activating factor. This process is also triggered when peripheral blood is exposed to thrombogenic agents at the site of blood vessel damage. Here agonists such as collagen present in the extracellular matrix, exposed in the subendothelium along with von Willebrand factor and fibrinogen produced at the wound site, initiate the cascade of events that leads to platelet aggregation and the formation of a platelet plug. In this process platelet-specific integrins act as receptor tyrosine kinases (GPIIbIIIa), which initiate the intracellular changes that mediate platelet activation and aggregation, and later binding to fibrin and clot retraction. Red blood cells amplify platelet responses.

Fig. 1 Cellular and molecular mediators of atherosclerosis. The arrows denote the production of factors and their principal cellular targets. (a) Endothelial cell: (i) Monocytes are recruited and adhere to the vascular endothelium, where extravasation and activation occurs. In the process of activation the monocyte is converted into the phagocytically active macrophage and produces numerous growth factors, growth inhibitors, and chemoattractants. (ii) T-lymphocytes undergo recruitment and activation. They secrete γ-interferon (IFNγ), transforming growth factor β (TGFβ), tumour necrosis factor α (TNFα), and interleukin-1 (IL-1). (iii) Platelet activation and adhesion is associated with coagulation cascade activation. Platelet degranulation and prostaglandin production occurs with release of (PDECGF), epidermal growth factor (EGF)/TGFα, TGFβ, thromboxane A and insulin-like growth factor I (IGF-I). (iv) Smooth muscle cells switch to a secretory phenotype and produce vascular endothelial cell growth factor (VEGF), IL-1, TNFα, TGFβ, collagen, elastic fibres, and proteoglycans. (v) Macrophages become phagocytically active. The scavenger receptor is induced with the engorgement of oxidized low-density lipoprotein (oxLDL) and foam cell formation. Activated macrophages produce VEGF, IL-1, TNFα, IFNγ. (b) Macrophage: (i) Endothelial cells become activated and dysfunctional. They secrete macrophage colony-stimulating factor (M-CSF)/granulocyte–macrophage colony-stimulating factor (GM-CSF), IL-1, TNFα, and produce oxLDL. (ii) Smooth muscle cells are recruited and may divide before switching from a contractile to a secretory phenotype. They secrete M-CSF/GM-CSF, heparin-binding epidermal growth factor (HB-EGF), VEGF, IL-1, TNFα, MCP-1, and produce oxLDL. (iii) T cells are recruited and secrete IFNγ, GM-CSF, and TNFα. Macrophage IL-2 is a potent agent for T-cell recruitment and activation. (c) Smooth muscle cells: (i) Platelets are activated and produce platelet-derived growth factor (PDGF), EGF/TGFα, TGFβ, TXA₂ and IGF-I. (ii) T lymphocytes become activated and produce (TFNγ), TGFβ, TNFα, and IL-1. (iii) Endothelial cells produce PDGF, basic fibroblast growth factor (bFGF), IL-1, TGFβ, prostaglandin I₂ (PGI₂), IGF-I, nitric oxide (NO), and oxLDL. (iv) Macrophage monocytes produce PDGF, bFGF, HB-EGF, TGFα, TGFβ, TNFα, IL-1, prostaglandin E (PGE), and oxLDL. (Based on Ross (1993).)

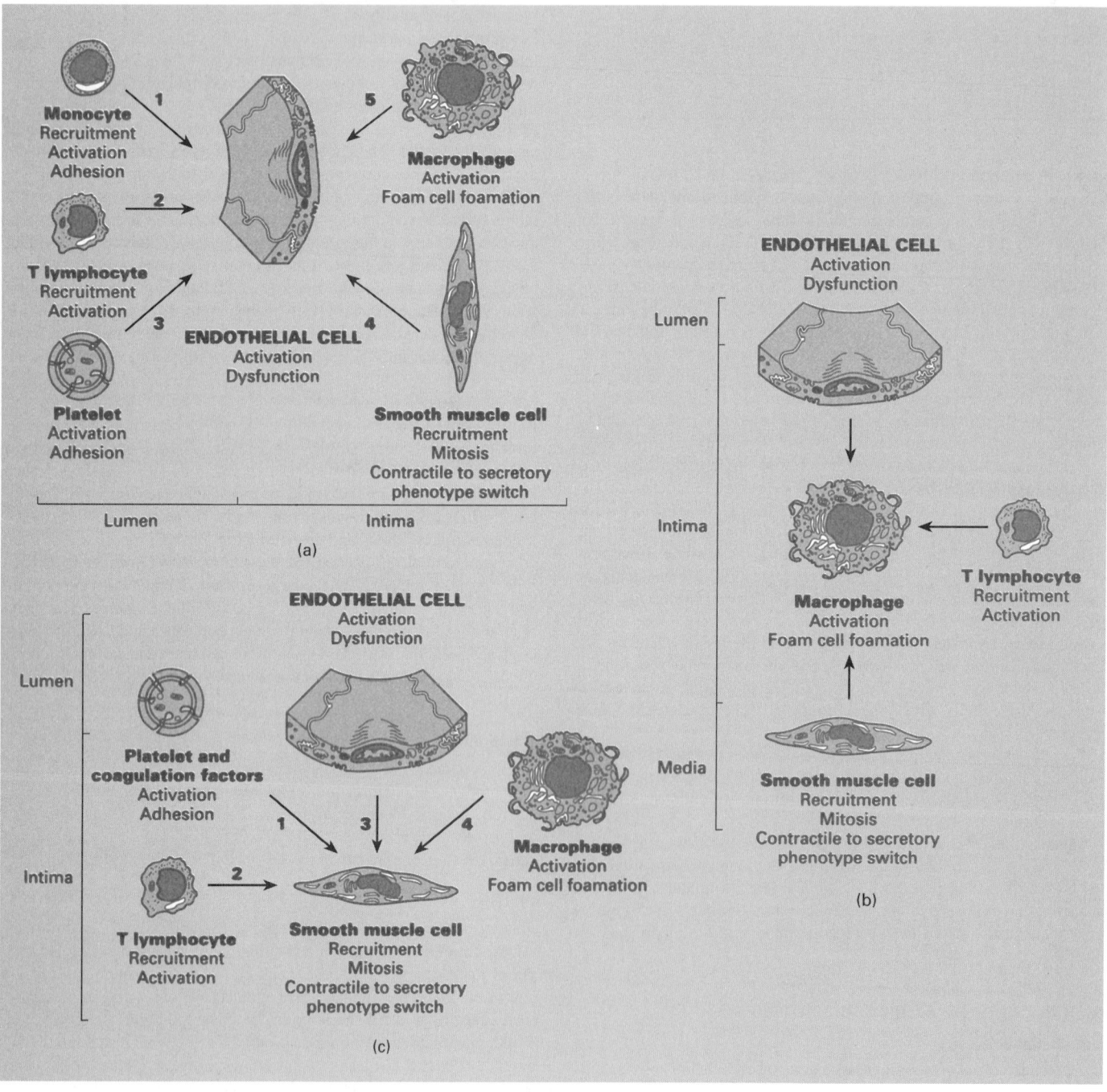

MOLECULAR INTERACTIONS

The formation of the atherosclerotic plaque is brought about by a complex series of cellular and molecular interactions. Substances expressed at the cell surface and secreted in response to cellular activation bring about these events. Growth factors generally promote mitosis or cellular hyperplasia, but can, in certain contexts, block cell growth. Cytokines are named because of their production from inflammatory cells and role in the generation of the inflammatory response. Many cytokines also act as mitogens and chemoattractants, and can inhibit cellular processes. Chemoattractants cause the movement of cells down a chemical gradient. Growth factors such as platelet-derived growth factor (PDGF) can also act as chemoattractants. Many of these substances are controlled by transcription factors, such as (NFKB), that respond to inflammation, and key promoter elements that respond to sheer stress and for which specific transcription factors exist. Molecular interactions are often local, having both autocrine and paracrine effects.

Growth factors

Much of what is known about the molecular interactions taking place in the arterial wall has been established in cell culture. A variety of substances affect the proliferation of smooth muscle cells *in vitro* and are implicated in the pathogenesis of the atherosclerotic plaque by the finding of their mRNA within the atherosclerotic lesion, but not in the normal artery wall.

Molecules that promote the proliferation of vascular smooth muscle cells *in vitro* are platelet-derived growth factor (PDGF), fibroblast growth factor (FGF), heparin-binding epidermal growth factor (HB-EGF), insulin-like growth factor I (IGF-I), interleukin-1 (IL-1), tumour necrosis factor α (TNFα), transforming growth factors α and β (TGF), thrombin, and angiotensin II.

PDGF was discovered in the platelet alpha (α) granule. Platelets also contain other growth regulatory substances, such as epidermal growth factor (EGF), TGFα, TGFβ, IGF-I, and thromboxane. The α-granule contents are released during platelet aggregation and activation. PDGF is also produced from activated endothelial cells, and smooth muscle cells with a secretory phenotype in response to the macrophage-derived cytokines IL-1, TNFα, and TGFβ. PDGF is derived from two genes that encode A and B chains, which may form both homo- and heterodimers. The PDGF receptor is a tyrosine kinase. It has two chains, which can similarly form homo- and heterodimers. PDGF is a potent mitogen for vascular smooth muscle cells *in vitro* and its mRNA can be demonstrated in the atherosclerotic plaque. Antibodies against PDGF block smooth muscle cell proliferation *in vitro* and in animal models of res-

tenosis after balloon angioplasty. PDGF also serves as a potent chemoattractant for vascular smooth muscle cells. PDGF is not normally a mitogen or chemoattractant for endothelial cells. Only in advanced lesions, where denuding injury takes place, does PDGF also come directly from platelets.

Apart from PDGF, FGF is the most potent mitogen for vascular smooth muscle cells. It also has mitogenic activity for endothelial cells. The FGFs are composed of nine structurally homologous proteins. The most important of these are acidic and basic FGF (a and b FGF). The FGFs are unusual in lacking a signal peptide, so they cannot normally be secreted from cells. However, bFGF becomes deposited in the extracellular matrix in association with heparin sulphate proteoglycans as well as with basement membrane proteins. This bFGF may be derived through an unusual secretory pathway or at sites of cell injury and necrosis and are released from endothelial and smooth muscle cells, both of which synthesize the protein. There are four homologous high-affinity tyrosine kinase receptors for FGF encoded by different genes, and there are numerous differentially spliced variants. These high-capacity receptors act in concert with low-affinity heparin sulphate proteoglycans, which serve to enhance their activity. Basic FGF and its receptor are dramatically induced by the events that surround vascular wall injury. It is likely that the FGFs have an important role in the chronic cycles of injury and repair that occur during atherogenesis.

HB-EGF is a much more potent growth factor for smooth muscle cells than either the closely related EGF or TGFα. This is because of the presence of a heparin-binding domain at its amino terminal. HB-EGF is also a potent chemoattractant for vascular smooth muscle cells. It has no activity against endothelial cells. It is induced in smooth muscle cells in response to serum, phorbol esters, and thrombin. It is also synthesized in endothelial cells in response to TNFα. This pattern of induction indicates an important role in vascular repair.

TGFβ is a multifunctional cytokine expressed along with its receptor system in many cell types, including vascular smooth muscle cells, endothelial cells, macrophages, and T lymphocytes. TGFβ is a potent inhibitor of smooth muscle cell mitosis. It also stimulates the elaboration of matrix proteins such as fibronectin and vascular collagen. TGFβ is secreted in a latent form that requires activation by trypsin-like serine proteases, such as plasmin. The proatherogenic role of lipoprotein(a) may operate through binding to the plasminogen receptor on vascular endothelial cells, thereby suppressing the formation of plasmin and inhibiting the activation of TGFβ. This would promote smooth muscle cell proliferation and plaque formation.

Vascular endothelial cell growth factor (VEGF) is a potent and specific mitogen for endothelial cells. It is also more potent than histamine in promoting permeability of small veins and venules, and has been called vascular permeability factor. It is homologous to PDGF. It binds with low affinity to heparin sulphate proteoglycans, which potentiates binding to tyrosine kinase receptors in the *fms* receptor family. VEGF is produced by endothelial cells and by macrophages. It acts as a potent chemoattractant for macrophages and induces endothelial cells to produce collagenase as well as urokinase-type plasminogen activator (uPA), tissue plasminogen activator (tPA), and their inhibitor plasminogen activator inhibitor-1 (PAI-1). Local production in response to vascular injury may be important in promoting vascular repair and stimulating angiogenesis.

A variety of other substances have mitogenic activity for cultured smooth muscle cells. These include IL-1, thrombin, and TNFα. They act indirectly by promoting the production of PDGF from endothelial cells and smooth muscle cells. IGF-I acts as a competence factor, which allows the progression of cells stimulated with PDGF. Angiotensin II is hypertrophic for vascular smooth muscle cells.

Cytokines

The cytokines IL-1, IL-2, TNFα, γ-interferon, and granulocyte–macrophage and macrophage colony stimulating factors (GM-CSF and M-CSF) are secreted from macrophages, T lymphocytes, activated endo-

Fig. 2 Oxidation of low-density lipoprotein (LDL). The figure shows the mechanisms by which oxidized LDL contributes to atherosclerosis. (1) Oxidized LDL is chemotactic for circulating monocytes. (2) Oxidized LDL inhibits the movement of resident macrophages out of the arterial intima. (3) Resident macrophages generate free radicals and contribute to production of oxidized LDL, leading to the generation of foam cells. (4) Oxidized LDL is cytotoxic and this leads to endothelial cell damage and loss of integrity. (Reproduced from Quinn *et al.* 1985, with permission.)

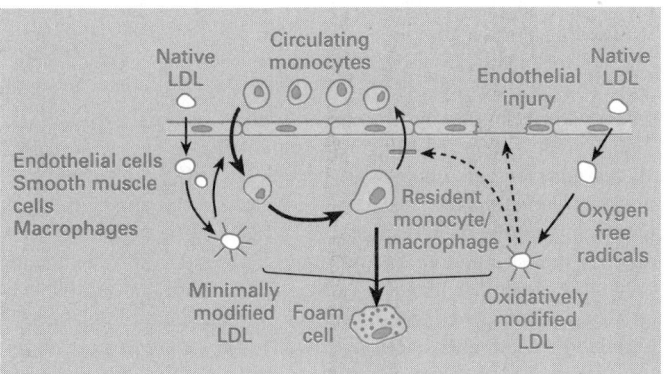

thelial cells, and smooth muscle cells with a secretory phenotype. IL-1, TNFα, and TGFβ induce endothelial cell activation, with the release of mitogens and chemoattractants for smooth muscle cells, and activate the coagulation cascade. Colony stimulating factors attract further inflammatory cells. Cytokines can also inhibit smooth muscle cell proliferation, and thus may either promote or retard atherogenesis. Their activity depends on the production of other substances with which they co-operate, as well as on their concentration and localization. Collectively they are regulated through the activity of the transcription factor, NFKB.

Chemoattractants

Proinflammatory monocytes and macrophages, and smooth muscle cells are recruited into the intima, and endothelial cells are attracted to repair the breached endothelium by chemotaxis. This is mediated by a variety of substances, some of which are also growth factors and mitogens. These include M-CSF and macrophage chemotactic protein 1 (MCP-1), and the lipid biproducts of oxidized LDL (oxLDL), all of which serve to attract monocytes and macrophages. PDGF is a chemoattractant as well as a potent mitogen for vascular smooth muscle cells, and operates in part through PDGF receptor modulation. This probably occurs through the down-regulation of PDGF receptors, as well as modulation of their activity through altered phosphorylation. Basic FGF is released from damaged smooth muscle cells and becomes associated with negatively charged proteins of the arterial matrix. It acts as a potent chemoattractant and mitogen for endothelial cells, as well as the growth factor for vascular smooth muscle cells.

Adhesion molecules

Dysfunctional endothelial cells undergo activation, with the production of cell surface proteins that mediate the adherence of inflammatory cells. This inductive process is mediated by cytokines produced by inflammatory cells and from the activated endothelium. The adhesion molecules induced include E-selectin, which is an endothelial cell specific membrane glycoprotein that mediates the adhesion of neutrophils. It is a member of the selectin gene family, which also includes L-selectin and P-selectin. These molecules are implicated in the initial 'rolling step' of leucocyte extravasation. The selectins have aminoterminal lectin domains capable of binding specific carbohydrate structures, such as sialylated Lewis X and related oligosaccharides. The selectins also contain EGF-like domains, which combine with the lectin domain to bind leucocyte cell-surface carbohydrates.

Vascular cell adhesion molecule 1 (VCAM1) is a member of the immunoglobulin gene superfamily. It is a mononuclear leucocyte-selective adhesion molecule induced on endothelial cells by IL-1 and TNFα. It is also induced by lipopolysaccharide and by oxidized LDL. VCAM1 binds cells expressing the integrins α4β1 (VLA4), such as monocytes and lymphocytes, but not neutrophils. Another cytokine-induced leucocyte adhesion molecule is intercellular adhesion molecule 1 (ICAM1), a receptor for the LFA-1 (αLβ2) and Mac-1 (αMβ2) integrins, which bind all leucocytes. Platelet endothelial cell adhesion molecule (PECAM) is another member of the immunoglobin family. PECAM exists at the tight junctions of endothelial cells and is required for the transmigration of neutrophils and monocytes and for platelet adhesion in these regions.

The time course of cytokine-induced expression of E-selectin, VCAM1, and ICAM1 indicates that these three endothelial cell adhesion molecules have distinct functions. In cultured human endothelial cells, E-selectin first appears on the cell surface within 1 to 2 h of cytokine treatment, with maximum expression at 4 to 6 h, and then rapidly declines even in the presence of cytokine. VCAM1 first appears at 4 to 6 h, peaks at 12 to 18 h, and gradually decays over days. In contrast, ICAM1 reaches its peak at 18 to 24 h and persists as long as cytokines are present. This time course is consistent with the role of E-selectin in transient adhesion, of VCAM in switching to more persistent adhesion and infiltration, and of ICAM1 in supporting transendothelial migration of leucocytes in collaboration with PECAM.

Matrix proteins

Connective tissue is a major constituent of the atherosclerotic plaque. It is produced from smooth muscle cells that have taken on a secretory phenotype. Matrix proteins produced from smooth muscle cells include fibronectin, laminin, and collagen types I, II, IV, and V, and glycosaminoglycans. The production of matrix proteins is controlled by IL-1, TNFα, and TGFβ, which mediate the switch between proliferative and secretory smooth muscle cell phenotypes.

Coagulation factors

The activation of endothelial cells initiates the cell-surface assembly of the prothrombinase complex and subsequent deposition of fibrin and platelet activation. As with clotting induced by the extravasation of blood, the process is initiated by plasma membrane expression of tissue factor, which activates factor VIIa and, in turn, factors IX and X. Thrombin is generated in the presence of endothelial cell factor V. Thrombin contributes to the inflammatory response by the induction of the adhesion molecule P-selectin and platelet activating factor, a biologically potent phospholipid molecule. Platelet arachidonic acid is released by the activity of phospholipase C and phospholipase A2. The enzyme cyclo-oxygenase generates platelet endoperoxides, and the enzyme thromboxane synthase generates thromboxane, which in turn increases phospholipase C activity and stimulates platelet activation and degranulation. Together these substances promote neutrophil and platelet adhesion. Thrombin also induces PAI-1, and increases tissue factor synthesis and PDGF expression. E-selectin is induced and serves as a site for leucocyte attachment. Thus the control of coagulation by cytokines closely mimics that of the inflammatory response and indicates the interdependence of the two processes.

Control mechanisms

Apart from the intrinsic processes required for biosynthesis and secretion of growth-regulating substances and their receptors, the molecules involved are controlled at various other levels. Many have short half-lives and may undergo amplification or attenuation by interaction with other molecules. PDGF, TGFβ, IL-1, IL-2, IL-6, and bFGF all become tightly associated with α_2-macroglobulin and this inhibits their activity. Heparin-like glycosaminoglycans bind PDGF, bFGF, HB-EGF, and TGFβ, and provide a reservoir for their action. Matrix proteins such as collagen, laminin, and fibronectin interact with cell-surface adhesion molecules, so that cell–cell and cell–matrix protein interactions may modulate the effect of growth factors, cytokines, and chemoattractants. For molecules that act locally, and which undergo rapid inactivation, the site of production and proximity to their target cells is most important.

Restenosis

The surgical treatment of arteries narrowed by atherosclerosis is by arterial or venous bypass grafting or by endarterectomy. Medical treatment is by percutaneous transluminal balloon angioplasty (PTCA). Immediate complications of this procedure are thrombosis and arterial wall dissection. There is also a high failure rate (30–40 per cent) due to restenosis of the arterial lumen. This is due to the adherence of platelets and inflammatory cells, and smooth muscle cell accummulation, which occurs in the days and weeks after the procedure. After 2 to 6 months the stenotic region becomes organized and consists of a maturing scar with foci of activated and quiescent smooth muscle cells, but little thrombus or lipid. Studies in animal models, such as the normal rat carotid subjected to balloon angioplasty, have demonstrated that PDGF and FGF are necessary for the early lesion. The receptors for these growth factors are upregulated in activated smooth muscle cells. The trauma of balloon angioplasty also removes heparin and TGFβ, which in the normal artery wall inhibit smooth muscle cell activity. The procedure of angioplasty exposes thrombogenic factors in the subendothelium and these contribute to local platelet aggregation and blood clotting. Thus the acute response to the PTCA mirrors the chronic processes, which lead to the development of atherosclerosis. Although antibodies against PDGF and FGF inhibit restenosis in the rat carotid model, satisfactory regimens for the treatment of restenosis in human subjects have yet to be established. With increased understanding of the molecular mechanisms that lead to restenosis, it is likely that new modalities of treatment, such as molecular atherectomy, will be developed, and that this important complication of PTCA will become treatable.

Future prospectives

The reduction in death rates from coronary heart disease in the latter part of the century can be attributed largely to improvement in lifestyle, particularly diet, exercise, and smoking. The prophylactic use of low-dose aspirin also helps to prevent thrombosis in those with atherosclerosis.

The response of the artery wall to injury, with the cascade of events that leads to the production of growth factors, adhesion molecules, and activation of the coagulation cascade, is now beginning to be understood. This understanding may suggest new ways in which treatment may be improved. An understanding of the central role of oxidized LDL and of the macrophage in the pathogenesis of atherosclerosis points to further improvement through dietary intervention and antioxidant supplementation. For established atherosclerosis, interventional approaches such as balloon angioplasty are plagued by a 30 to 40 per cent restenosis rate. An understanding of the trophic substances that control smooth muscle cell proliferation and recruitment and the process of re-endothelialization should provide tools that diminish this complication and further promote angioplasty for the treatment of atherosclerosis.

Already it is known that the management of risk factors can lead to the regression of atherosclerosis. Early interventions in those at risk should lead to an even more marked decrease in the prevalence of atherosclerosis and perhaps to its virtual disappearance. Simple measures such as the imaging of dysfunctional endothelium may point the way to such intervention.

REFERENCES

Altieri, D.C. (1993). Coagulation assembly on leukocytes in transmembrane signaling and cell adhesion. *Blood* **81**, 561.

Casscells, W., *et al.* (1993). Molecular atherectomy for restenosis. *Trends in Cardiovascular Medicine* **3**, 235.

Clark, E.A. and Brugge, J.S. (1993). Tyrosine phosphorylation in platelets: potential roles in intracellular signal transduction. *Trends in Cardiovascular Medicine* **3**, 218.

Collins, T., *et al.* (1993). A common theme in endothelial activation: insights from the structural analysis of the genes for E-selectin and VCAM-1. *Trends in Cardiovascular Medicine* **3**, 92.

Ferrara, N. (1993). Vascular endothelial growth factor. *Trends in Cardiovascular Medicine* **3**, 244.

Forstermann, U., *et al.* (1993). Nitric oxide synthases in the cardiovascular system. *Trends in Cardiovascular Medicine* **3**, 104.

Klagsbrun, M. and Dluz, S. (1993). Smooth muscle cell and endothelial cell growth factors. *Trends in Cardiovascular Medicine* **3**, 213.

Nachman, R.L. (1992). Thrombosis and atherogenesis: molecular connections. *Blood* **79**, 1897.

Quinn, M. T., *et al.* (1985). Endothelial cell-derived chemotactic activity for mouse peritoneal macrophages and the effects of modified forms of low density lipoprotein. *Proceedings of the National Academy of Sciences, USA* **82**, 5949–53.

Ross, R. (1993). The pathogenesis of atherosclerosis: a perspective for the 1990s. *Nature* **362**, 801–9.

Steinberg, D., *et al.* (1989). Beyond cholesterol: modifications of low-density lipoprotein that increase its atherogenicity. *New England Journal of Medicine* **320**, 915.

Wu, H., *et al.* (1992). Macrophage scavenger receptors and atherosclerosis. *Trends in Cardiovascular Medicine* **2**, 220.

15.9.2 Vascular endothelium, its physiology and pathophysiology

P. VALLANCE

A monolayer of endothelial cells lines the intimal surface of the entire vascular tree (Fig. 1). For many years it was assumed that this layer simply formed an inert physical barrier between the vessel wall and blood, but it is now becoming increasingly clear that endothelial cells are metabolically highly active and exert a profound influence on vascular reactivity, thrombogenesis, and the behaviour of circulating cells. Abnormalities of endothelial function have been implicated in a wide variety of diseases ranging from atheroma and hypertension to acute inflammation and septic shock (Table 1), and recent advances in endothelial research have led to the development of new therapies and re-evaluation of existing therapies. This chapter provides an introduction to the biology of the vascular endothelium and how endothelial dysfunction may contribute to cardiovascular disease.

Development of endothelium

During early development the endothelium forms the first layer of the circulatory system and extends to produce a network of interconnecting tubes. Later, these tubes differentiate into arteries, arterioles, capillaries, veins, and lymph vessels, and regional differences in function and structure evolve such that the properties of endothelial cells vary between arterial and venous beds, between micro- and macrovasculature, between organs and between different parts of individual organs. It is not known to what extent these differences reflect absolute differences in endothelial cells or differences in the local environment to which the cells are exposed. Heterogeneity of endothelial cells undoubtedly has implications for physiology, pathophysiology, and therapeutics, and some examples are discussed below. However, endothelial cells also have many features in common and a number of pathologies, including those causing premature vascular disease (Table 1), are associated with widespread endothelial dysfunction.

Anatomy of endothelium

Each endothelial cell is between 25 to 50 μm long, 10 to 15 μm wide, and up to 5 μm deep, and lies with its long axis aligned in the direction of the blood flow (Fig. 1). The underlying smooth muscle cells lie radi-

Fig. 1 Scanning electron micrograph of endothelium of human coronary vessel at a branch area (supplied by P.M. Rowles).

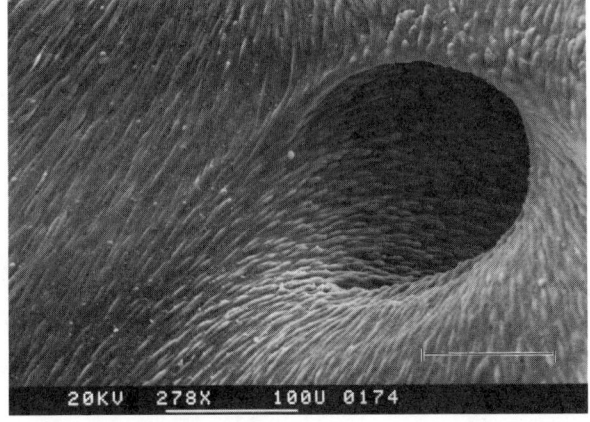

20KU   278X   100U 0174

Table 1 *Diseases associated with endothelial dysfunction. In certain diseases antiendothelial antibodies have been detected.*

Disease	Antiendothelial antibody
Hypertension	
Diabetes	Present
Hyperlipidaemia	
Atheroma	
Coronary and cerebral vasospasm	
Pulmonary hypertension	
Raynaud's disease	Present
Systemic sclerosis	Present
Kawasaki's disease	Present
Homocystinuria	
Haemolytic uraemic syndrome	Present
Vasculitides	Present
Transplant rejection	Present
Cyclosporin toxicity	
Malignant haemangioendothelioma	
Septic shock	

ally, are about 5 to 10 μm wide and taper at either end so that a single endothelial cell comes into contact with many smooth muscle cells and vice versa (Fig. 2). The endothelium also comes into intimate contact with circulating cells; the total area of the luminal surface of endothelium is in excess of 500 m². It is clear that these highly specialized cells are ideally placed to mediate communication between blood and the vessel wall, and this appears to be their major function. Endothelial cells detect signals in the lumen of the vessel and translate them into chemical messages understood by underlying smooth muscle or passing blood cells; the endothelium has been called the largest endocrine organ in the body. This thin layer of cells is particularly susceptible to injury and changes in endothelial cell morphology and turnover occurs in experimental hypertension, diabetes, and atheroma. Antibodies directed against endothelium can be found in a number of inflammatory and immune conditions (Table 1).

Control of vascular tone

Endothelium extracts and inactivates circulating hormones, converts inactive precursors into active products, and synthesizes and releases a variety of vasoactive mediators (Fig. 2). Vasoconstrictor and vasodilator mediators are produced and allow the vessel to respond to changes in the local milieu, but the predominant background influence of the endothelium is dilator with removal of the endothelium leading to vasoconstriction. Basal endothelium-dependent dilator tone seems to provide a physiological counterbalance to the continuous constrictor tone of the sympathetic nervous system.

Vasodilators

The endothelium produces at least three vasodilator mediators (Fig. 2).

NITRIC OXIDE

Production of nitric oxide is responsible for basal endothelium-dependent dilator tone. This simple gas is a potent vasodilator, which is synthesized from the semi-essential amino acid L-arginine and has a half-life of only a few seconds. Nitric oxide diffuses from endothelium into underlying smooth muscle, where it binds to the haem moiety of the enzyme guanylate cyclase; this interaction produces a conformational change that leads to enzyme activation. The subsequent increase in cyclic guanosine monophosphate relaxes the smooth muscle (Fig. 3). Nitric oxide is also released on the luminal surface where it inhibits platelet activation (see below and Fig. 3). However, contact with haemoglobin rapidly inactivates nitric oxide and this prevents any downstream effect.

The arterial circulation of animals and humans is vasodilated continuously and actively by endothelium-derived nitric oxide, and inhibition of nitric oxide synthesis with certain guanidino-substituted analogues of L-arginine, including N^G-monomethyl-L-arginine (L-NMMA), leads to vasoconstriction and hypertension. The precise physiological stimuli for the production of nitric oxide are not yet known, but probably include shear stress and platelet-derived mediators (Fig. 3). The nitric oxide produced in response to increased shear stress across the endothelial surface accounts for the phenomenon of flow-dependent vasodilatation, a response that may oppose myogenic autoregulation and optimize tissue perfusion. Endothelial cells also produce nitric oxide in response to aggregating platelets, causing vasodilatation and inhibition of further aggregation. This may be an important mechanism to protect against the potentially adverse effects of intravascular platelet activation (Fig. 3).

Nitric oxide synthesis is also stimulated by acetylcholine, bradykinin, and substance P. The physiological significance of these observations are not known, but in many vessels release of nitric oxide accounts for the vasodilator actions of these mediators, which are known as 'endothelium-dependent vasodilators'.

Veins differ from arteries and arterioles, and do not seem to be actively dilated by continuous release of nitric oxide. Venous endothelium releases nitric oxide when stimulated by acetylcholine or bradykinin, but not under basal conditions. Furthermore, human veins do not release much nitric oxide in response to platelet-derived mediators. Indeed, aggregating platelets constrict veins, due to the unopposed

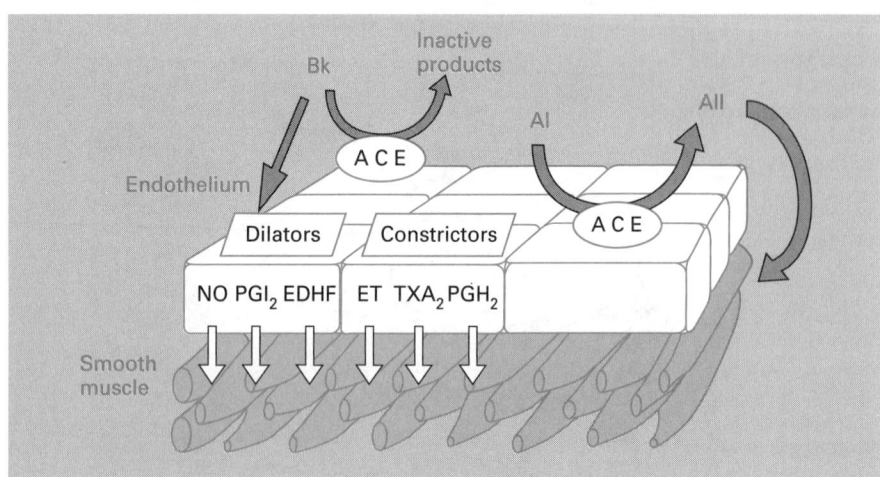

Fig. 2 Vasoactive mediators produced by endothelial cells. Dilator and constrictor mediators are synthesized and released. Angiotensin converting enzyme is located on the cell surface and converts angiotensin I into angiotensin II and metabolizes bradykinin to inactive products. Bradykinin stimulates the release of dilator mediators. Abbreviations: NO, nitric oxide; PGI_2, prostacyclin; EDHF, endothelium-derived hyperpolarizing factor; ET, endothelin; TXA_2, thromboxane A_2; PGH_2, prostaglandin H_2; Bk, bradykinin; AI, angiotensin I; ACE, angiotensin converting enzyme.

action of the mediators on vascular smooth muscle. The reasons for the arteriovenous difference in nitric oxide production are not fully understood, but one consequence is that the guanylate cyclase in venous smooth muscle is relatively up-regulated and veins respond to lower amounts of nitric oxide than do arteries or arterioles. This is of therapeutic relevance; nitric oxide is the active moiety of glyceryl trinitrate and other nitrovasodilators, and the low basal synthesis of endogenous nitric oxide by venous endothelium accounts, in part, for the venoselective action of these drugs.

It is now clear that vasoconstriction can arise from increased production of vasoconstrictors or loss of endogenous vasodilators, and diminished nitric oxide production has been implicated in a number of conditions associated with altered vascular reactivity including atherosclerosis, hypertension, and diabetes. In the coronary vasculature, loss of nitric oxide predisposes to vasospasm and may contribute to the onset of anginal symptoms. Atherosclerotic coronary arteries constrict in response to the platelet-derived mediator serotonin (5-hydroxytryptamine), whereas healthy vessels are stimulated to produce more nitric oxide and dilate (Fig. 3). Flow-dependent dilatation is also lost and the response to sympathetic stimulation is converted from dilatation to unopposed constriction. Endothelial dysfunction precedes the development of overt atheroma and there is a relationship between risk factors for ischaemic heart disease and impaired responsiveness of coronary arteries to endothelium-dependent vasodilators. Furthermore, hypercholesterolaemia, even in the absence of angiographic evidence of atheroma in large vessels, is associated with abnormal endothelium-dependent vasodilatation in coronary and peripheral arterioles. Modified low density lipoproteins appear to inhibit nitric oxide synthesis or speed its destruction, possibly by enhancing production of superoxide anion.

Basal endothelium-dependent dilatation is also impaired in patients with essential hypertension and the degree of impairment increases with blood pressure. However, it is not known whether the defect is a consequence or a cause of the raised pressure. Endothelial function appears to be restored by antihypertensive therapy and this argues in favour of dysfunction being a response to the raised pressure. Patients with diabetes show diminished endothelium-dependent dilatation and this defect does not reverse with treatment. Thus patients with uncontrolled hypertension, diabetes, and hypercholesterolaemia all display a similar defect

of nitric oxide mediated vasodilatation and this could provide a common mechanism of vascular dysfunction in these diseases. Inhibition of nitric oxide synthesis enhances atherogenesis in hyperlipidaemic animals and this effect can be reversed by dietary supplementation with arginine.

Overproduction of nitric oxide also contributes to cardiovascular disease. Bacterial endotoxin, and certain cytokines, including interleukin I and tumour necrosis factor, lead to expression of a second nitric oxide synthesizing enzyme in the endothelium, the vascular smooth muscle itself, and inflammatory cells in the vessel wall. Unlike the constitutive enzyme present in healthy endothelium, this inducible nitric oxide synthase is not regulated by calcium and produces large amounts of nitric oxide over long periods. In these quantities nitric oxide may contribute to tissue damage in addition to causing profound vasodilatation and hypotension. Overproduction of nitric oxide also mediates the vasodilatation associated with local inflammation. The therapeutic potential of inhibitors of nitric oxide synthase (e.g. L-NMMA) for the treatment of systemic or local vascular inflammation (including septic shock) is under investigation.

PROSTANOIDS

Nitric oxide appears to be the dominant vasoactive factor released from endothelial cells under basal conditions, but it is by no means the only mediator produced. The endothelium is also a rich source of prostanoids, including the vasodilators prostacyclin and the prostaglandins PGE_2 and PGD_2. However, whereas inhibition of nitric oxide leads to profound and widespread changes in vascular tone, inhibition of prostanoid synthesis with aspirin, or other non-steroidal anti-inflammatory drugs does not. Renal vasculature is an exception and dilator prostanoids do appear to be important in the regulation of basal renal blood flow; aspirin and other non-steroidal anti-inflammatories lead to vasoconstriction in the kidney, indicating tonic release of vasodilator prostanoids in this vascular bed. Furthermore, in the fetus and newborn, indomethacin leads to closure of the ductus arteriosus and a fall in cerebral blood flow suggesting a significant contribution of endothelium-derived prostanoids to cardiovascular control at this stage of development. Vasodilator prostanoids are also important in the vascular changes of inflammation, although whether the prostanoids derive exclusively from the endothelium is not known. A cytokine-inducible isoform of cyclo-oxygenase has been identified and this probably contributes to increased vascular prostaglandin synthesis in inflammation.

HYPERPOLARIZING FACTOR

An endothelium-derived hyperpolarizing factor (EDHF) has been identified in certain animal and human blood vessels. The chemical identity of endothelium-derived hyperpolarizing factor has not been clearly established, and its role as an endogenous dilator of human vessels remains to be determined. Preliminary data suggest a more prominent role for EDHF in childhood and early development.

Vasoconstrictors

Although the background influence of the endothelium is dilator, potent vasoconstrictor factors are also synthesized and released.

ENDOTHELIN

The endothelins are a family of potent vasoconstrictor peptides containing 21 amino acids that are closely related to the snake venom toxin of the Israeli burrowing asp. Three types of endothelin have been described, endothelin 1, 2, and 3; there are at least two endothelin receptors in human blood vessels: endothelin-A receptor and the endothelin-B receptor.

Endothelin-1 is synthesized from 'big endothelin' within human endothelial cells (Fig. 4), is a potent and long-lasting constrictor of

Fig. 3 Platelet-derived mediators, including adenosine diphosphate (ADP) and 5-hydroxytryptamine (5-HT; serotonin) stimulate endothelial cells to synthesize nitric oxide (NO) from L-arginine (L-arg). L-citrulline (L-cit) is the byproduct. Nitric oxide inhibits platelet adhesion and aggregation and relaxes vascular smooth muscle. These effects are mediated by cyclic guanosine monophosphate (cGMP); nitric oxide binds to the haem moiety (Hm) of guanylate cyclase (GC) and activates this enzyme, which converts guanosise triphosphate into cyclic guanosine monophosphate. The release of nitric oxide in response to activated platelets provides a negative feedback system to prevent activated platelets from causing vasospasm and further platelet adhesion and aggregation.

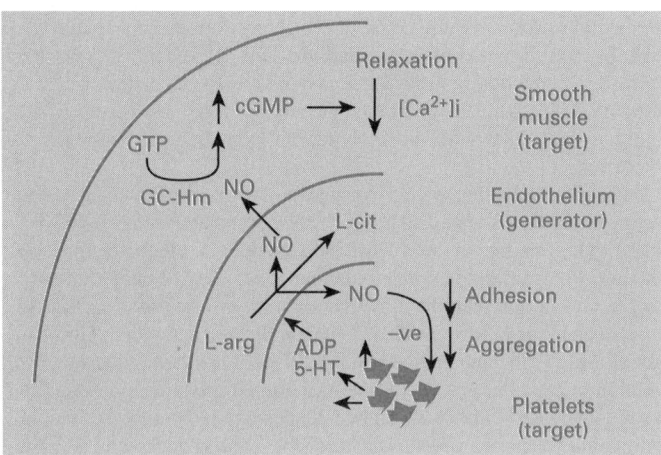

human blood vessels, and increases blood pressure when infused into healthy volunteers. Paradoxically, endothelin can also produce transient vasodilatation. However, the precise physiological role of endothelins remains uncertain. Their concentrations in circulating human plasma appear to be insufficient to vasoconstrict, and endothelin receptor antagonists seem to have little effect on resting vascular tone or blood pressure in healthy animals. Stimuli for the release of endothelins include hypoxia, thrombin, and transforming growth factor β (TGF-β), and it is possible that stimulated production of endothelins could have a local effect to increase vascular tone or enhance responses to other vasoconstrictors.

Increased production of endothelin has been implicated in a number of diseases associated with vasoconstriction. Elevated circulating levels of endothelin-1 occur in patients with myocardial infarction, hypertension, diabetes, and renal failure, and local increases in endothelin-1 are seen in the venous blood draining the hand of patients with Raynaud's disease and in coronary sinus blood of patients with coronary vasospasm. In some instances increased circulating levels reflect reduced renal clearance of the peptide rather than increased production, and in general the levels of endothelin detected appear to be too low to have a direct effect on vascular tone. However, hypotensive and vasodilator effects of endothelin antagonists have been reported in certain animal models of disease and an endothelin-A receptor antagonist dilates human resistance vessels *in vivo*. A slowly modulating background constrictor influence of endothelin seems to be present in certain vessels and a role for endothelin in the pathogenesis of vasospasm associated with subarachnoid haemorrhage and some types of renal ischaemia is suggested by results from experiments in animals. It seems likely that the precise role of endothelin in these diseases, and other vasospastic conditions, will become apparent as inhibitors of endothelin synthesis, and specific endothelin receptor blockers become available for use in man.

Increased production endothelin has been clearly implicated in the pathogenesis of a very rare form of secondary hypertension caused by malignant haemangioendothelioma, a vascular tumour characterized by intravascular proliferation of atypical endothelial cells. In this condition the degree of hypertension correlates with plasma levels of endothelin and when the tumour is removed blood pressure and plasma endothelin levels fall.

Fig. 4 Biosynthesis of the vasoconstrictor peptide endothelin-1. Endothelin-1 produces profound vasoconstriction, predominantly through activation of endothelin-A receptors. Inhibition of endothelin converting enzyme, or specific endothelin receptor antagonists may provide novel therapies for conditions associated with vasospasm or hypertension.

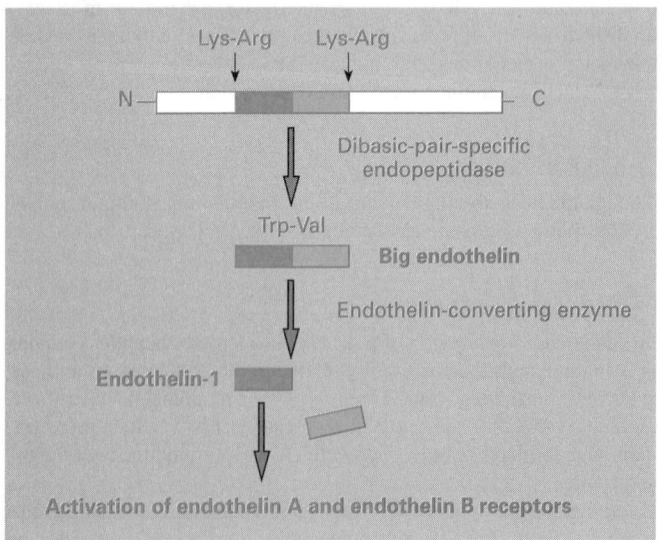

ANGIOTENSIN CONVERTING ENZYME

Angiotensin converting enzyme (ACE) is located primarily on the luminal surface of the endothelium. This enzyme converts angiotensin I to angiotensin II and also metabolizes bradykinin to inactive products (see Fig. 2). The pulmonary vasculature provides the largest area of endothelium, and is important in the regulation of circulating levels of angiotensin II. However, the activity of endothelial angiotensin converting enzyme in systemic vessels may be more important in determining the final concentrations of angiotensin II and bradykinin reaching the blood vessel wall. Furthermore, endothelial cells also have the ability to synthesize renin and its substrate and this raises the possibility that complete local renin–angiotensin systems are active in vessel walls.

The activity of the renin–angiotensin system is clearly important in cardiovascular diseases including hypertension and heart failure, but the relative importance of local compared with systemic regulation of angiotensin II production is not yet clear. Furthermore, the full clinical significance of bradykinin metabolism by endothelial angiotensin converting enzyme (see Fig. 2) has yet to be determined. It has been demonstrated that at least part of the vasodilator action of angiotensin converting enzyme inhibitors in isolated blood vessels is due to accumulation of bradykinin which stimulates nitric oxide synthesis.

PROSTANOIDS

The endothelium synthesizes thromboxane (TXA_2) and the unstable prostaglandin endoperoxides PGG_2 and PGH_2. Overproduction of constrictor prostanoids by the endothelium has been implicated in animal models of diabetes and hypertension but the significance of these findings to human disease remains uncertain.

Regulation of platelet function and haemostasis

The endothelium synthesizes and releases prothrombotic and antithrombotic factors. However, healthy endothelium presents a thromboresistant surface indicating that the antithrombotic factors predominate under basal conditions.

Platelets

Endothelial cells inhibit platelet aggregation and adhesion, and disaggregate aggregating platelets. Two mediators are of particular importance: nitric oxide and prostacyclin (or PGE_2 in microvascular endothelium). They act through different second messenger systems – cyclic guanosine monophosphate for nitric oxide and cyclic adenosine monophosphate for prostacyclin – and synergize to inhibit aggregation and promote disaggregation.

Thiols and sulphydryl-containing molecules react with nitric oxide to produce more stable adducts, including nitrosocysteine, nitrosoglutathione and nitrosoalbumin, some of which are formed *in vivo* and may enhance the antiplatelet effects of endothelium-derived nitric oxide. Furthermore, interaction between nitric oxide and tissue plasminogen activator (tPA) leads to the formation of nitroso-tissue plasminogen activator, a molecule with fibrinolytic, antiplatelet, and vasorelaxant properties.

Deficient production of nitric oxide has been implicated in a wide variety of cardiovascular diseases (see above) and abnormalities of prostanoid synthesis occur in experimental models of atherosclerosis and diabetes. Pharmacological manipulation of nitric oxide suggests that in the presence a quiescent healthy endothelium loss of basal nitric oxide alone does not lead to significant systemic platelet activation. However, loss of nitric oxide and prostacyclin at sites of endothelial damage, dysfunction or activation promotes the formation of platelet aggregates and may contribute to thrombosis and vessel occlusion. In animals, stenosed endothelium-denuded vessels lead to cyclical variations in flow as platelets stick to the vessel wall and release vasoactive and pro-aggregant mediators. If this also occurs in human vessels *in vivo* this might be an important mechanism of vasospasm and thrombosis.

Under basal conditions the endothelium inhibits platelet activation, but in response to certain stimuli, pro-aggregant, pro-adhesive mediators may be synthesized and released. Unstable prostaglandin endoperoxides activate platelets, platelet activating factor (PAF) may be produced, and von Willebrand factor (vWF), which is synthesized and stored within endothelial cells, increases platelet adhesion. These changes occur in response to inflammatory mediators and may also result from repeated endothelial 'injury'.

Coagulation

Heparan sulphate is a glycosaminoglycan closely related to heparin, and is found on the surface of endothelial cells. It possesses similar properties to heparin, but is less potent. Antithrombin III is expressed on the endothelial cell surface and, together with heparan sulphate, this provides a mechanism for binding and inactivating thrombin. In addition, endothelial cells participate in the activation of the anticoagulant protein C; protein S is secreted and thrombomodulin is found on the cell surface.

In the quiescent state, expression of anticoagulant factors predominates: however, if activated, the endothelium may promote coagulation; receptors for clotting factors appear on the endothelial surface, von Willebrand factor is secreted and tissue factor – the principal cellular initiator of coagulation – is expressed. Bacterial endotoxin, inflammatory cytokines, and glycosylated proteins activate the endothelium and shift the balance in favour of coagulation. This may occur in response to infection, inflammation, or endothelial injury. Circulating levels of von Willebrand factor are increased in certain patients with diabetes.

Thrombolysis

The endothelial cell surface has a fibrinolytic pathway. Urokinase and tissue plasminogen activator are secreted and there are specific binding sites for plasminogen activators and plasminogen. Thrombin, adrenaline, vasopressin and stasis of blood may be physiological stimuli for tissue plasminogen activator release from human endothelium.

Plasminogen activator inhibitor I (PAI) is also synthesized and bound by endothelium, providing a pathway for local inhibition of the fibrinolytic system. Under basal conditions fibrinolysis is dominant, but the balance may be altered by a variety of local and circulating factors, including inflammatory cytokines and the atherogenic particle lipoprotein (a), which inhibits plasminogen binding and hence plasmin generation. In the presence of atherosclerosis the fibrinolytic properties of endothelium are diminished.

Cellular adhesion

The resting endothelium prevents cells from adhering fully to the vessel wall but allows leucocytes to roll along its surface. The regulation of 'rolling', adhesion, and migration is governed largely by specialized glycoproteins known as cell adhesion molecules (CAMs), which are expressed in varying amounts on the endothelial cell surface and interact with complementary adhesion molecules on circulating cells. Endothelial–leucocyte adhesion molecule-1 (ELAM-1; also known as E-selectin), vascular adhesion molecule-1 (VCAM-1), intercellular adhesion molecule-1 (ICAM-1), and P-selectin (also known as GMP 140) are all expressed on cytokine-activated endothelium. The degree of expression and the type of adhesion molecules expressed determines the 'stickiness' of the endothelium for different cell types. Expression of adhesion molecules is an important mechanism of cellular adhesion during inflammation but is also important in recruitment of monocytes in atherosclerosis. Increased expression of endothelial-leucocyte adhesion molecule-1 is seen in coronary arteries of transplanted hearts and has

been implicated in the rapid development of atherosclerosis in these vessels. Nitric oxide and prostacyclin also inhibit the adhesion of white cells to endothelium and this effect may be mediated by changes in the expression or configuration of adhesion molecules.

Cell growth

The endothelium inhibits proliferation of the underlying smooth muscle. Endothelium-derived vasodilator, antiplatelet, and antithrombotic mediators tend to inhibit cell growth whereas vasoconstrictor prothrombotic mediators tend to promote it. Thus the basal state of the endothelium, in which dilatation and antithrombosis predominates, also prevents smooth muscle growth. The heparin-like molecules and TGFβ produced by endothelial cells seem to be particularly important in the prevention of cell growth, and molecules similar or identical to platelet-derived growth factor (PDGF) and fibroblast growth factor (FGF) are endothelium-derived growth promoters. The basal antiproliferative effects of the endothelium may retard the development of atherosclerosis and intimal proliferation.

Cytokines

Cytokines are released from activated leucocytes in response to infection and immunological stimulation and are also produced by the vessel wall itself; interleukins 1, 6, and 8, and colony stimulating factors are synthesized by endotoxin-stimulated endothelial cells, and tumour necrosis factor by human smooth muscle cells. A large number of cytokines alter endothelial functions, upsetting the balance of vasoactive mediators, and altering thrombotic activity and the expression of adhesion molecules. Interleukin-1 and tumour necrosis factor increase the synthesis of nitric oxide (see above) and a variety of prostaglandins; enhance the generation of thrombin, platelet activating factor, von Willebrand factor, and plasminogen activator inhibitor; alter endothelial permeability; increase expression of ICAM-1 and VCAM-1; and may also cause endothelial cell damage and death. These findings are of direct relevance to the vascular changes of inflammation and sepsis, but might also provide a link between chronic immunological stimulation and the development of cardiovascular disease.

Transport and metabolism

The endothelium presents a permeability barrier for molecules in the bloodstream. Transfer of molecules from the bloodstream into the vessel wall across the endothelium can occur by transport through the endothelial cells or between them. Transport between cells occurs when endothelial cells contract to leave intercellular gaps. This is an important mechanism of localized oedema formation. Transport through cells occurs by trancytosis and is an important mechanism for the passage of certain macromolecules, including insulin.

The endothelium is intimately involved in lipid metabolism. Lipoprotein lipase is located on the endothelial cell surface and receptors for low density lipoproteins (LDL) are present in varying amounts. In quiescent endothelium lipoprotein lipase is active but there are few low density lipoprotein receptors, indicating that healthy endothelium provides a barrier for entry of low density lipoprotein into the vessel wall. However, under conditions in which low density lipoprotein is taken into the endothelium, modification by oxidation occurs and this step may stimulate atherogenesis.

Signal detection by endothelial cells

It is clear that the endothelium has many functions and releases a wide variety of mediators. What is also clear is that it must also be able to respond to changes in its local environment. Indeed, endothelial cells act as signal transducers, responding to both chemical and physical stimuli and altering mediator release and enzyme activity accordingly. The endothelial cell membrane expresses a large number of receptors for circulating hormones, local mediators, and vasoactive factors released from blood cells, and can also sense local changes in pressure and flow; stretch of the cell membrane leads directly to opening of a cation channel permeable to calcium, and increased shear stress leads to opening of a potassium channel, which hyperpolarizes the cell. The precise mechanisms linking the various stimuli received to the messages produced by the endothelial cell have yet to be determined, but calcium is undoubtedly important. Receptor occupation, stretch, or shear stress all lead to changes in the concentration of intracellular free calcium, and the profile of change influences which endothelial functions are activated and therefore which message is produced by the cell.

Therapeutic implications

The balance of mediators produced by quiescent healthy endothelium promotes vasodilatation, inhibits activation of platelets and white cells, prevents thrombosis, and retards the growth of smooth muscle cells. However, the endothelium also has the capacity to constrict blood vessels, promote cellular adhesion, initiate thrombosis, and stimulate the growth of smooth muscle cells. Endothelial cells are of fundamental importance in the short- and long-term control of many aspects of cardiovascular function and it is hardly surprising that endothelial dysfunction has been implicated in the pathogenesis of a diverse list of diseases (see Table 1). Therapeutic implications of endothelial dysfunction are now emerging.

Certain therapeutic interventions cause endothelial damage. Antibodies directed against the endothelium are found after heart transplantation and endothelial dysfunction may contribute to the rapid development of coronary artery disease seen in transplant recipients. Balloon angioplasty leads directly to severe disruption of the endothelium and this has been implicated in the development of postangioplasty vasospasm, thrombosis, and restenosis due to smooth muscle growth. Venous coronary artery bypass grafts are more prone to occlusion than arterial grafts, and this may reflect differences between arterial and venous endothelium including reduced basal release of nitric oxide by venous endothelium or differential production of growth factors. Acute disruption of endothelial function may promote vasospasm, thrombosis, and occlusion and chronic changes enhance atherogenesis.

Drugs also affect endothelial function. Nitrovasodilators mimic an endogenous endothelium-derived relaxing factor; glyceryl trinitrate is metabolized to nitric oxide within the vessel wall while sodium nitroprusside liberates nitric oxide spontaneously. Like the endogenous mediator certain nitrovasodilators inhibit platelet activation and this may provide an additional mechanism to explain the beneficial effects of these drugs in coronary artery disease. Other drugs of benefit in acute coronary artery disease may also replace endothelial mediators, or restore the balance between mediators released by endothelium and bloodborne cells; heparin mimics heparans on the cell surface, plasminogen activators replace the endogenous molecule, and low-dose intermittent aspirin preferentially inhibits thromboxane synthesis in platelets while sparing endothelial prostanoid production. Furthermore, angiotensin converting enzyme inhibitors inhibit the breakdown of bradykinin (see Fig. 2) and this mediator stimulates the release of nitric oxide from endothelial cells. Recently it has been demonstrated that oestrogens modify endothelial function and enhance endothelium-dependent vasodilatation. A greater understanding of the normal protective functions of vascular endothelium and how these are altered by disease is bound to lead to therapies designed to modify endothelial function. New drugs based on nitric oxide, endothelin, adhesion molecules, and growth factors are in development and likely to enter clinical practice, and seeding of genetically altered endothelial cells on to blood vessels or genetic manipulation of the expression of endothelial mediators is an experimental possibility.

REFERENCES

Calver, A., Collier, J., and Vallance, P. (1993). Nitric oxide and cardiovascular control. *Experimental Physiology*, **78**, 303–26.

Clozel, M., Breu, V., Burri, K., *et al.* (1993). Pathophysiological role of endothelin revealed by the first orally active endothelin receptor antagonist. *Nature*, **365**, 759–61.

Furchgott, R.F., and Zawadzki J.V. (1980). The obligatory role of endothelial cells in the relaxation of arterial smooth muscle. *Nature*, **288**, 373–376.

Gerlach, H., Esposito, C., and Stern, D.M. (1990). Modulation of endothelial hemostatic properties: an active role in the host response. *Annual Review of Medicine*. **41**, 15–24.

Griffith, T.M., Edwards, D.H., Davies, R.L., Harrison, T.J., and Evans, K.T. (1987). EDRF coordinates the behaviour of vascular resistance vessels. *Nature*, **329**, 442–5.

Gryglewski, R.J., Botting, R.M., and Vane, J.R. (1988). Mediators produced by the endothelial cell. *Hypertension*, **12**, 530–548.

Hayden, M.R. and Reidy, M. (1995). Many roads lead to atheroma. *Nature Medicine*, **1**, 22–3.

Haynes, W.G. and Webb, D.J. (1993). The endothelin family of peptides: local hormones with diverse roles in health and disease. *Clinical Science*, **84**, 485–500.

Lorenzi, M., and Cagliero, E. (1991). Pathobiology of endothelial and other vascular cells in diabetes mellitus. *Diabetes*, **40**, 653–659.

Lüscher, T.F., Boulanger, C.M., Dohi Y., and Yang, Z. (1992). Endothelium-derived contracting factors. *Hypertension*, **19**, 117–130.

Masaki, T., Kimura, S., Yanagisawa, M. and Goto, K. (1991). Molecular and cellular mechanism of endothelin regulation. Implications for vascular function. *Circulation*, **84**, 1457–1468.

Mason, J.C. and Haskard, D.O. (1994). The clinical importance of leucocyte and endothelial cell adhesion molecules in inflammation. *Vascular Medicine Review*, **5**, 249–75.

Moncada, S., Palmer, R.M.J., and Higgs, E.A. (1991). Nitric oxide: physiology, pathophysiology and pharmacology. *Pharmacological Reviews*, **43**, 109–142.

Monatovani, A., Bussolino, F., and Dejana, E. (1992). Cytokine regulation of endothelial cell function. *FASEB Journal*, **6**, 2591–2599.

Petty, R.G., and Pearson, J.D. (1989). Endothelium – the axis of vascular health and disease. *Journal of the Royal College of Physicians of London*, **23**, 92–102.

Ross, R. (1993). The pathogenesis of atherosclerosis: a perspective for the 1990s. *Nature*, **362**, 801–9.

Zhihong, Y., Stulz, P., von Segesser, L., Bauer, E., Turina, M., and Lüscher, T.F. (1991). Different interactions of platelets with arterial and venous coronary bypass vessels. *Lancet*, **337**, 939–941.

15.9.3 Haemostatic variables in ischaemic heart disease

T. W. MEADE

Introduction

General recognition of the thrombotic contribution to arterial disease is a comparatively recent development. In some respects, clinical and preventive practice have altered substantially as a result of research stimulated by growing interest in thrombosis. In others, decisions for some years to come will still have to be based on only partial information from research.

Besides the structural effects of atheroma and thrombosis, the importance of functional influences on vasomotor tone have come into rapid prominence over the last few years, particularly the actions of nitric oxide and other endogenous mediators. The clinical implications of these advances are now being developed. This section concentrates on the coagulation and platelet determinants of thrombosis that either already have or may soon have practical implications in the primary and secondary prevention of ischaemic heart disease (IHD). The investigation and management of established thrombosis is considered in Chapter 15.26 and Section 22.

The term 'coronary thrombosis' was derived from clinical and pathological observations made many years ago (so that present interest in thrombosis is a reawakening rather than a discovery). When the growing epidemic of ischaemic heart disease led to concerted research after the Second World War, interest centred mainly on the lipid nature of the atheromatous plaque and on the contributions of dietary fat and of blood cholesterol levels to its initiation and development. The first randomized controlled trial suggesting the value of aspirin in the secondary prevention of myocardial infarction (MI) was reported in 1974, thus predating the clinical and pathological studies that resolved the debate as to whether thrombosis causes myocardial infarction or vice versa. By 1980, the advent of thrombolytic therapy and the need to establish the rationale for its use had led to angiographic studies demonstrating the involvement of total coronary occlusion in myocardial infarction. Even then, however, the place of thrombosis in sudden coronary death remained controversial and it was not until the mid-1980s that the almost universal occurrence of at least a degree of thrombosis in sudden coronary death was recognized. Thrombi associated with sudden coronary death may not occlude the arterial lumen as often as those causing transmural myocardial infarction because of the intense fibrinolytic activity accompanying sudden death, with the consequence that some thrombi, initially responsible for such episodes, are at least partially lysed by the time of autopsy.

Coronary artery thrombi are largely due to platelet aggregates and to the deposition of fibrin, in varying proportions. As interest in thrombosis and ischaemic heart disease developed, attention was directed initially towards the contribution of platelets and there is, of course, no dispute about the central role of platelets in arterial thrombosis. It is, however, fibrin which gives many developing thrombi their ultimate stability and volume and there is reason to believe that fibrin formation and platelet

Fig. 1 Summary of coagulation system showing interrelationships with platelets and the fibrinolytic system. Unbarred lines indicate activation, barred lines indicate inhibition. The scheme indicates the position of different factors, without distinguishing between inactive (zymogen) and active forms, e.g. conversion of factor X to activated X, Xa, by IXa, itself derived from factor IX. Non-coagulation cofactors, e.g. Ca^{2+}, also not shown.

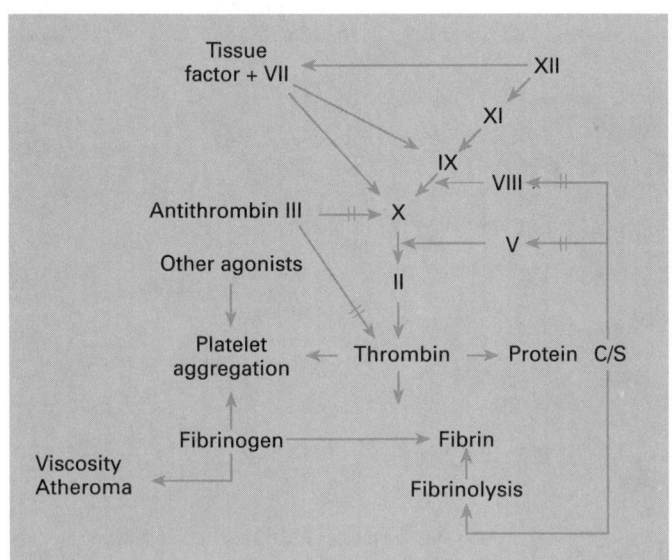

activation are equally important in the early hours of myocardial infarction, with the implication that the most effective approach to antithrombotic therapy may involve platelet-active agents and anticoagulants given simultaneously. Despite the obvious involvement of platelets in arterial thrombosis, however, it is studies of the coagulation system that have so far provided most information about particular constituents of the haemostatic system that may predispose to thrombosis. Figure 1 is a summary of the coagulation system, and also shows some of its interrelationships with platelets and the fibrinolytic system. The traditional distinction between the extrinsic and intrinsic coagulation pathways is an oversimplification. Thus, for example (and besides its contribution to atherogenesis), dietary fat intake probably influences coagulability through the activation of factor VII by factor XII. The factor VII activation of factor IX is another example. Different components of the haemostatic system may have several functions. Thus, thrombin—the main function of which is usually considered to be the conversion of fibrinogen to fibrin—is a potent platelet aggregating agent, leads to the activation of protein C and influences fibrinolytic activity, while platelets and platelet membranes also provide cofactors and surfaces for coagulation.

Factor VII and fibrinogen

Current interest chiefly centres on two clotting factors, factor VII and fibrinogen.

FACTOR VII

Factor VII mainly circulates in a single chain form. The activity of factor VII is due to the two-chain form which complexes with tissue factor to initiate thrombin generation. Activated VII itself can be derived through a pathway involving tissue factor and activated factor X or through the tissue factor—independent pathway of the contact or intrinsic system which can, in turn, be activated by lipoproteins. Both forms of factor VII have short circulating half-lives of under 5 h. It is increasingly clear that different factor VII activity assays are not equally sensitive to the two-chain form, a consideration of obvious clinical relevance if the relationship between VII and ischaemic heart disease is due to this more active form. Based on a biological activity assay system that is one of the more sensitive to the two-chain form, high factor VII levels were strongly associated with the subsequent incidence of ischaemic heart disease in the Northwick Park Heart Study, particularly in the case of fatal events. Several cross-sectional and prevalence studies also show higher factor VII levels in cases than controls. There is a direct relationship between the levels of factor VII and markers of thrombin generation, suggesting that factor VII activity is at least a valid index of the degree of coagulability. Whether the degree of factor VII activity itself contributes to the latter (as distinct from simply reflecting coagulability) is unresolved, although there is some evidence that it does directly influence coagulability. Factor VII concentrates successfully used in the management of haemophilia patients with antibodies to factor VIII probably work by activating factor X and thus the final common pathway. This observation does suggest that the factor VII level may have a direct effect on coagulability, although the concentrations used therapeutically in resistant haemophilia are very high and unphysiological. The general epidemiological features of factor VII are consistent with its involvement in ischaemic heart disease. Thus, increasing age, oral contraceptive use, the menopause, diabetes, obesity and (in particular—see below) high dietary fat consumption are all associated with raised factor VII levels.

Bearing in mind the difficulty of showing a relationship between habitual dietary fat intake and the blood cholesterol level within (as distinct from between) populations, the clear demonstration in both observational and experimental studies of a direct relationship between fat intake and factor VII activity is striking. One possibility is that large negatively charged and triglyceride-rich lipoproteins (e.g. chylomicrons and very low density lipoproteins) activate the intrinsic pathway which, in turn, activates factor VII. The effect of fat intake on factor VII is achieved in a matter of hours and may, along with effects on platelet function, be relevant to the diurnal variation in the onset of ischaemic heart disease. Incidence is greatest during the morning and could be partly explained by food intake the previous evening. The saturated fatty acid stearic acid is mainly responsible for the dietary fat activation of factor VII. Figure 2 illustrates the long-term, atherogenic effect of diet in ischaemic heart disease and its much shorter-term, thrombogenic effect. It is still often claimed that dietary intervention is unlikely to be effective in adults in whom significant atheroma has often already developed and that it is, therefore, only children and young adults who stand to benefit. If, however, dietary fat intake does have short-term, thrombogenic potential, this conclusion is largely misplaced and adults already affected by a significant degree of atheroma probably stand to benefit considerably.

FIBRINOGEN

High plasma fibrinogen levels are associated with the onset or progression of arterial disease at all major sites. Several prospective studies show an independent relationship between fibrinogen and the incidence of ischaemic heart disease. At face value, this relationship is of the same magnitude as for cholesterol, although because of the greater within-person variability in fibrinogen, the true relationship is probably rather stronger than for cholesterol. In the prospective studies with adequate numbers of older participants, there is also an association between high

Fig. 2 Diet and ischaemic heart disease: atherogenic and thrombogenic pathways.

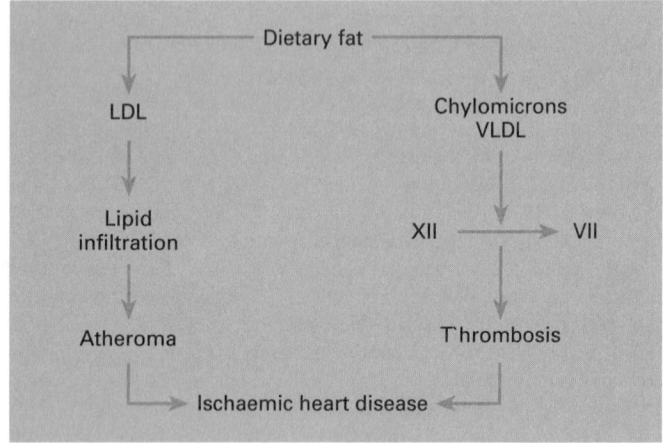

fibrinogen levels and the incidence of stroke in men that is of the same order as for ischaemic heart disease. As the association between cholesterol and stroke is probably not as clear as for ischaemic heart disease, the fibrinogen level may be a particularly useful index of the risk of major cardiovascular disease, defined as the sum of ischaemic heart disease and stroke. High fibrinogen levels also appear to predict the recurrence of ischaemic heart disease in those surviving a first episode. Only one of the prospective studies has included sufficiently large numbers of women, in whom high levels are also associated with ischaemic heart disease incidence though not very clearly with stroke (probably because of small numbers of events). High fibrinogen levels are undoubtedly associated with the progression of peripheral vascular disease in terms of worsening symptoms, loss of patency after vein grafting and of mortality from cardiovascular disease. It is also likely that fibrinogen levels influence the initial onset of peripheral vascular disease. Indications of the importance of fibrinogen in arterial disease are its equivalence with blood pressure in risk of stroke and, if anything, its greater contribution than smoking to the progression of peripheral arterial disease. Some of the prospective studies suggest there may be synergy between high fibrinogen levels and hypertension in the onset of ischaemic heart disease and stroke.

Fibrinogen is an acute phase protein. High levels might, therefore, simply reflect the underlying degree of arterial wall damage, bearing in mind that atheroma has many of the characteristics of an inflammatory response (although there is not much evidence for this explanation, and some that argues against it). Even if this were the full explanation for the association between fibrinogen and clinically manifest arterial disease, the strong and independent nature of the association still provides an opportunity for improved precision in identifying those at risk. The balance of evidence suggests, however, that—whatever their determinants—high fibrinogen levels are of direct, pathogenetic significance. It is useful to consider this important point in two stages.

1. Regardless of their origins, are high fibrinogen levels likely to predispose to thrombosis?
2. What are the origins of high levels?

Figure 3 summarizes the pathways through which high fibrinogen levels may predispose to thrombosis and clinical events and (considered in more detail later) the characteristics associated with high or low levels. The influence of fibrinogen on viscosity and the relationship, in turn, of viscosity to ischaemic heart disease is the pathway for which there is probably the strongest evidence at present—one of the prospective studies shows a strong association between plasma viscosity (as well as fibrinogen) and the incidence of ischaemic heart disease. Viscous drag exerted by the vessel wall on flowing blood determines how adjacent fluid layers move relative to each other. Viscosity is the ratio of shear stress to shear rate; shear stress is the force per unit area causing shear-

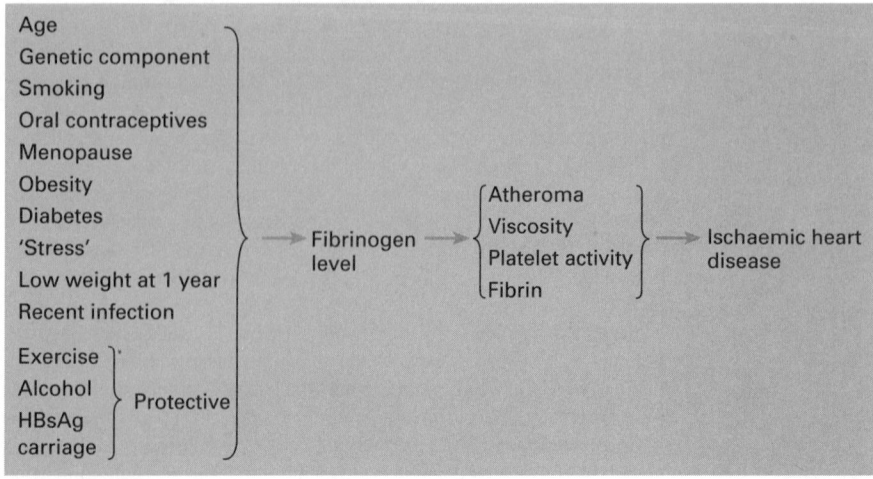

Fig. 3 Determinants and pathogenetic pathways of fibrinogen.

ing; and shear rate is the velocity gradient between adjacent fluid layers. Whole-blood viscosity is determined by plasma viscosity, the haematocrit, and the deformability and aggregation of red blood cells. The influence of different plasma proteins on plasma viscosity depends on their concentration, molecular size, and asymmetry. Thus, fibrinogen has a stronger effect than globulins and albumin, although the plasma hyperviscosity syndrome occurs when plasma viscosity increases as a result of a rise in immunoglobulins. Red cell deformability increases with shear stress, haematocrit, and plasma viscosity and thus partly offsets the increases in blood viscosity arising from haematocrit or plasma viscosity. The focal nature of atheroma may in part be explained by local increases in viscosity, which may also affect platelet behaviour and other prothrombotic influences at the arterial wall. Blood viscosity, mainly the plasma contribution, is associated with hypertension.

Until recently, perhaps the most controversial explanation for a causal role for fibrinogen in ischaemic heart disease was the postulated effects of high levels on fibrin deposition. It was argued that circulating levels of fibrinogen—usually between 2.0 and 3.0 g/l—exceed those required for haemostasis, although this observation does not in itself preclude the possibility that high levels may nevertheless predispose to the somewhat different process of thrombogenesis. However, these theoretical considerations have now been replaced by experimental results in animals and in studies using human plasma, which leave little doubt that when coagulation is initiated, the starting fibrinogen level directly influences the amount of fibrin deposited. There is consistent evidence that fibrinogen levels within the physiological range influence platelet aggregability though (see below) the extent to which tests of platelet function contribute to the prediction of ischaemic heart disease and other arterial events is still uncertain.

Finally, there is growing evidence for the involvement of fibrinogen in the onset and development of the atheromatous lesion itself.

In summary, therefore, there are several pathways through which high fibrinogen levels are likely to increase the risk of thrombosis, whatever their origins. Even if these include an acute or chronic phase contribution, this contribution is likely to be functionally significant. Figure 3 also shows the personal characteristics apparently influencing fibrinogen levels. One of the strongest is smoking, although it is important to recognize that fibrinogen is also strongly associated with ischaemic heart disease in non-smokers. The full return to non-smoking fibrinogen levels in those who discontinue smoking may take several years, paralleling the time course in the decline in the risk of ischaemic heart disease itself in ex-smokers. The extent to which fibrinogen levels are genetically determined, which may be substantial, represents a component of high levels that cannot be explained as a response to atheroma. In fact, fibrinogen levels are probably influenced by nearly all the major ischaemic heart disease risk factors—either adversely as with smoking, obesity, and diabetes or beneficially in the case of moderate alcohol consumption and strenuous physical activity. The one obvious exception is the absence of any apparent influence of diet, particularly dietary fat intake; although it is possible that fish oil lowers fibrinogen, the evidence on this point is equivocal. There is growing evidence that the clear relationship between recent infection and ischaemic heart disease may be partly mediated through increased fibrinogen levels.

High fibrinogen levels therefore appear to be a major channel through which likely determinants of ischaemic heart disease are translated into a number of pathways influencing thrombogenesis and clinically manifest disease. Besides the overall fibrinogen level, there is growing interest in the potential role of abnormal fibrinogens in thrombosis. Fibrinogen Dusart, for example, is a familial dysfibrinogenaemia causing recurrent venous thrombosis, probably through interference with fibrinolytic activity.

Other clotting factors

Evidence from prospective and cross-sectional studies and in haemophiliacs suggests that factor VIII may also be involved in ischaemic heart disease. Potential defence mechanisms against thrombosis include antithrombin-III and the vitamin K dependent anticoagulatory factors, protein C and protein S. Intuitively, it is low levels of the latter that seem likely to be associated with increased risk, and this is certainly true for the inherited thrombophilias leading to venous thrombosis. However, the relationships of antithrombotic factors to the risk of arterial thrombosis and thus of ischaemic heart disease often appear paradoxical. Both low and high antithrombin-III levels, for example, seem to be associated with an increased risk of arterial disease. These apparently contradictory findings could be partly explained by postulating that antithrombin-III levels tend not to be elevated in those at low risk and who do not therefore need to make an antithrombotic response. In those at high risk, on the other hand, levels may behave in one of two ways resulting in either low or high levels but each associated with increased risk:

1. Inability to increase antithrombin-III levels in some may directly contribute to subsequent events in which high procoagulatory clotting factor levels are involved.
2. Antithrombin-III levels in others may rise as a partial compensatory defence mechanism.

Fibrinolytic activity

There is prospective evidence that poor fibrinolytic activity is associated with the incidence of ischaemic heart disease and, in the case of high plasminogen activator inhibitor (PAI), with the recurrence of myocardial infarction. These associations appear particularly strong in younger individuals. The potential importance of fibrinolytic activity in ischaemic heart disease has of course been highlighted by the success of thrombolytic therapy in early myocardial infarction. Sequence homology between lipoprotein (a) and plasminogen has raised the suggestion that high levels of the former may increase the risk of ischaemic heart disease by competing with plasminogen for receptors on endothelium, thereby impeding plasmin generation. However, much of the evidence for this possibility comes from *in vitro* studies. In addition, initial interest in lipoprotein(a) as an independent risk factor for ischaemic heart disease is being tempered by further results that do not altogether support this view.

Platelets

The involvement of platelets in arterial thrombosis is obvious and beyond dispute. Furthermore (see below), there is no doubt about the value of antiplatelet measures in secondary prevention. Establishing any independent influence of platelet 'sensitivity' or 'aggregability' on ischaemic heart disease has so far been largely unproductive, for three main reasons.

1. The very great within-person variation in putative measures of aggregability, this variation being even greater than for clotting factors.
2. The distinct possibility that platelet adhesion and aggregability—though clearly involved in the pathogenesis of thrombosis—are determined at least as much by plasma influences such as fibrinogen and thrombin as by any intrinsic properties of the platelets themselves.
3. These considerations have so far made it difficult to establish clear associations between measures of platelet behaviour and the incidence of ischaemic heart disease.

Spontaneous platelet aggregation and platelet size are predictive of recurrent myocardial infarction although, once again, plasma influences such as fibrinogen may at least partly explain these associations.

In summary, the characterization of individuals at risk of ischaemic heart disease by measure of platelet sensitivity is not realistically possible at present. Attempting to identify those at subsequent risk should be distinguished from the investigation of thrombotic episodes, where the measurement of platelet specific proteins and of other platelet characteristics may be useful.

Practical implications

The practical implications of growing evidence on the role of haemostatic variables in thrombosis and arterial disease can be considered in relation to both investigation and management.

INVESTIGATION

Even with the addition of plasma fibrinogen to other indices, the case for prescriptive whole population screening for ischaemic heart disease (i.e. screening with the intention of intervening in those at high risk) is not strong, because sensitivity and specificity are still not sufficiently high. However, this is a controversial topic and, if prescriptive screening is considered justifiable, it is clearly valuable to include newer measures that make a substantial, independent contribution to predictive ability. Plasma fibrinogen meets these criteria and its measurement is not difficult. Less controversial is opportunistic screening, involving as it does only those who decide to consult their physicians who may then, in turn, select only some for further investigation. Here, whether in general or in hospital practice, there is a growing case for the measurement of fibrinogen as part of the routine investigation of those considered for other reasons to be a risk of thrombotic events, whether these are first events or recurrences. Two practical considerations arise.

1. Within-person variability of plasma concentrations of fibrinogen. This is appreciable, even in the absence of minor (let alone major) intercurrent illnesses that may lead to short term increases in concentration. More than one, and ideally three or four, estimations should be carried out to establish an individual's habitual level (a practice that should always apply to measurement of cholesterol and blood pressure, as well).
2. Differences between laboratories in methods for measuring fibrinogen and in the absolute levels of their reference ranges. In general, different methods for determining fibrinogen (clot weight, clotting time or immunological) give results that are highly correlated. Furthermore, associations with plasma fibrinogen—for example, according to current, previous or never smoking status—are remarkably consistent from one study to another. But absolute values may vary considerably.

To move towards the kind of standardization of cholesterol measurements that is now widely practised, an international standard for fibrinogen has recently been established and is likely to facilitate the comparison of results from different laboratories. For some time to come, however, clinical decisions will in many cases still have to be based on the different values and reference ranges in separate laboratories.

As already indicated, the practical value of factor VII activity measurements is currently limited by the rather different performance of the available assays and the probable need to consider assay systems sensitive to two-chain VII. In the general investigation of 'hypercoagulability' the measurement of activation peptides such as fragment 1.2 (F1.2, the activation peptide from prothrombin) or fibrinopeptide A, indicating the production and the action of thrombin respectively, is likely to be increasingly useful in establishing risk and in deciding about management. Similar considerations apply to the measurement of tissue plasminogen activator and plasminogen activator inhibitor, and of lysis time methods (e.g. euglobulin lysis) in assessing fibrinolytic potential.

MANAGEMENT

In contrast to the difficulty of predicting those at risk of arterial events on account of increased platelet aggregability (see above), the value of platelet-active agents in the secondary prevention of ischaemic heart disease (including unstable angina) and stroke is beyond dispute, the reduction in risk of further major cardiovascular events being about 25 per cent. Progress in demonstrating the value of aspirin after myocardial infarction had already been made before the relevant prostaglandin pathways had been elucidated, although when they were, the likelihood that quite low doses of aspirin might be as effective as conventional doses in reducing thromboxane production, while also sparing prostacyclin, provided a powerful incentive to investigating the preventive value of these lower doses. Currently, aspirin and streptokinase are mandatory (unless contraindicated) in the early stages of suspected myocardial infarction, and in the longer term aspirin is increasingly routine in the secondary prevention of further major episodes in those who have recovered from myocardial infarction or stroke, and in unstable angina. Although not formally tested in all these circumstances, there is increasing reason to believe that a dose of no more than 75 mg aspirin daily is effective, and lower doses are of course accompanied by less bleeding. Nevertheless, until there is further evidence to support low doses, the use of 325 mg daily or on alternate days is appropriate. The value of aspirin in the primary prevention of ischaemic heart disease (i.e. the prevention of a first episode) is, however, much less clear. Furthermore, it is possible, although not certain, that aspirin in this context may somewhat increase the risk of stroke, possibly because of an increase in cerebral haemorrhage. This uncertainty need not preclude the use of aspirin for primary prevention in those at particularly high risk and for whom a careful, considered decision has been reached. But on present evidence, the widespread use of aspirin in primary prevention is not justified.

The demonstration of a habitually raised fibrinogen level can already be acted upon in different ways. Of life-style modifications, much the most important is the avoidance or discontinuation of smoking although, once again, it is important to remember that levels in ex-smokers remain above non-smoking levels for several years, as does the risk of ischaemic heart disease itself, even though both start to fall fairly quickly. The advice to patients to stop is not, of course, dependent on knowledge of the fibrinogen level (and has other objectives besides preventing ischaemic heart disease) but it is probably justifiable to give special attention to those with raised levels, particularly younger subjects. The beneficial effect of strenuous exercise on fibrinogen now provides both doctors and patients with a further incentive towards prevention. Another approach is to use a high fibrinogen level as a marker of risk in helping to decide, for example, whether to prescribe aspirin, even though this has no effect on the fibrinogen level itself. Undoubtedly, definitive randomized controlled trials to establish how far ischaemic heart disease incidence can be reduced by fibrinogen lowering agents are now needed. Among the fibrates, clofibrate and bezafibrate reduce fibrinogen levels appreciably and the clinical benefit against ischaemic heart disease conferred by clofibrate may be due at least as much to this effect as to its effect on lipid levels (although the general use of clofibrate has not been adopted because of the possibility that it may increase mortality from cancer). Because these fibrates lower both fibrinogen and cholesterol levels, it may be difficult if not impossible to ensure how any benefits are actually conferred. Gemfibrozil, also effective in pre-

Fig. 4 Prevention of ischaemic heart disease: epidemiological and pathological implications.

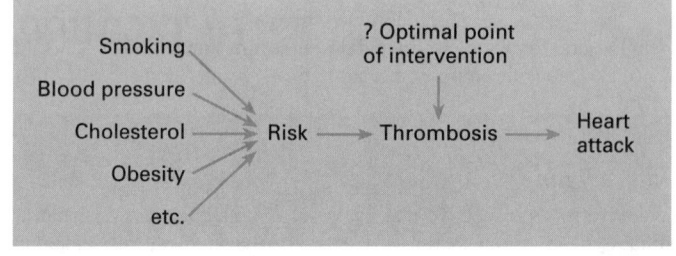

venting ischaemic heart disease, actually raises fibrinogen levels, an effect that is evidently offset by the decrease in thrombin production (resulting in less fibrinogen consumption) that it also leads to, as well as its lipid lowering properties. The defibrinating agent ancrod reduces the risk of thrombogenesis but can only be given by infusion and is therefore unsuitable for general use.

The last decade or so has seen a remarkable resurgence of interest in the potential value of oral anticoagulants in the secondary prevention of ischaemic heart disease. This is mainly due to a second generation of oral anticoagulant trials, from The Netherlands and Norway, that have taken advantage of requirements for satisfactory trials not fully appreciated during the earlier round of anticoagulant trials (although their results, too, left little doubt as to the value of oral anticoagulants in secondary prevention). The implications of the oral anticoagulant trials are by no means academic, even allowing the value and easier administration of aspirin in this context.

1. The indications are that oral anticoagulation may be slightly more effective than aspirin, although the extent to which the two regimens have been directly compared is at present limited. Even a small advantage in a condition as common as ischaemic heart disease may have substantial implications.
2. There is increasing, and so far very consistent, evidence from trials concerned with the management and prevention of venous thrombosis, the prevention of thromboembolism in atrial fibrillation, and in the management of patients undergoing heart valve surgery, that much lower than conventional intensity oral anticoagulation may be equally effective while carrying a lower risk of bleeding and also reducing the requirement for frequent blood testing and dose monitoring.
3. Recent trials also suggest that the simultaneous modification of platelet function and fibrin formation is substantially more effective than modifying either process on its own.

Contrary to general expectation, the concurrent use of aspirin and warfarin, particularly at low International Normalized Ratio (INR) values in carefully selected individuals, does not lead to an unacceptable increase in serious bleeding, although minor episodes (e.g. bruising and nose-bleeds) certainly do increase. At all events, several trials of combined aspirin and low intensity oral anticoagulation with warfarin are now under way and will determine the balance between additional benefits and hazards compared with single regimens. In specialist practice, the demonstration of 'hypercoagulability' as evidenced by persistently raised F1.2 or fibrinopeptide A levels is increasingly regarded as an indication for anticoagulation at an intensity determined by the response of these indices to treatment.

If the onset and progression of significant atheroma could be forestalled, there is no reasonable doubt that epidemic ischaemic heart disease would pass into history. Realistically, however, the extent to which this is likely in today's or tomorrow's affluent communities is debatable, even allowing for the welcome decline in ischaemic heart disease in some—though not all—communities. There will, therefore, be substantial interest in preventing the thrombotic complications of atheroma. If, as seems likely, thrombogenesis is the structural event immediately preceding and leading to major ischaemic heart disease, it may—as Fig. 4 suggests—be the optimal point for intervention, whether by lifestyle or pharmacological methods. This approach is of course entirely compatible with also trying to modify the risk factors and other pathways leading up to thrombosis.

REFERENCES

Antiplatelet Trialists Collaboration. (1994). Collaborative overview of randomised trials of antiplatelet therapy-1. Prevention of death, myocardial infarction and stroke by prolonged antiplatelet therapy in various categories of patients. *British Medical Journal*, **308**, 81–106.

Lowe, G.D.O. (1992). Blood viscosity and cardiovascular disease. *Thrombosis and Haemostasis*, **67**, 494–498.

Meade, T.W. (1993). Low-intensity oral anticoagulation. In *Thrombosis and its management* (eds. L. Poller and J.M. Thomson), Churchill Livingstone, Edinburgh.

Meade, T.W. (1994). The epidemiology of atheroma, thrombosis and ischaemic heart disease. In *Thrombosis and haemostatis* (3rd edn), (eds A.L. Bloom and D.P. Thomas), Churchill Livingstone, Edinburgh.

15.10 Ischaemic heart disease

15.10.1 Epidemiology and prevention

M. G. MARMOT AND J. I. MANN

Of all the chronic diseases, ischaemic heart disease (IHD) has been the object of the most detailed epidemiological study. There is now a substantial amount of information on possible causes of the disease and, with a reasonable degree of precision, it is possible to predict its future occurrence; that is, among an apparently healthy adult population we can distinguish those individuals with a high risk from those with a low risk of subsequently developing ischaemic heart disease. The highest risk group has more than 10 times the risk of the lowest risk group. We can also identify populations at differing risk. This epidemiological knowledge has provided the basis for efforts to prevent ischaemic heart disease. This chapter reviews the epidemiology and approaches to prevention, beginning with a consideration of the impact of the disease on the population. Current knowledge suggests that prevention may be possible both for the individual patient and in the community.

Occurrence of ischaemic heart disease

In most industrialized countries ischaemic heart disease is the most common cause of death. In England and Wales 30 per cent of all deaths among men and 22 per cent of all deaths among women are the result of ischaemic heart disease.

In recent years, in addition to the approximately 156 000 deaths every year in England and Wales, there have been, on average, 115 000 hospital discharges with the diagnosis ischaemic heart disease. It should be stressed that in 60 per cent of all fatal myocardial infarctions, death occurs in the first hour after the attack. Most ischaemic heart disease deaths, therefore, occur too rapidly for treatment to influence prognosis.

International differences

There are marked international differences in the rate of occurrence of ischaemic heart disease. For example, in one study in seven countries, among men aged 40 to 59 years initially free of ischaemic heart disease, the annual incidence rate (occurrence of new cases) varied from 15 per 10 000 in Japan to 198 per 10 000 in Finland. Mortality statistics show a similar picture. Table 1 shows that, even among the industrial-

Table 1 *Mortality from ischaemic heart disease, age standardized death rates, for ages 35 to 74; 1988*

Country	Men	Women
Northern Ireland	658	248
Scotland	625	262
CIS	596	273
Finland	557	172
'Czechoslovakia'	557	204
Hungary	496	191
England and Wales	490	178
Australia	374	143
Bulgaria	356	153
Poland	345	97
United States	339	140
'Yugoslavia'	232	90
Switzerland	225	62
Italy	201	61
France	137	37
Japan	62	26

ized countries, mortality rates vary considerably. Some of the variation between countries is undoubtedly due to differences in diagnostic practice and in coding of death certificates, but numerous studies using comparable methods have confirmed that real differences exist in the frequency of disease. In Europe there is almost a threefold difference between France, Italy, and Spain, on the one hand, and such countries as Finland and the United Kingdom on the other.

As shown below, these international comparisons have played an important part in the search for causes. The experience of migrants suggests that variations between countries are likely to be the result chiefly of environmental or behavioural differences. People who have migrated from a low-risk country (e.g. Japan) to a high-risk country (e.g. the United States) tend to have rates of ischaemic heart disease approaching that of the host country.

Time trends

In industrialized countries, ischaemic heart disease has emerged as the major cause of death in the twentieth century. This resulted both from a decrease in infectious disease mortality and an increase in the age-specific risk of ischaemic heart disease. The same process is now starting in many developing countries. The heart disease epidemic appears to have reached its peak, and is even declining in some countries. The current international picture is one of marked contrasts (Fig. 1). Many countries with traditionally high rates of ischaemic heart disease have now experienced declines: among these are the United States, Finland, and other countries of Western and Northern Europe. By contrast, countries of Central and Eastern Europe have shown marked increases in ischaemic heart disease rates over the last two decades. Singapore, which rapidly made the transition from a developing to a wealthy country, has experienced a dramatic increase in ischaemic heart disease rates. That an epidemic of ischaemic heart disease is not the inevitable consequence of a country growing wealthy is shown by Japan, which has experienced a 40 per cent decline in ischaemic heart disease over a 20-year period, starting from a low level.

Ischaemic heart disease is preventible

Three types of evidence suggest that ischaemic heart disease is, in principle, preventible. First, the time trends: the rapid change in ischaemic heart disease mortality is, in large part, likely to result from change in incidence rates. Therefore, factors determining the onset of disease must be able to change.

Second, the large international differences in ischaemic heart disease mortality, which are not fixed, as is shown by the experience of migrants. For example, Japan has high rates of stroke and low rates of ischaemic heart disease. Men of Japanese ancestry living in the United States have lower rates of stroke and higher rates of ischaemic heart disease.

Third, a great deal of knowledge has accumulated on causes of ischaemic heart disease with impressive evidence that: (1) some of these causes can be avoided; and (2) even though these causes exert their effect over decades, this effect is at least partially reversible in a few years.

It is often stated that the most important predictor of who gets ischaemic heart disease is who the individual's parents were. Family history of ischaemic heart disease is certainly a potent predictor of risk, but it is wrong to conclude that ischaemic heart disease rates are mainly determined by genetic endowment. The dramatic changes over time, and consequent on migration, suggest that there is an important environmental component, that interacts with genetic predisposition.

Risk factors for ischaemic heart disease

Causes, risk factors, and variations in occurrence

The term 'risk factor' is used in a variety of ways. It is worth making the following distinctions among risk factors for ischaemic heart disease: *inherent biological traits,* such as age, sex, and genetic endowment, which can not themselves be altered; *physiological characteristics* that predict future occurrence of ischaemic heart disease, e.g. blood pressure, serum cholesterol level, fibrinogen, weight/height^2, blood sugar; *behaviours,* e.g. diet, smoking, alcohol consumption, oral contraceptive use, that may be associated with ischaemic heart disease occurrence

Fig. 1(a) Change in age standardized mortality from IHD 1970–85; men and women aged 30 to 69. (b) Changes in coronary heart disease mortality (per cent) in Eastern Europe: 1970–85 age-standardized figures, men and women aged 30 to 69.

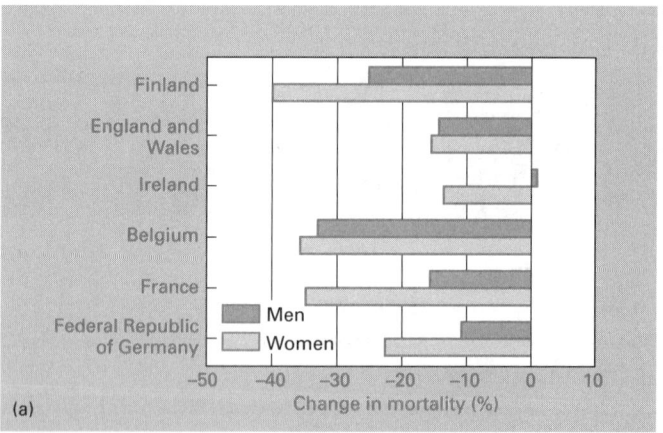

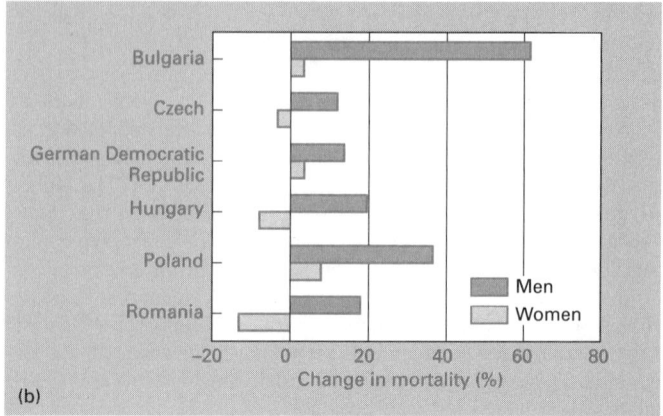

because of their links to characteristics such as blood pressure, or serum cholesterol, or may have other mechanisms by which they influence the risk of ischaemic heart disease; *social characteristics* such as social class or ethnic group, which mark out differences in rate of occurrence of the disease without telling us the reason, whether due to differences in behaviour, to other social and cultural factors or to genes; *environmental features* which may be physical (e.g. temperature), psychosocial, or biological.

The implications of these risk factors for prevention are different. A physiological characteristic such as blood pressure may be lowered by drugs regardless of the determinants of high blood pressure: or the intervention point could be in behaviour, as with diet affecting blood pressure, or smoking. If risk factors differ by social characteristic, then prevention should deal with the social distribution of risk factors. An appropriate response to an environmental cause, such as cold, will be to protect against it; the response to the psychosocial environment might be to change the environment.

AGE AND GENDER

The incidence of ischaemic heart disease increases exponentially with age. On a log scale, the increase is linear. This phenomenon is seen in all countries where figures are available. This has led to a point of view that atherosclerosis and consequent coronary heart disease are a normal part of ageing. This inference does not accord with the facts. Although the rise with age appears to be universal, the frequency with which ischaemic heart disease occurs varies widely among cultures. Therefore, a rise with age in a population where the age-specific rates are low, will have much less significance than where the rates are high.

Men have higher rates of ischaemic heart disease than women. The magnitude of the excess varies less among countries than do the absolute ischaemic heart disease rates. In middle age, the rate of ischaemic heart disease in men is 3 to 4 times that in women. The magnitude of the male excess varies with age. After the menopause, the male : female ratio narrows. This could either be due to loss of a protective effect in women, loss of a harmful effect in men, or even killing off of male susceptibles. The rise with age also differs between the sexes.

Risk factors at different ages

Most of the studies on the ability of risk factors to predict occurrence of ischaemic heart disease, have been in middle aged men. Because of the paucity of data, there had been doubts as to whether the same set of risk factors discussed below predicted in women and at different ages. It is now clear that they do. The magnitude of the association may vary. It is important to distinguish between relative and absolute risk. The relative difference in disease incidence between those exposed and those unexposed to a risk factor gives a measure of the aetiological force of that risk factor. The absolute difference in risk gives a measure of practical importance of the association: how much extra disease, in absolute amounts, can be attributed to the presence of the risk factor. For a number of risk factors the relative risk of ischaemic heart disease declines with age. Because the absolute risk of disease increases exponentially with age, the absolute risk attributed to a risk factor may increase with age. This suggests that using risk factors to identify people at subsequent risk of disease may continue to be useful at older ages.

Risk factors have also been assessed in children, among whom there is evidence of 'tracking.' If children are ranked according to their position on the distribution of, say, blood pressure, they tend to retain their position in the distribution upon remeasurement at a later age. Long term studies have not been done to show that this tracking continues from childhood to middle age. The importance of this is more for understanding aetiology and prevention than it is for treatment. There is, at the present, little justification for screening to detect 'abnormal' risk factors in children, except for the rare instances of a severe hereditary lipid abnormality in a family member. There are intriguing studies that suggest that some important influences on adult risks of ischaemic heart

disease may have their effect very early in life, raising the possibility of introducing further preventive measures at that early stage.

Physiological risk factors

LIPIDS AND LIPOPROTEINS

Total cholesterol and low density lipoprotein

No other blood constituent varies so much between different people as serum cholesterol. From New Guinea to east Finland the mean serum cholesterol ranges from 2.6 to 7.02 mmol/1 (100 to 270 mg/100 ml) when estimated by the same method in the same age and sex group. Mean levels tend to be similar in adult men and women, but this similarity hides the strikingly different age trends observed in cross-sectional studies. The extent to which total cholesterol explains the geographic variation of coronary heart disease varies in different studies. In the Seven Countries Study, mean cholesterol values were highly correlated with coronary heart disease death rates ($r = 0.8$), accounting for 64 per cent of the variance in coronary heart disease death rates amongst the cohorts. In the World Health Organization MONICA Study the classic risk factors (cholesterol, blood pressure, and smoking) accounted for a much smaller proportion of the variation in rates. However, more important is the fact that amongst individuals within populations the association is exceptionally strong. In over 20 prospective studies in different countries, total serum cholesterol has been shown to be related to the rate of development of coronary heart disease, the association being "dose" related, occurring in both sexes and being independent of all other measured risk factors. The association in the MRFIT (Multiple Risk Factor Intervention Trial) study is shown in Fig. 2. Risk of coronary heart disease varies over a fivefold range in relation to serum cholesterol levels found in an average American population. There is no discernible critical value, the risk tending to increase throughout the range. Whilst the absolute risk associated with any given cholesterol value varies in different parts of the world, within almost every population sampled, be it in the United States with high levels and high coronary heart disease rates or in China with low levels and low rates, the risk is greater in people with higher than lower levels. Multiple measurements of serum cholesterol in an individual improve the accuracy of appraisal of cholesterol mediated risk and predict an appreciably greater degree of risk

Fig. 2 Within-population relationship between plasma cholesterol and ischaemic heart disease and total mortality. From the study of > 360 000 men screened at entry to the MRFIT study.

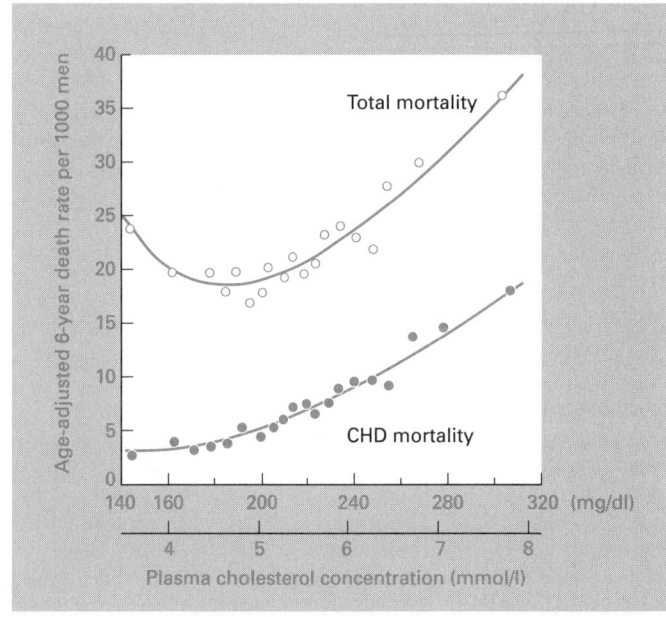

than single measurements. The association is apparent in older as well as younger people and although the relative risk associated with a particular cholesterol level may decrease with increasing age, the absolute risk may be greater because of the larger number of total events in older people. While cholesterol is an independent risk factor for coronary heart disease, the extent of the risk is magnified by the presence of other risk factors (see below and Fig. 7).

The association of total cholesterol with coronary heart disease morbidity and mortality appears to derive chiefly from the low density lipoprotein (LDL) fraction, with which it is highly correlated, and to some extent also intermediate density lipoprotein (IDL). Recent case control studies have suggested low density lipoprotein particle size may be a particularly important determinant of premature coronary heart disease risk. Small, dense, low molecular weight low density lipoprotein particles were more prevalent in men with premature coronary heart disease than controls, to the extent that these small particles (less than 225 Å) were associated with a threefold increase in risk of myocardial infarction.

Triglycerides and very low density lipoprotein

Increases in total triglycerides and levels of very low density lipoprotein (VLDL) are usually associated with increased coronary heart disease rates in prospective studies, though without the clear graded increase in risk seen for cholesterol. The extent to which the increased risk is independent of other measures of lipid metabolism has not been clearly established. A relatively recent analysis of the Framingham data suggests that raised levels of triglycerides are associated with coronary heart disease risk only in the presence of reduced levels of (HDL). Other studies support this, showing that raised triglycerides predict coronary heart disease in the presence of high low density lipoprotein:high density lipoprotein ratio. Case control studies suggest that 'abnormal' very low density lipoproteins (i.e. relative cholesterol-enriched very low density lipoproteins) may be important predictors of premature coronary heart disease. Thus measurement of total triglyceride and very low density lipoprotein undertaken in most of the prospective studies, may be insufficiently sensitive to determine the extent to which this component of the lipoprotein mediated risk predicts coronary heart disease. Further studies which include measurement of very low density lipoprotein composition may be required.

High density lipoprotein

High density lipoprotein has repeatedly been shown to be a protective factor against coronary heart disease in both case control and cohort studies. Women have higher levels of high density lipoprotein than men and there is little change with age. The protective effect seems more marked in women than men and some studies have shown the predictive value of low high density lipoprotein to be stronger than that associated with high low density lipoprotein in people over 50 years. Low high density lipoprotein may be associated with obesity, cigarette smoking, lack of physical activity, impaired glucose tolerance, or non-insulin dependent diabetes, as well as a genetic predisposition, and some prospective studies have found that the protective effect is not sustained when controlling for the effects of other risk factors. However, a recent analysis of four large American prospective studies suggests than an increment of 1 mg/100 ml (0.026 mmol/1) is associated with a 2 to 3 per cent reduction in coronary heart disease. The protective effect of high density lipoprotein appears to be mediated via the high density lipoprotein 2 subfraction.

Plasma apolipoproteins

Some patients with various clinical manifestations of atherosclerotic disease have reduced levels of apolipoprotein A_1, and high levels of apolipoprotein B. These two apolipoproteins form the major protein components of high density lipoprotein and low density lipoprotein, respectively, so that these observations are hardly surprising. However, because the association appears to be independent of plasma lipid levels, and has sometimes been noted in the absence of any elevation of them, it may be that such measurements, as well as those of apolipoprotein A_2 and apolipoprotein E, may be better predictors of the risk of coronary heart disease than measurements of total lipids. At present these observations have been based mainly on case controlled studies, and more information is required from large prospective trials before the true value of such measurements can be assessed.

Lipoprotein (a)

The protein and lipid composition of lipoprotein (a) is similar to that of low density lipoprotein, but the protein moiety consists of apolipoprotein A_1 linked to apolipoprotein B by disulphide bridges. Concentrations are not normally distributed and vary from near zero to more than 100 mg/100 ml. Case control studies suggest appreciably higher levels in those with various manifestations of atherosclerosis, and that high levels may help to differentiate those subjects with familial hypercholesterolaemia who develop coronary heart disease, from those who remain relatively free of this complication (Fig. 3). Lipoprotein (a) appears to retain its status as an independent risk factor after adjusting for the effects of low density lipoprotein-C on risk, but once again data from prospective studies are not available. Lipoprotein (a) may have thrombogenic as well as atherogenic effects. It is structurally similar to plasminogen and may compete with plasminogen for binding sites on endothelial cells and monocytes thus inhibiting fibrinolysis and promoting thrombus formation. There is also a strong correlation between concentrations of lipoprotein (a) in the serum and in arterial walls. No such correlation is apparent in the case of low density lipoprotein. This may be a reflection of the fact that lipoprotein (a) binds to glycosaminoglycans with an affinity which is several fold greater than that of low density lipoprotein.

ARTERIAL PRESSURE

Apart from intake of saturated fat and cholesterol levels, raised arterial pressure (both systolic and diastolic) was the only factor measured in the Seven Country Study which correlated in part with the geographic variation in ischaemic heart disease; it appeared to be responsible for about 40 per cent of the variance in the 10-year follow-up of ischaemic heart disease mortality.

Within populations, following defined cohorts, increased blood pressure has been shown consistently to be associated with a subsequent increase in ischaemic heart disease risk (Fig. 4). The relationship is linear and graded: the lower the pressure, the lower the risk. There is, therefore, no clear cut-off dividing 'hypertension' from normal pressure. The epidemiological data generally indicate that systolic blood pressure is as good a predictor of subsequent ischaemic heart disease as is diastolic. In middle aged men, it is estimated that 20 mmHg higher systolic blood pressure is associated with 60 per cent higher cardiovascular mortality and 40 per cent higher mortality from all causes combined.

Fig. 3 Frequency distribution of serum lipoprotein(a) concentrations among patients with familial hypercholesterolemia, who did and did not have coronary heart disease (reproduced from Seed *et al.* (1990) *New England Journal of Medicine*, **322**, 1494–9, with permission).

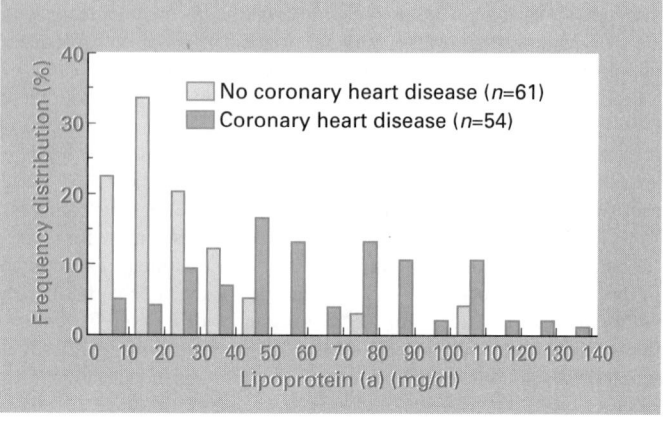

OVERWEIGHT

Long-term follow-up data of insured individuals have shown that obese men and women develop cardiovascular disease more frequently than the non-obese. Data from other prospective studies have continued this observation, the lowest risk occuring at a body mass index (BMI) (weight/height^2 in kg/m^2) of 23. However, there is no indication that obesity explains any of the geographic variations in ischaemic heart disease. Not all prospective studies support the finding of an association between overweight and ischaemic heart disease. This in part may be because they have 'adjusted' for the effects of other factors with which obesity is associated, such as hypertension and elevations of serum lipids.

More recent evidence has suggested a particular risk of ischaemic heart disease in those with a central distribution of obesity, best assessed by measuring the waist : hip ratio and associated with a characteristic pattern of metabolic disturbance. It has been shown that central adiposity, measured by increased waist : hip ratio, is related to ischaemic heart disease risk. The mechanism may be via a pattern of metabolic disturbance described by Reaven (see below).

GLUCOSE INTOLERANCE AND INSULIN RESISTANCE

Cohort studies provide strong evidence that people with both non-insulin dependent (NIDDM) and insulin dependent (IDDM) diabetes, or with impaired glucose tolerance (IGT), are at greater risk of coronary heart disease than those with normal glucose tolerance. There is no evidence for a linear association between plasma glucose and coronary heart disease, but fasting insulin and levels 2h after a glucose load do correlate with coronary heart disease risk, most strikingly in those with 2-h insulin levels in the top quintile of the distribution. It is difficult to disentangle whether increased concentrations of insulin contribute to risk of coronary heart disease directly, or by way of the association of hyperinsulinaemia with hypertension, hypertriglyceridaemia, low levels of high density lipoprotein cholesterol, glucose intolerance, and central obesity (the insulin resistance syndrome; IRS). High insulin levels appear to predict subsequent development of abnormalities of lipid and glucose metabolism as well as hypertension (in lean individuals). Reaven describes this cluster of metabolic derangements as 'syndrome X' and suggests the cause to be a defect in insulin mediated glucose uptake and compensating hyperinsulinaemia. It is difficult to define the prevalence of the condition because all of its clinical and metabolic characteristics are continuous variables. However, a Finnish study, using standard cut points, found that the full syndrome occurred more often in the elderly, reaching an overall prevalence of 5 per cent in men and 8 per cent in women by 65 to 74 years. A strong association has also been shown between plasma insulin levels and concentrations of plasminogen activator inhibitor 1 (PAI-1) in the 'normal' population, in obese subjects and in non-insulin dependent diabetes mellitus patients. PAI-1 appears to be an independent risk factor for myocardial infarction and it too may contribute to the association between insulin resistance and coronary disease.

Formal intervention studies have not yet tested the potential benefit of attempting to reverse the syndrome, but weight reduction and increased physical activity can usually improve most of its manifestation.

HAEMOSTATIC FACTORS

Most epidemiological research into the aetiology of ischaemic heart disease has concentrated on factors associated with atherogenesis and far less on those that might primarily increase the risk of thrombosis. It is now clear that most fatal and non-fatal myocardial infarcts are caused by coronary thrombosis and there is evidence of association between the long-term risk of ischaemic heart disease and measures of haemostatic function.

In the Northwick Park Prospective Heart Study, men who died of cardiovascular disease showed, at recruitment, significantly higher plasma levels of Factor VII, fibrinogen, and Factor VIII, than survivors. Associations with Factor VII and fibrinogen were at least as strong as that with cholesterol. Fibrinolytic activity was higher in survivors, but the difference was not statistically significant. Measures of platelet function were not suitable to show relationships in epidemiological studies. Other prospective studies have confirmed the link between fibrinogen level and risk of ischaemic heart disease.

Among the external factors related to haemostasis, smoking and diet stand out. Fibrinogen concentrations are strongly related to smoking and inversely to alcohol consumption. Dietary fat is related to Factor VII levels whilst n-3 polyunsaturated fatty acids from fish may be protective because they inhibit platelet aggregation.

Behavioural risk factors

Nutrition

The link between nutritional factors and coronary heart disease (CHD) has been investigated using a number of different epidemiological approaches (Table 2). The succeeding paragraphs describe the effects of individual nutrients but it is important to bear in mind that nutritional factors are closely inter-related and it may be difficult to disentangle separate effects.

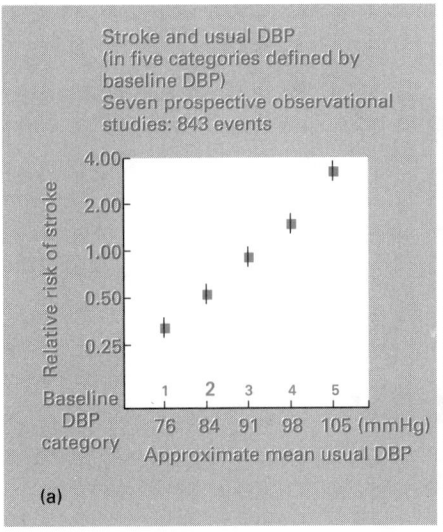

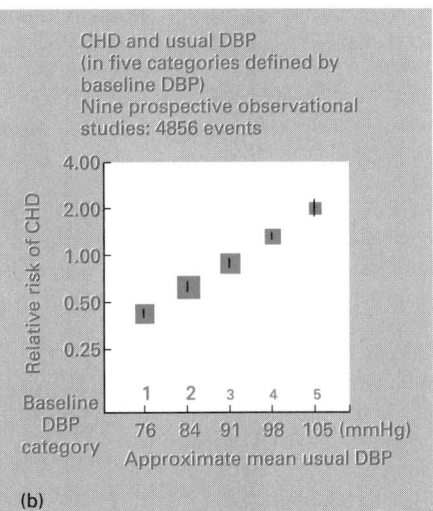

Fig. 4 Relative risks of stroke and ischaemic heart disease (CHD) estimated from combining the results of several studies. The solid squares represent disease risks in each category relative to risk in the whole study population. The sizes of the squares are proportional to the number of events in each diastolic blood pressure (DBP) category. The vertical lines represent 95 per cent confidence intervals.

Table 2 *The major dietary fatty acids and food sources from which they are derived*

		Common name	Food source(s)
Saturated fatty acids			
	C12 : 0	Lauric	Coconut oil
	C14 : 0	Myristic	Butter, high fat dairy products, coconut oil
	C16 : 0	Palmitic	Palm oil, lard, beef dripping, suet, butter
	C18 : 0	Stearic	Occurs in meat and many other foods
Monounsaturated fatty acids			
	C16 : 1	Palmitoleic	Present in small amounts in a wide variety of foods
	C18 : 1	Oleic	Olive oil, avocado, peanut oil, cashew nuts, almonds, hazelnuts, rapeseed oil (with low erucic acid content), sardines, tuna
	C22 : 1	Erucic	Rapeseed
Polyunsaturated fatty acids			
n-6	C18 : 2	Linoleic	Safflower oil, corn oil, wheatgerm oil, cottonseed oil, sunflower oils and seeds
n-3	C18 : 3	Linolenic	Widely distributed in foods but usually associated with C18 : 2
n-6 and n3	C18 : 2 and C18 : 3		Walnuts and walnut oil, soybean oil, wheatgerm oil, rapeseed oil (with low erucic acid)
n-3	C20 : 5	Eicosapentaenoic acid	Salmon oil, cod liver oil
	C22 : 6	Docosahexaenoic acid	Mackerel oil
Chemical notation:	C12 : 0	= 12 carbon atoms, no double bonds	
	C22 : 1	= 22 carbon atoms, one double bond	
	C18 : 2 (ω6)	= 18 carbon atoms, two double bonds; first double bond occurs at C6–C7.	

QUANTITY AND NATURE OF DIETARY FAT

The major dietary fatty acids and food sources from which they are derived are shown in Table 2. Intake of saturated fatty acids (SFA) has been shown to correlate with coronary heart disease rates in cross cultural comparisons and in studies which have examined changing coronary heart disease rates within countries. In the Seven Countries Study (in which food consumption was measured in 16 defined cohorts from countries with widely varying coronary heart disease rates) saturated fatty acid was the most important factor explaining the geographic variation in coronary heart disease. This study also demonstrated a more powerful relationship between cigarette smoking and coronary heart disease in the United States of America and Northern Europe (where intake of saturated fatty acid is high) than in Southern Europe where saturated fatty acid intake is relatively low (Fig. 5). Prospective studies of individuals within a single population have not shown an association between intake and coronary heart disease, but were based on a single point estimate of dietary intake, related to occurrence of coronary heart disease many years later. Several intervention studies have shown that reduction of dietary saturated fatty acid can reduce incidence of coronary heart disease events to an extent correlating to the fall in plasma cholesterol, but even these findings do not provide conclusive evidence for a causal role, as dietary intervention aimed principally at reducing saturated fatty acid, inevitably results in other potentially contributory dietary changes. Nevertheless, the effect of saturated fatty acid on atherogenic lipoproteins provides strong corroborative evidence. Low density lipoprotein (LDL) levels in the blood may be appreciably increased or decreased by raising or reducing dietary intake of myristic acid (C14 : 0). Palmitic (C16 : 0) and stearic (C18 : 0) acids do not appear to have an important effect on lipoprotein levels but animal studies suggest that high intakes may increase the risk of thrombosis.

Monounsaturated fatty acids (MUFA) found naturally in meats, olive

Fig. 5 The different risk of smoking for ischaemic heart disease in countries with different diets. The width of the bars is proportional to the number of men in each smoking class. Scales are the same for all three populations. The numbers above each bar indicate the number of IHD deaths per 10 000. The regression lines of death rate, Y, on smoking, are shown: 0, never smokes; 1, ex-smoker; 2, 2 to 10 cigarettes per day; 3, 10 to 19 cigarettes per day; 4, >20 cigarettes per day.

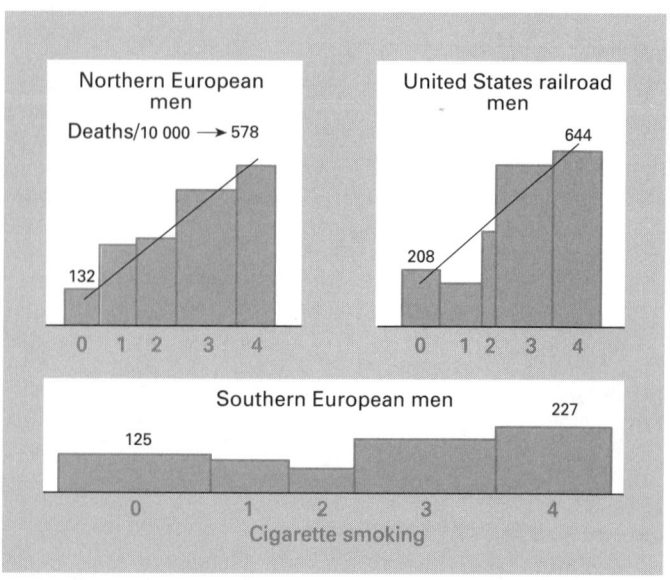

oil, low erucic acid rapeseed oil, avocados, and various nuts were previously believed not to affect the risk of coronary heart disease. However the low rates in Mediterranean countries suggest that some aspect of the Mediterranean diet might be protective. Olive oil, consisting largely of oleic acid (C18 : 1), has been a prime candidate. In the Seven Countries Study, intake of monounsaturated fatty acid was found to be negatively correlated with coronary heart disease rates. When olive oil replaces a proportion of dietary saturated fatty acid, low density lipoprotein levels fall without a concomitant decrease in high density lipoprotein (HDL). This is a potentially important attribute of monounsaturated fatty acid, since when saturated fatty acid are replaced by large quantities of other nutrients (e.g. carbohydrate or polyunsaturated fatty acids) the reduction of low density lipoprotein is accompanied by an unfavourable reduction in high density lipoprotein. There is also evidence that naturally occurring monounsaturated fatty acid can increase the resistance of low density lipoprotein to oxidative modification, thus reducing the atherogenicity of these lipoproteins. These beneficial attributes are seen only with naturally occurring monounsaturated fatty acid with a *cis* configuration. This may be modified in some manufacturing processes (e.g. in certain margarines) to a *trans* configuration, which also occur naturally in small quantities. *Trans* monounsaturated fatty acid increase low density lipoprotein and lower high density lipoprotein. And so at least in large quantities, is an unsuitable type of fatty acid.

Polyunsaturated fatty acids (PUFA) may have an *n*-6 or an *n*-3 configuration. The former are derived chiefly from plant and seed oils, the latter from fish oils and various nuts. Several prospective studies have linked low intakes of dietary *n*-6 polyunsaturated fatty acid with increased risk of subsequent coronary heart disease, confirming data from the Seven Countries Study suggesting that *n*-6 polyunsaturated fatty acid might protect against coronary heart disease.

Further supportive evidence comes from data relating fatty acid composition of plasma lipids, red cell membrane, and adipose tissue to coronary heart disease. Intervention studies have shown a reduced risk of coronary heart disease coincident with advice to increase these fatty acids, but it is not possible to determine the extent to which this was due to increased polyunsaturated fatty acid or decreased saturated fatty acid. A beneficial effect of *n*-6 polyunsaturated fatty acid could be mediated by lowered low density lipoprotein or by reduced platelet aggregation. In contrast to these, high levels of intake of *n*-6 polyunsaturated fatty acid have been associated with an increased risk of gallstones, reduced levels of high density lipoprotein-C, a possible increase in oxidation of low density lipoprotein and, in experimental animals, an increased risk of neoplasms.

The possibility that *n*-3 polyunsaturated fatty acid might reduce the risk of coronary heart disease started with the realisation that Greenland Eskimos have low rates of coronary disease despite consuming a diet high in cholesterol and total fat. This fat is derived almost exclusively from marine foods rich in *n*-3 fatty acids (eicosapentaenoate, C20 : 5 and decosahexaenoate, C22 : 6). In a large cross-sectional study in which levels of adipose tissue fatty acid were related to undiagnosed coronary heart disease, higher levels of C20 : 5 were associated with a reduced level of coronary heart disease risk. Regular fish intake has also been shown to be associated with reduced risk of subsequent coronary heart disease, perhaps in part due to the high *n*-3 polyunsaturated fatty acid content of certain fish. In one study in which men who had suffered a myocardial infarction were randomized to receive various dietary treatments, those advised to increase their intake of fish had a reduction in total mortality compared with the various other dietary treatment groups. A substantial body of evidence suggests that any protective effect of *n*-3 polyunsaturated fatty acid might be attributable to their anti-thrombogenic effects in inhibiting conversion of arachidonic acid to thromboxane A_2 and by facilitating the production of prostacycline PGI_3. The *n*-3 fatty acids also lower plasma triglycerides, but may on occasion increase low density lipoprotein. The optimal level of intake and the precise balance between *n*-3 and *n*-6 polyunsaturated fatty acid remains to be determined.

High intakes of dietary cholesterol are associated with elevations in low density lipoprotein, but there is controversy regarding the extent to which the relationship is a continuous one, or whether appreciable increases of low density lipoprotein are seen only with very high intakes. There is also a suggestion that some individuals may be hyper-responders to dietary cholesterol, whereas other show little change in total low density lipoprotein cholesterol in response to variations in intake. The extent to which dietary cholesterol influences low density lipoprotein cholesterol, and possibly also coronary heart disease, is influenced by the amount of saturated fatty acids in the diet; a low intake much reducing any adverse effect.

CARBOHYDRATE AND DIETARY FIBRE (NON-STARCH POLYSACCHARIDES)

Diets high in complex carbohydrate and dietary fibre (non-starch polysaccharide, NSP) have been shown to be associated with reduced risk of coronary heart disease in cross-sectional and prospective epidemiological studies. Such diets, which are also associated with low levels of low density lipoprotein are invariably low in saturated fatty acids and it is impossible to disentangle separate effects. Soluble forms of non-starch polysaccharide, found in barley, oat and rye products, lentils, chick peas, fruits high in pectin, and cooked dried beans, have a small effect on low density lipoprotein which is independent of the associated reduction in saturated fatty acid. Insoluble forms of non-starch polysaccharide do not influence lipid metabolism to any appreciable extent. There is no convincing evidence that sucrose or other simple sugars are associated with an increased cardiovascular risk.

PROTEINS

Vegetarians and vegans have been shown in prospective studies to have a decreased risk of coronary heart disease when compared with meat eaters. Early observations in Seventh Day Adventists in the United States have now been confirmed by British findings in more representative groups of vegetarians and controls. Vegetarians have lower levels of low density lipoprotein and factor VII suggesting that atherogenic as well as thrombogenic risk might be decreased. Despite the ability of soybean protein to reduce total and low density lipoprotein cholesterol when fed as a replacement for mixed animal protein, it has not been clearly established whether it is vegetable protein or some other attribute of the vegetarian diet which confers the protection against coronary heart disease. Indeed a recent analysis of Seventh Day Adventist data suggests that regular consumption of nuts was responsible for much of the protective effect of the diet consumed by this group.

DIET ANTIOXIDANTS

It is clear that the nature of dietary fat and other major recognised risk factors, do not alone account for the geographic variation in coronary heart disease seen in the WHO MONICA study. The French, for example, have much lower rates of coronary heart disease than would be expected from their intake of fat. The antioxidant hypothesis which suggests that antioxidants protect *in vivo* LDL lipids and apolipoprotein B against peroxidation, may account for some of the discrepancies, particularly when it is applied in conjunction with the lipid hypothesis. Fruit and vegetables are rich sources of antioxidant vitamins C, E, and beta-carotene. Differing intakes of these could explain the relatively low coronary heart disease rates in France, and partially account for the low rates in Mediterranean countries, the greater risk of coronary heart disease in men than women, the high coronary heart disease rates amongst Asians living in Britain, the predominance of coronary heart disease amongst the British working classes and some of the recently reported secular trends in coronary heart disease mortality. Such anecdotal observations are supported by at least two sets of epidemiological data. The

WHO MONICA project has involved the measurement of plasma concentrations of several vitamins and correlated them with incidence of coronary heart disease in 16 participating countries (Fig. 6). A strong inverse correlation was observed between plasma levels of vitamin E and coronary heart disease mortality. High calculated levels of vitamin E and betacarotene intake in the Nurses Health Survey, in the United States, were associated with a 30 to 40 per cent reduction in coronary heart disease risk. Animal experiments provide strong support for this hypothesis (chronic marginal dietary deficiency of these vitamins causes atherosclerosis-like lesions in rodents, pigs, and primates) but their value in the prevention or progression of atherosclerosis has yet to be firmly established. Trials involving clinical end points have been started. Amongst other antioxidant substances, attention has been given to selenium, an essential component of glutathione peroxidase, which has a protective effect against the damage caused by free radicals and hydroperoxides and could influence the metabolism of arachidonic acid and thrombogenesis. A single study from New Zealand, where selenium intakes are low, suggests that low levels of selenium and glutathione peroxidase activity may be important risk indicators for coronary heart disease in those who smoke. This is likely to be a major area of research in future years.

SODIUM INTAKE

Dietary sodium is likely to influence coronary heart disease risk via an effect on blood pressure. Two recent epidemiological contributions are particularly relevant. Twenty-four hour urinary sodium excretion provides the best available method of assessing sodium intake, and this method together with standardized blood pressures measurements were used in the 'INTERSALT' Study which collected data on over 10 000 people aged 20 to 59 from 52 centres and 32 countries. Populations with very low sodium excretion (less than 50 mmol/24 h) had low median rise of blood pressure with age but the overall association between sodium and median blood pressure or prevalence of hypertension were less striking. A recent series of meta-analyses of observational data, as well as intervention trials, suggested INTERSALT and many other studies might have appreciably underestimated the association between blood pressure and sodium intake. For example a 100 mmol/24 h reduction in sodium intake might be expected to reduce systolic blood pressure by about 10 mmHg. Were half such a reduction to be achieved, the calculated (but unproven) reduction in stroke incidence in a Western population might be 26 per cent and in coronary disease 15 per cent.

Reduction also in the amount of salt added to processed foods might also lower blood pressure by nearly twice as much, and might prevent as many as 70 000 deaths per year in Britain. Most antihypertensive drugs appear to be more effective when sodium intake is reduced. Views about the value of dietary sodium restriction are not unanimous.

OTHER NUTRITIONAL ISSUES RELEVANT TO DIET AND CORONARY HEART DISEASE

The importance of coronary heart disease as a major cause of premature morbidity and mortality has led to the subject becoming an emotive issue. The public has been bombarded with nutritional advice, some of which is valid, some without any justification, and some is based confusingly on half truths. A particular example is the recommendation to increase oatbran and niacin. Oatbran may reduce low density lipoprotein and nicotinic acid can certainly lower low density lipoprotein and very low density lipoprotein, but only in pharmacological doses. This diet, unless attention is paid to other more important determinants of cardiovascular risk, is likely to have a rather small overall beneficial effect. Similarly *n*-3 polyunsaturated fatty acid usually sold as concentrates in capsules are sometimes advertised as a useful means of lowering cholesterol as well as reducing coronary heart disease risk. While these preparations do have an effect on thrombogenesis and on very low density lipoprotein and may thereby reduce the risk of coronary heart disease, they do not have consistent effects on low density lipoprotein and total cholesterol except in pharmacological quantities. The safety of such preparations taken in large amounts has not been established and while it seems reasonable to recommend an increased intake of fish, it is inappropriate to be advising large amounts of these fatty acids in concentrated form until such safety has been established. On the other hand garlic has been used for medicinal purposes since at least 1550 BC. It now seems that garlic can favourably influence a whole range of cardiovascular risk factors. Popular interest appears to be greatest in Germany where garlic preparations have become the largest selling over-the-counter drugs.

From time to time there is a resurgence of interest in the association between coffee drinking, cholesterol levels and coronary heart disease. Data are not consistent but there is evidence suggesting that any hypercholesterolaemic effect of coffee may be related to method of preparation. Boiled coffee, which is most frequently drunk in the Nordic countries may be more hypercholesterolaemic than coffee prepared in other ways. This effect has not been sufficiently studied to justify the inclusion of advice concerning coffee drinking in relation to any risk of coronary disease.

Environmental influences in early life

The research of Barker and colleagues suggests that environmental influences in early life might influence later risk of coronary heart disease. Weights at birth and 1 year of males born during the period 1911 to 1930 were related to subsequent mortality. Men with the lowest weights at birth and 1 year had the highest death rates from coronary heart disease; the standardized mortality ratio (SMR) fell from 111 in men who weighed 8.2 kg or less at 1 year to 42 in those who weighed 12.3 kg or more. Subsequent levels of blood cholesterol and risk of developing diabetes have also been related to impaired growth and development in early life. It is possible therefore that measures which promote prenatal and post-natal growth may reduce the later risk of developing coronary disease in middle life; this is likely to be a fruitful area of future research.

Smoking

Several longitudinal studies in many countries have shown that people who smoke have a higher incidence of, and risk of dying from,

Fig. 6 Relationship between actual ischaemic heart disease mortality and that predicted for measurements of vitamins A and E, cholesterol, and diastolic blood pressure. Data from optimal interim study, the WHO MONICA project.

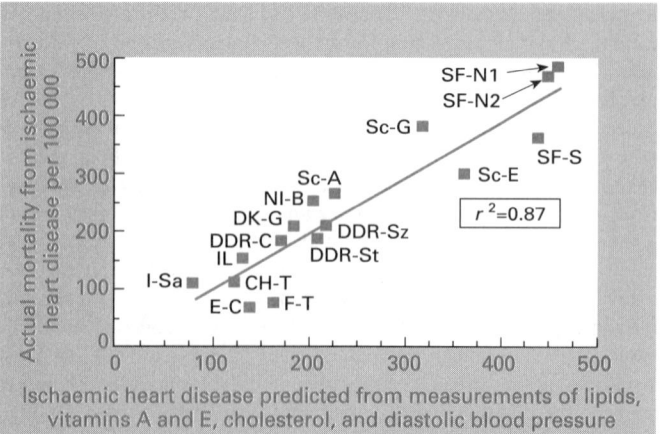

ischaemic heart disease than non-smokers. The relationship is that of dose response: the greater the number of cigarettes smoked, the higher the risk. Non-fatal myocardial infarction and sudden cardiac death are about equally related to smoking; angina pectoris is not. Of the several diseases that account for the excess morbidity and mortality among smokers in Northern Europe, North America and Australia, coronary heart disease is quantitatively the most important, because of its high frequency in the population. In countries where other risk factors are lacking and the overall level of coronary heart disease is low (e.g. in Japan) smoking appears not to increase the risk of coronary disease. The trend towards filter cigarettes in recent years appears to have made little impact on the risk of cardiovascular disease, but the risk of smoking cigars and pipes is lower than that for cigarettes, although Scandinavian studies suggest an increased risk for cigar smokers, possibly because they inhale.

It is not clear how smoking harms the cardiovascular system. Higher levels of carboxyhaemoglobin are not now believed to be the mechanism. Cigarette smoke has been shown to cause endothelial damage, and may affect platelet aggregation. A likely mechanism is through fibrinogen levels, which are higher in smokers. The demonstration of an association between smoking and ischaemic heart disease is not proof that smoking is a cause of the disease. Smokers may differ from non-smokers in other factors, which predispose them to ischaemic heart disease. The judgement that the smoking-heart disease relationship is causal is strengthened by: (1) the consistency of the relationship – it has been demonstrated in many studies in different countries; (2) its strength; a risk approximately three-fold greater among heavy smokers than among non-smokers; (3) its independence of other factors – in the presence of hypertension and elevated plasma cholesterol there is still a higher risk among smokers than among non-smokers; (4) the lower risk of ischaemic heart disease among ex-smokers – the greater the numbers of years as an ex-smoker, the closer the mortality risk to that of a life-time non-smoker; (5) the time relationship – for example, in England and Wales over the last 20 years, ischaemic heart disease has become more common in working class men than in middle and upper class men, and at the same time smoking has decreased in middle and upper class men to a greater extent than in working class men.

Multiplication of effect of risk factors

Plasma cholesterol level, blood pressure, and smoking each have independent and additive effects on ischaemic heart disease risk (Fig. 7). At each level of blood pressure and plasma cholesterol, smokers have a higher risk than non-smokers. Similarly, the effects of each of the other two risk factors are independent. Smoking leads to an approximate doubling of risk, but the absolute death rate from ischaemic heart disease in a smoker with diastolic pressure greater than 90 mmHg and in the highest quintile of plasma chosterol is about 13 times that of men in the lowest risk category.

Physical activity

In the Seven Countries Study physical inactivity did not appear to explain the geographic variation in ischaemic heart disease, but in several prospective studies vigorous exercise has been shown to protect. Initial evidence that physical activity might be protective against ischaemic heart disease came from Morris's observation that conductors on London's double-decker buses had half the ischaemic heart disease incidence of drivers; postmen a lower rate than sedentary clerks. As jobs involving aerobic exercise sufficient to ensure fitness have declined in number, attention has turned towards exercise in leisure time. From the beginning, the problem in interpreting these studies was 'selection': were the men who took regular exercise healthier to begin with, or of different constitution; hence their lower risk of ischaemic heart disease? Or was exercise truly protective? Long term follow up studies point to a likely protective effect of exercise, apparently independent of other major coronary risk factors and of bodily shape. There are a substantial number of plausible explanations for a beneficial effect: high density lipoproteins, triglycerides, insulin sensitivity, blood pressure, obesity and fibrinolytic activity are all influenced favourably by physical activity.

If exercise is genuinely protective, it is not clear how much is enough. In Morris's later studies of sedentary executive grade civil servants, he found no relation between total activity patterns and ischaemic heart disease; the protective effect was limited to vigorous aerobic exercise. Vigorous was defined as activity liable to reach peaks of energy expenditure of 7.5 kcal/min (31.5 kJ/min). Other studies, most notably in Harvard alumni, find no threshold of vigorous activity, but a graded effect: the more exercise, the greater the apparent protection. The evidence is not conclusive as to whether or not exercise such as long walks (the most convenient form of exercise for many) are truly protective.

Alcohol

Early reports suggested that alcoholics had excess mortality from ischaemic heart disease. Heavy drinking is associated with higher levels of blood pressure and possibly with stroke. The relation with ischaemic heart disease is less clear. Of greater concern have been several reports that non-drinkers have a higher mortality from ischaemic heart disease than people who consume a moderate amount of alcohol (up to three drinks per day). Data combining results from a large number of prospective studies are shown in Fig. 8).

This finding of higher ischaemic heart disease rates in abstainers, compared to moderate drinkers, has led some to argue that it is not alcohol that is protective, but that non-drinkers might differ from drinkers in other ways that put them at excess risk. They might, for example, have given up drinking because of illness or have higher levels of other risk factors. The evidence is not in favour of this view. The higher risk in non-drinkers is seen in life-time abstainers as well as in ex-drinkers; it is seen in people with no evidence of ill-health at the start of prospective studies; it persists after adjustment for the effect of other risk factors. The consistency of this finding in various studies, performed in different population groups from different cultures, makes it likely that a moderate intake of alcohol is truly protective against ischaemic heart disease.

Internationally, there is an inverse relationship between alcohol consumption and ischaemic heart disease mortality rates, perhaps one rea-

Fig. 7 Ischaemic heart disease death rate/1000 according to blood pressure, serum cholesterol level and smoking in males aged 35 to 57 screened for entry into the MRFIT study.

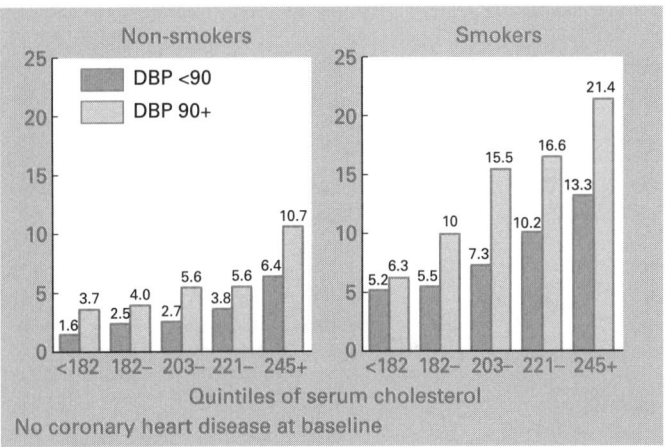

son why France, Switzerland, and other high alcohol-consuming countries of Southern Europe have lower ischaemic heart disease mortality than would be predicted from their fat intake. Although there has been much speculation that there is something specially protective about wine, the evidence does not at this stage suggest that one form of alcoholic drink is more protective than another.

Regular alcohol raises the level of plasma high density lipoprotein cholesterol and is associated with lower levels of plasma fibrinogen, possible mechanisms by which alcohol exerts its protective effect. It is also possible that moderate drinking is a successful way of dealing with stress.

Higher levels of alcohol consumption are associated with an increased risk of dying from non-cardiovascular disease – particularly from cancer. Above about two to three standard drinks (20 to 30 g alcohol) a day, blood pressure is increased and risk of death from other causes rises.

Steroid hormones

The excess of coronary disease rates in men compared to women has fuelled speculation that female hormones may be protective against ischaemic heart disease. There was a short lived vogue for giving such hormones to men who had already suffered a myocardial infarction, without evidence of net benefit. It was shown in the 1970s and 1980s that women who used oral contraceptives were at excess risk of ischaemic heart disease. If they also smoked, the absolute risk was further increased; and the absolute risk also increased with age. Studies are currently in progress to determine if newer low dose preparations of contraceptives give the same risk as the older formulations; and what the risk might be in women in Africa, Asia, and Latin America where other known risk factors are different from those in the United Kingdom and United States.

Hormone replacement therapy (HRT) decreases the risk of ischaemic heart disease by about 0.5 of the relative risk. There is a current tendency to prescribe hormone replacement therapy with progestogens as well as oestrogens because of the established problem of endometrial cancer with sole use of oestrogens. It is not known what this addition of progestogens will do to the cardioprotective effect of oestrogens. This question is the subject of current research.

Psychosocial risk factors

Ethnic differences

There are big differences in the rate of occurrence of ischaemic heart disease between countries. Rates change when people migrate, suggesting that international differences are likely to be related to lifestyle or environment rather than to genes. Although ischaemic heart disease rates do change in migrants, it takes up to a generation or more for this to happen. Different ethnic groups living in the same environment continue to have different rates of ischaemic heart disease. In the United States, Blacks once had low rates of ischaemic heart disease compared to whites, but this is less so now rates for blacks have increased compared to whites. Both groups have experienced a decline in ischaemic heart disease mortality in recent years.

In the United Kingdom, black immigrants from the Caribbean have low ischaemic heart disease rates compared to the average; by contrast immigrants from the Indian subcontinent have higher rates than the England and Wales average. Similarly, South Asians have higher rates than the local population in Trinidad, Fiji, Singapore, and South Africa. In the United Kingdom, it has been shown that South Asians have a high frequency of the metabolic syndrome of insulin resistance, low levels of high density lipoprotein cholesterol, high levels of plasma triglycerides, and central adiposity. This may underlie both their high rate of diabetes and of coronary disease. How much of this is genetic and how much environmental is not yet certain, although the observations suggest a strong genetic influence.

Socioeconomic

In general, ischaemic heart disease is more common in wealthy countries than in poor ones. Paradoxically, in wealthy countries it is the poorer groups who are most at risk. In England and Wales this is a change. In the past, ischaemic heart disease mortality was higher in higher status groups. Since the 1950s mortality from ischaemic heart disease in working class men has risen more steeply than in middle and upper class men, overtaking the latter by the 1960s. Between 1971 and 1981, ischaemic heart disease mortality declined among men in non-manual occupations, but not among those in manual jobs. Even among men in

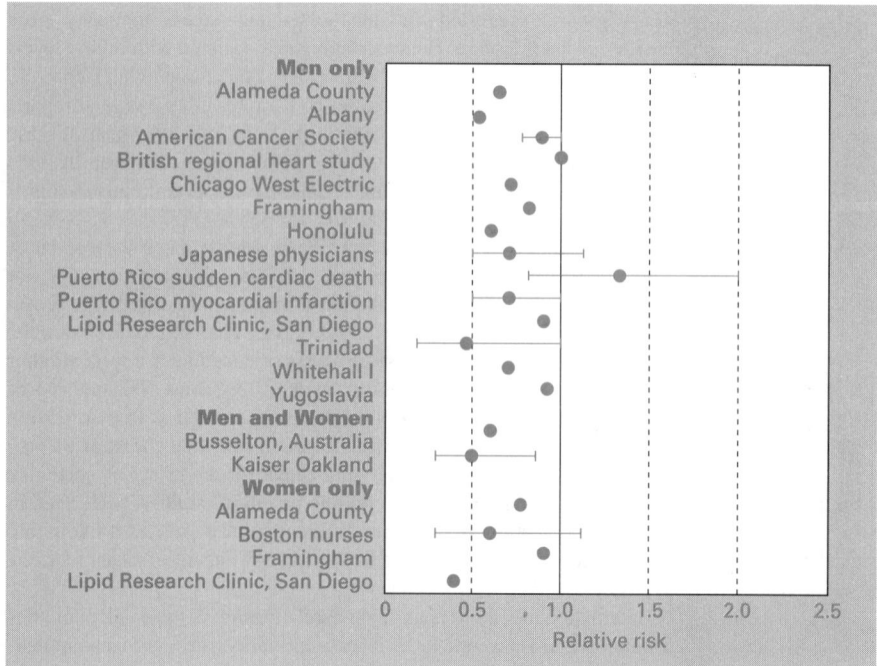

Fig. 8 Relative risk of ischaemic heart disease in moderate drinkers compared to non-drinkers in longitudinal studies. A relative risk of less than one means that moderate drinkers have a lower ischaemic heart disease risk than non-drinkers. The horizontal lines are 95 per cent confidence intervals, where available.

office based work, there is a steep social gradient. Figure 9 shows data from the Whitehall study of British civil servants: the lower the job grade the higher the mortality from ischaemic heart disease and other causes of death. In addition, more than one report shows a rise in unemployment to be followed by a rise in ischaemic heart disease mortality.

The reasons for the higher rates in lower income groups and for the change are not completely understood. Smoking has become relatively more common in working class men and women; they eat somewhat different diets including different amounts of fruit and vegetables (but not more fat); they tend to be more overweight; they have higher mean blood pressures; they report less leisure time physical activity. It is clear that there are other, as yet unidentified, factors which are also involved. Some of these may be psychosocial in origin.

Psychosocial

Many of the great clinicians of history believed that heart disease was related to psychosocial factors. William Harvey ascribed a patient's disease to the fact that he 'was overcome with anger and indignation which he yet communicated to no one'. John Hunter described his own angina pectoris as brought on by 'agitation of the mind . . . principally anxiety or anger'. Hunter reportedly died from an attack which was provoked by a particularly irritating hospital board meeting. Osler enquired after the cause of 'arterial degeneration in the worry and strain of modern life' and described the typical angina patient as the man 'the indicator of whose engine is at full steam ahead'.

These descriptions accord with much current clinical and lay feeling that an acute coronary event or angina pectoris may be precipitated by psychological factors. The difficulty has been to demonstrate this scientifically. Two main approaches have been taken: (1) to identify potentially stressful situations which may increase the risk of ischaemic heart disease; and (2) to identify a particular 'coronary prone' behaviour pattern.

Stressful situations

Much interest originally centred on the study of stressful life events. Widowers have a higher mortality from ischaemic heart disease in the 6 months following bereavement than married men of the same age. There is some other evidence that stressful life events may precipitate myocardial infarction.

In a chronic disease, it may be that long term stressful problems are of more relevance than acute events. There has been a good deal of research on the environment at work. Evidence from Scandinavia, the United States, and Britain support the hypothesis that jobs characterized by high demand and low perceived control are associated with increase in risk of ischaemic heart disease. Risk was further increased if there were low levels of social support at work. Other studies have also shown that low levels of social support outside work are associated with higher ischaemic heart disease death rates.

Coronary-prone behaviour patterns

The idea that there is a particular personality type, or behaviour pattern, that is associated with coronary disease received support from studies of the type A behaviour pattern. The type A individual is described as aggressive, striving, ambitious, restless, and excessively concerned with time and deadlines. This pattern of behaviour is particularly common where job stress is reported to be high. In longitudinal studies, type A individuals had been shown to have greater than twice the risk of developing ischaemic heart disease than individuals who do not show this behaviour pattern – type Bs. This increase in risk was independent of the other known coronary risk factors.

Much of the work on type A behaviour has come from the United States. Initially, European studies affirmed the importance of type A behaviour. The results of more recent studies have been equivocal. It has been proposed that the important component of type A behaviour is hostility. Increased hostility has been associated with ischaemic heart disease risk and with angiographically detected narrowing of the coronary arteries.

In summary, a wide body of research of varying quality has provided evidence that psychosocial characteristics are causally linked to the development of clinical ischaemic heart disease. The exact nature of this link remains to be elucidated, as does a definition of the type of social environmental situation which may increase the risk of disease. It is not known whether the risk of ischaemic heart disease can be altered by modifying the environment; more evidence is needed on the benefit or otherwise of individual changes in behaviour.

Geographic factors

In addition to the marked international differences, ischaemic heart disease rates vary geographically within countries. Part of this variation may be the result of differences in the risk factors reviewed above. There may also be environmental factors involved.

Climate and season

In England and Wales, the mortality from ischaemic heart disease varies with the season. It is consistently higher in winter months. This increase might be related to increased spread of infection and/or an increase in pneumonia leading to a greater risk of death in persons already suffering from ischaemic heart disease. It might also be related to ambient temperature itself. Throughout the year there is an inverse association between temperature and ischaemic heart disease; the lower the temperature the higher the mortality. Data from North America show that there is a rise in ischaemic heart disease deaths after heavy snowfalls. The suggestion has been made that the combination of cold and the unaccustomed physical activity entailed in shoveling snow place an acute burden on the heart.

Support for this association with climatic factors comes from a comparison of ischaemic heart disease mortality rates in different parts of Great Britain. There is a twofold variation in cardiovascular mortality (i.e. ischaemic heart disease, other heart disease and stroke) in Great Britain. The rate is high in Scotland, north-west England, and South Wales, and low in south-east England. The areas with high mortality rates in general have lower average temperatures and more rainy days than the low mortality areas. The regional differences in mortality are also negatively correlated with socioeconomic factors and water hardness. It is therefore difficult to disentangle their effects.

Fig. 9 Mortality in 10 years according to grade of employment in the Whitehall study of British civil servants. Administrators are the highest, 'other' the lowest grade.

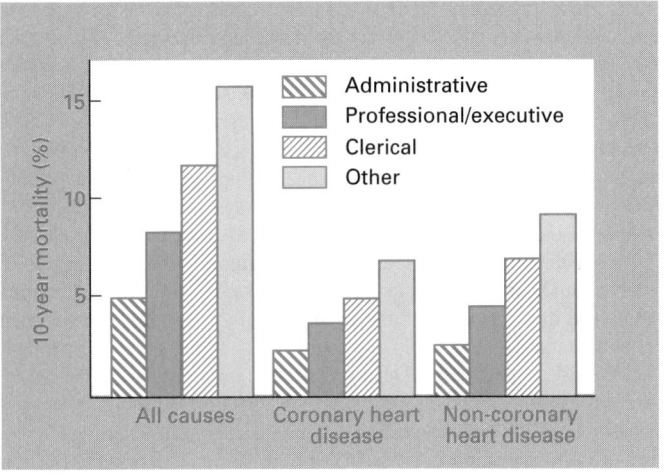

Water hardness

Studies in many countries have shown a negative association between water hardness and ischaemic heart disease mortality. The geographic differences in mortality in Great Britain are highly negatively correlated with water hardness: harder water, lower mortality. Adjustment for climatic and socio-economic differences between towns reduces but does not abolish the association with water hardness. To date there is no evidence that artificial softening of water increases the mortality from heart disease.

Socioeconomic factors

Geographic variation has also been studied in relation to socio-economic factors. Indices of social deprivation have been constructed using measures in the Census, such as home ownership, access to cars, crowding and unemployment rates. The small area variation in these measures of deprivation is correlated with ischaemic heart disease mortality: greater deprivation, higher mortality.

Prevention

Strategies of prevention

The high risk approach seeks to identify people at high risk of coronary disease or stroke and modify their risk by treatment or other means. This is the classic approach of preventive medicine. The population approach seeks to modify population levels of risk and, *pari passu*, to prevent high risk states from occurring. These two are complementary.

The population approach has the potential for delivering greater gains across the whole population. This is illustrated in Fig. 10 with data from the 350 000 white males screened for possible entry into the MRFIT (Multiple Risk Factor Intervention Trial). The excess deaths are calculated on the assumption that the mortality rate of men with a systolic blood pressure less than 110 mmHg is the basal rate. The higher death rates at higher levels of blood pressure can be 'attributed' to blood pressure. A high risk approach that sought to detect and treat those with casual systolic blood pressure of greater than or equal to 170 mmHg would potentially save only a small minority of excess deaths. The majority of deaths 'attributable' to a raised blood pressure come from the majority of the population with modest elevations of pressure. Only

Fig. 10 Ischaemic heart disease (CHD) death rates according to systolic blood pressure level. The histograms represent the number of excess deaths, at each blood pressure level, attributable to having a blood pressure above 110 mmHg. Although the death rate climbs sharply with blood pressure level, a large number of people with small elevations of pressure contribute more excess deaths attributable to raised pressure, than a small number of people with large elevations of pressure.

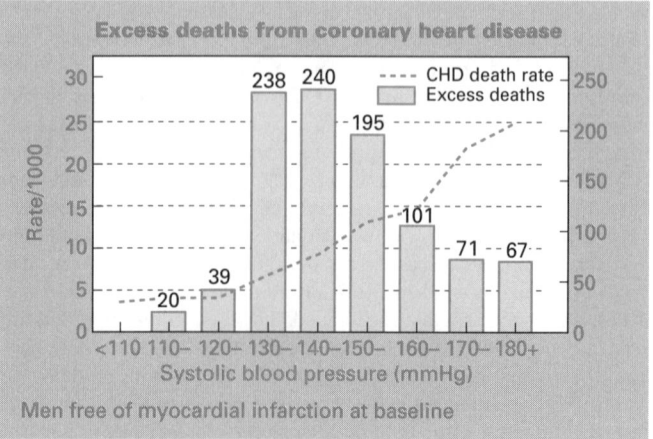

an approach that lowered average blood pressures of the population would be expected to reduce the majority of the deaths attributable to raised blood pressure.

Evaluating prevention

Two approaches have been used in studies to test the feasibility of preventing premature coronary heart disease. The earlier investigations were all aimed at modifying only one factor. There are at least three reasons why (with the knowledge of hindsight) these trials could not be expected to produce impressive results. First, the atheromatous process probably starts early in life. Consequently the ideal clinical trial should be started in young people. In fact, very few people under the age of 40 years have been entered into any of the studies and it should not be surprising if such studies fail to demonstrate striking benefit. Second, in a disease with multifactorial aetiology it might be expected that modification of only one factor would have little or no effect. Third, none of the trials was designed specifically to examine the effects of treatment on total mortality and *post hoc* attempts to do so (which are discussed below) have caused considerable confusion. Single factor intervention studies can, however, provide useful confirmatory evidence concerning aetiology: modification of a single factor in a randomised study, producing reduced frequency of coronary heart disease in comparison with a control group, is strong evidence that the association between the factor and coronary heart disease is causal.

More recently a multifactor approach to prevention has evolved. A pragmatic reason for this approach arises from the difficulty in changing only one factor at a time. For example, in one study (United States National Diet Heart Study) 50 per cent of the men who were asked to adhere to a special diet also reduced their cigarette consumption. Prevention trials may be either primary (carried out in individuals who at the outset have no clinical manifestations of coronary heart disease) or secondary where the subjects already have established disease.

Single factor intervention studies

CHOLESTEROL REDUCTION BY MEANS OF DIET AND DRUGS

The studies in which diet and drugs have been used to lower cholesterol have been considered in several recent reviews and meta-analyses which provide a helpful perspective, since the results of each of the trials, especially the smaller ones, are subject to a considerable margin of error. With regard to coronary events, the meta-analyses have shown a remarkably consistent effect; 1 per cent reduction in cholesterol may be expected to produce at least a 2 per cent reduction in total coronary events (ie, fatal and non-fatal coronary heart disease; Fig. 11). The effect is noted within 2 years of any fall in cholesterol and is more marked the longer the trial is continued. The beneficial effect is similar, regardless of the treatment used to lower cholesterol levels. Furthermore people at greatest risk, including those who have established disease, appear to derive greatest benefit. Angiographic studies involving the use of strict lipid lowering diets as well as hyperlipidaemic drugs suggest that reduction of low density lipoprotein cholesterol can produce regression of atherosclerosis over a relatively short time frame (1 to 5 years). The STARS study (St Thomas' Atherosclerosis Regression Study) involved computer-assisted assessment of coronary angiograms for quantifying atherosclerosis; differences between experimental and control groups are relevant to clinical practice. Ninety men, with coronary heart disease and a plasma cholesterol greater than 6.5 mmol/l, were randomized to receive usual care (UC), dietary advice (D), or diet plus cholestyramine (DC). The diet was comparable to that usually recommended for such patients (saturated and total fat 8 to 10 per cent and about 20 per cent total energy respectively). During the approximately 3-year follow-up period mean plasma levels were 6.9 mmol/l (UC), 6.2 mmol/l (D), and 5.6 mmol/l (DC). The proportions of patients showing overall progression of coronary stenosis were 46 per cent (UC), 15 per cent (D), and

12 per cent (DC). The mean absolute width of the coronary segments increased significantly in DC and to some extent in D, the changes being significantly correlated with the low density lipoprotein : high density lipoprotein ratio. This provides good evidence that reducing plasma cholesterol can favourably influence the pathological process underlying clinical coronary heart disease, as well clinical events. However, no study has yet demonstrated a reduction by interventions of fatal coronary events, and the potential for adverse effects of any treatment continued over a prolonged period must be considered. Some observational studies have suggested that those with the lowest levels of cholesterol have an increased mortality from non-cardiac causes, principally accounted for by deaths from cancers in the early years of follow up. This has led to the suggestion that low cholesterol levels may be a feature of undiagnosed cancer rather than being causally associated with an increased risk of malignant neoplasms. It has also been shown in a single study that low cholesterol levels may be associated with depression, but the observation applied only to the very old and the findings from only one study do not permit firm conclusions.

Several meta-analyses of the clinical trials of lowering cholesterol by diet and drugs have examined the finding in some individual studies that such lowering might increase deaths due to cancer or accidents, violence and suicide and suggestion that these untoward effects may offset any benefit resulting from reduced cardiovascular events. These analyses suggest that while dietary modification does not favourably influence total mortality, there is no evidence that any single cause of non-cardiac mortality is adversely influenced by dietary change along the lines currently recommended. However, in several of the drug trials there is a suggestion that, despite the benefits in terms of cardiovascular risk reduction, total mortality, and in particular death rates from accidents, violence and suicide may be greater in the experimental than the control groups. Again the implication is that these untoward effects may offset any benefits resulting from reduced cardiovascular events. This concern has not yet finally been resolved. Unfortunately most lipid lowering trials did not include sufficient subjects to address the effects of treatment on total or non-cardiac mortality. The sample sizes were calculated on the basis of determining whether reducing cholesterol level could reduce the risk of coronary events, a much more frequent end point. To be certain of the effect of any treatment on total mortality, or to be confident about the incidence of uncommon fatal end points, larger studies are needed and some are underway. For the present it can only be

Fig. 11 Overview of 22 trials of cholesterol lowering showing the percent reduction in ischaemic heart disease in treatment V's control groups. The three sets of histograms show: (a) periods of short and long duration; (b) trials achieving a 5 to 9 per cent reduction in plasma cholesterol and those achieving 10 to 15 per cent; (c) trials of primary and secondary prevention (reproduced from Peto *et al.* (1985) *Circulation,* **72,** 451, with permission).

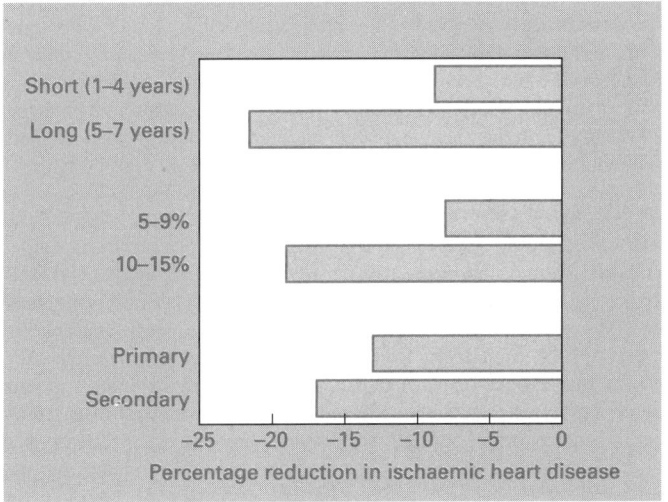

Table 3 *Major clinical events and mortality in the Oslo study*

Event	Intervention group (n = 604)	Control group (n = 626)
Coronary deaths (including sudden death)	7	17
Non-fatal myocardial infarction	18	28
Stroke	4	4
Total cardiovascular disease	29	49
Coronary bypass surgery	1	8
Total deaths	19	31

stated that an effect on increased mortality from non-cardiac causes in association with active cholesterol lowering treatment, has not been consistent or statistically significant in most individual trials. It has not been related to the extent of fall in cholesterol, is not in keeping with the epidemiological evidence and there are no established mechanisms. By contrast the benefit of lowering cholesterol on coronary heart disease is specific, highly statistically significant, proportional to the cholesterol lowering achieved, in keeping with the epidemiological evidence and is biologically plausible.

BLOOD PRESSURE REDUCTION

It is possible to lower blood pressure without drugs but it has not been shown whether reductions in blood pressure achieved by non-pharmacological intervention measures lead to reductions in ischaemic heart disease incidence.

There have been many trials of drug treatment of raised blood pressure in the prevention of cardiovascular disease. A meta-analysis of trials suggests that the fall in pressure achieved in the trials should correspond to a 20 to 25 per cent reduction in incidence of ischaemic heart disease and a 40 per cent reduction in stroke. The predicted reduction in stroke was achieved but the reduction in ischaemic heart disease was 14 per cent, about 60 per cent of that predicted.

Multiple risk factor intervention trials

The trials in which attempts have been made to modify more than one aspect of lifestyle provide more encouraging results. In the Oslo trial, men at high risk of coronary heart disease (as a result of smoking or having a cholesterol in the range of 7.5 to 9.8 mmol/l) were divided into two groups; half received intensive dietary education and advice to stop smoking, the other half served as a control group. An impressive reduction in total coronary events was observed (Table 3) in association with a 13 per cent fall in cholesterol and a 65 per cent reduction in tobacco consumption. The beneficial effect of intervention was reflected also in a significant improvement in total mortality; there were no significant differences between the two groups with regard to non-cardiac causes of death. Detailed statistical analysis suggests that approximately 60 per cent of the coronary heart disease reduction was attributable to change in serum cholesterol and 25 per cent to reduction in smoking.

In the MRFIT study over 12 000 men at high risk of coronary heart disease because of raised plasma cholesterol, smoking and high blood pressure, were randomized to special care or to usual care groups. Both groups tended to show a reduction in risk factor levels with a relatively small difference between the two groups. Nevertheless, after over 10 years of follow-up, mortality rates from coronary heart disease were 10.6 per cent lower in the special care group than in the usual care group. There was also a trend towards lower overall mortality as well as lower death rates from cancer and violence in the intervention group. In the European Collaborative Study, people working in factories in several

European countries were randomized to either receive advice aimed to modify a range of risk factors or to act as controls. The reduction in coronary heart disease was related to the degree of alteration in risk factors achieved in the various countries. In Britain there were only minimal changes in the intervention group and no reduction of coronary heart disease was observed.

SECONDARY PREVENTION TRIALS

Many of the early studies of diet and drug treatment in people with established coronary disease were small and results were inconclusive, though a recent meta-analysis has concluded that the findings support the suggestion that a multifactorial approach to risk reduction might lead to a significant reduction in further coronary events. One study warrants individual mention. The Diet and Reinfarction Trial (DART) involved randomization of over 2000 men who had survived myocardial infarction to receive or not receive advice on each of three dietary factors: a reduction in total fat and an increase in the ratio of polyunsaturated to saturated fatty acids; an increase in cereal fibre; and an increase in fatty fish intake. Within a 2-year follow-up period, the subjects advised to eat fatty fish had a nearly one-third reduction in all-cause mortality compared with those not so advised. The other two diets were not associated with significant differences in mortality, but as fat modification only achieved a 3 to 4 per cent reduction in cholesterol, it is conceivable that compliance with the fat modified and fibre diets may have been less than on the fish diet. Furthermore, diets aimed to reduce atherogenicity may take longer to produce a beneficial effect than those aimed to reduce thrombogenicity. The results are of particular interest.

PRACTICAL APPLICATION OF THESE FINDINGS

An approach involving attention to many potentially adverse factors in lifestyle appears to confer benefit even when started in middle age. Advice should therefore be offered to the population as a whole as well as to high-risk individuals. There would appear to be no adverse effects of such an approach, which should always be the first line of management of people with hyperlipidaemia. The main difficulty lies in persuading individuals of the need to change their way of life to the extent required. For the present it seems appropriate to conclude that lipid lowering drugs should be reserved for those at particularly high risk of coronary heart disease in whom other measures have failed to achieve an adequate change in plasma lipids. In such individuals any possible adverse effects are likely to be outweighed by the benefits of reduction in cardiovascular risk.

REFERENCES

Davey Smith, G., Song, F., and Sheldon, T.A. (1993). Cholesterol lowering and mortality: the importance of considering initial risk. *British Medical Journal*, **306**, 1367–73.
Grundy, S.M. and Denke, M.A. (1990). Dietary influences on serum lipids and lipoproteins. *Journal of Lipid Research*, **31**, 1149–72.

15.10.2 The pathophysiology of ischaemic heart disease

M. J. DAVIES

Atherosclerosis and ischaemic heart disease

Ischaemic heart disease is the clinical manifestation of coronary atherosclerosis. Atherosclerosis is a focal intimal disease best appreciated by viewing the inner surface of an involved artery opened longitudinally at autopsy. Numerous focal elevated lesions known as plaques can be seen.

The coronary arteries of young subjects of different ages who have died from accidental causes provide information on the development of plaques. The earliest lesions (fatty streaks) are flat yellow dots or streaks on the intima. Each is made up of lipid-filled (foam) cells of monocytic origin, which have accumulated beneath the intact endothelium. Extracellular lipid appears next, followed by smooth muscle cells and the production of increasing amounts of collagen. The process culminates in the formation of the advanced, or raised fibrolipid, plaque. Advanced plaques are the basis for the development of clinical symptoms.

The advanced plaque

MICROANATOMY

The microanatomy of the advanced plaque is fundamental to the development of ischaemic heart disease. In a coronary artery that has been distended at normal arterial pressures the lumen is circular. Many plaques are situated eccentrically, that is there is a residual arc of normal vessel wall opposite the plaque. The typical advanced plaque has a core of extracellular lipid (Figure 1), which is encapsulated by fibrous tissue produced by smooth muscle cells; a particularly vital part of the plaque is the fibrous cap separating the core from the lumen. The cap has considerable tensile strength due to high concentrations of collagen and elastin and is covered by endothelium on its luminal surface.

ADVANCED PLAQUES AND CLINICAL SYMPTOMS

Many advanced plaques cause no symptoms and are angiographically invisible. The insensitivity of angiography is due to vascular remodelling. The artery in this situation has responded to the presence of a plaque by increasing its external diameter, thus accommodating the plaque without compromising the lumen. However, the basic process of atherosclerosis (i.e. lipid accumulation, smooth muscle proliferation, and collagen production) may continue, and cause the individual plaque to increase in volume to a sufficient degree to overcome the remodelling process and cause focal narrowing of the lumen. The plaque now becomes angiographically visible, and when the lumen is reduced by more than 50 per cent by diameter, flow is limited when myocardial oxygen demand rises. This degree of stenosis cannot be compensated for by further falls in distal resistance to increase flow. The result is stable exertional angina.

A second mechanism for the production of clinical symptoms is that thrombosis complicates an advanced plaque, producing an acute reduction of blood flow and acute myocardial infarction or unstable angina. The third process involved in the production of the clinical symptoms is altered vascular tone. Normal coronary arteries dilate in response to an increase in blood flow; in atherosclerosis the arteries undergo paradoxical vasoconstriction. Such abnormal tonal responses are characteristic both of coronary segments with angiographic lesions, and adjacent segments which ostensibly look normal.

Progression of coronary atherosclerosis in man

Data on progression is derived from angiography performed at regular intervals. Despite the inherent insensitivity of angiography some facts are clear. Individual patients vary widely in the overall rate of progression; the rate of progression of individual stenoses is also variable. In general progression is episodic, and not at steady uniform rate. The lesions that appear between two angiograms often develop at points where the vessel previously appeared normal or minimally diseased. A significant proportion of these 'new' lesions are very high grade or even total obstructions and may appear without any overt signs of acute ischaemia.

Thrombosis in atherosclerosis

Two separate processes are responsible for thrombosis on plaques. In the first (superficial injury) there is endothelial denudation over the plaque. Subendothelial collagen is exposed and a platelet-rich thrombus forms over the surface of the plaque. In the second (deep intimal injury) the plaque splits or tears open through the cap. Blood enters the lipid core from the lumen and meets a very thrombogenic mixture of tissue factor, collagen, and lipid. A platelet-rich thrombus forms within the plaque, which may then extend into the lumen.

Superficial intimal injury

Studies of human atherosclerotic coronary arteries show that denudation of small groups of endothelial cells with the resultant formation of an ultramicroscopic monolayer of platelets is almost ubiquitous over advanced plaques. Thus the endothelial cells over many plaques are recently regenerated and cell turnover is increased. Approximately one in four of larger thrombi that occlude a coronary vessel are due to more severe degrees of superficial injury. A large lipid core is not a prerequisite for this form of thrombosis.

Deep intimal injury

A large lipid core is associated with cap tearing (fissuring) and plaque disruption. Plaque fissuring covers a wide spectrum of severity. At one extreme there are microfissures no more than a few hundred microns across, at the other extreme the whole cap may be torn open over a centimetre of the artery. When blood enters the lipid core, the formation of intraplaque thrombus, which distorts and increases plaque size, is inevitable. Thrombosis in the lumen, however, is not inevitable. Whether intraluminal thrombus occurs, and this is a major determinant whether acute clinical symptoms develops, depends on the interplay of many factors, including the systemic thrombotic and lytic state at the time, the size of the fissure and the amount of local flow. Markedly reduced flow, either because the plaque has been expanded from within or because of local spasm, will favour intraluminal thrombus formation.

PATHOGENESIS OF PLAQUE FISSURING

Plaque cap tearing reflects the imposition of increased mechanical stress on a tissue that is undergoing structural changes weakening its ability to withstand such stress. The stress on the cap is imposed by the systolic pulse. Circumferential wall stress is normally distributed evenly across the vessel wall but, being soft, the core cannot carry its share of the load, which must therefore be carried by another part of the vessel wall. Computer models show that the redistributed stress is carried by the cap. The larger the core, the greater the angle that the core subtends; the thinner the cap, the greater is the concentration of force on the cap in systole.

The cap tissue itself may also undergo changes reducing its mechanical strength. These changes include a loss of collagen and connective tissue mucins, a decrease in smooth muscle cell numbers, and an increase in the number of macrophages. Such changes reflect heightened macrophage and inflammatory activity in the plaque.

Evolution of thrombi

Thrombi invoke a rapid repair response in the arterial wall. The initial response is lysis but thrombus which is not removed invokes local smooth muscle proliferation and replacement by collagenous tissue (organization). Combinations of lysis and organisation mean that following coronary thrombosis a wide range of putative outcomes exist (see Fig. 1). These range from chronic total occlusion to restoration of a normal lumen. Study of subjects with coronary atherosclerosis but without ischaemic heart disease who die from accidents show that minor plaque fissures and intraplaque thrombi are not uncommon. Such data show that subclinical coronary thrombi are an important part in the episodic progression of coronary atherosclerosis.

The concept of stable and unstable plaques

With the realization that thrombosis was responsible for both acute clinical symptoms and silent progression of disease, the concept of unstable plaques has emerged. Vulnerable plaques are those with a high risk of thrombosis; unstable plaques are those actually undergoing thrombosis. Vulnerability is a reflection both of the amount of lipid present and the degree of inflammatory activity in the plaque. Regression of atherosclerosis by a variety of therapeutic means, in particular, that lowering plasma lipid levels is now being attempted. Animal models suggest that such manoeuvres will reduce plaque lipid and lead to a more solid fibrous plaque. This would increase plaque stability and, if it occurred in man, would reduce the frequency of new acute ischaemic events.

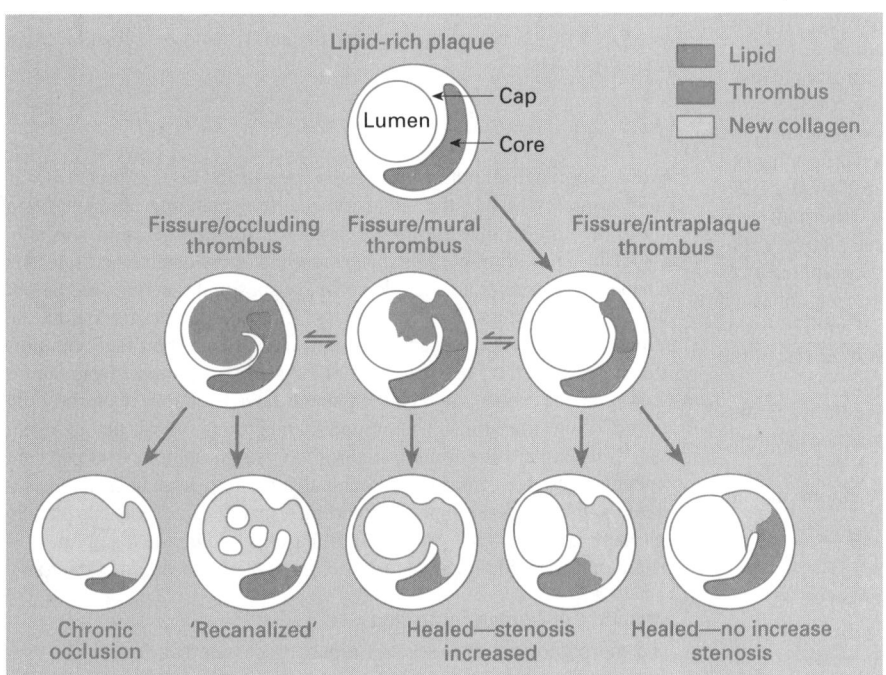

Fig. 1 Potential outcome of an episode of plaque disruption. A healing process is initiated with fibriolysis and followed by smooth muscle proliferation. This proliferation restabilizes the plaque and may often lead to an increase in the degree of stenosis.

The pathology of angina

Stable angina

Stable angina is caused by segments of stenosis of more than 50 per cent in diameter in one, two, or three of the major coronary arteries. The typical subject with stable angina has well preserved venticular function. The angiographic appearances of the stenoses are that of smooth regular narrowings (type I) and often remain unchanged for long periods, indicating stable plaques. The plaques show different combinations of certain morphological features. They may be concentric, i.e. involve the whole circumference of the vessel wall, or eccentric, i.e. leave a normal segment of vessel wall opposite the plaque. The importance of an eccentric plaque is that vascular tone in the residual normal arterial segment can alter the lumen size. The degree of stenosis thus may vary. Plaques may either be entirely fibrous, or have a lipid core. The lipid core may occupy up to 70 per cent of the entire plaque volume.

There is a very large subject to subject variability in the characteristics of plaques. Some subjects with stable angina have entirely fibrous concentric plaques; these may be those subjects whose disease remains stable for years. Others have a high proportion of lipid-rich plaques, and therefore a higher risk of an acute event. Most subjects with stable angina have a mixture of plaque types. Approximately 50 per cent of subjects with stable angina have potentially variable stenoses in series with fixed stenoses.

Autopsy studies show that up to 40 per cent of subjects with stable angina, even when there is no previous infarction, have a totally occluded artery at some point. At such a point the lumen may be occluded by fibrous tissue with extensive bridging collaterals in the adjacent adventitia, or there may be a number of new vascular channels within the original lumen. Both appearances indicate previous, clinically silent, occluding thrombus.

Unstable angina

Angioscopic and angiographic studies in life supported by necropsy studies show that in the crescendo type of unstable angina there is a non-occluding thrombus projecting into the lumen from an underlying plaque fissure. Angiography then reveals type II stenosis characterized by an irregular outline, eccentric indentation, overhanging edge, and intraluminal radiotransluscent thrombus, which is typical of the culprit lesion of unstable angina and reflects an unstable plaque undergoing thrombosis. The surface of such a plaque at autopsy is covered by platelet-rich thrombus, and distal embolization of small clumps of platelets occurs. These microemboli are associated with focal microscopic myocardial necrosis. The disrupted plaque is characteristic of the more severe cases of unstable angina and, as less severe cases are studied, the association with thrombosis becomes less certain. Altered or enhanced vascular tone at segments of eccentric stenosis is a substantiated alternative mechanism. Why such segments acquire this abnormal tonal behaviour is unclear. One possibility is that microscopic platelet deposition of insufficient magnitude to be recognized angiographically or angioscopically has occurred; another is that there has been enhanced inflammatory infiltration of the plaque itself, or in the adventitia. Endothelial dysfunction and altered tonal responses throughout the rest of the coronary vascular bed would potentiate any local spasm.

Examination of atherectomy samples taken from the causative lesions of unstable angina shows a significant increase of the presence of thrombus when compared to samples taken from subjects with stable angina. It is a consistent finding, however, that there are exceptions in both directions, i.e. no thrombus being found in unstable angina and thrombus present in stable angina.

Acute myocardial infarction

Infarction in heart muscle may be regional or diffuse. Regional infarction is further subdivided into transmural and non-transmural (sub-endocardial). Diffuse infarction usually consists of a circumferential necrosis of the subendocardial zone and the papillary muscle of the left ventricle. The causes of regional and diffuse infarction are very different. In regional infarction the cause lies in occlusion of the subtending artery, in the vast majority of cases by thrombosis in relation to an atherosclerotic plaque. Diffuse subendocardial infarction is due to a more general failure of myocardial perfusion; it often follows prolonged hypotension and is exacerbated by ventricular hypertrophy and high left ventricular diastolic pressure. Diffuse subendocardial infarction may be superimposed on regional infarction complicated by cardiogenic shock.

Animal models of infarction

Coronary artery ligation in the dog is a model of human regional infarction. The myocardium in the area supplied this ligated artery rapidly fails to contract normally. This is followed by a cessation of aerobic metabolism and the initiation of anaerobic glycolysis. Within the myocyte lactate accumulates, creatinine phosphate falls followed by a drop in adenosine triphosphate within 3 min. Detectable structural damage appears within 15 min and is heralded by breaks in the sarcoplasmic membrane of the myocyte. At this point cell death has occurred and the changes are not reversible. Survival for 8 to 12 h is required if light microscopy is to detect irreversible changes in structure of the myocyte. These changes include a local polymorphonuclear response, coalescence of myofibrils within the myocyte (coagulative necrosis) and nuclear disintegration. Myocyte disruption and a monocyte inflammatory reaction occur at 24 to 48 h, and invasion of the necrotic area of by fibroblasts and endothelial cells from adjacent viable myocardium can be seen from 48 h. Ultimately, a fibrous scar is formed.

The effect of restoring regional flow can be studied in animal models. Reperfusion alters the morphological appearance of damaged myocyte. In reperfused areas of infarction calcium pours into the myocyte, leading to the deposition of electron dense granules within mitochondria and a hypercontraction of myofibrils. The affected cells have deeply eosinophilic cross bands of shunted myofibrils (contraction band necrosis).

The lateral borders of the region of infarction are established at the time of cessation of flow and depend on the coronary artery anatomy. However, infarction spreads from the subendocardial zone to the epicardium over a period of 4 to 6 h. Restoration of flow within this time will prevent a transmural infarct. This gradient of vulnerability across the ventricular wall with the subepicardial myocytes having a greater resistance to necrosis depends to some degree on collateral flow, but possibly also on the greater energy demands made by subendocardial myocytes.

HUMAN MYOCARDIAL INFARCTION

Human regional infarction has similarities to the animal model but is more complex in that the occlusion of the subtending artery is often intermittent rather than abrupt. Regional transmural infarction is usually associated with thrombosis in the subtending artery on an atherosclerotic plaque. Rare exceptions include coronary spasm, dissection, and embolism. Three-quarters of all thrombi are due to a plaque disruption, the remainder being due to superficial intimal injury. The plaque fissures that underlie infarct-related thrombi range in magnitude from minor tears to major events in which the plaques have been torn open and lipid extruded into the lumen. This range of magnitude of the plaque event may well explain the failure of thrombolysis to achieve 100 per cent patency rates. Non-transmural regional infarction in man is also associated with thrombosis in the subtending artery due to events in a plaque, but there is a far higher proportion of cases in which the distal artery is patent and is filled either by restored antegrade flow or via collaterals.

Structure of human infarction

The morphological changes and repair processes that develop in man are no different in principle from those observed in animal models. Regional transmural infarction usually results in the changes of coagulative necrosis with uniform appearances throughout the infarcted zone. In contrast, many non-transmural infarcts appear to be built up by the coalescence of smaller focal areas of necrosis of different ages and contraction band necrosis indicating reperfusion. In the healed phase of human infarction, when fibrosis has replaced the dead tissue, strands and islands of surviving myocytes embedded in the scar are common.

The pathology of complications of human infarction

Sudden death due to ventricular arrhythmias during acute infarction is not directly related to infarct size and has a maximal risk in the first 24 h, when there are islands of ischaemic but still viable myocardium.

The incidence of cardiogenic shock is directly related to the proportion of the left ventricular muscle mass that has been lost. Because the left anterior descending coronary artery supplies up to 50 per cent of the left ventricular muscle mass, occlusions close to its origin have the highest risk of cardiogenic shock.

Cardiac rupture, responsible for 5 to 8 per cent of the mortality of acute infarction comes in two recognizable morphological forms. In the first, rupture occurs within 24 h and appears as a ragged tear at the margin of dead and viable myocardium. The infarct zone is only just developing the macroscopic features, which allow its recognition, and ventricular shape is not altered. In the second form rupture occurs later, and is through an infarct that has thinned and become aneurysmal. Ventricular septal defects complicating infarction have similar pathology, being examples of 'internal' rupture, which may be anteroseptal due to left anterior descending coronary occlusions or posteroseptal due to right coronary occlusion. Papillary muscle rupture is the rarest mechanical complication of infarction. The tear may involve one or several heads of either the anterolateral or posteromedial papillary muscle. While many such ruptures are associated with extensive free wall infarction, older people may have a very localized infarct of papillary muscle with resultant rupture caused by occlusion of the left marginal coronary artery.

Infarct expansion and remodelling

Following infarction, the ventricular shape may undergo very drastic changes. In the first 24 h after of the infarction the dead area may thin and stretch due to slipping and tearing of bundles of myocytes. When organization and repair by fibrosis occurs, the expanded shape of the infarct zone is retained permanently. Left ventricular cavity size is increased and the residual surviving myocardium may also undergo compensatory hypertrophy. This ventricular remodelling has long-term deleterious affects on function.

Infarct thinning and expansion is a complication of transmural and large regional infarcts; its predominant cause is proximal occlusion of the left anterior descending coronary artery. Survival of a rim of subpericardial muscle appears to prevent expansion, which is therefore not a complication of non-transmural infarcts. Ventricular aneurysms following infarction are closely related in many cases to infarct expansion. The aneurysmal bulge may be diffuse, with a very wide neck or more localized with a narrow neck. One form has a very narrow neck with the bulk of the aneurysm sac outside the ventricle itself. This is thought to result from partial rupture of the ventricle with the formation of a subpericardial haematoma. Because strictly speaking the wall is the pericardium these are often referred to as pseudoaneurysms.

Sudden ischaemic death

Clinical and pathological studies suggest that two mechanisms are involved in sudden cardiac death with a final common pathway of ventricular fibrillation or asystole. One mechanism is by way of a new acute ischaemic event due to coronary thrombosis or spasm; the other is of a fatal arrhythmia arising in a scarred and/or hypertrophied left ventricle. There is no agreement on the relative frequency of these two mechanisms, and differences in the literature are likely to depend on selection

of the cases examined and the proportion of patients with a previous known history of ischaemic heart disease or prodromal pain. This proportion varies between studies.

REFERENCES

Davies, M. (1990). A macroscopic and microscopic view of coronary thrombi. *Circulation*, **82**, 1138–1146.

Davies, M. (1992). Anatomic features in victims of sudden coronary death. *Circulation*, **85**, 1–19–1–24.

de Feyter, P., Serruys, P., Davies, M., Richardson, P., Lubsen, J. and Oliver, M. (1991). Quantitative coronary angiography to measure progression and regression of coronary atherosclerosis. Value, limitations, and implications for clinical trials. *Circulation*, **84**, 412–423.

Fuster, V., Badimon, L., Badimon, J., and Chesebro, J. (1992). Mechanisms of Disease: The pathogenesis of coronary artery disease and the acute coronary syndromes I. *New England Journal of Medicine*, **326**, 242–250.

Fuster, V., Badimon, L., Badimon, J., and Chesebro, J. (1992). The pathogenesis of coronary artery disease and the acute coronary syndrome II. *New England Journal of Medicine*, **326**, 310–318.

Glagov, S., Weisenberd, E., Zarins, C., Stankunavicius, R., and Kolettis, G. (1987). Compensatory enlargement of human atherosclerotic coronary arteries. *New England Journal of Medicine*, **316**, 1371–1375.

Jennings, R. and Reimer, K. (1991). The cell biology of acute myocardial ischaemia. *Annual Review of Medicine*, **42**, 225–246.

Lichtlen, P., Nikutta, P., and Jost, S. (1992). Anatomical progression of coronary artery disease in humans as seen by prospective, repeated, quantitated coronary angiography. Relation to clinical events and risk factors. *Circulation*, **86**, 828–838.

Mizuno, K., Miyamoto, A., and Satomura, K. (1991). Angiographic coronary macromorphology in patients with acute coronary disorders. *Lancet*, **337**, 809–812.

Richardson, P., Davies, M., and Born, G. (1989). Influence of plaque configuration and stress distribution on fissuring of coronary atherosclerotic plaques. *Lancet*, **ii**, 941–944.

Roberts, W. (1979). The coronary arteries and left ventricle in clinically isolated angina pectoris—a necropsy analysis. *American Journal of Medicine*, **67**, 792–799.

Ross, R. (1993). The pathogenesis of atherosclerosis—a perspective for the 1990's. *Nature*, **362**, 801–9.

Small, D. (1988). Progression and regression of atherosclerotic lesions. *Arteriosclerosis*, **8**, 103–129.

Stary, H. (1992). Composition and classification of human atherosclerotic lesions. *Virchows Archiv. Section A: Pathological Anatomy and Histology*, **421**, 277–290.

Weisman, H. and Healy, B. (1987). Myocardial infarct expansion, infarct extension and reinfarction—pathophysiologic concepts. *Progress in Cardiovascular Disease*, **30**, 73–110.

Witztum, J. (1993). Role of oxidised low density lipoprotein in atherogenesis. *British Heart Journal*, **69**, S12–S18.

15.10.3 Angina and unstable angina

R.H. SWANTON

On the 21 July 1768 William Heberden read to the College of Physicians his famous dissertation describing a symptom he called angina: There is a disorder of the breast marked with a strong and peculiar symptoms considerable for the kind of danger belonging to it and not extremely rare of which I do not recollect any mention among medical authors. The seat of it and sense of strangling and anxiety with which it is attended may make it not improperly be called Angina pectoris. Those who are afflicted with it, are seized, while they are walking, and more particularly when they walk soon after eating with a painful and most disagreeable sensation in the breast ... His description has never been equalled and remains as accurate today as then.

Stable angina

Angina is a symptom characterized by a heaviness in the centre of the chest induced by effort or emotional upset. The sensation has been variously described as squeezing, crushing, gripping, band-like, choking, throttling, or a vice-like grip. Patients describe it as a great weight on their chest. It is typically central and symmetrical. In its early stages it is a discomfort rather than a pain. The sensation may radiate up the neck and throat into the jaws and ears and down both arms to the wrists. It does not usually reach the fingers. It may spread round to the back and into the epigastrium and both subcostal regions. Occasionally it may present only as an ache in the jaw or the wrist and forearm, without chest symptoms but always the relation to effort is the clue. As in Heberden's description it is usually worse if exercise is taken after meals, in the cold weather, or against a strong wind. It is more troublesome at high altitude. Patients may find that they can walk through their angina and continue to exercise without getting it again. Angina may be precipitated by a variety of emotional stresses such as arguments, watching exciting television, waiting in traffic jams, or by sexual intercourse. Essentially stable angina is predictable and is always relieved by rest; patients can learn to avoid it by modification of lifestyle.

Nocturnal or decubitus angina is as a more serious symptom and may start as the patient's condition deteriorates. It may be precipitated by lying down in cold sheets, by tachycardia induced by dreaming, by alterations in coronary tone, or by the increase in wall stress of the left ventricle caused by an increase in end-diastolic volume when lying down. It may be partly related to the diurnal variation in blood pressure which starts to rise from about 4 to 5 a.m. It is relieved by sitting or standing up.

Atypical chest pain is characterized by a unilateral left submammary pain, sometimes sharp in quality, which radiates up to the left shoulder and left axilla. It does not bear a close relation to effort and may be sharp in quality. It is asymmetrical and often localised to a small area in the left chest. These symptoms are rarely anginal in origin.

Unstable angina

This term has taken over from crescendo angina, pre-infarction angina, acute coronary insufficiency, and intermediate coronary syndrome. Angina is said to be unstable when it occurs with increasing frequency and severity. The pain is more prolonged and is not quickly relieved by nitrates. It is no longer predictable and comes on at rest with no obvious precipitating factors. It is associated with ST segment depression and T wave inversion on the electrocardiograph. Other electrocardiographic changes may occur, such as the development of transient bundle branch block or ventricular arrhythmias. It may be the prelude to an acute myocardial infarction and is an indication for hospital admission, when differentiation from myocardial infarction may require measurement of cardiac enzymes, which should not exceed twice the upper limit of the normal range.

Variant angina

First described by Prinzmetal in 1959 this term refers to a rare form of angina induced by coronary spasm. The pain comes on at rest unpredictably and is associated with ST segment elevation on the electrocardiograph. The ST elevation indicates total coronary occlusion. It may cluster in the early morning and raised levels of endothelin have been found in the plasma in patients with Prinzmetal angina during pain. Spasm may not always be relieved by nitrates and can cause arrhythmias or myocardial infarction. In many cases of variant angina coronary spasm is associated with atherosclerotic lesions. Spasm in the presence of angiographically normal arteries is rare. The stimulus which causes spasm is completely unknown. The role of vasoactive substances in altering coronary tone is discussed below. Very occasionally patients appear to have a vasospastic tendency with a history of migraine and Raynaud's phenomenon.

Differential diagnosis

Pericarditis may cause symptoms very similar to those of angina. The pain is more prolonged, not related to effort and has two additional typical features. Pericardial pain is typically postural being relieved by sitting forward, and worse lying down. Second, a 'pleuritic' element is common; the pain being worse on deep breathing. The illness is usually associated with other systemic features and a fever.

Oesophagitis can be difficult to distinguish as its pain is also central, radiating up to the throat and back. However, it is often more burning in quality, brought on by stooping, lying down, heavy lifting, and straining. It is like the pain of drinking very hot fluids. It may be associated with acid reflux, a bitter taste in the mouth, and relieved by alkalis. It may start at night on lying down. It is uncommon for oesophageal pain to radiate down the arms. Patients may describe regurgitation and occasionally true dysphagia. Reflux may be induced by vigorous exercise which can make the distinction with angina more difficult. Diffuse oesophageal spasm produces quite severe sudden retrosternal pain which may be relieved by nitrates. This can cause particular diagnostic difficulty, but the pain is not effort-related.

Thoracic root pain is typically asymmetrical, affecting one side of the chest, radiating around from the back. The pain may only be felt at the front. It is made worse by twisting or lateral flexion of the thorax and is a continuous ache unrelieved by rest. It may be the cause of the atypical symptoms described above. If the thoracic root pain is due to wedge compression of a vertebra (e.g. osteoporosis or malignant disease) there will be associated localized pain over the relevant vertebral body.

Acute pulmonary embolism may cause pleuritic pain, dyspnoea, and haemoptysis if the embolus is small and peripheral. Involvement of the diaphragmatic pleura will produce shoulder tip pain. Large central pulmonary emboli result in extreme anguish, dyspnoea, hypotension, syncope, and a shocked patient, but pain is not a typical feature.

Dissecting thoracic aortic aneurysm produces a particularly severe sudden tearing pain in the central and left chest. It is continuous, unrelieved by rest or position, and often associated with shock. The pain may radiate into the neck, abdomen, and through to the back. Its sudden onset and its severity are its most typical features. A leaking aneurysm may occasionally produce pleuritic pain also, and dissection around a coronary ostium will induce true cardiac pain. The pain may migrate as the dissection extends.

The pain from peptic ulceration may sometimes be confused with angina; it is central, felt in the epigastrium and lower chest, radiating through to the back, may be worse after meals and wake the patient at night. Peptic ulcer pain is episodic, and generally relieved by alkalis. The relation to meals is much closer than anginal pain and ulcer pain is more protracted.

Very occasionally the pain of cholecystitis or pancreatitis may be confused with cardiac pain. The pain of cholecystitis is usually in the right hypochondrium with referred pain in the right shoulder tip. It is associated with nausea, vomiting, and a febrile illness. Acute pancreatitis produces a severe central and upper abdominal pain radiating through to the centre of the back which may be partially relieved by sitting hunched forward.

Pathophysiology of angina

Ischaemia develops if myocardial oxygen demand exceeds supply. Breakdown of high energy phosphates and of phosphocreatinine occurs first. An intracellular acidosis develops rapidly with the release of potassium ions, protons, and lactic acid from the cell. These changes precede

ST segment depression on the electrocardiograph, which in turn precedes angina. This sequence of events is sometimes referred to as the ischaemic cascade. ST segment depression without pain is termed silent ischaemia. Oxygen supply to cardiac muscle is increased by increasing coronary flow (autoregulation) rather than by increasing oxygen extraction from coronary arterial blood. Coronary arteriovenous O_2 difference remains relatively constant at about 11 ml per 100 ml of blood. Coronary venous blood (sampled from the coronary sinus) should not contain any excess of lactic acid, as the heart can use arterial lactate under normal conditions as a fuel. Abnormal myocardial metabolism is said to occur if fractional extraction of lactate from the arterial blood is less than 10 per cent.

The three prime determinants of myocardial oxygen demand (MVO_2) are heart rate, contractility, and wall stress. Wall stress is directly proportional to ventricular volume and ventricular pressure and inversely proportional to wall thickness. An increase in heart rate, contractility, ventricular volume or pressure will increase myocardial oxygen demand and may upset the supply/demand balance causing angina. Increased myocardial oxygen demand results in autoregulatory coronary vasodilatation and a consequent increase in coronary flow. The signal for this dilatation is probably adenosine released from the myocardial cell which acts on adjacent cells by a paracrine mechanism. This is the ideal messenger having a very short 2 to 10-s half-life. Adenosine deaminase on the surface of red cells rapidly converts adenosine to inosine. Adenosine is thought to be the cause of anginal pain when released from the ischaemic cell – acting as a self-protecting mechanism. Other metabolites released from the ischaemic cell cause vasodilatation, e.g. prostaglandin E series, lactate, bradykinin, hydrogen ions, and carbon dioxide. However, it is felt that adenosine is the essential dilating mediator.

Coronary flow depends on a pressure gradient between the aorta and the intramyocardial coronary arteriole which is determined by ventricular pressure. Systole compresses the intramyocardial coronary arteries and during the ejection phase of systole aortic and ventricular pressures are identical. Coronary flow is thus almost entirely diastolic, occuring when aortic diastolic pressure exceeds ventricular diastolic pressure. A reduction of this coronary gradient will reduce coronary flow and may result in angina. This occurs in aortic stenosis when aortic perfusion pressure is low and left ventricular diastolic pressure high. Tachycardia will shorten diastole relative to systole reducing the time for coronary flow. Thus even the normal patient may get angina in extreme paroxysmal tachycardia.

High intracavity left ventricular pressures such as occur in hypertension, aortic valve stenosis or hypertrophic obstructive cardiomyopathy result in high left ventricular wall stress and hence possible angina even in the presence of normal coronary arteries. Left ventricular hypertrophy which increases wall thickness cannot compensate for the increase in wall stress due to the high intracavity pressure. Angina may rarely occur in severe pulmonary hypertension with high right ventricular wall stress, a low cardiac output and low aortic perfusion pressure on exercise.

Oxygen supply will be reduced in anaemia with the resultant reduction in oxygen carrying capacity of the blood. When fully saturated, each gram of haemoglobin can carry 1.34 ml of oxygen. The normal oxygen carrying capacity of arterial blood is thus approximately 20 ml/100 ml, allowing for a small plasma correction factor. This will be directly proportional to the haemoglobin level and anaemia with levels of 7 to 8 g/100 g or less can provoke angina with normal coronary arteries as coronary arteriovenous O_2 difference remains constant.

Angina may be provoked by coronary obstructive lesions which reduce coronary flow and prevent the required autoregulatory increase on exercise. These may be atherosclerotic, embolic, or thrombotic. These usually involve the large epicardial coronary arteries. Microvascular angina is due to disease of the tiny intramural coronary arteries (less than 100 μm) invisible on the coronary angiogram and may account for the angina occuring in patients with seemingly normal coronary arteriograms but a positive exercise test (syndrome X).

Regulation of coronary tone

Coronary artery smooth muscle is under the influence of humoral and neurogenic control mechanisms. Minor alterations in coronary artery tone can have profound effects on coronary flow as flow is proportional to the fourth power of the radius. This is particularly important where coronary flow is already compromised by obstructive atherosclerotic lesions. The epicardial coronary arteries contain sympathetic ($\alpha > \beta1 > \beta2$), glucagon, dopamine, and histamine receptors. The coronary vascular endothelium itself also plays a vital role in controlling coronary tone. The four most important vasoactive substances produced by the endothelium are: endothelium derived relaxing factor (EDRF) now known to be nitric oxide, prostacyclin (PGI_2) which are both vasodilatory and balanced by the potent vasoconstrictors endothelin and thromboxane (TXA_2).

The presence of an intact endothelium is essential for the correct function of some vasodilators: acetylcholine and 5-hydroxytryptamine in the presence of an intact endothelium cause vasodilatation (via endothelium derived relaxing factor release) but, in the presence of a damaged or denuded endothelium, cause vasoconstriction. Some vasodilators are endothelium independent (e.g. organic nitrates and isoprenaline). There is a finely regulated balance between constriction and dilatation. The humoral and paracrine control mechanisms are more important than the neurogenic mechanisms. The short half lives of many of the messengers (endothelium derived relaxing factor, prostacyclin, adenosine) allows for immediate fine tuning of coronary flow. The role of peptides with longer half-lives, such as endothelin, remains incompletely understood. Table 1 summarizes the more important coronary tone regulators and the drugs involved. Figure 1 shows the main pathways by which agents cause vascular smooth muscle relaxation and vasodilatation.

Pathophysiology of unstable angina

The advent of coronary angioscopy has shed some light on why angina becomes unstable. Forrester and his colleagues have clearly demonstrated the presence of microthrombi at the site of a coronary stenosis. This was first demonstrated using the angioscope in theatre just prior to coronary bypass surgery in a patient with unstable angina. It is thought that the plaque becomes unstable and a tiny dissection occurs. This is followed by platelet activation, and the formation of microthrombi at the site of the dissection. As well as causing narrowing of the remaining lumen, platelet activation results in the release of vasoactive substances such as thromboxane A_2. The damaged endothelium fails to release its vasodilating peptides and endothelium derived relaxing factor, with resultant coronary constriction. The initial management of unstable angina depends on preventing the development of microthrombi and reversing any coronary spasm or constriction.

Silent ischaemia

It is now recognized that ST depression on the electrocardiograph, and demonstrable reductions in myocardial perfusion on thallium–201 scanning associated with this may occur in the absence of any cardiac symptoms. This can be documented on 24-h Holter monitoring using FM recording equipment or on exercise testing. Silent ST depression has been found in 2.5 per cent of the male population.

Silent ischaemia occurs in patients with chronic stable angina and up to 75 per cent of episodes of ST depression on 24-h Holter monitoring may be silent. Generally the more severe the ST depression the more likely it is to be felt by the patient as angina. The frequency of silent ischaemia on the 24-h tape parallels the exercise test result: the more positive the exercise test and the worse the exercise tolerance the greater the incidence of silent ischaemia.

Silent ischaemia on Holter monitoring occurs more commonly in the morning. This circadian rhythm is mirrored by the increased incidence

Table 1 *Regulators of coronary tone*

Vasoconstrictors

Mechanical	Systolic compression (intramural arteries)
	Muscle bridge (epicardial artery)
α-Adrenoceptor agonists	Noradrenaline
	Adrenaline
	High dose dopamine (> 15 μg/kg/min) via noradrenaline
	Ergotamine, ergonovine (partial α agonist and 5-HT$_2$ agonist)
Endothelium produced	Thromboxane A$_2$ (and from platelets)
	Endothelin
	Prostaglandin F series
Adventitial nerve plexus	Neuropeptide Y
Other hormones	Vasopressin
	Angiotensin II

Vasodilators

Mechanical	Diastolic relaxation
Metabolites from ischaemic myocardium	Adenosine, bradykinin, CO_2, H^+
α-Receptor antagonists	Prazosin, phenoxybenzamine
Angiotensin II antagonists	Captopril, enalapril
β-Receptor agonists	($\beta_1 - \beta_2$), e.g. dobutamine, isoprenaline
Dopamine receptor agonist	Low dose dopamine (<5 ug/kg/min)
Phosphodiesterase inhibitors	Papaverine, methylxanthines (aminophylline)
Voltage-dependent calcium channel blockers	Nifedipine, diltiazem, verapamil.
Potassium channel openers	Minoxidil, nicorandil, diazoxide
Purine receptor agonist	Adenosine (A$_2$ receptor)
Direct stimulator of intracellular cyclic GMP:	Nitrates, atrial natriuretic peptide
Endothelium produced	Endothelium derived relaxing factor: nitric oxide, prostacyclin (PGI$_2$)
	Calcitonin gene-related peptide (CGRP)
	Substance P
	Vasoactive intestinal peptide (VIP)
	Prostaglandin E series

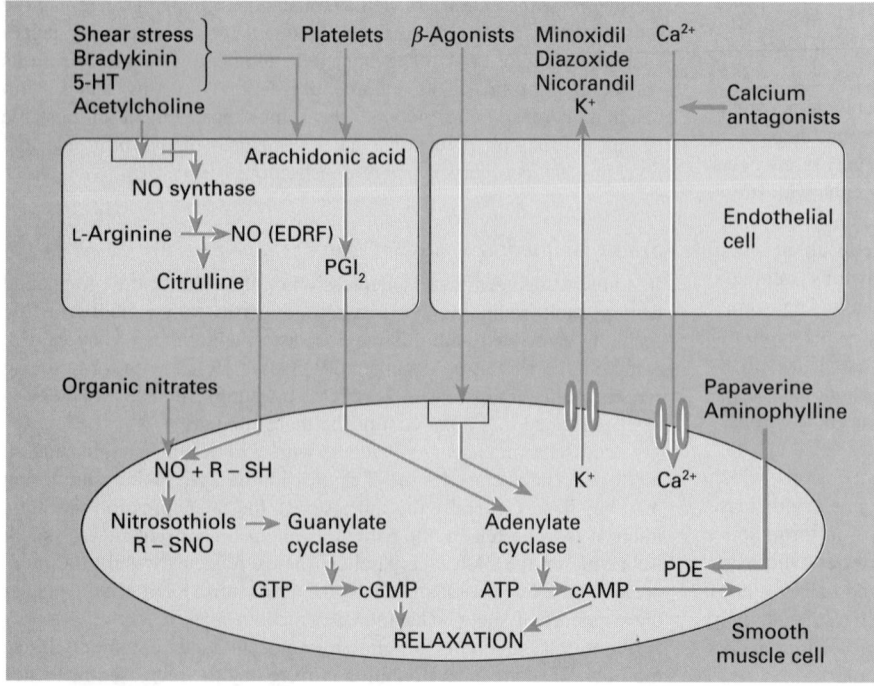

Fig. 1 Action of vasodilators on smooth muscle cell. Drug action may increase the activity of either guanylate cyclase or adenylate cyclase increasing intracellular cGMP or cAMP. Papaverine and aminophylline inhibit phosphodiesterase, which breaks down cyclic AMP. Calcium antagonists reduce influx of calcium ions and potassium channel openers increase potassium efflux hyperpolarizing the cell. cAMP, cyclic adenosine monophosphate; cGMP, cyclic guanyl monophosphate; EDRF, endothelial derived relaxant factor; NO, nitric oxide; PGI$_2$, prostacyclin; PDE, phosphodiesterase.

of myocardial infarction in the morning, and by the circadian increase in blood pressure in the early morning. It occurs in about 10 per cent of patients following myocardial infarction and has prognostic significance in this group.

Conventional treatment for stable angina reduces episodes of silent ischaemia. β-blockade reduces the early morning peak of ST depression. Episodes of profound silent ST depression should be investigated and treated as if they were episodes of painful ischaemia. Both represent reductions in myocardial perfusion and have the same prognostic significance.

Angina with angiographically normal coronary arteries

There is no doubt that there this a group of patients who give a history of angina but who on subsequent investigation appear to have normal coronary arteries angiographically. A few of these patients will turn out to have non-cardiac pain but many have genuine angina and respond to anti-anginal therapy. It is important to remember that frequent history taking by different doctors will educate the patient and the history may be changed unwittingly under the influence of leading questions, which must be avoided.

In addition a small number of patients who have had a myocardial infarction with demonstrable segmental abnormalities of left ventricular wall motion on left ventricular angiography appear to have normal coronary arteries angiographically. These are often young patients and may be heavy smokers; they may be women on the contraceptive pill. It is possible some of these cases have a thrombotic or procoagulable state and that their infarct was due to thrombus formation within the coronary artery. Spontaneous lysis may then have occured and on later coronary angiography the artery appears normal. Conditions which need to be excluded are polycythaemia, thrombocythaemia, antithrombin III deficiency, protein C or protein S deficiency, and the presence of the lupus anticoagulant. However even after a procoagulable state has been excluded no cause may be apparent. Table 2 summarizes the more common causes of angina with normal coronary arteries.

SYNDROME X

This term has been used since 1981 to describe a group of patients with angina, a positive exercise test, and a normal coronary arteriogram. The patients are often middle-aged women. They probably represent a heterogeneous group but the cause of their angina is unknown. There is evidence to suggest that the problem lies with the microvasculature (arterioles less than 100 μm in diameter) and that their angina is ischaemic. Vessels of this size cannot be seen on the coronary angiogram. There seems to be an abnormality of coronary flow reserve on effort: possibly due to a failure of dilatation or a diffuse fixed obstruction. Cardiac biopsies have shown abnormal intramural arteries and ischaemia has been shown in some studies with atrial pacing and coronary sinus lactate measurements. Perfusion abnormalities have been seen on thallium−201 scanning. On angiography, abnormally slow flow down the large epicardial coronary arteries is often seen. Abnormalities of both systolic function and diastolic function have been described with abnormal left ventricular filling rates and high end-diastolic pressures. Finally on cardiac biopsies abnormalities in the cellular ultrastructure have been noted with mitochondrial swelling.

It is important that patients with syndrome X are not dismissed as of no consequence. Their angina is genuine and merits treatment. Patients can be reassured that the prognosis is good.

Examination of the patient with stable angina

In the general examination it is important to exclude any possible precipitating factors such as anaemia, thyrotoxicosis, myxoedema, or rarely a high output state. Signs of hyperlipidaemia are sought: arcus senilis or xanthelasma in a young patient (under 40 years of age), tendon xan-

Table 2 *Causes of angina with normal coronary arteries*

Non-cardiac causes
  Bad history. No angina at all
  Musculoskeletal pain
  Anxiety and hyperventilation
  Thoracic root pain
  Cervical root pain
  Gastritis/peptic ulcer
  Oesophagitis
  Diffuse oesophageal spasm
  Anaemia
  Thyrotoxicosis

Cardiac causes
  Angiogram misinterpretation, e.g.
    ostial lesion
    lesion right at origin of a branch
    lesion masked by vessel overlap
  Coronary arteritis
  Coronary spasm
  Small vessel disease
  Coronary emboli, e.g. from:
    atrial myxoma
    mural thrombus
    valve vegetation
  Aortic valve stenosis
  Hypertrophic obstructive cardiomyopathy
  Syndrome X
  Procoagulable state

thomata, ear lobe crease, or orange palmar crease. Some types of hyperlipidaemia are associated with gout. It is important to exclude conditions which cause angina with normal coronary arteries: aortic valve stenosis, hypertrophic cardiomyopathy (with or without obstruction), and hypertension with a vigorous ventricle. Paroxysmal tachycardia may also produce angina and bursts of tachycardia during the examination should be pursued with a 24-h Holter monitor.

The blood pressure is taken in both arms after 5 min rest in the sitting patient. Hypertension may also be a feature of hypertrophic cardiomyopathy and aortic coarctation. Particular attention is paid to the arterial pulses. The brachial artery may appear thick, wiry, tortuous, and arteriosclerotic. The quality of the pulse is vital as an anacrotic carotid pulse is the most reliable sign of aortic stenosis. The upstroke of the pulse in hypertrophic cardiomyopthy is characteristically brisk and jerky. Sometimes there is a double pulse with a percussion wave followed by a large tidal wave. The carotid, femoral, and iliac arteries should be auscultated for bruits. Absent, weak, or delayed peripheral pulses are noted. An attempt should be made to feel the abdominal aorta and, if there is doubt about its size, ultrasound performed to check its transverse dimension. There may be a systolic thrill in the aortic area and the root of the neck in patients with aortic valve stenosis, and rarely a thrill at the left sternal edge in patients with hypertrophic obstructive cardiomyopathy.

The apex beat may yield some clues. Left ventricular hypertrophy occurs with hypertension and aortic stenosis at any level. Signs of left ventricular cavity enlargement suggest aortic or mitral regurgitation or left ventricular failure. The apex beat of an anteroapical left ventricular aneurysm is high and dyskinetic. A diffuse pulsation is felt at or above the left nipple. The apex beat of an inferobasal aneurysm is usually unremarkable. In hypertension, aortic stenosis and hypertrophic cardiomyopathy in sinus rhythm in thin patients a double apex can often be felt with an 'a' wave preceding the ventricular thrust.

Aortic stenosis is associated with an aortic systolic ejection murmur. The valve is usually calcified by the time the patient develops angina resulting in the disappearance of the aortic ejection click in a bicuspid valve and a very soft or absent aortic second sound. Angina is uncommon but not unknown in aortic regurgitation. Rarely angina in aortic regurgitation is due to syphilitic ostial stenosis. A history of angina in the presence of mitral regurgitation suggests an ischaemic origin for the mitral regurgitation (papillary muscle dysfunction).

The fundi are closely examined for signs of hypertensive or diabetic retinopathy. The urine is checked for protein and sugar.

Myocardial perfusion scanning

In some cases cardiac catheterization can be avoided by combining an exercise test with myocardial perfusion imaging using thallium−201 tomography. This increases the specificity of a positive exercise test and an entirely normal thallium scan makes it very likely that a positive treadmill tests was a false positive. Tomography increases the sensitivity of the test over planar imaging. This, and related techniques are discussed more fully in Chapter 15.4.4.

The value of thallium scanning in the diagnosis and management of angina is considerable. In younger patients with a low likelihood of coronary disease and no risk factors it may be the only investigation needed if the treadmill test is positive and the thallium scan is negative. A normal stress thallium scan makes it extremely unlikely that a patient has coronary disease, whatever the history and treadmill exercise test show. It may confirm that a patient has reversible ischaemia or has had an infarct when this cannot be shown on the electrocardiograph (e.g. in left bundle branch block, or with pre-excitation). In patients who have had coronary arteriography it may identify which lesion or lesions is likely to be the cause of the patients symptoms – the culprit lesion – which can be a very useful guide to the physician performing angioplasty or to the surgeon performing bypass surgery. The size of the defect(s) has prognostic implications: large defects or high lung uptake of thallium indicating a poor prognosis. Recently, reinjection of thallium may help to identify stunned myocardium which was initially thought to be dead scar tissue, but which may merit bypass grafting.

Unfortunately, thallium defects are not 100 per cent specific for coronary disease. They can occur in patients with normal coronary arteries angiographically in certain circumstances. Small defects may occur in left ventricular hypertrophy, hypertrophic cardiomyopathy, syndrome X, myocardial infiltration and even in left bundle branch block itself at high heart rates. Nevertheless it remains a most valuable diagnostic technique.

Management of stable angina

Once the diagnosis of angina has been made the first stage in management involves alteration of the patient's lifestyle, coupled with drug therapy. If, despite adequate drug therapy and modification of life-style, angina is still unsatisfactorily controlled, coronary angiography with a view to coronary angioplasty or coronary artery bypass surgery is the next step.

LIFESTYLE CHANGES

Modification of lifestyle is inevitable in patients who have angina and the physician can get an idea of how troublesome the symptoms are by what has had to be given up in order to control symptoms. Patients often report having to give up running, skiing, all sport, gardening, bed-making, and hoovering the house. With increasing symptoms, cycling, walking the dog, driving, sexual intercourse, and work are added to the list. With medical treatment it should be possible for patients to enjoy all these activities, with the exception of vigorous contact sports and squash, which should be prohibited. Advice should be given in the presence of a partner or close relative.

The patient must be strongly advised to give up smoking completely from the moment the diagnosis is suspected. Nicotine causes a tachycardia and may increase coronary tone. Increased levels of arterial levels of carbon monoxide in smokers reduce myocardial oxygen supply.

Patients often complain about weight gain on giving up smoking but the adverse effects of obesity are trivial in comparison to the benefits that can be expected from giving up smoking. Even so, every attempt should be made to control weight. Its loss often has a major effect on symptom control and improvement in exercise tolerance, as well as contributing to a reduction in serum concentrations of cholesterol and triglycerides. Very mild exercise after large meals may provoke angina. Once the lipid levels are known more specific dietary advice may be given. Generally a low saturated fat diet is recommended, with high fibre content and plenty of fruit and green vegetables. It is thought that vitamins C and E have an important antioxidant role and may help prevent the oxidation of low density lipoproteins in the arterial cell wall.

Alcohol can be continued in moderation but intake should not exceed more than two to three units per day, as more contributes to weight gain and large amounts may increase arterial pressure and can cause a dilated cardiomyopathy.

Work is the single greatest cause for anxiety. Some jobs will have to be given up at least temporarily by law: air-line pilots, air traffic controllers, divers, and heavy goods vehicle drivers. Coronary angiography is necessary for patients with these jobs, however mild their symptoms. Other jobs are clearly unsuitable: e.g. furniture removers, scaffolders, and miners. Redeployment must be considered for individuals with heavy physical jobs, but in the present economic climate this is often impossible. In some cases early retirement is necessary and grasped eagerly by patients with exacting jobs and bad symptoms. It may be a mistake to encourage early retirement for a patient whose angina may subsequently be completely relieved by angioplasty or surgery. It is generally better to defer any decision until after this.

Driving in a private car may be continued unless traffic induces angina. Flight as an airline passenger is not contraindicated provided the angina is only mild and and stable. With moderate or severe symptoms flying should be discouraged. The airline medical personnel should be informed, the patient should carry very little luggage and should be well insured for medical treatment abroad. An adequate supply of medication should be taken, with a reserve for any travel delays.

Vigorous competitive sports should stop. Regular daily exercise within the angina threshold should be encouraged with daily walks taking glyceryl trinitrate prophylactically. On cold or very windy days the walks should be postponed. Swimming is allowed if the angina is stable. The patient should not dive, never swim alone, and swim only in heated pools. Scuba diving is prohibited. Sexual intercourse should be discussed, as the subject is often avoided by an anxious patient. It should be encouraged provided that the angina is stable and exercise tolerance is reasonable (e.g. able to climb two flights of stairs without pain). Glyceryl trinitrate prophylaxis may be helpful but both anxiety and/or β-blockade may cause impotence.

Drug treatment

The most important types of drugs available for the treatment of angina are the nitrates, the β-adrenoceptor anatagonists, the calcium channel blocking agents, and potassium channel openers. Often agents from all groups are used together and their actions are complementary and synergistic. Additional diuretic or antihypertensive therapy may be needed. Patients should be warned about common side-effects on starting the medication, and compliance is often better if a small dose is started initially with relatively few side-effects.

NITRATES

The first drugs available for angina were introduced over a century ago, and Lauder Brunton's observations in 1867 as to the mode of action of amyl nitrite are still relevant today. Nitrates dilate both venous capacitance and arteriolar resistance vessels, but their action on the venous system is thought to be the more important. Nitrates cause coronary dilatation independant of endothelial cell function by increasing intracellular cyclic guanylate cyclase (cGMP), which results in smooth muscle relaxation. The release of the nitrite ion within the cell from organic nitrates requires tissue sulphydryl (—SH) groups. The formation of intracellular nitrosothiols results in stimulation of guanylate cyclase which increases cyclic guanylate cyclase synthesis. The exact mechanism whereby this induces relaxation of the contractile proteins is still not completely understood.

Nitrates reduce the preload by dilating the venous capacitance vessels in both systemic and pulmonary circuits. This reduces the ventricular diastolic pressure and volume, reducing diastolic wall stress in both ventricles. The arteriolar dilatation reduces arterial tone, reducing afterload, which in turn reduces systolic wall stress. A reduction in myocardial oxygen demand is the result. In addition there is a redistribution of coronary flow with an improvement in subendocardial flow partly due to the fall in intracavity pressure and partly due to a direct effect on reducing coronary tone particularly in collateral vessels. Overall coronary flow is increased in the normal heart but may not increase much in the ischaemic heart. Two cardiac effects, however, may be disadvantageous. The first is a reflex tachycardia due to a fall in arterial pressure, and the second is a reduction in coronary perfusion pressure as the aortic pressure falls slightly. The reduction in myocardial oxygen demand, however, usually greatly outweighs these disadvantages. Nitrates will, of course, also help relieve oesophageal spasm and biliary or renal colic. Overall they are of great value in the management of angina, and their haemodynamic effects on venous capacitance vessels makes them invaluable in the management of acute left ventricular failure.

Nitrates can be administered sublingually in tablet or spray form, beneath the upper lip in tablet form (buccally), orally, transdermally or intravenously.

Sublingual glyceryl trinitrate

This is given as a 0.5 mg tablet. The effect lasts about 30 min and often produces a transient headache and facial flushing, as well as relief of angina, with cerebral vasodilatation. This is its most limiting side-effect and often deters patients from using it. Some patients feel nauseated after taking it. Patients should be told to spit the tablet out as soon as their angina is relieved, as this will help curtail the headache; swallowing the tablet also inactivates it, as sublingual glyceryl trinitrate, unlike isosorbide preparations is rapidly converted to inactive inorganic nitrite in the liver.

Patients should also be told to renew their supply of sublingual glyceryl trinitrate every 6 months, and to keep the tablets in an air-tight container. Cotton wool or other drugs should not be put in the bottle. Glyceryl trinitrate tablets should produce a very slight burning sensation under the tongue. Patients should be told to take them prophylactically: one taken before exercise often prevents angina completely. They should be warned that taking too many in hot atmospheres will cause postural hypotension and syncope. If the angina is severe glyceryl trinitrate may be chewed to speed up buccal absorption. The tablets are not addictive and tolerance is not a problem in a drug with such a short half-life. Patients should be told that there is no need to limit their use of glyceryl trinitrate, but that they should keep a record of daily consumption. This is a valuable indication of change in the severity of symptoms. Generally not more than three glyceryl trinitrate tablets, or three metered squirts from the spray, should be taken at once. There is a theoretical risk of methaemoglobinaemia with very high nitrate consumption, but this is very rare in clinical practice.

Nitrates should be avoided if the angina is due to aortic stenosis. In aortic valve stenosis peripheral vasodilatation may provoke hypotension and syncope, and in muscular subaortic stenosis nitrates increase the outflow tract gradient. Care must also be taken in prescribing nitrates to patients with cerebral arteriosclerosis or severe carotid stenoses, as hypotension may provoke cerebral ischaemia. Similarly, nitrates will provoke hypotension in patients with severe mitral stenosis, and they are not indicated when the angina is due to anaemia.

Many patients prefer a glyceryl trinitrate spray to tablets. The spray (in metered doses of 0.4 mg) is quicker and easier to use. Less dexterity is needed in a hurry and the spray is absorbed quicker in the mouth than the tablet. The shelf-life of the spray is longer: about 3 years. A disadvantage for those with headache as a severe side-effect is that the spray cannot be spat out once the angina has been relieved.

Transdermal nitrates

A slow release transdermal nitrate preparation is popular with some patients; 5 or 10 mg patches are available and the patch applied once daily. They provide a continuous low plasma nitrate level (0.1 to 0.2 ng/ml), which helps prevent angina. The patches are waterproof. Patients should be instructed to take them off before going to bed to avoid nitrate tolerance (see below). Alternatively, the patch can be used only at night to help prevent decubitus angina. The patch should be applied to a different part of the skin each day to avoid erythemas. Skin sensitivity is uncommon. Dry, cracked, or ichthyotic skin should be avoided as absorption is then too rapid. If the patient has unpleasant side-effects the plaster is simply removed: a great advantage over oral preparations. The patches are also useful in causing local vasodilatation over peripheral veins to help obtain and maintain venous access for intravenous drips.

A 2 per cent nitrate ointment is also available and approximately 1.25 cm of ointment is applied to the skin (equivalent to 8.3 mg) and covered with a dressing. The ointment is rather more messy than the patch and exact dosing is impossible.

Buccal nitrates

A buccal form of glyceryl trinitrate is available (1 to 5 mg tablets). The tablet is placed between the gum and the upper lip and slowly dissolves. This can be used one to three times a day, but is particularly useful for preventing nocturnal angina.

Oral nitrates

Isosorbide preparations are available in the mononitrate or dinitrate form. Both should be swallowed and one then rapidly absorbed. First-pass metabolism in the liver of the dinitrate preparation produces the active mononitrate, but a clear advantage in using the mononitrate preparation to avoid this first pass effect has not been proved. Half-life of isosorbide dinitrate is about 4 to 6 h. The drugs can be given up to three times a day but patients should be told to try and take their last dose by 6:00 p.m. (provided they do not have decubitus angina) to allow for a nitrate-free period at night to avoid nitrate tolerance. Long-acting preparations are popular and may extend the drugs' action to 12 h. Typical dosing schedules are:

> Isosorbide dinitrate 10 to 20 mg b.d. or t.d.s. Retard preparations 20 to 40 mg o.d. or b.d.
> Isosorbide mononitrate 10 to 20 mg b.d. or t.d.s. Retard preparations 25 to 60 mg o.d. or b.d.

Intravenous nitrates

These are useful for the management of unstable angina and acute left ventricular failure. There is little to choose between isosorbide dinitrate (dose 2 to 10 mg/h IV) and glyceryl trinitrate (dose 10 μg/min to 400 μg/min). Both will cause hypotension, tachycardia, and headache. Restlessness, nausea, and retching may also occur. Both are incompatible with polyvinyl chloride (PVC) infusion bags or giving sets as the drug is adsorbed and up to 30 per cent of the potency may be lost. Polyethylene tubing is not a problem and a rigid plastic syringe with an infusion pump and a polyethylene tube is satisfactory. Intravenous nitrates are best avoided in pregnancy, hypotensive patients, patients with closed angle glaucoma, and those with severe cerebrovascular disease.

Nitrate tolerance

This remains one of the drugs chief drawbacks of oral nitrate therapy, but is not a problem with short-acting sublingual preparations. It is probably due to a depletion of sulphydryl (—SH) groups needed for the production of nitrite ions. It occurs quickly on starting oral therapy (within a few days). It has been shown that repletion of sulphydryl groups with *N*-acetyl cysteine may help prevent nitrate tolerance but this approach is too unpalatable to be clinically useful. It is preferable to avoid nitrates for a part of the day as described above.

Angiotensin converting enzyme inhibitors do not prevent nitrate tolerance so that nitrate activation of the renin–angiotensin system is unlikely to be the cause of nitrate tolerance.

β-ADRENOCEPTOR ANTAGONISTS

These drugs, commonly known as β-blockers, are the mainstay of treatment for angina and achieve their effect by reducing two prime determinants of myocardial oxygen consumption: heart rate and myocardial contractility. They also reduce systolic wall stress by reducing afterload and arterial pressure and reduce plasma concentrations of free fatty acids, which may favour myocardial glucose metabolism with relative conservation of adenosine triphosphate.

Contraindications to β-blockade in relation to angina

β-Blocking agents may provoke left ventricular failure in patients with borderline left ventricular function and thus increase diastolic wall stress as left ventricular diastolic volume increases. They are contraindicated in patients with a recent history of left ventricular failure, a large heart on chest radiograph or when a third heart sound is present. Blocking β-2 receptors in the lung will precipitate acute bronchospasm in those patients with asthma or chronic bronchitis. β-Blockers are generally contraindicated in this group but small doses of a highly cardioselective drug (e.g. bisoprolol or celiprolol) may be tried with the greatest care in patients with mild airways obstruction provided lung function is carefully monitored. Patients with a history of severe asthmatic attacks or chronic bronchitis should never receive β-blocking agents, whether selective or not. A common problem is the patient with angina and intermittent claudication. The angina may be improved by β-blockade but the claudication made worse as β-2 receptor blockade causes peripheral vasoconstriction and peripheral flow is reduced still further by the inevitable reduction in cardiac output caused by beta blockade. Once again a highly cardioselective agent should be tried. Clearly any β-blocker is unsuitable for patients who have peripheral rest pain or gangrene.

Diabetes mellitus is not an absolute contraindication to β-blockade, but great care must be used in patients who are likely to have hypoglycaemic attacks. β-Blockade prevents the sympathetic response to hypoglycaemia and muscle glycogenolysis is mediated via β-2 receptors. Thus hypoglycaemia may be prolonged and the reactions to it such as tachycardia and sweating may be masked. A cardioselective agent should be used in diabetic patients.

β-Blockade should be avoided in patients with second or third degree atrioventricular block or sinoatrial disease without permanent pacing cover. The drugs should also be avoided in patients with a definite diagnosis of coronary spasm (Prinzmetal's angina) as β-blockade leaves α receptors unimpeded. Patients with Raynaud's phenomenon should receive calcium antagonists rather than β-blocking agents.

Ancillary properties

The antiarrhythmic effects of β-blockade are discussed in Chapter 15.8.1.

β-Blocking agents have a wide variety of ancillary properties some of which are unimportant clinically. The two important ancillary properties are fat solubility and cardioselectivity (see Table 3). Drugs with intrinsic sympathomimetic activity (partial agonist activity) will be less likely to cause a bradycardia at rest. Drugs with strong intrinsic sympathomimetic activity will be less powerful as β-blocking agents. There is a mild reduction in platelet stickiness which is useful in all types of angina.

Fat-soluble agents such as propranolol are useful in the prophylaxis of migraine and are more useful when angina is associated with excessive anxiety. First-pass metabolism occurs with fat-soluble agents and patients with liver disease should be on lower doses of these drugs or switched to a non-fat-soluble agent such as nadolol or pindolol, which are primarily excreted by the kidneys. The dose of these water soluble drugs should be reduced in renal failure.

Cardioselective β-Blocking agents primarily block β-1 receptors, with a lesser effect on β-2 receptors. No drug is absolutely β-1 specific but newer agents are increasingly so. Patients with cool peripheries, peripheral vascular disease, diabetes mellitus, or mild bronchospasm who merit β-blockade should be started on a cardioselective β-blocker.

Side-effects

The most common side-effect is fatigue and a profound feeling of lethargy and listlessness. This is most apparent in the first few weeks of therapy as β-blockade results in up-grading of the β receptors. Fat-soluble drugs can produce bad dreams or nightmares, a lack of concentration, and some patients feel a fall in intellect, although this is rare. Patients with these symptoms should be given non-fat-soluble agents such as sotalol, atenolol, or nadolol. Limitation of exercise tolerance is to be expected, and prevention of the increase in cardiac output on effort results in legs feeling like lead. Cold peripheries are common even with cardioselective drugs. Impotence is common and one of the principle reasons for non-compliance. Exacerbation of bronchospasm, intermittent claudication, and Raynaud's phenomenon has been described above. Increasing dyspnoea on β-blockade may be due to bronchospasm or the development of left ventricular failure. Withdrawal of a β-blocking agent due to a side-effect may result in a brisk deterioration of the patient's angina.

Prescribing a β-blocking agent for angina

There are 15 oral β-blocking agents available on the United Kingdom market (Table 3) and choice will largely be governed by experience. The ancillary properties discussed above and specific additional conditions are taken into account in making a decision. Generally patients with angina will need β-blockade round the clock and once-a-day dosage is often inadequate, in contrast to the effectiveness of single doses in control of arterial pressure.

The elderly tolerate β-blockade poorly and small doses must be chosen initially, e.g. metoprolol 25 mg thrice daily. Asymptomatic resting bradycardia is not an indication to reduce the dose and patients may need reassurance in this context.

Care is needed in combination therapy. β-Blockade is best avoided in patients on verapamil as the combined negative inotropic effect of the two drugs may provoke left ventricular failure. β-Blockade synergizes well with other calcium antagonists whose negative inotropic effect is less. The elderly patient on a diuretic may be at risk from postural hypotension and β-blockade will reduce any residual sympathetic response with resulting worsening of symptoms.

Overdose

Overdosage of β-blockade is treated initially with 1 to 2 mg intravenous atropine. If this is not effective 10 mg intravenous glucagon may be given, but it may be necessary to infuse isoprenaline by drip, and refractory cases need temporary pacing.

CALCIUM ANTAGONISTS

This is the third group of drugs widely used for the management of angina. There are several cell membrane channels whereby calcium gets into the myocardial or smooth muscle cell. The three principal ones are the sodium–calcium exchange channel, the receptor-operated channel activated by β-1 agonists, and the voltage-dependent channel which opens only on cell depolarization. Calcium antagonists only act on the

Table 3 *Principal properties of β-blocking agents*

Drug	Fat-soluble	Cardio-selective	Half-life (h)	Elimination route	First oral dose	IV dose over 5 min
Acebutolol	Yes	Yes	3	Hepatic 60% Renal 40%	100 mg t.d.s.	10–50 mg
Atenolol	No	Yes	6–9	Renal only	50 mg o.d.	2.5–10 mg
Betaxolol	Yes	Yes	15–22	Renal	10 mg o.d.	-
Bisoprolol	Yes	Yes	10–12	Renal 50% Hepatic 50%	5 mg o.d.	-
Carteolol	No	No	6–9 renal	Mainly	2.5 mg o.d.	-
Carvedilol	Yes	No	6–7	Hepatic	12.5 mg o.d.	-
Celiprolol	Yes	Yes+ β-2	5–6	Hepatic and renal	200 mg o.d.	-
Labetalol	Yes	No	3–4	Hepatic 90%	100 mg t.d.s.	50 mg
Metoprolol	Yes	Yes	3	Hepatic and renal	50 mg t.d.s.	1–10 mg
Nadolol	No	No	16–24	Renal only	40 mg o.d.	-
Oxprenolol	Yes	No	2	Hepatic	40 mg t.d.s.	1–10 mg
Penbutolol	Yes	No	5	Hepatic	20 mg o.d.	-
Pindolol	No	No	3–4	Hepatic and renal	5 mg t.d.s.	-
Propranolol	Yes	No	3-6	Hepatic 95%	40 mg t.d.s.	1–10 mg
Sotalol	No	No	12–15	Renal only	80 mg b.d.	10–20 mg
Timolol	Yes	No	4–6	Hepatic and renal	10 mg b.d.	0.5–1 mg

voltage-dependent channel and reduce the slow calcium current by slowing the rate of calcium entry in phase 2 (the plateau phase) of the action potential. They are grouped into class IV of the Vaughan-Williams classification of antiarrhythmic drugs.

There are at least three types of voltage-gated calcium channel, labelled L, N, and T, by Tsien and colleagues. The main channel in vascular smooth muscle is the L channel. The N channel regulates neurotransmitter release. Exact knowledge of the channels structure is still fragmentary, but depolarization of the channel is thought to open gates in the cell membrane regulated by proteins: the 'h' and 'm' gates. Some form of voltage sensor must exist in the channel.

There are numerous calcium antagonist drugs with remarkably different structures, which emphasizes our ignorance about the channel's structure. The three most common types of drug in use are the dihydropyridine group (e.g. nifedipine, nitrendipine, nicardipine) the phenylalkylamines (e.g. verapamil, prenylamine, gallopamil) and the benzothiazepines (e.g. diltiazem). Modification of the molecules of these drugs has produced longer acting agents (e.g. amlodipine, felodipine, nisoldipine) and some more specific for particular vascular beds (e.g. nimodipine and the cerebral circulation).

Indications for calcium antagonists

Calcium antagonists can be used as monotherapy for angina and are particularly useful where β-blockade is contraindicated. They are also useful in the elderly, in whom β-blockade is not always well tolerated. They can be used in combination with β-blockade and synergize usefully with them – each drug tending to cancel out the other's side-effects. The exception is verapamil, which should not be used with β-blockade. Calcium antagonists are the drugs of choice in variant angina (Prinzmetal's angina) and in angina due to syndrome X – microvascular angina.

Drugs which act on peripheral vascular beds (e.g. the dihydropyridines) are helpful in hypertension and occasionally also in Raynaud's phenomenon. Verapamil, with its potent negative inotropic effect, is useful in patients whose angina is due to hypertrophic obstructive cardiomyopathy or hypertension. Nimodipine appears to be the drug of choice in the prevention of vasospasm following subarachnoid haemor-

rhage. Verapamil has potent effects on delaying conduction in the atrioventricular node. It can be used in the management of atrial tachycardias but its value has been superceded by the advent of adenosine which has a much shorter half life and no negative inotropic action. The newer agent bepridil has both class III and class IV antiarrhythmic actions but its value has yet to be established.

Side-effects

The vasodilating properties of calcium antagonists often produce a facial flush, and sometimes headache and dizzyness. These symptoms tend to decrease within the first few weeks of therapy. Postural hypotension is possible. Gravitational peripheral ankle and shin oedema is common and does not respond well to diuretics. Gum hyperplasia is a less common side-effect. All calcium antagonists cause constipation and this may be their limiting side-effect, particularly in the elderly. Pruritus can occur with any of the agents. Palpitation due to reflex tachycardia is to be expected in those patients on dihydropyridines unless they are also on β-blockade. Some patients notice a diuretic effect with nifedipine. Left ventricular failure may be precipitated by any calcium antagonist (particularly verapamil) if used in patients with poor left ventricular function.

Contraindications to calcium antagonists

These are few. These drugs should be avoided in patients with poor left ventricular function if possible, but in difficult cases diltiazem can be tried with care. They should also be avoided in hypotensive patients, in pregnancy and in porphyria. They are contraindicated in second or third degree atrioventricular block, digoxin toxicity, and sinoatrial disease unless covered by a pacemaker. In the management of tachycardias verapamil should not be used in wide complex tachycardia – in case this is ventricular – although it is useful for fascicular tachycardia if this can be diagnosed accurately. Verapamil should not be used in the acute or chronic management of Wolff–Parkinson–White syndrome as, like digoxin, it may rarely accelerate conduction through the accessory pathway. Nifepidine and other dihydropyridines should be avoided in patients with hypertrophic obstructive cardiomyopathy as peripheral vasodilatation will increase the subaortic gradient.

Table 4 *Principle properties of calcium antagonists*

Drug	Diltiazem	Nifedipine	Verapamil
Peripheral vessels	+	+ + +	+
Coronary vessels	+ + +	+ +	+ +
Heart	↑↓	↑↑	↑↓
Atrioventricular node refractoriness	↑	–	↑↑
Negative inotropic effect	+	+	+ + +
Protein binding (%)	80	90	90
Half-life (h)	4	5	3–7
Metabolism	Extensively deacetylated	90% in urine	90% first-pass hepatic
Starting dose for angina	60 mg t.d.s.	10 mg t.d.s.	80 mg t.d.s.
Slow release dose	90 mg b.d.	20 mg o.d.	120 mg o.d.
Intracoronary dose	–	0.2 mg IC	–
Intravenous dose	–	–	1–10 mg IV
Therapeutic concentration (ug/l)	30–130	25–100	15–100

Verapamil undergoes hepatic first-pass metabolism and should not be used in the presence of severe liver dysfunction.

Currently used calcium antagonists are all excreted in breast milk but, in the case of diltiazem and verapamil, the amount is considered too small to be harmful.

Choice of agent (Table 4)

There is little to choose between nifedipine, diltiazem, and verapamil in the management of angina. All three drugs are rapidly absorbed in the gastrointestinal tract, are heavily protein-bound and have similar half-lives requiring three times a day administration. Delayed release preparations are available for all three drugs for once or twice a day administration or alternatively there are different agents with longer half lives, e.g. amlodipine, nisoldipine, or felodipine.

Diltiazem is the most cardiospecific calcium antagonist and causes fewer peripheral side-effects than nifedipine. However, it can result in a pruritic rash which resolves when the drug is stopped. If angina is associated with hypertension or Raynaud's phenomenon then nifedipine is the drug of choice. A 10 mg capsule of nifedipine can be chewed for buccal absorption and quick relief of angina. Verapamil should be considered where angina is associated with a vigorous left ventricle or hypertrophic cardiomyopathy.

POTASSIUM CHANNEL OPENERS

Opening the potassium channel leads to relaxation of vascular smooth muscle (Fig. 1). Nicorandil, a new potassium channel opener, reduces preload and afterload in a similar way to nitrates, but without the problem of tolerance. It can be used in combination with other antianginal agents or as monotherapy. It is well absorbed, only slightly protein bound, with a half life of 1 h. Twenty per cent is excreted as metabolites in the urine.

The starting dose is 10 mg twice daily to a maximum of 30 mg twice daily. Headache is a common early side-effect. As with calcium antagonists flushing, dizziness, and a reflex tachycardia may occur, and the drug should be avoided in patients with poor left ventricular function.

Management of unstable angina

Patients with unstable symptoms should be admitted for complete bed rest to a quiet part of the ward with effective electrocardiograph monitoring facilities. They should be lightly sedated and visitors should be restricted. A β-blocking agent without intrinsic sympathomimetic activity, should be supplemented with soluble aspirin 150 mg daily. There is evidence from at least three trials that aspirin reduces the incidence of both fatal and non-fatal myocardial infarction in unstable angina.

There is no evidence that heparin confers any benefit over and above aspirin, although in patients whose pain is not settling heparin is usually started at 1000 u/h to aim to keep the thrombin time 2 to 4 times normal. Although there are doubts about calcium antagonists in this situation most physicians will prescribe one, e.g. diltiazem 60 mg thrice daily or nifedipine retard preparation 10 to 20 mg twice daily. Nifedipine should not be used in unstable angina unless the patient is also on β-blockade. β-Blockade is avoided if the unstable angina is thought to be of the Prinzmetal type. If the patient does not settle rapidly on this regimen, intravenous nitrates are started, for example isosorbide dinitrate 2 mg/h intravenously increasing up to 10 mg/h if necessary. Surprisingly, in spite of the angioscopic evidence of microthrombi at the site of lesions in unstable angina, thrombolytic agents have not yet been shown to have any beneficial effect. When the patient settles with no further rest pain coronary angiography should be performed.

If pharmacological methods fail to control the angina an intra-aortic balloon pump must be considered, as this can improve symptoms quickly. It is rarely used in unstable angina as most patients settle on medical treatment. Cardiac catheterization can easily be performed through the other leg with the intra-aortic balloon *in situ* as the angiographic catheters easily slip past the balloon. Occasionally the pain does not settle and angiography has to be performed as an emergency. Coronary angioplasty may be necessary for unstable symptoms but the procedure carries a slightly greater risk in the unstable situation as recurrent thrombus forming at the angioplasty site may be a particular problem, despite the use of intravenous heparin given after the procedure.

Coronary arteriography in unstable angina will show significant coronary disease in 90 per cent of patients (of whom about 10 per cent will have left main stem stenosis). Approximately 10 per cent will have angiographically normal arteries.

As platelet activation is thought to play such a vital role in precipitating unstable angina, and as aspirin is such an effective drug, research into other antiplatelet agents continues. Monoclonal antibodies to platelet glycoprotein IIb/IIIa have been developed and trials of these agents in unstable angina have started. The antibody (called at present C7E3) prevents platelet degranulation and the release of thromboxane A_2.

Aims of medical treatment

Medical treatment should aim at greatly improving the patient's quality of life and exercise tolerance. It may be necessary to advise changes to a lighter physical job, but every attempt should be made to keep the patient in work. Angina must be kept stable and patients should be able to complete Stage 2 of the Bruce protocol on the exercise treadmill. Failure to achieve these goals means that medical treatment is inadequate or has failed. In this situation the patient is already on maximum triple therapy and should be referred to a cardiothoracic centre for coronary angiography with a view to coronary angioplasty or bypass surgery.

The prognosis for medically treated patients is improving and the annual mortality for single vessel coronary artery disease managed medically is 2 per cent or less and approximately 4 per cent for two vessel disease. The recent ACME trial comparing angioplasty and medical treatment in patients with stable angina due to single vessel coronary disease showed that patients had better exercise tolerance following angioplasty but that there was no difference in survival over the short time (6-month follow-up) of the trial. The cost of angioplasty was greater and there were more cardiac events in the angioplasty group. Results of further randomized trials comparing the long-term results of angioplasty against medical treatment are awaited.

Patients should understand that medical treatment is not an inferior option in a world of high technology. For single and two vessel disease the prognosis is excellent on medical treatment and the quality of life is the determining factor in choosing to change to angioplasty or surgery. For patients with three vessel disease surgery is more likely to carry a long term prognostic benefit (as well as symptom relief) especially if left ventricular function is poor. Even clearer is the prognostic advance of coronary artery bypass grafting over medical treatment of those with significant left main stem vessel disease.

REFERENCES

Hamer, J. (1987). *Drugs for heart disease.* Chapman and Hall. London.
Nayler, W.G. (1988). *Calcium antagonists.* Academic Press Ltd, London.
Opie, L.H. (1990). *Clinical use of calcium channel antagonist drugs.* Kluwer Academic Publishers, Boston.
Opie, L.H. (1991). *Drugs for the heart.* W.B. Saunders Co.
Parisi, A.F., Folland, E.D., Hartigan, P. (1992). A comparison of angioplasty with medical therapy in the treatment of single vessel coronary artery disease. *N Engl. J. Med.* **326,** 10–16.
Patterson, (1987). *Angina pectoris.* D.L.H. Castle House Publications Ltd, Tunbridge Wells.
Pennel, D.J., Underwood, R., Costa, D.C., and Ell, P.J. (1992). *Thallium myocardial perfusion tomography in clinical cardiology.* Springer-Verlag, London.
Prinzmetal, M., Kennamer, R., Merliss, R., Wada, T., and Bor, N. (1959). Angina pectoris 1. A variant form of angina pectoris. *Am. J. Med.* **27,** 375–388.
Sherman, C.T., Litvack, F., Grunfest, W., Lee, M., Hickey, A., Chaux, A., Kass, R., Blanche, C., Matloff, J., Morgenstern, L., Ganz, W., Swan, H.J.C., and Forrester, J. (1991). Coronary angioscopy in patients with unstable angina pectoris. *N. Engl. J. Med.* **315,** 913–919.
Singh, B.N. (1988). *Silent myocardial ischaemia. Prevalence, prognosis and therapeutic significance.* Pergamon Press, New York.

15.10.4 Myocardial infarction

P. SLEIGHT

Introduction

Few areas of medicine have advanced more between two editions than that of myocardial infarction (MI).

These improvements have been the result of a remarkable explosion in our understanding of the pathology, epidemiology, genetics, and prevention of coronary heart disease, together with the development of large multicentre trials which have led to rapid acceptance of new therapies for reperfusion such as thrombolysis, aspirin, and primary angioplasty (PTCA). These have been accompanied by trials of prehospital care, and the widespread adoption of paramedic staffed ambulances equipped with defibrillators, and also capable of faxing domiciliary

electrocardiographs to the local coronary care unit. Treatment with a thrombolytic drug plus aspirin halves mortality in those treated within 4 h of onset of symptoms; if used during the first hour or so the attack may be aborted. Nevertheless the mortality of myocardial infarction remains high and there is plenty of room for further improvement.

This chapter should be read in conjunction with those on the pathology and prevention of myocardial infarction, together with that on unstable angina. In fact, this chapter might better be titled 'suspected acute myocardial infarction' as the real distinction between a definite myocardial infarction and an episode of unstable angina is often only possible retrospectively, based on the development of new Q waves on the electrocardiogram, and/or serum cardiac enzymes raised to more than twice the normal level. This distinction is somewhat arbitrary as the detection of raised enzymes has been shown to be dependent on the frequency of blood sampling. Nevertheless, this rough and ready practical distinction has some merit in that the mortality of unstable angina (including some small and undetected myocardial infarctions) is much less than that of acute myocardial infarction.

Historic aspects of myocardial infarction

Although myocardial infarction is often depicted as a modern disease it was clearly recognized before the modern era by Morgagni in 1761 and, more clearly, by Heberden (published posthumously in 1802). Caleb Parry, a physician in Bath, read a paper on coronary disease to the local medical society in 1788. An early personal description of myocardial infarction was given by John Hunter, surgeon to St George's Hospital London, who himself experienced what was probably a myocardial infarction in 1773. The description of his subsequent autopsy describes the scarred areas in his heart. Adam Hammer, a physician in Mannheim, is credited with the first antemortem diagnosis of coronary thrombosis 1878, with an autopsy showing a clot in a coronary artery. But it was James Herrick, a Chicago physician who, in 1912 in the *Journal of the American Medical Association,* described the clinical features of sudden obstruction of the coronary arteries. He also described survival after such an event, which belied the then current opinion that such an event was universally fatal.

The reason why, even then, myocardial infarction was not more generally recognized is probably because in the Victorian era the common cause of death was by infection, so that fewer people survived to the age of 50 and over, when coronary disease begins to take a serious toll. Furthermore, most of the population were too poor to suffer from this disease of affluence. In 1910 Sir William Osler delivered a lecture to the Royal College of Physicians, which noted that he had found the condition to be more common amongst his private or upper class patients than the poorer classes he saw at St Bartholomew's Hospital. He found this surprising, as he had expected that the stresses of life amongst the poor might have predisposed them to coronary thrombosis. Noting also the tendency for the disease to have a familial disposition he thus combined the modern aetiological theories of the interactions between environment and genetics.

Modern impact and public health importance

Coronary heart disease (CHD) has been correctly described as a modern epidemic in Western societies. In 1991 it accounted for 26 per cent of all deaths in the United Kingdom, 1 in 3 men and 1 in 4 women (Fig. 1). More than 1 in 15 men die of coronary heart disease before the age of 65 – accounting for more than one-quarter of all premature deaths. Women follow the same trend, but lag men by about 10 years (Figs. 2 and 3). This may be due to the protective effects of oestrogens before the menopause, but it is equally likely to be due to the previously low smoking rates in women compared with men. Young girls in many countries now smoke more than boys; it is already becoming clear that myocardial infarction in premenopausal women – a rarity 20 years ago – is now increasing. Myocardial infarction in premenopausal women is almost always associated with smoking, and in a few cases with familial hypercholesterolaemia.

Variation in coronary heart disease mortality within and between countries

Figure 4 shows the very great variability in coronary heart disease deaths in adults in different parts of the United Kingdom, as well as in a selection of other countries. It can be seen that Scotland and Northern Ireland have the dubious distinction of heading this league! These data are very striking. Although much of the variation, e.g. between Japan and the United Kingdom, can be explained by differences in serum cholesterol, this is not the whole story. For example, there is a striking increase in coronary heart disease deaths from South East England to Scotland and Northern Ireland, although the cholesterol values are much the same (deaths adjusted for other risk factors such as smoking, blood pressure, etc.). One factor that may be important is the level of antioxidants in the serum. This level is inversely related to the death rate from coronary heart disease, in keeping with the Steinberg hypothesis that it is oxidized low density lipoprotein-cholesterol, which is taken up by 'scavenger' receptors and macrophages as a 'foreign' substance, rather than normal low density lipoprotein-cholesterol which is taken up by liver cells. There are striking differences in diet between north and south, with less fruit and fresh vegetables eaten in Scotland. Similarly, other factors (such as alcohol intake), which are not generally included in risk factor

adjustment, may account for differences in coronary heart disease rates between, say, cities such as Lille (low coronary heart disease) and Belfast (high coronary heart disease), where the levels of cholesterol are similar. Other factors such as genetic make up are important between countries. Nevertheless, migrant studies both within and between countries suggest that individuals take up the coronary heart disease rates of the place where they live, so environmental factors are of great importance (see Chapters 15.10.1).

Although less developed countries have a low incidence of coronary heart disease, this rises sharply with increasing affluence, caused by a combination of diet, smoking, and other factors such as a lack of exercise. Asian populations may have an increased susceptibility to coronary heart disease when they develop Western habits. This seems to be related to metabolic factors such as diabetes and insulin resistance, in addition to rises in serum cholesterol.

Age is perhaps the greatest general predictor of risk of death from coronary heart disease. Although there is a less striking relation between cholesterol level and coronary heart disease incidence in the old compared with the young, the 'attributable' risk related to cholesterol is greater in the old because of the higher prevalence of the disease in the old. The case fatality rate is also very much greater in the old. Emergency room physicians generally get more excited (therapeutically) by myocardial infarction in a 40-year-old man than in a 75-year-old, although the former has a 5 week mortality risk of less than 5 per cent, whereas the risk of death for a 75-year-old is about 30 per cent (see Fig. 8).

Coronary artery thrombosis is the cause of myocardial infarction

For some years the relation between a thrombus in a coronary artery and a myocardial infarction was hotly debated. Some influential advocates held that the thrombus was a secondary phenomenon which followed a myocardial infarction. Fortunately these followers of the 'flat earth society' were seen off by the ugly facts of observation at acute surgery by De Wood and his colleagues. They showed that in the very early stages of myocardial infarction fresh thrombus was seen in over 90 per cent of cases. This fell progressively with time after the onset of pain, presumably as a result of spontaneous thrombolysis. This spontaneous lysis from endogenous tissue plasminogen activator was responsible for the pathological confusion, since postmortem studies at a later date showed myocardial infarction without any obvious fresh thrombus in the relevant coronary artery. Surgery and, more importantly, early angiography rectified this error and led to the modern era of reperfusion therapy with lytic agents or direct angioplasty (PTCA).

Fig. 1 Causes of death, United Kingdom 1991. Sources: OPCS and Government Statistics (from Coronary Prevention Group/British Heart Foundation database 1992, with permission).

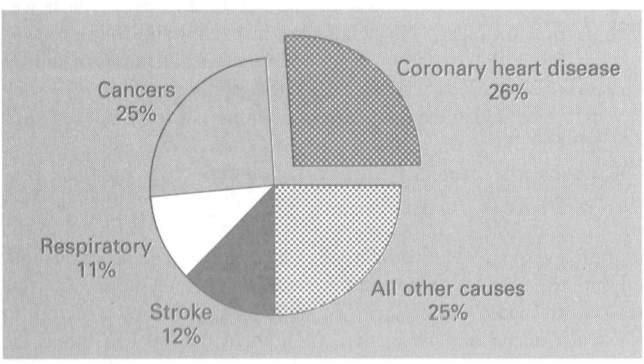

Fig. 2 Age related causes of death, United Kingdom 1991, men. Sources: OPCS and Government Statistics (from Coronary Prevention/Group/British Heart Foundation database 1992, with permission).

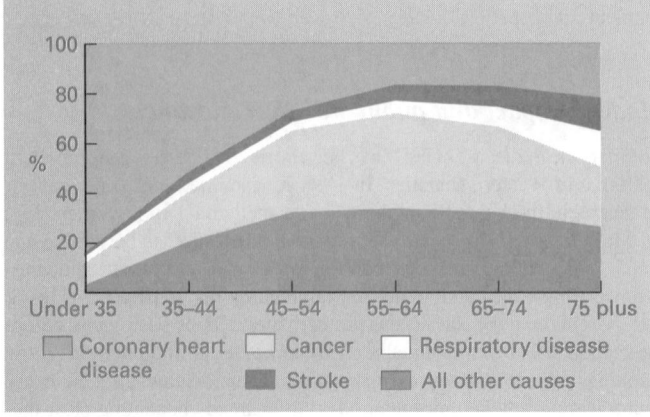

Fig. 3 Age related causes of death, United Kingdom 1991, women. Sources: OPCS and Government Statistics (from Coronary Prevention Group/British Heart Foundation database 1992, with permission).

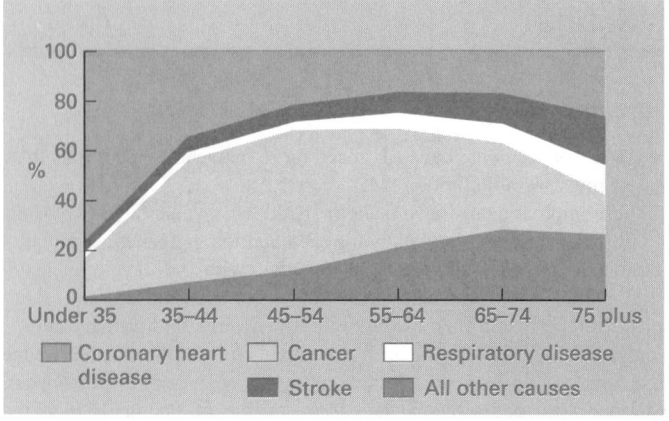

Pathology, precipitants, and time course of myocardial infarction

This is discussed in detail in Chapter 15.10.2. Briefly we now understand that myocardial infarction most commonly occurs as an acute platelet and fibrin thrombus provoked by a crack or rupture of a fatty plaque in a coronary artery. This rupture generally occurs at the edge of a plaque where there is a concentration of lipid laden macrophages which may, when they die, release protolytic enzymes which weaken the fibrous cap at the edge of a plaque.

The plaque which ruptures may only be a trivial bump which has not previously led to a critical stenosis. This is probably why thrombolysis has been such a successful intervention, since once the thrombus is lysed one may be left with a relatively unobstructed artery in about half the

cases of myocardial infarction. The so-called 'late remodelling' of the artery after lysis, described by Bertrand and his colleagues in Lille, is probably due to the consolidation and perhaps further lysis of residual thrombus; this residual thrombus exaggerates the stenosis seen during acute angiography. It is also now clear that the process of thrombosis and lysis is a dynamic balance; even in the absence of treatment there is a combination of lysis and simultaneous thrombosis following a plaque rupture. Maseri and his colleagues at the Hammersmith Hospital carried out serial angiography during evolving infarction and during treatment with intracoronary streptokinase. They found that there was repeated opening and closing of the artery with accompanying rapid electrocardiograph changes in ST segment elevation even during the infusion of the lytic agent (Fig. 5). We now know that during lysis the newly exposed thrombus is extremely attractive to platelets, hence the

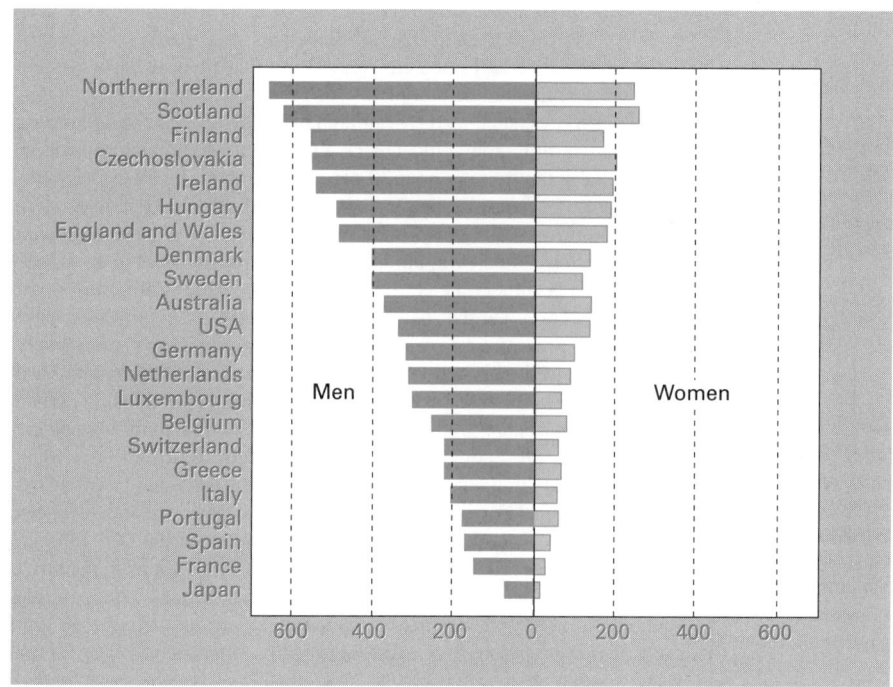

Fig. 4 Coronary heart death rates selected countries 1988 for men and women aged 35 to 74 years. Source: World Health Statistics annuals (from Coronary Prevention Group/British Heart Foundation database 1992, with permission).

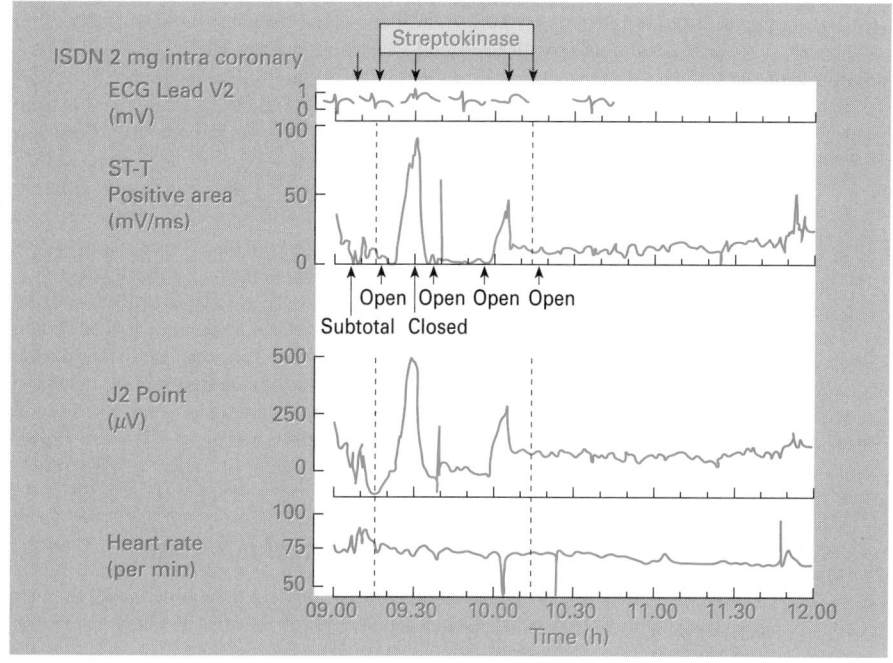

Fig. 5 Intermittent coronary opening and closing during streptokinase infusion in acute myocardial infarction, showing close correlation between angiographic patency or occlusion (arrows), computerized ST segment monitoring (ST&T, J Point) and lack of correlation with heart rate (from Hackett *et al.* (1987), *New England Journal of Medicine*, with permission).

great benefit of antiplatelet agents such as aspirin in the early phase of myocardial infarction.

The value of continuous registration of the electrocardiograph, especially the ST segment shift, has been explored by Krucoff and his colleagues during the TAMI-7 trial. In many cases this record gave a very good indication of vessel patency after lytic therapy. When the ST segments fell rapidly during lytic therapy this generally indicated successful reperfusion and vice versa (Fig. 6). However, the presence or absence of collateral vessels not unexpectedly confused the specificity of this finding. None the less, such methods may well be a useful marker of reperfusion or not, and so point to a need for further intervention when the ST segment remains high 2 to 3 h after attempted lysis. In parallel with the above observations of Maseri (Fig. 5), these continuous recordings of ST segment shifts also can demonstrate rapid rises and falls, illustrating that infarction in man does not always mimic the time course of ligation of a coronary vessel in animals – where cell death begins within minutes and may be complete by 20 to 30 min. This may occur with sudden occlusion of a major coronary artery such as the left anterior descending artery in a young man. More often the wave of necrosis is slower due to partial as opposed to total obstruction by a fresh thrombus and also due to intermittent occlusion when the cycle of lysis and thrombosis is occurring or when there is intermittent vasospasm. Necrosis is also delayed when collateral vessels are present. Such collateral vessels may become quite obvious by 2 to 3 h after a coronary occlusion, but may appear more rapidly when the patient has experienced ischaemia previously.

Time of occurrence of infarction

Large interventional studies such as those with propranolol (MILIS) and aspirin and streptokinase (ISIS-2) confirmed earlier suggestions that the time of onset of myocardial infarction shows a marked circadian rhythm with a peak onset in the early hours of the day, after waking, and a second peak after 5 p.m. In addition, there was an increasing incidence during the week to a peak on Friday and a weekend decline. It is likely that these peaks are related to a combination of factors caused by the increase in sympathetic tone on arousal and with excitement. These include platelet activation, rise in blood pressure with subsequent liability to plaque rupture, and increased susceptibility to arrhythmia, as

Fig. 6 Example of continuous ST segment monitoring in a patient with acute myocardial infarction. Note the peak at 1 h or so from the onset of monitoring, which then falls rapidly following thrombolysis indicating successful treatment. Also note the rather stuttering rise and fall in the first 30 min (From Krucoff *et al.* (1993), *Circulation* with permission).

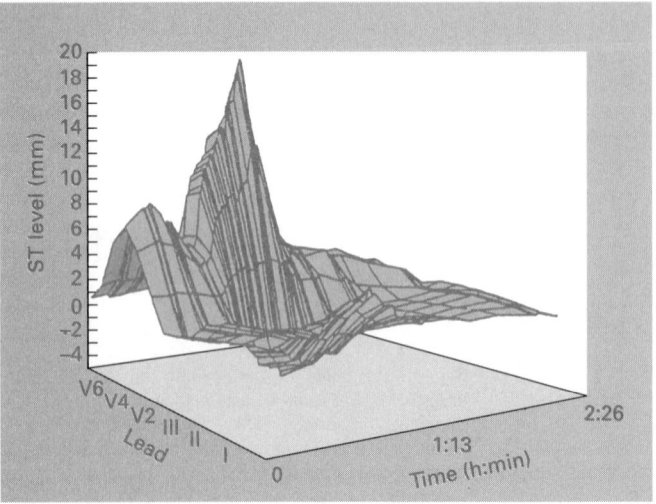

these peaks of infarction can be considerably lessened by either aspirin therapy or β-adrenoceptor blockade.

Presentation

Medical services, particularly those based in hospitals, have a distorted impression of the community impact of myocardial infarction. This is because around 40 per cent of deaths occur suddenly before contact with any level of medical or paramedic care. This fact above all should make us concentrate our efforts on prevention. Many of these very early deaths are arrhythmic – hence the importance of greater public education in closed chest cardiac massage and mouth-to-mouth resuscitation, pending arrival of defibrillation equipment.

The earlier the patient is seen during a myocardial infarction, the more difficult it may be to make the diagnosis correctly. This may be particularly so in older patients in which the symptoms or signs may be atypical. Lack of pain may be partly because of increasing autonomic neuropathy with age (especially in diabetics) and partly because of increasing numbers of collateral vessels, so that myocardial infarction in older patients may be completely or relatively painless. In epidemiological surveys, such as the Framingham study, Q wave infarction on the electrocardiograph could not be linked with a clinical episode of myocardial infarction in about 30 per cent of the population screened.

It has also been established from studies of the population of Western Washington State that up to one-third of patients who have been successfully resuscitated from an episode of sudden death have no subsequent evidence either on electrocardiograph or enzymes of a fresh myocardial infarction, i.e. the 'death' was arrhythmic.

Thus the presentation of acute myocardial infarction varies widely and is influenced mainly by the amount of pain or arrhythmia produced by the infarction. Large infarcts, due to the proximal occlusion of one of the main coronary arteries with few protective collateral vessels are major events, presenting either as sudden death or severe chest pain which demands immediate attention. Smaller infarcts due to occlusion of more peripheral vessels or of proximal vessels which have been bypassed by collateral vessels may be less painful particularly in older or diabetic patients and hence present later, say 4 to 12 h from the onset of pain or chest discomfort. Such smaller infarcts may, as stated, present without pain but with circulatory disturbances such as arrhythmia, syncope, and the new onset of heart failure. It is important to bear this in mind when assessing the results of clinical trials of the treatment of myocardial infarction. Great emphasis is rightly placed on early treatment, i.e. 1 to 4 h after the onset of the index symptoms. But patients who present very early (and have often been the patients included in clinical trials with restricted time windows, e.g. the recent GUSTO trials), differ markedly from the general run of patients admitted to ordinary hospitals. This must be borne in mind when extrapolating from such trials to normal clinical practice where the patients may be older, and delay more before getting to hospital.

In summary, myocardial infarction may present in many different ways, from sudden unheralded death, to the classic presentation with severe frightening chest pain. The presentation may mimic dyspepsia or oesophageal spasm, it may be painless and present as arrhythmia or new onset of breathlessness, or may present with cerebral or non-specific symptoms due to sudden hypotension. Finally, in patients in whom pain has not been prominent it may present with the sequelae of infarction: heart failure, a new murmur due to mitral incompetence secondary to papillary muscle ischaemia or rupture, an acquired ventricular septal defect, or embolization to the brain or elsewhere from a left ventricular mural thrombus.

Symptoms and signs of myocardial infarction

As stated earlier the attack may be completely unheralded, with the first manifestation being sudden death. However, when patients have been resuscitated from sudden death about three-quarters reveal that they have experienced some premonitory discomfort and may even have consulted a physician about this. It is important therefore to take such symptoms seriously and to begin prophylactic treatment with aspirin and β-blockade (if appropriate), pending more definitive investigation. New onset of angina, or a sudden deterioration of angina often indicates an evolving thrombus.

Before a myocardial infarction there are many patients who describe a non-specific prodromal phase of undue fatigue or shortness of breath. These symptoms are probably caused by a growing but subtotal thrombus which limits the cardiac reserve.

The pain of a typical myocardial infarction is usually central, felt deep behind the sternum as a tightness, crushing or bursting sensation. It is generally perceived to be serious or life-threatening. This can be a useful distinction from the equally severe pain of pericarditis, which does not usually generate the same anxiety. It is useful to ask the patient if they feel that the symptoms are so serious or threatening. The pain may also be felt in the back, between the scapulae, and sometimes only there; it may radiate down the arms to the wrists, most often in the left arm. Radiation to the jaws is also characteristic; this may be the only site of pain. Jaw pain of an oesophageal origin is unusual, and should always arouse suspicion.

The pain is often accompanied by nausea and sometimes vomiting, particularly with large transmural infarction., This has been attributed to stimulation of the Bezold–Jarisch reflex, which arises from receptors in the left ventricle, particularly in the inferior or right coronary region. This reflex gives rise to hypotension, bradycardia, and vomiting due to acute neurogenic gastric dilatation. The efferent arm is vagal, hence the bradycardia. The vagus also has a powerful negative inotropic effect on the left ventricle and it is this, together with the reflex bradycardia, which causes the dramatic fall in blood pressure; it is rapidly reversed by intravenous atropine, which can completely transform this picture of shock and circulatory collapse in the early hours of infarction. Sometimes the nausea and vomiting may misdirect the patient to the surgical side of casualty/emergency.

Because the ischaemic left ventricle becomes immediately stiff, patients may become short of breath due to the raised pulmonary venous pressure. This also produces subclinical (or occasionally clinical) pulmonary oedema, which results in arterial desaturation for up to 48 h.

The physical signs may be remarkably few at first so the diagnosis depends largely on the history. A third heart sound may be present, together with signs of autonomic dysfunction due to vagal reflexes as above, or due to sympathetic reflexes causing tachycardia and sweating. A very frequent sign (if looked for) is a raised venous pressure. Most commonly this results from increased sympathetic tone to the venous system from baroreceptor sensing of the lowered arterial pressure. It may also be the result of right ventricular infarction. In more severe and large infarctions there may be circulatory collapse, hypotension and shock. Because of the vasovagal reflex disturbances outlined above it is best to reserve the term shock to patients whose hypotension (< 90 mmHg systolic blood pressure), clammy sweating, pallor, oliguria, and mental obfuscation does not respond to atropine. True shock carries a very high mortality of around 80 per cent, whereas the transient shock like state from autonomic (vagal) dysfunction is not particularly dangerous.

Differential diagnosis

AORTIC DISSECTION

The differential diagnosis of myocardial infarction is extraordinarily wide because there are many causes of chest pain. Dissection of the aorta is of prime importance in view of the dangers for this of lytic treatment. Equally or even more painful than myocardial infarction, the pain is usually tearing, reaches an immediate peak and may travel outside the usual boundaries of true cardiac pain, e.g. into the abdomen. The patient can frequently describe the exact moment of onset, which may be precipitated by some sudden movement to pick up an object, or open a jammed door. Dissection may be suspected when the patient appears shocked but with a blood pressure at relatively normal levels. It is important to look for extravasation of blood, e.g. into the pleura, with the signs of effusion. Absent or unequal pulses are quoted in most books but are noted in fewer than 5 per cent of dissections. When seen later in its course aortic dissection usually gives rise to fever due to extravasation of large quantities of blood; this together with an aortic diastolic murmur (when the aortic root is involved) may lead to a mistaken diagnosis of bacterial endocarditis. (for helpful investigations see below under management)

PERICARDITIS

Pericarditis may pose a difficult differential diagnosis since it combines pain with ST elevation on the electrocardiograph. This ST elevation is usually more widespread than with myocardial infarction, but initially may also be limited to anterior chest leads. The pain of pericarditis is usually less threatening and characteristically is exacerbated by movement such as turning in bed or by swallowing; it may occasionally be felt in time with the heart beat. An echocardiogram may help if it shows an effusion together with no abnormalities of regional wall motion. Pericarditis may develop as a complication of myocardial infarction; it usually becomes clinically manifest 24 to 48 h after onset.

OESOPHAGEAL AND GASTROINTESTINAL PAIN

Oesophageal pain, from acid reflux, with or without spasm, may closely mimic the pain of myocardial ischaemia. The character and distribution may be identical. A glass of milk or antacid may give instant relief. Trinitrin may relieve both cardiac pain and oesophageal spasm, and so is less helpful as a diagnostic exercise.

Other gastrointestinal problems such as gallbladder disease and peptic ulcer may be confusing but are generally separable by an adequate history.

MUSCULOSKELETAL PAIN

Musculoskeletal pain may be identified by local tenderness or exacerbation on spinal or rib percussion. Costochondritis (Tietze's syndrome) is not often very confusing.

PULMONARY EMBOLISM

Pulmonary embolism may be a difficult differential diagnosis, especially in a postoperative patient who may be prone to both this and myocardial infarction. If not clear on the history, the electrocardiograph may be helpful if classic right ventricular strain and right axis deviation is present. Otherwise it may be identified by blood gas measures, serial cardiac enzymes, or by radionucleide pulmonary ventilatory/perfusion scans.

UNSTABLE ANGINA

Finally, the most obvious differential diagnosis is from unstable angina, or Prinzmetal angina due to spasm and/or a temporary platelet thrombus. Usually the pain of myocardial infarction lasts longer than 20 to 30 min. If it is accompanied by significant ST elevation (say > 1 to 2 mm in each of two limb leads or > 2 mm in two chest leads), then infarction is much more likely than unstable angina (where the occluding thrombus is usually subtotal). Where the electrocardiograph shows only T wave inversion or ST depression, the distinction is more difficult and is best achieved by the duration of an episode of constant pain, more than 30 min with myocardial infarction. Right ventricular chest leads should be done in all such cases (particularly if the ST depression is inferior) in order to rule out right ventricular infarction, which may easily be missed on a routine electrocardiograph. This carries a prognosis as grave as left ventricular infarction (Fig. 7). Prinzmetal angina is very uncommon; it may mimic myocardial infarction. The electrocardiograph may show such extreme ST elevation (anterior or inferior) that the QRS may appear bizarre and wide and be mistaken for extreme bundle branch block. The diagnosis is often clinched by a rapid response to intravenous or oral nitrates. Although the classic picture is rare, coronary vasospasm, perhaps related to vasoactive substances released from platelets, may be less rare but is hard to document.

Management of suspected myocardial infarction

Introduction

HOME OR HOSPITAL?

A few years ago, it was a reasonable option to consider treatment at home, particularly for elderly patients or for those seen late after the onset and when the condition appeared stable, provided that the home conditions were suitable. Indeed, a small trial was carried out in the south-west of England which appeared to show no more adverse outcome for home versus hospital care for such patients; but this trial enrolled a highly selected population. Even at the time of publication there was considerable controversy concerning the wisdom of home treatment, because of the inability totally to predict risk, particularly for arrhythmia.

Even without the stimulus of the results of thrombolysis the trend to hospital care has steadily increased. However, where other factors are present, such as other illness, poor quality of life, or clear contraindications to lytic treatment, then home treatment may still be a sensible option. Otherwise the trend in the treatment of myocardial infarction resembles modern obstetrics – hospital for the potentially hazardous early treatment, then home quickly, i.e. more people serviced by the same number of beds.

The combination of thrombolytic treatment and aspirin has completely transformed the management of acute myocardial infarction over the last few years. This therapy can halve the mortality of myocardial infarction and may even abort the infarction if begun within the first 60 to 90 min. Because it carries a small but definite risk of bleeding, particularly cerebral haemorrhage, it is of increasing importance to assess the risk of death from myocardial infarction in each patient presenting, and to do so quickly – ideally within 20 to 30 min of arrival in casualty. This means that in the majority of cases the decision has to be clinical and depend on the history, a rapid examination, and an electrocardiograph, which should be obtained simultaneously with the history.

The most immediate practical procedure, if this has not already been done, is to relieve the patient's pain with an adequate dose of intravenous morphine or diamorphine (5 to 10 mg), often given with an antiemetic. Even when such analgesia has been given out of hospital this is often overcautious and inadequate, so the first questions of the admitting physician should be about the severity of any residual pain. Relief of pain reduces sympathetic discharge and hence reduces cardiac work.

Oxygen will also have been given routinely in the ambulance and emergency room and should be continued for 24 to 48 h.

Initial assessment

Apart from the initial electrocardiograph, other investigations should be carried out later (if the electrocardiograph shows ST elevation characteristic of myocardial infarction), except where there are compelling reasons, e.g. for suspicion of aortic dissection.

Three particular types of ST segment elevation may cause confusion. First, where there has been a prior myocardial infarction with aneurysm formation ST elevation may persist over the dyskinetic area. It is usually accompanied by Q waves, which may help distinguish this from a recent myocardial infarction.

Second, ST segment elevation in leads V1 and V2 may follow a deep S wave as a normal variant and does not necessarily indicate infarction.

Third, pericarditis may cause ST elevation, but this is usually widespread and is often dome-shaped, i.e. convex upwards. An effusion on the echo together with a history of upper respiratory infection or malignancy may be helpful.

Routine tests such as a chest radiograph can normally wait until the lytic treatment has started. Aspirin (half to one tablet, 160 to 320 mg) should be chewed immediately the diagnosis is clear (it is rapidly absorbed, and reduces platelet reactivity in 20 to 30 min). Thrombolysis should also be started quickly, in the emergency room unless a coronary care bed is available immediately. Valuable hours are lost by the delays in clearing a bed. The reason for this haste is that time is crucial. Treatment within 1 h of onset of symptoms saves about 30 to 35 lives per thousand patients treated. By 2 to 3 h from onset this has dropped to 23/1000, at 4 to 6 h to 20/1000 and from 7 to 12 h to 17/1000 fewer deaths at 5 weeks, compared with routine treatment without thrombolysis. These figures are all highly significant and are derived from an overview of 99 per cent of the individual data (approximately 60 000 patients) available from the large trials of lytic therapy versus placebo or control (Fig. 8).

Thus a delay of 1 h during the initial 2 to 3 h may mean an increase in mortality of 5 to 10 patients per 1000 treated and with an inevitably more damaged ventricle. Even later on a 1 h delay imposes a penalty of 2 to 3/1000 extra deaths.

Causes of delay in treatment and how to lessen these

PATIENT DELAYS

Some delays are hard to influence. The longest delay is the time it takes for a patient to decide to call medical help. Initially it was thought that this could easily be reduced by education campaigns by the media. It became rapidly clear that such campaigns had very limited impact, which disappeared unless the effort was sustained and repeated at intervals, which is rarely done. Surprisingly patients who have previously

Fig. 7 Mortality rate and prevalence of major complications during hospitalization among 200 consecutive patients with acute inferior myocardial infarctions, according to the presence (solid bars) or absence (shaded bars) of ST-segment elevation of <0.1 mV in lead v_{4R}. The numbers above the bars are percentages of patients in each group. P values were determined by univariate analysis. (from Zehender et al. (1993), New England Journal of Medicine, with permission).

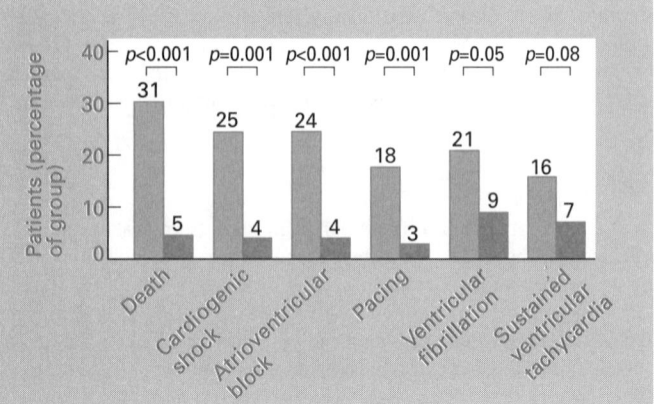

experienced an myocardial infarction take just as long to call for help on a second occasion. In my experience cardiologists with a myocardial infarction take longest of all!

However, individual patient counselling may help. It is important to warn patients with angina, who have experienced a previous myocardial infarction, or who are at high risk of myocardial infarction, that they should not delay calling for help if pain persists for 20 to 30 min and has not responded to trinitrin therapy. The procedure may be different in differing situations (see below). They should of course already be taking prophylactic aspirin (75 to 325 mg daily).

COMMUNITY PRACTICE DELAYS: PREHOSPITAL CARE

Surveys show that delays by general practitioners are generally surprisingly small. Delays in hospital are generally much greater unless special measures are taken. Ambulance delays are also generally small in Western and urbanized society, but may of course be appreciably more in rural areas with long distances from ambulance depot to patient, and from patient to hospital. In such cases initiation of thrombolytic treatment at the patients home has proven beneficial and safe. Where paramedics rather than general practitioners initiate domiciliary treatment this has usually been in conjunction with a hospital physician, who has received a transmitted electrocardiograph by phone or fax from the home or ambulance. The most striking result of trials of domiciliary versus hospital initiated lysis has been the great reduction in in-hospital delays!

This has led to the so-called 'fast track' admission for patients with suspected myocardial infarction. This has been shown in Edinburgh to reduce the time to treatment by 1 to 2 h at negligible cost. Under this system the ambulance crew simply obtains and reports on the domiciliary electrocardiograph and communicates the provisional diagnosis to the hospital. Paramedics may also insert an intravenous line and administer pain relief and aspirin.

All this needs local discussion between hospital, general practitioners, ambulance paramedics, and public health workers. They can then decide on what is the best plan for their practice. Some advocate that patients simply call a 24-h emergency number. This may not be satisfactory if the ambulance service is overstretched and cannot respond quickly.

Fig. 8 Absolute effects on fibrinolytic therapy on mortality during days 0 to 35 subdivided by age. The unstratified percentage dead during days 0 to 35 amongst all those allocated fibrinolytic therapy and all those allocated control in these trials. Fibrinolytic (F) and Control (C). The absolute numbers and percentage are given above the respective columns and the absolute benefit per thousand at the top. The horizontal lines divide deaths in days 0–1 (below) and 2–35 (above) (from Fibrinolytic Trialists Collaboration (1993), *Lancet*, with permission).

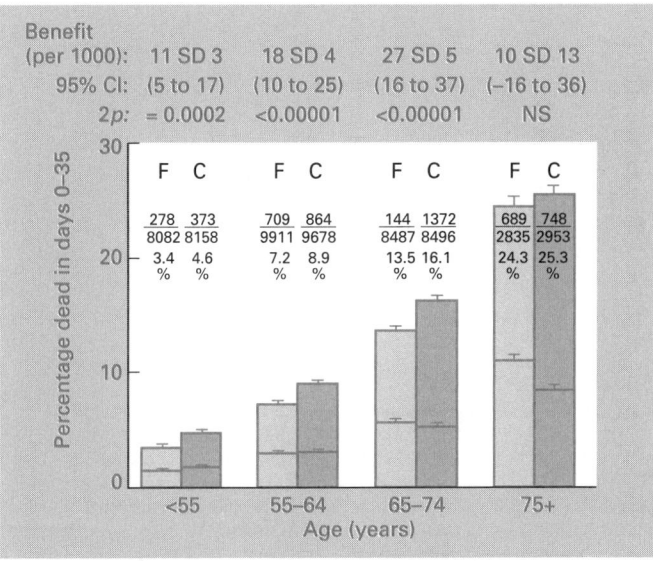

Some general practitioners resent that they are bypassed, and important medical and/or social data may not accompany the patient, quite apart from quicker and more effective pain relief. Perhaps the best plan is for the general practitioner to be called first. He or she can assess the probability of myocardial infarction on the phone and, if in doubt, call an ambulance before they leave their base. This of course means that the practice must be able to respond in this way at all hours. In countries with group practices this may be easy to organize; it is less so with single-handed practice in the middle of a busy session. In this case a direct call to an emergency number may be a better option.

HOSPITAL DELAYS

Given the complex patterns of a busy emergency department it is not difficult to understand how delays build on each other so that the 'door to needle' time may reach 2 h or longer. It has been clearly shown that these can be overcome, but this needs a great deal of coordination between cardiologists, emergency room physicians, and, most of all, nursing staff. In the case of myocardial infarction, a cardiologist may damage your health! It is better for the cardiologist to agree that the decision should be taken by the first (often junior) doctor who sees the patient. It is of course important to educate and also audit the results of this procedure, so that feedback can be given and bottlenecks identified. It is critical to realize that such simple organizational changes can make far greater improvements in the outcome for all patients with myocardial infarction than the differences between one thrombolytic drug and another.

Risk assessment early in myocardial infarction: simple clinical criteria suffice . . .

As we shall see below, although aspirin treatment has negligible risk, lytic treatment carries a risk of serious adverse effects, which approaches 0.5 per cent, so it is not sensible to treat patients if their immediate short term risk of death from the myocardial infarction is about 1 or 2 per cent only. This would be the risk from a small inferior myocardial infarction in a patient aged 45 to 50 with a stable circulation and no further pain. Overall, the mortality of acute myocardial infarction, for all comers, is about 8 per cent at 4 to 5 weeks but with wide variation with different baseline characteristics.

AGE

From the Fibrinolytic Therapy Trialists' (FTT) collaboration we now have reliable data on the risk of death for the control population in these trials, split by simple criteria. Age is far the most important predictor of risk. Infarction is not only much more common with increasing age but the case fatality increases greatly so that by 5 weeks after onset it is over 25 per cent for those over 75 years, over 15 per cent for 65 or older, about 10 per cent for 55 and less than 5 per cent for those under 45 years (see Fig. 8).

SEX

Women at present live longer than men and so are disproportionately over-represented in the older patients presenting with myocardial infarction. Even after matching for age, women have a case fatality more than 50 per cent higher than for males (Fig. 9). The reasons for this are not entirely clear. They appear to have more advanced disease at presentation, in smaller coronary arteries, and with a worse response to many treatments, including lytic therapy.

SIZE AND SITE OF INFARCTION

Anterior ST elevation carries about twice the risk of inferior myocardial infarction (5-week 13 per cent versus 7 per cent). The number of leads showing ST elevation and the sum of the ST segments (as a crude index of infarct size) is also a powerful indicator of risk. ST segment depression also carries a poor prognosis (approximately 15 per cent at 5 weeks), probably because it is often associated with multivessel disease and a history of prior infarction. The index infarction is often subendocardial and not localized as a result of a definitive large thrombus, which may explain why the evidence of benefit from lysis is less clear.

Bundle branch block (BBB) may be present on the initial electrocardiograph and so disguise the site of infarction and also make the assessment of the ST segment unreliable. Even if the age of the bundle branch block is uncertain (as it often is), the presence of right or left bundle branch block together with a suspicious history generally indicates a large myocardial infarction, and hence a poorer prognosis.

On the other hand, an initially normal hospital electrocardiograph in a suspected myocardial infarction carries a 5-week mortality risk of less than 2 to 3 per cent. Not unexpectedly, patients with a prior history of an earlier myocardial infarction, diabetes, or hypertension have an increase in risk about 50 per cent greater than those without.

Finally, patients who present with circulatory problems particularly a blood pressure below 100 mmHg and/or a tachycardia above 100/min have a poor prognosis. The risk of death approaches 60 per cent when both are present. If true shock is diagnosed (see above) the risk is over 80 per cent.

HEART FAILURE

Signs of pulmonary oedema, with the presence of substantial basal rales (more than one third of the chest height) and/or on the chest radiograph (even when transient) is a highly important predictor of future mortality. This is true regardless of the measured ejection fraction. This, however, is usually a sign which develops during the hospital course, rather than at entry. Pulmonary oedema at entry to the hospital carries a grave prognosis.

Other markers, e.g. presence of early primary ventricular fibrillation have a small but less important influence on prognosis.

Further investigations

EJECTION FRACTION

An echocardiogram should not delay treatment but can be an extraordinarily helpful tool, particularly if used as a simple portable device to assess left ventricular wall motion in the emergency room, in cases of diagnostic difficulty where the electrocardiograph is equivocal or where there is old infarction. Like the presence of heart failure a reduced ejection fraction is a powerful index of prognosis, but is not exactly concordant with clinical heart failure (Fig. 10). If both a reduced ejection fraction and signs of failure are present we can identify those patients with the worse prognosis.

CHEST RADIOGRAPH

This is generally carried out in the coronary care unit after or during the period of lytic therapy. Only if there is a real suspicion of aortic dissection should it be done before treatment. It is used to assess the presence of pulmonary congestion or diversion of blood to the upper lobes and to give a rough index of heart size (anteroposterior view), or the shape of the heart and aortic knuckle. Aortic dissection may be suspected if the upper mediastinal shadow is wide, although an unfolded aorta may also cause this. Irregularity of the outline of the knuckle, with a linear

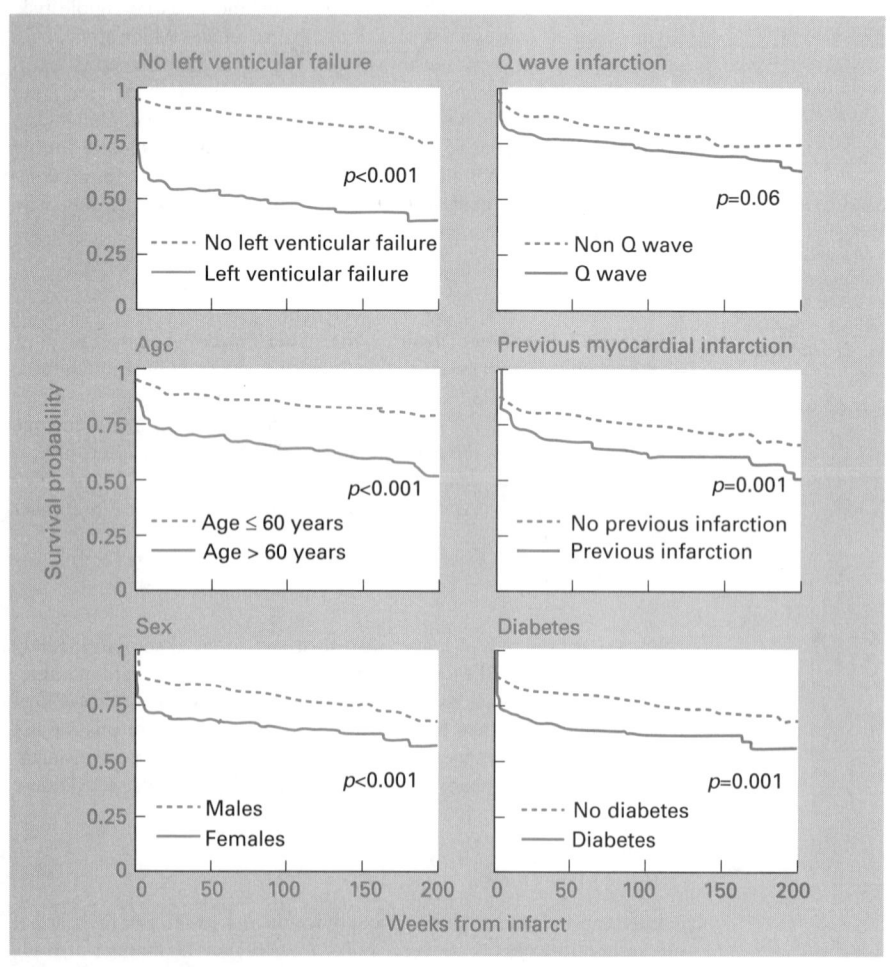

Fig. 9 Kaplan–Meier survival curves illustrating the effects on prognosis after infarction of left ventricular failure, Q wave infarction, age, sex, diabetes, and history of myocardial infarction; from 608 consecutive patients from one London general hospital (from Stevenson et al. (1993), British Medical Journal, with permission).

silhouette with angles, is particularly suspicious. Where suspicion is high magnetic resonance imaging (when available) is at present the most sensitive investigation compared with angiography or computerized tomography scanning.

BLOOD TESTS

As soon as possible after admission blood is drawn for routine tests including cardiac enzymes and cholesterol. Cholesterol levels fall rapidly after the onset of infarction and thus may be reassuringly low. The admission cholesterol (if taken) is usually a good approximate guide and worth recording. Otherwise it may be weeks or months before the patients usual cholesterol is reached.

Most laboratories record the serum glutamine oxaloacetic transaminase (SGOT or AST) and the serum creatinine kinase. The myocardial creatinine kinase (CKMB) form is specific to heart muscle and therefore more useful. A rise in the blood concentration of these enzymes usually occurs by 6 h from the onset, peaks at 24 h and falls to normal by 3 to 4 days. The height of the peak (which may be missed by infrequent sampling) is a good guide to the amount of myocardial necrosis. Serum lactic dehydrogenase (LDH) is released more slowly and persists longer (2 to 4 days). It is non-specific and may (like non-specific creatinine kinase) come from other sites of damage or injury (e.g. from liver, or from haemolysing red cells). The creatinine kinase enzymes can be fractionated further so that by comparing the ratio of MM and MB subforms it is possible to date the time of onset of infarction. Other, more sophisticated, enzyme tests measure serum myoglobin or troponin. These smaller molecules are released much earlier and may therefore be used

Fig. 10 Data from 1850 surviving AMI patients from the MPIP and MDPIT studies. Note the considerable overlap between different ejection fractions (LVEF) and the presence or absence of failure (PC = pulmonary congestion). Patients can still experience failure (and a poor prognosis) and yet have an ejection fraction which is relatively normal (from Gottleib *et al.* (1992), *American Journal of Cardiology*, with permission).

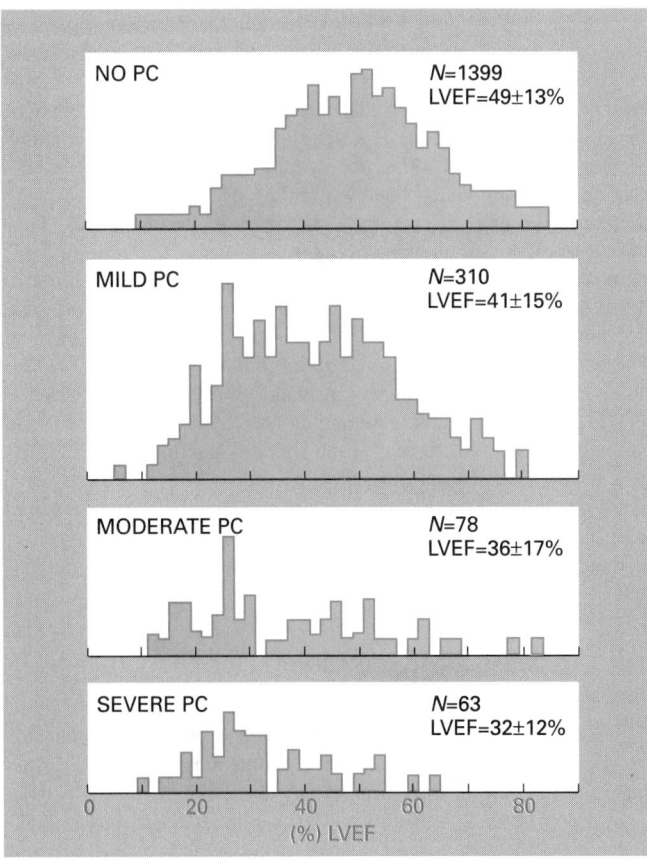

to identify infarction on admission when the electrocardiograph is equivocal.

IMAGING TECHNIQUES

For research purposes it is possible to use a γ-camera and radiolabelled monoclonal antibodies to myocardial proteins in order to delineate damaged cells. These methods are expensive, time consuming, and have now been superseded by improved measures of myocardial blood flow imaging using technetium-99m-sestamibi images of the initial area at risk and the final infarct size.

However, as stated above, the cheapest and most practical option is to use a simple portable bedside echocardiograph.

Treatment and subsequent course of acute myocardial infarction

General measures

As outlined above, the first priority is to relieve pain adequately. Surveys have shown that this is often only partially successful and deserves more care and attention. The use of oxygen has also been described above.

Coronary care units

These were developed mainly to ensure prompt treatment of life threatening arrhythmias, and to monitor the electrocardiograph continuously. There is now less emphasis on prophylactic drug treatment (see below) and more emphasis on prompt defibrillation with high voltage DC current when serious arrhythmia occurs, particularly ventricular fibrillation. Coronary care units also have facilities for temporary pacemaker insertion and for monitoring pressure, both in the pulmonary artery and pulmonary wedge (indirect left atrial pressure) via a Swan–Ganz catheter, or systemic arterial pressure. These methods are not free from morbidity and should be used only when the outcome and treatment is in doubt, and not routinely.

Clinical course

The patient is usually nursed in the semi-sitting position at about 45 degrees. Uncomplicated cases are mobilized progressively from the second day. An average length of stay in hospital is usually 5 to 7 days, but may be shorter when successful reperfusion by drugs or PTCA or, less commonly, surgery has limited the severity of the infarction. The length of stay in hospital has often been determined more by bed shortages or expense and subsequent pressure on the remaining beds, rather than by any clear medical decision. Nevertheless, early mobilization has been shown to be beneficial both physically and importantly, psychologically.

The uncomplicated patient may spend 1 to 2 days in the coronary care unit and then transfer either to an intermediate care unit (monitored) or to a general ward. Such studies as have been done throw some doubt on the usefulness of intermediate care units, which are expensive and technically demanding.

An approach to treatment of a routine case and possible complications is described later. Here we review more specific measures, first for the acute phase and then for post-hospital therapy aimed at secondary prophylaxis. There is a frighteningly large range of measures which have been shown in large clinical trials to reduce mortality and morbidity. Not all should be used in the same patient and some are not affordable in many health systems. The art of the physician is to tailor the proven therapies to particular patients. There is some room for manoeuvre since audit of current therapy reveals much inappropriate, unproven, and therefore irrational treatment.

Thrombolytic treatment

No field has better illustrated the need for adequate clinical trials. Streptokinase was first developed in the United States some 30 to 40 years ago. Small trials failed to demonstrate clear benefit but certainly did demonstrate clear risk of bleeding. Two large trials – GISSI-1 and ISIS-2 – were designed in conjunction. GISSI-1 (Gruppo Italiano per lo Studio della Sopravivenza nell'Infarcto Miocardico) studied streptokinase (SK) versus open control in over 11 000 patients with suspected myocardial infarction up to 12 h from the onset of symptoms. The results, published in 1986, showed a clear 18 per cent reduction in relative risk of death which was most evident in the first 6 h and particularly in the first hour when the risk reduction was 45 per cent (a retrospective analysis).

ISIS-2 (International Study of Infarct Survival) additionally was larger (over 17 000 patients) and also tested aspirin 160 mg daily for 1 month in a factorial double blind design with the same dose of streptokinase as GISSI-1 (1.5 million units intravenously over 1 h). The time window in ISIS-2 was up to 24 h from the onset of pain. In general this reinforced the GISSI result, showing a 25 per cent reduction in mortality with streptokinase, and a separate and striking 23 per cent reduction with aspirin. These results were approximately additive so that the quarter of the ISIS-2 patients who received both active agents had a 42 per cent reduction in the risk of dying (Fig. 11). In those randomized within 4 h streptokinase plus aspirin more than halved mortality. However, unlike GISSI there appeared to be significant benefit in those randomized between 4 and 24 h. In contrast to GISSI-1, the benefit seen in the prospectively specified group randomized within 1 h was less extreme.

Aspirin was without any severe side-effects. Not only was the effect of aspirin on mortality substantial and additive to streptokinase, but it also halved the increased reinfarction rate seen with streptokinase (from 4 per cent to 2 per cent) and also substantially reduced the risk of stroke.

These two trials together led to a substantial change in clinical practice. In the United Kingdom two separate surveys (in 1987 and 1989) of physicians responsible for the treatment of myocardial infarction found that between these surveys the percentage of physicians who routinely considered the use of thrombolysis increased from 4 per cent to

Fig. 11 Cumulative vascular mortality in days 0 to 35 in patients allocated to double-placebo, aspirin alone (160 mg daily for 1 month), streptokinase alone (1.5 million units intravenously over 1 h), or the combination. Note that aspirin has a similar effect on mortality whether or not streptokinase is present, but that the combination of streptokinase and aspirin is additive (from ISIS-2 Trial (1988), *Lancet* with permission).

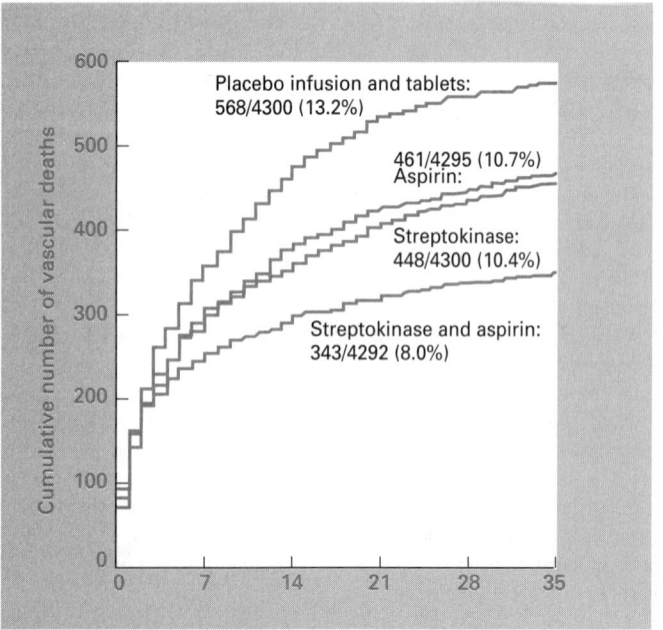

69 per cent, and of aspirin from approximately 10 per cent to 80 per cent. This same pattern could be seen worldwide in the almost 60 000 patients randomized into the ISIS-4 trial of various types of vasodilators in the acute phase of myocardial infarction. In ISIS-4 physicians were free to choose whether to use a lytic agent or not. The use of out-of-trial drugs was monitored, and thrombolytic use in these cases of suspected myocardial infarction ranged from around 50 per cent (Israel) to 89 per cent (United Kingdom).

However, there still remained some doubts about which type of patient benefits from thrombolysis. In this context a collaborative overview was set up of all the then available data on patients randomized to a lytic agent against placebo or control. Individual patient data on approximately 130 000 patients–99 per cent of the published data were obtained (FTT Collaboration).

HOW LONG AFTER THE ONSET OF MYOCARDIAL INFARCTION IS LYTIC THERAPY STILL USEFUL?

Because of differences in the results of GISSI-1 and ISIS-2 the time window for useful benefit was a matter of controversy, with many physicians limiting treatment to within 6 h from onset. However, the FTT overview makes clear that treatment is still beneficial up to 12 h from onset (Fig. 12). The earlier treatment is started the more impressive is the result. The MITI study of prehospital care of suspected myocardial infarction, carried out in the Seattle area, showed that patients treated (whether in the ambulance or hospital) within 60 to 90 min of onset had a strikingly lower mortality rate, a smaller infarct, and were less likely to develop a documented infarct than those treated later.

MECHANISMS OF LATE THROMBOLYSIS

Thrombolysis carried out after the first 2 to 3 h is unlikely to achieve much myocardial salvage, and therefore the initial reaction of cardiologists was one of disbelief at the benefits of thrombolysis seen in late treated patients in the ISIS-2 trial. As discussed above, these results have now been confirmed by the LATE trial, which randomized tissue plasminogen activator or placebo after 6 h, and the EMERAS trial, carried out in South America, which randomized streptokinase.

Further studies have shown that the mechanism of this late benefit from an open artery are: (1) less ventricular dilatation in the months after a myocardial infarction, probably by a combination of better scar formation and additionally, better 'splinting' of the ventricle when the vessels are open and stiffened by higher pressure perfusion; (2) better electrical stability and protection against serious arrhythmia; and (3) some possible myocardial salvage when the initial course of the infarction was stuttering, with intermittent occlusion and subsequent myocardial "stunning".

The most recently published large trial (Global Utilisation of Streptokinase and tissue plasminogen activator for Occluded arteries – GUSTO) compared streptokinase and an accelerated regimen of tissue plasminogen activator (see below) and similarly confirmed that patients treated within 2 h of onset (all agents pooled) had approximately half the early mortality of those treated within 2 to 6 h. GUSTO was remarkable in that within a time for randomization limited to 6 h from onset they managed to randomize a remarkable 54 per cent of the entered patients within 2 h.

WHAT ARE THE ELECTROCARDIOGRAPHIC CRITERIA FOR TREATMENT?

As indicated above, the first electrocardiograph taken is a good indicator of prognosis. The FTT overview shows that the most benefit from lysis occurs in those patients with suspected myocardial infarction who have ST elevation or bundle branch block on this initial electrocardiograph. Patients with other changes such as ST depression, T wave inversion, or a normal electrocardiograph had some harm (statistically not significant). This is understandable for smaller infarcts, as the hazards may balance any benefit in low risk patients. It is less easy to understand the apparent lack of benefit in patients with ST depression, since they are at high risk and certainly are mostly experiencing a myocardial infarction.

As stated above, it is wise to record VR chest leads so as not to overlook inferior infarction with ST depression. When the electrocardiograph does not show ST elevation it is reasonable to repeat the electrocardiograph at intervals and only use thrombolytics if ST elevation develops; some would treat immediately with lytics as the risk is high. At present there are insufficient trial data to be sure what is the correct procedure.

AGE

Both the incidence and the risk of myocardial infarction increases strikingly with age. Although the proportional benefit of lysis is less for older patients, their risk is much higher and so the absolute benefit of treating older patients is the same or greater than in young patients (see Fig. 8). Older patients (as well as patients treated late after onset) have a greater early hazard from lysis, of left ventricular failure, shock, and cerebral haemorrhage. Although the risk of haemorrhagic stroke is greater in older patients, particularly with tissue plasminogen activator (see below), there is a short fall of thrombotic and embolic stroke with streptokinase. The FTT overview also shows an increase in stroke with age in the control (non-thrombolysed) patients, so fear of stroke should not deter one from using thrombolysis in the old.

BLOOD PRESSURE AND OTHER PATIENT SUBGROUPS

Hypertension on arrival in hospital is a relative contraindication to lysis because of the increased risk of cerebral haemorrhage, but this risk should be assessed in comparison with the risk from the myocardial infarction. In the FTT overview patients with a history of hypertension derived benefit from lysis.

It is also clear that patients who present with low blood pressure (systolic blood pressure < 100 mmHg) also benefit. It is often said that hypotensive patients should not be treated with streptokinase because streptokinase itself causes hypotension, probably by the breakdown of other peptides to form vasodepressive kinins. The evidence from the FTT contradicts this opinion. Similarly, in the GUSTO trial hypotensive or shocked patients appeared to benefit more from streptokinase than tissue plasminogen activator.

DIABETES

Diabetics appear to benefit as much as non-diabetics. Although retinal haemorrhage from diabetic retinopathy is sometimes listed as a contraindication to thrombolysis, it is very little reported and must be an extremely rare event. I have never seen or heard of this complication personally, despite having seen thrombolysis used in many patients with retinopathy. On arrival in hospital, with pupils often contracted by morphine, and with the optic fundus not easy to see because of cataract, the chance of adequate retinoscopy by relatively junior residents is low! Diabetics have a higher risk and so most do get treated.

PREVIOUS INFARCTION: SEX

Patients who have had a prior myocardial infarction benefit somewhat less than those who are experiencing a first myocardial infarction, but should still be treated. Similarly, the FTT overview shows that women should be treated; although their proportional benefit is less than that of men, their age matched case fatality is higher than men.

HAZARDS OF THROMBOLYSIS

The most obvious risk of treatment is that of haemorrhage, particularly cerebral haemorrhage. Other hazards include a significant but small excess of death associated with impaired left ventricular function. It is not clear what causes this. It is possibly due to haemorrhage into necrotic myocardium in a completed infarction, since the risk of left ventricular dysfunction increases with delay in the time to treatment. A similar haemorrhagic infarction may be responsible for another risk of lysis, namely early cardiac rupture. In the non-thrombolysed patient the time to rupture is spread over the first few days, but in patients treated with thrombolysis rupture now occurs most commonly in the first 12 to 24 h. Whereas in randomized trials the risk of rupture appears less in patients treated by thrombolysis in less than 6 h from onset, it appears increased in those treated after 6 to 9 h, compared with control. This suggests that early treatment reduces infarct size and hence the risk of rupture. Despite the risk of rupture, later treatment appears to be beneficial, by mechanisms unrelated to myocardial salvage (see below).

Another possible cause for left ventricular damage could be excess calcium entry at reperfusion into cells damaged by ischaemia. Thrombolytic treatment may also cause damage to the collagen skeleton—another possible mechanism for rupture.

Finally, a small increase in cardiac arrest completes the excess mortality from lysis seen in the first few hours after treatment. Thereafter this early risk from haemorrhage, rupture, left ventricular dysfunction, and reperfusion arrhythmia is overcome by the later benefit.

It should be emphasized that these hazards of lysis are very uncommon–a total of about 5 to 10/1000 patients treated, but of course they are influenced by characteristics of the patient. Cerebral haemorrhage is strongly related to increasing age and blood pressure, and to the use of tissue plasminogen activator rather than streptokinase (see below). The early hazard is greater in patients who present late, when myocardial salvage is less likely. The physician has to bear in mind that for the vast majority of patients the short-term risk of their myocardial infarction

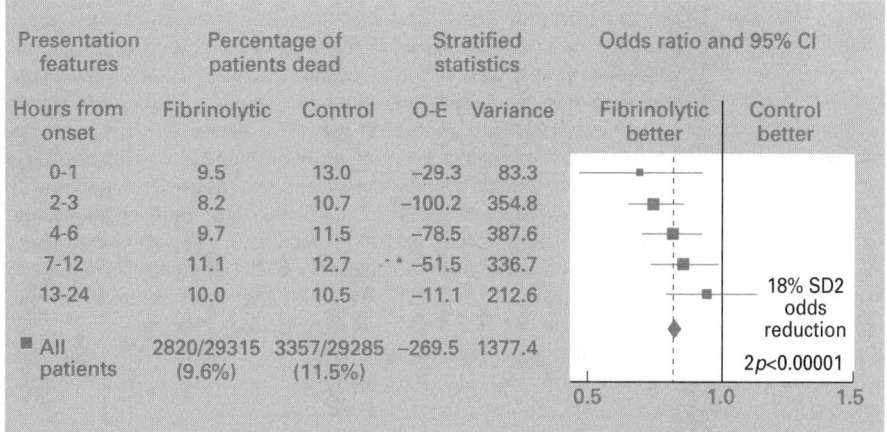

Presentation features	Percentage of patients dead		Stratified statistics		Odds ratio and 95% CI	
Hours from onset	Fibrinolytic	Control	O-E	Variance	Fibrinolytic better	Control better
0-1	9.5	13.0	−29.3	83.3		
2-3	8.2	10.7	−100.2	354.8		
4-6	9.7	11.5	−78.5	387.6		
7-12	11.1	12.7	−51.5	336.7		
13-24	10.0	10.5	−11.1	212.6		
■ All patients	2820/29315 (9.6%)	3357/29285 (11.5%)	−269.5	1377.4		18% SD2 odds reduction 2p<0.00001

Fig. 12 Benefit of thrombolysis versus control divided by hours from onset of myocardial infarction. Note that statistical benefit is clear up to 12 h from onset, but earlier treatment is more effective. The filled squares are proportional in size to the number of events for that particular comparison. The horizontal lines are the 95 per cent confidence limits (from FTT Collaboration, (1993), *Lancet,* with permission).

(up to 250/1000) is far greater than the risks from thrombolysis. A 25 per cent reduction in such a huge risk far outweighs these small risks of adverse events.

Choice of lytic agent: streptokinase, tissue plasminogen activator, or anistreplase (APSAC)

There will soon be a wider choice of thrombolytic agents and an even wider choice of regimens with which to use these different agents as attempts are made to improve the speed and degree of reperfusion. Despite the success of current thrombolysis, we should not be complacent, as recanalization is far from complete. Even with the aggressive regimen of 'front loaded' tissue plasminogen activator used in the GUSTO trial, full flow was only reached in about 50 per cent of patients at 90 min after starting treatment.

The three most tested drugs are streptokinase (a now much refined extract from the streptococcus); an ingenious derivative of streptokinase, anistreplase, which is given as a bolus over 3 to 5 min and releases streptokinase slowly from the anoysilated plasminogen streptokinase complex; and recombinant tissue plasminogen activator, which has the same amino acid sequence as human tissue plasminogen activator, but differs in its coating of sugars (in that the glycosylation pattern is derived from the hamster cells in which the tissue plasminogen activator is made). This may be the reason why the performance of tissue plasminogen activator has not been greatly different from streptokinase.

Both streptokinase and anistreplase suffer from their origin from the streptococcus – in that many patients already have antibodies as a result of previous infections. This necessitates a large dose. Both are highly allergic and so a big rise in antibodies follows after a few days and persists for years. The antibodies are capable of neutralizing a subsequent dose of streptokinase or anistreplase in vitro so for second time use it is preferable to use tissue plasminogen activator, which is not antigenic. However, in countries which cannot afford this a higher dose of streptokinase is an alternative. In ISIS-2 there seemed no advantage from the routine use of hydrocortisone as a prophylactic against anaphylactic shock. True anaphylaxis with streptokinase must be extremely rare. Most hypotension with streptokinase is due to the production of kinins rather than anaphylaxis. It may be protective in the avoidance of cerebral haemorrhage.

EFFECTS OF DIFFERENT AGENTS ON RECANALIZATION

The Thrombosis in Myocardial Infarction (TIMI-1) trial and the European Cooperative Study Group (ECSG) trial compared streptokinase and tissue plasminogen activator in their ability to recanalize arteries in acute myocardial infarction. In both trials patency at 90 min was better with tissue plasminogen activator than streptokinase. Ninety minutes was not chosen for any scientific reason, but rather as a compromise which allowed time for an effect to be seen, and also would not keep the patient in the catheter laboratory for too long. Full flow was designated TIMI-3 patency, partial flow TIMI-2, and minor improvement or no flow TIMI-1 and 0. It is now clear that mortality is least if full TIMI-3 flow can be achieved, and this is now the aim.

The GUSTO trial included a substudy of about 2400 patients in whom angiography was performed (in different subgroups) at 90 min, 3 h, 24 h, and 7 days. In this study four increasingly aggressive regimens were compared–streptokinase with subcutaneous heparin; streptokinase with intravenous heparin; and accelerated tissue plasminogen activator regimen in which tissue plasminogen activator (100 mg) was given in 90 min rather than the previous standard of 3 h; and a combination arm of less than 90 mg tissue plasminogen activator + 1 million units of streptokinase given over 1 h. Ninety-minute patency was slightly better with accelerated tissue plasminogen activator than the combination arm; both were better than the two streptokinase regimens, confirming the TIMI-1 data. However, all regimens showed similar effectiveness at 3 h, with

TIMI-2/3 patency slightly better with the combination arm than the others.

In this trial more than half the patients were entered in less than 2 h. More rapid lysis with accelerated tissue plasminogen activator was associated with a small reduction in mortality, but again a significant 3/1000 increase in stroke. Trials are now planned to evaluate the effects of streptokinase given within 30 min versus the current 60 min regimen.

MORTALITY COMPARISONS BY LYTIC AGENT

The FTT overview (which excludes GUSTO) compared the results of streptokinase versus tissue plasminogen activator (standard 3 h regimen) in about 66 000 patients, and found no difference in mortality overall, or in patients divided by age, by blood pressure or by time to treatment. As in the later GUSTO trial there was a significant excess of stroke with tissue plasminogen activator of 4/1000 treated. So, despite the theoretical advantage of recombinant tissue plasminogen activator being more clot-specific, and perhaps therefore having less risk of bleeding than the non-specific protease streptokinase, it has been difficult to demonstrate any great advantage in the context of mortality. The GUSTO trial did suggest a modest mortality advantage for tisuse plasminogen activator, but patient selection (and perhaps chance) may have exaggerated this (see below).

RISK DIFFERENCES: EXCESS STROKE WITH TISSUE PLASMINOGEN ACTIVATOR AND ANISTREPLASE

The reason why tissue plasminogen activator (100 mg) given over 3 h produces better patency at 90 min than streptokinase (1.5 million units) given over 1 h, yet produces no greater benefit in mortality may be because any small advantage of earlier recanalization is offset by a greater risk of cerebral haemorrhage with the more aggressive agent (Fig. 13). This excess risk of cerebral bleeding with tissue plasminogen activator is strongly related to the systolic pressure at the time, and to age. This excess with age is not seen, and the gradient related to pressure was much shallower with streptokinase. The reasons for these differences are not known, but may be because streptokinase lowers blood pressure by the formation of vasodilator kinins and this hypotension may be protective. Second, streptokinase may be less efficient and therefore be less likely to lyse old (and useful) clots in Charcot–Bouchard aneurysm in the cerebral white matter; these are of course strongly related to age and blood pressure.

The FTT overview shows that below a systolic pressure of 125 mmHg and an age of 55 the risk of cerebral haemorrhage is extremely low. The ISIS-3 and GISSI-2 trials, which contributed most of the data to the overview were criticized because they did not use full dose intravenous heparin. In these two very large trials, in addition to the thrombolytic comparisons (streptokinase versus tissue plasminogen activator (duteplase) versus anistreplase in ISIS-3, and streptokinase versus tissue plasminogen activator (alteplase) in GISSI-2, all patients were randomized to aspirin alone, versus aspirin + 12 500 units twice a day of subcutaneous heparin for 7 days. This subcutaneous high dose heparin regimen was felt by many physicians to be suboptimal, particularly for tissue plasminogen activator, which has a short half-life. However, the angiographic study in GUSTO showed that the simple subcutaneous heparin regimen used in ISIS and GISSI was equivalent to the carefully controlled intravenous heparin regimen used in three arms of the GUSTO trial. Clinical reinfarction was if anything less in the streptokinase with subcutaneous heparin arm than any of the three intravenous heparin arms. Comparing streptokinase with intravenous heparin versus streptokinase with subcutaneous heparin in GUSTO showed no mortality difference (each 7.2 per cent) but 2/1000 more cerebral haemorrhages with intravenous heparin added to aspirin and streptokinase.

Surprisingly, perhaps, the most aggressive arm of GUSTO (the combination of streptokinase and tissue plasminogen activator) showed no mortality benefit over the two streptokinase arms.

The GUSTO trial showed that the accelerated tissue plasminogen activator arm had nine fewer deaths per thousand and three more strokes per thousand than the ISIS/GISSI regimen of streptokinase with aspirin and subcutaneous heparin ($P = 0.04$); however, one of the strokes was fatal. On the other hand, interpretation of the subcutaneous heparin arm in GUSTO is complicated by the non-protocol use of intravenous heparin, particularly in the United States and Canada. In addition, the accelerated tissue plasminogen activator arm in this open trial was associated with an excess of 1 per cent emergency revascularization compared with streptokinase. These differences make it difficult to accept that the true advantage of tissue plasminogen activator (accelerated regimen) over streptokinase is as large as 9/1000 (or 8/1000 net clinical benefit if one counts the disabling strokes). Some have estimated the true result as 5 to 6/1000 (marginally significant) but balanced by 3/1000 excess of stroke (highly significant).

A reasonable interpretation is to accept that there is some marginal benefit for accelerated tissue plasminogen activator for the very early patient (seen within 2 to 3 h) with a severe myocardial infarction, who is not at risk of haemorrhagic stroke by reason of age (under about 60 years). Where cost is a relevant consideration the benefit of tissue plasminogen activator seems very marginal, as the difference in cost between tissue plasminogen activator and streptokinase is very large (about ten-fold at least). The excess cost per life saved by using tissue plasminogen activator is very high for the younger normotensive patient with little risk of cerebral haemorrhage with tissue plasminogen activator since such patients are at relatively low risk.

ANISTREPLASE

Anistreplase versus placebo was first tested in a large trial in the APSAC in myocardial infarction study (AIMS) study in patients with ST elevation less than 6 h from onset of symptoms. The resulting 42 per cent reduction in 30-day mortality was, at that time, the most promising of all agents tested. However, tested blindly, head to head with tissue plasminogen activator (duteplase) and streptokinase in the ISIS-3 study, anistreplase showed no mortality difference and was intermediate between streptokinase and tissue plasminogen activator with regard to safety, resulting in two fewer strokes/1000 than tissue plasminogen activator, and 2/1000 more than streptokinase.

Its main advantage, namely easier and simpler administration as a 30 mg bolus given over 3 to 5 min is somewhat reduced by the need (on present regulations) to keep it refrigerated. It is naturally more expensive than streptokinase but less costly than tissue plasminogen activator. Like streptokinase it is hypotensive and allergenic. Some find it convenient for emergency use by family doctor or paramedic, or in a general emergency department, as opposed to a coronary care unit.

OTHER THROMBOLYTIC AGENTS

Urokinase, extracted from urine as its name implies, is similar to streptokinase, but is not allergenic. It has not been tested in a large mortality trial. It is inexpensive and therefore a viable alternative to tissue plasminogen activator for second-time use. A recombinant version – single chain urokinase plasminogen activator (SCUPA)–has been cloned and is under development.

Other agents which appear promising are r-PA, a derivative of tissue plasminogen activator with a longer half-life, and staphylokinase (a derivative of staphylococci).

DOES HEPARIN ADD SIGNIFICANT ADVANTAGE TO FULL DOSE ASPIRIN (160 MG TO 250 MG DAILY) IN PATIENTS RECEIVING THROMBOLYSIS?

Considering the FTT overview, together with GUSTO, there seems no advantage for the routine use of any form of heparin added to streptokinase. It may be justifiable when there is high risk of, or existing ventricular mural thrombus, or continuing arrhythmia, or poor left ventricular function, when aspirin may not suffice. Otherwise the increased risk of cerebral haemorrhage does not seem justified, when there is no evidence of improvement in mortality.

For tissue plasminogen activator the evidence is totally inadequate to make a considered judgement. The only adequate trial of intravenous versus no heparin added to adequate aspirin during tissue plasminogen activator therapy was conducted by the ECSG. The trial was not large enough to assess mortality differences but showed a patency rate only 8 per cent higher for intravenous heparin versus no heparin (75 per cent versus 83 per cent). However, most physicians still use intravenous heparin added to aspirin after tissue plasminogen activator.

The GUSTO trial did show how difficult it is to ensure full heparinization in the important early phase of lytic therapy. Despite the avail-

Fig. 13 Cumulative percentage with any stroke (upper lines) and with definite or probable cerebral haemorrhage in hospital up to day 35 or prior discharge, from the ISIS-3 Trial of the Comparison of streptokinase, conventional 3 h/100 mg tissue plasminogen activator regimen, and APSAC. (a) All patients allocated aspirin plus heparin (thicker line) versus all allocated aspirin alone; (b) all patients allocated streptokinase (thicker line) vs all allocated APSAC; (c) all patients allocated streptokinase versus all allocated tissue plasminogen activator. The same excess risk of stroke with tissue plasminogen activator over streptokinase was also seen in GISSI-2 and in the GUSTO-1 trial (from ISIS-3, (1992), *Lancet,* with permission).

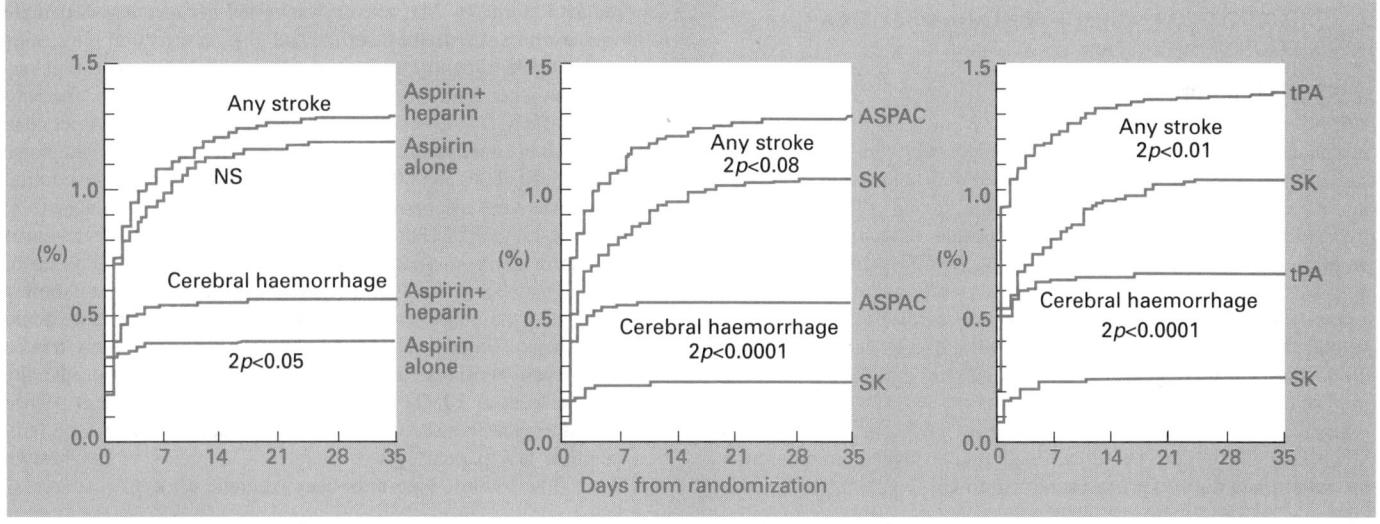

ability of bedside APTT estimations in GUSTO, only about half the patients were in the correct therapeutic range at 24 h. Newer agents such as the leech-derived hirudin or hirulog are now being tested; their efficiency in reducing reocclusion seems superior, but we await larger trials to assess the risk. Three such trials have now been stopped early because of an unacceptable rate of cerebral haemorrhage, underlining the fact that the quest for greater patency does have costs.

Heparin may induce a state of thrombocytopenia; less commonly there may be associated agglutination of platelets and paradoxical thrombosis, which can be arterial or venous. Both of these complications can be troublesome. Heparin should be withdrawn immediately if they are suspected, substituted if necessary by another anticoagulant. Platelet counts should be carried out during longer term (> 5 days) heparin therapy.

OTHER METHODS OF ACUTE REVASCULARIZATION IN MYOCARDIAL INFARCTION

Particularly in the United States, direct PTCA, i.e. coronary angioplasty without thrombolytic therapy, has become increasingly popular and surprisingly practical and available in the setting of community hospitals staffed by private physicians in generally prosperous communities. It has the advantage of avoiding the risks of bleeding from the lytic agent, but not those of intensive heparinization, which is always used in conjunction with angioplasty and which leads particularly to bleeding from the catheter entry site.

PTCA alone has recently been subjected to randomized trials in myocardial infarction, although only on a small scale. These trials have shown that in well organized units the time to opening the artery is very comparable to lytic agents, as the latter take 60 to 90 min to work, while PTCA takes about the same time to get the patient into a laboratory, but then the opening is very rapid. The other advantage of PTCA is that the resultant stenosis is generally less (than with lysis), with better flow. It may also lead to more rapid hospital discharge particularly in centres which advocate routine angiography after lysis (probably unnecessary).

All in all, PTCA may be a viable option in such well supplied communities, but it is certainly not an option for the majority of health care systems. Nor do we have enough information about the later restenosis rate, or about its safety in community settings with less experienced operators. Routine PTCA after lysis has been shown not to confer benefit (TIMI-2 and ECSG trials). Similarly, immediate coronary bypass surgery can, in experienced hands, be a safe option – a so-called 'one stop' alternative to the staged treatment of lysis, followed by PTCA and/or surgery.

OTHER AGENTS FOR THE ACUTE STAGE OF MYOCARDIAL INFARCTION

Immediate treatment: vasodilators

Nitrates

Sublingual trinitrin (0.4 mg) is almost universally administered in the acute stage of myocardial infarction, when it may help distinguish unstable angina or a prolonged attack of stable angina from an incipient myocardial infarction. It can be safely repeated on recumbent patients. On admission to hospital intravenous nitrate therapy is similarly in widespread use (5 to 10 mg/min initially). It is safe and very helpful in suppressing pain in unstable angina; it relieves cardiac risk by peripheral venodilation and reduction of venous return, and by reducing cardiac afterload as a result of arteriolar dilation. Nitrates may also have effects on platelets, reducing platelet aggregation.

Small scale trials suggest that nitrates may have beneficial long-term effects by reduction of ventricular dilation after myocardial infarction, but nitrates had not so far been subjected to large scale mortality trials

until recently. ISIS-4 and GISSI-3 have respectively tested oral isosorbide mononitrate (Imdur®-Astra), and intravenous nitrate followed by a skin patch. In neither ISIS-4 nor GISSI-3 was there any significant reduction in mortality. However, unlike the early small trials, physicians were allowed to use short-term intravenous or other nitrates in the first 24 to 48 h. So it is possible that ISIS and GISSI did not randomize those patients most likely to benefit. Certainly these trials show that nitrates do not need to be used in all patients, nor routinely for the 4 to 6 weeks after infarction.

The oral compounds are used either as sublingual trinitrin, buccal nitrate or nitrate pastes, or transdermal preparations. Nitrate tolerance rapidly develops (within 12 h) unless nitrate-free periods are introduced. With intravenous nitrates tolerance may be counteracted by increasing the dose over the first 24 to 48 h. With the other preparations it is best to stop the treatment for some hours by removing the patch at night, or in the case of the isosorbide preparations, developing a formulation which only lasts 14 to 18 h.

With all nitrate therapy headache is the major side-effect, but usually tolerance to this develops more readily than tolerance to the haemodynamic effects.

Angiotensin converting enzyme inhibitors

Angiotensin converting enzyme inhibitors are of great importance in the convalescent phase of myocardial infarction, where they have been shown to be particularly effective in patients who have had heart failure (even transiently) during the acute phase, or who have impaired left ventricular function on tests such as echocardiography or nuclear or conventional ventriculography.

Their place in the acute phase as routine treatment is now clear. The CONSENSUS-II trial tested immediate enalaprilat given intravenously, followed by oral enalapril in about 6000 patients and found no benefit.

ISIS-4 (58 000 patients – captopril) and GISSI-3 (about 20 000 patients – lisinopril) have now reported and show a small but highly significant reduction of about 5–6/1000 in 5-week mortality. This benefit doubles if one selects patients with larger infarcts, prior infarcts, or LV dysfunction. My preferred option is to start ACE inhibitors once the patient is clinically stable and not hypotensive and then reassess the need for long-term therapy by echocardiography at about 6 weeks. Others may prefer to target only high-risk patients initially.

Magnesium

Intravenous magnesium sulphate, about 80 milli-equivalents given intravenously over 24 h has been tested in several small trials in acute myocardial infarction, and in one remarkable larger trial of about 2300 patients in a single centre – Leicester (LIMIT-2).

LIMIT-2 found overall a 24 per cent decrease in mortality, but with very wide confidence limits, which ranged from no effect to over 40 per cent reduced mortality. Magnesium was tested because it was thought to have a useful antiarrhythmic effect and also an effect on prevention of excessive calcium entry during reperfusion. LIMIT, somewhat surprisingly found benefit in improved left ventricular function but no antiarrhythmic effect. If ISIS-4 had shown an effect as great as 24 per cent, it would have been terminated early. However, it continued to the finish and randomized about 58 000 patients between magnesium and control. The result was very disappointing. Mortality was slightly higher (NS) in the magnesium arm. Magnesium did reduce arrhythmia, but there was an increase in asystole, shock, and heart failure, just the opposite of LIMIT-2. It has been said that perhaps ISIS-4 was unable to show a benefit because the magnesium was given too late. However, we could not find a benefit in any subgroup examined, even very early treated patients, or patients (about 11 000) who did not receive lytic therapy (only 30 per cent of LIMIT-2 patients received thrombolysis). Hence intravenous magnesium should only be used in acute myocardial infarction in those few patients where there is a suspicion of magnesium deficiency (low sodium, long-term heavy diuretic use).

β-Adrenoceptor blockade

Two large trials, ISIS-1 (atenolol, 5 to 10 mg IV, 100 mg oral/day) and MIAMI (metoprolol 5 to 15 mg IV) have tested intravenous β-blocker followed by oral β-blockade in the acute phase of myocardial infarction. Both showed a similar 13 to 15 per cent reduction in hospital deaths, although only ISIS-1, which randomized over 16 000 patients (compared with about 5500 in MIAMI), reached statistical significance (Fig. 14).

Unlike lytic therapy almost all of the effect on mortality was immediate, in the first 24 to 36 h. One of the major reasons for benefit was reduction in the risk of cardiac rupture.

Also unlike lytic therapy the use of early intravenous β-blockade is very variable worldwide, with considerable use in the United States, and Australia, and with very little use in the United Kingdom and other European countries. As early cardiac rupture is one of the complications of thrombolytic therapy, β-blockade may be more relevant now than in the prethrombolytic era.

Because intravenous β-blockers can, and frequently do, cause hypotension (which, of course, may also protect against the risk of cerebral haemorrhage from thrombolytics), they worry inexperienced residents. Usually this hypotension responds to simple measures such as raising the foot of the bed.

Additional benefits include a very useful anti-arrhythmic effect with no pro-arrhythmic hazards, and rapid relief of pain by reduction in cardiac work.

Of course, they cannot be used where there is obvious circulatory collapse or hypotension. This means that in practice they can only be used in about 40 to 50 per cent of myocardial infarctions – the relatively good risk patients. A good clinical discriminator is to test the peripheral skin temperature – if the nose is warm the patient can usually tolerate intravenous β-blockers!

Calcium channel blocking agents

In contrast to the poor use of β-blockers, where there is good evidence for benefit, calcium blockers are used commonly despite considerable evidence for harm, and certainly no evidence for good in the early phase of myocardial infarction (first 48 h). Several trials have been negative or shown non-significant harm. Agents such as verapamil, or in some cases diltiazem, are useful in the convalescent and later phase provided the patient has not experienced heart failure or has poor left ventricular function (see below). The dihydropyridines, such as nifedipine, have no place in the acute or later phase of myocardial infarction except in the rather rare cases of coronary spasm. It is probably the undue theoretical emphasis on spasm in acute ischaemia which has led to the undeserved popularity of dihydropyridines.

Inotropic agents, shock, and surgical conditions

In theory, inotropes may increase infarct size by increasing cardiac work. Despite this they may be useful in temporarily supporting the circulation during shock and left ventricular failure. Low dose dopamine infusion (2 to 6 μg/min) may be particularly useful in promoting diuresis and protecting against renal shut down during hypotension. Dobutamine or adrenaline may also be useful if used with care. Anecdotal evidence suggests that acute angioplasty may be the most effective therapy for shock. This is often performed with the temporary use of circulatory support, e.g. with an intra-aortic balloon pump.

Finally, in all cases of shock it is important to consider a surgical diagnosis, particularly cardiac rupture (into the right ventricle or pericardium) or papillary or chordal rupture with torrential mitral regurgitation (which may be relatively silent). Prompt surgery may be life saving (again with temporary circulatory support).

ANTI-ARRHYTHMIC THERAPY

Ventricular fibrillation and tachycardia
Lignocaine

As noted above, early intravenous β-blockade may be useful in the prevention of arrhythmia. When coronary care units were first developed there was too great an emphasis on treatment of even minor arrhythmias, such as runs of ventricular tachycardia (usually with intravenous lignocaine).

The present attitude is towards avoidance of prophylactic use of anti-arrhythmic agents which generally have negative inotropic effects and also may be importantly pro-arrhythmic. This attitude of watchful waiting stemmed from the realization of these adverse effects, but particularly because an overview of all the randomized trials of the prophylactic use of lignocaine showed that although ventricular fibrillation was reduced significantly, asystole was similarly increased; the balance was an increase in mortality. Furthermore, effective prophylactic suppression of arrhythmia needed a high dose of lignocaine (3 to 4 mg/min), which produced a high incidence of side-effects such as light-headedness, confusion, and other neurological syndromes.

In a well run coronary care unit, ventricular fibrillation is satisfactorily and easily treated by DC shock, so the policy now is to avoid prophylactic treatment and use lignocaine only after a patient has experienced ventricular fibrillation. For recurrent ventricular arrhythmia (VF or VT) amiodarone is a useful agent (see below).

Atrial fibrillation and other supraventricular arrhythmias

For lesser but troublesome arrhythmias, such as atrial fibrillation, DC shock is not usually advised as there is a high likelihood of recurrence. Digitalis given intravenously may be toxic and oral digitalization is rather slow to control the rate. If the patient is not distressed it is often possible to wait a few hours for spontaneous reversion. Otherwise the treatment is a matter for individual choice based primarily on familiarity with the agent used, as there are no good trials and very little science to guide one. There are potential problems (pro-arrhythmia) in the use of agents such as quinidine, flecainide, and procainamide and agents with pronounced negative inotropic effects. Some would use a small intravenous dose of a β-blocker or intravenous verapamil. It may be best to give intravenous amiodarone 600 mg/day by a central venous line; it

Fig. 14 Mortality in days 0 to 7, re-infarction and ventricular fibrillation in hospital from all available randomized trials (in 1986) with early intravenous β-blockade in acute myocardial infarction. Hatched columns–intravenous β-blocker, open columns–control. The percentage of randomized patients affected by the various categories, figures above the bars are the absolute numbers of events, the proportional reduction in events in category is shown below the abscissa (from ISIS-1, (1986), *Lancet,* with permission).

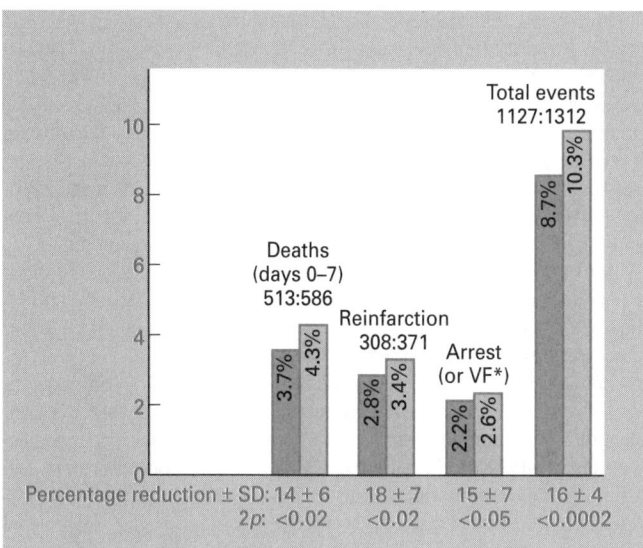

is probably the most effective agent available, is non-toxic in short-term use and is not noticeably depressant of left ventricular function. Indeed, a recent large trial of oral amiodarone (300 mg/day) carried out in Argentina in over 500 patients in class 3 to 4 heart failure was stopped early because of a 25 per cent reduction in mortality and a significant improvement in left ventricular function. Occasional instances of pro-arrhythmia (torsades de pointes) have been described. Amiodarone has also been tested after myocardial infarction in randomized trials from the United States, and from Poland, and found to be safe and effective (Fig. 15). It may be continued intravenously for the initial few days and then orally, aiming at a long-term dose of around 200 mg/day only in those patients in whom arrhythmia recurs.

HEART BLOCK

Heart block of any degree is more common with inferior than anterior infarction because the right coronary artery gives rise to the artery to the atrioventricular node and also because vagal reflexes are more likely from this area. It is often transient and does not necessarily imply a very large myocardial infarction. When heart block occurs with an anterior myocardial infarction it generally is associated with a very large myo-cardial infarction and the prognosis is grave. Temporary pacing is there-fore generally done only for symptomatic reasons where the low heart rate is clearly compromising the circulation. The prognosis is rarely helped by pacing as in most inferior myocardial infarctions the block is only transient and with anterior myocardial infarction is often fatal because of the size of the infarction, so pacing *per se* therefore makes little difference. Prophylactic pacing is not advocated for first or second degree heart block, as placing the wire may compromise lytic therapy; even without thrombolysis a central venous access via the subclavian vein has a significant morbidity from bleeding or pneumothorax.

PERICARDITIS

This is a quite common complication especially of anterior infarction. It is generally of nuisance value and rarely causes tamponade unless anticoagulant therapy leads to pericardial bleeding. It causes continued pain, which may worry the patient. If this is troublesome it may respond to non-steroidal anti-inflammatory agents or aspirin.

Rarely pericarditis may occur some 3 to 6 weeks, or even later, after myocardial infarction as part of an autoimmune process (Dressler's syn-drome). Steroids may be needed for recurrent attacks.

Fig. 15 Survival curve of 613 patients, who did not die of cardiac causes and were randomly allocated to treatment with amiodarone and placebo for 1 year after myocardial infarction (from Ceremyzinski *et al.* (1992), *Journal of the American College of Cardiology,* with permission).

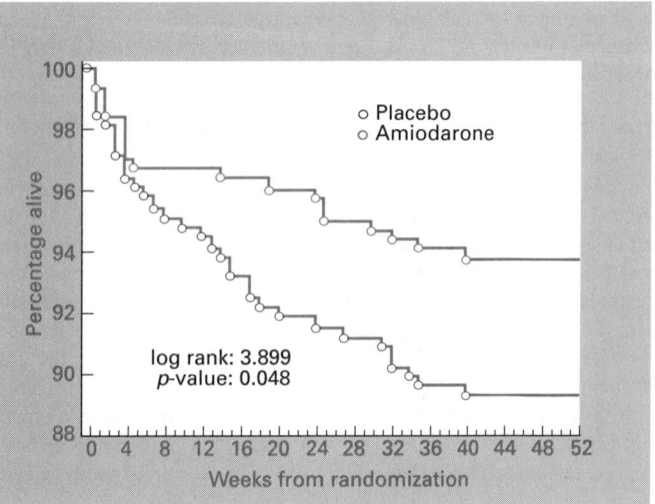

SHOULDER–HAND SYNDROME

This is a syndrome of rheumatism-like pain in the left shoulder, with restricted movement, which occurs in the weeks after myocardial infarc-tion. It usually subsides with symptomatic treatment and physiotherapy. It too may be an autoimmune phenomenon.

Risk assessment and treatment after myocardial infarction

Introduction

The reason for risk assessment is that many patients are at high risk of dying in the first few months after a myocardial infarction. Patients with left main stenosis and multiple vessel stenosis have the highest risk, particularly if there has been substantial ventricular damage and a reduced ejection fraction (< 40 per cent). Revascularization has been shown to be beneficial for such patients and may be beneficial for many others. On the other hand patients who have recovered from a small myocardial infarction, who have had an uncomplicated course, who have good exercise ability with no angina, and who are younger may have an excellent prognosis, i.e. 1 year mortality less than 1 to 3 per cent. The aim of risk assessment is to devise the most efficient and least expensive way of separating such good risk patients from those who may have a 1-year risk of mortality of 20 to 40 per cent. Overall, the first-year risk after myocardial infarction is about 10 per cent. Thereafter it flattens rapidly to a 3 to 5 per cent risk depending on age and left ventricular function.

There is a huge variation worldwide in the extent of investigation and treatment of patients who have survived a myocardial infarction. Even between the United States and Canada there are large differences in angiography and intervention rates, but with no obvious difference in mortality. It may seem desirable to know the exact coronary anatomy, but in uncritical hands this may result in interventions which carry mor-bidity and mortality risks but which are of little or no long term benefit.

Routine angiography or not?

One of the reasons why investigation and subsequent intervention is less rewarding than common sense would suggest is that the next myocardial infarction or ischaemic event is just as likely to take place at another innocent-looking plaque, as at the culprit plaque that caused the index myocardial infarction. This has been well studied in patients who happen to have had a prior angiogram and then later present with an acute ischaemic event. Of course, a residual stenosis which is very severe – say a 90 per cent diameter stenosis–is highly likely to occlude subse-quently. However, such an occlusion may not be so dangerous as might seem likely from simple consideration of the angiogram. The subtended myocardium distal to such a lesion might in fact be already necrotic, or equally, it might be supplied with new collateral vessels.

Another argument against early routine angiography is that the resid-ual stenosis seen at that time includes some thrombus, which is later absorbed so that the final lesion may look much less threatening.

A third reason for caution with regard to routine coronary angiogra-phy is that it may lead to what has been called the 'oculo-stenotic reflex'. It may be difficult to resist revascularization by PTCA or coronary artery bypass graft, even if it is not clinically useful.

A final and very compelling reason for caution is that the future prog-nosis for an individual patient is dominated by the state of the left ven-tricle, not by the number of anatomically narrowed vessels seen. A clas-sic study from Barcelona carried out routine coronary and left ventricular angiography on a series of patients after myocardial infarc-tion and showed that if the left ventricular ejection fraction was normal the 5-year survival was excellent, irrespective of the number of coronary stenoses found. Danish physicians are currently carrying out an interesting trial, randomizing patients after myocardial infarction to routine angiography versus angiography only if indicated on current clinical grounds.

Routine coronary angiography versus non-invasive risk

A number of non-invasive tests may be used to select out the patients with a poor prognosis from those who have a very low risk of a future event. Many of these can achieve this division when applied routinely to a series of patients, but it is critically important to decide what such tests really add to other simple and inexpensive clinical assessments. Relevant studies are rather few but those that have been done indicate that simple clinical markers should dominate any scheme of risk assessment. These markers are age, the presence of definite heart failure in the acute stage (however transient), continuing chest pain in the acute stage despite full medical therapy with nitrates, heparin, β-blockade and aspirin, a poor exercise ability, a clinically large infarction (electrocardiograph and enzymes) and the presence of serious arrhythmia on the coronary care unit, and later by Holter monitoring. Knowledge of the ejection fraction (by echo or radionuclide techniques) adds a little more.

EXERCISE (STRESS) TESTS

Formal exercise testing with monitoring of electrocardiograph ST segment and arrhythmia adds some further, but small, discrimination. The biggest discriminator, however, is whether the patient is actually able to take the test! The next is the length of time the patient can actually exercise. How quickly the ST segment depression develops and how long it persists during recovery are further, but relatively minor, discriminators. Another value of exercise testing is, importantly, to show patients what they can do safely, and so raise damaged morale. It is also useful to detect patients whose disability is psychological and who may derive particular benefit from rehabilitation.

The exercise test is also useful to identify whether the patient has residual angina and how severe it is; such angina is not (on its own) a marker for poor prognosis. Exercise-induced changes in the electrocardiograph are less useful when digitalis is being taken, or when the patient has a bundle branch block pattern. Drug treatment, particularly with β-blockers may also reduce sensitivity.

Exercise testing may also be combined with radio-isotope perfusion tests to identify reversible ischaemia (as opposed to scar tissue). In nonexpert hands such tests may have poor discrimination and also produce false positive results.

HOLTER MONITORING AND ELECTROPHYSIOLOGICAL TESTING

Sudden death from ventricular fibrillation or asystole can to some extent be predicted by these techniques, but not with any great sensitivity or specificity. Because of this there is now more emphasis on newer analyses such as of heart rate variability (including power spectral analysis and baroreflex sensitivity) to identify autonomic imbalance, measurement of late potentials on the signal averaged electrocardiograph, and most recently measurement of QT dispersion. This last is based on the fact that differing lengths of the cardiac cycle (particularly of repolarization) increase the chance of stimulation in the vulnerable period of the T wave and hence of ventricular fibrillation. Electrophysiological testing using repetitive ventricular stimuli can identify such an arrhythmic substrate. Unfortunately, drug treatment (apart from amiodarone) has been disappointing (see above). The alternative of implantation of a defibrillation device is effective but very expensive. The advantage of such devices over 'blind' amiodarone treatment is debatable, although drug treatment with amiodarone does carry a small but definite risk of serious toxicity. β-Blockers, where tolerated, are of proven benefit, as are some calcium blockers (see below).

These complex investigations should be used only when the above clinical indications suggest high immediate risk, or when the patient continues to have rest pain while on full medical therapy in hospital.

Conclusion

In high risk patients after a large infarction, or equally in patients who have settled down after a period of unstable angina or a small myocardial infarction, it is sensible to proceed directly to coronary angiography or, after an abnormal low level exercise test carried out before discharge.

For the others a full symptom-limited exercise test can be performed at about 4 weeks after myocardial infarction. Angiography with a view to revascularization should be considered if the test shows definite early and prolonged ischaemia, or if the patient can only manage a low level of exercise (less than 5 min on the Bruce protocol).

Complications and consequences of myocardial infarction: prophylaxis

As well as the problem of sudden death, patients are at risk of developing cardiac failure. This may follow from ventricular damage and scarring with subsequent ventricular dilatation or so called 'remodelling'. Such remodelling occurs not only in the scar, where it may lead to a ventricular aneurysm, but also in the non ischaemic myocardium. An associated risk is that of rupture (see β-blockade, above). This remodelling is important, leads to a worse prognosis, and can be prevented (see angiotensin converting enzyme inhibition, below).

Heart failure may also be due to surgically correctable conditions such as mitral incompetence, acquired ventricular septal defect, and aneurysm. Post-infarct patients are at risk of reinfarction, and of other vascular complications such as stroke, or peripheral vascular disease which are also preventable.

Prevention of reinfarction

β-BLOCKADE

Large trials with the β-blockers propranolol, metoprolol, and timolol against placebo have shown that β-blockade given for 2 to 3 years after myocardial infarction reduces the risk of reinfarction and of sudden death by 20 to 30 per cent, as well as being highly effective against other arrhythmia and against angina. A varying proportion of patients (around 50 per cent) cannot tolerate these agents because of precipitation or fear of heart failure, fear of exacerbation of asthma or bronchitis, or worsening of intermittent claudication. Verapamil or diltiazem may be useful and equally effective substitutes for these patients.

The mechanism of the reduction in sudden death is probably by prevention of ventricular fibrillation and partly by prevention of cardiac rupture. The mechanism of reduction in reinfarction is less clear. It might be simply by reduction in blood pressure, which would reduce the stress on an unstable plaque, or perhaps reduction in plasma angiotensin, a known growth factor for vascular smooth muscle.

CALCIUM ENTRY BLOCKADE

No calcium channel blocker has been shown to be beneficial in the first 48 h after myocardial infarction. Once the patient has stabilized, verapamil reduces the risk of reinfarction and sudden death (DAVIT-I and II trials) by about 20 to 25 per cent (Fig. 16). Verapamil had no overall beneficial effect on patients who had had heart failure in the acute phase– probably because, like diltiazem, it has some negative inotropic effect. The results of diltiazem treatment in the MDPIT trial were less impressive than of verapamil, possibly because of the simultaneous use of β-blockade in a large number of the patients in the MDPIT, but not in any in the DAVIT trials.

ANTITHROMBOTIC TREATMENT

Antiplatelet agents

As well as the use of aspirin in ISIS-2, an overview of the use of antiplatelet agents has shown that they are highly effective in prevention of recurrent myocardial infarction, stroke and other vascular events. The latest overview of antiplatelet trial shows a reduction in these events of 20 to 25 per cent in the first few years after the index event, and a reduction in all cause mortality of 13 per cent. The effective dose of aspirin is 75 to 160 mg/day; increasing the dose does not increase benefit but does increase side-effects and the risk of gastrointestinal haemorrhage; it is particularly effective in unstable angina.

In the few patients in whom low-dose aspirin is not tolerated, other agents, such as ticlopidine (expensive and more toxic) or dipyridamole, are effective. There is no evidence that dipyridamole added to aspirin gives any extra benefit.

In the short term, low-dose aspirin together with full anticoagulation with heparin or coumadins seems safe when the risk of thrombosis seems high. Longer term use of the combination is under evaluation.

Anticoagulation

Anticoagulation in acute myocardial infarction and after has had a varied history. Small trials were confusing. An overview of the randomized studies in the pre-aspirin era suggested a 20 per cent reduction in mortality. Long term trials of anticoagulation with coumarin derivatives added to low dose aspirin are awaited. Until the results of these are known it is probably wise to use the combination for no longer than 3 months after infarction, unless patients are considered at risk of thrombosis or thromboembolism, for instance with echo proven left ventricular thrombus, or in those with full thickness anterior myocardial infarction, particularly in the presence of heart failure and/or arrhythmia.

Angiotensin-coverting enzyme inhibition after myocardial infarction

Several recent large and well controlled trials have confirmed previous experimental work suggesting that angiotensin converting enzyme inhibition might reduce ventricular dilatation and hence preserve function after myocardial infarction.

The SAVE (Survival and Ventricular Enlargement) trial randomized patients with an ejection fraction below 40 per cent to receive captopril or placebo, beginning at an average of 11 days after myocardial infarction. There was a significant 19 per cent reduction in mortality and less readmission with heart failure in those who received the angiotensin converting enzyme inhibitor, but benefit was not seen until after about 6 months.

The more recent AIRE trial (active agent Ramipril) studied patients with clinical evidence of mild heart failure (even if only transient), e.g. with basal rales, or pulmonary congestion on the chest radiograph. Treatment was given early (beginning 48 h after infarction) and resulted in a 30 per cent reduction in mortality, substantial benefit being apparent as early as 30 days after the infarct. Severe heart failure was considered already an indication for ACE inhibition and such patients were not included in the trial. Both trials and the SOLVD (Studies Of Left Ventricular Dysfunction) trials showed a reduction in re-infarction in those treated. It is clear therefore that angiotensin converting enzyme inhibition is beneficial in patients with impaired left ventricular function after myocardial infarction. It is less clear at present to what extent all patients might benefit. It is clear that, provided patients with hypotension are avoided, and also provided that the dose is carefully titrated, it is safe to start ACE inhibition earlier, in the first 24 h. In GISSI-3 and ISIS-4 such a policy appears to avoid some very early deaths in the first 1 to 2 days.

Cholesterol reduction

As cholesterol is a major determinant of coronary risk it is logical to consider the potential value of reducing plasma cholesterol concentrations for secondary prevention. Many physicians take the attitude that it is too late to attempt such preventive measures after a myocardial infarction, particularly in patients who are over 65 years. This attitude may be mistaken, as several trials have shown remarkably rapid benefit of cholesterol lowering on cardiovascular risk, evident within 2 to 3 years. The mechanism may be due to an action on thrombotic processes as well as actions on the lipid content of plaques, rendering them more stable. Studies have shown that coronary stenoses may be reduced, but the reduction is not particularly impressive.

Whatever the level of cholesterol it is important to try to lower it further in a patient after a myocardial infarction. Diet may suffice in a well motivated patient but, if the cholesterol remains above 5.2 mmol/l there is a strong case for drug treatment with a statin or a fibrate.

A recent Scandinavian study (4S) showed a 30 per cent reduction in all cause mortality when simvastatin was given to middle-aged men after a myocardial infarction.

Lifestyle changes

Smoking cessation

Although changes in exercise activity and diet, and drugs such as aspirin, β-blockade, verapamil, angiotensin converting enzyme inhibitors, and cholesterol lowering drugs may reduce the risk of reinfarction, the degree of benefit is modest in comparison with that of stopping smoking. This reduces mortality by half within 1 to 2 years–the effect being seen remarkably quickly, suggesting that the mechanism may be by reduction in thrombotic factors, such as fibrinogen. It is very important to make this clear at the time of the infarct, talking to the patient and, importantly, to his or her family as well, as this is the ideal moment to persuade the patient of the absolute need to quit.

Rehabilitation after a myocardial infarction

It is difficult to conduct adequate trials of the benefit of regular exercise after myocardial infarction because the drop-out rate is high and moti-

Fig. 16 Cumulative mortality for verapamil 360 mg per day for 18 months, versus placebo in the DAVIT-2 trial in 1775 patients, after myocardial infarction. Note the significant reduction in mortality in patients without heart failure (bottom two lines) but little effect in those with heart failure (top two lines) (from DAVIT-2, (1990), *American Journal of Cardiology,* with permission).

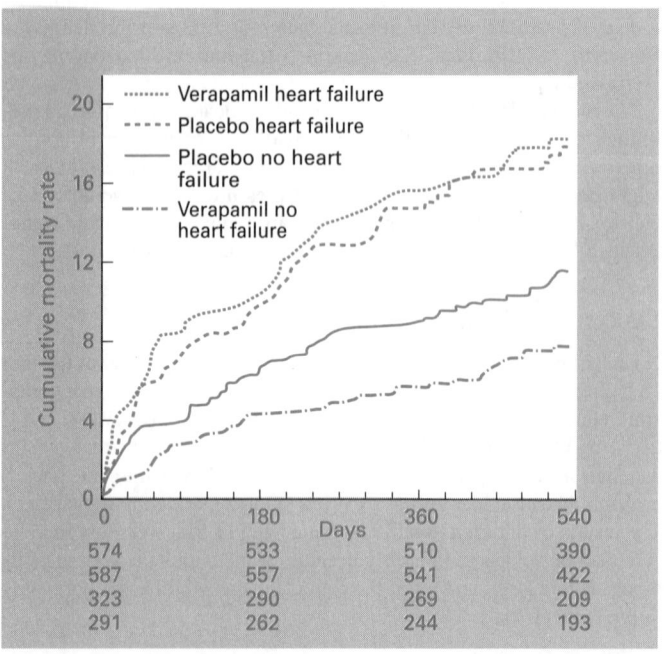

vation often low. Nevertheless, overviews of the available trials suggest that exercise does reduce the risk long term, albeit at the expense of a small increase in risk at the time of the actual exercise. Rehabilitation clinics are becoming increasingly popular, partly because they may reduce future risk but mostly because they improve the patient's confidence, and that of their families. They also provide an excellent vehicle to change lifestyles and smoking habits by means of group therapy. Such clinics fulfil an important and previously unmet need. After a myocardial infarction the patient and their family are full of apprehension, uncertainty, and self-doubt. They have many questions, which often go unanswered in a busy outpatient clinic or in the family doctor's surgery.

Conclusion

Although there have been major advances in the management of acute myocardial infarction, there is a need to streamline procedures for assessment and treatment. This means developing guidelines and agreeing protocols between the several groups involved–family doctors, paramedics and the ambulance service, the emergency or admission staff, the medical teams, the coronary care unit, and the cardiologists. Most important is to improve and apply more widely what we know of preventive measures, particularly the need to stop smoking.

REFERENCES

Fibrinolytic Therapy Trialists' (FTT) Collaborative Group. (1994). Indications for fibrinolytic therapy in suspected acute myocardial infarction: collaborative overview of early mortality and major morbidity results from all randomised trials of more than 1000 patients. *Lancet*, **343**, 311–22.

ISIS-4 (Fourth International Study of Infarct Survival) Collaborative Group. (1995). ISIS-4: a randomised factorial trial assessing early oral captopril, oral mononitrate, and intravenous magnesium sulphate versus control among 58 050 patients with suspected acute myocardial infarction. *Lancet*, in press.

Moss, A.J., Bigger, J.T., and Odoroff, C.L. (1987). Postinfarct risk stratification. *Progress in Cardiovascular Diseases*, **29**, 389–412.

Pfeffer, M.A., Braunwald, E., Moye, L.A., *et al.* (1992). Effect of captopril on mortality and morbidity in patients with left ventricular dysfunction after myocardial infarction. Results of the Survival and Ventricular Enlargement Trial. *New England Journal of Medicine*, **327**, 669–77.

2nd Antiplatelet Trialists' Collaboration. (1994). Collaborative overview of randomised trials of antiplatelet therapy. I: Prevention of death, myocardial infarction, and stroke by prolonged antiplatelet therapy in various categories of patients. *British Medical Journal*, **308**, 81–106. II: Patency by maintenance of vascular graft or arterial antiplatelet therapy. *British Medical Journal*, **308**, 159–68. III: Reduction in venous thrombosis and pulmonary embolism by antiplatelet prophylaxis among surgical and medical patients. *British Medical Journal*, **308**, 235–46.

Yusuf, S., Peto, R., Lewis, J., Collins, R., and Sleight, P. (1985). Beta blockade during and after myocardial infarction: an overview of the randomised trials. *Progress in Cardiovascular Diseases*, **27**, 335–71.

Yusuf, S., Sleight, P., Held, P., and McMahon, S. (1990). Routine medical management of acute myocardial infarction. Lessons from overviews of recent randomized controlled trials. *Circulation*, **82**(3) Suppl. II, 117–34.

15.10.5 Coronary angioplasty

D.P. DE BONO

The concept of dilating a narrowed channel, whether oesophagus, urethra, or uterine cervix, using mechanical dilators, or 'bougies', goes back to antiquity. Application of a similar technique to blood vessels narrowed by atheroma was pioneered by Dotter and Judkins in 1964. Their technique had the disadvantages of requiring a surgical operation to expose the vessel, and that dilatation by the passage of rigid tapered probes inevitably produced a longitudinal tearing force, which could itself cause damage to an atheromatous vessel. Gruntzig later invented the technique of dilatation using a non-compliant cylindrical balloon, which could be passed across a stenosis in a deflated state and would, on dilatation, apply a truly radial dilating force. The balloons were small enough to be passed through a 9 French gauge coronary guiding catheter and positioned under radiographic control, thus making 'percutaneous transluminal coronary angioplasty' (PTCA) practicable. Gruntzig's original balloons were of limited manoeuvrability; in an attempt to improve this, Harzler introduced a low-profile balloon formed around a guidewire. A more popular solution, however, was the introduction by Simpson and Roberts of a movable guidewire passed through a coaxial channel in the balloon. This enables the guidewire to be manoeuvred across the lesion first, followed by the balloon once the stenosis has been crossed. A further development of this theme, by Bonzel, is the monorail balloon, in which the channel for the guidewire is limited to the distal part of the catheter. This has the advantage that the guidewire can be positioned without the need for the balloon catheter to be loaded into the guiding catheter, and also that balloons of different sizes can be exchanged without a need to reposition or replace the guidewire (Fig. 1).

Technique of coronary angioplasty

All angioplasty balloons are made of plastic material with limited compliance. This is important to maintain the cylindrical shape of the balloon as it is inflated, and to prevent damage to the vessel by over dilatation.

Balloons are made in different diameters to allow for their use in coronary arteries of various sizes. The most commonly used diameters are 2.5, 3.0, and 3.5 mm. Some balloons are made slightly compliant to allow an extra 0.2 to 0.5 mm increase in diameter under very high pressure. The usual inflating pressure is about 5 bar (atmospheres) but most balloons are designed to withstand 10 to 12 bar. Inflation is performed using dilute radio-opaque contrast medium, using a hand syringe or mechanical inflation device. The equipment used in angioplasty is shown in Fig. 2, and stages in the dilatation of a coronary lesion in Fig. 3.

The effect of angioplasty on the vessel wall

Inflation of an appropriately sized angioplasty balloon in a normal artery causes fully reversible stretching of the vessel wall and minor endothelial damage. Gross overdistension of a normal vessel causes linear tears extending into the media. Knowledge of what happens when a balloon

Fig. 1 The evolution of coronary balloon angioplasty technology (not to scale).

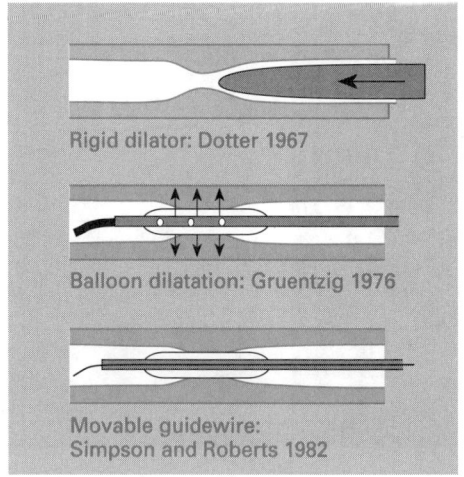

Rigid dilator: Dotter 1967

Balloon dilatation: Gruentzig 1976

Movable guidewire: Simpson and Roberts 1982

is inflated across an atheromatous lesion *in vivo* has been greatly advanced by studies using intracoronary two-dimensional ultrasound catheters. It is now clear that 'squashing' or displacement of atheroma is rare, and the usual mechanism of dilatation is the creation of one or more tears, either within the plaque, or quite often in the 'normal' vessel wall adjacent or opposite to it. Blood pressure within the lumen then distends the vessel and the stenotic appearance, and obstruction to flow, disappear (Fig. 4). Subsequent vessel wall remodelling usually preserves the new lumen, but sometimes, as discussed below, leads to restenosis.

Fig. 2 Diagram of angioplasty of a right coronary artery stenosis.

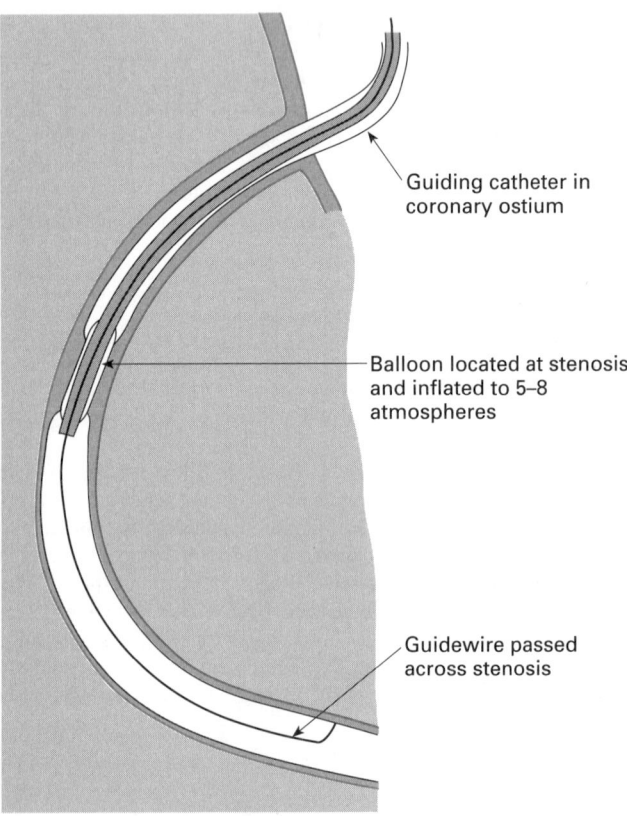

Guiding catheter in coronary ostium

Balloon located at stenosis and inflated to 5–8 atmospheres

Guidewire passed across stenosis

Complications of angioplasty

Patients are subject to the usual vascular and arrhythmia complications of cardiac catheterization, but these are rare. The most important immediate complication is abrupt vessel closure, and the most important long term complication is restenosis.

ABRUPT CLOSURE

This may be due to thromboembolism, coronary spasm, thrombosis *in situ,* or dissection of the vessel wall. Thromboembolism has become very rare with the universal use of aspirin pretreatment (150 to 300 mg daily), high-dose intravenous heparin (typically 10 000 units) during percutaneous transluminal coronary angioplasty, and careful attention to catheter flushing. Coronary spasm usually responds to nitrates or calcium antagonists. These can be given by direct intracoronary injection. Thrombosis *in situ,* either at the time of angioplasty or within the next 12 h, is frequently associated with percutaneous transluminal coronary angioplasty in the presence of pre-existing thrombus – either in unstable angina or following myocardial infarction. It is suggested that the intense thrombogenic stimulus of a fresh thrombus and a freshly disrupted atheromatous plaque, coupled with a reduced flow rate resulting from distal vasoconstriction induced by thrombin, thromboxanes, and platelet activating factor, may lead to thrombosis despite heparinization.

To some extent, coronary dissection is a feature of all angioplasty, but the formation of a large, unstable flap of intima obstructing the lumen is relatively rare. It is more common when angioplasty is performed for unstable angina or after myocardial infarction, in elderly patients or those with diffuse coronary disease, and at certain sites in the coronary tree, for example the proximal right coronary artery.

Dissections that do not compromise coronary flow may be treated conservatively, but the patient needs to be observed closely for 12 to 24 h, and urgent bypass grafting is indicated if ischaemic symptoms develop. Prolonged, low pressure balloon inflation, perhaps using a 'Stack' balloon, which allows flow to the distal vessel to be maintained, sometimes stabilizes the dissection. If it does not, the choice lies between emergency coronary bypass grafting or the use of an intracoronary stent. The risk of abrupt closure ranges from 2 per cent in elective angioplasty for stable angina to 8 to 10 per cent in emergency angioplasty for unstable angina or following thrombolysis. Abrupt closure

Fig. 3 Stages in coronary angioplasty: (a) preangioplasty angiogram; (b) balloon and guidewire across stenosis, balloon being inflated; (c) after inflation – guidewire and catheter removed.

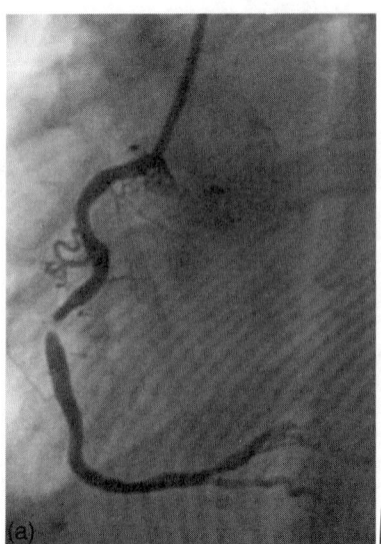

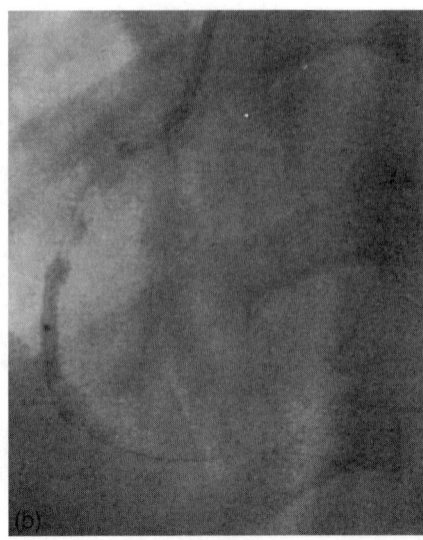

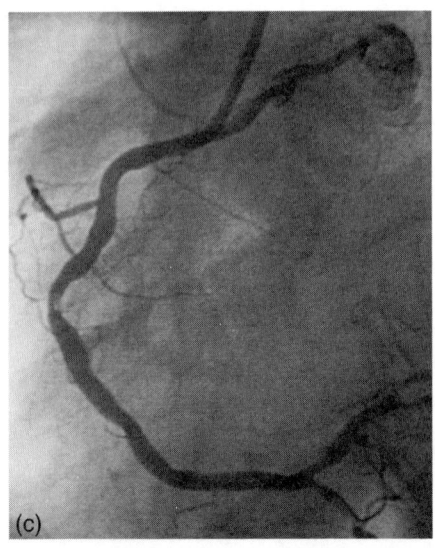

and subsequent infarction is responsible for most angioplasty-related mortality (overall mortality 0.5 to 0.8 per cent).

RESTENOSIS

Defined angiographically as a loss of more than 50 per cent of the improvement in lumen diameter produced by angioplasty, restenosis occurs in about 30 per cent of vessels treated by angioplasty. Histological studies suggest that about 40 per cent of cases of restenosis are associated with elastic recoil and 60 per cent with fibrovascular intimal proliferation: a distinctive lesion characterized by uniform, featureless proliferation of spindle-shaped cells derived from the tunica media.

Restenosis is likely if a patient has recurrent symptoms and a positive exercise test within 6 months of angioplasty. Neither symptoms nor a positive exercise test alone are reliable indicators of restenosis. Symptoms developing later than 6 months are more likely to be due to a new lesion.

Restenosis is more common in males, smokers, and left anterior descending lesions. No medication (e.g. aspirin, anticoagulants, calcium antagonists, fish oil, or angiotensin converting enzyme inhibitors) has consistently been shown to affect restenosis. The restenosed vessel may be redilated, with a risk of further restenosis of about 30 per cent. There is unconfirmed evidence that stent implantation could reduce restenosis risk to about 15 per cent at the cost of an increased risk of abrupt closure.

Indications and clinical results

STABLE ANGINA

Patients with stable angina and lesions suitable for angioplasty who are randomized to angioplasty rather than medical treatment are more likely to be angina free at 6 months, and have a better objective exercise tolerance, at the cost of increased risks of myocardial infarction and a need for coronary bypass grafting. Longer term follow-up data from controlled trials would be valuable, but are not currently available. In the United Kingdom, the majority of patients undergoing percutaneous transluminal coronary angioplasty have angina not adequately controlled by medical treatment and a more valid comparison is with coronary bypass grafting.

The RITA (Randomised Intervention Treatment of Angina Trial) randomized patients in whom equivalent revascularization could be achieved to either angioplasty or coronary bypass grafting. After 2 years of follow-up, mortality, non-fatal infarction, and angina status were similar in the two groups. Patients randomized to angioplasty were more likely to return to work early, but needed more subsequent interventions

Table 1 *Indications and contraindications for coronary angioplasty*

Major indications:
 Stable angina with accessible coronary lesions and symptoms
  refractory to medical treatment
 Unstable angina with accessible coronary lesions and
  continuing ischaemia despite medical treatment
 Recurrent angina after coronary bypass grafting with
  lesion(s) amenable to angioplasty
 Persistent or recurrent ischaemia after myocardial infarction
  (with or without thrombolytic therapy)

Other indications: (angioplasty may be indicated but benefit/
 risk ratio less clear and/or success rate lower)
 Stable angina, patient dislikes medical treatment
 Stable angina with long-standing occluded vessels

Contraindications:
 Unprotected left main coronary stenosis
 Absence of surgical backup facilities
 Extensive peripheral vascular disease preventing access
 Recent myocardial infarction treated with thrombolytic
  therapy, in the absence of evidence of persisting ischaemia

and were more likely to continue taking cardioactive medication. An economic analysis showed that the initial cost of angioplasty was about half that of bypass surgery, but after 2 years this increased to about 80 per cent because of the need for further interventions. Similar outcomes have been reported from other randomized trials in Germany and the United States of America.

The choice between angioplasty and coronary bypass grafting is frequently influenced by factors other than simple outcome measures. In particular, where surgical waiting lists are long, there is a tendency to perform angioplasty in all cases where the coronary anatomy is suitable and symptoms not adequately controlled by medical treatment. The current status of different indications for, and contraindications to, angioplasty is summarized in Table 1.

The definition of a 'lesion suitable for angioplasty' is flexible and continuously being updated in line with changes in technology and operator experience. It is generally accepted that patients with unprotected left main coronary stenosis are better managed by bypass grafting and that short, isolated proximal stenoses are usually very amenable to angioplasty. Angioplasty of the left main coronary artery is, however, acceptable if there is already a bypass graft to a distal branch of the vessel ('protected' left main). Calcification, angulated lesions, and lesions involving side branches are no longer regarded as major contraindications. The primary success rate of angioplasty is of the order of 90 to 95 per cent in experienced centres. Success rates are lower when segments which are completely occluded rather than stenosed (50 to 70 per cent), and success is even less likely if the occlusion has been present for more than 3 months. Coronary bypass grafts are suitable for angioplasty but the restenosis rate tends to be high and stenting may be indicated.

Over 80 per cent of angioplasty procedures in the United Kingdom are currently being done in patients with only a single significant coronary stenosis (single vessel disease), but the proportion of patients with two or three vessel disease is increasing. In several centres the ratio of patients referred for angioplasty and for coronary bypass grafting approaches parity.

UNSTABLE ANGINA

Patients with unstable angina which does not respond rapidly to medical therapy often have lesions suitable for coronary angioplasty. The success rate for angioplasty is high under these conditions, but the risk of abrupt closure is somewhat greater than for stable angina.

Fig. 4 Changes in the vessel wall during angioplasty.

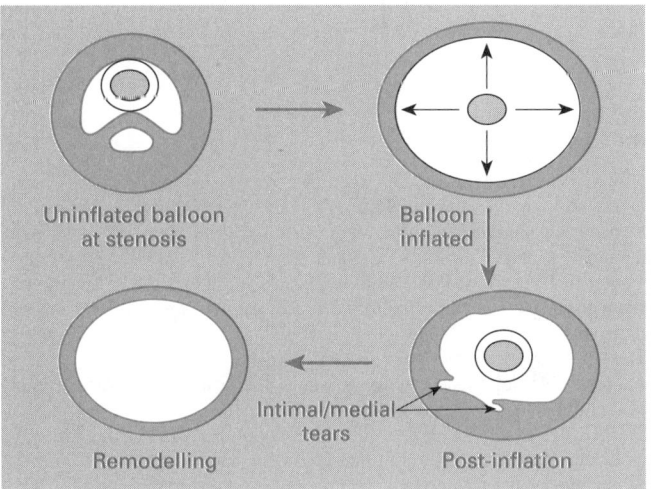

Uninflated balloon at stenosis

Balloon inflated

Remodelling

Post-inflation

Intimal/medial tears

MYOCARDIAL INFARCTION

Angioplasty as a primary treatment for coronary thrombosis requires the immediate availability of a catheterization laboratory and a skilled operating team. If these are available, patency rates at least as good as those of intracoronary streptokinase can be achieved, with the additional advantages of more rapid reperfusion and avoidance of the bleeding complications of thrombolysis.

Angioplasty as an adjunct to thrombolytic therapy has been examined in several randomized trials, which all agree that a blanket policy of angioplasty in any patient with a residual stenosis of greater than 70 per cent in an infarct related segment does not lead to any overall benefit in terms of survival, freedom from reinfarction or freedom from angina. The principal reason is that the increased rate of abrupt closure seen under these circumstances appears to outweigh potential benefit. This applies both to immediate angioplasty and to 'delayed elective' angioplasty after an interval of 48 h.

Angioplasty may however be indicated in patients with recurrent ischaemia presenting as unstable angina after initially successful thrombolysis or in patients who develop stable angina following infarction. Estimates of the 'need' for intervention (angioplasty or coronary bypass grafting) in the first year after myocardial infarction range from 20 to 42 per cent.

ANGIOPLASTY AS A SALVAGE PROCEDURE AFTER CORONARY BYPASS SURGERY

Angioplasty is frequently the treatment of choice for patients developing recurrent angina after coronary bypass surgery. The lesions responsible may be new stenoses of the native vessels or stenoses of the vein or internal mammary grafts. Vein graft stenoses are usually easily dilated, but stenoses in the midportion of the graft tend to recur, and may require stent implantation. Old vein grafts sometimes have a very friable intima, and dilatation may cause distal embolism of atheromatous material. Thrombosed vein grafts should be treated initially with a thrombolytic agent, to prevent distal displacement of thrombus.

ANGIOPLASTY IN PATIENTS WITH ANGINA AND SEVERELY IMPAIRED VENTRICULAR FUNCTION

Patients with significantly impaired left ventricular function often have multivessel disease and are best managed by bypass grafting to provide complete revascularization. Sometimes, however, a patient has severely impaired ventricular function but the only vessels available for revascularization are one or two arteries with stenoses amenable to angioplasty. Under these circumstances, angioplasty may be the treatment of choice provided temporary left ventricular support can be provided by intra aortic balloon pumping or percutaneous partial bypass. This is because balloon inflation in a single vessel crucial for myocardial perfusion tends to cause a fall in cardiac output and possibly irreversible hypotension.

ANGIOPLASTY IN THE ELDERLY PATIENT

Age in itself is not a contraindication to angioplasty. Older patients tend to have more extensive coronary disease and the proportion of patients suitable for angioplasty is lower than in younger age groups. The risk of vascular complications and of dissection tends to be higher.

Management of the pre- and post-angioplasty patient

Patients should be warned prior to angioplasty that in the unlikely event of abrupt vessel closure emergency surgery will be required, and that restenosis may occur in up to 30 per cent of patients.

Angioplasty is routinely performed under local anaesthesia; patients may be lightly sedated with diazepam or an opiate. Previous treatment with aspirin (150 mg daily) reduces the risk of abrupt vessel closure and supplements the heparin given at the time of the procedure. There is no evidence that nitrates or calcium antagonists given prior to angioplasty are any more effective than those given during the procedure. β-Blockers in theory increase the risk of coronary spasm and heart block; on the other hand they increase myocardial resistance to ischaemia and a relative bradycardia makes it easier to see the guidewire. Spasm can be relieved with nitrates and excessive bradycardia usually responds to atropine.

There is no evidence that prolonged administration of either heparin or nitrates after angioplasty improves outcome. A prolonged heparin infusion is sometimes used after a dissection or after reversal of abrupt closure. Aspirin is usually continued for at least a month; there is no evidence that it reduces restenosis. Some cardiologists stop all antianginal medication immediately after angioplasty, others tail it off a month later, once it is clear that symptoms have been relieved.

Patients with sedentary occupations may return to work within a few days of angioplasty. Regular isotonic exercise (walking, cycling, swimming) should be increased progressively within the limits of patient comfort. There are no data on the safety of vigorous isometric exercise (weight lifting) after angioplasty, but it would be prudent to avoid this for at least a month. In the United Kingdom, licensing to drive a large goods or passenger carrying vehicle may be permitted 3 or more months after successful angioplasty provided the driver can safely complete at least the first three stages of the standard Bruce protocol exercise test without symptoms or signs of cardiac dysfunction, having been off cardioactive mediation for at least 24 h.

No data are available on the efficacy of secondary prevention after angioplasty, but patients should be advised against smoking, and hyperlipidaemia should be treated vigorously.

New developments in angioplasty

These can be divided into new medications and new devices. Monoclonal antibody to platelet GPIIb/IIIa glycoprotein has been shown to reduce both the risk of abrupt closure and the risk of late symptom recurrence in high-risk angioplasty patients, but at the cost of increased bleeding complications. No medication has yet been shown to prevent restenosis. Stents – small tubes of metallic mesh positioned across the stenosis and expanded under balloon pressure or their own elasticity – now have an established niche in managing dissection, after dilatation of vein grafts, and perhaps in preventing restenosis. Various types of drill are under evaluation in helping to recanalize occluded vessels. Atherectomy, in which a small cutter excises slices of vessel wall into a removable container, may have a role in dissection, in ostial lesions, or in vein graft stenosis, but the restenosis rate has been disappointing. Laser devices, whether 'bare fibre' or working via a heated probe tip or balloon, have been rather disappointing and are not in routine clinical use.

REFERENCES

de Bono, D.P., McAreavey, D., Been, M., and Peterson, H. (1988). Long term follow up after coronary thrombolysis: the Edinburgh experience. In *Hyperlipidaemia and atherosclerosis* (ed C. de Groot), pp. 175–184. Academic Press, New York.

DeFeyter, P.J., Serruys, P.W., Van den Brand, M. et al. (1985). Emergency coronary angioplasty in refractory unstable angina. *New England Journal of Medicine*, **315,** 342–345.

Dotter, C.T. and Judkins, M.P. (1964). Transluminal treatment of arteriosclerotic obstruction: description of a new technic and a preliminary report of its application. *Circulation* **30,** 654–670.

Ellis, S.G., Debowey, D., Bates, E.R., and Topol, E.J. (1991). Treatment of recurrent ischaemia after thrombolysis and successful reperfusion for acute myocardial infarction: effect on in-hospital mortality and left ventricular function. *Journal of the American College of Cardiologists,* **17,** 752–757.

Feit, F., Mueeler, H.S., Braunwald, E. et al. (1991). Thrombolysis in Myocardial infarction (TIMI) phase II trial: outcome comparison of a ''conservative strategy'' in community versus tertiary hospitals. *Journal of the American College of Cardiologists* **17,** 1529–1534.

Gershlick, A.H. and de Bono, D.P. (1990). Restenosis after angioplasty. *British Heart Journal* **64,** 351–353.

Gruntzig, A.R. (1978). Transluminal dilatation of coronary artery stenosis. *Lancet* **i,** 263.

Gruntzig, A.R., Senning, A., and Siegenthaler, W.E. (1979). Nonoperative dilatation of coronary artery stenosis. *New England Journal of Medicine,* **301,** 61–68.

Hamm, C.W., Reimers, J., Ischinge, T., Rupprecht, H.J., Berger, J., and Bleifeld, W., for the German Angioplasty Bypass Surgery Investigators. (1994). A randomized study of coronary angioplasty compared with bypass surgery in patients with symptomatic multivessel disease. *New England Journal of Medicine,* **331,** 1037–43.

Hubner, P.J.B. (1990). Cardiac interventional procedures in the United Kingdom during 1988 *British Heart Journal,* **64,** 36–37.

Irvine, J., and Petch, M. (1994). Fitness to drive: updated guidelines for cardiovascular fitness in vocational drivers. *Health Trends,* **26,** 38–40.

King, S.B., Lembo, N.J., Weintraub, W.S., *et al.* for the Emory Angioplasty versus surgery trial (EAST). (1994). A randomised trial comparing angioplasty with coronary bypass surgery. *New England Journal of Medicine,* **331,** 1044–50.

Kohchi, K., Takebayashi, S., Block, P.C., Hiroki, T., and Nobuyoshi, M. (1987). Arterial changes after percutaneous transluminal coronary angioplasty: results at autopsy. *Journal of the American College of Cardiologists* **10,** 592–99.

Lincoff, A.M., Popma, J.J., Ellis, S.G., Hacker, J.A., and Topol, E.J. (1992). Abrupt vessel closure complicating coronary angioplasty: clinical, angiographic and therapeutic profile. *Journal of the American College of Cardiologists,* **19,** 926–935.

O'Neill, W., Timmis, G.C., Bourdillon, P.D. et al. (1986). A prospective randomised clinical trial of intracoronary streptokinase versus coronary angioplasty for acute myocardial infarction. *New England Journal of Medicine,* **314,** 812–815.

Parisi, A.F., Folland, E.D., and Hartigan, P. on behalf of the Veterns Affairs ACME investigators. (1992). A comparison of angioplasty with medical therapy in the treatment of single vessel coronary disease. *New England Journal of Medicine,* **326,** 10–16.

RITA Trial Participants. (1993). Coronary angioplasty versus coronary artery bypass surgery: the Randomised Intervention Treatment of Angina Trial. *Lancet,* **341,** 573–80.

Schatz, R.A., Goldberg, S., Leon, M., Baim, D., Hirshfeld, D., Cleman, M., Ellis, S., and Topol, E.J. (1991). Clinical experience with the Palmaz-Schatz Coronary Stent. *Journal of the American College of Cardiologists,* **17,** 143B–154B.

Sculpher, M.J., Seed, P., Henderson, R.A., *et al.* for RITA Trial participants. (1994). Health service costs of coronary angioplasty and coronary bypass surgery: the Randomised Intervention Treatment of Angina Trial. *Lancet,* **344,** 927–30.

Simoons, M.L., Arnold, A.E.R., Betriu, A. et al. (1988). Thrombolysis with tissue plasminogen activator in acute myocardial infarction: no additional benefit from immediate percutaneous coronary angioplasty. *Lancet,* **i,** 197–203.

SWIFT Trial Study Group. (1991). SWIFT trial of delayed elective intervention v conservative treatment after thrombolysis with anistreplase in acute myocardial infarction. *British Medical Journal,* **302,** 555–560.

The EPIC investigators. (1994). Use of a monoclonal antibody directed against the platelet glycoprotein IIb/IIIa receptor in high risk coronary angioplasty. *New England Journal of Medicine,* **330,** 956–61.

Waller, B.F. (1989). ''Crackers, breakers, stretchers, drillers, scrapers, shavers, burners, welders, melters'' – the future treatment of atherosclerotic coronary artery disease? A clinico-morphological assessment. *Journal of the American College of Cardiologists* **13,** 969–987.

Waller, B.F., Pinkerton, C., Orr, C.M., Slack, J.D., Van Tassel, J.W., and Peters, T. (1991). Morhological observations late (< 30 days) after clinically successful coronary balloon angioplasty. *Circulation,* **83** (suppl. I), I-28–I-41.

15.10.6 Coronary artery bypass grafting

T. Treasure

Since the first descriptions of a successful and reproducible operation to relieve myocardial ischaemia in the late 1960s, coronary artery bypass grafting has been performed in large numbers and subjected to more thorough evaluation then perhaps any other operation in the history of surgery. In the 1970s it became established as an effective means of relieving angina, and several large multicentre trials were initiated to define its role in protecting survival. During the 1980s the practice of coronary surgery continued to grow with the operation being performed in as many as 1000 patients per million of the population in the United States and between 300 and 600 per million in Europe and Australia.

In spite of its evident efficacy in relieving angina at relatively small risk and low mortality, the place of surgery in the management of patients with coronary artery disease has continued to be debated and is not easy to define. Coronary disease is extremely variable in its rate of progression and unpredictable in its manifestations. Primary and secondary prevention, medical therapy, and non-surgical interventions have evolved during the same time frame and the indications for surgery will vary as the place of newer treatments is established.

Selection of patients who will benefit from coronary surgery

In appropriately selected cases, surgical revascularization of the myocardium is effective both in relieving angina and in reducing the risk of myocardial infarction and death. In many cases both goals apply but it is useful to segregate the indications into those relating to symptoms and those influencing prognosis. The information required is summarized under the usual headings of history, examination, and investigations.

History

At the decision making stage the history must be reviewed or, better, retaken, in the light of facts available from investigations. The interview must focus on the severity of symptoms, the extent to which they are attributable to reversible myocardial ischaemia, and whether adequate attempts have been made to relieve them by medical measures. It is important to assess the extent to which the patient will benefit from the relief of angina because other disease or handicap may limit mobility and subjective well-being and then relief of exercise-related angina may make little contribution to health or the enjoyment of life. Risk factors should be reviewed, because although they may not alter the decision, they will reduce the duration of benefit of surgery if they continue unchecked. Those that can be influenced include smoking, diabetes, obesity, hypertension, hyperlipidaemia, and diet. It is also an opportunity to give advice to the family to reduce the risks for the next generation.

A history of transient ischaemic attacks, or stroke, is important in the risk benefit analysis.

Clinical examination

Availability and suitability of the long saphenous veins should be established. Varicosity or surgical removal of the saphenous system does not preclude coronary bypass surgery, but may make revascularization more difficult to achieve.

The suitability of the patient to undergo a major operation should be assessed at a general physical examination.

Specific investigations

Coronary angiography is performed in all cases. The anatomical extent of the disease, including the site and severity of stenoses, is a major determinant of prognosis. The operative plan depends on the anatomy and quality of the vessels, where grafts will be anastomosed, beyond the obstructive lesions.

The state of the left ventricle is important in defining prognosis and it may be judged by left ventricular cine angiography, echocardiography, or gated aquisition nuclear ventriculography. The poorer the left ventricular function, the worse is the natural history, and the greater the margin of benefit in survival terms, of surgical revascularization over medical management.

If there is doubt about the attribution of symptoms to myocardial ischaemia, or a need for objective evaluation of their severity, a graded exercise test, with continuous measurement of the electrocardiogram, should be performed at this stage if one is not already available. Myocardial perfusion scintigrams may help in very difficult cases to decide if there is an area of reversible ischaemia where a coronary bypass graft would be of use. This is sometimes helpful in assessing a case for repeat surgery.

INDICATIONS FOR OPERATION TO RELIEVE SYMPTOMS

Coronary artery bypass grafting is a highly effective means of relieving angina. The subjective sensations of tightness, choking, heaviness, or even 'breathlessness', may all be manifestations of ischaemia, encompassed by the diagnosis of angina pectoris, and can all be relieved by revascularization. 'Pain' is often not volunteered or may be denied by the patient. Atypical symptoms, provided there is convincing evidence that they are due to myocardial ischaemia, are as likely to be relieved. In contemporary practice over 90 per cent of patients are free of angina a year after surgery and this benefit is maintained in 80 per cent at 5 years and 60 per cent at 10 years.

As a general statement, operation should be considered to relieve angina in any patient where a reasonable expectation of activity or enjoyment of life is curtailed by angina despite a reasonable trial of medical treatment. The threshold at which operation is considered for symptoms will vary according to a realistic estimate of the risks—of death and morbidity—for the individual patient under consideration. On average the likelihood of leaving hospital alive is 97 per cent, a figure that will apply to the typical male, aged 55 to 60, with triple vessel disease and no worse than moderate impairment of left ventricular function. The estimate should be adjusted up or down according to the risk factors for the individual. It will also have to be modified as time goes by, depending on the available resources and success of medical measures or angioplasty.

INDICATIONS FOR OPERATION TO IMPROVE PROGNOSIS

This depends of estimates of three things for the individual under consideration:

(1) the natural history of that pattern of disease;
(2) the risk of operation in that case;
(3) and the probability of continued survival thereafter.

If the natural history is good (say 90 per cent probability of survival at 5 years) surgery cannot be justified on those grounds. The factors associated with a poor natural history are dangerous coronary anatomy, poor left ventricular function, and evidence of ischaemia at low work load, whether expressed as angina, or silent ischaemia documented on ambulatory monitoring by an exercise test. Dangerous anatomical patterns are left main stem stenosis, disease involving all three major vessels, and disease in the proximal segment of the left anterior descending coronary artery; the risks associated with these dangers can be largely neutralized by surgical revascularization. Patients with combinations of these risk factors can benefit from surgical revascularization as far as their prognosis is concerned.

Factors that adversely influence risk of the operation itself are:

(1) older age;

(2) female gender;
(3) obesity;
(4) respiratory disease.

Factors that unfavourably influence postoperative survival are:

(1) failure to use the internal mammary artery to the left anterior descending coronary artery;
(2) failure to achieve adequate revascularization;
(3) poor left ventricular function although, apart from patients whose ventricular function is extremely poor (for example an ejection fraction of approximately 10 per cent), the outlook is better with revascularization than without.

In summary, the more severe and extensive the coronary artery disease, the greater is the comparative benefit is the of operation over medical treatment, while the outlook is very similar for the two managements if the disease is less severe. The worse the left ventricular function, the greater the comparative benefit of surgical over medical management.

The coronary bypass operation

An understanding of the technical steps are of some importance for those who refer patients for surgery and supervise their care outside of the specialist unit. There are also several technical options, which may be employed according to preference, extenuating circumstances, or scientific evidence. Their implications are of considerable importance in the selection and follow-up of patients.

VASCULAR CONDUITS

The long saphenous vein

The most frequently used graft is still the long saphenous vein. This is taken from the leg, from the ankle to the groin, at the same time as the chest is being opened and while preparations are being made for the cardiac operation. The most common technique is to cut down through the skin and subcutaneous tissues, exactly over the vein, to avoid forming flaps which may necrose due to poor blood supply. The vein branches are tied or clipped and the veins stored briefly in heparinized blood. Appropriate handling of the vein at this stage, including avoidance of high distension pressures (> 300 mmHg) and unbuffered storage media, influences integrity of its endothelium and therefore may influence patency, not only in the short term but over subsequent years. The long saphenous vein may be unusable or unavailable due to varicose disease or its surgical treatment. Alternative veins are the short saphenous vein, which is a technically satisfactory conduit but surgically less accessible, and arm veins, which are fragile and more difficult to use.

There are no good data to suggest there is any difference in the results between these veins. The long saphenous vein is accessible, expendable, and convenient. As a group, vein grafts almost invariably deteriorate with time. There is an early phase of thickening over the first few months, when a new layer, derived from platelets, fibrin, and circulating cells, is formed concentrically on the intimal surface, thickening the wall. The attrition rate for vein grafts is about 2 per cent per annum with a high incidence of disease in the wall and occlusion from seven years onwards. Patency at 10 years is only about 50 per cent.

The internal mammary artery

The internal mammary artery is dissected off the chest wall with division of all its intercostal branches, but its proximal origin from the subclavian artery is left intact whenever possible. The artery can be divided and used as a free graft to extend its range and it is probable that its advantages still obtain. The pleura may be opened inadvertently, or deliberately. Both arteries can be used but sternal healing may be compromised, particularly in the obese and in diabetics. Increased operating time, a second pleural opening, and more opportunity for haemorrhage, all add to morbidity, and may exceed any advantage gained by two mammary artery grafts. Double internal mammary artery grafting is an attractive option in younger patients but is unproven, and the balance of risk and benefit should be in the surgeon's mind for older and high risk patients.

There is clear evidence that patients with a pedicled left internal mammary artery graft to the left anterior descending coronary artery are more likely to be alive, free from myocardial infarction, and free of angina at 10 years than those with a vein graft. Patency rate at 10 years can be as good as 95 per cent, and the artery can grow to accommodate the demands placed upon it by the size of its run-off.

Other arterial grafts

In the knowledge that there is an inevitable failure rate of vein grafts, and with more patients requiring repeat surgery, the right gastroepiploic artery (RGA) and the inferior epigastric artery have been used. The right gastroepiploic artery requires the peritoneum to be opened and a dissection of the artery off the greater curvature of the stomach. It is brought up, usually anterior to the pylorus, and provides a satisfactory arterial graft to the inferior surface of the heart.

Artificial conduits

In desperation surgeons may turn to synthetic grafts or glutaraldehyde fixed arterial tissue grafts. None has proved very satisfactory.

THE CARDIAC OPERATION

The chest is opened through a median sternotomy. In a large majority of cases the operation is performed on cardiopulmonary bypass, although it is possible to do a limited operation, particularly to the left anterior descending and to the main right coronary artery, on the beating and working heart. Cardiopulmonary bypass is established with drainage of systemic venous blood through a cannula inserted through the right atrial wall and, after artificial oxygenation, the blood is returned to the ascending aorta.

A range of techniques is in use to manage the heart during the performance of the coronary anastomosis. Vascular grafting is easier if the vessel is free of blood and immobilized, but, on the other hand, the myocardium is best protected if it has an adequate supply of arterial blood at 37°C. The chosen surgical management depends upon a compromise between these two requirements. Brief intermittent ischaemia or cardioplegic arrest are equally safe and effective and, in the routine case, it is a matter of surgical preference.

It is known that incomplete revascularization is a risk factor for premature death or recurrence of angina, so all blocked or significantly obstructed (> 50 per cent) vessels that are amenable to grafting by virtue of size and wall quality are grafted. Endarterectomy is performed if no better means of access to the system can be established. It is probably at least safe, if not ideal, in vessels already completely occluded. The distal patent segment of vessels in already infarcted territories are grafted, if only because they may be in communication with collaterals, but also because they may supply some viable myocardium and thus help in the relief of ischaemia. The typical operation includes three to five grafts.

RISK FACTORS FOR PERIOPERATIVE DEATH

The United Kingdom Cardiac Surgery Register provides an annual audit of mortality (in-hospital or 30-day) for all units, and therefore represents the true average risk for all patients and all hospitals, rather than selected series. During the early 1980s the falling death rate for coronary surgery levelled out and has remained remarkably consistent at between 2.5 and 2.7 per cent. The figure is comparable with worldwide Registry and Audit data and is in line with the observed increase in mortality figures in the United States as more exacting cases have been referred for operation, and perhaps as angioplasty has been used in the safer categories.

This average risk is applicable to the typical, representative patient who is male, aged around 60, has surgery for chronic stable angina, has had some previous ischaemic damage to the myocardium, has triple vessel disease, and has four grafts at an elective operation, including a mammary graft to the left anterior descending coronary artery. Factors that increase the perioperative risk of death compared with this typical patient are greater age, emergency operation, unstable angina, recent myocardial infarction, left main stem disease, worse distal vessels, worse left ventricular function, other disease, small stature, and female gender, in approximate order of importance. Elderly women undergoing emergency surgery for multivessel disease face a risk of 10 per cent or more. Conversely, the factors that are associated with lower risk are an undamaged left ventricle and fewer vessels diseased. A 50-year-old having a single graft has a risk of less than 1 per cent.

Perioperative morbidity

CARDIAC MORBIDITY

Perioperative infarction

Discrete, anatomically localized myocardial infarction, characterized by new Q waves or loss of R waves, occurs in about 2 per cent of cases. It is at least partly determined by surgical technique, and then results from occlusion of the grafted vessels or side branches of an artery where endarterectomy has been performed. More diffuse myocardial damage, detected by enzyme leakage and global deterioration of left ventricular function is more common but is less easy to define, and the wide range of estimates of its frequency reflect this. Methods of myocardial protection are designed to minimize myocardial ischaemia, and this is largely avoidable.

Low output state

This is usually seen in patients with poor preoperative left ventricular function, or those brought to theatre with evolving infarction. Treatment is supportive with intra-aortic balloon counterpulsation, afterload reduction with nitrates, and judicious use of inotropes. Techniques of myocardial reperfusion with substrate enhancement have something to offer in these cases and some will be supported temporarily with mechanical assistance of the left ventricle in the hope that there will be recovery of 'stunned myocardium' following surgical revascularization and reperfusion.

Cardiac arrhythmia

The most common arrhythmias after coronary surgery are atrial fibrillation and supraventricular tachycardia which occur in 20 to 30 per cent of all patients undergoing coronary surgery at about 2 to 5 days after operation. A wide range of prophylactic therapies have been suggested to reduce the incidence including digoxin, calcium channel blockers, β-blockers, magnesium, and maintenance of relative hyperkalaemia, but the incidence is essentially unchanged. The only important aetiological factors seem to be age and obesity, perhaps with hypoxia and left atrial distension being the proximate mechanisms. Treatment is equally diverse and the fortunately the complication is almost without exception benign, controllable, and does not recur after the perioperative period.

Heart block is seen immediately after surgery in about 5 to 10 per cent as a manifestation of an acute ischaemic event but persisting conduction abnormalities requiring permanent pacing are rare.

Acute ventricular arrhythmias, including ventricular fibrillation, are relatively uncommon but are usually evidence of perioperative ischaemia.

CENTRAL NERVOUS SYSTEM DAMAGE

Stroke

Discrete central nervous system damage is seen consistently after coronary surgery with an incidence of about 2 per cent. It is age related, increasing from 0.5 per cent for patients in their fifties, to 5 per cent in patients over 70 years of age. The most common cause is embolism of atherosclerotic debris from the ascending aorta. Some cases occur in patients who have had previous transient ischaemic attacks, but the presence of asymptomatic coronary artery disease is not predictive. Most cases are relatively mild and recover, but a minority have persisting severe disability. Stroke is sufficiently common, and the consequences so serious that the risk should be specifically mentioned prior to surgery, to the patient and family of those at particular risk.

Global cortical damage

Diffuse cerebral injury causing alteration in short-term memory and concentration is common but is only discernable by comparison of of carefully performed neuropsychological tests before and after surgery. It can then be identified in one-third of patients at 2 months after surgery, and persists at 1 year. Subjective complaints are a very poor guide to the presence of this form of cortical damage.

DAMAGE TO OTHER ORGANS

Cardiopulmonary bypass and major cardiac surgery are associated with damage to other organs including the lung, kidney, and gastrointestinal tract. These are, in general, more common with increasing bypass time, more severe disease and older age of the patient. They are rare in the routine elective case. In general, they are sufficiently rare and sporadic, that they are not included in the preoperative decision making process.

The outlook after coronary surgery

The probability of being alive 1 year after surgery is 95 per cent. Survival at 5 years is 88 per cent, and remains good at 10 years when 75 per cent can expect to be alive. At least half of the deaths are cardiac—due to myocardial infarction or heart failure—or, in the minority, occur suddenly. Death, infarction, and the return of angina are more likely with incomplete revascularization at operation and correlate with subsequent graft occlusion. Progression of disease in the native system is a major contributary factor and it is probable that thorough attention to risk factors will reduce the rate of progression of both graft and native vessel disease. Secondary prevention with low dose aspirin improves graft patency.

THE PROBLEM OF RECURRENCE OF ANGINA

Early return of angina is likely to be due to technical factors, either failure to bypass important stenoses, or early occlusion of the anastomosis.

Late recurrence occurs with increasing frequency beyond 5 years. Assessment is just as before, and the decision making progress is similar. Many cases have mild angina, which can be managed with medical therapy. If operation is considered, the decision process is along the same lines as for a first operation, but more weighted against surgery, allowing for an estimate of the increased risk and reduced likelihood of technical success at a second operation.

REFERENCES

Hammermeister, K.E., Burshfiel, C., Johnson, R., and Grover, F.L. (1990). Identification of patients at greatest risk for developing major complications at cardiac surgery. *Circulation*, **82**, (suppl. IV), IV-380–IV-389.

Kirklin, J.W., Akins, C.W., Blackstone, E.H. et al. (1991). ACC/AHA guidelines and indications for coronary artery bypass graft surgery. (A report of the American College of Cardiology/American Heart Association Task Force on Assessment of Diagnostic and Therapeutic Cardiovascular Procedures (Subcommittee on Coronary Artery Bypass Graft Surgery)). *Circulation*, **83**, 1125–1178.

Kirklin, J.W., Naftel, D.C., Blackstone, E.H., and Pohost, G.M. (1989). Summary of a consensus concerning death and ischemic events after coronary artery bypass grafting. *Circulation*, **79**, (suppl. I), I-81–I-91.

Loop, F.D., Lytle, B.W., Cosgrove, D.M., Stewart, R.W., Goormastic, M.,

Williams, G.W., Golding, L.A.R., Gill, C.C., Taylor, P.C., Sheldon, W.C., and Proudfit, W.L. (1986). Influence of the internal mammary artery graft on 10-year survival and other cardiac events. *New England Journal of Medicine*, **314**, 1–6.

Myers, W.O., Schaff, H.V., Gersh, B.J., Fisher, L.D., Kosinski, A.S., Mock, M.B., Holmes, D.R., Ryan, T.J., Kaiser, G.C. and CASS investigators (1989). Improved survival of surgically treated patients with triple vessel coronary artery disease and severe angina pectoris. A report from the CASS registry. *Journal of Thoracic and Cardiovascular Surgery*, **97**, 487–495.

Patterson, D.L.H. (1987). *The management of angina pectoris*. Castle House Publications, Tunbridge Wells.

Treasure, T., Smith, P.L.C., Newman, S., Schneidau, A., Joseph, P., Ell, P., and Harrison, M.J.G. (1989). Impairment of cerebral function following cardiac and other major surgery. *European Journal of Cardiothoracic Surgery*, **3**, 216–221.

Treasure, T. (1990). Surgery for coronary artery disease. *Current Opinion in Cardiology*, **5**, 490–195.

15.10.7 Vocational aspects of coronary artery disease

M. JOY

Introduction

About one-sixth of all patients presenting with ischaemic heart disease will do so by way of sudden cardiac death. As about one-quarter of the time of a fully employed individual is likely to be spent at work, such events are bound to occur in the workplace. Two-fifths of newly presenting ischaemic heart disease will do so as myocardial infarction and up to one-third of those so affected may die, half within 15 min of the onset of their symptoms. The occurrence of such events in the workplace has implications for safety, is likely to have a disturbing effect on the workforce, and will also have implications for the employer.

Attrition of the employed or potentially employable population by ischaemic heart disease is also caused by other manifestations of ischaemic heart disease, including angina pectoris, heart failure, and arrhythmias. The patient in whom coronary atheroma has been identified has 'impaired life' in insurance terms, and a prediction with regard to outcome can only be made following adequate assessment. All such patients therefore deserve investigation sufficient to enable accurate and confident advice to be given with regard to present and future health. Speculative diagnosis or incomplete review is unsatisfactory and may deny the substantial opportunities now available for symptomatic relief and improvement of prognosis. In occupations with statutory or non-statutory (i.e. advisory) fitness requirements this is essential.

Aspects of occupational medicine

Many large concerns run departments of occupational medicine, whose responsibilities include review of medical fitness for existing and potential employees, health education and, in the United Kingdom, advice on compliance with the various aspects of the Health and Safety at Work Act. Higher salaried employees may be offered regular health review. Regular medical fitness examinations, whether statutory or non-statutory, are often undertaken by such departments.

THE HEALTH AND SAFETY AT WORK ACT (1974)

In the United Kingdom the Health and Safety at Work Act (1974) enshrines much of the employment legislation that had been enacted in the preceding 100 years. It covers all employees apart from those in private domestic service. Under the Act, health policy in relation to employment is evolved by the Health and Safety Commission (HSC), while its requirements are monitored by the Health and Safety Executive (HSE). The Health and Safety Executive has an Executive in the form of the Employment Medical Advisory Service (EMAS), which provides, *inter alia*, advice on the development of occupational health services, on medical fitness for work, and on health standards for employees engaged in hazardous occupations.

Employers and employees both have duties under this act. The former are required to ensure the health and safety of the latter, while the latter are required to maintain health and safety in so far as it may impinge on others. Some industries are covered by statutory fitness requirements; in others there is an implied duty under the act to disclose any medical problem which may have safety implications. An employee, however, is not required to furnish their employer, even on request, with details of other aspects of health that are not relevant to safety issues.

STATUTORY AND NON-STATUTORY FITNESS REQUIREMENTS

Certain industries, such as transportation, have statutory, i.e. legally binding, medical fitness requirements which are the subject of local, national, or international agreement. An employee in such an industry has to demonstrate maintenance of the relevant fitness standard at regular intervals. Concern is not only restricted to the safety of the individual but is also directed towards the safety of those for whom he/she is responsible. A bus driver is an example.

If coronary artery disease is suspected or demonstrated, decisions have to be made which are likely to have a significant economic impact on the individual involved. This implies a need for both the standard and its application to be objective and fair. Even in those industries with non-statutory fitness requirements (such as the fire service) an adverse judgement will be disadvantageous. Such problems represent a challenge to occupational medicine and there has been an appropriate and increasing interest in the evolution of medical standards over the past decade or more.

Coronary artery disease

Almost 800 000 patients in the United States and at least 180 000 patients in the United Kingdom survive myocardial infarction each year. Nearly half of these will not have reached the age of retirement. In the United States about 330 000 coronary artery bypass grafts (CABG) are carried out each year and half of these are performed on people under the age of 65; some 300 000 American patients undergo percutaneous transluminal coronary angioplasty (PTCA) of whom two-thirds have not reached retiring age. The figures for Europe in general, and for the United Kingdom in particular are more modest; in the United Kingdom a total of some 18 000 coronary artery bypass procedures and 7300 percutaneous transluminal coronary angioplasty procedures were carried out in 1991.

Modern management has reduced the mortality of the coronary syndromes, thereby increasing the number of patients who might be returned to work, but after myocardial infarction only about three-quarters of those eligible do so and only half will still be in employment 5 years later. A 10-year renew by the Coronary Artery Surgery Study (CASS) has shown no difference in the work status between those treated surgically and those managed medically.

After uncomplicated percutaneous transluminal coronary angioplasty the majority of those in work remain in it, but recrudescence of angina pectoris is associated with a less favourable work outcome. In this context, within 30 months of the index event over one-third of those patients undergoing percutaneous transluminal coronary angioplasty in the Randomized Intervention in the Treatment of Angina (RITA(I)) study, had suffered recurrence of angina, further percutaneous transluminal coronary angioplasty, coronary artery bypass grafts, myocardial infarction, or death.

Recovery versus rehabilitation

In the last 10 years increasing attention has been paid to rehabilitation, with the aim of regaining, or perhaps improving, previous physical, social, emotional, and occupational status. This applies not only to patients who have suffered myocardial infarction but also to those with angina pectoris, heart failure, or following surgical intervention or angioplasty. A comprehensive approach starts in hospital and involves education with regard to risk factors, counselling, and emotional and psychological support. Exercise training has psychological value and helps the physiological deficit associated with the recumbency of illness: it may also reduce the risk of further coronary events or mortality.

A number of factors influence eventual return to work apart from the input of rehabilitation programmes. Adverse factors include age, the presence of significant symptoms, lower socioeconomic status, poor motivation, a perception of 'illness', and inadequate social support. Other considerations include the availability of welfare payment, preferment of governments to pay sickness rather than unemployment benefit, and a raft of other problems, which include a desire on the part of the employer to retire an individual on account of concern about his/her ongoing suitability to perform at a (previous) and appropriate level. To this may be added constructive dismissal in a disguised form. Finally, there is failure to meet the medical fitness requirements laid down for certain occupations.

In spite of mounting interest and a substantial literature on cardiac rehabilitation, its impact on lifestyle (including a sustained increase in physical activity), and in employment terms, has been more difficult to demonstrate. Meta-analysis of exercise rehabilitation programmes has suggested enhanced survival, but this benefit may not have been attributable solely to exercise. Rehabilitation is perhaps one of those happy specialist areas in which both the practitioners and the practised upon experience an improvement in the 'feel good' factor. Leaving aside, therefore, the philosophy of this approach and the pastoral care which is involved, the jobbing cardiologist, whilst not ignoring his or her responsibility towards rehabilitation, may be most often asked whether a patient has 'recovered from' an event and when he/she will be 'fit for work'.

Work and heart work

One of the striking changes which has taken place over the past four decades has been a reduction in the manual component of work with increased automation. The boilerman now pushes buttons rather than heaves the coal. This has led to a revolution in working practices and whereas a generation ago two-thirds of the population used to be involved in heavy manual work, the figure now is closer to one in twenty.

If aerobic capacity is measured in metabolic equivalents of oxygen consumption METs (1 MET (3.5 ml O_2/kg/min) represents a unit of oxygen uptake at rest), then the majority of occupations and professions are no more physically demanding than routine domestic chores about the home. Precise data are difficult to obtain about the demands of the workplace upon the cardiovascular system as a number of additional external influences are in play. These include mental and emotional activity (stress), and environmental factors – ambient temperature and noise as well as the energy expended as work. On the treadmill, the rate pressure product (systolic blood pressure × heart rate) quite closely mirrors oxygen uptake overall and also myocardial oxygen uptake (MVO_2). The heart rate is the best single variable to measure and reflects the myocardial oxygen uptake at higher workloads quite closely, although it is less reliable at lower workloads. For this reason in many occupations there is no close relationship between heart rate observed (i.e. at work) and the heart work on the treadmill. Table 1 illustrates the myocardial oxygen uptake of 142 subjects (including normal controls and patients with coronary artery disease) studied at work and calculated

Table 1 *Comparison of measured and equivalent oxygen uptake of 142 subjects with and without coronary heart disease*

Occupation	Number of patients	Measured oxygen uptake (ml/kg/ min)		V_{O_2}/heart rate equivalent of exercise ECG	
		Mean	Peak	Mean	Peak
Businessmen	15	5.1	5.9	7.2	22.0
Anaesthetists	26	5.2	5.5	5.8	10.9
Surgeons	39	5.3	6.0	11.3	16.5
Factory workers	63	5.3	6.3	13.5	18.6

Reproduced from Wenger, N.K. and Hellerstein, H.K. (eds.) (1992). *Rehabilitation of the coronary patient.* pp. 523–42. Churchill Livingstone, New York, with permission.

Table 2 *Mean and peak energy expenditure measured at work in subjects with and without heart disease*

Occupation	Energy expenditure (METs)	
	Mean	Peak
Clerical worker, electrician, garage attendant, painter	1.0–1.2	1.2–2.3
Anaesthetist, surgeon, tool maker, driver, light warehouse duties	1.3–1.6	1.6–3.3
Domestic work, machine operator, matron	1.6–2.0	1.8–3.4
Fireman, furnace worker, janitor, welder	2.0–2.5	2.5–5.4

Reproduced from Wenger, N.K. and Hellerstein, H.K. (eds.) (1992). *Rehabilitation of the coronary patient.* pp. 523–42. Churchill Livingstone, New York, with permission.

Table 3 *Canadian Cardiovascular Society classification of angina pectoris*

Class I	Symptom free for all normal activities; angina with strenuous or prolonged effort
Class II	Minor limitation. Symptoms with brisk effort on stairs, in the cold, or after meals
Class III	Significant limitation of ordinary activity. Symptoms with one flight of stairs or walking on the flat at a normal pace
Class IV	Any physical activity may provoke symptoms Angina at rest

Data from Campeau, L. (1976). Grading of angina pectoris. *Circulation,* **55,** 522–3.

Table 4 *New York Heart Association functional classification of symptoms*

Class I	Cardiac disease without symptoms on ordinary effort
Class II	Minor limitation of activity by symptoms
Class III	Marked limitation of activity by symptoms
Class IV	Symptoms at rest or on minimal exertion

Reproduced from the Criteria Committee of the New York Heart Association (1973). *Nomenclature and criteria for diagnosis for diseases of the heart and great vessels.* (7th edn.) New York Heart Association / Little, Brown Co., Boston, with permission.

oxygen cost equivalent derived from the same heart rate achieved on the treadmill.

Table 2 illustrates the differences in mean and peak energy expenditure in both normal controls and subjects with coronary artery disease in various occupations. In simple terms, advice on fitness for work in the presence of coronary artery disease requires two considerations. The first is the level of symptoms, if any; the second is the predicted outcome and any deleterious effect of continued employment. The severity of symptoms in terms of angina pectoris is best described using the Canadian Cardiovascular Society's classification (Table 3). Breathlessness may conveniently be described using the New York Heart Association (NYHA) classification (Table 4).

Outcome correlates well with the left ventricular ejection fraction; The lower the ejection fraction, the more guarded the prognosis. The extent of coronary artery disease also influences prognosis. The 5-year survival following myocardial infarction in a subject with little disturbance of myocardial function who can complete at least three stages of the Bruce protocol or equivalent (about 10 METs) without evidence of myocardial ischaemia may be as good as his/her uninvestigated peer. The same applies following coronary artery surgery and probably following angioplasty. Leaving aside issues of motivation, politics, economics, and employer strategy, there seems no reason why the majority of cardiovascular patients who are class I from the symptomatic point of view, who have been satisfactorily assessed, and in whom a management strategy has been evolved, should not be fit for work. An objective measurement might be the satisfactory completion of at least 7 to 8 min of the standard Bruce treadmill protocol.

Some occupations, however, have statutory or non-statutory fitness requirements which have to be fulfilled as criteria of ongoing employment. Employment under hazardous circumstances, such as in the offshore oil industry and fire fighting, are examples of this. The lifeboat service is a further example. The transportation industries (road, marine, aviation) and some recreational pursuits such as driving and flying are covered by statutory fitness requirements. Professional diving medical standards are the responsibility of the Health and Safety Executive in the United Kingdom whilst the railways have no statutory fitness standards in common with gliding, hang gliding, and amateur diving. The associated problems bear further consideration.

Coronary artery disease and transportation

ROAD

There are about one million holders of vocational driving licences in the United Kingdom. Three-quarters of a million hold large goods vehicle (LGV) licences and some 200 000, passenger carrying vehicle (PCV) licences. The present definition of an LGV is an unladen weight of greater than 7.5 tonnes, although this may be reduced to 4 tonnes under proposed European legislation. Passenger carrying vehicles are those designated as such by the Road Traffic Act and usually relate to vehicles with 20 seats or more. These two groups of (vocational) licences are now called group II while the ordinary driving licence (ODL) is now called the group I licence.

There are probably some 20 to 24 million holders of current group I licences. Although taxis carry passengers for hire and reward, only a group I licence is usually required. This also applies to emergency vehicles (of less than 7.5 tonnes). Their regulation, however, is the responsibility of individual municipal authorities, who may add additional medical standards up to and including those of the group II holders.

Although progress towards a common European driving licence has been made, discussion by an expert committee of European Economic Community (EEC) and European Society of Cardiology (ESC) representatives has not yet (1993) achieved agreement with regard to cardiological standards. As a result the responsible agency in the United Kingdom, the Driver and Vehicle Licensing Agency (DVLA), following the deliberations of its cardiological advisory committee promulgated a simplified standard for both group I and group II licences. These have appeared in two publications – DVLA CLE1111 and in the 'At a Glance' guide to current medical standards. As the majority of the population probably use some form of road transportation either to get to its place of work, or during the course of its occupation or recreation, these requirements are of some importance.

Motor vehicle licensing

In 1991 there was a total of nearly one-quarter of a million reportable road accidents from all causes in the United Kingdom. There were 4158 fatalities and 43 716 serious injuries. It is probable that no more than 1 in 1000 accidents are due to medical cause, and only one-tenth of these are likely to be due to cardiovascular disease. Extrapolating, therefore, it is likely that only some 25 accidents each year or so in the United Kingdom are attributable to cardiovascular events. This low figure is probably due to the fact that the majority of patients experience some prodromal symptom, and are able to pull into the side of the road. Large goods vehicles, on account of their greater mass and kinetic energy, are responsible for 70 per cent more fatal accidents than private motor vehicles and, for this reason, their drivers are required to be fitter than their non-vocational peers.

Group I licences

Group I drivers are legally required to notify the DVLA of any 'relevant' or prospective disability. Their medical attendants are also required to inform the patient if any bar to driving is thought to be present. This implies any condition which may lead to sudden impairment of consciousness or to sudden physical disability.

A group I licence permits driving 'Till 70' following which, subject to a medical declaration, a licence is issued for 3 years, or a shorter period as appropriate. The cardiological standards for group I are pragmatic and appropriate. Angina pectoris disbars only if particularly frequent or if it occurs at the wheel. It is optimistic to believe that such a circumstance is likely to be admitted readily. Following myocardial infarction the subject should not drive for a month; after which a return to driving depends on the absence of other disqualifying conditions. Successfully treated ventricular dysfunction (heart failure) does not disbar. Following coronary artery surgery the subject should not drive for at least a month whilst after coronary angioplasty a delay of only 1 week is required, provided that symptoms have not recurred.

Group II licences

Group II licence holders also require group I licences and are required to submit themselves to medical, but not electrocardiographic examination at entry, at age 45, 5-yearly until age 65, and then annually. The requirements for group II are necessarily more rigorous. Angina pectoris disbars whether or not freedom from the symptom can be achieved by medication. Likewise heart failure disbars on account of the greater like-

lihood of a sudden event implied by left (and/or right) ventricular dysfunction. Following myocardial infarction, coronary angioplasty and coronary artery surgery the requirements are broadly similar and rely upon the generally favourable prognosis that is associated with normal or near normal left ventricular function in the absence of demonstrable myocardial ischaemia. In practical terms this depends on the predictive power of the symptom limited exercise electrocardiogram, and notably in the duration of the walking time. The subject who, 3 months after the index event, can complete at least three stages of the standard Bruce protocol or equivalent, off all cardioactive treatment for 24 h, without electrocardiographic change which the investigating cardiologist would interpret as representing myocardial ischaemia, may, at the discretion of the Driver and Vehicle Licensing Agency, be considered for re-licensing. Further, annual review may be demanded. Failure to increase blood pressure or the emergence of significant rhythm disturbance during the exercise test is likely to disbar.

Coronary angiography *per se* is not required, but if it has been carried out there should be no reduction of the left ventricular ejection fraction below 40 per cent, overall: nor should there be reduction of the intra-luminal diameter of greater than 50 per cent in the proximal part of the left anterior descending coronary artery or in two or more major coronary vessels (greater than 30 per cent of the left main coronary artery). Like the group I holder, the group II licence holder is legally required to inform the Driver and Vehicle Licensing Agency of any relevant or prospective disability.

Motor racing

All motor racing drivers, whether amateur or professional, are required to have an ordinary driving licence. A competition licence is required for all competitive driving and this contains a medical declaration. The regulatory body in the United Kingdom is the Royal Automobile Club Motor Sports Association (RAC-MSA), which has its own medical advisory committee. It promulgates its own (national) medical standards, which are reviewed from time to time.

Motor sports may be divided three ways. In motor racing individuals compete together against one another, driving cars, trucks, and karts. The licence required may be national or international depending on the status of the event. Medical examination is required every 2 years until age 40 and annually above 40. Electrocardiography is required at 40 and 45 and beyond age 45 an exercise electrocardiogram is required as well. It is likely that kart drivers will require 2-yearly medical examinations only in future. Motor rallying requires only an ordinary driving licence and no special medical examination for competition is required. Speed events such as hill climbs, sprints, and drag racing, in which the competitor is competing against the clock rather than directly against another competitor likewise do not require medical examination. The medical standards for motor racing have been made more complicated by lack of international agreement. The Federation Internationale Sporte Automobile (FISA) promulgates its own standards which, in certain respects, are less rigorous than those of member nations. It has recently allowed insulin requiring diabetics to be permitted to drive. Notwithstanding this generous approach a driver is still required to fulfil the medical requirements of the country issuing his or her licence, leading to potential conflict. International agreement is wanting. Although the Cardiological Advisory Group to the medical committee of RAC-MSA has yet to define its requirements for motor racing, it is likely that these will be between the Driver and Vehicle Licensing Agency Group II (vocational licence) and that required for the Civil Aviation Authority (CAA) Class III (Joint Aviation Authority Class II) certificate.

AIR

The aeronautical environment is the only one in which standards of operation and of personnel licensing, including medical certification, are agreed by international statute. The responsible agency of the United Nations Organization is the International Civil Aviation Organization

(ICAO), based in Montreal. The International Civil Aviation Organization has seven regional offices, including one in Europe. Recently the European states, including the European Economic Community, in concert with the International Civil Aviation Authority, set up the European Civil Aviation Convention (ECAC) which will eventually become the European regional regulatory agency, as the Joint Aviation Authorities (JAA). At the present time the United Kingdom Civil Aviation Authority (CAA) is the responsible certificatory agency in the United Kingdom for the maintenance of the International Civil Aviation Authority (and the Joint Aviation Authority) standards should they diverge. The International Civil Aviation Authority medical standards are necessarily brief and are amplified in the International Civil Aviation Authority manual of Civil Aviation Medicine. This is now obselescent and the United Kingdom has taken a lead, with others, on an approach towards medical certification based on assessment of the probability of the event rather than an empirical statement of its likelihood. This material has been published in the proceedings of the First and Second United Kingdom and First European workshops in aviation cardiology.

The aviation environment

The world airlines now carry each year in excess of 1 billion passengers in some 16 000 aircraft flying for about 15 million hours. About 160 000 aircrew are involved. The average loss of life due to fatal accidents from all causes worldwide approximates 1000 in each year. This is less than one-quarter of the number of total road accidents in the United Kingdom alone. Almost all aircraft carrying passengers for hire or reward carry two crew and the required adequate operational training for the event of incapacity from any cause has reduced the fatal accident rate from such an event to negligible proportions. The last multicrew jet air transportation accident in which the cardiovascular system was implicated, but not the cause, was to the Hawker-Siddeley Trident 1 aircraft which crashed at Staines in 1972, 300 million flying hours ago.

In order to maintain this excellent record a number of reviews of cardiological problems in professional aircrew have been carried out to define with as much precision as possible acceptable latitude in standard fitness requirements. This is indicative of the importance licensing authorities attach to maintaining the licence to fly, if possible, in the highly skilled aircrew population. Use may be made of the 'waiver' clause by the licensing authority under International Civil Aviation Authority Annex I.2.4.8 with the application of an operational restriction to fly only 'as/with a co-pilot' if deemed necessary.

The 1 per cent rule

The United Kingdom and Europe have seen the emergence of the so-called 1 per cent rule. Any demonstrated abnormality should not carry a risk of 1 per cent or greater of any sudden adverse event/year. This is approximately the cardiovascular mortality of a 65-year-old male in north-western Europe. An 'event' in this context refers not only to sudden and total incapacitation, but also to symptoms which may cause subtle, rather than complete, impairment of function, for instance angina pectoris or rhythm disturbances. Professional aircrew with an unblemished record are given an unrestricted licence, those with less than 1 per cent risk of event an 'as/with co-pilot' endorsed licence and those with a risk greater than 1 per cent are not licensed. The United Kingdom Civil Aviation Authority Class I R (restricted) licence is almost equivalent to the Civil Aviation Authority Class III (Joint Aviation Authority Class II) or private pilot's licence.

There are some 15 000 professional licence holders in the United Kingdom and perhaps 35 000 private (i.e. recreational) licence holders. The medical standards required of the latter are less rigorous than of the former in sympathy with the lower construction, engineering, maintenance, and operating standards achieved in private aviation.

Symptomatic coronary artery disease disbars from all forms of certification to fly. In the United Kingdom with the agreement of the Civil Aviation Authority, recertification following myocardial infarction is possible subject to left ventricular function being normal or near normal,

to there being no demonstrable obstruction of the coronary circulation remote from the artery subtending the infarcted area greater than 30 per cent, and no evidence of myocardial ischaemia on symptom-limited exercise electrocardiography/scintigraphy. Class I (i.e. professional) certification in such a circumstance is subject to restriction to fly 'as/with or with a co-pilot'. No such restriction applies to a private pilot (Civil Aviation Authority Class III/Joint Aviation Authority Class II) who may be in sole command of an aircraft. No pilot, following a myocardial infarction, can expect unrestricted class I certification to fly an aircraft carrying passengers for hire or reward. The equivalance of the restricted Class I and the Class III (Joint Aviation Authority Class II) standard reflects the less rigorous overall requirements of the latter. Annual cardiological follow up with exercise electrocardiography is required.

Likewise, 9 months after coronary artery bypass procedures or successful percutaneous transluminal coronary angiography, an asymptomatic airman who has no demonstrable evidence of myocardial ischaemia as judged by exercise electrocardiography, and who has demonstrably patent coronary bypass grafts with satisfactory run-off, or, who has maintained the dilatation of a treated vessel (residual stenosis less than 30 per cent of the coronary lumen) at angiography immediately before recertification, may be considered for recertification on an annual basis, subject to satisfactory exercise electrocardiography. Further coronary angiography is required not later than 5 years later. Multivessel coronary angioplasty and angioplasty of coronary artery grafts is probably not acceptable.

SEA

Although general aspects of the regulation of activity at sea fall within the purview of the International Maritime Organization, individual nations are responsible for standards of construction, maintenance and of the operation of craft flying their national flag. In the United Kingdom medical standards for those going to sea are laid down in the Merchant Shipping (Medical Examination) Regulations (1983) following an advisory working party set up by the Faculty of Occupational Medicine of the Royal College of Physicians. The regulations have statutory authority. Medical examination of seafarers is carried out by medical examiners approved by the Department of Transport. Below the age of 18 all shall have an annual medical examination. Between the ages of 18 and 40 examination shall be not exceeding intervals of 5 years. After 40 the frequency shall be increased to 2 years. Those working on bulk chemical carriers may require more frequent examination and blood tests. There are five potential categories of fitness (or lack of it). Category A represents fitness for unrestricted service and category E fitness for restricted service. Category B relates to permanent unfitness for service at sea. Most cardiovascular problems including angina pectoris and myocardial infarction fall into category B. There are no explicit standards for recertification following coronary artery surgery or percutaneous transluminal coronary angiography such as exist in the aviation and road transport industries but the potential for a favourable decision may be present through a medical referee appointed by the Department of Transport.

Approved medical referees may use discretion, if appropriate. Consideration has to be given to the operational environment, which is often unfavourable and frequently involves long periods without skilled medical attention. Furthermore, although incapacitation of a crew member is unlikely to have the potentially serious effect that such an event may bring about in an aircraft, it may interfere with the efficient working of a ship and prejudice the health of the individual.

THE LIFEBOAT SERVICE

The lifeboat service in the United Kingdom is operated by a charitable foundation, the Royal National Lifeboat Institution (RNLI). The Institution is concerned with aspects of the design, construction, maintenance and operation of lifeboats which are not already covered by the existing maritime legislation. In general terms there are two categories of operation, inshore (rivers and estuaries) and offshore. The inshore craft are usually inflatable with outboard engines and carry a crew of two to three. The offshore lifeboats are of special construction to render them unsinkable and self-rightable. They may operate for several hours at a time in extremes of cold and wet and in high seas. The crews number five to six.

Medical examinations are carried out by appointed medical examiners on entry and 5-yearly thereafter. Age limits for service are 45 years for inshore operation and 55 years for offshore operation. In some cases an extension is granted, subject to annual medical examination. A recent expert advisory committee to the RNLI concluded that in view of the arduous nature of the tasks and the interdependence of the crew members, no lifeboatman in whom the diagnosis of coronary artery disease had been made, or was suspected, could serve. This is irrespective of whether treatment or intervention had been recommended or carried out. None the less, the possibility of expert review, following appeal, exists.

RAILWAYS

The responsibility for application of medical standards of railwaymen is vested, in the United Kingdom, in the Department of Transport. Railwaymen may be divided into footplatemen, who require a class F certificate, other (safety-related) staff, who require a class A certificate, and the remainder. There are some 25 000 footplatemen and there are very much larger numbers of other staff including signalmen, track workers, and some portering staff who have at least some safety responsibility and require the class A certificate. The frequency for medical examination for class F holders is at assimilation to the grade, 5-yearly until age 55, again at 57½ and 60, and 2-yearly thereafter. For class A, medical examination is carried out at entry, at age 30, 40, 45, and 5-yearly thereafter until 60, following which there is a further examination at age 63.

There is a Medical Advisory Committee to the Chief Medical Officer, British Rail, which is responsible for laying down advisory medical standards; these are unpublished. At present, all employees are reviewed at the appropriate time interval in ten designated centres in the United Kingdom. It is expected that this practice will cease with privatization but it is likely that the existing medical standards will be maintained, probably by the Health and Safety Executive. Medical fitness standards do not have statutory authority. Substantial inherent safeguards are present in railway operations with automatic track signalling and the employment of vigilance devices (formerly the dead man's handle) which should bring a train to a halt in the continued absence of input from the driver. Mainline trains travelling at less than 110 m.p.h. (170 k.p.h.) require one man in the cab; faster trains require two. There is normally another staff member on the train acting as a conductor or guard.

The presence of overt or suspected coronary artery disease denies certification to operate a locomotive on a main line. There is the possibility of recertificating individuals following a myocardial infarction or following revascularization of the myocardium at the discretion of the Chief Medical Officer. Such an individual, having been excluded from mainline operations, might find employment on a branch line. The operation of locomotives in marshalling yards and sheds is possible by railwaymen who are symptom-free on or off treatment for cardiovascular diseases.

DIVING

The standards of professional diving are the responsibility of the Health and Safety Executive in the British sector of the North Sea. Diving also takes place both inland and elsewhere in the world. Most divers are covered by the Diving Operations at Work regulations, 1981 (S11981 No. 399) Standards are laid down by a Diving Medical Advisory Committee to the Health and Safety Executive, which identifies five categories. The first three relate to the different gases in the inspired air while the fourth relates to air-breathing divers. The restricted fifth category relates to professional instructors teaching amateur divers.

Medical examinations are carried out anually by doctors approved by the Health and Safety Executive. Any history of ischaemic heart disease, whether symptomatic or not, debars from diving. This applies whether or not there has been myocardial infarction or revascularization of the myocardium. A diver found unfit or subject to limitation has statutory right of appeal to the Health and Safety Executive.

FIRE SERVICE

The standards for firemen in the United Kingdom are laid down by the Home Office and medical examinations are carried out annually by medical examiners appointed by individual fire brigades. Applicants have to be at least 18 years and under 31 years old and be fit for any manual work. The diagnosis of coronary artery disease, however presenting, whether or not there has been myocardial infarction and/or revascularization of the myocardium disbars from active duties. The possibility for a favourable decision in such a case is not necessarily ruled out but most brigades regard the presence of coronary artery disease as a reason for denial. Drivers of emergency vehicles greater than 7.5 tonnes are also required to fulfil the requirements of the Driver and Vehicle Licensing Agency Group II licence.

OTHER

The armed forces in the United Kingdom, and the police force, have their own medical standards. In the case of the armed forces these are applied by their integrated medical services; in the case of the police by appointed medical officers. Medical standards are similar to those of the civilian agencies. Individuals do not require civilian licences unless operating civilian equipment or service equipment in the civil area, such as on the roads. This does not apply to flying. Police officers in whom the diagnosis of coronary artery disease has been made may be retained at the discretion of the advising medical officer, the police being an equal opportunities employer.

Microlight flying and ballooning require a Civil Aviation Authority class D certificate embodying a short medical declaration and medical examination by a general practitioner. Microlight (and glider) instructors require a Civil Aviation Authority class III certificate with a medical examination carried out by an authorized medical examiner. The responsibilities for medical certification of glider and hang-glider pilots has been delegated by the Civil Aviation Authority to the British Gliding and the British Hang Gliding Associations.

Regulatory agencies

British Gliding Association, Kimberley House, Vaughan Way, Leicester, LE1 4SE, UK.
British Hang-gliding and Paragliding Association Ltd, The Old Schoolroom, Loughborough Road, Leicester, LE4 5PJ, UK.
British Sub-Aqua Club, Telford Quay, Ellesmere Port, The Wirral, Cheshire, UK.
Department of Transport, Shipping Policy Directorate, London, WC1V 6LP, UK.
FISA Medical Commision, Federation Internationale Sporte Automobile, 8 Place de la Concorde, 75008 Paris, France.
Health and Safety Executive, Information Centre, Broad Lane, Sheffield IS3 7HQ, UK.
Medical Advisory Branch, Driver and Vehicle Licensing Agency, Oldway Centre, Orchard Street, Swansea, SA99 1TU, UK.
Medical Branch, Civil Aviation Authority, Aviation House, South Area, Gatwick Airport, Gatwick, West Sussex, RH6 0YR, UK.
Medical Department, British Rail, Euston House, 24 Evershot Street, London, NW1 1DZ, UK.

RAC Motor Sports Association Ltd, Motor Sports House, Riverside Park, Colnbrook, Slough, SL3 0HG, UK.

Royal National Lifeboat Institution, West Quay Road, Poole, Dorset, BH15 1HZ, UK.

UK Offshore Operators Association, 3 Hans Crescent, London, SW1X 0LN, UK.

REFERENCES

De Busk, R.F. (1990). The Stanford University Cardiac Rehabilitation Programme. *Journal of Myocardial Ischaemia* 2, 28–36.

Dennis, C. Houston-Miller, R.N., Schwartz, R.G. et al (1988). Early return to work after uncomplicated myocardial infarction: results of a randomised trial. *Journal of the American Medical Association,* 260, 214–220.

Driver and Vehicle Licensing Agency (1993). *At a Glance Guide to Current Medical Standards of Fitness to Drive.* Driver and Vehicle Licensing Agency, Swansea.

Edmunds, F.C., McCallum, R.I, and Taylor, P.J. (1988). *Fitness for Work. The Medical Aspects.* Oxford University Press, Oxford.

Hedback, B. and Perk, J. (1987). Five year results of a comprehensive rehabilitation programme after myocardial infarction. *European Heart Journal,* 8, 234–242.

Hlatky, M.A., Harvey, T., Barefoot, J.C. et al (1986). Medical, psychological and social correlates of work disability among men with coronary artery disease. *American Journal of Cardiology,* 58, 911–915.

Holmes, D.R., Van Raden, M.J., Reeder, G.S. et al (1984). Return to work after coronary angioplasty: A report from the National Heart, Lung and Blood Institute/Percutaneous Transluminal Coronary Angioplasty Registry. *American Journal of Cardiology,* 53, 48C–51C.

Horgan, J., Bethell, H., Carson, P., *et al.* (1002). Working party report on cardiac rehabilitation. *British Heart Journal,* 67, 412–418.

Joy, M. (1992). First European Workshop in Aviation Cardiology. *European Heart Journal,* 13(Suppl. H), 1–175.

Joy, M. and Bennett, G. (1984). First United Kingdom Workshop in Aviation Cardiology. *European Heart Journal,* 5(Suppl. A), 1–163.

Joy, M. and Bennett, G. (1988). Second United Kingdom Workshop in Aviation Cardiology. *European Heart Journal,* 9(Suppl. G), 1–179.

O'Connor, G.T., Buring, J.E., Yusuf, S., Joldhager, S.Z., Olmstead, E.M., Paffenbarger, R.S., and Hennekens, C.H. (1988). An overview of randomised trials of rehabilitation with exercise after myocardial infarction: Combined experience of randomised clinical trials. *Journal of the American Medical Association,* 260, 945–950.

RITA Trial Participants (1993). Coronary angioplasty versus coronary artery bypass surgery: the Randomised Intervention Treatment of Angina (RITA) trial. *Lancet* 341, 573–580.

Rogers, W.J., Coggin, C.J., Gersh, E.J. et al (1990). Ten year follow up of quality of life in patients randomised to receive medical therapy or coronary artery bypass graft surgery. The Coronary Artery Surgery Study (CASS). *Circulation* 82, 1647–1658.

Russell, R.O., Abi-Mansour, P., and Wenger, N.K. (1986). Return to work after coronary surgery and percutaneous transluminal coronary angioplasty. Issues and potential solutions. *Cardiology* 73, 306–322.

Shenfield, S.B. (1990). Return to work after an acute myocardial infarction: a review. *Heart-Lung* 19, 109–117.

Walling, A., Tremblay, G.J., Jobin, J. et al (1988). Evaluating the rehabilitation potential of a large population of post myocardial infarction patients: Adverse prognosis for women. *Journal of Cardiopulmonary Rehabilitation,* 8, 99–106.

Wenger, N.K. and Hellerstein, H.K. (1992). *Rehabilitation of the Coronary Patient,* 3rd Edn. Churchill Livingstone, New York.

15.11 Peripheral arterial disease

P. J. MORRIS

The increase in the size of the elderly population in developed countries during the twentieth century, together with the great increase in cigarette smoking and possibly dietary changes, have led to many more patients presenting with clinical manifestations of peripheral arterial disease. Coincident with the growth of degenerative arterial disease has been the rapid expansion of arterial surgery as a speciality and, in particular, of the techniques of reconstructive surgery. Most arterial disease is due to atheromatous degeneration of the arterial wall, and this forms the bulk of the work of peripheral vascular clinics. Embolism, trauma, and vasospastic disorders are important, if less common, problems.

Atherosclerosis (see also Chapter 15.9.1.)

Atherosclerosis is a generalized degenerative disease and is found in all major arteries beyond middle age, and, indeed, if the fatty streak represents the first stage, then it is widespread even in childhood. The fatty streak is a reversible lesion, which may go on to the next stage of atherosclerosis, the fibrous plaque, which is rarely seen in children, and is unusual before the fourth decade. Fibrous plaques have a white appearance, are oval in shape, and are covered by endothelium. They are usually seen first in the lower aorta. Some become complicated, with calcification, ulceration, and thrombus formation on the ulcerated surface. It is this complicated lesion which is usually associated with clinical problems, for the enlarging plaques may gradually obstruct the lumen, reducing blood flow to a critical level. In contrast to this narrowing of the lumen, destruction of the media by the atheromatous process may lead to dilatation of the affected artery rather than occlusion. Although occlusive arterial disease is often considered a different entity to aneurysmal disease, because of the different clinical presentation, they each may represent different manifestations of the same process.

The distribution of atherosclerosis is peculiarly consistent in that plaques occur in large arteries with a high pressure, and at their bifurcation (for example carotid bifurcation, aorto-iliac bifurcation), or where there is kinking or external pressure on the artery, as in the adductor canal. At such points flow is disturbed, and the resulting unstable shear stresses may produce endothelial damage as the first stage in the development of atherosclerosis. Although many other factors must be important, this predilection of the lesions for the origin of branches or bifurcations in major arteries, the greater severity of lesions in the systemic arterial circulation in comparison to the pulmonary or venous circulation, and their greater severity in large arteries imply an important role in aetiology for haemodynamic or mechanical factors.

Following endothelial damage, which may also be accentuated in experimental models by hypertension, hypercholesterolaemia, high levels of carbon monoxide (comparable to those seen in heavy smokers), and in immune complex disease, the normal non-thrombogenic nature of the vessel wall is lost. This property of the vessel wall is maintained in part by the endogenous production of a prostaglandin, which inhibits platelet aggregation. The reparative process is characterized by platelet deposition and lipid infiltration into the area of the injury. This is followed by smooth muscle proliferation in the subendothelial layer of the wall. Collagen may also be produced by the smooth muscle cells, and so the fibrotic plaque has appeared. Further damage may produce a new cycle of plaque growth. Finally, with continuation of the process, calcification and ulceration of the plaque occur with further thrombus formation on the ulcerated surface (see Chapter 15.9.1). Although the process begins in the intima and subendothelial layer, it gradually extends from within out, and eventually may extend even into the adventitia.

Rish factors in peripheral arterial disease

Many risk factors can be identified in peripheral arterial disease, some certain, others less certain (Table 1). These are identical to those implicated in cardiovascular or cerebrovascular disease, but the risk attached to each may be different. For example, hypertension represents a greater risk for cardiovascular and cerebrovascular disease than for peripheral arterial disease, while smoking is by far the major risk factor in peripheral arterial disease but is possibly of minor importance in cerebrovascular disease. As might be expected, there is a cumulative increase in risk in the presence of more than one risk factor.

SMOKING

This is the major risk factor in peripheral arterial disease (Table 2). Although the mechanisms by which it produces atherosclerosis are uncertain, it is thought that the high level of carbon monoxide (CO) in the form of carboxyhaemoglobin is responsible for atherosclerosis. Endothelial damage can result from exposure to CO in experimental animals, and prostacyclin production by the endothelium may be depressed, allowing platelet deposition, especially in areas at risk for endothelial damage. Of particular relevance to the management of patients with peripheral arterial disease are the observations that cessation of smoking will result in fewer subsequent vascular incidents (e.g. myocardial infarction, stroke, amputation) than occur in those who continue to smoke, and also that the long-term success of arterial reconstruction (as judged by patency rates) is some fourfold greater in patients who give up smoking at the time of surgery than in those who continue to smoke (Fig. 1). Smoking is also the major risk factor in patients with Buerger's disease, a rare form of vasculitis in the Western world, and indeed smoking forms part of the recognized syndrome of this condition.

HYPERTENSION

Just as hypertension is an important risk factor in cardiovascular and cerebrovascular disease, so it is in the development of peripheral arterial disease. However, once severe occlusive arterial disease is evident, a moderate degree of hypertension may favour increased collateral blood flow around an obstructed artery.

DIABETES MILLITUS

Patients with diabetes mellitus provide a major part of any vascular clinic's work. Although predominantly presenting with small arteriolar occlusive disease, they are more likely to have occlusive atherosclerosis of major arteries than the normal population. The development of both forms of arterial disease is related to the quality of glucose control, but genetic factors play a role in the development of the small vessel disease (see Chapter 11.11).

HYPERLIPIDAEMIA

Although hypercholesterolaemia is associated with a greater risk of ischaemic heart disease, there is no clear evidence of its association with peripheral arterial disease, except in patients with familial hypercholesterolaemia. Similarly, hypertriglyceridaemia is not clearly established as a risk factor. However, there are reports, admittedly in a small number of patients, suggesting that reduction of a high serum cholesterol by diet can lead to regression of atheromatous plaques demonstrated on sequential angiograms.

Table 1 *Risk factors for peripheral arterial disease*

Smoking of cigarettes	Obesity
Hypertension	Physical inactivity
Diabetes mellitus	Stress
Hypercholesterolaemia	Family history
Hypertriglyceridaemia	

Table 2 *The relative risk of intermittent claudication (IC) associated with some of the risk factors in peripheral arterial disease*

Risk factor	Relative risk of IC
Systolic pressure > 160 mmHg	3.4
Diastolic pressure > 90 mmHg	3.2
Serum triglyceride ↑	2.0
Smoking > 15 cigarettes/day	8.8

Adapted from Hughson *et al.* (1978).

OTHER FACTORS

A number of other factors may be important in the development of peripheral arterial disease (Table 1) but their putative role as risk factors is based in the main on their known role as risk factors in ischaemic heart disease.

Clinical presentation

ACUTE ISCHAEMIA OF A LIMB

The patient with an acutely ischaemic limb presents clinically with a painful, pale, pulseless limb. Most commonly this is due either to acute thrombosis superimposed on an atheromatous stenosis or plaque, or to lodging of an embolus in a major artery to the limb. It should be stressed that there is no difference on clinical examination of the acutely ischaemic limb whatever the cause. A previous history of claudication in the ischaemic limb suggests that it may be due to acute thrombosis, while a history of a previous myocardial infarction, the presence of atrial fibrillation, rheumatic heart disease, or an abdominal aortic aneurysm would favour a diagnosis of embolism. However, only an angiogram will enable an accurate diagnosis of either embolism or thrombosis to

Fig. 1 Cumulative late patency rates for aortoiliac and femoropopliteal reconstructions based on the preoperative and postoperative smoking habits. Moderate smokers: 1–15 cigarettes/day; heavy smokers: more than 15 cigarettes/day. After operation smoking was assessed on the basis of smoking fewer than 5 or more than 5 cigarettes/day. (Reproduced from Myers *et al.* (1978). *British Journal of Surgery,* with permission of the publishers Butterworth and Co..)

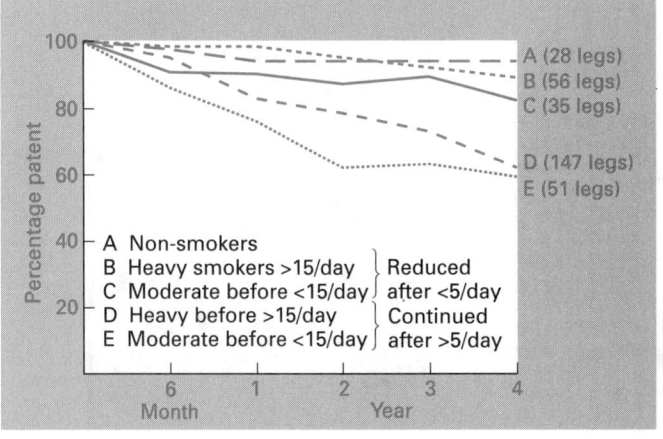

be made and the appropriate management instituted (Fig. 2). Arterial trauma, due to road-traffic accidents, knife wounds, or gunshot wounds, are becoming increasingly common, and so too is trauma following the insertion of intra-arterial catheters for diagnosis or therapy. In the presence of ischaemia of a limb following trauma immediate angiography is mandatory. A rare cause of acute ischaemia in the lower limb is phlegmasia cerulea dolens, in which massive thrombosis of all the major veins of the limb occurs with gross swelling causing obstruction of the arterial supply.

CHRONIC ISCHAEMIA OF A LIMB

The clinical manifestations of chronic ischaemia range from muscle pain on exercise relieved by rest (intermittent claudication), through rest pain and/or non-healing ulceration, to frank gangrene of the distal part of the limb. A relatively rare form of ischaemia in the Western world, but more common in South-East Asia, is Buerger's disease (thromboangiitis obliterans), which describes a syndrome of vasculitic disease in the medium-sized arteries of the lower limb, and less commonly in the upper limb, occurring almost always in young males who are heavy smokers and often associated with episodes of thrombophlebitis.

Clinical examination will reveal the absence of the appropriate pulses. Although the diagnosis of a severely ischaemic limb is usually quite apparent, that of intermittent claudication may present difficulties. Classically the patient will complain of a cramp-like pain, for example in the calf after walking 100 m at a constant pace, which disappears within minutes of resting, only to reappear again at the same distance as the patient walks again. Failure of the pain to disappear on resting or its reappearance at a shorter distance after each rest should draw the attention of the physician to a possible musculoskeletal cause of such symptoms, especially if distal pulses are present on examination. However, it should be remembered that pulses may be present in a limb distal to proximal disease, albeit weaker than the normal side, due to a good collateral flow, but in such cases exercise to the point of claudication will lead to disappearance of the distal pulses. Doppler pressures at the ankle at rest

will be lower than the brachial pressure, but will fall markedly after exercising for 1 min on a treadmill. Angiography is performed if reconstructive surgery is to be considered, but is not used as a diagnostic tool. A variety of conditions may mimic intermittent claudication (and are often grouped together under the heading pseudoclaudication). These include such disorders as spinal stenosis, and arthritis of the knee and hip.

ANEURYSMS

Abdominal aortic aneurysm

This is the most common aneurysm encountered in clinical practice and may present to the clinician in one of three ways:

1. Ruptured or leaking aneurysm: the patient classically presents with the triad of pain, hypotension, and a pulsatile mass in the abdomen. However, only 50 per cent of patients with a leaking aneurysm will present with all three features. The pain tends to be epigastric radiating through to the back, but may be situated in the loin or even in the testicle. Indeed, one of the most common misdiagnoses is renal colic. A pulsatile mass may be overlooked, especially in the obese patient, if an attempt is not made specifically to feel for it in a patient with an acute abdomen or shock. In general, femoral pulses will be present and the femoral arteries tend to be ectatic.

2. Symptomatic or expanding aneurysm: the patient presents with abdominal pain, usually epigastric, or with pain in the back of relatively recent onset, and is found to have a pulsatile mass on examination. Occasionally the presenting features are of ureteric obstruction when a fibrotic inflammatory reaction similar to retroperitoneal fibrosis has occurred around the aneurysm, or of an embolus of the lower limbs causing acute ischaemia.

3. Asymptomatic aneurysm: the patient is found to have a pulsatile mass on examination for some other condition, or an aneurysm is detected on a plain radiography or ultrasound of the abdomen, again performed for some other reason (Fig. 3).

Thoracic aortic aneurysm

Although syphilis was the most common cause of this type of aneurysm, this is no longer the case, the vast majority of cases today being due to atheroma, with a small but significant number resulting from previous

Fig. 2 A femoral angiogram showing the typical appearance of an embolus. Two emboli (arrows) can be seen in branches of the profunda femoris artery.

Fig. 3 A lateral plain film of the abdomen in a man found to have a pulsatile mass in his abdomen during an insurance examination, showing a large abdominal aortic aneurysm with calcification in the wall (arrow).

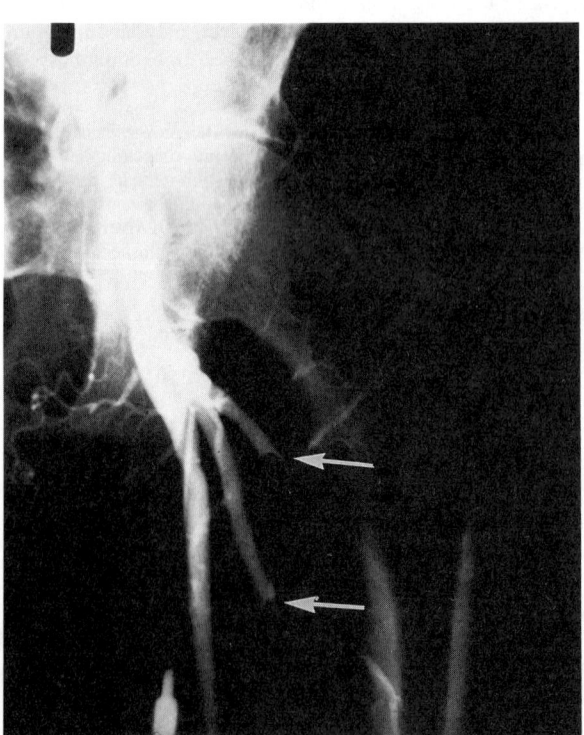

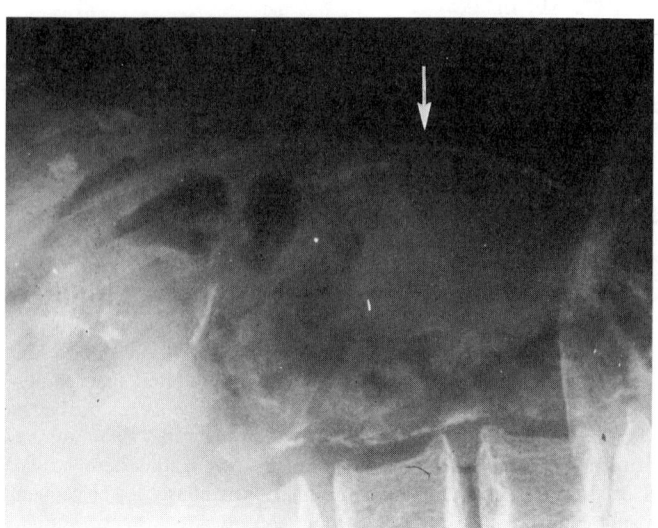

trauma. Although the syphilitic aneurysm usually involves the ascending aorta, the atheromatous aneurysm of the thoracic aorta is evenly distributed between the ascending aorta, the arch, and the descending aorta. Most thoracic aorta aneurysms are asymptomatic, and are detected on a chest radiography performed for some other reason. Very often the first presentation is due to rupture and sudden death. When these aneurysms are symptomatic they are usually large, anterior chest pain being the most common symptom, but other clinical features due to pressure, such as obstruction of the superior vena cava, dysphagia due to pressure on the oesophagus, or stridor due to pressure on the trachea, may be present. Aneurysms of the ascending aorta often involve the aortic valve, causing aortic insufficiency, and there may be obstruction of the orifices of the coronary arteries, causing myocardial ischaemia.

Dissecting aortic aneurysm

The thoracic aorta is the most common site of dissecting aneurysm, other arteries being involved by extension of the dissection. Dissection is associated with degeneration of the media of the aorta and most patients are hypertensive. In about 50 per cent of cases the dissection starts in the ascending aorta, the next most common site being just distal to the origin of the left subclavian artery. The arch of the aorta and the abdominal aorta are uncommon sites of origin. Pain, either substernal or in the upper back, is the most striking presenting feature, often with radiation to the neck or arms. An aortic diastolic murmur or a pericardial friction rub may be heard with a dissection of the ascending aorta, and there may be a significant diminution in the pulse and blood pressure in the right arm. A dissection of the descending thoracic aorta may extend into the abdominal aorta and involve all its major branches, thus being associated with acute renal failure, mesenteric ischaemia, or ischaemia of the lower limbs.

Popliteal aneurysms

These are not uncommon and are often associated with aneurysmal disease elsewhere. Although sometimes causing pain due to pressure on surrounding structures, they most commonly present as a pulsatile mass behind the knee or with ischaemia of the distal limb due to thrombosis or embolism.

Other aneurysms

Less commonly, aneurysms may occur in the iliac, femoral, carotid, splenic, renal, or one of the splanchnic arteries. With the exception of carotid or femoral artery aneurysms, which will usually present as a pulsatile mass, those elsewhere tend to be asymptomatic until they present as a major intra-abdominal bleed, more often fatal than not. Splenic artery aneurysms are the most common intra-abdominal ones apart from those of the aorta or iliac vessels, and are seen more frequently in younger women, in which case there is a marked tendency to rupture during pregnancy. Mycotic aneurysms (better called infected aneurysms) are rare, and usually are seen today as a complication of bacterial endocarditis due to impaction of an infected embolus at a bifurcation or perhaps in the vasa vasorum of the vessel wall (Fig. 4).

VASOSPASTIC DISORDERS

Inappropriate and symptomatic vasoconstriction of the arterioles and arteries of the limbs may be intermittent or persistent. Raynaud's syndrome is the most common vasospastic disorder. Less common and often not well-defined disorders are acrocyanosis, livedo reticularis, and cold sensitivity following cold injury or trauma.

Raynaud's syndrome

Raynaud's syndrome may be defined as intermittent vasospasm of the arterioles of the distal limbs following exposure to cold or emotional stimuli. Classical colour changes are observed, the extremities first becoming pale, then blue, and finally red as the attack passes. This condition may be associated with a variety of underlying diseases (Table

3), in which case it is known as Raynaud's phenomenon or secondary Raynaud's syndrome, or, on the other hand, no underlying condition can be detected, in which case it is known as Raynaud's disease or primary Raynaud's syndrome. True Raynaud's disease occurs mostly in young females, who have intermittent bilateral and symmetrical attacks in the absence of any organic arterial occlusion, and in the absence of severe trophic changes in the fingers or toes. Although upper and lower extremities may be affected, it is most common in the upper limbs.

Patients with Raynaud's phenomenon may not only present with vasospastic features in the hands or feet, but also with other clinical features due to the underlying disease. Trophic changes in the fingers or toes are common. Of all the disorders listed in Table 3, scleroderma is by far the most common (Chapter 18.11.4). It should be remembered, especially in scleroderma, that Raynaud's phenomenon may be the presenting clinical feature in many patients, other manifestations of the disease not being evident for several years. Investigations in patients with Raynaud's syndrome will be directed at the possibility of defining an underlying condition, and should include thoracic outlet radiographs, full blood examination, erythrocyte sedimentation rate, barium swallow, serum protein electrophoresis, cryoglobulins, cold agglutinins, antinuclear factor, anti-DNA antibody, rheumatoid factor, and perhaps angiography (Fig. 5).

Acrocyanosis

This condition virtually only occurs in women and is characterized by cold blue extremities, worse in cold weather but also present in warm weather. The symptoms are not episodic, and all peripheral pulses are present.

Livedo reticularis

This condition is characterized by persistent patchy reddish-blue mottling of the legs (occasionally involving the arms), and tends to be worse

Fig. 4 A mycotic aneurysm (arrow) at the bifurcation of the distal popliteal artery in a young woman with subacute bacterial endocarditis. Other aneurysms were present in the left iliac artery and the right profunda femoris artery.

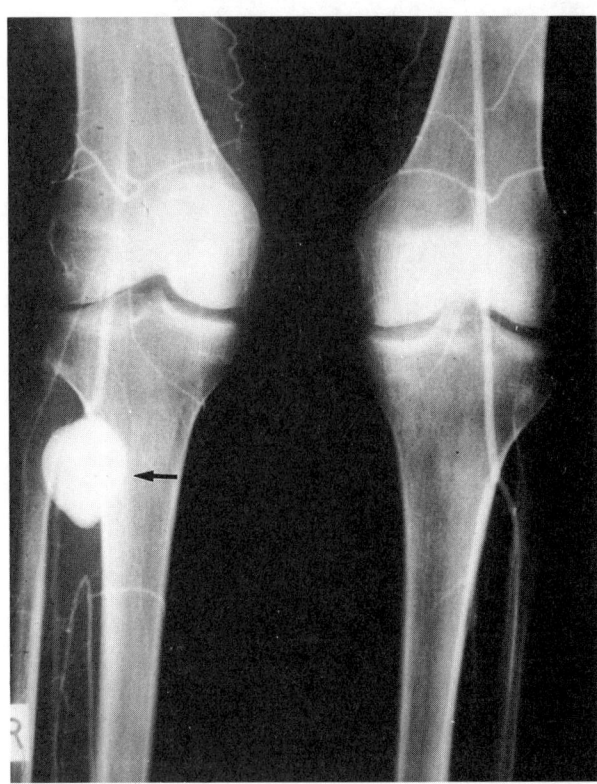

Table 3 *Underlying disorders which may give rise to Raynaud's phenomenon*

1 Collagen diseases
  Scleroderma; lupus erythematosus; rheumatoid arthritis; dermatomyositis
2 Neurogenic lesions
  Thoracic outlet compression; carpal tunnel syndrome; other nervous system diseases
3 Occupational trauma
  Chain-saw operators; pneumatic hammer operators; pianists
4 Occlusive arterial disease
  Atherosclerosis; thromboangiitis obliterans; embolism
5 Miscellaneous
  Cryoglobulinaemia; cold agglutinins; macroglobulinaemia; ergot intoxication

in cold weather (see also Section 23). It may sometimes be associated with chronic ulceration. It is due to random spasm of cutaneous arterioles, with secondary dilation of capillaries and venules. There may be an underlying vasculitis in some cases.

Cold hypersensitivity following cold exposure or trauma

A number of related conditions may be included under this heading, all presumably with a vasospastic aetiology, but following a variety of injuries to the limb or frost-bite. Pain is often a prominent feature of the clinical picture, especially when occurring after trauma (when it is usually known as causalgia). The limb is pale and cold, and often shows evidence of disuse atrophy.

Fig. 5 An arteriogram of the right upper limb in a patient with Raynaud's phenomenon due to scleroderma showing obliteration of most of the digital arteries.

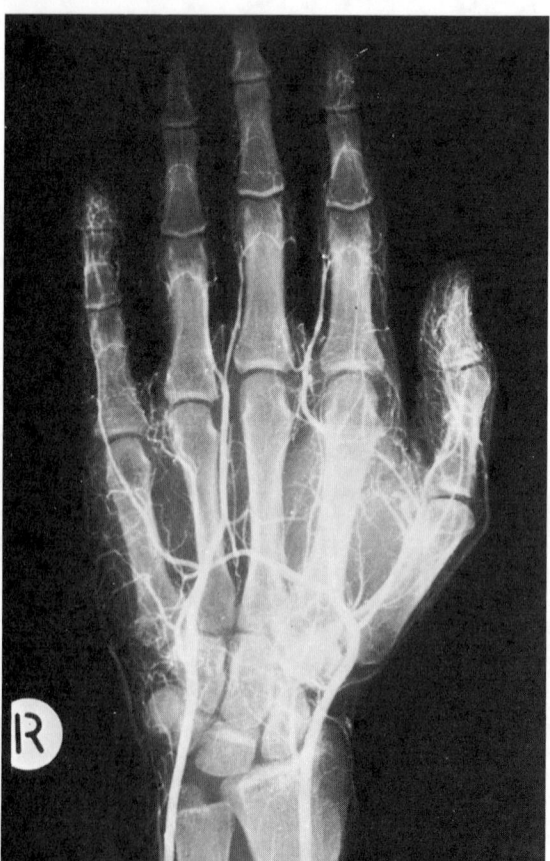

THORACIC OUTLET COMPRESSION

Compression of any one of the subclavian vein, subclavian artery, or the lower trunk of the brachial plexus, or all three structures, may occur due to a variety of anatomical abnormalities at the thoracic outlet. A cervical rib is perhaps the most easily recognized and so the most common cause of thoracic outlet compression; but compression of the above structures can occur despite normal anatomy as the structures cross the first rib into the axilla. In both instances the onset of symptoms tends to occur for the first time in early middle age, particularly in women, this being associated with poor posture. Patients may present predominantly with neurological symptoms such as pain which is usually poorly defined, or with paraesthesia in the C8–T1 distribution, or vascular symptoms due to either arterial obstruction or venous obstruction. Arterial obstruction may present as a unilateral Raynaud's phenomenon or pallor and pain in the hand when using the arm above the head, or at a later stage with distal emboli to the fingers from a post-stenotic aneurysm. Venous obstruction often presents in the younger person as a spontaneous axillary vein thrombosis (Fig. 6). Overall a neurological presentation is much more common than a vascular presentation in patients with thoracic outlet compression.

INTESTINAL ISCHAEMIA

Acute

Generally, patients presenting with acute intestinal ischaemia will be elderly, as are most patients with occlusive vascular disease, and will have evidence of generalized atheromatous disease. There may be a possible source of a peripheral arterial embolus, for example a previous myocardial infarction or atrial fibrillation. However, in addition to arterial thrombosis or embolism, acute intestinal ischaemia may be due to venous thrombosis, which is associated with portal hypertension, peritonitis, or a blood dyscrasia. Furthermore, in a significant number of patients with acute intestinal ischaemia, no major arterial or venous obstruction is found at laparotomy or autopsy, the ischaemia being presumed to be due to a low flow state in the bowel wall itself associated with cardiac failure or shock.

Fig. 6 Axillary venogram in a 25-year-old man with recurrent axillary vein thrombosis and a swollen right arm. Clinical evidence of thoracic outlet compression was evident. At operation the axillary vein was patent but compressed by a fibrous band as it crossed the first rib (arrow). Resection of the first rib relieved the symptoms.

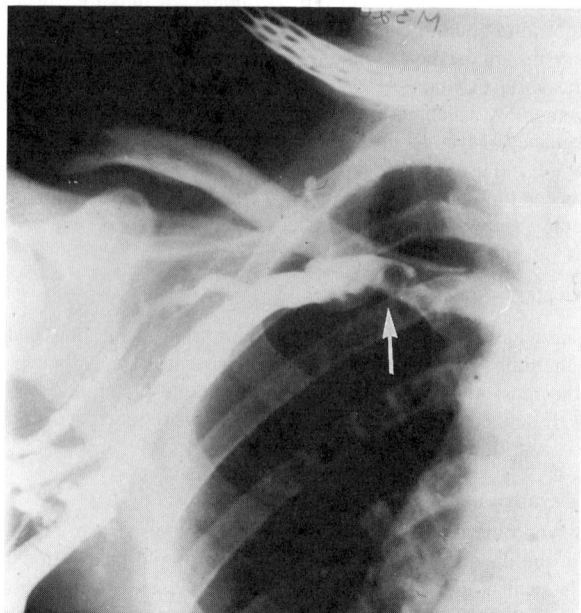

The patient presents with an acute abdomen and the features of bowel obstruction, namely colicky abdominal pain, and nausea and vomiting, but associated with tenderness in the early stages, while at a later stage there are all the signs of peritonitis. Diarrhoea is common, and is often bloody, especially with acute ischaemia of the large bowel. A peritoneal tap will reveal a serosanguinous aspirate containing leucocytes and, at a later stage, bacteria. A plain radiograph of the abdomen may show complete absence of gas shadows at an early stage, or fluid levels, sometimes localized to the ischaemic segment of small bowel, while a typical scalloped or fingerprinting appearance in the large bowel may be apparent on barium enema (Fig. 7). However, only an angiogram will confirm the obstruction of a major mesenteric artery with either an embolus or thrombus. Whether this is justified as an investigation of an acute abdomen in patients with possible intestinal ischaemia is debatable. Unless there is obstruction of at least one other major mesenteric artery by atheroma, severe ischaemia of the intestine is unlikely to occur. The mortality associated with acute intestinal ischaemia is high, of the order of 75 per cent, and only early diagnosis offers the patient a chance of survival.

Chronic

Patients with chronic intestinal ischaemia present with postprandial, central, colicky abdominal pain and weight loss. Usually two of the three main arteries supplying the bowel (coeliac, superior mesenteric, and inferior mesenteric) have to be obstructed for symptoms to result. Angiography with lateral views will define the vascular lesions but their presence does not necessarily mean that they are responsible for the symptoms.

Compression of the coeliac artery by an unusually low median arcuate ligament of the diaphragm is another postulated cause of chronic intestinal ischaemia, but the existence of this syndrome remains controversial. Indeed, it is really not known whether chronic mesenteric ischaemia is a relatively common cause of chronic abdominal symptoms, especially after eating, but probably it is rare. It should also be remembered that the bowel vasculature may be affected by a large number of diseases, for instance systemic lupus erythematosus, rheumatoid arthritis, or polyarteritis nodosa, as part of the generalized symptom complex of such disorders.

EXTRACEREBRAL VASCULAR DISEASE

Carotid artery ischaemia

Atheromatous disease of the origin of the internal carotid artery commonly presents as a transient neurological deficit (transient ischaemic attack), which by definition recovers within 24 h, or loss of vision (amaurosis fugax). The majority of transient ischaemic attacks are embolic in nature, arising from an ulcerated and/or stenosed origin of the internal carotid artery, but emboli may also arise from the heart, for instance from a diseased aortic valve. Some transient ischaemic attacks, especially in the presence of bilateral carotid artery disease, are haemodynamic in nature, rather than embolic. Disease of the internal carotid artery may present as a full-blown stroke, without the preceding warning of a transient ischaemic attack.

The neurological deficit is focal, often with loss of power or sensation in a limb, or speech disturbance, and recovery occurs usually within minutes to hours. Amaurosis fugax describes a unilateral loss of vision lasting only minutes, often resembling the sensation of a blind being pulled down over the eye. A bruit may be heard over the carotid bifurcation, but its absence does not exclude internal carotid artery disease. Examination of the fundus may reveal a platelet or cholesterol embolus in the retinal arterial circulation.

The initial investigation is a duplex scan of the carotids, which allows not only imaging of the carotid bifurcation but also measurement of the degree of stenosis. The gold standard remains carotid angiography (Fig. 8), and many vascular surgeons feel that if the patient is to have a carotid endarterectomy, it is mandatory. There is, however, a 1 to 4 per cent risk of a stroke following angiography, and for this reason it is appropriate to proceed with surgery on the basis of a technically satisfactory duplex scan without an angiogram, which is only performed if the duplex scan is unsatisfactory or if there is bilateral disease. A CT scan or MRI of the brain should always be performed to exclude other pathology and ascertain the presence of cerebral infarcts.

Vertebrobasilar ischaemia

The vertebrobasilar arterial system supplies the brain-stem, occipital lobes, and medial aspects of the temporal lobe, and hence ischaemia of this territory can produce a complex of symptoms. These include vertigo, ataxia, diplopia, dysphagia, dysarthria, and drop attacks. Tingling and numbness of the face and mouth, or indeed half the body, may occur,

Fig. 8 A carotid angiogram showing a severe stenosis of the origin of the internal carotid artery.

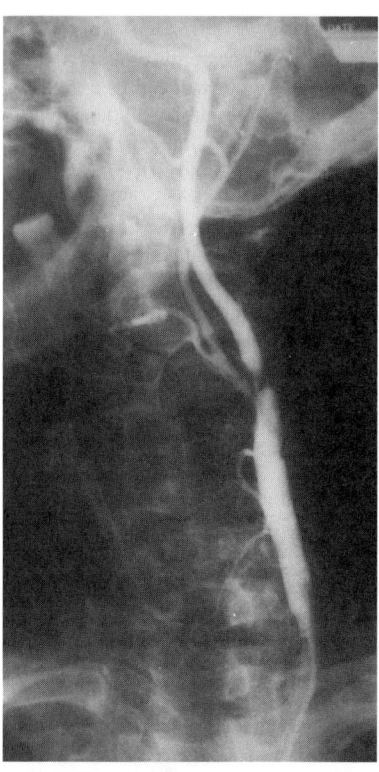

Fig. 7 Barium enema in a 68-year-old man with left-sided abdominal pain and positive occult bloods showing the typical appearance of an ischaemic colitis (arrow).

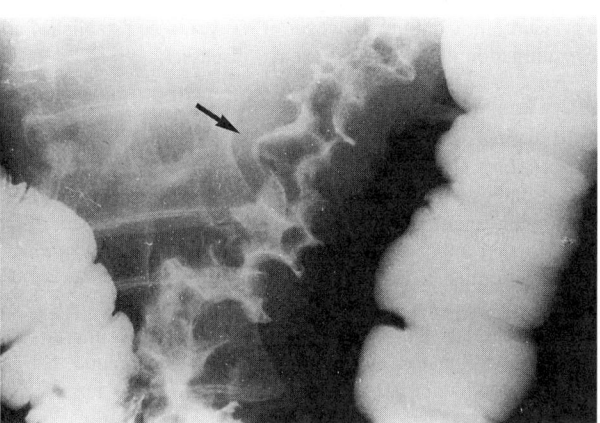

as also may transient hemiparesis. Episodes of visual impairment are common, varying from reduced vision in one half-field to impairment of vision on both sides.

In contrast to carotid artery transient ischaemic attacks, vertebro-basilar ischaemia is haemodynamic rather than embolic in origin. Bilateral disease of the vertebral artery origins may be responsible, but usually only in the presence of carotid artery disease or a non-intact circle of Willis. Rather uncommon, but more easily diagnosed, causes of vertebrobasilar ischaemia are the subclavian and innominate artery steal syndromes. In the former a stenosis or occlusion of the origin of the subclavian artery is associated with the steal of blood from the verte-brobasilar territory down the vertebral artery on the side of the occlusion, particularly while using that arm. In the latter there is a steal down both the vertebral and carotid arteries on the right side, again often associated with use of the right arm.

RENOVASCULAR DISEASE

The most common form of disease of the renal artery is renal artery stenosis, both atheromatous and non-atheromatous, but also included are renal artery aneurysm, arteriovenous fistula, and trauma to the renal artery. The majority of stenoses of the renal artery are atheromatous in origin (over 70 per cent), a much smaller proportion being due to one of several types of fibromuscular dysplasia, and rarely associated with non-atheromatous aortic aortitis.

Stenosis of the renal artery may present as renovascular hypertension with or without renal dysfunction. Characteristics of renovascular hypertension are that it may be seen in young patients, it may be poorly controlled, recent in onset, or associated with an acute presentation with pulmonary oedema. The prevalence of renovascular hypertension in the hypertensive population is between 1 and 5 per cent. The presentation and diagnosis of renovascular hypertension are discussed in detail elsewhere (Chapter 20.11).

Investigation of patients with arterial disease
DETECTION OF RISK FACTORS

Careful assessment of the blood pressure and a careful smoking history are most important, for these are two risk factors that can be corrected. Although generally non-rewarding, hypercholesterolaemia and hyper-triglyceridaemia should be excluded, especially in the younger patient. Polycythaemia, either vera or secondary, should not be overlooked, but although there is some evidence that hyperfibrinogenaemia with increased viscosity may be associated with peripheral vascular disease, the evidence is not sufficiently strong to warrant this investigation in most patients. Urine examination for glucose and a random blood glucose should be performed routinely in all patients with peripheral vascular disease.

NON-INVASIVE ASSESSMENT OF ARTERIAL DISEASE

Physiological measurements

The physiological dysfunction of arterial obstruction requires correction rather than the anatomical lesion. Hence efforts are directed at methods that attempt to measure, both qualitatively and quantitatively, this dysfunction of the anatomical lesion recognized by clinical examination and/or arteriography. They also provide a means of following the progress of arterial disease in patients after reconstructive surgery. The tests in common use comprise measurements of flow and pressure, and analysis of the changes in the flow or pressure patterns.

Peripheral blood flow can be measured relatively accurately and non-invasively by plethysmography. Radioisotope clearance or distribution provides a semi-invasive method of measuring flow, while, at operation, flow can be measured by the direct application of an electromagnetic or ultrasonic flow meter to the artery in question. However, flow at rest may be normal, and it is only by attempting to increase flow as a result of exercise, arterial occlusion, or by injection of papaverine directly into the artery (all of which produce peripheral vasodilation) that an abnormality may be recognized, for in the presence of arterial obstruction the expected increase in flow does not occur with peripheral vasodilation.

The measurement of pressures in the periphery is the most common of all the non-invasive techniques used by vascular units, as it is simple and reproducible. Generally, pressures are measured by the detection of the return of flow in an artery below a cuff using a Doppler ultrasonic velocity detector, although its sensitivity can be improved with the use of a mercury-in-silastic strain gauge or a photoplethysmograph. Measurement of pressure at the ankle is by far the most useful of the non-invasive measurements of peripheral arterial disease, since these measurements, both before and after exercise, provide an objective assessment of the degree of arterial obstruction. Normally the ankle pressure is expressed as a pressure index which is the ratio of the systolic pressure at the ankle to that in the brachial artery. Normal pressure indices at rest range from 0.9 to 1.2, while those in patients with intermittent claudication range from 0.4 to 0.9. In patients with severe ischaemia and rest pain the indices are below 0.4. After exercise or the production of reactive hyperaemia, the pressure, and hence the index, falls in the presence of arterial obstruction, the rate of recovery giving further information about the degree of ischaemia.

Pressure pulses can only be obtained invasively by intra-arterial catheters or needles, but flow pulses can be obtained not only by electromagnetic flow meters at operation but also non-invasively with an ultrasonic velocity detector. Volume pulses which reflect the arterial wall expansion in response to pressure can be detected with various types of plethysmography.

In most instances the non-invasive techniques described above provide an objective measurement of the clinical assessment of peripheral arterial disease, but in doubtful cases they can be extremely useful in excluding peripheral arterial disease as a cause of the symptoms.

Transcutaneous oxygen tension can now be measured using polarographic electrodes, but the information provided has not been particularly useful in determining the capacity for healing in the proposed skin flaps used for reconstruction after a below-knee amputation.

A more recent development in evaluating peripheral vascular disease is the application of magnetic resonance spectroscopy (MRS) which allows energy metabolism to be assessed in the legs of patients with intermittent claudication or rest pain, respectively. Spectra can be obtained from the calf muscles or extensor digitorum brevis in the foot, and in patients with claudication the fall in muscle phosphocreatinine and the acidosis after exercise recover much more slowly than in people without arterial disease. MRS provides a method of quantifying the metabolic changes associated with more proximal arterial obstruction, and does appear to relate more closely to patient symptoms than does Doppler ankle pressure, for example; however, it has yet to be established as a routine examination in peripheral vascular disease.

Non-invasive imaging techniques

Ultrasound imaging of large arteries, such as the abdominal aorta, is quick, cheap, and accurate. It allows the size of aneurysms and the presence of thrombus within the lumen to be determined, and is an ideal way of following small asymptomatic abdominal aortic aneurysms where surgery is not indicated. The advent of colour duplex ultrasound has increased the utility of this technique even further, and it has now become the technique of choice for investigating patients with putative carotid artery disease, as well as monitoring femorodistal vein grafts in the leg. Magnetic resonance angiography is another technique that is advancing rapidly and will replace conventional angiography in selected situations.

INVASIVE ASSESSMENT OF ARTERIAL DISEASE

Contrast angiography remains the most valuable diagnostic tool for the vascular surgeon, and has not been replaced to any great extent by non-invasive imaging techniques. Direct puncture techniques to inject contrast media have been replaced with retrograde catheter techniques, catheters being inserted via the femoral, axillary, or brachial arteries. The catheter techniques can be performed under local anaesthesia and allow lateral and oblique views to be obtained. Complications of arteriography, such as thrombosis due to intimal damage, clot embolism, or cholesterol embolism, are uncommon. However, angiograms are invasive and often unpleasant for the patient, and hence the drive for non-invasive techniques of determining arterial disease.

Digital subtraction angiography is a relatively simple technique in which contrast is injected intravenously, multiple images of the area in question are stored in a computer in digital form, and as the contrast passes through the area these multiple images are digitally processed, and subtracted from the background, leaving the arterial image. The resolution of digital subtraction angiography is inferior to that of a conventional angiogram, but can be enhanced by the intra-arterial injection of contrast. Furthermore, the area that can be shown is relatively restricted without repeated injections of contrast, which may reach levels capable of producing renal toxicity. Nevertheless, this technique has proven valuable in certain areas, such as the carotid bifurcation, the renal arteries, abdominal aortic, and peripheral arterial aneurysms, and in the sequential evaluation of known arterial lesions or of reconstructive surgery. It seems likely that it will be replaced in many instances by the rapidly advancing technology of duplex scanning and magnetic resonance angiography.

Management of the ischaemic limb

GENERAL MANAGEMENT

Careful attention must be paid to cleanliness of ischaemic feet or hands so as to avoid infection, and particular care must be given to the cutting of toe nails. In the elderly the nails of ischaemic feet are best trimmed by an assistant or a chiropodist so as to avoid laceration and infection, which may lead to gangrene.

Walking to the point of claudication several times during each day may improve collateral circulation in the patient with intermittent claudication, ultimately increasing the walking distance.

Reconstructive surgery, and so angiography, should not be considered in patients presenting with intermittent claudication until the symptoms have been present for at least 3 months and continue to interfere markedly with the patient's work or recreation. For it is distinctly possible that the claudication distance first noted by the patient will improve significantly over the succeeding months as collateral circulation develops. Obviously, the presence of rest pain and/or gangrene represents an indication for urgent investigation with a view to reconstructive surgery.

TREATMENT OF RISK FACTORS

Smoking is by far the most significant risk factor associated with occlusive arterial disease and every effort should be made to stop patients smoking. This edict applies equally well, but for different reasons, to patients with vasospastic disorders. It is just as important to stop patients smoking after reconstructive surgery, for even if patients have smoked for many years, the likelihood of a long-term successful outcome of surgery is fourfold greater in the patient who stops smoking (see Fig. 1). Furthermore, the incidence of other vascular events, such as myocardial infarction, is greater in patients with occlusive arterial disease who continue to smoke than in those who stop.

Diabetes must be controlled adequately, as should hypertension, although hypertension is not such a high-risk factor for peripheral arte-

rial disease as it is for cerebrovascular or coronary artery disease. Hyper-cholesterolaemia and hypertriglyceridaemia probably should be treated, although the evidence that these influence the progress of peripheral arterial disease is sparse and is based mostly on the known association of the various hyperlipidaemias with cardiovascular disease.

DRUGS

A variety of vasodilator drugs with different mechanisms of action have been used in the treatment of occlusive arterial disease but with virtually no improvement in any of the clinical features. At this time they have no place in management. Trials of treatment with prostacyclin have not been shown to be of value in the ischaemic limb.

Anticoagulants again have no place in the management of occlusive arterial disease, other than during reconstructive surgery, when heparin is administered either regionally or systemically before proximal arterial clamps are applied in the course of surgery.

Platelet disaggregators, especially aspirin and/or dipyrimadole, are being used more frequently after surgical reconstruction in the expectation of prolonging the patency of bypass grafts, especially distal prosthetic grafts. Recent evidence from controlled trials suggests that patency of infrainguinal grafts is prolonged by the prophylactic use of low-dose aspirin after reconstructive surgery.

RECONSTRUCTIVE ARTERIAL SURGERY

Aortoiliac reconstruction

Occlusive disease of the aortoiliac segment may be treated either by endarterectomy (in which the atheromatous plaque and approximately the inner two-thirds to one-half of the media are removed) or the insertion of a prosthetic graft. Either procedure may give satisfactory results, but endarterectomy is best restricted to relatively localized disease (Fig. 9), a graft being indicated for more extensive disease. Various prosthetic grafts are available, but a knitted Dacron graft remains the preferred graft by most vascular surgeons. This material best fits the requirements

Fig. 9 A translumbar aortogram in a 49-year-old woman with bilateral calf, thigh, and buttock claudication at 100 m, showing a localized obstruction of the aorta (arrow) with relatively normal vessels above and below. This lesion proved to be eminently suitable for an endarterectomy, but could have been treated equally well by angioplasty.

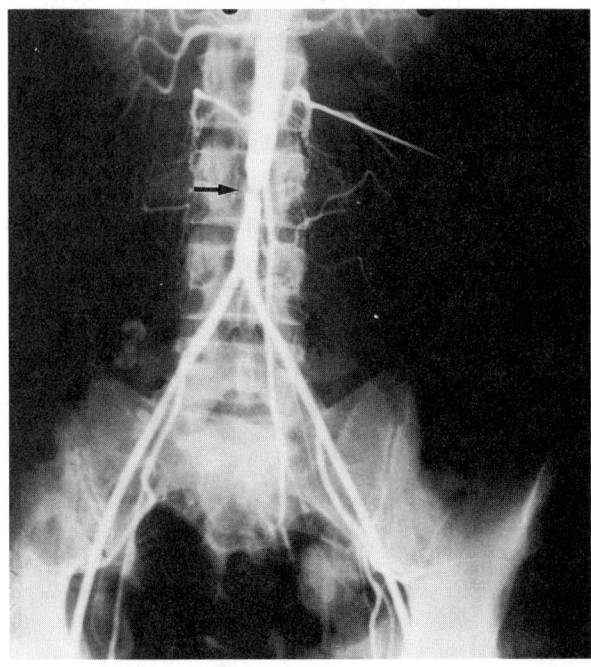

for a prosthetic graft, for it has an adequate porosity to allow ingrowth of fibroblasts to form a false but firmly attached neo-endothelium, it is non-toxic and non-allergenic, it is durable and does not deteriorate, and it is thin-walled and flexible. Usually a bifurcated graft is inserted, the proximal end being anastomosed end-to-end or end-to-side to the aorta above the disease and the two legs of the graft being anastomosed end-to-side to iliac arteries, or just as often to the common femoral arteries below the inguinal ligament if the iliac arteries are diseased. Both procedures give excellent results with patency rates of up to 70 per cent at 10 years being achieved in patients who do not die of cardiovascular or cerebrovascular disease. The long-term patency of bypass grafts appears superior to endarterectomy in the aortoiliac area, but endarterectomy does not preclude a subsequent graft. Recurrence of disease above or below endarterectomized segments of arteries or a prosthetic graft is common and further surgery for recurrence of symptoms may be required in such cases.

Reconstruction below the inguinal ligament

Femoropopliteal grafts are performed for occlusion of the superficial femoral artery, usually running from the common femoral artery to either the proximal popliteal artery above the knee or the distal popliteal artery below the knee. The ideal graft material is reversed or *in situ* autogenous saphenous vein, and if a suitable vein is not present in the operated leg, the vein is removed from the opposite side. If neither vein is suitable, then it may be possible to use the cephalic veins from the arm, as autogenous vein remains far superior to prosthetic grafts.

Prosthetic grafts below the inguinal ligament have a comparable patency rate to vein when used for above the knee bypass, but are markedly inferior to vein below the knee. At present three types of prosthetic graft are used below the inguinal ligament: expanded polytetrafluoroethylene (PTFE), glutaraldehyde-tanned umbilical vein supported by a polyester mesh, and double-velour knitted Dacron; PTFE is the most commonly used material.

Femorotibial grafts: where no popliteal artery is present but one of the three distal arteries is patent (anterior tibial, posterior tibial, or peroneal), it is possible to use one of these arteries for insertion of a graft arising from the common femoral artery. This type of procedure is only performed for limb salvage, and vein is always used if possible. *In situ* use of the saphenous vein is the preferred technique, where the vein is left in place and the valves are disrupted before anastomosing the vein proximally to the common femoral artery and distally to one of the patent run-off arteries, such as the posterior or anterior tibial or even the dorsalis pedis artery. The salvage rate in critically ischaemic limbs has been impressive, at least in the short term.

Profundaplasty: when a stenosis at the origin of the profunda femoris artery exists together with a block of the superficial femoral artery, profundaplasty, with or without a local endarterectomy, may significantly improve the circulation to the limb (Fig. 10). This is a simple procedure which can be performed under local anaesthetic and is ideal as a limb-salvage procedure in a poor-risk patient. Unfortunately, most patients do not have a significant stenosis at the profunda origin.

Extra-anatomical bypass grafts

Where aortoiliac disease exists but the patient is not considered well enough to undergo a major aortoiliac reconstruction, a prosthetic graft (Dacron or PTFE) can be brought subcutaneously from the axillary artery just below the clavicle down to the femoral artery on the same side, with another graft taken off this in the region of the iliac fossa to the opposite femoral artery.

Where one iliac artery only is obstructed, a prosthetic graft can be brought subcutaneously from the femoral artery on the side with a normal flow, just above the pubis, to the common femoral or profunda femoris artery on the obstructed side. This technique has proved to be so successful that it is the preferred technique now even in younger patients with unilateral iliac obstruction.

Extra-anatomical bypass grafts are being used more and more as a first-line reconstructive procedure in the more elderly patient rather than only in patients considered a poor risk for more major reconstructive surgery.

Factors influencing graft patency

Many factors influence graft patency. The site of the graft is important, for prosthetic grafts have a very high patency rate above the inguinal ligament, approaching that of vein grafts, whereas below the inguinal ligament they are to be avoided in favour of autogenous saphenous vein if at all possible. Both the inflow and outflow from a graft are important. This is so for all grafts, but especially for grafts below the inguinal ligament.

The continuation of existing risk factors obviously may influence not only the course of the arterial disease but also the patency of reconstructed arteries. None more so than smoking, for continued smoking decreases the likelihood of long-term patency in reconstructed arteries some fourfold. This is the most important factor to be corrected in the patient undergoing reconstructive arterial surgery. However, correction of other risk factors, such as hypertension, diabetes, and hyperlipidaemia, is just as important because of their prominence as risk factors for ischaemic heart disease.

Fig. 10 A femoral angiogram in a 75-year-old man with severe ischaemia of the leg, showing a complete block of the superficial femoral artery and a stenosis at the origin of the profunda femoris artery (arrow). As he had severe cardiac disease a profundaplasty was performed under local anaesthetic with relief of the symptoms.

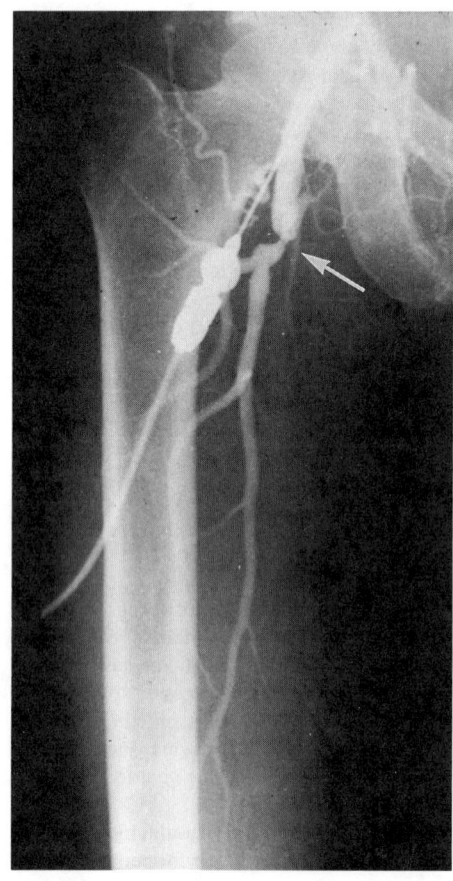

Complications of reconstructive surgery

Apart from those common to any major surgical procedure, the major complications that are seen after reconstructive arterial surgery are graft thrombosis, which is almost always due either to an unrecognized technical error or poor inflow and outflow, haemorrhage, and infection. Infection in the vicinity of an arterial anastomosis or a prosthetic graft represents one of the most serious complications that can occur in surgery, for it can lead to erosion of anastomoses and life-threatening haemorrhage. In the case of infected prosthetic grafts infection generally can be eradicated only by excising the graft, and replacing it with a new one, generally following an extra-anatomical path well away from the infected site. However, our own continuing experience with aggressive long-term antibiotic therapy and more conservative surgical management suggests that this may be an appropriate alternative approach to this dreadful problem.

Embolectomy

Where acute ischaemia of a limb is due to an embolus then the only treatment is embolectomy. With a Fogarty balloon catheter this is a simple procedure and can be performed under local anaesthetic even in the very poor-risk patient. Assuming the diagnosis is confirmed by angiography, embolectomy can be performed sometimes as long as 4 weeks after lodging of an embolus in a distal artery, provided of course that the limb is viable. There is no case for procrastination with anticoagulants in a patient with ischaemia of a limb due to an embolus. This is particularly so in the case of an embolus in the upper limb where it is unusual for the limb to be critically ischaemic and so treatment is often confined to anticoagulation or indeed no treatment is given. However, many patients so treated are left with residual claudication in the limb, which can only be prevented by early embolectomy performed under local anaesthetic.

Thrombolysis

Acute ischaemia due to embolism or thrombosis can sometimes be treated by thrombolysis. Infusion of streptokinase or tissue plasminogen activator through an intra-arterial catheter over several hours can lead to complete resolution of symptoms or permit balloon angioplasty of an underlying arterial stenosis. This has now become relatively common practice in vascular units with the appropriate expertise, for the initial management of the acutely ischaemic, but viable, limb. However, haemorrhage is a significant complication of this therapy, even in experienced centres.

Sympathectomy

In most instances of severe limb ischaemia due to occlusive arterial disease, the lower limb is affected. Where reconstruction is not possible, a lumbar sympathectomy may be performed either chemically or by operation. Although chemical sympathectomy by the paravertebral injection of phenol into the vicinity of the sympathetic chain is a simple procedure and can be performed in most poor-risk patients, it is not as effective as an operative sympathectomy in which the chain and the second and third ganglion are removed. However, as the results of sympathectomy in patients with severe ischaemia where reconstruction is not possible are not overly impressive, chemical sympathectomy is probably a reasonable approach provided some expertise in the technique is available, and especially in patients considered at high risk for any surgical procedure. It is certainly our preferred practice.

Percutaneous transluminal angioplasty

This is one of the major developments in recent years in the treatment of occlusive arterial disease, since the development by Gruntzig and Hopff in 1974 of a non-elastomeric double-lumen balloon catheter of polyvinyl chloride that could be expanded to a predetermined size, but no more. The catheter is introduced into the artery by the Seldinger technique and the balloon sited across the stenosis and distended. The actual mechanisms by which dilatation is produced is thought to be due to cracking of the intima and media adjacent to a plaque in an axial direction, allowing the media and adventitia to stretch and the lumen, therefore, to dilate as the plaque moves circumferentially. There may also be some crushing of soft atheromatous lesions. Technical improvements in the balloon itself are improving the success rate of dilation.

The indications for this technique are becoming clearer. The lesion for this treatment par excellence is the localized iliac artery lesion, not greater than 2.5 cm long, where over 90 per cent of dilatations are immediately successful with 2-year patency rates of around 80 per cent. Successful dilatation of localized stenoses or occlusions of the superficial femoral artery have been achieved with lesions of less than 10 cm, the immediate success rate being of the order of about 70 per cent. The use of dilatation is now being explored for limb salvage in blocks of the superficial femoral artery in patients considered at high risk for reconstructive surgery. In functional renal artery stenoses percutaneous transluminal angioplasty is becoming the first line of attack for most lesions, with surgery reserved for the failed dilatations.

The complication rate for this procedure is small in experienced hands and certainly less than for reconstructive surgery. Complications include distal embolization, significant groin haematomas, thrombosis, false aneurysm, and even death.

Percutaneous transluminal angioplasty has had a significant impact on the management of many patients with occlusive arterial disease and has expanded the criteria for angiography in the more elderly patient with claudication. However, for the most appropriate use of this technique it is essential that the vascular radiologists and vascular surgeons work closely together in the evaluation of the patient and the selection of the most appropriate treatment for a particular patient.

Amputation

Despite increasing skills in reconstructive surgery for salvage of severely ischaemic limbs, the rate of amputation in hospitals with a specialist vascular unit has not declined, presumably due to the increasing age of the patient population. The level of amputation is dictated both by the limb-fitter's requirements for an artificial limb and the likelihood of obtaining primary healing. In occlusive arterial disease there is no place for local amputations of gangrenous toes or even part of the foot, unless this is preceded by a successful graft restoring distal circulation. A definitive higher amputation must be performed. If possible, a below-knee amputation should be performed rather than above knee. No satisfactory method exists for determining whether the flaps of a below-knee amputation, especially the long posterior flap, have an adequate blood supply to achieve primary healing. Nevertheless with careful technique some 75 per cent of below-knee amputations will heal primarily or with a modest delay. This type of amputation allows a much more effective artificial limb to be fitted in an elderly patient, and allows more mobility without an artificial limb.

Rehabilitation of a patient after an amputation is of the greatest importance and must start as soon as there is recovery from the anaesthetic and continue until the patient is mobile on an artificial limb. This can take many months and is the special task of limb-fitting centres, but the vascular surgeon must pave the way by prior discussions and encouragement as well as providing a suitable stump. The number of amputees with peripheral vascular disease who are fully rehabilitated on an artificial limb remains depressingly low.

The diabetic foot

The diabetic with peripheral arterial disease not only has small artery disease but is more likely to have large artery disease as well. This possibility must be remembered when an infected or gangrenous toe or foot presents in the diabetic (see Chapter 11.11). If large artery disease exists, this should be dealt with on its merits, as reconstruction of an obstructed major artery will improve healing of the distal lesion even in the presence of small vessel disease. The results of reconstructive surgery are no worse in the diabetic than in the non-diabetic patient.

However, having excluded major artery disease, local amputations of gangrenous toes may be performed in the diabetic foot. Healing is slow, but often does occur with care and patience. If infection is present, the lesion must be laid open extensively with excision of any necrotic tissue or involved tendons. Furthermore, the diabetes itself can be difficult to control in the presence of diabetic gangrene, and is best achieved initially with insulin administered on a sliding scale based on blood glucose levels (BM stix), taken every 4 h.

Management of aneurysms

ABDOMINAL AORTA

Ruptured

This is a true surgical emergency, and when this diagnosis is made the patient should be taken immediately to the operating room where placement of a clamp on the aorta above the aneurysm should take preference over resuscitation and such procedures as radiography and the cross-matching of blood. Once the aorta is clamped above the aneurysm, resuscitation can begin. The results of surgery for ruptured aneurysm are poor; at best, about 50 per cent of patients survive. Not all patients should be operated on, but the decision not to operate may be difficult. However, as a general guideline, patients over 80 years of age who have been hypotensive for over 1 h have a poor prognosis in our experience.

After control of the aneurysm is achieved, the aneurysmal sac is opened, lumbar arteries controlled from within, and either a tube or bifurcated Dacron graft laid in the bed of the sac, the proximal end being anastomosed to the neck of the aneurysm and the distal end either to the lower end of the aorta or to the iliac or femoral arteries, depending on the extent of the aneurysmal dilation. Usually, a woven rather than knitted graft is used to reduce blood loss on restoring flow to the limbs.

Symptomatic aneurysm

In general, a symptomatic aneurysm should be operated on whatever its size, for if the symptoms are truly due to the aneurysm then rupture within weeks to months is very likely. However, severe cardiac or respiratory disease is sometimes a contraindication to surgery. In such patients there may be a place for aortic stenting (discussed below). In the past, tacking of a sheet of Dacron over the aneurysm, in the hope that this will be incorporated in a thick fibrous reaction around the aneurysm, hence preventing further dilatation, has sometimes appeared protective. The surgical procedure of aortic replacement is identical to that described for a ruptured aneurysm, and either a knitted or woven graft can be used.

Asymptomatic aneurysm

This may provide one of the more difficult management decisions. If the aneurysm is a large one (greater than 5 cm) then there is little doubt that it should be dealt with surgically, for there is good evidence that the likelihood of subsequent rupture of so large an asymptomatic aneurysm is high. In the case of the smaller aneurysms (less than 5 cm), two courses are available. Either the patient is followed regularly and the size of the aneurysm monitored by ultrasound, or surgery is advised provided that the patient's general health is reasonably sound. In the first instance an increase in size of the aneurysm or the development of symptoms would represent an indication for immediate surgery. The latter course can only be advised provided that a competent vascular surgeon is available and the patient's health is sound. For in the hands of an experienced vascular team, the hospital mortality associated with an elective replacement of an abdominal aortic aneurysm is around 2 per cent. Furthermore, it should be remembered that even patients with a small aneurysm show a decreased survival compared to an age- and sex-matched population without an aneurysm. This difference is due in

part to subsequent rupture of the aneurysm, but also in part to a higher death rate from cardiac and cerebral vascular disease, the aneurysm representing only a marker of the generalized atheromatous disease.

Attempts are now being made to develop techniques for inserting intraluminal stents within the aortic aneurysmal lumen. This appears promising and, if successful, would revolutionize the management of asymptomatic aortic aneurysms, both abdominal and thoracic, and in due course could be used in symptomatic abdominal aortic aneurysms as well.

POPLITEAL ARTERY

Aneurysms of the popliteal artery should always be bypassed or replaced after diagnosis, even though asymptomatic. For if a popliteal aneurysm presents with a severely ischaemic leg due to thrombosis or distal embolization, limb salvage is usually not possible. Either autogenous saphenous vein, Dacron, or PTFE can be used as a replacement graft, vein being the most satisfactory.

THORACIC AORTA

Rupture of thoracic aortic aneurysms is nearly always followed by sudden death, few cases surviving to reach an operating room, and in these few patients the chances of survival following surgery are remote.

Elective resection of aneurysms of the ascending thoracic aorta or aortic arch presents a formidable challenge to the surgeon because of the necessity to interrupt the cerebral circulation. Furthermore, the aortic valve may have to be replaced and coronary arteries reimplanted as part of the replacement of an ascending thoracic aortic aneurysm, while the innominate, left common carotid, and subclavian arteries need to be reimplanted after replacement of an aortic arch aneurysm. These procedures are performed under cardiopulmonary bypass together with bypass to the cerebral circulation. In addition, deep hypothermia may be employed to reduce cerebral damage.

Elective replacement of descending thoracic aortic aneurysms carries the risk of spinal cord ischaemia and renal ischaemia during the period of clamping of the aorta, and for this reason many surgeons employ extracorporeal bypass to perfuse the lower half of the body while the reconstruction is performed. However, if the anastomosis time can be kept to 30 min, then there is probably no need for an extracorporeal circuit.

Woven Dacron grafts are used for replacement of thoracic aortic aneurysms to diminish blood loss. Hospital mortality from the procedure is still high, especially in the case of aneurysms of the ascending aorta or arch, and is at least 10 per cent even in the most experienced hands.

DISSECTING ANEURYSM

The results of treatment of dissecting aneurysms of the thoracic aorta are poor, and there is no clearly defined plan of management. There are advocates of both surgical and medical treatment, and perhaps a combination of both provides the patient with the best chances of survival. Medical treatment is directed at reducing the blood pressure to normal or below normal levels (the patients inevitably being hypertensive), while surgical treatment is directed at resection of the aorta at the origin of the dissection, closure of the dissection proximally and distally, and replacement of the defect in the aorta by a dacron prosthetic graft. The problems of the surgical technique are the same as for aneurysms of the thoracic aorta.

Probably the most appropriate management of the patient with a dissecting aneurysm is first to stabilize the blood pressure and then, when the patient's condition is stable, to embark on surgical resection of the dissection in the most favourable circumstances. Mortality will still be high.

THORACOABDOMINAL AORTA

An aneurysm involving the thoracic as well as the abdominal aorta presents major technical problems as the coeliac, superior mesenteric, and renal arteries arise from the aneurysm. Virtually no patients have survived an emergency resection of such aneurysms, and the mortality of elective resections is still around 30 per cent. The most satisfactory approach is to insert a Dacron prosthetic graft from the thoracic aorta to the distal abdominal aorta, followed by implantation of the major intra-abdominal arteries before disconnecting the aneurysm. This inevitably results in prolonged ischaemia of the kidneys and bowel, which is largely responsible for the high mortality.

OTHER ARTERIES

Aneurysms of other arteries, such as the femoral splenic and renal arteries, should be excised and replaced with a graft if greater than 1.5 to 2.0 cm in diameter or if symptomatic, because the chances of rupture or other complications, although not really known, are probably higher with these relatively large aneurysms.

Extracerebral vascular disease

CAROTID ARTERY ISCHAEMIA

Management depends on the degree of stenosis of the internal carotid artery. Two large prospective randomized carotid surgery trials in Europe (ECST) and North America (NASCET) have resolved much of the controversy previously associated with carotid endarterectomy and transient ischaemic attacks. The two trials produced almost identical results. Patients with a tight internal carotid artery stenosis (greater than 70 per cent) showed a significant decrease in subsequent strokes after carotid endarterectomy compared to patients treated medically. These trials have established an unequivocal role for carotid endarterectomy in the treatment of a symptomatic tight internal carotid artery stenosis, but it must be stressed that the benefits of surgery depend on a combined rate of perioperative major stroke and/or death of less than 5 per cent. In the NASCET trial it was 2.1 per cent, in the ECST 3.8 per cent (and in Oxford it is 2.4 per cent).

For moderate internal carotid artery stenoses (30–70 per cent) the data are inconclusive and patients in this category continue to be entered into both trials. In the ECST trial, patients with a symptomatic mild stenosis (<30 per cent) were included, but here there was no benefit of surgery since the risk of a subsequent stroke with medical treatment alone was very small.

In patients with transient ischaemic attacks associated with mild or moderate stenosis of the internal carotid artery, treatment will consist of aspirin 300 mg daily and treatment of risk factors such as hypertension, hyperlipidaemia, and smoking. If aspirin is not tolerated because of dyspepsia, dipyridamole may be used. Continuing transient ischaemic attacks despite therapy may justify carotid endarterectomy, provided the patient's cardiac and respiratory status does not present an unacceptable risk for surgery. Patients undergoing carotid endarterectomy should continue on aspirin through surgery and thereafter, as well as having all the above-mentioned risk factors appropriately addressed.

Carotid endarterectomy requires meticulous performance and should be carried out in an experienced unit with associated expertise in anaesthetic management of these patients. The procedure is performed under local anaesthesia by some surgeons, to allow the immediate detection of any developing neurological deficit, but it is a long procedure and most in the United Kingdom prefer to use general anaesthesia. Intra-operative monitoring of middle cerebral artery flow is increasingly performed using transcranial Doppler. Shunts are used either routinely or selectively, depending on collateral flow from the contralateral side. Following completion of the endarterectomy an increasing number of surgeons will close the arteriotomy with a patch, in order to decrease the rate of recurrent stenoses. The major complications of surgery are perioperative stroke, or death as a result of a major stroke or cardiovascular disease.

VERTEBROBASILAR ISCHAEMIA

Surgical reconstruction of diseased vertebral arteries is now rarely performed. However, if there is associated significant internal carotid artery disease, carotid endarterectomy is often performed in the expectation that this will increase intracerebral circulation in general, thereby decreasing the likelihood of vertebrobasilar transient ischaemic attacks. The use of transcranial Doppler to evaluate the intracerebral circulation may help to define those patients who could benefit from this approach.

The subclavian steal syndrome is managed by an extra-anatomical bypass from the axillary artery on the non-affected side to the axillary artery on the affected side. The graft passes subcutaneously in front of the sternal notch and is associated with long-term patency. A graft may be inserted in the neck between the common carotid artery and the subclavian artery as another approach to this problem.

The innominate steal syndrome is usually dealt with by inserting a graft from the aortic arch to the distal innominate artery via a median sternotomy. This approach has tended to replace endarterectomy of the origin of the innominate artery.

Renovascular disease

Renal artery stenosis that is established as the cause of hypertension, with or without associated renal dysfunction, may be treated by transluminal angioplasty or open reconstructive surgery. Angioplasty will be the preferred option in virtually all cases of fibromuscular dysplasia, and the results of treatment are good. Angioplasty can be repeated if recurrent disease occurs. Atheromatous disease causing renal artery stenosis is often situated at the ostium of the renal artery and associated with a plaque in the aorta. In this position angioplasty is not often successful, and some radiologists suggest that with this type of lesion it is wiser to proceed straight to surgical reconstruction. Recurrence of atheromatous stenosis in the renal artery is common after angioplasty, but the procedure may be repeated.

Surgical reconstruction is the preferred approach in patients with ostial atheromatous lesions, in patients with recurrent stenosis after angioplasty, as well as in the rare instance of renal artery stenosis associated with a non-atheromatous aortitis. However, it must be remembered that surgical reconstruction is a major procedure, and as many of these patients are elderly with associated cardiac disease, there is a potential morbidity and mortality associated with the operative procedure.

There are several ways of reconstructing the renal artery, either for unilateral or bilateral disease. These include transaortic endarterectomy, aortorenal bypass graft with either saphenous vein or PTFE, splenorenal graft on the left side, and an autotransplant of the kidney. All these approaches have their place in a given situation and usually the final decision is made at the time of surgery.

The results of angioplasty are excellent for renal artery stenosis due to fibromuscular dysplasia but are poor when the stenosis is atheromatous. Atheromatous lesions have a better outcome with surgical reconstruction, both in terms of improvement in hypertension and in renal function. Nevertheless, the results of surgery in this group of patients is far from perfect. Roughly one-third of patients will be cured, one-third will have an improvement, with better control of hypertension, while one-third of reconstructions will not improve the hypertension at all. In patients with varying degrees of associated renal failure, surgical reconstruction is often of major benefit, with some 50 per cent of patients showing a significant improvement in renal function after a successful reconstruction.

Renal artery aneurysms, if greater than 1 cm in diameter, are best treated surgically. This usually requires removal and cooling of the kidney, with resection of the aneurysm and reconstruction of the vasculature on the bench, followed by reimplantation of the kidney as an autotransplant in the iliac fossa.

Management of vasospastic disorders

GENERAL MEASURES

The basis of all treatment initially should be advice on keeping warm and firm encouragement to stop smoking (Fig. 11). Warm clothing (gloves, hats, and boots for the outdoors) and well-heated houses are essential. Attention to such measures in the winter months will enable many patients to cope with their symptoms. Emigration to a warmer climate will be of benefit, but is not often a practical solution to the problem. Battery-warmed gloves are of value in severe cases.

DRUGS

Every vasodilator drug, each with its different mode of action, has probably had a trial of treatment in patients with Raynaud's syndrome, sometimes with occasional success but never consistently so. Usually the dosage necessary to produce relief of symptoms in the hands results in unpleasant side-effects. Reserpine is sometimes useful, and some striking claims for benefits of intra-arterial reserpine, at least in the short term, for patients with severe Raynaud's syndrome have been made. Nifedipine is the most commonly used drug for this condition at present. Another approach to severe Raynaud's syndrome, which does result in short-term beneficial effect, is a guanethidine block, the guanethidine being injected intravenously with a tourniquet on the proximal part of the limb. Plasmapheresis has also been used in some cases, with benefit. The use of prostacyclin infusion is discussed in Chapter 18.11.4.

SYMPATHECTOMY

This remains a satisfactory treatment in the short term but should be reserved for the patient with severe symptoms despite attention to general measures and drug treatment. Although most patients get an excellent result from sympathectomy in the early months after the operation, relapse of symptoms after 6 months to 2 years is common. Relapse occurs in about one-third of patients with Raynaud's disease, and in two-thirds of patients with Raynaud's phenomenon where the operation has been performed usually before the underlying disease has become evident. The results of sympathectomy are not so good once significant trophic changes have occurred in the hands or feet, because, usually, these are associated with organic changes in the digital arteries, which then play a more prominent role in the clinical features than the vasospastic element of the disorder. Thus the decision to perform a sympa-

thectomy should not be delayed too long in patients with severe symptoms.

In the upper limb the sympathetic chain is removed from and including the lower one-third of the stellate ganglion down to the third thoracic ganglion. This may be done as an open operation, either through the root of the neck or through the axilla, or endoscopically, which is now the more favoured approach to a cervical sympathectomy. The procedure is relatively free of complications, the two most distressing being Horner's syndrome if too much of the stellate ganglion is removed, and post-sympathectomy neuralgia. The latter begins some 10 days after the procedure and may result in such severe pain that opiates are necessary for relief. Fortunately, the neuralgia spontaneously disappears after several weeks.

In the lower limb the second and third lumbar ganglia and intervening chain are excised. The chain is approached retroperitoneally via a small anterior muscle-splitting incision in the abdomen. Again the major complication is a post-sympathectomy neuralgia. Rarely, failure to ejaculate in the male may follow excision of the second lumbar ganglion, but this is common only if the first lumbar ganglion is excised.

Management of intestinal ischaemia

ACUTE INTESTINAL ISCHAEMIA

Often the patient with acute intestinal ischaemia due to acute thrombosis or embolism presents late and with irreversible ischaemia of part of the small or large bowel, requiring immediate laparotomy and bowel resection. Nevertheless, if some patients are to benefit by embolectomy or reconstruction, then the possibility of this diagnosis must always be borne in mind in the patient with generalized atheromatous disease or a source of embolism who presents with an acute abdomen. Where this possibility exists, the diagnosis can only be established by angiography or, less reliably, at surgery.

At laparotomy there is usually a need for bowel resection, but if embolectomy or thrombectomy can be performed successfully, it not only

Fig. 12 Barium enema in the same patient as shown in Fig. 7, but 11 months later, at which time he presented with large-bowel obstruction, showing an ischaemic stenosis of the left transverse colon (arrow).

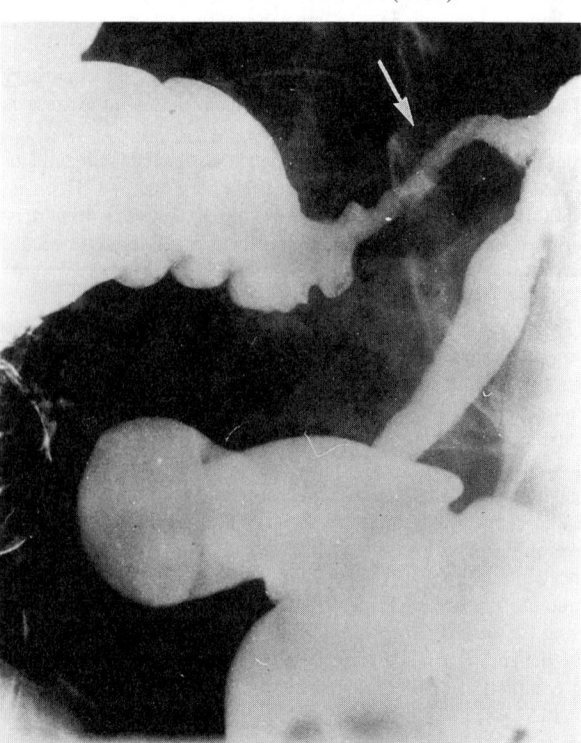

Fig. 11 An angiogram of the hand of a patient with Raynaud's disease, before and after smoking half a cigarette, showing the induced vasospasm of the small arteries of the hand.

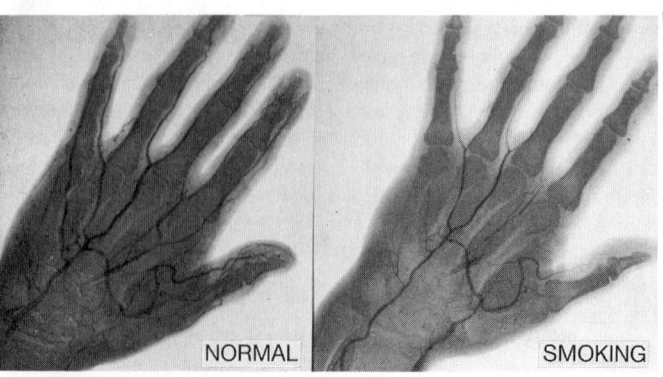

NORMAL   SMOKING

reduces the length of bowel that has to be resected but also enhances the healing of the anastomosis. This can be very important, for resection of most of the small bowel will lead to severe malabsorption after operation, often to a degree incompatible with life. If there is the slightest doubt about the viability of any bowel not resected, the abdominal wall should be loosely closed in a single layer and a second laparotomy performed after 24 h. Unfortunately, in at least 50 per cent of cases of small- and large-bowel ischaemia an obvious blockage of a main artery or venous thrombosis is not demonstrable. The ischaemic bowel presumably results from thrombosis of peripheral small vessels in the bowel due to a low-flow state accompanying some other catastrophe such as a myocardial infarction.

Ischaemia of the large bowel presents with a spectrum of clinical features ranging from mild abdominal pain to frank necrosis of the colon. Obviously the more severe examples will be managed by laparotomy and excision of the ischaemic bowel; preservation of large bowel is not nearly so critical as of small bowel. The less severe examples can be watched carefully, but with immediate laparotomy if any signs of peritonitis develop. These patients often present months to years later with an ischaemic stenosis and obstruction requiring resection of the stenosed segments (Fig. 12).

CHRONIC INTESTINAL ISCHAEMIA

If this diagnosis can be established, restoration of arterial flow beyond a stenosis can be achieved by a bypass graft from the aorta to the involved mesenteric artery, endarterectomy and patch plasty or transaortic endarterectomy for a lesion at the origin of the artery. In patients in whom a median arcuate ligament syndrome is defined, division of this abnormally low ligament to free completely the coeliac artery will result in cure. The results of reconstruction are excellent if the diagnosis of chronic intestinal ischaemia is correct, but the establishment of this diagnosis is extremely difficult.

Management of thoracic outlet compression

Patients with this syndrome may have demonstrable anatomical abnormalities at the thoracic outlet, but in many no such abnormality can be found. When a clearly defined anatomical abnormality accounts for the clinical features, surgical treatment is indicated, with correction of the abnormality, as for instance achieved by excision of a cervical rib. When no apparent abnormality exists, then exercises directed at strengthening the shoulder girdle muscles may be of benefit and should be the first approach to treatment. If no improvement follows, the most appropriate surgical procedure is excision of the first rib, which relieves most cases of thoracic outlet compression whatever the cause. This can be done through an axillary approach or an inferior clavicular approach.

If damage to the subclavian artery has occurred as a result of longstanding compression, a post-stenotic aneurysm may be present. As this is a source of emboli, resection of the artery and replacement with a graft is necessary. The most satisfactory approach for such a procedure is a joint approach from above and below the clavicle, without division of the clavicle.

REFERENCES

Bell, P.R., Jamieson, C.W., and Ruckley, C.V. (ed.) (1992). *Surgical management of vascular disease.* W.B. Saunders, Philadelphia.
Hands, L.J. and Morris, P.J. (1994). Renovascular hypertension. In *Oxford textbook of surgery,* (ed. P.J. Morris and R. Malt). pp. 435–43. Oxford University Press.
Hughson, W.G., Mann, J.I., and Garrod, A. (1978). Intermittent claudication: prevalence and risk factors. *British Medical Journal* **1**, 1379–81.
Kannel, W.B., Dawber, T.R., Skinner, J.J., McNamara, P.M., and Shurtleff, D. (1965). Epidemiological aspects of intermittent claudication – the Framingham Study. *Circulation* **32**, (Suppl. 2), 121–2.
Loberto, F.W., *et al.* (1977). A comparison of the late patency rates of axillo bilateral femoral and axillo unilateral femoral grafts. *Surgery* **81**, 33–8.
Loscalzo, J., Creager, M.A., and Dzaa, V.J. (1992). *Vascular medicine.* Little, Brown and Co., Boston.
McKusick, V.A. (1962). Buerger's disease: a distinct clinical and pathological entity. *Journal of the American Medical Association* **181**, 5–12.
Marston, A. (1977). *Intestinal ischemia.* Edward Arnold, London.
Morris, P.J. (1994). Extracerebral vascular disease. In *Oxford textbook of surgery* (ed. P.J. Morris and R. Malt). pp. 401–11. Oxford University Press.
Myers, K.A., King, R.B., Scott, D.F., Johnson, N., and Morris, P.J. (1978). The effect of smoking on the late patency of arterial reconstruction in the legs. *British Journal of Surgery* **65**, 267–71.
Roos, D.B. (1979). New concepts of thoracic outlet syndrome that explain etiology, symptoms, diagnosis and treatment. *Vascular Surgery,* **13**, 313–33.
Rutherford, R.B. (ed.) (1989). *Vascular surgery,* (3rd edn). W.B. Saunders, Philadelphia.
Smith, R.F., DeRusso, F.J., Elliott, J.P., and Sherrin, F.W. (1966). Contribution of abdominal aortic aneurysmectomy to prolongation of life. *Annals of Surgery* **164**, 678–99.
Spittell, J.A. (1983). Thromboangiitis obliterans – an autoimmune disorder. *New England Journal of Medicine* **308**, 1113.
Szilagyi, D.E., Rian, R.L., Elliott, J.P., and Smith, R.F. (1972). The coeliac artery compression syndrome: does it exist? *Surgery* **72**, 849–62.
Thompson, J.E. and Garrett, W.V. (1980). Peripheral arterial surgery. *New England Journal of Medicine* **302**, 491–503.

15.12 Cholesterol embolism

C.R.K. DUDLEY

Introduction

When atheromatous plaques ulcerate and become denuded of their endothelial covering, the underlying cholesterol-rich extracellular matrix may gain access to the arterial circulation and embolize. If the dislodged atheroma is sufficiently large, occlusion of a major systemic artery results in infarction of the organ or ischaemia of the limb supplied. This has been termed atheroembolism to distinguish it from cholesterol crystal embolism where more numerous smaller particles, composed principally of cholesterol crystals, lodge in a number of small arteries simultaneously. The presence of a collateral circulation usually prevents infarction, and the event frequently runs a subclinical course. However, with multiple showers of cholesterol emboli tissue damage results and becomes clinically apparent when a number of organs are involved. Because severe ulcerative atherosclerosis is most frequently present in the abdominal aorta, cholesterol embolism commonly affects the lower limbs, gastrointestinal tract, and kidneys. The clinical features are those of a systemic disorder with renal failure which can mimic vasculitis. The condition usually presents as a complication of vascular surgery or angiographic procedures when mechanical dislodgement of crystals from ulcerated plaques occurs. Anticoagulant use has also been implicated as a predisposing factor.

Epidemiology

The incidence of cholesterol crystal embolism found at post mortem is high: 77 per cent after aortic surgery, and 30 per cent and 25.5 per cent respectively when autopsies were performed within 6 months of aortography or cardiac catheterization. In contrast, the clinical syndrome of cholesterol crystal embolism is rare (complicating less than 2 per cent of cardiac catheterizations), suggesting that most cases are either unrecognized or run a subclinical course.

Since the condition occurs in patients with severe atheromatous disease, it is most frequently seen in older male patients with obvious risk factors (hypertension, diabetes mellitus, smoking) and overt vascular disease (ischaemic heart disease, abdominal aortic aneurysm, cerebrovascular disease). Although spontaneous cholesterol embolism may occur, it is much more common after vascular surgery or invasive radiology including aortography, angiography, and angioplasty. Under these circumstances direct trauma to the vessel may result in detachment of atheromatous material from a ruptured plaque or denude the endothelial lining of the vessel, exposing the underlying atheroma for subsequent embolization. Anticoagulant use has been associated with cholesterol embolism. It has been proposed that, by preventing thrombosis of ulcerating atheromatous plaques, anticoagulants favour the dissemination of atheromatous material from the plaques. However, a causal relationship is unproven and many patients with widespread atherosclerosis coincidently receive anticoagulants for a variety of reasons. Cholesterol embolism following the use of thrombolytic agents has been reported on rare occasions.

Clinical features

Symptoms are often non-specific with fever, weight loss, and myalgia. The clinical features are otherwise determined by the pattern of organ involvement, and are usually referable to the gastrointestinal tract, kidneys, and lower limbs. Bilateral skin changes over the lower extremities are the most common physical finding, and include livedo reticularis, 'trash feet', blue toes (acral cyanosis), and focal digital necrosis (Fig. 1). Ulceration, nodules, purpura, and petechiae have also been described. Despite these skin changes and the presence of calf claudication (or frank myositis), pedal pulses may be felt easily, emphasizing the fact that small vessels are occluded in this disorder. Carotid and femoral bruits are frequently heard, reflecting widespread and generalized atherosclerosis.

Abdominal pain, gastrointestinal bleeding, and pancreatitis may occur, and embolism to the stomach, small bowel, colon, gallbladder, and spleen have all been reported.

Because of their large blood supply and proximity to the abdominal aorta, the kidneys are commonly affected by cholesterol crystal embolism. Renal involvement usually manifests as a subacute stepwise deterioration in renal function over 2 to 6 weeks, invariably accompanied by a worsening of pre-existing hypertension which can be labile and difficult to control. Acute renal failure with necrotizing glomerulonephritis and crescent formation on renal biopsy has been described, but is rare. Thus a typical case is an elderly man presenting after angiography with progressive renal failure accompanied by livedo reticularis of the lower body and focal digital ischaemia of the toes.

Transient ischaemic attacks, amaurosis fugax, and strokes can occur when embolism is from the carotid arteries or aortic arch. Retinal cholesterol crystal emboli may be observed on ophthalmoscopy as bright refractile plaques within the retinal arterioles, particularly at their bifurcations. Spinal cord infarction has also been reported.

Investigations

Laboratory findings are non-specific but frequently include a raised erythrocyte sedimentation rate and leucocytosis. Transient eosinophilia is common and may be pronounced. In rare cases thrombocytopenia and disseminated intravascular coagulation result. Depending on the tissue involvement, elevated levels of creatine phosphokinase, amylase, lactate dehydrogenase, serum aspartate aminotransferase, and alkaline phosphatase may all be observed. Hypocomplementaemia, although firmly established in the literature, has been described by only one group in the last decade, and other factors including the use of contrast media may have accounted for the complement activation observed. Mild proteinuria is generally present and urine microscopy may be bland or reveal red cells, white cells (particularly eosinophils), hyaline, and granular casts. The non-oliguric nature of the renal failure and a urinary sodium which is frequently normal are unexpected features as hypoperfusion of the kidneys is presumed.

Histology

The definitive histological diagnosis of cholesterol crystal embolism can usually be made from biopsies of kidney, skin, or muscle (including

Fig. 2 Renal biopsy demonstrating the characteristic needle-shaped cholesterol clefts occluding a medium-sized renal arteriole with surrounding inflammatory cell infiltration, intimal proliferation, thickening and concentric fibrosis. There is extensive autolysis (postmortem sample).

Fig. 1 Livedo reticularis and vasculitic-like erythematous nodules on the leg of a patient in whom cholesterol crystal embolization occurred after coronary angiography.

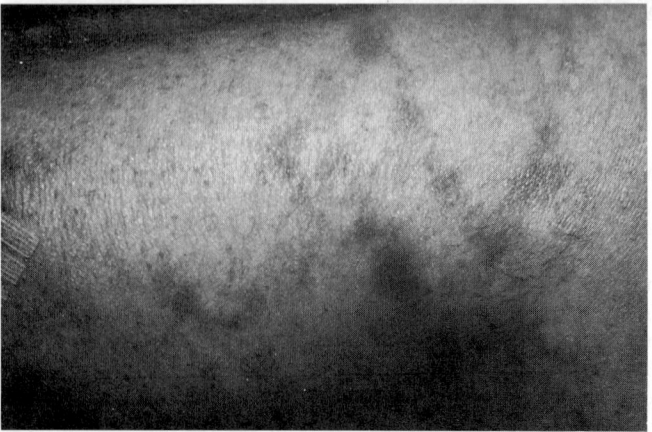

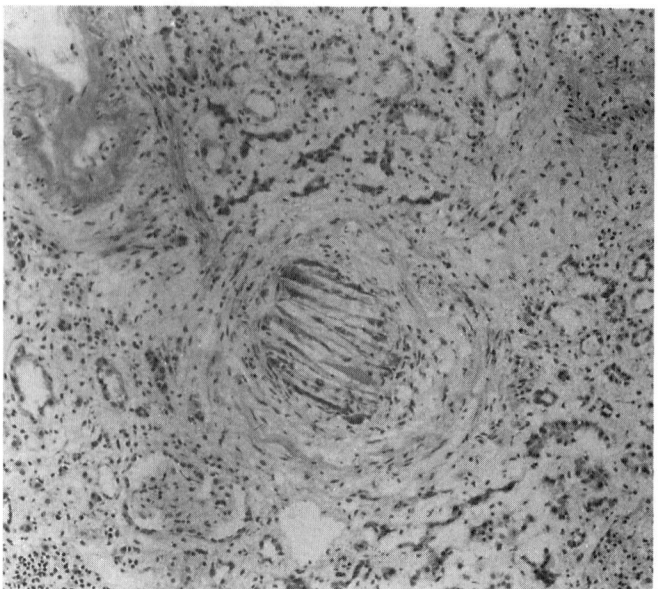

clinically uninvolved areas), although sampling error may miss the lesion owing to its patchy distribution. Ante-mortem histological diagnoses have also been made from other tissues including gastric biopsy, prostatic curettage, and bone marrow biopsy. The demonstration of characteristic biconvex needle-shaped cholesterol clefts within the lumen of arteries or arterioles, which remain after the crystals have dissolved during routine histological preparation, is diagnostic (Fig. 2). In fresh samples the crystals can be identified by birefringence under polarized light, and specific histochemical stains can be used to identify the cholesterol.

The presumed histological sequence of events is based on animal studies following the injection of atheromatous material and closely resembles the human disease observed at single time points. The presence of cholesterol crystals in the vascular lumen is believed to trigger a localized inflammatory and endothelial vascular reaction. An inflammatory cell infiltration (mainly macrophages and eosinophils) occurs, and multinucleated giant cells engulf the cholesterol crystals which, however, are resistant to the scavenger effects of macrophages and may remain in place for many months. The inflammatory phase is followed by marked intimal thickening with concentric fibrosis and occlusion of the vessel. Depending on the extent of organ involvement, these pathological changes result in ischaemia, infarction, or rarely necrosis of the distal tissue.

In the kidneys, small arteries and arterioles of diameter 150–200 μm such as the arcuate and interlobular arteries are occluded, resulting in patchy areas of ischaemia and small areas of infarction. Crystals may also be seen within the glomeruli. In chronic cases, ischaemia produces a wedge-shaped lesion involving all components of the renal cortex radiating towards the capsule. The glomeruli appear ischaemic and hyalinized and the tubules become atrophic and separated by interstitial fibrosis (Fig. 2). Grossly, the kidneys may be reduced in size with a rough granular surface and wedge-shaped scars.

Differential diagnosis

The diagnosis is frequently missed during life. Therefore a high index of clinical suspicion is required, particularly in elderly patients with evidence of atherosclerotic disease who develop renal failure after arteriography or aortic surgery. Spontaneous cholesterol crystal embolism associated with renal failure, fever, rash, and eosinophilia may not unreasonably be misdiagnosed as a vasculitic illness such as polyarteritis nodosa, Churg–Strauss syndrome, microscopic polyarteritis, Wegner's granulomatosis, or bacterial endocarditis. Under these circumstances a renal biopsy is required to make the diagnosis. Cholesterol embolism should be considered in the differential diagnosis of a multisystem disease in elderly patients.

Clinical course and management

Mortality is high owing to the occurrence of coexisting cardiac and vascular disease together with renal failure in elderly patients. Renal impairment frequently progresses and may require dialysis. However, partial recovery or stabilization in renal function has been reported even after several months of dialysis. The mechanism of this recovery is uncertain.

There is no effective therapy. Steroids, aspirin, dipyridamole, low-molecular-weight dextran, and sympathetic blockade have all been tried but without any clear effect. Anticoagulants are of no proven benefit and cannot be recommended given their potential role in the pathogenesis of the disorder.

Occasionally, a definitive source of cholesterol emboli (e.g. aortic aneurysm, localized plaque) can be identified in a young and otherwise fit patient. In this limited circumstance there may be a role for surgical replacement of the diseased vessel with a graft.

Generally, therapy is supportive only and is directed at control of hypertension and appropriate management of renal failure. Prevention is important, particularly with the increasing number of older patients submitted to invasive angiography. In patients with diffuse atherosclerosis, angiography should be strictly limited and careful attention must be paid to angiographic techniques including arterial approach (brachial instead of femoral for cardiac catheterization), use of softer and more flexible catheters, and reduced catheter manipulation.

REFERENCES

Case Records of the Massachusetts General Hospital (Case 30-1986). *New England Journal of Medicine*, **315**, 308–15.

Case Records of the Massachusetts General Hospital (Case 2-1991). *New England Journal of Medicine*, **324**, 113–20.

Case Records of the Massachusetts General Hospital (Case 34-1991). *New England Journal of Medicine*, **325**, 563–72.

Dahlberg, P.J., Frecentese, D.F., and Gogbill, T.H. (1989). Cholesterol embolism: experience with 22 histologically proven cases. *Surgery*, **105**, 737–46.

Fine, M.J., Kapoor, W., and Falanga, V. (1987). Cholesterol crystal embolization: a review of 221 cases in the English literature. *Angiology*, **38**, 769–84.

Hyman, B.T., Landas, S.K., Ashman, R.F., Schelper R.L., and Robinson, R.A. (1987). Warfarin-related purple toes syndrome and cholesterol microembolization. *American Journal of Medicine*, **82**, 1233–7.

Mannesse, C.K., Blankestijn, P.J., Man In 'T Veld, A.J., and Schalekamp, M.A.D.H. (1991). Renal failure and cholesterol crystal embolization: a report of 4 surviving cases and a review of the literature. *Clinical Nephrology*, **36**, 240–5.

Palmer, F.J. and Warren, B.A. (1988). Multiple cholesterol emboli syndrome complicating angiographic techniques. *Clinical Radiology*, **39**, 519–22.

Smith, M.C., Ghose, M.K., and Henry A.R. (1981). The clinical spectrum of cholesterol embolization. *American Journal of Medicine*, **71**, 174–80.

15.13 Takayasu's disease

K. ISHIKAWA

Takayasu's disease, a chronic inflammatory arteriopathy, occurs in humans the world over but is most frequently diagnosed in young Oriental women. It was first reported by a Japanese ophthalmologist in 1908. The main site of occurrence is the aorta and/or its main branches but the pulmonary artery is also often involved. Inflammatory changes in the affected vessels lead to occlusive changes in the lumina, often combined with dilation and secondary thrombus formation. Major complications attributed to the disease are Takayasu's retinopathy, secondary hypertension, aortic regurgitation, and aortic or arterial aneurysm. There are geographical variations in the clinical aspects of this disease. The following terms may be identical with what is known today as Takayasu's disease or arteritis: Takayasu's arteriopathy, occlusive thromboaortopathy, aortitis syndrome, and non-specific aortoarteritis.

AETIOLOGY

The cause of Takayasu's disease remains unknown. An autoimmune mechanism is possible, given the partial similarities in clinical systemic symptoms and laboratory findings between the early stages of this disease and systemic lupus erythematosus, and because there can be a good response to corticosteroid therapy during the inflammatory active stage of the disease. Attempts to demonstrate circulating antibodies against antigens of the arterial wall, however, have given both positive and negative results. Group A streptococcal infection, association with tuberculosis, hormonal imbalance, ethnic susceptibility, and genetic predisposition may be pathogenetic factors.

PATHOLOGY

The lesions in Takayasu's disease show a panarteritis of the aorta and its main branches and of the pulmonary artery. The lesions of the arterial wall begin with a mesoperiarteritis with subsequent fibrosis and are followed by fibrotic thickening of the adventitia and the vasa vasorum. These lesions lead to an intimal fibrosis, which progresses usually in marked thickening, often with thrombi. The destruction of the arterial wall leads to both stenotic and ectatic changes of the lumen, especially occlusion. These affected portions are clearly demarcated from the adjacent normal sites and segmental 'skipped' lesions are observed.

CLASSIFICATIONS

To evaluate the disease status and for a better understanding of the clinical profile in an individual patient, it is pertinent to clarify where the patient belongs according to the following three factors:

(1) inflammatory activity of the disease as determined by the erythrocyte sedimentation rate (ESR);
(2) sites of arterial lesions;
(3) complications attributed to Takayasu's disease.

Inflammatory activity

An erythrocyte sedimentation rate (ESR, Westergren) that is consistently over 20 mm/h or, more particularly, over 40 mm/h, suggests active inflammation, whilst less than 20 mm/h implies its absence.

Sites of arterial lesions

According to the location of arterial lesions, the disease is classified anatomically into three types:

(1) the arch type, which involves the aortic arch and its branches;
(2) the descending type, which involves the descending thoracic and abdominal aorta and its branches;
(3) the extensive type, which describes the combined arch and descending types (Fig. 1).

Pulmonary arterial involvement is sometimes added in the classification by location of this disease (Fig. 2).

Complications

Depending upon the presence and severity of the four complications attributable to the disease, it has been classified into four groups (groups I, IIa, IIb, and III).

Group I

Uncomplicated Takayasu's disease, with or without involvement of the pulmonary artery (Fig. 1).

Group II

Takayasu's disease with a single associated complication: (1) Takayasu's retinopathy (Plate 1); (2) secondary hypertension; (3) aortic regurgitation (Fig. 3); or (4) aortic or arterial aneurysm (Fig. 3). This group may be classified further, according to the severity of these complications, into group IIa (mild or moderate) and group IIb (severe complications).

Group III

Takayasu's disease with two or more associated complications (Fig. 3).

CLINICAL FEATURES AND DIAGNOSIS

Takayasu's disease has protean clinical features. There is often a long interval between the onset of symptoms, which usually begin at a young age, and the establishment of the diagnosis, which is usually made when patients are between the ages of 20 and 40 years. The disease is much more frequent in women. The symptoms and signs depend on the phase of the disease, the inflammatory activity, the involved site, and complications.

In general, patients in the early phase show evidence of active inflammation with an elevated erythrocyte sedimentation rate, increased levels

Fig. 1 Aortograms of an 18-year-old Japanese woman with Takayasu's disease in the active stage (erythrocyte sedimentation rate 88 mm/h), the extensive type, and in group I associated with mild pulmonary arterial involvement. (a) Arch aortogram. Note the segmental narrowing in both common carotid arteries, especially the left distal portion (arrow), but normal appearance of the carotid sinuses; also occlusion or severe narrowing of both subclavian arteries (mid portions). The vertebral arteries are spared. There is mild irregularity of the internal surfaces of the brachiocephalic trunk and the thoracic aorta. (b) Abdominal aortogram. Note moderate narrowing of the abdominal aorta (mid portion) and the right renal artery (proximal).

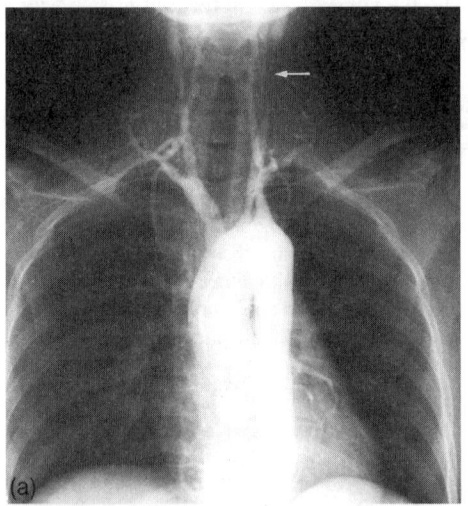

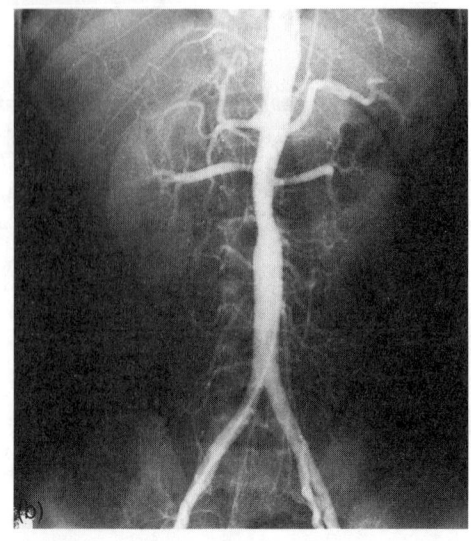

of C-reactive protein, increased α_2-globulin and gammaglobulin values, and slight normochromic anaemia. During this phase, most of the patients have general symptoms of malaise, headache, fever, easy fatiguability of the extremities, dizziness, transient visual disturbance, neck pain, mild palpitation and dyspnoea, arthralgia, stiffness of shoulders, and nausea. Syncopal attacks are not uncommon in this phase. Haemoptysis occurs rarely. Some patients, however, never suffer these symptoms. In them, the disease may present with its complications, for example pulselessness or hypertension. Some cases are picked up solely on investigation of a raised erythrocyte sedimentation rate, which is detected incidentally. The raised erythrocyte sedimentation rate varies in duration with each patient and is generally followed by a gradual return to a normal range. When the degree of narrowing of the involved arteries is advanced as in the late phase of the disease, cardiovascular symptoms and signs predominate. These include moderate or severe dyspnoea and palpitation on exertion, chest and back pain, recurrent syncopal attacks, intermittent claudication of the arms or legs, asymmetric pulses or pulselessness, bruits over the affected arteries, and high blood pressure.

It is vital, in making the diagnosis of Takayasu's disease, to think of it in the first place and to take a careful history, as often there are asymp-

tomatic periods during the course of the disease and a changing pattern of symptoms. With a careful bedside examination, patients can be broadly classified into one of the three types. It is useful to make a 'pulse–bruit–pressure' diagram, which shows the grade of palpability of arterial pulsations, bruits, and tenderness over the affected arteries, and values of blood pressure, including retinal arterial pressure, at various regions. Plain radiographs will often show widening of the aortic knuckle, aortic calcification, irregularity of the contour of the left lateral margin of the descending thoracic aorta, and focal areas of decreased pulmonary vascular shadowing. Perfusion lung scanning or pulmonary arteriography aid diagnosis; pulmonary hypertension is not uncommon (Fig. 2). Total aortography, however, is indispensable for the confirmation and differential diagnosis from congenital aortic coarctation at unusual sites, the aortitis of giant cell arteritis, and atherosclerosis alone. Sites most susceptible to the disease are bilateral mid-subclavian arteries. At the time of diagnosis the extensive type lesions, the group II complications, and pulmonary arterial involvement are present in about half the patients. Coronary arterial lesions attributed to this disease are rare.

TREATMENT AND PROGNOSIS

Medical

In general, patients with Takayasu's disease in the inflammatory active stage respond moderately well to corticosteroid therapy, although this therapy is not completely established for the disease. Not only are nonspecific symptoms reduced, but progression of arterial involvement during the active stage of the disease can be retarded or prevented. Arteriographic stenoses often improve. The recommended initial daily dose of corticosteroids is usually 30 to 50 mg of prednisolone per day, more often the latter. The dose is then reduced gradually, depending on response, but prolonged treatment (an average period of 9 years) is usually needed before the drug can be withdrawn completely. In selected patients unresponsive to steroid therapy alone, cyclophosphamide (2 mg/kg body weight) is sometimes added. All but a few patients in groups I and IIa, and especially the former group, are good candidates for medical treatment rather than surgery (see Fig. 1). Recently, percutaneous transluminal angioplasty has been used to dilate stenosed arteries present in the inflammatory inactive stage. However, the long-term results of such treatment are as yet unknown.

The inflammatory activity does not worsen during pregnancy, but various adverse cardiovascular events, including intrapartum cerebral haemorrhage, can occur. An evaluation of the disease before pregnancy, planning the mode of delivery according to both obstetric and non-obstetric indications, and intrapartum and anaesthetic considerations, with special reference to the control of blood pressure, are particularly important.

Surgical

Surgical treatments include reconstructive surgery of the aorta and its main branches, endarterectomy, aneurysmectomy, aortic valve replacement, and, rarely, coronary artery bypass grafting. Some surgical results are excellent, for instance in patients who have hypertension secondary to coarctation of the aorta but without significant bilateral lesions of the renal arteries or secondary to narrowing of one renal artery in the inactive stage of the inflammation. However, it is often difficult to decide on surgical indications for patients with Takayasu's disease, as the results of surgical treatments for those in the advanced phase are not always good. There are surgical problems specific to the disease. If the inflammation of the arterial wall is active, the possibility of suture failure or aneurysm formation, as well as occlusion of the graft, is higher than in the case of arterial disease of other causes; a healthy area of the arterial wall must be available and selected for the site of graft anastomosis. In general, in patients with this disease who have been selected for surgery, an increased erythrocyte sedimentation rate should be lowered by steroid therapy to a normal level (except in emergencies) before surgical treat-

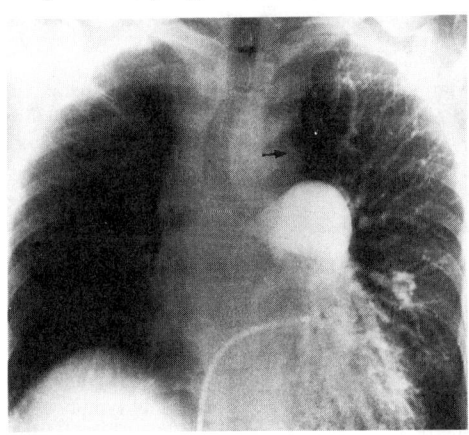

Fig. 2 Pulmonary arteriogram (right ventricular injection) in a 25-year-old Japanese man with Takayasu's disease in the active stage, the extensive type, and in group III. Note occlusion of the right pulmonary artery, and elevation of the ipsilateral diaphragm. There is calcification of the aortic knob (arrow).

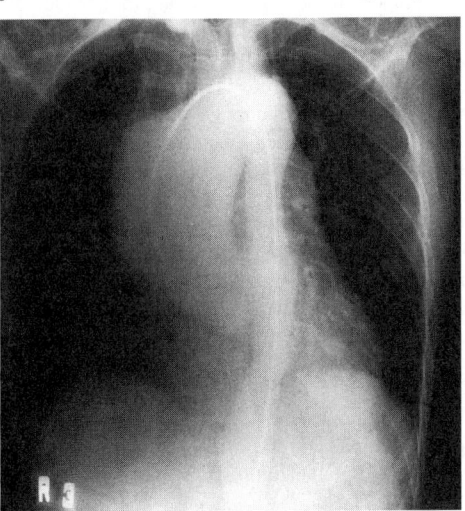

Fig. 3 Thoracic aortogram of a 25-year-old Japanese woman with Takayasu's disease in the active stage, the extensive type, and in group III associated with moderate pulmonary arterial involvement. Note the giant aneurysm of the ascending aorta and mild aortic regurgitation due to annulo-aortic ectasia, and severe irregularity of the internal surface of the entire thoracic aorta. The mid portion of both subclavian arteries are also gravely affected.

ment. A careful long-term follow up is required because of the surgical risks, including an increase of the inflammatory activity after operation.

In a large series of 120 patients, the 20-year overall survival rate after the diagnosis was established was nearly 83 per cent. The 15-year survival rates for patients in groups IIb and III combined, and for those in groups I and IIa combined were 66.3 and 96.4 per cent, respectively. Recently, the prognosis of patients with Takayasu's disease has improved. Among the major factors causing death or severe disability are congestive heart failure, cerebrovascular accidents, and blindness.

REFERENCES

Fiessinger, J.N., Tawfik-Taher, S., Capron, L., Laurian, C., Cormier, J.M., Camilleri, J.P., and Housset, E. (1982). Maladie de Takayasu: Critères diagnostiques. *La Nouvelle Presse Médicale*, **11**, 583–586.

Ishikawa, K. (1978). Natural history and classification of occlusive thromboaortopathy (Takayasu's disease). *Circulation*, **57**, 27–35.

Ishikawa, K. (1981). Survival and morbidity after diagnosis of occlusive thromboaortopathy (Takayasu's disease). *American Journal of Cardiology*, **47**, 1026–1032.

Ishikawa, K. (1986). Takayasu's disease. In *Extracranial cerebrovascular disease* (ed. F. Robicsek), pp. 387–394. MacMillan, New York.

Ishikawa, K. (1988). Diagnostic approach and proposed criteria for the clinical diagnosis of Takayasu's arteriopathy. *Journal of American College of Cardiology*, **12**, 964–972.

Ishikawa, K. (1991). Effects of prednisolone therapy on arterial angiographic features in Takayasu's disease. *American Journal of Cardiology*, **68**, 410–413.

Ishikawa, K. and Maetani, S. (1994). Long-term outcome for 120 Japanese patients with Takayasu's disease: clinical and statistical analyses of related prognostic factors. *Circulation*, **90** (in press).

Ishikawa, K. and Matsuura, S. (1982). Occlusive thromboaortopathy (Takayasu's disease) and pregnancy: Clinical course and management of 33 pregnancies and deliveries. *American Journal of Cardiology*, **50**, 1293–1300.

Kerr, G.S., Hallahan, C.W., Giordano, J., *et al.* (1994). Takayasu arteritis. *Annals of Internal Medicine*, **120**, 919–29.

Kumar, S., Mandalam, K.R., Rao, V.R.K., Subramanyan, R., Gupta, A.K., Joseph, S., Unni, M., and Rao, A.S. (1990). Percutaneous transluminal angioplasty in non-specific aortoarteritis (Takayasu's disease): Experience of 16 cases. *Cardiovascular and Interventional Radiology*, **12**, 321–325.

Liu Yu-Qing, and Du Jia-Hui. (1984). Aorto-arteritis: A collective angiographic experience in 244 cases. *International Angiology*, **3**, 487–497.

Lupi-Herrera, E., Sánchez-Torres, G., Marcushamer, J., Mispireta, J., Horwitz, S., and Vela, J.E. (1977). Takayasu's arteritis: clinical study of 107 cases. *American Heart Journal*, **93**, 94–103.

Nasu, T. (1982). Takayasu's truncoarteritis: Pulseless disease or aortitis syndrome. *Acta Pathologica Japonica*, **32** (suppl. 1), 117–131.

Shelhamer, J.H., Volkman, D.J., Parrillo, J.E., Lawley, T.J., Johnston, M.R., and Fauci, A.S. (1985). Takayasu's arteritis and its therapy. *Annals of Internal Medicine*, **103**, 121–126.

Suzuki, A., Amano, J., Tanaka, H., Sakamoto T., and Sunamori, M. (1989). Surgical consideration of aortitis involving the aortic root. *Circulation*, **80** (suppl. 1), I-222–I-232.

Takagi, A., Tada, Y., Sato, O., and Miyata, T. (1989). Surgical treatment for Takayasu's arteritis: A long-term follow-up study. *Journal of Cardiovascular Surgery*, **30**, 553–558.

Takayasu, M. (1908). A case with peculiar changes of the central vessels in the retina. *Acta Societatis Ophthalmologicae Japonicae*, **12**, 554–555 (in Japanese).

15.14 The cardiomyopathies

15.14.1 The cardiomyopathies, myocarditis, and specific heart muscle disorders

W. J. McKENNA

Cardiomyopathies

Introduction

Traditionally, heart muscle diseases have been classified as idiopathic or specific. The former, termed the cardiomyopathies, are classified as hypertrophic, dilated, or restrictive; this descriptive classification is useful in relation to natural history, treatment, and prognosis. A classification provides a bridge between ignorance and knowledge. Recent discovery of mutations in genes encoding sarcomeric contractile proteins in familial hypertrophic cardiomyopathy and a probable autoimmune pathogenesis of dilated cardiomyopathy indicates that knowledge of aetiology and pathogenesis will ultimately require a new classification of the 'idiopathic cardiomyopathies'. The term specific heart muscle disease incorporates myocardial involvement as part of a systemic disease (e.g. sarcoidosis, systemic hypertension) or when the mechanism of myocardial damage is recognized. (e.g. coronary ischaemia).

Myocarditis

DEFINITION

The literature is confusing because the term myocarditis has meant different things to different people. Clinicians have made a diagnosis of suspected myocarditis following the acute onset of heart failure, arrhythmia, or ECG changes, often in temporal association with viral infection in otherwise healthy, usually young, individuals. Pathologists have provided their own definitions based on varying criteria for myocyte necrosis and cellular infiltration. Does the presence of a few lymphocytes within the myocardium (a not uncommon autopsy finding) indicate myocarditis? The lack of appropriate accepted criteria for the histological diagnosis has hampered assessment of the incidence, natural history, treatment, and prognosis of myocarditis. In 1987 the Dallas criteria for the histological diagnosis from tissue obtained with endomyocardial biopsy were developed to test the hypothesis that immunosuppression would modify left ventricular dysfunction and prognosis of patients with idiopathic myocarditis. A major multicentre trial failed to provide conclusive results, in large part because only 200 of over 2000 patients with 'clinical suspected myocarditis' fulfilled the Dallas criteria (Table 1) and could be randomized. The finding of diagnostic histological changes in less than 10 per cent of patients with 'clinical myocarditis' is a function of several factors including variable clinical diagnostic criteria, restrictive histological criteria, endomyocardial biopsy sampling error, and reliance on histology alone for the assessment of inflammation.

A clinical diagnosis of 'suspected myocarditis' is not uncommon. Current criteria for the histological diagnosis according to the Dallas criteria requires demonstration of both myocyte necrosis and an inflammatory infiltrate. The fact that worldwide no myocardial tissue is obtained in most patients with suspected myocarditis reflects practical difficulties in the use of endomyocardial biopsy as well as a lack of demonstrated clinical utility in obtaining tissue. Information regarding the clinical entity of myocarditis must be seen in the context of these diagnostic and practical limitations. Future assessment of natural history, prognosis, and the role of immunosuppression will require clinical

Table 1 *Diagnostic categories of myocarditis*

First biopsy
- Active myocarditis (with or without fibrosis)
- Borderline myocarditis (not diagnostic and requiring further biopsy)
- No evidence of myocarditis

Subsequent biopsies
- Ongoing (persistent) myocarditis
- Resolving (healing) myocarditis
- Resolved (healed) myocarditis—this group may have the features of end stage dilated cardiomyopathy

Reproduced from Aretz, H.T. *et al.* (1987). *American Journal of Cardiology and Pathology,* **1**, 3–14, 1987, with permission.

and endomyocardial tissue diagnosis with evolution from reliance on stereological criteria to a broader evaluation of inflammation and viral involvement incorporating available immunohistochemical and viral hybridization techniques.

AETIOLOGY AND PATHOGENESIS

Myocarditis is usually idiopathic, with a probable infective cause documented in less than 20 per cent of cases. (Table 2). Different agents have regional predominance, for example *T. cruzi* in South America or Coxsackie B in North America and Europe. There are well-developed murine models for several of these agents including Coxsackie B3 and *T. cruzi*. In most AJ mouse strains the illness occurring after inoculation with Coxsackie B3 is self-limiting; however, some develop myocarditis followed by chronic cardiac failure resembling clinical dilated cardiomyopathy. Acute fulminant and fatal myocarditis following inoculation is rare. Most viral infections in man have multisystem involvement, and there is evidence to suggest that the heart is usually involved although without the development of symptomatic or significant clinical abnormalities. In animal models the size of the inoculum, the genetic strain, the age, and the activity (exercise) of the mice are determinants of the severity of myocardial involvement following systemic viral inoculation. The determinants in man are uncertain, although the young (aged less than 1 year) are prone to more severe illness. In Coxsackie-induced murine myocarditis there is an acute necrotic phase lasting less than a week with direct myocytolysis in the absence of an inflammatory infiltrate. Early in the disease (day 7–10) CD8 T lymphocytes are cytotoxic for virally infected cells; later (after the second week) they cause cytolysis of non-infected cells. The finding of ongoing myocytolysis associated with the development of cardiac-specific antimyosin antibodies and the absence of virus suggests the generation of autoimmune T-cell clones. These findings led to the development of an autoimmune murine model of myocarditis. Immunization of specific strains of AJ mice with cardiac-specific myosin induced histologically and immunologically similar disease to the murine Coxsackie myocarditis, whereas inoculation with cross-reactive myosin did not. Humoral and cellular transfer experiments demonstrated that the myocarditic process was transferable only with T cells and was inhibited by monoclonal antibodies binding to HLA class II molecules which disturbed antigen presentation to T-helper cells.

The pathogenesis of myocardial involvement with the causative agent of Chagas' disease *(T. cruzi)* has similarities with the murine models of myocarditis and dilated cardiomyopathy. The acute phase following infection is usually subclinical (more than 95 per cent of cases); however, a minority develop an acute febrile illness with myocarditis or pancarditis including endocardial thrombus formation and pericardial perfusion. The disease then enters a long latency period; 20 years after the initial infestation about 30 per cent of patients will have developed chronic Chagas' disease, but less than a third of these have parasitaemia.

Present evidence suggests postinfectious autoimmune pathogenesis. Macroscopic and histological changes are similar to dilated cardiomyopathy with atrial and ventricular dilatation, myocyte hypertrophy, extensive fibrosis, and chronic lymphomononuclear cell infiltrates.

CLINICAL PRESENTATION AND MANAGEMENT

Myocarditis is usually a subclinical illness but may cause minor symptoms (palpitation, atypical chest pain), ECG abnormalities (conduction, ST and T-wave changes), or arrhythmias (paroxysmal atrial fibrillation or ventricular arrhythmias) without demonstrable change in global or regional left or right ventricular function. Presentation with cardiac failure or arrhythmias is usually associated with cardiac chamber dilatation and/or impaired systolic performance. In the young, the elderly, and the debilitated, cardiac failure may be fulminant and fatal. Myocarditis and pericarditis often coexist (myopericarditis), and clinical presentation may resemble that of pericarditis in association with the symptoms and signs of cardiac failure.

There is no specific therapy for the management of either idiopathic or viral myocarditis. Heart failure and arrhythmias should be treated as appropriate, and there are no particular contraindications. The role of antiviral and immunosuppressive therapy will remain uncertain until more thorough characterization of individual cases in relation to viral and immune involvement provides a basis for appropriate clinical trials.

With the exception of the very young and the very old, prognosis of clinically suspected and/or biopsy-proven acute myocarditis is usually good. The determinants of acute myocarditis progressing to a chronic illness are discussed in the section on dilated cardiomyopathy.

The cardiac presentation of Chagas' disease resembles that of myocarditis and dilated cardiomyopathy. However, conduction disease and arrhythmias are particularly common and may precede the development of chamber dilatation and cardiac failure. The ECG findings are of increased chamber dimensions, and in many the findings are distinctive with left ventricular posterior wall hypokinesis and relatively normal interventricular septal motion. In advanced disease an apical aneurysm is common, and in asymptomatic patients 10–15 per cent have apical dyskinesis. Diagnostic confirmation requires previous geographical exposure and either a positive complement fixation test for the antigens of *T. cruzi* (Machado–Guerriero test which is highly sensitive and specific) or demonstration of parasites in the patient's blood by xenodiagnosis. Treatment with antiparasitic drugs (e.g. nifurtimox, benzimidazole) may reduce parasitaemia, but does not cure the disease or prevent progression.

Dilated cardiomyopathy

DEFINITION

Dilated cardiomyopathy is characterized by unexplained dilatation and impaired contractile performance of the left ventricle. For the diagnosis to be made, potential causes of ventricular dysfunction, particularly coronary artery disease and systemic hypertension, must be excluded. Typical angina pectoris, fluctuating ST- and T-wave changes, and regional abnormalities on two-dimensional echocardiography or thallium scintigraphy which reflect damage to a specific vascular territory suggest ischaemic heart disease. Renal and ocular hypertensive changes may provide a useful marker of previous systemic hypertension, but are often unremarkable in the decompensated phase in the normotensive patient. Calcific aortic stenosis may be overlooked as a cause of heart failure, particularly when the murmur is soft or absent. Specific heart muscle disorders should also be considered in differential diagnosis (Table 3). A primary cardiac presentation of diabetes mellitus, connective tissue disorders, and neuromuscular disease is rare, but arrhythmias or progressive conduction disturbance with mild left ventricular dysfunction may provide the earliest evidence of cardiac sarcoidosis. The definition of dilated cardiomyopathy provides a diagnosis of exclusion, and it is

Table 2 *Causes of acute myocarditis*

Infective group		Non-infective group	
Bacterial	Staphylococcal, streptococcal, gonococcal, or salmonella septicaemia *Corynebacterium diphtheriae* *Neisseria meningitidis* *Borellia burgdorferi* (Lyme disease) *Borellia recurrentis* *Brucella abortus* Bordetella pertussis, Bordetella persica, Bordetella pseudomallei	Immune-mediated	Idiopathic (lymphocytic, giant-cell myocarditis) Post-infectious: rhematic fever, chronic postviral, Chagas' disease, HIV Associated with autoimmune or immune-oriented disorders (rheumatoid arthritis, systemic lupus erythematosus, Churg–Strauss syndrome, scleroderma, polymyositis, myasthenia gravis, insulin dependent diabetes mellitus, thyrotoxicosis, sarcoidosis)
Protozoa	*Trypanosoma cruzi* *Toxoplasma gondii* *Entamoeba histolytica*		
Parasites	*Trichinella spiralis*		Hypersensitivity (serum sickness, tetanus toxoid, penicillin, sulphonamides, phenylbutazone, etc.)
Rickettsial	Coxiella *Rickettsia burnettii* (Q fever) *Rickettsia rickettsii* (Rocky Mountain spotted fever)		Transplant rejection
Viral	Picornaviruses: enteroviruses, such as Coxsackie, echo, polio, hepatitis A Orthomyxoviruses: influenza A, B, etc. Paramyxoviruses: respiratory syncytial viruses, mumps, measles Rubivirus: rubella Arboviruses: dengue, yellow fever Rhabdovirus: rabies Retrovirus: HIV Poxvirus: vaccinia Herpes virus: varicella zoster, cytomegalovirus, herpes simplex, Epstein–Barr Adenovirus	Toxins Metabolic Physical agents	Drugs: anthracyclines, cyclophosphamide, fluorouracil, lithium, catecholamines, phenothiazines, clozapine Heavy metals Anaesthetic agents Phaeochromocytoma, beri-beri Radiation, electric shock
Fungal	Opportunistic infection		

likely that such structural and functional abnormalities result from heterogeneous pathogenic processes.

In North America and Europe symptomatic dilated cardiomyopathy has an incidence and prevalence of 20 per 100 000 and 38 per 100 000 respectively and remains the commonest indication for cardiac transplantation. Pedigree analysis reveals familial disease in at least 25 per cent of cases and an additional cohort (10–20 per cent) with mild abnormalities of left ventricular performance who may have early presymptomatic dilated cardiomyopathy. Inheritance is most consistent with autosomal dominant and incomplete penetrance, although X-linked families have been reported.

PATHOGENESIS

By definition aetiology is unknown. Macroscopic examination of autopsy and explanted dilated cardiomyopathy hearts reveals dilated cardiac chambers, mural thrombi, and platelet aggregates with normal extra- and intramural coronary arteries. Histology shows features consistent with healed myocarditis with patchy perimyocyte and interstitial fibrosis and various stages of myocyte death, as well as myocyte hypertrophy and rare isolated inflammatory cells. These postinflammatory findings are non-specific and do not suggest a particular pathogenesis. The myocardial depressant effects of alcohol in normal and diseased myocardium are established. Alcohol, like pregnancy, may precipitate cardiac failure in predisposed individuals, but an additional specific aetiological or pathogenetic role remains uncertain. Viral involvement is supported by the progression of viral myocarditis to dilated cardiomyopathy in specific genetic strains of the murine model as well as in

isolated rare patients, an association with abnormal Coxsackie serology, and hybridization studies which show non-replicating enteroviral genome in a variable proportion (10–50 per cent) of myocarditis–dilated cardiomyopathy hearts. The potential for autoimmune pathogenesis is supported by the development of autoimmune murine myocarditis and the findings of a cardiac and disease-specific autoantibody in over 30 per cent of dilated cardiomyopathy patients and their first-degree relatives, inappropriate major histocompatibility complex class II expression on endothelial cells from cardiac tissue, and a weak HLA DR4 association. Pathogenesis of dilated cardiomyopathy remains controversial, and its resolution is hampered by clinical presentation at a stage when pathogenesis may be largely completed. A reasonable working hypothesis proposes an autoimmune pathogenesis with or without a viral trigger in genetically predisposed individuals.

DIAGNOSIS

Dilated cardiomyopathy has been described in Western, African, and Asian populations affecting both genders and all ages. Initial presentation is usually with symptoms of cardiac failure (fatigue, breathlessness, decreased exercise tolerance) but an arrhythmia (atrial fibrillation, ventricular tachycardia, atrioventricular block), a systemic embolus, or the finding of an ECG or radiographic abnormality during routine screening may prompt earlier diagnosis. Symptoms, physical signs, and chest radiographic changes are those of cardiac failure and depend on the stage of the disease. The recent recognition of the familial nature of dilated cardiomyopathy indicates that a correct diagnosis is of practical importance as there is now the potential to identify the disease at an early or

Table 3 *Systemic diseases associated with specific heart muscle disorders*

Metabolic/endocrine	Diabetes mellitus
	Gout
	Thyroid disease
	Acromegaly
	Phaeochromocytoma
	Morbid obesity
Infiltrating disorders	Sarcoidosis
	Amyloidosis
	Haemochromatosis
Systemic vasculitis	Systemic lupus erythematosus
	Scleroderma
	Polyarteritis nodosa
	Rheumatoid arthritis
	Wegener's granulomatosis
	Seronegative arthropathies
	Ankylosing spondylitis
	Reiter's disease
	Psoriatic arthritis
	Ulcerative colitis
	Crohn's disease
Malignancy	Metastatic
	Carcinoid
Infections	Rheumatic fever
	Tuberculosis
	Syphilis
	Infective endocarditis
Neuromuscular	Duchenne dystrophy
	Becker
	Fascioscapulohumeral
	Emery–Dreifuss
	Limb-girdle
	Distal myopathy
	Mitochondrial myopathies
	Oculopharyngeal
	Myotonic dystrophy
Drug use/dependence	Alcohol
	Cocaine
	'Ecstasy' (MDMA)
	Amphetamines

preclinical stage. Physical examination may be entirely normal or may reveal evidence of myocardial dysfunction with cardiac enlargement and signs of congestive heart failure. Systolic blood pressure is usually low with a narrow pulse pressure and a low volume arterial pulse. In patients with severe left ventricular failure, pulsus alternans may be present and the jugular veins may be distended with a prominent V-wave reflecting tricuspid regurgitation. In such patients the liver is often engorged and pulsatile, and there is usually peripheral oedema and ascites.

The precordium often reveals a diffuse and dyskinetic left ventricular impulse and occasionally a right ventricular impulse. The apical impulse is usually displaced laterally, reflecting ventricular dilatation. The second heart sound is usually normally split, but paradoxical splitting may be present when there is left bundle branch block, which occurs in approximately 15 per cent of patients. With severe disease and the development of pulmonary hypertension, the pulmonary component of the second heart sound may be accentuated. Characteristically, a presystolic gallop or fourth heart sound is present before the development of overt cardiac failure. However, once cardiac decompensation has occurred, ventricular gallop or third heart sound is often present. When there is significant ventricular dilatation, systolic murmurs are common, reflecting mitral and, less commonly, tricuspid regurgitation.

The development of unexplained cardiac failure during pregnancy or within the 3 months following birth is often labelled as peripartum cardiomyopathy. Unrecognized pre-eclamptic heart disease may also present with cardiac failure and should be excluded with careful examination of the antenatal records; this has a different prognosis and recurs with increasing severity during subsequent pregnancies unless prevented by monitored (uterine vascular resistance) aspirin treatment. In those with peripartum cardiomyopathy, antecedent cardiac evaluation is often absent and there is usually uncertainty whether the cardiac failure is acute (e.g. potentially myocarditis) or chronic and exacerbated by the haemodynamic stress of pregnancy and labour (e.g. dilated cardiomyopathy). When the heart failure is acute and there is persistence of left ventricular chamber dilatation or impaired systolic performance, the diagnosis of peripartum cardiomyopathy can legitimately be made. The mechanism and true natural history is uncertain, although it is highly probable that the adverse prognostic effect of subsequent pregnancies is less important than the literature would suggest, particularly in those with only mild residual abnormalities of left ventricular structure and function.

INVESTIGATIONS

Cardiological evaluation of patients with dilated cardiomyopathy is performed to confirm the diagnosis, to determine objective measurements of functional capacity as a guide to symptomatic treatment, and to assess risk of complications, particularly progressive deterioration, arrhythmias, and sudden death. By the time of diagnosis in a referral centre, a normal ECG is rare (less than 5 per cent) and most patients show features consistent with diffuse myocardial abnormalities. Twenty per cent are in established atrial fibrillation, and paroxysmal supraventricular and ventricular arrhythmias during 24 h ECG monitoring are common.

The perception by patients of functional limitation relates to many factors including the time course of the illness and is very variable. Maximal exercise testing, ideally with respiratory gas analysis, provides a simple reproducible measure of functional capacity and is also useful to exclude ischaemia and assess risk of arrhythmia. Similarly two-dimensional echocardiography is important, providing an easily repeated measure of cardiac cavity dimensions and systolic performance, and assessment of regional wall motion as well as mural and intracavitary thrombi. In the young the origins of the right and left main coronary arteries can often be visualized to exclude main-stem coronary anomalies as the cause of myocardial dysfunction. Symptoms, exercise testing, and two-dimensional echocardiography provide the basis for assessment of treatment and monitoring of disease progression.

Coronary arteriography should be performed if doubt remains regarding a potential ischaemic aetiology of left ventricular dysfunction. Cardiac catheterization is also warranted for measurement of pulmonary vascular resistance in those with very severe or rapidly progressive disease in whom cardiac transplantation may be required; however, if coronary artery disease can be confidently excluded and transplantation is not an imminent consideration, cardiac catheterization is not required for diagnosis or symptomatic management. Useful prognostic information regarding cardiac enlargement and systolic performance can be more readily provided from echocardiographic or radionuclide studies. Endomyocardial biopsy is warranted to exclude myocarditis and specific heart muscle disorders and to characterize patients for the presence of viral genome and markers of immune activation. Many of the systemic diseases which are associated with heart muscle disorders have typical clinical, immunological, and biochemical features. In the absence of evidence to suggest a systemic disease, a routine screen is probably not cost effective. However, there are several potential reversible secondary causes of heart muscle disorder which may simulate dilated cardiomyopathy, and basic screening tests should include serum phosphorus (hypophosphataemia), serum calcium (hypocalcaemia), serum creatinine and urea (uraemia), thyroid function tests (hypothyroidism), and serum iron/ferritin (haemochromatosis).

NATURAL HISTORY AND PROGNOSIS

The true natural history of dilated cardiomyopathy is uncertain because the diagnosis is usually not made until clinical features, which are late manifestations of the disease, become obvious. Symptoms develop when filling pressures rise or stroke volume diminishes sufficiently to cause salt and water retention and oedema. Once clinical symptoms of impaired ventricular performance are apparent, prognosis is poor and is related to the degree of left ventricular dilatation and impaired contractile performance. Data from adult and paediatric referral centres in the 1970s and 1980s indicate 50 per cent mortality from progressive heart failure or its complications in the 2 years following referral diagnosis. Undoubtedly, survival will be improved by recognition of asymptomatic family members as well as others with early or mild disease and by modern management including the early introduction of angiotensin-converting enzyme inhibitors, aggressive treatment of arrhythmias, and the availability of cardiac transplantation. Once symptoms develop, only a minority of patients (less than 25 per cent) will either stabilize or improve, with a reduction in cardiac dimensions and improvement in myocardial performance. Conventional evaluation of cardiovascular structure and function does not permit accurate prediction of outcome; indeed, there is an annual mortality of approximately 4 per cent, predominantly from sudden death, even in those who improve or stabilize.

TREATMENT

Treatment in dilated cardiomyopathy is aimed at improving symptoms, reducing left ventricular dilatation, and preventing complications, arrhythmia, and sudden death. Such non-specific therapy is unsatisfactory and will remain so until the aetiological triggers and pathogenesis of dilated cardiomyopathy are determined. Symptomatic therapy is the treatment of heart failure with reliance on digoxin, diuretics, and the early introduction of angiotensin-converting enzyme inhibitors. Vigorous exercise and significant alcohol intake are proscribed. The use of low dose β blockade with gradual dosage augmentation as tolerated over 3 to 6 months is often beneficial in dilated cardiomyopathy. Metoprolol (6.25–50 mg twice daily) and carvedilol (12.5–50 mg once daily) have proved beneficial in appropriate trials, but the mechanism of benefit remains uncertain; the up-regulation of β-receptors demonstrated with metoprolol was not seen with carvedilol. However, rapid administration of β-blockers or their withdrawal after chronic administration may precipitate rapid deterioration and they should be used cautiously. If sustained or symptomatic arrhythmias are documented during 24 h ECG monitoring or exercise testing, conventional treatment is warranted. 2Amiodarone (100–400 mg daily) has no negative inotropic effect and is effective in suppressing both supraventricular and ventricular arrhythmias; drugs which further depress left ventricular function are likely to be poorly tolerated.

Systemic and pulmonary emboli are common; in the retrospective series from the Mayo Clinic, 25 per cent of patients experienced a documented embolic event within 5 years. Precise guidelines for anticoagulation are not established. Patients with mural or intracavitary thrombi or with established or paroxysmal atrial fibrillation should be fully anticoagulated. Those with severe left ventricular dysfunction (ejection fraction below 20 per cent) or atrial dilatation (more than 40 mm) should be at least partially anticoagulated.

The other major complication is sudden death, which may occur in those who are stable or improving as well as in those who are deteriorating. The mechanism is probably a ventricular arrhythmia, although bradyarrhythmias may be more likely in patients with severe disease such as those awaiting cardiac transplantation. Conventional ECG monitoring and electrophysiological studies do not provide an accurate algorithm for identification of patients at particular risk of sudden death. The majority of patients have non-sustained ventricular tachycardia during ECG monitoring and inducible sustained ventricular tachycardia during programmed electrical stimulation, but both these investigations are notoriously insensitive for the detection of conduction disease. Management in relation to risk of sudden death remains unsatisfactory. New approaches to the identification of myocardial electrical instability are being evaluated, and the role of low dose amiodarone (200–300 mg daily) in the prevention of sudden death in heart failure is being examined in several multicentre studies. The practical, although unproven, therapeutic approach is to treat those with frequent episodes of asymptomatic non-sustained ventricular tachycardia during ECG monitoring, as well as those with symptomatic or documented ventricular arrhythmia.

Cardiac transplantation provides a lifeline in those with progressive deterioration. Results are best when surgery is performed as an elective procedure, and because of the inability to predict clinical course it should be considered as an eventual option in all patients with moderate to severe left ventricular impairment.

Hypertrophic cardiomyopathy

DEFINITION

Hypertrophic cardiomyopathy is defined as an idiopathic heart muscle condition characterized by a hypertrophied and non-dilated left and/or right ventricle in the absence of a cardiac or systemic cause. However, such a diagnosis of exclusion often presents problems. Does the patient with moderate systemic hypertension and 2 cm left ventricular hypertrophy have one or two diseases? Is 2 cm hypertrophy a physiological response in a highly trained athlete? The presence of other causes of left ventricular hypertrophy highlights a major limitation of the current definition of hypertrophic cardiomyopathy.

PATHOLOGY

Hypertrophic cardiomyopathy may involve the left, the right, or both ventricles. Hypertrophy in the left ventricle is usually asymmetric, involving the anterior and posterior septum and the free wall to a greater extent than the posterior wall. Right ventricular hypertrophy, which is usually symmetric, is seen in over 30 per cent of affected patients; isolated right ventricular hypertrophy is rare. Over 60 per cent of patients will have structural abnormalities of the mitral valve, including increased leaflet area, elongation of the leaflets, or anomalous papillary muscle insertion into the anterior mitral leaflet. Another common macroscopic finding is a patch of endocardial thickening just below the aortic valve which results from contact of the septum with the anterior mitral leaflet in patients with mitral leaflet abnormalities and/or reduced left ventricular outflow tract dimensions.

The histological findings in hypertrophic cardiomyopathy are distinctive (Fig. 1). Affected myocardium shows interstitial fibrosis with gross disorganization of the muscle bundles resulting in a characteristic whorled pattern. The cell-to-cell orientation of muscle cells is lost (disarray) and there is disorganization of the myofibrillar architecture within a given cell. Myocardial cells are wide, short, and often bizarre in shape. Foci of disorganized cells are often interspersed among areas of hypertrophied muscle cells that are otherwise normal in appearance. Such changes are not completely specific: congenitally abnormal hearts may also show fibre disarray, and some disarrangement is found at the junction of the septum with the anterior and posterior walls of the left ventricle in normal subjects. However, the extent of myocyte disarray in normal subjects rarely exceeds 5 per cent, while in hypertrophic cardiomyopathy up to 40 per cent of the myocardium may be involved. Occasionally, extensive myocyte disarray is found in macroscopically normal hearts in patients who experience typical clinical features. Such patients highlight the broader phenotype and suggest that hypertrophy may be a secondary rather than a primary abnormality.

Typically, left ventricular end-diastolic pressure, mean left atrial pressure, and mean pulmonary capillary wedge pressure are elevated as consequences of abnormal left ventricular diastolic filling and reduced compliance.

GENETICS

Hypertrophic cardiomyopathy is usually familial with autosomal dominant transmission and a high degree of penetrance. Gene penetrance is age related. Morphological and clinical features typically present during periods of childhood or adolescent growth; disease expression may not become apparent until adolescent growth has been completed. Variable expression of the disease is common, even within families bearing the same gene defect. Recently, mutations in the DNA encoding β cardiac myosin heavy chain (chromosome 14), α tropomyosin (chromosome 15), and cardiac troponin T (chromosome 1) have been identified in families with hypertrophic cardiomyopathy. Mutations in these genes have been found in over 50 per cent of pedigrees evaluated, and hypertrophic cardiomyopathy is emerging as a disease of sarcomeric contractile proteins. The majority of the mutations involve a single base pair change, which results in an amino acid substitution in exons encoding highly conserved regions of these contractile protein genes. Many of these mis-sense mutations alter the charge of the amino acid, which would be predicted to have a significant effect on the function of the encoded polypeptide. To date, the effect on sarcomeric assembly, stability, and function is not known. The strongest piece of evidence that they are causative of the disease comes from families in which a *de novo* myosin mutation, which was not present in the unaffected genetically proven parents, resulted in the disease phenotype with transmission of disease via the germline to subsequent generations. The incidence of spontaneous or *de novo* mutations of the myosin gene is uncertain.

Knowledge of the gene abnormality has the potential to aid identification and management of high risk individuals. Preliminary observations from families with myosin mutations reveals significantly worse prognosis in those with mutations which alter the charge of the encoded amino acid. However, the fact that there is marked heterogeneity of phenotypic expression and prognosis within a family indicates that other genetic and/or environmental factors are important.

PATHOPHYSIOLOGY

Disarray

Myocardial disarray and hypertrophy, hyperdynamic systolic function, and impaired diastolic function account for many of the clinical features of hypertrophic cardiomyopathy. The extent and distribution of myocardial disarray can only be determined postmortem. It is probable that the disorganized architecture with abnormal myofibre and myofibrillar alignment provides a substrate for electrical instability and contributes to diastolic abnormalities. The precise relation between myocardial disarray and spontaneous arrhythmia and the threshold for ventricular fibrillation have not been established.

Systole

Most young and some old patients have evidence of hyperdynamic systolic function with rapid, early, and near complete ventricular emptying. Approximately 30 per cent of patients with hyperdynamic systolic func-

Fig. 1 Transverse short-axis section through the ventricles from patients with cardiomyopathy. The upper left shows symmetrical left ventricular hypertrophy in hypertrophic cardiomyopathy. The upper right shows dense white fibrous tissue obliterating the apex of both ventricles in endomyocardial fibrosis. The lower left shows a globular dilated left ventricle in a child with dilated cardiomyopathy. The lower right shows a grossly dilated right ventricle with adipose infiltration of the right ventricular free wall in arrhythmogenic right ventricular dysplasia. (Reproduced with permission from M.J. Davies (1986). *Colour atlas of cardiovascular pathology,* Oxford University Press.)

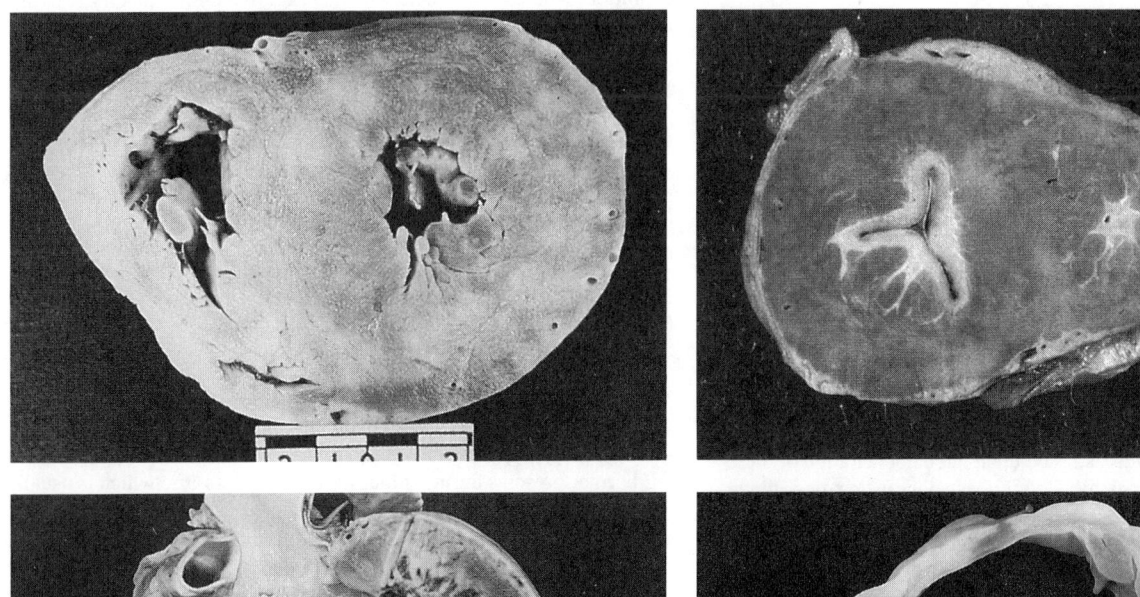
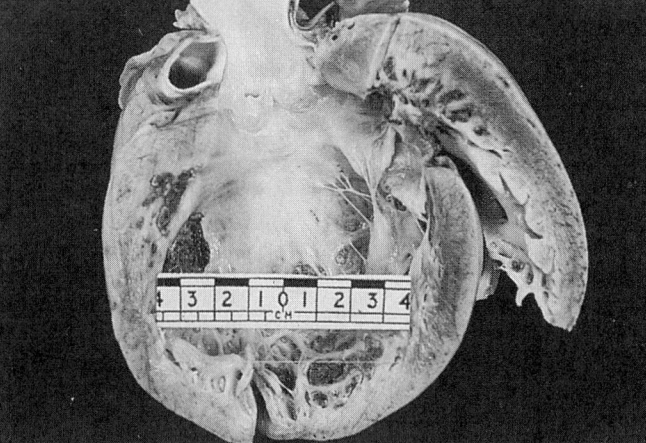
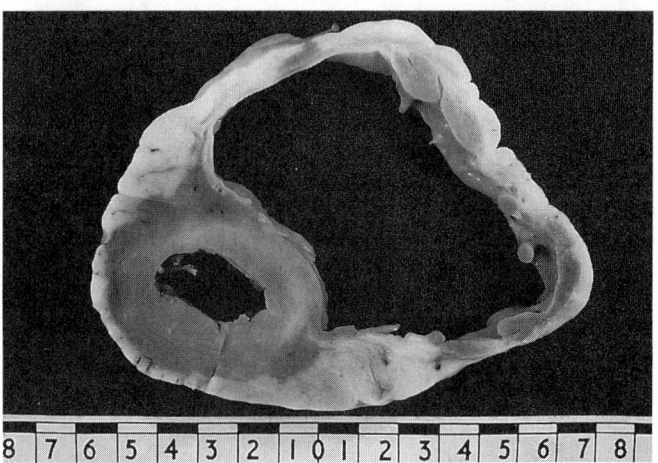

tion have recordable gradients at rest between the body and outflow tract of the left ventricle; an additional 20 to 25 per cent develop such a gradient following manoeuvres that increase myocardial contractility or result in a decrease in ventricular volume with reduced afterload or venous return. The presence and magnitude of a gradient is not only determined by systolic contractile performance, but is also a function of left ventricular outflow tract size and geometry which are determined by the extent of upper septal hypertrophy and mitral leaflet size and geometry. The most plausible proposed mechanism of the gradient is that venturi forces from increased ejection velocity in the narrowed out-flow tract draw the anterior and posterior mitral leaflets (which are often large and redundant) towards the septum. The significance of such gradients has been controversial. Many workers have claimed that the development of a left ventricular gradient in close temporal association with the development of systolic anterior motion of the mitral valve and a fall in peak aortic velocity represents impediment or obstruction to left ventricular emptying. Another interpretation of these findings is that they are generated by a dynamic left ventricle that has almost completely emptied. Assessment of the significance of a left ventricular gradient in an individual patient requires knowledge of the relative volume ejected by the onset of the gradient. In the majority of patients with resting left ventricular gradients, at least 70 per cent of stroke volume has already been ejected by the onset of the gradient.

Diastole

Diastolic abnormalities are common although variable. The period during which the heart is isovolumic (end systole and early diastole) is prolonged, filling is slow, and the proportion of filling volume that results from atrial systolic contraction (while still preserved) may be increased. Occasionally, there is rapid early filling with restrictive physiology which resembles the situation in patients with constrictive pericarditis or endocardial fibrosis. It is seldom possible to identify the predominant cause of altered diastolic function because most patients have myocardial hypertrophy, evidence suggestive of ischaemic and architectural abnormalities including myocardial disarray and fibrosis.

Ischaemia

Despite normal epicardial coronary arteries, myocardial ischaemia is common and is caused by several features which appear to relate to myocardial hypertrophy (Table 4). However, evidence of ischaemia is not limited to those with severe hypertrophy, and abnormalities of vasomotor behaviour may also be important.

DIAGNOSIS

Hypertrophic cardiomyopathy has been described in Western, African, and Asian populations. The precise prevalence is unknown, but is estimated to be between one per 1000 and one per 5000. The diagnosis of hypertrophic cardiomyopathy is based upon the demonstration of unexplained myocardial hypertrophy. This is best done using two-dimensional echocardiography where measurements of wall thickness should exceed two standard deviations for gender-, age-, and size-matched populations. These latter considerations may be important as myocardial mass increases with both age and size. In practice, the presence of a left ventricular myocardial segment of thickness 1.5 cm or more in an adult of normal size in the absence of a recognized cause is usually considered to be diagnostic. Isolated right ventricular hypertrophic cardiomyopathy is extremely rare. Less stringent criteria, which remain to be quantified, should be applied to first-degree relatives of an affected individual where the probability of carrying the disease gene drops from less than one per 1000 to one in two. Symptoms or minor ECG or echocardiographic abnormalities may represent disease expression when there is a 50 per cent chance of carrying the gene defect.

In children and adolescents the diagnostic features, particularly myocardial hypertrophy, often develop during growth spurts. A negative diagnosis made before adolescent growth has been completed must be

Table 4 *Potential causes of ischaemia in hypertrophic cardiomyopathy*

Increased muscle mass
Elevated diastolic filling pressures
Enhanced myocardial oxygen demand (increased wall stress)
Systolic compression of arteries
Adequate capillary density
Impaired vasodilatory reserve

tempered by the proviso of subsequent reassessment. However, the development of unexplained left ventricular hypertrophy *de novo* has not been reported in adults. Thus an asymptomatic adult with a completely normal ECG and two-dimensional echocardiogram does not have and is not at risk of developing hypertrophic cardiomyopathy, and does not need re-evaluation in this regard.

Problems in diagnosis often arise in highly trained athletes and patients with mild hypertension in whom the hypertrophic response appears greater than expected from the apparent stimulus. Competitive athletes normally have an increase in myocardial mass with a maximum increase of 2–3 mm in left ventricular wall thickness. The determinants of the hypertrophic response in a patient with hypertension are seldom known, but are at least in part racially determined; the African response is clearly greater than that of white subjects. In athletes and hypertensive subjects, the diagnosis or exclusion of hypertrophic cardiomyopathy is dependent on the total clinical picture. An athlete who has 1.7 cm left ventricular hypertrophy with either a small left ventricular cavity or a family history of hypertrophic cardiomyopathy probably does have the condition, whereas an athlete who has negative family history and normal left ventricular cavity dimensions probably does not. There is the potential for molecular genetic evaluation to provide a 'gold standard' when the clinical diagnosis is equivocal or when preclinical diagnosis may be of value in families where there have been multiple sudden deaths in children and adolescents. The identification of the remaining gene(s) will greatly increase the potential value of a DNA diagnostic test; at present the finding of a mutation in one of the identified contractile protein genes would confirm disease but its absence would not exclude it.

CLINICAL FEATURES

History

Symptomatic presentation may be at any age with breathlessness on exertion, chest pain, sustained palpitation, syncope, or sudden death. Occasionally, hypertrophic cardiomyopathy is found at autopsy in a stillborn or presents during infancy with cardiac failure which is usually fatal. In children and adolescents, the diagnosis is most frequently made during screening of siblings and offspring of affected family members. Paroxysmal symptoms or mild impairment of exercise tolerance are often present, but in the absence of a murmur may not elicit a diagnostic cardiac evaluation. Approximately 50 per cent of consecutive adult patient populations present with symptoms; in the remainder the diagnosis is made during family screening or following the detection of an unsuspected abnormality on physical, ECG, or echocardiographic examination.

Dyspnoea is common in adults (over 50 per cent) and is believed to be a consequence of elevated left ventricular diastolic, left atrial, and pulmonary venous pressures resulting from impaired ventricular relaxation and filling. Approximately 50 per cent of patients complain of chest pain which is exertional, atypical, or both in similar proportions of patients. Atypical pain may have no obvious precipitant; more commonly, it follows exercise or anxiety-related tachycardia when it persists for up to several hours after the stress has been removed without enzymatic evidence of myocardial damage. Approximately 15 to 25 per cent of patients have experienced syncopal episodes and in only a minority are there findings suggestive of an arrhythmia or evidence of overt conduction disease. In most patients, the mechanism cannot be determined. Rarely, patients present with symptoms attributable to left or right heart failure with paroxysmal nocturnal dyspnoea, cough, ascites, or peripheral oedema. Thus there is a wide spectrum of clinical presentation in hypertrophic cardiomyopathy, from severe cardiac failure in infancy to an incidental finding at any age.

Physical examination

In the majority of patients with hypertrophic cardiomyopathy, the physical examination is unremarkable and the detection of abnormalities is dependent on the elucidation of subtle physical signs. Most patients have a rapid upstroke arterial pulse, best felt in the carotid area, which reflects dynamic left ventricular emptying. In children and adolescents this pulse may be difficult to distinguish from normality, whereas in the elderly the normal pulse transmitted by non-compliant atheromatous vessels may appear to have a rapid upstroke. Most patients also have a forceful left ventricular cardiac impulse, best appreciated on full-held expiration in the left lateral position. In about a third of patients the jugular venous pulse may demonstrate a prominent 'a' wave reflecting diminished right ventricular compliance secondary to right ventricular hypertrophy. The first and second heart sounds are usually normal and, unless patients are in atrial fibrillation, there is either a loud fourth heart sound, reflecting increased atrial systolic flow into a non-compliant ventricle, or a palpable atrial beat reflecting forceful atrial systolic contraction which may or may not be associated with significant forward flow of blood. The most obvious physical sign in hypertrophic cardiomyopathy is an ejection systolic murmur present only in those patients (one-third) who have a resting left ventricular outflow tract gradient. This murmur starts well after the first heart sound and ends well before the second. It is best heard at the left sternal border radiating towards the aortic and mitral areas but not into the neck or the axilla. The intensity of outflow tract murmurs varies with changes in ventricular volume: it can be increased by physiological and pharmacological manoeuvres that decrease afterload or venous return (amyl nitrate, standing, Valsalva) and decreased by manoeuvres that increase afterload and venous return (squatting, phenylephrine). Occasionally, ejection systolic murmurs are associated with an ejection sound at their onset. The majority of patients with a left ventricular gradient also have mild mitral regurgitation which may be difficult to distinguish by auscultation. Doppler examination reveals that mitral regurgitation usually begins just before (30–40 ms) the onset of the gradient and continues for the duration of systole. Radiation of the systolic murmur to the axilla is often the best auscultatory clue to the presence of coexistent mitral regurgitation. Occasionally, mitral regurgitation may be moderate to severe either alone or in association with a left ventricular outflow tract gradient. A mid-diastolic rumble may occasionally result from increased transmitral flow in patients with severe mitral regurgitation; more commonly, it occurs in isolation, presumably reflecting inflow tract turbulence. Early diastolic murmurs of aortic incompetence may develop following surgical myotomy or myectomy or infective endocarditis involving the aortic valve. Although such murmurs are rare in the absence of such complications, they appear to occur more commonly than would be expected by chance and may reflect traction of the non-coronary cusp of the aortic valve by the septum. An ejection systolic murmur in the pulmonary area, reflecting right ventricular outflow tract obstruction, is also rare; when present, it is usually associated with severe biventricular hypertrophy and is more commonly seen in the young.

INVESTIGATIONS

Cardiological evaluation of patients with hypertrophic cardiomyopathy is performed to confirm or make the diagnosis, to characterize the functional and morphological features in order to guide symptomatic therapy, and to assess the risk of complications, particularly sudden death.

Electrocardiography

The 12-lead ECG is normal in 5 per cent of symptomatic patients and 25 per cent of asymptomatic patients, particularly the young. At the time of diagnosis, 10 per cent are in atrial fibrillation. The majority of patients have a intraventricular conduction delay, 20 per cent have left axis deviation, and 5 per cent have a right bundle branch block pattern; a complete left bundle branch block pattern is uncommon. It may develop following surgery and is occasionally seen in the elderly. ST-segment depression and T-wave changes are the most common abnormalities and are usually associated with voltage changes of left ventricular hypertrophy and/or deep S waves in the anterior chest leads V1–V3. Occasionally, giant negative T waves are seen. Repolarization changes alone or isolated voltage criteria for left ventricular hypertrophy are unusual. Approximately 20 per cent of patients have abnormal Q waves either inferiorly (2,3, and aVF) or, less commonly, in leads V1–V3. P-wave abnormalities of left and/or right atrial overload are common. The distribution of the PR interval is similar to that in the normal population, but occasionally a short PR interval may be associated with a slurred upstroke to the QRS complex, similar to that seen in the Wolff–Parkinson–White syndrome. In an electrophysiological study, such changes are not usually associated with evidence of pre-excitation, although patients with hypertrophic cardiomyopathy and accessory pathways have been described. Despite the many ECG abnormalities, there is no ECG which is typical of hypertrophic cardiomyopathy; a useful rule is to consider the diagnosis whenever the ECG is bizarre, particularly in younger patients.

The incidence of arrhythmias during 48 hour ambulatory ECG monitoring increases with age (Fig. 2). Non-sustained ventricular tachycardia is detected in 25 to 30 per cent of adults. Although this arrhythmia is invariably asymptomatic, its presence represents an approximately sevenfold increased risk of sudden death. Supraventricular arrhythmias in adults are also common. Sustained supraventricular arrhythmias (more than 30 s) are poorly tolerated unless the ventricular response is controlled; they carry an increased risk of embolism. In contrast, most children and adolescents are in sinus rhythm, and arrhythmias during ambulatory ECG monitoring are uncommon (Fig. 2). The increased incidence of supraventricular arrhythmias with age is not surprising as the

Fig. 2 The relation between arrhythmias and age in hypertrophic cardiomyopathy. SVT, supraventricular tachycardia; VT, ventricular tachycardia; AF, atrial fibrillation.

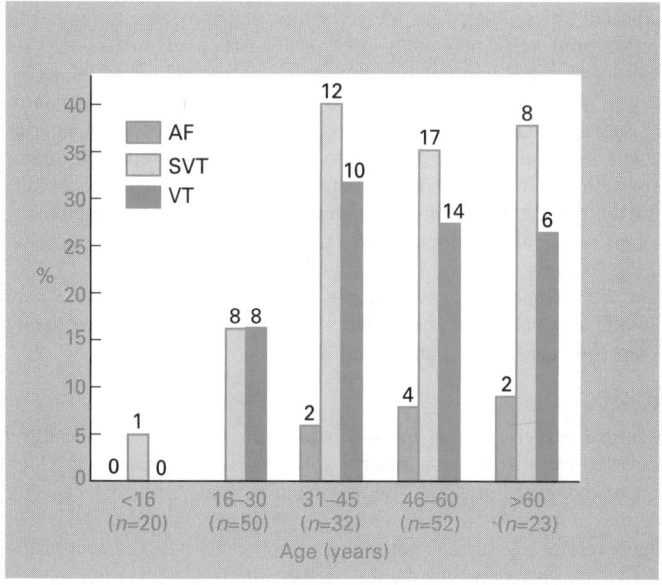

development of these arrhythmias is related to increased echocardiographic left atrial dimensions and increased left ventricular end-diastolic pressure, both of which increase with age. The aetiology of ventricular arrhythmias is not known, but may relate to myocyte necrosis and myocardial fibrosis which appear to be related to age. The occurrence of documented sustained ventricular tachycardia is uncommon.

Imaging

The chest radiograph may be normal or show evidence of left and/or right atrial or left ventricular enlargement; if left atrial pressure has been chronically elevated, there may be evidence of redistribution of blood flow to upper lung zones. Annular calcification of the mitral valve is not uncommon. The extent and severity of myocardial hypertrophy is best evaluated with two-dimensional echocardiography and Doppler studies. Left ventricular hypertrophy may be symmetric or asymmetric and localized to the septum or the free wall, but most commonly to both the septum and the free wall with relative sparing of the posterior wall. 'Apical' hypertrophic cardiomyopathy appears to be common in Japan; hypertrophy confined to the apex is rare, in the West although approximately 10 per cent of patients have left ventricular hypertrophy which is maximal in the distal ventricle from the level of the papillary muscle down to the apex. Approximately one-third of patients also have hypertrophy of the right ventricular free wall, the presence and severity of which is strongly related to the severity of left ventricular hypertrophy. Typically, left ventricular end-systolic and end-diastolic dimensions are reduced, and the left atrial dimension is increased. Indices of systolic function, such as ejection fraction and velocity of fibre shortening, are increased. Colour Doppler provides a sensitive method of detecting left ventricular outflow tract turbulence and, when combined with continuous-wave Doppler, the peak velocity (V_{max}) of left ventricular blood flow can be measured and left ventricular outflow tract gradients can be calculated.

Doppler-calculated gradients (pressure gradient (mmHg) = $4V^2_{max}$) are seen in 30 per cent of patients and correlate well with those measured invasively. Systolic anterior motion of the mitral valve is usually present when the calculated outflow tract gradient is more than 30 mmHg. Early closure or fluttering of the aortic valve leaflets and Doppler evidence of mitral regurgitation are often seen in association with systolic anterior motion of the mitral valve.

Cardiac catheterization

Two-dimensional echo and Doppler evaluation have replaced invasive haemodynamic measurements and angiography as the method of assessing left ventricular structure and function in hypertrophic cardiomyopathy. Cardiac catheterization is not necessary for diagnosis; it is rarely indicated unless symptoms are refractory, and direct measurement of cardiac pressures is potentially informative, particularly in assessing the severity of mitral regurgitation. Coronary arteriography may be necessary in patients above 40 years of age who have significant angina or ST-segment changes during exercise. Usually, the left coronary arteries have a large calibre. The left anterior descending and septal perforator arteries may demonstrate phasic narrowing during systole in the absence of fixed obstructive lesions; such changes do not relate to symptoms.

Left ventricular angiography is rarely indicated, but the recognition of the abnormally shaped ventricle which typically ejects at least 75 per cent of its contents in association with mild mitral regurgitation may provide a valuable diagnostic clue when hypertrophic cardiomyopathy is not suspected before catheterization.

Exercise testing

Maximal exercise testing in association with respiratory gas analysis provides useful functional and possibly prognostic information which can be monitored serially. The maximum oxygen ventilatory capacity Vo_2max is often moderately reduced even in patients who claim that their exercise tolerance is not limited. Continuous measurement of the blood pressure during treadmill exercise reveals that approximately one-third of younger patients have an abnormal blood pressure response with drops of 25–150 mmHg from peak recordings despite an appropriate increase in cardiac output. Such changes are usually asymptomatic, but preliminary observations suggest that they are likely to be of prognostic significance. The mechanism of the hypotensive response during exercise in hypertrophic cardiomyopathy is uncertain, but may relate to myocardial mechanoreceptor activation and altered baroreflex control of the systemic vasculature. ST-segment changes of 2 mm from baseline, which are associated with symptoms of angina, are documented in 25 per cent of patients. The relation of such changes to metabolic markers of ischaemia requires further evaluation and their prognostic significance has yet to be determined.

Electrophysiological studies

Electrophysiological studies may occasionally be necessary in patients with sustained rapid palpitation to identify associated accessory pathways or to aid management of sustained monomorphic ventricular tachycardia. Conventional programmed ventricular stimulation does not aid the identification of high risk patients. The prognostic significance of electrophysiological methods of measuring the inhomogeneity of intraventricular conduction is being examined.

NATURAL HISTORY

Patients with hypertrophic cardiomyopathy experience a slow progression of symptoms, a gradual deterioration of left ventricular function, and a significant incidence of sudden death which occurs at all ages. Data from referral centres reveal an annual mortality from sudden death of 2 to 3 per cent in adults and 4 to 6 per cent in children and adolescents. It is even greater in young patients with recurrent syncope or a family history of 'malignant' hypertrophic cardiomyopathy. Although the mortality figures from non-referral hospitals are lower, the risk of sudden death is still present. The annual mortality was approximately 4 per cent in two consecutive populations of apparent 'low risk' children and adolescents in whom the diagnosis of hypertrophic cardiomyopathy was made during routine family screening or who came to medical attention because of paroxysmal symptoms or an asymptomatic murmur.

Symptomatic deterioration is usually slow and associated with a gradual reduction in left ventricular systolic performance. Left ventricular hypertrophy is not progressive once growth is completed. However, severe symptoms may develop in association with progressive myocardial wall thinning, presumably reflecting myocyte necrosis and fibrosis, and severe reduction in left ventricular systolic performance and/or diastolic filling. Occasionally, patients who experience such a deterioration present with a clinical picture resembling restrictive cardiomyopathy with grossly enlarged atria, signs of right heart failure, and relative preservation of left ventricular systolic performance. The onset of atrial fibrillation has been considered an ominous development. A recent retrospective study revealed that 5 year survival in those with atrial fibrillation was similar to that of age and sex-matched patients who remained in sinus rhythm and, if the ventricular response was controlled, symptomatic status remained stable.

PROGNOSIS

The major problems in management are the identification of high risk patients and the prevention of sudden death. In adults, the finding of non-sustained ventricular tachycardia during ECG monitoring is associated with a sevenfold to eightfold increased risk of sudden death. It is the best single marker of the high risk adult, with a sensitivity of at least 70 per cent and a specificity of 80 per cent. However, the positive predictive accuracy of ventricular tachycardia as a marker is low (22 per cent), reflecting the fact that most patients with this condition do not die suddenly. Further risk stratification of this subgroup would be helpful because a policy of aggressive therapy may include patients at relatively lower risk. In adults, no other clinical feature, including symptoms, left ventricular wall thickness, filling pressures, or the presence of a left ventricular gradient, is associated with or predictive of sudden death. Children and adolescents who have experienced recurrent syncope and those who have two or more siblings with hypertrophic cardiomyopathy who have died suddenly are at increased risk. However, the majority of young patients who die suddenly have not experienced syncope nor do they have such a 'malignant' family history. The young pose problems in terms of both identification and therapy. Most are asymptomatic, many are athletic, and even those at apparently low risk have an annual mortality from sudden death of 3 to 4 per cent.

Identification of those at increased risk depends on understanding probable causes of sudden death. Possible initiating mechanisms include haemodynamic deterioration with reduced stroke volume following a physiological tachycardia or an arrhythmia as well as hypotension developing in the presence of a normal stroke volume but altered baroreflex control of vasomotor tone. The outcome (survival versus sudden death) is influenced by the underlying electrical stability of the myocardium which, it is reasonable to speculate, is related to the extent of myocardial disarray. In adults, non-sustained ventricular tachycardia is a marker of electrical instability; no such marker has been identified in younger patients.

MANAGEMENT

Symptomatic treatment

The aim of therapy is to improve symptoms and prevent complications, in particular sudden death. β-Adrenoceptor blockers, particularly propranolol, and calcium antagonists, especially verapamil, are the mainstay of symptomatic pharmacological therapy. Both drugs have several potentially beneficial actions including a decrease in the determinants of myocardial oxygen consumption and blunting of the heart rate response during exercise to provide increased time for filling at equivalent workloads in those with poor relaxation and slow filling. Both agents exert a negative inotropic effect, reducing hyperdynamic systolic function and left ventricular gradients; it is also claimed that they improve diastolic filling, verapamil by improving relaxation and propranolol by increasing compliance. The side-effects of propranolol are rarely serious; however, the suppressant effect of verapamil on impulse formulation and atrioventricular nodal conduction may cause problems in patients with unsuspected pre-existing conduction disease, and its vasodilatory and negative inotropic effects have resulted in acute pulmonary oedema and death. In practice, both drugs are effective but it is safer to use propranolol. If it is ineffective, verapamil can then be tried; in patients with conduction abnormalities, resting or provocable gradients, or impaired systolic function, verapamil should be started in hospital.

Surgery offers another therapeutic option with a reported experience of over 1500 patients. The conventional indication for surgery has been a resting left ventricular outflow tract gradient of more than 50 mmHg in patients refractory to medical therapy. The commonest operation has been to remove a segment of the upper anterior septum (myotomy/myectomy) via a transaortic approach. Transventricular approaches have also been used but are associated with a higher incidence of late complications, particularly cardiac failure. Despite this large experience, the operation carries a perioperative mortality of 3 to 10 per cent. Successful surgery confers symptomatic and haemodynamic improvement (reduced left ventricular gradient and filling pressures). It is not known which patients are at particular risk of perioperative complications; the optimal patient population for myotomy/myectomy has not been identified. Mitral valve replacement has also been advocated; excellent results have been achieved, particularly in elderly patients with severe mitral regurgitation. The role of DDD pacing for symptomatic management is being

evaluated. Alteration of the ventricular activation sequence with gradient reduction and optimization of filling characteristics in selected patients may result in reduction of gradients and filling pressures and improved symptoms.

Dyspnoea

Therapy depends on the predominant mechanism of dyspnoea. β-Blockers and verapamil are appropriate in patients with slow filling which continues throughout diastole. Conversely, those with rapid early filling may benefit from a relative tachycardia and do better without negative chronotropic agents. When dyspnoea is associated with significant obstruction, i.e. at least 50 per cent of stroke volume in the left ventricle at the onset of the gradient, β-blockers, disopyramide, and, failing this, myotomy/myectomy may be beneficial. Occasionally, dyspnoea is associated with severe mitral regurgitation and responds well to mitral valve replacement. Endocarditis is a rare complication; it occurs in patients with left ventricular outflow tract turbulence and/or mitral regurgitation. It may involve the mitral or aortic valve and is usually associated with increased dyspnoea. Antibiotic prophylaxis is important in appropriate patients.

Chest pain

When chest pain is severe, associated with significant ST-segment changes during exercise, or refractory to therapy, coronary arteriography is warranted. The results of coronary artery bypass grafting in hypertrophic cardiomyopathy are excellent even when additional procedures are performed (myectomy and mitral valve replacement). Exertional chest pain usually responds to therapy with propranolol or verapamil, but when it is refractory very high doses of these agents (propranolol 480 mg daily, verapamil 720 mg daily) have been beneficial. Atypical chest pain may persist long after the initial stimulus has been removed, presumably because a new dynamic situation has developed. Short-acting nitrates, diuretics, and high dose verapamil may be useful in selected patients, perhaps by reducing filling pressures and improving coronary flow to subendocardial layers.

Arrhythmia

Arrhythmias are a common complication of hypertrophic cardiomyopathy. Once atrial fibrillation is established, treatment with anticoagulants and digoxin with or without verapamil or β-blockers is appropriate. The aim of therapy is to control the ventricular response and prevent emboli. Most patients who develop atrial fibrillation during electrocardiographic monitoring are unaware of changes from sinus rhythm to atrial fibrillation as long as the ventricular response is well controlled. In a minority, the loss of atrial systolic contribution to filling volume is important; in these patients, electrical cardioversion can be facilitated by prior therapy (4–6 weeks) with amiodarone (300 mg daily) if pharmacological cardioversion does not occur first. Sustained (longer than 30 s) episodes of paroxysmal atrial fibrillation or supraventricular tachycardia occur and represent a risk of haemodynamic collapse and emboli. Amiodarone in low doses (1000–1400 mg weekly) is effective in suppressing such episodes and also provides control of the ventricular response should breakthrough occur. If episodes persist, the threshold for anticoagulation should be low as embolic complications are common even when atrial dimensions are only moderately increased. Non-sustained episodes of supraventricular arrhythmia are common, but are usually asymptomatic and poor predictors of the subsequent development of established atrial fibrillation. Antiarrhythmic therapy is not usually warranted. Episodes of non-sustained ventricular tachycardia are common but are rarely symptomatic, and therapy is warranted only if prognosis can be shown to be improved (see below).

Prevention of sudden death

The aim of management is to identify the high risk cohort and then to characterize those patients in relation to mechanisms of sudden death which are amenable to specific therapies (Table 5). In adults, there is a practical algorithm for management of those at increased risk of sudden death. The finding of non-sustained ventricular tachycardia during ECG monitoring identifies a high risk cohort; further risk factor stratification may identify a treatable mechanism. In those with non-sustained ventricular tachycardia and no identifiable treatable mechanism, the use of low dose amiodarone (maintenance 1000–1400 mg per week) is associated with improved survival when compared with well-matched historical control subjects. Serious side-effects are rare with plasma concentrations of amiodarone of less than 1.5 mg/l, although photosensitivity and sleep disturbance are common and may be troublesome. In the young, a practical management algorithm is complicated by the lack of sensitive non-invasive prognostic markers. The utility of altered vascular responses and evidence of ischaemia to aid identification of high risk young patients is under evaluation. As in high risk adults, young patients with established markers (syncope, adverse family history, out-of-hospital ventricular fibrillation) should undergo detailed evaluation to identify probable mechanisms for which targeted therapy can be administered. In the remaining high risk young patients, treatment is empirical with amiodarone, myectomy, or an implantable cardioverter defibrillator the principal options. The choice of which therapy to use will be influenced by clinical presentation and by the particular skills, financial resources, and biases of the individual centre. There is evidence to suggest improved prognosis for each of these therapies when they are selected for use in appropriate patients.

Young patients who do not have the recognized risk factors may none the less be at risk of sudden death; there is no evidence to suggest that symptomatic therapy with either β-blockers or calcium antagonists will prevent this. Preliminary evidence suggests that electrophysiological measurements of the inhomogeneity of ventricular conduction can predict the development of ventricular fibrillation. Until practical management guidelines are established, young patients with hypertrophic cardiomyopathy who are apparently at low risk should undergo assessment of possible mechanisms of sudden death at a specialist centre.

Restrictive cardiomyopathy

DEFINITION

Restrictive cardiomyopathy, the least common of the cardiomyopathies, is characterized by restrictive filling of one or both ventricles. This is usually caused by endomyocardial fibrosis. Two variants with similar pathology are recognized. Tropical endomyocardial fibrosis is more common and accounts for 10 to 20 per cent of deaths from heart disease in Africa. Endomyocardial fibrosis in temperate countries is rare, and typically is associated with hypereosinophilia (see Chapter 15.14.3). The pathology is similar in advanced cases with or without hypereosinophilia and both variants are considered to be different manifestations of the same disease process. Idiopathic myocardial restrictive cardiomyopathy occurs with and without myocardial fibrosis, but is rare. Myocardial infiltrative diseases (amyloidosis, sarcoidosis, Gaucher's disease), storage diseases (haemochromatosis, glycogen storage disease, Fabry's disease), and endomyocardial disease associated with malignancies (metastases, carcinoid, radiation, anthracycline toxicity) may also have a restrictive pattern of physiology and mimic restrictive cardiomyopathy.

PATHOLOGY

In endomyocardial fibrosis the cardiac pathology is distinctive, with endocardial fibrosis and overlying thrombosis involving the inflow tracts and apices, but sparing the outflow tracts of one or both ventricles. Necrotic, thrombotic, and fibrotic stages have been defined in patients with endomyocardial fibrosis and hypereosinophilia. In the necrotic stage there is an acute inflammatory reaction characterized by eosinophilic abscesses in the myocardium with associated necrosis and arteritis. The endocardium is often thickened and mural thrombi may

Table 5 *Identifiable and treatable mechanisms of sudden death in hypertrophic cardiomyopathy*

Paroxysmal atrial fibrillation	Amiodarone
Sustained monomorphic ventricular tachycardia	Amiodarone ± an implantable cardioverter defibrillator
Ischaemia	High dose verapamil
Conduction disease	Pacemaker
Accessory pathway	Ablation

develop. The thrombotic stage is characterized by endocardial thrombus formation which may be severe with massive intracavitary thrombosis causing restriction to ventricular filling and a low output state with high filling pressures. There is a risk of systemic emboli. During the necrotic and thrombotic stages the disease may mimic hyperacute rheumatic carditis. If the patient survives, healing by fibrosis with hyaline fibrous tissue occurs. There is no further evidence of inflammation, and the impact of the disease is caused by the effect of the dense fibrous tissue on ventricular filling volume and atrioventricular valve function.

CLINICAL FEATURES AND MANAGEMENT

Diagnosis and assessment

Disease onset is usually insidious. Clinical presentation relates to the degree of endomyocardial fibrosis; left-sided disease may present with symptoms of pulmonary congestion and/or mitral regurgitation, and right-sided disease with raised jugular venous pressure, hepatomegaly, ascites, and tricuspid regurgitation. Radiographic and ECG appearances are non-specific, showing evidence of raised left and/or right atrial pressure and cardiomegaly with left ventricular hypertrophy. Occasionally, pulmonary infiltrates, non-specific repolarization changes, and fascicular blocks may develop.

Two-dimensional echocardiography provides the best non-invasive means of confirming the diagnosis. This permits visualization of the structural abnormalities involving the endocardium and atrioventricular valves as well as demonstration of the abnormal physiology with restriction to filling. There may be intracavitary thrombus with apical cavity obliteration or bright echoes from the endocardium of the right or left ventricle with tethering of the chordae and reduced excursion of the posterior mitral valve leaflet. Typically, ventricular dimensions and wall thickness are normal whereas the atria are grossly enlarged. Left ventricular filling terminates early and is followed by a plateau phase coincident with the third heart sound.

The principal haemodynamic consequence of endomyocardial scarring is a restriction to normal filling. Early diastolic pressures are normal, but there is a rapid mid-diastolic rise (square-root sign) which reaches a plateau and is not associated with impairment of systolic performance. A similar functional haemodynamic abnormality is seen in pericardial constriction, but in the latter condition end-diastolic pressures within the two ventricles are usually very similar, whereas in endomyocardial fibrosis there is usually inequality of the end-diastolic pressures. Mitral and tricuspid regurgitation may be severe, and both ventricles appear abnormal in shape on angiography owing to obliteration of the apices. This may be particularly marked in the right ventricle in which the infundibulum is hypertrophied and hypocontractile. In addition, the fibrotic process results in smoothing of the internal architecture of the ventricle with loss of the normal trabeculae. The presence of intracavitary thrombi in the left ventricle may give rise to erroneous diagnosis of a cardiac tumour.

The structural and physiological abnormalities that can be demonstrated with two-dimensional echocardiography or during catheterization with angiography result from the thrombotic and fibrotic stages of the disease. During the early acute phase the appearances of the left and right ventricle are far less abnormal; at this stage the diagnosis can best be confirmed by endomyocardial biopsy. In later stages diagnosis should be apparent and the risk of biopsy is excessive.

Management

Medical treatment of advanced disease is not particularly effective and the prognosis is poor, with a 2 year mortality of 35 to 50 per cent. Congestive symptoms from raised right atrial pressure can be improved with diuretics, although too great a reduction in ventricular filling pressure will lead to a reduction in cardiac output. Arrhythmias are common, but their prognostic significance is uncertain and therefore they should not be treated unless they are sustained or associated with symptoms. Antiarrhythmic drugs which significantly slow the heart rate may be deleterious because of the small stroke volume. Digitalis glycosides may be helpful to control the ventricular response in atrial fibrillation, but they cannot be expected to improve congestive symptoms as systolic function is usually well preserved. Anticoagulants may help to prevent venous thrombosis and systemic emboli; both warfarin and antiplatelet drugs are advised.

Surgery with mitral and/or tricuspid valve replacement with or without decortication of the endocardium has been carried out in some patients. Good long-term symptomatic results have been obtained although there is a significant perioperative mortality (15–20 per cent).

Arrhythmogenic right ventricular dysplasia

DEFINITION

Arrhythmogenic right ventricular dysplasia or cardiomyopathy is a recently recognized heart muscle disorder of unknown cause. It is characterized pathologically by fibrofatty replacement of the right ventricular myocardium and by clinical presentation with arrhythmia and sudden death. The disease is often familial (approximately 30 per cent) with autosomal dominant inheritance and incomplete penetrance. The incidence is unknown. It occurs worldwide, but the high incidence of disease recognized in the Veneto region of Northern Italy raises the possibility of a founder effect. A cardiovascular cause, most commonly hypertrophic cardiomyopathy and arrhythmogenic right ventricular dysplasia, is identified in over 80 per cent of young athletes (aged below 25 years) who die suddenly.

AETIOLOGY AND PATHOGENESIS

Segmental disease is usual with involvement of the diaphragmatic, apical, and infundibular regions of the right ventricular free wall. Evolution to more diffuse right ventricular involvement and left ventricular abnormalities with heart failure have been described. The fibrofatty replacement of the myocardium may be focal or widespread, usually involves the subepicardial layer of the right ventricular free wall, and when severe may appear transmural. Two morphological patterns are recognized. Lipomatous replacement of the myocardium without fibrosis is usually seen with preservation of normal right ventricular free-wall thickness in the absence of an inflammatory infiltrate, while the fibrolipomatous pattern is characterized by replacement myocardial fibrosis with thinning and discrete bulges of the right ventricular free wall, often in association with lymphocytic infiltrates surrounding degenerating or necrotic myocytes. A potential inflammatory pathogenesis and the temporal relationship of these morphological patterns is under investigation. It remains unclear whether the genetic basis predisposes to a degenerative disease with atrophy and fibrofatty replacement of right ventricular myocardium or whether the inflammatory cells indicate an infectious or possibly genetically determined immune pathogenesis.

CLINICAL PRESENTATION AND MANAGEMENT

Clinical manifestations of the disease include structural and functional abnormalities of the right ventricle, ECG depolarization–repolarization changes, and presentation with sudden death or arrhythmias of right ventricular origin. Structural and functional evaluation of the right ventricle is problematic. There is no ideal method; reliance on invasive angiography, two-dimensional echocardiography, radionuclide angiography, computerized tomography, and/or magnetic resonance imaging will depend on local expertise and facilities. Quality imaging usually reveals segmental dilatation or localized aneurysm(s) of the right ventricular free wall with mild or no left ventricular impairment. The typical ECG presents inverted T waves in right ventricular precordial leads (V_1–$V_{3(4)}$) and ventricular postexcitation 'epsilon waves'. These waves are the surface ECG manifestation of late potentials that are found on the time domain signal-averaged ECG in 40 to 50 per cent of patients as a consequence of the inhomogenous and delayed right ventricular depolarization.

The disease usually presents with palpitation and/or syncope from sustained ventricular arrhythmia. These are of left bundle branch block morphology suggesting a right ventricular origin. Sudden death related to exercise may be the initial manifestation, particularly in young competitive athletes.

The diagnosis of right ventricular dysplasia is based on histological demonstration of fibrofatty replacement of right ventricular myocardium at either necropsy or surgery. Diagnosis based on right ventricular endomyocardial biopsy specimens is inherently difficult because the segmental nature of the disease causes false negatives, and because the amount of tissue obtained usually is insufficient to differentiate fibrofatty replacement from islands of adipose tissue which are not infrequently seen between myocytes in the right ventricle of normal subjects. Nevertheless, the positive finding of fibrofatty replacement of myocytes on biopsy can be a valuable diagnostic clue. Therefore diagnosis relies heavily on the clinical demonstration of structural, functional, and electrophysiological abnormalities that are caused by or reflect the underlying histological changes.

The natural history of arrhythmogenic right ventricular dysplasia is uncertain because published series are biased by necropsy patients and/or those presenting with sustained ventricular arrhythmias. In the absence of sustained ventricular arrhythmia most patients will be asymptomatic. Progression from localized (with no or minor symptoms) to more diffuse right ventricular involvement with symptoms of life-threatening ventricular arrhythmia or right ventricular failure has been reported. In long-standing disease, the left ventricle may be involved; differentiation from dilated cardiomyopathy with biventricular involvement may then be difficult.

The principal aim of management is to identify those at risk of sustained ventricular arrhythmia and to prevent sudden death. Assessment of asymptomatic patients should include exercise testing and Holter monitoring to detect occult arrhythmias. Antiarrhythmic treatment guided by electrophysiological studies is warranted in patients with palpitation or syncope and those with documented sustained ventricular arrhythmia, and should be considered in those with a markedly abnormal signal-averaged electrocardiogram who are at increased risk. The morphology of ventricular arrhythmia may vary, suggesting multiple sites of origin; arrhythmias are usually progressive and therapy, whether pharmacological, ablation, or surgical, is not usually definitive.

Specific heart muscle disorders

Cardiac manifestations of systemic vasculitis

INTRODUCTION

As in other organ systems, the cardiac manifestations of systemic vasculitis are subtle, complex, and difficult to diagnose (Table 6). Every anatomical structure may be involved, including coronary arteries, heart valves, myocardium, pericardium, and conducting tissue. There is usually no relation between the extent of systemic disease and cardiac involvement.

Table 6 *Cardiac manifestations of systemic vasculitis*

Disease	Cardiac manifestation
Systemic lupus erythematosus	Accelerated atherosclerosis Non-infective endocarditis Myocarditis Pericarditis Aortic valve lesions
Systemic sclerosis	Myocarditis Pericarditis Arrhythmias
Polyarteritis nodosa (Churg–Strauss syndrome)	Hypertension Pericarditis Arrhythmias
Wegener's granulomatosis	Constrictive pericarditis Atrioventricular block
Rheumatoid arthritis	Coronary arteritis Aortic and mitral regurgitation Pericarditis
Takayasu's syndrome	Aortic arch vasculitis Heart failure

Seronegative arthropathies
  Ankylosing spondylitis
  Reiter's syndrome
  Psoriatic arthritis
  Ulcerative colitis
  Crohn's disease
	Pancarditis
	Proximal aortitis
	Conduction disease

SYSTEMIC LUPUS ERYTHEMATOSUS

Clinical cardiac involvement is observed in 50 to 60 per cent of patients, while evidence of microvasculitis is found in almost all patients at autopsy. The clinical presentation is usually dominated by involvement of other organ systems. Pericarditis is the commonest cardiac lesion (60–75 per cent at autopsy) and is symptomatic in the majority. Other manifestations, particularly myocarditis and non-infective endocarditis of the mitral valve (Libman–Sachs endocarditis) are common but subclinical and rarely result in cardiac failure or significant regurgitation. Anticardiolipin syndrome, characterized by recurrent thromboses and abortions in association with antiphospholipid antibodies, occurs alone as well as with systemic lupus erythematosus; high antibody titres are associated with cardiac, particularly valvular, involvement. Arrhythmias are uncommon. Management is directed at control of hypertension and suppression of systemic vasculitis. Corticosteroids are useful in patients with coronary vasculitis and myocarditis, but may aggravate atherosclerosis and do not prevent constrictive pericarditis. Regular prophylaxis against infective endocarditis should be considered because of the predisposition to valvular disease. Death from cardiac complications of systemic lupus erythematosus is rare.

SYSTEMIC SCLEROSIS

Cardiac involvement is common in systemic sclerosis but is clinically not apparent until the skin disease is advanced. It is characterized by patchy myocardial fibrosis from gradual obliteration of small vessels. Pericarditis is common and congestive cardiac failure, which is seen in advanced disease, is progressive and carries a poor prognosis. The ECG may be normal despite cardiac involvement. Echocardiography typically shows features of dilated or restrictive cardiomyopathy. At present no therapy has been proved to alter the cardiac manifestations of scleroderma, although calcium antagonists and angiotensin-converting enzyme inhibitors may be of benefit.

RHEUMATOID ARTHRITIS

Rheumatoid arthritis is often associated with inflammation of the heart, particularly the pericardium, but clinically significant cardiac disease is uncommon and trends to correlate with the severity of the joint disease and the presence of rheumatoid nodules. Myocarditis has been reported in up to 20 per cent of patients postmortem and is associated with the presence of severe vasculitis or joint disease; however, such patients are not usually symptomatic and overt congestive cardiac failure is rare. Histological examination of valvular tissue often discloses non-specific inflammation and occasionally granulomas. Clinically significant aortic or mitral regurgitation requiring surgical intervention is rare. Evidence of pericarditis is often found in patients with rheumatoid arthritis but is rarely symptomatic; a pericardial rub can be heard in up to 30 per cent of patients, and a pericardial effusion can be identified echocardiographically in up to 50 per cent of patients. The commonest ECG abnormality is first-degree heart block, although complete heart block and left bundle branch block have also been described. Rheumatoid pericarditis is associated with a good prognosis (tamponade or constrictive pericarditis are rare) and usually responds to corticosteroid therapy although this treatment cannot prevent development of constrictive pericarditis. Coronary arteritis does occur but is rare.

SERONEGATIVE ARTHROPATHIES

Multisystem rheumatological diseases, including ankylosing spondylitis, Reiter's syndrome, psoriatic arthritis, and the gastrointestinal arthropathies, are associated with cardiac involvement. Their immunological hallmark is the absence of circulating rheumatoid factor, and these disorders are characterized by a combination of pancarditis, proximal aortitis, or aortic regurgitation (which may be clinically silent), and varying degrees of conduction disease including complete heart block; long-standing cardiac disease may result in amyloid deposition. Both aortic regurgitation and atrioventricular conduction block are more common in patients with peripheral joint involvement or disease of long duration, and patients occasionally present with aortic regurgitation prior to clinically evident joint disease. Management relies on appropriate surgical referral in the presence of deteriorating aortic regurgitation and insertion of a permanent pacemaker for atrioventricular conduction disease.

Neuromuscular disorders

Many individuals who present with cardiomyopathy also appear to have some evidence of skeletal myopathy, although this may be subclinical. This includes patients with hypertrophic cardiomyopathy who do not have overt cardiac failure. Conversely, many neuromuscular disorders (Table 7) show varying degrees of cardiac involvement. Molecular genetic approaches have begun to dissect these overlap syndromes.

It is important in the clinical management of these disorders to place any cardiovascular involvement in the overall context of the natural history of the particular disease. Thus, for example, the cardiac conduction system disease of Emery–Dreifuss muscular dystrophy is a significant cause of morbidity and mortality, whereas the heart muscle disease of Duchenne muscular dystrophy may be the cause of death but rarely dominates the clinical picture.

The assessment and treatment of cardiovascular involvement in these disorders is largely empirical and based on symptoms. Heart failure should be treated aggressively as the threshold for systemic desaturation may be low. Arrhythmias are common but only occasionally debilitating. Empirical therapy is usually sufficient. Permanent pacing is indicated in many instances, particularly in myotonic dystrophy and Emery–Dreifuss muscular dystrophy.

Table 7 *Cardiovascular abnormalities in neuromuscular disorders*

Condition	Transmission	CM	CD	Tachyarrhythmia	SD	CHF	Cardiovascular pathology	Genetic defect
Duchenne	XLR	+ Uncommon	−	−	−	+	Replacement fibrosis (posterobasal and lateral LV wall)	Xp21 absence of dystrophin
Becker	XLR	Common	−	−	−	+	Replacement fibrosis (posterobasal and lateral LV wall)	Xp21 altered size and/or quantity of dystrophin
Facioscapulohumeral	AD	−	+	−	−	−	Replacement fibrosis (conduction system)	Chr 4q35
Emery–Dreifuss	XLR	+	+	+	+	+	?	Xq28
Limb-girdle	AR/AD	+	−	+	−	+	?	Chr 15 (AR)
Distal myopathy	AD	−	+	−	−	−	?	None known
Mitochondrial myopathies	Cytoplasmic	+	+	−	−	−	?	Mitochondrial
Oculopharyngeal	AD	−	+	−	−	−	?	?
Myotonic dystrophy	AD	+ Uncommon	+	−	+	+ Uncommon	Fibrosis, fatty infiltration and atrophy of the conduction system	Chr 19 myotonin kinase

AD, autosomal dominant; AR, autosomal recessive; CD, cardiac disease; CHF, congestive heart failure; Chr, chromosome; CM, cardiomyopathy; LV, left ventricular; SD, sudden death; XLR, X-linked recessive; + present; − absent.

*Allelic forms of the same genetic defect

Up-to-date clinical and molecular references can be accessed from the online *Mendelian inheritance in man*.

Miscellaneous heart muscle disorders

SARCOIDOSIS

Cardiac sarcoid is clinically apparent in only 5 per cent of patients, usually young or middle-aged adults, but can be demonstrated at post-mortem examination in 20 to 30 per cent of patients, most of whom have generalized sarcoid. Many patients remain asymptomatic despite extensive cardiac involvement. Clinical presentation of cardiac involvement is usually with conduction disease or congestive cardiac failure, relating to either dilated or restrictive physiological changes. Palpitation and syncope related to tachyarrhythmia or conduction system disease are common cardiac presentations, but the heart is often normal on examination. The ECG is frequently abnormal with T-wave abnormalities and conduction abnormalities. Echocardiographic findings include a dilated and poorly contractile left ventricle, and occasionally abnormalities in the presence of regional wall motion which may be proximal in the left ventricle. The diagnosis is often made in patients with clinical or chest radiographic evidence of sarcoid who also have clinical, ECG, or echocardiography evidence of a myocardial disorder. Endomyocardial biopsy can confirm the diagnosis, but because of patchy myocardial involvement may only be positive in 50 per cent of affected cases. Thallium-201 imaging is useful to reveal perfusion defects which will reflect the extent of myocardial involvement. The management of this condition is difficult since arrhythmias are often refractory to drug therapy. The role of corticosteroids in prevention of both conduction disease and myocardial dysfunction is controversial in terms of both efficacy and the risk of causing left ventricular aneurysm. Premature sudden death occurs particularly in patients with more extensive myocardial involvement. Arrhythmias are often progressive and difficult to manage, and an implantable cardioverter defibrillator should be considered in appropriate patients.

AMYLOIDOSIS

Cardiac amyloid is found in 30 to 50 per cent of patients with primary amyloid, in whom it is the most common cause of death; post-mortem examination of these patients reveals widespread myocardial involvement. In contrast, cardiac disease is rare in patients with secondary amyloid and familial amyloidosis. However, senile amyloid may be associated with considerable ventricular involvement resulting in impairment of function. Pathology reveals biatrial dilatation and ventricular thickening associated with a loss of compliance. This is clinically manifested by changes reflecting restrictive physiology; the ventricular pressure pulse is characterized by a diastolic dip and plateau (the 'square-root sign') as a result of poor ventricular compliance. Presentation with clinical left ventricular dysfunction is ominous, and is associated with progressive heart failure and survival for less than 2 years. Patients occasionally present with postural hypotension as a consequence of autonomic neuropathy or infiltration of the adrenal glands. Physical examination may reveal signs of cardiac failure which is predominantly right-sided; systolic murmurs resulting from atrioventricular valvular regurgitation also occur. Chest radiography typically shows a normal cardiac silhouette with pulmonary plethora. The ECG is frequently abnormal, with small voltage complexes, loss of R-wave in the right ventricular leads, left-axis deviation, and conduction defects which are particularly common in patients with familial amyloidosis. Sustained arrhythmias, particularly atrial fibrillation, are common. Echocardiography is often abnormal, even in patients who are asymptomatic with biatrial dilatation, ventricular thickening, and impaired systolic and diastolic function. A characteristic granular texture may be present in the ventricular wall, and the degree of thickening may resemble hypertrophic cardiomyopathy. Pericardial effusion may be present but does not usually lead to cardiac tamponade. Clinical diagnosis is often made following biopsy of extracardiac tissue, such as abdominal fat aspirate or rectal tissue. If fat aspirate is negative then endomyocardial biopsy is often helpful. The management of these patients is difficult; diuretics and vasodilators provide symptomatic relief but can aggravate problems of hypotension. A permanent pacemaker may be useful in progressive conduction disease, but care must be taken with certain drugs, particularly digoxin and calcium antagonists, since these medications bind to amyloid infiltrates and cause enhanced sensitivity. At present no therapy has been proved to prevent progressive cardiac deposition of amyloid tissue or to prevent progressive deterioration and death.

THYROID DISEASE

Hyperthyroidism

Hyperthyroidism is more common in women and in the 30–40 age group, and there is a documented association with mitral valve prolapse. Cardiac symptoms include angina-like chest pain, fatigue, palpitation and exertional dyspnoea. Physical signs include tachycardia, systolic or diastolic hypertension, flow murmurs, and high output cardiac failure. The first heart sound and the pulmonary component of the second heart sound may be loud, and a third heart sound may be present. Elderly hyperthyroid patients may present with cardiac signs alone. Chest radiography may identify cardiomegaly in patients with cardiac failure; ECG reveals sinus tachycardia in 40 to 50 per cent of patients, particularly those in the younger age group, and up to 25 per cent of patients display symptoms of paroxysmal or sustained atrial fibrillation which may be the presenting feature. Conduction disease of varying degree including atrioventricular block is seen in approximately a quarter of patients. The clinical diagnosis is confirmed by the demonstration of elevated circulating levels of thyroid hormone. Specific management requires the restoration of the euthyroid state. In the intervening period it is necessary to treat any associated arrhythmia or cardiac failure. Atrial fibrillation is of concern since it may result in arterial embolization. Some patients, particularly the elderly, are resistant to digoxin; β-blockers should be used with caution in patients with cardiac failure but can be most effective in ameliorating many of the symptoms in the thyrotoxic patient.

Hypothroidism

Hypothyroidism can lead to a cardiomyopathy characterized by cardiac dilatation and fibrosis and altered capillary permeability. Cardiac symptoms are common in patients with hypothyroidism and include exertional breathlessness, fatigue, and ankle swelling. Although abnormal lipid metabolism and accelerated atherosclerosis are relatively common, the development of symptomatic coronary artery disease is rare. Physical examination usually reveals hypotension or, rarely, hypertension, bradycardia, non-pitting oedema, reduced heart sounds, and ascites. Overt congestive cardiac failure is rare. Pericardial effusion is present in up to a third of patients but cardiac tamponade is rare. The characteristic electrocardiographic features are sinus bradycardia and prolongation of the Q–T interval; reduction in P wave and QRS complex voltage is often seen in patients who have an associated pericardial effusion. The diagnosis is made by a combination of recognition of the typical features of hypothyroidism together with the detection of reduced circulating thyroid hormones. Echocardiography is a reliable method of differentiating pericardial effusion from ventricular dilatation. Management involves thyroid hormone replacement, which must be cautious in the elderly and those with documented coronary artery disease; such patients are best treated with increasing doses of tritium which has a short half-life. The detection and treatment of cardiovascular complications, particularly pericardial effusions, is of paramount importance. Effusions often resolve with thyroid hormone therapy.

REFERENCES

Myocarditis and dilated cardiomyopathy

Caforio, A.L.P., Bonifacio, E., Stewart, J.T., Neglia, D., Parodi, O., Bottazzo, G.F., and McKenna, W.J. (1990). Novel organ-specific cardiac autoantibodies in dilated cardiomyopathy. *Journal of the American College of Cardiology*, **15**, 1527–34.

Caforio, A.L.P., Keeling, P.J., Zachara, E., Mestroni, L., Camerini, F., Mann, J.M., *et al.* (1994). Evidence from family studies for autoimmunity in dilated cardiomyopathy. *Lancet*, **344**, 773–7.

Lieberman, E.B., Hutchins, G.M., Herskowitz, A., Rose, N.R., and Baughman, K.L. (1991). Clinicopathologic description of myocarditis. *Journal of the American College of Cardiology*, **18**, 1617–26.

Michels, V.V., Moll, P.P., Miller, F.A., Tajik, J.A., Chu, J.S., Driscoll, D.J., *et al.* (1992). The frequency of familial dilated cardiomyopathy in a series of patients with idiopathic dilated cardiomyopathy. *New England Journal of Medicine*, **326**, 77–82.

Rose, N.R., Herskowitz, A., Neumann, D.A., and Neu, N. (1988). Autoimmune myocarditis: a paradigm of post-infection autoimmune disease. *Immunology Today*, **9**, 117–20.

Tracy, S., Wiegand, V., McManus, B., Gauntt, C., Pallansch, M., Beck, M., and Chapman, N. (1990). Molecular approaches to enteroviral diagnosis in idiopathic cardiomyopathy and myocarditis. *Journal of the American College of Cardiology*, **15**, 1688–94.

Woodroof, J.F. (1980). Viral myocarditis: a review. *American Journal of Pathology*, **101**, 427–79.

Hypertrophic cardiomyopathy

Braunwald, E., Lambrew, C.T., Rockoff, S.D., Ross, J., and Morrow, A.G. (1964). Idiopathic hypertrophic subaortic stenosis. I. A description of the disease based upon an analysis of 64 patients. *Circulation*, **30** (Suppl. IV), IV-3–IV-119.

Goodwin, J.F. (1982) The frontiers of cardiomyopathy. *British Heart Journal*, **48**, 1–18.

McKenna, W.J., Oakley, C.M., Krikler, D.M., and Goodwin, J.F. (1985). Improved survival with amiodarone in patients with hypertrophic cardiomyopathy and ventricular tachycardia. *British Heart Journal*, **53**, 412–16.

Maron, B.J., Bonow, R.O., Cannon, R.O., Leon, M.B., and Epstein, S.E. (1987) Hypertrophic cardiomyopathy. Interrelations of clinical manifestations, pathophysiology, and therapy (1). *New England Journal of Medicine*, **316**, 780–9.

Seidman, C.E., McKenna, W.J., Watkins, H.C., and Seidman, J.G. (1994). Molecular genetic approaches to diagnosis and management of hypertrophic cardiomyopathy. In *Heart disease: a textbook of cardiovascular medicine. Update* (ed E. Braunwald), pp. 77–83. W.B. Saunders, Philadelphia, PA.

Spirito, P., Chiarella, F., Carratino, L., Berisso, M.Z., Bellotti, P., and Vecchio, C. (1989). Clinical course and prognosis of hypertrophic cardiomyopathy in an outpatient population. *New England Journal of Medicine*, **320**, 749–55.

Teare, D. (1958) Asymmetrical hypertrophy of the heart in young adults. *British Heart Journal*, **20**, 1–8.

Thierfelder, L., Watkins, H., MacRae, C., Lamas, R., McKenna, W., Vosberg, H-P., *et al.* (1994). Alpha-tropomyosin and cardiac troponin T mutations cause familial hypertrophic cardiomyopathy: a disease of the sarcomere. *Cell*, **77**, 1–20.

Watkins, H., Thierfelder, L., Hwang, D.S., McKenna, W., Seidman, J.G., and Seidman, C.E. (1992) Sporadic hypertrophic cardiomyopathy due to de novo myosin mutations. *Journal of Clinical Investigation*, **90**, 1666–71.

Wigle, E.D., Sasson, Z., Henderson, M.A., Ruddy, T.D., Fulop, J., Rakowski, H., and Williams, W.G. (1985). Hypertrophic cardiomyopathy. The importance of the site and the extent of hypertrophy. A review. *Progress in Cardiovascular Diseases*, **28**, 1–83.

Restrictive cardiomyopathy
See Section 14 C

Arrhythmogenic right ventricular dysplasia

Thiene, G., Nava, A., Corrado, D., Rossi, L., and Pennelli, N. (1988). Right ventricular cardiomyopathy and sudden death in young people. *New England Journal of Medicine*, **318**, 129–33.

Specific heart muscle disorders

Braunwald, E. (ed) (1992). *Heart disease: a textbook of cardiovascular medicine*. W.B. Saunders, Philadelphia, PA.

15.14.2 HIV-related heart muscle disease

N. A. BOON

The heart is involved in up to 50 per cent of patients with the Acquired Immunodeficiency Syndrome (AIDS) but heart disease currently causes symptoms in only 10 per cent, and death in less than 5 per cent, of all AIDS patients. The common lesions are listed in Table 1. Although

Table 1 *Cardiac lesions in AIDS*

Myocardial disease
    Myocarditis
        non-specific
        infectious
    Dilated cardiomyopathy
    Isolated right ventricular dilatation
    Neoplastic infiltration
        Kaposi's sarcoma
        Lymphoma
Pericardial effusion
    Sterile
    Infectious
    Neoplastic
Endocarditis
    Marantic endocarditis (non-bacterial thrombotic endocarditis)
    Infective endocarditis

tuberculous pericardial effusion is a major problem in Africa, left ventricular dysfunction due to myocarditis or dilated cardiomyopathy is the most important cardiac manifestation of AIDS in the Western world.

Myocarditis and dilated cardiomyopathy

Heart muscle disease usually occurs in the late stages of AIDS, and is likely to become an increasingly important cause of cardiac morbidity and mortality for two reasons. First, it has been estimated that by the year 2000 the human immunodeficiency virus (HIV) will have infected between 38 and 110 million people in the world. Second, success in combating opportunistic infections may mean that many patients who otherwise would have died of non-cardiac illnesses will now survive to develop heart muscle disease.

Postmortem and endomyocardial biopsy studies have demonstrated some form of myocarditis in approximately 40 per cent of patients with AIDS. Focal microscopic interstitial mononuclear infiltrates are common and may be accompanied by myocyte necrosis. The Dallas criteria for the diagnosis of active myocarditis are seldom satisfied but this might, perhaps, be expected in the presence of marked immunodeficiency.

Echocardiographic surveys have documented progressive global left ventricular systolic dysfunction in approximately 10 per cent of patients with AIDS. This tends to occur when there is advanced disease with CD4 counts of less than 100 cells/mm^3 and affects patients in all the major risk groups for HIV infection.

Pathogenesis

The pathogenesis of HIV-related heart muscle disease has not been established but is probably complex and multifactorial. Myocarditis may be the substrate for dilated cardiomyopathy and there are many potential aetiological factors:

OPPORTUNISTIC INFECTION

A huge variety of potentially cardiotoxic organisms including *Toxoplasma gondii, Aspergillus fumigatus, Cryptococcus neoformans,* and Cytomegalovirus have been isolated from the myocardium of patients with AIDS. However, in most cases of myocarditis there is no detectable causative organism.

DIRECT DAMAGE

The human immunodeficiency virus has been found in the heart and could damage the myocardium directly. The virus may also induce myocarditis by altering cell surface antigens, leading to immune recognition and autoimmune attack. Alternatively, a minority of infected cells within the myocardium, eg circulating immunocytes, could trigger an immune reaction which damages not only themselves but also the surrounding non-infected tissue. This so-called 'innocent bystander effect' may be mediated by the release of cytokines and has also been implicated in the pathogenesis of HIV encephalopathy.

MALNUTRITION

Many patients with HIV infection suffer from multiple nutritional deficiency states and may develop cardiac damage as a result of the increased oxidative stress associated with deficiency of specific micronutrients such as selenium, or high concentrations of circulating catecholamines.

ZIDOVUDINE

Zidovudine is widely used as an antiretroviral agent in HIV infection, has been shown to damage cardiac muscle in rats, and is known to cause a specific dose-related reversible skeletal myopathy by inhibiting mitochondrial γ-DNA polymerase. Moreover, there are reports of improved cardiac function following withdrawal of zidovudine in AIDS patients with heart failure. Nevertheless, dilated cardiomyopathy occurs in patients who have not received zidovudine and most clinical studies have failed to establish a link between this drug and HIV-related heart muscle disease.

Other potentially cardiotoxic drugs used in HIV infection include pentamidine (which may cause ventricular tachycardia), gancyclovir, and interferon α2a.

Clinical features

HIV-related heart muscle disease often presents with otherwise unexplained cardiomegaly. As the disease progresses the symptoms and signs of heart failure may appear. These are sometimes mistakenly attributed to anaemia or pulmonary infection and include breathlessness, fatigue, oedema, tachycardia, a high jugular venous pressure, gallop rhythm, and crepitations at the lung bases.

The differential diagnosis includes pericardial effusion (often tuberculous in Africa in this context), which may present with asymptomatic cardiomegaly or tamponade and sometimes accompanies heart muscle disease (Fig. 1).

Investigations

The electrocardiogram often shows non-specific ST segment and T wave changes, and may occasionally reveal left or right ventricular hypertrophy. Heart block and ventricular arrhythmias have also been described.

Although chest radiographs may reveal cardiomegaly and pulmonary venous congestion, the diagnosis usually depends on echocardiography, which can reliably detect pericardial effusion, chamber enlargement and ventricular dysfunction (Fig. 2).

Endomyocardial biopsy may occasionally reveal a treatable myocardial infection and should be considered in selected patients.

Treatment

Unless there is a myocardial infection that may respond to specific antimicrobial therapy treatment is palliative. The prognosis is very poor with few patients surviving more than 12 months; nevertheless, conventional treatments for heart failure are often worthwhile. In patients with severe heart failure zidovudine should be withdrawn but can be restarted if there is no demonstrable improvement in cardiac function within 4 to 6 weeks.

Isolated right ventricular dilatation

Dilatation of the right ventricle without any other demonstrable heart disease is a common finding in HIV patients, particularly intravenous

Fig. 1(a) Echocardiogram from a young man with AIDS, showing a dilated left ventricle and a coexisting pericardial effusion. The patient died of heart failure 3 months later. LA, left atrium; LV, left ventricle; MV, mitral valve; PE, pericardial effusion; RV, right ventricle. (b) Echocardiogram from an intravenous drug user with AIDS showing isolated right ventricular dilatation that was subsequently shown to be due to pulmonary embolism. AoV, aortic valve; IVS, interventricular septum; LA, left atrium; LV, left ventricle; RV, right ventricle.

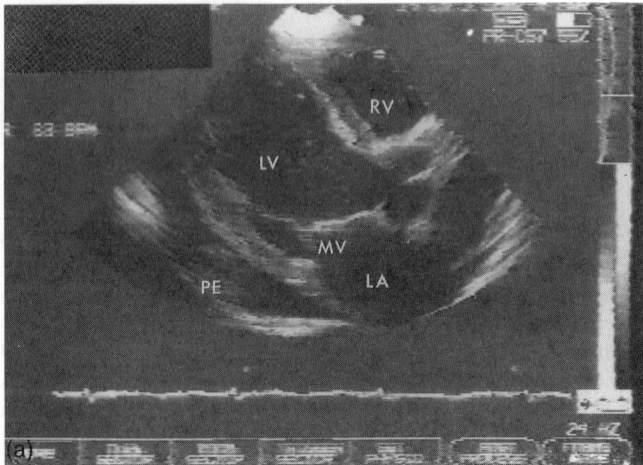

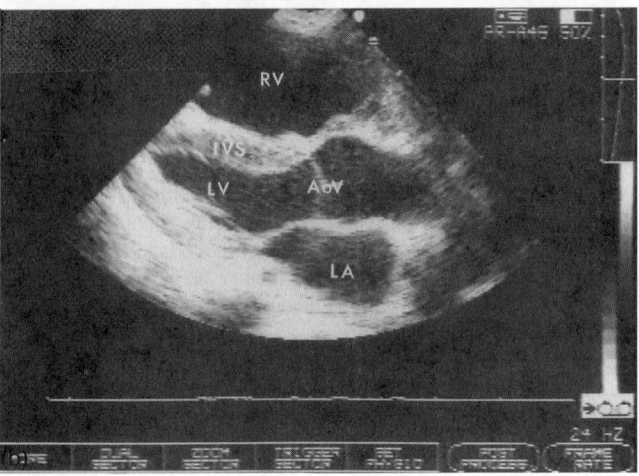

Fig. 2 2D and M mode echocardiogram from a 5-year-old girl with AIDS (acquired by vertical transmission from her mother) and heart failure. The left ventricle is dilated and contracts poorly. rv = right ventricle, lv = left ventricle

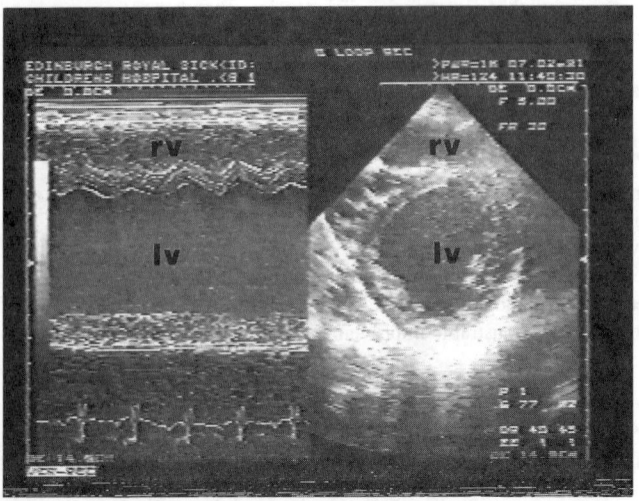

drug users. Whilst this may be the first sign of generalized heart muscle disease, it is usually due to pulmonary hypertension associated with repeated respiratory infections (when it may be transient), thromboembolic disease, or emboli acquired through intravenous drug use.

Neoplastic infiltration

Disseminated Kaposi's sarcoma may involve the heart, particularly the epicardium and subepicardial fat, and is the most common cardiac tumour in HIV disease. Although haemorrhagic pericardial effusion has been described, Kaposi's sarcoma in the heart seldom causes significant cardiac morbidity or mortality.

Cardiac malignant lymphomas are usually derived from B cells, may be focal or diffuse, and may cause pericardial effusion and tamponade, ventricular arrhythmias, heart block, and sudden death.

REFERENCES

Arnaudo, E., Dalakas, M.C., Shanske, S., Moraes, C.T., diMauro, S., and Schon, E.A. (1991). Depletion of muscle mitochondrial DNA in AIDS patients with Zidovudine-induced myopathy. *Lancet* **337**, 508–510.

Blanchard, D.G., Hagenhoff, C., Chow, L.C., McCann, H.A., and Dittrich, H.C. (1991). Reversibility of cardiac abnormalities in human immunodeficiency virus (HIV)-infected individuals: a serial echocardiographic study. *Journal of the American College of Cardiology*, **17**, 1270–1276.

Currie, P.F., Jacob A.J., Foreman A.R., Elton R.A., Brettle R.P., and Boon N.A. (1994). Heart muscle disease related to HIV infection: prognostic implications. *British Medical Journal*, **309**, 1605–7.

Herskowitz, A., Wu, T-C., Willoughby, S.B., *et al.* (1994). Myocarditis and cardiotropic viral infection associated with severe left ventricular dysfunction in late-stage infection with human immunodeficiency virus. *Journal of the American College of Cardiology*, **24**, 1024–32.

Himmelman, R.B., Dohrmann, M., Goodman, P., Schiller, N.B., Starksen, N.F., Warnock, M., and Cheitlin, M.D. (1989). Severe pulmonary hypertension and cor pulmonale in the acquired immunodeficiency syndrome. *American Journal of Cardiology*, **64**, 1396–1399.

Jacob, A.J., Sutherland, G.S., Bird, A.G., Brettle, R.P., Ludlam, C.A., McMillan, A., and Boon, N.A. (1992). Myocardial dysfunction in patients infected with HIV: prevalence and risk factors. *British Heart Journal*, **68**, 549–553.

Kaul, S., Fishbein, M.C., and Siegel, R.J. (1991). Cardiac manifestations of acquired immune deficiency syndrome: a 1991 update. *American Heart Journal*, **122**, 535–544.

Lewis, W. and Grody, W.W. (1992). AIDS and the heart: review and consideration of pathogenetic mechanisms. *Cardiovascular Pathology*, **1**, 53–64.

Lipshultz, S.E., Orav, E.J., Sanders, S.P., Hale, A.P., McIntosh, K., and Colan, S.D. (1992). Cardiac structure and function in children with human immunodeficiency virus infection treated with zidovudine. *New England Journal of Medicine*, **327**, 1260–1265.

15.14.3 The hypereosinophilic syndrome and the heart

C. J. F. SPRY

Introduction

The inner third of the heart is structurally and functionally distinct from other areas of the myocardium. This region – the endomyocardium – can be involved in a serious type of restrictive cardiomyopathy called endomyocardial fibrosis (EMF). In this disorder, a layer of fibrotic tissue develops within the endomyocardium. The stiff scar tissue lining the heart prevents it from relaxing or contracting properly. The fibrous tissue may be covered with thrombus, which reduces the size of the ventricular cavities.

There are two types of endomyocardial fibrosis, one of which is due to damage produced by eosinophils in patients with hypereosinophilia – eosinophilic endomyocardial fibrosis – and one that to pathologists appears identical, but is found principally in patients living 5° north and south of the Equator – tropical endomyocardial fibrosis. The cause of the tropical form of the disease remains unknown. It is discussed in Chapter 15.14.1.

In past years endomyocardial fibrosis was often rapidly fatal. Patients were diagnosed at a late stage when they were already in gross heart failure. They died suddenly from arrhythmias or massive emboli from the left or occasionally the right ventricle. Today, it is possible to diagnose the disease at an early stage. Medical treatment is designed to prevent its progression to the late fibrotic stage. When this occurs (about 50 per cent of patients with the disease present at the late stage), open heart surgery is now available in many centres to resect the fibrous tissue and replace the atrioventricular valves, which are usually also affected. In these patients the prognosis is often determined more by the cause of the underlying eosinophilia than by the heart disease itself. Recent work aimed at finding out the reasons why some patients in areas free from most parasitic diseases develop persistent eosinophilia is discussed in Chapter 22.5.7. This section describes the cardiological features of eosinophilic endomyocardial disease.

Aetiology

The mechanism of injury to the heart in patients with hypereosinophilia is now clear: eosinophil granules contain several proteins that can kill large parasites which invade tissues. When these are released in the heart, they damage the endocardium. The proteins that cause this damage are the eosinophil ribonucleases and eosinophil major basic protein. *In vitro*, these proteins can insert themselves into the sarcolemma and interfere with myocardial mitochondrial respiration by inhibiting pyruvate dehydrogenase. Large amounts of both are seen in cardiac biopsies from patients in whom the disease affects both ventricles. Damaged myocytes are replaced by extensive layers of scar tissue. As fibrosis progresses it distorts the shape and contractile functions of the inner third of the heart, and prevents normal operation of the atrioventricular valves. Thrombus can also form within the ventricular cavities. This restricts cavity filling even more. The rest of the myocardium responds by becoming hypertrophied. At a late stage in the disease much of the propulsive force of the heart is carried out by the infundibular region of the right ventricle and the outflow tract of the left ventricle, which are (fortunately) never damaged by the toxic eosinophil granule proteins.

It is not known why the endomyocardium should be singled out for eosinophil granule-mediated damage, or why the cardiac lesions develop in only a small proportion of patients with eosinophilia. Skeletal muscle is not affected in these patients. Despite the occurrence of persistent eosinophilia in most patients living in areas where there is dissemination of parasite eggs, the non-tropical form of eosinophil endomyocardial disease is virtually confined to temperate regions with higher standards of public health. The most common underlying disease is the 'idiopathic hypereosinophilic syndrome', although this can occur in patients with eosinophilia induced by malignant diseases. Eosinophilic endomyocardial fibrosis is very rare in women; 90 per cent of the idiopathic form of the disease occurs in men.

Symptoms and signs

The clinical features depend on the stage at which the disease is recognized. These are the early necrotic phase, the later thrombotic phase, and the late fibrotic stage. Patients in the first two stages may have no symptoms of heart disease, when it is often diagnosed by endomyocardial biopsy in patients at risk of the disease. Fifty per cent of patients in the larger clinics specializing in this disease present in the late fibrotic phase. They have symptoms related to the underlying hypereosinophilic disease and, in addition, are usually breathless, with peripheral oedema and decreased exercise tolerance. Unlike patients with the tropical form of the disease, they do not have periorbital oedema, and ascites is less common.

On examination in the late stage of the disease, the most striking features are a rapid pulse of 100 to 130 beats/min at rest, a markedly raised jugular venous pulse, rapid but jerky descent in diastole (rapid early filling comes to a sudden halt), a palpable praecordial pulse over the site of the outflow tract of the right ventricle without a discrete apex beat, and a range of sounds in diastole and systole, most of which are due to the abnormal pattern of blood flow in the ventricles. When the atrioventricular valves become incompetent (this is a very serious late stage complication in the disease) auscultation is dominated by the sounds of mitral incompetence. This is a sign that should promote an urgent decision about surgery and valve replacement.

Investigations

All patients with the hypereosinophilic syndrome (see also Chapter 22.5.7) should have an electrocardiogram, chest radiograph, and M mode and 2D echocardiograms to seek the presence of endomyocardial disease. When these are initially normal, it is sensible to repeat them annually, or possibly more frequently if the eosinophil count has increased. Abnormalities to look for in the electrocardiogram are T wave alterations, which can develop early, bundle branch block, and evidence of hypertrophy. The chest radiograph may be normal but, in the late stage, the cardiac silhouette is often increased, sometimes extending down and to the right with a notch. Pleural effusions are a late feature. The echocardiogram is diagnostic in many patients, and is helped by the stippled pattern of reflection produced by the areas of fibrosis. Early lesions can be detected only by cardiac biopsy, but this is usually reserved for patients who are at highest risk of developing the disease, and who might not otherwise be treated with steroids. Right ventricular cardiac biopsy in these patients should be done only by an experienced investigator, as the fibrotic tissue can be hard to grip with the bioptome forceps, and the infundibulum can be pierced if the catheter head is advanced too firmly beyond the area of fibrosis. Cardiac biopsy should be preceded by ventricular angiography, as thrombus is often more extensive than anticipated. It can be dislodged during the procedure, so particular care has to be taken when it is detected. Histopathologists have no difficulty in finding the characteristic alterations in biopsies of fibrotic or necrotic areas of endomyocardial disease containing degranulated eosinophils and their granule proteins, which can be detected by immunocytochemistry with antibodies to the eosinophil granule proteins. When the biopsy contains only thrombus or tissue from unaffected endomyocardium, the only abnormality that can be detected is the presence of hypogranular eosinophils, a sign that eosinophil degranulation may be taking place in other parts of the heart.

Treatment

Once patients have been found to have eosinophilic endomyocardial disease, the issues to consider are: Can the underlying eosinophilia be treated effectively? Will steroids prevent progression of the damage and scarring already present? Is the patient at risk of thrombotic and embolic lesions from the heart and how best can these be prevented? Is the heart damage so advanced that surgery is needed?

The last question is answered most easily. Surgery should not be delayed until patients are severely incapacitated. When it is carried out, special attention should be given to defining all the areas of scarring and ventricular restriction beforehand, as the endocardium may look relatively normal in the operating theatre, and it is important to remove as much of the scar tissue as possible. There is no consensus on how to treat this disease medically, but patients are usually given prednisolone 7.5 to 15 mg/day in the hope that this drug will reduce the amount of eosinophil granule proteins released into the heart. Often an attempt is made to prevent thrombus formation with the antiplatelet drugs dipyridamole (100 mg four times daily), or low dose aspirin. This is not always successful. If patients have a thrombus in the ventricle at diagnosis, it may be possible to assist its removal with streptokinase infusions. The presence of intracavity thrombus is not an indication for surgery, as thrombus can easily re-form over exposed cardiac muscle after resection of the fibrous tissue. Lifelong anticoagulation with warfarin is indicated for patients who have had valve replacements with endocardial resection, or who have had emboli from either ventricle.

Prognosis

The presence of endomyocardial disease in patients with hypereosinophilia has serious prognostic implications. Whereas 50 per cent of patients with uncomplicated hypereosinophilia live for more than 13 years from diagnosis, survival is probably less than 6 years for patients with heart disease. However, some patients can survive with a good quality of life for over 15 years, as the disease may become less aggressive or respond to treatment.

REFERENCES

Davies, J., Gibson, D.G., Foale, R., Heer, K., Spry, C.J., Oakley, C.M., and Goodwin, J.F. (1982). Echocardiographic features of eosinophilic endomyocardial disease. *British Heart Journal*, **48**, 434–440.

Davies, J., Sapsford, R., Brooksby, I., Olsen, E.G., Spry, C.J., Oakley, C.M., and Goodwin, J.F. (1981). Successful surgical treatment of two patients with eosinophilic endomyocardial disease. *British Heart Journal*, **46**, 438–445.

Davies, J., Spry, C.J., Sapsford, R., Olsen, E.G. de Perez, G., Oakley, C.M., and Goodwin, J.F. (1983). Cardiovascular features of 11 patients with eosinophilic endomyocardial disease. *Quarterly Journal of Medicine*, **52**, 23–39.

Davies, J., Spry, C.J., Vijayaraghavan, G., and De Souza, J.A. (1983). A comparison of the clinical and cardiological features of endomyocardial disease in temperate and tropical regions. *Postgraduate Medical Journal*, **59**, 179–185.

Parrillo, J.E., Borer, J.S., Henry, W.L., Wolff, S.M., and Fauci, A.S. (1979). The cardiovascular manifestations of the hypereosinophilic syndrome. Prospective study of 26 patients, with review of the literature. *American Journal of Medicine*, **67**, 572–582.

Spry, C.J. (1987). Eosinophils and endomyocardial fibrosis: A review of clinical and experimental studies 1980–86. In *Pathogenesis of myocarditis and cardiomyopathy: recent experimental and clinical studies* (eds C. Kawai and W.A. Abelmann), Cardiomyopathy Update, **1**, 293–310. University of Tokyo Press, Tokyo.

Spry, C.J., Davies, J., Tai, P.C., and Fattah, D. (1983). The pathogenesis of eosinophilic endomyocardial disease. In *Immunobiology of the eosinophil* (eds T. Yoshida and M. Torisu), pp. 229–244. Elsevier Biomedical, New York.

Spry, C.J. and Tai, P.C. (1990). Clinical studies on endomyocardial fibrosis in patients with hypereosinophilia: An historical review. In *Restrictive and electric disturbances in heart muscle diseases.* (ed M. Sekiguchi), Cardiomyopathy Update, **3**, 81–98. University of Tokyo Press. Tokyo.

Tai, P.C., Ackerman, S.J., Spry, C.J., Dunnette, S., Olsen, E.G., and Gleich, G.J. (1987). Deposits of eosinophil granule proteins in cardiac tissues of patients with eosinophilic endomyocardial disease. *Lancet*, **1**, 643–647.

Tai, P.C., and Spry, C.J. (1990). Eosinophil effector mechanisms: Studies on the ways in which eosinophils induce endomyocardial fibrosis. In *Restrictive and electric disturbances in heart muscle diseases.* (ed M. Sekiguchi), Cardiomyopathy Update, **3**, 99–107. University of Tokyo Press, Tokyo.

15.15 Congenital heart disease in adolescents and adults

J. SOMERVILLE

Introduction

The general physician, practitioner, casualty doctor, general surgeon, obstetrician, gynaecologist, and student health doctor are each likely to encounter the problems of congenital heart disease only when the patient has passed through childhood and paediatric care. Thus, in the context of internal medicine, it is appropriate to address the topic as it presents in adolescents and in adults. Each year this population in the United Kingdom increases by about 7 per cent because of the success of cardiac surgery in infants and children over the last 20 to 30 years. Survival depends on natural selection or the beneficial effects of surgery. Natural survivors comprise those with mild lesions that do not produce problems until after the second decade and others with more serious complex anomalies, inoperable or who escaped surgery during infancy and childhood, but whose circulatory physiology is compatible with survival. The majority (the 'unnatural'), amounting to about 75 per cent of the whole, are patients who have had cardiac surgery in infancy and childhood. Many live normal lives with few problems, but those with the complex lesions, however well they appear, need the help of an expert. Advice from a paediatric cardiologist will be useful but the problems that arise in adolescence and later are very different from those seen by the paediatrician.

Congenital abnormalities of the heart and cardiovascular system are reported in about 7 to 11/1000 live births. It is doubtful if all the trivial lesions are recognized in childhood and so the true incidence may be higher. During infancy, 50 to 60 per cent of these patients need medical and surgical help. In the first decade after infancy, a further 25 to 30 per cent require the skills of the cardiac surgeon to maintain or improve life.

Only 10 to 15 per cent survive without surgery to adolescence and adult life. Surveys from Liverpool, Switzerland, and the former Czechoslovakia suggest that some 80 per cent of patients with congenital cardiac lesions now reach adolescence or older age.

NATURAL SURVIVORS

Many congenital cardiovascular abnormalities that first come to light in adults have been mild and have caused little or no haemodynamic disturbance during childhood. These include bicuspid or mild aortic-valve stenosis, subaortic stenosis, mitral-valve abnormalities, small ventricular septal defects, atrial septal defects (more commonly secundum than primum), pulmonary-valve stenosis, persistent duct or fistulae, Ebstein's anomaly, and mild coarctation of the aorta. Symptoms develop later in life because of calcification in valves, progressive myocardial dysfunction, infective endocarditis, or the onset of arrhythmias. More serious lesions, such as one-ventricle hearts or large defects with the Eisenmenger reaction or Fallot's tetralogy for instance, will usually have caused symptoms in childhood, but survival without treatment will have resulted from the development of postnatal adaptive changes in the heart or pulmonary circulation. Such changes in form and function may be ultimately destructive, protective or beneficial.

This group of 'natural survivors' whose disease has been modified by time and not by man is small in comparison to the larger numbers of adults and adolescents who have had palliative or direct reparative surgery for congenital cardiac lesions in childhood and infancy. 'Total' correction is a much repeated hope but rarely a reality, at least in the more complex cases.

UNNATURAL SURVIVORS

This larger group is the result of medical progress in management over the last 30 years. These patients require continued medical care; many have residual lesions or cardiovascular disease, the result of the natural evolution of the original lesion. The problems of pregnancy, the genetic risk to offspring, the use or not of the contraceptive pill, the ability to drive a motor vehicle, employment, insurability, and adoption amongst others require expert advice from an informed physician. Although many of the complications suffered by today's survivors will not occur in the adolescents and young adults of 15 to 20 years hence, the problems of current survivors remain.

POSTNATAL ADAPTIVE CHANGES

An understanding of congenital heart disease in adolescents and adults requires knowledge of the adaptive mechanisms that change the form and function of the heart and pulmonary circulation over time. The heart at birth is not anatomically or functionally the same as the heart 10, 20, or 50 years later. A congenital structural defect may remain the same or may alter with time and the effects of disordered haemodynamic forces. The heart and blood vessels have few ways of responding to changes of their environment, but profound and progressive effects on function arise from the structural disorder of the heart and blood vessels, as follows.

1. Progressive hypertrophy of abnormally placed muscular bands may lead to obstruction to pulmonary blood flow as in acquired 'infundibular stenosis', bipartite right ventricle, and some forms of subaortic stenosis where there is abnormal muscle placed beneath the aortic valve, particularly when there is discordant ventricular arterial connection.

2. Deposition of endocardial fibrosis/elastic tissue may develop in architecturally abnormal outflows—for example, fixed subaortic stenosis or fixed infundibular stenosis. These lesions may calcify after 20 years; the same process occurs as a result of endocardial jet lesions, which produce no direct haemodynamic upset but provide a site for thrombus formation and infection.

3. Compensatory hypertrophy of ventricular myocardium in response to obstructive and/or regurgitant valvular lesions or increased peripheral resistance in the pulmonary and systemic circulations progresses with time to fibrosis and irreversible dysfunction.

4. Increasing pulmonary arteriolar disease, by raising pulmonary vascular resistance, reduces or reverses shunts through associated defects (see Chapter 15.24).

5. Spontaneous closure or diminution in size of ventricular septal defects and ducts can occur, through different pathological mechanisms.

6. Valves or outflow tracts may calcify, particularly abnormal semilunar valves or a right-ventricular outflow tract that is narrowed. Anterior calcification may be found lining the right outflow in patients with pulmonary atresia and intact septum, and less frequently when there is an associated ventricular septal defect; thus the tricuspid valve in severe pulmonary stenosis is often the site of annular calcification. Simple congenital valve lesions that have not caused sufficient haemodynamic disturbance to require surgical intervention before the age of 20 years are prone to develop calcification later. The most trivial obstruction caused by a bicuspid aortic valve may not declare itself until the seventh or eighth decades as calcific aortic stenosis. Atrioventricular valves also calcify when subjected to pressure loads imposed by distal obstructive lesions. The time taken for calcification to cause rigidity and increased obstruction depends on the initial degree of obstruction and generally occurs earlier in males. Other factors that determine the speed of calcification of congenitally abnormal valves and outflow tracts include infection, prolonged athletic activity, which may increase local trauma, and altered calcium metabolism.

7. Chordae tendinae of malformed, abnormally attached atrioventricular valves and valves subjected to unusual stresses may rupture. This complication usually causes severe regurgitation and tends to occur late in the natural history of complex anomalies such as univentricular hearts, tricuspid atresia, double-outflow right ventricle, classic transposition of the great arteries, and even with such simple lesions as bicuspid aortic-valve stenosis.

8. Aortic-valve cusps may prolapse into subarterial ventricular septal defects causing aortic regurgitation and signs of spontaneous diminution or closure of the defect.

9. The term myocardial dysplasia describes a malformation of cardiac muscle in which the functional polarity of cells does not follow the normal tensional alignment; myofibrils and groups of cells are related to each other in a bizarre, haphazard, criss-cross fashion. The histological pattern itself appears to be non-specific. Areas of dysplasia may change to cause disturbance of ventricular filling or ejection. The amount and site determines the clinical effects. Dysplasia is extensive in hearts with asymmetrical septal hypertrophy, which may manifest as hypertrophic obstructive cardiomyopathy, midventricular obstruction, diffuse hypertrophic cardiomyopathy, or inflow obstruction of either or both sides or the heart; occasionally it is limited to the apex, giving a very abnormal electrocardiogram.

   Myocardial dysplasia may be found in small areas of normal hearts, particularly in the ventricular septum, but is usually more extensive in the myocardium of patients with structural congenital cardiac anomalies. When dysplastic muscle is subjected to pressure strains from distal obstructions that normally lead to hypertrophy, such as aortic stenosis, coarctation or pulmonary stenosis, there is a disproportionate increase in local muscle mass, which in itself may contribute to obstruction to inflow or outflow, disturbance of normal ventricular contractile patterns, and other functional disorders not accounted for by the effects of simple, concentric ventricular hypertrophy alone.

The clinical manifestations related to the presence of excessive myocardial dysplasia occur in certain patients with congenital aortic-valve stenosis with disproportional septal bulging or late mitral-valve prolapse or dysfunction; they may also occur in patients with a small ventricular septal defect and an inexplicably large left ventricle, in pulmonary-valve stenosis, and in atrial septal defect with a strange-looking left ventricle and mitral regurgitation. These examples show that there is often more disease in the heart than the structural defect alone on which the clinician's attention tends to be focused. The importance for the physician is that congenital heart disease is often congenital cardiovascular disease and as such may manifest some unexpected, late, cardiovascular problems. The obvious example is in coarctation of the aorta, when despite correction there is much residual disease.

Changes in cardiac form that develop in response to disordered anatomy and physiology may be initially beneficial for survival but later the effects are excessive, leading to death in childhood, adolescence, or adult life. Changes in form require time to develop and this is the invariable factor that accounts for the differences between hearts in newborns and infants and hearts of adolescents and adults. It is likely that if structural lesions can be corrected early, many of these adverse adaptive changes will be prevented.

Morphological changes within the heart and vessels continue in patients who have had extracardiac palliative surgery that prolongs survival, a factor to consider when deciding the timing of more definitive surgery.

In this section, only the effects of congenital heart disease in adults and adolescents are emphasized. This selected group of patients does not include all lesions and has special features different from those described in paediatric cardiology textbooks. The vital role of cross-sectional echocardiography in diagnosis and management is discussed in Chapter 15.4.3.

CLASSIFICATION

For nomenclature of congenital heart diseases, a text on paediatric cardiology should be consulted.

No classification is entirely satisfactory, but for the clinician concerned with congenital heart disease what matters is not how had the lesion developed, but rather what effects has it produced. The segmental approach to the nomenclature of congenital heart disease has helped indexing and communication, particularly amongst those concerned with complex malformations. It is doubtful if it aids understanding for those who need an introduction to patient management.

One approach is to discuss anomalies of the heart according to the effects on the pulmonary circulation, that is by dividing conditions into those with increased, decreased, or normal pulmonary blood flow. This is unsatisfactory as, with the same basic lesion, it may change during the patient's life, so that the same anatomical defect in the heart could properly be classified in different groups at different points in the evolution of the disease.

Another possibility is to divide lesions into those that affect primarily the right or left sides of the heart, and leave the septal defects in a special category, separating them from lesions with anomalies of connection. When multiple lesions coexist, it is difficult to decide which is the prime abnormality and the correct categorization.

Recognizing that it is not ideal, lesions are here separated into cyanotic and acyanotic. Like the pulmonary blood flow, this can change but it is an easy starting place as the presence of cyanosis is easily recognized.

Cyanotic congenital heart disease

Central cyanosis is seen when the arterial oxygen saturation is below 85 per cent; lesser degrees of arterial desaturation are not obvious at the bedside. When the patient is anaemic, cyanosis may not be obvious despite reduced arterial oxygen saturation. If the presence of central cyanosis is doubtful at rest, exercise or warmth should make it obvious. It is associated with clubbing of the fingers and toes unless arterial desaturation has been established recently. Clubbing of the nails varies from mild heaping up and shininess of the nail beds seen first in the thumbs, to the classic 'drumstick' fingers and toes of severe chronic cyanotic heart disease. Extracardiac problems are found in adolescents and adults with cyanotic congenital heart disease. These need recognition as they may cause symptoms that are more or as troublesome as the symptoms from the basic cardiac defect.

POLYCYTHAEMIA

In a normal, nourished adult with cyanotic congenital heart disease who takes and absorbs adequate iron and vitamins, the compensatory polycythaemia should be proportional to the systemic arterial desaturation, but in adolescents and adults the haemoglobin and haematocrit are often extremely high. This causes increased blood viscosity and secondary symptoms: muzziness, headaches, and 'slowing up' as well as the tendency to spontaneous thromboses. Venesection, 500 to 750 ml, relieves such symptoms. The patient frequently knows when it is time for venesection. The ideal haemoglobin concentration is 17 to 18 g/dl but in patients in whom concentration regularly reach levels of 23 to 25 g/dl it is dangerous to reduce the level acutely to below 20 g/dl. In patients with values exceeding 20 g/dl there is a place for venesection and

replacement before cardiac or extracardiac surgery to prevent thromboses during or soon after the procedure.

Venesections should be done with the patient at rest for a period of hours. The volume removed must be replaced by a volume expander such as dextran or plasma; Haemocel is preferable to dextrose 5 per cent but is not ideal as it does not stay in the vascular compartment for long enough. More than 1000 ml of blood should not be removed at one session, and if this order of venesection is needed, it should be done on two separate occasions separated by at least 24 h. The common practice of venesection without fluid replacement is dangerous, particularly in patients with the Eisenmenger reaction, and should be abandoned. Patients feel weak for 5 to 10 days after excessive venesection, particularly if volume has not been replaced. The use of normal saline for replacement may precipitate thrombosis. Many cyanotic patients are made ill or anaemic by injudicious use of venesection without the correct volume replacement or because of excess zeal. Equally, if the procedure is done correctly, it will alleviate general symptoms.

GOUT

An elevated blood uric acid is common in cyanotic heart disease in both sexes, perhaps because of increased red-cell turnover and associated impaired renal function in adult cyanotic patients. There may be attacks of acute gout in classical sites in males and, less commonly, females. Wrong diagnosis of this complication is common and patients are often erroneously treated for chronic whitlows, paronychia, or traumatic arthritis. Thiazide diuretics may precipitate the problem but triamterene, spironolactone, and amiloride do not. Tophi have been reported in men with congenital heart disease but not yet in women. Surgical relief of cyanosis prevents polycythaemia and subsequent gout. Allopurinol and aspirin are useful. Indomethacin taken for too long (over 2 weeks) may precipitate deterioration in renal function, causing subsequent cardiac dysfunction. This is particularly dangerous in the otherwise well-compensated Eisenmenger patient.

RENAL PROBLEMS

The pathology of the kidney in the adult with cyanotic congenital heart disease is abnormal, with thickening of the glomerular basement membrane; the first signs of renal dysfunction are albuminuria and sometimes microscopic haematuria with a few casts. Later, creatinine clearance is reduced and oliguria, even anuria, may follow dehydration from any cause. This can be prevented by awareness and provision of adequate fluid intake by mouth and/or intravenously. Diuretics must not be given to maintain urine flow until fluid and electrolyte deficits have been adequately replaced. Patients with long-standing polycythaemia and reduced circulating plasma volume are at risk of an acute deterioration in renal function in relation to minor or major surgical procedures. Large doses of contrast media are known to provoke acute renal failure on occasion (see Chapter 20.16) and the risk is probably greater when patients are volume depleted. Hypertonic contrast media increase plasma osmolarity and may thereby cause cerebral or pulmonary oedema in patients with impaired renal function who cannot excrete the osmotic load.

Short periods of intermittent peritoneal haemodialysis or haemodiafiltration may be needed in some patients with cyanotic congenital heart disease, but they readily develop complications such as sepsis, thrombosis or paradoxical emboli, which are often fatal. Prevention of oliguria and anuria by early administration of fluid in 'at risk' patients helps prevent serious problems.

SKIN SEPSIS

Adolescents and young adults with cyanotic congenital heart disease frequently have serious, widespread, pustular acne that is more extensive than in the normal adolescent. Spontaneous systemic sepsis from this is unusual but wounds heal poorly with or without acne and stitches should be left in longer than in other patients. Systemic infection following surgery is common in these patients. Non-absorbent suture material or large knots in the subcutaneous layers should be avoided. The responsibility for wound closure should not be left to juniors unaware of such problems.

Attention to skin is vital before surgery and the advice of a dermatologist is useful. Improvement of the arterial oxygen saturation relieves the problem.

GUMS

Patients with long-standing polycythaemia and central cyanosis frequently have troublesome, bleeding, 'spongy' gums. Periodontitis and tooth loss occur prematurely, sometimes hastened by an associated enamel defect. Early and constant attention to oral hygiene is necessary.

THROMBOSIS AND BLEEDING

Spontaneous venous and, less commonly, arterial thromboses are a natural consequence of increased blood viscosity. Their occurrence is reduced by regular venesection and the avoidance of dehydration, prolonged immobilization, and oestrogen contraceptive pills. Low-oestrogen preparations have been associated with thromboembolism in patients with haemoglobin levels over 16 g/dl but can be prescribed with minimal risk in the mildly cyanosed with lower haemoglobin levels.

Any invasive procedure, including venepuncture or intravenous infusion, may precipitate venous thrombosis. This is dangerous because of the risk of paradoxical emboli causing strokes and cerebral abscess. Attacks of spontaneous cortical and cerebral venous thrombosis occur in those with very high haematocrits and mimic the symptoms of cerebral abscess; differential diagnosis can be made by computerized tomographic scanning or magnetic resonance imaging of the brain. Haemodilution is the first treatment.

In thrombotic lesions outside the brain, anticoagulants may be used, provided the patient is in hospital. The potential danger of haemorrhage is then always present because control is difficult, particularly in patients with irreversible pulmonary vascular disease (Eisenmenger reaction). Thus, long-term anticoagulation in outpatients are best avoided. If the clinical situation demands anticoagulants, for example when venous thrombosis is spreading in pulmonary arteries or systemic veins, or because of recurrent emboli (uninfected), small intravenous injections of heparin sufficient to prolong the bleeding time slightly above normal and measures to reduce platelet stickiness are recommended. Conventional doses of heparin are contraindicated because of the likely danger of catastrophic haemorrhage. Subcutaneous and intramuscular injections of heparin may cause large haematomas and should be avoided. If bleeding complicates anticoagulation, caution is required in reversing the anticoagulant effects, as thrombotic incidents develop readily. Particular care is needed after catheterization because of the risk of thrombosis in the vein used for access; transient strokes may occur in polycythaemic patients after catheterization.

Aspirin and/or dipyridamole are less hazardous and less effective than heparin but can lead to haemorrhage, particularly epistaxis and gastrointestinal. If aspirin is given it should be in the soluble buffered form, administered after meals.

Spontaneous bleeding, except from the gums, is uncommon except after trauma or surgery such as tonsillectomy, tooth extraction, or operations in which vascular adhesions are cut. Cyanotic patients with long-standing, severe polycythaemia often have multifactorial clotting defects and defective thromboplastin generation. Assessment of clotting function is needed before any surgery and fresh blood, plasma, and sometimes platelet transfusion should be available.

RELATIVE ANAEMIA

Paradoxically, it is possible for cyanotic patients to be relatively 'anaemic' even when the haemoglobin is above 14 g/dl. The haemoglobin concentration may then not be high enough for tissue oxygenation when cardiac function is impaired, or the red cells may not be the correct size and shape for optimum oxygen transport. In a very cyanosed patient a haemoglobin of 16 to 17 g/dl may represent important anaemia and, if long standing, may cause the heart to be larger than usual or even precipitate unexpected heart failure in sinus rhythm. The blood film may show signs of iron deficiency or macrocytosis but this is often not studied when the haemoglobin is normal, that is 14 g/dl or more. Iron, folic acid, or vitamin B_{12} replacement should be given when dietary deficiency has been demonstrated. Anaemia in cyanotic heart disease is uncommon unless there is dietary deficiency, as occurs in patients from developing countries, because of 'food fads', or after gastrectomy or repeated loss from menorrhagia or gastrointestinal lesions. Anaemia is one of the causes of malaise in cyanotic patients and is usually missed when the haemoglobin is above 14 g/dl. When the haemoglobin reaches appropriate levels for the arterial desaturation, iron therapy should be stopped to prevent excess polycythaemia, which readily occurs.

CEREBRAL ABSCESS

This diagnosis should be considered and excluded in any cyanotic patient with congenital heart disease who presents with stroke, new headache and vomiting, personality change, transient weakness or paraesthesiae, or unexplained low-grade fever and apathy. It may be a lethal complication in adult patients with the Eisenmenger reaction, probably because of circulatory disturbances induced by toxicity, anaesthesia, or secondary haemorrhage.

PREGNANCY

Patients with all forms of cyanotic congenital heart disease have difficulty in carrying a fetus to term. The main problem is the high incidence of spontaneous abortions between weeks 10 and 20. This may be caused by abnormality in the fetus or its death from hypoxia. Patients with moderate cyanosis (excluding Eisenmenger), and arterial saturation above 85 per cent, and with haemoglobin below 17 g/dl may carry to term without a problem, but there is a high incidence of premature and low birth-weight infants. Such patients need careful obstetric management, with rest, short labour, prevention of dehydration to minimize the fall in arterial saturation, and immediate attention to sepsis and to thrombotic or haemorrhagic complications. Pregnancy in patients with the Eisenmenger reaction exceptionally results in a live, normal child. It is a risk to the mother's life, may accelerate deterioration, and should be discouraged, ideally prevented. Unfortunately, termination carries risks but if done early these are less than those of pregnancy.

CONTRACEPTION

High-oestrogen contraceptive pills are absolutely contraindicated, and there is a small but definite risk of thrombosis and embolic complications in cyanotics taking low-oestrogen preparations. A randomized trial is needed but is impossible in view of the relatively small number of patients. Ill effects of contraceptive pills occur in the first 3 to 6 months of administration and patients should be warned to report any symptoms early and of the problems associated with taking the low-oestrogen pill. Progesterone-only pills have fewer risks but are not completely protective, may make the woman feel unwell, as well as having a bad effect on the skin. Sterilization may be the best solution if pregnancy is contraindicated or unwanted, but even this relatively minor operation has risks in patients with Eisenmenger reaction and should be done only in optimal circumstances.

ARTHRITIS

Adolescents and adults with chronic, cyanotic, congenital heart disease often complain of painful knees, ankles, and sometimes wrists. The periarticular tissues become thickened with severe long-standing clubbing and cyanotic heart disease. Occasionally the joint pains become acute, involving all joints including the spine. There is usually elevation of the plasma uric acid but the symptoms do not resemble gout and specific antigout treatment is not effective. Non-steroidal anti-inflammatory drugs may help but care must be taken because gastric bleeding occurs and fluid retention can precipitate right heart failure. Only relief of the cardiac condition will improve the joint stiffness but chronic thickening of the ankles and knees will persist in the affected adult. The ends of the long bones may become tender, as part of hypertrophic osteoarthropathy, when new bone formation can be seen on radiographs.

TUBERCULOSIS AND PULMONARY PROBLEMS

It used to be said that patients with a low pulmonary blood flow had a tendency to develop pulmonary tuberculosis. Tuberculosis was until recently a rare disease in the United Kingdom, except amongst immigrants, and it has therefore not been possible to substantiate this concept, but tuberculosis should always be considered when haemoptysis occurs in cyanotic patients. A more common cause of haemoptysis in these patients is thrombosis *in situ* causing infarction, and in the Eisenmenger reaction the thrombosis may be in a main right, or less commonly left, pulmonary artery.

CAUSES OF CYANOSIS IN CONGENITAL HEART DISEASE

The haemodynamic disturbances that lead to central cyanosis (systemic arterial desaturation) are:

1. Right-to-left shunt

The desaturated systemic venous blood can pass from the right side of the heart to the left with defects in the atrial, ventricular, or aortopulmonary septa, or a patent foramen ovale. Normally when a defect is present the shunt is from left to right. Shunt reversal occurs in special circumstances such as: (a) pulmonary vascular disease (Eisenmenger reaction); (b) pulmonary arterial stenosis or banding of the pulmonary artery; (c) pulmonary-valve stenosis or atresia; (d) abnormal function of the right ventricle without (a), (b), or (c); (e) tricuspid stenosis/atresia; (f) large Eustachian valve (sometimes called right-sided cor triatriatum) with atrial septal defect or patent foramen ovale. Cyanosis may be seen on exercise after complete repair of the Fallot's tetralogy when the patient foramen ovale remains open.

2. Complete mixing of systemic and pulmonary circulations

This occurs in single atrium, univentricular heart, and common trunk. The severity of central cyanosis depends on complications such as the degree of right ventricular obstruction (pulmonary infundibular or valve stenosis) or the degree of pulmonary vascular disease present; the more severe, the lower is the systemic arterial oxygen saturation.

3. Abnormalities of connection

These are (a) classic transposition of the great arteries when right ventricular blood is ejected directly into ascending aorta and left ventricular blood to the pulmonary artery; (b) inferior or superior vena caval drainage to the left atrium, a condition most unlikely to be seen in adolescents or adults; and (c) total anomalous pulmonary venous drainage, when some right-to-left shunt at atrial level is inevitable in order to maintain systemic blood flow.

4. 'Pulmonary' cyanosis

This occurs in pulmonary arteriovenous fistula and late after anastomosis of the superior vena cava to the pulmonary artery for treatment of tricuspid atresia (Glenn's operation) and other complex anomalies.

Note that (1), (2), and (3) often coexist in various combinations. These categories are not intended as a classification of cyanotic heart disease.

Specific disorders

Fallot's tetralogy

This anomaly consists of two basic abnormalities: (i) a large, subaortic, ventricular septal defect with cephalad borders formed by aortic-valve cusps; and (ii) abnormal, rotated infundibular bands, which can form infundibular stenosis. The pulmonary valve may be mildly stenosed, bicuspid, or normal. Occasionally a suprapulmonary-valve stenosis coexists and may be the main obstruction in Fallot's patients who survive to adult life. Pulmonary arterial anatomy is variable. It depends on the size of pulmonary blood flow, which in turn relates to severity, form of the obstruction, changes in the peripheral pulmonary arterioles, and any earlier attempts to improve pulmonary blood flow by 'shunts'. The other two classic features of the 'tetralogy', right ventricular hypertrophy and overriding aorta, are secondary to (i) and (ii).

In adults ('natural survivors') the pulmonary arteries are usually well developed, although exceptionally survival occurs with hypoplastic pulmonary arteries. The ventricular septal defect is often doubly committed subarterial (that is beneath both semilunar valves) in adults who have not required a shunt in childhood and is associated with part of the infundibular septum being missing, so there is no history of cyanotic attacks. Added problems in adults include calcification of the pulmonary valve (after 25 years), aortic regurgitation, and right ventricular failure after 40 years with extensive fibrosis of the myocardium.

SYMPTOMS AND PRESENTATION

Effort dyspnoea related to hypoxia is usual and there may be symptoms from polycythaemia. Rhythm disturbances include atrial fibrillation (after 40 years), supraventricular tachycardia, and spontaneous ventricular ectopics from the right ventricle. Right heart failure is uncommon below 40 years, but may be precipitated by pregnancy, rhythm disturbances, or chronic anaemia from non-cardiac causes and infection. Infective endocarditis occurs and involves the aortic valve, with jet lesions on the tricuspid valve from the contiguous aortic-valve cusp (right coronary); less frequently the mitral valve becomes involved but not the pulmonary valve or ventricular septal defect.

SIGNS

Clubbing and cyanosis occur in varying degrees depending on the severity of the right ventricular obstruction and age of the patient. Pulses are full and carotid pulsation is prominent. The aortic pulsation may be palpable in the suprasternal notch, often visible and even palpable to the right of the sternum with a right aortic arch; 'a' and 'v' waves are easily seen in the jugular venous pulse (often with a pronounced 'c' wave), which may be elevated with rapid 'x' descent if there is right heart failure. There is only a giant 'a' wave in the jugular venous pulse if there is an added obstructive lesion proximal to the ventricular septal defect, gross pulmonary regurgitation, or rare associated hypertrophic cardiomyopathy. The right ventricular impulse is palpable but not the left unless there is an additional lesion such as aortic regurgitation.

The clinical diagnosis of tetralogy of Fallot is characterized by a 'tetralogy' of signs—cyanosis, right ventricular hypertrophy, single second sound (aortic), and pulmonary ejection systolic murmur. Other similar lesions share these signs, which may be modified by age and severity of the obstruction.

The length and intensity of the ejection systolic murmur is related to the severity of the pulmonary stenosis. The murmur increases or remains unchanged on expiration and is maximal at the second or third left interspace, being conducted to the left and not to the right of the sternum. The milder the stenosis the more the pulmonary flow and the longer and louder is the murmur associated with thrill in the mildest cases. The student may meet patients considered to have 'acyanotic Fallot'. This term, used by Wood, refers to the condition of a large, subaortic, ventricular septal defect and moderate infundibular stenosis, which has allowed a normal or increased pulmonary blood flow initially; cyanosis appears later or after effort but is not always present at rest. The murmur is so loud and long that it sounds like the murmur of a ventricular septal defect and may be difficult to distinguish. With severe obstruction the murmur is very short, and is absent in pulmonary atresia. The systolic murmur diminishes with fever, hot weather, and inhalation of amyl nitrite or any other cause of vasodilation. No murmur arises from the ventricular septal defect in Fallot because it is so large.

Variable added signs include an ejection click from the dilated aorta, which is common in Fallot patients over the age of 20 years. There may be a late, delayed, diastolic murmur (after P2) when the pulmonary valve is calcified. Aortic regurgitation occurs through the right aortic cusp into the right ventricle causing an immediate diastolic murmur that may be associated with right heart failure and widening of pulse pressure. The venous pressure increases when regurgitation is severe because of reflux into the right as well as the left ventricle. When right heart failure develops, a pansystolic murmur appears low at the left sternal edge from tricuspid regurgitation. The left ventricle enlarges if there has been a previous functioning shunt or aortic regurgitation.

INVESTIGATIONS

ECG

Electrocardiographic features of Fallot's tetralogy are: (a) right atrial hypertrophy (moderate 3–4 mm P pulmonale); (b) right axis deviation; (c) right ventricular hypertrophy with mild ST depression or limited T inversion; (d) right bundle-branch block only in older patients with a dilated right ventricle; (e) good QR pattern in V_6 in adults but this is uncommon in children; and (f) the P–R interval can be lengthened in patients over the age of 40 years; it is not a feature in younger patients.

Radiology

The chest radiograph usually shows a normal-sized heart but there may be an increase after the age of 40 years, in pregnancy, chronic anaemia, or when there is added aortic regurgitation. There is evidence of right ventricular enlargement with a large ascending aorta and knuckle (Fig. 1); the aortic arch is right-sided in 15 per cent. The branches of the pulmonary artery are visible, the left usually larger than the right. Pulmonary blood flow is almost normal but may be diminished depending on severity. With very severe obstruction, uncommon in adults, there are small pulmonary arteries with a speckled appearance in the lungs, marked around the bronchi, due to acquired bronchopulmonary collaterals. There is a characteristic pulmonary 'bay' where the main pulmonary artery is normally seen. The infundibular chamber is often prominent and dilated on the left cardiac border. Dilatation of the main pulmonary artery is uncommon but may be seen in adults where there has been a raised pulmonary blood flow during infancy. Large (aneurysmal) pulmonary arteries are present when there is an associated 'absent' pulmonary valve. A left-sided superior vena cava is visible in 10 to 15 per cent.

Haemodynamic changes

Systolic pressures in both right and left ventricles are equal to those in the aorta; right and left atrial pressures are equal unless aortic regurgitation affects one ventricle more than the other. End-diastolic pressures increase after age 35 years and the 'a' wave of the venous pulse is prominent. There is evidence of a right-to-left shunt at ventricular level and sometimes at atrial level if there is an associated atrial septal defect. Systemic arterial oxygen saturation varies from 70 to 90 per cent, depending on the severity of the pulmonary stenosis. The pressure gradient may be present between the pulmonary artery and right ventricular body at infundibular (subvalve), valve, or pulmonary artery level, or a combination of these. The main pulmonary arterial pressure is 10 to 30 mmHg; those in whom the mean exceeds 20 mmHg have usually been through several years without cyanosis at rest and have acquired infun-

dibular obstruction later, having once had a significant left-to-right shunt. True elevation of the pulmonary vascular resistance may occur despite important pulmonary stenosis, so that pulmonary hypertension may be a problem even after radical repair.

Angiography

Right ventricular angiography shows a large, subaortic, ventricular septal defect and right ventricular outflow obstruction (Fig. 2(a,b)). Aortography shows a dilated aortic root and large, tortuous coronary arteries. Aortic regurgitation, generally in the region of the right sinus as well as centrally, may be directed into the right as much or more than into the left ventricle.

TREATMENT

Complete repair is the ideal treatment, euphemistically referred to as 'total correction'. If the haemoglobin exceeds 21 g/dl and there is near pulmonary atresia, there may be a place for a preliminary shunt procedure to reduce the red-cell mass and the early complications of polycythaemia; in cases so managed, complete repair should be done 6 to 12 months later.

Grown-up patients with Fallot's may have symptomatic benefit from late, radical, definitive repair but may require pulmonary-valve replacement and have a higher morbidity than in children from perioperative complications such as sepsis, haemorrhage, renal failure, persistent right heart failure, and prolonged low arterial Po_2.

ASSOCIATED CONGENITAL CARDIAC ANOMALIES

Other common associated congenital cardiovascular abnormalities are: (a) left superior vena cava in 15 per cent; (b) right aortic arch in 16 per cent; (c) coronary artery abnormality—a septal branch aberrantly crossing the right-ventricular outflow tract is the most important because it may prevent the ideal ventriculotomy and necessitate the use of a valved conduit to bridge the right ventricular obstruction; (d) atrial septal defects (secundum) in 8 per cent (pentalogy of Fallot); (e) aortic-valve

Fig. 1 Chest radiograph from a 25-year-old patient with Fallot's tetralogy showing normal heart size, pulmonary bay, small pulmonary arteries in the hila, and right aortic arch.

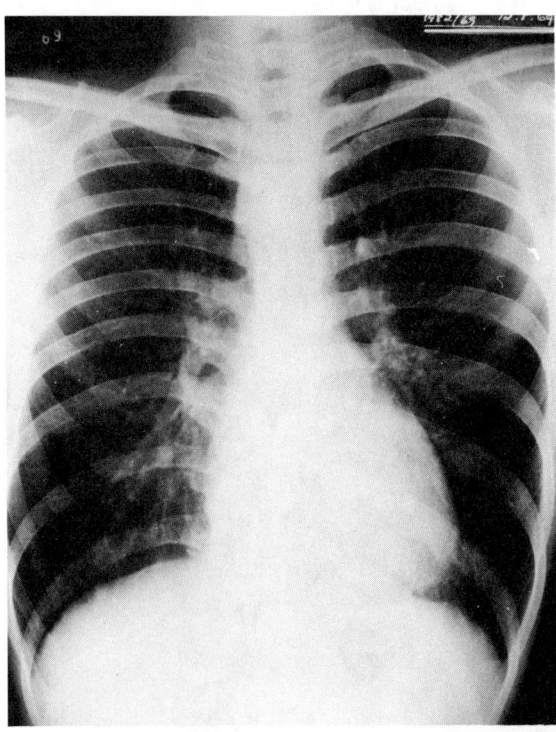

abnormality, fused or bicuspid in 3 per cent; (f) an additional ventricular septal defect in the muscular septum or an other site (5 per cent); (g) subaortic stenosis, which may form proximal to the septal defect either before operation or after a repair; (h) associated hypertrophic cardiomyopathy, which distorts the electrocardiogram and may produce associated mitral regurgitation or subaortic stenosis as part of diffuse cardiovascular disease.

VARIANTS OF FALLOT THAT CAN SURVIVE TO ADOLESCENCE OR ADULT LIFE

1. Absent pulmonary valve

In this syndrome, the pulmonary valve has failed to form. There may be little lumps of tissue at the site of the dilated valve ring. Usually this

Fig. 2 (a) Anteroposterior view of right ventricular angiogram from a patient with mildly cyanotic Fallot's tetralogy. This shows fixed infundibular stenosis (arrow) beneath a domed pulmonary valve. Medial to this the contrast peaks up beneath the aortic cusps above the large ventricular septal defect (not seen in this view). (b) Lateral angiogram from a patient with mildly cyanotic Fallot's tetralogy showing infundibular stenosis (lower arrow), domed pulmonary valve (upper arrow), and good-sized pulmonary artery (PA). Ao = aorta; VSD = ventricular septal defect.

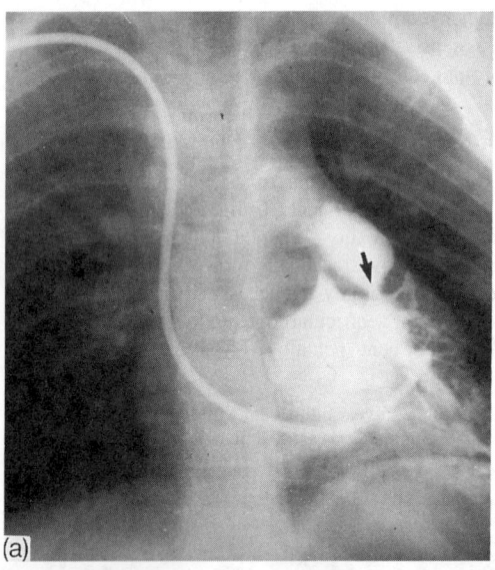

(a)

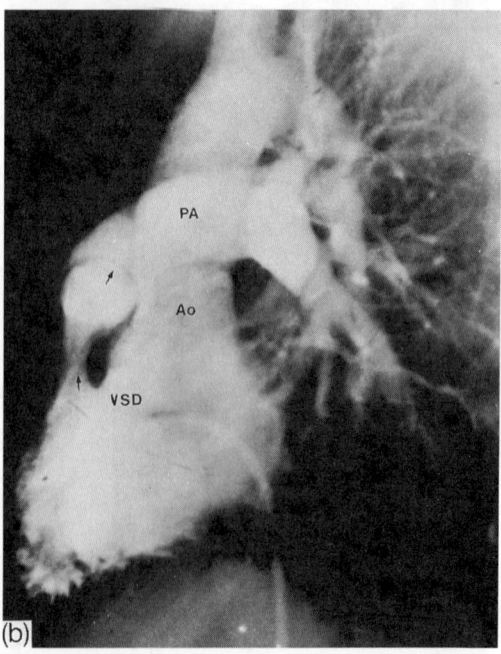

(b)

anomaly is associated with a subaortic ventricular septal defect and displaced infundibular bands that will, with time, form an infundibular stenosis. The patients then usually present as Fallot's tetralogy with atypical features such as an impressive diastolic murmur (pulmonary regurgitation)—surprisingly not always present—and the characteristic aneurysmal dilatation of the pulmonary arteries, sometimes with an absent pulmonary valve. A right aortic arch may coexist with stenosis in the main pulmonary artery contralateral to the aorta. Cyanosis is relatively mild, depending on the degree of pulmonary stenosis in the infundibulum or main-branch pulmonary artery. Patients tend to present in the neonatal period with obstructive emphysema and right heart failure, but if they survive this period and slowly acquire infundibular stenosis (which may cause 'spells') they can reach adolescence and even adulthood. Absent pulmonary valves may also occur without a ventricular septal defect, presenting as lone pulmonary regurgitation and right heart failure in adult life.

2. Absence of the body of the 'crista' or infundibular ventricular septal defect

Older patients with Fallot's tetralogy appear with this variant, in which the subaortic defect encroaches into the outflow tract beneath the pulmonary valve; the rotated septal band of the infundibulum (crista) is absent. The degree of cyanosis depends on the severity of pulmonary-valve stenosis; cyanotic attacks do not occur and this is an angiographic diagnosis to be distinguished from double-outlet right ventricle. It is important because there are special surgical problems.

DIFFERENTIAL DIAGNOSIS OF FALLOT

The quartet of cyanosis, right ventricular hypertrophy, ejection systolic murmur, and single second sound (aortic), which are the signs of Fallot, also occur with other lesions. Pulmonary stenosis with reversed interatrial shunt (closed ventricular septum) must be distinguished. The presentation of other anomalies with ventricular septal defects and pulmonary stenosis may also resemble Fallot; although the physiology is similar, anatomical complications and natural history differ so that accurate diagnosis is needed. Echocardiography is helpful in this context.

Below are summarized the cardinal clinical features of these conditions that more or less closely mimic Fallot.

1. One ventricle and pulmonary stenosis

This is compatible with longevity. The ventricle is of right ventricular morphology with a rudimentary chamber posteriorly or left ventricular morphology with an anterolateral rudimentary chamber, or indeterminate with no chamber. Those with pulmonary stenosis and 'left ventricle' have the best prognosis, influenced by the associated lesions. Those with 'right ventricle' can reach the early thirties irrespective of the type of palliation. The onset of atrial fibrillation and failure herald serious deterioration and have been seen in the sixth decade.

2. Corrected transposition

Atrioventricular discordance, ventricular arterial discordance with ventricular septal defect and pulmonary stenosis.

3. Double-outlet right ventricle with ventricular septal defect and pulmonary stenosis

In this, both great arteries arise from the right ventricle and the defect is usually subaortic in the few who reach adult life. There is aortic and mitral discontinuity (evident on echocardiography) and the aortic root 'points' anteriorly. Unless there is pulmonary stenosis the Eisenmenger reaction is to be expected.

4. Transposition of the great arteries

Associated with ventricular septal defect and pulmonary stenosis (atrioventricular concordance, ventricular arterial discordance) When the pulmonary valve stenosis is mild or moderate, these patients may reach adult life and can be expected to have pulmonary hypertension and vascular disease distal to the obstruction.

5. Atrioventricular defect plus pulmonary stenosis

6. Multiple ventricular septal defects or defects not in Fallot position

This is usually diagnosed on biventricular angiography, with infundibular stenosis or pulmonary-valve stenosis. When the septal defect is subtricuspid it may close spontaneously or become small so that the patient loses cyanosis and presents as with progressive, 'lone' infundibular stenosis.

7. Bipartite right ventricle with ventricular septal defect

In these patients there are anomalous muscle bundles that with time hypertrophy to create a 'low' infundibular stenosis dividing the small cavity of the right ventricular inflow below the tricuspid valve from the outflow. A ventricular septal defect may be in any position and when communicating with the right ventricular inflow will be associated with a right-to-left shunt. However, if it is in the inflow, distal to the obstruction, there may be a left-to-right shunt and pulmonary hypertension, particularly when this appears in adolescents or adults. The left ventricular muscle may also be abnormal and should be carefully investigated. The diagnosis of Fallot in the cyanotic patient with pulmonary stenosis must be questioned when:

1. The apex beat is not typical of right ventricular hypertrophy or 'nondescript'. This suggests the possibility of corrected transposition (atrioventricular discordance) or that only one ventricle is present. The tap of a loud first sound may be felt at the apex when there is one large (common) atrioventricular valve.

2. There is a palpable great artery and second sound in the pulmonary area. This occurs when the ascending aorta is anteriorly placed as in true classic transposition (atrioventricular concordance with ventricular arterial discordance) or corrected transposition (atrioventricular and ventricular arterial discordance).

3. The systolic murmur is conducted to the right rather than the left, suggesting that the pulmonary flow is preferentially directed to the right, which is characteristic when the pulmonary artery is posterior as in transposition or other abnormal relations of the great arteries.

4. There is a giant 'a' wave in the jugular venous pressure, which can only occur if the right ventricular pressure exceeds systemic indicating that a ventricular septal defect, if present, is small; or not there at all (intact ventricular septum); or there is a tricuspid obstruction or some unusual lesion on the left side should a large defect have been demonstrated. The giant 'a' is a feature of severe pulmonary valve stenosis with reversed interatrial shunt.

5. Very severe cyanosis and a long, loud, systolic murmur favours the diagnosis of transposition or malposition of the great arteries rather than Fallot, in which the louder the murmur the less is the cyanosis.

6. In the electrocardiogram, left axis deviation, a long P–R interval, right or left complete bundle-branch block (unless associated with Wolff–Parkinson–White syndrome), absent R waves in V_1, V_2, a QR in V_1, and S waves V_1–V_6 are all atypical for Fallot.

7. The chest radiograph has a narrow pedicle, a great artery making a straight shadow on the upper left mediastinal border to the level of the aortic knuckle due to an abnormally placed anterior aorta (Fig. 3). The presence of pulmonary venous congestion, enlargement of the left atrium or a small aortic knuckle signify complications with Fallot or another diagnosis. Any evidence of right or left isomerism (bilateral right or left bronchi) make the diagnosis of Fallot's tetralogy unlikely,

8. The demonstration of a left superior vena cava entering the left atrium or inferior cava entering azygos systems on left or right with situs ambiguus of abdominal viscera make Fallot unlikely.

FALLOT'S TETRALOGY AFTER SURGERY

Patients with Fallot's tetralogy mostly survive because of earlier palliative shunts for hypoxia and cyanotic attacks, or because of radical repair (usually referred to as 'total correction') with closure of the ventricular septal defect and removal of pulmonary stenosis. Only a few reach adult life without earlier surgery. Occasionally, older patients appear with only relief of pulmonary stenosis, either because the ventricular septal defect was left untouched or because it was not closed properly. Such patients have large hearts and are at risk of developing irreversible pulmonary vascular disease.

The aim of systemic-to-pulmonary arterial shunts is to increase pulmonary blood flow, which not only results in reduction of cyanosis but also causes a volume load on the left side of the heart leading to enlargement of both left atrium and left ventricle. Aortic regurgitation is common in such patients in whom shunts have been *in situ* for many years and should be searched for specifically in adolescents and adults who have had such surgery.

There are various types of shunt, named after the surgeon or physician who designed them. Residual pulmonary arterial stenoses often form when shunts have been surgically or naturally closed.

Blalock–Taussig

The subclavian artery is anastomosed to the right or left pulmonary artery. This with time and growth may cause upward kinking of the ipsilateral pulmonary artery. Endarteritis may occasionally develop, with aneurysm formation on the pulmonary artery side. Pulmonary vascular disease sometimes occurs if the shunt is large and left for too long before radical repair.

Subclavian autograft

A subclavian is joined to a pulmonary artery after transection at its origin and reimplantation lower in the descending aorta in order to prevent

Fig. 3 Chest radiograph from a patient with ventricular septal defect and pulmonary stenosis and 'corrected transposition' (ventricular inversion). The ascending aorta is anterior and to the left lying on left upper mediastinal border (arrow) making a longer shadow than a prominent pulmonary artery. Physiology is the same as in Fallot's tetralogy.

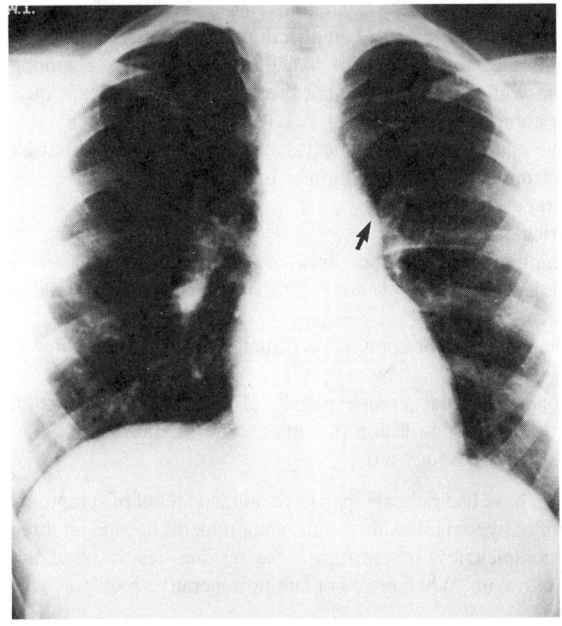

upward kinking of the pulmonary artery. Various modifications have been devised.

Modified Blalock

This technique involves the interposition of a 'Goretex' tube prosthesis between the subclavian artery and ipsilateral pulmonary artery; it has produced good results with less distortion of pulmonary arteries and maintained patency with ideal-sized shunts in infants and children. Such shunts last for 5 years or more but ideally should be removed at the time of definitive repair—when possible within 1 to 3 years. Results appear less satisfactory in adults. A possible complication is a 'seroma' from leakage of serum through the Goretex.

Waterston

Through a right thoracotomy a window is made between the ascending aorta and right pulmonary artery, sometimes referred to as Cooley's anastomosis. Although it provides good palliation, particularly in infants, it is associated with problems from anterior kinking of the right pulmonary artery, pulmonary vascular disease on the right, hypoplasia of proximal pulmonary arteries and overload of the left heart, early tamponade, and aneurysm of the right pulmonary artery; endarteritis occurs rarely.

Potts

Through a left posterolateral thoracotomy, an anastomosis is made between the descending aorta and the left pulmonary artery. Although it may initially relieve symptoms, it is a dangerous shunt, tending to be too large and often damaging the left pulmonary artery by kinking or stenotic occlusion, a frequent cause of irreversible pulmonary hypertension, and it may be difficult to close.

The complications which occur after palliative shunts are:

1. Increasing cyanosis from closure of the shunt or diminution in its size as the patient grows.

2. Acquired atresia of the infundibulum and/or the pulmonary valve.

3. Bronchopulmonary collateral development, particularly when the shunt is small or not patent. These vessels may be large, and when present are uncountable and can cause rib notching. There is a risk of major haemorrhage when adhesions are cut in an area where a previous thoracotomy has been done.

4. 'Subclavian steal': sometimes after a bilateral, long-standing, Blalock operation, the development of collaterals is so extensive that blood is 'stolen' by them from the vertebral artery; the patient may then develop faints on effort or other symptoms of vertebral insufficiency.

5. Cerebral abscess: this is a complication of having a right-to-left shunt, but not the consequence of a palliative anastomosis; among patients living with a man-made shunt there is also a significant incidence of this complication.

6. Infective endarteritis (on aortic valve or shunt), complicated by haemoptysis from aneurysm formation or infection on the shunt.

7. Aortic regurgitation.

8. Biventricular failure.

9. Shortening of an arm and smallness of the ipsilateral hand after an early Blalock has been in situ for over 8 to 10 years, having been done in the first decade.

10. Residual stenoses or complete obstruction in the ipsilateral pulmonary artery.

11. Pulmonary vascular disease (peripheral) related to size, duration in situ, and the underlying lesion (i.e. more common in double-outlet right ventricle and transposition).

Patients who have had radical repair have dramatic relief of symptoms from the relief of hypoxia. Residual signs and problems depend on three factors: the completeness of the repair, the residual lesions, and the duration of follow-up. Whether or not late postoperative problems will be different or reduced with earlier 'correction' in infancy remains to be seen. Certainly, the incidence and type of complications differ in those repaired in the 1970s compared to those in the 1980s.

Clubbing and cyanosis should disappear, but the jugular venous 'a' wave is larger than normal and the right ventricle may remain overactive and even with a palpable bulge if a patch has been used. A systolic ejection murmur is expected, with wide splitting of the second heart sound (related to the complete right bundle-branch block in 85–90 per cent) and a diminished but audible pulmonary component preceding a short diastolic rumble of pulmonary regurgitation. Exceptionally, the patient has no murmurs and a normal second sound. The heart on chest radiographs is usually larger than before operation, globular, with a prominence on the left border from the right outflow tract. Lung vascularity may be normal or may increase with a residual ventricular septal defect or be different in each lung if there is hypoplasia or obstruction in either pulmonary artery; the pulmonary bay fills out by the distended main pulmonary artery. The electrocardiogram should show sinus rhythm, variable patterns of right bundle-branch block, and variable electrical axis. T inversion may be restricted to V_1 or extend to V_5 and persist. T-wave inversion and wide Q waves may be found when there has been prolonged, intraoperative ischaemia.

Echocardiography is reliable for showing the large subaortic patch closing the defect, or any detachment, and for delineating the open outflow and increase in size of the pulmonary artery.

Complications after radical repair of Fallot's tetralogy are numerous and vary considerably according to the surgery performed:

1. Residual ventricular septal defect may be due to patch detachment or a separate lesion; some surgeons of the 1970s never closed the defect completely. Large defects produce right heart failure and should not be left without full investigation and surgical closure, preferably early. Small or moderate defects may do no harm except as a site for future endocarditis.

2. Residual pulmonary stenosis, which may be in a main branch at the site of a previous shunt, in the valve, its ring, or infundibular region. It does not increase in severity unless resection of outflow muscle has been inadequate or the patch edge protrudes into the outflow tract as can occur with double-committed, subarterial, ventricular septal defect.

3. Patent foramen ovale with shunt reversal on effort can occur early or with time, when the surgeon has not closed the foramen and right ventricular function is abnormal, or there is an associated abnormality of the tricuspid valve.

4. Rhythm disturbances are frequent and include: ventricular ectopic beats, which may increase on effort, paroxysmal ventricular tachycardia, and complete heart block, which is now uncommon. This may occur transiently intra- or perioperatively, or late, particularly if there has been transient block earlier in the perioperative period. Paroxysmal supraventricular tachycardia, most commonly atrial flutter or atrial fibrillation, may develop after 10 to 20 years. Residual lesions such as important pulmonary stenosis or regurgitation, or residual ventricular septal defect, may predispose; their presence causes serious symptoms with such arrhythmias. These rhythm disorders may then be related to cannulation, atrial incisions, particularly when transatrial closure of the defect has been used, or damage to the sinus node. Nodal tachycardias occur occasionally and usually are related to reoperation for closure of the defect, or its more posterior subtricuspid extension. Sinus arrest or bradycardias occur unexpectedly and late after repair, probably related to intraoperative damage of the nodes. These problems have been less common in the last decade with improved understanding of the anatomy of the sinus node and its arterial supply. The seriousness of atrial flutter cannot be overestimated. It should stimulate a search for haemodynamic causes, which may be removable, be recognized as a marker for possible sudden death, receive urgent therapy to cardiovert, and requires anticoagulation. The value of preventive medical therapy is an important consideration, but which of amiodarone, quinidine, digoxin or β-blocker might be most effective requires trial.

5. Infective endocarditis, which is uncommon after radical repair,

occurs with residual defects, open systemic-to-pulmonary shunts or on the aortic valve if already regurgitant, however slightly. There is little indication to protect patients after repair of Fallot with only pulmonary regurgitation/stenosis unless the other residual lesions are present and a prosthetic or biological valve has been used.

6. Right ventricular aneurysm, which occurs at the site of a large patch of pericardium in the right outflow tract either below or across the pulmonary valve ring, is uncommon without raised right-ventricular pressure (residual pulmonary stenosis). The aneurysm may increase in the first 1 to 2 years and then remains static, with calcium deposited in the wall. False aneurysms occur early, particularly if there has been sternal infection. Progressive increase in size, with or without elevation of the right ventricular pressure, requires surgical attention. Rupture is rare unless there is infection or a false aneurysm.

7. Pulmonary hypertension: when a large ventricular septal defect persists and there has been good relief of pulmonary stenosis, the patient develops pulmonary vascular disease 10 to 15 years later. Pregnancy can accelerate this process. Such a tragedy should be prevented by early reoperation on the residual defect. This is a more frequent complication after complete repair in adults.

8. Pulmonary regurgitation, which has been considered a benign complication but, when associated with a persistent defect or elevated pulmonary arterial pressure and residual pulmonary arterial stenoses, can cause chronic right heart failure. Without such complications, when severe, as with some transannular patches or excision of the pulmonary-valve cusps, progressive right ventricular dilatation occurs over a decade with ultimate right heart failure at the onset of atrial flutter or fibrillation. Pulmonary-valve replacement should be advised if cardiomegaly is shown to progress and should be done before the right ventricle shows signs of failure; the results of late surgery are not good—the heart remains dilated and prone to arrhythmias. These late effects of pulmonary regurgitation must raise concerns about the long-term future of infants who have received patches across the pulmonary annulus.

9. Aortic regurgitation, which may be iatrogenic or have been missed before the repair as it is common in adolescents and adult Fallot's, particularly when shunts have been established over several years; regurgitation occurs into the right ventricle as well as the left and leads to elevation of the venous pressure with right-sided congestion. Repair may be possible when the lesion is severe or progressive, but valve replacement is usually necessary as the aortic ring is so dilated at this stage.

10. Myocardial failure: patients appear in the first decade of follow-up with large or enlarging hearts without any structural lesion, appearing as dilated cardiomyopathy, related to myocardial damage at surgery either with a long ischaemic time or because myocardial protection was inadequate or unsuitable—a feature before the mid-1970s but uncommon in the 1980s. A line of subendocardial calcification may be visible in the left ventricle in affected patients. Only general measures for chronic congestive failure are useful, including ultimate consideration of cardiac transplantation. Myocardial dysfunction may occur if aberrant coronary arteries have been cut or damaged.

General state after radical repair of Fallot

Patients with well-repaired lesions mostly live normal lives. They may safely take the contraceptive pill, drive cars provided they have had no syncopal attacks, and have a low risk of infective endocarditis. They are also safe to undertake pregnancy in the context of their own health, but there is an increased risk of producing a child affected by congenital heart disease, particularly when the mother has had Fallot's tetralogy. All mothers with congenital heart disease, repaired or not, should undergo careful fetal echocardiography.

Pulmonary atresia with ventricular septal defect

The anatomy of the heart resembles Fallot, with a large, subaortic, ventricular septal defect that may encroach on the outflow tract (unlike Fallot); the right ventricular outflow is blind (atretic) and infundibular

bands are often absent or underdeveloped. The condition is wrongly but understandably referred to as pseudotruncus, as in some patients there is absence of the main pulmonary artery. Others refer to it as extreme Fallot because of the cardiac anatomy. The anomaly of pulmonary atresia and ventricular septal defect has specific problems in relation to the anatomy of the pulmonary artery and systemic blood supply to the lungs (Fig. 4) and therefore needs its own name for proper understanding and management. Patients born with large systemic collaterals to the lungs are referred to as 'complex pulmonary atresia'.

Central arteries may be small (hypoplastic)—characteristically taking the form of a seagull on angiography and frequently not supplying all segments of the lung (Fig. 5). This limits the effectiveness of a surgical shunt and often prevents total correction. Less frequently, and when supplied by a large duct or direct communication with a large systemic collateral artery, the pulmonary arteries are large and supply the majority of lung segments. Such cases have often undergone successful repair in childhood with closure of the defect and use of an homograft valve, which will calcify and degenerate after 15 to 20 years. A few patients reaching adolescence and adult life have no central pulmonary arteries.

In patients with pulmonary atresia and ventricular septal defect the systemic supply to the pulmonary circulation results from:

Fig. 4 Types of pulmonary artery development found with pulmonary atresia and ventricular septal defect. (a) Full set of central pulmonary arteries distal to valve atresia. (b) Right and left central pulmonary arteries without pulmonary trunk. May be confluent or disconnected. (c) One central branch pulmonary artery branching in hilum with absent branch on other side. (d) No central pulmonary arteries.

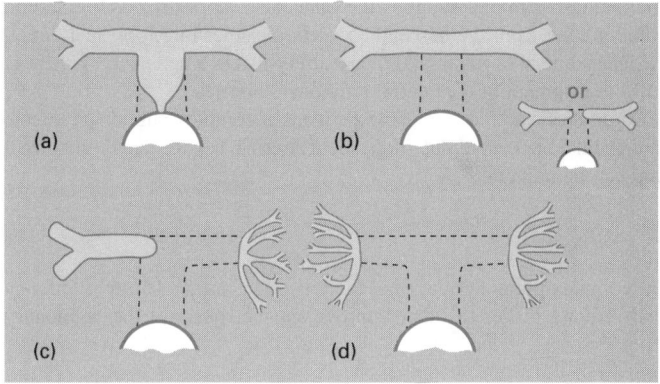

Fig. 5 Hypoplastic pulmonary arteries not supplying all segments of lung on right side from a patient with pulmonary atresia and ventricular septal defect.

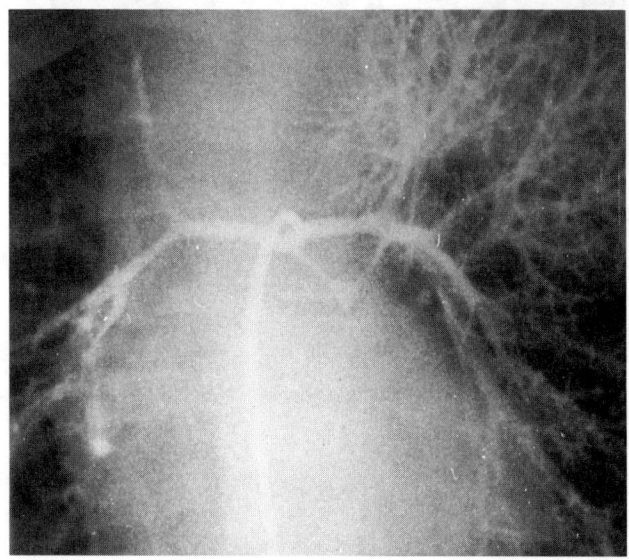

1. Ductus arteriosus: if this is the only supply, closure will lead to acute hypoxia as in the neonate. When the duct remains open in adults it may become aneurysmal with associated pulmonary hypertension.

2. Acquired systemic collaterals: these are multiple, uncountable, spidery, thin-walled, arising from mediastinal and intercostal vessels, and take time to develop; they increase after thoracotomy and account for improvement after a shunt has failed or closed. There is increasing evidence that coronary arteries make a contribution in adults and there may be 'steal' from the coronary circulation causing angina, which may appear after 20 years in some very cyanotic patients.

Patients with a duct or acquired collaterals usually have well-developed central pulmonary vessels, which if perfused and made to grow larger may allow radical repair.

3. Congenital systemic collaterals: when present the condition is referred to as 'complex pulmonary atresia'. These patients can and do survive to be adults, particularly if no earlier palliative or reparative surgery has been attempted. The collaterals usually arise from below the isthmus, exceptionally from the subclavian, and are large, tortuous, countable (1–6), and frequently stenosed at their origins or as they enter the lung from the hilar (Fig. 6). They communicate with the pulmonary arteries at hilar, lobar, or at small-artery level, or within the lung substance, sometimes forming vascular rings around bronchi. They take many forms, often bizarre, supply a lobe or segment or whole lung, or connect directly with pulmonary arteries. In 80 per cent of cases, central pulmonary arteries are 'hypoplastic', in 17 per cent they are large, and in 3 per cent they are absent.

One unusual form (1 per cent) is when a single artery arises from the midthoracic aorta, supplies all branches to the ipsilateral lung, crosses the mediastinum and supplies the other lung, appearing as a common trunk arising from the descending aorta. Another rare form is a direct, coronary artery-to-main pulmonary artery fistula where usually there is full development of the central pulmonary arteries.

Right aortic arch occurs in 45 per cent of complex pulmonary atresia and about 5 per cent of duct-dependent atresia when the duct is abnormal and can be bilateral.

SYMPTOMS

In 'complex pulmonary atresia' there is often cardiac failure in infancy and thriving difficulties that improve spontaneously as the pulmonary

Fig. 6 Large countable congenital systemic collateral arteries arising from the mid descending thoracic aorta in a patient with complex pulmonary atresia.

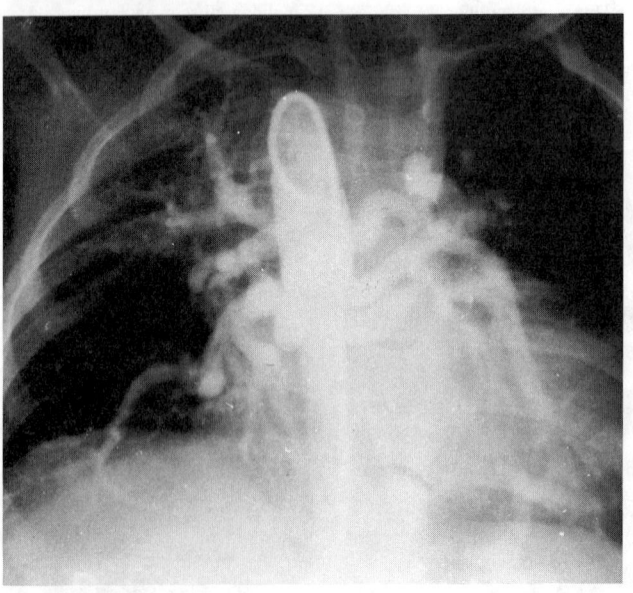

vascular resistance rises or stenoses on collaterals develop with growth, and cyanosis becomes more marked. Such patients have bulged, deformed chests with intercostal recession from reduced lung compliance. They are dyspnoeic from hypoxia due to high pulmonary vascular resistance, which may occur in the second decade but usually later on, with increasing stenoses, failed shunts or thrombosed collaterals. Haemoptysis may arise in adults or they may present with infective endocarditis on the aortic valve or aneurysm on a collateral. Severe kyphoscoliosis is a frequent complication. Those without congenital systemic collaterals share the same symptomatology as Fallot but without a history of cyanotic attacks because the right-ventricular outflow tract is permanently shut and cannot vary. Adults may appear with atrial fibrillation and right heart failure, contributed to by aortic regurgitation. Cerebral symptoms may result from abscesses or transient ischaemic attacks related to polycythaemia. Exceptionally, pulmonary atresia with ventricular septal defect and congenital coronary arterial fistulae may present late. Surgical treatment is then generally hazardous.

Rarely, patients with duct-dependent pulmonary atresia and ventricular septal defect, untreated and those with failed or without 'manmade' shunts, reach adolescence and adulthood. Such patients have severe disability and deep central cyanosis. They may have angina with minimum effort, and syncope or near syncope.

SIGNS

Pulses are full or collapsing. Cyanosis and clubbing are variable. Carotid pulsation is obvious. The aorta is palpable in the neck or, if right-sided (40 per cent), in the right upper chest. The second heart sound is loud and single (A_2). There are no intracardiac murmurs other than the occasional case with aortic reflux, but an aortic ejection click is constant. Continuous murmurs (inspiratory) from congenital systemic collaterals are audible at the back on either side or in the right or left upper chest. Murmurs are absent when there is one huge collateral without stenoses or when peripheral pulmonary vascular disease is severe, as is common in patients who survive beyond 30 years.

PULMONARY ATRESIA AFTER OPERATION

The complications of shunt surgery are the same as in Fallot. However, 'correction' of pulmonary atresia in patients with Fallot-type ventricular septal defect was made possible by the introduction of cadaver aortic homograft valves in 1966. Many patients with this treatment have reached adult life. They have late problems similar to those of Fallot patients but the homograft will require replacement, probably after 20 to 30 years. Calcification, which starts harmlessly in the graft aortic wall and only later affects the cusps, causes stenosis and/or regurgitation. Pulmonary regurgitation is likely to be severe when there is distal obstruction from stenoses. The speed with which valve degeneration develops depends on how it was sterilized (irradiation being disastrously destructive), the residual dynamics, conduit compression, and presence of pulmonary hypertension. The process is quicker in those youngest at the time of surgery.

Late infection of the homograft valves in this position is exceptional. Comparative 'valve survival' studies with other biological prostheses have shown the superiority in durability and lack of problems of the homograft in the right-ventricular outflow tract. Audibility of pulmonary-valve closure (P_2) provides evidence of good, pliable valve function and the loss of P_2 shows that the cusps are calcified.

More problems occur with the Dacron conduits used for extension, which develop intimal peel obstruction and calcification. Late pulmonary hypertension, right heart failure with pulmonary artery stenoses, and left heart failure from the chronic overload from systemic collaterals are more frequent than after Fallot repair.

Pregnancy is possible and the genetic risk to offspring appears no greater than in Fallot. A normal life and employment are possible.

Table 1 *Features which differentiate Fallot from pulmonary stenosis with reversed interatrial shunt*

	Fallot	Pulmonary stenosis with reversed interatrial shunt
Squatting	+ (in children)	−
Cyanotic attacks	+ (not present in adults or adolescents)	−
Giant 'a' wave	−	+
P_2 late, audible	Inaudible; A_2 single	±
Long SM to A_2 or later (late crescendo)	±	−
Palpable aorta	Sometimes	−
Extreme RVH, Steep T inv. V_1–V_4	−	+
Right bundle branch block	− (unless over 40 years)	+
P pulmonale > 5 mm	−	+
Right aortic arch	+ (16%)	−
Main pulmonary artery dilated	− (occasionally when mild)	+
Amyl nitrite ↑ cyanosis; ↓ murmur	+	−

Pulmonary-valve stenosis with reversed interatrial shunt

The cardinal signs of this and Fallot's tetralogy are similar; both appear in adolescents and adults. If the atrial septal defect is large the heart may not be enlarged but if it is small and the pulmonary stenosis is severe, the heart can be large with extreme right ventricular hypertrophy and dilatation.

For simplicity, the classical features that differentiate Fallot from pulmonary-valve stenosis with reversed interatrial shunt are shown in Table 1.

Pulmonary arterial stenoses

Multiple pulmonary arterial branch stenoses occur as part of a generalized congenital arteriopathy (see supra-aortic stenosis below). A single branch stenosis or multiple stenoses may coexist with septal defects, a combination that in adults presents with cyanosis and features of pulmonary hypertension. The wrong diagnosis of inoperable Eisenmenger is often made; the correct diagnosis is suggested by the finding of loud, long, widespread systolic murmurs with signs of pulmonary hypertension and even continuous murmur's which are audible in the anterior chest or axillae when the stenosis is severe but patent. The chest radiograph does not show huge central pulmonary arteries or peripheral pruning, but there may be some enlargement of the main pulmonary arteries with small, 'grape'-like dilatations around the hilum due to post-stenotic dilatations. The prognosis is better than in Eisenmenger reaction, as the obstruction does not progress in adult life whereas the pulmonary arteriolar disease worsens and increases the right-to-left shunt in the Eisenmenger syndrome.

Little is described about the natural history of these patients as multiple pulmonary arterial stenoses are uncommon. Apart from the problems of a chronic right-to-left shunt, they also suffer from right heart failure and supraventricular arrhythmias after 40 years. In addition, aneurysms may form in the thin-walled pulmonary arteries distal to the obstruction, causing haemoptysis, always to be regarded as a serious symptom and likely to herald disaster. Complete obstruction can occur in a large pulmonary artery, resulting in infarction, which is unusual as a collateral blood supply has generally developed; or chronic cough, lung infections, and increased dyspnoea and cyanosis, with the appearance of intense, speckled lung fields and even cavitation from infection on the side of the obstructed pulmonary artery.

Treatment is usually medical as the disease in the pulmonary arteries may be diffuse, often beyond the hilar vessels and therefore not amenable to surgical relief. Balloon dilatation may be helpful but the stenoses are elastic and usually recoil so 'stenting' is required to maintain relief. If the stenosis is in the main pulmonary arteries, surgery may be more successful. Paroxysmal supraventricular arrhythmias are frequent in adults and require control; right heart failure occurs after the age of 40 years. Patients may have associated systemic hypertension (see Supra-aortic stenosis, below) as this is part of diffuse congenital cardiovascular disease in conducting arteries.

Patients with a single branch stenosis and ventricular septal defect or atrioventricular defect or atrial septal defect occur. They show features of pulmonary hypertension, with an inspiratory continuous murmur over one side of the chest. The defect may be correctable by opening of the main branch stenosis but much depends on the state of the arterioles in the other lung.

Acquired pulmonary arterial stenoses in adult life may occur as a result of previous shunts and related distortions or in the left pulmonary artery where the duct closed, or where a pulmonary arterial band has been removed. These acquired lesions are usually amenable to balloon dilatation provided they have not been present for over 10 years as then the fibrous tissue may be hard to break without rupturing the pulmonary artery.

Defects with pulmonary hypertension

Eisenmenger reaction (syndrome)

Wood redefined the Eisenmenger complex as 'pulmonary hypertension at systemic level, due to a high pulmonary vascular resistance with reversed or bidirectional shunt through a large ventricular septal defect'. He pointed out that 'it matters little where the shunt happens to be', and suggested extending the definition of Eisenmenger syndrome to include all other defects associated with such pulmonary hypertension and pulmonary vascular disease. Patients have similar clinical features irrespective of the site of the defect through which the shunt reversal occurs. The syndrome may be found with the defects shown in Table 2.

Certain factors predispose to the establishment of early pulmonary vascular disease. These are associated Down's syndrome, birth at high altitude, associated left-sided lesions with other defects such as mitral stenosis or regurgitation, coarctation, congenitally abnormal lung arteries, multiple chest infections, chronic upper-airways obstruction, diaphragmatic hernia, and perinatal asphyxia. The role of vasoactive substances must be important and requires further study. Patients with atrial

Table 2 *Eisenmenger complex: associated defects*

Ventricular septal defect (VSD)*
Double outflow right ventricle (DORV)*
A–V canal
Truncus
Aortopulmonary defect
Duct (patent ductus arteriosus)*
Transposition of the great arteries (TGA) with VSD, duct, after shunts, rare with ASD
Double inlet ventricle (single, common, uni) ± mitral atresia*
Tricuspid atresia with large VSD
Atrial septal defect (ASD)
Ostium primum
Common atrium
Hemianomalous pulmonary venous drainage
Total anomalous pulmonary venous drainage (TAPVD)
Pulmonary atresia (complex) with large congenital systemic collaterals

*Rarely associated with coarctation which should NOT be operated on in adolescents/adults in this situation.

septal defect generally acquire pulmonary vascular disease later in adolescence or adult life than in the case of other defects when it usually dates from early infancy or childhood, below 2 years.

The prognosis is partly related to the site of the defect; more important is the medical care of the patient. Those with an Eisenmenger duct have the best prognosis and survival to the sixth or even seventh decade, although unusual, has been documented.

SYMPTOMS

Dyspnoea is related to the degree of hypoxia. Patients with a duct have 'blue' arterial blood shunted below the left subclavian artery at first and at this stage are not breathless. Symptoms appear when desaturated blood reaches the head, usually in adolescence with the duct; with the other defects, dyspnoea occurs earlier.

Effort syncope occurs, sometimes early in the disease when hypoxia is not severe. It is a more frequent symptom of primary pulmonary hypertension and is associated with a low fixed cardiac output. Sometimes angina of effort is experienced.

The cardiac reserve is relatively poor so that excess sinus tachycardia with palpitation occurs with exercise, heat or fright. After 35 to 40 years, paroxysmal supraventricular tachycardia is common, particularly with atrial septal defect. The onset of atrial fibrillation produces a rapid down-hill course.

There may be massive haemoptysis (pulmonary apoplexy), which is usually terminal when it is associated with rupture of capillaries or occasionally a pulmonary artery itself, as may happen after trauma, excitement, or anger. Smaller haemoptyses may occur as the result of infarction and thromboses *in situ*. The incidence of haemoptysis increases with age, starting late in the second decade. Haemoptysis before the age of 15 years in someone with the features of the Eisenmenger reaction should stimulate a search for added left atrial obstruction, which can be surgically treated. It is always a sinister symptom and often heralds the end; patients should be rested and only venesected if the haemoglobin exceeds 21 g. If there is evidence of pulmonary infarction, small doses of intravenous heparin by infusion and not in boluses can be given with caution. Antibiotics are indicated if there is evidence of secondary infection. With persistent fever and the development of a line of air around the pulmonary shadow, a mycetoma should be suspected and a search made for fungi in sputum and antibodies. The possibility of tuberculosis must not be forgotten.

Right heart failure develops after the age of 40 years in sinus rhythm or precipitated by supraventricular arrhythmias. Digoxin and diuretics

Table 3 *Causes of death in Eisenmenger complex*

Right heart failure
Sudden
Cerebral abscess
After surgery (cardiac or other)
Haemoptysis
Induction of anaesthesia
Haemorrhage (often anticoagulant-provoked)
Cardiac investigation and angiography
Pregnancy
Infective endocarditis (very rare)

may delay the distressing symptoms. The mechanisms by which death occurs are shown in Table 3.

PHYSICAL SIGNS

The signs of pulmonary hypertension are uniform with right ventricular hypertrophy, pulmonary systolic click, and loud pulmonary-valve closure. The patient may not be cyanosed at rest. With a duct, the toes are clubbed and more cyanosed than the hands—a sign that may be brought out by immersion in warm water; the left hand may be bluer and more clubbed than the right because the origin of the left subclavian is frequently opposite the duct. The behaviour of the second sound reveals the site of the defect, single with ventricular septal defect or single ventricle, normally split with aortopulmonary shunts, fixed with atrial septal defects (Fig. 7). As the right ventricle fails, the second sound becomes delayed and fixed. Murmurs do not arise from the defects themselves as they are too large to offer any turbulence. However, a pansystolic murmur may appear from tricuspid regurgitation when the right ventricle fails; this is the probable cause in Eisenmenger's original description.

Fig. 7 Physical signs diagram by Dr P. Wood to summarize auscultation in patients with Eisenmenger reaction and defects at different levels. EC = ejection click, VSD = ventricular septal defect.

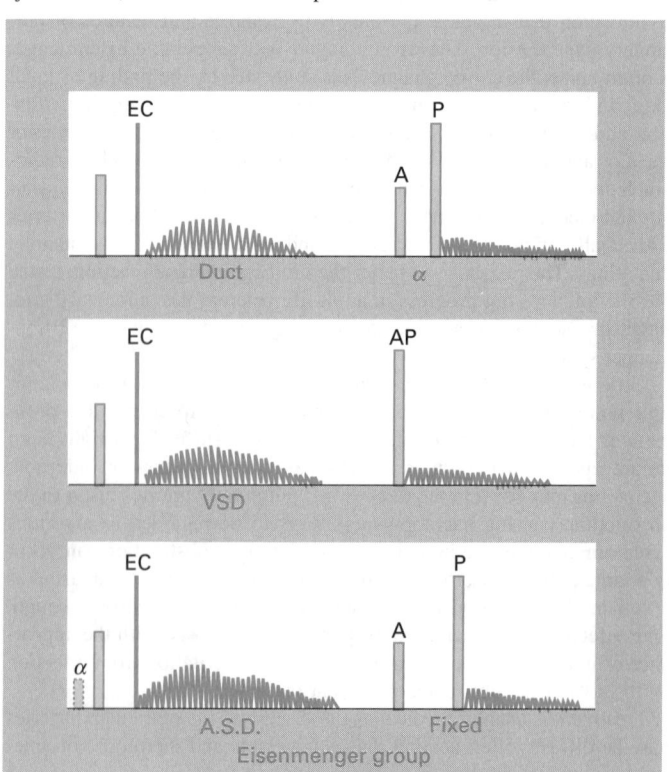

A high-pitched, long inspiratory, immediate diastolic murmur of pulmonary regurgitation is frequent and age related. The most extreme dilatation of the main pulmonary artery occurs earliest in patients with a duct, in whom a diastolic thrill may be palpable with delayed diastolic murmur at the right ventricular apex ('right-sided Austin Flint').

The chest radiograph shows large main pulmonary arteries and branches with peripheral pruning. Vessels are large in atrial septal defect and those patients where there was once a large pulmonary blood flow (Fig. 8). When high pulmonary vascular resistance dates from soon after birth the lungs have never carried an increased flow and pulmonary vessels (except for the main pulmonary artery) may be small, with lung fields looking oligaemic. In duct-and-trunk patients the aortic knuckle is prominent. Diagnostic calcification is seen in the duct after 35 years (Fig. 9) and may also appear in atheromatous plaques or thrombus after 40 to 45 years. When a double-inlet ventricle (single) fails, pulmonary venous congestion may appear with the onset of mitral regurgitation. Haemosiderosis with bone formation in the lungs can appear when there is mitral atresia or mitral stenosis.

The electrocardiogram shows varying degrees of right ventricular hypertrophy and axis shift in relation to the lesion and age of the patient.

DIFFERENTIAL DIAGNOSIS

Patients with Eisenmenger syndrome must be distinguished from those with acyanotic Fallot and transposition with pulmonary stenosis, conditions where the loud A_2 in the pulmonary area may be misinterpreted as a loud P_2. It is possible to differentiate which is A_2 by following the sound up to the base of the neck just below the left clavicle where it still is audible; P_2 disappears at this level.

A long praecordial systolic murmur suggests either diagnosis, and widespread systolic murmurs over the lungs suggest pulmonary arterial stenoses causing the pulmonary hypertension. In the presence of left atrial obstruction with a defect and secondary pulmonary hypertension, the diagnosis is suggested by a delayed diastolic murmur at the apex, P mitrale on the electrocardiogram, and an enlarged left atrium with prominent pulmonary venous shadows with haemosiderosis on the chest radiograph, together with history of early haemoptysis. An abnormal (underdeveloped) right ventricle with reversed interatrial shunt may be confused with Eisenmenger syndrome; a large 'a' wave, quiet right ventricle without murmurs, and a normal P_2 with normal or small pulmonary arteries on the chest radiograph should confirm this diagnosis.

MANAGEMENT

The general advice for care of adult patients with cyanotic heart disease should be followed for patients with the Eisenmenger reaction, whose circulation readily becomes unbalanced and in whom acute changes may lead to death. The systemic and pulmonary arterial pressures are the same or the systemic pressure may be lower with atrial septal defect. Any sudden change in volume from vomiting, diarrhoea, haemorrhage or trauma, or a vasovagal episode, may lead to death and should be prevented when possible. Patients should not go to high altitude above 1000 m. Flying is permissible but reduction in effort at the airports is more important than problems in the aeroplane. Oxygen should be available and used as the oxygen tension falls at high altitude. Long, transcontinental flights are a risk and it is important to avoid dehydration, alcohol consumption, and sitting for long periods. Ordinary driving licences can be issued provided there is no syncope. Employment should be encouraged when effort tolerance allows. Appropriate drug management of arrhythmias and heart failure should be instituted when indicated but it is important to remember that all drugs which may lower blood pressure should be avoided. Any change in cerebral state, new headaches or transient cerebral signs require exclusion of cerebral abscess. Indwelling intravenous lines are a potential source of systemic embolism and even expert nurses require special warning about avoidance of air bubbles, which carry a particular risk in the presence of right-to-left shunts.

A cerebral embolism may result from a local peripheral-vein thrombosis at the catheter site or a cerebral abscess may be the consequence of a minor skin infection. Catheterization and angiography carry the risks of complications and even death in Eisenmenger patients. Despite the risks of lowering arterial pressure there may, on occasion, be a strong indication for the use of vasodilators, usually in early cases without fixed pulmonary arteriolar disease, as occurs in young children.

Fig. 8 Chest radiograph from a 35-year-old woman with Eisenmenger atrial septal defect showing cardiomegaly, huge central pulmonary arteries with pruned vessels in periphery of lung, and small aortic knuckle.

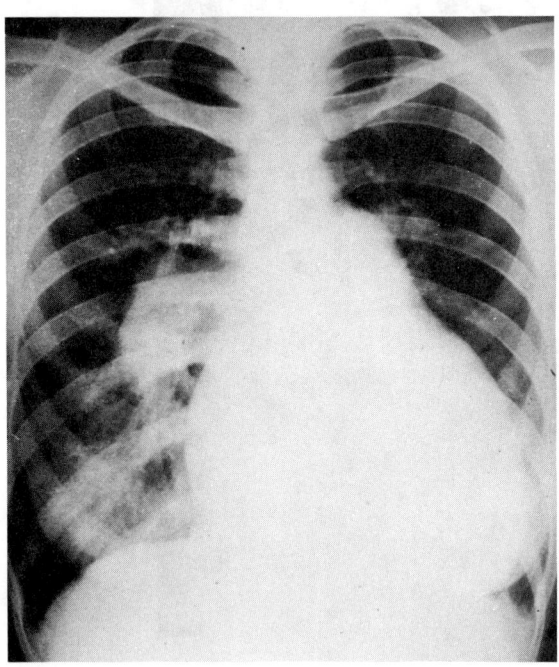

Fig. 9 Penetrated chest posteroanterior radiograph showing calcium in large duct (arrow).

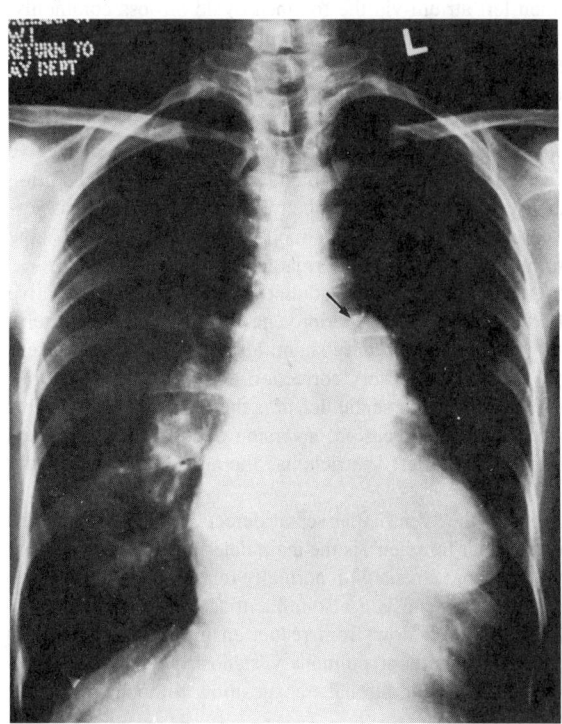

Heart/lung transplantation offers hope for some of these patients when they become severely disabled with hypoxia but without other organ dysfunction. It is important to ensure that the patient's existing prognosis and quality of life are not better than that offered by this radical surgical approach before referring the patient.

The physician must give special advice to patients about pregnancy and contraception. Pregnancy carries risks to mother and fetus. Maternal risk of death may still be of the order of 20 per cent but, with difficulty, it is possible to bring a patient with Eisenmenger through pregnancy to a satisfactory outcome, provided the oxygen saturation is above 85 per cent and she is young. Pregnancy should only be undertaken once the whole family, husband and his/her parents, understand every risk, as they may find themselves responsible for the child without a mother, or one who has deteriorated in health. There is a high incidence of spontaneous abortion and still births, premature births, low birth weight, and increased incidence of congenital heart disease in the fetus. If conception occurs, early termination in hospital, with cardiac intensive care, should be recommended. If termination is refused, the patient should be in hospital for most of the pregnancy, and early induction of labour or elective caesarian section advised. Any rise in blood pressure in the last weeks of pregnancy is a danger for added damage to the pulmonary arterioles and death. It is important to take steps to deliver the child should this start. Oxygen, as much as can be tolerated conveniently during the day and night, will help raise the oxygen saturation and the patient's well-being. There is no heart condition more demanding of the best cardiological care than the Eisenmenger in pregnancy.

The progesterone-only contraceptive pill can be used. Low-oestrogen pills carry a risk of thromboembolic complications during the first 6 months of administration as well as problems of fluid retention. An intrauterine device, with antibiotic prophylaxis at the time of insertion may be better, or the use of a diaphragm and condom. Laparoscopic sterilization may offer a better solution but should only be done where expert cardiac and anaesthetic care is available, as death is a known complication of all anaesthesia and surgery in such patients.

Tricuspid atresia

This anomaly is the result of a lack of development of the tricuspid valve. The direction of blood flow is then from venae cavae to right atrium and then left atrium via the foramen ovale or, less commonly, through a true atrial septal defect to left ventricle. From there, when the great arteries are normally related, the blood passes to the aorta and only to the pulmonary circulation via a ventricular septal defect and the right ventricle. The size of the right ventricle is then controlled by the size of the ventricular septal defect. The pulmonary infundibulum and valve stenosis further influence pulmonary blood flow, as does the condition of the pulmonary arteries. There may be transposition of the great vessels in some cases, accompanied by pulmonary-valve atresia and double outflow from rudimentary right or normal left ventricle.

Those who reach adolescence or adulthood will have had palliative surgery such as anastomosis of superior vena cava to pulmonary artery, systemic artery-to-pulmonary artery shunt, atrium-to-pulmonary artery or total caval-to-pulmonary artery correction. Rarely there is 'natural' survival when the ventricular septal defect is the ideal size and the pulmonary stenosis mild. On occasion, inversion of the ventricular morphology occurs when the left ventricle has the anatomy of that of the right.

The behaviour of the 'ventricular septal defect', sometimes referred to as 'bulboventricular foramen', is the main determinant of the clinical presentation of tricuspid atresia with normally related great arteries; the presence of pulmonary stenosis is also influential. Most patients have a reduced pulmonary blood flow from reduction in size of ventricular septal defect, with or without pulmonary stenosis, but if the defect remains large or there is additional transposition without pulmonary

stenosis, pulmonary hypertension with the Eisenmenger reaction may be present in adults.

With tricuspid atresia there may be:-

1. Patent foramen ovale (65–75 per cent); atrial septal defect, usually secundum.
2. A fleshy, large Eustachian valve looking like a right-sided cor triatriatum, which helps to prevent reflux back into the inferior vena cava.
3. Juxtaposition of the atrial appendages with ventricular inversion and double outflow giving a characteristic silhouette on chest radiograph (Fig. 10).
3. Unroofed coronary sinus as a rare cause of permanent cyanosis after Fontan with left superior vena cava draining into the coronary sinus or even left atrium.
4. Acquired subaortic stenosis may develop when the ventricular septal defect diminishes in size in association with transposition of the great arteries or with hypertrophy of muscle bands in the left outflow as the defect closes, causing angina and effort syncope.
5. Mitral-valve prolapse and regurgitation before or after the left ventricle dilates. Other congenital abnormalities of the mitral valve may be found at autopsy.

SYMPTOMS

Dyspnoea is related to hypoxia or left ventricular failure, the latter accelerated by shunts. Paroxysmal tachycardia, atrial flutter and fibrillation, or nodal rhythm occur after 15 years; complete heart block is unusual without atrial surgery. Haemoptysis may complicate pulmonary hypertension. Ventricular tachycardia may be the cause of fainting in adults. Angina, effort giddiness, and syncope appear, with progressive obstruction of conduits used in the modified Fontan procedure and with associated transposition of the great arteries. Right-sided congestion with a huge liver and ascites, and sometimes impending liver failure, occurs, with atrial fibrillation. When such patients present they may closely

Fig. 10 Chest radiograph from a patient with juxtaposition of the atrial appendages producing characteristic bulge on upper left cardiac border (arrow) from a patient with complex tricuspid atresia.

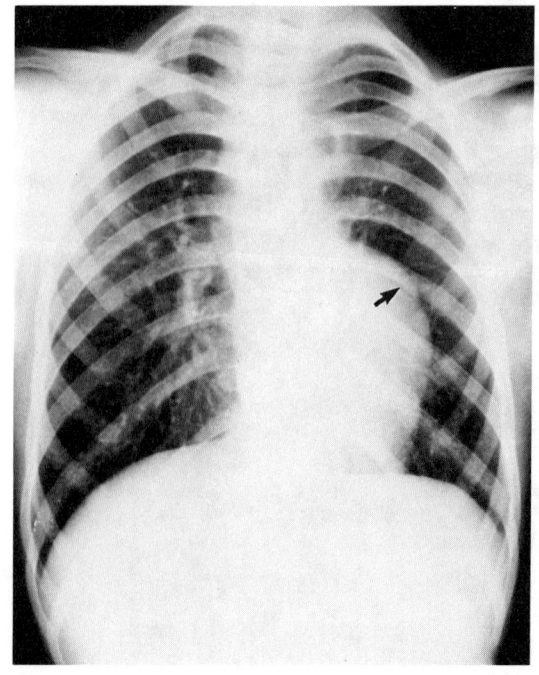

resemble those with a primary hepatic problem, when the urgent need to restore sinus rhythm may be ignored.

SIGNS (WITH NORMALLY RELATED AND CONNECTED GREAT ARTERIES)

Besides cyanosis and clubbing, a giant 'a' wave is characteristic, with a palpable left ventricle. Any systolic murmur is variable in length and intensity depending on the size of the ventricular septal defect and added pulmonary stenosis. There may be no systolic murmur if the defect is closed or pulmonary atresia is present, acquired or congenital. Signs are modified by earlier palliative procedures. Those with a Glenn anastomosis (superior vena cava to right pulmonary artery) lack pulsation in the venous pulse; an apical pansystolic murmur from mitral regurgitation is common in adults.

Electrocardiogram

This shows P pulmonale or P mitrale if there has been a successful shunt, left axis deviation or less commonly normal axis, varying degrees of left ventricular hypertrophy, and occasional Wolff–Parkinson–White with left bundle-branch block (8 per cent). Right ventricular hypertrophy or right axis deviation suggest an additional complication such as transposition of the great arteries, large ventricular septal defect with pulmonary hypertension, ventricular inversion or wrong diagnosis.

Chest radiograph

The right atrium surprisingly may not be prominent because there is no right ventricular inflow, particularly if a Glenn procedure has been done. The left ventricle is large. The pulmonary artery at the hila and size of peripheral vessels depend on pulmonary flow. In the lateral, there may be an anterior lung-(air-) filled space in front of the missing right ventricle.

DIFFERENTIAL DIAGNOSIS

Other anomalies may present with left ventricular hypertrophy associated with central cyanosis (Table 4) and must be distinguished from tricuspid atresia.

TREATMENT

This depends on the disability of the patient and degree of central cyanosis. A systemic–pulmonary artery shunt can be created at relatively low risk, but in adults shunts often thrombose. A form of atriopulmonary or caval pulmonary connection may succeed when pulmonary artery pressure is low (systolic below 20 mmHg) and the pulmonary vascular resistance is low, which is very difficult to determine with accuracy. Every effort to enter the pulmonary artery during catheterization to determine pressure and anatomy must be made if Fontan-type operations are considered. If there is doubt about a shunt, newer operations such as total caval–pulmonary connection or a bilateral Glenn alone have provided better short-term results, particularly with complex, double-inlet left and right ventricles or straddling atrioventricular valves. There is no surgical procedure for those with pulmonary hypertension; only heart-lung transplantation offers hope and heart transplantation for those with failed ventricles.

Patients may live with Glenn anastomoses (superior vena cava to pulmonary artery) for many years, but after 15 years or so fistulae at capillary level may form in the right lower lobe, which no longer oxygenates the blood; this is a cause of increasing cyanosis. Shunts, if ideally sized, may last many years but, unfortunately, left ventricular failure develops or they may lead to pulmonary hypertension. Equally, shunts with time can become inadequate, often leading to pulmonary arterial hypoplasia and stenoses. The late results of Fontan procedures and modifications made in early childhood are awaited. Unfortunately, irrespec-

Table 4 *Causes of left ventricular hypertrophy and central cyanosis*

Tricuspid atresia
Total anomalous systemic venous drainage
Inferior caval drainage to the left atrium
Double inlet ventricle of left ventricular morphology
Pulmonary atresia and intact ventricular septum (with small right ventricle)
Occasionally common atrium and A–V canal with pulmonary stenosis and/or small tricuspid valve
Ventricular septal defect and tricuspid stenosis
Double outlet right ventricle with tricuspid stenosis (hypoplasia)
Right ventricle hypoplasia with atrial septal defect
Absent tricuspid valve and blind right ventricle

tive of what is done, atrial arrhythmias causing congestion and low cardiac output are frequent and are associated with an embolic risk. It is vital to maintain sinus rhythm in tricuspid atresia. Attempts to revert atrial fibrillation should be made early with heparin cover and, if successful, be supplemented by an antiarrhythmic agent such as quinidine or amiodarone but not by drugs that are negatively inotropic. Heart block may follow the Fontan procedure, and should be managed by epicardial pacing; exceptionally, coronary sinus pacing is possible. Endocarditis is uncommon, except on shunts or on the mitral valve in adult patients.

Abnormal right ventricle and shunt reversal at atrial level

Ebstein's anomaly

For convenience this is discussed under cyanotic congenital heart disease but it is often acyanotic at rest, with mild cyanosis during exercise, rhythm disturbances, fever, and in pregnancy. Patients commonly survive to adult life, with or without cyanosis.

There are two interrelated basic disturbances: (i) the posterior and septal cusps of the tricuspid valve are 'prolonged' into the body of the right ventricle and originate from beneath the true atrioventricular ring, giving the appearance of an 'atrialized' part of the right ventricle; and (ii) there is abnormal thinning of right ventricular myocardium in the inflow (body), particularly in its anterior part.

The anterior cusp of the tricuspid valve is voluminous, ballooning out to close over the dilated tricuspid ring. Variable degrees of tricuspid regurgitation occur: indeed, the peculiar-looking valve may be competent in postnatal life. The right atrium is dilated and thin walled like the inflow of the right ventricle anteriorly; the right ventricular outflow is mildly hypertrophied. In 80 per cent the foramen ovale is open or defective (atrial septal defect), permitting a right-to-left shunt. Other associated abnormalities, such as pulmonary atresia or stenosis, ventricular septal defect, or mitral clefts, have been described but such patients do not reach adolescence. Rheumatic mitral stenosis has been found with Ebstein's anomaly, as has non-specific mitral-valve prolapse, probably secondary to left ventricular dysfunction, which is in various forms.

The severity and form of tricuspid-valve anomaly and right ventricular dysfunction vary. Indeed, it could be considered a primary right-ventricular myocardial problem acquired in fetal life, rather than a primary valvular problem. The right ventricular systolic pressure is low, with elevation of end-diastolic pressure; tricuspid regurgitation is usual, mild or severe depending on the rhythm, degree of myocardial dysfunction, and age of the patient. In adults, in sinus rhythm the right atrial pressure is normal until after age 40 years when it may rise. The jugular venous pressure rises with changes in rhythm at any age. Left-sided pressures are normal and there are no valvular gradients other than an occasional low subaortic one when the septum bulges into the small-cavity left ventricle and contacts the mitral valve. A right-to-left shunt causing central cyanosis on effort is present at rest in about 65 per cent of patients. The degree of desaturation depends on the degree of right ventricular myocardial dysfunction and the size of the atrial septal defect. Left ventricular function is often impaired in adults. Whether this is due to bulging of the dilated right ventricle and ventricular septum into the left ventricle (reversed Bernheim) causing abnormal contraction dynamics or to a diffusely abnormal myocardium is uncertain.

SYMPTOMS

Dyspnoea is proportional to hypoxia. Exceptionally a huge heart occupies most of the chest, displacing the lungs and reducing their volume with resultant dyspnoea and considerable limitation of activity. Right-sided congestion develops with onset of atrial arrhythmias. Paroxysmal supraventricular tachycardia may present with syncope because of a fall in an already low cardiac output. The natural history of Ebstein's anomaly is unpredictable; survival to 80 years of age is possible in those without cyanosis and it can appear as an incidental finding at necropsy. If the patient is severely cyanosed in childhood, survival into adulthood is unusual. In the mildly cyanosed or acyanotic, disability results from rhythm disturbances and subsequent heart failure. Infective endocarditis does sometimes occur and prophylaxis is advisable. Paradoxical emboli from peripheral venous thromboses or with atrial fibrillation occur. Haemoptysis is not a feature and if it occurs a search for tuberculosis or another cause should be initiated. Pregnancy is tolerated, but rest and increased diuretics are needed to prevent right heart failure.

SIGNS

The patient is characteristically slender, with peripheral cyanosis, cold hands and feet, and a malar flush. Central cyanosis is mild or moderate, rarely severe in adults. Clubbing is variable. Pulses are small, with a low to normal blood pressure. The jugular venous pulsation in sinus rhythm shows small flicking 'v' waves as the huge right atrium absorbs the effects of tricuspid regurgitation. Nodal rhythm or heart block lead to huge cannon waves. Atrial fibrillation or flutter increase the mean pressure, with large 'v' waves, a large pulsating liver, ascites, and oedema. The cardiac apex is displaced to the left and is gentle and diffuse. Pulsation is felt over the right ventricular outflow tract only.

Fig. 11 Typical chest radiograph from a cyanotic 40-year-old with Ebstein's anomaly. Shows gross cardiomegaly mainly from right atrial dilation, clear cardiac outline, and small pulmonary arteries.

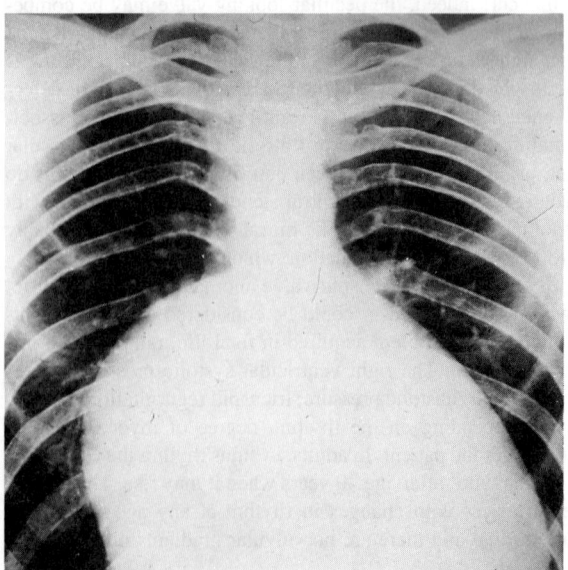

Abnormalities on auscultation increase on inspiration. The first sound is split, often widely, as is the second, with a normal pulmonary component. Atrial and third sounds are present if the P–R interval is prolonged or there is myocardial dysfunction. A short, delayed, scratchy diastolic with or without a pansystolic murmur is best heard at the lower left sternal edge.

Electrocardiogram

This shows variable right bundle-branch block patterns with low or normal-voltage V1–V$_3$. The axis may be right or leftward. Wolff–Parkinson–White conduction occurs in 9 per cent. V$_5$ and V$_6$ may be normal or QR patterns may be absent.

Chest radiograph

This usually shows globular cardiomegaly with right atrial and ventricular dilatation, a clear cardiac outline, clear underperfused lungs, and small (low) aortic knuckle (Fig. 11). The main pulmonary artery is not dilated, which helps distinguish the condition from pulmonary stenosis. Occasionally, the heart size is normal when the myocardium of the right ventricle is largely healthy and the tricuspid ring not dilated.

The left ventricle is bizarrely shaped and sometimes shows abnormal contraction patterns. The diagnosis is well shown by cross-sectional echocardiography.

MANAGEMENT

Rhythm disorders, supraventricular tachycardia, atrial flutter or fibrillation require cardioversion and suppressant medical therapy. Occasionally, complete heart block occurs, often preceded by Wenckebach phenomenon and prolongation of the P–R interval. Now that there are ways of repairing the tricuspid valve rather than replacing it, this approach should be undertaken earlier. Cardiomegaly alone, which may be static for many years, is not an indication for surgery.

The aim of surgery in Ebstein's anomaly is to stop hypoxic symptoms by closing the atrial septal defect (or foramen ovale), to restore a competent tricuspid valve by repair rather than replacement, and to improve right ventricular ejection by plicating the fibrotic anterior portion. Refractory rhythm disorders as part of the Wolff–Parkinson–White anomaly may precipitate the need for surgical help. Ablation of the abnormal pathway may obviate the need for surgery. If ablation fails, attempts should be made to cut the abnormal pathway as well as repair the basic lesions. The risks are 10 to 15 per cent, but excellent symptomatic benefit can result. Rhythm disturbances, including complete heart block and supraventricular tachycardia, may persist. The left ventricle often has functional abnormalities, which can be severe and cause death after operation from a low-output state. Whether the functional disorders are because the left ventricle is small, lying behind the dilated right ventricle, or also myopathic, is uncertain.

DIFFERENTIAL DIAGNOSIS

Ebstein's anomaly in adults must be differentiated from severe pulmonary stenosis in heart failure, pericardial effusion, Uhl's anomaly (in which the right ventricle is paper thin with a normally placed tricuspid valve), primary right-ventricular myocardial diseases such as the rare familial form of progressive fibrosis, abnormal right ventricle with reversed interatrial shunt, and arrhythmogenic right-ventricular dystrophy (dysplasia).

Echocardiography differentiates pericardial effusion with low voltage on the electrocardiogram from Ebstein's anomaly and the other right ventricular diseases. The presence of a significant pulmonary systolic murmur and a dilated main pulmonary artery extending to the left pulmonary artery supports the diagnosis of pulmonary stenosis. Primary right-ventricular dilatation as in Uhl's, or rare myopathies, may require angiography and the demonstration of a normally attached tricuspid valve in the correct position. Exceptionally, Ebstein's anomaly in adults may appear with a normal-sized heart and no tricuspid regurgitation.

Abnormal right ventricle with reversed interatrial shunt

This unusual condition appears in adolescents and adults, and may be familial. Central cyanosis appears in childhood or even infancy and slowly increases over the years. The right ventricle is described as hypoplastic, underdeveloped, thin, or containing aberrant bands and thickened endocardium. Symptoms are similar to those of Ebstein's anomaly but there is a large 'a' wave in the jugular venous pressure, a quiet, usually small, right ventricle, and often normal splitting of first and second sounds. The chest radiograph shows a normal-sized heart with prominent right atrium, with normal or diminished lung vascularity. The electrocardiogram shows peaked right-atrial P waves, a normal electrical axis without right ventricular hypertrophy, and left ventricular-lead dominance. An atrial septal defect is often seen on echo, with bulging of the septum to the left atrium, sometimes a small tricuspid ring or a dilated, poorly contracting right ventricle with normal left ventricle and no pulmonary stenosis. Cardiac catheterization confirms the unusual appearance and contraction of the right ventricle. A right-sided 'cor triatriatum' from a large Eustachian valve may be the cause of the problem and is obvious on echocardiography and angiography, causing a gradient between right atrium and ventricle.

MANAGEMENT

In those with primary right-ventricular pathology and mild symptoms, no treatment is necessary, but atrial rhythm disorders require therapy. If hypoxia is a problem, it is justifiable to close the atrial septal defect, now by a device, thereby preventing cyanosis; it may exchange cyanosis and dyspnoea for right-sided congestion. The decision to intervene is influenced by the size of the right ventricle cavity, which may be too small to permit safe closure of the defect. If there have been rhythm disturbances before operation, they will continue and can appear for the first time soon after operation. Early surgery is important in the patient with an obstructive Eustachian valve.

Abnormal connections of systemic and pulmonary veins

Inferior vena cava to left atrium

This rare anomaly, when isolated, may be found for the first time in adolescents and adults. Usually it is associated with common atrium, defects associated with isomerism, and less frequently with inferior vena caval or posterior type of atrial septal defect, when its presence is masked by the signs of the septal defect. If an isolated anomaly or iatrogenic following closure of an atrial septal defect, the diagnosis is easily missed. Patients present with breathlessness and cyanosis after exercise or during pregnancy. There may be a history of neonatal cyanosis that disappeared after the first 2 weeks when the pulmonary vascular resistance had fallen to normal.

The signs are of mild to moderate cyanosis with normal heart sounds, a flat right contour (from the small right atrium) of the normal-sized heart on radiographs, and a full left atrium, ventricle, and prominent aortic shadow. P mitrale may be found on the electrocardiogram. The condition should be suspected in any patient who becomes breathless on exercise after routine surgical closure of an atrial septal defect, yet retains a small heart shadow.

Treatment is by surgical redirection of venous drainage.

Superior vena cava to left atrium

This occurs as an isolated anomaly only very rarely. When present it is usually associated with common atrium, double-outflow right ventricle,

coronary-sinus atrial septal defect with unroofed or absent coronary sinus, and absence of the right superior vena cava. When isolated, features resemble inferior vena cava to left atrium but cyanosis is only induced by arm movements. Arterial oxygen saturation is 86 to 90 per cent and resting cyanosis may not be noted. Particular attention must be given to sepsis in upper limbs, face, and neck once the diagnosis is established, as cerebral abscess or other systemic embolic lesions may occur.

Total anomalous pulmonary venous drainage (TAPVD)

When all the pulmonary veins drain to the right atrium or a major systemic vein, the right side of the heart and pulmonary circulation become overloaded by the increased pulmonary blood flow. In order to maintain systemic flow, an obligatory right-to-left shunt occurs through the atrial septum, with or without atrial septal defect. Seventy-five per cent of patients die in the first year; 1 to 2 per cent may survive to late adolescence or adult life. A good prognosis (i.e. survival to childhood and adult life) usually depends on a large atrial septal defect, absence of obstruction in pulmonary venous pathways, drainage to the right atrium or left innominate vein, mild pulmonary-valve stenosis, and normal or only slight elevation of pulmonary vascular resistance. Adults with TAPVD generally appear deeply cyanosed, with the Eisenmenger reaction. These may have split sites of drainage, that is one lung to coronary sinus and another to right atrium. When one side has some obstruction to the pulmonary venous pathway and the other side drains freely, there is an obvious difference in the radiological appearance of both lungs, with a marked increase in flow and size of pulmonary vessels in the unobstructed lung. Exceptionally, obstructed TAPVD (even infradiaphragmatic) may appear in adults, with intense, speckly, haemosiderotic lungs and signs of pulmonary hypertension or added pulmonary-valve stenosis.

Adults with TAPVD develop atrial fibrillation, flutter or supraventricular tachycardia. Right heart failure occurs in sinus rhythm. The physical signs are those of atrial septal defect with central cyanosis. A continuous murmur—a venous hum—may be heard in the left upper chest, when pulmonary veins drain to the left innominate vein; or over the right chest when veins enter the azygos or right superior vena cava. The murmur is loud when there is mild obstruction at any venous site but such patients rarely survive to adolescence.

The electrocardiogram shows P pulmonale, a prolonged or normal P–R interval, right axis deviation, and right ventricular hypertrophy more severe than with atrial septal defect; Q waves are absent in V_6 and R waves are small. T inversion extending to V_1–V_4 or V_5 is usual.

When the pulmonary veins enter the right atrium or coronary sinus (exceptional in adults), the chest radiograph looks like that of a large atrial septal defect, with huge cardiomegaly and dilatation of the right atrium and pulmonary arteries with small left atrium and aortic knuckle. When connected to the left innominate, the enlarged upper systemic veins give the cardiac silhouette the appearance of a cottage loaf (or snowman) (Fig. 12).

Diagnosis is made by echocardiography and catheterization, which shows the abnormal channel of pulmonary venous return either after injection of contrast into the pulmonary arteries or more appropriately into an anomalous pulmonary venous channel. Some elevation of the pulmonary arterial pressure is expected and systemic and pulmonary arterial saturations are the same; sometimes the pulmonary arterial saturation exceeds that of the systemic by 5 to 7 per cent.

Differential diagnosis is from an unusually large atrial septal defect, cor triatriatum with two atrial septal defects, and the other causes of cyanosis coexisting with a left-to-right shunting atrial septal defect (Table 5). Treatment is surgical, with anastomosis of the common pulmonary vein to the left atrium and closure of the atrial septal defect provided that the pulmonary vascular resistance is not too high. Such treatment of the lesions in infancy and childhood has produced many adult survivors, often with residual pulmonary hypertension. Atrial arrhythmias or nodal rhythm are not uncommon after correction of the coronary sinus drainage type. Although a very serious lesion in infancy, the state of late survivors after surgery is excellent provided there is no residual obstruction at the site of anastomosis. Prophylaxis for endocarditis is not necessary in these patients.

Hemianomalous pulmonary venous drainage

This presents with signs of atrial septal defect (which often coexists), with slight central cyanosis and often modestly elevated pulmonary vascular resistance (see Atrial septal defect and cyanosis). If there is no significant atrial septal defect, the widely split second sound moves freely with respiration but does not close. The hemianomalous veins may enter the inferior vena cava/right atrial junction via a confluence of right pulmonary veins that descends to the drainage opening giving the classic 'scimitar' shadow on the chest radiograph (Fig. 13). However, it is more common for the hemianomalous veins to enter the right atrium, producing round, coin-like shadows seen end on in a penetrated view of right atrium, or to the left superior vena cava, which will appear dilated on the upper left mediastinal borders of the chest radiograph.

Partial anomalous pulmonary veins

See under Atrial septal defect.

Anomalies of arterial connection

Anomalies of the aortic and pulmonary artery connections to the ventricles have distinct entities such as transposition of the great arteries (classic), corrected transposition, corrected malposition, double-outlet right ventricle, and double-outlet left ventricle. Adolescents and adults with these conditions will usually have had palliation or radical surgery in infancy or childhood. There are a few who have survived without surgery because of an ideal degree of pulmonary stenosis restricting pulmonary blood flow or with the Eisenmenger reaction.

Fig. 12 Chest radiograph from patient with total anomalous pulmonary venous drainage into left ascending vein entering innominate. There is cardiomegaly, pulmonary plethora, and dilation of ascending innominate vein and right superior vena cava (arrows) giving 'snowman' appearance.

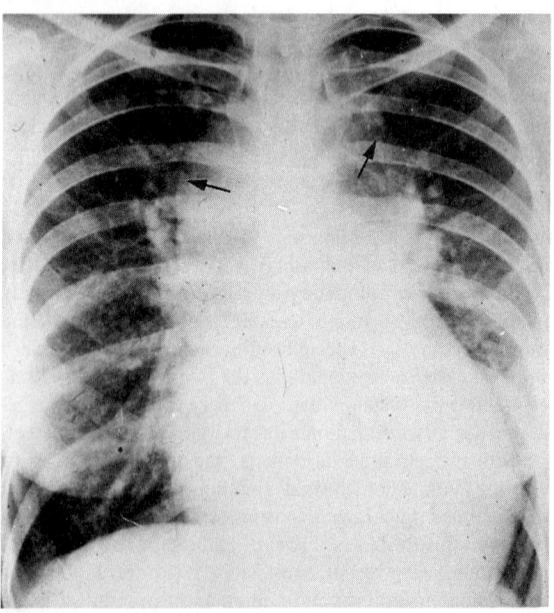

Table 5 *Causes of central cyanosis in atrial septal defect*

Total anomalous pulmonary venous drainage
Hemianomalous pulmonary venous drainage
Cor triatriatum + 2 atrial septal defects
IVC to left atrium
Huge atrial septal defect—common atrium
Abnormal right ventricle, i.e. Ebstein, fibrotic with age
Tricuspid stenosis/regurgitation
Atrial fibrillation
Mild right sided obstructive lesions
Bradycardia

Classic transposition of the great arteries (TGA, atrioventricular concordance, ventricular arterial discordance)

Classic transposition is an anomaly in which the right atrium opens to the right ventricle which connects to the aorta, usually positioned anterior to the pulmonary artery, but can be in any position. The left atrium empties into the left ventricle, which ejects into the (usually) posteriorly sited pulmonary artery. About 0.5 per cent of adult patients with TGA survive without surgery, depending on a large atrial septal defect, pulmonary stenosis with ventricular septal defect, or ventricular and atrial septal defect with Eisenmenger reaction. More often there has been palliative surgery either by shunt, banding of the pulmonary artery or with an intra-arterial baffle. There are some survivors of the 'Rastelli' operation in which the ventricular septal defect, large or enlarged, has been closed in such a way as to direct left ventricular blood to the aorta and the right ventricle connected to the posterior pulmonary artery by a valved conduit. In the palliated or natural survivors, symptoms depend on the degree of hypoxaemia (breathlessness) and on the development of right heart failure, often a problem after 15 to 20 years. Abnormally attached tricuspid valve chordae can rupture spontaneously. Infective endocarditis is uncommon but may occur on tricuspid and mitral valves, and on the ventricular septal defect if small. Atrial fibrillation and supraventricular tachycardia are seen in the third and fourth decades, and ventricular ectopic beats may cause symptoms. Experience of 30 patients who have survived over 20 years after intra-arterial baffle procedures (Mustard) shows that they may have near normal lives, even including successful pregnancy. Right heart failure will occur in 25 per cent by the age of 30. Late baffle obstruction causes ascites if sited in the inferior vena cava, and pulmonary oedema and haemoptysis when pulmonary veins become obstructed. Late tricuspid regurgitation with or without chordal rupture also causes acute pulmonary oedema.

SIGNS

Signs depend on associated lesions. All patients have clubbing and significant cyanosis. The neck veins show unusual pulsation. The right ventricle is palpable. When there is an atrial septal defect, the ejection murmur is short or absent. The aortic second sound is loud and single in the pulmonary area. The aorta is palpable. There is a danger of bronchial obstruction and pulmonary complications when the conduit is placed on the left side of the heart to avoid sternal compression. The heart is usually enlarged on chest radiographs, with a large pulmonary artery on the right side. Speckly shadows from bronchopulmonary collaterals are common in patients with severe pulmonary stenosis or an atrial septal defect. The vascular pedicle is narrow (Fig. 14) with the aorta anterior to the pulmonary artery; when the aorta is left sided it rises up to the knuckle on the left border.

The electrocardiogram shows severe right ventricular hypertrophy, awry axis, and large 'S' waves in the anterior chest leads. The association with ventricular septal defect and pulmonary stenosis produces signs resembling those of Fallot with a long systolic murmur conducted to the right and unexpectedly severe cyanosis for so long a murmur. The pulmonary valve may be calcified and thus visible on the lateral chest radiograph deep in the mediastinum. With ventricular or atrial septal defect and a patent duct the signs resemble those of Eisenmenger with huge pulmonary arteries and an unusual chest radiograph with an abnormal pedicle.

SURGICAL TREATMENT

Some patients with TGA and atrial septal defect may be suitable for intra-atrial baffle (Mustard or Senning procedure) in adult life but this depends on pulmonary vascular resistance. Those with TGA plus ventricular septal defect plus PVS do well with Rastelli procedure which is closure of the ventricular septal defect in a way which allows the left ventricle to eject through it into the aorta via the ventricular septal defect, ligation of the proximal pulmonary artery, and placing a valved conduit between the right ventricle and pulmonary artery distal to the ligature or transection of the pulmonary artery. Those patients with hyperkinetic pulmonary hypertension may be suitable for arterial switch, or a 'palliative switch' in which the ventricular septal defect is left open. Patients with TGA who survive to adolescence are likely to have a high pulmonary vascular resistance even with pulmonary stenosis.

Since 90 per cent of children born with TGA would die if untreated in the first year of life, survival to adolescence and adulthood usually depends on earlier surgery. Experience of 20 patients who have survived late after intra-atrial baffle shows that complex arrhythmias are common. Right heart failure causing pulmonary oedema is a problem over 20 years and haemoptysis from progressive pulmonary vascular disease occurs. Sudden death may occur despite careful monitoring of rhythm. Several people have lived normal lives in sinus rhythm, and pregnancy has been tolerated and produced a normal child. Late tricuspid regurgitation with and without chordal rupture may result in acute pulmonary oedema. Late results of Rastelli operation have been good, with few arrhythmias. The problems related to the fate and replacement of the valved conduit between right ventricle and pulmonary artery. There is a danger of bronchial obstruction and pulmonary complications when the conduit is placed on the left of the heart to avoid compression. There are no long-term results in adults of arterial switching yet but aortic (once the pulmonary valve) regurgitation can be expected in some.

Corrected transposition (atrioventricular discordance; ventricular arterial discordance; anterior aorta to the left)

Patients with the basic abnormality survive into the second decade without surgical treatment. Their survival depends on the associated lesions and the behaviour of the conducting tissue.

The right atrium empties through a bicuspid atrioventricular valve (mitral) into a morphological left ventricle which is connected to a posteromedial pulmonary artery. The left atrium receiving normal pulmonary venous drainage empties through a tricuspid valve, often abnormally formed and placed in a morphological right ventricle which ejects into an anterolateral aorta. Despite the strange anatomy, the circulation flows correctly – hence the name 'corrected' transposition. However, the conducting tissue takes an abnormal course, the coronary pattern is reversed, and the right ventricle and tricuspid valve support the systemic circulation, ill designed to face systemic arterial resistance rather than the usual pulmonary circulation. The associated anomalies are ventricular septal defect with and without pulmonary-valve stenosis, subpulmonary obstruction, which is not muscular, and Ebstein's anomaly of the left atrioventricular valve causing severe left atrioventricular valve regurgitation. A supravalve membrane close to the tricuspid valve gives signs of 'mitral' stenosis. Aortic stenosis, atrioventricular and atrial septal defect, common atrium, left superior vena cava, multiple ventricular septal defects and coarctation may coexist, as well as anomalies of situs.

Patients can present as ventricular septal defect with left-to-right shunt and hyperkinetic pulmonary hypertension; when pulmonary stenosis coexists they look like Fallot; or isolated left atrioventricular-valve regurgitation of varying severity; or late onset of left atrioventricular-valve regurgitation in the fourth decade; or arrhythmias that include sudden complete heart block or sudden death with bizarre supraventricular tachycardias, including atrial fibrillation. Complete heart block may date from birth or be acquired at anytime after. The ventricular rate tends to slow with age. Pacemaker implantation may be sufficient to control symptoms, particularly in adults who have well-compensated lesions.

The diagnosis depends on associated defects:

1. With pulmonary stenosis and ventricular septal defect (resembling Fallot). There is no history of cyanotic attacks since there are no infundibular bands (which are not part of a morphological left ventricle) to constrict the outflow tract. Cyanosis varies according to the severity of the pulmonary stenosis, which is usually valvar but occasionally subvalvar caused by fibrous tags or aberrant atrioventricular-valve tissue. The feel of the apex beat is non-specific, and arterial pulsation is felt in the pulmonary area due to the anterior aorta. There is a systolic murmur

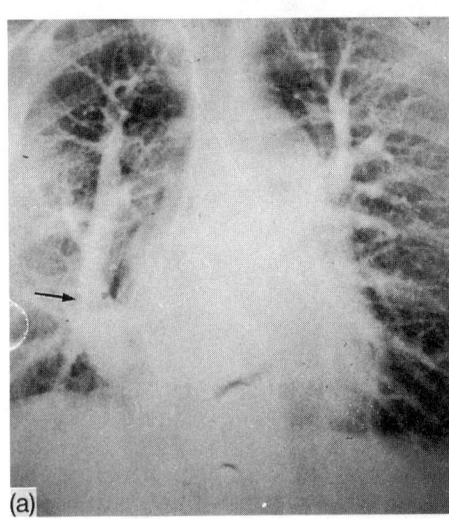
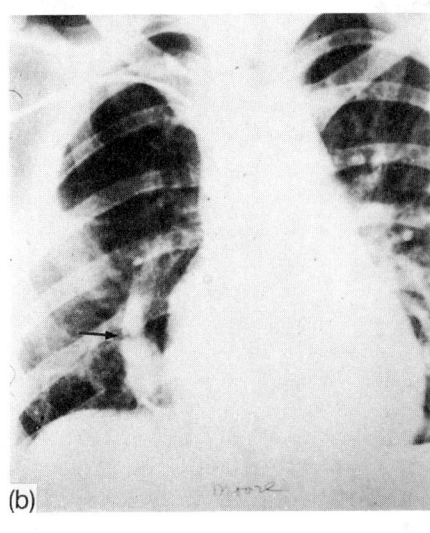

Fig. 13 (a,b) Angiogram and chest radiograph from patient with hemianomalous pulmonary veins entering the inferior vena cava/right atrial junction. The descending anomalous pulmonary vein is seen as a Scimitar on (b) the chest radiograph and (a) the angiogram (arrows). Left pulmonary veins are draining normally to left atrium.

maximal at the lower left sternal edge, A_2 is increased in the pulmonary area, and apical atrioventricular-valve regurgitant murmurs are frequent. The electrocardiogram shows a prominent QR pattern in II, III, and in V_1, with an rSR in V_6 and a VL. The Q wave is absent in the left chest leads even when the systemic ventricle is dilated. The chest radiograph shows a straight left aortic border with the right pulmonary artery higher and larger than the left. The left-sided ventricular outflow tract and aortic sinus may make a prominence on the left cardiac border in the region of and the appearance of a dilated left atrial appendage.

2. With ventricular septal defect and pulmonary hypertension. The chest radiograph and electrocardiogram are unusual for ventricular septal defect (Fig. 15), with no main pulmonary artery shadow and straight aorta on the left border, and an QR pattern of left ventricular overload in V_6.

3. With left atrioventricular regurgitation. Those with left-sided Ebstein rarely reach adult life but less severe anomalies of the left valve present often with atrial fibrillation, block or bizarre tachycardia precipitating pulmonary oedema. Diagnosis is made with the usual signs of mitral regurgitation, atypical electrocardiogram, and chest radiograph, with evidence of reversed ventricular morphology on two-dimensional echocardiography.

It is possible to have a normal lifespan with corrected transposition without defects or important left atrioventricular-valve regurgitation but this is rare as arrhythmias after 40 to 50 years cause trouble. The systemic ventricle of right morphology fails in the fifth decade and the tricuspid valve develops or increases its regurgitation, and the QT interval lengthens perhaps causally related to sudden unexpected deaths.

SURGICAL TREATMENT

It is technically possible to close associated ventricular septal defects and relieve pulmonary stenosis, but it may require a valved conduit because access is difficult and there are dangers of producing block or damaging the vulnerable right coronary artery. However, there is a high incidence of problems in relation to malignant arrhythmias, pacing problems for block, and progressive left atrioventricular valve regurgitation after closure of the defect.

Indications for surgical treatment are severe cyanosis and hypoxia, suprasystemic pressure in the right-sided ventricle, symptomatic hyper-

kinetic pulmonary hypertension with a large ventricular septal defect, and severe regurgitation in the left atrioventricular valve, which exceptionally will be repairable. Reoperation to replace the regurgitant atrioventricular valve may be needed in the first 5 years after the first 'corrective' operation.

Corrected malposition (atrioventricular concordance, ventricular arterial concordance, mitral/aortic discontinuity, anterior aorta)

This curiosity has features of corrected transposition, such as the position of the great arteries relative to one another, aorta to left and anterior-to-posteromedial pulmonary artery, but the morphology of right and left ventricles is not inverted. Subpulmonary and subaortic obstruction are common, as is ventricular septal defect, which may close spontaneously, or be large. Basically, the venous blood flows to the right side of the heart and the red blood is in the left heart of correct morphology. Complete heart block is not a special problem but mitral regurgitation may result, with resection of subaortic stenosis as part of definitive repair.

Double-outflow right ventricle

Both great arteries arise from the right ventricle and left ventricular ejection into the aorta is through the vital ventricular septal defect, which, when small, can become restrictive, causing subaortic obstruction; it can also be large, and this is the finding in most of those who reach adolescence. If patients have pulmonary stenosis they present like Fallot, and if not as pulmonary hypertensive, ventricular septal defects. Diagnosis is made by echocardiography and angiography showing mitral/aortic discontinuity with the aorta emerging from the right ventricle and pointing anteriorly. The electrocardiogram is not diagnostic.

Fig. 15 Chest radiograph from a patient with multiple ventricular septal defects, pulmonary hypertension, and corrected transposition showing unusual low bulge on left cardiac border (arrow) from aortic outflow beneath ascending aorta making the straight border up to the aortic knuckle, no obvious dilated main pulmonary artery despite intense pulmonary plethora and cardiomegaly.

Fig. 14 Chest radiograph from an adult with transposition of the great arteries, ventricular septal defect, and pulmonary hypertension. It shows narrow vascular pedicle, large branch pulmonary arteries, and 'absent' main pulmonary artery.

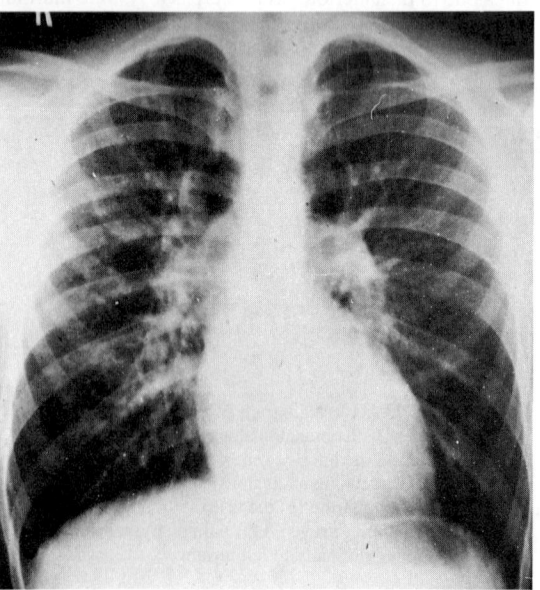

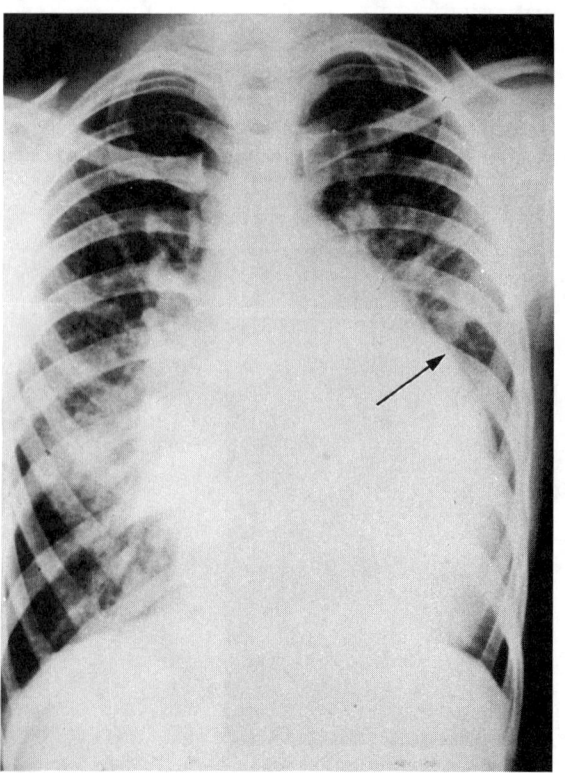

If there is subaortic obstruction due to muscle bands or a small ventricular septal defect, the carotid pulse may be delayed and with a thrill, the aortic sound may be delayed and diminished when it should be loud, and left ventricular hypertrophy is unexpectedly severe. Natural history and management relate to the site of the defect and the presence or absence or pulmonary stenosis, and to the competence of atrioventricular valves, which may develop chordal rupture in adults. Those with subpulmonary ventricular septal defects without pulmonary stenosis and with uncommitted defects or atrioventricular canals pose the greatest problems. The easiest to deal with are the most frequent, with subaortic defects. Those who survive without pulmonary stenosis usually have irreversible pulmonary vascular disease as adults and surgical treatment is likely to be ill advised. Late results of repaired double-outlet right ventricle in childhood may be good but there may be problems with aortic regurgitation, subaortic stenosis, ventricular arrhythmias or progressive pulmonary vascular disease. Tricuspid chordal rupture has been seen.

Double-outlet left ventricle

These are rare, presenting like Fallot, transposition or double-outlet right ventricle depending on associated lesions. The right ventricle is not normal, and failure is a likely problem in the adult after surgical repair.

Double-inlet ventricle (univentricular; single or common, ventricle)

Patients with one functioning ventricle with connections to both atria can reach adult life with or without surgery. Pulmonary-valve stenosis permits a normal or slightly increased blood flow and this may allow survival to the seventh decade, with final demise due to heart failure, often precipitated by atrial fibrillation. Subpulmonary obstructions usually progress to become atretic and calcified, but this may not occur until the second and third decades. Changes in morphology that affect presentation are acquired subaortic obstruction, subpulmonary stenosis, atrioventricular-valve regurgitation, and pulmonary vascular disease. The ventricle may be of left, right, or indeterminate morphology.

Systemic-to-pulmonary arterial shunts have an important place in those with pulmonary stenosis or atresia. Treatment is otherwise as for tricuspid atresia. Septating the ventricle has produced few long-term survivors and is no longer practised. It is not known how well are the few adult survivors.

Univentricular heart with mitral atresia

Patients with this combination may appear in adolescence, provided that the atrial septal defect is large. The ventricle is usually of right ventricular type with features of pulmonary hypertension and tricuspid regurgitation, and pulmonary venous congestion. Massive haemoptysis from capillary rupture occurs early, and atrial fibrillation in the second or third decade causes rapid deterioration and death.

Pulmonary arteriovenous fistula

Diffuse small or localized large isolated congenital pulmonary arteriovenous aneurysms may occur in the lungs. These patients have varying degrees of central cyanosis and inspiratory continuous murmurs if the fistula is large enough. The condition may be part of Babbington's disease (hereditary telangiectasia). Pulmonary angiography may confirm the diagnosis of single or multiple fistulae in the lung; some large ones can be treated by catheter embolization of the feeding vessel.

Acyanotic congenital heart disease in adults

More patients with acyanotic congenital heart disease than with cyanotic congenital heart disease survive to adult life. Many of the lesions are mild (for instance, bicuspid aortic or pulmonary valves, mitral-valve prolapse, and small atrial or ventricular septal defects). They may cause symptoms later, but when mild or small lead to little or no haemodynamic disturbance.

Right-sided obstructive lesions and other anomalies of the right side of the heart

The main anomalies are: (a) pulmonary-valve stenosis; (b) 'lone' infundibular stenosis; (c) bipartite right ventricle; (d) pulmonary arterial stenoses; (e) idiopathic dilatation of the pulmonary artery; and (f) Ebstein's anomaly.

Pulmonary-valve stenosis

Any grade of valve obstruction may be found in adolescents and adults. Severe pulmonary-valve stenosis is uncommon in adults unless there has been previous surgery. Patients with 'simple' pulmonary-valve stenosis may be cyanosed if severe, depending on the association with atrial septal defect or patent foramen ovale.

ANATOMY AND PHYSIOLOGY

The stenosed pulmonary valve may be bicuspid or tricuspid, a pliable dome, or the thick lumpy valve that is usual in patients with Noonan's syndrome and related syndromes. After 35 to 40 years of age, the valve calcifies and may become regurgitant. When right ventricular pressure is high (i.e. systemic or suprasystemic), calcification develops in the tricuspid-valve ring, sometimes involving a cusp. The effects of pulmonary-valve stenosis are to disturb right ventricular function. Right ventricular hypertrophy occurs when resting right-ventricular pressure exceeds 50 mmHg. The actual valve obstruction does not increase after the first decade but increasing infundibular hypertrophy may cause increasing obstruction and the effects on the hypertrophied right ventricle are progressive until fibrosis causes dilatation, failure, and tricuspid regurgitation, worsened or precipitated by atrial flutter and fibrillation.

SYMPTOMS

Fatigue, slight dyspnoea, and effort syncope occur with severe pulmonary-valve stenosis. Dyspnoea is more pronounced when there is cyanosis from a reversed intra-atrial shunt on effort. Acyanotic patients are usually symptom-free until the onset of atrial fibrillation or flutter and right heart failure, which lead to ascites and peripheral oedema. Adult patients with mild-to- moderate pulmonary-valve stenosis (right ventricular pressures 40–60 mmHg) may appear after the age of 50 years in right heart failure in sinus rhythm. Infective endocarditis on lone pulmonary-valve stenosis is unknown unless part of generalized septic process; routine prophylaxis is thus unnecessary.

SIGNS

The physical signs depend on the severity of the obstruction and the secondary effects on the right ventricular myocardium (Table 6). Pulmonary regurgitation occurs when the valve calcifies. Careful attention to physical signs allows a reliable assessment of severity to be confirmed by echocardiography: cardiac catheterization is not necessary unless as a part of therapeutic intervention.

In right heart failure, the pulse is small and irregular, the jugular venous pressure high with huge 'v' waves of tricuspid regurgitation, and there is a third sound that increases on inspiration. A loud pansystolic murmur, difficult to distinguish from the pulmonary ejection murmur, often occurs at the left lower sternal edge. In such cases, the ejection murmur at the pulmonary area is short.

Table 6 *Physical signs in pulmonary valve stenosis (PVS)*

	Mild	Moderate	Severe
Pulse	Normal	Normal	Small
Jugular venous pressure	Normal	Dominant 'a' wave on inspiration or exercise	Giant 'a' wave
Apex beat	RV palpable	RV++	RV++
Auscultation	Loud pulmonary ejection click, increases on expiration	Clock close to S_1 (absent if valve thick)	No click
	A_2/P_2 interval wide, increases on inspiration	A_2/P_2 interval wider, increases on inspiration	P_2 often very late, soft or not heard
	P_2 audible but late	P_2 audible but late	
	Grade 2 ejection murmur increases on inspiration, maximal 2nd left interspace	Grade 3 murmur + thrill	Loud murmur + thrill − late crescendo over A_2
Other			Mild clubbing (variable)
			Peripheral cyanosis
			Malar flush

Electrocardiogram

The degree of right ventricular hypertrophy depends on the severity of the obstruction and the length of time it has been present. Minimal changes are right axis deviation, increase in R wave in lead V_1 or splintered S in V_1. A more obvious increase in voltage in the right chest leads occurs in moderate stenosis with upright T in V_1 and S in V_6. In severe stenosis, increased R wave voltage and ST–T wave changes over right ventricular leads are seen. P pulmonale is usual and no true left ventricular complexes are recorded in V_6. A QR pattern in V_1 is occasionally seen. With increasing age and/or failure, complete right bundle-branch block can develop. In moderate stenosis with progressive cardiac dilatation, the T waves become progressively inverted across the right chest leads without increase in voltage of QRS.

Chest radiograph

In mild stenosis, the heart is normal in size. Pulmonary blood flow is normal. The main pulmonary artery and left pulmonary artery are dilated. In more severe cases, the heart may be slightly or grossly enlarged. The right atrium is dilated and poststenotic dilation of the pulmonary artery is present but not as marked as in moderate obstruction. The lung fields appear under-filled, with small peripheral vessels (oligaemic) in severe stenosis. The aorta is small, low, and left-sided. Calcification of the pulmonary valve should be expected after age 35 years, and is best seen on penetrated screening but can be documented by left lateral or anteroposterior views; it appears earlier if the patient is cyanosed and the obstruction is severe.

DIFFERENTIAL DIAGNOSIS

When stenosis is trivial it may be confused with mild aortic-valve stenosis or atrial septal defect but pulmonary artery dilation on radiographs and inspiratory murmurs should differentiate pulmonary-valve stenosis from aortic stenosis, which do coexist. To differentiate mild pulmonary-valve stenosis from modest atrial septal defect may be difficult and require catheterization in the adult, as echocardiography is unreliable. Other causes of a long systolic murmur at the left sternal edge include ventricular septal defect, infundibular stenosis, subaortic stenosis, and pulmonary artery stenosis.

Severe pulmonary-valve stenosis in failure with right ventricular dilation may be confused with Ebstein, pericardial effusion (no murmurs), or even ventricular septal defect with atrial fibrillation. The appearance of the dilated left pulmonary artery (in comparison to the right) on the radiograph a late soft P_2, and the 'a' wave if in sinus rhythm should distinguish pulmonary stenosis. It may be difficult to differentiate lone infundibular stenosis without invasive investigation.

PULMONARY VALVOTOMY

The late results of pulmonary valvotomy are excellent; 95 per cent of patients are relieved of any symptoms and endocarditis is not a risk. Murmurs persist and pulmonary regurgitation is common. Patients with lumpy, dysplastic valves can be left with serious pulmonary incompetence, particularly if cusps have been excised, and may have left-heart hypertrophic myopathy. Severe pulmonary regurgitation is not entirely benign long term and can lead, 15 to 20 years later, to progressive right ventricular dilatation, frank right ventricular failure with atrial flutter, and fibrillation. Pulmonary-valve replacement (with an aortic or pulmonary homograft) has been helpful in a few but the heart diminishes little in size once extreme dilatation has occurred—the tricuspid valve may also require surgery as it usually becomes grossly incompetent. This small group of patients requires careful watching—once the heart begins to show cardiomegaly, pulmonary-valve replacement should be done before frank failure or atrial fibrillation are established. Provided pulmonary-valve and annulus obstruction is relieved, infundibular stenosis should regress. Cyanosis and dyspnoea on effort may appear if the foramen ovale remains open and can be helped by closure: there are late problems arising when the right ventricle is fibrotic.

Coronary disease, with or without hypertension, can develop in older patients with unrelieved, important pulmonary-valve stenosis. This takes an insidious course, without left ventricular enlargement, as it is 'protected' by the pulmonary stenosis, which poses difficulties in management as relief of the pulmonary stenosis may then have catastrophic effects on the left ventricle. It may be that only coronary bypass grafting should be done in such unusual circumstances. Small experience of this confirms an unpredictable outcome.

There is evidence that in some patients the congenital cardiovascular disease is not limited to the pulmonary valve. There may be associated left ventricular disease, which may manifest early as pulmonary oedema with effusions after operation or later as myopathy—hypertrophic or dilated. The concept of more diffuse congenital cardiovascular disease in hearts with congenital structural defects applies to many other conditions besides pulmonary stenosis. It has wide implications for the future of many patients as there may be myocardial, coronary, and aortic abnormalities that are not caused by the obstruction or defect, but that may cause symptoms and signs which cannot be explained by the basic disorder.

'Lone' infundibular stenosis

ANATOMY AND PHYSIOLOGY

Fixed, right ventricular outflow-tract obstruction below the pulmonary valve is caused by muscle bands that are abnormally placed, at first causing slight obstruction and then slowly hypertrophying in postnatal life; the pulmonary valve may be normal, bicuspid, or minimally stenosed. The infundibular stenosis can appear as the only anomaly in the heart but careful searches should show evidence of a ventricular septal defect (subtricuspid or muscular) that has earlier closed spontaneously leaving only a scar. The speed with which infundibular obstruction develops relates to the stimulus from right ventricular hypertension, initially determined by the size of the ventricular septal defect, the degree of abnormal rotation, and size of the bands; probably also the amount of abnormal muscle within the displaced band. Slow enlargement/hypertrophy of bands may cause infundibular obstruction to become critical in adults and, by then, thickened endocardium in the outflow of the right ventricle covers the bands and contributes to the obstruction.

SYMPTOMS AND SIGNS

Murmurs may have been documented since early childhood. A click never precedes the long, pulmonary ejection systolic murmur, which is maximal in the third left interspace, sometimes resembling that of ventricular septal defect, and is conducted into the pulmonary area; it increases on inspiration. P_2, when audible, is delayed and diminished.

The chest radiograph resembles that of pulmonary stenosis without postobstructive dilatation of the main left pulmonary artery. A prominence on the left border of the cardiac shadow is due to a dilated infundibular chamber. Calcification in the endocardium of the outflow may be seen on the lateral chest radiograph as linear vertical shadows.

Bipartite right ventricle

This rare form of 'low' infundibular stenosis occurs in adults as well as children. Aberrantly placed muscular bands that divide the inflow portion of the right ventricle from the outflow cause obstruction with a fixed orifice in a muscular partition running from the apex of the right ventricle to the septum. Sometimes this is close to the tricuspid valve so that the inflow portion (body) of the right ventricle is small. If there is an associated subaortic ventricular septal defect, it may present as a Fallot variant or it may be missed when associated with an outflow ventricular septal defect large enough to cause a large pulmonary blood flow and pulmonary hypertension. Coexistent anomalies in the left ventricular muscle, or fixed subaortic stenosis, may also be found.

SYMPTOMS

These include tiredness and slight dyspnoea. Atrial rhythm upsets occur after 40 years of age.

SIGNS

The signs suggest a ventricular septal defect, with an intense pansystolic murmur at the lower left sternal edge, but an 'a' wave is visible and P_2 is delayed. The right ventricle is not obviously enlarged and may not be obviously hypertrophied on the electrocardiogram, although extensive T inversion in right chest leads suggests abnormality. The presence of left axis deviation makes the diagnosis more difficult. Echocardiography may reveal abnormal bands but is not diagnostic (except in retrospect). Catheterization with angiography is necessary but the high right-ventricular pressure cavity may be missed as it is shallow beneath the tricuspid valve. Angiography and careful searching will confirm the diagnosis. Left ventricular angiography should also be done as there may be a bulging ventricular septum, and aberrantly placed muscle lumps and papillary muscles.

TREATMENT

Treatment is surgical if there are symptoms and high right-ventricular pressure, as the lesion progresses to cause myocardial damage and dys-

function. The postoperative results are good; a raised venous pressure may persist.

DIFFERENTIAL DIAGNOSIS

Other causes of a long, loud systolic murmur at the left sternal edge are:

1. Ventricular septal defect: the murmur is pansystolic and increases on expiration. P_2 is not usually as delayed or diminished and the left ventricle is dominant.
2. Pulmonary-valve stenosis: the ejection click, large left pulmonary artery, and more obvious post-stenotic dilatation distinguish.
3. Subaortic stenosis: there is a soft aortic expiratory diastolic murmur, jerky pulse, a thrill in the suprasternal notch, delayed A_2, and left ventricular dominance.
4. Pulmonary arterial stenosis: the long inspiratory murmur is heard higher and is conducted to the lungs.

Idiopathic dilatation of the pulmonary artery

This condition has physical signs without symptoms and is compatible with a normal lifespan. In many, perhaps all, it is due to trivial pulmonary-valve abnormality—a bicuspid, open pulmonary valve—analogous to the floppy bicuspid aortic valve. Because patients do not die as a result of the condition, we do not know if these are always present. Gradients of 5 to 10 mmHg may be found. Sometimes it is found in patients with stigmata of Marfan's or Ehlers–Danlos syndromes and then it is due to pulmonary arterial dilatation. There is a late pulmonary ejection sound preceding a grade 1 murmur. A_2 and P_2 are normal. Pulmonary diastolic murmurs are frequent and increase on inspiration.

Left-sided obstructive lesions and other anomalies affecting the left side of the heart

The main anomalies causing left ventricular-outflow obstruction are aortic-valve stenosis, bicuspid aortic valve, aortic regurgitation, fixed subaortic stenosis, supra-aortic stenosis, and coarctation of the aorta. Kinked aorta (at isthmus), aorto–left ventricular tunnel, mitral anomalies, and left atrial obstruction may present exceptionally after childhood.

Aortic-valve stenosis

Minor congenital abnormality of the aortic valve (bicuspid, slight tricuspid fusion) is said to be the most common congenital lesion of the cardiovascular system. It is doubtful if it is truly more frequent than ventricular septal defect, but as it usually escapes detection in infancy when that defect is more evident, it is difficult to be sure.

Congenital aortic-valve stenosis can be critical at any age. When it has been moderate to mild, with gradients of 20 to 40 mmHg in childhood, it may become more significant around puberty during or after the period of rapid growth; less commonly, serious problems arise in the third and fourth decades. Isolated calcific aortic stenosis in patients over 60 years of age results from deposition of calcium on a congenitally abnormal valve. Valve calcification is less in the female and appears earlier and more floridly in males. In patients under 30 years with critical obstruction the valve remains pliable, with flecks of calcium in small myxomatous masses attached to the cusps. Severe calcification under 30 years seems only to occur after previous valvotomy, infection, or with a metabolic upset such as hypercholesterolaemic states or a hypercalcaemic state. The mildly congenitally deformed aortic valve (bicuspid, tricuspid, or rarely quadricuspid) may be regurgitant so that the patient is known to have had an immediate diastolic murmur since childhood.

The physical signs of established aortic-valve stenosis depend on severity and pliability. The condition should be differentiated from fixed subaortic stenosis as the management and surgical treatment are different.

In congenital aortic-valve stenosis the pathology may not be limited to the aortic valve. Patients can have an unusually disproportionally thick (>2 cm) ventricular septum (perhaps due to excessive myocardial dysplasia), secondary mitral-valve dysfunction, and aortic disease with systemic hypertension unmasked after aortic valvotomy or valve replacement, probably manifestations of diffuse cardiovascular disease in an apparently isolated congenital lesion.

Fixed subaortic stenosis

This is sometimes referred to as discrete congenital subvalvar obstruction. It is rarely discrete, is probably not truly congenital, but it does lie beneath the aortic valve. The following summarizes the muddled misconceptions about the disease.

The lesion is an accumulation of fibroelastic tissue in the form of a crescent or a complete ring. It may be close to the aortic valve, eccentric, and oblique or 1 to 2 cm beneath. It is never 'membranous' and is attached to a sheet of fibroelastic tissue overlying the bulging and usually excessively hypertrophic ventricular septum, depending on the age of the patient. It causes left-ventricular outflow obstruction, which is often only mild or moderate; when severe, as judged by a high gradient or gross left-ventricular hypertrophy, the myocardial septal hypertrophy contributes rather than the narrowing of the outflow tract by the subaortic ring or crescent. It can present in childhood at the age of 2 or 3 years but more commonly in adolescence and sometimes in an adult. Secondary aortic regurgitation occurs from jet lesions or associated congenital abnormalities; mitral regurgitation may also be an acquired complication.

There is increasing evidence that this is a lesion acquired in postnatal life as a result of some congenital abnormality of the left-ventricular outflow tract; whether this is a morphological or physiological abnormality is uncertain—probably both. Echocardiography provides an excellent way to observe its formation; it can be seen forming as a ventricular septal defect closes. Other congenital anomalies of the heart or cardiovascular system occur in 60 per cent, for instance duct, ventricular septal defect, aortic-valve stenosis (bicuspid or tricuspid), and coarctation. There is an interrelation between fixed subaortic stenosis and obstructive hypertrophic myopathy. In an adult over 30 years of age with signs of aortic stenosis and no radiological calcification, fixed subaortic stenosis should be the first diagnosis.

SYMPTOMS AND PRESENTATION

These are as for other forms of aortic stenosis. Left ventricular failure occurs after the age of 40 years. Infective endocarditis on the aortic valve is a lifelong risk.

SIGNS

Pulses are full and often slightly jerky, but they may be small and sharp when obstruction is severe, close to the aortic valve, or the ventricle is failing. There is a prominent 'a' wave in the jugular venous pulse if the ventricular septum is thick and encroaching on the right ventricular cavity, and a carotid thrill. The apex is left ventricular, powerful, and displaced to the left. There is an ejection systolic murmur not preceded by a click and maximal in the third left intercostal space, conducted to the apex and neck. This may be indistinguishable from, and associated with, a pansystolic murmur at the apex. The aortic second sound is usually audible but often delayed and splitting may be difficult to detect, or may be reversed. In adults a short, immediate diastolic murmur of aortic regurgitation is present.

Chest radiograph

This shows a left ventricular contour. The aorta is normal, but a low post-stenotic dilation may be seen within the heart shadow; more often there is no ascending aortic dilation. No calcification is evident.

Electrocardiogram

There is pure left-ventricular hypertrophy without large Q waves in the anterior chest leads; steep ST depression and T inversion are frequent. The axis may be left, normal, and sometimes inexplicably rightwards. Left bundle-branch block is common over age 45 years.

Echocardiography

M-mode may show premature closure of the aortic valve and a thick, abnormal ventricular septum. Cross-sectional echocardiography reveals the shelf protruding beneath the aortic valve, which may extend on to the anterior cusp of the mitral valve. A very thick, abnormal ventricular septum is commonly seen and abnormal movements of the mitral cusps are frequent. It can be difficult to differentiate from hypertrophic obstructive myopathy. It is vital to see the actual protruding shelf and not just the thickened septal endocardium. The aortic valve is thickened, regurgitant, and opens abnormally, with fixed subaortic stenosis.

INVESTIGATION

Catheter studies show a subvalvar gradient. Aortography shows minor aortic regurgitation unless there is cusp perforation. Thickened aortic-valve cusps open abnormally, with concavity outwards, but are not domed as with valve obstruction. Subvalvar obstruction may be seen as a linear defect, or a small indentation beneath the aortic cusps.

TREATMENT

The lesion should be resected when clinically producing obstruction. All the endocardial thickening attached to the shelf and overlying the ventricular septum must be completely removed. Whether it should be removed very early is disputed as there is a possibility, even when removed very early before any secondary effects or real obstruction occur (gradient over 25 mmHg), that it may reform and create 'tunnel' obstruction, particularly if resection has been incomplete in childhood or adolescence. Physiologically the left ventricular muscle often behaves as in hypertrophic obstructive cardiomyopathy following operation. A picture of congestive myopathy with progressive fibrosis may appear after age of 40 to 50 years.

The aortic valve has a lifetime risk of endocarditis, as jet lesions are usual and remain after resection.

The mortality of early resection is low but problems can return. Recurrence of subaortic obstruction is most likely in patients with persistent resting gradients above 25 to 30 mmHg immediately after operation, in association with a small aortic root, an irregular hypertrophic obstructive cardiomyopathy-like ventricle before operation, and isoprenaline-stimulated high gradients following operation. Asymptomatic patients with two or more of these features should be watched for electrocardiographic deterioration. Reoperation may be difficult and hazardous as tunnel obstructions present a formidable surgical problem. Total aortic-root/valve replacement may be necessary to provide real relief of obstruction. There appear to be two populations of patients with fixed subaortic stenosis: those with a simple shelf with little or no abnormal myocardial reaction or response and a normal-sized aortic root, who do not develop 're-stenosis'; and those with excessive muscular septal hypertrophy, a small root with a likelihood of requiring reoperation, and, in most extreme form, closely resembling severe hypertrophic myopathy.

Supra-aortic stenosis

Supra-aortic stenosis describes a narrowing above the aortic valve contiguous with the commissural attachments. It may be mild, appearing as a waist above the sinuses without causing a gradient, or a severe fibrous constriction above the coronary orifices. When well developed, the aortic cusps hang like a Marlin's nest; the cusps are usually thick and may be regurgitant. Surgical attention is focused on the stenosis and removal may be thought to cure the condition. Unfortunately, this is not so as the disease is not localized to the supra-aortic area. The central aorta beyond is grossly abnormal, often diffusely hypoplastic. Biopsy of the ascending aorta well beyond the supra-aortic narrowing shows a constant histological abnormality in the media termed 'higgledy-piggledy' in describing the disordered, disarrayed musculoelastic fibres. This is most severe in those with obvious aortic hypoplasia, where intimal changes may be found even in childhood. The same histological changes in the medial layers occur in those without apparent diffuse narrowing of the aorta and irrespective of whether the supra-aortic stenosis is part of the 'hypercalcaemic' syndrome with its characteristic facies and other features, familial with normal physical features, or sporadic with none of the known associations. This 'higgledy-piggledy' disorder, which extends throughout the major conducting arteries, appears in severely affected patients to fade out in the region of the common iliac arteries; at least this was found in the only two patients studied with the familial form. 'Higgledy-piggledy' changes are thus a non-specific result of arterial damage *in utero* from several causes. The actual supra-aortic stenosis is probably the result of more extensive damage at a vulnerable site in the conducting arteries, as are the other stenoses at origins of major arteries. These areas may not grow as do the rest of the arteries and so obstruction manifests years or decades later.

Important supra-aortic stenosis has not been found at birth or infancy and so it is doubtful if the lesion itself is truly congenital. It should, like subaortic stenosis, be regarded as acquired in postnatal life, occurring as part of a congenital arteriopathy. Stenoses occur at other sites, for instance carotid, innominate, mesenteric, sometimes renal, and peripherally in the pulmonary arteries in about 50 per cent of patients with supra-aortic stenosis.

If supra-aortic stenosis is relieved before growth of the patient has finished, an obstruction may develop distally in the aortic arch or other vessels later. Another abnormality is the degree and form of the left ventricular hypertrophy that often coexists; this appears to be disproportionate to the degree of outflow obstruction and is often associated with severe, irregular hypertrophy involving the septum, which causes cavity obliteration in the left ventricle resembling the appearance in hypertrophic cardiomyopathy. Perhaps the myocardium, particularly the ventricular septum, is abnormally disarrayed (dysplastic) as is the aorta, and when presented with distal obstruction or abnormally inelastic conducting arteries may hypertrophy erratically and irregularly as in other forms of left ventricular obstruction associated with excess dysplastic muscle. Certainly the conducting arteries in supra-aortic stenosis are thicker and less complaint, thus contributing to the systolic hypertension found in the majority of affected patients. Occasionally, the problem complicates other structural congenital heart anomalies such as pulmonary and aortic valve stenosis, duct, or ventricular septal defect.

SYMPTOMS

When supra-aortic stenosis occurs with the 'hypercalcaemic' facies, a history of early illness in infancy with failure to thrive, repeated infections, and constipation, all of which improve after the first year, are the result of infantile hypercalcaemia, which disappears. Cardiac symptoms are not present early. Angina occurs late as the coronary arteries are large and well perfused proximal to the obstruction but the walls are often pathologically thick and abnormal. Sometimes a stenosis at the origin of a coronary artery causes angina. Syncope may occur if there is marked septal hypertrophy together with atrial rhythm disturbances in older patients. Fits in adolescence are associated with severe systemic hypertension and carotid or innominate obstruction.

Dyspnoea occurs when the myocardium is grossly hypertrophied, with secondary mitral regurgitation. Infective endocarditis on the aortic

valve is a risk and leads to aortic regurgitation. Antibiotic prophylaxis is therefore essential. Supraventricular tachycardia may cause problems after age 30 years.

Supra-aortic stenosis is recognized by the following:

1. Signs of aortic stenosis (carotid systolic thrill, left ventricular hypertrophy).
2. Absence of an ejection click in young patients.
3. A murmur maximal at the right sternal edge.
4. A clear, loud aortic second sound.
5. Right arm and carotid pulses that are sharp and full unless obstructed at their origin. Left carotid and brachial pulses are usually less sharp. Femoral pulses are normal.
6. Systolic hypertension is usual, but diastolic hypertension is exceptional and may reflect renal-artery stenosis. If the supra-aortic stenosis is severe, the systolic hypertension is present only after operation.

In addition, there may be other long systolic murmurs in the neck, lungs posteriorly, axilla, or abdomen due to associated arterial stenoses. Hypertension should be expected and care taken to ensure that the true central aortic pressure is being accurately reflected by the peripheral measurements.

If the arteriopathy is part of the 'burnt-out' hypercalcaemic syndrome, the face is characteristic (Fig. 16), with prominent jaw and supraorbital ridges, large teeth, mental retardation, and exuberant personality, sometimes to the point of manic behaviour. Careful questioning may reveal a story of calcium injections or pills or vitamin D taken during the relevant pregnancy. Familial cases look normal, and siblings and parents should be examined when normal-looking patients present with supra-aortic stenosis.

Electrocardiogram

Left ventricular hypertrophy without large Q waves is usual. Severe ST–T wave changes occur exceptionally, usually late, and in association with a hereditary obstructive cardiomyopathy like ventricle. Right ventricular hypertrophy or right axis deviation coexist when pulmonary hypertension from pulmonary arterial stenosis is present.

Chest radiograph

The radiographic appearance resembles that of aortic stenosis, with a small aorta and low knuckle, but in milder cases there is high, postste-

Fig. 16 Classic face associated with supra-aortic stenosis (William's syndrome). Large ridged teeth, prominent jaw, and supraorbital ridges.

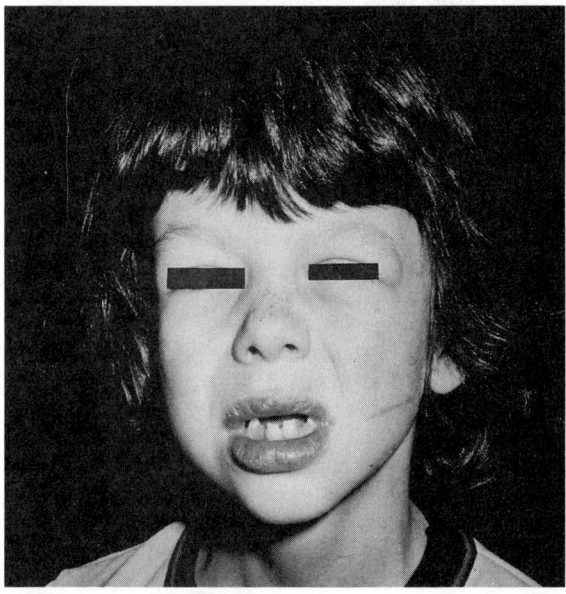

notic dilatation of the ascending aorta in adolescents and adults. Lung vascularity may be unusual and dilatation of the main pulmonary artery is obvious, with pulmonary arterial stenoses.

INVESTIGATIONS

Even when the signs suggest only aortic stenosis, a search for other arterial stenoses, including pulmonary, should always be made. Right-heart catheterization and angiography are necessary in the case of the pulmonary vessels; left ventricular angiography and ascending aorto-graphy are also mandatory and must include visualization of the origin of major vessels. Abdominal aortography should be included; unexpected vascular abnormalities are often revealed. Abdominal 'coarctation' may develop, particularly in relation to severe associated kyphoscoliosis.

TREATMENT

If the supra-aortic stenosis causes a gradient of over 50 to 60 mmHg, it should be relieved, particularly if there is evidence of abnormal left-ventricular and septal hypertrophy. This may be done by 'gusseting', but this can disturb aortic-valve function with resultant aortic regurgitation, which may progress to late cusp avulsion. The systolic blood pressure can reach 250 mmHg and requires therapy. Total aortic root and valve replacement with homograft and reimplantation of coronary arteries may be needed in severe or previously operated patients in order to relieve a diffuse root obstruction.

Coarctation of the aorta

This subject is addressed in Chapter 15.28.3.

Kinked aorta

This minor narrowing of the aortic isthmus looks like a mild coarctation angiographically. Gradients of 0 to 15 mmHg may be recorded. These are of no haemodynamic significance and require no treatment. In differential diagnosis from coarctation, there is no post-stenotic dilatation, nor any development of collateral vessels; femoral pulses are normal and hypertension is not a feature unless it be coexistent essential hypertension. Associated congenital aortic-valve abnormalities may need attention.

Aorto-left ventricular defect (tunnel)

This rare anomaly is a defect not a tunnel, between the right aortic sinus and left ventricular outflow tract. It presents as serious aortic regurgitation, documented in infancy or early childhood, and is characterized by a wide pulse pressure, loud systolic and diastolic murmurs (with thrill) at the left sternal edge, and loud aortic second sound as the aortic valve cusps are voluminous and pliable. The right aortic sinus is so dilated that it may be palpable at the upper left sternal edge and appear on the chest radiograph as a bulge above the right ventricular outflow; the ascending aorta is hugely dilated, as is the left ventricle. It can present in adolescence or young adults for the first time at routine examination or appearing as left ventricular failure.

The differential diagnosis is from other causes of gross aortic regurgitation in young people and a left coronary artery to left ventricular fistula. Treatment is by operation to close the defect and support the aortic root, which is weak and dilated. By adolescence, the aortic root is so dilated that the aortic valve remains incompetent after closure of the defect and valve replacement is necessary. The lesion should be treated early in childhood. If the physician meets this lesion in adult life, it is generally because the patient has persistent aortic regurgitation after earlier surgery and needs aortic root and valve replacement.

Mitral regurgitation (see Chapter 15.18)

Minor congenital lesions of the mitral valve such as cleft of the anterior cusp, redundancy of cusp tissue or chordal anomalies may become symptomatic in adults through infective endocarditis, chordal rupture or slow progression of the regurgitation. Diagnosis and treatment is the same as for other forms of mitral regurgitation.

Left atrial obstruction

When this is of congenital origin, that is mitral-valve stenosis/cor triatriatum or supramitral-valve membrane, the patients do not usually reach adult life without earlier surgical treatment. Occasionally a cor triatriatum with a wide hole in it presents as mitral stenosis in late adolescence. In contrast to mitral stenosis, the left atrial appendage does not enlarge unless there is added valve regurgitation. The echocardiogram should make the correct diagnosis but may be difficult to interpret. It is most important to exclude such lesions in patients presenting as primary pulmonary hypertension or apparent pulmonary venous disease.

Communications between systemic and pulmonary circulation (septal defects)

Atrial septal defect

Defects in the atrial septum are often not detected until they cause symptoms in adult life. There are two anatomical groups.

OSTIUM SECUNDUM DEFECTS

These do not border the atrioventricular valves and are named according to the site in the atrial septum. They may be in the sinus venosus or secundum septum, but are grouped together because of clinical similarity:

1. Oval fossa defects are central and the most common (75 per cent) consisting of fenestrations or true defects about 2 to 3 cm in diameter.
2. Inferior vena caval defects (7 per cent) are posteroinferior with no posterior rim of septal tissue. Particular problems of this defect are (a) anomalous or 'pseudo-anomalous' drainage of the right pulmonary veins, which enter the right atrium close to the midline where the posterior atrial septum is missing; (b) a large Eustachian valve, which can direct inferior vena caval blood into the left atrium through the defect thus causing unexpected cyanosis; and (c) the inexperienced surgeon may close the defect and redirect the inferior vena caval blood to the left atrium, resulting in a previously mildly or asymptomatic patient becoming breathless and mildly cyanosed with a small heart and absence of murmurs.
3. Superior vena caval defects (11 per cent) occur at the base of the superior vena cava and are associated with partial anomalous right upper and middle-lobe pulmonary veins, which enter the superior vena cava and/or right atrium/superior vena caval junction. The defect itself is usually smaller than other defects and the shunt is mostly contributed to by the anomalous pulmonary veins through which the pulmonary flow is greater than through the normally draining pulmonary veins.
4. Coronary-sinus defect. This is a rare form of atrial septal defect in the position of the coronary sinus, which is absent or unroofed and sometimes associated with a left superior vena cava entering the left atrium.
5. Other variants (7 per cent) include hemianomalous pulmonary venous drainage with or without atrial septal defect, and combinations of categories (1), (2), and (3). The whole atrial septum may be fenestrated.

Physiology

The presence of an interatrial hole permits a shunt of blood from left atrium to right atrium after the resistance to filling of the right ventricle lessens after the first weeks of life when the systemic resistance also rises to affect compliance of the left ventricle.

The effects of an established interatrial left-to-right shunt are: (a) increased volume load and dilatation of the right atrium and right ventricle; (b) increased pulmonary blood flow and enlarged pulmonary arteries; (c) increase in size of pulmonary veins (not upper lobes only as in left atrial obstruction); and (d) reduced flow to the left ventricle and aorta, which becomes smaller than normal with time.

The factors that influence the blood flow across an atrial septal defect are: (a) compliance of the right ventricle; (b) compliance of the left ventricle; (c) the size of the defect—least important because most defects are of similar size; and (d) atrioventricular-valve function. In sinus rhythm the left-to-right flow across the defect is mainly during diastole, but when atrial fibrillation occurs the shunt becomes systolic.

Increased blood flow across the defect is caused by left-sided lesions or by increased systemic resistance. The shunt is decreased by tricuspid-valve disease, impaired right-ventricular filling (myopathy, hypoplasia, fibrosis, pericardial effusion), by pulmonary stenosis, and pulmonary hypertension. Central cyanosis results from reversal of the shunt.

Symptoms/natural history

Infants with uncomplicated atrial septal defects are rarely symptomatic unless arrhythmias develop, which may occur in Holt–Oram syndrome with atrial flutter or slow nodal rhythm. There is also the exceptional infant which has developed recurrent chest infections, slightly elevated pulmonary vascular resistance, right heart failure, and difficulties in thriving; in these, early closure is advisable.

Symptoms from defects of the secundum type usually arise in adult life: in 10 to 20 per cent in the third decade, a few more in the fourth, and in the majority of those over the age of 40. By 50 years, 75 per cent have disability and heart failure, precipitated by atrial fibrillation; dyspnoea, bronchitis, palpitation, cyanosis, and chronic progressive failure continue, with haemoptysis. Patients over 60 years who remain in sinus rhythm may slip into right heart failure from chronic fibrosis in the stretched ventricle. Paradoxical emboli are rare but do occur, particularly with extracardiac surgery or trauma. Pulmonary hypertension occurs in about 8 per cent, producing massive cardiac enlargement, cyanosis, and severe failure. It is acquired (see Eisenmenger) in relation to thromboembolism, pregnancy, and life at high altitude. Patients with atrial septal defect over 50 years of age (or younger) can acquire ischaemic heart disease and essential hypertension, which may precipitate cardiac failure. When atrial fibrillation complicates a small atrial septal defect, this lesion may be missed as the heart may not be enlarged and the signs are subtle; the diagnosis must always be considered in the middle-aged female (the lesion is more common in them, 3:1) with atrial fibrillation without obvious cause. All such patients should undergo echocardiography and the transoesophageal route may be needed to show the anatomy of the atrial septum.

Signs

Girls with atrial septal defect are said to be slender ('gracile habitus'). If the defect is large or complicated, a malar flush may be present. Pulses are normal or small when complicated by mitral disease, or an unusually large shunt. Sinus arrhythmia is lost when the defect is large enough to allow equalization of atrial pressures unless the defect lies in the sinus venosus. Jugular venous pulsations are exaggerated, with easily distinguished 'a' and 'v' waves as in such high-output states as anaemia, thyrotoxicosis or pregnancy. Central cyanosis can be seen in association with a right-to-left shunt through the defect; some of the causes are shown in Table 5.

The right ventricle is overactive and dilated with gentle parasternal pulsation and the left ventricular impulse should be impalpable at the apex. On auscultation the first sound is loud (tricuspid-valve closure) and often split, sometimes widely. The second heart sound is widely split in inspiration and expiration. The time interval between A_2–P_2 is characteristically fixed to the ear but may widen on inspiration and not close on expiration when the defect is small or when partial anomalous pulmonary veins contribute more to the shunt than the atrial septal defect, or in the presence of anomalous caval drainage. The A_2–P_2 interval in adults is about 0.06 s. It becomes unusually wide with bradycardia, right ventricular failure, mild pulmonary stenosis, complete right bundle-branch block, and severe mitral regurgitation, which favours earlier closure of the aortic valve. Delay in A_2 makes the split narrower and can occur with left ventricular disease, aortic-valve stenosis, and left bundle-branch block as well as when inferior caval blood drains to the left atrium.

Pulmonary-valve closure (P_2) is loud in adults with atrial septal defect irrespective of pulmonary artery pressure. A pulmonary systolic click is common in adults over 40 years, suggesting pulmonary hypertension, which is not usually present; when it is coincident the click and P_2 are louder and associated with pulmonary regurgitation.

The classic auscultatory features of atrial septal defect are shown in Fig. 17. The diastolic murmur is not present in very small defects and in very large hearts with tricuspid regurgitation as the ring is too large to offer any resistance to the torrential flow. A pansystolic murmur occurs in patients in failure from tricuspid regurgitation. Apical murmurs from added mitral-valve dysfunction appear with advancing years and a pulmonary diastolic murmur is common over the age of 50 or in younger patients with pulmonary hypertension.

The chest radiograph of patients in sinus rhythm is typical (Fig. 18). The left atrium is usually not enlarged. The heart size slowly increases over decades, with dramatic increase once atrial fibrillation is established. Left atrial enlargement is then to be expected and upper-lobe pulmonary veins appear dilated; in the lower lobes, horizontal lines appear like 'Kerley lines', but thicker and often branching. Shadows of pulmonary infarction *in situ* are frequent. The pulmonary arteries can become aneurysmal, with calcification in atheromatous walls. In the patient with a small atrial septal defect who presents with atrial fibrillation and a normal-sized heart, a defect may be suspected from the large left pulmonary artery seen on the lateral view.

The electrocardiogram shows right axis deviation, sharp right-atrial P waves, slight prolongation of the P–R interval, partial right bundle-branch block, and absent QR in V_5–V_6. With increasing age there is prolongation of the P–R interval, an increase in the height of secondary R waves (right ventricular hypertension), increasing width of the QRS, and progressive T inversion across RV leads without necessarily increased voltage. Left axis deviation may be present in 7 per cent with secundum defects or can be acquired in middle life. P mitrale may develop when the P–R interval is greater than 0.20 s or because of a paroxysmal supraventricular rhythm disorder or associated mitral stenosis. Prolongation of the P–R interval above 0.20 s occurs in huge atrial septal defects, in patients over 40 years, sometimes in the Holt–Oram syndrome, and occasionally for no obvious reason. Over 40 years of age, pulmonary hypertension (systolic) may develop and results in right ventricular hypertrophy with large R waves in right chest leads.

Cross-sectional echocardiography should show the defect but sometimes in adults it is difficult to find a clear window to profile the atrial

Fig. 17 Auscultation in atrial septal defect. TDM = tricuspid diastolic murmur. (Reproduced by courtesy of Dr P. Wood.)

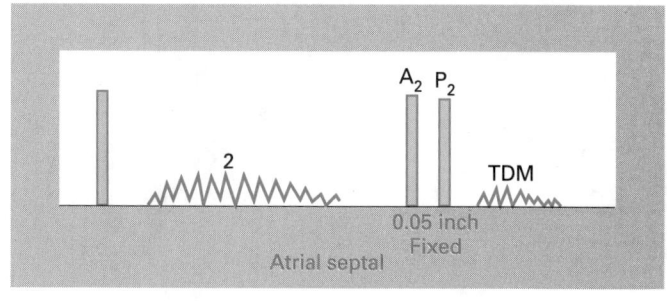

septum. Superior vena caval defects are the most difficult to see. Transoesophageal echocardiography gives important information and is mandatory if atrial septal defect is suspected but not seen with conventional echocardiography. Cardiac catheterization is required in older patients to exclude coronary disease and to assess the degree of pulmonary vascular disease.

Differential diagnosis

Differential diagnosis includes particularly mild pulmonary stenosis. In elderly patients with cardiomegaly and atrial fibrillation the condition

Fig. 18 Chest radiographs from patients with 'secundum' atrial septal defect showing cardiomegaly, pulmonary plethora, and small aorta. Special features are: (a) Dilated superior vena cava (arrow) because there is anomalous right upper lobe pulmonary vein entering it in association with superior vena cava defect. (b) Dilation of inferior vena cava opposite the uncommon inferior vena cava defect.

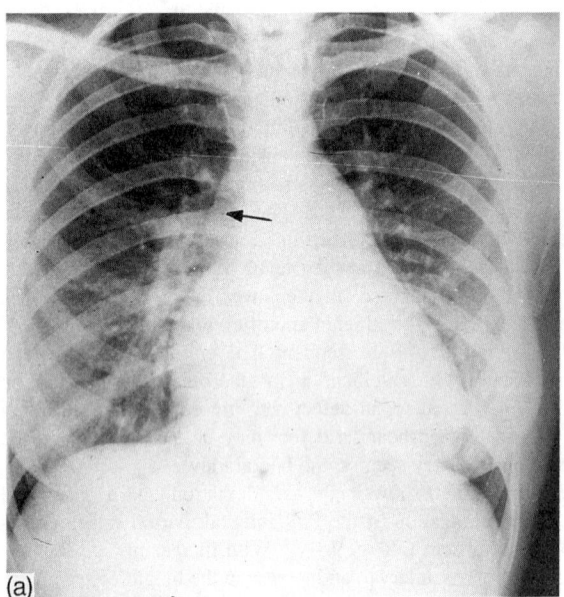

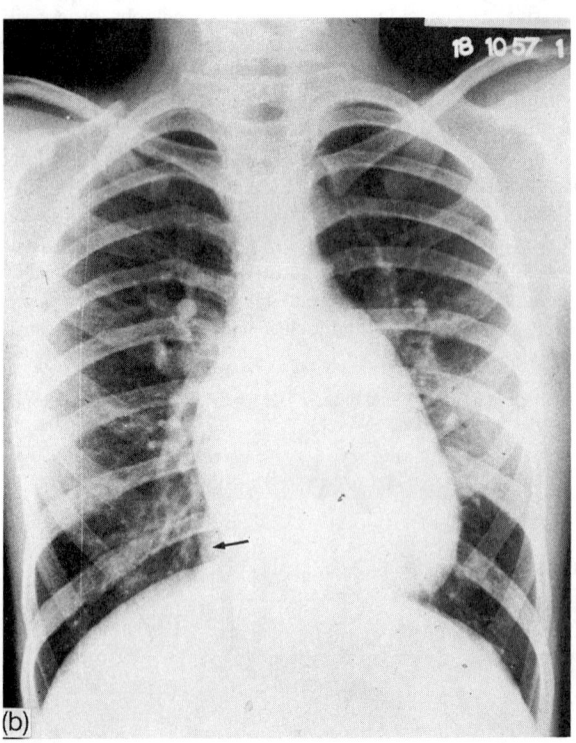

may mimic cor pulmonale, rheumatic mitral disease, and cardiomyopathy. The small atrial septal defect presenting with a paradoxical embolus is easy to miss unless sought by transoesophageal echocardiography.

Treatment

It is generally recommended that atrial septal defects large enough to give clear physical signs should be closed, but there are doubts in those diagnosed when over 50 years of age, as the risk of morbidity from surgery is then increased and atrial fibrillation tends to persist or recur. Echocardiography has resulted in earlier and more frequent diagnosis, many cases being discovered despite absence of classical signs and symptoms. In these, device closure is the best treatment; exceptions are when there is raised pulmonary vascular resistance and cyanosis due to Eisenmenger reaction, and in those over 65 years with only small shunts.

The adult of over 50 years may present difficulties in assessment as the pulmonary vascular disease appears more advanced than it really is because of the huge pulmonary artery, ejection click, and ringing P_2. Older patients with chronic failure and established atrial fibrillation do benefit but there is a higher morbidity from persistence of recurrent arrhythmias, mitral regurgitation, and persistent cardiomegaly.

Patients operated on in childhood and adolescence have excellent long-term results. They do not suffer from endocarditis unless there are left-sided valve problems. Mitral regurgitation occasionally appears. The heart size and electrocardiographic changes regress. Patients often retain an ejection click. Some adults 15 to 25 years after surgery suffer supraventricular rhythm disorders, sometimes nodal bradycardia, and rarely complete block. Whether these are due to surgical trauma or natural history is unknown. Preoperative rhythm disorders should not prevent physicians referring for surgery the asymptomatic or symptomatic young patients because the closure reduces not only the incidence but also the effects of rhythm disturbances. The operation can be considered as 90 to 95 per cent curative in young patients.

THE PATENT FORAMEN OVALE

Many normal adults (possibly 50 per cent) retain patency of the foramen ovale that causes no problem. However, there is the danger of paradoxical emboli, particularly in the presence of illness, necessitating surgery or prolonged bedrest. Device closure should be done in such cases but it is not practical to provide closure in the large number of asymptomatic patients in the population.

Atrioventricular defects

These account for about 5 to 10 per cent of atrial septal defects. The lesion has a sickle-shaped cephalad border sited in the lower (caudal) and anterior part of the atrial septum bounded by the anatomically abnormal atrioventricular valves below, which are also commonly structurally abnormal. Other shared anatomical abnormalities include mitral and tricuspid valves lying at the same level, an outflow of the left ventricle that is unusually long, and an upper border of the ventricular septum depressed caudally and frequently deficient. These features result in abnormal attachment of the mitral valve, which gives rise to diagnostic appearances on angiography and echocardiography.

The three main forms are:

1. Ostium primum (75 per cent): the anterior cusp of the mitral valve is cleft and 20 per cent also have abnormalities of the septal cusp of the tricuspid valve, which are probably of no clinical significance. The ventricular septum is functionally intact or deficient, filled by cusp and chordal tissue, an intermediate form between categories (1) and (2).

2. Common atrioventricular canal (20 per cent): there are functional atrial and ventricular defects with atrioventricular valve cusps draped like curtains across the defect, with and without formation of separate valve rings. These patients can survive to adult life with severe pulmonary vascular disease, for instance when cusp tissue blocks a ventricular septal defect or when there is mild pulmonary stenosis.

3. Common atrium (5 per cent): this is a special form of atrioventricular defect in which the atrial septum is completely absent or has a narrow and shallow posterior remnant with the atrioventricular valves and ventricular septum having the same pathology as described in (1) and (2), which makes the presentation similar. However, there are special features that give clues to the diagnosis, such as situs ambiguus, liver midline or to the right, bronchial isomerism, anomalous vena cavae, caval to coronary sinus, and absent or dual coronary sinus openings. A further complexity is that exceptionally the atrioventricular valves are normal, thus making it difficult to classify amongst atrioventricular defects.

OSTIUM PRIMUM DEFECT

The physiological disturbance is the same as in ostium secundum defects. Early pulmonary vascular disease is uncommon unless the defect is large, mitral regurgitation is severe, or there are added lesions such as supramitral-valve membrane, coarctation, or duct. Mitral regurgitation increases the left-to-right shunt and in many there is a left ventricular/right atrial shunt through the apex of the cleft. The natural history is worse than in ostium secundum atrial septal defect because of associated mitral regurgitation and the disturbance of conducting tissue. Behind the posterior edge of the defect is the atrioventricular node and beneath is the bundle of His, which may be stretched or damaged. Some patients can be symptomatic in childhood and with dyspnoea and failure of thriving problems in infancy, but many reach adolescence and adult life without problems, particularly if mitral regurgitation is mild or absent. Symptoms arise from arrhythmias, nodal bradycardia or tachycardia, complete block, and later atrial fibrillation or flutter. Infective endocarditis occurs uncommonly. Pulmonary vascular disease (Eisenmenger) develops in about 8 per cent. Patients with ostium primum defect can survive to the eighth decade but most die before 30 years. The symptoms are as in other atrial septal defects but with the addition of infective endocarditis and syncope from heart block. Signs are also similar to those of secundum patients but with the addition of a pansystolic murmur from an incompetent mitral valve in 75 per cent, which tends to increase with inspiration. The chest radiograph is also similar but the left atrium is enlarged in 20 per cent.

It is the electrocardiogram that distinguishes the atrioventricular defects from ostium secundum by the presence of left axis deviation in the standard leads associated with an rSR in V_1, and other features typical of atrial septal defect (Fig. 19). When severe right-ventricular hypertrophy coexists, the axis may be shifted to the right shoulder and the pattern of ventricular activation may be less easily recognized from the standard leads, which show SI, II, III dominance. This change of added right-ventricular hypertrophy may be caused by associated pulmonary stenosis, pulmonary hypertension, coarctation, and banding of the pulmonary artery. A normal electrical axis or right axis deviation may occur in unusually small ostium primum defects (2 per cent), in the presence of left bundle-branch block, and for no obvious reason. Fifty per cent have prolongation of the P–R interval, and P mitrale is common.

Diagnosis

The diagnosis of ostium primum should be made in a patient with the signs of atrial septal defect and mitral regurgitation, and an electrocardiogram showing left axis deviation or abnormal initial activation. Two-dimensional echocardiography shows the lesion clearly, as does left ventricular angiography, which demonstrates the abnormal outflow and characteristic attachment of the anterior cusp of the mitral valve.

Differential diagnosis

Ostium primum must be differentiated from ostium secundum with left axis defect, ostium secundum with associated mitral regurgitation, or separate ventricular septal defect. Echocardiography is diagnostic and catheterization is rarely required before decision about surgical closure.

Treatment

Closure of ostium primum defects and repair of mitral clefts causing regurgitation is recommended in all patients unless there is pulmonary vascular disease, a small shunt below 1.5:1 (pulmonary to systemic flow) or very abnormal mitral-valve anatomy. This is only to be done by surgery, device closure being contraindicated because of proximity of atrioventricular valves. However, if the patient is symptom free with evidence of tethered, deficient cusps with palisades of abnormal papillary muscles, it is worthwhile delaying surgery to prevent premature mitral-valve replacement; the latter has special risks and difficulties in atrioventricular defects because of the long abnormal outflow, which may be impinged upon and narrowed by a prosthesis thereby creating subaortic stenosis. Even elderly and middle-aged patients will benefit from closure if correctly selected.

Despite good anatomical 'correction' there may be late problems. Morbidity and mortality are caused by arrhythmias, particularly nodal and complete block, and mitral regurgitation, which progresses if originally moderate or severe. Endocarditis may develop on mitral valves and rarely subaortic stenosis may progress. There is therefore a need for continued informed supervision of these patients.

COMMON ATRIOVENTRICULAR CANAL

This is the most severe form of atrioventricular defect, with a significant ventricular component of the defect and frequently very abnormal atrioventricular valves or a common valve. Most patients die in infancy or childhood, but survival to adolescence or adult life over age 40 years is possible without prior surgery when the defects are small (5 per cent), in the absence of atrioventricular-valve regurgitation (15 per cent), or the presence of Eisenmenger reaction (common in Down's syndrome) or moderate pulmonary-valve stenosis. Older patients present with cyanosis, rhythm disturbances, haemoptysis, and respiratory infections and cerebral abscess. The physical signs vary according to whether the patient has the Eisenmenger reaction, pulmonary stenosis, or a small defect. The second sound is closely split or single according to the size of the ventricular septal defect, and there may be mitral regurgitation, which can be the dominant lesion with a small defect.

The heart is globular on chest radiographs, with a small aortic knuckle and large pulmonary artery. Radiographic features depend on the size

Fig. 19 Typical ECG from patient with ostium primum atrial septal defect (an atrioventricular defect) showing long P-R interval, left axis deviation, and an rSR in V_1.

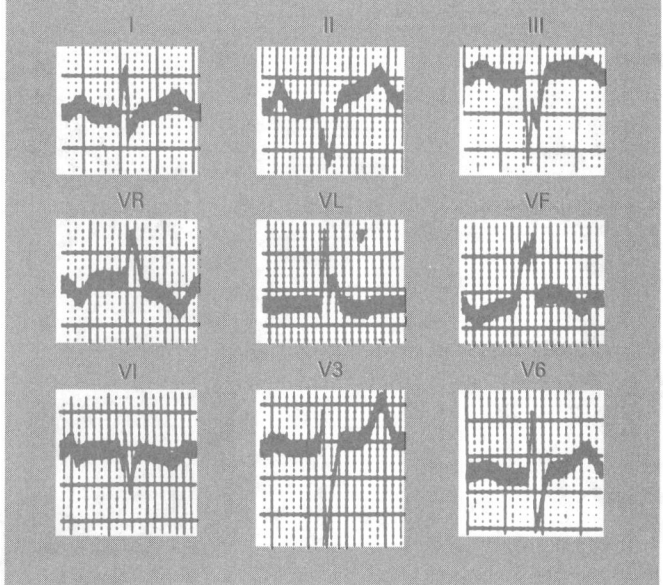

of the shunt and pulmonary blood flow. The left atrium is dilated unless the atrial component of the defect is large. The electrocardiogram shares typical features with the other atrioventricular defects such as left axis or modified left axis defects (SI, II, III patterns) and severe right ventricular hypertrophy with a large left-to-right ventricular shunt, and large equaphasic complexes in the anterior chest leads with evidence of left ventricular volume overload (QR V_5, 6_6) appear (Fig. 19). The P–R interval is prolonged in about 20 per cent.

Diagnosis

Diagnosis is confirmed by echocardiography and angiography. Problems tend to occur in the first 10 years after repair and are similar but more frequent than those found with repaired ostium primum defect, namely, rhythm disturbances, nodal and complete heart block, symptomatic mitral regurgitation; less frequently, mitral stenosis, chronic haemolysis, and effects of progressive pulmonary vascular disease. Left ventricular to right atrial and right ventricle to left atrial shunts as well as residual ventricular septal defects occur, predisposing to rhythm disturbances from atrial volume overload. Dramatic improvement in survival and quality of life is obtained in many survivors.

COMMON ATRIUM

This is found in 5 per cent of atrioventricular defects. Patients present with signs and symptoms of ostium primum defect or common atrioventricular canal. Few reach adolescence and young adulthood without earlier surgery. The diagnosis should be suspected when the patient has the features of an atrioventricular defect combined with any one or more of the following: (a) unexpected central cyanosis; (b) situs ambiguus (stomach on right, apex on left or vice versa); (c) abnormal inferior vena caval drainage to the left superior vena cava (via hemiazygos) or right superior vena cava (azygos), or both. The dilated inferior vena cava may be recognized when seen end-on as a coin-shaped shadow in the superior vena cava on the straight radiograph (Fig. 20). The inferior vena cava may also drain to the coronary sinus; (d) inverted P waves in standard leads or changing P waves and nodal rhythm; and (e) associated with Ellis van Creveld dwarfism.

The diagnosis is confirmed by cross-sectional echocardiography.

Surgical treatment

Partitioning of the atrium and repair of the mitral valve with closure of the ventricular septal defect as in other atrioventricular defects is advisable provided pulmonary vascular disease is not severe. Even then, the patient may benefit symptomatically when cyanosis and hypoxic symptoms are abolished. Estimating pulmonary vascular resistance in these patients is difficult in view of the mixing, which causes a right-to-left shunt increased by vena cavae entering to the left of the atrium and causing systemic streaming. Following operation, patients with septated common atrium have more problems with rhythm disorders than do those with other forms of atrioventricular defects. Progressive pulmonary vascular disease appears unexpectedly, particularly with residual mitral regurgitation when the new left atrium is small.

Ventricular septal defect

Ventricular septal defects occur at various sites. The natural history is therefore dependent not only on the size of the defect but also on its site. There is continued debate on the nomenclature of ventricular septal defects. The simple classification used here divides defects into subvalvar—relating the defect to the contiguous valve—or muscular—either apical central or posterior in the muscular septum. Defects may be single or multiple. Subvalvar defects are described as subaortic, subpulmonary, doubly committed subarterial, (both), subtricuspid and submitral (both inlet defects) (Fig. 21). Subaortic ventricular septal defects do not close spontaneously as the cephalad border is the aortic valve. In contrast, defects beneath the septal cusp of the tricuspid valve close spontaneously or become small and are the defects seen most frequently in adults; small, single, muscular defects also behave like this. Large subaortic or subarterial defects are found in adults, manifesting as the Eisenmenger syndrome or mild Fallot. Small subpulmonary or doubly committed subarterial defects in adults present with aortic regurgitation; indeed the prolapsed right aortic cusp may completely close the defect and even cause right ventricular obstruction. Inlet ventricular septal defects (subtricuspid and submitral) associated with left axis deviation are rarely found in adults except in those with Eisenmenger reaction.

Adults and adolescents with ventricular septal defects appear as follows: (a) small defects, without elevation of right ventricular pressure and a shunt below 2:1; (b) moderate-sized defects with slight elevation of right ventricular pressure and infundibular gradient, and shunts between 2 and 2.5:1; and (c) large ventricular septal defect in association with (i) advanced pulmonary vascular disease (Eisenmenger syndrome) or (ii) infundibular and/or mild pulmonary-valve stenosis.

SYMPTOMS

These relate to the size of the defect and complications. Patients present as follows:

1. Infective endocarditis, most commonly caused by *Streptococcus*

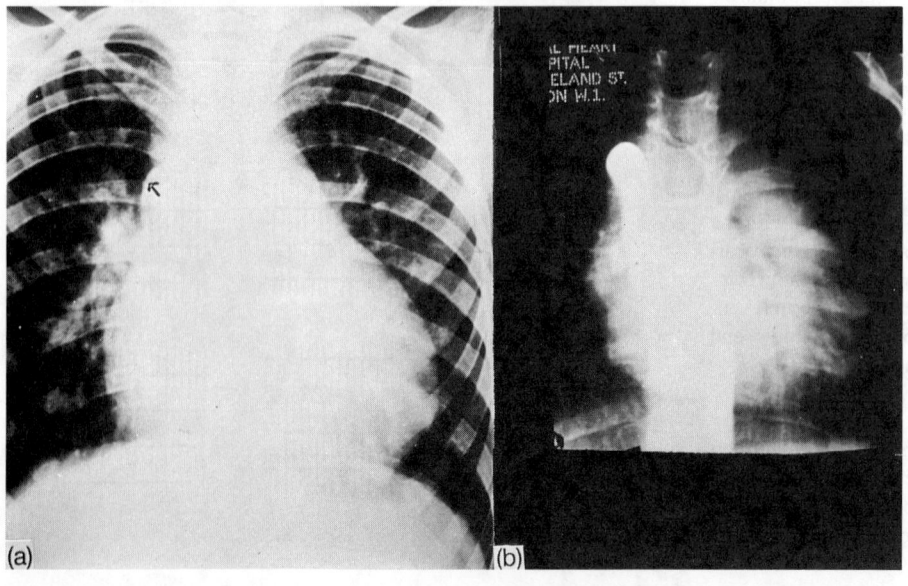

(a)   (b)

Fig. 20 Chest radiograph and venogram to show dilated azygos vein (arrow) which drains the inferior vena caval blood from a patient with common atrium. The inferior vena cava ascends on left and crosses the midline to enter the azygos.

viridans, tends to take an insidious course with low-grade fever, non-specific disability, and episodes of unexplained cough erroneously diagnosed as 'bronchitis', 'pleurisy' or pneumonitis; the true diagnosis is masked by injudicious use of short courses of antimicrobials handed out in the practitioner's surgery. These symptoms in a previously well patient with a pansystolic murmur demand immediate blood cultures and other investigations relevant to the diagnosis of endocarditis. The vegetations may appear on the tricuspid valve, jet lesions opposite or around the defect, or on the aortic valve; they may become large enough to obstruct the right ventricular outflow tract or tricuspid valve. Cross-sectional echocardiography provides an excellent method for following the size and behaviour of the vegetations. One attack of endocarditis is an indication for surgical closure of the defect and there is a place for removal of a large vegetation during the illness.

2. Atrial fibrillation after 30 years of age can precipitate right-sided congestion with tricuspid regurgitation and an apparent left ventricular to right atrial shunt. It may develop spontaneously or in association with pulmonary emboli or lung infections from other causes. The patient should be converted to sinus rhythm as soon as possible. It may be worthwhile closing the defect, however small, as the left ventricular to right atrial shunt can be surprisingly large, preventing maintenance of sinus rhythm.

3. Aortic regurgitation may develop with a small ventricular septal defect (outflow, subarterial) in adult life and progress to embarrass left ventricular function. Aortic regurgitation may also complicate larger subaortic defects but these are infrequent in adults unless part of Fallot. Aortic regurgitation may be acquired as the result of infective endocarditis on an abnormal aortic valve or through prolapse of an aortic cusp—usually the one associated with the right coronary. The signs of ventricular septal defect may disappear as the cusp blocks the small defect. There is usually a history of a murmur dating from infancy or childhood. The most common defects in adults are beneath the septal cusp of the tricuspid valve, already partially closed. In them, aortic regurgitation is acquired from spreading infection or primary abnormality of the valve.

The differential diagnosis of ventricular septal defect with aortic reflux is from causes of a continuous murmur, which include duct, fistulae, ruptured sinus of Valsalva aneurysm, and aortic—valve disease. The treatment is surgical and if the aortic regurgitation is due to prolapse, mild or moderate, it should be possible to conserve the aortic valve by repair. If the regurgitation is severe with aortic-root dilatation, the valve may need to be replaced to relieve the haemodynamic load on the left ventricle.

4. Aneurysm of the ventricular septum, which normally produces no

Fig. 21 Diagram to show simple classification of types of ventricular septal defect as seen from the right ventricle. 1–5, subvalvar; 1, inlet; 2, subtricuspid; 3, subaortic; 4, subarterial doubly committed; 5, subpulmonary; 6–8, muscular; 6, outlet; 7, central; 8, apical; MPM, medial papillary muscle.

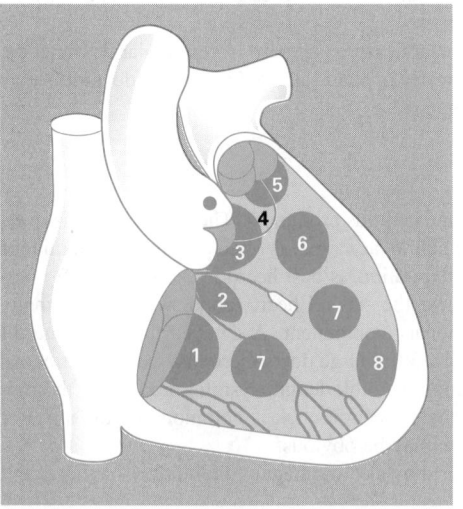

clinical problems: this is an acquired abnormality from spontaneous closure of a ventricular septal defect beneath the septal cusp of the tricuspid valve, which becomes adherent to the margins of the defect and forms an aneurysm that can be identified by two-dimensional echocardiography and left ventricular angiography. Sometimes there is a small hole in it where the defect has not completely closed. There is usually a fibrous reaction around these aneurysms and it is possible for this to invade the conducting tissue causing heart block or a change of electrical axis. If the tricuspid tissue is redundant or voluminous, the aneurysm can enlarge to cause pulmonary stenosis. It does not obstruct the tricuspid valve, as it distends in systole.

5. Large left ventricle disproportionate to the expected size for a small ventricular septal defect. There may be associated electrocardiographic and echocardiographic abnormalities. Either this is a residuum of the effects of a volume overload earlier in life or it is a manifestation of diffuse cardiovascular disease of which the small defect is one part. Prolapse of the mitral cusp may be found in these patients.

6. Spontaneous closure of a ventricular septal defect, which is most common in early childhood, can occur in adolescents and in adults.

DIAGNOSIS OF SMALL/MODERATE VENTRICULAR SEPTAL DEFECT

Pulses, venous pressure, and apex beat are normal. There is a pansystolic murmur, moderate or intense and associated with a thrill, maximal at the left sternal edge in the third or fourth interspace, and easily heard at the apex. The murmur is occasionally conducted to the right sternal edge. In a very small defect the murmur may be early systolic or late systolic, opened by a click from the tensing aneurysm of the ventricular septum, thus resembling the signs of a prolapsed mitral cusp. Sometimes P_2 is slightly delayed if there is associated hypertrophy of the infundibulum or right bundle-branch block. With larger defects the left ventricle is prominent and overactive, and a delayed diastolic murmur is present at the apex.

The chest radiograph can be normal or with prominence of the infundibulum. Pulmonary arteries are normal or slightly enlarged, and the aorta is normal. The left atrium is visible in some with shunts over 2:1, and the left ventricle may be prominent.

The electrocardiogram may be normal. The axis may be leftward or there may be true left-axis deviation. A mild form of rSr is frequent in V_1 with features of left ventricular dominance and upright T waves in V_5 and V_6. The addition of aortic regurgitation leads to features of left ventricular overload and even ST–T changes. The presence of added pulmonary stenosis shifts the axis to the right with added right ventricular hypertrophy shown in V_1. Diagnosis is confirmed by two-dimensional echocardiography or left ventricular angiography.

TREATMENT

Treatment (surgical closure) depends upon symptoms and complications. Without them none is necessary. The prognosis of a small ventricular septal defect is generally excellent if aortic regurgitation and endocarditis are excluded.

COMPLICATIONS

Many patients have now survived to adult life having had earlier surgical closure of a ventricular septal defect. Most are symptom-free. However, the following postoperative problems have required attention: (a) early and late heart block, which is now rare: (b) ventricular ectopics and ventricular tachycardia; (c) late sinoatrial problems; (d) myocardial damage and dysfunction manifesting as failure that relates to bypass technique or other complications; (e) tricuspid and mitral regurgitation, aortic regurgitation; and (f) progressive pulmonary hypertension leading to death or need for transplantation of the heart. Pulmonary vascular disease is uncommon when surgery for the defect has been done in infancy.

Unfortunately, some with large defects closed after the age of 2 years because of a left-to-right shunt are left with pulmonary artery pressures of 40 to 60 mmHg. Such pressures rise on exercise, and at or after puberty the resistance may rise to cause irreversible damage and ultimate right heart failure. Such patients should be identified, treated with calcium blockers such as nicardipine and prevented from doing sport in the hope of preventing or delaying a bad outcome. This course occurs after closure of large ventricular septal defects but has also been seen after large-duct ligation, aortopulmonary window, truncus operation, and Rastelli operation for banded transposition with ventricular septal defect. If there is doubt about the normality of the pulmonary arterioles, patients should be discouraged from mountaineering, living at high altitude, taking the contraceptive pill or slimming drugs, or indulging in athletics. The question of pregnancy requires careful judgement. Obstetric care must be optimal, with expert cardiological and intensive care available at delivery.

Residual ventricular septal defect despite surgery is common in patients operated on before 1974–75. Patients with residual defects or left-sided valve lesions should be protected from infective endocarditis and the defect closed early to prevent secondary problems.

Sinus of Valsalva aneurysm

Occasionally all three sinuses of Valsalva are aneurysmally dilated but this is usually due to acquired disease. One sinus of Valsalva may be aneurysmal due to deficiency or absence of local aortic media and this is congenital. Aneurysmal dilatation of a sinus may occur during endocarditis on the aortic valve, with the right aortic sinus most commonly affected. The lesions may be silent or enlarged to cause right ventricular obstruction or affect the conducting tissue causing heart block or left anterior hemiblock. Rupture into the right ventricle or right atrium occurs in men more than women. The patient may complain of a tearing sensation in the chest, becomes rapidly breathless, and soon develops congestive heart failure with hepatomegaly, ascites, and oedema. A loud continuous murmur is heard at the left or right sternal edge. The electrocardiogram may show a long P–R interval, right bundle-branch block, and mild voltage increase. The chest radiograph shows cardiomegaly and enlargement of the right atrium and right ventricle with mild pulmonary plethora. Sometimes linear calcification of the aortic sinus is seen.

Aortography and right heart catheterization delineate the site and source of the shunt. Surgical closure is urgently required, provided infection has been treated or excluded. It may be necessary to operate during active infection. The diagnosis is made from the acute history and finding of continuous murmur to the right or lower left of the sternum and heart failure with a jerky pulse. The condition must be distinguished from other causes of continuous murmur, dissection of the aorta and aortic regurgitation or other fistulae for example.

Coronary artery anomalies

Congenital anomalies of the coronary arteries are often symptomless but may cause premature angina, sudden death or persistent ventricular ectopics, or even underlie a cardiomyopathy. A left coronary artery arising from the pulmonary artery may be detected first in adult life but death is more usual in infancy or childhood. This may present with a continuous murmur with evidence of infarction (anterolateral wide Q waves) on the electrocardiogram, or with a left ventricular aneurysm in a young person, or mitral regurgitation with infarcted anterolateral wall, chronic failure, or as sudden death.

Treatment is surgical, with closure of the fistula and grafting of the left coronary artery into the aorta. This does nothing for previous infarction but may help angina and diminish chances of subsequent sudden death.

Single coronary arteries may be discovered in young patients with angina or a dilated left ventricle appearing as congestive myopathy or sudden death.

Coronary artery fistulae may cause a continuous murmur at the left sternal edge and enter the right ventricular outflow, the right atrium, or exceptionally the left ventricle. With long-standing fistulae they may 'steal' from the other coronary arteries and the myocardium, causing angina.

Calcification may develop in the orifice and in the coronary sinus, where clot may be laid down. Aneurysmal dilatation of the vessel and sinus often occur by the time the patient is adult and this may be visible on the chest radiograph. The electrocardiogram may reflect left ventricular volume overload, sometimes with anterior ischaemia. Normal resting T waves may invert or flatten on effort. Acquired coronary fistulae may occur following open heart surgery for ventricular septal defect and infundibular stenosis or Fallot, contributing to angina in the late survivor or a continuous murmur.

The fistulae should be closed from within the atrium or ventricle without damaging the normal coronary artery supply. This can now be done with coils and balloons placed through catheters so surgery is not necessary. Differential diagnosis is from a duct, if the continuous murmur is at the left sternal edge, other fistulae such as internal mammary, or ruptured sinus, which is usually associated with important symptoms and failure. Aortography and selective coronary angiography will make the diagnosis, together with oxygen saturation determination in the right heart.

Aberrant course of coronary arteries such as when the right arises from the left sinus or the left from a right sinus may lead to compression between aorta and pulmonary artery, particularly during circumstances that provoke systolic hypertension. This may cause angina, ischaemic signs on the electrocardiogram, and even cause sudden death. Rerouting of the coronary artery may be needed.

Aortopulmonary shunts

Persistent duct (ductus arteriosus)

When the duct remains open into the second decade and thereafter, a left-to-right shunt from just proximal to the aortic isthmus to the bifurcation of the pulmonary arteries occurs. The main pulmonary artery and branches dilate and may cause pulmonary regurgitation, the sound of which is difficult to separate from the continuous murmur. The pulmonary veins, left atrium, left ventricle, and aorta (ascending and arch) are dilated from accommodating the increased volume of blood. The pulmonary arterial systolic pressure may be moderately elevated and the diastolic pressure is low. The levels depend on the age of the patient, size of duct, and where the patient was born, that is at sea level or above 3000 m. The pulmonary and systemic pressures may be equal with a balanced or reversed shunt.

Symptoms include breathlessness if there is ventricular dysfunction. Atrial fibrillation may result in heart failure. Infective endocarditis may cause the first symptoms.

SIGNS

The pulse is jerky and the carotids prominent. The left ventricle is overactive and dilated. The pulmonary artery is often palpable. A continuous murmur, enhanced on expiration, is best heard in the second left intercostal space, loudest near the second heart sound, which is normally split with a loud pulmonary component. A delayed diastolic murmur may be heard at the apex. With large ducts there may be no continuous murmur; instead there is a variable-length systolic murmur in the pulmonary area. A pulmonary ejection click is common and the signs of pulmonary regurgitation may be obvious.

The chest radiograph shows cardiomegaly, pulmonary plethora, and large left atrium, pulmonary arteries, and aortic knuckle. Calcium is visible in the duct in many over 35 years of age and may be diagnostic when signs are atypical.

The electrocardiogram shows left ventricular dominance with large Q waves and increased voltage. Occasionally the T waves are flattened or depressed but if inverted may mean added aortic stenosis. The axis is usually normal, with exceptional left deviation. Right ventricular hypertrophy only occurs if there is serious pulmonary vascular disease. The features which should make the physician suspect that the patient with a long systolic and diastolic murmur does not have a duct, despite other suggested features, are shown (Table 7).

The differential diagnosis is from conditions such as ventricular septal defect with aortic regurgitation, aortic stenosis with regurgitation, or absent pulmonary valve with pulmonary regurgitation. Other diagnoses to consider include aortopulmonary defect, internal mammary or coronary fistulae, pulmonary arterial stenosis, pulmonary arteriovenous fistula, and left coronary artery arising from the pulmonary artery.

TREATMENT

Closure of all ducts that allow a left-to-right shunt is recommended. Many can now be closed by a device instead of surgery. Although a simple operation, the duct in an adult is treacherous as the tissue may tear or the aorta split.

Aortopulmonary window

This lesion is rare in children and even more uncommon in adults, when it presents with the Eisenmenger reaction. It then has the same features as a duct but more accentuated because the defect is larger and thus more likely to be associated with pulmonary hypertension and serious pulmonary vascular disease.

The diagnostic problems relate to distinguishing this lesion from a large duct or a large ventricular septal defect. A continuous murmur is exceptional—usually there is a long systolic murmur (not pansystolic) in those with a significant left-to-right shunt and features of pulmonary hypertension; there is often right ventricular hypertrophy.

Common trunk (truncus arteriosus)

Most patients with this lesion die in infancy or early childhood. When seen in adults the condition is complicated by pulmonary vascular disease (Eisenmenger) or rarely by pulmonary arterial stenosis.

A single trunk arises from the heart and gives off both pulmonary arteries from the ascending aorta. When the pulmonary arteries arise from descending aorta, the condition is almost always one of pulmonary atresia, with a 'blind' atretic right-ventricular outflow in front of the aorta. Beneath the common trunk is a large subtruncal ventricular septal defect and so blood from both ventricles is ejected into the trunk, the amount passing to the pulmonary circulation depending on the pulmonary arteriolar resistance. When pulmonary blood flow predominates, the pulses are full, even collapsing, with visible carotids and a palpable, enlarged, unfolded aorta, particularly obvious when there is a right arch (15 per cent). There is a long systolic murmur, single second sound, sometimes with several components caused by asynchronous closure of two to five cusps, together with an immediate diastolic murmur and delayed diastolic apical murmur from increased flow across the mitral valve. There is biventricular hypertrophy and left atrial enlargement, together with unusual high, large branches of the pulmonary artery on chest radiographs. A trace of cyanosis is usual, particularly after exercise. The electrocardiogram looks like that of ventricular septal defect.

Table 7 *Features that raise doubt as to whether a continuous murmur truly reflects a patent duct*

Central cyanosis
Continuous murmur:
  Not maximal
  Below left clavicle
  Increases on inspiration
Murmur 'to and fro':
  No crescendo around second sound
Second sound single
Important right-ventricular hypertrophy
Large wide Q waves in LV leads on ECG
Severe left ventricular hypertrophy with ST–T wave changes
  on ECG
Small aortic knuckle on chest radiographs

Large QR patterns in V_5–V_6 suggest volume overload of the left ventricle and the possibility of benefit from surgical repair. Diagnosis is confirmed by two-dimensional echocardiography and angiography.

SURGICAL TREATMENT

Patients with this lesion are probably inoperable by the second decade of life. They have survived because of raised pulmonary vascular resistance. Trunks have been repaired in adolescents with successful late results. Collapsing pulses, little or no cyanosis, a large left ventricle, and pulmonary plethora suggest suitability for operation. The principles of repair are to close the ventricular septal defect, leaving the trunk connected to the left ventricle, cutting the pulmonary artery origins from the trunk, and joining them to the right ventricle by a valved conduit and closing the hole in the trunk. Late results depend on what conduit had been used and the residual pulmonary vascular disease, which may advance, producing false or real aneurysm in distal suture line. Pregnancies are possible but with risk to mother, and the outcome depends on residual pulmonary vascular disease. Endocarditis can occur on aortic or truncal valves.

Hemitrunk

This is a condition where one pulmonary artery arises from the aorta and the other from the right ventricle or is absent. A ventricular septal defect with pulmonary valve stenosis or atresia may be associated. The physical signs present as a mixture of Fallot and truncus. The chest radiograph shows a marked difference in the perfusion and vascular pattern of the lungs. By the time adult life has been reached, irreversible damage to the lung supplied by the pulmonary artery arising from the aorta is likely. If the patient has pulmonary stenosis, it may be worthwhile relieving this or creating a systemic to pulmonary artery shunt on that side. Death from this condition is either from attempted surgery, massive haemoptysis or cerebral abscess.

REFERENCES

Roberts, W.C. (1979). *Congenital heart disease in adults*. Davis, Philadelphia.
Rosenthal, A. (1993). Adults with tetralogy or Fallot—repaired, yes; cured, no. *New England Journal of Medicine*, **329**, 655–6.
Somerville, J. (1979). Congenital heart disease—changes in form and function. *British Heart Journal*, **41**, 1–22.
Wood, P. (1958). The Eisenmenger syndrome. *British Medical Journal*, **2**, 701–9; 755–62.

15.16 The cardiac aspects of rheumatic fever

J. M. Neutze

Rheumatic fever is an illness of children and young adults, with major symptoms of arthritis and carditis, a prolonged course, and a tendency to recur. It is the result of abnormal immune reaction to an infection with a Group A β-haemolytic streptococcus. Despite decades of intensive study, the nature of this reaction remains obscure and, in many ways, rheumatic fever is still an enigma. Although the major cause of acquired heart disease in children, rheumatic fever declined dramatically in the Western world from the 1940s. In underdeveloped countries it remains a major problem, with annual incidence rates of 100 per 100 000 in the childhood age group, compared with fewer than 5 per 100 000 in most Western countries. In the 1980s an unexplained increased incidence was noted in a number of regions in the United States, but levels there are still well below those in underdeveloped regions.

Aetiology and pathogenesis

The streptococcus

An association between septic throats and rheumatic fever was noted in the nineteenth century, and in the 1930s there were many reports of outbreaks of rheumatic fever following tonsillitis or scarlet fever in closed communities. The development of serological tests for streptococcal infections established the role of the Group A β-haemolytic streptococcus. This was confirmed when penicillin treatment sharply reduced the incidence of rheumatic fever in epidemics of streptococcal infections, and effective prophylaxis came close to abolishing recurrences.

The way in which the streptococcus causes rheumatic fever is still only partly understood. Characteristics of the streptococcus are critical. The organism must be able to attach firmly to pharyngeal cells and produce a brisk antigenic response. Impetigo strains do not cause rheumatic fever. The properties of the streptococcus are described in detail in Chapter 7.11.2.

Streptococci do not persist in cardiac tissues in rheumatic patients. Both the peptidoglycan moiety of the cell wall and streptolysins O and S have produced cellular damage in experimental situations, but no animal model of rheumatic fever has been developed.

The host reaction

The latent period, the generally higher antistreptococcal titres in patients who develop rheumatic fever compared with those who do not, and the transient appearance of circulating immune complexes, point to an abnormal immune response to streptococcal antigens cross-reactive to mammalian tissues. There is now strong evidence for this, both at a humoral and cellular level, implying a genetically programmed predisposition. A monoclonal antibody to B cell surface antigens, called D8/17, has been found in over 90 per cent of patients with rheumatic fever but in only 10 per cent of healthy controls. Much needs to be done before these pieces of the jigsaw can be put together.

In some communities there is a high incidence of rheumatic fever in certain racial groups. In Britain, rheumatic fever is much more common in Asian immigrants, and in New Zealand it is eight times more common in the Polynesian than in the Caucasian population. Nevertheless, specific racial predilection has never been substantiated. Crowding, poor housing, poor hygiene, and inadequate medical care all contribute, overcrowding being the predominant factor. Increased rheumatogenicity of streptococci has frequently been demonstrated during epidemics. Possibly heightened rheumatogenicity occurs with repeated upper respiratory infections in crowded communities where there is an undue acceptance of symptoms of infection.

Pathology

The classic histological feature of rheumatic fever is the Aschoff nodule, a perivascular lesion with a central core of necrotic material surrounded by large cells with polymorphous nuclei and basophilic cytoplasm, and an outer layer of lymphocytes. Nodules have a widespread distribution in connective tissues, including those of joints, tendons, and blood vessels. In the heart they are found in myocardial tissue, most valvular lesions consisting of less organized collections of chronic inflammatory cells. The nodules heal by fibrosis, sometimes leading to extensive interstitial myocardial fibrosis.

The mitral valve leaflets become thickened, with impairment of closure exacerbated by ring dilation. Progressive distortion of the leaflets and subvalvar apparatus may lead to severe regurgitation. Leaflet and chordal fusion may lead to mitral stenosis, the structure of the valve becoming severely distorted by progressive fibrosis and eventually calcification. This process usually progresses slowly over many years, but proceeds rapidly in some children in developing countries. Similar but less severe changes occur in the tricuspid valve in up to 10 per cent of cases. In the aortic valve thickening of the leaflets is also seen, leaflet edges developing a rolled appearance. The dominant lesion is usually aortic regurgitation.

Clinical features

Rheumatic fever is rare under 4 years of age, most cases occurring in the 6- to 15-year age group. Some two-thirds of patients give a history of prior sore throat, usually 1 to 3 weeks before the development of rheumatic symptoms. Although there is considerable variation in the clinical presentation of rheumatic fever, most cases feature migratory polyarthritis, carditis, or both. Presentation may be abrupt, with fever and joint pains, or more gradual with a subacute course. In some cases no acute bout is recognized at all, the patient presenting with established rheumatic heart disease.

Arthritis (see Section 18)

Arthritis most commonly affects larger joints, especially wrists, elbows, knees, and ankles. Objective signs are usually limited to minor warmth and swelling, but pain may be excruciating, especially with pressure or movement. Characteristically one joint will be affected for 2 to 3 days and then the inflammatory process moves to another region, but two or more joints may be affected simultaneously to some degree.

Arthralgia without objective signs may occur in other joints or may be the only feature, symptoms varying from minor discomfort to severe pain. Untreated, joint pains usually settle over 1 to 4 weeks.

Carditis

This is the manifestation of rheumatic fever with permanent sequelae. When carditis occurs in the course of an acute illness, signs present in the first week in three-quarters of the patients. In patients with a subacute course, carditis may become manifest later in an illness featuring low grade fever, pallor, and joint aches.

VALVULITIS

The most common manifestation is the development of mitral regurgitation, consisting initially of a modest apical systolic murmur but sometimes progressing to a severe leak with an overactive and dilating heart, dyspnoea, and an increasing murmur. The appearance of an early diastolic murmur of aortic regurgitation may clinch the diagnosis of rheumatic fever. Aortic regurgitation may also progress rapidly to a severe leak. Echo Doppler studies have shown clear evidence of valve involvement when cardiac signs are restricted to a modest, innocent-sounding murmur. Our own group demonstrated 17 regurgitant lesions not diagnosed by careful clinical assessment in 34 patients with acute rheumatic fever. Lesions were detected in four out of ten patients with a possible clinical diagnosis of rheumatic fever, but none were found in 19 patients with a non-rheumatic acute febrile illness. With careful exclusion of trivial leaks demonstrable in many normal valves, echo Doppler has become an important diagnostic aid. Interestingly, significant regurgitation was seen quite commonly at the tricuspid and occasionally at the pulmonary valve.

RHEUMATIC MYOCARDITIS

Although some myocardial involvement probably occurs almost universally, severe impairment of ventricular function is relatively uncommon. When pulmonary venous congestion and heart failure develop, severe mitral (and sometimes aortic) regurgitation are usually present with modest reduction in myocardial contractility. As the heart dilates, stretching of the mitral valve ring exacerbates the leak, and dilation of the right heart secondary to left ventricular failure may produce severe tricuspid regurgitation.

PERICARDITIS

This may accompany myocarditis, sometimes presenting with upper abdominal or chest pain and characterized by the superficial scratchy sound of the pericardial bruit. A moderate pericardial effusion may develop.

CARDITIS

A third heart sound is commonly recorded, sinus tachycardia is usual, and supraventricular and ventricular ectopic beats may occur. The P–R and Q–T intervals may be prolonged on the electrocardiogram, but these findings alone are not usually enough to justify a label of carditis.

Carditis is thus diagnosed by the presence of new or changing murmurs, pericarditis, or heart failure. Careful monitoring and supervision are required, worsening failure and death being real possibilities in the presence of severe carditis.

Chorea

Once present in 50 per cent of patients, Sydenham's chorea is now recognized in about 5 per cent. It has a longer latent period than arthritis or carditis, from 1 to 6 months. It may occur in association with carditis, or as the only rheumatic manifestation – 'pure' chorea. In this case acute-phase reactants and streptococcal titres have frequently returned to base line levels. Chorea is characterized by jerky, purposeless movements, exaggerated by tension but disappearing in sleep. Clumsiness,

grimacing, emotional lability, and unclear speech may appear and, in severe cases, violent movements and progressive weakness develop. Occult chorea may be diagnosed by testing sustained hand grip. When the patient holds the observer's fingers, minor sudden movements and fluctuations in muscle tension can be detected.

Symptoms usually subside over 1 to 3 months but may persist for a longer period and occasionally recur over the following 2 years. They may occasionally reappear during the administration of oral contraceptives or during pregnancy.

Erythema marginatum and rheumatic nodules

These manifestations are seen much less frequently but may contribute to diagnosis. Erythema marginatum begins as a non-itchy, faint red macule, the erythema spreading outward while the centre returns to normal colour. The margin is often irregular in outline, and adjacent areas may coalesce. The rash usually fades in 24 h but may recur over a period of months. Carditis is usually present. Although most commonly associated with rheumatic fever, erythema marginatum also occurs in association with acute glomerulonephritis and drug reactions, and occasionally without recognized cause.

Rheumatic nodules usually appear in patients with long-standing carditis. They are firm, painless, 0.5 to 2 cm in diameter, and situated over tendons or bony prominences.

Other associated features

Other features are not specific enough to be diagnostic. Epistaxis is quite common, as is abdominal pain, particularly at the onset of an attack. Pleural effusions may occur, especially in association with pericardial effusions.

Diagnosis

Although diagnosis is easy in many cases, a number of factors may cause problems.

1. There is no single diagnostic test. The diagnosis is made on the basis of the clinical pattern with support from laboratory tests.
2. Many illnesses may mimic the clinical presentation. These include infective endocarditis and viral and other causes of polyarthritis, especially early rheumatoid arthritis. Monarthritides, including those of septic and traumatic origin, can cause initial confusion. Acute streptococcal infections may be followed by a period of mild fever, lethargy, malaise, and elevated erythrocyte sedimentation rate, sometimes lasting 2 to 3 weeks. These reactions may be difficult to distinguish from rheumatic fever but they do not show major rheumatic manifestations and generally have a briefer course. Rheumatic fever rarely settles in less than 2 months. It may continue for several months, particularly in patients with carditis where 2 to 4 per cent are still active at 6 months.
3. The murmur of a minor congenital cardiac lesion may first be noted during a viral infection. Even in expert hands the distinction of mild congenital aortic stenosis or prolapse of the mitral valve from a rheumatic lesion may be impossible. Changing murmurs and evidence of involvement of both aortic and mitral valves favour rheumatic fever.
4. The features of rheumatic fever may vary according to severity and time of presentation. With early presentation diagnosis may only be possible after a period of observation of clinical progress and laboratory tests. With late presentation some clinical and laboratory abnormalities may have subsided and the clinician may have to be content with a diagnosis of 'probable'

rheumatic fever. With a view to providing a basis for diagnosis and minimizing overdiagnosis, Duckett Jones published diagnostic criteria, subsequently modified by the American Heart Association with additional comments made by a World Health Organization working party (Table 1).

Laboratory tests

A throat swab should be taken although group A streptococci are isolated in only 15 to 20 per cent of cases. Blood cultures and other appropriate investigations are required to exclude infective endocarditis. Mild anaemia and leucocytosis are common.

ACUTE PHASE REACTANTS

The two most useful acute-phase reactants are the erythrocyte sedimentation rate and the C-reactive protein levels, which should be measured weekly. Where the patient presents in congestive heart failure the initial erythrocyte sedimentation rate may be high to normal, rising over the following 2 weeks as symptoms improve. C-reactive protein levels are not affected in this way. Later in the illness mild elevation of the erythrocyte sedimentation rate may persist after the C-reactive protein level has returned to normal. It may then be reasonably assumed that residual rheumatic activity is low grade, although the inflammatory process may not have completely subsided.

STREPTOCOCCAL SEROLOGY

Streptococcal titres should be measured on three occasions at 2-weekly intervals. Multiple tests are desirable, usually the streptococcal antistreptolysin O, anti-DNAse, and antihyaluronidase. A two-fold rise in titre may be considered diagnostic. Because of the late presentation, titres are usually convalescent and are considered positive when they exceed a given level – 250 for antistreptolysin O, 320 for anti-DNAse, and 300 for antihyaluronidase. Using these criteria, positive tests are obtained in over 90 per cent of patients with acute rheumatic fever. The inexpensive streptozyme test is often favoured but shows poor reproducibility and specificity.

Treatment of acute rheumatic fever

Admission to hospital is highly desirable for diagnosis and management, and for the education of patient and family. Following initial blood cultures, a (1.2 mega units) course of penicillin is given, either intramuscular benzathine penicillin or 10 days treatment with oral penicillin. Long-term prophylaxis should then be continued.

Rest

Rest remains the cornerstone of treatment. This recommendation has never been subjected to a controlled trial but is based on clinical observation that symptoms persist and carditis progresses in many patients who are not rested. Patients should remain on bed–chair rest until symptoms subside and acute-phase reactants have been normal for two successive weeks. It is likely that earlier mobilization will prove less important in patients who have had arthritis alone and, provided symptoms are settled and the C-reactive protein level is normal, gradual mobilization may be considered in those with a prolonged course even when the erythrocyte sedimentation rate remains mildly elevated. In patients with carditis, however, the period of rest should be strictly maintained. Once the acute phase reactants have settled, modest restriction of exercise activity is recommended for 2 weeks only. Measurement of phase reactants should be, however, continued at 2-weekly intervals for 2 months. With this regimen a rebound is unlikely in patients with arthritis alone, but may occur in patients with carditis, rarely requiring a further period of rest.

Table 1 *Revised Jones criteria for the diagnosis of rheumatic fever*

Major criteria
Carditis
Polyarthritis
Chorea
Erythema marginatum
Subcutaneous nodules
Minor criteria
Previous rheumatic fever or rheumatic heart disease
Arthralgia (included only in the absence of frank arthritis)
Fever
Raised erythrocyte sedimentation rate, positive test for C-reactive protein or leucocytosis
Electrocardiogram: prolonged P–R interval
Evidence of recent group A streptococcal infection
Raised antibody levels
Positive throat swab
Recent scarlet fever

Two major criteria, or one major and two minor criteria, make rheumatic fever very likely if supported by evidence of a preceding streptococcal infection.

The absence of a streptococcal infection should make the diagnosis doubtful, except in two situations in which rheumatic fever is first discovered after a long latent period from the antecedent infection: (1) Sydenham's chorea; (2) prolonged, insidious onset carditis. This is more common in developing countries with limited access to medical care.

In patients with established rheumatic disease the presence of only one major criterion, or of fever, arthralgia, or elevated phase reactants, suggests a presumptive diagnosis of a rheumatic recurrence. Evidence of a preceding streptococcal infection and exclusion of intercurrent illnesses including infective endocarditis are required.

Anti-inflammatory drugs

Treatment with anti-inflammatory drugs has naturally received intensive study. Joint pains and fever usually settle rapidly with aspirin or steroids. It is questionable, however, whether either drug has any effect on the duration of the illness or the extent of valve damage after the illness. Over 170 papers have failed to show that aspirin has either effect, despite suggestions of benefit in earlier uncontrolled studies.

In a controlled study in the 1960s, Feinstein showed that rheumatic activity may be prolonged by the use of steroids. Although studies without concurrent controls have suggested that the extent of valve disease may be reduced by steroid administration, this impression has not been confirmed by controlled studies. The Co-operative United Kingdom and United States study group and the United States Combined Rheumatic Fever study group found no benefit from adrenocorticotrophic hormone (ACTH) or prednisone in moderate or high doses. Claims have been made for the efficacy of combined steroids and aspirin but no adequately controlled studies exist.

One must conclude that, if there is any long-term benefit from the use of aspirin or corticosteroids, it is so small as to be unmeasurable. Despite this, steroid administration is often given to patients with moderate carditis, covering the withdrawal with aspirin because of the rather common rebound in symptoms. Such policies seem to reflect the desire of doctors to administer drugs rather than to allow nature to effect a cure. Aspirin should be given to control pain, the dosage tailored according to need. Prednisone may also be given for this purpose but can usually be reserved for the situation where aggressive carditis appears life-threatening. Steroids sometimes appear to help to arrest progressive heart failure. The required dose of prednisone is usually not more than 40 to 60 mg daily, and gradual reduction in dosage can usually start within 1 week. Three points should be noted.

1. Treatment should not be started until the diagnosis is secure.
2. When there is evidence of deteriorating cardiac output, dilation of the heart, and congestive heart failure, a severe valve lesion is usually present and valve replacement may give the only chance of survival.
3. Aspirin and prednisone depress acute phase reactants. The bout cannot be considered settled until the erythrocyte sedimentation rate and C-reactive protein levels have been normal in successive weeks, the first measurement being taken 2 weeks after stopping suppressive treatment.

Chorea

Treatment of chorea, other than with penicillin prophylaxis, is rarely required and does not influence the duration of symptoms. Bed rest is required only when chorea appears early and phase reactants are still positive, or in the rare case of extreme motor disturbance. For troublesome symptoms phenobarbitone, diazepam, or haloperidol are useful.

Recurrence of rheumatic fever and prophylaxis

Recurrence of rheumatic fever

In preantibiotic days recurrences of rheumatic fever were recorded in up to 70 per cent of patients. It was subsequently shown that a further streptococcal infection, often with a different strain, preceded each recurrence. The 'rheumatic' patient retains the tendency to develop rheumatic fever with further group A streptococcal infections. The risk of recurrence is highest in the first 3 years after the first attack, in young patients, and in patients with rheumatic heart disease. Carditis with a recurrence is more common in those patients in whom it was present in the first attack but it may occur in any patient. Recurrent attacks frequently lead to progressive deterioration in valvular and myocardial function. The need for meticulous prophylaxis in all patients is clear.

Prophylaxis

Fortunately the group A streptococcus remains uniquely sensitive to long-term, low-dose penicillin, which may be administered orally or parenterally. Regrettably, non-compliance can reach astonishing levels with oral prophylaxis. In the 1960s Gordis showed that 90 per cent of patients became non-compliant if they had four or more of the following characteristics: female, adolescent, large sibship, not admitted to hospital with acute attack, no activity restriction, or unaccompanied to clinic by parents. With rare exceptions treatment with benzathine penicillin is recommended. The injection is sometimes painful for 1 to 2 days but this may be eased somewhat by incorporating a low dose of local anaesthetic or procaine penicillin with the injection. The minimum treatment period for patients without carditis is often given as 5 years, or to 18 years of age, but recurrences beyond 5 years are by no means uncommon. Annual recurrence rates above 5 per cent were recorded in years 10 to 15 in the prepenicillin era. A minimum treatment period of 10 years is desirable. For patients with established heart disease more prolonged prophylaxis is mandatory and treatment is recommended to at least to the age of 45 years. Pressure may rise to change to oral prophylaxis after some years but this is recommended only in particularly reliable patients.

Recommended treatment programme

Benzathine penicillin. Under 9 years or 27 kg: 0.9 megaunits every 4 weeks. Over 9 years or 27 kg: 1.2 megaunits every 4 weeks. Penicillin VK or penicillin G 250 mg: 1 to 2 tablets daily.

OR *sulphadiazine.* Under 9 years or 27 kg: 0.5 g. Over 9 years or 27 kg: 1.0 g daily.

OR *erythromycin.* 250 mg twice daily for the rare patient allergic to both benzathine penicillin and sulphadiazine.

Blood levels 2 weeks after benzathine injections are extremely low and significant recurrence rates have been reported from some developing countries in patients receiving 4-weekly injections; 3-weekly injections are recommended for those with a recurrence. Although peak blood levels are low and unpredictable when oral penicillin is taken after a meal, total absorption is not much changed.

Anaphylaxis to penicillin occurs in approximately 1/10 000 with death in about 1/30 000 to 50 000 injections. The risk is greatest in patients with advanced heart disease. Adrenaline and a resuscitation protocol must always be available. The risks are very much lower than the risks of recurrent attacks of rheumatic fever.

Infective endocarditis

It must be remembered that prophylactic penicillin gives no protection against infective endocarditis and, in fact, induces tolerance to penicillin in the viridans streptococci in the buccal cavity. Prophylaxis against endocarditis with dental procedures therefore requires high-dose erythromycin or clindamycin, or a combination of a penicillin and an aminoglycoside. In patients with low-grade bacterial endocarditis, blood cultures may not become positive for 3 to 4 days after the last dose of oral penicillin, or 2 weeks or more after the last dose of benzathine penicillin.

Prevention of rheumatic fever

Early recognition and treatment of the streptococcal sore throat has been shown to reduce the incidence of rheumatic fever in closed communities and can play an important role, for example, in streptococcal epidemics in schools. Prevention of sporadic cases in a susceptible community is, however, extremely difficult, compounded by the fact that only a minority of patients seek medical care for a streptococcal sore throat. Education about the recognition, complications, and treatment of streptococcal pharyngitis is vital. Systems for taking throat swabs in school and family contacts in cases of acute rheumatic fever are cost effective. Clearly there is a major need in susceptible populations for a co-ordinated programme involving school and community health personnel. The tragedy is that, in the countries where rheumatic fever is the greatest problem, funds are often inadequate even to provide long-term penicillin for established cases. Some specific anti-M antisera have been developed but costs of production and the number of antigenic M types constitute formidable problems to a vaccination programme. This may become more practical as markers for the 'rheumatic' individual become more clearly defined. On the world scene, rheumatic fever is inextricably bound up with socioeconomic factors. Its elimination as a major health factor awaits abolition of poverty, overcrowding, and slum conditions.

REFERENCES

Abernethy, M., Bass, N., Sharpe, N., *et al.* Doppler echocardiography and the early diagnosis of carditis in acute rheumatic fever. *Australian and New Zealand Journal of Medicine* (in press).

Bisno, A.L. (1990). The resurgence of acute rheumatic fever in the United States. *Annual Review of Medicine*, **41**, 319–29.

Combined Rheumatic Fever Study Group (1965). A comparison of short-term, intensive prednisone and acetylsalicylic acid therapy in the treatment of acute rheumatic fever. *New England Journal of Medicine*, **272**, 63–70.

Feinstein, A.R., Spagnuolo, M., and Gill, F.A. (1961). *Yale Journal of Biological Medicine*, **33**, 259–78.

Gibofsky, A., Khanna, A., Suh, E., and Zabriskie, J.B. (1991). The genetics of rheumatic fever: relationship to streptococcal infection and autoimmune disease. *Journal of Rheumatology*, **August supplement,** 1–5.

Gordis, L., Markowitz, M., and Lilienfeld, A.M. (1969). Why patients don't follow medical advice: a study of children on long-term antistreptococcal prophylaxis. *Journal of Pediatrics*, **75**, 957–8.

Markowitz, M., and Gordis, L. (1972). *Rheumatic fever*, (2nd edn). Saunders, Philadelphia.

UK and US Joint Report (1960). The evolution of rheumatic heart disease in children: five year report of a cooperative clinical trial of ACTH, cortisone and aspirin. *Circulation*, **22**, 503–515.

Veasy, L.G., Wiedmeier, S.E., Orsmond, G.S., Ruttenbert, H.D., Boucek, M.M., Roth, S.J., Tait, V.F., Thompson, J.A., Daly, J.A., Kaplan, E.L., and Hill, H.R. (1987). Resurgence of acute rheumatic fever in the intermountain area of the United States. *New England Journal of Medicine*, **316**, 421–427.

15.17 Infective endocarditis

B. GRIBBIN AND D. W. M. CROOK

Definition and classification

Infective endocarditis is a condition characterized by a microbiological inflammation of the lining of the heart chambers, heart valves, and great vessels although endarteritis is a more accurate description of the last. The condition was first described in detail by Osler in 1885 at a time when it was considered universally fatal and great advances were being made in the understanding of the pathological basis of disease. The cases he described were of a 'malignant' form, a clinical description of severe constitutional symptoms and extensive valve lesions that would now be termed acute endocarditis with necrosis and abscess formation in the heart and other tissues of the body. In time it came to be recognized that this fulminant illness was likely to be caused by virulent organisms such as *Staphylococcus aureus,* often attacking normal heart valves, whereas a more indolent form of the disease could present as chronic ill health of weeks or months duration. Those patients usually had a pre-existing cardiac abnormality such as a bicuspid aortic valve and nominally less virulent organisms such as the *Streptococcus viridans* spp. were isolated from the blood. Thus the traditional classification of infective endocarditis into acute and subacute forms. However, over the last few decades it has been realized that the clinical effect of a given organism cannot be predicted and is modified by several other influences such as whether it is community or hospital acquired, previous use of antibiotics, the presence of prosthetic heart valves, and a history of intravenous drug abuse. In order to predict the prognosis of a given patient and to formulate a plan of management it is therefore best to classify infective endocarditis by the organism involved, the valves affected, whether native or prosthetic and with identification of other relevant clinical features; for instance *Staphylococcus aureus* endocarditis of a tricuspid valve in an intravenous drug user. (Also see section on Diagnosis of infective endocarditis.)

Incidence

Although the number of patients at risk in the community must be large, infective endocarditis is uncommon, with an estimated annual incidence of 22 cases per million population in England and Wales giving rather more than 1000 cases each year. There are no accurate figures, however, and this is almost certainly a considerable underestimation, particularly when a figure of 49 cases per million general population per year has been reported from the United States.

The pattern of the disease has changed considerably since antibiotics were introduced over 40 years ago. Once a disease mainly of young adults, there is now an increasing incidence in the over 60s, who are more likely to have degenerative valve disease such as aortic sclerosis or calcification of the mitral annulus and to be exposed to invasive investigation and therapy. Because of other diseases they may also be less able to mount an adequate resistance to bacterial infection. The fall in the incidence of chronic rheumatic heart disease, which was more common in women, has resulted in a current preponderance of males with infective endocarditis. Overall, mitral valve prolapse is the most common underlying abnormality, with the aortic valve affected more often in elderly people. Endocarditis has also emerged as a serious complication of valve surgery and intravenous drug abuse.

Microbiology

Infective endocarditis can be caused by many species of bacteria and some fungi, but streptococci and staphylococci are responsible for 60 and 25 per cent of cases, respectively. The majority of organisms causing infective endocarditis reside either in the mouth or on the skin; those originating in the gastrointestinal tract and genital tracts are a less likely cause. Chewing and tooth brushing result in a transient bacteraemia, which explains how oral organisms (e.g. streptococci) can enter the bloodstream. The source of staphylococci is mainly the skin, either by direct inoculation or secondary to a local cutaneous septic focus. A range of species-specific bacterial characteristics are important in determining which organisms cause endocarditis, relating to the tropism of organisms for heart valves and the type and course of the disease. For example, *Streptococcus mutans* is one 'oral' species that has high avidity for abnormal valves and when isolated from the blood should suggest infective endocarditis; the clinical disease caused by this organism is insidious and typical of 'subacute endocarditis'. In contrast, *Staphylococcus aureus* may infect normal valves and is characterized by a fulminant course with multiple systemic emboli and rapid valve destruction.

STREPTOCOCCI

Streptococci are the most frequent cause of infective endocarditis. In many parts of the world they account for 80 per cent or more of the cases. In the United States, the proportion of cases caused by streptococci has declined from 80 to just over 50 per cent over the past 30 years. Differences in epidemiology between countries and over time are related to local factors such as intravenous drug abuse, the age structure of the population, and the prevalence of rheumatic heart disease. The association of streptococcal blood isolates with infective endocarditis varies with the species; *S. mutans* bacteraemia is highly predictive of endocarditis whereas Group A streptococcal bacteraemia is not (Table 1).

Viridans streptococci

'Streptococcus viridans' is a group of α-haemolytic streptococci responsible for most cases of streptococcal endocarditis. They include *S. mitis, S. sanguis, S. angiosis,* (milleri), *S. salivarius, S. mutans,* and a distinct group of nutritionally variant streptococci. They usually inhabit the oropharynx, but S. bovis usually inhabits the bowel. A remarkable feature of endocarditis caused by this organism is that it is significantly associated with an underlying gastrointestinal lesion, usually an adenoma or carcinoma of the large bowel. Viridans streptococci are of low pathogenicity and produce a subacute clinical picture, although *S. milleri,* frequently causes metastatic septic foci. By contrast, *S. pneumoniae,* although considered a viridans streptococcus, infrequently causes endo-

Table 1 *The probability, in descending order expressed as a ratio, of a streptococcal species isolated from the blood being the cause of infective endocarditis*

Species	Probability ratio
S. mutans (*Dx*+)	14.2:1
S. bovis I (*Dx*+)	5.9:1
Dx+ *mitior*	3.3:1
S. sanguis	3.0:1
S. mitior	1.8:1
'Viridans'	1.4:1
E. faecalis	1:1.2
Miscellaneous streptococci	1:1.3
S. bovis II (*Dx*−)	1:1.7
S. milleri	1:2.6
Group G	1:2.9
Group B	1:7.4
Group A	1:32.0

Dx+, dextran positive; *Dx*− dextran negative.

Adapted from Parker, M.T. and Ball, L.C. (1976). *Journal of Medical Microbiology*, **9**, 284.

carditis. When it does, it may do so on normal valves with a fulminant course associated with rapid valve destruction and often a concominant pneumococcal meningitis.

β-Haemolytic streptococci

These organisms rarely cause infective endocarditis, but group A organisms can be responsible for fulminant disease and group C, G, and B streptococci may affect normal heart valves in adults, producing an acute form of infective endocarditis.

ENTEROCOCI

Enterococcus faecalis and *E. faecium* are the species in this genus, now separated from *Streptococcus spp.* that are most commonly encountered clinically. They form part of the normal faecal flora. Enterococci are of low pathogenicity, characteristically producing subacute disease comprising between 5 and 15 per cent of infective endocarditis in most series. These organisms are remarkable in that they are resistant to most classes of antimicrobials; the few groups of antimicrobials that are inhibitory only achieve bactericidal activity if used in combination with aminoglycosides. Cure depends on killing the organisms with a combination of an aminoglycoside and a penicillin or a glycopeptide (e.g. vancomycin).

STAPHYLOCOCCI

Staphylococci are the second most common cause of endocarditis after streptococci accounting for between 20 and 35 per cent of cases. Staphylococci are classified *S. aureus* if they coagulate serum. Coagulase-negative staphylococci consist of many species, 13 of which colonize man. The most important of these is *S. epidermidis (sensu stricto);* examples of other species are *S. warneri, S. cohnii, S. saprophiticus, S. haemolyticus, S. hominis,* and *S. lugdinensis.* The presentation of staphylococcal endocarditis varies depending on the infecting species and the route of infection.

Staphylococcus aureus

Staphylococcus aureus endocarditis usually presents in one of four settings. First, community-acquired, native-valve *Staphylococcus aureus* endocarditis, usually presenting acutely and following a fulminant course with a reported mortality in excess of 30 per cent. It affects mainly the left-sided valves and often arises without an obvious source of infection. Characteristically, there are multiple systemic emboli, rapid

valve destruction and central nervous involvement including meningitis in up to 20 per cent of cases. Secondly, patients may acquire endocarditis secondary to a removable device such as an intravenous line. They usually present with an acute febrile illness, which, untreated, may evolve into endocarditis indistinguishable from left-sided native-valve endocarditis described above. Third, prosthetic valves may become infected with *Staphylococcus aureus* and clinically present with fulminant disease as seen with community-acquired disease. Lastly, intravenous drug abusers present with endocarditis that affects mainly the right-sided heart valves. Although presenting with an acute febrile illness, these cases are relatively protected from the serious complications of multiple septic emboli, which instead lodge in the lung and produce impressive pulmonary infiltrates.

Coagulase-negative staphylococci

Coagulase-negative staphylococci are traditionally associated with prosthetic valve endocarditis and cause between 30 and 50 per cent of all such cases. They have also been recently recognized as an increasingly important cause of native-valve endocarditis, especially in elderly people. The presentation of the infection in both these categories is usually subacute, but a few cases may present with acute disease. *Staphylococcus lugdanesis,* in particular, appears to present with more acute features similar to those of *Staphylococcus aureus.*

GRAM-NEGATIVE BACTERIA

These comprise a heterogeneous collection of genetically unrelated bacteria conveniently grouped together by virtue of their Gram staining characteristics. They account for just under 10 per cent of all cases of endocarditis and a higher proportion of cases affecting prosthetic valves or related to intravenous drug abuse.

Pseudomonas spp.

Pseudomonas spp. and *P. aeruginosa* are leading causes of infective endocarditis in this group. Intravenous drug abusers account for a large proportion of these cases and present with right-sided disease indistinguishable from right-sided *Staphylococcus aureus* endocarditis. Left-sided disease caused by these organisms presents acutely and has a fulminant course characterized by multiple systemic emboli.

HACEK

A number of fastidious oropharyngeal Gram-negative organisms may cause endocarditis. The most commonly encountered of these species are referred to as the HACEK group, a term which (as explained under Pathology of complications) stands for *Haemophilus spp., Actinobacillus actinomycetemcomitans, Cardiobacterium hominis, Eikenella corrodens,* and *Kingella kingae.* These organisms cause an insidious infection with very large vegetations. As they may take as long as 3 weeks to grow in blood culture bottles, they may be missed when blood is cultured only for the routine period of 7 days.

Miscellaneous

In the pre-antibiotic era, *Neisseria gonorrhoea* accounted for as many as a quarter of cases of endocarditis. Enterobacteriaceae (e.g. *Salmonella* spp., *Escherichia coli, Klebsiella* spp. etc) are rare causes, despite the high frequency with which they cause bacteraemia. A range of other Gram-negative organisms, such as *Brucella* spp., *Yersinia* spp., *Pasteurella* spp., and *Neisseria* spp. may also infect heart valves.

UNUSUAL CAUSES OF BACTERIAL ENDOCARDITIS

A very wide range of organisms have been described as causing endocarditis, and consideration of them all is beyond the scope of this chapter. However a few of these bacteria deserve mention.

Coxiella burnetti, the cause of Q fever, can cause endocarditis. The organism both lacks a cell wall and is an obligate intracellular parasite and so is not culturable in standard media; recognition of this infection depends on serological tests. *Bartonella (Rochalimaea) quintana* was responsible for several recently reported cases of endocarditis in poor homeless men in Seattle and Marseilles. This organism would not be detected by routine blood culture but special methods are effective. *Mycoplasma* spp. and chlamydiae, two other genera lacking a cell wall, have also been described as causing endocarditis, as have the Gram-positive bacilli *Listeria monocytogenes, Corynebacteria* spp. (including *C. diphtheriae*), *Bacillus* spp., and *Propionibacterium acnes*. Anaerobic bacteria such as *Clostridium* spp and *Bacteroides* spp. are rare causes.

FUNGAL ENDOCARDITIS

This form of endocarditis is uncommon and accounts for approximately 1 per cent of all cases of endocarditis, but causes a greater proportion of the intravenous drug-abuse cases and prosthetic valve-associated endocarditis. Many fungal species have been reported to cause endocarditis, but *Candida* spp. and *Aspergillus* spp. account for the majority of cases. Large vegetations and the poor recovery of fungi (other than *Candida* spp.) from blood cultures often delays recognition. Histological examination and culture of emboli may be helpful in demonstrating a fungal aetiology.

CULTURE-NEGATIVE ENDOCARDITIS

Approximately 5 per cent of cases of endocarditis will fail to yield a positive blood culture. Some organisms such as obligate intracellular pathogens (e.g. *Coxiella burnetti*), filamentous fungi (e.g. *Aspergillus* spp.), fastidious organisms (e.g. HACEK) or nutritionally defective streptococci may not produce recognizable growth with standard culture techniques. In these cases, serological tests or histological examination of samples of vegetations may reveal the causative agent. Host factors such as renal failure, a chronic course, or right-sided disease may also reduce the yield of positive cultures. Some studies have also reported a lower incidence of positive blood cultures when endocarditis has affected prosthetic valves.

PATHOGENESIS

Attempts have been made to discover why some cardiac lesions are more susceptible to infection than others, how a blood-borne micro-organism manages to colonize the lining of the heart, and why some forms of micro-organism seem to be more adept at this than others. A sterile vegetation is thought to be the initial lesion and is composed of platelets, fibrin, and macrophages. Organisms adhere to this vegetation and multiply, and endocarditis ensues (Fig. 1). Vegetations are more common on the left side of the heart and on the free margins of incompetent valves, particularly on the atrial aspect in mitral reflux and the ventricular side in aortic reflux. They are also found on the right side of the ventricular septum in ventricular septal defects and distal to the constriction in coarctation of the aorta. Rodbard investigated the basis for this pattern and showed that when an aerosol containing bacteria was blown through a narrowing in an agar tube, most organisms settled immediately distal to the constriction. He then postulated that the ideal haemodynamic conditions for producing infective endocarditis consist of a high-pressure source forcing blood through a narrow orifice into a low-pressure chamber. Furthermore, if a defect allows a high velocity jet of blood to pass through it, as for example would be the case in valvular reflux, small ventricular septal defect or persistent ductus arteriosus, then endothelial damage occurs, not only at the site at which organisms would be expected to settle but also where the jet of blood impinges on the wall of the low-pressure chamber. The latter explains why satellite lesions may form on the left atrial wall in mitral reflux, on chordae tendineae in aortic reflux, and on the tricuspid valve and free right ventricular wall in ventricular septal defect; also why low-pressure haemodynamic forces such as exist in mitral stenosis, large ventricular septal defects, and atrial septal defects are unlikely to result in endocarditis.

The adherence of bacteria to the endothelial surface is crucial to the establishment of endocarditis. Animal studies have demonstrated that intact endothelium has a low affinity for circulating bacteria and is therefore resistant to endocarditis. However, injury to the endothelial surface, probably caused by turbulence, triggers the deposition of a non-bacterial vegetation, which has a high affinity for some bacteria. Adhesion of bacteria to the sterile vegetation is dependent on species-specific microbial factors. Dextran, which is produced by some species of oral streptococci, is strongly adhesive to the sterile vegetation. *Streptococcus sanguis, salivarius, mitans,* and *bovis* elaborate dextran. *Staphylococcus aureus* has been shown to have a receptor with high affinity for fibronectin, a glycoprotein component found in vegetations. It is believed that slime produced by *Staphylococcus epidermidis* plays a part in its adherence to sterile vegetations. These adhesive factors probably explain the high frequency with which these bacteria cause endocarditis. As the vegetation grows, organisms become incorporated and to some extent protected from defence mechanisms by layers of fibrin, and those in the depths of the vegetation may enter a resting phase with a very low metabolic rate. Valve tissue under the vegetation shows a variable amount of damage, ranging from attempts at healing and ingrowth of capillaries to perforation and necrosis.

Immunology

In infective endocarditis the persistent bacteraemia produces a sustained systemic antigenic stimulation of the host's immune system. The best-recognized effect is chronic, high-level antibody production by B lymphocytes. This humoral immune response may account for a number of associated features. The antibodies produced are of all classes and are both specific and non-specific.

The non-specific antibodies are associated with rheumatoid factor (present in 20–50 per cent of cases), antinuclear factor and cryoglobulins, and produce a generalized hypergammaglobulinaemia; all become pronounced once the infection has persisted beyond 6 weeks. The specific antibodies may be involved in a number of systemic effects. Tissue damage can result from the aggregation of excess circulating antigen and antibody into immune complexes, which may pass through capillary walls and be deposited in subendothelial tissues. In some instances these complexes may form *in situ* but, in either case, complement factors are then activated and acute inflammatory injury ensues. It remains controversial whether some of the peripheral manifestations of infective endocarditis are due solely to immune-complex deposition. Roth spots in the fundi, Osler's nodes, and petechial haemorrhages may have more than

Fig. 1 Scanning electron micrograph of a leaflet of a human aortic valve showing the normal surface covered by endothelial cells (E) adjacent to an area with a large vegetation (V). Inset: detail of the surface of the vegetation showing a group of bacteria (B) surrounded by strands of fibrin (arrows). (Micrograph by courtesy of D.J.P. Ferguson.)

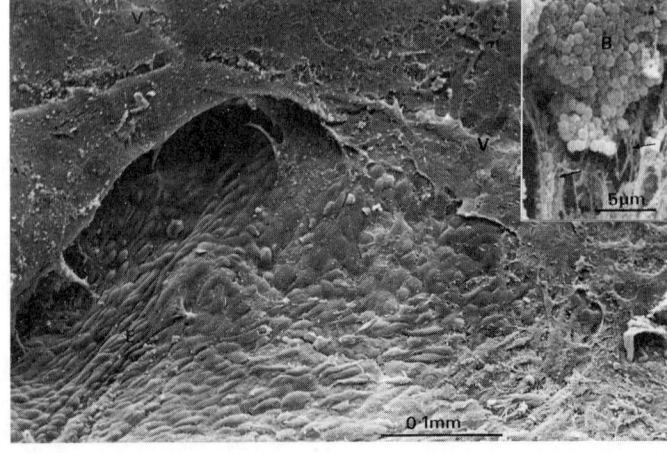

one cause, including immune-complex deposition, microembolization, and increased capillary permeability. Rarely, vasculitic skin lesions may occur with areas of haemorrhage and necrosis, and these too are likely to be manifestations of immune-complex deposition.

Infective endocarditis may also be complicated by renal disease. Embolism can lead to renal infarction but immune-complex deposition is thought to be responsible for the other main renal manifestations of the condition, focal glomerulonephritis, diffuse proliferative glomerulonephritis and, rarely, membranoproliferative glomerulonephritis. Renal biopsies have shown changes of glomerulonephritis in the majority of patients studied, although many with mild histological changes have no detectable abnormality of the urine or of renal function.

As a rule, improvement follows antibiotic treatment, with a rapid fall in the concentration of circulating immune complexes. Rarely the inflammatory changes progress and lead to irreversible renal failure. Immunofluorescent studies then show deposition of immunoglobulins and complement factors in the capillary walls of the glomerulus, along the basement membrane, and in the mesangium. Destruction of glomeruli is thought to result from the opsonic activity of complement, which leads to polymorphonuclear leucocyte infiltration and the release of enzymes that then injure vascular endothelium and the basement membrane.

Pathology

UNDERLYING HEART DISEASE

This may be rheumatic, congenital, degenerative (aortic sclerosis or stenosis, mitral annulus calcification), related to mitral valve prolapse, or absent. In the United Kingdom, underlying heart disease will not previously have been detected in some 40 per cent of patients with infective endocarditis. The kind of contributing heart disease has also changed considerably over the past three decades. At the beginning of this period (and still in certain parts of the world), chronic rheumatic heart disease accounted for 80 to 90 per cent of cases in adults, with the mitral valve most commonly involved, but now the proportion due to this is less than half. This follows a decline in the population at risk from rheumatic fever and also perhaps a greater awareness of non-rheumatic causes of valvular disease, such as mitral valve prolapse and age-related degenerative changes. Mitral valve prolapse is common: according to the Framingham study, 7.6 per cent of females and 2.5 per cent of males are affected to some degree. This high prevalence rather than extraordinary susceptibility explains the fact that the regurgitant mitral valve is the most frequent site for endocarditis, although aortic-valve infection in older men suggests that aortic sclerosis, which is common in this population, is the main lesion placing them at risk. Endocarditis also occurs in patients with hypertrophic cardiomyopathy made susceptible by mitral reflux or by the excessive turbulence caused by dynamic subaortic stenosis. Infection may also develop on mural endocardium in the region of a myocardial infarction or ventricular aneurysm.

Congenital heart disease is present in most children with endocarditis and in approximately 10 per cent of adults. The risk of infection increases over the second decade of life and again substantially over the age of 20 years. Most of the common congenital abnormalities predispose to infection, although it only occurs in patients with atrial septal defects if there is an associated mitral-valve abnormality, and involvement of a stenotic pulmonary valve is also very uncommon. A ventricular septal defect is an important predisposing state, with the risk of contracting endocarditis by the age of 30 years estimated at 9.7 per cent with a lifelong risk of about 12 to 13 per cent. This risk is increased further if there is associated aortic reflux. Early surgery has virtually abolished persistent ductus arteriosus (once commonly associated with endocarditis) and made it much less likely with ventricular septal defects and coarctation of the aorta. This is not the case, however, for aortic stenosis, in which the risk may actually increase after valvotomy perhaps because a measure of aortic reflux is frequently produced.

Cyanotic congenital heart disease in one form or another is still the most common underlying abnormality in children with endocarditis, and those who survive palliative or corrective surgery for the more complex abnormalities such as tetralogy of Fallot, pulmonary atresia, and tricuspid atresia now represent a new population at risk, not only by virtue of their continuing survival but also because of residual defects and the presence of prosthetic materials used in repair procedures. For example, there is a considerable risk of endocarditis in patients with tetralogy of Fallot or other cyanotic conditions treated by an aortopulmonary shunt, and to a lesser extent also in those who receive a valved conduit used to link the right atrium or right ventricle with the pulmonary arteries.

The presence of any foreign material in the heart increases the risk of infective endocarditis, although this is virtually non-existent for pacemakers.

PATHOLOGY OF COMPLICATIONS

Vegetations are a major feature of infective endocarditis. Some, for example in fungal and **HACEK** endocarditis (HACEK organisms are Gram-negative oropharyngeal species, comprising *Haemophilus* spp., *Actinobacillus actinomycetemcomitans, Cardiobacterium hominis, Eikinella corrodens,* and *Kingella kingae* can be very large, even sufficient to obstruct a valve orifice. With adequate treatment, healing of vegetations may occur. They shrink, become endothelialized and organized from the base, and at subsequent surgery may be recognized as small, fibrotic and calcified nodules on a distorted and leaking valve.

In some patients, erosive rather than proliferative lesions are prominent, leading to perforation of cusps, ruptured chordae, and severe valve reflux (Fig. 2). Local necrosis with abscess formation burrowing into adjacent tissue may occur. More commonly found around the aortic valve, this process can damage the conducting pathways of the heart and can weaken the aortic root so causing an aneurysm of a sinus of Valsalva. The area of continuity between the aortic and mitral valves may also be involved in aneurysm formation and fistulae, leading to shunting of blood into the pericardial sac, the left atrium or other adjacent chamber.

Multiple myocardial abscesses resulting either from direct spread or septic embolization into the coronary arteries are another complication, and evidence of myocarditis can be found in nearly all patients studied at autopsy.

Pericarditis can follow the direct spread of infection from a valve ring or myocardial abscess, and can also occur as a complication of coronary embolism and myocardial infarction. However, its presence is not

Fig. 2 Endocarditis on a bicuspid aortic valve showing vegetations and a perforation of one cusp.

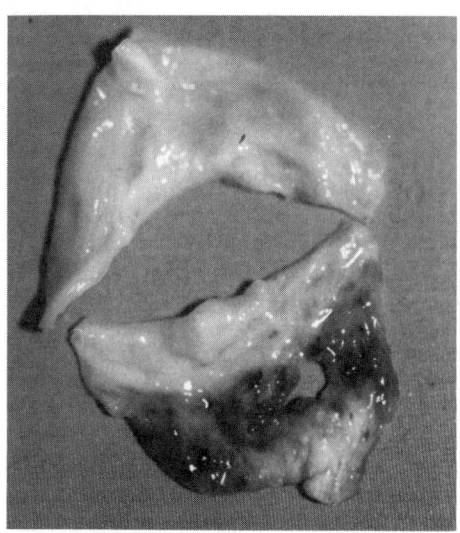

always serious, in that a sterile pericardial effusion can occur, presumably as an immunological phenomenon.

Systemic emboli are a serious threat and occur more commonly than can be detected clinically, although only too often a patient may develop the disabling features of a cerebral or coronary embolus. Knowledge about the relevance of vegetations to clinical management has been advanced by echocardiographic studies of left-sided, native-value endocarditis. Risk of a first embolism is related to the organism involved, with the greatest incidence found in patients with *Staphylococcus aureus* infection whether or not vegetations can be shown on echocardiography, whereas in *Streptococcus viridans* infection the risk is increased sevenfold if vegetations are found. There is no consistent evidence that unequivocally relates risk of embolism to the size of vegetations—at least for bacterial endocarditis. It appears that the threat from emboli falls quickly after starting antibiotic treatment. In ventricular septal defects and other forms of right-sided endocarditis, emboli pass into the pulmonary circulation and present clinically as pneumonia or pulmonary infarction.

Microemboli, too, are thought to be common and may be one of the causes of the peripheral stigmata of the condition such as Osler's nodes and the small petechial haemorrhages found in the skin and mucous membranes. They may also be responsible for an inflammatory myocarditis, the effect of which on overall myocardial function is usually difficult to judge.

Mycotic aneurysms, which can be multiple, are localized arterial dilatations caused by septic embolization of material from vegetations. In small peripheral arteries, impaction of such an embolus may be enough to weaken the adjacent wall structure but in larger vessels the initial injury can be best explained by microembolization of the vasa vasorum followed by inflammatory change in the wall, destruction of wall elements, and dilatation. Even if all infection is then eradicated, progressive dilatation may still occur, and eventually this may lead to rupture (Fig. 3).

Symptoms and signs of infective endocarditis

Many variables influence the clinical presentation, which is less likely nowadays to fall easily into acute or subacute types. The presentation may be atypical, especially in elderly individuals, and can cause diagnostic difficulties. For example, a patient may come under care initially with neurological or psychiatric disability or perhaps following sudden loss of vision due to occlusion of the central retinal artery. Awareness of these diverse manifestations of endocarditis allows the correct diagnosis to be considered and the relevant investigations done. More commonly the clinical features are characteristic of the condition, with fever, marked constitutional symptoms, and evidence of heart disease.

There is general agreement that the clinical course is governed by four main elements: first, the extent of cardiac damage; second, the risk and effect of systemic emboli; third, the degree of metastatic septic seeding; and fourth, the immunological response.

FEVER

This occurs at some time or another in nearly all patients and in most it is prominent and associated with sweats, chills, and occasionally rigors. The fever is often low grade in the subacute variety, falling to normal some time during a 24-h period, but spikes over 40 °C may occur. Elderly patients, those in congestive cardiac failure, and those in renal failure may have a blunted pyrexial response but even in them an elevated temperature can usually be recorded on several occasions.

CONSTITUTIONAL SYMPTOMS

These consist of malaise, with aches and pains, and are often summed up as 'flu-like'. In some, anorexia and weight loss are prominent, and in others, exhaustion. Aching joints and muscles and low back pain are common, headaches and arthritis less so and rarely severe. The low back

pain (febrile lumbago) may be disabling and if so may be the main presenting feature. Pleuritic chest pain and cough may be prominent in patients with right-sided endocarditis, the former also occurring in patients who develop a splenic infarct.

CARDIAC SYMPTOMS AND SIGNS

At the time of presentation most patients with endocarditis do not complain of newly acquired symptoms of heart disease. Of course, if endocarditis complicates a cardiac abnormality severe enough in its own right to cause effort dyspnoea or anginal chest pain, then the infection with its concomitant fever and anaemia is likely to cause further deterioration. Cardiac failure, however, is the most sinister complication and most common cause of death. Evidence of it should alert the physician to the possibility of acute aortic or mitral reflux, or to myocardial infarction caused by a coronary artery embolus.

Heart murmurs are detected in nearly all patients with a subacute presentation and in the majority of acute ones, although careful auscultation will often be required to make a diagnosis of mild aortic reflux in those thought to be free of valve disease. Some day-to-day variation in the intensity of murmurs is not uncommon and the importance of changing murmurs in infective endocarditis lies in the detection of progressive valve damage, for example, a louder and longer early diastolic murmur suggesting greater aortic reflux, or in the same patient a new, blowing systolic murmur at the apex suggesting secondary involvement of the mitral valve. Care should be taken to elicit confirmatory signs elsewhere, such as tachycardia, a hyperdynamic apex beat, and cardiac enlargement, or an increase in pulse pressure. A pericardial friction rub indicates the need to investigate further, perhaps by transoesophageal echocardiography, the possibility of infection tracking from a valve-ring abscess.

EXTRACARDIAC MANIFESTATIONS

Of these, only petechial haemorrhages are common. These are not specific for endocarditis but in the appropriate clinical context support the

Fig. 3 A mycotic aneurysm of the right femoral artery.

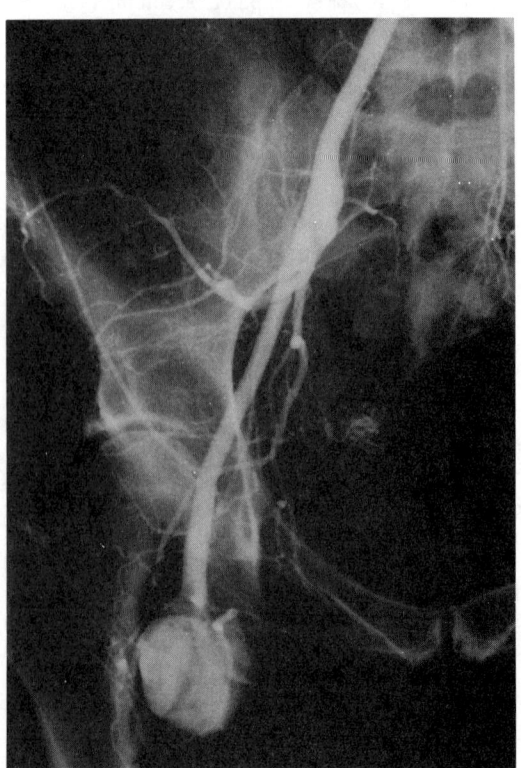

diagnosis if detected on the extremities and mucous membranes. Particular care should be taken when examining the eyes because small conjunctival haemorrhages are more significant than isolated splinter haemorrhages, which are found often under the fingernails of unselected hospital patients (Fig. 4). In this regard, lesions in the proximal portion of the nail bed are more likely to be due to endocarditis. Similar or slightly larger haemorrhages may be found in the fundi and some with central, pale areas have come to be called Roth spots, although different from the large exudates originally described by Roth in patients with septicaemia (Fig. 5). Osler's nodes are circumscribed, indurated, red, tender lesions that occur most frequently in the pulps of the fingers and toes but may also be found in the thenar and hypothenar eminences and on the sides of the fingers. Often their appearance is preceded by the sudden or insidious onset of a burning discomfort, although in some patients this may be no more than a sensation of heightened sensitivity. They may be multiple and usually disappear after a few days. Janeway lesions are rare, thought to be due to septic embolization, and are described as transient, non-tender, macular patches on the palms of the hands or soles of the feet, and occasionally the fingers and toes. Clubbing of the fingers is usually seen in patients with long-standing disease. Splenomegaly is variable, and although most likely to be prominent in those with a chronic illness, it may not be detected in patients with infection of considerable duration and yet be obvious in someone presenting with a 2-week history.

RENAL ABNORMALITIES

The pathogenesis of renal disease in endocarditis has been described above. Renal infarction may present with loin pain and haematuria. Glo-

Fig. 4 Conjunctival haemorrhages from a case of endocarditis.

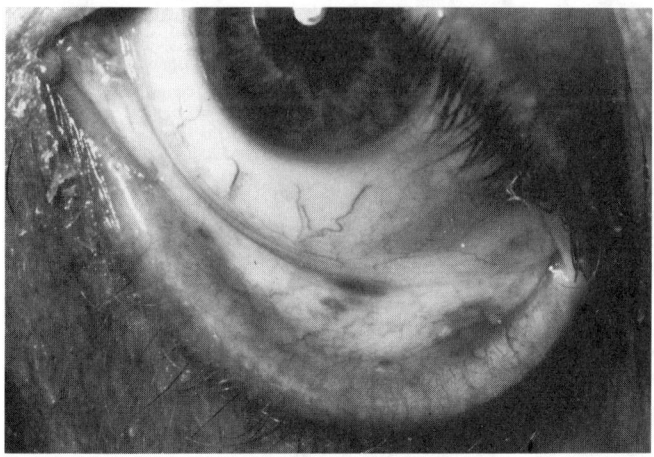

Fig. 5 Roth spot in the fundus of a patient with endocarditis.

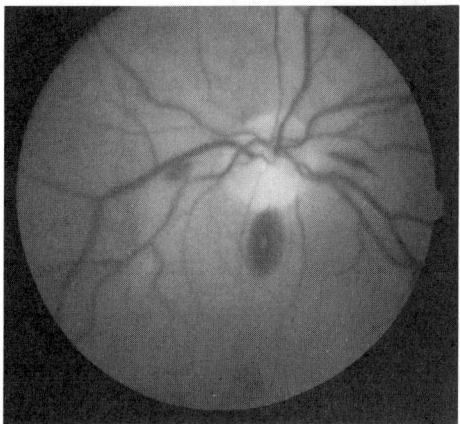

merulonephritis is seldom severe enough to cause endstage renal failure but more often function may be compromised sufficiently to justify close monitoring of potentially nephrotoxic drugs such as gentamicin. The urine may be normal, even in patients who have histological evidence of glomerulonephritis, but haematuria and proteinuria are not uncommon. These renal abnormalities usually disappear with effective antibiotic treatment. Rarely, a progressive rise in serum creatinine with haematuria and proteinuria can be caused by an acute interstitial nephritis, itself caused by penicillin or other antimicrobial, in which case the fever persists and there may be a coincident skin rash. Renal abscesses are rare.

NEUROLOGICAL ABNORMALITIES

These are common and may well be the mode of presentation, especially in elderly people. As in any severe infection a fluctuating confusional state with short-term memory impairment, disorientation, and behavioural changes may be prominent and yet is reversible with adequate antibacterial treatment. Presumably these changes are related to brain-cell damage, either through interference with normal metabolism or by more direct damage from microemboli or vasculitis. Cerebral emboli, mainly in the distribution of the middle cerebral artery, have been reported to occur in 17 per cent of cases of endocarditis and can lead to hemiplegia, sensory loss, and other focal abnormalities. It seems that haemorrhagic transformation of an ischaemic infarct caused by septic embolization is the most common cause of intracerebral haemorrhage. Similar features may follow rupture of a mycotic aneurysm, which tragically may occur up to 2 years after apparent cure of the infection. Most of these are in the territory of the middle cerebral artery and rupture leads to subarachnoid haemorrhage or intraventricular haemorrhage. Their presence should be suspected in any patient with endocarditis who develops a severe headache. In some cases, rupture of an aneurysm may be preceded by a clinically evident embolism to the same vascular territory.

Meningoencephalitis characteristically produces headache and neck stiffness. The cerebrospinal fluid is usually sterile but may show an increase in white cells. In *Staphylococcus aureus* endocarditis, purulent meningitis may be demonstrated, with the organism grown from the spinal fluid. Multiple cerebral abscesses are then the rule, whereas a single, large collection of pus is more typically a complication of endocarditis in children with cyanotic congenital heart disease. A study of natives in Alaska showed that *Streptococcus pneumoniae* endocarditis is another variety likely to be associated with a purulent meningoencephalitis—in these cases alcoholism was another feature.

Investigations

BLOOD CULTURE

This is the single most important investigation and should be done as soon as possible in any patient suspected of having endocarditis. Correct aseptic skin preparation and a no-touch technique should be used and normally three samples form different venepuncture sites are taken over a 24-h period. Seriously ill patients thought to have endocarditis should be started on antibiotics after two or three samples have been taken over 1 to 2 h. Conversely, it may be best to continue culturing for a few days in less severe cases, particularly when the patient has already had a short course of antibiotic treatment or if initial cultures are negative at 48 h. Serial sampling can also be a useful way of determining the relevance of an organism such as a coagulase-negative staphylococcus, which could be a skin contaminant if found in only one or two samples. Although the magnitude of bacteraemia in endocarditis is small, it does tend to be persistent and so it is not surprising that blood cultures are positive in about 90 per cent of cases; in nearly all of these the organism will be grown from the first sample.

With properly applied techniques, negative blood cultures should occur in less than 5 per cent of cases. They are said to be more common in patients with congestive cardiac failure and in those with renal complications, the explanation of which may be that if the patient has survived a low-grade disorder without adequate treatment for months, a high level of antibodies and other natural bactericidal factors might then sterilize the blood, although organisms persist in vegetations. Such a patient would be expected to develop immune-complex renal disease and cardiac failure. Patients with right-sided endocarditis may develop positive cultures only after seeding of the lung by infected pulmonary emboli.

Some negative results can be explained by poor culture techniques or by previous antibiotic treatment, although even under the latter circumstance organisms usually can be grown from the blood. Furthermore, it is not always realized that some organisms, for example the HACEK group, may require several weeks to grow in culture and advice should be sought about special culture techniques for anaerobes, microaerophilic organisms, nutritionally variant streptococci, and fungi. The HACEK group in particular may form large vegetations, which can be identified by echocardiography. *Coxiella burneti,* which causes Q-fever endocarditis, and *Bartonella quintana* (trench fever) should always be considered in culture-negative cases, as should fungi, and appropriate special culture techniques or serological testing may make the diagnosis. If prior antibiotic treatment is ruled out, one of the most common reasons for negative blood cultures is that the patient does not have endocarditis.

BLOOD TESTS

There is no set pattern of change in infective endocarditis. The haemoglobin concentration is likely to be well maintained in acute cases, whereas in subacute infections values below 10.5 g/dl occur in the majority; the anaemia is normochromic and normocytic. The white-cell count is variable, usually high with an acute presentation, perhaps as high as 20 000 to 30 000/mm^3 (predominantly polymorphonuclear leucocytes), and usually normal with the more subacute presentation caused by *Streptococcus viridans*. The erythrocyte sedimentation rate is elevated in 90 per cent of cases, as is the C-reactive protein. In subacute cases the concentration of immunoglobulins rises and the presence of autoantibodies can be inferred from a high titre of rheumatoid factors. Circulating immune complexes can be detected and in many the level seems to correlate directly with the duration of illness, the presence of extracardiac manifestations such as glomerulonephritis or skin changes, and inversely with serum complement values. Because effective treatment is followed by a fall in immune-complex levels and a rise in serum complement, with reversal of these changes in relapses, their assay may prove useful as a way of determining disease activity. In most hospitals, however, this is impractical and the C-reactive protein tends to be used as a way of following the clinical course.

Serological tests are useful in several instances. Q-fever endocarditis can be diagnosed by a rising or elevated titre of antibodies to *Coxiella burneti* phase-1 and -2 antigens. Likewise, the agent causing psittacosis, a rare cause of endocarditis, can be identified by a high titre of complement-fixing antibody. The place of serological tests in the diagnosis of fungal endocarditis will be discussed below.

ELECTROCARDIOGRAM

The electrocardiogram should be recorded early in the course of the illness because it adds to the information about the nature of the underlying heart disease, and serial records can show changes that imply extension of infection, myocardial damage, and haemodynamic deterioration. For example, new prolongation of the P-R interval in cases of aortic-valve endocarditis signifies likely extension of the infection from the aortic ring into the conducting tissue at the top of the intraventricular septum, and a similar suspicion can be raised if left bundle-branch block develops.

Prominent supraventricular or ventricular arrhythmias may be the

only indication of an extravalvular abscess or myocarditis. Changes of acute myocardial infarction due to embolization may provide an explanation for sudden clinical deterioration, and marked ST segment depression in someone with acute aortic reflux indicates poor subendocardial perfusion and unlikely survival with medical treatment alone. Pericarditis may be associated with the usual electrocardiographic changes.

ECHOCARDIOGRAPHY (SEE CHAPTER 15.4.3)

This plays an important part in the investigation of patients with endocarditis. It provides serial records of chamber dimensions and ventricular function as well as detecting evidence of pre-existing rheumatic or degenerative valve disease. By displaying premature closure of the mitral valve leaflets it can strongly support the diagnosis of acute aortic reflux and because of its ability to show vegetations it can support a clinical suspicion of endocarditis. Early reports describe vegetations as shaggy, irregular, mobile echoes, not restricting valve motion (Fig. 6). Two-dimensional echocardiography can detect vegetations as small as 2 to 3 mm, although it may not be easy to distinguish these from eccen-

Fig. 6 Two-dimensional echocardiogram showing vegetations (veg) on the aortic valve and the anterior leaflet of the mitral valve. LA, left atrium; AO, aorta; RV, right ventricle; LV, left ventricle.

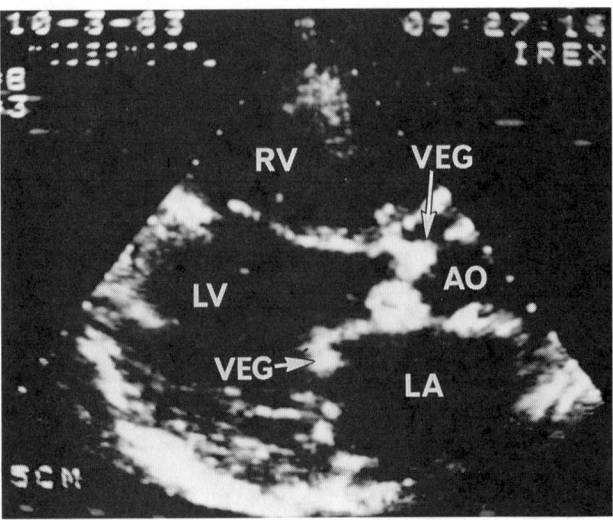

Fig. 7 Transoesophageal echocardiogram showing the aortic root with an abscess cavity at 2 o'clock. Ao, aortic root; LA, left atrium. (Published with the permission of Dr John Chambers.)

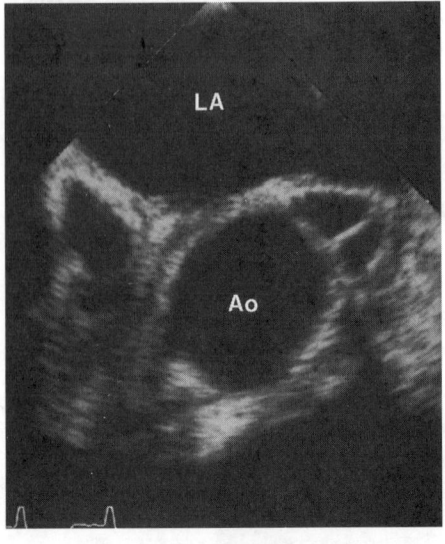

tric thickening of aortic cusps or the thick echoes seen in some cases of mitral-valve prolapse. Transoesophageal echocardiography, on the other hand, gives consistently high-quality pictures and can detect vegetations as small as 1 to 1.5 mm with a sensitivity and specificity of over 90 per cent. With colour-flow Doppler it has added enormously to the ability to detect other complications of endocarditis: it allows accurate scanning of prosthetic valves (difficult with the transthoracic approach), and can show perforations of valve leaflets, valve-ring abscesses (detected with a sensitivity of about 80 per cent), intracardiac fistulae, and aneurysms. (Fig. 7). Although the echocardiographic examination should always be considered along with the clinical features of the individual case and other investigations, a normal transoesophageal echocardiography study makes endocarditis unlikely.

Transoesophageal echocardiography should be considered for patients thought to have aortic-root infection, those with prosthetic-valve endocarditis, those who have persisting fever or other features of continuing infection despite appropriate antibiotic treatment, and those with negative blood cultures.

Other methods of imaging have made little impact in the investigation of the patient with presumed endocarditis. Magnetic resonance imaging can provide information about aortic-root infection but transoesophageal echocardiography is better and more easily applied.

Diagnosis of infective endocarditis

Because the diagnosis of endocarditis is often difficult, attempts have been made to establish criteria that allow a diagnosis to be made. The criteria are based on clinical, microbiological, echocardiographic and other investigational results that reflect the four main aspects of endocarditis: a predisposition, a persistent bacteraemia with organisms typically causing infective endocarditis, vascular phenomena, and evidence of endocardial involvement which may be found only by transthoracic or transoesophageal echocardiography. The clinical criteria proposed by the group at Duke University are outlined in Table 2. Definite endocarditis requires the presence of two major criteria or one major and three minor or five minor criteria.

Special clinical problems

AORTIC-ROOT INFECTION

Cardiac failure developing during endocarditis usually has its basis in severe and progressive valve damage with the aortic valve most often involved. Under these circumstances, acute aortic reflux is likely to be present, and if in addition there is electrocardiographic evidence of prolonged atrioventricular conduction or a pericardial friction rub is heard, then extravalvular extension of infection and an aortic ring abscess is a strong possibility and may be confirmed by transoesophageal echocardiography. If present, the subsequent course is likely to be one of sudden catastrophic cardiac failure brought about by further aortic-valve damage, rupture of a sinus of Valsalva aneurysm, or by secondary involvement of the mitral valve with leaflet perforation or rupture of chordae tendineae. Alternatively, a failing myocardium may be unable to sustain such a heavy haemodynamic load in the face of a reduced diastolic coronary-perfusion pressure and inflammatory changes. This state may be prevented in some patients if acute or progressive aortic reflux is diagnosed early enough, effective antibiotic treatment is started without unnecessary delay, and if it is realized that surgery often offers the best chance of survival. Early diagnosis rests on an awareness that the physical signs of acute aortic reflux may be misleading and quite different from those found in the more familiar situation of chronic reflux. In acute aortic reflux of more than moderate severity, a normal left-ventricular cavity suddenly receives a large volume in diastole so that left ventricular pressure increases abruptly from early diastole, to such an extent that it exceeds left atrial pressure and premature closure of the mitral valve occurs. Stroke volume hardly changes and cardiac output

is maintained by an increase in heart rate. Observation of such a patient will therefore reveal a tachycardia, a prominent but normally positioned apex beat, and a low systolic and diastolic blood pressure with perhaps some increase in pulse pressure. However, the peripheral pulses may not be collapsing in character. On auscultation the first sound is soft or absent, depending on the prematurity of mitral-valve closure, and the early diastolic murmur may be difficult to hear and limited to the very beginning of diastole. A low-pitched diastolic Austin–Flint murmur represents mitral flow passing through the valve as it is being forced shut by the high left-ventricular pressure. If the mitral valve is also infected and mitral reflux is present, then the protection afforded to the pulmonary circulation by early closure of the mitral valve is lost and pulmonary oedema may be uncontrollable.

The combination of the clinical features of an aortic-root abscess with valve reflux is generally accepted as an indication for surgery. An attempt is then made to replace the valve and excise as much necrotic and infected tissue as possible. The results of surgery are largely determined by preoperative left-ventricular function and are likely to be better in those patients referred before the onset of severe cardiac failure.

INFECTIVE ENDOCARDITIS IN CHILDREN AND ELDERLY PEOPLE

Endocarditis in children is uncommon, although there is some evidence of an increase especially affecting children after cardiac surgery and those with cyanotic congenital heart disease—in both cases an increasing population. In developing countries, acute rheumatic fever predisposes children to infective endocarditis, whereas in Western societies the majority of older children with the infection have congenital heart disease, most commonly tetralogy of Fallot, ventricular septal defect or a bicuspid aortic valve. Patients with ventricular septal defects have been estimated to run a risk of endocarditis of 9.7 per cent by the age of 30 years. In most instances the presentation is similar to that in adults, although in infancy it is usually one of generalized sepsis, underlying heart disease is infrequent, and mortality is high. Peripheral stigmata, such as Osler's nodes and petechial haemorrhages, are less common than in adults and severe constitutional symptoms with joint pains and splenomegaly more common. Right-sided endocarditis complicating tetralogy of Fallot or ventricular septal defect may present with pneumonia, pleuritic chest pain and haemoptysis, although with both these conditions the aortic valve may also be involved, with a subsequent risk of systemic emboli. Unfortunately, children with cyanotic congenital heart disease seem to have more dental caries and periodontal disease than do other children of similar age.

Elderly people are particularly at risk of developing endocarditis. There may be a number of reasons for this: they are more likely to have valvular disease, to have invasive investigations and procedures that cause bacteraemia, and they may be in a less fit state to combat incipient infection because of other conditions such as diabetes and heart failure. Enterococcal infection is more likely in elderly men who may have had instrumentation of the urinary tract. The clinical presentation is often atypical and it may be the relatives who seek advice because the patient has become confused, disorientated, and lethargic. Fever may not be evident and the physical signs unimpressive with perhaps a systolic murmur thought to be due to aortic sclerosis, although careful scrutiny may detect peripheral stigmata such as haemorrhages in the conjunctivae, the fundi, or the mucous membranes of the mouth.

PROSTHETIC-VALVE ENDOCARDITIS

The cumulative risk of this postoperative complication has fallen over the years and is considered to be about 2 to 4 per cent over the life-span of the valve. The first few months are the main danger period, although the patient remains vulnerable. This form of endocarditis accounts for 16 per cent of all cases of endocarditis treated in cardiac referral centres in the United Kingdom.

Table 2 *Diagnosis of infective endocarditis*

(a) Criteria for diagnosis of infective endocarditis

Definite infection endocarditis
    Pathological criteria
        Micro-organisms; demonstrated by culture or histology in a vegetation, *or* in a vegetation that
            has embolized, *or* in an intracardiac abscess, *or*
        Pathological lesions: vegetation or intracardiac abscess present, confirmed by histology
            showing active endocarditis
    Clinical criteria, using specific definitions listed below
        Two major criteria, *or*
        One major and three minor criteria, *or*
        Three minor criteria
Possible infective endocarditis
    Findings consistent with infective endocarditis that fall short of 'Definite', but not 'rejected'
Rejected
    Firm alternate diagnosis for manifestations of endocarditis, *or*
    Resolution of manifestations of endocarditis, with antibiotic therapy for 4 days or less, *or*
    No pathological evidence of infective endocarditis at surgery or autopsy, after antibiotic therapy
        for 4 days or less.

(b) Definitions of terminology used in criteria

Major criteria
    Positive blood culture for infective endocarditis
        Typical micro-organism for infective endocarditis from two separate blood cultures.
        Viridans streptococci, *Streptococcus bovis,* HACEK group, *or*
        Community-acquired *Staphylococcus aureus* or enterococci, in the absence of a primary
            focus, *or*
    Persistently positive blood culture, defined as recovery of a micro-organism consistent with
        infective endocarditis from:
        (i) Blood cultures drawn more than 12 h apart, *or*
        (ii) All of three or a majority of four or more separate blood cultures, with first and last
            drawn at least 1 h apart
    Evidence of endocardial involvement
        Positive echocardiogram for infective endocarditis
        (i) Oscillating intracardiac mass, on valve or supporting structures, *or* in the path of
            regurgitant jets, *or* on implanted material, in the absence of an alternative anatomic
            explanation, *or*
        (ii) Abscess, *or*
        (iii) New partial dehiscence of prosthetic valve, *or*
        New valvular regurgitation (increase or change in pre-existing murmur not sufficient)

Minor criteria
    Predisposition: predisposing heart condition *or* intravenous drug use
    Fever: $\geq$ 38.0°C (100.4°F)
    Vascular phenomena: major arterial emboli, septic pulmonary infarcts, mycotic aneurysm,
        intracranial haemorrhage, conjunctival haemorrhages, Janeway lesions
    Immunological phenomena: glomerulonephritis, Osler's nodes, Roth spots, rheumatoid factor
    Microbiological evidence: positive blood culture but not meeting major criterion as noted
        previously† *or* serological evidence of active infection with organism consistent with
        infective endocarditis
    Echocardiogram: consistent with infective endocarditis but not meeting major criterion as noted
        previously

HACEK = *Haemophilus* spp., *Actinobacillus actinomycetemcomitans, Cardiobacterium hominis, Eikenella* spp., and *Kingella kingae.*

*Including nutritional variant strains.

†Excluding single positive cultures for coagulase-negative staphylococci and organisms that do not cause endocarditis.

The condition has been conventionally classified as of early or late onset, with the dividing line at 2 months after surgery. When infection occurs early, the assumption is that organisms have gained entry during the perioperative period, perhaps from direct inoculation of the operation site, from wound infection or through seeding from intravenous or intra-arterial cannulation sites. Coagulase-negative staphylococci, predominantly *Staphylococcus epidermidis,* are the most common organisms isolated; approximately half of early cases can be attributed to this and *Staphylococcus aureus,* with Gram-negative bacilli, diphtheroids, and *Candida* spp. causing most of the remainder.

In early and late prosthetic-valve endocarditis the disease tends to produce circumferential necrosis of the valve annulus, which leads to separation of the sewing ring and the development of a periprosthetic leak. Abscesses may track into adjacent myocardium, particularly if staphylococci are involved. Less common, and mainly affecting the mitral valve, is functional stenosis caused by ingrowth of vegetations that obstruct the valve orifice and the free movement of the disc or poppet. Bioprosthetic valves are as susceptible to infection as mechanical ones, with retraction and perforation of leaflets another cause of valve reflux. The clinical picture may be one of persisting postoperative fever, although in time valve malfunction will be recognized, for example by an early diastolic murmur caused by an aortic periprosthetic leak. Mitral prosthetic-valve malfunction may be less easily detected and it is unwise to rely on auscultatory evidence of valve reflux. Unexplained cardiac failure in a postoperative patient with a prosthetic mitral valve must be assumed to be due to malfunction of that valve until proved otherwise.

Three other causes of persisting or recurrent postoperative fever should be borne in mind. The first is residual infection in the lung, urinary tract or healing wounds. The second is the postperfusion syndrome, in which fever occurs from 2 to 8 weeks postoperatively and is associated with 'flu-like' symptoms, splenomegaly, and a lymphocytosis with atypical lymphocytes. A virus infection transmitted from transfused blood is thought to be responsible and the cytomegalovirus antibody titre may be raised; recovery is usually uneventful over a 2-week period. The third condition is the postpericardiotomy syndrome, which can occur from 1 week to 2 months postoperatively and consists of fever, pericardial and pleuritic pain, often with effusions, and a high erythrocyte sedimentation rate. This responds to anti-inflammatory drugs but may recur.

The mortality of early prosthetic-valve endocarditis is high, although there may have been a decline in recent years from over 70 per cent to nearer 40 per cent. No doubt this reflects the increasing use of further surgery, which should be carefully considered in all patients, other than those with highly sensitive organisms, who are free of heart failure and in whom valve malfunction is apparently absent. Persisting fever on treatment, evidence of annular abscess formation, non-streptococcal aetiology, and heart failure are predictors of a high mortality.

Prevention is extremely important and consists of clearing septic foci preoperatively, routinely checking for contamination of equipment, and removing all intravascular cannulae and bladder drainage tubes as soon as possible. Prophylactic antibiotics are widely used to cover the perioperative period.

The microbiological profile of late-onset prosthetic-valve endocarditis is similar to that of native valve involvement, with streptococci assuming the predominant role. The clinical presentation is also similar, although systemic emboli appear to be more common and the importance of taking blood cultures from any patient with a prosthetic valve and unexplained fever cannot be overemphasized. Confirmation of valve malfunction can be provided by radiological screening to detect abnormal movement of the valve constituents, echocardiography, and very occasionally cardiac catheterization. The mortality of late prosthetic-valve endocarditis is now about 20 to 30 per cent despite surgical and medical treatment. Prevention is directed towards giving appropriate parenteral antibiotics for any manipulation or instrumentation likely to give rise to a bacteraemia. This is also recommended for any infection in which a bacterial cause can be assumed or proved. The details of antibiotic treatment for prosthetic-valve endocarditis are described below but one further therapeutic requirement may be anticoagulation. Evidence favours the view that the risks of stopping routine anticoagulation are greater than those of continuing this form of treatment.

Infective endocarditis in drug addicts

This merits separate discussion because it has emerged as a growing problem over the last decade or more and because its clinical presentation is often different from other forms of endocarditis. There is a predilection for the tricuspid valve and in general a good prognosis despite infection with virulent organisms such as *Staphylococcus aureus*, although community-acquired infection with methicillin-resis-

tant *Staphylococcus aureus* (**MRSA**) has been reported, perhaps as a result of self-administered antibiotics by addicts.

The annual risk of endocarditis for intravenous drug users is estimated at 2 to 5 per cent, with this being the main diagnosis in 5 to 8 per cent of drug addicts admitted to some hospitals in the United States. More recently, large American centres have found that admissions of intravenous drug users with endocarditis are now decreasing, perhaps as a result of the campaign to provide clean needles to addicts in order to reduce the risk of transmitting the AIDS virus.

Typically the patient is a young male addict without previously recognized heart disease and with a relatively short history of illness. Skin colonization with *Staphylococcus aureus* is common in this group and this organism accounts for more than half of cases, gaining entry from septic skin spots and superficial phlebitis. Enterococci and streptococci are more commonly isolated in left-sided disease and together make up about 20 per cent of cases with fungal endocarditis, usually left sided, occurring more often in the addict population. Double and even multiple infections are also more common in addicts than in the general population.

It is perhaps not surprising that the narcotic solution prepared and injected under unhygienic conditions carries the risk of infection. Although *Staphylococcus aureus* has the reputation of being able to infect normal valves, this risk is probably increased by the repeated injection of adulterants such as starch or lactose used to make up the solution. The intermittent injection of these contaminants may lead to right-heart endothelial damage, the development of a platelet nidus, and the ideal surface on which organisms can settle and multiply.

The clinical presentation of tricuspid-valve endocarditis owes much to the shedding of emboli into the pulmonary circulation. Apart from fever, chills and myalgias, dyspnoea, cough, haemoptysis, and pleuritic chest pain make up the typical features. Although examination may provide clear evidence of tricuspid-valve disease, this is not always the case and abnormal physical signs in the heart may be few, particularly if the patient presents early. The venous pressure is likely to be elevated but the absence of a large 'V' wave should not rule out the possibility of tricuspid reflux. A soft short systolic murmur, perhaps increasing with inspiration, may be present at the lower left sternal edge; in more florid cases the systolic murmur may be pansystolic and accompanied by a short mid-diastolic noise giving a to-and-fro quality. However, because of the inconstancy of these localizing signs, one should always consider right-sided endocarditis in mainline addicts who present with pneumonia. The chest radiograph can be very revealing and show pleural effusions and nodular densities, which may cavitate.

Staphylococcal infection of the tricuspid valve has a good prognosis if adequately treated with antibiotics, but if surgery is necessary because of persisting infection then valvulectomy may be the preferred option, with valve replacement deferred until after microbiological cure and only in the small proportion of patients who develop refractory right-heart failure. Gram-negative or fungal infections may only be controlled after surgical excision of the valve.

The presentation of left-sided endocarditis in addicts is usually acute, with rapid valve damage and early development of heart failure. Under such circumstances, valve replacement may be required and the risks of surgery are no greater than in non-addicts, although the long-term outlook is dismal with survival threatened by the patient's unwillingness to comply with medical advice.

Management

GENERAL PRINCIPLES

The purpose of treatment is to sterilize infected cardiac tissue and by so doing limit the extent of damage and prevent life-threatening complications such as systemic embolism and cardiac failure. In most instances, adequate antibiotic treatment is all that is required but in selected cases, usually patients in cardiac failure, surgery has an important part to play, sometimes early in the course. In order to devise a rational plan of management, which may cover a period of 4 to 6 weeks, it is important to have accurate identification of the organism involved, whether it is community or hospital acquired, and to know its sensitivity to various antimicrobials. To some extent the course of the illness can be predicted if, in addition, the nature and severity of the underlying heart disease are known. This exercise can be useful in deciding upon the degree of surveillance required for individual patients and in particular whether complications such as acute valvular damage are likely. An attempt should also be made to find the source of infection, because this too may require treatment, an obvious example being a periapical dental abscess, which would require drainage.

The principles of antibacterial treatment have been laid down as a result of experimental work in animals and clinical experience in man. In general the consensus is that bactericidal drugs should be used in preference to bacteriostatic, that parenteral treatment is indicated, and that bolus intravenous injections are preferable and possibly more effective than intravenous infusions or intramuscular administration. If indwelling intravenous needles are used, they should be changed every 2 days or at the first sign of local inflammation. In most cases a subcutaneous line tunnelled into the subclavian vein should be used and will allow drug administration over a 4- to 6-week period with very little risk of secondary infection.

Antimicrobial treatment

Identification of a micro-organism causing endocarditis and assessment of its susceptibility to antimicrobials is crucial in selecting optimal treatment. The best drug to give depends on the species as well as the results of sensitivity tests. For example, ampicillin is the preferred treatment of susceptible enterococci, whereas penicillin is preferred for susceptible *Streptococcus viridans*. The most important test to predict susceptibility reliably is a minimum inhibitory concentration (**MIC**). A number of standardized methods for performing the test are available. The role of routine bactericidal assays is more open to controversy. Measurement of the minimum bactericidal concentration (**MBC**), recommended by many authorities, is primarily used to identify tolerant organisms. Tolerance is defined as an MBC 32-fold or more greater than the MIC. However, other than for *Enterococcus* spp. which are intrinsically tolerant, no convincing data exist to suggest that for a given species, detection of a tolerant strain requires a different therapeutic approach than for non-tolerant organism. Enthusiasm for performing serum bactericidal titres is decreasing; the interpretation of the test is uncertain and there are no data to indicate that there is advantage in modifying treatment according to the result of such a test, the use and interpretation of which is largely individual and empirical. Measurement of serum bactericidal levels may, however, be a useful way of following drug concentrations in patients given an oral antimicrobial.

INITIAL THERAPY

In patients judged to be too ill to allow the delay of awaiting the results of blood cultures, the choice of empirical agent to be given (after three sets of cultures) depends on clinical features. For native-valve endocarditis with a subacute onset, the likely cause is *Streptococcus viridans* or *Enterococcus* spp., and ampicillin 2 g 6-hourly or penicillin 2.4g 4-hourly, together with, gentamicin 1 mg/kg 8-hourly should be given. If the presentation is acute, a penicillinase-resistant antistaphylococcal penicillin such as flucloxicillin or nafcillin should be given in a dose of 2 to 3 g 6-hourly. Empirical treatment of endocarditis of prosthetic valves should cover *Streptococcus* spp., *Enterococcus* spp., *Staphylococcus aureus,* and methicillin-resistant coagulase-negative staphylococci. Vancomycin or teicoplanin and gentamicin are a good choice. Treatment of intravenous drug-abuse cases should include cover for *Staphylococcus aureus* and Gram-negative bacilli, requiring an aminoglycoside, a penicillinase-resistant penicillin (e.g. flucloxacillin) and an antipseudomonal β-lactam (e.g. piperacillin).

In many cases it is better to await the isolation of the causative organism so that treatment can be adjusted according to its nature and susceptibility to antimicrobials.

TREATMENT FOR SPECIFIC ORGANISMS

Streptococcus and Enterococcus spp.

The presence of complications, risk of toxicity, and underlying medical conditions influence of choice of antimicrobial, which otherwise depends on laboratory tests of susceptibility and MIC. Although regimens described below are satisfactory for all streptococci, the greatest experience applies to *Streptococcus viridans* and enterococci and not to β-haemolytic streptococci and *Sreptococcus pneumoniae* (see Table 3).

Penicillin-susceptible (MIC ≤ 0.1 μ/ml)

In an uncomplicated infection, the most economical regimen consists of penicillin 1.2 to 2.4g i.v. 4-hourly with gentamicin 1mg/kg 8-hourly or streptomycin 7.5 mg/kg 12-hourly i.v. given for 2 weeks. An alternative is to give penicillin 1.2 to 2.4 g i.v. 4-hourly for 4 weeks. Either of these regimens will achieve about 99 per cent cure. The latter is preferred by many for the treatment of endocarditis caused by β-haemolytic streptococci or *Streptococcus pneumoniae*. In the patient allergic to penicillin either vancomycin 1 g i.v. 12-hourly (all types of allergy) or a first-generation cephalosporin (e.g. cephalothin) in high dose (2 g 6–8-hourly) can be used in patients with allergy of the non-anaphylactic type.

Moderately resistant to penicillin (MIC 0.2–0.4 μ/ml)

The following regimens also apply to patients who exhibit complications of infective endocarditis: penicillin 2.4 g i.v. 4-hourly for 4 weeks with gentamicin 1g 8-hourly or streptomycin 7.5 mg/kg 12-hourly given for the first two, or, in the penicillin allergic patient, vancomycin 1 g i.v. 12-hourly for 4 weeks combined with gentamicin or streptomycin in the above dosage for the first 2 weeks.

Penicillin resistant streptococci (MIC >0.5 μ/ml) and enterococcus spp.

The same antimicrobial regimen is appropriate for each of these conditions. Enterococci are inhibited by penicillin, ampicillin or vancomycin but these drugs used alone rarely cure endocarditis. However, when combined with streptomycin or gentamicin, they become bactericidal. The combination of one of these aminoglycosides with either a penicillin or vancomycin produces a cure in a majority of patients (over 80 per cent). Penicillin, 2.4 g I.V. 4-hourly or ampicillin 3 g I.V. 6-hourly are reasonable doses. In penicillin allergic patients or, if the isolate is resistant to ampicillin, vancomycin 1 g 12-hourly should be given and serum levels monitored. Gentamicin 1 mg/kg I.V. 8-hourly is the aminoglycoside of choice in combination with either of these regimens. Peak levels of gentamicin of 3 to 4 μg/ml are adequate and should cause less toxicity; Streptomycin at a dose of 7.5 mg/kg i.v. 12-hourly can be used as an alternative and the combination should be given for at least 4 and preferably 6 weeks, with regular monitoring for VIIIth nerve or renal toxicity. Cephalosporins have no role in the treatment of enterococcal infective endocarditis.

Isolates must be tested for resistance to either ampicillin or vancomycin, as these agents will then be predictably ineffective. Also, with the recent spread of serious aminoglycoside resistance in *Enterococcus* spp., isolates must be tested for this type of resistance, which results in failure of response to the above synergistic combination. There are now strains that exhibit combined resistance to ampicillin, vancomycin, and aminoglycosides. There is no effective antimicrobial treatment for these strains at present.

Staphylococcus spp.

Left-sided and prosthetic-valve infective endocarditis caused by *Staphylococcus aureus* is frequently fulminant and treatment is often both surgical and medical. Penicillin given in a dose of 2.4 g i.v. 4-hourly is

Table 3 *Antibiotic regimens used to treat infective endocarditis in adults*

Organisms[1]	Drug[2]/dose	Duration (weeks)
Streptococcus spp. and _Enterococcus_ spp.		
PENICILLIN MIC <0.1 μG/ML (HIGHLY SUSCEPTIBLE STREPTOCOCCI)	Penicillin G 1.2–2.4 g i.v. 4-hourly	4
	[or]	
	Penicillin G 1.2–2.4 g i.v. 4-hourly *[and]* Gentamicin 1 mg/kg i.v. 8-hourly (measure levels) *[or]* Streptomycin 7.5 mg/kg i.m. 12-hourly	2
Penicillin allergy: (highly susceptible streptococci) Non-anaphylactic type	Cephalothin 2 g i.v. 4-hourly *[or]* Cefazolin 1 g i.v. 8-hourly	4
All types of allergy	Vancomycin 30 mg/kg divided i.v. 12-hourly (measure levels)	4
PENICILLIN MIC ≥0.1 AND ≤0.5 μG/ML (RELATIVELY RESISTANT STREPTOCOCCI)	Penicillin G 2.4 g i.v. 4-hourly	4
	[and] Gentamicin 1 mg/kg i.v. 8-hourly (measure levels) *[or]* Streptomycin 7.5 mg/kg i.m. 12-hourly	2
PENICILLIN MIC >0.5 μG/ML (RESISTANT STREPTOCOCCI) AND ENTEROCOCCUS SPP.	Ampicillin 3 g i.v. 6-hourly *[or]* 2 g i.v. 4-hourly *[or]* Penicillin G 2.4 g i.v. 4-hourly *[and]* Gentamicin 1 mg/kg i.v. 8-hourly (measure levels) *[or]* Streptomycin 7.5 mg/kg i.m. 12-hourly	4–6
Penicillin allergy (applies to resistant and relatively resistant streptococci)	Vancomycin 30 mg/kg divided i.v. 12-hourly *[and]* Gentamicin 1 mg/kg i.v. 8-hourly (measure levels) *[or]* Streptomycin 7.5 mg/kg i.m. 12-hourly	4–6
Staphylococcus spp.		
PENICILLIN-SUSCEPTIBLE S. AUREUS AND COAGULASE-NEGATIVE STAPHYLOCOCCI	Penicillin G* 2.4 g i.v. 4-hourly	
PENICILLIN-RESISTANT AND METHICILLIN-SUSCEPTIBLE S. AUREUS	Flucloxacillin* Nafcillin* } 2 g i.v. 4-hourly Oxacillin	
Penicillin allergy: Non-anaphylactic type	Cephalothin* 2 g i.v. 4-hourly *[or]* Cefazolin* 1 g i.v. 8 hourly	4–6
All types METHICILLIN-RESISTANT S. AUREUS (MRSA) PENICILLIN- OR METHICILLIN-RESISTANT COAGULASE-NEGATIVE STAPHYLOCOCCI PROSTHETIC-VALVE COAGULASE-NEGATIVE STAPHYLOCOCCI INFECTION (GIVE APPROPRIATE ANTIMICROBIAL LISTED ABOVE)	Vancomycin* 30 mg/kg divided i.v. 12-hourly (measure levels)	
If susceptible add	Aminoglycoside (e.g. gentamicin 1 mg/kg i.v. 8-hourly)	2
	[and] Rifampicin 300-mg p.o. 8-hourly	4–6
HACEK[3]	Ampicillin 2 gm i.v. 4-hourly *[or]* Third-generation cephalosporin (e.g. ceftriaxone) i.v. *[and]* Gentamicin 1.5 mg/kg i.v. 8-hourly (measure levels)	4

Table 3 (*cont.*)

Organisms[1]	Drug[2]/dose	Duration (weeks)
Pseudomonas aeruginosa	Aminoglycoside (e.g. gentamicin) i.v. 8-hourly (measure levels) [and] Ceftazidime 2 g i.v. 8-hourly [or] Piperacillin 3 g i.v. 4-hourly [or] Imipenem 1 g i.v. 6-hourly	6
Enterobacteriacae	Aminoglycoside (e.g. gentamicin) i.v. 8-hourly (measure levels) [and] Third-generation cephalosporin (e.g. ceftriaxone) i.v. or Imipenem 1 g IV 6 hourly	4–6
Other penicillin susceptible Gram-positive organisms[5]	Penicillin 2.4-g i.v. 4-hourly [or] Ampicillin 2 g i.v. 4-hourly [and] Gentamicin 1 mg/kg i.v. 8-hourly (measure levels)	4
Other penicillin-resistant Gram-positive organisms and/or penicillin allergy[5]	Vancomycin 30 mg/kg divided i.v. 12-hourly (measure levels) [or] Cephalosporin i.v. (test MIC) [and] Gentamicin 1 mg/kg i.v. 8-hourly (measure levels)	4
***Neisseria* spp.**	Penicillin 2.4 g i.v. 4-hourly [or] Third-generation cephalosporin (e.g. ceftriaxone) i.v.	4
Fungal	Amphotericin B 1 mg/kg i.v. daily 2–3g total dose	4 weeks

[1]In cases of infective endocarditis caused by unusual organisms, further reference should be made to specialist literature.

[2]Organisms must be susceptible by MIC to the drugs used.

[3]HACEK, *Haemophilus* spp., *Actinobacillus actinomycetemcomitans, Cardiobacterium hominis, Eikenella corrodens, Kingella* spp.

[4]Other Gram-positive organisms, *Corynebacteria* spp., *Listeria* spp., *Propionibacteria* spp.,

*Combined with gentamicin (or other aminoglycoside to which the isolate is susceptible) i.v. for 3–5 days.

the agent of choice when the organism is susceptible, but penicillin-resistant, β-lactamase-producing strains must be treated with one of the penicillinase-resistant penicillins such as flucloxacillin, oxacillin or nafcillin in a dose of 3 g intravenously 6-hourly. Methicillin-resistant *Staphylococcus aureus* (MRSA) isolates should be treated with vancomycin 1 g intravenously 12-hourly initially, with further doses adjusted according to levels. In the penicillin allergic patient, vancomycin should be used, or if the allergy is not of the anaphylactic type a first-generation cephalosporin such as cephalothin can be used. Treatment must continue for 4 to 6 weeks. Right-sided infective endocarditis is perceived to be more responsive to treatment than left-sided disease, so that shorter courses and oral therapy have been used with satisfactory outcome. However, when practical, the above regimens remain the safest option.

Many practitioners are drawn to using combinations of antimicrobials for *Staphylococcus aureus* endocarditis; despite the lack of data to indicate an improved final outcome when combining one of the antimicrobials mentioned above with gentamicin, rifampicin, or fusidic acid. Monotherapy is well established as safe for this condition, but evidence of a slightly more rapid clearance of bacteraemia and fever when gentamicin is added to a penicillinase-resistant penicillin leads many clinicians to use an aminoglycoside for the first 3 to 5 days of treatment.

Antimicrobial treatment of infective endocarditis caused by coagulase-negative staphylococci depends on whether the disease involves native or prosthetic valves. Native-valve disease should be treated using the same approach outlined for *Staphylococcus aureus* above. The treatment of prosthetic-valve endocarditis is complicated: it often necessitates surgery and antimicrobial treatment calls for combinations of drugs. Unless penicillin susceptible, a combination of three drugs including vancomycin, rifampicin, and an aminoglycoside should be used. Penicillin should be used in place of vancomycin if the strain is penicillin susceptible. Limited studies indicate that such a combination may produce a better cure rate than does monotherapy or a two-drug combination. An aminoglycoside to which the strain is susceptible must be used and is only given for the first 2 weeks of a 6-week course. Rifampicin is inappropriate when organisms are resistant to it; in some parts of the world fusidin is then substituted empirically. There has been recent interest in using rifampicin in combination with a fluoroquinolone such as ciprofloxacin; initial data demonstrating efficacy of this regimen need to be confirmed before this regimen can be accepted as established for the treatment of prosthetic-valve endocarditis.

Other types of bacterial (infective) endocarditis

The efficacy of antimicrobial treatments for other causes of infective endocarditis (except in the case of *Pseudomonas aeruginosa*) comes from limited clinical experience and not from clinical trials. *Pseudomonas aeruginosa* endocarditis usually requires excision of the infected valve and a prolonged course of a combination of an aminoglycoside and a antpseudomonal β-lactam (see Table 3 for further details.)

Q fever and chlamydial and mycoplasmal endocarditis are relatively resistant to antimicrobial therapy. The mainstay of therapy is a tetracycline, usually combined with rifampicin. This regimen is bacteriostatic and experience suggests that prolonged and even indefinite treatment is need to control this form of endocarditis. Antimicrobial treatment combined with surgery may produce cure in some patients.

Culture-negative endocarditis should initially be treated with a combination of ampicillin and an aminoglycoside for 4 to 6 weeks. If the patient fails to respond, a further exhaustive search must be made for an aetiological agent or an alternative diagnosis.

Fungal

The treatment of fungal infective endocarditis requires combined surgical and medical treatment. Amphotericin B is the drug of choice and should be given for a prolonged course and in a total dose of 2 to 3 g. Two new triazole drugs, fluconazole and itraconazole, offer some promise, but remain to be evaluated adequately. Fluconazole has been administered indefinitely in cases of candida endocarditis when surgery was contraindicated. As itraconazole inhibits *Aspergillus* spp. it may offer a therapeutic option for endocarditis caused by this organism.

Once-a-day and outpatient treatment

The development of ceftriaxone, a β-lactam with a long half-life, has made possible effective treatment given once a day. Experience is also growing with the use of vancomycin and gentamicin i.v. once daily. Such regimens make self-administered home i.v. therapy possible. Successful experience with this approach in cases with uncomplicated infective endocarditis is rapidly growing, but as yet, no trials have shown the comparative efficacy of these once-a-day treatments compared to conventional regimens.

Oral therapy has been successfully used to treat uncomplicated, methicillin-susceptible *Staphylococcus aureus* right-sided and penicillin-susceptible *Streptococcus viridans* endocarditis, but such an approach should be considered only in unusual circumstances and then used with great caution.

SIDE-EFFECTS OF DRUGS

Hypersensitivity reactions can complicate treatment with virtually all the antibacterial drugs used in infective endocarditis. This is particularly the case for all forms of penicillin, which on occasions may cause an illness that mimics endocarditis itself, with persistent fever, aches, and pains, elevated erythrocyte sedimentation rate, and interstitial nephritis with red cells and protein in the urine. When penicillin is given in very large doses it may also cause convulsions, although this is unlikely to be a problem when doses of less than 18 g/day (30 Mu) are given to adult patients with normal renal function. The aminoglycosides are ototoxic and nephrotoxic, and plasma concentrations should be checked in all patients; notice should also be taken of the total dose of gentamicin administered because there is some evidence that this too may influence toxicity. Vancomycin can cause cochlear damage and again blood levels are required if the drug is to be given for more than 2 days.

SURGICAL TREATMENT

The surgical approach to the treatment of infective endocarditis began in 1940 when ligation of an infected persistent ductus arteriosus led to a cure. Because most deaths from endocarditis occur as a result of cardiac failure, itself a complication of aortic- or mitral-valve damage, it seems logical to attribute a prominent role to surgery in its management. However, suturing a prosthetic valve into a potentially infected site seems to go against basic surgical tenets and for that reason only those patients in gross cardiac failure were at first considered suitable. These were a group of patients that had an expected mortality with medical treatment alone of up to 89 per cent, and yet this was reduced to approximately 23 per cent by combined medical and surgical treatment. Moreover, it was found that the risk of developing infection of the prosthetic valve was low at 4 per cent, even when surgery was done before completion of the antibiotic course, and it is now accepted that surgery should be done in the presence of active infection if otherwise warranted. The main indications for surgery are presented in Table 4.

Postoperative survival is largely determined by the degree of preoperative left-ventricular failure; an attempt must be made therefore to recognize patients who may deteriorate rapidly. These include those with *Staphylococcus aureus* endocarditis characterized by rapid tissue destruction, those with evidence of aortic-root infection, and those with changing heart murmurs indicating further valve damage. The presence of valvular vegetations visualized by echocardiography is not by itself an indication for surgical referral but complications including emboli and heart failure appear more common in this group. The risk of emboli seems to be increased in patients with vegetations caused by streptococci and in those with *Staphylococcus aureus* endocarditis, and the size of the vegetations has little predictive value for risk.

Any patient with progressive cardiac failure should be referred early for a surgical opinion and even those with mild to moderate failure on medical treatment are best served by referral to a cardiac centre, where surgery can be done if necessary.

Surgery followed by antibiotic treatment may also be required in order to eradicate persisting infection with coagulase-negative staphylococci or Gram-negative organisms, and a combined surgical and medical treatment offers the best chance of cure in fungal endocarditis. Early-onset prosthetic-valve endocarditis is often caused by staphylococci or rather resistant organisms and for that reason surgery may be required, either because of persisting infection or valve malfunction. Late prosthetic-valve endocarditis is more likely to be due to sensitive organisms and may be cured by medical treatment alone, but close supervision is required to detect early evidence of dehiscence or mechanical derangement of the prosthesis.

Although valve replacement is the usual surgical procedure, abscess formation around the aortic root may have to be dealt with by means of root replacement with a conduit and valve. Excision of the tricuspid valve may be the surgical treatment of choice in intravenous drug addicts, and attempts are being made to conserve heart valves by means of debridement of large vegetations and repair—again mainly of the tricuspid valve.

Response to treatment

The patient's sense of well-being usually returns within a few days of starting effective antibiotic treatment and the fever often settles within 4 or 5 days. A retrospective study from the United States showed that 72 per cent of patients were afebrile within a week of starting treatment, although a British source gives a figure of only 50 per cent. With *Staphylococcus aureus* infection the elevated white-cell count should fall rapidly, although with all forms of infection the erythrocyte sedimentation rate may take weeks to return to normal, as may the anaemia and the serological abnormalities. The C-reactive protein concentrations will fall more quickly. New peripheral stigmata such as petechial haemorrhages can also occur during the first week or two of treatment, and splenic enlargement may take months to resolve.

PERSISTING FEVER IN A MEDICALLY TREATED PATIENT

Fever lasting for more than a week, or recurring after a period of defervescence, identifies a high-risk group with an increased mortality. There is an association with *Staphylococcus aureus* infection, peripheral stigmata such as petechial haemorrhages and Osler's nodes, and embolization of major vessels. These aspects should be self-evident but there is also the danger that extensive intracardiac infection, seen in a third of British cases, might be missed, and vigorous attempts should be made to detect the presence of valve-ring or myocardial abscesses. Otherwise the temptation to alter appropriate antibiotic treatment should be resisted, unless drug hypersensitivity is thought to be present, a diag-

Table 4 *Main indications for surgery in infective endocarditis*

- Cardiac failure due to valvular disease—moderate or severe
- Aortic reflux with progressive annular infection—abscess, aneurysm, fistulae
- Persisting infection despite optimal medical treatment
- Prosthetic-valve endocarditis caused by staphylococci or organisms relatively resistant to antibiotic
- An unstable or stenosed prosthetic valve
- Fungal endocarditis

nosis based on exclusion, often a low-grade fever with skin rashes and possibly eosinophilia.

Prognosis

The most common cause of death in patients with endocarditis is heart failure. Prognosis is influenced by many variables. It is worse in cases of prosthetic-valve endocarditis, especially of the aortic valve, and in elderly patients, and if diagnosis and treatment have been much delayed so that valve damage, cardiac failure, and cerebral and coronary emboli are more likely to have complicated matters. Major emboli, usually to the brain, can occur even after completion of antibiotic treatment, and late rupture of a mycotic aneurysm can tragically maim a patient who has apparently made a complete recovery. Overall mortality is quoted at about 20 per cent for native-valve endocarditis and a survey of endocarditis in the British Isles during 1981 and 1982 gives a mortality of 30 per cent for staphylococcal infections, 14 per cent for bowel organisms, and 6 per cent when sensitive streptococci are involved. Fungal infection carries a worse prognosis, which is improved by combined medical and surgical treatment. Of the survivors who achieve bacteriological cure, 20 per cent may have some incapacity caused by complications and some of them will require late valve replacement for cardiac failure. A 15-year follow-up of patients treated medically in a tertiary referral centre, and therefore possibly at higher risk, showed that 47 per cent required late cardiac surgery, most of them within the first 2 years.

The prognosis for patients undergoing surgery is largely determined by preoperative left-ventricular function, a fact that strengthens the view that surgery should be seriously considered in any patient with more than mild failure or evidence of impaired left-ventricular function in the setting of valvular disease.

Prevention

Many diagnostic and therapeutic procedures involving minor tissue trauma or the spillage of blood can produce bacteraemia; under these circumstances, susceptible patients must be at risk of developing infective endocarditis. However, when one considers the large number of patients having dental and other procedures, about 5 per cent of whom are susceptible, the risk must be small. For that reason it has not been possible to prove that antibiotic prophylaxis in man prevents infective endocarditis. Despite this, it has been generally accepted that prophylactic antibiotics should be used because experimental work in an animal model has shown that endocarditis can be prevented by prior administration of antibiotics and evidence is also available from clinical studies linking the onset of infective endocarditis with previous dental and other forms of instrumentation. Nevertheless, dental and medical procedures account for only a very small proportion of cases: one survey found that only 8 per cent of cases of endocarditis had undergone dental treatment within a month of the start of the illness. Poor oral hygiene leading to spontaneous bacteraemias may be a more important predisposing factor and the potential benefits of good dental care need to be emphasized to all. However, dental procedures do cause a transient bacteraemia and it is estimated that prophylactic antibiotics can provide a protective effi-

Table 5 *Recommendation for endocarditis prophylaxis in adults*

1. *Dental extractions, scaling, or periodontal surgery. Surgery or instrumentation of the upper respiratory tract*
   UNDER LOCAL OR NO ANAESTHESIA
   (a) *For patients not allergic to penicillin and not prescribed penicillin more than once in the previous month:*
   Amoxycillin 3 g as a single oral dose 1 h before the procedure
   (b) *For patients allergic to penicillin:*
   Clindamycin 600 mg as a single oral dose 1 h before the procedure
   UNDER GENERAL ANAESTHESIA
   (c) *For patients not allergic to penicillin and not given penicillin more than once in the previous month:*
   Amoxycillin 1 g i.v. or 1 g i.m. in 2.5 ml of 1% lignocaine hydrochloride just before induction plus amoxycillin 0.5 g by mouth 6 h later

   or

   Amoxycillin 3 g oral dose 4 h before anaesthesia followed by a further 3 g dose by mouth as soon as possible after the procedure

   or

   Amoxycillin 3 g together with probenecid 1 g orally 4 h before the procedure
   SPECIAL-RISK PATIENTS, WHO SHOULD BE REFERRED TO HOSPITAL
   (i) Patients with prosthetic valves who are to have a general anaesthetic
   (ii) Patients who are to have a general anaesthetic and who are allergic to penicillin or have had a penicillin more than once in the previous month
   (iii) Patients who have had a previous attack of endocarditis
   (d) *For those patients not allergic to penicillin and who have not had penicillin more than once in the previous month:*
   Amoxycillin 1 g i.v. or 1 g i.m. in 2.5 ml of 1% lignocaine hydrochloride plus 120 mg gentamicin i.v. or i.m. at the time of induction, then 0.5 g amoxycillin orally 6 h later
   (e) *For patients allergic to penicillin or who have had penicillin more than once in the previous month:*
   (i) Vancomycin 1 g by slow i.v. infusion over at least 100 min followed by gentamicin 120 mg i.v. at the time of induction or 15 min before the surgical procedure

   or

   (ii) Teicoplanin 400 mg i.v. plus gentamicin 120 mg i.v. at the time of induction or 15 min before the surgical procedure

   or

   (iii) Clindamycin 300 mg i.v. in 50 ml diluent over 10 min at the time of induction or 15 min before the surgical procedure, followed by 150 mg orally or i.v. in 25 ml diluent over 10 min 6 h later

2. *Genitourinary surgery or instrumentation*
   As for 1(d) or 1(e) above, directed against faecal streptococci

3. *Obstetric and gynaecology procedures*
   Cover is suggested only for patients with prosthetic valves or a previous attack of endocarditis and is as for 1(d), 1(e)(i), or 1(e)(ii) above, directed against faecal streptococci

4. *Gastrointestinal procedures*
   Cover is suggested only for patients with prosthetic valves or a previous attack of endocarditis and is as for 1(d), 1(e)(i), or 1(e)(ii) above directed against faecal streptococci

Copies of these recommendations are available from the British Heart Foundation, 14 Fitzhardinge Street, London W1H 4DH.

cacy of about 50 per cent for first-attack endocarditis occurring within 30 days of a procedure. It is logical, therefore, to offer antibiotic prophylaxis directed against streptococci to susceptible patients having any dental procedure that causes gingival bleeding. Instrumentation and surgery of the alimentary and genitourinary tracts are also potential sources of heavy bacteraemia involving group D streptococci and Gram-negative organisms, the former being more likely to cause endocarditis.

A vexed question is how to identify patients at risk. Almost 50 per cent cases of endocarditis have no recognized pre-existing cardiac abnormality and so prophylaxis will not have been offered to this group. Patients with known valvular disease should have antibiotic cover, as should those with a past history of rheumatic fever and those with a heart murmur, unless judged to be normal. Mitral-valve prolapse is associated with an increased risk and should be covered in the presence of a murmur of mitral reflux. Patients with congenital defects should be offered prophylaxis, as should postoperative patients if prosthetic materials have been used or if residual valve or septal defects persist. It is not necessary for patients with an atrial septal defect, ligated persistent ductus arteriosus, permanent pacemaker, or after coronary bypass surgery.

The risk of infective endocarditis is certainly greater in patients with prosthetic valves and in those with a previous history of endocarditis, and in them parenteral antibiotic cover should be given for any procedure that could conceivably cause a bacteraemia. This includes uncomplicated childbirth, which is otherwise not an indication for prophylactic treatment.

The drugs chosen must take into account the likely dominant organism gaining entry from a particular site, the nature of the underlying heart disorder, any history from the patient of hypersensitivity to antibiotics, and also the circumstances under which the drug will be given. Dental treatment is the most common indication for prophylaxis and any recommendation should take into consideration the fact that combination antibiotic treatment given parenterally is difficult to implement and has proved impractical in dental practice. The recommendations made by the British Society for Antimicrobial Chemotherapy should be followed and are presented in Table 5.

REFERENCES

Aronson, M.D. and Bohr, D. (1987). Blood cultures. *Annals of Internal Medicine*, **106**, 246–53.

Daniel, W.G. *et al.* (1991). Improvement in the diagnosis of abscesses associated with endocarditis by trans-esophageal echocardiography. *New England Journal of Medicine*, **324**, 795–800.

Durack, D. T., *et al.* (1994). New criteria for diagnosis of infective endocarditis: utilization of specific echocardiographic findings. *American Journal of Medicine*, **96**, 200–9.

Etienne, E. and Eykyn, S.J. (1990). Increase in native valve endocarditis caused by coagulase negative staphylococci: an Anglo-French clinical and microbiological study. *British Heart Journal*, **64**, 381–4.

Kaye, D. (1992). *Infective endocarditis*, (2nd edn). Raven Press, New York. An authoritative review of all aspects of endocarditis.

Petersen, L.R. and Shanholtzer, C.J. (1992). Tests for bactericidal effects of antimicrobial agents: technical performance and clinical relevance. *Clinical Microbiological Reviews*, **5**, 420–32.

Report of a Working Party of the British Society for Antimicrobial Chemotherapy (1985). Antibiotic treatment of streptococcal and staphyococcal endocarditis. *Lancet*, **ii**, 815–17.

Report of a Working Party of the British Society for Antimicrobial Chemotherapy (1990). Antibiotic prophylaxis of infective endocarditis. *Lancet*, **335**, 88–9. *See update:* Antibiotic prophylaxis and infective endocarditis. (Letter.) (1992). *Lancet*, **339**, 1292–3.

Steckelberg, J.M. *et al.* (1992). Emboli in infective endocarditis: the prognostic value of echocardiography. *Annals of Internal Medicine*, **114**, 635–40.

Tornos, M.P. *et al.* (1992). Long-term complications of native valve infective endocarditis in non-addicts. A 15-year follow-up study. *Annals of Internal Medicine*, **117**, 567–72.

15.18 Valve disease

D. G. GIBSON

Normal mitral valve

Anatomy

The normal mitral valve is a complex structure, consisting of leaflets, annulus, chordae tendineae, and papillary muscles. Its anatomy as studied at autopsy shows an unusual degree of variation between normal subjects. Of the two leaflets, the anterior one is the larger, both from base to margin, and also in its perimeter. It is attached to the root of the aorta and the membranous septum at the base of the heart, and is continuous with the chordae peripherally. It thus passes across the centre of the left ventricular cavity, dividing the inlet from the outlet portion. The posterior cusp is attached to the mitral ring and to the anterior cusp at both commissures. It is continuous with the posterior wall of the left atrium, and is divided into three portions by two scallops. The chordae arise from the ventricular margins of both cusps, and are inserted into the heads of the papillary muscles. There are multiple subdivisions in the chordae as they pass from papillary muscles to the cusps, which form an effective secondary pathway, additional to the main one between the cusps, for blood to enter the ventricle. There are two papillary muscles, one anteromedial and the other posterolateral. In general, the former is larger, and has a more uniform structure than the latter which may be double. Both may have up to six heads, giving rise to chordae. The papillary muscles are continuous with the trabecular and subendocardial layer of the ventricular wall. Both are supplied by a single end-artery. The mitral ring is an insubstantial structure whose function is to support valve cusps only. It is incomplete in the region of aortic root and the membranous septum. However, it is surrounded by a well developed circumferential ring of myocardium which supports it, and whose contraction during systole has the effect of significantly reducing the diameter of the valve orifice. Histologically, the normal valve cusp has a dense collagenous core, continuous with the valve ring, the valve fibrosa. This is covered on atrial and ventricular surfaces by a thin layer of loose connective tissue, and finally by endocardium.

Physiology

The normal mitral valve has a cross-sectional area of approximately 5 cm^2. This allows ventricular filling to occur at a peak rate of 500 to 1000 ml/s, with only a very small pressure drop across it. Left ventricular filling occurs mainly during early diastole, the rapid filling phase, and left atrial systole. During middiastole (diastasis), ventricular volume remains virtually constant, and the mitral valve itself almost closes. As heart rate increases during exercise, diastasis becomes shorter, while the duration of the rapid filling period remains virtually unchanged. At rest, approximately two-thirds of the stroke volume enters during early diastole, and the remaining one-third during left atrial systole. At rapid hearts rates, occurring at peak exercise, left ventricular filling time in normal subjects may fall to less than 100 ms. If stroke volume is taken as 100 ml, mean filling rate is of the order of 1 l/s, which is achieved with only a very small pressure difference between left atrium and left ventricle. This gives some indication of the effectiveness of normal mechanisms underlying left ventricular filling.

Mitral stenosis

Aetiology

Chronic rheumatic heart disease is by far the most common cause of mitral stenosis, though a number of other well defined pathological processes exist. Mitral stenosis may be congenital, when it is frequently associated with other lesions causing obstruction to left ventricular outflow, including aortic or subaortic stenosis or coarctation of the aorta. In such cases, the chordae are usually short, and the spaces between them obliterated. The leaflets are thick, with rolled edges. The insertion of the papillary muscles may be abnormal, being either directly from the free wall of the ventricle or from the septum. In parachute mitral valve, there is only a single papillary muscle. Congenital mitral stenosis may be associated with hypoplasia of the left ventricular cavity and the aorta, and also with endocardial fibroelastosis. Causes other than rheumatic acquired mitral stenosis are rare. It has been reported in occasional patients with calcified mitral valve ring, in infective endocarditis, when bulky vegetations may cause obstruction to flow or when granulomatous infiltration has occurred in association with eosinophilia. In nodular rheumatoid arthritis, thickening of the valve cusps has been observed, but true mitral stenosis does not result. However, in systemic lupus erythematosus, treatment of Libman–Sachs endocarditis with steroids may lead to fibrosis of the cusps with commisural fusion. The combination of ostium secundum atrial septal defect and mitral stenosis, Lutembacher's syndrome, is probably fortuitous.

Rheumatic mitral stenosis

INCIDENCE

The incidence of mitral stenosis varies considerably in different parts of the world, but approximately parallels that of acute rheumatic fever. It is much more common, and presents earlier, in the Middle East, the Indian subcontinent and the Far East than in the West. Accurate data about incidence in these countries are not readily available, but an approximate figure for chronic rheumatic heart disease is of the order of ten per 100 000.

PATHOLOGY

Rheumatic mitral stenosis is due to distortion of the normal mitral valve anatomy with fusion of the commisures. The cusps themselves are thickened, and frequently develop thrombus on their atrial surfaces. The sub-valve apparatus may also be affected, with thickening, fusion and contraction of the chordae tendineae. Finally, the valve cusps or ring may become calcified. The left ventricle is usually normal or small in pure mitral stenosis, but occasionally is greatly dilated. The left atrium is characteristically enlarged: its wall may be histologically normal, but sometimes, muscle fibres are disrupted. Mural thrombosis may be present, most commonly on the free wall just above the posterior mitral valve cusp (McCallum's patch). In long-standing cases, calcification of the left atrial wall may develop in plaques on its endocardial surface. Changes of pulmonary venous congestion, pulmonary hypertension, and haemosiderosis may develop in the lungs, with dilation and hypertrophy of the right ventricle and functional tricuspid regurgitation.

PATHOPHYSIOLOGY

The main disturbance in mitral stenosis is to left ventricular filling. When the mitral valve area is reduced to around 2.5 cm^2, ventricular filling rate falls and the normal period of diastasis is lost. This does not matter at rest when heart-rate is slow and filling period relatively long, but during exercise as the heart rate increases, flow can only be maintained by increasing the pressure difference between atrium and ventricle. If the valve area is smaller, the pressure difference is present at rest, and mean left atrial pressure rises. Patients with symptomatic mitral stenosis have a valve area of 0.75 to 1.25 cm^2, and a pressure drop as high as 20 to 30 mmHg across the valve during diastole. Cardiac output then falls and pulmonary vascular resistance usually increases. The stenosis may be either at valve level or below it, due to fusion of the chordae. The subvalvular apparatus may also interfere with left ventricular filling by restricting the wall movement, so reducing stroke volume and increasing left atrial pressure in the absence of any diastolic pressure drop across the valve itself. Left ventricular cavity size, usually normal in young patients, may be increased in the middle aged or elderly with mitral stenosis and the end-diastolic pressure may rise. A number of factors contribute to this left ventricular disease, including restriction of filling, coronary emboli, and distortion of the septum by right ventricular hypertrophy and overload. In addition, disturbed filling interferes in some way with systolic function, since after successful surgery, cavity size usually falls, as stroke volume increases. Chronic left atrial hypertension causes a corresponding rise in pulmonary capillary pressure; clinical evidence of pulmonary congestion appears when it reaches around 25 mmHg. Further lung disease may be caused by reactive pulmonary hypertension, repeated pulmonary emboli or chest infections, haemosiderosis, or even bone formation.

Clinical picture

SYMPTOMS

The symptoms of mitral stenosis usually appear insidiously, and may have been present for several years before the patient seeks medical attention. They may be apparent within 3 or 4 years of the attack of acute rheumatic fever, or be delayed by up to 50 years. Less frequently, the onset is abrupt with an attack of acute pulmonary oedema, systemic embolism, or the onset of atrial fibrillation. The most common manifestation of mitral stenosis is reduced exercise tolerance. In pure mitral stenosis, the major symptom is usually breathlessness and, less frequently, fatigue clearly related to exertion, or palpitation, due to an inappropriately rapid ventricular rate developing during exercise in patients in atrial fibrillation. Typical anginal pain may also occur, usually ascribed to previous coronary embolism, but sometimes apparently due to pulmonary hypertension and right ventricular hypertrophy. Late in the disease, nocturnal dyspnoea may be present. Episodes of florid acute pulmonary oedema are less frequent now than appears to have been the case some years ago, probably due to widespread treatment of virtually all patients with heart disease of whatever severity with powerful diuretics. Recurrent chest infection or winter bronchitis are very characteristic. They are associated with an increase in breathlessness, cough, and purulent sputum, with secondary fluid retention and pulmonary oedema. Haemoptysis is common, and caused by chest infections, pulmonary infarction, acute pulmonary oedema, or 'pulmonary apoplexy', the rupture of a small blood vessel within the lung. Massive or recurrent haemoptysis may be the presenting or only symptom of mitral stenosis. Systemic embolism from the left atrium is common in untreated mitral stenosis, particularly when atrial fibrillation is present.

Any organ may be affected, but the most common sites are cerebral, coronary, splenic, renal, mesenteric, or the arteries of the limbs. Pulmonary emboli may originate in the right atrium, and cause pulmonary infarction or progressive reduction in exercise tolerance due to an increase in pulmonary vascular resistance. Salt and water retention is common in untreated mitral stenosis, leading, initially, to nocturia as the normal diurnal rhythm of sodium excretion is reversed. Peripheral oedema, ascites, pulmonary oedema, and pleural effusion follow.

PHYSICAL EXAMINATION

Prolonged low cardiac output leads to weight loss and a malar flush. In pure mitral stenosis, the character of the pulse is normal, although its amplitude may be decreased and the rhythm irregular due to atrial fibrillation. All arterial pulses should always be checked in view of the possibility of previous arterial emboli. The venous pressure is normal unless tricuspid regurgitation is present. An 'a' wave in the venous pulse of a patient with what appears to be pure mitral stenosis should always raise the possibility of additional tricuspid stenosis or severe pulmonary hypertension. Palpation of the praecordium at the apex may reveal a palpable first sound, previously called a 'tapping apex' and, less frequently, a palpable opening snap. It may also be possible to feel pulmonary valve closure at the base of the heart if severe pulmonary hypertension is present. A left parasternal heave is usually due to right ventricular hypertrophy caused by pulmonary hypertension, but may also be due to tricuspid regurgitation, or increased prominence of a normal right ventricle secondary to an enlarged left atrium. In pure mitral stenosis, a sustained apex beat is unusual, but may be seen when the right ventricle is very considerably enlarged or more commonly, because of coexistent left ventricular disease. On auscultation at the apex, the classical findings are a loud first sound, preceded by a presystolic murmur if the patient is in sinus rhythm, an opening snap and a delayed diastolic murmur. An early systolic component to the first sound may be present in some patients with atrial fibrillation which has a superficial resemblance to a presystolic murmur. A loud first sound is less specific for rheumatic mitral stenosis than a palpable one, since it also occurs in high cardiac output states, such as hyperthyroidism. A soft or absent first sound in mitral stenosis strongly suggests that the anterior cusp of the mitral valve is calcified or immobile. An opening snap is a very characteristic physical sign. It is usually loudest at the lower left sternal edge, less commonly the apex or the base, and is absent if the valve structure is severely disorganized. The time interval between aortic valve closure and the opening snap depends on the diastolic drop gradient across the valve, being shorter when the left atrial pressure is high. This relation is not strong enough to be of any use in assessing individual patients, particularly those in atrial fibrillation in whom the interval varies from beat to beat. The delayed diastolic murmur starts after the opening snap, separated from it by an appreciable interval. It is low-pitched and persists for a variable period throughout diastole. If the stenosis is mild, the murmur is short, but if the murmur lasts throughout diastole at a normal ventricular rate, then the degree of stenosis is likely to be at least moderately severe. When the rate is rapid due to atrial fibrillation, the murmur may no longer be audible, although in these circumstances, the diagnosis can be suspected from the palpable first sound. However, there exists a group of patients in whom no delayed diastolic murmur is audible even when the heart-rate is controlled: so-called 'silent' mitral stenosis. These patients frequently, but not always, have severe pulmonary hypertension, and the valve itself is disorganized, often with significant involvement of the subvalve apparatus. The exact reason for the absence of the murmur is not clear.

CHEST RADIOGRAPH

The radiological appearances of mitral stenosis are characteristic (Fig. 1). The heart size may be normal or increased, but the most frequent abnormality is enlargement of the left atrium that is selective, i.e. proportionately greater than that of the heart shadow as a whole. This appears on the penetrated posteroanterior film as a double outline on the right side of the heart shadow, with elevation of the left main bronchus, and enlargement of the left atrial appendix which forms that part of the left heart border just below the main pulmonary artery. Apart from this, the cause of cardiac enlargement is hard to assess radiologically, as it may be due to an increase in size of any of the other three chambers or to the presence of a small pericardial effusion. Mitral valve calcification may be visible on the posteroanterior film just to the left of the spine, on the continuation of the shadow of the left atrium. In the lung fields, the upper lobe veins may be dilated with the patient in the erect position, indicating that left atrial pressure is raised, and the size of the main pulmonary artery may be increased due to pulmonary hypertension. Increased pulmonary vascular resistance causes upper lobe blood diversion: decreased prominence of the vessels to the lower zones, while those to the upper zones are normal or increased. When the left atrial pressure reaches approximately 25 to 30 mmHg, pulmonary oedema may deveop, with lymphatic lines, basal pleural effusions, generalized hazy shadowing, and finally obvious interstitial oedema. Longstanding left atrial hypertension may cause pulmonary haemosiderosis, or even bone formation, the latter causing dense nodules a few mm in diameter.

Electrocardiograph

The electrocardiograph is not very informative in mitral stenosis, but it allows atrial fibrillation to be confirmed. If the patient is in sinus rhythm, left atrial hypertrophy may be demonstrated by a bifid P wave in lead II and a dominant negative deflection in VI. Electrocardiographic evidence of right atrial hypertrophy suggests tricuspid stenosis in addition to mitral stenosis. The electrical axis is usually vertical: right ventricular hypertrophy, if severe, is shown by a dominant R wave in VI.

Echocardiograph

Echocardiography has totally changed the diagnosis and management of patients with mitral valve disease. The characteristic feature of rheumatic mitral valve disease on M-mode echocardiography is a reduced middiastolic closure rate of the anterior cusp of the mitral valve to less than 50 mm/s for mild mitral stenosis and to 0 to 20 mm/s for severe involvement (Fig. 2). Cusp fusion causes forward, rather than backward

Fig. 1 Chest radiograph from a patient with pure mitral stenosis. Heart size is normal, but the left atrial appendage is enlarged. The upper lobe vessels are dilated and there are Kerley lines at both bases.

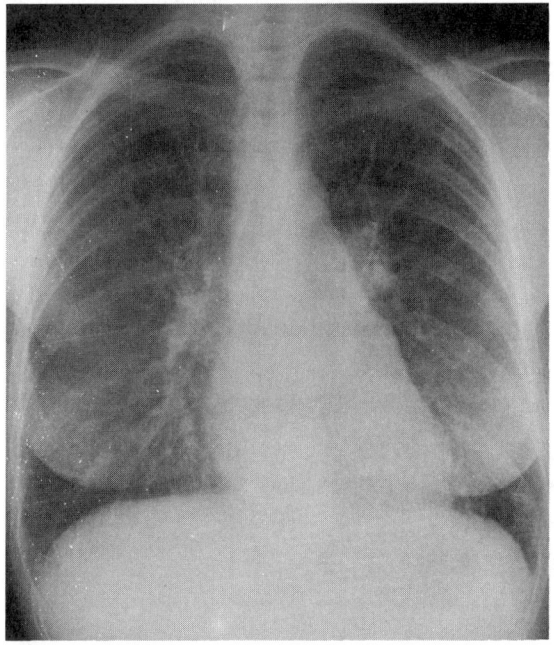

movement of the posterior cusp during diastole. On cross-sectional echocardiography, the mobility of the anterior cusp is reduced, particularly near its tip (Fig. 3(a)). Valve area can be estimated semiquantitatively from the parasternal minor axis view (Fig. 3(b)), provided that the cusps are not calcified. It is also possible to assess the degree of subvalve involvement. Occasionally atrial thrombus can be detected (Fig. 4). The diastolic pressure drop can be estimated by cross continuous wave Doppler, and valve area estimated from the pressure half time (p*). Peak right ventricular pressure is estimated from systolic velocities of tricuspid regurgitation. The aortic and tricuspid valves can also be checked.

Transoesophageal echocardiography is particularly useful for demonstrating thombus in the body of the left atrium or in the left atrial appendix. Spontaneous contrast within the left atrial cavity is probably due to stasis resulting from a combination of atrial fibrillation, low forward flow, and increased cavity size. It indicates an increased risk of thrombus formation. Finally, the degree of thickening and calcification of the cusps and the extent to which the subvalve apparatus is involved can be assessed particularly well from this approach.

Cardiac catheterization

This investigation is rarely necessary, either to make the diagnosis or to assess its severity. It is performed only to assess the state of the coronary arteries in older patients and as a prelude to balloon valvuloplasty, or in very occasional cases in whom diagnostic echocardiograms cannot be obtained.

DIAGNOSIS

The diagnosis of mitral stenosis is usually straightforward on the basis of history, physical signs, and chest radiograph, and can be confirmed rapidly by echocardiography. When the ventricular rate is rapid, the diastolic murmur may be inaudible, but becomes apparent when the rate is controlled by digoxin. Cases of silent mitral stenosis may present difficulties, and may mimic primary pulmonary hypertension. In such patients, mitral stenosis can often be excluded or confirmed only by echocardiography or direct measurement of left ventricular and left atrial pressures. Mitral stenosis should also be suspected as a source of systemic emboli and as a cause of unexplained atrial fibrillation, particularly in the elderly. In these circumstances, the valve lesion itself may be very mild, and the usual physical signs not be present, although the characteristic abnormalities can be demonstrated by echocardiography. One should always try to quantify the severity of the mitral stenosis as

well as diagnosing its presence. Probably the most reliable way to do this is still from the extent to which exercise tolerance is reduced, as judged from the history. The length of the mid-diastolic murmur gives some indication, as described above, although this is unsatisfactory when the ventricular rate is increased or the murmur inaudible.

Differential diagnosis

Left atrial myxoma

Left atrial myxoma may mimic all the physical signs of mitral stenosis including delayed diastolic and presystolic murmurs, loud first sound, and opening snap ('tumour plop', actually a modified third sound). It may lead to increasing dyspnoea and systemic embolization, and the length of the history may range from a single acute incident to one of many years' duration. There is often evidence of a systemic illness, and erythrocyte sedimentation rate and plasma proteins are frequently, but not invariably, abnormal. Variable murmurs are often described, but constant ones, or no abnormality at all on auscultation, are equally common. The only role of cardiac catheterization is to check the state of the coronary arteries in an older patient. Diagnosis depends on suspicion of

Fig. 3 (a) Two-dimensional echocardiogram from a patient with mitral valve disease, parasternal long axis view taken in mid-diastole. The anterior cusp (Aml) of the mitral valve is thickened, and fails to open normally. LA, left atrium; Se, septum; My, myocardial echoes; whose intensity is increased due to scarring of the subvalve apparatus; Pml, posterior mitral leaflet. (b) Rheumatic mitral valve disease, parasternal minor axis view during mid-diastole, at the level of the mitral valve orifice (MO). Other abbreviations as in (a).

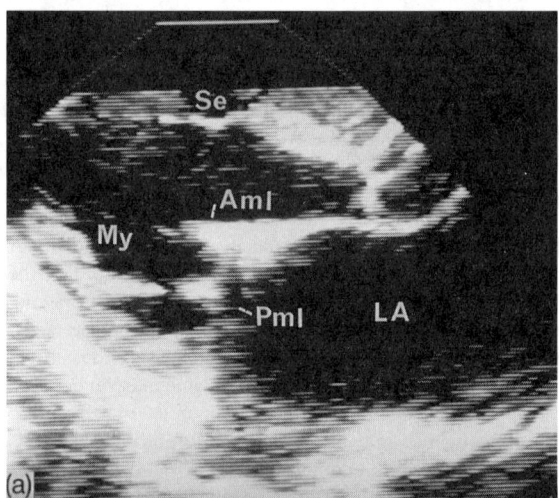

(a)

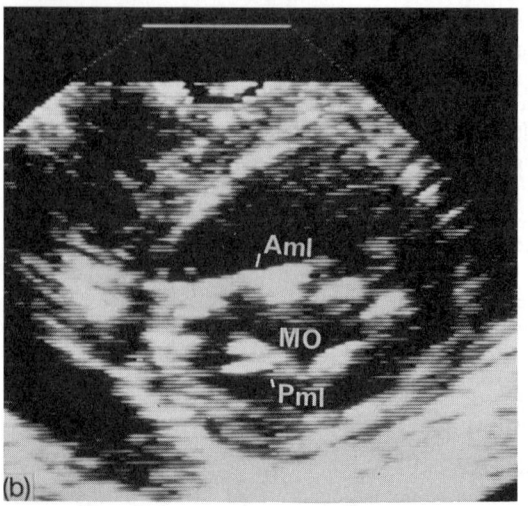

(b)

Fig. 2 M-mode echocardiogram from a patient with mitral stenosis. The anterior cusp (AML) is thickened, and its diastolic closure rate is reduced. The posterior leaflet (PML) moves forward during diastole. There is an opening snap on the phonocardiogram, coinciding with maximum forward motion of the anterior cusp.

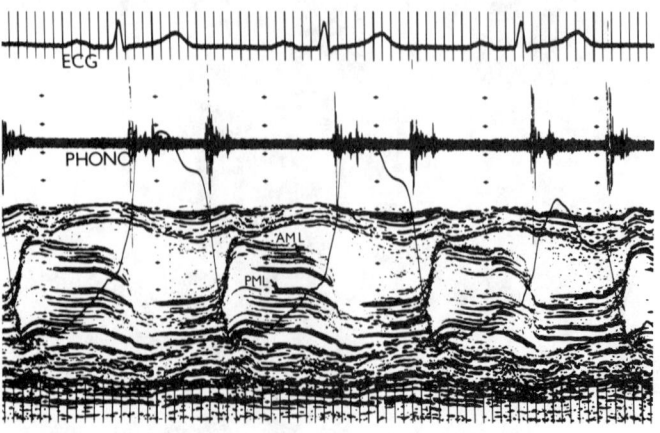

the condition, and performing echocardiography, which shows a characteristic mass of echoes behind the mitral valve during diastole.

Cor triatriatum (see Chapter 15.15)

This is a rare cause of obstruction to blood flow at left atrial level and may mimic mitral stenosis, particularly in childhood.

Pulmonary veno-occlusive disease

This may also present as silent mitral stenosis, often with a raised pulmonary wedge but a normal left atrial pressure.

Ostium secundum atrial septal defect (see Chapter 15.15)

Although the differential diagnosis between atrial septal defect and mitral stenosis is usually clear, in occasional cases it may become difficult on clinical grounds because of a loud tricuspid flow murmur, mid-diastolic in timing, and audible all over the precordium. Pulmonary valve closure is usually, but not always, delayed in atrial septal defect and, in occasional cases, the usual electrocardiograph pattern of partial right bundle branch block may be absent. The true diagnosis can be made by echocardiography. M-mode demonstrates a normal mitral valve and reversed septal motion. Cross-sectional echocardiography may demonstrate the defect on the subconstal view. A negative jet can be demonstrated by contrast echo, and abnormal flow across the defect demonstrated by colour flow mapping. Peak right ventricular pressure is assessed from the velocity of the tricuspid regurgitant signal.

Austin Flint murmur

In severe aortic regurgitation, a delayed diastolic murmur may be audible at the apex, though the mitral valve itself is quite normal. It may be accompanied by a loud first sound and a presystolic murmur. Unlike rheumatic mitral stenosis, though, the first sound is never palpable, and an opening snap is not present. The most satisfactory way of excluding rheumatic involvement of the mitral valve is by echocardiography, which demonstrates a high frequency fluttering on an otherwise normal anterior cusp echo.

TREATMENT

Medical treatment

1. In patients below the age of 21, penicillin prophylaxis against further attacks of acute rheumatic fever should be given.
2. Atrial fibrillation should be treated with a digitalis preparation to control the ventricular rate. Anticoagulant therapy should be given to reduce the risk of systemic embolism to all patients with atrial fibrillation, unless there are very strong contraindications. It is also advisable to consider giving this treatment to patients in sinus rhythm with mitral stenosis, particularly the middle-aged and elderly, as the incidence of embolism is not negligible in these patients, particularly at the onset of atrial fibrillation. The incidence of embolism is also high when an unanticoagulated patient with atrial fibrillation, is admitted to hospital with a rapid heart rate and pulmonary oedema. Intravenous heparin should thus be given until adequate anticoagulation with an oral agent has been established.
3. Fluid retention associated with mitral stenosis responds well to treatment with diuretics.
4. Chest infections should be treated promptly with appropriate antimicrobials. Patients should be given a supply of antimicrobial to take prophylactically at the start of a head cold. Chest infections often precipitate, or may be precipitated by fluid retention so that a diuretic is also often useful.
5. In all patients with valvular heart disease, prophylactic antimicrobial should be given for all dental manipulations and potentially septic hazards. This should preferably be amoxycillin, unless the patient is sensitive to penicillin, when cephaloridine or erythromycin should be used.

Mitral valvuloplasty

As rheumatic mitral stenosis results from fusion of the commisures between the two mitral cusps. This fusion is susceptible to rupture by inflating a catheter-mounted balloon across the valve orifice (Fig. 5). Mitral valvuloplasty has the great advantage over surgery of avoiding thoracotomy. A catheter is introduced through the inferior vena cava to the right atrium. The atrial septum is crossed, and the catheter stabilized across the mitral valve, usually by a guidewire, which is passed out through the aortic valve. The balloon itself may be single, often with a waist; less commonly, two balloons are placed simultaneously across the orifice. The balloon is inflated to a predetermined size for 20 s. Not all patients are suitable for valvuloplasty. There should be no more than minimal regurgitation. Ideally, the cusps should be pliable, with calcification in the commissures. The subvalve apparatus should not be scarred or contracted, and clot in the left atrial appendix should have been excluded by transoesophageal echocardiography. Using this procedure, a satisfactory fall in transmitral pressure difference is usually achieved, and maintained in the short and medium term. Embolism is unusual provided that clot in the left atrium has been excluded. Mitral regurgitation may be provoked, sometimes severe enough to require valve replacement on an elective or even an emergency basis. The

Fig. 4 Left atrial thrombus (Th) in a patient with mitral valve disease. LA, left atrium; LV, left ventricle; IAS, interatrial septum. The left atrium is considerably enlarged.

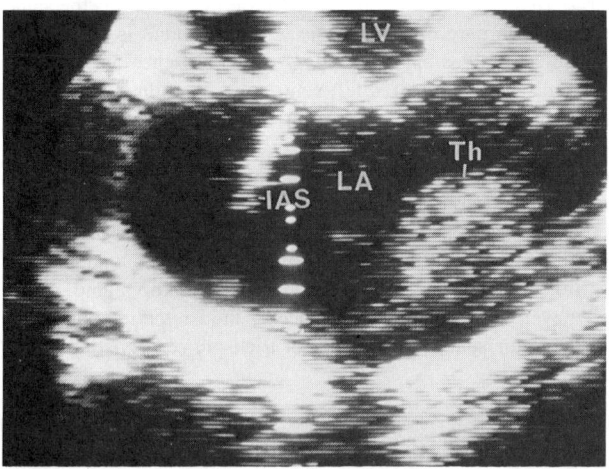

Fig. 5 The Inoue balloon catheter, as used for mitral valvuloplasty, partially (left) and completely (right) inflated.

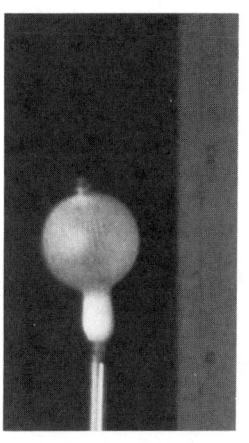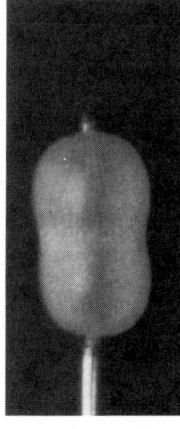

majority of patients are left with a small atrial septal defect at the site of passage of the catheter, but this is not of any haemodynamic significance.

Mitral surgery

A number of surgical procedures are available. These include mitral valvotomy, open or closed, and mitral valve replacement. The choice of operation depends on the anatomy of the mitral valve determined on the basis of the physical signs, the echocardiogram, the age of the patient, and the surgical resources available. Closed mitral valvotomy is a relatively simple procedure in terms of the resources that are required, although a satisfactory result presupposes considerable experience with the operation, experience that is now becoming rare in the developed world. This closed operation is particularly suitable in a Third World country, where the major radiographic and expensive disposables necessary for balloon valvuloplasty are not available. It is particularly appropriate in a young patient, in sinus rhythm, with evidence of a mobile anterior cusp. Symptom-free follow-up of 30 years or more occurs regularly after this procedure. Open valvotomy requires cardiopulmonary bypass but allows a more complete procedure to be undertaken and, in particular, the subvalvular apparatus can be inspected and adherent chordae divided. If the results of valvotomy are found to be unsatisfactory, then it is possible to proceed to valve replacement at the same operation. Mitral valve replacement will be required if the valve cusps are greatly thickened or calcified. This operation should not be considered in patients in whom the haemodynamic disturbance caused by the valve disease is mild, as the prosthesis causes a resting diastolic pressure drop across it, as well as interfering with systolic and diastolic left ventricular function. This is particularly the case if the left ventricular cavity is small, when a low profile prosthesis is preferred.

It is difficult to lay down hard and fast indications for intervention in a patient with mitral stenosis. If the clinical and echocardiographic evidence suggests that valvuloplasty is feasible, the presence of definite limitation of exercise tolerance is an adequate indication, particularly in a young person. Open valvotomy should be considered if there is any significant contraindication to valvuloplasty. Unless it is due to coronary artery disease, the presence of left ventricular disease is not a contraindication to operation, however severe it may appear to be in terms of increased cavity size or reduced amplitude of wall motion. Closed valvotomy is no longer available in most developed countries, but remains a most attractive possibility where medical and surgical resources are limited. In avoiding the use of either radiographic screening or cardiopulmonary bypass, valvotomy may be an attractive option for a patient who develops acute pulmonary oedema during pregnancy, provided that local surgical expertise is available. More severe symptoms require valve replacement. When there has been definite progression of symptoms in individual patients, the decision is not usually difficult. The problem of valve disease in pregnancy is discussed further in Chapter 13.4.

PROGNOSIS

In the absence of surgical treatment, mitral stenosis is usually a progressive disease, although the rate is unpredictable. Unfavourable features include a gradual increase in the severity of the valve disease with disorganization of its structure and superimposed calcification, an increase in pulmonary vascular resistance, and the development of functional tricuspid valve disease, with chronic elevation of the venous pressure leading to cardiac cirrhosis and impaired liver function. Surgical treatment has improved the prognosis considerably, although mitral valvotomy does not prevent progression of the rheumatic process, nor does it reduce the risk of infective endocarditis. It is still premature to assess the long-term prognosis of patients who have been treated by valvuloplasty. That of closed mitral valvotomy, which has been available for over 40 years, can be remarkably satisfactory, and it is not unusual to see a patient several decades after surgery still with effectively normal

flow velocities across the mitral valve. It has also become clear that the life of biological mitral valve substitutes, particularly the porcine xenograft, is limited to no more than 10 years in the majority of patients above the age of 21, and considerably less than this in children. The use of valves should thus be confined to the very elderly, and to young women who wish to undertake pregnancy knowing that repeat surgery will be needed. There are minor differences in the haemodynamic effects of the different types of mechanical valve substitutes, but in individual cases, these are of little consequence.

Mixed mitral valve disease

Mixed mitral valve disease, with both stenosis and regurgitation, is almost invariably rheumatic in origin. In these patients, the mitral regurgitation is not usually severe in terms of the volume load that it imposes on the left ventricle, but it is significant in so far as the increased stroke volume is associated with an increased mitral diastolic pressure drop and also because the presence of mitral regurgitation implies a more damaged mitral valve.

PATHOLOGY

The pathology of mixed mitral valve disease is similar to that of pure mitral stenosis, except that the disease process has frequently advanced further. The valve cusps are thickened and their edges everted so that the mitral valve orifice becomes fixed. The chordae tendineae are frequently shortened and thickened and the valve apparatus may become calcified. In addition, the patient may well have had a previous mitral valvotomy which led to symptomatic improvement for a number of years but which did not alter the progress of the disease.

CLINICAL PICTURE

Symptoms

As with pure mitral stenosis, the main complaint is of progressive reduction in exercise tolerance, although dyspnoea is frequently less prominent than fatigue or palpitation on exertion. Exacerbation of symptoms may result from chest infection or fluid retention, and systemic embolism remains a possibility.

Physical examination

Patients are usually in atrial fibrillation. The pulse character is normal unless additional aortic valve disease is present. The venous pressure may be raised due to increased right ventricular end-diastolic pressure, to tricuspid valve disease, or to obstruction to right heart filling due to massive enlargement of the left atrium. On palpation of the praecordium, a left parasternal heave is often present, whose mechanism is the same as in patients with pure mitral stenosis. The first sound is not usually palpable and a sustained apex beat suggests the presence of additional aortic valve disease or impaired left ventricular function. On auscultation the first heart sound is soft, reflecting thickening or calcification of the anterior cusp, rather than the degree of mitral regurgitation, as was once held, and the opening snap either soft or absent. Mitral regurgitation causes a pan systolic murmur which is loudest towards the axilla, because the posterior cusp is often fibrotic and retracted. The delayed diastolic murmur is not usually of full length, but may be loud, or even palpable, reflecting the increased left ventricular stroke volume. Ankle oedema or even ascites may be evidence of fluid retention, although these are rather unusual in the absence of tricuspid regurgitation.

Chest radiograph

This shows an enlarged heart with selective enlargement of the left atrium. In mixed mitral valve disease, the left atrium may be very large indeed with a volume of up to 3 litres ('giant left atrium') (Fig. 6). There may be calcification in its wall as well as in the mitral valve cusps. The lung fields show similar changes to those of pure mitral stenosis.

Electrocardiogram

This confirms atrial fibrillation and may shown voltage changes of left ventricular hypertrophy. As the patient is likely to be taking digitalis, it is not usually possible to comment on the T-wave changes.

Echocardiogram

A reduced diastolic closure rate with anterior movement of the posterior cusp during diastole confirms the presence of rheumatic mitral valve disease. Left ventricular cavity size may be increased due to valvular regurgitation or additional left ventricular disease. The extent of disease of the valve cusps and subvalve apparatus is apparent on the cross sectional display, and mitral regurgitation can be detected on the continuous (Fig. 7) and colour flow Doppler. Peak right ventricular pressure can be estimated from tricuspid regurgitation.

DIAGNOSIS

This is not usually in doubt. The severity of the overall lesion is best determined from the symptoms. Attempts to determine the relative importance of the stenosis and regurgitation are unhelpful, as the mitral regurgitation is seldom severe. It is much more important to establish the presence or absence of other valvular lesions, particularly of the aortic and tricuspid valves. A giant left atrium, although producing a striking radiographic appearance, is not necessarily evidence that the disease is severe, and its presence may actually improve the prognosis by damping the oscillations of the left atrial pressure. Similarly, the presence and severity of any pulmonary hypertension is not of major importance in determining the severity of the symptoms, nor in assessing the timing or risk of operation.

TREATMENT

This is on the same lines as for pure mitral stenosis, except that valvuloplasty is likely to be inappropriate, and operation will almost certainly involve mitral valve replacement. In a proportion of cases (the exact number depending on local surgical expertise and enthusiasm) the valve can be repaired.

Mitral regurgitation

AETIOLOGY

Unlike mitral stenosis, which is almost invariably due to chronic rheumatic heart disease, there are a number of causes of pure mitral regurgitation (Table 1).

The most common of these is the floppy mitral valve. This condition has been described under a number of names, based either on its pathology or on its clinical features. Thus it has been referred to as mucinous or myxomatous degeneration, or as a ballooning or billowing mitral valve. As described below, it is probably responsible for a significant proportion of patients described as having mitral valve prolapse, or the midsystolic click late systolic murmur syndrome. Floppy mitral valve, which is relatively common above the age of 50, is a non-inflammatory process which may affect either cusp, partially or completely. The most striking abnormality is an increase in cusp area, causing folding and upward doming into the left atrium during systole. The chordae may become elongated, tortuous, and thinned, predisposing to chordal rupture. The abnormal chordae can undergo fibrosis, as can the cusps, leading to an erroneous diagnosis of chronic rheumatic involvement. Ulceration of the cusps may also occur, predisposing to thrombosis on their surface, and also to infective endocarditis. The ring circumference may be normal or increased. The papillary muscles are normal. Histologically, the central valve fibrosa is abnormal with large areas in which fibrous tissue is either absent altogether, or where the collagen bundles are fragmented, coiled, or disrupted. These lie in pools of abnormal acid mucopolysaccharide. A dense layer of laminated collagen forms over the atrial surface of the cusp. There is no evidence of vascularization or of inflammatory cells in the absence of secondary infective endocarditis.

The cause of sporadic cases of floppy mitral valve is unknown. However, similar appearances may complicate Marfan's syndrome, pseudoxanthoma elasticum, Ehlers–Danos syndrome, and osteogenesis imperfecta. The incidence of the sporadic condition tends to rise with

Fig. 6 Chest radiograph from a patient with mixed mitral valve disease, showing gross cardiac enlargement, due mainly to dilation of the left atrium.

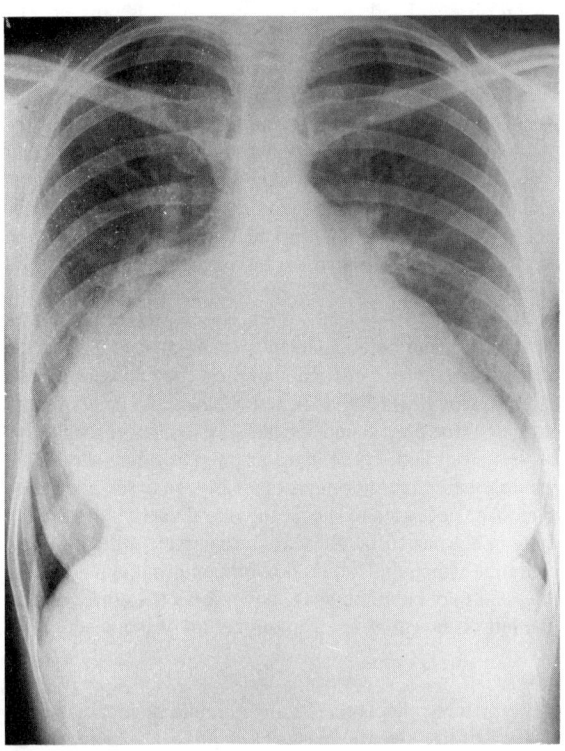

Fig. 7 Doppler cardiogram from a patient with mixed mitral valve disease, showing mitral regurgitation as a downward deflection during systole, and forward flow through the mitral orifice during diastole as an upward deflection. Peak diastolic velocity is increased due to mitral obstruction. (Gain increased for optimal recording of systolic flow velocity.)

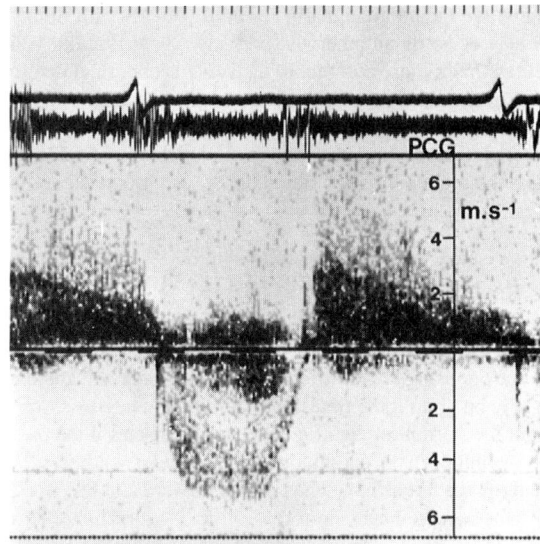

Table 1 *Common causes of pure mitral regurgitation*

Structure affected	Anatomical fault	Pathogenesis
Valve cusps	Congenital cleft	Primary atrial septal defect Isolated
	Redundant cusps	Floppy valve Marfan's syndrome
	Perforation	Infective endocarditis
	Scarring	Rheumatic
	Iatrogenic	
Chordae	Redundant	Floppy valve Marfan's syndrome Other CT diseases
	Rupture	Floppy valve Marfan's syndrome Other CT diseases Infective endocarditis Rheumatic
	Shortening	Rheumatic EMF
Papillary muscle	Dysfunction	Ischaemic heart disease Cardiomyopathy
	Prolapsing cusp	Various
	Rupture	Acute myocardial infarction
Valve ring	Dilatation	Severe LV disease
	Calcification	Various

CT, connective tissue; EMF, endomyocardial fibrosis, LV, left ventricular.

age, and individual case histories suggest that it can be a very benign and chronic process.

Infective endocarditis is an important cause of mitral regurgitation, which may affect the valve directly or be secondary to an infection on the aortic valve. Vegetations developing on the cusps vary from small nodules along the line of apposition to large, friable masses up to 10 mm or more in diameter, which are especially common when then organism is a fungus. Lesions on the anterior cusp of the mitral valve may occur in association with aortic endocarditis, usually involving the right coronary cusp. These 'jet lesions' may appear as localized aneurysms, or perforate the cusp causing mitral regurgitation severe enough to need valve replacement. Rarely, mitral vegetations may be large enough to cause mitral valve obstruction: much more commonly, the haemodynamic disturbance is of pure regurgitation. Infective endocarditis may also involve the chordae, particularly in patients with floppy mitral valve. It may occur on an otherwise normal valve, particularly in the old or debilitated, but more commonly the valve is abnormal due to minor congenital abnormality, previous rheumatic involvement, floppy mitral valve, hypertrophic cardiomyopathy, or calcification of the mitral valve ring. Mitral prostheses, or xenografts are also liable to be infected by endocarditis, which may either be blood borne, or introduced at the time of operation.

PATHOPHYSIOLOGY OF MITRAL REGURGITATION

Pure mitral regurgitation is associated with a large increase in left ventricular output. As the pressure in the left atrium is lower than that in the aorta, the force opposing left ventricular ejection is reduced, and the stroke volume may be up to three times normal. Ejection begins almost immediately after the start of left ventricular contraction, and at the time of aortic valve opening, up to one-quarter of the stroke volume may already have entered the left atrium. The relative forward and backward flows depend on the relative opposing forces in the two directions. This has therapeutic significance in the treatment of severe mitral regurgita-

tion. Left atrial pressures are therefore increased, with the V wave sometimes reaching 50 to 60 mmHg. These high pressures shorten the phase of isovolumic relaxation and greatly increase the velocity of early diastolic left ventricular filling. Left ventricular end-diastolic cavity size is not greatly increased, particularly when the history is short, but end-systolic size is considerably smaller than normal due to the low force opposing ejection. Left ventricular output is also maintained by a sinus tachycardia, which is nearly always associated with significant non-rheumatic mitral regurgitation.

CLINICAL PICTURE

The clinical picture of pure mitral regurgitation is very variable, depending on the underlying pathology, the severity of the regurgitation and whether or not the left ventricle is diseased. These clinical patterns will be described separately, recognizing that there is some overlap between them and that the relation between the clinical picture and the underlying aetiology is not fixed.

Ruptured chordae tendineae

The ruptured of a chorda is often associated with severe mitral regurgitation. The onset of symptoms is usually gradual but, in a minority of cases, may be so sudden that patients are able to describe exactly what they were doing at their onset. In these latter cases, the symptoms are most severe at their onset, and improve over the next few weeks, as the ventricle adapts to the volume load. Even in this more compensated phase, though, exercise tolerance may be severely limited by breathlessness or fatigue. A murmur has often been heard in the past, often many years previously and described at the time as 'innocent' or 'benign'. The most severe cases may present in intractable pulmonary oedema and require immediate intermittent positive pressure ventilation. On the other hand, when the regurgitation is only moderately severe it is remarkably well tolerated for many years with minimal symptoms.

Clinical examination

Patients are usually in sinus rhythm until late in the course of the disease if the mitral regurgitation is non-rheumatic. As tachycardia is frequent, the pulse is 'jerky', implying that its amplitude is normal although the upstroke is rapid. The venous pressure is normal unless severe pulmonary hypertension or associated tricupsid regurgitation is present. The precordial impulse at the apex is prominent and sustained, and may be double due to a palpable third sound. A systolic thrill may also be present. A left parasternal heave is frequently apparent with severe regurgitation, and usually reflects the presence of systolic expansion of the left atrium or of left ventricular disease, rather than right ventricular hypertrophy. The first sound is not palpable. On auscultation, the first sound is normal or reduced in intensity and the most prominent features are a loud pan systolic murmur and a third heart sound. The third sound may be rather more high-pitched than that associated with left ventricular disease, reflecting the considerable early diastolic inflow velocity, and may be confused with the second sound. The murmur may thus be mistimed. This mistake can be avoided by starting auscultation at the base of the heart where the true second sound can be appreciated, and 'inching' the stethoscope towards the apex, when it can be heard to bury itself in the murmur as the third sound appears. If the mitral regurgitation is very severe, left atrial and left ventricular pressures equalize before the end of systole, so that the murmur stops early. In cases presenting with acute pulmonary oedema and shock, the mitral valve is effectively absent, and there is no murmur at all. Unlike rheumatic mitral regurgitation, the position at which the amplitude of the murmur appears maximal is variable, and may be at the apex, down the left sternal edge, at the back, to the left of the spine, or even on the top of the head.

Chest radiograph

The radiographic picture reflects the haemodynamic disturbance (Fig. 8). Most characteristically, overall heart size is normal or only moderately increased, with selective enlargement of the left atrium, although not to the same extent as in rheumatic mitral valve disease. The appearance of the pulmonary vasculature reflects the increase in mean left atrial pressure. A chest radiograph taken soon after the onset of severe mitral regurgitation may show a characteristic picture of pulmonary oedema with a normal-sized heart. If the condition is severe and long-standing, considerable cardiac enlargement may develop due to coexistent left ventricular disease.

Electrocardiograph

The electrocardiograph usually shows sinus rhythm with only moderate left ventricular hypertrophy. There may, in addition, be evidence of left atrial hypertrophy. Frequent ventricular ectopic beats are characteristic of mild or moderate mitral regurgitation.

Echocardiogram

On the M-mode, the mitral valve echo may be abnormal, showing prolapse, with cusp remnants visible in the left atrium during systole. Early in the natural history of the condition, the large left ventricular stroke volume is mediated by a small end-systolic volume. As the left ventricle adapts, so the end-diastolic dimension increases. Finally, when irreversible left ventricular disease supervenes, there is progressive increase in end-systolic left ventricular cavity size. The left ventricular filling rate may be very rapid indeed. Cross-sectional echocardiography confirms the presence of very active left ventricular wall motion and allows a clearer view of the extent of systolic cusp prolapse into the left atrium; the affected cusp is also recognized more reliably. Regurgitation can be confirmed by continuous wave Doppler (Fig. 9) and the jet mapped within the left atrium by colour flow. Apparent jet area, whether or not normalized to left atrial cavity size, has proved a disappointing measure of the severity of the regurgitation. Transoesophageal echo may give more information about valve anatomy, allowing small vegetations to be detected. If the regurgitation is severe, retrograde flow can be detected in the pulmonary veins.

Cardiac catheterization

This is not usually necessary to make the diagnosis when the clinical features and echocardiography are typical, though many surgeons require views of the coronary arteries in older patients.

Papillary muscle dysfunction

Normal mitral closure depends on the integrity of the myocardium as well as that of the valve apparatus itself. In part, the position of the cusps is maintained during systole by contraction of the papillary muscles as the left ventricular cavity gets smaller. This mechanism may be disturbed in a number of ways. The papillary muscles themselves may be affected by ischaemic or other left ventricular disease, so that their ability to contract is impaired. If left ventricular cavity size is greatly increased, the relation between wall movement and papillary muscle shortening becomes abnormal. In hypertrophic cardiomyopathy, the greatly hypertrophied papillary muscles and abnormal cavity shape may contribute to the characteristic forward movement of the whole mitral valve apparatus during systole, which is associated with a pressure drop between the left ventricular cavity and the aorta as well as with significant mitral regurgitation. Finally, the mitral ring itself is supported in systole by circumferentially arranged myocardium at the base of the heart.

Mitral regurgitation associated with left ventricular disease, and a structurally intact valve apparatus, is usually referred to as papillary muscle dysfunction, although this has not be confirmed directly in humans. The mitral regurgitation itself is usually mild, though in a minority it may be as severe as that due to ruptured chorda. Even when mild, though, its duration may be considerable, particularly when left bundle branch block is present, so that it limits the time available for ventricular filling when the heart rate is rapid. The clinical picture, therefore, is usually dominated by the left ventricular disease. The presence of mitral regurgitation is demonstrated by either a late or a pansystolic murmur, which often varies in its intensity and timing from day to day, and which becomes softer with successful treatment of the underlying condition. In addition, there is evidence of left ventricular disease, usually cavity dilatation with reduced anmplitude of wall motion. Echocardiography is thus informative, when it demonstrates a large cavity with poor wall movement, quite different from the picture seen in severe mitral regurgitation. The mitral regurgitation itself can be detected by continuous wave and colour flow Doppler. Hypertrophic cardiomyop-

Fig. 8 Chest radiograph showing acute pulmonary oedema due to acute mitral regurgitation resulting from ruptured chordae tendineae.

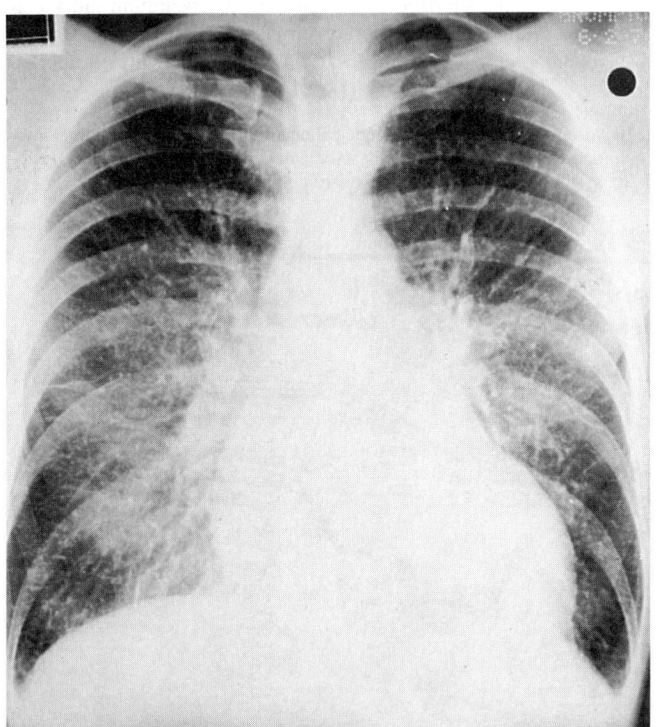

Fig. 9 Doppler cardiogram from a patient with pure mitral regurgitation, showing regurgitant flow as a downward deflection during systole. Diastolic flow velocity pattern is normal, with peak velocity coinciding with the third heart sound (III) on the phonocardiogram (PCG).

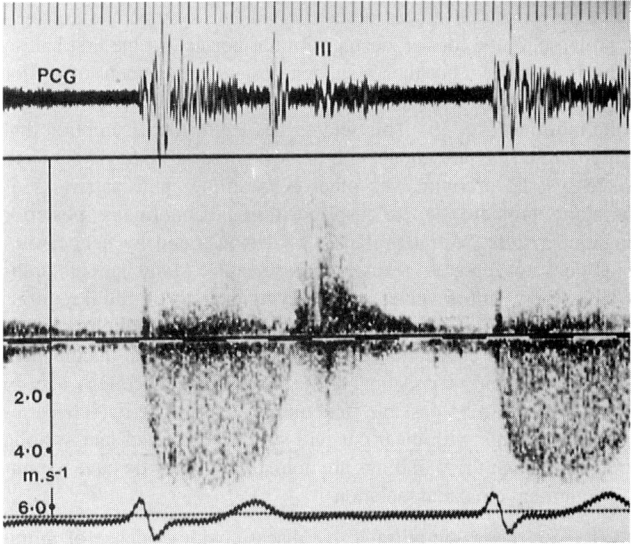

athy can be recognized. Cardiac catheterization confirms the presence of a raised left atrial pressure, secondary to a corresponding elevation of the left ventricular end-diastolic pressure. Left ventricular angiography shows a dilated and poorly functioning left ventricle with reflux of contrast into the left atrium where it tends to accumulate here due to poor forward flow. Coronary artery disease as the underlying cause can only be confirmed or excluded by coronary arteriography.

Ruptured papillary muscle

This is a rare complication of acute myocardial infarction, causing a sudden deterioration in the patient's clinical condition. Complete rupture of a papillary muscle may occur, or less commonly, only a single head may be involved. Complete rupture usually occurs 2 to 5 days after the infarct, and is rarely associated with survival for more than 24 or 48 h without very prompt surgical intervention. Death is due to cardiogenic shock and pulmonary oedema. A pansystolic murmur may sometimes be audible at the apex. Partial rupture, i.e. loss of one of the heads, occurs rather later after the infarct and, like complete rupture, causes a striking deterioration in clinical state, along with the development of a pansystolic murmur, but in this case more prolonged survival is possible. The posteromedial papillary muscle is involved more frequently than the anterolateral, by both partial and complete rupture. When complete rupture occurs, death usually occurs before definitive treatment can be undertaken, but partial rupture can be diagnosed by cross-sectional echocardiography and potentially treated by early mitral valve replacement, once the haemodynamic situation has been stabilized. The prognosis, however, is significantly worse than that after chordal rupture due to severe left ventricular disease.

Mitral prolapse

Prolapse of the mitral valve cusps into the left atrial cavity during systole is a non-specific finding that may occur in many different types of mitral valve disease, trivial or severe. Such prolapse can be documented in a number of ways, the most satisfactory being direct inspection at the time of operation. Alternatively, it may be detected by left ventricular angiography or echocardiography. Unfortunately, these various methods do not agree about the presence and severity of mitral prolapse in individual patients. In ostium secundum atrial septal defect, for example, left ventricular angiography frequently shows evidence of mitral prolapse, although the valve is usually quite normal to inspection at the time of operation. Similarly, echocardiography and angiography may disagree, particularly in patients with coronary artery disease, when only the former method shows mitral prolapse to be present.

The ability to demonstrate abnormalities of mitral valve movement by echocardiography once led to considerable preoccupation with prolapse and, unfortunately, to confusion. Two echocardiographic patterns of valve movement have been demonstrated, late systolic and holosystolic prolapse. In the former, cusp position is normal for the first half to two-thirds of systole, but then a sudden posterior movement of one or both cusps occurs, often accompanied by a mid-systolic click and late systolic murmur (Fig. 10). This finding has led to the assumption that mitral prolapse is synonymous with the syndrome of mid-systolic click and late systolic murmur. The other echocardiographic pattern is of holosystolic prolapse, when cusp position is abnormally posterior throughout systole. Mitral prolapse, as demonstrated by echocardiography, does not represent a single disease entity. Many patients probably have floppy mitral valves, with varying degrees of mitral regurgitation. In others, the primary abnormality may be cardiomyopathy. However, identical echocardiographic findings have been documented in up to 21 per cent of presumably normal females of college age. In addition, it may not be possible to demonstrate prolapse by echocardiography in patients with clear-cut mid-systolic click and late systolic murmur. Although these findings are non-specific, they do have a number of important cinical associations.

1. Non-rheumatic mitral valve disease, with evidence of mitral prolapse, is a significant cause of infective endocarditis. It is likely that such patients have floppy mitral valves. Nevertheless, all patients in whom minor mitral valve abnormalities are suspected should have prophylactic antimicrobials for dental manipulations and other potentially septic hazards.

2. Young people with evidence of mitral prolapse have a significantly increased risk of cerebral embolism. This again appears to result from non-bacterial thrombotic vegetations due to cusp ulceration. This complication is unusual, and there is no indication to treat all patients with evidence of mitral prolapse with long-term anticoagulants.

3. A minority of patients develop chest pain. This may be characteristic of angina pectoris, or more commonly, it is 'atypical'. It is often associated with inferior T wave changes on the resting electrocardiogram. Left ventriculography may show regional abnormalities of wall motion, particularly affecting the inferior wall. Coronary arteriography is normal, in typical cases showing neither fixed disease nor spasm. The condition thus overlaps that described as 'syndrome X' (Chapter 15.10.3).

4. Ventricular ectopic beats are common with mild mitral regurgitation of any cause. Much less frequently, recurrent ventricular arrhythmias may occur; very rarely these may be life threatening. It is these unusual cases that appear to be the basis of a small number of reports of sudden death in this condition. Approximately half of these cases had a history of syncopal or presyncopal episodes. A late systolic murmur was common, but a mid-systolic click was unusual. The resting electrocardiogram almost invariably showed T wave abnormalities and ectopic beats. Left ventriculography, when it was performed, characteristically demonstrated severe mitral prolapse. The autopsy appearances were those of floppy mitral valve. However, in the absence of severe left ventricular hypertrophy, mitral valve abnormalities are a very unusual cause of sudden death in the general population. Mitral prolapse should not therefore be regarded as a single disease entity, but a non-specific finding. Mitral regurgitation and other associated abnormalities should be treated on their own merits.

Endomyocardial fibrosis

This is a disease characterized by fibrosis of the endocardium and underlying myocardium of either or both ventricles. It is common in Uganda and surrounding countries in East Africa where it accounts for approx-

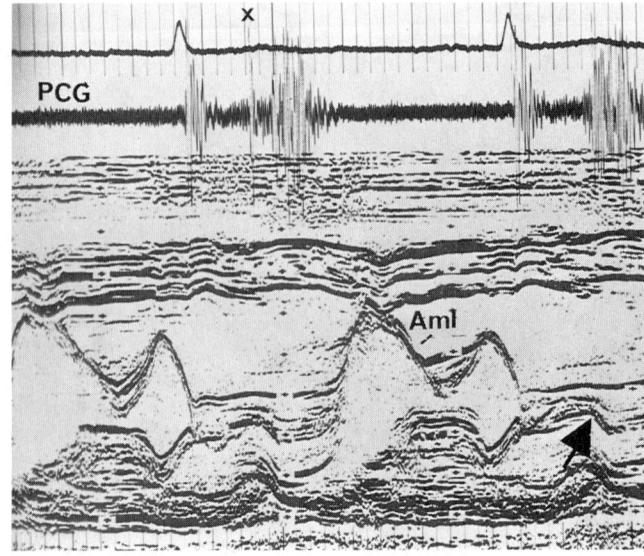

Fig. 10 Mitral valve prolapse, M-mode echocardiogram. Mid-systolic prolapse occurs, marked by the arrow. This is associated with a mid-systolic click (x) and late systolic murmur on the phonocardiogram (PCG).

imately 10 per cent of hospital admissions with heart disease, and in Nigeria in West Africa. It also occurs, less commonly, in South India and Sri Lanka. Occasionally, it is seen in Europeans who have lived in affected areas and very rarely in those who have never been to the tropics. When the right ventricle is involved, fibrosis starts at the apex and spreads upwards towards the tricuspid valve, involving the papillary muscles and chordae, but sparing the outflow tract. In the left ventricle, the inflow tract, apex, and lower part of the outflow tract are characteristically involved, and also the posterior mitral valve cusp and its papillary muscle. 'Skip' areas of normal endocardium on the inflow tract have been described. In both ventricles there is involvement of the underlying myocardium, and mural thrombosis. The aetiology of the condition is not known, but it does not appear to be related to rheumatic fever, malnutrition, or any vector-borne virus. The clinical picture is of progressive mitral or tricuspid insufficiency of insidious onset, together with restriction of ventricular filling by subendocardial scarring. When the tricuspid valve is mainly involved, there is gross fluid retention, whereas mitral or combined involvement leads to pulmonary oedema. Embolic incidents from the right or left ventricle are common.

TREATMENT

Medical treatment consists of high doses of diuretics and vasodilators if valvular regurgitation is severe. Decortication of the ventricular cavities may be possible surgically, along with replacement of mitral or tricuspid valve.

Mitral ring calcification

Heavy calcification of the mitral valve ring is a disease of the elderly, and is particularly common in females. Although it appears to be a degenerative condition, it occurs more frequently when the resistance to left ventricular ejection is increased, such as with aortic stenosis or hypertension. It usually causes no symptoms, being detected incidentally by the presence of calcification in the mitral ring on chest radiography or on echocardiography. Yet it is not a totally benign condition. It is a potential source of systemic emboli, and a focus for infective endocarditis. Approximately half the patients have abnormalities of conduction, including high-grade atrioventricular block, sinus node disease or bundle branch block. Mild mitral regurgitation is common, but rarely is it severe enough to need valve replacement. Very occasionally it has been reported as causing mitral stenosis with diastolic gradients of up to 20 mmHg. The diagnosis is usually made from the plain chest radiography, and confirmed by echocardiography, which shows heavy calcification in the valve ring. The central fibrous body may also be involved, with calcium spreading down the anterior cusp. In the absence of complications, no treatment is required other than prophyllaxis against infective endocarditis. Complications are treated on their own merits.

DIAGNOSIS OF MITRAL REGURGITATION

The diagnosis of mitral regurgitation is usually straightforward on the basis of the physical signs. These may be atypical when the regurgitation is severe enough to cause the pressures in left atrium and left ventricle to equalize by end-ejection, so that the murmur ends prematurely. In very severe cases, it may be absent altogether. Such patients may present with pulmonary oedema of sudden and unexplained onset with a chest radiograph showing a normal sized heart shadow. Echocardiography demonstrates very active left ventricular wall movement, showing that the poor peripheral blood flow is due to valvular regurgitation rather than left ventricular disease, and in addition, may show abnormal mobility of one or both mitral valve cusps. Doppler may be atypical, showing an abbreviated regurgitant flow signal of low velocity. In patients who present with more typical signs, the main diagnostic problem is to decide the relative contributions of the valvular regurgitation and left ventricular disease to the overall clinical state. This may be difficult and even after full investigation, the final decision may not be clear cut.

Differential diagnosis

Ventricular septal defect

A congenital ventricular septal defect may persist into adult life and cause a pansystolic murmur maximal at the lower left sternal edge (maladie de Roger). However, such a ventricular septal defect is invariably small, with no haemodynamic consequences and thus does not cause cardiac enlargmement, limitation of exercise tolerance or abnormality on the chest radiograph. Acquired ventricular septal defect, due to septal perforation, may present as a pansystolic murmur developing in the first few days or weeks after a myocardial infarction. Unlike the small congenital ventricular septal defect described above, its presence may be associated with a large left to right shunt. In addition, it is situated in the muscular, rather than in the membranous septum, so that the physical signs to which it gives rise, are significantly different. The differential diagnosis from mitral regurgitation is an important one since either condition may require surgical treatment. This distinction cannot reliably be made clinically or on the basis of the chest radiograph or electrocardiograph. The presence of a ventricular septal defect can be diagnosed at the bedside from a simple right heart catheter, by demonstrating a left to right shunt at right ventricular level. It may be possible to see the abnormality itself with two-dimensional echocardiography, from either an apical or a subcostal view. Either may show a defect in the muscular septum, with impaired movement of its apical segment. The diagnosis can be confirmed by colour flow Doppler, which may also demonstrate associated mitral regurgitation. These findings are confirmed by contrast left ventriculography performed at the same time as coronary arteriography. In individual patients, the main problems are to decide the relative contribution of valvular regurgitation, the septal defect, and left ventricular disease to overall clinical state, and on the optimal timing of operation. These decisions may be difficult.

Aortic valve disease

The ejection systolic murmur of aortic valve disease is frequently audible at the apex, where it may be louder than at the base, and have a slightly different quality. However, this is not an adequate basis for diagnosing additional mitral regurgitation and it is essential to establish that the timing of the murmur is pansystolic, either from its relation to the second heart sound, or in aortic regurgitation, from its relation to the start of the early diastolic murmur.

Tricuspid regurgitation

The pansystolic murmur of tricuspid regurgitation may be mistaken for that of mitral regurgitation, particularly when the right ventricle is greatly enlarged. The presence of tricuspid regurgitation can be suspected from an elevated venous pressure with systolic waves, and confirmed by Doppler echocardiography. In severe mitral regurgitation, however, additional tricuspid regurgitation may be present and the distinction between the two becomes academic.

Treatment

Mild or moderately severe mitral regurgitation is well tolerated and does not require treatment apart from prophylactic antimicrobial for all dental manipulations and potentially septic hazards. Such patients should be followed up at annual intervals, as mitral regurgitation, particularly when due to degenerative disease, may be progressive. When mitral regurgitation is due to papillary muscle dysfunction, treatment is that of the underlying condition, which usually means administering a diuretic and a vasodilator. Mitral regurgitation due to hypertrophic cardiomyopathy does not require specific treatment. Severe mitral regurgitation, which causes significant symptoms in spite of medical treatment, is best managed by mitral valve surgery. This will involve either mitral valve replacement, or in suitable cases, mitral valve repair. After acute chordal rupture, it is often possible to treat the patients medically with rest, diuretics, and vasodilators for 1 to 2 weeks, while the left ventricle enlarges to compensate for the increased volume load. Clinical improvement may be striking, so that surgery becomes a less hazardous procedure than an emergency operation in the acute stage would have been. Very severe mitral regurgitation may require emergency treatment on account of intractible pulmonary oedema or a low output state. Such pulmonary oedema is best treated by intermittent positive pressure respiration. The most effective means of managing a low cardiac output state associated with mitral regurgitation is not to administer drugs with a positive inotropic effect, such as isoprenaline or dobutamine, but rather to use a vasodilator. This reduces the peripheral resistance, and thus increases the volume of blood entering the aorta at the expense of that going back into the left atrium. Sodium nitroprusside, by continuous intravenous infusion, at a dose of 20 to 200 μg/min as a 0.01 per cent solution is the agent most frequently used. This requires that arterial pressure, and preferably pulmonary wedge pressure and cardiac output are measured at frequent intervals in order to control the infusion rate. Vasodilators, with or without intermittent positive pressure respiration may make it possible for the cardiac state to be stabilized long enough to allow the underlying diagnosis to be confirmed and cardiac surgery arranged. Vasodilators are also very effective in patients with papillary muscle dysfunction associated with severe left ventricular disease where their use may lead to a temporary, but nevertheless, useful symptomatic improvement.

Aortic stenosis

Aortic stenosis is the consequence of a fixed obstruction to left ventricular ejection. The obstruction is most commonly at the level of the valve itself, but may also be immediately above the sinuses or within the left ventricle.

Aetiology

Types of valvar aortic stenosis are summarized in Table 2.

Valvar aortic stenosis

Valvar aortic stenosis is an important cause of cardiac disability and, though it is most common in the elderly, it may present at any time of life. Congenital aortic stenosis, due to a valve with only a single commissure is most frequent in infancy or childhood. A much more common abnormality, the congenital bicuspid valve, consisting of fusion of one of the three commissures, may be detected as an incidental finding early in life, but does not usually give rise to significant haemodynamic abnormality unless it becomes calcified or involved by infective endocarditis. Rheumatic aortic stenosis develops as the result of commissural fusion in a tricuspid valve and may subsequently become calcified. Senile or degenerative aortic stenosis results from deposition of calcium in a tricuspid valve in the absence of any inflammatory process. Very rarely, vegetations in infective endocarditis, or lipid deposits occurring in hyperlipidaemia may be bulky enough to cause significant left ventricular outflow tract obstruction.

Pathophysiology

The presence of aortic stenosis leads to the development of a systolic pressure drop between the left ventricular cavity and the aorta, which in symptomatic cases, may be greater than 50 to 70 mmHg at rest, and reach over 200 mmHg on exertion. The resistance is a fixed one, and so differs from the increased peripheral vascular resistance of systemic hypertension, which falls during exercise. As a result of the increase in stroke work, left ventricular hypertrophy develops, with the thickness of the wall increasing, although the cavity size is normal or even reduced. This hypertrophy and associated fibrosis causes the diastolic stiffness of the myocardium to increase so that the end-diastolic pressure may rise causing pulmonary congestion. Increased left ventricular wall thickness also predisposes to ventricular arrhythmias. Late in the disease, when left ventricular involvement is severe, the cavity becomes dilated and more spherical in shape. In the majority of cases, calcification is confined to the aortic valve, but in a minority it may spread to

Table 2 *Types of aortic stenosis*

Valvular
Congenital
Fused commissure 'bicuspid'
Rheumatic
'Senile' (calcified tricuspid valve)
Infective endocarditis (rare)
Hyperlipidaemia (rare)
Fixed subaortic
Membrane
Tunnel
Supravalvular

involve the anterior cusp of the mitral valve or the atrioventricular node, and thus give rise to a prolonged P-R interval or even to complete heart block. Finally, aortic stenosis is most common in a population of patients in whom the incidence of ischaemic heart disease is high, so that obstructive coronary artery disease may contribute, coincidentally, to the symptoms or the impairment of left ventricular function.

CLINICAL PICTURE

Symptoms

The three characteristic clinical features of aortic stenosis are breathlessness, chest pain, and syncope. Breathlessness in aortic stenosis is frequently associated with an elevated left ventricular end-diastolic pressure and it occurs at first on exercise, but later at rest. Paroxysmal nocturnal dyspnoea is common in late stages of the disease. The length of the history of breathlessness from its onset until it becomes severe is usually only of the order of 1 to 2 years, and thus considerably shorter than that of mitral stenosis. Angina occurring in aortic stenosis is clinically indistinguishable from that due to coronary artery disease, and indeed, in many cases, this is the underlying cause. However, typical anginal pain can occur in aortic stenosis in patients in whom the large and medium-sized coronary arteries are normal. The mechanism for this is uncertain, but may represent the effect of abnormal myocardial relaxation in left ventricular hypertrophy on coronary flow. Syncope in aortic stenosis probably reflects a number of different types of disturbance. In some patients, it is clearly related to exertion and appears to be due to hypotension resulting from the combination of exercise-induced vasodilation and a fixed cardiac output. In other cases, it results from transient complete atrioventricular block due to involvement of the atrioventricular node by calcification, carotid sinus hypersensitivity, or even from short periods of ventricular tachycardia or fibrillation. Exactly similar mechanisms may underlie the increased incidence of sudden death in these patients.

Clinical examination

The physical signs of aortic stenosis are very characteristic. The carotid pulse is slow rising with a reduced amplitude and an early notch on the upstroke, followed by a thrill. The venous pressure is usually normal until late in the disease, but a small 'a' wave is frequently present. This cannot be taken as evidence of pulmonary hypertension, but appears to be related in some way to the presence of left ventricular hypertrophy (Bernheim 'a' wave). The apex beat is sustained and is often double, due to the presence of an additional left atrial impulse. On auscultation, the first sound is normal or soft, and may be preceded by a fourth heart sound. The second sound is single when the valve is calcified, due to lack of the aortic component. In younger patients with mobile aortic valve cusps, aortic valve closure may be audible, but delayed, so that splitting of the second sound is reversed. When left ventricular disease is severe, pulmonary valve closure is accentuated. The characteristic ejection systolic murmur is maximal at the base of the heart, and is also audible over the right common carotid artery. It may seem longer than the ejection systolic murmur of, for example, anaemia or thyrotoxicosis due to prolongation of ventricular systole and delay in aortic valve closure. An additional short, soft early diastolic murmur is nearly always present, although this does not imply haemodynamically significant aortic regurgitation.

Chest radiograph

Heart size is normal in uncomplicated aortic stenosis. If it is increased, the underlying cause is likely to be unsuspected aortic regurgitation, left ventricular cavity dilatation, or very severe left ventricular hypertrophy, when the cavity may be normal in size, but the myocardium up to 50 mm in thickness. Increased left ventricular filling pressure may cause left atrial hypertension and thus dilatation of the upper lobe vessels as well as selective enlargement of the left atrium in the absence of organic mitral valve disease. The aortic root is nearly always dilated and the aortic valve calcified in older patients, which is best seen on the lateral chest radiograph or with screening.

Electrocardiogram

Electrocardiography characteristically shows changes of left ventricular hypertrophy, although it may be entirely normal, even in the presence of severe aortic stenosis. Left atrial hypertrophy is shown by a bifid P wave in lead II or a dominant negative deflection in V1. Conduction disturbances include left axis deviation, left bundle branch block, prolonged P-R interval, or complete heart block. Poor progression of R waves across the chest leads is common, and may be caused by septal hypertrophy rather than anterior myocardial infarction.

Echocardiogram

If the aortic valve is calcified, disruption of the normal anatomy can be demonstrated by M-mode, but in younger patients, it may appear entirely normal, even when severe aortic stenosis is present. Two-dimensional echocardiography is very useful for demonstrating abnormalities in the left ventricular outflow tract. Thickening and reduced mobility of the valve cups can nearly always be demonstrated (Fig. 11). In young patients with a bicuspid valve, doming of the cusps during systole can be seen, while in older patients, a calcified aortic valve appears as an immobile mass. The pressure drop across the outflow tract can be reliably measured by continuous wave Doppler. Additional aortic regurgitation can also be detected. Left ventricular anatomy and function, both in terms of the extent of hypertrophy and cavity size and ejection fraction can be studied. The hypertrophy itself may be concentric, or may involve the septum to a much greater extent than the posterior wall, resembling the pattern seen in hypertrophic cardiomyopathy. Late in the disease, the left ventricle becomes enlarged and its ejection fraction falls to values commonly seen in dilated cardiomyopathy.

Fig. 11 Aortic stenosis, two-dimensional echocardiogram from apical four-chamber view, showing left ventricle (LV) and heavily calcified aortic valve (Ao). Se, septum.

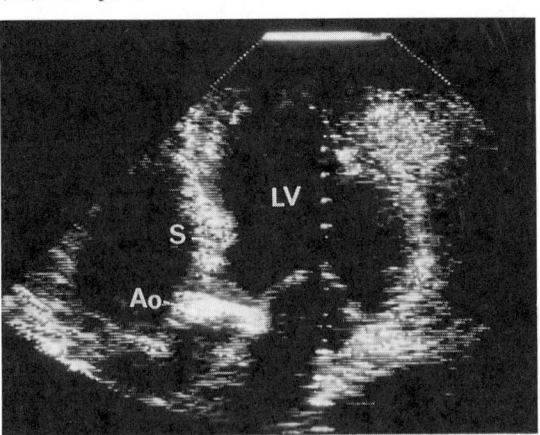

Cardiac catheterization

The abnormal haemodynamics of aortic stenosis and associated left ventricular disease can usually be completely demonstrated by echocardiography. The role of cardiac catheterization is thus to confirm the pressure drop across the valve in the minority of cases in whom this is not possible for technical reasons using continuous wave Doppler, and to display coronary artery anatomy.

Diagnosis

A complete diagnosis of aortic stenosis depends not only on establishing the anatomical abnormality but also on its severity and the degree of associated left ventricular disease. Mild aortic stenosis is associated with a normal carotid pulse and a short systolic murmur, which stops well before the second sound, as a pressure difference between the left ventricular cavity and the aorta is present only during the first part of systole. In addition, both components of the second heart sound are audible and splitting is normal. An uncalcified bicuspid aortic valve causes mild stenosis, with an ejection click and systolic murmur, often followed by a short early diastolic murmur. Unless the aortic stenosis is very long standing and accompanied by severe left ventricular disease, the upstroke of the carotid pulse is slow. Left ventricular hypertrophy can be diagnosed from an apical impulse which is characteristically sustained, although not necessarily displaced, as the heart size is normal. A double impulse due to a palpable left atrial contraction is further evidence of left ventricular hypertrophy, and its presence correlates with an increase in the contribution of left atrial systole to overall stroke volume. A raised left ventricular end-diastolic pressure can be deduced from accentuation of pulmonary valve closure, which forms the only component of the second sound. The severity of left ventricular disease does not necessarily parallel that of aortic stenosis, and it is not uncommon to see mild aortic stenosis in association with severe left ventricular disease.

Differential diagnosis

Hypertrophic cardiomyopathy (see Chapter 15.4.1)

Patients with hypertrophic cardiomyopathy frequently have a history of dyspnoea, chest pain, and syncope, which may be very similar to valvular aortic stenosis, although it may have lasted for longer. On physical examination the carotid pulse is normal or jerky, rather than slow rising, and the systolic murmur, when present, tends to be louder down the left sternal edge, or even at the apex rather than at the base of the heart and over the carotid arteries. The definitive diagnosis is made by echocardiography or left ventricular angiography, which shows obliteration of the apical part of the left ventricular cavity at end-systole. In some patients with valvular aortic stenosis, the pattern of left ventricular hypertrophy may resemble that seen in hypertrophic cardiomyopathy, and which may persist postoperatively. This should probably be regarded as a manifestation of severe secondary left ventricular hypertrophy rather than as the coexistence of two independent conditions.

Fixed subaortic stenosis

This condition usually presents in asymptomatic children and young adults, but in whom a systolic murmur is found at routine examination. The physical signs differ from those of aortic valve stenosis in the same age group in that an ejection click is absent, and a short early diastolic murmur is usually present. As with valvar aortic stenosis, there is clinical and cardiographic evidence of left ventricular disease which may be very severe. Two-dimensional echocardiography usually demonstrates the site of obstruction to left ventricular outflow, and is capable of distinguishing between a discrete membrane or a more extensive, tunnel stenosis. M-mode echocardiography may show mid-systolic closure of the aortic valve, which is not specific to this condition, but is none the less rather suggestive of its presence. The diagnosis can also be confirmed by left ventricular angiography which demonstrates the presence of a small chamber immediately under the aortic valve.

Congestive cardiomyopathy (see Chapter 15.6.1)

Patients with long-standing aortic stenosis may present with severe breathlessness, a large heart on radiography, a small volume pulse with a normal upstroke, a third heart sound, and pansystolic murmur due to papillary muscle dysfunction. This clinical picture represents one possible outcome of patients with untreated aortic stenosis. The diagnosis is suspected from the presence of calcification in the aortic valve on lateral chest radiography and can be confirmed by demonstrating a pressure drop across the valve. Values as low as 30 to 40 mmHg are common in these circumstances, even when the stenosis is severe, so that It is thus necessary to allow for the small forward stroke volume, and calculate the valve area; Values of less than 0.7 cm^2 indicate severe stenosis. If the clinical state can be improved by medical management, then the typical physical signs of aortic stenosis reappear.

Heart block

Patients with aortic stenosis may develop complete heart block and, with the slow heart-rate and corresponding increase in stroke volume, the slow-rising pulse may not be apparent, so that the condition can mimic uncomplicated complete heart block. The combination should be suspected when the systolic blood pressure is low or normal, since it is raised in uncomplicated heart block with a slow ventricular rate. The true diagnosis becomes apparent when pacing is instituted.

Treatment

Medical treatment has little to offer in aortic stenosis because, in mild cases it is unnecessary, and in severe ones ineffective. However, it is essential that all patients with aortic stenosis, of whatever severity, have prophylactic antimicrobials for any potentially septic hazard. Patients with severe left ventricular disease and fluid retention will benefit from a period of bed rest and treatment with a diuretic before operation is contemplated, but it must be remembered that the primary abnormality is a mechanical one, which cannot be significantly modified by altering renal sodium handling by diuretic agents. Prolonged treatment of such patients with large doses of powerful diuretics merely induces potassium depletion with a corresponding increase in the risk of postoperative rhythm disturbances.

Severe aortic stenosis requires intervention. Unfortunately, aortic balloon valvuloplasty, though satisfactory in infants and children, is almost uniformly ineffective in adults in whom the cusps are calcified, and the procedure has been largely abandoned for this age group. Aortic valve replacement, however, is an extremely effective operation. In uncomplicated cases, it can be carried out with low mortality and morbidity, and thus should be considered in all patients in whom the disease causes significant symptoms. It is likely to relieve breathlessness, angina, and syncope, whether due to ischaemic heart disease or to the aortic stenosis itself. Associated coronary artery disease is usually treated with bypass grafting at the same operation. This combined approach implies that all patients should be studied with coronary arteriography preoperatively, and increases the length of the operation itself. It is possible that left ventricular function can be improved, or that mortality reduced still further by this means, but it has still to be proved. Aortic valve replacement is also effective when significant aortic stenosis is complicated by severe left ventricular enlargement. Although the risks of surgery are greater, so are the benefits, and the remarkable improvement in both symptoms and prognosis that may follow surgery for this combination of valve and ventricular disease is amongst the most gratifying in cardiology. At the other extreme is the patient who is asymptomatic, but who is found to have a systolic murmur and evidence of significant aortic stenosis at routine examination. Although a decision will clearly be influenced by local surgical facilities and the preferences of the patient, it should be remembered that in the absence of symptoms or limitation of exercise tolerance such patients have an excellent prognosis, so that operation can safely be delayed. Clearly, though, they would be kept under review.

Aortic stenosis and incompetence

Aetiology

The combination of aortic stenosis and regurgitation usually results from chronic rheumatic heart disease, but may also be caused by infective endocarditis on a previously stenotic valve. As with mixed mitral valve disease, the additional regurgitation may not be severe enough to constitute a significant volume load on the left ventricle, but nevertheless, increases the systolic pressure drop across the valve during systole. In addition, the increased cavity size which accommodates the larger stroke volume is not usually associated with extreme values of wall thickness sometimes seen in pure aortic stenosis, which reduces diastolic stiffness.

Clinical picture

The clinical features of mixed aortic valve disease do not differ significantly from those of pure aortic stenosis, except that breathlessness is usually the most prominent symptom. On examination, uncomplicated cases remain in sinus rhythm until late in the disease, and atrial fibrillation suggests the presence of additional rheumatic mitral valve disease. A subgroup of patients, in whom the mitral valve is normal, however, should be recognized in whom left ventricular end-diastolic pressure is greatly raised, and who resemble those with rheumatic mitral valve disease by developing atrial fibrillation, selective left atrial enlargement, and severe pulmonary hypertension. The character of the carotid pulse is modified in mixed aortic valve disease, being bisferiens, a term that describes the presence of a notch half way up the upstroke. As in pure aortic stenosis, left ventricular hypertrophy is shown by a sustained apical impulse, with or without a palpable left atrial contraction. The diagnosis is confirmed by aortic systolic and diastolic murmurs, maximal down the left sternal edge. If the patient is in atrial fibrillation, evidence of additional rheumatic mitral valve disease should be sought, particularly a palpable first heart sound, an opening snap, and a mid-diastolic murmur.

Chest radiography shows moderate cardiac enlargement and, in older patients, evidence of aortic valve calcification. Selective enlargement of the left atrium suggests the presence of additional mitral valve disease. Electrocardiography confirms left ventricular hypertrophy. Echocardiography can be used to measure left ventricular cavity size and thus to gain some idea of the severity of the regurgitation from the stroke volume. The technique can also be used to confirm or exclude the presence of rheumatic mitral valve disease. The pressure drop across the aortic valve is estimated by continuous wave Doppler, and colour flow mapping can give some idea of the extent of regurgitation.

Diagnosis and treatment

The main differential diagnosis is from pure aortic stenosis, or regurgitation, though it is not very useful to try and assess the relative importance of stenosis and regurgitation. The indications for surgery are similar to those for pure stenosis or regurgitation.

Aortic regurgitation

Aortic regurgitation is an important form of valvular heart disease, and may result from a number of pathological mechanisms which are summarized in Table 3.

Pathology

Chronic rheumatic involvement leads to the characteristic appearance of a tricuspid valve whose cusps are thickened, with rolled edges, and whose commissures are fused. There may be superimposed calcification or thrombosis. Infective endocarditis may lead to cusp destruction or perforation and may spread to involve the sinus of Valsalva, the atrioventricular node and the interventricular septum, where abscess formation may occur. Organisms may also be carried to the anterior cusp of the mitral valve, where they cause 'jet lesions', localized aneurysms,

Table 3 *Causes of aortic regurgitation*

Cusp
    Distortion
        Rheumatic
        Rheumatoid
    Perforation
        Infective endocarditis
        Traumatic
Ring
    Dilatation
        Dissecting aneurysm
        Marfan's syndrome
        Syphilis
        Ankylosing spondylitis
    Reiter's syndrome, ulcerative colitis
Loss of support
    Subaortic ventricular septal defect

or perforations. Dilatation of the aortic ring may cause aortic regurgitation with normal cusps. This can result from a 'flask-shaped' aneurysm of the ascending aorta, complicating Marfan's syndrome, or isolated medionecrosis. Syphilitic aortitis causes dilatation of the valve ring, with aneurysm formation of the ascending aorta and involvement of the coronary ostia. Dilatation of the ring may occur on its own or with a connective tissue disease such as ankylosing spondylitis, rheumatoid arthritis, Reiter's syndrome, or relapsing polychondritis. Dissecting aneurysm involving the aortic root may separate the cusps from the valve ring; and the presence of a high ventricular septal defect or Fallot's tetralogy may leave the cusps unsupported from below.

Pathophysiology

Aortic regurgitation is associated with an increase in left ventricular stroke volume with a corresponding increase in left ventricular cavity size. Ventricular mass is therefore increased, although wall thickness is usually within normal limits. In moderately severe aortic regurgitation, the stroke volume is twice normal, and when it is severe, up to three or even four times normal. The characteristics of ejection are altered in that the end-diastolic pressure in the aorta is low, so that the resistance to ejection of blood by the left ventricle is reduced. This, together with the large stroke volume, explains the characteristic rapid upstroke and large volume pulse. Additional peripheral vasodilatation may be present, which also contributes to the large forward stroke volume. In long-standing cases, left ventricular cavity size increases out of proportion to the stroke volume, with loss of the normal myocardial architecture, so that the cavity becomes more spherical in shape, the walls stiffer, and the end-diastolic pressure increased.

Clinical picture

Patients with aortic regurgitation remain asymptomatic for many years. When symptoms develop, they are those of left ventricular disease, with breathlessness the most prominent one. This usually occurs on exercise, but the presenting symptom may be nocturnal dyspnoea, or an attack of acute pulmonary oedema precipitated by severe exertion. Chest pain may also be a prominent symptom resulting from a low coronary perfusion pressure during diastole, coexistent coronary artery disease, or ostial involvement in syphilitic aortitis. A rather similar retrosternal pain, aggravated by exertion, may develop in patients with aneurysms of the ascending aorta in whom the coronary arteries are normal, which seems to originate from the aortic root itself. Aortic dissection may also cause severe central chest pain.

The physical signs of aortic regurgitation are characteristic. The carotid pulse has a large amplitude and a rapid upstroke, the latter feature beng described as 'collapsing'. Significant aortic stenosis is excluded by the presence of visible arterial pulsation in the neck (Corrigan's sign).

Other physical signs which depend on a large pulse volume and peripheral vasodilation include capillary pulsation, visible in the nail beds, and de Musset's sign, nodding of the head in time with the heart beat. Durosiez's sign, which is of greater clinical value, is elicited by compression of the femoral artery and listening proximally with the stethoscope for a diastolic murmur. It implies retrograde flow in the femoral artery due to aortic regurgitation that is at least moderately severe. The peripheral pulses should always be checked to exclude the presence of coarctation of the aorta. The venous pressure is normal until late in the course of the disease, although the venous pulse may show a Bernheim 'a' wave. The left ventricular impulse is sustained indicating the presence of hypertrophy: a palpable 'a' wave is much less common than in aortic stenosis, and when present usually denotes additional left ventricular disease. On auscultation, the characteristic finding is an early diastolic murmur, maximal down the left sternal edge: less commonly, it is loudest at the apex or even in the left axilla (the Cole–Cecil murmur). An ejection systolic murmur is nearly always present, due to increased flow across the valve, and not necessarily to additional stenosis. Aortic valve closure is not usually audible, but pulmonary hypertension due to a raised left atrial pressure may increase the volume of the pulmonary second sound. At the apex, a third heart sound may be present, if the left ventricular cavity is dilated but, more commonly, a delayed diastolic murmur may be audible, indistinguishable from that of mitral stenosis (Austin Flint murmur). This may continue throughout diastole, and be associated with presystolic accentuation and even a loud first heart sound, though the last is never palpable. In addition, there may be a mitral pansystolic murmur due to dilatation of the valve ring. These classical signs of aortic regurgitation may be modified in number of circumstances. If infective endocarditis has caused cusp perforation, the early diastolic murmur may have a high pitched musical quality (a 'seagull murmur'). In the presence of severe left ventricular disease or, less commonly, of rheumatic mitral stenosis or severe pulmonary hypertension, the collapsing pulse and other evidence of aortic regurgitation may be lost, although the aortic diastolic murmur persists. It is worth noting, however, that Durosiez's sign frequently remains positive in these circumstances if the regurgitation is moderate or severe. It is very important to recognize severe aortic regurgitation of rapid onset, usually due to infective endocarditis affecting the aortic valve. The patient presents with a low cardiac output state, normal or reduced pulse volume, sinus tachycardia and, on auscultation, the main abnormality is a loud, low-pitched early diastolic sound, due to a very short period of forward flow across the mitral valve. A short early diastolic murmur may be audible, though Durosiez's sign is usually positive.

Chest radiograph

Significant aortic regurgitation nearly always causes cardiac enlargement on chest radiography (Fig. 12). The aortic root is often dilated, but the aortic valve not necessarily calcified. The pulmonary vessels remain normal until severe left ventricular disease develops.

Electrocardiograph

This usually shows left ventricular hypertrophy on voltage and T wave criteria, with left atrial enlargement. Left bundle branch block may develop, and indicates the presence of left ventricular disease. A long P-R interval in association with aortic regurgitation is very suggestive of disease of the aortic root.

Echocardiogram

Left ventricular cavity size can be measured by echocardiography and stroke volume estimated (Fig. 13). The anatomy of the aortic valve and root can be determined. Dissection can sometimes be detected, vegetations on the aortic valve are well seen Fig. 14, and sometimes aortic root abscess can be detected (Fig. 15). When infective endocarditis is suspected, transoesophageal echo may give further useful information. It is also the means of choice for demonstrating aortic root aneurysms. In acute aortic regurgitation, mitral valve movement is very abnormal, showing premature closure (Fig. 16). This results from severe regurgitation into a relatively non-compliant left ventricle causing the pressure to rise, and thus closing the mitral valve in mid-diastole. The rise in ventricular diastolic pressure causes difference from aortic pressure to fall to 20 mmHg or less. This figure is an important one, as it represents the pressure supporting coronary flow, which may therefore be compromised.

Cardiac catheterization

It is not usually necessary to resort to cardiac catheterization to make the diagnosis of aortic regurgitation. Although an aortogram may give

Fig. 12 Chest radiograph from a patient with chronic aortic regurgitation showing cardiac enlargement and dilation of the ascending aorta.

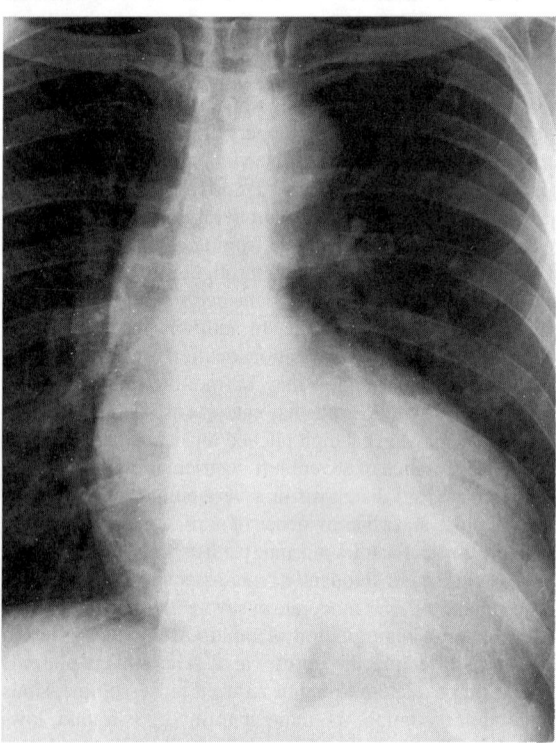

Fig. 13 Chronic aortic regurgitation, M-mode echocardiogram, showing 'flutter' on the anterior cusp of the mitral valve, marked by the arrow. PCG, phonocardiogram.

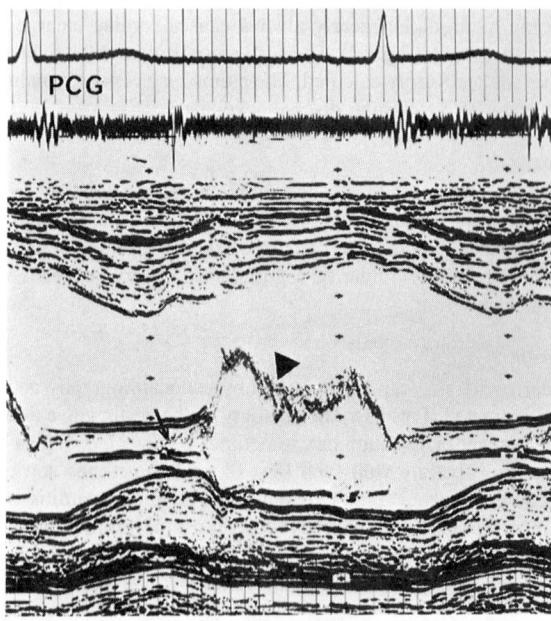

Fig. 14 Two-dimensional echocardiogram, parasternal long axis view, of a patient with aortic endocarditis, showing vegetation (Veg) on aortic valve. Amv, anterior mitral valve cusp; Se, septum; Ao, aortic root.

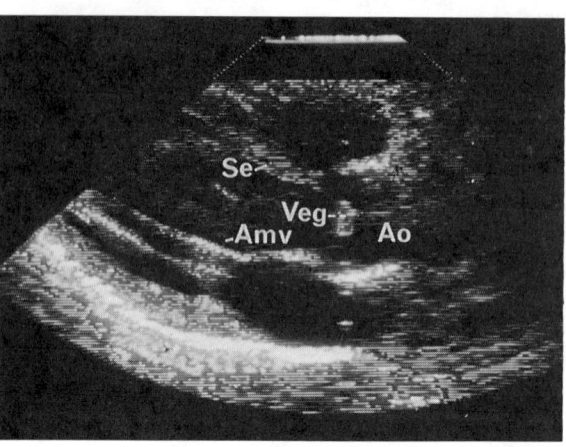

Fig. 15 Parasternal long axis view of aortic root (Ao) showing an abscess cavity (Ab) containing a vegetation (Veg), bulging into the left atrium (LA). LV, left ventricle.

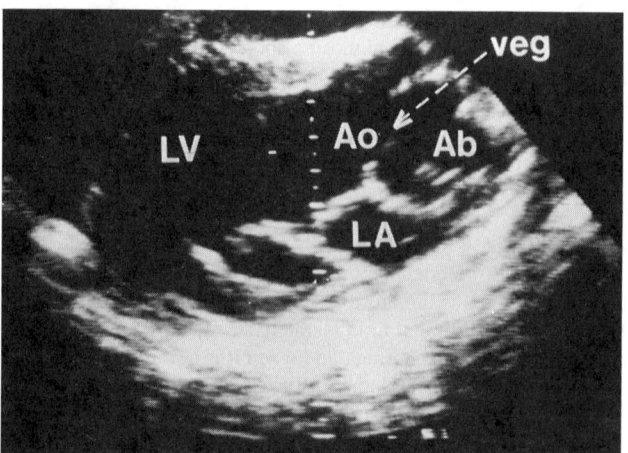

Fig. 16 M-mode echocardiogram showing premature mitral valve closure (arrow) in a patient with acute aortic regurgitation due to infective endocarditis.

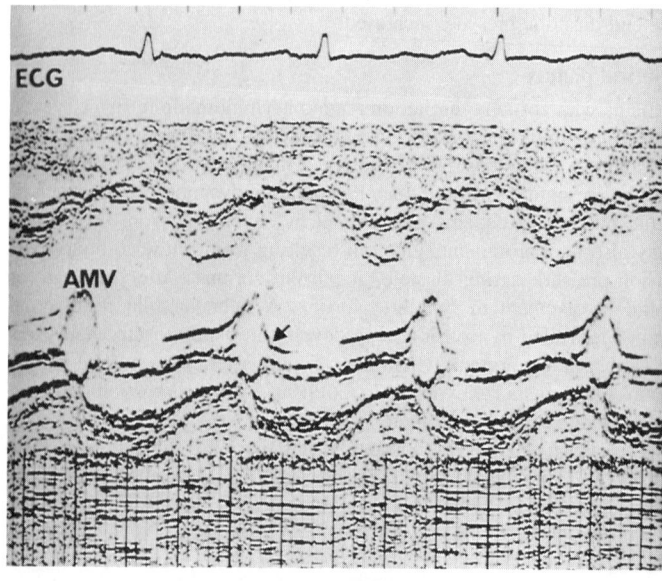

useful information, it should be avoided in seriously ill patients because radiographic contrast medium expands the plasma volume and depresses ventricular function, but many surgeons require coronary arteriography to be performed even in the absence of clinical evidence of significant coronary artery disease.

Diagnosis

As with aortic stenosis, it is not enough to establish the presence of aortic regurgitation; its severity must be estimated and the state of the left ventricle assessed. In uncomplicated cases, the severity can be judged indirectly from the carotid pulse and from the heart size on chest radiography, but direct measurement of left ventricular cavity size and stroke volume by echocardiography or angiography is a much more satisfactory method. Left ventricular disease can be suspected clinically from accentuated pulmonary valve closure, and from chest radiography by the presence of pulmonary vascular congestion and inappropriate cardiac enlargement, but again, left ventricular function is most satisfactorily assessed by echocardiography or angiocardiography, the characteristic feature being enlargement of end-diastolic, and in particular, end-systolic cavity size out of proportion to stroke volume so that ejection fraction falls. Acute aortic regurgitation may present difficulties in diagnosis when the classical physical signs are modified, but it should be suspected in any patient with severe systemic infection, low cardiac output state, and a normal or sightly collapsing pulse, with pulmonary congestion on chest radiography. Echocardiography is particularly useful in making a definite diagnosis non-invasively, demonstrating aortic vegetations, a large stroke volume, and premature mitral valve closure. It is also important to confirm or exclude other types of valve disease. Coexistent aortic stenosis is often diagnosed on the basis of an ejection systolic murmur, but this does not constitute adequate evidence, and in order to confirm its presence clinically, a bisferiens pulse should be present. Additional rheumatic mitral stenosis is best confirmed or excluded by echocardiography, although the presence of atrial fibrillation, a palpable first sound, or an opening snap makes its presence very likely on clinical grounds. Mitral regurgitation leads to an additional pansystolic murmur at the apex, which may sound continuous with the early diastolic murmur across the second sound. It is usually caused by a dilated valve ring in the absence of organic mitral valve disease, and thus indicates considerable left ventricular enlargement. It is usually unnecessary to establish the exact aetiology of the aortic regurgitation, although it is important to exclude infection and investigate the presence of disease of the aortic root. This should be suspected if there is a history of chest pain that is not clearly anginal in nature, and also from excessive dilatation of the ascending aorta on chest radiography or a long P-R interval on electrocardiography.

Differential diagnosis

In the presence of severe pulmonary hypertension, the pulmonary artery may dilate, causing functional pulmonary regurgitation and a soft early diastolic murmur (Graham–Steell murmur). The carotid pulse is normal. Difficulty in diagnosis usually arises when the patient has pulmonary hypertensive mitral valve disease, and an early diastolic murmur. In these circumstances, aortic regurgitation may not necessarily cause an abnormal carotid pulse. In many cases, the differential diagnosis can only be made by Doppler echocardiography, but on clinical grounds, pulmonary incompetence is more likely when there is other evidence of severe pulmonary hypertension, and in particular, when chest radiography shows the main pulmonary artery to be appreciably dilated. Aortic regurgitation should also be distinguished from other causes of aortic run-off, which include persistent ductus arteriosus, ruptured sinus of Valsalva aneurysm or coronary arteriovenous fistula. These all cause an increase in pulse pressure, and a continuous murmur down the left sternal edge, which may be confused with the combination of aortic regurgitation and mitral regurgitation. Additional abnormalities which may give rise to confusion are the combination of aortic regurgitation and a ventricular septal defect, and finally, the rare anomaly of aortic-left ventricular tunnel, in which the haemodynamic disturbance is identical to

that of aortic regurgitation. This differential diagnosis can usually be established by Doppler echocardiography, but contrast angiography may sometimes be needed.

Treatment

Mild or moderately severe aortic regurgitation is well tolerated and requires no treatment other than prophylactic antimicrobial to prevent infective endocarditis. Severe aortic regurgitation should be treated by aortic valve replacement. If the patient is symptomatic, the decision as to timing of the operation is not difficult. In an asymptomatic patient with severe disease, this may depend on local facilities, and the views of the patient must be taken into account. In general, however, evidence of left ventricular disease, aortic root disease, increasing heart size on chest radiography, or cavity size on echocardiography, or a history of infective endocarditis, are all indications for early operation. To depend on the results of any single investigation, convenient as it may seem, is inflexible in practice and not recommended. However, the patient must be kept under regular review, since severe left ventricular disease may become apparent over a period as short as 1 to 2 years in the absence of significant symptoms, increasing the risk of operation and reducing the functional improvement postoperatively. Acute aortic regurgitation is a surgical emergency. As it is nearly always due to infective endocarditis, blood cultures should be taken so that the organism can be isolated retrospectively and antibiotics strated preoperatively. One of the most useful single criteria for emergency aortic valve replacement has proved to be the presence of premature mitral valve closure on the M-mode echocardiogram. When emergency surgical facilities are not available, the haemodynamic state can sometimes be stabilized with vasodilator treatment as with severe mitral regurgitation. However, the patient should be transferred as soon as possible to a centre capable of performing open heart surgery, if progress is not maintained. A prolonged preoperative course of antibiotics is contraindicated in such patients, since the valve is rarely sterilized, and the delay causes further deterioration in left ventricular function.

Acquired tricuspid valve disease

Tricuspid stenosis

Although functional tricuspid stenosis may occur with a large flow through the right heart such as occurs in an atrial septal defect, organic tricuspid stenosis is almost invariably due to chronic rheumatic heart disease. Except in occasional cases with congenital heart disease and raised right ventricular systolic pressure, rheumatic tricuspid stenosis coexists with mitral valve disease, although its incidence is about one-tenth. The two conditions are similar both with respect to their pathology and to the functional disturbance that they cause. The valve cusps become thickened, and the commissures fused, so that the cross-sectional area of the orifice is reduced. The subvalvar apparatus, though, is not usually involved. The primary functional abnormality is obstruction to right ventricular filling associated with a diastolic pressure drop across the valve. In clinically severe tricuspid stenosis, however, this drop is smaller than it would be with mitral stenosis, and is usually within the range of 3 to 10 mmHg. This causes a corresponding increase in right atrial pressure, which leads to fluid retention, manifesting itself as ascites and peripheral oedema.

CLINICAL PICTURE

The clinical problem is to recognize the presence of additional tricuspid stenosis in a patient known to have mitral and possibly also aortic valve disease. This is not always possible on clinical grounds, but a number of indications may be sought. There are no specific findings in the history. If the patient is in sinus rhythm, tricuspid stenosis is often associated with an 'a' wave in the venous pulse and with evidence of right atrial hypertrophy on electrocardiography. These findings are unusual in the presence of pulmonary hypertension and mitral stenosis alone. The venous pulse is usually otherwise unremarkable. On auscultation, a separate tricuspid delayed diastolic murmur may be audible. This is similar in timing to a mitral one, but it is higher in pitch, resembling an aortic diastolic murmur in this respect. It is maximal down the left sternal edge or in the epigastrium. A tricuspid opening snap may also be present; it is later than a mitral one and its timing with respect to pulmonary valve closure varies with respiration. Chest radiography may be suggestive, as right atrial enlargement causes the heart shadow to enlarge to the right of the midline. These appearances, however, are non-specific, and may be present with functional tricuspid regurgitation, or even a giant left atrium. Echocardiography can be used to give a specific diagnosis. Cross-sectional echocardiography shows doming of the tricuspid valve into the right ventricle during systole (Fig. 17), in the apical four chamber view. The diastolic pressure drop can be estimated by continuous wave Doppler. Cardiac catheterization is now rarely performed to diagnose tricsupid stenosis, but it may show a small diastolic pressure drop across the valve. Cases of organic tricuspid stenosis may still reach operation without the diagnosis having been made. When they do so, the previously undiagnosed tricuspid stenosis may be unmasked by successful mitral valve surgery, which allows cardiac output to increase. This causes a corresponding increase in the tricuspid diastolic pressure drop, which leads to salt and water retention, so that a patient thought to have had a satisfactory operation develops striking ascites or peripheral oedema.

TREATMENT

Medical treatment is not very satisfactory, and consists of diuretic administration to control fluid retention. Prolonged administration of inappropriately large doses leads to potassium depletion. Definitive treatment is surgical consisting of either valvotomy or tricuspid repair, at the time that the other valve lesions are dealt with. Isolated tricuspid stenosis, developing after mitral valve surgery can be dealt with by balloon valvuloplasty if the anatomy is suitable. Tricuspid valve replacement is avoided whenever possible, because of the importance of the pressure drop in diastole across all normally functioning prostheses. An additional procedure on the tricuspid valve also increases the operative risk of mitral valve surgery due to the greater postoperative incidence of jaundice and arrhythmias.

Fig. 17 Rheumatic tricuspid stenosis, apical four-chamber view showing doming and thickening of the tricuspid valve during diastole (arrows). LA, left atrium; LV, left ventricle; RA, right atrium; RV, right ventricle.

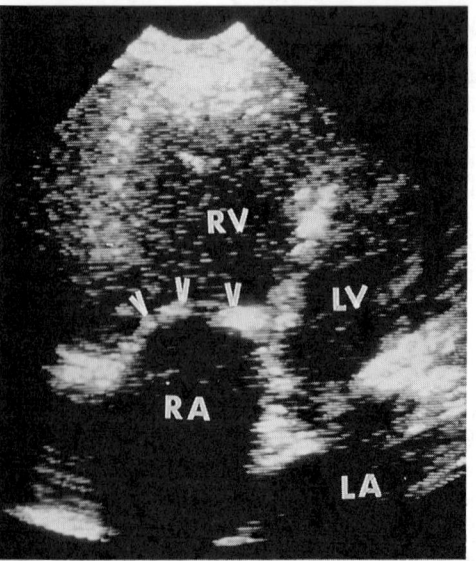

Table 4 *Causes of tricuspid regurgitation*

Organic
Rheumatic
Infective endocarditis
Ebstein's anomaly
Atrioventricular defect
Carcinoid syndrome
Cirrhosis of the liver
Endomyocardial fibrosis
Prolapsing cusp
Functional

Tricuspid regurgitation

As with mitral regurgitation, a number of different pathological processes may cause tricuspid regurgitation (Table 4). It is frequently functional, occurring in association with dilatation of the right ventricular cavity. It is particularly common in patients with pulmonary hypertensive mitral valve disease, but may also occur with primary pulmonary hypertension, or in the terminal stages of many types of congenital heart disease, particularly those with a significant left to right shunt. The tricuspid valve is much more liable to develop functional regurgitation than the mitral valve. Severe, non-rheumatic tricuspid regurgitation is being increasingly recognized as occurring late after mitral valve replacement, in the absence of significant left-sided disease or pulmonary hypertension. Its cause is not clear, but there is no evidence of disease of the valve cusps or subvalve apparatus.

Organic tricuspid regurgitation may be congenital, as an isolated abnormality, or associated with Ebstein's anomaly. A cleft right-sided atrioventricular valve may also occur in ostrium primum atrial septal defect. Acquired, organic tricuspid regurgitation may be rheumatic in origin, or result from infective endocarditis of a previously normal valve, which occurs particularly commonly in intravenous drug users. Right-sided endomyocardial fibrosis causes progressive obliteration of the right ventricular cavity with scarring and distortion of the tricuspid subvalvular apparatus. The carcinoid syndrome is associated with severe tricuspid regurgitation, and similar findings may occur after methysergide therapy, and in longstanding hepatic cirrhosis. Midsystolic prolapse of the tricuspid valve can occur in exactly the same way as that of the mitral valve, and is common in Marfan's syndrome. Organic tricuspid regurgitation has been described as a long term consequence of radiotherapy to the thorax, when it may be associated with features of pericardial constriction or restrictive myocardial disease, making its diagnosis difficult.

Clinical picture

The clinical features of tricuspid regurgitation are those of severe and chronic elevation of the venous pressure, often in association with disease on the left side of the heart. The symptoms are non-specific, although, when tricuspid regurgitation supervenes in a patient with mitral stenosis, it is often associated with an increase in the prominence of fatigue as a factor limiting exercise tolerance instead of breathlessness. Symptoms may also be related to the development of oedema or ascites: hepatic enlargement may be associated with nausea and upper abdominal or epigastric pain aggravated by exercise. The main physical sign of tricuspid regurgitation is a raised venous pressure with a prominent systolic wave, which is almost a *sine qua non* for the diagnosis. The mean venous pressure may be very high, greater than 15 cm, with pulsations visible in the retinal vessels or palpable in the femoral veins. The high venous pressure is also responsible for the protein-losing enteropathy that sometimes occurs in the same way as with constrictive pericarditis. In approximately two-thirds of patients, there is associated systolic expansile pulsation of the liver which may be considerably enlarged and tender. In long-standing cases, hepatic fibrosis develops so that this physical sign is no longer evident. Hepatic dysfunction may also be associated with mild jaundice, which with increased skin pigmentation, gives these patients a very characteristic appearance. In approximately one-third of cases, a tricuspid pansystolic murmur is present, which is audible down the left sternal edge. Although it is said to increase in intensity during inspiration, this physical sign is difficult to demonstrate in individual patients, so that the murmur is usually indistinguishable from that of functional mitral regurgitation. The findings on chest radiography depend mainly on other cardiac disease present, but, as with tricuspid stenosis, there may be enlargement of the heart shadow towards the right. Electrocardiography may show right atrial hypertrophy in isolated tricuspid regurgitation if the patient is in sinus rhythm, but otherwise is dominated by other cardiac disease present. Echocardiography is the best way of making the diagnosis. Cusp disease and right ventricular function are assessed by the cross-sectional technique, while the extent of the regurgitation can be measured by continuous wave and colour flow Doppler. The nature and extent of left-sided disease and pulmonary hypertension can also be documented. Cardiac catherization is thus rarely necessary to make the diagnosis.

Treatment

Medical treatment with diuretics deals with associated fluid retention, and may even allow right ventricular cavity size to decrease restoring competence to the tricuspid valve. Isolated tricuspid incompetence, unless very severe, or accompanied by right ventricular disease, is reasonably well tolerated so that surgical treatment is avoided if possible. When tricuspid regurgitation occurs in association with rheumatic heart disease involving the left side of the heart, it may subside spontaneously after the latter has been dealt with surgically, although there is a case for routine tricuspid valve plication or repair to prevent tricuspid regurgitation developing postoperatively. If the regurgitation is very severe, and the fluid retention requires doses of diuretics large enough to cause significant metabolic consequences, then intervention may be considered. Unfortunately, repair and relacement of the tricuspid valve are unsatisfactory operations; the former does not usually control the regurgitation and the latter leads to a very significant diastolic pressure drop between right atrium and right ventricle. In addition, the risks of surgery are high in these patients, and postoperative jaundice is very common.

Carcinoid heart disease

A characteristic form of heart disease develops in patients with metastatic carcinoid disease affecting predominantly the right heart, with thickening of the tricuspid and pulmonary valves and enlargement of the right ventricular cavity. The left side of the heart is rarely involved, unless a septal defect is present. Microscopically, the thickening is due to deposits of fibrous tissue, but there is no evidence of inflammation. Not all patients with carcinoid disease develop cardiac manifestations, but when they are present they may progress, even after removal of the tumour.

Clinical picture

Patients may demonstrate the well-recognized manifestations of the carcinoid syndrome of flushing, telangiectasia, bronchoconstriction, and intestinal hypermotility. The venous pressure is raised, due partly to tricuspid valve disease and partly to right ventricular fibrosis manifestations, which dominate the clinical picture from the cardiac point of view. Chest radiography shows cardiac enlargement. ECG findings are non-specific but include low-voltage QRS complexes and evidence of right ventricular hypertrophy. Echocardiography may show very considerable enlargement of the right ventricular cavity, often to a degree unusual in acquired heart disease. Tricuspid regurgitation, which may be very severe, can be demonstrated by continuous wave Doppler. The systolic pressure drop across the valve is low, and if the valve cusps are effectively absent, the flow may be laminar. The prognosis of the underlying disease varies greatly between patients, but in some long term survival after valve replacement has been reported.

Pulmonary valve disease

Acquired pulmonary valve disease is unusual. The most common form is that associated with severe pulmonary hypertension and dilatation of the pulmonary valve ring, causing mild regurgitation. This commonly occurs in association with pulmonary hypertensive mitral valve disease, causing a soft early diastolic murmur (the Graham–Steell murmur), but an identical picture may be present with severe pulmonary hypertension from any cause. Although the murmur itself is early diastolic in timing, there is no associated abnormality of the carotid pulse as would be expected in aortic regurgitation. Nevertheless, the differential diagnosis on clinical grounds may be difficult when the mitral valve disease is severe. Mild pulmonary regurgitation is effectively a normal finding on colour flow Doppler; a more extensive jet in a patient with pulmonary hypertension is thus required to confirm the diagnosis. Aortic regurgitation can be confirmed or excluded by Doppler. Rheumatic pulmonary regurgitation is extremely rare, although it has been reported in populations exposed to considerable altitudes. Even when present, though it contributes little to overall disability. Pulmonary regurgitation may also form part of the carcinoid syndrome, or be iatrogenic, following pulmonary valvotomy for pulmonary stenosis. It is associated with short early diastolic murmur, and may contribute to the elevated venous pressure that may persist for a variable period after pulmonary valvotomy. It is then of no clinical consequence and requires no specific treatment.

Management of patients with valve prostheses

Valve replacement has been a major advance in the treatment of patients with valvular heart disease. Large numbers of patients have been treated in this way over the past 25 years since the operation was introduced with very significant improvement in their quality of life. Valve prostheses may be mechanical or biological. Mechanical prostheses inserted over the last 10 years are likely to be either the ball and cage type, of which the commonest example is the Starr-Edwards (Fig. 18(a)), the tilting disc (Fig. 18(b)), or the bileaflet. The first has the advantage of a 30-year follow-up and remarkable reliability. Both the latter have a

Fig. 18 Thrombosed Star–Edwards prosthesis, removed at emergency operation.

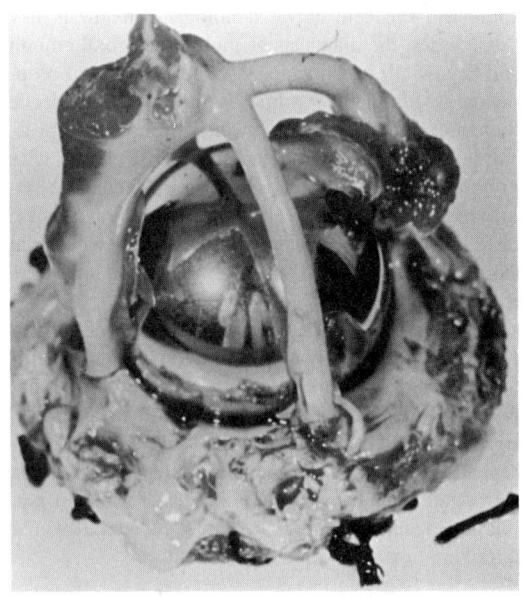

larger effective orifice area in relation to the size of the ring. Biological prostheses consist of a plastic stent on which cusps made from some biological material are mounted. The cusps may be derived from porcine aortic valve (Fig. 18(c)) or pericardium. In a class of its own is the aortic homograft, which is not mounted on a plastic stent, but on a ring of native aortic root. Minor differences in performance exist between these various valve substitutes are of little clinical significance. All fall short of their natural counterpart *in vivo*. Under normal working conditions, pressure differences are present across mitral prostheses, which range from 4 to 5 mmHg for the Starr–Edwards to 2 to 4 mmHg for the others. In addition, all mitral valve substitutes have a rigid mitral ring which interferes with ventricular function. Apart from the homograft, whose performance is very similar to that of the native valve, systolic gradients across aortic prostheses are in the range 10 to 25 mmHg at rest, increasing on exercise. The main factors guiding choice of one or other of them is the durability of the prosthesis and the likely incidence of thrombotic complications. Unfortunately it has become clear that in spite of the great improvement in outlook, patients with valvular prostheses are at significantly increased risk of cardiac complications and death in comparison with matched normal controls. Present operative mortality is in the region of 3 to 5 per cent for single valve replacement and approximately 10 per cent for double valve replacement. Long term survival studies have shown that 10-year survival after single valve replacement is approximately 50 to 55 per cent, and after double valve replacement 35 to 45 per cent. For reoperation, mortality is higher, the exact figure depending on the circumstances in which surgery is performed.

Late complications of valve replacement
Thromboembolism

This is a major complication associated with all mechanical prostheses. Long term anticoagulant therapy with a drug of the warfarin type is thus essential in all patients in whom these prostheses have been inserted, and even with satisfactory control an incidence of significant events, including transient weakness, dysphasia or visual disturbances of 1 to 2 per cent per annum can be expected. At the same time, anticoagulant therapy itself causes bleeding complications severe enough to require admission to hospital with an incidence of approximately 1 per cent per annum. In a small minority of patients, emboli are much more frequent in spite of good anticoagulant control. Initially, such cases should be given an antiplatelet agent such aspirin or dipyridamole, and the anticoagulant dose adjusted accordingly. The possibility of some other cause for the neurological manifestations must always be considered, such as cerebrovascular disease. However, frequent embolization may be associated with thrombosis of the prosthesis, and if it cannot be suppressed medically, reoperation and replacement with a biological prosthesis may be necessary. In such cases, the diagnosis of multiple cerebral emboli must be established beyond all question because the mortality of reoperation is significantly greater than for a first operation. The incidence of thromboembolic complications is much lower with biological prostheses, so that long-term anticoagulant therapy can be dispensed with in patients in sinus rhythm after aortic or mitral valve replacement; however, many surgeons recommend a short course of 2 to 3 months in such patients while suture lines become endothelialized. Patients with atrial fibrillation and mitral valve replacement will require standard long-term anticoagulant therapy.

In developing countries, mitral replacement may have to be performed in children under the age of 15, in whom biological valves are unsuitable. The use of a mechanical prosthesis might seem appropriate, but facilities for regular prothrombin estimations may not be available, while uncontrolled administration of standard doses of warfarin are associated with unacceptable risk of haemorrhage. This therapeutic dilemma is, at present, unsolved, although the use of small doses of warfarin, e.g. 2 mg daily, without anticoagulant control has been advocated. It would seem that clinical trials in this area would be justified.

Limited prosthetic function

In a minority of patients, valve replacement may give rise to severe haemodynamic disturbances, so that in extreme cases, the condition of the patient may be worse after the operation than before. This usually arises when the valve ring or the ventricular cavity is very small, so that it proved necessary to insert a correspondingly small prosthesis. In the mitral position resting diastolic pressure differences as high as 20 mmHg may be present, or of 50 mm across the aortic valve on this basis. A second, related problem is the insertion of a prosthesis that is too large, particularly of the ball and cage type. In the mitral position, the cage may impinge on the septum, and obstruct the left ventricular outflow tract, causing subaortic stenosis, while in the aortic position, obstruction may develop between the ball and the aorta. Normally, such complications are avoided by the use of a low profile prosthesis, such as a Bjork–Shiley. They are sometimes referred to by the sonorous description of 'valve prosthesis-patient mismatch'.

Infection

Patients with prostheses – mechanical or biological – are at greatly increased risk of infective endocarditis. The infecting organism may have been introduced at the time of operation, when it usually manifests itself within 2 months of surgery; later infections are blood borne. It is thus essential that all patients receive full antimicrobial prophylaxis for dental manipulations and other potentially septic hazards in a course lasting for at least 48 h, rather than in the single dose currently recommended for routine dental prophylaxis. Infective endocarditis in this situation is a very serious complication, and rarely responds to antimicrobial therapy alone. A second valve replacement is nearly always required, often in a seriously ill patient in whom the valve ring may be infected and friable.

Prosthetic dysfunction

This is an important cause of morbidity in patients who have undergone valve replacement. There may be structural damage to the prosthesis itself, which is uncommon in mechanical valves, though occasional batches may undergo strut fracture due to metal fatigue, a well known example being the concavoconvex Bjork–Shiley valves inserted in the late 1970s. Malfunction is much more common with biological prostheses, when cusps may become calcified, perforated, or detached. Calcification of porcine bioprostheses regularly occurs within 1 to 2 years in children under the age of 15. This complication takes much longer to develop in the aortic homograft, usually 10 to 15 years. Mechanical prostheses are subject to thrombosis. This may take two forms. Deterioration in function may be insidious over a period of several months or years due to ingrowth of organized clot (pannus) usually from the atrial side (Fig. 18). This may be associated with an increased incidence of emboli in spite of adequate anticoagulant therapy. Alternatively, the prosthesis may clot acutely; this is particularly likely to occur with the Bjork–Shiley in the mitral position, and represents a surgical emergency. It can often be recognized clinically, the patient presenting with pulmonary oedema or in a low cardiac output state, and the closing click of the prosthesis no longer audible. Operation is required as soon as possible, as deterioration may occur within hours. If the condition of the patient is so poor as to preclude anaesthesia, then intravenous streptokinase should be given, at a dose of 500 000 u immediately, followed by 100 000 units hourly, though a risk of systemic embolism must be accepted. Such treatment may be associated with improvement within a few hours; the streptokinase is then neutralized, and surgery undertaken.

Finally, paraprosthetic regurgitation may develop. In the aortic position, this may have been present since the original operation, because heavy calcification of the original valve extended into the valve ring. Paraprosthetic regurgitation suddenly appearing always raises the possibility that the prosthesis might have become infected. Mitral paraprosthetic regurgitation usually results from part of the valve sewing ring tearing away. Again, infection should always be considered, but regurgitation is well documented in its absence.

Recognizing prosthetic dysfunction

Stenosis or regurgitation associated with a prosthesis does not have the same physical signs as the corresponding lesion of the native valve. In general, it presents as deterioration in cardiac state, whose progress may be acute or chronic. The patient complains of reduced exercise tolerance, followed by orthopnoea. On examination, the venous pressure is raised, the liver enlarged, and chest radiography shows that the heart has enlarged and pulmonary congestion appeared. When a mitral prosthesis is involved, there are characteristically no murmurs, other than those of tricuspid regurgitation; an aortic systolic murmur may be present, but its intensity and timing differs little from that of a normally functioning prosthesis. The clinical picture may thus be indistinguishible from that of ventricular disease or 'heart failure'. It is essential, therefore, that the possibility of a prosthesis related complication is considered in all such patients. This requires echocardiography, Doppler, and possibly cardiac catheterization by an experienced operator. All patients presenting in this way should thus be referred to a unit where these investigations can be reliably performed, and emergency surgery, if necessary, can be undertaken.

Haemolysis

All mechanical prostheses are associated with increased intravascular haemolysis. This rarely gives rise to clinical problems when the prosthesis is functioning normally, and anaemia does not occur. The extent of haemolysis can be estimated from a peripheral blood film, which shows fragmented forms, from depression or absence of serum haptoglobin, and from an increase in lactic dehydrogenase levels. Haemolysis may become significant with a normally functioning prosthesis when the patient has a compensated haemolytic state of some different aetiology, such as congenital spherocytosis or thalassaemia minor. In these circumstances, there is a risk of the extent of haemolysis becoming severe. Mild paraprosthetic regurgitation, whose severity is insufficient to give rise to any haemodynamic complications, may cause clinically significant haemolysis. In such cases, it may be undesirable to expose the patient to the risk of reoperation, particularly if the original valve leak was due to some predictable cause such as heavy calcification of the valve bed, and so likely to recur. Provided that haemolysis is not severe, such cases can usually be treated medically on maintenance therapy with iron and folic acid. A requirement for transfusion, however, is a strong indication for reoperation.

Left ventricular disease

This is now a major cause of morbidity and mortality after valve replacement. There is no single cause. In many patients, severe left ventricular disease was present preoperatively, and though some improvement frequently occurs with correction of the valve disease, function never returns to normal. Operation itself causes additional damage. Methods of myocardial preservation during the period of cardiopulmonary bypass have improved very considerably over the last 20 years with the general introduction of cold blood cardioplegia, but before then ischaemic arrest appears to have been associated with myocardial damage that may take several years to become manifest. Postoperatively, the prosthesis itself may interfere with ventricular function. This is particularly the case if there is any disparity in size with the site at which it is inserted. A rigid mitral ring invariably leads to abnormal function, and there is increasing evidence that section of the papillary muscles may have the same effect. Coronary emboli may arise from the prosthesis. Many patients are of an age to have additional coronary artery disease; there is no evidence to suppose that routine bypass grafting at operation affects the development of ventricular disease. Left ventricular disease presents after valve replacement presents its usual clinical features. There is progressive limitation of exercise tolerance and breathlessness due to reduction in cardiac output and pulmonary congestion. Venous pressure becomes raised, and the earliest clinical evidence may relate to right rather than left ventricular disease, with elevated venous pressure, fluid retention, and hepatic congestion. Auscultatory signs may be modified, and in particular third and fourth heart sounds are not audible in patients with mechanical mitral prostheses. Chest radiography shows an increase in heart size and pulmonary congestion. Electrocardiography may show Q waves, but their absence is of no significance. The differential diagnosis of ventricular disease after valve replacement is thus with prosthetic dysfunction, and it is essential that a comprehensive diagnosis is established in any patient who fails to progress, or whose improvement after operation is not maintained. Echocardiography has proved of great value in such patients, since it allows the very active left ventricular wall motion that accompanies a paraprosthetic leak to be distinguished from the dilated cavity and poor shortening fraction of left ventricular disease. Continuous wave Doppler can be used to detect significant gradients across biological valves. However, unless the diagnosis is clear from non-invasive investigation cardiac catheterisation is required to settle the diagnosis beyond doubt. The prognosis once clinically apparent left ventricular disease has developed is poor, usually being of the order of 1 to 2 years, so it is essential that no remediable cause is overlooked.

Follow-up of patients after valve replacement

It is clear, therefore, that after valve replacement, patients require regular follow-up. This must be for life, and after recovery from the operation itself, should be at a minimum of 6-monthly intervals, with regular chest radiography and electrocardiography. It is also very helpful if echocardiography is performed early, not only to detect immediate postoperative complications such as a pericardial fluid collection, but also to establish a baseline to detect future change. Dental prophylaxis is essential. Deterioration must be detected early, and investigated in detail so that life-threatening complications are not missed, and essential treatment implemented early when it has the greatest chance of success. Only in this way will the maximum benefits of valve replacement surgery be realized.

REFERENCES

Ball, C.J.D., Williams, A.W., and Davies, J.N.P. (1954). Endomyocardial fibrosis. *Lancet* 1, 1049–1040.

Barnett, H.J.M., Boughner, D.R., Taylor, D.W., Cooper, P.E., Kostuk, W.J., and Nichol, P.M. (1980). Further evidence relating mitral valve prolapse to cerebral ischemic events. *New England Journal of Medicine*, **302**, 139–144.

Benjamin, E.J., Plehn, J.F., D'Agostino, R.B., et al. (1992). Mitral annular calcification and the risk of stroke in an elderly cohort. *New England Journal of Medicine*, **327**, 374–379.

Blackstone, E.H. and Kirklin, J.W. (1992). Recommendations for prophylactic removal of heart valve prostheses. *Journal of Heart Valve Disease*, **1**, 3–14.

Bulkley, B.H. and Roberts, W.C. (1976). The heart in systemic lupus erythematosis, and change induced in it by corticosteroid therapy. *American Journal of Medicine*, **58**, 243–264.

Cohen, D.J., Kuntz, R.E., Gordon, S.P.F. et al. (1992). Predictors of long-term outcome after percutaneous balloon mitral valvuloplasty. *New England Journal of Medicine*, **327**, 1329–1335.

Davies, M.J., Moore, B.P., and Braimbridge, M.C. (1978). The floppy mitral valve. Study of incidence, pathology, and complications in surgical, necropsy and forensic material. *British Heart Journal*, **40**, 468–481.

Fowler, N. and van der Bel-Kahn, J.M. (1979). Indications for surgical replacement of the mitral valve with particular reference to common and uncommon causes of mitral regurgitation. *Americal Journal of Cardiology*, **44**, 157.

Groves, P.H. and Hall, R.J.C. (1992). Late tricuspid regurgitation following mitral valve surgery. *Journal of Heart Valve Disease*, **1**, 80–86.

Jeresaty, R.M. (1976). Sudden death in the mitral prolapse click syndrome. *Americal Journal of Cardiology*, **37**, 317–318.

Leatham, A. and Brigden, W. (1990). Mild mitral regurgitation and the mitral prolapse fiasco. *American Heart Journal,* **99,** 659–664.

Oakley, C.M. and Burkhardt, D. (1993). Optimal timing of surgery for chronic mitral or aortic regurgitation. *Journal of Heart Valve Disease,* **2,** 223–229.

Rahimtoola, S.H. (1983). Valvular heart disease; a perspective. *Journal of American College of Cardiology,* **1,** 199–215.

Roberts, W.C., Hehoe, J.A., Carpenter, D.F., and Golden, A. (1968). Cardiac valvular lesions in rheumatoid arthritis. *Archives of Internal Medicine,* **122,** 141–146.

Roberts, W.C., Morrow, A.G., McIntosh, C.L., Jones, M., Epstein, S.E. (1987). Congential bicuspid aortic valve causing severe, pure aortic regurgitation without superimposed infective endocarditis. *Americal Journal of Cardiology,* **47,** 206–209.

Ruttley, M.S.T. (1992). The chest radiograph in adult heart valve disease. *Journal of Heart Valve Disease,* **2,** 205–217.

Selzer, A. (1987). Changing aspects of the natural history of aortic stenosis. *New England Journal of Medicine,* **317,** 91–98.

Smith, N., McAnulty, J.H., and Rahimtoola, S.H. (1978). Severe aortic stenosis with impaired left ventricular function and clinical heart failure: results of valve replacement. *Circulation* **58,** 255–264.

Smith, H.J., Neutze, J.M., Roche, A.H.G., Agnew, T.M., Barratt-Boyes, B.G. (1976). The natural history of rheumatic aortic regurgitation and the indications for surgery. *British Heart Journal,* **38,** 147–154.

Vaughton, K.C., Walker, D.R., and Sturridge, M.F. (1979). Mitral valve replacement for endocarditis caused by Libman Sachs endocarditis. *British Heart Journal,* **41,** 730–733.

Vijayaraghavan, G., Cherian, G., Krishnaswami, S., Sukamar, I.P., John, S. (1977). Rheumatic aortic stenosis in young patients presenting as combined aortic and mitral stenosis. *British Heart Journal,* **39,** 294–298.

Vijayaraghavan, G., Cherian, G., Krishnaswami, S., Sukamar, and John, S. (1977). Rheumatic aortic stenosis in young patients presenting as combined aortic and mitral valve disease. *British Heart Journal,* **39,** 294–298.

Vlodaver, Z. and Edwards, J.E. (1977). Rupture of ventricular septum or papillary muscle complicating myocardial infarction. *Circulation* **55,** 815–822.

Waller, B.F., Morrow, A.G., Maron, B.J., et al. (1982). Etiology of clinically isolated, severe, chronic pure mitral regurgitation: analysis of 97 patients over 30 years of age having mitral valve replacement. *American Heart Journal,* **104,** 276–288.

Wood, P. (1954). An appreciation of mitral stenosis. Part 1. Clinical features. *British Medical Journal,* **1,** 1051–1063.

Wood, P. (1954). An appreciation of mitral stenosis. Part II. Investigations and results. *British Medical Journal,* **1**: 1113–1124.

15.19 Cardiac myxoma

T. A. TRAILL

Cardiac myxomas are lobulated, gelatinous, amber-coloured masses, almost always attached by a peduncle to the atrial septum. They are not common, but they are important because they can present in a number of ways to general physicians, and because the majority are easily and permanently removed by heart surgery. They are easily demonstrated by conventional transthoracic echocardiography, and it is usually the echocardiographer who first suspects and then confirms their presence; seldom has the patient been referred with this diagnosis in mind. Estimates of the prevalence of such a rare condition are necessarily approximate and range from 1 to 5 per 10 000 in autopsy series, or 2 per 100 000 in the general population, with a sex ratio of 2 : 1 in favour of women. Most develop in the left atrium, and only a few, much larger ones in the right. As a cause of left atrial obstruction, myxomas are 200 to 400 times less common than mitral stenosis. The majority of patients are between 30 and 60 years, but there are reports of tumours occurring in infants and in the elderly.

Myxomas are not the only cardiac tumours. Other benign tumours found in adults are the papillary fibroelastoma, usually attached to the leaflet of one of the left-sided valves, and lipoma. The latter may arise in the atrial septum but seldom grows into the lumen of the cardiac chambers. Malignant cardiac tumours include angiosarcoma, fibrosarcoma, malignant fibrous histiocytoma, leiomyosarcoma, and secondary deposits. There are reports of some of these being resected, with a few short-term survivors, but in general malignant cardiac tumours are rapidly fatal.

Most myxomas are sporadic, unassociated with other diseases. However, there is at least one syndrome involving myxoma, variously named the Carney complex, LAMB syndrome, NAME syndrome, and Swiss syndrome. This syndrome, which is referred to here as Carney's syndrome, is characterized by lentiginosis, multiple myxomas (most of them cardiac), and various kinds of endocrine overactivity. These have included Cushing's syndrome caused by pigmented adrenocortical hyperplasia, acromegaly, and Sertoli cell tumour. Unlike the usual kind of atrial myxoma, myxomas in Carney's syndrome may arise anywhere in the heart, are commonly multiple, and frequently recur. Inheritance

of this rare disease is as an autosomal dominant, with centrofacial freckling as the most obvious outward marker of the phenotype.

Pathology

Cardiac myxomas are benign. Local invasion is unknown and metastatic growth is exceptional, despite the lesions' situation in the bloodstream. They take the form of polypoid masses arising from a stalk, ranging in size from 3 cm to as much as 10 cm or more, with a smooth or lobulated surface and gelatinous consistency. They are frequently covered with more or less adherent thrombus. More than 75 per cent occur within the left atrium, with the base of the pedicle arising from the fossa ovalis or its rim. Occasionally they arise from the base of the mitral valve leaflets, from the posterior part of the left atrium, or from within the right atrium. Sometimes they grow in both atria, in the form of a dumb-bell. Ventricular myxomas are exceptional, seen almost exclusively as part of Carney's syndrome. Left atrial tumours, being freely mobile, descend into the mitral orifice during ventricular filling, and may thus acquire an indentation on the circumference corresponding to the atrioventricular valve ring. Because they are in the systemic circulation, left atrial myxomas usually draw attention to themselves at a size smaller than those on the right side.

The histology is that of a loosely woven, sparsely cellular connective tissue tumour, with very infrequent mitotic figures. Several cell types are identifiable, including undifferentiated stellate and polygonal cells, as well as smaller numbers of fibroblasts, smooth muscle cells, and endothelial cells. Among these are found macrophages and plasma cells. Other mesodermal tissues, including bone, may occasionally be found. Cytogenic studies fit with the general presumption that these indolent masses are indeed neoplastic, but immunohistochemical studies of differentiation markers do not clearly define their histogenesis. It is suggested that the source is a primitive multipotential mesenchymal cell, and that the predilection of these tumours for the atrial septum reflects the abundance of such cells in this region. There are also suggestions, based on finding Schwann cell and neuroendocrine markers in some tumours, that the tumour may originate in cardiac sensory nerve tissue. The abundant myxoid stroma contains large amounts of an acid mucopolyaccharide similar to chondroitin C, as well as glycoprotein and variable numbers of collagen and elastic fibres.

Clinical features

PRESENTATION

Although the present wide availability of echocardiography has made the diagnosis of atrial myxoma quite straightforward, it remains true that the prerequisite for recognizing this rare lesion is to include it in the differential diagnosis of patients presenting with symptoms and signs of much more common conditions. Left atrial myxomas may mimic mitral stenosis, and cause left atrial obstruction. They may be the source of emboli to the systemic circulation, and occasionally they may present as an obscure constitutional illness with fever. Right atrial myxomas seldom cause symptoms until they are very large, when they cause right atrial obstruction with elevated systemic venous pressure, splanchnic congestion and oedema.

Left atrial obstruction

In about 50 per cent of cases the history and physical examination suggest mitral stenosis, with left ventricular inflow obstruction as the chief pathophysiological change. Thus the presenting symptoms include progressive breathlessness, orthopnoea, paroxysmal nocturnal dyspnoea, fluid retention, and atrial arrhythmias. Examination suggests rheumatic heart disease and, before the routine use of ultrasound, a few such patients were referred for mitral valvotomy and the lesion was first diagnosed at surgery. Some patients may develop pulmonary hypertension before the diagnosis becomes apparent.

Systemic embolism

Systemic emboli occur in about 40 per cent of patients and are frequently the first manifestation of disease. In contrast to mitral stenosis such emboli often occur while patients are in sinus rhythm. They may be sizeable, for example large enough to occlude the aortic bifurcation, and besides thrombus they frequently contain tumour material, so that histological examination may be diagnostic. Thus, when systemic emboli are removed from patients they should always be sent to the pathology laboratory. When emboli occur in young people, patients in sinus rhythm or where there is no obvious source, even in the absence of abnormal cardiological signs, they should be referred for echocardiography.

Constitutional effects

The constitutional effects of the neoplasm predominate in about one-quarter of patients. These effects include fever, weight loss (which is more conspicuous than in mitral stenosis and often occurs without severe left atrial obstruction), Raynaud's phenomenon, finger clubbing (both of which are rare), a raised erythrocyte sedimentation rate, which is present in about 60 per cent of patients, and abnormal serum proteins with elevated immunoglobulin levels. These changes are usually attributed to abnormal proteins secreted by the tumour, although the nature of these has not been determined. Other haematological abnormalities include anaemia (which may be due to mechanical haemolysis), polycythaemia (associated particularly with right atrial tumours), leucocytosis, and thrombocytopaenia. Such constitutional changes may lead to an initial diagnosis of infective endocarditis in patients who have heart murmurs, or to the suspicion of collagen vascular disease or occult malignancy.

Physical signs

Specific cardiovascular signs of myxoma are inconspicuous or absent in many patients. In others they vary from a prominent first heart sound to obvious changes similar to those of mitral valve disease. These include apical systolic murmurs, somewhat more common than diastolic rumbles, and occasionally signs of pulmonary hypertension with accentuated pulmonary closure and tricuspid regurgitation. Some patients have an audible 'tumour plop' in early diastole, analogous to a mitral opening snap, but this is often heard best only after echocardiographic diagnosis. On combined echocardiographic and phonocardiographic recordings the plop is seen to coincide with the end of the tumour's downward movement into the ventricle, usually a short time after mitral valve opening; similarly the accentuated first heart sound occurs at the end of the early systolic movement of the mass into the atrium, and may be identified graphically as a notch on the upstroke of the apex cardiogram. A rare but specific feature of the condition is variation of the auscultatory findings with change in posture; this may be particularly obvious in right atrial tumours.

INVESTIGATIONS

The chest radiograph and electrocardiogram do not help to distinguish myxoma from mitral valve disease. Left atrial enlargement is common but seldom marked and signs of pulmonary venous hypertension are infrequent. Calcification within the tumour is rarely demonstrable.

Echocardiography

While the first account of left atrial myxoma diagnosed during life was not until 1951, it is now exceptional for the diagnosis to be made first at autopsy. This is chiefly attributable to the wide availability of echocardiography, which has proved itself both reliable and specific for recognizing these tumours. The characteristic pattern of left atrial myoma is easily recognized, and it is no accident that the echocardiographic appearance of these lesions was among the first clinical reports by ultrasonographers, in 1959. Figure 1 illustrates a typical two-dimensional echocardiogram from a patient with left atrial myxoma. This 'four-chamber view' shows the characteristic dense mass of echoes from the tumour lying just above the mitral valve orifice. The video recording demonstrates the mobility of the mass as it flops to and fro within the atrium, restrained only by its peduncle. Transoesophageal echocardiography affords the opportunity to examine the tumour and its attachment with great precision; generally this extra clarity is unnecessary, but on occasion the transoesophageal technique is helpful if there is difficulty differentiating tumour from an atrial thrombus.

Differential diagnosis of left atrial myxoma is seldom difficult. Large masses may occasionally be difficult to distinguish from left atrial ball

Fig. 1 Echocardiograph in the four-chamber view showing a myxoma occupying much of the left atrium.

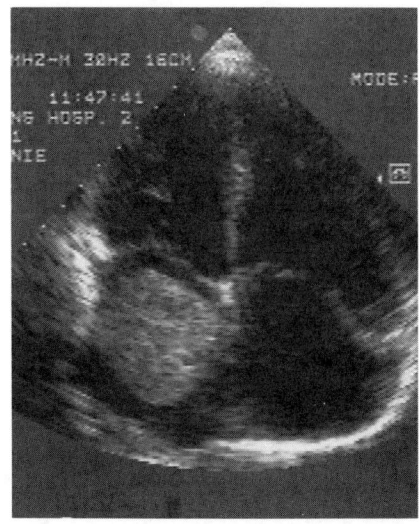

thrombus, a lesion which is today probably even rarer than myxoma. Smaller left atrial masses may be papillary fibroelastomas or infective vegetations caused by endocarditis. These can usually be distinguished by their clinical context. Masses in the right atrium may also represent thrombus, sometimes propagated from the inferior vena cava, or occasionally venous extension of abdominal cancers, for example hypernephroma. In a few patients abundant strands of the Chiari network of right atrial trabeculation may give rise to similar echocardiographic appearances.

Cardiac catheterization

The echocardiographic appearance is so characteristic that angiography no longer has a role in diagnosis of myxoma. The only time to undertake it is in an older patient in whom there is fear of occult coronary artery disease.

Treatment and prognosis

Atrial myxoma is treated by urgent surgical removal with its pedicle. Except in patients with severe pulmonary hypertension, or those with profound debility from the constitutional effects of their disease, the risk is low—comparable to that of surgery for mitral valve disease. It is important to ensure complete removal of the base by excising a full thickness button of the atrial septum. The resulting defect is repaired with a small patch.

Functional results of surgery are good. Some patients are left with mitral regurgitation but this is seldom severe. Recurrence is uncommon, provided excision has been complete, except in Carney's syndrome. In these patients regular echocardiographic follow-up is required, at intervals of 6 months. The rare occurrence after excision of the usual kind of myxoma usually occurs within the first 2 years; thereafter follow-up can safely be infrequent.

REFERENCES

Carney, J.A., Gordon, H., Carpenter, P.C., Shenoy, B.V., and Liang, V. (1985). The complex of myxomas, spotty pigmentation, and endocrine overactivity. *Medicine*, **64,** 270–283.

Greenwood, W.F. (1968). Profile of atrial myxoma. *American Journal of Cardiology*, **21,** 367–375.

Krikler, D.M., Rode, D., Davies, M.J., Woolf, N., and Moss, E. (1992). Atrial myxoma: A tumour in search of its origins. *British Heart Journal*, **67,** 89–91.

Markel, M.L., Waller, B.F., and Armstrong, W.F. (1987). Cardiac myxoma. A review. *Medicine*, **66,** 114–125.

Murphy, M.C., Sweeney, M.S., Putnam, J.B. et al. (1990). Surgical treatment of cardiac tumors: A 25-year experience. *Annals of Thoracic Surgery*, **49,** 612–618.

15.20 Pericardial disease

D. G. GIBSON

Anatomy of the pericardium

The normal pericardium consists of serous and fibrous components. The fibrous pericardium is thick and unyielding, separating the heart from surrounding organs. It fuses with the central tendon of the diaphragm below and with the great vessels above, 1 to 2 cm beyond their origins. The serous pericardium, in which the heart is invaginated, itself has two layers, a parietal layer, which lines the fibrous pericardium, and a visceral layer (sometimes called the epicardium), which covers the surfaces of the heart and the origins of the great vessels. The pericardial cavity is thus a potential space normally containing only a few ml of fluid, but with considerable capacity where fluid may accumulate.

Physiology of the pericardium

The normal pericardium is not essential to life – the pericardial space is often obliterated after open heart surgery and both layers may be removed in patients with constrictive pericarditis without apparent ill effect. Normal pericardial pressure has not been measured directly in man, although there is evidence to suggest that its value may be several mmHg negative to atmospheric. In man, pericardial pressure increases during isovolumic contraction, is maintained during ejection, and falls to its lowest value during isovolumic relaxation. It is possible, though unproved, that the normal pericardium may limit stroke volume during exercise in humans, thus preventing inappropriate ventricular distension. Whether restraint by the normal pericardium is of any pathophysiological importance as a mechanism limiting stroke volume in disease, or as a cause of raised ventricular filling pressures when the cavity is dilated again remains uncertain.

Congenital abnormalities of the pericardium

Congenital abnormalities of the pericardium are uncommon with an incidence of 1 to 2 per 10 000 autopsies. Congenital absence of the pericardium may be partial or complete. A partial defect, involving the left side of the pericardium is about four times as common as the complete form. About one-third of cases of either type may be associated with additional congenital anomalies, including Fallot' tetralogy, atrial septal defect, or sequestered pulmonary segments. Clinical features include non-specific chest pain and sinus bradycardia, with an electrocardiograph showing right axis deviation. Chest radiography is characteristic, with a shift of the heart to the left and prominence of the main pulmonary artery. Heart size is increased and the lower border of the cardiac shadow ill-defined. Echocardiography shows increased right ventricular size and reversed septal motion, as occurs in atrial septal defect. If the defect is partial, the left atrial appendix may herniate through it, and may even strangulate, leading to a clinical picture suggesting acute pericarditis. If the defect is larger, the left ventricle may herniate and undergo torsion. Alternatively lung may become trapped in the pericardial space. These complications are treated surgically by enlarging the defect.

Pericardial cysts

These are rare. They have a variety of embryological origins, and may be continuous with the pericardium or separate from it. They do not usually cause symptoms, but are discovered by routine chest radiographs. Their nature becomes obvious with a computerized tomography scan, but the exact diagnosis is often established only when they are removed surgically.

Mulibrey nanism

Mulibrey (**mu**scle, **li**ver, **br**ain, **ey**e) nanism is an autosomal recessive disorder characterized by growth failure, a triangular face, often with a hydrocephaloid skull, hypotonia, a peculiar voice, a large liver, and yellowish dots and pigment dispersion in the optic fundi. The majority of cases have cardiac constriction due to congenital thickening of the pericardium, and this may be responsible for many of the clinical features. Histologically, the pericardium shows simple fibrosis. Considerable improvement follows pericardiectomy.

Acquired pericardial disease

Diseases of the pericardium may be considered from two points of view. The first is aetiological as, in common with other serous membranes, the pericardium is affected by a number of disease processes. The second is in terms of the physiological and clinical disturbances that result. There is no fixed relation between the two, so that an account will be given of the different diseases affecting the pericardium and then of the three main syndromes: acute pericarditis, pericardial tamponade, and pericardial constriction.

Aetiology

Diseases affecting the pericardium are given in Table 1.

ACUTE IDIOPATHIC PERICARDITIS

Acute idiopathic pericarditis is a disease occurring, usually sporadically, in young adults. Prospective studies have suggested a viral basis for around half. Coxsackie B virus is most commonly involved, but others, including ECHO type 8, rubella, hepatitis B, mumps, and influenza may also be identified. Epidemics may occur, with approximately equal numbers of patients developing pericarditis and myocarditis. The most common clinical feature is chest pain, but 'flu-like symptoms, palpitations, orchitis, encephalitis, and radiographic appearances of pneumonitis or pleural effusion have all been reported. The condition is usually self-limiting, but a minority of cases follow a relapsing course over the succeeding 6 to 12 months. The virus may be identified from paired blood samples taken 2 weeks apart, or recovered from throat or rectal swabs. However, in many cases, no clear cause is identified, and positive virology is not necessary for the diagnosis.

PYOGENIC INFECTION

Pyogenic infection of the pericardium is much less common. It is usually due to blood-borne infection of a previously sterile pericardial effusion, or the result of direct spread from the lungs or pleural space. The organisms most commonly involved are staphylococci, pneumococci, or streptococci. Bacterial infection of the pericardium is not usually an isolated event, but occurs more commonly in an immunonologically compromised patient.

TUBERCULOUS INFECTION

Tuberculous infection is an important cause of pericardial disease, particularly in the Third World, where it is often associated with HIV infection. It may take the form of acute pericarditis, pericardial effusion or constriction. Acute pericarditis appears to be a 'primary' response, and can be regarded as an exudative lesion whose main basis is allergic. Chronic pericardial effusion and constriction both reflect granulomatous disease, often with fibrosis and calcification in the late stages. Both parietal and visceral layers of the pericardium may be involved, and spread of the disease to the myocardium follows. In the first instance treatment is with antituberculous drugs. In both effusion and constric-

Table 1 *Diseases affecting the pericardium*

Acute idiopathic pericarditis
Infections:
   viral
   bacterial (including tuberculosis)
   toxoplasmosis
   amoebiasis
   histoplasmosis
   actinomycosis
   nocardiosis
   echinococcal
Other inflammatory:
   postcardiotomy
   Dressler's syndrome
In association with systemic disease:
   connective tissue disorders (rheumatoid arthritis, systemic
     lupus erythematosus, systemic sclerosis, rheumatic fever,
     polyarteritis nodosa, Churg–Strauss syndrome, giant cell
     arteritis)
   uraemia
   hypothyroidism
Neoplastic:
   primary or secondary
Physical agents:
   radiotherapy
   blunt trauma
Haemorrhage:
   trauma
   aortic dissection
Drug-induced chylopericardium

tion, adding steroids for the first 11 weeks reduces the need for pericardiectomy, increases the rate at which heart rate and venous pressure fall to normal, and expedites return to work. In the absence of specific contraindication, therefore, steroids should be added to standard antituberculous chemotherapy.

FUNGAL PERICARDITIS

Fungal pericarditis is uncommon, but infection with actinomycosis, coccidioidomycosis and histoplasmosis have all been recorded, the last leading to constriction and calcification. Pericardial calcification by hydatid disease is increasingly recognized in areas where the disease is endemic, and may require surgical treatment if cardiac compression occurs.

MYOCARDIAL INFARCTION

Evidence of acute pericarditis may be found in up to 15 per cent of patients in the first 24 to 72 h after acute myocardial infarction. This may take the form of a friction rub, implying that the infarction was transmural. It seldom gives rise to symptoms other than a dull retrosternal pain, which differs from that due to the infarction itself by varying with posture and respiration. Not surprisingly, patients with pericarditis have more extensive ST segment changes on electrocardiography, and a slightly higher risk of supraventricular arrhythmia. There is no evidence to suggest any increased risk of complication with thrombolysis. Echocardiography may demonstrate a small pericardial effusion, but this is unlikely to require treatment.

Pericardial involvement is an important component of the postcardiotomy syndrome. This is an acute febrile illness occurring up to 1 year after cardiac surgery. The onset is usually sudden, with pleural or precordial pain and a pyrexia of up to 40°C. Chest radiographs may show an enlarged heart shadow or a pleural effusion; the electrocardiograph is unaffected. The condition is usually self-limiting, but may recur. Diagnosis is by excluding, in particular, infective endocarditis or cytomegalic inclusion disease from blood transfusion. Treatment is with aspirin or indomethacin. Occasionally, a large pericardial effusion may develop, requiring surgical drainage. Dressler's syndrome is a related condition, seen 2 to 4 weeks after acute myocardial infarction, in 3 to 4 per cent of cases. It also presents as a self-limiting febrile illness, accompanied by pericardial or pleural pain, and by pneumonitis in more severe cases. Like the post-cardiotomy syndrome, it responds to aspirin, indomethacin, or, if necessary, to steroids.

RHEUMATIC FEVER

A small pericardial effusion accompanies virtually all cases of acute rheumatic fever, where it is associated with epicardial inflammation. Less commonly, the effusion may be large enough to cause cardiac enlargement on chest radiograph, and so to suggest myocardial disease. It may cause acute pericarditis; it has also been invoked as a cause of subsequent constriction. Healing is virtually complete, although rheumatic pericarditis may be responsible for adhesions found at the time of subsequent valve replacement. The diagnosis is made echocardiographically, and the condition must be distinguished from myocarditis or severe valve disease.

RHEUMATIC DISORDERS

Pericardial involvement may be a major manifestation of rheumatoid disease, particularly in male patients with positive serology. Transient pericardial pain, symptomatic pericardial effusion, and particularly pericardial constriction may all occur. Pericardial involvement is also common in systemic lupus erythematosus, whether spontaneous or precipitated by drugs such as procainamide or hydralazine. Pericardial pain, asymptomatic effusion, and chronic constriction have also been reported. Pericardial effusion may also be seen in association with systemic sclerosis, polyarteritis nodosa, and the Churg–Strauss syndrome, when it may accompany myocardial involvement and functional mitral regurgitation.

URAEMIA

The pericardium is often involved in untreated or inadequately treated chronic renal failure. It usually presents as pericardial pain and a rub, both of which subside if a pericardial effusion develops. The most common manifestation is fibrinous pericarditis, associated with bloody pericardial effusion. Tamponade is common in untreated cases. Collagenous thickening of the epicardium is less common, but may give rise to myocardial constriction. Either of these complications may need surgical relief. The incidence of these pericardial complications is greatly reduced by adequate treatment of the underlying renal failure, by dialysis or renal transplantation.

HYPOTHYROIDISM

Pericardial effusion is common in untreated hypothyroidism, leading to an enlarged heart shadow on chest radiography, although clinically silent. The effusion itself has a high cholesterol content, which may produce an unusual secondary pericarditis with cholesterol deposits, which have a 'gold paint' appearance. The pericardial effusion does not need to be treated in its own right, and subsides when thyroid replacement therapy is given.

MALIGNANCY

Malignant involvement of the pericardium may be due to a primary tumor, or much more commonly to secondary involvement. The least rare primary tumours are mesothelioma or myosarcoma. Clinical manifestations of malignant involvement include supraventricular arrhythmias or atrial fibrillation as well as pericardial tamponade or constriction. Malignant effusion is a common cause of tamponade, which requires drainage. Definitive diagnosis is best made by a limited surgical approach, which allows open biopsy and the fashioning of a window into the pleural cavity to prevent recurrence.

IRRADIATION

Pericarditis may be caused by irradiation. It is usually asymptomatic, and a rub is unusual, but transient cardiac enlargement and minor electrocardiograph changes occur. A small pericardial effusion can be demonstrated by echocardiography. In a minority of cases, though, the effusion may be clinically significant. It may occur at the time of the irradiation or at any time over the succeeding years, and may be large enough to require drainage. At operation, the pericardium is found to be thickened with fibrosis and dense adhesions. This clinical picture must be distinguished from recurrence of the original malignancy. In a small minority of patients, pericardial constriction may develop up to 40 years after the original irradiation.

HAEMORRHAGE

Haemorrhage into the pericardium is an important cause of tamponade. It may occur with aortic dissection involving the ascending aorta. If the leak is large, it causes pericardial tamponade and death, but a small volume of blood is not uncommon with dissection. It can be detected by echocardiography, and may be responsible for ST segment changes on the electrocardiograph. Pericardial haemorrhage may be the result of stab wounds or blunt injury, or may occur after cardiac surgery. It may be induced by excessive anticoagulant therapy, or may follow invasive procedures such as myocardial biopsy or pacemaker insertion. Symptoms may occur at the time of bleeding, or may be delayed by 2 to 3 weeks, possibly because autolysis of blood clots increases the volume of fluid within the pericardial space. Delayed tamponade causes a characteristic syndrome of elevated venous pressure, fluid retention, and a low cardiac output, which resembles myocardial disease. Haemorrhage into the pericardial space may also be the basis of delayed pericardial constriction which can occur up to 10 years after open heart surgery.

Clinical syndromes associated with pericardial disease

Acute pericarditis

CLINICAL FINDINGS

There are three main components to the clinical syndrome of acute pericarditis: chest pain, pericardial rub, and electrocardiograph changes. The pain is usually retrosternal, continuous, and sharp or 'raw' in character. It is frequently aggravated by sudden movements or deep inspiration, and is relieved by sitting up. Less commonly it may resemble angina pectoris, or may be mild and 'atypical'. Painful breathing causes dyspnoea. The onset of the pain is usually sudden, but in idiopathic pericarditis, it may have been preceded by several days' malaise or other non-specific symptoms.

On examination, the main abnormality is a pericardial rub, audible in any position over the precordium. In patients in sinus rhythm it has two components, corresponding to atrial and ventricular systole. Rubs are frequently evanescent, and may vary with posture. They are often louder in inspiration. An irregular pulse due to supraventricular ectopic beats is common, particularly in patients with renal failure or after cardiac surgery. Atrial fibrillation or flutter are also seen.

The third clinical feature of the syndrome of acute pericarditis is an abnormal electrocardiograph. Symmetrical elevation of the ST segments by 1 mm or more in all leads other than aVr is seen in over 90 per cent cases in whom the diagnosis is confirmed. Early in the illness, the T waves are upright, but over the next 2 to 3 weeks they become flattened and inverted as the ST segment changes regress. These T wave changes are variable in incidence, direction, and extent. They usually resolve completely, but a minority of patients may be left with minor non-specific abnormalities, only to be detected many years later at a routine electrocardiograph.

Chest radiography is usually uninformative. It may show cardiac enlargement, but it is not possible to tell whether this is due to pericardial fluid, an increase in wall thickness or enlargement of one or more cardiac chamber.

ECHOCARDIOGRAPHY

Echocardiography is the method of choice for detecting pericardial effusion. Cross-sectional echo may also detect pericardial adhesions that are responsible for the rub. Acute pericarditis, however, can occur without demonstrable pericardial effusion.

DIAGNOSIS

Diagnosis is usually straightforward, although it is possible that either the late systolic murmur of mitral prolapse or the systolic 'scratch' of Ebstein's anomaly may be mistaken for a pericardial rub. An underlying cause for acute pericarditis should always be sought, though it may not be found; a final diagnosis of idiopathic pericarditis is probably the most common in such patients. In all cases, though, it is important to examine the possibility that additional myocarditis may be present, and if so, to attempt to quantify its severity.

TREATMENT

Idiopathic acute pericarditis is usually self-limiting, requiring simple analgesics only. As additional myocarditis is possible, the patient should rest until the pain has subsided. Pericarditis due to Dressler's or the postcardiotomy syndrome responds well to aspirin, or if more severe, to a non-steroidal anti-inflammatory drug. When symptoms are severe, repeated, or prolonged, moderate doses of steroids may be given. Associated pericardial effusion is treated on its own merits: only rarely does it need to be drained. Supraventricular arrhythmias are treated in the standard way. Pericarditis is often part of a generalized disease, which should be treated appropriately.

Pericardial tamponade

Pericardial tamponade is a complication of pericardial effusion, in which pericardial pressure is high enough to interfere with ventricular filling. The volume of fluid needed to cause tamponade varies considerably between patients. If the fluid has collected slowly, 1 to 2 litres may be present, but if it has collected rapidly, or the pericardium is rigid, much less may cause tamponade.

When pericardial pressure is raised, right and left atrial pressures rise to maintain a normal transmural pressure across the ventricular walls during filling. Sinus tachycardia is present, as filling occurs only in early diastole. Stroke volume is therefore small and fixed, and an adequate cardiac output depends on a rapid heart rate. Peripheral resistance increases to maintain arterial pressure in the presence of reduced flow. Patients with cardiac tamponade therefore present with clinical evidence of a low cardiac output. The skin is cold, the pulse volume small and urine flow reduced. Sinus tachycardia is usually present, although systolic arterial pressure may be above 100 mmHg. Arterial 'pulsus paradoxus' is a very important physical sign when arterial pressure falls with inspiration, and is very characteristic of advanced pericardial tamponade. Its presence indicates that the circulation is considerably embarrassed. Arterial pressure normally falls a little with inspiration because the intrathoracic pressure drops. This fall is also more obvious in patients with obstructive lung disease. Arterial paradox is thus an accen-

tuation of the normal response and not, in fact, paradoxical. What is abnormal is the extent to which the arterial pressure falls. In the absence of asthma, the upper limit for the normal fall with inspiration is 10 mmHg. In severe tamponade, the reduction in pulse pressure can readily be palpated at the radial artery, and, with critical circulatory embarrassment, the pulse may disappear altogether with inspiration. In milder cases, arterial paradox is sought using the sphygmomanometer.

The mechanism of pulsus paradoxus is still uncertain. Direct measurement of the pericardial pressure shows it to rise during inspiration, probably because the cavity is distorted by downward motion of the diaphragm. This increase is accompanied by a corresponding rise in right atrial and central venous pressure. There is no corresponding increase in pulmonary venous pressure on the left side of the heart, and pressure may fall to very low levels compared with that in the pericardium. Left ventricular filling first becomes compromised: this can be shown on the Doppler transmitral flow pattern; isovolumic relaxation time becomes prolonged, early diastolic filling velocity drops, and that during atrial systole increases. Overall stroke volume falls, and the interventricular septum shifts from right to left. Right ventricular stroke volume is thus maintained only by almost complete obliteration of the left ventricular cavity during inspiration. Finally, as pericardial pressure rises, there is diastolic collapse of right atrium and right ventricle.

Abnormal right ventricular filling is reflected in the venous pulse. The pressure is always raised: if it is not the diagnosis of tamponade must be questioned. Usually, it is very high, and it may be difficult to see the top. If a central venous line is in place, a further increase occurs with inspiration (Kussmaul's sign). This is a non-specific finding and merely reflects the inability of the right heart to deal with an increase in stroke volume, so it is seen in a variety of conditions including right ventricular disease and pulmonary hypertension. Although 'x' and 'y' descents are visible, their amplitude is small, reflecting the main disturbance of elevation of the mean venous pressure. Unlike pericardial constriction, therefore, abnormalities of the venous pulse are not particularly helpful in making the diagnosis. The precordium is quiet, and added heart sounds are absent, an important finding because if the clinical picture were due to ventricular disease, a loud third sound or summation gallop would be expected.

Chest radiography shows a large globular heart (Fig. 1), similar to that seen in dilated cardiomyopathy. More useful in making the diagnosis, therefore, is the absence of any evidence of pulmonary congestion, which would be expected if myocardial disease were the main abnormality. Pulmonary oedema is most unusual in tamponade.

The electrocardiograph shows tachycardia, often with low voltage QRS complexes, but without Q waves or conduction disturbances. If the effusion is large, electrical alternans is present. The alternate QRS complexes show differing morphology (Fig. 2), with the heart swinging to and fro in a large, and therefore usually malignant effusion.

ECHOCARDIOGRAPHY

Echocardiography is an important investigation because it allows rapid and unequivocal diagnosis of pericardial effusion, which is usually large (Fig. 3). Evidence for circulatory embarrassment is diastolic collapse of the right ventricle or right atrium (Fig. 4), and a striking increase in the amplitude of septal motion with respiration. If electrical alternans is present, motion of the heart within the pericardium can be confirmed. Arterial pulsus paradox can be confirmed or excluded from a simultaneous trace of respiration and peripheral arterial Doppler (Fig. 5). The nature of the circulatory embarrassment occurring with pericardial effusion varies in its exact nature between different cases. 'Tamponade' does not therefore represent a uniform diagnosis. In the small minority of cases in whom an echocardiographic diagnosis of pericardial effusion cannot be made for technical reasons, some other imaging method such as computerized tomography or magnetic resonance imaging may have to be used. Cardiac catheterization is no longer necessary.

DIFFERENTIAL DIAGNOSIS

The main step in the differential diagnosis of pericardial tamponade is to think of it in a patient presenting with clinical evidence of a low cardiac output. The condition must be distinguished from severe ventricular disease, massive pulmonary embolism, hypovolaemia, or overwhelming sepsis. Hypovolaemia is ruled out by a high venous pressure, while the absence of added heart sounds and pulmonary congestion makes severe ventricular disease unlikely. Massive pulmonary embolism is accompanied by a right ventricular third sound and characteristic electrocardiograph abnormalities. Clearly, an echocardiogram should be obtained early in all such patients; if there is a large pericardial effusion, the diagnosis becomes very likely. It is essential for the occasional echocardiographer to distinguish pericardial effusion from pleural effusion. This is done by locating the high intensity echo from the fibrous pericardium posterior to the left ventricle on the left parasternal view. A pericardial effusion is inside this structure, and a pleural effusion outside. Rarely, a large pleural effusion may compress the heart and cause a clinical picture very similar to tamponade in the absence of any pericardial fluid. It seems to occur when the pleural effusion is under pressure, and haemodynamics rapidly return to normal with pleural drainage.

TREATMENT

Pericardial tamponade is a medical emergency. It needs urgent treatment, particularly if there is obvious arterial paradox, or if the effusion is of recent onset and fluid is collecting rapidly. In a shocked patient cardiac output can be improved or maintained by infusion of saline or colloid to increase right ventricular filling pending urgent aspiration of the effusion. This should preferably be done in an area where resuscitation facilities are available. It is helpful to perform an echocardiogram immediately before the start of the procedure to determine the safest spot to insert the needle, and to get some idea of the best direction to aim it. The subcostal or apical routes may be used. The former is more satisfactory if the heart is accessible in this way, as damage to the anterior descending coronary artery is possible from the apex. The depth of the pericardial fluid can usually be confirmed when the local anaesthetic is inserted. A larger needle or a polythene cannula should then be inserted, and up to 500 ml of fluid removed; this will relieve the haemodynamic problem. Continuous drainage should then be instituted. Many pericardial effusions, particularly malignant ones, are heavily bloodstained, and may be indistinguishable from blood when they are withdrawn. These can be distinguished from puncture of a chamber by their colour, because they are very desaturated, and by their failure to clot, because they are defibrinated. If necessary, the haematocrit of the fluid can be compared with that of blood taken simultaneously.

Pericardial aspiration is necessary when there is any suspicion of tamponade. It should also be considered in any patient with a large pericardial effusion, even in the absence of specific evidence of circulatory embarrassment, since exercise tolerance is commonly limited before overt tamponade develops. Aspiration is not the best way of managing pericardial effusion definitively. It does not always prevent recurrence, and it is often not possible to make a diagnosis from analysis of the pericardial fluid alone. The most satisfactory line of treatment, therefore, is to undertake limited thoracotomy, either through the fifth interspace, or subcostally. The latter operation is possible with local anaesthetic. This allows an adequate specimen of pericardium to be removed for histology, and assures drainage of the pericardial space by making a window to the pleura. It is also possible to deal with a loculated effusion and to remove blood clots whose presence can give rise to delayed tamponade.

Pericardial constriction

Pericardial constriction causes a haemodynamic disturbance in which ventricular filling is seriously limited by the diseased pericardium. The pericardium itself is usually, but not always, thickened. The myocardium may also be involved, particularly in its subepicardial layers, by atrophy and fibrosis. Constriction usually affects both ventricles symmetrically, but in rare cases it may be more localized. The majority of cases, particularly in the developed world, show no evidence of inflammation, acute or chronic, so it is better to call it 'pericardial constriction' rather than 'constrictive pericarditis'.

PATHOPHYSIOLOGY

Pericardial constriction prevents cardiac filling in late diastole. Early diastolic ventricular pressure is thus normal, but as the pericardium is effectively indistensible, a normal or reduced stroke volume causes a striking increase in filling pressure. Right and left atrial filling are equally compromised because the two sides of the heart are usually affected symmetrically. End-diastolic pressures are thus equal to within 1 to 2 mmHg in all four cardiac chambers. This persists with respiration and even with fluid loading, and is the main criterion on which the invasive diagnosis of constriction is based. The ventricular pressure trace during filling is also characteristic. It rises rapidly in early diastole,

Fig. 1 Posteroanterior chest radiograph of a patient with a large pericardial effusion. The heart shadow is greatly enlarged and globular in configuration. The lung fields are normal.

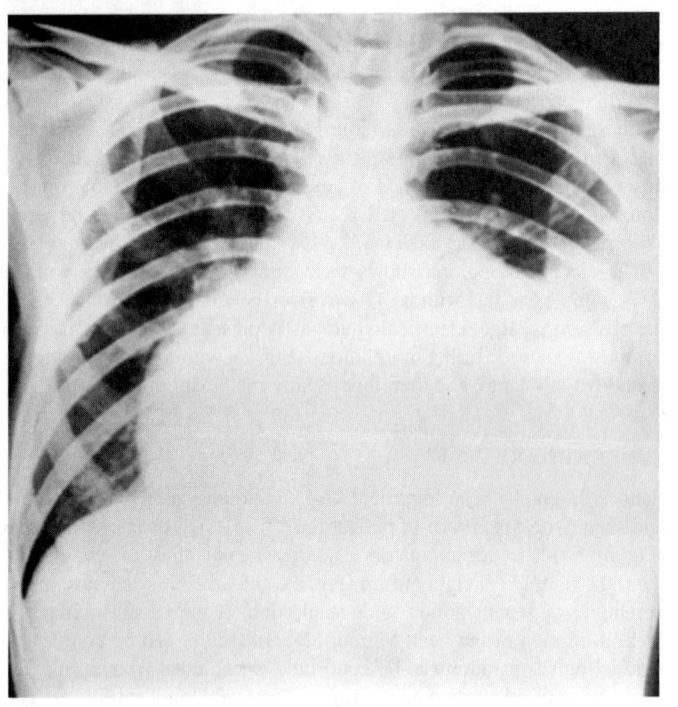

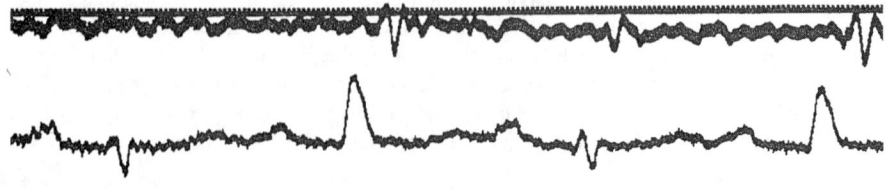

Fig. 2 Electrocardiogram from a patient with massive malignant pericardial effusion showing electrical alternans. Note that all are sinus beats with the same PR interval, but that the QRS axis alternates.

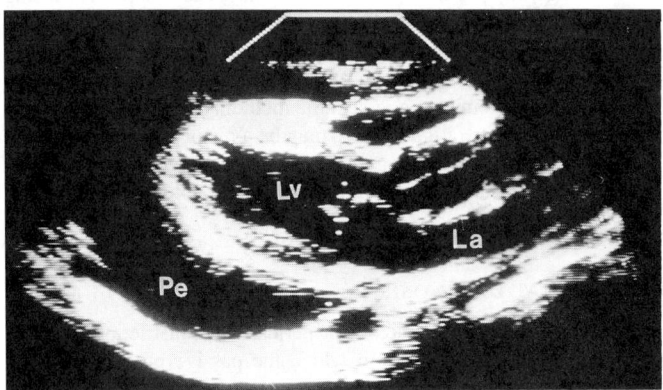

Fig. 3 Two-dimensional echocardiogram, parasternal long axis view, showing a large pericardial effusion (Pe) posterior to the left ventricle (LV). LA, left atrium.

Fig. 4 M-mode echocardiogram showing diastolic collapse of the right ventricle (marked by arrow) in a patient with a large pericardial effusion. Note that minimum dimension of the right ventricle occurs at the end of diastole. PE, pericardial effusion; RV, right ventricle; Se, interventricular septum; A2, aortic valve closure on phonocardiogram; LV, left ventricle (time marker = 200 ms).

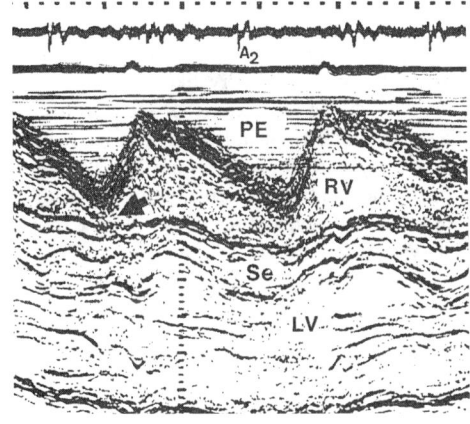

then stops abruptly, often with a slight rebound, it then remains constant for the remainder of diastole. This pattern is often referred to as the 'square root sign' from a fanciful resemblance to the mirror image of the mathematical symbol for a square root. Abnormal early diastolic filling is also reflected in the transmitral Doppler trace, which shows a rapid early diastolic deceleration, and reduced or absent flow across the valve during atrial systole. The jugular venous pulse is also characteristic. Overall pressure is raised, with the dominant descent during systole, the X descent (Fig. 6). This systolic descent is independent of right atrial systole, occurring later in the cardiac cycle than the A wave. Flow towards the heart in the superior cava is also systolic, meaning that right atrial volume must be increasing at this time. This rather unexpected combination of an increase in right atrial volume with a fall in right atrial pressure is caused by the increase in right atrial capacity as the tricuspid ring moves towards the apex of the right ventricle as it ejects. In pericardial constriction, ventricular filling is largely maintained by such AV ring motion, which, of course, is not affected by the pericardium. In all cases of constriction of clinical significance, the mean venous pressure is raised, and the inferior cava is dilated. Stroke volume is reduced, so that tachycardia or atrial fibrillation are common. Fluid is retained leading to peripheral oedema and ascites.

It has been suggested, largely on the basis of experimental data, that the normal pericardium may restrict ventricular filling, particularly when the ventricular cavity is dilated. On this basis, a high left ventricular end-diastolic pressure is not the result of a high transmural pressure difference; the pressure difference is normal or even low, but pericardial pressure itself is raised. This increase is also thought to limit right ventricular filling, and thus be a major cause of elevation of the jugular venous pressure. These ideas are based mainly on acute animal experiments, or observations in patients in the period immediately after open heart surgery when pericardial pressures can be measured directly. Although constriction by the normal pericardium remains a possibility, filling pressures are usually widely different in the two ventricles in these circumstances. Pericardial constriction does not therefore appear to be the major cause of increased filling pressure in patients with ventricular disease.

CLINICAL FINDINGS

The clinical picture of pericardial constriction is dominated by obstruction to right ventricular filling. In well developed cases, venous pressure

Fig. 5(a) Arterial Doppler, respiration, and phonocardiogram recorded from a patient with a large pericardial effusion. Note that peak arterial velocities drop to approximately half their peak values with inspiration. Art Dop, arterial Doppler; insp, inspiration. (b) The same patient after aspiration of the pericardial effusion. Note that the arterial pulse no longer varies with respiration (time marker = 100 ms).

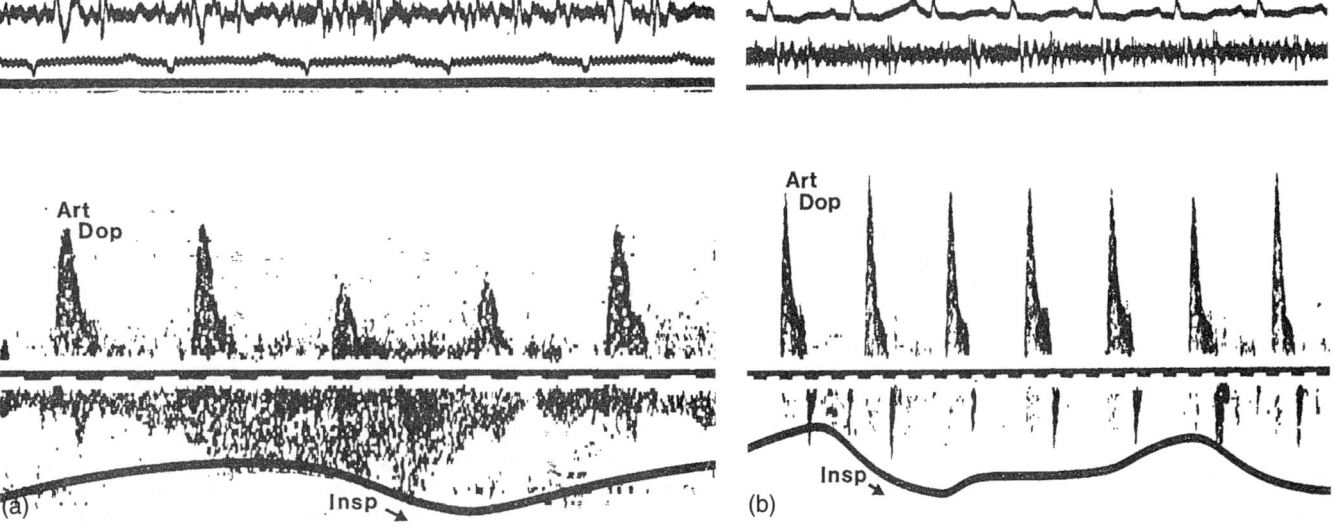

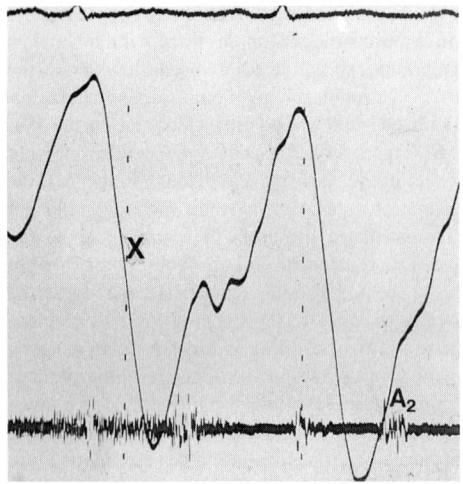

Fig. 6 Jugular venous pulse recording showing a dominant X descent in a patient with pericardial constriction. A2, aortic valve closure (time marker = 500 ms).

is raised by 15 cm or more, showing abrupt systolic and, to a lesser extent, early diastolic descents. The mechanism of the systolic or X descent does not depend on atrial systole, so it is also present in atrial fibrillation. The precordial impulse is not usually palpable, and on auscultation, the heart sounds are soft. There may be an early diastolic sound, whose timing corresponds to the end of rapid filling, and which should therefore be classified as a third, though it is sometimes referred to as a ventricular 'knock'. It is often heard earlier than the classic third heart sound, because the acceleration phase of rapid filling ends earlier in constriction than in uncomplicated ventricular disease. The liver is enlarged and, in patients with long-standing disease, there may be wasting and jaundice. Ascites is often more prominent than peripheral oedema, particularly when the patient has been treated with large doses of diuretics.

Chest radiograph

The heart may be normal in size or enlarged, but the lung fields are clear. An important finding is pericardial calcification, which may be present as multiple plaques or more frequently, as a rim covering the diaphragmatic and anterior surfaces of the heart. In a minority of cases, the chest radiograph is entirely normal.

Electrocardiograph

The electrocardiograph often shows atrial fibrillation, low voltage QRS complexes and non-specific T wave abnormalities. There are no diagnostic features.

Computed tomography and magnetic resonance imaging

Computed tomographic scanning or magnetic resonance imaging can demonstrate the extent and distribution of pericardial thickening. While this does not make the diagnosis of constriction, it is often very useful to know that the pericardium is, in fact, abnormal in a patient in whom this diagnosis is suspected. M-mode and cross-sectional echocardiography are unhelpful in making the diagnosis of constriction, but Doppler may be useful in demonstrating abnormalities of ventricular filling.

Cardiac catheterization

Unless the diagnosis is very obvious, cardiac catheterization is still usually performed. The diagnostic finding is equal end-diastolic pressures in the two ventricles, persisting with respiration and fluid challenge.

ALTERNATIVE CLINICAL PRESENTATIONS

A number of less common clinical presentations have been described.

1. Localized constriction may compress the outflow tract of the right ventricle or may mimic mitral or tricuspid stenosis.
2. A greatly raised venous pressure may lead to a protein-losing enteropathy, or to a classic nephrotic syndrome.
3. The possibility of occult pericardial constriction has been raised. In these patients, the venous pressure is normal, and the symptoms are non-specific including mild loss of exercise tolerance or fatigue. There may be a history of previous acute pericarditis. The diagnostic haemodynamic changes of constriction can then be unmasked by rapid volume expansion by infusion.

DIFFERENTIAL DIAGNOSIS

The main differential diagnosis of pericardial constriction is from restrictive myocardial disease, in which the passive properties of the myocardium itself are abnormal, usually as the result of fibrosis or infiltration. Exactly as in constriction, therefore, ventricular early diastolic pressure is normal, but that at end-diastole is greatly increased. The haemodynamics are thus very similar in the two conditions. The differential, however, is an important one because both are debilitating and life-threatening conditions; constriction can be treated effectively by surgery whereas restrictive myocardial disease cannot. In an individual case, it may be very difficult to distinguish between these two conditions and severe tricuspid regurgitation. However, there are a number of approaches:

1. *Anatomical.* If the pericardium is thickened or calcified, this makes a diagnosis of constriction very likely. Similarly, if echocardiography shows the characteristic appearances of amyloid, and these are confirmed histologically, then it is very likely that restrictive myocardial disease is present. The same applies when only one ventricle is greatly dilated with a reduced ejection fraction. In typical restrictive disease, however, ventricular systolic function is well maintained. Tricuspid regurgitation severe enough to lead to a clinical picture resembling condition can readily be diagnosed by echocardiography.
2. *Haemodynamics.* Raised ventricular filling pressures, with a square root sign on the pressure pulse, increased early diastolic filling velocities and shortened early filling periods do not distinguish between the two. The most useful ventricular haemodynamic feature is equalization of diastolic pressures within the heart, persisting with fluid challenge. A dominant systolic (X) rather than (Y) descent on the jugular venous pulse is also very characteristic.
3. *Clinical progress.* The venous pressure in patients with restrictive myocardial disease usually drops with diuretic treatment, albeit at the cost of causing fatigue and hypovolaemia. It is very rare to be able to bring the venous pressure down to normal in a patient with constriction. In a minority of cases, it is necessary to perform an exploratory thoracotomy in order to make the diagnosis. This enables the diagnosis of constriction to be made and treated accordingly, or to be excluded definitively, so that the patient can be reconciled to medical treatment, unsatisfactory as it may be.

Pericardial constriction must also be distinguished from other causes of raised venous pressure. Superior caval obstruction is excluded by the presence of venous pulsation. Right ventricular inflow may be obstructed by tricuspid stenosis or, very rarely, by a right ventricular tumour. Elevation of the venous pressure is also a feature of selective right atrial compression by blood clot occurring in the postoperative period. Severe tricuspid regurgitation may occur on its own, or because of right ventricular disease. It seems to be becoming increasingly common as a long term complication following mitral valve replacement.

These possibilities can all be excluded by echocardiography, and by recording the venous pulse.

TREATMENT

Mild pericardial constriction can usually be managed by diuretics. Although the venous pressure does not fall to normal, the fluid retention can often be contained. However, if fluid retention persists, or if an excessive dose of diuretic is needed, as shown by an increase in blood urea, or impaired exercise tolerance due to fatigue, then surgery should be considered. The thickened pericardium must be removed from the anterior and inferior surfaces of the heart, and from the atrioventricular sulci. Cardiopulmonary bypass is usually needed to expose the heart satisfactorily. The operation is often a long and difficult one, particularly when the pericardium is calcified, and when there is fibrosis of the myocardium. In many patients, the venous pressure is as high after the operation as it was before, though the X descent is lost and the Y descent becomes dominant. However, with digitalis and diuretic treatment, the pressure gradually falls over the succeeding weeks, as the condition of the patient improves.

Other manifestations of pericardial disease

Postoperative pericardial disease

A modified type of pericardial tamponade occurs after open heart surgery due to blood clots within the pericardium. This is most common after cardiac surgery, but may also occur with trauma or uraemia. It is often due to clot behind the left atrioventricular sulcus. Clinically, it presents as a fall in urine flow and cardiac output, a reduction in skin temperature and finally hypotension. The atrial pressures may normal or raised, and the classic arterial and venous pulse abnormalities are absent. Chest radiography and electrocardiography show no specific abnormality, and transthoracic echocardiography shows no abnormality, though transoesophageal echo may be useful, if it is available. The condition is suspected in a patient who may have bled rather heavily after operation, and the suspected diagnosis is contained by reopening the chest and removing the blood clots.

Clot may also compress the right atrium. This characteristically occurs towards the end of the first postoperative week, after the chest drains have been removed, when the patient is being mobilised. The main clinical features are fluid retention and elevation of the venous pressure. The diagnosis can usually be made by transthoracic echocardiography, which demonstrates distortion of the right atrial cavity by blood clot, and sometimes increased right atrial filling velocities. If the precordial window is poor, transoesophageal echocardiography is required. Treatment is by drainage.

Pericardial constriction as a long-term complication of open heart surgery is being increasingly recognized, and may occur in 1 to 2 per cent of patients. Minor degrees are probably rather more common. It presents as chronic elevation of the venous pressure, and is often diagnosed as postoperative 'heart failure'. The diagnosis is made from a recording of the venous pulse, which shows a dominant X descent on the pressure and Doppler records, and by the absence of any intracardiac cause of the syndrome of heart failure. It can usually be controlled by a small dose of diuretic, but in a minority of cases, pericardial surgery may be needed.

Recurrent acute pericarditis

Recurrent acute pericarditis is an uncommon, though clinically demanding, form of pericardial disease to manage. It occurs any time up to 10 years after an apparently uncomplicated episode of acute pericarditis of any aetiology: idiopathic, infective, postoperative, or postinfarction. Its most common manifestation is chest pain, although occasionally it may present as recurrent pericardial effusion. Electrocardiographic changes and echocardiographic evidence of effusion occurs in about half the patients. As with the original attack, immunological studies are likely to be indecisive. The clinical problem is that the repeated episodes may become debilitating to the patient, particularly as they occur after what was represented as a self-limiting disease. Constriction appears to be a most uncommon complication, as does the development of significant myocardial disease. Management thus consists of maintaining a positive outlook and controlling the manifestation of acute pericarditis. Simple analgesia with aspirin is the most satisfactory means, but this may not always be adequate. Non-steroidal anti-inflammatory agents or corticosteroids may thus be required, the latter often in doses large enough to lead to cushingoid manifestations. There is no evidence to suggest that other immunosuppressive agents have a therapeutic role. Pericardiectomy may be necessary, but it is not necessarily effective, presumably because all the pericardium cannot be removed. The overall prognosis of the condition is good.

Tuberculous pericardial constriction

In the Third World, tuberculous pericardial constriction runs a very different course from that seen in developed countries. It occurs early in the disease and may be the presenting feature, or may supervene after an effusion has been drained. Patients present with sinus tachycardia rather than atrial fibrillation, a very high venous pressure, ascites, and weight loss. The venous pressure often does not show the characteristic pattern of systolic dip. A third heart sound is present in about half the patients. Radiography shows a normal sized heart, but characteristically a 'shaggy' left heart border. There is no pericardial calcification. Electrocardiography shows sinus tachycardia and non-specific T wave abnormalities. Cross-sectional echocardiography is very helpful showing the two layers of pericardium separated by amorphous echoes, often with small loculated pockets of fluid (Fig. 7). This pattern is sometimes referred to as 'effusive-constrictive pericarditis'. The amplitude of ventricular wall motion is reduced, and the pericardial surface shows a very characteristic 'frozen' appearance. Treatment is by antituberculous chemotherapy. Added steroids make clinical improvement significantly more rapid, with heart rate and venous pressure returning more rapidly to normal. Adjuvant steroids also reduce the risk of death and the incidence of operation. When possible, fluid retention should be controlled by diuretics because, during the early subacute phase, surgery is demanding and not wholly satisfactory. However, surgery may be

Fig. 7 Cross-sectional echocardiogram showing effusive-constrictive pattern of pericardial involvement (marked with arrow) in a patient with tuberculous pericarditis.

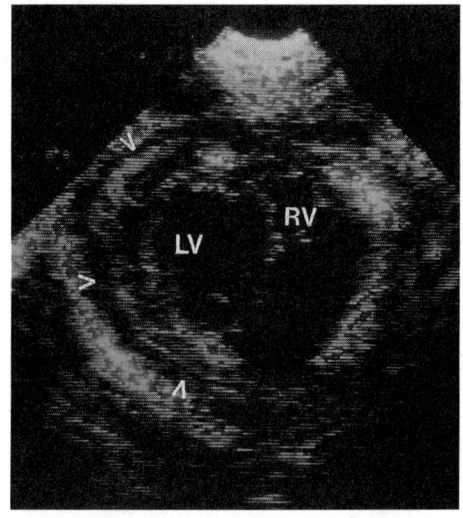

needed in a minority of seriously ill cases who cannot be held on medical treatment. The ultimate prognosis of patients surviving the initial attack, whether treated medically or surgically, is excellent, being indistinguishable from that of the population at large.

REFERENCES

Baldwin, J.J. and Edwards, J.E. (1976). Uremic pericarditis as a cause of tamponade. *Circulation* **53**, 896–901.

Caird, R., Conway, N., and McMillan, I.K.R. (1973). Purulent pericarditis followed by early constriction in young children. *British Heart Journal,* **35**, 201–203.

Carty, J.E., Deverall, P.B., and Losowsky, M.S. (1975). Retrosternal pain, widespread T wave inversion and collapse of left lower lobe with effusion, Strangulated atrial appendix. *British Heart Journal,* **37**, 98–100.

Dressler, W. (1959). The post-myocardial infarction syndrome. A report of 44 cases. *Archives of Internal Medicine,* **103**, 28–30.

Fowler, N.O. and Gabel, M. (1985). The hemodynamic effects of cardiac tamponade: mainly the result of atrial, not ventricular compression. *Circulation* **71**, 154–157.

Fowler, N.O. and Harbin, III A.D. (1986). Recurrent acute pericarditis: follow-up study of 31 patients. *Journal of Americal College of Cardiology,* **7**, 300–305.

Hatle, L.K., Appleton, C.P. and Popp, R.L. (1989). Differentiation of constrictive pericarditis and restrictive cardiomyopathy by Doppler echocardiography. *Circulation* **79**, 357–370.

Kahn, A.H. (1975). Pericarditis of myocardial infarction. *American Heart Journal,* **90**, 788–794.

Martin, R.G., Ruckdeschel, J.C., Chang, P., Byhardt, R., Bouchard, R.J., and Wernick, P.H. (1975). Radiation induced pericarditis. *American Journal of Cardiology,* **35**, 217–220.

Mounsey, P. (1955). Annular constrictive pericarditis. *British Heart Journal,* **21**, 325–320.

Perheentupa, J., Autio, S., Leisti, S., Raitta, C., and Tuuteri, L. (1973). Mulibrey nanism, an autosomal recessive syndrome with pericardial constriction. *Lancet* **2**, 351–355.

Spodick, D.H. (1974). ECG in acute pericarditis. *American Journal of Cardiology,* **40**, 470–474.

Strang, J.I.G. (1984). Tuberculous pericarditis in Transkei. *Clinical Cardiology,* **7**, 667–670.

Tubbs, O.S. and Yacoub, M.H. (1968). Congenital pericardial defects. *Thorax* **23**, 598–607.

Vaitkus, P.T. and Kussmaul, W.G. (1991). Constrictive pericarditis versus restrictive cardiomyopathy: a reappraisal and update of diagnostic criteria. *American Heart Journal* **122**, 1431–1441.

Wood, P. (1961). Chronic constrictive pericarditis. *American Journal of Cardiology* **7**, 48–55.

15.21 Cardiovascular syphilis

B. GRIBBIN AND D.W.M. CROOK

Introduction

Cardiovascular syphilis is no longer a prominent cause of heart disease, and even in specialized cardiac units it is now a rarity. Natural history studies have shown that about 12 per cent of untreated syphilitic patients will eventually develop cardiovascular complications. Although gummata can occur in the pericardium, myocardium, and endocardium, and have been the cause of Stokes–Adams attacks caused by their presence in the atrioventricular node or the bundle of His, the characteristic lesion is an aortitis. This follows spirochaetal infection of the aortic wall and leads to an endarteritis and periarteritis of the aortic vasa vasorum, initially in the adventitia and subsequently in the media. Lymphocytes and plasma cells surround these small feeding vessels and obliterative changes result in the loss of medial smooth muscle and elastic fibres, occasionally with frank necrosis and eventually with fibrous tissue replacement. This causes scarring of the aortic wall and weakening of its structure. Macroscopically the intima becomes thickened in a gelatinous patchy fashion and fibrosis produces an irregular linear thickening which has been termed the tree-bark appearance. Intimal scarring may involve the ostia of the coronary arteries which are susceptible to further narrowing by accelerated and superimposed atheroma. The ascending aorta is involved in about half of all cases, the arch is next in frequency, and the descending aorta in only 10 per cent, with changes virtually limited to that part of the vessel lying above the renal arteries. As the aortic wall structure weakens so dilatation occurs, resulting in aneurysm formation, which in turn leads to further dilatation and the risk of rupture. The major branches of the aorta may also be affected, especially the innominate artery.

Enlargement of the aortic root and separation of the cusp commissures causes aortic reflux, and although thickening and retraction of the leading edges of the cusps also occurs, this is thought to be a secondary change due to abnormal turbulence rather than a consequence of direct syphilitic involvement of cusp tissues.

Clinical features

Because cardiovascular syphilis may take up to 40 years after primary infection to become apparent, most patients are middle aged or elderly, with men more often affected. Patients with aortitis can present in four main ways: asymptomatic aortitis, aneurysm formation, aortic reflux, and lastly as the result of coronary artery ostial stenosis. The last three are not mutually exclusive and aortic reflux plus ostial stenosis may coexist with aneurysm formation.

Aortitis in asymptomatic patients is usually diagnosed as the result of radiographic findings of a dilated ascending aorta with calcification in the wall (Fig. 1). Although aortic calcification is common particularly in the elderly and hypertensive population, it is then virtually limited to the aortic knuckle and descending aorta. When visible in the ascending aorta, syphilitic aortitis should come to mind and supporting evidence, such as mild aortic reflux, may be noted. Serology is in such a case likely to be positive.

Aortic aneurysms tend to be saccular rather than fusiform and occur most commonly in the ascending aorta, also in the arch, and with increasing rarity down the descending aorta. This is in contrast to atherosclerotic aneurysms, which tend to involve the distal aorta below the renal arteries. The clinical features vary depending on the site of the aneurysm, its size, and whether or not compression and even erosion of adjacent structures occurs. A large aneurysm may cause no symptoms, but pain can be a prominent feature, often sustained and boring in nature, influenced by position, and exacerbated by impending rupture. Pain due to ascending aortic aneurysms is felt in the upper chest wall to the right of the sternum, and with large aneurysms a bulge may appear at this site and erosion of ribs and even sternum may be apparent on radiographs. Aneurysms of the arch produce pain over the upper sternum and occasionally in the throat and there may be visible arterial pulsation in the root of the neck with tracheal deviation. Pressure on upper mediastinal structures can produce superior vena caval obstruction, dysphagia, stridor, and a tracheal tug in time with the pulse. Involvement of the upper descending aorta causes pain between the scapulae or to the left of the spine, and there is a risk of hoarseness from pressure on the left recurrent laryngeal nerve and complications arising from compression of the left main bronchus. Rupture can occur into the bronchus, into the left pulmonary artery or the left pleural space, and erosion of vertebrae may result in chronic and debilitating pain.

Syphilitic aortic reflux may have a number of features to help distinguish it from the more usual varieties. Radiographic or clinical evidence of aneurysmal dilatation of the ascending aorta is one, and explains the fact that the early diastolic murmur may be heard best at the right, rather

Fig. 1 Posteroanterior and lateral radiographs showing evidence of syphilitic aortitis. A line of calcium (arrowed) is visible in the wall of the dilated ascending aorta.

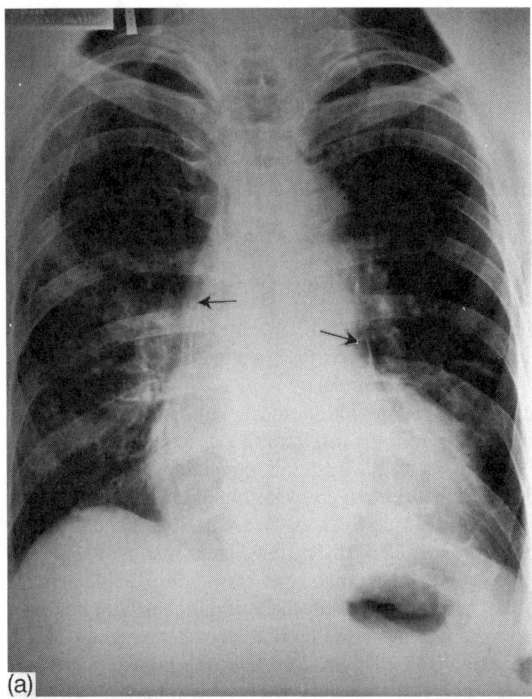

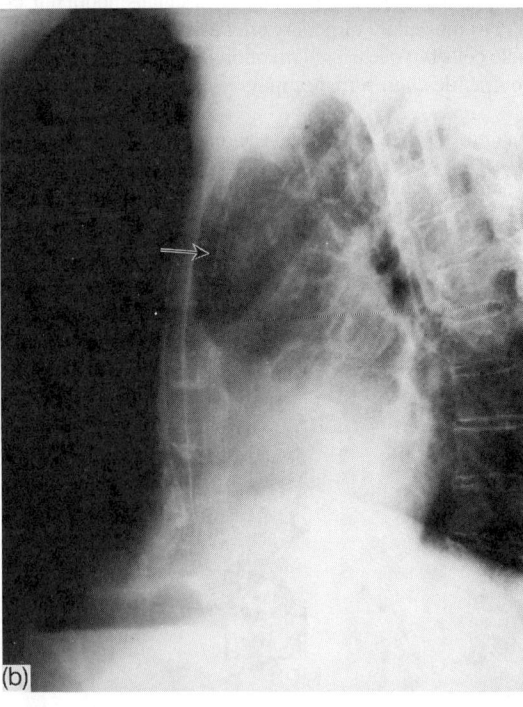

than the more usual left, sternal edge position. Furthermore, an ejection click may be audible and probably occurs as a result of sudden distension of the dilated aortic root by the large stroke volume. However, these auscultatory signs are not entirely specific and may be found in patients with annulo-aortic ectasia, now a more common condition characterized by a flask-like dilatation of the proximal ascending aorta. Even severe aortic reflux may be well tolerated for years, but eventually the volume overload of the left ventricle leads to cardiac failure which carries a poor prognosis without, and sometimes despite, surgical intervention.

Coronary ostial stenosis is not restricted to cases of syphilitic aortitis and may occur as a variant of the more usual atheromatous coronary artery disease. It presents as angina, the true cause of which may be missed unless a thin line of calcification is noted in the ascending aorta or there is other evidence of syphilitic disease in the cardiovascular system or elsewhere. Myocardial infarction may occur as a further complication.

Diagnosis

The diagnosis of cardiovascular syphilis is usually made by detecting a positive serum antibody test in a patient who may give a history of past syphilitic infection, and who has evidence of aortitis or one of its complications. It is also important to note that 10 to 25 per cent of patients with cardiovascular syphilis also have central nervous system involvement.

Non-specific antibody tests such as the Venereal Diseases Research Laboratory (VDRL) test may be negative in cardiovascular syphilis, but specific tests such as the fluorescent treponemal antibody absorption test (FTA-ABS) remain positive, even after treatment. For more detailed information see Chapter 7.11.34.

Treatment

Patients with cardiovascular syphilis who have not received effective antibiotic treatment in the past should be treated. The drug of first choice is benzylpenicillin, 2.4 g given intravenously 4 hourly for 3 weeks. For patients known to be allergic to penicillin some practitioners desensitize and then use penicillin, and others use a tetracycline such as doxycycline (200 mg orally twice a day for 3 weeks). More recently ceftriaxone has been used in a dose of 1 to 2 g given intravenously or intramuscularly once a day for 3 weeks. In those patients with a positive VDRL test, effective treatment should be followed by a fall in titre over a 1 to 2 year period. In all cases the cerebrospinal fluid should be examined and, if antibody tests are found to be positive, further cerebrospinal fluid examinations should be performed after treatment to demonstrate a similar fall in titre. Although it is generally accepted that antibiotic treatment is indicated, there is no evidence that the severity of aortitis is in any way altered, and indeed there has been concern that provocation of a Jarisch–Herxheimer reaction might lead to inflammatory swelling of the aortic wall with the risk of rupture or further critical narrowing of ostial stenosis. However, large numbers of patients with cardiovascular syphilis have been given penicillin without untoward effects, and whereas the Jarisch–Herxheimer reaction can occur rarely, it has never been shown to cause life-threatening changes in the aortic wall.

Surgery may be required to deal with the complications of aortitis. Symptoms of ischaemic heart disease caused by severe ostial stenosis have been relieved successfully by endarterectomy of the coronary orifices, and also by coronary bypass grafting. Aortic valve replacement has been carried out successfully for severe aortic reflux. Saccular aneurysms have been excised and scarred aortic tissue replaced by grafts. Indications for the latter form of surgery are based on the need to relieve pain, to prevent rupture, the risk of which is considerable when the aneurysm reaches 6 to 7 cm in diameter, and the need to decompress adjacent organs such as the left main bronchus, pulmonary artery, or oesophagus.

REFERENCES

Heggtveit, H.A. (1964). Syphilitic aortitis. A clinicopathologic autopsy study of 100 cases, 1950 to 1960. *Circulation* **29**, 346–55.

Rimsa, A. and Griffith, G.C. (1957). Trends in cardiovascular syphilis. *Annals of Internal Medicine* **46**, 915–24.

15.22 The pulmonary circulation in health and disease

J. S. PRICHARD

This chapter describes the structure and functional behaviour of the pulmonary circulation in the healthy adult lung. It is intended to be read in conjunction with those that follow on cor pulmonale, pulmonary hypertension, pulmonary oedema, and pulmonary embolism, to help the reader to spot the various malfunctions responsible for the clinical manifestations and to understand therapy, prognosis and differential diagnosis.

The role of the pulmonary circulation: general considerations

The whole of the cardiac output passes through the lungs, giving the pulmonary circulation a unique opportunity to alter the composition of the blood. The most obvious way in which this is achieved is by gas exchange but, in addition, there is a host of metabolic and immunological functions of the endothelium of the 'lesser' circulation, which have a profound affect upon physiology and pathophysiology. The main functions that have been identified are:

1. Gas exchange by diffusion.
2. Release of carbon dioxide from plasma bicarbonate.
3. Metabolism of hormones and biogenic amines.
4. Metabolism of xenobiotic substances.
5. Phagocytosis of particulate matter by endothelium and intravascular macrophages.
6. Filtration of blood to remove the small venous thromboemboli which are probably a normal phenomenon in healthy people.

Of these, the overwhelmingly important need to sustain efficient gas exchange over a wide range of ventilation and blood flows imposes the greatest constraints, and these are reflected in four important requirements of physiology:

1. The passage time for individual red blood cells through the alveolar capillaries is long enough for complete oxygen exchange by diffusion.
2. Regional blood flow is regulated to match local variations in regional ventilation.
3. Increase in blood flow through the capillaries is achieved without any great increase in the capillary hydrostatic pressure.
4. Fluid exchange in the region of the alveoli is highly regulated to prevent disruption of gas exchange.

The physiological constraints set by the non-gas-exchange functions are less stringent and depend mainly depend upon the endothelium having a huge surface area. The endothelium can, broadly, be regarded as as a monolayer of metabolically active cells whose surfaces possess the requisite molecules to to process substrates constantly delivered by flowing blood, to sustain a non thrombogenic and immunologically privileged surface and to maintain a permeability barrier.

Morphology

The structure of the pulmonary vasculature differs quantitatively from that of the systemic vessels. The difference applies throughout the system to include the large and small pulmonary arteries and veins, whose media are poorly developed compared with comparable vessels in the systemic circulation.

THE PULMONARY ARTERIAL SYSTEM

The pulmonary arterial system can be divided into four structural regions as it passes from hilum to periphery: (1) elastic; (2) muscular; (3) partially muscular; and (4) non-muscular.

The elastic arteries are, by definition, those with five or more elastic laminae and they extend from the origin of the system down to vessels of 2000 μm. Compared with the systemic circulation, the pulmonary arteries are thin-walled with relatively wide lumina (Fig. 1). Thus, the pulmonary trunk is about half as thick as the aorta. Both it and the other elastic arteries are normally very distensible. Their media contain few smooth muscle fibres and consist mainly of elastic fibrils, collagen and an acid mucopolysaccaride ground substance continuous with the basement membrane of the intima—itself composed of endothelial cells.

As the system extends deeper into the lung the number of elastic laminae steadily decreases, so that those vessels with between two and five laminae have a relatively greater quantity of vascular smooth muscle and are referred to as muscular pulmonary arteries. The majority of cells are smooth muscle cells but occasional myofibroblasts, which have both secretory and contractile characteristics may be encountered.

Fig. 1 Comparison of (a) a systemic (prostate) and (b) a pulmonary artery. The pulmonary artery is a thin-walled vessel with a limited capacity for vasomotion. (Photomicrograph kindly given by Professor D. Heath.)

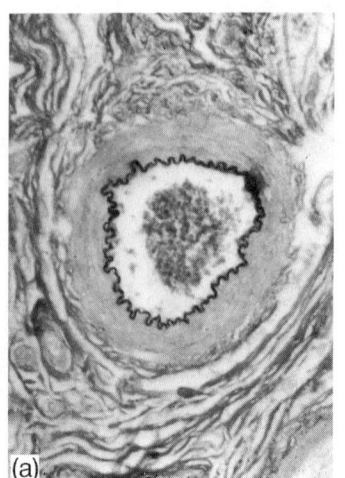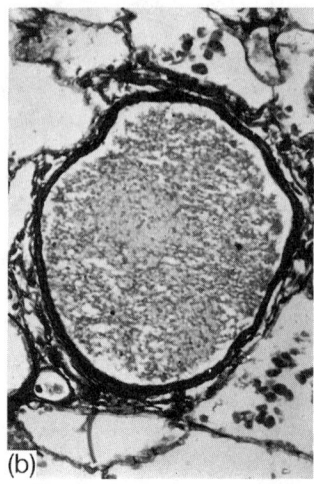

(a)   (b)

Below about 100 to 150 μm the muscle fibres within the artery become discontinuous and finally disappear when the diameter is less than about 50 μm. Vessels from 100 μm to the capillaries (< 15 μm) are referred to as non-muscular arteries or pulmonary arterioles. These have a single internal elastic lamina resting upon a basement membrane applied to the intima. Pericytes and intermediate cells are encountered at this level of the system. These cells are stellate, lie in the elastic laminae of the vessel, and occasionally actin and myosin filaments can be identified within them. Their importance lies more in their developmental potential in pathological conditions than in normal physiology. The scanty adventitia of the non-muscular arteries consists of collagen interspersed with elastic fibres, but this adventitia is continuous with the connective tissue of the lung parenchyma and thus radial traction provides a mechanism for maintaining patency of these thin walled vessels during periods—such as expiration—when intrathoracic pressure may be above atmospheric.

The relationship of the smaller arteries and arterioles to the terminal bronchioles, respiratory bronchioles and alveoli is shown in Fig. 2.

THE PULMONARY CAPILLARIES

The human lung contains approximately 300×10^6 alveoli, each surrounded by a mesh of capillaries so short that they resemble a fenestrated 'sheet' through which blood is transported as a fine film (Fig. 3). The mean capillary length is 9 to 13 μm and their density 118 to 237×10^2/ cm² alveolar wall. This is too short to allow development of Poiseuillian flow. Erythrocytes need only remain within the capillaries for 0.3 s for gas exchange so, despite an estimated 70 m² area available for capillary gas exchange, the lung capillary volume is as little as 150 to 200 ml. Most of the capillary bed is comprised of the alveolar capillary sheet. It is therefore susceptible to alveolar gas pressure. However, some capil-

laries are located at the angles of the alveoli in the deformable extra-alveolar connective tissues joining contiguous alveoli. These vessels are not directly susceptible to alveolar pressure and remain patent even when alveolar gas pressure exceeds capillary hydrostatic pressure. They are probably also the vessels that remain open during the 'pleating' of alveolar walls, which occurs during expiration below functional residual capacity.

The tissue and fluid layers that lie between the gas-filled lumen of the alveolus and the blood-filled capillary constitute the alveolar–capillary blood–gas barrier. In many regions the vascular endothelium and alveolar epithelium are so closely juxtaposed that the two basement membranes fuse and no connective tissue is interposed. The geometric mean thickness of the barrier is approximately 0.5 μm, which offers little resistance to gas diffusion (Fig. 4).

Fig. 3 Lung capillaries. The pulmonary capillaries are arranged as a meshwork around the alveoli.

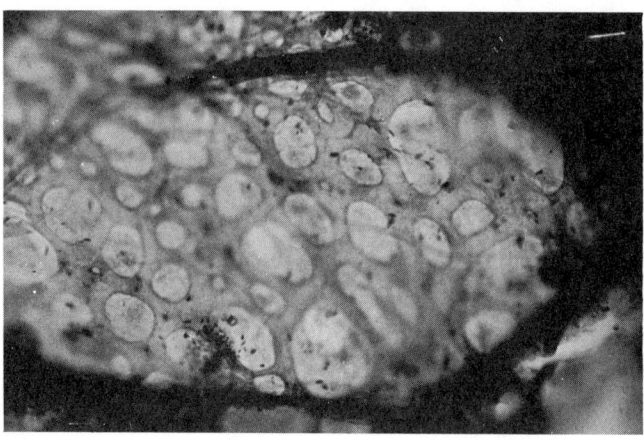

Fig. 2 Diagrammatic representation of the pulmonary arterial pathway. By light microscopy (top diagram) the artery is first seen to be muscular, partially muscular and then non-muscular (elastic, arterial). Electron microscopy (second diagram) shows that in the muscle free region of the wall pericytes (P) are found and in the partially muscular portion, intermediate cells (I). These are precursor smooth muscle cells. E = endothelial cells; M = smooth muscle cells. (Reproduced from Reid, L., *et al.* (1986). In *Abnormal circulation. Contemporary issues in pulmonary disease* (ed. E.M. Bergofsky). Vol. 4, p. 221, with permission).

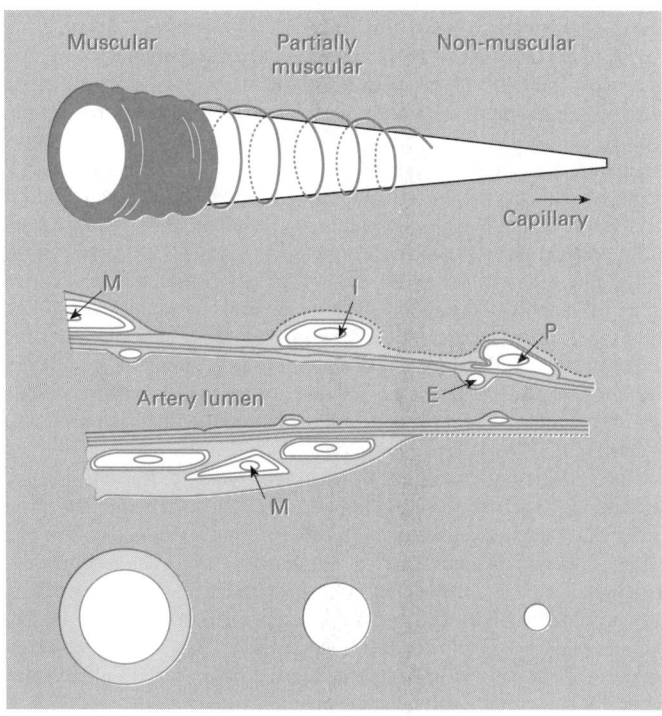

Fig. 4 The pulmonary microcirculation and blood–gas barrier. EC, endothelial cell; AS, alveolar space. (Reproduced by courtesy of Dr E. Schneeberger.)

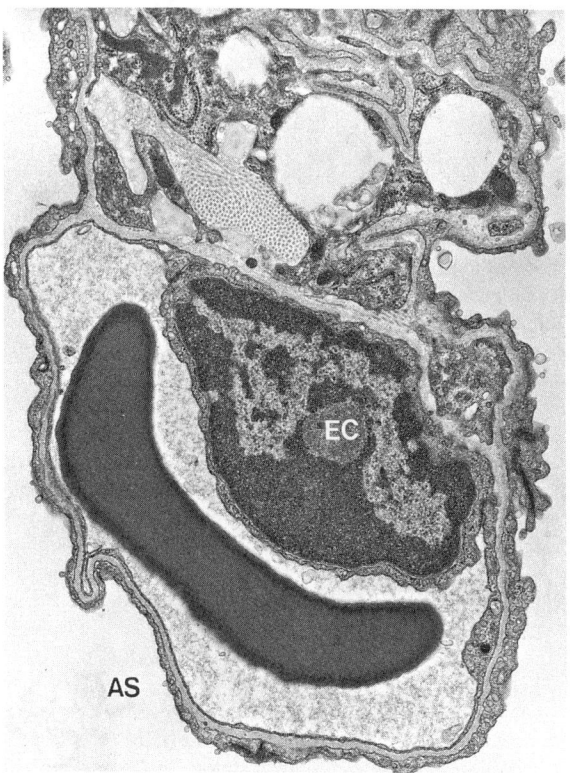

THE PULMONARY VENOUS SYSTEM

Pulmonary venules are virtually indistinguishable from arterioles. Commencing near the bronchioles, they pass into the connective tissue septa between secondary lobules to become pulmonary veins, which lie separated from the bronchi. Their media consists of irregularly arranged circular and oblique smooth muscle fibres, interspersed with collagen.

The large extraparenchymal pulmonary veins that lie in the loose tissue of the mediastinum and that connect the lung to the left atrium are largely composed of collagen with some elastic fibres.

THE LUNG LYMPHATICS

The lymphatic capillaries are relatively large, blindly ending vessels formed from a thin irregular endothelium with a poorly developed basement membrane. The individual cells are only weakly attached to each other by feebly developed adhesions and often adjacent cells may be separated by gaps as large as 1 to 10 μm. They are not present in alveolar walls but begin at the respiratory bronchioles. Thus fluid that enters the alveolar interstitium is first contained within the interstitial space and moves through this to the lymphatics. The vessels run centrally to the hila, coalescing as they do so. One group forms the right lymphatic duct. Another group unites to form the tracheobronchial duct, which joins the thoracic duct just before it enters the venous system. A third group of posterior mediastinal lymphatics runs through the caudal mediastinal node and also joins the thoracic duct.

Drainage of fluid by the lymphatics is continuous but can be enhanced by three factors:

1. The basement membrane is attached by fibres to the surrounding connective tissues so that any tissue swelling opens and holds patent the vessels.
2. Lymphatic vessels in the lungs, like those elsewhere, are actively pulsatile. This pulsatility, together with endolymphatic valves, forms an active pumping system.
3. Lung movements, working in conjunction with the endolymphatic valves, form a second pumping system analogous to the muscle pump in the systemic lymphatic system.

Normally total lung lymph flow is less than 10 ml/h but, in diseases leading to increased transcapillary water filtration, lymph flow may increase several fold, as in chronic venous pulmonary hypertension of mitral stenosis.

THE PULMONARY ENDOTHELIUM

When the pulmonary blood vessels are examined in section by simple light microscopy, so attenuated is the endothelial cell cytoplasm that the very existence of the cells is inferred largely from identification of the nuclei, which bulge into the vessel lumen. However, scanning and transmission electron microscopy, together with such specialized techniques as freeze fracture, reveal a complex system of endothelial cells that has many more functions than merely acting as a barrier.

The surface of the cells is covered by a thin glycocalyx composed of glycoproteins and glycolipids, which is locally interrupted by thin membranes covering the openings of the plasmalemmal vesicles. The endothelium when viewed from the surface shows a 'cobble-stone' appearance as a result of the intraluminal bulging of the nuclei but, at a more detailed level, this surface is shaggy with numerous irregular cytoplasmic projections, which frequently fuse to give a network of finger-like projections. It has been surmised that these produce locally turbulent flow and thereby facilitate metabolic and transport functions of the endothelial cells.

The endothelial cell cytoplasm contains a variety of organelles in addition to the usual nucleus and mitochondria. These include rough endoplasm reticulum, microtubules, microfilaments, 'rod-shaped organelles', and micropinocytotic vesicles. In addition, there are caveolae intracellulares, which may be micropinocytotic vesicles at the stage where they are still adherent to the cell membrane and opening into the lumen of the vessel.

The extent of intracellular organelles varies systematically through the pulmonary circulation. Organelles are few in the capillary endothelial cells but are found in considerably greater numbers in both the arteriolar and venular vessels.

Pulmonary endothelial cells are joined by 'tight' junctions which consist of continuous interconnected rows of particle-to-groove adherences. There are also numerous 'gap' junctions—both between endothelial cells and occasionally between endothelial and smooth muscle cells—allowing cell to cell communication. As in the case of intracellular organelles, there are considerable quantitative differences between junctions at the capillary, venular and arteriolar levels. In the arterial circulation the tight junctions usually consist of two to six rows of adherences and there are few gap junctions. In the capillaries there are rarely more than three rows of tight junction particles and no gap junctions. In the venous endothelium the number of particle rows are similar to the arterial but gap junctions are few.

NERVE SUPPLY OF THE PULMONARY BLOOD VESSELS

The arterial system, but not the venous system, is adequately supplied with sympathetic (adrenergic) and parasympathetic (cholinergic) fibres. The innervation is highest in the elastic arteries and diminishes towards the periphery, and this has been interpreted as suggesting that neural control is of vessel stiffness rather than of resistance. Peptidenergic fibres (non-adrenergic, non-cholinergic; NANC) are also present but their role is unknown. In spite of this, the normal lung circulation has low inherent reflex vasomotor activity.

Biological functions of the pulmonary endothelium

METABOLIC FUNCTIONS

The pulmonary endothelial cells possess carbonic anhydrase as a surface enzyme and this probably plays a minor part in carbon dioxide transport. However, more important, as long ago as 1969, Vane pointed out that the strategic position of the pulmonary circulation, its exposure to the whole of the cardiac output and its extensive surface area gave it the opportunity to exert a powerful effect upon the composition of blood entering the systemic circulation.

One of the most important functions may be the continuous provision of a major substrate for regulation and maintenance of systemic blood pressure—pulmonary endothelial cells form a huge area of tissue containing angiotensin converting enzyme, which hydrolyses the inactive circulating decapeptide angiotensin I to the highly vasoconstrictive octapeptide angiotensin II. In contrast, the vasoactive peptide bradykinin is removed from the blood by the pulmonary endothelium—to the extent of 80 per cent during each passage.

The role of the endothelium in the disposal of circulating vasoactive amines is important, and all cells have the capacity rapidly to take up, by active sodium carrier linked cotransport, the vasoactive biogenic amines 5-hydroxytryptamine and noradrenaline. Adrenaline, a circulating hormone, is not taken up, nor are histamine or dopamine. The absorbed amines are broken down by catechol-O-methyl-transferase (COMT).

The endothelium has phosphohydrolytic activity for the adenine nucleotides, adenine triphosphate (ATP), adenine monophosphate (AMP), and adenine diphosphate (ADP). So rapid is the metabolism that when a tritiated nucleotide and an intravascular dye, such as blue dextran, are injected simultaneously into the pulmonary artery, the washout curves of radioactivity and dye are indistinguishable—despite the fact that the phosphorylated nucleotide has been 90 per cent converted to adenosine. The site of the 5-nucleotidase appears to be the caveolae intracellulares of the endothelial cells.

Carboxypeptidase N (synonyms: kininase I, sereine carboxypeptidase

B, anaphylotoxin inactivator A) is distributed widely over the luminal endothelial surface and has the capacity to cleave the C-terminal basic amino acids of kinins—anaphylotoxins, fibrinopeptides, and enkephalins. This activity suggests a considerable endothelial potential for regulating and modulating inflammatory reactions within the lung in diseases such as Adult Respiratory Distress Syndrome and disseminated intravascular coagulation.

Pulmonary endothelial cells have the ability to produce, release, transport, and degrade a number of eicosanoids. This may allow a powerful regulatory function over vascular resistance, endothelial permeability, and endothelial adhesiveness. The most clearly identified activity is the production (from endogenous arachidonic acid) and release (in response to shear stress) of the strongly vasodilator prostaglandin I_2 (prostacyclin, PGI_2). The production of other arachidonic acid derivatives is less certain, although there is evidence for the synthesis of 11, 12, and 15, hydroxyeicosotetraenoic acids (HETEs), and this could be a method of inhibiting neutrophil leukotriene production while these cells are adhering to the endothelium. Carrier-mediated uptake and selective degradation of the prostaglandins of the D, E, and F series by pulmonary endothelium is documented but its role is unknown.

ENDOTHELIAL–VASCULAR SMOOTH MUSCLE INTERACTIONS—AMPLIFICATION AND MODULATION OF STIMULI

Acetylcholine, substance P, bradykinin, Ca^{2+}-ionophore, and arachidonic acid all relax a precontracted isolated pulmonary artery, provided the endothelium is intact. If the endothelium has been ablated, the effect is abolished. The responsible mediator—endothelium-derived relaxation factor (EDRF)—which may be involved in hypoxic pulmonary vasoconstriction, is probably identical to that in the systemic circulation and one of its components is likely to be nitric oxide.

Another product is the vasoconstrictor peptide endothelin. As its production can be stimulated by hypoxia it too could be a mediator of hypoxic constriction.

Prostaglandin I_2 (PGI_2) produced by the pulmonary endothelium is a powerful vasodilator of constricted pulmonary smooth muscle and is liberated in response to shear stress applied to endothelial cells. A feedback role in control could easily be envisaged. On the other hand, any role for another endothelial eicosanoid product—platelet activating factor (PAF)—remains obscure. It can act as a pulmonary vasodiator but although it is produced by systemic endothelial cells its production by pulmonary endothelium is uncertain.

In summary, although it is probable that pulmonary endothelium has a pivotal role in instigating, modulating, and controlling pulmonary vasomotor activity the overall pattern is, as yet, far from clear.

CELLULAR ADHESION PROPERTIES OF THE ENDOTHELIUM—MODULATION OF THE INFLAMMATORY PROCESS

Pulmonary endothelial cells have specific receptors that allow the direct adhesion of white cells. Both the selectins and the intracellular adhesion molecules (ICAMs) of the immunoglobulin superfamily are present.

Both E-selectin (CD62) and P-selectin (ELAM-1) are on the endothelial surface and, by interaction with the L-selectin of the leucocyte, allow immediate capture of rolling neutrophils from flowing blood. The intracellular adhesion molecule endothelial receptors subsequently react with the neutrophil integrins (CD11/CD18) to stabilize the captured cell and to promote migration through the endothelium.

The expression of endothelial adhesion molecules can be altered. Intracellular adhesion molecule expression is increased by interleukin 1, and upregulation occurs during inflammation. Conversely, selectins are probably downregulated once the inflammatory process has started.

Neutrophil adhesion and interaction with the endothelium may also be promoted indirectly. Such indirect action is modulated by the endothelial receptors for C1q (a component of the macromolecular first component of complement). C1q is bound to endothelial cells by a saturable, concentration-dependent mechanism that binds the collagenous tail and leaves free the immunoglobulin G (IgG) binding areas to promote both adhesion and binding of immune complexes, and to promote but localize complement activation. The pulmonary endothelial cells probably do not express receptors for the anaphylotoxins (complement) C5A and C3A constitutionally but C3b receptors do appear after the cells have been injured.

ANTI- AND PROCOAGULANT ACTIVITY OF THE ENDOTHELIUM

Intact, healthy endothelium does not support blood clotting. This observation originally led to the idea that the endothelium was largely an inert layer separating the clotting mechanism of blood from the coagulation activators of the subendothelial tissues. However, the endothelium has a more active role and can express both anticoagulant and procoagulant function.

Under normal conditions the anticoagulant functions predominate and pulmonary endothelial cells possess marked fibrinolytic activity due to their ability to secrete plasminogen activators. These are narrow-spectrum serum proteases, which cleave the plasma protein plasminogen to yield the broad-spectrum protease, plasmin. If, as has been surmised, the pulmonary circulation acts as a filter for small thromoemboli formed continually in the systemic venous circulation, this lytic function would be a defence against inappropriate local coagulation and preventing microvascular occlusion and damage.

Exposure of endothelial cells to endotoxin or to interleukin-1 changes the situation considerably, so that procoagulant activity is expressed. This is due to increased synthesis of thromboplastin (synonyms: tissue factor, factor III), which can initiate coagulation by either the intrinsic or extrinsic pathways. At the endothelial surface, the former is probably the more important and conversion of factor IX to activated IXa occurs.

RETICULOENDOTHELIAL AND PHAGOCYTIC FUNCTION WITHIN THE PULMONARY CIRCULATION

Pulmonary intravascular macrophages (PIMs) are recently identified cells of the reticuloendothelial system. They are distinct from circulating blood monocytes and they reside in the lung where they are adherent to the alveolar capillaries. They are anchored by specialized adhesion plaques and they phagocytose both cellular and non-cellular matter. Both lipoxygenase and cyclo-oxygenase products are produced when the cells are exposed to ionophore and these cells may be the major source of pulmonary thromboxane, which has vasoconstrictor effects in addition to any role in modulation of clotting. Other appropriate functions such as antigen presentation have not yet been documented.

It is possible that endothelial cells themselves also have some phagocytic capacity. This can certainly be shown in tissue culture where endothelial cells have been shown to phagocytose both inert particulate matter and bacteria. Bacterial uptake is mediated by C1q receptors and leads to a respiratory burst and subsequent expression of fragment, crystallizable (Fc) receptors. However the significance of these *in vitro* observations remains unknown.

Circulatory dynamics

PRESSURES, VOLUMES, AND RESISTANCE IN THE PULMONARY CIRCULATION

The pulmonary circulation receives the entire output from the right ventricle. In the adult this ranges from 5 to 8 l/min at rest up to 25 to 30 l/min during exercise. Despite the large blood flow, the system operates at a low pressure of approximately one-fifth that of the systemic pressure because the pulmonary vascular resistance is itself low (Table 1).

Table 1 *The pulmonary circulation: representative normal adult values*

Intrapulmonary blood volume	900 ml
Pulmonary capillary blood volume	100–200 ml
Pulmonary artery pressure	25/15 mmHg
Pulmonary capillary pressure*	7 mmHg
Pulmonary vascular resistance**	20–120 dyne/s/cm⁵
	1–4 mmHg/l/min
Pulmonary venous pressure	5 mmHg

*Calculated value for the midpoint of the upright lung.

**There is considerable debate as to what units should be used to measure pulmonary vascular resistance. Dynes have largely dropped out of scientific use. The appropriate SI unit – $N/s/m^5$ – does not seem to have become accepted. The original units of mmHg/l/min have the advantage of emphasizing that resistance is a derived variable relating pressure and flow.

The longitudinal distribution of pressure within the pulmonary circulation differs from the systemic bed, where the arterioles are the major resistance vessels. In the lungs, resistance is fairly evenly distributed. Probably about 40 per cent lies in the arteries and arterioles with further 40 per cent and 20 per cent contributions from capillaries and veins, respectively. This distribution of resistance suggests a fairly even pressure drop throughout the system. Calculations give a mean capillary pressure of about 7 mmHg at the midpoint of the upright lung.

The amount of blood in the pulmonary circulation is important because variations in its volume may influence venous return to the left heart, efficiency of gas exchange, and the mechanical behaviour of the lungs. Furthermore, the vertical distribution of the volume of blood in the upright lung is responsible for the characteristic radiological appearances in health and disease. The normal pulmonary blood volume between the pulmonary valve and left atrium is approximately 900 ml, of which only 150 to 200 ml are in the gas-exchanging lung capillaries. However, the distensibility of the pulmonary circulation and its reserve unperfused capacity in the upright position is such that the central blood volume may increase by as much as 500 ml when changing from the upright to the lying position. This may be of little consequence in health but, when the pulmonary vascular pressures become elevated by heart failure, the shift may cause further pressure rise and precipitate pulmonary oedema.

When upright, the distribution of blood volume in the lung increases vertically from apex to base. This parallels the regional distribution of blood flow which shows an eight-fold increase from top to bottom of the lungs (see below). Ventilation is also heterogeneous—increasing from top to bottom of the lungs but less steeply than does blood flow. Both the distribution of ventilation and of blood flow are partly determined by the anchorage of the blood vessels at the hilum, as well as by gravitational effects. Because of gravity, lower regions are relatively compressed by the weight of lung above them. In the upright position, vessel diameters increase from the top to the bottom of the lung as a result of gravitational increase in hydrostatic pressure unopposed by any baroregulatory mechanism.

The obstacle to blood flow presented by the pulmonary circulation is usually quantified as the pulmonary vascular resistance. Resistance is a concept derived from the rheology of laminar, non-pulsatile flow of a Newtonian liquid in tubes of invariant dimension, which are relatively long in relation to their cross-sectional area. In the lung, flow is pulsatile, frequently turbulent, and, in relation to the dimensions of the capillary bed, the particulate nature of blood makes its behaviour far from Newtonian. So, use of this term in the pulmonary circulation is a gross simplification but it is practically useful—particularly in conditions such as pulmonary hypertension where the high pressures make the errors arising from simplification less significant. The calculation of vascular impedance is a more correct theoretical approach but its greater complexity limits its usefulness.

Pulmonary vascular resistance is calculated as the pressure drop between the pulmonary artery and left atrium divided by the blood flow:

$$R = (P_{pa} - P_{la})/Q$$

where P_{pa} is the mean pulmonary artery pressure, Q is pulmonary blood flow, R is the pulmonary vascular resistance, and P_{la} is the mean left atrial pressure, although this is not usually measured directly. More usually, the pulmonary wedge pressure is measured by advancing a catheter into the circulation until it 'wedges' in a small artery. This wedging occludes blood flow in the vascular segment and, provided the catheter is in a part of the lung which is in a zone 3 condition (see below), produces a static column of fluid from the tip of the catheter to the pulmonary veins. Under these conditions the 'wedge' pressure is a measure of pulmonary venous pressure. Approximate normal values for pulmonary vascular resistance in adult humans at rest are 1 to 4 mmHg/l/min.

THE FACTORS DETERMINING BLOOD FLOW THROUGH AND WITHIN THE PULMONARY CIRCULATION (TABLE 2)

Because the lung blood vessels are so frugally supplied with smooth muscle, pulmonary arterial resistance to blood flow is low and vasomotion is relatively weak. The distribution of blood to the capillary bed and its variation are thus largely determined by passive factors and as we shall see, these can explain the following:

1. Perfusion varies systematically from region to region within the lung. This phenomenon is a reflection of the interaction between the low hydrostatic pressure in the pulmonary circulation and the physical dimensions of the human lung – particularly in the upright position.
2. Pulmonary vascular resistance varies with lung volume and in phase with respiration.
3. The pulmonary circulation can permit great changes in total blood flow with little change in inflow pressure.
4. Changes in central venous return – from such factors as posture – change right ventricular output and alter the quantity of blood and mean pressure in the pulmonary vessels.
5. Flow in pulmonary capillaries is pulsatile.
6. Flow in pulmonary veins is also pulsatile but whereas, *in vivo*, the wave form at the capillary end is in phase with the capillary pulse, at the atrial end this is not so.

Although passive changes dominate the pulmonary circulation, active regulation does play an important part and it is local vasomotion, induced by hypoxia and hypercapnoea in the smaller divisions, of the pulmonary circulation, which allows each small region of the lung to achieve an optimal ventilation/perfusion balance. On the other hand, whereas a large number of humoral and neural factors are known to affect the overall pulmonary vascular resistance – both *in vivo* and under experimental conditions – so far, no coherent homeostatic role has emerged.

Passive changes and adaptations in the pulmonary circulation

REGIONAL PRESSURE-FLOW RELATIONSHIPS: THE BEHAVIOUR OF THE PULMONARY ARTERIAL AND ALVEOLAR CAPILLARY SYSTEMS

Flow, per unit volume of the upright, resting lung is about eight times greater at the base than at the apex, which is barely perfused at all. There is also a second, independent distribution of blood flow in which flow diminishes with distance from the hilum.

The mechanism of inhomogeneous vertical flow distribution depends upon the pulmonary microvessels behaving as a vertical stack of 'Star-

Table 2 *Major factors affecting lung capillary blood flow*

Physical factors		
Pulmonary arteries	Compliance × resistance = $K(t)$	Stabilize capillary inflow conditions over wide pulmonary arterial pressure range
Capillary relationships	'Waterfall effect' Gravity-dependent and centrifugal zones with added 'tidal' effects	Hydrostatic capillary recruitment regulates pulmonary arterial pressure and allows optimal capillary gas exchange
Pulmonary veins intraparenchymal veins large extraparenchymal veins	Behaviour still obscure Indistensible but collapsible – combined capacity equivalent to right ventricular stroke volume	Lung capillaries 'decoupled' from left atrium Pulsatile capillary flow preserved 'Venous reservoir' provided for left heart
Chemical and reflex responses		
Hypoxia, hypercapnia, pH	Local action	Powerful peripheral hypoxic arteriolar vasoconstriction homoeostatic control of ventilation/perfusion Less active in large pulmonary arteries
Neurological	Reflex action	Weak peripheral constriction More powerful constriction of larger arteries – homeostatic role not known

ling resistors' within the lung (Fig. 5). A Starling resistor is a thin-walled collapsible tube through which fluid flows, and which is surrounded by a pressure reservoir. In the lung, the pressure reservoir is the alveoli. The collapsible tubes are the capillaries. Their arteriolar inflow and venular outflow pressures are determined by the pressures in the pulmonary artery and left atrium, respectively, minus the gravitational hydrostatic pressure caused by the vertical height of the resistor above the pulmonary valve and left atrial ostium.

The height of the vertical human lung is approximately 30 cm. Normally, pressure in the pulmonary outflow tract rises to approximately 30 cmH$_2$O only during the peak of systole. Thus, at the very top of the lung in normal erect humans (West: zone 1) the reservoir pressure (alveolar pressure) will be atmospheric, but its vascular inflow pressure will only approach this level for a brief period during systole. Venular outflow pressure in zone 1 will be subatmospheric throughout the cardiac cycle because the normal left atrial pressure rarely exceeds 12 to 15 cmH$_2$O. Thus, under resting conditions in zone 1, there is little or no blood flow through the lung capillaries except during part of systole.

Further down the lung (West: zone 2) arterial pressure will be greater than alveolar pressure (which is again atmospheric) but alveolar pressure

will still be greater than venous pressure. Under these conditions flow is determined by the difference between alveolar and arterial pressure, and not by the arterial to venous pressure difference. As the mean vascular pressures increase progressively down the zone while the alveolar pressure remains constant, there is a steady increase in perfused capillary volume as well as total blood flow down zone 2.

In zone 3, both the arterial and the venous pressures are greater than alveolar pressure and each is augmented by the same gravitational amount as the zone is descended. In zone 3 all capillary systems are recruited for perfusion because their intracapillary hydrostatic pressure exceeds alveolar pressure. The rate of blood flow through the region depends on the mean arteriovenous pressure difference, modulated in a pulsatile fashion throughout the cardiac cycle as a result of the pressure events taking place in the right ventricle. A small increase both in regional perfusion volume and flow occurs with descent through the zone, probably because of a gravitational increase in overall hydrostatic pressure in vessels below the heart, which in turn causes their distension, thereby lowering resistance to flow.

There is probably a fourth zone (zone 4) at the extreme base of the lungs where regional blood flow diminishes despite the continued rise

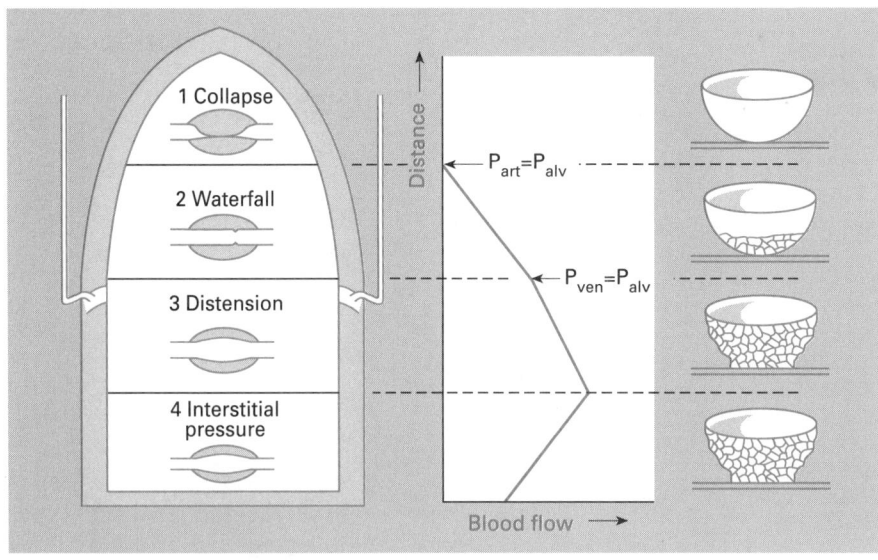

Fig. 5 The upright human lung as a vertically stacked pile of 'Starling resistors'. In zone 1 there is no blood flow (except through 'angular' vessels) because alveolar pressure is greater than both arterial and venous pressure. In zone 2, arterial pressure is greater than alveolar pressure which in turn exceeds venous pressure. Here flow is determined by the arterial–alveolar pressure difference and increases progressively as the lung is distended. In zone 3 both arterial and venous pressures are greater than alveolar pressure, so that flow is determined by arterial–venous pressure difference. This is constant and independent of height so that the increase in flow may be due to increasing calibre of the vessels as pressure within distends them. There is some doubt about the existence of zone 4 where flow may be restricted by perivascular cuffing. On the right is indicated the pattern of alveolar perfusion within each zone. (After Fishman). In zone 3 the natural inflation of the lung leads to the alveolar wall being undulated and not pleated; all alveolar capillaries are open and their cross-sections have rounded profiles. In zone 2 there is some pleating of the alveolar wall and there are patches of completely closed capillaries. In zone 1 there is considerable pleating of the alveolae and no blood flow apart from that through the angular capillaries.

in intravascular pressure. One explanation of this has been that the perialveolar interstitium in the lowermost areas is subject to greater hydrostatic transcapillary fluid transfer than elsewhere. The resulting reduction in interstitial distensibility could increase capillary vascular resistance in the area. An alternative possibility is that it results from the superimposition of a hilar–fugal gradient upon the vertical one. In the hilar–fugal gradient, blood flow decreases with distance from the hila – probably as a result of increasing vascular resistance offered by progressively longer vascular paths.

THE PULMONARY CIRCULATION IN EXERCISE AND POSTURAL CHANGE

Pulmonary arterial pressures increase surprisingly little when the cardiac output rises with exercise (Fig. 6). This is usually taken to mean that pulmonary vascular resistance decreases as flow goes up although, because of the uncertainty introduced by using a steady-flow measure to describe a pulsatile system, the point has been disputed.

The limitation of arterial pressure rise minimizes the work of the right ventricle. It results from the gravitationally determined gradient of perfusion, which gives unused capacity in the apical parts of the vascular bed at rest. As pulmonary artery pressure tends to rise with exercise there is increasing vertical recruitment from base to apex, accompanied by increasing evenness of blood flow throughout the lung. As a result, pressures rise much less than would have been the case if the system had maintained a fixed volume. However, once recruitment is complete, further increase in pulmonary blood flow will then be accompanied by a rise in arterial pressure.

Alveolar capillary recruitment augments the available capillary surface for gas exchange, so diffusing capacity increases. It also preserves optimal kinetics for gas exchange for, despite the overall increase in blood flow, red cell velocity through individual units remains remarkably constant.

In a normal individual, a change from standing to lying causes an increase in pulmonary blood volume of up to 500 ml. The mechanism is as follows. Hydrostatic factors increase central venous pressure (CVP) directly and this increase is sustained by fluid mobilisation from the periphery. Raised central venous pressure increases right ventricular end diastolic volume and stroke volume. But an increase in left ventricular stroke output can only occur after the increased intrapulmonary blood

volume has led, through small increases in pressure, to increased pulmonary venous pressure. Until the Starling mechanism has brought the outputs of the two ventricles back into balance intrapulmonary blood volume continues to increase.

PULMONARY CAPILLARY BLOOD FLOW: THE NATURE OF ITS PULSATILITY

The physical behaviour of the pulmonary arterial and alveolar capillary systems together determine that lung capillary blood flow is pulsatile. This has been demonstrated by study of gas exchange, both in the lying and upright positions, using body plesythmography (Fig. 7). In the upright position this pulsatile flow interacts with the normal vertical gradient in an interesting way. During peak ejection by the right ventricle, the systolic input pressure from the pulmonary artery to the capillaries will temporarily exceed the alveolar gas pressure in all lung zones. As a result, capillaries from the bottom to the top of the lungs will accommodate flowing blood. When diastole ensues, the pulmonary arterial pressure and blood flow velocity both begin to fall, so blood flow will first cease in the uppermost alveolar capillary systems as the input pressure from the pulmonary artery to the capillaries drops below alveolar gas pressure in that zone. Only in the more dependent parts of the lung where both pulmonary arterial and venous pressures exceed alveolar gas pressure will the capillaries continue to conduct at a rate determined by the arteriovenous pressure difference between them. Thus, during each cardiac cycle, a tidal rise and fall of distributed blood flow takes place up and down the lungs during systole and diastole respectively.

Pulsatile capillary blood flow persists even in arterial hypertension. This is surprising because the rise in pulmonary arteriolar resistance might have been expected to damp out such pulsation. However, when the pulmonary arterial resistance (R) rises, there is a reciprocal fall in compliance (C) proximal to the site of increased resistance. As a result, the time constant (kt) of the arterial system as a whole remains constant ($R \times C = kt$) so that lung capillary flow pulsatility is largely unaffected.

Fig. 7 The effect of pulsatile lung capillary flow upon oxygen and carbon dioxide exchange. Pulmonary capillary blood flow, estimated from the rate of N_2O uptake, is compared with the rate of flow of O_2 into and CO_2 out of the lungs, measured by the body plethysmograph. (Reproduced from Bosman *et al.* (1965). *Clinical Science,* **28,** 295–300, with permission).

Fig. 6 Pressure flow curves from exercising humans. The pressure gradient across the pulmonary vasculature (mean pulmonary arterial pressure (P_{pa}) minus the mean wedge pressure (P_{pw}) is plotted against cardiac output (Q). Cardiac output was varied by exercise. In these normal subjects the pressure flow curve is quite flat (from Ekelund and Holmgren (1987). *Circulation Research,* **20,** 1–33, with permission).

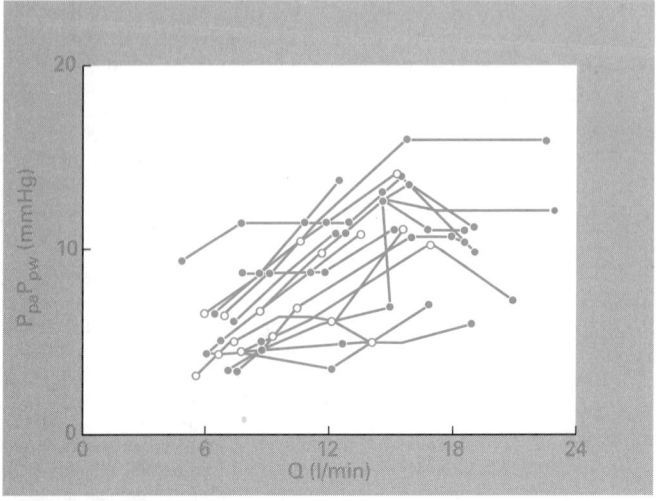

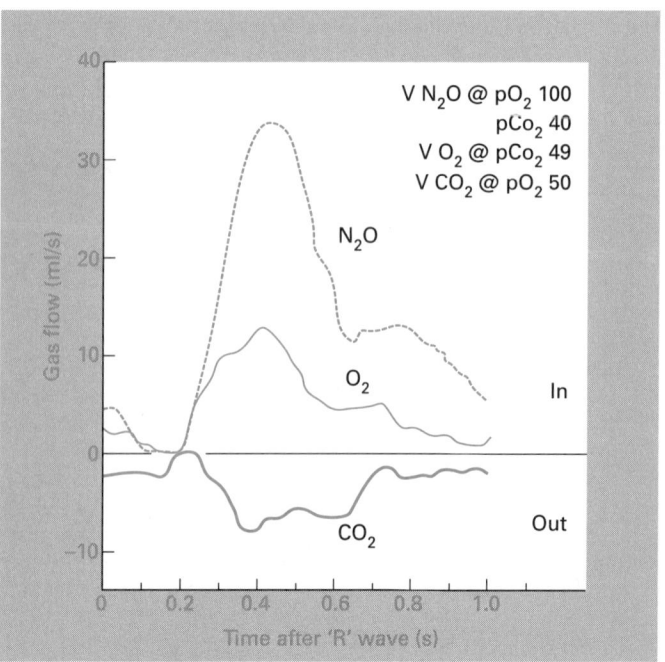

THE ROLE OF THE PULMONARY VEINS

The pulmonary venous system is 'designed' to protect the autonomy of lung capillary blood flow from pressure perturbations from the left atrium despite the absence of valves in the pulmonary veins. Lung capillary pulsatility remains unchanged, even when large pressure transients are generated in the left atrium for example, from cannon waves in complete heart block.

When blood flow is measured in the large pulmonary veins outside the lungs near the left atrium it is found to be pulsatile, but its pattern is different from that in the capillaries; its wave form is virtually a mirror image of left atrial pressure. However, when pulmonary vein flow is isolated from the left atrium, its wave form resembles the capillary flow pulse. These observations might suggest that some component of the pulmonary venous system is highly compliant, so that it can absorb left atrial pressure waves and prevent them from reaching the lung capillaries. However, human postmortem studies reveal that the pulmonary veins are largely indistensible and non-compliant. Instead, the large extraparenchymal pulmonary veins, lying in the loose areolar tissue of the mediastinum, are highly collapsible and their cross-section changes

from a cylindrical, fully filled shape to one of complete collapse over a narrow pressure range (Fig. 8). Their combined volume, when full, is about the same as one stroke volume of the heart.

The extraparenchymal pulmonary veins thus provide a variable volume reservoir that decouples venous outflow from the lungs from left atrial events and allows preservation of capillary pulsatility. At normal left atrial pressures, during ventricular systole, the veins collapse as they empty into the left atrium. As left atrial pressure rises, particularly during the 'a' and 'v' waves, the veins refill and their cross-sectional dimensions become circular once more (Fig. 9). These events take place from 0 to 16 mmHg transmural pressure. Thereafter the veins are capable of only slight distension.

Within the lungs themselves, the behaviour of the veins connecting the capillary bed to the large extraparenchymal pulmonary veins remains obscure. However, their histology suggests that they have relatively little distensibility so they probably add little further protection to capillary outflow.

Fig. 8 (a) Stress–strain relationships obtained from circumferential strips of human pulmonary artery and pulmonary vein, postmortem. The pulmonary artery is highly distensible. The pulmonary vein is virtually inelastic. (Reproduced from Banks *et al.* (1978). *Clinical Science*, **55**, 477–81, with permission). (b) Schematic diagram showing how the extraparenchymal pulmonary veins behave as collapsible tubes whose cross-sectional dimensions change over a narrow range of transmural pressure.

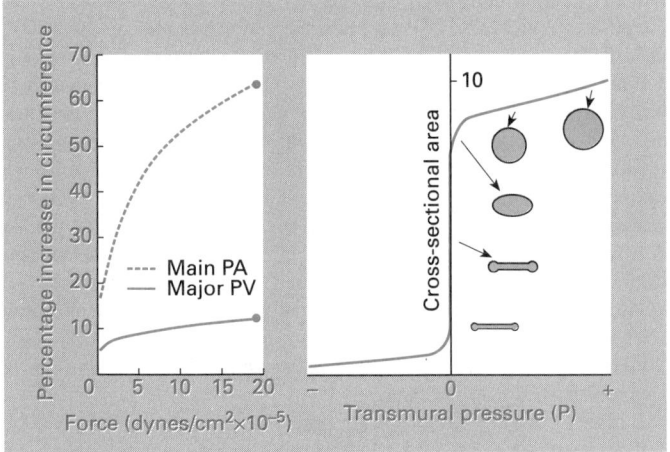

Vasomotor activity in the pulmonary circulation

LOCAL VASOMOTOR EFFECTS: HYPOXIC PULMONARY VASOCONSTRICTION (SEE CHAPTER 15.25)

The pulmonary circulation differs from the systemic in its physiological reaction to hypoxia. Whereas systemic vascular beds dilate, the pulmonary circulation constricts. This is the most clearly documented vasomotor activity of the pulmonary circulation, and the only one for which a homeostatic role has been demonstrated. It consists of the vasoconstriction of small muscular arteries and arterioles in response to local hypoxia and is a mechanism for fine tuning ventilation/perfusion balance at the infundibular level, and possibly even within the infundibulum, at the alveolar level (Fig. 10). An additional role is the redistribution of blood flow away from locally diseased areas of the lung to more normal areas for gas exchange as in centrilobular emphysema or lobar pneumonia.

Although the phenomenon was first clearly demonstrated as long ago as 1946 by von Euler and Lillestrand who showed a vasoconstrictive reaction of whole lung to hypoxia, the mechanism has so far eluded description. The reaction occurs at every level of progressive subdivision of the lung and is always locally confined. It is independent of an intact nervous system and, in experimental studies, of the perfusing fluid. At the level of the smooth muscle, the contraction appears to be associated with membrane depolarization, increased intracellular con-

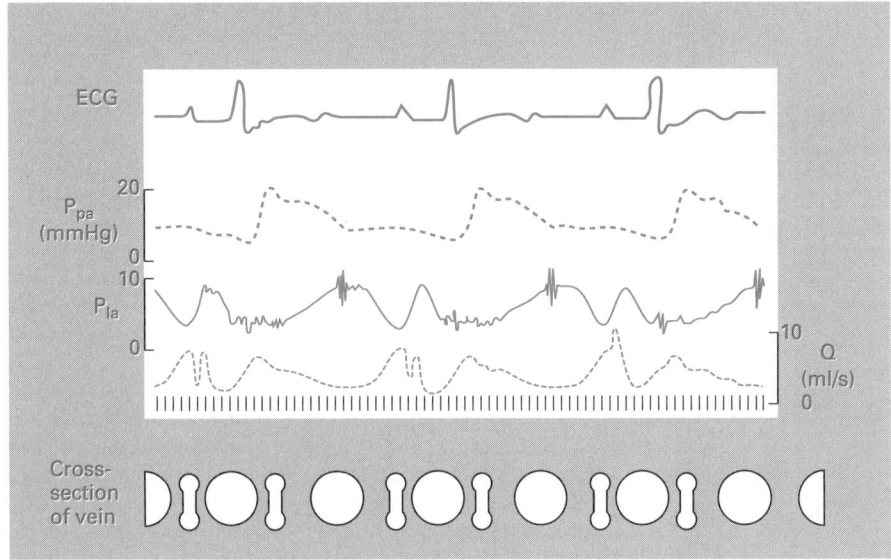

Fig. 9 The pulmonary veins. The relationship between pulmonary artery pressure (P_{pa}), left atrial pressure (P_{la}), pulmonary venous outflow (Q) and pulmonary venous distension in the dog. Note that the left atrial pressure events dominate Q; when P_{la} is high Q is low and *vice versa*; pulmonary veins are distended at high P_{la} and collapsed at low P_{la}. However, despite this relationship pulmonary capillary pulsatility does not follow pressure events in the left atrium (see text) (from Rajagopalan *et al.* (1979). *Cardiovascular Research*, **13**, 684–92, with permission).

centrations of calcium ions, and increased intracellular cyclic guanidine triphosphate (cGTP) levels. Four possible mechanisms – none of which are mutually exclusive – have been investigated as possible links between the initiating local hypoxia and the final events in the contracting smooth muscle:

1. Direct action upon smooth muscle – possibly modulated through conformational change of an oxygen sensitive molecular receptor leading, through depression of a calcium ion-dependent potassium channel, subsequent membrane depolarization, and calcium ion entry into the cell, to contraction.

2. Extravascular release of mediators. Over many years, mast cells, neuroepithelial bodies, and autonomic nerve endings have all been proposed and the suggested mediators have included histamine, serotonin, and eicosanoids, but none has been substantiated and this hypothesis is not now greatly favoured.

3. Mediators released from the endothelium. In experiments, hypoxia has been shown to reduce the endothelial liberation of endothelium derived relaxant factor. If it could be shown that continuous production of an endothelium derived relaxant factor (EDRF) were responsible for maintaining the normoxic pulmonary arteriolar system in sustained relaxation, hypoxic pulmonary vasoconstriction could result from the suppression of its secretion leading to reduction in small vessel calibre. However, hypoxia has also been shown to stimulate the production of the vasoconstrictor peptide endothelin and, from this observation, an alternative hypothesis could be constructed. The two local mediators could, of course, act in a coupled fashion and only further experiments will confirm or refute the suggestion.

4. Direct endothelial to smooth muscle communication through gap junctions is a worthwhile suggestion but has, as yet, no experimental support.

GENERAL VASOMOTOR EFFECTS: REFLEX AND HUMORAL

Experimentally, many features of the pulmonary circulation make it technically difficult to demonstrate physiologically relevant vasomotor effects. These include very large species differences, the pulsatile nature of blood flow, the low hydrostatic pressure (causing both considerable 'noise' and the need for sensitive instruments), and the extent of confusion from passive responses. Additionally, there is little evidence of any resting vasoconstrictor tone in the pulmonary circulation so that, to identify vasodilators, preconstriction by various, probably unphysiological methods is usually necessary. Finally, recent data that demonstrate the modulatory effect of the endothelium in pharmacological effects, which were originally thought to affect smooth muscle directly, has added a further layer of confusion!

Fig. 10 Hypoxic pulmonary vasoconstriction as a homeostatic mechanism. At the alveolar or infundibular level ventilation perfusion balance (V_A/Q) is determined by alveolar ventilation (V_A) and blood flow (Q). V_AQ determines alveolar oxygen tension (P_AO_2) which in turn regulates local flow.

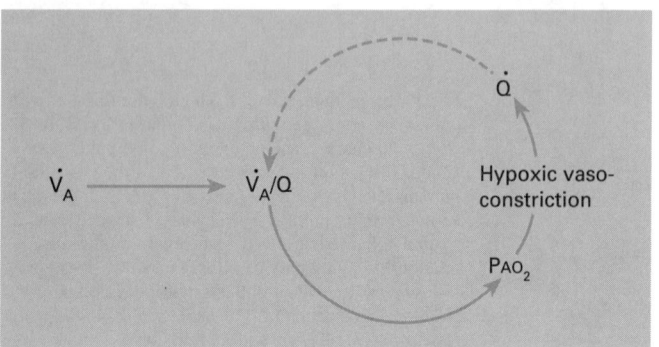

Despite the difficulties, a large number of factors have been identified which affect the overall pulmonary vascular resistance although, usually, the effects are small.

Activation of α-adrenoreceptors, whether by the sympathetic nervous system or by circulating catecholamines, appears to cause vasoconstriction. In contrast, activation of β-receptors, acetylcholine, and parasympathetic activity are vasodilator to preconstricted vessels. The 'classic' prostaglandins, PGF_2, PGE_2, and PGD_2, are all vasoconstrictor. By contrast, prostaglandin I_2 relaxes the constricted pulmonary circulation. Leukotrienes have weak vasoconstrictor effects of doubtful significance. Bradykinin, in contrast to its effect upon the systemic circulation, appears without effect in the pulmonary circulation. Angiotensin II is a pulmonary vasoconstrictor.

Direct stimulation of the sympathetic nerves can either increase or decrease pulmonary vascular resistance, depending upon the initial state of the vessels and whether an α or β effect predominates. Efferent vagal stimulation usually produces vasodilation in the constricted circulation and this is blocked by atropine. Interestingly, afferent stimulation of the cut vagus appears to cause increased pulmonary vascular resistance, but this potentially important phenomenon has received little attention. Stimulation of carotid baroreceptors, at least in dogs, causes pulmonary vasoconstriction but an effect from the aortic receptors has not been shown. Reflexes from the upper airways, possibly from chemoreceptors, seem to be vasoconstrictive, but the effects are not yet fully disentangled from the hypoxia that often occurs during these experiments. Stimulation of the aortic chemoreceptors appears to constrict pulmonary veins, while reactions from the carotid chemoreceptors are also constrictive, but to the pulmonary arterioles. Hypothalamic stimulation causes an increase in pulmonary vascular resistance, which is mediated via sympathetic pathways but, so far, no brain-stem centre analogous to the 'vasomotor centre' affecting the systemic circulation has been identified.

Despite this large number of effects upon the pulmonary circulation none, apart from hypoxic pulmonary vasoconstriction, has been shown to have a homoeostatic role. Even if we invoke teleology, it is difficult to see in what way generalized reactions would be helpful – unless it were an arterial constriction to 'protect' the alveolar capillary circulation during periods of high cardiac output and thereby to reduce the chances of development of pulmonary oedema.

Amongst vasoactive drugs, nitrates and inhaled nitric oxide appear to be the most potent in relaxing any existing pulmonary vasocontriction. Similar, but less powerful, effects have been noted with calcium channel antagonists such as nifedipine.

Figure 11 shows many of these interrelationships and indicates the active or passive nature of each. The peripheral pulmonary arteries and venules appear more sensitive to chemically induced vasomotion than to reflex effects, while the larger conducting radicals of the pulmonary arterial system appear to respond more to reflex stimulation than to hypoxia or catecholamines.

Transvascular and interstitial fluid dynamics

FLUID AND IONIC BALANCE AT THE ENDOTHELIAL AND EPITHELIAL SURFACES

The arterial and venous systems impart a largely autonomous fluid dynamic status upon the capillary gas exchange units, which form a gravity dependent, variable volume vascular bed largely independent of active vasomotor control.

Fluid exchange between the intravascular and interstitial compartments is determined by the balance of forces first described by Starling in 1896. The pressure for outward water filtration from the capillary results from the sum of its own hydrostatic pressure and the subatmospheric interstitial tissue pressure. This is almost, but not quite, balanced by the reabsorption pressure caused by the gradient of colloid osmotic pressure between interstitial fluid and interstitium. The small net excess pressure results in a continuous flux from capillary to interstitium which is balanced by removal as lymph by the lymphatics, pumping against an interstitial pressure which is normally subatmospheric and estimated to be in the order of − 7 mmHg (Fig. 12).

To sustain the system, the capillaries must be freely permeable to water and small ions but must present a significant barrier to plasma proteins, which generate oncotic pressure. Physiological studies show that this is so and electron microscopy demonstrates that the capillary endothelial cells are joined by discontinuous adhesions giving small aqueous pathways of macromolecular dimensions which join intravascular and interstitial spaces.

The negative interstitial hydrostatic pressure results from the chemical nature of the glycoproteins which make up most of the interstitial space.

These giant molecules, more than 10^6 Da in weight, contain large numbers of mucopolysaccharide chains, each of about 50 000 Da, bound to a central core of protein and hyaluronic acid. The side-chains are all strongly anionic and mutually repulsive. This mutual repulsion is translated into a hydraulic force by chemical interaction between water and the macromolecular side-chains so that the whole of the interstitial space may be likened to a sponge avid to imbibe water under conditions of deranged fluid balance.

The colloid osmotic pressure (oncotic pressure) of the interstitial fluid is high partly due to the transcapillary leak of plasma proteins and partly due to the influences of what has been termed the interstitial 'exclusion volume' for water. Analysis of interstitial fluid shows that its protein concentration is only about half what should be expected from oncotic

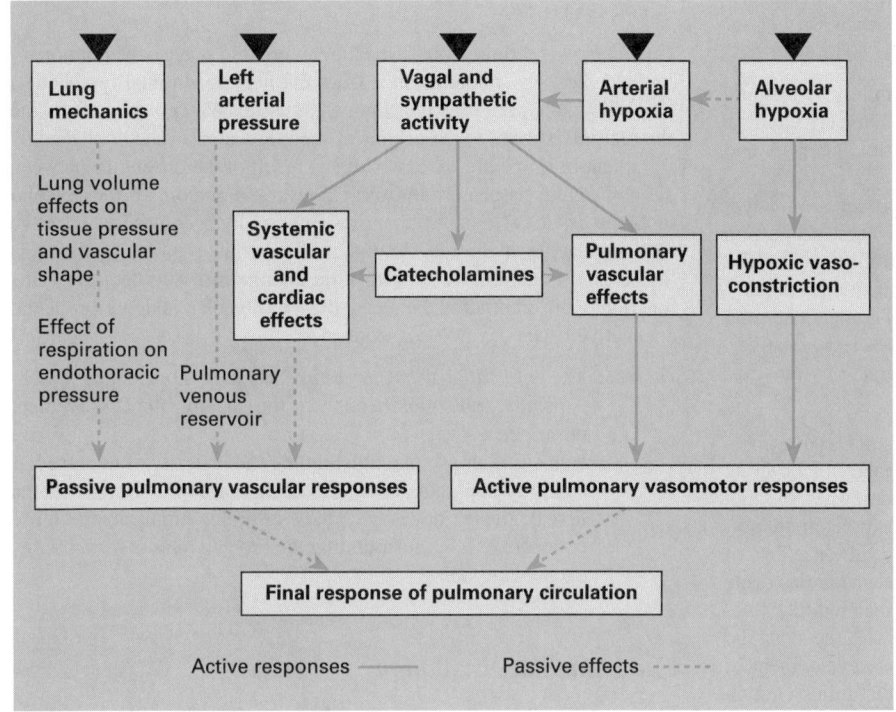

Fig. 11 Active and passive effects in the pulmonary circulation.

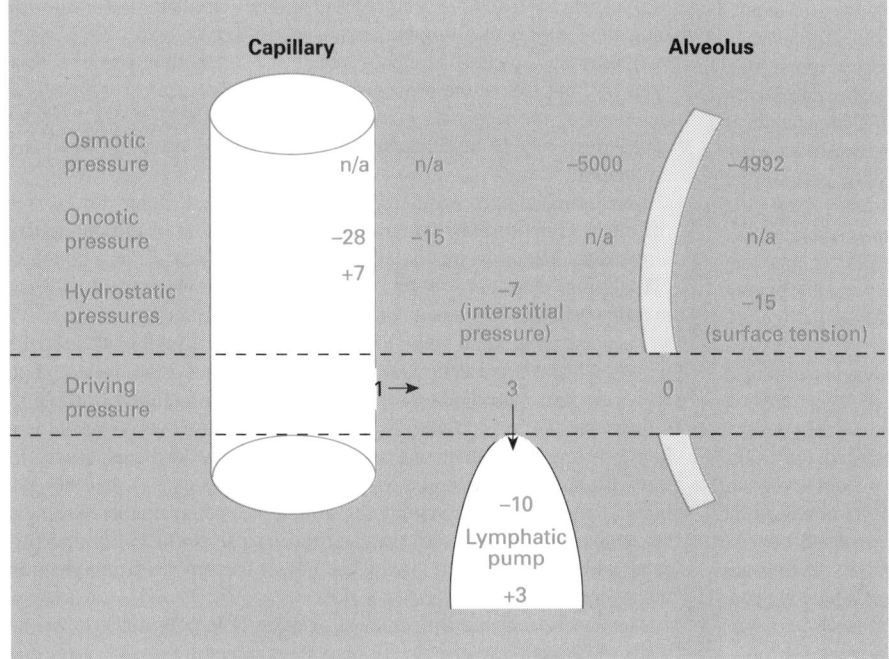

Fig. 12 Pressures causing fluid movements between lung water compartments (expressed as mmHg. n/a = non-applicable). The capillary endothelium is leaky to crystalloids but restricts the movement of macromolecules. Therefore only oncotic (colloid osmotic) pressure is exerted. The net pressure driving fluid into the interstitium is about 1 mmHg. The permeability of the alveolar membrane is much lower and movement of both colloids and crystalloids is restricted. Therefore true osmotic pressure can be exerted. The surface tension exerted by the alveolar fluid (probably about −15 mmHg) reflects both the acute radii of curvature at the alveolar angles and the effect of surfactant. The pressure causing water movement across the alveolar epithelium is probably very small as full humidification of the air phase has occurred higher up the respiratory tract. Interstitial pressure is subatmospheric but fluid can be removed from the interstitial space because the lymphatic system is actively pulsatile and has valves.

pressure estimations. This discrepancy can be explained if 50 per cent of the interstitial water has had protein 'excluded' from it because that water is entrapped within the confines of the mucopolysaccharide gel, whose interstices are too small to allow macromolecules, such as albumin, to enter.

The alveolar epithelium has tight junctions. It is largely impermeable to macromolecules, and even relatively small ions and molecules such as sodium and glucose cross relatively slowly. It can therefore act as a semipermeable membrane and crystalloids can exert osmotic pressure across it. The forces acting to maintain fluid balance are: surface tension of alveolar fluid; negative interstitial pressure; a small osmotic differential which balances the net hydrostatic pressure. Quantitative aspects are shown in Fig. 12.

Efficient gas exchange depends upon the alveolar capillary interstitium being capable of limiting increased inward wall flux and/or disposing of an increased water load without swelling whenever should capillary pressure rises. Four mechanisms enable this:

1. Macromolecular sieving. Increasing transcapillary hydrostatic pressure increases water flux but not protein permeability. Consequently, the ratio of water to protein flux increases and the interstitial fluid oncotic pressure falls.
2. Increased water entry into the interstitium produces a relative diminution of the 'excluded' volume. So a larger proportion of the interstitial water will be available to macromolecules and this will further reduce the interstitial oncotic pressure.
3. An increased interstitial water content raises the interstitial hydrostatic pressure, which therefore becomes less negative.
4. Lymph flow increases in response to the increase in transcapillary water flux.

Further protection against fluid overload of the interstitial space probably comes indirectly from the pulsatile nature of capillary blood flow. Because capillary blood flow is pulsatile, it is only during systole that high hydrostatic pressure can cause movement of osmotic fluid outwards. During diastole hydrostatic pressure will fall so the net flux of water will be reversed. At rest, the diastolic period of each cardiac cycle is longer than the systolic, so the tendency will be to maintain the alveolar capillary interstitium in a dry state. With exercise, the diastolic period becomes shorter and shorter. This results in the development of a greater outward flux of water from capillary to interstitium. Though small in total volume, the alveolar interstitial gel is avid for water, as already explained. As the interstitium becomes charged with water the alveolar walls become turgid and less compliant. Strategically located within the interstitium at the corners of the alveoli are afferent vagal nerve endings, termed J (juxta-alveolar) receptors. These respond maximally when lung interstitial compliance is reduced; they excite breathlessness. As a result of the breathlessness, the individual stops exercising, the heart rate returns to normal, the duration of the diastolic period of the cardiac cycle once more exceeds that of the systolic period, fluid present in the alveolar interstitium returns to the capillaries, interstitial compliance returns to its resting state, and the sensation of breathlessness disappears. Normally the breathlessness of exercise occurs long before alveolar flooding takes place, although extreme exercise beyond the point of endurance can lead to acute pulmonary oedema, particularly at altitude.

Capillary pulsatility in the lung appears to have other benefits also. Its preservation in diseases leading to pulmonary venous hypertension, such as mitral stenosis or left ventricular dysfunction, imparts protection over and above that possible if steady flow conditions existed. For example, with mean pulmonary venous presure elevated to a level approaching plasma osmotic pressure (approximately 30 mmHg), provided the heart rate is within normal limits, there will still be a considerable period during diastole when the pulmonary venous and capillary hydrostatic pressures fall below the osmotic equilibrium level. Consequently, good therapeutic control of heart rate is an important requirement when managing patients liable to hydrostatic pulmonary oedema.

Diseases leading to pulmonary arterial hypertension do so as a result of medial hypertrophy in the peripheral arteries and arterioles leading to increased peripheral arterial resistance to blood flow into the capillaries. This effectively downregulates their mean hydrostatic pressure towards osmotic pressure level, or even lower. Details of these diseases will be found in subsequent chapters. However, as already explained, the concomitant reduction in pulmonary arterial compliance that accompanies the increased peripheral arterial resistance in such circumstances, effectively preserves pressure and flow pulsatility into the capillaries even at mean pulmonary arterial pressure levels as high as 70 mmHg, with the protective advantages regarding fluid homeostasis already described in the case of pulmonary venous hypertension.

FLUID MOVEMENTS WITHIN THE PULMONARY INTERSTITIUM

The major site of fluid input to the lung interstitial space – the pulmonary capillary bed – is some distance from the nearest terminal lymphatics, which lie in the peribronchial connective tissue. Water passage from the alveolar interstitium to the origins of the lymphatics is accomplished by a gradient of tissue pressure, which is a result of the difference between the connective tissues around the airways and alveoli. In the alveolar septa the tissue is 'tight', so that pressure rapidly becomes less negative with increasing hydration. In the peribronchial region the tissue is 'loose' and is able to swell with little change in tissue pressure. This functional differentiation between the perialveolar and peribronchial connective tissue has two consequences:

1. The interstitial tissue pressure becomes more negative centripetally, and this leads to the steady fluid movement described above.
2. It is a further provision defending the integrity of the alveolar capillary apparatus for gas exchange, for when lung oedema first begins to develop it does so preferentially in the loose connective tissue surrounding the bronchi remote from the gas exchanging areas.

The bronchial circulation

There are usually three or four bronchial arteries, which originate from the aorta. Before they reach the lung they anastomose extensively with the oesophageal, thymic, and thyroid arterial circulations. Within the lung they supply the bronchi, major plumonary blood vessels (vasa vasorum) and pleura; branches reach the interstitial tissue. Those branches that follow the bronchi cease to be a distinct set of vessels at the level of the respiratory bronchioles, where they form a mesh of capillaries, which anastomose with capillaries of the pulmonary circulation.

The bronchial microvasulature has a structure that, when viewed with the electron microscope, is quite different from that of the pulmonary circulation. The bronchial capillaries are of the 'visceral' type and their cytoplasmic extensions show numerous fenestrations as well as pinocytotic vesicles. Cytoplasmic fibrils are often prominent.

The contribution to total lung blood flow is usually taken to be between 1 and 3 per cent, although some estimates have been as high as 8 per cent. Vasomotor properties are quite different from the pulmonary circulation and, in particular, hypoxia causes vasodilation by a locally acting mechanism that can be blocked by cyclo-oxygenase inhibitors. By analogy, the structure of the capillaries suggests that they are highly permeable, but quantitative estimates are not available. However, autocoids, such as histamine, appear to increase permeability dramatically when studied by following the transit of particles using electron microscopy.

The function of the bronchial circulation is largely nutritive to the walls of bronchi, larger pulmonary vessels, interstitium, and interstitial pleura. However, in the vessels that anastomose with the pulmonary circulation, it has an important component, relevant in disease. This enlarges in conditions leading to cyanosis from ineffective alveolar blood–gas exchange, such as in chronic lung disease and congenital heart disease with right-to-left shunts. Under these circumstances the bronchial circulation may contribute a large fraction of the total blood flow to the alveoli, effectively becoming a reperfusion system to boost gas exchange.

There is a further beneficial effect from the increased precapillary bronchopulmonary anastomosis in localized chronic lung disease. The bronchial arterial pressure, being at systemic level and thus greater than pulmonary arterial pressure, tends to deflect pulmonary arterial blood flow away from the disease areas to more normally ventilated areas, thus helping ventilation/perfusion relationships to remain as normal as possible.

REFERENCES

Editorial (1978). Imbalanced ventricles and cardiac failure. *British Medical Journal*, **i**, 324.
Fishman, A.P. (1990). *The pulmonary circulation: Normal and abnormal.* University of Pennsylvania Press, Philadelphia.
Guyton, A.C., Jones, C.E., and Coleman, T.G. (1973). *Circulatory Physiology: Cardiac output and its regulation.* W.B. Saunders and Co., Philadelphia.
Harris, P. and Heath, D. (1986). *The human pulmonary circulation.* Churchill Livingstone, Edinburgh.
Hasleton, P.S. and Gibbs, A.R. (1994). Exploration of the pulmonary circulation. *Thorax*, **49**, suppl. S2–S62.
Lee, G. de J. (1983). The pulmonary circulation in health and disease. In *Scientific foundations of cardiology* (eds P. Sleight and J.V. Jones), Heinemann, London.
Mathew, R. and Altura. (1990). Physiology and pathophysiology of the pulmonary circulation. *Microcirculation, Endothelium and Lymphatics*, **6**, 211–252.
Prichard, J.S. (1982). *Edema of the lung.* Charles C. Thomas, Springfield, Illinois.
Rabinovitch, M. (1989). Structure and function of the pulmonary vascular bed. *Cardiology Clinics*, **7**(4), 895–914.
Versprille, A. and Jansen, J.R.C. (1992). Pulmonary circulation: Pressure, flow and vascular resistance. In *Adult respiratory distress syndrome* (eds A. Artigas, F. Lemaire, P.M. Suter and W.M. Zapol), pp. 229–249. Churchill Livingstone, Edinburgh.
Will, J.A., Dawson, C.A., Weir, E.K., and Buckner, C.K. (1987). *The pulmonary circulation in health and disease.* Academic Press, London.

15.23 Pulmonary oedema

J. S. PRICHARD

Acute fulminant pulmonary oedema is a terrifying but fortunately uncommon event in which patients literally drown in their own body fluids. Much more commonly, the clinician is called to treat pulmonary oedema in its less acute form, for breathlessness disturbs the patient long before serious alveolar flooding has begun.

Because pulmonary oedema is so commonly seen as a manifestation of left-sided heart disease – where its relief by diuretics is so effective – there is a temptation to forget the very wide range of other causes. Indeed, it is prudent to make the diagnosis of hydrostatic pulmonary oedema of cardiac origin only when other manifestations of heart disease are present and to consider wider possibilities in all other circumstances despite apparent relief from diuretics.

Pulmonary oedema has many possible causes and these occur in combination more often than is usually recognized. Only by careful and clear analysis of clinical and pathophysiological data can the contributing factors be identified and the clinical situation fully understood.

Physiological and experimental aspects of pulmonary oedema

FLUID BALANCE BETWEEN THE CAPILLARIES AND THE INTERSTITIAL SPACE

The continuous movement of water from the lung capillaries into the interstitium is regulated by the permeability of the endothelium to water and protein and by the imbalance of hydrostatic and osmotic forces across the membrane. The Starling hypothesis suggests that perturbation of any one of five factors could lead to oedema (Figs 1 and 2). These are capillary hydrostatic pressure, (P_{cap}), interstitial tissue pressure (P_{int}), plasma colloid osmotic (oncotic) pressure (Π_{cap}), endothelial permeability (expressed by κ and σ), and lymphatic function. Abnormalities in the first four will cause oedema by increasing water entry to the

interstitial space, whilst impaired function of the last will diminish drainage. Interstitial colloid osmotic pressure (Π_{int}) has not been included as an independent variable as it is generally considered to be entirely determined by plasma protein concentration and endothelial permeability.

Experimentally, the development of pulmonary oedema may be characterized by the relationship between tissue water and microvascular hydrostatic pressure (Fig. 3). In the normal lung, water content rises only slowly until capillary pressure reaches 25 to 30 mmHg. Thereafter, rise is rapid. The curve is shifted leftwards by decreased interstitial pressure, increased endothelial permeability, decreased plasma oncotic pres-

Fig. 1 (a) The lung endothelial membrane is permeable to water and electrolytes but less permeable to macromolecules. (b) The Starling equation: $Q_1 = K(P_{cap} - P_{int}) - K\sigma(\pi_{cap} - \pi_{int})$ where Q_1 is the net fluid filtration rate, K is the filtration coefficient, σ is the reflection coefficient, ($P_{cap} - P_{int}$) is the hydrostatic pressure gradient from the capillary lumen to interstitial space and ($\pi_{cap} - \pi_{int}$) is the oncotic pressure difference across the capillary membrane.

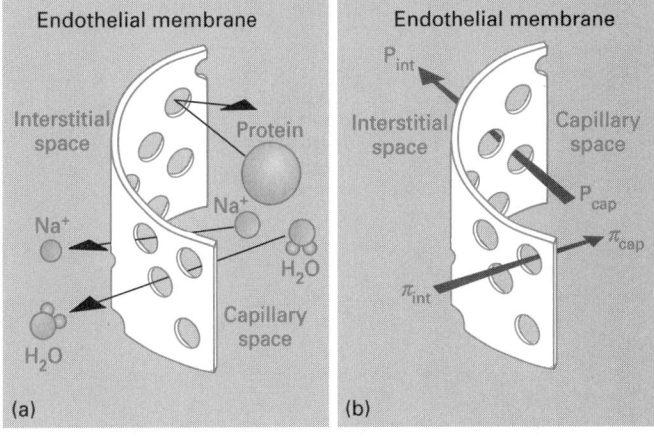

sure, or impaired lymphatic drainage. Figure 3 illustrates the interactions between these factors for, at low and normal hydrostatic pressures, changes in oncotic pressure, permeability, and lymphatic drainage do not readily cause oedema but, at higher hydrostatic pressures, their effect is much more dramatic.

The striking feature is that, in a normal lung, pulmonary capillary pressure may be raised to 25 to 30 mmHg before there is any significant accumulation of water. This 'safety factor' is multifactorial, but a component common to all forms of pulmonary oedema arises primarily from the behaviour of the lymphatic system. In response to faster transcapillary water flux from whatever cause (see below) the lymphatic system can increase its activity so much that flow accelerates to between three and ten times basal before the drainage becomes overwhelmed. The situation in which lung water content has increased only little whilst transcapillary and lymph fluxes have increased considerably emphasizes that pulmonary oedema is a dynamic phenomenon – in which tissue swelling is but the end stage reached when lymphatic drainage capacity is exceeded. Only then does fluid accumulation begin – slowly at first in the interstitial space, but then rapidly as alveolar flooding begins.

Fig. 2 The initiation of pulmonary oedema and the sequence of development.

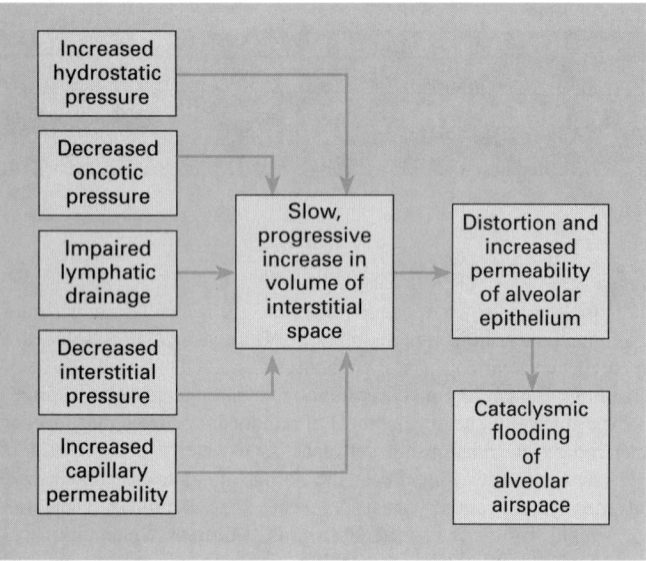

Fig. 3 Lung water content and capillary pressure. In the normal lung tissue, the water content does not begin to increase until capillary pressure is approximately 30 mmHg. Where colloid osmotic pressure (e.g. plasma protein concentration) is reduced, endothelial permeability is increased or the lymphatic pump is impaired, the whole curve is shifted to the left. (Reproduced from Prichard, J.S. (1982). *Edema of the lung*. Charles C. Thomas, Springfield, Illinois, with permission.)

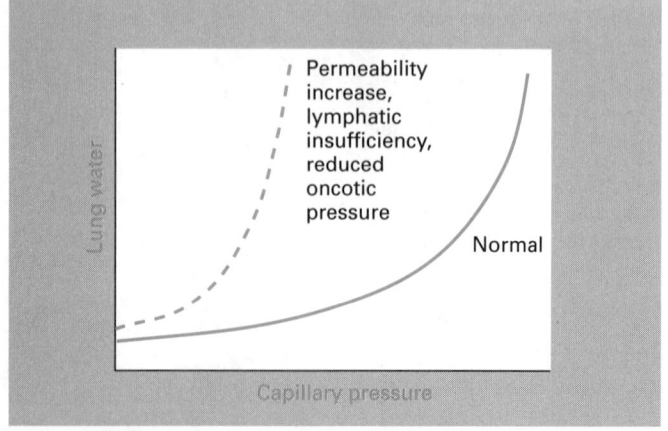

HYDROSTATIC PULMONARY OEDEMA

Any increase in capillary hydrostatic pressure, whether from cardiac failure, fluid overload, or pulmonary venous occlusion, speeds the rate of water flow into the interstitium. Provided the increase in pressure is not too great, this process will be self-limiting. Thus, molecular sieving, by allowing water to enter the interstitial space more readily than macromolecular solutes will reduce Π_{int}. Increased interstitial water increases the interstitial hydrostatic pressure P_{int} and decreases the macromolecular exclusion volume – again increasing Π_{int}. So, as long as lymphatic pumping can keep pace, the tissue water will expand only slightly. However, once the capacity of the lymphatic drainage is exceeded, accumulation of an oedema fluid with a low protein content begins. This starts in the lower parts of the lung (because it is here that hydrostatic pressures are greatest) and is associated with a characteristic redistribution of blood flow away from the lung bases.

The activity of lung lymphatics is critical in determining the onset and extent of hydrostatic oedema, and therefore it is not surprising to find that, in conditions where pulmonary vascular pressures are chronically elevated, the lymphatics undergo hypertrophy as a protective mechanism. Consequently, acute elevations of pulmonary vascular pressure will produce acute life-threatening oedema at levels that, when reached chronically, cause little distress and are registered clinically only by the characteristic radiological changes of lymphatic hypertrophy.

HIGH PERMEABILITY PULMONARY OEDEMA

Endothelial damage speeds water flux into the interstitial space. But, unlike hydrostatic oedema, there is also an increase in protein flux so that the oedema fluid has a high protein content. This has four consequences:

1. The oncotic pressure of the interstitial fluid increases and one of the major mechanisms for limiting the progress of oedema becomes unavailable.
2. Much of the protein reaching the tissue and alveoli is fibrinogen, which coagulates. Initially, the damage from interstitial coagulation is limited by fibrinolysis by plasminogen but this defence is soon exhausted and mobilization of the coagulum ceases.
3. The residual coagulum impairs lymphatic drainage.
4. The residual coagulum becomes the skeleton on which lung fibrosis develops.

There are many causes of permeability oedema (Table 1) but broadly they appear to fall into two major groups – those in which damage appears to result from a misdirection or perturbation of the normal defense mechanisms and those in which it is caused directly by toxic substances.

The first group is exemplified by septic shock and the mechanisms can partly be understood by realizing that the processes involved are very similar to those of the acute inflammatory response. For instance, when appropriately mounted against invading organisms, such as the pneumococcus, a cascade of reactions takes place, which results in phagocytosis by macrophages and granulocytes and destruction of the organisms by activated lytic enzymes and free oxygen radicals. Immune proteins and complement are also mobilized rapidly to the site of invasion via the alveolar and endothelial cell junctions, whose permeability is greatly augmented.

These cascades are of particular importance in relation to pulmonary oedema because they result, when inappropriately or uncontrollably activated, in the life-threatening clinical syndrome of adult respiratory distress syndrome (ARDS), in which pulmonary oedema is the consequence of changes in permeability. Three different, interacting mechanisms may be involved (Fig. 4).

Table 1 *Causes of pulmonary oedema*

Hydrostatic pulmonary oedema
Pulmonary venous hypertension – cardiogenic. Left ventricular failure; mitral stenosis and regurgitation; left atrial thrombosis; left atrial myxoma; cor triatriatum; loculated pericarditis
Pulmonary venous hypertension – non cardiogenic. Veno-occlusive disease; congenital pulmonary venous stenosis; mediastinal granulomata, fibrosis, masses; neurogenic
Pulmonary arterial hypertension. Hyperkinetic states (extreme exercise, left–right shunts, hypoxia, anaemia, thyrotoxicosis); pulmonary emboli; high altitude

Permeability oedema
Drugs and circulating toxic substances. Hydrochlorthiazide; phenylbutazone; aspirin; methylsalicylate; nitrofurantoin; hydralazine; bleomycin; heroin; morphine; methadone; dextropropoxyphene; paraquat; alloxan; α-naphthylthiourea; coral snake venom; silver nitrate; ammonium chloride; ammonium sulphate; chelating agents; oleic acid (fat embolus); diltiazem; iodine containing contrast media; interleukin 2
Immunological. Goodpasture's syndrome; antilung serum; Stevens–Johnson syndrome
Radiation.
Viral infection.
Aspirated toxic substances. Fresh water; salt water; stomach contents
Inhaled toxic substances. Smoke; nitrogen oxides; ozone; chlorine; cadmium oxide; oxides of sulphur; carbonyl chloride; phosgene; lewisite; oxygen
Metabolic. Hepatic failure; renal failure
Mechanical endothelial disruption. ?Neurogenic pulmonary oedema
Mechanical epithelial disruption. ?Pulmonary hyperinflation
Other causes of permeability oedema: adult respiratory distress syndrome. Particularly: shock lung; septicaemia; pancreatitis; burns; fat embolism; cardiopulmonary bypass; banked unfiltered blood; amniotic fluid embolism

Reduced alveolar septal tissue interstitial pressure
Upper airway obstruction, acute. Laryngospasm; epiglottitis; laryngotracheobronchitis; spasmodic croup; foreign body; tumour; upper airway trauma; strangulation; peritonsillar abscess; Ludwig's angina; angio-oedema; near drowning; ?asthma
Upper airway obstruction, chronic. Obstructive sleep apnoea; adenoidal, tonsillar, or nasopharyngeal mass; thyroid goitre; acromegaly

Reduced plasma colloid osmotic pressure
Rare as sole cause. Contributes to oedemas of adult respiratory distress syndrome, hepatic and renal failure, fluid overload, myocardial infarction. Important when hypoproteinaemia occurs with other oedemogenic conditions

Failure of lymphatic clearance
Lymphangitis carcinomatosa; mediastinal obstruction; lung transplant; contributes to oedema in adult respiratory distress syndrome, malaria, silicosis

1. The complement–neutrophil cascade, by which, under normal circumstances, activated complement causes granulocytes to localize in the lung so as to kill bacteria.
2. Coagulation–fibrinolysis imbalance – leading to inappropriate deposition of fibrin and damage by split products (the fibrinogen cascade).
3. Local aggregation of macrophages.

An important step in inappropriate activation may be complement-induced leucocyte aggregation in the pulmonary capillaries. Experimentally, infusion of activated complement into sheep with chronic pulmonary lymphatic fistulae leads rapidly to an increased flow of a lymph with a high protein concentration. This is considerably reduced if the animal has previously been rendered agranulocytic and the procedure is thought to be a good animal model of the early phase of adult respiratory distress syndrome. This is because:

1. Many of the factors that induce adult respiratory distress syndrome (such as endotoxin, proteases, or prolonged contact of blood with foreign surfaces) are also known to activate complement in man.
2. There is correlation between the appearance of circulating complement components C5A and C3A and the development and intensity of adult respiratory distress syndrome.
3. Pathological studies show considerable granulocyte adherence to endothelium and capillary blockage in the early phase of the syndrome.

It is uncertain whether activation of complement occurs directly or indirectly by release of cytokines and eicosanoids from macrophages and endothelial cells. In the case of activation by endotoxin there is evidence that tumour necrosis factor (TNF) may be the earliest mediator while interleukins 1, 6, and 8, together with platelet activating factor (PAF) also all appear at a very early stage.

Complement activation may have effects in addition to causing granulocyte adhesion. Complement fragments can themselves stimulate eicosanoid production from endothelium and increased levels of thromboxane A_2 and prostaglandin E_2 have been observed in human adult respiratory distress syndrome. The former, in conjunction with platelet activating factor, could be responsible not only for the vasoconstriction that has been observed, but also for platelet aggregation.

The adherent neutrophils themselves amplify the process by positive feedback by producing their own mediators, in particular leukotriene B_4,

Fig. 4 Endothelial damage in adult respiratory distress syndrome and permeability oedema. The diagram emphasises the role of complement activation and tumour necrosis factor (TNF) in causing damage. Macrophages may be responsible for TNF production. Neurophils damage endothelium by superoxide production and, possibly proteases. Leukotriene B_4 (LTB_4) amplifies neutrophil chemotaxis, activation, and adherence. The process of damage is intensified by activation of the coagulation cascade—caused by the first phase of endothelial damage. PAM = pulmonary alveolar macrophage. PIM = pulmonary intravascular macrophage.

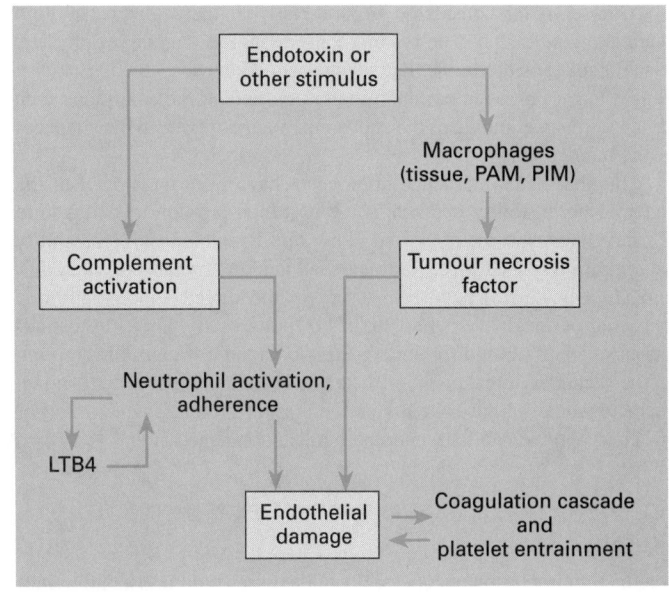

which cause further migration. Adherence is progressively promoted by the appearance of endothelial leucocyte adhesion molecules (ELAMs) and intercellular adhesion molecules (ICAMs) adherence molecules on the endothelial cells.

A large number of the identified early mediators – including tumour necrosis factor, platelet activating factor, and thromboxane A_2 – all increase endothelial permeability but, after granulocytic adherence, there is release of toxic oxygen metabolites such as superoxide anion and hydrogen peroxide. These can damage the vascular endothelium directly – by peroxidation and enzyme alteration – and can also alter the balance of local eicosanoid production towards metabolites that increase permeability and cause vasoconstriction. Proteolytic enzyme released by the adherent granulocytes may also play a part in damage.

The suggestion that the coagulation cascade is inappropriately activated comes from the observations that disseminated intravascular coagulation is common in adult respiratory distress syndrome, fibrin often appears in pulmonary capillaries and *in situ* microthrombosis is a frequent occurrence. However, although fibrin degradation products such as fragment-D can both damage capillaries and induce an adult respiratory distress syndrome-like syndrome in experimental animals, the evidence for a primary involvement of coagulation–fibrinolysis imbalance in the pathophysiology of adult respiratory distress syndrome is uncertain, because although early mediators such as tumour necrosis factor and interleukin 1 have procoagulant activity, neither heparin anticoagulation nor platelet or fibrin depletion prevents the onset of the syndrome.

Macrophages play an important role both in the inflammatory cascade by providing a number of key initiating and amplifying mediators, such as tumour necrosis factor, interleukins 1 and 6, and platelet activating factor, and also as cells that can cause physical endothelial damage, because they contain the same range of enzymes for lysis and generation of free oxygen radicals as neutrophils. The relative roles of circulating, tissue, and pulmonary intravascular macrophages is, as yet, unclear.

Although these three different mechanisms and cascades are clearly involved in initiating and sustaining adult respiratory distress syndrome, they do not act in isolation; for considerable cross-links are known. For instance, virtually any of the tissue destruction products arising as a result of neutrophil of macrophage action will activate Hageman factor and the complement cascade.

The mechanisms of damage so far discussed all involve systems that are primarily intravascular and blood-borne. However, lung oedema may also result from damage to the airspace epithelium from inhaled and aspirated liquids and gases or from mechanical trauma such as stretching. The mechanisms of these causes of oedema necessarily differ from those so far considered – particularly in the sequence of fluid accumulation. In many it is commonly assumed that direct physical tissue damage is the immediate mechanism. However, alveolar macrophages may often be important initiators, particularly in conditions such as aspiration pneumonia or the appearance of endotoxins in the airspaces of the lung.

A number of experimental approaches have been developed in the study of permeability oedema, some of which are now evolving into clinical diagnostic methods that allow the distinction of permeability oedema from other forms. Radiolabelled markers (notably serum albumin and transferrin) have been used for the direct demonstration of increased permeability, while studies of pulmonary lymph (by cannulation), interstitial fluid (by microaspiration), and alveolar fluid (relying on the secondary breakdown of the alveolar membrane) have all shown characteristically high contents of the plasma proteins, which are not present when the capillary endothelium is undamaged.

PULMONARY OEDEMA AND REDUCED PLASMA ONCOTIC PRESSURE

A reduction in plasma oncotic pressure increases fluid transudation into the lung and leads to pulmonary oedema at lower hydrostatic pressures than would otherwise be expected. Although this is readily demonstrable experimentally, it is frequently overlooked in clinical practice, where it may be of importance following myocardial infarction, after transfusion of crystalloids, and in adult respiratory distress syndrome. A useful clinical guide to the danger is the difference between pulmonary wedge pressure (measured by a Swann–Ganz catheter) and colloid osmotic pressure (the COP–PAW gradient). The normal lower limit of this index is about -12 mmHg, but at levels below -9 mmHg the risk of oedema is considerably enhanced. A practical problem in applying this method has been the difficulty in standardizing and maintaining protein oncometers. The alternative of using serum protein measurements is valuable but slower.

LYMPHATIC OEDEMA AND THE ROLE OF THE LUNG LYMPHATICS

The lymphatic system provides the lung with its major 'safety factor'. It is capable of increasing the tissue clearance rate at least ten-fold before becoming overwhelmed. In chronic venous and capillary hypertension, as in mitral stenosis, even larger lymph flows occur because of lymphatic hypertrophy.

Oedema soon develops when lymphatic drainage is occluded experimentally. This has clinical relevance for patients with lung transplants, whose lung lymphatic pathways are severed and in whom initial alveolar flooding is common. Lymphatic oedema also plays a part in pulmonary oedema from lymphangitis carcinomatosa and in facilitating oedema in patients with silicosis and malaria.

REDUCED INTERSTITIAL PRESSURE AND PULMONARY OEDEMA

Tissue pressure within the interstitial space is one of the determinants of transendothelial fluid movement. It can be altered independently of intravascular events by changes in intrapleural pressure. Thus when extreme negative intrapleural pressures occur, the interstitial perialveolar tissue pressure can fall considerably below its normal subatmospheric level and accelerate the rate of fluid movement into the interstitium. Oedema will appear if the rate of fluid entry exceeds the rate at which it can move through the interstitium and be removed by the lymphatics.

THE SEQUENCE OF OEDEMA ACCUMULATION

When oedema fluid begins to accumulate in lung tissue – irrespective of the underlying cause – it does so first around fissures, blood vessels, and airways because these tissues are 'loose' and swell easily without great change in tissue pressure. When this 'sump' has become near maximally dilated, swelling and thickening of the alveolar wall begin. Finally, after a phase of progressive alveolar wall thickening, fluid begins to accumulate in the alveoli themselves. This final phase begins at a point where total lung water has increased by about 30 per cent (Fig. 5).

At first, the fluid in the alveoli is confined to the alveolar angles. Subsequently, complete flooding of individual alveoli occurs. A striking feature of the microscopic appearance at this stage is the way in which alveoli are either completely filled with fluid or else have only minimal accumulation in the angles. There are no half-filled alveoli and flooding is a 'quantal' event, so that flooded alveoli are scattered at random throughout the affected area. During the process, although the volume of each alveolus is smaller when fluid-filled than when air-filled, atelectasis is uncommon and air is rarely trapped.

The quantal nature of alveolar flooding arises from the interaction of surface and tissue forces (Fig. 6). The immediate precipitating factor is probably an increase in alveolar epithelial permeability – caused by the distortion and swelling of the alveolar wall. This allows water to flood from the interstitium into the air space. An alternative, less likely, hypothesis is that fluid entry occurs via pores in the epithelium of the terminal airways. Irrespective of the route, the ease of fluid entry now makes the relationship between pressure and volume inverse and unstable. There are two reasons for this:

1. In an alveolus filling with fluid, the area of the liquid surface is considerably diminished. At these low dimensions, surfactant cannot produce its characteristic effect by which surface tension is directly proportional to area. The surface tension becomes constant and independent of area.

2. As fluid movement across the alveolar wall now takes place with ease – without increasing transepithelial osmotic pressure and without tissue distortion – elastic and osmotic forces play no part. Overall, the relationship between air volume and pressure in the alveolus with a damaged epithelium is that of a gaseous bubble in liquid where pressure and volume are inversely related (i.e. $P = 2T/R$ where P is the luminal pressure, R is the alveolar radius, and T is the (now constant) surface tension). This unstable situation is only resolved when the alveolus has flooded.

THE RESOLUTION OF PULMONARY OEDEMA

The extent and rapidity of resolution of pulmonary oedema depend upon cause. Hydrostatic and oncotic oedema can resolve completely and rapidly but this is rarely the case with permeability oedema, where slow disappearance and permanent lung damage are the rule.

Resolution of hydrostatic oedema occurs in two phases – return of the capillary pressure towards normal and then lymphatic and osmotic resorption of tissue and alveolar fluid. In cardiac failure, the shift of blood from the pulmonary circulation to the systemic by sitting up is the most powerful method of reducing capillary pressure, but other mechanisms have also been suggested, including:

1. Progressive hypovolaemia (from fluid extravasation into the lung).
2. Increasing plasma oncotic pressure from the relatively greater transendothelial loss of water than of plasma protein.
3. Hypoxic vasoconstriction of the muscular pulmonary arteries causing a fall in capillary pressure.
4. Exhaustion of sympathetic neurotransmitter in the systemic circulation with reduction in venomotor tone and left heart afterload.

The first three are all known to occur but quantitatively their contributions are uncertain. The fourth is conjecture.

In hydrostatic oedema, once hydrostatic pressure has been reduced, fluid is removed from the interstitial space by lymphatic drainage, which, experimentally, can be increased for as long as 24 h after an acute episode. In addition, oncotic resorption into the circulation can

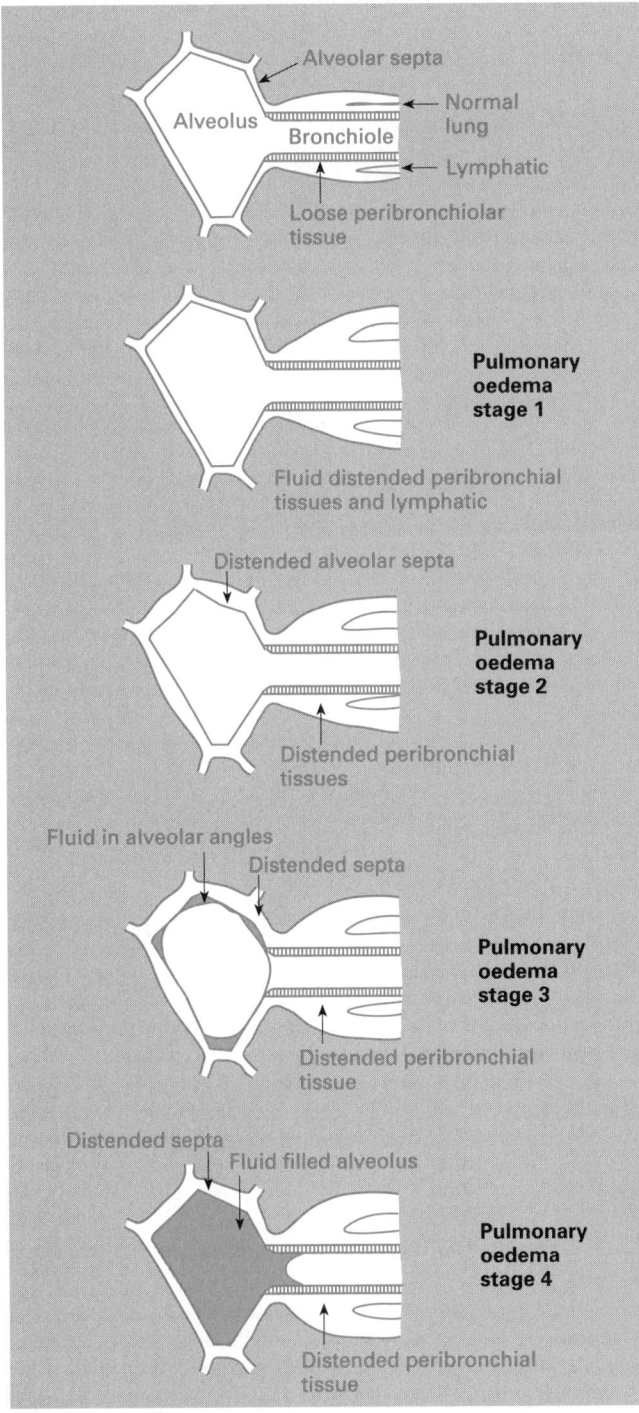

Fig. 5 Stages in the development of pulmonary oedema. Stage 1: peribronchial swelling; stage 2: distended alveolar septa; stage 3: limited accumulation of fluid in alveolar angles; stage 4: alveolar flooding. (Reproduced from Prichard, J.S. (1982). *Edema of the lung.* Charles C. Thomas, Springfield, Illinois, with permission.)

Fig. 6 Pressure–volume relationships in the alveolus. Phase 1 represents the normal alveolus lined by surfactant. Tissue elasticity, osmotic balance, and the presence of surfactant combine to produce a direct, mechanically stable relationship between pressure and volume. Phase 2 represents the situation in which alveolar permeability has increased. Any influx of fluid into the alveolus decreases the overall surface area. At these lower dimensions, surfactant is inoperative and surface tension is independent of area. The relationship between volume and pressure is that of an air bubble in liquid ($P = 2T/R$) and is unstable. The air volume therefore shrinks as air is expelled until phase 3 is reached. Here the remaining air is a 'bleb' at the bronchiolar orifice.

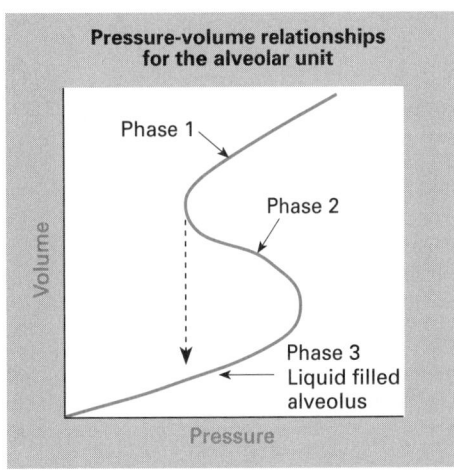

Table 2 *The multifactorial nature of pulmonary oedema*

	Hydrostatic pressure increase	Oncotic pressure decrease	Endothelial permeability increase	Lymphatic drainage impairment	Reduced interstitial pressure	Reduced alveolar surfactant
Shock lung	From therapy	Yes	Yes	Yes		(Yes)
Hepatic failure		Yes	Yes			
Renal failure	Yes	(Yes)	Yes			
Neurogenic oedema	Yes		Yes			
Fluid overload	Yes	(Yes)				
Pulmonary emboli	Yes		Yes			
Myocardial infarction	Yes	(Yes)				
Carcinomatosis		Yes		Yes		
High altitude	Yes		Yes			
Re-expansion			(Yes)		Yes	(Yes)
Airway obstruction	(Yes)				Yes	

Parentheses indicate minor contributions.

play a significant part because no endothelial damage has occurred. However, the mechanism of alveolar clearance is not well understood. A considerable amount of fluid is removed by coughing and ciliary drainage but, for final clearance and re-establishment of normal fluid balance, restoration of the normal (low) alveolar epithelial permeability is first necessary. Once it has occurred, final resorption seems to occur as a result of active sodium ion transport, although it is uncertain whether this takes place in the alveolar or terminal airway epithelium.

The clearance mechanisms in permeability oedema are considerably less efficient than in hydrostatic oedema because fibrin has coagulated in the interstitium, lymphatics, and alveoli and because the endothelium and epithelium have been damaged. The coagulum retracts and expels serum but endothelial damage prevents osmotic absorption and lymphatic drainage is impeded. The problem in the alveoli is compounded by the inactivation of surfactant by fibrin and continuing high permeability of the alveolar epithelium. Removal of the retracted coagulum is rarely complete because fibrinolysis fails as plasminogen and fibronectin become exhausted. Finally, the incompletely removed coagulum acts as a skeleton for fibrosis because the action of macrophages is rarely sufficiently prompt to avert this.

Reconstruction of epithelium and endothelium is frequently necessary in the permeability oedemas. In the case of the alveolar epithelium, cell replacement is by transdifferentiation from type II pneumocytes and this is rarely complete. Whether the transdifferentiated cells are able to play an efficient part in active transport and fluid removal is unknown.

Clinical aspects

CAUSES OF PULMONARY OEDEMA

Table 1 lists the main causes of pulmonary oedema classified according to the predominant pathophysiological mechanism. However, the clinician should never forget that more than one cause may be operating (Table 2), and must not neglect one remediable factor at the expense of another, or allow therapy itself to intensify the problem. For example, overvigorous fluid replacement following pulmonary endothelial damage may be the very factor that accelerates water and protein flow into the interstitium and provokes oedema.

Descriptions of the clinical manifestations and management of the more common diseases listed in Table 1 are provided elsewhere. But certain aspects need particular comment.

Pulmonary oedema in heart failure

This common form of pulmonary oedema is well known, but two features deserve comment. The first is the symptom of orthopnoea in which the oedema either first appears or, if already present, intensifies after a period of lying down. The cause is a shift of blood from the systemic circulation to the pulmonary, which occurs because of the change in posture. This leads to an increase in intracapillary hydrostatic pressure, which in turn triggers oedema. The symptom is at its most dramatic in paroxysmal nocturnal dyspnoea (see below). The second feature – and one that frequently causes confusion because it is contrary to expectation – is the tendency of the blood pressure to rise as patients progress into left heart failure. The cause is probably increasing sympathetic activity and circulating catecholamines, which lead to intense systemic arterial and venous vasoconstriction, thereby increasing after load and central venous pressure inappropriately and so intensifying the development of oedema.

Loculated constrictive pericarditis

Loculated constrictive pericarditis, predominantly involving the left ventricle, can occur in patients with chronic renal failure undergoing dialysis. Echocardiography is helpful in diagnosis, which may be difficult because the characteristic signs of pericardial tamponade may be missing. When located posteriorly, the fluid is difficult to aspirate percutaneously, but open drainage is rarely necessary because strict attention to fluid regulation during and between dialyses usually leads to resolution.

Pulmonary venous thrombosis

This is a rare condition and is difficult to diagnose. It may be idiopathic or may be a subsidiary manifestation of conditions such as polyarteritis nodosa, other vasculitic disorders, and occult neoplastic disease. More common in middle-aged women, symptoms of increasing lassitude and breathlessness, sometimes with low grade fever, are the presenting symptoms. Ultimately, gross effort dyspnoea and pulmonary oedema, usually with pleural effusions, develop. The signs of pulmonary hypertension are present but proof of diagnosis is difficult. Difficulty in obtaining a clear pulmonary artery wedge pressure tracing and normal left atrial pressure (measured directly by the transseptal route) should alert suspicion. Pulmonary artery angiography should demonstrate poor segmental drainage in the regions affected by thrombosis. Open lung biopsy will confirm the diagnosis but is dangerous and should be undertaken only when there is real fear of missing an alternative cause of the oedema.

Left atrial myxoma, ball thrombus of the left atrium, and cor triatriatum

These are rare, but must not be missed as they are remediable by surgery. Their clinical presentation may be very similar to that of pulmonary venous thrombosis because the characteristic episodic mitral diastolic murmurs that occur with left atrial myxoma and ball thrombus may be missed. All three conditions also enter into the differential diagnosis of tight mitral stenosis. Echocardiography is the key investigation.

High altitude oedema

Some apparently normal people who ascend rapidly to high altitudes experience acute pulmonary oedema. The condition is a particular instance of the oedema that occurs in severe hypoxia and develops only in that minority of individuals who have an exaggerated acute pulmonary arterial pressor response to hypoxia and who develop pulmonary hypertension at high altitude. The oedema may result from transarterial fluid leakage at high pressures but alternatively could be due to inhomogeneity of vasoconstriction and consequent extreme hyperperfusion of those areas not vasoconstricted. A further contribution may arise from the effects of vasoactive amines on the contractile filaments of endothelial cells leading to separation of endothelial junctions.

Pulmonary oedema with pulmonary arterial hypertension

Occasionally, pulmonary arterial hypertension secondary to high output states, such as large shunts, can be associated with pulmonary oedema (possibly from transarterial leakage) especially following exercise. This is usually avoided because acute breathlessness is such a prominent early symptom.

Pulmonary oedema following acute intracranial lesions

A large variety of intracranial lesions may occasionally be associated with acute pulmonary oedema. It is probable that damage to the nucleus of the tractus solitarus and the hypothalamus lead to severe systemic vasoconstriction ('sympathetic storm'), which shifts blood to the pulmonary circulation, causing an extreme paroxysm of pulmonary hypertension – reaching 410/200 in one recorded case. In addition, there is evidence to suggest that pulmonary venoconstriction also occurs, thus causing a rise in pulmonary capillary pressure even in excess of that which would have been predicted from the pulmonary arterial pressure measurements. The extreme high blood pressure in the capillaries first induces hydrostatic oedema and if sufficiently severe also damages the endothelium leading to a less easily resolved permeability oedema.

Pulmonary thromboembolism

This may occasionally lead to florid pulmonary oedema and two hypotheses have been proposed. (1) local overperfusion caused by diversion of blood flow away from the occluded site; and (2) humoral alteration of permeability. It is possible that both mechanisms may play a part and also that the causes may be different in micro- and macroemboli. In favour of the permeability change is the observation that the lymphatic fluid following experimental microembolization is of high protein content – even when the microemboli are pharmacologically inert glass microspheres. The clotting cascade may be involved, as prior heparinization prevents the oedema. Conversely, evidence for the first mechanism originates with experiments in which balloon occlusion of the major pulmonary vessels leads to oedema and increased flow of a low protein lymph from the areas. As in altitude oedema, the site fluid transudation is unclear and the arterial vessels have been proposed, but without any strong positive evidence.

Expansion pulmonary oedema

The incidence of pulmonary oedema after expansion of a collapsed lung is low. It is more likely when the lung (or lobe) has been collapsed for some time, but can occur after quite short periods. The occurrence may be reduced by ensuring that the negative pressures in the pleural space during re-expansion do not exceed 10 cmH$_2$O, that the procedure is terminated if cough develops and that not more than 1500 ml are aspirated at any one time when collapse is related to an effusion. The mechanism is uncertain. Permeability change is likely as high protein oedemas have been found in both clinical and experimental situations. The mechanism of damage may be from toxic oxygen radicals, as in cardiac reperfusion injury. Additional contributing factors could be loss of surfactant during the period of collapse and increased negativity of interstitial pressure during re-expansion.

Postobstructive pulmonary oedema

The initiating event is a markedly negative intrapleural pressure generated by forceful inspiratory effort against an obstructed upper airway. This is then transmitted to the pulmonary interstitial space. During normal breathing, intrapleural pressures rarely fall below − 5 cmH$_2$O but, in upper airway obstruction the value may be as low as − 50 cmH$_2$O. Postobstructive oedema should therefore always be suspected wherever there is the rapid onset of dyspnoea, cyanosis, frothy pink sputum production, and radiological pulmonary infiltrates after the rapid relief of upper airway obstruction. The onset is usually immediate but, occasionally, delays of up to 2 h have been reported. The chronic form occurs in patients with obstructive sleep apnoea, in whom negative intrapleural pressures as low as − 100 cmH$_2$O have been recorded.

Lymphatic oedema and lymphatic obstruction

Although, in one sense, all pulmonary oedema can be thought of as lymphatic failure, surprisingly little is known of pulmonary lymphatic failure in clinical practice. Lymphatic occlusion underlies the oedema and dyspnoea of lymphangitis carcinomatosa. In cases where cardiac failure and pneumoconioses coexist it has been found that oedema develops at lower capillary pressures than would be expected and this has been attributed to lymphatic blockage. Mechanical lymphatic disruption is probably a contributing factor to the ease with which immediate posttransplant lungs develop oedema.

Disorders of capillary permeability

Many of the conditions associated with adult respiratory distress syndrome can also be associated with less dramatic degrees of oedema. It is a good rule always to consider the possibility that a permeability abnormality might exist as an associated cause in all cases of pulmonary oedema. The history can be particularly helpful, particularly with regard to possible infections, use of drugs and occupational chemicals. The possibility of oxygen toxicity should be borne in mind for all patients in intensive care.

Unilateral oedema

This frequently causes diagnostic confusion. Unilateral oedema on the same side as pre-existing lung abnormalities (ipsilateral oedema) may arise from posture (lying on one side during oedema development), increased perfusion of one lung secondary to a systemic to pulmonary shunt, unilateral venous occlusion (either from unilateral veno-occlusive disease or from extrinsic compression), or unilateral lymphatic pathology such as lymphangitis carcinomatosa. Contralateral oedema is seen where the pre-existing pathology protects that lung. Instances include congenital unilateral pulmonary artery, Swyer-James–McLeod syndrome, unilateral thromboembolism, and unilateral fibrosis causing unilateral hypoxia and vasoconstriction.

THE DIAGNOSIS OF PULMONARY OEDEMA

The diagnosis of pulmonary oedema is by clinical observation and chest radiograph.

The characteristic symptom of pulmonary oedema is breathlessness – probably generated by an inappropriate awareness of respiratory effort and by firing of 'J' (juxta-alveolar) receptors. This dyspnoea comes on more or less acutely in the first instance, often following exercise. Later, paroxysmal nocturnal dyspnoea develops because of postural hydrostatic factors. Only then are signs of diminished breath sounds at the bases and fine lung crepitations found. The crepitations (crackles) characteristic of pulmonary oedema are intermittent explosive sounds lasting less than 20 ms. They are probably caused by the sudden opening of a succession of small airways, the acoustic wave being produced either by equalization of downstream and upstream pressures or by sudden alterations in the tension of the airway walls. They thus relate to the 'all-or-none' features of alveolar flooding observed physiologically. The rhonchi (musical sounds) that are sometimes heard, and that may cause considerable diagnostic confusion in the dyspnoeic patient, can arise either from bronchiolar wall oedema or from vagally mediated reflex bronchospasm.

Although it is important to remember that pulmonary oedema is never a static condition, but is always either developing or regressing, the observations of Altschule who, nearly 40 years ago, recorded the sequence of events as a patient progressed into ever greater left heart failure, are worth recalling.

1. *Premonitory*: anxiety, pallor, tachycardia, raised blood pressure, cold sweaty skin.
2. *Interstitial oedema*: dyspnoea, orthopnoea, cyanosis, congested neck veins, wheezing and rales.
3. *Intra-alveolar oedema*: crackling rales progressing to general bubbling. Cough, sputum – becoming frothy then blood-stained.
4. *Shock*: clouding of consciousness.
5. *Terminal*: cardiac and respiratory arrhythmias.

The clinical features of the non-haemodynamic oedemas are not dissimilar but are generally less florid.

The chest radiograph is a sensitive and easily available tool for spotting early pulmonary oedema (Figs 7 and 8). The majority of studies of radiographical studies have been made during cardiogenic oedema where necessarily, changes of oedema are superimposed on other circulatory alterations. Three successive and overlapping phases can be identified.

Pre-oedema

This reflects cardiac and circulatory changes and the increased flow of fluid which occurs through the lymphatics before swelling of the tissue takes place. Usually, the cardiothoracic ratio on a posteroanterior film is >0.5 (>0.57 for an anteroposterior film is standard when geometry is preserved). Distension and engorgement of blood vessels occur – particularly in the upper zone with inverse changes at the bases leading to reversal of the usual pattern. Subsequently distended lymphatics become identifiable. Septal lines, perilobular lines, and rosettes all represent engorged lymphatics. Septal lines were originally identified by Kerley: type A lines are ragged, unbranched, and run centripetally

Fig. 7 Radiological signs and pulmonary pathophysiology. Kerley lines are a particularly useful radiological sign as they occur at a stage where lymph flow and transinterstitial water flow have both increased but where appreciable tissue swelling has not yet appeared. (Reproduced from Prichard, J.S. (1982). *Edema of the lung*. Charles C. Thomas, Springfield, Illinois, with permission.)

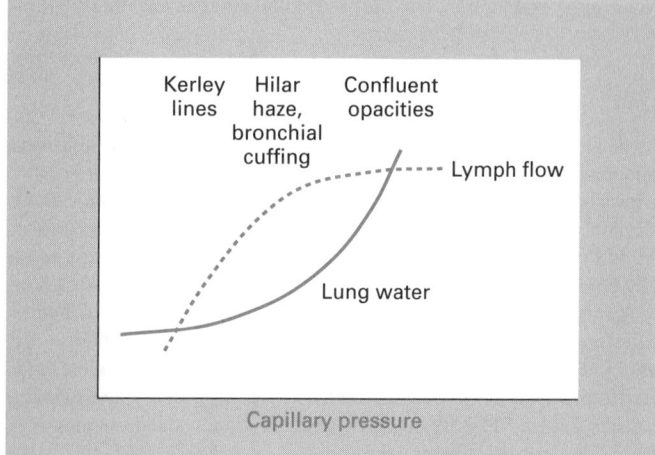

towards the hilum; type C lines are fine, interlacing, and seen most easily in the central and perihilar regions; type B lines are the best known and most commonly seen. They are short, sharp, horizontal, and found in the costophrenic angles. They occur most often in pulmonary oedema due to chronic pulmonary venous hypertension. Indeed there is excellent correlation between the density of Kerley B lines and left atrial pressure in mitral stenosis. The lines are rarely seen below a mean left atrial pressure of 13.5 mmHg, are commonly found in the region of 22 mmHg and are invariably present when the left atrial pressure exceeds 30 mmHg. Perilobular lines and rosettes are found on close inspection in about 3 per cent of radiographs and probably represent the lymphatics running around the respiratory acini.

Interstitial oedema

This first appears in areas of 'loose' connective tissue when wedge pressure begins to rise above 15 mmHg (see sequence of oedema accumulation, above). Visible interlobar and accessory lung fissures are the first manifestations. They are followed by perivascular and peribronchial cuffs, which contribute respectively to the homogeneous circular shadows formed by the already distended vessels and to the 'ring' shadows around bronchi seen close to the hilum. Micronoduli consist of small round densities < 3 mm arising from accumulation of fluid around the smaller blood vessels. Blurring and hazing of the hilar regions represent the beginning of true alveolar septal interstitial oedema and, in hydrostatic oedema begin at wedge pressures of around 20 mmHg. A diffuse increase in lung density (clouding) represents the final phase.

Alveolar oedema

This starts when wedge pressure reaches 25 to 28 mmHg. It is seen as a 'fluffy' loss of lucency. This can be either around the hila in a 'butterfly' or 'batswing' pattern, or predominantly in the lower zones – usually reflecting a 'gravitational' distribution. Associated changes are the development of effusions and a loss of lung volume caused by a fall in lung compliance.

Radiologically, the permeability oedemas follow the pattern of the hydrostatic except that: (1) the distribution of alveolar oedema tends to be patchy; and (2) the characteristic vascular and cardiac changes are not present.

The presence of pre-existing lung disease – particularly chronic obstructive pulmonary disease – may modify the radiological appearance of pulmonary oedema considerably. Hyperinflation may render the silhouette of a large heart unremarkable; with the onset of interstitial oedema, a hyperinflated lung may shrink to normal size; the distribution of oedema shadowing may be patchy and only evident where parenchyma is sufficiently preserved; Kerley lines may be difficult or impossible to identify.

Fig. 8 Characteristic radiological appearances in interstitial oedema (see text). (Reproduced from Prichard, J.S. (1982). *Edema of the lung*. Charles C. Thomas, Springfield, Illinois, with permission.)

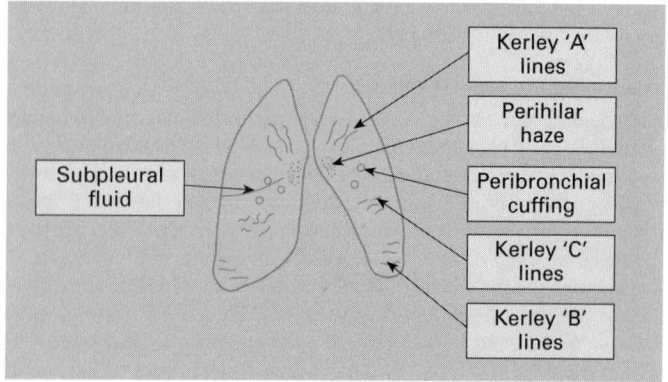

CT scanning is not necessary for the diagnosis of pulmonary oedema but the appearances are characteristic. Thickening and increased visualisation of interlobular septa and associated thickening of subpleural and peribronchial interstitial spaces. Alveolar oedema leads to varying degrees of alveolar consolidation. As in the plain radiograph, there may be associated heart and vascular changes and pleural effusions.

The detection of endothelial damage was originally by lymphatic cannulation in experimental models of adult respiratory distress syndrome. This technique obviously has no direct clinical applicability but it led to the validation of methods using radioactively labelled intravenous markers such as albumin or transferrin. The marker is injected intravenously and over the following hours, external radioactivity from the lung is measured at the surface of the chest (Fig. 9). Simultaneously, the radioactivity of blood is assessed either directly or by external counting over a blood pool such as the heart. From the lung, a gradual increase in counts takes place due to the labelled marker leaving the plasma compartment to enter the interstitium. The rate of rise of radioactivity in the chest relative to that in the blood is then an indication of capillary permeability. The faster the relative rise in chest counts, the greater will be the permeability of the capillaries in the underlying lung.

Epithelial permeability

This can be assessed by measuring the rate of clearance of submicron aerosols of technetium-99m-diethylenetriamine penta-acetic acid ($^{99}Tc^{m}$-DPTA).

Aspiration of bronchioalveolar fluid

This procedure, during bronchial toilet in the intensive care ward, allows assessment of endothelial epithelial function. Changes in capillary permeability may be assessed from sizing analysis of the proteins present, for even if the alveolar epithelium has not been damaged directly it will have been disrupted by the presence of interstitial oedema. Generally, in cardiac oedema, the protein content is low as the vascular endothelium

is intact. In permeability oedemas, the protein content of alveolar fluid may approach that of plasma itself.

PULMONARY FUNCTION IN OEDEMA OF THE LUNG

The oedematous lung shows a mixture of restrictive and obstructive defects, although the former dominate. The restrictive component arises from a decreased compliance, which is a result of vascular congestion (in cardiogenic and fluid overload oedema), interstitial oedema, and surfactant washout. Of these, the interstitial oedema contributes surprisingly little, so that, to start with, restrictive changes are indicative of an engorged vascular system and later, of alveolar flooding.

Sometimes, airflow resistance may cause easily audible rhonchi and a reduction in forced expiratory volume in 1 s and forced vital capacity (FEV_1/FVC) but, more usually, it is difficult to detect by simple methods because it occurs predominantly in the small airways of 1 to 2 mm diameter, which contribute relatively little to overall resistance. There are a number of causes for this airflow obstruction. In the preoedematous phase of heart failure the smallest airways may be compressed by distension of adjacent vessels in the bronchovascular bundle. In frank interstitial oedema it has been suggested that perivascular cuffing could have the same effect but recent research has not substantiated this. However, submucosal oedema and vagally mediated reflex bronchoconstriction are substantiated and are probably responsible for the majority of the effect. Restriction and obstruction may combine to reduce vital capacity and serial measurements of this can be a good index of severity of and recovery from pulmonary oedema.

Tachypnoea is a prominent feature of all forms of pulmonary oedema. Although it is associated with a low tidal volume, total ventilation (V_E) – both at rest and during exercise – is high relative to the prevailing level of carbon dioxide consumption. But the high total ventilation is expended mainly in deadspace ventilation and, unless the patient is progressing into severe alveolar oedema (see below), he or she remains normocapnic. The mechanism underlying this tachypnoea is uncertain. Hypoxic effects upon the central carbon dioxide chemostat do not appear to be an explanation and recent evidence using perialveolar local anaesthetic suggests that the 'J' (juxta-alveolar) receptor – an unmyelinated nerve ending in the vicinity of the alveoli, which responds to interstitial swelling and distension – is only involved at more severe levels of oedema. Respiratory muscle fatigue is a possibility but one which has not been significantly investigated in heart failure and early oedema.

In acute, severe oedema the usual blood gas abnormalities are hypocapnia and hypoxia. The hypoxia is a result of ventilation/perfusion mismatching. The hypocapnia is accounted for by the reflex tachypnoea leading to an increased alveolar ventilation, which more than compensates for the increased pulmonary deadspace (volume of deadspace/volume of tidal air ratios V_D/V_T ratio). However, in about 20 per cent of severe cases, hypercapnia (with respiratory acidosis) is seen, even when no chronic airflow disease coexists. A number of mechanisms have been proposed and include uncontrolled oxygen administration accompanied by low central carbon dioxide sensitivity, respiratory muscle fatigue, and severe ventilation perfusion imbalance. In acute oedema blood gas abnormalities are usually accompanied by a mild metabolic acidosis but occasionally the base excess may exceed -15 mmol/l. This frank metabolic acidosis is most likely in patients with severe oedema who already have carbon dioxide retention.

In the more chronic permeability oedemas – as in adult respiratory distress syndrome – the overwhelming problem is continuing severe hypoxaemia. Three mechanisms have been proposed: (1) diffusion impairment; (2) low ventilation/perfusion ($\dot{V}_A/\dot{Q}$) values; and (3) shunt ($\dot{V}_A/\dot{Q} < 0.005$). Using both the arterial oxygen response to changing fractional inspired oxygen concentration (FiO_2) and the inert gas technique, it has been shown that diffusion impairment plays little part. Shunt and ventilation/perfusion mismatch are more important, but their contribution varies greatly from patient to patient.

Fig. 9 Pulmonary vascular permeability change demonstrated by surface counting in the dog. The heart to lung ratio is shown following the injection of ^{99}Tc-HSA (human serum albumin). Initially the macromolecular marker penetrates slowly into the lung tissue. After injection of oleic acid, vascular permeability increases and penetration is extremely rapid. (Reproduced from Sugarman *et al.* (1982). *Journal of Trauma*, **22**, 179–85, with permission.)

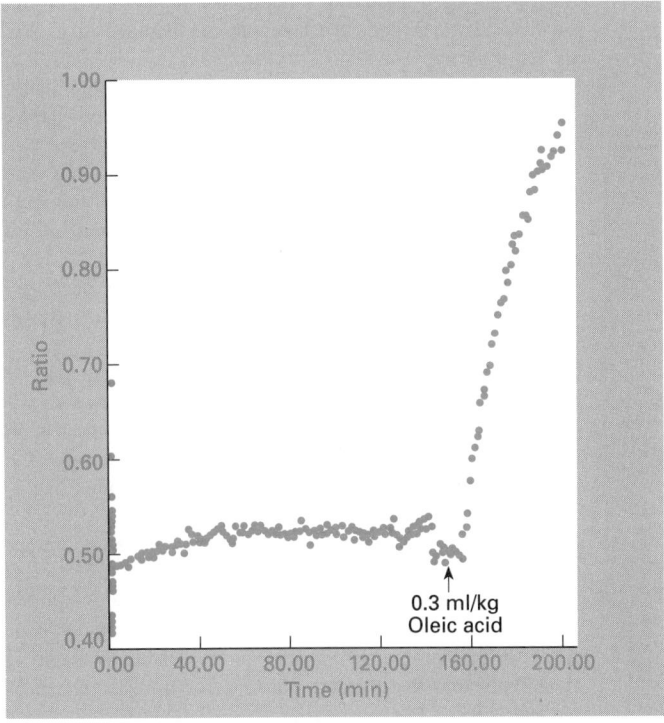

Treatment of pulmonary oedema

Pulmonary oedema may result from increased microvascular hydrostatic pressure, decreased tissue interstitial pressure, decreased plasma colloid oncotic pressure, increased microvascular permeability, or impaired lymphatic drainage. Treatment of each form should try to include measures specifically to reverse the specific cause. However, with the exception of reduction of elevated hydrostatic pressure and relief of upper airway obstruction, these are rarely available and the clinician has to rely upon general supportive measures combined with meticulous attention to fluid balance and monitoring of plasma oncotic pressure.

ACUTE CARDIOGENIC AND FLUID OVERLOAD PULMONARY OEDEMA

By far the most common causes are acute and chronic left-sided heart disease – although overenthusiastic use of intravenous fluid regimes containing normal saline are frequently an additional factor. The patient is most comfortable in the 'trunk up, legs down' position to help pool blood in the dependent parts and reduce central venous pressure. Morphine, diuretics, and oxygen are the fundamentals of current treatment. Thigh cuffs inflated to occlude venous return can help as a form of a bloodless phlebotomy and venesection and removal of 200 to 500 ml of blood is still an effective treatment when other measures are not available.

Morphine acts centrally to relieve the distress of dyspnoea. It also vasodilates the systemic venous system. This reduces venous filling pressure to the heart and performs 'pharmacological phlebotomy' by shifting blood from the lesser to the major circulation. It is best administered by slow intravenous injection in a total dose of 2 to 10 mg at a rate of 2 mg/min.

A bolus dose of frusemide (or other loop diuretic), administered intravenously, is usually given. This acts both by 'pharmacological phlebotomy' and as a diuretic. Diuretics are at their most valuable where pulmonary oedema is a component of congestive cardiac failure and where the volume of extracellular fluid is generally increased. When left ventricular failure has come on acutely, significant fluid retention has not occurred and the pulmonary oedema is a result of fluid shift from the systemic circulation. Over-vigorous use of diuretics then runs the risk of causing hypovolaemia. If the patient is in extremis or heavily sedated, it is wise to catheterize the bladder for, as a result of the diuresis, bladder distension may induce intense reflex systemic vasoconstriction leading, on occasion, to disastrous cardiac overload.

Hypoxia is relieved with a standard face mask or nasal prongs delivering oxygen at relatively high flow rates – up to 10 l/min – providing an inspired concentration of about 60 per cent. If the patient's arterial oxygen tension continues to fall, and/or hypercapnia develops, tracheal intubation and intermittent positive pressure ventilation will be needed.

Aminophylline was once commonly used. As it has diuretic, bronchodilator, cardiac inotropic, and respiratory muscle inotropic effects, its use would still seem logical but it is now scarcely ever used. If it is to be used, administration of 250 to 500 mg should be given intravenously in not less than 20 min because of its capacity to induce arrythmias.

The use of digoxin needs thought. If the patient is already receiving this it may best to discontinue it, at least temporarily, to avoid digitalis toxicity from potassium loss, particularly if large amounts of diuretics are being administered. But if the cardiac failure is associated with fast atrial fibrillation or other supraventricular tachyarrhythmias, these must be controlled and other antiarrythmic drugs, with the exception of amiodarone are negatively inotropic.

The patient who becomes refractory to digoxin and to diuretics often progresses to a state in which a low cardiac output, low blood pressure, oliguria, intense peripheral vasoconstriction, and pulmonary oedema all coexist. In such a state, reduction in left ventricular afterload by means of vasodilators is required. Acutely, sodium nitroprusside infusion may be used to reduce both afterload (by arteriolar vasodilatation) and preload (by venodilatation – 'pharmacological phlebotomy').

Any further improvement in left ventricular function demands the use of inotropic agents such as dopamine or dobutamine which require facilities for careful haemodynamic monitoring.

MANIPULATION OF OSMOTIC AND ONCOTIC PRESSURES

A reduction in oncotic pressure may contribute to pulmonary oedema, as in crystalloid fluid overload, hepatic failure, or nephrotic syndrome. In fluid overload, the most appropriate therapy is the use of diuretics for these not only reduce the extracellular and blood volumes but also return osmotic pressure towards normal.

It is more difficult to be certain about therapy in true hypo-oncotic states. Even where there is no evidence of endothelial damage, the effects of salt-free albumin and plasma concentrate are disappointing. They may even be counter productive when the condition is combined with permeability damage as in the adult respiratory distress syndrome (see below).

MANAGEMENT OF HIGH PERMABILITY PULMONARY OEDEMA

The best form of management would be to block the inappropriate activation and progress of the cascades which are responsible for the condition. Unfortunately there is no therapy which allows this at present and glucorticoids, which used to be recommended, are not now thought to be beneficial.

For the specific treatment of Gram-negative shock (which has as one of its components adult respiratory distress syndrome) use of HA-1A human monoclonal antibody against endotoxin showed initially encouraging results but later observations have not confirmed the early data and this substance has now been withdrawn.

Other possible specific therapies are only at an experimental stage but include:

1. Suppression of the neutrophil superoxide dependent and supplementary calcium–xanthine oxidase dependent cell-destructive mechanisms using phosphodiesterase inhibitors. Pentoxifilline has been shown to reduce lung injury and improve survival after mechanical and endotoxin damage in experimental models.
2. The injection of free radical scavengers and antioxidants. Some very preliminary pilot studies using N-acetylcysteine have suggested that its use in adult respiratory distress syndrome can lead to improved radiological clearing and improved lung compliance. Superoxide dismutase and catalase, although available, have practical problems which limit their potential use.
3. Use of desferrioxamine to chelate the iron that is necessary for hydrogen peroxide cell damage. Benefit has been shown in animal models.
4. Inhibition of the metabolic pathways of arachidonic acid by non-steroidal anti-inflammatory substances. This has a significant effect in ameliorating lung damage in animal models. In the clinical situation, pilot studies have shown that ibuprofen can reduce manifestations of septic shock but no other data is available at present.
5. Use of monoclonal antibodies against cytokines; tumour necrosis factor and interleukin 8 are candidates.
6. Prevention of the adherence of neutrophils to endothelium. No method for this is available at present because, although monoclonal antibodies against adhesion molecules are available, it is unlikely that these are responsible for the first phase of sequestration.

As direct therapy of permeability oedema is at present uncertain, the only treatment available which is not purely supportive is to limit transendothelial fluid flow. Placement of a Swan–Ganz catheter is a first step for this allows monitoring of pulmonary vascular pressures in order to:

1. Optimize fluid replacement.
2. Control a reduction of pulmonary capillary pressure using diuretics. Unless the pressure is already raised, this manoeuvre will be limited by hypovolaemia particularly in patients undergoing positive pressure ventilation.

The role of oncotic pressure management is uncertain. Low oncotic pressures are a feature of many cases of adult respiratory distress syndrome and permeability oedema but, as the endothelium is damaged, any supplementally administered colloid such as human serum albumin will not only enter the interstitial space but will also be unable to exert oncotic pressure. These are probably the reasons why trials have so far been quite inconclusive.

Supportive therapy

This initially consists of oxygen administration. This is given at as high a fractional inspired oxygen concentration as is necessary to keep the arterial partial pressure of oxygen near to the normal level – and no more – because, in permeability oedema: (1) high oxygen levels may lead to absorption atelectasis in areas of low ventilation/perfusion; (2) oxygen toxicity may become a problem where prolonged administration is often necessary. If oxygen administration at normal, airway pressure cannot maintain the arterial partial pressure of oxygen, continuous positive pressure during spontaneous breathing may be tried and may obviate intubation and mechanical ventilation.

Positive pressure ventilation

This allows the buying of time for healing or improvement of the underlying disease. The aim is, most often, to improve arterial oxygenation but, on occasions, because of a high volume of deadspace/volume of tidal air ratio, the technique may also be used to achieve adequate alveolar ventilation. Both intermittent and continuous positive pressure ventilation are used – the choice depends upon the severity of the disease. Neither has been shown to reduce the mortality of adult respiratory

distress syndrome in a formal trial, but so great is the immediate benefit of ventilation in respiratory failure that such an investigation would probably be unethical at this stage.

Extracorporeal respiratory support

This has been attempted using both extracorporeal membrane oxygenation (ECMO) and extracorporeal support with carbon dioxide removal (ECCO$_2$). So far, neither technique has been shown to promote lung healing or improve prognosis.

REFERENCES

Anonymous (1986). Adult respiratory distress syndrome. *Lancet,* **i,** 301–303.
Anonymous (1986). The enigma of breathlessness. *Lancet,* **i,** 891–892.
Artigas, A., Lemire, F., Suter, P.M., and Zapol, W. (1992). *The Adult Respiratory Distress Syndrome.* Churchill Livingstone, Edinburgh.
Bone, R.C. (1991). The pathogenesis of sepsis. *Annals of Internal Medicine,* **115,** 457–469.
Donnelly, S.E. and Haslett, C. (1992). Cellular mechanisms of acute lung injury: Implications for future treatment in the adult respiratory distress syndrome. *Thorax,* **37,** 260–263.
Egan, E.A. (1983). Fluid balance in the air filled alveolar space. *American Review of Respiratory Disease,* **127,** 37–39.
Guyton, A.O. and Lindsey, A.W. (1959). Effect of elevated left atrial pressure and decreased plasma protein concentration upon the development of pulmonary oedema. *Circulation Research,* **7,** 649.
Morgan, P.W. and Goodman, L.R. (1991). Imaging of diffuse lung diseases: Pulmonary oedema and adult respiratory distress syndrome. *Radiologic Clinics of North America,* **29,** 943–963.
O. Brodovich, H. (1990). When the alveolus is flooding, it is time to man the pumps. *American Review of Respiratory Disease,* **142,** 1247–1248.
Prichard, J.S. (1982). *Edema of the lung.* Charles C. Thomas, Springfield, Illinois.
Simon, R.D. (1993). Neurogenic pulmonary edema. *Neurologic Clinics,* **11** (2), 309–23.
Szidon, P.S. (1989). Pathophysiology of the congested lung. *Cardiology Clinics,* **7,** 39–48.
Trimby, J., Reid, C., Zeilender, S., and Glauser, F.L. (1990). Mechanical causes of pulmonary oedema. *Chest,* **98,** 973–979.
Wiedemann, H.P. and Matthay, M.A. (eds) (1990). Adult respiratory distress syndrome. *Clinics in Chest Medicine,* **11,** (4), 575–811.

15.24 Pulmonary hypertension

J. S. PRICHARD

Introduction

Pressures within the normal pulmonary circulation alter surprisingly little with change in blood flow. Sustained high blood pressure in the pulmonary circulation therefore indicates that functional and structural changes have taken place. Most commonly these are an indirect result of events elsewhere, such as hypoxia from lung disease or high blood flow through the lung generated by cardiac shunts, and the pulmonary hypertension is a secondary phenomenon. Occasionally this is not so and the immediate problem is in the pulmonary vasculature itself. Under these, rarer, circumstances primary pulmonary hypertension is said to be present.

Probably in every individual with pulmonary hypertension two functional changes are present simultaneously. The first is constrictive vascular disease, in which the rise in resistance is a consequence of smooth muscular contraction or spasm. The second is restrictive vascular dis-

ease, in which structural, non-contractile re-modelling of the pulmonary vascular system has reduced the capacity and increased the resistance to blood flow in the system. The balance between these components varies greatly from case to case but generally, the milder the hypertension, the less the restrictive component.

Because such a wide range of events and circumstances can lead to constrictive and restrictive changes, it might be assumed that each caused these through a different mechanism. Until recently most investigators would indeed have thought this to be the case. But, more recently, the hypothesis has emerged that damage to the endothelial cell represents a final common pathway through which each of the initiating events calls into play first the vasoconstriction and subsequently the structural remodelling which underly pulmonary hypertension. This exciting new idea, which could unify much thinking about a hetrogeneous subject, will be discussed at the end of the chapter.

The diseases that initiate secondary pulmonary hypertension are

Table 1 *Pulmonary and systemic circulations – representative values*

	Normal pressures		
	Systolic (mmHg)	Diastolic (mmHg)	Mean (mmHg)
Right atrium	'a' 7 'v' 5	'x' 3 'y' 3	5
Right ventricle	25	pre 'a' 3 post 'a' 7	N/A
Pulmonary artery	25	15	18
Left atrium (direct or wedge)	'a' 12 'v' 10	'x' 7 'y' 7	10
Left ventricle	120	pre 'a' 7 post 'a' 12	N/A
Aorta	120	80	90–95
Cardiac index			2.8–4.2 l/min^2
Systemic vascular resistance			10–20 mmHg/l/min
Pulmonary vascular resistance			< 2.0 mmHg/l/min

described elsewhere: here, only the features in the pulmonary circulation will be set out. On the other hand, primary pulmonary hypertension will be described in detail.

The identification and measurement of pulmonary hypertension

The definition of pulmonary hypertension depends upon what limits are put on normality (Table 1). Usually, it is said to be present when the systolic pulmonary arterial pressure at rest exceeds 30 mmHg or the mean arterial pressure 20 mmHg.

Although we measure pulmonary arterial pressure and use the term 'pulmonary hypertension' as though this were itself a disease, the fundamental physiological abnormality is the increased obstacle to blood flow presented by the pulmonary circulation and an important point is how this should be quantified. In a normal individual, use of the term pulmonary vascular resistance is potentially misleading, because the concept of resistance applies to the Pouiseillian flow of a Newtonian liquid through a system of vessels whose dimensions are independent of pressure and whose lengths are great in comparison to their diameters. As most of these conditions do not apply in the normal pulmonary circulation, the situation is better analysed by the calculation of impedance.

However, in considering pulmonary hypertension, use is made of the simpler concept. Not only, at high pressures, are the approximations less distorting, but the very large increases in resistance seen are an order of magnitude greater than any improvements in accuracy that would result from a more sophisticated approach using impedance. For the remainder of this chapter the simple concept of resistance will be used to quantify pulmonary hypertension.

Classification of pulmonary hypertension

Pulmonary hypertension can be classified either by aetiology or by the histopathological changes in the lung blood vessels. Unfortunately, the two classification systems overlap and this can cause confusion.

Classification by aetiology (Table 2) recognizes that pulmonary hypertension may be either primary or secondary. However, the term 'primary' can cause confusion because in some accounts it is used synonymously with 'idiopathic', whilst in others it is used to imply that the disease originates in the pulmonary vessels, even though the cause (such as a toxin or collagen vascular disease) may have been identified. In this

Table 2 *Pulmonary hypertension – aetiology*

Idiopathic
    Primary pulmonary hypertension
    Pulmonary veno-occlusive disease
    Pulmonary haemangioendotheliomatosis

Secondary to:
    Persistently increased pulmonary blood flow (pre-tricuspid
        and post-tricuspid shunts)
    Left atrial hypertension
    Chronic hypoxia*
        chronic lung disease
        thoracic musculoskeletal disease
        dwellers at high altitudes
    Pulmonary embolism.
        thromboembolism
        foreign body embolism from intravenous drugs
        amniotic fluid embolism
    Collagen and autoimmune diseases
    Pulmonary vascular toxins – including:
        drugs (aminorex, ?oral contraceptives, ?phenformin),
        plants (*Crotolaria* and *Senecio* spp.), denatured rape-seed
        oil (oleoanilide)

Parasitic lung disease

Hepatic cirrhosis

Altered blood rheology (sickle-cell disease)

*Causes of cor pulmonale are set out in more detail in Chapter 15.25.

chapter, following the World Health Organization report of 1973, the term 'primary' is used to describe those diseases in which the cause is quite unknown. These include primary pulmonary hypertension itself, the rare pulmonary veno-occlusive disease, and pulmonary haemangioendothelioma. In the West, the most common causes of secondary hypertension are persistent hypoxia from chest disease and high pulmonary blood flow from cardiac shunts; other causes are quite uncommon.

If pulmonary hypertension is classified by histopathological changes a slightly different pattern emerges. All forms of chronic pulmonary hypertension show medial hypertrophy of the muscular arteries and proliferative intimal lesions but, in addition, certain characteristic patterns are recognized. These are:

1. *Plexogenic pulmonary vasculopathy*. Primary pulmonary hypertension, hypertension from increased pulmonary blood flow, hepatic cirrhosis, and certain types of toxic pulmonary hypertension share a common characteristic abnormality—plexogenic arteriopathy—and no parenchymal lung disease is present.

2. *Hypoxic pulmonary vasculopathy*. Characteristic vascular changes emerge in long term hypoxia, irrespective of whether there are associated parenchymal lung changes (e.g. in chronic airways disease or fibrosis) or not (e.g. high altitude dwellers, thoracic deformity).

3. *Congestive pulmonary vasculopathy*. Venous outflow obstruction and pulmonary oedema lead to distinctive parenchymal changes and pulmonary haemosiderosis in addition to non-plexogenic vascular changes.

4. *Embolic pulmonary arteriopathy*. Thromboembolism can usually be identified by fresh or organizing thrombus. However, the presence of eccentric intimal fibrosis of muscular arteries in early primary pulmonary hypertension can occasionally make the distinction between primary disease and microthromboembolic disease extraordinarily difficult.

5. In parasitic disease (such as pulmonary schistosomiasis or echinococcosis (hydatid disease)), tumour, amniotic fluid embolus, collagen disease and foreign body embolism, morphological changes are closely, if not uniquely, associated with the particular aetiology.

Necrotizing vasculitis is a terminal feature of all types of pulmonary hypertension and is not particular to any. Similarly, dilatation, atherosclerotic change, and aneurysm in the larger elastic arteries are secondary results common to all syndromes where high pressure has been persistent and severe.

Pulmonary hypertension associated with high pulmonary blood flow

Histological changes

Congenital cardiac septal defects subject the pulmonary circulation to continuous haemodynamic stress. In post-tricuspid shunts, such as ventricular septal defects, the pulmonary vasculature is exposed to a high level of pressure from birth, whereas in pretricuspid shunts, such as atrial septal defects, the onset of pulmonary arterial hypertension occurs later in life. However, although such hypertension may emerge at different times in the two types of shunt, and although the progress may be at different speeds, both run a similar course—the sequence of histological changes of which were originally identified by Heath and Edwards in 1958. Six stages are recognized:

1. *Muscularization*. Scanning electron microscopy demonstrates that the normal delicate endothelial ridges running in the direction of flow disappear and, instead, the surface of the endothelial cell becomes irregular and disorganized. Arterioles are easily visible and instead of the normal elastic tissue, circularly disposed muscles can be seen in the media. Hypertrophy occurs in the muscular arteries. Not all the muscle is circularly orientated and a certain proportion of the hyperplasia in the outer part of the media occurs with the fibres parallel to the axis of the vessel.

2. *Cellular intimal proliferation*. The newly muscularized arterioles show proliferation of intimal cells. Initially this was thought to be endothelial. However, it is probably from myofibroblasts which, as they proliferate, progressively reduce the size of the blood vessel lumen.

3. *Progressive fibrous vascular occlusion*. Following the proliferation of myofibroblasts, fibroblasts appear and lay down collagen fibres. These lie within intervening ground substance to produce an 'onion skin proliferation' (Fig. 1). Elastic fibres are then laid down and progressive fibroelastosis eventually causes complete occlusion.

4. *Appearance of complex 'dilation lesions'*. The process leads onward to the formation of a number of different 'dilatation lesions' (Fig. 2). There are three types:

   (a) Plexiform lesions consist of complex distensions of the smallest pulmonary arteries to form thin wall sacs with connections to the alveolar capillaries. Endothelial proliferation and thrombosis often occur within them. The cells which line the plexiform lesion resemble plump endothelial cells. However, it is more likely that they have partly differentiated from mesenchymal cells for they lack a basal lamina, micropinocytotic vesicles or caveolae. Their cytoplasm often contains numerous microfilaments arranged in whorls.

   (b) Vein-like branches of hypertrophied muscular arteries emerge from parent arteries proximal to a point of obstruction. They act as collateral channels to the alveolar capillaries.

   (c) Angiomatoid lesions are usually only seen in association with ventricular septal defect. They arise in small pulmonary arteries just proximal to points of fibrotic occlusion.

5. *Chronic vascular dilation with haemosiderosis*. The fragile dilation lesions allow diapedesis of erythrocytes and rupture easily. Foci of haemosiderin laden macrophages appear.

6. *Necrotizing arteritis (fibrinous vasculosis) of the muscular arteries* is found only in extreme cases. Disruption of the endothelium allows fibrinogen to diffuse into the intima where the extrinsic cascade produces fibrin. Initially, the intima and inner elastic lamina form a barrier which prevents macromolecular penetration into the media. However, as the condition develops, deficiencies appear in this barrier which allow deep penetration of fibrinogen. At this stage the characteristic

Fig. 1 Transverse section of a small muscular pulmonary artery from a woman of 26 years with a aortopulmonary septal defect and pulmonary hypertension. There is pronounced concentric intimal proliferation ('onion skin proliferation'). (Reproduced from Harris P. and Heath D. (1986). *The Human pulmonary Circulation*, p. 252 Livingstone, Edinburgh, with permission. Micrograph kindly supplied by Professor D. Heath.)

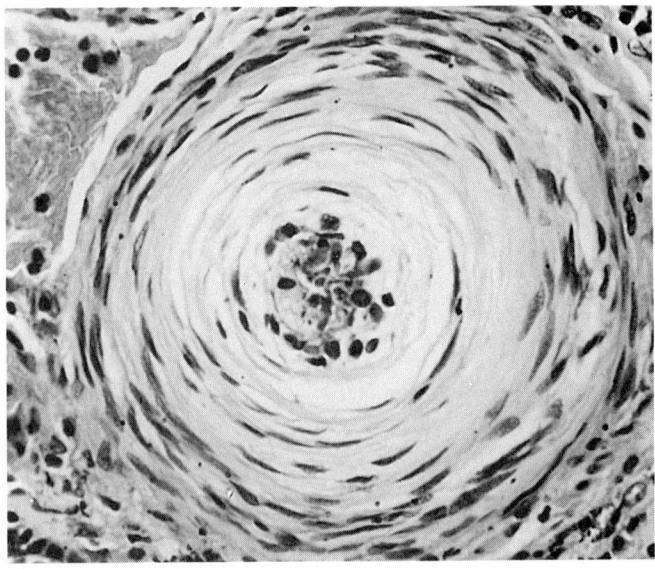

appearances of 'fibrinoid necrosis' occurs. Although the classic term implies cell death, this is not the case and there is no evidence that cells die. Thus, the term fibrinous vasculosis is preferable.

The effect of persistent hypertension on the structure of elastic pulmonary arteries

Sustained pulmonary hypertension causes structural changes in the large pulmonary vessels.

In the media there is proliferation of muscle cells and the development of additional elastic tissue. Where high pulmonary blood flow is present from birth the increased elastic tissue—when compared with a normal individual—retains a fetal orientation with long firm longitudinal elastic bundles linked by cross fibres at 90° to the main direction. When pulmonary hypertension develops late in life the quantity of elastic tissue increases but the normal adult disposition of an irregular network of fragmented elastic fibrils is retained. In addition there is also a significant expansion in ground substance due to the extra production of proteo-

Fig. 2 Diagram to show the origin and probable connections of small thin walled blood vessels in the lung in grade 5 hypertensive pulmonary vascular disease. 1 = dilated muscular pulmonary artery with thin media and intimal fibrosis: this is part of the generalized dilation proximal to the site of vascular occlusion. 2 = hypertrophied muscular pulmonary artery arising as a side branch of 1 with a heaped up intimal fibrous tissue at the site of origina. 3 = terminal muscular pulmonary artery totally occluded by fibrous tissue: the media may be thick, as shown, or abnormally thin. 4 = terminal dilated pulmonary arteriole. 5 = capillaries in alveolar wall arising from pulmonary arteriole. 6 = dilated thin walled, vein-like branch of hypertrophied parent muscular pulmonary artery. 7 = localized 'dilation': an angiomatoid lesion. 8 = capillaries in alveolar walls arising from dilation lesions. 9 = dilated thin wall vessel in submucosa of small bronchus. 10 = small bronchial artery in fibrous coat of small bronchus giving rise to thin wall branches as shown as 11. A = bronchopulmonary anastomosis at capillary level. B = anastomosis between capillaries arising from parent muscular pulmonary artery and from 'dilation lesions'. C = possible anastomosis between thin wall vessels derived from pulmonary artery and those derived from pulmonary vein. (Reproduced from Harris, P. and Heath, D. (1986). *The Human pulmonary circulation*. p 255. Churchill Livingstone, Edinburgh, with permission.)

glycans by the smooth muscle cells. These areas of media tend to become cystic and the term 'cystic medial necrosis' is applied. It is yet another misnomer, as necrosis forms no part of the process!

Initially, the endothelium reacts to hypertension and high blood flow by elongation of the cells themselves and by their more obvious longtitudinal orientation. Subsequently, the major reaction is the development of atheroma. Occasionally the effects may be so severe as to cause aneurysm formation.

Pathophysiology of high-flow pulmonary hypertension

Pulmonary arterial pressure and vascular resistance rise in parallel with histological severity of both post- and pretricuspid shunts (Fig. 3) although, grade for grade, tend to be higher in the post-tricuspid. In the post tricuspid shunts, if infants are excluded, the majority of patients of Grade 1 to 3 histological severity have a total pulmonary resistance of less than 9 mmHg/l/s, whereas most patients with Grade 5 lesions have a total pulmonary resistance that exceeds 18 mmHg/l/s.

One of the problems has been to distinguish between the contributions to increased resistance of vasoconstriction and fixed stenosis. A number of studies have tried to distinguish by measuring resistance whilst the patient is breathing 100 per cent oxygen or, more recently, other vasodilators. In patients with Grade 1 lesions, such procedures often lower the pulmonary vascular resistance to normal levels. With increasing grades of abnormality, they still cause a fall in resistance but cannot reduce it to normal. Thus, Heath and his colleagues found that patients with Grade 5 lesions maintain a resistance of more than five times normal even during the inhalation of 100 per cent oxygen. The general conclusion, therefore, is that whereas in the lowest grades of abnormality the dominant effect is vasoconstriction of hypertrophied muscle, as the disease progresses the relative contribution of restrictive, fixed stenosis becomes progressively greater.

Pulmonary hypertension associated with pulmonary venous hypertension

Pathological changes

The lung is engorged with blood and veins and capillaries are distended.

In the veins there is intimal fibrosis and medial hypertrophy of the smooth muscle. At the alveolar capillary wall there is an increase in the

Fig. 3 Relation between grade of plexogenic pulmonary arteriopathy (PPA) and total pulmonary resistance in 13 patients with pretricuspid shunts. (Reproduced from Harris P. and Heath D. (1986). *The Human pulmonary Circulation*. p. 299 Livingstone, Edinburgh, with permission.)

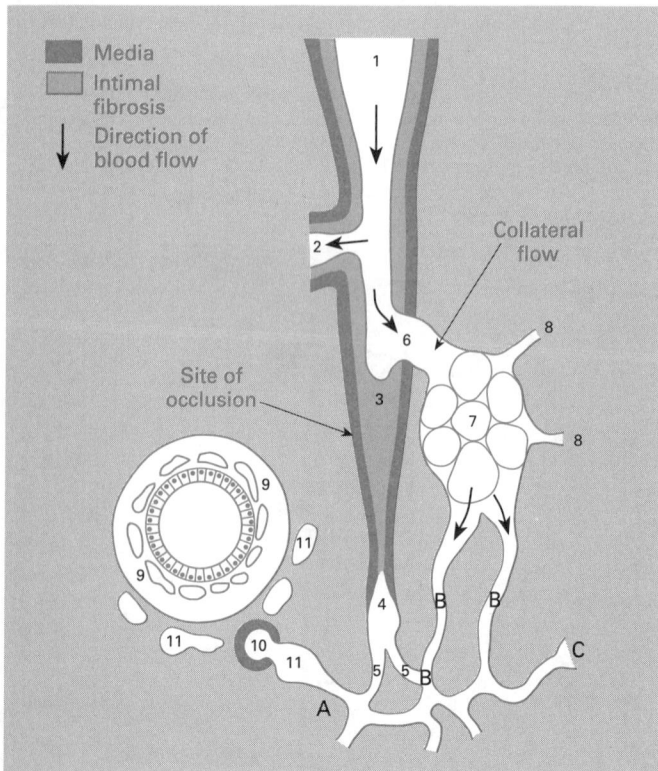

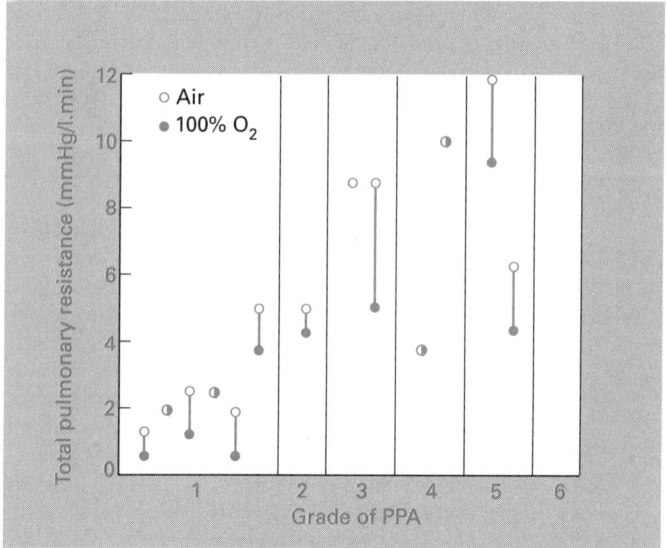

basement membrane which enlarges from its normal thickness of 8 to 10 nm to between 15 and 30 nm. Frequently, there is a subendothelial infiltration of hyaline mucopolysaccharide. The endothelial cells themselves may become oedematous so that their cytoplasm, seen by the electron microscope, is swollen and abnormally lucent. However, the endothelial junctions remain intact. Over wide areas, membraneous type 1 pneumocytes are lost and replaced by granular type 2 pneumocytes.

Interstitial oedema appears as lucent areas in the alveolar wall and these cause wide separation of cells and fibrils. With persistence of oedema there is proliferation of reticular and elastic fibrils so that the alveolar capillaries become embedded in connective tissue. Red blood cells pass through capillary walls, split the basement membranes and subsequently disintegrate. They are ingested by macrophages which group together to give pulmonary haemosiderosis. Mast cells appear as a secondary response to the haemosiderosis. Occasionally, microlith—and even bone—formation may occur.

The arterial changes are the first three stages of plexogenic arteriopathy. However, although fibrinous vasculosis may occasionally also be seen in very severe cases, dilatation and, in particular, plexiform lesions do not develop.

The distribution of changes in the lung follows a gradation from base to apex. Thus, the muscular pulmonary arteries and pulmonary veins in the lower lobes are more severely hypertrophied than those of the apices. Pulmonary haemosiderosis, congestion, oedema, and the dilatation of lymphatics are maximal in the posterior part of the upper lobe where the arterial hypertrophy has not been so great, and this might suggest that the arterial changes have a protective effect for the capillary circulation.

Pathophysiological changes

The pathophysiological changes of pulmonary hypertension caused by a rise in venous pressure have been most extensively studied in mitral valve disease where pulmonary arterial pressure increases more rapidly than wedge pressure (Fig. 4). Resistance is thus increasing as a result of pulmonary vascular changes and, arguing teleologically, it has been suggested that this protects the capillaries and delays the onset of

Fig. 4 The relationship between mean pulmonary arterial (A) and mean wedge (W) pressure in 27 patients with mitral stenosis. The dotted straight line represents the relation which would be expected if resistance remained constant. (Reproduced from Harris P. and Heath D. (1986). *The human pulmonary circulation*. p. 347. Churchill Livingstone, Edinburgh, with permission.)

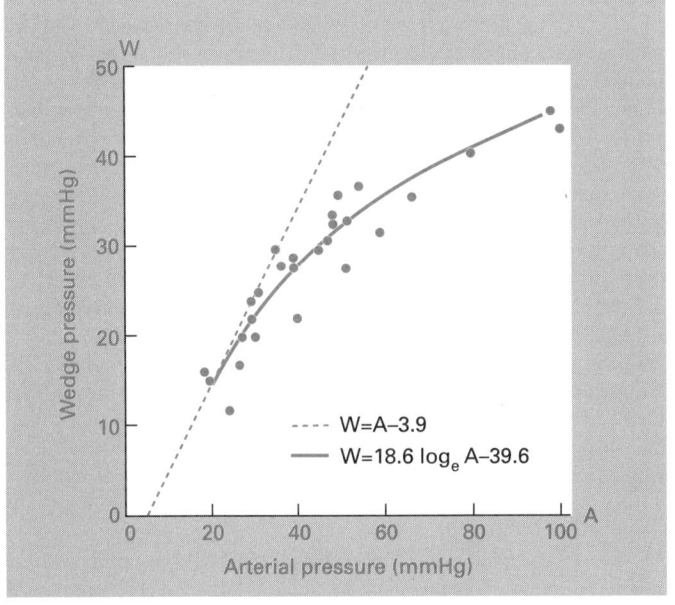

oedema. A second abnormality is the redistribution of perfusion. Under normal circumstances perfusion increases progressively from the apex of the lung towards the base in the upright position at rest. When pulmonary venous hypertension is present there is a redistribution of blood flow so that the upper portions of the lungs become more perfused than the bases. This reversal may be caused partly by structural changes in the vessels, as indicated above. However, there is an additional component from vasoconstriction demonstrable by the administration of vasodilators such as acetylcholine and oxygen, both of which lessen the apex to base gradient. A further demonstration of active vasoconstriction can be seen in the effect of lying alternatively on the right and left sides in patients with mitral stenosis. Within 10 min of lying on the right side, blood flow to the left lung is increased and that to the right lung diminished. Reversal of the dependent side reverses the flow.

Pulmonary hypertension following long-term hypoxia

Chronic hypoxia from any cause stimulates the formation of smooth muscle bundles arranged longitudinally within the intima and media of the muscular pulmonary arteries extending proximally. Muscularization of the arterioles between their internal and external elastic laminae also occurs. In addition, there is destructive loss of lung parenchyma if chronic lung disease is present.

Tropical disease and pulmonary arterial hypertension

Severe sickle-cell disease, particularly in the young, may be associated with sequestration crises. Red cell sequestration in the lungs with resulting increased viscosity, vascular stasis, and even complete blockage of the microvasculature may occur leading to local areas of infarction and acute pulmonary hypertension. Recurrent episodes can lead to microvascular destruction, fibrosis and chronic hypertensive changes.

Tropical parasitic infestations excite complex, partially immune, inflammatory responses with the formation of granulomata in the lungs—as in schistosomiasis from *Schistosoma mansoni* but less commonly from *Schistosoma japonica*. The early symptoms are allergic with attacks of asthma and mild fever. Severe pulmonary hypertension develops slowly, leading to chronic right heart failure within a few years.

Particularly in the Far East, filariasis and tropical eosinophilia associated with helminth infestations other than filariasis produce both an allergic and granulomatous response to the larvae with scattered lesions in the lung substance, liver, and sometimes the lymph glands. Again, attacks of asthma, often with purulent blood-streaked sputum, are the presenting symptoms. Gradually the insidious symptoms of fatigue and breathlessness herald the development of pulmonary hypertension. A careful history should alert the clinician to the possibility of tropical parasitic exposure, particularly if associated with a high eosinophil count.

Pulmonary hypertension associated with hepatic disease

Pulmonary hypertension is a rare association of liver disease—most frequently cirrhosis or portal hypertension. This is surprising as the common pulmonary abnormalities in hepatic disease are intrapulmonary arteriovenous shunts and a blunting of the hypoxic vasoconstrictor response. Where pulmonary hypertension does occur it evolves into the plexogenic form.

The aetiology is obscure. The slightly increased pulmonary vascular flow and hypertension commonly seen in liver disease seem too mild to be of significance. Thromboemboli entering the lung through the portapulmonary anastomoses, which develop in portal hypertension, are an unproved alternative explanation. Dietary factors in association with portapulmonary venous anastomoses (which by-pass normal detoxification mechanisms) fit with the observation that pulmonary hypertension has not been induced by production of even severe cirrhosis in animal models.

Pulmonary hypertension and collagen vascular diseases

Collagen vascular diseases can induce secondary pulmonary hypertension by their ability to damage lung parenchyma and cause hypoxaemia. However, particularly in systemic lupus erythematosus, polymyositis, dermatositis, systemic sclerosis, rheumatoid arthritis, and juvenile rheumatoid arthritis, pulmonary hypertension has been reported where there was no apparent pulmonary parenchymal disease. Histological examination has revealed an obliterative vascular disease which has on occasions shown a plexogenic pattern. The situation is further confused by the fact that positive antinuclear antibody (ANA) serology (titre > 1 : 80) occurs in about 50 per cent of patients with primary pulmonary hypertension. When this figure is compared with other conditions (e.g. normal individuals—20 per cent; discoid lupus—40 per cent; rheumatoid arthritis—50 to 60 per cent; systemic sclerosis—70 per cent; systemic lupus erythematosus—90 per cent; dermatositis–polymyositis—95 per cent) the suggestion of a link between primary pulmonary hypertension and the collaganoses becomes strong.

A group of patients with collagen diseases who have pulmonary hypertension without obvious parenchymal disease have been studied at the National Institutes of Health (NIH) registry and compared with primary Pulmonary hypertensives. They are more likely to be female, to have restrictive lung disease (demonstrated by lung function testing despite absence of clinical features) and to show Raynaud's phenomenon. Life expectancy was very short in these cases, with a mean survival of only 471 days.

Clinical features common to secondary pulmonary hypertension

In secondary pulmonary hypertension, the raised pulmonary arterial pressure is merely one component in the pathophysiology. The clinical features are not seen by themselves but are embedded within—and have to be distinguished from—those of the initiating disease. Nonetheless, it is often important to identify and note them for two reasons:

(1) their intensity may allow assessment of the severity of the pulmonary hypertension;
(2) their character may assist in the differential diagnosis

Intense fatigue, breathlessness even at rest, and faintness on exertion, often culminating in syncope, are all symptoms of severe pulmonary hypertension. Chest pain resembling angina of effort may arise as a result of the high right ventricular workload, right ventricular hypertrophy, and reduced coronary blood flow from low cardiac output. As the disease progresses the right ventricle fails to cope with the increased afterload and the patient will complain of the symptoms of right heart failure, including ankle swelling, abdominal pain from liver distension, and, eventually, abdominal distension from ascites.

Episodes of pleural pain with haemoptysis suggest recurrent pulmonary embolism. Haemoptyses without pain occur in severe pulmonary venous hypertension and also in the late states of plexogenic arteriopathy.

On examination, a small volume pulse, peripheral vasoconstriction, cool extremities, and peripheral cyanosis all reflect the low cardiac output state. Except in hypoxic pulmonary hypertension, central cyanosis is not a notable feature unless there has been reversal of a previous left-to-right intracardiac shunt or unless recurrent pulmonary emboli is a likely diagnosis.

The severity of pulmonary hypertension can be assessed clinically. Significant, long-standing pulmonary hypertension will lead to right ventricular hypertrophy, a palpable right ventricular heave and the presence of an increasingly prominent right atrial 'a' wave in the neck veins,

because of the increased force of the right atrial systolic contraction needed to overcome the elevated end-diastolic right ventricular pressure. Atrial fibrillation will develop at some stage, but is often quite a late manifestation.

As pressure rises further, the pulmonary valvular component of the second heart sound is accentuated. The high diastolic pressure leads to forceful closure with an accentuated, often palpable sound at the apex. Also during expiration, the closer the pulmonary second sound approaches the aortic component, the higher the pulmonary artery pressure is likely to be, provided right bundle branch block is not present.

As the disease progresses, a right ventricular third heart sound, often with an atrial fourth sound superimposed, leads to a summation gallop. The presence of a third heart sound heralds the onset of right heart failure and, as the ventricle fails to overcome the ever-increasing afterload, the central venous pressure rises, with subsequent fluid retention and peripheral oedema. Dilatation of the right ventricle and stretching of the valve ring leads to the systolic murmur of tricuspid incompetence which increases during inspiration and to a ventricular 'v' wave in the jugular venous pulse. Tricuspid incompetence accelerates right heart failure and to the peripheral oedema may be added pulsatile swelling of the liver and eventual cardiac cirrhosis and ascites. The pulmonary valve may become incompetent in severe pulmonary hypertension, leading to a basal early diastolic murmur, which may become louder on inspiration. An early pulmonary systolic ejection sound or even a short murmur may be heard when there is significant dilation of the main pulmonary trunk and this can sometimes be confused with the tricuspid systolic murmur.

Where pulmonary arterial hypertension has developed secondary to obstruction of the pulmonary venous outflow, the additional sign of basal lung crepitations under stable resting conditions may indicate significant pulmonary venous hypertension.

Functional investigations in secondary pulmonary hypertension

The chest radiograph

The appearances are frequently dominated by primary pathology, such as chronic obstructive airways disease, pulmonary fibrosis, or pulmonary embolism. The cardiac silouhette may suggest various congenital or acquired heart diseases.

None the less, various features that result from pulmonary hypertension itself will frequently be detectable. Enlargement of the main pulmonary trunk is usual but variable. It causes a prominent convexity of the upper left mediastinum between the aortic knuckle and the upper left border of the heart (left ventricle and left atrial appendage). The left and right main pulmonary arteries and their proximal branches are also enlarged. In contrast, in severe pulmonary hypertension, the peripheral pulmonary arteries appear pruned so that they are much narrower than normal. This leads to increased radiological translucency peripherally.

The size of the peripheral arteries also helps decide whether there is a high pulmonary blood flow. Thus, patients with large septal defects and hyperdynamic pulmonary hypertension show plethoric lung fields with engorged peripheral vessels, whereas patients who are developing a low output state from pulmonary hypertension associated with severe vascular changes will show conspicuous peripheral vascular pruning, as in congenital septal defects with the Eisenmenger syndrome.

Where pulmonary venous hypertension is present, evidence of increased pulmonary venous and capillary hydrostatic pressures is also obtained from the chest radiograph if redistribution of the venous vascular shadows from base to apex, perihilar haze, presence of Kerley lines or other features of pulmonary oedema are found.

Radioisotope lung scan

This investigation helps in distinguishing thromboembolic disease from primary pulmonary hypertension. Its value in reported series probably results from the fact that primary hypertension occurs in relatively young people where other confounding pathologies such as pulmonary emphysema are not present.

The electrocardiogram

Irrespective of the effects of the primary pathology, pulmonary hypertension itself is likely to cause development of the pattern of right ventricular hypertrophy with right axis deviation (more than + 120° in the limb leads, dominant R and T inversion in the right precordial leads and a dominant S wave in the left precordial leads). Right atrial hypertrophy is shown by tall, often peaked P waves in right precordial leads and in the inferior leads.

The pattern may be modified when both pulmonary venous and pulmonary arterial hypertension are present (as in mitral stenosis), for the associated dilation and hypertrophy of the left atrium will lead to the development of bifid P waves and a negative terminal deflection in lead V_1.

If both left and right ventricular hypertrophy are present, as in large ventricular septal defects with pulmonary hypertension, then tall R waves will be found in the left precordial leads with large biphasic RS complexes in the midprecordial leads, indicating biventricular hypertrophy. In cor pulmonale, or where emphysema coexists with some other cause of pulmonary hypertension, the electrocardiograph is insensitive in the diagnosis of right ventricular hypertrophy because the increased lung volume leads to diaphragmatic depression so that the heart hangs vertically and rotates clockwise. This may be recognized by inversion of both the right and left unipolar limb leads associated with deep S waves in both.

Right bundle branch block is common in all forms of pulmonary hypertension and, in pulmonary hypertension from congenital atrial septal defects, it is present from birth. In septum secundum defects the terminal portion of the QRS complex will be orientated anteriorly (producing an rsR in V1) and rightward (producing a permanent S wave in lead 1). Left axis deviation in a young patient with a right ventricular conduction defect, pulmonary hypertension, and a tendency to cyanosis with exercise suggests the presence of an ostium primum atrial septal defect.

The echocardiograph

This has two useful roles. First, it assists in assessing the severity of the pulmonary hypertension. The pulmonary valve echo tends to show a reduced 'a' wave excursion, an increased 'b' to 'c' slope, a prolonged right ventricular pre-ejection period and a midsystolic notch. However, echocardiographic visualization of the pulmonary valve is notoriously difficult and the findings, when obtained, show poor correlation with the severity of the pulmonary hypertension. Assessment of right ventricular cavity size and right ventricular wall thickness is also somewhat unreliable because it is often difficult to obtain clear chamber definition. This is because of interference from overlying lung tissue, particularly in patients with emphysema.

The second major use of echocardiography is in finding the underlying cause of the pulmonary hypertension. Thus, in venous pulmonary hypertension, it helps to verify the presence and severity of mitral stenosis and to exclude rarer conditions such as left atrial myxoma and cor triatriatum. In hyperdynamic pulmonary hypertension, particularly when used with contrast enhancement, echocardiography is a remarkably precise non-invasive tool for localizing and defining the size of intracardiac septal defects.

Cardiac catheterization and pulmonary angiography

Catheterization gives direct evidence of the presence and severity of pulmonary hypertension. It allows assessment of whether arterial, venous, or mixed hypertension is present. It permits pressures and flows to be related so that pulmonary vascular resistance can be calculated. These measurements, combined with pulmonary angiography (which has the risk of precipitating acute right heart failure or ventricular fibrillation from sudden pump overload from the injectate), may be essential if accurate diagnosis is needed in difficult cases of unexplained severe pulmonary hypertension.

Arterial blood gas analysis

Arterial blood gas analysis is useful in the differential diagnosis of intracardiac shunts, in assessing the likelihood of hypoxic cor pulmonale and in detecting ventilation–perfusion abnormalities. The analyses should be undertaken both at rest and under exercise.

Primary pulmonary hypertension

Primary pulmonary hypertension is a synonym for unexplained or idiopathic pulmonary hypertension. Clinically the condition was characterized over 40 years ago but the number of patients is so small (approximate incidence 1 to $2/10^6$) that good descriptions have remained few. However, the situation has improved since the establishment of the United States National Registry on Primary Pulmonary Hypertension at the National Institutes of Health in 1981 and, more recently, of the European International Primary Pulmonary Hypertension Study.

Histopathology

The histopathological features are those of plexogenic pulmonary arteriopathy and, both in the larger and smaller vessels, are indistinguishable from those in pre- and post-tricuspid shunts. However, it has never been formally demonstrated that the changes are progressive and the grading system is best not used.

Clinical features

The disease most often presents between 20 and 45 years and is twice as common in women as in men. Occasionally (in about 7 per cent) it may be familial and due to an autosomal dominant inheritance with incomplete penetrance.

The initial clinical manifestations are diverse and the presenting symptoms include (in approximate order of frequency), dyspnoea (60 per cent), fatigue (20 per cent), chest pain (10 per cent), palpitations, and syncope and swollen ankles. Often diagnosis is delayed for between 1 and 2 years both because of the ill-defined nature of symptoms and because of the paucity of physical signs in the early stages.

On examination, the major features are the presence of third and fourth right heart sounds with, less frequently, pulmonary ejection and regurgitant murmurs. Tricuspid incompetence is often present and right ventricular hypertrophy may be detected. Clubbing is not a feature and Raynaud's phenomenon is only slightly more common than in an age- and sex-matched population. A degree of arterial hypoxia is found but this is rarely sufficient to cause cyanosis at the time of diagnosis.

Investigations

The blood count and erythrocyte sedimentation rate are unremarkable, but immunological tests may occasionally be abnormal so that in about 30 to 50 per cent of cases antinuclear antibodies can be detected in the blood despite the fact that there are no other features—immunological or clinical—of collagen disease. Abnormalities in one or more of various non-invasive physiological tests are present in about 90 per cent of patients but none is diagnostic:

1. *The radiograph* almost invariably shows enlargement of the main and hilar pulmonary arteries with pruning of the peripheral vasculature.
2. *Perfusion scans* are almost equally distributed between those that show segmental abnormalities and those in which the perfusion remains homogeneous.
3. *The electrocardiogram* shows right axis deviation, right ventricular hypertrophy and right ventricular strain to a degree corresponding to the hypertension. The rhythm is almost invariably sinus and the atrial fibrillation, which is such a common feature of cor pulmonale, is not often seen.

4. *Echocardiography* demonstrates a small or sometimes normal-sized left ventricle but, at diagnosis, right ventricular enlargement is present in 75 per cent of patients.
5. *Pulmonary function* shows a mild restrictive disease with reduced diffusing capacity and mild arterial hypoxaemia.
6. *Cardiac catheterization.* By the time of diagnosis, mean pulmonary arterial pressure is usually increased about three-fold (to approximately 60 mmHg), although right atrial pressures are not greatly elevated. Wedge pressure is normal and cardiac index is marginally reduced. Resistance is usually in the range 15 to 25 mmHg/litre/min/m². There are correlations between the severity of dyspnoea and: (1) reduction in cardiac index; and (2) right atrial pressure, suggesting that right ventricular performance may be the main determinant of severity of symptoms. There is surprisingly little relationship between the duration of symptoms and the haemodynamic abnormalities at the time of diagnosis—suggesting that the rise in pulmonary vascular resistance may perhaps be a rapid initial phenomenon in the disease.

Differential diagnosis

The diagnosis of primary pulmonary hypertension is by exclusion. By far the most difficult alternative to exclude is progressive thromboembolic disease and, on occasions, this may not even be eliminated by angiography (see below).

Prognosis and natural history

Data from various clinical series and, in particular from the United States National Prospective Registry shows that the outlook, if untreated, is very poor. The median survival is slightly less than 3 years from diag-

Fig. 5 Assessment and treatment of the patient with primary pulmonary hypertension (Dr L. Rubin, personal communication).

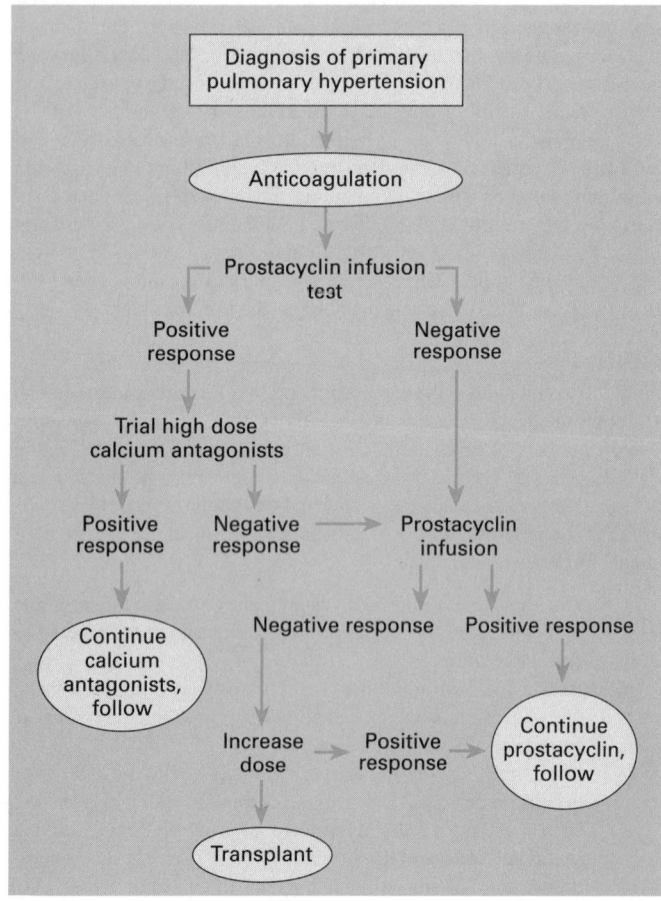

Table 3 *Relevant possibilities in the differential diagnosis of pulmonary hypertension of uncertain origin*

Conditions leading to pulmonary venous hypertension
Mitral valve disease
Left atrial myxoma
Left atrial thrombus
Pulmonary veno-occlusive disease
Venous thrombosis secondary to neoplastic disease

Conditions leading to pulmonary arterial hypertension
Recurrent thromboembolism
Tumour emboli
Amniotic fluid embolism – late sequelae
Foreign body embolism (intravenous drug abuse)
Primary pulmonary hypertension

Unrecognized direct effects upon the endothelial cell
Toxic substances
Collagen diseases

nosis (mean 2.8 years; 95 per cent confidence 1.9 to 3.7 years) and the mode of death involves progressive right heart failure, pulmonary thromboembolism, pneumonia, and sudden death. Survival is negatively correlated with pulmonary artery pressure and with right atrial pressure, and positively with cardiac index. The first of these presumably relates to the severity of the underlying disease, while the latter two reflect the importance of right ventricular function. Other factors indicating poor prognosis include dyspnoea, the presence of Raynaud's phenomenon and decreased lung diffusing capacity for carbon monoxide.

Treatment

Two worthwhile treatment strategies have evolved during the last decade. These are the reduction of pulmonary vascular resistance by vasodilators and the use of anticoagulants.

In 1980 it was shown that hydralazine reduced pulmonary vascular resistance in primary pulmonary hypertension. Many other systemic vasodilators have the same effect. Unfortunately, at conventional doses, the effects did not seem to be sustained. However, there is now evidence that calcium channel blockers, when used in high dosage, not only produce sustained haemodynamic improvement but also have a dramatic effect on survival. Most recently, continuous prostacyclin infusion by portable pump has also been shown to reduce pulmonary vascular resistance and the effects are sustained for up to 18 months. Inhalation of nitric oxide and use of thromboxane A₂ synthesis inhibitors are even newer approaches.

Two lines of evidence point to the use of anticoagulation in primary pulmonary hypertension:

1. In 1984 a retrospective Mayo Clinic study suggested that, in 120 patients who had unexplained pulmonary hypertension, survival was significantly better if anticoagulants had been given—irrespective of whether subsequent pathology was plexogenic or thromboembolic. A similar result appeared in a recent extensive study of the long-term benefit of high dose calcium channel antagonists.
2. Going back to the 1950s, there are case reports of patients whose primary pulmonary hypertension regressed during anticoagulant treatment.

These clinical data fit well with recent evidence of raised fibronectin levels in primary hypertension and the inability of clinical (and occasionally even pathological) methods to distinguish between primary and microthromboembolic disease—both of which suggest an important role for deranged local thrombotic mechanisms amenable to anticoagulant treatment.

A plan for assessment and for evolving a treatment strategy is shown in Fig. 5.

Table 4 *Major investigations used in identifying the aetiology of newly discovered pulmonary hypertension*

Collagen vascular screen	Eliminate atypical presentations of collagen diseases
Liver function tests	Eliminate unsuspected hepatic cirrhosis
Chest radiograph; CT-scan	Eliminate pulmonary and mediastinal disease
Pulmonary function tests	Eliminate/identify pulmonary disease
Arterial blood gases	Assess whether hypoxia (if present) is sufficient to cause hypoxic pulmonary hypertension
Ventilation/perfusion scan	Identification of thromboembolic disease
Angiography	Identification of thromboembolic disease
Echo; echo Doppler	Identification of left heart disease. Assessment of right heart function
Cardiac catheterization	Direct measurement pressures, calculation of vascular resistance, assess haemodynamic responses to pulmonary vasodilators.
Lung biopsy (open)	Dangerous. May be of limited value as histological appearances 'converge' and overlap

Once heart failure has developed, diuretics assist in the control of systemic oedema. The patients's breathlessness, of reflex origin and rarely associated with cyanosis, is not particularly relieved by oxygen—either continuous or intermittent—although its effect in relieving vasoconstriciton makes long term use theoretically sensible. Palliative relief of breathlessness at rest, particularly to assist sleep at night in terminal cases, may require opiates.

Experience of combined heart–lung transplantation is as yet small but in selected patients has had success. Single lung transplantation may offer a further means of treatment but, so far, remains unevaluated.

The differential diagnosis of pulmonary hypertension

Pulmonary hypertension is usually one stage in an already-recognized disease, such as mitral stenosis or an intracardiac shunt. Occasionally, however, cause is not evident and, theoretically, any cause in Table 1 could be a possibility. However, the main conditions that cause actually cause difficulty are listed in Table 3, and appropriate investigations are given in Table 4.

Clues may occasionally be obtained from the history. Some examples illustrate this. The slimming drug aminorex fumarate was probably the cause of one outbreak of pulmonary hypertension and adulterated rape seed oil (oleoanilide) of another. Phenformin has been suggested as a rare cause, as have some early oral contraceptives. Dietary pulmonary hypertension is so well known in animals that, even in patients, the possibility cannot be neglected. Herbs such as Crotolaria and Senecio (ragweed), which contain pyrrolizidine alkaloids, are suspect and can occasionally be found in health stores. Pulmonary hypertension may also occasionally develop as a late sequel postpartum, following the complication of amniotic fluid embolism and the time-lapse can cause confusion. Foreign body emboli in intravenous drug users are another rare, but increasing, cause.

Mitral valve disease can be difficult to diagnose because, as it becomes more severe, the cardiac output drops and the murmur diminishes. However, it should be identified by a combination of echocardiography and cardiac catheterization. The same investigations should also establish the rare diagnoses of left atrial myxoma and left atrial thrombus.

Recurrent systemic venous thromboembolism is relatively easy to diagnose when it occurs as recurrent attacks of breathlessness often with pleuritic pain, haemoptysis and characteristic changes on the ventilation/perfusion scan. But the characteristics of microthromboembolic disease are its insidious onset with unexplained breathlessness and fatigue. Pulmonary angiography or even lung biopsy – with its attendant dangers – may be necessary. Even then, in the presence of eccentric intimal fibrosis, the diagnosis may be in doubt but, as thrombosis may contribute to primary pulmonary hypertension, and as anticoagulation may be used

in its treatment of this disease, the distinction between these two forms of pulmonary hypertension may not be as important as was once thought.

Pulmonary hypertension may be a manifestation of autoimmune diseases, including connective tissue disorders, Goodpasture's syndrome, polyarteritis nodosa, and fibrosing alveolitis, so that an autoimmune screen should be part of the investigations. However, the situation is somewhat confused by the fact that up to 50 per cent of cases of primary pulmonary hypertension may show titres of antinuclear antibodies of greater than 1 : 80 (see above).

Biopsy has an important but restricted place in diagnosis. Generally, fibreoptic bronchoscopy biopsy specimens are unsatisfactory. Open biopsy, from several different sites, is needed for accuracy; this inevitably imposes risks. Lung biopsy should therefore be reserved only for those cases where there is deep doubt about the aetiology of the pulmonary hypertension and serious apprehension that a remediable cause is being missed, such as sarcoidosis or polyarteritis nodosa or recurrent pulmonary embolism. Even here it could be argued that a therapeutic trial of drugs such as steroids or immunosuppressants combined with oral coagulants is a less hazardous course.

When every other cause has been ruled out the cause of the hypertension must be considered to be either primary pulmonary hypertension or pulmonary veno-occlusive disease. The clinical features of veno-occlusive disease are the same as those in severe primary pulmonary hypertension though there are often, in addition, pulmonary oedema and pleural effusions. Cardiac catheterization reveals an elevated pulmonary artery pressure but also difficulty in obtaining a clearly transmitted left atrial pressure wave from a pulmonary artery wedge pressure tracing. The left atrial pressure measured directly by the trans-septal route will be normal.

Pathogenesis of primary and secondary pulmonary hypertension

The occurrence of similar changes in the early stages of diseases as diverse as primary pulmonary hypertension, hypoxic cor pulmonale, and ventricular septal defect has always provoked the speculation there may be a common aetiology. Most theories have assumed that the immediate cause is raised intravascular pressure caused by increased flow in shunts, by cardiac failure in other cases, and by hypoxic vasoconstriction in cor pulmonale. Two hypotheses have been put forward to link the raised intravascular pressure with structural changes.

The myogenic theory developed from the observation that pulmonary smooth muscle appears to react to stretch (from increased intravascular pressure) by contraction. It suggests that repeated or continued contraction eventually causes the muscle to hypertrophy. When the hypertrophied muscles are subjected to further stress their response changes to become one of proliferation, synthesis, and secretion. Such a hypothesis could also fit cor pulmonale, as there is evidence that pulmonary vascular smooth muscle can react directly to hypoxia by contraction. It is unhelpful when dealing with primary hypertension.

The endothelial hypothesis provides more wide-ranging possibilities. It considers that damage to, or abnormality of, the endothelial cell is the common pathway through which hypertension is initiated and it has the potential for linking a wide range of diseases (Fig. 6). There is considerable general evidence in support of this hypothesis:

1. A close association exists between endothelial damage and the development of hypertension. Thus, in toxic or immunologically caused diseases it is a very early event. In high-flow hypertension, endothelial surface changes are always present at an early stage.

2. Endothelium has the capacity to secrete a wide range of vasoconstrictors and vasodilators. Many of these, including endothelium-derived relaxation factor, endothelin and prostacyclin have been described in Chapter 15.22. Their production can be modulated by stimuli that appear highly relevant such as shear stress (prostacyclin), hypoxia (endothelium-derived relaxation factor) and superoxide damage (adult respiratory distress syndrome – endothelin). In addition to direct production, the endothelium can entrain platelet metabolism to cause local production of vasoconstrictor thromboxane A.

3. The endothelium can interact with both the blood clotting system and blood platelets in a way that could explain the involvement of thrombosis and fibrin deposition in pulmonary hypertension from many causes.

4. Endothelial and associated cells posess the ability to produce a wide range of substances that can induce the migration and replication of smooth muscle cells and their precursors. These include polypeptide growth factors (such as platelet derived growth factor (PDGF); fibroblast growth factor (FGF); insulin like growth factor 1 (IGF1); epidermal growth factor (EGF); transforming growth factor α (TGF-α) and transforming growth factor β (TGF-β)) and a number of cytokines.

Although the growth of new knowledge is generous in granting possibilities, some specific evidence is now also emerging. In hypoxic hypertension, it has been found that inhibition of endothelium-derived relaxation factor production – either non-specifically by methylene blue or more specifically by the nitric oxide synthetase inhibitor L-N^G-nitroarginine methyl ester; L-NAME leads, in experimental animals, to pulmonary hypertension and suggests that the endothelium maintains the pulmonary circulation in a continually vasodilated state. On the other hand, endothelium-derived relaxation factor production by pulmonary endothelium, when monitored by measuring exhaled nitric oxide, is found to diminish in hypoxia. Finally, nitric oxide, which is a component of natural endothelium-derived relaxation factor, inhibits hypoxic vasoconstriction.

More broadly, in patients with both primary and a wide range of secondary causes of pulmonary hypertension, there is common perturbation of eicosanoid metabolism. Increased production of metabolites of thromboxane A (a pulmonary vasoconstrictor) is accompanied by decreased production of prostacyclin (prostaglandin I$_2$ – a vasodilator). Similarly, pulmonary artery endothelial cells from calves with pulmonary artery pressures raised by rearing at high altitude show a reduced capacity for prostacyclin synthesis. Finally, as a link to recent evidence of the capacity of the endothelial cell to modulate clotting, it has been shown that fibrinopeptide A levels are elevated in patients with primary pulmonary hypertension.

The concept that emerges is of a metabolically and immunologically competent endothelial cell, which can modulate the physiological activity and growth of vascular smooth muscle in a host of ways and which must be a prime candidate for the post of conductor of the pulmonary hypertensive orchestra!

REFERENCES

D'Alonzo, G.E. *et al.* (1991). Survival in patients with primary pulmonary hypertension. *Annals of Internal Medicine*, **115**, 343–349.

D'Alonzo, G.E., Gianotti, L., and Dantzker, D.R. (1986). Non-invasive assessment of haemodynamic improvement during chronic vasodilator therapy in obliterative pulmonary hypertension. *American Review of Respiratory Disease*, **133**, 380–384.

Fishman, A.P. (1990). *The pulmonary circulation: Normal and abnormal.* University of Pennsylvania Press, Philadelphia.

Fuster, V., Steele, P.N., Edwards, W.D. *et al.* (1984). Primary pulmonary hypertension: Natural history and the importance of thrombosis. *Circulation*, **70**, 580–587.

Harris, P. and Heath, D. (1986). *The human pulmonary circulation.* Churchill Livingstone, Edinburgh.

Hasleton, P.S. and Gibbs, A.R. (1994). Exploration of the pulmonary circulation. *Thorax,* **49**, Supplement, S1–S56.

LeRoy, E.C. (1991). Pulmonary hypertension: The *bete noir* of the diffuse connective tissue diseases. *American Journal of Medicine*, **90**, 539–540.

Loscalzo, J. (1992). Endothelial dysfunction in pulmonary hypertension. *New England Journal of Medicine*, **327**, 117–119.

Packer, M. (1989). Is it ethical to administer vasodilator drugs to patients with primary pulmonary hypertension? (editorial). *Chest*, **95**, 1173–1175.

Palvesky, M.I. and Fishman, A.P. (1991). The management of primary pulmonary hypertension. *Journal of the American Medical Association*, **265**, 1014–1018.

Rich, S. and Brundage, B.H. (1987). High dose calcium channel-blocking therapy for primary pulmonary hypertension. *Circulation*, **76**, 135–141.

Rich, S., Kaufmann, E., and Levy, P.S. (1992). The effect of high doses of calcium channel-blockers on survival in primary pulmonary hypertension. *New England Journal of Medicine*, **327**, 77–81.

Rubin, L.J. *et al.* (1990). Treatment of primary pulmonary hypertension with continuous intravenous prostacyclin. *Annals of Internal Medicine*, **112**, 485–491.

Will, J.A., Dawson, C.A., Weir, E.K., and Buckner, C.K. (1987). *The pulmonary circulation in health and disease.* Academic Press, London.

Fig. 6 The endothelial cell as the initiator of pulmonary hypertension.

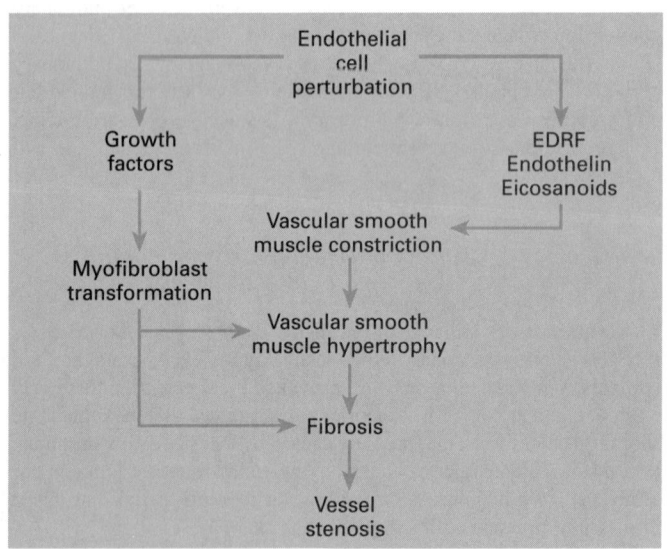

15.25 Cor pulmonale

J. S. PRICHARD

Introduction

The term 'cor pulmonale' denotes structural or functional right heart changes caused by diseases of the lung, thoracic cage, or respiratory control mechanisms. The association has been recognized since the middle of the nineteenth century and a variety of expressions such as 'pulmonary heart disease', 'emphysema heart', and 'black cardiacs' has been used. However, from the time of the introduction of the term 'cor pulmonale' in the 1950s, there have been attempts to emphasize hypertrophy of the right ventricle rather than actual cardiac failure, as in the World Health Organization definition of 1961, which was 'hypertrophy of the right ventricle resulting from diseases affecting the function and/or structure of the lung, except where these pulmonary alterations are the result of diseases that primarily affect the left side of the heart'.

The view adopted here is that right heart hypertrophy and eventual failure are consequences of a high afterload produced by pulmonary hypertension, and that the hypertension is itself a result of physiological and anatomical changes in the lung caused by the primary disease. It is necessary to distinguish:

1. *Pulmonary arterial hypertension*, which is the initiating event and which creates the high afterload against which the ventricle must work.
2. Subsequent *hypertrophy and dilatation of the right ventricle* – cor pulmonale – which is adaptive to the hypertension and allows normal cardiac output despite the raised afterload.
3. Eventual *right heart failure*, which occurs when the hypertrophied ventricle is no longer able to compensate for the hypertension and venous pressure becomes elevated.

Throughout discussion of cor pulmonale a continuing problem is the use of the term 'right heart failure'. 'Cardiac failure' is a term usually used to denote an inappropriate relationship between venous filling pressure and output which, in cardiac disease, arises from intrinsic damage to the heart. In cor pulmonale, on the other hand, there is no evidence of intrinsic abnormality of the heart; the problem is increased right ventricular afterload and there may even be sufficient functional reserve for the cardiac output to increase in response to hypoxia and exercise.

Pathological changes

The lungs

Cor pulmonale may be secondary to many diseases (Table 1) and the features of one or more of these will be present. Marked pulmonary pathology may be seen in diseases of the parenchyma and airways, but where the problems are those of the thoracic cage, of neuromuscular disease, or of the respiratory control mechanisms, lung damage may be very slight.

However, a common pattern of abnormalitites of the smaller pulmonary blood vessels can be found wherever cor pulmonale has developed. These changes were first and most clearly identified in chronic obstructive airflow disease, but have been noted in all conditions characterized by chronic hypoxia including kyphoscoliosis, the obesity–hypoventilation syndromes, and persistent residence at high altitudes:

1. There is development of longitudinal muscle in the intima of

Table 1 *Diseases associated with cor pulmonale*

Diseases of the lung parenchyma and intrathoracic airways
    Chronic obstructive lung disease
    Asthma (severe, recurrent, or chronic)
    Bronchiectasis (including cystic fibrosis)
    Pulmonary interstitial fibrosing and granulomatous diseases

Occlusive pulmonary vascular disease*
    Multiple pulmonary emboli
    Schistosomiasis
    Filariasis, tropical eosinophilia
    Sickle-cell disease

Disorders of the thoracic cage
    Kyphosis (particularly when deformity angle > 100°)
    Scoliosis (particularly when deformity angle > 120°)
    Thoracoplasty
    Pleural fibrosis

Neuromuscular disease
    Poliomyelitis
    Myasthenia gravis
    Amyotrophic lateral sclerosis
    Myopathies and muscular dynstrophy

Disturbance of respiratory control
    Idiopathic hypoventilation syndrome
    Obesity–hypoventilation syndrome
    Cerebrovascular disease

Obstruction of extrathoracic airways*
    Tonsils and adenoids in children

*These causes of cor pulmonale are not discussed in this chapter.

pulmonary arterioles and muscular pulmonary arteries. This appears to arise by differentiation of myofibroblasts and as the disease progresses, it is succeeded by elastosis and eventually by fibroelastosis.

2. A distinct media of circular muscle forms in the pulmonary arterioles. This can frequently be seen as a layer between the internal and external laminae. Although there may be some medial hypertrophy in the muscular pulmonary arteries this is far less pronounced than in other forms of pulmonary hypertension.

Of these changes, muscularization of the arterioles is the lesion most closely associated with the development of pulmonary hypertension and, certainly in the early phases of the disease, is mainly responsible for the increase in pulmonary vascular resistance.

The right ventricle

Right ventricular hypertrophy is the hallmark of cor pulmonale but its extent varies greatly. Increases in weight range from slightly above normal (60 g) to as high as 200 g, whilst the ratio of left ventricular weight (plus septum) to that of the right ventricle may fall below 2.5 and the right ventricular wall thickness may become greater than 0.5 cm.

The left heart

The left ventricle becomes slightly hypertrophied in patients with cor pulmonale even where there is no valvular or systemic vascular disease. This may be a response to hypoxia and/or erythrocytosis.

The carotid body

The carotid body is enlarged by an increased number of chief cells. The clinical significance of this is not known.

The pathogenesis of cor pulmonale

As the majority of cases of cor pulmonale occur in chronic obstructive lung disease, the view was put forward by Budd in 1840 that emphysematous destruction of lung parenchyma led to obstruction of pulmonary blood flow because of anatomical reduction of the pulmonary capillary bed. This view held until the 1960s, although it was never able to take into account the dynamic nature of changes in pulmonary artery pressures and it produced no explanation for cor pulmonale in diseases where severe lung damage was not a feature. Finally, when methods of quantification of lung pathology became available, it was found that there was little correlation between degree of emphysema, internal lung area or any other index of parenchymal damage and right ventricular hypertrophy.

Evidence now suggests that hypoxia is the initiating event common to all forms of cor pulmonale (Fig. 1). This leads to pulmonary vasoconstriction, which causes pulmonary hypertension and increased afterload. The hypoxia acts synergistically with vasoconstriction and raised intravascular pressures to induce smooth muscle hypertrophy. Constriction of the hypertrophied muscle and subsequent intimal fibrosis produce sustained hypertension and right heart failure follows. The following evidence supports this hypothesis:

1. The inhalation of a gas with a reduced oxygen content so that arterial oxygen tension falls below 7 kPa raises pulmonary vascular resistance in isolated perfused lungs, in experimental animals, in 60 to 70 per cent of normal individuals, and in patients with lung disease. This phenomenon of pulmonary hypoxic vasoconstriction differentiates the pulmonary from the systemic circulation. The response arises within lung tissue and is independent of perfusing fluids and the autonomic nervous system. The mechanism remains unclear but it may be mediated either by the pulmonary endothelium, which can produce autocoids able to cause both constriction and relaxation of smooth muscle or by a direct effect upon oxygen-sensitive potassium channels in smooth muscle. The endothelial autocoids include endothelial-derived relaxing factor (EDRF – nitric oxide), endothelin (a vasoconstrictive peptide), and prostaglandin I_2 (prostacyclin – a potent vasodilator). The most likely hypothesis is that, under normoxic conditions, the continuous release of endothelium-derived relaxation factor maintains the vascular smooth muscle in a state of relaxation. Hypoxia suppresses production and constriction follows.

2. Long-standing hypoxia is associated with increased muscularization of the pulmonary blood vessels. Hypoxia in experimental animals leads to remodelling similar to that seen in human cor pulmonale. Thymidine labelling has shown this to start with pericyte and intermediate cell proliferation. Subsequently these cells lay down fibrin and elastin and develop into smooth muscle cells. Hypoxia can have similar effects in appropriate tissue cultures and therefore probably acts directly. However, as vascular change also occurs wherever there is pulmonary hypertension – irrespective of hypoxia – mechanical factors may also play a part. In some experiments hypertrophy appears to have been prevented by blocking vasoconstriction using Ca^{2+} channel antagonists. In others fibroblast proliferation has been stimulated directly by the vasoconstrictor endothelin and vascular remodelling has been blocked by ligustrazine, which does not block the acute response.

3. Experimentally induced pulmonary hypertension in animals leads rapidly to right ventricular hypertrophy.

4. Patients with established cor pulmonale are inevitably hypoxaemic and late in the disease there is a reasonable correlation between the degree of hypoxaemia and that of right ventricular hypertrophy.

5. Long-term relief of hypoxia will cause some lowering of even a chronically raised pulmonary vascular resistance.

A problem in accepting this logical chain of events has always been the fact that the pulmonary vascular resistance is often not raised early in cor pulmonale (except during exacerbations) and right heart hypertrophy may be present before many attacks of decompensation have occurred. Observations upon arterial oxygen saturation during sleep may provide an explanation. At night, oxygen saturation is not stable and large and rapid changes occur (Fig. 2). Episodes of desaturation are particularly likely during rapid eye movement (REM) sleep and, in turn, these are associated with elevated pulmonary arterial pressure and vascular resistance. Not only is each episode of desaturation accompanied by a period of pulmonary hypertension but a stepwise progression of pulmonary artery pressure takes place with each successive episode.

Hypoxic vasoconstriction, whether from alveolar hypoventilation, ventilation/perfusion imbalance, or reduced environmental oxygen is thus the major cause of the pulmonary hypertension which invokes cor pulmonale. However, other factors can play a part:

1. Erythrocytosis may be present as a response to hypoxia and, where the haematocrit exceeds 0.55, increased resistance to flow and red cell clumping can become significant.

2. Where arteritis is present, as in some collagenoses (particularly systemic sclerosis and disseminated lupus erythematosus) this may in itself be a factor increasing pulmonary vascular resistance and, in the calcinosis-Raynaud's-sclerodactyly-telangiectasis (CRST) variant of systemic sclerosis, myxomatous change in the small and medium-sized pulmonary arteries may have a similar effect.

3. In chronic obstructive lung disease, high expiratory intraveolar pressure may be an additional factor, and this may be particularly important during the increased ventilation and intraalveolar pressures that occur during exercise.

4. Although, as we have seen, it is not the primary cause, physical

Fig. 1 Pathogenesis of cor pulmonale.

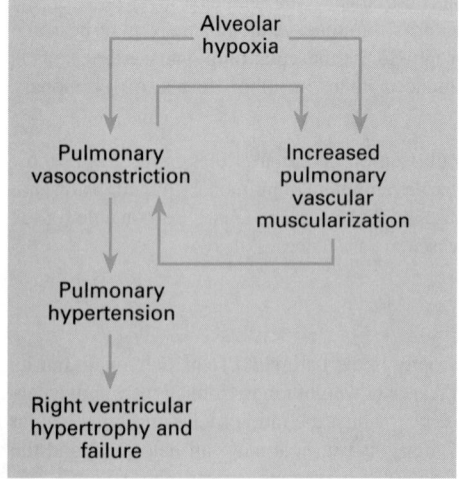

destruction of the vascular bed may also contribute. Experimental studies show that two-thirds occlusion of the pulmonary vascular bed causes significant hypertension and, in advanced chronic obstructive airways disease, fewer than 20 per cent of the capillaries and small vessels remain. This reduction may also explain the extreme pressure changes which result from small increases in cardiac output.

Pathophysiology in cor pulmonale

Experimentally, after the acute induction of pulmonary hypertension, right ventricular output is maintained by the Starling mechanism of increased end diastolic volume and central venous pressure. Subsequently, hypertrophy occurs and contractility improves so central pressure returns to normal. In cor pulmonale where hypertension usually develops steadily, this presumably leads to a virtually simultaneous progressive right ventricular hypertrophy, which sustains a normal central venous pressure despite the increased afterload. However, the compensatory process is eventually overwhelmed and, although cardiac output may be maintained, central venous pressure (CVP) rises. Subsequently, oedema develops – most extensively when hypercapnia coexists with hypoxia.

The retention of sodium and water, which accompanies the raised central venous pressure and thereby allows the progressive development of oedema, appears to result from:

1. Decreased renal blood flow – possibly as a result of increased renal autonomic nervous activity secondary to or amplified by hypercapnia.
2. Increased secretion of renin, angiotensin, and aldosterone.
3. Circulating antidiuretic hormone concentrations, which are high in relation to prevailing plasma osmolality.

Interestingly, variations in atrial naturetic peptide (ANP) secretion do not appear to play any great immediate role. Levels are increased during the period when patients with cor pulmonale have oedema and increase yet further in response to further salt loading. This suggests that the atrial naturetic peptide feedback loop is itself responding normally to changes in total body fluid, but that its ability to compensate for the primary perturbing factors has been compromised.

However, sodium and water retention may not be the only cause of oedema for, in some cases, although body weight falls as expected during treatment it frequently returns to the pretreatment levels in convalescence without reappearance of oedema. Two interrelated factors may be responsible. First, much of the oedema may be due to a shift of fluid from the intracellular to the extracellular compartment, possibly exacerbated by the need for extracellular buffering where hypercapnia is present. The increase in weight during convalescence may then be due to increased synthesis of body tissue, a suggestion that is supported by a considerable decrease in total body potassium observed during acute attacks.

The hypoxia that initiates pulmonary vasoconstriction also restricts potential oxygen supply to the tissues. Many patients with cor pulmonale have been found to have low coefficients of oxygen delivery – showing that cardiac output has not been able to increase in order to compensate for the low oxygen content of arterial blood. Generally, a low coefficient of oxygen delivery has been found to correlate well with a subnormal mixed venous oxygen saturation.

Clinical features

Natural history

Cor pulmonale occurs in patients in whom there is long-standing hypoxia from disease of the lung parenchyma, airways, thoracic cage, or respiratory control mechanisms (see Table 1). None is invariably associated with the condition which only develops in the more severe cases in which hypoxia is prominent.

The natural history consists first of a period during which right ventricular hypertrophy and strain are developing but frank failure has not yet occurred. Subsequently, the first attack of right heart decompensation appears and is frequently triggered by an episode of pulmonary infection. The age at which the signs and symptoms first appear is determined largely by the underlying primary pathology, and may stretch from adolescence to old age. Similarly, the period of hypoxia and pulmonary arterial hypertension that precedes the onset of cor pulmonale may also vary very greatly from months to years. The right heart failure is usually treated satisfactorily at first but relapses occur with increasing frequency and with less response to treatment until eventually death results. Little is known of the mode or mechanisms of death, except that it most frequently occurs during a period of heart failure unresponsive to treatment.

In the Western world, the most common cause is undoubtedly chronic obstructive airways disease but even in this disorder fewer than 50 per cent of patients will ever develop right heart hypertrophy and failure. These are usually men presenting in their late 50s and, as might be expected, the disease is more common amongst the hypoxic 'blue bloaters' than amongst the emphysematous 'pink puffers'. Overall, the incidence of cor pulmonale is largely determined by the prevalence of chronic obstructive lung disease and is most common where smoking is widely practised and air pollution heavy. In industrial cities in Britain,

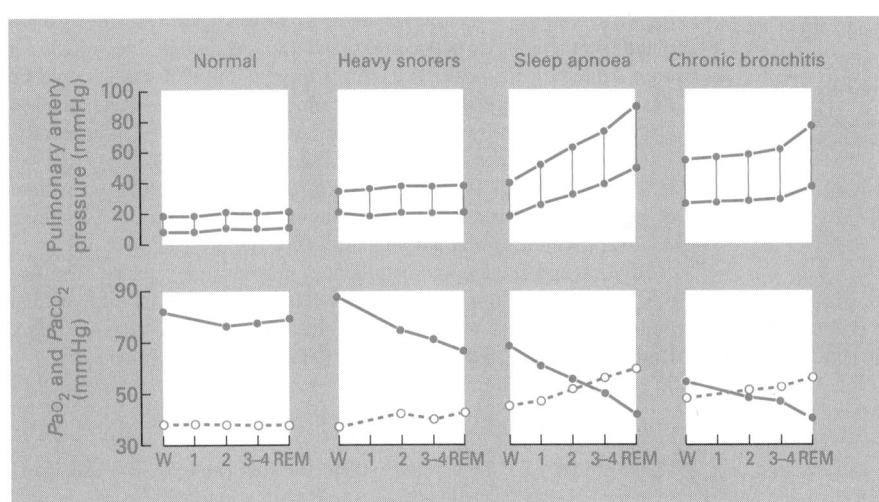

Fig. 2 The effect of different levels of sleep upon arterial oxygen (P_aO_2) (•———•), carbon dioxide ($PaCO_2$) (o----o), and pulmonary arterial pressure. W = waking; REM = rapid eye movement sleep. Hypoxia develops with increasing sleep level in smokers, patients with sleep apnoea, and in chronic bronchitits. In the apnoeic and bronchitic patients pulmonary artery pressure also rises. (Reproduced from Harris, P. and Heath, D. (1986). *The Human pulmonary circulation* (p. 541 redrawn from Lugaresi *et al.*), Churchill Livingstone, Edinburgh, with permission.)

30 to 40 per cent of heart failure a decade ago arose from this cause, whilst comparative figures from Delhi in India were 15 per cent and for the United States 6 to 7 per cent.

In the progress of pulmonary disease, the onset of pulmonary hypertension, and subsequent right heart failure carries a particularly bad prognosis. In the period from 1950 to 1980, various studies suggested a mortality of 50 to 70 per cent in the 3 to 5 years from the onset of clinically recognizable cor pulmonale. The situation may be improving as a result of alterations in therapy but, outside controlled studies on limited numbers of patients (see for instance below the studies of long term oxygen therapy), large-scale data are not available. However, within the group of patients with cor pulmonale, there are differences in prognosis such that recent studies suggest that those patients who can adapt to persistent tissue hypoxia by developing increased cardiac output fare better than those who either cannot or who develop polycythaemia.

In the 1960s and 1970s between 50 and 60 per cent of patients with chronic obstructive airways disease and cor pulmonale died within 3 years of the onset of cardiac failure, but most authors are agreed that survival now is probably somewhat longer.

Clinical signs

Apart from the primary disease, the clinical signs are associated with:

    (1) pulmonary hypertension;
    (2) right ventricular hypertrophy;
    (3) right heart failure.

These three constitute a chronological sequence but merge imperceptibly into each other.

In the thorax, the enlarged right ventricle may produce a sternal heave (unless masked by deformity or distortion of the chest wall), while cardiac pulsation may also be felt in the epigastrium. The heart beat may be rapid or irregular for arrhythmias may develop (see below). An emphasis on the pulmonary component of the second heart sound, a pulmonary valvular click, and (unless bundle branch block is present) shortening of the interval between the components of the second heart sound all denote pulmonary hypertension. Frequently, when frank right heart failure is present, the systolic murmur of tricuspid incompetence can be heard and a right ventricular third heart sound develops. More rarely, the diastolic murmur of pulmonary incompetence may occur.

Outside the thorax no signs are present until the right heart begins to fail. Then the central venous pressure becomes raised. It is usually visible as an elevated jugular venous pressure in the neck and, if tricuspid incompetence has developed, a 'v' wave can be seen. An enlarged and often tender liver becomes palpable and, in the presence of tricuspid incompetence, may be pulsatile. Oedema commonly forms in the legs and/or sacrum but appears later in the non-hypercapnic than in the hypercapnic forms of cor pulmonale. Ascites and pleural effusion are relatively rare. Hepatic dysfunction may result but, acutely, this is usually only detectable biochemically. If the heart failure persists, hepatomegaly, cardiac cirrhosis, and splenomegaly may eventually result. In extreme and chronic cases persistently elevated venous pressure may lead to renal dysfunction, proteinuria and, rarely, nephrotic syndrome.

Routine investigations

BLOOD GAS OXYGEN TENSIONS

These are usually in the range 6 to 7 kPa (45 to 53 mmHg) or lower: arterial carbon dioxide tensions are more variable. If the primary disease is associated with alveolar hypoventilation, hypercapnia is present with carbon dioxide tensions raised to between 8 and 9 kPa (60 to 68 mmHg) (or higher). On the other hand the interstitial lung diseases are associated with hyperventilation and carbon dioxide tensions are below normal. As noted above, mixed venous oxygen saturation could be used as an indicator of oxygen delivery to the tissue, but this is not usually a practicable investigation. Haematocrit is frequently raised, often above 55 per cent.

Table 2 *Electrocardiograph changes in cor pulmonale*

Right axis deviation of mean QRS vector
R/S ratio in V1 > 1
R/S ratio in V6 < 1
S1, Q3 or S1, S2, S3 patterns
Clockwise rotation
P Pulmonale (increased P wave amplitude in II, III, aVl)
Isoelectric P wave in I or right axis deviation of P vector

The presence of chronic obstructive lung disease and deformity of the chest wall and thoracic cage may confuse electrocardiogram interpretation considerably.

Arrhythmia and conduction defects are not included.

RADIOLOGICAL APPEARANCES

These are often dominated by the primary pathology and, particularly where emphysema is present, diaphragmatic descent and increased thoracic diameters may disguise cardiomegaly. When the right ventricle becomes detectable, the left cardiac border is displaced laterally but the apex gives the appearance of pointing upward. In the lateral view, the upward displacement of the right atrium gives an increased density in the upper anterior part of the heart shadow. The central pulmonary arteries are prominent and it has been suggested that, on the standard posteroanterior radiograph a diameter of more than 16 mm for the right pulmonary artery and more than 19 mm for the left pulmonary artery may be diagnostic of pulmonary hypertension. The more peripheral vessels show rapid tapering. If frank right ventricular failure is present, the superior venacaval and azygos vein shadows may be enlarged.

ELECTROCARDIOGRAM CHANGES

These arise from hypertrophy of the right ventricle (particularly the crista supraventricularis) and dilation of the right atrium. The basic changes are set out in Table 2 but may often be partially masked by the primary disease. Thus, where obstructive lung disease is present, the diaphragm is depressed, the anteroposterior diameter of the chest increased and the electrical conductivity of the lungs changed. The heart becomes more vertical and rotated left so that the right atrium and right ventricle lie more anteriorly, while the apex is more posterior. These features affect the electrocardiogram by causing clockwise rotation, low QRS voltage and, occasionally, large Q or QS waves in the inferior and/or mid-precordial leads reminiscent of healed myocardial infarction. Similarly, in diseases associated with deformity of the chest wall and thorax, problems arise from alterations in the anatomical position of the heart. Over the spectrum of cor pulmonale, correlation of ECG changes with autopsy proven right ventricular hypertrophy (particularly in the presence of chronic obstructive airways disease) is closest with a frontal plane mean QRS axis between 90° and 180°. Although this produces a high degree of diagnostic accuracy a large number of cases would be missed if this were the only criterion used and assessment of each electrocardiograph by reference to a number of features is necessary. Usually about 20 per cent of patients show p-pulmonale (a p-wave >2 mm in standard lead II) whilst between 70 and 80 per cent have a pattern of right ventricular strain (with a dominant R in V1 or V3 and/or a dominant R in a Vr and a dominant S in V5).

Rhythm and conduction disturbances may also be detected. The former are mainly supraventricular and paroxysmal atrial tachycardia, nodal rhythms, and wandering pacemakers are not infrequently seen. Right bundle branch block is the commonest conduction defect.

PULMONARY HAEMODYNAMICS

These are assessed by cardiac catheterization (Table 3). The usual pattern seen is of a normal cardiac output with a markedly increased pulmonary arterial pressure. At rest, the pressure does not increase linearly

Table 3 *Pressure and flows in the pulmonary circulation in cor pulmonale*

	Normal individual	Phase I pulmonary hypertension	Phase II right ventricular hypertrophy	Phase III frank cardiac failure
Pulmonary artery pressure (mmHg)	18–20	30–40	40–50	40–50
Pulmonary wedge pressure (mmHg)	6–8	6–8	6–8	6–8
Right ventricular end diastolic pressure (mmHg)	4	4	8–10	14–15
Cardiac output (l/min)	6	6	6	6 (variable)

with flow but the slope of the relationship becomes less steep at high flows. This implies that those vessels that are the chief sites of resistance (the muscularized arterioles) are narrower than normal at normal flow but distend readily as flow increases. In exercise the pressures increase markedly and the pressure-flow relationship is displaced from that seen at rest. The most likely explanation is that increased intra-alveolar pressure – itself a result of raised airway resistance and increased alveolar ventilation – is compressing the arteriolar and capillary beds (Fig. 3). Radionuclide studies, including thallium-201 imaging and first pass angiocardiography may be used to assess right ventricular size and ejection fraction. Right ventricular ejection fraction (RVEF) is almost invariably found to be reduced. Echocardiography may also assist but its application is frequently frustrated by emphysema. Doppler echocardiography has an increasing role in assessing the function of the pulmonary and tricuspid valves.

BODY WEIGHT

This reflects a complex interplay of fluid retention and tissue loss and, because of these two factors, may not in itself be of great value in following the course of the disease.

PLASMA ELECTROLYTE CONCENTRATIONS

These are usually normal, although persistent hyponatraemia may occasionally be seen.

ASSESSMENT OF PULMONARY HYPERTENSION NON-INVASIVELY

No simple non-invasive method has so far emerged which allows the degree of pulmonary hypertension to be assessed. However, there has been considerable progress in the application of discriminate and multivariate analysis to a wide range of measurements so as to provide a prediction of the presence of pulmonary hypertension. In men, sensitivity and specificities of above 80 per cent have been achieved by combining measures of pulmonary artery diameter, forced expiratory volume in one second (FEV_1), arterial oxygen tension at rest and age.

SLEEP STUDIES

Continuous transcutaneous oximetry can help in studying patients who have mild hypoxia whilst awake but in whom there is doubt about the cause of pulmonary hypertension.

THE DIFFERENTIAL DIAGNOSIS OF COR PULMONALE

In many patients, right heart failure, hypoxia, and respiratory disease coexist. The question then arises 'Is this cor pulmonale?' To answer may be difficult, for respiratory diseases are common and the non-respiratory causes of pulmonary hypertension all eventually lead to secondary hypoxia. The differential diagnosis usually consists of:

1. Cor pulmonale itself.
2. Pulmonary hypertension from unrecognized left heart failure or pulmonary veno-occlusive disease.
3. Pulmonary arterial occlusive disease from emboli.
4. Primary pulmonary hypertension.

The diagnosis of cor pulmonale requires demonstration: (1) that the respiratory disease is sufficiently severe to generate the necessary degree of hypoxia; and (2) that no other cause of pulmonary hypertension is present.

In the first instance, the severity of respiratory disease will be evaluated clinically but detailed pulmonary function tests and blood gas measurements will also be needed. For cor pulmonale, the minimal degree of hypoxia required is an arterial partial pressure of oxygen (PaO_2) below 9.0 kPa (approximately 68 mmHg) but this is only a very rough guide, as the vasoconstrictive response to hypoxia is very variable. Furthermore, the recent recognition of the various sleep apnoea syndromes suggests that studies of oxygen tension during sleep may be necessary to establish the diagnosis in patients where waking oxygen tensions are only mildly lowered.

In the elimination of cardiac causes of pulmonary hypertension, left heart failure can usually be identified by clinical examination, but mitral stenosis and shunts may present problems that require echocardiography, radionuclide studies or catheterization for their solution. In per-

Fig. 3 The relationship between flow and pressure across ($P = P_{pa} - P_{pw}$) in the pulmonary circulation at rest (○) and during exercise (●). Measurements were made upon flow in the left lung and alterations in flow were achieved by transient occlusion of blood flow to right lung. During exercise the flow–pressure curve is displaced probably as a result of increased intra-alveolar pressure. (Reproduced from Harris, P. and Heath, D. (1986). *The Human pulmonary circulation* p. 526. Churchill Livingstone, Edinburgh, with permission.)

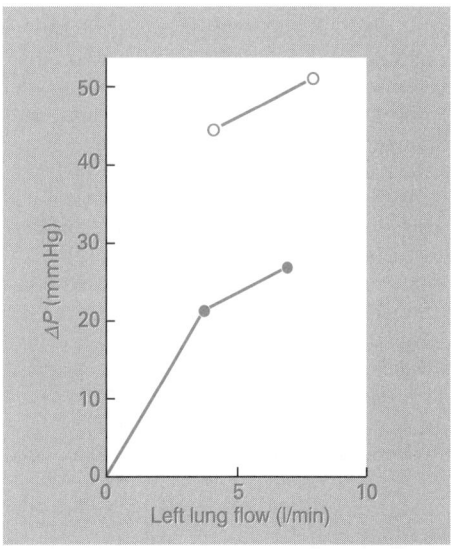

plexing cases, measurement of wedge pressure may be particularly valuable as a normal study eliminates both left heart failure and pulmonary veno-occlusive disease.

Large pulmonary emboli may frequently be identified by a clinical history aided by ventilation/perfusion scanning and, if necessary pulmonary angiography. On the other hand, insidious, recurrent small emboli may be extraordinarily difficult to diagnose. If the diagnosis is considered, a search for a cause should be made and pulmonary angiography performed However, it may be impossible to identify small emboli even by angiography, particularly where the pulmonary circulation is already damaged by some other process such as emphysema.

The diagnosis of primary hypertension can only be made when all other causes have been eliminated and, in the case of differentiation from multiple emboli, this may be all but impossible.

Treatment of cor pulmonale

The object of treatment of cor pulmonale is reduction of the work-load of the right ventricle by lowering of pulmonary vascular resistance and pulmonary arterial pressure. To this end success depends upon:

1. Treatment of the primary disease to relieve respiratory failure.
2. Use of supplemental oxygen to reduce hypoxia and pulmonary vascular resistance.
3. Reduction of oedema by use of diuretics and fluid restriction.

More controversial are:

4. Venesection.
5. Use of digoxin to obtain an inotropic effect on the right ventricle.
6. Reduction of pulmonary arterial pressure by pulmonary vasodilators.

As yet very uncertain is:

7. Diminution of intrapulmonary ventilation–perfusion imbalance by use of almitrine bismesylate.

TREATMENT OF PRIMARY DISEASE

The condition most commonly responsible for cor pulmonale is chronic obstructive lung disease, and the episodes of frank heart failure commonly first appear during infective exacerbations. At this time, there is an acute deterioration of pulmonary function, an increase in ventilation–perfusion imbalance and heightened hypoxia. Therefore, the more rapidly and effectively the exacerbation can be overcome the less the strain on the right heart. The essentials of treatment are a combination of physiotherapy and appropriate antibiotics.

Also, chronic obstructive lung disease (whether or not a result of underlying asthma) may be associated with reversible airways obstruction. In these cases, whether by use of steroids or bronchodilators, the relief of airways obstruction will reduce the work of breathing, will reduce intra-alveolar pressures, and will aid the clearance of lung secretions and infection. Irrespective of the bronchodilator used, however, the immediate result of bronchodilation will be increased hypoxia due to increased ventilation–perfusion imbalance and it is essential that supplemental oxygen should also be given.

The same principles apply to treatment of bronchiectasis but other lung conditions causing cor pulmonale are more difficult to treat. In the fibrosing diseases and pneumoconioses there is an increased tendency to pulmonary infections, which should be treated promptly; otherwise the mainstay of treatment is supplemental oxygen. Deformation of the spine and chest wall have been treated surgically but the effects upon pulmonary function and pulmonary vascular physiology have been disappointing.

In the hypoventilation syndromes – of whatever cause – various arti-

ficial methods for sustaining ventilation have been attempted. Where the problem is mild, and particularly where upper airway dynamic obstruction is present, nasal continuous positive alveolar pressure (nasal CPAP) has been shown to be effective in sustaining arterial oxygen tensions but more severe cases may require extrathoracic cuirasses or phrenic nerve pacemakers. Patients with obesity–hypoventilation syndrome frequently improve greatly after weight reduction and, for all these groups, sublingual methoxyprogesterone or protriptyline may be a suitable respiratory stimulant.

Supplemental oxygen

Supplemental oxygen has been used in the treatment of acute exacerbations of chronic obstructive airways disease since the development of controlled titrated administration by Campbell and his colleagues in the early 1960s. The oxygen is used to maintain cerebral function, to reduce pulmonary artery pressure and to aid the resolution of oedema.

Long-term oxygen treatment is particularly interesting in view of the fact that, in experimental animals, structural vascular changes induced by hypoxia are reversible. For long-term oxygen therapy (LTOT) in humans, results suggest that oxygen must be given in low dose (2/l/min) or low concentration (24 per cent) for long periods each day. In trials, mortality, morbidity, and frequency of hospital admissions are reduced and pulmonary arterial pressure and haematocrit may fall (Fig. 4). The oxygen must be taken continuously for at least 12 to 15 h each day; continuous use for 24 h has a greater benefit than for the shorter period; patients with hypercapnia may benefit most; in men, although morbidity may be reduced by 50 per cent after 3 to 4 years there is a lag of about 18 months before benefit becomes apparent; in women, the effects are more immediate.

The results have considerable consequences when the high incidence of chronic obstructive disease and the cost (at least £1200 per year) of providing oxygen are considered. A system of patient selection proposed by the (United Kingdom) Department of Health suggests that the patient should fall into one of three groups: (1) cor pulmonale; (2) chronic hypoxic bronchitis and emphysema; and (3) hypoxic lung disease requiring palliation. For the first two groups the patient should be stable when assessed and have on two occasions an arterial oxygen pressure $(Pao_2) < 7.3$ kPa (55 mmHg), an arterial carbon dioxide pressure $(Paco_2) > 6.0$ kPa (45 mmHg), and a forced expiratory volume of < 1.5 litre. Oxygen may be provided by compressed gas, oxygen concentrator, or liquid oxygen systems. Delivery is by mask, nasal prongs or transtracheal catheters. The last, though the most difficult to insert has cosmetic advantages and is economical of oxygen.

Early results suggested that long-term oxygen therapy would confer

Fig. 4 Overall mortality of patients with chronic obstructive lung disease treated with continuous (○) or noctural only (●) oxygen therapy. (Reproduced from Nocturnal Oxygen Therapy Trial Group. (1980). *Annals of Internal Medicine*, **93**, 391, with permission.)

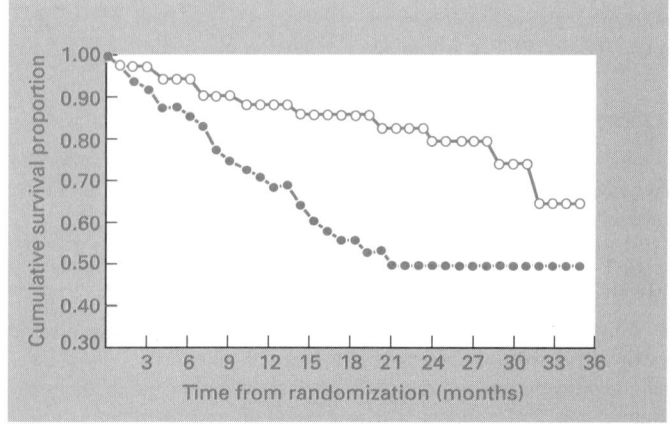

up to 5 years additional survival in hypoxic chronic obstructive airways disease. However, recent evaluations show that, in general use, this is not being achieved. Many patients comply poorly with the regimen and is seems that the apparatus is largely being used for near-terminal patients, in whom little benefit would be expected.

Diuretics

In cardiac failure, by the time frank oedema has developed, the accumulation of fluid and increased central venous pressure are no longer adaptive responses to increased afterload. The use of diuretics reduces oedema, improves peripheral circulation, allows improved ventricular contractile efficiency by reducing intravascular volume, and may also improve gas exchange in the lung if pulmonary extravascular water has increased.

Usually, powerful loop diuretics such as frusemide are used. There is no evidence that any one diuretic is more effective than others but in resistant cases combinations may be necessary. The addition of spironalactone is logical in view of the raised aldosterone levels. Finally, fluid restriction to 1000 to 1500 ml/day may be tried.

There is an important relationship between oxygen treatment and diuretic therapy. It has frequently been observed that the administration of oxygen alone will improve cardiac failure and lead to diuresis. Consequently, the dose of diuretic required may be less when supplemental oxygen is being given. Also, once the acute exacerbation that led to the frank heart failure has been treated satisfactorily, pulmonary vascular resistance and diuretic requirement may both fall. Where this happens, failure to reduce the dose of diuretic can lead to hypovolaemia, hypotension, and prerenal failure.

A final complication of diuretic therapy may be metabolic alkalosis in the presence of potassium deficiency. This is a particular problem in chronic obstructive airways disease for the alkalosis may reduce yet further the carbon dioxide sensitivity of the medullary centres. To avoid this, potassium chloride supplements should be given, or potassium sparing diuretics (such as spironalactone or triamterene) added.

Venesection

The increase in haematocrit in chronic hypoxia is initially an adaptive response to reduced oxygen saturation. As the haematocrit rises progressively above 50 per cent, blood viscosity increases significantly and this increase, together with thrombosis and sludging in the pulmonary circulation, adds to right ventricular strain. Thus, the disadvantages of the increased red cell mass begin to outweight the advantages of the increased oxygen-carrying capacity and venesection has been advocated. Haemodynamic studies have shown that optimal benefit is obtained by reduction of haematocrits above 60 per cent to values in the mid or low 50s, and that this should be achieved by exchange transfusion with low molecular weight dextran solutions. It is not clear that there are any long term benefits and, overall, phlebotomy should be reserved as adjunctive therapy in acute situations.

Digoxin

It is doubtful if digoxin is therapeutically effective in cor pulmonale unless atrial fibrillation needs to be controlled. In the absence of fibrillation, evidence that its administration improves pulmonary haemodynamics or right ventricular performance is lacking. On the other hand, it is certainly known that in hypoxia and potassium depletion, digoxin is potentially more liable to cause cardiac arrhythmias.

Pulmonary vasodilators

A large number of drugs including hydralazine, the nitrates, nifedipine, verapamil, uradabil (α-adrenergic blocker), captopril (angiotensin converting enzyme inhibitor), and prostaglandins I_2 and F_2, have all been shown to act as vasodilators in the hypoxic pulmonary circulation. Unfortunately, the clinical benefit is not proven and, although many have beneficial cardiovascular effects, these are often largely negated by the adverse effects of: (1) systemic hypotension; (2) diminished arterial oxygen saturation (Sao_2). The first problem relates to the fact that each pulmonary vasodilator has a greater affect upon the major circulation than upon the pulmonary circulation. The second problem arises from the fact that each also causes an increased intrapulmonary ventilation/perfusion imbalance. In general, pulmonary vasodilators cannot yet be recommended but, in the situation where all else has failed, if, by invasive investigation, it can be demonstrated that the vasodilator reduces pulmonary vascular resistance by more than 20 per cent, yet at the same time does not diminish cardiac output, reduce pulmonary arterial pressure or reduce systemic blood pressure, then a trial is worth while.

The most recent assessments have been of inhaled nitric oxide – the rationale being to replace hypoxia-suppressed intrinsic production of endothelium-derived relaxation factor. The effects have been encouraging and pulmonary haemodynamics have improved without any deleterious effect upon ventilation/perfusion balance and shunt.

Almitrine bismesylate

This reduces ventilation–perfusion imbalance in the diseased lung. It has been shown to improve arterial oxygenation in patients with severe chronic obstructive airways disease but its role in cor pulmonale remains doubtful as it may induce pulmonary hypertension.

Lung transplantation

A limited number of severe lung diseases that cause hypoxia and cor pulmonale may be treated satisfactorily by lung transplantation.

REFERENCES

Anonymous (1985). Long term domiciliary oxygen therapy. *Lancet*, **ii**, 365–357.

Baudoin, S.V., Waterhouse, J.C., Tahtamouni, T., Smith, J.A., Baster, J., and Howard, P. (1990). Long term domiciliary oxygen treatment for chronic respiratory failure reviewed. *Thorax*, **45**, 195–198.

Department of Health and Social Security (1986). *Introduction of oxygen concentrators to the domiciliary oxygen therapy service*. Department of Health and Social Security, London.

Elliott, M.W., Mauvey, D.A., Moxham, J., Greene, M., and Branthwaite. (1991). Domiciliary nocturnal nasal intermittent positive pressure ventilation in COPD: Mechanisms underlying changes in arterial blood gas tensions. *European Respiratory Journal*, **4**, 1044–1052.

Grover, R.F. (1990). Chronic hypoxic pulmonary hypertension. In *The pulmonary circulation: Normal and abnormal* (ed. A. P. Fisman), University of Pennsylvania, Philadelphia.

Harris, P. and Heath, D. (1986). The pulmonary vasculature in emphysema. In *The human pulmonary circulation* (eds P. Harris and D. Heath), Churchill Livingstone, Edinburgh.

Harris, P. and Heath, D. (1986). Pulmonary haemodynamics in chronic bronchitis and emphysema. In *The human pulmonary circulation* (eds P. Harris and D. Heath), Churchill Livingstone, Edinburgh.

Hasleton, P.S. and Gibbs, A.R. (1994). Exploration of the pulmonary circulation. *Thorax*, **49**, Supplement, S2–S62.

Heath, D., Brewer, D., and Hicken, P. (1968). *Cor pulmonale in emphysema*, Charles C. Thomas, Illinois.

Higgenbottam, T., Otulana, B.A., and Wallwork, J. (1990). Transplantation of the lung. *European Respiratory Journal*, **3**(5), 594–605.

Howard, P. and de Haller, R. (1991). Domiciliary oxygen – by liquid or concentrator? *European Respiratory Journal*, **4**, 1284–1287.

Howard, P. and Waterhouse, J.C. (1992). Mortality and its prevention in COAD. *European Respiratory Review*, **2**, 203–207.

Palevsky, H.I. and Fishman, A.P. (1990). Chronic cor pulmonale. *Journal of the American Medical Association*, **263**, 2347–2351.

Schulman, D.W. and Matthay, R.A. (1992). The right ventricle in pulmonary disease. *Cardiology Clinics*, **10**, 111–135.

Whyte, K.F. and Flenley, D.C. (1988). Can pulmonary vasodilators improve survival in cor pulmonale due to hypoxic chronic bronchitis and emphysema? *Thorax*, **43**, 1–8.

Wiedemann, H.P. and Matthay, R.A. (1990). Cor pulmonale in chronic obstructive pulmonary disease. *Clinics in Chest Medicine*, **11**, 523–545.

15.26 Pulmonary embolism

J.G.G. LEDINGHAM AND D.J. WEATHERALL

The vast majority of pulmonary emboli, whether detected clinically or at post-mortem examination, consist of thrombi which have originated in the deep veins of the legs and pelvis, although the embolic material may on rare occasions arise from malignant tumours, from amniotic tissue, from fat and even from aggregations of parasites that have invaded the venous system. Attention has been drawn to the importance of detecting emboli from choriocarcinoma, which can closely mimic the syndrome of thromboembolism, because the condition can be detected by inappropriately high concentrations of human chorionic gonadotrophin (hCG) in blood or urine and can then be treated sometimes effectively by chemotherapy.

Incidence

The incidence of pulmonary thromboembolism remains high, although precise figures are difficult to come by and estimates have varied widely depending on the population studied and whether the diagnosis (usually on death certificate) has been made on clinical grounds without investigation, after investigation, or in a proportion at postmortem.

Quoted figures for pulmonary embolism as a cause of *death* in hospital patients range from 20 000 to 50 000 per annum in the United States, or more recently up to 200 000 when deaths in nursing homes, hospitals for the chronic sick, and at home are taken into account.

An analysis of death certificates in England and Wales in 1967 revealed 4981 reports in which pulmonary embolism was the suspected primary cause of death but the number increased to 21 000 when more than one cause had been recorded. Many patients die *with* rather than *from* emboli, particular the elderly with malignant disease or chronic cardiac or lung disease.

The frequency of detected thromboembolism in the lungs at post mortem examination depends on the care with which they are sought. There is evidence for a 12 per cent incidence in routinely performed examinations; this increases to 52 per cent when the lungs had been inflated before fixation and then examined meticulously. However, embolism was considered to be the *sole* cause of death in only 7 per cent of adults dying in a busy district general hospital, with a contribution made towards death in another 7 per cent. Other similar, or higher figures, have been reported. The incidence may truly be higher now because patients in hospital are substantially older and less mobile than they were in the 1960s, when the original work was performed.

It has been suggested that some 300 000 to 600 000 patients suffer a pulmonary embolism in the United States each year, with a mortality of 30 per cent, if untreated, and some 3 to 8 per cent dying despite treatment, either from recurrent embolism or more often with embolism complicating an underlying fatal disorder.

Deep vein thrombosis

Unfortunately, the occurrence of a pulmonary embolus may be the first and often the only indication of venous thrombosis. However, in order to try to prevent this serious condition it is essential that clinicians are aware of the symptoms and signs of venous disease when they are present, and that they are aware of the clinical situations in which it is more likely to occur. The pathogenesis, and management of venous thrombotic disease with anticoagulants, is described in Section 22. Here, we describe the major clinical features of venous disease and outline the background in which it is most often seen.

Major risk factors

Venous thrombosis giving rise to the risk of pulmonary embolism occurs postoperatively in some 50 per cent of major orthopaedic operations, in some 20 to 30 per cent after other major surgery and in 30 per cent of medical patients and 60 per cent of surgical ones at postmortem.

The major risk factors for venous thrombosis, particularly of the lower limbs and pelvis, apart from recent surgery, are immobility for more than 3 or 4 days, age over 40 years, previous venous thrombosis and/or embolism, presence or suspicion of malignant disease, sepsis, obesity, and varicose veins. The risk of venous thrombosis, and therefore of resultant pulmonary embolism, is increased in pregnancy, in the puerperium, in young women taking the oral contraceptive pill, and in the nephrotic syndrome. Rarer conditions that increase the risk of venous disease include paroxysmal nocturnal haemoglobinuria, homocystinuria, and Behçet's disease. It is important to screen for a lupus anticoagulant, for a deficiency of antithrombin III or proteins C and S and for resistance to activated protein C, especially in younger patients who have sustained deep venous thrombosis and/or pulmonary embolism without a precipitating cause, in those who have recurrent episodes, or where there is a family history. Deficiencies of antithrombin III or proteins C and S are rare, being found in only some 10 per cent of patients with unexplained recurrent venous thromboembolism, but resistance to activated protein C is probably much more common and has been reported in between 20 and 60 per cent of patients in some series. These conditions are described further in Section 22.

There are still many areas of uncertainty in the epidemiology of venous thrombotic disease. For example, in clinical practice it is not uncommon to encounter patients with deep venous disease of the legs who have recently completed a long journey by air. It is assumed that this can occur in otherwise normal people following immobility associated with dehydration exacerbated by alcohol. Curiously, however, apart from anecdotal reports a recent review of the literature suggests that there is no evidence that air travel is a major risk factor in venous thrombotic disease. There are similar gaps in our knowledge about the risk of long car journeys or cigarette smoking.

Clinical features

As emphasized earlier, deep venous disease may be completely silent. Venous thrombosis involving the hepatic venous system is described in Section 14 and cerebral sinus thrombosis in Section 22. Here we will consider only the clinical features of venous disease involving the limbs and pelvis.

VENOUS THROMBOSIS OF THE LEGS AND PELVIS

The cardinal features of venous thrombosis of the legs and pelvis are pain and swelling. The pain is usually described as deep, and boring involving the calves or thigh muscles. It is usually, but not always, associated with swelling of the legs. In venous disease that is restricted to below the knees the swelling can be demonstrated by the measuring the mid-calf diameter, whereas if the disease involves the femoral and pelvic venous systems the mid-thigh diameter will also be increased. It is important to make these measurements from a fixed point below and above the knee and to make a clear mark so that serial measurements can be made. An increase in diameter of more than 1 cm at either level should raise the possibility of a venous thrombosis. It is essential to repeat the measurement of the diameter of the calves and thighs at frequent intervals. What starts as a swollen calf may, later, involve the thighs, suggesting spread of the disease to the femoral and pelvic venous systems. There may also be muscle tenderness and pain on extending the foot, Homan's sign; both are non-specific and may occur in many other conditions.

Additional signs of venous thrombosis of the legs include an increased temperature on the affected side, cyanotic discoloration of the limb, and engorgement of the superficial veins. The legs should be examined both in the vertical and horizontal position. It should be remembered that superficial varicose veins are almost always emptied after lying down; if they remain engorged it is likely to be due to impaired venous return due to thrombotic disease.

It is important to palpate the arterial pulses in the feet at regular intervals, particularly in old patients with grossly swollen legs. Tense venous oedema may cause arterial compression and the rare syndrome of venous gangrene.

The clinical diagnosis of venous disease of the legs is not easy. Conditions which may mimic it include simple muscle strain, infection involving the skin or muscle, a ruptured Baker's cyst or plantaris tendon, and many other traumatic conditions. Streptococcal infections of the skin of the lower limbs are very common in old people, and may closely mimic venous disease. It is essential, therefore, to confirm the diagnosis by venography or, if expert facilities are available, by Duplex Doppler ultrasound. The latter is particularly useful for identifying a ruptured Baker's cyst or a muscle haematoma.

THROMBOSIS OF THE VENA CAVA

This rare condition is associated with gross swelling of the legs and the signs of deep venous disease which are outlined in the previous section.

AXILLARY VEIN THROMBOSIS

This is also a rare condition, which may be due to obstructive lesions in the axilla but, more often, occurs without any apparent cause. Although embolic disease is said to be rare, it does occur; more information is required about this risk. The physical signs are characterized by swelling of the arm, dilatation of the superficial veins over the arm and anterior chest wall, and a cyanotic hue.

SUPERFICIAL THROMBOPHLEBITIS

This is a common condition which may involve any of the superficial venous systems. It is usually seen in patients with varicose veins of the legs but may accompany some of the prethrombotic states described in detail in Section 22, including malignant disease. It is characterized by a painful swelling along the course of the superficial veins. Over a period of a week or two the pain gradually subsides and leaves hard thrombotic cords, which can be felt along the course of the veins. It is rarely associated with deep venous disease and does not seem to be a risk factor for pulmonary emboli.

Management

Deep venous disease of the legs and arms should be managed by a short period of rest and early mobilization as soon as the pain has diminished. In most cases, heparin should be administered and warfarin started at the same time. Heparin should be continued until adequate anticoagulation has been obtained. If there are no remaining risk factors it is current practice, based on the results of several trials, to continue with oral anticoagulants for 6 to 12 weeks after the episode. If there is extensive above-knee or pelvic vein involvement, or gross swelling of the arm due to an axillary vein thrombosis, and provided there are no contraindications, fibrinolytic therapy should be used to try to reduce the severity of the post-thrombotic syndrome. Severe venous disease of the legs may result in an abnormally swollen leg and the danger of recurrent varicose ulceration.

There is still considerable controversy about whether it is necessary to anticoagulate every patient with venous thrombotic disease which is confined to below the knees. Pulmonary embolic episodes seem to be extremely rare and anticoagulant therapy has important side-effects. More information is required on this question.

Full details of the ways of administering anticoagulants, monitoring progress, and the management of complications, are given in Section 22.

The syndrome of pulmonary embolism

Symptoms and signs of pulmonary embolism vary from none (perhaps the most common) to the life-threatening collapse which follows an acute, massive blockage of the pulmonary circulation. Diagnosis is most difficult when the clinical setting does not raise suspicion and when symptoms and signs are minimal. A chronic syndrome of repeated small pulmonary emboli may be particularly difficult, but equally important to detect. The clinical syndromes may conveniently be reviewed under a somewhat arbitrary classification of acute minor pulmonary embolism, acute massive pulmonary embolus, moderate pulmonary embolism and chronic repeated pulmonary embolism, the latter often leading to pulmonary hypertension.

Acute minor pulmonary embolism

When emboli are small and have impacted in terminal pulmonary arteries or arterioles it is likely that there will be no symptoms or signs, although dyspnoea is the most common single symptom of pulmonary embolism. Small emboli give rise to only very minimal local inflammatory response, because the dual blood supply to the lungs from both the pulmonary and bronchial arteries protects against infarction. Involvement of tissue immediately adjacent to the pleura may, however, cause pleuritic chest pain with or without an audible rub. In most cases there are no visible changes on the chest radiograph but some 24 h after the event there may develop an initial area of non-specific pulmonary shadowing, followed sometimes by a characteristic linear scar, but more often resolving without trace. There may also be a small effusion at the base of the lung, which is often bloodstained.

Haemoptysis is uncommon and was reported in only 30 per cent of 327 subjects with proven pulmonary emboli of various degrees of severity analysed in the urokinase–streptokinase pulmonary embolism trial, whereas breathlessness was recorded in 84 per cent and pleuritic pain in 74 per cent. When haemoptysis does occur it does so some three to seven days after the initiating event. Many minor pulmonary emboli must go undetected.

Massive pulmonary embolism

At the other end of the spectrum, and much rarer, is the life-threatening sequence of events accompanying a massive pulmonary embolism. When preceding cardiopulmonary function has been normal the syndrome requires acute obstruction of at least 50 per cent of the pulmonary vascular tree, but lesser degrees of obstruction produce the same effects in the presence of previous cardiac dysfunction.

HAEMODYNAMICS

The immediate haemodynamic consequences of impaction of these large emboli, usually arising from clot in the ileofemoral veins, follow only partly from the direct anatomical effects of the occlusion of the major vessels. More important are a number of secondary effects arising from neurogenic reflexes and local release of vasoactive substances, 5-hydroxytryptamine and thromboxane released from accumulated activated platelets, for example. Reflex effects include vasoconstriction of both pulmonary and coronary arteries and, on occasion, marked vasodilatation of peripheral systemic vessels. The importance of these latter events is illustrated by the observation that ligation of a main pulmonary artery in the course of surgical pneumonectomy has no major adverse circulatory consequences.

The acutely increased right ventricular afterload results in a sudden rise in end-diastolic pressure, consequent elevation of the jugular venous pressure, considerable dilatation of the right ventricle often with tricuspid regurgitation and a rise in pulmonary artery pressure. The latter does not exceed 40 to 50 mmHg unless there has been preceding right ventricular hypertrophy. The delayed emptying of the right ventricle and coincident fall in left ventricular stroke volume may be detectable in widening of the interval separating the sounds of aortic and pulmonary valve closure but the pulmonary component is not increased in volume. Third and fourth heart sounds are commonly heard and may summate to produce a true gallop rhythm because of the associated increase in heart rate. A combination of a reversed Bernheim effect (displacement of the interventricular septum into the left ventricular cavity) and the reduced pulmonary blood flow result in a substantial fall in systemic stroke volume. This and peripheral arterial vasodilatation combine to cause a substantial fall in systemic arterial pressure.

CLINICAL FEATURES

The cardinal features of a massive pulmonary embolism are collapse associated with an acute onset of severe breathlessness. In addition, there may be central chest pain resembling angina.

Fig. 1 (a) Angiogram of the pulmonary artery demonstrated clot at its bifurcation. (b) Pulmonary artery shown in (a) but 2 h after clot lysis by tPA. (By courtesy of Drs E.W.L. Fletcher and B. Gribbin.)

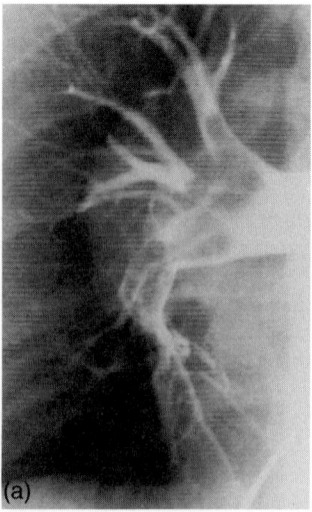
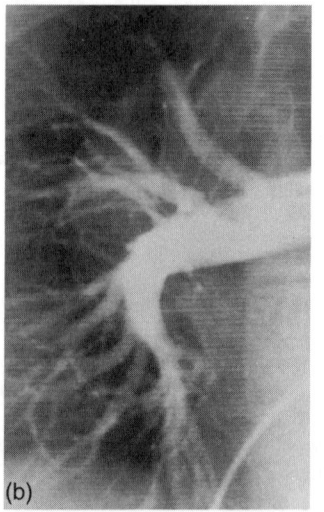

In assessing a patient in this critical state it is essential to identify the cardinal clinical signs of a massive pulmonary embolus and to try to rule out other causes of sudden collapse and dyspnoea, particularly acute left ventricular failure. Patients who have had a massive pulmonary embolus are equally dyspnoeic in the prone and upright positions and are not relieved by sitting up, as in the case with acute left ventricular failure. There is usually marked jugular venous engorgement which, of course, occurs in both conditions. The most striking differences are on auscultation of the chest; despite the acute dyspnoea which accompanies pulmonary embolus, there are no abnormal breath sounds, or added sounds, and this is the most valuable way of distinguishing it from acute left ventricular failure in which there are showers of crepitations. After a large pulmonary embolus there is marked hypotension and, often, some degree of pulsus paradoxus. As mentioned earlier, there may be a gallop rhythm. If the embolus breaks up and moves to the periphery there may be pleuritic chest pain, a pleural rub, and, later and a blood-stained pleural effusion.

Chronic repeated pulmonary emboli

Repeated episodes of pulmonary embolism, silent, producing trivial symptoms or unrecognized by the physician, may result ultimately in pulmonary hypertension and the clinical manifestations of cor pulmonale. This condition is usually insidious in its clinical course and when established has a very poor prognosis (see Chapter 15.24). The source of emboli is, again, usually the veins of the legs or pelvis but renal vein thrombosis complicating chronic nephrotic states (particularly membranous glomerulonephritis) may be an occult source. Pulmonary artery pressures may be very high and even exceed systemic pressures in this condition with associated gross right ventricular hypertrophy. The major symptoms are breathlessness and syncope on exertion. Signs are those of right ventricular hypertrophy, and a loud pulmonary second sound. Right ventricular failure develops later.

Diagnosis

When a minor embolism is suspected, the diagnosis may be made on clinical grounds alone when circumstances render it highly probable; for instance, when pleuritic pain or transient acute breathlessness have occurred 10 to 14 days after major surgery or injury. It is sometimes justified to treat by anticoagulation without investigation, especially if the perceived risks of potential ill effects of such treatment appear minimal. Most commonly, however, it is important to seek a source of embolism in the legs, pelvis or renal veins by venography or ultrasound techniques and evidence of occlusion of pulmonary vessels by ventilation perfusion scanning or angiography.

The methods for detecting a source of embolism from venous thromboses are discussed in Section 22. The most accurate method of proving pulmonary embolism is angiography, but most clinicians prefer to use less direct methods unless massive embolism is suspected when this technique is obligatory if surgery is envisaged. Less definitive investigations may also be used to aid diagnosis.

ARTERIAL BLOOD GASES

Hypoxemia and hypocapnoea are common after major pulmonary embolism and may also be found after more minor events. Absence of these phenomena, on the other hand, by no means excludes embolism and their presence is non-specific. In suspected minor embolism this investigation is, at best, only of marginal value. The precise stimulus to hyperventilation is unknown and there is also difficulty in understanding the reasons for hypoxaemia when it is present.

CHEST RADIOGRAPH

Chest radiographs are nearly always normal in acute minor pulmonary embolism. In more major cases vascular shadows may be reduced in the oligemic area, often in a patchy pattern. Other signs of major embolism include prominence of the hilar shadow of the affected main pulmonary artery at the site of enlargement of a large clot. Inflammatory changes resulting from a moderate-sized emboli may also be visible, or there may be a small pleural effusion.

ELECTROCARDIOGRAPH

Electrocardiographic changes do not occur as a result of minor pulmonary embolism and for practical purposes are confined to those who have suffered a major acute event or who have 'packed' multiple small emboli chronically, resulting in pulmonary hypertension and right ventricular hypertrophy. Even after major pulmonary emboli with obvious haemodynamic disturbance, changes on the electrocardiograph occur in only 80 per cent of cases. These include the classic S1, Q3, T3 pattern in the limb leads, T wave inversion in the right ventricular chest leads, and, on occasion, right bundle branch block.

D-DIMER IN PLASMA

Concentrations in plasma of this cross-linked fibrin derivative may be raised for some 2 to 3 days after pulmonary embolism, but also after venous thrombosis without embolism, after myocardial infarction and indeed in any event in which fibrin deposits in the circulation, as for instance when there has been disseminated intravascular coagulation. In one series of 171 patients with possible pulmonary embolism the diagnosis was confirmed in 55 and in 54 of these plasma levels of D-dimer were in excess of 500 µg/l. In this series the sensitivity of the test was 98 per cent but the specificity only 39 per cent. In general clinical practice neither this, nor estimation of concentrations fibrin degradation products are very much used.

VENTILATION PERFUSION SCANNING

A perfusion scan is the most commonly used screening test for the investigation of a suspected acute minor pulmonary embolism. Indeed a normal scan makes any but the smallest embolism unlikely. In the event of an abnormal perfusion scan radiologists currently report results as showing a low, moderate or high probability of an embolism, an approach which reflects the lack of certainty with which this investigation can be interpreted.

Low probability scans

These are reported when perfusion scans without ventilation images have revealed subsegmental defects, or when larger defects have been matched with coincident ventilation defects.

Moderate probability

This is suggested by segmental or larger perfusion defects without any information about ventilation; or by scans revealing many subsegmental defects with normal ventilation patterns.

High probability

This exists when segmental or larger defects are accompanied by normal ventilation of the unperfused areas of lung.

The presence of pre-existing lung disease makes for difficulty when mismatched areas coincide with areas of previously existing abnormality on the chest radiograph.

Studies in the 1980s correlating the results of lung scans with those of pulmonary angiography have demonstrated angiographic evidence of embolism in some 60 to 85 per cent of those whose scans were designated 'high probability', in some 15 per cent of those with 'low probability' and intermediate numbers in the other categories. The Prospective Investigation of Pulmonary Embolism Diagnosis (PIOPED) study analysed data from six centres from which 755 of 1493 thought to have had an embolism had had angiography and 931 scintigraphy. Taking

scintigraphy alone, the overall sensitivity of the technique was 98 per cent but specificity only 10 per cent. Of the 116 patients with high probability scans 102 (88 per cent) had angiographic lesions whilst only 33 per cent of 322 patients with a moderate probability scan had had an embolism demonstrable by angiography. The figure for low probability scans was 12 per cent. Even when the clinical setting was taken into account a number of emboli detected by angiography were missed by scanning and results were particularly difficult to interpret in the presence of pneumonia, bronchospasm, or when there had been a previous episode of pulmonary embolism. Whilst only 2 per cent of subjects with high probability scans had not suffered an embolism, 59 per cent of all angiographically detected emboli were 'missed' if a report of high probability was taken as the only diagnostic criterion.

This study, then, confirms pulmonary angiography as the gold standard of investigation but the data also demonstrate that the combination of a low probability scan and an unconvincing clinical case makes embolism unlikely and a completely normal scan very unlikely indeed.

PULMONARY ANGIOGRAPHY

In the PIOPED study in which 1111 patients underwent angiography, the mortality was 0.5 per cent, there were major complications in 1 per cent and minor in 5 per cent. Thirteen subjects developed renal dysfunction, requiring dialysis in some, a complication more common in the elderly. The deaths occurred only in very ill patients many of whom had not had an embolism. High pulmonary artery pressures, a large volume of injected contrast and the presence of an embolism were not factors thought to have affected outcome but allergy to contrast material is a potential hazard and there are dangers in performing angiography with conventional contrast media when right ventricular end-diastolic pressure exceeds 20 mmHg. This problem is reduced somewhat by the use of newer media of lower osmolality.

Pulmonary angiograms require expert interpretation and a diagnosis of embolism can only be made with certainty when a filling defect in the arterial tree can be seen to outline the presence of the embolus itself. Lesser indices of embolism such as areas of reduced vascularity, prolongation of the arterial phase or late venous filling can also occur in asthma, left ventricular failure or severe mitral stenosis.

INDICATIONS FOR PULMONARY ANGIOGRAPHY

A normal perfusion scan can be taken as good evidence that a pulmonary embolism has not occurred and a high probability scan is so likely to indicate an embolism that an angiogram is unnecessary. It is when the clinical circumstances are uncertain and the scan of only moderate probability that an angiogram has most to offer. In this situation the physician must weight the value of the procedure against its ill effects and costs and the overall clinical situation. Often the decision will be made to anticoagulate without angiography, but if there are seen to be hazards of such treatment to be weighed against the risks of a further more serious event, the finding that 30 per cent of positive angiograms in the PIOPED series occurred in those whose scans showed only moderate probability strengthens the case for an angiogram.

Treatment

ACUTE MINOR PULMONARY EMBOLISM

Unless there are serious concerns about ill effects of anticoagulation it is common and sensible practice to begin treatment with intravenous heparin with the intention of withdrawing anticoagulation if subsequent investigations persuades the physician that an embolism has not occurred.

The aim of heparin therapy is to prevent further venous thrombosis and thereby reduce the risk of further embolism. A loading dose followed by constant intravenous infusion is commonly the preferred pattern of administration, but there is no firm evidence that continuous intravenous infusion is any better than intermittent intravenous or high dose subcutaneous administration. A reasonable regimen is to give a loading dose of 5000 units, followed by a total of 30 000 to 40 000 per 24 h, the precise amount dictated by regular measurements of the activated partial thromboplastin time (APTT) which should be kept between 1.5 and 2.5 times the control value.

The risk of significant haemorrhage complicating this approach has been assessed at around 7 per cent. There may be advantage in those judged to be at particular risk in using one of the low molecular weight heparin products derived from enzymatic or chemical hydrolysis of the original substance. A number of studies of these compounds using daily or twice daily subcutaneous injection have compared anticoagulant efficacy and the haemorrhagic complications with traditional intravenous heparin regimens in a variety of thrombo-embolic conditions. Anticoagulant efficacy of low molecular weight heparin appears to be no less good, and perhaps better, than with traditional treatment with perhaps also a lesser risk of haemorrhagic complication. Further evaluation, including comparative analyses of costs, are required before firm recommendations can be made.

Heparin therapy, however given, is generally required for an initial 4 to 5 days before being replaced by oral anticoagulants.

Coumarin anticoagulant drugs are the ones most commonly used and they are introduced at least 48 h before it is planned to withdraw heparin. Dosage is adjusted to achieve an internationally normalized ratio (INR) two- to three-fold that of controlled samples. The value of assaying native prothrombin antigens as a possibly better way of monitoring Coumarin therapy is yet to be determined.

FIBRINOLYTIC DRUGS IN ACUTE MINOR TO MODERATE EMBOLISM

In 1973 the Urokinase Pulmonary Embolism Trial comparing treatment by heparin alone with heparin plus urokinase provided evidence for more rapid improvement in lung scans among patients given urokinase, but there was no difference in the occurrence of repeated emboli or in mortality between the two groups. More recently there have been a number of studies of the efficacy of recombinant tissue plasminogen activators given with heparin compared with standard therapy. There is some evidence from these that right ventricular function and lung perfusion improves more rapidly after thrombolysis. Whether or not this approach truly reduces the risks of further embolism, reduces mortality, or reduces the already minimal risk of later morbidity related to long term pulmonary hypertension is uncertain and requires a large scale controlled clinical trial. A single embolism probably never causes cor pulmonale. In cases in which there is an apparent association of a single recognised embolism with chronic pulmonary hypertension and right ventricular dysfunction there are also likely to have been a number of repeated previous events and breathlessness will have been a feature before the acute episode.

ACUTE MAJOR PULMONARY EMBOLISM

The diagnosis of an acute major pulmonary embolism will only be entertained if the patient is in an unstable haemodynamic state, ranging from a moderate degree of hypotension at best to profound hypotension and cardiac arrest at worst. Immediate resuscitation and the application of conservative measures to maintain cardiac output and reduction of hypoxaemia to a minimum are essential first steps. Apart from standard resuscitation procedures it is essential to maintain right ventricular filling pressure to a level that maximizes cardiac output and maintains arterial pressure. Vasodilatory drugs and diuretics are particularly to be avoided, and plasma expanding solutions should be infused to maintain blood pressure and organ perfusion, even when central venous pressure is already raised substantially.

The immediate question, once the patient has been resuscitated and

Table 1 *Contraindications to thrombolytic treatment*

Preceding stroke
Recent (7 to 14 days) head injury or neurosurgery
Active bleeding from the gastrointestinal tract
Severe diabetic retinopathy
Major surgery
Cardiopulmonary resuscitation
Postpartum

the diagnosis established, is to decide between medical and surgical treatment and in the medical option whether to give heparin alone or thrombolytic drugs followed by heparin.

When haemodynamic disturbances are easily controlled by routine measures heparin treatment, as for minor emboli, is commonly effective, even though it does not lyse emboli so that occluding lesions cannot be cleared by natural fibrinolysis for seven to ten days.

When the circulatory state, as judged by the pulse and blood pressure, remains precarious, or worsens, it is a moot point whether to continue heparin and await improvement or to proceed to surgery or thrombolysis (Fig. 1). Much will depend on the local availability or otherwise of an experienced surgical team. In a centre regularly accustomed to embolectomy the results of surgery appear very similar to those of thrombolysis. But there is no case for the occasional pulmonary embolectomy when thrombolytic therapy is feasible and physicians will have become thoroughly familiar with such treatment in its regular use in the management of acute myocardial infarction. A determining factor may be the presence of a major contraindication to thrombolysis (Table 1). A compromise approach, recently suggested, is to break up emboli which have lodged in major pulmonary vessels, dispersing the fragments to more distal sites using the guide wire and/or catheter itself introduced in the course of pulmonary angiography. There are favourable reports of good results from this relatively simple procedure in some 30 to 40 patients at the time of writing.

The principles of thrombolytic therapy are described in Section 22. Streptokinase is given intravenously with a loading dose of 250 000 i.u. given over 45 to 60 min followed by 100 000 i.u./hour for the first 24 h. The equivalent regimen for urokinase is 4400 i.u./kg over 10 to 15 min, followed by a further 4400 i.u./kg/h for a total of 24 h. Heparin, without the usual loading dose, follows when the thrombin time has fallen to about twice the normal duration.

Complications of thrombolytic therapy, apart from local oozing at venepuncture or arterial puncture sites, include gastrointestinal and retroperitoneal bleeding, and most serious, of intracranial haemorrhage, which may occur in as many as one or two per thousand patients treated. Such complications require immediate cessation of the lytic therapy and when bleeding itself appears life threatening restoration of clotting factors by the use of fresh frozen plasma or cryoprecipitate.

PULMONARY EMBOLECTOMY

In most centres this procedure will only be undertaken when thrombolysis is contraindicated and shock and hypotension cannot be relieved by plasma volume expansion and other conservative measures for maintaining arterial pressure. In one major series of 139 patients treated in a specialist unit between 1964 and 1986 the mortality of this procedure was around 30 per cent.

Duration of treatment

Recurrent embolism is rare while patient are adequately anticoagulated but the question arises of how long to continue such treatment in each case. When there has been a readily recognized precipitating event such as recent surgery or injury, a 3 month period is commonly advocated after venous thrombosis, and 6 months or more if there has been an embolism in addition. However, it has also been suggested that a period of 3 weeks might suffice in such cases, even after pulmonary embolism and the British Thoracic Society currently recommends 4 weeks in this situation. These recommendations do not apply to patients with persistent risk factors for further thromboembolism nor to those whose emboli were sufficiently large to result in thrombolytic or surgical treatment. In them the choice lies between long-term anticoagulation (3 to 6 months) or treatment for life.

The risk of further embolism if anticoagulation is withdrawn must be balanced against the haemorrhagic consequences of long-term treatment. An analysis of 171 separate studies of long-term anticoagulants for a variety of causes, reveals a total incidence of haemorrhagic complication of 23 per cent and of major bleeding of 8 per cent in those treated for thromboembolism. However no fatal cases were reported in these series. The risk was substantially higher when the internationally normalized ratio was kept between 3 and 4.5 rather than between 2 and 3.

Ultimately decisions must be made on the perceived balance of advantage versus disadvantage reached jointly between the physician and the patient.

REFERENCES

Bauer, K.A. (1994). Hypercoagulability—a new co-factor in the Protein C anticoagulant pathway. *New England Journal of Medicine*, **330**, 566–7.

Bounameaux, H., Cirafici, P., DerMoerloose, P., Schneider, P.-A., Slosman, D., Reber, G. and Unga, P.-F. (1991). Measurement of D-dimer in plasma as a diagnostic aid in suspect pulmonary embolism. *Lancet* **337**, 196–200.

Bradey, A.J.B., Crake, T., and Oakley, C. (1991). Percutaneous catheter fragmentation and distal dispersion of proximal pulmonary embolus. *Lancet* **338**, 1186–1189.

Carson, J.L., Kelly, M.A., Duff, A., *et al.* (1992). The clinical course of

pulmonary embolism. *New England Journal of Medicine, **326**, 1240–1245.

Dalen, J.E. and Alpert, J.S. (1975) The natural history of pulmonary embolism. *Progress in Cardiovascular Disease*, **17**, 259–70.

Goldheber, S.Z. and Braunwald, E. (1988). Pulmonary embolism. In *Heart Disease – a textbook of cardiovascular medicine* (ed. E. Braunwald). pp. 1577–1593. WB Sanders & Co. Philadelphia.

Goldheber, S.Z., Haire, W.D., Feldstein, M.L. *et al.* (1993). Alteplase versus heparin in acute pulmonary embolism: Randomised trial assessing right ventricular function and pulmonary perfusion. *Lancet* **341**, 507–511.

Gray, H.H., Morgan, J.M., Paneth, M, and Miller, G.A.H. (1987). Pulmonary embolectomy: Indications and Results. *British Heart Journal*, **57**, 572.

Hirsh, J. (1991). Drug therapy—heparin. *New England Journal of Medicine*, **324**, 1565–1574.

Levine, M.N., Raskob, J., and Hirsh, J. (1989). Hemorrhagic complications of long term anticoagulant therapy. *Chest* **95**, Supplement 26s–36s.

The PIOPED Investigators (1990). Value of the ventilation-perfusion scan in acute pulmonary embolism. Results of the prospective investigation of pulmonary embolism diagnosis (PIOPED). *Journal of the American Medical Association*, **263**, 2753–2759.

Routledge, P.A. and West, R.R. (1992). Low molecular weight heparin. *British Medical Journal*, **305**, 906.

Salzman, E.W. (1992). Low molecular weight heparin and other new antithrombotic drugs. *New England Journal of Medicine*, **326**, 1017–1019.

Seckl, M.J., Rustin, G.J., Newlands, E.S., Gwyther, S.J., and Bomanji, J. (1991). Pulmonary embolism, pulmonary hypertension and choriacarcinoma. *Lancet* **338**, 1313–1315.

Stein, P.D., Athanasoulis, C., and Alavi, A. et al (1992). Complications and validity of pulmonary angiography in acute pulmonary embolism. *Circulation* **85**, 462–468.

Svenson, P.J. and Dählback, B. (1994). Resistance to activated protein C as a basis for venous thrombosis. *New England Journal of Medicine*, **330**, 517–22.

The Urokinase Pulmonary Embolism Trial Study Group. (1974). The urokinase–streptokinase embolism trial: Phase 2 results. *Journal of the American Medical Association*, **229**, 1606–1613.

15.27 Essential hypertension

J.D. Swales

Definition

Blood pressure, like height and weight, is a biological characteristic of the individual. Like these other characteristics, blood pressure shows a wide interindividual variability. The blood pressure of some individuals lies above the mean, while others have a blood pressure below the mean. The distribution curve is slightly asymmetrical with a tail to the right, which becomes particularly pronounced with age.

The analogy with height and weight is a close one. The spread of values reflects the influence of genetic and environmental factors. It is rare for a single disorder to result in a subject being grossly overweight or markedly hypertensive. Such secondary obesity or secondary hypertension is sufficiently uncommon that it does not produce a discrete group at the upper end of the body weight or blood pressure distribution curves. The shape of the blood pressure distribution curve was the basis for the well-known Platt–Pickering controversy in the 1950s and the 1960s. Platt noted an apparent bimodality of blood pressure distribution in a clinic population and claimed that the upper mode was due to a disease of hypertension transmitted as a mendelian autosomal dominant characteristic. The apparent bimodality of blood pressures in Platt's report is now regarded as an artefact due to small populations, observer bias, and selected population samples. Ironically, more recent sophisti-

cated analysis of blood pressure in families has provided evidence for detectable single gene effects, but these do not modify the basic conclusion that high blood pressure is, in most, cases a multifactorial condition. Essential hypertension may therefore be defined as sustained high blood pressure not attributable to a single cause but reflecting the interaction of multiple genetic and environmental influences. In Pickering's phrase it is a 'quantitative deviation from the mean'. The diagnosis of essential hypertension is thus one of exclusion.

Prevalence of hypertension

Because the blood pressure distribution curves are smooth and unimodal the selection of a criterion for 'hypertension' is an arbitrary process. The lower the criterion selected the higher the apparent prevalence (Fig. 1). Further, blood pressure normally falls with repeated measurements as patients become habituated to the procedure. Thus, definition of hypertension using a single initial blood pressure measurement will yield a much higher apparent prevalence rate than an average blood pressure taken over several occasions. The apparent prevalence of hypertension can be more than halved by taking the average of blood pressures on the second or third occasion of measurement.

The apparent prevalence is also influenced by age. Population studies of men and women in Western societies have shown that systolic pressure rises steadily until the seventh decade in men and the sixth in women. The relative increase in systolic blood pressure in men up to the age of 25 is greater than the increase in women. Acceleration of the rise in women then leads to a cross-over in systolic blood pressure between the ages of 45 and 60. Diastolic blood pressure rises in both sexes until the end of the sixth decade, when it begins to fall. The United States Joint National Committee on Detection, Evaluation and Treatment of High Blood Pressure recommended as a criterion for the diagnosis of hypertension an average of two or more blood pressure readings of 140/90 mmHg or more confirmed on two subsequent occasions. This has the advantage of establishing that blood pressure elevation requires to be sustained for the diagnosis of essential hypertension to be made. Nevertheless, using this criterion the prevalence of essential hypertension is still very high (33 per cent of white men and 38 per cent of black men in the United States in an age range 18 to 74 years). The longer-standing World Health Organization criteria are often used in recruiting patients for trials but consist of single readings only (systolic blood pressure of 160 mmHg or more and diastolic blood pressure of 95 mmHg or more). Such definitions and prevalence figures are of little clinical or scientific value. Much more relevant are the blood pressure levels at which treatment is initiated. As this threshold varies in different countries even this figure has only limited practical value.

gested that American Blacks evolved a tendency to retain sodium which gave them an evolutionary advantage in a hot climate, but thereby rendered them more prone to hypertension. Whilst this theory has provoked a great deal of interest there is no evidence for sodium retention or volume expansion in American Blacks: neither does it explain the absence of excessive hypertension in blacks of Caribbean origin.

Some rural populations have lower blood pressures at all ages and show very little rise in blood pressure with age. Such populations have been described in Africa, South American, India, and Australia. It seems likely that environmental factors account for these differences because in several cases it has been shown that when individuals migrate to an urban environment blood pressure rises. A change in blood pressure can occur within a few weeks under these circumstances. Unravelling the factors responsible for the blood pressure change presents formidible problems. Clearly diet and social stress are the major candidates. Whilst most of the rural populations have a low salt intake (see below) other dietary factors may be important in determining the blood pressure response. When, for instance, Australian aborigines return from an urban to a rural mode of life a substantial fall in blood pressure is associated with reduced body mass and alcohol intake, and with improved glucose tolerance and serum lipids. The clinical importance of population differences in blood pressure lies in demonstration of the feasibility of modifying environmental factors to produce a reduction in population blood pressure which could have substantial public health benefits.

Ethnic and population differences in blood pressure

Adult Blacks in the United States have higher blood pressures than Whites. This difference is not observed in the United Kingdom, where Blacks of Caribbean origin and Asians have similar blood pressures to Whites of similar social background. The blood pressures of the original Caribbean population still residing in the West Indies also do not differ from a matched White population. Social factors are very important in these comparisons. Thus, there is an inverse relationship between educational achievement and blood pressure in both Blacks and Whites. However, this does not appear to account wholly for the difference in blood pressure between American Blacks and Whites. It has been sug-

Intraindividual blood pressure variation

Blood pressure shows great variability. Exposure to pain, mental stress, exercise, or sexual intercourse give rise to rapid elevation of pressure. Blood pressure also changes over the 24-h period, reaching its nadir during the early hours of the morning and reaching a maximum on rising (Fig. 2). This is not an endogenous circadian rhythm and is clearly dependent upon environmental factors. Thus, when workers change from a day to a night shift the circadian rhythm changes immediately. Circadian rhythm is not observed in immobilized patients, patients with autonomic dysfunction (e.g. diabetics) patients with pre-eclamptic toxaemia and cardiac transplantation, and in a minority of elderly hypertensive subjects. In the latter group the absence of the normal nocturnal fall in blood pressure is associated with a high incidence of atherosclerotic disease. Whether vascular disease is a cause of this phenomenon or a consequence of it is unknown.

The long-term changes in blood pressure with age also show impor-

Fig. 1 Effect of different cut off points on apparent prevalence of blood pressure, based upon single blood pressure measurements in a healthy population (reproduced from Swales *et al.* 1991, with permission).

Fig. 2 Changes in blood pressure (measured by intra-arterial cannula) over 24 h (reproduced from Swales *et al.* 1991, with permission).

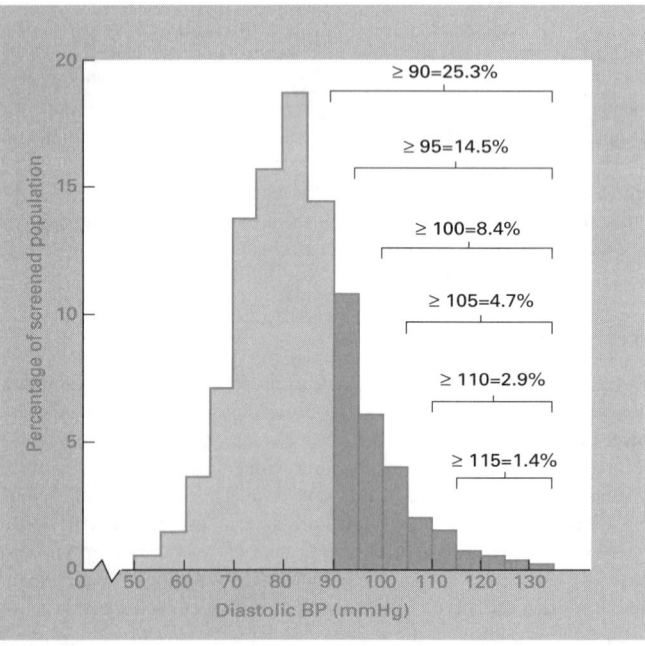

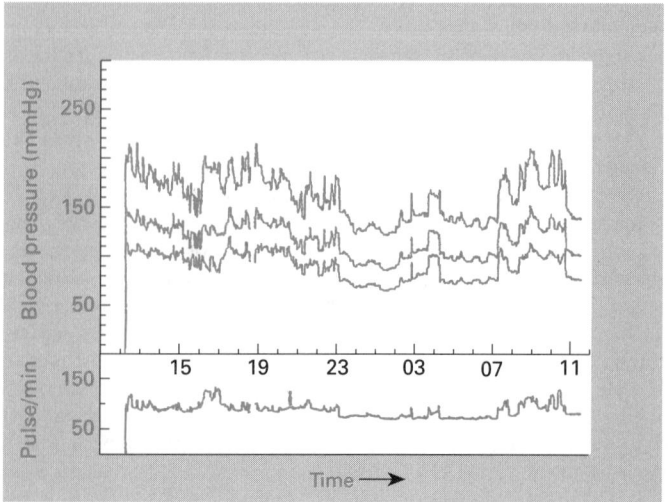

tant individual characteristics. Thus, young adults whose blood pressure lies in the upper part of the population blood pressure distribution tend to remain there (Fig. 3). This phenomenon is referred to as tracking and applies equally to subjects whose blood pressures lie in the lower part of the population range. As a result of tracking, high normal blood pressures in young adults are good predictors of those whose blood pressure will later cross any arbitrary threshold for the diagnosis of hypertension.

Pathogenesis

The interaction of genetic and environmental factors in determining blood pressure is just as complex as it is in determining weight or height. Unravelling these factors is a formidible task and, although progress has been made in recent years, there are still fundamental uncertainties. There are two important reasons for this. First, because hypertension is a multifactorial disorder, any individual factor may make a comparatively small contribution to overall blood pressure. For instance, if five genes contribute equally and independently to blood pressure and if genetic factors contribute, as seems likely, less than one-third to blood pressure variance, each gene is likely to account for only a 2 mm or a 3 mm difference in blood pressure between a moderately hypertensive and normotensive subject. The second major difficulty is that environmental and genetic factors are not independent of each other. Blood pressures tend to be higher in social classes IV and V. Diet, alcohol intake, ethnic mix, and probably social stress all differ between different social classes. Identifying cause and effect under these circumstances is fraught with difficulty. Nevertheless, important progress has been made in disentangling genetic and environmental factors that determine blood pressure level.

Genetic factors

Blood pressures of members of the same family tend to be correlated. This relationship is independent of whether propositi are diagnosed conventionally as hypertensive or normotensive. Likewise, blood pressures in relatives of hypertensive prepositi do not segregate out into normotensive and hypertensive populations. This, of course, supports Pickering's original hypothesis that blood pressure is a quantitative deviation from the population mean rather than a discrete disease, and emphasizes the multifactorial nature of hypertension. Thus, if only one or two genetic loci gave rise to hypertension there would be a discontinuity amongst those relatives who had inherited the disorder and those who had not. In fact, relatives show a complete spectrum of blood pressure from high to normal levels, although as a group they have higher blood pressures than relatives of normotensive controls. Although this relationship has been observed in many studies from different parts of the world, the correlation between blood pressures in blood relatives of hypertensives is relatively weak and certainly of little clinical value in screening programmes. Thus, the average correlation coefficient when blood pressures are corrected for age and sex is only of the order of 0.2. This suggests that the influence of the underlying genetic mechanisms is diluted by environmental factors and blood pressure variability. Adoption studies provide the possibility of determining the correlation between blood pressures of genetically distinct individuals under similar environmental circumstances. The largest of these studies (the Montreal Adoption Survey) showed a correlation between parents and natural children that was approximately twice as great as the correlation between parents and adoptive children (Fig. 4). A similar relationship was observed for the correlation between siblings. However, environ-

Fig. 3 Upper and lower percentile blood pressures in a healthy population. Patients tend to remain in the same percentile groups as they become older (reproduced from Swales J.D. (1979). *Clinical hypertension.* Chapman and Hall, London, with permission).

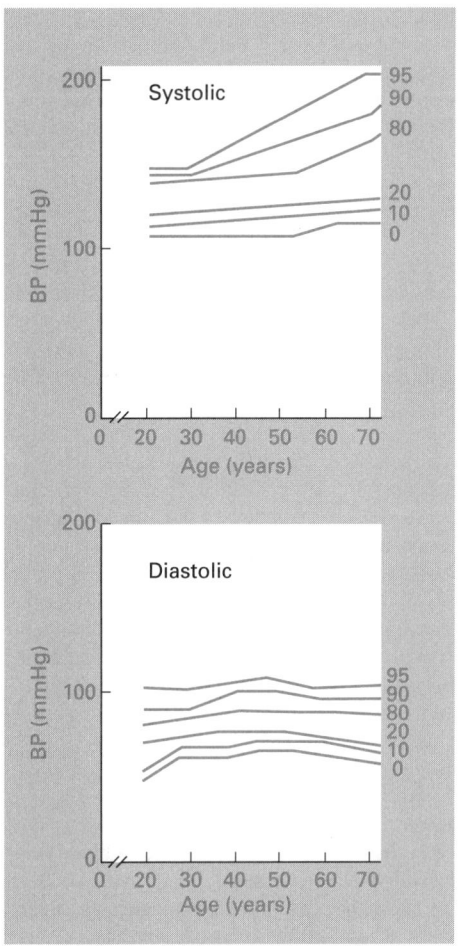

Fig. 4 Correlation of systolic and diastolic blood pressures in the Montreal Twin Study. Note the closer associations between blood relatives compared with adoptive relatives (reproduced from Swales *et al.* 1991, with permission).

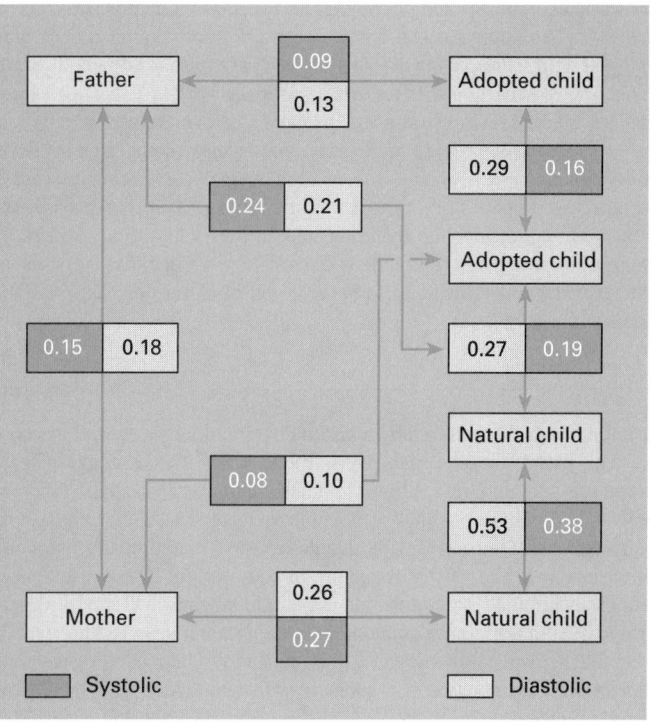

mental influences were clearly important because the correlation of blood pressure between adoptive siblings was approximately twice as great as that between parent and adoptive child. Twin studies suggest a rather higher genetic contribution. However, it is likely that greater environmental similarity for monozygotic twins produces an overestimation of the genetic contribution. Overall these various studies suggest that genetic factors contribute about 30 per cent to blood pressure variance, when blood pressure is measured under screening conditions.

The importance of genetic factors has been confirmed by breeding strains of rat with genetic hypertension. It has been calculated that, in the most frequently used strain (the spontaneously hypertensive rat bred in Kyoto, Japan), four to five genes contribute to blood pressure although recent evidence suggests that this may be an underestimate. Environmental factors can be important even in this situation, however. Thus, if genetically hypertensive rats are protected from environmental stimulation their blood pressure rises much less compared with animals subjected to noise and competitive stress.

The genes that contribute to human essential hypertension have not been identified. There is a family linkage with the angiotensinogen gene however. There are, also, phenotypic associations with blood pressure that may provide a clue about some of the underlying genes. Thus, high blood pressure is associated with a high body mass index, insulin resistance, and hyperlipidaemia. There is also an association with an erythrocyte sodium transport system (sodium–lithium countertransport) and a negative association between blood pressure and urinary kallikrein excretion. We can only speculate at present about the causal chain that gives rise to these associations. In some cases they may be the result of high blood pressure.

Environmental factors

Diet and stress are the two groups of environmental influences which contribute significantly to blood pressure.

Nutrition

Several components of the diet may change blood pressure. This has been shown by direct intervention trials, i.e. changing the diet under controlled conditions and observing the effect on blood pressure. There are also population associations between different components of diet and blood pressure. Taken in isolation, such associations do not indicate causality. A particular diet reflects a particular way of life, which may elevate blood pressure quite independently. Nevertheless, population associations may provide important clues. Thus, some studies have shown that subjects with a lower birth weight and higher placental weight have higher blood pressures in middle age. This has been interpreted as suggesting that maternal malnutrition may be an important cause of hypertension (and indeed other cardiovascular disease) in later life. However, it is difficult to separate out malnutrition, deprivation, and social stress.

Obesity

'Central' obesity measured by waist to hip circumference correlates better with blood pressure than overall body mass. The association with blood pressure may reflect humoral factors and perhaps genetic linkage. However, longitudinal studies in humans have shown that change in body weight is correlated with change in blood pressure, and intervention trials have shown that reduction in body weight is associated with reduction in blood pressure. This is quite independent of any effect of arm width circumference on blood pressure measurement (cuff artefact). The mechanism is unknown, although there is some evidence that dietary weight reduction is associated with a reduction in sympathetic nervous system activity.

Alcohol intake

High alcohol intake (more than six units a day, where one unit equals half a pint of beer, one measure of spirits, or a glass of wine) has been shown to be associated with elevated blood pressure in a large number of studies. The relationship is independent of body mass index, age, or social class. In some investigations the relationship has been J-shaped, i.e. the lowest incidence of hypertension occurs with a modest alcohol intake of two to three drinks a day. Although some researchers therefore claim a protective effect, this could be due to artefacts created by higher risk patients abstaining from alcohol totally as a result of previous cardiovascular disease or by heavy drinkers claiming to be total abstainers. The relationship between alcohol intake and blood pressure is causal as reduction in alcohol intake in heavy drinkers lowers blood pressure.

Sodium and potassium intake

A number of studies where different cultures are compared (intercultural studies) have shown a positive association between sodium intake and blood pressure and a negative association between potassium intake and blood pressure. By combining the two into a sodium–potassium ratio a closer correlation with blood pressure has been observed. The largest of these, the Intersalt Study reported data from over 10 000 subjects from 52 different cultures. The relationship between sodium and blood pressure was weak and partially attributable to other factors, such as body weight and alcohol. However, there was a stronger relationship between the rise in blood pressure with age and sodium intake. By contrast, analysis of electrolyte intake and blood pressure within a single culture has failed in most cases to show a significant association, although such studies have been able to demonstrate an association between body mass, alcohol intake, and blood pressure relatively easily. Intervention studies in which sodium intake is restricted or potassium intake increased have shown modest effect in hypertensive subjects but only very small effects in normotensives. Only if sodium intake is restricted to extremely low levels (less than 10 mmol per day), as in the Kempner rice–fruit diet, has blood pressure been lowered substantially. On current evidence the contribution of excessive sodium intake or inadequate potassium intake to hypertension in Western society is small.

Other electrolytes

Some population studies have suggested that subjects with a low calcium or magnesium intake have higher blood pressures. Controlled intervention trials have either failed to show any effect or shown minimal effects when dietary intake of these electrolytes was increased. It seems likely that the population association is therefore spurious.

Vegetarian diet

Vegetarians have lower blood pressures at all ages than omnivores. When omnivores change to a vegetarian diet blood pressure falls in both normotensives and hypertensives by a few mmHg. Despite intensive research it has been impossible to attribute this phenomenon to differences in calorie, electrolyte, or protein intake. One possibility is that unsaturated vegetable fats lower blood pressure. Some studies have shown small effects with oleic acid, although linoleic acid is inert in this respect. Saturated (ω-3) fish oils have been shown to lower blood pressure in several studies, although clearly these are not relevant to a purely vegetarian diet.

Stress

Ambulatory monitoring has demonstrated the major rise in blood pressure which can be produced by acute pain, tension, or mental stress. It is much more difficult to show that chronic stress produces sustained elevation of blood pressure. There are two particular problems. First, the difficulty in measuring stress and second, individual variability in the response to external stress. Animal experiments illustrate some of these difficulties. Mice that have to compete for food ultimately develop severe fatal hypertension, whilst rats and primates are extremely resistant to stress-induced hypertension. While there are clear social differences in human blood pressure these are not necessarily related to occupation or stress. However, it has been possible to demonstrate an association between 'job strain' and blood pressure. The former is characterized by high psychological demand and low levels of control over the work process. Body mass and alcohol intake appear to have additive effects to job strain confirming the popular impression of the hypertensive as an individual working under heavy pressure, overeating, and overdrinking. Such studies should be interpreted with care. The elevation of blood pressure in subjects exposed to job strain was only a few mmHg. Whether chronic job strain leads to progressive increase in blood pressure as some animal studies of stress would suggest is still uncertain.

Mechanisms of hypertension

Multiple genetic and environmental factors therefore produce an integrated sustained elevation of blood pressure in certain otherwise healthy individuals. The final common pathway in this respect appears to be the vessels that maintain peripheral resistance, as cardiac output is normal in chronic hypertension although increased cardiac output has been described in some young subjects with mild hypertension. How is this increase in peripheral resistance brought about? The resistance vessels (i.e. the smaller arteries and arterioles) in patients with hypertension show a reduction in luminal diameter associated with an increase in wall thickness. These structural changes can readily be demonstrated functionally in the form of reduced maximal vasodilatation (in response to warmth and pharmacological vasodilators) and a steep vasoconstrictor dose–response curve resulting in enhanced constrictor response to a given dose of vasoconstrictor agent such as angiotensin II or noradrenaline (Fig. 5). Whether there is an actual increase in mass of the resistance vessel or whether it is remodelled to reduce the lumen without any increase in mass is still a matter of controversy. There is a close relationship between resistance vessel wall to lumen ratio and blood pressure in essential hypertension, although this appears to be secondary. Where vessels are protected against increased blood pressure structural changes are not in general seen. This has led to the hypothesis that the causes of elevated high blood pressure lie elsewhere, but increased pressure on the resistance vessels leads to structural changes, which maintain blood pressure. This does not entirely exclude a role for genetic factors modulating resistance vessel structure. An increased resistance vessel structural response to pressure might amplify other blood pressure elevating mechanisms. Some of the rat genetic models of hypertension show enhanced smooth muscle growth and proliferation in tissue culture. So far there is no evidence for an abnormality of smooth muscle growth in man, however. There is one other possible genetically regulated structural mechanism. Overall resistance would be elevated if the number of resistance vessels were decreased. Such rarefaction has been demonstrated in some tissue beds in both in animal models of hypertension and in human hypertension. This seems to be a likely contributor.

Autonomic nervous system

The autonomic nervous system carries out a central role in blood pressure regulation and it would be surprising if it failed to play a role in upwards resetting of blood pressure. Indeed, in the absence of any central resetting mechanism, other influences upon peripheral resistance and blood pressure would tend to be opposed by compensatory autonomic responses. Essential hypertension in young subjects is associated with slightly elevated circulating noradrenaline and increased pulse rate and cardiac output. The changes are small in each case and there is extensive overlap with values obtained from normotensive subjects, but the degree of autonomic change needed to produce modest hypertension is small and the markers of increased autonomic activity are relatively insensitive. Genetically preconditioned autonomic overactivity and social stress probably play important complementary roles.

Autonomic resetting of blood pressure could occur as a result of changes in the baroreceptors or centrally. The latter is the more probable. Although baroreceptor sensitivity is reduced in hypertensive patients this is probably the result of structural changes in the walls of the large arteries on which the baroreceptors are situated causing them to become more inelastic. Rendering baroreceptors totally insensitive by denervation increases blood pressure variability but does not cause sustained increases in blood pressure.

Sodium

In certain clinical situations blood pressure is wholly sodium dependent, e.g. in the bilaterally nephrectomized subject. Sodium restriction produces a modest fall in blood pressure in patients with essential hypertension (see above). This response is variable and it has been claimed that there is a discrete group of subjects with essential hypertension who are 'sodium sensitive'. Very few data have been published on the reproducibility of this phenomenon and there is no evidence to believe that sodium is the cause of blood pressure in these individuals. If sodium sensitivity is indeed a genuine reproducible characteristic of certain individuals it is more likely that the fall in blood pressure produced by sodium restriction reflects impaired protective cardiovascular responses. Essential hypertensives as a group show no increased sodium intake, no impairment of sodium excretion, and no increased body sodium content. At most, dietary sodium may amplify other blood pressure raising mechanisms and contribute secondarily to the rise in blood pressure with age.

Other humoral mechanisms

A number of humoral systems are capable of influencing blood pressure. The most important of these is probably the renin–angiotensin–aldosterone system, but the kallikrein–kinin, atrial natriuretic peptide, prostaglandin, and renomedullary lipid systems may also play a role under some circumstances. There is no persuasive evidence to associate any of these systems with essential hypertension in man, but this may simply reflect the difficulty of detecting small effects. For instance, in some

Fig. 5 Response of resistance vessels from hypertensive and normotensive patients to vasoconstrictor stimuli (such as noradrenaline). Note steeper curve, displaced upwards in hypertensives. This is due to the increased wall to lumen ratio (reproduced from Swales *et al.* 1991, with permission).

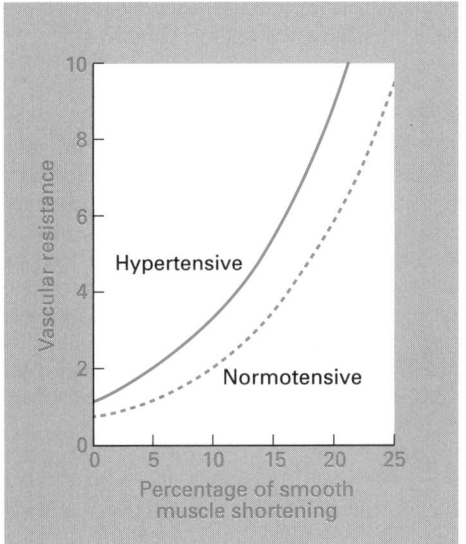

genetically hypertensive strains of rat a particular renin gene allele has been shown to be associated with blood pressure but contributes only 5 to 20 per cent of the difference in blood pressure between normotensive and hypertensive strains. This association has not been detected in human essential hypertension, but this may simply reflect the difficulty in detecting small effects in the face of much more important environmental factors. The negative correlation between urinary kallikrein and blood pressure is impressive but could be explained by high blood pressure suppressing kallikrein excretion. Genetic analysis in large populations may help to resolve these issues over the next few years.

Natural history

There are probably more data on the prognosis of hypertension than any other clinical condition. This information comes from two sources: (1) the insurance industry, which has compiled data on very large groups of relatively healthy subjects; and (2) long-term epidemiological studies such as that carried out at Framingham, Massachusetts, which has provided information not only on the life-expectancy of hypertensive patients but also on specific morbidity and mortality.

Mortality

Experience of North American insurance companies has been pooled to provide information on the life expectancy of several million subjects. These data show progressive increases in relative mortality with increasing systolic and diastolic blood pressures (Fig. 6). This relationship is continuous, i.e. there is no break in the mortality curve below which blood pressure ceases to be a risk factor. As a result those individuals with blood pressure below the population mean have a relative mortality less than the population average. The second important point to emerge from the life insurance statistics is that systolic and diastolic blood pressures are independent risk factors, i.e. for a given diastolic blood pressure a progressive rise in systolic pressure is associated with increasing mortality and vice versa. Although life insurance data have the strength of enormous numbers, they are deficient in some respects. Thus, they provide no information on the prognosis of elderly subjects. Longitu-

Fig. 6 Standardized mortality ratios in a healthy population. Note that systolic and diastolic pressures are independent risk factors. Risk progressively increases throughout the 'normal blood pressure range' (reproduced from Swales *et al.* 1991, with permission).

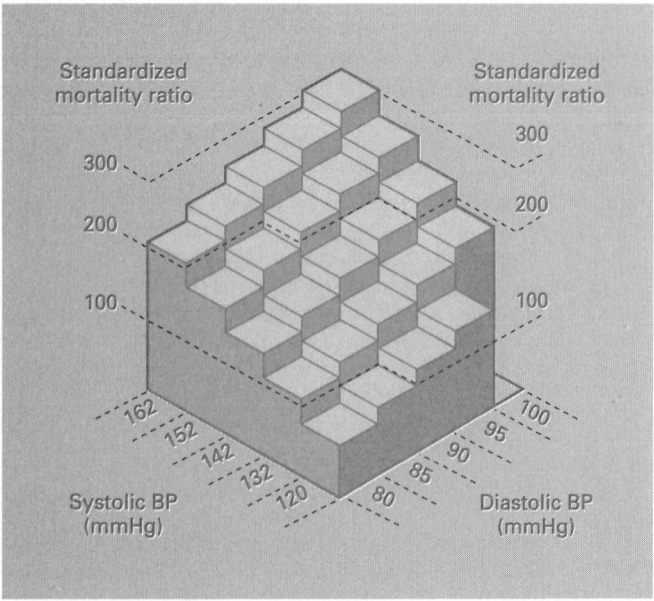

dinal studies, however, indicate that systolic blood pressure continues to be an important risk factor for cardiovascular death in elderly subjects. Cardiac deaths are increased two- to threefold in patients with isolated systolic hypertension (i.e. systolic blood pressure over 160 mmHg, diastolic blood pressure below 95 mmHg). Diastolic blood pressure, however, becomes less important as an independent risk factor and is only marginally related to life expectancy.

Mild hypertension and prognosis

As a consequence of the bell-shaped blood pressure distribution curve the mildest degrees of blood pressure elevation are the most frequent. This carries important consequences. First, the mildly hypertensive patient is a much more common clinical problem than moderate or severe hypertension in unselected clinical practice. It should not be forgotten, however, that even modest elevation of blood pressure impairs prognosis substantially. Thus, the life expectancy of a 35-year-old man with a casual blood pressure of 150/100 is reduced from 41.5 to 35 years; at 55 the relevent figures are 23.5 years and 17.5 years. The preponderance of mild over severe hypertension also has important public health consequences. Approximately half the hypertensive deaths in the Framingham population occurred in patients with blood pressures of 140 to 160/90 to 95 mmHg. Few clinicians would use antihypertensive drugs in these subjects. Non-pharmacological methods have to be identified which are safe and can be used in large populations.

Prognosis in severe and malignant hypertension

Individual risk increases markedly and life expectancy decreases sharply in individuals with moderate and severe hypertension (i.e. blood pressures in excess of 160/110 mmHg). The presence of malignant hypertension as shown by fundal changes (see below) greatly worsens prognosis because it indicates life-threatening vascular damage. Before effective antihypertensive medication was available malignant hypertension was associated with a 1-year life expectancy of only 10 to 20 per cent. This has now been radically altered, particularly when effective treatment is begun early. Thus, some specialist centres have reported 5-year survival rates in excess of 80 per cent amongst patients who were free of significant renal impairment at presentation.

Specific morbidity of hypertension

The predominant causes of death in hypertensive patients are cerebrovascular disease and coronary heart disease. Hypertensive patients are also at risk from peripheral arterial disease and renal failure.

Cerebrovascular disease

In the Framingham study hypertensive patients were six times more likely to develop a stroke than normotensive controls. Epidemiological studies have not hitherto differentiated between cerebral haemorrhage and cerebral infarction. It seems extremely probable that the risk of cerebral haemorrhage is more closely related to blood pressure than the risk of cerebral infarction. However, a high proportion of strokes (70 to 80 per cent) in unselected populations are due to cerebral infarction and there is no doubt that hypertension is a risk factor for cerebral infarction as well as cerebral haemorrhage. Cerebral haemorrhage is probably associated with more severe degrees of hypertension than cerebral infarction.

Cardiac disease

In the Framingham study patients with hypertension (defined as blood pressure equal to or more than 160/95 mmHg) were three times more likely to develop coronary heart disease and chronic heart failure than normotensive people. In large-scale longitudinal studies, such as the Pooling Project and the MRFIT Screening Programme, there is a smooth relationship between diastolic and systolic blood pressure on the one hand and cardiac mortality on the other. This extends right through the blood pressure range, so that patients with the lowest pressures were at least risk. Adding together the three major risk factors for coronary heart disease, i.e. blood pressure, cholesterol, and smoking, it was possible to account for 55 to 70 per cent of the total coronary risk in the Pooling Project. The remaining risk may be due to the presence of additional unassessed risk factors or to inadequate assessment of the role of these three major risk factors. It seems unlikely that the initial measures reflected precisely an individual's exposure over the period of observation.

Peripheral arterial disease

Peripheral artery disease is twice as common in hypertensive patients than normotensive controls. Smoking as a risk factor greatly outweighs blood pressure, although the two risks are additive.

Renal failure

In most cases renal failure only occurs when essential hypertension enters the malignant phase. The effectiveness of antihypertensive treatment has rendered advanced renal failure as a consequence of essential hypertension very uncommon, as control of blood pressure makes progression of renal disease in severe hypertension much less likely. However, hypertension is reported as the cause of renal failure in about 25 per cent of patients entering renal replacement programmes. Uncontrolled hypertension also exacerbates renal failure in patients with primary renal disease such as chronic pyelonephritis or chronic glomerulonephritis. The difficulty in distinguishing renal failure due to primary hypertension and primary renal disease and the rarity of hypertensive renal failure explain the paucity of epidemiological data, although it has been estimated that only one in 10 000 deaths in the United States is due to hypertensive renal failure.

Deterioration in renal function in non-malignant hypertension may be due to progressive nephron loss due to nephrosclerosis or to progressive renal arterial atheroma. The former represents an acceleration of a process which occurs normally with ageing.

Pathology

Sustained high blood pressure is associated with changes in the exposed vessels as well as secondary changes in the heart, brain and kidneys.

Blood vessel changes

LARGE ARTERIES

Hypertension produces medial thickening in the aorta and large arteries associated with disruption and uncoiling of elastic fibres and increase in the relatively inelastic collagen. Calcium is deposited secondarily. These changes are, of course, associated with ageing as well as with hypertension: the two processes are additive so that loss of elastic reservoir function of these vessels (the Windkessel vessels) occurs at an earlier age in hypertensive than in normotensive subjects. The decrease in arterial compliance allows the pressure wave generated during systole to be transmitted throughout the arterial tree in a less dampened form thereby increasing pulse pressure. The shape of the arterial wave form is also altered as a result of early return of the reflection wave from the periphery. This boosts the arterial pressure wave in late systole in both hypertensive and elderly patients and so increases the stress on the arterial wall. The clinical significance of this potentially important change

in arterial wave form and peak systolic blood pressure is unknown: it is not of course evident on conventional sphygmomanometry of the brachial artery.

Decreased compliance of the large arteries also has an important effect on the carotid and aortic baroreceptors which normally buffer rapid changes in blood pressure. The baroreceptors become less sensitive. As a result, circulatory adaptation to rapid changes in posture may be impaired. This is only usually seen in elderly hypertensive subjects, as age and blood pressure have additive effects on vessel compliance. Clinically these effects may be manifest as postural hypotension, most commonly seen when blood pressure is reduced too rapidly in elderly hypertensive patients.

ATHEROMA IN HYPERTENSION

There is a close association between the development of atheroma and blood pressure. The local mechanical consequences of increased pressure and turbulence on the arterial wall are of prime importance in this relationship. Thus, atheroma is not usually seen in the pulmonary arterial tree in essential hypertension unless pulmonary hypertension is also present. Other risk factors have additive effects. Atheroma cannot usually be produced in hypertensive rabbits unless their lipid levels are raised by feeding cholesterol. Atheroma can be induced in the proximal part of the aorta in monkeys fed a high cholesterol diet: although a low cholesterol diet prevents the development of atheroma at this site. These observations are particularly important clinically as there is an association between elevated cholesterol and triglycerides and essential hypertension. The risks of hypertension *per se* are thus amplified. The key process in atherogenesis in the hypertensive patient is probably increased endothelial permeability arising as a result of local stress. This allows exposure of the subendothelial arterial wall to growth factors derived from endothelium, macrophages, and platelets. Migration and proliferation of smooth muscle cells in the intima and accumulation of lipid-laden macrophages produce the characteristic atheromatous plaque.

Resistance vessel changes

The characteristic change in resistance vessels is an increase of the wall to lumen ratio. This causes important functional changes characterized by an increased reactivity to pressor agonists (see above). The major histological change is growth and remodelling of the medial smooth muscle cells. Increased wall mass can be demonstrated in some experimental models: this is due in some cases to increase size of smooth muscle cells (hypertrophy) and in other cases due to increased number (hyperplasia). There is no evidence for hyperplasia of smooth muscle cells of resistance vessel smooth muscle cells in essential hypertension. The increased wall to lumen ratio may be rearrangement (remodelling) and perhaps hypertrophy although the evidence for this is controversial.

Specific organ changes in hypertension

The heart

Angina and myocardial infarction in the hypertensive patient are usually due to coronary atheroma. In a minority of patients anginal pain occurs in the absence of significant coronary atheroma ('syndrome X'). Functional studies of the coronary vascular tree in these patients have shown an impaired response to vasodilators (reduced coronary flow reserve). A possible explanation of this is that it is caused by the increased wall to lumen ratio of smaller coronary vessels demonstrated in other tissue beds. Other explanations which have been put forward are increased vasomotor tone (although this has never been convincingly shown in other vascular beds) and increased wall pressure causing some endocardial ischaemia (this has not been directly demonstrable). Impaired endothelial derived relaxation has been demonstrated in the coronary vascular bed and may be of major importance.

Left ventricular hypertrophy occurs as a result of an increase in the size of cardiomyocytes, which are associated with increase in intercellular matrix. Two processes occur in the hypertensive patient: (1) increase in left ventricular mass; and (2) dilatation. The major trophic stimulus is unquestionably left ventricular load. It has been suggested, however, that the response to pressure may be amplified by activation of the renin–angiotensin–aldosterone system or increased sympathetic nerve activity. The bad prognosis carried by left ventricular hypertrophy in the hypertensive patient could have several explanations. It could simply reflect integrated exposure of the circulation to raised pressure. Alternatively the increased risk may be due to ischaemia produced by the increased muscle mass or the increased prevalence of simple and complex ventricular arrhythmias, which can be demonstrated in left ventricular hypertrophy. The decrease in ventricular compliance produced by increased left ventricular mass also probably predisposes patients to left ventricular failure.

Cerebral blood vessels

Cerebral infarction in a hypertensive patient is usually attributable to atheroma of one of the larger cerebral arteries (usually the middle cerebral artery). Intracerebral haemorrhage is usually the result of rupture of a small intracerebral degenerative aneurysm (Charcot–Bouchard aneurysm). These lesions develop in the small perforating arteries in the region of the basal ganglia, thalamus, and the internal capsule. There is hyaline degeneration in the aneurysmal wall and a defect in the media at the neck of the aneurysm. The incidence of Charcot–Bouchard aneurysms is closely correlated with age and blood pressure, the two factors acting additively so that lesions are rarely if ever seen in younger normotensive people.

Hypertensive encephalopathy

The cerebral resistance vessels usually constrict in the face of increased pressure and dilate in the face of decreased pressure to maintain a constant flow (autoregulation). Resistance vessel hypertrophy seems to have a protective function in this respect so that the autoregulatory range is raised in long-standing hypertension. When blood pressure rises above the autoregulatory range, however, focal areas of vasodilatation and localized oedema occur. In particular, haemorrhages, localized ischaemia, and infarction may result, giving rise to the clinical picture of encephalopathy. Reduction of blood flow below the autoregulatory range reduces cerebral blood flow and may precipitate cerebral infarction. As the autoregulatory range is raised in long-standing hypertension, patients with essential hypertension are particularly at risk when sudden therapeutic reductions in blood pressure are produced (see below).

The kidney in essential hypertension

In non-malignant hypertension glomerular filtration rate is well preserved so that filtration fraction (ratio of glomerular filtration rate to renal plasma flow) is increased. This results from a relative increase in efferent as opposed to afferent glomerular resistance so that intracapillary pressure is increased. The renal vascular changes are associated with arteriolar wall thickening, thus reducing luminal diameter. Hyaline degeneration is particularly observed in the afferent arterioles of the kidney. The lesion consists of a patchy hyaline eosinophilic thickening of the whole vessel wall beginning in the subendothelial region and extending to the media. Progressive hyalinization of nephrons accounts for the slow decline in glomerular filtration rate with age which is observed in normotensive subjects. The rate of this loss is increased in essential hypertension. Effective blood pressure control probably reduces the rate of nephron loss.

Blood vessels in malignant hypertension

The malignant phase of hypertension occurs when blood pressure rises rapidly. In more long-standing hypertension (such as that occurring in coarctation of the aorta, where malignant hypertension is very rare) hypertrophy seems to be protective. The characteristic pathological change in malignant hypertension is fibrinoid necrosis (necrotizing arteriolitis). The normal structure of the vessel wall is lost and replaced with fibrin-like material. A variable cellular-like reaction occurs. Fibrinoid necrosis is usually associated with focal areas of vasodilatation and increased permeability. These changes appear to be primarily a mechanical effect. The endothelium of the dilated segments is disrupted and the vessel wall becomes permeable to particles as large as colloidal carbon. This increased permeability permits exudation of plasma into the media and local tissue destruction. The intima may become massively thickened by concentric collagenous rings until the lumen is almost obliterated. This trophic response probably results from exposure of subendothelial tissues to growth factors in an analogous way to the trophic changes which are seen in the atheromatous plaque. Changes in the glomerular vessels lead to rapidly progressively renal failure associated with increased glomerular permeability, proteinuria, and haematuria: in the cerebral vessels cerebral haemorrhage occurs. Without effective antihypertensive treatment the lesions of malignant hypertension result in death of 90 per cent of patients within 1 year, largely from renal failure.

The clinical features of essential hypertension

Symptoms

Elevated blood pressure is usually asymptomatic until organ damage occurs. Most patients are not aware of this and as a result attribute most concurrent complaints to high blood pressure. In some cases the knowledge that a patient has high blood pressure creates a fertile soil for the growth of functional symptoms. Thus, patients who have been told that they are hypertensive have a much higher incidence of headache than hypertensive patients who are unaware of the fact. In some studies 'labelling' a patient as hypertensive has led to an increased absenteeism from work, although target organ damage had not occurred. It is a common lay fallacy that a patient can recognize when their blood pressure is elevated usually on the basis of such symptoms as plethoric features, palpitations, dizziness, or a feeling of tension. A screening survey carried out in the United States examined the frequency of such symptoms as headache, epistaxis, tinnitus, dizziness, and fainting in healthy subjects. None of these symptoms was more prevalent in subjects with diastolic blood pressures over 100 mmHg. However, higher levels of blood pressure may be associated with symptoms even in the absence of obvious target organ damage.

HEADACHE

The classic hypertensive headache is present on waking in the morning, situated in the occipital region of the head, radiating to the frontal area, throbbing in quality and wearing off during the course of the day. Most headaches in hypertensive patients are tension headaches not directly related to blood pressure at all. Nevertheless, treatment of hypertension reduces the prevalence of headache. How far this is a specific consequence of blood pressure lowering and how far it is due to reassurance is uncertain. Morning headaches in obese hypertensives may be due to nocturnal sleep apnoea.

EPISTAXIS

Whilst epistaxis it not particularly associated with mild hypertension, it is more common in moderate to severe hypertension. Where patients present with epistaxis and high blood pressure it is important to dissociate hypertension as a cause of epistaxis from a pressor response to the episode.

NOCTURIA

This is one of the most frequent consequences of blood pressure elevation resulting from reduction in urine concentrating capacity.

Symptoms associated with target organ damage

CARDIOVASCULAR SYSTEM

Effort dyspnoea and orthopnoea suggest cardiac failure. Increase in left ventricular mass is associated with decreased compliance and an impaired cardiac output response. This may be manifest as decreased effort tolerance. Angina of effort or claudication suggests superimposed atheromatous vascular disease.

Symptoms associated with the central nervous system

Scotomata suggest fundal haemorrhages or exudates whilst blurring of vision is associated with papilloedema. Failure of concentration and memory is most often a reflection of depression or centrally acting medication. Less commonly it is due to hypertensive cerebrovascular disease. Strokes may be due to cerebral haemorrhage, occlusion of large vessels (atherothrombotic brain infarction) or lacunar infarctions giving rise to minor strokes. Occasionally a lacunar state may be associated with hypertension characterized by progressive pseudobulbar palsy and dementia.

Renal system

Haematuria or haematospermia, if associated with hypertension, is usually seen only in the malignant phase. Renal failure is a late and fortunately now rare complication.

Clinical examination

The objective of physical examination is to assess blood pressure and any consequences of its elevation.

Measurement of blood pressure

Blood pressure can be measured directly from a cannula inserted into an artery. Portable recording devices enable continuous arterial blood pressure measurements to be made with this technique. These are the 'gold standard' for blood pressure measurement and have demonstrated minute-by-minute blood pressure variability and the usual nocturnal fall in blood pressure. However, the invasive nature of this method has confined it to research studies. Routine clinical assessment relies wholly therefore upon indirect techniques, which do not require arterial cannulation. The manual auscultatory method is still the technique universally used. Based upon the sounds described by Korotkoff in 1905, and using the air-filled inflatable cuff described by Riva–Rocci in 1897, it has remained fundamentally unchanged for 90 years. The brachial artery is occluded by inflating the cuff above the pressure at which the radial pulse disappears to palpation. Pressure in the cuff is estimated either by a mercury or aneroid manometer. Pressure is then lowered through the valve on the inflating bulb. The point at which sounds return (Korotkoff phase I) is taken as the systolic blood pressure. As the pressure is further lowered the sounds suddenly become muffled (Korotkoff phase IV) and shortly afterwards disappear (Korotkoff phase V). Both Korotkoff phase IV and Korotkoff phase V sounds have been used as estimates of diastolic pressure. Although so frequently employed, auscultatory measurement of blood pressure is often carried out badly: inter- and even intraobserver variability is often unacceptably high. There are a number of important precautions which have to be taken.

BLADDER AND CUFF

The inflatable bladder has to be long enough and wide enough to achieve adequate occlusion of the brachial artery when the pressure within the cuff equals arterial pressure. If the cuff is too small (usually as a result of an obese arm) inadequate pressure will be applied and blood pressure will be overestimated. The length of the bladder should be at least 80 per cent and the width of the bladder at least 40 per cent of the circumference of the arm. Minor overlap of the ends of the bladder does not significantly influence readings.

MANOMETERS

Mercury manometers should be vertical and should read zero when no pressure is applied to the cuff. The diameter of the reservoir must be at least ten times that of the vertical tube. Aneroid manometers require regular calibration (at least yearly) by comparison with a mercury manometer.

BULB AND TUBING

These require checking for significant leaks (i.e. more than 1 mmHg per second) and for smooth working of the valve and inflation systems.

TECHNIQUE OF BLOOD PRESSURE MEASUREMENT

Patients should be comfortable either in a seated or supine position and additionally standing when postural change in blood pressure is a possibility. The arm should be held horizontal and supported at midsternal level. Tight or restrictive clothing should be removed from the arm. An appropriate sized cuff should be applied so that its midpoint lies over the position of maximal pulsation of the brachial artery. Blood pressure should be recorded in both arms on initial examination and the arm found to have the higher pressures subsequently used. Systolic blood pressure is initially determined by palpation and then the stethoscope is lightly placed over the brachial artery and the cuff pressure raised to approximately 30 mm above the point at which the radial pulse disappears and then released at the rate of 2 to 3 mm per second. Both systolic and diastolic blood pressure should be read to the nearest 2 mm mark. The point of disappearance of sounds (phase V Korotkoff) is preferable to the point of muffling (phase IV). The reasons for this advice are: (1) direct arterial blood pressure measurements indicate that the phase of muffling is 5 to 10 mmHg higher than actual diastolic blood pressure; (2) there are fewer observer errors in identifying the disappearance of sounds; and (3) most of the epidemiological data and multicentre trials of treatment in hypertension use phase V as the criterion for diastolic blood pressure. In some clinical situations where blood flow through the brachial artery is high (immediately after exercise, in hyperthyroidism in children, in pregnant women, and in anaemic patients) sounds can be detected down to zero cuff pressure. Under these circumstances the fourth phase has to be used.

Indirect ambulatory blood pressure monitoring

Indirect monitoring can be carried out either by patient-triggered blood pressure measurement (e.g. the Remler) or automatic blood pressure measurement with cuff inflation at regular intervals (e.g. SpaceLabs or the Oxford System). The recording device is suspended on a belt or sling and the record subsequently subject to computer analysis. Ambulatory monitoring has demonstrated major divergences between casual blood pressure in the clinic and blood pressure levels outside the clinic. In most cases clinic measurements are higher than levels outside the clinic environment. In some cases dramatic elevations of blood pressure occur when measurements are carried out by a doctor (white coat hypertension) (Fig. 7). Although the evidence is by no means conclusive it seems probable that average blood pressures measured by ambulatory monitoring are better predictors of cardiovascular risk than clinic measurements. Certainly, left ventricular mass is more closely correlated with ambulatory blood pressure measurements than it is with clinic blood pressures. Apart from its use in diagnosing white coat hypertension however, ambulatory blood pressure monitoring is still fundamentally a research tool. The reason for this is that all the trial data and epidemiological data which we have are based upon clinic blood pressure measurements and the true clinical significance of a particular set of ambulatory measurements cannot therefore be assessed.

Fundal examination

Fundal appearances provide vital information on vascular pathology and prognosis in hypertension. The Keith Wagener classification is still the one generally used clinically although it has some serious shortcomings; most important of these are that grade I and II changes are produced by ageing as well as hypertension.

GRADE 1

The light reflex from the arterial wall is increased as a result of thickening.

GRADE 2

The arterial light reflex is wider still and gives rise to a homogenous silver wire appearance. Nipping of the retinal vein occurs largely as a result of the optical effect of the thickened arterial wall preventing visualization of the column of blood within the vein. Thus, the vein appears to taper until it disappears before it is actually crossed by the artery. The vein may also be displaced posteriorly or laterally. Venous obstruction is much less common. Generalized reduction in arterial diameter with a

consequent reduction in arterial-to-venous ratio is probably the most sensitive, early phase of elevated blood pressure. Focal arterial narrowing is seen less often usually when an acute rise in blood pressure has occurred.

GRADE 3

Lesions may occur singly or in combination.

Haemorrhages

Flame-shaped haemorrhages are more superficial and owe their character to constraints imposed by nerve fibres. Dot and blot haemorrhages are deep to the nerve fibres and so are not limited in the same way. Haemorrhages usually disappear after a few weeks of effective blood pressure control.

Exudates

These are of two types. Hard or waxy exudates represent the end results of fluid leakage into the fibre layers of the retina from damaged vessels often with associated nerve vessel damage. Fluid is resorbed leaving a protein–lipid residue which is slowly removed by macrophages. Soft exudates or cotton-wool patches are aetiologically and ophthalmoscopically quite different. They are usually larger than hard exudates and have a woolly, ill-defined edge. They are not true exudates but nerve fibre infarcts caused by hypertensive vascular occlusion. Unlike hard exudates these lesions disappear within a few weeks of establishing adequate antihypertensive therapy.

GRADE 4

Papilloedema is associated with raised pressure in the disc head secondary to severe vascular damage. Venous distension is followed by increased vascularity of the optic disc, which has a pink appearance with blurring of the disc margins and loss of the optic cup. Raising of the optic disc with anterior displacement of the vessels occurs later. The surrounding retina often shows oedema, small radial haemorrhages, and cotton-wool exudates.

Grade III and IV changes are considered diagnostic of the malignant phase, requiring urgent assessment and treatment. Attempts were once made to discriminate between accelerated (grade III) and malignant (grade IV) hypertension. It is now clear that the prognosis does not differ

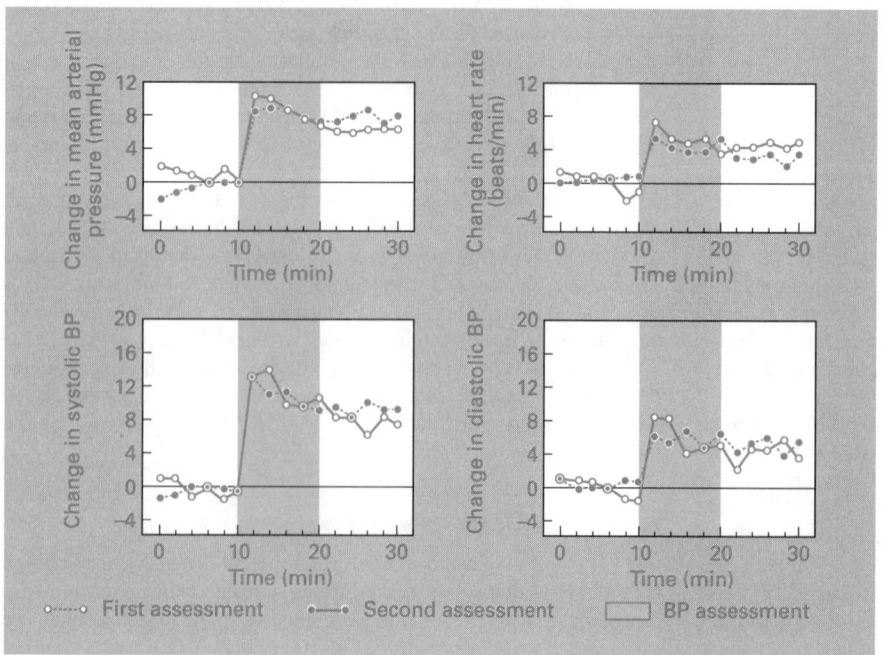

Fig. 7 White coat hypertension measured by an intra-arterial cannula on two occasions. Note the rise in blood pressure when a doctor approached the patient (reproduced from Swales et al. 1991, with permission).

between these two grades, so that each retinal appearance should be treated with the same degree of urgency, and the terms 'accelerated' and 'malignant' can be considered synonymous. The presence of significant renal failure carries a much worse prognosis.

OTHER PHYSICAL SIGNS

Clinical evidence of left ventricular hypertrophy and a loud aortic second sound usually indicate moderate or severe hypertension. Other physical signs indicate target organ damage to the cardiovascular, renal, or central nervous systems.

Investigations

Concentrations of urea, electrolytes, and creatinine are usually normal in essential hypertension unless secondary renal damage has occurred. Severe hypertension, particularly in the malignant phase, may be associated with elevated plasma renin and aldosterone levels, which may give rise to a modest hypokalaemic alkalosis. Serum sodium is usually low normal or low under these circumstances. This is an important differentiating point from primary aldosteronism, in which hypokalaemic alkalosis is usually associated with a high or high normal serum sodium concentration.

Urinary casts, haematuria and proteinuria usually indicate that hypertension has entered the malignant phase, or reflect primary renal disease.

Electrocardiographic left ventricular hypertrophy indicates the presence of moderate or severe hypertension and is important prognostically when present.

Echocardiography is much more sensitive in detecting the early changes of left ventricular hypertrophy and provides the best independent measure of severity in mild to moderate hypertension.

Management of essential hypertension

Management has three components, assessment, advice (including non-pharmacological therapy) and drug therapy.

Assessment

The initial assessment of the hypertensive patient has three objectives: (1) to establish the diagnosis, i.e. to exclude secondary hypertension; (2) to evaluate the effects of hypertension; and (3) to assess the presence of concurrent disease.

ESTABLISHING THE DIAGNOSIS

History and examination will provide few positive features. The usually-quoted age of presentation is 35 to 55 years, but this, of course, simply reflects the arbitrarily selected threshold for diagnosis. Hypertension first observed outside this age range, particularly when it is severe, suggests a secondary cause, although more often than not previous blood pressures are not documented. The presence of hypertension in siblings or parents is of modest value. Often a negative family history simply reflects ignorance or failure to diagnose hypertension, particularly in the previous generation. In addition of course a positive family history can often be obtained fortuitously for a condition of very high prevalence, such as hypertension. Positive indications of a cause for hypertension are of more value, e.g. history of oestrogen-containing contraceptive pill exposure, previous renal disease, or features suggestive of phaeochromocytoma, primary aldosteronism, etc. Where there is no clinical suspicion of secondary hypertension, extensive investigation for a primary cause is unnecessary, because the prevalence of secondary hypertension is so low under these circumstances. Measurement of serum urea, sodium, potassium, and creatinine, urinary microscopy, and dip stick

measurement of protein are sufficient. More intensive investigation for renal or adrenal causes should be reserved for situations where there is a clinical suspicion.

ASSESSMENT OF THE EFFECTS OF HYPERTENSION

This provides important information for the evaluation of prognosis and the urgency of treatment. The presence of heart failure, secondary renal failure, grade III or IV fundal changes all indicate the need for urgent treatment. A history of stroke or ischaemic heart disease is not necessarily an indication for urgent treatment but may influence timing and selection of therapy. Thus, it is dangerous to attempt to reduce blood pressure to normal in a patient who has sustained a stroke within the previous few days: a history of recent myocardial infarction (in the absence of cardiac failure) would favour the use of β-blockade, as this class of drug has the additional advantage of reducing the risk of secondary infarction. Examination of the fundi and clinical examination for evidence of left ventricular hypertrophy provide the best evidence of severity of hypertension. Clinical signs of cerebrovascular, coronary artery, or peripheral vascular disease are not necessarily measures of the severity of hypertension: they may reflect duration and presence of other risk factors. Fundal changes or left ventricular hypertrophy where present exclude the possibility of white coat hypertension unless another cause for abnormalities can be identified. Unfortunately, neither of these signs is particularly sensitive and the large majority of patients with essential hypertension will show neither unequivocal fundal changes nor clinical left ventricular hypertrophy.

CONCURRENT DISEASE AND RISK FACTORS

The presence of other diseases and risk factors may play an important role both in the decision to treat and on the selection of treatment. A history of smoking, the presence of glucose intolerance or diabetes, and hyperlipidaemia increase the cardiovascular risks of hypertension and may tip the balance in favour of active treatment, as well as requiring management in their own right. A history of obstructive airways disease contraindicates the use of β-blockers and non-insulin dependent diabetes usually contraindicates thiazide diuretics in the management of hypertension.

Advice and non-pharmacological treatment

The hypertensive patient may present in one of three ways:

1. As an asymptomatic individual whose blood pressure has been measured at routine examination for employment, insurance, or as a result of screening.
2. As a patient presenting with an unrelated disorder.
3. As a result of symptoms caused by hypertension.

Clinicians who deal with hypertension, therefore, are at a great disadvantage with the majority of their patients. While treatment of most conditions leads to subjective improvement of a clinically unwell patient, drug treatment of hypertension often creates unpleasant symptoms in an individual who was previously, to the best of his knowledge, perfectly well. It is essential therefore to explain the significance of high blood pressure at the earliest opportunity. It is important to point out that in most cases it does not have a single cause. Many patients find difficulty in grasping the concept of blood pressure variability. Often they are alarmed at single high readings. Discussion of a simple plan for assessment, which involves evaluation of blood pressure on repeated measurement and explanation that treatment will not necessarily improve subjective symptoms, encourages a realistic approach by patients.

Except for patients who present as hypertensive emergencies, repeated measurements of blood pressure should be carried out before drug therapy is considered.

This period of assessment can be combined with advice and non-pharmacological treatment of blood pressure. There are two reasons for repeated measurement of blood pressure:

1. Habituation to blood pressure measurement results in a fall in pressure from initially higher readings. Making a decision to treat on the basis of these initial readings will therefore result in gross overtreatment.
2. Average blood pressures over a period of time reflect the risk better than single blood pressure measurements.

The duration of the period of observation and the number of blood pressure measurements that need to be carried out before a decision about drug therapy is made depend upon the severity of hypertension. A period of 3 to 6 months observation with measurements every 2 to 4 weeks is consistent with the recommendations of the Joint National Committee of the National High Blood Pressure Education Program in the United States and the British Hypertension Society for the treatment of mild hypertension (diastolic blood pressure less than 110 mmHg) without advanced retinopathy. This period should probably be curtailed for diastolic blood pressures of 110 mmHg or more unless a marked 'white coat' response is suspected. It is unwise to initiate drug therapy without at least three blood pressure readings carried out on separate occasions unless the patient has grade III or IV retinopathy, hypertensive, cardiac, or renal failure.

White coat hypertension

Suspicion of this diagnosis should be raised by high blood pressure levels in the absence of any evidence of target organ damage, divergent readings (particularly when the divergence occurs between recordings taken by a nurse and a doctor), or by the presence of clearcut evidence of tension during blood pressure measurement. Where this diagnosis is suspected the simplest initial approach to diagnosis is to seek evidence of left ventricular hypertrophy on echocardiographic left ventricular dimensions. Where the diagnosis is still entertained and there is no change in echocardiographic left ventricular dimensions, non-invasive ambulatory monitoring of blood pressure should be carried out.

Non-pharmacological treatment

The period of blood pressure assessment and advice should also be used for the deployment of other measures of lowering blood pressure which do not require the use of drugs.

Non-pharmacological measures include dietary and behavioural methods. Dietary methods include weight reduction, alcohol withdrawal, sodium restriction, and potassium supplementation. Behavioural methods include physical training, biofeedback and relaxation.

WEIGHT REDUCTION

The epidemiological relationship between weight and blood pressure is reflected in a number of trials, which have shown that dietary weight reduction in obese subjects produces a useful fall in arterial pressure. Even a weight loss of 3 kg on average produces a fall in blood pressure of 7/4 mmHg. Most studies have been carried out in overweight individuals. It has still not been established whether weight reduction in patients close to the ideal weight lowers blood pressure.

ALCOHOL WITHDRAWAL

The elevated blood pressures shown by heavy drinkers (more than 6 units of alcohol per day) are lowered by withdrawal. This is not related to changes in weight or electrolyte intake. This useful clinical effect has to be differentiated from the pressor response sometimes exhibited by chronic alcoholics on abstension from alcohol. Blood pressure elevation

in this case is associated with increased sympathetic nervous system activity.

SODIUM RESTRICTION

The average intake of sodium in Westernized cultures is 120 to 180 mmol per day. Severe sodium restriction (to less than 10 mmol a day) produces substantial blood pressure lowering but is not feasible. Moderate sodium restriction (to 70 to 80 mmol a day) can be achieved by abstaining from adding salt at the table, avoiding salt in cooking, and avoiding heavily salted processed foods. Such moderate salt restriction enhances the blood pressure lowering action of angiotensin converting enzyme inhibitors, β-blockers, and diuretics. Curiously it seems to be ineffective in patients treated with calcium antagonists. As sole therapy, moderate salt restriction has a modest blood pressure lowering action in some patients (particularly in the older age groups). Whilst claims have been made for specific 'salt sensitivity' in a minority of hypertensive patients, there is no evidence that such patients form a discrete group. Nevertheless, the individual response to moderate salt restriction is variable and it is worth a therapeutic trial during the period of assessment if the patients are willing to undergo the substantial change in life style that is involved.

POTASSIUM SUPPLEMENTATION

Potassium intake is about half that of sodium on the normal Western diet. Doubling potassium intake (i.e. supplementing it by about 80 mmmol a day) has a modest blood pressure lowering action of the same approximate order of magnitude as moderate sodium restriction. Indeed, the natriuresis produces by potassium loading may contribute to the blood pressure reduction observed. There is no justification for potassium supplementation as an independent form of treatment for essential hypertension. Advising patients to consume liberal quantities of fruit and vegetables may be justified on general grounds but is likely to have only a very small influence upon blood pressure.

OTHER DIETARY MANOEUVRES

Several studies have shown that fish-oils (ω-3 fatty acids) lower blood pressure in hypertensive patients. The effect only appears to be seen in those whose consumption of fish is low. Olive oil has been shown to have a very small blood pressure lowering effect in some studies but there is little evidence to support a therapeutic effect of other unsaturated fatty acids. Claims have been made for calcium and magnesium supplementation but these are not persuasive and have no place in clinical practice.

PHYSICAL EXERCISE

Repetitive isotonic exercise produces a useful fall in blood pressure independently of any fall in weight. Initial trials employed fairly severe protocols, i.e. those that demand oxygen consumption of more than 60 per cent maximum. These produced falls in arterial pressure which, in some cases, exceeded those which would have been expected with a single class of antihypertensive drug. Training exercises of this order of magnitude are clearly not feasible in most hypertensive patients. More moderate exercise in the form of daily jogging or brisk walking is probably sufficient to have a useful effect in lowering blood pressure, as well as improving well-being. All patients should be encouraged to undertake it where this is practical.

BEHAVIOURAL THERAPY

There is some evidence that biofeedback and relaxation exercise can effectively lower blood pressure in hypertensive patients. This is not, perhaps, surprising in view of the likely reduction in sympathetic nervous system activity and alerting response produced by relaxation. There are, however, two problems with this innocuous approach to treatment. First, if patients are to be instructed adequately, training is extremely costly in terms of labour. Second, unless regularly reinforced, the effects of behavioural treatment tend to diminish with the passage of time, reflecting the considerable demands which their maintenance places upon patients as well as doctors. For instance, follow-up of patients who initially showed a response has shown disappointing results at 1 year.

There is now support for the view that the effect of some of these manoeuvres at least is additive. Combined dietary manoeuvres and advice about physical exercise may enable clinicians not only to avoid drug treatment in many patients but also to reduce the amount of medication in patients who do require drugs.

Antihypertensive drug treatment

The decision to control hypertension with medication has major implications, not only for the patient, who will probably require lifelong therapy, but also for the agencies which will have to pay for treatment and its supervision. Important decisions have to be made in selecting appropriate patients for drug therapy, choosing the most suitable treatment for them and in monitoring the effectiveness of treatment.

Selection of patients

The British Hypertension Society recommend that drug therapy should be given if diastolic blood pressure averages 100 mmHg or more over the assessment period. The Joint National Committee of the National High Blood Pressure Education Program in the United States suggested a slightly lower threshold of diastolic blood pressure in excess of 94 mmHg over a 3- to 6-month period. They added, however, that 'some experts believe that drug therapy should be initiated in these patients if the diastolic blood pressure remains above 90 mmHg'. Joint recommendations from the International Society of Hypertension and World Health Organization recommended treatment in patients whose diastolic blood pressure remained at 95 mmHg or above after 3 months of observation. Although the differences between these varying recommendations seem small they have important implications for the number of patients treated. For instance, 25.3 per cent of patients at the Hypertension, Detection and Follow-Up Program Screening Study had a blood pressure equal to or more than 90 mmHg, 14.5 per cent had a value equal to or more than 95 mmHg, and only 8.4 per cent had diastolic blood pressures equal to or more than 100 mmHg. Taking average blood pressures over a period of time reduces these figures of course, but it still probably remains true that reducing the threshold of treatment from 100 to 95 mmHg increases the number of patients eligible by 73 per cent. At some point the costs of treatment and the potential adverse effects outweigh the benefits. This balance differs substantially from patient to patient, and also depends upon the treatment employed. Ideally we should attempt to identify the patients at high risk so that we can avoid unnecessary treatment of those at low risk. Analysis of the Australian Therapeutic trial showed that an average diastolic reading of 100 mmHg or more over the period of the trial was associated with a much higher incidence of trial endpoints (such as strokes or myocardial infarctions). Below the average of 100 mmHg there was little relationship between blood pressure and endpoints. For this reason the British Hypertension Society selected a slightly higher criterion for treatment than other bodies that have made recommendations in this area. Other risk factors (smoking, hyperlipidaemia, left ventricular hypertrophy, and glucose intolerance) increase the risk to the individual patient substantially, and when they are present the threshold treatment should therefore be reduced to 95 or even (in the presence of several risk factors) to 90 mmHg.

The effect of drug treatment

The aim of treating hypertension is to reduce complications (particularly cerebrovascular and cardiac disease). Unless a very high-risk population is tested, trials of endpoint efficacy require large numbers of patients, as the incidence of overt cardiac or cerebrovascular disease is relatively low in those with moderately elevated blood pressures. Most of the trials designed to detect the threshold of benefit have required collaboration between a large number of centres and have extended over several years. Patients recruited have differed, and in particular some trials have confined recruitment to elderly subjects. In addition, drug regimens and protocols have shown marked divergences. Nevertheless, the conclusions have shown an impressive degree of concordance. Meta-analysis of the data has demonstrated that for a drug-induced fall in diastolic blood pressure of only 5 mmHg, the incidence of strokes was reduced by 38 per cent and coronary heart disease by 16 per cent in patients with mild hypertension (Fig. 8). Epidemiological observations indicate an excess risk for stroke of 40 per cent for an increase of 5 mmHg, so that at least over the period of the trial the risk of stroke attributable to hypertension was totally reversed. This does not of course imply that drug treatment abolishes the lifelong risk of stroke, but it does indicate that pharmacological lowering of blood pressure reduces the short-term risks both of atherothrombotic and haemorrhagic strokes, as the majority of strokes in mild hypertension will be due to infarction rather than haemorrhage. The impact of treatment on coronary events is more difficult to interpret. Although pooling of trials does indicate a significant impact this probably falls short of complete reversibility of the risk attributable to hypertension. The reasons for this are still controversial (see below).

Selection of therapy

Treatment is normally begun with a single agent (monotherapy). While combination tablets are widely available, they are less desirable as initial therapy because it is more difficult to attribute adverse effects to a particular component. An exception to this rule is the combination of thiazide and potassium sparing diuretic, which is widely employed. Five classes of agent are widely used as first line therapy. A sixth class, i.e. the centrally acting agents (methyldopa and clonidine) are not now recommended as first line therapy because of the relatively high incidence of central side-effects (particularly sleepiness and depression).

THIAZIDE DIURETICS

Thiazide diuretics lower arterial pressure and were used in several of the endpoint trials which demonstrated efficacy at least as far as stroke prevention is concerned. The major concern in their use relates to metabolic adverse effects. These include increased total cholesterol, impairment of glucose tolerance, and hypokalaemia. It has been suggested that these undesirable effects may oppose the beneficial consequences of lowering blood pressure, and thus account for the failure of therapy to have a greater effect on the incidence of myocardial infarction. This is certainly not the case in elderly subjects, among whom diuretics have been associated with a greater reduction in cardiac events than β-blockers in endpoint trials (Fig. 9). Comparison of β-blockers and diuretics in younger subjects has given rise to more equivocal findings in this context. Two large trials (the MRC and HAPPHY trials) failed to show any difference in outcome between diuretics and beta blockers. However, total infarction in the MRC Trial (i.e. silent plus clinical myocardial infarction) was decreased by β-blocker treatment only and the MAPPHY trial comparing a cardioselective β-blocker with diuretics showed a better cardiac outcome in the β-blocker-treated group. The dose of diuretic used may be an important factor. The earlier trials used very high doses, although the blood pressure dose–response curve of thiazides is flat, so that little antihypertensive efficacy is lost through use of low doses. Metabolic disturbances are, however, minimal or nonexistent at low doses (e.g. bendrofluazide 2.5 mg a day). There is no justification for exceeding this, or an equivalent dose.

In summary, low-dose thiazide diuretics are probably preferred first line treatment in elderly hypertensive subjects. An incidental advantage may be the reduction in osteoporosis that has been demonstrated in some

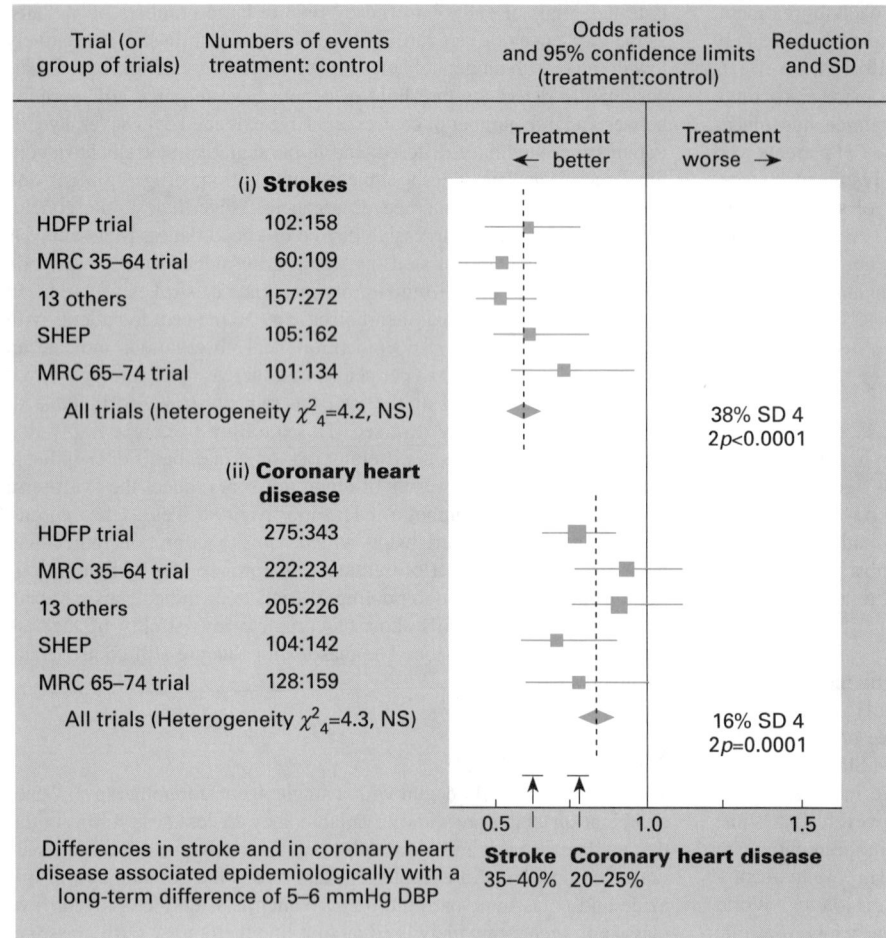

Fig. 8 Meta-analysis of end point trials in the treatment of mild hypertension. Results from the 13 smaller trials are pooled together and the larger trials listed separately. (Reproduced from Collins, R. and Peto, R. (1994). In *Textbook of Hypertension* (ed. J.D. Swales) Blackwell Scientific Publications, Oxford with permission.)

Fig. 9 Meta-analysis of the five trials of treatment in the elderly. Whilst the impact upon stroke was significant in most cases, the impact on coronary heart disease appeared to be better with diuretics ('D') than with β-blockers (B.B), where data on the two were presented separately.

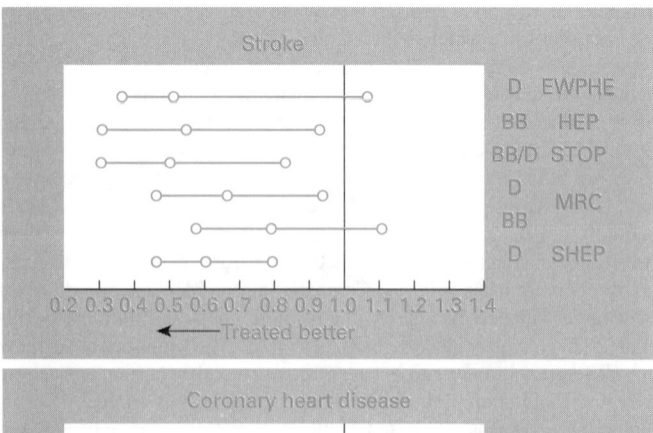

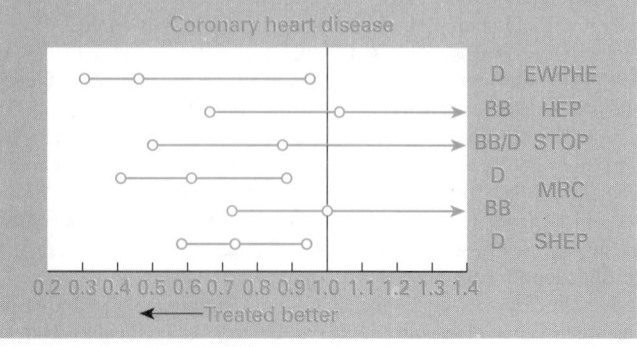

open trials. These agents are contraindicated in non-insulin dependent diabetes mellitus and in gouty patients (Table 1).

β-BLOCKERS

β-Blockers were also used in some of the multicentre trials which demonstrated the benefits of treating hypertension. They too have potentially adverse metabolic effects, producing an increase in serum triglycerides and a decrease in high density lipoprotein cholesterol. These effects are seen less with cardioselective agents and not at all in agents with intrinsic sympathomimetic activity. β-Blockers have the additional advantage of well-demonstrated efficacy in reducing the incidence of a second myocardial infarction in patients who have already sustained one previously. However, their efficacy in primary prevention is still controversial (see above).

β-Blockers probably remain first line therapy in younger patients (i.e. below the age of 65) who do not suffer from obstructive airways disease, peripheral vascular disease, or cardiac failure. Their role in diabetic hypertensives is also questionable, as they may mask clinical symptoms of hypoglycaemia and impair recovery by blunting compensatory mobilization of glucose. This particular problem is less evident with cardioselective agents.

ANGIOTENSIN CONVERTING ENZYME INHIBITORS

These drugs are well tolerated, apart from the relatively high incidence of chronic dry cough (15 per cent). There are two serious side-effects, but these are rare in carefully screened patients.

Hypotension following the first dose of angiotensin converting

Table 1 *Drugs and dosages in the treatment of hypertension*

Drug class	Drug	Dosage and regime
Diuretics	Bendrofluazide	2.5 mg o.d.
	Chlorthalidone	12.5 mg o.d.
	Amiloride	5 mg o.d.
	Triamterene	150–250 mg o.d.
β-Blockers	Propranolol*	80–160 mg b.d.
	Oxprenolol*	40–160 mg t.d.s.
	Pindolol	15–30 mg o.d.
	Sotalol	80–200 mg o.d.
	Timolol	10–30 mg o.d. or b.d.
	Acebutolol	200–400 mg o.d. or b.d.
	Atenolol	25–100 mg o.d.
	Bisoprolol	5–20 mg o.d.
	Metoprolol	100–200 mg o.d. or b.d.
	Celiprolol	200–400 mg o.d.
Calcium-channel blockers	Nifedipine (Retard)	10–40 mg b.d.
	Nicardipine	20–40 mg b.d. to t.d.s.
	Isradipine	2.5–10 mg b.d.
	Felodipine	5–20 mg o.d.
	Acidipine	2–6 mg o.d.
	Amlodipine	5–10 mg o.d.
	Verapamil	120–240 mg b.d.
Angiotensin-converting enzyme inhibitors	Captopril	12.5–50 mg b.d. or t.d.s.
	Enalapril	2.5–40 mg o.d.
	Fosinopril	10–40 mg o.d.
	Lisinopril	2.5–40 mg o.d.
	Perindopril	2–8 mg o.d.
	Quinapril	5–40 mg o.d.
	Ramipril	1.25–10 mg o.d.
α-Blockers	Prazosin	0.5–10 mg b.d.
	Doxazosin	1–16 mg o.d.
	Terazosin	1–20 mg o.d.
	Indoramin	25–100 mg b.d. or t.d.s.
Combined α-β	Labetalol	100–400 mg b.d.
Central	Alpha methyl dopa	250 mg–1 g b.d. or t.d.s.
	Clonidine	0.05–0.4 mg t.d.s.
Vasodilators	Hydralazine	25–100 mg b.d.
	Minoxidil	2.5–25 mg b.d.
	Diazoxide	50–500 mg b.d.

a preferential effect in causing arteriolar vasoconstriction in the efferent glomerular vessels, therefore maintaining intraglomerular filtration pressure. Blocking formation of angiotensin II removes this compensatory effect, resulting in a drastic fall in glomerular filtration caused by the fall in transglomerular capillary hydraulic pressure.

There are no large endpoint trials of the use of angiotensin converting enzyme inhibitors in uncomplicated essential hypertension. Claims have been made that their usage might have a greater impact than those of other agents on coronary events as a result of beneficial effects upon cardiac mass, insulin resistance and on the basis of an absence of effect on serum lipids. These arguments are theoretical and must be recognized as such. As yet, angiotensin converting enzyme inhibitors cannot be considered routine first line treatment of uncomplicated hypertension. Their major role is in those patients in whom the preferred first-line agents cannot be used or when they have proved unacceptable. Angiotensin converting enzyme inhibitors are, however (together with diuretics), particularly indicated when hypertension is associated with compromised cardiac function, when the evidence for their contribution to an improved prognosis is very strong.

CALCIUM ANTAGONISTS

These agents are effective and, like β-blockers, have added advantages in patients with ischaemic heart disease. The major disadvantage of the earlier dihydropyridine calcium antagonists was sympathetic nervous system activation with headache, sweating, palpitation, and a burning sensation in the skin. Longer-acting agents and slow release preparations have reduced the incidence of these side-effects, although all the dihydropyridine calcium antagonists may give rise to significant oedema. The phenylalkylamine calcium channel blocker verapamil is free from autonomic adverse effects and oedema, but has a significant action upon gastrointestinal smooth muscle, which may cause severe constipation. Verapamil is also contraindicated in hypertensive patients with cardiac conduction disturbances.

This class of drug, like the other newer agents is best considered an alternative to diuretics or β-blockers when these cannot be used, or are ineffective.

α-ADRENOCEPTOR BLOCKERS

These agents are less extensively used as first line therapy than the other four major classes of drug. The reasons for this are probably historical. The first widely used member of this class (prazosin) gave rise to serious hypotension following the first dose, attributable at least in part to the excessive dose recommended. The longer acting α-blockers (doxazosin and terozasin) are better tolerated although occasional postural hypotension is still seen. Unlike any other class of antihypertensive, α-blockers have a beneficial action upon plasma lipids producing a slight increase in high density lipoprotein cholesterol and a reduction in low density lipoprotein cholesterol. How far this can be translated into reduced incidence of ischaemic heart disease is unknown. α-Blockers provide a reasonable alternative treatment to the preferred first line agents (Table 2).

Vasodilators

The direct acting vascular smooth muscle relaxant hydralazine was once extensively used as part of the recommended stepped care regime. The main disadvantages were autonomic activation and the development of a lupus-like syndrome in patients with the slow acetylator genotype. This disadvantage, together with the need for multiple daily doses has resulted in the replacement of hydralazine by other agents.

Minoxidil and diazoxide are extremely potent vasodilators which are reserved for patients whose blood pressure is resistant to other medication. The major disadvantages with both these drugs are severe oedema and hair growth, which is a particular problem in dark-haired

enzyme inhibitors is occasionally observed in patients with high levels of renin in plasma, usually as a result of previous intensive diuretic therapy. Hyper-reninaemia can also occur in severe and malignant hypertension. In any of these circumstances, if an angiotensin converting enzyme inhibitor is to be given it is essential to start with the lowest available dose and to monitor blood pressure closely for several hours. In patients who have been on low dose diuretic therapy and there is no other reason to suspect major stimulation of the renin–angiotensin system, it is probably sufficient to instruct them to take the first dose before retiring at night.

Acute renal failure may follow the use of angiotensin converting enzyme inhibitors in patients with critically reduced renal blood flow, i.e. bilateral tight renal artery stenosis or renal artery stenosis to a single kidney. Under these circumstances, and when cardiac output is low enough to produce comparably poor renal perfusion, angiotensin II has

Table 2 *Selection of different classes of drugs in different clinical situations*

	Diuretics	β-Blockers	ACE inhibitors	Calcium blockers	α-Blockers
< 60 years healthy		+			
> 60 years healthy	+				
Ischaemic heart disease		+			
Previous infarction		+			
Cardiac failure/dilatation	+	−	+		
Blacks	+			+	+
Diabetics			+	+	+
Contraindications to or poor tolerance of other therapy	+	+	+	+	+

women. In addition, T wave changes have been observed in electrocardiograms performed during the initiation of treatment with these drugs. This may be due to an increase in cardiac work as a result of generalized vasodilatation. Diazoxide has the added disadvantage of causing glucose intolerance and diabetes in over half of patients treated long term. For this reason it is now rarely used as an oral preparation.

COMBINATION THERAPY

When a single drug does not control blood pressure there is a simple choice to be made between substituting another class of drug or adding a second agent. Both are legitimate manoeuvres, although the latter is more generally favoured because it is more likely to produce early effective blood pressure control. The principle is to add a second drug of a different class while maintaining optimal dosage of the first drug. Certain combinations are logical and particularly effective. These include adding a β-blocker or an angiotensin converting enzyme inhibitor to a diuretic or adding a calcium channel blocker to a β-blocker. α-Blockers can be combined with any other class of agent. The combination of a β-blocker and angiotensin converting enzyme inhibitor or a diuretic and calcium channel blocker appear to be less effective and these combinations are not normally used unless there are other indications for the component drugs.

Target blood pressure

The objective of treatment should be to maintain diastolic blood pressure in the range 80 to 90 and systolic blood pressure below 160, except in the case of diabetes mellitus, when evidence would suggest lower target pressures. Open studies of clinic populations have suggested that when diastolic blood pressure is reduced below 80 to 85 mmHg there is increased mortality in patients with pre-existing ischaemic heart disease. As the major trials excluded such patients trial data does not help here. It is possible that low blood pressures in patients with established heart disease are markers for greater severity of heart disease. From the practical point of view however, the benefits of reducing diastolic blood pressure below 80 are minimal.

Isolated systolic hypertension

Systolic blood pressure is a better predictor of adverse cardiovascular events in the elderly than is diastolic blood pressure. Nevertheless, most of the large trials on which recommendations for treatment are based recruited patients on the basis of diastolic blood pressure. However, the Systolic Hypertension in the Elderly Program (SHEP) recruited patients with systolic blood pressure of 160 mmHg or more and diastolic blood pressures of 90 mmHg or less. This demonstrated that treatment (based upon a diuretic as initial therapy) significantly reduced both strokes and myocardial infarctions. It is difficult to extrapolate with confidence from this study to younger patients with systolic hypertension in whom

increased sympathetic nervous activity rather than increased arterial rigidity may be the cause. However, as an increase in systolic blood pressure adds risk in both groups it should be treated equally as vigorously as diastolic hypertension. It is often difficult, however, to reduce systolic pressure in these patients, and in some an excessive fall in diastolic pressure may be a limiting factor.

Resistant hypertension

Clinic blood pressures may remain high despite potent therapy. The reasons for this are:

(1) poor patient compliance;
(2) 'white coat' hypertension;
(3) genuinely resistant hypertension.

COMPLIANCE

Poor compliance is often difficult to detect. Clues are provided by an initial reluctance to take medication, absence of expected pharmacological effects of medication (e.g. bradycardia with β-blockers), or evidence of failure to consume tablets as revealed by tablet counts or prescription frequency. In some cases it may be necessary to admit a patient to hospital and supervise administration of treatment. Where compliance is obviously poor a number of manoeuvres can help to improve it. These include ensuring that the regimen is as simple as possible, discussion of treatment with adequate feedback of blood pressure levels and the provision of adequate information about rationale for treatment.

WHITE COAT HYPERTENSION

The pressor response to stress is preserved despite drug treatment, although the absolute increase may be blunted. Diagnosis may require ambulatory monitoring, although the absence of target organ damage and left ventricular hypertrophy despite apparent poor control provide a clue.

GENUINE REFRACTORY HYPERTENSION

Blood pressure may not respond to usual combination therapy in a minority of patients. On occasions, previously well controlled blood pressure may escape from control. Under these circumstances enquiries should be made about other pharmacological agents which may be inhibiting the response such as sodium retaining drugs (particularly nonsteroidal anti-inflammatory agents), sympathomimetics, antidepressants, and adrenal steroids. In other cases alcohol excess may be the reason. Patients who develop renal failure may become resistant to antihypertensives because of sodium retention. Another possibility is renal ischaemia due to atheroma superimposing renovascular on essential hypertension. Where none of these explanations can be demonstrated more potent regimes may be required. The combination of calcium channel blocker, angiotensin converting enzyme inhibitor and diuretic is particularly effective. Alternatively a combination of minoxidil with a β-blocker and diuretic will control blood pressure in the large majority of cases. Probably the most potent combination of all is minoxidil, an angiotensin converting enzyme inhibitor and diuretic. This combination carries a significant risk of serious hypotension.

Malignant hypertension

Hypertension associated with grade III or grade IV retinopathy requires immediate treatment, but parenteral therapy is normally contraindicated because of the risk that an over-rapid reduction in pressure at a time when autoregulation of cerebral blood flow is compromised carries the risk of acute cerebral or retinal infarction. Oral therapy producing a gradual fall in blood pressure over 3 to 4 days is normally sufficient. Some clinicians use a 20 mg nifedipine capsule, bitten to release its contents. This produces a more rapid fall in blood pressure, occurring over an hour or two. Treatment can then be continued with a β-blocker, diuretic combination adding a third class of drug if necessary. Parenteral treatment is required in the presence of encephalopathy and, on occasion, when there is associated left ventricular failure.

Hypertensive encephalopathy

Clinically this is manifest by fluctuating neurological signs associated with high blood pressure and usually advanced retinopathy. The critical feature is the fluctuation of signs. If the neurological deficit is present for several hours, or slowly becomes more dense or more extensive, a cerebrovascular accident is more likely. Encephalopathy is more common in patients whose hypertension has developed over a relatively short period of time and who have not therefore had the opportunity to develop protective vascular hypertrophy. Encephalopathy, therefore, is particularly seen in hypertension of pregnancy, in association with renovascular hypertension, in scleroderma, renal crisis, or in acute nephritic syndromes.

Blood pressure must be reduced immediately. The agent of choice is sodium nitroprusside although other vasodilators such as diazoxide, hydralazine, or nitroglycerine can be given parenterally. Sodium nitroprusside has the advantage that overtreatment, with excessive lowering of blood pressure, can be immediately reversed by discontinuation. The major danger is precipitation of cerebral infarction through an excessive fall in blood pressure. 'Excessive' in this situation may include restoration of blood pressure to apparently normal levels (see above). It is therefore inadvisable to lower diastolic blood pressure in the first 24 to 48 h below 100 to 115 mmHg. In some patients with relatively acute hypertension (particularly pregnant women) in whom encephalopathy may occur with modest elevations of blood pressure (110 to 115 mmHg), however, pressures may need to be reduced to normal levels nevertheless.

Essential hypertension in the elderly

The elderly present some particular problems as a result of the changed physiology of ageing. Thus:

1. Arterial wall rigidity is associated particularly with systolic hypertension and with impaired baroreflex sensitivity. This results in increased risk of orthostatic hypotension with treatment.
2. Renal conservation of sodium and fluid in the face of depletion is impaired. Elderly patients are therefore more subject to dehydration as a result of diuretic therapy or dietary restriction. Loop diuretics are particularly dangerous in this respect.
3. Clearance of drugs and their active metabolites is often de-

creased as a result of impaired hepatic and renal function. The incidence of adverse drug reactions is much higher in the elderly.
4. Cardiac compliance and reserve are reduced and patients are more likely to develop cardiac failure.
5. Communication and compliance are more difficult.

Despite these important considerations there is no fundamental difference in the mode of treating an elderly patient. However, drug regimens should be as simple as possible and dosages increased more gradually. The greatest danger is in lowering arterial pressure excessively. Unless contraindicated thiazides are the first choice.

Hypertension in black patients

With optimal care the prognosis in black patients is as good as other ethnic subgroups. Indeed, in some studies it has been somewhat better as hyperlipidaemia is less common in black subjects. Renin activity in plasma is often low in these patients and this probably accounts for the relatively poor response to β-blockade or angiotensin converting enzyme inhibition. First line therapy should therefore be with diuretics with calcium antagonists or α-blockers as alternatives.

Hypertension in children

Although secondary hypertension is more common in children, no specific cause is found for hypertension in the majority of adolescents. The criteria for drug treatment, however, have to be modified because of lower blood pressures. The American Joint National Committee recommends that blood pressures above the 99th percentile for the patients age require treatment.

REFERENCES

British Hypertension Society Working Party. Management guidelines in essential hypertension: report of the second working party. (1993). *British Medical Journal*, **306**, 983–7.

Collins, R., Peto, R., MacMahon, S., *et al.* (1990). Blood pressure, stroke and coronary heart disease. Part 2, short-term reductions in blood pressure: overview of randomised drug trials in their epidemiological context. *Lancet* **335**, 827–838.

Joint National Committee on Detection, Evaluation and Treatment of High Blood Pressure. (1986). Non-pharmacological approaches to the control of high blood pressure. *Hypertension* **8**, 444–467.

Joint National Committee on Detection, Evaluation and Treatment of High Blood Pressure (1993). The Fifth Report. *Archives of Internal Medicine*, **153**, 154–83.

Kaplan, N.M. (1994). *Clinical hypertension.* Williams and Wilkins, Baltimore.

MacMahon, S., Peto, R., Cutler, J. *et al.* (1990). Blood pressure, stroke and coronary heart disease. Part 1, prolonged differences in blood pressure: prospective observational studies corrected for the regression dilution bias. *Lancet* **335**, 765–774.

Medical Research Council Working Party. (1985). MRC trial of treatment of mild hypertension: principal results. *British Medical Journal*, **291**, 97–104.

SHEP Cooperative Research Group. (1991). Prevention of stroke by antihypertensive drug treatment in older persons with isolated systolic hypertension. Final results of the Systolic Hypertension in the Elderly Program. *Journal of the American Medical Association*, **265**, 3255–3264.

Swales, J.D., Sever, P.S., and Peart, S. (1991). *Clinical atlas of hypertension.* Gower Medical Publishing, London.

Swales, J.D. (1994). *Textbook of hypertension.* Blackwell Scientific Publications, Oxford.

WHO/ISH. (1993). Mild hypertension liason committee. Guidelines for the management of mild hypertension: memorandum from a World Health Organization/International Society of Hypertension meeting. *Journal of Hypertension*, **11**, 905–18.

15.28 Secondary hypertension

15.28.1 Renal and renovascular hypertension

A.E.G. RAINE AND J.G.G. LEDINGHAM

Introduction

The great majority of patients who are found to be hypertensive, whether in the hospital clinic or in general practice, will have essential hypertension. Nevertheless, a close watch must always be maintained for patients in whom hypertension is caused by an underlying disorder, and this possibility should be considered in the initial evaluation of any new hypertensive patient. Despite their relative rarity, such cases deserve particular attention both because of the importance of establishing the underlying diagnosis, and because in some cases surgery may be curative.

This need for vigilance is especially true in cases where hypertension is suspected to be due to primary renal or renovascular disease. Detection of raised blood pressure or of incidental proteinuria often gives the first clue to underlying renal disease, and in these patients adequate investigation and effective treatment may lessen the progression to end stage renal failure and the need for renal replacement therapy. Greater awareness of the likelihood of renovascular hypertension, especially in the elderly, has led to increased recognition that this condition is frequently part of the spectrum of atherosclerotic disease that so commonly affects the coronary, cerebral, and peripheral vasculature.

Frequency of renal and renovascular hypertension

Although essential hypertension is very common, only a small proportion of hypertensive patients have underlying renal or renovascular disease. Different series have indicated that the prevalence of renal parenchymal disease is 3 to 4 per cent in unselected hypertensive populations, and that the incidence of renovascular disease varies between 5 per cent and less than 1 per cent. Estimates of this kind are inevitably affected by the degree of selection of the group of subjects studied and, in particular, the strictness of the criteria and investigations employed to confirm or exclude underlying renal or renovascular disease, and the vigour with which these are pursued.

Viewed from the reverse perspective, how frequently does hypertension accompany renal or renovascular disease? This question is difficult to answer precisely in the case of renovascular disease because of a relative dearth of large-scale studies that have routinely employed renal angiography, but there is no doubt that patients with mild or moderate renal arterial narrowing frequently remain normotensive. However, virtually all patients with severe renal impairment become hypertensive. When renal failure is a complication of diseases such as diabetes or systemic sclerosis, in which microvascular pathology is prominent, hypertension is frequent and develops early in the course of the renal disease. Hypertension also commonly accompanies glomerulonephritis, especially mesangiocapillary glomerulonephritis, focal glomerulosclerosis and immunoglobulin A nephropathy. It is relatively less common when renal failure arises from tubulointerstitial disease, but is an early

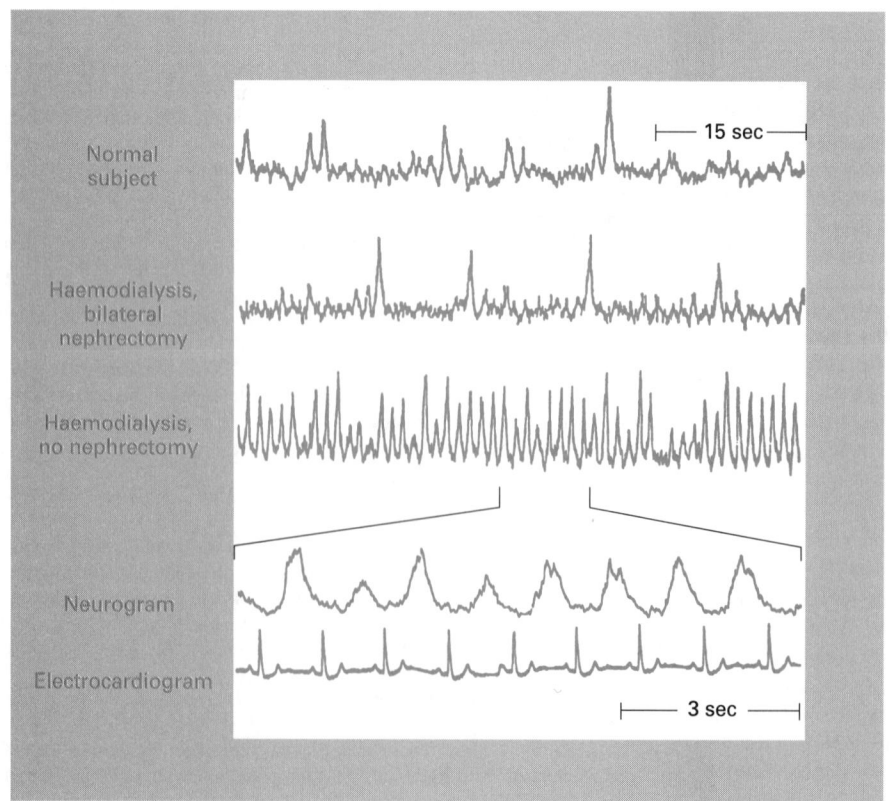

Fig. 1 Recordings of sympathetic nerve discharge obtained from the peroneal nerve in a normal subject and in two haemodialysis patients, one with and one without bilateral nephrectomy. (Reproduced with permission from Converse *et al.* (1992).)

feature in polycystic kidney disease, often developing when renal function remains normal.

Aetiology

RENAL HYPERTENSION

The frequency with which hypertension occurs in renal disease has assumed added importance because of the large body of evidence now available that shows that development of hypertension creates a vicious circle, hastening the progression of renal failure (see Chapter 20.11). Although much of the evidence has come from experimental studies, retrospective clinical reviews have confirmed that the rate of progression of renal insufficiency is greater when diastolic pressure is above rather than below 90 mmHg, even in those patients receiving antihypertensive therapy.

It is commonly assumed that hypertension in renal disease is due primarily to salt and water retention as renal function declines. Inadequate excretion of sodium and water, resulting in intravascular hypervolaemia, undoubtedly provides a simple rationale for hypertension in renal disease, but it is also likely that the increase in body sodium content that occurs in renal failure also promotes hypertension through other, more subtle, mechanisms, such as stimulation of increased production of endogenous inhibitors of the sodium–potassium adenosine triphosphatase pump. Another frequent finding in patients with renal disease and hypertension is that plasma renin levels are inappropriately high, especially when assessed in relation to hypervolaemia and sodium retention. This probably arises because the normal feedback suppression of renin secretion from juxtaglomerular cells is impaired in the diseased kidney.

It could therefore be argued that hypertension in renal disease may be virtually completely accounted for by a combination of volume overload and inappropriate renin system activation. The reality is more complex than this; many uraemic patients show no relationship between blood pressure and blood volume, plasma renin activity, or the product of the two. Evidence from direct recording of efferent sympathetic nerve outflow now indicates that sympathetic activity is increased in hypertensive dialysis patients, and has suggested also that the abnormal sympathetic drive may be triggered by an afferent reflex arising in the scarred failing kidneys, as sympathetic tone is normal in nephrectomized patients (Figure 1). Abnormalities of the vasodilator nitric oxide pathway may also contribute to renal hypertension, a possibility supported by observations that up to nine-fold increases in circulating levels of endogenous inhibitors of nitric oxide synthesis occur in uraemic patients.

Renovascular hypertension

The initiating factor in renovascular hypertension is the development of stenosis of one or both renal arteries, the two most common causes being atheromatous disease and fibromuscular dysplasia. Other much rarer causes of renovascular hypertension include dissecting aneurysm of the aorta, renal arterial thrombosis or embolism, abdominal trauma, neurofibromatosis, postradiation fibrosis and Takayasu's arteritis.

Hypertension in renovascular disease arises because underperfusion of the kidney leads to activation of the renin–angiotensin system, which in turn causes the initial elevation of pressure. Animal models involving renal artery clipping (Goldblatt hypertension) suggest that when there is stenosis of a sole functioning kidney, hypertension subsequently becomes dependent on volume and sodium retention, and plasma renin may then return to normal or low levels. When there is moderate unilateral stenosis, plasma renin levels may gradually decline towards normal, but they remain elevated when the stenosis is severe. In established human renovascular hypertension basal peripheral plasma renin is elevated in most patients, though by no means in all.

Table 1 *Factors in the clinical history which support a diagnosis of renal or renovascular hypertension*

Known history or family history of renal disease
Hypertension under 30 years of age
Loss of blood pressure control in previously stable hypertensive
Accelerated phase hypertension
Polyuria or nocturia
Dysuria
Gross haematuria
Coexisting vascular disease; cardiac, cerebrovascular, or peripheral
Deterioration in renal function after converting enzyme inhibitor therapy

Table 2 *Findings on physical examination suggesting renal or renovascular hypertension*

Renal
    Peripheral or pulmonary oedema
    Palpable kidneys
    Uraemic features
    Bladder enlargement

Renovascular
    Abdominal bruit
    Carotid or femoral bruits
    Reduced or absent leg pulses
    Severe grade *iii–iv* hypertensive retinopathy

Clinical diagnosis of renal and renovascular hypertension

DEFINITION

Most discussions of hypertension in renal disease avoid the question of the definition of hypertension in this setting; such definitions are notoriously arbitrary in any context. The current World Health Organization recommendations give the threshold for drug treatment of essential hypertension as 160/95 mmHg. This cut-off for hypertension is simple and easily applicable, though clearly it cannot take account of factors such as the variation of blood pressure with age, the effect of the observer on measured blood pressure, and the presence or absence of other risk factors for cardiovascular disease. An alternative operational approach is to define hypertension as the blood pressure above which morbidity and mortality are unequivocally increased over time. Although controlled trials of the benefit of treatment of hypertension in renal disease are still awaited, there is a strong case for regarding blood pressures of above 140/95 mmHg or even 140/90 mmHg as being too high.

The normal nocturnal fall in blood pressure, or 'dipper' pattern is also often lost in patients with renal hypertension. Consequently, the overall 24-h blood pressure 'load' may be increased disproportionately in relation to the daytime blood pressure reading.

CLINICAL ASSESSMENT

What clinical findings in a hypertensive subject should raise the suspicion that there may be an underlying renal cause? This may be either a primary renal disease or a renovascular disorder, and it is not usually possible to make the distinction on initial clinical assessment. Particular features to look for in the clinical history are given in Table 1, and those to assess on physical examination are given in Table 2. The presence of any of these indicates the need for further assessment and investigation, although the predictive value of any one alone is low. For example, abdominal bruits are often absent in patients with known renovascular disease, and are often heard in patients with generalized atherosclerotic disease, but are not necessarily due to specific renal arterial narrowing.

HISTORY

When taking the history a background of familial renal disease, especially adult polycystic kidney disease, Alport's syndrome or other hereditary nephropathy should be specially confirmed or excluded. Symptoms suggestive of active renal or urinary tract disease, such as gross haematuria, urine frothing (proteinuria), or dysuria may have been noticed. Those due to progressive chronic renal failure, such as polyuria and nocturia, are of limited use, as patients normally become aware of these only when renal function has declined to less than 50 per cent of normal. Presentation with hypertension in an adolescent or young adult should always arouse the suspicion of underlying renal disease, or another form of secondary hypertension such as adrenal adenoma or phaeochromocytoma. Equally, hypertension arising over a short space of months in late middle age in a patient known to have been previously normotensive should bring to mind the possibility of acquired atherosclerotic renovascular disease.

These considerations apply also to previously well-controlled patients with essential hypertension, in whom blood pressure becomes more severe or refractory to treatment. Essential hypertension is a risk factor for vascular disease and acquired secondary renovascular disease is a relatively frequent complication. Life-long cigarette smokers are especially prone to these renovascular complication of essential hypertension, as for other forms of vascular disease. It is also well known that angiotension converting enzyme inhibitors such as captopril, enalapril, and lisinopril may cause an acute deterioration in renal function when severe renovascular disease is present. The basis of this response and its diagnostic use are discussed further under the investigation of renovascular disease, but the occurrence of a significant (> 50 μmol/l) increase in serum creatinine within 7 to 14 days of commencing converting enzyme inhibitor therapy should always bring to mind the possibility of occult renovascular disease.

PHYSICAL EXAMINATION

It is unusual on general physical examination to obtain evidence of underlying renal disease. Occasionally large kidneys may be palpated, indicating polycystic disease or possibly hydronephrosis. Features of systemic disease, such as systemic lupus erythematosus, may be obvious. Nephropathy is a late complication in diabetes, and it is therefore unlikely that renal impairment in a hypertensive patient will be due to undiagnosed diabetes. Occasionally, hypertensive patients present with evidence of gross obstructive uropathy or with the pallor, foetor, and anaemia of advanced uraemia, making the diagnosis obvious.

Careful evaluation of the cardiovascular system is essential when renal or renovascular hypertension is suspected, or is known to be present. Clinical assessment of intravascular (elevated jugular venous pressure) and extravascular (pulmonary and peripheral oedema) hypervolaemia is obligatory, because of the importance of salt and water retention in the pathogenesis of renal hypertension. A relatively detailed examination for evidence of major vessel vascular disease is also required, in view of the frequency with which renovascular disease is associated with coronary artery disease, peripheral vascular disease or both. This should include careful palpation of peripheral pulses and carotid, abdominal and femoral ausculation for vascular bruits.

An abdominal or epigastric systolic bruit is itself of low predictive value for renovascular disease, as such bruits are relatively common over the age of 50 or 60 years. Continuous or systolic–diastolic abdominal bruits, on the other hand, are rare but when present strongly indicate renovascular hypertension. In the Indianapolis experience, such a bruit was heard in only 0.5 per cent of patients with essential hypertension, but in 39 per cent of patients with renovascular hypertension.

A further reason for careful cardiovascular assessment is the frequency with which cardiovascular complications arise in both renal and renovascular hypertension. Careful optic fundoscopy is necessary to assess the severity of microvascular disease. The degree of left ventricular hypertrophy requires equally careful assessment; this should be by echocardiography rather than electrocardiogram, if possible, in view of its greatly enhanced sensitivity in quantifying left ventricular dimensions.

INITIAL INVESTIGATIONS

The importance of simple first-line investigations cannot be overemphasized (Table 3). Dipstick testing at the initial assessment will show whether or not proteinuria or haematuria are present. The presence of either makes it essential to perform urine microscopy to look for granular or cellular casts, which if present indicate underlying renal disease. Urine should be cultured to exclude intercurrent infection as a cause of proteinuria or haematuria. Blood biochemistry is routinely performed, and may show elevation of urea and creatinine concentrations. Many cases of hypertension arising secondary to underlying renal disease are first detected in this way. Full blood count may show a normochromic anaemia if renal impairment is well established.

Twenty-four-hour urine collection, apart from enabling determination of creatinine clearance, gives reasonably accurate quantitation of protein excretion. Although proteinuria is quite common in moderate and severe essential hypertension, it rarely exceeds a total of 1 g in 24 h. Proteinuria is virtually always present in renal or renovascular disease. In bilateral renovascular disease up to 3 or 4 g in 24 h may be found, but heavy proteinuria, greater than this level, usually indicates underlying glomerular disease and may be accompanied by an overt nephrotic syndrome.

When the clinical history and initial investigations in a newly diagnosed hypertensive patient have raised the suspicion of an underlying renal cause, further investigations must be carried out to confirm or rule out this possibility, and to enable a specific diagnosis. Renal ultrasound, the first of these, should be performed whether the provisional diagnosis is of renal parenchymal or renovascular disease. Thereafter, the more specialized investigations and the principles of management of these two forms of renal hypertension differ. Those for intrinsic renal disease will be considered first, and those for renovascular hypertension subsequently.

Investigation of renal hypertension

RENAL ULTRASOUND

Renal ultrasound is rapid, readily performed, non-invasive and generally available, and should be the first specific test performed in any patient with suspected renal hypertension. It may give a firm diagnosis of polycystic kidney disease or obstructive uropathy. It will show whether the kidneys are reduced in size or have parenchymal thinning, suggesting established chronic renal disease. In addition, it will show whether the two kidneys are of unequal length, increasing the likelihood of renovascular disease. If an inequality of more than 1.5 cm in length is found, or there are other strong pointers to renovascular disease such as a continuous abdominal bruit or evidence of atheromatous disease elsewhere, further investigations for renovascular disease are indicated.

INTRAVENOUS UROGRAPHY

Rapid sequence intravenous urography has been the traditional screening test to confirm or exclude renal causes of hypertension. The physiological basis of its application in renovascular disease is the delay which the stenosis imposes on the rate at which the contrast dye reaches

Table 3 *Initial investigations in hypertension*

Urine
> Dipstick urinalysis for blood, protein, glucose
> Microscopy for casts, red or white blood cells
> Culture for infection

Blood
> Full blood count, erythrocyte sedimentation rate
> Urea and creatinine
> Uric acid
> Electrolytes
> Fasting glucose
> Fasting lipids

Radiology
> Chest radiograph for heart size; pulmonary oedema
> Electrocardiogram and echocardiography for left ventricular
> hypertrophy

Table 4 *Renal diseases causing hypertension*

Common
> Diabetic nephropathy
> Chronic glomerulonephritis
> Chronic interstitial nephritis
> Adult polycystic kidney disease
> Renovascular disease

More rare
> Analgesic nephropathy
> Renal vasculitis
> Systemic vasculitis
> Systemic lupus erythematosus
> Systemic sclerosis
> Obstructive uropathy
> Renal amyloidosis
> Renal tuberculosis
> Haemolytic–uraemic syndrome
> Thrombotic thrombocytopaenic purpura
> Postpartum renal failure
> Myeloma
> Other causes of chronic renal failure

the tubules, and the increased tubular reabsorption of water and electrolytes occurring in the ischaemic kidney. Pictures taken at 1-min intervals for 5 min show a delay in first appearance of the nephrogram, and subsequent increased density of the pyelogram phase, together with asymmetry of kidney size. The sensitivity and specificity of the test are imperfect, being 80 per cent and 85 per cent, respectively, for unilateral renovascular disease and less if bilateral disease is present. For these reasons it is increasingly being replaced by isotope renography or newer imaging techniques for the initial investigation of renovascular disease, though whether or not these offer a true advance in diagnostic sensitivity remains controversial.

The intravenous urogram remains invaluable in the diagnosis of chronic pyelonephritis with renal scarring, which is the most common cause of hypertension in patients aged under 20, and it is also essential when renal ultrasound has shown dilated pelvicalyceal systems, indicating obstructive uropathy. Plain abdominal films taken in conjunction with the intravenous urogram will show the presence of nephrocalcinosis or of renal stone disease, which may lead to unilateral obstruction and hypertension.

RENAL BIOPSY

Renal biopsy is an invasive investigation with appreciable morbidity and mortality, and it should be undertaken only in those patients with hypertension and suspected renal disease who have proteinuria, and in whom renal size is within normal limits but renal function is impaired. Moreover, there should be a genuine likelihood that confirmation of a specific histological diagnosis will enable improved management. Biopsy is not indicated when a diagnosis has already been made by alternative means such as the intravenous urogram.

Renal biopsy is often invaluable in determining whether renal impairment in patients with accelerated phase hypertension is a consequence of damage from malignant hypertension itself, or whether an underlying primary renal disease is the precipitant of the accelerated phase. This distinction has a major bearing on outcome; in a Japanese survey of 69 patients presenting with accelerated hypertension and renal impairment, renal survival was 60 per cent after 5 years in patients with underlying essential hypertension, and only 4 per cent over 18 months in patients with chronic glomerulonephritis.

Any of the many different forms of specific renal disease may cause secondary renal hypertension, and do so in some cases before renal function is appreciably impaired. These diseases are shown in Table 4. Five are common: the most common cause of all of severe renal impairment leading to endstage disease is now diabetic nephropathy, which is the diagnosis in 34 per cent of all patients undergoing dialysis treatment or transplantation in the United States, and it is becoming as frequent

in the larger European countries. The other major causes of progressive renal failure and of renal hypertension are chronic glomerulonephritis, chronic pyelonephritis and interstitial nephritis, polycystic kidney disease, and bilateral renovascular disease, including microvascular ischaemic nephropathy associated with essential hypertension. The many other causes shown in Table 4 are all much rarer.

Treatment of renal hypertension

Early and effective treatment of renal hypertension is essential, both because hypertension will accelerate progressive renal disease and because of the high risk of later cardiac and vascular complications in these patients. In practice, optimal control of hypertension may be very difficult to achieve. Patients with renal failure are often particularly resistant to antihypertensive therapy and may require a combination of several different agents to achieve even passable blood pressure control. Antihypertensive therapy in renal failure is also complicated by the possible risks of drug accumulation, and by an increased incidence of adverse effects when clearance is primarily by renal excretion.

The treatment of renal hypertension is addressed further in Chapter 20.17.1.

Hypertension in acute renal disease

The majority of cases of acute renal failure arise when hypotension secondary to shock, sepsis, or another insult results in sudden and severe renal hypoperfusion, leading to acute tubular necrosis. Hypertension is not a feature of established acute tubular necrosis, even in patients who have developed sodium retention and hypervolaemia. However, it can develop in any acute intrinsic renal disease which may lead to uraemia, such as acute interstitial nephritis or rapidly progressive glomerulonephritis. Why hypertension should be so prominent a feature of acute glomerulonephritis when it is absent in other causes of acute renal failure is not known. It may develop early in the course of the disease, which is characterized by gross haematuria, oliguria, and peripheral and periorbital oedema. The increase in blood pressure may be rapid and severe, sufficient to cause the malignant phase or the neurological manifestations of hypertensive encephalopathy, with mental slowing, coma and generalized seizures. Acute glomerulonephritis is now relatively rare in the United Kingdom and occurs mainly in children. Complete recovery is usual, and the long-term outlook for renal function and blood pressure is good, but a significant proportion of older children and adults who develop acute nephritis progress to chronic renal failure and persistent hypertension.

Renin-secreting tumours

Benign haemangiopericytomas (reninomas) in the kidney may contain cells resembling those of the juxtaglomerular apparatus, and are a very rare cause of potentially curable hypertension. Renin secreted from the tumour results in increases in plasma renin, angiotensin II, and aldosterone with an accompanying hypokalaemic alkalosis. Hypertension is often severe, and most frequently arises in the second to fourth decade, affecting males and females equally. The tumours are usually small, and are easily missed on angiography. Diagnosis of this extremely rare condition may be supported by demonstration of elevated renin activity in the renal venous blood on the affected side. The response to surgical removal of the tumour is excellent.

A similar syndrome may result from hypersecretion of renin from Wilms' tumour (nephroblastoma), from renal cell carcinoma or from extrarenal tissues such as pancreatic, pulmonary, hepatic, or fallopian tube carcinoma. The incidence of hypertension in patients with renal cell carcinoma ranges from less than 10 per cent to 50 per cent. Measurement of peripheral plasma renin or renal venous renin ratios have proved of little help in predicting blood pressure response to surgery in these cases.

Renovascular disease

The likelihood that renovascular disease may be the underlying cause should be considered in a patient with suspected secondary hypertension whenever one or more of the relevant features given in Tables 1 and 2 are observed. Of these, evidence of generalized atherosclerotic disease (suggesting atheromatous renal arterial disease) or of onset of hypertension in an otherwise fit young female without a family history of hypertension (pointing to renal arterial fibromuscular dysplasia) tips the provisional diagnostic balance towards renovascular rather than renal parenchymal hypertension.

ATHEROMATOUS DISEASE OR FIBROMUSCULAR DYSPLASIA?

It is not difficult to obtain an unambiguous answer from renal angiography as to whether or not renovascular disease is present, and to determine whether it is due to atheroma or to fibrous dysplasia. In the former group, who comprise 65 to 75 per cent of all cases of renovascular hypertension, patients are generally over 50 years old, are often smokers, there is usually evidence of vascular disease elsewhere, and abdominal and renal angiography show extensive aortic atheromatous disease, together with atheromatous narrowing of one or both renal arteries. The lesions are usually located at or near the junction of the renal artery and the aorta, and quite frequently there is total occlusion of one renal artery as a result of the atheromatous process (Fig. 2).

In contrast, the aorta appears normal in fibromuscular dysplasia and the lesions occur in the distal two-thirds of the renal arteries, often extending into the intra renal branches. The radiological appearance resembles a string of beads (Fig. 3), and is caused by alternating areas of stenosis (due to medial fibrosis) and aneurysmal dilatation in areas where the internal elastic lamina and vascular smooth muscle are deficient. These lesions may affect one or both renal arteries, and may also occur in the carotid, coeliac axis, and mesenteric and iliac vessels, although involvement of these sites rarely leads to symptoms or to complications. Fibromuscular dysplasia is much more common in women than in men, and occurs predominantly in the third and fourth decade.

Although demonstration of these anatomical abnormalities is relatively straightforward, the questions of difficulty in assessing renovas-

cular disease are, first, deciding what criteria should be fulfilled to justify proceeding to invasive renal angiography, and second, determining whether or not such lesions, even if anatomically demonstrable, are functionally significant? Many patients with essential hypertension develop mild atheromatous renal vascular disease, without compromising renal perfusion significantly. Even when moderate or severe renal

Fig. 2 Aortography in a 65-year-old man with severe atheromatous disease, with extensive aortic atheroma, total occlusion of the right renal artery, and a tight stenosis of the left renal artery (arrow).

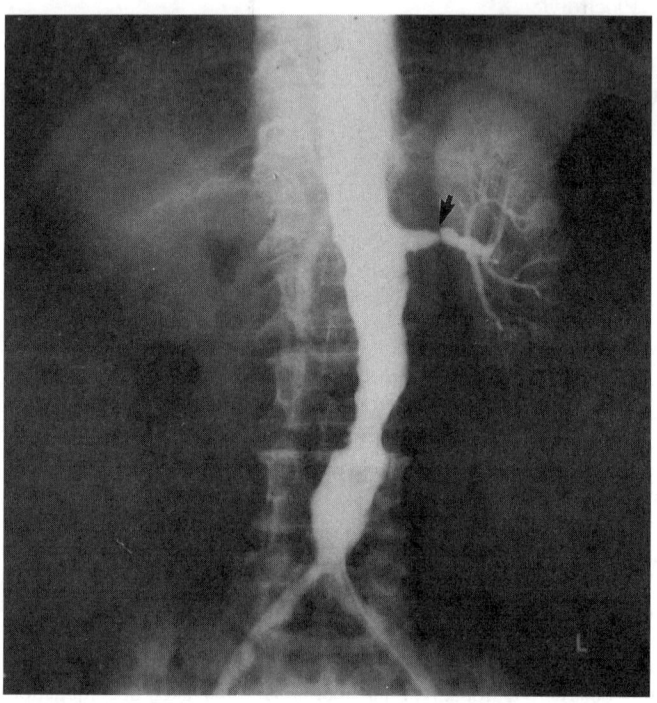

Fig. 3 Selective right renal angiography in a patient with hypertension due to fibromuscular dysplasia.

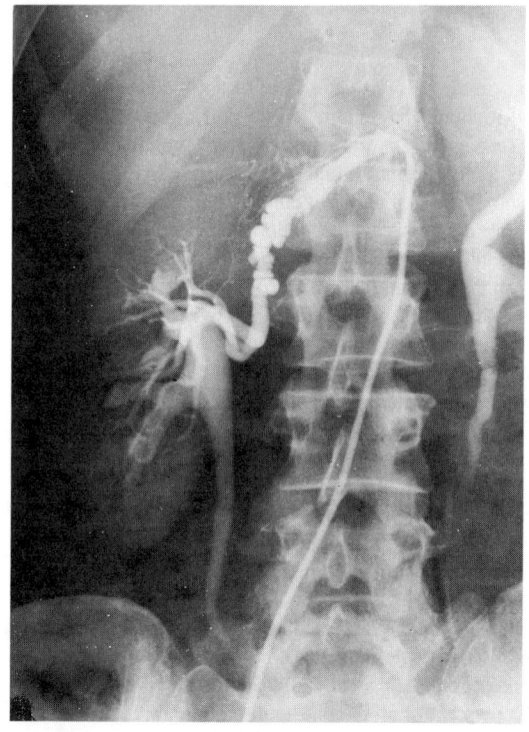

arterial stenosis is present, it may not be relevant; in a Scandinavian series half of a group of 450 patients undergoing angiography for peripheral vascular disease had severe renal arterial disease, including total occlusion, yet 20 per cent of these patients remained completely normotensive. Positive proof that a stenotic lesion is functionally important requires demonstration of an improvement in hypertension or in renal function after correction of the stenosis by angioplasty or surgery. Operational definitions such as these are of value and widely used in clinical investigations, but clearly are of little help for the making of decisions in the case of a particular patient.

Investigation of renovascular disease

Both the invasive nature of renal angiography and the difficulty in assessing the pathophysiological importance of stenotic lesions have encouraged the search for widely applicable non-invasive diagnostic investigations. Just how far to pursue these in an individual case depends very much on the age and general fitness of the patient, the severity of hypertension and degree of renal impairment, and the likelihood that the patient will be suitable for a corrective procedure if a lesion amenable to intervention is ultimately detected.

Most non-invasive diagnostic tests for renovascular disease are based on the impaired and delayed renal perfusion and the activation of the intra renal renin angiotensin system caused by the stenosis. The rapid sequence intravenous urogram, already discussed, may yield useful information, showing a delayed and dense nephrogram on the affected side, but its sensitivity and specificity are limited, necessitating renal angiography in any cases of uncertainty.

RENAL VEIN RENIN RATIO

A number of screening tests for renovascular disease have depended on the assumption that there should be an increase in renin secretion from the affected kidney, or that there should be functional effects of activation of the intrarenal angiotensin system within the stenosed kidney. For many years renal vein renin concentration has been measured both to aid diagnosis of renovascular hypertension and to attempt to predict the outcome of surgery. The technique is invasive, involving bilateral catheterization and sampling from each renal vein, and the adjacent vena cava above and below the origin of the vein. A renal vein renin ratio of 1.6 or greater is taken to be positive, and diagnostic accuracy may be improved by sodium restriction or captopril administration, thereby increasing renin secretion. Although this test, in one form or another, has shown a specificity of 90 to 95 per cent in different series, it has poor sensitivity, as between 30 and 60 per cent of patients with renal vein renin ratios below 1.6 have been found to benefit from invasive treatment. Further difficulties arise when the renovascular disease is bilateral, or when segmental areas of renal ischaemia are present. This approach has now fallen into relative disfavour, with the advent of non-invasive tests employing captopril stimulation of the renin system, together with improved methods of imaging of the renal vasculature.

CAPTOPRIL CHALLENGE TEST

This test is based on observations that blocking the renin–angiotensin system in renovascular disease by the angiotensin II analogue saralasin or by converting enzyme inhibition causes an exaggerated increase in peripheral plasma renin activity. The mechanism of this effect is not defined, but it may be a response to an acute fall in distal tubular sodium and chloride delivery to the macula densa. The test is simple, involving measurement of plasma renin activity before and 60 min after oral administration of 50 mg captopril. Initial experience involving retrospective analysis in 246 patients claimed remarkable sensitivity of 100 per cent and specificity of 98 per cent. The test was considered to be valid in bilateral renovascular disease, but inaccurate when renal func-

tion was impaired. Subsequent prospective evaluations of the captopril test have had mixed success, confirming a high sensitivity, but a limited specificity of 80 to 90 per cent.

ISOTOPE RENOGRAPHY

Captopril renography is an alternative and increasingly widely used approach to diagnosis of renovascular hypertension. Original renographic techniques employing ^{131}I-hippuran to compare renal blood flow in affected and unaffected kidneys gave a high incidence of false positive results in patients who were subsequently proven to have essential hypertension. Hence, for a time isotopic renography fell out of favour. Renewed interest in this approach arose from observations that acute administration of a converting enzyme inhibitor caused an often dramatic fall in glomerular filtration in the stenosed kidney, presumed to be secondary to loss of angiotensin II-dependent efferent arteriolar vasoconstriction, together with a compensatory increase in filtration on the contralateral side. These opposing effects may be clearly demonstrated by split renal function isotopic studies.

To perform captopril renography, ^{99}Tc^{m}-diethylenetriaminepenta-acetic acid (DTPA) uptake, a measure of glomerular filtration rate, and/or ^{123}I-hippuran uptake, a measure of renal blood flow, are documented before and 60 min after a 25 mg oral dose of captopril. When functionally significant stenosis is present, diethylenetriaminepenta-acetic acid uptake is decreased, indicating a fall in glomerular filtration rate, whereas hippurate secretion is delayed, seen as a prolongation of mean parenchymal transit time. With use of a variety of diagnostic criteria, an impressive specificity of 100 per cent combined with a sensitivity of 80 per cent have been reported with captopril renography for identification of functionally significant stenosis, defined by a hypotensive response to subsequent dilatation of the stenosis by angioplasty, together with correction of the renogram abnormality.

Despite the high specificity and reasonable sensitivity reported for these tests in experienced hands, their acceptance is by no means universal. The low prevalence of renovascular disease in the unselected hypertensive population means that the tests are unsuitable for general screening. With a sensitivity even as high as 95 per cent, only one unselected hypertensive patient in ten or more undergoing arteriography as a result of positive captopril renography would prove to have renovascular disease. For these reasons screening of all patients is not recommended. The predictive value of these dynamic tests is improved considerably if they are reserved for patients with clinical clues suggesting renovascular disease; even so, it may be argued that in such cases the only means of obtaining an unequivocal answer as to whether or not renovascular disease is present is to perform angiography.

RENAL ANGIOGRAPHY

Renal angiography will identify and localize renal arterial lesions and is currently the only way of determining whether they appear anatomically suitable for angioplasty or reconstructive surgery. It cannot predict whether there will be a functional improvement after intervention. The aorta and its branches should be visualized, as well as the renal vasculature. Good quality images are usually obtained by employing intra-arterial digital subtraction angiography; those obtained by intravenous digital subtraction angiography (DSA) often do not yield sufficient detail.

Renal angiography carries a risk of radiocontrast-induced acute renal failure (contrast nephropathy), those at most risk being patients who are volume-depleted or have diabetic nephropathy. There is also a significant morbidity from local haemorrhage, and mortality may approach 0.1 per cent. For these reasons, newer non-invasive imaging techniques, at present still under evaluation, may prove of great use in the future. The two most promising are spiral computerized tomographic scanning of the renal arteries, after prior intravenous contrast injection, and magnetic

Table 5 *Progression of untreated atherosclerotic renovascular disease*

No. of patients	Initial degree of luminal narrowing (%)	Stenosis unchanged (%)	Progression without occlusion (%)	Progression to total occlusion (%)
78	<50	69	26	5
30	50–75	53	37	10
18	75–99	61	0	39

Adapted from Schreiber *et al.* (1984).

resonance imaging of the renal vasculature, which is totally non-invasive.

Treatment of renovascular disease

PROGRESSION OF UNTREATED RENOVASCULAR DISEASE

The decision whether or not to attempt to correct a stenosis will be influenced by the likelihood that the lesion is functionally important, and by the probable pattern of progression if left untreated. In the majority of patients with a renal arterial stenosis of 75 per cent or greater, hypertension is improved by correction of the stenosis, although not necessarily cured. Currently minor stenoses of less than 50 per cent are usually treated conservatively, but the practice of preventative correction of even these lesions is increasing. The purpose is primarily to minimize the future risk of ischaemic renal failure. This risk is significant, as the natural history of untreated atherosclerotic disease is one of continuing progression. The Cleveland clinic series (Table 5) showed that nearly 40 per cent of patients with a 75 per cent to 99 per cent stenosis developed complete occlusion within a mean period of 2 years of follow-up. Progressive disease was even found in a third of patients who had stenosis of less than 50 per cent. Development of progression was, predictably, related to deterioration in renal function and reduction in kidney size, but effective antihypertensive therapy had little effect on rate of progression. Progression of this degree of severity is much less of a problem in fibromuscular disease, though it has been observed in half or more of patients in some series, with occasional total occlusion.

Although it is not possible to predict which patients are at greatest risk of progressive stenosis and occlusive disease with loss of renal function, useful additional information on the potential antihypertensive benefit of intervention may come from the therapeutic response to converting enzyme inhibition. Several series have shown that the long-term (6 to 8 weeks) hypotensive response to these drugs in patients with renovascular disease may be predictive, as it was closely correlated with the subsequent blood pressure fall in response to correction of the stenosis by reconstructive surgery or by percutaneous renal angioplasty.

WHEN SHOULD SURGERY OR ANGIOPLASTY BE ATTEMPTED?

There is no universally agreed approach to management of patients with renovascular hypertension, and no prospective trials comparing medical and invasive treatment, or reconstructive surgery and angioplasty have been completed. Attitudes to invasive correction of stenoses have changed appreciably in the past decade, with angioplasty now being available and practised in many centres. Surgical approaches have also been refined, and increasingly good results are reported, with acceptable mortality.

Nevertheless, renal vascular surgery should be undertaken only in specialized centres, and even in these the overall expectation of cure of hypertension by surgery is unlikely to be more than 50 per cent. Features favouring an attempted corrective approach include the presence of fibromuscular disease, relative youth and absence of severe extra renal

vascular disease, a positive result on predictive tests such as captopril renography or a documented long-term blood pressure response to converting enzyme inhibition, and, especially, a lesion or lesions which appear suitable for intervention, together with a relative absence of distal small vessel intrarenal atherosclerosis.

SURGICAL TREATMENT

Nephrectomy is rarely appropriate treatment in renovascular hypertension, and is indicated only when the affected kidney is contributing 10 per cent or less of total function and, at the same time, has been established to be the probable cause of the hypertension. A number of surgical reconstructive techniques are in use, including endarterectomy, aorto-renal bypass employing the saphenous vein, arterial autograft or Dacron graft bypass, arterial resection and reanastomosis, autotransplantation to the iliac fossa, and 'bench' repair of the kidney. Particularly encouraging results have recently been reported with splenorenal bypass and hepato-renal bypass. In bilateral disease, postoperative acute renal failure is common, whatever approach is used, often necessitating temporary support by dialysis.

PERCUTANEOUS TRANSLUMINAL RENAL ANGIOPLASTY

This technique is now established as an effective and relatively safe method of correction of renal vascular stenosis. The procedure involves catheterization of the involved artery by the Seldinger technique, followed by use of a guidewire to traverse the stenosis, and placement of the balloon dilatation catheter, which is then inflated for 30 s to 1 min. Access to the renal vasculature is usually via the femoral route, although an axillary arterial approach may sometimes be necessary if there is severe disease of the lower abdominal aorta or iliac vessels. Balloon inflation achieves dilatation not from compression of the plaque, but by splitting and fracture of the plaque involving intima and media. A postoperative angiogram will show clearly the degree of immediate success of the procedure (Fig. 4).

The decision whether or not to attempt angioplasty of a unilateral lesion depends largely on technical feasibility, but the appropriate approach to bilateral stenoses often involves considerable debate. The relative contribution of each kidney to overall renal function must be evaluated by prior isotope renography. Unless it is effectively non-functioning, the decision usually is made to tackle the smaller, more tightly stenosed kidney first, with subsequent angioplasty of the contralateral kidney. Excellent results may be obtained from bilateral angioplasty in appropriately selected patients (Fig. 5). Ostial lesions, which occur frequently in atheromatous disease, are usually least suitable for angioplasty. Complications of the procedure occur in up to 15 per cent of patients, the most severe being renal artery dissection, occlusion or perforation, and cholesterol embolism to the renal or lower limb vasculature.

The results reported for angioplasty vary widely. The procedure is technically successful in 70 to 100 per cent of cases reported, and rates for improvement of hypertension range from 10 to 75 per cent. Restenosis is common, occurring in 20 per cent or more of patients at up to 2 years follow-up. The results for fibromuscular disease are better than those for atherosclerotic disease, both for technical success, blood pressure outcome, and re-stenosis rate.

MEDICAL TREATMENT

If reconstructive surgery or angioplasty is not considered appropriate, treatment with antihypertensive agents is required. Diuretics should be used with caution in these patients, as in unilateral disease volume depletion with accompanying hyponatremia and hypokalaemia is not uncommon, as a consequence of pressure natriuresis in the unaffected kidney. Calcium entry blockers have been established to be safe and reasonably effective treatment in renovascular hypertension; β-blockers are an acceptable alternative, unless there is associated severe peripheral vascular disease.

RENAL FUNCTION IMPAIRMENT ASSOCIATED WITH CONVERTING ENZYME INHIBITORS

Converting enzyme inhibitors should be used with caution in patients with renovascular disease. They are very effective in reducing blood pressure (through their suppression of angiotensin II formation) but they carry the risk of causing a marked fall in glomerular filtration rate. The mechanism, already discussed, is commonly attributed to acute loss of glomerular filtration pressure, which is dependent on efferent arteriolar vasoconstriction when renal perfusion is impaired. It is now widely recognized that deterioration in renal function may occur with converting enzyme inhibition when severe macroscopic disease is present. It is less well known that these drugs may cause similar acute renal dysfunction in renal microvascular disease, such as hypertensive nephrosclerosis, even when major vessel disease is absent.

The risk of this complication is increased by volume depletion or excessive diuretic therapy, and *irreversible* loss of renal function has been described in 15 per cent of a group of patients with hypertension or congestive cardiac failure and intrarenal arteriosclerosis in whom renal function declined in association with converting enzyme inhibitor therapy. Animal studies have also suggested that, when renal perfusion is impaired by arterial clipping, long-term converting enzyme inhibition may lead to renal atrophy. These concerns can lead to major difficulties in the management of patients with ischaemic cardiomyopathy and severe congestive failure, for whom converting enzyme inhibition is the treatment of choice, but who also have renal impairment from accompanying atherosclerotic renovascular disease.

PROGNOSIS OF RENOVASCULAR DISEASE

The overall prognosis for patients with renovascular disease remains relatively poor, despite the advances achieved in both invasive and medical management. With increasing acceptance of elderly patients for maintenance dialysis treatment, the detected frequency of renovascular disease as a cause of endstage renal failure has increased, and it is at present reported as the underlying disease in between 8 and 14 per cent of patients commencing dialysis. In a proportion of these cases, patients had been receiving long-term converting enzyme inhibitor therapy, emphasizing again the need for regular monitoring of renal function after initiating treatment with these drugs.

The outlook for patients with endstage renal failure due to renovascular disease is especially poor, and in one series 5-year survival was less than 10 per cent, half that of dialysis patients with diabetic nephropathy and one-sixth that of patients with glomerulonephritis. These depressing figures undoubtedly reflect the attrition due to severe gen-

Fig. 5 (a) Aortography in a 45-year-old patient with type II diabetes showing bilateral atheromatous renal artery stenoses (arrows). (b) Appearances after successful bilateral angioplasty. (Reproduced by permission of Dr J. Dacie.)

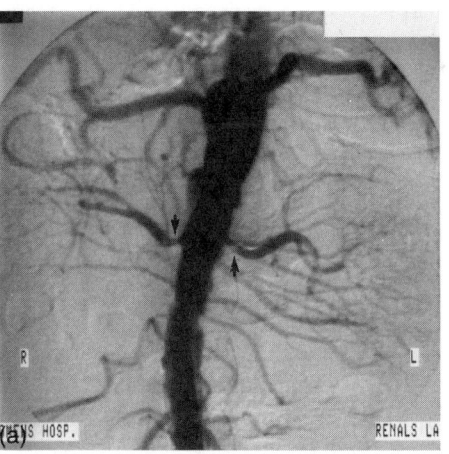

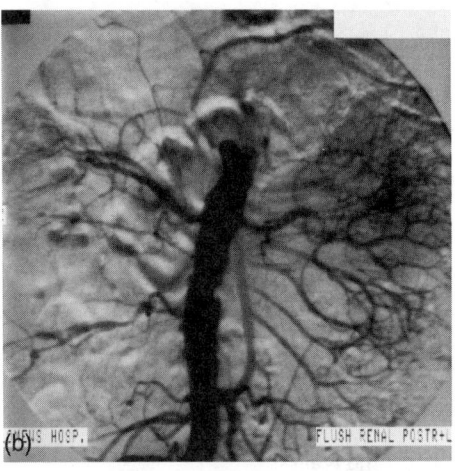

Fig. 4 Selective left renal angiography in the patient shown in Fig. 2, demonstrating appearances after successful angioplasty. (Reproduced by permission of Dr J. Dacie.)

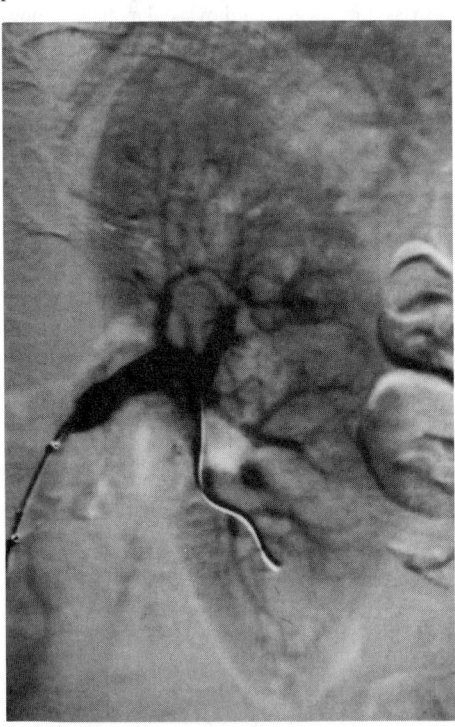

eralized atherosclerosis. Patients with atheromatous bilateral renovascular hypertension are also at high risk of recurrent severe pulmonary oedema. This complication is probably related to the volume expansion, which is known to accompany bilateral renal artery stenosis, and it may be effectively eliminated by successful renal revascularization.

Unilateral renal parenchymal disease

Unilateral renal parenchymal disease is, overall, a rare cause of secondary hypertension, but it assumes relative importance in children and young adults. The common unilateral parenchymal diseases which may give rise to hypertension are shown in Table 6. Pyelonephritic scarring from reflux or dysplasia of a single kidney are the most common causes; reflux nephropathy accounts for over 60 per cent of cases of severe childhood hypertension. The mechanism by which hypertension comes about in these patients is not clear. It has been suggested that it is due to renal ischaemia arising from parenchymal scarring, with activation of the renin angiotensin system, but this ignores the finding that in many cases hypertension arises after some years of known scarring, with no increase in the scars and no obvious other precipitating factor.

Improvement in blood pressure after nephrectomy is reported in the majority of cases in published series, although measurement of renal venous renin ratios or the response to captopril challenge tests have proved of little value in predicting the response to surgery. Clearly, careful assessment of divided renal function is essential before decisions concerning partial or total nephrectomy of the affected kidney are made. If there is appreciable remaining function in the affected kidney, surgery specifically designed to relieve hypertension should only be undertaken when blood pressure is uncontrolled, despite maximal tolerated doses of combinations of antihypertensive drugs, including converting enzyme inhibitors, minoxidil, and calcium channel blockers.

Hypertension also occurs in association with unilateral hydronephrosis in 10 to 20 per cent of cases. The mechanism remains uncertain but may in part involve loss of renal medullary vasodepressor factors (medullipin). The response of hypertension to surgical correction of hydronephrosis is variable, generally disappointing, and appears to depend in part on the duration of the obstruction to urine outflow.

Hypertension and cardiovascular mortality in renal disease

In addition to accelerating the progression of renal impairment, hypertension in patients with renal failure is of major importance because it

Fig. 6 Cumulative survival in 91 patients with endstage renal disease, according to echocardiographic left ventricular hypertrophy. (Reproduced with permission from Silberberg *et al.* (1989).)

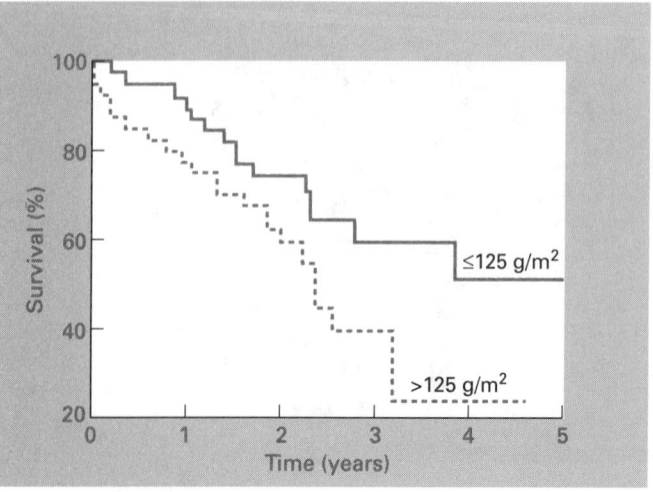

Table 6 *Unilateral renal parenchymal disease causing hypertension*

Chronic pyelonephritis
Reflux nephropathy
Dysplastic kidney
Segmental hypoplasia (Ask–Upmark kidney)
Obstructive uropathy
Tuberculosis
Trauma
Radiation fibrosis
Simple renal cysts

Table 7 *Survival in long-term dialysis patients in relation to treated blood pressure*

No. of patients	Mean arterial pressure (mmHg)	Percentage patient survival (years)			
		5	10	15	20
222	<99	93	85	67	53
223	≤99	81	65	43	–

Adapted from Charra *et al.* (1992).

increases their susceptibility to cardiovascular disease. The absolute death rate from cardiovascular complications, in particular ischaemic heart disease, in these patients is many times higher than in the general population. In young patients receiving renal replacement therapy by dialysis or transplantation in the United Kingdom, for example, the excess risk of death from myocardial infarction is over 90 times that of the age- and sex-matched general population. Mortality from ischaemic heart disease is three-fold higher again in diabetic than non-diabetic dialysis and transplant patients.

The reasons for this high rate of cardiovascular mortality have not been fully clarified, but it is certainly relevant that patients with renal failure have many of the risk factors for cardiovascular disease now well-defined for the general population, including disordered lipid metabolism and in particular hypertension and left ventricular hypertrophy. Although large-scale epidemiological data relating these risk factors to outcome in patients with renal failure are lacking. observations from single centres have confirmed their importance. As Fig. 6 shows, in one such study, left ventricular hypertrophy in patients with endstage renal disease was associated with particularly poor survival.

Left ventricular hypertrophy is very common in renal disease; echocardiographic studies show that more than 50 per cent of patients with even mild renal impairment have significant hypertrophy, which is usually asymmetrical in pattern. It is present in the great majority of dialysis patients and resolves only partially after renal transplantation. Many factors are believed to contribute, but the most important are renal anaemia and especially the high prevalence of hypertension, often poorly controlled, which these patients suffer.

The prime importance of blood pressure itself as a determinant of survival in renal disease is emphasized by long term follow up of dialysis patients in Tassin, France, (Table 7). Twenty-year survival of patients with a mean blood pressure of 99 mmHg or less (roughly equivalent to a blood pressure of 140/80 mmHg) was virtually the same as that of the general population. In contrast, no patients whose blood pressure was above this level survived for 20 years. Data such as these emphasize the need for early detection and effective management of hypertension in renal disease. The aims are two-fold – optimal preservation of renal function, and the reduction as far as possible of the burden from cardiovascular complications in later life.

REFERENCES

Baldwin, D.S. and Neugarten, J. (1985). Treatment of hypertension in renal disease. *American Journal of Kidney Disease*, **5**, A57–A70.

Bell, P.E., Hossack, K.F., Gabow, P.A., *et al.* (1988). Hypertension in autosomal dominant polycystic kidney disease. *Kidney International* **34**, 683–90.

Boer, P., Koomans, H.A. and Dorhourt Mees, E.J. (1987). Renin and blood volume in chronic renal failure: a comparison with essential hypertension. *Nephron* **45**, 7–13.

Brazy, P.C., Stead, W.W. and Fitzwilliam, J.F. (1989). Progression of renal insufficiency: role of blood pressure. *Kidney International* **35**, 670–4.

Bridoux, F., Hazzan, M., Pallot, J.L., *et al.* (1992). Acute renal failure after the use of angiotensin-converting-enzyme inhibitors in patients without renal artery stenosis. *Nephrology, Dialysis and Transplantation* **7**, 100–104.

Brunner, H.R. (1992). ACE inhibitors in renal disease. *Kidney International* **42**, 463–479.

Charra, B., Calemard, E., Ruffet, M., *et al.* (1992). Survival as an index of adequacy of dialysis. *Kidney International* **41**, 1286–1291.

Converse, R.L., Jacobsen, T.N., Toto, R.D., *et al.* (1992). Sympathetic overactivity in patients with chronic renal failure. *New England Journal of Medicine* **327**, 1912–1918.

Corvol, P. (1984). Tumour-dependent hypertension. *Hypertension* **6**, 593–596.

Harding, M.B., Smith, L.R., Himmelstein, S.L., *et al.* (1992). Renal artery stenosis: prevalence and associated risk factors in patients undergoing routine cardiac catheterization. *Journal of the American Society of Nephrology*, **2**, 1608–1616.

Jacobson, H.R. (1988). Ischaemic renal disease: an overlooked clinical entity? *Kidney International,* **34**, 729–743.

Kalra, P.S., Mamtora, H., Holmes, A.M., and Waldek, S. (1990). Renovascular disease and renal complications of angiotensin-converting enzyme inhibitor therapy. *Quarterly Journal of Medicine,* **282**, 1013–18.

Klahr, S., Schreiner, G., and Ichikawa, I. (1988). Mechanism of disease: the progression of renal disease. *New England Journal of Medicine,* **318**, 1657–66.

Lewis, E.J., Hunsickler, L.G., Bain, R.P., and Rohde, R.D. (1993). The effect of angiotensin-converting-enzyme inhibition on diabetic nephropathy. *New England Journal of Medicine* **329**, 1456–62.

Pickering, T.G., Devereux, R.B., James, G.D., *et al.* (1988). Recurrent pulmonary oedema in hypertension due to bilateral renal artery stenosis: Treatment by angioplasty or surgical revascularisation. *Lancet* **3**, 551–552.

Schreiber, M.J., Pohl, M.A., and Novick, A.C. (1984). The natural history of atherosclerotic and fibrous renal artery disease. *Urology Clinics of North America* **11**, 383–392.

Silberberg, J.S., Barre, P.E., and Prichard, S.S. (1989). Impact of left ventricular hypertrophy on survival in end-stage renal disease. *Kidney International* **36**, 286–290.

Vallance, P., Leone, A., Calver, A., *et al.* (1992). Accumulation of an endogenous inhibitor of nitric oxide synthesis in chronic renal failure. *Lancet* **339**, 572–575.

Weidmann, P., Beretta-Piccoli, C., Steffen, F., et al. (1976). Hypertension in renal failure. *Kidney International* **9**, 294–301.

Wilcox, C.S. (1993). Use of angiotensin-converting-enzyme inhibitors for diagnosing renovascular hypertension. *Kidney International* **44**, 1379–1390.

15.28.2 Phaeochromocytoma

M. BROWN

Incidence and importance

Phaeochromocytoma is a rare tumour. Most doctors are unlikely to meet more than one patient with the condition in their lifetime. A large general hospital will admit only one patient on average each year. *In vivo* estimates of incidence are unreliable because none has been undertaken in an unselected group of patients. It is safe to say that the incidence is less than 1 per cent and more than 0.1 per cent of hypertensives. In the past 3 years, we have screened 27 000 healthy subjects in general practice, selected only for the absence of known hypertension or vascular disease. Only 0.7 per cent (~200) were found to have hypertension, defined as a diastolic blood pressure above 90 mmHg after three readings over 3 months. Two of these patients, with previously unidentified hypertension, had a phaeochromocytoma, giving an incidence of 1 per cent of hypertensives. On the other hand, of 550 patients referred over 6 years by family doctors following their own diagnosis of hypertension, before initiation of treatment, only one has been found to have a phaeochromocytoma, giving an incidence of under 0.2 per cent.

Despite its rarity, phaeochromocytoma justifies the disproportionate interest and awareness of the condition that exists among physicians. Like a few other rare conditions which share this position, such as infective endocarditis or Addison's disease, phaeochromocytoma combines the potential for being lethal if not diagnosed and treated, and for cure in most patients if diagnosed. The diagnosis of phaeochromocytoma offers the best chance of a cure of all the secondary causes of hypertension (especially those presenting in the second half of life), and avoidance of the need for lifelong antihypertensive therapy.

The need for maintaining a high awareness of the condition is emphasized by the small number of deaths each year, in both anaesthetic and obstetric practice, due to undiagnosed phaeochromocytoma.

Catecholamine biochemistry

An understanding of the tests used to diagnose phaeochromocytoma requires reference to an outline of both the synthetic and degradative pathways of catecholamine metabolism. The term catechol refers to a phenyl ring with hydroxyl groups at adjacent carbons (conventionally, the 3′ and 4′ positions). The precursor essential amino acid, phenylalanine, is not itself a catechol; neither is tyrosine which has only the 3′ hydroxyl. This amino acid is the substrate for the rate-limiting step in the biosynthetic pathway, tyrosine hydroxylase, which yields L-dopa, the first catechol and still an amino acid. Decarboxylation of L-dopa yields the first catecholamine in the pathway, dopamine. Occasionally this can be the principal catecholamine secreted by phaeochromocytomas, or more often by childhood neuroblastomas. But usually in the chromaffin tissue from which phaeochromocytomas originate dopamine is further hydroxylated, in the side-chain bearing the amine group, to noradrenaline. The final step in the biosynthetic pathway is the N-methylation of noradrenaline to adrenaline (the prefix 'nor' is used for substances which are N-demethylated, a common step in degradative metabolism). This N-methylation usually occurs in only two sites in the body: the adrenal medulla and certain hindbrain nuclei involved in blood pressure control. The enzyme, phenylethanolamine-N-methyltransferase (PNMT), may differ between these sites, as outside the central nervous system it is dependent for induction on glucocorticoids, which are provided in the adrenal through the portocapillary circulation. The clinical importance of this is threefold. First, extra-adrenal phaeochromocytomas rarely produce adrenaline, most of the reports to the contrary being in older literature when the methodology was less satisfactory for separating adrenaline and noradrenaline. Second, the normal adrenal produces mainly adrenaline, and accounts for less than 2 per cent of circulating noradrenaline concentrations. Third, when a tumour is present in the adrenal, the disruption of the portocapillary circulation causes a reversal of the normal adrenaline to noradrenaline ratio. The relevance of these to the clinical features and diagnosis of phaeochromocytoma will become apparent.

The metabolic breakdown of catecholamines is due to two principal enzymes, monoamine oxidase (MAO) and catechol-O-methyltransferase (COMT). The metabolism of catecholamines is different from normal in phaeochromocytoma in that adrenaline and noradrenaline are liberated directly into the bloodstream rather than mainly into the synaptic gap around sympathetic nerve endings. Noradrenaline released from these is largely recaptured by neuronal and extraneuronal uptake, and metabolized before any free amine escapes into the bloodstream. Consequently, the proportion of parent amine to metabolite is usually higher in blood and urine in the presence of a phaeochromocytoma than in any other cause of elevated catecholamine production.

The most abundant product of the action of monoamine oxidase and catechol-O-methyltransferase (acting in sequence, in either order) is vanillylmandelic acid (VMA). Normetanephrine and metanephrine are produced by catechol-O-methyltransferase from noradrenaline and adrenaline, respectively. The products of monoamine oxidase alone are less often used in diagnosis, but in specialized laboratories the ratio of one of these, dihydroxyphenylglycol (DHPG) to noradrenaline is a useful clue to the origin of noradrenaline, as dihydroxyphenylglycol arises mainly intraneuronally, and relatively little is therefore formed from noradrenaline liberated directly into the bloodstream as in phaeochromocytoma.

ANALYSES

Most routine laboratories should be able to undertake one of the screening tests on 24 h urine samples; of these, measurements of metabolites are most appropriate because they offer an integrated measure of total catecholamine release over this period; vanillylmandelic acid is the product least prone to interference, L-dopa being the only drug which can cross-react in measurement through its equivalent metabolite, homovanillic acid. Although, for the reasons discussed, quantitation of vanillylmandelic acid is less sensitive than other measures, it remains very rare that a patient with a secreting phaeochromocytoma has a 24-h vanillylmandelic acid result that is entirely normal. The problem is more that of distinguishing a true positive among the relatively large number of hypertensive patients with results in the grey zone. Metanephrines are arguably more sensitive than vanillylmandelic acid, but their assay is more prone to interference by drugs, especially by β-blockers.

The measurement of free catecholamines is a more specialized procedure. Assays can be made in plasma or urine. The former is generally more accurate, and also allows variation in secretion to be assessed because of the very short half-life in plasma of catecholamines, of around 1 min. The assay used in most of the specialized laboratories is based on high performance liquid chromatography separation of the catecholamines followed by electrochemical or fluorometric detection. However, this technique does not eliminate the possibility of interference, especially in the adrenaline peak, and it is necessary to be particularly suspicious of any result showing a higher adrenaline than noradrenaline concentration. A few centres still undertake the gold-standard radioenzymatic assay in which the catecholamines are converted to their [³H]-methylated derivative in the presence of catechol-O-methyltransferase and a [³H]-methyl donor; a double-isotope technique is usually used to ensure accurate quantification.

Apart from the catecholamines, most phaeochromocytomas also secrete one or more neuropeptides, especially neuropeptide (NPY), which is a normal cotransmitter of noradrenaline and adrenaline. Much rarer, but essential to detect preoperatively, is adrenocorticotropic hormone which may cause a coexisting ectopic adrenocorticotropic hormone syndrome; a particular catch is that the excess secretion of catecholamines may suppress release of other peptides until treatment with α-blockade is initiated. For instance, secretion of somatostatin may exaggerate the episodic nature of catecholamine discharge by inhibiting its own (and the catecholamine) release as soon as a discharge starts.

Pathology

Phaeochromocytomas arise in chromaffin tissue, and their anatomical distribution closely parallels the sites where this tissue is present at the time of birth. These tumours, like the normal sympathoadrenal tissue, are of neuroectodermal origin. The term phaeochromocytoma reflects the dusky colour of the cut surface of the tumour, whereas the term chromaffin refers to the brownish colour caused by contact with dichromate salts, which oxidize the catecholamines. Much has been written about pathological differences between extra-adrenal phaeochromocytomas at various sites, but this is not relevant to clinical practice except as a possible explanation for the failure of some head and neck phaeochromocytomas to accumulate the noradrenaline analogue used as a radionuclide in scanning, as discussed later.

The pathogenesis of phaeochromocytomas is not known, but in some patients, mainly those with associated abnormalities such as the multiple endocrine neoplasia (MEN) type 2 syndrome or in von Hippel Lindau syndrome (VHL), the tumour is familial. The genes for both these disorders have been identified and may shed light also on the origin of sporadic phaeochromocytoma. If the analogy with some other endocrine tumours is correct, it is to be expected that a mutation or genetic recombination leads to an oncogene being driven by a catecholamine activated promoter.

Most phaeochromocytomas are benign. However, the pathologist can rarely provide a clear distinction between benign and malignant phaeochromocytomas. On the one hand, benign tumours can appear to be invading the capsule of the tumour, which is often ill-defined, whilst on the other, malignant tumours may show no mitoses because of their slow rate of division.

Clinical features

Hypertension is the most common form of presentation of phaeochromocytoma in clinical practice, but other presentations include unexplained heart failure or as part of multiple endocrine neoplasia, or other rarer associated genetic diseases. In the last groups of patients, the diagnosis is made by screening of patients with or without specific clinical features of a phaeochromocytoma. In the hypertensive patients, a spontaneous history or direct enquiry will usually reveal at least one of a group of characteristic symptoms. The most common are headache, sweating, and palpitations. Less frequent are episodes of pallor, a feeling of 'impending doom', and paraesthesiae. Examination rarely reveals useful signs, but an exception is a Raynaud's-type of discoloration over the extremities and the larger joints in the limbs. This is due to ischaemia and occasionally progresses to atrophic ulceration over pressure points.

Occasionally phaeochromocytomas can present with a dangerous syndrome, due to acute haemorrhage and infarction of the tumour. This gives rise to a unique combination of the features of retroperitoneal haemorrhage and intermittent hypertension, which is pathognomonic but even prompt recognition of the diagnosis is not always sufficient to save patients presenting with this particular crisis. At the other extreme, it should be emphasized that not all patients with a phaeochromocytoma, even those with quite large tumours causing severe hypertension, have any specific symptoms, and we advocate screening, therefore, of all patients presenting in one of the ways listed above.

Many of the symptoms of phaeochromocytoma can be readily ascribed to the expected effects of the catecholamine excess, and disappear rapidly on initiation of appropriate treatment. Some remain more difficult to explain, including the sweating whose control in healthy subjects is usually ascribed to cholinergic sympathetic innervation. Because large tumours secrete principally noradrenaline, even when arising within the adrenal gland, tachycardia is usually only modest, and can be replaced altogether by reflex bradycardia when episodes of hypertension are triggered by release of noradrenaline alone. I have once treated a 'cardiac arrest' with phentolamine when the arrest call was for an episode of apparent asystole that was in reality severe sinus bradycardia triggered by an arterial pressure of over 300/160. In a few patients, catecholamine excess can cause myocardial necrosis which is probably due to a mixture of α-receptor mediated vasoconstriction and a β-receptor direct toxic effect on the cardiomyocytes. These are rare presentations and it is important to recognize that clinical features are usually less impressive than expected, possibly because the adrenoceptors have been down-regulated by years of exposure before the diagnosis is first entertained. Indeed, hypertensive patients who complain of symptoms suggestive of excess catecholamines are more likely to be found suffering side-effects of a vasodilator drug activating the baroreflex than to have a phaeochromocytoma.

Diagnosis

The diagnosis is usually not difficult once the possibility has been entertained, but it is important to exclude the diagnosis in patients who have clinical and/or biochemical features of catecholamine excess, due to sympathetic overactivity and not a phaeochromocytoma. There are two distinct questions to ask when considering the diagnosis. The first is, 'Does the patient have a phaeochromocytoma?'; the second is, 'Where is it?'. The tests required to answer the first question are mainly biochemical, whereas the second is answered by radiological investigation. A golden rule, which saves countless false positives and negatives, and therefore a large number of unnecessary investigations and sometimes operations, is that the first question should be answered before proceeding to the second. No single radiological investigation is sufficiently accurate to detect more than 80 to 90 per cent of phaeochromocytomas, whilst computed tomography scanning in particular is sufficiently sensitive to detect small non-functional adenomas in the adrenal gland that should not lead to further investigation in the absence of biochemical abnormalities.

The symptoms of a functioning phaeochromocytoma are remarkably variable and maybe absent; to avoid missing the diagnosis, therefore, it is reasonable to screen many patients presenting with hypertension, a few with unexplained heart failure, and even fewer of those with the MEN or VHL syndromes. Although the diagnosis is often postulated in other patients with isolated features of catecholamine excess, e.g. patients without hypertension but complaining of palpitation, headaches, sweating, or panic attacks, the chance of such patients having a phaeochromocytoma is very, very small. In a 15-year period during which I have investigated more than 100 phaeochromocytomas, and investigated more than a thousand patients referred with a possible phaeochromocytoma, none has proven to have phaeochromocytoma in the absence of the three conditions listed at the start of this paragraph.

The next question is how screening should be performed. There is no single perfect or 'best' test. It is important to recognize the diversity of analyses in use, quite different from the position for most standard endocrine analyses, and reflecting the difficulty of achieving an entirely reliable method in routine laboratories. The specialized laboratories tend to be those which carry out a large number of catecholamine estimations for research studies. Our own practice is to use 24 h urine vanillylmandelic acid as the initial screen in most patients, supplemented when necessary with the specialized catecholamine analyses. An advantage of a 24-h urine screen is that a single plasma measurement can miss the very occasional phaeochromocytoma with truly episodic secretion, whereas 24-h urine samples integrate the products of secretion over 24 h. An entirely normal 24-h urine vanillylmandelic acid measured in a good hospital laboratory is most unlikely in the presence of a phaeochromocytoma; indeed, the normal urinary vanillylmandelic acid probably reflects the incompetence of the laboratory rather than failure of the phaeochromocytoma. Conventionally, patients are asked to avoid vanilla containing foods during the collection, for assay of vanillylmandelic acid and to undertake three collections in order to exclude the diagnosis of phaeochromocytoma. Both of these precautions are unnecessary in the majority of patients. Because patients with phaeochromocytoma have become relatively insensitive to the effects of catecholamines, a patient with 'significant' hypertension (diastolic BP > 100 mmHg) requires a several-fold elevation of catecholamine secretion to develop hypertension. Although the vanillylmandelic acid is not proportionally elevated, for the reasons discussed earlier, the elevation is still sufficient to ensure an abnormal vanillylmandelic acid result provided this is correctly measured. A vanilla-free diet is unnecessary because the dietary contribution to vanillylmandelic acid excretion is small compared to that derived from noradrenaline, and is unlikely to push the vanillylmandelic acid excretion into an abnormal range.

Vanillylmandelic acid results which are less than twofold above the upper limit of normal cannot usually be considered pathognomonic of phaeochromocytomas. Most patients whose urine contains more than this will prove to have a phaeochromocytoma, and a threefold elevation is almost always diagnostic. The patients therefore who need further biochemical analyses are those with less than twofold elevation of vanillylmandelic acid excretion, of whom only a very small proportion (less than 5 per cent) will have a phaeochromocytoma. Here, the single most helpful investigation is the plasma catecholamines. In most patients with a phaeochromocytoma, the plasma noradrenaline will be at least twofold elevated, whereas in most without a phaeochromocytoma, a single resting plasma noradrenaline will often be normal.

SUPPRESSION TESTS

If the urinary vanillylmandelic acid analysis, together with assay of resting plasma noradrenaline does not resolve, whether or not the patient has a phaeochromocytoma, there are two further useful investigations. The most widely used is a pharmacological suppression test, in which physiological elevations of noradrenaline release are temporarily suppressed by administration of either the ganglion-blocking drug, pentolinium, or centrally acting α_2-agonist, clonidine. The former is more widely used in the United Kingdom and has three advantages: (1) it is most effective at suppressing noradrenaline release in the problem patients — namely those with elevated sympathetic nervous activity but without a phaeochromocytoma; (2) it suppresses also release of adrenaline from the adrenal medulla; and (3) it has a short half-life (of approximately 20 min) so that the test can be completed in the outpatient clinic. Clonidine has the supposed advantage of suppressing release of noradrenaline even when the basal level is normal, but in practice when this is the case a suppression test is rarely necessary; the exception is in patients being screened for phaeochromocytoma because of associated tumours (usually medullary carcinoma of the thyroid) in the multiple endocrine neoplasia syndrome; even here, pentolinium is more helpful, as a characteristic of these patients is that the only plasma catecholamine to be elevated may be adrenaline, whose secretion is very sensitive (in non-phaeochromocytoma patients) to pentolinium but not to clonidine.

The protocol for the pentolinium test requires that patients' renal function is ascertained prior to the test, as pentolinium is entirely excreted by the kidneys. We have not used pentolinium in patients with a serum creatinine level greater than 150 μmol/l. Patients should rest supine for 15 to 30 min before the test. Plasma catecholamines are measured in two samples taken 5 min apart from an intravenous cannula, and in two further samples taken 10 and 20 min after an intravenous bolus of pentolinium 2.5 mg. They should remain supine for a further 60 min, and their erect arterial pressure should be checked before they are allowed to leave the clinic. A normal response to pentolinium is a fall of both plasma noradrenaline and adrenaline concentrations into the normal range or by 50 per cent from baseline. It should be noted that, since ganglion-blocking drugs are less effective at low rates of sympathetic nerve discharge, there may be little fall in plasma catecholamine values when the basal levels are already within the normal range.

It is helpful to measure plasma catecholamines even in patients with unequivocal elevation of their 24-h urine vanillylmandelic acid as the adrenaline level is a most useful clue to the location of the phaeochromocytoma. Modern assays have established that it is exceptional for extra-adrenal phaeochromocytomas to secrete adrenaline (because of the lack of cortisol stimulation). Most adrenal phaeochromocytomas do secrete adrenaline, although the proportion of noradrenaline to adrenaline is reversed from that in normal subjects. The plasma sample may also be assayed for dihydroxyphenyl glycol, the deaminated metabolite synthesized principally in sympathetic nerve endings. It has been shown that the ratio of dihydroxyphenyl glycol to noradrenaline is reversed from normal (more dihydroxyphenyl glycol than noradrenaline) in patients with phaeochromocytoma, allowing an alternative method to a suppression test for distinguishing patients with borderline noradrenaline results.

LOCALIZATION OF PHAEOCHROMOCYTOMAS

Although a major clue can be provided by measurement of plasma adrenaline, CT scanning is the method of choice, as 90 per cent of phaeochromocytomas arise in the adrenal (Fig. 1). This form of imaging has revolutionized localization of phaeochromocytoma because the adrenal is easy to visualize as it is so well differentiated from its surrounding fatty tissue. In addition, the type of abnormality in the adrenal will influence the Hounsfield units of the adrenal image, permitting the radiologist to distinguish cortical tumours such as a Conn's tumour from medullary tumours. Phaeochromocytomas are also usually larger than Conn's tumours, and may appear non-homogeneous because of areas of haemorrhage and infarction. These differences should, however, be regarded as largely academic as diagnostic mistakes will be made if the differentiation between these tumours is attempted radiologically rather than biochemically. It should also be emphasized that both these tumours account for a minority of adrenal tumours identified by computerized tomography, the majority of which are non-functional adenomas of no significance.

While modern computed tomography is capable of whole body imaging at high resolution, it is preferable to withhold computerized tomography for extra-adrenal phaeochromocytomas until the radiologist can be given some clue as to where to concentrate. In about 85 per cent of patients, this can be achieved by radioisotope scanning, using the iodinated analogue of noradrenaline, m-iodobenzylguanidine. This may carry either an [^{123}I]- or [^{131}I] label. The former is more sensitive but also more expensive, and may be misinterpreted if users are unaware that normal adrenal glands also accumulate m-iodobenzylguanidine. There is a case for undertaking m-iodobenzylguanidine scanning in addition to computed tomography, even for patients found to have an adrenal phaeochromocytoma, to identify extra-adrenal secondary deposits when tumours are malignant, and because there may be coexisting adrenal and extra-adrenal phaeochromocytomas.

If these investigations fail to localize a phaeochromocytoma diagnosed by biochemical assays, the next step is to undertake selective venous sampling. In this procedure, about 25 samples of blood are collected under fluoroscopic guidance from various sites in the vena cava and the veins which drain into it, for estimation of catecholamine concentration. An arterial sample taken at the end of the procedure is invaluable for interpreting the results, as it enables sites with a positive venoarterial difference to be readily detected. Albeit invasive in the strict sense, venous sampling is free of significant hazard and it is not necessary to monitor the arterial pressure or pulse rate during the procedure. It is important, however, that the radiologist is not tempted to undertake a venogram of the phaeochromocytoma, since this can cause immediate infarction of the tumour with release of the stored catecholamines and catastrophic consequences. The procedure is more helpful in the diagnosis of phaeochromocytoma than of other endocrine tumours because of the very short half-life of catecholamines in the circulation (about 1 min) such that most is removed during one passage round the circulation, and the concentration at the tumour site is usually several fold greater than concentrations elsewhere. This procedure should not usually be used for adrenal phaeochromocytomas because the concentration of catecholamines is much higher than elsewhere in veins draining normal adrenals and because computed tomography scanning should have already rendered their imaging unnecessary.

The place of angiography has been much diminished but not entirely removed by computed tomography scanning. As phaeochromocytomas are vascular tumours, they provide a good tumour blush, and angiography should resolve equivocal computed tomography scans. This procedure in contrast to that of venous sampling can provoke an outpouring of catechols. Patients must be fully α-and preferably also β-blocked prior to angiography, and their blood pressure pulse rate and ECG monitored during the procedure with phentolamine and practolol readily available to treat sources of arterial pressure or tachycardia.

In some centres, magnetic resonance imaging may be tried before angiography to determine the nature of lesions of doubtful significance on computed tomography. However, the semi-infarcted nature of some phaeochromocytomas can make it difficult to interpret magnetic resonance scans, and in our experience magnetic resonance has so far helped only with a few head and neck phaeochromocytomas which were not detected by m-iodobenzylguanidine or computed tomography scanning.

OTHER INVESTIGATIONS

It is important to check blood glucose in every patient as there may be α mediated inhibition of insulin release prior to effective treatment. All patients should be screened for an associated medullary carcinoma of the thyroid by a plasma calcitonin estimation. There is no need routinely to measure other neurotransmitters which may be cosecreted with the catecholamines. However, unusual symptoms may indicate the measurement of a gut peptide screen.

The very rare patient who cosecretes adrenocorticotropic hormone will be detected by measurement of plasma electrolytes revealing the characteristic from the typical gross hypokalaemia of the ectopic adrenocorticotropic hormone syndrome; because adrenocorticotropic hormone release may be inhibited by noradrenaline prior to initiation of α-blockade, it is important to re-check the electrolytes after a few days of α-blocking treatment.

Treatment

The definitive treatment is surgical removal of the tumour or tumours. Even the small number of phaeochromocytomas which can be recognized to be malignant preoperatively (e.g. by the presence of bone or liver metastases) may still benefit from resection of the primary tumour. The task for the physician is to make the surgery safe. The mainstay of medical treatment is α-blockade, but not all patients – especially those without elevated plasma adrenaline levels – require β-blockade. The objective of this treatment is not solely control of blood pressure but also the expansion of blood volume, which is always reduced in phaeochromocytoma patients. The α-blocker of choice is phenoxybenzamine. The principal reason for this choice is that it is an irreversible blocker,

Fig. 1 CT scan of right adrenal phaeochromocytoma. The phaeochromocytoma has the typical non-homogeneous appearance due to areas of haemorrhage and infarction. The normal left adrenal has the typical tricornuate appearance with concave borders.

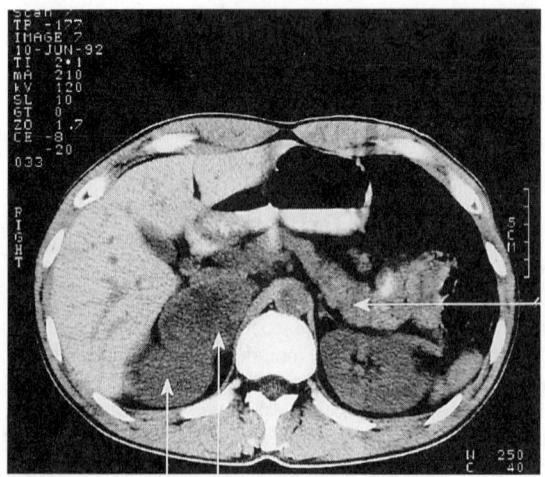

Normal adrenal

Kidney   Phaeochromocytoma

which actually destroys the α-receptor by alkylation. More modern α-blockers, such as prazosin, doxazosin, and the mixed α- and β-blocker, labetalol, cause competitive blockade, which can be overcome by a surge of noradrenaline release from the tumour. An additional advantage of phenoxybenzamine is that it will block both α_1- and α_2-receptors. Blockade of the latter is considered disadvantageous in essential hypertension since the main α_2-receptors outside the central nervous system are presynaptic and may serve a useful role in damping neuronal release of noradrenaline, whereas in phaeochromocytoma patients α_2-receptor blockade may be advantageous because a small population of extrasynaptic α_2-receptors mediate direct vasoconstriction by circulating (non-neuronal) catecholamines. The diabetogenic effect of catecholamines is also an α_2-mediated response.

The starting dose of phenoxybenzamine is 10 mg twice daily. The effect of irreversible antagonists is cumulative, and the effect of the drug – and each subsequent dose increment – takes several days to reach maximum. It is reasonable to aim for a diastolic blood pressure between 90 and 100 mmHg during treatment, and to admit patients for 5 days preoperatively, during which time the dose is increased until there is at least a 10 mmHg postural fall in blood pressure and little if any variability in arterial pressure.

The need for β-blockade is indicated by tachycardia, which may become apparent only after treatment with phenoxybenzamine. Lower doses of β-blocking drugs are necessary than generally used in the treatment of hypertension. It is usually better to use a selective β_1-selective agent so that the peripheral vasodilatation mediated by β_2-receptors is not affected. The reason for using as low a dose as possible is that immediately upon removal of the phaeochromocytoma, there may be a period of hypotension despite the preoperative preparation that has been outlined. This hypotension is due to the withdrawal of any α-mediated vasoconstriction, and should normally be offset by the ability to mount a tachycardia. It is important to note that if hypotension does occur, it should not be treated with pressor agents; the correct treatment is by volume replacement, supplemented if necessary by β-agonists and, extremely rarely, by angiotensin as a vasoconstrictor.

The treatment of malignant phaeochromocytomas remains uncertain and unsatisfactory. As is the case for many endocrine cancers, the rate of growth is usually slow. The prognosis for affected individuals can, however, vary between the extremes of local recurrence at intervals of many years, and rapid demise sometimes precipitated by surgery. These tumours are not particularly sensitive either to chemotherapy or to radiotherapy, although the variability of response may still make a course worth trying. There has been interest in the use of therapeutic doses of *m*-iodobenzylguanidine, as a means of targeting high doses of radioactivity to the tumour, and some patients show considerable regression after such treatment. Long-term results are less certain. If the primary tumour has been removed or debulked, it is rare for the pharmacological effects of the tumour to be the principal problem. High doses of phenoxybenzamine are greatly preferable to α-methyltyrosine, which is occasionally used as an inhibitor of noradrenaline synthesis, but which also depletes noradrenaline in the brain, causing sedation and depression.

Prognosis

Ninety per cent of phaeochromocytomas are benign. For adrenal phaeochromocytomas, the proportion is probably even higher, whereas extra-adrenal phaeochromocytomas have a greater than 10 per cent likelihood of proving malignant. Because, however, of the difficulties already described in ascertaining malignancy, all patients with a phaeochromocytoma should be followed indefinitely with at least an annual measurement of arterial pressure and analysis of one of the indices of catecholamine secretion.

The removal of a phaeochromocytoma in the majority of patients cures their hypertension, especially in younger patients. In only 13 out of a personal series of 76 patients with phaeochromocytoma was the blood pressure greater than 140/85 at 6 and 12 months postoperatively (compared with an average 172/114 at presentation), and these 13 were all aged over 50 (compared with an average age of 37 for all 76 patients).

REFERENCES

Allison, D.J., Brown, M.J., Jones, D.H. and Timmis, J.B. (1983). Role of venous sampling in locating a phaeochromocytoma. *British Medical Journal* **286**, 1122–1124.

Bravo E.L. and Gifford R.W., Jr. (1984). Current concepts. Pheochromocytoma: diagnosis, localization and management. *New England Journal of Medicine,* **311**, 1298–303.

Brown, M.J., Jenner, D.A., Allison, D.J., Lewis, P.J. and Dollery, C.T. (1981). Increased sensitivity and accuracy of phaeochromocytoma diagnosis achieved by use of plasma adrenaline estimations and a pentolinium suppression test. *Lancet* **i**, 174–177.

Manger, W.M. and Gifford, R.W. (1977). *Pheochromocytoma.* Springer Verlag.

Sisson J.C., Frager M.S., Valk T.W. et al (1981). Scintigraphic localization of pheochromocytoma. *New England Journal of Medicine,* **305**, 12–17.

15.28.3 Coarctation of the aorta as a cause of secondary hypertension in the adult

N. A. BOON

Although a congenital narrowing may occur at any point in the thoracic or abdominal aorta, most coarctations are found beyond the left subclavian artery and either above or just below the ductus arteriosus.

Preductal coarctation usually presents with heart failure in infancy and is commonly associated with a patent ductus arteriosus (which allows blood to enter the lower aorta from the pulmonary artery) and a variety of other cardiac defects, particularly ventricular septal defect and malformation of the mitral valve. Postductal coarctation tends to be less severe and approximately 20 per cent of cases are diagnosed for the first time in adolescents or adults.

Coarctation of the aorta is more common in males and is sometimes a feature of Noonan's and Turner's syndromes. There is a bicuspid aortic valve in at least 50 per cent of patients and this may lead to aortic valve disease in later life. The condition is also associated with cerebral artery aneurysm.

Partial obstruction of the aorta in coarctation has several important consequences. First, there is progressive elevation of the arterial pressure in the proximal vasculature. Second, a collateral circulation develops; this allows blood to enter the lower aorta from the subclavian and axillary arteries through the internal mammary, scapular, and intercostal arteries. Collateral vessels grow slowly but are usually evident after the first few years of life and may eventually become enormous. Third, there may be aneurysmal dilatation of the aorta immediately before or after the stenosis.

The pathogenesis of hypertension in coarctation involves more than simple mechanical obstruction. The exact mechanism is disputed but resetting of the baroreceptors, decreased aortic wall compliance and generalized vasoconstriction due to increased renin–angiotensin or sympathetic nervous activity have all been implicated. This may explain why the blood pressure sometimes remains high following surgical correction, particularly if this is carried out late in life.

Clinical features

PRESENTATION

In young adults coarctation of the aorta is usually asymptomatic and the first clue to the diagnosis is often the discovery of hypertension or an abnormality on a routine chest radiograph. Occasionally the condition presents with a serious complication such as infective endocarditis, which may occur at the site of the coarctation or, more commonly, on an associated bicuspid aortic valve. Cerebral haemorrhage may be due to rupture of a cerebral artery aneurysm or uncontrolled hypertension.

Older patients may present with heart failure attributable to aortic valve disease, hypertension, or premature coronary disease. Aortic dissection and aortic aneurysm are also recognized features and may reflect generalized arterial disease or intrinsic fragility of the ascending aorta. These complications account for the substantial reduction in life expectancy observed in untreated coarctation of the aorta (Fig. 1).

PHYSICAL SIGNS

Hypertension in the upper limbs is almost invariable in adults and there is often a greatly exaggerated rise in blood pressure during exercise. The lower limbs are sometimes underdeveloped and the femoral pulses are absent or weak and delayed. Occasionally there is a strong femoral pulse due to well developed collaterals, but even then it is usually possible to detect radiofemoral delay by simultaneous palpation of the radial and femoral pulses.

Collateral vessels in the back muscles are often palpable and may even be visible. The apex beat is forceful due to left ventricular hypertrophy and there may be a systolic thrill in the suprasternal area.

Auscultation may reveal an ejection systolic click if there is an associated bicuspid aortic valve, accentuation of the aortic component of the second heart sound due to hypertension, and an atrial or fourth heart sound due to the presence of left ventricular hypertrophy.

Murmurs may arise from the aortic valve, the coarctation itself, or arterial collaterals and it may be difficult to distinguish one from another. There is often an ejection systolic murmur over the base of the heart reflecting turbulence at the aortic valve, and occasionally aortic regurgitation (due to severe hypertension or associated aortic valve disease) gives rise to an early diastolic murmur at the left sternal edge. Turbulence at the coarctation produces a widespread systolic murmur that is often best heard over the back, where there may also be systolic or continuous bruits arising from the collateral vessels.

Investigations

The electrocardiogram may show left ventricular hypertrophy but is of little help in diagnosis. In contrast, the chest radiograph usually shows subtle but pathognomonic changes (Fig. 2). Dilatation of the aorta on either side of the coarctation gives the aortic knuckle a characteristic '3' configuration. Notching or erosion of the inferior margins of the posterior ribs is caused by progressive dilatation of the intercostal arteries and is usually visible in older children and adults.

Fig. 1 Comparative survival, excluding deaths in the first year of life, of the general population and patients with repaired and unrepaired coarctation of the aorta (redrawn, with permission, from Bobby *et al.* (1991)).

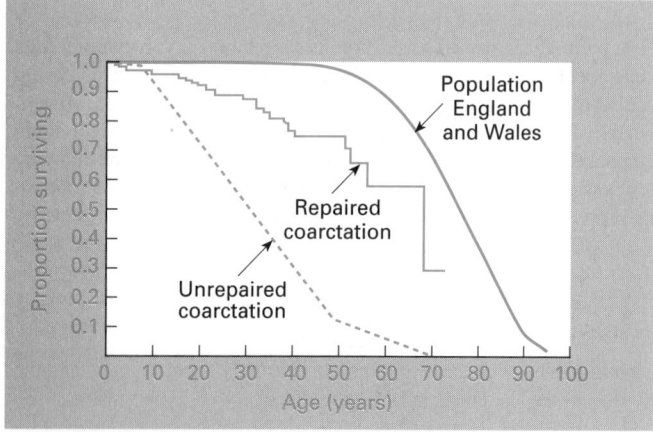

The coarctation and associated pre or post stenotic dilatation of the aorta may be visualized by two-dimensional echocardiography (from the suprasternal notch), angiography (Fig. 3), computerized tomography scanning or magnetic resonance imaging (Fig. 4). Echocardiography is also a valuable means of evaluating any associated aortic valve disease. The pressure gradient across the stenosis can be measured by Doppler echocardiography or catheterization but is critically dependent on the degree of collateral flow into the lower aorta and must therefore be

Fig. 2 Chest radiograph from a patient with hypertension and coarctation of the aorta showing an abnormal aortic knuckle (the '3' sign) and bilateral rib notching (arrowheads).

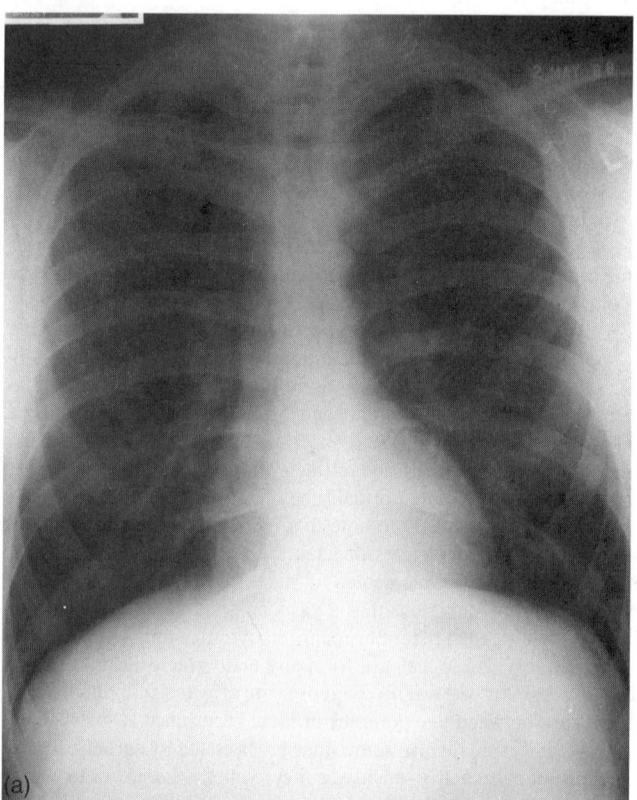

(a)

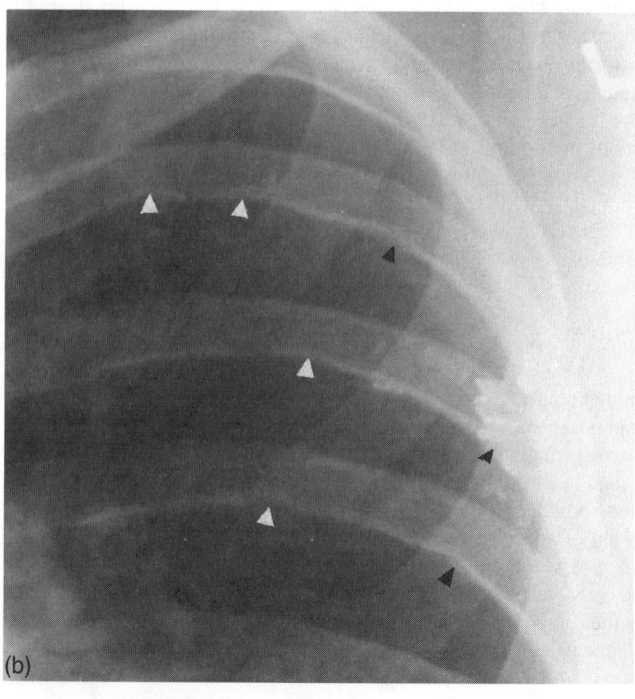

(b)

Fig. 3 Digital aortogram from an adolescent showing a typical coarctation of the aorta. (b) A later frame showing marked dilatation of the internal mammary arteries due to increased collateral flow.

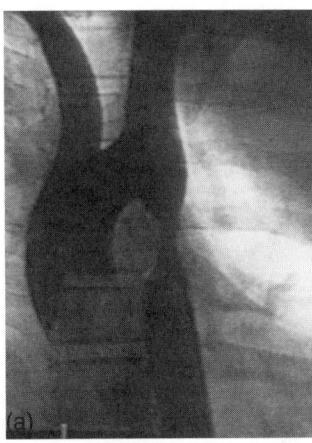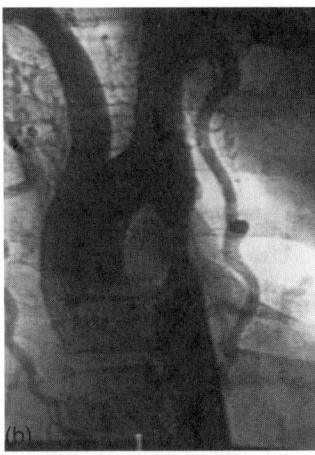

Fig. 4 Sagittal spin echo magnetic resonance image scan showing a well defined coarctation (arrow) in the typical position.

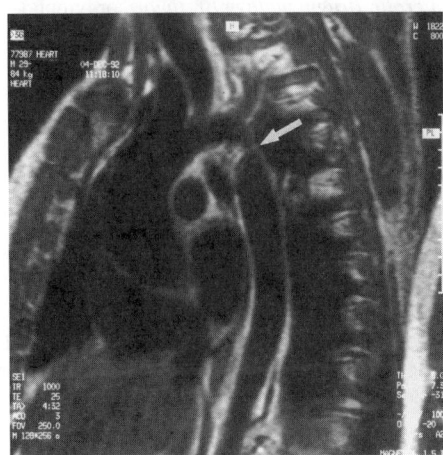

interpreted in conjunction with the relevant clinical and anatomical information.

Treatment

Surgical repair (resection with end-to-end anastomosis or subclavian flap aortoplasty) has been shown to improve life expectancy and reduce blood pressure and is usually advisable in all patients with significant coarctation. Early postoperative complications include paradoxical hypertension, mesenteric ischaemia and paraplegia due to infarction of the spinal cord. The perioperative mortality for elective surgery in adults is less than 1 or 2 per cent in most centres.

Balloon angioplasty is a safe and effective alternative treatment for both native coarctation and recoarctation. However, the long-term results of balloon dilatation are unknown and there is concern that angioplasty may be followed by a high incidence of recoarctation and aneurysm formation.

Patients who have undergone coarctation repair require careful medical surveillance because they may encounter significant cardiovascular morbidity and mortality in later life (see Fig. 1). The long-term prognosis appears to be inversely related to the extent and duration of preoperative hypertension; hence early repair is usually advisable.

Residual or recurrent hypertension is common after repair and may require drug therapy. Exercise testing is a useful means of evaluating blood pressure control in these patients. Relapse is due occasionally to recoarctation, which requires further intervention. Premature death is frequently due to rupture of an aortic or cerebral aneurysm, or heart failure (related to persistent hypertension, recoarctation, aortic valve disease, or coronary artery disease).

All patients with coarctation remain at risk of developing infective endocarditis and therefore require appropriate antibiotic prophylaxis (see Chapter 15.17).

REFERENCES

Bobby, J.J., Emami, J.M., Farmer, R.D.T., Newman, C.G.H. (1991). Operative survival and 40 year follow up of surgical repair of aortic coarctation. *British Heart Journal,* **65,** 271–276.

Campbell, M. (1970). Natural history of coarctation of the aorta. *British Heart Journal,* **32,** 633–640.

Lindsay, J. (1987). Coarctation of the aorta, bicuspid aortic valve and abnormal ascending aortic wall. *American Journal of Cardiology,* **61,** 182–184.

Nanton, M.A., Olley, P.M. (1976). Residual hypertension after coarctectomy in children. *American Journal of Cardiology,* **37,** 769–772.

Rao, P.S., Chopra, P.S. (1991). Role of balloon angioplasty in the treatment of aortic coarctation. *Annals of Thoracic Surgery,* **52,** 621–631.

15.29 Lymphoedema

J. G. G. LEDINGHAM

INTRODUCTION

On occasion, local oedema can be caused predominantly by inadequacy of lymphatic drainage of extracellular fluid. Such inadequacy may be related to hypoplasia of lymphatic vessels or to structural change related to trauma, surgery, inflammation, fibrosis, or neoplasm.

ANATOMICAL CONSIDERATIONS

Lymphatic vessels permeate the extracellular spaces of the body. The smallest of them, lymphatic capillaries, are thin-walled, blind-ended structures found especially around collecting venules. They are lined by a layer of endothelial cells with a discontinuous basement membrane. Anchoring filaments, attached laterally, probably alter the size of intercellular clefts. Vesicles within the endothelial cells probably undertake pinocytosis of proteins, macromolecules, and cell debris taken up by the highly permeable lymphatic vessels. Numbers of lymphatic capillaries from the superficial and deeper networks join to form the collecting lymphatics of larger dimension, lined also by a layer of endothelium, but now with a continuous basement membrane, a layer of smooth-muscle cells, valves retarding retrograde flow, and adrenergic innervation. Collecting lymphatics themselves merge to form larger vessels, which tend then to aggregate along veins.

The largest lymphatic trunks ultimately join either the right lymphatic duct or the thoracic duct, which empties into the junction of the jugular and subclavian veins in the thorax.

NORMAL PHYSIOLOGY

Interstitial fluid is derived from net filtration across capillary membranes, dependent on the forces described by Starling in 1896. These are the intracapillary hydrostatic pressure opposing that of the interstitial fluid, and the plasma and tissue colloid oncotic pressures. The formation of interstitial fluid is determined by these forces and by the coefficient of ultrafiltration of the relevant capillary wall. Capillary filtration pressure on the arteriolar side is regulated by the precapillary arteriolar sphincter as well as by gravitational forces, whereas on the venous side there is no such sphincter to 'protect' from high venous pressures. On passive standing therefore, arterial and venous pressures in the legs increase in parallel, so that the arteriovenous gradient is not altered; but absolute hydrostatic pressure increases according to the vertical distance of the capillary in question below the heart. The capillary pressure in the feet on quiet standing has been measured and reaches some 125 cm of water. The normal plasma oncotic pressure is some 33 cm of water. Not surprisingly, therefore, the volume of the feet increases rapidly over some 2 to 3 min on quiet standing, and after 10 to 15 min, swelling continues steadily at a rate of some 20 to 30 ml/h. The mechanisms preventing more rapid capillary transudation and therefore oedema in such a situation are threefold. Much the most important is precapillary vasoconstriction, which attenuates the rise in capillary hydrostatic pressure and may, by reducing the area of functional perfused capillaries, reduce the coefficient of ultrafiltration. Extreme ultrafiltration of the much reduced blood flow results in only modest changes in hydrostatic and oncotic pressure in the extracellular fluid, but a marked increase in intracapillary oncotic pressure. Venous blood draining a foot passively dependent for some 30 to 40 min may contain protein up to a concentration of over 9 g/l with a haematocrit as high as 52 per cent at a time when the haematocrit in the forearm venous blood is at 42 per cent. This rise in oncotic pressure, mediated in part by reduced flow, is critical to the limitation of the formation of tissue fluid. The colloid oncotic pressure depends not only on the protein concentration but also on charge and ionic strength. On quiet standing, colloid osmotic pressure may rise from around 33 to as much as 60 cm of water in 30 to 40 min. Such an increase allows local plasma oncotic pressure to balance the increased hydrostatic pressure with resultant filtration equilibrium.

A change in interstitial tissue-fluid pressure, postulated at one time to be an important factor in limiting tissue fluid formation, is no longer considered to be so. Some tissue fluid is reabsorbed at the venous end of the capillaries, but the remainder by the lymphatic system.

Increased rates of formation of tissue fluid are known to occur in dependent limbs when heat or other vasodilatory influences relax precapillary arteriolar tone; when there is fluid overload; and when venous pressure is increased by obstruction. Rates are decreased by vasoconstriction, particularly when there is a deficit of blood volume.

LYMPHATIC FLOW

Lymphatic valves resemble functionally those of the venous system. Local fluid accumulation results in considerable dilatation of the lymphatic vessels, mediated at least in part by the physical action of the attached fibrils such that distension of the extracellular fluid space pulls on the walls to increase the lumen. Although tissue-fluid formation is increased in dependent limbs, there is no corresponding increase in lymphatic flow in the absence of muscular activity. Passive or active exercise does, however, increase lymphatic flow very considerably.

The lymphatic vessels normally return some 2 to 4 litres of extracellular fluid to the circulating blood volume each 24 h, half of this coming from the splanchnic tissues. Apart from the important influence of muscular exercise on lymphatic flow, the passage of lymph within the thorax into the subclavian veins is considerably influenced by the intrathoracic pressure, with a marked increase observed to accompany hyperventilation.

Protein in lymph

Capillaries leak protein, some of which is returned to the circulation by way of lymphatic uptake and transport, while little or none is reabsorbed by way of the vascular capillaries. In the limbs at rest, lymphatics contain proteins in the concentration some 15 to 20 per cent of that in blood, an amount much reduced by exercise and increased by lymphatic obstruction.

Lymphatic oedema

Congenital lymphatic hypoplasia may induce local oedema from earliest infancy. Familial oedema (Milroy's disease), coming on at any age or in either sex but mostly at puberty and in girls, is also due to lymphatic hypoplasia, as can be demonstrated by lymphangiography. Sporadic as well as familial cases are well recognized.

Structural damage to the lymphatic systems sufficient to cause local oedema may be the consequence of neoplastic infiltration, of scarring from trauma or irradiation, or chronic lymphangitis from such infective organisms as *Wucheria bancrofti, Brugia malayi, Br. timori,* or lymphogranuloma venereum.

Obstructed lymphatic vessels dilate, rendering valves incompetent, and the walls become thickened. Stagnation of tissue fluid stimulates local interstitial inflammation and ultimately fibrosis. The swelling of lymphatic oedema is usually asymmetrical, painless, pits readily initially, and subsides at night. With time, however, fibrosis develops in the interstitial tissues of the affected limb, such that the oedema resolves much less easily with posture and becomes 'brawny' (firm and non-pitting). The skin may then become considerably thickened and pigmented. Indolent ulcers tend to develop at sites of pressure. The skin of a chronically oedematous area is abnormally susceptible to bacterial infection, particularly with the streptococcus.

Lymphatic oedema fluid contains a higher concentration of protein than is the case with the oedema of cardiac renal or hepatic origin.

TREATMENT

Treatment is unsatisfactory. The affected part should be elevated above the heart whenever possible, and at other times supported externally by firm elastic bandage or appropriate graded elastic stockings, applied after a period of postural drainage. Devices designed to massage the affected part through the night or at other times of rest can be helpful.

Prevention of skin sepsis, or its prompt treatment, are important in their own right and to prevent further lymphatic insufficiency.

REFERENCES

Kinmonth, J.B. and Taylor, G.W. (1954). The lymphatic circulation in lymphoedema. *Annals of Surgery,* **139,** 125–36.

Kinmonth, J.B. (1982). *The lymphatics,* (2nd edn). Edward Arnold, London.

Landis, E.M. (1946). Capillary permeability and factors affecting the composition of capillary filtrate. *Annals of the New York Academy of Science,* **46,** 713–31.

Michel, C.C. (1979). Fluid movement through capillary walls. In *Handbook of physiology: the cardiovascular system,* (2nd edn), Vol. IV, pp. 375–409. American Physiological Society, Washington DC.

Mortimer, P. and Regnard, C.F.B. (1986). Lymphostatic disorders. *British Medical Journal,* **293,** 347–48.

Ryan, T.J. (1989). Structure and function of lymphatics. *Journal of Investigative Dermatology,* **93,** 18–24s.

Wolfe, J.H.N. (1984). The prognosis and possible cause of severe primary lymphoedema. *Annals of the Royal College of Surgeons of England,* **66,** 251–7.

Section 16 *Intensive care*

16 Intensive care

R. D. Bradley and D. F. Treacher

Intensive care does not exist as a medical speciality. It is a form imposed upon present-day medicine by what is technically possible on the one hand and economic necessity on the other. The following account attempts to add comments upon disease from the very special point of view of its management within an intensive care unit. The experience upon which the comments rest was gained from over 20 000 patients in a single unit with very diverse commitments encompassing coronary care, pacemaking, postoperative cardiac surgical care, the haemofiltration of patients with both renal failure and circulatory problems, head injuries, respiratory failure, circulatory failure, diabetes with serious metabolic disturbance, intoxications, and major trauma including burns.

The general philosophy of the unit has been to provide the space, equipment, and staff necessary for the performance of medical as opposed to surgical operations not possible in a normal ward.

The practical management of the patients has to be a blend of the expertise of the permanent staff of the unit with that of the physicians and surgeons under whose care the patients were initially admitted to the hospital. Success depends not only upon special competence of the unit staff with the very sick, but also their ability to communicate and cooperate with the entire hospital staff.

At best, the special competence with the very sick is not merely confidence born of familiarity, but the ability to clarify situations that are often very muddled. This depends partly upon techniques for the investigation of patients who may well be deemed too sick to be investigated. A few measurements in such situations are worth a deal of conjecture.

There is a logical difficulty in the management of some very sick patients, which is not widely appreciated. The dilemma that faces the physician is that, on the one hand, diagnosis must come before treatment, and on the other that the physical signs upon which the diagnosis depends tend to disappear as the patient approaches death. A grossly hypotensive patient with an intestinal perforation may have few abnormal abdominal physical signs; partial restoration of the patient's circulation with a volume expander will restore the abdominal physical signs.

The solution to this seeming impasse depends upon arriving at a diagnosis in stages, each stage allowing some supportive manoeuvre that will not obscure the diagnosis.

Major acute derangements of the circulation

The word shock is commonly used to describe all major acute circulatory disturbances. The term has the value of brevity but little else to recommend it. It is imprecise, cannot be measured, and is applied to circulatory states that differ profoundly when analysed. The gravest disadvantage of the idea of shock as a physiological entity is the pervasive quest for some form of treatment that might be universally applicable.

The human circulation may deteriorate to the point of death in many different ways. Reversal of the process of deterioration can only be undertaken in a logical fashion if the diagnosis is known and the adjustments most likely to produce optimum performance of the circulation under those circumstances are understood.

The ensuing account describes in broad terms how the diagnosis may be pursued, and the manipulations appropriate to most acute circulatory disorders, based upon their abnormal physiology.

A systematic approach to patients with major acute circulatory dis-

turbances of an unknown nature is outlined in Figs. 1 and 2. Most of the measures and the order in which they are undertaken require no further comment. The early elimination of the possibility that the patient has a tension pneumothorax is required because the condition does not belong in either of the main groupings in the subsequent system of diagnosis. There is usually little difficulty in the diagnosis of a tension pneumothorax, provided that its existence is considered. It should be remembered that a relatively shallow pneumothorax, in the presence of emphysema, is potentially lethal and extremely difficult to diagnose from the physical signs, or the chest radiograph. With any life-threatening pneumothorax the venous pressure will appear raised.

The central venous pressure

It will be seen that assessment of the venous pressure occupies a critical position in the diagnostic scheme, and this should be measured with a catheter advanced to lie within the thorax. Introduction of the catheter through the internal jugular vein has the advantage that its position does not require radiographic confirmation. The subclavian approach carries a small risk of producing a pneumothorax.

Fig. 1 A systematic approach to patients with acute circulatory disturbances.

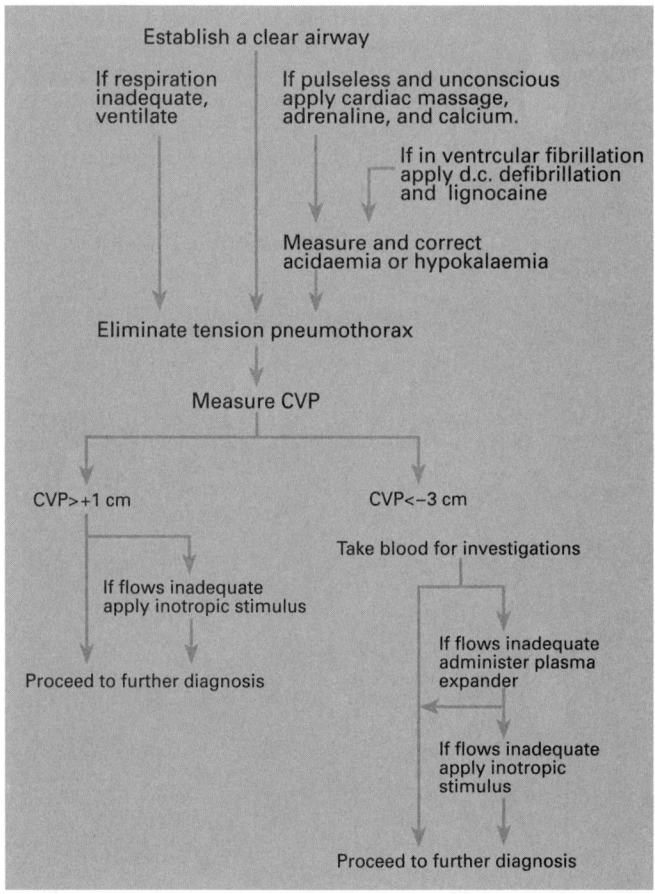

Pressures within the circulation must be measured relative to some fixed point. The sternal angle is convenient and does not pose the uncertainties of mid-chest if the patient is unable to lie flat. It is to the sternal angle that all the figures quoted in this Section are related. The range of normal venous pressures may be from $+3$ to -5 cm of water.

It is possible in practice to divide patients suffering from major acute circulatory derangements into a group with central venous pressures above $+1$ cm and a group below -3 cm. Should a patient present with an obvious profound circulatory disturbance and a filling pressure lying between the limits described above, dual pathology is the likely explanation. Acute myocardial infarction and diabetic ketoacidosis are a relatively common combination and serve as a reminder that it is possible to have heart failure without a raised venous pressure.

Once the height of the venous pressure is known, a decision has to be made in the light of the patient's condition, for if this is deteriorating there is now information upon which to base logical first-stage supportive therapy without risk of concealing the diagnosis.

In the high filling-pressure group, the rapid provision of support requires the administration of an inotropic agent that preferably should not raise systemic resistance: dopamine in doses up to 5 μg/kg per min supplemented by dobutamine, if greater dosage is required. If this regimen fails to restore a urine output of 0.5 ml/kg per hour, or if the arterial systolic pressure remains below 80 mmHg, adrenaline should be added, and the dose adjusted to between 0.01 and 0.4 μg/kg per min to produce acceptable levels of blood pressure and perfusion. If the initial level of systolic arterial pressure is less than 60 mmHg, it is likely that adrenaline will be required. In the presence of sepsis, doses as high as 7 μg/kg per min may stabilize the circulation. In cases where the heart rate is slow, the inotropic agent of choice is isoprenaline in a dose of 0.007 to 0.07 μg/kg per min.

Should supportive intervention be required at this juncture in the low filling-pressure group, blood should be taken for haematology (haemoglobin, or haematocrit, white-cell count, platelet count, blood grouping, and serum for possible cross-matching), and chemistry (electrolytes, urea, sugar, and plasma proteins). Only then should the filling pressure of the right heart be restored toward normal with a plasma expander. If a normal right-atrial pressure fails to produce an adequate circulation there must also be something amiss with the heart, and an inotropic agent should be administered in addition to the plasma expander.

Fig. 2 The approach to patients with circulatory insufficiency when the central venous pressure is low.

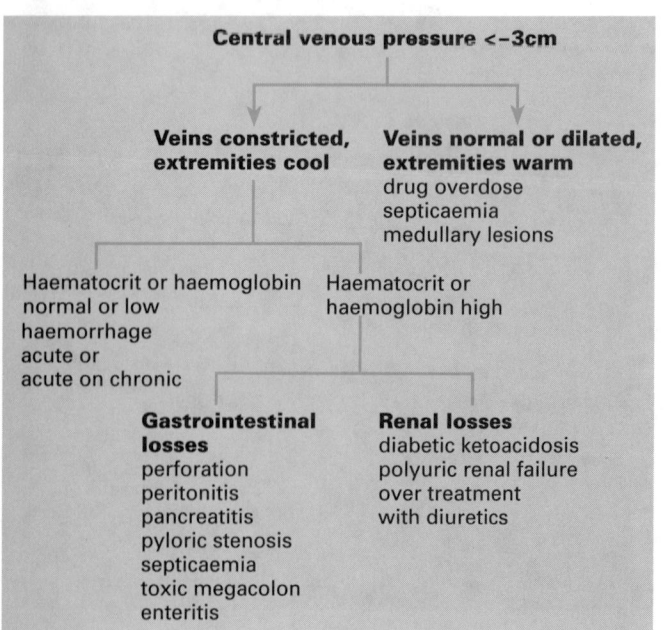

Low venous-pressure group (-3 cm or below)

Further logical separation of patients in this diagnostic group is not usually a matter of great difficulty, and depends, as is indicated in Fig. 2, on clinical observation of the state of the peripheral circulation and the haematocrit.

Low venous-pressure – low venous-tone group

If the cause of the fall in venous pressure is a drop in venous tone, as may occur in barbiturate and opiate intoxication, certain brain-stem lesions, and in some patients with septicaemia, then the limb veins will appear to be of normal calibre or even dilated, and the limbs will be of normal temperature or warmer than normal.

These patients may retain a moderate cardiac output with arterial pressures as low as 50 to 60 mmHg because the systemic resistance is also low. They may even produce urine normally when hypotensive. The general circulatory treatment, as opposed to specific treatment aimed at the cause, should be to raise the central venous pressure toward normal with a plasma expander. Restoration of a normal venous pressure in these patients will only partially restore the arterial pressure, because of the low systemic vascular resistance. Attempts to raise the arterial pressure to normal by raising the venous pressure to high positive values are a common iatrogenic cause of pulmonary oedema.

Low venous-pressure – high venous-tone group

If oligaemia is the cause of a low venous pressure, the normal vascular reflexes will produce venoconstriction and cold extremities. If the haematocrit or haemoglobin are normal, the probable cause is acute haemorrhage. Should the haematocrit be high, renal or gastrointestinal loss of fluid, electrolyes, and plasma proteins should be sought. Common causes of gastrointestinal loss of this nature are gastrointestinal perforations, peritonitis, pancreatitis, dysentery, toxic megacolon, and septicaemia. The loss may be into the lumen of the gut, the peritoneal cavity or both. Renal losses on this scale occur in diabetic ketoacidosis, the polyuric phase of acute tubular necrosis, and certain 'salt-losing' chronic renal disorders (Section 20). The diagnostic scheme just described will, of course, break down should patients having chronically severe anaemia, in becoming oligaemic by loss of salt and water, raise their low haematocrit to normal. Although the diagnosis of acute haemorrhage will be incorrect, the conclusion that the oligaemia should be treated initially with whole blood remains true.

Ideally, oligaemia should be treated by the replacement of whatever fluid has been lost. This may have to be modified by considerations such as the changes in blood viscosity that occur with oligaemia, and the changes in the circulation that may have occurred during the period of oligaemia.

Blood viscosity changes

As blood flow rate falls, viscosity rises disproportionately, and as the haematocrit increases, viscosity rises exponentially. Also it has been shown that, after injury, red-cell dispersion is abnormal for at least 3 days, perhaps because of an increase in fibrinogen levels. All of these changes increase the chance of intravascular sludging. Moderate haemodilution is probably of advantage in countering these changes. There is evidence that tissue oxygen requirements may be met by an increase in perfusion associated with the lowering of the haematocrit. The theoretical optimum level of haematocrit in the presence of poor flows may be as low as 30 per cent.

Much has been made of the microcirculatory effects of low molecular-weight dextrans, although their capacity to make any measurable difference to blood fluidity, beyond that due to dilution, has been difficult to demonstrate in the concentrations obtained clinically. These solutions are hyperosmolar and will transfer fluid from other compartments into the circulation.

Volume and rate of circulatory-fluid replacement in oligaemia

It might be thought that the volume of the replacement should equal the volume which has been lost from the circulation, and, although this is probably ultimately true, it is not a particularly helpful concept. The volume lost is not usually known, and although the remaining circulating volume can be estimated with isotopic techniques, replacements based upon measurements of volume in this way may cause serious circulatory problems. The reason for this apparent anomaly is the variability in the capacity of the vascular bed. There are few more powerfully constrictive influences upon the systemic capacity vessels than oligaemia. The events which occur in that part of the circulation during haemorrhage and transfusion can be illustrated diagrammatically. In Fig. 3, the central venous pressure is plotted on the ordinate, and the change of volume of blood in the systemic venous capacity vessels on the abscissa. Each broken line represents a line of constant venous tone (an isophleb) ranging from maximum on the left to diminished venous tone on the right. During haemorrhage, volume is lost from the venous bed, but initially the drop in venous pressure is very small as the veins constrict upon the shrinking volume; the changes are described by the line A, B, C, D, E in Fig. 3. Only latterly is there a sharp fall in the venous pressure and with it the cardiac output and arterial pressure.

In ideal circumstances during transfusion the opposite path is retraced. Events may not follow this simple course. A low cardiac output, coldness, pain, apprehension, and possibly acidaemia and hypoxia may all cause the venous system to remain tightly constricted. If the venous system remains constricted in the face of transfusion, the patient may take the path E, F, G in Fig. 3, and the venous pressure may rise to undesirably high levels before the volume of blood that was lost from the system has been replaced. The fact that the heart must generate its own blood supply causes a circulatory disturbance of a compound nature. Oligaemia and low filling pressures cause a normal heart to produce a reduced cardiac output. If these changes are gross and sustained, the impairment of coronary flow will add the complication of a failing heart with an impaired ability to generate work at any given filling pressure, especially if there is pre-existing coronary artery disease. Recognition of this compound disturbance depends upon the observation that restoration of the venous pressure to normal levels fails to restore the peripheral circulation.

Fig. 3 As blood is removed from the circulation the venous pressure falls slowly initially, but later more steeply, as the patient proceeds to lines of greater venous tone. With retransfusion the patient should follow the path EDCBA; return via EFGA may produce pulmonary oedema.

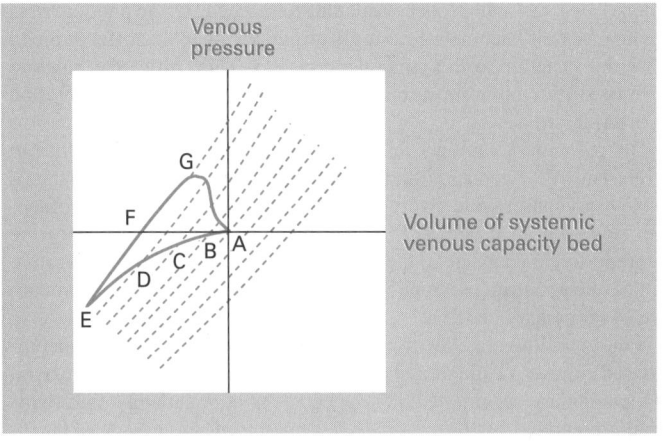

Resolution depends upon the correction of acidaemia or hypoxia, and the administration of an inotropic stimulus. Plainly inotropic drugs given during a period of coronary underperfusion may produce myocardial damage. The damage will be reduced by breaking out of this circulatory disturbance with the minimum of delay.

Where there is reason to believe that the pulmonary basement membrane has been damaged, these exclusively circulatory considerations may be forced to take second place, if the condition of the lungs is already life threatening. The principal consideration then has to be the avoidance of anything that may worsen gas exchange, and under these circumstances it may be preferable to leave the circulation underfilled, and increase the flows by the use of inotropic agents. Damage to the capillary basement membranes anywhere in the circulation causes a leakage of both water and protein at the site of damage, and this leakage is worsened by the addition of fluid of any nature. The lungs and brain are the organs in which the process is most obvious when it occurs, but it almost certainly occurs in other tissues. Once fluid has been deposited at such sites it cannot be removed until the activity of the basement membrane has been restored, because only then will the normal physical laws governing the distribution of fluid apply. Only the avoidance of fluid administration will prevent a deterioration in lung function in this situation.

High venous-pressure group (+ 1 cm or above)

The diagnosis of patients with profound circulatory disturbance in the high venous-pressure group is commonly achieved by clinical examination and inspection of the electrocardiogram and chest radiograph. In the event that it is not possible to make the diagnosis in this way or if the diagnosis requires substantiation because of the nature of the treatment to be undertaken, left and right heart catheterization and angiography are possible at the bedside within the unit. Ready availability of these facilities not only provides a lower threshold to investigation, but also allows measurements to continue to be made over a longer time course than would be possible in a catheter laboratory.

Immediate supportive measures

The immediate supportive measures available in this group are the correction of any acidaemia or hypoxaemia, positive pressure ventilation, and inotropic stimulation.

It has been shown that if all other variables are held constant the contractility of an isolated papillary-muscle preparation varies linearly with change in pH. The correction of severe degrees of acidaemia would therefore seem to be mandatory. However, recently both in vitro and animal experiments have been used to suggest that the treatment of severe acidaemia with bicarbonate is harmful. This because it causes a rise in carbon dioxide concentration and leads to an initial fall in intracellular pH, because carbon dioxide passes into the cells much more rapidly than bicarbonate.

A paradoxical intracellular acidosis was induced by this mechanism as a result of the addition of bicarbonate to platelets suspended in a bicarbonate-free buffer. Repetition of such experiments using white blood cells, which have similar systems to myocardial cells for the regulation of their intracellular pH, suspended in a more physiologically appropriate buffer system, and starting from a position of intracellular acidosis instead of the normal resting pH, produced diametrically opposite results.

The published clinical trials of bicarbonate administration do not show any adverse effect, they merely fail to show any advantage. Most concern patients with only mild to moderate metabolic disturbance, and none relates to those with extremes of circulatory disturbance. It would be formidably difficult to design a trial that might be applied to the problem of cardiac arrest.

There can be no doubt that alkalinization affects the oxygen-carrying capacity of blood adversely, and the 8.4 per cent solution of bicarbonate given in large amounts inevitably carries the penalties of a heavy sodium load and the risks of hyperosmolarity and hypernatraemia. However, there are few pharmacological agents that are not harmful if given in excess.

Nevertheless, it would be difficult for anyone who has witnessed the response of a severely acidotic, adrenaline-driven, exposed, beating heart to the administration of bicarbonate to doubt the necessity for its use in such circumstances. On the present evidence it seems unreasonable not to give bicarbonate if the pH is less than 7.1, given that underventilation, which often seems to be ignored, is dealt with as vigorously as circumstances allow.

Repeatedly in this text, it will be found that the actions required in dealing with very sick patients involve the resolution of opposing constraints. Always the solution has to centre on identifying the disturbances that are most likely to kill the patient, and the avoidance of their aggravation. The requirement to minimize hypoxia in the presence of a seriously impaired circulation needs no comment. The value of positive-pressure ventilation in low cardiac-output states has long been recognized intuitively, but there is now substantial experimental evidence, both animal and human, that circulatory performance and survival rates are both improved if the energy required for the performance of ventilation is supplied by a machine.

Diagnosis, pathological physiology, and management of patients in the high venous-pressure group

The notes that follow about the conditions in this group are peculiar to the management of these problems in an intensive care unit, but the principles can be applied without elaborate facilities for measurement.

The treatment of the acute phases of myocardial infarction with aspirin and thrombolytics in the absence of any contraindications is well accepted, and frequently takes place in the setting of the intensive care unit. Also, although angioplasties have been performed in the unit in the acute phase of myocardial infarction, the cardiac laboratory is a more appropriate place for such manoeuvres because of the quality of the radiographic screening. These topics and the management of dysrhythmias and heart block are therefore more appropriately dealt with under the heading of cardiology (Section 15).

The complications of acute myocardial infarction requiring consideration here are pulmonary oedema and impairment of cardiac output of sufficient severity to require the circulatory or ventilatory support available within an intensive care unit.

Diagnosis

In the great majority of cases this follows from the history and the electrocardiogram, and later confirmation is provided by an appropriate rise in enzymes.

Pathological physiology

The venous tone is high, and the compliance of the venous system can be measured by observing right-atrial pressure (**RAP**) change in relation to rapid removal of volume from the circulation. In acute myocardial infarction, measurements of compliance made in this way vary from 50 ml/mmHg change in RAP to 150 ml/mmHg: the least values relate in general to patients with lower values of cardiac output.

The relation between the filling pressure of the two sides of the heart and the flows generated is illustrated in Fig. 4. The equations of stroke volume versus filling pressure in the first three cases (a), (b), and (c) are of the pattern most commonly seen in acute anterior or lateral myocardial infarction. The wide separation of the equations occurs because, although both ventricles are damaged, the left ventricle is affected disproportionately.

Failure of a ventricle, or an increase in the resistance against which it ejects, will move its equation downward and to the right, and inotropic stimulation or a reduction in the resistance faced by the ventricle will move its equation upward and to the left, making the gradient steeper.

For these reasons, worsening left ventricular performance or an increase in systemic vascular resistance separates the equations of the right and left heart, and conversely worsening right ventricular function or an increase in pulmonary vascular resistance approximates the equations.

Most commonly, in acute inferior or diaphragmatic myocardial infarction, both ventricles are involved with the emphasis on right ventricular damage. This results in close approximation of the left- and right-sided equations, as shown in the examples in Fig. 4(d) and (e).

The equations shown in Fig. 4(f) are from a case of inferior myocardial infarction with papillary muscle dysfunction resulting in acute mitral regurgitation.

Systemic vascular resistance is the difference between mean arterial pressure and mean right atrial pressure in mmHg divided by the cardiac output in l/min. In a normal person this gives a value of 18 units ($(90 - 0)/5$). These are the units described by Paul Wood and can be converted into $dyn/s/cm^5$ by multiplication by 79.9. In cases of acute infarction this value may range from normal to values as high as 60 units.

Pulmonary vascular resistance is the difference between mean pulmonary artery pressure and mean left-atrial pressure in mmHg divided by the cardiac output in l/min. In a normal person this gives a value close to 1 unit ($(10 - 5)/5$). In acute myocardial infarction, the pulmonary vascular resistance may be less than normal where the left atrial pressure is high and the volume of blood in the pulmonary circuit increased. In some patients with acute infarction, who have been treated with β-blockade, the pulmonary resistance may be grossly increased to 10 or 12 units. (In the measurement of pulmonary vascular resistance it is sometimes acceptable to use pulmonary wedge pressure or left ventricular end-diastolic pressure instead of the left atrial pressure.)

Management

In any case of heart failure there are two entirely separate issues to be considered: impairment of the cardiac output and pulmonary oedema. It is important to consider them separately, for measures that improve one may make the other worse.

Pulmonary oedema

Pulmonary oedema is potentially lethal and must be treated or death will ensue from failure of ventilation due to enormous increases in the work of breathing and failure of gas exchange.

The formation of pulmonary oedema occurs as pulmonary capillary pressure rises above a critical value. The critical value is approximately $0.57 \times$ the plasma albumin level in g/l. The rate at which the oedema forms is proportional to the amount by which this value is exceeded. Once formed the rate at which pulmonary oedema will reabsorb is related principally to the amount by which the pulmonary capillary pressure is reduced below the critical value, and also partly to the level of pressure in the subclavian veins; this is because the lymphatic drainage of the lungs is into the innominate and subclavian veins.

As pulmonary capillary pressure rises, breathlessness may occur before levels that will produce oedema are reached. As the pressure rises the lung vessels become increasingly turgid, owing to a transfer of blood from the systemic to the pulmonary system. This causes the lungs to become stiffer and in most, but not all, patients produces the sensation of breathlessness.

The pulmonary capillary and left atrial pressure are likely to rise to levels that will engender pulmonary oedema when the pattern of damage to the heart causes wide divergence of the equations of ventricular function (Fig. 4(a, b, c, and f)). In the example shown in Fig. 4(b) the disproportionate damage to the left ventricle is so extreme that negative values of right atrial pressure correspond to left atrial pressures productive of pulmonary oedema.

If the equations are close together, as is commonly the case in uncomplicated inferior or diaphragmatic myocardial infarction (Fig. 4(d and e)), pulmonary oedema will not appear, even at remarkably high right-atrial pressures.

The reversal of pulmonary oedema requires that the pulmonary capillary and left atrial pressures be reduced below the critical pressure (24 mmHg if the albumin level is 42 g/l) by a sufficient margin to produce a useful rate of reabsorption. The ratio of slopes of the equations for the left and right heart determine the degree of reduction in right atrial pressure necessary to produce the required fall in left atrial pressure. In acute anterior infarction the ratio of slopes varies from the normal 2 : 1 to as high as 8 : 1. A fall in left atrial pressure of 10 mmHg will be brought about by reducing the right atrial pressure between 1 and 5 mmHg depending upon the ratio in the individual case.

The reduction in circulating volume needed to depress the right atrial pressure depends largely upon the systemic venous tone, which is raised, and, as was stated, the compliance of the system is such that removal of between 50 and 150 ml of volume are required for each mmHg fall in right atrial pressure.

Water is distributed between the plasma space and the extracellular space in a ratio dependent upon the concentration of the plasma proteins. If the protein concentration is normal, reduction of the circulating space by 100 ml implies a removal of about 450 ml from the combined plasma and extracellular spaces.

Although the pathological physiology of anterior and lateral myocardial infarction makes the complication of pulmonary oedema likely to occur, it also makes it very sensitive to treatment by the removal of relatively small volumes of salt and water, for the reasons given above.

Treatment of pulmonary oedema by removal of volume from the circulation inevitably causes a reduction in cardiac output, which in its turn may be as threatening as the original pulmonary oedema. The reduction in cardiac output occurs because the ventricles generate less work as their filling pressures are reduced and because the removal of volume from the circulation increases the resistance of the systemic and pulmonary circulations. The treatment of pulmonary oedema by infusion of solutions of either glyceryl trinitrate or sodium nitroprusside does not carry this penalty. The diminution in venous tone that they produce reduces the right and left atrial pressures and ventricular stroke work, but this is offset by a fall in systemic and pulmonary resistance and a modest increase in heart rate. The penalty is a lower arterial pressure and diminished coronary perfusion pressure; in the case of nitroprusside a consequent increased mortality has been demonstrated.

Fig. 4 (a–c) Equations of stroke volume in acute myocardial infarction showing wide separation of the equations and consequent susceptibility to pulmonary oedema. (d–e) From cases of acute inferior infarction: the relation between left and right atrial pressures preserves the patient from pulmonary oedema, and reduction of the right atrial pressure will only diminish the stroke volume. (f) Inferior infarction complicated by inferior papillary dysfunction and mitral regurgitation, producing separation of the equations similar to that seen in anterior infarction.

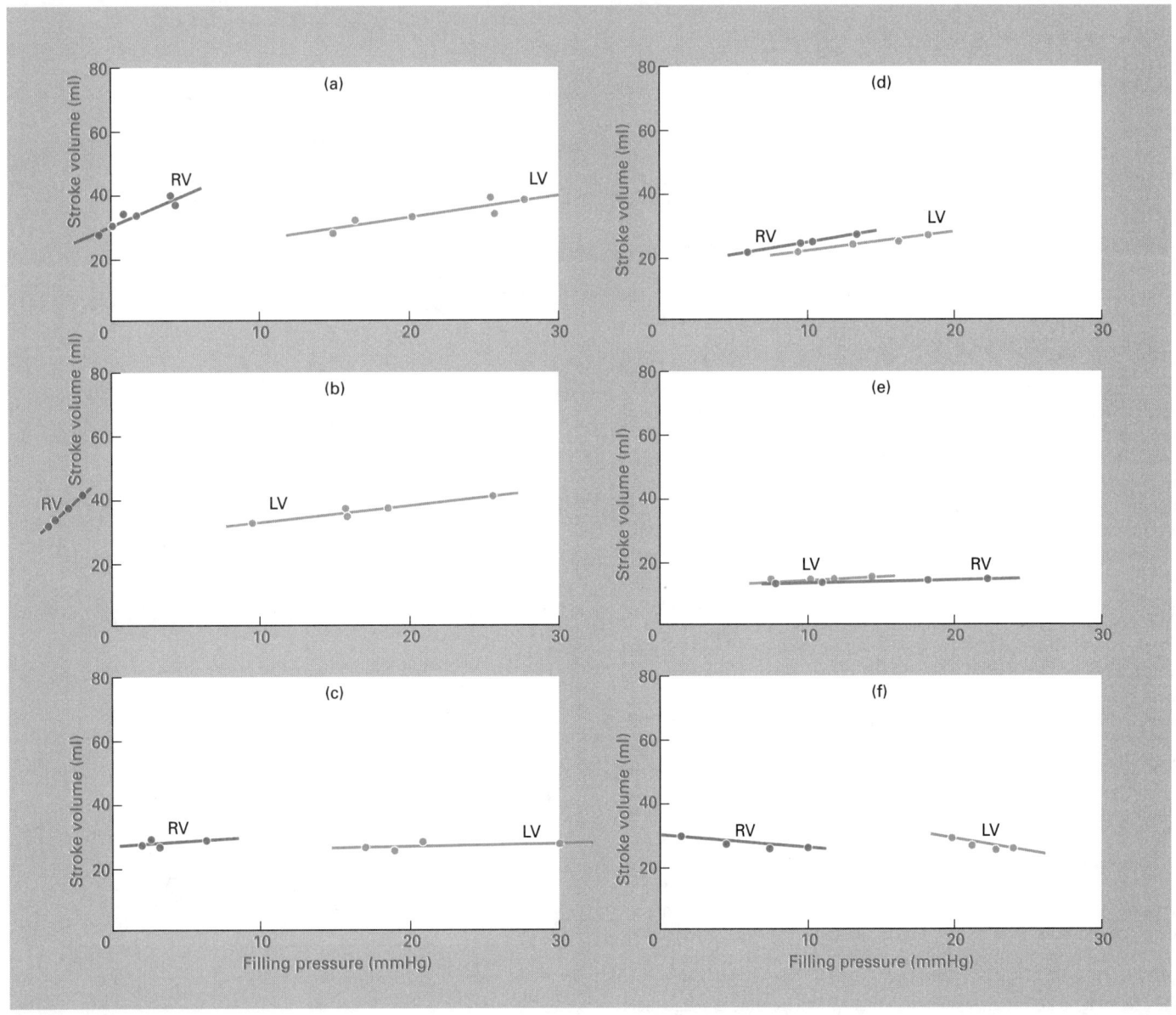

Positive-pressure ventilation and the sedation that accompanies it produce similar circulatory changes to those of sodium nitroprusside, with the reservation that the changes in pulmonary vascular resistance are variable and difficult to interpret. This approach to treatment has considerable advantage in the presence of a marginal cardiac output; the greatly increased work of ventilation no longer has to be provided by the patient. Patients with papillary muscle dysfunction (Fig. 4(f)) may be responsive to any measure that reduces left ventricular volume. The negative sloping equations of stroke volume in response to a diminution in atrial pressures seen in this case as a result of removal of volume from the circulation are only explicable either as errors of measurement or that each of the points obtained must lie on a separate equation with a positive slope, which increases as volume is removed.

Positive-pressure ventilation and sedation have certainly proved very effective in relieving the acute mitral regurgitation in these patients. The physical signs change with dramatic speed, the left atrial pressure falls and the stroke-volume equations move together again into the configuration most commonly seen in diaphragmatic myocardial infarction. Provided that the papillary muscle does not rupture, these patients can be weaned from the ventilator as their infarct matures, using vasodilators to continue the afterload reduction. It is important that they be kept relatively well sedated at the time of removal from the ventilator, in contrast to normal practice. If the papillary muscle ruptures it is sometimes possible to contain the pulmonary oedema with positive-pressure ventilation, sedation, and vasodilators. If these manoeuvres fail, the afterload reduction can be augmented by balloon counterpulsation. The aim is to support the patient for long enough from the time of infarction for surgical replacement of the mitral valve to be possible.

Impairment of cardiac output

There are five approaches to increasing a cardiac output critically impaired by myocardial infarction.

Firstly, the heart rate can be increased with atropine or with atrial pacing; the latter is more easily controlled and can be continued over many days. In practice it is found that in badly failing hearts with relatively flat performance equations, cardiac output rises linearly with heart rate up to rates just over 100/min, but diminishes at higher rates. Myocardial oxygen consumption is very closely related to the proportion of time spent in systole, and therefore to rate.

Secondly, the cardiac output can be increased by raising the filling pressures of the two sides of the heart. This is of least value when most needed, because the equations relating filling pressure to stroke volume become flatter as the damage to the ventricles increases. In the worst cases, the gain is negligible. This manoeuvre produces the most strikingly beneficial results in those whose hearts still have useful positive-sloping equations, but whose cardiac outputs have been reduced to grossly inadequate levels with diuretics. The case of inferior myocardial infarction illustrated in Fig. 5(a) has a cardiac output of 1.9 l/min at a right atrial pressure of 6 mmHg, rising to 2.4 l/min at a right atrial pressure of 13 mmHg. This very high level of right atrial pressure is tolerable because the corresponding left-sided filling pressure is 18 mmHg. The configuration of the left- and right-sided equations most commonly associated with acute inferior myocardial infarction protects them from pulmonary oedema. If there is no pulmonary oedema, treatment of a high venous pressure with diuretics is harmful because it will reduce the cardiac output. If the filling pressures of the left and right heart are raised with a plasma expander, the expansion of the systemic and pulmonary beds will also reduce their resistance. In the case of the overdiuresed, small-volume circulation this is a very important effect.

Thirdly, an inotropic stimulus may be given, which will increase the work generated by the ventricles at any given filling pressure. Examples of agents that have this action are calcium, adrenaline, isoprenaline, dopamine, dobutamine, and digoxin (Section 15). Some of these agents are more powerful than others; Fig. 5 illustrates the relative effects of digoxin and isoprenaline. It is a general truth that the worse the performance of the heart, the less its response to any inotropic agent; this is shown in Fig. 6 and relates to the fact that with increasing damage there

is less surviving muscle to respond. Acidaemia and hyperkalaemia impair the response to these agents, which all have the disadvantage that they are likely to increase the extent of an existing infarction by increasing myocardial oxygen demand.

There are some patients who, following infarction, have sufficient potentially viable myocardium to survive, but whose cardiac output and coronary perfusion are temporarily reduced to levels which will not allow that survival. This often follows an acute dysrhythmia that has either reverted spontaneously or with treatment. Inotropic agents are the only rapidly effective method of breaking out of this circle, which exists

Fig. 5 (a) The effect of digitalization contrasted with (b) stimulation with isoprenaline in patients with acute myocardial infarction. Isoprenaline produces a greater shift of the equations upwards and to the left.

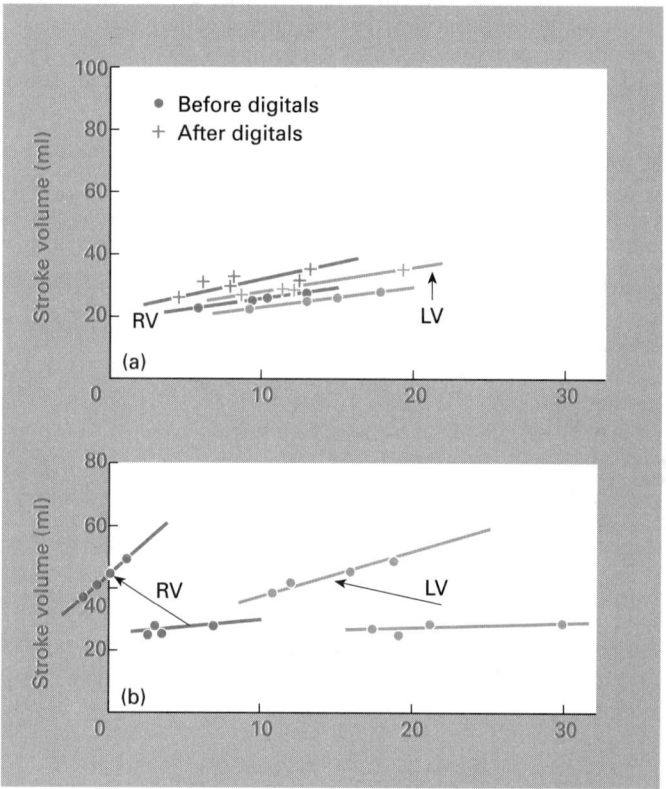

Fig. 6 With extreme impairment of function the stroke volume equations (●) are flat, so that stroke volume cannot be increased by adjustment of the filling pressures. Digitalization (○) produces no change, and isoprenaline (+) a very modest elevation of the equations.

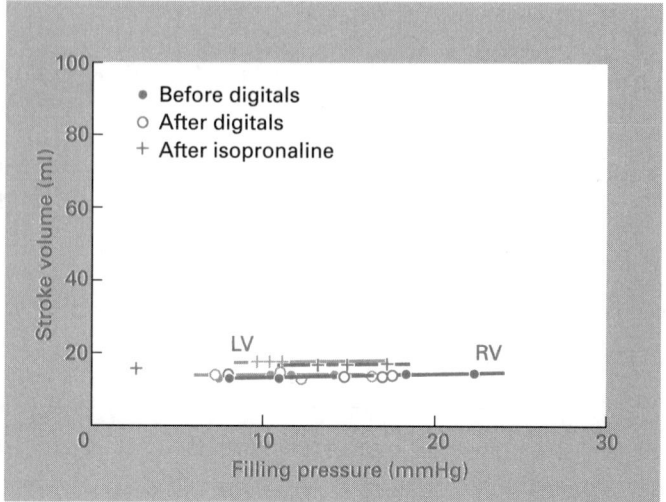

because the heart must generate its own blood supply. The inotropic agents undoubtedly cause damage, but without them the patient will not survive.

At the other extreme there are patients with insufficient heart muscle to permit survival however they are treated. Between these two groups there is an area of uncertainty where the use of inotropic agents may, in spite of their known harmful effects, prevent patients entering a cycle from which they cannot escape because of inadequate perfusion.

Fourthly, cardiac output can be increased by diminishing the resistance of the pulmonary and systemic circuits. It should be remembered that the physiological concept of increasing flows by diminishing the ventricular afterload assumes that the filling pressure of the ventricle is kept constant. If vasodilators such as sodium nitroprusside are used to increase flows in contradistinction to the control of pulmonary oedema, it should be remembered that they are also venodilators, and a plasma expander will be required to maintain the right and left atrial pressures; this combined therapy minimizes the drop in coronary perfusion pressure. As already pointed out, a volume expander will enhance the reduction of systemic and pulmonary resistance; this effect is especially marked if the resistance values are very high or where the circulating volume is small.

Sodium nitroprusside and the longer-term orally administered drugs prazosin and captopril all markedly reduce myocardial oxygen consumption, and are particularly valuable in the presence of a dilated left ventricle, their hypotensive effect being then less marked.

Fifthly, cardiac output may be increased by counterpulsation with an intra-aortic balloon. This technique might be grouped with agents operating by reduction of afterload. Like those agents it produces a marked drop in myocardial oxygen consumption, but in addition some of the energy required to drive blood around the systemic circulation is derived from the filling of the balloon. The physiological changes produced by counterpulsation both in the internal and external economy of the heart are all beneficial producing an increase of cardiac output of the order of 0.5 l/min at a considerably lower myocardial oxygen consumption. Yet the application of the technique in the field of acute myocardial infarction has been of limited value.

Experience has shown that the majority of patients suffering acute infarction who are unable to survive without counterpulsation cannot be weaned from its support. Moreover, those few with massive myocardial damage who have been supported and weaned from counterpulsation have a very limited prognosis (Section 15).

There are two relatively rare complications of acute myocardial infarction in which balloon counterpulsation is of value in supporting the patient until surgical treatment can be undertaken. These are papillary muscle rupture (already considered in this section) and rupture of the interventricular septum. Counterpulsation is effective in reducing the run-off into the left atrium or the right ventricle, and increasing the proportion of left ventricular ejection that goes to the aorta.

Massive acute pulmonary embolism (see also Section 15)

Many patients die with pulmonary emboli present in their lungs, but relatively few die due to pulmonary embolism. The incidence of life-threatening embolism is relatively small.

DIAGNOSIS

The diagnosis of pulmonary embolism can only be made with certainty by pulmonary angiography. Isotopic scanning techniques may be suggestive of the diagnosis but do not offer the degree of certainty necessary before embolectomy can be undertaken.

Pulmonary angiography can be accomplished very rapidly at the bedside using a portable image intensifier and a video-recording system. Catheterization of the pulmonary artery through a sheath placed in the internal jugular vein by Seldinger's technique has the advantage of ease of manipulation of the catheter to the pulmonary artery, compared to the more conventional approach through the femoral vein, which may harbour a further clot.

PATHOLOGICAL PHYSIOLOGY

The venous tone is very greatly raised, probably as a response to the gross impairment of cardiac output. The compliance of the system may be as little as 30 ml volume change/mmHg-change in the right atrial pressure.

The relation between the filling pressure of the two sides of the heart and the flows generated is illustrated in Fig. 7. A considerably raised pulmonary vascular resistance and a reduction in right ventricular stroke work in relation to filling pressure conspire to move the right ventricular equation relating stroke volume to filling pressure so far downward and to the right from its normal position that it moves through the left ventricular equation and comes to lie upon its far side. This has consequences of the greatest importance.

The depression of right ventricular stroke work is related to an acute change in ventricular diameter that interferes with the generation of tension in the wall of the ventricle in a manner which might be expected from the application of Laplace's law.

The pulmonary vascular resistance in the presence of an acute life-threatening pulmonary embolus is usually in the range 12 to 16 units. Higher values up to 25 units can be sustained with chronic, packed pulmonary emboli because the right ventricle is hypertrophic.

The systemic vascular resistance is raised to values between 25 and 50 units, with the result that the systemic arterial pressure is better preserved than the cardiac output. The fact that the blood pressure may be only moderately reduced should not militate against the diagnosis nor should it be allowed to engender a false sense of security.

The doubling of systemic resistance is a reflex response probably triggered by the very considerable impairment of cardiac output. There is some evidence that the increase in pulmonary resistance to values over 10 times normal is in part reflexly engendered, and not entirely related to obstruction of the vessels by emboli.

MANAGEMENT

There is evidence that the administration of heparin (15 000 u intravenously) acts to reverse that part of the rise in pulmonary vascular resistance due to vasospasm, and heparinization is logical to prevent further clot formation.

Patients with acute pulmonary embolism in whom the right atrial

Fig. 7 The equations of stroke volume in acute pulmonary embolism are laterally transposed.

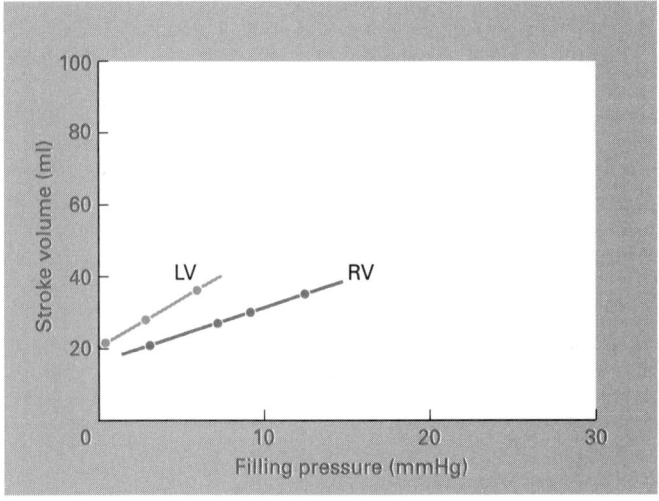

pressure is found to be in excess of 15 mmHg are in an unstable circulatory state that can only be controlled with sufficient rapidity by pulmonary embolectomy. Provided that cardiopulmonary bypass can be instituted before cardiac arrest occurs, there is a very good chance of success.

The threat to life in massive pulmonary embolism depends upon the reduction of cardiac output that follows obstruction of the pulmonary circulation, and the circulation can be manipulated to diminish the degree of obstruction without surgical removal of the embolus. The essence of this manipulation is the expansion of the remaining pulmonary vascular bed with a volume expander such as plasma. This manoeuvre will reduce considerably the very high pulmonary vascular resistance that is the central problem. Two effects are involved: the raising of the right atrial pressure from 3 to 12 or 15 mmHg increases the work output of the right heart (see Fig. 8), and, more importantly, distribution of some of the administered plasma into the pulmonary circulation reduces the pulmonary vascular resistance by as much as one-half. As will be seen from Fig. 7 the elevation of right atrial pressure produces a considerable increase in cardiac output without the production of pulmonary oedema because the left atrial pressure is very much lower than the right. Oedema may subsequently appear when flow is restored, in that part of the pulmonary circulation which was obstructed. This is probably due to damage to the basement membrane, for it occurs at low pulmonary capillary pressures.

The administration of inotropic agents will increase the work output of the heart and improve flows. Their use increases the importance of minimizing hypoxaemia and acidaemia. Digitalization is a valuable insurance against the appearance of atrial flutter or fibrillation, which are common in pulmonary embolism.

Volume expansion, inotropic stimulation, and oxygen may be sufficient to stabilize the patient's circulation whilst the natural process of thrombolysis takes place. Where there is no risk of provoking haemorrhage the thrombolytic process can be accelerated with streptokinase or urokinase. When taking the decision to use these thrombolytic agents, it should be remembered that there is no evidence that they increase survival. The existing evidence only shows an increased rate of clearance of clot demonstrated by angiography.

Equally important in the management of these patients is the avoidance of measures having the opposite physiological effects. Sedation, diuretics, haemorrhage, the induction of anaesthesia, vena caval ligation, and the administration of contrast material during angiography may all precipitate the patient's death by reducing the right atrial pressure. The sequence of events is as follows: the fall in right atrial pressure decreases the stroke volume pumped into the lungs; the matching fall in stroke volume from the left heart only occurs when there has been a net transfer of blood out of the pulmonary circulation, causing the left atrial pressure

to fall. The loss of volume from the pulmonary bed causes a further sharp rise in its resistance, which, with the diminished right-ventricular stroke work, still further reduces the right ventricular output. Unless this chain of events is interrupted it must end in circulatory arrest. The changes can be prevented by maintaining the right atrial pressure with volume expanders and the stimulation of venous tone with α-agonists such as phenylephrine. For similar reasons it is important to avoid drugs that have a negative inotropic effect, including those that reduce the patient's own catechol secretion.

The measures described above do not detract from the need for heparinization and venous ligation to diminish the chances of further embolization.

Cardiac tamponade (see also Section 15)

The critical physiological disturbance that appears with tamponade is impairment of cardiac output by interference with the filling of the heart.

DIAGNOSIS

The clinical physical signs of restlessness, oliguria, breathlessness, and hypotension stem from the diminished cardiac output. The systolic descent in the venous pressure is due to a fall in pressure in the pericardial sac at the time of ventricular ejection. Pulsus paradoxus, which is not paradoxical but an exaggeration of a normal phenomenon, when it appears in tamponade, is principally due to failure of transmission of the intrathoracic pressure swings to the left atrium. During inspiration the fall in intrathoracic pressure is transmitted to the pulmonary veins; if this fall is not also transmitted to the left atrium it will produce a diminution in the effective filling pressure of the left heart, and a fall in arterial pressure. The absence of pulsus paradoxus does not exclude the presence of tamponade; neither does the presence of a pericardial rub exclude a large pericardial effusion.

Echocardiographic confirmation of a pericardial effusion, although usually correct, is not always so, whereas a right atrial angiogram is a definitive investigation if the patient has a large enough pericardial volume to produce tamponade.

PATHOLOGICAL PHYSIOLOGY

The venous tone is high. The equations of function of the left and right heart move together and eventually are coincident as tamponade worsens, and the systemic vascular resistance is high.

MANAGEMENT

Until the effusion is drained, cardiac output can only be sustained by maintaining high right and left atrial pressures. In the limiting case these may both be as high as 15 mmHg.

The safety of the procedure of tapping the pericardium has been much enhanced by not attempting to drain the fluid through the needle with which the puncture is made, but by replacing the needle with a soft catheter over a Seldinger guidewire. The catheter should have multiple side holes, and it is possible by the use of dilators and sleeves in conjunction with the Seldinger guidewire to introduce a drain of appreciable size.

If because of clotting it is impossible to remove the pericardial fluid in the above manner, or if it is probable that an actively bleeding vessel requires to be controlled, a surgical approach is necessary.

Overtransfusion (see also Section 22)

The critical lesion that appears in overtransfusion is pulmonary oedema. The diagnosis depends principally upon the realization that sufficient fluid may have been administered.

Fig. 8 The equations of stroke work in acute pulmonary embolism.

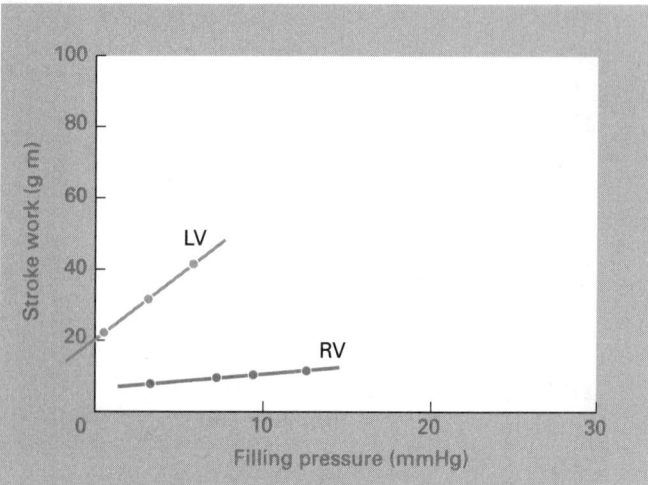

PATHOLOGICAL PHYSIOLOGY

Initially the circulation may be characterized as follows:

1. The venous tone is low and the compliance of the system may be as great as 300 to 350 ml volume change/mmHg right-atrial pressure change. The venous pressure is moderately raised in spite of this because of the very large circulating volume.
2. The equations of function of the two sides of the heart are normal (Fig. 9) and the cardiac output greatly raised in response to the raised filling pressures.
3. The pulmonary and systemic vascular resistance are reduced.
4. The rate at which pulmonary oedema appears in the lungs is proportional to the amount by which the critical pulmonary capillary pressure has been exceeded. The critical pulmonary capillary pressure is related to albumin concentration (0.57 × plasma albumin in g/l), which may well have been greatly reduced, depending upon the nature of the transfusional insult.

If the pulmonary oedema is allowed to accumulate unchecked this pattern changes so that the venous tone rises, driving the right atrial pressure to values as high as 25 mmHg, and the equations of function of both sides of the heart move towards those of extreme failure (Fig. 10) and the cardiac output dwindles from its previous elevated levels to grossly impaired values.

MANAGEMENT

In the initial phase described, the pulmonary oedema will probably be brought under control by lowering the left atrial pressure by 12 mmHg. The relative slopes of the equations of a normal heart imply that this will be achieved by a fall of half this magnitude in the right atrial pressure. The compliance of the system is such that this will entail removal of approximately 2 litres from the circulation. If the distribution of fluid between the circulation and extracellular space were normal this would necessitate the removal of as much as 6 or 7 litres of fluid from the combined spaces. A diuresis of this size takes time to accomplish, and for this reason if the situation is threatening, rapid control can be obtained by removing 1.5 to 2 litres of blood from the circulation. This can be stored in order that the red cells and albumin can be returned to the patient as the matter is brought in hand by diuresis. The volume and nature of the fluid to be removed and its distribution between the body compartments will vary with the nature of the infused fluid that caused the problem.

If the insult has reached the physiological stage at which the right atrial pressure is inordinately high, the patient should be ventilated, inotropic agents infused, and the left-sided filling pressure (pulmonary wedge pressure or left ventricular end-diastolic pressure) controlled by circulatory volume adjustment at a level that will allow the reabsorption of the pulmonary oedema.

The circulatory failure associated with obstructive airways disease (see also Section 17)

The term cor pulmonale is not used because this may be taken to include pulmonary embolism, which creates a different pattern of physiological disturbance.

The critical lesion in asthma and chronic bronchitis is obstruction of the airways and adjustment of the circulation should be directed toward relief of the obstruction.

DIAGNOSIS

The diagnosis is made from the obvious physical signs of obstructive airways disease in the presence of a raised arterial carbon dioxide tension and lowered arterial oxygen tension, whilst the patient is breathing air.

PATHOLOGICAL PHYSIOLOGY

Patients in a stable circulatory state with obstructive airways disease show the following features:

1. The venous tone is very much less raised than in severe pulmonary embolism, the compliance of the system being of the order 150 ml volume change/mmHg change in right atrial pressure. The raised venous pressure is principally due to water and salt retention. This contrast with acute pulmonary embolism may relate to the passage of sufficient time to allow the water retention to occur.
2. The important features of the performance of the heart in obstructive airway disease are illustrated by the equations in

Fig. 9 Equations of stroke volume in relation to filling pressure for the left and right heart of a patient with a normal heart.

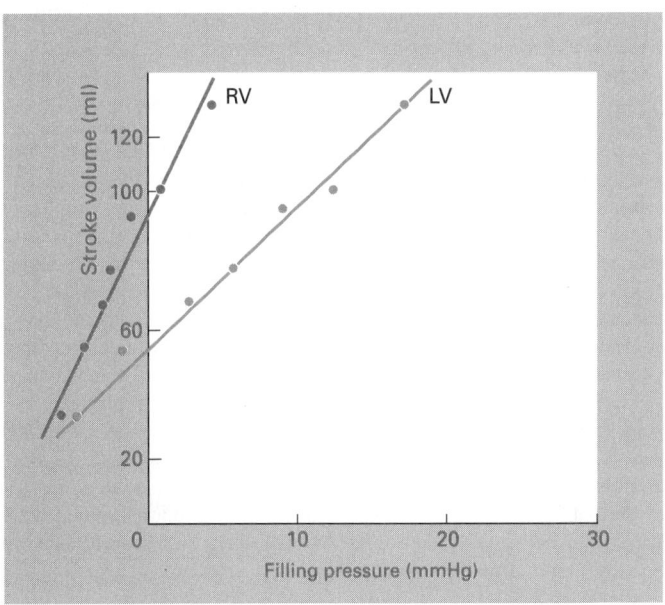

Fig. 10 Stroke volume equations of a case of extreme pump failure compared with those of a normal heart.

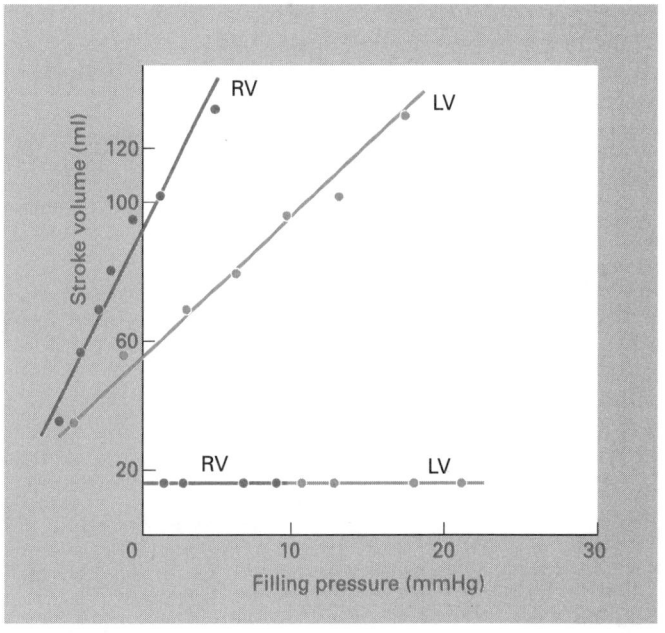

Figs. 11 and 12. In contrast to pulmonary embolism the cardiac output generated is normal or raised, depending upon filling pressure. The equations of stroke volume of the right and left heart are moved into close apposition. That of the right heart is moved to the right by the combined influences of a raised pulmonary vascular resistance and right ventricular dilation and that of the left heart is moved to the left by a lower than normal systemic vascular resistance. The consequences of these changes are a relatively good cardiac output and immunity from pulmonary oedema over a wide range of filling pressures.

3. The pulmonary vascular resistance is moderately elevated to values of the order four to eight times normal, and the systemic resistance reduced (14 to 16 units), perhaps due to hypercapnia.

The above circulatory state may be destabilized by a number of events, which are probably most commonly precipitated by extremes of hypoxaemia. The obvious signal that the patient has entered this unstable state and is likely to die within a few hours is coldness of the limbs.

Fig. 11 Equations of stroke volume in a case of severe chronic bronchitis. Corresponding values of atrial pressure are close together due to the coincidence of a raised pulmonary vascular resistance (PVR 4 u) and a low systemic resistance (SVR 15 u), in the presence of normal stroke-work equations (Fig. 12) for both sides of the heart. The important difference between this patient and cases of pulmonary embolism is the very much higher values of stroke volume.

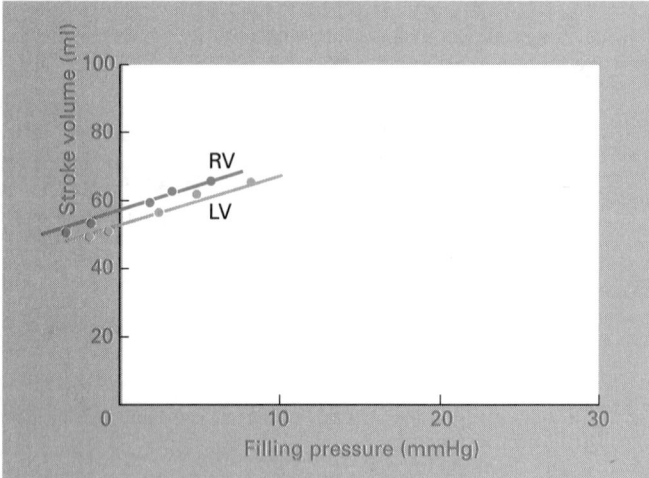

Fig. 12 The stroke-work equations for the left and right heart of a patient with severe chronic bronchitis.

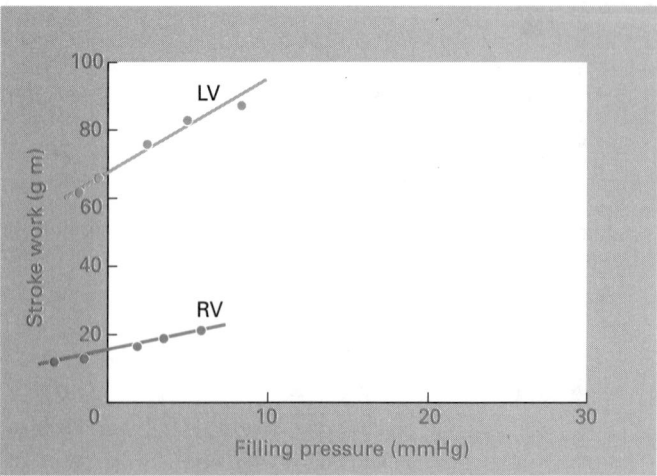

The physiological nature of this change is that terminally the patient's heart is failing and its equations of performance are falling.

MANAGEMENT

In the stable state described above, the optimal conditions are achieved by reducing the patient's atrial pressures to values around zero. Although cardiac output will be less at these values than at the naturally occurring values of between 5 and 10 mmHg, circulatory flows are not the major problem, and the airway obstruction, which is critical, is improved by reducing the atrial pressures. The improvement in airway resistance may be due to a reduction of the pressure in the system into which the lymphatics from the bronchial mucosa drain.

The relative compliance of the venous system, and the distribution of the retained salt and water, imply that a relatively large diuresis is required; − 3.5 l to lower the right atrial pressure by 7 mmHg.

The avoidance of treating such patients with high concentrations of oxygen in the inspired air in order to preserve their ventilatory drive has been greatly stressed. It is no less important to avoid the extremes of hypoxaemia, which, by raising pulmonary vascular resistance and depressing ventricular function, are likely to induce the unstable circulatory state discussed above. Once the patient enters this cycle of depression of cardiac function, evidenced by coldness of the limbs, reversal of the trend can only be induced by positive-pressure ventilation and inotropic stimulation. The decision to adopt such measures must depend upon judgements of the degree of reversibility of the patient's airway disease.

The artificial ventilation of patients with airway obstruction of this degree presents special difficulties essentially because any further rise in functional residual capacity of the lungs produces a sharp rise in pulmonary vascular resistance. This will be discussed in the section of this chapter dealing with positive-pressure ventilation.

Septicaemia and the circulation

The most important feature of circulatory derangement due to sepsis is the intense variability of the nature of the disturbances produced, not only between different patients but often in the same patient as a function of time. Therapy that is at one moment beneficial may become harmful, and logical treatment can only be applied upon a background of continuing analysis of the circulation.

DIAGNOSIS

The diagnosis should be suggested by the occurrence of hypotension in the presence of any infective process (see Section 7).

PATHOLOGICAL PHYSIOLOGY (SEE ALSO CHAPTER 7.5)

The venous pressure is determined by the interaction of the venous tone and the volume contained within the circulation, and in the presence of sepsis the venous tone may be abnormally high or low, the compliance of the system may be as little as 50 ml or as great as 350 ml volume change/mmHg change in right atrial pressure. Similarly the circulating volume may be disturbed in either direction. Oligaemia may be produced by the loss of fluid containing albumin into the peritoneal cavity or distended loops of bowel. Oliguric renal failure and over-generous intravenous therapy are common causes of an opposite volume change.

The heart may be normal or may fail in the sense that it produces less work from both ventricles in relation to their filling pressure. A normal ventricle will show a moderate diminution in stroke work in response to afterload reduction, but the impairment of stroke work seen in many of the patients with sepsis has been massive. In contrast, others with sepsis in whom the systemic vascular resistance has been reduced to one-third of normal have retained normal stroke-work equations. It seems reasonable to conclude that in some the heart muscle is affected, and in others not. This assessment is the only arbiter of heart failure in these circumstances; the significance of the venous pressure is often in doubt because of the many influences described.

The systemic vascular resistance may be as low as 2 units or may be considerably raised, and the pulmonary vascular resistance may be altered in either direction.

The venous tone and systemic vascular resistance do usually vary in the same direction, and when both are raised in association with depressed ventricular stroke work, produce all the accepted physical signs of heart failure: a high venous pressure, deficient cardiac output, and sometimes a high enough left atrial pressure to generate pulmonary oedema.

The fact that the heart is failing may be obscured where deficient ventricular function is associated with a low venous tone and systemic vascular resistance, because the venous pressure is not raised and the cardiac output may be as high as 10 or 12 l/min. These relatively high flows are generated by a defective heart because the resistance to flow may be as little as one-tenth of normal.

Pulmonary oedema may occur in sepsis because of a raised left atrial and pulmonary capillary pressure, or because of damage to the capillary basement membrane in which case the oedema appears at normal pulmonary capillary pressures and has a protein content approximating to that of the plasma. Very commonly, pulmonary oedema is iatrogenic, stemming from unavailing attempts to restore the arterial blood pressure to normal in the face of a grossly reduced systemic vascular resistance.

Perhaps the most bizarre of all the unpredictable changes observable in the presence of sepsis is the breakdown of the normal distribution of blood flow to individual organs. Aortography of a patient with sepsis showed the vessels of the coeliac axis and the renal arteries to be so constricted that they did not fill with contrast medium in spite of a seemingly more than adequate cardiac output of 7 l/min. The patient was anuric at the time of the investigation, and at autopsy all the vessels in question appeared normally patent. These focal abnormalities of distribution of flow can be observed to change very much with time, and are perhaps responsible for the generation of severe degrees of metabolic acidosis that appear in sepsis in the presence of more than adequate values of cardiac output.

Any of these changes may be further compounded by the appearance of a consumptive coagulopathy.

MANAGEMENT (SEE ALSO SECTION 7)

The one therapeutic manoeuvre of unequivocal value is the administration of appropriate antibiotics in adequate dosage without delay. Delay is important because of the rate at which bacteria multiply; it may be much reduced if a stock of blood culture medium is readily available.

Life-threatening septicaemia may be due to a single organism, as is commonly the case with pneumococcal, meningococcal, streptococcal, and staphylococcal infections. If these are strongly suspected or proven, treatment with a single, appropriate antibiotic is allowable. This is not the case with septicaemias secondary to intestinal perforations, where, although blood cultures may yield a single organism, there are likely to be multiple organisms and contamination of the circulation is likely to be continued. It is illogical to accept that failure to grow an organism excludes its presence; anaerobic organisms were the cause of septicaemia before techniques were available for their culture.

In the absence of a clear indication that a single organism is involved, broad-spectrum antibiotic cover is required and should only be changed if an insensitive organism is grown. Negative blood cultures are not a logical reason for changing or stopping antibiotic therapy in a patient with the circulatory hallmarks of sepsis; rather they are an indication of some measure of control being achieved with the existing therapy.

Oligaemia due to loss of protein-containing fluid from the circulation is best treated with plasma, but the addition of any fluid to the circulation has to be tentative until it is clear this is not causing lung function to deteriorate. A worsening of gas exchange in these circumstances suggests that the pulmonary basement membrane is leaking. Under these circumstances it is apparently less damaging to the lungs to maintain the pressures and flows in the circulation by using the vasoconstrictive and inotropic properties of adrenaline. It is difficult to understand why the maintenance of similar pulmonary pressures with volume loading should be more harmful to the lungs.

It is very important to realize that once the lungs are no longer abnormally leaky, the volume deficit that has been masked by adrenaline will have to be replaced.

Heart failure manifested by an inability to generate normal amounts of work in relation to filling pressure is very commonly present in severe sepsis, and is best treated with inotropic agents. It goes unrecognized clinically because the venous pressure may not be raised, for the reasons already discussed. If, as is most frequently the case, the sepsis has also caused a major reduction in the systemic vascular resistance, an inotropic agent that will raise the resistance (adrenaline) should be used. In the rare cases where the systemic resistance is found to be raised, then an inotropic agent that is also a dilator (such as dobutamine) should be used. Dopamine in doses up to 5 µg/kg per min is a useful adjunct to either of these strategies, for the support of renal function, as well as its inotropic effect. Where adrenaline is the appropriate choice, the rate of intravenous infusion is adjusted to provide a mean arterial pressure in excess of 75 mmHg, and the range of dosage (0.07 to 7 µg/kg per min) that has been found to be effective in these circumstances is very much greater than in any other situation.

Noradrenaline has no inotropic effect; it is purely a vasoconstrictor. Its use in sepsis must be confined to patients whose hearts are still able to generate normal amounts of work in relation to filling pressure, but who have a grossly reduced systemic resistance. In contrast to its action in a normal individual, by raising the systemic vascular resistance from perhaps one-third of normal to half normal values, noradrenaline can restore urine flow and perfusion of the extremities. Noradrenaline in the presence of poor cardiac performance produces disastrous failure of perfusion with massive necrosis of the extremities.

There is much current enthusiasm for increasing oxygen delivery to the tissues by expanding the circulation. This will only be effective if the function of the heart remains sufficiently good that it will respond to a rise in filling pressure, and also if the fluid load in the presence of a potentially leaking pulmonary basement membrane does not nullify the whole process by interfering with gas exchange.

Renal failure requiring support by haemofiltration may well add to the problems of those with profound circulatory disturbance associated with sepsis. It is important that those who also have a lactic acidosis or who are unable to metabolize the lactate provided as the buffer in commercially available replacement fluids should be given a fluid buffered with bicarbonate instead.

Corticosteroids in high dosage were said to improve the distribution of blood flow, and to stabilize damaged capillary endothelia, reducing leakage of plasma from the vascular compartment. A large, multicentre, double-blind, randomized trial showed steroids to be of no benefit, and to be associated with a higher mortality in the syndrome of severe circulatory derangement due to sepsis. Provided that the atrial pressures are controlled, steroids have no effect on cardiac output, systemic vascular resistance or arterial pressure. On the present evidence, corticosteroids should not be used in this condition.

The theoretical advantages of using anticytokine agents such as centoxin suggest that these should have made a very considerable impact on the treatment of serious sepsis, inasmuch as they ought to deal in an absolutely specific way with the damaging effects of such infection. It is therefore very surprising that the results of the trials that have so far been published have not yielded very much more clearly favourable results. Nevertheless, in the present state of knowledge, centoxin administration is probably mandatory in cases of meningococcal septicaemia. It is very important that the use of centoxin apparently makes no difference in nature or amount to the requirements for circulatory support that have already been described. In those who are seriously compromised with sepsis that has a high probability of being due to Gramnegative organisms, and who have failed to respond to the other measures, the use of centoxin is debatable and has to be further evaluated.

Acute dissections of the thoracic aorta (see also Section 15)

The important possible circulatory consequences of aortic dissection are obstruction of any of the branches of the aorta, aortic regurgitation, and haemorrhage into the pleural or pericardial space; the last may result in cardiac tamponade.

DIAGNOSIS

The history of a sudden agonizing pain in the chest or abdomen may be associated with symptoms or signs relating to obstruction of any of the aortic branches. The chest radiograph may show a widened mediastinal shadow or pleural effusion, but definitive diagnosis depends upon transoesophageal echocardiography, CT scanning, or aortic angiography. The last of these has the advantage that it may reveal the site of origin of the intimal tear. Angiography is possible with relatively little disturbance to a well-sedated patient, as a bedside manoeuvre. Catheterization of the true aortic lumen may entail the use of unusual approach sites such as the axillary arteries, and confirmation that the catheter lies in the true aortic lumen depends upon retrograde passage across the aortic valve to the left ventricle (Fig. 13).

PATHOLOGICAL PHYSIOLOGY

The angular shearing forces that act to extend an existing fault or tear in the aortic lining are related to the wavelength of the harmonics that go to make up the pressure pulse propagated along the aorta by the heart. The shorter the tear and the greater the length of the pulse wave the less likely it becomes that the tear will extend.

MANAGEMENT

Medical treatment is directed toward control of the hypertension that is so often an antecedent factor in the causation of aortic dissection, and the attenuation of the pulse wave by interference with the rate of ventricular ejection by β-blockade. The trials of medical treatment suggest

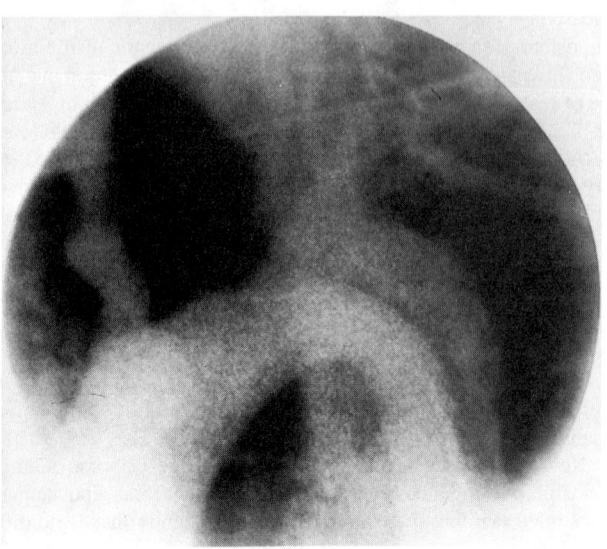

Fig. 13 Aortic angiogram of an acute aortic dissection obtained with portable equipment at the bedside.

that the systolic arterial pressure should be reduced to 100 mmHg, provided the patient continues to pass more than 30 ml urine per hour.

Intense β-blockade with propranolol and hypotensive agents that are effective in the recumbent posture provoke water and salt retention, which in turn may make control of the hypertension more difficult. Minoxidil may achieve control when other agents fail but is particularly prone to produce fluid retention. Physical considerations suggest that depression of the rate of ventricular ejection is the most important factor.

A recent trial of medical and surgical treatment demonstrated that, for dissections originating in the ascending aorta, surgical treatment had a considerable advantage. For aortic dissections originating in the region of the left subclavian artery, medical and surgical treatment offered a very similar mortality. Failure of perfusion of a major organ or limb is always an indication for a surgical approach.

Adult respiratory distress syndrome (see also Section 17)

The term 'adult respiratory distress syndrome' (**ARDS**) implies a diffuse lung injury caused by a variety of different underlying conditions and characterized by shortness of breath, tachypnoea, hypoxaemia, impaired lung compliance, pulmonary hypertension, and infiltrates seen on the chest radiograph. Because it has many causes, the most common of which are shown in Table 1, the statement that a patient has ARDS is not a particularly useful diagnostic label as it does not describe the primary underlying pathology and cannot therefore predict the appropriate treatment, or management, or the prognosis. In these regards it is no more specific than the phenomenon of disseminated intravascular coagulation: it might have been less misleading if Ashbaugh and Petty had used a less grandiose label such as 'the leaky lung syndrome'. Furthermore, the defining constellation of symptoms, signs, and physiological derangements is similar to that found in both atypical pneumonia and pulmonary oedema and it may be difficult to make the distinction. Although the term is now entrenched in the literature, it is very important for the clinician to remember that nothing specific with regard to either treatment or prognosis has been achieved by bestowing this label.

The reason for the similar clinical and pathophysiological picture produced by the many different causes of ARDS is that the lung has a limited number of responses to injury. The damage starts at either the alveolar epithelium, as with inhalational injury, or at the pulmonary capillary endothelium, as in the indirect or blood-borne causes. Wherever the primary insult occurs the capillary and endothelial cell linings and their basement membranes are damaged, resulting in the development of oedema and the passage of proteins and cells into the interstitial and alveolar spaces at normal pulmonary capillary hydrostatic pressures. Measurement of the left atrial or 'wedge' pressure may be necessary, but the distinction from hydraulic pulmonary oedema may prove more difficult in practice, due to the timing of the measurement. A patient with symptoms and signs compatible with ARDS, but which were in reality generated by an elevated left-atrial pressure, may already have received treatment effective in lowering the left atrial pressure by the time the measurement is made, allowing the erroneous supposition that the patient has non-hydraulic oedema. Time and observation are of the essence in this situation, because if the left atrial pressure remains normal, the patient will improve and the radiographic changes will resolve more rapidly than is likely with ARDS. Also, subsequent surges in left atrial pressure are likely to reveal the true cause of the oedema.

PATHOLOGY

The neutrophil appears to play a crucial part in initiating the pulmonary capillary endothelial damage. Macrophages and cytokines both activate the neutrophils and promote their adhesion to the endothelium, resulting in the release of a range of inflammatory mediators including cytokines

Table 1 *Common conditions causing adult respiratory distress syndrome*

Inhalational injury
Aspiration of gastric contents
Toxic gases
Oxygen toxicity
Near drowning
Trauma
Pulmonary contusion
Blood-borne injury
Sepsis
Necrotic tissue (bowel infarction)
Burns
Pancreatitis
Drugs (heroin, barbiturates, salicylates)
Toxins
Major blood transfusion, or reaction
Anaphylactic reactions
Cardiopulmonary bypass
Eclampsia
Carcinomatosis

(tumour necrosis factor, interleukins), prostaglandins, leukotrienes, complement and coagulation proteins, platelet-activation factors, and vasoactive peptides. This 'soup' of mediators and enzymes destroys the pulmonary capillary endothelium and basement membrane, allowing the leak of fluid and cells into the interstitial and alveolar spaces, and promotes blockage of the pulmonary capillaries with fibrin and cellular debris, leading to the development of pulmonary hypertension. Type 1 alveolar cells are readily destroyed, leaving an exposed alveolar basement membrane, which, if the process persists, will be recovered by proliferating type 2 alveolar cells. Proteins, fibrin, and cellular debris coalesce to form hyaline membranes and the failure of production of pulmonary surfactants causes alveolar collapse. If the underlying cause is not successfully treated, following the initial oedematous phase that occurs over 24 to 48 h, cellular proliferation and then interstitial fibrosis will occur.

The extent to which different patients will develop the described pathological changes varies greatly. Why one patient should respond to a given insult by a transient and minimal derangement of pulmonary function while another should develop severe changes with inexorable progression to irreversible pulmonary fibrosis remains unclear. The changes that occur at the pulmonary capillary membrane are not organ specific and it is both to be expected, and has been demonstrated, that other organs suffer similar endothelial damage. Myocardial biopsies taken in patients with severe sepsis show the development of oedema now believed to be central to the observed impairment of the function of the heart. The emphasis on the lung, rather than damage to other organs, is probably due to the fact that radiographic imaging, arterial blood-gas analysis, and compliance measurements are very sensitive detectors of the pulmonary pathology. It is of great interest that similar blood-borne insults are capable of producing different patterns of organ failure that cannot simply be explained by the site or nature of the initial insult.

LUNG FUNCTION

The increased alveolar–arterial oxygen gradient is, in the early stages, due to both an increase in the extravascular lung water, and the alveolar collapse consequent upon surfactant loss. Both result in intrapulmonary shunting. If the process progresses, microemboli and *in situ* thrombosis, and the development of fibrosis with reduced gaseous diffusion, further impair gas exchange. The oedema and lung collapse produce a reduced functional residual capacity and lung compliance, and result in increased airway and intrathoracic pressures that in turn cause secondary pulmo-

nary and circulatory complications (pneumothorax, increased right-ventricular afterload, reduced cardiac output.)

TREATMENT

The appropriate treatment is that of the underlying condition (Table 1) and this should be as early as possible if progressive lung injury and damage to other organs is to be avoided.

If treatment is delayed or ineffective, the progression in the lung injury, with its increased metabolic demands, will invariably result in the patient requiring artificial ventilation both to remove the increased work of breathing (due to the reduced lung compliance) and to allow correction of the hypoxaemia. The aim of ventilation should be to achieve the minimum inspired oxygen concentration and airway pressures that allow adequate oxygen delivery. Each ventilatory manoeuvre carries its own benefit and disadvantages, which will vary between patients and, with time, in an individual patient. There is very little substitute for making repeated assessments and alterations to achieve the maximum clinical benefit.

In general terms the ventilatory settings will initially be for volume-controlled ventilation with reversed inspiratory to expiratory ratio and the addition of positive end-expiratory pressure to a level that produces maximum lung compliance. The end-expiratory pressure may have to be reduced if the cardiovascular effects are unacceptable, or if a pneumothorax develops. It may be necessary to accept increased levels of $Pa\text{CO}_2$, even in excess of 60 mmHg (8 kPa), so-called permissive hypercapnia, so that the effects of excessive lung volumes and resultant barotrauma are minimized. If the lung lesion progresses, pressure-regulated ventilation and variation of the patient's position should be tried. It is remarkable, and not yet fully explained, that in some patients turning from the conventional supine to a prone position produces a dramatic improvement in gas exchange. This cannot be simply a gravitational effect on the extravascular lung water or the drainage of retained lung secretions. The inspired oxygen concentration ($F\text{IO}_2$) should be kept as low as possible provided that the arterial oxygen saturation is maintained above 90 per cent. If the $F\text{IO}_2$ does not exceed 80 per cent, progressive lung damage from oxygen toxicity is unlikely, but levels above 80 per cent for significant periods of time increase the likelihood of the lung lesion progressing to irreversible fibrosis.

For most patients with severe ARDS, paralysis is appropriate, both to prevent them 'fighting' the ventilator and to avoid any increase in metabolic requirements from skeletal muscle activity. Other measures that reduce metabolic requirements and therefore the demands on pulmonary gas exchange include active cooling to reduce core temperature below 38.0°C, adequate analgesia and sedation, and where possible, minimizing the use of drugs that increase metabolic rate, particularly inotropic agents with β-agonist activity.

The appropriate circulatory management in ARDS is disputed. Studies suggesting that oxygen consumption is delivery dependent have led to the practice of increasing oxygen delivery to supranormal levels (greater than 600 ml/min per m²) to correct any covert tissue oxygen debt. It is recommended that this should be attempted initially by aggressive volume loading to left atrial pressures in excess of 15 mmHg. Whether this practice is beneficial where the pulmonary capillary membranes are intact is uncertain, but in the presence of damaged membranes, excessive volume loading, whether with crystalloid or colloid, results in an increase in extravascular lung water and a deterioration in gas exchange. This cannot then be corrected by the removal of a similar volume of fluid from the intravascular space. Another fallacy in the logic of this approach is that many of the patients, particularly those with sepsis, have markedly impaired myocardial contractility with flat myocardial function curves, so that the gain in stroke volume and hence cardiac output is minimal. This therefore results in all the disadvantages of volume loading in exchange for trivial improvements in oxygen delivery. Clinical experience has confirmed the folly of exuberant volume loading in such patients.

Pragmatically, it appears that better results are achieved by keeping the patient as 'dry' as possible during the phase at which the lungs are leaking, and maintaining the flows and therefore oxygen delivery, by driving the circulation with inotropic agents. The economy with added volume has to stop short of causing collapse of the tissue microcirculation. The recent introduction of the gastric tonometer may provide a means of assessing the adequacy of the microcirculation. The use of pulmonary vasodilators to reduce the pulmonary hypertension in ARDS has proved disappointing, largely because of unacceptable systemic hypotension, and also the potential for increasing the ventilation–perfusion mismatch, with a consequent further deterioration in gas exchange. A promising new strategy is the use of inhaled nitric oxide. This offers pulmonary vasodilation, with reduction in right ventricular afterload, without any effect on the systemic circulation. Furthermore the inhaled nitric oxide promotes increased blood flow to the ventilated parts of the lungs, improving gas exchange and arterial Pao_2. The outcome of studies to prove whether this will improve matters in ARDS is awaited.

Extracorporeal-membrane oxygenation has been shown to improve outcome in carefully selected patients with ARDS when compared to conventional techniques alone. The technical problems of maintaining an extracorporeal circuit for many days and even weeks without encountering the many serious complications make this and other techniques for replacing or augmenting lung function a form of therapy that will be limited to very few specialist centres.

It had been hoped that the recent development of human antibodies to various cytokines (endotoxin, tumour necrosis factor, interleukin 1) involved in the early stages of capillary endothelial damage would provide a new approach that would prevent the development of ARDS or at least arrest its progression. The results of several clinical trials have not, however, been encouraging and almost certainly a more targeted approach is required to prevent inappropriate adhesion of neutrophils to the vascular endothelium.

Despite intensive research the mortality of patients who develop ARDS remains depressingly high, ranging in various series from 20 to 80 per cent: ultimately the mortality will be that of the underlying condition. Although some exciting new approaches are now available for the treatment of the acquired lung lesion, it must not be forgotten that the rapid identification and treatment of the underlying problem remains the mainstay of management.

Positive-pressure ventilation

Positive-pressure ventilation has been in use in the treatment of ventilatory failure for over 30 years. The effectiveness of the technique increased very considerably when valves that allow the pressure in the system to be maintained at a level above atmospheric throughout the ventilatory cycle became available.

The mechanical arrangements of ventilators differ; those that are volume cycled inflate the lungs by the volume selected, whereas pressure-cycled ventilators achieve a tidal volume that is the resultant of the compliance of the patient's lungs and chest wall on the one hand and the pressure to which the ventilator is set to inflate them on the other.

Both types of ventilator, and various subdivisions within each group, can be manipulated by the physician to achieve the same end in terms of the amount of ventilation delivered and the manner of its delivery. The matching of the pattern of ventilation delivered, and the disturbance of the patient's pulmonary physiology, is therefore largely independent of the type of ventilator which is used.

Indications for mechanical ventilation

The indications for the employment of positive-pressure ventilation embrace all those conditions that may cause ventilatory failure. Delay

in its institution commonly adds the problems of renal failure and cerebral oedema because widespread damage has usually occurred before ventilatory failure causes cardiac arrest.

The headings under which the indications for positive-pressure ventilation may conveniently be considered are respiratory, circulatory, neurological, and musculoskeletal, post-traumatic and postoperative.

Respiratory indications

Patients suffering from pneumonia, pulmonary oedema, asthma, chronic bronchitis, pulmonary fibrosis, massive atelectasis, the leaking lungs associated with septicaemia, or any of the other listed causes of lung damage described under the heading of ARDS can almost always be prevented from dying from ventilatory failure by the use of a mechanical ventilator. Patients with pneumonia may still die from the toxic effects of the infection on other organs, but inability to maintain ventilation at a level that will sustain life is most unusual with modern ventilators suitably adjusted to match the patient's disease.

The judgement that the patient's condition has deteriorated to a level that justifies mechanical ventilation is complex. It depends not only upon the observation that, with appropriate measures short of positive-pressure ventilation, the patient is unable to ventilate the arterial blood adequately and that there is a worsening trend in the arterial blood-gas tensions; equally important is the observation that the patient's own respiratory efforts are inducing a state of increasing physical exhaustion, which is likely to be irreversible. Implicit within the judgement of the level of exhaustion that can be tolerated is an appreciation of the patient's general state of fitness and the adequacy of systems other than the patient's lungs. The physician must also consider the reversibility or otherwise of the patient's underlying condition, before embarking upon treatment that may be viewed as the medical equivalent of a surgical operation. Broadly this will depend upon an estimate of the proportion of the pulmonary disorder that is reversible.

Circulatory indications

The value of positive-pressure ventilation in states of low cardiac output has long been recognized, but Macklem's group have now provided substantial experimental evidence that circulatory performance and survival rates are both improved if the energy required for the performance of ventilation is supplied from an external source. For these reasons a cardiac output of less than 2 l/min in a 70 kg patient or a cardiac index of less than 1.2 l/m² per min is of itself an indication for mechanical ventilatory support. The sharp increase in the ventilatory workload occasioned by pulmonary oedema, in addition to its interference with pulmonary gas exchange, make this condition particularly susceptible to treatment with positive-pressure ventilation when it cannot be contained sufficiently rapidly by manipulation of the circulation.

Neurological and musculoskeletal indications

Weakness of the respiratory muscles occasioned by acute infective polyneuritis, poliomyelitis, myasthenia gravis, or rarely multiple sclerosis may be sufficiently severe to make ventilatory assistance necessary. In general such assistance will be required when the patient's vital capacity falls below 1 litre because the patient will then be incapable of generating a cough of sufficient force to maintain a clear airway. The possibility that any of these conditions may be complicated by bulbar weakness may dictate that the ventilatory assistance is provided as positive-pressure ventilation via an endotracheal tube. Where it is clear that there is no bulbar weakness and that this will not appear, ventilatory support may be provided either from a positive-pressure ventilator through a well-fitting face mask, or by other techniques more appropriate to chronic weakness such as tank ventilators, cuirasses, or rocking beds. The face mask may be of the nasal type or may cover both nose and mouth. Success with these masks will depend to a great extent upon the care with which they are fitted to ensure comfort over a relatively long period of time. Also, they tend to inhibit coughing and do not provide the access to the airway for the removal of secretions, so that they must be removed from time to time to allow clearance.

Following traumatic head injuries and in cases of brain damage secondary to asphyxiation or periods of cardiac arrest, an initial period of partial neurological recovery is not infrequently followed by neurological death due to cerebral oedema. There is evidence that the occurrence of this cerebral oedema may be prevented by hyperventilation. Reduction of the arterial carbon dioxide tension to values between 25 and 30 mmHg (3.3 and 4.0 kPa) acts by reducing cerebral blood flow to control the development of the oedema. Ideally, ventilation undertaken for these reasons should be monitored by extradural measurement of intracranial pressure, as premature withdrawal of the treatment may be followed by overwhelming cerebral oedema which is irreversible by the time that signs of upper midbrain compression appear.

Respiratory depression of a central nature due either to drug overdose or the action of anaesthetic agents may necessitate a period of mechanical ventilation.

Underventilation due to kyphoscoliotic deformities may require treatment with a mechanical ventilator but the results are poor unless undertaken to deal with an acute episode of ventilatory insufficiency precipitated by a potentially reversible pulmonary infection, or to provide support during a postoperative period when the patient's ventilatory capacity is further reduced temporarily.

Post-traumatic and postoperative indications

Patients who have sustained traumatic chest injuries may be best treated with a period of positive-pressure ventilation, either because a segment of the chest wall is moving paradoxically secondary to fracture of the rib cage at more than one point on its circumference, or as an adjunct to the management of pain, or in the treatment of respiratory failure due to contusion of the lung.

An uncontrolled flail segment of the chest wall is inevitably complicated by collapse and consolidation of the underlying segment of lung and also impairs ventilatory capacity by its paradoxical movement. These complications can be prevented either by wiring the rib fractures, or by positive-pressure ventilation. Pain can be controlled either by epidural anaesthesia or by sedation and positive-pressure ventilation, which is the obvious treatment of choice where the three problems of paradoxical movement, lung contusion, and pain coexist. The chest wall usually becomes stable and the pain occasioned by the patient's own respiratory effort becomes tolerable within a period of 10 days.

Following cardiac operations for the circulatory reasons already discussed, and following abdominal operations where for some reason the abdomen remains either distended or acutely painful, an elective period of positive-pressure ventilation is an effective means of avoiding pulmonary complications.

Extensive burns involving the chest wall may impose a remarkable degree of restriction upon the chest wall, which is best treated by escharotomies and positive-pressure ventilation.

Technical considerations involved in the institution of positive-pressure ventilation

By face mask

As has already been stated, it is possible to provide positive-pressure ventilation either intermittently over a long period of time, or with only short pauses, for a period of a few days, through a well-fitting face mask. These devices can only be used if bulbar function and the entire swallowing mechanism are intact. They are of two types: those that encase the nose, and those that cover both nose and mouth. They are held in place with a head harness, and to be tolerated at all require very careful fitting, especially at likely pressure points such as the bridge of the nose. Ventilation provided in this manner is often very successful for some hours, but then fails because the patient's airway fills with uncleared secretions. A degree of cooperation is required of the patient and so the system is not of value in those who are unconscious or very sick.

The short-term ventilatory support required in some patients with acute pulmonary oedema suggests the use of this technique, but the difficulty with secretions and the sense of claustrophobia induced by the tight-fitting mask have limited its applicability.

Endotracheal intubation

Where positive-pressure ventilation through a mask is either inappropriate or has failed, it is necessary to intubate the trachea by either the oral or nasal route, or through a tracheostomy. The details of technique are all directed toward the minimization of laryngeal and tracheal damage.

A tube diameter of 9.5 mm in an adult male and 8.5 mm in a female leaves a small space between tube and trachea that can be sealed by minimal inflation of the cuff. The cuff should be inflated until the leak, audible with a stethoscope over the trachea, just disappears. Tracheal damage is occasioned by the use of tubes of small diameter because high cuff pressures are then necessary to produce an air seal.

Oral endotracheal tubes are preferred because, although nasal endotracheal tubes may be marginally less uncomfortable for the patient, the fact that smaller tubes have to be used because of the diameter of the nasal airspace increases the likelihood of tracheal damage, and also makes aspiration of the airway with catheters more difficult.

The factors that increase the chance of laryngeal abrasion from an endotracheal tube are the shape of the female larynx, oedema of the head and neck, and of greatest importance, movement of the tube relative to the patient, due to restlessness, hiccupping, or respiratory efforts. Where all these factors are reduced to a minimum an oral endotracheal tube can be used for a maximum of 2 weeks. Except in children, a longer period of ventilation requires the formation of a tracheostomy. The recently introduced technique of percutaneous tracheotomy seems a considerable advance. It allows the procedure to be performed within the unit, and has diminished the incidence of haemorrhage and local infection.

Plastic tubes should be used in preference to rubber because they produce less tissue reaction. The length of the tube should be adjusted before insertion so that the connector at the proximal end of the tube buttresses the tube as it lies between the patient's teeth, to prevent severence or compression of the tube. The distal end of the tube must lie well above the carina. Inadvertent intubation of the right main bronchus is manifested by diminished movement of the left chest. The correct positioning of the tube should be confirmed radiologically after insertion.

In small children, nasotracheal tubes are preferred to oral because the most important consideration is stability of the tube. Stability is difficult to ensure because the distance between the larynx and carina is small, and the tolerance between an ideally placed tube halfway between these points and inadvertent extubation is correspondingly small. These problems are best countered by anchorage of a nasal tube to a wire frame secured to the child's forehead with adhesive pads.

The nasal endotracheal tubes used for small children are non-cuffed and the tube diameter selected is such that there is a modest leak of 0.5 to 1 l of gas per minute between the tube and the trachea. The leak is compensated for by augmentation of the minute volume and forms a non-traumatic cushion between the tube and trachea. The tube should be changed to the other nostril at least each week or more frequently if it becomes part obstructed with inspissated secretions, but this arrangement can be used for long-term ventilation if necessary. Tracheostomy should be avoided in small children.

Matching the ventilator settings with the patient's disease

The matching of the ventilator to the patient's physiological disturbance is made at a number of levels.

The first approximation

With the notable exception of patients suffering from obstructive airways disease, the minute volume is adjusted to bring the arterial carbon dioxide tension to a level between 30 and 35 mmHg (4 and 4.7 kPa). This mild degree of overventilation increases the patient's tolerance of the ventilator by diminishing the ventilatory drive. In an adult the minute volume required to achieve this is likely to lie between 6 l/min if the patient has normal lung function and 22 l/min with extremes of pulmonary disorder. An estimate is made of the patient's degree of disturbance, and the ventilator adjusted to deliver a minute volume related proportionately to this estimate of dysfunction. The oxygen concentration of the inspired gas is adjusted with the aim of producing an arterial oxygen tension between 100 and 150 mmHg (13 and 20 kPa). The desired end is achieved by a process of successive approximation by measurement of the arterial blood gases and adjustment of the ventilator.

Oxygen toxicity

Inspired oxygen concentrations in excess of 75 per cent are undesirable because they engender pathological changes in the lung. Animals ventilated with 100 per cent oxygen show changes in the alveolar basement membrane after 10 h and after 2 days there is an intense fibroblastic reaction in the lungs. Inspired oxygen concentrations in excess of 75 per cent are therefore only acceptable for a very short period where the arterial oxygen tension is below 50 mmHg (6.6 kPa) in spite of mechanical ventilation.

Detailed matching of disease and ventilator

Patients requiring ventilation who have normal lungs, pneumonia, pulmonary oedema, or atelectasis are best ventilated at a slow rate, with an inspiratory time as great as 30 per cent of the respiratory cycle and with a pause in full inspiration. Theoretically, an inspiratory pause allows redistribution of gas from overventilated to underventilated alveoli. In practice, it is difficult to demonstrate that the introduction of a pause makes any measurable difference to the efficiency of ventilation. Its practical importance is that it allows the pressure within the airway to be measured under conditions of no gas flow.

In an adult a respiratory rate of 15/min is more efficient than more rapid rates. In children a suitable rate is determined, once the required minute volume is known, by holding the minute volume constant and varying the rate until the observed excursion of the child's chest wall seems appropriate to its size.

Patients in this respiratory group all benefit very considerably from being ventilated with an end-expiratory pressure raised above atmospheric pressure unless cardiac output is severely impaired. The application of a positive end-expiratory pressure (**PEEP**) has been an important advance in the technique of mechanical ventilation. PEEP valves allow gas to escape freely from the airway during expiration down to a selected pressure between 0 and 20 cmH₂O. Their closure at a pressure above atmospheric has the effect of inflating the lungs to a greater functional residual capacity over the course of a few breaths. Once equilibrium is re-established between the inspired and expired gas volume, the patient continues to be ventilated with the original values of tidal and minute volume, but with the lungs held inflated to a larger functional residual capacity, so that their volume in inspiration and in expiration are both increased by the same amount.

Experimental evidence suggests that the optimum value of PEEP, from both respiratory and circulatory points of view, is that end-expiratory pressure at which the compliance of the lungs is greatest. This can be determined by measuring the excursions in airway pressure occurring between end-expiration and the inspiratory pause. The ideal value of PEEP is that at which the pressure swings are the minimum for the same applied tidal volume.

PEEP is contraindicated in low cardiac-output states for the reason that it further lowers the cardiac output, and in obstructive airways disease, where its application worsens lung compliance and raises the pulmonary vascular resistance.

The pattern of mechanical ventilation required by patients with severe asthma or major obstructive airways disease for any other reason is unlike that for any other disease. In essence it entails deliberate underventilation, avoidance of any measure that might further increase the already large functional residual capacity and, in the case of acute asthma, intense humidification.

The inception of positive-pressure ventilation, unless correctly managed, can prove lethal in these patients. The lungs should be oxygenated from a face mask and an isoprenaline or salbutamol infusion started before anaesthesia is induced for the placement of an endotracheal tube. The patient should then be intubated under general anaesthesia, ideally with halothane because of its bronchodilator properties, and underventilated with a gas mixture containing 75 per cent oxygen. No attempt should be made to reduce the arterial carbon dioxide tension from the high levels that it will have attained in such patients before they are subjected to ventilation. Ventilation of an adult with 6 l/min in such circumstances may well correspond with an arterial carbon dioxide tension of 70 mmHg (9.3 kPa) or more. An increase in minute volume will produce an increase in both functional residual capacity and pulmonary vascular resistance, with a deleterious effect upon the circulation. If the patient's deterioration before ventilation was rapid, the respiratory acidosis will not have been offset by the retention of bicarbonate, and this should be administered to bring the arterial pH toward normal.

The underventilation and consequent high arterial carbon dioxide tension make it necessary to continue the anaesthesia and muscle relaxation. Pancuronium should be avoided because it causes histamine to be released. For the same reason that halothane was the best anaesthetic because of its dilating effect on the bronchial tree, ketamine has some advantage for sedation in this situation.

A slow ventilatory rate and an inspiratory phase as short as 5 per cent of the cycle allow greater time for expiration. An inspiratory pause theoretically allows redistribution of gas from overventilated to underventilated alveoli, but makes little demonstrable difference to the efficiency of ventilation.

A positive end-expiratory pressure is absolutely contraindicated in patients whose disease has already raised their functional residual capacity beyond the point at which the compliance of their lungs improves. In the severe asthmatic, PEEP constitutes a threat to life by increasing the pulmonary vascular resistance.

The use of an expiratory choke to limit the rate of emptying of the lungs has been advocated to prevent premature closure of small airways, so allowing more complete alveolar emptying. The pattern of emptying is converted from an exponential to a linear form. The improvement in the arterial gases so obtained is usually modest, and the benefit is probably outweighed by the potentially very dangerous threat posed by minor maladjustment of this control, limiting the expiratory rate sufficiently to cause an increase in functional residual capacity.

Humidification and warming of the air delivered to the patient is important whatever the nature of the disease that has occasioned treatment by mechanical ventilation. In the case of acute asthma, the eventual dislodgement of viscid bronchiolar casts, which intense humidification produces after about 10 h, is central to successful treatment. As the airways are cleared of this material, the pulmonary abnormalities diminish, allowing the alveolar ventilation to be increased.

Patients with restrictive abnormalities either of the lungs or chest wall, as may occur in fibrosing alveolitis or kyphoscoliosis, require modification of the ventilatory pattern in the sense of a smaller tidal volume and higher respiratory rate. The optimal rate can be found in each case by measurement of the arterial blood gases whilst the minute volume is held constant and the respiratory rate raised. A fall in the optimal rate will be found where it has been possible to reverse a fibrotic change.

Where ventilation has been undertaken with the object of reducing or preventing cerebral oedema, it might be expected that PEEP would have the effect of raising intracranial pressure by transmission of the raised intrathoracic pressure to the theca through the rich plexus of veins around the vertebral bodies within the thorax. Direct measurement of the intracranial pressure in a very limited number of cases suggests that this may not be so.

Management of the ventilated patient

Once patient and machine have been matched according to the nature of the disease process, there are details of management that relate to all ventilated patients.

The effect of gravity is paramount and the optimum drainage of secretions from the airway is achieved with the patient lying horizontal, and alternating from side to side so that a coronal plane through the chest is truly vertical. This ideal may be rendered impossible by multiple injuries or may require to be sacrificed in some degree by the greater importance of nursing a patient threatened with cerebral oedema in a steeply head up position. Similarly, where the greatest threat to life is circulatory instability, patients must remain flat on their backs.

Aspiration of the airway is necessary with a frequency related to the amount of the secretions. This should be done with catheters as aseptically and atraumatically as possible.

When soiling of the airway with secretions is heavy in spite of normal toilet with small quantities of saline and aspiration with catheters, it is very important to clear the airway bronchoscopically perhaps three or four times in each 24-h period. The results have been found to vary very much with the care and time that the operator is prepared to devote to the task, but are of enormous value in limiting the damage to lung function produced by discharging lung abscesses.

Atelectasis can usefully be treated by manual inflation of the chest with an anaesthetic bag. A series of hyperinflations of the lungs is followed by sudden disconnection of the endotracheal tube simulating a cough, followed by aspiration of the airway. This process should not be employed indiscriminately and is contraindicated in the presence of a precarious circulation and in severe obstructive airways disease.

Restlessness in a ventilated patient should never pass unheeded, and makes the measurement of the arterial blood gases obligatory. The most common cause is underventilation, the basis for which should be determined and the ventilation increased. Circulatory inadequacy may be manifested by restlessness without any demonstrable change in the respiratory status, and the deterioration of any ventilated patient must always suggest the possible occurrence of a pneumothorax. It is almost always possible to continue ventilating a patient despite the presence of a pneumothorax, but an adequate chest drain must be inserted.

The requirement of patients with oral endotracheal tubes for sedation is immensely variable and must be adjusted to the individual. Restlessness in spite of adequate ventilation and sedation is an indication for either curarization or early conversion to a tracheostomy.

Bronchoscopy on the intensive care unit

A fibreoptic bronchoscope should be readily available on an intensive care unit to allow the prompt and effective management of upper airways obstruction. In the patient with respiratory distress and clinical evidence of proximal airway obstruction (stridor, reduced lung volumes and chest wall recession), it will both confirm the diagnosis (Table 2) and may provide the means of treatment.

Intubation will normally be required to secure the airway and if conventional intubation is difficult, an endotracheal tube may be introduced over the bronchoscope. A similar bronchoscopic 'Seldinger' technique may be used to change tracheostomy tubes in difficult cases.

In the intubated patient, proximal displacement of inspissated secretions into an already partially occluded tube following turning, coughing, suction or physiotherapy may produce sudden proximal obstruction and a dramatic deterioration in gas exchange. These episodes, characterized by an inability to introduce the suction catheter satisfactorily, may initially be brief but, if repeated, warrant early bronchoscopy to

Table 2 *Common causes of upper airways obstruction*

Epiglottitis
Laryngeal oedema
Bilateral vocal-cord paralysis
Narrow, misplaced or occluded tube
Tracheobronchial disruption
Foreign body
Mucus plug
Blood clot
Tumour

relieve the problem and assess the need for tube replacement. In situations where an inspissated mucus plug, situated in the lower trachea or in the tube itself, cannot be removed via the bronchoscope or with a directed suction catheter it may be necessary to remove the tube, reintubate and repeat the bronchoscopy. The adequacy of patient hydration and humidification of the inspired gas should be reviewed.

Haemoptysis following overenthusiastic suctioning in a patient with a coagulopathy, or from a bronchial tumour or lung infection (particularly from an abscess, bronchiectasis or tuberculosis) may threaten the patency of proximal airways and requires urgent bronchoscopy to provide toilet and to control and localize, if possible, the source of the bleeding. It is, however, notoriously difficult to identify the culprit orifice when the bleeding site lies beyond the range of the scope and there has been extensive prior soiling of the entire bronchial tree. It should, however, be possible to localize the bleeding to one side and the patient should then be positioned with that side dependent to prevent further soiling of the 'good' lung. If haemostasis is achieved with tolerable gas exchange, fresh thrombus should be left undisturbed and the temptation to investigate further resisted, at least until cardiorespiratory stability has been restored. Even massive haemoptysis can usually be controlled with a wide-channel flexible bronchoscope but occasionally it may be necessary to resort to a rigid bronchoscope to control the bleeding. Persisting bleeding may be temporarily controlled and the offending lobe identified by inserting a Fogarty catheter via the bronchoscope into the orifice and inflating the balloon. Although described as a method for continuing control after removal of the bronchoscope, it is extremely difficult to keep the inflated balloon appropriately positioned. Recently, fibrin glue has been successfully used to occlude a lobar orifice, and proved both durable and relatively easy to apply using catheters introduced via the bronchoscope.

Bronchoscopy is also indicated in persisting lung collapse/consolidation to exclude proximal obstruction from mucus, pus or tumour and to obtain more representative microbiological samples in patients with an undiagnosed pneumonia. The collection of specimens using a protected brush technique has been shown to improve the microbiological yield, predominantly by reducing the false-positive rate from upper airways contamination. Washings and brushings for cytological examination may confirm the diagnosis of *Pneumocystis carinii* pneumonia and help in the diagnosis of diffuse pulmonary infiltrates of unknown aetiology. The role of transbronchial biopsy in this latter situation is more controversial because of the risk of pneumothorax and haemorrhage in a patient population who will almost by definition have markedly impaired gas exchange. The use of a portable image intensifier during the biopsy procedure provides a three-dimensional perspective and reduces the risk of pneumothorax.

In cases of thoracic trauma, particularly deceleration injuries, fibreoptic bronchoscopy should be used early to exclude tracheobronchial disruption, which may not be clinically apparent initially; failure to make an early diagnosis increases the risk of stricture formation and associated complications. In cases of inhalation injury, bronchoscopy is indicated to assess the extent of upper airway oedema and probable need for intubation and to perform bronchial toilet to remove sloughed mucosa and carbonaceous debris.

Although an invaluable instrument on an intensive care unit, complications may arise if the operator is inexperienced and if the preparation and precautions taken are inadequate. As aspiration of thick secretions is often necessary, a wide-channel bronchoscope (≥ 2.3 mm i.d.) is preferable but this will require an endotracheal/tracheostomy tube of ideally ≥ 8 mm i.d. The smaller the tube the higher will be the peak airway pressures, with a consequent loss of minute volume that will be further exacerbated by over vigorous suctioning. The inspired oxygen should be increased before starting the procedure, if necessary to 100 per cent, and the adequacy of arterial saturation continuously monitored by pulse oximeter. Adequate sedation and topical anaesthesia are important to prevent cardiovascular complications. Instrumentation of the upper airway may produce a profound bradycardia and bronchoconstriction in those with an asthmatic tendency. If reported to occur with routine suctioning alone, prophylactic treatment with an anticholinergic and inhaled β_2-agonist is prudent and any saline used for lavage should be warmed to body temperature.

Weaning from the ventilator

A period of mechanical ventilation may either be terminated abruptly or by gradual transfer of the ventilatory workload from machine to patient. In either case the factors that govern the possibility of the patient's independence of the ventilator fall under three headings: the adequacy of pulmonary function, the likely work cost of spontaneous ventilation, and the patient's capacity to sustain such a workload.

The simplest measure of adequacy of pulmonary function, which is available in any ventilated patient, is the relation of the minute volume and inspired oxygen concentration, supplied through the ventilator, to the arterial blood-gas tensions that they engender. An arterial carbon dioxide tension between 30 and 35 mmHg (4.0 and 4.7 kPa) in response to a minute volume of 6 litres is likely to be associated with substantially normal lungs. If the minute volume required to produce this level of alveolar ventilation is in excess of 12 litres for a 70-kg patient who has been ventilated, it is unlikely that the patients' own ventilatory efforts will sustain them other than briefly. Between these limits there is a range of respiratory dysfunction that may be compatible with a reversion to spontaneous ventilation, necessitating a judgement of the balance between the implied workload, and the patient's competence to undertake this.

Patients whose pulmonary pathology is best treated with PEEP during mechanical ventilation should not be weaned from positive pressure as a prelude to weaning from the ventilator. The very considerable benefits of PEEP are best maintained in order that the lungs are in the best possible condition at the moment of separation from the ventilator.

An estimate of the likely workload is provided by the size of the minute volume and of the pressure swings in the airway generated by the conjunction of patient and ventilator. Although neither value may remain unchanged once the patient is divorced from the ventilator, both are good indicators.

Estimation of the patient's ability to support the workload requires examination of the cardiovascular system, the nervous system, and the abdomen.

Withdrawal of ventilatory support in the presence of a cardiac output that is less than half the normal resting value is likely to lead to further circulatory deterioration. An elevated left-atrial pressure or any residual pulmonary oedema will increase the work of breathing by stiffening the lungs. A pulmonary vascular resistance greater than 10 units is a contraindication to the removal of ventilatory support for at least 48 h after cardiopulmonary operations, and for longer periods if the pulmonary vascular resistance is higher. Premature removal of support probably causes death by provoking a sharp rise in pulmonary vascular resistance, which is not reversed by reventilation. If this is the mechanism, infusion of acetylcholine into the pulmonary artery might be effective where reventilation fails.

Lungs that have been flooded with pulmonary oedema as a result of insults to the capillary basement membrane, rather than for hydraulic reasons, require to be ventilated for a minimum of 4 days following the insult. Premature cessation of ventilation results in extensive atelectasis. It seems possible that the surfactant mechanism is destroyed and requires time to regenerate. The pulmonary oedema in such cases has the same appearance as the patient's plasma and the same albumin concentration.

Central nervous depression whether organic or metabolic in origin, and, most important, the integrity of the patient's brain-stem and spinal-cord function, together with any damage to the phrenic and intercostal nerves, may all make adequate spontaneous ventilation impossible. Wasting and weakness of the respiratory muscles have the same effect, and in this context the atrophy of the muscles that results from prolonged periods of artificial ventilation is of particular importance. The sensory nervous system is also involved, in as much as pain is commonly a transcending respiratory depressant.

Abdominal distension and tenderness interfere with diaphragmatic movement and are of especial relevance to the patient's ability to cough. A vital capacity of at least 1 litre and the apposition of the vocal cords are necessary for the production of an effective cough, without which an initially adequate ventilatory capacity is likely to deteriorate.

Whilst any of these circulatory neuromuscular or abdominal considerations may offer a clear contraindication to the discontinuation of mechanical ventilation, the requirement for fine judgement in cases of doubt is obviated by allowing the patient to breathe a high flow of a suitable gas mixture from an anaesthetic bag, whilst still intubated. This manoeuvre will very quickly make any deficiencies of drive or neurological integrity obvious from the movements of the chest wall and the movements of the diaphragm inferred from those of the abdomen. It also allows a judgement to be made of the likelihood that the patient will become unduly exhausted. The deficiencies of this trial are the increased airway resistance presented by the endotracheal tube and the intolerance of the tube, which some patients show after the withdrawal of sedation. A brief trial of this nature also leaves in doubt the patient's longer-term independence of the ventilator.

The problems of sedation are to some extent overcome by the replacement of all other forms of sedation with nitrous oxide for a period of hours to allow excretion of the other agents. The effects of nitrous oxide wear off very rapidly allowing a brief time for the trial assessment and a decision, if all seems well, to remove the endotracheal tube. Nitrous oxide is not suitable for long-term sedation because of bone marrow changes and after 24 h, neutropenia. Propofol can be used in a similar fashion for short-term sedation. Expense limits its use for longer periods.

Careful observation of the patient in the first hours after the removal of ventilatory support will confirm or confound the decision. The most important indications for reventilation are those of respiratory distress, a rising respiratory and pulse rate, and the appearance of such effort being required as can only end in increasing exhaustion. From the circulatory point of view the most favourable response is a fall in right atrial pressure and a small rise in arterial pressure. A rise in both venous and arterial pressure suggests that apprehension or pain require treatment with mild sedation or analgesia. A rise in right atrial pressure, a fall in arterial pressure, a diminished hourly urine output, and cooling limbs suggest that ventilatory support should be restored.

Evidence of underventilation in the sense of a rising carbon dioxide tension is not of itself an indication for reventilation unless it is extreme (over 65 mmHg or 8.6 kPa), or unless it is due to weakness rather than the unwanted persistence of sedation, for which small doses of respiratory stimulants are effective.

If exhaustion is evident, the patient should be restored to the ventilator before serious derangement of the arterial blood gases occurs. For this reason these measurements are of less importance than is commonly believed in the solution of this problem.

Laryngeal obstruction following removal of an endotracheal tube is suggested by the appearance of wheeze that is predominantly inspiratory rather than expiratory, and not associated with overinflation of the chest. This may well respond to intravenous hydrocortisone. If this is not effective, it is necessary to pass through the intermediate steps of reintubation and conversion to a tracheotomy. The breathing of helium mixtures is not of value, because the gas flow through the restriction breaks down and becomes turbulent rather than laminar.

The weaning of the tracheostomized patient from the ventilator presents few of these problems, because the tube is tolerated without sedation and should be left in place until the process is successfully completed.

Because a tracheostomy makes it possible to separate the patient from the ventilator intermittently for gradually increasing periods of time, if necessary over the course of many days, this is the method of choice where the respiratory muscles have been subject to wasting. Most chronic bronchitics can only be weaned from a ventilator in this manner, when the oedema of the airway and the infective process in their lungs has been reduced to the absolute minimum. Tracheostomy in these patients has the added advantage of allowing continued aspiration of the airway.

Underventilation of chronic bronchitic patients prior to their removal from the ventilator decreases rather than increases their ventilatory drive in accord with changes in intrathecal pH, and is not of value. The inspired oxygen concentration should of course be limited during weaning, in contradistinction to the requirements at the initial inception of ventilation in such patients.

Tracheostomies are best closed by allowing them to shrink down around uncuffed metal tubes that are daily decreased in size. A flap valve allows the patient to talk and provide a more effective cough than is possible with no occlusion. When sufficient shrinkage has occurred, the tube can be replaced with an occlusive dressing.

Minitracheostomies can be fashioned as a relatively minor procedure. Their insertion is much less likely to be accompanied by troublesome haemorrhage if this is done by Seldinger's technique, starting with a small needle and guidewire, followed by a series of dilators of increasing size, and eventually the insertion of the tube. Prior topical anaesthesia by transtracheal injection of 3 to 5 ml of cocaine hydrochloride reduces the problem of coughing, and makes the procedure more tolerable for the patient. These small tracheostomy tubes allow the airway to be cleared by intermittent aspiration with sterile catheters, but are not suitable for connection to positive-pressure ventilators, although they can be used with high-frequency jet ventilators. They are of great value where the patient's problem is an inadequate cough and the inability to keep the airway clear because of large amounts of sputum. Their limitations are that, in contrast to a formal tracheotomy with a cuffed plastic tube, they neither provide protection of the airway from the aspiration of pharyngeal contents, nor do they allow an exhausted patient respite from the work of ventilation.

Renal failure within the intensive care unit

The most common form of renal failure met with in the intensive care unit is established acute tubular necrosis, resulting from a period of inadequate renal perfusion. At its beginning there is always the possibility that renal function may be restored if the circulation can be repaired by taking the measures already described for its support. The vital points are the exclusion of oligaemia, support of a failing heart with dopamine and other appropriate inotropic agents, and the realization that some patients require a greater than normal blood pressure for the maintenance of their renal function. The rapidity and vigour with which this is done may ultimately save weeks of renal replacement therapy, but the window of opportunity is always small.

The possibility that the renal failure may be obstructive should always be excluded, especially if there is complete anuria, or a history of trauma or any surgical intervention in the abdomen or pelvis.

Myoglobinuria as a cause of renal failure is usually preventable if treated early enough. Damage to muscles from either crush injury, ischaemia, hypo- or hyperthermia, or from lying unconscious and therefore motionless for a long enough period, should raise the possibility

that myoglobin may have been released into the circulation. The urine passed before the proximal tubules become obstructed with the protein has a pink or brownish colour. With haemoglobinuria, the plasma will also be found to be stained pink, but if the plasma is of normal colour, it is likely that the pigment in the urine is myoglobin.

If a high rate of urine flow can be established in the proximal tubules by giving mannitol with a loading dose of up to 25 g followed by an infusion of 2 g/h before they become obstructed with myoglobin, the kidneys will usually continue to function in spite of the continued passage of considerable quantities of myoglobin, sometimes for many days. The mannitol should, of course, be continued until the pigment disappears from the urine. Simultaneous alkalinization of the urine by the intravenous infusion of isotonic sodium bicarbonate will also help to prevent the precipitation of myoglobin.

Acute renal replacement therapy

Acute renal replacement provided within the intensive care unit at one time encompassed haemodialysis, peritoneal dialysis, and haemofiltration. With experience, haemofiltration has come to occupy a very dominant position. The reasons for this are principally that it causes less disturbance to the other systems, particularly the circulation, than either form of dialysis. It makes possible the solution of many chemicophysiological problems with extraordinary economy of effort, and it can be operated by the normal staff of the intensive care unit with safety.

The original haemofiltration systems were arteriovenous, and dependent therefore on the patient's arterial blood pressure. They also suffered from the disadvantage that accidental disconnection could result in serious haemorrhage. Currently, pumped venovenous systems are used, and with the larger filter sizes (1.4 m^2) and good access filtration rates of 120 ml/min may be achieved. Such high rates are totally unnecessary for the management of acute renal failure once any hyperkalaemia has been dealt with. Filtration rates of 20 to 30 ml/min, which can be achieved with a 0.4 m^2 filter, will remove nitrogenous waste, and 4 litres of water could be removed in each 24-h period with a filtration rate of only 3 ml/min.

Access is usually provided as a double-lumen tube in either an internal jugular, subclavian or femoral vein. It is very unusual for there to be any difficulty in the provision of adequate blood flows. The process will allow the removal of very substantial quantities of salt and water from the patient where this is necessary, without noticeable disturbance of the circulation. This also makes it very easy to provide the necessary 'space' for intravenous nutrition or blood products. The replacement fluid contains appropriate quantities of sodium, chloride, calcium, and magnesium, but no phosphate. Usually after 48 h of haemofiltration, phosphate supplements are needed to keep the plasma level above 0.6 mmol/l.

The concentration of potassium in the replacement fluid can be adjusted so that reasonable blood levels are maintained. The concentration of any ion may be manipulated in the same way. Hypernatraemia may be managed with great security by using a sodium concentration in the replacement fluid only 10 mmol less than the level in the patient's plasma so that the level is 'clamped' and can only fall 10 mmol in 24 h, while at the same time the patient's total water balance may be regulated completely independently. Hyponatraemia can obviously be dealt with in like manner, and the system has been used in the authors' unit to control hypercalcaemia.

The buffer used in the commercially available replacement fluid is lactate. If a patient with a lactic acidosis or an inability to metabolize lactate is filtered using this fluid, bicarbonate will be removed and a rapidly progressive acidaemia will develop with disastrous circulatory consequences. Such patients can be filtered very successfully using a replacement fluid, which can be varied as necessary. Usually a ratio of 90 mmol/l of chloride to 50 mmol/l of bicarbonate is appropriate.

Haemofiltration has proved sufficiently reliable and effective in the control of acute renal failure that the prognosis is now effectively that of the underlying disease. The survival rate in the 302 patients who have undergone haemofiltration for acute renal failure in this unit in the course of the last 10 years, many of them with multiorgan failure, has risen from 20 per cent to a current figure of 67 per cent for the last 150 patients. The survival rate in those who also required mechanical ventilation was 42 per cent.

Diagnosis and management of the unconscious patient

Much of the substance of this section is taken from the work of Posner and Plum, whose contribution to this topic marked such an advance in the neurological assessment of the unconscious patient. The eventual management of such a patient will vary according to the diagnosis, but the need for a clear airway, adequacy of both ventilation and circulation, and the elimination of hypoglycaemia transcend all else, if the patient is not to be exposed to further needless brain damage.

The first approximation to the diagnosis depends upon the history and physical signs. The patient's inability to give any history must not preclude enquiry being made of relatives or witnesses concerning the mode of onset of the coma.

Any injury to the head, the appearance of either blood or cerebrospinal fluid in the auditory meati, or nose, or bleeding into the orbits, or the presence of meningism are of obvious significance. The neurological assessment of the unconscious patient depends upon observation of responses to a relatively small number of manoeuvres, some of which are not applicable to a conscious patient. There follows a relatively detailed account of these manoeuvres and the information they may yield.

Brain-stem function

Consciousness probably depends upon interaction between the reticular formation in the midbrain and pons and hemispheric structures, and may be interfered with by damage to any of these areas. In the case of the hemispheres the damage must be bilateral to produce loss of consciousness.

The brain-stem is accessible to moderately detailed examination even in the absence of consciousness. This assessment depends upon:

(1) the pupillary responses;
(2) abnormalities of resting gaze of the eyes;
(3) observation of eye movements induced by stimulation of the patient's vestibular apparatus, either in response to movement of the head or by caloric stimulation;
(4) the corneal reflexes;
(5) the presence of a jaw jerk;
(6) the ability of the patient to swallow and gag;
(7) the pattern of any spontaneous respiratory movements that may be present;
(8) the ciliospinal reflex.

As will be seen when they are considered in detail, these responses may be interfered with by depression of brain-stem function or damage to the cranial nerves. In practice it is not usually difficult to discern where the problem lies.

The pupils (see also Section 24)

The localization of lesions to the optic nerve, optic tract, and either the pretectal or oculomotor nuclear region of the midbrain is most succinctly summarized by the diagram in Fig. 14.

Tectal midbrain lesions produce mid-position (4 mm) or widened (5–6 mm) pupils that are unreactive to light but may spontaneously fluctuate in size (hippus) and dilate in response to a painful stimulus to the skin of the neck (ciliospinal reflex). Lesions of the oculomotor nuclear region of the midbrain interrupt both sympathetic and parasympathetic supply to the eye, producing mid-position pupils that do not react to any stimuli and are often non-circular in outline and slightly unequal in size. Pontine lesions produce bilaterally small pupils. Lateral medullary lesions produce a Horner's syndrome, but do not interfere with the response to light. Third-nerve lesions produce pupillary dilation and, if the lesion is complete, are accompanied by an oculomotor palsy producing downward and outward gaze of the affected eye.

Fixed, dilated pupils following a cardiac arrest may be due to cerebral damage but the pupils will also dilate in response to adrenaline and atropine, and, although in these circumstances they may still respond to

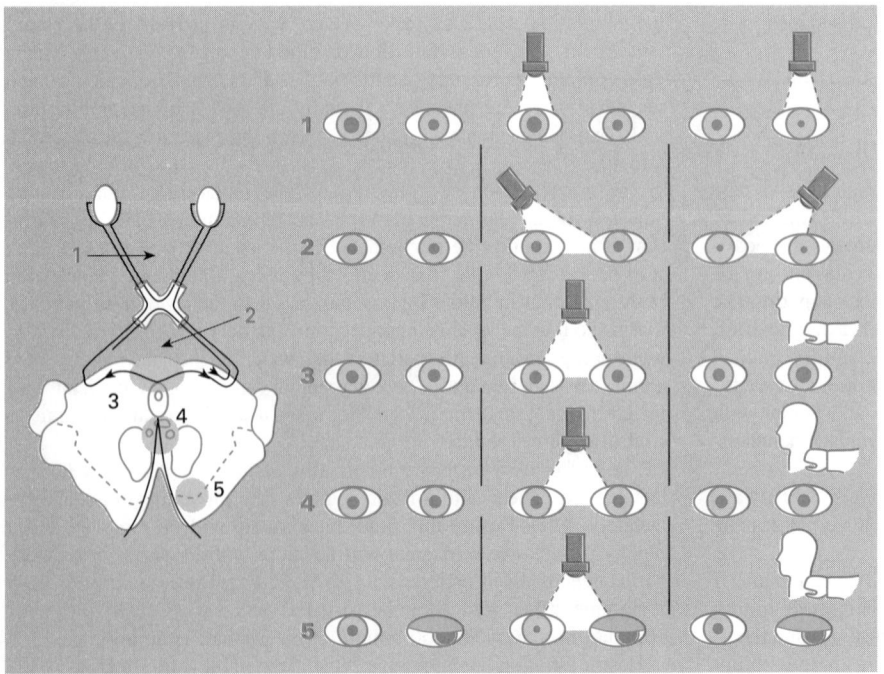

Fig. 14 Pupillary responses associated with various lesions: 1, optic nerve; 2, optic tract: 3, midbrain pretectum; 4, midbrain oculomotor nucleus; 5, emerging IIIrd nerve fibres in midbrain. (Reproduced from Plum and Posner. (1966). *The diagnosis of stupor and coma*. 1st edn. F.A. Davis, Philadelphia, with permission.)

light, it is often difficult to detect the response. Because intense sympathetic stimulation and the administration of these drugs are common accompaniments of a cardiac arrest, it is wise to be guarded about the significance of such pupils following an arrest.

Metabolic depression of the brain-stem produces even depression of all the brain-stem functions with the important exception that the pupillary light response is preserved.

Eye movements and disorders of gaze

The resting position of the eyes, and their response to movement of the head or caloric stimulation of the vestibular apparatus, are potentially more revealing than any other bedside observation that may be made about an unconscious patient.

Most conjugate gaze disorders in comatose patients are the result of destructive lesions because compression and metabolic disturbances affect the supranuclear oculomotor pathways symmetrically. Conjugate deviation of the eyes away from the side of a hemiplegic arm and leg has the same significance as a hemianopic field defect toward the arm and leg; the lesion is hemispheric. Conjugate deviation of the eyes toward the paralysed arm and leg may occur in the early, irritative stages of a hemispheric lesion, but is otherwise the result of a lateral pontine lesion.

Disconjugate lateral deviation of both eyes may be the result of a nuclear lesion in the midbrain; if this is the cause, the pupils will not react to light. Metabolic depression can produce a similar deviation, but the pupils react and stimulation of the patient commonly causes the eyes to assume a central position.

The oculocephalic responses are elicited by holding the eyelids open and rotating the patient's head rapidly to one or other side, and then holding the head still. (This should be done with a light touch, and the response to flexion may only be tested when it is clear that there is no question of a neck injury.) If the patient is unconscious the eyes will initially be 'left behind', but will subsequently 'catch up' with the movement of the skull, and come to occupy their original resting position in relation to the skull. The movements so elicited are called 'doll's head eye movements'. These movements will only occur if the overriding influences controlling eye movement from the hemispheres are suppressed, and the oculomotor and vestibular components and the connections between them in the brain-stem are still functioning.

The caloric responses are elicited, provided that the tympanic membrane is intact, by slow irrigation of the auditory canal with at least 50 ml of ice-cold water. The patient's head should be positioned 45 °, head up, with the eyelids held open. In an unconscious patient with an intact brain-stem, both eyes will deviate toward the irrigated ear. In a patient feigning loss of consciousness the manoeuvre is extremely unpleasant and will produce nystagmus with the slow component toward the irrigated side and possibly vomiting. If the vestibular and oculomotor components or the connections between them in the brain-stem are nonfunctioning as a result of either a focal lesion or severe, generalized, metabolic depression, the eyes will not move in relation to the skull.

In metabolic and drug-induced coma the oculocephalic and caloric responses are present at first because of the removal of the overriding hemispheric influences, but disappear later as brain-stem function is depressed. Caloric stimulation provides a much stronger stimulus than head turning and may therefore still produce a response when the doll's head eye movements have already been lost.

Both manoeuvres will demonstrate a VI nerve palsy by absence of lateral movement of the affected eye and make the oculomotor consequences of a IIIrd nerve palsy very obvious because the affected eye remains turned laterally and downward whilst the other moves in relation to the skull. Failure of either eye to move to the nasal side of the midline is evidence of an internuclear lesion in the brain-stem. The presence of doll's head eye movements is good evidence that the patient is unconscious, except in the presence of blindness or lesions affecting the connections between the motor eyefields on the frontal cortex and

the oculomotor nuclei. These exceptions may seem to render this test of unconsciousness of little value, but in practice patients who have doll's head eye movements for these reasons are usually obviously conscious.

The transition from unconsciousness to consciousness is usually heralded by the appearance of small, quick, conjugate movements of the eyes interspersed within the doll's head movements. Oddly, these rapid movements, which represent the beginnings of the ability to fixate, always precede the reappearance of any response to menace.

Relatively rapid jerking movements of both eyes commonly occur during grand-mal seizures. Retraction nystagmus due to the simultaneous contraction of all the extraocular muscles is associated with mesencephalic lesions, and caudal pontine lesions produce a repetitive and very distinctive rapid downward movement of the eyes followed by a slow upward return to the mid-position. This phenomenon is known as ocular bobbing and is very specific to lesions in this area.

The jaw jerk and corneal responses

The presence of an abnormally brisk jaw jerk signals a bilateral, upper motor neurone lesion above the motor nucleus of the Vth cranial nerve, and always suggests the possibility of a pseudobulbar palsy. The corneal reflexes test the integrity of the Vth and VIIth cranial nerves and a small pontine section of the brain-stem and will be depressed with bilateral hemispheric damage.

Swallowing and the cough reflex

The total reliability of the swallowing mechanism should always be mistrusted in any unconscious patient. Overflow of saliva from the mouth is simple evidence of an inability to swallow, but the fact that the patient does not cough when fluid is instilled into the mouth is no guarantee of the continence of the swallowing mechanism unless the cough reflex has been demonstrated to be intact by laryngeal stimulation with a suction catheter.

Any patient who cannot guard their airway should ideally be positioned on their side, slightly head down and without a pillow, so that one corner of the mouth is at a lower level than any other part of the upper airway. This requirement may well conflict with the need to position the patient steeply head up to limit the generation of cerebral oedema. Should this conflict arise, it is a clear indication for the placement of a cuffed endotracheal tube to isolate the airway from the pharynx.

The respiratory pattern

Distortions of the normal respiratory pattern may assist in the localization of the neurological disturbance. The characteristic patterns associated with lesions at various levels are illustrated in Fig. 15.

The respiratory patterns in Fig. 15((a) and (d)) are both examples of Cheyne–Stokes breathing. In Fig. 15(d), where the lesion is at the junction of pons and medulla, Cheyne–Stokes breathing will occur in the presence of a normal lung to brain circulation time of approximately 8 s, and a respiratory cycle length of 16 s measured from apnoea to apnoea. In this case the periodic respiration appears because the mechanism that turns ventilation on and off is damaged, analogous to a sticky thermostat switch. In long-cycle Cheyne–Stokes breathing, where the respiratory cycle length may be from 30 to 200 s, the essential lesion is not neurological but a prolonged lung to brain circulation time, occasioned either by a diminished cardiac output or an expanded central blood volume or commonly both. The system exhibits periodicity in this case because blood that has been relatively hyper- or hypoventilated in the lungs takes an abnormally long time (always half the respiratory cycle length) to reach the brain-stem and exert its moderating influence. This form of Cheyne–Stokes respiration is frequently revealed by the administration of opiates, which probably act in the same non-specific way as the deep-seated hemispheric lesions in Fig. 17(a) by removing hemispheric influences that otherwise conceal the abnormal respiratory pattern.

Abnormal hyperventilation (Fig. 17(b)) may be associated with focal, usually destructive, lesions in the midbrain and pons, and an apneustic respiratory pattern (Fig. 17(c)) with similar lesions in the pons (see also Section 24). The apneustic pattern always betokens a neurological lesion, but hyperventilation is only rarely due to focal brain-stem damage and the diagnosis is only tenable in the presence of other evidence of midbrain or pontine damage, and in the absence of a metabolic cause.

Ataxic irregular patterns of respiration (Fig. 17(e)) shading into apnoea are associated with medullary depression occurring for any reason.

Frequently it is necessary to inspect the respiratory pattern of a patient who is already being ventilated. To prevent hypoxia during the period that the patient is left to his or her own respiratory devices, the lungs should be washed out with 100 per cent oxygen from an anaesthetic bag. Whilst the patient remains apnoeic the arterial carbon dioxide tension will rise at a rate of approximately 2 mmHg/min, and the spontaneous respiratory pattern may not emerge until the carbon dioxide level has risen considerably, but with the preoxygenation described, this should be possible without hypoxaemia.

The ciliospinal reflex

The ciliospinal reflex is a homolateral pupillary dilation evoked by pinching the skin of the neck. It probably depends upon both active sympathetic stimulation, and inhibition of the parasympathetic outflow from the Edinger–Westphal nucleus. It is enhanced by depression of hemispheric function, but its principal significance is to indicate that there are functioning long tracts passing through the entire length of the brain-stem.

The motor responses of the limbs

The cerebral hemispheres are more sensitive to hypoxia, malperfusion, and metabolic depression than is the brain-stem. In an unconscious patient, if the brain-stem can be shown to be intact to the system of testing already described, then the responses of the limbs to noxious stimuli can be used as a test of hemispheric and spinal cord function. The noxious stimulus may be applied as pressure in the region of the stylomastoid foramina, supraorbital pressure, tracheal suction, vigorous cutaneous stimulation over the sternum or pressure applied to the nail beds. The responses of the limbs are graded as in the Glasgow coma scale (Section 24) from, at best, an attempt to remove the stimulus, to localization of the site of stimulation, to flexion and external rotation of the arms coupled with extension, internal rotation, and plantar flexion of the legs (decorticate rigidity), to extension and internal rotation of the arms with hyperpronation of the hands and powerful extension of the legs (decerebrate rigidity) and finally, at worst, a failure to produce any movement of either arm or leg.

These responses clearly involve the sensory elements of the nervous system as well as the motor and require that the long tracts in both brainstem and spinal cord are intact. Decerebrate rigidity is associated experimentally with brain-stem disorders and commonly appears with damage at this level, but it is also seen in the absence of other brain-stem signs with widespread hemispheric damage such as occurs after hypoxia where the anatomical changes have been confined to hemispheres.

The motor responses together with the limb reflexes and the plantar responses may make it possible to determine that one hemisphere is disproportionately affected, suggesting a focal lesion.

There are two clinical syndromes associated with expanding, supratentorial mass lesions that must be recognized. Symmetrical supratentorial expansion interferes with the midbrain structures from above downwards. Initially it produces bilaterally unresponsive, mid-position pupils, and loss of upward gaze of the eyes in response to head flexion followed by loss of the lateral component of the doll's head eye movements. Usually, if the signs have progressed to the stage of loss of the lateral eye movements, the damage is irretrievable, and will be followed in order by signs of pontine and hindbrain destruction. Asymmetrical supratentorial expansion (the uncal syndrome) produces progressive dilation of the pupil on the same side as the lesion, followed by an oculomotor palsy as the IIIrd nerve is progressively stretched by herniation of the uncal portion of the temporal lobe downwards between the edge of the tentorium and the midbrain. This is followed by dilation of the other pupil to the mid-position and loss of the doll's head eye movements due to midbrain compression or sometimes wide dilation of

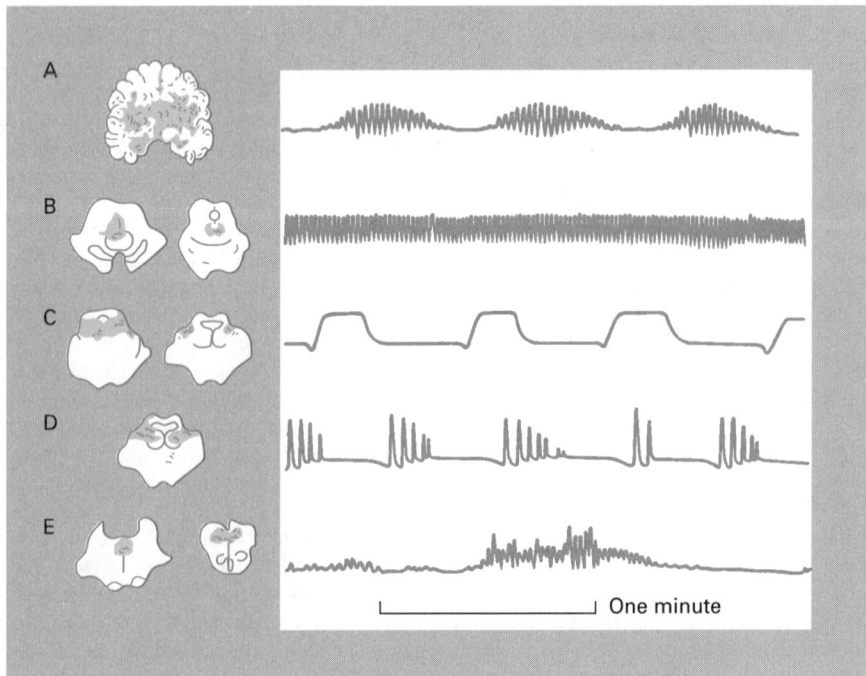

Fig. 15 Abnormal respiratory patterns associated with pathological lesions (shaded) at various levels of the brain. Tracings by chest–abdomen pneumograph, inspiration reads up. (A) Cheyne–Stokes respiration. (B) Central neurogenic respiration. (C) Apneusis. (D) Cluster breathing. (E) Ataxic breathing. (Reproduced from Plum and Posner. (1966). *The diagnosis of stupor and coma*. 1st edn. F.A. Davis, Philadelphia, with permission.)

the other pupil perhaps due to stretching of the other IIIrd nerve as a result of the further distortion of the midbrain.

The ocular fundus

Subhyaloid haemorrhages tend to be associated with either subarachnoid or intracerebral haemorrhage, and obvious diabetic changes may establish that the patient has long-standing diabetes. Perhaps the most important fact of which the physician should be aware is that patients presenting with acute coma and who have raised intracranial pressure very rarely have papilloedema. In patients who succumb as a result of overwhelming cerebral oedema, angiography reveals total obstruction of the cerebral circulation, probably due to compression of the cerebral capillaries, but the circulation through the retinal vessels is preserved, consonant with the observation that these patients do not have papilloedema.

Investigations

The techniques of examination that have been described are all possible in an unconscious patient and an intelligent analysis of the patient's responses should make it possible to determine whether the patient has a focal or generalized disturbance affecting the brain-stem or hemispheres, and whether the disturbance is progressing for better or worse and at what rate.

If the patient is unconscious and has focal signs, the most useful investigation is likely to be a computerized tomographic (**CT**) scan. If a CT scan is not available, decisions about further investigation in this group of patients will depend upon the direction and rate of change of the signs. If there is improvement, it is reasonable to delay angiography, but if there is deterioration at a rate which allows it, angiography should be undertaken seeking a treatable space-occupying lesion. If deterioration is rapid the patient should be transferred directly to theatre for exploratory bur holes if there is any possibility that the signs are due to an extradural haematoma.

If the patient is unconscious and does not have focal signs, but has meningism, a lumbar puncture should be made, seeking evidence of subarachnoid haemorrhage or meningitis. If the history is very strongly suggestive of subarachnoid haemorrhage and CT scanning facilities are readily available, a scan is the preferred investigation, as it is thought that lumbar puncture may further destabilize patients with subarachnoid haemorrhage. It should be borne in mind that some patients with meningitis, especially those who are very ill, may not have menigism, so that other signs of infection in combination with unconsciousness are an indication for lumbar puncture. The prognosis of those with meningitis who are unconscious before the institution of treatment is so bad that the outcome may not be influenced by diagnosis or treatment.

The remaining group of patients who are unconscious, and who have neither focal signs nor meningism, are likely to be suffering from generalized brain contusion, anoxic damage, the postictal stage following a fit, metabolic coma, or drug intoxication. The metabolic causes of coma, hepatic or renal failure, carbon dioxide narcosis, and hyperglycaemia are usually very obvious on other clinical grounds, and hypoglycaemia should always be tested for at a very early stage in the examination of any unconscious patient. The metabolic cause that is sometimes missed is that due to porphyria. Drug intoxication can only be proved by appropriate chemical testing and most laboratories require guidance as to the drugs they should be seeking. There are, in the United Kingdom, a number of poisons centres from which advice may be sought. Intoxication due to carbon monoxide may be missed; its neurological manifestations in the acute phase are identical to those of hypoxia, and the half-time for its clearance from the blood is 250 min if the patient is breathing air, and is reduced to 50 min if the patient breathes 100 per cent oxygen. There may therefore be little of the gas remaining in the blood by the time that its presence is sought.

Management of the unconscious patient

It is inappropriate to detail here the treatment of space-occupying lesions, subarachnoid haemorrhage, meningitis, and the various causes of metabolic coma and intoxications considered in the section on investigation. It is the general aspects of management, and those appropriate to an intensive care unit that will be considered.

Immediate measures

The clearance and maintenance of the airway takes precedence over all else. How this is achieved depends upon the setting in which the patient is first seen and what apparatus is to hand. Gravity is always available and it may be sufficient to position the patient on his or her side with no pillow under the head so that one corner of the mouth is the lowest part of the upper airway. It is important to avoid flexion or extension of the neck until cervical injury has been excluded.

In the early management of an unconscious patient in hospital, the placement of a cuffed endotracheal tube has so many advantages that it is perhaps easier to separate those patients who may be safely managed without this intervention; essentially those who can be demonstrated to cough in response to laryngeal stimulation, and who will swallow without coughing if a small quantity of water is instilled into the mouth. Such patients will usually be sufficiently reactive that they will not tolerate endotracheal intubation. The important advantage of intubation is the ability to clear the major airways and protect them from any further obstruction or soiling, especially if gastric lavage is necessary. Also, there is freedom to position the patient optimally in response to either neurological or circulatory requirements, and the option that the patient may be ventilated mechanically. If there is any doubt as to the adequacy of of spontaneous ventilation, the patient must be ventilated. The practical disadvantage of intubation is that it may be necessary to use anaesthetic agents or muscle relaxants, which will obscure the trend of neurological events. Agents with the briefest duration of action should be used, ideally perhaps only suxamethonium chloride.

The autoregulatory nature of the cerebral circulation tends to preserve the perfusion of the brain against circulatory inadequacy, but any such inadequacy must be dealt with appropriately. Similarly, cerebral metabolism must be protected by rigorous treatment of any hypo- or hyperglycaemia. It has been demonstrated that close control of blood sugar concentrations so that they lie between 4 and 8 mmol/l offers better eventual preservation of function in cases of both hypoxic and traumatic brain damage.

When the integrity of the cerebrospinal fluid compartment has been breached, usually because of a fracture of the base of the skull, it is normal practice to give augmentin.

Measures for the control of intracranial pressure

After damage to the brain, from whatever cause, it is common to observe a trend of improvement in the function of the nervous system followed, usually after a period of between 10 and 72 h by a rapid and often catastrophic deterioration. Given that an expanding intracranial haematoma has been excluded in the manner outlined in the section on investigation, this deterioration follows a rise in intracranial pressure and an increase in intracranial water. CT scanning suggests that the water is distributed both intravascularly and as oedema fluid. The view has been expressed that once damage of a certain severity has occurred the outcome is inevitable and that the excess intracranial water is not instrumental in the destruction of the brain, but the fact that the patient's nervous system may improve to function at levels approaching normal consciousness after the insult and yet be overwhelmed subsequently is very persuasive evidence to the contrary. The angiographic evidence suggests that the increase in fluid obstructs the cerebral circulation by compression at capillary level and that the intracranial venous system and the retinal circulation are not obstructed, explaining the absence of

Table 3 *Complications of malnutrition*

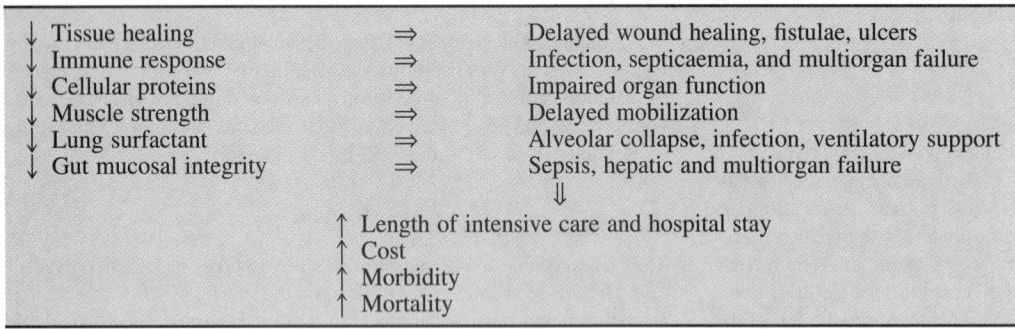

↓ Tissue healing	⇒	Delayed wound healing, fistulae, ulcers
↓ Immune response	⇒	Infection, septicaemia, and multiorgan failure
↓ Cellular proteins	⇒	Impaired organ function
↓ Muscle strength	⇒	Delayed mobilization
↓ Lung surfactant	⇒	Alveolar collapse, infection, ventilatory support
↓ Gut mucosal integrity	⇒	Sepsis, hepatic and multiorgan failure

⇓

↑ Length of intensive care and hospital stay
↑ Cost
↑ Morbidity
↑ Mortality

papilloedema in the presence of gross rises in measured intracranial pressure.

If the inferences drawn from the above observations are correct, it becomes very important to limit the rise in intracranial pressure by every possible means. It is neither possible nor desirable to measure the intracranial pressure of every unconscious patient, but where it is known that there has been a profound cerebral insult and there is evidence of a good initial recovery, there is a strong case for such monitoring. The pressure may be measured intradurally or extradurally; both approaches are effective in that they warn of a rise in intracranial pressure, although they may not yield the same values. The intradural system, because of the risks of infection, can only be used for 48 h, which in many cases is too brief a period. Experience with monitoring in selected cases has demonstrated that the single, most effective measure for the reduction of intracranial pressure is to position the patient as steeply head up as possible, in the sitting position. This may compromise the ideal management of the lungs or circulation, but may have to take precedence. Intracranial-pressure measurement also offers a solution to the dilemma that, on the one hand, it would be beneficial to sedate the patient whose restlessness will drive the intracranial pressure up still further, yet on the other, the sedation will obscure changes in the neurological signs. Pressure measurement gives much earlier warning of change that requires intervention than do the signs of midbrain compression, which only appear when the damage to the brain-stem is near to irreversible.

Experimental evidence suggests that dexamethasone is only effective in the limitation of cerebral oedema if it is given before the cerebral damage occurs, or in the control of the oedema associated with abscesses or cerebral tumours. It is currently accepted practice to use hyperventilation to an arterial carbon dioxide tension of between 25 and 30 mmHg, posture, and precise control of the blood sugar (4–8 mmol/l) in patients at risk from cerebral oedema. Perhaps the best evidence that these measures may be effective comes from the observation that cessation may produce a sharp rise in intracranial pressure in some patients for as long as 10 days after the initial cerebral insult, and that their reintroduction returns the pressure to its original level.

Both osmotic and renal tubular diuretics can be used effectively in the control of intracranial pressure. Mannitol as a bolus is very effective if used as a temporary measure to allow time for surgical intervention, but has the disadvantage that after about 4 h it causes the intracranial pressure to rise. This problem can be circumvented by continuous infusion, but if a sustained effect is required it is probably simpler to use frusemide. It must be remembered that, although a low right-atrial pressure and a strongly negative water balance will reduce oedema formation wherever it is occurring, diuresis must not be taken to the point at which the circulation is jeopardized.

Two further measures aimed at reducing brain damage may conveniently be considered at this point, although they operate by reducing cerebral metabolism rather than by acting directly on oedema formation, i.e. the administration of barbiturates in high dosage and cooling of the patient to 31°C. Although both are effective in reducing cerebral metab-

olism, recent evidence from three controlled trials failed to show any advantage for the use of barbiturates after head injury, or anoxic brain damage. The use of corticosteroids following traumatic head injury tested by comparison of predicted outcome between centres also failed to show any difference.

Nutritional support

The importance of early nutritional support for critically ill patients is now well recognized. After the brief, metabolically quiescent period (24–48 h) that may follow the initial insult, a hypercatabolic state develops such that, in the absence of an exogenous supply of protein, energy, vitamins and trace elements, a rapid loss of muscle protein occurs and the patient becomes progressively more susceptible to the complications of malnutrition (Table 3).

Virtually all patients appropriately admitted to intensive care for more than 3 days should receive nutritional support, preferably by the enteral route. Severe injury, surgery, and sepsis comprise the majority of admissions where prompt nutritional support is necessary to limit the extent of the negative nitrogen balance. It is important to assess the baseline nutritional and fluid balance status on admission and to review both fluid and calorie requirements daily.

Assessment

Assessment requires a thorough medical and nutritional history as well as details of recent weight change and calorie and fluid intake. Examination should assess the extent of any weight loss, muscle wasting, and evidence for specific nutrient deficiencies. Precise monitoring of body weight is extremely difficult in intensive care and the decision concerning the appropriate fluid balance for the forthcoming 24 h will rely on the bedside assessment of not only intravascular volume but also the cellular and interstitial components of the extravascular space. From the clinical signs it should be possible to decide whether or not the patient's current fluid balance lies within 5 per cent of a putative ideal state and hence the appropriate goal for the next 24 h may be decided. There are relatively few blood tests of much value in assessing nutritional status or the response to treatment. However, in the absence of specific haematological conditions, the absolute lymphocyte count is a useful guide, with a count of less than $1000 \times 10^9/l$ indicating marked nutritional impairment. Serum albumin is the most commonly quoted biochemical index of nutritional status but there is no useful correlation with nitrogen balance in the critically ill and its long half-life (in excess of 10 days) means that it cannot reflect rapid changes. A single value merely reflects the net effect of production, breakdown, excretion and infusion and the rate of fall is a better guide to requirements: if greater than 1 g/l per day there is urgent need for nutritional support. Transferrin, prealbumin, and retinol-binding protein are more sensitive tests but generally less readily available.

Table 4 *Nitrogen–calorie requirements in different catabolic states*

Energy output (kcal)	Nitrogen losses (g)	Metabolic state	Energy input (kcal)	Nitrogen input (g)	E/N ratio (kcal/g)
500–1000	4–6	Starvation	1500–2000	6–8	200–250
1500–2000	8–12	Normal	1500–2000	8–12	165–200
2000–3000	15–25	Catabolic + +	2000–2500	12–15	150–180
> 3000	> 25	Catabolic + + +	2500– > 3000	18–20	125–150

1 kcal is approx. 4.2 kJ.

Total nitrogen losses may be determined from direct measurement of urinary nitrogen excretion and estimation of other losses, particularly from the gastrointestinal tract. Energy expenditure may be calculated by indirect calorimetry from measurements of carbon dioxide production and oxygen consumption. Such measurements are obviously necessary for research studies and provide a precise statement about the metabolic state of the patient. However, the metabolic constraints in critically ill patients mean that, despite a markedly hypercatabolic state, frequently only relatively modest amounts of nitrogen and energy can be efficiently handled and there is an obligatory negative nitrogen and energy balance. Further increases in the amount of nitrogen provided will produce complications rather than benefit, resulting in excessive urea production and increased urinary nitrogen output but no improvement in nitrogen balance. Similarly, it is now realized that excessive energy provision with either fat or carbohydrate is not beneficial but causes hyperglycaemia, glycosuria, fatty liver, futile substrate recycling, increased oxygen consumption and carbon dioxide production, and adverse effects on platelet and pulmonary capillary basement-membrane function.

Consequently, irrespective of measurements of nitrogen loss and energy consumption, the practical and appropriate prescription for nitrogen will usually lie between 0.15 and 0.25 g/kg body weight and for calorie requirements between 25 and 40 kcal/kg body weight according to an 'end-of-the-bed' assessment of metabolic state and as specified in Table 4. The energy should be supplied as carbohydrate and fat in energy-equivalent amounts, although in patients with serious hepatic or pulmonary complications, rather less fat is given. The appropriate energy/nitrogen ratio varies from 250 : 1 to 125 : 1 as the metabolic state changes from simple starvation to hypercatabolic.

Timing and route of feeding

The urgency to start feeding depends on the underlying diagnosis, the pre-existing nutritional state, the metabolic state, and the anticipated clinical course. To avoid delay in starting enteral feeding in patients who are already malnourished with upper gastrointestinal lesions, insertion of a feeding gastrostomy or jejunostomy should be considered at laparotomy.

During the initial 48 h of an admission to intensive care, most patients will receive 5 per cent dextrose as the only source of energy, and even for those admitted following major surgery or trauma this will be quite appropriate as it coincides with the metabolically quiescent period. If a nasogastric tube has been passed and there are no surgical contraindications, enteral feed at 20 ml/h may be started within the first 24 h. If after 48 h there is no immediate prospect of resuming a normal oral diet, a nasogastric or nasoenteral tube should be passed and enteral feeding commenced. If full enteral feeding cannot be established over the next 2 to 3 days, parenteral nutrition will be necessary.

Enteral feeding

Provided there is no absolute surgical contraindication or significant risk of lung aspiration, enteral feeding is always preferable to parenteral nutrition. It is unnecessary to await the return of bowel sounds or passage of flatus per rectum, as these traditional signs may be absent despite normal small bowel function. After confirming a satisfactory tube position, a standard tube feed should be started at 20 ml/h and progressively increased until the required volume of feed per day is achieved. There is no evidence that starting with half-strength feeds is of any benefit in establishing enteral feeding. Four-hourly aspiration should be done with return of the aspirate provided it does not exceed 100 ml for the extubated patient at risk of aspiration, or 300ml for the intubated patient with a protected airway. It is important not to aspirate too frequently and discard the aspirate, as gastric motility is often impaired in intensive-care patients and a relatively large 'end-gastric volume' is necessary to promote emptying.

Early attention to bowel habit forestalls later problems. Regular lactulose or a suitable bulking agent should be started early, rectal examination made and suppositories/enemata given if appropriate. If unsuccessful, a cathartic agent such as senna may be used, provided mechanical obstruction has been excluded; sodium docusate is preferable for patients with renal failure because it has a lower potassium content.

Continuing problems with large aspirates should prompt a check of the tube position and an attempt to stop drugs that impair motility such as opiates, muscle relaxants and dopamine. Attempting to pass the tube beyond the pylorus using radiographic screening, and nursing the patient with a 'head-up' tilt, may also help. Addition of fibre to the feed promotes normal bowel function and there is evidence that it provides additional mucosal protection.

The pattern of feeding is also an important consideration. Continuous feeding is widely practised but reduces gastric acidity, favouring bacterial colonization, and may promote nosocomial infection. Bolus feeding to simulate normal behaviour often causes regurgitation and diarrhoea. The ideal pattern may be to allow several periods of 3 to 4 h during which feeding is stopped to allow a normal acid pH to be restored thereby limiting bacterial overgrowth.

Enteral feeding is safe, more physiological, easy to administer, requires less medical and nursing expertise, and avoids both the risks and cost of parenteral nutrition. Recent evidence also suggests that it helps to maintain gut mucosal integrity by stimulating gut blood flow, encouraging motility, and by providing a luminal supply of glutamine, which is the major energy source of the gut mucosa. These effects may reduce the endotoxin and bacterial load gaining access to the portal venous blood, thereby protecting against the development of hepatic dysfunction and multiorgan failure.

It should be possible to establish enteral feeding in the majority of patients: the need to start parenteral nutrition in more than 20 per cent of patients in a general medical/surgical intensive care unit suggests a failure of gut care and/or the enteral feeding protocol and should prompt a review of unit policy.

Parenteral nutrition

Depending on the case mix in the intensive care unit, total parenteral nutrition will be required in approximately 10 per cent of patients. It requires suitable central access and safe prescription, preparation, and delivery. There have been considerable advances in all these areas, particularly the development of the 'all-in-one-bag', which is prepared in the pharmacy sterile unit, contains the entire nutritional requirements for 24 h, and provides the advantage of simultaneous rather than sequential delivery of the nutrients. The volume is usually prescribed to the nearest 500 ml on the basis of the overall daily fluid requirements, typically ranging from 1500 to 3000 ml/day (65–125 ml/h). Unless direct measurements are made the nitrogen and energy requirements are calculated according to Table 4.

Glucose is the preferred carbohydrate because it is physiological, relatively inexpensive, and blood concentrations are easily monitored. It is available in 5, 10, 20, 40, and 50 per cent concentrations and provides from 200 (5 per cent) to 2000 (50 per cent) kcal/l. Earlier enthusiasm for using alternative carbohydrate sources has subsided because there are no significant benefits; lactic acidosis may complicate the use of fructose, sorbitol and ethanol while xylitol increases urate and oxalate production.

Fat is available for intravenous use as an oil-in-water emulsion containing soybean extract, egg phospholipids and glycerol ('intralipid'), produced in 10, 20, and 30 per cent strengths that provide 1000, 2000, and 3000 kcal/l, respectively. Their advantage is that they are only slightly hyperosmolar with a neutral pH and provide high levels of the essential fatty acids, linoleic and linolenic acids. However, with impaired hepatic clearance or if given in excess they may impair liver and platelet function and exacerbate existing lung damage through coating the pulmonary endothelial membrane and stimulating prostaglandin synthesis.

Clearance of fat from the plasma is reduced in both sepsis and carnitine deficiency and should be assessed by inspecting the plasma for a turbid, lipaemic appearance persisting 30 min after the infusion of parenteral nutrients has been stopped. Early in the hypercatabolic phase of an illness, fat should be given in relatively small amounts (20 g/day) sufficient to supply the essential fatty acids and to act as a vehicle for the fat-soluble vitamins.

The necessary vitamins, minerals, and trace elements are provided in commercially available ampoules containing the appropriate daily or weekly requirements. It is important to remember that excessive administration may be more harmful than relative deficiency. Phosphate con-centrations should checked regularly and maintained above 0.6 mmol/l; typically, with normal renal function, 30 to 40 mmol are required daily.

REFERENCES

Aubier, M., Trippenbach, T., and Roussos, C. (1981). Respiratory muscle fatigue during cardiogenic shock. *Journal of Applied Physiological Respiration and Environmental Exercise Physiology*, **51**, 499–508.

Barber, R.E., Lee, J., and Hamilton, W.K. (1970). Oxygen toxicity in man: a prospective study in patients with irreversible brain damage. *New England Journal of Medicine*, **283**, 1478–84.

Bell, J.A., Bradley, R.D., Jenkins, B.S., and Spencer, G.T. (1974). Six years of multidisciplinary intensive care. *British Medical Journal*, **ii**, 483–488.

Bihari, D., Smithies, M., Gimson, A., and Tinker, J. (1987). The effects of vasodilatation with prostacyclin on oxygen delivery and uptake in critically ill patients. *New England Journal of Medicine*, **317**, 397–403.

Bradley, R.D. (1973). Shock. In *Recent advances in surgery*, (ed. S. Selwyn Taylor), pp. 275–96. Churchill Livingstone, Edinburgh.

Bradley, R.D. (1977). *Studies in acute heart failure*. Edward Arnold, London.

Bradley, R.D. (1978). Intensive care. In *Progress in clinical medicine*, (eds A.R. Horler and J.B. Foster), pp. 303–19. Churchill Livingstone, Edinburgh.

Bradley, R.D., Jenkins, B.S. and Branthwaite, M.A. (1970). The influence of atrial pressure on cardiac performance following myocardial infarction complicated by shock. *Circulation*, **42**, 827–37.

Branthwaite, M.A. (1980). *Artificial ventilation for pulmonary disease*. Pitman, London.

Braunwald, E., Covell, J.W., Maroko, P.R., and Ross, J., Jr. (1969). Effects of drugs and of counterpulsation on myocardial oxygen consumption. Observations on the ischaemic heart. *Circulation*, **40** (suppl. 4), 220–8.

Bryan-Brown, C.W. and Ayers, S.M. (ed.) (1987). *Oxygen transport and utilisation*. Society of Critical Care Medicine, Fullerton CA.

Burn, J.M.B. (1970). Design and staffing of an intensive care unit. *Lancet*, **i**, 1040–1043.

Chamberlain, D.A., Leinbach, R.C., Vassaux, C.E., Kastor, J.A., De Sanctis, R.W., and Sanders, C.A. (1970). Sequential atrioventricular pacing in heart block complicating acute myocardial infarction. *New England Journal of Medicine*, **282**, 577–82.

Chatterjee, K., Parmley, W.W., Ganz, W., Forrester, J., Walinsky, P., Crexells, C., and Swan, H.J.C. (1973). Haemodynamic and metabolic responses to vasodilator therapy in acute myocardial infarction. *Circulation*, **28**, 1183–93.

Cohn, J.N., Guiha, N.H., Broder, M.I., and Limas, C.J. (1974). Right ventricular infarction, clinical and haemodynamic features. *American Journal of Cardiology*, **33**, 209–14.

Cournand, A., Motley, H.L., Werko, L., and Richards, D.W. (1948). Physiological studies of the effects of intermittent positive pressure breathing on cardiac output in man. *American Journal of Physiology*, **152**, 162–174.

Guyton, A.C. and Lindsey, A.W. (1959). Effect of elevated left atrial pressure and decreased plasma protein concentration on the development of pulmonary oedema. *Circulation Research*, **7**, 649–657.

Guyton, A.C. (1963). *Circulatory physiology: cardiac output and its regulation*, pp. 380–3. Saunders, Philadelphia.

Lee, H.A. and Venkat Raman, G. (ed.) (1970) *A handbook of parenteral nutrition* (1970) Chapman and Hall, London.

Macklem, P.T. and Roussos, C.S. (1977). Respiratory muscle fatigue. A cause of respiratory failure? *Clinical Sciences*, **53**, 419–22.

Miller, G.A.H., Sutton, G.C., Kerr, I.H., Gibson, R.V., and Honey, M. (1971). Comparison of streptokinase and heparin in the treatment of isolated acute massive pulmonary embolism. *British Medical Journal*, **ii**, 681–684.

Mueller, H., Ayres, S.M., Gianelli, S., Conklin, E.F., Mazzara, J.T., and Grace, W.J. (1972). Effect of isoproterenol, L-norepinephrine and intra-aortic counterpulsation of haemodynamics and myocardial metabolism in shock following acute myocardial infarction. *Circulation*, **45**, 335–52.

Pontoppidan, H., Geffin, B., and Lowenstein, E. (1972). Acute respiratory failure in the adult: *New England Journal of Medicine*, **287**, 690–8; 743–52, 799–806.

Poole-Wilson, P.A. and Langer, G.A. (1975). Effect of pH on ionic exchange and function in rat and rabbit myocardium. *American Journal of Physiology*, **229**, 570–81.

Replogle, R.L., Meiselman, H.J., and Merrill, E.W. (1967). Clinical implications of blood rheology studies. *Circulation*, **36**, 148.

Ritter, J.M., Doctor, H., and Benjamin, M. (1990). Paradoxical effect of bicarbonate on cytoplasmic pH. *Lancet*, **335**, 1243–6.

The urokinase pulmonary embolism trial. A national co-operative study. (1973). *Circulation*, **47** (suppl. 2).

Vincent J.L. (ed.) (1990). *Update in intensive care and emergency Medicine 10*. Springer Verlag, Berlin.

Weissman, C., (ed.) (1987). Nutritional support. *Critical Care Clinics*, **3**, 1–238.

Wheat, M.W. and Palmer, R.F. (1968). Dissecting aneurysms of the aorta: present status of drug versus surgical therapy. *Progress in Cardiovascular Diseases*, **11**, 198–210.

Yatsu, F.M. (1986). Cardiopulmonary–cerebral resuscitation. *New England Journal of Medicine*, **314**, 440–1.

Section 17 *Respiratory medicine*

17.1	Introduction	2591

17.2	Structure and function	2593
	17.2.1 Functional anatomy of the lung	2593
	17.2.2 The upper respiratory tract	2609

17.3	Lung defences and responses	2612
	17.3.1 Non-immune defence mechanisms of the lung	2612
	17.3.2 Inflammation and the lung	2616

| 17.4 | Pathophysiology of lung disease | 2628 |

| 17.5 | The clinical presentation of chest diseases | 2642 |

17.6	Investigation of respiratory disease	2652
	17.6.1 Thoracic imaging	2652
	17.6.2 Tests of ventilatory mechanics	2666
	17.6.3 Microbiological methods in the diagnosis of respiratory infections	2675
	17.6.4 Diagnostic bronchoscopy and tissue biopsy	2678
	17.6.5 Histopathology and cytology in diagnosis of lung disease	2685

17.7	Respiratory infection	2691
	17.7.1 Upper respiratory tract infection	2691
	17.7.2 Acute lower respiratory tract infections	2692
	17.7.3 Suppurative pulmonary and pleural infections	2704
	17.7.4 Chronic specific infections	2707
	17.7.5 Respiratory infection in the immunosuppressed	2708

17.8	The upper respiratory tract	2714
	17.8.1 Allergic rhinitis ('hay fever')	2714
	17.8.2 Upper airways obstruction	2719

17.9	Airways disease	2724
	17.9.1 Asthma	2724
	(a) Basic mechanisms and pathophysiology	2724
	(b) Clinical features and management	2729
	(c) Occupational asthma	2742
	17.9.2 Cystic fibrosis	2746
	17.9.3 Bronchiectasis	2755
	17.9.4 Chronic obstructive pulmonary disease	2766

17.10	Diffuse parenchymal lung disease	2779
	17.10.1 Introduction	2779
	17.10.2 Cryptogenic fibrosing alveolitis	2786
	17.10.3 Bronchiolitis obliterans	2795
	17.10.4 The lung in collagen-vascular diseases	2796
	17.10.5 Pulmonary vasculitis and granulomatosis	2800
	17.10.6 Pulmonary haemorrhagic disorders	2803
	17.10.7 Pulmonary eosinophilia	2804
	17.10.8 Lymphocytic infiltrations of the lung	2806
	17.10.9 Extrinsic allergic alveolitis	2809
	17.10.10 Sarcoidosis	2817
	17.10.11 Pulmonary histiocytosis X (eosinophilic granuloma of the lung) and lymphangiomatosis	2832
	17.10.12 Pulmonary alveolar proteinosis	2833
	17.10.13 Pulmonary amyloidosis	2835
	17.10.14 Lipoid (lipid) pneumonia	2837
	17.10.15 Pulmonary alveolar microlithiasis	2838
	17.10.16 Pneumoconioses	2839
	17.10.17 Toxic gases and fumes	2847
	17.10.18 Radiation peneumonitis	2848
	17.10.19 Drug-induced lung disease	2848
	17.10.20 Adult respiratory distress syndrome	2852
	17.10.21 Lung disorders in genetic syndromes	2861

| 17.11 | Pleural disease | 2863 |

| 17.12 | Disorders of the thoracic cage and diaphragm | 2872 |

17.13	Neoplastic disorders	2879
	17.13.1 Tumours of the lung	2879
	(a) Lung cancer	2879
	(b) Pulmonary metastases	2893
	17.13.2 Pleural tumours	2893
	17.13.3 Mediastinal tumours and cysts	2895

17.14	Respiratory failure	2901
	17.14.1 Definition and causes	2901
	17.14.2 Sleep-related disorders of breathing	2906
	17.14.3 The management of respiratory failure	2918
	(a) Acute respiratory failure: intensive care	2918
	(b) Chronic respiratory failure	2925
	17.14.4 Lung and heart-lung transplantation	2933

17.1 Introduction

J. M. HOPKIN and D. J. LANE

The lungs, as the portal of entry into the body of the oxygen needed for tissue respiration, almost imperceptibly shift in excess of 10 000 litres of air a day. Inevitably inhaled at the same time are noxious chemicals in various forms, allergens, and microbes. Yet for most individuals the lungs remain clear and healthy. Only excessive 'pollution' or faults (that may include 'exuberant' response) in the normally robust defence mechanisms of the lungs will result in lung damage and disease. Whatever technological advantages occur in the future, those concerned with respiratory health, as well as disease, will need to be alert to dangers in the air we breathe. Infections, industrial and personal pollution, and allergens are all known hazards—what is yet to come?

Epidemiological trends in the pattern of respiratory diseases can be an early warning system as well as a tool for investigating causes. The association between smoking and lung cancer raises one of the most notable contributions in the field of respiratory medicine.

At least one-third of the population in developed countries continue to smoke cigarettes and lung cancer and disabling chronic airflow obstruction will remain prevalent in the foreseeable future. Tobacco manufacturers have launched a major and cynical advertising campaign in developing countries.

Infection will continue to play a major role in respiratory disease and human health. In developing countries where living conditions and nutrition are poor, measles, whooping cough, and infection by *Haemophilus influenzae* and the pneumococcus cause more than 5 million deaths annually in children under the age of 5. Tuberculosis causes 3 million deaths annually worldwide. This mortality is principally in the developing countries, but there are strong indications that the prevalence of tuberculosis is increasing in North America and Europe in the wake of the acquired immunodeficiency syndrome (AIDS) epidemic, and that multiply resistant drug strains are being increasingly encountered. There is an epidemic of pneumonia due to the opportunistic fungal pathogen *Pneumocystis carinii* in the AIDS population, in whom it is a leading cause of illness and death.

Asthma affects at least 5 per cent of most populations; it is the commonest chronic disease of children, causing more absence from school than any other condition in many countries. It is a heterogeneous disorder resulting from the interaction of genetic and environmental factors. There has been a significant increase in its prevalence over the past 20 years; the reasons for this are unclear, except that they must be 'environmental' changes of some kind.

Respiratory medicine will need to meet the challenge of new disease as well as to deal with existing pathology by increased research effort. Here, advances in molecular medicine and investigative techniques, and novel therapeutic approaches offer new hope.

Molecular advances

The application of powerful molecular genetic techniques in research is beginning to yield rewards. The gene locus and defects that underlie the development of cystic fibrosis have been identified. Deletion of a trinucleotide (ΔF 508) in the gene on chromosome 7 for the transmembrane chloride regulator (CFTR) is the commonest mutation underlying cystic fibrosis (Fig. 1) in Caucasian populations. Preliminary trials have been launched on the delivery of normal CFTR gene to respiratory epithelium in cystic fibrosis.

The structure, function, and interactions of various cytokines involved in inflammatory response in the lung are becoming increasingly documented. These advances offer opportunities for the development of improved prevention and treatment of disease for the future. The molecular mechanisms underlying the genetics of atopy and asthma and the biology of cancer are also subjects of intensive current investigations.

Molecular techniques are becoming increasingly applied in the practical diagnosis of respiratory infection. DNA amplification (by the polymerase chain reaction) offers a powerful, swift and specific diagnostic method and is becoming increasingly applied to viral infections, Pneumocystis pneumonia (Fig. 2), and tuberculosis.

Investigative methods

Computerized tomography (CT) of the thorax and lungs is becoming a standard investigation for the diagnosis and staging of lung cancer. High

Fig. 1 DNA sequence of exon 10 of the cystic fibrosis gene, showing the normal sequence and that of a patient homozygous for the ΔF508 mutation (deletion of CTT, resulting in the loss of phenylalanine at amino acid 508). (By courtesy of S. Shackleton and A. Harris.)

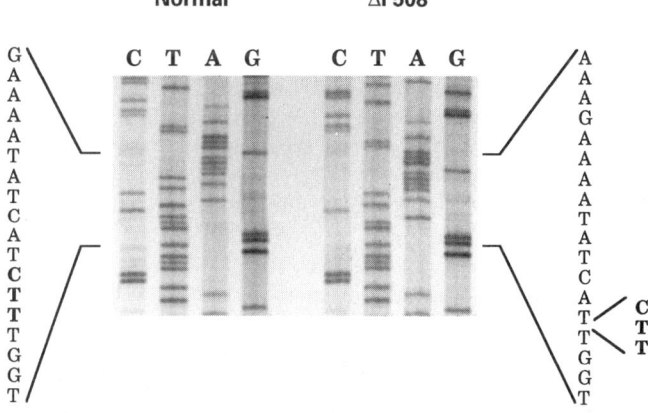

Fig. 2 DNA amplification for the specific diagnosis of *Pneumocystis carinii* from induced sputum. A diagnostic band (345 bp) is seen on electrophoresis after simple ethidium staining and UV light transillumination.

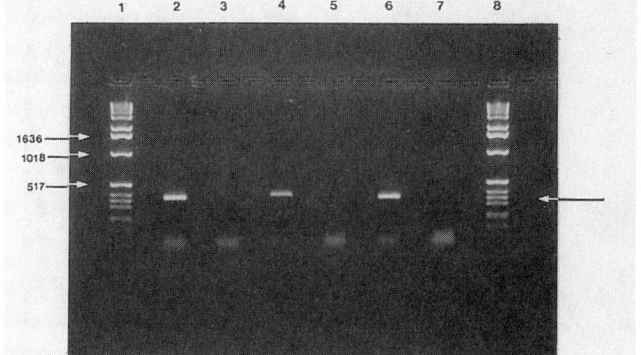

resolution CT provides accurate imaging also for bronchiectasis and inflammatory parenchymal lung disease (Fig. 3). Adjunctive percutaneous biopsy can be accurately targeted on pulmonary or pleural lesions.

Pulse oximetry has emerged as an easy non-invasive, but accurate, bedside or clinic method for measuring and monitoring oxygen saturation. Similar ease of measurement of CO_2 tensions is still just out of reach. Techniques for non-invasive ambulatory recording of lung function, particularly in airflow obstruction, have so far failed to be robust enough for clinical use, but will be developed.

Fibreoptic thoracoscopy is being increasingly developed; its potential applications include accurate pulmonary and pleural biopsy sampling, the closure of air leaks, pleuroadhesis and pleurectomy, and the excision of peripheral pulmonary tumours.

Therapy

Orally active antibiotics with significant anti-Gram-negative effects, including activity against Pseudomonas, have been developed as in the form of the 4-quinolones.

Cytotoxic chemotherapy is becoming increasingly established as a valuable palliative measure in small-cell lung cancer. Single-agent treatment, for example with oral etoposide, can achieve significant medium-term remission and palliation, although reliable bio-availability after oral administration has yet to be fully developed. There is little prospect of curative chemotherapy with current approaches.

The increasing recognition that asthma is an inflammatory disorder, often based on atopic response in children and young adults, has led to increasing emphasis on the use of inhaled locally active steroids for the control of asthma. β-Adrenergic agents remain best in the relief of symptoms, but significant concerns have emerged about potential ill effects when they are used on a regular basis. New insights into the biology of asthma will lead to fundamentally different approaches.

Developments in automatic ventilation have been significant. Nocturnal positive-pressure nasal ventilation can significantly improve daytime performance status and hypoxaemia in patients with chronic respiratory failure due to muscular or skeletal disorder; the method may find application in severe chronic airflow obstruction. In acute respiratory failure and acute lung injury, the need to minimize the barotrauma and haemodynamic disturbance caused by positive pressure ventilation is recognized; methods that include 'permissive hypercapnia', very high

Fig. 3 High resolution CT scan showing an air bronchogram traversing a small area of eosinophilic consolidation in a patient with atopic asthma and systemic vasculitis (Churg–Strauss syndrome).

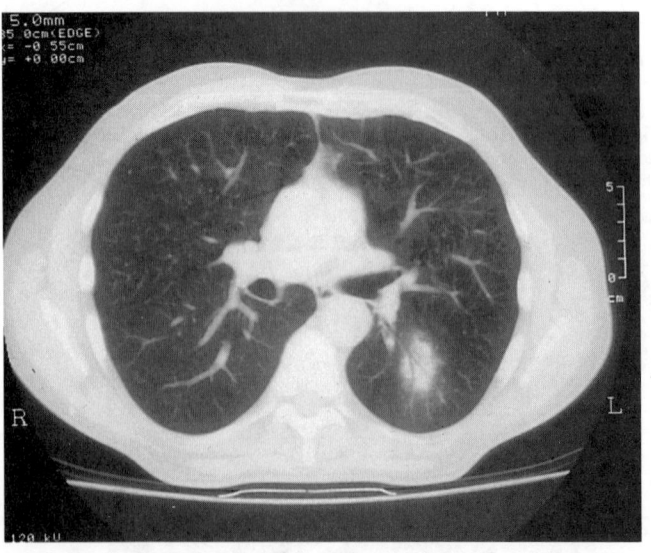

frequency ventilation, and intravascular and extraporeal gas exchange devices are being increasingly tested.

Transplantation of lungs or heart and lungs is being performed for endstage patients with cystic fibrosis, pulmonary hypertension, airflow obstruction due to α_1-antitrypsin deficiency, and other disorders. One and two year survival rates approach 80 per cent in centres with most expertise, but progressive obliterative bronchiolitis, as part of allograft rejection in the later term, remains a significant problem. The supply of human lungs is limited, so that the results of pioneering research into the use of lungs (and other organs) from transgenic pigs is eagerly awaited.

REFERENCES

Barnes, P.F., Bloch, A.B., Davidson, P.T., and Snider, D.E., Jr. (1991). Tuberculosis in patients with human immunodeficiency virus infection. *New England Journal of Medicine*, **324,** 1644–50.

Bousquet, J., Chanez, P., Lacoste, J.Y., *et al.* (1990). Eosinophilic inflammation in asthma. *New England Journal of Medicine*, **323,** 1033–9.

Calverley, P.M.A. (1992). Domiciliary ventilation in chronic obstructive lung disease. *Thorax*, **47,** 334–6.

Christensson, B.A., Nilsson-Ehle, I., Ljungberg, B., Lindbald, A., Malmborg, A.S., Hjelte, L., and Strandvik, B. (1992). Increased oral bioavailability of ciprofloxacin in cystic fibrosis patients. *Antimicrobial Agents and Chemotherapy*, **36,** 2512–17.

Clark, J.S., Votteri, B., Ariagno, R.L., *et al.* (1992). Non-invasive assessment of blood gases. *American Review of Respiratory Diseases*, **145,** 220–32.

Comis, R.L. (1992). Oral etoposide in oncology: an evolving role. *Annals of Oncology*, **3,** 63–7.

de Hoyos, A.L., Patterson, G.A., Maurer, J.R., Ramirez, J.C., Miller, J.D., and Winton, T.L. (1992). Pulmonary transplantation: early and late results: the Toronto Lung Transplant Group. *Journal of Thoracic and Cardiovascular Surgery*, **103,** 295–306.

Flotte, T.R., Afione, S.A., Solow, R., Drumm, M.L., Markakis, D., Guggino, W.B., *et al.* (1993). Expression of the cystic fibrosis transmembrane conductance regulator from a novel adeno-associated virus promoter. *Journal of Biological Chemistry*, **268,** 3781–90.

Goble, M., Iseman, M.D., Madsen, L.A., Waite, D., Ackerson, L., and Horsburgh, C.R.Jr. (1993). Treatment of 171 patients with pulmonary tuberculosis resistant to isoniazid and rifampicin. *New England Journal of Medicine*, **328,** 527–32.

Goldstraw, P. (1992). Endoscopy assisted micro-thoracotomy. *Thorax*, **47,** 489.

Heckmatt, J.Z., Loh, L., and Dubowitz, V. (1990). Night-time ventilation in neuromuscular disease. *Lancet*, **335,** 579–82.

MacKay, J. (1991). Tobacco: the third world war. *Thorax*, **46,** 153–6.

Marcy, T.W. and Marini, J.J. (1992). Modes of mechanical ventilation. In: *Current pulmonary*, (13th edn.) (ed D.H. Simmons and D.F. Tierney) pp. 43–90. C.V. Mosby, St. Louis, MO.

Mennie, M.E., Gilfillan, A., Compton, M., Curtis, L., Liston, W.A., Pullen, I., *et al.* (1992). Prenatal screening for cystic fibrosis. *Lancet*, **340,** 209–10.

Riordan, J.R., Rommens, J.M., Kerem, B., *et al.* (1989). Identification of the cystic fibrosis gene: cloning and characterization of complementary DNA. *Science*, **245,** 1066–73.

Salmeron, S., Guerin, J.C., Godard, P., *et al.* (1989). High doses of inhaled corticosteroids in unstable chronic asthma: a multicenter, double-blind, placebo-controlled investigation. *American Review of Respiratory Diseases*, **140,** 161–71.

Sears, M.R., Taylor, D.R., Print, C.G., *et al.* (1990). Regular inhaled beta-agonist treatment in bronchial asthma. *Lancet*, **336,** 1391–6.

Standiford, T.J. and Morganroth, M.L. (1989). High-frequency ventilation. *Chest*, **96,** 1380–9.

Swensen, S.J., Aughenbaugh, G.L., Douglas, W.W., and Myers, J.L. (1992). High resolution CT of the lungs: findings in various pulmonary diseases. *American Journal of Roentgenology*, **158,** 971–9.

Wakefield, A.E., Guiver, L., Miller, R.F., and Hopkin, J.M. (1991). DNA amplification on induced sputum samples for diagnosis of *Pneumocystis carinii* pneumonia. *Lancet*, **337,** 1378–9.

17.2 Structure and function

17.2.1 Functional anatomy of the human lung

E. R. WEIBEL and C. R. TAYLOR

Overview

In heavy exercise, when an average adult requires about 2.5 litres of oxygen every minute to fuel the energy needs of his or her muscles, gas exchange in the lung must be achieved in a fraction of a second. This clearly asks for a high level of bioengineering design of the pulmonary gas exchanger, mainly by establishing a high diffusion conductance. The chief design features of the lung are that the surface of air–blood contact is very large (almost the size of a tennis court) and that the tissue barrier separating air and blood is extraordinarily thin (50 times thinner than a sheet of airmail stationery).

This poses a number of problems that must be solved by appropriate design. First, the large area of the air–tissue interface must be made stable against the prevailing surface forces, despite the minimal amount of tissue available for support. Second, the thin tissue barrier must be vital, i.e. made of cells, in order to control the fluid balance between blood, tissue, and alveolar space, and to allow the tissue some capacity for repair and reaction to small and large insults. Third, the large surface must be ventilated and perfused with blood as evenly and as well matched as possible to ensure efficient gas exchange.

In this chapter we shall address these issues and then ask to what extent the lung is designed to meet the needs of the body. This will lead us to consider the lung as part of the respiratory system that extends from the lung through the circulation of blood to the mitochondria, the organelles that generate ATP, the energy currency of the cells, through oxidative phosphorylation. We shall ask whether all the structures involved are designed to serve the overall functions of the system well.

The cells of the gas exchange barrier

Although the gas exchange barrier is very thin, it must be composed of three tissue layers: an endothelium lining the capillaries, an epithelium lining the air spaces, and an interstitial layer to house the connective tissue fibres. The guiding principle in designing these cells must evidently be to minimize thickness and maximize extent. However, there is a limit to this, which is set by the need to make the barrier and its constituent cells strong enough to resist the various forces that act on it—capillary blood pressure, tissue tension, and surface tension in particular. Furthermore, the barrier must remain intact for a lifetime, and this requires continuous repair and turnover of the cells and their components.

Squamous cells line the barrier

The major part of the barrier surface is lined, on both the air and the blood side, by simple layers of squamous cells (Fig. 1(a)). This histological description is sufficient for the endothelium whose cell population is uniform. However, the epithelium is a mosaic of different cell types, and therefore a small fraction of the total surface (a few per cent) (Table 1) is occupied by secretory cells. The squamous lining cells are

usually called type I, and the secretory cells are called type II alveolar cells or pneumocytes. A rare third cell, the brush cell, is also found in some specific regions near the terminal bronchiole; its function is as yet unknown.

The capillary endothelium and the type I epithelial cells show rather similar design features (Fig. 1(b)). They are simple cells with a small compact nucleus which is surrounded by a thin rim of cytoplasm containing only a few small mitochondria and some cisternae of endoplasmic reticulum, characteristics of a quiescent cell with little metabolic activity.

At the edge of the perinuclear region a very attenuated cytoplasmic leaflet emerges (Fig. 1(a)), essentially composed of two plasma membranes with a very small amount of cytoplasmic ground substance interposed; it spreads out broadly over the basal lamina. Terminal bars are formed where the cytoplasmic leaflets of epithelial cells, or of endothelial cells, meet (Fig. 1(c)). In this respect there is a notable difference between these two linings: the tight junction between the epithelial cells constitutes a powerful seal of the intercellular cleft, whereas that in the endothelium is rather leaky, allowing an almost uninhibited exchange of water, solutes, and even some smaller macromolecules between the blood plasma and the interstitial space.

The two basically similar lining cells differ in size. Although the capillary surface is some 10 to 20 per cent smaller than the alveolar surface, the capillary endothelial cells are about four times more numerous than type I cells; this means that the surface covered by one type I

Fig. 1 (a) Alveolar septum with capillary (C) containing erythrocytes (EC). The tissue barrier is lined by type I alveolar epithelial (EP1) and capillary endothelial cells (EN) whose nuclei (N) are surrounded by a small amount of cytoplasm which extends as thin leaflets with intercellular junctions (J). The interstitial space contains fibroblast processes (Fb) and bundles of collagen and elastic fibres (F) in the thick part of the barrier. (b) A portion of the minimal barrier with fused basement membranes (BM) and the four plasma membranes of epithelium and endothelium with some pinocytotic vesicles. (c) The intercellular junctions (J) which are long and tight in the epithelium and short and 'leaky' in the endothelium. Scale markers: (a) 2 μm; (b), (c) 0.2 μm.

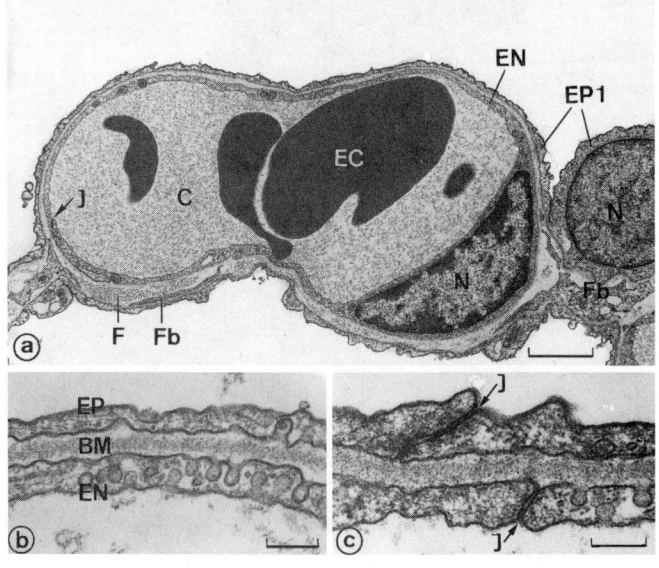

Table 1 *Morphometric characteristics of cell population in human lung parenchyma*

Cell population	Percentage of total cell number*	Average cell volume (μm^2)	Average apical cell surface (μm^2)
Alveolar epithelium			
Type I	8	1764	5098
Type II	16	889	183
Endothelium	30	632	1353
Interstitial cells	36	637	—
Alveolar macrophages	10	2492	—

*Total cell number in human lung, 230×10^9.

Data from Crapo, Barry, Gehr, Bachofen, and Weibel, *American Review of Respiratory Diseases*, **125**, 332, 1983.

epithelial cell must be about four times larger, namely 4000 to 5000 μm^2 compared with about 1000 μm^2 for endothelial cells (Table 1).

Scanning electron micrographs of the surface of the alveolar epithelium (Fig. 2) show that the patches covered by single type I cells are variable in size, and that even the largest are much smaller than the 4000–5000 μm^2 given above. One finds that type I cells are not simple squamous cells, but rather branched cells that extend to both sides of the septum where they form multiple apical faces (Fig. 3).

The alveolar secretory cell produces surfactant

Although it is often called the 'large alveolar cell', the type II cell is, in fact, relatively small with a mean volume less than half that of the type

Fig. 2 Scanning electron micrograph of the alveolar wall surface in the human lung reveals a mosaic of alveolar epithelium made of type II cells (asterisk), and broad type I cells whose cytoplasmic leaflet (boundary outlined by arrows) extends over many capillaries (C). Note the interalveolar pore of Kohn (K). Scale marker: 10 μm.

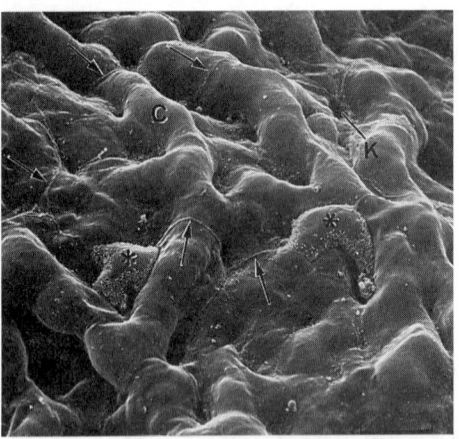

I cell (Table 1). Its shape is cuboidal and it has no cytoplasmic extensions (Figs 2–4). The apical cell surface bulges toward the lumen and is provided, mostly around its periphery, with a tuft of microvilli.

The type II cell shows a wealth of cytoplasmic organelles of all kinds (Fig. 4): mitochondria, substantial endoplasmic reticulum with ribosomes, and a well-developed Golgi complex surrounded by a set of small lysosomal granules among which so-called multivesicular bodies (membrane-bounded organelles containing a group of small vesicles) stand out (Fig. 4(c)). In addition, one finds the characteristic lamellar bodies—larger membrane-bounded organelles which contain a dense stack of phospholipid lamellae which stain black with osmium.

These structural properties are directly related to the principal function of the type II cell: the synthesis, storage, and secretion of surfactant, a complex of phospholipids and proteins that spreads in a thin film on the alveolar surface and drastically lowers the surface tension at the air–tissue interface.

The main surfactant phospholipid of the lung, dipalmitoylphosphatidylcholine (DPPC), lowers the surface tension at an air–water interface by spreading on the surface as a monomolecular film with the hydrophilic polar groups immersed in the water and the two hydrophobic palmitic acid residues sticking out. Additional components are phosphatidylglycerol and some cholesterol which modulate surfactant properties. It is well established that the type II cells synthesize DPPC, store it in the lamellar bodies, and secrete it into the thin fluid layer that covers the alveolar epithelium.

Despite a large number of biochemical studies, it is less certain how the type II cells synthesize DPPC. The most common biochemical pathway for the synthesis of lecithins or phosphatidylcholines, the so-called Kennedy pathway, results in phosphatidylcholine where at least one of the two fatty acids is unsaturated; the final synthesis of DPPC, where both fatty acid chains are fully saturated palmitic acids, involves reacylation.

Biochemical and autoradiographic studies support the notion that the primary site of DPPC synthesis within the type II cells is the endoplas-

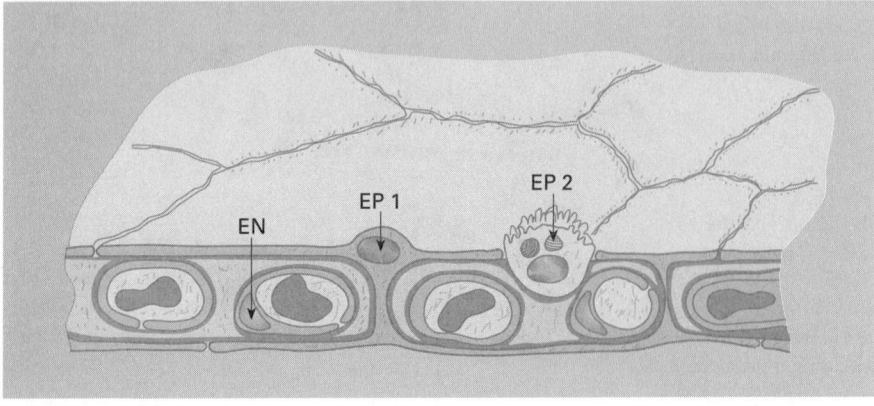

Fig. 3 Diagram of the alveolar wall showing the complexity of a type I epithelial cell (EP1) and its relation to a type II cell (EP2) and endothelial cells (EN).

Fig. 4 (a) Cuboidal type II epithelial cell from human lung contains osmiophilic lamellar bodies (LB) and a rich complement of organelles which are shown at higher power in (c): mitochondria (m), endoplasmic reticulum (ER), Golgi complex (G), lysosomes (Ly), and multivesicular bodies (mv). The plasma membrane shows microvilli on the surface towards the alveolus (A). (b) The apical part of a type II cell from rabbit lung with lamellar bodies (LB); one of these is seen in the process of being secreted into the surface lining layer with tubular myelin (TM) and a thin black film of DPPC (arrow) at the surface. Scale markers: (a) 1 µm; (b), (c) 0.5 µm.

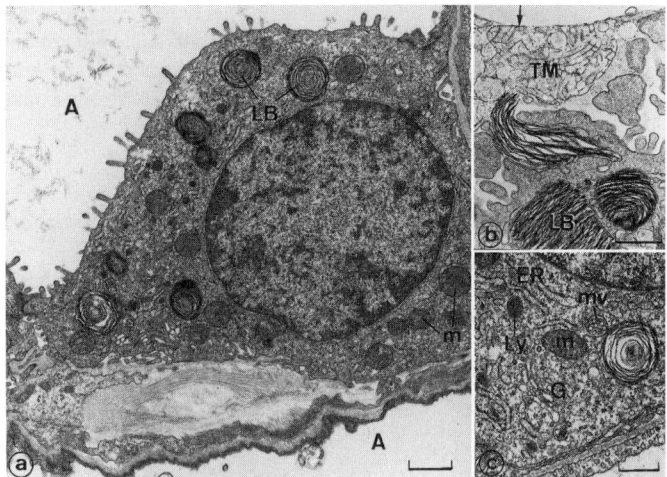

mic reticulum; from there the product is transferred to the Golgi apparatus and then to the multivesicular bodies that deliver it to the lamellar bodies (Fig. 4(c)). These organelles are arranged in a kind of complex (Fig. 5) and thus could establish a spatial sequence for the intracellular processing of phospholipids. It is possible that all sites are involved in one step or another of the complex pathway leading to DPPC.

Pulmonary surfactant also contains a significant fraction of specific proteins—the surfactant apoproteins SP-A, SP-B, and SP-C of different size and function which partly depend on their degree of hydrophobicity. The major protein is SP-A which makes up about 3 to 4 per cent of the total mass of isolated surfactant; its gene, which is located on chromosome 10, is expressed in the endoplasmic reticulum of type II cells and is regulated developmentally, partly through glucocorticoids. Apoproteins seem to be delivered in part to the lamellar bodies, but also partly discharged directly through microvesicles (Fig. 5).

The content of lamellar bodies is eventually secreted onto the alveolar surface by exocytosis: the granule membrane fuses with the apical plasma membrane and the content is discharged (Fig. 4(b)). In the alveolar lining layer the once densely packed phospholipid lamellae unravel and become associated with the apoproteins (Fig. 5). Within the lining layer this lipoprotein complex now forms a new pattern of regular array (Figs 5 and 4(b)), the so-called tubular myelin, which spreads on its free surface as a monomolecular film.

Turnover of pulmonary surfactant is rather rapid. Therefore continuous synthesis must be coupled with regulated removal, for which sev-

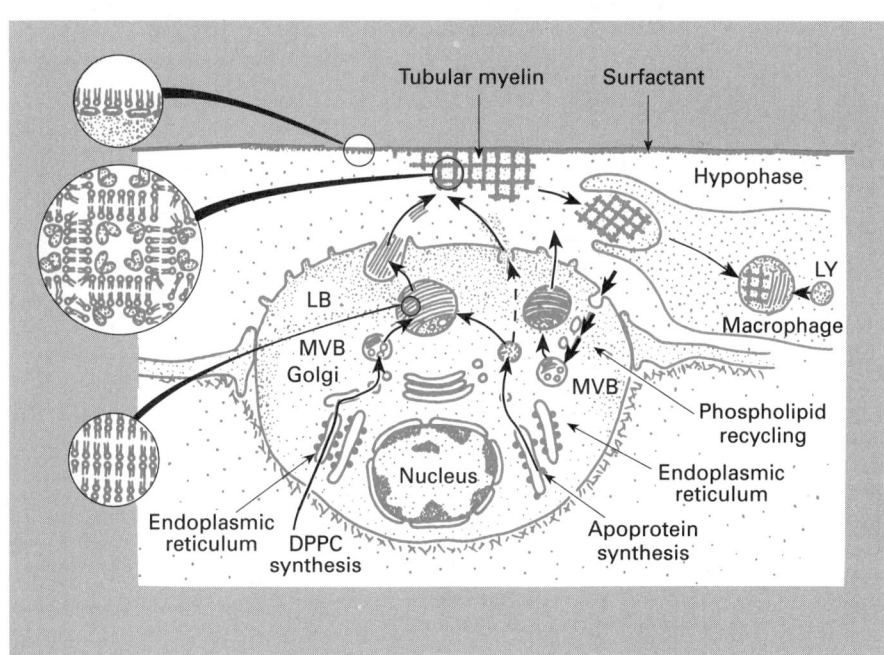

Fig. 5 Schematic diagram of a type II cell with pathways for synthesis and secretion of surfactant DPPC and apoproteins and for their (partial) removal by macrophages, as well as their recycling through epithelial cells. Multivesicular bodies (MVB) appear as precursors of lamellar bodies (LB). Note the arrangement of phospholipids and apoproteins in the lamellar bodies, in tubular myelin, and in the surface film.

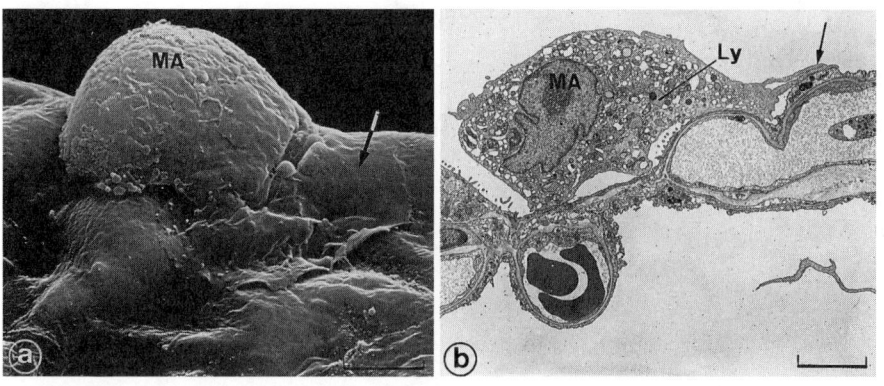

Fig. 6 (a) Scanning electron micrograph of an alveolar macrophage (MA) sitting on the epithelial surface of human lung. Note the cytoplasmic lamella (arrow) which represents the advancing edge of the cell. (b) The same type of cell in thin section to reveal the cytoplasmic lamellae (arrow) that serve as advancing edge for cell movement and as 'lips' for phagocytosis. Note the rich complement of lysosomes (Ly) in the cytoplasm. Scale marker: 5 µm.

eral pathways are known. Recent evidence indicates that an appreciable part of surfactant is recycled through the type II cells (Fig. 5). Some surfactant leaves the alveolar region over the surface of terminal bronchioles, from where it is removed by the mucociliary escalator; another part is engulfed by alveolar macrophages (Fig. 5) and broken up in their lysosomes which are known to contain, in addition to their usual complement of acid hydrolases, the enzyme phospholipase A2 that cleaves fatty acids from phosphatidylcholine.

Surfactant synthesis and turnover are tightly regulated both developmentally and in the mature lung. 'Neurohumoral' pathways have been postulated, but nothing very precise is known as yet. On the one hand, local regulatory effects must be postulated because it is known that surfactant production becomes stimulated by increased ventilation. However, it is possible that this increased surfactant production is the result of neural effects, since it can also be brought about by stimulation of the vagus nerve and by some neurotransmitters, mainly beta-adrenergic agonists. The problem with respect to neural control is that the lung parenchyma contains very few nerve fibres and they have not been shown to be related to type II cells.

There is reasonably good evidence that the potential for surfactant synthesis develops under the effect of some hormones, particularly glucocorticoids. This plays a major role during fetal lung development when, between the 18th and 25th gestational week in humans, surfactant begins to be secreted into the lung fluid. Sufficient quantities of surfactant have usually been produced by the 28th gestational week to allow stable expansion of alveoli, although birth normally takes place at about the 40th week.

Lung cells cope with vulnerability of the delicate tissue

The surface lining layer which carries the surfactant film overlays the alveolar epithelium and thus separates it from the air; it will intercept any fine particulate matter (dust, bacteria, etc.) that may reach the alveoli and become deposited on their wall. This fluid layer houses the alveolar macrophages (Fig. 6), which are large mobile cells with phagocytic activity and a rich complement of lysosomal elements in their cytoplasm. Alveolar macrophages constitute the first cellular defence line of the gas exchange tissue. They remove any unwanted materials, from foreign particles to surfactant wastes, from the surface lining layer. They cooperate in their defence activity with interstitial macrophages or histiocytes, mast cells, and leucocytes which are, however, rare in the normal septum, occurring mostly near lymphatics in the peripheral connective tissue sheaths of acini. Blood leucocytes have a tendency to be slowed in their passage through the lung, which suggests that they may exercise some of their defence functions in the capillaries, but this may sometimes have deleterious effects, leading to damage to the endothelial and epithelial cells. In some species, the capillaries contain a special class of intravascular macrophages, similar to Kupffer cells of the liver, but these cells seem to be missing in human lungs.

Among the tissue components of the alveolar septum, the alveolar epithelium is particularly vulnerable; this is because each of the very thin type I cells is exposed to air over a much larger surface than any other cell and, owing to the scarcity of organelles, has only a limited potential for repairing membrane defects. Furthermore, type I cells are not capable of mitosis, neither during lung growth when more cells are needed to coat the expanding alveolar surface, nor upon damage in the adult lung when cells need to be replaced. In both instances new type I cells are made by mitotic division and transformation of type II cells which form squamous extensions and lose their potential for surfactant synthesis, a process which takes about 2 to 5 days.

A syndrome of severe catastrophic respiratory failure develops when this normal repair mechanism cannot cope with excessive damages. One condition for this to happen is when the lung becomes diffusely damaged by toxic fumes, and here it is noteworthy that breathing pure oxygen over a prolonged period is also highly toxic to lung cells, but it also

occurs in shock, for example upon severe blood loss or as a consequence of multiple bone fractures, possibly mediated by blood leucocytes that rapidly settle in the lung capillaries. In such patients one finds that large parts of the type I cell lining of the alveolar surface are destroyed; as a consequence, the barrier has become leaky and the alveoli fill with alveolar oedema, so that they can no longer take part in gas exchange.

Even if alveolar oedema is resolved by proper medical care, gas exchange often does not improve immediately. The repair of the severely damaged alveolar epithelium requires many new cells made by division of type II cells. These form a rather thick cuboidal lining of the barrier surface which offers a high resistance to oxygen flow. Several weeks are required for the thin barrier to be restored by transformation of the cuboidal cell lining into delicate type I cells.

Organization of tissues in the pulmonary gas exchanger

Alveoli and capillaries structure the air–blood contact

In order to establish a very large area of contact between air and blood, alveoli are formed in the wall of all airways within the acinus, i.e. in the gas exchange units derived from the first-order respiratory bronchiole (Figs. 7 and 8). It is estimated that there are about 1.5×10^5 acini and 3×10^8 alveoli in the human lung, so that each acinar unit contains,

Fig. 7 Model of airway branching in human lung from trachea (generation $z = 0$) to alveolar ducts and sacs (generations 19–23). The first 14 generations are purely conducting; transitional airways lead into the acinus.

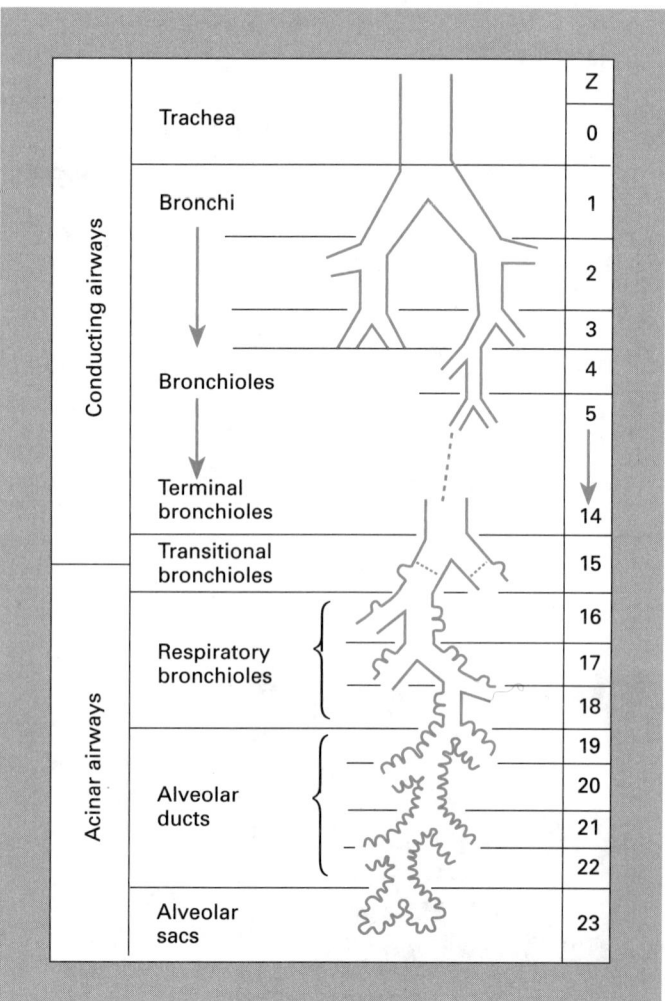

on average, about 2×10^3 alveoli connected to about six to eight generations of acinar airways, respiratory bronchioles, and alveolar ducts.

The alveoli are so densely packed that they occupy the entire surface of alveolar ducts; they are separated from each other by delicate alveolar septa which contain a single capillary network. About half the space of the septum is occupied by blood which is thus exposed to the air in two adjacent alveoli (Fig. 9).

The capillary network is continuous through many alveolar walls, probably at least throughout the entire acinus, if not for greater distances. It forms dense meshworks made of very short segments (Fig. 9(c)), and is so dense that it has been described as a sheet bounded by two flat membranes, the air–blood barrier, connected by numerous 'posts'.

The barrier separating air and blood is extremely thin because the two cell layers lining the alveolar and capillary surfaces are very much attenuated over the largest part of the surface, as we have seen above. To make the barrier very thin the interstitium must also be reduced to the minimum required (Fig. 1); it contains very few cells, mostly thin fibroblasts with long extensions and fine bundles of contractile filaments.

A fibre continuum supports the parenchymal structures

The reduction of the tissue mass in the alveolar septa to a minimum introduces a number of major problems with respect to maintaining the capillary bed expanded over a very large surface, a task which is made difficult because surface forces that act on the complex alveolar surface would tend to collapse alveoli and capillaries. This requires a very subtle economic design of the fibrous support system.

The solution of this problem is ingenious. The lung is pervaded by a system of fibres that extend from the hilum to the visceral pleura. It forms a three-dimensional fibrous continuum that is structured by the airway system and is closely related to the blood vessels (Fig. 10). First we find that all airways, from the main-stem bronchus that enters the lung at the hilum out to the terminal bronchioles and beyond, are encased in a strong sheath of fibres which constitute the axial fibre system; they form the 'bark' of the tree whose roots are at the hilum and whose branches penetrate deep into lung parenchyma, following the course of the airways. A second major fibre system is related to the visceral pleura which is made of strong fibre bags that encase all lobes from where connective tissue septa penetrate into lung parenchyma, separating units of the airway tree. We call these fibres the peripheral fibre system because they form the boundaries between the hierarchical units of respiratory lung tissue, segments, lobules, and finally acini.

The construction of the acinus, the functional unit of the lung parenchyma, deserves detailed description. The airway that leads into the acinus, the first-order respiratory bronchiole, continues branching within it for about six to ten additional generations (Figs 7 and 8). These intra-acinar airways, called respiratory bronchioles and alveolar ducts, carry in their walls relatively strong fibres of the axial fibre system that extend to the end of the duct system. However, since the wall of intra-acinar air ducts is densely populated by alveoli, these fibres are reduced to a network whose meshes encircle the alveolar mouths (Fig. 8(b)). These fibre rings serve as anchoring cables for the network of finer fibres that spread within the alveolar septa. The other end of these fibres is attached

Fig. 8 (a) Scanning electron micrograph of the lung shows branching of a small peripheral bronchiole (BL) into terminal bronchioles (T) from where the airways continue into respiratory bronchioles and alveolar ducts (arrows). Note the location of the pulmonary artery (a) and vein (v). (b) An alveolar duct (D) in cross-section surrounded by alveoli (A) and outlined by axial fibre tracts (arrow heads). Scale markers: (a) 0.5 μm; (b) 100 μm.

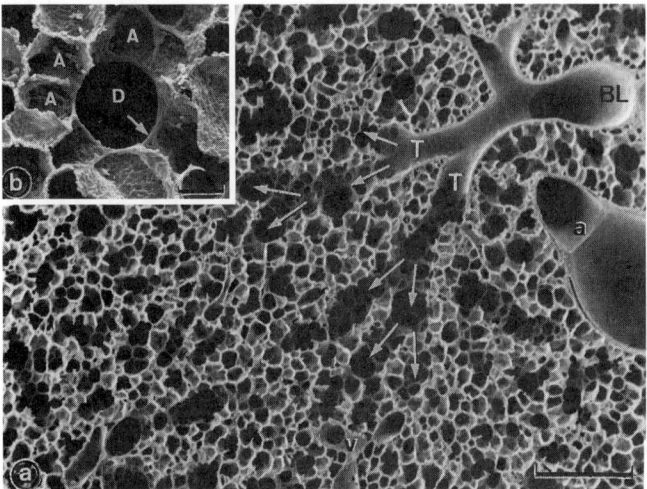

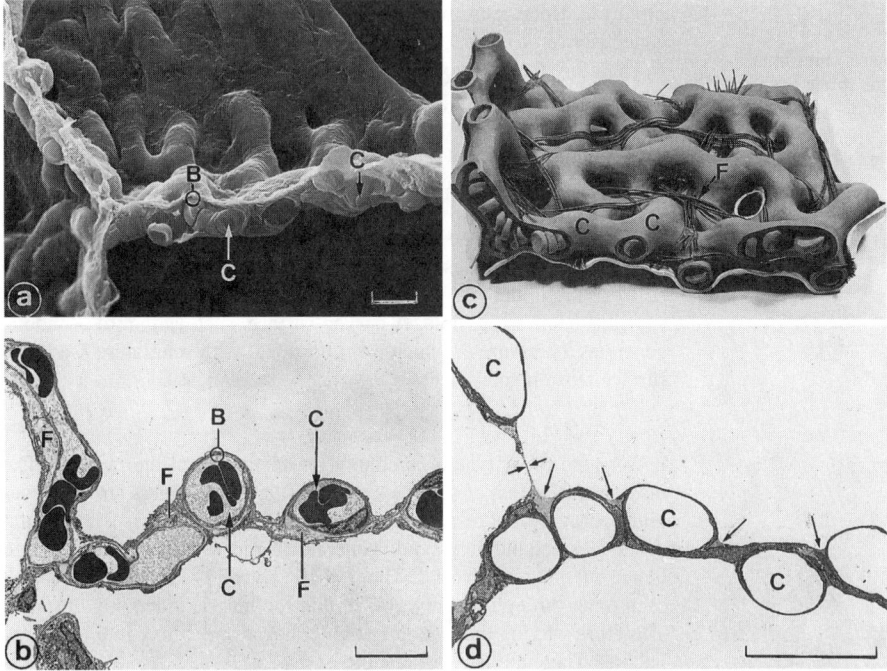

Fig. 9 In alveolar walls from the human lung, shown in (a) a scanning electron micrograph and (b) a thin section transmission electron micrograph, the capillary blood (C) is separated from the air by a very thin tissue barrier (B). (c) The model shows the capillary network to be interwoven with the meshwork of septal fibres (F) which occur on only one side of each capillary as seen in (b). (d) Similar septum from rabbit lung fixed by vascular perfusion to retain the surface lining layer which forms pools between bulging capillaries (arrows) and extends across an alveolar pore (paired arrows). Scale marker: 10 μm.

to extensions of the peripheral fibres that penetrate into the acinus from interlobular septa (Fig. 11).

The septal fibre meshwork is interlaced with the capillary network; Figs 9(b) and 9(c) show that, when the fibres are taut, the capillaries weave from one side of the septum to the other. This arrangement has a threefold advantage: (1) it allows the capillaries to be supported directly on the fibre strands; (2) it causes the capillaries to become spread out on the alveolar surface when the fibres are stretched; (3) it optimizes

Fig. 10 Scheme of the fibre tracts of the lung which are divided into axial fibres along the airways, peripheral fibres connected to the pleura, and septal fibres in the alveolar septa.

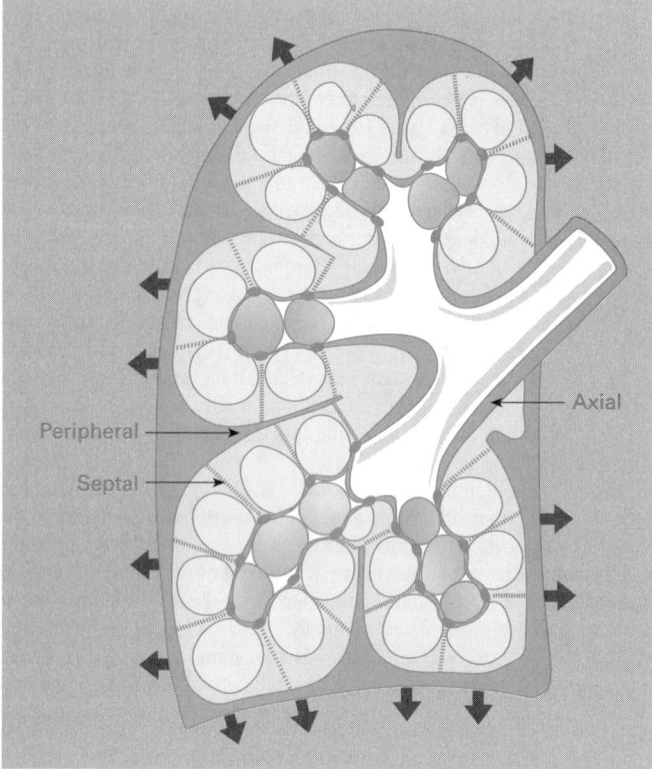

Fig. 11 Model of the disposition of axial, septal, and peripheral fibres in an acinus showing the effect of surface forces (arrows). Note the strong positive force on the free edge of alveolar septa supported by axial fibres.

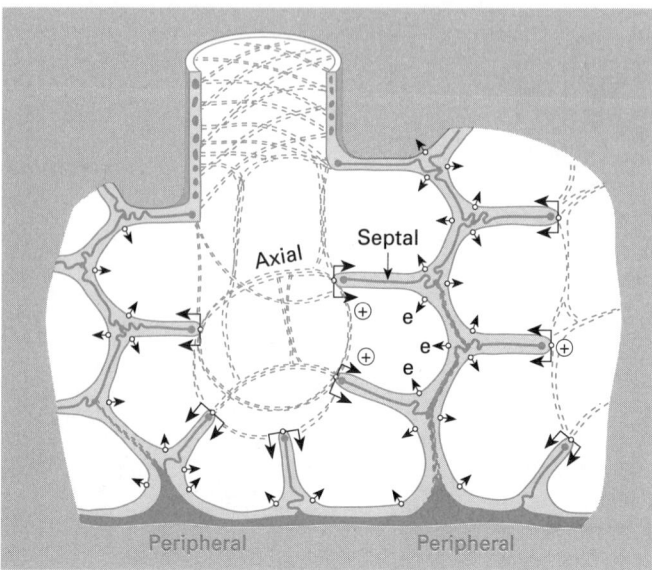

the gas exchange conditions by limiting the presence of fibres, which must interfere with oxygen flow, to half the capillary surface. An interstitial space with fibres and fibroblasts exists only on one side of the capillary, whereas on the other the two lining cells, the endothelium and the epithelium, become closely joined with only a single common basement membrane interposed (Fig. 1(b)). Therefore over half the surface the capillary blood is separated from the air merely by a minimal tissue barrier made of epithelial and endothelial cytoplasmic sheets with their basement membranes fused (Fig. 1(a)).

The formation of minimal barrier portions is a particularly important feature with respect to avoiding ill effects of interstitial oedema. Indeed, the differential permeability of endothelial and epithelial cells noted above makes it likely that fluid leaks from the plasma into the interstitial space but is prevented from leaking into the alveolar lining layer. However, this fluid will be limited to those parts of the interstitium that contain fibres and excluded from the minimal barrier portions where the basement membranes are fused (Figs 1 and 9(b)). Thus, even if some interstitial oedema forms, half the capillary surface can function normally as a gas exchanger. Furthermore, fluid which accumulates in the free interstitial spaces around the fibres can be drained away towards the lymphatics in the peripheral fibre system following the drainage pathways along the tracts of the fibre continuum.

In many respects, the fact that the pulmonary fibre system forms a continuum is an essential design feature of the lung. Its importance for the mechanical integrity of the gas exchanger becomes evident in pulmonary emphysema. When some fibres are disrupted they cannot be kept under tension; the broken fibres will retract and larger air spaces will form in the process of rearranging the fibre system in the surroundings of the damage.

Tissue design and surface tension determine parenchymal mechanics

The connective tissue fibres of the lung are a composite of collagen and elastic fibres. The practically inextensible collagen fibres have a very high tensile strength, whereas the elastic fibres have high extensibility but much lower tensile strength. In the relaxed composite fibre collagen fibres are longer than the elastic fibres, so that upon stretching the fibres elongate up to the point where the collagen fibres are taut, but from there on they resist stretching very strongly, protecting the fibre system from rupturing. Upon relaxation the elastic fibres shorten the fibres as homogeneously as possible.

Therefore the question is whether the fibre system is responsible for the recoil of the lung upon expiration when the distensive force of the chest wall is relaxed. It turns out that, at physiological inflation levels, the retractive force generated by the fibre system amounts to no more than a few millibars; the recoil force of the air-filled lung is appreciably higher, but this is due to surface tension rather than to fibre elasticity.

Surface tension arises at any gas–liquid interface because the forces between the molecules of the liquid are much stronger than those between the liquid and the gas. As a result the liquid surface will tend to be as small as possible. A curved surface, such as that of a bubble, generates a pressure P_s which is proportional to the curvature K and the surface tension coefficient γ:

$$P_s = 2\,\gamma K = 2\,\gamma/r. \tag{1}$$

In a sphere the curvature is simply the reciprocal of the radius r. The most critical effect of surface tension is that it endangers air-space stability because a set of connected bubbles of different sizes is inherently unstable: small bubbles should generate a larger pressure and empty into larger bubbles that expand. The 3×10^8 alveoli are all connected with each other through the airways, so that the lung is inherently unstable. Therefore why do the alveoli not all collapse and empty into one large bubble? There are two principal reasons.

The first reason concerns tissue structure. The alveoli are not simply soap bubbles in a froth, but their walls contain an intricate fibre system, as we have seen (Fig. 11). Thus, when an alveolus tends to shrink, the fibres in the walls of adjoining alveoli are stretched and, to a certain extent, this prevents the alveolus from collapsing. It is said that alveoli are mechanically interdependent and that this stabilizes them.

The second reason is related to the fact that the alveolar surface is lined by surfactant (Fig. 12), which has unusual properties in that its surface tension coefficient γ is variable. From a large volume of evidence it is now established that surface tension falls as the alveolar surface becomes smaller and rises when the surface expands, a feature which is due to the phospholipid nature of alveolar surfactant. Combined with interdependence, this property of surfactant allows the complex of alveoli to remain stable.

In the normal air-filled lung, surfactant properties and interdependence due to fibre tension both contribute to stabilizing the complex of alveoli and alveolar ducts. Interdependence is established by the continuum of axial, septal, and peripheral fibres (Fig. 11). Surface tension exerts an inward pull in the hollow alveoli where curvature is negative. However, over the free edge of the alveolar septa, along the outline of the duct, the surface tension must push outwards because there the curvature is positive; however, this force is counteracted by the strong fibre strands, usually provided with some smooth muscle cells, that we find in the free edge of the alveolar septum. Thus interdependence is an important factor in preventing the complex hollow of the lung from collapsing. However, its capacity to do so is limited and requires low surface tensions, particularly on deflation when the fibres tend to slack. If lungs are depleted of surfactant, the axial fibre system is not able to support the free edges of the alveolar septa and the alveoli collapse.

Micromechanics of the alveolar septum

The fibre network of the alveolar septum serves as a platform for spreading the capillary network on the alveolar surface (Fig. 9). When the fibres are stretched the capillaries bulge alternately to one side or the other, and this will cause pits and crevices to occur in the meshes of the capillary network. This irregular surface is to some extent smoothed out by the presence of an extracellular layer of lining fluid which is rather thin over the capillaries but forms little pools in the intercapillary pits (Fig. 12). This lining consists of an aqueous layer of variable thickness, called the hypophase, topped by the surfactant film.

The configuration of the alveolar septum results from the moulding effect of the various forces that must be kept in balance: tissue tension, surface tension, and capillary distending pressure. The fibres of the alveolar septum are under varying tension; owing to fibre elasticity this causes the capillaries to be shifted to one side of the septum or the other (Figs 9(b) and 13). The wall of the capillaries is exposed to the vascular distending pressure which causes the thin barrier of the capillary opposite the fibres to bulge outward. This is counteracted by the force generated by surface tension, which is positive over bulging capillaries and negative over pits (Fig. 13).

The alveolar septum achieves a stable configuration when all these interacting forces are in balance. Combined forces tend to squash the capillary flat; this happens at high levels of lung inflation when the fibres are under high tension and the surface tension coefficient of surfactant reaches its highest value due to expansion of the surface (Fig. 14(a)). On deflation the fibres are relaxed and surface tension falls drastically; the capillary distending pressure now exceeds both the tissue and the surface forces, with the result that the slack fibres allow the capillaries to bulge slightly toward the air space, giving the surface a 'crumpled' appearance (Figs 9(d) and 14(b)).

Fig. 13 Interaction of the micromechanical forces of surface tension, tissue tension, and capillary distending pressure that shape the alveolar septum.

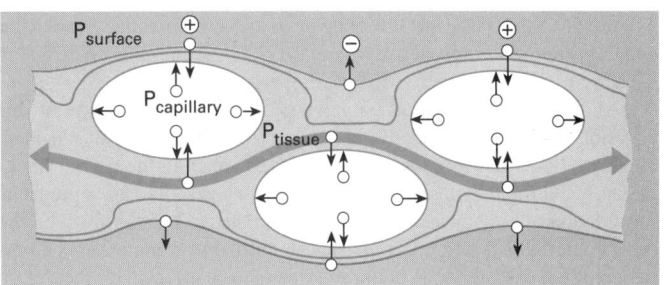

Fig. 14 (a) When surface tension exceeds capillary distending pressure at high levels of lung inflation (tissue fibres taut) the capillaries (C) become slit-like in the septum but remain open in the corners (C*). (b) At low inflation levels surface tension is very low and capillaries bulge towards the alveolar surface which has a 'crumpled' appearance. Scale marker: 20 μm. (Scanning electron micrographs from Bachofen, Weber, Wangensteen, and Weibel. (1983). *Respiration Physiology*, **52**, 41–52.)

Fig. 12 Alveolar lining layer (LL) topped by surfactant film which appears as a fine black line (arrows) and forms pools in crevices between capillaries (C). Note the type II cell with lamellar bodies and the fold in the thin tissue barrier (bold arrows). Alveolar septum of human lung fixed by perfusion through blood vessels. Scale marker: 2 μm.

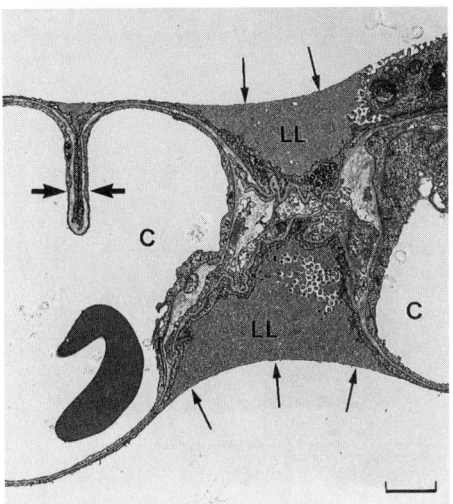

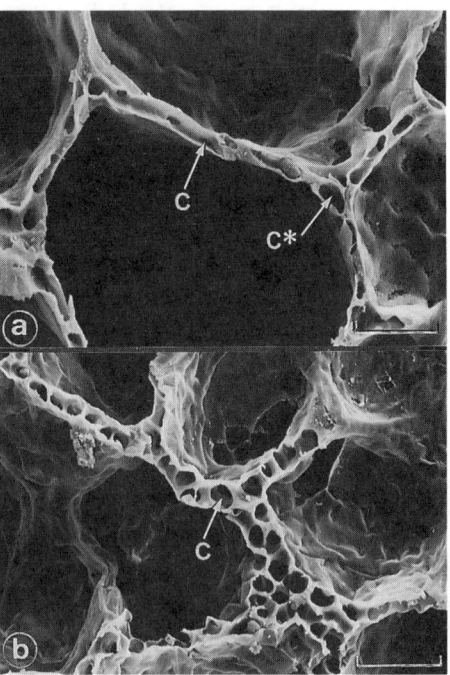

The alveolar capillary network forms such a dense meshwork that some people believe that blood flows through the alveolar walls like a sheet rather than through a system of interconnected tubes. Although this sheet-flow concept oversimplifies the actual structural conditions, it does provide a useful description of the pattern of blood flow through the alveolar walls and explains why blood flow is not interrupted when some parts of the capillary bed become squashed flat at high inflation levels (Fig. 14(a)); the capillaries which remain open in the corners are simply some channels of this broad sheet.

Design and function of the gas exchanger

The purpose of setting up a complex fibre system to support a dense capillary network in the alveolar wall, in lining the thin tissue barrier with live cells, and in garnishing it with surfactant which has dynamical properties is to establish a stable structural framework for efficient gas exchange between air and blood. We now need to ask how well this structure serves the gas exchange function.

In the pulmonary gas exchanger the oxygen flow rate is determined by the Bohr equation:

$$\dot{V}O_2 = (PAO_2 - Pco_2)DLO_2 \qquad (2)$$

where PAO_2 and Pco_2 are the oxygen partial pressures in alveolar air and capillary blood respectively, and DLO_2 is the pulmonary diffusing capacity or conductance for diffusion of oxygen.

It should be noted that all parameters on the right-hand side of this equation may be significantly affected by design features. We have already pointed out that the alveolar surface area and the barrier thickness affect diffusive oxygen uptake; we now need to find an appropriate formulation of how these features may be related to DLO_2. However, the oxygen partial pressure difference is established by ventilation and perfusion of the gas exchange units, and this may be affected by the design of the airway and vascular trees, particularly by their quantitative properties.

Airways and vessels are branching trees

The millions of gas exchange units that constitute lung parenchyma are all arranged around the terminals of several generations of a meticulously designed system of branching airways which serve to conduct the inspired air from the upper airways to the alveolar ducts and sacs (Figs 7 and 8).

The pattern of airway branching can be studied on resin casts. Consistently, each branch is seen to divide into two smaller branches, i.e. to undergo dichotomous branching so that the number of airways in each generation z is

$$N(z) = 2^z. \qquad (3)$$

The two daughter branches from the same parent often differ in diameter and/or length: hence, dichotomy is irregular. Within each generation, the lengths and diameters of the branches have a characteristic range of sizes, but the mean diameter of the conducting airways (to about generation 16) decreases systematically following a simple law (Fig. 15):

$$d(z) = d_0 \times 2^{-z/3}. \qquad (4)$$

where $d(z)$ is the mean diameter of airways in generation z and d_0 is the diameter of the trachea. This equation shows that with each generation the airway diameter is reduced by the cube root of the branching ratio 2, a law that is well known in hydrodynamics as it defines an optimal design of a branched system of tubes which minimizes the work of transport. From an engineering point of view, the airways of the lung are well designed. The total volume of the conducting airways down to generation 14 (the anatomic dead space) is about 150 ml; it is rapidly flushed by simple gas flow in the course of inhaling 500 ml of fresh air

during quiet inspiration. Therefore, for the larger airways, optimization of flow and its distribution to peripheral units is the essential condition for good design.

Figure 8 shows peripheral airways at the transition from terminal bronchioles that serve as conducting tubes to respiratory bronchioles and alveolar ducts. These terminal airways also branch by dichotomy. Figure 15 shows that the diameters of the most peripheral airways (generations 15–23) do not follow the law of reduction by the cube root of 2, but change very little with each generation. Does this imply a less than optimal design? On the contrary, the 'cube root of 2 law' relates to optimizing the mass flow of air. In the most peripheral airways, diffusion of oxygen in the air phase is more important, and this is best served by establishing as large an interface as possible between residual air and the fresh air that flows in from the trachea. In fact, since the airway diameter falls very slowly, the total airway cross-section almost doubles with each generation beyond generation 16 (Fig. 16). This causes a rapid fall of air flow velocity along the airway tree; at rest the mean flow velocity on inspiration is about 1 m/s in the trachea and less than 1 cm/s in the terminal airways. This suggests that in the small airways the transport of oxygen by mass air flow is slower than by diffusion.

The design of the airway tree has some basic features in common with fractal trees. This is significant in two ways. First, it means that the proportions between successive airway generations are maintained and this is in the interest of homogeneous ventilation of all lung units. Second, the pathlength from the entrance to the airways to the acini or even the alveoli is of the same order of magnitude for central and peripheral parenchymal units, although there is considerable variation in individual path lengths.

The pulmonary arteries form a tree which is basically very similar to that of the airways. Arteries follow the airways to form jointly the axis of the bronchoarterial units; they are of about the same diameter and length as their associated airways. Towards the periphery, particularly as they approach and penetrate into the acini, pulmonary arteries show additional 'supernumerary' branches which lead blood into adjacent parts of the gas exchanger. Accordingly, we find that arteries branch over about 28 generations of dichotomous branching, on average, compared with 23 generations for the airways. The close matching of arterial diameter to that of the airways suggests that the rule of optimized design for mass flow, noted above for conducting airways, also applies to the arteries; indeed, it can be shown that in the arteries the 'cube root of 2 law' for diameter reduction applies all the way out to the arterioles. This

Fig. 15 Average diameter of airways in the human lung plotted by generations of regularized dichotomous branching. (From Haefeli-Bleuer and Weibel. (1988). *Anatomical Record*, **220**, 401–14.)

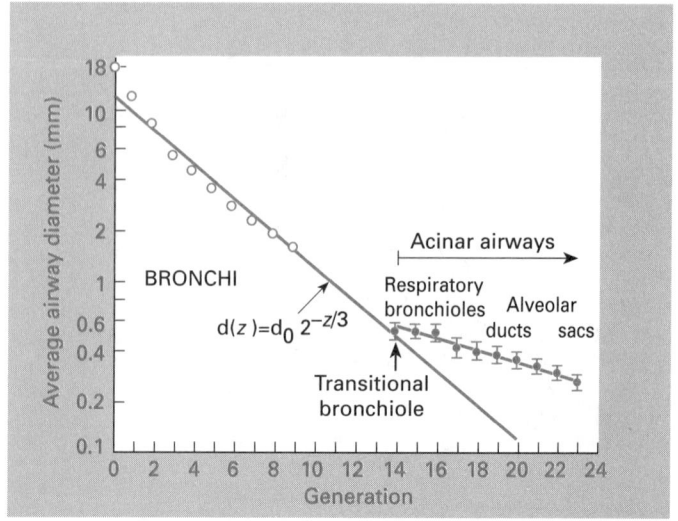

close match between airway and arterial design suggests that the lung is constructed to ensure as good a match as possible between ventilation and perfusion of the millions of gas exchange units.

Pulmonary diffusing capacity depends on design

One of the parameters of the Bohr equation (equation (2)), the pulmonary diffusing capacity $D\text{LO}_2$, depends crucially on the design properties of lung parenchyma, mainly on the area of contact between air and blood and on the barrier thickness. We now wish to work out precise and quantitative relationships between these design features and the gas exchange function in a morphometric model for $D\text{LO}_2$.

MORPHOMETRIC MODEL FOR PULMONARY DIFFUSION CAPACITY

As oxygen diffuses from the air in an alveolus to the haemoglobin in a red blood cell, it crosses a series of barriers which act as resistances to flow (Fig. 17): (1) the tissue barrier (t), consisting of alveolar epithelium, interstitium, and capillary endothelium, (2) the plasma barrier (p) separating the capillary endothelium from the red blood cell, and (3) the erythrocyte (e) through which oxygen must diffuse to reach haemoglobin molecules. The total diffusion conductance $D\text{LO}_2$ of the gas exchanger is obtained as the sum of the resistances offered by these barriers which are the reciprocals of the respective conductances:

$$D\text{LO}_2{}^{-1} = D\text{tO}_2{}^{-1} + D\text{pO}_2{}^{-1} + D\text{eO}_2{}^{-1}. \tag{5}$$

The two conductances for tissue and plasma are pure diffusion conductances and are commonly combined into the 'membrane' diffusing capacity $D\text{MO}_2$, such that

$$D\text{MO}_2{}^{-1} = D\text{tO}_2{}^{-1} + D\text{pO}_2{}^{-1}. \tag{6}$$

Each of these conductances is composed of a physical coefficient and some structural parameters that can be quantified morphometrically.

The tissue and plasma barriers are sheets of thickness τ which separate two compartments over an area S; thus, in principle, Fick's law determines oxygen flow across each of these barriers:

$$\dot{V}\text{O}_2 = D\text{O}_2 \Delta P\text{O}_2 = K\text{O}_2(S/\tau)\Delta P\text{O}_2 \tag{7}$$

where $K\text{O}_2$ is Krogh's permeation coefficient for oxygen (3.3×10^{-8}

cm²/min/mmHg) and $\Delta P\text{O}_2$ is the pressure head for diffusion across the barrier. Therefore the diffusion conductance of the barrier is

$$D\text{O}_2 = K\text{O}_2(S/\tau) \tag{8}$$

This also applies for the tissue and the plasma barriers, and for the 'total' diffusion barrier which is the same as the 'membrane' diffusing capacity.

The tissue barrier is a complex structure. Its two bounding surfaces are not perfectly matched and the thickness of the barrier varies considerably. It appears reasonable to use the mean $[S(\text{A}) + S(\text{c})]/2$ of the two surface areas as an estimate of the effective gas exchange surface. The effect of varying the barrier thickness is that the oxygen conductance will vary from point to point; in fact, it will be approximately inversely proportional to the local thickness so that the relevant estimate of barrier thickness is its harmonic mean τ_{ht}, i.e. the mean of the reciprocal local thicknesses. This turns out to be quite important, for we find that the value of the harmonic mean thickness of the pulmonary air–blood barrier is consistently about three times smaller than the arithmetic mean thickness $\bar{\tau}_t$; in humans, for example $\bar{\tau}_{ht}$ is about 0.6 µm compared with 2.2 µm for $\bar{\tau}_t$. This difference is the result of design features which must optimize various functional requirements. Thus we need fibres to support the capillaries, but it suffices to have them in only half of the barrier, keeping the other half very thin. Or, the barrier needs cell bodies with bulky nuclei to maintain the cell linings alive, but these can be tucked away into the meshes of the capillary network (Figs 1, 2, and 17). Barrier thickness becomes highly irregular, but this turns out to be an advantage in that it allows the diffusion-effective mean thickness to be three times smaller than a barrier of the same total mass but regular thickness—a remarkable finding!

On the basis of these arguments we find that the conductance of the tissue barrier is

$$D\text{tO}_2 = K\text{tO}_2[S(\text{A}) + S(\text{c})]/2\tau_{ht}. \tag{9}$$

The morphometric variables $S(\text{A})$, $S(\text{c})$, and τ_{ht} can all be measured on electron micrographs of lung sections using stereological methods provided that the micrographs are obtained by proper statistical random sampling.

The plasma barrier forms a sheet of highly variable thickness. Much of the surface of the red blood cells is 'hidden' from the capillary surface by neighbouring red cells (Fig. 17), so that the red-cell surface 'accessible' for diffusion of oxygen is found to be similar to the capillary surface. Thus the conductance of the plasma barrier is

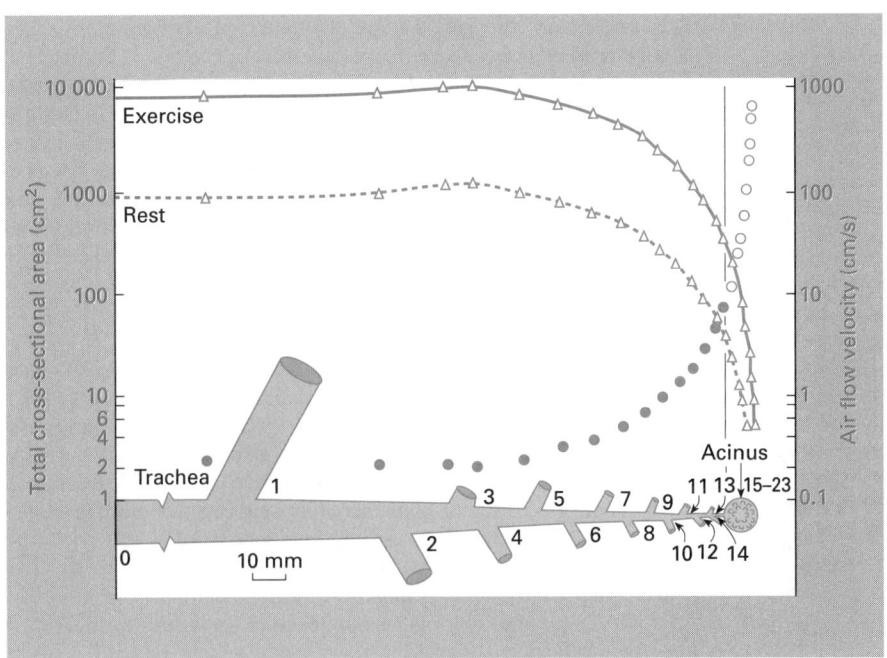

Fig. 16 As the total airway cross-section increases with the generations of airway branching, the mass flow velocity of inspired air decreases rapidly as it enters the acinus, eventually falling below the molecular velocity of oxygen diffusion in air.

$$Dpo_2 = Kpo_2S(c)/\tau_{hp}. \tag{10}$$

The permeation constants Kpo_2 and Kto_2 for plasma and tissue are approximately the same.

A number of arguments can be advanced in favour of combining tissue and plasma barriers into a single barrier of diffusion conductance Dmo_2. One is that the permeability coefficients are about the same for tissue and plasma, and another is that the plasma barrier thickness cannot be reliably estimated because some parts are so very thin. If the harmonic mean thickness τ_{hb} of the total barrier is estimated as the harmonic mean distance between the alveolar surface and the erythrocyte membrane, then we can estimate Dmo_2 directly as

$$Dmo_2 = Ko_2[S(A)/\tau_{hb}]. \tag{11}$$

The erythrocyte conductance De is of a different nature in that it involves two coupled events: diffusion of molecular oxygen and oxyhaemoglobin within the red blood cell, as well as the chemical reaction of oxygen with haemoglobin. Roughton and Forster developed a simplified expression based on an empirical measure of the rate θo_2 at which oxygen is bound to whole blood:

$$Deo_2 = \theta o_2 V(c) \tag{12}$$

where $V(c)$ is the total capillary blood volume, which again can be estimated on sections by stereological methods.

The coefficient θo_2 causes problems for two reasons: the measured values reported in the literature are variable, and it is not really a constant but depends on haematocrit and the degree of oxygen–haemoglobin saturation since the oxygen binding rate varies non-linearly as the oxygen saturation of haemoglobin increases. It should also be noted that θo_2 is different for different species. Thus when calculating De, one should use a value for θo_2 that has been determined on the appropriate species, normalize it to the haemoglobin concentration that is observed in the individual, and account for the venous and arterial oxygen–haemoglobin saturation. For many purposes one may have to be content with an approximate estimate of θo_2 as a 'constant'. There is no consensus yet what the 'good' value of θo_2 is for human blood, but a value of 1.5 ml O_2/ml/min/mmHg is a 'reasonable' estimate, or better still [3.3 × (haematocrit)] ml O_2/ml/min/mmHg.

THE HUMAN PULMONARY GAS EXCHANGER

Estimation of the diffusing capacity of the human lung on the basis of the model given above requires the morphometric data listed in Table

Fig. 17 Alveolar capillary from human lung showing the different steps in the pathway for oxygen molecules diffusing from alveolar air (A) to haemoglobin in erythrocytes (C). Calculation of diffusing capacity requires estimates of the morphometric parameters indicated in the figure and discussed in the text. Scale marker: 2 μm.

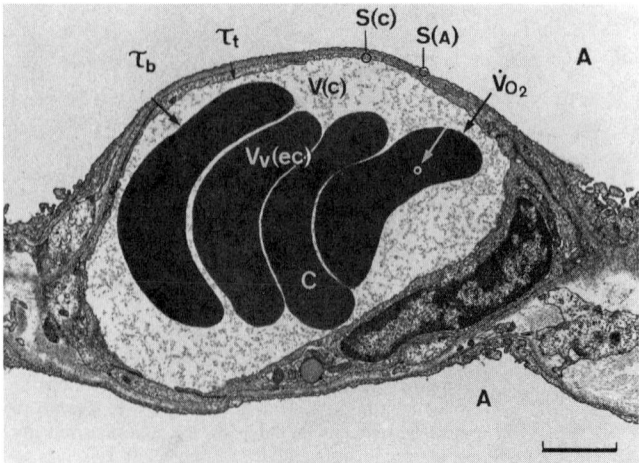

Table 2 *Morphometry of the human lung and estimate of* Dlo_2

Body mass (kg)	74 ± 4kg
Body length (cm)	177 ± 3cm
Alveolar surface (m²)	130 ± 12m²
Capillary surface (m²)	115 ± 12m²
Capillary volume (ml)	194 ± 30ml
Tissue barrier thickness (μm)	0.62 ± 0.04μm
Total barrier thickness (μm)	1.15 ± 0.01μm
Diffusing capacity (Dmo_2 from eqn (11))	
Dmo_2	349 ml O_2/min/mmHg
Deo_2	289 ml O_2/min/mmHg
Dlo_2	158 ml O_2/min/mmHg

Original data from Gehr, Bachofen, and Weibel, *Respiration Physiology*, **32**, 121, 1978.

2. These data, obtained by electron microscopic morphometry on seven young adults, reveal that the alveolar surface area is 130 m² and the capillary surface area is about 10 per cent less. These values are higher than those generally quoted in textbooks and derived from light microscopy studies which did not adequately resolve the alveolar surface texture. The harmonic mean thickness of the tissue barrier is 0.6 μm and the total barrier thickness is 1.15 μm. The capillary volume is estimated at about 200 ml. Using these data we calculate Dlo_2 for the adult human lung to be about 150–200 ml O_2/min/mmHg, with the variation depending mostly on the choice of θo_2 and on whether we use the total barrier thickness or the tissue and plasma thickness separately in calculating Dmo_2.

Using these data we can also determine how the resistance to oxygen diffusion is distributed between the diffusion barrier and the red cells. Table 2 shows that the diffusion conductance of the 'membrane' is some 20 per cent larger than that of the red cells, which means that the resistance to oxygen uptake is almost equally divided between the membrane and the red cell, perhaps being somewhat higher in the erythrocytes.

These theoretical estimates of the diffusing capacity are based on model assumptions that are considered reasonable. The test of their validity must be to compare them with physiological estimates. The standard physiological value of Dlo_2 of a healthy adult at rest is about 30 ml O_2/min/mmHg, which is considerably less than our determination on the basis of morphometric estimates. However, this is not a valid comparison because under resting conditions we take up only one-tenth of the amount of oxygen that our lungs are capable of absorbing under conditions of heavy work. There have been a number of estimates of Dlo_2 in exercising humans, and these have yielded values of the order of 100 ml O_2/min/mmHg. This estimate should come closer to the 'true capacity' of the oxygen transfer to the blood in the lungs than the value obtained at rest. The fact that it is about half to two-thirds the morphometric estimate is not disturbing, for we do not know whether the 'true diffusing capacity' is completely exploited even in heavy exercise. For example inhomogeneities in the distribution of ventilation and perfusion would limit the degree to which 'true' Dlo_2 can be exploited.

TESTING THE MORPHOMETRIC MODEL FOR Dlo_2

The apparent discrepancy between the morphometric and physiological estimates of Dlo_2 in humans could, of course, be due to the fact that morphometric and physiological estimates were obtained in independent studies. In order to test whether the two estimates measure the same thing, some years ago we performed a combined physiological and morphometric estimation of pulmonary diffusing capacity on four species of canids with body masses ranging from 4 to 30 kg.

The physiological estimation of Dlo_2 is based on the Bohr equation (equation (2)). Since it is impossible to estimate mean capillary Po_2 reliably, most physiological measurements of the diffusing capacity use carbon monoxide as a tracer gas. Carbon monoxide binds so avidly to haemoglobin that for practical purposes P_{bCO} is zero so that it suffices to measure carbon monoxide uptake and alveolar carbon monoxide concentration. It is also possible to revise the morphometric model of diffusing capacity to estimate the conductance for carbon monoxide instead of oxygen by appropriately changing the permeability coefficients and the rate θ_{CO} of carbon monoxide binding to erythrocytes, whereas the morphometric parameters are not changed. In the study on dogs and other canids the calculated morphometric value of D_{LCO} was found to be larger than the physiological estimate by about a factor of 1.5 to 2, depending on which model was used, thus confirming the observation made with respect to human lungs.

Therefore we conclude that the pulmonary gas exchanger is designed with a certain amount of redundancy or excess capacity, but this is by no means unreasonable from an engineering point of view. Indeed, designing the pulmonary gas exchanger with a degree of redundancy may make a lot of sense. The lung forms the interface to the environment and thus its functional performance will depend on environmental conditions, such as the prevailing oxygen partial pressure which falls on going from sea level to higher altitudes. It has been shown that goats, whose D_{LO_2} is about twice as large as seemingly required, can maintain their maximal level of exercise-induced $\dot{V}_{O_2}$ even under moderate hypoxia, and that the redundancy apparent under sea-level conditions then disappears. It has also been suggested that human athletes exercising at high altitude may fully exploit their D_{LO_2}. This suggests that the apparent redundancy in D_{LO_2} may be a safety factor to ensure the good functioning of the pulmonary gas exchanger even when environmental conditions are not optimal.

Design of the respiratory system as a whole

Can we test for a match between structure and function?

Intuitively, it seems reasonable to expect that the structural design of the lung is matched or optimized to meet the oxygen needs of the body, which are set by the energetic demands of the cells and their mitochondria when these produce ATP by oxidative phosphorylation to allow the cell to do work. The flow of oxygen from the lung to the cells required to maintain this function proceeds along the respiratory system through various steps (Fig. 18): into the lung by ventilation, to the blood by diffusion, through the circulation by blood flow, and from the blood capillaries by diffusion to the cells and mitochondria where it disappears in the process of oxidative phosphorylation. A number of basic features characterize this system:

1. Under steady state conditions the oxygen flow rate $\dot{V}_{O_2}$ is the same at all levels, i.e. oxygen uptake in the lung is equal to oxygen consumption in the tissues;
2. The basic driving force for oxygen flow through the system is a cascade of oxygen partial pressure which falls from inspired P_{O_2} down to near zero in the mitochondria.
3. The oxygen flow rate at each step is the product of a partial pressure difference and a conductance which is related to structural and functional properties of the organs participating in oxygen transfer. For example, it can be shown that the oxygen flow rate into the oxygen-consuming step in the cells is directly related to the amount of mitochondria that perform oxidative phosphorylation.

The highest levels of overall oxygen consumption are found in exercise. Thus, when the upper limit of oxygen consumption is reached, most of the oxygen is consumed in working muscles as they produce ATP by oxidative phosphorylation. Therefore, to a first approximation, we could propose the hypothesis that the lung is designed according to functional needs if D_{LO_2} is matched to $\dot{V}_{O_2}$ under conditions of maximal work, i.e. when the limit of oxygen supply to the working muscles is reached.

Clearly, each step in the cascade shown in Fig. 18 could be limiting $\dot{V}_{O_2}$, but in a well-designed system we should expect all steps to reach their functional limit at about the same level; in other words, no step

Fig. 18 Model of the respiratory system from lung to cells. The oxygen flow rate at each level is determined by the P_{O_2} difference as the driving force, multiplied by a conductance which depends in part on morphometric parameters. The conductances of airways and circulation are convective (G_A, G_B), those of the pulmonary and tissue gas exchangers are diffusive (D_L, D_T), and that in the mitochondria (G_{mi}) depends on enzyme kinetics.

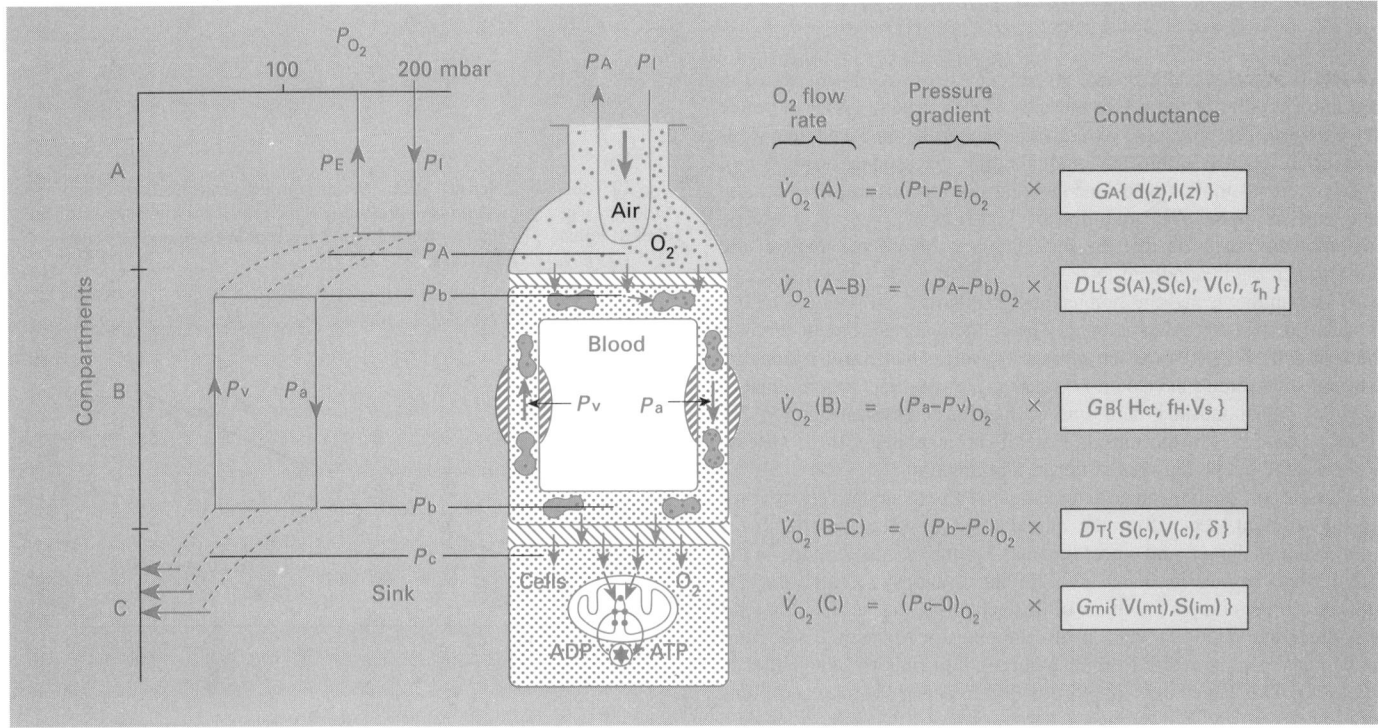

should have an excess capacity for oxygen flow. We have called this 'common-sense' hypothesis of economic design 'symmorphosis'. Testing the validity of this hypothesis is a demanding task. The complexity of the system and the interdependence of the various steps make it impossible to approach it directly. Therefore we have chosen a comparative approach, exploiting the large variations in maximal oxygen consumption between different species of the animal kingdom.

The basic strategy of the approach is to compare differences in maximal oxygen consumption $\dot{V}O_2$max with differences in the structural parameters that determine oxygen flow through each of the steps of the oxygen pathway, such as the diffusing capacity of the lung. We shall focus on the lung, but it is evident that all steps of the respiratory system must enter our considerations.

The procedure for measuring $\dot{V}O_2$max under steady-state conditions consists in measuring the oxygen consumption of a subject as a function of exercise intensity, i.e. speed or work rate. Oxygen consumption increases linearly with exercise intensity up to a maximal rate $\dot{V}O_2$max. It does not increase beyond this point with further increases in exercise intensity, and the additional energy required to sustain these higher intensities is supplied by anaerobic glycolysis. Lactate, an end-product of anaerobic glycolysis, accumulates, limiting the duration of exercise.

Large differences in $\dot{V}O_2$max occur between animals of different size (about six-fold between cows and mice on a per gram basis), between species of the same size adapted for different levels of athletic endurance (e.g. two- to threefold between goats and dogs or cows and horses), and even between individuals of the same species (e.g. more than 1.5-fold between sedentary individuals and highly trained athletes). $\dot{V}O_2$max can be increased simply by exercise training. It takes only a few weeks of relatively intense training—exercising at 70 per cent of $\dot{V}O_2$max for 20 min every day—to achieve a 20 to 35 per cent increase. This indicates an important feature which has now been demonstrated for both humans and animals, namely that the respiratory system is adaptable to functional needs in that the limit for oxygen supply to the working muscles can be pushed to higher values of $\dot{V}O_2$max when the energetic demands imposed on the muscles are increased.

We can now use these large variations in $\dot{V}O_2$max to test symmorphosis at the various steps of the respiratory system.

Do mitochondria and capillaries limit oxidative metabolism?

During heavy physical exercise, 90 per cent of oxygen is consumed in the mitochondria of the active muscles as they produce ATP to power the exercise. The process of oxidative phosphorylation occurs in a well-controlled manner within the mitochondria: the production of 6 mol ATP requires 1 mol oxygen. The fact that $\dot{V}O_2$ reaches a limit ($\dot{V}O_2$max) and that additional ATP required by higher work loads is produced anaerobically suggests that the mitochondria themselves may set the limit to aerobic metabolism.

This can be tested in humans by comparing individuals whose $\dot{V}O_2$max differs by a factor of 2. The mitochondrial content of their muscle cells (Fig. 19) can be measured using small muscle biopsies. Several such studies have demonstrated an almost direct proportionality between mitochondrial volume and $\dot{V}O_2$max, as demonstrated in Fig. 20. Thus, at the level of the muscle's metabolic machinery, there appears to be a good match between structure and function.

This proportionality can be demonstrated more quantitatively by comparing different species from the animal kingdom where the differences in $\dot{V}O_2$max are larger, and where the total volume of mitochondria in the muscles can be measured instead of relying on biopsy samples of a few muscles. If we compare animals of different size, we find that the total volume of mitochondria scales in direct proportion to $\dot{V}O_2$max in a group of animals ranging in size from 20 g mice to 500 kg horses and bullocks (Fig. 21). This same strict proportionality between $\dot{V}O_2$max and mito-

chondrial volume is also observed when comparing pairs of mammals of the same body mass but with widely differing energy requirements, such as dog and goat, or horse and cow (Table 3). When the animals exercise at $\dot{V}O_2$max, each millilitre of mitochondria consumes about 4 to 5 ml of oxygen per minute, irrespective of size or adaptation.

Humans appear to be the exception to the general rule; they possess twice as many mitochondria as quadrupeds relative to their $\dot{V}O_2$max. It seems likely that this is a result of their bipedal gait; they use only about half their muscles to reach $\dot{V}O_2$max when running or cycling, and the mitochondria in these muscles appear to operate at the same maximum rate of 4 to 5 ml O_2/ml/minute as in other species. The difference appears to be that humans can reach $\dot{V}O_2$max with only a fraction of their total musculature.

At the level of the mitochondria the results are simple and consistent with the hypothesis; the limit on oxygen consumption is directly related to the quantity of mitochondria which can perform oxidative phosphorylation. If a muscle needs more oxidative capacity, it builds more mitochondria.

The second structural factor which determines O_2 flow in the muscles is the capillary network which must maintain an adequate supply of

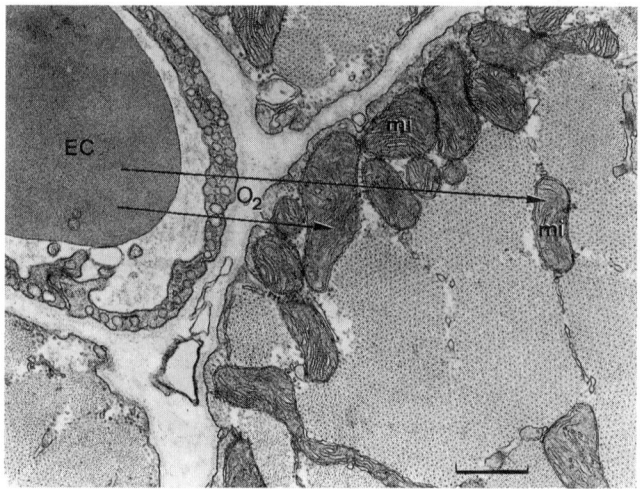

Fig. 19 Electron micrograph showing the spatial relationship between a capillary and its adjacent muscle fibres with their mitochondria (mi) that are often concentrated towards the fibre surface. Arrows mark the pathway for oxygen supply from the erythrocyte (EC) to the mitochondria (mi). Scale marker: 0.5 μm.

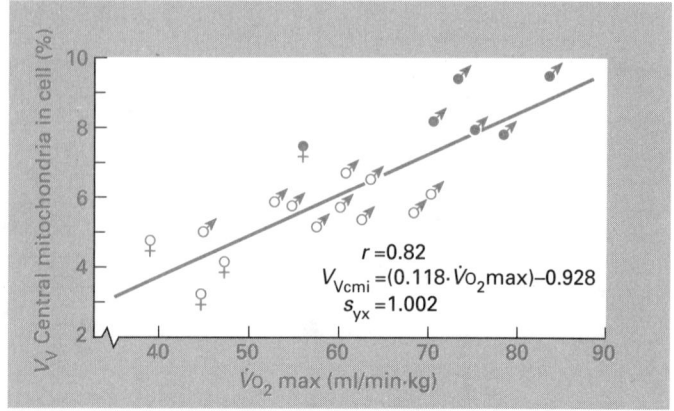

Fig. 20 The volume density of mitochondria in leg muscle cells is proportional to $\dot{V}O_2$max in a population of untrained (open circles) and highly trained (full circles) humans. (From Hoppeler, Lüthi, Claassen, Weibel, and Howald. (1973). *Pflügers Archiv*, **344**, 217–32.)

Table 3 *Differences in morphometric and physiological parameters of muscle mitochondria and capillaries, and of heart, blood, and lung with variation of* $\dot{V}O_2max$ *in three pairs of athletic and sedentary species.*

Design Function	$\dot{V}O_2max/M_b$ (ml/min/ kg)	Mitochondria $V(mt)/M_b$ (ml/kg)	Capillaries $V(c)/M_b$ (ml/kg)	Blood V_V(ec)	Heart f_H (min^{+1})	Heart VsM_b (ml/kg)	Lung D_{LO_2}/M_b (ml/sec/mmHg/kg)
25–30 kg							
Dog(D)	137.4	40.6	8.2	0.50	274	3.17	7.08
Goat(G)	57.0	13.8	4.5	0.30	268	2.07	4.80
D/G	2.4	2.9	1.8*	1.68*	1.02*	1.53*	1.48*
150 kg							
Pony(P)	88.8	19.5	5.1	0.42	215	2.50	4.74
Calf(C)	36.6	9.2	3.2	0.31	213	1.78	3.00
P/C	2.4	2.13	1.6*	1.35*	1.02*	1.40*	1.57*
450 kg							
Horse(H)	133.8	30.0	8.3	0.55	202	3.11	6.48
Bullock(B)	51.0	11.6	5.3	0.40	216	1.52	3.24
H/B	2.6	2.6	1.6*	1.4*	0.94*	2.1*	2.0*
Ath/Sed†	2.5	2.5	1.7*	1.5*	1.0*	1.7*	1.7*

†Overall ratios of athletic to sedentary species.

*Ratios significantly different from that for $\dot{V}O_2max$.

After Weibel, Taylor, and Hoppeler. (1991). *Proceedings of the National Academy of Sciences USA*, **88**, 10 357.

oxygen to the muscle cells (Fig. 19). The capillaries form more or less dense networks between the muscle cells (Fig. 22), and the oxygen flow rate will depend on design features such as the distance from the capillary to the mitochondria and on the volume of blood available for unloading oxygen. The hypothesis predicts that capillary volume, like the mitochondrial volume, should vary directly with $\dot{V}O_2max$.

This is exactly what we find when we compare animals of different size. The length of capillaries in the muscle is directly related to $\dot{V}O_2max$ (and to the volume of mitochondria that they supply with oxygen) over a range of body size from mice to horses (Fig. 23). We can calculate that there are about 3 μm^3 of mitochondria for every cubic micrometre of capillary blood! Surprisingly, athletic species have a relatively smaller capillary volume than sedentary animals of the same size (Table 3); however, on closer examination the athletic species are found to have a higher haematocrit, so that the volume of oxygen-carrying red cells per volume of mitochondria remains constant. In this case two structures are modified to match oxygen delivery to demand: the quantity of capillaries, and the concentration of red cells in the capillary blood. By shared effort the match becomes nearly perfect.

Thus it appears that, in the muscle, the oxygen consumer—the mitochondria—and the oxygen supplier—the capillaries and their red blood cells—are directly related to $\dot{V}O_2max$, and therefore that both can be considered to contribute equally to the limitation of oxygen flow.

Does the heart set the limit?

Oxygen is transported from the capillaries in the lung to the capillaries in the muscle by the circulation. This convective step is often considered the limiting step in oxygen transport during strenuous exercise. The transport of oxygen by the circulation depends on the properties of the heart as a pump and of the blood as an oxygen carrier. Cardiac output increases directly with maximal oxygen uptake over the size range of animals where data are available (Fig. 24). This suggests a structure–function match as predicted by symmorphosis. However, in this instance the match does not appear to be achieved by adjusting a structural variable as we found to be the case with mitochondria and capillaries. Cardiac output is the product of heart frequency f_H and stroke volume V_s. On average, the heart makes up the same fraction of body mass over the size range of animals from mice to cows, about 0.58 per cent. Furthermore, it pumps the same volume per gram of heart (about 43 per cent) under rate-limiting conditions. Haemoglobin concentration and oxygen capacity of the blood are also about the same over the entire size range of mammals; 13 g haemoglobin and 17.5 ml oxygen per 100 ml of blood. This evidence taken together suggests that the two structural parameters determining oxygen delivery at this step, V_s/M_b and oxygen content of the blood, are invariant with size. A functional variable, heart frequency, accounts entirely for the adjustment, as shown in Fig. 24.

It is interesting that maximal heart frequency appears to be closely linked to body size. Our pairs of athletic and sedentary animals of the same size, dogs versus goats, ponies versus calves, and bullocks versus

Fig. 21 $\dot{V}O_2max$ and whole-body mitochondrial volume $V(mt)$ plotted as a function of body mass M_b in logarithmic coordinates: open symbols, sedentary species; full symbols, athletic species.

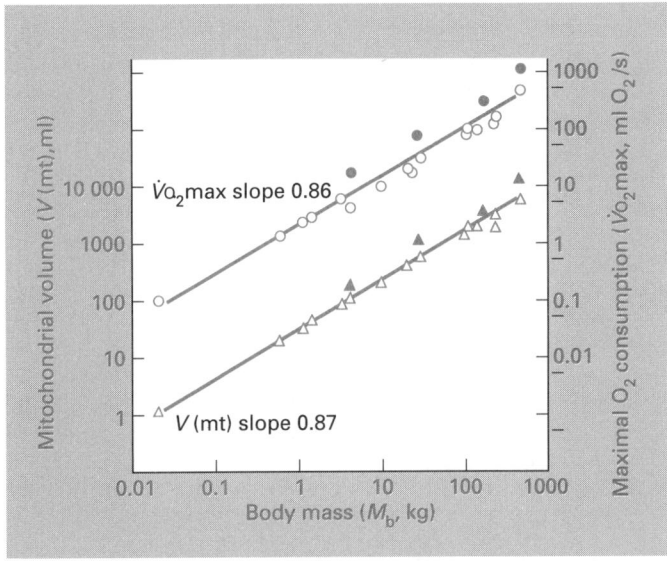

horses, have the same rate despite the two- to threefold difference in maximal oxygen uptake (Table 3). In this case a match is achieved entirely by building more structure. Two structures are involved, just as we observed with the capillaries, namely red-cell volume and size of the heart. Both structures contribute almost equally to the match (Table 3).

Is the pulmonary diffusing capacity matched to the body's oxygen needs?

Is the lung's gas exchange capacity adjusted to the body's oxygen needs? A number of early comparative and experimental studies suggested this. A particularly striking case was that of the Japanese waltzing mice: their well-known hyperactivity results in rates of oxygen consumption which are about 60 per cent higher than in normal laboratory mice. A morphometric study of their lungs revealed that their alveolar surface area and the diffusing capacity were also larger, about in proportion to the elevated oxygen needs. Some of this difference may have been genetic, but a subsequent experiment showed that the same proportionality between $\dot{V}_{O_2}$ and D_{LO_2} occurred in mice in which a waltzing syndrome was induced by drug treatment during early growth. This suggested that D_{LO_2} is adapted to $\dot{V}_{O_2}$. In several subsequent experiments attempts were made to induce a chronic increase in the oxygen needs of the body, either by exercise training or by cold environment, in view of testing the hypothesis that the lung's gas exchanger will

increase its diffusing capacity in response to elevated demand. However, the results of these studies were not consistent, perhaps because the degree of experimental $\dot{V}_{O_2}$ increase achieved was insufficient to trigger a response. In contrast, some studies have shown convincingly that the lung may adapt to changes in the oxygen partial pressure. Animals raised at high altitude develop a larger gas exchange surface than those raised at sea level; however, chronic hyperoxia leads to a reduction in D_{LO_2}. An important type of experiment asks whether the lung can compensate for gas exchange capacity lost as a consequence of partial pneumonectomy, a question of evident clinical significance. Experiments performed on growing rats revealed that the remaining lung expands in volume and alveolar surface area so as to compensate fully the lost diffusing capacity. This is achieved by proliferation of cells and tissue. When pneumonectomy was performed in adult dogs the result was different. Upon removal of the left lung, or 45 per cent of the gas exchanger, the remaining right lung expanded to fill the available space in the chest cavity; in the process, the alveolar surface became stretched, but this was accompanied by only a very modest proliferation of capillaries and tissue so that the diffusing capacity was not fully compensated. As a consequence, the pneumonectomized dogs did not regain their normal $\dot{V}_{O_2}$max. However, removing the right lung, or 55 per cent of the gas exchanger, appears to trigger proliferative processes and the diffusing capacity becomes compensated to a higher degree. We conclude from these experimental studies that the lung cannot easily make new gas exchanger tissue, so that its possibility to respond by adjustment of its diffusing capacity to elevated oxygen needs is very limited.

Another line of study which suggested adjustment of the lung's gas exchange capacity to the body's oxygen needs was the observation that very small mammals that have a high metabolic rate also have very small alveoli, and this should give them a relatively large diffusing capacity. For instance, the Etruscan shrew weighs only 2 g and has the highest metabolic rate of all mammals; its alveoli have a diameter of only about 20 μm so that several hundred shrew alveoli fit into one human alveolus. This suggested that the allometric variation of metabolic rate could be matched by a similar allometric regression of D_{LO_2}.

The studies that had suggested some kind of relationship between D_{LO_2} and the rate of oxygen consumption suffered from two shortcomings: (1) they were more anecdotal case studies rather than systematic tests of a hypothesis, and (2) they were often based on some ill-defined level of $\dot{V}_{O_2}$ rather than on a measure of the limit to oxidative metabo-

Fig. 22 Capillaries (arrows) in muscle show a preferred longitudinal orientation parallel to muscle fibres. Scale marker: 200 μm.

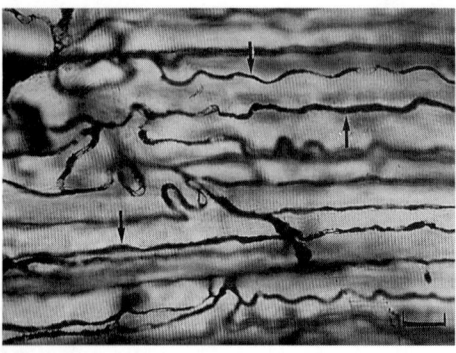

Fig. 23 $\dot{V}_{O_2}$max and whole-body muscle capillary volume $V(c)$ plotted as a function of body mass M_b in logarithmic coordinates: open symbols, sedentary species, full symbols, athletic species.

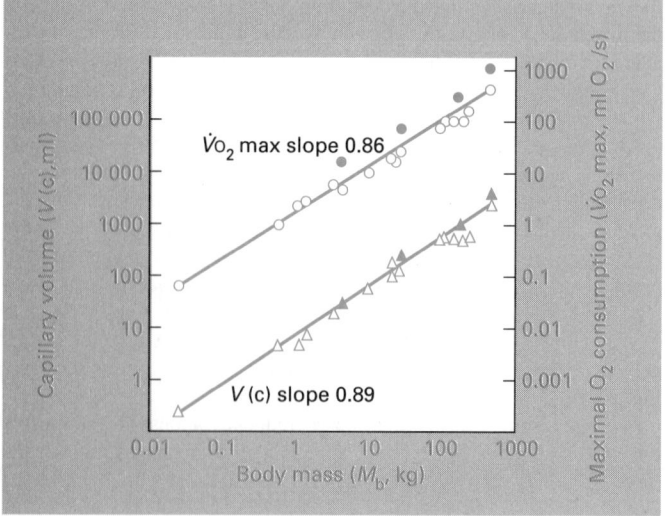

Fig. 24 $\dot{V}_{O_2}$max and cardiac output $\dot{Q}$ plotted as functions of body mass M_b in logarithmic coordinates: open symbols, sedentary species; full symbols, athletic species. The broken lines show the regressions for the two factors of cardiac output: heart frequency f_H which decreases with size, and stroke volume V_s which is directly proportional to body mass.

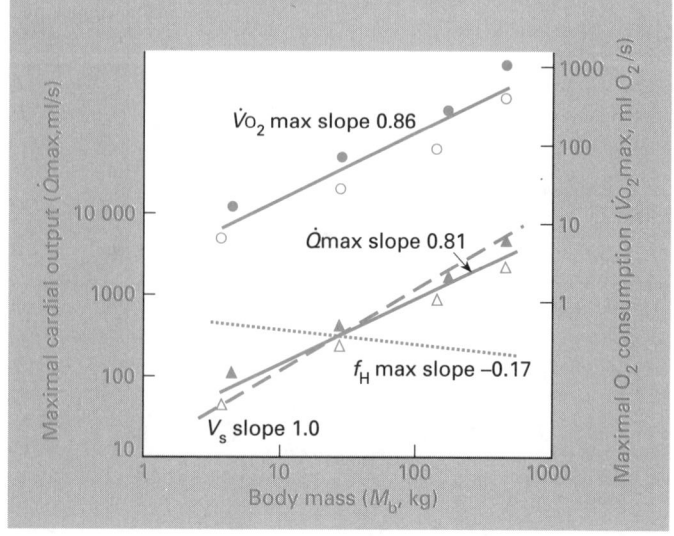

lism $\dot{V}_{O_2}$max. Therefore we have undertaken a systematic study of the variation of the pulmonary diffusing capacity and its morphometric parameters using our comparative approach to obtain large differences in $\dot{V}_{O_2}$max. The specific hypothesis, derived from the general hypothesis of symmorphosis, predicts that $D_{L_{O_2}}$ estimated by morphometry varies in parallel with $\dot{V}_{O_2}$max both across animal size and between athletic and sedentary species, or that the ratio $D_{L_{O_2}}/\dot{V}_{O_2}$max is invariant under both modes of variation.

We find that this hypothesis is not supported. When we compare athletic and sedentary species of about the same body mass we find that the athletic species have a $D_{L_{O_2}}$ which is about 1.7 times larger than that in the sedentary species, but this is clearly not matched to the 2.5-fold greater $\dot{V}_{O_2}$max (Table 3). The higher $D_{L_{O_2}}$ is the result of both an enlargement of gas exchange surface and the increased haematocrit that we have already noted in the muscle capillaries.

Fig. 25 $\dot{V}_{O_2}$max and morphometric pulmonary diffusing capacity $D_{L_{O_2}}$ plotted as function of body mass M_b in logarithmic coordinates. Athletic species (full symbols) have higher diffusing capacities than sedentary species of the same size (open symbols).

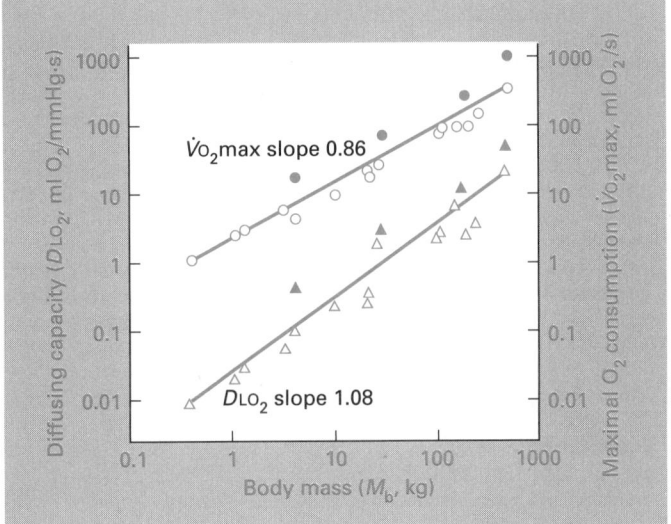

In extensive studies on species ranging from shrews and mice to horses and cows we found that $D_{L_{O_2}}$ increases more rapidly than $\dot{V}_{O_2}$max with body mass (Fig. 25). The consequence of these different slopes is that, on average, a 30-g animal, like a mouse, has the same amount of diffusing capacity per unit body mass as an animal weighing 300 kg, like a cow, but it has to accommodate an oxygen flow rate which is six times greater. As a consequence, the driving force for oxygen uptake, the alveolar–capillary P_{O_2} difference, must be much larger in the smaller animal. A recent re-evaluation of these data suggests that the regressions in Fig. 25 may be somehow distorted by the fact that athletic species occur only in the larger size classes. If we exclude the athletes and take the sedentary animals as the 'normal' species, then we find that, on a per gram basis, $D_{L_{O_2}}$ of the mouse is about 2.5 times greater than that of the cow. This means that $D_{L_{O_2}}$ is partially (about halfway) adjusted to the six-fold difference in $\dot{V}_{O_2}$max, a result similar to that observed between athletic and sedentary species.

The mismatch between $D_{L_{O_2}}$ and $\dot{V}_{O_2}$max observed in the studies reviewed above leads to the conclusion that the driving force for oxygen diffusion from air to erythrocytes is variable. This driving force has two components: the alveolar P_{O_2} as the pressure head and the mean capillary P_{O_2}. The latter parameter depends crucially on gas exchange itself because the mean capillary P_{O_2} is the integrated mean of the instantaneous P_{O_2} along the capillary, which ranges from the mixed venous to the end-capillary or arterial P_{O_2}. The gradual increase in P_{O_2} along the capillary depends on the membrane diffusing capacity and on the rate of oxygen binding by haemoglobin; it can be calculated by combining the physiological and morphometric data that we have obtained. Two examples are shown in Fig. 26, comparing the profiles of P_{O_2} change along the capillary path at rest and at $\dot{V}_{O_2}$max. We first note that the transit time becomes shorter as $\dot{V}_{O_2}$ increases; it falls from 1.5 s at rest to about 0.3 s in the dog and 0.47 s in the goat at $\dot{V}_{O_2}$max. Accordingly, loading oxygen into the blood at rest is completed well before the blood leaves the capillary in both dogs and goats. At $\dot{V}_{O_2}$max, however, the dog uses most of its capillary length for oxygen uptake with its blood reaching the P_{O_2} of arterial blood shortly before it exits from the lung (Fig. 26). In contrast, the goat arterial P_{O_2} utilizes only about half the capillary path for oxygen uptake even at $\dot{V}_{O_2}$max (Fig. 26).

If these calculations for the goat are correct, then it should be possible to decrease the pressure head for diffusion of oxygen drastically without reducing oxygen flow across the lung. In fact, using the morphometric

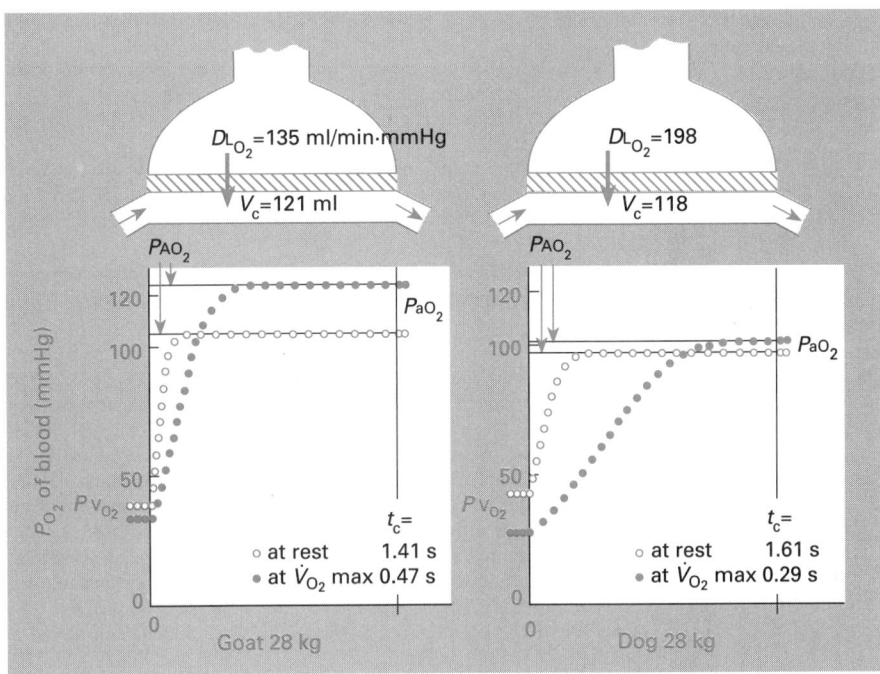

Fig. 26 Bohr integrals of P_{O_2} for blood passing through lung capillaries in goat and dog at rest and in maximal aerobic exercise respectively.

value for $D_{L}O_2$, it can be predicted that there will be excess diffusing capacity for oxygen across the lung until alveolar P_{O_2} is reduced to approximately 40 mmHg. When this prediction was tested it was found that $\dot{V}_{O_2}max$ was not decreased until alveolar and arterial P_{O_2} dropped to approximately 40 mmHg; at this P_{O_2} capillary blood equilibrated with alveolar air just prior to leaving the lung. Hence, the redundancy built into the pulmonary gas exchanger was fully exploited to allow goats to maintain their maximal work capacity even in severe hypoxia. It can be predicted that this would not be possible in dogs or horses which use most of their $D_{L}O_2$ at $\dot{V}_{O_2}max$, and indeed it appears from several studies that, in hypoxia, these species must reduce their level of aerobic exercise since their oxygen consumption is nearly limited by pulmonary diffusing capacity, even under normoxic conditions. This is apparently also the case in the highly trained human athlete.

Therefore we must conclude that the design of the pulmonary gas exchanger is not quantitatively matched to the body's oxygen needs at the limit of aerobic metabolism measured by $\dot{V}_{O_2}max$. In most species we find that a certain redundancy is maintained, but this redundancy is variable. Therefore the lung deviates from the pattern of coadjustment of structure and function noted in the other steps of the respiratory system. What could the reasons be? We do not know, but several arguments can be advanced. First, lung structure and size could be genetically determined and the target reached during development and growth, i.e. long before the lung can 'feel' the oxygen needs of the body. This is important in the light of the observation that the lung is almost unable to up-regulate its diffusing capacity by making new gas exchange structure in later life. This limited malleability of lung structure may be related to mechanical design constraints of the parenchyma; it may be difficult to add new alveolar septa without disrupting the continuity essential for maintaining integrity of the alveolar complex. Second, the ideal gas exchange conditions that we have supposed to exist when setting up the model for $D_{L}O_2$ may not exist *in vivo*; functional heterogeneity in ventilation–perfusion matching may allow the design-determined $D_{L}O_2$ to be exploited only to a certain degree, and there may well be species differences in this factor. Finally, the lung forms the interface to the environment so that its structure must not only be adjusted to internal requirements, but must also be capable of accounting for possible variations in the external boundary conditions of gas exchange, one of these being the prevailing ambient P_{O_2}.

Conclusions from the test

The question as to whether the lung's design is commensurate to its main functional task, the uptake of oxygen from the air at the rate required by the body, has been asked for a long time, and it has usually been answered in the positive. Some of our own findings seemed to lead to the same conclusion, but this did not stand up to a more refined test. It now appears that the hypothesis of symmorphosis applies to all parts of the respiratory system except the lung.

To reach these conclusions we have used as the overall functional reference parameter the aerobic capacity measured by $\dot{V}_{O_2}max$. This may not be totally adequate because an animal will very rarely, if ever, experience $\dot{V}_{O_2}max$. A more suitable reference parameter might be the sustained metabolic rate $\dot{V}_{O_2}sus$, which is the time-averaged rate of oxidative metabolism that an animal can maintain in free life, which is usually about two to five times the basal metabolic rate and thus up to about half $\dot{V}_{O_2}max$. When measuring $\dot{V}_{O_2}max$ we were, in fact, estimating the 'break-point' of the system when all reserves or safety factors have been called upon. We found that this break-point is reached at the same level of $\dot{V}_{O_2}$ in all steps of the respiratory system from the heart to the mitochondria, so that these structures are coadjusted to the function they serve with about the same safety factors. That the lung is designed with an additional safety margin may indeed be regarded as a sign of good design for at least two reasons. First, its limited structural malleability upon altered functional stress requires excess capacity at

this initial step of the respiratory system in order to allow malleability of the subsequent steps. Second, as explained above, the lung is at the interface with the environment; it must ensure high levels of oxygen uptake even if ambient P_{O_2} is low, and it may well be designed to cope with external stresses of various kinds.

REFERENCES

General

Crystal, R.G., West, J.B., Barnes, P.J., Cherniack, N.S., and Weibel, E.R. (1991). *The lung: scientific foundations*. Raven Press, New York.

Dejours, P. (1981). *Principles of comparative respiratory physiology* (2nd edn). North-Holland, Amsterdam.

Schmidt-Nielsen, K. (1984). *Scaling: why is animal size so important?* Cambridge University Press.

Weibel, E.R. (1963). *Morphometry of the human lung*. Springer-Verlag Berlin, and Academic Press, New York.

Weibel, E.R. (1984). *The pathway for oxygen. Structure and function in the mammalian respiratory system*. Harvard University Press, Cambridge, MA.

Weibel, E.R. and Taylor, C.R. (1988). Design and structure of the human lung. In: *Pulmonary diseases and disorders* (2nd edn), Vol. 1. (ed A.P. Fishman), pp. 11–60. McGraw-Hill, New York.

Cells and tissues

Bachofen, M. and Weibel, E.R. (1977). Alterations of the gas exchange apparatus in adult respiratory insufficiency associated with septicemia. *American Review of Respiratory Disease*, **116**, 589–615.

Bachofen, M. and Weibel, E.R. (1988). Sequential morphologic changes in the adult respiratory distress syndrome. In: *Pulmonary diseases and disorders* (2nd edn), Vol. 3 (ed A.P. Fishman), pp. 2215–22. McGraw-Hill, New York.

Burri, P. (1991). Postnatal development and growth. In: *The lung: scientific foundations*, Vol 1 (ed R.G. Crystal, J.B. West, P.J. Barnes, N.S. Cherniack, and E.R. Weibel), pp. 677–87. Raven Press, New York.

Weibel, E.R. (1985). Lung cell biology. In: *Handbook of physiology. Section 3: The respiratory system* (ed A.P. Fishman), pp. 47–91. American Physiological Society, Bethesda, MD.

Lung mechanics

Clements, J.A., Hustead, R.F., Johnson, R.P., and Gribetz, I. (1961). Pulmonary surface tension and alveolar stability. *Journal of Applied Physiology*, **16**, 444–50.

Hawgood, S. (1991). Surfactant: composition, structure and metabolism. In: *The lung: scientific foundations*, Vol. 1 (ed R.G. Crystal, J.B. West, P.J. Barnes, N.S. Cherniack, and E.R. Weibel), pp. 247–61. Raven Press, New York.

Hitchcock, K.R. (1980). Lung development and the pulmonary surfactant system: hormonal influences. *Anatomical Record*, **198**, 13–34.

Mead, J. (1961). Mechanical properties of lungs. *Physiological Reviews*, **41**, 281–330.

Weibel, E.R. (1986). Functional morphology of lung parenchyma. In: *Handbook of physiology. Section 3: The respiratory system*, Vol. III, Part 1 (ed P.T. Macklem and J. Mead), pp. 89–111. American Physiological Society, Bethesda, MD.

Weibel, E.R. and Bachofen, H. (1987). How to stabilize the pulmonary alveoli: surfactant or fibers? *News in Physiological Sciences*, **2**, 72–5.

Gas exchange

Forster, R.E. (1964). Diffusion of gases. In: *Handbook of Physiology, Section 3: Respiration*, Vol I, pp. 839–72. American Physiological Society, Bethesda, MD.

Fung, Y.C. (1984). *Biodynamics: circulation*. Springer-Verlag, New York.

Hsia, C.C.W., Carlin, J.I., Ramathan, M., Cassidy, S.S., and Johnson, R.L., Jr. (1991). Estimation of diffusion limitation after pneumonectomy from carbon monoxide diffusing capacity. *Respiration Physiology* **83**, 11–22.

Hsia, C.C.W., Herazo, L.F., Fryder-Doffey, F., and Weibel, E.R. (1994). Compensatory lung growth occurs in adult dogs after right pneumonectomy. *Journal of Clinical Investigation*, **94**, 405–12.

Weibel, E.R. (1991). Design of airways and blood vessels considered as branching trees. In: *The lung: scientific foundations*, Vol. 1 (ed R.G. Crystal, J.B. West, P.J. Barnes, N.S. Cherniack, and E.R. Weibel), pp. 711–20. Raven Press, New York.

Weibel, E.R., Federspiel, W.J., Fryder-Doffey, F. *et al.* (1993). Morphometric model for pulmonary diffusing capacity. I. Membrane diffusing capacity. *Respiration Physiology*, **93**, 125–49.

Weibel, E.R., Taylor, C.R., O'Neil, J.J., Leith, D.E., Gehr, P., Hoppeler, H., *et al.* (1983). Maximal oxygen consumption and pulmonary diffusion capacity: a direct comparison of physiologic and morphometric measurements in canids. *Respiration Physiology*, **54**, 173–88.

West, J.B. and Wagner, P.D. (1977). Pulmonary gas exchange. In: *Bioengineering aspects of the lung* (ed J.B. West), pp. 361–457. Dekker, New York.

Respiratory system

Hoppeler, H. (1990). The different relationship of $\dot{V}_{O_2}$max to muscle mitochondria in humans and quadrupedal animals. *Respiration Physiology*, **80**, 137–46.

Hoppeler, H., Lüthi, P., Claassen, H., Weibel, E.R., and Howald, H. (1973). The ultrastructure of the normal human skeletal muscle. A morphometric analysis on untrained men, women, and well-trained orienteers. *Pflügers Archiv*, **344**, 217–32.

Taylor, C.R., and Weibel, E.R. (1991). Learning from comparative physiology. In: *The lung: scientific foundations*, Vol. 2 (ed R.G. Crystal, J.B. West, P.J. Barnes, N.S. Cherniack, and E.R. Weibel), pp. 1595–1607. Raven Press, New York.

Taylor, C.R., Karas, R.H., Weibel, E.R., and Hoppeler, H. (1987). Adaptive variation in the mammalian respiratory system in relation to energetic demand. *Respiration Physiology*, **69**, 1–127.

Weibel, E.R., and Taylor, C.R. (1981). Design of the mammalian respiratory system. *Respiration Physiology*, **44**, 1–164.

Weibel, E.R., Taylor, C.R., and Hoppeler, H. (1992). Variations in function and design: testing symmorphosis in the respiratory system. *Respiration Physiology*, **87**, 325–48.

17.2.2 The upper respiratory tract

J. R. STRADLING

The upper respiratory tract extends conventionally from the anterior nares to the larynx. This part of the respiratory tract has to cope with specific problems, mainly because of its exposure to the incoming air and because it has to double as the entry to the digestive system. This has led to specific evolutionary adaptations which are not always perfect.

The nose

The anterior nares, which includes the nasal valve just inside the nose, is usually the narrowest part of the respiratory tract and accounts for about 40 to 50 per cent of the total respiratory resistance. In normal subjects the resistance in the lower airways is small (less than 25 per cent) compared with the larynx and nose. This anterior nasal resistance is actively controlled by the levator alae nasi and procerus muscles, which flare the nostrils, and the compressor naris muscle, which narrow the nasal valve further. During mild exercise these muscles (combined with sympathetic nasal mucosal vasoconstriction) can halve the nasal resistance and allow minute ventilations up to 30 l/minute before conversion to oral breathing is necessary. These muscles receive a phasic inspiratory signal, to brace open the nares with each breath, just in advance of diaphragmatic activity.

Occasionally, owing to deformity of the anterior nasal cartilages, the anterior nares are very narrow and limit inspiration, particularly during sleep when the dilator muscle activity is reduced. This is one of the causes of snoring which is amenable to treatment. The main function of the nose is as the first-line defence against problems with the incoming air. In this respect it acts as a coarse particle filter and a conditioner (temperature and humidity) of the air, and the sense of smell helps to detect noxious substances which are best avoided.

The turbinates in the nose present a large surface area onto which large inhaled particles will precipitate. Thus pollen grains and house dust mite faecal particles will be retained with the potential for an allergic response producing allergic rhinitis. Debris arriving on the mucosal surfaces is wafted backwards to be swallowed eventually. Without this so-called 'mucociliary carpet' there is decreased resistance to infections (usually a generalized respiratory problem and not just in the nose) with pooling of mucopurulent material. This mucociliary function can be tested by placing a saccharine tablet on the anterior floor of the nasal cavity and timing the period that elapses before it can be tasted in the oral cavity. The normal interval is about 15 to 20 min, but when ciliary defects exist this can extend to an hour or more.

The turbinates fill such a large proportion of the nasal cavity that minor swelling produces large changes in nasal airflow resistance (Fig. 1). The degree of mucosal swelling is controlled by the rich blood supply from the sphenopalatine branch of the maxillary artery to several vascular beds at different depths in the mucosa. The venous drainage passes back into the cavernous sinus around the carotid artery. This is an interesting arrangement, and in some animals (e.g. the desert camel) it allows cooling of the blood flowing to the brain (a countercurrent system) and helps keep the brain temperature down, particularly during exercise in

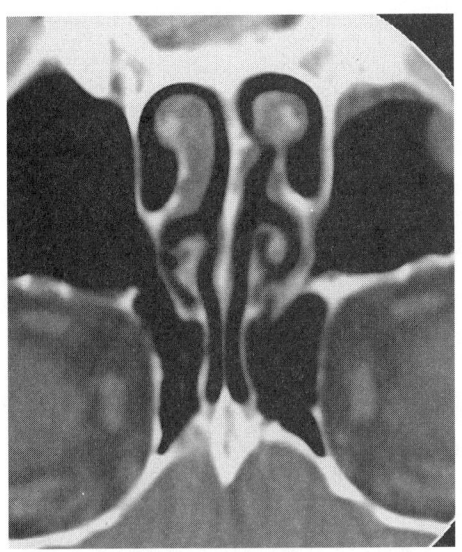
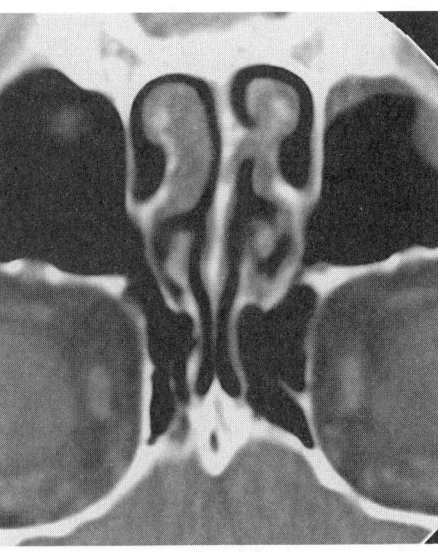

Fig. 1 Coronal sections of human maxillary sinuses and the turbinates in the nose. The second view is taken after ephedrine drops and shows the mucosal shrinkage. This consequent small increase in the lumina was attended by a large increase in maximum nasal airflow. (By courtesy of Dr F. Gleeson.)

hot climates. The volume of fluid in the nasal mucosal vascular bed is controlled via the vidian nerve (containing sympathetic vasoconstriction and parasympathetic vasodilation) acting on both arterioles and venules. The overall blood flow and total volume of blood in the sinusoids determines the degree of mucosal congestion and undergoes a cyclical reciprocal change across the two sides of the nose over 2 to 4 h, i.e. as one side is congesting the mucosa of the other side is shrinking. This nasal cycle is usually only obvious to individuals with already narrowed nasal passages when blockage occurs as part of the cycle. This cycling can be interrupted by a reflex, initiated through lying down on one's side and mediated by pressure on the side of the thorax or axilla. Thus the upper nostril becomes clearer and the lower more congested, with the two sides swapping within a minute or two of turning on to the other side. The purpose of this nasal cycle is not known, but using the upper rather than the lower nostril when lying on one's side may lessen the chance of inhaling particulate matter. In addition to this effect, there is a general increase in nasal congestion on lying down owing to a hydrostatic rise in capillary pressure.

This rich vascularization over a large surface area warms and humidifies incoming air. The volume of fluid needed to do this is considerable, but is reduced by condensation of some of this moisture back onto the cooler nasal mucosa during exhalation. Of course, this conditioning is lost during oral breathing, which has important implications for exercise-induced asthma which is due to cooling and drying of intrathoracic airways.

Nasal secretions come mainly from submucosal glands which are stimulated by parasympathetic (cholinergic) fibres. There is some evidence that sympathetic activity can also stimulate secretions, but of higher viscosity.

The sensory fibres from the nose travel in the maxillary nerve (mainly the ophthalmic branch) and are the afferent part of some interesting reflexes. Airflow is sensed and can itself influence breathing pattern. Nerves containing substance P in the epithelium seem to be responsible for sensations leading to sneezing. Sneezing is like coughing in that an explosive expiration is generated in an attempt to expel foreign matter. Coughing involves closure of the larynx until pressure builds up, whereas sneezing involves closure of the pharynx. Unlike coughing, sneezing is never voluntary. Sensory fibres from much of the upper airway, nose, and face are also involved in the diving reflex. This reflex is of great importance to diving mammals when the combination of facial stimulation by cold water, apnoea, and hypoxaemia produce intense peripheral, splanchnic, renal, and muscular vasoconstriction.

This diverts blood mainly to the brain and conserves oxygen (producing a heart–lung–brain circulation which prolongs diving time), with the rise in blood pressure limited by a marked vagally induced bradycardia. This vestigial reflex in humans can be utilized in the control of some cardiac arrhythmias, when a brisk increase in vagal tone can be produced by applying ice-cold water to the face.

Nasal irritation can lead to either bronchoconstriction or bronchodilation. The bronchoconstriction can be prevented by atropine and is presumably vagally mediated. This reflex may be important in provoking bronchospasm in some asthmatics.

Negative pressure in the nasal cavities can also be sensed, producing a reflex increase in upper airway dilator action (see the following section on the pharynx).

Olfaction depends on recognition of different molecular shapes by mucosal receptors at the very top of the nose. These olfactory cells have central axons that pass through multiple tiny holes in the skull (cribriform plate) to the brain. At this point they are very vulnerable to shearing forces during a blow to the head, leading to anosmia (loss of ability to smell).

The pharynx

The pharynx is conventionally divided into the nasopharynx, oropharynx, and laryngopharynx or hypopharynx—behind the soft palate, the back of oral cavity down to the tip of the epiglottis, and the tip of the epiglottis down to the cricoid cartilage respectively. Thus the top end is level with the base of the skull and the bottom end is about level with the sixth cervical vertebrae, giving an overall length of about 12 cm. When being used to breathe through, the pharynx has to be a rigid tube (like the trachea), but during swallowing it has to be a collapsed tube capable of peristalsis (like the oesophagus). This conflict of functions is achieved by having a muscular tube that can constrict to propel food, but also has external muscles whose function is to brace open the pharynx when required. Figure 2 shows the enormous complexity of the pharyngeal musculature, supplied mainly by the hypoglossal nerve (XII). The pharyngeal constrictors (superior, middle, and lower) are the main peristaltic muscles; the lower part of the inferior constrictor also functions as a sphincter to the top of the oesophagus, preventing air entry during inspiration. Most of the other pharyngeal muscles work in concert to hold open the pharynx. For example, the genioglossus pulls forward the tongue, the geniohyoid together with the strap muscles (ster-

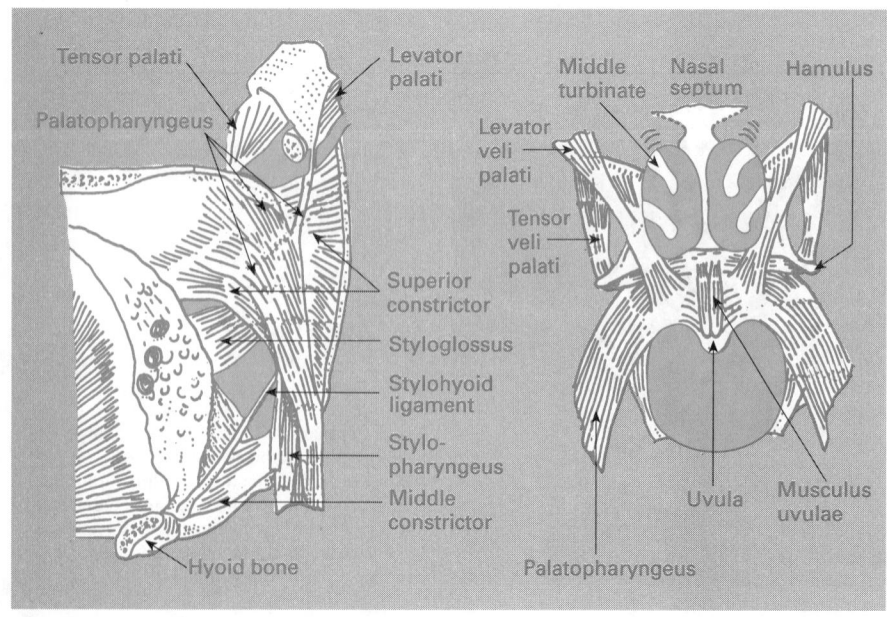

Fig. 2 Two views of the pharyngeal muscles: from inside the pharynx looking laterally, and from high up on the posterior pharyngeal wall looking anteriorly. These muscles act in concert and the physical effect of their contraction depends on which other muscles are simultaneously activated.

nothyroid, thyrohyoid, etc.) pulls forward the hyoid (enlarging the oropharynx), and the stylopharyngeus probably pulls sideways on the lateral pharyngeal walls. The palatopharyngeus will hold open the pharynx if supported by the levator palati, but will also pull forward the palate to open the nasopharynx. The upper pharyngeal muscles (tensor palati and levator palati) also close off the nasal cavity during swallowing to prevent regurgitation of fluids into the nose. To prevent aspiration, closure of the larynx and the false cords above is coordinated with swallowing. Some of these actions require sensory information about the exact location and consistency of any food being swallowed, carried via the glossopharyngeal and vagus nerves (IX and X). Sensory branches of these nerves also supply the ear, which explains why pharyngeal lesions may provoke pain in the ear.

Given the complexities of pharyngeal function, it is not surprising that severe swallowing difficulties with aspiration of food and drink are often seen following cerebrovascular accidents in the brain-stem involving the control of pharyngeal muscles and the sensory pathways.

Powerful mechanisms are available to maintain patency of the pharyngeal airway during breathing. As with the alae nasi, the pharyngeal dilator muscles receive a respiratory input in time with diaphragm activation. The diaphragm receives a gradually increasing level of phrenic activity to overcome elastic recoil as tidal volume increases, whereas the pharyngeal activation follows more of a 'square wave'. This makes teleogical sense since the collapsing force is dependent on inspiratory flow and this is roughly constant throughout inspiration. In addition, if pharyngeal patency is threatened, the dilator activity increases. Figure 3 shows the increase in genioglossus tone in response to a fall in intrapharyngeal pressure. This negative pressure will pull in the pharyngeal walls, and there are thought to be 'distortion' receptors of some kind mediating this reflex. Snoring occurs when the pharynx narrows enough to vibrate, and there is some evidence that this vibration itself can also activate pharyngeal dilators, thus warding off full collapse. The factors predisposing to pharyngeal collapse during sleep are discussed in the section on sleep-related disorders of breathing.

Sets of lymphoid tissue (Waldeyer's ring), comprising the adenoids, the palatine tonsils, and the lingual tonsils (back of tongue), are situated in the pharynx. These subepithilial collections of lymphoid tissue are ideally suited to process inhaled and swallowed antigens. Unfortunately, if they hypertrophy too much in response to recurrent infections, they are also ideally situated to obstruct the airway. This is usually first apparent during sleep, but may become severe enough to provoke inspiratory stridor, even while awake. Adenoidal enlargement, by blocking nasal airflow, will force mouth breathing which, if it occurs early enough (perhaps under 18 months of age), retards development of the lower jaw (the so-called 'adenoidal facies'). This probably leads to overcrowding of the teeth and a narrower retroglossal space (this is further discussed in the section on sleep-related disorders of breathing).

The larynx

The larynx (Fig. 4) has three important functions: communication, protection of the airway, and dynamic control of lung volume.

A minority of the intrinsic and extrinsic muscles of the larynx (e.g. cricothyroid, posterior cricoarytenoid) open (abduct) or brace the vocal cords, whereas the majority (e.g. thyroarytenoid, transverse and oblique arytenoids) close (adduct) the cords. The recurrent laryngeal nerve (from the vagus) supplies all the muscles apart from the cricothyroid (supplied from the superior laryngeal nerve, which is also a branch of the vagus). The left recurrent laryngeal nerve comes off the vagus and passes under the aortic arch before running up close to the thyroid gland to the larynx. This means that it can be damaged by a tumour at the left hilum and surgically during a thyroidectomy. The right recurrent laryngeal nerve passes under the right subclavian artery where it can be damaged by a right-sided apical lung tumour.

Complete paralysis of the recurrent laryngeal nerve gives permanent

hoarseness of the voice, and the affected cord assumes a position midway between full abduction and adduction. The cord is floppy and can be moved passively very easily; for example it will be 'sucked' towards the mid-line during inspiration and blown open during expiration. If paralysis of the recurrent laryngeal nerve is incomplete, the affected cord

Fig. 3 Response of the genioglossus muscle in a conscious human to a sudden fall in intrapharyngeal pressure. The time delay (about 50 ms) is too short to be due to a cortical response and is presumably a spinal cord reflex. (Reproduced with permission from Horner (1991).)

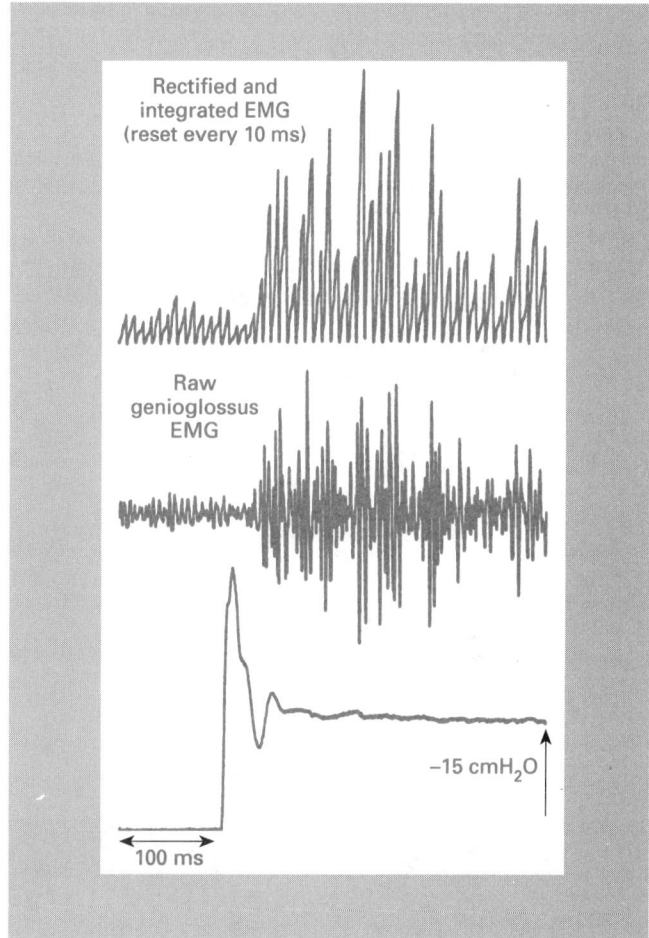

Fig. 4 Bronchoscopic view of the larynx from above. The top of the picture is the posterior (By courtesy of Dr P. Stradling.)

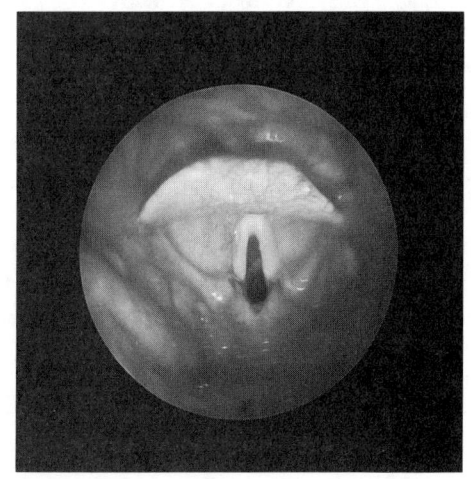

may take up the adducted position, presumably because fibres running to the abductors are damaged first.

When there is bilateral damage to the recurrent laryngeal nerves, loss of powerful abduction causes inspiratory stridor as the cords are passively drawn together.

As mentioned earlier, there are reflexes initiated by supralaryngeal sensory fibres (mainly via the internal branch of the superior laryngeal nerve) designed to protect the airway. Fluid or food landing on or near the vocal cords will provoke coughing and/or laryngeal closure. During sleep, irritation of the cords tends to produce apnoea, and coughing occurs only when wakefulness supervenes.

One of the less well-known functions of the larynx is to brake expiratory flow and thereby control lung volume. In some species, and in neonates, laryngeal expiratory braking is very important, acting rather like positive end-expiratory pressure. In adults there is no good evidence that the rate of expiration is particularly under active control, although this mechanism may come into action again during respiratory illnesses (such as pneumonia) especially if there is marked hypoxaemia.

Of course, this laryngeal braking of expiration will be bypassed by a tracheostomy or intubation. In newborn animals this expiratory braking maintains end-expiratory lung volume above the passive functional residual capacity, thus preventing atelectasis. If the upper airway is bypassed, then other mechanisms come into play to maintain the end-expiratory lung volume, such as postinspiratory contraction of the diaphragm (thus delaying expiration) and shortening of expiratory time (thus starting inspiration again before lung volume has fallen too far). Figure 5 is from a tracheotomized dog with areas of atelectasis. This shows how once laryngeal braking is denied to the animal, expiration proceeds faster, lung volume falls, and expiratory time is shortened to produce tachypnoea. This reflex was not present when the areas of atelectasis had resolved.

The clinical correlate of this is sometimes seen as an expiratory grunt in babies who have a respiratory illness. Intubation may worsen gas exchange in this situation unless positive end-expiratory pressure is also used.

Fig. 5 Recorder tracings in a dog with atelectasis showing the effect of switching from upper airway to tracheostomy breathing (arrow at (a)) and from tracheostomy to upper airway breathing (arrow at (b)). The signal is from an inductive plethysmograph measuring movement of both the ribcage and abdomen which represents lung expansion and contraction.

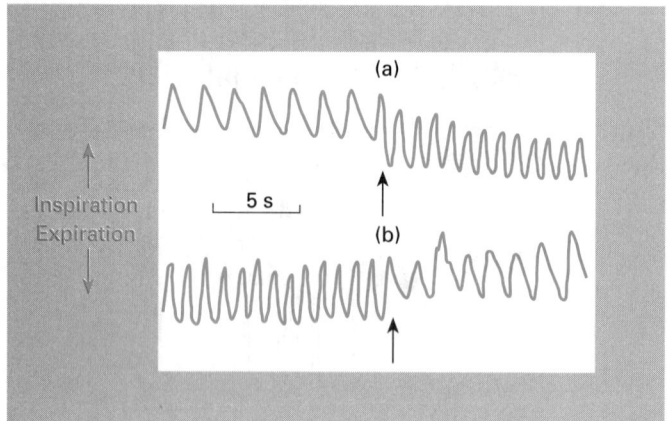

REFERENCES

Brouillette, R.T. and Thach, B.T. (1979). A neuromuscular mechanism maintaining extrathoracic airway patency. *Journal of Applied Physiology*, **46**, 722–29.

Gautier, H. (1973). Control of the duration of expiration. *Respiration Physiology*, **18**, 205–21.

Horner, R.L. (1991). Evidence for reflex upper airway dilator muscle activation by sudden negative airway pressure in man. *Journal of Physiology*, **436**, 15–29.

Matthew, O.P. and Sant 'Ambrogio, G.S. (1988). Respiratory function of the upper airway. In: *Lung biology in health and disease*, Vol. 35. Marcel Dekker, New York.

Remmers, J.E. and Bartlett, D. (1977). Reflex control of expiratory airflow and duration. *Journal of Applied Physiology*, **42**, 80–87.

17.3 Lung defences and responses

17.3.1 Non-immune defence mechanisms of the lung

C. HASLETT

The respiratory tract is protected by different mechanisms at its various levels. Broadly speaking, in the large airways physical mechanisms, including cough, are particularly important. The lower airways are protected by complex mucociliary clearance mechanisms, and the gas exchange units at the alveolar level are protected by surfactant and by 'patrolling' alveolar macrophages. The lung lining fluids (mucus in the airways and surfactant in the gas exchange units) contain a variety of proteins that are particularly important in host defence. Therefore in this chapter we shall consider physical defences, mucociliary clearance mechanisms, surfactant, and the important defensive proteins in the lining fluid of the lung.

Physical defences

The nose makes an important contribution to the physical defences of the upper airway. It is comprised of a stack of fine aerodynamic filters of respiratory epithelium arranged over the turbinate bones. These remove most large particles from inspired air. Their filtering effect is greatly enhanced by fine hairs in the anterior nares and by mucociliary action which, apart from a small area anterior to the inferior turbinates, is directed posteriorly such that trapped particles are swallowed or expectorated. The larynx acts as a sphincter during cough and expectoration, and is an essential protective mechanism for the lower airways during swallowing and vomiting.

Particles of size greater than 0.5 μm which survive passage through the nose will be trapped by the lining fluid of the trachea and bronchi, and will be cleared by the mucociliary clearance mechanism (which has also been called the 'mucociliary escalator').

Mucociliary clearance

The mucociliary escalator works by a complex interaction between cilia, which are a series of projections on the bronchial epithelial cells, and mucus. The mucus forms a 'raft' on top of the cilia which then sweep it in a cephalic direction. The combined effect of this interaction can readily be appreciated by scanning electron microscopy (Fig. 1). There are about two hundred cilia on each of the pseudostratified columnar epithelial cells lining the bronchi, and it has been calculated that they can carry weights of up to 10 g/cm without slowing. They work with a ciliary beat frequency of 12–14 beats/s. Their motility depends upon the contraction of longitudinal fibrils which contain the contractile protein tubilin arranged as nine outer and two central microtubular pairs. The effectiveness of the cilia in sweeping mucus in the cephalic direction is enhanced by small 'claws' in the tip which penetrate the overlying mucus sheet. The actual driving mechanism of the cilia is uncertain, but involves dynein, an ATPase protein which forms a major part of the cilium. Dynein appears to derive energy from ATP along the cilium. It is then converted into the forces which are generated by the contractile proteins.

Ciliary function can be assessed in a number of ways, facilitated by the fact that cilia can survive freezing for up to a month and may beat for several hours after the death of the host. Thus it is possible to assess their motility directly in cytological specimens from nasal and bronchial brushings and to perform detailed photometry and enumerate ciliary beat frequency in epithelial specimens sampled by biopsy. Cilial structure can also be assessed by electron microscopy. In a simple and practical clinical test, the time taken for saccharine placed in the anterior nares to cause a sweet taste in the mouth (normally around 11 min) can be used as a convenient clinical measure of ciliary function, which is informative because in most examples of ciliary disease the nasal cilia are also affected. Other more complex methods of assessing mucociliary clearance *in vivo* include cine-bronchography and assessment of the rate of clearance of radioaerosols.

Mucus is secreted by the goblet cells and submucosal glands of the first several bronchial generations. Secretion is under the control of a variety of chemical mediators. Neuropeptides including substance P, vasoactive intestinal peptide (VIP), and bombesin, in addition to vagal stimulation and acetylcholine, will cause discharge. In health, mucus is composed of 95 per cent water, the mucus glycoproteins or mucins, and a variety of other proteins (see below) which, although present in low concentration, probably play an important part in the defence of the bronchial tree. The function of mucus is to trap and clear particles, to dilute noxious influences, to lubricate the airways, and to humidify respired air. The viscoelastic or rheological properties of mucus are probably controlled by the concentration of different mucins and are probably critical in determining adequate mucociliary transport.

A number of external factors may reduce mucociliary clearance by interfering with ciliary function or by causing direct ciliary damage. These include pollutants, cigarette smoke, local and general anaesthetic agents, bacterial products, and viral infection. It is thought that in severe asthma eosinophil products, including major basic protein, may have detrimental effects on ciliary function. Thus there are a number of diseases in which mucociliary clearance may be adversely affected in a secondary fashion. There is also an autosomal recessive condition (occurring with a frequency of about one in 30 000 population), called primary ciliary dyskinaesia, in which defects in cilial dynein may be associated with male infertility and situs inversus (Kartagener's syndrome). Primary ciliary dyskinesia is associated with repeated sinusitis and respiratory infections which often progress to persistent lung suppuration and severe bronchiectasis, thus underlining the importance of cilia in antibacterial lung defences.

There is now a great deal of interest in abnormal properties of mucus and deranged mucociliary clearance in cystic fibrosis. In this condition mucus is abnormally viscous with grossly altered rheological properties resulting in markedly retarded mucociliary clearance (see Chapter 17.9.2).

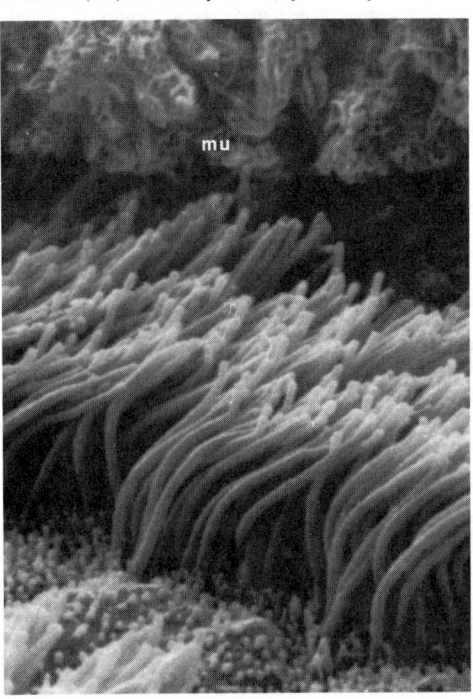

Fig. 1 Scanning electron micrograph of the 'mucociliary escalator' of the bronchial epithelium (magnification 14 000×). The cilia and the overlying raft of mucus (mu) are clearly seen. (By courtesy of Dr P.K. Jeffery.)

Surfactant

As is discussed in more detail in Chapters 17.2 and 17.4, surfactant is a complex surface-active material that lines the alveolar surface to reduce surface tension and prevent the lung from collapsing at resting transpulmonary pressures. It also provides a simple mechanism for alveolar clearance since, at end-expiration, surface tension decreases and the surface film moves from the alveolus towards the bronchioles, thus carrying small particles, damaged cells, etc. towards the mucociliary transport system.

Surfactant is synthesized and secreted by the alveolar type II pneumocytes. It comprises phospholipids, neutral lipids, and at least three different specific proteins—surfactant proteins A, B, and C. It is now recognized that, in addition to promoting the surface-active properties of surfactant, these proteins have important roles in host defence. There are several studies showing that surfactant from normal lungs exerts a variety of influences on alveolar macrophages, including chemotaxis and enhancement of phagocytosis and killing of microorganisms. Surfactant protein A is the most abundant protein, accounting for 3 mg of protein per 100 mg phospholipids of surfactant. On ultrastructural examination it closely resembles the complement component C1q and interacts with the C1q receptor (or collectin receptor). It has been shown to enhance alveolar macrophage phagocytosis of micro-organisms including *Staphylococcus aureus*, and may also be important in HIV and Pneumocystis recognition. It adheres to pollen grains and enhances FcR- and CR1-mediated phagocytosis of a variety of particles opsonized with IgG or C3b respectively. Surfactant proteins may be involved in local immunoregulation as well as bacterial defence. Experiments have shown that surfactant proteins can suppress certain lymphocyte and macrophage functions, including endotoxin-stimulated release of interleukin-1 (IL-1), tumour necrosis factor, (TNF) and interleukin-6 (IL-6). The *in vivo* significance of these observations is as yet uncertain.

Other protective proteins of the lining fluid of the respiratory tract

These may be derived from plasma (e.g. albumin, transferrin, antiplasmin, α_2-macroglobulin), by secretion from local epithelial cells, macrophages, or inflammatory cells (e.g. lysozyme, lactoferrin, and other defensins), or by selective epithelial transport (e.g. IgA). Clearly, the local availability of plasma-derived proteins will increase greatly during the exudative phase of any inflammatory process, thus adding more complement, antiproteinases, immunoglobulins, and proteins including cytokines derived from inflammatory cell secretion (see Chapter 17.3.2).

DEFENSINS AND OTHER BACTERIOSTATIC OR BACTERIOCIDAL PROTEINS

Defensins are a family of cytotoxic cationic peptides secreted mainly by leucocytes. Their antibacterial effects correlate with charge, which is determined by the arginine content. Defensins kill a variety of Gram-positive organisms, fungi, and viruses *in vitro*. Lactoferrin is an iron-binding protein, the antibacterial action of which is in part related to competition with iron which is an essential growth factor for certain bacteria. Lysozyme is a highly cationic protein which can disrupt bacteria which contain susceptible cell-wall peptidoglycans.

IMMUNOGLOBULINS

Normal lung secretions contain all the immunoglobulins present in plasma, but in different proportions. IgA is greatly in excess, and there are only small contributions from IgG and IgM. In the absence of disease, immunoglobulins are produced by local lung tissues. It is thought that B lymphocytes and plasma cells are particularly important in producing secretory IgA in the upper airways by a collaborative mechanism involving the epithelial cells. Dimeric IgA is assembled in the plasma cells from two monomeric IgA molecules and joined by another protein, the J chain. Dimeric IgA binds to the secretory component on the surface of epithelial cells, forming a dimeric IgA–secretory component complex which is pinocytosed, transported through the epithelial cell, and released from its luminal surface into the airways. The secretory component appears to protect IgA from enzymic attack during bacterial infection and inflammation in the host. IgA is produced in very high concentrations in the upper airways and probably serves a number of important roles, not all of which been fully elucidated. IgA deficiency is associated with local defects in immunity.

IgG concentrations in lung secretions are quantitatively similar to plasma IgG concentrations, and may be particularly important in the lower airways where IgG may act as a very effective opsonin and activator of complement. IgG deficiency is associated with recurrent respiratory tract infection, suggesting that it provides an important local defence mechanism.

COMPLEMENT PROTEINS, PROTEINASE INHIBITORS, ETC.

Most of the proteins involved in the complement system have been identified in lung secretions. The majority are probably derived by plasma exudation during inflammation, and C3a, C3b, and C5a may be secreted by alveolar macrophages. Patients with C3 deficiency have recurrent upper and lower respiratory tract infections, particularly with *Streptococcus pneumoniae* and *Haemophilus influenzae*. C3 is likely to play a key role in opsonization (via C3bi) of bacteria.

Lung secretions also contain a variety of antiproteinases, including the large molecules α_2-macroglobulin and α_1-antiproteinase as well as moieties of lower molecular weight, such as systemic leucoproteinase inhibitor. These agents are probably secreted in larger concentrations by local epithelial cells and alveolar macrophages during inflammatory and injurious processes, at which time there will be additional contributions to local defences from leakage of plasma-protein-derived antiproteinases. It is likely that these antiproteinases play an important part in the antiproteinase 'shield' which is necessary to protect the healthy local tissues against damage from the release of proteinases by inflammatory cells.

The alveolar macrophage and other alveolar cells

Alveolar macrophages are highly differentiated cells which have matured in the lung from blood-borne monocytes derived from bone marrow. They normally 'patrol' the alveoli (Fig.2) where they exist with a half-life of several weeks. The technique of bronchoalveolar lavage, whereby fluid is instilled into the small airways via a fibreoptic bronchoscope and fluid and harvested cells (normally more than 95 per cent alveolar macrophages in healthy individuals) are returned by suction, has greatly facilitated the *ex vivo* study of the various functions of these versatile cells. It was quickly recognized that alveolar macrophages possessed marked phagocytic ability, with the capacity to ingest and destroy pathogenic bacteria, but their capacity to generate mediators of central importance in the initiation of inflammation and to present antigen in the initiation of the immune response has been fully recognized only recently. The alveolar macrophage could be considered as a 'microcomputer', sampling and sensing the external environment in the alveolar spaces via a vast array of receptors (see Table 1) and subsequently determining whether and to what degree inflammatory or immune responses should be generated. It is also likely to assist the inflammatory monocyte-derived macrophages in the scavenging roles required during the aftermath of infections and the resolution of inflammation, and may play a further important role in the processes whereby inflammatory tissue injury is repaired, since it can produce a number of proteins involved in tissue repair processes and can generate a variety of cytokines that influence fibroblast function (see Table 2 for macrophage secretory products).

PHAGOCYTOSIS AND BACTERIAL KILLING

Macrophages can recognize and ingest opsonized (via their surface CR3 or FcR) or non-opsonized particles by a variety of receptors (see Table 1). Within the phagolysosome, ingested particles are subjected to the combined destructive forces of reactive oxygen intermediates generated via the metabolic burst and a wide range of degradative enzymes which have the capacity to digest proteins, lipids, and carbohydrates. It appears

Fig. 2 Scanning electron micrograph showing alveolar macrophages (arrow) 'patrolling' the alveolar airspaces (magnification 350×). A single alveolar macrophage adhering to the alveolar lining (arrows) is shown in section on the transmission electron micrograph in the insert. (By courtesy of Dr P.K. Jeffery.)

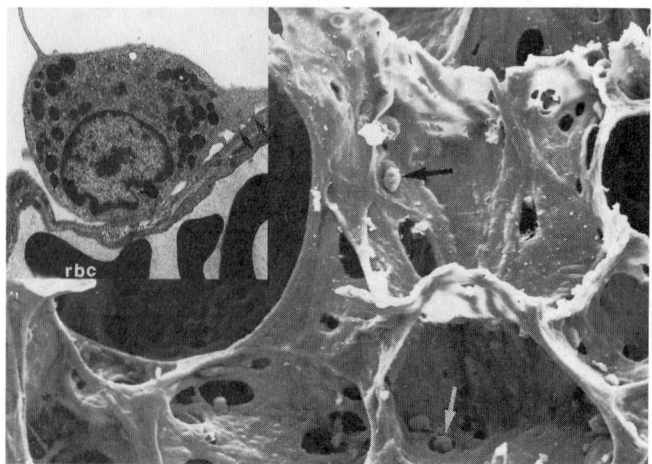

Table 1 *Some receptors on and molecules binding to macrophages*

Complement components
C1q, C3b, C3bi, C3d, C5a

Immunoglobulins
IgG, IgA, IgE

Growth factors and cytokines
IFN-α/β, IFNα, CSF-1, GMCSF, TNF-α
IL-1, IL-2, IL-3, IL-4, IL-6

Adhesion molecules and phagocytic receptors
LFA-1, MAC-1, p150/95, ICAM-1, α v β_3 (VnR), CR-1, CR-3,
    FcR

Glycoproteins and carbohydrates
Mannosyl fucosyl receptor
Mannose 6-phosphate
Heparin
Advanced glycosylation end-products

Proteins and hormones
Fibronectin, laminin, transferrin, fibrin, lactoferrin, calcitonin
Oestrogen, insulin, parathormone, progesterone

Peptides and small molecules
Adenosine, bombesin, bradykinin, adrenaline
Dexamethasone, glucagon, histamine
Tachykinins, PAF, serotonin, substance P
VIP

Lipids and lipoproteins
Leukotrienes C, D_4, B_4, E_2
LDL, β-VLDL, modified LDL

Table 2 *Some secretory products of macrophages*

Cytokines and growth factors
IFN-α/β/γ, IL-1, IL-6, TNF-α
IL-8, GRO α, MCP-1
TGFβ, PDGF, FGF, IGF, GM-CSF, G-CSF
Erythropoietin, lactoferrin

Enzymes
Elastase, collagenase, lysozyme
Phospholipase A_2, amylase
Hyaluronidase, acid hydrolases
β-galactosidase, β-glucuronidase
Nucleases, ribonucleases, acid phosphatases
Sulphatases, cathepsins

Enzyme inhibitors
α_1 Antiproteinase, α_2-macroglobulin
Lipomodulin, α_1-antichymotrypsin
Inhibitors of plasminogen and plasminogen activator

Reactive oxygen intermediates
O_2, H_2O_2, OH, hypohalous acid

Reactive nitrogen intermediates
NO, NO_2, NO_3

Complement components etc.
C_1, C_4, C_2, C_3, C_5, factor B, factor D, properdin

Lipids
Leukotrienes B, C, D, E, PGE, $PGF_{2\alpha}$
PAF, prostacyclin, thromboxane A_2

Matrix proteins
Fibronectin, thrombospondin, proteoglycans

Coagulation factors
Factor X, factor IX, factor V, factor VII, tissue factor,
    prothrombin, thromboplastin

that the local generation of nitric oxide is an important defence mechanism against a variety of micro-organisms. Activated macrophages form nitrite (NO_2), nitrate (NO_3), and nitric oxide (NO). *In vitro* experiments suggest that these products, particularly NO and the peroxynitrite anion, contribute to the antifungal, antiparasitic and tumouricidal activity of macrophages. Macrophages may 'call in antibacterial reinforcements' of other phagocytic cells including neutrophils, monocytes (which mature into inflammatory macrophages), and eosinophils by the generation of specific chemotaxins (see below). They may also generate a local immune response by presenting antigen and producing a variety of lymphokines.

Despite the availability of such powerful mechanisms, it is clear that not all phagocytosed particles are effectively destroyed. For example, asbestos, silica, and a number of micro-organisms, including tuberculosis, some strains of *H. influenzae,* and trypanosomes at various stages of their life-cycle, are able to resist destruction within macrophages.

GENERATION OF THE INFLAMMATORY RESPONSE

Macrophages can secrete a number of chemotactic proteins from the chemokine family as well as mediators in the 5-lipoxygenase and cyclooxygenase pathways, all of which can exert profound proinflammatory effects. Neutrophil chemotaxins include IL-8, leukotriene B_4, and NAP-2. Peptides which are chemotactic for monocytes include MCP_1 and MIP_1. Other macrophage-derived cytokines may have important secondary proinflammatory effects through their influences on other cells. For example, TNF and IL-1 act not only on endothelium to stimulate the expression of the adhesive molecules necessary for inflammatory cell emigration, but may also act on local fibroblasts to produce IL-8 which exerts neutrophil chemotactic effects. Thus macrophages not only generate chemoattractants for inflammatory cells, but can also recruit other local cells such as fibroblasts to help in the initiation of inflammation, thereby governing graded levels of amplification of the inflammatory response.

GENERATION OF THE IMMUNE RESPONSE

Alveolar macrophages are effective antigen-presenting cells and can display partially degraded antigens on their surface to interact with recirculating T and B cells, generating clonal expansion and initiating the immune response.

TISSUE REMODELLING AND REPAIR

Alveolar macrophages can secrete proteins, including fibronectin, vitronectin, and laminin which are important in tissue repair. Macrophages can also produce a number of cytokines including platelet-derived growth factor, transforming growth factor β, and IL-1 which can influence the behaviour of other cells, particularly fibroblasts which are critically involved in the repair process (see Chapter 17.3.2).

The pulmonary marginated pool of neutrophils

The neutrophil is the archetypal acute inflammatory cell, equipped with a variety of mechanisms (Table) which make it a very effective agent in host defences against bacteria such as Streptococci. After release from the bone marrow, mature neutrophils exist in the vascular compartment with a half-life of about 6 h. Unlike red blood cells, up to half of the neutrophils in the vascular compartment do not circulate at any given time but form a 'marginated pool' which is in dynamic equilibrium with the 'circulating pool' of vascular neutrophils. The marginated pool can be released into the circulating pool by exercise or adrenaline. The vascular beds of the lung and spleen appear to make the most important contribution to the marginated pool, which may serve as source of rapidly releasable neutrophils in times of stress or injury. The presence of large numbers of neutrophils in the pulmonary microvascular bed is likely to increase the mobilization and effectiveness of local lung defences in response to their inevitable exposure to inhaled micro-organisms or toxins. The mechanisms underlying the formation of the marginated pool in the lung are uncertain. It could be formed as the result of low grade adhesive interactions between neutrophils and lung capillary endothelial cells. However, it is likely that the rheological properties of neutrophils in pulmonary capillaries are more important in the physiological margination of neutrophils in the lung. The mean diameter of the pulmonary capillary is 5.5 μm, whereas that of the neutrophil is 7.5 μm. Thus neutrophils are normally required to squeeze through the pulmonary capillaries, and minor changes in their deformability or alterations in the fluid pressure gradient across the lung capillary bed would be expected to have a marked influence on the size of the pulmonary marginated pool. The existence of this pool of neutrophils in the lung may have advantages for host defence, but, paradoxically, it could also partly explain why the lung appears to be such an important target in conditions such as the adult respiratory distress syndrome, which may result from systemic or distant insults (e.g. Gram-negative septicaemia, multiple trauma, or pancreatitis).

REFERENCES

Adams, D.O. and Hamilton, (1992). Macrophages as destructive cells in host defence. In: *Inflammation: basic principles and clinical correlates* (2nd edn) (ed J.I. Gallin, I.M. Goldstein, and R. Snyderman), Chapter 31. Raven Press, New York.

Clarke, S.J. (1995). Physical defences of the lung. In: *Respiratory medicine* (ed Brewis and Geddes), in press.

Klebanoff, S.J. (1992). Oxygen metabolites from phagocytes. In: *Inflammation: basic principles and clinical correlates* (2nd edn) (ed J.I. Gallin, I.M. Goldstein, and R. Snyderman), Chapter 28. Raven Press, New York.

Stockley, R.S. (1995). Humoral and cellular mechanisms of lung defence. In: *Respiratory medicine* (ed Brewis and Geddes), in press.

17.3.2 Inflammation and the lung

C. HASLETT

Historical and other general considerations

The external signs of acute inflammation have been recognized since the time of Celsus when the cardinal features *calor* (heat), *rubor* (redness), *tumor* (swelling), *dolor* (pain), and *functio laesa* (loss of function) were recorded. In the eighteenth and nineteenth centuries physiologists and pathologists, including Conheim, Virchow, and Metchnikoff, made the classical observations which underpin our present understanding of the vascular and cell biology of inflammation. Throughout the centuries, inflammation was perceived as an entirely beneficial response of the body to injury or infection. From his experiences on the battlefields of Europe, John Hunter asserted 'Inflammation is itself not to be considered as a disease but as a salutary operation consequent either to some violence or to some disease', and Metchnikoff, the father of modern inflammatory cell biology, emphasized this concept in his writings. The inflammatory response, which is now recognized as a complex interplay between constitutive cells (e.g. microvascular endothelium), multiple biochemical mediator cascades, and migratory cells from the bloodstream, evolved as a highly effective component of the 'innate' immune response of the host. One of the best examples of a 'beneficial' inflammatory response in the lungs is provided by the massive acute inflammatory cellular response in streptococcal pneumonia. Full-blown streptococcal 'lobar' pneumonia was very common in the preantibiotic era,

Table 1 *A short list of lung diseases in which inflammation plays an important part of the mechanism*

Chronic bronchitis and emphysema
Asthma
Adult respiratory distress syndrome
Neonatal respiratory distress syndrome
Bronchopulmonary dysplasia
Complicated pneumonias
   Staphylococcal pneumonia
   Klebsiellae pneumonia
Lung transplant rejection
Fibrosing alveolitides
Pneumoconioses
Extrinsic allergic alveolitides

yet most patients survived because of the effectiveness of local inflammatory responses.

Over the last two or three decades, however, it has become clear that this complex response may also contribute to a variety of diseases which have assumed importance in the developed world. A limited list of examples from the lung is presented in Table 1. These diseases are characterized by the persistent accumulation of inflammatory cells, which in many examples is associated either with tissue destruction or with the development of a fibrogenic (scarring) response.

In a simplistic model of pulmonary function, gases are transferred by small airways to the alveolar units where exchange of oxygen and carbon dioxide occurs across fine membranes comprised of the capillary endothelial cell, basement membranes, a small amount of interstitial matrix, and the alveolar epithelial cell layer. Inflammation and its consequences can exert detrimental effects on lung function at all levels.

1. In asthma it is thought that inflammation causes microvascular leak of protein-rich fluid which contributes to mucus plugging and submucosal oedema. These are major contributory factors to the airways obstruction which underlies the disorders of gas exchange (Fig. 1(a)).
2. In emphysema there is major loss of the surface area available for gas exchange (Fig. 1(b) (ii) as compared with normal lung (1(b)(i)). It is now thought this pathological process results from smoking-induced persistent low grade inflammation which causes the local release of destructive proteolytic enzymes from neutrophils and other inflammatory cells.
3. Inflammatory oedema, proteinaceous exudate, and hyaline membranes can cause marked widening of the interstitial spaces of the capillary gas exchange membranes in the adult respiratory distress syndrome (Fig. 1(c)).
4. The interstitium can also be widened on a more chronic basis with scar tissue comprised of proliferating fibroblasts and matrix proteins (Fig. 1(d)) as exemplified by the fibrosing alveolitides.

Diffuse interstitial oedema or fibrosis markedly reduces the capacity of the lung for oxygenation. Unlike the skin where the extravascular exudate and oedema of inflammation, and even secondary scarring, may result in little more than undesirable cosmetic effects, these processes occurring diffusely in the lung have catastrophic consequences for lung function and cause serious morbidity and mortality.

Inflammation in the lung can have other consequences. Inhibition of the mucociliary transporter process may occur through inflammatory damage to ciliary function or bronchiectasis, gross thickening of the peripheral lung parenchyma and pleura with chronic inflammation and scar tissue results in detrimental mechanical effects on lung inflation and deflation, and the function of the diaphragm and intercostal muscles may be disrupted in systemic myositis and other connective tissue diseases.

Because of these potentially detrimental effects of inflammation, much research effort has been targeted at the events involved in initiation and amplification of lung inflammation. However, it is important to recognize our current lack of understanding of mechanisms responsible for the normal resolution processes of inflammation. The potential power of such resolution mechanisms is well illustrated by pneumococcal pneumonia. Radiological and pathological descriptions from the preantibiotic era clearly demonstrate that, in the majority of patients, the massive accumulation of neutrophils, inflammatory macrophages, and fluid and protein exudate was effectively cleared, with less than 2.5 per cent of cases progressing to fibrosis. This is remarkable when we consider what is now known of the destructive, proinflammatory, and pro-

fibrotic capacity of the cell and mediator cascades involved. Why an acute inflammatory response in the lung may sometimes resolve (e.g. pneumococcal pneumonia) but in other circumstances (e.g. Klebsiella and staphylococcal pneumonia) progress to tissue destruction and scarring remains a mystery, the solution of which may provide important insights into the pathogenesis of inflammatory diseases of the lung and other organs. Some inflammatory lung diseases, such as fibrosing alveolitis, may not present clinically until the pathogenetic processes have progressed far beyond the early initiation stages, and it is reasonable to suggest that improving our understanding of how inflammation normally resolves may provide new insights into the pathogenesis of persistent inflammatory states and lead to therapies directed at promoting those mechanisms favouring resolution.

Therefore this chapter will comprise a discussion of the mechanisms

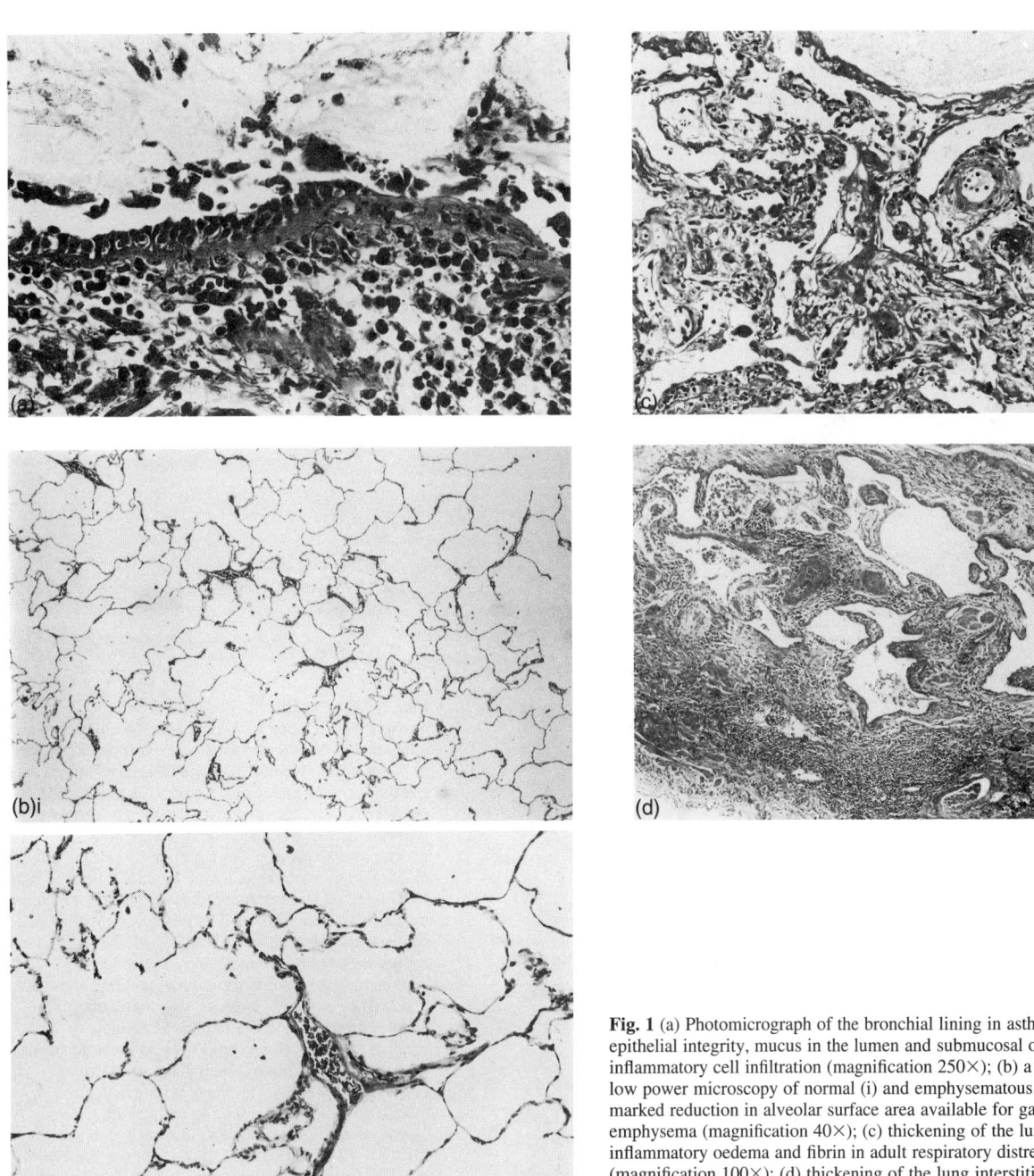

Fig. 1 (a) Photomicrograph of the bronchial lining in asthma showing loss of epithelial integrity, mucus in the lumen and submucosal oedema with inflammatory cell infiltration (magnification 250×); (b) a contrast between the low power microscopy of normal (i) and emphysematous (ii) lung, showing marked reduction in alveolar surface area available for gas exchange in emphysema (magnification 40×); (c) thickening of the lung interstitium by inflammatory oedema and fibrin in adult respiratory distress syndrome (magnification 100×); (d) thickening of the lung interstitium by inflammatory infiltrates and scar tissue in fibrosing alveolitis (magnification 40×). (Figures 1 (a–d) by courtesy of Dr D. Lamb.)

which are likely to be involved in the processes of evolution and resolution of lung inflammation, how these may relate to the pathogenesis of inflammatory lung disease, and the relationship between inflammation and scarring. Finally, we shall speculate on how recent knowledge of underlying mechanisms suggests novel mechanism-driven anti-inflammatory therapies.

Initiation of the inflammatory response

In this section we will consider the generation of a simple inflammatory response such as might be expected to occur following deposition of bacteria in the lung alveolus. In most acute inflammatory responses neutrophils can be observed in the extravascular tissues from about 2 h after the initial stimulus or insult, with neutrophil emigration from the local microvessels reaching a peak at 4 to 6 h. Monocyte emigration into the tissues begins at around 4 to 6 h and reaches a peak 12 to 18 h later. Neutrophils migrate rapidly through the tissues to the 'scene of the crime' where they ingest and destroy bacteria. Extravasated monocytes mature into inflammatory macrophages at the inflamed site where they have important controlling roles in the later phases of inflammation, particularly scavenging, resolution, and repair.

Emigration of neutrophils and monocytes from the capillaries

In most organs other than the lung it is likely that the site of neutrophil emigration is the postcapillary venule, but it is now generally agreed that the bulk of neutrophil emigration in the lung occurs in the capillaries themselves. These events involve a complex interplay between the local tissue cells, which generate the mediators driving neutrophil chemotaxis, and the expression of adhesive molecules on the surface of neutrophils and capillary endothelial cells. This sets in train sequestration of neutrophils in the capillaries, adhesion between the neutrophil and capillary endothelial cell surfaces, and finally the complex process of capillary transmigration whereby the neutrophil undergoes diapedesis between endothelial cells and migration through the capillary endothelial basement membrane. In the past few years there has been intense interest in this area of inflammatory vascular biology since the processes are common to the initiation of inflammatory diseases in all organs, and the explosion of knowledge of the molecular mechanisms of chemotaxin generation and the adhesive mechanisms whereby inflammatory cells interact with endothelial cells has provided specific targets for manipulation of the inflammatory response at the earliest stages of its evolution.

LOCAL GENERATION OF THE INFLAMMATORY RESPONSE

Bacteria may release agents such as chemotactic formylated peptides, for example formyl-methionyl-leucyl-phenylalanine (fMLP), and may activate the complement cascade to produce the chemotactic complement peptide C5a. When injected into tissues many inflammatory agents lead to neutrophil emigration, but the number of true chemotactic peptides, i.e. agents which cause directed migration via ligation of specific surface receptors, is likely to be quite restricted. True chemotaxins include C5a, leukotriene B_4 (LTB_4), and fMLP, and recent information suggests that chemoattractive cytokines ('chemokines') such as interleukin 8 (IL-8) also act via specific surface receptors. Agents like inter-

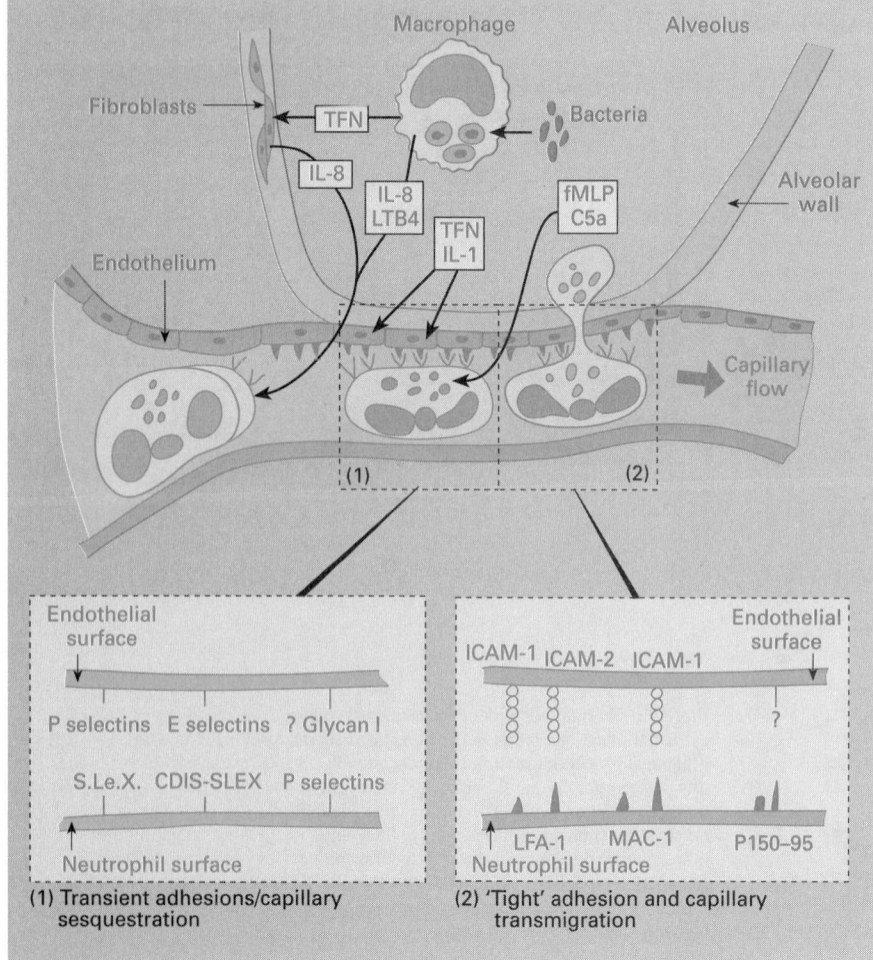

Fig. 2 Diagram depicting probable events involved in neutrophil emigration from pulmonary capillaries to an inflammatory stimulus caused by deposition of bacteria in the adjacent alveolus. Bacteria themselves may release chemotactic factors (e.g. fMLP), activate the complement cascade producing the chemotaxin C5a, or provoke macrophage secretion of a variety of agents which promote neutrophil emigration by causing direct up-regulation of neutrophil-adhesive molecules (LTB_4, GRO-α, IL-8) and neutrophil chemotaxis. Macrophages may also produce TNF or IL-1 which act on other local cells to generate IL-8 and stimulate endothelial expression of adhesive molecules. Reduction of neutrophil deformability caused by the direct effect of C5a, fMLP, or the chemokines also contributes to the initial sequestration of neutrophils in pulmonary capillaries. Exploded box (a) shows adhesive molecules involved in the initial transient phase of neutrophil–endothelial adhesion. This stage is dominated by members of the selectin family linking with their carbohydrate ligands (e.g. sialyl Lewis X antigen (SLEX)). Exploded box (b) shows adhesive molecules involved in the second phase of 'tight' adhesion and endothelial transmigration. The leucocyte integrins, particularly LFA-1 and endothelial ICAM-1, are critically involved in this stage.

leukin 1 (IL-1) and tumour necrosis factor (TNF), which themselves are not specifically chemotactic *in vitro*, exert indirect chemoattractant effects *in vivo* by inducing the release of specific chemotaxins from other cells in the microenvironment (Fig. 2). It is likely that the alveolar macrophage plays a key role in this respect by releasing chemotactic and other pro-inflammatory mediators in response to local tissue pertubation or exposure to bacteria. It can release a number of specific chemotactic peptides, including interleukin-8 (IL-8) and leukotriene B$_4$ (LTB$_4$), in addition to agents such as IL-1 and TNF which have further effects on neutrophil emigration by acting upon capillary endothelial cells to activate them and induce the expression of adhesive molecules which are essential for neutrophil adhesion and capillary transmigration. In the lung it appears that, while the local generation of C5a may not be a major factor in neutrophil emigration, IL-8 is particularly important. This chemokine is an extremely powerful neutrophil chemoattractant and can be produced in large concentrations by lung macrophages.

While alveolar macrophages are of undoubted importance in sensing the need for an inflammatory response and initiating recruitment of inflammatory cells, it is now also clear that other resident lung cells (including airway epithelial cells and interstitial fibroblasts) have the capacity to generate agents such as IL-8, IL-1, and TNF which are centrally involved in the initiation of inflammation. Local paracrine effects, such as macrophage-derived TNF acting on local fibroblasts and epithelial cells to induce their release of IL-8 (Fig. 2), may also be brought to bear, with multiple opportunities for rapid amplification of signals leading to the local recruitment of inflammatory cells.

Until recently it was thought that the sequential emigration of neutrophils followed by monocytes was likely to result simply from their different rates of response to a common chemotactic factor such as C5a. However, it is now clear that chemotactic factors relatively specific for neutrophils or monocytes can be generated at the inflamed site and that monocytes may use different components of the repertoire of adhesive molecules (such as the VLA$_4$–VCAM-1 axis) than the neutrophil for the processes of endothelial adhesion and transmigration (see below). Since VCAM-1 tends to be expressed later than E-selectin (an endothelial adhesive molecule which interacts with neutrophils) on the surface of stimulated endothelial cells, sequential emigration of leucocytes may also be influenced by the time course of endothelial cell adhesion molecule expression.

INFLAMMATORY CELL SEQUESTRATION

The arrest of neutrophils in pulmonary capillaries is a necessary prelude to capillary transmigration, and is likely to result from the combination of a reduction in neutrophil deformability and the expression/activation of neutrophil surface adhesive molecules which interact with counter-receptors on the surface of activated endothelial cells. As has been discussed above, the neutrophil is normally required to deform and squeeze through the pulmonary capillary, and hence any reduction in its ability to deform would lead to its prolonged sequestration in the capillary. Agents such as C5a, bacterial products, and exposure to cigarette smoke cause marked reduction in neutrophil deformability in a fashion which correlates directly with its sequestration in pulmonary capillaries.

Adhesion between neutrophils and capillary endothelial cells is a complex process. Under the conditions of shear stress which accompanies blood flow in postcapillary venules, it appears that molecules of the selectin family (particularly L-selectin) are important in the first phase of transitory adhesion ('rolling'), whereas neutrophil surface molecules of the integrin family are involved in the second phase of tight adhesion ('sticking') which is required for capillary transmigration. Whether these general observations made in postcapillary venules of the systemic circulation hold true for the pulmonary microvascular capillaries (the major site of neutrophil emigration in the lung) remains to be established.

The *in vivo* importance of the leucocyte integrins, and more recently the selectins, has been underlined by accidents of nature in which

patients with genetic deficiencies of these receptors suffer from recurrent infections associated with the inability of neutrophils to migrate effectively to the inflamed site (these are considered in more detail below), and there are now intriguing suggestions that inflammatory processes in different organs, and even different infective processes within the same organ, may utilize different components of the adhesive molecule repertoire. For example, Doerschuk and her colleagues have shown that monoclonal antibodies directed against CD18, the common beta chain of the leucocyte integrins, will inhibit neutrophil emigration to sites of streptococcal infection in the skin but will not block neutrophil emigration to streptococcal pneumonia. Furthermore, anti-CD18 antibodies will inhibit neutrophil emigration to experimental pneumonia caused by *Escherichia coli* or endotoxin. These observations allow us to speculate that it may be possible to develop specific therapeutic strategies directed at blocking neutrophil emigration to tissues involved in a particular pathological process while permitting neutrophils to enter other organs in order to provide the necessary defences against infection. A large number of adhesive molecules, which are important in adhesion and transmigration, have now been identified on the surface of neutrophils and microvascular endothelial cells. They have broadly been divided into molecules of the integrin, selectin, and immunoglobulin supergene families. Counter-receptors have been identified for most, but by no means all, of the adhesion molecules so far characterized (Table 2).

The integrins

The leucocyte integrins are part of a family of phylogenetically ancient molecules which have important functions in the morphogenesis and tissue organization of insects and vertebrates. The term 'integrin' was used to describe the nature of these membrane glycoproteins and their possible role as a link between the cell cytoskeleton and extracellular matrix, implying an important role as potential regulators of cellular responses to the microenvironment. They are heterodimeric transmembrane glycoproteins, each with an alpha and beta subunit. At least seven beta units have now been cloned and sequenced. Single beta units have the capacity to associate with different alpha units, and the description of subfamilies has been based on the subunit associations. Most of the 'beta-1' family are involved with cell matrix interactions, although some in this family including the 'very late antigens' VLA-1 and VLA-4 are expressed on lymphocytes. The only beta-1 integrin of relevance to this discussion is VLA-4, a monocyte ligand for the endothelial vascular cell adhesion molecule VCAM-1 which may be important in the capillary emigration of monocytes and eosinophil granulocytes. There has been much recent interest in the role of the beta-2 subfamily or the 'leucocyte integrins' LFA-1, CR3 (Mac-1), and P150.95. Monoclonal antibodies defining the subunits of the leucocyte integrins have been designated by the leucocyte typing workshops using the following nomenclature: CD11a (LFA-1 alpha subunit), CD11b (CR3 alpha subunit), CD11c (P150.95 alpha subunit), and CD18 (common beta subunit).

The fundamental importance of the leucocyte adhesion integrins was underlined by an experiment of nature which is now called 'leucocyte adhesion deficiency'. In the 1970s there were a number of reports of patients suffering from recurrent bacterial infection which appeared to be the result of impaired neutrophil function, including reduced adhesiveness, reduced phagocytosis, chemotaxis, and metabolic burst in response to phagocytosis of opsonized zymosan particles. This autosomal recessive trait was shown by several groups to be the result of a deficiency of surface glycoproteins now recognized as the leucocyte integrins. Clinical features include delayed umbilical cord separation, repeated infections throughout life, and destructive ulceration of the skin with poor wound healing and dystrophic scars. It was noted that neutrophils failed to migrate from local blood vessels to these ulcers and infected sites. Such examples clearly demonstrate the *in vivo* importance of these molecules for neutrophil emigration.

Individual leucocyte integrin receptors may serve a number of functions and may combine with different ligands on endothelial cells (Table 2). LFA-1 is involved in the binding of leucocytes to a number of cell

Table 2 *Some cell-surface adhesion molecules important in leucocyte endothelial adhesion and transmigration*

Receptor	Other names/cluster designation	Distribution	Induced by	Ligand/counter receptor	Promotes adhesion of
Integrin family					
LFA-1	CD11a/CD18	All leucocytes		ICAM-1, ICAM-2, ICAM-3	Endothelial cells
Mac-1/ CR3	CD11b/CD18	Monocytes, granulocytes, natural killer cells, lymphocytes		ICAM-1, Factor X, LPS, C3bi, Factor B	Endothelial cells Phagocytic particles
P150.95	CD11c/CD18	Monocytes, granulocytes		?	Endothelial cells
Immunoglobin superfamily					
ICAM-1	CD54	Endothelial cells, epithelial cells, fibroblasts, mast cells	TNF IL-1 LPS } 2–4 hours	LFA-1 MAC-1 ?CD43	All leucocytes
ICAM-2		Monocytes, lymphocytes, endothelium	Not induced	LFA-1	All leucocytes
ICAM-3		All leucocytes, not endothelium			
VCAM-1	INCAM-110	Activated endothelium	IL-1 TNF IL-4 } 2–4 hours	VLA-4	Monocytes ?Eosinophils
Selectin family					
E-selectin	ELAM-1	Endothelium	LPS TNF IL-1 } 30 minutes	Sialyl Lewis X (CD15) CD66 express sialyl? CD67 CD15	Neutrophils Memory T cells
P-selectin	GMP-140 CD62 PADGEM	Endothelium, platelets	Thrombin PAF Histamine } 5 minutes	Sialyl Lewis X	Neutrophils
L-selectin	LECAM-1 LAM-1 Leu 8 Mel 14 gp90 Dreg 56	Neutrophils, monocytes, lymphocytes	Rapidly shed on activation	?E-selectin ?P-selectin Gly-CAM-1	Endothelium

types, including endothelial cells, epithelial cells, keratinocytes, and fibroblasts. The intercellular adhesion molecule ICAM-1, a member of the immunoglobulin supergene family, was first demonstrated as a ligand for LFA-1 but subsequent observations showing that LFA-1-dependent adhesion to endothelial cells was not fully inhibited by monoclonal antibodies against ICAM-1 led to the discovery of ICAM-2 and ICAM-3 (see below). As well as being important in the phagocytosis of particles opsonized by the complement component iC3b, CR3 is also involved in the interactions whereby stimulated neutrophils bind to endothelial cells. This occurs via a site on endothelial ICAM-1 distinct from that recognized by LFA-1. P150.95 has also been implicated in neutrophil endothelial interactions, but the endothelial ligands have not yet been identified.

In the two-stage model of neutrophil binding to microvascular endothelial cells (see above) the leucocyte integrins appear to be critically involved in the 'tight' second stage of the adhesive interaction which precedes and is a prerequisite for capillary transmigration. The attachment and detachment processes which must occur during capillary transmigration implies regulation of integrin function and at least the need for 'on–off' switching. Regulation of integrin function is likely to occur at a number of different levels. These include both ligand regulation, for example local expression and cell surface distribution of ICAM-1 can be modulated by cytokines in a fashion which could markedly alter interactions with LFA-1, and receptor regulation, whereby fine tuning of inflammatory cell adhesion and the potential for leucocyte-integrin-bearing cells to remain unresponsive in the presence of abundant ligand or to hyper-respond to low levels of ligand require regulation of the leucocyte integrin itself. This is not likely to occur simply as the result of expression of different receptor numbers, but at the level of more

sophisticated regulation of avidity and affinity of the receptors themselves.

The selectins

The selectins, including E-selectin and P-selectin on the endothelial surface and L-selectin on the leucocyte surface, are a family of cell surface glycoproteins that may have a particularly important role in the earliest stages of leucocyte–endothelial interaction. They were so named because of their amino-terminal C-type lectin domain which appears essential for their adhesive properties.

E-selectin (previously known as ELAM-1) is expressed on vascular endothelial cells after their activation *in vitro* with endotoxin or cytokines including IL-1 and TNF-α. This occurs within 30 min, peaks at 2 to 4 h, and returns to basal levels within 24 h. *In vitro* it mediates neutrophil adhesion to endothelium. E-selectin may also have a role in eosinophil adhesion *in vivo*, since E-selectin antibodies block pulmonary granulocyte influx in an experimental model of asthma. The counter-receptor on neutrophils for E-selectin is a surface glycoprotein termed the sialyl Lewis X antigen.

P-selectin (previously termed GMP-140) is a cell surface glycoprotein which may be of great importance in the early adhesion of neutrophils to endothelial cells in inflammation since it is rapidly transferred from the Weibel Palade bodies of endothelial cells to the surface where it is then thought to interact with sialylated carbohydrate on the neutrophil surface.

L-selectin (previously known as LAM-1) is expressed by lymphocyte subsets (where it is known as the 'peripheral node homing receptor'), but is also present on the surface of neutrophil granulocytes and monocytes. Surface L-selectin is shed from the neutrophil once this cell has been activated and is adherent to the endothelium. L-selectin appears to be particularly important in the transient neutrophil adhesion to endothelial cells which occurs under conditions of blood flow in the phase of the adhesive process before integrins assume a dominant role. The endothelial counter-receptor for L-selectin may be glycam-1, but under some circumstances it can also bind to E- and P-selectins.

A further genetic abnormality has recently been described which provides direct support for an *in vivo* role for selectin molecules in neutrophil emigration. A clinical syndrome of repeated infections and failure of neutrophil emigration resembling leucocyte adhesion deficiency was described in two boys who had a common distinctive facial appearance, mental retardation, and short stature, but retained CD18 integrins. However, sialyl lewis X (NEUACα2, 3Galβ1.4(FUCα1.3), Glc-NAC) deficiency and a failure of the neutrophils to adhere to E-selectin expressed on activated endothelial cells was demonstrated. It has been suggested that this genetic abnormality should be called 'leucocyte adhesion deficiency type II'.

The immunoglobulin supergene family

This family, which possesses a common amino acid chain originally described in the constant and variable regions of immunoglobulin light and heavy chains, now includes a diverse range of surface molecules including T-cell receptors (CD4, CD8, CD3, major histocompatibility complex class I, and major histocompatibility complex class II) and also a range of adhesive molecules such as the neural cell adhesion molecule (NCAM). Those of direct relevance for leucocyte endothelial interaction are ICAM-1, ICAM-2, ICAM-3, and VCAM-1 on the surface of endothelial cells. ICAM-1 is the major ligand for LFA-1, but lack of complete inhibition of binding in the presence of anti-ICAM-1 monoclonal antibodies led to the discovery of ICAM-2. This is also a member of the immunoglobulin superfamily, but in contrast with the five extracellular domains of ICAM-1 has two Ig-like domains. The combination of monoclonal antibodies to ICAM-1 and ICAM-2 failed to block CD18-dependent adhesion mechanisms completely, suggesting the presence of a third moiety ICAM-3.

ICAM-1 has a wide distribution, including many cells of great relevance to the generation of inflammatory responses. It is highly expressed on 'stimulated' vascular endothelium, where it is involved in the transendothelial migration of T cells, and is also implicated in neutrophil emigration from microvessels. It is particularly important in the second phase of tight neutrophil adhesion and transendothelial migration where it interacts with LFA-1 and MAC-1, expressed on neutrophils. However, it seems not to be effective under conditions of shear stress or to be involved in the transient initial phase of neutrophil adhesion. The use of anti-ICAM-1 monoclonal antibodies in experimental models of allergic asthma indicate a role of ICAM-1 in eosinophil migration into the lung. ICAM-1 is constitutively represented on the surface of all endothelial cells, but is strongly upregulated in the presence of cytokines such as TNF-α, IL-1 and platelet-activating factor (PAF). In contrast, ICAM-2 does not appear to be as responsive to cytokine induction. Injection of IL-1 or TNF-α into tissues causes a gradual increase in ICAM-1 expression: 50 per cent at 6 h, reaching a maximum at 24 h with continued expression for 24 to 72 h. This further suggests that ICAM-1 may have a particularly important role in the later phases of neutrophil emigration from blood vessels rather than at the initiation of neutrophil emigration. Corticosteroids have a powerful inhibitory effect on ICAM-1 induction by cytokines. ICAM-1 is clearly a centrally important molecule in the control of the inflammatory and immune responses.

There are two forms of VCAM-1, one with six extracellular Ig-like domains and one with seven. The seven-domain form is found on vascular endothelial cells. VCAM-1 is activated by IL-1 TNF-α, and lipopolysaccharide, with maximum up-regulation taking several hours to occur. VCAM-1 binds to monocytes and eosinophils in a CD11/CD18 independent fashion and it is thought that the adhesive interaction is mediated through the beta-1 integrin VLA-4. It has been suggested that this may be part of the mechanism for selective eosinophil emigration in allergic conditions such as asthma, but this is by no means established *in vivo*.

Contemporary thinking can be summarized as follows. Neutrophil emigration is initiated by the release of local mediators and cytokines from resident tissue 'sensing cells'. These act on neutrophils in the microvasculature and on the capillary endothelial cells to generate a complex sequence of adhesive processes involving at least two stages. The first stage is one of temporary adhesion or sequestration which occurs through activation of the selectin molecules, particularly L-selectin on the neutrophil surface and P-selectin on the endothelial surface. Thereafter there is a second phase of tight adhesion involving the integrin molecules on the neutrophil surface and ICAM-1 on the endothelium. This step must be carefully controlled by mechanisms including 'on–off' regulation of the integrins to permit the neutrophil to take part in the process of capillary transmigration.

CAPILLARY TRANSMIGRATION

Since Addison's classical light microscope observations in 1843 and Lord Florey's detailed electron microscope work, it has become clear that emigrating neutrophils can 'squeeze' between endothelial cells by a process of diapedesis. However, the complex intercellular signalling processes that must be required are obscure at present. The next barrier to neutrophil emigration is the capillary basement membrane, the transgression of which probably involves some inevitable degradation of matrix proteins. Some intriguing recent experiments by Weiss have suggested the plausible hypothesis that the endothelial cells themselves play a key role in the local degradation and re-formation of the capillary basement membrane during neutrophil transmigration.

In the example of a neutrophil migrating to an inflamed focus within a lung airspace, the neutrophil must then broach the epithelial cell layer which, unlike endothelial cells, is formed by cells attached via a number of complex intercellular adhesive mechanisms including 'tight junctions'. Neutrophils can be induced to migrate between epithelial cells *in vitro* without causing cell injury or loss of electrical resistance of the epithelial monolayer. The mechanisms which permit broaching and resealing of the epithelial tight junctions without causing increased permeability or even loss of electrical resistance across the monolayer are intriguing, but are entirely obscure at present. Nevertheless, it is also true that, even in acute 'beneficial' inflammation such as streptococcal pneumonia, there is usually evidence of significant injury to endothelial and epithelial cell layers. Therefore it seems likely that this stage of inflammation represents a pivotal point where any loss of local control mechanisms could greatly amplify inflammatory tissue injury, and it may also be relevant that many inflammatory lung diseases are characterized by evidence of excessive endothelial and epithelial injury and persistent microvascular fluid and protein exudation.

Neutrophil chemotaxis, activation, and phagocytosis

After penetration of the resident cellular 'barriers', neutrophils undergo directed migration, or chemotaxis, towards the inflammatory focus. Chemotaxins take effect by binding to specific receptors. The receptors for fMLP and C5a have now been cloned and are identified as members of the G-protein-linked receptor superfamily. During the remarkable and complex process of chemotaxis, neutrophils are able to sense across their length (around 5.5 μm) the tiny changes in concentration of chemotaxins that form the chemotactic concentration gradient. Chemoattractant receptors are highly mobile and appear to be swept back from the leading edge of the cell, internalized, then recycled. Ligation of chemotactic receptors causes generalized activation of the cell together with the actin polymerization and cytoskeletal rearrangement which are necessary for locomotor responses. The broad details of chemotactic receptor ligation, activation of the cell, and changes in the cytoskeleton are becoming better understood (Fig. 3). However, the fine details of the sensing mechanisms and discrete motor mechanisms necessary for the localized protrusive and retractive movements that are necessary for locomotion through tissues remain obscure. Neutrophil chemotactic responses and activation appear to be mediated through common receptor-driven mechanisms, causing rapid formation of the intracellular signalling molecules inositol (1,4,5)-trisphosphate and diacylglycerol, and a marked increase in free intracellular calcium $[Ca^{2+}]_i$. The modulating effects of guanine triphosphate and the inhibitory effects of certain bacterial toxins indicate a role for a guanine–nucleotide binding protein (G-protein) in this process. Stimulation of the receptor G-protein complex activates phospholipase C which hydrolyses phosphatidylinositol (4,5)-bisphosphate into inositol trisphosphate and 1,2 diacylglycerol. Newly formed inositol trisphosphate causes a rapid release of Ca^{2+} from intracellular stores and may contribute to the subsequent influx of Ca^{2+} from the extracellular environment. Diacylglycerol activates protein kinase C which initiates a series of protein phosphorylation events which are critical to cell locomotion and degranulation. These general processes are also intimately associated with membrane-associated NADPH oxidase which converts O_2 to O_2^- in the metabolic burst. Although the same general pathways are activated by many chemotaxins, there are finer levels of control for individual agents and for specific neutrophil functions such as degranulation, superoxide production, and motility. For example, LTB_4 is a good chemotaxin but a poor secretagogue. This may be related to the observation that, unlike other chemotaxins, LTB_4 stimulation does not cause the later rise in $[Ca^{2+}]_i$. Similarly, a degree of cell activation and alteration in the cytoskeletal framework is necessary for maximal effect of the adhesive receptors in capillary transmigration, but the full-blown activation associated with the respiratory burst and the maximal secretory response would not be desirable until a much later stage when the neutrophil has recognized and phagocytosed bacterial agents which, when secure in the phagolysosome, could receive the full, direct force of these mechanisms.

One of the earliest physical events in the stimulated neutrophil is a change of shape from its normal spherical state to a polarized form. This is associated with a reduction in cell deformability and the mechanical changes which precede locomotion and phagocytosis. Actin polymerization plays an important role in these cytoskeletal changes. When neutrophils are in a resting state about half their complement of actin is insoluble and forms a branching network under the cell membrane which extends into and controls the formation of microvillae and other conformational changes. The network is composed of actin monomers (G-actin) which are polymerized to form actin filaments (F-actin). These in turn are cross-linked into a web structure by another protein, actin-binding protein. The remaining 50 per cent of actin is maintained in a soluble form by agents which inhibit polymerization, thus providing the opportunity for considerable amplification of the actin framework upon cell activation. Further controls are exerted by profilin, which appears to sequester G-actin, whereas gelsolin binds to the end of actin preventing polymerization. Gelsolin has an additional inhibitory effect by cleaving binding sites between actin filaments, further restraining the formation of an insoluble actin web. These proteins in turn are controlled by second messengers generated during generalized neutrophil activation. For example, the affinity of profilin–actin is reduced by inositol phosphates. Gelsolin is under dual control: Ca^{2+} promotes its effect in cleaving actin filaments and blocking monomer addition, whereas inositol phosphates inhibit these effects. Once formed, the actin web can be induced to contract by myosin which is activated locally by the action of a Ca^{2+}-calmodulin-dependent myosin light-chain kinase. Although the control mechanisms are poorly understood, the mechanical responses critical for most neutrophil functions are centrally linked to early events in signal transduction. However, the nature of gel–sol changes and membrane conformational changes which need to be regulated locally in a very precise fashion for such complex events as phagocytosis and degranulation are poorly understood as yet.

The functional states of neutrophils in tissues

Until quite recently the neutrophil was thought of as an unsophisticated cell which migrated to the inflamed site where it killed bacteria and disgorged its enzyme contents before dying and disintegrating. However, it is now clear that granulocytes can exist in tissues in relatively quiescent states, that the presence of neutrophils within tissues is not synonymous with tissue injury, and that neutrophils themselves can secrete a number of important inflammatory cytokines including GM-CSF, IL-8, and IL-1. Furthermore, not all inflammatory mediators exert identical effects on neutrophil granulocytes; some important mediators, (e.g. the chemotaxins, C5a, LTB_4, and IL-8) are powerful secretagogues which stimulate neutrophils to release superoxide granule enzymes etc., whereas others (e.g. LPS, TNF, or PAF) are only moderately effective as secretagogues even at high concentration. However, these latter agents may have profound effects in 'priming' or modulating neutrophils to release enhanced quantities of potentially injurious agents upon subsequent stimulation with known secretagogues such as C5a. Priming agents appear to exert population effects whereby cells are recruited to form a pool which are then in an enhanced 'state of readiness'. The molecular mechanisms of priming are as yet poorly understood, but $[Ca^{2+}]_i$ is likely to play a central role. In order for us to understand the prolonged or excessive secretory states that may be associated with exacerbated tissue injury in relation to inflammatory diseases, it will be important to understand fully the underlying mechanisms of priming and activation, particularly since, during the priming process, a number of other important neutrophil functions are modulated. These include increased adhesiveness, reduced deformability, and reduced chemotaxis, the combination of which might be expected to lead to excessive and prolonged vascular sequestration of actively secreting neutrophils in direct contact with capillary endothelial cells.

Phagocytosis, degranulation, and the respiratory burst

Bacterial and other foreign particles are phagocytosed most effectively when coated with an opsonizing IgG or with opsonic components of

Fig. 3 Diagram showing a simplified version of the early intracellular events following ligation of the chemotaxin receptor. PLC, phospholipase C; PIP_2, phosphatidyl inositol (4,5)-bisphosphonate; IP_3, inositol triphosphate; DAG, 1,2-diacylglycerol; PKC, protein kinase C.

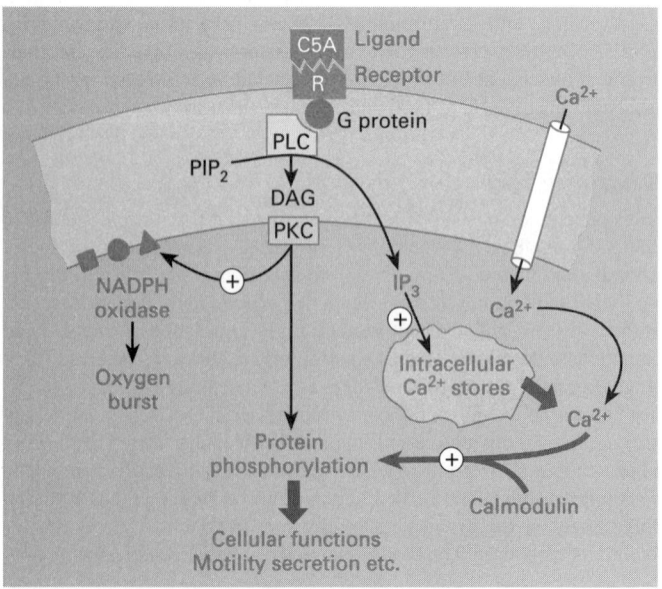

C3. Particles coated with IgG are recognized by the Fc receptors of the neutrophil, and particles coated with opsonic complement components such as C3b and C3bi are recognized by complement receptors type I (CR1) and type III (CR3) respectively. Engulfment of particles is accompanied by a movement of granules or lysosomes (Fig. 4 and see Table 3) to the site of phagosome formation, where they fuse with the phagosome forming a phagolysosome into which they discharge their enzymic contents. It appears that specific and azurophil granules may be under different control mechanisms, with specific granules being the first to accumulate and degranulate. Some external secretion of granule enzymes inevitably appears to occur as a consequence of this process, but it is uncertain how significant this is quantitatively and what its mechanisms and purposes are. However, since a large variety of neutrophil granule proteins are not only damaging to bacteria, but may also be histotoxic to surrounding host tissues, it is important to understand these mechanisms in terms of their control and their relevance for inflammatory disease processes. Mobilization and translocation of granules to the phagolysosome are likely to be effected by cytosolic or cytoskeletal contractile proteins and appear to be triggered by the rapid rise in $[Ca^{2+}]_i$ which occurs during neutrophil activation. A variety of reactive oxygen intermediates are also generated in response to phagocytosis. It is likely that all the associated events occur within the membrane of the phagosome with an electron transport chain generating a variety of highly toxic reactive oxygen intermediates including superoxide anion, hydrogen peroxide, hydroxyl radical, singlet oxygen, and hypohalous acids. While some of these agents may be highly toxic to bacteria, they may also exert important effects in the pathogenesis of inflammatory diseases (Table 3). The respiratory burst may also play an important role by acidifying the phagolysosome microenvironment, thus facilitating the action of some of the degradative acid hydrolyses from the azurophil granules which have a low optimal pH.

Monocyte emigration and maturation into inflammatory macrophages

Compared with resident macrophages, inflammatory macrophages are larger and contain more lysosomes and mitochondria. They have a greatly increased pinocytotic rate and increased phagocytic ability, in addition to a greater capacity to secrete enzymes and reactive oxygen

Fig. 4 Electron micrography of neutrophil granulocytes showing the multilobed nucleus and large numbers of intracytoplasmic granules. (magnification *c.* 11 000).

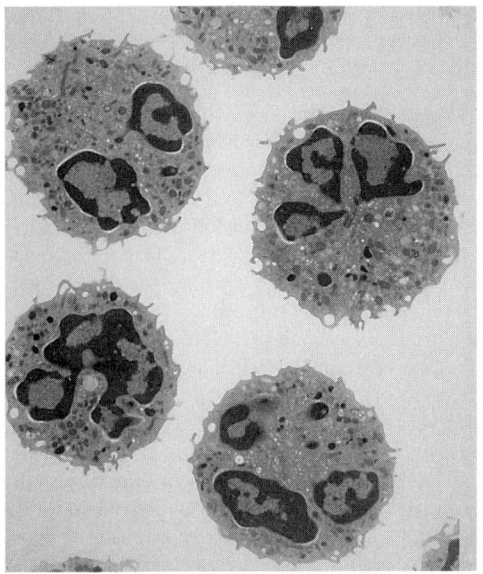

species. The inflammatory macrophage population is generally considered to be derived from monocytes which migrate to the inflamed site, and achieve their full potential by a combination of maturation and activation under the upregulating influences of local cytokines. Monocytes take several days to mature into macrophages *in vitro*, but *in vivo* it is likely that this process occurs over a 24 to 48 h period. Monocyte emigration is even less well understood than neutrophil emigration from blood vessels. It follows neutrophil emigration sequentially, and there is some evidence to suggest that monocyte emigration may actually depend upon prior neutrophil emigration. The temporal sequence of neutrophil emigration followed by monocytes may be explained by a combination of responsiveness to specific monocyte chemokines (e.g. MCP-1, MIP-1) and the monocyte's use of different components of the adhesive molecule repertoire (e.g. VLA_4/VCAM-1 versus IL-8, and leucocyte integrins/ICAM-1) that are utilized by the neutrophil. Monocyte maturation into macrophages with characteristics of inflammatory macrophages can be studied *in vitro*. A variety of changes occur, including loss of membrane cyclic nucleotides, increased pinocytosis, the expression of functional complement receptors, increased content of some lysosomal enzymes, and the potential for greatly increased release of reactive oxygen species and lysosomal enzymes. Of great relevance to the resolution of inflammation, monocyte-derived macrophages gain the capacity to recognize and ingest senescent neutrophils. They also gain the capacity to recognize a range of altered and damaged proteins and altered, damaged, and senescent cells including red blood cells.

Termination of acute inflammation

In his treatise on acute inflammation, Hurley considered that it may terminate by development of chronic inflammation, suppuration (abscess formation), scarring, or by resolution. It is reasonable to suggest that all the alternatives to resolution are 'non-ideal' and are likely to contribute to disease processes, particularly in organs like the lung whose function depends on the integrity of delicate gas exchange membranes. In fact, in most of the diseases of the lung considered in other chapters it is widely thought that persistent inflammation contributes to permanent architectural damage (e.g. emphysema) or the deposition of scar tissue (e.g. fibrosing alveolitis).

Resolution of lung inflammation

It is clear that circumstances must exist whereby even massive inflammatory cellular reactions in the lung can resolve completely. However, in contrast with the mechanisms of initiation and amplification, there has been comparatively little research into the processes responsible for the resolution of inflammation and many of the underlying processes are as yet poorly understood. For tissues to return to normal, all the events occurring during the evolution of inflammation must be reversed including removal of the inciting stimulus, dissipation of mediators generated, cessation of granulocyte emigration from blood vessels into tissues, return of normal microvascular permeability, limitation of granulocyte secretion of potentially histotoxic and proinflammatory agents, cessation of the emigration of monocytes from blood vessels and their maturation into inflammatory macrophages. Finally the removal of extravasated fluid, proteins, bacterial and cellular debris, neutrophils and macrophages must occur.

MEDIATOR DISSIPATION

For inflammation to cease, inflammatory mediators must be removed, inactivated, or otherwise rendered impotent. This can occur by spontaneous decay, for example thromboxane A_2 and endothelial-derived relaxing factor (nitric oxide) are evanescent factors which are spontaneously unstable. PAF and C5a are inhibited *in vitro* by inactivating enzymes, and reduction of mediator efficacy might also occur by reduc-

Table 3 *A short list of neutrophil contents and products*

Azurophil granules	Specific granules	Lipids	Oxidants and reductants
Lysozyme	Vitamin B_{12} binding protein	PAF	Hydrogen ion (H^+)
Peroxidase	C3bi receptor	Arachidonic acid	Superoxide anion (O_2)
Acid phosphatase	fMLP receptor	Thromboxane B_2	Hydroxyl radical (OH.)
Neuraminidase	Lactoferrin	Leukotriene B_4	Singlet oxygen ($^1O_2$)
β-Glucosaminidase	Cytochrome B	5-HETE†	Hydrogen peroxide (H_2O_2)
α-Fucosidase	Lysozyme		Hypochlorous acid (HOCl)
Esterase	Collagenase		
Cathepsin G			
Cathepsin D			
Elastase			
Histonase			
Defensins			
BPI*			
Glycosaminoglycans			
Chondroitin sulphate			
Heparin sulphate			

*Bacterial/permeability inducing protein.

†5-Hydroxyeicosatetraenoic acid.

tion in concentration due to dilution in inflammatory oedema fluid or by reduction in target-cell responsiveness as exemplified by the down-regulation of receptors which occurs during desensitization of neutrophils to a variety of inflammatory mediators. There may also be local generation of factors exerting negative influences (e.g. neutrophil immobilizing factor and adenosine) which would tend to counteract the effects of chemotactic peptides at the inflamed site. Thus a complex function such as neutrophil chemotaxis in response to peptides such as C5a would be influenced by a number of factors, including the concentration of mediators and their inhibitors or inactivators, possible desensitization mechanisms, and the effect of negative influences. At this point it is worth noting that the inflammatory response has a variety of redundant mechanisms, perhaps best exemplified by the plethora of mediators with similar effects. Thus it is important to consider how a variety of important mediators may act in concert at an inflamed site and to attempt to appreciate the integrated impact of negative and positive stimuli on the dynamic events of the inflammatory response *in situ*. Therefore the overall propensity for inflammation to persist would be expected to wane when the balance of mediator effects tips towards the inhibitory rather than the stimulatory. A final requirement for the success of most of the above mechanisms is that the production of mediators must cease.

CESSATION OF NEUTROPHIL AND MONOCYTE INFLUX

In human lobar pneumonia and its experimental models, neutrophil emigration ceases very early in the evolution of the pathological process. This early 'switch off' of cellular accumulation would obviously greatly limit further addition to the load of neutrophils in tissues and could represent an important early resolution mechanism. In contrast, in inflammatory models such as bleomycin injury which progresses to scarring, neutrophil influx may persist for many weeks. As with the accumulation of inflammatory cells, cessation of emigration must be considered at the chemotaxin level and at the adhesive molecule level, both being necessary for the specific accumulation of cells. There has been little study, as yet, of mechanisms responsible for loss of the chemotactic response, but chemotactic factor inhibitors may be generated locally and could inactivate neutrophil chemotactic factors. Desensitization of extravasated neutrophils may play a role, and negative feedback loops might operate whereby neutrophils that have already accumulated exert an influence that prevents more neutrophils emigrating from the blood stream. Alternatively, cessation of neutrophil emigration may simply result from dissipation or removal of chemotactic factors at the inflamed

site. The cell layers (both endothelial and epithelial) through which neutrophils can emigrate during the initiation could alter to form a 'barrier' preventing further neutrophil emigration. There has as yet been no detailed research on neutrophil or endothelial adhesion molecule expression *in situ* during the termination of inflammation, but it is clear that the inflamed site can respond to a second inflammatory stimulus by permitting a further wave of neutrophil emigration. Therefore any 'barrier' to cell adhesion or transmigration existing at the time of cessation of neutrophil emigration must be readily reversible, presumably by the further generation of inflammatory cytokines which would induce renewed expression/activation of endothelial adhesive molecules at the same time as activating neutrophil locomotion and inducing renewed expression/activation of neutrophil-surface-adhesive molecules. Thus it is reasonable to suggest that the identification of mechanisms controlling the local generation and dissipation of agents which promote chemotaxis and adhesive function of neutrophil and endothelial cells are central to our understanding of the processes of termination and persistence of inflammatory cell accumulation at inflamed sites. Much less is understood of the control of monocyte emigration, although similar principles are likely to be applicable in defining the factors involved in the cessation of their emigration.

RESTORATION OF NORMAL MICROVASCULAR PERMEABILITY AND ENDOTHELIAL/EPITHELIAL 'REPAIR'

Classical ultrastructural studies by Lord Florey and others have demonstrated that neutrophil emigration to inflamed sites is not necessarily associated with overt endothelial injury. Nevertheless, even in examples of acute 'beneficial' inflammation including lobar streptococcal pneumonia there is morphological evidence of endothelial and epithelial injury ranging from cytoplasmic vacuolation to areas of complete denudation resulting in marked fluid leakage into alveolar spaces. However, the cell sheets must retain their capacity for repair or renewal as pneumonia resolves. Although the underlying processes are poorly understood, repair is likely to occur by a combination of local cell proliferation to bridge gaps and the recovery of some cells from sublethal injury. Endothelial and monolayers deliberately 'wounded' *in vitro* have a remarkable capacity to re-form. Little is known of how endothelial cells recover from sublethal injury, but epithelial cells *in vitro* appear to recover from hydrogen-peroxide-induced injury by a mechanism which requires new protein synthesis. These cytoprotective mechanisms have received little study, but their definition may provide 'natural approaches' to boosting local defences against excessive inflammatory injury.

CONTROL OF INFLAMMATORY CELL SECRETION

In order to understand how tissue injury is normally limited at inflamed sites, the mechanisms controlling secretory behaviour of neutrophils, macrophages, and other inflammatory cells must be defined. Although much is known of how phagocyte secretion is stimulated *in vitro*, mechanisms whereby secretion is down-regulated or terminated *in vivo* have received little study. As with chemotaxis, inflammatory cell secretion *in situ* is likely to be modulated by the balance between stimulatory and inhibitory mediators. The simplest mechanism for termination—the cell having exhausted its secretory potential—is unlikely to be responsible since cells isolated from inflamed sites retain the capacity for further secretion on stimulation. Other factors which may contribute to down-regulation or termination of secretion are the exhaustion of internal energy supplies, receptor down-regulation, dissipation of stimuli, and finally death and removal of the cell itself. In a short-lived cell like the neutrophil granulocyte, which has a half-life in the blood of about 6 h, the death of the cell could itself represent an important mechanism in the final irreversible down-regulation of its secretory function (see below).

CLEARANCE PHASE OF INFLAMMATION

Once the inflammatory cells have completed their tasks in host defence and the inciting influences (e.g. bacteria) have been effectively destroyed), the site must be cleared of fluid, proteins, antibodies, and bacterial or cellular debris, and finally the key cellular players (neutrophils and inflammatory macrophages) must be removed before tissues return to normality.

Clearance of fluid, proteins, and debris

Lymphatic drainage and phagocytosis and pinocytosis by inflammatory macrophages are key processes in this phase. Most fluid is probably removed via the lymph vessels, although reconstitution of normal haemodynamics may contribute by restoring the balance of hydrostatic and osmotic forces in favour of net fluid absorption at the venous end of the capillary. Proteolytic enzymes from plasma exudate and inflammatory cell secretions are likely to break down any fibrin clot at the inflamed site, and products of this digestion are drained by lymphatics which become widely distended as the removal of fluids and proteins increases. The macrophage may also play an important role in this phase. It can remove fluids, which may contain a variety of proteins, by pinocytosis which in activated inflammatory macrophages can be amplified to the point at which the macrophage turns over 25 per cent of its cell surface per minute! Inflammatory macrophages have been shown to develop surface receptors for a wide range of altered and damaged proteins. The critical role of macrophages in the clearance phase of inflammation was first recognized by Metchnikoff more than a century ago, and we are now just beginning to elucidate the molecular mechanisms of some of his seminal observations.

Clearance of extravasated neutrophils

There is little evidence to suggest that extravasated neutrophils return to the bloodstream or that lymphatic drainage provides an important disposal route, and it is generally agreed that neutrophils meet their fate *in situ*. It had been widely assumed that neutrophils inevitably disintegrate before their fragments are removed by local macrophages. If this were the rule, healthy tissues would inevitably be exposed to large quantities of disgorged neutrophil contents. However, since Metchnikoff's observations more than a century ago, there has been evidence of an alternative injury-limiting fate whereby intact senescent neutrophils are removed by macrophages. Over the intervening decades there have been a number of sporadic reports which described intact neutrophils located

within macrophages, but the probable role of this process in the control of inflammation only became apparent recently. It is now clear that aging granulocytes (both neutrophils and eosinophils) have the capacity to undergo apoptosis, or programmed cell death.

Apoptosis was first described in situations where large numbers of unwanted cells are removed in a 'programmed' or physiological fashion. These include thymus involution, gut crypt cell turnover, and embryonic tissue remodelling. It can be recognized by characteristic ultrastructural features (Fig. 5(a)) and a pattern of DNA fragmentation indicative of internucleosomal cleavage. In contrast with cell necrosis, large numbers of cells can be removed by apoptosis without causing local tissue injury or inciting an inflammatory response. Neutrophil apoptosis leads to recognition of the intact senescent cell by macrophages which utilize a novel surface phagocytic receptor mechanism which is highly efficient in clearing the cells, but which fails to provoke a proinflammatory macrophage response. These observations suggest that apoptosis may indeed represent an injury-limiting alternative fate to necrosis which would tend to promote resolution rather than persistence of the inflammatory response. There is now clear evidence that this process occurs at acutely inflamed sites in human arthritides, neonatal lung injury, and resolving pneumonia (Fig. 5(b)). This is not to suggest that granulocyte necrosis fails to occur at acutely inflamed sites, but it is reasonable to speculate that the balance between the proportion of neutrophils disintegrating and those being removed by apoptosis may be an important factor in limiting the degree of local tissue injury and determining whether inflammation progresses or resolves.

Fig. 5 (a) An electron micrograph of a neutrophil showing the classical ultrastructural features of apoptosis, including chromatin condensation and prominence of the nucleolus in the nucleus, and marked dilatation of the endoplasmic reticulum. The cell membrane is intact and there are large numbers of apparently normal granules in the cytoplasm. (b) An apoptotic neutrophil which has been phagocytosed by a scavenging macrophage. This electron micrograph is of streptococcal pneumonia during the resolution phase.

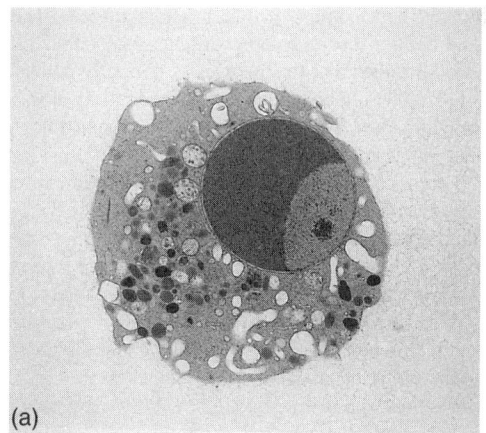
(a)

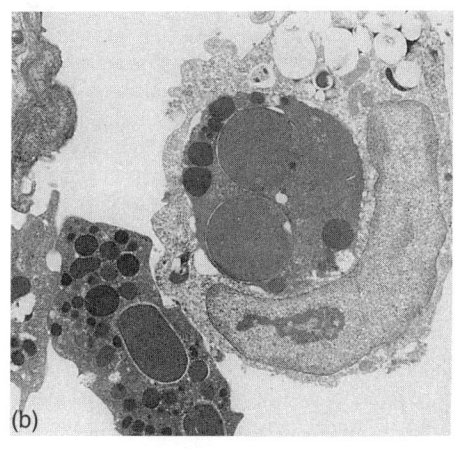
(b)

Clearance of inflammatory macrophages

The fate of the inflammatory macrophage during the resolution of inflammation remains a mystery, but there is some preliminary evidence to suggest that, unlike the granulocyte which meets its fate 'in situ', the inflammatory macrophage may emigrate from the inflamed site and subsequently be removed in draining lymph nodes by currently obscure processes.

A paradox—beneficial versus detrimental effects of inflammation

It is reasonable to speculate that in 'beneficial inflammation' potentially injurious events are tightly controlled so that inflammatory tissue injury is limited and inflammation ceases promptly. Therefore the following would be expected.

1. Neutrophil emigration is rapid and contact time between neutrophil and endothelial or epithelial cells is minimal, possibly with the neutrophils in a non-secretory state during this phase.
2. Essential matrix degradation necessary for cell emigration is localized and tightly controlled.
3. Neutrophil release of granule enzymes and reactive oxygen intermediates during phagocytosis, and digestion of bacteria, is minimal.
4. Neutrophil emigration ceases promptly and extravasated neutrophils (mostly intact apoptotic cells) are removed rapidly.
5. Local injury to epithelial and endothelial cells is minimal and is rapidly repaired.
6. Fibrosis would not be expected to be present except for the tiny amounts necessary for effective repair.

Although the mechanisms controlling many of these events are poorly understood, it is likely that any loss of their efficiency could tip the balance towards excessive tissue injury and development of chronic inflammation and scarring, key features of inflammatory disease. The fact that endothelial and epithelial injury do occur, even in 'beneficial' self-limited inflammation, implies that this balance is normally precarious, and that endothelial and epithelial cells may be particularly at risk in poorly controlled inflammation, a concept supported by the histological appearance of many inflammatory and allergic diseases.

The mechanisms whereby neutrophils may cause excessive injury to host cells are coming under more rigorous scrutiny. Firstly, it is likely that both priming and activation are required for the cell to achieve its maximum injurious potential. Secondly, very close apposition between the neutrophil and the target cell is necessary for injury. This may be mediated by surface-adhesive molecules, but in vascular beds like the lung capillary factors reducing neutrophil deformability could also promote cell–cell contact. Intercellular adhesion is a dynamic event *in vivo*, and the kinetics as well as the degree of intercellular adhesion are likely to be important since prolongation of cell–cell contact would obviously increase the potential for injury. Close and prolonged contact (between actively secreting neutrophils and endothelial cells (for example) is thought to favour injury by more than one mechanism. Firstly, the intercellular microenvironment creates an exclusive domain in which the local concentrations of histotoxic agents would reach very high levels, and inhibitors and scavengers, particularly those of high molecular weight, would tend to be excluded. Secondly, the highly reactive nature of oxygen intermediates inevitably limits their range of activity in tissues. Therefore this may be enhanced in circumscribed areas of cell–cell contact. Furthermore, potentially injurious neutrophil enzymes may be present in very high local concentrations on the neutrophil surface which makes contact with the endothelial cell.

A difficult problem at present is to identify which of the plethora of potentially injurious inflammatory cell products (Table 3) are centrally involved in mediating tissue injury in disease processes. Many of these, even if secreted in small amounts, may prove highly toxic if presented on the surface of adherent neutrophils. In the last decade much attention has been centred on a primary role for reactive oxygen intermediates. However, the most toxic intermediates are so ephemeral and reactive that they are likely to be rapidly inactivated, and it has been suggested more recently that reactive oxygen intermediates could exert a more important indirect role by damaging antiproteinases, some of which are very prone to being rendered ineffective by low concentrations of oxidants. Neutrophil elastase is now widely believed to play a prominent role in neutrophil-mediated tissue injury. It is capable of digesting a variety of proteins in addition to elastin and is a highly cationic molecule. It is certainly toxic to cells *in vitro*, but whether its toxic effects are mediated by its enzymic activity or by other properties remains unclear.

Lung inflammation and scarring

While the inflammatory response in streptococcal pneumonia characteristically resolves completely without scarring, other types of pneumonia (e.g. Klebsiella and staphylococcal pneumonias) are often associated with persistent inflammation, tissue destruction, and massive scarring responses. In most examples of inflammatory lung disease (even asthma) there is evidence that persistent accumulation of inflammatory cells is associated with tissue scarring responses.

A causal link between inflammation and the scarring response has been suspected for many years. In many inflammatory diseases (e.g. fibrosing alveolitis and rheumatoid arthritis) an acute inflammatory phase appears to precede chronic inflammation and scarring. While this is likely to be generally true, scarring may occur very early in adult respiratory distress syndrome, and even in 'endstage' fibrosing alveolitis there is often clear evidence of continued emigration of acute inflammatory cells, including neutrophils, as well as monocytes and lymphocytes which characterize chronic inflammation. Lung injury by cytotoxic agents such as bleomycin (see p.), which in humans can cause a chronic inflammatory scarring lung disease indistinguishable from chronic fibrosing alveolitis, is a useful paradigm since in experimental animal models it causes phases of acute inflammation and chronic inflammation which merge with the development of lung scarring, and provides an opportunity to study underlying *in situ* mechanisms in more detail.

Whether or not there has been a critical level of epithelial injury in the primary inflammatory damage to the lung seems to be a key factor determining whether excessive scarring occurs. Most pathologists now believe that the lung can tolerate a certain degree and extent of injury to type I epithelial cells without the necessity for excessive scarring. It is thought that gaps in the epithelium are repaired by the division of type II epithelial pneumocytes to form a new monolayer of type I cells. However, if there is extensive disruption of the epithelium, and particularly if the basement membrane is severely damaged and loses its architectural integrity, a scarring response appears more likely to result. The inflammatory response can impinge at two levels on the scarring process (Fig. 6(a)): first, on the degree of epithelial injury caused by the inflammatory process, and second, through inflammatory cell products which can induce fibroblasts to proliferate and deposit scar tissue matrix proteins.

Granulation tissue (the precursor of scar tissue) is a very cellular and dynamic tissue, particularly in the lung. It contains proliferating fibroblasts which lay down scar tissue matrix proteins such as collagen. Collagen production by fibroblasts is normally a highly regulated process with controls being exerted at several levels (Fig. 6(b)). All but 30 per cent of the extracellularly secreted collagen is normally degraded, mainly by the effect of fibroblast-derived collagenase. The effect of collagenase is under a further internal control mechanism whereby it is kept in check by enzyme inhibitors, e.g. tissue inhibitor of metalloproteinases (TIMP). Fibroblast activity is also under the control of external factors including cytokines and growth factors, many of which can be secreted in large quantities by local cells, particularly inflammatory macrophages. Most of these factors including PDGF, TGFβ, FGF, and IGF have been shown to exert permissive or stimulatory effects on fibroblast growth and secretion. External factors exerting negative influences must also exist. Although these have received less attention, PGE$_2$ represents a good example of a factor with mainly inhibitory effects on fibroblast function.

The fibroblast is now recognized as a complex and multipotent cell which is not only important in the control of tissue architecture and matrix assembly but is also capable of generating a number of important cytokines, including IL-8, IL-1, and TNF-α, which are likely to play important roles in the initiation of inflammation. Furthermore, it now appears that subpopulations of fibroblasts exist with different phenotypic features, some of which appear to be important in lung diseases associated with persistent inflammation and scarring.

New opportunities for anti-inflammatory therapy—and possible pitfalls

Non-specific anti-inflammatory agents including corticosteroids have been useful in many inflammatory diseases, but in some, such as fibrosing alveolitis, results are disappointing or associated with serious adverse effects from chronic use of the medications themselves. With the recent explosion of knowledge of the cellular and molecular mechanisms of inflammation it is likely that novel and specific therapeutic strategies will be developed. These might include the following:

(1) agents which specifically inhibit the mediators which initiate inflammation;
(2) agents directed against specific cell–cell adhesion molecules;
(3) inhibitors of certain secretion mechanisms;
(4) agents directed against injurious products such as neutrophil elastase or reactive oxygen intermediates.

Nevertheless, these exciting possibilities should not distract us from the knowledge that any really effective anti-inflammatory therapeutic strategy will have to take on board the problems associated with the paradox of inflammation, i.e. the mechanisms that appear to be involved in tissue injury and in inflammatory diseases are legion and many may be identical with those used in host defence. This raises at least two immediate problems.

First, the efficacy of the inflammatory response in host defence lies,

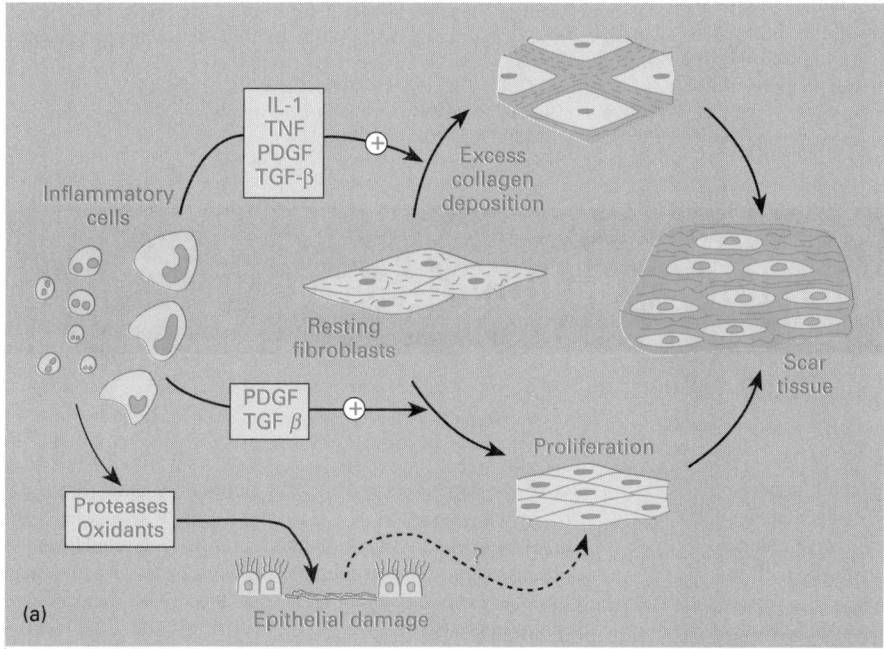

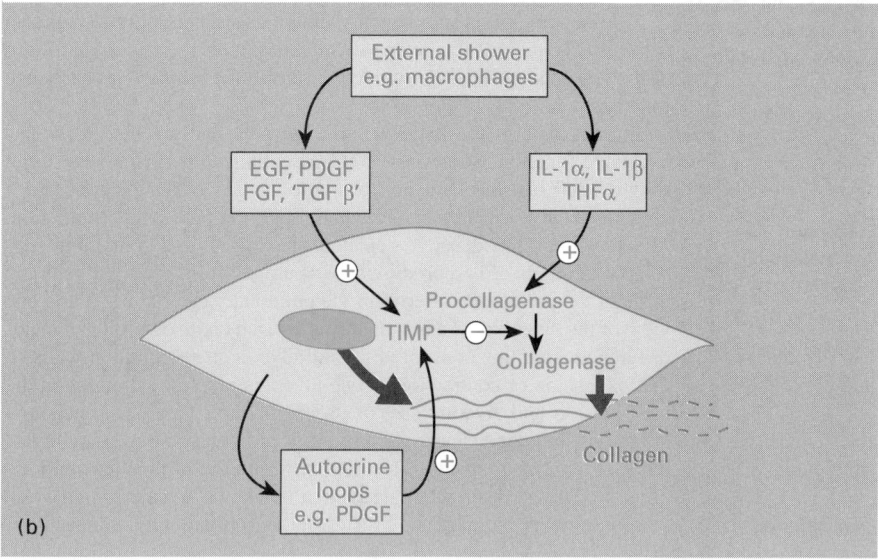

Fig. 6 (a) A diagram showing possible relationships between inflammation and scarring. Products of inflammatory cells, particularly macrophages, may release agents which promote both proliferation and secretion of scar tissue matrix proteins by fibroblasts. (b) A diagram showing some of the levels at which fibroblast secretion and reabsorption of collagen may be controlled, and the influence of some inflammatory mediators.

at least in part, in the redundancy of many of its mechanisms. Thus the inhibition of a single mediator, or possibly of a single cell type, is not likely to render the whole response ineffective. For example, several members of the PF-4 family of cytokines (e.g. IL-8, ENA-78) may initiate neutrophil emigration, but components of other important inflammatory cascades (e.g. C5a and leukotriene B$_4$) as well as the bacterial products themselves are also chemotactic for neutrophils. The spider's web provides a useful analogy, since unless the 'key strand' can be identified, the removal or loss of other less important strands is not likely to attenuate the overall effectiveness of the response. This redundancy is obviously of great advantage in providing an effective host defence, but when the principle is turned against the host in inflammatory disease the development of rational therapeutic strategies becomes a formidable task. However, it may be possible to identify key groups of mediators which could be rendered ineffective with limited 'cocktails'.

The second problem is that effective anti-inflammatory strategies are likely to weaken host defences critically, particularly against bacterial infection. While it may be possible to identify mainly detrimental mechanisms, the more we learn about inflammatory diseases the clearer it becomes that many of the cellular and molecular mechanisms are identical with those employed in host defence. Therefore, it is likely that powerful new mechanism-based anti-inflammatory strategies will require to be applied during 'windows of opportunity' when the inflammatory mechanisms are more critical to the evolution of the disease process than they are to the general defence of the host, while at the same time it will be necessary to employ other strategies to prevent infective complications during the therapeutic periods.

Alternatively, it may be possible to promote mechanisms which favour resolution of inflammation rather than progression, or to boost local defence mechanisms by, for example, promoting local genetic expression of antiproteinases, antioxidants, or other agents responsible for anti-inflammatory cytoprotection.

REFERENCES

Baggiolini, M., Dewald, B., and Walz, A. (1992). Interleukin 8 and related chemotactic cytokines. In: *Inflammation: basic principles and clinical correlates* (2nd edn) (ed J.I. Gallin, I. Goldstein, and R. Snyderman). Raven Press, New York.

Bauman, H. and Gauldie, J. (1994). The acute phase response. *Immunology Today*, **15**, 74–81.

Bevilacqua, M.P. (1993). Endothelial–leukocyte adhesive molecules. *Annual Reviews of Immunology*, 767–805.

Downey, G.P. (1994). Mechanisms of leukocyte motility and chemotaxis. *Current Opinions in Immunology*, **6**, 113–25.

Haslett, C. (1993). Neutrophils. In: *Allergy illustrated* (ed S.T. Holgate and M.K. Church). Gower, London.

Haslett, C. (1992). Resolution of acute inflammation and the role of apoptosis in the tissue fate of granulocytes. *Clinical Science*, **83**, 639–48.

Henson, P.M., Henson, J.E., Fittschen, C., Bratton, D.L., and Riches, D.W.H. (1992). Degranulation and secretion by phagocytic cells. In: *Inflammation: basic principles and clinical correlates* (2nd edn) (ed J.I. Gallin, I. Goldstein, and R. Snyderman). Raven Press, New York.

Postlethwaite, A.E. and Kang, A.H. (1992). Fibroblasts and matrix proteins. In: *Inflammation: basic principles and clinical correlates* (2nd edn) (ed J.I. Gallin, I. Goldstein, and R. Snyderman). Raven Press, New York.

Weiss, S.J. (1989). Tissue destruction by neutrophils. *New England Journal of Medicine*, **320**, 365–76.

17.4 Pathophysiology of lung disease

P. D. WAGNER

The term pathophysiology implies the relationship between lung structure and lung function, particularly in disease. If one can understand how the structural changes in disease lead to subsequent functional derangement, rational management of disease can be enhanced. However, before embarking on a survey of the pathophysiology of a variety of disease groups, one must set the stage by briefly reviewing the key structure–function relationships of the normal lung. For excellent and fundamental textbooks the reader is referred to *Pulmonary pathophysiology–the essentials* and *Respiratory physiology—the essentials* by J. B. West.

Structure and function in the normal lung

The primary function of the lungs is to exchange those amounts of oxygen (and carbon dioxide) used (and produced) by the metabolizing tissues of the body. Additional 'housekeeping' non-exchange functions of the lung are required to maintain its integrity.

1. Surfactant synthesis and release to maintain low alveolar surface tension. This reduces alveolar collapse and also opposes the development of pulmonary oedema.
2. Particulate and immune defence at the alveolar and airway levels to prevent and react to inflammatory pathological reactions and infections.
3. Fluid clearance (of the water and protein that normally moves out of the capillaries and into the pulmonary interstitium) to prevent lung oedema.
4. Airway and blood vascular smooth muscle tone regulation, of dubious origins but considerable significance to lung function.
5. Pulmonary capillary endothelial regulation of some hormones such as angiotensin.

At least some of these secondary functions are necessary to make up for normally present (or potential) weaknesses in the structural design of the lung that would otherwise compromise the primary gas exchange function.

The structure of the lungs is well, but not ideally, suited to its gas exchange function. Some 300×10^6 essentially spherical alveoli, each roughly 300 μm in diameter, constitute the gas exchange zone. Each alveolus receives fresh inspired gas through the process of ventilation. Mixed venous blood partly depleted of oxygen (and containing substantial amounts of carbon dioxide) is pumped from the right ventricle through the pulmonary arteries to the pulmonary capillaries. While one view of the alveoli is as a bunch of grapes each on its own stalk, a major difference from this concept is that all alveoli share common walls so that expansion or contraction of one alveolus has a direct effect on the wall tension and alveolar size of its neighbours. This phenomenon is known as interdependence and primarily promotes volume stability of the vast number of alveoli. This, together with the surface-tension-lowering properties of surfactant, leads to efficiency of exchange that could otherwise never be imagined in a cluster of so many tiny air spaces.

Ventilation—the dead space

It is well known that, for inspired air to reach and inflate an alveolus, its molecules must first flow from the mouth through some 17 branched generations of airways (before traversing up to six more generations of alveolated airways) that are constructed purely as conducting plumbing without significant oxygen–carbon dioxide exchange ability (Fig. 1). After giving up to the blood part of its oxygen and receiving an approximately similar volume of carbon dioxide from the blood, the alveolus deflates to some extent and the gas must return in the reverse direction through the very same airways to reach the mouth again. These 17 conducting airway generations collectively form the dead space of the lung and immediately create (potential) problems for gas exchange. Thus the volume of air to be inhaled must be increased by an amount equal to the volume of the dead space of every breath to provide effective ventilation. This is a trivial concern in the normal lung but a major concern in some lung diseases, particularly those causing airways obstruction (see below). The volume of the 17-generation dead space approximates 1 ml per pound of body weight. Impedance to air flow, which is normally inconsequential, may be greatly increased to the point of causing respiratory muscle fatigue in obstructive airways diseases (often due to chronic inflammatory changes in those airways). A major problem is encountered by physiologists and physicians attempting to understand the relationships between gas exchange and airway function because it is generally considered that the proximal conducting airways dominate gas flow impedance, while the peripheral conducting and subsequent gas exchange segments control distribution of gas among gas exchange units and thus play a role in gas exchange.

Ventilation—gas flow

Transport mechanisms responsible for moving gas between the mouth and the alveoli are exceedingly complex and consist of a linked series of convective (or bulk flow) processes and diffusive gas mixing steps that occur together in varied relative importance at all generations of airways from the mouth to the alveoli. Detailing these components is beyond the scope of this chapter (see Chapter 17.2.1). Despite the theoretical potential for major disruption of inspired gas distribution on the basis of the airway structures referred to above and the complexity of gas flow regimes, it remains remarkable that in normal subjects overall distribution of inspired gas is relatively uniform, as implied by gas exchange that is trivially less than perfect.

How much gas an alveolus receives depends not only on the resistance of conducting airways interposed between it and the mouth, but also on its intrinsic elastic properties. It is well known that, in a healthy subject, the volume of an alveolus can increase about fivefold from minimal to maximal lung volume due to elasticity, much like a toy balloon. Pathological changes in the alveolar wall such as fibrous connective tissue deposition, cellular inflammation, and oedema fluid accumulation reduce the distensibility (i.e. compliance) of the alveolus; changes such as collagen/elastin dissolution by proteolytic enzymes increase compliance. Compliance is also low at both low and high levels of lung expansion. Thus changes in regional resistance and/or compliance are common in disease and have much potential for disrupting the distribution of ventilation and hence interfering with oxygen and carbon dioxide exchange. Such changes also have the potential for inducing respiratory muscle fatigue because of the associated increase in the work of breathing.

Diffusion

Gases move between the alveolar gas space and the intracapillary red cell (Fig. 2) by passive diffusion along a partial pressure gradient. The diffusion pathway is generally very short; in fact, the blood–gas barrier (Fig. 2) is of the order of 0.5 μm thick. This barrier, which separates blood and gas, must be thin enough to permit adequate rates of gas diffusion (gas flux by diffusion is inversely proportional to barrier thickness) but strong enough to withstand transmural pressures of 30 mmHg or more (which develop during exercise) without mechanical disruption that would cause alveolar flooding by red cells and plasma. The barrier contains a thin surfactant layer (dissolved and thus not seen in Fig. 2 because of the method of processing the tissue) and then the alveolar epithelium, the interstitium, and the capillary endothelium as marked in the figure. Finally, there is the plasma space and intracapillary red cell containing the haemoglobin molecule, the ultimate destination of oxygen taken up from the lungs. It is also remarkable that this composite barrier poses essentially no problem to gas diffusion, but this is the case in resting normal man. It has been calculated that diffusive movement of oxygen is complete within about 0.25 s (at rest), whereas the average red cell spends 0.75 s in the capillary—a considerable margin of safety.

There is even more of a safety net than this, however, owing to the shape of the oxygen–haemoglobin dissociation curve (Fig. 3). Because the normal balance between oxygen uptake and ventilation sets alveolar (and hence arterial) blood P_{O_2} at about 13.3 kPa (100 mmHg), it can be seen from Fig. 3 that even if there were a substantial reduction in blood P_{O_2} to 9–10 kPa, for example, the concentration of oxygen in arterial blood would be barely reduced (by only 5 per cent in this example). Thus arterial oxygen saturation of haemoglobin, which is normally 98 per cent, would fall to about 93 per cent (of available oxygen binding sites), a level that is generally inconsequential to cellular metabolism and clinically unnoticeable.

Fig. 1 Plastic cast of the human tracheobronchial tree. The trachea divides into the two main-stem bronchi, which continue subdividing for another 15 generations of conducting airways. Thereafter the respiratory or gas exchange region of small airways and alveoli continues for another six orders of branching. Because of their small size, these branches have been lost during preparation of the cast so that only the conducting airways are shown. (Reproduced with permission from West 1990.)

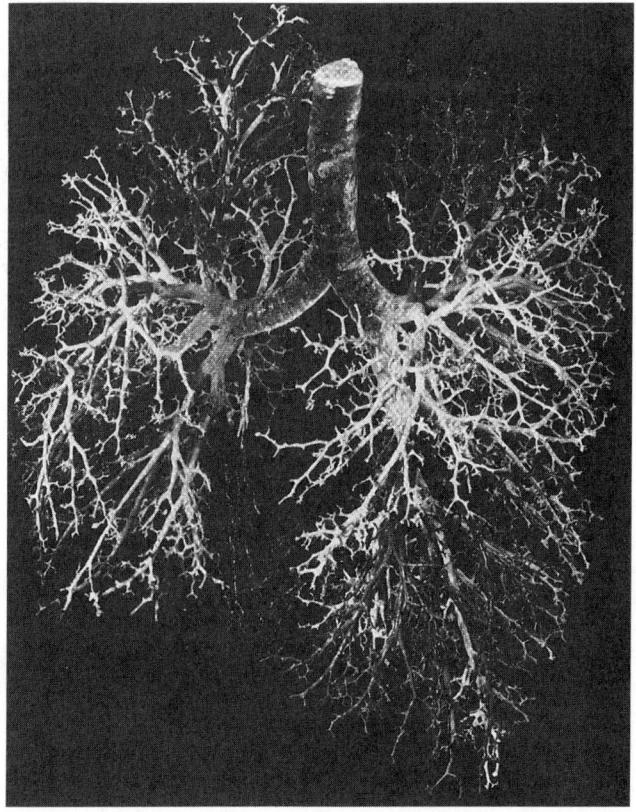

Perfusion and oxygen transport in blood

Oxygen is transported by convection from the pulmonary capillaries in flowing blood. Normally, more than 98 per cent of the oxygen in arterial blood is haemoglobin bound, leaving less than 2 per cent physically dissolved in the blood. Even breathing 100 per cent oxygen, with a normal arterial PO_2 of more than 80 kPa, about 90 per cent of the oxygen per cent in arterial blood is haemoglobin bound and only about 10 per cent is carried as dissolved oxygen. The concentration ($[O_2]$) of oxygen in blood can be expressed as the sum of that bound to haemoglobin ($[Hb]$) and that physically dissolved:

$$[O_2] = 1.39[Hb] \times SO_2 + 0.003PO_2 \qquad (1)$$

where SO_2 is the fractional oxygen saturation of haemoglobin binding sites and PO_2 is blood partial pressure. The constant 1.39 is the number of millilitres of oxygen that can be carried per gram of haemoglobin at standard temperature and pressure and 0.003 is the solubility coefficient of oxygen in blood, expressed as $ml/dl^1/mmHg^{-1}$. When $[Hb]$ is in g/dl and PO_2 mmHg, $[O_2]$ is in ml/dl.

The concept of oxygen transport by blood flow ($\dot{Q}O_2$) from the lungs to the body tissues is of increasing importance, particularly in intensive care. Globally, this is simply the product of cardiac output $\dot{Q}_T$ and arterial $[O_2]$. Thus

$$\dot{Q}O_2 = \dot{Q}_T \times [O_2] \text{ arterial} \qquad (2)$$

This equation is also applicable to any individual organ (or smaller tissue unit), in which case $\dot{Q}_T$ is replaced by the corresponding value for organ (or tissue unit) perfusion rate. Of course, arterial $[O_2]$ is uniform throughout the normal vascular system.

It is convenient and generally acceptable to disregard the amount of dissolved oxygen when using equation (2) clinically. Under such conditions, for the entire body

$$\dot{Q}O_2 = 1.39[Hb] \times SaO_2 \times \dot{Q}_T \qquad (3)$$

where SaO_2 is the saturation of arterial blood with haemoglobin-bound oxygen.

The special attraction of this form of the equation is that it quantifies the convective oxygen flux via the vascular system to the body tissues as the product of three variables that reflect (1) the oxygen transport capacity of the blood (1.39 $[Hb]$), (2) the pulmonary gas exchange function (SaO_2), and (3) the cardiovascular function ($\dot{Q}_T$). Clearly, many permutations of these three variables could combine to produce similar levels of oxygen transport. The clinical relevance of such computations of total oxygen transport is presently under investigation. In intensive care, patients with adult respiratory distress syndrome often demonstrate a linear dependence of metabolic rate $\dot{V}O_2$ on oxygen transport which, when eventually understood, may have major therapeutic implications (this remains quite unclear at present).

While the above discussion focuses on the importance of total pulmonary blood flow (or cardiac output) on systemic oxygen transport, the well-known observation that the intrapulmonary distribution of blood flow is non-uniform even in health is of major importance. This may become even more important in diseases of the lungs, with serious consequences for arterial oxygenation. The reasons for, and consequences of, such non-uniformity are discussed below in the context of each disease.

Causes of hypoxaemia

There are four classical primary causes of hypoxaemia. One is incomplete equilibration, by diffusion, of oxygen between alveolar gas and pulmonary end-capillary blood. Such diffusion limitation does not occur in normal man at rest. It is seen during maximal exercise in many normal

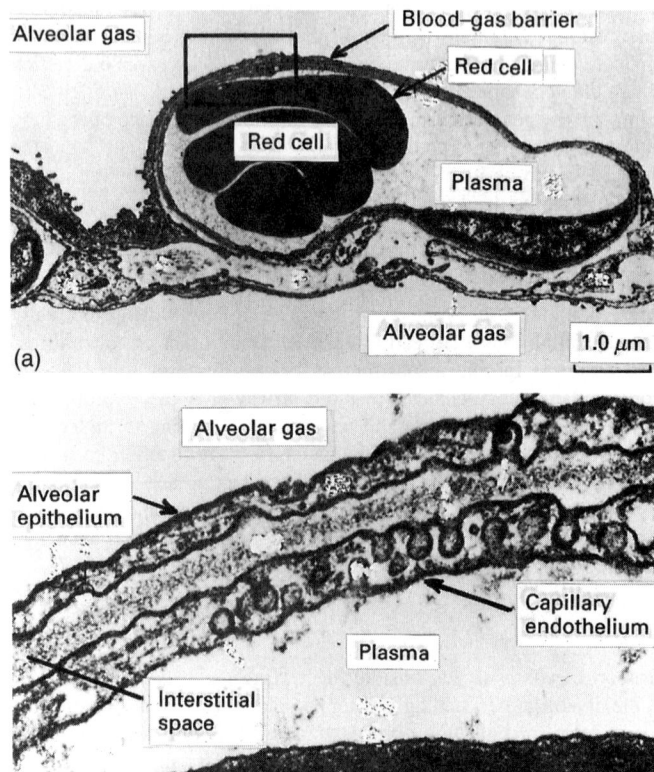

Fig. 2 (a) Low power electron micrograph of the normal alveolar wall; (b) higher-power micrograph of enclosed area of (a). Structures and scales are indicated on the figures. In this preparation the thin layer of alveolar surfactant normally present on the surface of the alveolar epithelium is not seen for technical reasons. The distance from the alveolar epithelial surface to the red blood cell surface is very short, and the combination of alveolar epithelium, interstitial space, and capillary endothelium is well under 0.5 μm. (Reproduced with permission from Weibel (1984).)

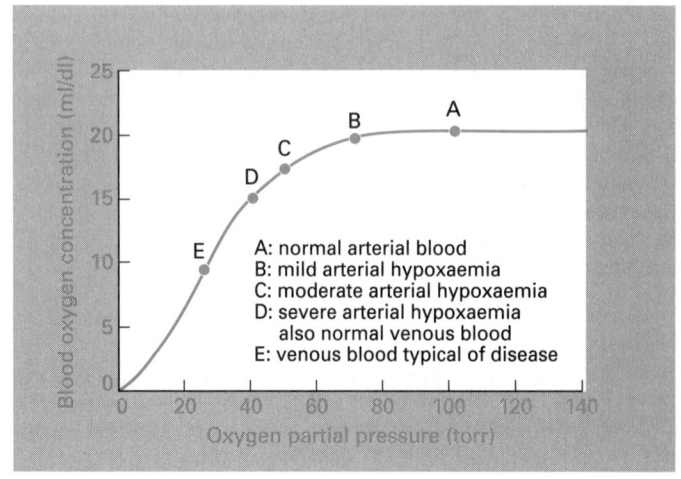

Fig. 3 A standard equilibrium binding curve between haemoglobin and oxygen, showing the oxygen concentration of normal whole blood as a function of oxygen partial pressure.

subjects and is universally present in normal subjects exercising at altitude. It has been shown that diffusion limitation rarely occurs in human lung diseases (even if the measured diffusing capacity D_{LCO} for carbon monoxide is reduced). The exception is in diffuse interstitial fibrosis where D_{LCO} is so greatly impaired that diffusion limitation does occur, particularly on exercise.

The second cause of hypoxaemia is reduced ventilation. The following equation shows the simple mass conservation equation that relates the volumes of oxygen inhaled and exhaled per minute and the difference between them, which must reflect that amount of oxygen transferred by the lungs from the air to the arterial blood:

$$\dot{V}_{O_2} = \dot{V}_I \times F_{IO_2} - \dot{V}_A \times F_{AO_2} \tag{4}$$

In this equation, $\dot{V}_{O_2}$ is minute oxygen uptake (i.e. the metabolic rate set by the tissues), $\dot{V}_I$ and $\dot{V}_A$ are respectively the inhaled and exhaled volumes of gas per minute, and F_{IO_2} and F_{AO_2} are respectively the fractional concentrations of oxygen in the inspired gas and in the exhaled alveolar gas. The same considerations, using corresponding terminology and neglecting the inconsequential concentration of carbon dioxide in air, lead to the following equation for carbon dioxide:

$$\dot{V}_{CO_2} = \dot{V}_A \times F_{ACO_2} \tag{5}$$

From equations (4) and (5) and the further reasonable assumption that inspired and expired minute volumes are virtually the same, it becomes very clear that hypoventilation (a drop in $\dot{V}_I$ and thus $\dot{V}_A$) at fixed metabolic rate will cause F_{ACO_2} to rise and F_{AO_2} to fall. Arterial P_{CO_2} and P_{O_2} will follow these alveolar concentrations closely. Hence hypoventilation from any cause produces hypoxaemia (reduced P_{aO_2}) but must also cause hypercapnia (increased P_{aCO_2}). Manipulation of equations (4) and (5) (with the greatly simplifying assumption that $\dot{V}_I = \dot{V}_A$ in equation (4)) allows expression of F_{AO_2} in terms of the other variables, and subsequent multiplication by total dry gas pressure converts these fractional concentrations to more familiar partial pressure terms:

$$P_{AO_2} = P_{IO_2} - P_{ACO_2}/R \tag{6}$$

where $R = \dot{V}_{CO_2}/\dot{V}_{O_2}$ is the respiratory exchange ratio. Equation (6) is a good approximation to a much more complicated equation that can be derived if one wishes to be more rigorous and not make the assumption that $\dot{V}_I = \dot{V}_A$. For clinical purposes, equation (6) is quite satisfactory and is used to predict a hypothetical mean alveolar P_{O_2} from the other three variables. In practice, a further assumption is made that P_{ACO_2} (alveolar) = P_{aCO_2} (arterial); this is often but not always reasonable, particularly in diseased lungs. With this assumption and the measurement of arterial P_{O_2} and P_{CO_2}, equation (6) is used to compute the difference (A − a)P_{O_2} between alveolar and arterial P_{O_2}:*

$$(A - a)P_{O_2} = P_{AO_2} - P_{aO_2} = P_{IO_2} - P_{ACO_2}/R - P_{aO_2} \tag{7}$$

Because the assumptions $P_{ACO_2} = P_{aCO_2}$ and $P_{AO_2} = P_{aO_2}$ are reasonable in normal lungs, simple hypoventilation, while causing often severe hypoxaemia and hypercapnia, does not cause an increase in (A − a)P_{O_2}. Furthermore, even in severe hypoventilation, the hypoxaemia is easily rectified (without restoring ventilation) simply by administering an elevated concentration F_{IO_2} of inspired oxygen. Since 1 per cent of an atmosphere is about 7 mmHg, each 1 per cent increase in F_{IO_2} will raise arterial P_{O_2} by about 7 mmHg if the only cause of hypoxaemia is hypoventilation.

*There is no universal agreement about the symbol for the difference between the alveolar (A) and the arterial (a) oxygen tensions. In line with the nomenclature P_{aO_2} and P_{aO_2}, it should probably be $P(A-a)O_2$. This is seldom used. The editors have opted for (A-a)P_{O_2} for clarity. Many still use (A-a)D_{O_2}, but D (for difference) suffers from not signifying in a unit. Expressions which have used A-a without brackets are mathematically incorrect and should not be used.

The third cause of hypoxaemia is a shunt, which is the passage of blood from the systemic venous to the systemic arterial side of the circulation without ever encountering alveolar gas and thus absorbing oxygen or releasing carbon dioxide. Shunt can occur between cardiac chambers (in many combinations) or as a result of perfusion of lung regions that are completely unventilated. Such lack of ventilation will occur in lung regions that are collapsed, in alveoli that are non-compliant from pathological changes, and in alveoli that are filled with oedema fluid or cellular debris (pneumonitides of many types). Owing to the absence of ventilation in such units, blood flowing through them joins the systemic arterial blood while still at venous oxygen concentrations, causing venous admixture and reducing P_{aO_2}. In general, arterial P_{CO_2} is unaffected by shunt until it reaches very high values (around 50 per cent of the cardiac output). Consequently, alveolar P_{O_2} calculated from equation (6) is usually near normal. Correspondingly, (A − a)P_{O_2} is often markedly increased. Furthermore, the hypoxaemia is often refractory to added inspired oxygen, again because of the complete failure of contact between inspired gas and blood in the affected regions.

The fourth cause of hypoxaemia is inequality between ventilation $\dot{V}_A$ and perfusion $\dot{Q}$. This means that the ratio of alveolar ventilation to blood flow in small regions of the lung is not the same everywhere. Such variance in the local $\dot{V}_A\dot{Q}$ ratio occurs in health, but its effects on gas exchange are trivial. In diseases of the lung it becomes a major cause of impaired gas exchange. It is not difficult to understand why heterogeneity of local $\dot{V}_A\dot{Q}$ ratios causes hypoxaemia. First, in any small region of the lung, steady state mass balance considerations show that local alveolar P_{O_2} is dictated by the local $\dot{V}_A\dot{Q}$ ratio (for any given values of inspired and venous P_{O_2}). A lung without heterogeneity, operating at a normal overall $\dot{V}_A\dot{Q}$ ratio of about unity, produces alveolar (and arterial) P_{O_2} values of about 100 mmHg. A lung with $\dot{V}_A\dot{Q}$ heterogeneity, which has some regions whose $\dot{V}_A\dot{Q}$ ratios are greater than unity and some whose $\dot{V}_A\dot{Q}$ ratios are less than unity (due to increases or decreases in local $\dot{V}_A$ or local $\dot{Q}$), produces a corresponding array of local P_{O_2} values: less than 100 when $\dot{V}_A\dot{Q} < 1$ and greater than 100 when $\dot{V}_A\dot{Q} > 1$. When one then considers that areas of low $\dot{V}_A\dot{Q}$, which are necessarily hypoxic, must by definition be relatively overperfused in relation to ventilation, the final mixed arterial blood is more heavily weighted by blood from these hypoxic regions than by the relatively lower contribution from areas of high $\dot{V}_A\dot{Q}$ ratio (with relatively lower perfusion). The result is hypoxaemia, no matter what the cause of the $\dot{V}_A\dot{Q}$ inequality in pathological terms, and an increase in (A − a)P_{O_2}. However, because by definition all alveoli are ventilated at least to some extent, breathing 100 per cent oxygen will fully correct the hypoxaemia. This is a theoretically and clinically important difference from the gas exchange consequences of a shunt discussed above.

While the above constitute the four primary causes of hypoxaemia, it is of major importance to understand the modulating role played by cardiac output in the determination of P_{aO_2} in patients with hypoxaemia due to shunt, $\dot{V}_A\dot{Q}$ inequality, or diffusion limitation. Specifically, when cardiac output is reduced, oxygen extraction generally increases to compensate in order to preserve tissue metabolic rate $\dot{V}_{O_2}$. Consequently, venous P_{O_2} falls. This in turn reduces the alveolar and end-capillary P_{O_2} in all lung units, particularly when the local $\dot{V}_A\dot{Q}$ ratio is low or zero, and this consequently aggravates the hypoxaemia, sometimes substantially as in heart failure. The converse is equally important clinically. When cardiac output is elevated, oxygen extraction may fall; venous P_{O_2} then increases and this serves to improve arterial P_{O_2} (unless at the same time there has been some offsetting consequence of the higher cardiac output such as disproportionate redistribution of blood flow to lung regions which already have a low $\dot{V}_A\dot{Q}$ ratio). Asthma is a good clinical example of the beneficial effect of an often increased cardiac output on arterial P_{O_2}.

With this brief review of the major elements of lung structure and function, the pathophysiological hallmarks of common pulmonary disease states can be described and understood.

Pathophysiology of syndromes of diffuse airway obstruction

Chronic obstructive pulmonary disease

As usually defined, this disease complex represents a mixture of pathologies consisting predominantly of alveolar emphysema and chronic airway inflammation in varying degrees.* Relatively few patients appear to have emphysema only or airway disease only, but those who do have served as valuable models to separate the effects of these two different components on lung function. Clinically, such patients have been traditionally been grouped as type A and type B respectively. It was held that, in type A, clinical features of lung hyperexpansion, relatively mild hypoxaemia, lack of carbon dioxide retention, high minute ventilation, and increased lung compliance were associated with evidence of emphysema. The classical type B features of more severe hypoxaemia, carbon dioxide retention, pulmonary hypertension, and absence of increased ventilation were thought to be associated with chronic bronchiolitis (small airways disease). Further study has shown that both clinical features and pathology are much more likely to be mixed in any one patient. Despite this, understanding of the pathophysiology of chronic obstructive pulmonary disease is well served by examining the effects of the two pathological processes separately.

EMPHYSEMA

Emphysematous changes involve enzymatic degradation of collagen and elastin in the alveolar walls and are scattered throughout the lung, such that there are areas of normal tissue interspersed with regions of emphysema (abnormally enlarged alveolar spaces due to alveolar septal degeneration (Fig. 4)) in varying degrees. However, gravitational influences modulate this distribution of pathology. In the common form of emphysema caused mainly by cigarette smoking, there is often greater lung damage at the apex of the lung and in the uppermost regions of each lobe. This is probably because the mechanical stress on upper lung regions is higher than for other areas owing to the weight of the remaining lung below. However, in the much less common form of emphysema caused by inherited α_1-antitrypsin deficiency, this pattern of disease is essentially reversed. Thus most of the emphysematous changes are seen in the dependent lung regions. This is presumably explained by the higher blood flow of these regions and the absence of the antiprotease molecule α_1-antitrypsin in the blood.

MECHANICAL PROPERTIES OF THE LUNG

Enzymatic degradation of collagen and elastin in alveolar walls leads to two major effects on the mechanical properties of lung airways. First,

*Readers should be aware of differences that exist in the use of terms for chronic obstructive pulmonary disease. Alternatives for this term are chronic obstructive lung disease, chronic obstructive airways disease, chronic airways obstruction, and chronic airflow limitation. At least two types of pathological process lead to this syndrome: (1) a destructive lesion in the alveoli (emphysema); (2) irregular inflammation and fibrotic narrowing of small airways. There may also be a third pathology: (3) mucous gland hyperplasia in large airways. In this chapter the term 'chronic bronchiolitis' is used to describe the small airways pathology ((2) above), whereas others might call it chronic obstructive bronchitis or more simply small airways disease. The author of this chapter has chosen the term chronic bronchitis to describe inflammatory airways disease from the trachea down to the small bronchioles. To the east of the Atlantic, the term 'chronic bronchitis is understood to mean the clinical syndrome of cough with mucoid sputum (present for 3 months of the year in at least 2 consecutive years and not due to other pathology); the causative pathology is mucous gland hyperplasia ((3) above). This lesion is not necessarily associated with airflow obstruction and can occur without the other lesions, even though all three are most likely to be due to the effects of tobacco smoking. The editors have chosen the term 'chronic bronchiolitis' to describe the small airways disease that is an integral part of chronic obstructive pulmonary disease; see Chapter 17.9.4 for further discussion).

alveolar walls disappear in the affected regions, causing confluence of alveoli, the generation of enlarged parenchymal air spaces, and a loss of the normal elastic recoil of the lungs (Fig. 4). Thus lung compliance is increased. Second, many of the normal attachments between alveoli and the airways are broken. Loss of these attachments, which normally exert radial traction and help to maintain airway patency, leads to greater susceptibility of airways to compression and collapse, impeding air flow.

Loss of elastic recoil alters the balance of forces between the chest wall (which, over most of the range of lung volume, tends to spring outward) and the lungs (which, over the entire range of lung volume, tend to collapse due to elastic recoil). With less collapsibility, the equilibrium volume of the lungs (at which volume these opposing forces are in balance) must increase. By definition, the equilibrium volume is called the functional residual capacity (FRC), so that an increased FRC is one hallmark of emphysema.

Loss of radial traction, the second major effect of emphysema on the airways, causes particular problems to the small peripheral conducting airways that are devoid of cartilaginous support—the small bronchioles. They are easily compressed during expiration, and to such an extent that lung emptying to normal minimal (i.e. residual) volume does not occur. Consequently, residual volume is increased.

While increases in residual volume and FRC are highly characteristic and quite early manifestations of emphysema, vital capacity is relatively well maintained until late in the course of disease. Consequently, maximal (total) lung capacity is often also increased.

Changes in mechanical properties of the airways explain not only the changes in lung volume, but also changes in inspiratory and expiratory flow rates. In particular, the loss of radial traction on non-cartilaginous peripheral airways makes them highly susceptible to compression during expiration, and this limits expiratory flow rates to a major extent (Fig. 5). This mechanism of air flow obstruction is an accentuation of normal control of maximal expiratory air flow rates in that dynamic compression limits flow during much of maximal expiration even in healthy subjects; normal radial traction on airways caused by intact alveolar attachment opposes compression in health, but this stabilizing mechanism is greatly reduced in emphysema. During normal quiet breathing in health, dynamic compression does not limit flow, but this is generally not the case in emphysema. Thus expiratory flow rates in emphysema are not improved by additional respiratory muscle effort and one often sees a greater degree of compression during a maximal vital capacity exhalation than when the same manoeuvre is performed with less volitional

Fig. 4 (a) Microscopic and (b) macroscopic views of the parenchyma of a normal lung contrasted with similar views ((c), (d)) of a lung showing emphysematous changes. The alveoli have coalesced into large spaces with considerable loss of alveolar wall surface and of capillaries. (Reproduced with permission from West (1987).)

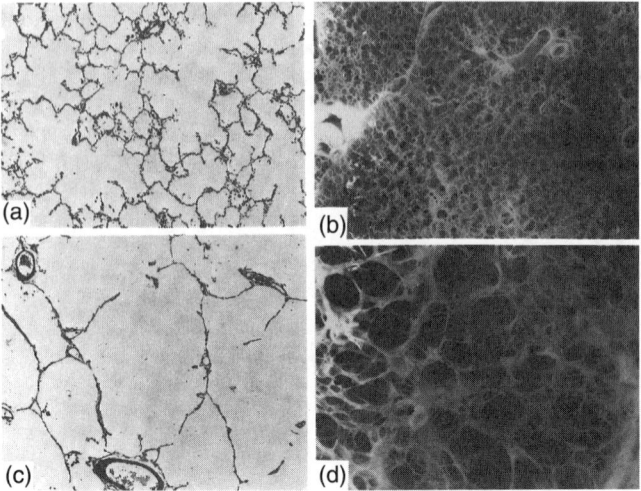

effort. This results in a discrepancy between the forced vital capacity (FVC) recorded during maximal effort and the relaxed vital capacity (VC) (i.e. VC > FVC), which is referred to as gas trapping.

Dynamic compression is clearly the major cause of air flow obstruction in pure emphysema. Other potential factors such as bronchoconstriction (airway smooth muscle contraction), luminal obstruction due to secretions, mucosal oedema or hypertrophy, and distortion of airways are much less prominent. Evidence supporting this conclusion is that in the absence of small airways disease, inspiratory air flow rates are generally well preserved in emphysema. This is precisely what would be expected since dynamic compression is not seen in inspiration. The other possible causes of airway obstruction would, if present, clearly exist throughout the respiratory cycle and thus impede flow during both inspiration and expiration.

When the flow–volume curve is measured in normal subjects, dynamic compression limits expiration in such a manner that flow decreases essentially linearly as lung volume falls. This in turn implies an essentially single-exponential fall in flow rate with time, as would be expected from a virtually homogeneous lung emptying under such conditions. In emphysema the greater degree of dynamic compression does not merely reduce flow magnitude at any given lung volume. There is a change in the shape of the flow–volume curve. Early in expiration, flow may be relatively high, but it usually falls rapidly and persists at low rates for most of the expiratory manoeuvre. This creates a 'scalloped-out' appearance to the curve and is probably the result of non-uniformity in the process of alveolar emptying due to corresponding non-uniformity of the emphysematous process.

PULMONARY CIRCULATION

The structural changes occurring in emphysema also affect the pulmonary vasculature. The loss of alveolar walls characteristic of emphysema also implies loss of pulmonary capillaries. Consequently, pulmonary vascular impedance is increased. However, because the vasculature of the normal lung is sufficient to accommodate the entire cardiac output at low pressures without requiring blood flow in all capillaries, considerable alveolar destruction can occur without clinically significant increases in pulmonary artery pressure or right heart work. Consequently, clinical evidence of right heart failure is uncommon in pure emphysema until late in the course of the disease. Other potential contributions to increased vascular impedance exist. Thus (1) capillary

stretching due to increased FRC, (2) distortion of blood vessels from uneven distribution of emphysematous changes, and (3) active hypoxic vasoconstriction may affect vascular impedance, but are probably relatively unimportant until late in the disease.

GAS EXCHANGE

For all gases, diffusional conductance between the alveolar gas and the capillary blood is typically reduced in emphysema. This is explained by the reduced capillary surface area in the lung which, as previously mentioned, is the result of alveolar wall degradation by the emphysematous process. Thus, the diffusing capacity D_{LCO} (otherwise known as the transfer factor) for carbon monoxide is classically reduced. Despite this finding, there is generally sufficient time for oxygen and carbon dioxide exchange in the lung so that this reduced diffusional conductance does not contribute to any hypoxaemia or hypercapnia. This is explained by the roughly threefold reserve in capillary transit time that exists in the normal lung at rest, such that large reductions in diffusional conductance can be accommodated without any consequence for gas exchange.

The distribution of both ventilation and blood flow is abnormal in emphysema. Surprisingly, the airway obstruction caused by dynamic compression does not appear to produce reductions in local ventilation and thus areas of abnormally low ventilation-to-perfusion ratio are usually absent. This is probably explained by the relative preservation of inspiratory flow rates (see above) which allows local inspiratory ventilation to be sustained. Then, despite dynamic compression causing expiratory obstruction, adequate expiration can occur if sufficient time is available. Patients take advantage of this scenario by reducing inspiratory time and increasing expiratory time.

Topographically, the distribution of ventilation is irregularly abnormal with some areas, presumably those subject to emphysema, having some reduction in flow. However, these areas are probably also just those subject to alveolar wall destruction and thus have substantial reduction in local perfusion as well. The net effect of a modest reduction in ventilation and a greater reduction in blood flow is an increase in local ventilation-to-perfusion ratios. The existence of such areas is indeed reported in emphysema, as is the general absence of areas of subnormal ventilation-to-perfusion ratio. True shunts, i.e. the continued perfusion of completely unventilated areas, are also rare in emphysema, which is consistent with the pathological effects described above.

Despite the increased work of breathing, most patients with emphysema maintain an elevated total minute ventilation, generally some 50 per cent greater than for a normal resting individual of the same size. It is this, together with the specific changes in ventilation-to-perfusion ratio distribution noted above, that accounts for the often remarkably well-preserved levels of arterial P_{O_2} and P_{CO_2}. Arterial P_{O_2} is commonly above 9 kPa (73 mmHg), while P_{CO_2} is normal or even slightly reduced (4.5–5.3 kPa (33–40 mmHg) is common). The relationships of oxygen and carbon dioxide exchange to ventilation, blood flow, and their distribution is as follows. Absence of severe hypoxaemia is explained by absence of shunt and of areas of abnormally low ventilation-to-blood flow ratio together with the above-normal total minute ventilation. Hypercapnia is prevented by the increase in minute ventilation which compensates for the dead-space-like effect of areas with high ventilation-to-perfusion ratios. Thus the high total ventilation sustains normal levels of alveolar ventilation in those portions of the lung carrying most of the blood flow (and hence responsible for most of the carbon dioxide exchange). Without such an increase in total ventilation, alveolar ventilation of these regions would be abnormally low (because of the diversion of inspired gas to the areas of high ventilation-to-perfusion ratio). This in turn would lead to an increase in arterial P_{CO_2}.

Thus all the typical physiological manifestations of the purely emphysematous patient are readily explained by the pathological changes caused by the disease. Owing to the irreversible nature of these changes, it is clear that, other than potential lung transplantation, little can be done therapeutically to address the disease process directly. Thus current

Fig. 5 Typical flow–volume curves obtained during maximal expiratory and inspiratory efforts in a normal subject, in a patient with emphysema, and in a patient with fibrosis.

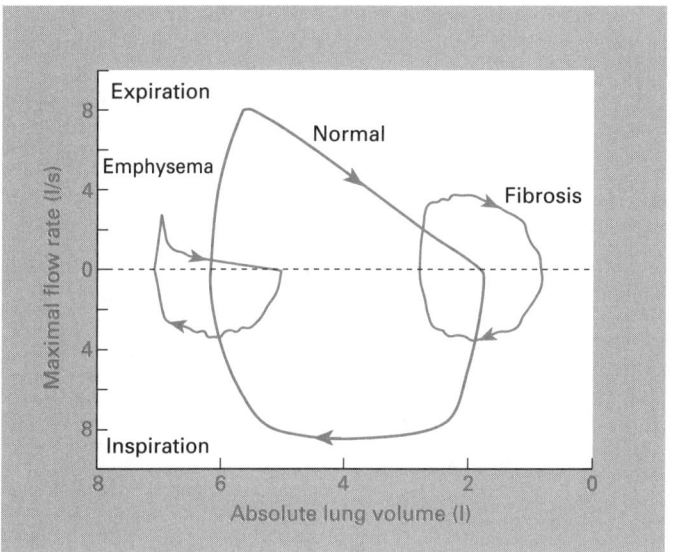

therapeutic strategies have their pathophysiological rationale in either avoiding disease progress (e.g. smoking cessation, avoidance of respiratory infection), enhancing ancillary physiological processes (e.g. using bronchodilators even when bronchoconstriction is not the principal problem), or offering rehabilitational therapy to improve life-style (unfortunately, no effect on pulmonary structure occurs).

CHRONIC BRONCHIOLITIS

Chronic bronchitis without coexistent pathological changes of emphysema is relatively common in the early stages of smoking-related lung disease, although clinically the effects of emphysema and chronic bronchiolitis overshadow those of simple bronchitis as the disease evolves. Effects of chronic airways inflammation *per se* are discussed in the following; to the extent that a given patient also has emphysema, the preceding discussion of that entity applies.

The principal site of disease in chronic bronchitis is in the major conducting airways from the trachea down, and in chronic bronchiolitis it is in the smallest (terminal) bronchioles. Repeated chemical inflammatory insults from the content of cigarette smoke (and occasionally other inhaled gases, vapours, or particles) give rise to a pathological response typical of chronic inflammation.

Airways become obstructed by (1) secretions of mucus, (2) luminal encroachment caused by mucosal gland hypertrophy and mucosal oedema, (3) variable amounts of airway smooth muscle contraction (bronchoconstriction), and (4) fibrotic airway distortion due to uneven distribution of the disease process (Fig. 6).

Chronic chemical inflammation not only increases the volume of

Fig. 6 Structure of the bronchial wall in (a) a normal subject and (b) a patient with chronic bronchitis. In chronic bronchitis, the mucous glands are increased in number, thickening the submucosa as shown. There is also chronic inflammatory cellular infiltration. (Reproduced with permission from West (1987).)

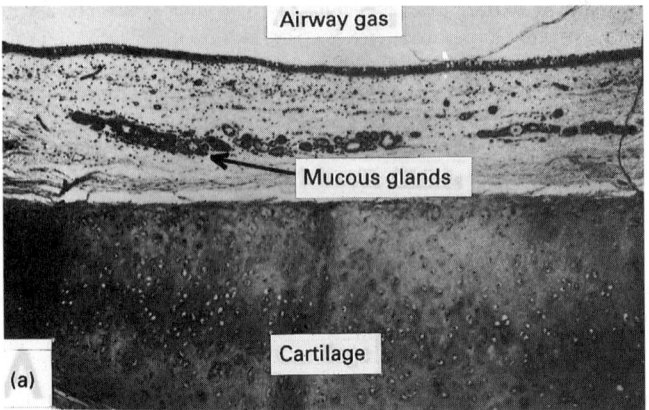

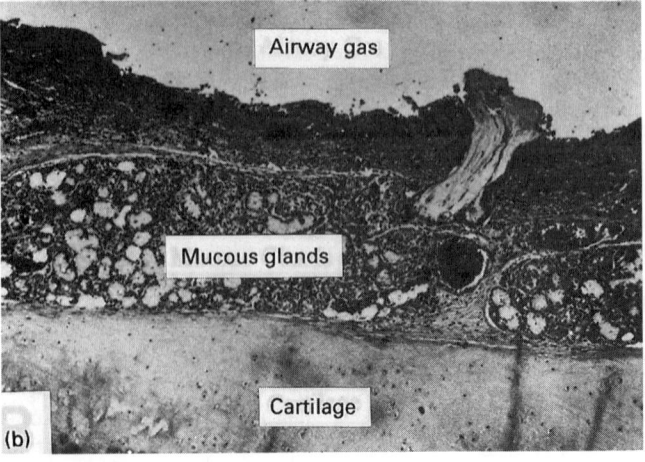

mucus secreted into the airway, but also impairs the normal mode of clearance of this mucus—the mucociliary escalator. Thus more mucus is produced than in normal subjects and its clearance is impaired. Coughing then becomes a major mechanism for mucus elimination, and the expectorated mucus is manifest as sputum, sometimes in volumes exceeding a cup per day. The increased sputum production noticed particularly in the morning on awakening from sleep is explained by inadequacy of the mucociliary system to clear the secretions accumulated during sleep.

MECHANICAL PROPERTIES OF THE LUNG

Inflammatory changes in large airways cause minimal obstruction. The principal effect on lung mechanical properties is caused by bronchiolitis. Total lung resistance to air flow is considerably increased, usually symmetrically in both inspiration and expiration, since the causes of obstruction are relatively fixed and present throughout the respiratory cycle. The tactic that may preserve ventilation of air spaces distal to obstruction in emphysema, namely shortening inspiratory times to allow prolonged expiration (see above), is not particularly effective, so that areas of abnormally low ventilation, and hence of low ventilation-to-perfusion ratio, are commonly seen. Obstruction may be so severe in some lung regions that it may become complete and give rise to pulmonary shunts.

The increase in FRC and residual volume typical of emphysema is not so common or severe in chronic bronchiolitis, presumably because elastic recoil *per se* is not reduced (unless emphysema is also present). Early airway closure during a forced expiration can occur to some extent due to the luminal encroachment described above in combination with dynamic compression (which may not be very abnormal *per se*). Expiratory flow rates are usually considerably reduced in chronic bronchiolitis owing to luminal encroachment, but so are inspiratory flow rates, in contrast with the purely emphysematous patient.

PULMONARY CIRCULATION

Pulmonary circulation is more severely affected in chronic bronchiolitis than in emphysema. There are several reasons for this, even if emphysematous destruction of capillaries does not occur. Thus, irrespective of total minute ventilation, hypoxic poorly ventilated areas exist due to airways obstruction, and this hypoxia results in sustained pulmonary vasoconstriction. In addition, many patients with chronic bronchiolitis hypoventilate, so that even in relatively unaffected areas alveolar P_{O_2} is low and P_{CO_2} is high, producing further vasoconstriction. Chronic hypoxaemia stimulates erythropoietin release from the kidneys which, over time, produces polycythaemia in many patients with chronic bronchitis. The associated increase in blood viscosity contributes to increases in pulmonary artery pressure and the work of the right heart. Finally, parenchymal distortion due to uneven disease distribution adds to the vascular impedance.

Not surprisingly, pulmonary hypertension and failure of the right heart are fairly common. If emphysema is also present, the additional capillary destruction can only worsen the haemodynamic situation.

GAS EXCHANGE

The diffusional conductance of gases moving between the alveoli and the capillaries (and $D_{L_{CO_2}}$ in particular) may be relatively well preserved in chronic bronchiolitis. Lack of destruction of pulmonary capillaries (and thus preservation of an adequate gas exchange surface area) is probably the principal reason. Thus, despite often marked hypoxaemia, the low arterial P_{O_2} is not the result of impediments to diffusion of oxygen, just as for emphysema.

As in emphysema, the distribution of both ventilation and blood flow within the lung is abnormal. The principal phenomenon is local reduction in ventilation due to airways obstruction. While this can occur in any lung region, the lung bases are particularly vulnerable for gravitational reasons. While some degree of reversible hypoxic vasoconstriction can be demonstrated, it is not sufficiently strong to prevent considerable levels of continued perfusion of these obstructed regions. Consequently, considerable portions of the lung are severely underventilated and somewhat underperfused, but the net result is areas of abnormally low ventilation-to-perfusion ratio. Unless there is coexistent emphysema, areas of high ventilation-to-perfusion ratio (typical of emphysema) are rarely, if ever, seen. Areas of low ventilation-to-perfusion ratio may be multiple, small, and scattered throughout the lung, or there may be confluent areas of disease, but the effects on gas exchange are similar. Severe obstruction may cause shunt by completely cutting off ventilation of associated alveoli.

Total ventilation in patients with chronic bronchiolitis may be reduced despite moderately severe hypoxaemia and hypercapnia that would normally stimulate breathing. Reasons for failure of the ventilatory response system are still speculative, but may include inherent genetic differences in chemoreceptor sensitivity to altered P_{O_2}, P_{CO_2}, and pH, as well as factors related to the high energy cost of breathing due to airway obstruction.

The presence of significant regions with low or zero ventilation-to-perfusion ratios accounts for the often severe hypoxaemia typical of chronic bronchiolitis. The potential efficacy of normal or increased ventilation in restoring arterial P_{O_2}, so evident in emphysema (see above), is reduced in the presence of areas of extremely low (or zero) ventilation-to-perfusion ratio. This is because even if this ratio (typically 0.01–0.05 in affected regions) could be doubled, it would still be so low that alveolar P_{O_2} would be only minimally improved (Fig. 7). Lung regions with less abnormal ventilation-to-blood flow ratio, which also contribute to hypoxaemia when total ventilation is low, would be significantly improved by an increase in total ventilation.

Thus, to restore arterial P_{O_2} effectively (without increasing F_{IO_2}) in such patients, one would have to clear any airways obstruction and restore total ventilation (in those patients with low ventilation to begin with); neither tactic alone would be sufficient.

Arterial P_{CO_2} is commonly elevated in chronic obstructive pulmonary disease. This is due predominantly to reductions in total ventilation rather than to the presence of lung regions of very low ventilation-to-perfusion ratio. Owing to the different slopes and shapes of the binding curves for oxygen and carbon dioxide in blood, oxygen exchange is much more severely affected by areas of zero and low ventilation-to-perfusion ratios, while carbon dioxide exchange is more strongly affected when high ventilation-to-blood flow areas develop or when total

ventilation is reduced. Thus arterial P_{CO_2} often readily returns to normal when ventilation is returned to normal levels.

While the effects of chronic bronchiolitis on the conducting airways offer reasonable explanations for the pathophysiological changes described, the difficulty in establishing the extent of coexisting emphysema often results in rather confusing conglomerations of clinical findings. Thus, as mentioned at the beginning of this section, both processes—emphysema and chronic airways inflammation—are present simultaneously in most patients. The clinical picture becomes an amalgamation of the consequences of both processes, with some dependence on their relative preponderances.

Asthma

Asthma is also an obstructive lung airway disease and is generally chronic in that a given patient may well show manifestations of the disease over many years. While the progression of chronic obstructive pulmonary disease is inexorable (in the continued presence of cigarette smoking), that of asthma is generally quite different. The clinical course is usually typified by acute exacerbations followed by remissions. The severity and frequency of exacerbations as well as the completeness of functional recovery in remissions is subject to great variability over time, both within a single patient and between patients.

Unlike chronic obstructive pulmonary disease, most cases of which are clearly the result of cigarette smoking, asthma has no well-defined cause beyond obvious genetic influences. In particular, exacerbations can be provoked by a variety of stimuli—immunological (allergic), inflammatory (infective), physical (cold, dry air), and emotional. The fundamental defect remains obscure.

The primary pathophysiological disturbance in asthma is airways obstruction which can develop in seconds to minutes. Its basis is a combination of excessive smooth muscle airway contraction, secretion of increased amounts of particularly tenacious mucus into the airway lumen, and airway wall inflammation causing oedema and luminal encroachment. These phenomena take place throughout the conducting airway system from the trachea down to the smallest bronchioles containing smooth muscle and bronchial epithelium. The biology of these airway changes is discussed in Chapter 17.9.1, where current knowledge of the roles of muscle contraction, inflammatory mediators, and neural modulation as contributors to the processes causing obstruction is discussed.

Pathological changes are not prominent and reflect smooth muscle contraction, luminal secretions, and inflammatory changes (cells and oedema) in and around the airway walls. Alveoli remain microscopically normal.

MECHANICAL PROPERTIES OF THE LUNG

These changes lead to predictable effects on the mechanical properties of the lung that have similar outcomes as in chronic bronchitis. Thus air flow resistance is increased and maximal expiratory flow rates are decreased. The disease is patchy in distribution, and the consequent spectrum of locally different degrees of airways obstruction results in a scalloped-out flow–volume curve just as in chronic obstructive pulmonary disease. There may be a small reduction in lung elastic recoil, but the reasons are obscure. Just as for chronic obstructive pulmonary disease, these effects have the potential for increasing both residual volume and FRC (due to early airway closure from obstruction and altered lung–chest wall equilibrium respectively). This hyperinflation is particularly prevalent in children, perhaps related to their more elastic (or 'springy') chest wall. While vital capacity may be reduced, the major spirometric manifestations are those of airways obstruction, i.e. reduced maximum flow rates.

It is important to discuss the basis of an important potential disparity between clinical features and spirometric findings. Thus, while spirometric findings are dominated by obstruction of the larger central air-

Fig. 7 The effect of local ventilation-to-perfusion ratio on local alveolar P_{O_2}. When the ventilation-to-perfusion ratio of a lung region is less than about 0.1, alveolar P_{O_2} is very close to that of mixed venous blood. Above this value, alveolar P_{O_2} rises rapidly with ventilation-to-perfusion ratio, approaching that of inspired gas as shown.

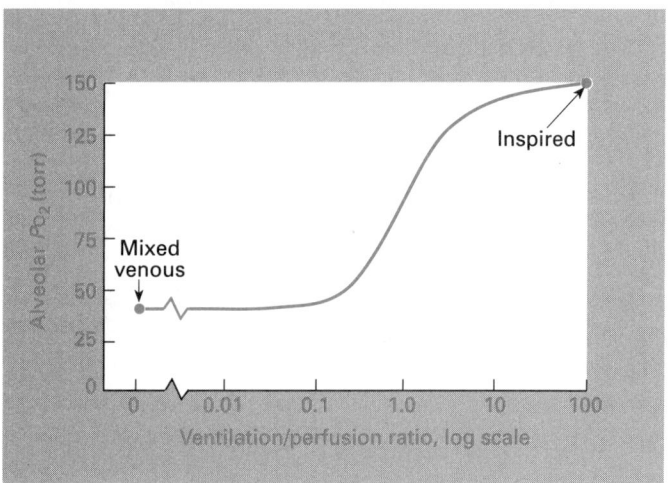

ways due to their normally smaller total cross-sectional area, some clinical findings may be more causally related to obstruction in the small peripheral airways which, owing to their large number, still possess a large total cross-sectional area, even in asthma. To the extent that in a particular patient obstruction occurs principally peripherally rather than centrally, clinical abnormalities may seem greater than expected for the spirometric changes. The converse occurs when airways involvement is primarily central.

PULMONARY CIRCULATION

Just as in most lung diseases, even those appearing to be dominated by airways involvement, the pulmonary circulation may be abnormal in asthma. This should not be surprising because the pulmonary arteries (1) lie beside the airways, and so may be influenced by neural and humoral factors that affect airways, and (2) contain contractile smooth muscle as do the airways. Thus there is evidence of locally increased vascular tone in affected lung regions. While this is due in part to local hypoxic vasoconstriction, it is also due partly to the effects of vasoconstrictive mediators released during the asthmatic process. However, frank pulmonary hypertension and right heart failure are very uncommon, and are usually seen only in a few patients with severe intractable asthma in endstage circumstances.

In contrast, in many patients the pulmonary circulation accommodates an above-normal cardiac output without significant pulmonary hypertension. Several factors probably contribute to this including a β_1-stimulatory effect of sympathetic agonists used as bronchodilator therapy. Such agents can be absorbed systemically, even when inhaled, and when used too frequently cause tachycardia and an elevated cardiac output. Other contributing factors are the anxiety of acute illness often prominent in asthma and possibly arterial hypoxaemia causing further sympathetic stimulation. All these factors not only raise cardiac output, but overall they promote pulmonary vascular dilatation.

GAS EXCHANGE

Diffusional conductance of gases across the blood–gas barrier is, if anything, increased in patients with asthma. This is difficult to explain, particularly in the presence of ventilatory inequality that would tend to reduce $D_{L}CO$, but the reason may be an increase in average pulmonary capillary volume and thus surface area. Such changes could be the result of the mechanical consequences of airways obstruction causing more negative intrapleural pressures than normal.

As might be predicted, the distribution of ventilation is typically abnormal, just as in chronic bronchitis, as described more fully above, and for similar reasons. Thus airways subject to obstruction receive abnormally little ventilation and lead to alveoli of low ventilation-to-perfusion ratio. However, areas of high ventilation-to-perfusion ratio are not seen, at least in adults. Completely unventilated regions are rarely seen, and when present are due to segmental or lobar atelectasis. This in turn is due to obstruction of large airways by inspissated mucus or occasionally to pneumothorax that may occur spontaneously.

The distribution of blood flow is less affected than that of ventilation, but regional reduction in blood flow accompanies that of ventilation due to local vasoconstriction. This does not usually compensate fully for reduced ventilation, and thus areas of low ventilation-to-perfusion ratio remain prominent in most patients, as mentioned.

Hypoxaemia occurs in asthma, but is often mild despite the existence of occasionally severe ventilation-to-perfusion inequality and the presence of areas of low ventilation-to-blood flow ratio. In order not to underestimate clinical severity, it is important to recognize that the mildness of hypoxaemia does not necessarily indicate a correspondingly mild degree of ventilation-to-blood flow inequality. The reasons for the relative preservation of arterial P_{O_2} are as follows: (1) local vasoconstriction due to hypoxia and/or vasoconstriction mediators that buffers the

fall in local ventilation; (2) elevated cardiac output (see above) that in turn elevates mixed venous P_{O_2} above that which would otherwise occur, thus permitting a higher arterial P_{O_2} due to higher P_{O_2} of the blood from poorly ventilated regions, causing less venous admixture; (3) often elevated total ventilation, despite the high work of breathing entailed, which helps to maintain alveolar and thus arterial P_{O_2}.

Arterial hypercapnia is rare in asthma uncomplicated by other disease states or by sedative medications that reduce the drive to breathe. In general, patients hyperventilate and arterial P_{CO_2} is lower than normal, often between 4 and 5 kPa (30–37 mmHg). It is felt that an arterial P_{CO_2} of conventionally normal values (i.e. 5.3 kPa (40 mmHg)) is an indication of impending respiratory muscle fatigue and ventilatory failure, requiring close observation with immediate provision for assisted ventilation. When arterial P_{CO_2} exceeds 5.5 kPa (in patients known not to be chronically hypercapnic between exacerbations), this warning is even more imperative.

Acute administration of sympathomimetic bronchodilators poses a special problem in understanding response to therapy in asthma. While there may be quite evident and dramatic relief of obstruction of upper (central) airways by such agents, peripheral airways obstruction from mucus or oedema is not ameliorated. Systemic effects of such bronchodilators serve to increase total cardiac output to some extent and the relative perfusion of hypoxic vasoconstrictive areas in particular. Consequently, there is simultaneous improvement in spirometric indices (and symptoms of airways obstruction) with deterioration in indices of gas exchange. Whether the latter has played a role in the recent apparent upswing in asthma-related deaths in some countries continues to be debated.

Finally, it should be pointed out that, irrespective of bronchodilator therapy, the relationships amongst clinical symptoms, spirometric indices of airways obstruction, and pulmonary gas exchange are extremely loose. The major reasons have already been given: central airways obstruction by bronchoconstriction dominates spirometry, while peripheral airways obstruction in part due to mucus and oedema more heavily influences gas exchange. It has proved impossible to predict arterial P_{O_2} from spirometric defects, not only in individual subjects but even in groups of subjects. It thus remains a clinical leap of faith to assert that an asymptomatic asthmatic with (nearly) normal air flow rates is in remission.

Airways obstruction by tumours or aspiration of a foreign body

An extrinsic tumour mass or hilar lymph node can cause local, sometimes complete, obstruction of a single bronchus, often at the lobar level, by compression of the airway. A tumour growing in the airway wall can do the same, and any inhaled foreign objects, such as aspirated food particles, have the potential for causing similar complete obstruction.

Should this occur, there will probably be no symptoms of the more usual forms of airways obstruction dealt with above, because functional deletion of a single lobe is easily tolerated at rest owing to the large reserve in normal lung function.

Severe but incomplete lobar obstruction often produces localized rhonchi (i.e. wheezing or whistling sounds) during breathing owing to altered airflow patterns in the region of the obstruction. There may well be some hypoxaemia because ventilation of the alveoli distal to the site of obstruction is considerably reduced, but blood flow continues. Thus a relatively large confluent region of low ventilation-to-perfusion ratio is created, which explains the hypoxaemia.

Complete obstruction of a lobar airway will result in gradual atelectasis of the lobe as alveolar gas is absorbed into the capillary blood over a period of several hours to days. Again, this will probably not produce symptoms related to pulmonary mechanical changes, but hypoxaemia will be seen due to the unventilated but perfused nature of the affected lobe, i.e. a shunt develops.

Diffuse interstitial fibrosis

In contrast with syndromes of airways obstruction, those due to interstitial fibrosis produce an entirely different pathophysiological picture. Interstitial fibrosis is the end result of any of a very large number of inflammatory processes which, rather than resolving, go on to chronic pathological change characterized by the extensive deposition of collagen in alveolar walls throughout the lungs. The following does not deal with the acute inflammatory phases that precede fibrosis, nor does it distinguish amongst the many initiating causes of fibrosis, because, no matter what the aetiology, the pathophysiological consequences are very similar for all.

Figure 8 shows the typical thickening of the alveolar walls due to laying down of collagen. Parenchymal distortion, loss of gas volume, alveolar wall rigidity and microvascular destruction are all readily apparent consequences of the fibrosis. The oxygen diffusion distance between alveolar gas and the intracapillary red cells is considerably increased and, although not evident in Fig. 8, alveolar attachments to airways and blood vessels tend to maintain patency of these large structures to a greater extent than normal owing to the contracted nature of collagenous scar tissue. Thus radial traction on conduit vessels is greater than normal.

Mechanical properties of the lung

The major effect on mechanical properties of the lung is an increase in elastic recoil. Lung compliance is considerably reduced, and the work of breathing is necessarily increased owing to the greater elastic recoil. Because of (1) the volume occupied by the fibrous tissue and (2) the increased elastic recoil, there is loss of gas volume. Thus all commonly measured volume parameters (residual volume, functional residual capacity, total lung capacity, and vital capacity) are below normal. In general, the percentage reduction of each of these indices is similar for a given patient. A 30 per cent reduction (below predicted normal values) reflects moderate disease, while reduction of 50 per cent or more signals severe fibrosis.

When based on the reduced lung volumes actually present, maximal expiratory flow rates are not only well preserved but classically exceed predicted values. Wording becomes confusing here and so a numerical example is presented for clarification. For a normal person whose forced vital capacity (FVC) is 5.0 litres and whose forced expiratory volume 1 second (FEV_1) is 4.0 litres, the ratio FEV_1/FVC, expressed as a percentage, is 80 per cent. Simple reduction of all volumes and flows by 50 per cent would reduce FVC to 2.5 litres, and FEV_1 to 2.0 litres but leave the FEV_1/FVC ratio unchanged. However, in diffuse interstitial fibrosis, the increase in airway radial traction resulting from increased elastic recoil stabilizes the airways and reduces the degree of airway dynamic compression during expiration. Typically, if FVC has been reduced by 50 per cent to 2.5 litres as in the above example, FEV_1 for the same hypothetical individual would be greater than 2.0 litres and may in fact equal FVC (implying completion of the forced expiratory manoeuvre within 1 second). If $FEV_1 = 2.25$ litres, the FEV_1/FVC ratio would be 90 per cent, and if $FEV_1 = 2.5$ litres, FEV_1/FVC would be 100 per cent, i.e. both values are in excess of the normal value of 80 per cent. In summary, absolute lung volume and flow rates are both reduced, but volumes are reduced more than flow rates, resulting from less dynamic compression than normal.

The flow–volume curve usually reflects the above and in particular shows the lessening of dynamic compression. In the healthy subject, dynamic compression is responsible for the failure to maintain maximum expiratory flows throughout expiration, thus explaining the linear fall in flows throughout expiration. In fibrosis, flows are relatively well maintained at lower lung volumes, and the flow–volume curve is more rectangular (Fig. 5).

Pulmonary circulation

Collagen deposition not only affects the alveolar mechanical properties, but also results in gradual loss of the alveolar wall capillary network as shown in Fig. 8. This is the principal reason for perhaps the most devastating consequence of interstitial fibrosis—increased pulmonary vascular impedance and ultimately right heart failure. Other factors contribute to the increase in pulmonary vascular impedance: many regions of the lung are hypoxic owing to inadequate local ventilation, and hypoxic pulmonary vasoconstriction will occur. In addition, the distortion produced by shortening of irregularly distributed collagen fibres further impedes blood flow and increases the work of the right heart. While the effects of interstitial fibrosis on ventilation and lung mechanics are obvious and easily measured, those on the pulmonary circulation and the right heart are essentially silent until severe pulmonary hypertension results in right heart failure. Consequently, the importance of right heart compromise must not be underestimated simply because bedside examination fails to disclose evident right heart failure. Right heart failure signifies a poor prognosis; ventilatory compromise from fibrosis, while clearly producing symptoms of dyspnoea that may be distressing, rarely results in carbon dioxide retention (raised arterial P_{CO_2}), except perhaps terminally.

Fig. 8 Typical parenchymal structure in a patient with diffuse interstitial fibrosis. The alveolar walls are greatly thickened, and very few alveolar capillaries are visible. Those that can be seen are often located deep within the thick alveolar septa. The long dimension of this figure is approximately 1000 μm. (Reproduced with permission from Hinson 1970.)

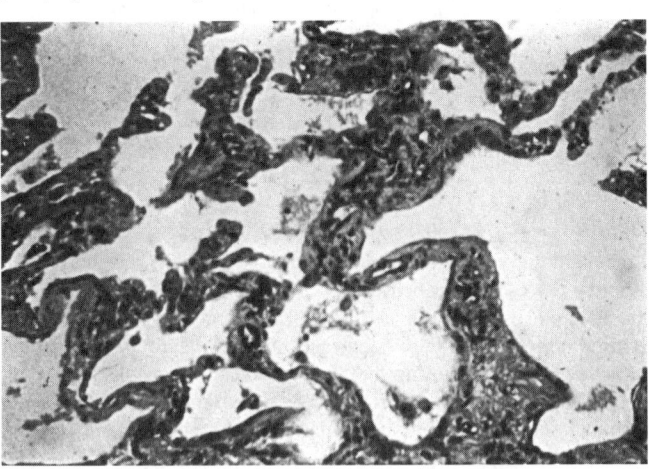

Gas exchange

Not surprisingly, diffusing capacity, which is usually measured for carbon monoxide and denoted D_{LCO}, is reduced in fibrosis. As a rule, percentage reduction of D_{LCO} exceeds that of lung volumes throughout the disease process. Several factors contribute to the reduction in D_{LCO}.

1. Increased thickness of the blood–gas barrier owing to interstitial deposition of collagen: the blood–gas barrier widens from about 0.5 μm to as much as 10–20 times this value.
2. Reduced volume of capillary blood due to capillary destruction: because D_{LCO} depends in part on the number of red cells in the microvasculature (as a result of limited carbon monoxide–haemoglobin binding reaction rates), reduced capillary volume leads to reduction in D_{LCO}.
3. Overall capillary wall surface area, another factor contributing to D_{LCO}, is also reduced as a consequence of capillary destruction and contributes to the low D_{LCO}.
4. As described below, distribution of inspired gas is non-uniform with respect to alveolar blood flow. Such non-uniformity impedes overall pulmonary uptake of all gases and CO is no exception.

The distribution of ventilation and blood flow are abnormal in interstitial fibrosis. Reduced compliance in those areas most subject to collagen deposition reduces local ventilation considerably so that, despite simultaneous local vascular compromise, local ratios of ventilation to blood flow are reduced. These sometimes reach very low values, often about 1 per cent of normal. Uneven ventilation and blood flow are seen topographically using radioactive tracer techniques, with the abnormalities paralleling the distribution of collagen deposition. Areas of abnormally high ventilation-to-blood flow ratio do not develop, presumably because fibrosis in a region reduces ventilation more than blood flow. Some alveolar wall blood vessels function as true shunts, with their end-capillary P_{O_2} values remaining at venous levels. Whether this represents absent convective ventilation of the affected alveoli owing to reduced compliance or failure of significant diffusive movement of oxygen across a greatly thickened alveolar wall is not clear, but it is not important from a clinical perspective.

As would be expected, the abnormalities described in ventilation, blood flow, and their distribution interfere considerably with pulmonary gas exchange. However, while hypoxaemia is often severe (resting room air arterial P_{O_2} is frequently 40 to 50 mmHg), arterial P_{CO_2} is generally normal or low (30–35 mmHg is common). These seemingly paradoxical observations reflect the following three principal factors and are readily explained on their basis: (1) total ventilation is generally greater than normal, despite the high work of breathing; (2) cardiac output, even at rest, is somewhat reduced owing to the high pulmonary vascular impedance, so that mixed venous P_{O_2} is correspondingly low (3–4 kPa (23–30 mmHg) rather than the normal value of 5.3 kPa); and (3) between 10 and 20 per cent of the pulmonary blood flow usually passes through alveoli with very low or zero ventilation (relative to blood flow). Hyperventilation is a very effective mechanism for reducing arterial P_{CO_2} even in disease, owing to the virtually linear nature of the carbon dioxide dissociation curve, and this accounts for the low arterial P_{CO_2}. For oxygen exchange in the presence of a 10 to 20 per cent shunt, hyperventilation is of little benefit; unventilated regions do not respond at all, very poorly ventilated regions respond minimally, and well-ventilated regions enjoy almost no improvement in end-capillary oxygen concentration owing to the shape and slope of the oxygen dissociation curve. The severity of hypoxaemia when only 10 to 20 per cent of the total pulmonary blood flow is shunted past ventilated alveoli is accounted for by the low cardiac output and the resulting low venous P_{O_2}. This is because, for a given shunt fraction, hypoxaemia worsens as venous P_{O_2} is reduced owing to increasing venous admixture of such blood with that leaving well-ventilated lung regions.

Nowhere in the preceding paragraph is mention made of diffusion limitation as a cause of hypoxaemia in interstitial fibrosis. Although D_{LCO} is typically reduced, and to a considerable degree, as pointed out earlier there is a large transit time reserve in the normal resting lung. With an available mean transit time of about 0.75 s, and only 0.25 s required for diffusive equilibration, D_{LCO} would have to be reduced considerably before diffusion limitation significantly contributed to hypoxaemia at rest. Current experimental evidence suggests that patients with advanced interstitial fibrosis are at the borderline of becoming diffusion limited at rest, and that if this mechanism of hypoxaemia is present, it is a relatively small contributing factor to resting hypoxaemia.

The reason why arterial P_{CO_2} is so commonly below normal, reflecting hyperventilation, is not clear. In patients with severe hypoxaemia, hypoxic ventilatory drive via the carotid chemoreceptors is one probable factor. In less hypoxaemic patients, this explanation does not hold since there is relatively little influence of P_{O_2} on ventilation until it falls below 8 kPa (60 mmHg). There is evidence that juxtacapillary or J sensory receptors are activated in fibrosis, possibly because of the associated alveolar distortion from shortening of collagen fibres, and that this drives ventilation. Whatever the mechanism, as for asthmatic patients, the significance is that a normal or mildly elevated arterial P_{CO_2} should be taken as a serious warning signal of impending ventilatory failure.

Exercise deserves a special mention in a discussion of the pathophysiology of interstitial fibrosis. Exercise tolerance is extremely low in advanced fibrosis, yet when ventilation and blood gases are measured there is little or no evidence of inadequate ventilation or elevation of arterial P_{CO_2} despite the high cost of breathing caused by the increased elastic recoil. Once again, evidence points to the importance of the cardiovascular complications of fibrosis in exercise limitation. Thus, just as at rest, cardiac output during exercise is subnormal for the metabolic rate encountered and mixed venous P_{O_2} values drop precipitously to values of 1.5 to 2.5 kPa (11–18 mmHg) even at modest oxygen consumption rates of less than 1 l/min. In the continued presence of a 10 to 20 per cent shunt, arterial P_{O_2} often falls dramatically during exercise, and the reduced venous P_{O_2} is the major reason. A second contributing factor to the fall in arterial P_{O_2} during exercise is the appearance of diffusion limitation of oxygen transfer in the lungs which is seen in essentially all patients. This in turn is the result of the reduction in capillary transit time that must accompany even a small increase in cardiac output through a pulmonary circulation that is so compromised by fibrosis as to possess little or no capillary recruitment reserve. Thus the normal mechanism buffering reduced capillary transit times in exercise, i.e. recruitment of unperfused capillaries to increase pulmonary blood volume, is not available in fibrosis . As might be expected, pulmonary artery pressure generally rises dramatically in exercise in these patients, as further testimony to the severe effects of fibrosis on the pulmonary circulation.

Diseases characterized by alveolar filling

In addition to diseases characterized by airflow obstruction or by interstitial fibrosis, a number of other syndromes can affect the lungs leading to well-defined pathophysiological consequences. One such group is characterized by the filling of alveolar gas spaces by cellular debris or oedema fluid. Most of these disease states are acute processes of one kind or another and a large number of aetiological agents may be involved. Alveolar filling with cellular debris is commonly the result of pneumonias caused by infection. The classical example is streptococcal pneumonia causing intense packing of all alveoli of one or more lobes by inflammatory cells and their debris. More diversely distributed forms of non-streptococcal pneumonia showing local areas subject to similar changes are more common than lobar pneumonia since the advent of penicillin. Oedema is the other major category of alveolar-filling disease where largely cell-free collections of fluid, transudative or exudative, collect in and thus fill alveoli, usually more in the dependent than the non-dependent lung regions. Such oedema may be the result of left heart failure or pulmonary capillary permeability increases due to any of a variety of cytokine-associated inflammatory processes. High pulmonary vascular pressures causing oedema may occur in previously healthy lungs, as for example in high altitude and neurogenic forms of pulmonary oedema. However, this is not the place to classify the alveolar-filling defects but to point out that such syndromes, irrespective of their aetiology, produce a generally similar pathophysiological picture. However, this collection of syndromes does not include the much more severe and disastrous complex that constitutes the adult respiratory distress syndrome. This syndrome requires special discussion because of the almost routine requirement of assisted mechanical ventilation and the associated additional pathophysiological consequences.

Mechanical properties of the lung

To maintain the same sequence of discussion as for the obstructive and restrictive diseases described earlier, the mechanical properties of the lung should be discussed first. However, most patients with acute alveolar-filling diseases, be they due to pneumonitis, heart failure, or other causes, are not studied using tools that elucidate the mechanical properties of the lung. Effects on respiratory system mechanics are usually clinically minor unless respiratory muscle fatigue, and hence respiratory failure, has developed. Moreover, the mechanical consequences are conceptually clear, and the focal points in treatment are not closely related to changes in lung volumes, flow rates, or elastic recoil. Basically, alveolar filling eliminates alveolar ventilation of the affected regions, reduces lung volumes accordingly, and increases elastic recoil. In this manner, alveolar filling produces the same qualitative effects as interstitial fibrosis described above. However, there is often perivascular and/ or peribronchial cuffing with oedema fluid, and this has the potential for impairing delivery of ventilation or blood flow distal to the cuffed vessel locations. Thus an element of airway obstruction may develop, but this *per se* is not likely to be clinically significant. Such airway and blood vessel compression potentially alters distribution of ventilation and/or blood flow and this may contribute to ventilation–perfusion mismatch.

Pulmonary circulation

There are relatively few effects of alveolar-filling diseases *per se* on the pulmonary circulation, with no evidence of direct involvement from intravenous thrombosis, in contrast with what is often seen in adult respiratory distress syndrome (see below). Because affected areas of the lung are unventilated, or at best very poorly ventilated, local alveolar hypoxia develops and this elicits local pulmonary hypoxic vasoconstriction. This helps to limit the blood flow in the abnormal areas, and this in turn limits the degree of right-to-left shunting and associated hypoxaemia. There is rarely clinically significant pulmonary hypertension observed from such vasoconstriction, and thus little concern for right heart failure in alveolar-filling diseases of non-cardiac origin unless the patient has pre-existing heart disease unrelated to the current alveolar filling process. However, if alveolar filling is due to left heart failure producing pulmonary oedema, pulmonary hypertension and right heart failure may well ensue.

Gas exchange

Ventilation–perfusion mismatch is the important consequence of alveolar-filling diseases. As expected, the filling of the alveoli and/or peripheral airways produces areas of reduced or completely absent ventilation. Perfusion of these alveoli generally continues, but at a reduced rate due to the activation of pulmonary hypoxic vasoconstriction (which follows the local hypoxia caused by local ventilatory reduction). This is the major cause of inequality; perivascular or peribronchial cuffing may further modify distribution of blood and gas.

D_{LCO} is not generally measured in such patients; it is expected to be reduced owing to loss of accessible surface area for gas exchange, and its measurement would offer nothing to disease management.

Hypoxaemia is the important consequence of the ventilation–perfusion mismatch referred to above, and its severity generally parallels that of the clinical extent of the disease. It is due to poorly ventilated or unventilated alveoli that still retain perfusion, just as in interstitial fibrosis. However, the magnitude of the hypoxaemia can be modified by the cardiac output response. For example, when alveolar filling is due to pneumonia, cardiac output may be elevated due to associated fever, and this will improve arterial P_{O_2} (other factors, such as metabolic rate, being equal). In contrast, alveolar filling with oedema fluid from left heart failure is often associated with a reduced cardiac output. As for several diseases already discussed above, this will worsen the hypoxaemia because of the concomitant fall in mixed venous P_{O_2}.

Despite hypoxaemia, carbon dioxide retention is rarely seen and arterial P_{CO_2} is usually normal or reduced. As for interstitial fibrosis, reasons for hyperventilation are not clearly established but may include a component of hypoxic ventilatory stimulation and also ventilatory drive via the J (juxtacapillary) receptors that appear to respond to interstitial pulmonary oedema.

An interesting and unique question posed by bacterial pneumonias that cause alveolar filling is whether the alveolar contents (cells and bacteria) consume significant volumes of oxygen and thus possibly contribute to the arterial hypoxaemia. Evidence both for and against this phenomenon exists such that this question remains open at present.

An almost universal therapeutic approach to patients with oedema or pneumonia is to supplement the inspired gas with oxygen via a face mask or nasal prongs. The improvement in arterial P_{O_2} is quite variable. In part this is due simply to the poorly controlled nature of such mask/ nasal catheter systems whereby the actual mean inspiratory oxygen concentration can vary greatly for the same level of flow from the oxygen source. However, another factor is the extent to which alveolar filling partly reduces rather than fully eliminates local alveolar ventilation. Partial ventilatory reduction will lead to greater improvement in arterial P_{O_2} than if complete reduction of ventilation had occurred. Therefore it is not possible to predict accurately how much additional oxygen to administer to a given patient, and a trial and error approach is required to optimize this aspect of therapy.

Adult respiratory distress syndrome

Adult respiratory distress syndrome encompasses a group of severe, often lethal, clinical syndromes with varied initiating causes but a relatively similar set of consequences. Initiating factors include systemic or pulmonary infection, trauma, and major surgery. Consequences for the lung include respiratory failure (hypoxaemia with or without hypercapnia), hypoxaemia poorly responsive to added inspired oxygen, pulmonary vascular obstruction, alveolar filling with oedema fluid and cellular debris, loss of surfactant function with propensity to alveolar collapse, and respiratory fatigue which, together with the need for added inspired oxygen, necessitates assisted ventilation. In many respects, adult respiratory distress syndrome is not distinctly different from the alveolar-filling processes discussed above. What sets it apart is the severity of the pulmonary abnormalities, such that ventilator support is required, and the fact that adult respiratory distress syndrome often progresses to involve other critical organs, resulting in multiple organ failure.

Patients with adult respiratory distress syndrome may recover completely. More often, some residual pulmonary structural changes and corresponding functional deficits are observed in survivors. All too often, the disease is fatal (40–50 per cent mortality in the United States) and this outcome statistic has not been improved significantly by aggressive supportive therapy and years of research.

The pathophysiological findings in adult respiratory distress syndrome reflect this diversity of possible outcomes, and also depend on when in the course of disease observations are made.

Mechanical properties of the lung

The mechanical properties of the lung can be severely disrupted in adult respiratory distress syndrome. Although the processes are qualitatively similar to those of oedema/alveolar filling discussed above, there comes a time when so much of the lung is full of exudate or debris from the inflammatory processes that only a small portion remains available for ventilation and to support gas exchange. It is then that the mechanical properties deteriorate seriously. Specifically, when most of the lung is refractory to expansion owing to alveolar filling, wall oedema, or fibrosis, what little lung that remains becomes overdistended with each breath, usually at moderately high inflation pressures. These normal regions lose their compliance due to overdistension and in addition capillaries in the alveolar wall become compressed. This causes distribution of perfusion away from these few normal regions to oedematous regions of poor gas exchange, and thus may interfere with gas exchange. Perhaps even more importantly, overinflation of normal regions leads to their susceptibility to trauma from high wall stresses. This may produce local inflammation that eventually leads to changes similar to these of emphysema due to protease release from white cells.

The fluid- or debris-filled alveoli cause problems because they resist inflation yet remain perfused with blood. Strategies for opening collapsed alveoli are a focus of treatment in patients with adult respiratory distress syndrome, and the most common has been the application of positive end-expiratory pressure. This strategy is designed to prevent airway or alveolar collapse with each expiration by maintaining pressure at the end of a breath sufficient to keep the alveoli open. It is clearly of no value if applied to a lung where alveoli are never open in the first place, or at levels that do not prevent the unwanted expiratory collapse. Moreover, positive end-expiratory pressure compounds the problem of damaging normal alveoli from overinflation. This is because of the distributed nature of the lesions in adult respiratory distress syndrome; it is not possible to apply positive end-expiratory pressure to the fluid-filled alveoli only.

Positive end-expiratory pressure and other ventilatory strategies have another negative influence on cardiopulmonary function in patients with adult respiratory distress syndrome—they reduce systemic venous return and thus cause a fall in cardiac output. Cardiac work is increased and systemic oxygen delivery to critical organs may be reduced as a result. This can happen even if some alveolar inflation has occurred from positive end-expiratory pressure, eliminating some of the shunt and improving the arterial PO_2.

Thus the extreme degree of the process of adult respiratory distress syndrome (rather than fundamental qualitative differences from less severe alveolar-filling diseases) produces serious therapeutic dilemmas traceable to fundamental pathophysiological principles—the need for assisted ventilation balanced by the intrinsic negative effect of this on the mechanical properties of the lung. No adequate solution to this dilemma exists despite years of research into the details of different modes of ventilator support. Perhaps as a result of this frustrating situation, a growing number of investigators are studying a completely different ventilatory strategy in adult respiratory distress syndrome. Thus, rather than be aggressive in optimizing lung mechanics and gas exchange with little improvement and substantial risk of iatrogenic lung damage, the opposite track is taken. Ventilation is kept at much lower levels to reduce ventilator-related lung injury, and techniques such as partial right heart bypass with extracorporeal gas exchange are introduced to augment oxygen and carbon dioxide exchange. Hypercapnia is allowed to develop; the concept is that allowing the lungs to heal by pulling back on aggressive ventilator strategies will ultimately be beneficial. Long-term results are not yet available but will be of considerable interest.

Pulmonary circulation

While most attention in patients with adult respiratory distress syndrome focuses on alveolar filling and ventilator strategies, the pulmonary circulation represents a site of potentially major involvement. Pulmonary hypertension is commonly observed in such patients and histopathological studies have revealed multiple platelet and white-cell thrombi in small pulmonary arteries. Presumably these could represent either migration of peripheral venous thrombi or *in situ* thrombus formation on injured endothelium. Whatever the pathogenesis of those vascular problems, their pathophysiological effects are predictable and will depend on how extensively the pulmonary circulation is obstructed. Right heart function may be compromised by the associated increase in heart work required. Delivery of oxygen to the myocardium may be impaired by hypoxaemia and left ventricular dysfunction, which can also occur in adult respiratory distress syndrome, and such a situation leads to a worsening of the oxygen supply–demand situation of the right ventricle, ultimately causing right heart failure. Pulmonary arterial thrombi also impede local perfusion and cause local areas of extremely high ventilation-to-perfusion ratio. If this occurs in well-ventilated areas of the lung, the associated local ventilation participates negligibly in total oxygen and carbon dioxide exchange. While not a true effect of altered lung mechanics *per se*, this problem is interwoven with those described above, compounding the issue of maldistribution of ventilation and blood flow and further interfering with gas exchange.

Gas exchange

It is very clear that gross abnormalities in oxygen and carbon dioxide exchange can be found in adult respiratory distress syndrome. As with most other diseases, oxygen exchange suffers earlier and to a greater degree than carbon dioxide exchange. Hypoxaemia is due to continued perfusion of unventilated and poorly ventilated alveoli. Carbon dioxide retention, when present, is due to inadequate ventilation of those lung regions receiving the bulk of the blood flow, which in turn may be the result of the aggressive ventilatory strategies and/or pulmonary thromboembolism.

Because the majority of the pathological effects of adult respiratory distress syndrome involve complete alveolar filling, and thus venous shunting, arterial PO_2 is often poorly responsive to high oxygen concentrations in inspired gas (high FIO_2). To the extent that areas of low ventilation-to-perfusion ratio do exist from partial alveolar filling, there will be more response of arterial PO_2 to increased FIO_2. More importantly, when such patients are maintained at relatively high values of FIO_2 (about 0.5 is common), a variable fraction of regions with low ventilation-to-perfusion ratio will be well oxygenated. While this is therapeutically useful to the patient, the physician will not be able to quantify the presence of such regions precisely because, at the elevated FIO_2, they do not contribute to venous admixture. Consequently, monitoring of arterial PO_2 in such patients requires careful interpretation and is inherently prone to underestimating the prevalence of inadequately ventilated regions.

This problem is compounded by another cause of uncertainty in the interpretation of arterial PO_2 and adult respiratory distress syndrome. It has been mentioned previously that as cardiac output varies, so too will mixed venous PO_2 (in the same direction). Thus arterial PO_2 may change due to changes in cardiac output alone rather than to changes in pulmonary damage. This uncertainty is easily resolved if mixed venous PO_2 or saturation is measured together with arterial values, but this requires a pulmonary artery catheter, itself a contentious issue.

Yet another interpretative problem, also related to changes in cardiac output, exists for understanding arterial PO_2 in adult respiratory distress syndrome. In both human disease and animal models of adult respiratory distress syndrome, as pulmonary blood flow is acutely manipulated, the computed shunt fraction parallels the directional changes in total blood flow. This occurs rapidly (within minutes), reversibly, and in virtually all circumstances in which it has been studied. As Fig. 9 shows, it is not a trivial phenomenon. Its rapid reversibility all but completely dispels the notion that there is a sudden increase in the extent of lung damage

Fig. 9 An example of how the shunt (i.e. perfusion of unventilated regions of the lung) varies with total pulmonary blood flow. The 11 data points were all obtained for a single patient and show a remarkable threefold change in shunt as pulmonary blood flow is increased. (Reproduced with permission from Lemaire *et al.* (1985).)

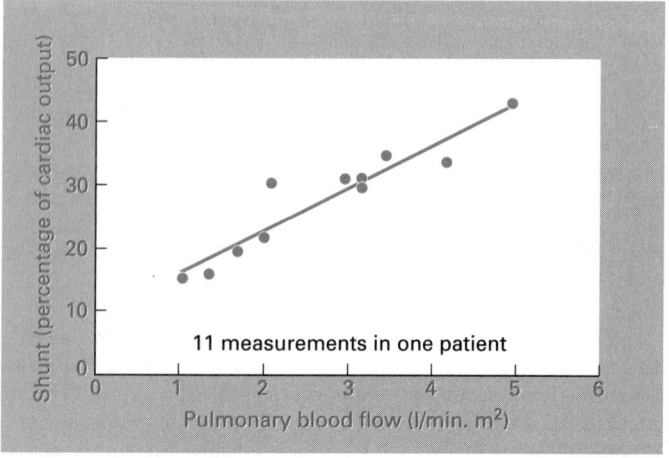

when blood flow is increased, and a more plausible explanation is redistribution of intrapulmonary blood flow. In this scenario, as total blood flow rises so too does the fraction perfusing unventilated lung regions. This is probably related to interactions between mechanical factors and reactive vascular muscle tone in response to blood flow changes, but research studies have so far failed to establish the site of redistribution definitely. However, the clinical implications are evident: when pulmonary blood flow is increased, an increase in shunt fractions is to be expected and may not represent an increase in lung pathology *per se*. Similar problems may occur when vasoactive drugs are given to patients with adult respiratory distress syndrome, i.e. a change in shunt fraction without a true change in lung damage.

The major point arising from the preceding paragraphs is as follows: the causes of hypoxaemia in adult respiratory distress syndrome are well known and easy to understand. Measures of arterial oxygenation necessary to infer adequate arterial levels from the therapeutic standpoint are easy to gather and to interpret for that purpose. However, if arterial blood gas data are to be interpreted quantitatively as indicators of change of lung pathology, the user must be aware of the factors that alter arterial P_{O_2} in the absence of any changes in lung damage *per se*.

Pulmonary vascular diseases

This group of diseases is characterized by obstruction of the pulmonary vascular tree, mostly by particulate material, which over time is usually compounded by reactive hypertrophy of the pulmonary arteries. The most common type is that due to thromboembolism where blood clots formed in peripheral veins migrate to and lodge in the pulmonary vasculature. There are many other causes of vascular obstruction, including emboli consisting of air, fat, foreign matter from intravenous drug abuse, microorganisms, tumour cell clumps, septic collections of cells and bacteria, and amniotic fluid. As with many pulmonary diseases, the pathophysiology is in general primarily due to the event common to all causes (here vascular obstruction), with secondary differences due to specific aetiologies. Such secondary factors include processes such as tumour cell growth or abscess formation from septic emboli, and are beyond the scope of this section. A distinct entity in this general group is the rare disease of primary pulmonary hypertension. The following discussion pertains particularly to the best-studied syndrome of thromboembolism.

Mechanical properties of the lung

Thromboembolism produces two major pathophysiological consequences—increased pulmonary vascular impedance and ventilation–perfusion inequality. In contrast, effects on the mechanical properties of the lungs are mild or even absent. However, when such effects occur in humans, the most common is diffuse bronchoconstriction. This rarely causes severe obstruction requiring specific intervention. Rather, it is a source of diagnostic confusion in those who may be unaware that wheezing or rhonchi reflecting such bronchoconstriction may be a sign of thromboembolism. Whether this represents effects of specific mediators, released by interaction of the embolus with the pulmonary vascular endothelium, or of airway hypocapnia in the embolized areas of the lung with a high ventilation-to-perfusion ratio (see below) is unknown at this time.

Pulmonary circulation

The chance of pulmonary vascular obstruction causing rapidly developing right heart failure depends mostly on the amount of the pulmonary circulation that has been obstructed. Other factors are also important, such as the pre-existing health of the right ventricle and arterial P_{O_2} subsequent to the embolus. Depending on these factors, there may be no discernible pulmonary hypertension at one extreme, but circulatory collapse and sudden death from overwhelming right heart failure could

occur at the other extreme, with any intermediate level of response between these ends of the spectrum possible. With severe embolic obstruction, systemic hypotension and hypoxia may occur together and impede oxygen delivery to the left ventricle sufficiently to cause typical ischaemic myocardial pain, rather than the classical pleuritic chest pain so often described. It is rare to see the development of frank pulmonary oedema in thromboembolism, even though one could argue for its logical development as non-embolized elements of the pulmonary circulation are forced to endure high vascular pressures.

Gas exchange

While the lethal effects of embolism as described above are due to right heart failure, thromboembolism classically alters the distribution of blood flow within the lung, and possibly also that of ventilation. The primary mechanism of altered blood flow distribution is mechanical, with flow distributed away from affected regions toward those that are unaffected. Whether secondary humoral factors further modify perfusion distribution, and if so in what manner and for how long after the acute thromboembolic episode, is unclear in humans. However, in experimental animals, heparin pretreatment, for example, reduces pathological damage and thus such factors could play a role in humans, but this will be difficult to elucidate.

While perfusion distribution is rapidly changed in a major fashion, the distribution of ventilation changes little, and sometimes not at all. When changes are seen, they reflect some reduction in ventilation of the embolized regions, probably the result of low local airway P_{CO_2} values (causing local bronchoconstriction). Reduction of local P_{CO_2} is the expected result of reducing blood flow and the resulting development of regions where the ventilation-to-perfusion ratio is high.

It is of academic and possible also of clinical importance that the embolized regions in both human disease and animal models reveal some residual perfusion, rather than absolutely no blood flow. Whether this is due to continued bronchial arterial blood supply of the embolized region or simply to incomplete pulmonary arterial obstruction is not known. However, the end result is a ventilation-to-perfusion ratio distribution that consists of two major populations of lung units—unaffected areas with normal to slightly reduced ratio and embolized areas with extremely high ratio. The small degree of perfusion that remains, while of essentially no use to overall gas exchange, may be important in maintaining the viability of the embolized region.

Studies have shown the increasing development of areas of scattered atelectasis and the corresponding development of shunts in many patients with the passage of time following the initial thromboembolic event. These may well represent the effects of retained secretions obstructing peripheral airways and thus causing absorption atelectasis. In the presence of pleuritic chest pain, which is common in embolism owing to pleural inflammation from a region of pulmonary infarct, coughing may be suppressed, contributing to retention of secretions. In addition, embolized areas are known to exhibit reduced surfactant activity, which also predisposes to atelectasis. Surfactant activity is abnormal, probably because of the marked local alkalosis caused by the greatly reduced P_{CO_2} explained above. Occasional patients exhibit large shunts weeks or months after recovery from the acute episode of embolism, and in the absence of radiological evidence of atelectasis one can only surmise that a patent foramen ovale exists, or that large arteriovenous anastomoses have opened up in the lungs secondary to prolonged pulmonary hypertension.

From the above, it should be apparent that there are several reasons to expect hypoxaemia after an embolus: ventilation—perfusion mismatching from the acute, largely mechanical, event and perhaps subsequent shunting from atelectasis. There is evidence to rule out other putative factors such as rapid red-cell transit through remaining pulmonary capillaries causing oxygen diffusion limitation and, for the most part, arteriovenous anastomoses. Observed ventilation–perfusion mismatch satisfactorily accounts for the measured hypoxaemia in those human studies conducted to date, and it should no longer be considered a mystery as to why hypoxaemia occurs following embolism. However, many patients exhibit no blood-gas abnormalities after episodes of documented thromboembolism. This also has a straightforward explanation, at least in theory, although substantiating data are not available. If one assumes absence of any shunting from atelectasis and a normal ventilatory system in such patients, a modest increase in total ventilation can compensate for that 'wasted' portion still delivered to embolized alveoli and allow the remaining non-embolized portion of the lung to function with normal overall levels of both ventilation and blood flow. Physiological dead-space measurement would reveal high values, but absolute levels of arterial P_{O_2} and P_{CO_2} would be entirely normal.

REFERENCES

Fishman, A.P. (1988). *Pulmonary diseases and disorders*, (2nd edn). McGraw-Hill, New York.

Heard, B.E. (1969). *Pathology of chronic bronchitis and emphysema*. Churchill, London.

Hinson, K.F.W. (1970). Diffuse pulmonary fibrosis. *Human Pathology*, **1**, 275–88.

Lemaire, F. *et al.* (1985). Oxygen exchange across the acutely injured lung. In: *Acute respiratory failure* (ed W.M. Zapol and K.J. Falke), p. 540. Dekker, New York.

Rahn, H. and Fenn, W.O. (1955). *A graphical analysis of the respiratory gas exchange. The O_2–CO_2 diagram*. American Physiological Society, Washington, DC.

Weibel, E.R. (1963). *Morphometry of the human lung*. Academic Press, New York.

Weibel, E.R. (1984). *The pathway for oxygen. Structure and function in the mammalian respiratory system*. Harvard University Press, Cambridge, MA.

Weiss, E.B., Segal, M.S., and Stein, M. (1985). *Bronchial asthma. Mechanisms and therapeutics*, (2nd edn). Little, Brown, Boston, MA.

West, J.B. (1987). *Pulmonary pathophysiology—the essentials*, (3rd edn). Williams & Wilkins, Baltimore, MD.

West, J.B. (1990). *Respiratory physiology—the essentials* (4th edn). Williams & Wilkins, Baltimore, MD.

17.5 The clinical presentation of chest diseases

D. J. LANE

The presenting symptoms of chest diseases are few, but the structural and functional disturbances which these symptoms reflect are numerous and the underlying disease entities are very many. It is a useful starting point to consider the symptoms of lower respiratory tract disease under just three headings: cough, breathlessness, and chest pain.

Cough may or may not produce sputum. Patients occasionally report the expectoration of sputum while denying that they have cough. This seems to be a socially determined separation of the act of 'clearing the throat', to expel sputum, from a non-productive cough which, perhaps because it appears to have no purpose, is regarded as more sinister. Breathlessness itself is a complex symptom. Wheezing and stridor, which are audible accompaniments to the act of breathing, are rarely reported without breathlessness and so will be considered with it. Discussion of the third member of the triad, chest pain, will include mention of chest tightness.

In the analysis of symptoms it is important to recognize and differentiate between the pathology or disordered physiology likely to be responsible for the symptoms, and the clinical diagnoses associated with that symptom. The investigation of mechanism, although superficially of little clinical relevance, can be the key to symptomatic treatment, creating opportunities for relief when the underlying condition is untreatable. Knowledge of the clinical significance of symptoms is largely empirical but forms the essential diagnostic base of clinical medicine. Thus research into the mechanisms of breathlessness, for example, will continue to be a proper concern of clinicians as long as disabling and irreversible conditions such as chronic airways obstruction exist. In contrast, knowing the mechanism of dyspnoea in pleural effusion is unimportant compared with knowing how to relieve the dyspnoea by draining the effusion and being able to diagnose the clinical condition causing it.

Cough

Coughing is a defensive reflex designed to clear and protect the lower respiratory tract. The act of coughing is essentially a forced expiratory effort against a transitorily closed glottis, which then opens allowing a sudden expulsion of air from the lungs. Except perhaps when the cough arises from laryngeal irritation, there is an initial deep inspiration which presumably allows the respiratory muscles to act to greater mechanical advantage. However, this could draw the offending material deeper into the bronchial tree. The pressure which builds up behind the closed glottis can reach as much as 40 kPa and, if often repeated in a sequence of coughs, can seriously impede venous filling of the heart. The consequent drop in cardiac output is responsible for the well-described 'cough syncope'.

Mechanism

The cough reflex can be initiated by the stimulation of irritant receptors in the larynx, trachea, and major bronchi. These receptors respond to mechanical irritation by intraluminal material such as mucus, dust, or foreign bodies, and to chemical irritation by fumes and toxic gases such as sulphur dioxide. Mechanical events within the thorax, such as sudden and large changes in airway calibre or lung collapse, can also stimulate cough receptors. The afferent fibres run in the branches of the superior laryngeal nerve and the vagus to the medulla, where the resultant efferent activity of virtually the whole of the respiratory musculature is coordinated. The explosive action of the respiratory muscles produces laryngeal air velocities which can approach the speed of sound and is accompanied by laryngeal and bronchial constriction, mucus secretion, and a transient systemic hypertension.

Causes of cough

An epidemiological analysis of cough would reveal acute viral upper respiratory tract infection affecting the pharynx, larynx, or postnasal space as the most common cause of short-lived cough over all ages, with smoking being the major aetiological factor in chronic cough in adults. A quarter of those smoking 10 cigarettes a day and half of those smoking 20 cigarettes a day, can expect to have a persistent cough. Children exposed to passive smoking from their parents are twice as likely to cough as children in non-smoking families. Asthma is the next commonest cause at all ages with chronic upper or lower respiratory tract infection also important. Tuberculosis heads the list in the developing world. Of the more sinister causes, carcinoma of the lung is the most important. It remains the commonest neoplasm in men and is second only to carcinoma of the breast in women, and must feature high in the differential diagnosis of a new presentation of cough or a change in the character of cough in a middle-aged smoker. Less usual causes are endobronchial sarcoidosis and pulmonary fibrotic conditions. Although rare, inhaled foreign body and drug therapy must not be forgotten because of the potential for cure. Both β-blockers and angiotensin-converting enzyme inhibitors (captopril, enalapril, etc.) can cause an irritating and persistent cough.

Clinical features

The clinical description of cough relies on its sound, its timing, and whether or not there is expectoration. A dry cough with an irritative barking quality, short and often repeated, is heard in inflammatory conditions of the pharynx, tracheobronchitis, and early pneumonia. With laryngitis the sound is harsh and hoarse ('croup'). The long inspiratory sound that gives whooping cough its name is also produced by tracheal and laryngeal inflammation. Abductor paralysis of the vocal cords creates a cough that is prolonged and lowing like the sound of cattle, and hence is described as 'bovine'. The usual cause is pressure on the left recurrent laryngeal nerve by lesions in the thorax: carcinoma of the bronchus or oesophagus, enlarged (usually neoplastic) hilar nodes, or, now very rarely, aortic aneurysm. If similar lesions press on the trachea but spare the nerve, the cough has a hard metallic quality described as 'brassy'. Unilateral abductor palsy of the larynx does not affect the voice, and even with additional abductor palsy the voice often remains good. Complete paralysis of both cords give aphonia and a weak ineffectual cough. Weakness of the thoracic muscles, as in polyneuritis or the muscular dystrophies, will lessen the expulsive force in coughing, as will the general weakness of prostration, toxaemia, or the deeper states of unconsciousness. Cough may be suppressed when there is severe thoracic or upper abdominal pain.

Certain aspects of the timing of coughing may give useful diagnostic clues. A cough that awakens the patient in the small hours of the night suggests asthma; wheezing need not be evident. Cough with expectoration on rising in the morning is characteristic of chronic bronchitis, although it may also be reported by asthmatics. A bout of coughing with food or when lying down after a meal points to oesophageal, pharyngeal, or neuromuscular disease, causing aspiration into the lungs. Changes of posture can also set off coughing in the bronchiectatic; the free expectoration of sputum at any time of day is common in these patients. A dry cough which persists over many weeks can signify a neoplasm, but a non-productive barking cough that has lasted for years is more likely to be a nervous habit often perpetuated by psychogenic factors.

A cough may fail to produce expectoration because there is nothing to produce, because the secretions are swallowed, as is almost universal in children; because there is complete obstruction of the airway, because of weakness as outlined above, or because the secretions are too viscid. In the last four instances the sound quality of the cough differs from that of a dry cough in the sense that secretions can be heard moving in the major airways. This type of cough and the cough productive of sputum can be described as 'moist' or 'loose'.

Phlegm and sputum

Phlegm, the secretions of the lower respiratory tract, is admixed with nasal and pharyngeal secretions as well as saliva to give expectorated sputum. It has been very difficult to study the natural secretions of the healthy tracheobronchial tree in man, for only about 100 ml is produced daily and most of this is swallowed. In disease the quantity of secretions is often sufficient to swamp contamination in the upper respiratory tract,

so that valid observations can be made, but in clinical medicine, no less than in research, it is important to obtain expectorated material that has actually come from the lungs.

Mucus is viscoelastic. Its viscosity or stickiness influences the effect of forces applied to it in coughing. Initially it resists flow and then as increasing force is applied it becomes more and more liquid, returning to its original state when flow stops, rather like a dripless paint. The elasticity of sputum appears to alter with the rate of application of stress to it, and may be important in relation to the rate of beating of the bronchial epithelial cilia. Intrabronchial mucus appears to exist in two layers, one of low viscosity and high elasticity touching the cilia, and above this a more viscous layer which, in disease, carries globules of mucus.

Airway mucus is 95 per cent water and it derives its distinctive physical characteristics from its glycoprotein content, although cystic fibrosis (Chapter 17.9.2) is a clear example of how low water content can have major consequences on the physical properties of airway mucus. Two components in these glycoproteins, sialic acid and sulphate, enable airway mucus to be chemically analysed and identified *in situ* in histological sections. At least four glycoproteins have been identified in human bronchial mucus and are found to be produced in various combinations from different mucous cell types. Serous fluid is produced from other cells in the bronchial glands, and with water, lipids, and proteins makes up a transudate component of sputum that can be separated from the glycoproteins. Although bronchial secretions do not show diagnostically distinctive changes in disease, there is, for example, a shift towards greater glycoprotein production in chronic bronchitis and greater transudate formation in asthma. In infection both components increase and the breakdown of leucocytes and of bronchial mucus increases the DNA content of sputum, making it less viscid. The accumulated debris of cells and microorganisms imparts a yellow colour to infected sputum, and the subsequent action of verdoperoxidase derived from leucocytes gives a green colour.

The distinction between infected and non-infected sputum is one of the most obvious descriptive features of sputum that is relevant in clinical medicine. Non-infected mucoid sputum is variously described as clear, white, or like jelly like. Exceptionally viscid mucoid sputum is sometimes seen in asthma, and the patient may report seeing pellets or even branching plugs of mucus that are presumed to be casts of small bronchi. In bronchopulmonary aspergillosis similar pellets or casts have a dark brown colour. In city dwellers and those in dusty occupations mucoid sputum can be various shades of grey. Coal miners may produce jet black sputum (melanoptysis) if an area of fibrosis breaks down and is expectorated.

In most lower respiratory tract infections pus is admixed with mucus to produce mucopurulent sputum. Pure pus can be expectorated from a lung abscess or from stagnant bronchiectatic cavities. An offensive smell to the sputum, particularly in these last two conditions, often comes from infection with anaerobic organisms. A rarely seen but distinctive brown discoloration ('anchovy sauce') comes from the pus from an amoebic lung abscess (usually secondary to hepatic amoebiasis).

Apart from its appearance, the only other macroscopic attribute to sputum is its quantity. Excessively large quantities of sputum are found in bronchiectasis, particularly where this is widespread, as in cystic fibrosis, and in the rare alveolar cell carcinoma where large quantities of watery mucus may occasionally be produced. The amount of sputum in both chronic bronchitis and asthma is very variable, but can be excessive. Briefly, pulmonary oedema leads to the production of a large quantity of frothy sputum.

Haemoptysis

Patients rightly regard the presence of blood in the sputum as of sinister significance. Despite this, a definite cause of haemoptysis is only found in about half of the cases in most series. In the assessment of haemoptysis it is important to establish first that the blood-stained material has come from the chest and not from the gastrointestinal tract. Some patients find this difficult. Haemoptysis is produced with a 'cough' not a 'retch'. Accompanying features of an appropriate disease are usually present, but it is worth remembering that in haemoptysis there is usually froth due to admixed air, and the blood is bright red and not dark brown. Gastric contents should be acid; bronchial contents should be alkaline. Another trap for the unwary is contamination with blood from the nose or upper respiratory tract.

It is unwise to attribute haemoptysis simply to 'bronchitis' or infection. In bronchiectasis, however, haemoptysis not uncommonly mixes with mucopurulent sputum. In the early stages of pneumococcal pneumonia a 'rusty' staining of mucoid sputum is quite characteristic. In tuberculosis, frank blood in otherwise mucoid sputum is well recognized. Sudden haemoptysis is a hallmark of pulmonary embolism with infarction. In bronchial neoplasia there may be streaking of the sputum with blood or more substantial bleeding with clots, often observed daily. Recurrent blood-staining of the sputum is seen in idiopathic pulmonary haemosiderosis and also, although usually over a shorter time span, in Goodpasture's syndrome, which are both uncommon conditions. Cardiac conditions associated with blood in the sputum are pulmonary oedema, with pink frothy sputum, and mitral stenosis. The recurrent haemoptyses of the latter condition are infrequently seen today. In a general context, it may be necessary to consider thoracic trauma, endometriosis, or a blood coagulation disorder as causes of haemoptysis.

In the investigation of haemoptysis the chest radiograph will often indicate a probable diagnosis, for example an apical tuberculous infiltrate or a neoplastic hilar mass, but this must be backed up by appropriate microbiological or cytological examination of the sputum. Old, presumably healed and calcified, tuberculous lesions may be a sufficient cause for haemoptysis simply due to local bronchiectasis though reactivation, and invasion by mycetoma must be considered. However, bronchiectasis and pulmonary infarction may not be evident on a plain radiograph. Both should give a suggestive history. High resolution CT is increasingly used to diagnose bronchiectasis, and ventilation–perfusion scanning is of great value in diagnosing pulmonary embolism. If examination of the sputum and radiology (plain or specialized) yields no obvious cause for the haemoptysis, then bronchoscopy must be considered. After a single haemoptysis in a young person, this can be deferred for a month. If there has been no recurrence and radiology is normal, no further action need be taken. A recurrence of haemoptysis or a single episode in an older person, particularly a smoker, are indications for early bronchoscopy, not omitting a careful look at the pharynx and larynx. Selective bronchography through the bronchoscope may be useful in delineating areas of unsuspected bronchiectasis, although CT scanning is increasingly favoured as the technique of choice for detecting this condition.

Laboratory examination of sputum

Expectorated sputum should be subjected to microscopic and microbiological investigation as appropriate (see Chapter 17.6.3). Sputum eosinophilia is a good guide to airway allergy. The cytological examination of sputum for malignant cells can only be done by an expert, but in skilled hands it is invaluable and time saving.

Investigating cough

The cause of cough of recent onset will usually be obvious enough. Infection tops the list. Carcinoma must be excluded in the smoker. In the case of persistent cough without apparent cause in a non-smoker, occult asthma should be eliminated first. Hence an assessment of airflow variability using either diurnal peak flows or a histamine reactivity test are first-line investigations (see also Chapter 17.9.1(b)). It is worth looking for chronic sinonasal infection or allergy and then for gastro-oeso-phageal reflux before proceeding to bronchoscopy which statistically is not very rewarding in the context of cough as a lone symptom.

Treatment

The investigation of a patient with cough very often reveals a recognizable cause. This may well be treatable, even if the only appropriate advice is to stop smoking. If the condition is not treatable or if no cause can be found, symptomatic measures need to be considered. Two lines of approach are open: to suppress the cough or, accepting the cough as inevitable, to make expectoration easier.

All cough suppressants in common use act centrally. Most are opiate derivatives. Codeine and pholcodeine have a weak antitussive action, but when made into a sweet syrup they seem to have a soothing effect. Methadone and the stronger opiates are more powerful in suppressing cough, but they depress respiration and also cause constipation. In terminal bronchial carcinoma they are invaluable. Attempts to suppress cough by a peripheral action on bronchial afferent receptors have not been conspicuously successful. Inhaled local anaesthetic may be helpful, and its effect on cough may long outlast its anaesthetic action; it may perhaps break a vicious cycle in which cough leads to throat irritation and hence further stimulus to coughing. Drugs which act on the production of bronchial mucus will lessen cough if its purpose is the expectoration of that mucus. Atropine is used to this end preoperatively, but rarely in disease. Corticosteroids can diminish mucus production in alveolar cell carcinoma and in asthma. In the latter condition disodium cromoglycate will have a similar effect.

Water is said to be the most effective expectorant. Certainly, dehydration causes a drying of the bronchial secretions. However, there are a multitude of agents which are claimed to increase sputum quantity or accelerate its expectoration. The volatile oils such as menthol probably act as direct irritants. The inorganic salts such as potassium iodide probably have to cause vomiting if they are going to assist expectoration. The movement of particles up the mucociliary escalator of the bronchial tree has been charted using radio-isotope techniques and shown to increase under the influence of ingested guiaphenesin (present in several 'cough medicines'), inhaled β-adrenergic agonists and hypertonic (1.2 M) saline.

Attempts to decrease the viscosity of sputum using mucolytic agents have been clinically disappointing, despite definite in vitro evidence of activity. These strictures apply to both bromhexine, now discontinued, and orally administered cysteine derivatives. Inhaled acetylcysteine works more convincingly as a mucolytic but has the great disadvantage of inducing bronchoconstriction.

Most patients with haemoptysis require no more than treatment appropriate to their underlying condition, but occasionally haemoptysis is massive and life-threatening. The recorded mortality of 50 per cent with haemoptysis of 200 ml or more includes patients with initially poor respiratory reserve, as well as those who asphyxiate. At bronchoscopy it may be difficult to locate the source of bleeding, but local endoscopic measures may be applicable (topical adrenaline application, balloon tamponade, and cold saline lavage). An open surgical approach (lobectomy or pneumonectomy) carries a mortality of up to one-third, and if operative intervention is contemplated bronchial arteriography should be considered. The source of bleeding is from the bronchial arteries, so that embolization of the appropriate bronchial artery has been successfully used to control massive haemoptysis in a high proportion of actively bleeding patients. However, its effect is temporary.

Breathlessness

This major symptom of pulmonary, cardiovascular, and other systemic diseases suffers much because it is so frequently referred to by physicians as dyspnoea. Whilst patients sometimes speak of difficulty in breathing, they more frequently use the terms 'breathlessness', 'short of breath', 'out of breath', or even more colloquially 'puffed'. It is usually only on direct questioning that specific features or associations of breathlessness, such as the effect of position, reveal clues that are likely to be useful clinically. Despite the often quoted statement of Comroe that dyspnoea is not tachypnoea, hyperpnoea, or hyperventilation, but difficult, laboured, or uncomfortable breathing, patients are quite unaware of these fine distinctions. Rapid breathing, the necessary increase in ventilation in response to exercise, and ventilation in excess of metabolic requirements are all at times described by patients as breathlessness. Just what degree or quality of awareness of respiratory movement deserves to be called breathlessness is probably indefinable; awareness undoubtedly varies from patient to patient and even within the same subject from time to time. However, the implication of most terms used by patients to describe this type of pulmonary sensation is that in some way the performance of the respiratory apparatus ('breath-') is not meeting ('-less') a demand placed on it.

Pathophysiology

Any attempt to understand breathlessness from the standpoint of disordered physiology must start with a brief description of the appropriate features of the performance of the respiratory apparatus. The respiratory muscles are supplied by motor nerve fibres from cervical and thoracic anterior horn cells, from C3 to T12. Like all other anterior horn cells, the respiratory motor nerve cells are served by pyramidal fibres from the motor cortex in the precentral gyrus. Directives from the cortex enable respiratory movement to be modulated to serve such functions as talking, singing, holding the breath, voluntary hyperventilation, and the performance of lung function tests. This pathway will also be responsible for the conscious, and perhaps unconscious, transmission of anxiety or a calming influence on respiratory performance. However, to an extent that is unparalleled in other mammalian skeletal muscle, the respiratory motor neurones are under dual control, the second component being the motor output from the brain-stem respiratory centres responsible for involuntary or automatic respiratory movement. This is the movement necessary to satisfy metabolic requirements for oxygen supply and carbon dioxide removal.

For the purposes of understanding breathlessness, respiratory centre activity, which is explained in more detail in Chapter 17.9.4, can be seen as being under the influence of chemical and neurogenic stimuli. The chemical stimuli of hypoxia and acidaemia are relevant to the breathlessness of high altitude and diabetic coma. This is not to say that the hyperventilation induced by these means is the sole cause of breathlessness, but to deny that it plays a part is quixotic. The general traffic of neurogenic stimuli impinging on the reticular formation from all sources maintains a certain level of activity in the medullary respiratory neurones irrespective of more specific stimuli. The modest quietening of this activity in sleep is associated with a small drop in minute ventilation, and the dramatic curtailment of spinal ascending information that sometimes occurs following high spinal tractotomy (usually for intractable pain) can completely abolish automatic medullary respiratory activity. There is no clear-cut association between increased reticular formation activity causing hyperventilation and states of breathlessness, but the increase in ventilation at the very onset of exercise is thought to be neurogenic in origin, possibly quite specifically originating from the exercising muscles.

The respiratory centre receives information from the lungs through the vagus nerve. This originates in bronchial epithelial irritant receptors, luminal stretch receptors, and interstitial J receptors within the alveolar and capillary network. Stimulation of all these receptors will produce reflex effects amongst which, for example, tachypnoea might easily make up a component of breathlessness in an appropriate setting. Whether the afferent information travelling up the vagus itself reaches the sensorium, or whether it merely modulates some other afferent pathway, is not clear. Afferent information that undoubtedly reaches consciousness is that concerning the rate and degree of thoracic cage movement and, quite accurately, a sense of lung volume (degree of lung inflation/deflation). This information presumably comes from joint, tendon, and muscle receptors in the chest wall, and for sense of movement (of air) perhaps also from the oropharyngeal mucosa. It seems evident that information from these latter sources is part of natural and healthy sensation; it also seems likely that the same channels will signal increased rate or depth of movement which, if excessive (in some way fairly specifically for that individual), will be described as breathlessness. In exercise the description 'breathless' often comes at the point where the smooth linear relation between ventilation and oxygen consumption is disturbed. Ventilation becomes excessive for metabolic requirements. How this becomes described as a shortness or loss of breath is not at present clear.

Two 'unnatural' respiratory sensations that can only be inadequately mimicked in a healthy individual are those associated with abnormal lung mechanics (e.g. in airways narrowing) and muscle paralysis. An obvious parallel for the first is breathing through an external resistance. This technique has been widely used by those investigating dyspnoea. The useful finding that may have some bearing on the clinical situation is that in resistance breathing the ability to detect an increased load depends not on the absolute magnitude of the load, but on the ratio of that load to the basal, i.e. pre-existing, loading of the system. Thus a given absolute increase in airways resistance will be much more obvious to an individual with near normal airways function than to one already suffering a considerable increase in resistance due to airways narrowing. The sensations of those few normal individuals who have undergone muscle paralysis (usually curarization) for experimental purposes include phrases such as 'choking' and 'I would give anything to be able to take one deep breath'. These are similar to the reported symptoms of patients with paralytic diseases affecting the respiratory muscles. The element of inadequate performance is stressed. Whether this sensation can be at all simulated by the voluntary withholding of respiratory movement, as in breath-holding, is very doubtful. This much studied experimental. model undoubtedly gives sensations most of which probably arise from the diaphragm twitching ineffectually. It is difficult to see where this fits into a clinical setting.

If any common thread can be drawn between these examples, it is at the level of an interaction between the drive to breathing and achievement—a drive that fails to achieve because of poor performance or mechanical loading of the respiratory system. The neurophysiological implications of this hypothesis are that there should be monitoring systems for both drive and performance. It is obviously feasible for the brain to assess and in some way sum the various drives to breathing, but suggestions have also been made that there may be a monitoring system for motor output. The muscle spindle has been proposed as the probably detector of achievement, but several objections exist to this proposal, not least that there are relatively few muscle spindles in the diaphragm, which is the most important muscle of respiration.

When it comes to the application of these principles to disease, some parallels are obvious, but an example from one common condition—acute bronchial asthma—will illustrate that the situation is not straightforward and is frequently multifactorial. In acute asthma there may be excessive drive from bronchial irritant receptors, and there is often cortical drive expressing itself in anxiety, even panic, as well as hyperventilation. There is clearly poor performance on account of the increased resistance of narrowed airways, but in addition it seems likely that the respiratory muscles will act at a mechanical disadvantage on account of lung hyperinflation.

The clinical analysis of breathlessness

Whilst bearing these neurophysiological points in mind when it comes to devising symptomatic measures for the relief of breathlessness, the

Table 1 *Conditions causing breathlessness classified by rate of onset*

1. Dramatically sudden: over minutes
   Pneumothorax
   Pulmonary embolism
   Pulmonary oedema
2. Acute: over hours
   Pneumonia
   Acute pulmonary infiltrations, e.g. allergic alveolitis
   Asthma
   Left ventricular failure
3. Subacute: over days
   Pleural effusion
   Bronchogenic carcinoma
   Subacute pulmonary infiltrations, e.g. sarcoidosis
4. Chronic: over months or years
   Chronic airflow obstruction
   Diffuse fibrosing conditions
   Chronic non-pulmonary causes, e.g. anaemia,
       hyperthyroidism
5. Intermittent: episodic breathlessness
   Asthma
   Left ventricular failure

Table 2 *The Medical Research Council breathlessness scale*

1. Troubled by shortness of breath when hurrying on level
   ground or walking up a slight hill
2. Short of breath when walking with other people of own age
   on level ground
3. Have to stop for breath when walking at own pace on level
   ground

Table 3 *A classification of acute breathlessness by grade of severity (based on the Jones index)*

Grade I	Able to do housework or job with difficulty
Grade IIa	Confined to chair/bed but able to get up with moderate difficulty
Grade IIb	Confined to chair/bed and only able to get up with great difficulty
Grade III	Totally confined to a chair or bed
Grade IV	Moribund

clinician must still largely rely on an empirical approach to the analysis of this symptom. Such an analysis will rely on four characteristics of breathlessness: its quality, its timing, its severity, and the circumstances which precipitate or relieve it.

QUALITY

Breathlessness is difficult to describe. Most patients can go no further than saying that they are 'short of breath'. The asthmatic will generally recognize the quality of wheeze and, contrary to the opinion of physiologists, usually finds it more difficult to breathe in than out. An asthmatic who develops more persistent breathlessness between attacks often recognizes this as 'different from my asthma'. A sense of suffocation is a feature of massive pleural effusions and of pulmonary oedema. Phrases such as 'I can't fill my lungs properly' and 'I need to take a big breath' suggest the possibility of psychogenic breathlessness, but muscle weakness must be carefully excluded.

TIMING

Of the greatest value in separating out conditions likely to be associated with breathlessness is noting its rate of onset. There are five categories.

Breathlessness may be of dramatic onset (over minutes), acute onset (over hours), subacute onset (over weeks), or chronic onset (over months or years), or it may be intermittent. Table 1 gives a guide to conditions falling into these categories. The subdivisions are not rigid. Asthma again provides an example. About half of all acute attacks of asthma build up in less than 24 h, but some asthmatics slowly deteriorate over a week or so and occasionally, when they are anaphylactoid features perhaps with laryngeal spasm as well, they can be transformed from an asymptomatic state to desperate breathlessness and unconsciousness within 15 min. Of course, asthma is also intermittent although some patients have chronic exertional breathlessness as well. Likewise, left ventricular failure, although usually developing over hours, may be dramatic in, for example, aortic valve rupture or more persistent in long-standing hypertension. The pattern of breathlessness in certain disorders depends on the stage of the disease and the structural or functional changes that it causes. Thus in early sarcoidosis diffuse infiltration of the lungs can cause the quite rapid development of breathlessness over several days or a week or so; in contrast, the late fibrotic stage of sarcoid will be associated with relentlessly progressive breathlessness as pulmonary reserve diminishes. Breathlessness in a condition such as carcinoma of the lung will be determined by the pattern of structural change—whether there is, for example, bronchial stenosis, collapse, or pleural effusion.

SEVERITY

The severity of breathlessness is gauged traditionally on scales relating to activity. Two such scales (one from the Medical Research Council chronic bronchitis questionnaire and the other the Jones index for acute asthma) are shown in Tables 2 and 3. Many other scales have been devised. All have two faults. The first is that there is a temptation to assume that the grading system with which one is familiar is universally known; it is not and thus it is usually preferable to describe the amount of exercise limitation. Secondly, no scale suggests a convention for dealing with variable breathlessness. Very few patients have a consistent level of severity of breathlessness, but any attempt to introduce a range of severity will have to be accompanied by some assessment of the time extent of each grade, which is an almost impossible task.

A refinement of the scaling technique can be used to record the degree of breathlessness during exercise. During a standard exercise test a record is made of breathlessness on a visual analogue scale concurrently with minute ventilation. The sort of data produced can be used to assess the benefits of therapeutic intervention (Fig. 1). The Borg scale (Table 4) can be adapted similarly and has been used with simpler exercise tests. Caution needs to be expressed about popular tests such as the distance walked in a specified time (e.g. 6 or 12 minute walk). Apart from the effects of training and motivation, patients may differ in their approach to a treatment benefit. One might walk no further and be relieved to achieve the same distance with less breathlessness, whereas another might extend the walking distance by being prepared to become just as breathless as before.

OCCURRENCE

The circumstances under which breathlessness is experienced can give important diagnostic clues. Only psychogenic breathlessness bears no relation to exertion or is experienced only at rest, although many patients with organic diseases are breathless at rest as well as on exertion; this is an expression of the severity of their breathlessness. Breathlessness made worse by lying flat (orthopnoea) is characteristic of left ventricular failure and is also experienced by patients with diaphragmatic paralysis. Nocturnal awakening with suffocating breathlessness and frothy sputum production (paroxysmal nocturnal dyspnoea) is a more serious manifestation of left ventricular failure and can be relieved by sitting or standing up. The asthmatic also awakens in the small hours of the night with breathlessness accompanied by coughing and wheezing, or these symp-

Table 4 *Modified Borg Scale**

Number	Verbal description
10	Severe
9	
8	Moderately severe
7	
6	
5	Moderate
4	
3	
2	Slight
1	
0	None

*Modified from Borg, G.A.V. (1982). Psychological basis of perceived exertion. *Medical Science of Sports and Exercise*, **14**, 377-81.

toms may be delayed until the normal awakening hours. Any sputum produced by the asthmatic under these circumstances is likely to be sticky and mucoid. Postexertional breathlessness and the immediate triggering of an episode of wheezing breathlessness by non-specific irritants (dust and fumes) or specifically allergic stimuli (pollen, animal danders, etc.) also characterize the asthmatic. In occupational asthmas breathlessness will bear a temporal and circumstantial relation to the working environment. In byssinosis the first day at work is characteristically troublesome (Monday morning tightness). Patients with type III hypersensitivity reactions such as bronchopulmonary aspergillosis (Chapter 17.9.1(b)) or extrinsic allergic alveolitis (Chapter 17.10.9) will notice breathlessness 4–6 hours after exposure. An intercurrent respiratory tract infection will worsen breathlessness in patients with any form of diffuse airway or parenchymatous lung disease.

Spontaneous improvement occurs in most breathless patients with rest or the removal of trigger factors; the postexertional breathlessness of the asthmatic is an important though temporary exception. Patients with pulmonary hypertension, even with severe exertional breathlessness, improve dramatically quickly immediately they sit down.

Fig. 1 Mean relationships between breathlessness and ventilation for six healthy subjects during identical periods of submaximal graded exercise. Increasing breathlessness during exercise is shown in the panel on the left, and decreasing breathlessness during recovery is shown on the right. (Reproduced from Stark, R.D. (1988). Dyspnoea: assessment and pharmacological manipulation. *European Respiratory Journal*, **1**, 280–7, with permission.)

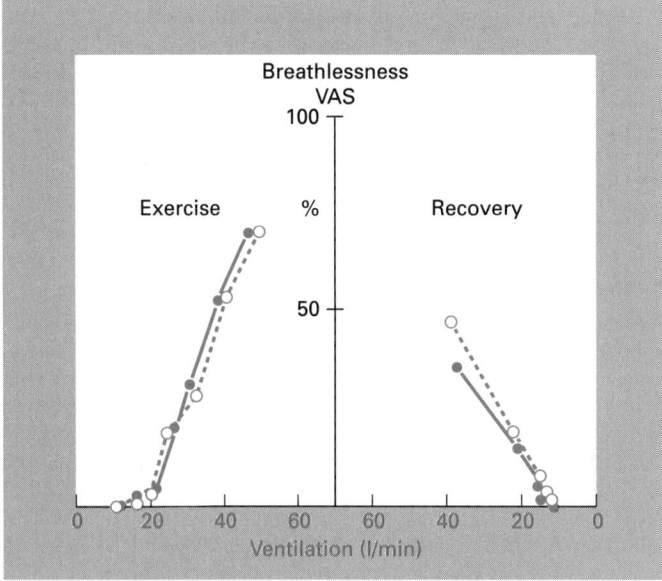

Breathlessness as an isolated symptom is likely to be due to diffuse parenchymal lung disease such as emphysema or diffuse fibrosis, pulmonary hypertension, or to extrathoracic conditions.

The investigation of the breathless patient

The clinical history may immediately suggest a probable cause. Beyond this the two most helpful pointers are simple lung function tests and chest radiology. Spirometric testing will define three groups; normal, an obstructive pattern, and a restrictive pattern (see Chapter 17.6.2). The chest radiograph will be of most value in furthering the diagnosis in conditions giving a restrictive pattern. The further investigation of the patient with airflow obstruction is dealt with in Chapters 17.9.1(b) and 17.9.4.

Breathlessness in a patient with normal spirometric testing and a clear chest radiograph presents special problems. Four categories should be considered. Is there intermittent disease? Are the tests being used too crude to pick up significant abnormalities? Is there extrathoracic disease? Is this psychogenic breathlessness?

Many asthmatics reviewed in a clinic will have normal lung function. The value of serial recordings of lung function over several days in these patients cannot be overemphasized. Conditions affecting the heart and pulmonary circulation may also be intermittent, but more often the problem is that conventional tests of lung function do not seem to demonstrate significant abnormalities when there is quite considerable dyspnoea. Pulmonary embolism is a good example of this. Tests for muscle power and the integrity of the pulmonary vascular bed are required to diagnose early neuromuscular conditions weakening respiratory movement and the easily missed pulmonary hypertension. The hyperventilation of acidosis as in uraemia or diabetic coma is not often described by patients as breathlessness and is otherwise easily diagnosed. However, hyperthyroidism and anaemia should not be forgotten as causes of breathlessness. It is said that 60 per cent of patients with a haemoglobin level of less than 8 g/dl will have this symptom.

Psychogenic breathlessness is a diagnosis by exclusion, although there may be clues in the history and examination. The quality of the breathlessness has been described above. The sighing and irregular breathing will be readily noticeable to a keen observer (Fig. 2). Associated complaints directly related to the hyperventilation are paraesthesiae in the hands and perhaps feet, tetany, dizziness, and collapse. Apparently non-specific features such as fatigue, insomnia, muscle weakness, or vague chest pains may all be part of the syndrome. Depression and anxiety may both be aspects of the underlying psychiatric state. By definition, in pure psychogenic breathlessness, the chest radiograph and lung function are normal. However, some patients may develop

Fig. 2 Patterns of breathing . Upper trace, normal. Lower traces: patients with psychogenic breathlessness.

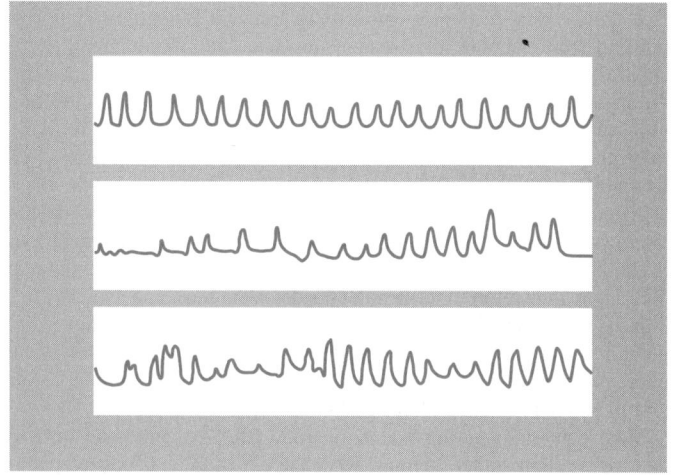

breathlessness because they have been told that they have a 'shadow on the lung' or through anxiety exhibit a degree of breathlessness disproportionate to a mild functional abnormality. The latter patients tend to have an obsessional personality or may be looking for compensation for supposed 'lung damage' due to injury or to their occupation. The obverse of this situation—the patient with a severe lung function abnormality, usually airflow obstruction, who is little distressed by breathlessness—is discussed on Chapter 17.14.1.

Treatment

The relief of breathlessness is best achieved by treating the underlying condition. This may mean the removal of 'mass' lesions (pneumothorax, pleural effusion) or the treatment of pneumonia or alveolitis. In airflow obstruction useful reversibility often follows appropriate treatment. Loss of muscle power is occasionally treatable, as in myasthenia gravis, or may recover spontaneously. An approach to breathlessness through these channels must not be neglected even when the underlying condition is untreatable (pleural effusion in carcinoma of the bronchus, or a reversible steroid-responsive component in a patient with chronic airflow obstruction).

The symptomatic treatment of breathlessness is far from satisfactory. It may be usefully considered along the lines of disordered physiology. An excessive drive may be dampened, for example oxygen for the hypoxic. A direct approach to the vagal afferent system has met with little success; local anaesthetic to the airways gives a short-lived effect and may itself be irritant. In a select few with intense breathlessness due to diffuse infiltrative disease, vagotomy in the thorax has given some relief. Psychogenic breathlessness may be helped with β-blockers (but asthma must be excluded with absolute certainty). Dihydrocodeine reduces breathlessness in chronic obstructive lung disease but is very constipating and, like the more powerful opiate sedatives, can dangerously depress respiration. There has been a sad failure to find opiate derivatives with a more selective action on breathlessness. Diazepam and promethazine have given subjective relief to some patients disabled by breathlessness from severe emphysema. The use of rehabilitation measures is considered on Chapter 17.14.3(b).

Chest pain

The greater part of the lower respiratory tract is insensitive to pain. Most parenchymal lung disorders proceed to an advanced state without pain. However, the parietal pleura is exquisitely sensitive to painful stimuli and unpleasant sensations can arise from the tracheobronchial tree.

Pleurisy

Typical pleural pain has a sharp stabbing and knife-like character and is accentuated by respiratory movement. Hence it is aggravated by respiration and coughing, thus leading to rapid shallow breathing and a suppressed cough. That it is less obvious during expiration than inspiration is one reason for now believing that the pain is not due to friction between the two roughened inflamed surfaces. The pain is more likely to be due to stretching of the inflamed parietal pleura and can be relieved by splinting the chest wall.

Afferent pain fibres from the rib cage pleural surface pass up the intercostal nerves. Those from the central portion of the diaphragm run in the phrenic nerve to the cervical cord (C3/4). Central diaphragmatic pleurisy is thus referred to the lateral side of the neck and shoulder tip; indeed, local anaesthesia to the shoulder trigger area can relieve diaphragmatic pleurisy. The outer portions of the diaphragm are served by intercostal nerves (T7–12), causing referred pain to be felt in the lower thorax, lumbar region, and upper abdomen.

Most conditions giving rise to pleuritic pain are acute and inflammatory in origin: either infective when there is usually associated pneu-monia (pleurisy is particularly common in pneumococcal pneumonia) or infarctive as in pulmonary embolism. The immunologically based pleurisies (as in systemic lupus erythematosus or rheumatoid disease) give pain rather less frequently. Recurrent pleurisy at the same site should suggest bronchiectasis; at different sites it suggests embolism or bronchopulmonary aspergillosis.

If pleurisy progresses to pleural effusion, the sharp pain largely disappears and is replaced by a dull and more constant ache or heaviness, quantitatively roughly proportional to the amount of fluid. Pleural fibrotic disease is rarely painful, but pleural neoplasia frequently is. The severity and quality of pain depends on the degree of pleural inflammation and the extent of the tumour, particularly outside the chest. A superior sulcus tumour of bronchial origin (Pancoast's tumour) infiltrating the brachial plexus gives very severe and persistent pain in the shoulder and in the distribution of C8, T1, and T2. Later complications are wasting down the inner side of the arm and Horner's syndrome from involvement of the cervical sympathetic trunk.

Pain from the chest wall

Chest-wall pain can mimic pleurisy, and conditions in the chest wall provide its most important differentials. Pain due to strain or tearing of thoracic muscles can be quite sharp, and since it may be caused by coughing and may cause shallow respiration, it can easily be confused with pleurisy. However, there is always local tenderness over the affected muscle and none of the ancillary investigations for pleurisy prove positive. Patients with persistent cough or distressing breathlessness, particularly due to asthma, may complain of muscular pain around the lower rib cage.

Epidemic myalgia or Bornholm disease (see Section 7) is a bothersome manifestation of Coxsackie B infection giving fever and recurrent muscle pain. If the intercostal muscles are involved (pleurodynia), the associated breathlessness and tachypnoea can exactly mimic pleurisy, as can the pre-eruptive stage of thoracic herpes zoster which gives a stabbing pain in the distribution of the affected nerve. Costal cartilage pain is generally not inflammatory. In Tietze's disease there is a painful protuberance of one or more costal cartilages, usually the second to fourth, probably due to asymmetrical growth of the rib cage. Osteoarthritis and dislocation of the costosternal joints can give chronic pain. Rib fractures rarely present diagnostic problems; cough fracture in osteoporotic bone should be remembered. Thrombophlebitis of chest-wall vessels after surgery or trauma gives anterior chest pain and a tender palpable vascular cord. Most primary chest-wall tumours are not painful, but the more common metastatic disease of bone frequently is, and may be symptomatic before radiological change is evident.

Fleeting transient chest pains are often part of chronic somatized anxiety states, and when this is the case tend to be accompanied by tachycardia, palpitations, and features indicating hyperventilation. Perhaps the commonest chest pain of all is left inframammary pain. This is a transitory sharp but quite severe pain, felt over the apex of the heart at rest or on mild activity. It lasts up to a few minutes and may cause a catching of the breath or shallow breathing. Its cause is unknown but it seems to be totally benign.

Central chest pain

Sensations arising from the tracheobronchial tree are less easy to characterize as painful, although some are exceedingly unpleasant. Instrumentation of the trachea causes pain referred to the anterior chest wall. This is usually abolished by vagotomy and is most likely to be perceived from irritant receptor discharge. Tracheal inflammation, as in infective tracheobronchitis or following the inhalation of toxic vapours, causes a raw painful sensation retrosternally. It is difficult to say how much or how often sensations arising from the main airways are describable as pain. There is often a component of what is described by the patient as tightness. This sensation is a common complaint of patients with generalized airflow obstruction, although it is probably naive to think that the sensation is a direct appreciation of airways narrowing. Further complicating the interpretation of sensation in these conditions is the almost universal association with coughing which, if persistent, can itself lead to soreness in the upper airways and trachea.

Finally, the mediastinal structures of the thorax are responsible for a multitude of pains, the majority of which are dealt with elsewhere in the sections on cardiology and gastrointestinal disease. Myocardial ischaemia, pericarditis, pulmonary embolism, aneurysm, oesophagitis, and referred abdominal pain will all need to be considered in the differential diagnosis of central chest pain. Most have distinctive features that will rarely lead to confusion with the few central pulmonary lesions likely to give mediastinal pain. As well as pain due to inflammatory conditions of the trachea, only neoplasia is a common culprit. A central bronchial carcinoma or hilar nodes associated with it can be responsible for a deep dull aching pain in the centre of the chest. A similar pain may occasionally be recorded in the early stages of sarcoidosis with hilar lymphadenopathy and in lymphoma.

Other pulmonary symptoms

Patients or their relatives on their behalf may complain of noisy breathing, generally using the word 'wheeze'. A harsh inspiratory wheezing sound arising from obstruction in the larynx or major airways is termed stridor. There may be accompanying hoarseness or features of intrathoracic disease. Wheeze is the externally audible counterpart of the sounds heard with the stethoscope in asthma and obstructive bronchitis. It is a term frequently used by asthmatic patients to describe their respiratory symptoms.

When airflow obstruction is suspected, specific enquiries should be made for the features of bronchial irritability. In response to changes in atmospheric conditions (particularly temperature) or to the inhalation of dusts, fumes, or vapours, the patient with irritable bronchi will respond with a variety of symptoms: cough, tightness in the chest, wheeze, or breathlessness.

Rarely, patients may complain that they are cyanosed, although their carers may do so more often. This and finger clubbing are more often elicited as physical signs (see below).

General history in the patient with pulmonary disease

A full history is essential, emphasizing the following features: (a) the cardiovascular system for features which might indicate cardiac disease as a cause or aggravating factor in breathlessness; (b) the legs for fluid retention (ankle oedema) as a result of lung disease or any suggestion of deep venous thrombosis; (c) the upper respiratory tract for infective allergic or vasculitic disorders; (d) the skin for a history of eczema, urticaria erythema nodosum, or vasculitis; (e) the locomotor system or elsewhere for the features of rheumatoid or collagen-vascular disease; (f) the nervous system for the effects of respiratory failure or neuromuscular disease that might impair ventilatory control; (g) many systems for pointers to metastatic spread or the non-metastatic manifestations of malignant disease.

The past history may reveal atopy or other allergic disease, tuberculosis, or other serious infective disease particularly in childhood. It is always worth asking about previous chest radiographs which may be obtainable for comparison.

Note must be made of smoking history because of its influence as an aetiological factor and alcoholism because of its effects on antibacterial defences. Steroid and immunosuppressive therapy will also depress defences, and a detailed drug history is essential because of the wide variety of toxic effects on the lungs which are now recognized (see Chapter 17.10.19).

A complete occupational and environmental history is of the utmost importance. Whilst the mining industries will be obvious, many other occupations which create dusts of both inorganic and organic materials are now recognized as presenting hazards to the chest (see Chapter 17.10.16). Certain working environments may lead to exposure to organisms likely to cause pulmonary infection: *Chlamydia psittaci* from contact with domestic or wild birds, *Coxiella burnetti* in slaughterhouses and amongst cattle, and tuberculosis through working with immigrants or vagrants.

Finally certain disorders have a familial predisposition. These include asthma and other atopic diseases (see Chapter 17.9.1(b)), cystic fibrosis (see Chapter 17.9.2), Kartagener's syndrome, familial fibrocystic pulmonary dysplasia (a form of fibrosing alveolitis) (see Chapter 17.10.2), pulmonary lymphangiomyomatosis (see Chapter 17.10.8), and alveolar microlithiasis (see Chapter 17.10.15). A family or personal contact history of tuberculosis should be noted, as should any record of previous tuberculin testing or BCG.

Physical signs in pulmonary disease

Inspection of the chest

The pattern of breathing and the configuration of the chest must be observed. The normal respiratory rate when the subject believes himself to be unobserved is around 10 to 14 per minute. Higher rates than this are commonly recorded in the healthy, but a rate above 20 per minute is abnormal. Pneumonia, many interstitial lung disorders, and abnormal drives to breathing, including anxiety, will increase rate. If the chest is free to move, the tidal volume will also increase, but this is not the case with restrictive disease or painful conditions of the thoracic cage or upper abdomen. An abrupt stop to inspiration when there is pain can be seen. The frequency of deep sighs, normally 8 to 10 per hour in quiet breathing, is greatly increased in psychogenic breathlessness when there may be a quite irregular breathing pattern including phases of rapid breaths or relative apnoea. A regular alternation of apnoeic periods of 5 to 30 s with a period of increasing and then decreasing ventilation characterizes Cheyne–Stokes respiration. This and several other irregular breathing patterns are usually associated with brain-stem or cerebral lesions but can also be a feature of severe heart failure.

In observing respiratory movement, particular attention must be paid to expansion. Poor movement of the chest on one side only always indicates pathology on that side. Generally poor expansion is seen in the hyperinflated chest of the patient with severe airflow obstruction and in the fixed thoracic cage of advanced ankylosing spondylitis. In airflow obstruction two other features may be observed: an indrawing of intercostal spaces during inspiration (reflecting the negative intrapleural pressure necessary to draw air into the lungs) and abnormal movement over the lower chest. Normally, the lower chest moves outwards during inspiration. In gross hyperinflation the diaphragm is flat and its contraction merely causes the lower thoracic cage to move inwards. In the same patients the anterior abdominal wall may move inwards during inspiration instead of outwards. This asynchrony of movement carries a poor prognosis.

Abnormalities of the shape of the chest are well recognized. An increased anteroposterior diameter to give a 'barrel chest' is as often a sign of the kyphosis that accompanies senile osteoporosis as it is of the hyperinflation of emphysema and chronic airflow obstruction. Pectus carinatum (pigeon chest), an outward protuberance of the sternum, may reflect severe attacks of asthma in childhood when it may be accompanied by bilateral indrawing of the anterior portions of the lower ribs (Harrison's sulci); it is now rarely due to rickets. The opposite, pectus excavatum (depressed sternum), is a congenital anomaly (see Chapter 17.12). Scoliosis of skeletal origin is of importance because of the severe impairment of respiratory movement that it causes, and it can lead to respiratory failure (see Chapter 17.12). Localized collapse and fibrosis may draw in the adjacent rib cage (which will also move poorly) and, if severe, unilateral fibrosis of the whole lung can cause a scoliosis with its curvature towards the affected lung.

Palpation of the chest

Palpation is used to confirm the observed patterns of chest expansion and to identify the position of the trachea and apex beat. The trachea should be localized in the suprasternal notch with the index finger. With the patient looking directly forwards, any deviation of the trachea from the mid-line should be assessed using a combination of touch and vision. Deviation of the trachea to one side is due to either apical fibrosis pulling it to the affected side or a mass in the neck (e.g. goitre) or upper mediastinum pushing the trachea across to the opposite side. As with the trachea, the position of the apex beat can reflect pressure against or traction on mediastinal structures, but due consideration must be given to displacement of the apex beat due to intrinsic cardiac disease.

The detection of the transmission of vocal sounds by the placing the palm of the hand on the chest (vocal fremitus) should be abandoned in favour of vocal resonance (listening with the stethoscope for voice sounds), except for simultaneous comparison of the two sides of the chest.

Percussion of the chest

In properly performed percussion the examiner listens for the pitch and loudness of the percussed note, and both listens and feels for the post-percussive vibrations which give the note its resonance. The sides of the chest must be compared from identical sites. A dull note lacks resonance and is higher in pitch and softer than a normal percussion note; it signifies the presence of solid tissue or fluid underneath the percussed area. 'Stony' dullness with a complete lack of any vibrations coming back from the lung is heard over pleural effusions. It is important to delineate the surface markings of the dullness. Pneumonic consolidation and collapse will follow the distribution of the affected lobe, whereas the upper limit of a pleural effusion will be determined by the effects of gravity. It requires a fine ear to pick up Ellis's S-shaped line—a slightly higher level of dullness in the axilla when the patient is in the sitting position. Large effusions which displace mediastinal contents may produce an area of dullness at the opposite base close to the mid-line (Grocco's sign).

A hyper-resonant note is lower in pitch and louder than normal, and occurs over hyperinflated lung as in emphysema or an air-filled space, i.e. a large bulla or a pneumothorax. It is more difficult to be certain about hyper-resonance than dullness, particularly in thin subjects.

Auscultation of the chest

Three types of sound can be heard coming from the lung: breath sounds, adventitious sounds, and voice sounds.

BREATH SOUNDS

Normal breath sounds are better termed 'normal' rather than 'vesicular'. They are certainly not generated in the vesicles or alveoli of the lung where air flow is too low, but probably reflect turbulent flow in major bronchi. The pattern and intensity of breath sounds reflects regional ventilation. Thus in the normal upright lung breath sounds are loudest at the apex in early inspiration and at the bases in mid-inspiration. Breath sounds are quietened over areas of atelectasis. During expiration normal breath sounds rapidly fade out, probably due to decreasing air flow rate. Bronchial breathing is heard over airless lung as in consolidation, atelectasis, or dense fibrosis. There is some resemblance to the sounds heard over the normal trachea, but, by comparison with normal breath sounds, bronchial breathing is higher in pitch and more blowing in quality. It does not have to be loud. Bronchial breath sounds are classically heard throughout both inspiration and expiration. Very quiet breath sounds are heard over hyperinflated lungs as in emphysema or when breath sounds are prevented from reaching the chest wall by a layer of air or fluid (pneumothorax, pleural effusion, malignancy).

ADVENTITIOUS SOUNDS

The terminology of adventitious sounds is confused. This arises because, whereas Laennec originally used the term râles (rattle) to embrace all added sounds, Latham, introducing the classification dry and moist sounds in 1876, applied râle exclusively to the former and rhonchi to the latter. Until recently the established convention in the United Kingdom was to drop râle altogether and to call interrupted non-musical sounds crepitations and continuous musical sounds rhonchi. The move to replace the term crepitations with crackles and the term rhonchi with wheezes has now gained widespread acceptance. Crackles may be coarse or moist when they are due to the movement of sputum in large airways, or fine when they are probably created by small airways snapping open as pressure equalizes in the distal lung compartment. Coarse early inspiratory and expiratory crackles are often heard in respiratory tract infection, particularly in patients with chronic obstructive lung disease, whilst fine late inspiratory crackles are characteristic of pulmonary oedema and fibrosing alveolitis. Occasionally a single mid to late inspiratory 'squawk' is heard in patients with a variety of pulmonary fibroses.

Wheezes signify obstruction in airways. A sound of single pitch (monophonic) in inspiration and/or expiration, which cannot be altered by coughing to shift mucus, signifies localized obstruction in a major airway. Several sounds of varying pitch (polyphonic) heard randomly in inspiration and expiration are typical of the widespread airways obstruction of asthma and chronic obstructive bronchitis. A polyphonic wheeze on forced expiration signifies diffuse airflow obstruction and can be a useful sign when tidal breathing is free of added sounds.

A pleural rub is the diagnostic added sound of pleurisy. It is a superficial grating or rasping sound synchronous with late inspiration and early expiration, best heard at the bases and rarely at the apices. A soft friction rub may be mistaken for crepitations but is not altered by coughing; it can be made louder by pressure with the stethoscope. Inflammation of the pleura close to the heart can give a friction rub that synchronizes with the heart beat but will cease if the breath is held.

VOICE SOUNDS

A long sound such as 'ninety-nine' is favoured for detecting voice sounds which are transmitted by normal lung, but not by air space or fluid, and pass through solid lung with undue clarity, even allowing whispered sounds to be heard (whispering pectoriloquy). Certain physical characteristics of solid lung allow low frequency sounds to be filtered out, leaving a sound of bleating or nasal quality (aegophony); this is particularly noticeable over collapsed lung adjacent to a pleural effusion.

The relevance of the general examination in respiratory disease

Clues to the diagnosis of respiratory disease and critical extrathoracic manifestations of primary lung conditions must be sought in the general examination.

OVERALL APPEARANCE

Obesity places an added burden on the respiratory system, sometimes sufficient in itself to cause a degree of exertional breathlessness and potentially a cause of obstructive sleep apnoea (see Chapter 17.14.2). Truncal obesity with moon facies and skin bruising is an unfortunate complication of oral corticosteroid therapy which may have to be given for several pulmonary diseases.

Weight loss is a feature of emphysematous obstructive lung disease and, of course, malignancy, with the late stages of bronchial carcinoma and pleural mesothelioma often being characterized by a distressing cachexia. Malabsorption can result in weight loss in cystic fibrosis if inadequately managed.

Body habitus can alert to possible respiratory complications, particularly the more severe degrees of kyphoscoliosis, which can lead to hypoventilation, and also rarer disorders such as Marfan's syndrome (associated with pneumothorax) or ankylosing spondylitis.

CYANOSIS

Cyanosis is the blue discoloration imparted to the nail beds, lips, and tongue by hypoxaemic blood. Peripheral cyanosis due to a sluggish peripheral circulation as in cold weather will leave the tongue still pink, whereas in central cyanosis the tongue will be blue and the peripheries blue yet often warm. The frequently repeated statement that 5 g of reduced haemoglobin is required before cyanosis can be detected is false. Most patients with a saturation of 90 per cent or less will appear cyanosed. This represents just 1.5 g of reduced haemoglobin if the total haemoglobin is 15 g. Cyanosis is less marked in severe anaemia and more obvious in polycythaemia. The curious phenomenon of orthocyanosis (due to hypoxia occurring only in the upright position) is generally associated with pulmonary arteriovenous malformations.

THE SKIN AND EYES

Eczema and urticaria point to an atopic diathesis and hence possible asthma. Erythema multiforme can accompany mycoplasma pneumonia, rarely other pneumonias, and pulmonary blastomycosis. Erythema nodosum, tender nodules fading to a bruised purple on the shins and occasionally the forearms, is a classical presentation of sarcoidosis, frequently associated with hilar lymphadenopathy and less often with pulmonary infiltrates. It may also be found in primary tuberculosis and rarely in other chest infections.

Several other dermatological, ocular, arthritic, and internal manifestations may also alert to the diagnosis of sarcoid. Skin and eyes are also the site of lesions in Wegener's granulomatosis, systemic lupus erythematosus, systemic sclerosis, and dermatomyositis, each of which has potential pulmonary manifestations.

Patients with diffuse neurofibromatosis and tuberous sclerosis can both develop a severe pulmonary fibrosis with late-stage destructive emphysema. Rarely, hereditary haemorrhagic telangiectasia with its characteristic lesions on the lips, face, and mouth can extend to the lungs with pulmonary haemangiomas which give haemoptysis as well as the more commonly found gastrointestinal lesions. The latter give anaemia, and this, whatever its cause, can cause breathlessness and so must be checked for, as must jaundice in looking at the eyes.

The skin is the site of secondary deposits from carcinoma of the lung in a small percentage of cases, although usually late in the disease when the diagnosis is all too obvious. Other carcinomas may spread to skin and lungs, and Kaposi's sarcoma is a cutaneous manifestation of disseminated HIV infection (see Chapter 17.10.29).

CLUBBING OF THE FINGERS

Loss of the natural angle between the nail and the nail bed in a properly manicured finger, and a boggy fluctuation of the nail bed are cardinal signs of clubbing (Fig. 3). An increased curvature of the nail and enlargement of the end of the finger develop later. The toes may also be affected. The differential diagnosis of clubbing of the fingers includes many extrathoracic conditions but, as far as the lungs are concerned, three categories deserve consideration: (a) suppurative disease, particularly bronchiectasis of long standing and also, acutely, lung abscess and empyema but not uncomplicated bronchitis; (b) fibrosing alveolitis and asbestosis, but rarely other diffuse fibrotic diseases; (c) malignant disease, particularly carcinoma of the bronchus and also pleural malignancy. If finger clubbing is associated with hypertrophic pulmonary osteoarthropathy, a painful osteitis of the distal ends of the long bones of the lower arms and legs, there is associated malignancy in 95 per cent of cases.

There is no totally satisfactory explanation for clubbing and hypertrophic pulmonary osteoarthropathy. Pathologically, there is abnormal vascularity and new bone formation in the peripheries, and evidence of abnormal bronchopulmonary anastomoses in the lungs. The latter may be under vagal control since vagotomy has sometimes abolished clubbing in lung cancer patients. These intrathoracic channels may allow substances normally detoxified by the lungs, which could be responsible for the peripheral changes, to enter the systemic solution. There is evidence to support a role for reduced ferritin in this respect.

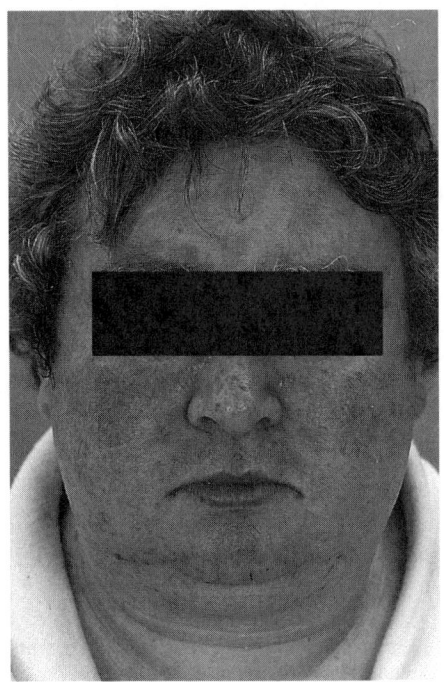

Fig. 4 Local extension of central bronchogenic carcinoma, causing superior vena-caval obstruction.

Fig. 3 Clubbing of the fingers.

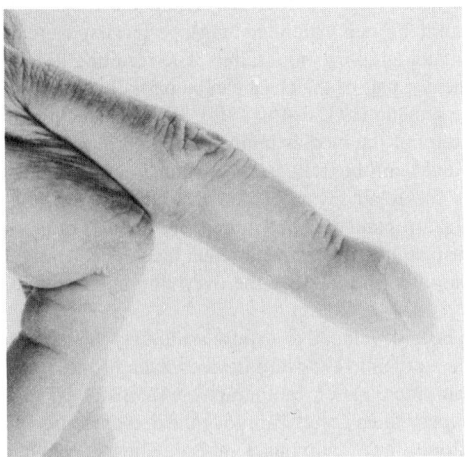

HEAD AND NECK

Signs of upper respiratory tract disease are relevant in pointing to a site and source of infection that could track down to the lungs, and for the ways in which they signify allergy. Furthermore, neurological disease of the pharynx or structural abnormalities of the larynx encourage aspiration and repeated respiratory tract infection. A short thick neck, retrognathia, and a large uvula can all predispose to sleep apnoea. A goitre may be large enough to compress the trachea and cause stridor. It could be associated with hyperthyroidism and so breathlessness, hypothyroidism, and hence hypoventilation, or even be a source of a carcinoma which could metastasize to the lungs. Even more important are signs in the neck that represent primary intrathoracic malignancy. Hard enlarged cervical lymph nodes are a well-recognized metastatic site for carcinoma of the lung, but can signify lymphoma or primary cancer from elsewhere (stomach, breast). The local extension of central bronchogenic carcinoma gives superior vena caval thrombosis. There is fixed elevation of jugular venous pressure, a large neck, a congested face and head, and, in severe cases, exophthalmos and impaired vision (Fig. 4).

CARDIOVASCULAR SYSTEM

The pulse is of poor volume in pulmonary hypertension, bounding and full in hypercapnic respiratory failure, and waxes and wanes in acute severe airflow obstruction (pulsus paradoxus). In the last of these the pulse can actually disappear at the height of the negative intrapleural pressure swing (mid to late inspiration). The pulmonary hypertension that accompanies sever hypoxic cor pulmonale is manifested on physical examination by a raised jugular venous pressure with a prominent A wave, peripheral pitting oedema, and cardiac signs of right ventricular heave, a loud P_2 wave, and, in failure, a gallop rhythm. Oedema alone should raise differential diagnoses such as liver or renal disease, both of which can have pulmonary manifestations, and, it must be remembered, can occur with truncal obesity and skin bruising in patients treated with oral corticosteroids for their lung disease.

Miscellaneous

A detailed general examination will also pick up lymph node enlargement which can signify bronchial cancer or intrathoracic lymphoma, or be due to benign disease such as infection or sarcoidosis.

Rheumatoid arthritis has several intrathoracic manifestations, as has ankylosing spondylitis. An acute arthritis occurs with sarcoid, and non-specific arthropathies can be a non-metastatic manifestation of malignancy.

Occasionally radiological abnormalities may be the presenting feature of respiratory disease rather than a part of the assessment of a patient with respiratory symptoms. Two appearances which are particularly likely to be detected on routine or coincidental chest radiology are the solitary pulmonary nodule and diffuse widespread radiological change (Chapter 17.6.1).

Finally, although the presentation of chest disease may be with a single feature such as cough, breathlessness, or chest pain, it is often a combination of symptoms with physical signs and radiology that leads to the recognition of well-defined syndromes such as respiratory tract infection, diffuse or localized airways obstruction, pleural effusion, pneumothorax, consolidation, atelectasis, and fibrosis, which are considered in detail in subsequent chapters of this book.

17.6 Investigation of respiratory disease

17.6.1 Thoracic imaging

D. M. HANSELL

Despite recent technological advances, chest radiography remains the cornerstone of thoracic imaging. The chest radiograph is justifiably regarded as an integral part of the examination of the patient in respiratory medicine. Because of the wealth of information available from chest radiography, careful interpretation of the chest radiograph remains a necessary clinical skill. Advances in cross-sectional imaging have had a great impact in improving the diagnosis of thoracic pathology, not only for the assessment of mediastinal disease but also in the evaluation of patients with suspected diffuse lung disease. Never the less, a chest radiograph should always be obtained and looked at carefully before submitting a patient to more sophisticated imaging techniques. In the case of computed tomography, the expense and radiation burden is an important consideration.

Techniques in thoracic imaging

Chest radiography

The first chest radiograph was taken nearly a hundred years ago and is now the most frequently requested radiological investigation worldwide. The technique of chest radiography has changed surprisingly little over the years, although digital technology has recently been used to overcome some of the shortcomings of conventional film-based radiography.

TECHNICAL CONSIDERATIONS

An ideal chest radiograph is taken with the patient standing erect, suspending respiration at total lung capacity, and with the X-ray beam traversing the thorax from back to front (the posteroanterior or frontal view). Because of the wide range of densities within the chest (soft tissues of the mediastinum through to aerated lung), perfect exposure of every part of the chest radiograph is impossible. The resulting suboptimal exposure of the denser part of the chest can be partially overcome with a high kilovoltage technique (120–150 kVp). With this technique there is greater penetration of the mediastinum which improves visualization of the trachea and main bronchi. A disadvantage of high kilovoltage radiography is the relatively poor demonstration of calcified structures, so that rib fractures and calcified pulmonary nodules or pleural plaques are less conspicuous. Even with optimal technique, nearly a third of the lungs is partially obscured by the overlying mediastinum, diaphragm, and ribs.

Newer devices have been developed to expose accurately the various parts of the chest using automatic exposure devices. One of these, the advanced multiple beam equalization radiography (AMBER) system, produces chest radiographs which greatly improve the demonstration of both mediastinal anatomy and pulmonary abnormalities. Another approach to this problem is phosphor plate computed radiography which uses digital technology; this is ultimately expected to replace conventional film radiography. A phosphor plate is handled in a conventional cassette (which does not contain film) and is exposed in the normal way. The energy of the incident X-ray beam is stored as a latent image. The phosphor plate is then scanned with a laser beam and the light emitted from the excited latent image is detected by a photomultiplier. Thereafter this signal is processed in digital form. The digital image can be viewed on a television monitor or laser-printed on to film. The advantage of phosphor plate computed radiography is that it can retrieve an image of diagnostic quality from an imperfect exposure which would result in a non-diagnostic conventional film radiograph. Manipulation or processing of the digital image data can enhance certain features of the radiograph to improve diagnosis.

STANDARD RADIOGRAPHIC VIEWS OF THE CHEST

The posteroanterior projection is the standard view. The patient is positioned with the anterior chest wall against the film cassette and the arms are abducted to rotate the scapulae away from the posterior chest. Chest films in the anteroposterior projection are usually taken when the patient is too ill to stand for a formal posteroanterior radiograph. A consequence of this view is that the heart is magnified because it lies further from the film. Moreover, the shorter X-ray tube-to-film distance which is inevitable when a portable anteroposterior radiograph is taken causes further magnification which must be taken into account when assessing the heart size on an anteroposterior chest radiograph.

A lateral chest radiograph is often taken in addition to the posteroanterior film when a patient first presents with a respiratory problem; a lateral film at follow-up is usually unnecessary. The lateral radiograph is obtained by placing the patient at right angles to the film cassette. In practice, whether the film is a left or right lateral is unimportant. The lateral projection provides the third dimension and helps to determine the site of a lesion identified on the posteroanterior projection (although it is surprising how often an opacity clearly seen on the posteroanterior radiograph is invisible on the lateral radiograph). As well as allowing accurate localization of lesions, the lateral radiograph may reveal cryptic abnormalities which lie behind the heart or diaphragm. Furthermore, with some experience, evaluation of the hilar structures and major airways is aided by the lateral radiograph (see section on the anatomy on the lateral chest radiograph).

Over the years a number of supplementary projections have been developed to provide information about areas which are not easily seen on the standard posteroanterior and lateral radiograph. With the advent of cross-sectional imaging, notably computed tomography (CT), many of these extra views have become obsolete. However, even with access to CT, some of these views supply extra anatomical detail readily and inexpensively, and these will be considered briefly.

The lateral decubitus projection is sometimes useful for the demonstration of small pleural effusions: for this view the patient lies on his side with the side in question downwards. The film is positioned behind the patient and the X-ray beam traverses the patient horizontally. This view will demonstrate small quantities of pleural fluid (50–100 ml) tracking up the lateral chest wall; such small effusions are not detectable on a posteroanterior chest radiograph. However, ultrasonography is increasingly being used as a reliable technique for demonstrating small pleural effusions.

Other supplementary projections, for example apical and lordotic views, used to improve visualization of the lung at the extreme apices are now less commonly performed; CT is much more effective at showing pathology in these difficult areas. For the same reason, linear tomography which merely blurs out structures which overlie the area of interest has now been supplanted by CT.

The technique of screening the patient with fluoroscopy has the advantage of allowing 'real-time' radiographic examination of the patient. It allows localization of lesions by the use of unusual oblique projections, for example distinguishing a small pleural plaque from an intrapulmonary nodule. Fluoroscopy is also the quickest method of evaluating diaphragmatic movement and diagnosing air-trapping in a child with suspected inhalation of a foreign body.

Ultrasonography

High frequency sound waves do not traverse air and are completely reflected at interfaces between soft tissue and air. The use of this technique in the chest is therefore limited because of normally aerated lung. However, fluid can be readily detected and the main use of ultrasound is for the localization of small or loculated pleural effusions. Furthermore, ultrasound can differentiate between pleural fluid and pleural thickening in cases in which radiography cannot make this distinction. Ultrasonography is an extremely useful technique for guiding percutaneous needle biopsy of masses arising from the chest wall or pleura, or peripheral pulmonary masses or consolidation, and for aiding the accurate placement of a chest drain within a pleural collection. Ultrasonography may show numerous septations within an exudative pleural effusion (Fig. 1), in which case simple percutaneous drainage of the effusion is unlikely to be successful. Ultrasonography of the upper abdomen may reveal abnormalities in a patient with primarily pulmonary disease, for example hepatic metastases from a bronchial carcinoma.

Computed tomography

CT depends on the same basic principle as conventional radiography, namely the differential absorption of X-rays by tissues of disparate densities. However, CT has much greater sensitivity to differences in attenuation of X-rays by various tissues. The image display of CT is fundamentally different from the projectional (shadow) image of a chest radiograph. A CT machine consists of an X-ray source and an array of detectors which surround the patient. The X-ray source rotates around the patient and the resulting attenuated beam is measured by the detectors. The signals from the detectors are used to construct an image by a mathematical technique. The reconstructed images are transverse (axial) cross-sections of the patient and are viewed as if from the feet of the patient (i.e. on the image the patients's right side is to the viewer's left). Each CT section is a matrix of three-dimensional elements (voxels) containing a measurement of X-ray attenuation, arbitrarily expressed as Hounsfield units (HU): water measures 0 HU, air measures 1000 HU (so that lung parenchyma is approximately −600 HU), fat measures −80 HU, soft tissue measured 40–80 HU, and bone measures 800 HU. If a voxel is completely occupied by a tissue of uniform density (most

Fig. 1 Ultrasonography showing a pleural effusion. Fibrinous septations traverse the pleural space.

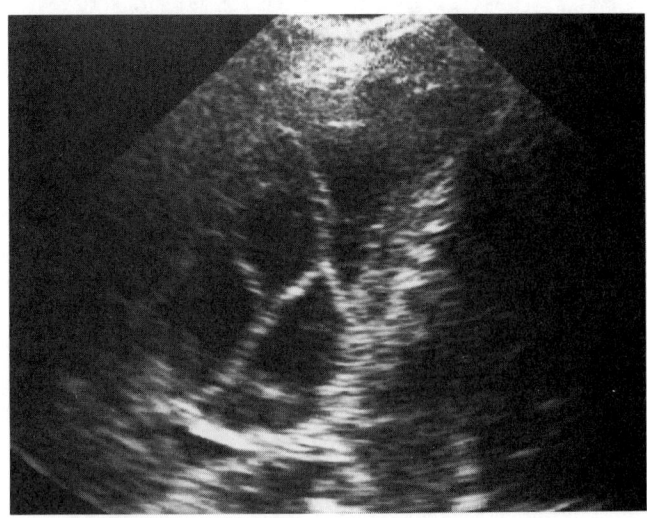

frequently the case with narrow sections), then the attenuation will be truly representative of that tissue. However, if the section contains tissues of two different densities (more likely with thicker sections), for example half lung and half dome of diaphragm, then the attenuation value will be a weighted average of the two components; this is known as the 'partial volume' effect.

Because of the cross-sectional nature of CT it can accurately localize lesions seen on only one view on chest radiography. The superior contrast resolution of CT gives exquisite detail of the various components of mediastinal anatomy (e.g. lymph nodes and vessels) and density differences (e.g. calcifications within a pulmonary nodule). Different image settings are needed to view the soft tissue structures of the mediastinum and the aerated lung parenchyma respectively (Fig. 2). A recent refinement is high resolution CT which produces highly detailed sections of the lung parenchyma. Submillimetre structures can be resolved with this technique, and the complex morphology of interstitial lung diseases can be shown with great clarity (Fig. 3).

The disadvantages of CT are its relatively high cost and the increased radiation exposure to the patient, particularly compared with chest radiography. For these reasons, CT should not be regarded as a routine investigation and examinations should always be tailored to solve ques-

tions not answered by less sophisticated investigations. The commonest indications for thoracic CT are summarized in Table 1.

Magnetic resonance imaging

The physical principles of magnetic resonance imaging (MRI) are very different from those governing CT scanning. A magnetic resonance image is obtained by placing an individual in a strong magnetic field which polarizes some of the ubiquitous hydrogen protons (which can be thought of as behaving like randomly orientated bar magnets) in the body so that they have the same alignment. The application of radiofrequency wave pulses of specified lengths and repetition (pulse sequences) displaces the protons, and some of this transmitted energy is absorbed by them. With the cessation of the radiofrequency pulse, the protons return to their initial alignment and in so doing they emit, as a weak signal, some of the energy that they have absorbed; this signal is received, amplified and handled in digital form, and subsequently reconstructed into an image.

The advantages of MRI include its ability to obtain sections in any plane (Fig. 4), the improved contrast resolution between different soft tissues compared with CT scanning, and the use of special sequences which give functional information (e.g. the velocity of blood flow). An important advantage of MRI is the lack of any known hazard to the patient, in contrast with CT scanning with its small attendant risk from ionizing radiation. Disadvantages of MRI include the long scan time (although this is continually being shortened), reduced spatial resolution compared with CT, the inability to image calcium, reduced acceptability to patients because of the claustrophobic bore of the magnet, and its limited availability.

In many respects the imaging of the mediastinum by CT scanning and MRI are comparable. However, magnetic resonance images of the lungs are currently markedly inferior to CT scanning. This is because of the very low water (and therefore proton) content of the lungs; thus the signal produced by normal lung is small and so is not visualized by conventional sequences. However, further developments are likely which will increase the application of MRI for both mediastinal and lung imaging.

Radionuclide imaging

Ventilation–perfusion radionuclide scanning is an effective non-invasive method of providing both anatomical and physiological information

Fig. 2 CT section through the mid-thorax. The window settings have been adjusted to show details of (a) the lungs and (b) the soft tissues of the mediastinum.

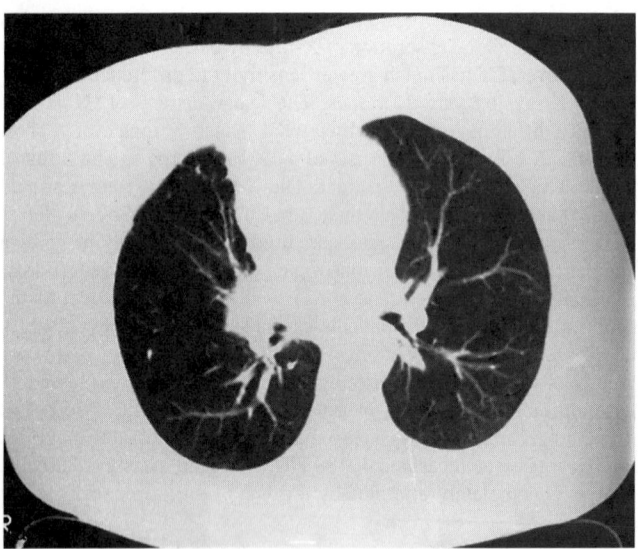

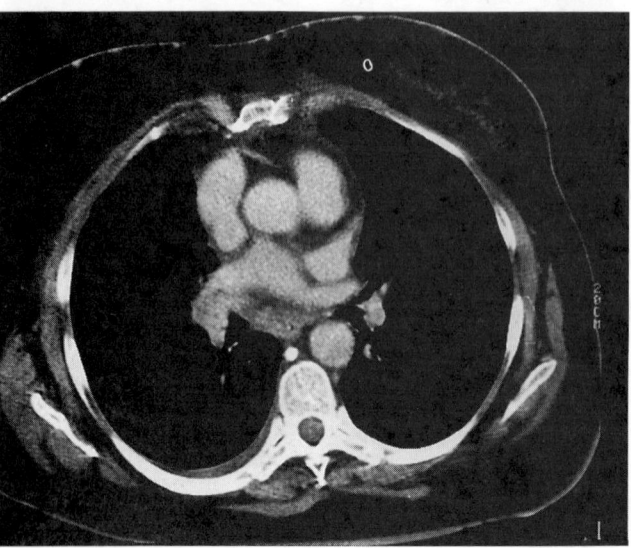

Fig. 3 High resolution CT of a patient with cryptogenic fibrosing alveolitis. The peripheral distribution of the disease and the fine detail of the small cystic air spaces in the destroyed fibrotic lung are clearly shown.

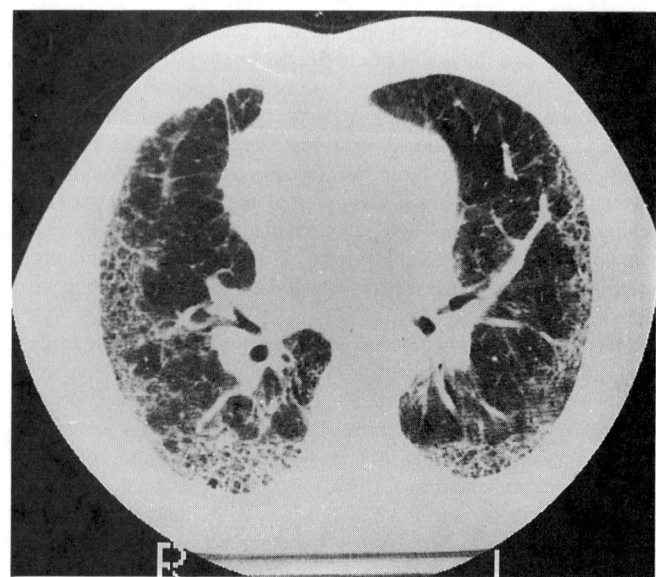

Table 1 *Indications for CT of the thorax*

1. Elucidation of an abnormal mediastinal or hilar contour on chest radiography
2. As part of the staging procedure in the evaluation of a patient with known lung cancer (the findings on CT must be interpreted in conjunction with other investigations)
3. Detection of pulmonary disease in the face of a questionably abnormal chest radiograph (notably diffuse interstitial disease and bronchiectasis)
4. Investigation of a patient with haemoptysis in whom chest radiography and bronchoscopy are normal
5. Assessment of complex pleural or chest wall pathology when chest radiography does not adequately show the extent of disease
6. As a means of guiding the percutaneous needle biopsy of centrally placed pulmonary lesions, mediastinal masses, or chest wall pathology

about the lung. It is the most common radionuclide study of the lungs and is most frequently used to confirm or exclude the diagnosis of suspected pulmonary embolism.

Regional pulmonary capillary perfusion can be assessed following the intravenous injection of a bolus of particles which have been labelled with technetium-99m. The minute particles are microspheres or macroaggregates of human albumin (between 15 and 70 μm in diameter). These particles are evenly dispersed by the time that they reach the pulmonary circulation and they become temporarily lodged in a very small fraction (less than 0.5 per cent) of the precapillary arterioles and capillaries of the lungs. There is a small theoretical risk of compromising the pulmonary vascular bed in patients with severe pulmonary hypertension, although this is not an absolute contraindication to the examination. The distribution of gamma-ray emission from the technetium-labelled particles is directly proportional to the regional pulmonary flow and a significant defect in perfusion is usually readily detected. It is important to appreciate that such defects may be due to a variety of conditions other than pulmonary embolism, including any cause of hypoxic vasoconstriction such as an area of subsegmental collapse or space-occupying lesions not supplied by the pulmonary circulation. However, in these cases the affected area of lung will be neither ventilated nor perfused, in contrast with acute pulmonary embolism in which there is

no corresponding defect of ventilation. Thus ventilation scintigraphy is usually performed at the same time as perfusion scanning to improve the specificity of the diagnosis of pulmonary embolism.

Evaluation of ventilation of the lungs depends on filling the distal air spaces with a gamma-ray-emitting radionuclide. The radionuclides suitable for inhalation are the inert gases xenon-133 and krypton-81m or a technetium-99m aerosol (Technegas). Although Krypton-81m gives the highest quality images, Technegas is increasingly being used because of its ready availability. The characteristic abnormality of pulmonary embolism is the so-called mismatched defect in which a regional defect in perfusion is not matched by a defect in ventilation (Fig. 5). However, the picture in pulmonary embolism may not always be clear cut, particularly when pulmonary infarction has occurred when there will be a matched defect of both ventilation and perfusion. Because of the importance of establishing a correct diagnosis of pulmonary embolism, ventilation–perfusion scans should always be interpreted in the light of current chest radiographs and clinical information; even then, a substantial proportion of ventilation–perfusion scans remain indeterminate, and in doubtful cases pulmonary arteriography may be necessary to confirm or exclude pulmonary embolism.

Pulmonary and bronchial arteriography: superior vena cavography

Currently, the most accurate means of identifying emboli within the pulmonary arteries is by the injection of a contrast agent into the main pulmonary artery or its branches (Fig. 6). Pulmonary arteriography requires the catheterization of an antecubital, jugular, or femoral vein;

Fig. 5 A ventilation–perfusion radionuclide study (oblique views). The perfusion scan (a) shows a defect in the left mid-zone which is not matched on the corresponding view of the ventilation scan (b). The so-called mismatched defect is characteristic of a pulmonary embolus.

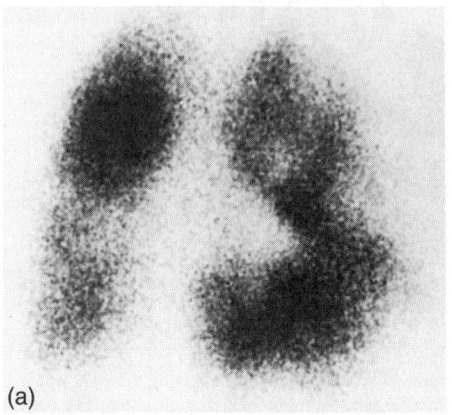

(a)

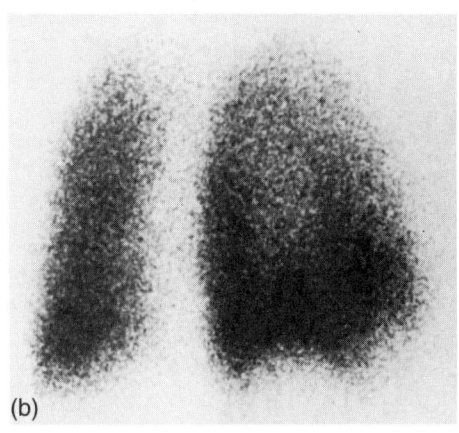

(b)

Fig. 4 Magnetic resonance image (coronal section) showing the relationship of an apical bronchial carcinoma to the chest wall and adjacent mediastinum. There are enlarged subcarinal lymph nodes and a metastatic deposit in the right adrenal gland (by courtesy of Dr P. Goddard).

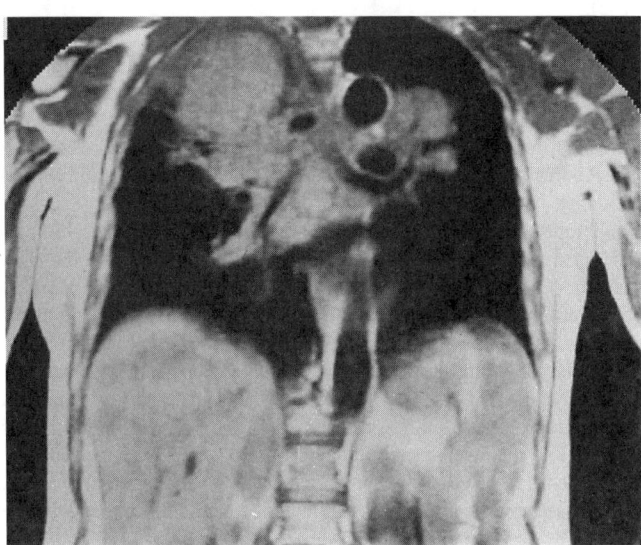

the catheter is guided through the right heart under fluoroscopic control. While the complication rate is low, it is a time-consuming procedure which requires a experienced angiographer.

The bronchial arteries which supply the airways become hypertrophied in chronic inflammatory pulmonary disease, notably bronchiectasis. Rupture of these vessels can cause severe and life-threatening haemoptysis. The bronchial arteries are selectively catheterized by the passage of a catheter via the femoral artery and aorta. Once the abnormally hypertrophied bronchial arteries have been identified (Fig. 7), they can be therapeutically embolized. This technique is usually successful in abating a massive haemoptysis in patients not able to undergo immediate surgical treatment for the cause of haemoptysis.

Superior vena cavography is usually performed to evaluate the exact site of narrowing in patients with symptoms of obstruction of the superior vena cava (Fig. 8); it is not generally required to confirm the diagnosis which is usually evident from the clinical signs alone. Patients with symptoms of superior vena cava obstruction, most frequently due to neoplastic involvement of adjacent mediastinal lymph nodes, may be successfully palliated by radiotherapy or the insertion of an expandable metallic wire stent at the site of the narrowing.

Percutaneous lung biopsy

Percutaneous needle biopsy of a pulmonary lesion or mediastinal mass is usually performed in patients in whom a bronchoscopic biopsy has failed to produce a histological specimen or if a thoracotomy to resect

Fig. 6 A digital subtraction pulmonary arteriogram showing abrupt termination of the vessels supplying the right upper lobe caused by a pulmonary embolus.

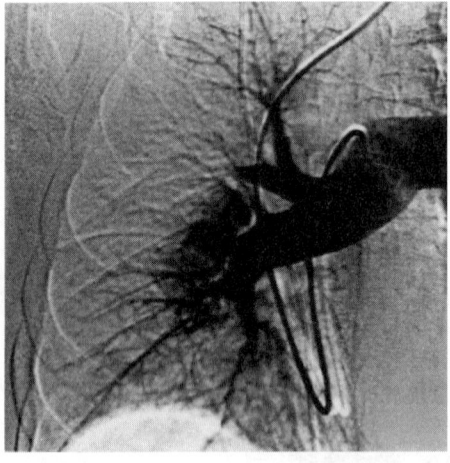

Fig. 7 Abnormally hypertrophied bronchial arteries supplying the right upper lobe shown on a selective digital subtraction bronchial arteriogram. The patient had cystic fibrosis and had had a massive haemoptysis; these bronchial arteries were subsequently embolized.

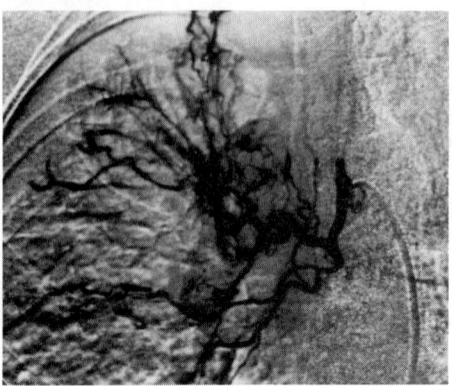

the lesion is deemed inappropriate. It should not be regarded as a routine procedure in the investigation of all solitary pulmonary nodules, and should only be performed after considering the risks to the patient and whether the information forthcoming from the procedure will direct management.

Many different types of needles have been developed and the frequency of complications, mainly pneumothorax and haemoptysis, is in part related to the diameter of the needle. Percutaneous biopsy is performed under local anaesthesia with fluoroscopic guidance; CT-guided biopsy of small intrapulmonary lesions is more time consuming and often less successful. However, CT guidance is mandatory for the biopsy of centrally placed masses adjacent to large vessels, and is ideal for pleural and chest wall lesions. Contraindications to the procedure include any patient with poor respiratory reserve who is unable to withstand a pneumothorax and pulmonary arterial hypertension.

Normal radiographic anatomy

The mediastinum

On a posteroanterior chest radiograph (Fig. 9) the mediastinal structures are superimposed on one another and thus cannot be distinguished individually. The mediastinum is conventionally divided into superior, anterior, middle, and posterior compartments: the practical use of these arbitrary divisions is that specific mediastinal pathologies show a definite predilection for individual compartments (e.g. a superior mediastinal mass is most frequently due to intrathoracic extension of the thyroid gland, and a middle mediastinal mass is usually due to enlarged lymph nodes). However, it should be borne in mind that the position of a mass within one of these compartments is no guarantee of a specific diagnosis nor do these boundaries preclude disease from spreading from one compartment to the next.

Because only the outline of the mediastinum and the air-containing trachea and bronchi are clearly seen on a posteroanterior chest radiograph, the mediastinal anatomy will be considered in more detail in the description of CT anatomy. On a chest radiograph, the right superior mediastinal border is formed by the right brachiocephalic vein and superior vena cava. The mediastinal border to the left of the trachea above the aortic arch represents the sum of the left carotid and left subclavian arteries together with the left brachiocephalic and jugular veins. The left cardiac border comprises the left atrial appendage which merges inferiorly with the left ventricle. The cardiac silhouette is always sharply outlined; any blurring of the border denotes replacement of the adjacent aerated lung, usually by collapse or consolidation (see description of the silhouette sign in the section on common radiological signs of disease).

The density of the cardiac shadow to the left and right of the vertebral column should be identical, and any difference signals pulmonary pathology (e.g. consolidation in a lower lobe). A density with a convex lateral border is often seen through the right heart border on a well-penetrated film; this apparent mass is due to the confluence of the pulmonary veins as it enters the left atrium and is of no pathological significance.

The trachea and main bronchi are visible through the upper and middle mediastinum. The trachea is rarely straight and is often to the right of the mid-line at its mid-point. In elderly patients, the trachea may appear dramatically displaced by a dilated aortic arch. The angle of the carina is usually somewhat less than 80°. Splaying of the carina is a sign of gross disease, either in the form of massive subcarinal lymphadenopathy or a markedly enlarged left atrium. A more sensitive sign of a subcarinal mass is obliteration of the azygo-oesophageal line which is usually visible on a well-penetrated chest radiograph. The origins of the lobar bronchi, where they are projected over the mediastinal shadow, can usually be made out, but the segmental bronchi within the lungs are not generally seen on plain radiography.

The hilar structures

The hilar shadows on a chest radiograph are a complex summation of the pulmonary arteries and veins with virtually no contribution from the overlying bronchial walls or normal-sized lymph nodes. The hila are approximately the same size and the left hilum always lies between 0.5 and 1.5 cm above the level of the right hilum. The size and shape of the hila in normal individuals show remarkable variation, so that subtle abnormalities are difficult to detect. At least as important as an abnormal contour in detecting a mass at the hilum, is a discrepancy in density between the two hila: both hilar shadows, at equivalent points, will be of equal density and a mass at the hilum (or an intrapulmonary mass projected over the hilum) will be evident as increased density of that hilum.

The pulmonary fissures, vessels, and bronchi

The lobes of each lung are surrounded by visceral pleura; the upper and lower lobes of the left lung are separated by the major (or oblique) fissure. The upper, middle, and lower lobes of the right lung are separated by the major (or oblique) and minor (horizontal or transverse) fissures. The minor fissure is visible in about 60 per cent of normal posteroanterior chest radiographs. In normal individuals, this fissure runs horizontally and any deviation from this course represents loss of volume of a lobe. The major fissures are inconstantly identifiable on lateral radiographs. Other fissures are occasionally seen; for example in the left lung a minor fissure can occur which separates the lingula from the remainder of the upper lobe.

All the branching structures seen within the lungs on a chest radiograph represent either pulmonary arteries or veins. The larger pulmonary vessels can be traced back to the hila and mediastinum. The pulmonary veins can sometimes be differentiated from the pulmonary arteries; the superior pulmonary veins have a distinctly vertical course, but in practice it is often impossible to distinguish arteries from veins in the outer two-thirds of the lung. On a chest radiograph taken in the erect position, there is a gradual increase in the diameter of the vessels, at equidistant points from the hilum, travelling from lung apex to base; this is a grav-ity-dependent effect and is abolished if the patient is supine or in cardiac failure.

The lobes of the lung are divided into segments, each of which are supplied by their own segmental bronchi. The walls of the segmental bronchi are rarely seen on the chest radiograph, except when lying parallel to the X-ray beam when they are seen end-on as ring shadows measuring up to 8 mm in diameter.

The diaphragm and thoracic cage

The interface between aerated lung and the domes of the diaphragm is sharp, and in general the highest point of each dome is medial to the mid-clavicular line. The right dome of the diaphragm is up to 2 cm higher than the left in the erect position unless the left dome is temporarily elevated by air in the stomach. Laterally, the diaphragm dips steeply downwards to form an acute angle with the chest wall. Filling in or blunting of these costophrenic angles usually represents pleural disease, either pleural thickening or an effusion.

Localized humps on the dome of the diaphragm are common and represent minor weaknesses or defects of the diaphragm. Similarly, interposition of the colon in front of the right lobe of the liver is a normal variant which is frequently seen.

Deformities of the thoracic cage may cause distortion of the normal mediastinum and so simulate disease. One of the commonest deformities is pectus excavatum which, by compressing the heart between the depressed sternum and vertebral column, causes displacement of the apparently enlarged heart to the left and blurring of the right heart border.

High kilovoltage chest radiographs often allow the vertebral bodies to be seen through the cardiac shadow. However, with this technique the ribs, and particularly their posterior parts, are often rendered invisible.

Anatomy on the lateral chest radiograph

It is useful to become accustomed to viewing a lateral film (Fig. 9) in the same orientation whether it is a right or left lateral projection. Famil-

Fig. 8 (a) A cavagram showing obstruction of the superior vena cava (in this case due surrounding malignant lymphadenopathy) just below the level of the azygos vein (arrow). Palliative radiotherapy gave the patient temporary relief. (b) Following balloon dilatation and insertion of a metallic stent, venous blood flow is restored with normal flow into the pulmonary circulation.

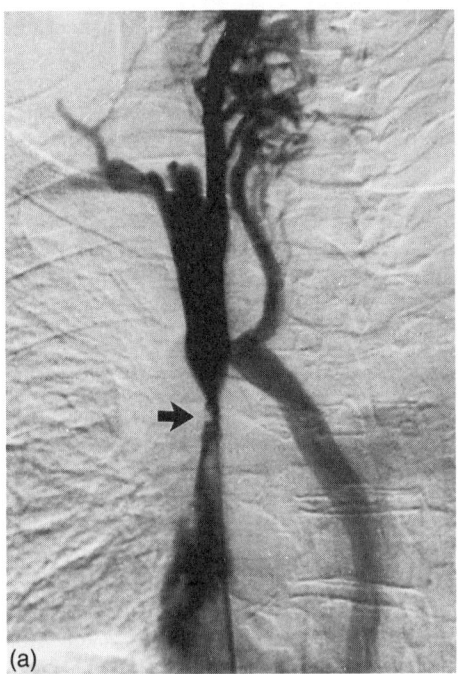

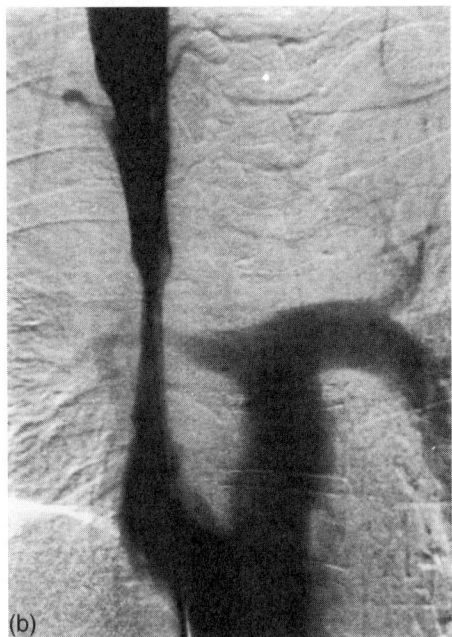

(a)

(b)

iarity with the same orientation improves the viewer's ability to detect deviations from normal.

The trachea is angled slightly posteriorly as it runs towards the carina, and the posterior wall of the trachea is always visible as a fine stripe. Furthermore, the posterior walls of the right main bronchus and the right intermediate bronchus are outlined by air and are also seen as a continuous stripe on the lateral radiograph. The spines of the scapulae are invariably seen running almost vertically in the upper part of the lateral radiograph and should not be confused with intrathoracic structures. Further spurious shadows are formed by the soft tissues of the outstretched arms which are projected over the anterior and superior mediastinum. Although the carina is not visible on the lateral radiograph, the two transradiancies projected over the lower trachea represent the right main bronchus (superiorly) and the left main bronchus (inferiorly).

More lung is obscured by overlying structures on a lateral radiograph than on the posteroanterior view. The unobscured lung in the retrosternal and retrocardiac regions should be of the same transradiancy. Furthermore, as the eye travels down the dorsal spine, the viewer should be aware of a gradual increase in transradiancy. The loss of this phenomenon suggests the presence of disease in the posterobasal segments of the lower lobes (sometimes not visible on the frontal radiograph).

The two major fissures are seen as diagonal lines, often incomplete and of hair's breadth, running from the upper dorsal spine to the anterior surface of the diaphragm. Care must be taken not to confuse the obliquely running edges of ribs with fissures. The minor fissure extends horizontally from the mid-right major fissure. It is often not possible to distinguish the right from the left major fissures with confidence. Similarly, although the two hemidiaphragms may be identified individually (particularly if the gastric bubble is visible under the left dome of the diaphragm), the distinction between the right and the left is often not possible. A helpful sign is the relative heights of the two domes; the dome furthest from the film is usually higher because of magnification.

The summation of both hila on the lateral radiograph generates a complex shadow. However, there are some generalizations which aid the interpretation of this difficult area. The right pulmonary artery lies anterior to the trachea and right main bronchus, whereas the left pulmonary artery hooks over the left main bronchus so that a large part of it lies posterior to the major bronchi. As a result, any mass identified on a posteroanterior and lateral radiograph that lies anterior to the left hilum or posterior to the right hilum is not vascular in origin and is most likely to represent enlarged hilar lymph nodes.

A band-like opacity is often seen along the lower third of the anterior chest wall behind the sternum. This represents a normal density and occurs because there is less aerated lung in contact with the chest wall as the space is occupied by the heart; it should not be confused with pleural disease.

Fig. 9 Normal radiographic anatomy. (a) posteroanterior chest radiograph: (1) trachea: (2) aortic arch; (3) left main pulmonary artery; (4) right main pulmonary artery; (5) right atrial border; (6) left atrial appendage; (7) left ventricular border; (8) right ventricle; (9) right dome of diaphragm; (10) costophrenic angle; (11) breast shadow. (b) Lateral chest radiograph; (1) trachea; (2) scapulae; (3) anterior aortic arch; (4) right pulmonary artery; (5) left pulmonary artery; (6) right ventricle; (7) breast shadows; (8) gastric bubble under the left hemidiaphragm; (9) left main bronchus.

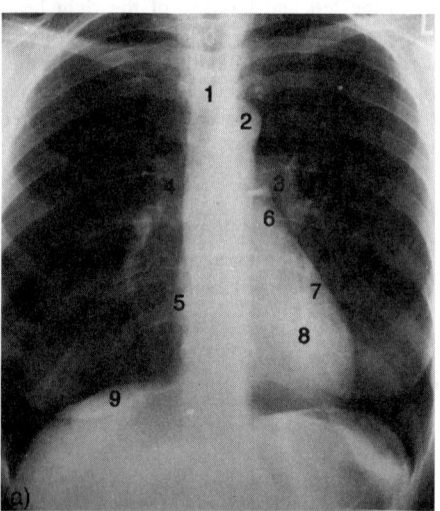

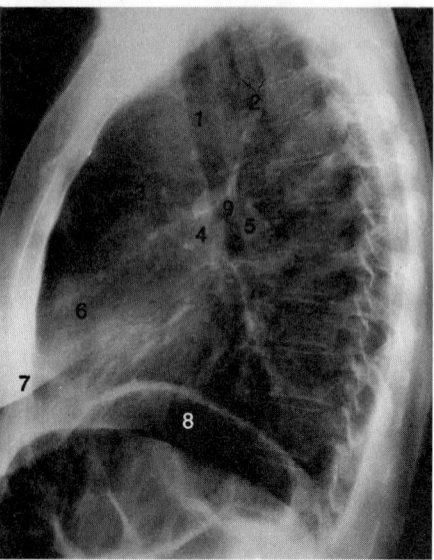

Normal CT anatomy of the mediastinum

CT provides unique information about the anatomy of the mediastinum and is often used to provide further detail about abnormalities which are seen merely as a deformity of the mediastinal contour on chest radiography. The normal structures that are always identified on a CT of the mediastinum are the blood vessels (which make up the bulk of the superior mediastinum), the major airways, the oesophagus, the heart, and mediastinal fat. An appreciation of the relationship of these structures to each other is crucial for the correct interpretation of CT scans; four important levels are shown in Fig. 10.

Normal lymph nodes surrounded by fat can be identified throughout the mediastinum. Many schemes have been devised to map their precise locations, but they can be broadly divided into (1) anterior mediastinal, (2) posterior mediastinal, and (3) tracheobronchial. The latter can be further subdivided into the following regions: (a) right and left paratracheal, (b) subaortic, (c) pretracheal and (d) subcarinal. It is important to appreciate that the absolute size of lymph nodes identified on CT (or by direct inspection at mediastinoscopy) should not be regarded as a foolproof criterion for significant disease, particularly in the context of lung cancer. Although markedly enlarged lymph nodes (greater than 2 cm in diameter) almost invariably signify pathology, moderate enlargement of mediastinal lymph nodes may represent reactive hyperplasia of little clinical significance. Conversely, small volume lymph nodes or lymph nodes not identified by CT may sometimes contain micrometastases from a distant primary neoplasm.

The thymus gland occupies a large part of the anterior mediastinum in children. In adult life the remnants of the normal thymus are normally inconspicuous on CT.

Points in the interpretation of a chest radiograph

Even when there is an obvious radiographic abnormality, there is much to recommend a careful and systematic method in reviewing a chest radiograph. Such an approach will allow an appreciation of normal variations of anatomy to be built up with time. With increasing experience an appreciation of deviation from normal appearances becomes more rapid, and this quickly leads to a directed search for related abnormalities.

Before interpreting a chest radiograph, it is vital to establish whether there are any previous radiographs for comparison; the sequence and pattern of change are often as important as the identification of a radiographic abnormality. Information gained from preceding radiographs, particularly the lack of serial change, will often prevent needless further investigation. Demographic details, particularly the age and racial origin of the patient, should be noted since this information may increase the probability of a diagnosis which is based on the radiographic findings alone.

A quick check that the radiograph is of satisfactory quality includes an estimation of the radiographic exposure, depth of inspiration, and position of the patient. As a general rule, the intervertebral disc spaces of the entire dorsal spine should be visible on a correctly exposed radiograph; the mid-point of the right hemidiaphragm lies at the level of the

anterior end of the sixth rib if the patient has taken a satisfactory breath in. The patient is axially rotated if the medial ends of the clavicles are not equidistant from the spinous process of the cervical vertebral body at that level.

The order in which the structures on a chest radiograph are analysed is unimportant. A suggested sequence is to start with a scrutiny of the position of the trachea, the mediastinal contour (which should be sharply outlined in its entirety), and then the position, outline, and density of the hilar shadows. Only then are the lungs examined, taking into account their size, the relative transradiancy of each zone, and the position of the horizontal fissure (and any other indirect signs of volume loss—see later section on lobar collapse). Pulmonary vessels are seen as far as the outer third of the lung and the number of vessels should be roughly symmetrical on the two sides. Next, the position and clarity of the hemidiaphragms should be noted, followed by an assessment of the ribs and soft tissues of the chest wall. Special care should be taken to identify pleural thickening along the lateral chest walls which may be easily overlooked.

Fig. 10 CT with contrast enhancement to show the normal anatomy at four levels through the mediastinum: (1) trachea; (2) superior vena cava; (3) brachiocephalic artery; (4) left common carotic artery; (5) left subclavian artery; (6) oesophagus; (7) aortic arch; (8) azygos vein; (9) ascending aorta; (10) descending aorta; (11) main pulmonary artery; (12) right pulmonary artery; (13) left pulmonary artery; (14) right main bronchus; (15) left main bronchus; (16) left atrium; (17) left inferior pulmonary vein; (18) segmental bronchi of the left lower lobe; (19) right atrium; (20) right ventricular outflow; (21) left ventricle.

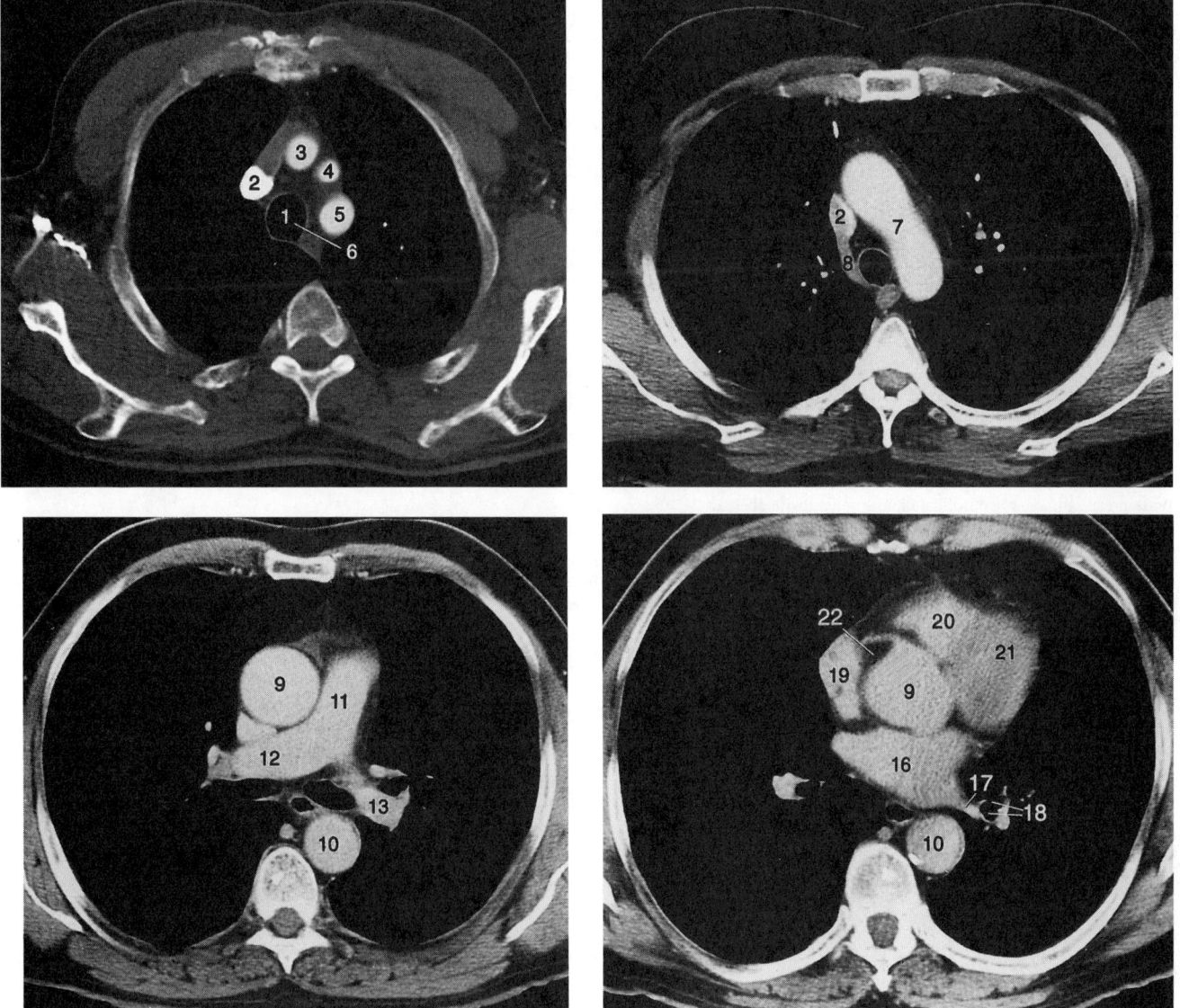

Before assigning normality to a chest radiograph, it is worth reviewing areas which are either poorly demonstrated on chest radiography or often misinterpreted. These include (a) the central mediastinum where even a large mass may be barely visible on the posteroanterior view, (b) the areas behind the heart and hemidiaphragms, (c) the lung apices, which are often obscured by overlying clavicle and ribs, and (d) the lung and pleura just inside the chest wall.

Once a radiographic abnormality has been detected, it should be considered in terms of gross pathology. Both the site and the radiographic characteristics of the lesion will allow the observer to proceed to, at the very least, a generic diagnosis. A precise histopathological diagnosis can only rarely be achieved from the radiographic appearances alone, if clinical context is not known.

Common radiological signs of disease

Pulmonary consolidation

Consolidation is a pathological description of the state of the lungs when the normal air-filled spaces, distal to the bronchi, are occupied by the products of disease (e.g. water, pus, or blood). The most important radiographic signs of pulmonary consolidation are (a) an area of increased opacification in the lungs which obscures the underlying blood vessels and has a poorly defined margin, unless it is bounded by a fissure, (b) an 'air bronchogram', and (c) the 'silhouette sign' (Fig. 11). The air bronchogram is a distinctive and certain sign of intrapulmonary pathology and is seen as a radiolucent (grey) branching structure of the bronchi against a more opaque (white) background of airless lung. Although an air bronchogram is seen almost invariably in consolidation, lung which has become collapsed and airless, for example due to a large surrounding pleural effusion, may also show an air bronchogram. The silhouette sign is seen when the normally clear border of a structure is lost because the air-filled lung outlining the border is replaced by fluid or a mass. Recognition of this sign can help to localize the area of abnormality within the lungs; for example consolidation in the lingula will make the left heart border indistinct. As with the air bronchogram sign, the silhouette sign may be seen in either pulmonary consolidation or collapse. For example loss of a clear right heart border may be due to right middle lobe consolidation with or without lobar collapse; the common feature is loss of normal aeration of the affected lung. The causes of widespread pulmonary consolidation are numerous but can be broadly divided into the five categories shown in Table 2.

Fig. 11 Widespread pulmonary consolidation in a patient with alveolar proteinosis. The right heart border is obscured, confirming that a large part of the consolidation is in the right middle lobe (the silhouette sign).

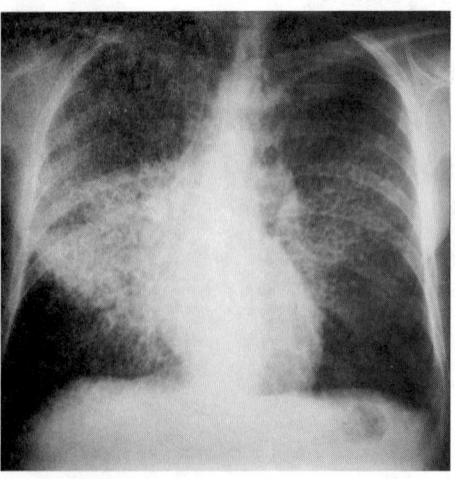

Table 2 *Causes of widespread pulmonary consolidation*

Pulmonary oedema
Cardiogenic/fluid overload
Adult respiratory distress syndrome
Inhalational injury (noxious gases)
Drug abuse
Neurogenic (raised intracranial pressure or head injury)
Renal disease
Traumatic (fat embolism)

Exudate
Infective consolidation
Eosinophilic lung disease
Collagen vascular disease
Cryptogenic organizing pneumonia
Radiation pneumonitis

Neoplasm
Bronchioloalveolar cell carcinoma
Lymphoproliferative disorders

Blood
Contusion
Infarction
Idiopathic pulmonary haemorrhage (Goodpasture's syndrome)

Other
Sarcoidosis
Alveolar proteinosis

Pulmonary collapse

Pulmonary collapse is the term used to describe loss of aeration and therefore inflation in part or all of a lung. Depending on the cause, collapse may occur at any level from small subsegmental areas of lung through to an entire lung. Small areas of subsegmental collapse occur very commonly in debilitated and postoperative patients, where they are seen as linear, usually horizontal, opacities. At the other end of the spectrum, collapse of an entire lung, usually due to an endobronchial lesion or inhaled foreign body, has a dramatic radiographic appearance with complete opacification of the affected lung and loss of volume of that hemithorax. At the lobar level, the signs of collapse of an individual lobe are characteristic but, depending on the lobe, may be very subtle. Recognition of the collapse of individual lobes is important, and these are described in detail.

Collapse of individual lobes

Right upper lobe On the frontal radiograph there is elevation of the minor fissure and of the right hilum. If the collapse is complete the non-aerated lobe is seen as a density alongside the superior mediastinum (Fig. 12). On the lateral view the minor fissure moves upwards and the major fissure usually moves forwards. The retrosternal area becomes progressively more opaque, and the anterior margin of the ascending aorta becomes obscured.

Right middle lobe On the frontal radiograph the lateral part of the minor fissure usually moves down. There is blurring of the normally sharp right heart border and this may be a subtle abnormality which is easily overlooked (Fig. 13). On the lateral view the minor fissure moves downwards and lower half of the major fissure moves forwards, giving rise to a triangular shadow with its apex at the hilum and the base behind the lower sternum.

Right lower lobe There is an increase in density overlying and obscuring the medial portion of the right hemidiaphragm and the right hilum is displaced inferiorly on the frontal radiograph (Fig. 14). In contrast with right middle lobe collapse, the right heart border usually remains sharply defined since this is in contact with the aerated right middle lobe. On the lateral view the major fissure moves backwards and downwards; with increasing collapse there is a loss of definition of the posterior part of the right hemidiaphragm as well as increased density overlying the lower dorsal vertebral column.

Left upper lobe The main finding on the frontal radiograph is a veil-like increase in density without a sharp margin (quite unlike right upper lobe collapse), spreading outwards and upwards from the elevated left hilum (Fig. 15). The outlines of the aortic knuckle, left hilum, and left heart border become ill defined. As the collapse increases, the lobe moves centrally and the apical segment of the left lower lobe expands to fill the space left by the collapsed upper lobe; this is the cause of the relatively transradiant lung apex. With complete collapse of the left upper lobe, a sharp border may return to the aortic arch because it is surrounded by the hyperinflated apical segment of the lower lobe. On the lateral view the major fissure moves superiorly and anteriorly while remaining relatively vertical and roughly parallel to the anterior chest wall.

Left lower lobe On the frontal radiograph there is a triangular density behind the heart with loss of the medial part of the left hemidiaphragm (Fig. 16); even on a properly exposed radiograph it may be difficult to appreciate the collapsed lobe behind the heart. Supplementary signs include inferior displacement of the left hilum, loss of volume, and increased transradiancy of the left hemithorax. On the lateral view there is posterior displacement of the major fissure. As with right lower lobe collapse, there is increased density over the lower dorsal vertebral column and the posterior part of the left hemidiaphragm is effaced.

Complete opacification (or white-out) of a hemithorax is generally due to either collapse of a lung or the presence of a large pleural effusion or tumour. Shift of the mediastinum to the affected side implies that volume loss, i.e. collapse of the lung, has occurred. In contrast, a pleural effusion or soft tissue mass which is large enough to cause complete opacification of a hemithorax will almost invariably displace the mediastinum away from the side of the opacified hemithorax. An important exception is an advanced mesothelioma which may encase one lung and 'freeze' the mediastinum, preventing contralateral mediastinal shift. Occasionally, when there is no obvious shift of the mediastinum, it is

Fig. 14 Right lower lobe collapse.

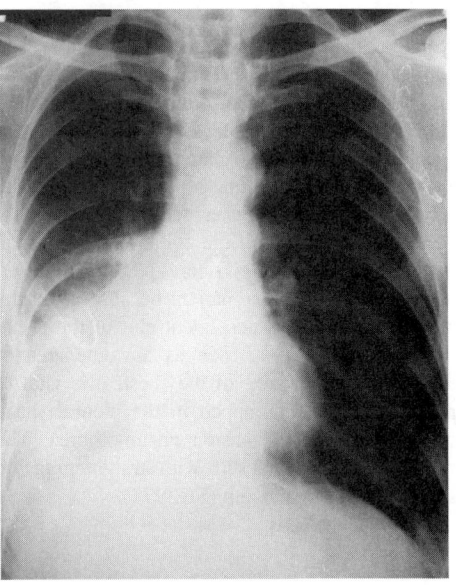

Fig. 12 Right upper lobe collapse.

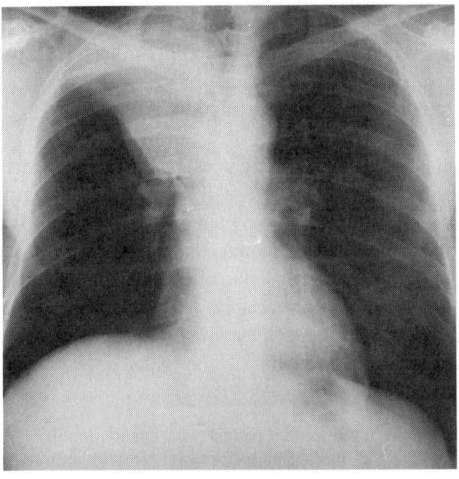

Fig. 15 Left upper lobe collapse.

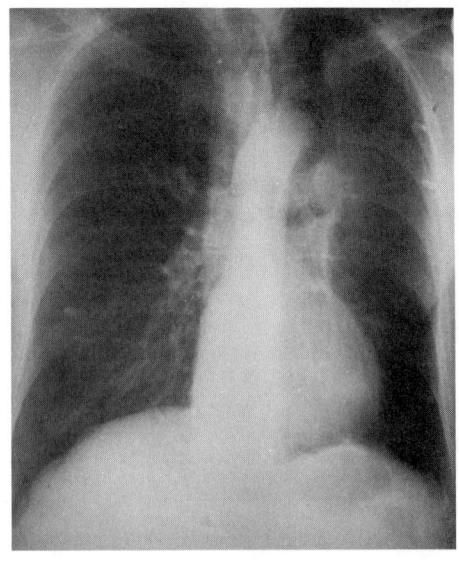

Fig. 13 Right middle lobe collapse.

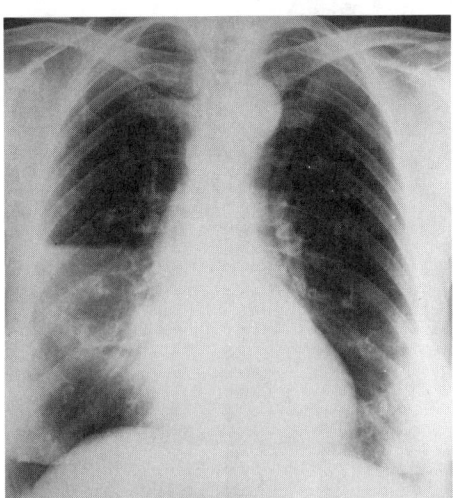

surprisingly difficult to differentiate between these two completely different causes of an opacified hemithorax. In such instances, ultrasonography and CT allow the distinction to be made with confidence and may give further information about the underlying disease.

Increased transradiancy of a hemithorax

There are many causes of increased transradiancy (darkening) of one lung, ranging from a loss of soft tissues of the chest wall (e.g. mastectomy) through to reduced perfusion of one lung due to hypoxic vasoconstriction resulting from underventilation of the lung (e.g. because of an inhaled foreign body or a tumour in a main bronchus). It is surprisingly easy to overlook this important radiographic abnormality, particularly when the density difference between the two lungs is slight; a subtle discrepancy in density between the two hemithoraces is more readily appreciated by viewing the radiograph from a distance of at least 1.5 metres. The commonest causes of a relatively transradiant hemithorax are shown in Table 3. Close scrutiny of the chest radiograph will usually indicate which of the categories of causes is responsible for this radiographic sign. If there is any clinical suggestion that the cause of the increased transradiancy is due to an obstructing lesion in a central airway, a chest radiograph taken in full expiration will accentuate the increased transradiancy and will show that the lung fails to empty.

Once it has been established that the difference in density of the lungs is not due to a technical problem (e.g. rotation of the patient), points to look for are (a) loss of symmetry of the soft tissues of the chest wall, (b) discrepancy in the volumes and vascular pattern between the two lungs, and (c) a visceral pleural edge (denoting a pneumothorax). The identification of a pneumothorax on an erect chest radiograph is usually straightforward because of the appearance of the collapsed lung which is clearly demarcated by the fine edge of the visceral pleura. However, such an edge is often not seen in the supine patient because air in the pleural space drifts anteriorly to the least dependent part of the chest. In this situation, a pneumothorax is only seen as a vague area of increased transradiancy over the lower zone of the chest. It is vital to recognize when the pressure of the air trapped in the pleural space exceeds alveolar pressure—the so-called tension pneumothorax. The typical signs are of contralateral mediastinal shift with straightening and flattening of the ipsilateral dome of diaphragm (Fig. 17).

The pulmonary mass

Many pulmonary masses are discovered incidentally on a chest radiograph. Whenever possible, previous films should be obtained so that the growth rate of the lesion can be estimated. The growth rate is a more reliable indicator of the probable nature of a pulmonary mass than any one of its radiographic features: if a lesion doubles in volume (increases

Fig. 16 Left lower lobe collapse (an AMBER chest radiograph which improves exposure in the mediastinal region).

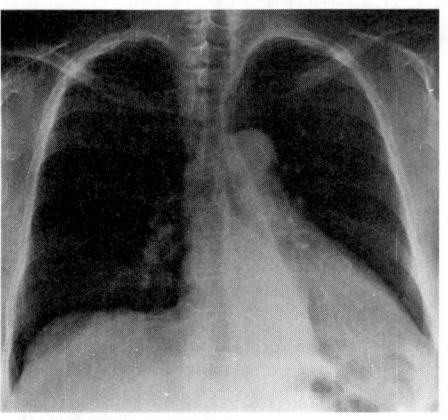

Table 3 *Causes of increased transradiancy of one hemithorax*

Technical	Rotation of the patient
Chest wall	Loss of soft tissues, most commonly due to a mastectomy
Pneumothorax	Particularly in supine patients
Compensatory overinflation	Postlobectomy Overlooked lobar collapse (e.g. left lower lobe)
Reduced pulmonary perfusion	Hypoxic vasoconstriction due to underventilation caused by an inhaled foreign body or endobronchial tumour Following childhood viral infection (MacLeod's syndrome) Recurrent pulmonary emboli (rarely unilateral)

in diameter by approximately 25 per cent on serial chest radiographs) in less than a week or more than 18 months, it is very unlikely to be malignant. The doubling time of most malignant lesions is between 1 and 6 months.

Over the years much importance has been attached to the radiological characteristics of a solitary pulmonary mass in an attempt to make the crucial distinction between benign and malignant lesions. With the possible exception of heavy calcification within the lesion (most commonly seen in ancient granulomas), no radiological appearance will reliably differentiate a benign from a malignant mass. Although generalizations can be made that, for example, bronchial carcinomas have irregular and spiculated margins whereas benign lesions are more likely to have smooth outlines, in the individual patient it is not safe to rely on these radiographic features alone to make the distinction between a benign and a malignant lesion.

After the discovery of a pulmonary mass on chest radiography, further imaging and other investigations of a patient will depend on the symptomatology, age, and smoking history of the patient. CT is valuable in evaluating the extension of a central mass into the mediastinum (Fig. 18), for demonstrating the presence or absence of enlarged mediastinal lymph nodes which may, but do not invariably, indicate local tumour spread, and for the detection of distant metastases, for example to the contralateral lung, adrenal glands, and liver. It is usually the overall

Fig. 17 A left-sided tension pneumothorax in a patient with cystic fibrosis. The mediastinal shift and straightening of the left hemidiaphragm should be noted.

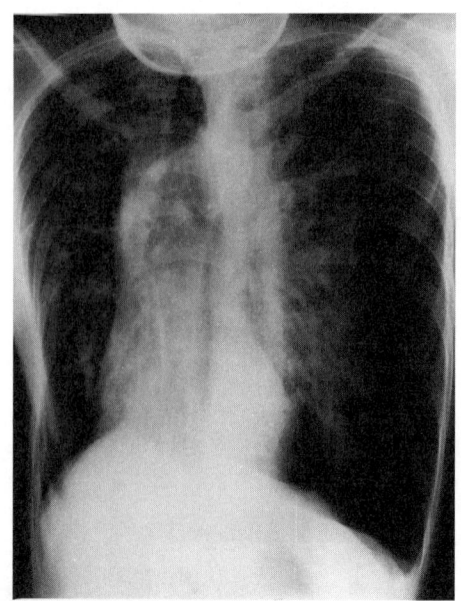

pattern and extent of disease on a staging CT examination, rather than any single abnormality, which indicates whether a patient with bronchial carcinoma, who is otherwise fit, is likely to be suitable for surgical resection. Local invasion of the chest wall by an adjacent bronchial carcinoma may not always be demonstrated by CT, and MRI may be useful because of its ability to image in different planes. When surgery is not indicated and a histological diagnosis is needed, percutaneous needle biopsy of central lesions can be performed safely under CT guidance. Similarly, smaller peripheral lesions that are not accessible by bronchoscopy may be biopsied, usually under fluoroscopic control.

Cavitating pulmonary lesions

The radiological definition of cavitation is a lucency, representing air, within a mass or area of consolidation. The cavity may or may not contain a fluid level or an intracavitary body and is surrounded by a wall of variable thickness. The two most likely diagnoses in an adult presenting with a cavitating pulmonary mass on chest radiography are bronchial carcinoma (central, large, and often squamous in type) (Fig. 19) or a lung abscess (usually peripheral and sometimes multiple). Cavitation is recognized in a variety of bacterial pneumonias, particularly those due to tuberculosis, Staphylococcus, anaerobes, and Klebsiella.

Less commonly, cavitation is seen within pulmonary infarcts and in areas of pulmonary contusion due to trauma. Long-standing cavities in lungs scarred by previous tuberculosis predispose to the formation of mycetomas; once these fungus balls occupy most of the cavity, a characteristic translucent 'air-crescent sign' can be seen between the upper surface of the fungus ball and the margin of the cavity on chest radiography (Fig. 20).

Multiple pulmonary nodules

Many conditions are characterized by multiple small pulmonary nodules (Fig. 21). Only by combining the relevant clinical information with a precise description of the size and distribution of the nodules can the differential diagnosis be narrowed. In the United Kingdom, metastatic deposits are by far the commonest cause of multiple pulmonary nodules of varying sizes in an adult. In some parts of the southern United States, histoplasmosis is endemic and multiple granulomatous nodules are more common than those due to disseminated malignancy. In the absence of a known malignancy and when clinical findings and laboratory investigations are inconclusive, biopsy of one of the nodules may be the only means of establishing a diagnosis.

A myriad of small nodules, less than 5 mm in diameter, produces a

Fig. 18 CT of a central cavitating bronchial carcinoma showing direct extension of the tumour into the subcarinal region of the mediastinum.

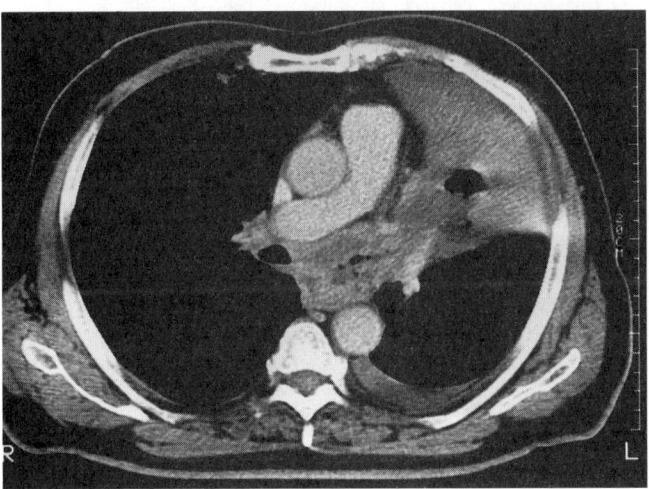

Fig. 20 An air crescent (arrow) around a fungus ball at the left apex. This had developed in a tuberculous fibrotic cavity.

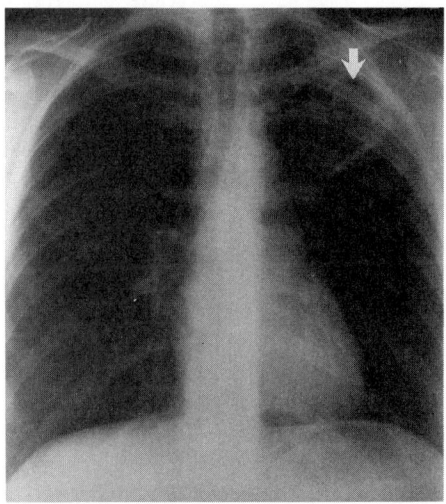

Fig. 19 Chest radiograph of a large cavitating squamous-cell bronchial carcinoma adjacent to the right hilum. The right hemidiaphragm is raised because of phrenic nerve invasion by the tumour.

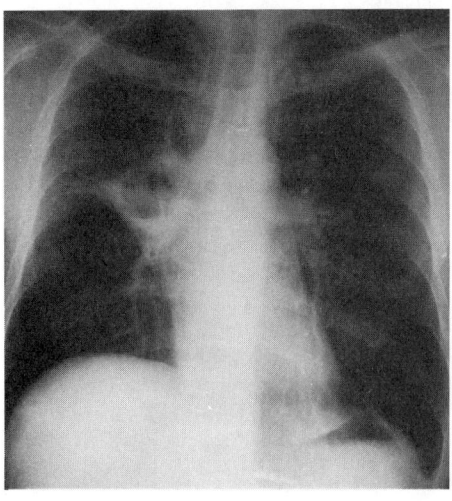

Fig. 21 Multiple pulmonary nodules of varying sizes typical of metastatic disease.

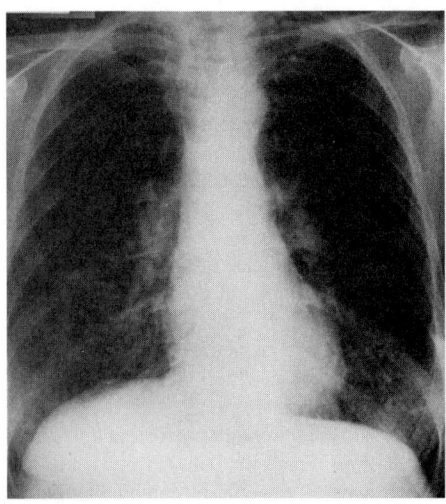

Table 4 *Differential diagnosis of widespread fine nodular (0.5–3 mm in diameter) shadowing*

Miliary tuberculosis
Fungal diseases
Metastatic disease
Pneumoconiosis
Sarcoidosis
Extrinsic allergic alveolitis
Idiopathic pulmonary haemorrhage

pattern which is often described as miliary. A list of causes of miliary shadowing is given in Table 4. An important diagnosis to consider in any patient with this radiographic pattern is miliary tuberculosis. Other differential diagnoses in an asymptomatic patient with numerous pulmonary nodules include sarcoidosis, metastatic disease, or, if there is a relevant occupational history, pneumoconiosis. As always, comparison with previous radiographs will give invaluable information about the rate of progression and thus the probable nature of the pulmonary nodules. To a lesser extent the distribution of nodules is a consideration in refining the differential diagnosis of multiple pulmonary nodules; for example, the small nodules of pulmonary sarcoidosis tend to be midzone and perihilar, whereas haematogenous metastases are generally of varying sizes and have a predilection for the lower lobes (probably because of increased blood flow to these regions).

The density of nodules sometimes provides conclusive evidence that the nodules are of benign aetiology, for example the heavily calcified nodules which are seen following histoplasmosis or chickenpox (varicella) pneumonia. The majority of multiple pulmonary nodules are of soft tissue density, and it may be extremely difficult to judge whether small nodules are of calcific or soft tissue density because their apparent density depends so critically on the radiographic technique used.

Numerous poorly defined nodules of low density of approximately 8 mm in diameter can be seen around areas of pulmonary consolidation. In other areas they may be confluent and so make up a larger poorly defined opacity; occasionally these nodules will be uniformly distributed throughout the lungs. At a pathological level these nodules correspond to individual acini which are full of the products of disease such as pulmonary oedema, an inflammatory exudate, or haemorrhage.

Radiographic features of specific diseases

Pleural and chest wall disease

Because of the two-dimensional nature of a posteroanterior chest radiograph, abnormalities arising from the pleura or chest wall are often difficult to assess. The appearance of a pleural mass on chest radiography depends on whether it is face-on or tangential to the X-ray beam. Generally, a pleural mass will produce a rounded opacity with a sharp medial border and a less well-defined lateral margin (Fig. 22). Although abnormality of an adjacent rib will usually indicate that an apparent 'pleural' mass is of chest wall origin, the distinction between a pleural and chest wall mass often cannot be made from a chest radiograph alone.

With extensive pleural pathology it may be difficult to distinguish between a pleural effusion, chronic pleural thickening, or even a neoplasm of the pleura such as a mesothelioma. In such cases a lateral decubitus film will distinguish between pleural fluid or thickening by demonstrating redistribution of the shadowing if it is due to an effusion. Ultrasonography is also useful in identifying pleural fluid. CT will show even more precisely the site and extent of an abnormality which is apparently 'pleural' on a chest radiograph. Furthermore, CT will reveal subtle abnormalities not shown on a plain chest radiograph, for example flecks of calcification within the wall of a chronic empyema (Fig. 23) or underlying rib abnormalities in the case of a neoplastic tumour. Similarly,

masses arising from the chest wall which give the appearance of a 'pleural' mass, such as an intercostal neurofibroma or lipoma, are most accurately assessed by CT.

Chronic obstructive airways disease

The majority of patients with chronic obstructive airways disease show remarkably little radiographic abnormality despite often considerable symptoms. Of the two principal components falling under the heading of chronic obstructive airways disease, emphysema, when it is severe, can be detected on chest radiography whereas chronic bronchitis is a clinical diagnosis with no specific radiographic features.

Whilst emphysema is correctly regarded as a pathological diagnosis, the destruction of alveolar walls distal to the terminal bronchial results in certain radiographic features in more advanced cases; overinflation of the lungs causes flattening of the domes of the diaphragm, which may have a scalloped appearance; a lateral chest radiograph may show striking translucency of the enlarged retrosternal and retrocardiac regions. The pattern of the pulmonary vasculature is deranged, with the smooth tapering of the vessels replaced by an abrupt change in calibre from the larger proximal pulmonary arteries to the spindly and attenuated peripheral vessels, giving a so-called pruned appearance. Depending on the aetiology of the emphysema, there may be an upper zone (e.g. smokers)

Fig. 22 The typical features of a mass of pleural origin (a left mesothelioma): a sharp medial border which fades into a less well-defined lateral border.

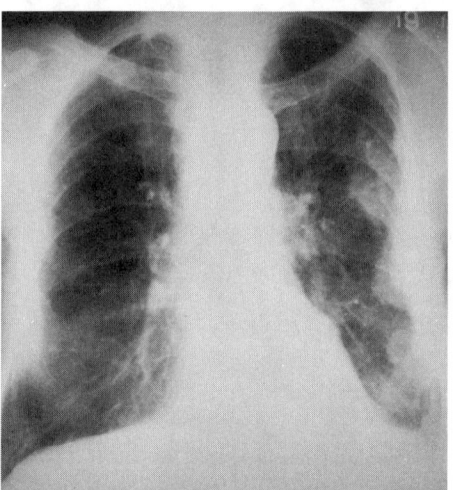

Fig. 23 CT of a chronic tuberculous empyema. The wall of the collection is thick and typically contains calcifications. The chronic empyema has caused contraction of the right hemithorax.

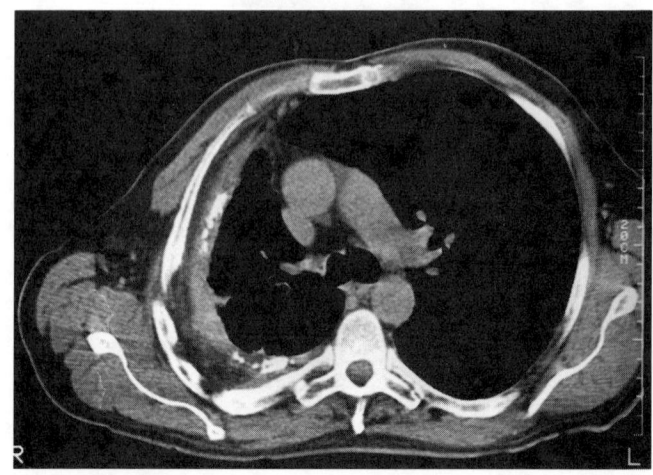

or a lower zone (e.g. α_1-antitrypsin deficiency) predominance; the relatively spared lung often shows a prominent vascular pattern due to blood diversion to these areas. Bullous emphysema is characterized by cystic air spaces bounded by extremely thin walls. They may become extremely large and occupy a large part of the lung. A fluid level within a bulla represents either infection or haemorrhage. Another complication is a pneumothorax which may be chronic and is sometimes difficult to distinguish from a large bulla. CT is far more sensitive than chest radiography in the detection of emphysema, and in some early cases will show evidence of emphysema before lung function tests become abnormal.

Bronchiectasis

Bronchiectasis is defined as damage to the bronchial wall causing irreversible dilatation of the bronchi, whatever the aetiology. The diagnosis of bronchiectasis is rarely made with certainty from the chest radiograph alone, unless the disease is extensive and severe. On a chest radiograph the abnormal bronchi may be visible as either ring shadows and curvilinear shadows, which represent thickened bronchial wall seen end-on, or as parallel thin lines or 'tram-lines', particularly in the lower lobes; this latter sign can be very subtle and may be more obvious on the lateral chest radiograph. Other radiographic signs of bronchiectasis include round or oval nodular opacities and sometimes band shadows representing grossly dilated fluid-filled bronchi.

High resolution CT has supplanted bronchography as the imaging technique of choice in the investigation of patients with suspected bronchiectasis. Abnormally dilated and thickened bronchi are readily identified on high resolution CT (Fig. 24); a normal bronchus is of approximately the same diameter as its accompanying pulmonary artery. In addition to allowing a confident diagnosis of bronchiectasis to be made, often in the face of a normal chest radiograph, high resolution CT will show whether one or more lobe is involved, which may be an important consideration in deciding on medical or surgical management.

Chronic diffuse lung disease

Many conditions are characterized by diffuse shadowing of the lungs on a chest radiograph. The lung has few ways of responding to injury (capillary leak, cellular infiltration, or interstitial fibrosis), and the resulting spectrum of radiographic patterns is correspondingly limited. It is important that reproducible terms are used in the description of widespread pulmonary shadowing; vague terms which may convey a patho-

Fig. 24 High resolution CT showing thickened and dilated subsegmental airways characteristic of severe bronchiectasis.

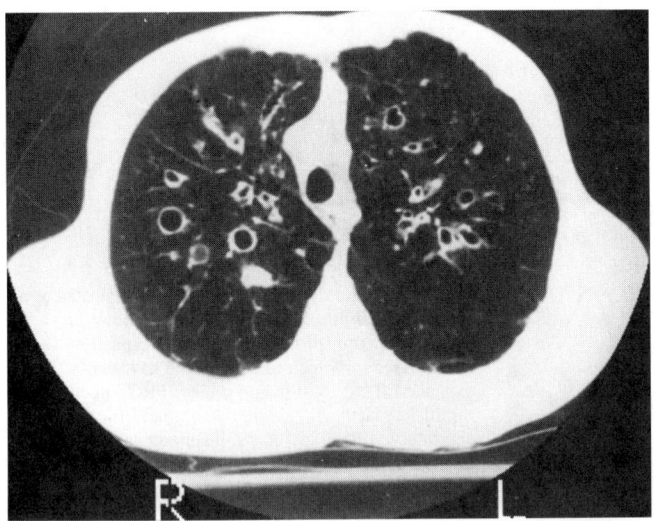

logical meaning (which in fact cannot be inferred from the gross signs of disease on a chest radiograph), for example 'inflammatory shadowing', should not be used. Instead, descriptions of the radiographic pattern should be limited to strictly morphological terms such as reticular (a fine network), nodular (small dots of a specified size), linear (fine lines which are not vessels), ground-glass (a greying-out of the lungs which makes the vascular markings indistinct), and air-space shadowing or consolidation (opacification of the lungs in which an air bronchogram may be visible). These descriptors are more reproducible and are preferable to the wide range of imprecise and whimsical terms that have been coined in the past.

An analysis of the distribution of the disease is often at least as important as defining the radiographic pattern in reaching a differential diagnosis. This involves an assessment of whether the disease involves all parts of the lung uniformly, or whether there is a zonal predominance (upper, mid, or lower; central or peripheral). The perihilar, mid-zone, and upper-zone distribution of the reticulonodular pattern in sarcoidosis is quite different from the lower-zone peripheral distribution of cryptogenic fibrosing alveolitis; these differences in distribution are even more obvious on cross-sectional CT images. The differential diagnosis can be further refined by assimilating other radiographic abnormalities, for example the presence of pleural disease in the case of asbestosis or enlarged hilar lymph nodes in the case of sarcoidosis or lymphangitis carcinomatosa.

Only when the radiographic findings of a patient with diffuse lung disease are taken in conjunction with the clinical features should a working diagnosis be attempted. Many pieces of information contribute to the final diagnosis, as can be seen from the following example. A middle-aged female, known to have systemic sclerosis, has become increasingly short of breath over a period of 8 months. She has questionable finger clubbing and inspiratory crackles at the lung bases; a chest radiograph shows small-volume lungs and a reticular pattern predominantly in the lower zones with an area of consolidation in the left lower lobe. The patient has developed fibrosing alveolitis, an association of systemic sclerosis. A subsequent barium swallow showed free gastro-oesophageal reflux and an aperistaltic oesophagus, suggesting that the consolidation in the left lower lobe was due to aspiration. In the context of diffuse lung disease, the chest radiograph should be considered as only one part of the clinical jigsaw since a specific diagnosis can rarely be achieved with complete confidence from the radiographic findings alone. In addition to the non-specific appearances of many diffuse lung diseases, the sensitivity of chest radiography is less than ideal, with up to 15 per cent of patients with biopsy-proven diffuse lung disease having a normal chest radiograph. Conversely, a less than perfectly exposed chest radiograph, particularly of an obese patient, may misleadingly raise the spectre of diffuse lung disease.

In the last 10 years the development of high resolution CT has changed the radiological approach to the diagnosis of diffuse lung disease. High resolution CT images of the lung correlate closely with the macroscopic appearances of pathological specimens, and high resolution CT represents a substantial improvement over chest radiography in terms of sensitivity, specificity, and diagnostic accuracy. Furthermore, CT samples a far greater volume of lung than even the most generous lung biopsy, making it less prone to errors of sampling. Nevertheless, despite the increased confidence with which a specific diagnosis of diffuse lung disease can be made with high resolution CT, open-lung biopsy is still required to achieve a definitive histological diagnosis in difficult cases. The extent of diffuse lung disease can be precisely estimated on high resolution CT and, when a biopsy is indicated, the distribution of disease will indicate whether a transbronchial biopsy or an open-lung biopsy is more likely to obtain a representative specimen.

REFERENCES

Armstrong, P., Wilson, A.W., Dee, P., and Hansell, D.M. (1994). *Imaging of diseases of the chest* (2nd edn). Mosby Year Book, St Louis, MO.

Aronchick, J.M. (1990). CT of mediastinal lymph nodes in patients with non-small cell lung carcinoma. In: *Lung cancer, The Radiologic Clinics of North America* (ed J.H. Woodring), Vol. 23, pp. 573–82. W.B. Saunders, Harcourt Brace Jovanovich, New York.

Fleischner Society. (1984). Glossary of terms for thoracic radiology: recommendations of the nomenclature committee of the Fleischner Society. *American Journal of Roentgenology*, **143**, 509–17.

Freundlich, I.M. and Bragg, D.G. (1992). *A radiologic approach to diseases of the chest*. Williams & Wilkins, Baltimore, MD.

Heitzmann, E.R. (1988). *The mediastinum: radiologic correlations with anatomy and pathology* (2nd edn). Springer-Verlag, Berlin.

Mathieson, J.R., Mayo, J.R., Staples, C.A., and Müller, N.L. (1989). Chronic diffuse infiltrative lung disease: comparison of diagnostic accuracy of CT and chest radiography. *Radiology*, **171**, 111–16.

Müller, N.L. (1991). Clinical value of high resolution CT in chronic diffuse lung disease. *American Journal of Roentgenology*, **157**, 1163–70.

Naidich, D.P., Zerhouni, E.A., and Siegelman, S.S. (1991). *Computed tomography and magnetic resonance of the thorax* (2nd edn). Raven Press, New York.

Proto, A.V. and Speckman, J.M. (1979). The left lateral radiograph of the chest. In: *Medical radiography and photography*. Eastman Kodak, Rochester, NY.

Reed, J.C. (1991). *Chest radiology: plain film patterns and differential diagnoses* (3rd edn). Mosby Year Book, St Louis, MO.

Wilson, A.G. (1992). Interpreting the chest radiograph. In: *Diagnostic radiology, an Anglo-American textbook of imaging* (2nd edn) (ed R.G. Grainger and D.J. Allison), pp. 149–61. Churchill Livingstone, Edinburgh.

17.6.2 Lung function testing

N. B. PRIDE

Tests of ventilatory mechanics

Static lung volumes (Fig. 1)

VITAL CAPACITY

Vital capacity (VC) is the volume expired from full inflation (total lung capacity (TLC)) to full expiration (residual volume (RV)) and can be measured by a spirometer or by integrating expired flow at the mouth. A reduction in vital capacity can occur with a reduction in TLC (as in lung fibrosis or inspiratory muscle weakness) or an increase in RV (as in emphysema, asthma, and other forms of intrapulmonary airway disease). Measurement of TLC and subdivisions distinguishes between these two possibilities.

FUNCTIONAL RESIDUAL CAPACITY AND TOTAL LUNG CAPACITY

In normal lungs resting breathing volume (functional residual capacity (FRC)) is about 50 per cent of the fully expanded volume of the lung (TLC).

FRC can be measured by either gas dilution or whole-body plethysmography. In the gas dilution methods a known volume and concentration of a relatively insoluble foreign gas (usually helium) is allowed to mix with resident intrapulmonary gas, the volume of which is measured from the difference between the initial and final concentrations of marker gas. In normal lungs a single breath test provides a reasonable estimate of lung volume, but multibreath methods lasting more than 5 min may be required to achieve mixing in patients with intrapulmonary airway obstruction. In the whole-body plethysmograph method the subject makes panting efforts against a closed shutter while seated in a large air-tight chamber. As mass movement of gas is prevented, changes in alveolar volume during this manoeuvre are due to compression and rarefaction of alveolar gas. Once change in alveolar volume and pressure are known, the alveolar volume can be calculated using Boyle's law. The volume inspired during a maximum inspiration or expiration from FRC can then be measured with a spirometer to derive TLC or RV. The plethysmographic method often gives higher values than the gas dilution method for FRC in severe intrapulmonary airway disease. Some of this difference occurs because plethysmography measures intrathoracic gas which barely communicates with the airway (bullae and other very poorly ventilated areas). An accurate estimate of thoracic volume can also be obtained from planimetry of standard posteroanterior and lateral chest radiographs taken at full inflation. Corrections have to be made for tissue and vascular volumes of the lungs so as to estimate gas volume.

In normal subjects FRC is passively determined by the balance between the inward recoil of the lungs and outward recoil of the chest wall. Reductions in VC in lung fibrosis, respiratory muscle weakness and chest wall deformity are accompanied by decreases in TLC and FRC. In obesity there is a reduced FRC. Intrapulmonary airway disease consistently leads to a rise in RV and FRC, while TLC is either normal or, in some subjects with emphysema, increased. When TLC is increased, the accompanying increase in RV is almost always greater so that there is still a decreased VC. When airway obstruction is severe, FRC may be considerably greater than the volume determined by lung and chest wall recoil. This reflects continuing inspiratory muscle activity

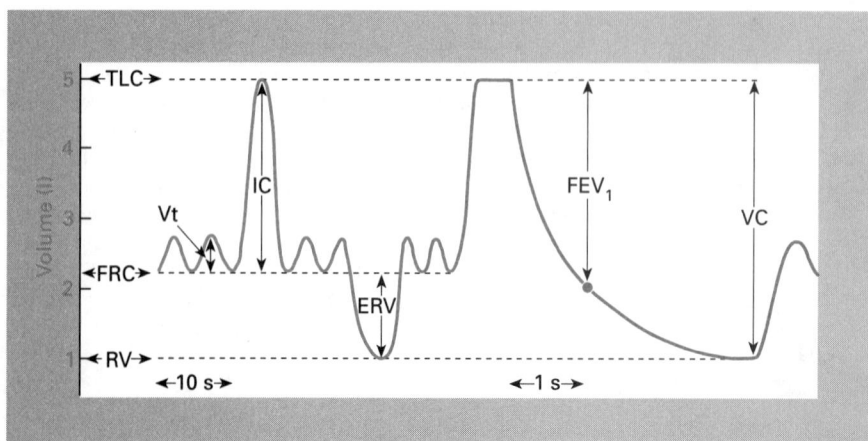

Fig. 1 Static and dynamic lung volumes indicated as a record of tidal breathing against time, followed by expiratory and inspiratory forced vital capacity manoeuvres for which the time scale has been expanded. TLC, total lung capacity; FRC, functional residual capacity; RV, residual volume; FEV$_1$, forced expiratory volume in 1 s; IC, inspiratory capacity; Vt, tidal volume; ERV, expiratory reserve volume; VC, vital capacity.

through expiration and slowing of tidal expiratory flow. The alveolar pressure at the end of expiration, which is normally equal to atmospheric pressure, is then positive ('intrinsic' positive end-expired pressure) and provides a threshold load which has to be overcome by the inspiratory muscles before inspiratory flow can begin.

Tests of forced expiration and inspiration

The volume expired in the first second of a forced expiration commenced from TLC (forced expiratory volume in 1 second (FEV_1)) (Fig. 1) was originally introduced because it was found to relate well to the maximum voluntary ventilation that could be sustained over 15 seconds both in subjects with normal lungs and in the presence of many lung diseases. The physiological basis of these tests depends on the development of plateaux of expiratory flow at any particular lung volume once a certain minimum expiratory pressure is achieved. Provided that flow plateau conditions are achieved, the values obtained do not depend on the pressure applied but only on the mechanical characteristics of the lungs and airways. In contrast, tests of forced inspiration are much more dependent on the applied inspiratory pressures. Both forced expiration and inspiration can be analysed as change in volume versus time (by spirometry) (Fig. 1) or as change in instantaneous flow rate (usually measured by a pneumotachograph) versus change in lung volume (maximum flow–volume curve) (Fig. 2). Standard spirometric measurements are the FEV_1 and the VC; the latter can be obtained from forced expiration (forced vital capacity (FVC)) or from a separate slower full expiration. In airway disease FVC may be considerably less than the slow VC. Normally, FEV_1 is more than 70 per cent of VC. Two patterns of spirometric abnormality can be distinguished: 'obstructive' in which, although there is usually some reduction in FVC, FEV_1 is reduced even more so that the ratio FEV_1/FVC is low, and 'restrictive', in which a small FVC is associated with normal or even accelerated emptying on forced expiration and a normal or increased FEV_1/FVC ratio. The maximum flow–volume curve (Fig. 2) shows that, on expiration, flow normally rapidly rises to a peak value and then declines in an approximately linear fashion. Peak expiratory flow (PEF) can also be measured with a peak flow gauge. The most effort-dependent part of expiration is close to full inflation, and therefore in measuring PEF the subject must take a full inspiration and make a rapid and forceful start to the subsequent full expiration. Provided that subject cooperation is obtained and gross expiratory muscle weakness is not present, a reduction in maximum expiratory flow usually indicates intrinsic airway disease or reduction in lung recoil. For clinical assessment of ventilatory function, FEV_1 and VC (or FVC) are usually adequate, although these tests will not pick up mild airway disease. In asthma the value of PEF is closely related to the value of FEV_1, and because PEF can be measured by simple meters which can be used by patients in the home or at work, this measurement is particularly useful for identifying asthmatic episodes and their response to treatment. The maximum flow–volume curve cannot be used to distinguish different mechanisms of intrapulmonary airway narrowing, but distinctive curves are found when obstruction is extrathoracic (Fig. 2).

Airways resistance

Airways resistance is the ratio of driving pressure (difference between alveolar and mouth pressures) to instantaneous gas flow. Alveolar pressure can be obtained non-invasively with a body plethysmograph or derived from oesophageal pressure obtained via a balloon-catheter system. During quiet tidal breathing via the mouth about one-third of the total resistance is in the extrathoracic airway, about one-third is in the central intrathoracic conducting airways, and the remaining one-third is in the peripheral airways of less than 2 to 3 mm internal diameter. Although resistance is measured during resting breathing, its precise value varies according to the lung volume at which it is measured, the

Fig. 2 Characteristic patterns of maximum flow–volume curves for normal subjects, and patients with intrathoracic and extrathoracic airway obstruction. (a) Normal subjects. Left: simultaneous record of maximum expiratory flow vs volume (MEFV, upper curve) and expired volume versus time (spirogram, lower curve) during a forced expiration in a healthy normal subject. The volume expired in first second (forced expiratory volume in one second, FEV_1) is indicated. Right: maximum expiratory and inspiratory flow-volume (MEFV, MIFV) curves in another normal subject. Note the different shape of the MEFV curve in the two normal subjects. PEF, peak expiratory flow; TLC, total lung capacity; RV, residual volume: FVC, forced vital capacity. (b) Intrathoracic airways obstruction. Left: mild obstruction. Despite preservation of a normal peak expiratory flow the MEFV curve shows marked convexity to the volume axis in contrast to the linearity or concavity to the volume axis in normal subjects. Right: severe obstruction with gross reduction on both the flow and volume axis and convexity to the volume axis. Reduction in flow on MEFV curve considerably greater than on MIFV curve. (c) Extrathoracic airways obstruction. Left: fixed obstruction pattern as seen in tracheal stenosis with reduction in flow on MEFV and MIFV curves and a distinctive plateau of flow on MEFV curve. Right: variable obstruction with inspiratory narrowing of the upper airway but preservation of a normal MEFV curve in a patient with severe obstructive sleep apnoea.

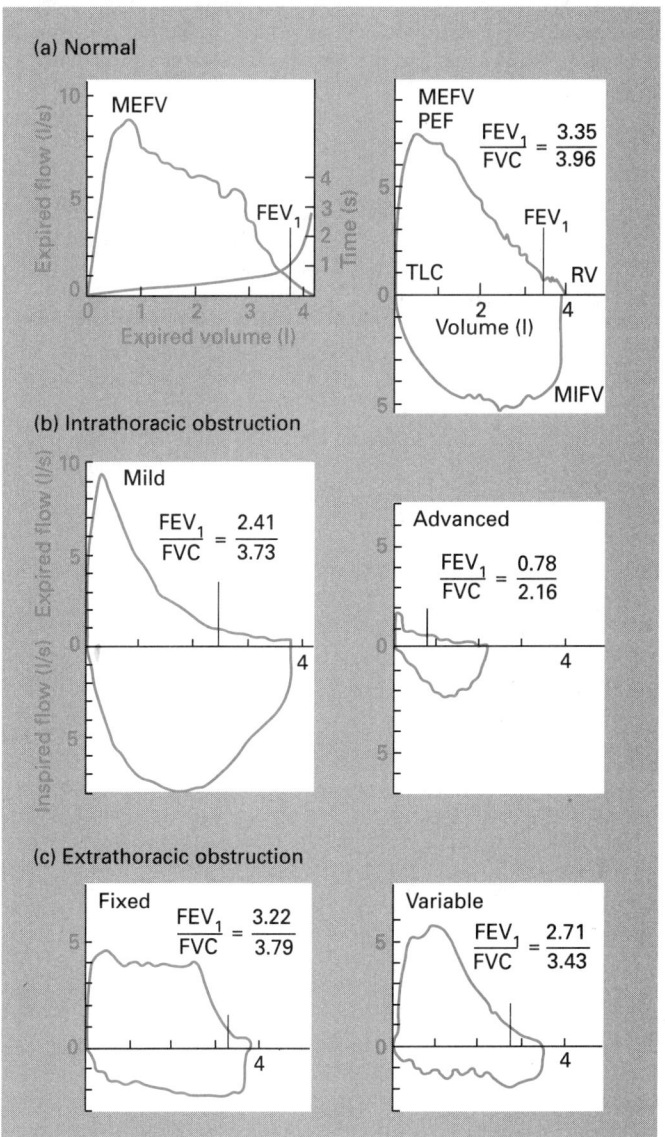

phase of respiration (inspiration or expiration), the size of the laryngeal aperture, and the flow rate. Consequently, the measurement is used more for research into airway pharmacology than for routine clinical assessment.

Lung recoil pressure and compliance

Lung recoil pressure is the difference between alveolar and pleural pressure. Pleural pressure is estimated from the pressure measured by a balloon-tipped catheter placed in mid-oesophagus. The relation between lung recoil pressure and volume is obtained by interrupting inspiration and expiration during vital capacity manoeuvres when mouth pressure will equal alveolar pressure. The change in volume for unit change in recoil pressure is the static lung compliance. Analysis of lung recoil and compliance helps in examining mechanisms of airflow obstruction and also in determining whether a reduction in TLC is due to extrapulmonary causes (when there is a low recoil pressure at TLC and low compliance). A low recoil pressure and a high static compliance are found in emphysema. Lung compliance measured during ordinary or accelerated tidal breathing reflects the effects of airway disease as well as the static elastic properties of the lung. The effective dynamic compliance of the lungs is reduced below static compliance when there is peripheral airway narrowing. Airway pressure during the end-inspiratory pause is often used to assess compliance in patients on assisted ventilation in the intensive care unit; this indicates the total compliance of lungs and chest wall which is normally about half that of the lungs alone.

Tests to define the site and mechanism of airflow obstruction

An increased airways resistance or reduced maximum expiratory flow is produced by primary disease at any site along the tracheobronchial tree or may be secondary to a loss of airway distension as occurs in emphysema.

The role of loss of airway distending forces can be assessed by relating maximum expiratory flow or resistance to the corresponding lung recoil pressure, rather than to lung volume. If airway obstruction is extrathoracic, distinctive maximum flow–volume curves may be obtained (Fig. 2). Owing to the serial distribution of airway geometry, values of PEF and airways resistance reflect mainly the dimensions of large airways in normal subjects, but this cannot be assumed to apply in airway disease which inevitably distorts the serial distribution of airway dimensions. Comparing measurements of resistance or maximum expiratory flow breathing air or a mixture of 80 per cent helium and 20 per cent oxygen gives some information on the serial site of narrowing: improvement on helium–oxygen breathing is present when narrowing is in the central airway and absent when it is in peripheral airways. An immediate improvement in airway function after bronchodilators is assumed to be due to reduction in bronchial muscle contraction.

Tests to detect minor peripheral airway disease

Minor changes in the peripheral airways, which commonly develop in smokers, cannot be detected by standard spirometric tests or by measuring airways resistance, but lead to reduced maximum flow in the last 25 per cent of FVC, a fall in dynamic lung compliance as respiratory frequency is increased, and an abnormal single-breath nitrogen test (see below). Once airway disease becomes sufficiently advanced to lead to changes in standard spirometry, these additional tests provide little further information.

Airway responsiveness

In subjects with asthma there is an increased tendency for airways narrowing to occur in response to a whole range of stimuli (e.g. exercise,

hyperventilation, breathing cold air, hypo- or hyperosmolar aerosols, constrictor drugs such as histamine or cholinergic agonists, or mediators such as bradykinin or leukotrienes). This responsiveness can be quantified using an incremental dose–response technique. Histamine or methacholine is generally used as the stimulus and the dose is increased until a 20 per cent fall in FEV_1 is produced. Airway responsiveness is often increased in smokers with chronic airflow obstruction, when it may reflect altered airway geometry and increased thickness of the airway wall.

Other aspects of airway function

The sensitivity of the cough reflex can be assessed by inhaling sequential small doses of capsaicin; other stimulants sometimes used are citric acid, hypo- or hyperosmolar solutions, or mediators such as bradykinin. Capsaicin cough sensitivity is normal in most patients with productive cough, such as that due to chronic bronchitis, and is usually normal in asthma. Sensitivity is enhanced in persistent non-productive cough such as may occur with angiotensin-converting enzyme inhibitor drugs, variant asthma, following acute respiratory tract infection, or associated with gastro-oesophageal reflux. Mucociliary function can be assessed by inhaling radionuclide-labelled microspheres and following their clearance from the airways after impaction. Ciliary beat frequency can be assessed *in vitro* on specimens obtained by brushing at bronchoscopy. Defects in mucociliary clearance are common in smokers with chronic bronchitis, in cystic fibrosis, and in rare syndromes where there are immotile, or more commonly dysmotile, cilia. Epithelial permeability has been assessed by following the clearance of inhaled radio-aerosols of diethylenetriamine penta-acetate (DTPA), but it is uncertain how much of the clearance is via bronchiolar epithelium and how much via alveolar epithelium. Clearance is greatly accelerated in smokers and rapidly slows after stopping smoking.

Respiratory muscle function

The simplest test of respiratory muscle function is to measure mouth pressure when maximum inspiratory or expiratory efforts are made against a closed valve. Portable meters for bedside use are now available. Properly performed, this test indicates the overall strength of inspiratory or expiratory muscles, but low values may be due to poor technique. Bilateral paralysis of the diaphragm can be suspected if there is orthopnoea and paradoxical inspiratory indrawing of the abdominal wall (particularly in the supine position). The pressure developed across the diaphragm during maximum inspiratory efforts can be measured by placing balloon catheters in the oesophagus and stomach, and further measurements of diaphragm function can be made using bilateral electrical stimulation of the phrenic nerves in the neck. A reduction in VC in the sitting position is often found in respiratory muscle weakness; a further fall of 25 per cent or more in VC on adopting the supine position is said to be characteristic of diaphragmatic weakness. Serial measurements of maximum effort mouth pressures (or, failing this, PEF or VC) may be useful in monitoring conditions where muscle strength varies rapidly (e.g. myasthenia gravis).

Respiratory muscle function is often impaired in generalized muscle disease and motor neurone disease and can then be the most important factor determining prognosis. Weakness is also common in polymyositis, some connective tissue disorders, notably systemic lupus erythematosus, and cachexia from whatever cause. Respiratory muscle function should be checked when there is unexplained restrictive lung disease or hypercapnia. Weakness of the respiratory muscles can be a limiting factor preventing weaning from assisted ventilation in the intensive care unit and is related to such factors as cachexia, muscle catabolism, electrolyte disturbance, and corticosteroid treatment, as well as the underlying lung disease.

An important factor compromising inspiratory muscle function is hyperinflation associated with severe airways obstruction. This may be found in acute severe asthma (when the respiratory muscles are normal or even 'trained') as well as in severe chronic obstructive pulmonary disease where there may be associated loss of muscle mass. Because of the abnormal lung and airway mechanics, the inspiratory muscles have to produce larger pressures to maintain a normal minute ventilation; in practice, because of the associated inefficiency of pulmonary gas exchange, minute ventilation at rest is usually increased. The raised FRC shortens the initial length of the inspiratory muscles so that they operate on a suboptimal part of their force–length curve and expend more energy to generate a given inspiratory pleural pressure. All these mechanisms stress the inspiratory muscles and increase their oxygen consumption. In normal subjects the oxygen consumption of the respiratory muscles is very small even during exercise but, with disease, particularly airflow obstruction, they may account for a significant proportion of the total oxygen consumption.

The mechanical work of breathing can be calculated from changes in oesophageal pressure and volume during tidal breathing, but the oxygen consumption of the respiratory muscles can only be measured in the research laboratory.

Tests of pulmonary gas exchange

Distribution and mixing of inspired gas

Inequalities of ventilation and inefficient gas mixing may be either between regions or within regions. The topographical distribution of ventilation can be examined by placing counters over the chest wall and detecting the distribution of inhaled radionuclides such as xenon-133 or krypton-81m. The lung volume at which airways begin to close (closing volume) can be measured by asking the subject to inhale a small quantity of a foreign gas (argon, helium, or xenon-133 have all been used) at the beginning of an inspiration from RV. Because of basal airway closure this foreign gas is preferentially distributed to the lung apices. During the subsequent expiration an abrupt rise in concentration of the foreign gas at the lips indicates that gas is now coming preferentially from the apices due to closure of airways at the bases. Closing volume in the upright position is well below FRC in young non-smokers, but rises with age when it may occur within the tidal breathing range. Increases in closing volume occur in many smokers at an early stage in the development of airway disease.

In normal subjects much of the inequality in ventilation is on a regional basis; in the upright posture ventilation is greater in the dependent basal zones. In most diseases of the lung, however, inequalities within a region are of greater importance than inter-regional differences. This applies even in diseases like asthma and emphysema, where obvious inequalities of ventilation are easily demonstrated by radioactive gas methods. These inequalities may be detected by tests which follow gas mixing by sampling expired air at the mouth. A simple single breath test measures the expired nitrogen concentration at the mouth after a preceding vital capacity breath of 100 per cent oxygen. The rate of rise of expired nitrogen over the middle part of the expiration indicates the unevenness of ventilation: towards the end of the breath there may be a sharp rise in nitrogen concentration which corresponds to closing volume. Other techniques are based on the rate of equilibration when helium is washed in or nitrogen washed out of the lung to measure FRC, and on the difference between the volume measured by a single-breath test using a foreign gas and that obtained from multibreath techniques or body plethysmography.

The major use of the single-breath nitrogen test is as a sensitive indicator of early lung damage as with smoking or occupational lung disease.

Regional ventilation scans are most widely used in conjunction with regional perfusion scans to diagnose pulmonary embolism by the presence of 'unmatched' perfusion defects. They are also useful in assessment of bullous emphysema, unilateral transradiancy, and suspected inhalation of foreign bodies. In bronchial carcinoma, defects in regional ventilation (and perfusion) are very often more severe than suspected from the chest radiograph. Using a combination of preoperative spirometry and regional ventilation scans quantifying the contribution of each lung, a reasonably accurate prediction of postoperative spirometry after pulmonary resection can be made. Because there is usually close concordance between ventilation and perfusion defects in bronchial carcinoma, the preoperative regional distribution of blood flow can also be used to make this prediction.

Transfer factor (diffusing capacity) for carbon monoxide

The transfer of carbon monoxide across the alveolar–capillary membrane and into combination with haemoglobin within the red blood corpuscle mimics the uptake of oxygen. By measuring carbon monoxide transfer at two or more levels of alveolar P_{O_2} it is possible to obtain separate values for transfer across the alveolar–capillary membrane and transfer into the haemoglobin within the red blood corpuscle and so derive pulmonary capillary blood volume. Values of carbon monoxide transfer are reduced if there is anaemia, but correction can be made for haemoglobin level.

In normal lungs carbon monoxide transfer can be used to define a true diffusing capacity of the lungs, which depends on the diffusivity of the gas and the available area and thickness of the alveolar–capillary membrane. The technique is extremely simple: the subject inhales a full breath of a gas mixture containing a very low carbon monoxide concentration and the gas transferred during breath-holding for 10 s at TLC is measured. The physiological significance of this measurement in lung disease is less clear cut as carbon monoxide transfer is affected by inhomogeneities within the lungs as well as by a true loss of area or increase in thickness of the membrane, and for this reason the term carbon monoxide transfer factor has been adopted in Europe to emphasize that a low carbon monoxide transfer does not indicate that a true diffusion defect is present or allow a prediction of maximum oxygen uptake.

Despite these theoretical limitations, values of carbon monoxide transfer (particularly when expressed per litre alveolar volume (transfer coefficient)) provide a test of peripheral lung function which is useful in differential diagnosis (Table 1). Apart from the major reductions found in severe emphysema and fibrosing alveolitis, smaller reductions are found in systemic sclerosis, chronic renal disease, graft versus host disease, pulmonary oedema, *P. carinii* pneumonia, pulmonary toxicity due to amiodarone, lymphangitis carcinomatosa, and a host of other conditions where the alveoli are involved with disease. However, the carbon monoxide transfer coefficient is also greatly influenced by pulmonary blood volume. An increase in blood volume per unit alveolar volume probably accounts for slightly increased values for the carbon monoxide transfer coefficient found with lung volume restriction in respiratory muscle weakness or after pneumonectomy. Values tend to be below normal in primary pulmonary hypertension, but increased when there is a right-to-left shunt in atrial septal defect. The avidity of carbon monoxide uptake by haemoglobin is utilized to make serial measurements of carbon monoxide transfer to monitor the number of haemoglobin binding sites (intra- and extravascular) accessible in the lungs in intrapulmonary haemorrhage.

Assessment of arterial hypoxaemia and hypercapnia

Arterial P_{O_2} (Pa_{O_2}) and P_{CO_2} (Pa_{CO_2}) are determined by the interaction between the efficiency of the lungs as gas exchangers and extrapulmonary factors (oxygen in the inspired air, total ventilation, cardiac output, and oxygen consumption). Despite gravitational differences in the distribution of ventilation and blood flow, normal lungs are very efficient gas exchangers. This efficiency can be assessed by measuring the alveolar–arterial P_{O_2} difference; mean alveolar P_{O_2} (PA_{O_2}) can be estimated if the arterial P_{CO_2} and P_{O_2} in the inspired air (PI_{O_2}) are known and a normal respiratory exchange ratio R is assumed. Then

Table 1 *Examples of the value of carbon monoxide transfer coefficient in differential diagnosis*

	Reduced	Normal or increased
Airway obstruction	Emphysema	Asthma
Chronic restrictive lung disease	Fibrosing alveolitis	Often remains normal in sarcoidosis; may be slightly increased when restriction is due to respiratory muscle weakness
Acute pulmonary infiltration	Pulmonary oedema	Intrapulmonary haemorrhage

Table 2 *Determinants of arterial P_{O_2} and P_{CO_2}*

Intrapulmonary abnormalities
Impaired diffusion
Ventilation-perfusion mismatch
Alveolar shunt†

Extrapulmonary modifying factors
Inspired O_2 concentration/pressure
Total ventilation/breathing pattern (influence alveolar P_{O_2} and CO_2 excretion)
Cardiac output/whole body metabolism (influence mixed venous P_{O_2} and P_{CO_2})

*All characterized by an increased alveolar–arterial P_{O_2} difference.

†Extrapulmonary shunts (e.g. right-to-left intracardiac shunts) also lower arterial P_{O_2} and increase alveolar–arterial P_{O_2} difference.

$$P_{A_{O_2}} = P_{I_{O_2}} - (1.2 \times P_{a_{CO_2}}).$$

When breathing room air at sea level $P_{I_{O_2}}$ is 20 kPa (150 mmHg) and the upper limit for alveolar–arterial P_{O_2} difference is 2.5 kPa (18.5 mmHg) in normal young subjects but 4.7 kPa (35 mmHg) in subjects aged 60 to 70 years. Average values are considerably lower. Unfortunately, for a given inefficiency of pulmonary gas exchange, values of alveolar–arterial P_{O_2} difference increase as absolute values of $P_{A_{O_2}}$ rise, and so serial measurements can only be used to assess trends in pulmonary gas exchange if $P_{I_{O_2}}$ and $P_{a_{CO_2}}$ remain constant. With changing inspired oxygen, the arterial-to-alveolar P_{O_2} ratio or the ratio of $P_{a_{O_2}}$ to fractional concentration of inspired oxygen should remain approximately constant if the efficiency of pulmonary gas exchange remains the same.

The three types of abnormality in the lungs which impair pulmonary gas exchange (Table 2) are all characterized by an increased difference between mean alveolar and arterial P_{O_2}. Most evidence suggests that, at least at rest, diffusion limitation is not important in the hypoxaemia of lung disease, and so resting alveolar–arterial P_{O_2} difference can be assumed to be due to either shunt or to ventilation–perfusion imbalance chiefly due to units with very low ventilation-to-perfusion (V/Q) ratios. The contribution of these low V/Q units to hypoxaemia can be estimated by calculating the proportion of total blood flow (effective shunt) which would have to bypass the ventilated lung completely (i.e. $V/Q = 0$) and so act as venous admixture to mixed arterial blood to produce the same alveolar–arterial difference. A simplified calculation can be based on arterial oxygen saturation % ($S_{a_{O_2}}$) when breathing air at rest, assuming an arterial–mixed venous saturation difference of 25 per cent and that blood leaving a ventilated alveoli has a saturation of 98 per cent. Then

effective shunt (percentage cardiac output)
$$= (98 - S_{a_{O_2}})/98 - (S_{a_{O_2}} - 25) \times 100.$$

This calculation includes extrapulmonary shunt (usually about 2 per cent of cardiac output), areas of intrapulmonary shunt ($V/Q = 0$), and areas of low V/Q ratio.

The distinction between ventilation–perfusion mismatch and shunt is of considerable practical importance, because the former can readily be corrected by modest increases in inspired oxygen concentration, while this is not the case with shunt. Attempts to distinguish shunt from low V/Q areas by measuring the alveolar–arterial P_{O_2} difference while breathing 100 per cent oxygen are unreliable because the high inspired oxygen leads to loss of volume in low V/Q units and their conversion to unventilated units. By using a research method which follows the excretion and arterial retention of several infused inert gases, ventilation–perfusion mismatch and alveolar shunt can be distinguished during spontaneous breathing without the need to give 100 per cent oxygen. This technique has shown that increase in alveolar shunt is rare even in severe airways obstruction (due to chronic obstructive pulmonary disease (COPD) or asthma), and is only present in the most severe exacerbations of disease requiring assisted ventilation in the intensive care unit. This indicates that, despite presumed airway occlusions by secretions and mucosal swelling, the subtended alveoli are receiving some fresh inspired gas, presumably via collateral ventilation through patent adjacent airways. The practical consequence is that $P_{a_{O_2}}$ in patients with severe exacerbations of airway disease can almost always be raised to safe levels with modest rises in inspired oxygen concentration, thus minimizing the risk of worsening hypercapnia. Ventilation–perfusion mismatch is the most important cause of hypoxaemia in pulmonary vascular disease and in severe fibrosing alveolitis at rest, as well as in airways obstruction.

In contrast, hypoxaemia due to shunt is relatively difficult to correct with modest rises in inspired oxygen concentration. Shunt is found with permanent anatomical defects in the heart or with pulmonary arteriovenous malformations. However, effective shunts develop with acute lung diseases which lead to extensive fluid filling of alveoli, such as pulmonary oedema, severe pneumonia, and adult respiratory distress syndrome. Increases in inspired oxygen to levels which carry a risk of causing pulmonary toxicity are often required, but oxygenation can be assisted by applying positive end-expired pressure to expand the resting lung volume and recruiting additional alveolar surface area for gas exchange.

Extrapulmonary factors play a large part in modifying the effects of impaired pulmonary gas exchange on the arterial blood gases. The alveolar P_{O_2} ($P_{A_{O_2}}$) depends on $P_{I_{O_2}}$ and the total ventilation. A low $P_{I_{O_2}}$ occurs at altitude owing to the reduced total atmospheric pressure. A reduced minute ventilation is an unusual cause of a low alveolar and arterial P_{O_2} and is accompanied by a rise in alveolar and arterial P_{CO_2}. Apart from acute crises such as asphyxia due to obstruction of the upper airway or cardiorespiratory arrest, reduced total ventilation is only found with sedation induced by anaesthesia or drugs, with paralysis or gross weakness of the respiratory muscles, or with rare breathing disorders such as Ondine's curse where the central control of breathing is abnormal. In most patients with lung disease, including chronic obstructive pulmonary disease with hypercapnia, there is some increase in total ventilation above normal, which plays an important part in minimizing the effects of impaired pulmonary gas exchange.

The effects of cardiac output and body oxygen consumption are reflected chiefly in the mixed venous P_{O_2} and P_{CO_2}. Thus, if there is significant shunt, a lower cardiac output and mixed venous P_{O_2} will result in a fall in PaO_2. When body oxygen consumption is increased (as most obviously on exercise), ventilation and cardiac output normally rise in parallel. However, in severely compromised patients in the intensive care unit increases in basal oxygen consumption due to fever, parenteral nutrition, or extra mechanical work during weaning may play a significant role in reducing PaO_2.

The interaction between intra- and extrapulmonary factors is particularly important in determining $PaCO_2$ because, when there is impaired pulmonary gas exchange, a small increase in total ventilation is more effective in maintaining a normal $PaCO_2$ than a normal PaO_2. Ventilation–perfusion mismatch impairs carbon dioxide as well as oxygen exchange in the lungs and leads to mean alveolar PCO_2 being lower than arterial PCO_2. However, whereas units with low V/Q ratios chiefly cause hypoxaemia, units with high V/Q ratios have most effect on the efficiency of carbon dioxide elimination. The effect of high V/Q units can be calculated as the proportion of the tidal breath V_t which would have to act as dead space V_d, completely avoiding contact with pulmonary blood ($V/Q = \infty$), to produce the same effect on the efficiency of carbon dioxide elimination:

$$V_d/V_t = (PaCO_2 - \text{mixed expired } PCO_2)/PaCO_2.$$

This equation gives the physiological dead space V_d, which at rest is normally 30 per cent or less of the tidal volume but may rise to 50–60 per cent in lung disease. This calculation includes the inspired gas which only penetrates as far as the conducting airways and is subsequently expired (anatomical or series dead space). The difference between anatomical and physiological dead space is sometimes called alveolar (or parallel) dead space.

Arterial PCO_2 is determined by the relation between metabolic carbon dioxide production and alveolar ventilation. Conventionally, alveolar ventilation is calculated from the difference between total ventilation and the dead space ventilation:

$$\text{alveolar ventilation (l/min)} = \text{total ventilation} \times (1 - V_d/V_t).$$

This calculation defines alveolar ventilation as the volume of gas leaving the alveoli each minute which has $PCO_2 = PaCO_2$. Since the mixed alveolar PCO_2 is much lower than arterial $PaCO_2$ in the presence of ventilation–perfusion mismatch, alveolar ventilation defined in this way is always lower than the true volume of gas leaving the alveoli per minute, and the terms 'alveolar' hypoventilation and hyperventilation merely indicate that the arterial $PaCO_2$ is above and below normal respectively and so can be a source of confusion.

A raised arterial $PaCO_2$ is found when total ventilation is reduced below metabolic needs (as occurs with sedation, asphyxia, paralysis, or gross weakness of the respiratory muscles, and rarely with a severe metabolic alkalosis). In all these conditions, mean alveolar PCO_2 is increased, pulmonary gas exchange is usually normal, and there is true alveolar hypoventilation with a modest fall in alveolar and arterial PO_2. When chronic hypercapnia is associated with intrapulmonary disease and ventilation–perfusion imbalance, arterial PCO_2 is considerably higher than mean (mixed) alveolar PCO_2. If the efficiency of CO_2 excretion is decreased by ventilation–perfusion imbalance and the V_d/V_t ratio is increased, a normal arterial PCO_2 can be maintained at first by a modest increase in total ventilation. However, as the ventilation–perfusion imbalance progresses, this compensation fails to prevent the development of chronic hypercapnia. The pattern of breathing also has an influence as the V_d/V_t ratio is higher with small tidal volumes. Patients with chronic obstructive pulmonary disease and a raised PCO_2 tend to breathe with a small tidal volume. The precise reasons why some patients with severe COPD maintain a normal $PaCO_2$, while others with equally severe obstruction develop chronic hypercapnia are uncertain, but may be related to differences in control of breathing and inspiratory muscle strength. Apart from severe COPD, the only group of patients who commonly develop chronic hypercapnia are those with respiratory muscle weakness and/or chest wall deformity. Chronic hypercapnia leads to a considerable rise in plasma bicarbonate so that arterial pH stabilizes close to 7.40 (see Chapter 17.14).

OXYGEN DELIVERY TO THE TISSUES

The ready availability of measurements of PaO_2 and oxygen saturation enable the efficiency of the lungs to be assessed satisfactorily. However, the supply of oxygen to the tissues depends on the total cardiac output, its correct distribution to the different organs, the total amount of haemoglobin available for oxygen carriage (reduced by anaemia or occupation of haemoglobin by carbon monoxide as in smokers), and the position and shape of the oxygen dissociation curve. At rest, about 20 to 25 per cent of the oxygen delivered to the tissues is usually metabolized, so that there is a considerable safety margin before the oxygen supply becomes limiting. This accounts for the good response to modest increases in inspired oxygen concentration and PaO_2 in acute-on-chronic respiratory failure; in a hypoxaemic patient increasing inspired oxygen to 24.5 per cent from the 20.9 per cent in room air in the presence of a normal cardiac output may increase tissue oxygen delivery by about 200 ml/min which is close to the resting metabolic need. However, this increment is critically dependent on the maintenance of cardiac output, which is rarely assessed. Patients with chronic hypoxaemia develop compensatory mechanisms such as polycythaemia and possibly changes in tissue capillary density which enable them to tolerate levels of arterial PO_2 which, if acutely imposed on normal subjects, would lead to unconsciousness. Hence the adequacy of oxygenation has to take into account not only the arterial PO_2 or oxygen saturation but the probable cardiac output and preceding adaptation to chronic hypoxaemia.

Pulmonary circulation

Disorders of the pulmonary circulation usually result in modest reductions in PaO_2 and carbon monoxide transfer with normal or slightly reduced lung volumes and airway function. Alterations in carbon monoxide transfer presumably reflect changes in effective pulmonary capillary blood volume. Modest reductions are found in primary pulmonary hypertension, chronic heart failure, pulmonary vasculitis (in the absence of recent intra-alveolar haemorrhage when carbon monoxide transfer is increased) and in pulmonary embolism; surprisingly, reductions are also found when there is vascular dilatation as in pulmonary arteriovenous malformations and in rare hypoxaemic patients with cirrhosis. Increased carbon monoxide transfer may be found in patients with intracardiac right to left shunts.

Conventional lung function testing provides little information on the pulmonary circulation and does not contribute usefully to the diagnosis of pulmonary embolism, which rests on abnormalities in the regional distribution of pulmonary blood flow after venous injection of radiolabelled microspheres. Similar to ventilation, in normal subjects pulmonary blood flow is greatest in the dependent zones of the lungs. Pulmonary embolism also leads to an increase in total ventilation and V_d/V_t ratio, and a reduction in PaO_2; the mechanism of the reduction in PaO_2 has not been clarified. However, all these changes may be mimicked by chronic lung disease; indeed, local perfusion defects can only be interpreted as evidence of embolism if there are no 'matched' defects in the ventilation scan.

Non-invasive methods of assessing the right ventricle and pulmonary circulation in chronic lung disease such as echocardiography–Doppler studies and radionuclide assessment of right ventricular ejection fraction and wall thickness have not come into widespread use because of technical limitations; therefore direct measurements of pulmonary vascular pressure are still used for assessing the response to drugs, oxygen, or exercise. It is useful to measure PaO_2 during studies of pulmonary vasodilator drugs, as these may worsen the ventilation–perfusion balance by preferentially dilating vessels supplying low V/Q areas which may be sites of hypoxic vasoconstriction.

Detecting small increases in extravascular lung water before frank alveolar oedema appears is also difficult. None of the research methods developed have proved to be both simple and accurate. However, comparisons with the research methods have shown that abnormalities in the chest radiograph appear with a surprisingly small increase in extravascular water.

Control of ventilation

Measuring ventilation at rest has played a surprisingly small part in clinical assessment, except in the intensive care unit. This is because methods that require breathing via a mouth-piece with the nose clipped are not well tolerated by breathless patients, always add some dead space, and generally increase minute ventilation. Less obstructive methods, in which pneumographs or magnetometers are used to measure expansion of rib cage and abdomen, have shown that minute ventilation in healthy subjects at rest is less than previously believed—commonly about 5 to 6 l/min. Unfortunately, methods which monitor chest-wall expansion are influenced by postural changes and, even with careful calibration, it is difficult to achieve an accuracy better than ± 10 per cent, but they are particularly valuable for detecting irregularities in pattern of breathing, as during sleep.

Increased ventilation occurs in normal subjects during pregnancy, probably in response to increases in progesterone, and in response to the hypoxaemia of altitude, when the effect is mediated via stimulation of the carotid chemoreceptors. It is also a feature of aspirin poisoning and conditions which cause metabolic acidaemia, such as renal failure, diabetic ketosis, and lactic acidosis; acidaemia probably stimulates both peripheral and central chemoreceptors. Hyperventilation is a feature of many cardiorespiratory diseases, notably asthma, severe pneumonia, pulmonary embolism, and pulmonary oedema, and is associated with a respiratory alkalaemia; some of the increase in ventilation may be explained by hypoxaemic stimulation of the carotid chemoreceptors, but stimulation of vagal afferent receptors within the lungs also plays a part. Most of the conditions associated with hyperventilation are easily recognized; when there is no obvious cause the differential diagnosis often lies between pulmonary vascular disease and psychogenic hyperventilation. Psychogenic hyperventilation may be associated with dizziness, tetany, chest pain, and paraesthesia, but settles during sleep. Reduced total ventilation (hypoventilation) is much less common and is usually due to sedative drugs or neuromuscular disease, although occasionally it occurs with brain-stem disease or severe metabolic alkalosis. In most patients with chronic obstructive pulmonary disease, minute ventilation is slightly above normal values; as discussed above, this reduces the effect of ventilation–perfusion mismatch on Pa_{CO_2} and, to a lesser extent, Pa_{O_2}. Even in episodes of acute respiratory failure, ventilation is usually greater than normal. Relatively small variations in the pattern of breathing can influence the development of hypercapnia in such patients.

Most studies of ventilatory control have examined the ventilatory response to imposed hypoxia or hypercapnia when the extra stimulus outweighs confounding cortical influences which are important at rest. These techniques are most useful when lung and respiratory muscle mechanics are normal, as in studies of the effects of drugs or anaesthesia in normal subjects, Pickwickian patients with obesity, or unusual patients with abnormal central control of breathing due to brain-stem pathology. Impaired responses to hypoxia and hypercapnia are also found in many patients with chronic airflow obstruction, but when there are abnormalities of ventilatory mechanics, a given neurological output inevitably results in less ventilation than in a normal subject. A better idea of neurological output may be obtained by measuring oesophageal pressure throughout the breath or mouth pressure during a transitory 0.1 s occlusion at the start of a breath. Recent studies with these techniques have generally reduced the role of decreased central drive and emphasized the role of impairment of respiratory muscle and lung mechanics in limiting the ventilatory response in such patients. There is a similar problem in assessing the respective roles of central control mechanisms and impairment of ventilatory muscle function in assessing hypercapnia in patients with respiratory muscle weakness.

Exercise capacity

Breathlessness on exercise is one of the major symptoms of lung disease, and exercise tests play an important part in quantifying effort intolerance, investigating its cause, and monitoring progress and response to treatment and rehabilitation programmes. They are also used for confirming a diagnosis of exercise-induced asthma and ischaemic heart disease. The mechanisms responsible for increasing ventilation in parallel with the increase in metabolic load and oxygen consumption are still not well understood. An increased ventilation in relation to oxygen consumption is found at high work loads in normal subjects when blood lactate begins to rise. In lung disease increased ventilation is particularly found with fibrosing alveolitis and primary pulmonary hypertension; some of this increase may be due to stimulation of peripheral chemoreceptors by a fall in arterial Po_2 during exercise, but mechanoreceptor stimulation has also been implicated since increasing inspired oxygen does not restore exercise ventilation to normal values.

In chronic airflow obstruction and fibrosing alveolitis, exercise tolerance appears to be limited by the impaired ventilatory capacity and there is often a considerable fall in oxygen saturation, which in fibrosing alveolitis is due to impaired diffusion.

Quantitative exercise tests usually involve either a treadmill or a bicycle ergometer. Many clinical problems can be investigated by a simple progressive work load test on a bicycle ergometer measuring ventilation, heart rate, electrocardiogram, and oxygen consumption. This will often indicate whether exercise is limited by the cardiac response or by ventilation, and will give an objective measurement of maximum oxygen consumption. More elaborate measurements, including arterial blood gases and cardiac output, may occasionally be required. These tests indicate cardiopulmonary fitness and exercise capacity. Exercise tolerance (the amount of work a patient is prepared to achieve) can be assessed by the distance walked on the flat in 6 or 12 min in patients with more severe disability. In such patients walking distance tests correlate well with disability in daily life; they evaluate motivation as well as cardiopulmonary status.

Clinical applications of lung function testing

Bedside monitoring of respiratory function in acute illness

Currently, outside the intensive care unit, this is usually confined to continuous monitoring of oxygen saturation with oximetry and frequent but intermittent use of arterial blood gases to measure Pa_{O_2}, Pa_{CO_2}, pH, and PEF to monitor airway function crudely. Transcutaneous electrodes can indicate trends in P_{CO_2} with a rather slow time constant; values are considerably higher than Pa_{CO_2}. Often it would be useful to follow minute ventilation, for instance in acute respiratory failure or severe asthma, but although chest-wall movements (rib cage and abdomen) can be detected by pneumographs or magnetometers, these devices are very sensitive to changes in the position of the subject and therefore only provide qualitative information. The best solution at present is to place a portable pneumotachograph at the mouth for about 30 s. Fortunately, PEF remains a valid measurement in distressed patients with severe asthma as the expiratory effort to achieve true PEF is less in acute

Table 3 *Standard aspects of lung function assessed in lung function laboratories*

Function	Available techniques	Applications
Airway function, including response to dilator and constrictor agents	Spirometry, peak expiratory flow Maximum flow–volume curves Body plethysmograph (airway resistance and flow–volume curves)	Airflow obstruction due to asthma, emphysema, chronic obstructive pulmonary disease, and extrathoracic airways obstruction Tests can all be repeated after bronchodilators or bronchoconstrictor challenges (such as histamine, methacholine, exercise, cold air, specific allergens, etc.) Constrictor tests are useful for diagnosis of asthma, when initial airway function is normal
Lung volumes and distensibility	Multibreath gas equilibration using helium Body plethysmography (thoracic gas volume) Lung compliance using oesophageal intubation	Hyperinflation in airflow obstruction Diagnosis of restrictive lung disease Distinguish cause of restrictive lung disease
Respiratory muscle function	Mouth pressures during maximum inspiratory and expiratory efforts	Systemic muscle disease Unexplained ventilatory failure or restrictive lung disease Severe hyperinflation
Pulmonary gas exchange	Single-breath CO transfer coefficient Pulse oximetry PaO_2 and $PaCO_2$ with simultaneous collection of expired gas: response to increasing inspired oxygen, etc.	Reduced with emphysema or interstitial lung disease Increased with intrapulmonary haemorrhage, asthma Detection of inefficiency in pulmonary gas exchange for O_2 or CO
Exercise capacity	Treadmill, cycle, or step ergometry with measurement of work, O_2 consumption, heart rate, ventilation (O_2 saturation, PaO_2, $PaCO_2$) Simple tests of walking distance against time	Integrated performance of cardiorespiratory–muscular system Assessment of response to treatment or training programmes Assess disability in severe disease

asthma than in the absence of airway obstruction; underestimates occur if PEF measurement is not preceded by a full inflation. In gross weakness of the respiratory muscles (crises of myasthenia gravis, Guillain–Barré syndrome), the vital capacity gives a better indication of respiratory reserve than PEF. Portable meters are now available for bedside measurement of mouth pressures developed during maximum inspiratory efforts (made at resting breathing level) and maximum expiratory efforts (made at full inflation) against a closed airway, and these provide a direct measurement of respiratory muscle strength.

In patients requiring assisted ventilation in the intensive care unit, a more detailed assessment of respiratory mechanics can be obtained with modern ventilators. Carbon monoxide transfer coefficient can be measured in intubated patients with a rebreathing technique. Lung water and endothelial and epithelial integrity can be assessed using radionuclide techniques and external counting.

Use of lung function tests in evaluating stable disease

During the last 20 years arterial blood gas analysis, oximetry, regional ventilation and perfusion scans, and PEF monitoring have moved from the lung function laboratory to general hospital use. The standard tests widely available in lung function laboratories and their applications are summarized in Table 3. These tests are most useful for assessing patients with airways obstruction and restrictive lung disease. More elaborate methods are needed to evaluate breathing problems during sleep, function of the diaphragm, the central control of breathing, and the pulmonary circulation (Table 4), and these are not so widely available.

Physiological variation in lung function

BODY SIZE, GENDER, AND ETHNIC DIFFERENCES

Lung size is generally related to body size and particularly to height. Height is used to predict expected values of TLC and the subdivisions of lung volume, FEV_1, and PEF, and the carbon monoxide transfer factor. The difference in lung function between men and women partly reflects differences in body size but, at a given height, TLC is about 20 per cent greater in men than in women. Similarly there are ethnic differences, apart from those explained by height; lung volumes are about 15 per cent larger in Caucasians than in Asians.

GROWTH AND AGEING

Lung function is fully developed by about 18 to 20 years and probably remains constant (at least in non-smokers) until about 30 years old. After this age, many aspects of lung function slowly deteriorate even when there is no exposure to tobacco or environmental pollution. Thus FEV_1, VC, carbon monoxide transfer factor, and exercise capacity all fall with

Table 4 *Additional aspects of respiratory function assessed in some lung function laboratories*

Function	Available techniques	Applications
Disturbance of breathing, oxygenation, and upper airway occlusion during sleep	Monitoring oxygenation (oximeter) and chest wall movements during sleep Additional measurements to detect snoring, movement, EMG, EEG, heart rate, and transcutaneous P_{CO_2} may be used	Investigation of daytime somnolence, narcolepsy, unexplained respiratory failure or polycythaemia Adequacy of oxygen or other therapy in patients with COPD or respiratory muscle weakness
Diaphragm function	Transdiaphragmatic pressure, EMG of diaphragm and other muscles, electrical stimulation of phrenic nerves or magnetic stimulation of cervical nerve roots	Suspected diaphragm disease Further investigation of low mouth pressures with maximum voluntary efforts
Control of breathing	Ventilatory response to induced hypoxia or hypercapnia Non-invasive monitoring of chest-wall movements (pneumographs or magnetometers)	Investigation of unexplained hypoxia or hypercapnia Disorder of breathing rhythm
Pulmonary circulation Haemodynamics	Right-heart catheterization, echocardiogram–Doppler studies	Evaluation of pulmonary hypertension, resistance, and response to O_2 or vasodilator drugs
Epithelial/endothelial function	Clearance of injected or inhaled* (e.g. radio-aerosol of DTPA) markers	Progress of adult respiratory distress syndrome Lung damage after inhalation injury Interstitial lung disease
Regional lung function	Distribution of ventilation with radiolabelled gas or aerosols Distribution of blood flow with radiolabelled microspheres	Pulmonary embolism Assessment of suitability for pulmonary resection or bullectomy (plus tests of overall lung function)
Cough responsiveness	Response to increasing doses of inhaled capsaicin or citric acid	Unexplained non-productive cough
Mucociliary transport	Clearance of radiolabelled inhaled particles from the lungs	Investigation of recurrent bronchopulmonary infections, Kartagener's syndrome, etc.
Detection of mild lung damage	Single-breath nitrogen test	Occupational and environmental lung disease
Exposure to cigarette smoke	Concentration of CO in expired air	Confirmation of smoking habit

*May also reflect airway epithelial function.

increasing age. Forced lung emptying slows, and because FEV_1 falls more than VC, FEV_1/VC also drops. Loss of lung recoil leads to increase in FRC and RV with age, while increased ventilation–perfusion imbalance leads to a larger difference between alveolar and arterial P_{O_2} and a fall in arterial P_{O_2}. Aspects of lung function that do not change with increasing age are TLC, arterial P_{CO_2}, pH, and airways resistance.

POSTURE, SLEEP, AND DIURNAL VARIATION

A number of physiological factors potentially impair lung function at night in healthy subjects. End-tidal lung volume (FRC) is lower in the supine position than when sitting or standing; in older subjects this may lead to airway narrowing, and even closure of airways in dependent regions of the lungs, and to a reduction in Pa_{O_2}. Ventilation becomes more dependent on the diaphragm and total intrapulmonary blood volume increases. During sleep, total ventilation falls and there is a small fall in Pa_{O_2} and a rise in Pa_{CO_2}. There may also be a disproportionate reduction in the inspiratory activation of tongue, palatal, and pharyngeal muscles, leading to partial obstruction of the airway and snoring. Finally, the circadian rhythm of airway tone peaks in the early hours of the morning.

In patients with cardiopulmonary disease many of these effects may be amplified and account for the frequency of problems with breathing and oxygenation at night. Thus in subjects with daytime hypoxaemia due to ventilation–perfusion imbalance, the usual small fall in ventilation and Pa_{O_2} when asleep causes much larger falls in oxygen saturation and delivery to the tissues. In some obese men, the mechanisms normally responsible for snoring may be exaggerated, particularly after alcohol, leading to repeated episodes of complete obstruction of the airway and hypoxaemia at night. In patients with active asthma, the amplitude of the circadian rhythm in airway function is greatly increased compared with normal subjects, leading to the common symptom of wheezing in the early hours of the morning.

ENVIRONMENT, SMOKING, AND POLLUTION

The most obvious environmental factor is altitude which reduces inspired and arterial P_{O_2}: ventilation is stimulated so that Pa_{CO_2} is also reduced. Smoking has both immediate and long-term effects. The carbon monoxide in the blood occupies up to 10 per cent of the haemoglobin-binding sites which would otherwise be used to carry oxygen. Some compensation is achieved by an increase in red-cell mass in smokers. Inhalation of cigarette smoke also produces immediate increases in air-flow resistance and minute ventilation. Regular cigarette smokers show deterioration in many aspects of lung function—notably in FEV_1 and other tests of maximum expiratory flow, tests of unevenness of ventilation, and carbon monoxide transfer factor. Subtle differences in lung function between smokers and non-smokers can be detected in subjects in their twenties; although these changes are sometimes reversible in the early years of smoking, in middle age and beyond they usually persist indefinitely after stopping smoking. In Western countries, the effects of smoking on lung function are now quantitatively more important than general environmental pollution. This may not be the case in some Third World countries, for instance in societies where domestic cooking and heating fuels generate extremely polluted air in confined living quarters.

REFERENCES

Braun, N.M.T., Arora, N.S., and Rochester, D.F. (1983). Respiratory muscle and pulmonary function in polymyositis and other proximal myopathies. *Thorax*, **38**, 616–23.

Clark, J.S., Votteri, B., Ariagno, R.L., *et al.* (1992). Non-invasive assessment of blood gases. *American Reviews of Respiratory Diseases*, **145**, 220–32.

Cotes, J.E. (1993). *Lung function*. 5th edn. Blackwell Scientific Publications, Oxford.

Forster, R.E. and Ogilvie, C.M. (1983). The single breath carbon monoxide transfer test 25 years on: a reappraisal. *Thorax*, **38**, 1–9.

Gibson, G.J. (1984). *Clinical tests of respiratory function*. MacMillan, London.

Gibson, G.J. (1989). Diaphragmatic paresis: pathophysiology, clinical features and investigation. *Thorax*, **44**, 960–70.

Laroche, C.M., Moxham, J., and Green, M. (1989). Respiratory muscle weakness and fatigue. *Quarterly Journal of Medicine*, **71**, 373–97.

Pride, N.B. and Macklem, P.T. (1986). Lung mechanics in disease. In *Handbook of physiology*: Section 3. *The respiratory system* (ed. P.T. Macklem and J. Mead), Vol III. Mechanics of Breathing. Ch. 37, pp. 659–92. American Physiological Society, Bethesda.

Sue, D.Y. and Wasserman, K. (1991). Impact of integrative cardiopulmonary exercise testing on clinical decision making. *Chest*, **99**, 981–92.

Wagner, P.D. and Rodriguez-Roisin, R. (1991). Clinical advances in pulmonary gas exchange. *American Reviews of Respiratory Diseases*, **143**, 883–8.

West, J.B. (1990). *Respiratory physiology—the essentials*. 4th edn. Williams and Wilkins, Baltimore.

17.6.3 Microbiological methods in the diagnosis of respiratory infections

D. W. M. CROOK AND T. E. A. PETO

Introduction

A wide range of bacteria, viruses, fungi, and parasites colonize or infect the airways, lung, and pleura. The choice and interpretation of laboratory tests for the isolation or detection of these organisms present clinicians with a demanding challenge. It is important to appreciate that the diagnosis of pneumonia, or respiratory tract infection, can only be made clinically. The role of the microbiology laboratory is only to provide some clues as to the likely causative organism. Unfortunately, in many cases, the causative organism wil never be isolated with certainty.

Micro-organisms causing respiratory infection gain access to the lung or pleura via the airway or, occasionally, the blood. These infections are caused by both nasopharyngeal colonizers and non-colonizers. The organisms which usually colonize the nasopharynx (e.g. *Streptococcus pneumonia*, *Haemophilus influenzae*) may spread to the lung and cause mucopurulent exacerbations of chronic bronchitis or pneumonia. However, for every case of true infection there are many more nasopharyngeal carriers. The pathogens which do not colonize the nasopharynx include *Mycobacterium tuberculosis*, *Legionella pneumophila*, *Histoplasma capsulatum*, and the respiratory viruses. They may be airborne and settle directly in the lung or spread to the lung haematogenously

where they form an infected focus. The distinction between nasopharyngeal colonizers and non-colonizers is critical for the interpretation of microbiological tests of respiratory tract secretions, fluids, or tissues.

Samples for microbiological testing

1. Expectorated sputum is the most readily available sample of respiratory secretions. It is a particularly attractive specimen for analysis as it can be obtained simply, at low cost, and without risk to the patient. However, it is liable to be contaminated with upper respiratory tract colonizers. 'Induced' sputum is considered a valuable sample for the detection of some respiratory pathogens in patients who otherwise fail to expectorate sputum.

2. Transtracheal aspiration provides samples of respiratory secretions which are largely free from nasopharyngeal contamination. This procedure is useful when bronchoscopy is not available, but is unpleasant for the patient.

3. Bronchoscopy specimens can be obtained by bronchoalveolar lavage, protected specimen brush, or biopsy of lung tissue. Samples obtained by this technique are relatively free of contaminating upper respiratory tract flora; therefore microbiological test results should be reliable. However, this procedure is complicated to perform and expensive. There is a risk from bleeding and hypoxia which can sometimes require mechanical ventilation of a patient.

4. Lung fluid for examination can be aspirated from the lung parenchyma using a fine needle. This technique is conventionally used to aspirate fluid from peripherally located intrapulmonary cavities (abscesses). It has also been used in the investigation of childhood and adult pneumonia. There are risks of pneumothorax, haemorrhage, and occasional sudden death; therefore in most centres there is little enthusiasm for using this technique for the investigation of pneumonia.

5. Open-lung biopsy samples provide the most informative specimens, but biopsy is too invasive to be performed routinely.

6. Pleural fluid or pleural biopsy specimens obtained by percutaneous needle provide reliable samples free from contamination with nasopharyngeal colonizing organisms.

7. Pleural fluid samples obtained from a chronically draining chest tube are not reliable, since chest drains rapidly become colonized with potential pathogens after insertion.

8. Blood cultures provide highly reliable results and should be performed in ill patients suspected of infection. Approximately 10 to 28 per cent of pneumococcal pneumonias are associated with bacteraemia. Other organisms that cause pneumonia, such as *H. influenzae*, *Staphylococcus aureus*, *Klebsiella pneumoniae*, can be cultured from the blood of patients.

Microbiological examination of samples

Microscopy of unstained sputum

This examination is rarely made, but may be helpful in a few circumstances. On adding potassium hydroxide, yeasts or hyphae can be seen. The experienced microscopist is able to recognize yeast forms which are sufficiently characteristic to be highly predictive of an infection by a specific species of fungus (e.g. *Blastomyces* spp) (Table 1). Hyphal elements in bronchoalveolar lavage fluid are suggestive of a filamentous mould fungal infection, and in the setting of fever, neutropenia, and pulmonary infiltrates are highly predictive of *Aspergillus* spp. invasive disease. In patients from endemic foci of paragonomiasis, the diagnosis can be made by finding the typical opuculated eggs in unstained sputum.

Table 1 *Bacterial, viral, and fungal respiratory pathogens*

Colonizing organisms
Hospital-acquired pneumonia
　Pseudomonas aeruginosa
　Escherichia coli
　Klebsiella pneumoniae
　Staphylococcus aureus
　Enterobacter spp.
　(many other *Enterobacteriacae* spp.)
　Candida spp.
　Aspergillus spp.
　Cytomegalovirus (latent virus)
Community-acquired pneumonia
　Streptococcus pneumoniae
　Haemophilus influenzae
　Moraxella catarrhalis
　Staphylococcus aureus
Lung abscess
　Mixed oropharyngeal flora, e.g.
　　Prevotella spp. (anaerobes)
　　Streptococcus spp.
　　Eikenella corrodens

Non-colonizing organisms
　Legionella spp.
　Nocardia spp.
　Chlamydia spp.
　Mycoplasma pneumoniae
　Mycobacteria tuberculosis
　Blastomyces braziliensis
　Coccidioides immitis
　Histoplasma capsulatum
　Cryptococcus neoformans
　Respiratory syncytial virus
　Influenzae A and B
　Parainfluenza virus

Table 2 *Antigen tests*

Bacterial
　Chlamydia spp.
　Streptococcus pneumoniae
　Legionella pneumophila (serogroup I)
Fungal
　Cryptococcus neoformans

Direct examination of stained samples

An early aetiological diagnosis of the cause of a respiratory infection can be achieved by specific staining techniques and microscopic examination of various samples (Table 2). Gram staining has been extensively studied as a test for the early identification of the causative agent in pneumonia. Gram stain and visualization of organisms in bronchoalveolar lavage fluid is highly predictive of pyogenic bacterial pneumonia in patients with community-acquired, hospital-acquired, or ventilator-associated pneumonia. Cases of community-acquired pneumonia who have Gram-positive diplococci, pleomorphic Gram-negative coccobacilli, or Gram-positive cocci in clusters in their bronchoalveolar lavage fluid are likely to have pneumococcal, *H. influenzae* or *Staph. aureus* pneumonia respectively. It has been commonly considered that microscopy of Gram-stained expectorated sputum is helpful in the identification of the bacterial agent causing pneumonia. Although it is widely held that a sputum sample with less than 10 squamous cells and more than 25 neutrophils per low powered field (100×) is predictive of an aetiological agent on examination of a Gram stain, this is not supported by published data. Some studies, which have attempted to confirm this, have mainly focused on the identification of pneumococci in the sputum of patients with suspected community-acquired pneumonia. Although sputum Gram stain appears useful in these patients (with a positive predictive value of 70–80 per cent), this can be largely attributed to the high prevalence (60–80 per cent) of a pneumococcal aetiology in cases of community-acquired pneumonia. Also, the probability of excluding pneumococcal pneumonia (negative predictive value) by sputum Gram stain may be as low as 64 per cent. There are no good data supporting the value of Gram stain in identifying the aetiology of pneumonia caused by other colonizing organisms. In nosocomial and ventilator-associated pneumonia, Gram-stain examination of expectorated sputum or endotracheal aspirates is poorly predictive of the aetiology of pneumonia. However, when more than 7 per cent of cells in bronchoalveolar lavage fluid from a ventilated patient contain stainable intracellular organisms, the probability of pneumonia caused by these organisms is high (70–80 per cent). Gram staining of pleural fluid is a useful test for examining pleural fluid. The presence of many neutrophils suggests an empyema, and organisms can be seen in up to 80 per cent of these cases.

Ziehl–Neelsen or rhodamine auramine staining of respiratory secretions or tissue for the detection of acid-fast organisms is useful in the examination of all respiratory samples. The presence of acid-fast organisms is more than 90 per cent specific for mycobacteria; therefore in the correct clinical setting it is highly predictive of mycobacterial disease. Unfortunately, the sensitivity of the test is relatively low (20–78 per cent for sputum and less than 10 per cent for pleural fluid). Therefore a negative test result does not reliably exclude mycobacterial pulmonary or pleural disease.

Direct fluorescent antibody testing is commonly used to detect respiratory syncytial virus and occasionally *Legionella* spp. The test is both specific and sensitive. In children with suspected respiratory syncytial virus infection, the most accessible specimen is a nasopharyngeal aspirate. *Legionella* spp can occasionally be detected in sputum or bronchoalveolar lavage fluid.

Pneumocystis carinii in respiratory secretions is highly predictive of pneumocystis pneumonia. Induced expectorated sputum has been used in AIDS patients with a yield of 80 per cent in cases with pneumocystis pneumonia. Examination of bronchoalveolar lavage fluid or lung tissue stained with methenamine silver is highly sensitive (90 per cent) and is specific (more than 95 per cent) for *P. carinii*.

Direct histological examination of stained lung or pleural biopsy material can be helpful in making an immediate aetiological diagnosis of respiratory infection. Granulomas with specific features strongly suggest tuberculosis. In pulmonary schistosomiasis, eggs characteristic of the parasite may be seen. Fungi with characteristic features, such as *Aspergillus* spp., *Rhizopus* spp. *Coccidioides immitis*, *H. capsulatum*, and *Blastomycosis braziliensis*, may be seen and establish the diagnosis of invasive pulmonary fungal disease. Also, characteristic histological changes are found in cases of cytomegalovirus pneumonia or measles pneumonia (giant-cell pneumonia).

Detection of antigens

Detection of specific antigen is another direct test which gives rapid results (Table 2). Pneumococcal antigen can be detected by either latex agglutination or counter-current immunoelectrophoresis. The test is highly specific when used on reliable samples such as blood, pleural fluid, bronchoalveolar lavage fluid, or urine. The sensitivity is known to be high (80 per cent) for testing pleural fluid, but is unacceptably low for testing blood or urine. It has been suggested that the presence of pneumococcal antigen in sputum, as detected by latex agglutination in patients with pneumonia, is highly predictive of a pneumococcal aetiology. However, as with Gram staining, the high predictive power of pneumococcal antigen testing is related to the high probability of a pneumococcal aetiology in cases of community-acquired pneumonia and its utility in cases of diagnostic difficulty is disappointing.

Legionella antigen testing of urine is both sensitive and specific for legionellosis. However, at present the test only detects cases caused by serogroup 1, the most common pathogen. Cryptococcal antigen testing of serum has high sensitivity and specificity for cryptococcal disease and therefore is a useful test for investigating possible pulmonary cryptococcosis.

Culture

The isolation from sputum of respiratory pathogens that frequently colonize the upper respiratory tract does not reliably predict the aetiology of pneumonia or lung abscess. However, isolation of non-colonizing organisms is strongly associated with infection caused by these pathogens.

The isolation of more than 10^3 or more than 10^5 organisms from a protected specimen brush sample obtained bronchoscopically or by bronchoalveolar lavage respectively predicts the cause of pneumonia. This approach would seldom be desirable in cases likely to have pneumococcal pneumonia which is sensitive to routine empiric antibiotic treatment. However, it has been found to be particularly useful in investigating cases with suspected ventilation-associated pneumonia. The isolation of mixed oral flora (both aerobic and anaerobic organisms) from reliable specimens such as bronchoalveolar lavage or lung aspirate suggests an aspiration or suppurative pneumonia. The culture of *Aspergillus* spp. in bronchoalveolar lavage fluid in neutropenic patients has been shown to be predictive of invasive disease, but in hosts with normal neutrophil counts its growth is of less certain significance. Cytomegalovirus can be grown from respiratory secretions, but the sensitivity, specificity, and predictive value of a number of culture methods for this organism have not been reliably determined. The 'gold standard' test for this condition remains biopsy and the visualization of characteristic histological changes. The growth of organisms from pleural fluid suggests a pleural infection. The presence of pyogenic organisms (*Staph. aureus*, *Strep. pneumoniae*, oral streptococci, anaerobes, etc.) suggest an empyema. Although an insensitive test (30 per cent), isolation of tuberculosis establishes the diagnosis of tuberculous pleurisy.

Culture of an organism such as *Strep. pneumoniae*, *H. influenzae*, or *Staph. aureus* from blood in a patient with community-acquired pneumonia is highly predictive of its aetiology. Positive blood cultures in ventilated patients with the adult respiratory distress syndrome and multiorgan failure are a less reliable predictor of the aetiology or presence of pneumonia.

Serological tests

Pulmonary infection by a range of respiratory pathogens can be predicted late in the infection or retrospectively by a range of serological tests. (Table 3) The presence of IgM antibodies is predictive of recent or active infection. This test has been most useful in testing for mycoplasma and cytomegalovirus infectious disease. The usual approach to making a serological diagnosis is the measurement of a fourfold rise in antibody levels between an acute and convalescent serum sample. This form of serodiagnosis is useful for viral, mycoplasma, chlamydial, TWAR (which refers to the first two laboratory isolates TW-183 and AR-39 or *Chlamydia pneumoniae*), Q fever, and *Legionella* spp. infections. Serological tests for a number of infections, such as histoplasmosis, coccidioidomycosis, filariasis, and echinococcus, have been used. In these infections, the presence of antibody suggests the presence of active infection by these organisms.

Detection of specific DNA sequences

The amplification of species-specific DNA sequences using the polymerase chain reaction offers an attractive new approach to detecting the presence of a pathogen. This technique should be highly sensitive as five or less target sequences should be detectable. Therefore, when used

Table 3 *Valuable serological tests*

Viral
    Cytomegalovirus
    Influenza virus

Bacterial
    Legionella spp.
    Mycoplasma pneumoniae
    Coxiella burnettii (Q fever)
    Chlamydiae psitticae

Fungal
    Blastomyces braziliensis
    Coccidioides immitis
    Histoplasma capsulatum

as a test of respiratory infection, its potential is limited to infections caused by organisms which are not associated with colonization of the upper respiratory tract. Also, slow growing or non-culturable organisms may be detected more rapidly using this test. Many studies are under way evaluating this technique in the diagnosis of tuberculosis and pneumonia caused by *P. carinii*, *Mycoplasma pneumoniae*, and *L. pneumophila*. Many other respiratory pathogens are suitable for detection using this approach. However, it may be many years before the polymerase chain reaction or other DNA amplification techniques are routinely and widely used in the diagnosis of respiratory infectious disease.

Choice of samples

Samples of respiratory secretions obtained by techniques which avoid nasopharyngeal contamination (e.g. bronchoalveolar lavage or protected specimen brush) are the most reliable specimens for analysis. However, these are obtained at increased risk to the patient. The aetiology of pneumonia caused by colonizing organisms, such as *Strep. pneumoniae* or *Pseudomonas aeruginosa*, would be most reliably established using samples obtained by these higher-risk invasive techniques. However, in most cases of community-acquired pneumonia, where empirical antibiotics of low toxicity are predictably effective, there is little need to obtain reliable respiratory samples (e.g. by bronchoalveolar lavage). Furthermore, the bacterial aetiology can be determined by taking blood cultures in as many as 20 per cent of these cases. In contrast, nosocomial pneumonia, particularly in ventilated patients, is caused by more antibiotic-resistant colonizing organisms for which empirical antibiotic treatment is less reliably effective than in community-acquired pneumonia. In these cases, the identification of the pathogen enables susceptibility testing and the choice of appropriate antibiotic treatment. Therefore the increased risk of obtaining reliable samples using invasive techniques is worthwhile.

The detection of non-colonizing organisms (e.g. Mycobacteria) in samples liable to contamination, such as sputum, is highly predictive of infection caused by these organisms. For example, examination of nasopharyngeal swabs has proved helpful in the detection of respiratory syncytial virus and *Bordetella pertussis*. However, the value of examining sputum for many of these pathogens is limited by the low sensitivity of tests for these organisms. Improvement in sensitivity can be achieved by using more invasive techniques such as lung biopsy to detect Mycobacteria or fungi (e.g. *H. capsulatum*).

Infection caused by a range of non-colonizing organisms may only be detected routinely by indirect tests. Cryptococcal pneumonia or legionellosis may be recognized by antigen detection using serum or urine respectively. Serum can also be used to detect antibodies to a variety of respiratory pathogens (Table 3).

In cases with possible pleural infection, pleural fluid should be analysed. In cases of suspected tuberculous pleurisy, pleural biopsy provides a reliable sample for microscopic examination and culture.

Interpretation of microbiological tests

The interpretation of a microbiological test is similar to the interpretation of any test in medicine. The clinician must form an opinion of the probable range of causative organisms before the test is performed. Knowledge of the prevalence of the disease and the sensitivity and specificity of any test allows the particular predictive value (and therefore the false-positive and false-negative rates) of the test result to be determined. Although attempts can be made to estimate this precisely using Bayes theorem, many clinicians do this intuitively. In general, diagnostic tests for colonizing organisms have low specificity and therefore have a high false-positive rate, especially in circumstances when the chance of infection by a pathogen in a particular patient under study is low. The same tests for non-colonizing organisms have much higher specificity, and therefore the false-positive rate is low even when the chance of a patient having the disease is considered to be low. The main example of this is in the diagnosis of tuberculosis, where a positive sputum culture is considered significant even if it is unexpected. In general, samples obtained directly from the lung, either bronchoscopically or via open-lung biopsy, are less likely to be contaminated and therefore are more specific. The specificity and sensitivity of all indirect tests vary according to the test used and the particular organism identified. The interpretation of these tests varies according to the test used and to the particular organism identified. Thus these tests must be interpreted with great care.

The microbiological investigation of patients with pneumonia—one approach

The rational approach to making a microbiological diagnosis of a pulmonary infection rests on balancing the risk of the procedure to obtain reliable samples against the risk of treating empirically without defining the cause of a respiratory infection. There are empirical antibiotic regimens (e.g. cefuroxime and erythromcyin) which have negligible side-effects and adequately cover the majority of likely pathogens in community-acquired pneumonia (e.g. *Strep. pneumoniae*, *H. influenzae*, *Mycoplasma*, etc.). However, such an approach is inadequate if the patient is too ill to risk a poor response to a therapeutic trial. In such patients, bronchoscopic examination may be justified even if the patient subsequently requires mechanical ventilation. In less severely ill patients, bronchoscopy is justified if tuberculosis or rarer pathogens resistant to empiric treatment such as fungi, parasite, or multiresistant bacterial infection are suspected.

REFERENCES

Barrett-Connor, E. (1971). The nonvalue of sputum culture in the diagnosis of pneumococcal pneumonia, *American Review of Respiratory Disease*, **103**, 845–8.

Bartlett, J.G., Ryan, K.J., Smith, T.F., and Wilson, W.R. (1987). In: *Cumitech 7A. Laboratory diagnosis of lower respiratory tract infections* (ed. J.A. Washington II). American Society for Microbiology, Washington, DC.

Davidson, M., Tempest, B., and Palmer, D.L. (1976). Bacteriologic diagnosis of acute pneumonia. *Journal of the American Medical Association*, **235**, 158–63.

Mackowiak, P.A. (1982). The normal microbial flora. *New England Journal of Medicine*, **307**, 83–94.

May, J.R. (1953) The bacteriology of chronic bronchitis, *Lancet*, **12**, 534–7.

O'Neill, K.P., Lloyd-Evans, N., Campbell, H., Forgie, I.M., Sabally, S., and Greenwood, B.M. (1989). Latex agglutination test for diagnosing pneumococcal pneumonia in children in developing countries, *British Medical Journal*, **298**, 1061–4.

Pugin, J., Acukenthaler, R., Mili, N., Janssens, J.P., Lew, P.D., and Suter, P.M. (1991). Diagnosis of ventilator-associated pneumonia by bacteriological analysis of bronchoscopic and nonbronchoscopic "blind" bronchoalveolar lavage fluid. *American Review of Respiratory Disease*, **143**, 1121–9.

Research Committee of the British Thoracic Society and the Public Health Laboratory Service. (1987). Community-acquired pneumonia in adults in British hospitals in 1982–1983: a survey of aetiology, morality, prognostic factors and outcome. *Quarterly Journal of Medicine*, **62**, 195–220.

Thorsteinsson, S.B., Musher, D.M., and Fagan, T. (1975). The diagnostic value of sputum culture in acute pneumonia, *Journal of the American Medical Association*, **233**, 894–5.

Venkatesan, P. and MacFarlane, J.T. (1992). Role of pneumococcal antigen in the diagnosis of pneumococcal pneumonia. *Thorax*, **47**, 329–31.

Wilson, S.M., McNerney, R., Nye, P.M., Godfrey-Faussett, P.D., Stoker, N.G., and Voller, A. (1993). Progress toward a simplified polymerase chain reaction and its application to diagnosis of tuberculosis, *Journal of Clinical Microbiology*, **31**, 1007–8.

Wimberley, N., Leendert, J.F., and Bartlett, J.G. (1979). A fibreoptic bronchoscopy technique to obtain uncontaminated lower airway secretions for bacterial culture. *American Review of Respiratory Disease*, **119**, 337–43.

17.6.4 Diagnostic bronchoscopy and tissue biopsy

M. F. MUERS

Diagnostic bronchoscopy and tissue biopsy are an integral part of the investigation of respiratory disease, but should be regarded as complimentary to, rather than substitutes for, simpler diagnostic tests.

Bronchoscopy

In the last 15 years the development of fibreoptic bronchoscopy and its associated techniques of transbronchial lung biopsy and bronchoalveolar lavage have revolutionized the practice of respiratory medicine worldwide. In contrast, rigid bronchoscopy, although essential in some circumstances, has become less common.

Indications (Table 1)

In practice, bronchoscopy is mainly used to investigate the possibility of carcinoma and/or to obtain histological or cytological confirmation of a clinical diagnosis. It may also be used to assess operability. Some bronchial abnormalities may present in ways which do not immediately suggest endobronchial disease, such as recurrent chest infections or breathlessness with a normal radiograph. Diagnosis at bronchoscopy is not confined to visible lesions; the simultaneous use of flexible sampling instruments and fluoroscopy allows biopsy of distal bronchi or lung parenchyma.

Techniques

FIBREOPTIC BRONCHOSCOPY

Fibreoptic bronchoscopy using flexible instruments 4.5–6.5 mm in diameter is usually a day-case procedure carried out under local anaesthesia and light sedation. A posteroanterior and a lateral chest radiograph, together with spirometry, are required beforehand. Any cardiac abnormalities need to be assessed and arterial blood gases estimated if spirometry is poor. Patients with coagulopathies or on anticoagulants need clotting studies, and corrective treatment is required if biopsies are to be done.

Instruments should be carefully cleaned as there have been many instances of cross-infection. They should be dismantled and all parts washed in neutral detergent before immersion for several minutes (routine) or 60 min (immunocompromised patients) in 2 per cent alkaline glutaraldehyde. Immediately before use bronchoscopes should be rinsed and wiped with sterile water or 70 per cent alcohol. The combination

Table 1 *Indications for bronchoscopy*

Diagnosis
    Suspected malignancy
    Unexplained localized or diffuse radiographic opacity (e.g.
       'persistent pneumonia')
    Unexplained respiratory symptoms (particularly haemoptysis,
       wheezing)
    Microbiological sampling (e.g. ? tuberculosis but no sputum;
       ? *Pneumocystis carinii* pneumonia in AIDS)
    Bronchoscopic bronchogram
Therapy
    Removal of secretions—foreign body
    Palliation of carcinoma symptoms by laser, diathermy,
      cryotherapy, endobronchial radiotherapy

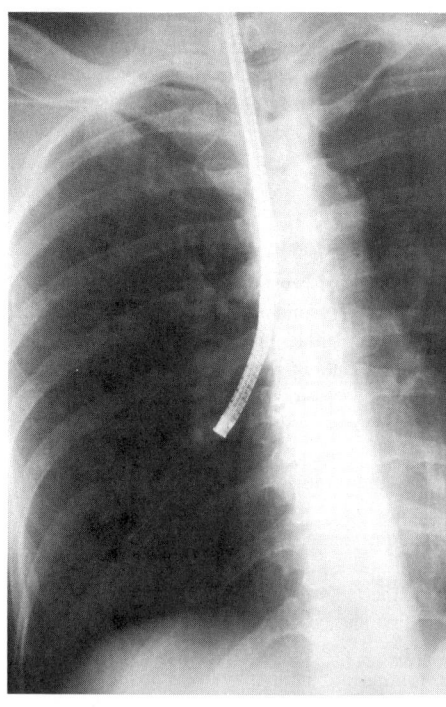

Fig. 1 Fibreoptic bronchoscopy: a brush biopsy has been taken from the right middle lobe.

of these three procedures will reduce the possibility of cross-infection to very low levels and should be routine. Bronchoscopists and their assistants should be gowned and gloved; consideration should also be given to the wearing of masks and goggles to minimize the risk of HIV transmission, particularly in high incidence areas.

Patients are usually fasted for at least 4 h, and lightly sedated either by preoperative intramuscular atropine and papaveretum or, more commonly, by perioperative intravenous diazepam, midazolam, and/or fentanyl. Deep sedation is not required. The procedure can be undertaken without sedation, particularly in the elderly or in patients with marked respiratory impairment, provided that local anaesthesia is adequate. Supplemental oxygen by nasal cannulae at 2 l/min prevents the desaturation which the procedure entails, and higher-risk patients should have their transcutaneous oxygen saturation monitored.

The nares and oropharynx are sprayed with 4 per cent or 10 per cent lignocaine. The bronchoscope is usually inserted by the nasal route because this provides easier access to the larynx and over-free movement of the instrument is restricted. The vocal cords are anaesthetized either by a previous transtracheal injection of 2–5 ml of 4 per cent lignocaine or 5 per cent cocaine, or by the injection of 2 ml aliquots of 2 per cent or 4 per cent lignocaine through the bronchoscope. Anaesthesia of the bronchial tree is obtained similarly.

With due care fibreoptic bronchoscopy should be regarded as a safe procedure. A survey of practice in the United Kingdom during 1983 revealed a complication rate of 0.12 per cent and a mortality rate of 0.04 per cent from 40 000 bronchoscopic procedures, 96 per cent of which were performed using the fibreoptic bronchoscope. The major cause of morbidity in this series was the problem of respiratory depression due to inappropriate sedation.

RIGID BRONCHOSCOPY

Indications for this technique are similar to those for fibreoptic bronchoscopy, but in addition rigid bronchoscopy is useful if previous fibre optic bronchoscopy has failed to make a diagnosis owing to inadequate biopsies or anxiety about uncontrolled bleeding from vascular lesions. It is also better when operability is being assessed, when foreign body removal is being contemplated, and in children. Rigid bronchoscopy is performed under general anaesthesia and oxygen venturi ventilation. Overnight stay in hospital is usually required.

Bronchoscopic diagnosis (Figs. 1 and 2)

With a standard 5-mm diameter fibreoptic bronchoscope it is possible to inspect all lobes to the subsegmental level, and the smaller paediatric bronchoscopes extend this range of vision although they cannot be used for biopsies.

Diagnosis at bronchoscopy often does not depend just on tissue sampling, since many abnormal appearances are characteristic. Examples are lack of movement of the left vocal cord due to recurrent laryngeal

Fig. 2 Endobronchial appearances at bronchoscopy: (a) A normal right upper lobe: the mucosa is smooth and the airways patent. (b) Bronchial carcinoma: samples can be taken by brush and forceps biopsy, and a limited 'bronchial wash'. (By courtesy of Dr Peter Stradling.)

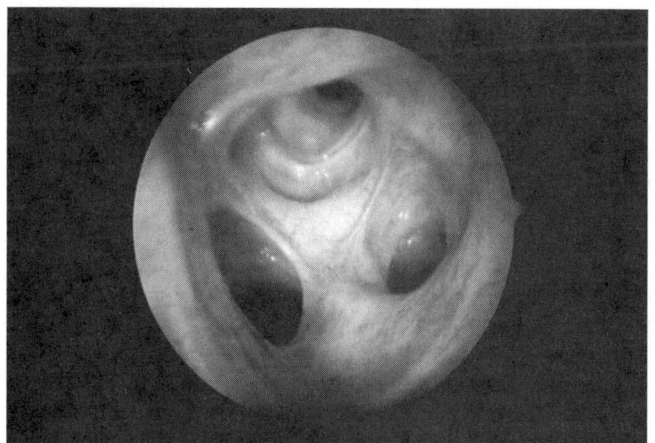

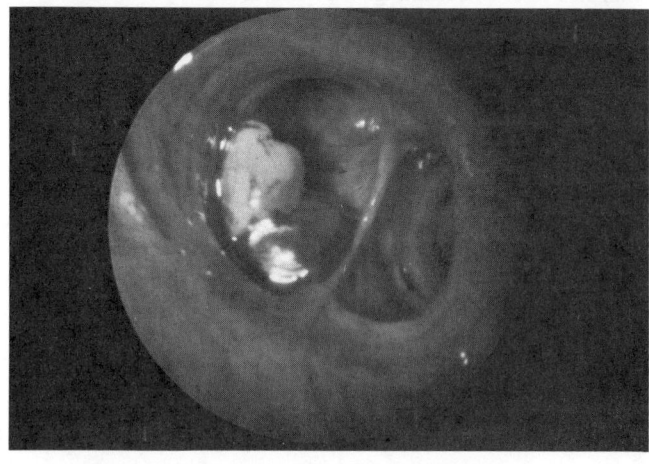

nerve palsy, endobronchial pus from infected segments, endobronchial distortion due to lung collapse or metastatic carcinoma, or endobronchial tumours. Approximately 70 per cent of bronchial carcinomas are within visible and sampling range of fibreoptic bronchoscopes, and these have a particular advantage over the rigid instruments with respect to examination of the upper lobes and the apical segments of the lower lobes.

Bronchoscopic biopsy techniques

ENDOBRONCHIAL SAMPLING

The majority of endobronchial lesions are carcinomas, and these are best investigated by a combination of brushing or catheter samples for cytology, forceps biopsy for histology, and a bronchial 'wash' for cytology. Sheathed nylon brushes can safely be applied to most tumours through the 2-mm instrument channel of the fibreoptic bronchoscopes, and the resulting specimens rubbed on to slides and air or ethanol fixed for cytology. Suction specimens using polythene catheters provide similar samples. Flexible biopsy forceps provide adequate samples from most endobronchial tumours, and up to four or five biopsies are advisable from a single lesion. For a bronchial wash, 20 to 40 ml of normal saline is injected over an endobronchial lesion into the peripheral lung. The residual fluid is aspirated into a trap. When this is done in addition to brush and forceps biopsy, the yield for malignancy is increased. It is sensible to perform a brush first and proceed to forceps biopsy and then wash if profuse bleeding is not seen.

Simple aspiration of secretions into a trap may likewise provide material for cytology, but in practice this technique is more useful for microbiological tests for bacteria, fungi, or mycobacteria. It is not sensitive as a lone investigation for neoplasm where a formal wash is better.

BRONCHOALVEOLAR LAVAGE

Although the aspirated trap specimens of small volume bronchial washes are adequate for the diagnosis of malignancy, a larger sample of cells from peripheral lung tissue is needed for the investigation of diffuse lung disease and often for research purposes. For bronchoalveolar lavage, the bronchoscope is wedged into the chosen segment of lung and three to five aliquots of 20 to 60 ml buffered normal saline at 37°C are instilled using gentle pressure on a syringe. Continuous suction is applied after each aliquot to obtain the specimens, and the average return is approximately 60 per cent of the injected volume.

Transient pyrexia lasting 4 to 8 h may occur after about 10 per cent of lavages, and the transient hypoxaemia during bronchoalveolar lavage requires prophylactic oxygen treatment and postoperative oxygen for about 2 h. Formal large volume bronchoalveolar lavage is contraindicated with a forced expiratory volume in 1 second (FEV_1) of less than 1.5 litres, and patients with evidence of asthma should have pretreatment with nebulized bronchodilators.

These bronchoalveolar lavage samples are suitable for cytological examination after cytocentrifugation when absolute yields and differential cell counts as well as functional studies can be made (Table 2). Lavage in normal non-smoking subjects shows a preponderance of pulmonary alveolar macrophages, with less than 20 per cent of the cells being lymphocytes, polymorphs, and eosinophils. Cell counts are increased approximately fourfold in smokers. Many diffuse lung diseases, such as sarcoidosis or allergic alveolitis, change the cell counts. Although characteristic profiles are recognized, their lack of specificity is a major problem, and in routine clinical practice they provide supportive evidence only for most diagnoses. However, the role of bronchoalveolar lavage in the immunocompromised patient is quite different (see below).

TRANSBRONCHIAL BIOPSY

This technique enables specimens of lung parenchyma to be examined. Under fluoroscopic screening, closed bronchial biopsy forceps are advanced to within 1 cm of the pleura, and are then opened and moved gently backwards and forwards two or three times before being advanced more firmly peripherally (Fig. 3). At this point the patient is asked to breathe out and the forceps are closed and withdrawn, usually with a perceptible 'tug'. Specimens, of volume approximately 1–2 mm³, are placed in formol saline for histology and others can be taken dry or in normal saline for culture. Normal lung tissue floats, but consolidated lung or abnormal tissue sinks.

Multiple biopsies are advisable. A minimum of three or four should be taken from diffusely abnormal lung, and up to five or six from localized lesions provided that significant bleeding or a pneumothorax does not occur. Bleeding can be controlled by injecting 1 to 5 ml of 1:10 000 adrenaline through the bronchoscope. Bilateral sampling is necessary in the assessment of post-lung-transplant rejection, but in other circumstances it is not advised. Complications are more common in immunocompromised patients or in the presence of coagulopathies. Overall, significant bleeding occurred in 0.5 per cent and pneumothoraces in 2.1 per cent of the 3500 procedures reported in a United Kingdom survey in 1983. The use of fluoroscopic screening significantly reduces the incidence of pneumothorax. It is possible, but usually inadvisable, to carry out biopsies in patients on intermittent positive pressure ventilation, and under these circumstances bronchoalveolar lavage alone or an open-lung biopsy is probably safer.

TRANSBRONCHIAL NEEDLE ASPIRATION

This technique utilizes a sheathed needle which, when in position, is pushed out through the instrument channel of the bronchoscope into and

Table 2 *Normal cellular constituents of bronchoalveolar lavage*

Cells	Non-Smoker	Smoker
Total ($\times 10^4$/ml)	13	42
Pulmonary alveolar macrophages (%)	80–95	85–98
Lymphocytes (%)	<15	10
Neutrophils (%)	<3	<5
Eosinophils (%)	>0.5	<3

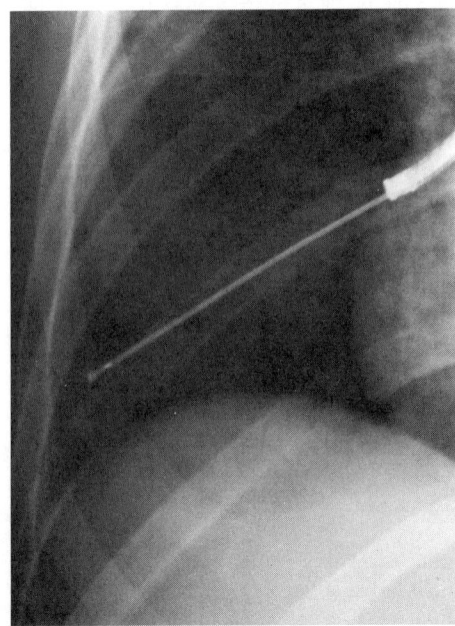

Fig. 3 Transbronchial lung biopsy through the fibreoptic bronchoscope. Flexible forceps can be seen sampling peripheral lung tissue in the right lower lobe. The bronchoscope had been wedged in a lobar bronchus. The diagnosis: miliary tuberculosis in a renal transplant patient.

through the bronchial mucosa to sample deeper tissue up to 1 cm from the surface. Steady suction is applied to the proximal end, while the needle tip is advanced and withdrawn several times. Aspirated tissue is expressed on to slides for cytological examination. This technique can sample subcarinal and paratracheal nodes, particularly those on the right side, by sampling from the posterior wall of the right main bronchus. When applied as a routine technique in the assessment of carcinoma, the yield is low, although on a few occasions it may obviate the need for formal mediastinal sampling. The same technique can be used to sample peripheral coin lesions when it is combined with peripheral brush biopsy or transbronchial biopsy, all performed under fluoroscopic guidance. The technique may be particularly useful in the diagnosis of endobronchial tumours which produce distortion of the bronchial mucosa without large endobronchial lesions, as these are difficult to biopsy with forceps. Small-cell carcinoma often presents in this way.

BRONCHOSCOPIC BRONCHOGRAMS

Bronchographic contrast medium can be injected either directly through the suction channel of a fibreoptic bronchoscope or through a narrow polythene catheter, and segmental or lobar bronchograms or full unilateral or bilateral bronchograms of good quality can be obtained (Fig. 4). This is a useful complementary investigation when endobronchial appearances are normal and the problem under investigation is, for example, haemoptysis or a chronic productive cough with a normal chest radiograph, or perhaps persistent unexplained lobar or segmental shadowing. Fluoroscopy is necessary. In these circumstances, and particularly in patients over the age of 40, a selective bronchogram may reveal unsuspected bronchiectasis or, less commonly, stricture due to endobronchial sarcoidosis or tumour for example. The advent of high resolution CT has led to a reappraisal of the use of bronchograms for the routine investigation of possible bronchiectasis, and it is now probably the diagnostic method of choice where it is available.

Percutaneous lung biopsy

Percutaneous fine-needle aspiration biopsy

Needle aspiration of the lung was first used by Leyden in 1883 to diagnose pneumonia, and in recent years has been increasingly used to sample peripheral lesions, particularly where malignancy is suspected. Large immediately subpleural lesions can be targeted using plain posteroanterior and lateral radiographs with skin markers, but all other lesions need to be examined under screening control. This is usually either

Fig. 4 A selective bronchogram using the fibreoptic bronchoscope. Diagnosis: tubular bronchiectasis in the left lower lobe.

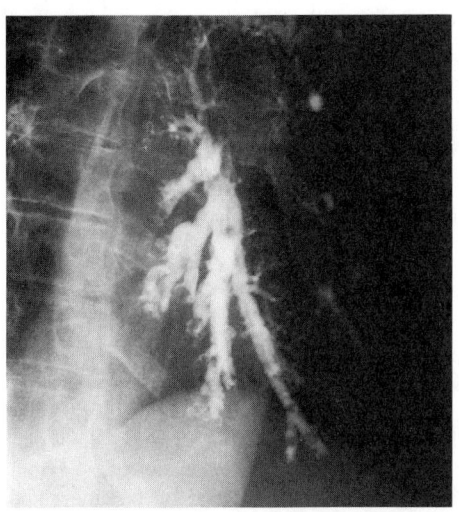

biplane or C-arm fluoroscopy, although now CT, or real time ultrasonography if the lesion is subpleural, is often preferred. Patients are examined either supine or prone, and a fine aspiration needle (0.5–1.0 mm, 25–17 gauge) or a rotex screw needle is advanced perpendicular to the skin under local anaesthesia into the lesion. Suction is applied and the needle is passed several times within the lesion. Aspirated material is expressed on to slides for cytological examination. Small needles, single passes, and lesions within 2 to 3 cm of the pleura are associated with a pneumothorax rate of approximately 8 per cent, but this rises substantially with larger needles, multiple passes, and deeper sampling. Slight haemorrhage may occur in 1 to 10 per cent of cases but is rarely severe. Contraindications are untreated coagulopathies, severe coexisting lung disease, and suspicion of a vascular malformation.

Percutaneous cutting-needle biopsy

Whereas fine-needle aspiration biopsy produces samples suitable for cytological examination only, the use of cutting needles allows histological examination of lung tissue. The Trucut biopsy needle is now favoured over the previous Silvermann needle, and automated systems such as the Biopty now make sampling easier. The sampling technique is similar to fine-needle aspiration biopsy, but repeated attempts to sample are accompanied by a much higher complication rate. Pneumothorax is likely to occur in 20 per cent of cases, with perhaps half of these requiring aspiration or tube drainage. Haemorrhage appears to occur in about 15 per cent. Theoretically, cutting needles can sample diffuse lung disease, but the complication rate appears to be greater still when this is done and transbronchial biopsies are probably safer.

A percutaneous drill biopsy technique has been refined by Steele. A compressed air drill rotates at high speed driving a 2.5 mm cutting trephine which can sample 3 to 4 cm subpleurally. The technique needs experience, and there is scanty literature to support its widespread use apart from Steele's own series. It has not found favour, probably because of this, and there is a relatively high complication rate. However, the histological samples are substantial.

Open-lung biopsy

Introduced by Klassen in 1949, the sampling of lung tissue under direct vision through a small (7–10 cm) thoracotomy under general anaesthesia is the final arbiter in difficult cases, particularly of diffuse lung disease. A pneumothorax requiring intubation occurs in approximately 4 per cent of cases. Bilateral diffuse lung disease is best sampled by a right submammary incision when samples can be taken from all three lobes. Sampling from the upper lobes, particularly the apical segments, requires a much larger incision. Surgeons are advised not to sample simply the most visibly affected areas, but also the less abnormal where active pathology is often more likely to be found. Directed biopsy is possible, usually after CT scanning. Adequate material for histology is always obtained, and appropriate diagnosis should follow in more than 90 per cent of cases. However, the indications for open-lung biopsy are decreasing following the advent of transbronchial biopsy and high resolution CT.

Mediastinal sampling

Mediastinal sampling is required when the clinical problem is either the diagnosis of a mediastinal mass or assessment of the operability of lung cancer.

Needle biopsy of the mediastinum

Mediastinal masses can be diagnosed by percutaneous needle biopsy. The techniques used are similar to those described above for pulmonary sampling. Biopsy under fluoroscopy was introduced in the late 1970s but has now largely been superseded by ultrasound, which allows screening of anterior and posterior mediastinal masses, or CT scanning, which allows any mediastinal mass to be sampled. With fluoroscopy, and including cases requiring lung puncture, a complication rate of more than 10 per cent due to pneumothorax or bleeding can be expected. However, the complication rate is very much lower if sampling is done under CT or ultrasound, and the needle track avoids the lung. As with pulmonary lesions, fine-needle aspiration biopsy is both sensitive and highly specific for the diagnosis of cancer, but much less satisfactory if the prebiopsy diagnosis is considered likely to be a benign lesion, a cyst, lymphoma, or a thymic tumour. Fine-needle aspiration biopsy has a sensitivity of approximately 85 per cent for any malignancy, but allows accurate histological classification of only about 60 per cent in such cases. However, when fine-needle aspiration biopsy is combined with cutting-needle biopsy, sensitivity approaches 90 per cent with an accurate histological diagnosis in a similar percentage of cases.

Surgical mediastinal sampling

This is required for assessment of operability, sampling of hilar lesions, and for cases where needle biopsy has failed to produce an accurate diagnosis.

Mediastinoscopy, which was introduced by Carlens in 1959, is an endoscopic examination under general anaesthesia through a small cervical incision with a rigid instrument passing beneath the pretracheal fascia. It allows sampling of tissue or nodes within the superior mediastinum as far as the carina. Mediastinotomy involves a short transverse incision in the second intercostal space on either side. Exploration under direct vision is extrapleural, and is particularly useful in assessment of tumours arising in the left upper lobe. Complications, including bleeding and pneumothorax, are rare if the surgeon is experienced occurring in less than 1 per cent of cases.

Pleura and pleural fluid sampling

Large pleural effusions can be sampled using the physical signs and the chest radiograph to direct the sampling needle into the intercostal space above the area of maximum dullness to percussion. However, it is best to direct the needle into small effusions under ultrasound guidance. For routine aspiration a 21-G venepuncture needle on a 20 to 50 ml syringe should be used. Local anaesthesia is sometimes an advantage. Diagnostic information is obtained from the appearance of the fluid (e.g. blood-stained or chylous), the protein content (transudates contain less than 30 g/l), cytology, and microbiological examination. Pleural fluid pH, glucose and amylase, immunological tests (apart from LE cells or ANF), and tumour markers are all much less useful. Simple aspiration cytology has a diagnostic sensitivity of about 60 per cent for primary or secondary malignant pleural effusions, and the yield rises to about 75 per cent with repeated aspirations.

Pleural biopsy

Percutaneous pleural biopsy using the Abram biopsy needle should usually be done at the same time as the aspiration of pleural fluid, if a pleural effusion is being investigated and local pulmonary or pleural disease, as opposed to organ failure, is suspected as the cause. Strict asepsis and adequate local anaesthesia down to the pleural surface are mandatory, as is verification of the presence of a pleural effusion by prebiopsy needle aspiration. A small incision with a fine scalpel blade allows the punch biopsy needle to be introduced into the pleural space. Multiple samples, avoiding the inferior surface of the rib above, are taken and examined histologically, and in appropriate cases sent for culture including mycobacteria. The technique is not easy, although samples are highly specific for tuberculosis and malignancy. However, if repeated fluid cytology is negative, routine biopsy increases the diag-

nostic yield for neoplasia by only about 10 per cent overall. False-negative biopsies are particularly common in mesothelioma.

The Trucut needle is more appropriate than the Abram needle when a pleural mass is present, and in experienced hands compares favourably with the Abram needle for routine use.

Thoracoscopy

Many exudative pleural effusions remain undiagnosed even after pleural aspiration and needle biopsy. If further histological specimens are required, thoracoscopy is necessary. This involves the inspection and sampling of the visceral and parietal pleura, usually using a rigid 9-mm thoracoscope. Under general anaesthesia, or a combination of sedation and local anaesthesia, the pleural space is entered through a small stab incision, pleural fluid is drained, and 200 ml of air is introduced to collapse the lung and allow the pleural surfaces to separate. The use of a fibreoptic bronchoscope with a rigid introducer under local anaesthesia has been described. The technique, which needs an experienced operator, allows wide inspection of the pleural surface and multiple biopsies. Complications are rare and deaths from the procedure are extremely uncommon. The technique has a sensitivity of greater than 90 per cent for pleural malignancy and tuberculosis, although mesothelioma remains difficult to diagnose. After thoracoscopy, a pleural drain is needed until aspirated air has been removed but it can then be withdrawn.

Special cases

Children

Both rigid and fibreoptic bronchoscopy need to be performed under general anaesthesia. The 3.5-mm diameter paediatric fibre bronchoscopes do not easily allow biopsy, although 1-mm forceps are now available. Other sampling techniques are similar to those for adults, although greater recourse has to be made to open surgical sampling.

The elderly

With appropriate attention to sedation and oxygenation, fibreoptic bronchoscopy and the other biopsy techniques are safe and effective in the elderly.

Novel techniques

Video-assisted minimally invasive techniques have recently been introduced into thoracic surgery. Using three small incisions in the chest wall, it is possible to take 1 cm^3 specimens of peripheral lung tissue using a stapler, and also to take samples from the pleura and pericardium. It is likely that this approach will eventually replace conventional open-lung biopsy and thoracoscopy in some cases.

Clinical applications

The use of the techniques described above to assist in the diagnosis and management of different common respiratory conditions is discussed in this section.

Perihilar lesions

In modern adult practice the most common and important diagnosis is lung cancer. If simple investigations are inconclusive, fibreoptic bronchoscopy should then be considered unless there are technical contraindications or good clinical reasons why further information is not required. The advantage of bronchoscopy over information derived from radiology is that a tissue diagnosis may be obtained, operability can be assessed, and specific anticancer therapy such as chemotherapy may be given, for example if a small-cell tumour is diagnosed. More than 70 per cent of all primary lung neoplasms are within the field of view of the fibreoptic bronchoscope and the diagnostic sensitivity for tissue sampling is about 90 per cent for visible lesions. This sensitivity is increased by another 10 per cent or so if, as is recommended, brush biopsy is followed by tissue biopsy and bronchial wash. It must be remembered that the differential diagnosis of primary lung cancer at bronchoscopy includes adenomas, metastatic deposits, and, more rarely, tuberculosis or sarcoidosis.

If a perihilar lesion is present but the bronchoscopy is entirely normal, percutaneous needle aspiration sampling, a mediastinotomy, or even a thoracotomy is probably necessary, usually after further imaging such as a CT scan. If endobronchial lesions are seen but biopsy is unhelpful, repeat examination with transbronchial needle aspiration and multiple biopsies is suggested. An alternative is a rigid bronchoscopy allowing larger samples.

Circumscribed peripheral lung lesions (the 'coin' lesion)

The first point to consider is whether such lesions need to be biopsied, or whether, if the probability of a primary lung cancer is high, it is not better to proceed directly to thoracotomy. In a few cases a policy of observation is justified, but commonly even these eventually come to removal. The possibility of solitary metastases, particularly from renal or adrenal primaries, must be carefully borne in mind, and a prebiopsy upper abdominal ultrasound scan is recommended. Whatever the diagnosis, lesions less than 2 cm in diameter are difficult to sample accurately either at bronchoscopy or by fine-needle aspiration biopsy.

The sensitivity of bronchoscopic sampling of lesions of dimensions greater than 2 cm but which are not visible is only about 50 per cent. However, this is a sensible approach if the patient is thought to be unable to tolerate a pneumothorax or if percutaneous biopsy is not available. Fluoroscopy is necessary and brushings, forceps biopsies, and saline lavage should all be done.

For all other cases, if biopsy is required, percutaneous fine-needle aspiration should be considered first. This is particularly so if the likely diagnosis is malignancy, since the specificity of this examination is nearly 100 per cent. However, cell typing is less accurate, perhaps 80 per cent. In cases where fine-needle aspiration biopsy has failed to demonstrate malignancy, or a benign diagnosis is thought to be probable, cutting-needle biopsy should be preferred. Specificity for a benign diagnosis approaches 80 per cent with excellent specificity for malignancy and typing. Lesions should not be biopsied if they are deeper than 8 cm from the pleural surface.

If the working clinical diagnosis is vasculitis, even cutting-needle biopsies are inappropriate and open-lung biopsy is recommended. A trephine drill should not be used for localized lesions.

Diffuse parenchymal lung disease (pulmonary infiltrates and/or interstitial shadowing)

Widespread bilateral, interstitial, or alveolar shadows, and also similar shadows confined to one lobe or segment of the lung, e.g. 'persistent pneumonia', are included under this heading.

The role of tissue biopsy in the diagnosis and management of patients with these shadows is one of the most perplexing problems in thoracic medicine. The published series do not give adequate answers to the questions of when and how the lung should be biopsied since there are unquantifiable biases of patient selection and it is often uncertain how the achievement of precise tissue diagnosis has benefited the patients or altered their management. Furthermore, even with adequate tissue sampling a proportion of all reported series have shown non-specific interstitial changes which are impossible to classify nosologically with present histological techniques.

Practical points are as follows.

1. Biopsy should not be considered until simpler non-invasive procedures have been exhausted. Nowadays, these may include a high resolution CT scan. Pathognomonic CT appearances such as those in cryptogenic fibrosing alveolitis or lymphangitis carcinomatosa may complement simple clinical data and render a tissue diagnosis unnecessary in many cases.
2. Biopsy should not be considered if a tissue diagnosis will not result in any change of treatment, or will not allow more accurate prognosis to be made. For example, if a patient has clinical evidence of a well-established non-progressive alveolar fibrosis, the benefit to the patient of a biopsy may be small.
3. Biopsy should be performed by experienced operators, or under their immediate supervision, and the safest techniques should be preferred.
4. Biopsy should not be performed if the occurrence of a complication, particularly a pneumothorax, in the presence of a reduced respiratory reserve will endanger the patient.

The techniques to be considered are transbronchial biopsy with or without lavage, transcutaneous cutting-needle biopsy, and open-lung biopsy. Most physicians faced with this problem and requiring a tissue diagnosis would first attempt transbronchial biopsy under fluoroscopic control. Multiple biopsies provide acinar tissue in 90 per cent of cases and diagnostically useful specimens in about 80 per cent. The disadvantage of these biopsies is their small size (1–2 mm³) and crush artefact. Transbronchial biopsies are particularly indicated if the working diagnosis is sarcoidosis, allergic alveolitis, diffuse malignancy such as lymphangitis or alveolar-cell carcinoma, or diffuse infection such as disseminated tuberculosis or pneumocystis. However, if the prior probability of these is low, and rarer diseases such as leiomyomatosis, histiocytosis X, or a vasculitis are considered more likely, open-lung biopsy is necessary since the small samples from transbronchial biopsies are much less likely to yield a specific diagnosis. Bronchoalveolar lavage alone only occasionally produces pathognomonic evidence. Two examples are alveolar proteinosis (lipoproteinaceous material) and idiopathic pulmonary haemosiderosis where iron-laden macrophages may be seen.

If the probable diagnosis is a fibrosing alveolitis, the situation is even more complex. If all that is required is a confirmation of interstitial alveolar fibrosis and the exclusion of, for example, malignancy or granulomata, transbronchial biopsies may suffice although the proportion of negative or unsatisfactory specimens may be high. If a more detailed histological assessment is required, even after CT scanning, an experienced operator may choose a cutting-needle biopsy, but otherwise the physician should advise an open biopsy. For the generality of other cases, the author would advise transbronchial biopsy first, proceeding to open biopsy if no diagnosis was achieved. On balance, this is a better and probably safer approach than the use of cutting-needle biopsies with their higher complication rates.

It must be recognized that in all circumstances a proportion of investigations will not yield diagnostically useful information and patients should be informed of this beforehand.

External masses and pleural disease

If the reason for enlarged supraclavicular nodes is thought to be carcinoma, the preferred investigation is fine-needle aspiration biopsy. This has a 96 per cent sensitivity for malignancy and is also highly specific. It is much harder to diagnose lymphoma or tuberculosis in this way, and excision biopsy is better. Subcutaneous masses—usually due to tumour—can be considered similarly. The Trucut needle provides adequate tissue from larger masses if fine-needle aspiration biopsy is negative or more accurate histology is required.

Most pleural effusions can be diagnosed confidently with a combination of basic clinical information and needle aspiration. This should always be the first approach. For the remainder, the usual problem is to decide whether or not a persistent exudative effusion is due to malignancy. If simple aspiration fails to diagnose malignancy, it should normally be repeated with Abram's punch biopsies and at least one sample should be sent for mycobacterial culture at the same time. Failure to reach a diagnosis at this point is usually an indication for thoracoscopy. However, bronchoscopy is usually unrewarding if the only radiographic abnormality is a small to moderate effusion.

Matters are different if a pleural effusion occurs in the presence of apparently diffuse pleural thickening. In industrialized countries in patients over 50, mesothelioma must be carefully considered alongside diffuse peripheral adenocarcinoma. Mesothelioma is notoriously difficult to diagnose. Multiple pleural aspirations and punch pleural biopsies may be negative. The reason for this is that the malignant cells may be surrounded by a thick dense fibrous stroma. In the author's experience thoracoscopy occasionally helps in this situation. Whether to proceed to an open pleural biopsy is a difficult question and needs to be very carefully considered since there is then a high incidence of tumour seeding in the skin. Biopsy solely for medicolegal purposes is usually not advisable.

Tuberculosis

Fibreoptic bronchoscopy, particularly utilizing brush biopsies for slide preparations, and a limited bronchoalveolar lavage from the affected lung segments is recommended for cases where tuberculosis is suspected but sputum specimens are negative, and further information is thought necessary before treatment begins. It is also useful in cases of obscure shadowing where tuberculosis is a possible, but not likely, diagnosis. Fifty-three of 134 such patients (40 per cent) from three series had positive microscopic examination of bronchial brushings or transbronchial biopsies and a further 36 per cent were positive on culture.

Tuberculosis is an important differential diagnosis for large pleural effusions not only in the younger patient where primary disease is likely but also in the older patient where reactivation may have occurred. Pleural fluid sampling is less satisfactory than pleural biopsies. Multiple samples need to be taken both for histological examination and, importantly, for culture.

Mediastinal disease

PREOPERATIVE ASSESSMENT IN LUNG CANCER

Mediastinal assessment is a prerequisite before surgery. After confirmation of the diagnosis, usually at fibreoptic bronchoscopy, potentially operable lesions require a CT scan of the thorax. Inoperability may be indicated by evidence of mediastinal invasion or mediastinal lymphadenopathy. If mediastinal invasion is seen on the CT scan, usually no biopsies are appropriate and inoperability should be accepted. Enlarged nodes need sampling, since the sensitivity of CT scanning is only 50 per cent, because many large nodes are reactive and not malignant, particularly if the primary is a squamous carcinoma.

For enlarged mediastinal nodes, if the operator is experienced and the plain radiographs or CT scans show paratracheal or subcarinal nodes only, bronchoscopic needle aspiration biopsy may suffice. In all other cases, mediastinal sampling by a surgeon is recommended. This will involve mediastinoscopy or anterior mediastinotomy or a combination of the two. Fine-needle sampling of involved nodes is not appropriate.

MEDIASTINAL MASSES

Sampling under CT control is best if it is available. Ultrasound is equally good if the masses are anterior or posterior. If the prior working diagnosis is carcinoma, fine-needle aspiration biopsy is recommended. If this test is negative (no malignant cells) or there is indication on the smear that the diagnosis may be thymoma or lymphoma, or if the prior working diagnosis is either of these two diseases, then a cutting-needle biopsy should be performed. It is unwise to diagnose thymoma or lymphoma on the results of fine-needle aspiration. In all other cases, open surgical biopsy is required usually at mediastinotomy or mediastinoscopy.

Diagnosis in the immunocompromised host

A precise diagnosis is required when pulmonary complications occur in the immunosuppressed. This often demands invasive sampling.

Therapeutic bronchoscopy

Suction and saline lavage through either a fibreoptic bronchoscope or a rigid bronchoscope can be used to relieve bronchial obstruction due to secretions. Rigid bronchoscopy is necessary if these are inspissated or very tenacious as in many cases of non-asthmatic mucous impaction in the elderly.

Carcinoma

Bronchoscopic treatment of stenosing carcinomas, which often cause distressing stridor or breathlessness can be performed by using cryotherapy, diathermy, or more commonly laser therapy. In this technique, a plastic catheter containing the optical fibre is passed through the instrument channel and directed at the tumour. Pulses of high energy light, usually from a neodymium:YAG laser, will cause superficial vaporization and charring of the tumour tissue while small blood vessels are sealed, providing a relatively dry field. Palliation is satisfactory in about 60 per cent of operated cases. Most units now prefer to do this using a modified rigid bronchoscope and general anaesthesia, although for smaller lesions a fibreoptic bronchoscope can be used.

Brachytherapy (endobronchial radiotherapy) utilizes a fibreoptic bronchoscope to place a catheter alongside an endobronchial tumour with the tip wedged peripherally. This is left in place while the bronchoscope is withdrawn and then, using a remote control device, a radioactive source is subsequently advanced through the catheter delivering a high dose of radiotherapy endobronchially (10 Gy at 1 cm). This single procedure produces symptomatic and functional benefit as primary therapy for inoperable lung cancer, although its major role is likely to be for the relief of recurrent symptoms after a first course of external beam radiotherapy.

Several units have now reported the use of expandable Silastic or stainless steel lattice stents for the immediate relief of symptoms due to airway narrowing by inoperable tumour. The lattice stents are easier to insert, and to date their placement has entailed rigid bronchoscopy and general anaesthesia. These specialized techniques require considerably more practice than routine bronchoscopy.

REFERENCES

Brewis, R.A.L., Gibson, J.G., and Geddes, D.M. (eds) (1990). *Respiratory medicine*. Ballière Tindall, London.

Flower, C.D.R. and Schneerson, J.M. (1984). Bronchography via the fibreoptic bronchoscope. *Thorax*, **39**, 260–3.

Flower, C.D.R. and Verney, G.I. (1979). Percutaneous needle biopsy of thoracic lesions—an evaluation of 300 biopsies. *Clinical Radiology*, **30**, 215–81.

Fulkerson, W.J. (1982). Current concepts: fibreoptic bronchoscopy. *New England Journal of Medicine*, **311**, 511–15.

Harrison, B.D.W., Thorpe, R.S., Kitchener, P.G., McCann, B.G., and Pilling, J.R. (1984). Percutaneous Trucut lung biopsy in the diagnosis of localized pulmonary lesions. *Thorax*, **39**, 493–9.

Harrow, E.M., Oldenburg, F.A. Jr, Lingenfelter, M.S., and Marshall-Smith, A. (1989). Transbronchial needle aspiration in clinical practice. A five-year experience. *Chest*, **96**, 1268–72.

Hetzel, M.R. and Smith, S.G.T. (1991). Endoscopic palliation of tracheobronchial malignancies. *Thorax*, **46**, 325–33.

Klech, H. and Hutter, C. (ed) (1990). Clinical guidelines and indications for bronchoalveolar lavage (BAL): Report for the European Society of Pneumonology. Task Group on BAL. *European Respiratory Journal*, **3**, 937–74.

Klech, H. and Pohl, W. (1989). Technical recommendations and guidelines for bronchoalveolar lavage (BAL). Report of the European Society of Pneumonology. Task Group on BAL. *European Respiratory Journal*, **2**, 561–85.

Loddenkemper, R. (1981). Thoracoscopy results in non-cancerous and idiopathic pleural effusions. *Poumonologie-coeur*, **37**, 261–6.

Simpson, F.G., Arnold, A.G., Bellfield, P.W., Muers, M.F., and Cooke, N.J. (1986). Postal survey of bronchoscopic practice by physicians in the United Kingdom. *Thorax*, **41**, 311–17.

Stradling, P. (1976). *Diagnostic bronchoscopy* (3rd edn). Churchill Livingstone, Edinburgh.

Yu, C.J., Yang, P.C., Chang, D.B., Wu, H.D., Lee, L.N., Lee, Y.C., *et al.* (1991). Evaluation of ultrasonically guided biopsies of mediastinal masses. *Chest*, **100**, 399–405.

17.6.5 Histopathology and cytology in diagnosis of lung disease

M. S. DUNNILL

Routine biopsy procedures are a well-established method of diagnosis in renal and gastrointestinal disease. The kidney and the entire alimentary tract are easily accessible to needle or punch biopsy procedures. Furthermore, small biopsy specimens from kidney, gut, or liver are nearly always representative of the whole organ. The situation in the lung is more complex. Direct needle biopsy carries with it the risk of pneumothorax and haemorrhage. Many pulmonary conditions are focal in distribution, and there is a fair chance that tissue obtained may not include a diseased focus although admittedly use of CT-guided biopsy has reduced this risk.

Tissue diagnosis of pulmonary diseases is initially dependent on non-invasive procedures. Cytological examination of sputum and lavage fluid is the key to diagnosis in some infections and neoplasms. Bronchial biopsy and transbronchial biopsy may often yield diagnostic results in disorders affecting large airways and hilar regions of the lung. For peripheral parenchymal lesions fine-needle aspiration cytology may provide sufficient material for diagnosis, but if this fails open-lung biopsy may be needed. In order to obtain the best results from all these procedures it is essential that considerable care is taken in handling the material obtained. It is negligent to submit a patient to the hazards of, say, an open-lung biopsy and then to treat tissue so obtained in a manner which renders it of little value for diagnostic purposes.

Sputum and bronchioloalveolar lavage specimens

Disappointment in the results of sputum examination in diagnosis of bronchial tumours is almost always attributable to inadequate collection of the sample and delay in transmission to the laboratory. It is essential that sputum is of the 'deep cough' or aerosol-induced variety, and samples collected on three separate days are examined. Because sputum collection and examination are free from the albeit minor hazards of more invasive investigations, its importance in diagnosis needs emphasis. Examination of bronchioloalveolar lavage fluid has resulted in an increased diagnostic yield and is most suitable for peripheral parenchymal lesions.

Benign conditions

In chronic bronchitis the findings are non-specific but, in addition to inflammatory cells and goblet cells, metaplastic squamous cells are frequently detected. It is important to distinguish the latter from carcinoma cells. Sputum from patients with asthma is characterized by the presence of eosinophils, diamond-shaped Charcot–Leyden crystals, and often coiled masses of inspissated mucus known as Curschmann's spirals.

One outstanding pathological feature of asthma is desquamation of bronchial mucosa followed by regeneration in the form of metaplastic squamous epithelium. As a consequence of this, clusters of epithelial cells, often referred to as Creola bodies, are a constant finding in sputum and it is important not to confuse these with adenocarcinoma cells.

The importance of direct examination of sputum, and subsequent culture, for bacterial organisms in pneumonia is self-evident, but in viral pneumonias desquamation of bronchial mucosa with subsequent regeneration occurs with changes in the sputum similar to those seen in asthmatics but with more marked cellular fragmentation and less well preserved cilia. In many instances characteristic viral inclusions can be seen and cytomegalovirus, respiratory syncytial virus, and herpes simplex virus infections all have characteristic cytological features (e.g. nuclear inclusion bodies, syncytial masses with basophilic cytoplasmic inclusions, and multinucleate cells with eosinophilic nuclear inclusions) pointing to the correct diagnosis.

Identification of infecting organisms by direct examination of sputum is of prime importance in tuberculosis and fungal infections, e.g. aspergillus, *Candida albicans*, cryptococcus, coccidioidomycosis, and especially *Pneumocystis carinii*, particularly in the increasing number of patients with immunodeficiency.

In industrial lung disease sputum examination may reveal the presence of ferruginous bodies in asbestosis and can be of value in establishing the diagnosis of malignancy in this condition. In alveolar proteinosis sputum, or more often lavage fluid, yields amorphous material which is positive to periodic acid–Schiff reagent and resistant to diastase digestion, which is typical of the condition. Examination of this material by electron microscopy should show the typical laminated bodies derived from type 2 pneumocytes.

It is in the diagnosis of malignant bronchial tumours that sputum examination is most often employed in clinical practice. While there are no absolute criteria for distinguishing carcinoma *in situ* from invasive carcinoma, in practice experienced cytologists can make a firm diagnosis of squamous carcinoma in many cases. It is notable that accuracy of diagnosis increases markedly with the number of specimens examined. In bronchial carcinoma examination of a single specimen results in diagnosis in approximately 50 per cent of cases, but this increases dramatically to up to 90 per cent if multiple samples are examined. In small-cell undifferentiated carcinoma sputum cytology is usually diagnostic and the same is true in adenocarcinoma, although it is more unusual to harvest malignant cells in the latter condition owing to the peripheral nature of the tumour. Bronchioloalveolar cell carcinoma may give rise to numerous exfoliated tumour cells that can be difficult to distinguish from adenocarcinoma, although in the latter cells tend to be more clustered in groups. In carcinoids and adenocystic carcinomas sputum examination, and even cytological examination of bronchial brushings, may not always yield diagnostic results as these tumours often lie beneath intact bronchial mucosa with the result that tumour cells are not exfoliated.

Bronchioloalveolar lavage

Many conditions mentioned in preceding paragraphs can be diagnosed using sputum samples alone. However, examination of lavage fluid is of particular value in parenchymal infiltrates, particularly in immunocompromised patients. In these patients rapid diagnosis of *P. carinii* pneumonia, fungal infections, and tuberculosis can be established and is of great value (Fig. 1).

Differential cell counts on lavage fluid obtained from normal non-smoking subjects reveals that over 50 per cent of the cells are macrophages and less than 1 per cent are neutrophils, with the remainder being lymphocytes. In smokers up to 5 per cent neutrophils may be found, but in those with idiopathic fibrosing alveolitis neutrophil and eosinophil counts may be much higher. In patients in the early stages of sarcoidosis the lymphocyte count is greatly raised. This lymphocytic infiltrate may not be entirely diagnostic as occasionally it is found in other conditions.

Fine-needle aspiration cytology

This form of investigation is being used with increasing frequency in combination with CT in the diagnosis of peripheral lung lesions. It is essential that the pathologist is present when the procedure is undertaken if good preparations of diagnostic value are to be obtained. Samples may be taken via the percutaneous route or at fibreoptic bronchoscopy. Although of value in some inflammatory conditions, the procedure is of most use in tumour diagnosis and in particular in distinguishing secondary tumour deposits in patients in whom there are multiple opacities in the chest radiograph. It is important to emphasize that negative findings on fine-needle aspiration specimens do not exclude a diagnosis, that general architecture of tumours and other lesions cannot be assessed, and finally that classification of malignant tumours is often not feasible. Specific diagnosis is rarely possible in benign lesions. The procedure has a definite complication rate with pneumothorax and local haemorrhage occurring in a small percentage of cases.

Pleural fluid

Examination of pleural fluid is well established in investigation of effusions. In general there is a much better diagnostic yield than with pleural biopsy. Cell preservation is excellent provided that the sample is correctly handled. The fluid should be placed in a sterile universal container with an anticoagulant and taken to the laboratory immediately.

Distinction of benign from malignant effusions should not prove difficult in experienced hands. In reactive effusions found in heart failure or the nephrotic syndrome mesothelial cells and macrophages are present in variable numbers. In pyogenic empyemas there are degenerate neutrophils and organisms with few mesothelial cells, whereas in tuberculous effusions neutrophils are absent except in the very early stages, lymphocytes predominate, and acid alcohol-fast organisms may be found on examination of a centrifuge deposit. Multinucleated epithelioid cells are not present, in contrast with certain effusions described below.

Effusions found in some connective tissue disorders may have a characteristic cytology. Thus in rheumatoid disease epithelioid cells, some of which may be multinucleated, are seen together with degenerate polymorphs, plasma cells, and macrophages. In systemic lupus classical lupus erythematosus cells may be found in the effusion which contains a large number of neutrophils.

In malignant disease the pleural fluid does not invariably contain sufficient cells for a firm diagnosis. However, in many instances sufficient

Fig. 1 A group of *P. carinii* organisms stained by the Grimelius method in bronchioloalveolar lavage fluid.

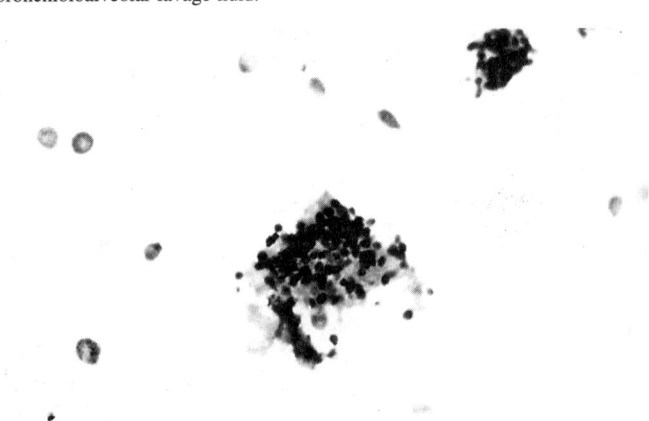

numbers are present which are easily distinguishable from the normal population of mesothelial cells. Identification of the cell type is facilitated by use of modern immunocytochemical methods, although in most cases Papanicolau and Giemsa preparations suffice. Squamous carcinoma of the bronchus seldom gives rise to effusions with malignant cells, whereas in adenocarcinoma such cells, often adhering together in clusters, are seen and special stains readily demonstrate mucin secretion. Small-cell undifferentiated carcinoma cells also have a typical appearance in effusions with pleomorphic nuclei, much nuclear moulding, and apparently absent cytoplasm.

Mesotheliomas of the pleura appear with increasing frequency, but diagnosis of the condition from examination of pleural fluid may be difficult. Distinction from reactive mesothelial cells presents problems in well-differentiated tumours, but the malignant cells are larger, show more frequent multinuclear forms, and exhibit polyploidy. Furthermore, increasingly sophisticated immunocytochemical preparations are serving to distinguish malignant mesothelioma from adenocarcinoma; thus at least 85 per cent of mesotheliomas are negative to carcinoembryonic antigen but are positive when stained for low molecular weight intermediate filament keratin. Epithelial membrane antigen is said to be positive on mesothelioma cells but negative on benign mesothelial cells, and the antibody EP4 which reacts with epithelial cells does not produce a positive result with mesotheliomas. It must be emphasized that no immunocytochemical test is absolutely diagnostic.

Pleural biopsy

Owing to difficulty in obtaining adequate samples, pleural biopsy is often less helpful in diagnosis than examination of pleural fluid. The biopsy needs to be taken by an experienced operator as all too often all that the laboratory receives is a crushed portion of striated muscle. Difficulty encountered with the blind biopsy technique can be overcome if tissue is obtained at thoracoscopy but, although popular in some European centres, this procedure has not found general favour. Examination of pleural tissue is of most value in the diagnosis of effusions due to tuberculosis, mesothelioma, carcinoma and lymphomas. It has the advantage over cytology, provided that the sample is adequate, of revealing the general tissue architecture essential in the diagnosis of many tumours.

Bronchial biopsy

Since the advent of the flexible fibreoptic bronchoscope, biopsy of endobronchial masses has become a relatively simple procedure. The flexible bronchoscope has the added advantage of being able to penetrate to more distal airways than the rigid instrument. The disadvantage of biopsies taken by this method is that they are extremely small and may not include the main lesion, particularly if it is submucosal. The use of this instrument is not restricted to visible tumours as biopsy forceps can be extended beyond the visual field to sample more peripheral lesions and use of transbronchial biopsy forceps allows tissue to be obtained from extrabronchial pulmonary parenchymal tissue near the hilum. Thus diagnosis of diffuse parenchymal diseases such as sarcoidosis is possible. However, the results in pulmonary vasculitides and in fibrotic conditions are poor, and open-lung biopsy is often needed for a firm diagnosis. The importance of obtaining a diagnosis in tumours before undertaking a lobectomy or pneumonectomy needs no emphasis. Occasionally, if the diagnosis is not established a lung may be completely or partially removed for a benign condition such as an endobronchial lipoma or hamartoma. In malignant bronchial tumours a very good indication of the main cell type can be obtained from examination of bronchial biopsy material, but it must be remembered that examination of the entire tumour following lobectomy or pneumonectomy may often reveal a more heterogeneous appearance.

Open-lung biopsy

On many occasions investigations of the type described above fail to give a firm diagnosis and in such cases it is best to obtain an open-lung biopsy. This is not an operation to be undertaken without careful thought as it does carry some risk of morbidity. A persistent air leak, whether or not a drain is placed in the pleura, occurs in some 5 per cent of cases. There is an appreciable mortality, but this is often due to patients being severely ill and is an argument for carrying out the biopsy at an early stage of the disease rather than as a final effort to establish a tissue diagnosis. As with other methods of obtaining pulmonary tissue, an open-lung biopsy requires the services of a skilled and experienced thoracic surgeon. It is essential that the lung is carefully palpated and that an adequate sample of affected tissue is obtained, not necessarily just the most accessible piece of lung.

Handling of open-lung biopsy specimens

The specimen, fresh and unfixed, should be sent immediately in a sterile container, to the laboratory where small portions should be taken from the cut surface for microbiological and virological investigations. Where possible, further pieces should be diced and placed in glutaraldehyde for electron microscopy and, if sufficient tissue is available, a further small portion can be frozen and stored at −70°C for immunological study.

Fig. 2 Open-lung biopsy which has not been fixed by distension with fixative. It is not possible to make out the alveolar architecture.

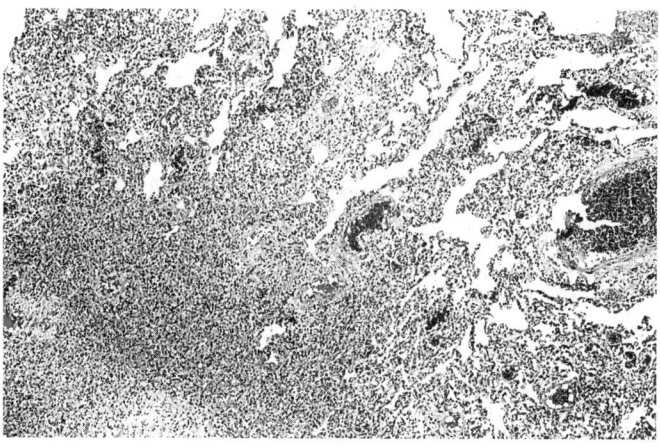

Fig. 3 Open-lung biopsy which has been prepared by inflation with fixative. The alveolar architecture and relationship of the alveoli to alveolar ducts and bronchioles is easily appreciated.

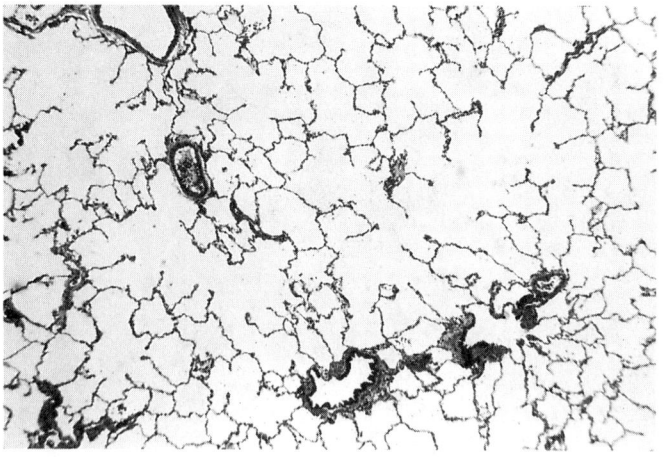

The greater part of the specimen must be retained for routine histology. If a good opinion is to be given on the architecture of the lung it is essential that it is inflated with fixative (Figs. 2 and 3). This is readily achieved by using a syringe, filled with formol saline, and a fine needle. The needle is inserted into the cut surface and formalin is gently injected into the lung tissue. The lung will then gradually inflate to assume a volume comparable with that during inspiration. If an entire lobe or lung is removed, then inflation with formol saline via the bronchus is a simple matter. The bronchus is connected via a plastic tube to a tank of formalin 60 cm above the specimen and the lung is inflated by gravity drainage. It is unnecessary to tie the bronchus once the lung is inflated. The inflated specimen can then be placed in formalin overnight and the following morning divided into appropriate blocks of tissue 0.5 cm thick for processing and paraffin embedding.

Frozen sections on open-lung biopsy material are of limited value except in the case of some neoplasms as the tissue is often so collapsed that no opinion can be given on the general architecture. With modern processing machines a paraffin section can be produced in 4 h if necessary.

Conditions amenable to diagnosis by open-lung biopsy

It is in investigation of peripheral solitary 'coin' lesions that open-lung biopsy is often essential in order to establish a diagnosis, particularly when fine-needle aspiration cytology has failed to give a satisfactory result.

Peripheral lung carcinomas can often only be diagnosed by removal of the affected portion of lung. Yet difficulty in distinguishing primary from metastatic neoplasms may be encountered here. This is particularly true in the case of adenocarcinomas. Differentiating primary adenocarcinoma of the lung from metastatic deposits, particularly from the colon, ovary, and pancreas, can prove difficult. All may show mucus production, have a papillary pattern, and also often contain psammoma bodies. Furthermore, many metastatic tumours have a tendency to grow along alveolar walls in a manner reminiscent of alveolar cell carcinoma. In secondary tumours satellite lesions, not visible on chest radiography, are more frequent than in primary neoplasms, whereas hilar lymph node metastases are seen more frequently in primary lung tumours. It is worth noting that many primary peripheral adenocarcinomas also originate in a scar. The use of electron microscopy in distinguishing metastatic colorectal carcinoma was thought to be of considerable value at one time, but has in fact proved disappointing. Distinction from the tubulopapillary form of mesothelioma may be aided by the fact that most pulmonary adenocarcinomas contain mucus, which is negative to periodic acid–Schiff reagent and resistant to diastase, and also carcinoembryonic antigen, which can be detected by the immunoperoxidase method, whereas most mesotheliomas do not show these two reactions.

The rare mixed epithelial and connective tissue pulmonary neoplasms (e.g. carcinosarcoma, pulmonary blastoma, and teratoma) can only be diagnosed reliably by open-lung biopsy and lobectomy is usually required.

In patients found to have diffuse miliary mottling on the chest radiograph only a small and limited quantity of lung tissue is usually needed to establish a diagnosis. This procedure is of particular value where the clinical picture may point to interstitial fibrosis or sarcoidosis but in fact the lesion is one of diffuse lymphatic permeation by tumour cells (Fig. 4).

Peripheral carcinoids are rare but easily diagnosed on biopsy, not only by the strikingly uniform appearance of their cells with small darkly staining central nuclei, but also by their characteristic argyrophilia and immunocytochemistry. Ultrastructural examination reveals typical neuroendocrine granules. It is notable that bone may occasionally be found in the stroma of these tumours which may be revealed on the chest radiograph.

Kaposi's sarcoma involving the lung is becoming increasingly frequent owing to its association with acquired immunodeficiency. The diagnosis is usually made on clinical grounds, but occasionally lung biopsy is needed where skin manifestations are minimal or absent and the pulmonary features predominate. Histological diagnosis in the absence of relevant clinical information may prove difficult in these cases. Multiple nodules are found in the lung, and these are composed of spindle cells resembling fibroblasts and endothelial cells with variable numbers of plasma cells, usually distributed along lymphatic pathways in interlobular septa and pleural surfaces. This infiltrate, in which the cells themselves may not appear malignant, extends into the walls of bronchi. In one form inflammatory cells predominate and there is a relative lack of spindle cells, and here biopsy diagnosis is extremely hazardous in the absence of relevant clinical and serological information.

Benign tumours presenting as coin lesions are best approached through open-lung biopsy as removal of the lesion is the only method of being certain of the diagnosis. The most frequently encountered tumour is the chondroma or chondroid hamartoma. These are usually single, measure up to 3 cm in diameter, are encapsulated, and are quite benign. Leiomyomas, benign clear-cell tumours, and nerve sheath tumours are all rare benign lesions lending themselves to diagnosis by excision biopsy.

Certain inflammatory conditions in the lung parenchyma, so-called pseudotumours, may be confused clinically and radiologically with neoplasms, and need biopsy to establish the true diagnosis. Prominent among such lesions is the plasma-cell granuloma or histiocytoma which may be found as an isolated asymptomatic peripheral pulmonary nodule at any age. They are sharply demarcated and are usually about 3 cm in diameter, although they may be much larger. Histological examination shows them to be made up of cellular fibrous tissue mainly infiltrated by plasma cells and histiocytes. Their aetiology is unknown, but in some cases there is a history of repeated respiratory infections.

One of the many manifestations of rheumatoid disease is the isolated necrobiotic pulmonary nodule. This may be quite large and be indistinguishable from a tumour on the chest radiograph. Histology of the excised nodule reveals typical areas of necrosis surrounded by palisaded histiocytes, plasma cells, and giant cells. This may be confused with an isolated tuberculous lesion, but no acid alcohol-fast bacilli are isolated and satellite granulomas of the type so often seen in tuberculosis are absent.

Restrictive lung disease

One of the most frequent indications for open-lung biopsy in patients with this form of functional defect occurs when there is generalized reticular shadowing on the chest radiograph. In the majority of cases the lesion is an idiopathic fibrosing alveolitis but biopsy is of value in excluding more specific disease. Thus asbestosis may give rise to a similar clinical picture and pathological appearance, but the presence of ferruginous bodies will point to the correct diagnosis. Prominent among such restrictive diseases is extrinsic allergic alveolitis (farmer's lung) which in its early stages has small granulomas without necrosis, often in the region of respiratory and terminal bronchioles with consequent mucosal ulceration (Fig. 5). Giant cells may be prominent and contain needle-shaped clefts. There is oedema and lymphocytic infiltration of alveolar walls. Distinction from sarcoidosis may be difficult or impossible on purely histological criteria, but the granulomas in general are smaller and less well defined in extrinsic allergic alveolitis and interstitial inflammation is not usual in sarcoidosis where the granulomas are often very discrete, perivascular, or peribronchiolar in location and seldom give rise to mucosal ulceration. In the chronic stages both conditions progress to diffuse interstitial fibrosis.

Pulmonary involvement may occur in isolation in histiocytosis X and lung biopsy may be the only method of confirming the diagnosis. Microscopically there are typical eosinophilic granulomas in the interstitial tissues, but it is the identification of groups of Langerhans cells that clinches the diagnosis. Electron microscopy is the most reliable method for identifying these cells which contain characteristic pentalaminar inclusions, (Birbeck granules) in their cytoplasm. In any patient where the diagnosis is suspected it is important to obtain tissue for electron microscopy. Immunocytochemistry is rather less specific, but Langerhans cells stain for S100 protein and the T6 antigen.

Another rare disorder in which there are widespread pulmonary lesions is lymphangioleiomyomatosis. A history of repeated pneumothoraces may give a clue to the diagnosis. There is a diffuse or focal proliferation of immature smooth muscle cells in the walls of alveoli and bronchioles with surrounding areas of focal emphysema. Involvement of pulmonary vessels and, in particular, pulmonary veins is common with consequent veno-occlusive disease. Smooth muscle proliferation may also surround and occlude lymphatics, giving rise to chylothorax.

The vast majority of biopsies taken from patients with restrictive lung disease reveal changes which are labelled cryptogenic fibrosing alveolitis. In most such cases the aetiology is obscure, yet in some there is evidence of drug-induced disease but there is nothing specific in the histological appearances to distinguish such cases from the idiopathic form, as the lung has a limited number of responses to noxious stimuli. Two distinct forms of pulmonary fibrosis have been recognized, namely organizing pneumonia and bronchiolitis obliterans. The distinction may be of some therapeutic importance as it is claimed that there is a favourable response to steroids in those patients where bronchiolitis obliterans

Fig. 4 Secondary tumour deposits from a primary carcinoma of the breast in perivascular lymphatics in the lung (open-lung biopsy).

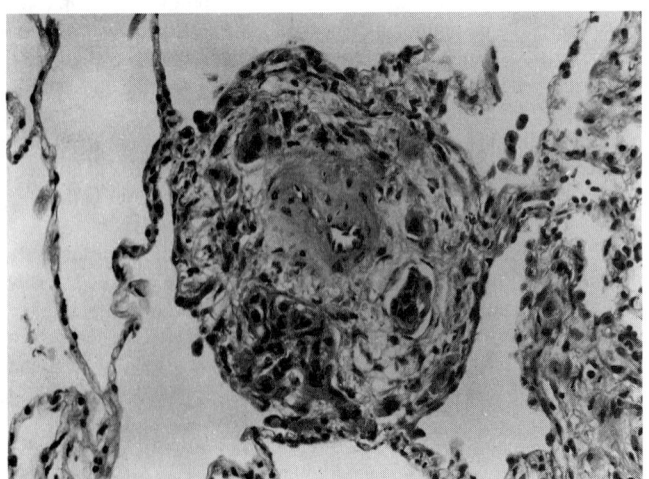

Fig. 5 A granulomar ulcerating bronchiolar mucosa in extrinsic allergic alveolitis.

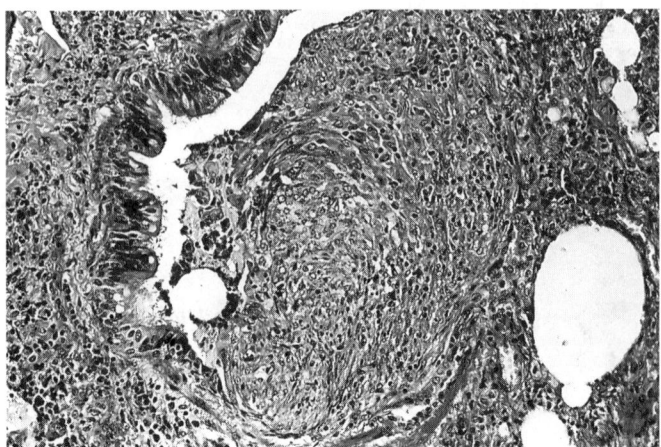

predominates. The histological criteria for these two types of lesions are fairly clear cut, but it must be emphasized that both are present to a greater or lesser degree in most biopsy specimens.

Bronchiolitis obliterans is characterized by the presence of oedematous granulation tissue, sometimes covered with a thin layer of fibrin, within alveoli and the lumen of bronchioles (Fig. 6). Alveolar walls may show oedema and chronic inflammatory cell infiltration.

In early stages of cryptogenic fibrosing alveolitis there is oedema, inflammatory cell infiltration, and fibrosis of alveolar walls (Fig. 7), often accompanied by the presence of many intra-alveolar macrophages—so-called desquamative interstitial pneumonia. Later, there is architectural disorganization with marked fibrosis replacing the alveolar structures resulting in cyst formation, giving rise to the 'honeycomb lung'. The irregular cystic spaces which replace the normal alveolar tissue are often lined by cuboidal or bronchiolar type epithelium and have walls formed by dense collagen, changes which are largely irreversible.

Infection

The use of open-lung biopsy in pulmonary infections is limited, but on occasion it may be of value in certain opportunistic conditions such as

Fig. 6 Lung biopsy from a patient with bronchiolitis obliterans. Oedematous granulation tissue is growing in the lumen of alveolar ducts and respiratory bronchioles. Adjacent tissue is the seat of collapse and fibrosis.

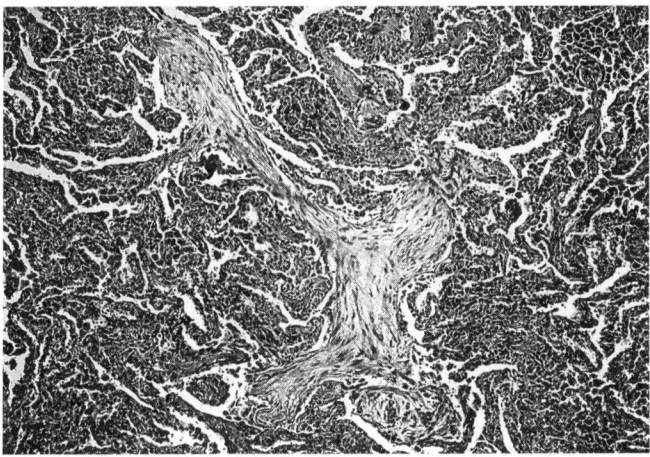

Fig. 7 Early cryptogenic fibrosing alveolitis with oedema and inflammatory cell infiltration in the walls of the air spaces. The spaces themselves contain macrophages—so called desquamative interstitial pneumonitis.

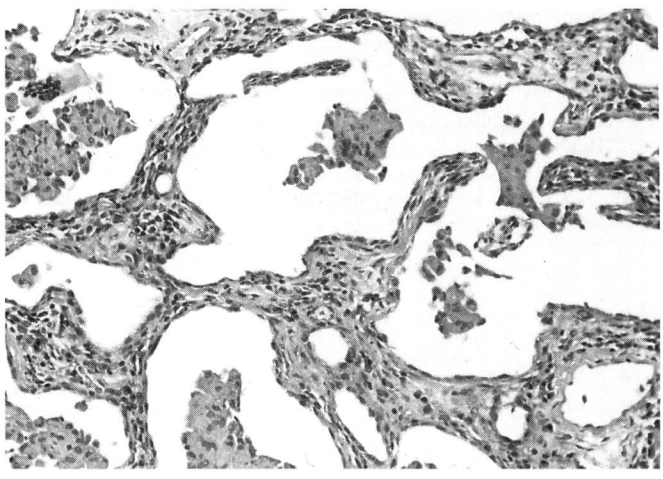

P. carinii pneumonia where the organism has not been isolated from sputum or bronchioloalveolar lavage washings. Actinomycosis may be present within a localized pulmonary mass, and in such cases it is important to examine multiple blocks of tissue as there may be very extensive inflammation and fibrosis as a reaction to an extremely small quantity of fungus. In all cases where inflammatory nodules are found on biopsy it is worth using special stains, notably Gomori's methenamine silver and the periodic acid–Schiff reagent method, for fungal spores which may not be readily observable in routine haematoxylin and eosin sections. The role of biopsy in viral infections is limited, though sometimes typical cytomegalovirus inclusions are found in tissue removed from immunosuppressed patients.

Pulmonary vascular disease

Indications for open-lung biopsy in order to arrive at a precise diagnosis in pulmonary vascular disease are few. However, in many patients with congenital or acquired cardiac defects who are undergoing corrective cardiac surgery a routine biopsy of the lung is taken in order to assess and grade the degree of vascular change. Lung biopsy may also be of value in those few cases with unexplained pulmonary hypertension where examination of lung tissue may reveal a precise diagnosis such as, for instance, in unsuspected pulmonary schistosomiasis. Pulmonary veno-occlusive disease provides another example of this category of patient where the occluded or narrow veins can be seen in oedematous interlobular septa after careful examination of a well-prepared inflated lung biopsy of adequate dimensions. Direct examination of pulmonary tissue is also of value in patients with congenital cardiac shunts and pulmonary hypertension where severity of the vascular lesions needs to be ascertained in order to decide whether or not corrective cardiac surgery is likely to be of benefit. The presence of severe concentric intimal fibrosis, numerous dilatation lesions, fibrinoid necrosis, or plexiform lesions may all be taken as indication that surgery is unlikely to relieve the pulmonary hypertension.

Pulmonary granulomatoses and angiitis

In the variety of conditions that give rise to granulomatous and vasculitic pulmonary lesions accurate diagnosis is dependent on findings at lung biopsy. The most distinctive of these conditions is Wegener's granulomatosis. In its classical form there is involvement of the upper respiratory tract and kidneys as well as the lung. However, the disease may occur in a limited pulmonary form and may then be mistaken for a tumour. It is sometimes stated that it never occurs in the upper lobes, but this is not true and when these are involved the condition can on occasion be mistaken for tuberculosis. There are nodules of varying size which may show cavitation. On microscopy there is fibrocaseous necrosis which has a serpiginous outline, often referred to as 'geographical'. Epithelioid cells and Langhans' giant cells surround the necrotic lesions and are accompanied by lymphocytes, plasma cells, and neutrophils, but eosinophils are not unduly prominent. The vasculitis which is typical of the disease affects pulmonary arteries, veins, and capillaries, and is well demonstrated in preparations stained for elastic tissue where the cellular infiltrate can often be seen breaching the elastic laminae in muscular arteries (Figs. 8 and 9). In a rare form of the disease diffuse pulmonary haemorrhage is found and may cause confusion with Goodpasture's syndrome—a problem which is resolved by detection of circulating antiglomerular basement membrane antibody.

The Churg–Strauss syndrome is a rare form of allergic angiitis and granulomatosis which may be confused with Wegener's granulomatosis. However, the clinical setting is entirely different as this syndrome occurs in asthmatics with a history of atopy. There is a profound peripheral eosinophilia and in many patients there is evidence of a peripheral vasculitis. The pulmonary nodules seldom cavitate. There are yellowish necrotic zones surrounded by a cellular infiltrate in which eosinophils predominate though epithelioid histiocytes and giant cells are also present. Charcot-Leyden crystals and eosinophilic debris are found in such areas of necrosis.

Sarcoidosis and rheumatoid disease, already referred to above, are granulomatous disorders with a vasculitic component but are usually easily diagnosed from their clinical setting and their distinctive histological appearance. Classical sarcoid with its discrete well-circumscribed granulomata cannot be easily mistaken for Wegener's granulomatosis. Confusion may arise with the rare disorder known as necrotizing sarcoid granulomatosis. Here there is usually less necrosis than in Wegener's granulomatosis and there is invasion of bronchial and bronchiolar walls. Vascular involvement is often extensive, with granulomas invading the adventitia, media, and intima of pulmonary arterial vessels. The precise nature of this rare disorder is not understood, but although it is considered by some to be a variant of sarcoid it should be noted that there is a frequent lack of hilar lymphadenopathy and a neg-

Fig. 8 A granulomatous reaction with giant cells surrounding and obliterating a small pulmonary vessel in Wegener's granulomatosis.

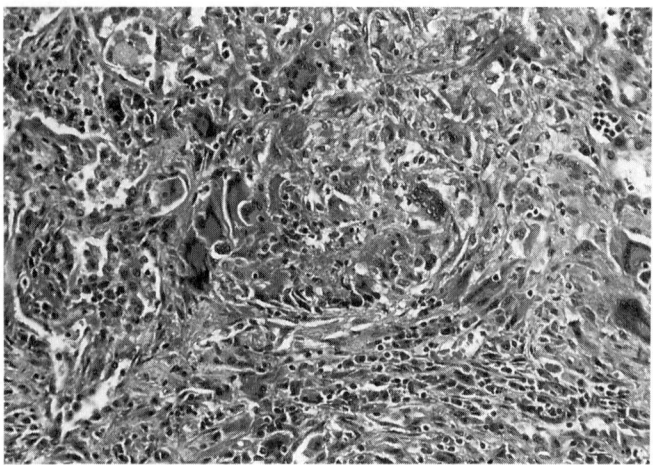

Fig. 9 An elastic tissue preparation showing breaching of the wall of a pulmonary vessel in Wegener's granulomatosis.

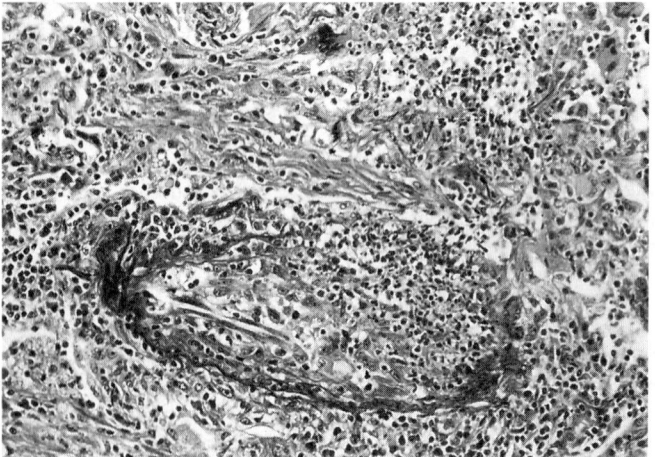

ative Kveim reaction, and in many instances the serum angiotensin-converting enzyme levels are not raised. The degree of necrosis is also much more extensive than in sarcoidosis.

There are a wide variety of lymphoproliferative disorders having a vasculitic component which, when confined to the lung, may only be diagnosed confidently by looking at lung biopsy material. These range from benign lymphocytic angiitis through lymphomatoid granulomatosis to large-cell angiocentric lymphoma and Hodgkin's disease. It is likely that all these disorders are varieties of pulmonary lymphoma.

In benign lymphocytic angiitis there is a focal but dense infiltrate of mature round lymphocytes, together with a few plasma cells, effacing normal alveolar architecture and characteristically infiltrating small pulmonary arterioles and venules. Necrosis is seldom if ever present. Its distinction from well-differentiated small-cell lymphoma is unclear, but it is said to respond to chlorambucil.

Lymphomatoid granulomatosis of the lung is an angiocentric disorder which was originally described before the concept of extranodal lymphoma was fully recognized. It is now accepted that most cases are a manifestation of malignant lymphoma with initial pulmonary involvement. The chest radiograph may reveal dense opacities, often with cavitation. and Diagnosis depends upon the findings at lung biopsy as fine-needle aspiration cytology is unlikely to yield useful results. The lesions may be multiple and, though often small, in some instances may be as large as 10 cm in diameter. Histologically the main features are centred on pulmonary arteries and veins which are surrounded and invaded by a polymorphic infiltrate in which atypical and bizarre lymphoid cells predominate. Initially this infiltrate is in the perivascular lymphatics and the lymphatics in the interlobular septa. Invasion of vessels may be of such severity that its true extent can only be appreciated in elastic preparations which reveal the outline of obliterated arteries and veins. Cytology of the abnormal lymphoid cells and the scarcity of Langhans' giant cells serve to differentiate the condition from Wegener's granulomatosis. Furthermore, immunocytochemical studies reveal many of these cases to be T-cell lymphomas, although occasionally even B-cell lymphomas and Hodgkin's disease may masquerade under the title of lymphomatoid granulomatosis.

Isolated pulmonary large-cell high grade lymphoma may not be distinguishable from the above conditions clinically or on chest radiograph, but on biopsy the cytology of the infiltrate will reveal the diagnosis. There are numerous large lymphoid cells with a high nuclear cytoplasmic ratio and bizarre mitotic figures. The nuclei are vesicular and often possess numerous nucleoli.

Involvement of the lung with Hodgkin's disease is usually a late phenomenon, but when it occurs it is easily recognized owing to the presence of typical Reed–Sternberg cells and the polymorphic nature of the infiltrate which shows a predilection for bronchial associated tissue. Indeed, it is one of the disorders that can often be diagnosed by bronchial biopsy.

REFERENCES

Corrin, B. (1990). The lungs. In: *Systemic pathology*, Vol. 5 (ed W.St.C. Symmers). Churchill Livingstone, London.
Dail, D.H. and Hammar, S.P. (1987). *Pulmonary pathology*. Springer Verlag, New York.
Dunnill, M.S. (1987). Pulmonary pathology (2nd ed). Churchill Livingstone, London.

17.7 Respiratory infection

Infection of the respiratory tract is a leading cause of illness and death worldwide.

Epidemics of influenza continue because of the difficulties in maintaining appropriate vaccines in the face of antigenic shift and drift of the virus and in implementating vaccination programmes. Measles, the pneumococcus, and *Haemophilus influenzae* cause annually some 5 million deaths in young children in the developing countries where vaccination programmes and the use of simple antimicrobials are not adequately provided for in poor, often rural, populations.

Tuberculosis causes 3 million deaths in the developing countries annually and, in the wake of the AIDS epidemic, notification rates are rising in North America and Europe where multiply resistant strains are being increasingly reported.

The immunosuppressed population—organ transplant recipients—and oncology groups, as well as AIDS patients, is subject to infection by pathogens but also by effective opportunistic organisms including, in particular, *Pneumocystis carinii*, cytomegalovirus, and the mycobacteria.

The clinical syndromes of respiratory infection are described here, but detailed accounts of specific infections, including tuberculosis, are given in the section on infectious diseases.

17.7.1 Upper respiratory tract infection

J. M. HOPKIN

Upper respiratory tract clinical syndromes include rhinitis (coryza, the common cold), pharyngitis, laryngitis, and laryngotracheal rhonchitis. In any illness, these syndromes may occur in combination or be accompanied by a lower respiratory tract infection. Viruses (Table 1) are the principal cause of upper respiratory tract infection. The various respiratory DNA or RNA viruses may be transmitted by small droplet aerosol, as a result of sneezing or coughing; in this way adenovirus and influenza A and B (Section 7) can be transmitted over reasonable distances and infect many individuals to cause epidemics. In addition, respiratory syncytial virus and rhinoviruses can be spread by direct contact with infected secretions, hand to hand, or involving an intermediate fomite.

A specific diagnosis may be established by culture of the virus on suitable cell culture media, by direct detection of virus DNA from respiratory secretions, or by serology retrospectively. The chief value of these techniques is in delineating the epidemiology of infections rather than clinical management.

Most upper respiratory illnesses are self-limiting, but may be complicated by significant secondary bacterial infection, usually *H. influenzae* or pneumococcus.

The common cold

The common cold syndrome is caused principally by rhinovirus and coronavirus infections. Respiratory syncytial virus and parainfluenza viruses may also cause the syndrome in adults, whereas they cause principally lower respiratory tract disease, either as bronchiolitis or pneumonia, in infants and toddlers (Table 1).

Table 1 *Viruses causing respiratory infection by frequency*

Upper respiratory infection	Lower respiratory infection
Rhinovirus	Respiratory syncytial virus
Coronavirus	Influenza A + B
Adenovirus	Parainfluenza
Parainfluenza	Measles
Echovirus	Adenovirus
Respiratory syncytial virus	Rhinovirus
Coxsackie A	Coronavirus
Influenza A and B	

The array of virus subtypes, notably rhinovirus, ensures that no long-lasting immunity occurs, and adults continue to suffer between one and six coryzal illnesses annually. The familiar features of the common cold begin with nasal or nasopharyngeal stinging, progressing to variable nasal blockage and watery nasal discharge. In contrast with influenza, there is relatively little constitutional disturbance. Potential complications, due to secondary bacterial infection, include sinusitis (manifest as facial pain and nasal tenderness with purulent nasal discharge or retropharyngeal drip), middle-ear infection (with pain and deafness), or tracheobronchitis (with cough producing purulent sputum).

These secondary complications require antibiotic treatment appropriate for *H. influenzae* or pneumococcal superinfection, such as amoxycillin or cotrimoxazole. Uncomplicated rhinitis requires no specific therapy, although large sums of money are spent by sufferers on 'over the counter' relief medications of marginal efficacy.

Croup

Croup represents one clinical form of laryngotracheal bronchitis in young children. It is characterized by a bark-like cough and respiratory stridor. Most episodes are caused by parainfluenza virus. The illness starts with cough, hoarseness, and fever. Croup symptoms follow and are typically worse at night. There may be accompanying signs of wheeze and there is usually hypoxaemia. Humidification of inspired air and oxygen supplementation are necessary supportive treatments. Nebulized epinephrine and systemic corticosteroids are used by many clinicians, and there is some trial evidence of efficacy. A recent study of nebulized budesonide suggests significant benefit for children with mild to moderate croup.

Acute epiglottitis

Croup must be distinguished from acute infective epiglottitis, another febrile syndrome showing features of upper airflow obstruction. In this syndrome, often caused by *H. influenzae* infection, there is severe throat pain, painful dysphagia, and often the need to sit upright with jutted chin in an effort to maintain a patent airway. If the diagnosis is suspected, then expert laryngoscopy is essential when a nasally introduced endotracheal intubation may be required. Antimicrobial therapy, effective against local strains of *H. influenzae*, is essential.

REFERENCES

Klassen, T.P., *et al.* (1994). Nebulized budesonide for children with mild to moderate croup. *New England Journal of Medicine*, **331**, 285.

Knight, G.J., Harris, M.A., Parbari, M., O'Callaghan, M.J., and Masters, I.B. (1992). Single daily dose ceftriaxone therapy in epiglottitis. *Journal of Paediatric and Child Health*, **28**, 220–2.

Pisareva, M., Bechtereva, T., Plyusnin, A., Dobretsova, A., Kisselev, O. (1992). PCR amplification of Influenza A virus specific sequences. *Archives of Virology*, **125**, 313–8.

Tibballs, J., Shann, F.A., and Landau, L.I. (1992). Placebo-controlled trial of prednisolone in children intubated for croup. *Lancet*, **340**, 745–8.

Waisman, Y., Klein, B.L., Boenning, D.A., Young, G.M., Chamberlain, J.M., O'Donnell, R., and Ochsenschkager, D.W. (1992). Prospective randomized double-blind study comparing L-epinephrine and racemic epinephrine aerosols in the treatment of laryngotracheitis (croup). *Paediatrics*, **89**, 302–6.

17.7.2 Acute lower respiratory tract infections

J. T. MACFARLANE

Acute infections of the respiratory tract are one of the commonest illnesses to affect humans, whether healthy or debilitated by other disease. In this chapter we discuss acute lower respiratory tract infections, adopting a practical and clinical approach. Further details of specific pathogens and individual syndromes can be found in other parts of this textbook.

Bronchial infections

Acute bronchitis in previously healthy people

This very common condition is often preceded by an upper respiratory infection and the feeling that 'the cold has gone to the chest'. It is usually believed to be caused by viral infections, particularly adenovirus, rhinovirus, or influenza virus in adults, and respiratory syncytial virus or parainfluenza virus in children and the elderly. Recent studies have suggested that secondary bacterial infections with *Streptococcus pneumoniae* and *Haemophilus influenzae* are not infrequent. Atypical infections with *Mycoplasma pneumoniae*, *Chlamydia pneumoniae*, and *Chlamydia psittaci* sometimes present as acute bronchitis in young adults. Thus the aetiological agents are very similar to those causing more severe infection, such as community-acquired pneumonia.

Symptoms include mild general malaise, retrosternal soreness, and initially a dry tickly cough. Sputum may be produced, initially mucoid but becoming mucopurulent. Associated upper respiratory tract symptoms, including sore throat and runny nose, are common. The patient does not look ill and the chest is clear. Investigations are not normally required; the white blood count will be normal and the chest radiograph clear. The C-reactive protein may be raised in the presence of bacterial infection. Sometimes the virus can be cultured from a nasopharyngeal swab, or a bacterial pathogen can be cultured from sputum.

Treatment is symptomatic, and the decision to use antibiotics will be based on various considerations including duration of history, social factors, pointers to bacterial infection such as purulent sputum, and pre-existing medical conditions. Compound cough mixtures may be helpful at night, largely owing to their sedative properties.

Acute exacerbations of chronic bronchitis

PRESENTATION

Chronic bronchitis is characterized by persistent production of excess bronchial mucus. Those affected by this syndrome are liable to suffer repeated acute exacerbations characterized by an increase in sputum purulence and worsening cough that lasts for 48 h or more. In addition, there may be general malaise, a mild fever, increased breathlessness, increased sputum volume or thickness, and increased difficulty in expectoration. Such exacerbations are more common in the winter months.

AETIOLOGY

Identifying the supposed role of acute bronchial infection in such exacerbations can be difficult. Over three-quarters of patients with stable chronic bronchitis have *H. influenzae* present in their sputum, and *Strep. pneumoniae* is also found in a third. Therefore the culture of these pathogens during an exacerbation is not necessarily informative. Long-term studies of patients with chronic bronchitis suggest that, although the incidence of positive sputum cultures for *H. influenzae* and *Strep. pneumoniae* does not rise during exacerbations, the actual numbers of bacteria (particularly pneumococci) do increase. *Moraxella catarrhalis* is the third commonest bacterial pathogen isolated from the sputum of patients with acute exacerbations of chronic bronchitis. Regarding non-bacterial causes, viruses have been associated with 40 to 60 per cent of acute exacerbations, particularly in the winter months, and the reported incidence of *Mycoplasma pneumoniae* infection (proven on serological testing) is 1 to 8 per cent. *Mycoplasma* species can colonize the lower respiratory tract in chronic bronchitics, but their role in acute exacerbations is unclear.

CLINICAL FEATURES

The clinical features reflect both the infection itself and the effect on the underlying lung disease and lung function. Sputum usually changes in quantity and consistency, and becomes mucopurulent. Variable wheezes and scattered coarse crepitations may be heard on auscultation. Radiographically the chest is usually clear, although some peribronchial thickening or subsegmental infiltration may be noted. The occurrence of dyspnoea, cor pulmonale, and changes in lung function will be determined by the degree of underlying chronic airflow obstruction.

MANAGEMENT OF ACUTE EXACERBATION

Routine sputum culture is unnecessary during the exacerbation unless the patient is seriously ill, the presentation is unusual, or there is a known high prevalence of pathogens with altered antibiotic susceptibility in the locality. Except for the mildest of exacerbations, antibiotics are indicated and hasten recovery. Studies have shown equally good response with ampicillin, amoxycillin, co-trimoxazole, and erythromycin, even though the latter has poor activity against *H. influenzae*. The choice of antibiotic depends more on side-effect profile, patient acceptability, and cost. Tetracycline, previously widely used in this setting, is uncommonly prescribed now because of side-effects and increasing bacterial resistance, particularly amongst common strains of *H. influenzae* and also some *Strep. pneumoniae*.

Treatment is traditionally given for 7 to 10 days, but is guided by patient improvement and resolution of sputum purulence. The associated problems of airflow obstruction, ventilatory failure, and cor pulmonale can be precipitated or aggravated by an acute infective exacerbation in a severe chronic bronchitic, and these aspects will require vigorous treatment when present.

PREVENTATIVE MEASURES

The place of measures to prevent acute exacerbations in patients with chronic bronchitis is unclear. Antibiotic prophylaxis with such agents as daily tetracycline or weekly long-acting sulphametopyrazine has been shown to be helpful, but only in patients with very frequent exacerbations and at the expense of side-effects and are rarely used. An influenza vaccination in the autumn is helpful. There is no evidence that pneumococcal vaccination protects the individual from the whole spectrum of pneumococcal infection. However, as patients with chronic lung disease are at risk of severe life-threatening pneumococcal pneumonia, they fall into the group where pneumococcal vaccination is recommended. As non-capsulated strains of *H. influenzae* are implicated in exacerbations, haemophilus vaccination is ineffective.

Acute bronchial infections and asthma

Adults with asthma frequently date the start of their condition from an attack of acute bronchitis. Acute infective bronchitis, particularly due to viral infection, can lead to a state of airways hyper-reactivity. This explains the persistence of cough and wheeze for several weeks after an acute bronchitic illness. In certain susceptible people this appears to initiate the development of true asthma.

It is very important to identify such patients as the treatment and prognosis of asthma is very different from that of a simple infective bronchitis. Persisting cough and wheeze, particularly at night, together with a reduced peak expiratory flow rate point to the development of asthma. All too often such patients receive repeated and inappropriate courses of antibiotics, whereas they really need bronchodilators or even corticosteroids.

In patients with established asthma, bacterial infections are an unusual cause of acute exacerbations and antibiotics have little place in the routine management of acute asthma. Similarly, viral infections have been implicated in only 10 to 20 per cent of acute exacerbations.

Bacterial superinfection following acute viral respiratory infection

Bacterial infection is not infrequently preceded by a primary viral illness. This is of greatest clinical importance when a secondary bacterial pneumonia develops and is considered later in this chapter.

Pneumonia

History

Pneumonia has been recognized for many centuries. 'Peripneumonia' was described by Hippocrates in the fourth century BC. The erroneous concepts of anatomy and physiology which prevailed up to the last century hampered any real understanding of the nature of pneumonia, although it was regarded as some sort of inflammation of the lung. Treatment included leeches, cupping, and stupes applied to the chest, together with emetics, tonics, and purges to draw the inflammation away from the chest. Vigorous blood-letting was popular, particularly in Britain.

In 1834 Laennec paved the way for our modern understanding of lobar pneumonia by describing the three stages of consolidation that are still recognized today. Pathologically, these include a first state of engorgement: the lung, when cut, is wet, oedematous, and congested. In the second stage of red hepatization, the lung is dry, red, friable, and solid like liver. Thirdly, grey hepatization occurs with softening of the cut lung and exudation of yellow purulent fluid which denotes resolution. Laennec also perfected the use of the stethoscope and described the crepitous rattle (crepitation) as a pathognomonic sign of the first stage of peripneumonia. Red hepatization was heralded by the development of bronchial breathing, and resolution by the return of crepitations (rhonchus crepitous redux).

Towards the end of the nineteenth century the cause of pneumonia became a matter of hot debate, with some expounding atmospheric conditions and others infection as the cause. Friedlander, between 1881 and 1884, first found bacteria in the lungs of fatal cases of pneumonia using the staining techniques of his colleague Gram, and Fraenkel, in 1884, first isolated an organism which he called 'pneumoniemikroccus' (pneumococcus) from a 30-year-old man dying of pneumonia. The identification of the pneumococcus rapidly led to a realization of its importance as a cause of pneumonia and to the production of specific antisera for treatment. By the early twentieth century microbiologists had become expert and quick at typing and isolating pneumococci as a guide to specific serum therapy.

With the discovery of penicillin and other antibiotics the problem of pneumonia seemed to be conquered and interest in the condition waned. However, it was recognized that there was a group of pneumonias, which did not behave like lobar pneumococcal pneumonia, in that they were generally not severe and did not respond to penicillin. These 'atypical' pneumonias were subsequently identified as being caused by *Chlamydia psittaci* (psittacosis), *Coxiella burnetii* (Q fever), and *Mycoplasma pneumoniae* (Eaton's agent).

The next major event in the history of pneumonia was the first outbreak of legionnaires' disease in Philadelphia in 1976. This was followed just a few years later by the increasing recognition of unusual and opportunistic lung infections in patients with AIDS, and the increasing importance of pneumonia in patients receiving immunosuppression therapy for inflammatory disease and cancer, and following organ transplantation.

The most recent event has been the description, in 1986, of a pneumonia caused by a new atypical pathogen *Chlamydia pneumoniae*. In contrast with psittacosis, this *Chlamydia* species has man as its only host and appears to be a significant cause of sporadic and epidemic lower respiratory infections. These changes have generated an increasing awareness that pneumonia of all types is still a common cause of morbidity and mortality, even in the days of readily available antibiotics.

The continuing importance of pneumonia

Pneumonia is one of the leading causes of death in both the United Kingdom and North America. Around 30 000 patients died of pneumonia in England and Wales in 1991. Pneumonia accounts for about ten times as many deaths in the United Kingdom as all other infectious diseases together. The mortality in those admitted to hospital with pneumonia ranges from 6 to 24 per cent, with rates between 10 and 50 per cent being reported for patients with pneumococcal bacteraemia.

Pneumonia is the most common cause of hospital attendance for both adults and children in developing countries, and it is estimated that 5 million children under the age of 5 years die of pneumonia each year. The impact on health service resources is also substantial. Respiratory infections are the commonest reason for general practitioner consultation, with the incidence for adult lower respiratory infections being around 40 per 1000 population per year and 2 to 3 per 1000 for community-acquired pneumonia. Pneumonia acquired in hospital ranks as the third most common nosocomial infection, has a considerable mortality and morbidity, and considerably prolongs hospital stay and costs.

Classification of pneumonia

The traditional divisions of pneumonia are by radiological appearance or microbiological cause. Neither is of much practical help to the clinician. The radiological description of pneumonia as lobar pneumonia, lobular pneumonia, segmental pneumonia, and bronchopneumonia does not help in either diagnosis or management as there is much overlap of changes, none of which is unique to a single pathogen. Similarly, grouping under aetiology presupposes that the clinician knows the cause of the pneumonia when the patient first presents—a theoretically ideal but, in practice, very unusual situation.

A useful classification of the types of pneumonia includes reference to the clinical circumstances under which the pneumonia is acquired and to the clinical background of the particular patient. A practical classification that helps to guide investigation, management, and therapy is outlined in Table 1.

In this chapter we concentrate mainly on community-acquired pneumonia, nosocomial pneumonia, and aspiration pneumonia. Pneumonia in the immunocompromised patient and in the patient with HIV infection are special examples of secondary pneumonia that are increasingly

Table 1 *Classification of pneumonia*

Community-acquired pneumonia
Hospital-acquired (nosocomial) pneumonia
Aspiration and anaerobic pneumonia
Pneumonia in the immunocompromised host
AIDS-related pneumonia
Geographically restricted pneumonias
Recurrent pneumonia

important and are dealt with in Chapter 17.7.5. Pneumonia peculiar to specific geographical areas of the world is discussed briefly in this chapter, but more details of the specific infections are described in Chapter 7.11.3. Recurrent pneumonia is defined as three or more separate attacks of pneumonia in the same patients and is discussed at the end of this chapter.

Community-acquired pneumonia

INTRODUCTION

Community-acquired pneumonia continues to be a common cause of acute hospital admission. There are few studies of the incidence in the community of patients not requiring hospital admission, but studies in a large group health practice in Seattle suggested an annual rate of 10 to 15 cases per 1000 population of all ages with the highest rates in the very young and the very old. Only 16 per cent of cases required hospital admission. Community studies in Nottingham suggest that a general practitioner will see about eight to ten cases of pneumonia each year in adults between 16 and 79 years, and will manage three-quarters of them at home. Those with pneumonia constitute only about 6 per cent of all the patients that they treat for respiratory infections with antibiotics. In the United Kingdom around 30 million prescriptions for antibiotics are written each year for new episodes of respiratory illness (all ages). Therefore a substantial number of patients are being treated for pneumonia and chest infections in the community. Pneumonia is twice as common in the winter months. It has been suggested that winter air of low humidity dries the nasopharyngeal mucosa and impairs local defences. Viral respiratory infections prevalent in the winter also increase the risk of secondary bacterial pneumonia.

TYPES OF COMMUNITY-ACQUIRED PNEUMONIA

Community-acquired pneumonia can occur in a number of different settings that are important to consider as they affect the likely cause and severity of the infection.

Pneumonia can affect the previously healthy individual or the patient with underlying disease, particularly chronic lung disease. The latter is associated with increased colonization of the respiratory tract with pathogenic bacteria together with impaired local defence mechanisms.

Infection can result either from bacteria already colonizing the upper airways or by direct spread from other infected individuals (e.g. droplet transmission of respiratory viruses), animals (e.g. Q fever, tularaemia, psittacosis), or infected water droplets (e.g. legionella infection). The age of the patient will also influence likely pathogens.

The term 'atypical pneumonia' is used widely but can be confusing. It is best used to describe the community-acquired infections, including *M. pneumoniae*, *Chlamydia* species, *Legionella* species, and *Coxiella burnetii*, which respond to macrolides or tetracycline but not to β-lactam antibiotics. *Legionella* species can also be a cause of nosocomial pneumonia.

AETIOLOGY

Before the introduction of antibiotics, the predominance of pneumococcal infection as a cause of pneumonia emerged very clearly. Reports on over 14 000 cases of lobar pneumonia by Cecil in 1927 and Heffron in 1939 found pneumococcal infection in over 95 per cent. After the discovery of antibiotics and their subsequent widespread use, the pattern appeared to change. There have been numerous recent hospital studies of adults admitted from the community with pneumonia in the United Kingdom, Europe, and elsewhere which have produced a broad agreement on the current causes of community-acquired pneumonia (Table 2), although the relative frequency of some of the pathogens is affected by where, how, and when the study was performed. This is particularly true for legionella pneumonia and Q fever where wide geographical variations are reported.

Antibiotics given before admission to hospital reduce the ability to culture common pathogens from sputum, blood, and body fluids, and this is one reason for disappointing microbiological results. In some studies no pathogen has been identified in up to half the cases. Pneumococcal infection may still be the cause in many of these undiagnosed cases because pneumococcal antigen can be detected by countercurrent immunoelectrophoresis in many, even after antibiotic therapy. The detection of bacterial antigen is much less affected by prior antibiotics or delay in specimen collection (see Chapter 17.6.3). Some viral and atypical pneumonias are also underdiagnosed because both acute and follow-up serological samples are needed to identify such infections.

The main conclusion from these studies is that community-acquired pneumonia is caused by a limited number of organisms. *Strep. pneumoniae* is the principal pathogen. Other bacteria are uncommon but include *H. influenzae* and *Staphylococcus aureus* (particularly in association with influenza virus infection). In some areas legionella pneumonia is a significant problem, but in the United Kingdom it accounts for around 3 per cent of pneumonia cases overall. Although *H. influenzae* is usually seen in those with chronic lung disease, it can sometimes be a primary pathogen in previously fit adults. Infections with the Gram-negative coccal bacteria, *Neisseria meningitidis* group Y and *Moraxella catarrhalis* have been reported infrequently, but Gram-negative bacillary infections are very unusual. Viral and atypical pneumonias, particularly *M. pneumoniae* infection, form a sizeable group. Viral infections, of which influenza virus is the commonest followed by parainfluenza and respiratory syncytial virus infection, are usually associated with superadded bacterial pneumonia. These conclusions have important implications for deciding on antibiotic treatment.

In contrast, some community acquired pneumonia studies in the United States report much more frequent Gram-negative, anaerobic, and staphylococcal infections than in the United Kingdom. This is probably because debilitated patients, alcoholics, and drug abusers form a larger proportion of patients with pneumonia in such studies from centres in North America, and pathogens associated with such patients are similar to those encountered in nosocomial infection.

The causes of community-acquired pneumonia cases not requiring hospital admission have been studied less extensively. Surveys from Plymouth, Sweden, and Seattle found mycoplasma pneumonia in 15 to 20 per cent of cases and viral infection in only 5 to 7 per cent. Legionella pneumonia was found in 1 per cent of cases in Seattle. A community study in Nottingham has helped to clarify the role of bacteria in this situation. Pathogens were identified in 53 per cent of 236 adults with pneumonia including *Strep. pneumoniae* in 78 (33 per cent), *H. influenzae* in 24 (10 per cent), tuberculosis in three, *Staph. aureus* in two, and *Legionella pneumophila* in one. In addition, viruses were found in 30 cases and atypical pneumonia in six. This pattern is very similar to hospital-based studies, except that legionella and staphylococcal infections more commonly cause an illness severe enough to require hospital admission.

Table 2 *Causes of adult community-acquired pneumonia (CAP) found in 10 hospital-based studies performed in the last 10 years**

	CAP(%) (range (%)) (2679 patients)	Severe CAP (%) (233 patients)
No cause found	36 (3–50)	33
Strep. pneumoniae	25 (9–79)	27
Influenza virus	8 (5–8.5)	2.3
M. pneumoniae	7.2 (2–18)	2.3
Legionella spp.	7 (2–18)	17
H. influenzae	5.4 (2–11)	5
Other viruses	5 (1–10)	8†
Psittacosis/Q fever	3 (0–6)	1
Gram-negative enteric bacilli	2.7 (0–8)	2
Staph. aureus	2 (0–3)	5

*Severe CAP data from various studies based on intensive care units (overall mortality 39 per cent) are also included.

†Four of these patients had varicella pneumonia.

EPIDEMIOLOGY

Many respiratory pathogens have characteristic epidemiological features, a knowledge of which can be of value to the clinician (Fig. 1). Seasonal peaks vary from year to year, but bacterial infections, including pneumococcal, moraxella, and staphylococcal pneumonia, are much commoner in the first quarter of the year at the time of increased influenza virus activity. Haemophilus infections peak both during this period and in the last quarter of the year. In contrast legionella infection is commoner in the summer months, sometimes related to foreign travel, hotel stays, and exposure to air conditioning and other water systems. Respiratory syncytial virus occurs in major epidemics in late autumn and early winter, affecting the very young and the very old. Parainfluenza virus 3 has a peak in late summer, in contrast with types 1 and 2 which are more usually seen in the winter.

Whooping cough and mycoplasma have a much longer periodicity. Mycoplasma occurs in large epidemics every 3 to 4 years throughout the world, when suspicion will be heightened. The last epidemic was in 1990–1991 (Fig. 2). Enquiry should be made about recent contact with pet birds or fowl at home or work (possible psittacosis), contact with farm animals (Q fever), recent foreign travel or stays in large hotels or hospitals (legionella pneumonia), or contact with others with pneumonia, influenza, or chicken pox.

CLINICAL FEATURES

It is not possible to guess the cause of pneumonia correctly from the history and signs on presentation as no pathogen has an unique pattern.

Symptoms

Males are affected more commonly than females in a ratio of 2–3 to 1. General symptoms include those of any febrile illness—malaise, anorexia, sweating, aches and pains, and headache. There may be a preceding history of upper respiratory tract symptoms, particularly with viral and mycoplasma infections. Respiratory symptoms are variable, but classically include cough, sputum, dyspnoea, pleural pain, and, less commonly, haemoptysis (Table 3).

Sputum is usually mucoid, scanty, or absent early on in the illness, particularly with legionella and atypical pneumonias. Purulent sputum develops later, and can be pinkish coloured in classic pneumococcal infection.

Non-respiratory symptoms sometimes dominate the picture and mask the diagnosis. Lower-lobe pneumonia may present with abdominal pain, rigidity, and ileus, and should be excluded in anyone with an 'acute' abdomen. Marked confusion may also be seen in patients with any severe pneumonia, and it is a feature of legionella pneumonia in less seriously ill patients. Meningitis, hypoxia, and metabolic upset must also

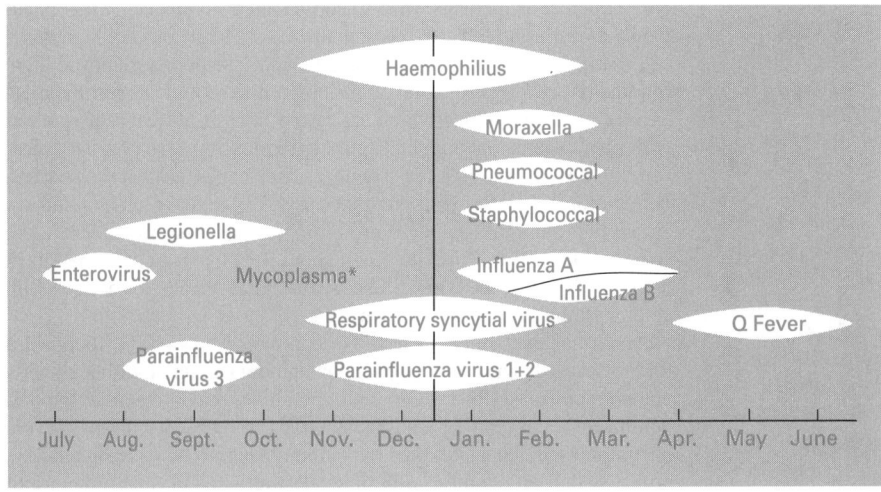

Fig. 1 Seasonal peaks in respiratory medicine. Respiratory pathogens usually occur throughout the year but many have seasonal peaks as well. (Adapted from R. A. L. Blewis, J. Gibson, and D. M. Geddes, eds. (1990). Figure 21.1.3. Balliere Tindall, London, with permission).

be considered in the confused patient. Severe headache, cerebellar dysfunction, memory loss, and myalgia also occur with legionella pneumonia. Vomiting and diarrhoea are prominent in some cases, although they may be the result of initial antibiotic therapy.

The duration of symptoms before hospital presentation varies with the severity of the illness, but is usually 3 to 7 days. However, 10 to 14 days is not unusual with atypical pneumonia, particularly mycoplasma infection, and patients will often have received a course of a β-lactam antibiotic without improvement. Pneumococcal and staphylococcal pneumonias may present abruptly with fever, rigors, cough, and pleural pain. Adults with influenza or chickenpox who develop lower respiratory symptoms may deteriorate quickly, and should be assessed and treated as a matter of urgency.

Physical signs

The patient usually looks flushed and unwell with tachypnoea and a tachycardia. High temperatures (greater than 39.5°C) and rigors occur in young people, particularly with pneumococcal, staphylococcal, and legionella pneumonia. Elderly or debilitated patients may have little or no rise in temperature; the main sign is a raised respiratory rate. Herpes labialis is a particular feature of pneumococcal infection, and is found in a third of cases. Examination of the chest will show reduced movement of the affected side, particularly if pleural pain is prominent, and the patient may splint that side by shallow breathing and hand holding of the chest. Classic signs of lobar consolidation are uncommon and bronchial breathing occurs in less than a quarter of cases; inspiratory crepitations are the commonest focal sign. A pleural rub may be heard even in the absence of pleural pain. On occasion, chest examination appears normal and the extent of radiographic shadowing comes as a surprise, a feature said to be more common with atypical and viral pneumonias.

Signs outside the chest may be found. Upper abdominal tenderness and confusion are not uncommon in more severely ill patients. A rash is unusual with community-acquired pneumonias, but has been reported with mycoplasma and psittacosis pneumonia. More commonly, a rash is a reaction to antibiotic therapy.

It is important to emphasize that respiratory symptoms may not be elicited even in the presence of extensive pneumonia. This is particularly the case in the very young, elderly, or debilitated patient, and the diagnosis may be missed without careful chest examination and a chest radiograph.

Fig. 2 Laboratory reports of *Mycoplasma pneumoniae* infections, England and Wales demonstrating the 3- to 4-year epidemic cycles preceded by smaller peaks. (Reproduced from the Communicable Disease Report with permission of the Editor.)

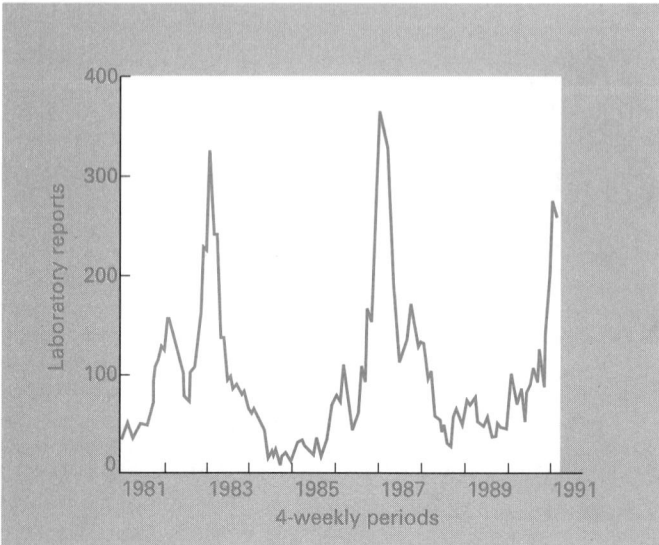

Table 3 *Symptoms in 127 consecutive adults with community-acquired pneumonia*

Symptom	Percentage
Fever	86
Headache	55
Muscle aches	44
Nausea/vomiting	48
Diarrhoea	24
Sore throat	19
Dyspnoea	67
Pleural pain	62
Cough	92
New sputum production	54
Haemoptysis	15

Source: Macfarlane, unpublished data.

Table 4 *Initial total white cell count in 329 patients with different types of community-acquired pneumonia*

	$10.0 \times 10^6/dl$ or less	(11–15) $\times 10^6/dl$	More than $15 \times 10^6/dl$
Pneumococcal (n = 93)	15%	32%	53%
Legionella (n = 78)	53%	36%	11%
Mycoplasma (n = 85)	61%	28%	11%
Psittacosis (n = 12)	58%	42%	0%
Staphylococcal (n = 61)	36%	23%	41%

INVESTIGATIONS

Investigations are performed for a number of reasons and should be tailored to fit the individual clinical situation. Investigations are necessary to assess the severity and cause of the infection, to identify complications, and sometimes for epidemiological purposes.

General

The total white cell count is over $15.0 \times 10^6/dl$ in the majority of patients with pneumococcal pneumonia, with the differential showing a neutrophila (Table 4). However, in legionella pneumonia the total white cell count is usually not above $15.0 \times 10^6/dl$ and sometimes there is a lymphopenia. In patients with uncomplicated atypical or viral pneumonia a near normal white cell count is usual. A low or very high white cell count can be found in the very ill and is a poor prognostic sign. Marked red cell agglutination on the blood film should suggest the presence of cold agglutinins which are raised in over 50 per cent of cases with mycoplasma pneumonia. Cold agglutinin titres are normally measured in the laboratory, but a screening test can be useful at the bedside. A few drops of fresh blood are mixed with the same volume of sodium citrate (as found in a standard prothrombin tube) and this is left in the refrigerator for 2 to 3 min to reach about 4°C. Coarse agglutination of the blood, seen as the cooled tube is rotated, is usually associated with cold agglutinin titres greater than 1:64.

Abnormal liver function tests are common, and may be found in a third of patients with pneumococcal pneumonia and half with legionella pneumonia. Raised blood urea and creatinine, hyponatraemia, hypoalbuminaemia, proteinuria, and haematuria can be seen with any severe pneumonia (see later). Marked hypoalbuminaemia can develop quickly, probably due to a combination of sequestration of plasma protein into the lung and generalized increased vascular permeability from toxaemia.

Patients ill enough to require hospital admission will often be hypoxic, and sometimes acidotic. Hypercapnia denotes the onset of ventilatory failure. Signs of multisystem involvement are less usual with mycoplasma or viral pneumonia.

Specific

Many patients with mild pneumonia, treated successfully in the community, will not need any investigations, except for a chest radiograph after clinical recovery to confirm resolution. For patients who are ill enough to require hospital treatment, the aim is to identify the cause of the pneumonia and the severity of the infection as soon as possible. Blood, any pleural fluid, and sputum, if possible, should be collected for culture before antibiotics are started because a single dose can interfere with the culture of common pathogens such as *S. pneumoniae* and *H. influenzae*. However, antibiotic treatment should not be delayed if sputum cannot be obtained quickly, as a third of patients will not be able to produce sputum in the early stages.

Gram staining of sputum (and pleural fluid) sometimes gives a quick and accurate indication of the pathogen if predominant numbers of one pathogen are seen in a good sputum specimen. Although the specificity of the Gram stain is high, the sensitivity is low. Predominant numbers of Gram-positive diplococci on Gram stains are seen in only 10 to 20 per cent of patients with pneumococcal pneumonia. If more than 10 squamous epithelial cells are seen in each low-powered field, the specimen is probably of oropharyngeal origin and is of little use. Because the bacterial flora of sputum represents a mixture of organisms from the lower respiratory tract and those acquired during passage through the mouth, isolation of a pathogen may not reflect what is occurring in the lung itself. The specificity of the culture may be improved by washing or diluting the sputum. Even then sputum culture is a relatively insensitive method of diagnosis for bacterial pneumonia. Less than half of patients with untreated bacteraemic pneumococcal pneumonia have pneumococci isolated from their sputum. Isolation of a pathogen from blood (or pleural fluid) culture provides certain evidence of its importance and identifies those bacteraemic patients who have a worse prognosis.

The commonest practical problem is that over half the patients have received an antibiotic before hospital admission and this greatly reduces the usefulness of Gram stain and culture of secretions and body fluids. The detection of bacterial antigen can partially overcome this problem and is particularly helpful in pneumococcal infection (see Chapter 7.11.3).

The diagnosis of non-pneumococcal bacterial pneumonia raises similar problems to those encountered with pneumococcal pneumonia. Potential pathogens like staphylococci, meningococci, and streptococci can be part of the normal respiratory flora. *H. influenzae* can be cultured in mucoid sputum in over half of patients with chronic bronchitis. Over a quarter of patients in hospital may carry Gram-negative organisms in their upper respiratory tract, particularly if they are receiving broad-spectrum antibiotics. There are no tests available for detecting antigens from these other bacteria, and serological testing for bacterial precipitating antibodies is of no value in diagnosing acute infections.

The major limitation of diagnostic virology is the length of time required for isolating and identifying a particular virus. The direct fluorescent antibody staining technique for detecting viral antigens in respiratory secretions has been useful in the rapid diagnosis of respiratory syncytial virus bronchiolitis in children, producing a sensitivity of 90 per cent or over, and is being developed for other respiratory viruses, including influenza, parainfluenza types 1 and 3, and adenoviruses. Recently, similar techniques have been successfully used for detecting chlamydial antigens in respiratory secretions of patients with culture-proven *Chlamydia pneumoniae* pneumonia. Of the organisms causing 'atypical' pneumonia, only *M. pneumoniae* can be grown with any ease, although even here growth may take several weeks despite using a special diphasic medium.

To diagnose viral and atypical pneumonias by serological methods, blood should be collected early in the illness and again 10 to 14 days later or during convalescence. A fourfold or greater change in specific antibody titre is accepted as evidence of recent infection. Unfortunately, the result often arrives too late to influence the management of the patient. A single sample taken late in the illness showing a high titre does not distinguish between a recent or past infection. The detection of a raised specific IgM antibody by the indirect fluorescent antibody test can overcome this problem, and is also used for the early detection of *M. pneumoniae* infection.

The majority of cases of legionella pneumonia are diagnosed serologically by repeat indirect fluorescent antibody testing. Only about 10 to 15 per cent are identified in the acute phase of the illness by culture of the organism or by direct fluorescent antibody staining for organisms in lower respiratory secretions or lung biopsy material. About a third of cases will have detectable antibody levels (titres above 16) on admission, and this may be a pointer to the diagnosis in populations with a low background of seropositivity, such as in the United Kingdom. Diagnostic seroconversion can be very slow and a proportion of cases of legionella infection, proven by culture of the organism, never seroconvert. Detection of legionella antigen in concentrated urine has proved a valuable early diagnostic tool in some epidemic outbreaks and this technique should be more widely available for clinical use.

Invasive techniques for investigating pneumonia

Two problems inhibit further advances in sputum diagnosis. Contamination of sputum by oropharyngeal organisms has already been mentioned. In addition, about a quarter to a third of patients with pneumonia cannot produce sputum for testing. Therefore, various invasive techniques have been developed to overcome these problems. They are usually reserved for patients with severe infection. Close liaison between the clinicians and the microbiologist is essential at this stage so that the correct specimens are collected in the optimum manner and transported rapidly to the laboratory where they are processed immediately.

Induced sputum

Although not strictly 'invasive', induced sputum has proved valuable in experienced hands for the early diagnosis of infection, particularly pneumocytic pneumonia in AIDS patients. Inhalation of a 3 per cent saline mist from an ultrasonic nebulizer can induce coughing and good specimens of bronchoalveolar material.

Percutaneous lung aspiration

This technique was first used in 1920 to follow the clearance of pneumococci from the lungs of patients with lobar pneumonia. More recently it has been used extensively to investigate pneumonia in children in whom sputum is often not available and tracheal aspiration is difficult. The small samples of 'lung juice' obtained can be examined by Gram stain, culture, direct fluorescent antibody staining (e.g. for *L. pneumophila*), and countercurrent immunoelectrophoresis for bacterial antigen. Pneumothorax can occur in up to 10 per cent but the need for drainage is unusual; significant haemoptysis is rare. The use of slim 25-gauge needles reduces any risk of complications and the technique can be performed at the bedside. In one study from Barcelona in Spain, transthoracic needle aspiration produced a specificity of 100 per cent and a sensitivity of 57 per cent in 173 cases of community-acquired pneumonia. It is contraindicated in patients with assisted ventilation.

Bronchoscopy

Fibreoptic bronchoscopy will provide bronchial secretions, bronchoalveolar lavage fluid, and transbronchial biopsies from specified areas of the lung. Some contamination of equipment by passage through the nasopharynx is inevitable. Protected specimen brush catheters partially overcome this problem (Fig. 3). Bronchoscopy is rarely needed for patients with community-acquired pneumonia, except to exclude a bronchial obstruction, but is increasingly used for investigating nosocomial and ventilator associated pneumonia and pneumonia in the immunocompromised patient. Protected brush specimens cultured with a quantitative method produce the best results in ventilator-associated pneumonia. A high diagnostic yield is reported from bronchoalveolar lavage (Fig. 4) in patients with lung infections and AIDS, particularly from those with pneumocystis pneumonia.

Transtracheal aspiration

This technique, first described by Pecora in 1963, is rarely used now owing to the availability and acceptability of bronchoscopy. A needle is inserted through the cricothyroid membrane and a sterile catheter is passed through it towards the carina. Uncontaminated lower respiratory secretions can then be aspirated. Small quantities of sterile saline are sometimes injected first to obtain a better sample. The technique is useful for diagnosing anaerobic infection. Local neck emphysema and haemoptysis are not uncommon. Significant side-effects such as large bleeds and mediastinal emphysema are rare. Occasional deaths are reported, usually in patients with bleeding disorders. Often a saline injection with a small 21-gauge needle and syringe through the cricothyroid membrane (without recourse to catheters etc.) will be enough to produce a deep cough specimen of respiratory secretions, and this is a simple and safe technique.

Open-lung biopsy

This is certainly the most effective biopsy method for diagnosing the cause of both infection and non-infective lung shadowing, and acts as the 'gold standard'. A specific diagnosis can be made in over three-quarters of cases, although the risks of the procedure have to be weighed against the likelihood of discovering a diagnosis that would affect management. It is rarely used for investigating community-acquired pneumonia, but has a part to play in the investigation of lung shadowing in the immunocompromised host if bronchoscopic techniques have been unhelpful (see Chapter 7.17.3). The advent of video assisted thoracoscopic lung biopsy has reduced the morbidity of 'open' biopsy.

Radiographic features

The initial radiographic pattern is not particularly helpful in differentiating types of community-acquired pneumonia. Homogeneous lobar or

Fig. 3 Chest radiograph taken during a bronchoscopy in a patient with right lower lobe pneumonia. A protected specimen brush (*) has been extended deep into the lobe to obtain uncontaminated specimens for quantitative bacterial culture. (Reproduced from J. T. Macfarlane, R. G. Finch, and R. E. Cotton. (1992). *Colour Atlas of Respiratory Infections*. Chapman and Hall, London, with permission.)

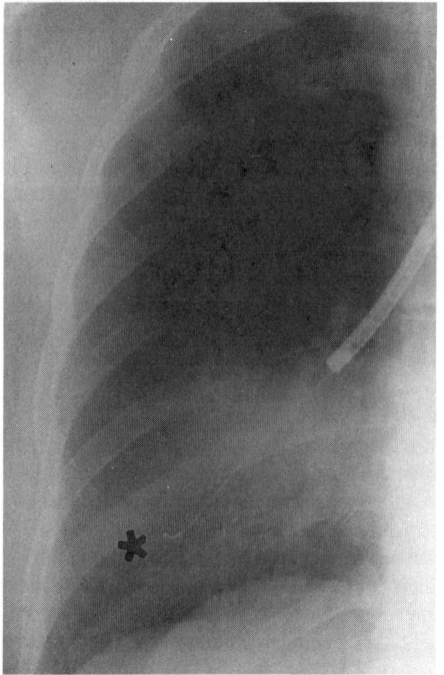

segmental shadows are more common than patchy shadows in bacterial pneumonia (Fig. 5), but they are also seen in over half the patients with atypical pneumonia. Multilobe involvement is common with severe infection. The lower lobes are most often affected in all types of pneumonia. Pleural effusions are seen in about a quarter of all cases, and more will be revealed by lateral decubitus films. Although some degree of pulmonary collapse should raise the possibility of an endobronchial obstruction (e.g. tumour, foreign body, mucus plug), it occurs in a quarter of otherwise uncomplicated cases of community-acquired pneumonia. Hilar lymphadenopathy is seen with mycoplasma pneumonia and occasionally in psittacosis. Lung cavitation is unusual except with staphylococcal and pneumococcal serotype 3 pneumonia or in immunosup-

Fig. 4 Chest radiograph demonstrating a bronchoalveolar lavage. Alveolar filling can be seen even with an injection of only 30 ml of radio-opaque fluid into a subsegment of the right middle lobe. (Reproduced from J. T. Macfarlane, R. G. Finch, and R. E. Cotton. (1992). *Colour Atlas of Respiratory Infections*. Chapman and Hall, London, with permission.)

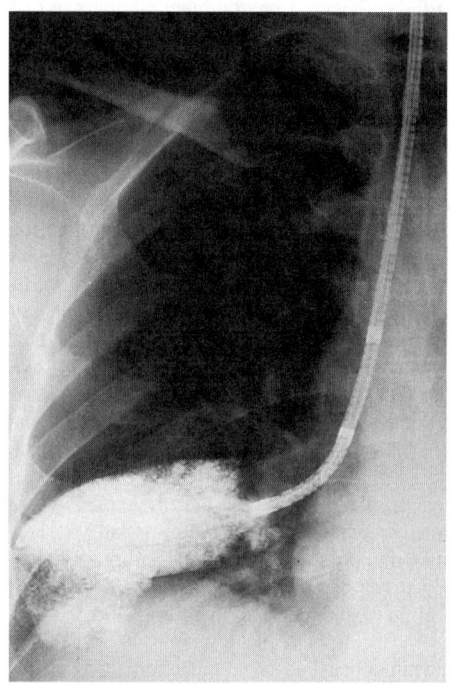

Fig. 5 Chest radiograph of a 54-year-old man with pneumococcal pneumonia demonstrating homogeneous segmental consolidation in the right upper lobe.

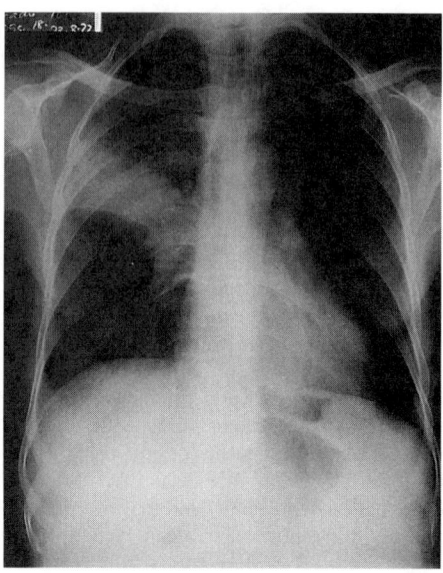

pressed patients. Pneumatoceles are only seen with staphylococcal infection (Fig. 6). An intense inflammatory and exudative response may produce a swollen lobe with a displaced interlobar fissure. This is said to be a feature of klebsiella pneumonia but is also seen with other severe infections.

The rate of radiographic resolution can be surprisingly slow, and lags considerably behind clinical recovery. It is related to the cause of the pneumonia, the age of the patient, and the presence of any underlying chronic lung disease (Fig. 7). Atypical pneumonias clear quickly. In the majority of cases radiographs return to normal within 2 months following mycoplasma pneumonia. At the other extreme, radiographs may not clear for several months after legionella and bacteraemic pneumococcal pneumonia.

DIFFERENTIAL DIAGNOSIS

When there is a classic history of fever, malaise, sweats, cough, discoloured sputum, pleural pain, and dyspnoea, together with the clinical and radiographic signs of lung consolidation, a diagnosis of pneumonia is usually obvious. The commonest diagnostic confusion is with pulmonary infarction or atypical pulmonary oedema. A source of pulmonary

Fig. 6 Lateral chest radiograph of a child with staphylococcal pneumonia revealing a tense pneumatocele (arrow) and surrounding consolidation in the apical segment of the left lower lobe.

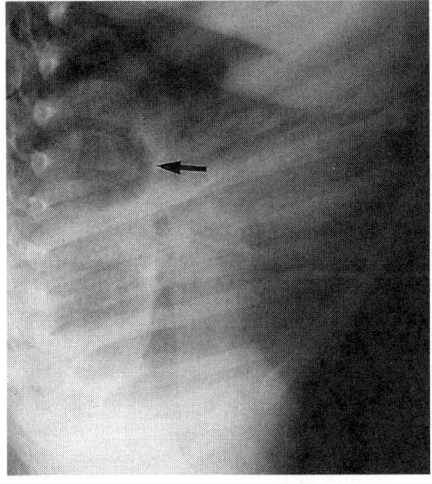

Fig. 7 Rate of radiographic clearance for different types of adult community acquired pneumonia. (Adapted from Macfarlane, J. T. *et al.* (1984). *Thorax*, **36**, 566–70, with permission of the editor of *Thorax*.)

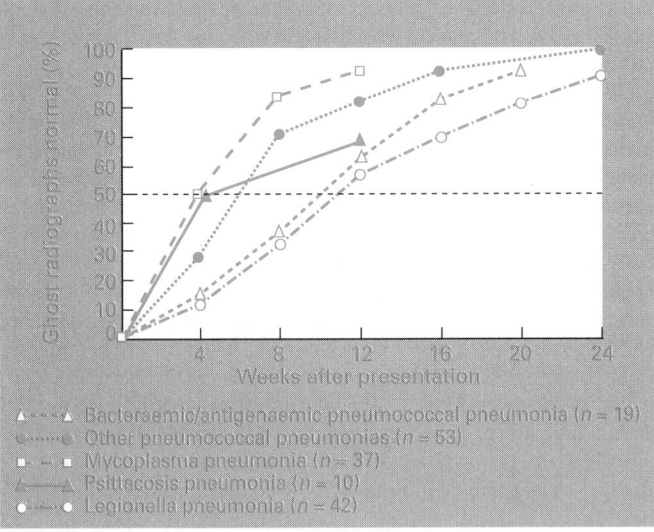

emboli or evidence of valvular disease or cardiac failure should be sought by physical examination. On occasions the distinction is very difficult, and treatment may have to be given for more than one condition until the true diagnosis becomes clearer. Less common conditions that enter the differential diagnosis include alveolitis, pulmonary eosinophilia, cryptogenic organizing pneumonitis, bronchoalveolar lung tumours, and more chronic lung conditions (Fig. 8). Subdiaphragmatic conditions such as subphrenic or hepatic abscess or acute pancreatitis may present like lower-lobe pneumonia, often with an accompanying pleural effusion. Ultrasound examination can be very helpful in such conditions.

SECONDARY PNEUMONIAS ACQUIRED IN THE COMMUNITY

Some circumstances require careful consideration in the context of community-acquired pneumonias because of their influence on clinical presentation, likely pathogens, and antimicrobial therapy. These include the occurrence of pneumonia during an influenza epidemic, pneumonia in patients with chronic lung disease, and pneumonia at extremes of age.

Bacterial pneumonia with influenza

Since influenza virus A was first isolated in 1933, a link between viral and subsequent bacterial infection has been recognized. Secondary bacterial pneumonia with *Strep. pneumoniae*, *Staph. aureus*, or *H. influenzae* is now the most common pulmonary complication of influenza. Rarely, the influenza virus itself causes pneumonia.

The pattern of bacterial infection varies. Necropsy studies have shown that the principal bacterial pathogen during the 1918–1919 influenza epidemic was *H. influenzae*, whereas during 1957 it was *Staph. aureus* and in 1969–1970 it was *Strep. pneumoniae*. Data from recent studies, where the relationship between influenza and bacterial superinfection was detailed, revealed *Strep. pneumoniae* in 34 cases, *H. influenzae* in seven cases, *Staph. aureus* in six cases, and others in six cases.

There are several reasons why viral infection may promote explosive bacterial superinfection. There is increased susceptibility of the respiratory tract to bacterial adherence and colonization which is most evident about a week after the onset of the viral infection. The ciliated epithelium of the bronchial tree is destroyed by virus invasion and therefore mucociliary clearance is reduced. There also appears to be suppression of the activity of the alveolar macrophages and reduction in lysozyme activity—other essential features of the lung defences.

Usually the patient experiences the typical symptoms of influenza, starts to improve, and then 3 to 7 days later suddenly deteriorates with rigors, chest pain, dyspnoea, and cough with discoloured or blood-stained sputum. In approximately a third of cases, the pulmonary symptoms blend with the influenza. Pregnant women and those with chronic cardiac or respiratory diseases are particularly at risk. Influenza virus and staphylococcal infections are often a lethal combination.

Fig. 8 This 72-year-old woman presented with a 4-week history of night sweats, anorexia, cough, and increased sputum production. The chest radiograph showed homogeneous shadowing of the right upper lobe and right lower lobe with air bronchograms. There was no improvement with antibiotics and a transbronchial lung biopsy demonstrated alveolar cell carcinoma.

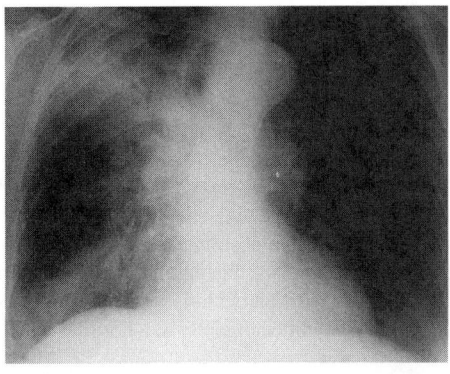

Complications vary with the nature of the bacterial organism (see Section 7), but overall prognosis is not good. The mortality of postinfluenza bacterial pneumonia remains high, at 20 to 25 per cent, even in young people, who were previously well.

Bacterial pneumonia in patients with pre-existing chronic obstructive lung disease

It is not easy without a chest radiograph to determine whether parenchymal lung infection is present in the chronic bronchitic or emphysematous patient suffering an acute infective exacerbation. Symptoms will resemble those described above for the acute bronchitic infection, although the addition of pleuritic chest pain suggests pneumonia as does a generally rather sick patient. New focal chest signs point to the presence of pneumonia.

Radiographic features are less likely to be a classic lobar consolidation than to reveal patchy infiltrates and peribronchial thickening. Emphysematous bullae may form cystic areas with surrounding consolidation, mimicking cavitation, and occasionally a cyst may partially fill with infected fluid.

Whilst Strep. pneumoniae, H. influenzae, and sometimes M. catarrhalis will still be important organisms in these pneumonic consolidations, consideration will also have to be given to staphylococci and Gram-negative enteric bacilli, including pseudomonas, particularly if the patients patient has associated bronchiectasis or has received repeated courses of antibiotics.

COMMUNITY-ACQUIRED PNEUMONIA AT EXTREMES OF AGE

The causes of pneumonia in the very young and the elderly show important differences. In neonates, infections are usually contracted from the mother's genital tract during delivery and include Staph. aureus, H. influenzae type B, streptococci, Gram-negative enteric bacilli, and Chlamydia trachomatis. In children under 2 years, the major respiratory pathogen is respiratory syncytial virus. At school age mycoplasma and pneumococcal infections are most usual, although H. influenzae infection is still occasionally seen.

Acute pneumonia in the elderly is common and carries a high mortality ranging up to 30 per cent. Reports from the United States record Strep. pneumoniae to be common, Staph. aureus to occur in up to 10 per cent of cases, and Gram-negative enteric bacilli to account for 6 to 36 per cent of infections, with the last of these being commoner in the debilitated elderly living in nursing homes. The occurrence of these pathogens in community-acquired bacterial pneumonias in the elderly can be partly explained by previous antibiotic exposure, ageing infection defences, and aspiration of oropharyngeal contents in debilitated patients.

In the United Kingdom, recent studies of the elderly admitted from their own homes have reported a pattern of pathogens very similar to that in younger adults, apart from a higher incidence of H. influenzae (usually associated with chronic lung disease).

Atypical infections are uncommon in the very young and the elderly, and usually occur in older children and adults of working age. Legionella pneumonia is mainly associated with adults in the working years.

MANAGEMENT OF COMMUNITY-ACQUIRED PNEUMONIAS

General measures

Patients with acute pneumonia should be in bed. Fever and pleuritic pain can often be relieved by regular analgesia. Adequate hydration is essential. For patients managed at home, the severity of the illness and the need for hospital admission should be assessed regularly (see discussion of prognostic factors below). On occasions this will be influenced by psychological and social factors. Pneumonia developing in someone with influenza or chickenpox is particularly worrying. Patients with severe pneumonia should be admitted urgently to a hospital which

has facilities for assisted ventilation. For patients ill enough to be in hospital, correction of fluid balance and hypoxia is very important. An arterial oxygen tension of 8 kPa or less on added inspired oxygen or rising arterial carbon dioxide is an indication of severe pneumonia, and assisted ventilation may well be required for advancing respiratory failure. This can be life-saving and should be started early. Therefore patients with severe pneumonia are best managed in an intensive care unit or similar high dependency area where they can be carefully monitored. Although the outlook of patients with pneumococcal and staphylococcal pneumonia who require assisted ventilation is poor, those with legionella infection, atypical pneumonia, and varicella pneumonia have a recovery rate of over 50 per cent. Chest physiotherapy and postural drainage are rarely helpful in the acute stage, and may exhaust a toxic and ill patient. When there is increased sputum production during recovery, physiotherapy can be useful. In patients with severe infection and those in whom recovery is slow and prolonged, adequate enteral or parenteral nutrition is important.

Specific measures
Antibiotics

The cause of the pneumonia is not usually known when the patient is first seen and therefore lists of pathogens matched to ideal antibiotics are of little help. In practice, a 'best guess' antibiotic choice has to be made, depending on the type of patient, severity of infection, and any aetiological clues from the clinical picture. The small number of likely causes of community-acquired pneumonia makes this relatively easy.

Mild or moderate pneumonia. In most previously fit patients with mild pneumonia the most likely infecting agent is the pneumococcus or, less commonly, an atypical organism. Therefore the choice lies between a β-lactam antibiotic, such as a penicillin, and erythromycin. An aminopenicillin such as oral amoxicillin is well tolerated, cheap, and effective. Erythromycin is appropriate for penicillin-allergic individuals or during a mycoplasma epidemic or if an atypical infection is suspected. Gastrointestinal intolerance is less of a problem with the newer macrolides. Tetracycline, although helpful for atypical organisms, is often no longer effective for the pneumococcus.

In those with chronic lung disease an antibiotic which is also effective against H. influenzae is required. Amoxicillin is usually suitable. However, around 10 per cent of H. influenzae are ampicillin resistant in the United Kingdom, with higher figures being reported from some countries such as Spain and some parts of the United States. If the patient has failed to respond to amoxicillin or is moderately ill, β-lactamase-stable alternatives include co-amoxiclav, co-trimoxazole (but beware of skin rashes and blood dyscrasias in the elderly), newer generation cephalosporins, and chloramphenicol. Currently available quinolones, such as ciprofloxacin, are highly effective against H. influenzae, M. catarrhalis, and some atypical pathogens, but their expense and questionable activity against the pneumococcus argues against their routine use as first line agents.

Severe pneumonia. The physician needs to be on the alert for any signs of deterioration (see discussion of prognostic factors below). Severe pneumonia can evolve rapidly even in previously fit people, and the mortality remains high despite apparently effective antibiotics. Antibiotics should be given parenterally without delay, and must cover all likely pathogens. Any antibiotic must provide effective cover against pneumococcal infection. Penicillin-resistant pneumococci are a significant problem in only a few countries so far but this worrying situation is changing progressively. Other likely causes of severe community-acquired pneumonia include L. pneumophila, Staph. aureus (particularly during influenza epidemics), H. influenzae (particularly in those with chronic lung disease), and occasionally atypical and varicella pneumonias (Table 2). High doses of intravenous ampicillin (500 mg–1 g 6 hourly) or cefuroxime (750 mg–1.5 g 8 hourly) together with erythromycin (as erythromycin lactobionate 500–1000 mg 6 hourly) provide good initial cover for all these pathogens. Patients allergic to penicillins can be given erythromycin alone in high doses or combined (cautiously) with a cephalosporin such as cefuroxime which has the advantage of being β-lactamase stable. Phlebitis at the cannula site with intravenous erythromycin can be reduced by a slow dilute infusion. During a period of influenza, or where there is a chance of secondary staphylococcal pneumonia, flucloxacillin should be used as well. The antibiotics are adjusted appropriately as soon as investigations identify a specific pathogen.

Duration of antibiotic therapy

Patients with uncomplicated pneumonia are usually treated with anti-biotics for 7 to 10 days. This may be unnecessarily long in some cases. Studies in Africa have shown equally good results when treating pneumonia for 1, 3, and 7 days. The duration of therapy for those with more severe pneumonia is judged on clinical response. In the presence of lung cavitation, treatment may be needed for 3 to 4 weeks.

Identifying prognostic factors

Prognosis is related to the pathogen, the host, and the interplay between the two. A positive blood culture is a bad prognostic sign in bacterial pneumonias; the mortality of bacteraemic pneumococcal pneumonia is 25 to 33 per cent compared with 5 per cent for non-bacteraemic cases. There were around 2500 reported deaths for pneumococcal pneumonia in England and Wales in 1991, but many were probably not reported. Pulmonary infections with *Staph. aureus*, *H. influenzae*, or Gram-negative bacilli carry a poor prognosis. However, patients with atypical pneumonia generally do well. The mortality of community-acquired legionella pneumonia is 5 to 15 per cent.

Mortality and morbidity rise with increasing age of the patient and the presence of coexisting chronic illness (such as cardiac or respiratory disease or diabetes). Other factors associated with a poor prognosis for pneumonia are summarized in Table 5 and can be used for early identification of those with severe disease.

Failure to improve

The majority of patients will improve quickly a few days after starting treatment. If recovery is unsatisfactory the causes shown in Table 6 should be considered.

Intrathoracic complications

Pleural effusions are the commonest intrathoracic complication and a sample should always be aspirated to exclude an empyema. Usually these effusions are clear straw-coloured sympathetic exudates with a high protein content and sparse neutrophils, and are sterile. The fluid can be tested for bacterial antigen. Empyemas occur in up to 5 per cent of pneumonias, although the incidence is higher with some pathogens such as *Staph. aureus*, streptococci, and anaerobes.

Following a severe pneumonia, some degree of pulmonary fibrosis may occur with a resulting restrictive lung defect. Persistent intrapulmonary streaky opacities may be seen on the chest radiograph. Abnormalities in lung function and tracheobronchial clearance have been reported many months after apparent recovery from mycoplasma pneumonia.

Prevention of pneumonia

Better housing and working conditions and better community health have contributed greatly to the reduced incidence of community-acquired pneumonia.

Vaccination has been helpful in specific instances and may have a greater role to play. Post-measles pneumonia, a common occurrence in children in developing countries, can be reduced by a measles vaccination campaign, and pertussis immunization reduces the frequency of respiratory complications of whooping cough. Pneumococcal vaccination has been shown to be effective in reducing serious pneumococcal

Table 5 *Simple clinical features associated with severe pneumonia*

Clinical features	Laboratory features
Confusion*	Blood urea > 7 mmol/l*
Respiratory rate < 30/ min*	White cell count < 4 × 10⁹/l or > 30 × 10⁹/l
Diastolic blood pressure < 60 mmHg*	Arterial oxygen < 8 kPa
New atrial fibrillation	Serum albumin < 25 g/l Multilobe involvement on chest radiograph

*Three recent studies have found a large increase in chance of death if at least two of these features are present.

pneumonia. It is recommended in patients who are particularly liable to severe pneumococcal infection, such as those with chronic respiratory and cardiac disease or sickle-cell disease, and in those due to have a planned splenectomy. Some authorities recommend its use in all adults over the age of 60 years. Influenza vaccination in the autumn gives some protection to patients who are debilitated and in whom an attack of influenza or its complications could be serious.

Nosocomial pneumonia

INTRODUCTION

Nosocomial pneumonia is a new episode of pneumonia developing more than 48 h after a patient has entered hospital for whatever reason. The infection is usually identified by the development of fever, purulent respiratory secretions, elevated white cell count, and a new pulmonary infiltrate on the chest radiograph. Nosocomial respiratory infections have been estimated to occur in 0.5 to 5 per cent of patients in hospital and to rank third behind urinary infections and wound infections in the frequency of hospital-acquired infections.

PATHOGENESIS

The infection usually arises from aspiration of nasopharyngeal contents, inhalation of bacteria from contaminated equipment, or, rarely, by haematogenous spread.

Some aspiration of nasopharyngeal secretions is common even in healthy people, particularly during sleep. The normal lung copes easily with this, both because the bacteria are relatively non-pathogenic and because the local pulmonary defences are working normally. However, colonization of the nasopharynx with Gram-negative bacilli occurs in 30 to 40 per cent of patients in hospital. The frequency can be even higher in patients receiving broad-spectrum antibiotics or those who are seriously ill. These bacilli arise by the direct contamination of the nasopharynx from the hospital environment and from the patient's own gastrointestinal tract.

Patients who are ill, bed-bound, have impaired consciousness from their illness or from drugs, or who have neurological disease will be more likely to aspirate such pathogens. Reduced ability to clear bronchial secretions after a general anaesthetic and impaired coughing after thoracic or abdominal surgery are further risk factors, and occasionally impaired general antimicrobial defences contribute to the development of these infections. The presence of malignancy and the prior use of antibiotics, steroids, or cytotoxic drugs increase the risk of nosocomial pneumonia.

The risk of postoperative pneumonia is associated with increasing age, smoking habit, obesity, the presence of chronic illness, long preoperative stay, prolonged anaesthesia, use of intubation, and thoracic and upper abdominal operations.

Inhalation of bacteria from contaminated respiratory equipment such

Table 6 *Factors to consider when a patient with pneumonia is responding poorly to initial therapy*

Factor	Action
Improvement expected too soon	Continue—review again (improvement slow in elderly and debilitated)
Diagnosis of pneumonia wrong (pulmonary infarction/oedema?)	Review history, examination, and data
Organism resistant to antibiotic/unexpected organism involved	Review history: travel abroad? avian contact?
	Review microbiological data
	Consider alternative or invasive investigations
Complicating pulmonary disease (e.g. bronchial obstruction, bronchiectasis)	Review chest radiograph; consider bronchoscopy
Local intrathoracic complications (e.g. empyema, lung abscess)	Repeat chest radiograph
	Aspirate any pleural fluid
Secondary complications (e.g. deep venous thrombosis, intravenous cannula infection)	Detailed clinical examination
Metastatic infective complication (e.g. arthritis, endocarditis, meningitis)	Detailed clinical examination
General factors (e.g. dehydration, hypoxia)	Treat appropriately
Allergic reaction to antibiotic (usually after several days therapy)	Take allergic history; look for rash; consider stopping/changing antibiotic

as ventilators, nebulizers, intubation and suction equipment, humidifiers, and nasogastric tubes is a particular problem in ventilated patients. Spread of pathogens via the hands of the personnel must be remembered.

Pneumonia caused by haematogenous spread of infection from a distant site is uncommon, but may arise after intra-abdominal infection or as a result of infected pulmonary emboli. Intravenous cannulae left *in situ* for long periods are a potential source of bloodstream infection.

PATHOGENS IMPLICATED

The spectrum of pathogens encountered in nosocomial pneumonia is much wider and more varied than that for community-acquired pneumonia. Gram-negative bacilli comprise about half of all isolates and Gram-positive bacteria, of which *Staph. aureus* is the commonest, less than a quarter. Specific circumstances may make one particular infection more likely. Patients who develop pneumonia shortly after an elective operation are usually infected by their own community-acquired respiratory flora such as *Strep. pneumoniae* and *H. influenzae*, particularly in the presence of chronic lung disease. Respiratory equipment harbours pseudomonas, and klebsiella, the presence of bowel or urinary tract infection favours *Escherichia coli* and proteus-type organisms, *Serratia marcescens* can survive in certain disinfectant fluids, and any situation which encourages aspiration from the oropharynx can produce a pneumonia due to klebsiella, pseudomonas, or a whole range of anaerobes including Gram-negative bacilli of bacteroides and fusobacterium species, Gram-positive cocci, and various Gram-positive clostridial species. The potential list of pathogens causing nosocomial pneumonia in the immunocompromised host is even more varied (see Chapter 7.17.3). Outbreaks of nosocomial legionella infection have been caused by colonization of hospital heating and water systems. Mists generated by contaminated cooling towers and ward showers have also been implicated. Debilitated and immunosuppressed patients are most at risk.

DIAGNOSIS

The diagnosis of a pneumonia is not usually difficult provided that the patient is carefully examined. Sometimes the diagnosis will only be suspected after a chest radiograph is performed in a patient who has deteriorated for no obvious cause.

Identifying the pathogen is more difficult. Colonization of the oropharynx by a variety of hospital-acquired pathogens means that sputum examination is generally unhelpful. If blood, sputum, or pleural fluid cultures are negative, invasive techniques may be required to obtain lower respiratory secretions (see above). Bronchoscopy provides a convenient way of obtaining samples in ventilated patients. Serological tests for legionella infection should be considered.

TREATMENT

A mild early postoperative pneumonia in a previously fit person can usually be treated like a community-acquired infection. Because of the variety of potential pathogens in other types of nosocomial pneumonia, it is advisable to use broad-spectrum or combination antibiotics as initial therapy, pending the results of tests. These may include a broad-spectrum third-generation cephalosporin such as cefotaxime with or without an aminoglycoside such as gentamicin. If there is a high probability of pseudomonas infection, an appropriate penicillin derivative such as azlocillin or ticarcillin or a cephalosporin such as ceftazidime should be used. For suspected anaerobic infection, penicillin and metronidazole, or clindamycin, will have advantages. Newer antibiotics such as the quinolones are likely to have an expanding role in nosocomial infections. Physiotherapy aids the clearance of infected secretions and, used postoperatively, may help to prevent nosocomial pneumonia. Despite therapy the mortality is high, ranging from 25 to 50 per cent, largely dictated by the underlying condition of the patient, and in survivors there is a considerable prolongation of hospital stay.

PREVENTION

The frequency of nosocomial respiratory infection can be reduced by such measures as prevention of smoking preoperatively, early postoperative mobilization, hospital staff hygiene, scrupulous care of respiratory equipment, and infection control in high risk areas such as intensive care units. Selective decontaminations of the gastrointestinal tract and direct applications of antimicrobial agents to the respiratory tract have been used with some success to prevent Gram-negative colonization of the respiratory tract and pneumonia in the intensive care unit.

Aspiration and anaerobic pneumonia

The most frequent conditions associated with aspiration pneumonia are impaired consciousness and dysphagia. The resulting insult to the lung can involve gastric acid, particulate matter, and contamination of the lower respiratory tract with a complex bacterial flora.

Anaerobes from the oropharynx and teeth crevices usually predominate in community cases, and these are mostly penicillin sensitive. In contrast, in hospital-acquired infections aerobic bacteria, particularly Gram-negative enterobacteriaceae and *Pseudomonas aeruginosa* related to nasopharyngeal colonization, become increasingly important.

Anaerobic infection in the lung is usually caused by two or more bacteria acting synergistically and result broadly in four syndromes including anaerobic bacterial pneumonia, necrotizing pneumonia (Fig. 9), lung abscess, and empyema.

The diagnosis of anaerobic infection is difficult, but there should be a clue from likely predisposing factors such as poor dental hygiene, aspiration, or impaired consciousness. Foul smelling and purulent sputum appears only once necrosis occurs, when multiple cavities will be seen on the chest radiograph. The presence of multiple Gram-positive cocci and Gram-negative bacilli in the sputum that are negative on aerobic culture is suggestive.

A parenteral penicillin with or without metronidazole, or clindamycin, is appropriate for community-acquired cases. Gram-negative bacillary cover obtained by adding a third-generation cephalosporin, an aminoglycoside, or a quinolone is necessary for hospital-acquired cases. Quinolones alone have no anaerobic activity. Prolonged therapy is usually necessary.

Geographically restricted pneumonia

A number of respiratory infections are geographically restricted to the tropics and subtropics, or in the case of some mycoses to the Americas, and will only be seen in other parts of the world as a result of travel. The worldwide panic about the potential spread of infection by air travellers following the outbreak of pneumonic plague in India in 1994 is a graphic example of a potential problem.

Examples of bacterial disorders which can involve the lung include tularaemia, typhoid pneumonia, glanders, melioidosis, pulmonary anthrax, and brucellosis. Paragonimiasis is an example of a helminthic respiratory pathogen which is largely limited to the Far East and Indian subcontinent.

A number of fungal diseases are geographically restricted. Amongst these, the dimorphic fungi causing histoplasmosis (mainly found around the Ohio and Mississippi river basins of North America), blastomycosis (south and east central United States), coccidioidomycosis (southwestern United States and central America), and paracoccidioidomycosis (South America) present an interesting spectrum of disease in which the lung may or may not be the primary target. Cryptococcosis, which is most prevalent in the United States and Australia, can affect normal people but is increasingly recognized in those with impaired immunity.

Details of all these pathogens are given elsewhere in this textbook.

Recurrent pneumonia

In patients with a history of three or more episodes of pneumonia, several possibilities need to be considered.

LOCALIZED RESPIRATORY DISEASE

Recurrent pneumonia in the same part of the lung raises the possibility of a bronchial or pulmonary abnormality. Localized bronchiectasis or bronchial obstruction are the commonest reasons. Obstructions may be intraluminal (e.g. foreign body), intramural (e.g. bronchial stenosis, adenoma, or carcinoma), or due to compression from outside (e.g. by lymph nodes). Intrapulmonary sequestration may present as recurrent basal pneumonia. This is a development abnormality where a portion of the lung has an arterial supply from the systemic circulation and little or no normal bronchial architecture. The disorder may be discovered by chance on a radiograph or because of recurrent infection in early adult life.

GENERALIZED RESPIRATORY DISEASE

When pneumonia recurs in different sites, a more generalized disorder is likely. The commonest is chronic obstructive lung disease, perhaps with some bronchiectasis. Rarely, the problem is one of impaired pulmonary defences as in the immotile cilia syndrome. Chronic sinusitis can lead to recurrent lower respiratory infections due to aspiration of infected material.

NON-RESPIRATORY PROBLEM

Aspiration of pharyngeal or oesophageal contents may be caused by neuromuscular conditions such as muscular dystrophy, motor neurone disease, multiple sclerosis, strokes, or disorders of oesophageal motility in achalasia and scleroderma. Rarely, pharyngeal diverticulae, tracheo-oesophageal fistula, or gastro-oesophageal reflux can be implicated.

Alcoholics, drug abusers, and epileptics are liable to recurrent aspiration and anaerobic pneumonia during episodes of depressed consciousness.

Immune deficiency states are an uncommon cause of recurrent pneumonia, but their recognition is important because of the availability of replacement therapy in antibody-deficient syndromes.

REFERENCES

American Thoracic Society. (1993). Guidelines for the initial management of adults with community acquired pneumonia. *American Reviews of Respiratory Disease*, **148**, 1418–26.

Anon. (1994). Lower respiratory tract infections. *Medical Record Bulletin* **5**, 5–8.

Ausina, V. (1989). Rapid laboratory diagnostic methods in respiratory infections. *Current Opinion in Infectious Diseases*, **2**, 541–6.

British Thoracic Society, Public Health Laboratory Service. (1987). Community acquired pneumonia in adults in British hospitals in 1982–83: a survey of aetiology, mortality, prognostic factors and outcome. *Quarterly Journal of Medicine*, **239**, 195–200.

British Thoracic Society. (1993). Guidelines for the management of community acquired pneumonia in adults admitted to hospital. *British Journal of Hospital Medicine*, **49**, 346–50.

Glynn, J.R. and Jones, A.C. (1990). Atypical respiratory infections, including *Chlamydia TWAR* infection and legionella infection. *Current Opinion in Infectious Diseases*, **3**, 169–75.

Kauffman, R.S. (1988). Viral respiratory infections. *Current Opinion in Infectious Diseases*, **1**, 575–9.

Fig. 9 Chest radiograph of a 27-year-old alcoholic admitted with a cavitating right upper lobe pneumonia. Pus aspirated at bronchoscopy from the right upper lobe grew mixed anaerobic bacteria and he improved with a month of clindamycin therapy.

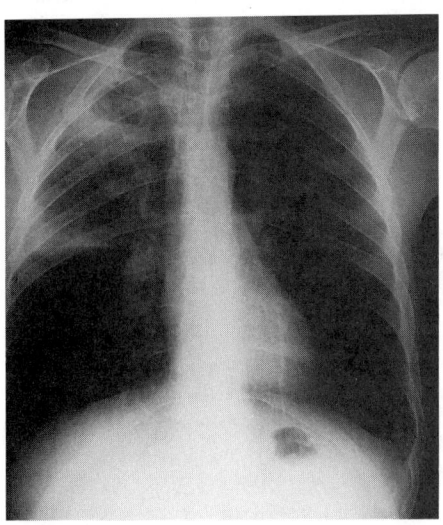

Macfarlane, J.T. (1991). Community acquired pneumonia. In: *Recent Advances in Respiratory Medicine*, Vol. 5, (ed D M Mitchell), Chapter 7, pp. 109–24. Churchill Livingstone, London.

Macfarlane, J.T. (1994). An overview of community acquired pneumonia with lessons learned from the British Thoracic Society Study. *Seminars in Respiratory Infections*, **9**, 152–64.

Macfarlane, J.T., Colville, A., Guion, A., Macfarlane, R.M., and Rose, D.H. (1993). Prospective study of aetiology and outcome of adult lower respiratory tract infections in the community. *Lancet*, **341**, 511–14.

Manresa, F. (1989). Rapid clinical diagnostic methods in respiratory infections. *Current Opinion in Infectious Diseases*, **2**, 536–40.

Marrie, T.J. (ed.) (1994). Community acquired pneumonia. *Seminars in Respiratory Infections*, **9**, 129–219.

Marrie, T.J., Durant, H., and Yates, L. (1989). Community acquired pneumonia requiring hospitalisation: 5 years prospective study. *Reviews of Infectious Diseases*, **11**, 586–99.

Noah, N.D. (1989). Cyclical patterns and predictability in infection. *Epidemiology and Infection*, **102**, 175–90.

Niederman, M.S., Sarosi, G.A., and Glassroth, J. (1994). *Respiratory infections. A scientific basis for management*. W.B. Saunders, Philadelphia.

Pennington, J.E. (ed) (1989). *Respiratory infections: diagnosis and management*. (2nd edn.) Raven Press, New York.

Santoro, J. (1984). Nosocomial respiratory tract infections. In: *The pneumonias* (ed M.E. Levison). John Wright, Boston, MA, pp. 182–96.

Sorensen, J., Forsberg, P., Hakanson, E. *et al.* (1989). A new diagnostic approach to the patient with severe pneumonia. *Scandinavian Journal of Infectious Diseases*, **21**, 33–41.

Torres, A. (1991). Accuracy of diagnostic tools for the management of nosocomial respiratory infections in mechanically ventilated patients. *European Respiratory Journal*, **4**, 1010–19.

Verghese, A., and Berk, S.L. (1983). Bacterial pneumonia in the elderly. *Medicine (Baltimore)*, **62**, 271–85.

Woodhead, M.A. (1992). Management of pneumonia. *Respiratory Medicine*, **86**, 459–69.

17.7.3 Suppurative pulmonary and pleural infections

J. M. HOPKIN

Lung abscess

Lung abscess describes suppurative infection with necrosis of lung which is seen typically as a cavitating, usually rounded, pneumonic opacity on the chest radiograph. The underlying causes are listed in Table 1.

The commonest cause is pulmonary aspiration of debris or fluid, with anaerobic bacterial contamination. Oropharyngeal secretions may contain up to 10^8 anaerobes per millilitre even in health, and higher concentrations are present with oropharyngeal sepsis. Normal individuals aspirate to some small extent during sleep, but this is cleared by the mucociliary escalator and coughing. These defences can be overwhelmed during spells of impaired consciousness, as in general anaesthesia, alcoholism, drug overdosage, epilepsy, or cerebrovascular accident. The incidence of lung abscess has significantly diminished following increased standards of anaesthesia and postoperative care. Other risk factors include oropharyngeal or periodontal sepsis. The dominant organisms are anaerobes, including fusiforms, *Bacterioides* species, and anaerobic cocci. In hospital, colonization of the mouth and upper airways by Gram-negative bacteria and staphylococci may make these organisms important. Aspiration lung abscesses occur at typical sites, influenced by gravity and bronchial geometry. Most form in the right lung which continues in a more direct line from the trachea than the left. Aspiration in the supine position leads to disease in the apical segment of the lower lobe or posterior segment of the upper lobe.

Bronchial obstruction due to bronchial carcinoma and leading to infection of retained sputum is an increasingly common cause of lung abscess. Foreign body is an important cause in childhood. One or more lung abscesses may result from vascular embolization of infected material to the lung as in septicaemias of diverse origin, right-sided endocarditis, infected intracours cannulae, and 'mainline' drug abuse. The organisms implicated include *Staphylococcus aureus* and *Streptococcus milleri*. Extension of a subphrenic abscess or hepatic amoebic abscess may lead to formation of a secondary abscess in the right lower lobe. Necrosis of the lung can occur as a complication of severe pneumonia without significant aspiration or obstruction, (e.g. *Staph. aureus* and *Klebsiella pneumoniae*).

Progression across interlobar fissures and into the pleural space to produce a secondary empyema can occur. The cavity of the abscess is composed of debris, pus cells, and organisms with a wall of granulation tissue with fibrosis. Nearby pulmonary arteries may show marked inflammation and minimal fibrosis.

CLINICAL FEATURES

The illness generally begins with shivers, fever, cough, and pleuritic chest pain. At some stage, not usually earlier than a week, the abscess discharges into a bronchus resulting in large amounts of bloodstained purulent sputum. The patient appears toxic and febrile. There may be only a local area of crepitation, rarely progressing to so-called 'amphoric' breathing. Finger clubbing can develop rapidly. Empyema ensues in 20 to 30 per cent.

A chronic course is well recognized in which less severe symptoms progress over weeks or months, punctuated with brief improvements following short courses of antibiotics when the diagnosis has not been suspected.

When one or more lung abscesses are secondary to a bacteraemic or septicaemic illness, the clinical picture may be dominated by the latter.

DIAGNOSIS

When purulent sputum or fever imply infection, the diagnosis of abscess is suggested by the radiographic appearances of a pneumonic opacity

Table 1 *Causes of lung abscess*

Condition	Micro-organisms
Pulmonary aspiration	Often anaerobes, *Actinomyces* species
Bronchial obstruction	Mixed organisms
Bacteraemia/septicaemia	*Staphylococcus aureus*, *Streptococcus milleri*, others
Spread from subphrenic or hepatic abscess	Coliforms, *Streptococcus faecalis*, *Amoeba histolytica*
Primary infection with cavitation	*Mycobacterium tuberculosis*
	Klebsiella pneumoniae, *Nocardia asteroides*
Immunosuppression (AIDS, leukaemia, chronic granulomatous disease)	Unusual organisms can be encountered, e.g. *Rhodococcus equi*, *Lactobacillus casei*

with a cavity in which a fluid level may be seen. An abscess in the apical segment of the lower suggests or the posterior segment of the upper lobe raises the possibility of aspiration (Fig. 1). At other sites the possibility of an obstructing bronchial carcinoma has to be considered and bronchoscopy performed. Lung abscess in the right lower zone may be due to spread from a subphrenic or hepatic abscess. Multiple abscesses suggest a bloodborne source of infection.

The differential diagnosis for a solitary cavitated lesion includes tuberculosis, fungal infection such as coccidioidomycosis, a cavitating squamous-cell carcinoma, pulmonary infarct, and pulmonary vasculitis.

Blood cultures should be taken. Sputum should be examined by microscopy and culture for bacteria including anaerobes, mycobacteria, and fungi. Fibreoptic bronchoscopy is valuable in excluding bronchial obstruction, and may be useful in providing deep specimens for accurate microbiological assessment (Fig. 1) particularly in the immunosuppressed (Table 1).

MANAGEMENT

The most important aspect of treatment is effective antimicrobial therapy. The organisms in aspirational disease are generally anaerobes, and unless aerobic Gram-negative organisms or staphylococci are recovered from early cultures, treatment should be based on benzylpenicillin, 2–3 MU four times daily initially, changing to oral therapy once there has been clinical improvement and resolution of fever. Treatment in general should be continued for 4 to 6 weeks. When there are laboratory or clinical doubts about the sensitivity of the anaerobe to penicillin, addition of metronidazole is appropriate. Postural drainage with vigorous percussion aids the clearance of pus. Ultimately, recovery occurs in 70 to 80 per cent.

If there is failure to resolve, bronchoscopy to allow the clearance of pus from the relevant bronchus and assessment of malignant and other microbiological possibilities (Table 1) is required before considering surgical resection. The presence of a carcinoma requires definitive management in its own right; an accompanying distal abscess is not a contraindication to surgery. The presence of an obstructing carcinoma makes abscess resolution by medical means less likely, and so encourages surgical intervention depending on the general state of the patient and the staging of the tumour.

In single or multiple lung abscesses secondary to bacteraemia or septicaemia the antibiotics of choice should be dictated by blood culture results, but in practice a combination of antibiotics is given parenterally to cover a broad spectrum of bacteria.

Empyema

Empyema describes a purulent pleural effusion; the excess of white cells present denotes active intrapleural infection. A number of underlying causes are recognized (Table 2).

Empyema usually follows a pulmonary infection in the form of pneumonia, lung abscess or bronchiectasis, but may occur after septicaemia, thoracic surgery, or penetrating chest wounds, or following transdiaphragmatic extension from a subphrenic or hepatic abscess. Tuberculous empyema, once a complication of advanced pulmonary disease and of artificial pneumothorax, is now uncommon in developed countries. Lowered resistance to infection, which is multifactorial in origin and which occurs in chronic disorders such as rheumatoid disease, results in an increased risk of empyema.

Infection in the pleural space results in the production of an inflammatory exudate with varying numbers of pus cells and, depending on the organism involved, the production of fibrinous adhesions between visceral and parietal pleura which may cause loculation of the fluid. The presence of a bronchopleural fistula will result in a pyopneumothorax. Failure to resolve rapidly results in the sequential deposition of layers of fibrin with trapped cellular debris on both pleural surfaces, particu-

Fig. 1 Chest radiographs (posteroanterior and right lateral) of a 50-year-old man with treated acute myeloid leukaemia, cough, and unremitting fever, showing an abscess in the right upper lobe. Microbiology on sputum was non-contributory, but specimens taken at bronchoscopy showed numerous Gram-negative rods which were found to be the anaerobe *Bacteroides bivius* on culture. An excellent clinical and radiological outcome followed treatment with metronidazole.

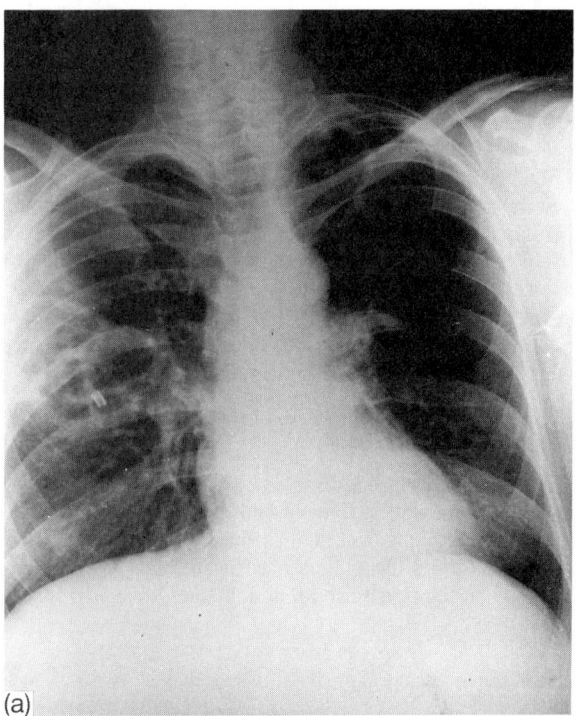
(a)

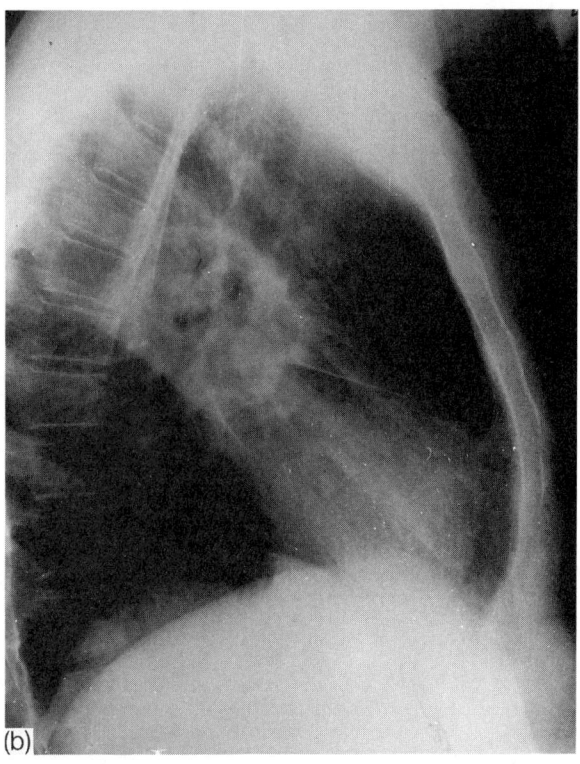
(b)

Table 2 *Causes of empyema*

Underlying condition	Micro-organism
Acute pneumonia	*Streptococcus pneumoniae*, others
Bronchiectasis, lung abscess	Mixed organisms, *Actinomyces* species
Post-thoracic surgery	Various organisms including late *Aspergillus fumigatus* infection
Bronchial obstruction, e.g. carcinoma	Mixed organisms
Penetrating injury	Various organisms including *Clostridium welchii*
Oesophageal perforation	Mixed organisms
Debility, e.g. rheumatoid disease	Mixed organisms
Spread from subphrenic abscess	Coliforms, *Streptococcus faecalis*, *Amoeba histolytica*
Primary infection	*Mycobacterium tuberculosis*, *Nocardia asteroides*

larly the parietal. Progressive fibrosis leads to markedly impaired pulmonary expansion and chest wall deformity.

The organisms implicated depend on the underlying cause of the empyema. Following simple pneumonia, a single organism (e.g. *Streptococcus pneumoniae*) may dominate. Mixed growths are common otherwise. Following extension from a subphrenic abscess, faecal organisms are likely to be present. Spread from an hepatic abscess may be due to amoebic disease (Chapter 7.13.1). *Aspergillus fumigatus* may produce an empyema years after surgery or artificial pneumothorax or pneumonectomy. Overall, the organisms most frequently implicated have been anaerobes, staphylococci, and Gram-negative organisms.

CLINICAL FEATURES AND DIAGNOSIS

Empyema occurring as an acute disorder complicating the course of pneumonia generally presents as failure of this pneumonia to resolve or as a recurrence of symptoms and signs some days after an apparent recovery. Clinical features include malaise, fevers, and pleuritic pain. Leucocytosis may be found and careful examination reveals an area of stony dullness.

Chronic empyema usually results from failure to diagnose or treat adequately an acute empyema, but may arise from chronic infection, as in tuberculosis, or from an underlying carcinoma or chronic pulmonary sepsis. Chronic empyema may result from retention of an intrapleural foreign body following surgery or trauma. The features of chronic empyema are continuing malaise, pain, sometimes purulent sputum and progression to normochromic anaemia, weight loss, finger clubbing, and chest wall deformity.

The chest radiograph shows signs of effusion (which might be loculated) or a pleural mass (Fig. 2). The presence of a fluid level implies a leak of air from a previous pleural aspiration, a bronchopleural fistula, or, more rarely, the presence of gas-forming organisms (e.g. *Clostridium welchii* in post-traumatic empyema). The development of bronchopleural fistula often leads to a foul odour on coughing or to the expectoration of large amounts of purulent sputum. The diagnosis of empyema is confirmed by the demonstration of purulent fluid on pleural aspiration; a wide-bore needle is used to ensure extraction of thick pus.

The fluid aspirated needs careful microscopy and culture for aerobic and anaerobic bacteria, together with studies for tuberculosis and fungi. In tuberculous empyema, the organism is usually visible on Ziehl–Neel-

Fig. 2 Chest radiographs taken before and after treatment of a 51-year-old man with a chronic empyema and associated glomerulonephritis with renal impairment and the nephrotic syndrome. Microbiology on the pleural pus produced a growth of the Gram-negative *Morganella morgani*. Successful treatment of the empyema with surgery and appropriate systemic antibiotics also led to complete resolution of the renal lesion.

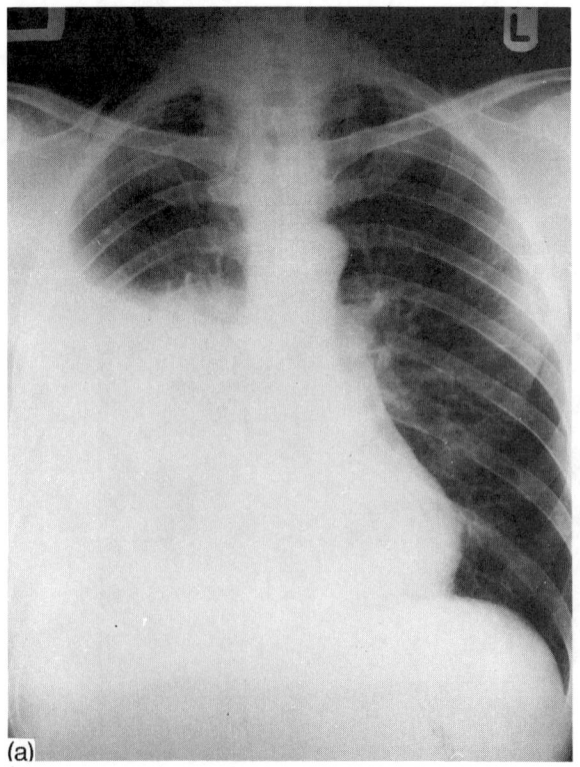
(a)

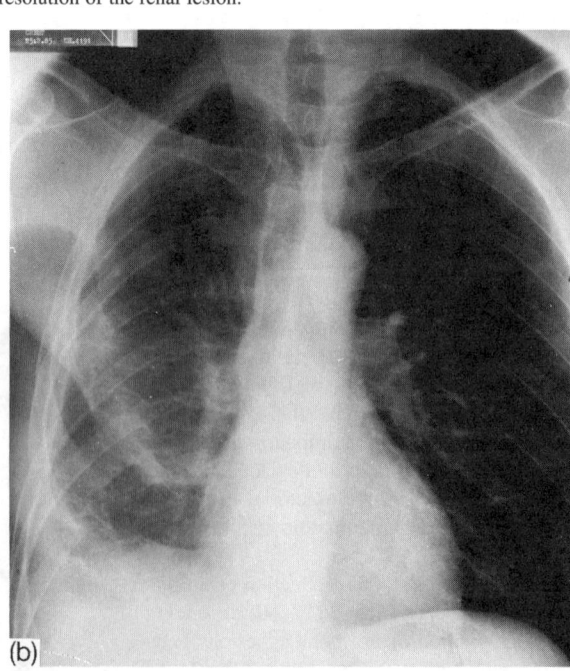
(b)

Fig. 3 CT scan of the thorax demonstrating empyema with an indwelling slim drainage tube. Large-bore cannulae are commonly used for the drainage of empyema, but slim tubes flushed regularly with saline can also be effective.

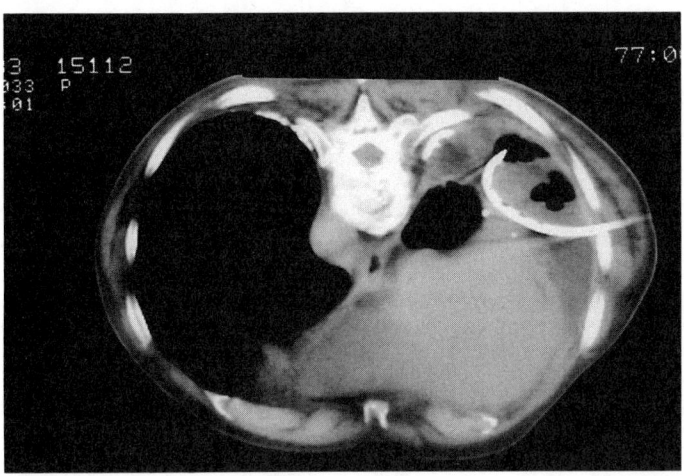

sen staining of the pus; in contrast with non-purulent tuberculous effusions, pleural biopsy is not required. All specimens, irrespective of odour, should be taken to the laboratory rapidly in a syringe from which air bubbles have been expressed to allow culture for anaerobes. Methods such as countercurrent immunoelectrophoresis for pneumococcal antigen and gas–liquid chromatography for volatile fatty acids from anaerobes may be helpful, particularly if antibiotics have already been used. In amoebic disease, microscopy of temporary wet mounts of pleural fluid or sputum may identify the trophozoites. Pleural fluid cytology may be helpful in excluding malignancy, but bronchoscopy is required in unexplained disease or when there is clinical suspicion. Ultrasound or CT scan (Fig. 3) helps with assessment and the search for predisposing subphrenic or hepatic abscess, bronchiectasis, or obstructing bronchial tumour.

TREATMENT

Effective treatment of an empyema requires prompt drainage combined with appropriate antibiotics. Clinical circumstances resulting in the development of an empyema may give a clue to the infecting organism. The initial choice of antibiotics is usually made without microbiological guidance and should offer cover against a broad range of Gram-positive and Gram-negative organisms. The regimen should be revised in the light of clinical response and subsequent laboratory findings. Ampicillin (in high dosage) or cefuroxime will eliminate the more common anaerobic organism and can be combined with metronidazole if resistant species are suspected.

Antibiotic treatment alone will be ineffective and must be combined with pleural drainage, but there is no clear consensus as to the best approach. Repeated aspiration through a wide-bore needle can be used, particularly if loculated collections can be identified with ultrasound guidance. A more conventional approach is to insert an intercostal drain, but even here prejudice abounds. There is increasing evidence that correct placement of the tube is of greater importance that the size of the intercostal drain. Catheter drainage using a soft 12 French gauge catheter (e.g. Van Sonenberg) is considerably more comfortable for the patient than the traditional large-bore tube. It is effective unless the pus is exceptionally thick and viscid when a larger-bore catheter may be required. Regular saline flushing of the slim catheter is necessary. The use of intrapleural urokinase (100 000 IU) has been advocated to help break down loculi and allow free drainage.

Empyema may fail to resolve because of unextractable thick pus, extensive loculation, the development of bronchopleural fistula, or the presence of gross fibrin and debris deposition on the pleura. If available, surgical thoracoscopy to allow breakdown of adhesions and septae or

placement of a fresh tube can be curative. If it is not, formal surgery for the clearance of the pleural space and decortication of the lung or closure of a bronchopleural fistula is essential. The results of surgical treatment are good, and failure to achieve adequate drainage by aspiration or indwelling tube should lead to prompt consultation with a thoracic surgeon. Antibiotic treatment should be continued for 2 to 3 weeks following successful surgery.

REFERENCES

Bartlett, J.G. and Finegold, S.M. (1974). Anaerobic infections of the lung and pleural space. *American Review of Respiratory Disease*, **110**, 56–77.

Brock, R.C. (1952). Lung abscess. Oxford University Press.

Delikaris, P.G., Conlan, A.A., Abramor, E., Hurnitz, S.S., and Studi, R. (1984). Empyema thoracis—a prospective study on 73 patients. *South African Medical Journal*, **65**, 47–9.

Storm, H.K., Krasnik, M., Bang, K., and Frimodt-Moller, N. (1992). Treatment of pleural empyema secondary to pneumonia: thoracocentesis regimen versus tube drainage. *Thorax*, **47**, 821–4.

Wells, F.C. (1990). Empyema thoracis: what is the role of surgery? *Respiratory Medicine*, **84**, 97–9.

17.7.4 Chronic specific infections

J. M. HOPKIN

Bacteria, fungi, protozoans, and helminths can all cause pulmonary disease of slow evolution that results in chronic illness or death. Detailed accounts of these are given in the section on infectious diseases. Geographical variation is significant.

Effective diagnosis often depends on clinical suspicion. Chest radiographs, which can now be supplemented in many centres by CT scanning, provide useful diagnostic pointers (Figs 1, 2, and 3). Formal diagnosis demands careful microbiological examination, with appropriate stains and culture methods, of appropriate samples—sputum, cutaneous masses, pleural fluid, and bronchoscopic bronchoalveolar samples if needed.

Tuberculosis is the leading cause of specific chronic respiratory infection worldwide. Notification rates are rising again in the wake of the AIDS epidemic and the increasing recognition of resistant strains is of great concern. Atypical mycobacteria cause cavitating apical disease, which is radiographically indistinguishable from *Mycobacterium tuber-*

Fig. 1 Bilateral cavitating apical tuberculosis in a 60-year-old unemployed Briton who drank and smoked to excess.

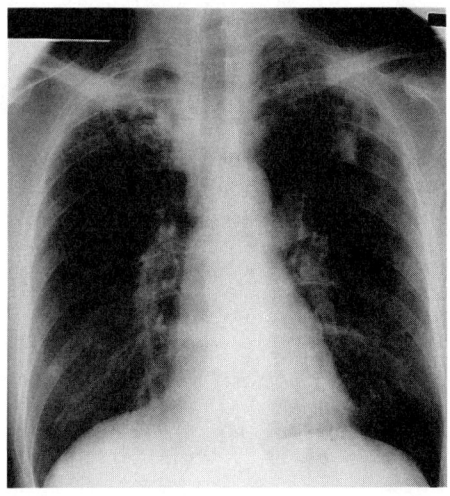

Fig. 2 Miliary tuberculosis (with small right pleural effusion) in a 20-year-old HIV-negative Ugandan man.

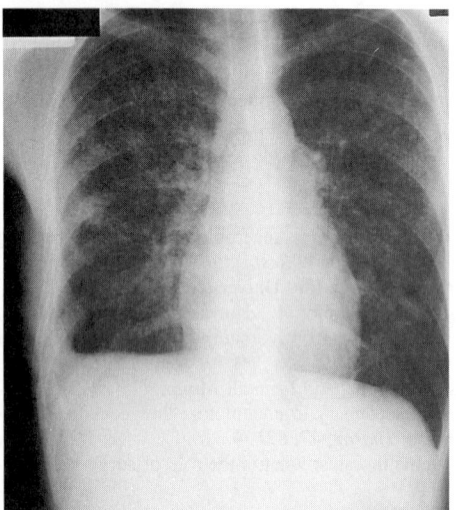

Fig. 3 Infiltrating and nodular shadows of South American blastomycosis scattered through the middle and lower zones in a 50-year-old Brazilian agricultural worker. (By courtesy of Dr CC Fritscher.)

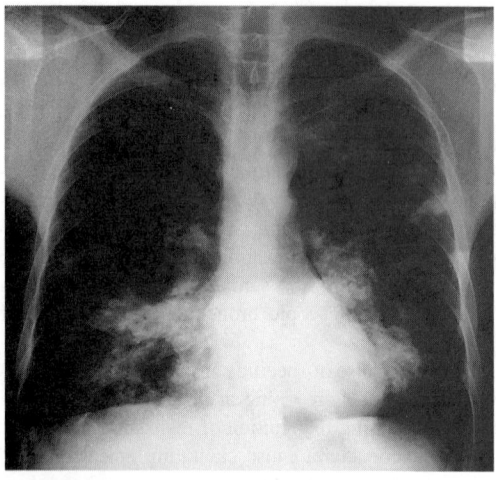

Fig. 4 CT scan showing an Aspergillus mycetoma (or fungal ball) within a right apical lung cavity.

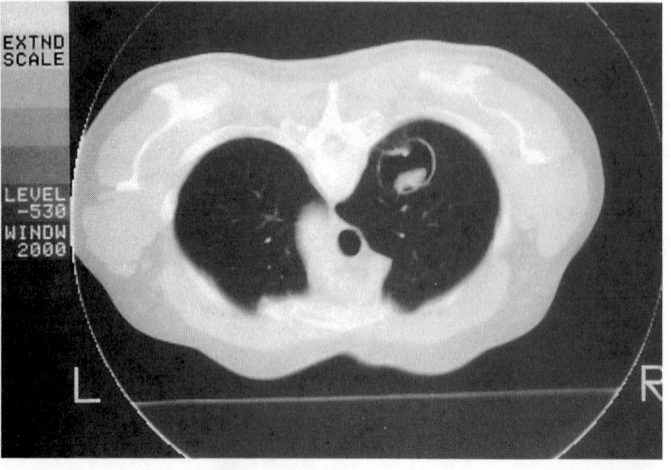

culosis, in normal and debilitated hosts, such as the elderly or those with severe diabetes mellitus or rheumatoid disease.

Actinomyces species (true *Actinomyces* and *Arachnia* species) are oral cavity anaerobes which, after aspiration, produce indolent pulmonary infection that can spread to mediastinum, pleura, and thoracic wall. *Nocardia asteroides*, a saprophytic soil bacterim, causes chronic pulmonary infection that can disseminate in immunosuppressed and normal subjects.

Aspergillus fumigatus is a ubiquitous fungus that causes a range of respiratory syndromes: allergic bronchopulmonary aspergillosis, in which its antigens trigger intense bronchial inflammation in some atopic asthmatic individuals (Chapter 17.9.1(b)); mycetoma (Fig. 4) in which the fungus colonizes a cavity within the lung, scarred by old tuberculosis or sarcoidosis for example, and cause variable haemoptysis; invasive pneumonitis in immunosuppressed subjects (e.g. on oncology or transplant programmes (Chapter 17.7.5)); chronic empyema, often after surgery or trauma.

Other fungi, often of soil origin, are important causes of acute and chronic pulmonary infections in defined geographical regions: histoplasmosis, coccidioidomycosis, blastomycosis, paracoccidioidomycosis (or South American blastomycosis (Fig. 3)), and cryptococcosis.

Helminths cause pulmonary eosinophilia syndromes. Because of the deposition of larvae in the pulmonary circulation with ensuing intense inflammation and fibrosis, schistosomiasis can cause pulmonary hypertension and cor pulmonale. *Echinococcus granulosus* (hydatid disease) produces space-occupying rounded masses and cysts in the lung.

Amoebiasis of the liver can spread through the diaphragm, causing empyema or abscess/pneumonitis over or within the right lower lobe of the lung.

REFERENCES

Foley, N.M. and Miller, R.F. (1993). Tuberculosis and AIDS: is the white plague up and coming? *Journal of Infection*, **26**, 39–43.

Glassroth, J. (1991). Tuberculosis in the United States. *American Review of Respiratory Disease*, **146**, 278–9.

Grzybowski, S. (1991). Tuberculosis in the third World. *Thorax*, **46**, 689–91.

17.7.5 Respiratory infection in the immunosuppressed

J. M. HOPKIN

Defence of the lungs against infection depends upon (a) effective laryngeal and cough reflexes, (b) the mucociliary escalator and secretory IgA of the airways, (c) the scavenging macrophages of the alveolar spaces supported by neutrophils, and (d) specific immunity conferred by T- and B-lymphocyte responses.

Defects in these defences are various and can produce characteristic syndromes of infection. This chapter focuses on respiratory infection complicating severe deficiency of immunity that may occur as congenital disease but which is most commonly seen amongst patients on cancer chemotherapy and organ transplantation programmes, in those with the acquired immunodeficiency syndrome (**AIDS**), and in those receiving immunosuppressive agents for inflammatory disorders (e.g. vasculitis). Amongst such patients, pneumonia is a leading cause of disease and death.

The pulmonary complications seen in the immunosuppressed may be due to (a) infection with pathogenic organisms, (b) infection with opportunistic organisms of medium to low pathogenicity (Table 1), and (c) non-infective complications of various types (Table 2). These different

Table 1 *Opportunistic respiratory infection in the immunosuppressed*

Defect	Infections
Neutropenia (e.g. treated leukaemia)	Bacteria (particularly Gram-negative and *Staphylococcus aureus*), (*Aspergillus fumigatus*, *Mucor* spp.)
Immunoglobulin deficiency (e.g. multiple myeloma, inherited defects)	Encapsulated bacteria (*Streptococcus pneumoniae*, *Haemophilus influenzae*)
T-lymphocyte deficiency (e.g. AIDS, organ transplant recipients, treated malignancy)	Fungi (particularly *Pneumocystis carinii*, *Cryptococcus neoformans*), cytomegalovirus, *Mycobacteria* (tuberculous and atypical), bacteria (including *Legionella pneumophila*, *Nocardia asteroides*)

Table 2 *Non-infectious complications in the immunosuppressed*

Pulmonary oedema
Pulmonary haemorrhage
Pulmonary embolism
Tumour (solid tumour, lymphoma and leukaemia, Kaposi's sarcoma)
Drug-induced pneumonitis
Radiation pneumonitis
Alveolar proteinosis
Leucagglutinin reaction

entities often have overlapping clinical and radiographic features, and therefore pose diagnostic and therapeutic difficulties. Making a precise diagnosis, often with resort to invasive investigation, allows the use of highly specific and effective treatment, with the minimum of side-effects. This significantly improves the likelihood of survival.

An effective diagnostic approach requires knowledge of the potential pulmonary complications in the patient under care, a thorough clinical and radiographic assessment, and a strategy for further investigation.

Patterns of pulmonary complication

Although knowledge of the limb of immune defence disrupted provides guidelines to the likely causes of infection (Table 1), the type of immunosuppression can be mixed in any particular patient and may vary with the stage of their underlying disease and treatment.

Cancer chemotherapy programmes

Patients undergoing aggressive cytotoxic chemotherapy for leukaemia and lymphoma have a high risk of fatal respiratory infection that threatens their ultimate survival, despite control of their malignancy.

Profound neutropenia is a common occurrence during the early phases of treatment; therefore Gram-negative pneumonia is a special risk, and fungal pneumonia, particularly caused by *Aspergillus fumigatus*, is possible if the neutropenia is severe and prolonged. Later during the course of the illness, T-lymphocyte immune deficiency develops and with it the risk of pneumocystis pneumonia which, before the introduction of specific chemoprophylaxis, produced an annual attack rate of 18 per cent in the childhood leukaemia population.

Non-infectious complications are various, but include diffuse pneumonitis as a drug reaction to cytotoxic agents and the rare, but well described, leucagglutinin reaction of the lung in which diffuse radiographic change and hypoxaemia may follow white-cell transfusion.

Organ transplantation

RENAL

Bacterial pneumonias, due to *S. pneumoniae* and Gram-negative bacteria including Legionella, may occur at any stage after transplantation.

Mycobacterial disease, particularly tuberculosis, is a high risk for individuals with a past history of tuberculosis or of likely past infection because of their ethnic origin or country of origin. The disease may take a rapid and disseminated pulmonary form (Fig. 1).

Cytomegalovirus (**CMV**) pneumonia presents as a diffuse pneumonitis of mild to moderate severity 4 to 6 weeks after transplantation. The most severe form occurs in CMV-serology-negative recipients of a CMV-positive donor kidney.

Fungal infections are significant, particularly by *Pneumocystis carinii*; without chemoprophylaxis the annual attack rate for pneumocystis is 20 per cent. The disease typically occurs 1 to 6 months after transplantation when immunosuppression is at its zenith, and presents with a rapidly progressive diffuse pneumonitis that is fatal unless specific treatment is initiated quickly. Other fungal pneumonias can be caused by *As. fumigatus*, *Mucor* spp., *Fusarium* spp., and *Trichosporon* species and, in some parts of the world, by *Coccidioides immitis* and *Histoplasma capsulatum*.

Non-infectious complications are frequent and include pulmonary oedema (the result of impaired renal salt and water excretion, cardiac dysfunction, or fluid overload) and thromboembolism. The original renal-destroying disease may recur in the lung, for example in Wegener's granulomatosis or Goodpasture's syndrome.

LIVER

The infective risks are similar to those listed for renal transplantation. Because of the prolonged surgery intubation, non-infectious complications include postoperative collapse and effusion, particularly at the right base, and postoperative adult respiratory distress syndrome (Chapter 17.10.20).

HEART–LUNG

Infective complications are caused by the organisms listed for renal transplantation, but there is also disease due to *Nocardia asteroides* and the protozoan *Toxoplasma gondii*, both of which may be transmitted with the donor heart. Non-infectious complications include collapse of the left lower lobe and paralysis of the left diaphragm, often due to phrenic nerve cold injury. Pulmonary oedema, due to heart failure, and adult respiratory distress syndrome (postpump syndrome) are not rare. A common late complication after lung transplantation is the development of obliterative bronchiolitis as a manifestation of organ rejection (Chapter 17.10.3).

BONE-MARROW TRANSPLANTATION

Profound neutropenia makes Gram-negative pneumonia a special risk. Cytomegalovirus pneumonia, occurring at 6 to 12 weeks, is particularly common, is progressive, and carries a high mortality despite initiation of treatment (Chapter 7.10.6). Non-infectious complications include early pulmonary oedema due to large-volume donations of intravenous fluid or the cardiotoxicity of cytotoxic drugs. An often fatal interstitial pneumonitis, which is probably due to the direct pulmonary toxicity of the preparative irradiation and methotrexate therapy, is particularly common and fatal.

Acquired immunodeficiency syndrome (AIDS)

Although many forms of pulmonary infective complication are documented, a small number are predominant. Bacterial pneumonia due to pneumococcal infection, as well as *S. aureus,* coliforms, and Legionella as nocosomial infections, occurs frequently. The development of chronic bronchial suppuration associated with *Haemophilus influenzae* or other infection, with or without acquired bronchiectasis, is documented. Lung abscesses due to unusual organisms like *Rhodococcus equi,* have been reported.

Mycobacterial disease is significant. Infection due to *M. avium intracellulare* complex usually takes a systemic form, without pulmonary preponderance, and in the later stages of HIV disease. Tuberculosis is becoming an increasing problem during the earlier phases of HIV infection as well as in AIDS. Thus the AIDS population is becoming a poten-

Fig. 1 Chest radiographs of two renal transplant recipients with tuberculosis showing (a) miliary and (b) nodular/confluent consolidative changes. In both the radiographs advanced to these appearances over 16 to 20 days. The diagnosis was established at alveolar lavage by Ziehl–Neelsen staining, and subsequently confirmed on culture as *Mycobacterium tuberculosis.*

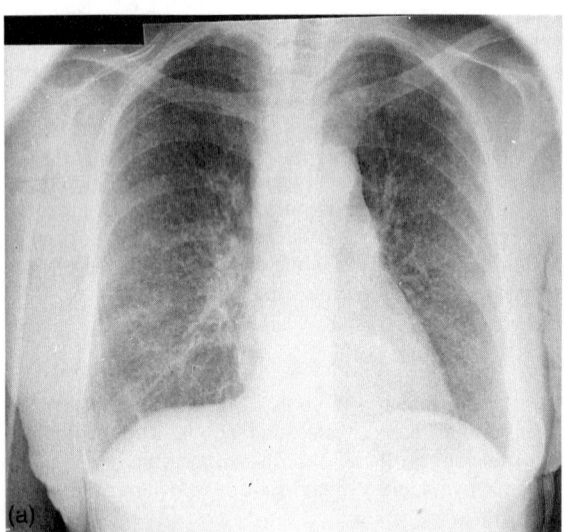

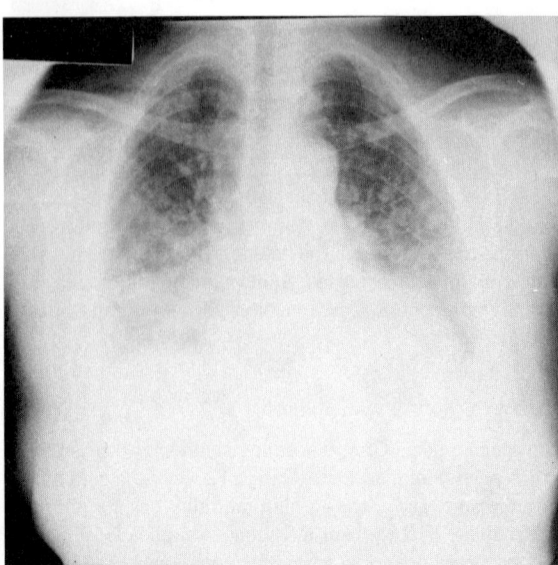

tial source of infection within the community at large, and multiple drug-resistant strains are becoming increasingly documented in the United States. Mantoux test negativity, accompanying extrapulmonary disease and atypical basal bilateral nodular radiographic features, is frequent.

Fungal infections in AIDS are dominated by the occurrence of *P. carinii* pneumonia (Fig. 2) which has shown an annual attack rate of 70 per cent for AIDS subjects not receiving chemoprophylaxis. Pneumocystis pneumonia in AIDS is often of gradual onset and progression, often of some weeks; if left untreated, the diffuse pneumonitis causes increasing hypoxaemia and death. Histoplasmosis and coccidioidomycosis pneumonias are increasingly documented; they cause diffuse fibronodular radiographic change. Cryptococcal infection generally presents with meningeal disease, but pulmonary disease or pleural effusion may be significant.

Non-infectious pulmonary complications of AIDS include a diffuse, usually non-aggressive, pneumonitis which in one form is characterized by an excess of CD8 lymphocytes in bronchoscopic alveolar lavage samples. In some subjects, such reactions can be attributed to drug reactions or, more rarely, alveolar proteinosis. Tumour in the lung is well recognized as either non-Hodgkin's lymphoma or Kaposi's sarcoma. Kaposi's sarcoma presents in the lung, usually after the development of extrapulmonary disease, particularly in the skin, and can present with focal bronchial disease, pulmonary change, hilar lymphadenopathy, or pleural effusion.

Hypogammaglobulinaemia

Hypogammaglobulinaemia may be due to a variety of congenital and acquired causes and may be global or confined to subclass deficiency in IgA, IgG, or IgG_4. Pulmonary complications can take the form of recurring bronchial infection, the development of bronchiectasis, or bacterial pneumonias due to encapsulated pneumococci or *H. influenzae*. Pneumococcal disease is particularly common in the marked dysgammaglobulinaemia that accompanies multiple myeloma.

Clinical features

The first requirement is thorough clinical and radiographic review in which account must be taken of the various potential infectious and non-infectious pulmonary problems and the clues that are available from the

Fig. 2 Chest radiograph, showing extensive bilateral consolidation radiating from both hila in Pneumocystis pneumonia.

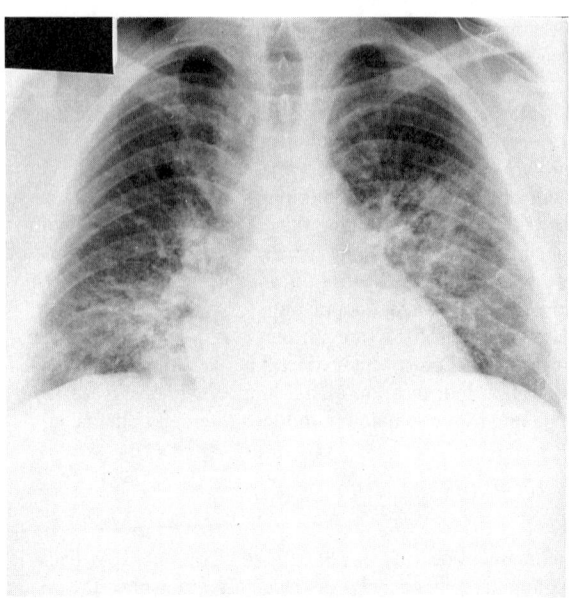

history, examination, review of fluid charts, drug schedules, and chest radiography. Pulmonary capillary wedge pressure measurements, pulmonary angiography, and ventilation/perfusion lung scanning may be required to establish the diagnosis of pulmonary oedema or embolism that may frequently complicate organ transplantation.

In some instances, the respiratory illness may simply be an episode of acute bronchitis with cough and purulent sputum following a coryzal illness, with little constitutional disturbance and no clinical or radiographic signs of pulmonary consolidation.

The more important clinical problem is the patient with breathlessness or radiographic consolidation accompanied by fever, for whom the differential diagnosis is broad and includes non-infectious disease. Fever itself, particular when it is high and associated with chills, suggests infection, although some non-infectious conditions such as drug reactions may also cause high fever.

The patient's background, the underlying disease, and the type of immune deficiency provide useful pointers in the differential diagnosis. Gram-negative sepsis and fungal disease are particular risks in the profound neutropenia seen in the early vigorous treatment of leukaemias and lymphomas; pneumocystis pneumonia is a possibility at a later stage; cytomegalovirus complicates organ transplantation, usually at about 2 months, and may be severe and fatal in bone marrow transplantation whereas it is relatively milder after renal transplantation. Geographical factors may be relevant; infection with, or reactivation of, fungal disease such as coccidioidomycosis or histoplasmosis occurs in North America, and disseminated strongyloidiasis is seen in patients particularly from the West Indies and Far East. Tuberculosis may be reactivated in patients from many developing countries, but particularly the Indian subcontinent and southeast Asia.

Physical examination should search for tumour or bleeding at extrapulmonary sites. Skin disease may be present in graft versus host disease, and cutaneous lesions may provide diagnostic clues to systemic vasculitis. Signs of intracerebral infection are a principal feature of cryptococcal disease and may complicate Aspergillus and nocardial infections. Arthropathy and biochemical evidence of hepatitis occur frequently in cytomegalovirus disease. Haemoptysis may be part of an infective syndrome but also raises the possibility of pulmonary embolism or haemorrhage. Pleurisy with pleural pain and pleural rub is not a feature of either infection with pneumocystis or of cardiogenic pulmonary oedema or alveolar haemorrhage. In pneumocystis pneumonia, fever and breathlessness may precede definite radiographic changes; absence of auscultatory physical signs in the chest is characteristic.

Radiology and lung sampling

The chest radiograph usually provides definitive evidence on the presence of pulmonary consolidation, its extent, distribution, and character, and the presence or absence of other features including those of cardiac failure (cardiomegaly, pulmonary venous congestion, and Kerley B lines) or pleural disease (Fig. 3). The lateral chest radiograph is valuable in localizing lesions for further investigation by bronchoscopy. CT scanning can provide more detailed anatomical information for targeting of sampling procedures. There are few microbe-specific radiographic changes; there can be a good deal of overlap between the radiographic features or *Pneumocystis*, mycobacterial, and cytomegalovirus infection. However, confluent segmental or lobar consolidation accompanying a very acute clinical illness strongly suggests bacterial pneumonia.

Sputum, if expectorated, provides a valuable sample for preliminary microbiological assessment. It may be induced by the inhalation of nebulized hypertonic (3–6 per cent) saline; and such samples have proved useful in the diagnosis of pneumocystis pneumonia in AIDS subjects.

Open-lung biopsy provides the best sample of pulmonary tissue but may precipitate the need for assisted ventilation or be complicated by pneumothorax or wound sepsis. Percutaneous lung biopsy or fine-needle aspiration, carrying the risk of bleeding or pneumothorax (proportion-

ately related to the calibre of the needle), offers rather unpredictable sampling, but is useful for examining peripheral nodules. Fibre optic bronchoscopy, with alveolar lavage but with or without transbronchial biopsy, is being increasingly used in the immunosuppressed and has produced diagnostic rates of 70 to 80 per cent or better. Alveolar lavage produces a large sample from the alveolar space with 10^4 cells/ml and provides a good specimen for microbiological assessment by staining, the application of monoclonal antibodies and DNA probes, and culture (Fig. 4). Cytological examination of the fluid may diagnose pulmonary haemorrhage and malignant infiltrates.

Bronchoscopic lavage does not produce bleeding or pneumothorax, and provides a bedside test with good diagnostic results and little mor-

Fig. 3 Chest radiograph showing pulmonary oedema in an immunosuppressed renal transplant recipient. Characteristic Kerley B lines are not visible, but pleural fluid is evident on the right and the patient was markedly orthopnoeic.

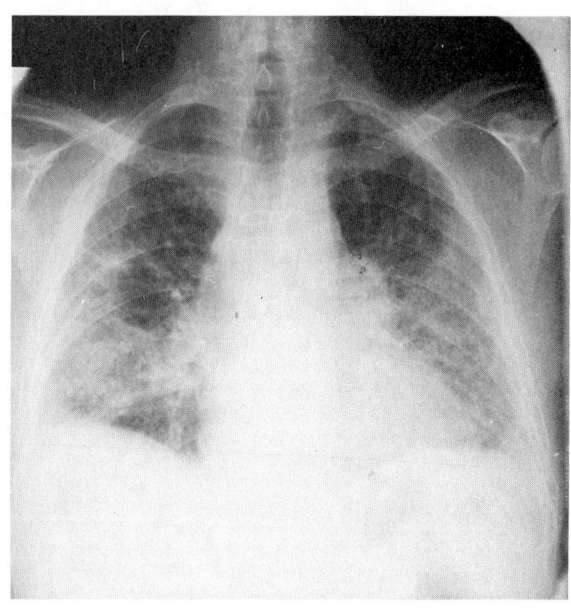

Fig. 4 Laboratory analysis of bronchoscopic alveolar lavage.

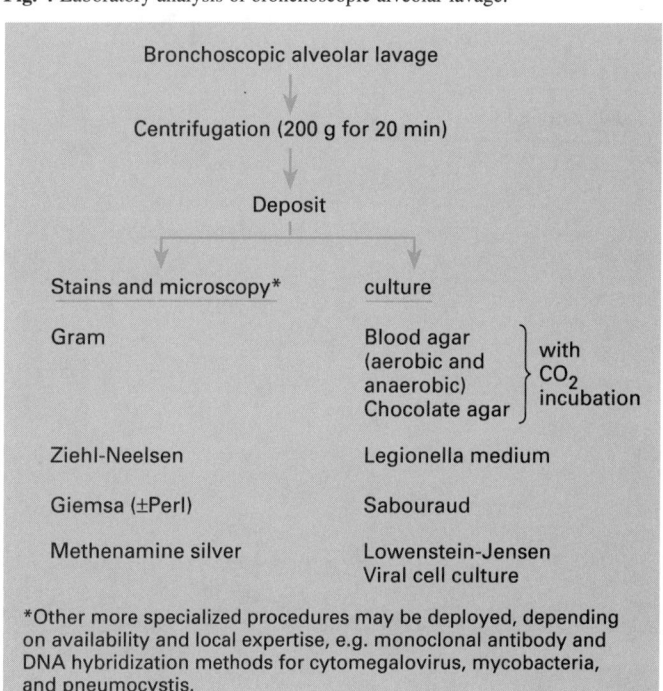

Bronchoscopic alveolar lavage

Centrifugation (200 g for 20 min)

Deposit

Stains and microscopy*	culture
Gram	Blood agar (aerobic and anaerobic) Chocolate agar } with CO₂ incubation
Ziehl-Neelsen	Legionella medium
Giemsa (±Perl)	Sabouraud
Methenamine silver	Lowenstein-Jensen Viral cell culture

*Other more specialized procedures may be deployed, depending on availability and local expertise, e.g. monoclonal antibody and DNA hybridization methods for cytomegalovirus, mycobacteria, and pneumocystis.

bidity, which is now the first investigation of choice in many centres. It cannot provide definitive information on drug-induced lung disease or other non-infective inflammatory alveolitides. In such cases a broncho-scopic transbronchial lung biopsy is required.

A practical approach to management (Fig. 5)

Episodes of bronchitis are typified by prominent cough producing puru-lent sputum but no clinical or radiographic evidence of consolidation. After sputum has been obtained for study, these episodes should be treated with an antibiotic effective against the likely pathogens *H. influenzae* and *Streptococcus pneumoniae*. β-Lactamase-producing strains of *H. influenzae* occur (15 per cent of cases), but treatment with oral ampicillin or tetracycline is usually highly effective.

Pneumonia of abrupt onset and progress, with accompanying seg-mental or lobar radiographic shadowing, strongly suggests bacterial infection. It is then appropriate to start antibiotic treatment promptly after swift and simple microbiological investigation based on blood, urine, natural or induced sputum, and, if available, pleural fluid sam-plings. Treatment should be an intravenously administered antibacterial regimen providing broad antibacterial activity against the pneumococ-cus, *H. influenzae*, *Staphylococcus aureus*, and many other Gram-neg-ative bacteria. A suitable combination is cefuroxime and gentamicin.

When the pace of the illness is less acute or when the chest radiograph shows more diffuse or scattered change the differential diagnosis enlarges. Sputum or induced sputum should be examined by micros-copy, but if this does not provide a prompt diagnosis, a decision needs to be made about further diagnostic techniques. Percutaneous fine-nee-dle aspiration for cytology and microbiology is appropriate for periph-erally placed nodules. Open-lung biopsy is the only technique that will give totally reliable information on inflammatory alveolitis of non-infec-tive origin. Both carry significant morbidity.

For infiltrative or pneumonic changes on radiographs when infection is the primary suspicion, many investigators proceed to fibre optic bron-choscopy with alveolar lavage. If there is some suspicion of autoimmune or drug-induced alveolitis, transbronchial lung biopsies should also be taken at bronchoscopy. The procedure can be completed in 15 min and can be performed in hypoxaemic patients using local anaesthesia and concurrent oxygen supplementation. Chest radiographs allow localiza-tion of the pneumonia and the accurate direction of the 5 mm flexible bronchoscopy to this site. In diffuse disease, the middle lobe may be chosen and the bronchoscope is impacted firmly there. Three or four 50-ml aliquots of sterile saline are instilled singly and 30 to 60 per cent of the fluid is recovered by suction into a trap. Some of this sample is centrifuged and slides made from the deposit for diagnostic microscopy. The remainder is used for culture. Semiquantitative techniques improve accuracy in diagnosing bacterial disease. The use of monoclonal anti-bodies facilitates the counting of CMV-positive alveolar macrophages. Silver staining of alveolar lavage for *P. carinii* has been shown on cor-relative postmortem studies to have a sensitivity and specificity approaching 100 per cent. Mycobacteria can be efficiently screened for by fluorescent microscopy with Auramine stains as well as by the Ziehl–Neelsen method. Giemsa stains are used to assess haemorrhage or malig-nant infiltration. Many results should be available within 4 h, and simple cultures within 36 h.

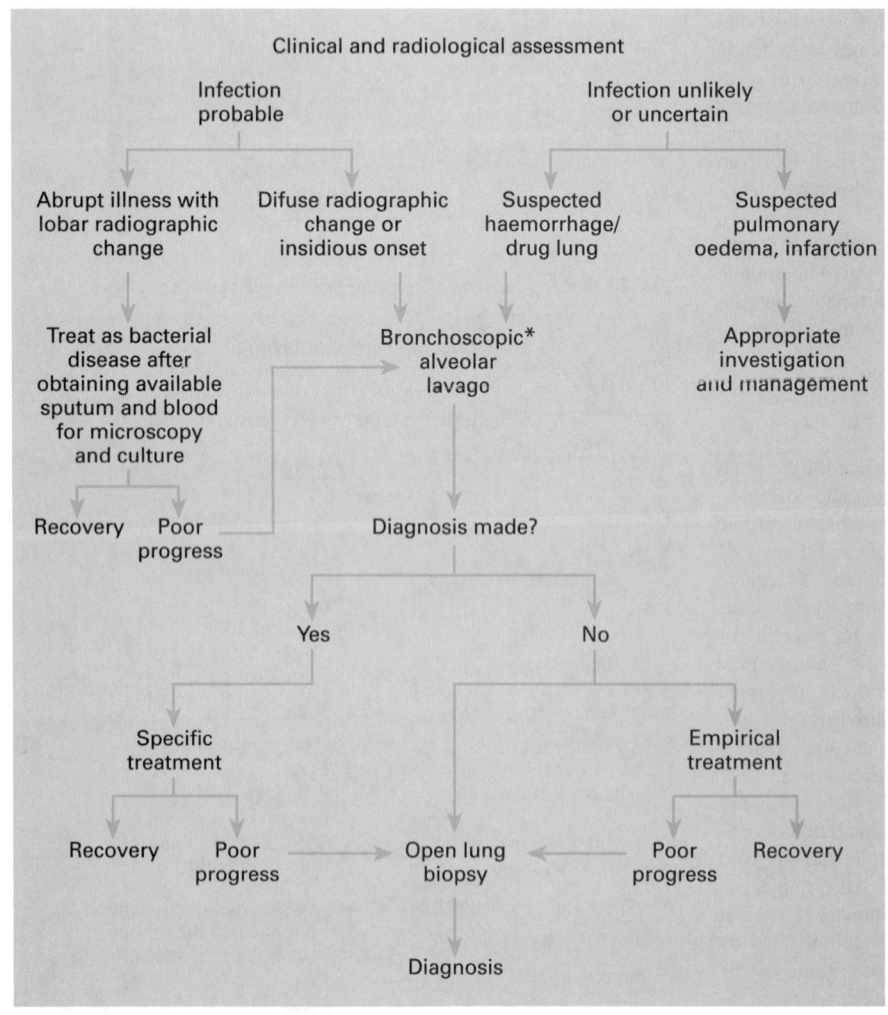

Fig. 5 An algorithm showing one approach to the investigation and management of pneumonia in the immunosuppressed. *Transbronchial biopsy should also be taken if drug-induced alveolitis is suspected. Percutaneous needle aspiration is an alternative diagnostic procedure for discrete pulmonary nodule(s).

If bronchoscopic lavage provides no diagnosis in a patient with declining state, then open-lung biopsy offers definitive sampling.

Results and treatment

With the exception of acute onset lobar pneumonia, antimicrobial therapy is best started when a specific diagnosis has been made. The details for the different forms of infection are recorded elsewhere in this volume.

In Pneumocystis pneumonia, the first-line treatments are high dosage cotrimoxazole or pentamidine. In the AIDS population, the rate of side-effects to these agents is high; reactions which include fever, rash, and renal impairment often demand change of therapy to the alternative agent or to other agents, including trimethoprim, dapsone, or naphthoquinone, to allow the necessary 3 weeks treatment to be completed. There is little evidence that changing regimens because of failure of the pneumocystis pneumonia to respond is useful, but there are data supporting the coadministration of corticosteroids particularly to AIDS patients.

Despite the severity of the disease, recovery is frequently seen in aspergillus pneumonia treated vigorously with amphotericin. The side-effects of this agent may be limited by formulation of the drug with liposomes or lipid emulsion. Preliminary studies suggest that oral itraconazole may become an effective but less toxic alternative.

The standard chemotherapeutic regimens should be used for tuberculosis, although increasing rates of drug resistance to agents that include isoniazid and rifampicin are being documented in cities in the United States.

Cytomegalovirus pneumonia is treated with the guanine analogue gancyclovir. The addition of intravenous immunoglobulin should be considered in severe disease.

In many instances, the severe hypoxaemia accompanying many of these pneumonias may demand a period of automatic ventilation, high concentrations of inspired oxygen, and the use of positive end-expiratory pressure. However, the outlook for AIDS patients with disease of such severity is grim, and most centres recognize that humane terminal care is more appropriate.

In transplant patients and oncology patients still receiving immunosuppressive chemotherapy, it may be necessary to taper the dosage of such agents to allow recovery from pneumonia.

Prevention

Prevention of pneumocystis pneumonia is dependent upon chemoprophylaxis with either thrice-weekly oral cotrimoxazole or monthly inhaled pentamidine. Such prophylaxis is a routine part of leukaemia chemotherapy in childhood, organ transplantation schedules, and the management of AIDS patients, provided that the agent can be tolerated.

Chemoprophylaxis is also important in the prevention of tuberculosis. Daily oral isoniazid over 1 year can be used at the initiation of immunosuppressive chemotherapy (e.g. in the transplant group) if there is a past history of tuberculosis or if the patient is from a geographical location where the disease is prevalent.

Cytomegalovirus disease is most severe in transplant patients who are seronegative and who receive seropositive blood products or transplant. Avoidance of a positive organ is advised, if possible, but many centres now administer live attenuated CMV vaccine to potential transplant recipients who are CMV seronegative since it offers protection against cytomegalovirus disease of moderate to severe severity.

In general, the risk of any opportunistic pneumonia is increased by the number and dosage of immunosuppressant agents used, and therefore clinicians and investigators should use the lowest dosages of such agents, compatible with achieving underlying goals for suppressing inflammatory vasculitis, maintaining organ transplant, or eradicating treatable tumour.

REFERENCES

Bermejo, A., Veeken, H., and Berra, A. (1992). Tuberculosis; incidence in developing countries with high prevalence of HIV infection. *AIDS*, **6**, 1203–6.

Bigby, T.D., Margolskee, D., Curtis, J.L., et al. (1986). The usefulness of induced sputum in the diagnosis of *Pneumocystis carinii* pneumonia in patients with the acquired immunodeficiency syndrome. *American Review of Respiratory Disease*, **133**, 515–18.

Broaddus, C., Dake, M.D., Stulbarg, M.S., et al. (1985). Bronchoalveolar lavage and transbronchial biopsy for the diagnosis of pulmonary infections in the acquired immunodeficiency syndrome. *Annals of Internal Medicine*, **102**, 747–52.

Chaisson R.E., Slutkin G. (1989). Tuberculosis and HIV infection. *Journal of Infectious Diseases*, **159**, 96–100.

Como, J.A. and Dismukes, W.E. (1994). Oral azole drugs as systemic antifungal therapy. *New England Journal of Medicine*, **330**, 263–72.

Ettinger, N.A. and Trulock, E.P. (1991). Pulmonary considerations of organ transplantation. *American Review of Respiratory Diseases*, **143**, 1382–1405; **144**, 213–23, 433–51.

Grosset J.H. (1992). Treatment of tuberculosis in HIV infection. *Tuberculosis and Lung Diseases*, **73**, 378–83.

Guillon, J.M., Autran, B., Denis, M., et al. (1988). Human immunodeficiency virus-related lymphocytic alveolitis. *Chest*, **94**, 1264–70.

Hamilton, P.J. and Pearson, A.D.J. (1986). Bone marrow transplantation and the lung. *Thorax*, **41**, 497–502.

Hopkin, J.M. (1988). Respiratory infection in the immunocompromised patient. In *Advanced medicine* (ed. M.C. Sheppard), pp. 104–17. Baillière Tindall, London.

Hopkin, J.M., Turney, J.H., Young, J.A., et al. (1983). Rapid diagnosis of obscure pneumonia in immunosuppressed renal patients by cytology of alveolar lavage fluid. *Lancet*, **ii**, 299–301.

Kovacs, J.A., Ng, V.L., Masur, H., et al. (1988). Diagnosis of *Pneumocystis carinii* pneumonia: improved detection in sputum with use of monoclonal antibodies. *New England Journal of Medicine*, **318**, 589–93.

Masur, H. (1992). Prevention and treatment of pneumocystis pneumonia. *New England Journal of Medicine*, **327**, 1853–60.

Maxfield, R.A., Sorkin, I.B., Fazzini, E.P., et al. (1986). Respiratory failure in patients with the acquired immunodeficiency syndrome and Pneumocystis carinii pneumonia. *Critical Care Medicine*, **14**, 443–9.

Montgomery, A.S., Luce, J.M., Turner, J., et al. (1987). Aerosolised pentamidine as sole therapy for *Pneumocystis carinii* pneumonia in patients with acquired immunodeficiency syndrome. *Lancet*, **ii**, 480–3.

Murray, J.F. and Mills, J. (1990). Pulmonary complications of human immunodeficiency virus infection. *American Review of Respiratory Disease*, **141**, 1356–72, 1582–98.

Reed, E.C. (1991). Treatment of cytomegalovirus pneumonia in transplant patients. *Transplantation Proceedings*, **23** (Suppl. 1), 8–12.

Savic, V. (1992) Evaluation of polymerase chain reaction, tubercular stearic acid analysis and direct microscopy for the detection of *Mycobacterium tuberculosis* in sputum. *Journal of Infectious Diseases*, **166**, 1177–80.

Smiley, M.C., Wlodavier, C.G., Grossman, R.A., et al. (1985). The role of pretransplant immunity in protection from CMV disease following renal transplantation. *Transplantation*, **41**, 157.

Thorpe, J.E., Baughman, R.P., and Frame, P.T. (1987). Alveolar lavage for diagnosis of acute bacterial pneumonia. *Journal of Infectious Diseases*, **155**, 855–61.

Wakefield, A.E., Millar, R.M., Guiver, L., and Hopkin, J.M. (1991). DNA amplification for the diagnosis of pneumocystis pneumonia from induced sputum. *Lancet*, **i**, 1378–80.

Winston, D.J., Ho, W.G., and Lin C.H. (1987). Intravenous immunoglobulin for prevention of cytomegalovirus infection and interstitial pneumonia after bone marrow transplantation. *Annals of Internal Medicine*, **106**, 12–18.

Young, J.A., Hopkin, J.M., and Cuthbertson, W.P. (1984). Pulmonary infiltrates in immunocompromised patients: diagnosis by cytological examination of bronchoalveolar lavage fluid. *Journal of Clinical Pathology*, **37**, 390–7.

17.8 The upper respiratory tract

17.8.1 Allergic rhinitis ('hay fever')

S. R. DURHAM

Introduction

Although frequently trivialized, allergic rhinitis remains a common cause of morbidity and social embarrassment. Estimates have suggested that 10 to 15 per cent of the population of the United Kingdom may be affected. Furthermore, the prevalence of hay-fever in the United Kingdom appears to be increasing. One recent survey revealed a fourfold increase in the number of consultations with general practitioners for summer hayfever (Table 1).

The reasons for this increasing prevalence are unclear, and it cannot be explained by changes in diagnostic fashion or a greater awareness of the condition alone. In recent years there have been major advances in our understanding of the basic mechanisms involved in the pathogenesis of allergic rhinitis. These advances have been paralleled by important developments in the diagnosis and management of the condition. The lining of the nose and paranasal sinuses is in continuity with the lower respiratory tract. Frequently, diseases of the upper and lower airways coexist. The nose provides an accessible 'window' for study of allergic disorders and other diseases which may also affect the lower airways. Nasal disease is also important since it may reflect the presenting features of a multitude of systemic diseases.

Recent developments in the understanding of the aetiology and pathogenesis of allergic rhinitis are described in this chapter. This is followed by a practical section on the diagnosis of allergic rhinitis in the context of other nasal and systemic disease. Finally, recent advances in treatment of allergic rhinitis are considered, including how improvements of our knowledge in basic mechanisms may lead to novel strategies for future therapy.

Aetiology

Seasonal allergic rhinitis

Pollens of importance include tree pollens in the spring and grass pollens during the summer. Weed pollens and mould spores predominate in the latter part of the summer and early autumn (Fig. 1). Allergy to grass pollen allergens is by far the most common cause of seasonal allergic rhinitis in the United Kingdom. Permanent grassland contains many species of grass, with the most common being perennial rye-grass (*Lolium perenne*), timothy grass (*Phleum pratense*), cocksfoot (*Dactylis glomerata*), and meadow grass (*Festuca pratensis*). Grasses are flowering plants whose pollens are dispersed by the winds. Pollen grains are 10 to 20 μm in diameter, ideal for being 'trapped' in the conjunctiva, nasal hairs, and anterior nares where they produce typical immediate symptoms of itching, sneezing, congestion, watery rhinorrhoea, and conjunctivitis. Warm dry conditions trigger pollen release, whereas rainfall reduces pollen counts. Although grass pollen release is maximal mid-morning and during the afternoon, maximal pollen counts occur in the evening and night. This is because as the air cools, pollen grains fall, thereby elevating pollen counts at ground level. This accounts for the increase in hay-fever symptoms during the evening and at night. Pollen counts above 50/mm³ are considered high and represent the level at

Table 1 *Consultations with general practitioners for hay fever (per 1000 population in the United Kingdom)*

1955–1956	5.1
1981–1982	19.8

Adapted from Fleming and Crombie 1987.

which most hay fever sufferers experience symptoms. The grass pollen season extends from the last week in May until the end of July, with the peak season corresponding to 'Wimbledon fortnight'.

Paradoxically, the increase in prevalence of hay fever has occurred in the face of falling pollen counts, at least in London and southeast England. One factor of possible importance may be pollution from car exhaust fumes. These include high levels of sulphur dioxide and nitrogen dioxide which may damage the nasal mucosa. Studies from Japan have indicated that increases in hay fever are confined to urban polluted districts. Diesel particulates have been shown to absorb major pollen allergens and also to be adjuvant for antibody production *in vivo*.

Perennial allergic rhinitis

By far the commonest cause of perennial allergic symptoms is the house dust mite (*Dermatophagoides pteronyssinus*, *Dermatophagoides farinae*, and *Euroglyphus maynei*). Mites are found in almost every home where they live in dust that accumulates in carpets, bedding, fabrics, and furniture. They live on shed human skin scales and thrive in temperatures of 15–20°C and a relative humidity of 45 to 65 per cent, which corresponds to conditions typical of many modern centrally heated

Fig. 1 Calendar of common seasonal aeroallergens. (By courtesy of Professor A.B. Kay.)

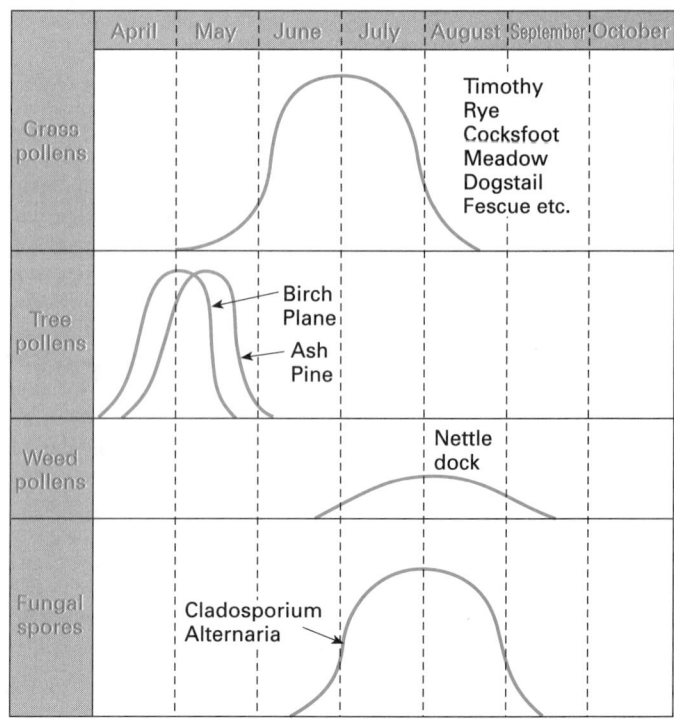

homes. The major allergen of the house dust mite (Der p 1) has been identified as a digestive enzyme (cysteine protease) which is present in high concentrations in the faeces. Mite faecal pellets are approximately the same size as grass pollen particles and become airborne when room air is disturbed.

Domestic pets are the second important cause of perennial allergy, identifiable in up to 40 per cent of children with asthma and/or rhinitis. The major cat allergen (Fel d 1) is a salivary protein which is preened on to the fur during grooming. Fel d 1 is found throughout the home in dust from floors and soft furnishings, in the air, and even on walls. This distribution, wider than mite allergens, is because Fel d 1 is present on very small particles (less than 2.5 μm in diameter) which readily become airborne. This small particle size may explain why a sensitized person may experience symptoms almost immediately upon entering a home containing a cat without being directly exposed to the animal. Dog allergens are less well characterized, although recently Can F 1 has been described. In the United States a major allergen from cockroaches has been characterized and related to the prevalence of asthma and rhinitis in inner city areas.

Occupational rhinitis refers to rhinitis caused by an agent inhaled in the workplace. Like other causes of seasonal and perennial rhinitis, occupational rhinitis may also be associated with bronchial asthma. Occupations at risk include laboratory animal handlers (rats, guinea pigs, mice), bakers (flour), agricultural workers (cows, pollens, fungal spores), solderers (colophony), and users of rubber gloves, particularly surgeons (latex).

Pathophysiology

Immediate symptoms of allergic rhinitis occur as a consequence of the interaction between solubilized allergen and IgE on the surface of mast cells in the nasal mucosa (Coombs classification type 1 immediate hypersensitivity). Mast-cell degranulation results in the release of a wide range of mediators, including histamine and tryptase, and the generation of bradykinin. IgE-dependent activation of mast cells also results in the release of newly formed membrane-associated mediators derived from arachidonic acid. These include the leukotrienes C4, D4, and E4, and prostaglandin D2. Platelet-activating factor is a further potent lipid mediator. The biological properties of these mediators may account for the majority of immediate symptoms which occur following allergen exposure. For example, vasodilation, vascular engorgement of nasal venous sinusoids, and increased vascular permeability cause nasal congestion and blockage. Watery and mucus discharge result in rhinorrhoea. Induced neural reflexes result in itching and sneezing. These mediators have been found in nasal secretions during natural disease and following local allergen provocation. However, confirmation of their biological relevance depends upon the clinical efficacy of specific antagonists. For example, histamine is obviously an important mediator, as reflected by the value of antihistamines for hay fever. Leukotriene antagonists and lipoxygenase inhibitors have also recently been shown to have some effect, although this requires confirmation. Similarly, the role of bradykinin will be put to the test with the recent availability of specific bradykinin antagonists.

In patients with allergic rhinitis, eosinophils are prominent in nasal washings and in biopsies of the nasal mucosa. Eosinophils produce leukotrienes (predominantly leukotriene C4 which is a potent mucus secretagogue), platelet-activating factor, and a range of toxic basic proteins which are contained within intracytoplasmic granules. These include major basic protein and eosinophil cationic protein, which are known to be toxic to human respiratory epithelium. The mechanism of this tissue eosinophilia is largely unknown. Chemotactic factors released following mast-cell activation may play a role. However, recent evidence suggests that peptide messengers (cytokines) released predominantly from T lymphocytes may be important. Helper (CD4+) T lymphocytes may be subdivided according to their profile of cytokine release. 'TH$_1$-type' cells produce predominantly IL-2 and γ-interferon, whereas 'TH$_2$-type' cells produce mainly IL-4 and IL-5. Both TH$_1$ and TH$_2$ cells produce IL-3 and granulocyte–macrophage colony-stimulating factor. This functional dichotomy, originally described in murine studies, has recently been shown to apply to T lymphocytes isolated from the peripheral blood of human donors.

The biological properties of TH$_2$-type cytokines suggest their involvement in allergic rhinitis. For example, IL-4 is the major cytokine responsible for switching B-cell immunoglobulin production from IgM and IgG to predominately IgE. IL-3 is a growth factor for mast cells. IL-3, IL-5, and granulocyte–macrophage colony-stimulating factor are important in the proliferation of eosinophils from bone marrow precursors and their maturation, activation, and prolonged survival in tissues. IL-5 promotes the selective adhesion of eosinophils to vascular endothelium prior to diapedesis.

Recent *in vivo* studies provide strong evidence for a role for TH$_2$-type cytokines during human allergic rhinitis. For example, nasal biopsies were obtained 24 h after local nasal allergen provocation and following a control challenge in the same subjects. Specific immunostaining demonstrated an increase in CD4+ T lymphocytes, an increase in 'activated' CD25+ (IL-2 receptor bearing) cells (presumed T lymphocytes), and an increase in eosinophils. Parallel *in situ* hybridization studies of nasal biopsies were performed using gene probes directed against mRNA for specific interleukins. There was a marked increase in mRNA expression for IL-3, IL-4, IL-5, and granulocyte–macrophage colony-stimulating factor. In contrast, no change in IL-2 or γ-interferon was observed (Figs. 2 and 3). A close correlation was found between the number of eosinophils in the nasal mucosa and the number of cells expressing mRNA for TH$_2$-type cytokines, particularly IL-5. These changes were associated with the development of late nasal responses 6–24 hours after allergen provocation. These studies suggest that TH$_2$-type cytokines may be important in the local regulation of IgE and tissue eosinophilia during chronic ongoing allergic rhinitis (Fig. 4).

Fig. 2 Autoradiographs of cryostat sections of human nasal mucosal biopsies taken 24 h after exposure to (a) allergen and (b) control solution. Sections were labelled with a ^{35}S-labelled antisense probe for IL-5. Sections from allergen-challenged sites hybridized with (c) antisense and (d) sense (control) IL-4 probes. Cellular infiltration by 'activated' (EG2 positive) eosinophils at (e) allergen-challenged sites compared with (f) control sites after challenge with allergen diluent. Positive cells stain red. (Reproduced with permission from Durham *et al.* (1992). *Journal of Immunology*, **148**, 2390–4. Copyright 1992. *The Journal of Immunology*.)

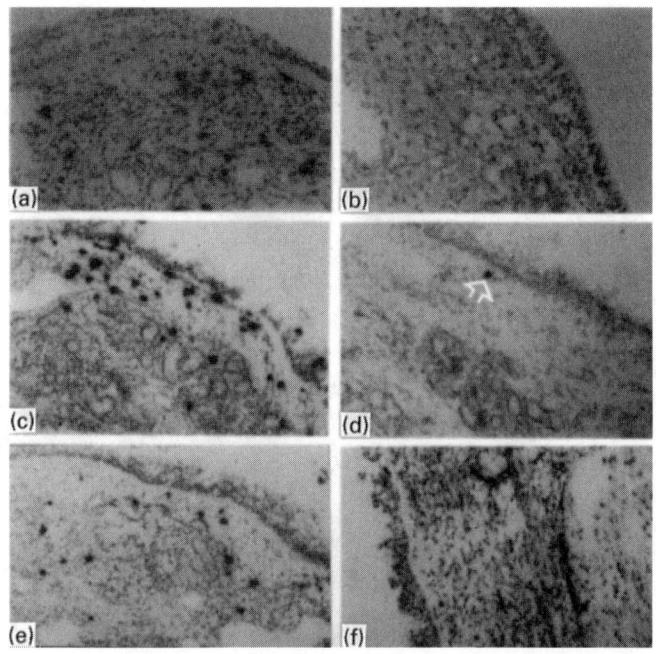

Clinical diagnosis

History

In clinical terms allergic rhinitis can be defined as symptoms of nasal itching, sneezing, discharge, or nasal blocking which occur for more than 1 h on most days. A careful history is essential both to establish the diagnosis and to assess the severity of symptoms in individual patients. An allergic aetiology is suggested by dominant itching, sneezing, and watery discharge. Associated eye or chest symptoms (asthma) point to an allergic cause, and a history of potential allergic triggers should be sought. The diagnosis of allergic rhinitis is often straightforward. However, it should be remembered that allergen exposure, in addition to provoking immediate nasal symptoms, may also result in late symptoms several hours after exposure when an allergic aetiology may be missed. A history of potential allergic triggers includes enquiry into

the seasonality of symptoms and whether symptoms are work related (i.e. occur at work or in the evening following work, with improvement at weekends and during holiday periods). The home environment, including the presence of domestic pets or birds, fitted carpets, central heating, or non-synthetic bedding, should be established. A personal or family history of atopy is extremely common in patients with allergic rhinitis. There are many alternative causes of rhinitic symptoms. Different causes may coexist. Therefore it is always important to consider the differential diagnosis (Table 2).

The presence of facial pain, fever, systemic upset, and mucopurulent discharge suggests an infective aetiology. Nasal obstruction which alternates with the nasal cycle is common to both allergic and infective causes. Nasal crusting and/or bleeding may occur in granulomatous disorders, atrophic rhinitis, or, rarely, tumour (particularly if associated with persistent unilateral symptoms). Impaired taste and/or smell may

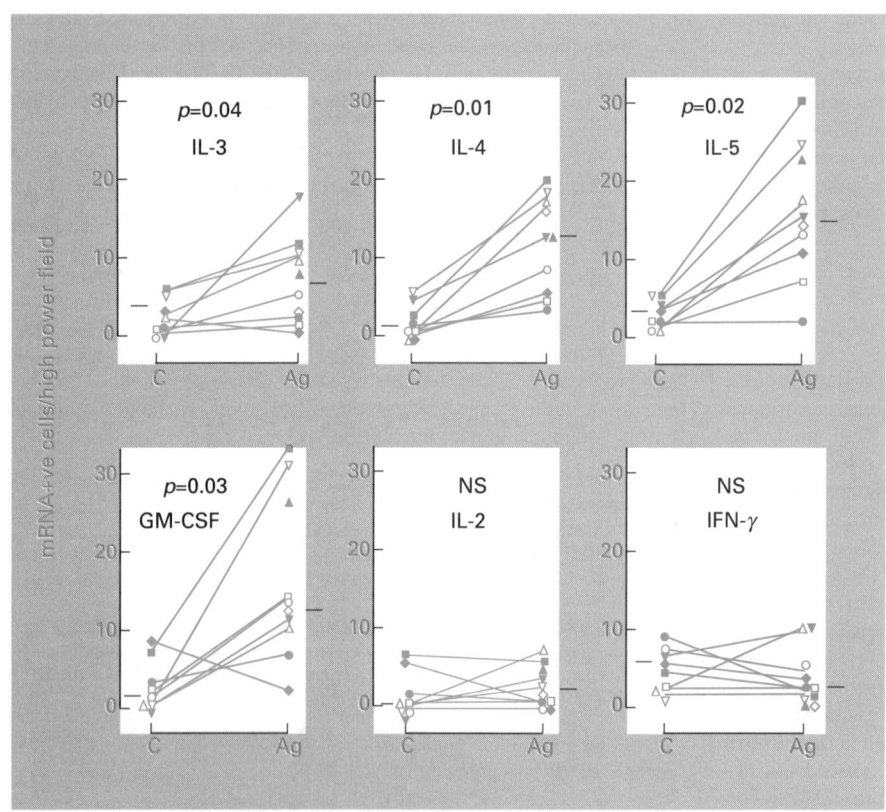

Fig. 3 Cytokine mRNA expression for TH$_2$-type cytokines (particularly IL-4 and IL-5) in the nasal mucosa 24 hours after local allergen challenge (Ag) and following a control challenge (c) using the allergen diluent in the same patients. (Reproduced with permission from Durham *et al.* (1992). *Journal of Immunology,* **148,** 2390–4. Copyright 1992. *The Journal of Immunology.*)

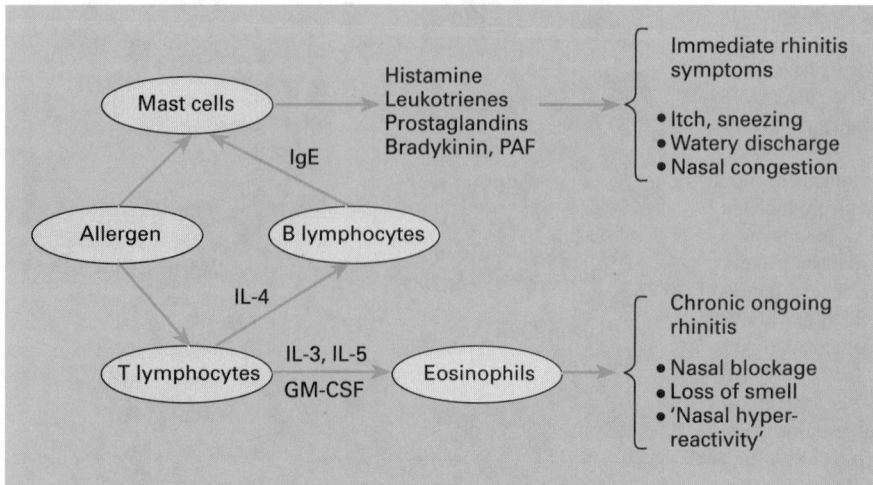

Fig. 4 Hypothesis: pathogenesis of allergic rhinitis.

Table 2 *Differential diagnosis of rhinitis*

Allergic
Seasonal
Perennial
Occupational

Non-allergic
Infective (acute, chronic)
Autonomic
Hormonal
Structural
Drugs
Mucociliary abnormalities
Sarcoidosis
Connective tissue diseases
Immune deficiency syndromes
Tumours
Atrophic
Idiopathic

Table 3 *Advantages of skin-prick tests*

- They diagnose atopy—the underlying predisposition to develop allergic disorders
- They provide helpful supportive evidence (positive or negative) for the clinical history
- They are essential when potentially expensive and time-consuming environmental control measures, the removal of a family pet, or a change of occupation are involved
- They have educational value, providing a clear illustration to the patient which may reinforce verbal advice.

occur with many forms of rhinitis. It is particularly common with nasal polyposis and may occasionally follow trauma (olfactory nerve damage). Enquiry regarding associated chest disease is important. Rhinitis and asthma coexist, and recognition and appropriate treatment of rhinitis may improve asthma control. The presence of infertility and recurrent respiratory infections (including bronchiectasis) should raise the possibility of abnormalities of mucus (Young's syndrome or cystic fibrosis) or ciliary dysfunction (primary ciliary dyskinesia, Kartagener's syndrome). Recurrent respiratory infections or a history of chronic rhinosinusitis should also raise the possibility of immune deficiency states including hypogammaglobulinaemia and acquired immune deficiency syndrome (AIDS). Hormonal imbalance (premenstrual symptoms, pregnancy, hypothyroidism, or acromegaly) may be associated with rhinitis. A history of trauma or previous nasal surgery should be sought. The efficacy, frequency, and regularity of previous treatments should also be established.

Examination

Local examination may be performed with a head mirror and speculum. Alternatively, an ophthalmoscope with an auroscope attachment may be used. Allergic rhinitis is accompanied by a pale bluish 'boggy' appearance of the nasal mucosa only if the patient has current symptoms. A red inflamed appearance with pus suggests an infective cause. A granular appearance with fine pale nodules is diagnostic of sarcoidosis. Enlarged turbinates may be confused with polyps by the unwary. If doubt exists, further examination with rigid and/or flexible endoscope should be performed. The identification of structural abnormalities such as polyps, deflected nasal septum, or enlarged turbinates is important since surgical treatment may be indicated. A major advance has been the development of techniques of minimally invasive endoscopic sinus surgery. Examination of the nose should also include tests of smell and examination of the ears, eyes, mouth, and throat. Examination of the chest and a general examination should also be performed in view of common associations with chest and systemic diseases.

Investigations

Skin-prick tests

In the presence of a clear history, particularly seasonal hay-fever symptoms, skin-prick testing is not essential. However, skin-prick tests are useful for several reasons (Table 3).

Skin-prick tests should only be interpreted in conjunction with the

clinical history. False-positive responses are common. Skin-prick tests should not be performed when the patient is taking antihistamines, if 'dermographism' (wealing in response to pressure) is present, or in the presence of severe eczema. In these circumstances measurement of serum IgE antibodies by radioallergosorbent test (RAST) or enzyme-linked immunosorbent assay (ELISA) is occasionally indicated. A useful basic skin-prick testing kit should include the following:

(1) a positive control (histamine 10 mg/ml);
(2) negative control (allergen diluent solution);
(3) house dust mite (*D. pteronyssinus*);
(4) grass pollen;
(5) cat fur;
(6) *Aspergillus fumigatus*.

Skin-prick tests should be performed with a sterile 23 gauge needle or lancet which is lightly inserted through the epidermis without inducing bleeding. Responses are recorded as mean weal diameter at 15 min. A positive prick test is defined as a weal diameter 2 mm or more greater than that of the negative control test.

Treatment

The mainstay of treatment for allergic rhinitis involves the avoidance of provoking allergens where possible and the use of topical corticosteroids and oral H₁ selective antihistamines (Table 4).

Allergen avoidance

It is not possible to avoid pollens, although sensible advice includes wearing sunglasses and keeping car windows tightly shut. All windows should be kept closed, particularly in high buildings. Walking in parks and wide open spaces should be avoided during the late afternoon or evening when pollen counts are at their highest. A holiday by the sea or abroad during the peak pollen season may be helpful. House dust mite control and avoidance measures should be undertaken in the homes of sensitive individuals with disease. Precise advice concerning the bedroom can be provided, with avoidance of non-synthetic bedding, restriction of soft toys, which should be washable, the use of mattress covers, changes to vinyl or cork flooring, and thorough vacuum cleaning and damp dusting at least once weekly. A leaflet entitled *House dust mites: avoidance measures for allergy sufferers* is available from the British Allergy Foundation, St Bartholomew's Hospital, West Smithfield, London EC1A 7BE. At present, it is possible to recommend that treatment for adults should be concentrated on the bedroom and living room, while measures for sensitive children should be extended to all parts of the home. Measures to eradicate mites and allergens should be undertaken only following proper diagnosis and with appropriate medical supervision. At present there is no firm evidence to recommend the additional use of air conditioners, air ionizers, or acaracides. Where animal exposure is relevant, there is frequent resistance to advice to remove a family pet. However, patients can be advised to avoid replacing animals, to

Table 4 *Treatment of allergic rhinitis*

- Allergen avoidance (house dust mite, animal danders, occupational causes)
- Topical corticosteroids; check technique and place emphasis on regular use even when symptoms are absent
- Non-sedative antihistamines provide helpful combination treatment
- Sodium cromoglycate is useful for eye symptoms and is first choice in children
- Immunotherapy retains a place in pollen-sensitive patients unresponsive to the above measures
- If patient fails to respond, review diagnosis and treat any associated conditions (e.g. antibiotics for infection, surgery for structural problems).

confine them where possible, and to avoid contact with animals or contaminated clothing. Recent evidence suggests that washing the cat is extremely effective in reducing cat allergen exposure!

Pharmacotherapy

A major advance in the treatment of allergic rhinitis in recent years has been the introduction of corticosteroid nasal sprays with high topical potency and a low potential for systemic side-effects. Topical corticosteroids are effective in 70 to 90 per cent of hay fever sufferers. Beclomethasone (Beconase) and budesonide (Rhinocort) are now both available in Freon propellant and aqueous formulations. Aqueous formulations are better tolerated and have a better local distribution in the nose. Side-effects are minor. The importance of regular treatment even when symptoms are absent should be emphasized. The drug should also be commenced before the hay fever season for maximal effect. Attention should be paid to the technique of inhaler use and the regularity of use. Systemic effects are virtually absent at conventional doses, although care should be exercised when concomitant inhaled corticosteroids are used for asthma and/or cutaneous application of steroids for eczema. Recently, fluticasone propionate has been shown to be effective compared with placebo and has the advantage of a once daily dosage. Topical corticosteroids are effective for all symptoms of allergic rhinitis, including nasal blockage.

A further advance has been the availability of potent specific histamine H_1 receptor antagonists with a low potential for anticholinergic side-effects and a low sedative profile. Antihistamines are particularly effective for sneezing, itching, and rhinorrhoea, although, unlike topical corticosteroids, they have little effect on nasal blockage. They have the additional advantage of being effective for eye and throat symptoms. The best tried and tested antihistamine available is probably terfenadine (60 mg twice daily or slow-release formulation 120 mg daily). There is little interaction with alcohol, although a rare important complication is prolongation of the QT interval on the ECG. This only occurs when doses in excess of those recommended are employed, or in the presence of hepatic impairment or concomitant use of ketoconazole or erythromycin which modify the hepatic metabolism of terfenadine. Alternatives include astemizole which is effective, although it has the disadvantage of an extremely long half-life (several weeks). Acrivastine, loratadine, and cetirizine have all been shown to be effective in placebo-controlled trials, although few comparative trials have shown additional benefit to justify their increased costs. Acrivastine has a shorter half-life and may be useful when only occasional episodic symptoms occur. Cetirizine is probably more potent, although may occasionally cause drowsiness. Ideally, all these drugs should be avoided during pregnancy.

Sodium cromoglycate is available as a topical nasal spray for use four times daily. It is less effective than topical corticosteroids, although it

is the first choice in children. Topical cromoglycate eye drops (Opticrom) are effective for allergic eye symptoms in the majority of patients.

In a small proportion of patients whose symptoms are not controlled by the above measures, there is a place for a short course of prednisolone (20 mg daily for 5 days). This approach may also unblock the nose, thereby improving access for topical corticosteroids which may then be more effective. Topical decongestants (oxymetazoline) are effective in treating nasal blockage, although they should only be used for short periods (no more than a few days) in view of the risk of tachyphylaxis and rebound persistent nasal blockage (rhinitis medicamentosa).

Immunotherapy

In patients with sole grass pollen allergy unresponsive to topical corticosteroids and antihistamines, immunotherapy (hyposensitization) retains a place in treatment. Immunotherapy is widely practised in the United States and Europe, although its use has largely disappeared from the United Kingdom following a report from the Committee on Safety of Medicines in 1986. This report questioned the efficacy of immunotherapy and quite rightly expressed concern about occasional deaths in asthmatics from severe bronchospasm and anaphylaxis. The Committee also recommended that injections should be given only where facilities for cardiopulmonary resuscitation are immediately available and that patients should be kept under medical observation for at least 2 h following injections. The Committee's ruling was generally welcomed because it highlighted the potential dangers of immunotherapy, particularly in asthmatic patients. Nevertheless the 2-h waiting period has made this treatment impracticable for both patients and doctors. Several recent controlled studies have confirmed the efficacy of immunotherapy for patients with grass-pollen-induced summer hay fever. It may be considered in those who fail to respond adequately to conventional drug treatment. However, patients should be carefully selected and chronic asthmatics specifically excluded. The procedure should only be performed in specialized centres with access to resuscitative measures.

REFERENCES

Anonymous (1986). CSM Update. Desensitising vaccines. *British Medical Journal*, **293**, 948.

Anonymous (1990). Three new antihistamines—worth staying awake for? *Drugs and Therapeutics Bulletin*, May.

Bascom, R., Pipkorn, U., Lichtenstein, L.M., and Naclerio, R.M. (1988). The influx of inflammatory cells into nasal washings during the late response to antigen challenge: effect of glucocorticoid pretreatment. *American Review of Respiratory Disease*, **138**, 406–12.

Colloff, M.J., Ayres, J., Carswell, F., Howarth, P.H., Merrett, T.G., Mitchell, E.B., *et al.* (1992). The control of allergens of dust mites and domestic pets: a position paper. *Clinical and Experimental Allergy*, **22**, (Suppl. 2), 1–28.

De Blay, R., Chapman, M.D., and Platts-Mills, T.A.E. (1991). Airborne cat allergen (Fel d I): environmental control with the cat *in situ*. *American Review of Respiratory Disease*, **143**, 1334–9.

Durham, S.R., Sun Ying, Varney, V.A., Jacobson, M.R., Sudderick, R.M., Mackay, I.S., *et al.* (1992). Cytokine messenger RNA expression for IL-3, IL-4, IL-5 and granulocyte/macrophage-colony-stimulating factor in the nasal mucosa after allergen challenge: relationship to tissue eosinophilia. *Journal of Immunology*, **148**, 2390–4.

Fleming, D.M. and Crombie, D.L. (1987). Prevalence of asthma and hay-fever in England and Wales. *British Medical Journal*, **294**, 279–83.

Howarth, P.H. (1989). Allergic rhinitis: a rational choice of treatment. *Respiratory Medicine*, **83**, 179–88.

Muranaka, M., Susuki, S., Koizumi, C., Takafuji, S., Miyamoto, T., Ikemori, R., and Tokiwa, H. (1986). Adjuvant activity of diesel exhaust particulates for the production of IgE antibodies in mice. *Journal of Allergy and Clinical Immunology*, **77**, 616–23.

Mygind, N. and Naclerio, R.M. (eds). (1993). *Allergic and non-allergic rhinitis*. Clinical Aspects Munksgaard, Copenhagen.

Naclerio, R.M., Proud, D., Togias, A.G., *et al.* (1985). Inflammatory mediators in late antigen-induced rhinitis. *New England Journal of Medicine* **313**, 65–70.

Pollart, S.M., Smith, T.F., Morris, E.C., Gelber, L.E., Platts-Mills, T.A.E., and Chapman, M.D. (1991). Environmental exposure to cockroach allergens: analysis with monoclonal antibody-based enzyme immunoassays. *Journal of Allergy and Clinical Immunology*, **87**, 505–10.

Varney, V.A. (1991). Hayfever in the United Kingdom. *Clinical and Experimental Allergy*, **21**, 757–62.

Varney, V.A., Gaga, M., Aber, V.R., Kay, A.B., and Durham, S.R. (1991). Usefulness of immunotherapy in patients with severe summer hayfever uncontrolled by antiallergic drugs. *British Medical Journal*, **302**, 265–9.

Varney, V.A., Jacobson, M.R., Sudderick, R.M., Robinson, D.S., Irani, A.-M.A., Schwartz, L.B., *et al.* (1992). Immunohistology of the nasal mucosa following allergen-induced rhinitis. Identification of activated T lymphocytes, eosinophils and neutrophils. *American Review of Respiratory Disease*, **146**, 170–6.

Wierenga, E.A., Snoek, M., De Groot, C., Chretien, I., Bos, J.D., Jansen, H.M., and Kapsenberg, M.L. (1990). Evidence for compartmentalisation of functional subsets of CD4+ T lymphocytes in atopic patients. *Journal of Immunology* **144**, 4651.

World Health Organisation/International Union of Immunological Societies Working Group (1989). Current status of allergen immunotherapy. Shortened version of a WHO/IUISWG report. *Lancet*, **i**, 259–61.

17.8.2 Upper airways obstruction

J. R. Stradling

Definition

The trachea and carina are usually included in discussions of upper airways obstruction. This is because many of the conditions that can completely block off the main airway can affect the trachea, presenting in a similar way to those affecting the larynx and pharynx. For convenience, the causes of upper airways obstruction are divided into acute (within minutes or hours) and non-acute, although there is not quite such a clear distinction in clinical practice. Many of the causes of upper airways obstruction (particularly infection) are more common in children, but this section deals with the problem mainly from an adult physician's perspective.

At resting levels of minute ventilation the main airway can be reduced to 3 mm or so before respiratory distress and stridor occur. Thus not much more obstruction is required to precipitate complete asphyxia. When upper airways obstruction is suspected, assessment of severity, diagnosis and treatment must be regarded as a medical emergency.

Causes (Table 1)

Acute

The most acute obstruction is caused by inhaling foreign bodies, although acute oedema of the upper airways (angio-oedema, thermal injury) can develop rapidly (within minutes). Infections of the upper airways (pharyngitis, tonsillitis, epiglottitis, retropharyngeal abscess, croup) may also present with a dramatic onset, although prodromal symptoms will usually have been present. Haemorrhage is a rare cause, and iatrogenic causes, such as incorrect placement of endotracheal tubes, may occur.

Non-acute

The most important non-acute causes of upper airways obstruction are tumours. These are often misdiagnosed as asthma or chronic airways obstruction. The trachea can be narrowed by intrinsic stenosis (postintubation or following tracheostomy closure), by external compression,

Table 1 *Causes of upper airways obstruction*

Acute	Non-acute
Inhaled foreign body	Tumours

Oedema
  Allergy
  Angioneurotic oedema
  Smoke burns
	Tracheal stenosis
	  Postintubation
	  Post-tracheostomy

Infections
  Pharyngitis
  Tonsillitis
  Epiglottitis
  Retropharyngeal
  abscess
  Croup
	Tracheal compression
	  Tumour
	  Thyroid
	  Aneurysm

	Tracheal abnormalities
	  Tracheomalacia
	  Tracheobronchiomegaly
	  Tracheobronchopathia-
	   osteochondroplastica

	Recurrent laryngeal nerve palsy
	Laryngeal dysfunction

or by abnormalities of the trachea itself such as tracheomalacia, scabbard trachea, and relapsing polychondritis. Laryngeal abnormalities (other than tumours) include recurrent laryngeal nerve damage and laryngeal dysfunction from a variety of other causes.

Diagnosis

Diagnosis of upper airways obstruction requires a high degree of awareness. Not all that wheezes is asthma. If upper airways obstruction develops non-acutely, then it is most likely to be misdiagnosed as asthma or chronic airways obstruction, particularly if, for example, a carcinoma of the trachea coexists with chronic airways obstruction, which is quite likely since both are usually due to smoking. Clues in the history will be a shorter onset than might be expected for chronic airways obstruction and no previous history of a similar problem. The progression is usually relentless without fluctuations. At first stridor or noisy breathing will only be heard on exercise, but it will gradually appear at lower and lower levels of activity. Sometimes the patient is well aware that the blockage is 'somewhere in the neck' and such a complaint should be taken seriously, as should associated haemoptysis. A non-productive cough is often present also. A change in the voice in association with shortness of breath should also alert one to obstruction at the laryngeal level. Sometimes upper airways obstruction is more symptomatic on lying down.

Examination

In pure upper airways obstruction the noisy breathing will localize to the airway and tend to be monophonic and stridulous. Stridor may be absent if there is a long segment of obstruction. The only sound at the periphery on auscultation of the chest will be the transmitted noise of the stridor. However, as mentioned above, there may be lower airways obstruction as well, which should not discourage further investigation of a suggestive history.

If the upper airways obstruction is extrathoracic, the stridor will tend to be worse on inspiration, and the converse may be true when the lesion is intrathoracic. The reasons for this are discussed below.

Lung function

During a forced expiration from total lung volume down to residual volume there is a progressive fall in expiratory flow rates which is largely due to the fact that the airways are becoming narrower as the lungs become smaller, and this progressively restricts maximum flow rates regardless of the effort made. This can be displayed graphically as a plot of expiratory flow against the volume exhaled from total lung capacity down to residual volume, the so called 'flow–volume' plot or loop (Fig 1(a)). This fall-off in maximal flow rates with falling lung volume is called 'volume dependence of flow'. However, if a fixed resistance is introduced (such as tracheal stenosis), then the maximal flow rate possible is independent of the lung volume. Instead of the normal triangular appearance of the flow–volume plot, it has more of a square appearance with the high flows (normally seen at larger lung volumes) severely clipped. At lower lung volumes the normal intrinsic airways resistance may again exceed the abnormal upper airways resistance so that the flow–volume plot may once again follow the normal path (Fig. 1(a)).

Even if the apparatus required to measure flow–volume plots or loops is not available, a peak expiratory flow (**PEF**) meter and spirometry plot may be useful. Because the fixed extra expiratory resistance clips the high flow rates predominantly, then the PEF rate will be reduced disproportionately to the forced expiratory volume in 1 s (**FEV$_1$**). This is because the FEV$_1$ is a measure over a longer time period, which includes lower flow rates because of the falling lung volume. This gives rise to a simple index of upper airways obstruction; FEV$_1$ (ml) divided by the PEF rate (l/min). Normally this index will be less than 10, but as the PEF rate is preferentially clipped (which does not happen when there is increased diffuse airways obstruction such as asthma) it may rise above 10. An index of less than 10 does not exclude upper airways obstruction because the lesion may not be rigid and, if it is intrathoracic, it may also narrow a little as lung volume falls.

The other clue from spirometry is the shape of the FEV$_1$ curve. Normally this is a gentle ever-flattening curve because flow rates (the slope of the curve) are falling. Because of the fixed flow rate of upper airways obstruction this line will tend to become straighter (Fig. 2(a)).

If flow–volume plotting apparatus is available, inspiratory patterns can also be examined. The normal inspiratory limb of the flow–volume loop is almost semicircular (Fig. 1(b)). This is because at residual volume the airways are small and limit flow; towards total lung capacity

Fig. 1 (a) Expiratory flow volume loop. The subject exhales with maximum effort from total lung capacity (TLC) until residual volume (RV) is reached. Normally, maximum flow (vertical axis) is reached early on and the flow falls almost linearly with lung volumes thereafter. In lower airways obstruction (e.g. asthma) all flows are reduced, but particularly at lower lung volumes. In upper airways obstruction the maximum flow is clipped and roughly constant across most of the manoeuvre. (b) Inspiratory volume loop. The subject inhales maximally from residual volume (RV) up to total lung capacity (TLC). Normally, maximum flow is reached at about half-way when there is the best combination of airways size and muscle strength (see text). In upper airways obstruction maximum flow is determined by the size of the remaining orifice and is roughly constant across the manoeuvre.

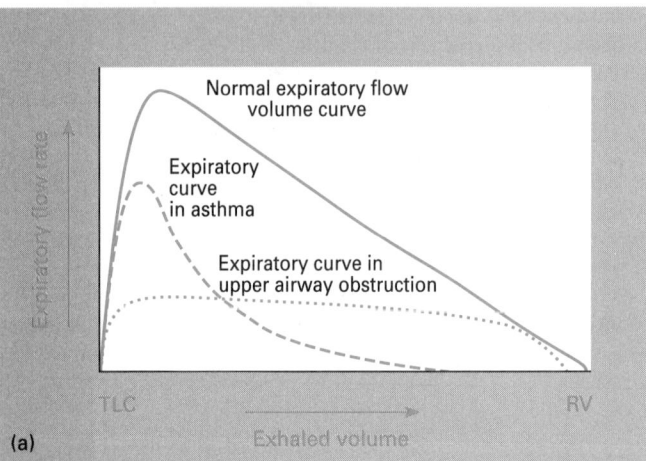

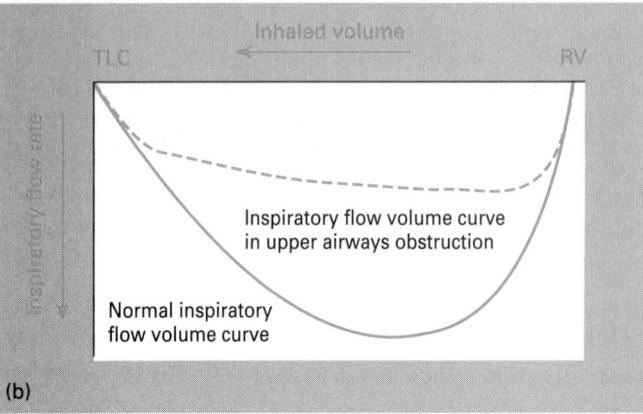

Fig. 2 (a) Curves of forced expiratory volume (FEV) against time. Normally exhalation is rapid, and more than 75 per cent of the final volume (vital capacity (VC)) is exhaled in 1 s (FEV$_1$). In lower airways obstruction, flows are slower and thus less air is exhaled in 1 s; the line is still curved because flows are falling. In upper airways obstruction, because flows are roughly constant at a low level set by the remaining orifice, the line is nearly straight and FEV$_1$ is also low. (b) Following a forced exhalation manoeuvre into a spirometer, a forced inhalation can be made. Normally inspiration is fast and the forced inspiratory volume in 1 s (FIV$_1$) is almost the vital capacity (VC). If there is upper airways obstruction, particularly extrathoracic such as at the vocal cords, then inspiration will be very limited and FIV$_1$ will be small.

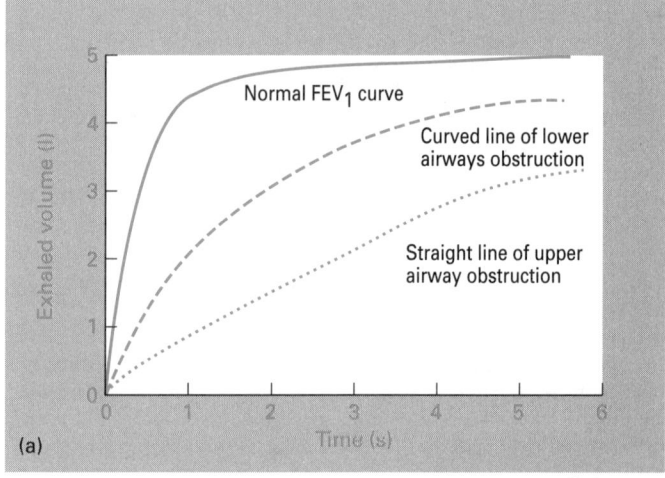

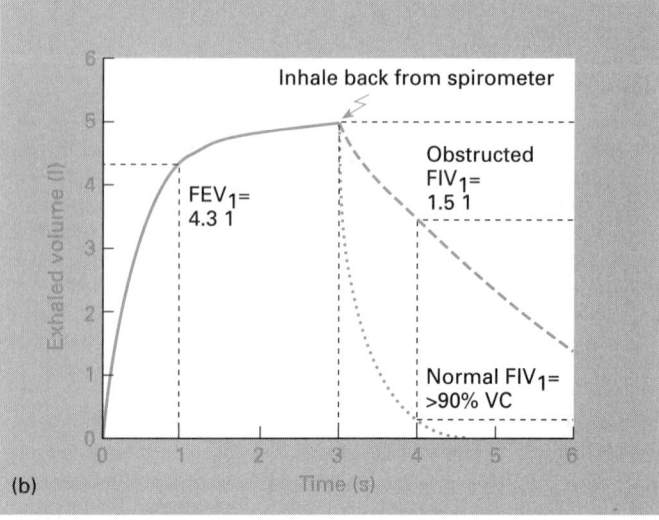

the inspiratory muscles are reaching their full contraction and power is falling off. Hence maximum flows are achieved in the mid-range of lung volume (Fig. 1(b)). Again, if upper airways obstruction is present, this pattern may be replaced by a squarer shape owing to the imposition of a lower maximum flow rate by the fixed resistance (Fig. 1(b)).

A comparison of the inspiratory and expiratory limbs may also give some clues as to the location of an upper airways obstruction. If the lesion is extrathoracic and has any variability to its lumen, it will tend to be narrowest during inspiration (walls sucked together) and widest during expiration (blown apart). Conversely, an intrathoracic lesion will tend to be squashed on expiration by the raised intrathoracic pressures, thus presenting a higher resistance than during inspiration when it will tend to be pulled open. Although in theory these statements are correct, in practice flow–volume loops are not always sufficiently characteristic to allow a confident diagnosis about the exact site and presence of an upper airways obstruction. They may be more useful as a tool to follow changes, such as in response to treatment.

Vocal cord paresis due to bilateral recurrent laryngeal nerve damage is often very much worse on inspiration. Simple spirometry can be diagnostic here. The expiratory tracing will be normal as the cords are blown apart. If the patient immediately inhales back from the spirometer (make sure that a new in-line filter is present first) the inspiratory rate will be tortuously slow (Fig. 2(b)). The forced inspiratory volume in 1 s (FIV_1) will often be much smaller than the FEV_1, whereas normally the reverse is true (Fig. 2(b)).

The effect of breathing a low density gas mixture such as 21 per cent oxygen in helium (Heliox) on airways resistance has also been used to try to differentiate lower from upper airways obstruction. Flow in small airways is largely laminar and not affected by the density of the intraluminal gas. However, flow at a tight stenosis will be turbulent, and then becomes dependent on the gas density. Thus airflow resistance will fall on breathing Heliox if the obstruction is in the upper airways, but will remain unchanged when the increased resistance is due to peripheral airways narrowing. This test may be particularly useful when there is evidence of both lower and upper airways obstruction, but proof of a significant contribution from an upper airways lesion is required before considering any intervention.

For simple monitoring of progress, once the diagnosis is known (e.g. during treatment), the PEF rate is probably adequate.

Bronchoscopic and radiological findings are discussed in the following sections.

Specific causes

Acute

ASPIRATION

Aspiration of an object sufficiently large to cause acute upper airways obstruction is usually due to its lodging in the larynx, since this is the narrowest portion of the airway until two or three divisions down the bronchial tree. The object is usually a piece of food, and thus this condition has been colourfully called the 'café coronary'. The patient will suddenly become distressed, be unable to talk, and apparently unable to breathe. He may point to his throat trying to indicate the problem. Inspiration may not be possible to provide the air necessary for a good expulsive cough. Indeed, lung volume may 'ratchet' down to residual volume.

The Heimlich manoeuvre was invented for this circumstance. If the patient is still upright then the helper stands behind with his arms clasped around the upper abdomen. A very forceful pull, backwards and upwards, will drive the diaphragm upwards and should provide enough expired air to shift the aspirated food off the cords (Fig. 3). The manoeuvre can be repeated, of course, but a forceful first try is likely to be the most successful. The principles of this manoeuvre can and should be taught to first-aid workers. If the Heimlich manoeuvre fails, then it may

be possible to dislodge the lump of food with a finger once the patient has become unconscious. The only alternative is an emergency cricothyrotomy which requires a hole to be made in the cricothyroid membrane just below the Adam's apple of the thyroid cartilage and above the cricoid cartilage. Even a small hole (2 mm or so) will allow sufficient ventilation to keep the patient alive. Emergency cricothyroidotomies have been attempted with everything from penknives to ballpoint pens: special large-bore curved-needle kits are available for the purpose and are safer than an unskilled attempt at a tracheostomy.

OEDEMA

Acute oedema of the larynx or pharynx is usually either due to allergy (atopic or non-atopic), a hereditary abnormality in the complement pathway, or inhalation of noxious gases.

Episodes of upper airways and facial oedema sometimes have no known cause and appear without warning. Often there will be an atopic history with a specific allergy. Some allergic reactions are not based on atopy and IgE, but may occur through IgG or direct activation of other inflammatory pathways. Allergies to nuts, strawberries, etc. may involve this latter mechanism rather than IgE. Insect stings usually produce pharyngeal and glottic oedema via IgE mechanisms.

Treatment of these allergic causes of upper airways obstruction consists of subcutaneous (or intramuscular) adrenaline (1 ml of 1:1000) with antihistamines and steroids. Aerosolized adrenaline may also be useful, using 10 ml of 1:10 000 in an ordinary nebulizer. Desensitization to insect stings is possible, but should be carried out with facilities for resuscitation nearby because of the occasional severe anaphylactic reactions to the injections.

Hereditary angio-oedema is due to a deficiency (true or functional) of plasma C1 esterase inhibitor. There are also similar acquired forms of angio-oedema due to activation by a paraprotein. The absence of C1 esterase inhibitor means that the enzyme activating the first component of the complement pathway is unchecked, thus allowing greater activation of the whole pathway and its vasoactive products. This abnormality is often first manifest in infancy and there is usually a family history, as it is an autosomal dominant condition. Colicky abdominal pain due to intestinal oedema is an alternative presentation when the

Fig. 3 The Heimlich manoeuvre for the emergency treatment of acute pharyngeal or laryngeal obstruction due to a bolus of food. Two or three sharp thrusts in the direction of the arrow may cause the food to be ejected (Reproduced with permission from Flenley 1990.)

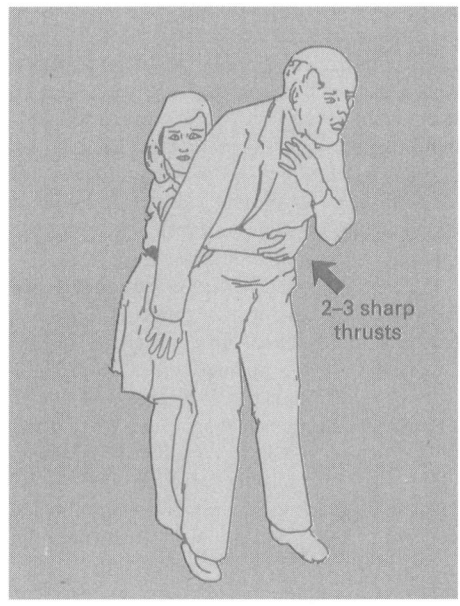

2–3 sharp thrusts

pooling of fluid in oedematous bowel may be sufficient to cause hypotension and shock.

Diagnosis hinges on the clinical presentation, a positive family history, and low levels of C1 esterase inhibitor. In the form where normal amounts of inactive C1 esterase inhibitor are present, it is necessary to demonstrate low C4 levels during an attack. An episode of swelling is often precipitated by local trauma, such as a tooth extraction or a blow to the face, and lasts about 48 to 72 h. The skin manifestations do not itch in the way that allergic oedema does.

Mortality in this condition is such that about 25 to 30 per cent of sufferers will eventually die from asphyxia if adequate treatment is not available. Treatment of the acute attack consists of adrenaline and steroids, although the response is much less satisfactory than in allergic oedema. Emergency tracheostomy or cricothyrotomy may be necessary. Purified C1 esterase inhibitor is available, but takes time to work. Fresh-frozen plasma is reported to work sometimes, although it will also contain more C4 and C2 which may provide more substrate and hence provoke more oedema.

Prophylaxis of hereditary angioneurotic oedema is possible in several ways. Danazol (or other androgenic steroid) raises C1 esterase inhibitor levels within a few weeks. The mode of action of this drug is not fully understood, but it probably increases hepatic synthesis. ϵ-Aminocaproic acid will prevent most attacks, mainly by inhibiting plasmin. If episodes such as tooth extractions are triggers, then C1 esterase inhibitor can be given on the preceding day.

Inhalation of hot smoke can burn the upper airways and contributes significantly to deaths due to fires. Upper airways obstruction due to heat injury and mucosal swelling usually develops within 24 h of exposure, but stenosis due to scarring can develop later. A hoarse voice, stridor, severe conjunctivitis, burnt nasal hairs, and falling peak flow all suggest significant upper airways damage. Bronchoscopy is then the best tool to establish whether there is significant oedema or mucosal ulceration obstructing the airways.

Management usually consists of simple measures such as elevating the head of the bed and inhaling cool moist air with added oxygen. If peak flow continues to fall, then transfer to an intensive care unit and bronchoscopy with the capability to perform an intubation, guided by direct vision, is the correct approach.

INFECTIONS

Upper airways infections rarely cause obstruction in adults, but can do so in infants and young children. Streptococcal pharyngitis, tonsillitis, and retropharyngeal abscesses are amongst the most important. Croup (due to para-influenza and other viruses) is very common, with narrowing of the subglottic trachea, sometimes with a thick purulent coating over the larynx and trachea; respiratory syncytial and parainfluenza viruses are the usual cause. Treatment consists of cool mist and supplemental oxygen, with careful monitoring of upper airways function.

Although again more common in children, acute epiglottitis, usually due to *Haemophilus influenzae*, can affect adults. Pyrexia, drooling, hoarse voice, difficulty in breathing, intense sore throat, and stridor are the usual presenting symptoms. Compared with croup, there is usually a faster onset and course. The diagnosis may be missed initially but lateral neck radiographs show swelling of the epiglottis (Fig. 4). Attempts to examine the back of the throat may precipitate further obstruction, particularly in children. Even tipping the head back for a lateral neck radiograph may be disastrous. Thus, if there is evidence of breathing difficulty with stridor and the clinical diagnosis is epiglottitis, then the usual management for children is immediate transfer to intensive care and intubation for 48 to 72 h whilst the infection is controlled by ampicillin or chloramphenicol. In adults, close monitoring in intensive care is probably adequate and prophylactic intubation is not routinely practised.

General use of *H. influenzae* vaccines should make this problem increasingly rare.

Non-acute

TUMOURS

Laryngeal, and less commonly tracheal, tumours are usually seen in smokers. The dominant cell type is squamous. Spread of a primary bronchial carcinoma into the base of the trachea is probably the commonest cause of upper airways obstruction in pulmonology practice.

Laryngeal tumours nearly always present with hoarseness, or voice change, and cough. Large airways tumours are commonly undiagnosed until far advanced. This is because they mimic lower airways obstruction, as mentioned earlier, and chest radiography is often normal. Tumours may also respond to asthma therapy, showing temporary shrinkage with steroids, which may further mask the real diagnosis.

If history, examination, and lung function tests suggest an upper airways obstruction, then some form of imaging is required. CT is the least invasive approach and therefore least likely to disturb the airway and make matters worse, but of course will provide no histology. Plain films (posteroanterior and lateral) may show tracheal narrowing but they can be very deceptive. Direct visualization is usually necessary for diagnosis and to aid future therapy.

There is some disagreement as to whether fibreoptic or rigid bronchoscopy should be the investigation of choice. Rigid bronchoscopy requires anaesthesia and sometimes this precipitates acute obstruction; then the bronchoscope has to be passed quickly and forced through the obstructing tumour. This 'core-out' may reduce tumour bulk with control of haemorrhage possible under direct vision. This improvement in the airway will buy time while other treatments such as radiotherapy are employed. Flexible fibreoptic bronchoscopy may be possible without disturbing the tumour, although any coughing and increased secretions can precipitate complete occlusion. Direct application of adrenaline may help as an initial emergency treatment, and in theory cocaine (a vasoconstrictor) would be preferable to lignocaine as a local anaesthetic. If the stenosis is less than 4 mm or so, it is probably best left alone during flexible bronchoscopy and certainly should not be biopsied (Fig. 5). Alternatively, the flexible bronchoscope can be introduced with

Fig. 4 Lateral neck radiograph of a child with epiglottitis. Note the swollen epiglottis overlying the glottis.

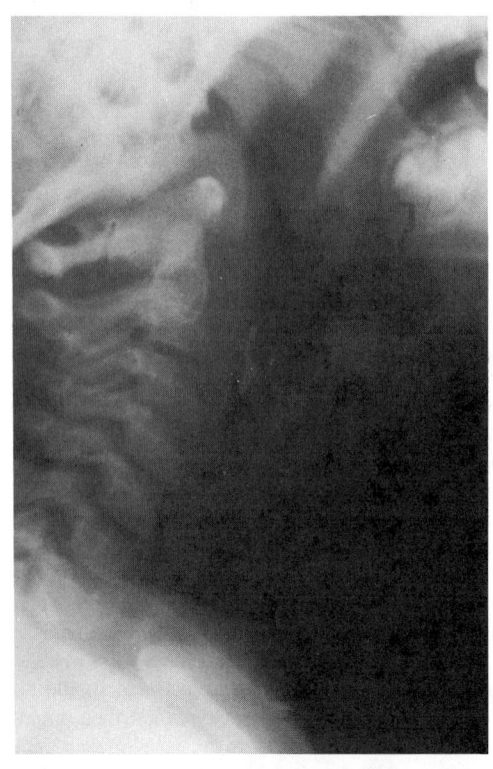

an endotracheal tube passed over it first. This allows a guided intubation in an emergency, using the bronchoscope as a guidewire.

Whilst waiting for other treatments to work or be organized, dexamethasone (12 mg daily), nebulized adrenaline (10 ml of 1:10 000 up to six times daily), humidification of inspired air, and breathing Heliox (21 per cent oxygen in helium) are all that is really available.

Improvement in the airway may be achieved by treatment of the tumour with chemotherapy or radiotherapy. Sometimes there is an initial swelling of the tumour so that steroids are usually prescribed first, with emergency treatments kept close to the patient (Heliox, adrenaline). If these therapies do not help, then palliation can be achieved with the use of bronchoscopically guided laser therapy literally to burn away tumour tissue with a low incidence of serious haemorrhage. This is a laborious procedure, currently only available in a few specialist centres. It is only of use with intraluminal tumours and cannot be applied when the narrowing is due to external compression. Another approach is the use of silicon or metal endobronchial stents. Some of these stents can be inserted bronchoscopically and others require surgery. The stents are particularly useful when external compression is present. It is rarely appropriate to 'debulk' a malignant tumour at thoracotomy in an attempt to improve large airway patency.

Unfortunately, in many cases upper airways obstruction from a tumour becomes a terminal event. Powerful sedation is indicated because the patient should be made unaware that he or she is asphyxiating and choking to death.

There are some rare non-malignant tumours that can obstruct the trachea, and rarely granulomatous conditions such as sarcoid and Wegener's granulomatosis may mimic tumour.

TRACHEAL STENOSIS

Tracheal stenosis usually develops either following prolonged intubation or after a tracheostomy has been allowed to close following tube removal (Fig. 6). This scarring may appear some time after the initiating event. Again, radiology or bronchoscopy will usually confirm the diagnosis, already strongly suspected from the history. Temporary treatment may be possible by dilating the stricture at rigid bronchoscopy. Definitive treatment involves resection of the stenosed portion and reanastomosis.

TRACHEAL COMPRESSION

Tracheal compression (Fig. 7) may be due to malignant or non-malignant conditions. External compression by malignant tumour (primary or secondary) has essentially been covered in the previous section. Non-malignant causes include thyroid enlargement, aortic aneurysm, scle-

rosing mediastinitis, mediastinal neurofibroma, and Castleman's disease. If definitive treatment is not possible, then stenting the airway is the only treatment possible. When thyroid enlargement leads to tracheal obstruction, surgical removal may not solve the problem completely. Prolonged pressure on the trachea can lead to tracheomalacia so that a tracheal wall, now unsupported by the thyroid, will collapse. Temporary use of an endotracheal silicone stent is then appropriate.

TRACHEAL ABNORMALITIES

Tracheomalacia may be secondary to prolonged external compression (see above) or a primary abnormality that presents in childhood. It is essentially a weakness or deficiency of the supporting cartilages. It is sometimes seen secondary to a long history of chronic airways obstruction. Normally the anteroposterior diameter of the trachea decreases by up to about 10 per cent during a cough. In tracheomalacia, collapse during coughing is over 50 per cent and sometimes is complete. The symptoms of this are usually stridor, shortness of breath, and paroxysms of coughing. In addition, there can be an inefficient cough with recurrent pneumonia and bronchiectasis.

A 'scabbard trachea' is said to be present when the lateral dimensions of the trachea are significantly narrower than the anteroposterior dimensions. This deformity is usually present along the whole intrathoracic trachea and is normally associated with chronic airways obstruction. It rarely causes severe upper airways obstruction and on a plain chest radiograph there is obvious tracheal ring calcification.

Fig. 6 Bronchoscopic view of a post-tracheostomy tracheal stricture. The remaining hole is about 2–3 mm in diameter. (By courtesy of Dr P. Stradling.)

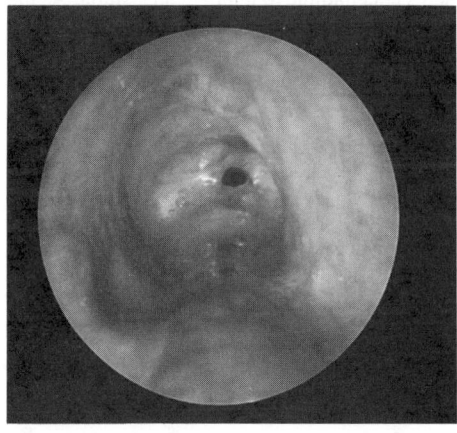

Fig. 7 Bronchoscopic view of external tracheal compression by right-sided paratracheal malignant nodes. (By courtesy of Dr P. Stradling.)

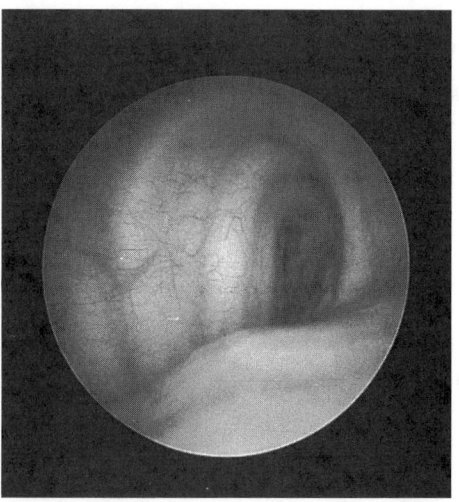

Fig. 5 Bronchoscopic view of a tracheal carcinoma blocking most of the lumen. (By courtesy of Dr P. Stradling.)

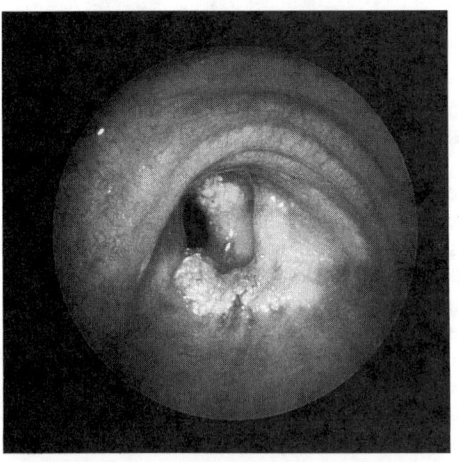

Tracheobronchiomegaly (or Mounier–Kuhn disease) is probably an inherited structural abnormality of the trachea presenting in adult life as apparent chronic airways obstruction. The trachea is dilated from the larynx to the second- or third-generation airways. There is atrophy of both cartilage and muscle. This condition is usually misdiagnosed as chronic airways obstruction; the presence of prolonged but ineffectual coughing and harsh upper airway sounds should lead to lung function tests which then show evidence of an expiratory (intrathoracic) upper airway resistance. Radiological examination will show the dilated airways.

Tracheobronchopathia osteochondroplastica is a very rare condition characterized by cartilaginous and bony excrescences growing into the large airway lumina. This can lead to significant upper airways obstruction, but is more often a postmortem finding which is unsuspected in life.

Relapsing polychondritis is an 'autoimmune' systemic disorder affecting cartilage all over the body (ribs, trachea, ear lobes, nose, joints) and is associated with systemic lupus erythematosus, Wegener's granulomatosis, and cryptogenic liver cirrhosis. Large airways involvement is a frequent cause of death in this condition. There is irregular narrowing of the trachea and main airways with some flaccidity which allows marked collapse on expiration. The clinical picture should be clear, with involvement of other cartilaginous sites. Treatment requires steroids and other immunosuppressive therapy.

LARYNGEAL DYSFUNCTION

Damage to one recurrent laryngeal nerve usually causes a weak voice that improves a little with time as the opposite cord 'learns' to compensate and move slightly across the midline to improve apposition. As the recurrent laryngeal nerve is invaded or compressed (usually by tumour at the left hilum), differential effects on abductors and adductors may be seen. For example, unapposed adduction may occur prior to complete paralysis. Bilateral recurrent laryngeal nerve paralysis produces flaccid cords that lie passively midway between full abduction and adduction, whereas damage to the superior laryngeal nerves supplying the cricothyroid (a vocal cord tensor) causes only a weak voice with speech still possible because the main adductors still function. Because there is very poor abduction with bilateral recurrent laryngeal nerve paralysis, rapid inspiration will draw the cords together and produce stridor, thus limiting exercise tolerance. Because of the general decrease in muscle tone during sleep, any residual laryngeal abductor activity will tend to decrease. Thus inspiratory stridor may initially be present only at night. Although this may be labelled as snoring, careful questioning of a witness will identify whether snoring or the machinery-like screech of inspiratory stridor is present (particularly if the physician can imitate the two noises).

The usual clinical history is of a voice change following thyroidectomy some years before. This may have been quite subtle, such as difficulty in singing but with speech relatively unaffected. Then over the following years nocturnal stridor develops with a reduction in exercise tolerance. Eventually the obstruction at night may be sufficient to produce obstructive apnoea and respiratory failure. This late progression may be due to involvement of the previously damaged recurrent laryngeal nerves in scarring at the thyroidectomy site. Sometimes bilateral paralysis can occur for no apparent reason, and it is assumed that the aetiology is similar to Bell's palsy or the diaphragmatic palsy of neuralgic amyotrophy.

Laryngeal surgery would be possible to prevent inspiratory cord closure, but at the expense of the voice. Thus a tracheostomy with speaking tube is the usual approach. However, if the night-time obstruction is the main problem (with sleep disruption and daytime sleepiness), nasal continuous positive airway pressure therapy will usually keep the cords apart during sleep.

Apart from laryngeal paralysis, laryngeal destructive conditions such as rheumatoid arthritis can lead to poor abduction with inspiratory stridor, particularly at night. In Parkinson's disease with autonomic involvement (Shy–Drager syndrome) or more generalized brain atrophy (multisystem atrophy) there can be a fairly specific wasting of the laryngeal abductors. This also presents with inspiratory stridor (or apnoea) at night and can progress to respiratory failure.

Functional laryngeal abnormalities, with narrowing during either inspiration or expiration, can occur. These may be due to psychological problems, but the syndrome blends with reflex laryngeal dysfunction in patients with asthma. Some patients with asthma develop expiratory laryngeal wheezing. This may occur, even when the asthma is well controlled, in response to emotional pressures or be part of worsening asthma. In this situation the laryngeal component of the increased airways resistance can be considerable. Inhalations of histamine can sometimes mimic this and therefore may be due to a reflex originating from afferent receptors. Why this should happen is not clear, but it may be activation of the laryngeal braking mechanism to help raise functional residual capacity.

Functional inspiratory stridor is not particularly related to asthma, but may follow a respiratory tract infection. There is some evidence that techniques used by speech therapists can help with this problem.

REFERENCES

Empey, D.W. (1972). Assessment of upper airways obstruction. *British Medical journal*, **3**, 503–5.
Flenley, D.C. (1990). *Respiratory medicine*. Baillière Tindall, London.
Fraser, R.G., Paré, J.A.P., Paré, P.D., Fraser, F.S., and Genereux, G.P. (1990). *Diagnosis of diseases of the chest*, Vol. 3. W.B. Saunders, Philadelphia, PA.
Goldman, J. and Muers, M. (1991). Vocal cord dysfunction and wheezing. *Thorax*, **46**, 401–4.

17.9 Airways disease

17.9.1 Asthma

(a) Basic mechanisms and pathophysiology

A. J. FREW and S. T. HOLGATE

Introduction

Bronchial asthma is a common clinical condition which affects individuals at almost any age and is an important cause of respiratory morbidity and mortality. Recent epidemiological surveys suggest that the prevalence of asthma is steadily increasing, while death rates attributed to asthma have remained stable or have slightly increased over the past 30 years. The cause of these temporal trends in asthma prevalence is unclear: in part they represent changes in diagnostic labelling, but there does appear to have been a real increase in prevalence. A number of explanations have been proposed, including increased environmental pollution from motor vehicles, dietary changes associated with affluence, and the increased use of bottle feeding with cow's milk in infancy. Increased mortality rates from asthma may also be partly due to changes in diagnostic labelling, but the widespread use of β-adrenergic agonists has also been implicated. Much new information on the pathophysiology of asthma has been obtained in the past 15 years, and the recent advent of fibreoptic bronchoscopy as a research tool has allowed detailed examination of the respiratory tract in mild asthma. This has led to a fundamental reappraisal of the pathophysiological mechanisms of this disease and has provided a firm scientific basis for treatment strategies in this condition.

Causes of asthma

Asthma can arise at any age, but there are peaks of onset in childhood and in middle life. Childhood asthma is usually associated with atopic allergy, whereas adult onset asthma often (but not always) arises in non-atopic individuals. Both allergic and non-allergic asthma appear to have significant inherited components.

The inheritance of asthma *per se* does not obey simple Mendelian laws, and family studies suggest that genetic and environmental components are required before asthma becomes evident. Several lines of evidence suggest that the ability to make large amounts of IgE which is directed against environmental allergens (atopy) is genetically controlled. IgE responses to highly purified allergen fragments are often restricted to individuals bearing a particular major histocompatibility complex (**MHC**) class II haplotype, but IgE responses to more complex allergens (e.g. house dust mite and animal danders) are not MHC restricted. Correspondingly, there are no clear associations of atopic asthma with particular HLA types. Genetic linkage studies have suggested that atopy (defined as one or more skin tests to a common aero-allergen, clinical asthma, rhinitis, or conjunctivitis) is strongly linked through direct maternal transmission to the gene for the β chain of the FcεRI molecule on the long arm of chromosome 11 in some families; further studies of this are in train. It is important to recognize that development of atopy is not sufficient to cause allergic asthma since many individuals have allergic rhinitis or allergic conjunctivitis without clinical asthma or any evidence of increased bronchial irritability. Nevertheless, atopic allergy is an important cause of asthma and is an important inducer of episodic symptoms in those who are already sensitized to airborne allergens.

When asthma arises in adult life, it may represent reactivation of childhood asthma, in which case atopic allergy is usually demonstrable. Asthma arising *de novo* in adulthood is less frequently associated with atopy. The serum IgE concentration is usually within the normal range and skin tests to common airborne allergens are negative. Many individuals with late-onset asthma appear to develop the condition for the first time following upper respiratory tract infections. Rhinovirus infection has been linked with the development of asthma on both clinical and epidemiological grounds. Moreover, most individuals with asthma experience acute exacerbations when they develop upper respiratory tract infections. Respiratory viruses are also important in childhood asthma, and an epidemiological survey of asthma in schoolchildren found virus infection in nearly 80 per cent of exacerbations when sensitive isolation techniques based on the polymerase chain reaction were used (Fig. 1).

Occupational asthma is an important cause of ill health in the workplace. A wide range of organic and inorganic materials have been implicated as causes of occupational asthma. These can be loosely divided into high molecular weight and low molecular weight agents. High molecular weight occupational agents (e.g. rat urinary protein) cause asthma through the same mechanisms as other airborne protein allergens such as grass pollen and house dust mite antigens. IgE is usually demonstrable and there is strong association with atopic status. In contrast, occupational asthma due to low molecular weight agents (isocyanates, acid anhydrides, platinum salts, plicatic acid) is less clearly linked to IgE, except in the case of platinum salts, and pre-existent atopy is not a risk factor for low molecular weight occupational asthma.

While withdrawal from exposure often leads to clinical improvement, it is quite common for occupational asthma to persist despite cessation of exposure, and in these cases the clinical picture gradually comes to resemble intrinsic asthma.

Bronchial hyper-responsiveness

Asthma is characterized by marked variation in the calibre of the intrapulmonary airways over short periods of time. In addition, asthmatic individuals often report acute episodes of asthma on exposure to non-specific irritants such as cold air, inorganic dusts, cigarette smoke, perfumes, paint, etc. These are not allergic responses, but are exaggerated responses of the airways to the non-specific irritant. This phenomenon is termed non-specific bronchial hyper-responsiveness and can be formally documented by the response to the non-specific bronchoconstrictors methacholine or histamine.

In experimental studies, a wide range of non-specific stimuli have been used to induce bronchospasm in asthmatic patients; some agents

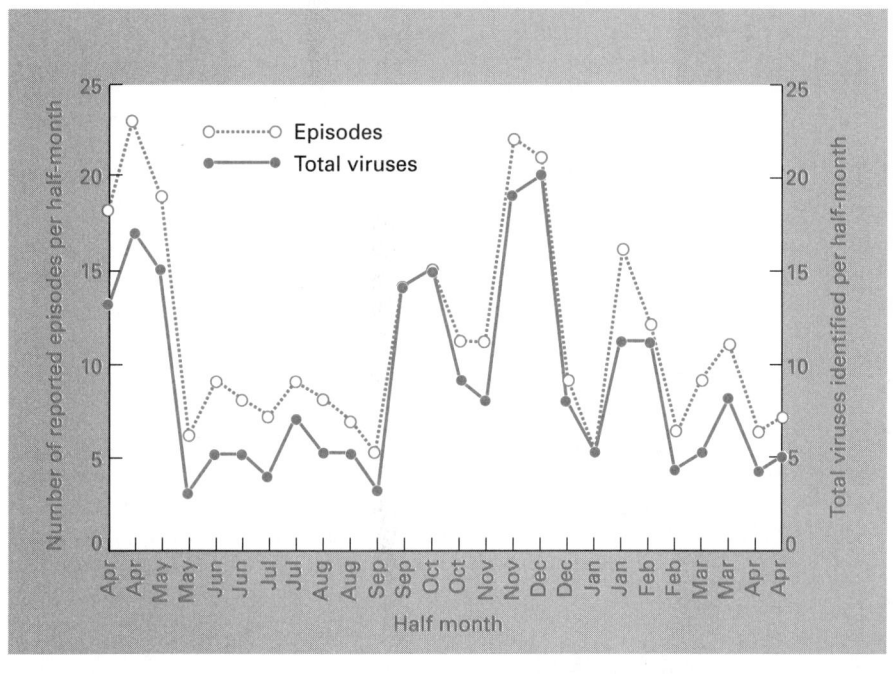

Fig. 1 Relationship of exacerbations of asthma to episodes of viral infection in a group of schoolchildren with respiratory symptoms. (Reproduced with permission from Dr S.L. Johnston.)

act directly on the airways smooth muscle (histamine, methacholine, etc.), while others act indirectly either by inducing the release of mast cell mediators (adenosine etc.) or through neural reflex mechanisms. Some of these agents will also induce bronchoconstriction in non-asthmatic individuals, but this increased non-specific responsiveness is characteristic of asthma and correlates with disease severity (Fig. 2). Other pharmacological agents have no direct bronchoconstrictor effect but increase bronchial responsiveness by increasing epithelial permeability or increasing postreceptor sensitivity of smooth muscle. Several mechanisms have been proposed to explain bronchial hyper-responsiveness. Originally it was thought that the abnormality might lie in the bronchial

Fig. 2 Schematic representation of the relationship between response to methacholine and severity of asthma (non-specific bronchial hyper-responsiveness).

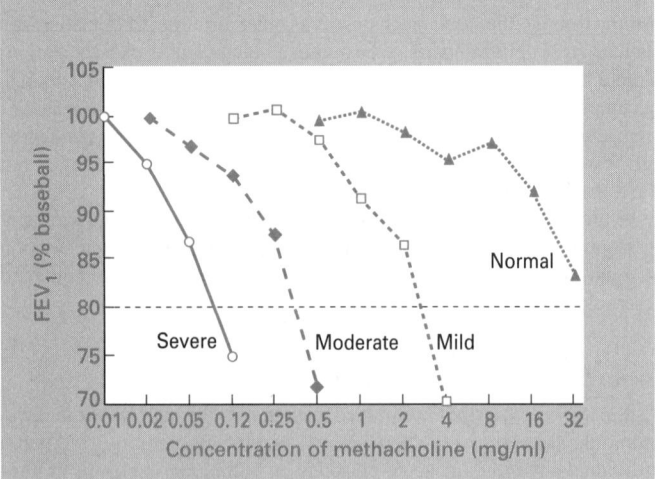

Fig. 3 Influence of airways geometry on bronchial responsiveness to a fixed dose of a non-specific bronchoconstrictor.

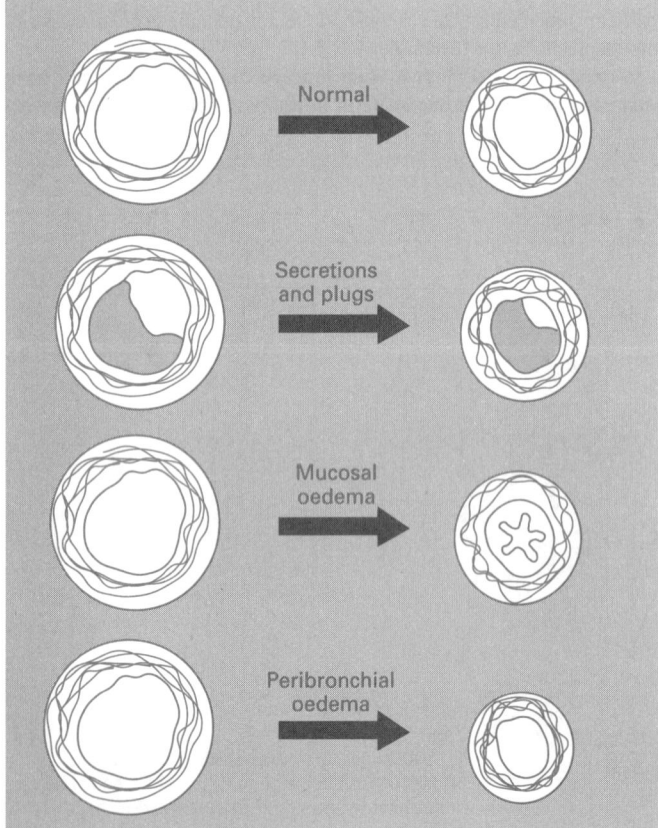

smooth muscle, but the accumulated evidence indicates that bronchial smooth muscle behaves no differently in asthmatics than in normal subjects when studied *in vitro*. Current thinking emphasizes the importance of changes in the geometry of the airways in the response to broncho-constriction (Fig. 3). Thickening of the airways mucosa due to inflammation and oedema has little influence on baseline airways resistance, but when the bronchial smooth muscle contracts the swollen mucosa continues to occupy the same absolute volume and thus the airways lumen is decreased by a much greater proportion than if the mucosa was not swollen. Since resistance is inversely proportional to the fourth power of the radius (Poiseuille's law), a small increase in the thickness of the airways mucosa will have a marked effect on airways resistance in response to a given contraction of the bronchial smooth muscle. Intraluminal secretion of mucus and cells will also narrow the lumen and, like mucosal swelling, will have a disproportionate effect on airways resistance when the bronchial smooth muscle contracts. Finally, peribronchial oedema reduces the elastic recoil of the airways and this in turn allows a greater degree of airways narrowing to a given dose of a bronchoconstricting agonist.

There is more to bronchial asthma than bronchial hyper-responsiveness, but symptoms such as exercise-induced asthma, nocturnal asthma, cough, and variability of peak flow measurement are largely manifestations of different types of bronchial hyper-responsiveness. Measurements of bronchial hyper-responsiveness by inhalation challenge have been widely used in epidemiological studies of asthma but are not usually required in clinical management, except in cases where there is doubt about the diagnosis of asthma or in the assessment of occupational asthma. Finally, it is worth noting that β-adrenergic agonists have no effect on bronchial responsiveness, while inhaled corticosteroids significantly reduce hyper-responsiveness when used regularly over 4 to 6 weeks.

The pathology of asthma

Until quite recently, virtually all the available information on the histology of asthma was based on postmortem studies. When individuals die from acute severe asthma, their lungs show widespread obstruction of the small airways with mucus plugs containing fibrin and eosinophils. Death in such cases is primarily due to asphyxiation secondary to endobronchial plugging rather than bronchoconstriction. The bronchial epithelium is often damaged and may be shed into the airway. The basement membrane is thickened with subepithelial fibrosis and there is bronchial inflammation with oedema, vasodilatation, and a mixed cellular infiltrate consisting of eosinophils, neutrophils, and T lymphocytes. Ten years ago, it was thought that these changes reflected severe fatal asthma and were not present in milder forms of the disease.

This view has radically changed following a series of studies which have used fibreoptic bronchoscopy to obtain biopsies from asthmatic airways for histological examination. It turns out that bronchial biopsies from mild asthmatics show inflammatory changes similar to those found in asthma deaths, with fragility of the bronchial epithelium and subepithelial fibrosis with deposition of types III and V collagen. Light and electron microscopy reveal mast-cell degranulation and infiltration by eosinophils and mononuclear cells (Figs. 4 and 5). The eosinophils present in such biopsies are activated as shown by monoclonal antibody staining for the secreted form of eosinophil cationic protein on their surface.

The lymphocyte content is slightly increased in bronchial biopsies from asthmatic subjects but the principal difference from control subjects is that the T lymphocytes present in asthmatic biopsies are activated as shown by expression of the IL-2 receptor (CD25) and the presence of mRNA for the cytokines IL-5 and granulocyte–macrophage colony-stimulating factor. These changes are clinically relevant in that there is an association between eosinophil infiltration, T-cell activation, and the degree of bronchial hyper-responsiveness. Treatment with inhaled corticosteroids for 4 weeks leads to a reduction in all inflammatory parameters, which parallels the reduction in non-specific bronchial responsiveness. These findings have led to the reclassification of asthma as an inflammatory disorder of airways mucosa, with bronchial hyper-responsiveness and other associated features being viewed as consequences of inflammation rather than primary phenomena.

Histological studies of intrinsic non-allergic asthma and occupational asthma show very similar findings to the biopsy appearances of allergic asthma. In fact, eosinophil and lymphocyte activation are, if anything, rather more prominent in intrinsic asthma, emphasizing the importance of cellular inflammation as a common feature of all forms of asthma and raising the possibility that intrinsic asthma may represent a form of autoimmune disease.

Inflammatory events in the bronchial mucosa

In patients with allergic asthma, exposure to a relevant allergen causes degranulation of mast cells present in the airway lumen and airway mucosa. This leads to the release of histamine and a range of newly formed mediators (Table 1) which induce bronchoconstriction, oedema, mucus secretion, and vasodilatation. Acute bronchospasm due to allergen exposure usually resolves within 1 to 2 h, but 3 to 12 h after allergen exposure there may be a recurrence of bronchoconstriction which is much more persistent and much more difficult to reverse with bronchodilating drugs than the acute asthmatic response to allergens. This late-phase asthmatic response is associated with an increase of non-

Fig. 4 Histology of bronchial epithelium in asthma. The normal appearance to the left and disruption to the right with desquamation and thickening of basement membrane due to sub-basement membrane collagen deposition should be noted. (By courtesy of Dr R. Djukanovic.)

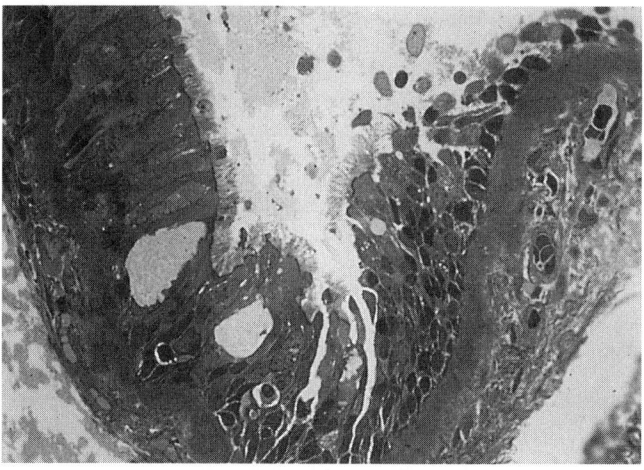

Fig. 5 Histology of asthma: activated eosinophils (stained by immune operoxidase for eosinophil cationic protein) below and above the basement membrane in a biopsy from a mild asthmatic patient. (By courtesy of Dr R. Djukanovic.)

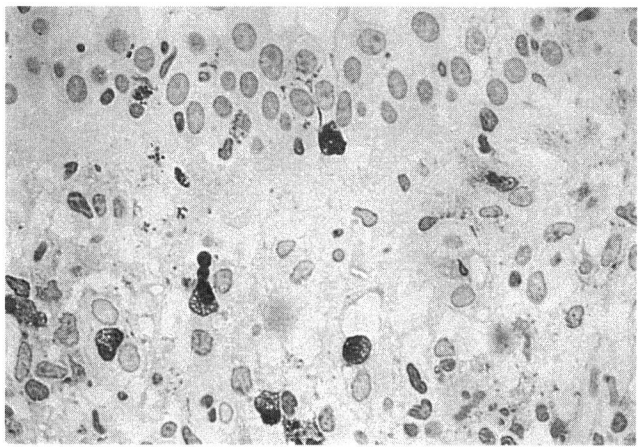

specific bronchial responsiveness and with the accumulation of neutrophils, eosinophils, and other leucocytes. Eosinophils are a characteristic feature of asthmatic inflammation and are capable of causing considerable damage to the bronchial epithelium. They contain several basic proteins (major basic protein, eosinophil cationic protein, eosinophil-derived neurotoxin, and eosinophil peroxidase) which induce detachment of the bronchial epithelium in experimental models and which can induce degranulation of mast cells directly (Fig. 6). Mast-cell and eosinophil-derived growth factors can induce the proliferation of myofibroblasts which in turn are probably responsible for the deposition of interstitial collagens beneath the basement membrane. In addition to their effect on epithelial growth and integrity, the eosinophil basic proteins may damage the epithelium by direct effects on the basement membrane which may in turn alter the ability of the epithelium to regulate the water and ion content of the fluid lining the bronchial tree. Exposure of autonomic nerve endings beneath and within the epithelium appears to enhance the inflammatory response through the release of the neuropeptides substance P, neurokinin A, and calcitonin-gene-related peptide.

Eosinophil growth and differentiation are controlled by the cytokines IL-3, IL-5, and granulocyte–macrophage colony-stimulating factor. These cytokines are principally produced by T lymphocytes, but mRNA for granulocyte–macrophage colony-stimulating factor can also be identified in macrophages and bronchial epithelial cells. Colabelling studies have demonstrated that the mRNA hybridization signals for IL-3, IL-5, and granulocyte–macrophage colony-stimulating factor in bronchial lavage cells are confined to T cells. Consequently, there has been considerable interest in the role of T lymphocytes in atopic allergy. T cells have long been implicated in the regulation of IgE production, principally through the production of IL-4, which promotes isotype switching of B cells to IgE and facilitates differentiation into IgE-producing plasma cells. Interestingly, IL-4 protein has been localized to mast cells in bronchial biopsies using immunocytochemical methods. This may reflect *de novo* synthesis or storage of IL-4 produced by other cells.

While regulation of IgE induction is clearly important in the development of asthma, it appears to be less relevant to the pathophysiology of established disease. It has been clearly demonstrated that allergen challenge of the skin or airways leads to recruitment of CD4+ T cells. This process has mainly been studied in the skin where it is easier to control the allergen dose and to obtain serial samples. In the skin model, the recruited T cells are mainly of the CD45RO+ ('memory') phenotype and, as the reaction develops over 12 to 24 h, activated T cells can be identified by increased expression of the IL-2 receptor (CD25) and production of the cytokines IL-3, IL-4, IL-5, tumour necrosis factor-α, and granulocyte–macrophage colony-stimulating factor as shown by *in situ* hybridization. Histological studies of allergen challenge in asthmatic airways have been less detailed, but are broadly consistent with the skin model. Based on these patterns of cellular recruitment and activation, the T cells recruited after allergen exposure appear to be the human homologue of the murine T_H-2 cell. Other studies have demonstrated an excess of T_H-2 cells in the blood of atopic individuals and preferential activation of T_H-2 cells on exposure to allergens as compared with non-allergenic proteins. T cells in BAL and bronchial biopsies are generally of the CD45RO+ 'memory' subset phenotype and are more often 'activated' than peripheral blood T cells, as shown by increased expression of the IL-2 receptor CD25. To date there has been no convincing evidence that T cells in asthmatic airways mucosa differ in their T-cell antigen receptor family usage, although there are some preliminary data which suggest that there may be a reduced usage of T-cell receptor V; n-α gene families in asthmatic lungs.

Further evidence supporting the importance of eosinophils and T cells in the pathogenesis of asthma comes from histological studies performed before and after a course of inhaled corticosteroids. This form of treatment is very effective for most forms of asthma, and reduces both non-specific bronchial responsiveness and airways inflammation. When given over a 6-week period, beclomethasone dipropionate substantially reduces the numbers of eosinophils and activated T-cells present in asth-

Table 1 *Actions of mediators released from mast cells*

	Leukotrienes	Histamine	PAF	Prostaglandins
Bronchoconstriction	$LTD_4 > C_4 > E_4$	+++	++	PGD_2, $PGF_{2\alpha}$
Mucosal oedema	LTC_4, D_4	+++	++	PGE_2
Mucus secretion	LTC_4, D_4		++	
Chemotaxis and cellular activation	LTB_4		++++	
Increased NSBR (duration)	LTB_4 transient	No effect	+++ prolonged	PGD_2 30 min only

matic airways. Additional evidence comes from a 6-month double-blind placebo-controlled clinical trial of cyclosporin A (a specific inhibitor of T-cell activation) which showed a clear beneficial effect on spirometric measures in patients with chronic severe asthma.

Interest in the mechanisms of cellular recruitment in asthma has also directed attention towards the vascular endothelium as a potential site for therapeutic intervention. Allergen exposure leads to upregulation of ICAM-1, E-selectin, and VCAM-1, and it seems highly likely that these endothelial changes are important in inducing the influx of inflammatory cells to the site of allergic reactions. In a primate model of asthma, administration of a monoclonal antibody directed against ICAM-1 has been shown to attenuate the development of bronchial responsiveness on subsequent exposure to allergen. This area is now the subject of intense research with a view to modulating cellular recruitment in human asthma.

Physiology of asthma

In the presence of airways inflammation and bronchial irritability, a wide range of specific and non-specific insults lead to transient smooth muscle contraction. More prolonged bronchoconstriction and airflow obstruction arise when a chronic inflammatory process is set in train, with mucosal oedema, mucus secretion, and epithelial damage. These changes in airways calibre affect both large and small airways and lead to an overall increase in airflow resistance. Because of the relative numbers of large and small airways and the relationship of resistance of flow to airways diameter, most of the airways resistance in health and disease is due to small airways. Thus it is principally the obstruction of small bronchioles which leads to increased airflow resistance in asthma. Measures of expiratory flow rates (forced expiratory volume in 1 s (FEV_1)

and peak expiratory flow rate) are decreased and disturbed airflow patterns are clinically audible as wheeze. Air is trapped in the lungs, leading to an increase in functional residual volume, usually without any change in total lung capacity. As a direct consequence of the increase in airways resistance the work of breathing is increased, leading to the subjective sensation of breathlessness. Arterial blood gases are usually normal in stable asthma. In acute exacerbations, some bronchioles become completely obstructed by mucus plugs, leading to ventilatory perfusion mismatch and hence to arterial hypoxaemia. To compensate the patient hyperventilates; this blows off carbon dioxide but is unable to restore a normal PaO_2. In very severe exacerbations, the patient may eventually fail to sustain the increased respiratory effort, and will then present with a relatively quiet chest, hypoxaemia, and a normal or rising $PaCO_2$. This represents a life-threatening deterioration and requires urgent treatment and ventilatory support, otherwise respiratory arrest and death by asphyxiation will follow.

In summary, asthma is a chronic inflammatory condition of the airways which has a complex aetiology (Fig. 7). There is undoubtedly a genetic component, but the inheritance pattern is not simple. Development of asthma appears to require a susceptible airway, upon which one or more environmental inciting agents act to induce a chronic mucosal inflammation, characterized by eosinophil and T-cell infiltration. Once established, this chronic inflammatory process leads to the development of the clinical symptoms of asthma. This inflammation allows a wide variety of non-specific irritants to cause bronchoconstriction (bronchial hyper-responsiveness). Acute episodes of asthma may be precipitated by mast-cell degranulation via sensitizing IgE antibody. Once established, the airways of all asthmatics, mild or severe, show chronic inflammatory changes with a characteristic infiltration by eosinophils

Fig. 7 Overview of the mechanisms of asthma.

Fig. 6 Interaction of eosinophils, mast cells, and fibroblasts.

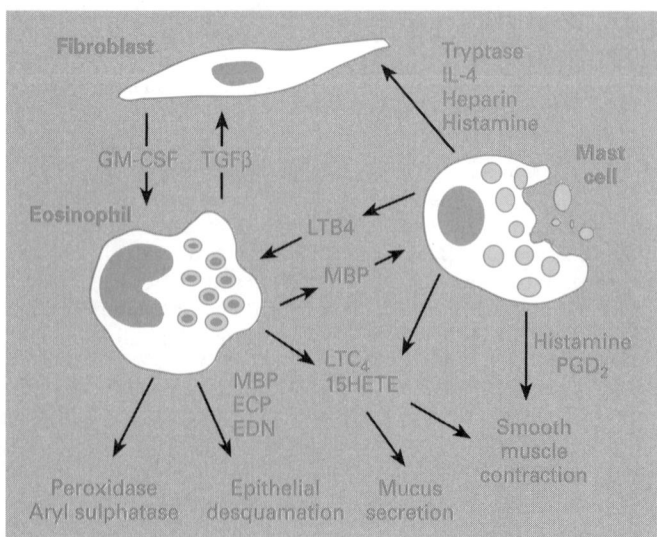

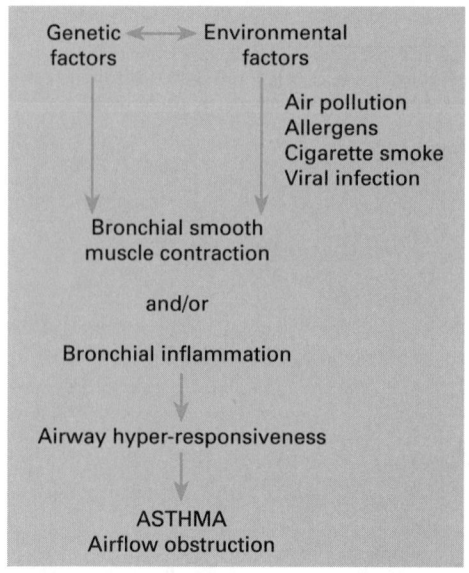

and T lymphocytes. Unlike classical delayed-type hypersensitivity, the T cells present express cytokines of the T_H-2 subset which are probably important in perpetuating the eosinophilic tissue response and may contribute to the continued induction and production of IgE. Chronic asthma is associated with the continued influx of inflammatory leucocytes (particularly eosinophils and T cells) and further damage to the bronchial epithelium. Recognition of the inflammatory basis of asthma has led to a reappraisal of treatment strategies in asthma and to the identification of several possible future therapeutic targets. The current rationale of treatment is to try to suppress the inflammatory component of asthma using prophylactic anti-inflammatory drugs. Direct-acting bronchodilators retain an important role as first-aid relief for smooth muscle spasm but do not influence the inflammatory process and therefore should not be regarded as first-line maintenance treatment. Acute exacerbations of asthma are associated with increased inflammatory changes and mucus plugging of the airways; these require systemic anti-inflammatory therapy as inhaled medication will not be able to penetrate the blocked airways and reach the affected site.

With this new understanding of the cellular and molecular mechanisms of asthma, there is also the potential for the development of novel therapeutic interventions. Such treatments may not replace conventional medication for the majority of patients but might relieve those who are not helped by current treatments.

REFERENCES

Alexander, A.G., Barnes, N.C., and Kay, A.B. (1992). Cyclosporin A in corticosteroid-dependent chronic severe asthma. A randomized double-blind placebo-controlled crossover trial. *Lancet*, **339**, 324–8.

Bardin, P.G., Johnston, S.L., and Pattemore, P.K. (1992). Viruses as precipitants of asthma symptoms. I. Physiology and mechanisms. *Clinical and Experimental Allergy*, **22**, 809–22.

Barnes, P.J. (1986). Neural control of human airways in health and disease. State of art. *American Review of Respiratory Disease*, **134**, 1289–1314.

Chan-Yeung, M. and Lam, S. (1986). Occupational asthma—state of the art. *American Review of Respiratory Disease*, **133**, 688–703.

Corrigan, C.J. and Kay, A.B. (1992). T cells and eosinophils in the pathogenesis of asthma. *Immunology Today*, **13**, 501–7.

Djukanovic, R., Roche, W.R., Wilson, J.W., Beasley, C.R.W., Twentyman, O.P., Howarth, P.H., *et al.* (1990). Mucosal inflammation in asthma. State of the art. *American Review of Respiratory Disease*, **142**, 434–57.

Frew, A.J. and Kay, A.B. (1990). Eosinophils and T-lymphocytes in late phase allergic reactions. *Journal of Allergy and Clinical Immunology*, **85**, 533–9.

Frigas, E. and Gleich, G.J. (1986). The eosinophil and the pathophysiology of asthma. *Journal of Allergy and Clinical Immunology*, **77**, 527–37.

Morton, N.E. (1992). Major loci for atopy. Editorial. *Clinical and Experimental Allergy*, **22**, 1041–3.

Ninan, T.K. and Russell, G. (1992). Respiratory symptoms and atopy in Aberdeen schoolchildren: evidence from two surveys 25 years apart. *British Medical Journal*, **304**, 873–5.

Sandford, A.J., Shirakawa, T., Moffat, M.F., *et al.* (1993). Localisation of atopy and β-subunit of high affinity IgE receptor (FceRI) on chromosome 11q. *Lancet* **341**, 332–4.

17.9.1(b) Clinical features and management

D. J. LANE

Introduction

Episodic breathing difficulties were recognized and labelled as asthma long before the anatomy of the airways had been described or their function elucidated. From Hippocratic times onwards much emphasis was placed on the 'thick and viscid humours' that prevented the proper movement of air in and out of the lungs in asthma. Willis and Floyer, English physicians of the seventeenth century who were themselves asthmatic, vividly described the condition, distinguishing a 'convulsive or periodic' type of intermittent wheezing asthma (curiously often mistaken for or allied to epilepsy) from a 'pneumonic' type in which mucus production predominated.

With increased understanding of physiology in the twentieth century, it became evident that the fundamental functional abnormality which caused the symptoms of asthma was airways narrowing, and this became embedded in the first generally acceptable definition of the condition: '. . . widespread narrowing of the intra-pulmonary airways which varies either spontaneously or in response to treatment'. Such a definition allowed informed investigation of the phenomenon, but suffered from a lack of precision in terms of 'how variable' (both degree and time-scale). Furthermore, since this was essentially a description of a functional syndrome, it was unclear how many 'diseases' in which such a functional change occurred should be included. The word 'asthma' continued to be used both for the syndrome of variable airways narrowing and for diseases in which the syndrome was part, causing such confusion that a CIBA Symposium in 1951 on the identification of asthma decided that 'on the evidence available' asthma could not be defined.

The introduction of the term 'inflammatory disease of the airways' into current definitions of asthma has served to highlight an important aspect of the pathological anatomy of the condition, encouraged a shift in treatment, and offered some clarification of the nature of the asthmatic process. Yet the underlying dilemma of how best to use the term asthma still remains and has not been properly resolved.

The recognition of asthma

The cardinal symptom of asthma is generally thought to be wheezing (see Chapter 17.5). However, a few asthmatics say that they never wheeze, and many describe other airways symptoms such as cough with or without sputum production, chest tightness, or simply shortness of breath.

Asthmatic wheezing is polyphonic, is present on inspiration as well as expiration, and is often not detectable at rest and therefore only heard on exercise or forced expiration. It is produced by vibrations set up in small airways that are almost closed off. Most asthmatics sense that it is coming from the lower respiratory tract. Although there is plenty of noise to be heard with the stethoscope over the central airways, this is transmitted sound. Just as wheeze signifies narrowing of the airways, so does the sensation of tightness. It is not a pain and so should be distinguishable from angina pectoris and oesophageal spasm, both of which may be described by patients as tightness. In asthma, the sensation partly reflects the effort required to breathe and partly arises from the central airways, with those deeper in the lungs being devoid of sensation. Asthmatics generally find it more difficult to breathe in than out, although doctors usually assume that the reverse is true.

Exertional shortness of breath for the asthmatic has both a variable component, which tallies with the waxing and waning of their airways narrowing, and a persistent more fixed component. Indeed, patients will sometimes comment, 'It's not my asthma: I'm just short of breath'.

Cough is insufficiently emphasized as a symptom of asthma. However, it is one of the commonest symptoms of asthma in children and can be a lone symptom of the condition in adults. Whilst asthmatic cough may be non-productive, it is frequently accompanied by the expectoration of mucoid sputum. At times this may be quite frothy and liquid, although more often it is sticky and difficult to expectorate. The asthmatic's sputum may contain cylindrical or branched casts in the shape of the small airways from where they are presumed to have originated.

The physical signs of asthma are those described for airways obstruction in Chapter 17.5 with special features (described below) that reflect severity in the acute severe attack. Objective confirmation of airways narrowing in asthma can be carried out using any of the tests of airways function described in Chapter 17.6.2. In practice, because of its simplicity of use, portability, and reliability, the device generally used in clinical practice is a peak expiratory flow rate meter (Fig. 1). The test results reflect changing levels of airflow obstruction with ease and accuracy, can be a more subtle indicator of change than symptoms, and are nearly always more reliable than chest physical signs.

All the features described so far are commonplace in cardiorespiratory disease. Therefore what aspects of them suggest asthma? It is chiefly their variability, pattern, and timing. First, there is a classic diurnal pattern with symptoms awakening sufferers in the small hours of the morning (3–5 a.m.) or, if sleep is not broken, being most obvious on awakening at the natural time. Improvement follows later in the day, with late afternoon often being the most trouble-free time, with possibly some hint of deterioration again late in the evening. This diurnal pattern is disrupted by episodic attacks of asthma, initiated by triggers which are described more fully below. Some will act transiently over minutes, others set up a wheezy attack lasting for an hour or so, and yet others create a more prolonged deterioration lasting for days on end. Conversely, asthmatic symptoms, both diurnal and episodic, can be abolished with effective treatment.

This pattern of symptomatic variability is reflected in a parallel variability in serial peak expiratory flow measurements. Thus diurnal variability gives a sawtooth pattern over several days (Fig. 2), whereas a triggered attack produces either a short-lived deterioration in function over minutes or hours, or a much more prolonged episode if there is a severe attack (Fig. 3).

An appropriate history backed up by characteristic serial lung function measurements will enable asthma to be recognized in many, but not all, individuals. For the diagnosis of asthma in these other cases and for a better understanding of asthma as a whole, it is necessary to examine how the mechanisms underlying the bronchial pathophysiology of asthma detailed in the last chapter translate themselves into the clinical features of this disorder.

The clinical relevance of bronchial hyper-responsiveness

The cardinal feature of the functional behaviour of asthmatic airways is that they respond by narrowing to a whole variety of circumstances that leave healthy airways unaffected. The structural basis of this narrowing, as described earlier, is complex: bronchial smooth muscle contraction, submucosal inflammation, mucosal swelling, and intraluminal mucus accumulation all contribute. Some components of this airways narrowing, for example muscle contraction and mucosal swelling, are clearly transitory. Others, such as mucus impaction in an inflamed airway, can easily lead to complete airway blockage which will be much more permanent. The different time courses of these pathological changes are likely to be the basis of recognizable patterns of symptoms, for example those following environmental change, allergen exposure, infection, etc., although it is not necessarily easy to match symptoms with pathology.

It is possible and instructive to rank asthmatic responses by time course.

Deep inspiration

Deep inspiration is the shortest lived. Following a deep inspiration to total lung capacity and a relaxed expiration, there is a very transient increase in airways resistance that begins in less than 1 min and is over

Fig. 1 The mini-Wright peak expiratory flow meter.

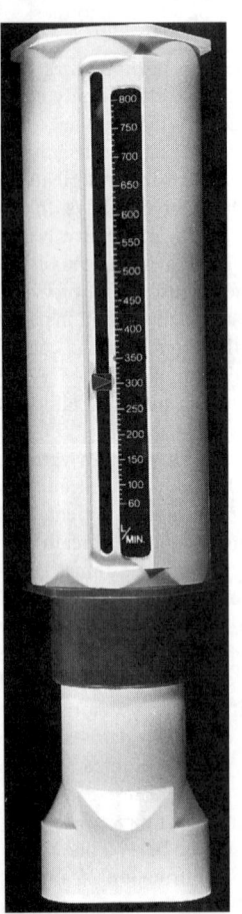

Fig. 2 Serial peak expiratory flow rates in a patient with nocturnal asthma.

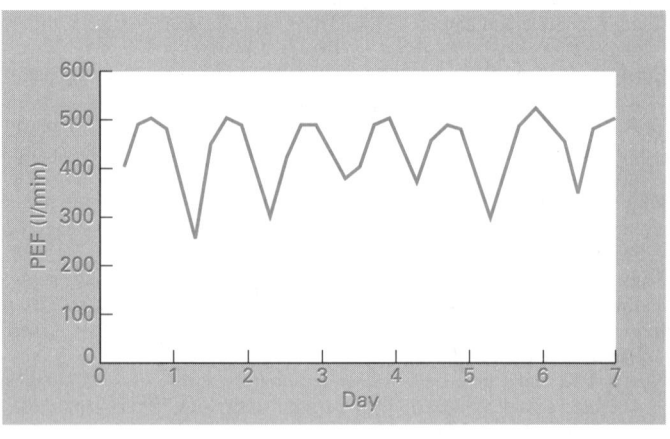

Fig. 3 Serial peak expiratory flow rates in a patient developing and recovering from an acute attack of asthma.

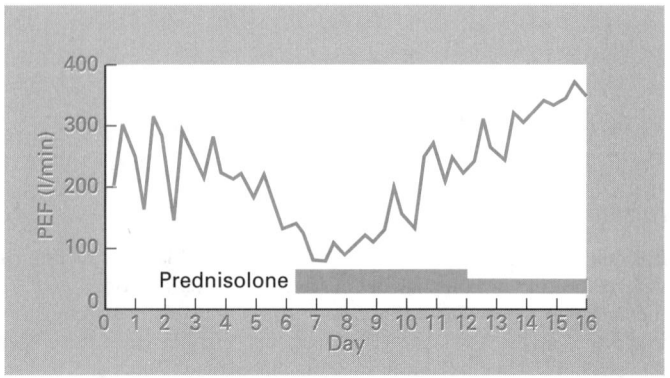

in 3 min. This type of reactivity, presumably entirely due to reflex bronchial muscle contraction, may well be why asthmatics notice increased wheeziness after laughter or coughing. It can influence lung function testing. Some asthmatics will always give a best result on the first of the recommended three blows when performing tests of forced expiration.

Environmental change

Clinically, the asthmatic frequently notices bronchial hyper-reactivity as tightness, cough, or wheeze in response to environmental events. Temperature change, particularly to cold, smoke inhalation, perfumes, irritant gases, dusts, etc. cause an immediate reaction that settles over a space of a few minutes, provided that the provocation is not sustained. This phenomenon also seems likely to be a reflex bronchoconstriction presumably initiated via bronchial wall irritant receptors.

Exercise-induced asthma

This well-described and intensively investigated phenomenon is not a special and separate type of asthma, but an integral part of asthmatic symptomatology. Almost universally present in children and teenagers, it would probably be reported much more frequently in adults if they were inclined and fit enough to undertake sufficient exercise. Exercise-induced asthma is not just the curtailment of exercise because the asthmatic becomes short of breath or wheezy. It is a highly characteristic worsening of symptoms after exercise has finished. Serial peak expiratory flow (PEF) measurements show a trough which may represent a drop to as little as half the initial value and which is maximal 5 to 10 min after the end of exercise, with gradual recovery over the next hour unless treated (Fig. 4).

The magnitude of the response is related to the level of ventilation achieved, and indeed a response can be induced by hyperventilation alone without exercise. Breathing moist humidified air during exercise will greatly reduce the degree of exercise-induced asthma, but conversely exercise in very cold weather (when the air will also be very dry) can induce airways narrowing in hitherto normal individuals. Indeed, any deviation of the tonicity of inhaled fluids from normal (either hypertonicity or hypotonicity) can upset airways function, so that it is generally thought that airways osmolality and fluid transport are more important than temperature change in producing exercise-induced asthma. However, it is far from being as simple as that. Prevention of cold weather exercise-induced asthma in healthy athletes by prior inhalation of an anticholinergic suggests that a vagal reflex may be involved, and prevention of exercise-induced asthma with disodium cromoglycate (see below) points to the importance of mediator release. A clear refractory period of 2 to 4 h after one challenge has produced exercise-induced asthma before exercise will again induce asthma supports the mediator theory. The important message for patients is that exercise-induced asthma can almost always be prevented immediately by using either disodium cromoglycate or a β_2-agonist, and that longer-term control over the asthma with steroid aerosols will be effective after 3 to 4 weeks of treatment.

Nocturnal asthma

Like exercise-induced asthma, nocturnal asthma is an integral part of asthmatic symptomatology. Indeed, it is so characteristic of the untreated condition that asthma should not be diagnosed if it is absent. Symptomatically, the subject awakes around 3 to 5 a.m. with cough, chest tightness, or wheezing. Objectively, there is increased airflow limitation at this time which is reflected in reduced PEF and other tests of airway calibre. Even if sleep itself is not disturbed, lung function at the natural awakening time 2 or 3 h later will still be abnormal—the morning dip (see Fig. 2). Likewise, asthmatic symptoms are most likely to be troublesome on awakening. Improvement follows during the day, so that better lung function and freedom from symptoms are most likely to prevail at 4 p.m.

This phenomenon, which is so dramatic in the asthmatic, is an exaggeration of a natural circadian rhythm detectable even in normal subjects if sufficiently sensitive tests of airways function are used. It is related to sleep itself. An asthmatic shift worker changing from day to night duties will shift the trough in lung function by 12 h within one sleep cycle. The change in function most closely parallels changes in circulating sympathomimetic amines rather than corticosteroids, but there may also be cyclical changes in β-receptor sensitivity.

Why this diurnal rhythm is so exaggerated in the asthmatic is less clear. It is not related to baseline function (which can be quite normal in the middle of the day) but more to the degree of airways hyper-responsiveness, which in its turn reflects the extent of airways inflammation. Histamine reactivity (see below) and diurnal lung function variability run parallel with each other. It has been suggested that heightened exposure to dust mites in bedding is important, but whilst this could certainly increase bronchial hyper-responsiveness in those allergic to the mite, it hardly serves to explain the morning dip in asthmatics who are not. Likewise, acid reflux from the stomach, although a common phenomenon when recumbent and curiously linked with asthma (see below), is far from being universal. Effective treatment of asthma is accompanied by abolition of nocturnal attacks.

The causes of bronchial hyper-responsiveness

The phenomena so far described are indicative of an existing state of bronchial hyper-responsiveness, but they are not capable of initiating that state in the first place. Three further triggers are now described which not only set off an attack of asthma when bronchial hyper-responsiveness has already been established, but can create that state *de novo*. They are allergic reactions, infections, and pollutants.

Allergic bronchial hyper-responsiveness

The capacity to develop atopic allergic reactions is inherited. When individuals with this inherited allergic diathesis are exposed to allergens in appropriate concentrations and probably at appropriate times (in the evolution of their immune system), they will develop allergic disease. If these allergens are inhaled into the lungs, local IgE receptors will become sensitized and on further challenge the clinical result will be asthma.

Fig. 4 Exercise-induced asthma: fall and recovery of FEV_1 as a percentage of basal value.

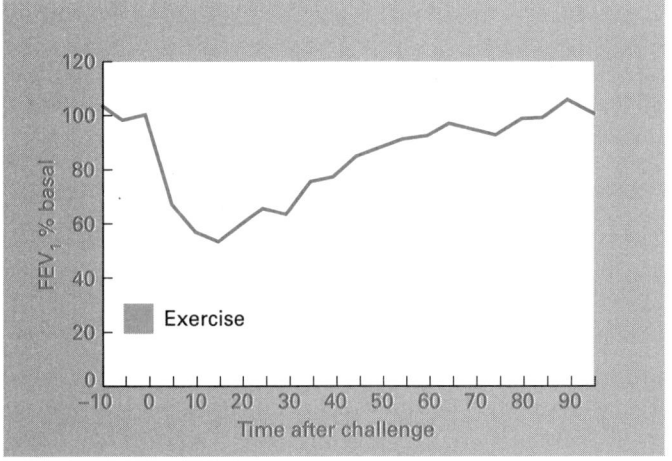

The changes which follow allergen challenge have been studied in great detail over the last few decades. As in all challenges, symptoms tend to run parallel to lung function changes and the latter are used as the benchmark for studying allergic asthma. Following inhalation challenge, two time courses are defined: (1) an immediate reaction beginning within minutes of exposure and reaching a peak in 5 to 15 min; (2) a late reaction with its onset some 4 to 6 h after exposure which lasts for up to 24 h (see Fig. 5). Antigen challenge may give rise to an immediate reaction alone, a dual reaction with return of function to normal in an asymptomatic period of an hour or so, or occasionally a lone late reaction.

In immediate reactions, it seems likely that mucosal oedema and bronchial muscle spasm are the chief components of airways narrowing. If a late reaction is to follow, there is increasing cellular infiltration, particularly with eosinophils, and an intense inflammatory reaction is seen.

Immediate reactions can be prevented by the inhalation of disodium cromoglycate or a β_2-agonist prior to allergen exposure, but these do not necessarily prevent a subsequent late reaction. However, steroids have no obvious effect on the immediate reaction but abort the late reaction.

Several observations signify that this allergic inflammatory reaction has created a state of bronchial hyper-responsiveness. First, if histamine reactivity testing (see below for details) is carried out during the course of a dual-response allergen challenge, it is found to increase (i.e. become more reactive) during the interval between the early and late reactions, and remain abnormal after the late reaction has recovered (Fig. 5). Second, patients followed for several days after a late reaction may complain of nocturnal awakening with asthmatic symptoms; there will be an associated series of 'morning dips' in lung function (Fig. 6). Finally, pollen-sensitive asthmatics will not only show increased histamine reactivity during the appropriate season but, in addition, may complain of worsening exercise-induced asthma.

Bronchial hyper-responsiveness resulting from infection

The time course, pathology, and mechanisms of infection-induced asthma are far from being clearly defined. In previously healthy individuals an acute viral respiratory tract infection will create a state of bronchial inflammation during which chemical airways reactivity is increased. This lasts for 3 to 6 weeks. Something similar must occur in asthmatics, but no experiments to test this hypothesis have been considered ethical. Bacterial infection may act similarly, but again has not been seriously studied.

The factors determining the evolution of infection-induced wheezing into something more like persistent asthma are complex and ill-understood, but on *a priori* grounds as well as clinical experience there is little doubt that infection can and does initiate persistent asthma in hitherto apparently healthy individuals. Several mechanisms have been postulated to explain how viruses might initiate asthma. They cause severe epithelial damage. This could create excessive irritant receptor discharge or lead to local release of inflammatory mediators and/or sensory neuropeptides as in allergen-induced asthma.

Since respiratory tract infection is exceedingly common and quite clearly does not inevitably lead to asthma, one must ask what additional features are necessary. Clearly, genetic predisposition is one possibility: nothing is known of this. The type of infecting organism may be important. Respiratory syncytial virus is an example. Some 25 per cent of children who had documented respiratory syncytial virus in infancy were found to have evidence of airways obstruction of asthmatic type when examined 5 to 8 years later. Children who were atopic, particularly those who had existing atopic illness (e.g. eczema, rhinitis), featured prominently, and it may be that the infection was no more than a secondary feature acting on airways already primed to become hyper-responsive.

It is recognized that certain bacteria (particularly *Haemophilus*

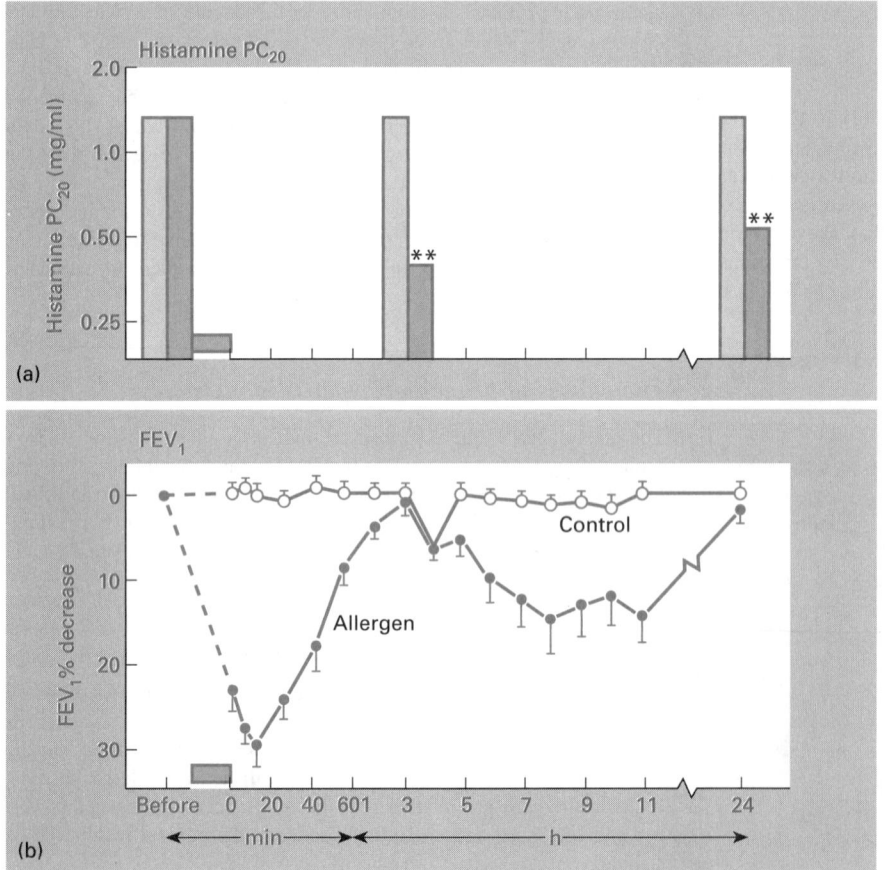

Fig. 5 Allergen (●) challenge producing a dual response with control (○) for comparison. (a) changes in PC_{20} for histamine. (b) Percentage change in FEV_1.

influenzae) release histamine, which could increase bronchial hyper-reactivity. There is also the possibility that there is an interaction between atmospheric pollution and infection. The children of smoking mothers are prone to both respiratory tract infection and asthma.

Once bronchial hyper-responsiveness has been established, respiratory tract infection will trigger exacerbations of symptoms. About a half of asthmatics with an identified infection will have an exacerbation of symptoms, although only 10 to 20 per cent of all exacerbations seem to have a viral trigger. None the less these can be amongst the most serious and prolonged of asthma attacks, with slow recovery after the episode apparently the rule.

Environmental pollution and bronchial hyper-responsiveness

Cigarette smoking creates hyper-reactive airways as assessed by histamine and methacholine challenge. Is this asthma? In the sense that there is increased reactivity, diurnal variation in airways function, and response to bronchodilators, the answer must be in the affirmative. However, in most smokers the fixed component is, or becomes, so dominant in their clinical symptomatology that it overwhelms the picture of reversible airways obstruction and disallows the use of the term asthma.

Much interest has been shown recently in the possibility that other atmospheric pollutants, particularly nitrogen dioxide and ozone, might initiate asthma. Good experiments attest to the fact that there is a positive interaction between these pollutants and allergens. In inhalational challenge studies prior inhalation of ozone, for example, at a concentration that causes no reaction will enhance reactivity to an allergen to which that subject has been sensitized. Similar enhancement occurs with nitrogen dioxide.

What is less clear is whether exposure to such environmental pollutants can create *de novo* a state of bronchial hyper-responsiveness manifest in terms of diurnal or postexercise swings in peak flow, without interaction with allergens. In an occupational setting (see Chapter 17.10.16), whilst it is generally supposed that small sensitizing molecules combine with host proteins to form haptens which then act as allergens, there is clear evidence that certain pollutants (e.g. sulphur dioxide and chlorine) are capable of creating a state of bronchial hyper-responsiveness which did not exist in that individual prior to the exposure.

TESTING REACTIVITY IN CLINICAL PRACTICE

Formal assessment of hyper-reactivity could be carried out with deep inspiration, exercise, or allergen challenges, but these procedures are less reliable and more difficult to standardize than inhalation challenges with pharmacologically active chemicals. Histamine and methacholine are the most frequently used. The former is presumed to imitate preformed mediator release and the latter imitates cholinergic mechanisms of airways narrowing. Testing involves the inhalation of logarithmically increasing doses of the challenge until bronchial narrowing occurs which is of sufficient degree to reduce standard tests of airflow obstruction (PEF and forced expiratory volume in 1 second (FEV_1) by 20 per cent (Fig. 7). The dose of inhaled histamine or methacholine which produces a 20 per cent deterioration in function (PD_{20}) is the quoted index of reactivity. For histamine challenge a PD_{20} of more than 8 mg/ml is normal; figures down to 2 mg/ml are found in mild asthma, and lower values are obtained in moderate and severe asthma.

The clinical use of reactivity testing is confined to the diagnosis of the difficult or confusing case, research into mechanisms, and population epidemiological studies.

A diagnostic algorithm for asthma

A clinical suspicion of asthma based on the symptoms described above in conjunction with challenge tests or spontaneous variations in function can describe a diagnostic pathway suitable for subjects who present when their function is normal or nearly so (Fig. 8). If significant airways narrowing is already present, however, it is unpleasant (even dangerous) to create more airflow obstruction by using a challenge test. The alternative way of demonstrating variability of obstruction is to correct existing narrowing therapeutically. A β-agonist is chosen first, followed by an oral corticosteroid trial (Table 1) if this fails. Again a 20 per cent change is sought. This cut-off is as arbitrary for a therapeutic test as for a challenge, but if used sensibly it allows most cases to be logically categorized.

The asthmatic disorders

If asthma is regarded as a syndrome of reversible airflow obstruction, then it becomes necessary to describe the disorders of which it is a clinical feature.

Extrinsic atopic (allergic) asthma

Rackemann was the first to distinguish extrinsic asthma, which is characterized by a clear provocation by recognized allergens, from intrinsic asthma, in which such a provocation is lacking. He noted that such allergic individuals were generally young ('less than 30 years') and that other allergic disorders besides asthma may coexist. The concept of atopy had been formulated by Coca some decades earlier as a grouping

Fig. 6 A series of nocturnal dips following a single allergen challenge in a patient sensitive to formalin. (Reproduced from Hendrich, D.J. and Lane, D.J. (1977). Occupational formalin asthma. *British Journal of Industrial Medicine*, **34**, 11–18, with permission.)

Fig. 7 Percentage fall in FEV_1 during challenge with histamine and methacholine in a normal subject and a moderately severe asthmatic.

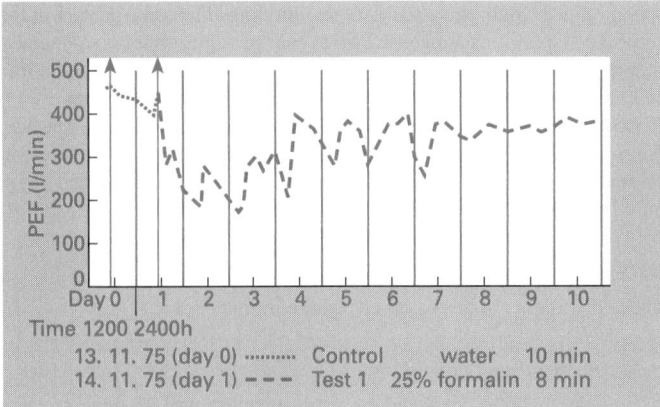

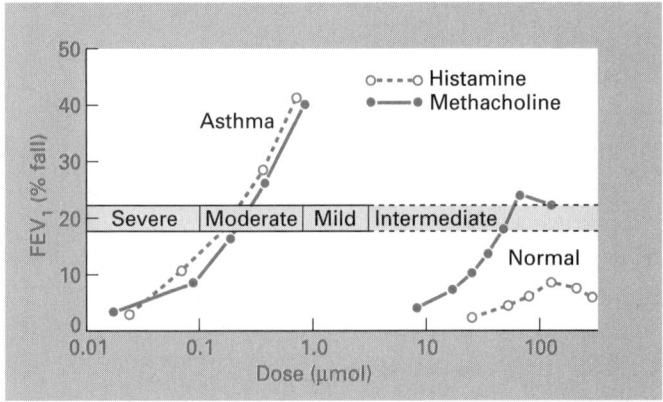

for individuals with infantile eczema, urticaria, allergic rhinitis ('hay fever'), asthma, or any combination of these disorders. He also initially included migraine and hypertension, but these were dropped later. As well as having these clinical features in common, it later emerged that atopic individuals have raised serum levels of IgE (total and/or specific to certain allergens) and positive skin-prick tests (a weal and flare reaction 15 min after the intradermal inoculation of a solution of allergen). The capacity to develop atopic allergy is inherited, and in some 60 per cent of United Kingdom individuals, the mode of inheritance is dominant with a gene carried on chromosome 11q (see also Chapter 17.9.1(a)).

Intermittent exposure to allergens produces episodic attacks of asthma with or without rhinitis in atopic individuals who are appropriately sensitized. A good example would be a young girl allergic to cats who becomes symptomatic each time she visits a friend's house where there is a cat. There is always an immediate reaction (type I) but this can be followed by a late reaction (type III) some 6 to 8 h later and possibly recurrent nocturnal wheezing for several nights. In contrast, continuous exposure produces more continuous asthma. A good example here would be allergy to the house dust mite *Dermatophagoides pteronyssinus*. Exposure is likely all the time that the victim is in a domestic environment, but particularly at night, since mite concentration in bedding is particularly high, and after vacuuming carpets, when clouds of mite particles are whirled up into the atmosphere. Exposure is greatly reduced out of doors, in a scrupulously clean environment, or at a sufficiently high altitude (house dust mite does not survive above 4000 m), and so are asthmatic symptoms.

In some individuals, particularly from the teenage years onwards, asthmatic symptoms are confined to a particular season of the year. It seems from skin-prick and radio-allergosorbent testing that these individuals are responding to pollens released into the atmosphere by flowering trees and plants. During the pollen season sensitized individuals will have symptoms that are very often in the upper respiratory tract with coryza and watering of the eyes as well as wheezing. Non-specific hyper-responsiveness to histamine as well as exercise-induced asthma and nocturnal awakening are all enhanced during the appropriate pollen season.

Inhaled allergens are far more important than ingested allergens in

Fig. 8 A diagnostic protocol for asthma.

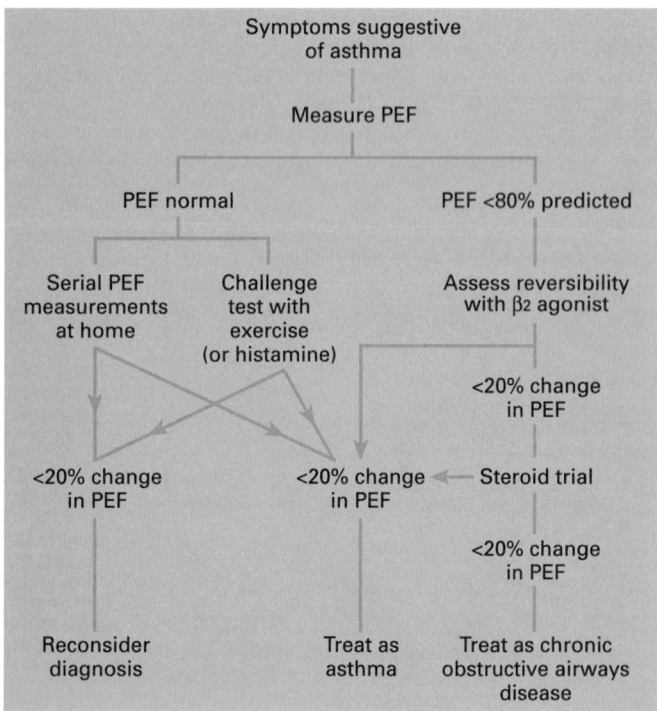

Table 1 *Protocol for oral steroid trial*

- Instruct in use of mini PEF meter
- One week's measurement of twice daily PEF at home noting daily requirement for relief bronchodilator
- Give prednisolone 15–20 mg twice daily for 1 week whilst continuing to record serial PEF readings
- Positive response is 20% improvement in morning, evening or mean PEF
- If <20% improvement after 1 week, trial can be continued for 2nd week
- Replace oral steroids with appropriate dose of inhaled steroids. Oral steroids can be stopped abruptly after 2 weeks

causing asthma in atopic individuals, but notable examples exist. Most are obvious from the history, and it is seldom an exclusively asthmatic response. In addition, there is often urticaria, angio-oedema, gastrointestinal upset, and even full-blown anaphylaxis. Fruits, nuts, and shellfish are notorious for causing such symptoms in sensitized individuals. Asthmatic responses to allergens in frequently ingested foods such as milk, cereals, and eggs are more often reported than objectively confirmed. Strict blinded dietary challenge will confirm the rare case; skin and radio-allergosorbent tests are unreliable.

Extrinsic non-atopic allergic asthma

Pepys coined this term describing individuals with asthma who show allergic airways responses often characterized by a late asthmatic reaction alone, but sometimes a dual reaction, yet who are not atopic. The best examples come from occupational asthma and are described in Chapter 17.10.16.

Allergic bronchopulmonary aspergillosis

Airways disease due to *Aspergillus fumigatus* spores has sufficiently distinctive features to separate it from other extrinsic asthmas. The allergen is ubiquitous; it is found in garden compost, decaying matter in soil, and damp houses. Spores are released into the atmosphere in the autumn and early winter, making this a predominantly seasonal asthma. Symptoms are often straightforward at first but increasingly there are attacks with non-wheezing breathlessness and a tendency to increased sputum production with the description given of bronchial casts and brown pellets. Chest radiographs in attacks show transient infiltrates which, when they have been examined pathologically, are found to be areas of eosinophilic pneumonitis and collapse. The latter is due to severe mucus impaction in a central airway. Fungal elements can be seen in, and grown from, these mucus plugs. The reaction within the airways is more violent than that with other asthmas and after repeated attacks there is an obvious proximal saccular bronchiectasis. An excessive reaction initiates granuloma formation (see bronchocentric granulomatosis, Chapter 17.10.5). Challenge tests are not to be encouraged, but both an early and late reaction would be produced. Eosinophilia is marked and total, and specific IgE is high; there are also precipitating antibodies present in the serum to Aspergillus antigens. Two to four precipitin lines are generally found. More than that number generally signifies mycetoma. One line or lines present only on concentrating the serum are non-specific.

Oral and high dose aerosol steroids are needed for the acute episode. Antifungals, of which itraconazole is probably the best and safest at present, will reduce the fungal load and can be recommended for 3 months or so during the fungal sporing season.

Asthma with parasitic disorders

These disorders are discussed elsewhere in this book.

Infective asthma

As indicated above, viral and bacterial infection will *de novo* create a state of bronchial hyperreactivity in previously healthy airways. This can be evident clinically as audible wheeze and functionally with abnormalities (usually minor) in tests of airways function. Such a state of bronchial hyper-reactivity usually recedes in 3 to 6 weeks. The factors determining the evolution of this into something more like a persistent asthmatic state are complex and ill understood. Infection seems responsible for many episodes of wheezing in neonates and infants. The illness is distressing, generally responds poorly to available treatment (although this may be no more than technical problems of delivering aerosols to very small airways), and carries a good prognosis. Many individuals with this disorder will be non-atopic. Persistent asthma at follow-up 5 to 10 years later is not the rule.

Many adult smokers with early chronic obstructive pulmonary disease suffer infections; there is often wheeze in these bronchitic illnesses. It is reversible to a degree with antibiotics and bronchodilators (particularly anticholinergics), and is of sufficient degree to warrant the diagnostic label 'asthma'. Some of these individuals are atopic or have had asthma as children. Since both asthma and smoking are common, a concurrence of the two is quite frequent.

'Psychogenic' asthma

At one time it was thought that asthma was 'all in the mind'. Osler included it among the hysterical disorders. This view has now been expunged from all reputable texts, but to deny that psychological factors play a part in asthma flies in the face of clinical experience.

Suggestion can certainly alter airways calibre—narrowing if an innocent inhaled solution is presented as a bronchoconstrictor, and vice versa. Protection with atropine implicates parasympathetic pathways. Panic sufficient to produce acute hyperventilation can initiate airways narrowing by drying the airways, or worsen an evolving attack due to other causes. Chronic stress, at a clinical observation level, can cause persistent asthma which can be quite resistant to conventional therapy.

However, it seems singularly unlikely, that stress or emotional stimuli can initiate asthma in the absence of an underlying cause such as allergy or infection. The importance of psychological factors as a potential reason for the persistence of asthma should always be remembered, since appropriate attention to stress factors can sometimes bring unexpected therapeutic rewards.

Asthma and gastro-oesophageal reflux

Gastric distension is uncomfortable for asthmatics, and the acute aspiration of gastric contents into the airways during anaesthesia (or other states of unconsciousness) can give intense airways narrowing as well as pneumonic consolidation (Mendelsohn's syndrome).

Considerable interest has centred on the concept of a direct link between oesophageal disease and asthma, particularly during the last two decades. It seems beyond doubt that acid reflux into the oesophagus can cause immediate airways narrowing. How often this is a cause of what otherwise might be called asthma is hotly contested. Symptoms of reflux are reported in 50 per cent or more of asthmatics in some series as well as in those with lone asthmatic-type nocturnal cough. The association is not confined to adults or the non-atopic.

Diagnosis is not easy. Barium studies are not considered a reliable guide and the gold standard is held to be intra-oesophageal pH monitoring. To establish the association, acidity must run parallel to lung function deterioration. Neither antacids nor H_2 blockers, alone or combined, help consistently, but omeprazole (a proton pump inhibitor) will help in most instances. Surgery is advocated by enthusiasts, but long-term success rates are poor.

Proposed mechanisms are microaspiration into the airways or a vagal reflex to account for asthma arising from acid reflux. The situation is not straightforward, however, since both repeated coughing and the use of methylxanthines, or even β_2-agonists in the treatment of asthma can

lead to gastro-oesophageal sphincter inadequacy and hence reflux as a consequence, rather than a cause, of the asthma.

Intrinsic asthma

Rackemann in his working classification of asthma stated, 'when asthma begins after age forty, it should be considered as due to factors other than allergy until proved otherwise' (Rackemann 1921). Such patients included those in whom infection, psychosocial stress, malnutrition, and erroneous diagnosis seemed responsible for their wheezing, but there remained a group in whom no recognizable cause of asthma could be determined. These are intrinsic asthmatics.

By definition total IgE is normal and skin tests or specific radioallergosorbent tests are negative. However, eosinophilia is not absent from either sputum or, less commonly, blood. Histology of the airways epithelium is similar to that of asthma due to other causes. The clinical course is more likely to be progressive with persistent wheeze and eventual dependence on oral corticosteroids.

Such patients undoubtedly exist and, although they are more likely to be older adults, can be young; a small number will be children. It must be presumed that the inflammatory process is triggered by some mechanism that is not allergic, infective, or environmental. The designation 'intrinsic' should be used sparingly and only after all potential mechanisms, particularly occupation- and drug-induced, have been excluded.

Drugs and asthma

The varied pulmonary reactions that can be attributed to drugs are fully described elsewhere (Chapter 17.10.19). However, it is necessary in the context of asthma to emphasize the potentially dire consequences of administering β-blockers, even in the form of eye drops, to asthmatics. The earlier non-specific blockers (e.g. propranolol) were more likely to cause problems, but it is unwise to use any β-blockers except under careful supervision and when other alternative therapies have been rejected.

Some 2 per cent of asthmatics react adversely to aspirin compounds and/or non-steroidal analgesics. Samter described a diagnostic triad of asthma, nasal polyps, and aspirin use. Symptoms of streaming coryza followed by intense wheezing develop 10 to 20 min after ingesting the drug. The nasal polyps grow after repeated attacks. Although attempts to desensitize affected subjects with initially minute and then progressively larger doses of aspirin have been tried, success is not ensured and the best policy is strict avoidance. The NSAIDs and certain dyes and colourings (e.g. tartrazine, benzoic acid) should also be avoided by these individuals, although cross-reactivity is not universal and sensitivity can be found to one agent and not others.

The postulated mechanism for aspirin is that the inhibition of the metabolic pathway to prostaglandin production allows more arachidonic acid to be converted to leukotrienes which trigger the asthma. The situation must be a good deal more complex than this, however. First, aspirin-sensitive asthmatics are highly reactive (rather than hyporeactive) to prostaglandin challenge and, second, prostaglandins in the airways are a complex mixture of bronchodilators as well as bronchoconstrictors. Indeed, in the occasional patient (about 0.1 per cent of asthmatics) aspirin and related drugs will relieve or prevent asthma.

Asthma at different ages

Half of those who ever develop asthma will do so before the age of 10 and many before the age of 5. The first onset of asthma in adults then occurs fairly evenly across the age bands with a slight increase in the forties and fifties and rather fewer beyond 70, although asthma can certainly begin for the first time in the elderly. Once asthma has begun, it generally persists for some years. In children it will last for longer the earlier it begins. Many children have a remission of symptoms in the teens, but in at least 50 per cent there will be a recurrence, sometimes early in adult life but more often somewhat later. Remission is less frequent if asthma begins later in life.

Boys predominate over girls early in life with sex ratios of three or four to one in infants (male to female). Later in life the sex ratio is around unity with females predominating in the elderly.

Most children who are asthmatic are also clearly atopic, yet early in life their asthma does not bear a close relation clinically to allergen exposure. Viral infections are a more likely trigger, particularly in the early years. More specifically allergen-induced attacks occur with exposure to pets and pollens, and the ubiquitous house dust mite is undoubtedly responsible for much of the background allergic airways responsiveness of the young. As activity increases during the school years exercise-induced asthma becomes a troublesome interference with activity. Nocturnal sleep disturbance by wheeze or even just cough can be enough to interfere with school work and cause much concern to parents. Despite the now well-described symptoms of asthma in school children, only half those identified as asthmatic in epidemiological studies will have been formally diagnosed and appropriately treated.

By the teenage years many children will notice an easing of symptoms, although the highly atopic, particularly those with marked eczema, suffer persistent symptoms that may not ease until later in life. Exercise-induced asthma can remain a serious hindrance in the athletic, and those foolish enough to smoke cigarettes lay down the foundations of subsequent decline into chronic airways obstruction.

Women may notice a distinct worsening of symptoms just before or during each menstrual cycle. The pattern of asthma in pregnancy is unpredictable. In many it remains stable: some feel much better, but others feel worse, although an attack during labour is virtually unknown.

The worsening, or first appearance, of asthma in young adults should prompt enquiry about occupation and the changing of place of work or working practices. As Rackemann described, asthma in middle life is less likely to be atopic in origin. Apart from occupation, infection remains a potent initiator, particularly in the presence of tobacco smoking, but also in other potentially hazardous environments. The part played by stress in adult asthma should not be overemphasized, but neither should attention to this trigger be neglected. Some adults appear to have true intrinsic asthma for which no clear cause can be identified. It seems preferable to identify mechanisms as far as possible rather than to lump all these new or relapsed cases together under the somewhat meaningless terms of late or adult-onset asthma.

Asthma is probably as inadequately recognized in the elderly as it is in schoolchildren. The causes and triggers are as described for younger adults, but there is a sad tendency to dismiss increasing breathlessness as simply the effect of age or smoking. Asthma is worth diagnosing because it is treatable. Drugs increasingly prescribed for a variety of complaints in the elderly should be screened as possible causes of asthma. Allergy is a rare cause, but should not be forgotten.

Acute severe asthma

The most dramatic attacks are very rapid in onset, the victim being transformed from a state of relative well being to one of intense life-threatening asthma in less than 30 min. These attacks may be brought on by a recognizable allergic trigger, and seem to differ in aetiology from the severe attack which evolves over several days of worsening symptoms, and is more likely to be associated with infection.

In the attack, the patient is desperately breathless, unable to move or complete more than a few words in one breath. Respiratory rate is rapid ($\geq$ 25/min) and there is a trachycardia ($\geq$ 110/min). Children attain much higher rates. Wheeze is usually readily audible, and a silent chest is a warning of extremely severe obstruction. Life-threatening features

are bradycardia, hypotension, reduced respiratory effort, exhaustion, and coma.

It is difficult to give precise guidelines on peak expiratory flow rate. A figure of 33 per cent or more of normal would certainly qualify (as suggested in the current guidelines), but if 'normal' is 150 l/min a drop to 90 l/min (60 per cent) could be sufficient to be life threatening. Oximeter saturations below 90 per cent are likely in severe attacks, representing on blood gas analysis a PaO_2 of below 8 kPa. Hyperventilation usually lowers the $PaCO_2$, and any rise in $PaCO_2$ or a low pH are grave prognostic features.

Investigations in asthma

Lung function tests

These tests are mandatory and determine the degree of functional disturbance. A single set of tests, however complex, provides only a snapshot of a rapidly moving target. Repeated tests are essential and therefore should be simple. Measurement of PEF using a portable meter satisfies these aims. Qualitative evaluation of peak flow charts (Fig. 2 and 3) provides almost all the information required. Quantitative evaluation with respect to predicted values based on height, age, and sex is important. Care needs to be taken in recording percentage change. In a patient with a predicted PEF of 600 l/min, a figure of 400 l/min represents a value 33 per cent below that predicted, whereas improving that same patient's peak flow from 400 to 600 l/min using a bronchodilator is a 50 per cent change. A series of PEF values recorded over a period of time may be analysed as an overall mean, mean values morning and evening, or a 7-day running mean.

There is little need for more complex tests. Serial $FEV_1 \pm FVC$ (functional vital capacity) readings are possible with recently introduced miniaturized electronic spirometers, but add little to the information given using the PEF meter. Plethysmographic and flow volume loop measurements of airflow obstruction add more sensitivity when lung function is only minimally disturbed, and lung volume measurements add a dimension to understanding of the nature of the functional disturbance. Breathing at high lung volumes is uncomfortable whatever the degree of airflow obstruction. These types of assessment are only applicable to short-term challenge or therapeutic trial situations.

Chest radiology

Chest radiology reveals nothing of asthmatic airways *per se* and is frequently normal in asthma. Its use is confined to patients presenting diagnostic problems, usually for the exclusion of other disorders. In an acute attack, beyond reflecting the hyperinflation secondary to severe airflow obstruction, the plain radiograph will pick up a pneumothorax and segmental or lobar collapse or consolidation.

Evaluating mechanisms

Atopic status is evaluated using skin-prick tests, total IgE, and specific IgE (radio-allergosorbent tests). Such tests would be essential if defining atopic status influenced therapeutic decisions. However, it rarely does although if safe desensitization procedures were reintroduced, this would be different. As an adjunct to influencing decisions on inhaled allergen avoidance, specific allergen tests can be valuable.

In the difficult chronic asthmatic, particular circumstances would dictate the need to follow particular lines of investigation: Aspergillus precipitins for those with transitory pulmonary infiltrates, tests of gastro-oesophageal function where positional cough and wheeze suggest possible reflux, or quantitative immunoglobulins where there are recurrent infective episodes. A peripheral eosinophilia of the order of 5 to 10 per cent ($0.4–1.0 \times 10^9$/l) is not uncommon in both extrinsic and intrinsic asthma, but counts higher than this range should alert to the possibility of vasculitis (see Chapter 17.10.7) or intestinal parasites causing the asthma.

Differential diagnosis

It is rightly said that 'all that wheezes is not asthma', but equally all that is asthma need not wheeze. Therefore there is a differential diagnosis to be considered.

In childhood the most worthwhile differential is inhaled foreign body. Wheezing is more likely to be monophonic and localized over the appropriate airways. Radiology may reveal pneumonitis behind the obstruction, failure of the lobe to deflate on expiration, and, in a few cases, the foreign body itself if it is radio-opaque.

There is an increased prevalence of atopy in cystic fibrosis (Chapter 17.9.2), and in the early stages of the disease recurrent infection may present as wheezing episodes.

In older age groups single airway obstruction is more likely to be due to benign or malignant tumours, although uncommonly infiltrative disorders of the airways such as sarcoid and amyloid can be confusing. Diffuse airways obstruction in smokers and bronchiectatics is occasionally sufficiently reversible to deserve the label asthmatic (and, conversely, endstage asthma can end up as irreversible chronic airways obstruction).

Organic upper-airways obstruction (trachea, larynx, pharynx) can trap the unwary, but it is as important to recognize functional upper-airways obstruction. This is a syndrome of variable, usually laryngeal, obstruction in which the vocal cords can be seen to be tightly adducted. Wheeze is intense and distress all too obvious. The appearances have all the hallmarks of acute severe asthma and this is how it is usually treated, even to the extent of ventilation and high dose steroid therapy, both with their attendant dangers. However, response, particularly to sedation, is uncharacteristically rapid, and a certain 'belle indifference' eventually alerts attendants to the essentially psychological nature of the disorder. There is a predominance of young females and an excess of health care workers amongst sufferers. Some have a past, even present, history of mild genuine asthma, making the diagnosis of the acute (apparently) life-threatening attack that much more difficult. Psychotherapy and speech therapy help most individuals.

Other diffuse pulmonary diseases, particularly the vasculitides, may present with asthmatic features. The carcinoid syndrome from hepatic metastases needs to be remembered, and, in the cardiovascular system, left-ventricular failure and very occasionally pulmonary emboli can present in a very similar manner to acute asthma.

Treatment

Although asthma can, and often does, remit spontaneously in individuals, there is no known way of enhancing or encouraging this process, except for instances where a recognized allergen entirely responsible for the asthma can be eliminated from the environment. Even so, allergen avoidance must remain a primary principle in management strategies for asthma. Control of the condition by effective prophylactic medication follows next, and relief of symptoms is required when other measures have failed.

Allergen avoidance

The best examples come from occupational asthma (Chapter 17.9.1(c)), where adaptation of the environment to contain or eliminate the allergen is often possible or, failing that, the affected individual can be removed to a safer environment. An essentially occupational phenomenon sometimes has secondary effects on the population at large. A fascinating and still unfolding story relates to epidemics of acute asthma encountered in the Spanish city of Barcelona in recent years. Careful epidemiological research revealed that high admission rates for acute asthma

Table 2 *Precautions against exposure to house dust mites*

1. Cover, having first replaced if possible, pillows and mattresses with occlusive covers
2. Cut down soft furnishings and carpets to a minimum
3. Use synthetic fibre furnishings in preference to those of plant or animal origin
4. Clean sheets etc weekly on a 'hot wash'
5. Vacuum only with a cleaner with a powerful filter
6. Keep heat and humidity low

coincided with days on which soya bean was being unloaded at the port into one particular silo and when the wind was blowing towards the city. IgE antibodies to soya bean were detected in the blood of affected individuals, making this seem like a typical atopic asthma. The age distribution suggested the possibility of an interaction with cigarette smoking.

In the common forms of extrinsic atopic asthma, much effort has been expended in devising methods for reducing the load of *D. pteronyssinus* in household dust. That these efforts are ultimately worthwhile is illustrated by work showing good symptomatic relief and reduced bronchial hyper-reactivity in individuals housed in dust-free environments. Half-hearted measures are of no value. Vacuum cleaners without an efficient filter are worse than useless. Care needs to be taken with certain acaracides (agents which kill mites) which can be harmful to humans. Various programmes have been devised. One that embodies measures which are known to reduce dust load and yet not require superhuman devotion to implement is given in Table 2.

Domestic pets should be banished if possible, but, failing that, weekly washing combined with antidust measures will help the sufferer but perhaps not be appreciated by the animal! Items of food that give obviously violent allergic reactions are easy enough to avoid, but elaborate diets which aim to eliminate common foodstuffs such as milk, eggs, wheat, etc. should be avoided unless rigorous double-blind elimination trials have proved positive. No asthmatic should take a β-blocker by any route (including eye drops). Aspirin and NSAIDs should be treated with caution, but many asthmatics are unaffected by these drugs. Safe drugs for simple analgesia in asthmatics are paracetamol and usually trilisate.

Asthmatics should not smoke tobacco actively or passively and have the right of a smoke-free environment at work. Asthma is twice as common in the children of smoking parents as it is in those from non-smoking households, and smoking aggravates the harmful effects of many occupational causes of asthma.

Prophylaxis

The foundation of present-day treatment of asthma is prophylactic regular therapy to control symptoms. A scheme is outlined in Table 3. Treatment is begun simply and built up until satisfactory control is achieved. Control means freedom from symptoms, particularly nocturnal awakening, lung function within the normal range and varying by less than 20 per cent within 24 h, and normal quality of life. The attainment of these aims is limited by treatment side-effects and patient compliance. Maintenance oral corticosteroids give well-recognized side-effects, but even aerosol corticosteroids are not free from toxicity. At doses of inhaled beclomethasone or budesonide of 1000 μg or more daily, skin bruising is common, bone density may be reduced and hypothalamus–pituitary–adrenal axis function can be impaired. Taking regular treatment is demanding and can appear unrewarding when it gives no immediate benefit. Patients resent relying on medication, and may have real or imagined fears about it or culturally determined resistance to taking inhaled drugs. All these concerns must be met if prophylactic therapy is to achieve clinically all that it promises pharmacologically, and in the end the level of treatment accepted will be a mutually agreed compromise between benefit, side-effects, and acceptability.

Table 3 *Management guidelines for asthma*

Avoidance of allergens and stopping smoking where appropriate
Step 1 Occasional use of relief bronchodilators
Step 2 For regular or persistent symptoms, night-time awakening or daily use of relief bronchodilators: low dose inhaled steroid, e.g. beclomethasone 100–400 µg twice daily[1]
Step 3 High does inhaled steroid, e.g. beclomethasone 500–1000 µg twice daily. OR[2] low dose inhaled steroid + additional bronchodilator, e.g. inhaled salmeterol 50 µg twice daily, inhaled ipratropium, or oral methylxanthine
Step 4 High dose inhaled steroids and regular bronchodilators
Step 5 Intermittent courses[3] or maintenance corticosteroids[4]
Step down: review progress regularly and reduce to minimum necessary to maintain control
[1] Alternative preventive therapy, e.g. DSCG 20 mg four times a day or nedocromil 8 mg twice daily suitable for young, atopic asthmatics
[2] The author favours this alternative using inhaled long-acting β_2 agonist
[3] One course may dampen airway inflammation sufficiently to allow other preventive therapy to work more effectively
[4] Seek specialist advice before taking this step

Alternative prophylactics

The choice of inhaled prophylactics is not wide and can essentially be divided into steroids and non-steroids. In children, in young atopic adults, in those with mild disease, and in those with an aversion to steroids, disodium cromoglycate (Intal) or nedocromil (Tilade) should be tried first. Disodium cromoglycate needs to be given four times a day, at least initially, which is an impediment to compliance, and at full dose (20 mg on each occasion). This is best achieved with the Spincaps: the metered dose inhaler contains only 5 mg per puff. Nedocromil is recommended for twice daily dosage, but needs to be at a quantity of 8 mg each time.

If, after a 2 to 3 month trial, response is inadequate, a change should be made to a steroid inhaler. The current standard beclomethasone and budesonide are being challenged by the new generation of inhaled steroids which are absorbed even less and rapidly metabolized. Fluticasone is the first on the market. All steroid aerosols can be given in a patient-friendly twice daily regimen.

Devices for inhaled therapy

One central feature of asthma treatment is route and method of delivery. The inhaled route is preferred whenever possible. The device chosen should be that which the individual can use most effectively. Figure 9 illustrates the types of device available. It will remain usual to try the metered dose inhaler first (at least until it becomes unacceptable to use chlorofluorocarbons (CFCs) even in medication). The technique needs to be taught carefully and checked regularly, and an alternative device prescribed if use of the metered dose inhaler cannot be mastered. Large spacer devices (Fig. 10) reduce local side-effects in the mouth because the aerosol is no longer forced into the back of the throat, reduce systemic side-effects because less drug is deposited on the buccal mucosa, allow the propellant to evaporate in the spacer, and overall deliver a greater percentage dose to the lungs. Dry powder devices are generally more expensive, more complex to use, and still suffer from problems of deposition in the oropharynx, but do not use CFC propellants. Nebulizers should be reserved for patients who require larger doses, cannot use any other device, or are likely to need unexpected emergency treatment for an acute attack. Because delivery from a nebulizer is very wasteful

and much solution is left in the chamber, side-effects dose for dose are significantly less than those with the metered dose inhaler.

Oral bronchodilators

Inhaled β_2-agonists are so effective that there should be minimal need to use the larger doses required for the oral route with their attendant systemic side-effects. Methylxanthine bronchodilators, such as theophylline and aminophylline, cannot be given by inhalation, but have a time-honoured place in asthma therapy. Their mechanism of action is complex, probably involving adenosine pathways as well as phosphodiesterase inhibition. Taken long term they may have additional advantageous immune-modulating activity. Slow-release preparations allow these drugs to be administered twice daily. They are widely favoured in North America but are less popular in the United Kingdom, where British stomachs seem unduly prone to the gastrointestinal disturbance (nausea, dyspepsia, and even vomiting) which is their chief use-limiting side-effect. They also relax the lower oesophageal sphincter, and so should not be used when reflux is thought to be present, and they cause cerebral stimulation and wakefulness in some individuals.

Oral corticosteroids

Short courses of oral corticosteroids are indicated in asthma as a diagnostic test, to gain good control when initiating treatment in more severe cases, when inhaled treatment proves unsatisfactory, and when intercurrent infection or allergen exposure produces a sharp decline in function. Prednisolone is the standard steroid prescribed. The daily dose required varies from 20 mg/day in a child or small female to 40 mg/day in a heavy muscular male. Larger doses are not infrequently used and become more necessary as the disease becomes more chronic due to fixed inflammatory airways narrowing. The duration of the course depends on clinical and functional indices of recovery. The once favour-

Fig. 9 A collection of inhaler devices.

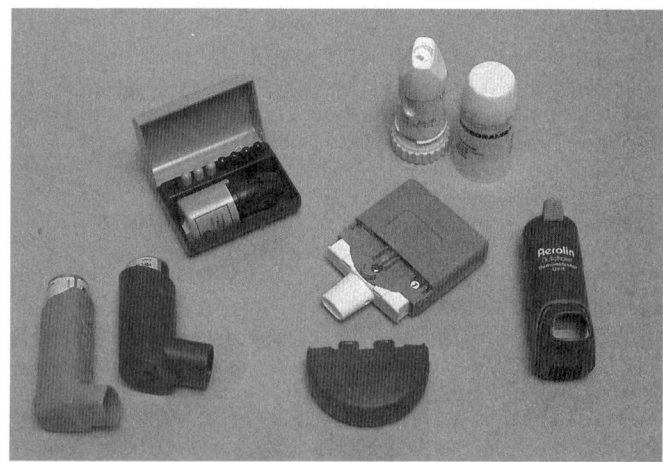

Fig. 10 A large-volume spacer (the Nebuhaler).

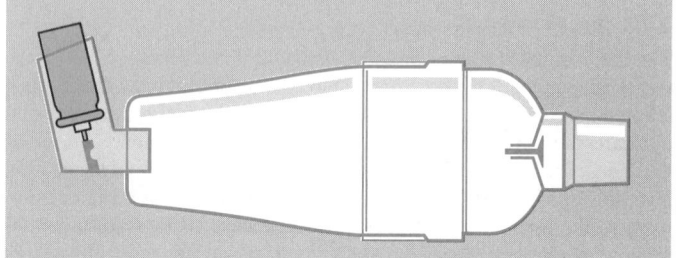

ite regimen of 30 mg on the first day, followed by 5 mg less on each of five subsequent days, had no good trials to support its use. A simple recommendation suitable for many cases is to maintain the starting dose until previous or best function is restored, and then to give half that dose for an equal number of days. Individuals will differ in their responses, however, and side-effects may prevent a predetermined plan from being carried through. Aerosol steroids should not be stopped during a course of prednisolone, and should be kept at a higher dose than before the oral drug was used until continued good control signifies that it can be reduced.

Maintenance oral corticosteroid therapy should be avoided whenever possible. Long-acting inhaled bronchodilators (the β_2-agonist salmeterol and the anticholinergic oxitropium), slow-release methylxanthines (theophylline and aminophylline SR), and antihistamines (including the more broadly antiallergic agent ketotifen) should all be given a trial before taking this step, despite considerations discussed below about the possible dangers of regular bronchodilator therapy. Once maintenance steroid therapy is started, every effort should be made to keep the dose below 10 mg of prednisolone a day and to use an alternate day regimen if this proves clinically satisfactory. Patients should be monitored for long-term side-effects, particularly remembering diabetes and osteoporosis. In postmenopausal women on maintenance oral corticosteroids, cyclical diphosphonates (e.g. etidronate 200 mg daily for 2 weeks in 13) and calcium supplements (for the remaining 11 weeks of the 13) may halt the progress towards osteoporosis, but it is not known whether this treatment is equal to or could be supplemented with oestrogen hormone replacement therapy.

In those instances where prednisolone is required in a dose of more than 10 mg, daily consideration should be given to trials of other immunosuppressive agents. Those under study at present include methotrexate 10 mg weekly and cyclosporin; other cytotoxic immunosuppressives such as cyclophosphamide and azathioprine have also been tried, as has intramuscular gold. All these agents carry their own side-effects which must be balanced against those of the corticosteroid; most give a degree of steroid sparing, but rarely allow prednisolone to be withdrawn altogether.

Relief of symptoms

Even with the best control, asthmatic symptoms occur spontaneously or in response to challenge. Inhaled β_2-agonist bronchodilators give the most immediate relief (detectable improvement in airways calibre within a minute). The more selective β_2-agonists (e.g. salbutamol and terbutaline) should be used from a metered dose inhaler or dry powder device. The dose can be repeated within 10 min if required or it can be increased. High doses can be achieved either by using multiple actuations (10–12) in a large spacer or with prepacked nebulizer solutions. Both devices minimize side-effects. Failure at this point means that therapy for an acute attack should be instituted (see Table 4).

The acute attack

The approach to the acute attack is therapeutically simple but managerially complex. In essence therapy consists of adequate doses of β_2-agonist bronchodilators, systemic steroids, and oxygen. Only a few attacks will fail to respond to this scheme. For those that do, additional tactics include additional bronchodilators and ventilatory support.

Some attacks are dramatically sudden in onset and seem to include an element of anaphylaxis with laryngeal as well as bronchial narrowing so that a rapidly acting non-selective β-agonist is indicated. Subcutaneous adrenaline (0.5–1.0 ml of 1:1000 solution) is advised. It is available in a prepacked syringe as Mini Jet adrenaline, and in this form can be used directly by patients or carers. Nebulized anticholinergics (250–500 μg ipratropium) can speed recovery in the first 24 h if given (up to 4 hourly) with β_2-agonists. The position of the methylxanthines is inse-

Table 4 *Treatment of a severe asthmatic attack*

Immediate treatment in all patients
- Oxygen—highest concentration available (CO_2 retention is rarely a problem)
- Prednisolone 30–60 mg orally, or hydrocortisone 200 mg IV if $Pa\mathrm{CO_2}$ is raised or there is any doubt about tablet absorption, or both
  - Salbutamol 2.5–5 mg } via a nebulizer
    or   } (driven by O_2 in hospital)
  - Terbutaline 5–10 mg

Table 5 *Acute severe asthma*

Indications for intensive care
Patients with following features always require intensive care
- Hypoxia ($Pa\mathrm{O_2}$ < 8kPa) despite receiving 60% inspired oxygen
- Hypercapnia ($Pa\mathrm{CO_2}$ > 6kPa)
- Onset of exhaustion
- Confusion or drowsiness
- Unconsciousness
- Respiratory arrest

cure. Once a mainstay of treatment (it was commonplace to give an intravenous bolus of 250 mg of aminophylline), they fell out of favour because of reported acute cardiovascular toxicity, even deaths, with the effect being enhanced in those already taking slow-release oral methylxanthines. For the difficult attack or in the rare patients sensitive to β-agonists, they can be given effectively as a slow intravenous infusion (0.5 mg aminophylline/kg body weight/hour). Gastrointestinal upset, as well as tachycardia and dysrhythmias, limit the use of higher doses. An intravenous infusion for fluid replacement (caused by hyperventilation and being too breathless to drink) is important in severe attacks, to which potassium should be added to counteract the metabolic effects of high dose β-agonist therapy.

Ventilatory support is rarely needed, but the indications for its use (Table 5) should be clearly recognized by any physicians who handle acute asthma.

Failure to respond to therapy

Despite following recommended guidelines, some asthmatics fail to respond as might be expected. Several reasons for this should be explored.

Whilst it is always worth reconsidering the diagnosis, remembering that individuals may have more than one condition and asking whether allergen avoidance could be stepped up, the fault usually lies with therapy. The commonest is poor technique in using inhaled therapy. Many patients still fail to grasp the skills necessary to use the metered dose inhaler most effectively. A spacer device or a dry powder inhaler will ensure adequate delivery for most subjects, and a nebulizer is rarely necessary. Special attention needs to be paid to the arthritic or partially sighted.

Secondly, the dose of the inhaled medication may be wrong—usually too low a dose of inhaled steroid although rarely too high a dose of bronchodilator. The balance of prescribed therapy may be wrong—over-reliance on relief bronchodilators when prophylactic inhalers are more appropriate.

Equally, the patient may be neglecting to use therapy even though it has been prescribed correctly. Patients are still afraid of steroids, even in inhaled form, and much patience and time is needed to overcome prejudices that arise from folklore, family pressure, or erroneous media reporting. Sometimes side-effects are real, and this issue also needs addressing.

Although the majority of patients respond to treatment in a way that seems pharmacologically correct, we should be aware that individuals are allowed to differ from the norm. Recognized examples are truly steroid-unresponsive asthma and paradoxical bronchoconstriction, particularly to some anticholinergic bronchodilators, which is only partly explained by adverse reactions to the vehicle conveying the active drug.

Desensitization

The concept of desensitization for allergic disease was introduced about 1910 at a time when immunization for infectious diseases was becoming popular. The allergen thought to be responsible for the patient's symptoms is injected intramuscularly in increasing concentration. So-called 'blocking antibodies' are generated, but how and whether they prevent responses to inhaled allergens has not been properly determined. Clinical trials support some benefit in allergic rhinitis, but very little in asthma. Greater success is recognized in the treatment of those hypersensitive to bee and wasp stings, and this is attributed to the use of highly purified antigen solution. Unfortunately, when similar purified preparations of house dust mite antigen were studied in asthma, there were some deaths. This led to very stringent restrictions being placed on the use of desensitizing injections in the United Kingdom where this form of treatment is now seldom used. Such is not the case in North America or most of Europe where continued research is now beginning to yield data that suggest that this form of treatment will have a part to play in future strategies of asthma management.

Organization of care

Broader management strategies for acute asthma must recognize events before the application of the therapies outlined above and plans that must be made afterwards which aim to prevent further acute attacks. In any recorded series of asthma deaths, there are always some that by all accounts seem to have been so dramatically sudden in onset that no form of intervention could have been life-saving. However, there are others where errors of judgement on the part of the sufferer, the carers, or the medical attendants seem to have been at least partly responsible for the death. It is here that improved care programmes, action plans, and education should pay dividends.

Each asthma attack initiates a chain of events. An essential prerequisite is that both asthmatics and their carers recognize that an attack is likely or has already begun. Simple guidelines include exposure to conditions previously recognized as dangerous, failure of normal doses of bronchodilator to give relief, progressive deterioration over several days with worsening nocturnal awakening, and reduction in PEF below a level previously determined as critical. The action taken at this point should be based along lines previously agreed, and in terms of seeking help could mean either calling primary care services or going directly to hospital. The latter course of action will usually mean just going to an accident and emergency department, although some chest services offer open access for those asthmatics recognized as having severe and brittle asthma. The important issues as far as education is concerned are that the patient (carer) knows what to do and when to do it, and that the services that they contact are competent and skilled in handling acute asthma.

Important steps can be taken when patients emerge from an attack to try to prevent further acute attacks. The efficient chest unit will explore with the patient any correctable causes of the attack and give instruction in asthma management, ensuring that the reason for and the actions of prescribed therapy are understood. No patient should be discharged without prophylactic therapy or knowledge of how to proceed in the next acute attack.

It is becoming evident that asthma is a condition, like several other chronic disorders, where it is appropriate that patients take a leading role in managing their own illness. This involves a thorough understanding of the need for regular therapy, self-checking of inhaler technique, and self-monitoring. The peak flow meter (now prescribable on the National Health Service drug tariff) is the key to the latter. The life of the asthmatic is often not smooth. They should have a clear action plan, which is written down and is specific to their needs. It should describe how to recognize deterioration, when to take bronchodilator treatment, how much to take and how often to take it, when to start or change the dose of corticosteroids, and when to call for or seek out help. Instructions should indicate not only how symptoms influence these decisions but also take into consideration changes in home-monitored peak flow. One example of such a management plan is listed in Fig. 8. This information can be provided by general practitioners or hospital doctors, but increasingly it is being supplied by highly trained and sympathetic practice nurses who run asthma clinics from general practitioners' health centres.

On a wider level, there is a need for consistent and well-organized training and education about asthma for sufferers, carers, and professionals. The National Asthma Campaign, the national charity for asthmatics in the United Kingdom, has taken a lead in patient education providing literature, a telephone help line (0345 01 02 03), and support groups. Nurse training is expertly provided at the Asthma Training Centre in Stratford-upon-Avon, chiefly for practice nurses but also for school nurses. The pharmaceutical companies are active in the educational field, at the same time promoting their products so that there is inevitable bias. The nationally agreed guidelines for the treatment of asthma devised by a widely representative group from the British Thoracic Society, National Asthma Campaign, Royal College of Physicians, and Kings Fund, and subsequently an audit of practice, show that there is resolve within the profession to set standards.

Death from asthma

Osler incorrectly taught that death does not occur in the attack. However, it does. In the United Kingdom just over 2000 deaths per annum are certified as due to asthma. Trends in mortality over the last 30 years are illustrated in Fig. 11. The data raise several interesting issues. First, despite major innovations in the treatment of asthma, there has been no overall improvement in the mortality situation for many decades. Second, there was a sharp increase in mortality in the late 1960s which was seen in the United Kingdom as well as in many, but not all, Westernized countries; it was confined to young people (10–40 years). Finally, there has been a drift upwards in mortality, most marked in the elderly, in the past 20 years which has now reached a plateau.

Fig. 11 Mortality statistics: deaths from asthma in England and Wales by age band. (Source: OPCS.)

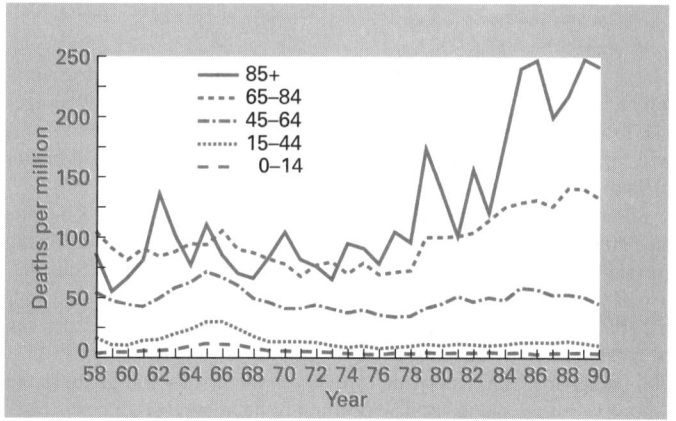

Various explanations exist for these trends, and it is likely that the reasons are multifactorial. First, there have been changes in international classifications for disease; these can and have been catered for in recent statistics, and the last change took place in 1978. What cannot easily be removed are physicians' habits in diagnostic labelling. With an increasing awareness of the benefits of treatment which can reverse airways obstruction, more adults, particularly elderly adults, are being labelled as asthmatic. They would previously have been certified as dying from chronic obstructive lung disease.

Second, there is now good evidence that the recorded prevalence (and even incidence) of asthma is on the increase. Among children, diagnosed asthma is now present in 5 to 6 per cent and probable asthma in 10 to 12 per cent, and 20 per cent or more are often found to have wheezed at some stage in their first decade. Surveys conducted in the same place by the same team using the same methods on more than one occasion 5 to 20 years apart are showing that prevalence figures are on the increase, sometimes amounting to a doubling over 20 years. Similar trends have been noted in other European countries, Australasia, and North America. If increased prevalence covers all degrees of severity, it is clear that mortality figures would also rise.

Yet there are other explanations that point to problems with treatment and the organization of care for asthmatics. An upsurge of asthma deaths in New Zealand in the 1980s has been linked with the use of the somewhat non-selective β_2-agonist fenoterol and a study from Canada incriminated all β_2-agonist treatment, giving risk ratios of 2.4 to 5.4. Great care has been exercised in choosing controls in these retrospective studies, but the doubt must exist that there could be some factor other than the treatment that they were taking which distinguished those who died in the acute attack from those who survived.

Concern over β_2-agonists and asthma deaths led inevitably to the investigation of these drugs in relation to asthma morbidity. Surprisingly, it was found that continued regular use of drugs that are prescribed to give relief of asthmatic symptoms led to worsening morbidity. In a double-blind placebo control study of the β_2-agonist fenoterol in New Zealand, patients on regular fenoterol four times daily scored less well on all counts than those on placebo.

In a separate study from The Netherlands, a rather more mixed group of subjects with both asthma and bronchitis were followed over 2 years with serial lung function measurements. Those on regular bronchodilator treatment showed a faster rate of decline of FEV_1 than those using on demand bronchodilator. The effect was seen with both β_2-agonists and anticholinergics. Anecdotal evidence has also suggested that reducing very high doses of inhaled bronchodilators can improve symptomatology.

How can these observations be explained? Probably no single factor is wholly responsible. Most concern has concentrated on the development of tachyphylaxis or adverse effects on bronchial reactivity from repeated regular doses of β_2-agonists. Some preparations have contained preservatives or are dissolved in vehicles that can themselves cause bronchoconstriction. It has been argued that bronchodilatation allows antigens greater access to distal airways and that the dextro-isomer of the racemic mixture that makes up β_2-agonist preparations causes serious side-effects. Whatever the reason, these studies have reinforced the primacy of regular prophylactic therapy in the management of asthma which is aimed to achieve good control with the use of bronchodilators just for occasional relief.

Epidemiological studies in asthma, apart from producing statistics on deaths and prevalence that raise more questions than they answer, play an important role in charting change and indicating clues to the cause of asthma.

There is a striking tendency for asthma to be more common in urban than in rural communities. A good example comes from Zimbabwe, where the prevalence of reversible airways obstruction was 5.8 per cent in high socioeconomic class urban children from northern Harare, 3.1 per cent in lower-class urban children from southern Harare, and only 0.1 per cent in rural Zimbabwean children. In addition, when there is movement of a population group from a rural to an urban environment, the prevalence of asthma (and often of other atopic disorders) increases. For example, this effect was observed, in Tokelau islanders moving to towns in New Zealand following an environmental disaster in their home islands. It seems most likely that these trends are explained in terms of changes in exposure to environmental allergens. Urban houses are more likely to provide the warm humid well-furnished environment that encourages dust mites. A corollary of this was the probable introduction of dust mites into rural populations in Papua New Guinea by the introduction of Western made materials. Although dietary allergy is generally not thought to be of great significance, urban living favours the use of pre-prepared food and drink containing colourings and additives and is associated with a move away from infant breast-feeding, and so a loss of potentially protective maternal antibodies. Salt may also be higher in urban diets, and in some subgroups of asthmatics this is associated with a higher prevalence of asthmatic symptoms and greater bronchial hyperreactivity. Environmental pollution is greater in cities. Industrial pollution from the burning of coal is certainly much less now in countries with advanced economies but remains a problem in eastern Europe and Asia. Current concern is with exhaust fumes from internal combustion engines. As described earlier, ozone and nitrogen dioxide interact with allergens to increase bronchial reactivity, and this effect will be more obvious in an urban environment.

Epidemiological methodology is also suited to investigating local epidemics of asthma as described in certain places (e.g. the Barcelona soya bean story, or more locally in occupational asthma) or at certain times. There are well-recognized associations between outbreaks of acute asthma and thunderstorms, probably caused by the sudden release of fungal spores with heavy rainfall. At other times weather changes appear to trap pollutants near the ground which, alone or in combination with allergens, trigger asthma.

The future

A combination of increased awareness enabling the early recognition of the disorder, sensible application of excellent prophylactic therapies, and education to ensure that management is optional has succeeded in reducing much of the terror of the condition and has made it controllable in most sufferers. However, it cannot be cured. Although remissions occur, relapse is also frequent and continuous treatment over many years is a sentence for many. The genetic approach offers a hope for novel forms of treatment, but success is some way over the horizon and at present can only be envisaged for atopic asthmatics. There are so many potential mediators of asthmatic inflammation that it seems a forlorn hope that a single mediator blocker will be found that will prove therapeutically successful alone. However, research into inflammatory and other mechanisms, must remain an essential ingredient of future endeavour. Clinicians have been lulled into a sense of security with the successes of current therapy, and this has stifled any interest in dissecting out different forms of asthma and hence tailor-made types of treatment. The epidemiological approach is ideally placed to solve outbreaks traced to industrial processes or specific pollutants, but if it reveals that rising prevalence is related to living conditions and/or more general pollution, such as that due to car exhaust, it will require great personal and political resolve to turn the tide.

REFERENCES

Anderson, S.D., Schoeffel, R.E., Follet, R., Perry, C.P., Daviskas, E., and Kendall M (1982). Sensitivity to heat and water loss at rest and during exercise in asthmatic patients. *European Journal of Respiratory Disease*, **63**, 459–71.

Anonymous (1993). Guidelines on the management of asthma. *Thorax*, **48**(2), Supplements.

Anto J., Sunyer J., Rodriguez-Roison, R., Suarez-Cervera, M., and Vazquez,

L. (1989). Community outbreaks of asthma associated with inhalation of soya bean dust. *New England Journal of Medicine*, **320**, 1097–1101.

Burr, M. L., Charles, T. J., Roy, K., and Seaton, A. (1979). Asthma in the elderly: an epidemiological survey. *British Medical Journal*, **i**, 1041–4.

Burr, M.L., Butland, B.K., King, S., and Vaughan-Williams, E. (1989). Changes in asthma prevalence: two surveys 15 years apart. *Archives of Disease in Childhood*, **64**, 1452–6.

CIBA Foundation Guest Symposium (1959). Terminology, definitions and classification of chronic pulmonary emphysema and related conditions. *Thorax*, **14**, 286–99.

Clark, T.J.H. and Hetzel, M.R. (1977). Diurnal variation of asthma. *British Journal of Diseases of the Chest*, **71**, 87–92.

Cookson, W.O.C.M., Craddock, C.E., Benson, M.K., and Durham S.R. (1989). Falls in peripheral eosinophil counts parallel the late asthmatic reaction. *American Review of Respiratory Diseases*, **139**, 458–62.

Gaynard, P., Orehek, J., Grimaud, C., and Charpin C. (1975). Bronchoconstrictor effects of a deep inspiration in patients with asthma. *American Review of Respiratory Diseases*, **111**, 433–9.

Goldman, J. and Muers, M. (1961). Vocal cord dysfunction and wheezing. *Thorax*, **46**, 401–4.

Grainger, J., Woodman, K., Pearce, N., Crane, J., Burgess, C., Keane, A., and Beasley, R. (1991). Prescribed fenoterol and death from asthma in New Zealand 1981–7: a further case–control study. *Thorax*, **46**, 105–11.

Hill, R.A., Standen, P.J., and Tattersfield, A.E. (1989). Asthma, wheezing and school absence in primary schools. *Archives of Diseases of Children*, **64**, 246–51.

Keeley, D.J., Neill, P., and Gallivan, S. (1991). Comparison of the prevalence of reversible airways obstruction in rural and urban Zimbabwean children. *Thorax*, **46**, 549–53.

Molfino, N.A., Wright, S.C., Katz, I., Tarlo, S., Silverman, F., McClean, P.A., *et al.* (1991). Effect of low concentrations of ozone and inhaled allergen responses in asthmatic subjects. *Lancet*, **338**, 199–203.

Page, C.P. (1991). One explanation of the asthma paradox: inhibition of natural anti-inflammatory mechanism by beta$_2$-agonists. *Lancet*, **337**, 717–20.

Platts-Mills, T.A.E., Tovey, U.R., Mitchell E.B., *et al.* (1982). Reduction of bronchial hyperreactivity during prolonged allergen avoidance. *Lancet*, **ii**, 675–8.

Rackemann F.M. (1921). A clinical classification of asthma. *American Journal of Medical Science*, **162**, 802.

Sears, M.R., Taylor, D.R., Print, C.G., Lake, D.C., Li, Q., Flannery, E.M., *et al.* (1990). Regular inhaled beta-agonist treatment in bronchial asthma. *Lancet*, **336**, 1391–6.

Sontag, S.J., O'Connell, S., Khandelwal, S., Miller, T., Nemchausky, B., Schnell, T.G., and Serlovsky, R. (1990). Most asthmatics have gastro-oesophageal reflux with or without bronchodilator therapy. *Gastroenterology*, **99**, 613–20.

Spitzer, W.O., Suissa, S., Ernst, P., Horwitz, R.I., Habbick, B., Cockcroft, D., *et al.* (1992). The use of beta-agonists and the risk of death and near death from asthma. *New England Journal of Medicine*, **326**, 501–6.

Sterk, P.J. (1993). Virus-induced airway hyperresponsiveness in man. *European Respiratory Journal*, **6**, 894–902.

Young, R.C., Bennett, J.E., Vogel, C.L. *et al.* (1970). Aspergillosis: the spectrum of the disease in 98 patients. *Medicine*, **49**, 147–73.

van Schayck, C.P., Dompeling, E., van Herwaarden, C.L.A., Folgering, H., Verbeek, A.L.M., van der Horgen, H.J.M., and van Weel, C. (1991). Bronchodilator treatment in moderate asthma or chronic bronchitis: continuous or on demand? A randomised controlled study. *British Medical Journal*, **303**, 1426–31.

Welliver, R.C., Sun, M., Rinaldo, D., and Ogra, P.L. (1986). Predictive value of respiratory syncytial virus-specific IgE response for recurrent wheezing following bronchiolitis. *Journal of Paediatrics*, **109**, 776–80.

17.9.1(c) Occupational asthma

A. J. NEWMAN TAYLOR

Occupational asthma is asthma induced by an agent inhaled at work. Agents inhaled at work can aggravate pre-existing asthma, but the term occupational asthma is usually restricted to asthma initiated or induced by such agents.

Asthma may be initiated or 'switched on' either by respiratory irritants inhaled in toxic concentrations—so-called reactive airways dysfunction syndrome (**RADS**)—or as the outcome of an acquired specific hypersensitivity response. Hypersensitivity-induced occupational asthma occurs considerably more commonly than RADS and is important to recognize because in the majority of cases it improves or resolves with avoidance of further exposure. Furthermore, the earlier further exposure is avoided the more probable is complete resolution of the asthma. Recognition and avoidance of the specific occupational cause provides one of the few opportunities to cure asthma in adult life by identification and avoidance of its specific cause.

Causes

The described causes of RADS are relatively few and include well-recognized respiratory irritants, such as chlorine and ammonia, as well as others such as toluene di-isocyanate inhaled in toxic concentrations. However, any respiratory irritant inhaled in concentrations toxic to airways epithelial cells is a potential cause of RADS.

In contrast the number of reported causes of hypersensitivity-induced occupational asthma is considerable, and with the rapid development of biotechnology and the continuous introduction of newly synthesized organic chemicals is likely to increase. The causes described include proteins of animal, vegetable, and microbiological origin, naturally occurring organic chemicals, synthetic chemicals, and inorganic chemicals, particularly metal salts. Some of the more important are listed in Table 1.

Importance of occupational causes of asthma

The contribution of asthma of occupational cause to the prevalence of asthma in the community is not known. A voluntary reporting scheme for new causes of occupational lung disease (SWORD) seen by respiratory and occupational physicians, which started in January 1989, provides a potentially valuable source of information. Occupational asthma was the most common single disease, accounting for about a quarter of the reported cases. The most frequently reported causes of asthma were isocyanates, grain and flour, wood dusts, colophony, and laboratory animals. The estimated incidence of occupational asthma in the working population in 1989 was 22 per million and varied from 114 per million in industries processing metal and electrical materials and those engaged in painting, assembly, and packing to less than 10 per million in professional, management, clerical, and selling occupations (Table 2).

Determinants of hypersensitivity induced occupational asthma

Three major factors have been found to contribute to the development of occupational asthma: exposure, and for agents which induce an IgE associated response, atopy and tobacco smoking. In general, the incidence of sensitization and asthma (1) increases with increasing intensity of exposure to the initiating cause; (2) is greatest during the first 1 to 2 years of exposure; and (3) is increased among atopic individuals and tobacco smokers. Although influenced by host factors such as atopy and cigarette smoking, the incidence of the disease seems primarily determined by exposure to its cause; reduction of disease incidence will be primarily achieved by reducing exposure rather than by the identification and exclusion of 'susceptible' individuals. Although the exclusion of atopics is a tempting approach to reduce incidence of occupational asthma, atopy as a pre-employment test, even in circumstances such as work with laboratory animals where the risk to atopics may be fivefold greater than for non-atopics, is poorly discriminating and is associated both with false negatives and a high false positive rate.

Table 1 *Some important causes of occupational asthma*

	Proteins	Low-molecular-weight chemicals
Animal	Excreta of rats, mice, etc; Locusts Grain mites	
Vegetable	Grain and flour Castor bean Green coffee bean Ispaghula	Plicatic acid (Western red cedar) Colophony (pinewood resin)
Microbial	Harvest moulds *Bacillus subtilis* enzymes	Antibiotics (e.g. penicillins, cephalosporins)
'Minerals'		Acid anhydrides Isocyanates Complex platinum salts Polyamines Reactive dyes

Table 2 *Incidence of occupational asthma in high risk occupations*

Occupational group	Cases	Population	No./million/ per year
Welders/solderers/electronic assemblers	35	220 068	159
Laboratory technicians and assistants	26	127 478	204
Metal-making and treating	14	56 270	249
Plastics making and processing	27	66 005	409
Bakers	29	70 839	409
Chemical processors	31	73 189	424
Coach and spray painters	35	54 737	639
Other painters	21	201 225	104

Pathology and pathogenesis

The pathological changes in the airways of patients with asthma of occupational cause are not in any important way different from those in patients with asthma of other or unknown cause: a desquamative eosinophilic bronchitis, with infiltration of the airway wall by eosinophils and lymphocytes accompanied by desquamation of bronchial epithelial cells.

In common with asthma caused by allergy to proteins encountered in the general environment, hypersensitivity-induced occupational asthma is probably the outcome of TH_2 lymphocyte stimulation, and the pathological features observed are primarily the consequence of TH_2 lymphocyte–eosinophil interaction. The evidence for TH_2 lymphocyte stimulation is in part direct, but primarily comes from evidence of specific IgE antibody to many, although not all, of the causes of occupational asthma. In a few cases specific IgG antibodies can also be detected. These seem to reflect exposure, whereas IgE is more closely associated with disease. In general, specific IgE has been identified with the protein causes of occupational asthma but only with a minority of the non-protein causes. While it is likely that the majority of the low-molecular-weight chemicals which cause occupational asthma do so by binding to body proteins and acting as haptens, the difficulties of preparing the relevant hapten–protein conjugate *in vitro* have limited demonstration of this process, other than with chemicals such as acid anhydrides and reactive dyes which form stable conjugates with human serum albumin.

Clinical features

IRRITANT-INDUCED ASTHMA (RADS)

Asthma caused by the inhalation of an irritant chemical in toxic concentrations is usually one manifestation of the general tissue injury to exposed mucosal surfaces—eyes, nose, throat, and bronchial airways.

The onset of symptoms follows a single identifiable exposure to a toxic chemical. Running, swelling, and discomfort of the eyes, running and obstruction of the nose, and painful throat usually occur within minutes of the exposure, and symptoms of asthma (shortness of breath, wheezing, chest tightness, and cough) develop within a few hours—certainly within 24 h—of inhalation of the chemical in toxic concentrations. Respiratory symptoms often have the characteristic circadian pattern characteristic of asthma: they are more severe during the night and on waking than during the daytime. In the majority of cases asthma resolves spontaneously within a few weeks, but occasionally can persist for several years, if not indefinitely.

HYPERSENSITIVITY-INDUCED ASTHMA

In the more frequently occurring cases of hypersensitivity-induced occupational asthma respiratory symptoms develop insidiously and do not follow a single identifiable exposure to its cause. Asthma develops after an initial symptom-free period of exposure, commonly within 1 year of starting a new job or changing duties at work, although in some cases asthma may not develop until several years of exposure have elapsed. The onset of asthma may have been preceded or be accompanied by 'hay-fever'-like symptoms of the nose and eyes. Characteristically, symptoms become increasingly severe during the working week and improve during absences from work during holidays and at weekends. However, the relationship between their respiratory symptoms and work may not be appreciated by patients. This is particularly the case when symptoms develop during the second half of the day and are most severe, as is characteristic of asthma, in the evenings, during the night, and on waking in the morning. Asthmatic symptoms can also persist for several days after avoidance of exposure when appreciable symptomatic improvement at weekends does not occur; improvement is usually sufficient to be appreciated by the end of a 2-week holiday or deterioration to be recognized on return to work. With continuing exposure asthma can become chronic and the relationship between symptoms and periods at work less clear, although even in these circumstances it is usual for some symptomatic improvement to occur on avoidance of exposure, although this may take several weeks.

The findings on clinical examination depend upon the severity of asthma at the time of the examination. If seen when away from exposure, no abnormal findings may be found. During a period of symptomatic exposure the patient will have signs of airflow limitation, with breathlessness on minimal exertion (e.g. undressing), tachycardia, pulsus paradoxus, expiratory and inspiratory wheezes, and reduced breath sounds.

Diagnosis

The diagnosis of occupational asthma should be considered in any adult who develops asthma or whose asthma has deteriorated in working life. In the case of RADS the association of the onset of asthma with inhalation of a toxic chemical is usually clear. The association of asthma caused by a specific hypersensitivity reaction is often less apparent, and the diagnosis is based on the following.

1. Exposure to a sensitizing agent at work.
2. Characteristic history of:
   (a) onset of asthma after an initial symptom-free period of exposure;
   (b) deterioration in symptoms during periods at work and improvements during absence from work.
3. Results of objective investigations:
   (a) lung function tests
   (b) immunological tests
   (c) inhalation tests.

Objective investigations

LUNG FUNCTION TESTS

The most commonly used criterion for diagnosing asthma—improvement in airflow limitation (usually measured as forced expiratory volume in 1 second (FEV_1) or peak expiratory flow (**PEF**)) after inhalation of bronchodilator—is often not present in cases of occupational asthma because lung function may be normal when the patient is seen away from work and, if present, does not identify a work relationship. The measure of lung function most commonly used to identify work related asthma is serial self-recorded PEF. A patient with suspected occupational asthma is asked to record his PEF at intervals of 2 to 3 h for a month from waking to sleeping, and at night if awoken, both during periods at and absences from work. The results can be summarized in a graphical display which records the best, worst, and average values for each day, allowing comparison of PEF during days at work with days away from work (Fig. 1). The diagnostic value of the test depends on the reproducibility of the patients' forced expiratory manoeuvres and their honesty and compliance. Concurrent treatment can influence the results, particularly when treatment is systematically increased during periods at work and reduced during absences from work. When possible treatment should be kept constant during the period of testing and at a minimum recorded. Comparisons with the results of inhalation testing as the 'gold standard' have shown that serial self-recorded PEF measurements are a sensitive and specific index of work-related asthma. Patients who did not show evidence of asthma on PEF records (i.e. less than 20 per cent within-day variability) did not react in inhalation tests unless they were not exposed to the cause of asthma at work during the period of peak flow measurement. The patients with evidence of work-related asthma on PEF records reacted on inhalation testing to a specific agent inhaled at work and had occupational asthma. The major diagnostic difficulties were patients with evidence of asthma on PEF records without a work relationship, of whom a proportion were eventually shown to have occupational asthma; the commonest reason for this false-negative response was insufficient time away from work for significant improvement to have occurred.

IMMUNOLOGICAL TESTS

The presence of specific IgE antibody, identified either by immediate skin test response to a soluble protein extract or a hapten–protein conjugate or by immunoassay in serum (usually radio-allergosorbent testing) is evidence of sensitization to a specific agent. The diagnostic value of a positive test depends upon its predictive value in cases of asthma among those exposed to the specific agent. Specific IgE can be identified in most, if not all, protein causes of occupational asthma, and in a small number of low-molecular-weight chemical causes of asthma, notably complex platinum salts, acid anhydrides, and reactive dyes. No reliable immunological test has been developed for sensitivity to the other important causes of asthma such as isocyanates and colophony. The diagnostic value of a positive test has been formally examined for few of the causes of occupational asthma, and in these cases has been found to be significantly associated with asthma caused by both proteins and low-molecular-weight chemicals inhaled at work.

INHALATION TESTING

The objective in an inhalation test is to expose the individual under single-blind conditions to the putative cause of his asthma in circumstances which resemble as closely as possible the conditions of exposure at work. The different test methods used depend upon the physical state of the test material, which can be water soluble (most proteins) and inhaled in solution, a volatile organic liquid inhaled as a vapour, or a dust. Any change in lung function in both airways calibre (usually measured as FEV_1 or PEF) and airways responsiveness to inhaled histamine or methacholine, measured as PC_{20}, is compared with results on appropriate control days. The patterns of airways response provoked by specific inhalation tests have been distinguished by their time of onset and duration. Immediate asthmatic responses occur within minutes of the test exposure and usually resolve spontaneously within 1 to 2 h (Fig. 2). Late asthmatic responses develop 1 h or more after the test exposure and can persist for 24 to 36 h (Fig. 3). Late asthmatic (but usually not immediate) responses are accompanied by an increase in non-specific

Fig. 1 Serial PEF results in a baker sensitive to flour. The best, worst, and average value are plotted for each day. Shaded areas are periods at work; unshaded areas are periods away from work. Peak flows are consistently worse in each work period and improve during each period away from work.

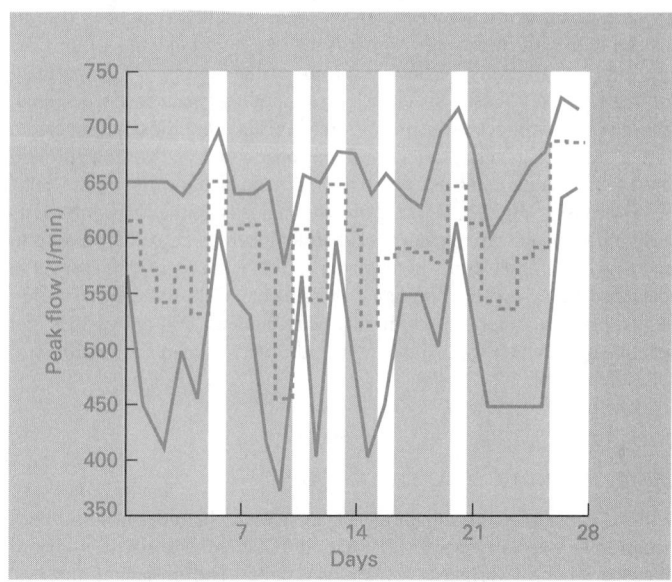

airways responsiveness 3 h and, less reliably, 24 h after the test inhalation. An immediate response followed by a late response has been called a dual response.

Inhalation testing allows the investigation of specific causes of asthma in individuals exposed to them. Provided that the agent being tested is not a non-specific mucosal irritant and does not provoke an immediate asthmatic response in patients with hyper-responsive airways, such as sulphur dioxide, histamine, or exercise, the provocation of an asthmatic response by an occupational agent implies that it is a cause of asthma. This causal relationship is strengthened if the agent reproducibly provokes a late asthmatic response and increases non-specific airways responsiveness.

There are four major indications for inhalation testing in the diagnosis of occupational asthma:

(1) where the agent considered responsible for causing asthma has not previously been reliably shown to do so;

(2) Where an individual with occupational asthma is exposed at work to more than one potential cause which cannot be distinguished by other means;

(3) where asthma is of such severity that further uncontrolled exposure at work is unjustifiable;

(4) where the diagnosis or cause of occupational asthma remains in doubt after other investigations, including serial PEF and immunological tests where applicable, have been completed.

Inhalation tests should be undertaken only for clinical purposes, to provide information important for future management advice. Inhalation tests undertaken solely for medicolegal purposes are not justified.

Differential diagnoses

The diagnosis of occupational asthma requires the following differentiation of asthma:

(1) from other causes of the similar respiratory symptoms, in particular chronic airflow limitation and hyperventilation;

(2) of occupational from non-occupational cause;

(3) initiated by an agent inhaled at work from pre-existing or incidental asthma aggravated by non-specific provocative stimuli encountered at work such as sulphur dioxide, exercise, and cold air.

Prognosis

Asthma initiated by an agent inhaled at work which either is caused by toxic damage to the airway epithelium (RADS) or is the outcome of a hypersensitivity response may become chronic and persist for several years, if not indefinitely. Chronic asthma induced by a hypersensitivity response has been reported most frequently in cases caused by low-molecular-weight chemicals such as isocyanates, colophony, plicatic acid from Western red cedar, and acid anhydrides. Continuing asthmatic symptoms and airways hyper-responsiveness have been reported in 50 per cent or more of patients several years after avoidance of exposure to the initiating cause. Chronic asthma has also been reported in snow crab process workers in Canada in whom airways responsiveness improved during the first 2 years of avoidance of exposure but subsequently reached a plateau.

The only important determinant of developing chronic asthma identified to date has been the duration of symptomatic exposure to the initiating cause after the onset of asthma: those who remain exposed to the cause are more likely to develop chronic asthma.

Fig. 2 Immediate asthmatic reactions in a radiographer provoked in inhalation tests of 3 and 5 min with X-ray fixative material, but not by control test.

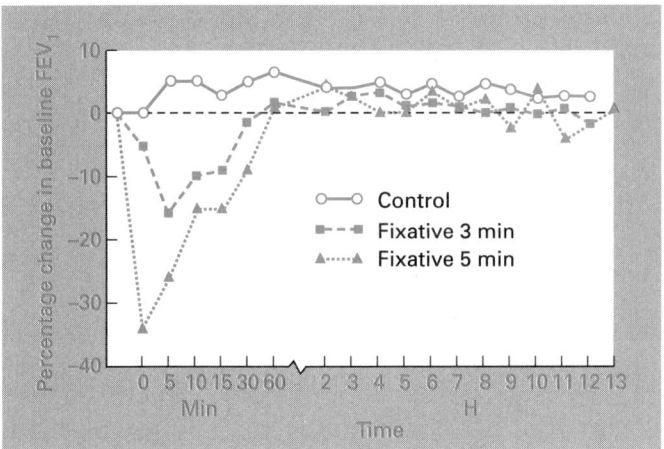

Management

Patients who develop occupational asthma in whom a specific cause is identified should be advised to avoid further exposure to that cause. This seems particularly important where low-molecular-weight chemicals, such as isocyanates, plicatic acid, or anhydrides, are the cause, as continuing symptomatic exposure to these is particularly associated with the development of chronic asthma and airways hyper-responsiveness.

Avoidance of further exposure may require a change or loss of job which, for social or financial reasons, may not be possible. A change of occupation can be particularly difficult for highly trained individuals, such as experimental scientists whose livelihood depends on their knowledge and experience of working with laboratory animals. Such individuals and others sensitized to biological dusts who are unable to change their job, at least in the short term, should be advised to minimize exposure to the cause of their asthma and to wear adequate respiratory protection, most conveniently laminar-flow equipment, when in contact with the organic dust. In addition, background prophylaxis such as sodium cromoglycate can minimize the risk of the provocation of asthma by indirect allergen contact, such as dust on colleagues' clothing. None the less, it should be emphasized that such measures are temporary, and in the long term means should be sought to avoid exposure to the cause of asthma.

When an individual does remain in employment exposed to the cause

Fig. 3 Late asthmatic reaction in a platinum refiner provoked by exposure to the complex platinum salt ammonium hexachloroplatinate in a concentration of 10 mg but not 1 mg in 250 g of lactose (the control material).

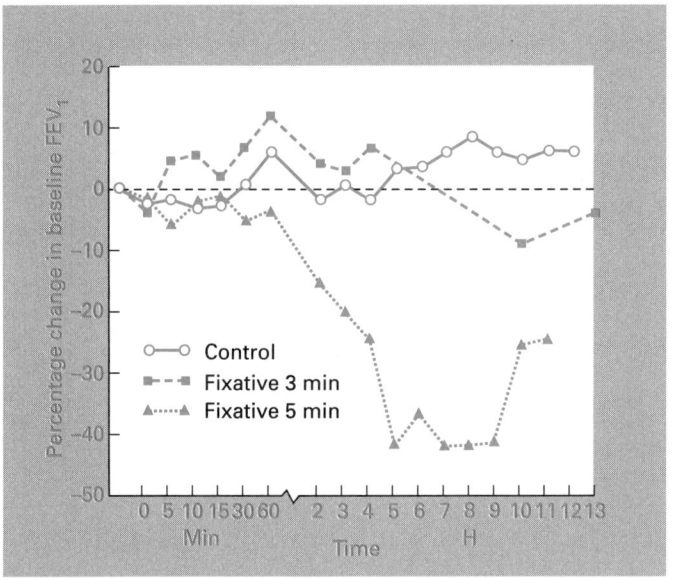

of his asthma, either directly or indirectly, the effectiveness of relocation or of respiratory protection needs to be monitored. This can be conveniently done by serial self-recordings of PEF to determine whether or not asthma is continuing and, if so, whether it is work related.

Compensation

STATUTORY COMPENSATION IN THE UNITED KINGDOM

Occupational asthma is a prescribed disease for 'employed earners'. The terms of prescription have recently been broadened considerably. They now include asthma caused by exposure to 22 specified groups of agents as well as a z category, which specifies 'any other sensitising agent inhaled at work'.

The current terms of prescription are as follows.

Disease	Occupation
Asthma	Exposure to:

(a)   isocyanates;
(b)   platinum salts;
(c)   acid anhydride and amine hardening agents;
(d)   fumes arising from the use of rosin as a soldering flux;
(e)   proteolytic enzymes;
(f)   animals including insects and other arthropods or their larval forms used for the purposes of research, education, in laboratories, pest control, or fruit cultivation;
(g)   dusts arising from barley, oats, rye, wheat or maize, or meal or flour made from such grain;
(h)   antibiotics;
(i)   cimetidine;
(j)   wood dusts;
(k)   ispaghula;
(l)   castor bean dust;
(m)   ipecacuanha;
(n)   azodicarbonamide;
(o)   glutaraldehyde;
(p)   persulphate salts or henna arising from their use in the hairdressing trade;
(q)   crustaceans or fish or products arising from these in the food processing industry;
(r)   reactive dyes;
(s)   soya bean;
(t)   tea dust;
(u)   green coffee bean dust;
(v)   fumes from stainless steel welding;
and
(z)   any other sensitising agent inhaled at work.

Byssinosis

Byssinosis is a disease which in United Kingdom occurs most commonly in cotton mill workers. It is probably a response to agents inhaled in the cotton bract. It is characterized by chest tightness on the first day of the working week, which usually develops some 3 to 4 h after the start of a work shift. Typically, the chest tightness improves on subsequent working days, despite continuing exposure to cotton dust. Byssinosis usually develops after some 20 to 25 years of exposure to cotton dust. The symptoms are often, although not always, accompanied by changes in lung function and the majority of cases of byssinosis have hyper-responsive airways. Cotton dust also provokes acute airway narrowing in about one-third of persons exposed to an extract of cotton bract for the first time; this reaction is probably an important contributory factory in the high turnover in the early months of employ-

ment in cotton mills. Whether byssinosis causes long-term respiratory impairment and disability remains controversial. Several studies have failed to find an increase in mortality from respiratory causes, which has been interpreted as suggesting that exposure to cotton dust does not cause chronic lung disease. However, in one survey of a community, which included ex-cotton workers, a reduction in FEV_1 of between 2 and 8 per cent was observed in the ex-cotton textile workers and a loss of lung function in those with 15 years heavy exposure to cotton dust which was equivalent to that observed in light and ex-smokers.

Byssinosis should probably be considered as a form of occupational asthma: the characteristic symptoms are associated with acute reductions in FEV_1 and patients with byssinosis commonly have hyper-responsive airways.

REFERENCES

Bernstein, I.L., Chan Yeung, M., Malo, J.-L., and Bernstein, D.I. (ed) (1993). Asthma in the Workplace. Marcel Dekker, New York.

Durham, S.R., Graneek, B.J., Hawkins, R., and Newman Taylor, A.J. (1987). The temporal relationship between increases in airway responsiveness to histamine and late asthmatic responses induced by occupational agents. Journal of Allergy and Clinical Immunology, **79**, 398–406.

Fishwick, D. and Pickering, C.A.C. (1992). Byssinosis—a form of occupational 'asthma.' Thorax, **47**, 401–3.

Malo, J.-L., Cartier, A., Ghezzo, J., Lafrance, M., McCante, M., and Lehrer, S.B. (1988). Patterns of improvement in spirometry, bronchial hyper-responsiveness and specific IgE antibody levels after cessation of exposure in occupational asthma caused by snow crab processing. American Review of Respiratory Diseases, **138**, 807–12.

Meredith, S., Taylor, V.M., and McDonald, J.C. (1991) Occupational respiratory disease in United Kingdom 1989: a report to the British Thoracic Society and the Society of Occupational Medicine by the SWORD project group. British Journal of Industrial Medicine, **48**, 292–8.

Venables, K.M., Topping, M.D., Nunn, A.J., Howe, W., and Newman Taylor, A.J. (1987). Immunologic and functional consequences of chemical (tetrachlorophthalic anhydride) induced asthma after 4 years of avoidance of exposure. Journal of Allergy and Clinical Immunology, **80**, 212–18.

17.9.2 Cystic fibrosis

D. J. LANE

Introduction

Cystic fibrosis is the commonest potentially lethal autosomal recessive disorder in Caucasians: a disease frequency of one in 1600 live births is matched by a carrier frequency of one in 22. The recent discovery of the precise genetic abnormality in cystic fibrosis, after a period of research of almost unprecedented intensity, has been a triumph for molecular medicine. The precise functional damage caused by the defect is now under active investigation, and the race is on for means of correcting the fault.

Cystic fibrosis was distinguished from other wasting diseases of childhood in the late 1930s and is characterized as a condition combining pancreatic insufficiency with repeated respiratory tract infections associated with salty sweat. The latter led to the first diagnostic test and one that remains a cornerstone of clinical diagnosis.

Genetics and biochemistry

The gene in which mutations give rise to cystic fibrosis lies on the long arm of chromosome 7. It spans about 250 kb of DNA and can be divided into 27 exons (protein coding regions). The protein for which this gene codes has been titled the cystic fibrosis transmembrane conductance regulator (CFTR). Inferences drawn from the characteristics of the gene so far defined allow a three-dimensional picture of the protein to be drawn. It emerges as a transmembrane protein with a hydrophobic region (the membrane-spanning domain) linked to two nucleotide-binding domains (NBF1 and NBF2), between which lies, intracellularly, the R domain which binds phosphokinase enzymes (Fig. 1).

The first abnormality described, and still the commonest, involves a deletion within the first nucleotide binding domain (NBF1). Since it occurs at position 508 on the amino acid sequence, where a phenylalanine molecule (designated F) has been lost, the abnormality is designated Δ F508 (Fig. 2). Current analyses reveal that some 54 per cent of north European and American cystic fibrosis patients are homozygous for Δ F508 and another 20 per cent carry one copy of this abnormality. Some 170 other mutations have now been identified, many in only a few individuals. As a result, 82 per cent of cystic fibrosis patients in the United Kingdom have a pair of recognizably abnormal genes, which leaves 18 per cent with clinical disease but either just one or no identified abnormal gene to account for it. Across Europe there is a clear northwest to south-east gradient for the prevalence of Δ F508 from 100 per cent in the Faroe Islands to 26 per cent in southern Yugoslavia and Turkey. Other mutations are quite varied. Some, like Δ F508, lie within a similar area of one of the nucleotide binding fractions, but others seem to occur in areas of the protein molecule associated with phosphorylation and intracellular transport.

Cystic fibrosis as a disease affects epithelial cell membranes, and physiological research throughout the 1980s pointed to an abnormality in chloride transport. The discovery of the CFTR protein and its cloning has substantially supported this hypothesis. Inserted into a lipid membrane, CFTR can be shown to transport chloride ions. It appears that CFTR regulates the function of a bicarbonate chloride exchanger. How mutations which occur in areas of the gene involved with phosphorylation influence chloride transport is as yet uncertain. The biochemical consequences of defective chloride transport are deficient water transport into, and deficient sodium reabsorption from, mucus secretions. These viscid low water content secretions cause 'clogging' of the ducts of various exocrine glands, particularly those in the lungs and the pancreas.

Significant anomalies exist in correlating genetic abnormalities with disease patterns. As far as lung function is concerned, there appears to be no discernable or consistent correlation between the pulmonary disease and the presence of either the Δ F508 abnormality or indeed any other. With pancreatic disease the situation is a little clearer. Those homozygous for Δ F508 are much more likely to have pancreatic insufficiency (defined as requiring pancreatic enzyme supplements and likely to signify destruction of up to 90 per cent of the pancreas); only 4 per cent of this group have normal pancreatic function. However, when only one gene carries the Δ F508 mutation, there is no correlation with pancreatic disorder. Liver disease fails to show any pattern of genetic change.

Other anomalies that await explanation lie in the area of the tissue localization of CFTR identified through the *in situ* staining of messenger RNA. The protein is easily identified in the apical regions of the pancreas duct glands, intestinal crypts, and salivary glands, but very little can be picked up in the lungs where an abundance might be expected. In contrast, CFTR is strongly expressed in renal tissue where the only clinical abnormality is unduly rapid excretion of certain antibiotics.

Fig. 1 Schematic representation of the domains of CFTR.

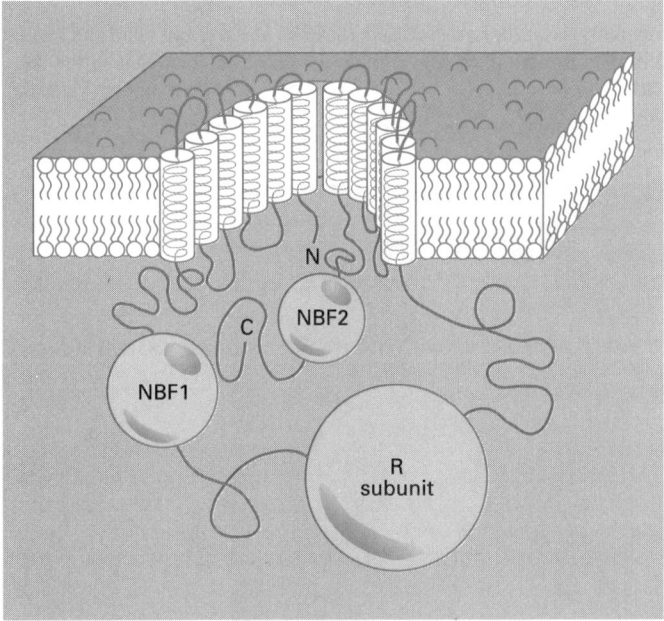

Fig. 2 Autoradiograph of a normal and cystic fibrosis chromosome: the latter shows a trinucleotide deletion that removes phenylalanine from position 508 of the CFTR (△ F508).

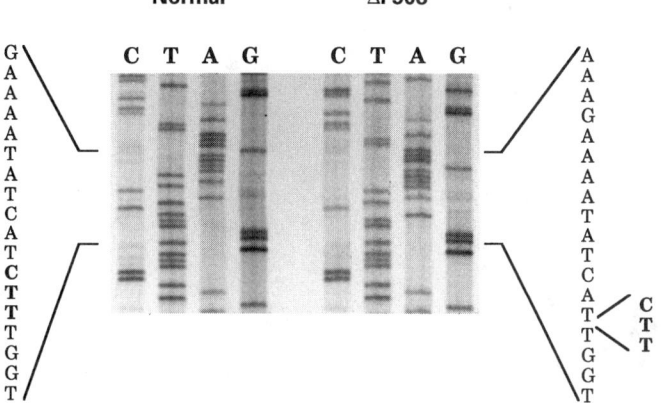

Pathology

Gastrointestinal tract

Both the small intestine and the pancreas demonstrate histological abnormalities *in utero*. Early in the neonatal period, the precipitation of proteinacious material within the pancreatic ducts leads to occlusion, resulting in local inflammation which leads on to fibrosis of the acinar portion of the gland. The destruction of the exocrine glands results in failure of their enzyme secretion. The consequence of this is poor digestion of ingested fat and hence steatorrhoea.

The lung

Infants with cystic fibrosis who die of meconium ileus have normal lung histopathology. The earliest visible pathological change is probably mucous gland hyperplasia with areas of pneumonitis appearing in acute infections. Airways plugging leads to local organizing pneumonia, focal atelectasis, and mucocoele formation. Damaged airways dilate to give areas of cystic bronchiectasis and the lung is eventually all but destroyed. There is no systemic host antimicrobial defence abnormality. Airways infections, particularly with *Staphylococcus aureus* and *Pseudomonas* species, are clearly critical in the evolution of airways damage, and it seems likely that the altered luminal electrolyte and water content produces a mucus which encourages bacterial growth. Breakdown of alveolar macrophages and neutrophils, releasing damaging oxidants and enzymes, combined with the inability of immunoglobulins to penetrate the alginate coating of *Pseudomonas* species predispose to local tissue damage. It has also been suggested that surges of proteolytic enzymes from the damaged pancreas create focal areas of non-infective inflammation in the lungs.

Clinical features

Early life

Three types of presentation should alert to the possibility of cystic fibrosis. The most characteristic, occurring in 10 to 15 per cent of infants, is meconium ileus, i.e. intestinal obstruction with vomiting and abdominal distension due to delayed passage of particularly tenacious meconium. No other diagnosis needs considering. Meconium ileus is the commonest cause of neonatal death in cystic fibrosis. Secondly, cystic fibrosis should be considered in the child who fails to gain weight despite good to excessive food intake. Fatty offensive stools point to malabsorption and pancreatic insufficiency. The lungs are to all appearances normal at birth but, if intestinal disorders do not point to the diagnosis, will eventually suggest the condition on account of recurrent respiratory tract infections. This is the most difficult presentation; the lungs are often clear initially and whooping cough or asthma may be diagnosed. Well-recognized but much rarer presentations are rectal prolapse, neonatal jaundice, and salt depletion.

The respiratory tract

Initial symptoms are cough, with vomiting of swallowed secretions in the young child and, rarely, expectoration. Repeated respiratory tract infections then begin. Only as the child learns to expectorate will it be seen that the secretions are mucopurulent. Before this stage the chest radiograph may give more clues with patchy areas of pneumonitis and sequential collapse running parallel to episodes of fever and intensified cough. Between exacerbations, the sputum is at first mucoid, but even with the control of clinical signs of infection, mucopurulence does not clear from the sputum and the features become more and more those of bronchiectasis. The mucopus is yellow-green in colour, excessive in quantity, and unpleasant in taste and smell. Blood-staining or frank haemoptysis are not infrequent.

Microbiology

Early colonizing bacteria are conventional—pneumococci and *Haemophilus influenzae*. Staphylococci are to be feared in young children since they seem to hasten progress towards bronchial wall damage. Even more serious is the appearance of *Pseudomonas* species in sputum cultures. This organism should never be regarded as a mere commensal in the cystic fibrosis patient. Hopefully, it is not seen until the teenage years but can appear in the first decade. *Pseudomonas aeruginosa* is the most common, but other species are increasingly being isolated; *Pseudomonas cepacia* is particularly dangerous because of its antibiotic resistance and its greater ability to pass between individuals. Many other organisms, of which Klebsiella, *Escherichia coli,* Proteus, and anaerobes deserve mention, can and do cause infective exacerbations.

Pseudomonas antibodies can be detected in the serum and may be a more reliable index than sputum culture of progressive invasion by the organism. The test is not widely available.

Physiology

Physiological abnormalities are those that reflect airways disease and lung destruction. Tests of small airways obstruction become abnormal first with a raised ratio of RV to total lung capacity (TLC), changes in the flow–volume curve at low lung volume, and increases in the $P(\text{A-a})o_2$ gradient. As airways disease progresses, flow rates on forced expi-

ration are reduced and the airways resistance, measured plethysmographically, increases. Unlike diseases characterized by pure airways obstruction, however, TLC does not increase and indeed becomes smaller as the lung destruction progresses, as does the vital capacity. The $P(\text{A-a})o_2$ gradient also widens, and eventually arterial CO_2 rises with other tests of gas exchange also becoming abnormal at this stage.

Bronchial hyper-reactivity to methacholine is sometimes increased and those cystic fibrosis patients with an asthmatic tendency will show other features of asthmatic bronchial irritability including exercise-induced asthma.

Tests of physical fitness and exercise capacity, though somewhat limited in validity, none the less can be shown to be abnormal in cystic patients.

Radiology

After the stage of non-specific pneumonitis, the plain chest radiograph becomes characteristic of bronchiectasis with ring shadows and tramlining appearing in the upper lobes and progressing to involve all areas eventually (Fig. 3). The thickened airways, associated fibrosis, and patchy emphysema are horrifyingly emphasized on CT scans (Fig. 4).

Respiratory complications

Haemoptysis has been mentioned. It can be massive and fatal, and comes from overgrowth of vessels with arteriovenous connections in the sub-

Fig. 3 Posteroanterior plain chest radiograph in an adult patient with cystic fibrosis.

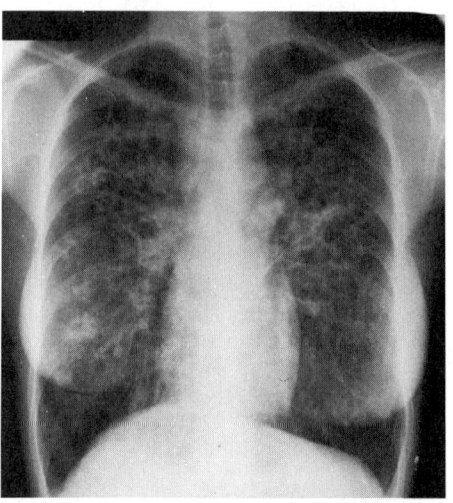

Fig. 4 CT scan from a patient with cystic fibrosis showing thickened bronchi, areas of pneumonitis, and an encysted pleural effusion.

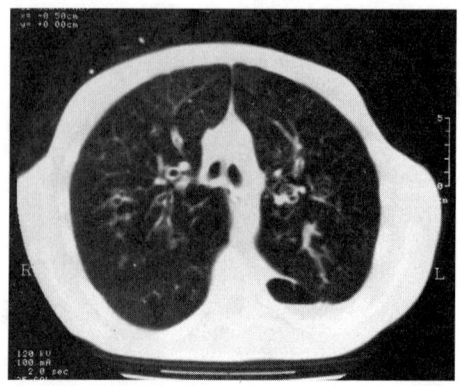

mucosa of heavily infected bronchiectatic areas of lung. Pneumothorax occurs in up to 20 per cent of patients. The clinical features are typical, but when it occurs in patients with an already diminished respiratory reserve the effect on function can be devastating. A persistent pneumothorax can easily become infected, leading to an empyematous hydropneumothorax, which is a serious and potentially fatal complication.

Fibrotic cicatrization between bronchiectatic areas can lead to fixed airways obstruction, but in addition there is variable obstruction related to increasing airways reactivity due to both infection and concurrent asthma. Atopy is seen in a high proportion of cystics (88 per cent compared with 36 per cent of control subjects in one study) and is associated with the usual immunological features (positive skin-prick tests, increased total and specific IgE) as well as with clinical asthma.

The destruction of lung tissue together with airways obstruction eventually leads to ventilatory failure with hypoxaemia and carbon dioxide retention. The pattern follows that seen in any other form of chronic progressive airways disease, but occurs at a tragically early age. Cor pulmonale accompanies the respiratory failure, and in this state many cystic fibrosis patients will die.

Upper respiratory tract

The mucosa of the nose and sinuses shows the same pathological and functional abnormalities that afflict the remainder of the respiratory tract. Recurrent infections lead on to chronic inflammatory damage and bacterial colonization (including *Pseudomonas* species). The nose is unduly susceptible to polyp formation, which is partly but not totally explained by atopy. As in other disorders, surgical treatment of polyps is successful, although only temporarily. The polyps removed are invaluable for *in vitro* studies of cystic fibrosis and its treatment, as is the intact nasal mucosa.

Gastrointestinal tract

STEATORRHOEA

The cardinal gastrointestinal feature of cystic fibrosis is malabsorption due to pancreatic insufficiency. None the less a few individuals (up to 15 per cent) appear to have no such problem. Classically the stools are pale, bulky, and offensive in odour. The fat content makes them difficult to flush away. If left untreated, the malabsorption results in weight loss and eventual cachexia with hypoproteinaemia. Fat-soluble vitamins are lost in the stools, and in the severest cases there have been examples of visual disturbance due to vitamin A deficiency and osteomalacic rickets due to vitamin D deficiency. None of these complications need arise since treatment is simple and effective (see below).

RECTAL PROLAPSE, VOLVULUS, AND INTUSSUSCEPTION

Occasionally a presenting symptom of this disorder, these bowel complications are only likely to occur in young children. Proper attention to correcting the malabsorption helps greatly, but surgical intervention may be needed and should be successful for volvulus and intussusception.

DISTAL INTESTINAL OBSTRUCTION SYNDROME

Known at one stage as meconium ileus equivalent, this syndrome of small intestinal obstruction can be fatal, particularly in its acute form when it presents with vomiting, abdominal pain, distension, and complete constipation. Less severe attacks with subacute obstruction can be a recurrent feature; in some series they affect one in five of adult cystic fibrosis patients.

Episodes last 1 to 2 days and may be precipitated by a large meal or insufficient pancreatin. An abdominal mass is usually palpable in the attack, and dilated loops of small bowel are visible on plain abdominal radiography. The pathogenesis of distal intestinal obstruction syndrome is unclear. Although the bowel is blocked by firm sticky material, this is not like meconium. There appears to be no true ileus. The abnormal intestinal contents appear to consist of poorly digested fat and protein, the latter perhaps precipitated by the altered acidity of the bowel contents owing to the known electrolyte abnormalities of cystic fibrosis.

Surgical treatment of the distal intestinal obstruction syndrome should be avoided, except as a life-saving measure. Intravenous hydration and parenteral, rather than oral, feeding are needed. The tenacious bowel contents can be persuaded to break up and move on with the use of full doses of pancreatic enzymes and H_2 blockers (cimetidine or ranitidine) by mouth and acetylcysteine. Acetylcysteine can be given by mouth, but if it is not tolerated by this route it can be delivered directly to the bowel via a nasojejunal tube. The dose is 800 mg three times daily, although in severe cases up to 18 g per day has been used and has been well tolerated.

Liver and biliary tract

Hepatic disease in cystic fibrosis has long been described. A fatty liver is common but asymptomatic, except rarely in infancy where there can be massive hepatic steatosis. Likewise, focal biliary fibrosis is silent at its onset, but as it progresses the liver first enlarges and then shrinks in typical cirrhotic style. This pathognomonic lesion appears to be due to blockage of the intrahepatic bile ducts with lipid and bile pigment. A surrounding inflammatory reaction leads to fibrosis and, later, to nodular regeneration. At this stage the lesion will not remain undetected for long because of the development of portal hypertension resulting in splenomegaly, oesophageal varices, which declare themselves through haemorrhage, and ultimately hepatic encephalopathy.

Older patients with cystic fibrosis are liable to develop cholesterol gallstones and the gall bladder itself is often small in size. Acute presentation with bile duct obstruction is recognized but rare.

Diabetes

Diabetes is an increasingly common feature with the ageing cystic fibrosis population, being present in about one in 10 as a clinical disorder, although 50 per cent may have abnormal glucose tolerance tests towards the end of life. Pancreatic islet cells do not appear abnormal to light microscopy, and the concept that the fibrotic exocrine pancreas is strangling the endocrine function is not really tenable. Treatment is along conventional lines with oral hypoglycaemics or insulin.

Miscellaneous clinical manifestations

ARTHROPATHY

A severe episodic inflammatory arthropathy has been documented in some 10 per cent of older children and young adult cystic fibrosis patients. There may be associated fever and erythema nodosum. Its origin is uncertain. In some cases it seems to be a toxic or allergic reaction, perhaps to toxins released from invading bacteria, perhaps to antibiotic therapy. Spontaneous remission is usual. Non-steroidal anti-inflammatory drugs (NSAIDs) give symptomatic relief. A few adults may also have considerable disability from severe hypertrophic pulmonary osteoarthropathy.

VASCULITIS

This condition, like the arthropathy which may accompany it, giving a Henoch–Schönlein-like picture, is uncommon. The lesions are usually on the lower limbs, particularly around the ankles. Antinuclear cytoplasmic antibody (cANCA) is reported to be positive in some 40 per cent of these cases, but the test is non-specific as it is also positive in other cystic fibrosis patients, generally when heavily infected. Oral corticosteroids are indicated, but NSAIDs may also be effective.

AMYLOIDOSIS

As in other disorders where there is long-standing suppurative disease, secondary amyloidosis can develop.

SYNDROME OF INAPPROPRIATE SECRETION OF ANTIDIURETIC HORMONE (SIADH)

Inappropriate secretion of antidiuretic hormone, most commonly in respiratory disease associated with small-cell carcinoma of the lung, may occur with respiratory infection, and hence has been reported in isolated patients with cystic fibrosis.

INFERTILITY

Over 90 per cent of males with cystic fibrosis are infertile. There is obstructive azoospermia, giving a close resemblance to Young's syndrome (obstructive azoospermia) in which there can also be bronchiectasis. Although there is diminished fertility in female patients, women with cystic fibrosis can have and have had children. In a National Institute of Health survey one in four of 129 pregnancies were terminated by spontaneous or therapeutic abortion. Most women do not attempt pregnancy because of the severity of their lung disease by the time that they have reached childbearing age, but with steady improvement in the management of the disease this stricture will apply less and less. Each child will carry one cystic fibrosis gene and, if the patient is unfortunate enough to have chosen a heterozygous partner also carrying a cystic fibrosis gene (a one in 20 chance), then 50 per cent of the offspring will have cystic fibrosis.

Psychological consequences of cystic fibrosis

For the most part children with cystic fibrosis succeed in adapting to their disease and make light of their disability, which enables them to survive psychologically. This is not so true of adolescent and adult patients, although the numbers who suffer are remarkably low considering the devastating nature of the disease with which they have to cope.

The inexorable progression of cystic fibrosis, with the almost inevitable outcome of death for the vast majority of patients, naturally induces a degree of anxiety and depression, particularly in acute illnesses. At other times patients are particularly sensitive to any change in their physical state that might herald such an acute physical decline. In social adaptation patients with cystic fibrosis are often isolated and stigmatized as a group, and sufferers are disadvantaged in employment, not just because of their physical disability but because of the impression that the public at large has of the disorder. Close contact with family members, essential for their physical support, means that patients with cystic fibrosis do not make many social contacts outside the family or fellow sufferers. Family dynamics can be seriously upset by a child with cystic fibrosis, reflecting itself in psychological illness in the parents, particularly the mother. Fathers tend to distance themselves from the problem, and there is an increased divorce rate amongst the parents of children with cystic fibrosis.

Marriage and its contemplation are particularly stressful areas for adults, with males realizing for the first time the true significance of their almost certain infertility and women ill at ease with the thought of the consequences on their physical health of embarking on pregnancy. Having said this, adult patients with cystic fibrosis are generally remarkably robust and learn to cope extremely well with their distressing illness. They are capable of adjusting well to their social environment and

gain much support from contact with fellow sufferers (for example through the Adult Cystic Fibrosis Trust).

Diagnosis

The sweat test

The concentrations of both sodium and chloride in apocrine gland secretions are substantially raised in patients with cystic fibrosis. Two values of 70 mmol/l or more for sodium can be considered diagnostic. Normal sweat sodium and chloride are both below 50 mmol/l. Careful attention has to be paid to technique in performing the test, which relies on quantitative pilocarpine iontophoresis. Pilocarpine stimulates sweating, but its penetration into the skin needs to be enhanced by the use of a galvanic current (iontophoresis). The sweat is collected on a piece of filter paper fixed to the forearm. At least 100 mg of fluid is required for reliable analysis.

Neonatal screening

Various tests have been devised to detect the presence of the gastrointestinal effects of cystic fibrosis very early in life, for example high albumin content in the meconium or low faecal trypsin. Immunoreactive trypsin can be detected in serum and blood (even dried blood), and would be expected to be low. The latter test is more reliable than the others, which give a false negative rate of up to one in four, but all these tests depend on the severity of the pancreatic abnormality which can be mild or absent even in genuine cystic fibrosis.

Prognosis

Until 1965 the median age at death of children with cystic fibrosis was 2 years with the 75th centile only about 8 years. In 1993, 50 per cent of cystic fibrosis patients are still alive at the age of 25 years (Fig. 5). Furthermore, those born with cystic fibrosis in the early 1990s are likely to survive to about 40 years and may have their lives further prolonged if gene therapy proves successful. In most cohorts, there is a small but rapid attrition rate in the neonatal period, after which survival is usually good until the teens. At most ages boys seem to fare slightly better than girls. Survival in longer in children from social classes with non-manual occupations, and there are (within the United Kingdom at least) striking and unexplained regional differences (by a ratio of up to 2.67). The development of recurrent or permanent Pseudomonas colonization is a poor prognostic feature.

There is no suggestion that the incidence of the disease is increasing,

Fig. 5 Current survival rates for United Kingdom cystic fibrosis cases, years 1986–1987 by sex. (Reproduced from Dodge *et al.* (1993), with permission.)

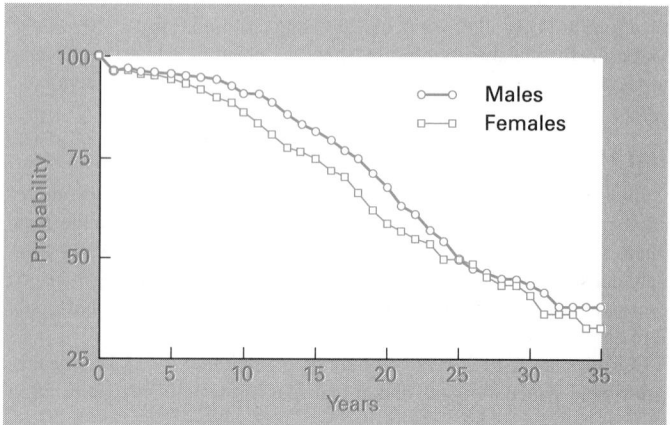

and although population screening could theoretically reduce the number of new cases, the improved prognosis offsets the necessity for screening to lead to abortion. Therefore the implication of the prolonged survival of patients with cystic fibrosis is a steady increase in the numbers of adult cystic fibrosis patients; current statistics (1991) reveal some 6100 patients with the disease in the United Kingdom, compared with 2820 in 1971.

Treatment

Nutrition

DIET

With the development of effective pancreatic enzymes, restriction of dietary fat is no longer necessary for the cystic fibrosis patient. A full diet with high energy and calorie content relative to assessed metabolic requirements is to be encouraged, and the aim should be to keep the body mass index within, and preferably towards, the upper part of the normal range. In those who are underweight, nutritious snacks and compound dietary supplements, which include glucose, essential fatty acids, and protein, can be used to supplement normal meals.

Depending on the variety and nature of the natural diet it is necessary to supplement the diet of the more seriously affected cystic fibrosis patients with both vitamin A and vitamin D. The use of vitamins E and K is more controversial, but many units would prescribe them. Cystic fibrosis patients should not need other vitamins unless tests have shown that they are deficient. Likewise, it is controversial as to whether cystic fibrosis patients should be given zinc and selenium. Iron will only be necessary if that has also been shown to be deficient on straightforward blood testing.

FURTHER NUTRITIONAL SUPPORT

With progressive pulmonary disability, there is often a regrettable decline in appetite and loss of weight which dietary encouragement and liquid food supplements cannot combat. The simplest way to support nutrition is to give the same food supplements that seem unacceptable by mouth via a thin nasogastric feeding tube, often through the night. If this is inadequate or not well tolerated, there are two alternatives. A spell of intravenous parenteral feeding is a worthwhile short-term measure that can restore well-being for many months or prepare the patient for some necessary surgical intervention. A gastrostomy is a more serious intervention which warrants consideration in selected cases and need not always be permanent. Exercise tolerance improves significantly when nutritional status is improved in these ways.

PANCREATIC ENZYME REPLACEMENT

Enteric-coated granules or tablets of mixed pancreatic extract have been to a great extent now being replaced by specific pancreatic enzyme mixtures made up of varying combinations of lipase, amylase, and protease (Table 1). Two strengths are available in both brands that are prescribable in the United Kingdom, and the larger capsules have been successful in reducing the excessive numbers of capsules required before each meal. A regimen is devised for each individual which is distributed in amount according to the probable intake at a given meal. Reports that high concentration capsules may be associated with intestinal obstruction have led to a return to lower strength schedules. The situation is being actively monitored.

Additional help with steatorrhoea can be obtained by adding cimetidine, although this should not be necessary with the newer preparations of pancreatic enzymes because they are protected during their passage through the stomach.

Diabetes, liver disease, and the other non-pulmonary complications

Table 1 *Pancreatic enzyme replacement therapy*

	Enzyme content (units/capsule)		
	Protease	Lipase	Amylase
Creon	210	8 000	9 000
Creon '25 000'	1 000	25 000	18 000
Nutrizym 10	500	10 000	9 000
Nutrizym GR	650	10 000	10 000
Nutrizym 22	1 100	22 000	19 800
Pancrease	330	5 000	2 900
Pancrease HL	1 250	25 000	22 500

are treated according to standard guidelines which are described elsewhere in this book.

Treating bronchopulmonary disease in cystic fibrosis

PROTECTION FROM INFECTION

It is unfairly restricting to insist on rigid isolation of patients with cystic fibrosis from friends and contacts with infectious respiratory tract illness, but sensible precautions should be encouraged in early life with the hope of delaying colonization of the respiratory tract with bacteria. Adult patients with *P. cepacia* infection should be kept from close contact with others who have not been so colonized. No such restriction seems to be necessary for *P. aeruginosa*.

It seems sensible to immunize cystic fibrosis patients fully against the usual childhood illnesses, particularly pertussis and measles since these infections can damage the lungs. Likewise, influenza vaccination seems a wise precaution, particularly in epidemic years. Trials of a polyvalent vaccine for *P. aeruginosa*, which appears safe and capable of raising appropriate IgG antibodies, are now under way.

Throughout the 1960s and 1970s there was a vogue for using prophylactic antistaphylococcal antibiotics almost continuously. This usually meant a daily dose of 500 mg or more of flucloxacillin. Much of the success in improving prognosis at this time was attributed to this approach. However, there were no good trials to support the concept of continuous prophylaxis, although some physicians still use it and are convinced of its value.

PRINCIPLES OF THE USE OF ANTIMICROBIAL AGENTS

Symptoms and signs of respiratory tract infection must always be taken seriously in cystic fibrosis patients. Because of the range of organisms which invade their lungs, it is wise to culture the sputum at the onset of an obvious infective exacerbation and request sensitivities. This basic rule applies to infection in most illnesses, but in cystic fibrosis the necessity for repeated courses of antibiotics predisposes to the eventual emergence of resistance in the micro-organisms, so that accurate antibiotic sensitivities are important in guiding therapy. Chronic colonization with *Pseudomonas* species can lead to multiple, even total, resistance as assessed in the laboratory. This desperate situation may still be containable for, notwithstanding laboratory results, antimicrobial therapy will still sometimes be clinically effective (see below).

In addition, there are important pharmacokinetic factors to consider. First, antibiotics penetrate poorly into the infected recesses of the bronciectatic cavities, and the alginate coating of Pseudomonas provides the microbe with fearsome protection; second, there may be interference with drug metabolism if there is liver disease; third, the rapid renal clearance of many antibiotics (including penicillins and aminoglycosides) means that larger than usual doses have to be given in cystic fibrosis.

There is an increased tendency for patients with cystic fibrosis to develop sensitivity reactions to antibiotics. These may take the form of rashes, which can be severe and widespread, a curious perineal pain (with intravenous penicillins), or airways narrowing when using inhaled antibiotics. However, toxic reactions (e.g. damage to cranial nerve VIII with aminoglycosides) may be less often encountered than with other patients because of rapid renal excretion.

In the early stages infecting organisms are usually conventional (e.g. Pneumococcus, *H. influenzae*) and will respond to oral antibiotics. *Staphlococcus aureus* should be regarded with more respect. Flucloxacillin by mouth will often be effective; fusidic acid, macrolides, or cephalosporins are alternatives which can be used if resistance has developed. Two antimicrobial agents should be used together if there is any suggestion of persistent colonization. Intravenous antibiotics are rarely required for this type of infection.

Pseudomonas infection, as already hinted, is an event of serious import for the patient with cystic fibrosis. A vigorous attack on the organism when it is first isolated may sometimes eradicate it for months, even years, on end, and is to be advocated. There is then debate as to whether a semiprophylactic approach should be used, with regular treatment every 3 months, or whether the organism should only be tackled when shown to be present on sputum culture. Trials are under way to try to adjudicate on these different approaches.

ANTIMICROBIALS FOR PSEUDOMONAS

Oral agents

The four quinolones, ciprofloxacin, and ofloxacin are the only oral agents against *Pseudomonas* species that are commercially available. The dose of ciprofloxacin should be at least 500 mg twice daily, (preferably 750 mg twice daily and occasionally 1000 mg twice daily). These antimicrobial agents have an excellent clinical effect, but resistance emerges all too readily. Side-effects are uncommon, with gastrointestinal disturbance and cerebral dysfunction (unpleasant dreams, disorientation) being the most probable. It is a pity that the drug has been used so widely for respiratory tract infection in non-bronchiectatic patients in the community, for this has undoubtedly contributed to the emergence of resistant strains of Pseudomonas.

Inhaled agents

The concept of using the inhaled route, so successful for the treatment of obstructive diseases of the airways with bronchodilators, has been an important step in the evolution of treatment of respiratory tract infection in cystic fibrosis. Three classes of antibiotic have been used with success. The first tried were the penicillins, particularly carbenicillin. However, a number of patients complained of sensitivity reactions in the airways, and there is less use of this group by the inhaled route now. Aminoglycosides, particularly gentamicin, have been more successful and less trouble. There has been nervousness about exploring high doses even though absorption seems minimal and renal elimination brisk. There is always the fear of damage to cranial nerve VIII with aminoglycosides, but it seems extraordinarily uncommon even with repeated courses. None the less since the mode of nerve VIII damage may well be by interfering with cilial function, increasing the doses delivered to the airways may bode ill for cilial function there.

Colomycin (a polymyxin antibiotic) has been the most successful inhaled agent for the long-term treatment of bronchopulmonary Pseudomonas infection in cystic fibrosis. Even in doses of 2 MU daily or more, there is no evidence of absorption sufficient to give side-effects and the incidence of bacterial resistance is very low.

Intravenous agents

Many minor Pseudomonas infections can be dealt with successfully with oral ciprofloxacin and an inhaled agent, but there is an increasing trend towards intravenous therapy. The agents used and commonly recommended doses are listed in Table 2.

It is common practice when Pseudomonas is first isolated to use a

Table 2 *Antimicrobial agents for Pseudomonas infection in cystic fibrosis*

Oral	
Ciprofloxacin	750 mg twice daily
Ofloxacin	400 mg twice daily
Inhaled*	
Colistin	1 MU twice or three times daily
Gentamicin	80–160 mg twice or three times daily
Intravenous injection	
Azlocillin	2–5 g three times daily
Piperacillin†	2–4 g three times daily
Ticarcillin†	2–5 g three times daily
Ceftazidime	2–3 g three times daily
Aztreonam	1–2 g three or four times daily
Imipenem with cilastatin	0.5–1 g three or four times daily
Gentamicin‡	80–160 mg three times daily
Netilmicin‡	100–200 mg three times daily
Tobramycin‡	80–160 mg three times daily

*The antipseudomonal penicillins have also been given by inhalation.

†Both also available with clavulanic acid.

‡High doses of aminoglycosides can be tolerated but check levels. Reduce to twice daily or daily if renal function is impaired. May be given at 80 per cent total daily dose as a single daily injection.

single intravenous antipseudomonal antibiotic with an inhaled or oral drug. As the disease advances and the Pseudomonas infection becomes more difficult to treat, two intravenous antibiotics become the rule, often accompanied by inhaled colistin. By this stage microbial resistance to ciprofloxacin is all too likely. Chronic colonization eventually leads to the need for almost continuous use of intravenous treatment and the increasing likelihood of development of resistance, even to intravenous drugs. It is helpful if the organism can be allowed to evolve, at least for a short while, without continuous attack. If the patient cannot manage without an antibiotic, a useful strategy is to ignore the culture result and treat with large doses of antibiotics which have no recognizable effect on Pseudomonas. The logic is that other Gram-positive and Gram-negative organisms may well be present, contributing to the persistent inflammatory state, which are being swamped out in culture plates by Pseudomonas. Antibiotics which have been used successfully in this way are chloramphenicol (no more than 500 mg four times daily), amoxil (3 g twice daily), and the newer macrolides (e.g. clarithromycin). The cephalosporins seem to be less successful in this respect.

VENOUS ACCESS

It is customary to use a Venflon or similar device in the early stages of intravenous therapy in this as in other disorders. Because of the likely repeated use of veins, great care must be taken to ensure that as little damage is done as possible. This means careful insertion, meticulous attention to sterile technique, and full flushing after use. Whilst studies have suggested that normal saline is as effective in keeping veins patent as saline heparin mixtures, many cystic fibrosis centres prefer to use the heparinized solution on the grounds of caution. Longer venous lines inserted through the forearm will ensure delivery of the drug into a faster stream of venous blood and are used at some stage in many patients, but the time eventually comes when most of the veins in the arm are thrombosed and those that remain are fragile. The repeated resiting of an intravenous cannula during a course of therapy is distressing as well as inconvenient. The next step is a more permanent venous access. The Hickman lines used for cancer chemotherapy are one option, but many centres now prefer a completely buried venous access port of the Portacath or Vascuport type (Fig. 6). The major disadvantage of this approach is that the port needs to be inserted surgically, preferably with a general anaesthetic, although in a patient with very poor respiratory reserve it is, of course, possible to complete the operation under local anaesthesia. The port is usually placed under the skin of the anterior chest wall with the line passing through a tributary into the subclavian vein. The earlier practice of putting the venous line into the external jugular meant that the catheter turned back on itself, and fractures of the catheter at this point have been reported. Again, flushing is vitally important to prevent the port from silting up. In this respect, both for arm and for port venous access, it is important that the antibiotics should be diluted according to the manufacturer's instructions. Some, such as the aminoglycosides, can be given in a relatively small volume of fluid but others, particularly imipenem, require a considerable volume of fluid (up to 200 ml) and have been known to precipitate out in the catheter system.

One of the greatest advances in the general management of cystic fibrosis patients has been self-management of venous lines. With children the parent takes on the responsibility; with adults it is done by the patients themselves. They are taught to care for the catheter, draw up their own drugs, inject them, and flush the system afterwards. Of course, this has greatly decreased the number of inpatient days or hospital visits and has allowed cystic fibrosis patients to remain active and at work despite needing intravenous antibiotics.

Newer devices have recently been introduced that allow even greater convenience to the patient. The antibiotics are pre-prepared in portable delivery devices which automatically deliver the antibiotic slowly over a preset time. The device itself can be sited in a pocket. It seems likely that these devices will come into greater use, but it is hoped that, with time, they will become cheaper than they are at present.

Other therapeutic approaches

REDUCING THE VISCOSITY OF SPUTUM

Acetylcysteine has been given by inhalation but frequently causes bronchospasm. Carbocysteine attempts to achieve the same effect—breaking down the disulphide bonds in sticky mucus—via the oral route. There is so little evidence for benefit in straightforward obstructive airways disease that it has been withdrawn as a prescribable drug. However, it is sometimes of benefit in cystic fibrosis.

Trials of DNA-ase are under way at present, and there are more encouraging signs that this can liquefy sputum, allow its more effective expectoration, and improve lung function.

Fig. 6 Portacath venous access system.

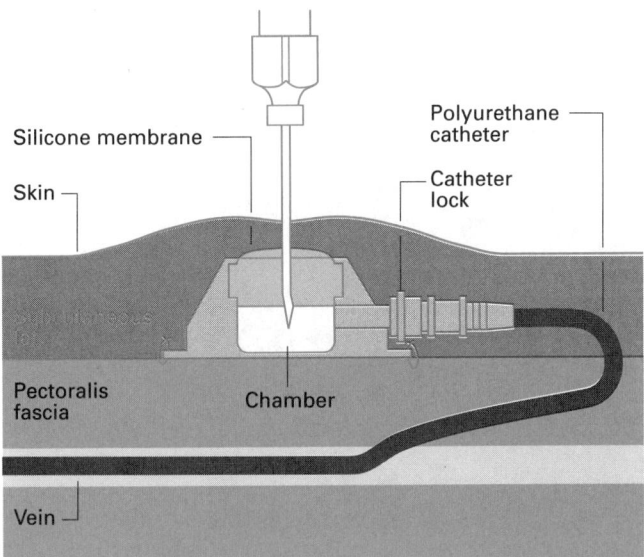

Silicone membrane

Skin

Polyurethane catheter

Catheter lock

Pectoralis fascia

Chamber

Vein

AMILORIDE

This potassium-sparing diuretic has been tried by the inhaled route in an attempt to improve chloride transport and so correct the basic biochemical defect in cystic fibrosis. Single doses of 3 ml of 10^{-3} mol solution improve mucociliary clearance as measured with labelled technetium, and this effect can be maintained over a 3 week period with repeated doses (twice or three times daily). Clinically, the effects are not dramatic, but individual patients seem to derive considerable benefit.

α_1-ANTITRYPSIN

On the grounds that bronchial inflammatory damage in cystic fibrosis results from locally released neutrophil elastase, α_1-antitrypsin by inhalation has been investigated experimentally. In a preliminary 1 week trial it restored some of the antipseudomonal properties of bronchial epithelial lining fluid.

Physiotherapy

The management of cystic fibrosis without a central role for physiotherapy cannot be contemplated. The bronchial secretions cannot simply be 'coughed up'; they must be helped. The techniques which the physiotherapist uses and teaches are as follows.

- Postural drainage: placing the patient in such a position that gravity aids the movement of secretions, first into the central airways and then up through the trachea. Foam wedges help when lying on a flat bed or floor, or tipping beds with one end of adjustable height, are used.
- Percussion and vibration: cupped hands alternately, firmly but gently, percuss the chest with shaking vibration to assist the movement of secretions down the airways.
- Forced expiration (huffing): forcibly breathing out from a position of moderate inspiration, is effective in shifting secretions and is self-administered.
- Controlled breathing, between short spells of using the above techniques, allows relaxation and time for expectoration.

The amount of time devoted to physiotherapy will vary from patient to patient, but there are very few who can dispense with physiotherapy altogether. Physiotherapists can use their skills and close rapport with patients to help with inhalation therapy, oxygen use, and exercise training.

The treatment of respiratory complications

HAEMOPTYSIS

The immediate treatment of excessive haemoptysis is rest. Adrenaline inhalations may help, and vasopressin or desmopressin have been used successfully. In the most serious cases, where the bleeding is threatening to cause exsanguination, arterial embolization with metal coils has halted the bleeding, as in other disorders with excessive lung haemorrhage (e.g. haemangiomas).

PNEUMOTHORAX

This is treated along conventional lines with early recourse to surgery. The use of sclerosing agents is discouraged in cystic fibrosis because of the damage done to the pleural surface which may preclude later lung transplant. If the pneumothorax does not seal spontaneously, then the best surgical approach is to use a thoracoscopic technique.

AIRWAYS OBSTRUCTION

To the extent that this is atopically mediated in some patients, it should be treated along the lines of asthma in any other patient. In addition, some of the airways obstruction is due to the inflammatory process within the airways rather than mucopus in their lumen. This has encouraged the use of corticosteroids to reduce the inflammatory process, and such treatment has met with some success. It should be reserved for patients with seriously disabling airflow obstruction associated with cystic fibrosis, when there is little doubt that significant improvements in lung function and reduction in disability can be achieved.

ASPERGILLUS COLONIZATION

The damaged airways of the patient with cystic fibrosis are vulnerable to colonization with *Aspergillus fumigatus*. This ubiquitous fungus causes several pulmonary disorders, most of which can be seen in cystic fibrosis (for details see Chapter 7.12.1). Atopic asthma and allergic bronchopulmonary aspergillosis are the most likely, but mycetomas can form and if the fungus spreads to the pleural cavity say during surgical procedures, generalized spread of infection can be devastating and even fatal. Steroids and antifungal agents such as itraconazole should be used.

RESPIRATORY FAILURE

This is treated conservatively along the lines described elsewhere in this chapter. Ventilatory support should be reserved for those patients who have a good prospect of benefiting from heart–lung transplant.

Heart–lung transplant

The success of heart transplants prompted surgeons to begin a programme of lung transplantation in the late 1970s. For technical reasons combined heart and lung transplant became the favoured procedure. Because of their young age and the invariably fatal outcome, patients with cystic fibrosis have become attractive propositions for this procedure. Their hearts can often be used for other patients. However, there has been an unfortunate tendency to regard heart–lung transplant as a cure rather than the life-saving procedure that it really is.

Up to mid-1993 some 200 heart–lung transplants for cystic fibrosis have been carried out in the United Kingdom, mainly in two centres (London and Cambridge). There is a significant perioperative mortality, which is not surprising in view of the serious nature of the disease, but the subsequent attrition rate is slower. The 3 year survival is currently around 65 per cent and the 5 year survival is just over 50 per cent, although few patients have lived this long so far. None the less, when death is an imminent prospect and life is a 24 h toil of physiotherapy and intravenous antibiotics, even these statistics represent a chance worth taking.

Patients are selected on the grounds of poor lung function (spirometric values less than one-third of the predicted value), arterial desaturation on exercise, and deteriorating quality of life. Patients need to have a stable background, a robust attitude, and strong home support to survive the rigors of postoperative monitoring. Prognosis is adversely affected by malnutrition, other organ failure, previous thoracic surgery, and preoperative intermittent positive-pressure ventilation. Rejection is dealt with along conventional lines. Obliterative bronchiolitis afflicts one in five patients after about the first year and is usually fatal.

Management strategies for cystic fibrosis

The highly specialized nature of the care that is necessary for the treatment of patients with cystic fibrosis has prompted strong moves to create cystic fibrosis centres (Table 3). Such centres need to be regionally based, and offer multidisciplinary care as well as assessment facilities for pulmonary and gastrointestinal systems. The obvious advantages that such centres offer in terms of skills and economies of scale are to some extent offset by the reduced availability of such services near the patient's home and the lack of the personal touch that smaller units are often so expert at providing. However, highly specialized centres seem

Table 3 *The role of regional centres for cystic fibrosis*

- Clinical care should be supervised according to the individual patient's needs and wishes; in most cases this would entail regular attendances at the cystic fibrosis centre together with shared care with the general practitioner and, where appropriate, with the local hospital
- Ideally, regional cystic fibrosis centres would care for both children and adults, but sometimes the local organization of hospital services dictates that paediatric and adult care are in different hospitals; joint clinics between adult physicians and paediatricians are desirable to facilitate transfer of care at around the age of 16 years
- The centre would be responsible for coordination with the local genetic services of DNA analysis, prenatal diagnosis, neonatal screening, and counselling
- Clinical links should be developed between the regional cystic fibrosis centre and centres providing more specialized forms of care (e.g. transplantation)
- The centre should be responsible for keeping records of all cystic fibrosis patients within the region and for coordinating clinical research
- Staffing requirements for a clinic with 50 adult patients: consultant physician with a major commitment to, and experience of, cystic fibrosis; junior medical staff, including a clinical fellow; specialist full-time nurse/coordinator; physiotherapists (two whole-time equivalents); dietitian (part-time); full-time social worker; part-time secretarial support
- Expert advice will be needed from many specialists, such as gastroenterologist, diabetologist, thoracic surgeon, microbiologist, radiologist, clinical geneticist, etc.
- Facilities for inpatient treatment should include the provision of three to four beds for each 50 patients

to be the best option until such time as a simple and easy preventative regimen with gene therapy is widely available and proven to be effective.

Prevention: the future

Families with an affected child require genetic counselling. The risk of a further affected child is one in four; the risk of a carrier unaffected child is two in four. Parents should understand that accurate antenatal diagnosis of an affected child is possible. Genetic linkage analysis using polymorphic DNA markers can effectively complement direct mutation

Fig. 7 Polyacrylamide gel electrophoresis of polymerase chain reaction products of the △ 508 region showing a normal homozygote (1, 2, 7), a heterozygote carrier for △ 508 (3, 4, 5, 8), and homozygote △ 508 with cystic fibrosis (6).

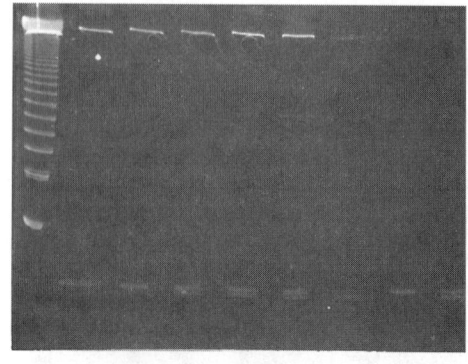

1   2   3   4   5   6   7   8

analysis (Fig. 7) to achieve this. Therefore termination of pregnancy, based on accurate diagnosis, could be offered within 16 weeks of gestation.

Female cystic fibrosis sufferers can be fertile, and the risk of an affected child is relatively low at one in 44 (if the partner is also a carrier the risk is one in 2).

Prevention of cystic fibrosis in the general population by antenatal diagnosis and termination of pregnancy presents problems of a different order. The limitations of current readily available mutation screens, defining up to 12 mutations and recognizing 90 per cent of cystic fibrosis chromosomes, are significant. The issues of cost and effectiveness, personal confidentiality, and acceptability of termination on a large scale have not been seriously addressed.

The future

One major hope for the future lies with gene therapy. In a mouse model of cystic fibrosis in which the murine CFTR gene has been ablated, inhalation of the gene restores the chloride channel function to normal. The way is open for preliminary human studies.

Two vectors for conveying the gene into human airways—respiratory viruses and liposomes—have undergone preliminary trials. The former are favoured in the United States but doubts exist as to long-term safety. Liposomes, as used in the mouse experiments, are easy to make, cheap, safe, non-immunogenic, and non-toxic to humans. They deliver DNA to epithelia effectively and work in the mouse model. Initial single-dose studies have involved nasal epithelia and surgically removed tissue (nasal polyps and lungs at transplantation). So far results have been encouraging rather than spectacular, but this work could lead to single-dose studies involving installation of DNA into the airways followed by long-term clinical studies, possibly with nebulized DNA-impregnated liposomes.

REFERENCES

Al-Jader, L.N., Meredith, A.L., Ryley, H.C., Cheadle, J.P., Maguire, S., Owen, G., et al. (1992). Severity of chest disease in cystic fibrosis patients in relation to their genotypes. Journal of Medical Genetics, 29, 883–7.

Andersen, D.H. (1938). Cystic fibrosis of the pancreas and its relation to coeliac disease. A clinical and pathological study. American Journal of Diseases of Children, 56, 344–99.

Anonymous (1992). Editorial Screening for cystic fibrosis. Lancet, 340, 209–10.

App, E.M., King, M., Helfsrieder, R., Köhler, D., and Matthys, H. (1990). Acute and long term amiloride inhalation in cystic fibrosis lung disease. American Review of Respiratory Diseases, 141, 605–12.

Britton, J.R. (1989). Effects of social class, sex, and region of residence on age at death from cystic fibrosis. British Medical Journal, 298, 483–7.

Cheng, S.H., Gregory, R.J., Marshall, J., Paul, S., Souza, D.W., White, G.A., et al. (1990). Defective intracellular transport and processing of CFTR is the molecular basis of most cystic fibrosis. Cell, 63, 827–34.

Cleghorn, G.J., Fortstner, G.G., Stringer, D.A., et al. (1986). Treatment of distal intestinal obstruction syndrome in cystic fibrosis with a balanced intestinal lavage solution. Lancet, i, 8–11.

Cohen, L.F., di Sant'Agnesse, X., and Friedlander, J. (1980). Cystic fibrosis and pregnancy: a national survey. Lancet ii, 842–4.

Dixey, J., Redington, A.N., Butler, R.C., Smith, M.J., Batchelor, J.R., Woodrow, D.F., et al. (1988). The arthropathy of cystic fibrosis. Annals of Rheumatic Diseases, 47, 218–23.

Dodge, J.A., Morison, S., Lewis, P.A., Coles, E.C., Geddes, D., Russell, G., et al. (1993). Cystic fibrosis in the United Kingdom, 1968–1988: incidence, population, survival. Paediatric and Perinatal Epidemiology, 7, 157–66.

Elborn, J.S. and Shale D.J. (1990). Lung injury in cystic fibrosis. Thorax, 45, 970–3.

Finnegan, M.J., Hinchcliffe, J., Russell-Jones, D., Neill, S., Sheffield, E., Jayne, D., et al. (1989). Vasculitis complicating cystic fibrosis. Quarterly Journal of Medicine, 72, 609–21.

Heeley, A.F., Heeley, M.E., King, D.N., Kuzemko, J.A., and Walsh M.P. (1982). Screening for cystic fibrosis by dried blood spot trypsin analysis. Archives of Diseases of Childhood, 57, 18–21.

Hodson, M.E., Mearns, M.B., and Batten, J.C. (1976). Meconium ileus equivalent in adults with cystic fibrosis. British Medical Journal, ii, 790–1.

Hyde, S.C., Gill, D.R., Higgins, C.F., Trezise, A.E., MacVinish, L.J., Cuthbert, A.W., et al. (1993). Correction of the ion transport defect in cystic fibrosis transgenic mice by gene therapy. Nature, London, 362, 250–5.

Kerem, B., Rommens, J., Buchanan, J., Markiewich, D., Cox, T., Chakravarti, A., et al. (1989). Identification of the cystic fibrosis gene: genetic analysis. Science, 245, 1073–80.

LiPuma, J.J., Dasen, S.E., Nielson, D.W., Stern, R.C., and Stull, T.L. (1990). Person-to-person transmission of Pseudomonas cepacia between patients with cystic fibrosis. Lancet, 336, 1094–6.

McElvaney, N.G., Hubbard, R.C., Birrer, P., Chernick, M.S., Caplan, D.B., Frank, M.M., and Crystal, R.G. (1991). Aerosol alpha₁ antitrypsin treatment for cystic fibrosis. Lancet, 337, 392–4.

Penketh, A.R.L., Knight, R., Hodson, M.E., and Batten J.C. (1982). The management of pneumothorax in adults. Thorax, 37, 850–3.

Pinkerton, P., Duncan, F., Trauer, T., Hodson, M.E., and Batten, J.C. (1985). Cystic fibrosis in adult life: a study of coping patterns. Lancet, ii, 761–3.

Skeie, B., Askanazi, J., Rothkopf, M.M., Rosenbaum, S.H., Kvetan, V., and Ross, E. (1987). Improved exercise tolerance with long term parenteral nutrition in cystic fibrosis. Critical Care Medicine, 15, 960–2.

Smyth, R.L., Higenbottam, T., Scott, J., and Wallwork, J. (1991). Cystic fibrosis 5—The current status of lung transplantation for cystic fibrosis. Thorax, 46, 213–16.

Thanasekaraan, V., Wiseman, M.S., Rayner, R.J., Hillier, E.J., and Shale, D.J. (1989). Pseudomonas aeruginosa antibodies in blood spots from patients with cystic fibrosis. Archives of Diseases of Childhood, 64, 1599–1603.

Tobin, M.J., Maguire, O., Reen, D., Tempany, E., and Fitzgerald, M.X. (1980). Atopy and bronchial reactivity in older patients with cystic fibrosis. Thorax, 35, 807–13.

Tsui, L.C. (1992). The spectrum of cystic fibrosis mutations. Trends in Genetics, 8, 392–8.

17.9.3 Bronchiectasis

R. A. STOCKLEY

Introduction

Bronchiectasis is a condition in which there is chronic dilatation of the bronchi. The condition is usually suspected when patients present with a long history of persistent or intermittent sputum production in the absence of other known causes, such as asthma or smoking. In practice, the condition may coexist with these other causes.

Although the condition has been recognized since the early nineteenth century, there is a general impression that it is now less frequent or at least less severe than previously. This may reflect changes in socioeconomic conditions, the introduction of vaccination, and the use of antibiotics. The true incidence is unknown, since this would require extensive population screening by CT scanning or bronchography; the estimate of prevalence is mainly based on ordinary chest radiograph changes which are far less sensitive. Between the mid-1940s and late 1950s several reports suggested that the incidence ranged from as high as 1.3 per 1000 population to one new case each year per million children.

However, these figures may reflect a low index of suspicion, a tendency to attribute symptoms to other causes, and failure to refer patients for specialist assessment when the symptoms are deemed to be irremediable or the patient learns 'to live with' the problem. Nevertheless, when the condition is sought the number of cases in specialist clinics gradually rises.

Pathology

The best description of the pathology of bronchiectasis was provided by Whitwell (1952) in a review of 200 resected specimens published in 1952. Gross inspection reveals the dilated bronchi that are pathognomonic of the disease (Fig. 1). The airways are inflamed, often tortuous and collapsible, and often contain secretions which may cause occlusion. There is a varying degree of parenchymal damage with scarring and fibrosis (Fig. 2). The condition is usually widespread, but may be localized to the upper lobes if it is due to tuberculosis or related to an area distal to bronchial obstruction or the site of a previous lobar pneumonia.

Microscopically there is a varying degree of damage to the bronchial epithelium (Fig. 2). There may be areas of ulceration, and the columnar ciliated epithelium is replaced patchily by squamous epithelium. There is goblet cell and mucus gland hyperplasia and the peribronchial connective tissue is often damaged or lost (leading to dilated but collapsible airways). There may be microabscesses in the bronchial wall and evidence of pulmonary vascular dilatation, occlusion, or hypertension. There is usually extensive inflammatory cell infiltration which consists of neutrophils (predominantly in the lumen) and mononuclear cells (in the bronchial wall). There is also a variable degree of tissue oedema and fibrosis.

Individual specimens show a wide range of severity which is in keeping with the wide range of clinical features (see later).

Whitwell described three major types of bronchiectasis based on pathological features, although the distinctions are often unclear.

1. Saccular bronchiectasis: this is less common today but is associated with the most severe damage and large saccular dilatation with loss of bronchial subdivisions.
2. Atelectatic bronchiectasis: this is usually lobar or segmental in distribution and occurs in the absence of other forms. This type of bronchiectasis is usually related to proximal bronchial distortion or occlusion, and inflammatory changes are less marked histologically.

3. Follicular bronchiectasis: this is the most commonly encountered form of bronchiectasis. It is characterized by the formation of multiple lymphoid follicles which may distend and project into the bronchial tree. They are associated with extensive loss of elastic tissue in the bronchial wall. The follicles themselves contain activated lymphocytes which are predominantly CD8 positive cytotoxic/suppressor T cells. In addition, there is an increase in B lymphocytes in the bronchial wall. At present it is known that many of these produce the IgA1 and IgA2 subclasses of immunoglobulins. It is unknown whether B lymphocytes producing the IgG subclasses are also increased in number, but there is evidence of the local production of the IgG subclasses 1 to 4.

Pathogenesis

The pathogenesis of bronchiectasis is only partly understood at present. The symptoms often date from childhood and may be related (by the patient) to a single event described as 'pneumonia'. Indeed, several epidemiological studies have noted that bacterial pneumonia or more specified infections (whooping cough and measles pneumonia) may relate to the onset of symptoms in 30 to 60 per cent of patients. Unfortunately, most of the information is collected in retrospect, and its validity has been questioned since patients often like to relate their illness to a specific event. Nevertheless, some infections, including tuberculosis,

Fig. 2 Histological sections of bronchial wall in bronchiectasis highlighting some of the features (arrowed). Section (a) shows the epithelial damage with loss of ciliated epithelium (1), dilated sub mucosal blood vessels (2), and increased interstitial collagen (3). These features are seen at higher magnification (section (b)) together with submucosal inflammatory cell infiltrate (4).

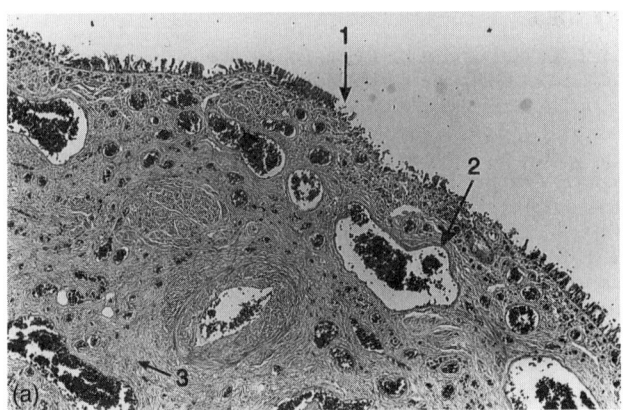

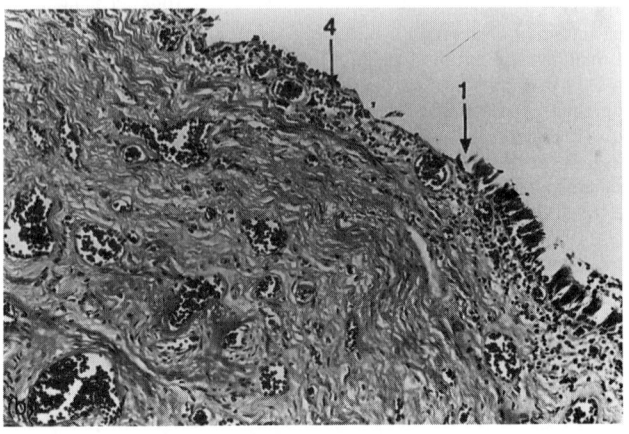

Fig. 1 Macroscopic appearance of extensive bronchiectasis of the lung. Dilated bronchi are arrowed (1). The remaining architecture is distorted and large white areas of fibrosis (arrow 2) are seen.

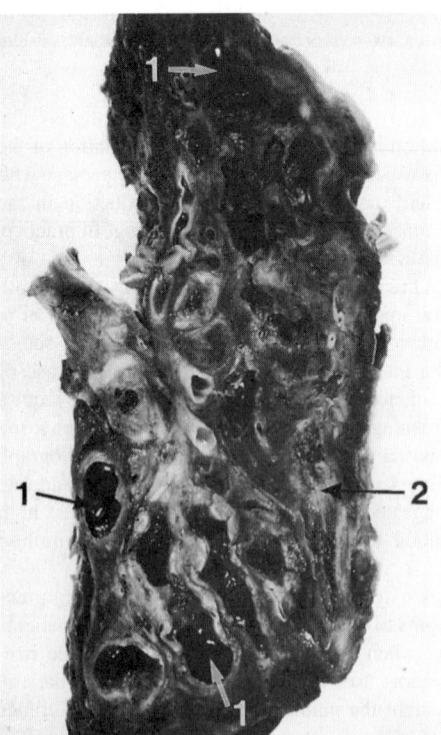

whooping cough, adenovirus infections, and mycoplasma infections, have undoubtedly been linked to bronchiectasis. An animal model of bronchiectasis has been described following *Mycoplasma pneumoniae* infection. Circumstantial evidence also supports the concept that infection plays a role. The reduction in the incidence and severity of bronchiectasis seen since the introduction of antibiotic therapy and immunization regimens suggests an infective aetiology in many patients. Nevertheless, only a proportion of subjects who have these infections in childhood develop bronchiectasis. This suggests a susceptibility of some individuals to develop sufficient tissue damage during an infection leading to bronchiectasis. This is supported by the occasional family history of the disease and the association with abnormalities of the α_1-antitrypsin gene (see Chapter 17.9.4). This gene codes for a plasma protein (2 g/l) which is a major inhibitor of proteolytic enzymes, including neutrophil elastase which is released by activated neutrophils and may cause extensive tissue damage (see later). α_1-Antitrypsin protects the lung against damage by neutrophil elastase and its concentration increases (two-fold or more) during episodes of inflammation, thereby increasing the protection when it is needed.

Severe deficiency of α_1-antitrypsin is associated with bronchiectasis, probably because of an inability to protect the lung from neutrophil elastase during infective episodes. Although this deficiency is a relatively rare cause of bronchiectasis, more subtle defects can occur in approximately 20 per cent of unselected patients. Kalsheker and colleagues found an abnormality in one of the control sequences for the α_1-antitrypsin gene which would interfere with the increased production during episodes of inflammation.

The role of infection in the development of bronchiectasis is also highlighted by the association with identified defects in host defence (Table 1). Recurrent infections and bronchiectasis have been described in subjects who have defects in the humoral and cellular components of the lung defence system. In addition, factors that influence the non-specific clearance of organism (ciliary beating, mucus production, and airways patency) all play a key role in lung defence, and defects are associated with bronchiectasis. Indeed, the most useful animal model of bronchiectasis is produced by the instillation of live bacteria into an area of lung that has had its physical clearance mechanism impaired by partial ligation (analogous to obstruction by tumour, nodes, fibrosis, or a foreign body in humans).

However, other toxic processes, including aspiration of gastric contents or inhalation of toxic chemicals such as ammonia, also lead to bronchiectasis. These processes result in extensive airways inflammation and this may be the common pathway of most causes of bronchiectasis. Inflammation is associated with tissue damage and repair, and if this occurs in the lung and the repair process is inadequate, resulting in loss of supporting structures and scarring, the airways may become distorted and dilated (both of which are features of bronchiectasis).

Clinical features

The patients show a broad spectrum of clinical disease. The least affected subjects may have no symptoms or signs between clinical exacerbations. During these episodes they develop cough with the production of purulent sputum associated with fever, occasional chest pain (localized to the area of the disease), a variable degree of breathlessness, and occasional haemoptysis. Clinical signs are non-specific, but localized medium to coarse crackles or wheeze may suggest the diagnosis, particularly if symptoms date back to childhood or a severe acute respiratory illness (see later).

In more severely affected subjects sputum production becomes continuous (often large volumes) and varies from mucoid (clear) to frankly purulent, often changing during episodes of acute exacerbations. However, some patients continuously produce purulent secretions, and these usually have the most extensive disease in terms of bronchial dilatation and regions of the lung affected.

Table 1 *Conditions associated with bronchiectasis*

Host defence defects
Immune defects
   Immunoglobulin deficiency (primary and secondary)
   Complement deficiency
   Phagocyte defects
   Chronic granulomatous disease
   Chediak–Higashi disease
   Leucocyte adherence deficiency
Hyperimmune states
   Allergic bronchopulmonary aspergillosis
   Following lung transplant
Mucociliary clearance defects
   Immotile cilia
   Kartagener's syndrome
   Young's syndrome
   Cystic fibrosis
   Bronchial obstruction (tumour or nodes)

Infection
Tuberculosis
Measles pneumonia
Whooping cough
Adenovirus 21, 3, and 7
M. pneumoniae
Pneumococcal pneumonia
AIDS

Other inflammatory disease
Gastric aspiration
Ammonia inhalation
Heroin
Inflammatory bowel disease
Rheumatoid arthritis
Vasculitis

Miscellaneous
Inhalation of foreign body
Pulmonary fibrosis
Absence of bronchial cartilage
α_1-Antitrypsin deficiency
Yellow nail syndrome
Primary lymphoedema
Treated lymphoreticular malignancy

There is often a history of symptoms dating from a previous childhood illness or acute or chronic lung injury (see pathogenesis). Specific questioning may reveal a positive family history, suggesting a genetic or social predisposition (although this is rare), or symptoms of an associated disease (Table 1), although occasionally bronchiectasis may precede these conditions. Infertility may indicate a disorder of mucociliary clearing, particularly the primary ciliary dyskinesias such as immotile cilia syndrome and Kartagener's syndrome.

Patients often have symptoms of disease throughout the respiratory tract and may suffer from chronic or recurrent otitis and sinusitis. Indeed postnasal drip, which occurs in approximately 75 per cent of patients, was thought to be important in the pathogenesis of bronchiectasis, although it may also reflect the same condition in both the upper and lower respiratory tract. Between 30 and 40 per cent of patients have chronic purulent sinusitis.

Clinical signs

There are no specific signs for bronchiectasis. The patient may have a productive cough, signs of an associated disease (rheumatoid arthritis, lymphoedema, etc.), and finger clubbing (patients with persistent purulent bronchiectasis). The remaining signs may be minimal and confined

Table 2 *Investigation of bronchiectasis*

Blood tests
Biochemistry
  α_1-Antitrypsin
  Aspergillus precipitins
  Immunoglobulins (subclasses)
  Complement components
Neutrophil function
  Superoxide production
  Bacterial killing
  Chemotaxis
  Adherence assays
  Neutropenia

Genetic studies
α_1-Antitrypsin gene
Cystic fibrosis gene and/or sweat chloride test

Mucociliary clearance
Ultrastructural studies
Functional
  Nasal clearance
  Lung clearance

Radiology
Sinus radiography
Chest radiography
CT scan
Barium swallow

Electrocardiography
Echocardiography
Right heart catheter

Lung function
Arterial blood gases
Exercise capacity
Static lung volumes
Dynamic flow rates/reversibility
Sleep studies

Sputum culture
Gram stain
Aerobic
Anaerobic
Selective medium

Table 3 *Radiographic abnormalities in bronchiectasis*

Tramline shadows
Cystic lesions (often fluid filled)
Volume loss with crowding of vessels
Areas of atelectasis
Evidence of previous tuberculous infection
Fibrosis
Evidence of previous heart surgery

deficiency, and IgG2 with IgG4 deficiency have been highlighted as causative. However, IgA deficiency is common (one in 700) and most subjects are well, suggesting that it may not be the cause even when present. Furthermore, the establishment of other subclass deficiencies usually depends upon identifying values that are more than two standard deviations below the 'normal' mean for a healthy population. More recently, it has become clear that the 'normal' range is wide and true deficiency (outside the normal range) is rare, being present in only 1 to 2 per cent of patients. Despite this low incidence, immunoglobulin deficiency can affect management (see later) and thus its identification is important.

More extensive studies of immunoglobulin subclasses are currently

Fig. 3 Bronchograms of left lower lobe from two patients. (a) demonstrates marked saccular dilatation usually seen as cystic lesions on plain chest radiograph. (b) demonstrates long nontapering bronchi characteristic of fusiform bronchiectasis that may demonstrate tram-line shadows on plain chest radiograph.

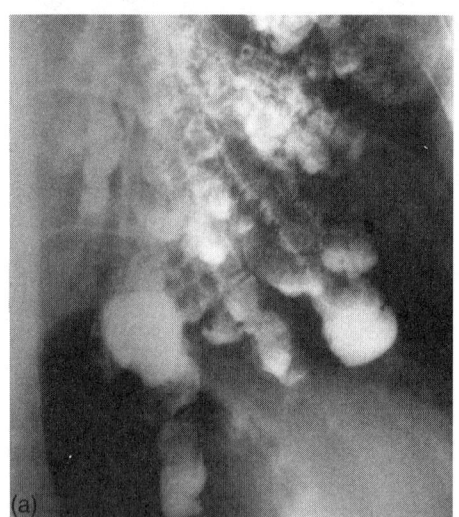

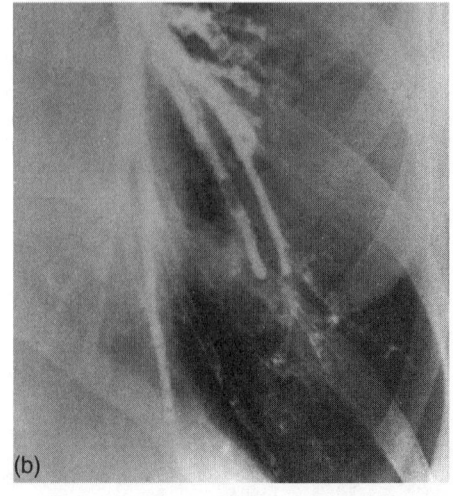

to the chest, consisting of localized or widespread medium to coarse crackles, with or without wheeze. The most severely affected patients may have signs of cor pulmonale (parasternal heave, loud pulmonary second sound, or features of overt right heart failure) or respiratory failure (cyanosis or signs of carbon dioxide retention).

Investigations

Many of the investigations are designed to assess the severity of the disease in order to establish a baseline for long-term monitoring of any progression. In a few instances investigations may provide evidence of the underlying cause, although this rarely affects management of the individual patient. The investigations that may reveal a cause are outlined in Table 2 and most are covered elsewhere in the text or in other sections. However, a few are worthy of further discussion at this point.

IMMUNOGLOBULINS

Panhypogammaglobulinaemia predisposes to infection and is known to be associated with bronchiectasis. However, it is only a rare cause, and more subtle defects of the immune system have been sought. In some series, deficiencies of immunoglobulin subclasses have been found in a significant proportion of patients. In particular, IgA deficiency, IgG2

under way. In most patients the levels are increased, but it is unknown whether the antibody is effective in bacterial killing and more common subtle defects (antigen-specific abnormalities) may yet emerge.

NEUTROPHIL FUNCTION

Tests of neutrophil function are not widely available. Where this has been studied, defects are rarely found in the circulating neutrophil. However, conditions like chronic granulomatous disease (failure to produce superoxides), Chediak–Higashi disease (lack of chemotactic response), and leucocyte adhesion deficiency (failure of cells to adhere to the endothelium and hence migrate into tissues) all predispose to bronchiectasis. More recently, secondary defects due to cleavage of the complement receptor (C3bi), which impairs bacterial killing have been identified in lung neutrophils. This latter abnormality may have significant implications for treatment (see later in this chapter). Finally, neutropenia may be associated with exacerbations of bronchiectasis, particularly if it is related to treatment for lymphomatous malignancies.

MUCOCILIARY CLEARANCE

Primary ciliary dyskinesia is autosomal recessive with incomplete penetrance and is believed to occur with a frequency of one in 15 000 to 30 000. The cilia appear grossly normal, but ultrastructural defects leading to partial or total loss of the outer dynein arms are associated with the disorder, although other rarer defects may be seen. The condition is associated with abnormal rotation of the archenteron, resulting in dextrocardia or situs inversus in 50 per cent of cases. This may result in the triad of situs inversus, sinusitis, and bronchiectasis, first described by Kartagener in the 1930s.

The function of mucociliary transport can be assessed by clearance of an inhaled radionuclide from the lung or the nasal saccharine test. In the latter procedure a small tablet of saccharine is placed on the inferior turbinate and the time taken to sense the taste is recorded. However, it should be noted that acquired mucociliary defects (loss of ciliated epithelium, excess viscous mucus, and toxic damage to cilia) will also affect these tests. Indeed, ultrastructural abnormalities may also occur following recent viral infections causing additional confusion.

RADIOLOGY

Radiographic examination of the chest has usually been the major diagnostic procedure in bronchiectasis. However, many of the abnormalities seen are suggestive rather than diagnostic (Table 3). Collapse of the lung as indicated by atelectasis or 'crowding' of pulmonary vessels indicate an area of damage and consolidation that may become infected, leading to bronchiectasis. 'Tramline shadows' suggest bronchial wall oedema, and cystic lesions (particularly if fluid filled) suggest saccular bronchiectasis.

The bronchogram (Fig. 3) has long been considered the 'gold standard' in the diagnosis of bronchiectasis. Radio-opaque contrast medium is either injected via a needle through the cricoid ligament or introduced through a fibre optic bronchoscope. However, high resolution CT scanning is now replacing the bronchogram. Although gross abnormalities (Fig. 4) can also be seen on routine chest radiographs, the sensitivity is increased for minor lesions (although specificity is reduced) and this non-invasive technique can be used to monitor progress. At present all chest imaging should be regarded as complementary and used in conjunction with clinical features.

Occasionally barium studies are indicated. Recurrent aspiration due to oesophageal reflux has been implicated in bronchiectasis and it may be subclinical. Although the bronchiectasis cannot be reversed, its symptoms and perhaps progression can improve with appropriate management of the reflux.

CULTURES OF RESPIRATORY SECRETIONS

Bacteria are usually cultured from the secretions of patients with bronchiectasis even at the end of successful antimicrobial therapy. Indeed, it is often possible to identify and culture three or more different organisms from the same sample, provided that this is done carefully using aerobic and anaerobic techniques as well as a selective medium. Many of these organisms are found colonizing the oropharynx and may be reported as 'normal mouth commensals' or 'upper respiratory tract flora' in sputum samples that have been expectorated via the oropharynx. Indeed, when it is necessary to identify infecting organisms, direct aspiration of secretions using a transcricoid needle or fibre optic broncho-

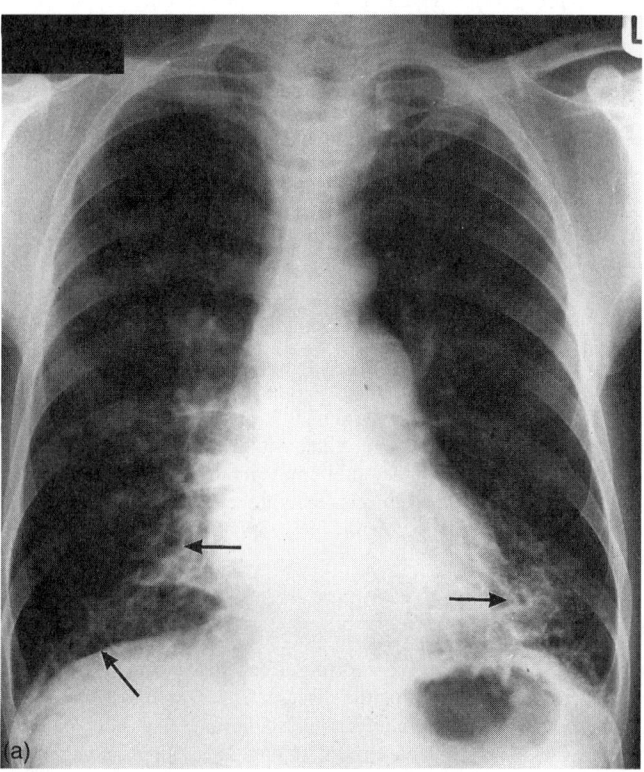

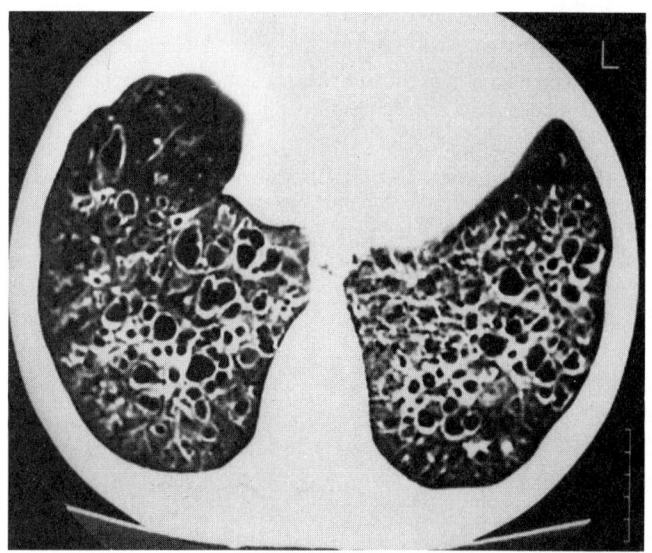

Fig. 4 Cystic lesions arrowed on the chest radiograph (a) indicate the presence of saccular bronchiectasis demonstrated clearly on the corresponding CAT scan (b).

scope has been recommended. However, the organisms isolated with these selective sampling techniques are usually the same as those obtained from sputum, and such invasive methods are rarely indicated.

The interpretation of sputum cultures requires collaboration between clinician, physiotherapist, and bacteriologist. It is important that the sample is sputum rather than saliva, and this can be facilitated with the help of an experienced physiotherapist and the use of postural drainage. The sample should then be analysed as soon as possible since standing or storage in the refrigerator may affect the culture of more fastidious organisms.

Gram stain is often useful for identifying the presence of significant numbers of organisms (Fig. 5) and partially characterizing them. This information may help the initial choice of antibiotic and determine the significance of subsequent culture. For instance large numbers of Gram-negative bacilli may indicate the predominance of *Haemophilus influenzae*, whereas culture may yield a heavy growth of *Pseudomonas* species (a far less fastidious organism). However, with careful culture techniques, and particularly the simultaneous use of selective medium to suppress bacterial overgrowth, it is possible to identify most organisms present, after which the significance of each isolate needs to be determined. It is possible that all play a role by adding to the total bacterial load, or that the appearance or an increase in the number of one of the organisms is the most important factor. These issues are often difficult to resolve and are currently the subject of clinical studies.

Some organisms of low pathogenicity are regularly identified and presumed to be clinically important in the compromised lung. These organisms rarely cause invasive infections but colonize the airways and elicit an inflammatory response. The organism most commonly isolated (if selective media are used) is *H. influenzae* (present in approximately 75 per cent of samples). The organism is unencapsulated (and hence cannot be typed), unlike *H. influenzae* type B which has a polysaccharide capsule and which causes invasive infections such as meningitis. Other organisms identified include *Streptococcus pneumoniae*, *Moraxella catarrhalis* (previously known as *Branhamella catarrhalis*), and *Pseudomonas aeruginosa* (mucoid type), which is more commonly a feature of severely affected patients where multiple courses of antibiotics have been used. In addition, a variety of anaerobic β-lactamase-producing organisms are often present, which may influence the choice and dosage of antibiotic used (see later).

Complications

The most common complication of bronchiectasis is an acute exacerbation. Episodes with worsening of symptoms may vary from once every few years to several times each year. Despite the frequency in some patients, the exact cause of an exacerbation remains uncertain on many occasions. An increase in symptoms (sputum volume, breathlessness, or chest pain), as well as the appearance of new symptoms (haemoptysis and temperature), are all included in the definition of an exacerbation. Thus such episodes may reflect natural fluctuations in symptoms, sputum retention, and increased airflow obstruction, as well as 'infective' exacerbations. Clearly, the regular presence of bacteria in the bronchial secretions tends to result in the assumption that they play a role in most exacerbations and hence broad-spectrum antibiotics are often prescribed (see later).

More careful history-taking and assessment may help clarify the cause. For instance, if the sputum is generally clear and remains so, it is unlikely that a bacterial infection is the cause of the deterioration and evidence of increased airflow obstruction with reversibility should be sought. Furthermore even a change in sputum colour to purulent may indicate airflow obstruction as the cause of an exacerbation if the cells in the sputum are eosinophils rather than neutrophils. The picture becomes more confusing when the sputum is usually purulent and symptoms worsen. A proportion of these episodes are also likely to represent increased airflow obstruction, and evidence for this should still be sought and treated appropriately.

Nevertheless, many exacerbations are infective in origin. Features such as pyrexia, systemic symptoms (particularly if associated with a rise in erythrocyte sedimentation ratio and/or acute-phase proteins such as C-reactive protein) and new changes on the chest radiograph suggest infection. A proportion of these infective episodes (probably up to 30 per cent) are probably viral in origin, and the remainder are presumed to be bacterial. Nevertheless, antimicrobial therapy is appropriate for such episodes whether presumed to be viral or bacterial, since the former can result in a secondary bacterial 'infection'.

HAEMOPTYSIS

Transient haemoptysis occurs frequently in exacerbations of bronchiectasis. In an individual patient this may vary from occasional streaks of blood to frank haemoptysis, and from a single episode to recurrence with every exacerbation. The episodes are usually self-limiting and resolve with the exacerbation. Occasionally, the haemoptysis can be severe and life-threatening, and may require intervention (see later).

EXTRAPULMONARY SPREAD OF INFECTION

This complication is now rarely seen owing to the prompt use of effective antibiotics. Classically, brain abscesses occurred as a result of vascular dissemination of organisms from the lung. Abscesses do not occur at other sites in the absence of any known host defence defects. Empyema has also become rare in bronchiectasis in recent years although, paradoxically, it can occur in poorly treated lobar pneumonias, resulting in the subsequent development of bronchiectasis.

AMYLOIDOSIS

Secondary amyloid has been recognized as a complication of bronchiectasis, although again it is now rare. It is presumed that most of the amyloidosis is caused by protein A deposition, as with amyloidosis in other chronic disorders, although it may represent immunoglobulin light-chain disease in some subjects receiving replacement therapy since many of the early immunoglobulin preparations were fragmented and contained free light chains.

JOINT DISEASE

A seronegative arthropathy has been described in bronchiectasis, particularly during exacerbations of the disease. The symptoms may settle with appropriate antibacterial therapy, suggesting that it is directly related to the lung problem. Recent studies have suggested that the

Fig. 5 Gram stain of sputum smear from a stable patient with bronchiectasis. Streaks of mucus can be seen with several neutrophils. There are large numbers of Gram-negative diplococci typical of *Moraxella catarrhalis* (arrowed) which were subsequently identified following primary culture.

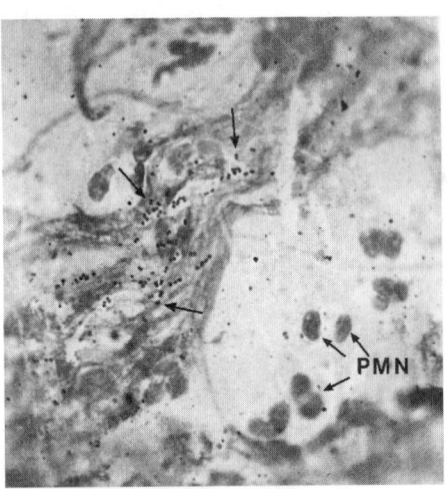

arthropathy may be the result of immune complexes formed between high levels of circulating immunoglobulin and bacterial antigens.

VASCULITIS

Cutaneous vasculitis has been described in severe bronchiectasis with and without cystic fibrosis. Again, the cause is thought to be circulating immune complexes which may be deposited in peripheral vessels.

RESPIRATORY FAILURE AND COR PULMONALE

A small proportion of the most severely affected patients deteriorate progressively and develop respiratory failure with clinical signs of hypoxia and carbon dioxide retention. Cor pulmonale will develop in some of these, eventually resulting in right heart failure. These complications are less common than previously, presumably as a result of improved management of the disease in its earlier stages.

Management

The majority of patients with bronchiectasis have minimal or undiagnosed disease; they have few symptoms most of the time and require or tolerate little or no medical intervention. Many of the symptoms (cough and sputum production) are often regarded as no more than a nuisance or a 'fact of life'. It is only when these symptoms become sufficient to interfere with life that medical advice is sought, and even then intervention may not alter them significantly.

Surgery

In the past surgery was considered to be the main way of curing the disease. Resection of the affected area should result in cure; however, in most cases such radical intervention was far from effective. The disease was rarely localized to a single lobe or even lobes, although the severity in individual areas may have varied at the time of surgery. In addition, the underlying cause of the disease (immune deficiencies etc.) still persisted in some patients. Furthermore, extensive chest surgery itself often led to atelectasis in the remaining lung during the postoperative phase, resulting in further lung damage. For these reasons many of the patients still attending specialist clinics with bronchiectasis have had previous surgery aimed at 'curing' the disease. Thus elective surgery has largely been eliminated as a therapeutic option. In a few limited cases, including bronchiectasis following foreign body inhalation or severe lobar pneumonia, surgery may still be considered as an option in patients with persistent ill health.

However, surgery also remains an option for persistent and extensive haemoptysis. Although most cases of even major haemoptysis will settle spontaneously, this complication can still be life-threatening. In such cases localization of the bleeding to a single lobe or segment by bronchoscopy can result in a curative operation. However, more recently bronchial artery embolization has also proved effective, particularly when there is difficulty in identifying the lobar source of the bleeding or lung function is poor, thereby precluding surgery.

PULMONARY SEQUESTRATION

Intralobar pulmonary sequestration is a malformation in which a segment of lung derives its blood supply from the aorta, or one of its branches, and which does not normally communicate with the bronchial tree. Usually placed within a lower lobe and covered by the lobe's visceral pleura, the sequestered segment has cystic dilated spaces and presents with recurrent infection at the site and may therefore mimic bronchiectasis. Doppler techniques and magnetic resonance imaging often suggest the diagnosis. Aortography is definitive and is currently undertaken before surgical resection.

Some sequestered segments cause significant aortal–ventricular shunting, may be associated with other cardiac anomalies, and may present as cardiovascular disease in infancy.

Deficiency status

At present our understanding of deficiencies in the immune system is relatively superficial. Although gross deficiency states can be recognized (hypogammaglobulinaemia, IgA deficiency, complement deficiencies, and neutrophil chemotactic defects), most cannot be treated. Furthermore, there may be many more subtle defects (epitope-specific IgG defects) that have yet to be identified. Thus at present most patients with identified immune deficiencies have to be treated conventionally (see later).

Replacement therapy is available for immunoglobulin deficiency. Panhypogammaglobulinaemia, selective IgG and IgM deficiency, and IgG subclass (usually IgG2) deficiency may respond to immunoglobulin replacement therapy. This has been given as weekly intramuscular injections which are painful and often ineffective (normal immunoglobin levels may not be achieved). More recently, intravenous replacement has been shown to be more effective and certainly more acceptable to the patient than intramuscular therapy. It is important to confirm that the intravenous preparation is functional and capable of opsonizing antigens for phagocytosis prior to embarking upon an extended trial period. Preliminary studies are being conducted with immunoglobulin inhalation which may prove both effective and more acceptable to the patient.

Seletive IgA deficiency is not usually amenable to replacement therapy because the patient may have or develop IgA-specific antibodies. Thus therapy may lead to anaphylaxis or immune complex deposition.

α_1-Antitrypsin deficiency is associated with bronchiectasis. Replacement therapy as a weekly or monthly infusion has been approved in the United States for patients with emphysema. Whether such therapy would be helpful in deficient subjects with bronchiectasis is unknown, but augmentation therapy with α_1-antitrypsin has been shown to reduce lung elastase activity in cystic fibrosis patients.

Other specific causes

Few of the other known causes of bronchiectasis respond to specific therapy with consequent improvement of the lung problem. Prompt therapy in allergic bronchopulmonary aspergillosis should prevent further development of bronchiectasis. Treatment of chronic rhinosinusitis and gastro-oesophageal reflux may improve respiratory symptoms. Some cases of bronchiectasis associated with conditions like rheumatoid arthritis may improve if the primary condition is treated adequately, perhaps because of an effect of the therapy upon lung inflammation itself (see later).

Physiotherapy

Postural drainage has long been considered a cornerstone of the management of bronchiectasis. Because of the reduced mucociliary clearance and excess mucus production, the secretions tend to accumulate in dependent areas of the lung until expectorated. Some have assumed that such accumulation is harmful and that assistance in clearance of these areas may be beneficial, but there is little evidence to support this assumption. No long-term studies of the effect of postural drainage on morbidity have been conducted. The volume of secretions expectorated is not altered over a 24-h period, although physiotherapy does increase the volume of sputum produced immediately after the procedure.

With these reservations many patients and doctors still advocate regular twice daily postural drainage, designed to allow the affected areas to be cleared at least temporarily. This does have the advantage of a marginal improvement in lung function (probably due to airways clearing) and a reduction in the frequency of cough and expectoration between episodes. Nevertheless, despite this, patient compliance (when assessed) has been shown to be poor.

Formalized and supervised physiotherapy during acute exacerbations, particularly when mucus expectoration becomes more difficult, can be helpful in relieving symptoms of chest discomfort and improving ventilation–perfusion mismatching, which may be of critical importance in patients with respiratory failure. Steam inhalations can also occasionally prove beneficial by facilitating expectoration, but mucolytic therapy has largely fallen out of favour. Perhaps with the recent development of human recombinant DNAse further studies will clarify the role of agents in the liquefaction of tenacious mucus.

Drug therapy

At present, therapy is predominantly targeted at the management of any airflow obstruction or infection that may be playing a critical role in the disease morbidity. However, as the pathogenesis of the condition becomes clarified, alternative strategies are being considered and some have been assessed (see below).

AIRFLOW OBSTRUCTION

Although many patients with bronchiectasis have relatively normal lung function some develop a degree of obstructive or restrictive lung disease. Indeed, with the degree of inflammation, tissue damage, and repair (by fibrosis) that occurs, it is surprising that lung function remains well preserved in most subjects. Nevertheless, a proportion do develop some physiological abnormality and in a few this can progress towards respiratory failure (see later). Thus, it is important to assess baseline lung function in all patients and review this every 6 to 12 months, particularly in those with most severe or persistent disease, in order to determine whether abnormalities are present, developing, or progressing.

Those with airflow obstruction should be investigated appropriately and treated for any reversibility. A proportion will have demonstrable reversibility and benefit from treatment regimens appropriate for non-complicated asthma. This will involve a combination of inhaled β_2-agonists and corticosteroids, as well as appropriate oral therapy including theophylline. However, before embarking upon continuous therapy with such agents, it is important to be sure that they are having the desired effect. This is particularly true of β_2-agonists which are conventionally prescribed following demonstrable improvement of airflow obstruction. Expectoration itself can improve lung volumes and forced vital manoeuvres (forced expiratory volume in 1 s (FEV_1), forced vital capacity (FVC), and peak flow rate (PFR)), can often facilitate expectoration (as can inhaled β_2-agonists) and thus it is wise to perform all short-term reversibility tests after vigorous postural drainage.

The aetiology of any asthmatic component is uncertain (in the absence of allergic bronchopulmonary aspergillosis), although asthma itself is a common condition and could coexist by chance in patients with bronchiectasis. Nevertheless, it has been suggested that airways inflammation as a result of bacterial colonization may result in the development of irritable airways. Appropriate antibiotic therapy (see below) can reduce asthmatic symptoms in some patients.

AIRWAYS INFECTION

As mentioned previously, the airways of patients with bronchiectasis are often persistently colonized with viable bacteria. This does not represent invasive infection as the organisms are of low pathogenicity and systemic symptoms are usually absent. However, in many patients these organisms are associated with a host response leading to inflammation in the airways and persistent recruitment of neutrophils from the circulation, resulting in purulent secretions (Fig. 5).

The role of these organisms in bronchiectasis has been debated, but the mortality from bronchiectasis has undoubtedly changed with the introduction of antibiotics. Prior to the antibiotic era, approximately 70 per cent of patients died before the age of 40, whereas more recently the proportion of patients dying at an early age is much lower. Over a 14-year period up to 1981 approximately 20 per cent of patients treated medically died of their disease at an average age of 53. The incidence

of severe complications such as amyloidosis, respiratory failure, and cor pulmonale has decreased, suggesting that the course of the disease has been altered. There is a general impression that the disease is less prevalent. Although this may reflect a change in management and referral patterns, it may also be due to prompt antibiotic therapy in childhood, reducing the incidence and severity of pneumonic illness that could lead to the development of bronchiectasis.

There have been few long-term studies of the role of antibiotic therapy in bronchiectasis, but the Medical Research Council (MRC) trial in 1957 demonstrated that prophylactic therapy could prevent exacerbations and improve morbidity.

INDICATIONS FOR ANTIBIOTIC THERAPY

Antibiotic therapy in bronchiectasis can be divided into short courses for exacerbations, prophylactic therapy to prevent or modify exacerbations, and continuous therapy. In general terms the use of antibiotics should go through each of these three stages, with clinical response and observation determining whether one should proceed to the next step.

Acute exacerbation

Although many acute infective exacerbations (up to 30 per cent) may be self-limiting or even viral in origin, it seems appropriate to prescribe a course of antibiotic therapy. Furthermore, patients with bronchiectasis often develop an exacerbation following an upper respiratory tract infection and, if this is bacterial and not an acute episode of airflow obstruction, it may well be appropriate to start such patients on therapy prior to the development of lower respiratory tract infection.

Recurrent exacerbations

Initially, it is probably appropriate to treat each recurrent exacerbation in its own right. However, once a pattern is established and it is known that several exacerbations will occur each year the role of prophylactic therapy has to be considered. This may be confined to the winter months or given throughout the year, depending on the clinical pattern. Just when prophylactic therapy is introduced remains a value judgement based upon frequency of exacerbation or the morbidity associated with each episode. A reasonable guideline would be episodes occurring more than every 2 months, particularly if the patient is unable to carry out his or her normal daily routine for 2 or more weeks on each occasion.

More recently the threshold for the introduction of preventative therapy has been reduced as the potential pathogenic role of such episodes has become clearer (see below).

Persistent infection

Some patients with bronchiectasis persistently produce purulent secretions that contain numerous neutrophils. Although such patients remain reasonable well and appear to be clinically stable, this state indicates a continuous host response in the lung to the organisms colonizing the airways. A small proportion of patients with bronchiectasis deteriorate, and these usually have extensive disease with persistently purulent lung secretions. This has led to a series of investigations to determine the role of bacteria and the host response in the progression of lung damage in some subjects.

The vicious circle of destructive lung disease

The presence of large numbers of bacteria within the airways results in mobilization of the host defence system. In most subjects this will be sufficient to sterilize the airways. However, if the host response fails to clear the organisms it may persist and even become self-generating. In some patients with bronchiectasis this situation is undoubtedly present with a heightened immune response, lymphocytic infiltration, and continued recruitment of neutrophils to the airways. This combination of bacterial colonization with an exuberant host response has been implicated in the progressive deterioration seen in some patients.

A key factor is believed to be the release of proteinases, particularly elastase, from the neutrophils recruited to the lung. The enzyme neutrophil elastase has been shown to have several potentially harmful effects.

1. It can damage ciliated epithelium and reduce the cilia beat frequency.
2. It stimulates mucus secretion and, when combined with effect 1, will reduce mucociliary clearance, thereby promoting bacterial proliferation.
3. It can interfere with host defence by cleaving (and thereby inactivating) immunoglobulins and damaging the C3bi receptor on neutrophils, thus reducing bacterial phagocytosis and killing. These effects will also facilitate the survival and proliferation of bacteria in the airway and thus perpetuate the host chemotactic response to recruit more neutrophils.
4. It is directly responsible for the degradation of lung connective tissues, leading to further damage. However, the fragments released by this degradation also attract neutrophils, resulting in further recruitment.
5. It causes epithelial cells to secrete IL-8, another major chemoattractant, once again perpetuating neutrophil recruitment.

The neutrophil may not be the sole agent involved in the persistent cycle of lung damage. Bacteria release toxins that can damage ciliated epithelia, thereby reducing mucociliary clearance further. In addition, activated lung lymphocytes may themselves cause damage to host cells by a process of antigen-dependent cell cytotoxicity.

These concepts are more complex because a multitude of cytokines and cell–cell interactions will also be involved in this chronic inflammatory process. An outline of the broad principles involved in this destructive self-perpetuating sequence of events is shown in Fig. 6. It is possible to break this sequence by successful antibiotic therapy. Studies

Fig. 6 Summary of the general concept of self-perpetuation of lung damage in bronchiectasis. Following an initiating event that leads to the development of bronchiectasis, the tissue damage impairs mucociliary clearance resulting in sputum retention and bacterial proliferation. The subsequent recruitment of phagocytes may persist if the organisms are not cleared and a state of chronic inflammation is established. These various factors may amplify other steps in the sequence resulting in a failure of host defences and perpetuation of lung damage.

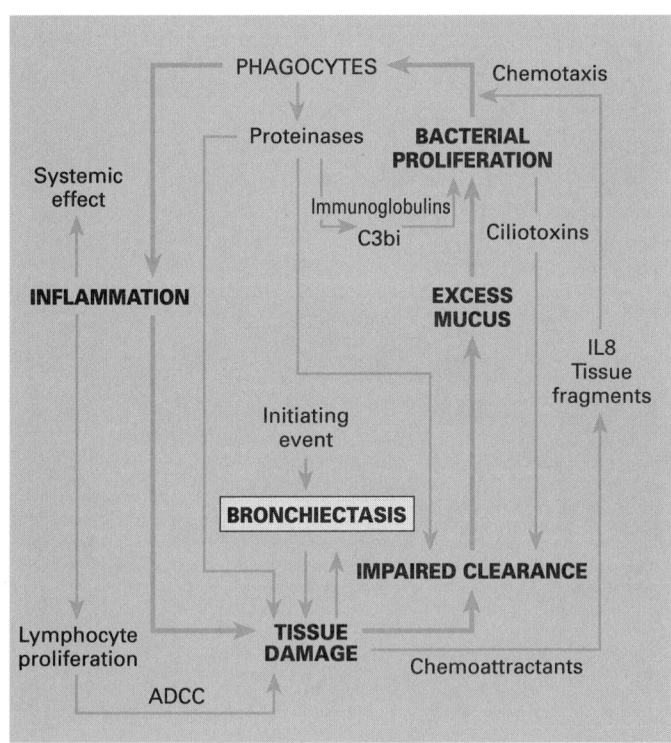

have shown that neutrophil recruitment is reduced, the chemotactic activity in the lung is reduced, and the damaging neutrophil enzymes disappear. However, the effect is usually short-lived, and it is becoming accepted that continuous therapy with antibiotics is important in patients who show evidence of this perpetuating process.

Choice of antibiotic

Several factors influence the choice and efficacy of the antibiotic used to treat patients with bronchiectasis. First, the sensitivity of the organism or organisms involved will be crucial. Second, the lungs are often scarred in bronchiectasis, and the antibiotic must be able to penetrate the airways and secretions where the organisms reside. Finally, the antibiotic may need to be resistant to degradation by enzymes such as β-lactamase that may be present in some secretions. With these factors in mind it is clear that no standard regimen can be applied to all patients. However, it is possible to establish some general guidelines based upon the patient's clinical status.

THE ORGANISMS

Although many organisms can be identified in bronchiectatic secretions there are several that predominate. The most commonly isolated is *H. influenzae* (75 per cent) with *Strep. pneumoniae* and *M. catarrhalis* making up most of the rest. In a small proportion of patients (particularly the most severely affected) *P. aeruginosa* may become a persistent pathogen. These organisms show good sensitivity to many orally administered antibiotics, although a degree of resistance is developing to some.

H. influenzae is usually sensitive to ampicillin, although recent surveys in the United Kingdom have shown that approximately 13 per cent of all isolates are resistant, often because of the presence of β-lactamase production. However, the incidence varies from country to country, and up to 30 per cent resistance has been reported in Spain. Resistance to erythromycin is higher than that to ampicillin in the United Kingdom (19 per cent), although resistance to tetracycline (1–2 per cent) and cephaclor (2 per cent) is lower and most organisms remain sensitive to co-trimoxazole and chloramphenicol.

Strep. pneumoniae is still relatively sensitive to ampicillin, although some resistance is emerging. Again, however, erythromycin resistance is high whereas cephaclor resistance is negligible.

M. catarrhalis usually produces β-lactamase and thus is resistant to ampicillin, although erythromycin and cephaclor are still effective *in vitro*.

ANTIBIOTICS

The antibiotics most commonly used for exacerbations of bronchiectasis are those with a broad spectrum of activity that are effective when administered orally; precise choice may be dictated by local data on microbial sensitivities. The initial choice (based upon the probable organism sensitivity outlined above) usually rests between ampicillin/amoxycillin or some other antibiotic (e.g. tetracycline, co-trimoxazole, or cephaclor) for penicillin-sensitive patients. Amoxycillin probably remains the most effective at present because it is easily tolerated, is fully absorbed from the gastrointestinal tract, and penetrates lung secretions well. However, as the ampicillin resistance of *H. influenzae* increases and Moraxella becomes more important, the initial choice may alter.

The role of newer antibiotics including the quinolones (e.g. ciprofloxacin) needs to be carefully established, and they should probably be reserved at present for specific indications such as Pseudomonas infection requiring oral therapy.

ACUTE EXACERBATION

The management of an acute exacerbation depends upon the preceding clinical state of the patient. If the patient usually has no symptoms or the sputum is usually mucoid, an infective exacerbation is indicated by the production of purulent sputum. This usually responds to a short course (7–10 days) of amoxycillin or a similar alternative in conventional doses (e.g. 250–500 mg amoxycillin three times daily). At the end of the course the sputum production either ceases or returns to its former mucoid state.

However, management is less clear if the patient usually produces mucopurulent or purulent secretions. These patients already have a significant bacterial load in the lung, resulting in neutrophil recruitment during the stable state. If the symptoms suggest an infective exacerbation, it is still advisable to prescribe an antibiotic course although the response may appear less impressive. Mucopurulent sputum often becomes clear, but may return to its pretreatment state within a few weeks although the symptoms of the exacerbation may not return. Patients with purulent sputum may notice no change in sputum colour unless high concentrations of antibiotics are used (3 g amoxycillin twice daily), although symptoms may settle. If the sputum clears, it may be only for 2 to 4 days, suggesting that the organisms responsible may have only been suppressed temporarily.

The failure of sputum colour to clear or the development of rapid relapse has implications for long-term management (see below). The antibiotic regimen may need to be reviewed within 1 to 2 days depending on the results of antimicrobial culture, although some studies have indicated that patients often respond to therapy (symptoms settling and sputum clearing) despite the presence of apparently resistant organisms. Such responses may indicate that the episode was self-limiting anyway or that the antibiotic was altering other organisms present rather than the assumed major pathogen.

Failure to respond despite the presence of an apparently sensitive organism may suggest that the antibiotic is not reaching the lung in concentrations that remain high enough to be effective. This is particularly true of patients who persistently produce purulent secretions where conventional therapy may not alter the nature of these secretions. In these patients increasing the dosage may be all that is required. The effect is to overcome any blood–lung barrier due to scarring of the tissues and in particular to overcome any production of β-lactamase by anaerobic 'bystanding' organisms that may degrade the antibiotic *in situ* before it can be effective against the true pathogen.

For severe exacerbations where oral therapy has failed, or may not be appropriate, it is usual to embark upon broad-spectrum intravenous therapy, particularly to cover the less common organisms. In this instance an initial Gram stain may help but often therapy remains empirical. Many agents can prove effective in individual cases, including gentamicin, carbenicillin, and tobramycin (when Pseudomonas is expected) or imipenin with or without ampicillin and metronidazole. Choice and dosage will depend upon individual hospital policy and local resistance patterns.

PROPHYLAXIS

Prophylactic therapy is indicated in patients who have frequent exacerbations and can usually be achieved with oral therapy. In the original MRC trial (1957) the agent used was tetracycline given twice a week. However, there is no reason to believe that the same effect cannot be achieved with other oral agents, particularly since tetracycline resistance of some of the organisms is becoming more prevalent.

More recently, prophylactic therapy has also been advocated for patients who persistently produce purulent secretions for the reasons outlined above in an attempt to break the vicious circle. Although such patients appear to be clinically stable, studies have shown that continuous antibiotic therapy can improve well-being and reduce plasma acute phase proteins, suggesting that the presence of purulent sputum alone is associated with a systemic response, albeit low grade.

Again, the choice of regimen can be influenced by the patient's clinical state prior to therapy. Those with mucopurulent (pale yellow or pale green) secretions usually respond to conventional doses of antibiotic given orally. However, patients whose secretions are usually purulent (dark green) rarely respond to conventional therapy and may require high dosage orally (e.g. amoxycillin 3 g twice daily) or even nebulized drug (e.g. amoxycillin 500 mg twice daily). The response (clearance of secretions) can be maintained with such a regimen (Fig. 7). Clinical experience suggests that patients treated in this way have few clinical exacerbations and, despite obvious concern, the emergence of resistant organisms is unusual provided that therapy is maintained.

Clinical exacerbations in patients treated prophylactically require careful sputum assessment and often short courses of parenteral therapy before returning to the usual regimen. Some patients treated successfully with prophylactic therapy may remain well (with mucoid sputum) if treatment is stopped after 4 to 6 months. Thus it seems sensible to attempt withdrawal of therapy at this stage, but early relapse would indicate that prophylactic therapy should then become long term.

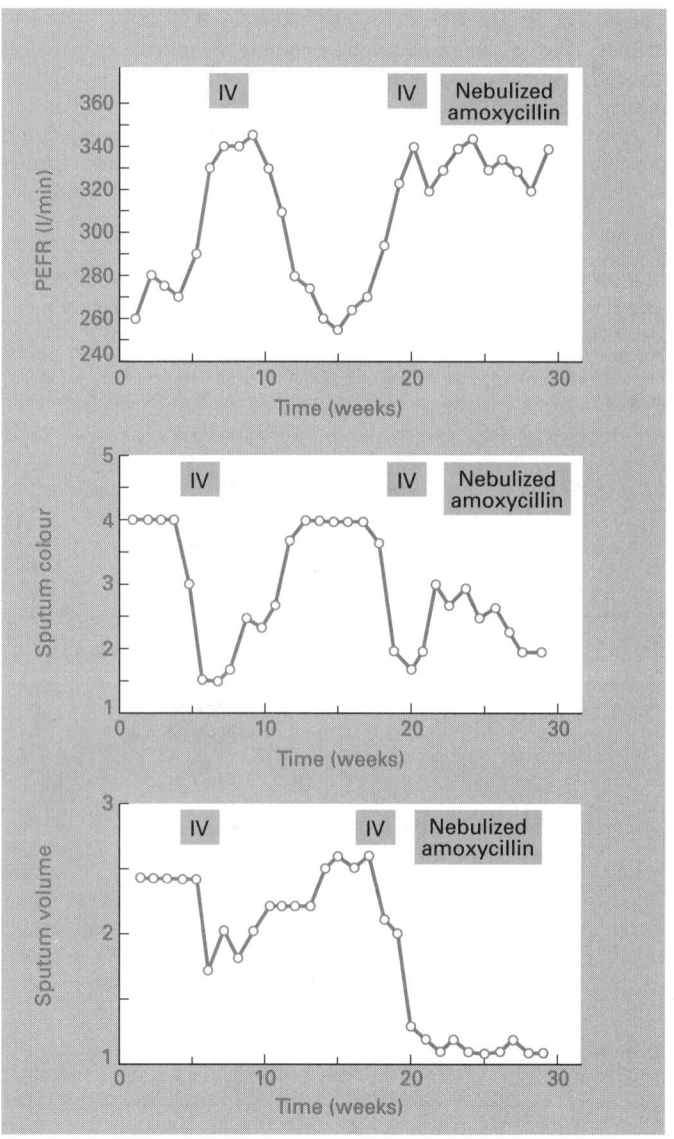

Fig. 7 Flow chart of PEFR and sputum characteristics of a patient with bronchiectasis. Sputum colour and volume are given as arbitrary units. High values for colour reflect the degree of purulence (1 = mucoid) and for volume a value of 1 reflects little or no sputum/day. Following a 2-week course of intravenous therapy (IV), PEFR increases, sputum colour improves (becoming mucoid), and sputum volume decreases. However there is a gradual return to the pretreatment state and a further course of IV therapy followed by regular nebulized antibiotic improves and maintains the lung function and sputum values.

A general summary of these principles and guidelines is indicated in Fig. 8.

VACCINATION

The role of vaccination in bronchiectasis is uncertain. As with other forms of chronic obstructive pulmonary disease there is a tendency to consider immunization against influenza virus prior to the winter. However, there have been no formal studies of its efficacy which depends upon cross-reactivity with the prevalent strain in the respective year. Nevertheless, it may have a role in the most severely affected patients where severe influenza infection could precipitate respiratory failure and death.

Immunization with bacterial antigens is even more contentious. The immunodominant antigens for *H. influenzae* and *Strep. pneumoniae* have yet to be characterized. Polyvalent vaccines are unlikely to benefit the patient since they are usually persistently exposed to the antigens of the bacteria which already colonize the airways. If patients are unable to develop their own immune response naturally, it is unlikely that they will do so when these are administered artificially. Furthermore, patients usually have excessive antibodies to bacterial antigens both locally (in the lung) and systemically. The administration of bacterial antigen may potentially lead to immune complex generation. For these reasons immunization with polyvalent bacterial vaccines would be inappropriate in most patients with bronchiectasis.

ALTERNATIVE THERAPY

As the pathogenic processes involved in bronchiectasis have become clarified, interest has increased in alternative ways of intervening in the vicious circle at other stages.

Immunosuppressive therapy

The lung shows many features of an overexuberant immune response, some of which may be directed against autoantigens. Thus immunosuppressive therapy may have a role in some patients. The major concern

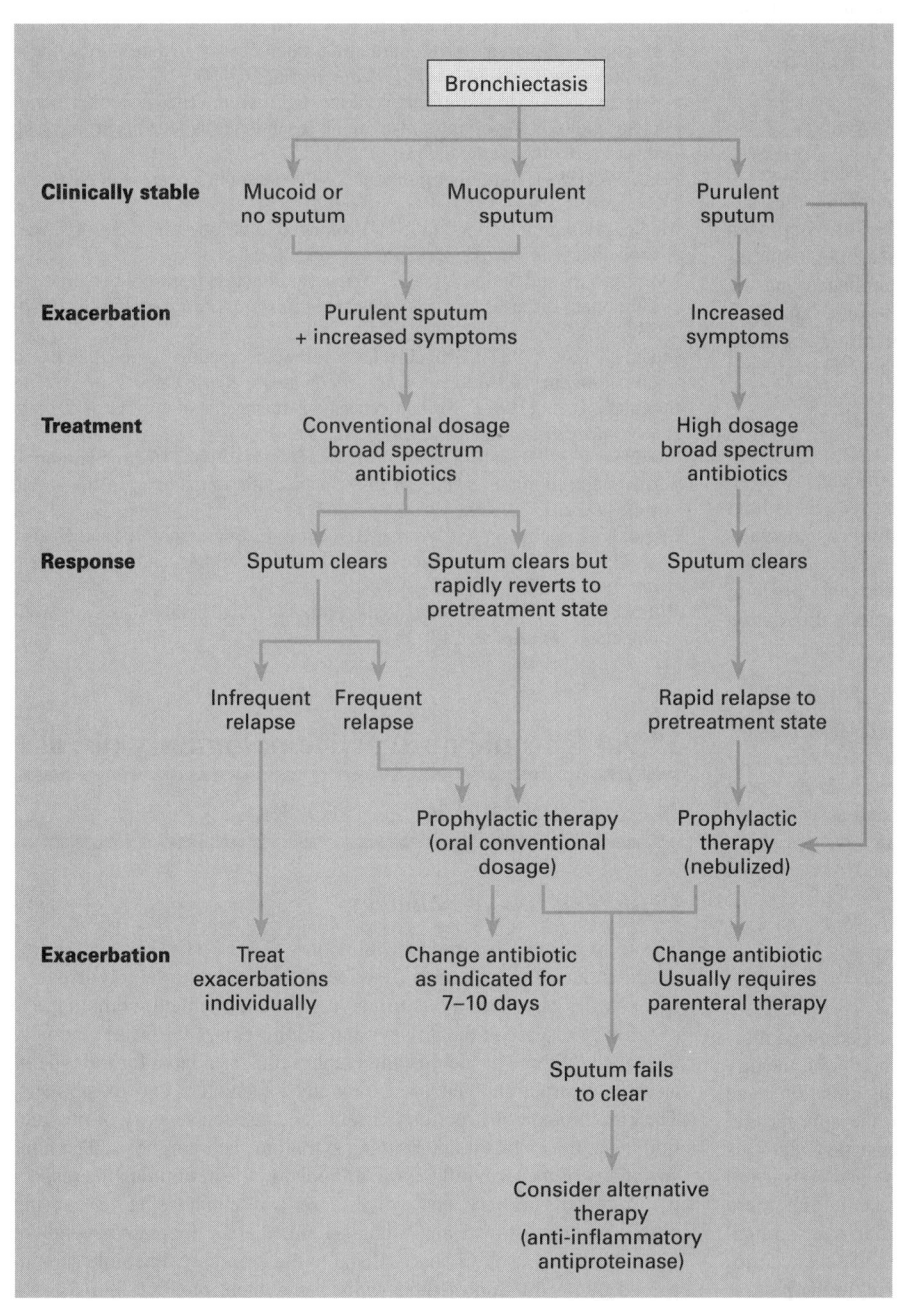

Fig. 8 Flow chart for the management of bronchiectasis, indicating treatment protocols. Note patients are assessed sequentially as indicated by symptoms with the exception of those who persistently expectorate purulent sputum where a strong case can be made for prophylactic therapy from the start.

is whether this approach would result in an increase in bacterial proliferation if the host defence is reduced. However, this may be a theoretical rather than a practical problem. Corticosteroids have been used successfully in patients with severe endstage bronchiectasis in cystic fibrosis (40 mg daily) and a similar effect might be obtained in patients without cystic fibrosis. Some patients with bronchiectasis associated with rheumatoid arthritis have shown dramatic improvement in their lung symptoms following aggressive immunosuppressive therapy for their joint disease.

Future studies will clarify the role of such therapy. At present it should be reserved for the most severely affected patients where conventional therapy has failed. Patients on such therapy should be carefully monitored to ensure a positive clinical response with no detrimental effect occurs.

Neutrophil modulation

As recruitment of neutrophils to the lung results in release of harmful proteinases, it may be possible to modulate their response. Several agents used in immunosuppressive therapy (including steroids and cyclosporin A) have been shown to alter neutrophil chemotaxis and may have a role via this mechanism. Alternatively, non-steroidal anti-inflammatory agents can also reduce neutrophil responses and should be considered in the management of severely affected patients.

Antiproteinases

Proteolytic enzymes may play a key role in many of the pathogenic processes in the lung, and thus the role of inhaled antiproteinases has been investigated. At present it is not known whether this approach affects the clinical features and progression of the disease, but the studies have shown that the elastase activity is reduced or abolished and the release of the chemoattractant IL-8 from epithelial cells and damage to the C3bi receptor on neutrophils (reducing its bacterial killing potential) are abrogated. More formal trials of such therapy should be considered for selected patients.

Transplantation

Lung and heart–lung transplantation is being undertaken successfully in cystic fibrosis patients with severe endstage lung disease with or without cor pulmonale. A similar approach may be indicated in bronchiectasis without cystic fibrosis. However, the time course of the disease is longer in the absence of cystic fibrosis and respiratory failure is more likely to occur in middle to late middle age, if at all. Nevertheless, this option should be considered for any severely affected younger patient.

Respiratory failure and cor pulmonale

As with other causes of chronic obstructive pulmonary disease, patients may develop respiratory failure, sleep apnoea syndromes, secondary polycythaemia, and cor pulmonale leading to heart failure. These patients may benefit from long-term oxygen therapy and assisted ventilatory support (such as nasal continuous positive airways pressure). Occasionally repeated venesection may be helpful, and conventional therapy for right heart failure should be used.

Prognosis

The natural history of bronchiectasis has changed, with decreased mortality and probably morbidity, since the 1940s when antibiotic therapy became available. Recent longitudinal studies of lung function have shown little or no progression in general, supporting the concept that prognosis is generally good. Other studies have shown that vigorous antibiotic therapy increases well-being in patients who had considered themselves clinically 'well' for many years, suggesting that these patients had become used to general ill health, regarding it as normal. A small proportion of patients undoubtedly deteriorate and die of cardiorespiratory failure. However, these patients have proved, in the past, to

be resistant to conventional therapy. Perhaps as the pathogenesis of the disease becomes clearer, newer therapeutic approaches may improve their prognosis.

REFERENCES

Amitani, R., Wilson, R., Rutman, A., *et al.* (1991). Effects of human neutrophil elastase and *Pseudomonas aeruginosa* proteinases on human respiratory epithelium. *American Journal of Respiratory, Cell and Molecular Biology*, **4**, 26–32.

Cole, P. (1984). A new look at the pathogenesis and management of persistent bronchial sepsis: a vicious circle hypothesis and its logical connotations. In: *Strategies for the management of chronic bronchial sepsis* (ed R.J. Davies), pp. 1–16. Medicine Publishing Foundation, Oxford.

Doyle, A.J. (1992). Demonstration of blood supply to pulmonary sequestration by MR angiography. *American Journal of Roentgenology*, **158**, 989–90.

Hill, S.L., Morrison, H.M., Burnett, D., and Stockley, R.A. (1986). Short term response of patients with bronchiectasis to treatment with amoxycillin given in standard or high doses orally or by inhalation. *Thorax*, **41**, 559–65.

Hill, S.L., Burnett, D., Hewetson, K.A., and Stockley, R.A. (1988). The response of patients with purulent bronchiectasis to antibiotics for 4 months. *Quarterly Journal of Medicine*, **66**, 163–73.

Kalsheker, N.A., Hodgson, I.J., Watkins, G.L., *et al.* (1987). Deoxyribonucleic acid (DNA) polymorphism of the α_1-antitrypsin gene in chronic lung disease. *British Medical Journal*, **294**, 1511–14.

Kent, M. (1991). Intralobar pulmonary sequestration. *Progress in Pediatric Surgery*, **27**, 84–91.

Medical Research Council (1957). Prolonged antibiotic treatment of severe bronchiectasis. *British Medical Journal*, **2**, 255–9.

Murphy, T.F. and Sethi, S. (1992). Bacterial infection in chronic obstructive pulmonary disease. *American Review of Respiratory Disease*, **146**, 1067–83.

Stockley, R.A. (1987). Bronchiectasis—new therapeutic approaches based on pathogenesis. *Clinics in Chest Medicine*, **8** (3), 481–94.

Stockley, R.A. (1988). Bronchiectasis—a management problem? *British Journal of Diseases of the Chest*, **82**, 209–19.

Stockley, R.A., Hill, S.L., and Morrison, H.M. (1984). Effect of antibiotic treatment on sputum elastase in bronchiectatic outpatients in the stable state. *Thorax*, **39**, 414–19.

Sugio, K., Kaneko, S., Yokoyama, H., Ishida, T., Sugimachi, K., and Hasuo, K. (1992). Pulmonary sequestration in older children and adults. *International Surgery*, **77**, 102–7.

Whitwell, F. (1952). A study of the pathology and pathogenesis of bronchiectasis. *Thorax*, **7**, 213–39.

17.9.4 Chronic obstructive pulmonary disease

N. B. PRIDE and R. A. STOCKLEY

Definitions and terminology

The term chronic obstructive pulmonary disease (**COPD**) was introduced about 30 years ago to describe individuals with largely irreversible airways obstruction due to varying (but unspecified) combinations of intrinsic disease of the airways and emphysema. COPD has gradually displaced 'chronic bronchitis and emphysema' as a label for the type of airways obstruction seen predominantly in smokers and ex-smokers. The emphasis on obstruction is useful, because the severity of obstruction is the major factor determining symptoms and prognosis. The nonspecificity of the term reflects the difficulty in life of defining the respective roles of primary airways disease and emphysema in causing obstruction to airflow. Emphysema—defined as an 'increase beyond the normal in the size of air spaces distal to the terminal bronchiole accompanied by destruction of their walls and without obvious fibrosis'—is only detected reliably in life by imaging and lung function tests when it is relatively severe. In contrast 'chronic bronchitis', which is a synonym for chronic mucus hypersecretion, is easily diagnosed by the presence of chronic cough and expectoration not attributable to other lung disease. Thirty years ago it was thought there was a direct connection between 'chronic bronchitis' and the development of airways narrowing. This has not proved to be the case; the pathological changes responsible for chronic mucus hypersecretion are predominantly in the central conducting airways which are not significantly narrowed by the accompanying gland hyperplasia and mucosal inflammation. The airways disease which contributes to the obstruction to airflow is in the smaller airways (Table 1). Both processes are strongly related to smoking, but many smokers have chronic cough and expectoration without significant airways obstruction, while perhaps 25 per cent of smokers with obstruction of the peripheral airways do not have chronic expectoration. Hence, while the definition of 'chronic bronchitis' remains internationally accepted and is used widely by epidemiologists, it has become a source of confusion in clinical practice.

COPD is a diagnosis of exclusion. By convention it is only applied to a widespread obstruction of the intrathoracic airways. Obstruction of the extrathoracic airway is excluded, as are less widespread causes of airways obstruction such as scarring and distortion following tuberculosis or sarcoidosis. Conventionally, other specific causes of diffuse obstruction of the intrathoracic airways such as cystic fibrosis and rarer causes of obstruction of the small airways are excluded (Table 2). The main exception is α_1-antitrypsin deficiency which is usually regarded as a subcategory of COPD, perhaps because the pulmonary effects are clearly accelerated by smoking and emphysema is a predominant feature, which is not the case for the other disorders listed.

The most troublesome aspect of COPD is the overlap with chronic incompletely reversible asthma, a common alternative diagnosis in middle-aged and older patients. This distinction has never been clarified precisely; almost all patients with COPD show some short-term improvement after using bronchodilators, although this is usually less than 15 per cent of predicted forced expiratory volume in 1 second (FEV_1). Overlap terms such as 'chronic asthmatic bronchitis' are commonly used because of this difficulty. From the point of view of current therapy the distinction between COPD and chronic asthma is irrelevant (provided that a trial of corticosteroids is made in all severely obstructed patients) because the same drugs are used in asthma and COPD, but this may not be the case in future (specific treatments for α_1-antitrypsin deficiency and cystic fibrosis are already being developed). However, the two conditions have a very different prognosis for progression and mortality (much worse in COPD), and probably a different pathogenesis, so that the distinction is of critical importance for investigators and epidemiologists.

Epidemiology

Prevalence

The high prevalence of chronic cough and expectoration in the United Kingdom was recognized long before cigarette smoking was widely adopted, but only became a subject for medical research after the smog disasters in London in the 1950s. At that time 20 to 30 per cent of middle-aged men had chronic cough and phlegm; with the reduction in active smoking and environmental SO_2 and particulate pollution, this had dropped to about 15 to 20 per cent of middle-aged men and about 8 per cent of middle-aged women by the late 1980s.

COPD is the commonest cause of impaired spirometry in the population; by middle age about 18 per cent of male and 14 per cent of female smokers have FEV_1 values more than two standard deviations below the mean predicted values, in contrast with rates of about 7 per cent in men and women who have never smoked. These rates are probably somewhat higher than those observed in the United States.

Table 1 *Serial distribution of airways resistance*

	Normal (cmH$_2$O/l/s) (% of total)	Severe COPD (cmH$_2$O/l/s) (% of total)
Extrathoracic airway	0.5 (33)	0.5 (8)
Major intrathoracic conducting airways	0.5 (33)	1.0 (17)
Peripheral airways (< 3 mm diameter)	0.5 (33)	4.5 (75)
Total	1.5 (100)	6.0 (100)

The values are for a typical patient with severe COPD during tidal breathing via the mouth. Extrathoracic resistance would be at least 1.0 cmH$_2$O/l/s when breathing through the nose.

Table 2 *Some 'specific' causes of chronic airflow obstruction*

Cystic fibrosis
α_1-Antitrypsin deficiency
Hypogammaglobulinaemia

Obstructive bronchiolitis
    Irritant gas inhalation
    Virus infections
    Connective tissue disorders
    Following lung or bone marrow transplant
    Mineral dust inhalation

Bronchiectasis (Kartagener's syndrome)
Bronchopulmonary dysplasia
Byssinosis

Although the rates for spirometric impairment are broadly similar to those for chronic cough, as already discussed, both changes are not necessarily found in the same individual smokers.

Mortality

Since about 1970 male mortality from COPD in the United Kingdom has steadily fallen in all except men aged more than 75 years. The total mortality in women is about one-third of that in men, but there is some upward trend over the same period, presumably reflecting increased smoking by women since the Second World War. Other countries, including the United States, report increasing mortality from COPD over the same period, mainly in elderly men. Because cigarette smoking has declined more dramatically in the United States than in the United Kingdom, this is somewhat surprising; one factor may be that COPD was underdiagnosed in the United States in the period before 1970. In many countries the expansion of cigarette smoking is relatively recent and, as with lung cancer, the peak of COPD mortality probably has not been reached. Reliable international comparisons are sparse, but it appears that death rates from COPD are particularly high in the United Kingdom and Eastern Europe and low in Southern Europe, Scandinavia, and Japan.

Within the United Kingdom mortality is higher in conurbations than in rural areas, and there are considerable regional variations with the lowest rates in south-east England. In part this may reflect the importance of poor socioeconomic status in determining mortality. Although cigarette smoking is now most prevalent in persons of low socioeconomic status, the mortality trend was evident at a time when cigarette smoking was relatively independent of this factor. Indeed, downward trends in overall mortality for chronic respiratory disease in the United Kingdom cannot all be explained by improvements in air pollution or reduction in cigarette smoking, and may reflect changes in social conditions and nutrition in early life.

Natural history

Clinically significant COPD is believed to arise following many years of a moderately accelerated decline in lung function in those smokers who are particularly susceptible to the effects of cigarettes (Fig. 1). Although there is an effect of cumulative lifetime smoking history, there is a very large spread of individual rate in decline of lung function within a group of subjects with similar exposure. Much research in recent years has sought to establish the factors which determine this varying susceptibility of smokers.

On stopping smoking, chronic cough and expectoration usually cease or reduce within a few months. In younger smokers there may be a small improvement in FEV_1 and other aspects of lung function, but this is less obvious in older ex-smokers for whom the main benefit is that subsequent rates of decline in FEV_1 revert to close to the average value in healthy never-smokers. Overall FEV_1 at any given time in an individual represents the cumulative effect of the total smoking history, and it is difficult to distinguish between smokers and ex-smokers until smoking cessation has been sustained for many years.

Aetiology (Table 3)

The major risk factor in Westernized countries is cigarette smoking, but there is a wide variation in the susceptibility of individual smokers to develop progressive airflow obstruction, suggesting that other important risk factors remain to be identified. In the United States, mortality rates for COPD in cigarette smokers are at least 10 times those in never-smokers at all ages below 80 years; COPD is estimated to cause about 15 per cent of smoking-related deaths compared with 28 per cent attributed to lung cancer. Smoking promotes inflammation in the periphery of the lung; it is uncertain whether this is a direct toxic effect of tobacco smoke (e.g. oxidants) or is due to smoke recruiting neutrophils and other inflammatory cells into the airways and airspaces. α_1-Antitrypsin deficiency, a rare genetic disorder, is the strongest single risk factor. Occupational risks have been a subject of much controversy, particularly in coal miners. It has been difficult to distinguish changes due to dust exposure and to smoking. In general, many dusty occupations cause

Fig. 1 Development of impairment of FEV_1 in a susceptible smoker as proposed by Fletcher and Peto. In practice there will be a range of rates of decline in FEV_1 in susceptible smokers. On stopping smoking there is no improvement in FEV_1 but the subsequent loss of FEV_1 is similar to that in healthy never-smokers. (Reproduced with permission from Fletcher and Peto 1977.)

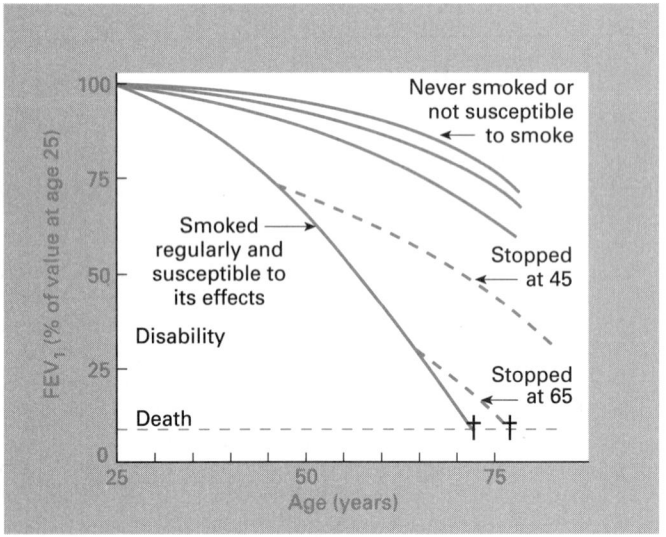

mucus hypersecretion, but few have been proven to lead to airways obstruction. In some countries domestic environmental factors may be of great importance; for instance in New Guinea household pollution due to heating and cooking within a small space is important, and COPD is more common in women than men. The established risk factors shown in Table 3 only account for a small part of the variability in the susceptibility of smokers to develop COPD. Two popular hypotheses are that repeated bronchopulmonary infections lead to permanent airways damage and hence to COPD (British hypothesis), and that the susceptible smoker has a pre-existing asthmatic constitution with airways hyper-responsiveness which accentuates the effects of smoking (Dutch hypothesis). Both are entirely reasonable; neither has been proven.

Pathophysiology

Morbid anatomy

Changes are found throughout the tracheobronchial tree and lungs. In the central conducting airways, there is enlargement of submucosal glands and an increase in surface goblet cells which also extend into more peripheral airways than in normal subjects. There is often some evidence of persistent airways inflammation even during the interval between acute airways infections, but loss of surface epithelium is less common than in asthma although ciliary function is impaired. There may be some increase in airways smooth muscle.

In the smaller bronchi and bronchioles there are inflammatory changes, increased intraluminal mucus, thickening of all elements of the airway wall (although less marked than in asthma), fibrosis, and stenosis. These changes are the major source of the increased resistance to airflow in COPD (Table 1).

Emphysema is classified by its location: confined to the centre of a lobule (centrilobular, syn. centriacinar), diffuse throughout the lobule (panlobular, syn. panacinar) or paraseptal, a variety occurring around the periphery of lobes and associated with very little disturbance to lung function. Centrilobular emphysema is surrounded by macroscopically normal lung, tends to be more obvious in the upper lobes, and is not well identified by *in vivo* imaging. Opinions vary as to whether panlobular emphysema is a more advanced stage of centrilobular emphysema, but most authorities do not believe this. There is usually evidence of active inflammation in centrilobular emphysema but this is less obvious in panlobular emphysema, although conventional teaching is that emphysema is the end result of an alveolar inflammatory process. Consequences of the emphysematous destruction of airspace walls are loss of pulmonary capillary bed and loss of attachments between alveolar and bronchiolar walls; these attachments are responsible for the normal increase in bronchiolar diameter as the lung expands, and so their loss may contribute to the airways obstruction. Overall, the relative contributions of airspace destruction and 'intrinsic' disease of the airway wall to the development of airways obstruction remains uncertain. The problem is that quantitative morphometry of airways and airspaces is extremely time consuming and should be combined with functional assessment. The consequence is that there remains an extreme diversity of views on the importance of emphysema. There are good grounds for supposing that the major effect of macroscopically visible emphysema is functionally to remove areas of the lung, because these areas receive little ventilation or blood flow. The importance of recognizing macroscopic emphysema may well be that it is associated with lesser degrees of airspace enlargement in the remaining macroscopically normal and still functioning lung.

In advanced COPD there are also changes in the heart and pulmonary circulation (thickening of the walls of pulmonary arteries (particularly vascular smooth muscle in the media), right ventricular hypertrophy) and enlargement of the carotid body. These changes are probably secondary to alveolar hypoxia and are non-specific. There is controversy

Table 3 *Risk factors for the development of chronic obstructive pulmonary disease*

Increasing age	Ventilatory impairment reflects cumulative lifetime smoking history
Smoking habit	Some relation to number of cigarettes smoked per day; risk not reduced by reduction in tar content
Gender	After standardizing for smoking, men are probably more at risk than women
Environmental pollution	Greater urban than rural death rates; historically linked to particulate rather than photochemical pollution
Socioeconomic status	More common in individuals of low socio-economic status
Diet	High fish and antioxidant intake may reduce risk in smokers
Occupation	Cadmium workers probably have increased risk of emphysema, and coal and gold miners, and cotton and grain dust workers of chronic airways obstruction; many other inorganic dusts cause mucus hypersecretion but in most cases obstruction is mild or absent
Genetic factors	Severe serum α_1-antitrypsin deficiency is the strongest single risk, but is rare
Birthweight and childhood respiratory infections	Mortality related to weight at birth and at 1 year; chest infections in early life predict adult COPD

about the effect of advanced COPD on the mass of the diaphragm, but this muscle certainly shares in the general loss of skeletal muscle mass that frequently occurs in advanced disease.

Evolution of pathophysiology

Early changes in the evolution of smoking-related COPD are the development of cough (associated with hypertrophy of mucous glands and mucus hypersecretion) and inflammatory changes in the respiratory bronchioles. These changes may develop in young adults early in their smoking history. In never-smokers spirometry shows little change in early adult life; age-related decline begins at about 30 years. In many smokers, however, some decline in FEV_1 occurs through the twenties. Early changes in lung function are due to inflammatory and occlusive changes in the peripheral airways. By middle age the FEV_1 may be significantly reduced (this is often associated with hyper-responsiveness of the airways to inhaled histamine and other agents) and the early changes of emphysema are developing, functionally revealed by reductions in lung recoil and carbon monoxide transfer coefficient. Because of the enormous total cross-sectional area of the peripheral airways, breathlessness on exertion does not develop until there is considerable pathological change and FEV_1 may be 50 per cent or less of the expected values. As the disease advances ventilation becomes uneven, reducing the efficiency of the lungs as gas exchangers and leading to falls in PaO_2 and increasing ventilatory requirements on exercise. To overcome the airway narrowing the resting end-tidal volume (functional residual capacity) increases; although this widens the airways it increases the work of the inspiratory muscles, which are less able to generate inspiratory pressures because of their shorter length at the start of inspiration. Until FEV_1 drops below about one-third of predicted values there is hypoxaemia but not hypercapnia; this is because the inefficiency of the lungs as gas exchangers for carbon dioxide is overcome by a modest increase in resting ventilation. In advanced disease, this compensation is insufficient and hypercapnia often develops; this is related to a combination of the severity of airways obstruction and impaired ability of the inspiratory muscles to generate pressure. With advanced disease, moderate rises in pulmonary artery pressure are found; the precise contributions of loss of pulmonary vascular bed, hypoxaemia, structural changes in the pulmonary vessels, and increased blood viscosity associated with a high haematocrit are uncertain.

Airways obstruction and impaired gas exchange in patients with advanced COPD result from varying combinations of obstructive changes in the peripheral conducting airways (intrinsic airways disease) and destructive changes in respiratory bronchioles, alveolar ducts, and alveoli (emphysema). Many attempts have been made to characterize different patterns of clinical presentation or pulmonary function in COPD and to relate them to the presence and severity of emphysema.

The best established contrast is between 'pink and puffing patients' (type A, 'fighters'), who are underweight with severe breathlessness, relatively normal blood gases, and without oedema, and 'blue and bloated' patients (type B, 'non-fighters') with severe hypoxaemia and hypercapnia, polycythaemia, and oedema, but without such severe breathlessness. Type A was originally thought to be associated with severe emphysema but this has not been confirmed in subsequent studies; retained ventilatory responsiveness to hypoxia is now thought to be a more important factor. There are distinct functional changes associated with emphysema which all reflect the airspace changes: an enlarged total lung capacity, a severely reduced carbon monoxide transfer coefficient, and loss of lung recoil. The enlargement in total lung capacity is responsible for the low flat position of the diaphragm on full-inflation chest radiographs.

Cellular and molecular events

Our concepts of the molecular and cellular processes involved would be far from clear except for two important observations in the early 1960s. The most critical was the identification of five subjects with a deficiency of the α_1 protein band seen on paper electrophoresis of serum. Three of these five subjects had severe emphysema (Fig. 2) at a relatively young age suggesting an association. Subsequent studies confirmed that the missing band was responsible for most of the antitryptic activity of the blood (Fig. 3). Thus the α_1 band contained a proteinase inhibitor which was called α_1-antitrypsin (also known more recently as α_1-proteinase inhibitor since it will inhibit enzymes other than trypsin).

A year later details of the first animal model of emphysema were published, demonstrating that a proteolytic enzyme (papain) could produce airspace enlargement. These two observations were clearly complementary, and it was concluded that emphysema occurred in subjects with α_1-antitrypsin deficiency because an enzyme, normally controlled by the inhibitor, was able to digest lung tissues unopposed. This concept forms the basis of the proteinase–antiproteinase theory of the pathogenesis of emphysema and other destructive lung diseases.

Over the next 10 years other animal models were developed and studies showed that only enzymes with the ability to digest elastin produce emphysematous change. Eventually a human enzyme with this ability was identified in the neutrophil (neutrophil elastase) and was also shown to produce emphysema when instilled into the lungs of experimental animals. Furthermore, α_1-antitrypsin is the most potent inhibitor of this enzyme and hence neutrophil elastase became accepted as the most likely mediator of chronic lung damage.

The enzyme is produced during neutrophil differentiation, and is packaged and stored in the azurophil granules prior to release of the cells from the bone marrow. Neutrophil elastase is a serine proteinase (serine at the active site) with a broad range of substrate specificities, many of which are important in the lung. First and foremost, it can degrade elastin; hence its ability to produce emphysema. However, it is also capable of digesting several other lung connective tissues including type IV collagen and fibronectin. Furthermore, the enzyme can damage ciliated epithelium *in vitro*, reduces the beat frequency of cilia, induces mucus gland hyperplasia *in vivo*, and is an important secretogogue for mucus glands *in vitro*. Thus neutrophil elastase may be an important mediator of the bronchial damage, reduced mucociliary clearance, and excess mucus production seen in smokers in addition to emphysema itself. Furthermore neutrophil elastase can also degrade immunoglobulins and the C3bi receptor on neutrophils that is responsible for phagocytosis and bacterial killing, and hence it can reduce the efficiency of several other lung host defences. Finally, it has also recently been shown to increase IL-8 production by bronchial epithelial cells, and since this cytokine is also a potent neutrophil chemoattractant it provides a mechanism to continue to recruit neutrophils which contain neutrophil elastase capable of stimulating even more IL-8. These factors, which are summarised in Fig. 4, can result in a sequence of events which perpetuate themselves, leading to progressive lung damage.

The proteinase–antiproteinase theory of COPD

As can be seen above, proteinases (particularly neutrophil elastase) have the potential to damage many lung proteins and tissues but to do so the enzymes need to remain functionally active. The lung and plasma contain inhibitors which can inactivate these enzymes and hence protect the lung from this effect. Thus it has become accepted that a balance must exist between the enzymes and the inhibitors which inactivate them. Inflammatory damage occurs when the enzyme activity exceeds the capacity of the inhibitors to inactivate them. Provided that the inhibitors dominate, lung damage is limited. This concept is the basis of the proteinase–antiproteinase theory of COPD.

Over the last 20 years or more there has been extensive research activity into mechanisms that disturb this balance, thereby leading to lung damage. In broad terms there are three possible ways that this may occur.

Fig. 2 Thin-layer section of whole lung of patient with emphysema related to α_1-antitrypsin deficiency. Emphysematous 'holes' are seen throughout the lung parenchyma.

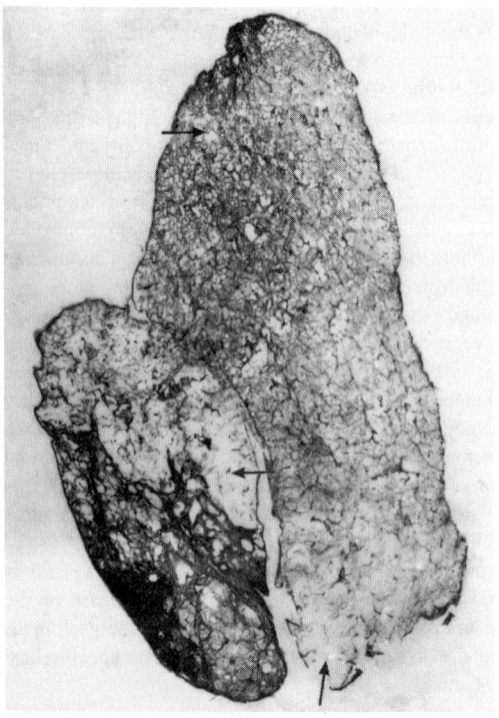

(1) decrease in protective inhibitor (as with α_1-antitrypsin deficiency);
(2) increase in enzyme load (as with excess neutrophil recruitment);
(3) a combination of (1) and (2).

DECREASED INHIBITOR

A reduction in the protective inhibitor within the lung would effectively lower the threshold for inflammatory damage by proteolytic enzymes. Most of the current research in the field of proteinases and antiproteinases has concentrated on factors that reduce the protective screen in the lung. This could be the result of either a primary or secondary defect, i.e. an absolute deficiency of the proteinase inhibitors or a relative deficiency due to inactivation of the protein present, thereby reducing its functional capacity. Evidence exists for both kinds of 'deficiency'.

α_1-ANTITRYPSIN DEFICIENCY

Most of our current concepts of the pathogenesis of COPD depend upon the association of α_1-antitrypsin deficiency with lung disease. Indeed, the early studies confirmed that both COPD (and emphysema) and bron-

Fig. 3 Paper electrophoresis of plasma from a patient with α_1-antitrypsin deficiency (upper) is shown next to that of a normal subject (lower). The antitryptic activity of fractions from each protein band is shown, confirming that most of the activity is in the α_1 band. (Reproduced with permission from Eriksson 1964.)

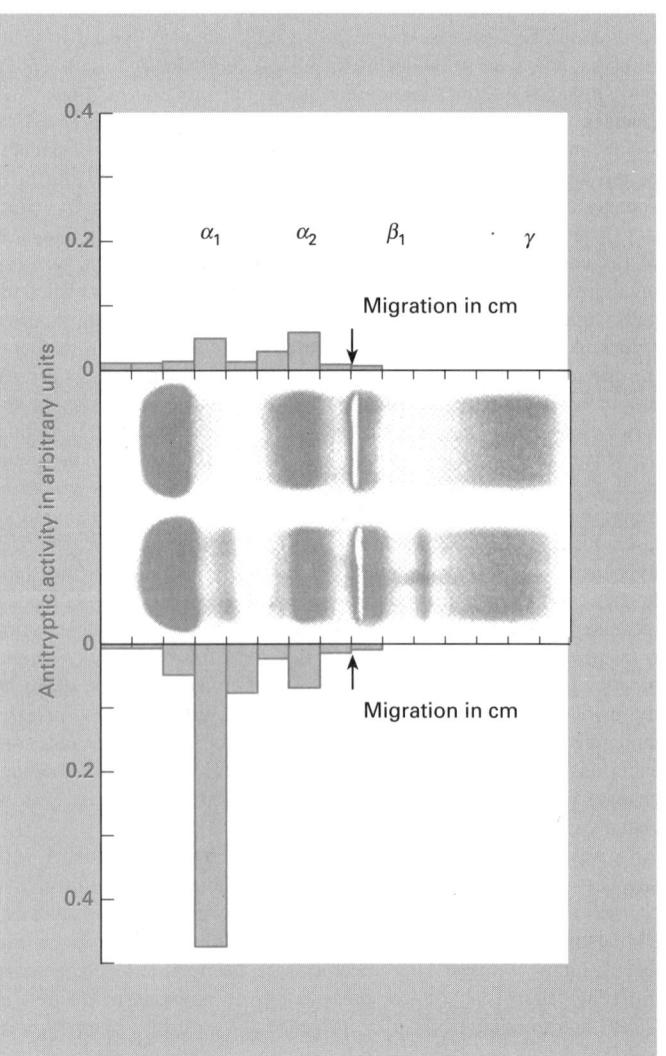

chiectasis were common associations with this protein deficiency. The emphysema itself was often described as panlobular and predominantly localized to the lung bases with an onset of symptoms below the age of 40. However, it is becoming clearer that, although such young patients may have an increased incidence of α_1-antitrypsin deficiency (up to 50 per cent in some series), the spectrum of disease and age range is wide.

Early studies confirmed that α_1-antitrypsin deficiency was inherited, and subsequent studies demonstrated that the protein showed wide electrophoretic (charge-related) polymorphism. This led to the Pi system of classification of α_1-antitrypsin, and over 70 phenotypes are now recognized. The gene is located on chromosome 14 and both alleles are expressed. The most common variant is the M allele (subdivided into M_1, M_2, M_3, etc.) which codes for about 1 g/l of the protein in plasma. About 85 per cent of the population have the phenotype MM, and the 'normal' concentration of plasma α_1-antitrypsin is about 2 g/l although a wide range exists (approximately 1.4–2.7 g/l). Furthermore, it is an acute-phase protein and its concentration may rise to 4 g/l or more.

The commonest deficiency allele associated with COPD is the Z variant. This is due to a single amino acid change at position 342 of the protein chain caused by a point mutation in the codon for glutamic acid (*GAG*) resulting in replacement by lysine (*AAG*). Recent studies have shown that this single mutation results in a change in the tertiary structure of the protein leading to polymerization of the protein in the rough endoplasmic reticulum. Thus, although the gene is transcribed normally and translated into protein, this polymerization results in secretion of only 10 to 15 per cent of the α_1-antitrypsin. The accumulation of protein in hepatocytes is seen as PAS-positive 'bodies' which are characteristic on liver biopsy.

The Z phenotype can occur with any other phenotype or even itself. The common combinations are thus MZ, SZ, or ZZ, and the α_1-antitrypsin concentrations are typically 1–1.1 g/l, 0.7 g/l, or 0.2 g/l respectively. These phenotypes can be identified clearly by their migration pattern on isoelectric focusing (Fig. 5).

Other causes of α_1-antitrypsin deficiency have now been identified by a combination of protein measurement, isoelectric focusing, and gene sequencing (Table 4). Abnormalities range from non-functional protein ($M_{mineral\ springs}$), reduced secretion (Z variant), increased catabolism (S variant), to absent product (null variants). A range of defects are outlined in the table. Many of these are rare; the commonest deficiency phenotypes in the United Kingdom are MS (6 per cent), MZ (3 per cent), SS (3 per cent), SZ (0.02 per cent), and ZZ (0.03 per cent).

Studies have suggested that there is a threshold below which α_1-antitrypsin deficiency is a significant risk factor for emphysema. There is controversy concerning whether MZ (60 per cent, normal α_1-antitrypsin) is a true risk factor, but SZ (40 per cent) seems to be and this has implications for therapy (Fig. 6).

RELATIONSHIP OF α_1-ANTITRYPSIN DEFICIENCY TO COPD

Early studies suggested that α_1-antitrypsin deficiency was associated with severe airflow obstruction and emphysema in approximately 80 per cent of cases. The life expectancy of PiZ individuals (both male and female) was reduced, particularly if they smoked, indicating an additive effect. However, many of these early studies relied upon identifying a patient with established disease and then screening family members for other cases. This may have biased the data since an effect of other familial and environmental factors could not be excluded. Indeed, one study carried out at the Johns Hopkins Hospital, Baltimore, in 1975 showed that the incidence of COPD was increased in a family related to an α_1-antitrypsin-deficient subject irrespective of the α_1-antitrypsin

Fig. 4 Diagrammatic representation of some of the pathways involved in the perpetuation of features of COPD by neutrophil elastase. Development of lung damage alters lung defences, and destruction of tissues may perpetuate neutrophil recruitment leading to further damage.

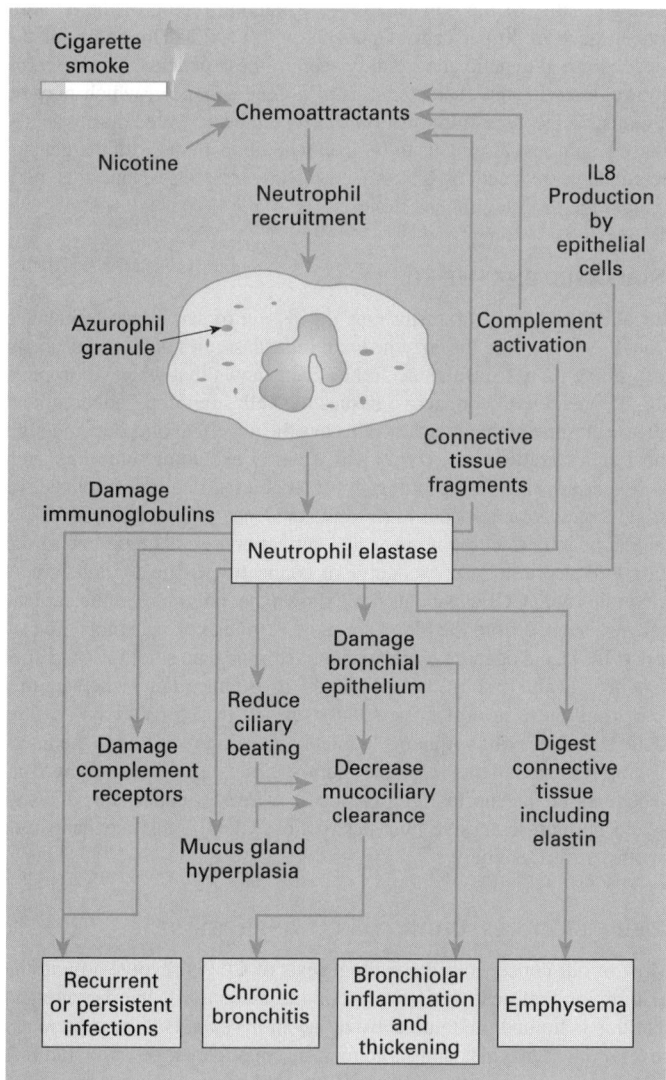

Fig. 5 Isoelectric focusing of α_1-antitrypsin from three subjects (PiM, PiMZ, and PiZ). The M and Z specific bands are indicated by arrows (+ marks the most constant bands). Gel kindly supplied by E.J. Campbell (University of Utah, USA).

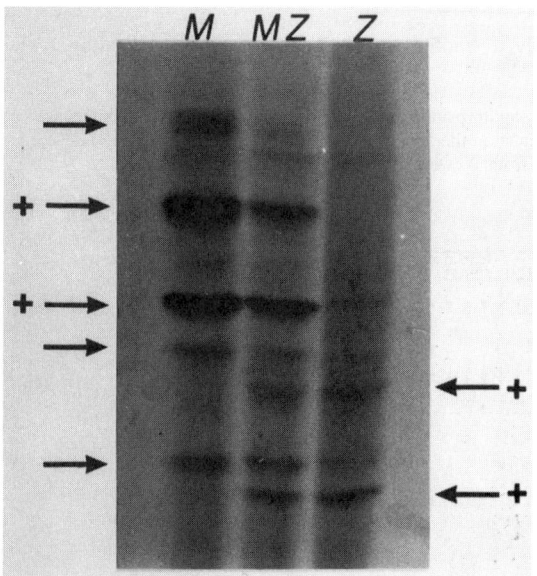

Table 4 *Summary of some of the mechanisms involved in α_1-antitrypsin deficiency*

Allele	Genetic defect	Effect on α_1-antitrypsin
Z	Point mutation Glu^{342}GAG-Lys AAG	Spontaneous polymerization and reduced secretion
S	Point mutation Glu^{264} GAA-Val GTA	Increased intracellular catabolism
NULL$_{isola\ de\ procida}$	Gene deletion Deletion of 10 kb of the gene	No transcription
NULL$_{Bellingham}$	Point mutation Lys^{217}AAG-STOP TAG	mRNA degraded; no α_1-antitrypsin is made
NULL$_{granite\ falls}$	Frameshift nucleotide deletion Tyr^{160} TAC delete C- 5' shift STOP^{160} TAG	mRNA degraded; no α_1-antitrypsin is made
NULL$_{mattawa}$	Frameshift nucleotide insertion Leu^{353} TTA-insert T- Phe^{353} TTT-3' shift-STOP^{376} TAG	No α_1-antitrypsin made
M$_{mineral\ springs}$	Point mutation Gly^{67} GGG-Glu GAG	Secretion of a non-functional protein

phenotype. More recently it has been recognized that some subjects with α_1-antitrypsin deficiency (even smokers) may live to old age with relatively preserved lung function. Furthermore, random population screening has confirmed that α_1-antitrypsin deficiency is compatible with normal health. Presumably, in these subjects the elastase burden is low or other inhibitors provide additional protection (see later).

COPD IN SUBJECTS WITH 'NORMAL' α_1-ANTITRYPSIN

It is clear that most patients develop COPD against the background of normal concentrations of α_1-Antitrypsin with the normal (PiM) phenotype. However, normal concentration does not necessarily mean normal function and there have been extensive theoretical, as well as practical, *in vitro* and *in vivo* studies of this possibility. α_1-Antitrypsin can be inactivated as an antielastase by previous complexing with enzymes, cleavage at or near the active site, and oxidation of the active-site methionine. Although all three inactive forms have been identified in the lungs of COPD patients, most studies have concentrated on the role of oxidation of the active-site methionine. This amino acid can be oxidized directly by cigarette smoke or indirectly by superoxide radicals released by lung macrophages obtained from smokers. These two observations suggest a simple mechanism whereby smoking itself can reduce lung α_1-antitrypsin function either directly or indirectly. Indeed, an early study showed that α_1-antitrypsin from the lungs of healthy smokers was partially inactive, and a supporting study showed that increased oxidized methionine residues were present. Thus it seemed logical that this biochemical inactivation would upset the α_1-antitrypsin–elastase balance, resulting in emphysema. However, this would not explain why most smokers do not develop severe airflow obstruction and emphysema, and the results showing a reduction in lung α_1-antitrypsin function in smokers compared with non-smokers have not been reproduced by other workers.

More recently, α_1-antitrypsin purified from the lungs of healthy smok-

Fig. 6 Plasma α_1-antitrypsin levels in subjects with α_1-antitrypsin deficiency receiving augmentation therapy: —— the susceptible threshold. (Reproduced with permission from Wewers *et al.* 1987.)

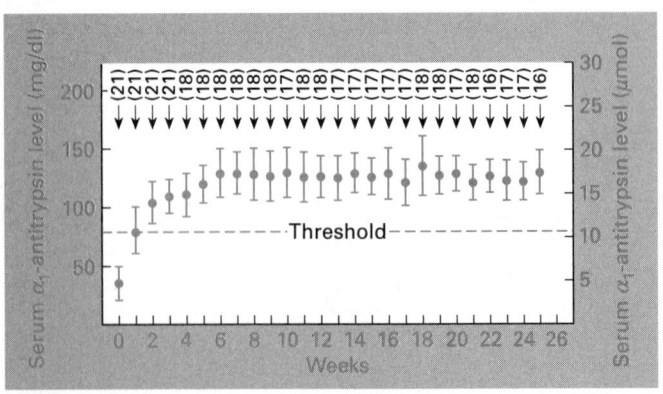

ers was shown to have a slightly reduced association rate constant for elastase. Theoretically, this should double the time required to inhibit the enzyme. The biological importance of this has yet to be determined but, again, despite this change most smokers do not develop COPD, suggesting that it may be of little importance in the pathogenesis of the disease.

A further 'functional' defect of α_1-antitrypsin that may be of importance relates to the acute-phase nature of the inhibitor. During inflammation the concentrations of α_1-antitrypsin rise and this has to be regulated. If the rise does not occur or is damped, an imbalance could occur during such episodes. Studies of the acute-phase response have not been carried out in patients with COPD. However, recent work has identified an abnormality of the downstream (3') flanking region of the α_1-antitrypsin gene in 20 per cent of patients with COPD. This is by far the most common genetic abnormality seen in these patients. The defect is in a region with the characteristics of a gene enhancer, which may be responsible for gene amplification and would be activated during acute-phase responses. It remains to be seen whether patients with the genetic defect have reduced or absent acute-phase responses, but this may explain the disease in these subjects.

INCREASED ENZYME LOAD

An alternative way of disturbing the α_1-antitrypsin–elastase balance would be to increase the enzyme load. Indeed, studies of this mechanism may prove more fruitful, since it has been shown that when neutrophils are in contact with connective tissues the cells are tightly adherent and release elastase at the interface. This has the net effect of producing high local concentrations of enzyme whilst partly excluding inhibitors such as α_1-antitrypsin. This privileged site enables a degree of connective tissue degradation to occur even in the presence of α_1-antitrypsin. Thus factors which affect the number and activation of cells recruited to the lung will also influence the degree of connective-tissue degradation.

Studies with COPD patients have shown that polymorphonuclear leucocytes isolated from the blood are more responsive to chemotactic factors (Fig. 7) and degrade more connective tissue than smoking- and age-matched healthy subjects. Although it is uncertain whether this represents cause or effect, the results suggest that, for a given chemotactic stimulus, polymorphonuclear leucocytes are recruited to the lungs of emphysema patients in greater numbers and can degrade more connective tissue than normal. If this process were continuous, the net result would be more extensive lung destruction. Clearly, this mechanism is worthy of further study.

OTHER ENZYMES, INHIBITORS, AND PROTEINS

Most of our concepts of the pathogenesis of COPD revolve around the assumption that neutrophil elastase is the mediator of the damage and that this is limited predominantly by α_1-antitrypsin. However, there are several other enzymes and inhibitors that may play a direct or indirect role. For instance, enzymes from the macrophage and bacteria have been shown to inactivate α_1-antitrypsin as an inhibitor of neutrophil elastase and may disturb the elastase–antielastase balance by this mechanism. However, there are reasons to implicate other enzymes more directly.

For example, proteinase 3, another enzyme from the neutrophil, has also been shown to produce emphysematous lesions in an animal model. This enzyme is also a serine proteinase and would be controlled *in vivo* by the same inhibitors (including α_1-antitrypsin) that control neutrophil elastase. Furthermore, a cysteine proteinase (cathepsin B) has also been shown to produce emphysema and bronchial damage when instilled into the lungs of hamsters. This enzyme is not inactivated by α_1-antitrypsin and would cause damage independently of this inhibitor, and cathepsin B activity has been identified in the lung secretions of COPD patients.

In addition, if enzymes with the ability to degrade lung elastin play a central role in the pathogenesis of emphysema, then a metalloproteinase (dependent upon metal ions for activity) with elastolytic activity (macrophage elastase) and another cysteine proteinase (cathepsin L) have been identified in the macrophage. Finally, bacteria may play a role, and a metalloelastase has been isolated from *Pseudomonas aeruginosa*. Whether these other enzymes cause emphysema is unknown at present.

Just as other enzymes are being identified with the capability of causing lung damage, so several more enzyme inhibitors are being identified in the lung. These include other inhibitors of neutrophil elastase including the serum inhibitor α_2-macroglobulin, although its size (750 kDa) largely restricts its diffusion into, and hence its role in, the lung. The secretory leucoprotease inhibitor, which is made locally in the lung, is likely to be of more importance in the control of neutrophil elastase. This inhibitor, which is made by the serous glands, is the dominant neutrophil elastase inhibitor in the bronchi. However, it is also present in Clara cells in the peripheral airways and has been identified in association with lung elastin. Indeed, this inhibitor is far more effective than α_1-antitrypsin in inhibiting neutrophil elastase that has become attached to elastin. Thus, in most patients, its role may turn out to be more critical

than that of α_1-antitrypsin in the protection of lung elastin. Finally, an inhibitor of metalloproteinases (TIMP) is made by macrophages and has also been identified in lung secretions, as have cystatins which inhibit cysteine proteinases. These inhibitors will play a role in limiting lung damage by their respective enzyme classes. At present the role of these and other enzymes and their inhibitors has received little attention in the study of the pathogenesis of COPD.

Although there is uncertainty concerning which enzymes and inhibitors determine the pathogenesis of COPD, it is clear that emphysema is related mainly to the destruction of lung elastin. However, this connective tissue is also regulated with some degradation and remodelling (albeit slowly) in health. Indeed, even in elastase-induced emphysema in animal models the initial loss of elastin leads to regeneration as the pathological changes evolve. Furthermore, prevention of normal elastin fibre cross-linking during this regeneration phase worsens the pathological changes. Thus it seems likely that disorders of elastin itself may play a role in the development of emphysema in some subjects. Indeed, emphysema is a recognized feature of cutis laxa where defects of the expression of the elastin gene have been identified. Further studies will clarify the role of elastin defects in other patients with emphysema.

FUTURE MANAGEMENT

These extensive biochemical, cellular, and genetic studies have clarified the general mechanisms involved in the pathogenesis of COPD. They also lay the foundation for new approaches to the prevention and treatment of COPD. Identification of α_1-antitrypsin deficiency in patients and relatives should lead to added efforts to avoid or stop smoking. Preliminary studies of the replacement of α_1-antitrypsin in deficient individuals are in progress.

Clinical features

Symptoms

Patients may present either with chronic productive cough and recurrent bronchial infections, or with insidious breathlessness on exercise, or a combination of the two types of symptoms.

The tendency to bronchial infections is associated with impaired mucociliary clearance and chronic bacterial colonization of the normally sterile tracheobronchial tree. Diagnosis of chronic bronchitis requires a normal chest radiograph which effectively excludes tuberculosis, bronchiectasis, neoplasms, and many other lung diseases which cause cough. Other possibilities such as postnasal drip, aspiration, asthma, and immune deficiency may have to be excluded by appropriate investigations. Although lung function deteriorates during acute infections and takes several weeks to recover, there is no evidence that the progression of airways obstruction is related to the occurrence of recurrent infections in otherwise healthy smokers.

Airways obstruction leads to breathlessness on exertion and the insidious development of a reduced exercise capacity. A temporary exacerbation due to infection often triggers seeking medical advice. Some patients first present at a very advanced stage and give a short history, but prospective population studies have failed to identify subjects who show rapid and catastrophic falls in FEV_1.

Examination

There are no abnormalities on clinical examination in the earlier stages; diagnosis then depends on spirometry. With progression of the disease signs of hyperinflation (barrel-shaped chest, low position of the laryngeal prominence, loss of cardiac dullness, and lowering of hepatic dullness) develop and there may be increased frequency of breathing, use of accessory muscles, loss of the normal outward movement of the abdomen during inspiration, and wheeze, particularly in the second half of

Fig. 7 Diagram of the steps involved in differentiation and recruitment of neutrophils to the lung. Intervention therapy is possible at the stages indicated in the boxes and may lead to a reduction in lung destruction. In general, this could involve modification of the destructive potential of the cell or specific blocking of individual steps necessary for the migration of the cell into the lung and its release of proteinases.

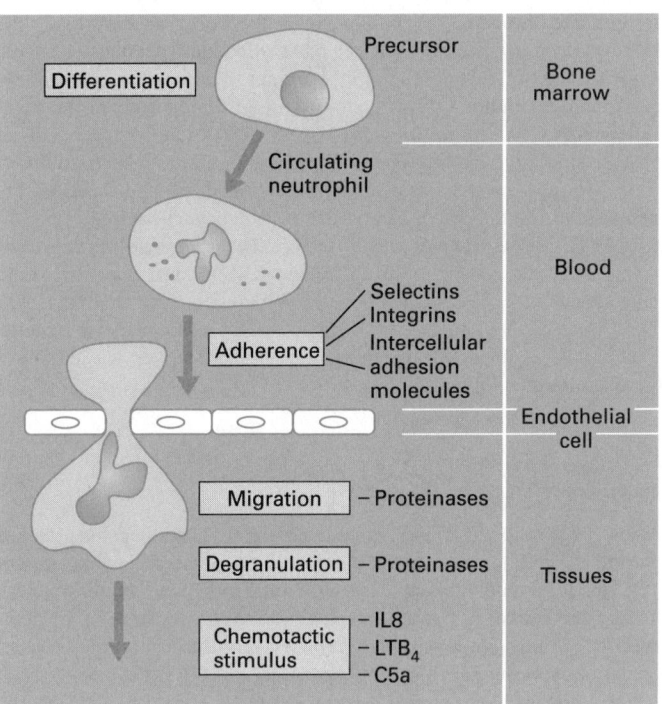

expiration. At the most advanced stage there is often pursed lip breathing, cyanosis (detected reliably only when oxygen saturation is below 85 per cent), and indrawing of the lateral rib cage (Hoover's sign) on inspiration. Clubbing is not a feature. Ankle oedema may develop, often without any detectable abnormality of the heart or pulmonary circulation. A few patients develop gross cardiac enlargement, gallop rhythm, signs of tricuspid incompetence, raised jugular venous pressure, and hepatic engorgement. Signs of advancing respiratory failure (apart from cyanosis) are restlessness and confusion, a coarse tremor, and warm peripheries. In hypercapnic ventilatory failure, papilloedema occasionally develops if diagnosis and treatment are grossly delayed.

Investigations

Thoracic imaging

The chest radiograph is a relatively insensitive indicator of COPD; it is possible to die from COPD with a normal chest radiograph. The most striking changes are those due to enlargement of total lung capacity, which is found with emphysema but not usually when obstruction is due to intrinsic airway disease. The domes of the diaphragm are then low with loss of the normal curvature (often seen best on the lateral radiograph); with severe hyperinflation the insertions of the diaphragm into the ribs may be revealed due to loss of the normal area of apposition between diaphragm and rib cage at total lung capacity. A further sign of hyperinflation is an increased retrosternal airspace. Generalized emphysema is often difficult to diagnose with confidence; local differences in transradiancy and paucity of medium-size vascular markings, such as the characteristic bilateral basal transradiancy of α_1-antitrypsin deficiency, are more obvious. Bullae and panlobular emphysema are

Fig. 8 CT of the thorax showing emphysematous destruction of the lung.

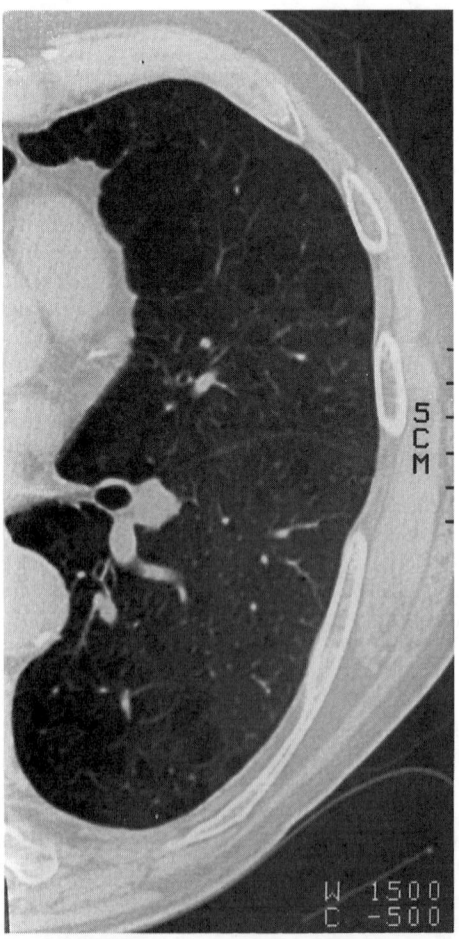

detected more easily than centrilobular emphysema. Signs of airway disease are few; airway wall thickening is not obvious, but a few patients with recurrent infections with COPD may have bronchiectatic changes.

Secondary effects on the circulation may develop with advanced disease, resulting in upper-zone prominence of medium-size pulmonary vessels, enlargement of the main branches of the pulmonary arteries (a standard measurement is right main descending artery more than 16 mm in diameter), and eventual enlargement of the heart.

Computerized tomography (Fig. 8) has significantly improved the ability to diagnose generalized emphysema and bullae compared with conventional chest radiographs.

Scans of regional ventilation and perfusion become patchily abnormal with the development of relatively mild airways obstruction. The coarse moth-eaten defects seen are usually 'matched', affecting ventilation and blood flow similarly, but inevitably make it more difficult to detect additional vascular defects due to pulmonary embolism.

Heart

Electrocardiographic signs of right heart disease are usually modest, probably in part because they are masked by hyperinflated lung. Right-bundle branch block and P pulmonale in leads 2, 3, and aVf are common but do not bear a close relation to pulmonary artery and right-ventricular pressures. Evidence of right-ventricular hypertrophy is uncommon. Atrial fibrillation is the commonest arrhythmia. Echocardiographic assessment is also impeded by the hyperinflation, but some indirect estimate of pulmonary artery pressure and of the ejection fraction of the right ventricle can be achieved.

Blood examination

The major change is a raised haematocrit (secondary polycythaemia) in hypoxaemic patients. Smokers have about a 25 per cent rise in all elements of the white blood cell count; a rise in the percentage of eosinophils suggests an asthmatic component. Biochemical tests show a raised venous bicarbonate level in patients with established hypercapnia.

Sputum examination

Many physicians believe that sputum culture is redundant unless the patient fails to respond to a course of antibiotics. Three main bacteria are cultured: *Haemophilus influenzae, Streptococcus pneumoniae*, and *Moraxella catarrhalis*. At present most infections respond to a wide range of antibiotics, but ampicillin-resistant *H. influenzae* is becoming increasingly common (15 per cent or more in some areas). So far, penicillin-resistant *Strep. pneumoniae* is very rare (less than 1 per cent) in many countries, including the United Kingdom, but isolated multiple-antibiotic-resistant organisms have been found in New Guinea, the Republic of South Africa, and Spain. After repeated courses of antibiotics *Pseudomonas* species may be predominant. *Staphylococcus aureus* is important during epidemics of influenza. The commonest organism causing a lobar pneumonia is *Strep. pneumoniae*, but smokers with COPD are at increased risk of *Legionella pneumophila* infections. Tuberculosis is relatively common in the elderly smoker, particularly if there is also alcohol abuse.

Respiratory function tests

SPIROMETRY

A low FEV_1 and FEV_1/VC ratio are essential to the diagnosis; values of both depend on age, gender, and height. If the result is not clear cut (e.g. low FEV_1 and vital capacity (VC) without reduction in FEV_1/VC), finding convexity to the volume axis of the expiratory limb of the maximum expiratory flow–volume curve is useful because this change occurs early in the development of obstruction (Fig. 9).

The response to an inhaled β-adrenoceptor agonist and/or muscarinic antagonist should also be measured; a large increase immediately raises the prospect of a reversible ('asthmatic') component. Absence of an immediate bronchodilator response, while disappointing, should not prevent a full trial of corticosteroid treatment (see below).

Once the diagnosis is established, peak expiratory flow can be used to monitor progress and to assess diurnal variation, which is relatively small in typical COPD, but because peak expiratory flow is better preserved than FEV_1 in COPD, an initial assessment with full spirometric tests is essential.

Other tests of airways function, such as airways resistance measured by body plethysmography and tests of the inequality of airways narrowing (single breath N_2 test), are useful adjuncts but not central to diagnosis.

CARBON MONOXIDE TRANSFER COEFFICIENT

Reduction in this simple test, particularly when expressed per litre of lung volume (carbon monoxide transfer coefficient), gives an indication of the extent of generalized emphysema. A normal or even increased transfer coefficient is found in asthma; therefore finding a high or normal value in a patient with chronic airways obstruction should encourage persistence with antiasthma treatment.

STATIC LUNG VOLUMES

In COPD the reduction in VC indicates that the residual volume (volume at the end of a full expiration) is increased. An increase in total lung capacity (TLC) indicates probable emphysema. However, the most important static lung volume is the volume at the end of a tidal expiration (functional residual capacity (FRC). In healthy subjects, FRC is about 0.5 TLC, rising slightly above this ratio beyond middle age. In severe COPD the FRC/TLC ratio may be 0.7 or 0.8; as a result during tidal breathing the inspiratory muscles have to generate inspiratory pressure from a shortened length at which their pressure-generating capacity is reduced.

RESPIRATORY MUSCLE STRENGTH

The maximum inspiratory pressure developed at FRC is reduced in severe COPD. The major factor is probably the muscle shortening due to the increased FRC. Indeed, some studies indicate that, allowing for hyperinflation, patients with COPD can generate slightly greater inspiratory pressures than normal subjects at equivalent lung volumes, suggesting the development of some compensatory mechanisms in the mus-

cles. In advanced COPD there is often loss of weight and muscle bulk; the diaphragm and other respiratory muscles share in this loss of mass, and this is a further factor reducing the pressures generated on both maximum inspiratory and maximum expiratory efforts.

BLOOD GASES

Resting PaO_2 falls as airways obstruction increases. Oximetry has made it easy to monitor oxygen saturation during outpatient visits and to assess the need for long-term oxygen at home. Hypercapnia can be suspected from elevation of venous blood bicarbonate. $PaCO_2$ is usually normal until FEV_1 is reduced below 1.2 litres. The chronicity of any elevated $PaCO_2$ can be judged from the pH, which tends to remain at about 7.40 in the steady state, particularly when the patient is on diuretics.

EXERCISE CAPACITY

Simple walking tests, such as the distance covered in 6 or 12 min, provide a useful summary of the patient's disability and can be supplemented by monitoring oxygen saturation with oximetry.

Management of chronic stable disease

Disability and prognosis in COPD are dominated by the severity of airways obstruction. While symptoms can be ameliorated by a large variety of treatments, radically improved prognosis is unlikely unless obstruction can be relieved or at least future decline aborted. Generally available options are to stop smoking and to be certain that the reversible component of airways obstruction is adequately recognized and treated.

Stopping smoking

In young smokers with minor airways obstruction there may be an improvement in FEV_1 on stopping smoking, but in middle age the major effect is to slow subsequent decline in FEV_1, nearly to that of healthy never-smokers. In advanced COPD it is less certain that further decline in FEV_1 is slowed, so that there is a strong case for early intervention. Stopping smoking consistently results in a reduction in cough, expectoration, and acute respiratory infections, but patients should not expect improvement in breathlessness. Low tar cigarettes are associated with less cough but any slowing of decline in FEV_1 is slight. The benefits of stopping smoking on the subsequent development of cardiovascular dis-

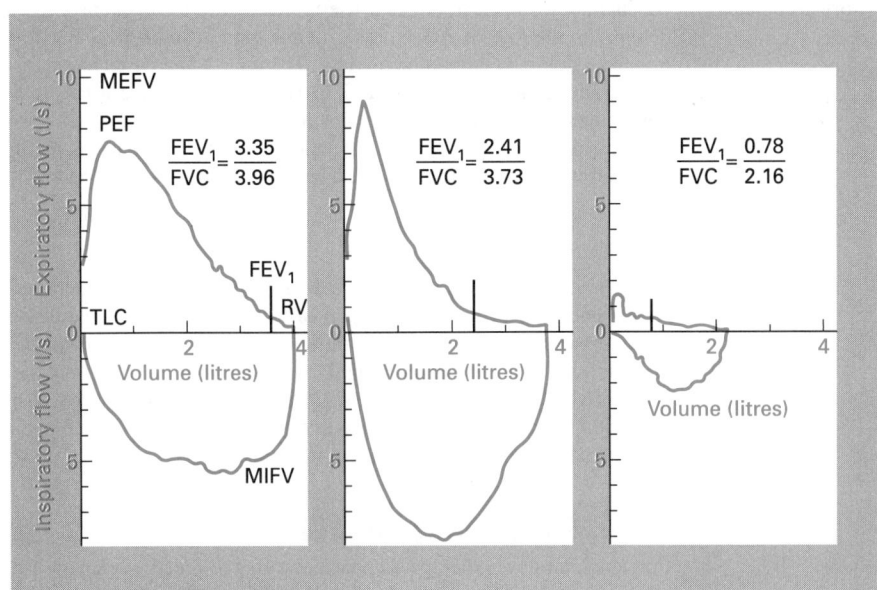

Fig. 9 Maximum expiratory and inspiratory flow–volume (MEFV and MIFV) curves in a normal subject (left), a smoker with mild intrathoracic airways obstruction (centre), and a patient with severe airways obstruction (right): PEF, peak expiratory flow; RV, residual volume; FVC, forced vital capacity; TLC, total lung capacity. With developing airways obstruction the earliest distinctive change is development of convexity of the flow signal to the volume axis (centre); in this subject peak expiratory flow and the MIFV curve were normal. In severe obstruction there are gross reductions on both the flow and volume axes.

ease and lung cancer apply equally to patients with COPD as to the rest of the population.

Response to bronchodilator and corticosteroid treatment

Virtually all patients with chronic airways obstruction show some immediate response to treatment with β-adrenergic agonists, muscarinic antagonists, and theophylline, but these improvements are usually small. If the response is large, the possibility of further improvement with corticosteroids is evident. The patient at risk of undertreatment is the heavy smoker with a small immediate bronchodilator response, particularly if there is evidence of emphysema. Conventional management is to make a 2 to 3 week trial of 30 to 40 mg of prednisolone daily, monitoring peak expiratory flow daily and spirometry at least at the beginning and end of a trial. In the great majority of 'responders', improvement can be sustained subsequently by inhaled corticosteroids. If there is a large improvement in airways obstruction, the prognosis should be dramatically improved.

A more difficult question is whether long-term treatment is beneficial even when immediate effects are negligible. Several large-scale trials of inhaled corticosteroids are currently in progress to see if these can attenuate the progression of airways obstruction in subjects with mild to moderate COPD. Five years of treatment with an inhaled muscarinic antagonist failed to attenuate decline in FEV_1 in a large North American Study. Trials of continuous versus on-demand treatment with β-agonists are also being made to exclude the possibility of deleterious effects of continuous treatment. In the meantime it seems reasonable to decide the usage of all these drugs on the basis of short-term benefit.

In contrast with asthma, where β-agonists are clearly superior to muscarinic antagonists as bronchodilators, muscarinic antagonists are overall as effective as β-agonists in COPD. A combination of two or three types of bronchodilators is commonly used, but addition of effects is uncertain. Patients with severe COPD often claim more sustained relief from use of β-agonists and muscarinic antagonists via home nebulizers instead of conventional metered dose inhalers. Whether this is because of the increased dosage (there can be a 10-fold difference between the doses given by conventional inhalers and by nebulizers), the sequential inhalation, the more impressive mode of treatment, or the mimicry of crisis management in accident and emergency departments is uncertain, but several studies have suggested reduced hospital admissions in disabled patients.

Apart from relaxation of airways smooth muscle, β-agonists may have some anti-inflammatory effects, aid ciliary clearance, and increase mucus secretion; they are pulmonary vasodilators and modulate cholinergic neurotransmission. Theophyllines also have anti-inflammatory actions, increase ciliary clearance, and are mild ventilatory stimulants and diuretics; their ability to improve respiratory muscle performance is disputed.

Other drugs

Mucolytic drugs have been shown to reduce slightly the number and length of bronchopulmonary infections. Trials of long-term antibiotics in the 1960s, admittedly with small doses and less effective drugs than now available, failed to attenuate decline in FEV_1. Trials of $α_1$-antitrypsin replacement, either intravenously or by inhalation, are under way for patients with severe deficiency. Oral ventilatory stimulants (such as medroxyprogesterone, carbonic anhydrase inhibitors, or almitrine) can improve PaO_2 and $PaCO_2$ by 0.5–1.0 kPa but are not widely used.

Sedative drugs should almost always be avoided, although they may have a place under carefully monitored conditions in a few patients with distressing dyspnoea. β-Blocker drugs, even when relatively cardioselective or given as eye drops, can worsen airways obstruction.

Immunization

Immunization against influenza and pneumococcal infection seems sensible, although the protective effect in patients with COPD may be less than in the general population.

Long-term oxygen treatment

When oxygen is administered for more than 15 of each 24 h to hypoxaemic patients with advanced disease, survival is enhanced and hospital admissions are reduced. The precise reasons are unclear; the treatment was introduced in the expectation that it would reduce pulmonary hypertension but this is not achieved consistently. Present United Kingdom guidelines recommend long-term home oxygen when PaO_2 is less than 7.3 kPa (55 mmHg) in the chronic stable state, but it is arguable that earlier intervention could be useful. Only a small proportion of potential subjects in the United Kingdom receive this treatment. Spirometry is unchanged and exercise capacity remains very limited during long-term oxygen treatment, but there is no evidence that it damages the lungs or precipitates hypercapnic ventilatory failure. Portable oxygen therapy has a place in improving exercise tolerance—for instance allowing a patient to walk the distance between home and car—but logistic difficulties limit its use. Intermittent use of home oxygen in patients not on long-term oxygen is commonly used for relief of short breathless episodes.

Venesection

An increase in haematocrit is a useful adaptation to maintain oxygen delivery in the face of arterial hypoxaemia (and in smokers occupation of haemoglobin by carbon monoxide). The price is increased blood viscosity, and a haematocrit above 0.55 is believed to have a net unfavourable effect. Small improvements in symptoms have followed venesection or erythropheresis, but most patients with such high haematocrits are severely hypoxaemic and should be on long-term oxygen treatment.

Nutrition

Many patients with advanced COPD lose weight. There is an increased resting energy expenditure, only part of which can be attributed to the increased work of the respiratory muscles. Skeletal and diaphragmatic mass and strength are related to body weight, so that cachexia reduces the ability of the muscles to deal with the requirements of exercise. In contrast with these trends, a subgroup of patients with COPD are overweight and may develop obstructive sleep apnoea.

Physical therapy and rehabilitation

Conventional physiotherapy emphasizes trying to breathe at a slow frequency and with a large tidal volume, but patients with advanced COPD

Fig. 10 Relation between mean daytime and mean nocturnal oxygen saturation SaO_2 in 99 patients with severe COPD: ○ Oxford patients; ● Edinburgh patients. (Reproduced with permission from Connaughton et al. 1988.)

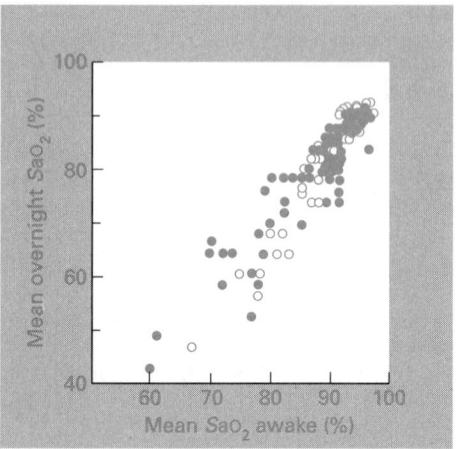

often cannot breathe with a normal tidal volume because of expiratory flow limitation. Assistance for the respiratory muscles can be obtained by leaning forward and leaning on the elbows to allow use of the pectoral and shoulder girdle muscles. Training programmes may aim to increase general exercise performance or specifically increase the strength and endurance of the respiratory muscles by regular periods of breathing through a resistance at the mouth. Undoubtedly, some patients benefit considerably, particularly those who are depressed and feel that their problems are neglected and intractable. Recently there have been attempts to provide non-invasive ventilatory support either at night or during the day with nasal positive pressure ventilation or pressure support with nasal continuous positive airways pressure; the precise benefit and selection of patients is not yet established.

Surgical treatment

Some patients with large bullae can be improved by surgical obliteration. Lung transplantation, usually of a single lung, can provide dramatic relief of symptoms and improvement in lung function for patients with advanced COPD; shortage of donor organs effectively confines this option to a few patients who develop advanced disease at a relatively young age, often with bullous emphysema or α_1-antitrypsin deficiency.

Acute increases in breathlessness

It is not always easy to diagnose the cause of an acute increase in breathlessness in patients with more severe COPD, and often they are treated with a combination of increased bronchodilators (and possibly corticosteroids), antibiotics, and diuretics.

Acute respiratory infection

This is the most commonly diagnosed cause if there is an exacerbation associated with some evidence of infection (raised temperature, infected sputum, abnormal chest radiograph, and raised C-reactive protein) and wheeziness. Treatment with bronchodilators and antibiotics is obviously appropriate, but the use of systemic corticosteroids is more controversial, particularly in a patient known to have had an earlier negative elective trial of prednisolone or other tablet corticosteroids. Some evidence suggests that initial improvement in airways function over the first few days is faster in patients given a course of corticosteroids, but the effect is small. Whereas in the stable outpatient state inhaled muscarinic antagonists (ipratropium, oxitropium) are as good as (and some would maintain better than) β-agonists as bronchodilators, in acute exacerbations there is no evidence that muscarinic antagonists can add to the bronchodilatation produced by β-adrenergic agonists alone.

Pneumothorax

COPD is the commonest cause of spontaneous pneumothorax in older patients. Detection by clinical examination may be difficult in the presence of hyperinflated lungs and because the degree of lung collapse is often modest. The threshold for inserting an intrapleural drain is lower than normal in patients with COPD, both because of the greater significance of a small further loss in function when baseline function is compromised and because the lung does not readily collapse, so that the increase in pleural pressure cannot be estimated from the degree of collapse. Sustained re-expansion is often slow, requiring prolonged pleural intubation and the hazards of relative immobilization in elderly subjects.

Pulmonary embolism

This is also more difficult to detect in patients with COPD, but is common at autopsy. The usual presentation is with an unexplained increase in breathlessness. The most useful investigations are ventilation and perfusion scans; the common abnormality in stable COPD is matched ventilation and perfusion defects. Perfusion defects in areas that are still ventilated are more likely to be due to pulmonary embolism than to emphysema. Relative immobility, development of leg oedema, and high haematocrit all predispose to venous thrombosis in advanced COPD, but no studies provide useful guidance on whether anticoagulants should be routinely used long term in such patients in sinus rhythm.

Left ventricular failure

This is also common in COPD and is particularly dangerous because the ability of such patients to survive with low arterial P_{O_2} depends on maintaining at least a normal and preferably a high normal cardiac output. The coincidence of two common conditions may simply reflect that smoking is a major risk factor for both ischaemic heart disease and COPD, but other suggestions have been that left ventricular function may be compromised by arterial hypoxaemia or hypertrophy of the interventricular septum.

Other complications

Oedema and right heart failure

The mechanism of oedema formation in COPD is controversial; while it is associated with severe airways obstruction and often a raised Pa_{CO_2}, it can occur with only modest rises in pulmonary artery pressure and without conventional evidence of heart failure. It responds to treatment with diuretics alone. Some patients with severe COPD do develop more severe pulmonary hypertension, right ventricular dysfunction, and tricuspid incompetence (cor pulmonale). Increasing inspired oxygen is important in treating resistant oedema; most physicians reserve digoxin for patients with atrial fibrillation or flutter because of the risks of toxicity in patients with chronic hypoxaemia. Calcium-channel blockers and angiotensin-converting enzyme inhibitors may reduce pulmonary artery pressures but can worsen pulmonary gas exchange or have undesired effects on the systemic circulation.

Acute ventilatory failure

The management of this complication is discussed in Chapter 17.14.3(a).

Sleep-related hypoxaemia

Patients with COPD show greater than normal falls in oxygen saturation at night and there is a close association between daytime Sa_{O_2} and mean Sa_{O_2} at night (Fig. 10). Because Pa_{O_2} during wakefulness is reduced and close to the steep part of the dissociation curve, the usual small fall in ventilation during sleep leads to a much greater fall in oxygen saturation. Obstructive sleep apnoea may coexist, but is probably related to obesity and alcohol usage (see Chapter 17.14.2).

Special categories of COPD

Bullous emphysema

Bullae (thin-walled intrapulmonary airspaces more than 1 cm in diameter) may occur as isolated lesions in otherwise normal lungs or in lungs where there is accompanying airways obstruction and generalized emphysema.

In the former case there are often no symptoms and the diagnosis may be fortuitous on a routine chest radiograph; alternatively, presentation may be with a spontaneous pneumothorax. The aetiology is obscure; bullae may be found in early middle age when common forms of generalized emphysema are unusual. If there are large bullae occupying a third or more of a hemithorax, surgical obliteration improves lung function. However, the necessity for and timing of any surgical intervention is often difficult to assess in patients with no or few symptoms.

When bullae are associated with more severe airways obstruction the problem is to decide whether their presence is playing a significant part in a patient's breathlessness. This requires detailed anatomical and physiological assessment. Anatomical assessment is made by CT of the thorax. Functional assessment is more difficult. Uncommon patients who have significant ventilation of a bulla can be detected by scans of regional ventilation. In the remaining patients bullae act solely as space-occupying lesions and the problem is to assess the degree of interference by bulla(e) with the surrounding lung and the ability of the surrounding lung to expand into the space provided in the hemithorax following surgical obliteration. If bullae are not ventilated, tests of overall lung function indicate the function of non-bullous lung. There is no doubt that some patients with generalized airways obstruction can be helped by obliterative surgery, at least if bullae occupying one-third or more of a hemithorax can be obliterated. The consensus is that the chance of useful sustained postoperative improvement in symptoms, spirometry, and Pao_2 is less when there is evidence of generalized emphysema (as judged by CT or functional criteria such as low carbon monoxide transfer factor or loss of lung recoil). Nevertheless, bullectomy in patients with accompanying airways obstruction can lead to a useful improvement in disability which may last for some years and is a worthwhile palliation of a distressing condition; an alternative in younger patients is single-lung transplantation.

Bronchopulmonary dysplasia

This has become an important cause of chronic airways obstruction in childhood. It follows premature delivery and ventilation for respiratory distress of the newborn and may be associated with lack of full lung development during growth. Although the airways obstruction and impairment of lung function is usually mild, children with bronchopulmonary dysplasia tend to have enhanced airways responsiveness to non-specific stimuli and may prove to be at particular risk of smoking-related damage in adult life.

Unilateral transradiancy of the lung (Swyer–James or Macleod's syndrome)

This is an uncommon condition in which there is unilateral airways obstruction, hyperinflation, and small central and medium-size pulmonary arteries. Because the contralateral lung is normal there may be few symptoms and the diagnosis may be made when a chest radiograph is taken for other reasons. The pathogenesis is believed to be a severe unilateral bronchiolitis (not always recognized at the time) followed by impaired lung growth. The diagnosis can be suspected from physical signs and the standard chest radiograph and is confirmed by obtaining expiratory radiographs (the affected lung shows only a small decrease in volume and so may cause mediastinal shift), scans of regional ventilation and perfusion, and a characteristic 'two-compartment' maximum expiratory flow–volume curve. No treatment is required, but contraindications to smoking are amplified by the lower reserves of lung function. Occasionally the condition can be mimicked by asymmetrical development of emphysema or by compensatory overexpansion of the remaining lobes when there is complete collapse of a lobe.

REFERENCES

Afford, S.C., Burnett, D., Campbell, E.J., Cury, J.D., and Stockley, R.A. (1988). The assessment of a₁-proteinase inhibitor form and function in lung lavage fluid from healthy subjects. *Hoppe-Seyler's Zeitschrift für Biologische Chemische*, **369**, 1065–74.

Anthonisen, N.R., Connett, J.E., Kiley, J.P. *et al.* (1994). Effects of smoking intervention and the use of an inhaled anticholinergic bronchodilator on the rate of decline of FEV_1. The Lung Health Study. *Journal of the American Medical Association*, **272**, 1497–1505.

Barker, D.J.P., Godfrey, K.M., Fall, C., Osmond, C., Winter, P.D., and Shaheen, S.O. (1991). Relation of birth weight and childhood respiratory infection to adult lung function and death from chronic obstructive lung disease. *British Medical Journal* **303**, 671–5.

Becklake, M.R. (1989). Occupational exposures: evidence for a causal association with chronic obstructive pulmonary disease *American Review of Respiratory Disease*, **140**, S85–91.

Begin, P. and Grassino, A. (1991). Inspiratory muscle dysfunction and chronic hypercapnia in chronic obstructive pulmonary disease. *American Review of Respiratory Disease*, **143**, 905–12.

Belman, M.J. (1993). Exercise in patients with chronic obstructive pulmonary disease. *Thorax*, **48**, 936–46.

Boudier, C., Pelletier, A., Pauli, G., and Bieth, J.G. (1983). The functional activity of alpha₁-proteinase inhibitor in bronchoalveolar lavage fluids from healthy human smokers and non smokers. *Clinica Chimica Acta* **132**, 309–15.

Burrows, B. (1990). Airways obstructive diseases: pathogenetic mechanisms and natural histories of the disorders. *Medical Clinics of North America*, **74**, 547–59.

Burrows, B. (1991). Predictors of loss of lung function and mortality in obstructive lung diseases *European Respiratory Review*, **1**, 340–5.

Burrows, B., Bloom, J.W., Traver, G.A., and Cline, M.G. (1987). The course and prognosis of different forms of chronic airways obstruction in a sample from the general population. *New England Journal of Medicine*, **317**, 1309–14.

Calverley, P.M.A. and Pride, N.B. (eds.). (1995). *Chronic obstructive pulmonary disease*. Chapman and Hall, London.

Campbell, E.J., Senior, R.M., McDonald, J.A., and Cox, D.W. (1982). Proteolysis by neutrophils. Relative importance of cell-substrate contact and oxidative inactivation of proteinase inhibitors *in vitro*. *Journal of Clinical Investigation*, **70**, 845–52.

Carp, H., Miller, F., Hoidal, J.R., and Janoff, A. (1982). Potential mechanisms of emphysema: α₁-proteinase inhibitor recovered from lungs of cigarette smokers contains oxidised methionine and has decreased elastase inhibitory capacity. *Proceedings of the National Academy of Sciences of the United States of America*, **79**, 2041–5.

Cherniack, N.S. (ed) (1991). *Chronic obstructive pulmonary disease*. W.B. Saunders, Philadelphia, PA.

Cohen, B.H., Ball, W.C., Bias, W.B., *et al.* (1975). A genetic-epidemiologic study of chronic obstructive pulmonary disease. *Johns Hopkins Medical Journal*, **137**, 95–104.

Connaughton, J.J., Catterall, J.R., Elton, R.A. Stradling, J.R. and Douglas, N.J. (1988). Do sleep studies contribute to the management of patients with severe chronic obstructive pulmonary disease? *American Review of Respiratory Disease*, **138**, 341–4.

Crystal, R.G. (1989). The α₁-antitrypsin gene and its deficiency states. *Trends in Genetics*, **5**, 411–7.

Douglas, N.J. and Flenley, D.C. (1990). Breathing during sleep in patients with obstructive lung disease. *American Review of Respiratory Disease*, **141**, 1055–70.

Eriksson, S. (1964). Pulmonary emphysema and alpha₁-antitrypsin deficiency. *Acta Medica Scandinavica*, **175**, 197–205.

Eriksson, S. (1965). Studies in alpha₁-antitrypsin deficiency. *Acta Medica Scandinavica*, **177**, (Suppl. 432), 197–205.

Fletcher, C. and Peto, R. (1977). The natural history of chronic airflow obstruction. *British Medical Journal*, **i**, 1645–8.

Fletcher, C.M. and Pride, N.B. (1984). Definitions of emphysema, chronic bronchitis, asthma and airflow obstruction: 25 years on from the CIBA Symposium. *Thorax*, **39**, 81–5.

Gadek, J., Fells, G.A., and Crystal, R.G. (1979). Cigarette smoking induces functional antiprotease deficiency in the lower respiratory tract of humans. *Science*, **206**, 1315–16.

Gould, G.A., MacNee, W., McLean, A., Warren, P.M., Redpath, A., Best, J.J.K., *et al.* (1988). CT measurements of lung density in life can quantitate distal airspace enlargement—an essential defining feature of human emphysema. *American Review of Respiratory Disease*, **137**, 380–92.

Gross, P., Pfitzer, E.A., Tolker, E., Babyok, M.A., and Kaschak, M. (1964). Experimental emphysema. Its production with papain in normal and silicotic rats. *Archives of Environmental Health*, **11**, 50–8.

Hogg, J.C., Macklem, P.T., and Thurlbeck, W.M. (1968). Site and nature of airway obstruction in chronic obstructive lung disease. *New England Journal of Medicine*, **278**, 1355–60.

Janus, E.D., Phillips, N.T., and Carrell, R.W. (1985). Smoking, lung function and alpha₁-antitrypsin deficiency. *Lancet*, **i**, 152–4.

Kalsheker, N.A., Hodgson, I., Watkins, G.L., White, J.P., Morrison, H.M., and Stockley, R.A. (1987). Deoxyribonucleic acid (DNA) polymorphism of the alpha₁-antitrypsin (AAT) gene in chronic lung disease. *British Medical Journal* **294**, 1511–14.

Laurell, C.-B. and Eriksson, S. (1963). The electrophoretical alpha₁-globulin pattern of serum in alpha₁-antitrypsin deficiency. *Scandinavian Journal of Clinical and Laboratory Investigation*, **15**, 132–40.

Lomas, D.A., Evans, D.Ll., Finch, J.T., and Carrell, R.W. (1992). The mechanism of Z α₁-antitrypsin accumulation in the liver. *Nature, London*, **357**, 605–7.

MacNee, W. (1994). Pathophysiology of cor pulmonale in chronic obstructive pulmonary disease. (Part One and Part Two). *American Journal of Respiratory and Critical Care Medicine*, **150**, 822–52.

Murphy, T.F. and Sethi, S. (1992). Bacterial infection in chronic obstructive pulmonary disease. *American Review of Respiratory Disease*, **146**, 1067–83.

Peto, R., Speizer, F.E., Cochrane, A.L., Moore, F., *et al.* (1983). The relevance in adults of air-flow obstruction, but not of mucus hypersecretion, to mortality from chronic lung disease. *American Review of Respiratory Disease*, **128**, 491–500.

Peto, R., Lopez, A.D., Boreham, J., Thun, M., and Heath, C., Jr (1992). Mortality from tobacco in developed countries: indirect estimation from national vital statistics. *Lancet*, **339**, 1268–78.

Postma, D.S., Peters, I., Steenhuis, E.J., and Sluiter, H.J. (1988). Moderately severe chronic airflow obstruction. Can corticosteroids slow down obstruction? *European Respiratory Journal*, **1**, 22–6.

Rochester, D.F. and Braun, N.M.T. (1985). Determinants of maximal inspiratory pressure in chronic obstructive pulmonary disease. *American Review of Respiratory Disease*, **132**, 42–7.

Snider, G.L., Kleinerman, J., Thurlbeck, W.M., and Bengali, Z.H. (1985). The definition of emphysema. Report of a National, Heart, Lung, and Blood Institute, Division of Lung Diseases Workshop. *American Review of Respiratory Disease*, **132**, 182–5.

Stone, P., Calore, J.D., McGowan, S.E., *et al.* (1983). Functional alpha₁-protease inhibitor in the lower respiratory tract of smokers is not decreased. *Science*, **221**, 1187–9.

Thurlbeck, W.M. (1976). *Chronic airflow obstruction in lung disease*. W.B. Saunders, Philadelphia, PA.

U.S. Department of Health and Human Services (1984). *The health consequences of smoking—chronic obstructive lung disease. A report of the Surgeon General*. Public Health Office, Office on Smoking and Health, Rockville, MD.

Wewers, M.D., Casolaro, M.A., Sellers, S.E., *et al.* (1987). Replacement therapy for alpha₁-deficiency associated with emphysema. *New England Journal of Medicine*, **316**, 1055–62.

Wright, J.L., Cagle, P., Churg, A., Colby, T.V., and Myers, J. (1992). Diseases of the small airways. *American Review of Respiratory Disease*, **146**, 240–62.

17.10 Diffuse parenchymal lung disease

17.10.1 Introduction

R. M. DU BOIS

Diseases of the parenchyma, or functioning gas exchanging regions, of the lung are often called interstitial lung diseases. In most of the disorders embraced by this label, major pathological change is present within the lung interstitium on histological examination; however, histological examination also demonstrates coexistent disease, usually inflammatory or infiltrative, in the alveoli, terminal bronchioles, and/or the pulmonary capillary. Such damage in all regions distal to the terminal bronchiole, and not just the interstitium, is responsible for producing the radiographic appearances which are considered to be 'interstitial lung disease'. Therefore the term 'diffuse parenchymal lung disease' will be used here.

Many of the processes which are included within this broad subsection of pulmonary disease are chronic and therefore have persistent radiographic abnormalities. Some, such as fibrosing alveolitis, asbestosis, and alveolar proteinosis, are often progressive in the absence of treatment, whereas others, such as sarcoidosis, extrinsic allergic alveolitis, and pulmonary eosinophilia run a more chronic relapsing–remitting course, sometimes with episodes of spontaneous remission. This variability in natural history mirrors the different mechanisms underlying the pathogenesis of individual diffuse parenchymal lung diseases; the pattern of each diffuse parenchymal disease is dependent upon the nature of the stimulus, the site at which it acts within the peripheral air spaces, the host's predisposition to show a pathological response, and the nature of that pathological response, with particular importance being attached to whether the initiation of disease triggers an immunological response or produces non-immunogenic injury. To produce disease in the peripheral regions of the lung, initiating factors such as organic or inorganic dust which reach the lung through inhalation must be of a size (1–3 μm) which can reach the periphery. Other triggers are likely to be blood-borne. Individuals appear to have variable degrees of predisposition to

disease; not all budgerigar owners or asbestos workers develop disease. This predisposition is likely to involve complex and multiple factors which include major histocompatibility complex gene haplotype expression and other genes which impact on immune response.

The clinician's role is to determine the nature of the diffuse parenchymal lung disease at a stage when it is most important for the patient, i.e. before sufficient respiratory reserve has been lost such that the patient will never be restored to significant health, so that appropriate management can be introduced early. Persistent inflammatory triggers can produce severe tissue injury with fibrosis (honeycomb lung), a point at which clinical and functional features cannot discriminate between the initiating processes. It is only by identifying the specific nature of the problem during the evolution of the disease that precise diagnoses can be made, and of course this is relevant where avoidance of exposure and suppression of inflammation may protect the lung from further injury and subsequent fibrosis. Good examples include extrinsic allergic alveolitis and occupational lung diseases in which removal of the patient from exposure to causative organic antigens, such as avian proteins in bird fancier's lung and cobalt in hard metal disease, is a crucial component of management.

An approach to patients with diffuse parenchymal lung disease

At the outset, producing a specific diagnosis may appear to be a daunting task because more than 180 causes of diffuse parenchymal lung disease have been described (Table 1). However, an ordered logical approach to the problem almost inevitably results in a relatively manageable short list from which the final diagnosis can be made. The aim of this chapter is to provide a series of signposts which allow these many entities to be differentiated and to focus particularly on disorders producing persistent abnormality. The approach is summarized in Table 2.

The approach can be considered in two phases. Phase 1 consists of clinical evaluation, which includes a complete history and examination,

Table 1 *Diffuse parenchymal lung diseases*

Unknown causes	Known causes

With interstitial fibrosis
  Cryptogenic fibrosing alveolitis
  Systemic sclerosis
  Polymyositis
  Sjögren's syndrome
  Rheumatoid arthritis
  SLE
  Ankylosing spondylitis
	Organic dusts
	  Avian e.g. pigeon antigens
	  Fungal e.g. aspergillus
	  Chemical e.g. diisocyanates

With granulomas
  Sarcoidosis
  Wegener's granulomatosis
  Langerhans' cell histiocytosis
  Eosinophilic granulomatosis (Churg–Strauss syndrome)
  Lymphomatoid granulomatosis
  Bronchocentric granulomatosis
	Pneumoconiosis
	  Fibrogenic inorganic dusts (e.g. asbestos, silica, hard metal alloy, beryllium, coal)
	  Inert inorganic dusts (e.g. iron, barium, tin)

Inherited disorders
  Tuberous sclerosis
  Neurofibromatosis
  Hermansky–Pudlak syndrome
  Lipid storage disorders
  Familial fibrosing alveolitis
	Infection
	  Viruses (e.g. cytomegalovirus)
	  Bacteria (e.g. tuberculosis)
	  Fungi (e.g. histoplasmosis)
	  Protozoa (e.g. Toxoplasma, Pneumocystis)
	  Helminths (e.g. Ascaris, filaria)

With vasculitis
  Wegener's granulomatosis
  Microscopic polyarteritis
  Rheumatic diseases (e.g. SLE, rheumatoid arthritis)
  Hypersensitivity vasculitis (e.g. response to drugs)
	Drugs
	  Producing lung injury (e.g. cytotoxic/chemotherapeutic, illegal opiates)
	  Producing immunogenic lung injury (e.g. anti-inflammatory, cardiovascular)
	  Causing eosinophilia (e.g. antibiotics, anti-inflammatory, anticonvulsant, cytotoxic)
	  SLE-like responses (e.g. hydrallazine)
	  Organizing pneumonia (e.g. acebutalol, gold, sulphasalazine)

Individual pathology
  Cryptogenic pulmonary eosinophilia
  Idiopathic pulmonary haemosiderosis
  Pulmonary veno-occlusive disease
  Lymphangioleiomyomatosis
  Lymphocytic interstitial pneumonia
  COP (BOOP in the United States)
    Known causes: amiodarone, sulphasalazine, acebutalol
    Unknown cause: idiopathic
  Alveolar proteinosis
  Alveolar microlithiasis
  Amyloidosis
	Neoplasia
	  Lymphangitis carcinomatosa
	  Lymphoma
	  Alveolar cell carcinoma
	
	Miscellaneous
	  Radiotherapy
	  Gases (e.g. mercury vapour, high oxygen concentrations)
	  Chemical (e.g. paraquat)
	  Associated with chronically elevated left atrial pressure, uraemia
	  Multiple pulmonary emboli
	  Post-ARDS

SLE, systemic lupus erythematosus; COP, cryptogenic organizing pneumonia; BOOP, bronchiolitis obliterans organizing pneumonia; ARDS, adult respiratory distress syndrome.

Table 2 *Approach to diffuse parenchymal lung disease*

History, examination, blood tests, chest radiography, lung function

THEN

Bronchoalveolar lavage + transbronchial biopsy if bronchocentric disease suspected

OR

CT proceeding to open-lung biopsy if
  diagnosis not clear
  transbronchial biopsy unhelpful
  disease staging needed (fibrosing alveolitis)

baseline blood tests, lung function studies, and chest radiography from which a short list of differential diagnoses can be constructed. Phase 2 requires a decision on which more detailed investigations, particularly bronchoalveolar lavage, high resolution CT, and biopsy, are needed to make a precise diagnosis. These will be determined by the results of phase 1 evaluation. These tests can also help to stage certain diseases.

In cryptogenic fibrosing alveolitis, where the relative degrees of cellularity and fibrosis seen on histological examination are important guides to prognosis and response to treatment, and rheumatological disorders such as systemic sclerosis and rheumatoid arthritis, where again precise histological information can provide invaluable guidelines to management of the lung complications of the condition, high resolution CT and lung biopsy can be predictive of disease progression and therefore a guide to management.

History

A full and detailed history is vital to the process of establishing a precise diagnosis in diffuse parenchymal lung disease. A history of breathlessness is a common presenting symptom which is usually chronic and progressive. Wheeze is uncommon but may be a feature of diffuse parenchymal diseases such as Langerhans' cell histiocytosis which impact significantly upon the airways. Presentation with acute breathlessness is less common but can be a feature of extrinsic allergic alveolitis or alveolar haemorrhage. A pneumothorax complicating chronic disease may be the presenting problem.

Cough, particularly a dry cough, is relatively common in patients with fibrosing alveolitis and also in patients with airways inflammation in association with diffuse parenchymal lung disease. This may occur with Sjögren's syndrome and rheumatoid arthritis, which commonly have airways inflammation as part of the systemic disorder, and also in the chronic phases of bronchocentric diseases such as sarcoidosis, Langerhans' histiocytosis, and extrinsic allergic alveolitis.

Regular sputum production is not usually a feature of diffuse parenchymal lung disease and suggests primary airway disease. At late stages of diffuse parenchymal lung disease recurrent infection may be a problem and can be mistaken for bronchiectasis when the radiographic appearance of honeycomb lung may be indistinguishable from severe bronchiectasis. Haemoptysis is uncommon in uncomplicated diffuse parenchymal lung disease, although it is a prominent symptom in small-vessel disorders such as Wegener's granulomatosis, idiopathic pulmonary haemosiderosis, and other forms of pulmonary vessel disease which may give rise to alveolar haemorrhage.

Pleural disease can be present in several diffuse parenchymal lung diseases: pleuritic chest pain may be a presenting feature of the rheumatological diseases, asbestos exposure, or Churg–Strauss syndrome. However, the presence of pleural disease should dissuade the clinician from making a diagnosis of cryptogenic fibrosing alveolitis or extrinsic allergic alveolitis in which pleural disease is rare and should suggest other diagnoses.

A history of cigarette smoking can be discriminatory. Granulomatous diseases such as sarcoidosis and extrinsic allergic alveolitis are associated with a low incidence of cigarette smoking, whereas pulmonary Langerhans' cell histiocytosis almost never occurs in non-smokers; diffuse pulmonary fibrosis in cryptogenic fibrosing alveolitis, asbestosis, and fibrosing alveolitis in rheumatoid arthritis are also associated with a high prevalence of cigarette smoking. Smoking also increases the risk of lung malignancies of all histological types in patients with pulmonary fibrosis; these include alveolar cell carcinoma which may have a diffuse appearance on chest radiography, may be bilateral, and therefore may mimic more benign diffuse lung disease.

A history of symptoms outside the respiratory system, such as joint stiffness in the rheumatological diseases, dysphagia and Raynaud's phenomenon in systemic sclerosis, and skin rashes or haematuria in systemic vasculitis, provide important clues to the aetiology of the pulmonary problem.

Occupation

A detailed occupational history is mandatory to exclude occupational-induced lung disease. A history of all occupations since leaving school must be taken, because disease may only become manifest after an interval as in asbestosis or chronic berylliosis. Other inorganic dust exposures such as coal-miner's pneumoconiosis, siderosis, and talcosis produce radiographic changes which persist long after exposure has ceased. The medicolegal aspects of occupationally induced lung disease are highly relevant to the patient, particularly if employment has been lost because of ill health, and the importance of a full occupational history cannot be understated.

Hobbies

In addition to the organic and inorganic dusts to which an individual may be exposed in the workplace, domestic exposure may be relevant. Budgerigars are a common household pet and bird fanciers, particularly pigeon fanciers, are numerous. Less common hobbies such as mushroom growing should be elicited. It often requires skill to unearth this aspect of the history. Bird fanciers seem particularly reticent to divulge their hobby because not infrequently the birds have become an important part of their owners' lives and if there is any suspicion that the birds may have caused their problem, patients may suppress this relevant information.

Associated conditions

All the rheumatological diseases can produce diffuse parenchymal lung disease. In rheumatoid arthritis, associated intrathoracic pathology includes fibrosing alveolitis, lymphocytic interstitial pneumonia, follicular bronchiolitis, pulmonary vasculitis, pleural effusions and thickening, rheumatoid nodules, and bronchiectasis. Other rheumatic diseases such as Sjögren's syndrome and systemic lupus erythematosus have a similarly broad range of potential pulmonary manifestations, added to which are the myopathies associated with polymyositis and systemic lupus erythematosus which give the appearance of small lungs on chest radiography (and therefore are mistaken for fibrotic lungs) because of muscle weakness. Treatment for the rheumatic diseases may include drugs which can produce diffuse parenchymal lung disease. Important examples of these include gold and methotrexate which are used in the treatment of rheumatoid arthritis. Immunosuppression for rheumatological disease increases the risk of opportunistic infection.

A history of previous malignancy, including lymphoma and leukaemia, is important to establish for three reasons. The majority of cytotoxic drugs are capable of producing diffuse parenchymal lung damage. Furthermore, patients receiving treatment for malignant processes are at risk from opportunistic infection. Lastly, malignant processes may recur within the lung, and thus the differential diagnosis of diffuse parenchymal lung disease in the presence of past or current malignancy is wide.

The emergence of HIV disease must always be considered in an individual presenting with a diffuse parenchymal lung problem, and appropriate serology performed if the patient is at high risk of having contracted HIV infection.

Examination

As in any other clinical situation a full examination is necessary, but particular attention should be paid to the identification of abnormality indicative of more systemic disease—lymphadenopathy in lymphoma, skin lesions or mononeuritis multiplex vasculitis, joint abnormalities in the rheumatological disorders, or eye changes in sarcoidosis or vasculitis. Digital clubbing is an important sign which occurs in approximately 70 per cent of all patients with cryptogenic fibrosing alveolitis and fibrosing alveolitis associated with rheumatoid arthritis, but almost never in sarcoidosis or the fibrosing alveolitis associated with systemic sclerosis. It is also usually present in chronic berylliosis. It is rare in Langerhans' cell histiocytosis, is less commonly a feature of other diffuse parenchymal lung diseases, and never occurs in extrinsic allergic alveolitis unless the end-stage of the process has been reached.

Clinical examination of the chest reveals fine end-inspiratory basal crackles as the characteristic feature of fibrosing alveolitis whatever its cause. Other aspects of the examination may identify cor pulmonale, but this is a reflection of chronicity and severity rather than type of lung disease process.

Investigations

Blood tests

Routine haematological and biochemical investigations are usually of little help in the differential diagnosis of diffuse parenchymal lung disease. Peripheral blood eosinophilia (above 1500/mm³) is a prerequisite for diagnosis of pulmonary eosinophilia. IgE concentrations can help to discriminate between the types of pulmonary eosinophilia. IgE levels are elevated in proportion to the eosinophilia in allergic causes such as helminthic infection and drug hypersensitivity, whereas disproportionately high eosinophil counts with a much more modest elevation in serum IgE are seen in cryptogenic pulmonary eosinophilia. Specific IgE measurements will confirm the identity of a suspected cause. Similarly, identification of precipitating antibodies to organic allergens will confirm exposure to suspected causes of extrinsic allergic alveolitis. Measurements of antineutrophil cytoplasmic antibodies (**ANCA**) are helpful if vasculitis is suspected, and cANCA positivity is highly suggestive of Wegener's granulomatosis. Autoantibodies such as rheumatoid factor and antinuclear antibody, together with more specific autoantibodies such as anticentromere antibody (limited systemic sclerosis), anti-DNA topoisomerase-1 (Scl-70) (diffuse systemic sclerosis) anti-amino-acyl t-RNA synthetase antibodies such as Jo1, PL-7, and PL-12 (polymyositis and other myositic diseases associated with fibrosing alveolitis), anti-SS-A and anti-SS-B (Sjörgen's syndrome) and anti-double-stranded DNA antibodies together with C3 and C4 complement component levels (systemic lupus erythematosus) will help to define the rheumatological diseases. It is important to consider looking for the presence of these autoantibodies in all patients with diffuse parenchymal lung disease because the lung manifestation of the systemic disorder may antedate evidence of disease elsewhere. In rheumatoid arthritis, for example, the lung problem may occur 4 to 5 years before other abnormalities including arthropathy. Angiotensin-converting enzyme levels may be elevated in sarcoidosis, but this test is not specific and may be normal in progressive sarcoidosis.

Lung function tests

In the majority of patients with diffuse parenchymal lung disease, lung function tests reveal a restrictive pattern of ventilatory defect with reduced gas transfer (D_{LCO}). Arterial oxygen tensions (Pa_{O_2}) may be normal or low and (Pa_{CO_2}) may also be normal or low. In more subtle disease with normal gas transfer at rest, exercise tests can unmask abnormality: Pa_{O_2} falls and the alveolar–arterial oxygen gradient (A–a gradient) widens, indicating abnormalities of gas exchange. These investigations of pulmonary function can confirm the presence of disease but cannot discriminate between the different causes.

In disorders in which an airway component is associated with the diffuse parenchymal disease a mixed obstructive–restrictive ventilatory defect is observed. This occurs in Langerhans' cell histiocytosis and advanced sarcoidosis, both of which are bronchocentric disease processes. Combined pathologies may coexist; in patients with fibrosing alveolitis who have been heavy cigarette smokers a mixed obstructive–restrictive process is present. This can be a very valuable discriminating observation because pure fibrosing lung disorders such as asbestosis and cryptogenic fibrosing alveolitis do not produce an obstructive pattern, and alternative explanations must be sought.

Chest imaging

Both standard chest radiography and radionuclide imaging may be of value in diffuse parenchymal lung disease.

CHEST RADIOGRAPHY

Chest radiography is one of the most important keys to differentiating one diffuse parenchymal lung disease from another. Five important features should be noted:

(1) lung size;
(2) distribution of abnormalities;
(3) size and nature of nodular and reticular abnormalities;
(4) presence of confluent shadows;
(5) presence of pleural disease or lymphadenopathy.

Lung size

Patients with fibrosing lung diseases will generally show small lungs on radiography. Provided that the patient has taken a full inspiration and that neuromuscular and other extrathoracic reasons for an inability to take a full inspiration are excluded, small lungs almost always mean

fibrosing lung disease, particularly in the presence of abnormal shadowing. If other clinical features have suggested a diagnosis of fibrosing alveolitis, normal or large-size lungs indicate the coexistence of emphysema and fibrosing alveolitis; lung function tests can confirm this by showing a mixed obstructive–restrictive ventilatory defect but with a disproportionate reduction in gas transfer measurement because both diseases damage the pulmonary vascular bed.

Other causes of large or normal-sized lungs on radiography in the presence of nodular or reticular shadowing include Langerhans' cell histiocytosis (Fig. 1), lymphangioleiomyomatosis (a disorder involving smooth muscle which occurs only in females during the childbearing years), tuberous sclerosis, and neurofibromatosis. Chronic sarcoidosis can also feature large lungs, but this is usually associated with fibrosis in the upper zones which is discriminating (Fig. 2). Bronchiectasis with or without cystic fibrosis can also be mistaken for diffuse parenchymal lung disease, but the history of regular sputum production and the presence of clearly thickened bronchial walls and bronchial dilatation usually allows a firm alternative diagnosis to be made.

Distribution of abnormalities

The distribution of the abnormalities in diffuse parenchymal lung disease is always helpful. Fibrosing alveolitis occurring alone, in associa-

Fig. 1 Chest radiograph of a patient with pulmonary Langerhans' cell histiocytosis. The large-volume lungs and cystic changes, particularly in the mid-zones, should be noted.

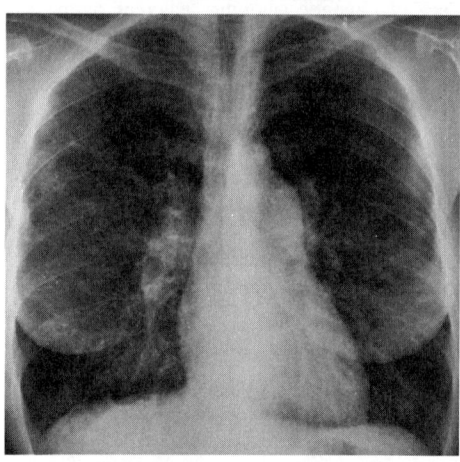

Fig. 2 Chest radiograph of a patient with chronic sarcoidosis. The upper-zone contractions and prominent pulmonary vessels consistent with secondary pulmonary hypertension should be noted.

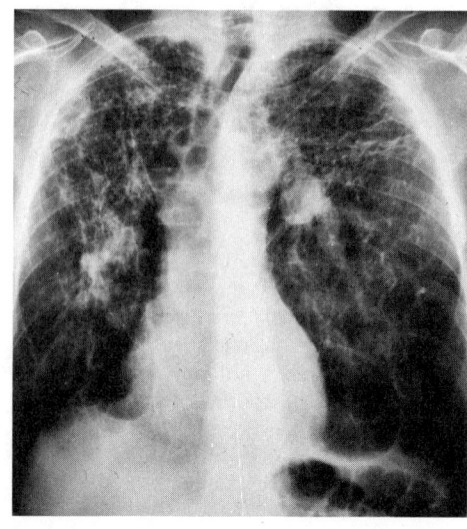

tion with rheumatic diseases, or due to asbestos exposure produces a nodular or reticulonodular abnormality predominantly in the basal zones but also visible to the critical eye in the periphery of the lung, obscuring the diaphragm and the right and left heart borders. Predominantly upper-zone disease, particularly that involving loss of lung volume with an upward shift of the hilar shadows denoting upper zone fibrosis, occurs in chronic sarcoidosis and tuberculosis, extrinsic allergic alveolitis in its chronic stage, bronchopulmonary aspergillosis (almost always in the presence of asthma), ankylosing spondylitis, and occasionally may be the residual pattern in Langerhans' cell histiocytosis.

Many occupationally induced lung diseases such as silicosis, siderosis (iron dust), stannosis (tin), and baritosis (barium) have a predilection for the upper zones. Sarcoidosis, extrinsic allergic alveolitis in its acute and subacute forms, and Langerhans' cell histiocytosis occur in a predominant mid-zone distribution.

Size and nature of nodular and reticular abnormalities

In disorders in which there is a nodular or reticular pattern of abnormality, the size of the abnormalities and their shape are helpful pointers. These can be scored in a more formal grading system devised by the International Labour Office which seeks to categorize the size and shape of opacities and their profusion. More simply, very small 'granular' nodules less than 1 mm in size are seen in conditions such as idiopathic pulmonary haemosiderosis, miliary tuberculosis, and alveolar microlithiasis. Nodules up to 5 mm in diameter are seen in more commonly encountered disorders such as sarcoidosis, extrinsic allergic alveolitis, and silicosis, and larger shadows (greater than 5 mm) are present in Wegener's granulomatosis, rheumatoid arthritis, lymphoma, and other malignancies. Nodules of varying size and shape are highly suggestive of metastatic malignancy, and nodules which cavitate should make the clinician suspect Wegener's granulomatosis, necrotizing tumours (usually of the squamous-cell type), rheumatoid nodules, or multiple staphylococcal abscesses. Lower-zone reticular opacification is the hallmark of fibrosing alveolitis occurring alone or in the context of rheumatological disease and asbestosis.

Confluent shadowing

Confluent shadowing denotes air-space opacification, and the presence of air bronchograms is a supporting sign. Conditions which have a predominant alveolar filling component as part of the disease process may manifest with confluent pneumonic-like shadowing. Such disorders include pulmonary alveolar proteinosis, alveolar haemorrhage, pulmonary eosinophilia, in which the shadowing is often typically peripheral producing a reverse bat's wing pattern (Fig. 3), cryptogenic organizing pneumonia, and opportunistic infections, notably Pneumocystis and cytomegalovirus.

Pleural disease and lymphadenopathy

Pleural disease is uncommon in sarcoidosis and should suggest alternative diagnoses if Pneumocystis, fibrosing alveolitis, or extrinsic allergic alveolitis are suspected. These exceptions apart, pleural disease may be seen in most forms of diffuse parenchymal lung disease, particularly those associated with rheumatological conditions, the granulomatous vasculitides (Churg–Strauss syndrome and Wegener's granulomatosis), and asbestos exposure.

Hilar lymphadenopathy if symmetrical is almost always due to sarcoidosis. Tuberculosis and lymphoma (and other malignancies) must always be considered, and these diagnoses are more likely if the changes are unilateral. Lymphadenopathy is rarely observed in other diffuse lung diseases, with the notable exception of silicosis.

RADIONUCLIDE IMAGING

Gallium scanning may be helpful in determining the presence of lung disease when there is doubt, but is not specific, it is time consuming, it produces a considerable radiation burden, and quantitation is imprecise.

Other techniques of imaging are $^{99}Tc^m$-DTPA scanning which measures epithelial permeability, ^{111}In-transferrin labelling which assesses microvascular leak, ^{111}In-neutrophil labelling to identify neutrophil traffic, and positron emission tomography in association with radiolabelled carbohydrate administration which indicates local increases in metabolic activity. All these tests are promising as specific indices of early inflammation and are likely to be important in the future, but their present role is still being defined.

More specific investigation

Once phase 1 tests have been completed, appropriate confirmatory investigations are performed.

BRONCHOALVEOLAR LAVAGE

Once heralded as the alternative to lung biopsy as a diagnostic test in diffuse parenchymal lung disease, bronchoalveolar lavage is now viewed more circumspectly. However, useful information can be obtained from patients with almost all forms of diffuse parenchymal lung disease, but sample collection and storage must be carried out in such a way that specialist tests can be performed if necessary (e.g. glutaraldehyde fixation for electron microscopy, snap freezing for fluorescent antibody studies). Diagnostic material is obtained in some diseases (Table 3). Examples of this include the lipoproteinaceous material obtained from patients with alveolar proteinosis, the Langerhans cells of Langerhans' cell histiocytosis identified by specific stains such as S-100 or the characteristic electron microscopic appearances of cells containing Birbeck granules, electron microscopy of lipoproteinaceous material in alveolar proteinosis (Fig. 4); the bizarre multinucleate giant cells obtained from patients exposed to the alloy hard metal, and the iron-laden macrophages which are present in profusion in patients who have been exposed to iron ores (siderosis) or those who have had repeated intrapulmonary haemorrhage as part of a pulmonary vasculitic syndrome or idiopathic pulmonary haemosiderosis. Asbestos bodies indicate asbestos exposure, and proliferative responses of lung lymphocytes to beryllium are diagnostic of chronic berylliosis. Energy-dispersive X-ray analysis of cytospin slide preparations of lung cells can identify the presence of elements within the cells by analysing X-ray emissions by these elements in response to electron bombardment (Fig. 5). Suspected infection in patients who are immunosuppressed because of either their disease or its therapy can be identified reliably with bron-

Fig. 3 Chest radiograph of a patient with pulmonary eosinophilia. The bilateral peripheral pattern of consolidation should be noted.

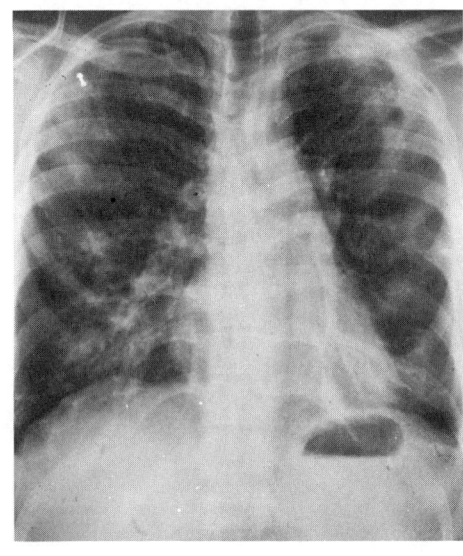

Table 3 *Bronchoalveolar lavage in diffuse parenchymal lung disease*

Diagnostic
 Opportunistic infection
 Alveolar haemorrhage
 Alveolar proteinosis
 Langerhans' cell histiocytosis
 Occupational disease

Indicative
Lymphocytosis
 Sarcoidosis
 Berylliosis
 Tuberculosis
 Extrinsic allergic alveolitis
 Drugs
Granulocytosis
 Fibrosing alveolitis
 Adult respiratory distress syndrome
 Infection

choalveolar lavage provided that a minimum of 100 ml of saline is instilled (usually in aliquots). Combining such techniques with novel methods of immunofluorescent staining or polymerase chain reaction amplification of DNA provides highly sensitive identification of opportunist infections such as *Pneumocystis carinii*, mycobacterial infections, and viral infections, particularly cytomegalovirus infection in which the detection of early gene protein products in infected cells can be identified within hours of lavage using a fluorescence assay. This has obvious advantages over conventional viral cytopathic culture methods in terms of time saved before commencing treatment; in the case of *P. carinii*, the organism cannot be cultured.

Differential cell counts of material obtained by bronchoalveolar lavage can also provide a useful signpost in differential diagnosis. An excess of lymphocytes occurs in disorders which are characterized by granuloma formation, particularly sarcoidosis, extrinsic allergic alveolitis, and tuberculosis, and also in disorders which are provoked by drugs such as methotrexate or gold. An excess of neutrophils is obtained from patients with diffuse fibrosing lung disorders such as cryptogenic fibrosing alveolitis, asbestosis, fibrosing alveolitis in association with rheumatological diseases, and adult respiratory distress syndrome. Increases in neutrophils also occur in infection. In contrast, an excess of eosinophils, although not present in infected individuals, may also be observed

Fig. 4 Electron microscopy of lavage material from a patient with alveolar proteinosis demonstrating the bilamellar 'whorls' of phospholipid (left, magnifications EM 9000 ×; right, magnification 45 000 ×).

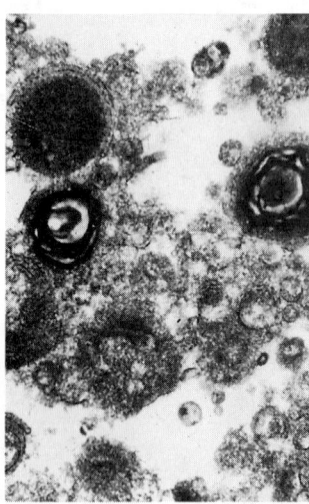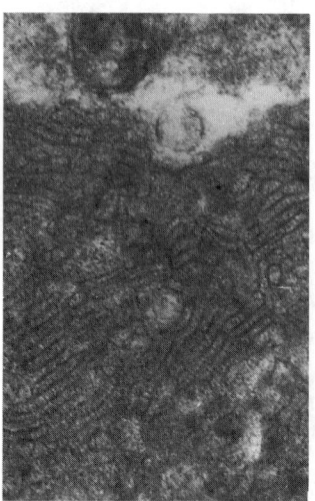

in fibrosing lung conditions. Increases in eosinophils are also present in lavage material obtained from patients with asthma and pulmonary eosinophilia, but differentiation from fibrosing lung disease is usually obvious from the clinical picture.

This differentiation of diffuse parenchymal diseases into those with a preponderance of either lymphocytes or granulocytes was initially promising, but further studies revealed that lymphocytes were not always present in granulomatous disorders; lymphocytes may be present at the earlier stages of fibrosing lung disorders and heralded a good response to therapy, and neutrophils are present in the lungs of patients recently exposed to the antigens which provoke extrinsic allergic alveolitis and also emerge when diseases such as sarcoidosis enter a more fibrotic phase. Therefore, in these circumstances, bronchoalveolar lavage cannot be considered to be diagnostic but rather is a helpful indicator of the sort of disease process with which the clinician is dealing. The test can also be of value where initial investigations have suggested one disease (e.g. fibrosing alveolitis) but a very high percentage of one cell type (e.g. lymphocytes) would force the physician to reconsider the suspected diagnosis.

COMPUTED TOMOGRAPHY

CT of the lungs of patients with diffuse parenchymal lung disease has increased the role of imaging in differential diagnosis and is more sensitive and specific than chest radiography in differential diagnosis. One of the major advantages of CT is that the whole of the lung is sampled and in certain circumstances may provide more detailed information than might be available from the small sample obtained at open-lung biopsy. Fine-section (1–3 mm) thickness images in conjunction with appropriate computer software can produce images of extremely high resolution. By 'sampling' lung at 1 cm intervals, the burden of radiation is approximately half that of a standard thoracic CT examination. A second advantage of high resolution CT is that it can demonstrate abnormality before conventional chest radiography, and in certain instances before standard pulmonary physiology has become abnormal. The pattern of abnormality may be pathognomonic in certain diffuse parenchymal lung diseases and may obviate the need for biopsy confirmation (Table 4). This is particularly useful when the patient has little pulmonary reserve when biopsy would be hazardous.

In fibrosing alveolitis, the pattern of high resolution CT also differ-

Fig. 5 Energy-dispersive X-ray analysis of lung lavage cells obtained from a patient exposed to iron ores. The peak of activity corresponding to iron (Fe) should be noted.

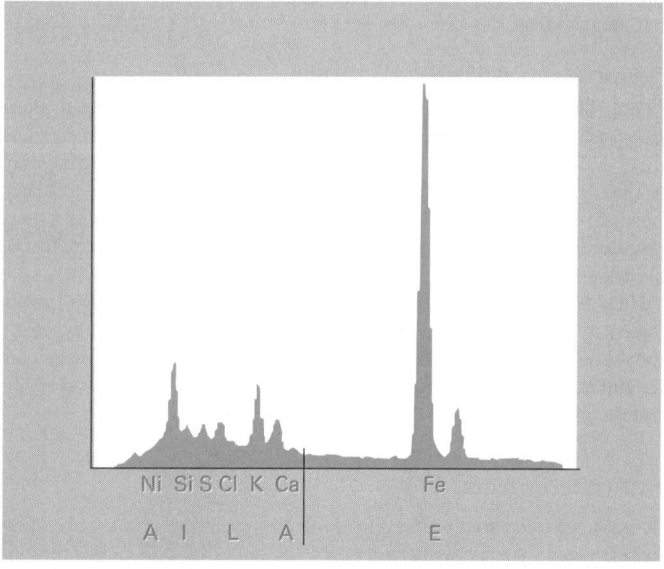

Table 4 *Conditions showing characteristic features in high resolution CT*

Fibrosing alveolitis
Sarcoidosis
Extrinsic allergic alveolitis
Langerhans' cell histiocytosis
Lymphangioleiomyomatosis
Lymphangitis carcinomatosa

Table 5 *Choice of biopsy procedure*

Transbronchial	
Sarcoidosis	
Extrinsic allergic alveolitis	Granulomatous
Berylliosis	or
Tuberculosis	bronchocentric
Lymphangitis carcinomatosa	processes
Open-lung (or thoracoscopic)	
Fibrosing alveolitis	
Rheumatological disease	
Other diffuse fibrosing lung disease	
Pulmonary vasculitis	
Neoplasia	
Lymphangioleiomyomatosis	
Langerhans' cell histiocytosis	

entiates between a more cellular inflammatory disease process (ground-glass appearance) and the more fibrotic disease stage (reticular pattern). An assessment of the relative amounts of ground-glass opacification and reticular changes may prove to be of value in prognosis and assessment of response to therapy.

Finally, high resolution CT can be used to guide the surgeon to sites for biopsy when the disease process is more patchy, and this will increase the biopsy yield.

LUNG BIOPSY

Because of the large number of potential causes of diffuse parenchymal lung disease, it is imperative in most cases to establish the diagnosis firmly before embarking on therapy. The advantage of having a firm diagnosis is that appropriate and rational therapy can be commenced. The alternative of treating empirically may result in the patient's deteriorating while on therapy, developing side-effects due to that therapy in the face of no improvement in the disease process, at which stage the risks of biopsy are increased.

However, it is important to weigh up the relative risks of a biopsy procedure. In an elderly individual with poor respiratory reserve, particularly one in whom the other clinical features and high resolution CT have confirmed the diagnosis beyond reasonable doubt, biopsy is superfluous. However, in younger patients who may need to be treated for a prolonged period reasons should be sought for not performing a biopsy, rather than subject the patient to prolonged potent treatment with potentially major side-effects without the security of knowing precisely what process is being treated.

The type of biopsy procedure is determined by a consideration of the most probably diagnosis following initial investigations (Table 5). In diseases which are either bronchocentric or granulomatous (often both), transbronchial biopsy together with bronchoalveolar lavage will provide diagnostic material in more than 80 per cent of instances. This procedure can now be performed safely without screening. Transbronchial biopsy may result in pneumothorax or haemoptysis in a small number of

patients, but these are uncommon complications provided that the patient is able to cooperate with the procedure and has no underlying problem with haemostasis. Therefore it is imperative to check the patient's platelet numbers and clotting status prior to the transbronchial procedure.

Trephine percutaneous drill sampling can provide good biopsy specimens. This technique carries the risks of pneumothorax and haemorrhage, particularly in non-expert hands and is no longer recommended.

Open-lung biopsy has traditionally been the 'gold standard' biopsy technique for fibrosing alveolitis and where diagnosis remains uncertain after the full evaluation outlined above. In these circumstances, the transbronchial approach is inadequate because the samples are small, often unrepresentative, and do not provide critical information regarding relative degrees of cellularity and fibrosis in fibrosing alveolitis or the spatial relationships of inflammatory responses which help determine the nature of individual diseases. Therefore open-lung biopsy is the procedure of choice in these conditions.

Recently, lung biopsies have been undertaken through the thoracoscope. This technique has the advantages of requiring much smaller skin incisions, more rapid procedure times, and a shorter stay in hospital. It is too early to say whether complication rates will be improved by this technique, but it is possible that this procedure may supersede open-lung biopsy in certain situations.

Treatment

Treatment strategies for individual diseases are detailed in subsequent chapters, but four general points about treatment need to be made. Firstly, disease must be identified early before lung injury has progressed to such a degree that functional improvement cannot be achieved. This requires an increased awareness of early symptoms or radiography changes which require further evaluation. Secondly, if treatment is given to patients with early relatively asymptomatic disease, reliable predictors of probable disease progression and response to therapy need to be developed. At present high resolution CT and ^{99}Tc^m-DTPA assessment show promise as indices of progression and probable response to treatment in fibrosing alveolitis, but further studies are needed to improve the definition of the role of these newer technologies used in this and other diffuse parenchymal diseases. Thirdly, the relative risks of treatment (side-effects) must be balanced against the probability of improvement on treatment. In this regard, the presence of advanced disease merits caution in the use of potentially toxic drugs. If a trial of therapy is considered to be acceptable, this must be carefully controlled and clear outcome measures must be defined. To await the presence of significant and progressive symptomatology before treating is to risk irreversible lung function loss. Finally, newer approaches to therapy are needed. These will target specific mechanisms involved in the inductive phases of diseases, attacking the basic mechanisms of aetiology. Molecular and cellular biological methods are rapidly improving our knowledge of these mechanisms and will give direction to developing drugs which inhibit important components of inflammation such as T-cell triggering, granulocyte traffic and activation, and fibrogenesis.

REFERENCES

Baughman, R.P. (1992). *Bronchoalveolar lavage*. C.V. Mosby—Year Book, St Louis, MO.
Corrin, B. (1990). *Systemic pathology*, Vol. 5, *The lungs*. Churchill Livingstone, London.
Crystal, R.G. and West, J.B. (1991). *The lung. Scientific foundations*. Raven Press, New York.
Daniele, R.P. (1988). *Immunology and immunologic diseases of the lung*. Blackwell, Boston, MA.
Lynch, J.P., III, and DeRemee, R.A. (1991). *Immunologically mediated pulmonary diseases*. J.B. Lippincott, Philadelphia, PA.

Reed, J.C. (1991). *Chest radiology: plain film patterns and differential diagnoses*. C.V. Mosby—Year Book, St Louis, MO.

Thurlbeck, W.M., Miller, R.R., Muller, M.L., and Rosenow, E.C., III. (1991). *Diffuse diseases of the lungs: a team approach*. Dekker, New York.

17.10.2 Cryptogenic fibrosing alveolitis

R. M. DU BOIS

Definition

Fibrosing alveolitis is defined as a condition which is characterized by inflammation and fibrosis of the pulmonary peripheral air spaces and interstitium. 'Cryptogenic' indicates that no cause has been identified. It is known as idiopathic pulmonary fibrosis in the United States. Although this definition is based on histological examination of lung tissue, there are a number of clinical, physiological, and radiographic features which will suggest the diagnosis before confirmatory histology is obtained.

Since the entity was first described in 1907 as 'interstitial pulmonary fibrosis', a number of different terms have been used to describe the same disorder and the literature is replete in confusing terminology. One of the earlier terms which has endured is 'Hamman–Rich' syndrome. The four cases to which this eponym refers ran a much more rapid course than in the majority of patients with fibrosing alveolitis, although the histological features bore a number of similarities.

Later, subclassification of the 'interstitial pneumonias' into five groups was made on the basis of histological appearance (Table 1). In 'usual interstitial pneumonia', variable degrees of interstitial and air-space cellularity and fibrosis coexist. The second group, 'desquamative interstitial pneumonia', was defined by an almost exclusively cellular biopsy, with very little evidence of fibrosis; this appearance was associated with a much better prognosis. These subdivisions have caused some confusion, largely because it is not clear whether desquamative interstitial pneumonia should be considered as a disease quite distinct from usual interstitial pneumonia with different clinical features and response to therapy. The majority of patients with fibrosing alveolitis have disease which is of the usual interstitial pneumonia pattern but with variable amounts of cellularity and fibrosis.

It is less confusing to consider cryptogenic fibrosing alveolitis (and thus idiopathic pulmonary fibrosis) as comprising a spectrum of disease consisting mainly of usual interstitial pneumonia with different relative amounts of cellularity and fibrosis but with desquamative interstitial pneumonia being at the cellular terminus of this spectrum. This is a more practical classification than to consider desquamative interstitial pneumonia and usual interstitial pneumonia as two distinct entities, which ignores the important variability of disease which can be classified under usual interstitial pneumonia. This concept is discussed further in the section on pathology.

Therefore it is clear that under the 'umbrella' of a diagnosis of cryptogenic fibrosing alveolitis there are almost certainly a heterogeneous group of patients whose disease has been triggered by a variety of different factors and whose disease course, including response to treatment, is variable.

Aetiology

EPIDEMIOLOGY

Fibrosing alveolitis may occur in any decade of life, but is most commonly seen between the ages of 50 and 60. The male-to-female ratio is 1 : 1, provided that associated rheumatological diseases are excluded. The disease is more common in patients who have a history of cigarette smoking. There have been no studies of the prevalence or incidence of the disease. It is estimated that approximately five per 100 000 of the population of the United Kingdom may be affected. Disease incidence appears to be increasing based on evidence of mortality statistics for England and Wales: in 1990, 2728 patients died from fibrosing lung disease and of these 775 had fibrosing alveolitis. Studies of the accuracy of death certification have revealed that fibrosing alveolitis is under-diagnosed in life and misnotified at death, and therefore the real prevalence is likely to be higher than previously estimated; true United Kingdom mortality figures are likely to be close to 1500 per annum.

There have been no properly controlled prospective epidemiological studies addressing the aetiology of the disease, and suggestions of possible aetiological factors are at present only speculative.

POSSIBLE TRIGGER FACTORS

As in most chronic inflammatory disorders, multiple factors are likely to be involved in triggering and amplifying cryptogenic fibrosing alveolitis, although there is by definition no known single cause. Similarities with other diseases of known cause which result in lung damage and fibrosis (Table 2) have stimulated the search for trigger factors. Viral infections have been implicated but never proved. In one series of 13 patients with fibrosing alveolitis, antibodies to Epstein–Barr virus (10 patients) and IgA against viral capsid antigen (13 patients) were observed. These circumstantial data suggesting viral triggers of fibrosing lung disease are consistent with some patient histories which include a disease onset described as an 'influenza-like illness', although conclusive proof of a viral trigger has never been obtained.

More recently, a pilot study has reported an excess of exposure to metal dusts and wood fires in patients with fibrosing alveolitis compared with controls.

IMMUNOGENETICS

A number of studies support the concept that inherited factors play a role in the pathogenesis of fibrosing alveolitis. In disorders which are known to be inherited, such as neurofibromatosis and the Hermansky–Pudlak syndrome (a condition characterized by oculocutaneous albinism and abnormal platelets), fibrosing alveolitis may coexist, suggesting that these patients have increased susceptibility to fibrosing alveolitis.

HLA studies have been inconclusive, perhaps because incomplete analyses have been performed and inadequate numbers of homogeneous groups of patients have been studied. In contrast, in systemic sclerosis, a rheumatological condition in which fibrosing alveolitis is commonly seen, the presence of pulmonary fibrosis is associated with the presence of a class II major histocompatibility complex haplotype DR3/DR52a and/or the presence of the anti-DNA topoisomerase I antibody Scl70.

There is no family history of fibrosing alveolitis in the majority of patients, but a familial pattern is observed in a small subgroup. The inheritance pattern is unpredictable, and therefore it is probable that transmission involves variable penetrance.

Gene linkage disequilibrium studies using α_1-antitrypsin phenotype and immunoglobulin polymorphisms have suggested that, at least in the family studied, genetic loci on chromosome 14 may be involved in the pathogenesis of cryptogenic fibrosing alveolitis.

In one study of 17 individuals from three families in whom more than one member had fibrosing alveolitis, evidence of inflammation within the lower respiratory tract was observed (abnormal neutrophil numbers, enhanced production of macrophage proinflammatory cytokines, or abnormal gallium scan) in eight subjects, even though clinical examination, chest radiography, and pulmonary function studies were normal.

Therefore it seems likely that individuals are predisposed in one or more ways to developing fibrosing lung disease and that disease onset occurs in response to one of a number of potential triggering factors. In this regard, support comes from studies of asbestosis in which not all individuals exposed to equivalent amounts of asbestos dust develop lung

Table 1 *Histopathological classification of 'interstitial pneumonias'*

	Major histological features	Disease
Usual interstitial pneumonia	Interstitial fibrosis Interstitial cellular (mainly mononuclear) infiltrate Type II cell hyperplasia Lung injury	Fibrosing alveolitis
Desquamative interstitial pneumonia	Uniform airspace and interstitial cellular infiltrate Minimal fibrosis No necrosis	Fibrosing alveolitis
Bronchiolitis obliterans with usual interstitial pneumonia	Granulation tissue within distal air spaces	COP (BOOP in United States)
Lymphoid interstitial pneumonia	Widespread thickening of interstitium with lymphocytes, monocytes, plasma cells	Rheumatoid arthritis Sjögren's syndrome Lymphoma HIV
Giant-cell interstitial pneumonia	Bizarre multinucleate giant cells in air spaces (macrophage derived) and epithelium (type II cell derived)	Hard metal disease

COP, cryptogenic organizing pneumonia; BOOP, bronchiolitis obliterans organizing pneumonia.

Table 2 *Known causes of lung disease which may mimic fibrosing alveolitis*

Extrinsic allergic alveolitis (chronic stage)
Occupational lung disease
   Asbestosis
   Hard metal disease
Drug therapy
   Cytotoxic (e.g. bleomycin, busulphan, BCNU, methotrexate)
   Antibacterial (e.g. nitrofurantoin, sulphasalazine)
   Cardiological (e.g. amiodarone, tocainide)
   Rheumatological (e.g. gold, D-penicillamine)
   Analgesics (e.g. heroin)
   Anticonvulsants (e.g. diphenylhydantoin)
Inhaled agents
   Mercury vapour
   Nitrogen dioxide
Ingested agents
   Paraquat
Irradiation

fibrosis. It would seem that inherited factors are important in this situation, but they have yet to be identified.

Pathology

In typical cases, histological examination of biopsy material demonstrates the presence of varying amounts of connective tissue matrix cells, their products (including collagen), smooth-muscle cells, proteoglycans, and variable numbers of inflammatory cells within the interstitium and bronchioloalveolar air spaces. The pathological processes are restricted to the acinar regions of the lung, i.e. distal to the terminal bronchiole.

In 1975, the interstitial pneumonias were subdivided into five groups based upon histological appearance. Included in the five groups are usual interstitial pneumonia and desquamative interstitial pneumonia, which can be seen in cryptogenic fibrosing alveolitis. In usual interstitial pneumonia, there is damage to, and loss of, alveoli, inflammatory cells are present within the lung interstitium (mainly lymphocytes and plasma cells, but also neutrophils and eosinophils) and air spaces (mainly macrophages), interstitial fibrosis is present and may extend into the alveoli, and type II alveolar cells proliferate. At later stages, honeycombing due to extensive lung injury is present.

Desquamative interstitial pneumonia, in contrast, is characterized by the striking absence of fibrosis and the uniform infiltration of interstitium and alveolar spaces with mononuclear phagocytes.

The other three groups of interstitial pneumonias have distinctive pathological features and are not forms of fibrosing alveolitis, although they may mimic fibrosing alveolitis clinically (Table 1).

A different and more functional way of subdividing cryptogenic fibrosing alveolitis into groups on the basis of the histological patterns involves an assessment of the relative degrees of cellularity and fibrosis. A cellular pattern of disease is characterized by the intra-alveolar accumulation of macrophages; infiltration with mononuclear cells, granulocytes, plasma cells, and mast cells is present in the interstitium together with a variable degree of fibrosis, but with the predominant abnormality being cellular. In the fibrotic pattern, dense interstitial infiltration with collagen and other connective tissue matrix cells and proteins is observed with a tendency to lung injury and air-space dilatation, resulting in honeycombing. Small numbers of mononuclear cells may still be present, but the injury and fibrosis predominate. In the majority of biopsies obtained from patients with cryptogenic fibrosing alveolitis cellularity and fibrosis coexist within the usual interstitial pneumonia group of histopathological appearances, and it is the relative proportions of each process which are of most importance in predicting prognosis and response to therapy. A semiquantitative approach can be applied to the determination of the relative amounts of each pathological process by scoring independently the extent of fibrosis and cellularity within the interstitium, air-space cellularity, type II cell hyperplasis, loss of architecture, bronchiolization of the alveoli, and vascular changes. A conclusion about the relative amounts of each process can then be derived from the scores, and in practice this provides more information than does a categorization of 'usual interstitial pneumonia' alone.

The evaluation of relative amounts of cellular and fibrotic pathological change is the most important reason for undertaking lung biopsy because a predominantly cellular biopsy is a good predictor of response to treatment, and therefore survival. Degrees of cellularity and fibrosis differ widely between patients, between different biopsies from the same patient, and, strikingly, between different regions of the same biopsy. Therefore the pathological process is patchy and inflammation at different sites of the lung is not always at the same stage of the pathological process. An overall assessment of the biopsy is required to provide an accurate assessment of fibrosis and cellularity, and this is the main reason why transbronchial biopsies are of such limited value in this condition — the small size precludes an accurate measure of the extent of the different pathological components.

In association with these changes of inflammation and fibrosis, a typical lung biopsy will show prominent lymphoid follicles. Immunohistological analysis of these follicles has shown that they contain true germinal centres and therefore that they are secondary follicles, responding locally to antigen triggers. This highlights the role of immunological mechanisms in pathogenesis.

Ultrastructural examination of areas of lung biopsy material which are normal to light microscopy has revealed that the earliest stages of the pathological process are characterized by the presence of injury to both epithelial and endothelial cells (cell swelling, electrolucence), exposure of basement membrane, and loss of basement membrane structure.

CLINICOPATHOLOGICAL CORRELATIONS

Correlations between clinical and physiological indices of disease and lung biopsy appearances have generally proved to be disappointing. This is probably a reflection of the fact that biopsy samples a small area of the peripheral (and most involved) part of the lung, whereas other indices reflect the function of the whole of both lungs. Despite this, it has been shown that the degree of fibrosis within the lung interstitium is correlated with the $P(\text{A-a})O_2$ gradient, changes in exercise PaO_2, and lung compliance.

A detailed system of assessing clinical status has been devised more recently. This involves scoring clinical features, pulmonary physiology, and radiographic appearance, from which a clinical–radiographic–physiological (**CRP**) score is derived. It has been shown that the CRP score at the time of biopsy correlates with an independent index of overall pathological abnormality, and the score after therapy for 6 months correlates with the degree of fibrosis observed in the pretreatment biopsy.

Pathogenesis

The lung has a limited repertoire of response to injury, and the appearance at the most advanced stages of any of the parenchymal lung diseases may be identical i.e. 'honeycomb lung'. What identifies individual disease processes at earlier stages of pathogenesis and makes them distinctive is the nature of the initiating agent, the pathological response to that agent, and the distribution of this response within the peripheral lung. The nature of the triggering factor, and in particular whether it is capable of raising an immunological response, is a critical early determinant of pathogenesis of individual parenchymal lung disease. Much has been learned about the pathogenesis of parenchymal lung disease by the studies of the processes which produce cryptogenic fibrosing alveolitis.

The pathogenesis of cryptogenic alveolitis can be considered under four headings:

    (1) initiating factors;
    (2) immunological mechanisms;
    (3) inflammatory response;
    (4) fibrogenesis.

INITIATING FACTORS

The evidence from ultrastructural observations in man and animal models of lung fibrosis support the concept that lung injury is the first event in the pathogenesis of the disease, although the nature of the initiating factor is not known. In predisposed individuals, this initial injurious process is followed by an influx of acute and chronic inflammatory cells which are responsible for initiating and maintaining immunological and inflammatory responses, and for producing progressive disease.

IMMUNOLOGICAL MECHANISMS

Evidence for the involvement of immunological processes in the pathogenesis of cryptogenic fibrosing alveolitis comes from studies of lung biopsies, bronchoalveolar lavage cells, epithelial lining fluid (sampled by bronchoalveolar lavage), and peripheral blood.

Histological examination of lung biopsies shows the presence of lymphoid follicles within the interstitium (not just associated with the bronchi) and abundant lymphocytes and plasma cells. Immunohistochemical studies have clarified the nature of the lymphoid aggregates which have the morphological and immunohistochemical features of secondary follicles with true germinal centres (i.e. as seen in reactive lymph nodes). Within the interstitium of the lung, macrophages express the phenotype of inflammatory cells and lymphocytes are predominantly CD4+ helper/inducer subset cells with variable numbers of CD8+ suppressor/cytotoxic cells present. Many of the T cells express markers of activation, and the majority of T cells have the surface phenotype of antigen-primed memory T cells (CD45RO+). The deposition of IgG and complement has been observed within alveolar walls and capillaries in some studies, but they are not found in the majority of cases and are rarely identified under the electron microscope. The epithelial cells express HLA-DR class II major histocompatibility complex molecules.

In samples obtained by bronchoalveolar lavage, a subset of patients has an excess of lymphocytes within the lower respiratory tract, and patients within this group are more likely to respond better to corticosteroid therapy than patients in whom granulocytes predominate. Lung lavage cells, evaluated using reverse haemolytic plaque assay, have been shown to be actively secreting immunoglobulins. In addition, lung lavage cells secrete more B-cell growth factor than control populations, and epithelial lining fluid contains high levels of immunoglobulin, particularly IgG and immune complexes.

Increases in one or more classes of immunoglobulins in the peripheral blood, are usually seen in fibrosing alveolitis, and approximately 45 per cent of patients have non-organ-specific autoantibodies in their serum (antinuclear antibodies or rheumatoid factor). In one series, antibodies to DNA topoisomerase II were found in 37 per cent of patients.

Taken together, the immunological data are consistent with immune mechanisms being important components of disease pathogenesis. There are many immunopathological features which are shared with autoimmune diseases at other sites, but at present there is no clear evidence that cryptogenic fibrosing alveolitis is an autoimmune disease restricted to the lung.

INFLAMMATORY RESPONSE

Macrophages

Mononuclear phagocytes are present in abundance within the lungs of patients with fibrosing alveolitis. Macrophages obtained by bronchoalveolar lavage spontaneously synthesize and secrete a lipid chemotactic factor for neutrophils which is uncharacterized but may be LTB4. More recent studies have shown that the expression of IL-8, a potent member of the chemokine family, is enhanced in patients with fibrosing alveolitis. Tumour necrosis factor α and IL-1 are produced by alveolar macrophages from patients with fibrosing alveolitis, and both these molecules may exert important effects on the vascular endothelium by increasing the expression of the adhesion molecules ICAM-1, E-selectin, and VCAM-1, all of which enhance the traffic of other inflammatory cells to disease sites.

The first and perhaps best-defined group of macrophage products which are believed to play important roles in the pathogenesis of fibrosing alveolitis are the growth factors. Spontaneous synthesis and secretion of fibronectin, platelet-derived growth factor, and insulin-like growth factor 1 provide the local environment for stimulation of resting (G_0) fibroblasts to proceed through the G_1, S, and G_2 phases of growth to cell division.

Granulocytes

Neutrophil polymorphonuclear leucocytes, through their packaged proteolytic enzymes, particularly neutrophil elastase and collagenase, and

Table 3 *Diseases associated with fibrosing alveolitis*

Rheumatological diseases
　Systemic sclerosis
　Rheumatoid arthritis
　Polymyositis/dermatomyositis
　Sjögren's syndrome
　Systemic lupus erythematosus
Chronic liver disease
　Chronic active hepatitis
　Primary biliary cirrhosis
Chronic inflammatory bowel disease
Renal tubular acidosis

their capacity to generate potent oxygen radicals, are capable of producing host tissue damage and there is evidence for their involvement in fibrosing alveolitis. They are present in increased numbers (up to 15-fold, particularly in smokers) in lung lavage samples, although they are less prominent in lung tissue, suggesting that there may be a chemotactic gradient such that neutrophils which have migrated from the vascular compartment proceed through the interstitium and into the air spaces. Epithelial lining fluid glutathione, a potent naturally occurring scavenger of oxygen radicals, is present in a predominantly oxidized form, and this is believed to be due largely to the generation of neutrophil oxygen radicals in the lower respiratory tract. The presence of neutrophil collagenase and myeloperoxidase in epithelial lining fluid would support the concept of neutrophil-induced damage playing a role in pathogenesis.

The role of eosinophils and mast cells is less clear, but both are present in increased numbers in the lung interstitium and are capable of inducing lung injury through release of their secretory products, particularly eosinophil cationic protein and vasoactive amines.

Fibrogenesis

Excess collagen is present within the lungs of patients with fibrosing alveolitis. Immunohistochemical studies have shown that this is predominantly type I and type III collagen, and that the presence of excess type III collagen (as opposed to type I) is associated with a more active disease process which is more amenable to therapy. Precise control of fibroblast and other connective tissue matrix cells and their secretory products almost certainly involves finely tuned cellular interrelationships involving cell–cell contact and cytokine production in the local microenvironment. A mediator which has received increasing attention recently is transforming growth factor β, which exists in a number of isoforms which are emerging as potent fibroblast chemotactants and stimulators of fibrogenesis.

Although injury and subsequent loss of lung tissue are irreversible, deposition of collagen is not an end stage process. There is clear evidence that collagen turnover takes place in both humans and animals; in animal models, approximately 10 per cent of lung collagen is turned over every day. Therefore it is relevant to concepts of therapy in humans to consider that control of collagen synthesis could result in an overall diminution in total lung collagen content and improved lung function.

Clinical features

HISTORY

A typical patient with cryptogenic fibrosing alveolitis will have a history of progressive breathlessness on exertion in the absence of wheeze. A dry cough may be present, but it is unusual for sputum to be produced until the later stages of the disease. Haemoptysis is uncommon and should suggest the development of lung malignancy which occurs with a 14-fold excess frequency by comparison with the general population. Chest pain is uncommon. Constitutional symptoms such as weight loss and lethargy are recognized.

A full occupational history (from school-leaving) is necessary to exclude inorganic dusts as the cause of fibrosing alveolitis. In particular, exposure to asbestos and hard metal can produce a disease which is indistinguishable from cryptogenic fibrosing alveolitis. Causes of extrinsic allergic alveolitis due to avian or fungal antigens, for example, should be sought; the chest radiography of the subacute (fibrosing) form of extrinsic allergic alveolitis can be confused with fibrosing alveolitis. It is important to obtain a history of other diseases, particularly the rheumatological disorders, because the prognosis of fibrosing alveolitis in the context of rheumatological disease is different from that of fibrosing alveolitis occurring alone (Table 3). Previous or current malignancy must be noted, particularly when cytotoxic therapy has been used. A full therapeutic drug history is required to exclude drug causes of fibrosing alveolitis (Table 2).

EXAMINATION

Digital clubbing is present in approximately 70 to 80 per cent of patients. In the respiratory system, the most striking observation is the presence of very fine crepitations, best heard at the lung bases or in the mid-axillary line, which occur at the end of inspiration in early cases but become paninspiratory in more advanced disease. The characteristic 'shower' of crepitations, typical of fibrosing alveolitis, is quite distinctive and, once heard, never mistaken. In the presence of more subtle disease, the crackles may disappear as the patient leans forward but usually persist in the mid-axillary line.

At more advanced stages of disease, central cyanosis may be evident, and the signs of right ventricular hypertrophy, pulmonary hypertension and cor pulmonale with parasternal heave, gallop rhythm, loud pulmonary second heart sound, raised jugular venous pressure, and ankle oedema may be present.

Examination may also reveal features that are consistent with other disease; in rheumatological disorders, arthropathy or the skin changes of systemic sclerosis or systemic lupus erythematosus may be observed. Full examination may also disclose features which would suggest that a provisional diagnosis of fibrosing alveolitis may be incorrect and another diffuse lung disease should be considered. Examples of this are the presence of mononeuritis multiplex or skin vasculitic lesions in necrotizing vasculitis, the presence of lupus pernio or erythema nodosum in sarcoidosis, or the occurrence of Kaposi's sarcoma together with a diffuse opportunistic lung infection in AIDS.

The key clinical and laboratory features of fibrosing alveolitis are shown in Table 4.

Investigations

RADIOLOGY

Chest radiography

A typical chest radiograph of a patient with cryptogenic fibrosing alveolitis is characterized by small lung fields and reticulonodular shadowing particularly at the periphery of the lung and at the bases, obscuring the right and left heart borders and making the diaphragmatic surfaces irregular (Fig. 1). This distribution of radiographic abnormality should suggest the diagnosis, even in more subtle examples of fibrosing alveolitis. In more advanced cases, all lung zones are involved, at which point evidence of honeycomb shadowing may be present.

Rarely, the chest radiograph may be normal or present a diffuse 'ground-glass' pattern. This pattern is highly suggestive of a more cellular pathological process, and is the typical finding in the desquamative interstitial pneumonia form of diffuse parenchymal lung disease. Lymphadenopathy is rarely observed with chest radiography, and the presence of pleural disease should suggest an alternative diagnosis. Cardiomegaly and prominent pulmonary arteries indicate secondary pulmonary hypertension.

Table 4 *Key clinical and laboratory features of fibrosing alveolitis*

Physical examination
    Digital clubbing
    Fine mid- to end-inspiratory crackles
Radiographic
    Chest radiograph: small lung volumes; peripheral, basal
       reticulonodular shadowing
    CT: peripheral, subpleural increase in attenuation
Physiological
    Restrictive ventilatory defect
    Reduced gas transfer
    Reduced lung compliance
    Low/normal Pao_2 at rest
    Low/normal $Paco_2$ at rest
    Widening of A-a gradient and fall in Pao_2 on exercise
Bronchoalveolar lavage
    Excess numbers of eosinophils and/or neutrophil
       polymorphonuclear leucocytes

High resolution computed tomography

The use of high resolution CT has revolutionized the approach to diffuse parenchymal lung disease over the last 5 years. The pattern of abnormality may be characteristic in a number of diffuse parenchymal lung diseases and is virtually pathognomonic in cryptogenic fibrosing alveolitis. Typical early changes are of a peripheral rim of increased attenuation present posteriorly at the bases. In more cellular disease this assumes a ground-glass pattern (Fig. 2), but in more fibrotic destroyed lung the pattern is reticular (Fig. 3). As disease becomes more extensive, these changes are observed in the other lung zones and more centrally.

Fig. 1 Chest radiograph of a patient with advanced fibrosing alveolitis. The small lung fields with obscured right and left heart borders and both hemidiaphragms should be noted.

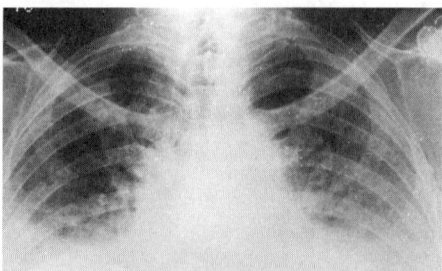

Fig. 2 High resolution CT of the lungs of a patient with fibrosing alveolitis. The widespread ground-glass opacification, denoting a more cellular histopathological pattern of disease, should be noted.

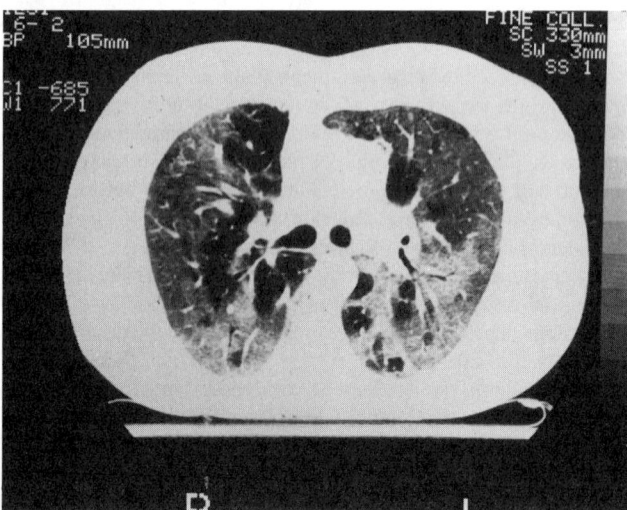

CT confirms that pleural disease is not present in fibrosing alveolitis but, in contrast with the observation on plain chest radiography, mediastinal lymphadenopathy is commonly present.

In more subtle cases, it is important to perform both prone and supine scans to exclude the contribution of gravity to the radiographic appearances due to vascular and interstitial pooling in the dependent areas.

RADIONUCLIDE IMAGING

Ventilation–perfusion scans

Ventilation–perfusion scans show mismatching of perfusion and ventilation in fibrosing alveolitis, probably reflecting damage to the pulmonary vascular bed. This means that ventilation–perfusion imaging is completely unreliable in excluding thromboembolic disease in fibrosing alveolitis. This is important because there is an increased incidence of pulmonary embolus in this disease, and therefore the diagnosis of pulmonary embolus will rely on the clinical features, identification of the venous source of emboli, and in some instances pulmonary angiography to identify proximal embolic lesions.

Gallium scanning

Gallium scanning is a useful technique for identifying the presence of subtle parenchymal lung disease when routine chest radiography is normal. It is a highly sensitive test but is not specific, as it is positive in a wide range of diffuse processes which involve macrophage activation. However, in the presence of defined disease gallium scanning adds nothing to the information obtained using other tests.

In attempts to measure degrees of activity, there have been reports of quantification of gallium uptake into the lungs in parenchymal lung disease. However, these measures are not universally reliable, and the test involves an expensive isotope and requires the patient to visit the hospital on two occasions (one visit for intravenous isotope administration and a second visit 2 to 3 days later to scan the lungs). Therefore the technique should be restricted to patients in whom other tests have failed to confirm a pulmonary problem but in whom disease is still suspected. It is not recommended for established fibrosing alveolitis.

Other radionuclide techniques

Other techniques of radionuclide imaging are the subject of research. Of these the clearance from the lung of inhaled $^{99}Tc^m$-DTPA may prove to be of value, not just in identifying early disease but also in identifying a group of patients whose disease will run a more stable non-progressive course, i.e. those with normal clearance. The clearance of isotope is dependent upon the integrity of the epithelial barrier and therefore anything which disrupts this, either inflammation or fibrosis, will increase the rate of clearance. It is highly sensitive; cigarette smoking will pro-

Fig. 3 High resolution CT of the lungs of a patient with fibrosing alveolitis. The predominantly peripheral abnormality should be noted. In the left lung the disease process is more extensive and has a reticular pattern indicative of a more fibrotic disease process.

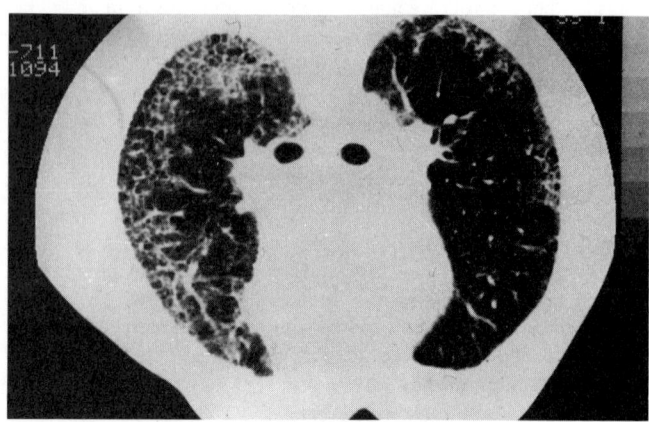

duce increased clearance rates, and therefore the test is only of value in non-smokers or those who have given up smoking for at least a month prior to assessment. However, the role of DTPA in routine clinical management needs to be further defined.

Imaging with ^{111}In-labelled neutrophils is being used in research studies to demonstrate neutrophil traffic to the lungs. ^{111}In-labelled transferrin is also being explored as a measure of pulmonary vascular leak. Positron emission tomography has been used to identify increased metabolic activity within the lung in fibrosing alveolitis. The role of magnetic resonance imaging in identifying early inflammation in the lung is also being investigated. All these techniques hold immense promise and may establish themselves in the future as routine investigations in fibrosing alveolitis. At present, however, they should be reserved for research studies.

LUNG FUNCTION TESTS

Fibrosing alveolitis is characterized by a restrictive ventilatory defect of mechanical function, resulting in reduced pulmonary compliance, vital capacity, and total lung capacity. Residual volume is usually decreased unless there is coincident airflow obstruction due to cigarette smoking and lung recoil pressure is increased.

Carbon monoxide transfer factor (a measure of diffusion capacity) is reduced and may be the only abnormality in early disease. In the majority of patients the gas transfer measurement adjusted for alveolar volume is also reduced, indicating that the total gas transfer depression is not purely attributable to decreased lung volumes but, rather, indicates that the capacity to exchange gas is impaired even in the remaining lung.

Typical blood gas measurements will reveal a reduced PaO_2 value with a normal or low $PaCO_2$ measurement. In more advanced cases, $PaCO_2$ will be reduced because of the increase in ventilatory drive in a patient with more severe lung stiffening due to fibrosis, but in terminal stages carbon dioxide may arise. The low PaO_2 is largely attributable to ventilation–perfusion mismatching. On exercise, hypoxaemia is exacerbated and a widening of the alveolar–arterial (A-a) gradient is observed. Infrequently, these are the only physiological abnormalities observed, but usually there is already some abnormality in the gas transfer measurement at rest by the time that the patient seeks advice.

In a small percentage of patients, there is evidence of airflow obstruction on routine lung function assessment. This is usually due to the coexistence of emphysema due to cigarette smoking—a common habit in patients with fibrosing alveolitis. A clue to the presence of dual pathologies is the chest radiograph which generally reveals relatively preserved lung volumes in the face of a disproportionately depressed gas transfer measurement. Gas transfer is reduced by both the emphysematous and the fibrosing processes, whereas lung volumes will tend to be increased by emphysema but reduced by fibrosis, and these two opposing influences result in relatively normal-sized lungs radiographically.

Lung function measurements should be made sequentially to assess the progression of the disease process. Vital capacity and gas transfer measurements will usually suffice, and it is generally unnecessary to perform exercise tests as monitors of change in disease. It is often sensible to plot serial lung function studies in order to visualize more gradual change which may be missed if results are compared only with the previous set of measurements.

BLOOD TESTS

Blood tests are of little value in the diagnosis of fibrosing alveolitis. In severe cases, secondary polycythaemia may be observed and a high neutrophil count may indicate superadded infection. Corticosteroid therapy will elevate the total white count to $(13-14) \times 10^9/l$.

Elevations may be seen in one or more classes of immunoglobulins, particularly IgG and IgM, and rheumatoid factor or antinuclear antibody may be present in abnormal titres in approximately 45 per cent of patients, but neither of these immunological assessments is specific. It is noteworthy that the titres of autoantibodies rarely approach those seen in the acute rheumatological diseases. Interestingly, in one study the presence of anti-DNA topoisomerase II was found in over a third of patients, but the significance of this is unclear at present.

It is helpful to perform precipitin tests against the fungal antigens which produce diseases such as farmer's lung or the avian antigens which can provoke budgerigar or pigeon fancier's lung in cases where there is a history of significant antigen exposure or where there may be doubt about relevant exposures.

BRONCHOALVEOLAR LAVAGE

Bronchoalveolar lavage has been used for almost 20 years to sample cells and non-cellular material from the lower respiratory tract in the evaluation of parenchymal lung disease. Initial hopes that this would provide an alternative to lung biopsy with high specificity for diagnosis have not been realized. However, there is still a place for bronchoalveolar lavage in the evaluation of parenchymal lung disease. The presence of abnormal numbers of granulocytes, particularly neutrophils and eosinophils, is typical for a patient with cryptogenic fibrosing alveolitis or rheumatoid lung disease, asbestosis, and the adult respiratory distress syndrome. Excess lymphocytes are associated with granulomatous diseases and drug-induced causes of lung disease. Therefore the predominant inflammatory cell provides a useful indication of the nature of the underlying disease process, particularly when the diagnosis is not clear. It can also alert the physician that a provisional diagnosis may be erroneous if the lavage produces a high percentage of cells not normally found in that condition.

The prognostic value of bronchoalveolar lavage findings is uncertain. The presence of excess granulocytes, as opposed to lymphocytes, may be associated with a poorer response to treatment and prognosis. The use of serial bronchoalveolar lavage as a monitor of disease is unhelpful and should be reserved for research purposes.

In a typical patient with fibrosing alveolitis, bronchoalveolar lavage would produce an increase in total cell returns of three- to sixfold (up to 6×10^5/ml of fluid return) and up to 20 per cent may be neutrophils or eosinophils. Excess lymphocytes may be found (up to 20 per cent of the total cells) and an increase in mast cells may be observed in a small percentage of patients.

LUNG BIOPSY

The only lung biopsy technique which provides useful information is open-lung biopsy through either minithoracotomy or video-assisted thoracoscopic biopsy. Transbronchial biopsy is generally unhelpful. Adequate samples are obtained in only about 35 per cent of instances using this technique. They are small, and do not allow an assessment to be made of the relative degrees of cellularity and fibrosis which is important in assessing the probable response to treatment. A trephine drill biopsy technique has been used in the past in some units, but this has now fallen into disuse. A Trucut biopsy is hazardous as it carries the risk of uncontrolled haemorrhage and air leak.

The more open approaches have the advantage of sampling lung which is clearly abnormal, and the specificity of this approach can be improved when CT is used to guide the surgeon to the relevant sites. The surgeon may sample one or more sites and the biopsy can be divided into parts which will be stored, if necessary, for immunohistochemical, molecular, and electron microscopic analysis in addition to the more routine histological evaluation.

Management

No specific treatment or prevention will be available for cryptogenic fibrosing alveolitis until its cause and pathogenesis are understood. Until then the most important issues with regard to management are as follows.

1. Should lung biopsy confirmation of the diagnosis be obtained before treatment is started?
2. When should treatment be commenced?
3. Which drugs should be used?
4. How long should treatment continue?

SELECTION OF PATIENTS FOR TREATMENT

By the time that a patient presents with an increase in breathlessness, a considerable proportion of lung functional capacity has already been lost. Diseases affecting the acinar regions of the lungs produce piece-meal reductions in lung function which may not be perceived by the patient because there is considerable pulmonary reserve capacity. Lungs which are capable of producing adequate gas exchange to run marathons are not put to this test by the average patient who therefore presents to the physician only when normal daily activities are impeded by breath-lessness. By the time that this stage has been reached, it may not be possible to improve function because the disease involves injury and fibrosis which are essentially irreversible. In this situation, the best that can be achieved is often only stabilization of the disease.

Detection of early disease at a time when symptoms are trivial or absent would provide the opportunity to prevent the disease advancing to the stage of symptoms, but treatment at this stage would only be justifiable if reliable predictors of disease progression could be developed to justify the use of potentially toxic drugs at a stage before the onset of symptoms. It is now being shown that the appearance of the lungs on high resolution CT scanning can predict the degree of the inflammatory (and therefore potentially reversible) component in lung biopsies, and this may prove to be of help in deciding whether to start treatment. Other imaging techniques, including ^{99}Tc^m-DTPA scanning, are being explored for their value as predictors of disease progression and show promise.

The author's present policy is to start treatment if the patient is symptomatic or shows evidence of disease progression without symptoms. Prospective clinical trials will be needed to confirm whether the presence of a particular pattern on CT (ground-glass, suggesting inflammatory histology, or reticular, suggesting more fibrotic histology) is sufficiently predictive of active disease to justify commencing therapy. Similar studies of the predictive value of ^{99}Tc^m-DTPA will be needed but preliminary work has suggested that a reticular CT together with a normal ^{99}Tc^m-DTPA clearance may be predictive of stable disease, in which situation an expectant policy can be followed with more confidence. However, awaiting the development of progressive symptoms before treating the patient often allows the disease to advance to a stage at which improvement in symptoms cannot be achieved.

THE NEED FOR OPEN-LUNG BIOPSY

A decision to perform open-lung biopsy depends upon assessment of the individual case. A patient over the age of 65 with poor lung function, particularly with hypoxia at rest, is at high risk of any operative procedure. Under these circumstances, it is reasonable to make a clinical diagnosis, particularly with the more sensitive imaging provided by CT. However, with a younger patient, for whom prolonged treatment with potentially toxic drugs is being considered, it is important to establish a clear diagnosis before treatment is commenced. It is often argued that the treatment options will be the same with or without biopsy confirmation of the diagnosis and therefore that biopsy changes little. This policy would be acceptable if empirical treatment always produced an improvement, but when the reverse is the case the next step in management is more difficult. This is made worse if drug-induced side-effects have developed, particularly those related to high dose corticosteroid therapy. A clear diagnosis, confirmed by biopsy, allows the clinician and patient to discuss fully the implications of the disease process, to develop a clear treatment plan, and to weigh up the advantages and disadvantages of treatment.

Treatment

ESTABLISHED DRUG REGIMENS

There is now extensive experience of three regimens of therapy in fibrosing alveolitis, but there have been few coordinated clinical trials of treatment. Therefore data on the efficacy of therapy are derived largely from individual series.

Corticosteroids

An objective response to corticosteroid therapy, defined as an improvement in chest radiography or lung function tests, occurs in only a quarter of all cases reported in the literature. A subjective improvement is obtained in just over 50 per cent of treated individuals, but this is generally short lived. The factors which predict a good response to corticosteroids include a patient with less dyspnoea, less radiographic abnormality, better Pao_2 at presentation, an excess of lymphocytes obtained by bronchoalveolar lavage, and a more cellular open-lung biopsy. All these features would suggest early disease.

Treatment is generally commenced at a dosage of 1 mg/kg/day to a maximum of 80 mg/day. This should be continued for 6 weeks. If the disease has either stabilized or improved, dosage can be reduced by 5 mg/day every 7 days, aiming to hold the patient at 20 mg of prednisolone every other day for a minimum of 1 year before contemplating further dosage reduction. These high doses over prolonged times can only be tolerated in younger patients. Side-effects limit the use of prednisolone in the elderly, and an alternative regimen including other drugs is preferred.

If there is no response to corticosteroids or if deterioration occurs during dosage reduction, treatment should be replaced with a combination of prednisolone and an immunosuppressant. Treatment with pulses of methyl prednisolone have been used in some cases, but the value of this approach is unproven.

Corticosteroids and cyclophosphamide

Two regimens are being used with some success in fibrosing alveolitis. A combination of prednisolone 20 mg on alternate days with cyclophosphamide (up to 125 mg/day depending upon body weight) has been tested in a prospective controlled study comparing this regimen with high dosage corticosteroids. Objective response was found in approximately 20 per cent of patients, which is a similar response rate to that with corticosteroids alone. However, a small percentage of those who failed to respond to corticosteroids showed a response to the corticosteroid–cyclophosphamide regimen. The mortality at 5 years was not significantly different between the two treatment groups—approximately 50 per cent. A placebo group was not included.

If disease is stabilized or improved by prednisolone 20 mg on alternate days plus cyclophosphamide 125 mg daily, this regimen should be continued for 1 year. Maximum improvement may not be seen until after 6 months of treatment. Cyclophosphamide toxicity should be monitored by weekly full blood counts and dipstick urine testing for haematuria for the first month, following which the interval between blood counts can be extended. Urine testing should continue weekly. A small number of patients will develop abnormal liver function tests, sometimes associated with dyspeptic symptomatology which resolves on discontinuing therapy.

If the disease has become stable or improved at the end of 1 year's treatment, consideration should be given to discontinuing cyclophosphamide by a stepwise reduction of 25 mg every 2 to 3 months.

Pulsed cyclophosphamide has been tried in an attempt to stabilize disease, but has not been shown to provide better response than oral regimens.

Corticosteroids with azathioprine

A recent study has suggested that a combination of azathioprine with prednisolone conferred better response, defined as physiological improvement (gas exchange) and improved survival, than prednisolone alone, although the small numbers in the study prevented these differences from reaching statistical significance. The dosages used were high: prednisolone was commenced at 1.5 mg/kg/day and increased to a maximum of 100 mg/day for the first 2 weeks followed by a taper every 2 weeks to a maintenance dosage of 20 mg/day. Azathioprine was administered at 3 mg/kg/day up to a maximum of 200 mg/day. A lower dosage combination of prednisolone 20 mg on alternate days with azathioprine up to 150 mg/day has been reported, more anecdotally, to improve the disease in some patients.

Other treatment regimens

Other drugs which have been used to treat fibrosing alveolitis include penicillamine and cyclosporin. There are no good data to support the clinical efficacy of penicillamine.

However, it is a logical approach to attempt to improve lung function by using a drug which blocks collagen cross-linking, thereby inhibiting the deposition of collagen with high tensile strength. Occasional individual responses to this drug would support this logic but most patients do not respond.

Cyclosporin A, which blocks T-cell activation by inhibiting IL-2 gene upregulation, is an attractive option in view of the known involvement of the immune system in pathogenesis. A pilot study of a small number of patients has recently been reported, and this confirms that cyclosporin up to 7 mg/kg/day given with a small dosage of prednisolone improves patients with a more cellular disease process. This drug has not been the subject of more extensive clinical trials.

TRANSPLANTATION

Single-lung transplantation is now the organ replacement therapy of choice for end-stage fibrosing alveolitis. The procedure has not been used for a sufficiently long period to provide information about long-term survival, but approximately 60 per cent of all patients are alive at 1 year. A major complication of lung transplantation is the development of progressive obliterative bronchiolitis, and if this complication can be controlled it would seem likely that survival figures will improve considerably.

At present the shortfall in organs precludes many patients from being considered for transplantation, and with the majority of patients with fibrosing alveolitis presenting between the ages of 50 and 60 this reduces the numbers of patients for whom transplantation is likely to be an option.

SUPPORTIVE THERAPY

When all treatment options have failed, supportive therapy is necessary. Supplemental oxygen may be required and this can be provided in the home through oxygen concentrators. Diuretics may be necessary and infection should be treated promptly. In the more terminal phases, small dosages of opiates have been shown to suppress the sensation of extreme breathlessness which occurs as the lungs become much less compliant.

MONITORING OF TREATMENT

Patients should be seen 2 to 3 months after commencing treatment. At present treatment response is assessed using a measure of change of symptoms together with changes in chest radiograph and lung function tests. Some centres perform exercise lung function studies, but these add little to a full series of lung function tests at rest provided by a laboratory with good quality control. This applies particularly to measurement of gas exchange which must be assessed together with blood gases at each visit because the measurement of lung volumes alone may fail to identify change (improvement or progression). Simple spirometry is certainly not sensitive enough to be used as a monitor of disease. Of the three indices of change (symptoms, chest radiography, and lung function test-

ing), changes in lung function are the most reliably quantifiable and when measures of volume or gas transfer have improved or deteriorated by 15 per cent this provides unequivocal evidence of disease response or progression. The situation in which there is a change in lung function measurements by less than this percentage coupled with equivocal radiographic change is more difficult. In this situation the clinician does not know whether the disease has been stabilized by therapy or has not been affected by therapy and was already in a stable phase. Under these circumstances, in the absence of a 'run-in' period before treatment was commenced which would provide information about the progression of the disease, it is safest to assume that treatment has produced a stabilizing effect and to continue therapy unless the presence of significant side-effects precludes this approach. Newer indices of disease may enhance our ability to detect change. In this regard CT is a more sensitive radiographic modality than chest radiography, and it is likely that it will be possible to determine change in disease extent more definitively by comparison of equivalent CT sections obtained before and after treatment than by using chest radiography alone. CT has yet to be established as a monitor of parenchymal lung disorders, however, and controlled studies will be needed to see whether it has a role in monitoring disease progression.

Other indices which have been used to try to assess response to therapy have included gallium scanning and bronchoalveolar lavage. Gallium scanning quantification can be difficult to achieve, and for this reason and the reasons mentioned above this technique is no longer used in most centres. Monitoring changes in differential counts of cells removed by bronchoalveolar lavage has proved to be unhelpful in most patients. However, in some patients the percentage of neutrophils has been shown to fall after treatment, but this only occurs in those who have unequivocal chest radiographic or physiological measurement evidence of response to treatment. Neutrophil percentages can remain abnormal but unchanged in patients whose other indices have remained stable. It is possible that newer indices of cell activation using cellular and molecular biological approaches may enhance the utility of serial lavage as a monitor, although this has yet to be proven. In general, these other indices provide no information over and above that obtained by radiographic imaging and lung function testing.

DURATION OF TREATMENT

The optimal duration of treatment of fibrosing alveolitis has yet to be defined. It can be argued that the most logical approach is to try and achieve disease stability, maintain that stability on a dosage of therapy which is acceptable for a period of a year, and then to discontinue treatment if disease stability is maintained. However, it is known that the cessation of therapy may result in a rebound of activation of disease in some patients which then does not come under control even with the recommencement of therapy which had previously been shown to be efficacious. In practice, therefore, attempts are made to reduce the prednisolone dosage to 15 or 10 mg on alternate days and to continue this indefinitely.

Prolonged use of immunosuppressant therapy has been associated with the development of malignancy, although this has not been proved in the context of treating fibrosing lung disease. None the less, this potential complication should encourage the clinician to try and withdraw immunosuppression after a year provided that the disease is stable; corticosteroids should be continued. It is encouraging, in this regard, to note that patients who have had to discontinue immunosuppressant therapy because of side-effects usually maintain the improvement produced by this therapy after the drug had been stopped provided that the maintenance corticosteroid dosage is continued.

SUGGESTED TREATMENT PLAN

The main lines of treatment of fibrosing alveolitis (Table 5) are prednisolone up to 80 mg/day for 6 weeks, prednisolone 20 mg on alternate

Table 5 *Treatment of fibrosing alveolitis—first-line options*

Drug(s) dosage	Length of initial treatment	Taper regimen
Prednisolone 1 mg/kg/day (max. 80/mg)	6 weeks	5 mg/week until 20 mg on alternate days
Prednisolone 20 mg on alternate days AND cyclophosphamide 100 mg/day (< 65 kg) 125 mg/day (>65 kg)	6–12 months	Cyclophosphamide 25 mg reductions every 2–3 months
Prednisolone 20 mg on alternate days AND Azathioprine 2.5 mg/kg/day (max. 150 mg)	6–12 months	Azathioprine 25 mg reductions every 2–3 months

days plus cyclophosphamide 2 mg/kg/day up to a maximum of 125 mg/day, or prednisolone 20 mg on alternate days plus azathioprine 2.5 mg/kg/day up to a maximum of 150 mg per day.

The final decision on first-choice treatment depends upon a number of factors.

1. The potential for side-effects. In an obese diabetic hypertensive patient high dose prednisolone may provoke unacceptable side-effects, and a combination regimen would be preferable. In contrast, for an individual of childbearing years, high dosage prednisolone may be preferred in view of the risk of inhibition of ovulation by cyclophosphamide, a side-effect which is often irreversible. The regimen best tolerated is generally prednisolone and azathioprine.

2. The speed of response. Prednisolone will produce a maximum improvement approximately 6 weeks after the start of therapy, whereas the combination therapy may require 3 to 6 months to see the maximum effect. If the deterioration in the patient's condition is rapid, high dose prednisolone would be the treatment of choice.

3. The patient's opinion. The pros and cons of all treatment options must be discussed with the patient and his or her views taken into account before a final decision is made.

If first-line treatment fails to produce an improvement or results in deterioration, one of the alternative options should be tried. If one form of combination therapy fails, it is worth trying the other combination because occasionally a response is seen with one immunosuppressant when treatment with the other has failed. If all three options fail, a decision must be made about transplantation, and if this is not realistic because of complicating disease in other organs or other contraindications, supportive therapy, including social support, must be provided.

Prognosis

In all series, 50 per cent of all patients are dead within 5 years of presentation despite therapy. In the United Kingdom, death rates from fibrosing alveolitis are increasing and are now approaching 1500 per annum. Improved survival is determined largely by those factors which predict good response to therapy. If prognosis is to be improved, new management strategies need to be devised. For the reasons indicated, the detection of early disease is important. Furthermore, disease which is regarded as 'trivial' on chest radiography still merits further investigation using more sensitive techniques even in asymptomatic patients. In this regard more sensitive investigations such as CT and radionuclide imaging are likely to play an increasing role because it is now well

recognized that symptoms and chest radiography are not sensitive indices of disease extent or prognosis. If early detection can be combined with good indicators of progression, a much more logical approach to treatment will be achieved using currently available drugs given at an earlier time point or newer more targeted treatments as they become available.

REFERENCES
Clinical overview

Carrington, C.B., Gaensler, E.A., and Coutu, R.E. (1978). Natural history and treated course of usual and desquamative interstitial pneumonia. *New England Journal of Medicine*, **298**, 801–9.

Crystal, R.G., Fulmer, J.D., and Roberts, W.C. (1976). Idiopathic pulmonary fibrosis. *Annals of Internal Medicine*, **85**, 769–88.

Panos, R.J. and King, T.E., Jr. (1991). Idiopathic pulmonary fibrosis. In: *Immunologically mediated pulmonary diseases* (ed J.P. Lynch III and R.A. DeRemee), p. 1. J.B. Lippincott, Philadelphia, PA.

Turner-Warwick, M., Burrows, B., and Johnson, A. (1980). Cryptogenic fibrosing alveolitis: clinical features and their influence on survival. *Thorax*, **35**, 171–80.

Pathology

Corrin, B. (ed). (1990). *Systemic pathology*, Vol. 5, *The lungs* (3rd edn), p. 201. Churchill Livingstone, London.

Hamman, L. and Rich, A.R. (1944). Acute diffuse interstitial fibrosis of the lungs. *Bulletin of the Johns Hopkins Hospital*, **74**, 177–212.

Liebow, A.A. (1975). Definition and classification of interstitial pneumonias in human pathology. In: *Progress in respiratory research*, Vol. 8, *Alveolar interstitium of the lung* (ed H. Herzog), p. 1. Busel, Karger.

Scadding, J.G. and Hinson, K.F.W. (1967). Diffuse fibrosing alveolitis (diffuse interstitial fibrosis of the lungs). *Thorax*, **22**, 291–304.

Pathogenesis

Crystal, R.G., Ferrans, V.J., and Basset, F. (1992). Biologic basis of pulmonary fibrosis. In: *Lung injury* (ed R.G. Crystal and J.B. West), p. 271. Raven Press, New York.

Turner-Warwick M. (1978). *Current topics in immunology series*, No. 10. *Immunology of the lung*, p. 216. Edward Arnold, London.

Imaging

Hansell, D.M. and Kerr, I.H. (1991). The role of high resolution computed tomography in the diagnosis of interstitial lung disease. *Thorax*, **46**, 77–84.

Muller, N.L., Miller, R.R., Webb, W.R., Evans, K.G., and Ostrow, D.N.

(1986). Fibrosing alveolitis: CT pathologic correlation. *Radiology*, **160**, 585–8.

Bronchoalveolar lavage

Haslam, P.L., Turton, C.W.G., Lukoszek, A., Salsbury, A.J., Dewar, A., Collins, J.V., *et al.* (1980). Bronchoalveolar lavage fluid cell counts and cryptogenic fibrosing alveolitis and their relation to therapy. *Thorax*, **35**, 328–9.

Weinberger, S.E., Kelman, J.A., and Elson, N.A. (1978). Bronchoalveolar lavage in interstitial lung disease. *Annals of Internal Medicine*, **89**, 459–66.

Treatment

Johnson, M.A., Kwan, S., Snell, N.J.C., Nunn, A.J., Darbyshire, J.H., *et al.* (1989). Randomized controlled trial comparing prednisolone alone with cyclophosphamide and low dose prednisolone in combination in cryptogenic fibrosing alveolitis. *Thorax*, **44**, 280–8.

Raghu, G., DePaso, W.J., Cain, K., Hammar, S.P., Wetzel, C.E., *et al.* (1991). Azathioprine combined with prednisolone in the treatment of idiopathic pulmonary fibrosis: a prospective double blind randomized placebo controlled clinical trial. *American Review of Respiratory Disease*, **144**, 291–6.

Prognosis

Turner-Warwick, M., Burrows, B., and Johnson, A. (1980). Cryptogenic fibrosing alveolitis: response to corticosteroid treatment and its effect on survival. *Thorax*, **35**, 593–9.

Watters, L.C., King, T.E., and Schwartz, M.I. (1986). A clinical, radiographic and physiologic scoring system for the longitudinal assessment of patients with idiopathic pulmonary fibrosis. *American Review of Respiratory Disease*, **133**, 97–103.

Wells, A.U., Hansell, D.M., Corrin, B., Harrison, N.K., Goldstraw, P., Black, C.M., and du Bois, R.M. (1992). High resolution computed tomography as a predictor of lung histology in systemic sclerosis. *Thorax*, **47**, 738–42.

17.10.3 Bronchiolitis obliterans

J. M. HOPKIN

Obliteration by abnormal tissue of bronchiolar lumina was observed as a histological entity as long ago as 1901, but useful clinical observations and correlates emerged only in the 1970s. Despite some controversy

Fig. 1 Cryptogenic organizing pneumonia (or bronchiolitis obliterans with organizing pneumonia): photomicrograph of tissue from an open-lung biopsy shows fibrous tissue and inflammatory cell infiltration obliterating the bronchioles and extending to the alveoli.

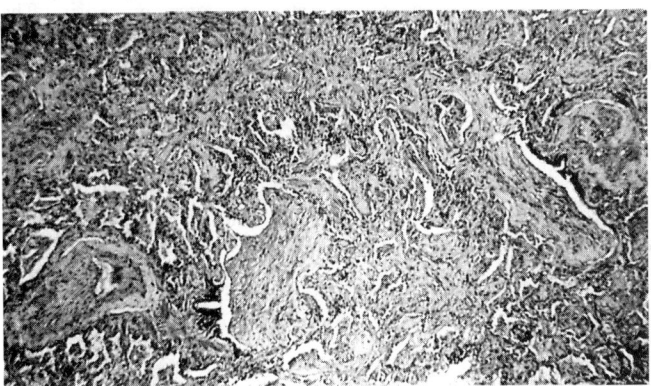

over clinicopathological clinical correlates and classifications, bronchiolitis obliterans is now recognized to occur in two distinct syndromes.

1. Bronchiolitis obliterans with organizing pneumonia (BOOP), otherwise known as cryptogenic organizing pneumonia (COP): in this, the bronchiolitis obliterans is part of a more major process affecting the alveoli and interstitium and the characteristic ventilatory defect is restrictive.
2. Constrictive bronchiolitis obliterans: in this the histological changes are confined to the small airways and are associated with a progressive obstructive ventilatory defect.

Bronchiolitis obliterans with organizing pneumonia or cryptogenic organizing pneumonia

In this syndrome buds or polyps of fibrous tissue, occurring patchily in the bronchioles and causing partial obstruction, extend into the alveolar sacs and are associated with a variable degree of interstitial inflammation and fibrosis (Fig. 1). Inflammatory cells, including lymphocytes, plasma cells, and also some neutrophils and eosinophils, aggregate within the fibrous tissue buds and tracts.

Such pathological features have been recorded with a variety of pul-

Fig. 2 Cryptogenic organizing pneumonia (or bronchiolitis obliterans with organizing pneumonia): (a) plain chest radiograph and (b) CT of the thorax showing scattered peripheral pneumonic changes in an 80-year-old man who presented with influenza-like illness, cough, and dyspnoea. There were scattered crackles, a restrictive ventilatory defect, and hypoxaemia. No response followed antibiotic regimens over 1 month, but oral corticosteroids produced prompt, sustained improvement.

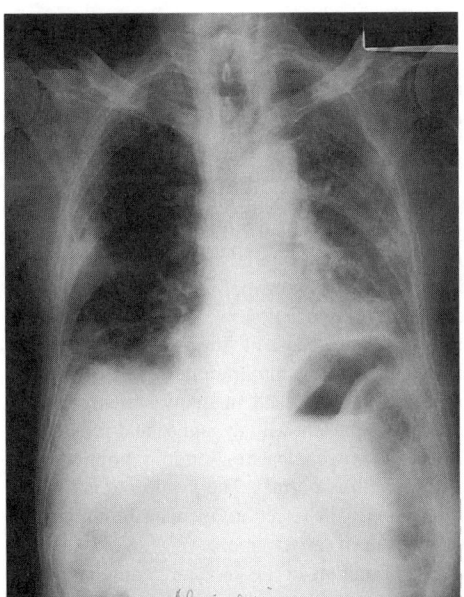

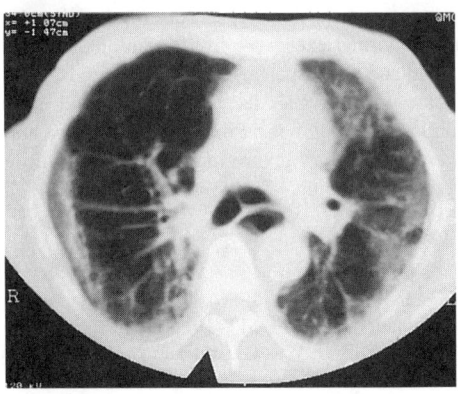

monary insults or disorders including adult respiratory distress syndrome, organizing infections (e.g. *Pneumocystis carinii*, *Mycoplasma pneumoniae*, and viral infections), inhalation of toxic agents, and extrinsic allergic alveolitis. The distribution of the disease may be focal or diffuse, and in some instances the histological changes may be seen as a 'reaction' adjacent to a lung abscess, area of pulmonary vasculitis, infarct, or other conditions.

Idiopathic bronchiolitis obliterans with organizing pneumonia or cryptogenic organizing pneumonia is a well-recognized syndrome that often appears to follow an upper respiratory tract infection and presents as a subacute influenza-like illness with variable fever and malaise, cough, and dyspnoea. Crackles are audible on auscultation in most cases, and there is a restrictive pulmonary ventilatory defect with hypoxaemia. Chest radiograph abnormalities are typically multiple and may be fleeting, but local and diffuse changes are also well recognized; in half the cases CT of the thorax shows a strikingly peripheral distribution of changes (Fig. 2). There is no response to antibiotics. Indeed, this failure of response of an apparently infective illness is often the first clinical clue to the diagnosis of cryptogenic organizing pneumonia. Peripheral blood eosinophilia and autoantibodies are absent; there are no diagnostic 'blood test' abnormalities. Response to corticosteroids is good, and these can be slowly tapered over 6 to 12 months. Therefore the initial dilemma is whether to introduce corticosteroids for what clinically appeared to be an infective illness. It is generally recommended that fibreoptic bronchoscopic lavage, to allow culture of deep lung samples, is the minimum needed to exclude continuing bacterial infection. Most physicians proceed to a diagnostic open-lung biopsy. The long-term outlook is good, but over-rapid tapering of the corticosteroid dosage can lead to relapse.

Constrictive bronchiolitis obliterans

In this syndrome, there is chronic bronchiolar inflammation with concentric bronchiolar luminal narrowing, submucosal fibrous thickening, and mucostasis. These features may also be seen in response to a range of pulmonary insults, but the chief clinical associations of constrictive bronchiolitis obliterans are rejection of a pulmonary allograft, as a complication of rheumatoid disease, as a result of viral infection in childhood (particularly by adenovirus), and following inhalation and injury from gases that include nitrogen dioxide, ammonia, and chlorine. In some cases there is no evident cause or association.

Bronchiolitis obliterans is a major cause of illness and death on current lung and heart–lung transplantation programmes. Half of patients develop the syndrome after 3 months, and in many series mortality approaches 50 per cent. Patients present with dyspnoea and progressive airflow obstruction; arterial oxygen haemoglobin saturations are reduced, but the chest radiograph is normal. The syndrome is thought to be due to chronic or repeated graft rejection; increased immunosuppression may occasionally result in improvement.

Constrictive bronchiolitis obliterans occurs as a rare complication of rheumatoid disease often in women of 50 to 60 years of age; presentation is with dyspnoea. Lung function tests show typical obstructive changes and the chest radiograph is normal except for hyperinflation. The disorder is usually progressive and not responsive to corticosteroids.

Although the syndrome in postviral disease in childhood may improve or remit, the outlook is often poor. Progressive dyspnoea and airflow obstruction towards respiratory failure may develop with little or no useful response to corticosteroids.

REFERENCES

Burke, C.M., Baldwin, J.C., and Morris, A.J. (1986). Twenty-eight cases of human heart-lung transplantation. *Lancet* **i**, 517–19.

Davison, A.G., Heard, B.E., McAllister, W.A.C., and Turner-Warwick, M.

(1983). Cryptogenic organizing pneumonitis. *Quarterly Journal of Medicine*, **52**, 382–94.

du Bois, R.M. and Geddes, G.M. (1991). Obliterative bronchiolitis, cryptogenic organizing pneumonitis, and bronchiolitis obliterans or bronchiolitis obliterans organizing pneumonia: three names for two different conditions. *European Respiratory Journal*, **4**, 774–5.

Epler, G.R. (1988). Bronchiolitis obliterans and airways obstruction associated with graft-versus-host disease. *Clinics in Chest Medicine*, **9**, 551–6.

Epler, G.R., Colby, T.V., McLoud, T.C., Carrington, C.B., and Gaensler, E.A. (1985). Bronchiolitis obliterans organizing pneumonia. *New England Journal of Medicine*, **312**, 152–8.

Geddes, D.M. (1991) BOOP and COP. *Thorax*, **46**, 545–7.

Geddes, D.M., Corrin, B., Brewerton, D.A., David, R.J., and Turner-Warwick, M. (1977). Progressive airway obliteration in adults and its association with rheumatoid disease. *Quarterly Journal of Medicine*, **46**, 427–44.

Gosink, B.B., Friedman, P.J., and Liebow, A.A. (1973). Bronchiolitis obliterans, roentgenologic–pathologic correlation. *American Journal of Roentgenology*, **117**, 816–32.

Liebow, A.A. and Carrington, C.B. (1969). The interstitial pneumonias. In: *Frontiers of pulmonary radiology* (ed M. Simon, E.J. Potchen and M. LeMay), pp. 102–41. Grune and Stratton, New York.

Wright, J.L., Cagle, P., Churg, A., Colby, T.V., and Myers, J. (1992). Diseases of the small airways. *American Review of Respiratory Disease*, **146**, 240–62.

17.10.4 The lung in collagen–vascular diseases

R. J. SHAW

Pulmonary involvement can be prominent in the systemic collagen–vascular diseases.

Rheumatoid arthritis

Rheumatoid arthritis is a symmetrical inflammatory polyarthropathy with a female preponderance. The cause is unknown, but the disease is associated with autoantibody production. In at least two-thirds of adults IgM is directed against the Fc region of IgG, the so-called IgM rheumatoid factor. The clinical course varies from a chronic disease in 75 per cent of patients to the severe progressive condition in 15 per cent. Although the majority of the symptoms come from the joint disease, three-quarters of the patients have extra-articular manifestations. These are more common in those with aggressive disease characterized by erosive lesions on radiographs, high rheumatoid factor titre, and circulating immune complexes. The underlying pathogenesis of these extra-articular manifestations is believed to involve vasculitis, and the presence of these complications indicates a worse prognosis. The extra-articular manifestations include subcutaneous nodules, eye disease, pericarditis, lymphadenopathy, splenomegaly, Felty's syndrome, cutaneous ulceration, and pleuropulmonary disease.

The different ways in which rheumatoid arthritis may affect the lung are listed in Table 1. Fortunately, these complications occur in severe form in less that 5 per cent of patients.

Cricoarytenoid arthritis

This is manifested by ear pain, dysphagia, and the sensation of a foreign body in the throat. In severe cases there is dyspnoea stridor and evidence of upper airways obstruction.

Table 1 *Pleural pulmonary manifestations of rheumatoid arthritis*

Upper airways dysfunction—cricoarytenoid arthritis
Pleural disease
Nodules (necrobiotic and Caplan's syndrome)
Interstitial lung disease
Bronchiolitis obliterans without or with organizing pneumonia
Others (infection including mycobacterial infection and
    bronchial sepsis, vascular disease, apical fibrobullous
    disease, thoracic cage immobility, drug-induced lung
    disease)

Pleural disease

Although over 40 per cent of patients have evidence of pleurisy at autopsy, only 5 per cent of patients have clinically evident pleural effusions. These effusions may give rise to no symptoms or be associated with mild dyspnoea and pleuritic chest pain. Typically, the fluid is an exudate with high protein and high lactate dehydrogenase levels. Often the glucose and pH of the fluid are reduced, mimicking an infectious or malignant process. The cells in the fluid are predominantly lymphocytes. A large number of polymorphonuclear cells may be present in the setting of either a sterile or septic empyema. Typically, the pleural effusion either resolves spontaneously or remains for months or years without requiring any specific treatment. Development of an empyema is very rare, but will require appropriate drainage.

Rheumatoid nodules

Rheumatoid nodules fall into two types: necrobiotic nodules and Caplan's syndrome. Both types are generally asymptomatic. The necrobiotic nodule can pose a difficult diagnostic problem in a patient with rheumatoid arthritis who has a solitary nodule on the chest radiograph which gives rise to a differential diagnosis with malignancy. The nodules may also cavitate, leading to a differential diagnosis with tuberculosis. Cavitation of a subpleural nodule may cause a spontaneous pneumothorax. Since percutaneous needle aspiration of a necrobiotic nodule is usually unrewarding, with the material having no specific features, radiographic observation or open biopsy is indicated. The difficult clinical problem occurs when one is faced with a patient with a solitary nodule and a strongly positive rheumatoid factor, and one has to decide whether to proceed to an open-lung biopsy with the attendant morbidity or risk waiting and watching serial chest radiographs for signs of enlargement of the nodule.

Caplan's syndrome was first described as the development of either single or multiple nodules in Welsh coal miners with rheumatoid arthritis. However, they can occur in other dust-exposed occupations. They may also occur in the absence of appreciable background pneumoconiosis. These nodules appear rapidly and often cavitate. Histologically, they are similar to necrobiotic nodules with the additional feature of dust-laden macrophages.

Interstitial lung disease

Histological evidence of interstitial inflammation and fibrosis is common in rheumatoid arthritis. It is more uncommon for it to be an important clinical problem. When it occurs, interstitial lung disease is more common in men with rheumatoid arthritis. The clinical manifestations resemble cryptogenic fibrosing alveolitis–idiopathic pulmonary fibrosis, and include progressive dyspnoea initially on exertion and later at rest. Tachypnoea and bibasilar fine crepitations are common and many patients develop clubbing. It is interesting to note that, although pulmonary symptoms usually follow the arthritis, simultaneous onsets may occur or pulmonary disease may precede joint manifestations. As a rule

joint and lung symptoms tend to develop within 5 years of each other. In severe disease physiological abnormalities are identical to cryptogenic fibrosing alveolitis–idiopathic pulmonary fibrosis with a restrictive defect, i.e. reduced lung volumes and carbon monoxide transfer. The arterial P_{CO_2} is low or normal; the arterial P_{O_2} is normal or near normal but falls with exercise. In mild disease there may be little in the way of physiological impairment. Many patients also have evidence of chronic obstructive airways disease. The chest radiograph of early disease shows bibasilar patchy alveolar infiltrates. In more severe disease a reticular nodular pattern supervenes with progression to honeycombing. In 20 per cent of cases there is associated pleural disease which may prove useful in differentiating patients with collagen vascular disease associated interstitial lung disease from those with lone cryptogenic fibrosing alveolitis.

In routine clinical practice, bronchoalveolar lavage may be used to document an increase in total cell number and an increase in a variety of other inflammatory markers but provides little extra clinically useful information.

Is it necessary to perform a lung biopsy to identify the nature of the interstitial lung disease in a patient with rheumatoid arthritis? This question is still unresolved. In routine clinical practice when dealing with disabled patients with clear-cut disease it is often necessary to make a diagnosis in the absence of histology. The lung histology is often nonspecific, with evidence of inflammation in the perivascular peribronchial regions and interstitium with infiltration by lymphocytes, plasma cells, and macrophages. There is evidence of fibrosis and, in advanced cases, of honeycomb lung. A predominant lymphocytic infiltration with germinal follicles adjacent to the airways of vessels (termed follicular bronchitis or bronchiolitis), rheumatoid nodules, pleural fibrosis, or adhesions suggest interstitial lung disease associated with rheumatoid arthritis as opposed to lone cryptogenic fibrosing alveolitis.

There are few data on the prognosis of lung fibrosis in association with rheumatoid arthritis, but it is probably similar to that of cryptogenic fibrosing alveolitis. A proportion of patients have progressive disease while others have stable chronic disease. A median interval from diagnosis to death is probably around 5 years. Similarly, there is conflicting evidence of the benefits of corticosteroid treatment and whether prognosis is improved by the addition of immunosuppressants such as cyclophosphamide. It is thought more likely that these agents will be more useful in those with early predominantly inflammatory disease than in those with established fibrosis.

Bronchiolitis obliterans

Bronchiolitis obliterans without organizing pneumonia occurs when small airways are infiltrated by inflammatory cells, become occluded, and are converted into a fibrous strand. This appears more commonly in smokers and presents as rapidly progressing dyspnoea. Lung function reveals marked airflow obstruction (peak expiratory flow rate and forced expiratory volume in 1 second decreased) with air trapping (functional vital capacity decreased and respiratory volume increased), but little change in carbon monoxide transfer and normal compliance, indicating no destruction of lung architecture. The chest radiograph shows hyperinflated lung fields. As an *aide-memoire*, the clinical picture is similar to a rapid onset of emphysema without the reduction in carbon monoxide transfer or destruction of lung architecture. The prognosis of bronchiolitis obliterans is poor.

Other pulmonary complications of rheumatoid arthritis

Respiratory tract infection is common in patients with rheumatoid arthritis. Infectious agents include *Mycobacterium tuberculosis* and nontuberculous mycobacteria (Fig. 1). Acute vasculitis as seen in systemic lupus erythematosus is not a feature of rheumatoid arthritis, although pulmonary hypertension in the absence of lung fibrosis is reported. Apical fibrobullous disease similar to that in ankylosing spondylitis is reported, and some patients experience problems associated with thoracic cage immobility. Differentiating rheumatoid arthritis from drug-induced lung disease can pose a problem since the drugs used for rheumatoid arthritis, namely gold salts, penicillamine, and methotrexate, have all been associated with the development of pulmonary fibrosis. Withdrawal of the suspected drug may be indicated.

Systemic lupus erythematosus

Systemic lupus erythematosus is a common autoimmune disorder which affects women 10 times more frequently than men. It has a complex mix of clinical manifestations. In the absence of another clear cause, four or more of the following satisfy the American Rheumatism Association Criteria for diagnosis of systemic lupus erythematosus:

(1) malar rash;
(2) discoid rash;
(3) photosensitivity;
(4) oral ulcers;
(5) arthritis;
(6) serositis (pleuritis and pericarditis);
(7) renal disorder (persistent proteinuria, high urea, or cellular urinary casts);
(8) neurological disorder (seizures or psychosis);
(9) haematological disorder (haemolytic anaemia, leucopenia, lymphopenia, or thrombocytopenia);
(10) anti-DNA antibody or anti-Sm antibody or false-positive syphilis serology or positive lupus erythematosus cell preparation;
(11) antinuclear antibody.

The different ways in which systemic lupus erythematosus can affect the lung are listed in Table 2.

Pleural disease

Pleural disease is common in systemic lupus erythematosus, with one in three patients initially presenting with pleurisy. Pleuritic pain is a common symptom indicating pleurisy. Pleural effusions are common at autopsy, when pleural thickening or effusions are present in over 90 per cent of cases. The pleural effusions may be bilateral and are usually

Fig. 1 Chest radiograph showing cavitating consolidation at the L apex in a 65-year-old man with aggressive rheumatoid disease. (Caused by *M. kansasii*.)

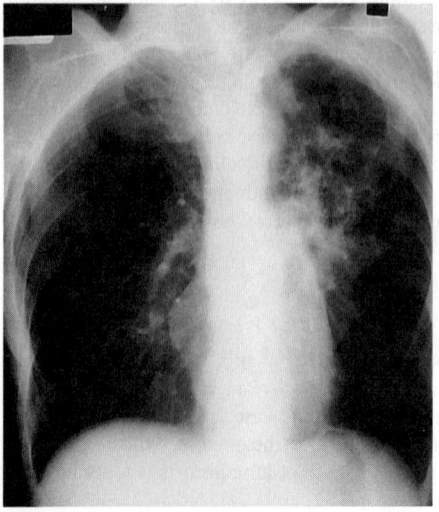

Table 2 *Pleuropulmonary manifestations of systemic lupus erythematosus*

Pleuritis with or without effusion
Diaphragmatic dysfunction or shrinking lung
Acute lupus pneumonitis with or without pulmonary haemorrhage
Opportunistic infection in the setting of immunosuppressive drugs used in treatment
Thromboembolism
Other

small. The fluid is an exudate and tends to have a higher glucose and pH than that in rheumatoid arthritis. Antinuclear antibodies, anti-DNA antibodies, and lupus erythematosus cells may be found in the fluid. Complement levels in the fluid may be reduced, suggesting local immune activation in the pleural space.

Diaphragmatic dysfunction or shrinking lung

This syndrome presents with dyspnoea and loss of lung volume. On the chest radiograph there are small but clear lungs with high diaphragms bilaterally. This syndrome has been termed 'the shrinking lung syndrome'. One hypothesis is that it is due to diaphragm dysfunction, as these patients have a reduction in transdiaphragmatic pressures. (Two simple clinical tests which suggest diaphragmatic weakness are (a) reduction in the vital capacity by 25 per cent or more when recumbent, and (b) a reduction in maximum inspiratory mouth pressure.) An alternative hypothesis is that vasculitis in the lung causes small infarcts with consequent reduction in lung volumes.

Acute lupus pneumonitis with or without pulmonary haemorrhage

Acute lupus pneumonitis is a dramatic and severe complication of systemic lupus erythematosus. It often accompanies a generalized exacerbation of the disease. The syndrome consists of fever, dyspnoea, and hypoxaemia. Examination reveals tachypnoea, and fine or coarse crackles may be present. There are diffusive pulmonary infiltrates on the chest radiograph which may progress to give a picture similar to adult respiratory distress syndrome. Pathologically, there is diffuse alveolar damage with inflammation, vasculitis, and pulmonary haemorrhage. (Haemoptysis is a surprisingly rare symptom.) A clinician faced with a patient in respiratory failure and white lung fields on the chest radiograph, in the setting of an exacerbation of systemic lupus erythematosus already on treatment with immunosuppressant agents, may find differentiating acute lupus pneumonitis and severe opportunist infection—a critical but difficult decision. Classically, the erythrocyte sedimentation rate and C-reactive protein are elevated in acute infection whereas the C-reactive protein is not elevated to the same extent in acute lupus. An elevated carbon monoxide transfer may also suggest pulmonary haemorrhage. However, the carbon monoxide transfer may also be low in acute lupus pneumonitis owing to the widespread alveolar damage. Bronchoalveolar lavage may help to identify infectious organisms, or in acute pulmonary haemorrhage show haemosiderin laden macrophages. Open-lung biopsy is the definitive investigation, if it can be tolerated by the patient. Treatment of acute lupus pneumonitis requires large doses of corticosteroids or immunosuppressant agents. The mortality is about 50 per cent.

Other pulmonary complications of systemic lupus erythematosus

Upper airway disease due to inflammation of the upper airway structures has been documented but is rare. Atalectasis is recorded in systemic lupus erythematosus but it is rarely clinically significant. Bronchiolitis obliterans and other causes of small airways dysfunction can occur in systemic lupus erythematosus. Interstitial lung fibrosis is rare in systemic lupus erythematosus. Restricted lung function tests have been documented but changes tend not to progress.

Systemic sclerosis and CREST

Systemic sclerosis is a syndrome comprising of inflammation and fibrosis of skin and internal organs. CREST (calcinosis, Raynaud's disease, (o)esophageal dismotility, sclerodactyly, and telangiectasia) is considered to be a more benign variant. There are four main pulmonary complications.

Recurrent bacterial infection

Poor oesophageal mortality predisposes to recurrent aspiration pneumonias which may contribute to lower-lobe fibrosis or bronchiectasis.

Pulmonary fibrosis

The majority of patients with scleroderma will develop pulmonary fibrosis over time. This has similar symptoms, signs, lung physiology, and chest radiograph changes to cryptogenic fibrosing alveolitis and is largely uninfluenced by treatment. In a proportion of patients the disease may remain static for many years. Some non-invasive measures such as DTPA clearance may provide a method of identifying those who are likely to progress and thus allow therapy to be targeted to the group at risk. Treatment is similar to that for cryptogenic fibrosing alveolitis, with corticosteroids and possibly cyclophosphamide.

Pulmonary hypertension

Pulmonary hypertension occurs in 25 to 50 per cent of patients with systemic sclerosis and two-thirds of those with CREST, where it may occur in the absence of pulmonary fibrosis. Affected patients complain of dyspnoea in the presence of clear lung fields on the chest radiograph. The pathology is similar to that in the peripheral vessels, with intimal proliferation medial hyperplasia and perivascular hyperplasia. There is debate as to whether appreciable vascular reactivity of the pulmonary vessels to cold contributes to the condition.

Other reported pulmonary complications of systemic sclerosis include pleuritis, pneumothorax, pulmonary haemorrhage, and scar carcinoma.

Polymyositis and dermatomyositis

Polymyositis and dermatomyositis are characterized by muscle pain and weakness. There are a number of pleural and pulmonary complications.

1. Aspiration pneumonia may occur due to diminished cough reflex or weak pharyngeal muscles.
2. Respiratory muscle weakness may lead to loss of lung volumes and basal atelectasis. This may progress to hypoventilation and respiratory failure.
3. Fibrosing alveolitis is a rare complication of both diseases. In the case of polymyositis the presence of anti-JO-1, which is an antibody to the enzyme histidyl-tRNA-synthetase is associated with the development of pulmonary fibrosis.
4. Dermatomyositis is associated with underlying malignancy. The lung is a common site of primary malignancy.

Sjögren's syndrome

Sjögren's syndrome, comprising keratoconjunctivitis sicca and xerostomia, commonly occurs as part of other collagen vascular diseases. In its own right it may give rise to dryness and atrophic changes in the upper airways, leading to atrophic rhinitis, xerostomia (dry mouth), and xerotrachea. Xerotrachea or bronchitis sicca is perhaps the most common condition. It presents as an unremitting non-productive cough. There is debate as to the contribution of poor quality of airway secretions to the chronic bronchitis, recurrent infections, atelectasis, and obstructive airways disease which occur in these patients. A proportion of patients develop one of a spectrum of diseases ranging from lymphocytic interstitial pneumonitis to pseudolymphoma (see below).

Mixed conective tissue disease

Mixed conective tissue disease combines features of systemic lupus erythematosus, systemic sclerosis, Sjögren's syndrome, and polymyositis. These patients have antibodies to an extractable nuclear antigen comprising protein and RNA. The major component of this antigen is soluble ribonucleoprotein. Patients with mixed connective tissue disease commonly have evidence of interstitial lung disease; as many as 80 per cent may have impairments in lung function. In the majority this is subclinical, although a proportion progress to fibrosing alveolitis and behave as patients with systemic sclerosis. The proportion with pulmonary hypertension is similar to that in systemic sclerosis.

Ankylosing spondylitis

Ankylosing spondylitis classically affects males under 40. Pulmonary complications occur in under 2 per cent of patients.

Apicofibrobullous disease has the chest radiograph features of bilateral progressive upper-zone fibrosis with cavitation. Patients may complain of cough, sputum production, and dyspnoea, or may be asymptomatic. The differential diagnosis includes tuberculosis. In advanced cases the cavities can be infected by aspergillus or atypical mycobacteria.

Skeletal deformity

The fusion of vertical bodies may cause reduced rib movement which may result in loss of lung volume (functional vital capacity, total lung capacity). This may lead to a 'frozen thorax'. However, it usually causes little ventilatory impairment, presumably because of the large contribution of the diaphragm to ventilatory function.

Behçet's disease

Behçet's disease is characterized by orogenital ulcers, relapsing iritis, joint manifestations, thrombophlebitis, migraine, erythema nodosum, and mengingoencephalitis. The lungs may also be affected. Those affected may have haemoptysis, pleuritis, fleeting chest radiograph shadows, and pulmonary artery aneurysms. The Hughes–Stovin syndrome, which includes venous thrombosis and pulmonary aneurysms, may be a manifestation of Behçet's disease.

REFERENCES

Banks, J., Banks, C., Cheong, B., Umachandran, V., Smith, A.P., Jessop, J.D., and Pritchard, M.H. (1992). Epidemiological and clinical investigation of lung function and symptoms in rheumatoid arthritis. *Quarterly Journal of Medicine*, **85**, 795–806.

Constantopoulos, S.H. and Moutsopoulos, H.M. (1986). Respiratory involvement in patients with Sjögren's syndrome: is it a problem? *Scandinavian Journal of Rheumatology (Suppl.)*, **61**, 146–50.

Efthimiou, J., Johnston, C., Spiro, S.C., and Turner-Warwick, M. (1986). Pulmonary disease in Behçet's syndrome. *Quarterly Journal of Medicine*, **58**, 529.

Eisenberg, H., Dubois, E.L., Sherwin, R.P., and Balchum, O.J. (1973). Diffuse interstitial lung disease in systemic lupus erythematosus. *Annals of Internal Medicine*, **79**, 37–45.

Frazier, A.R. and Miller, R.E. (1974). Interstitial pneumonitis in association with polymyositis and dermatomyositis. *Chest*, **65**, 403–7.

Geddes, D.M., Corrin, B., Brewerton, D.A., Davies, R.J., and Turner-Warwick, M. (1977). Progressive airway obliteration in adults and its association with rheumatoid disease. *Quarterly Journal of Medicine*, **46**, 427–44.

Gibson, G.J., Edmonds, J.P., and Hughes, G.R. (1977). Diaphragm function and lung involvement in systemic lupus erythematosus. *American Review of Respiratory Medicine*, **63**, 926–32.

Hunninghake, G.W. and Fauci, A.S. (1979). Pulmonary involvement in collagen–vascular diseases. *American Review of Respiratory Medicine*, **119**, 471–503.

Owens, G.R. and Follansbee, W.P. (1988). Cardio-pulmonary manifestation of systemic sclerosis. *Chest*, **91**, 118–27.

Rosenow, E.C., III, Strimlan, C.V., Muhm, J.R., and Ferguson, R.H. (1977). Pleuropulmonary manifestations of ankylosing spondylitis. *Mayo Clinic Proceedings*, **52**, 641–9.

17.10.5 Pulmonary vasculitis and granulomatosis

D. J. LANE and J. M. HOPKIN

Introduction

Although various forms of systemic vasculitis were well described in the nineteenth century, notably by Schonlein and Kussmaul, syndromes which include a prominent pulmonary component were not well defined before about 1930. Klinger noted an association of pulmonary lesions with polyarteritis in 1931, and this was followed in 1939 by Wegener's description of the granulomatous vasculitis that bears his name. Churg and Strauss described allergic granulomatosis in 1951. The classic paper by Liebow in 1973 divided the pulmonary granulomas into five types on morphological grounds.

Classification

Classification of these disorders remains unsatisfactory. The reasons for this are complex, partly explained by our lack of knowledge about aetiology, by the wide variation in the size and distribution of vessels involved, and by the variable clinical picture. Positive antineutrophil cytoplasmic bodies (ANCA) are present in Wegener's granulomatosis, most cases of Churg–Strauss syndrome, and microvasculitic polyarteritis nodosa, but are not present in systemic lupus and allied disorders in which hypocomplementaemia and anti-DNA antibodies are typical.

The vasculitides can be divided into three categories as shown in Table 1. The granulomatous vasculitides, in which the lungs are prominent sites of pathology, form the subject matter of this chapter. The hypersensitivity vasculitides, in which the lungs are occasionally involved as part of a systemic disease and the pulmonary vascular and granulomatous manifestations of the connective tissue disorders are described in Section 18.11.

Pathogenesis

Little is known about the aetiology of these disorders; the biology of autoimmunity is discussed in Section 5. Modest HLA associations are known for certain connective tissue disorders. If the conditions are acquired, there seems no pattern of consistent association with external agents. There are specific examples of associations between polyarteritis nodosa and either drug therapy (e.g. sulphonamides) or infections (specifically hepatitis B). Recently, mycobacterial DNA has been detected

Table 1

Granulomatous vasculitides
Allergic granulomatosis and angiitis
Classic Wegener's granulomatosis
Limited Wegener's granulomatosis
Lymphomatoid granulomatosis
Necrotizing sarcoidal granulomatosis
Bronchocentric granulomatosis
Hypersensitivity vasculitis
Anaphylactoid purpura
Mixed cryoglobulinaemia
Vasculitis associated with malignancy, infection, drugs
Pulmonary vasculitis with connective tissue diseases
Rheumatoid disease
Systemic lupus erythematosus
Systemic sclerosis
Dermatopolymyositis
Mixed connective tissue disease

in some pulmonary vasculitic lesions, but these observations need replication and clarification.

Churg–Strauss syndrome: allergic granulomatosis

Churg and Strauss described a group of young adults with a history of asthma who developed evidence of systemic vasculitis in association with a marked peripheral eosinophilia. The condition is not common (154 cases have been cited in the English literature), and it seems likely that other examples of the condition have been described as polyarteritis nodosa, eosinophilic pneumonia, or Loeffler's syndrome.

CLINICAL FEATURES

The sex ratio shows a slight preponderance of males and the age of diagnosis is usually late in the fourth decade. Preceding this there will have been a history of rhinitis and then asthma, although the onset of these is usually in early adult life rather than in childhood. Peripheral eosinophilia then becomes marked and there may be eosinophilic infiltrates in various organs, particularly the lungs. The appearance of vasculitis in the middle to late thirties should alert the physician to the true diagnosis. The overall clinical course can be acute and rapidly fatal with heart failure, but it is more usually subacute and relapsing.

Therefore the diagnostic triad is asthma, eosinophilia, and systemic vasculitis. Pulmonary infiltrates accompanying the asthma are patchy and transient, not particularly favouring any lobe or zone; hilar lymphadenopathy, pleural effusion, and both fine small and large (non-cavitating) nodules are described in some cases. The eosinophilia is greater than 1.5×10^9/l unless reduced by therapy, and so is greater than that seen in conventional atopic asthma but less than that found in the hypereosinophilic syndrome. Vascular lesions affect the body widely. A mononeuritis multiplex is perhaps the most common, being seen in some two-thirds of patients; other neurological abnormalities are infrequent, perhaps an optic neuritis or, rarely, involvement of other cranial nerves. Abdominal pain is a frequent complaint, reflecting vascular lesions in the bowel which resemble those in eosinophilic gastroenteritis in causing mass lesions with the potential for intestinal obstruction, and also ulceration leading to haemorrhagic diarrhoea. Vasculitis of the skin vessels causes a variety of maculopapular, urticarial, or purpuric rashes, and there may also be subcutaneous granulomatous nodules. Whilst a focal segmental glomerulonephritis may occur, this is not common and rarely dominates the clinical outcome. The upper respiratory tract features usually remain simply 'allergic' in type with congestion and polyposis rather than vasculitic or granulomatous lesions.

LABORATORY FINDINGS

There is eosinophilia; a normochromic normocytic anaemia is not uncommon and the erythrocyte sedimentation rate (ESR) is usually high. Skin-prick tests are often positive for common environmental allergens, reflecting the atopic status, as does the elevated IgE. Antineutrophil cytoplasmic antibody is usually found.

Eosinophils dominate the histological picture with a dense infiltrate of these cells in almost all lesions together with foci of eosinophilic necrotic material and Charcot–Leyden crystals. Immunocytochemical studies reveal the presence of large amounts of potentially toxic compounds secreted by the activated eosinophils. Of these, both eosinophil cationic proteins and eosinophil protein X can be shown to be toxic to cardiac muscle and other cells. It seems likely that these products are responsible for the development of the damaging lesions of this syndrome. Necrotizing vasculitis can usually be demonstrated in vessels in and around the lesions, but granulomas have been found in less than half the cases examined at autopsy.

PATHOGENESIS

The disorder may just represent an unusual progression of allergic disease in a subset of predisposed atopic individuals or an allergic response to an unusual undetected antigen. There is a disturbing report of six atopic patients who developed systemic vasculitis after hyposensitization treatment.

TREATMENT

One fortunate aspect of the disease is that corticosteroids are almost universally successful, transforming a previously poor prognosis into one in which death is now uncommon. Cytotoxics are rarely needed. Hypertension can be a problem, particularly since steroid therapy may need to be maintained for months or years.

Wegener's granulomatosis

The classic triad of upper and lower respiratory tract granulomas combined with necrotizing focal glomerulonephritis make this syndrome the best known and most easily identified of the pulmonary granulomatous vasculitides. Involvement of two of the three sites is said to be sufficient to make the diagnosis, but lack of glomerulonephritis makes the disease less than 'classical'; alternatively there may be vasculitic lesions elsewhere.

CLINICAL FEATURES

The disease can develop at any age though it is most common in the fifth decade, with predominance in men. Pulmonary involvement can cause haemoptysis and some chest pain, but often the radiology seems out of proportion to the symptoms and paucity of physical signs, and may be the only manifestation of pulmonary involvement in a patient who presents with renal disease. The chest radiograph can show changing pulmonary opacities which frequently cavitate but may regress spontaneously. Nodules reach up to 9 cm in size and are usually multiple and bilateral (Fig. 1). Other pulmonary features include more widespread 'pneumonic' or reticulonodular shadows, bronchial obstruction leading to atelectasis, and pleural involvement giving effusion, pneumothorax, and even bronchopleural fistula. Lymphadenopathy is uncommon.

In the upper respiratory tract granulomas in the nose may produce little more than coryza with epistaxis and some nasal crusting, but extensive destruction is possible leading to nasal septal perforation and saddle nose, or there may be ulcerative lesions of the sinuses, palate, or pharynx.

The third component of the classical disease is necrotizing glomerulonephritis, which is often asymptomatic but sometimes acute and fulminating (occasionally accompanied by pulmonary haemorrhage such that Goodpasture's syndrome is suggested). Hypertension is rare.

Beyond these features there is often malaise, fever, and arthralgia. Vasculitic lesions can affect the skin (papular, vesicular, or bullous), the nervous system (uveitis, orbital pseudotumour, peripheral neuropathy), the cardiovascular system (pericarditis and coronary arteritis), and infrequently elsewhere. There may be a normochromic normocytic anaemia with an elevated ESR. Antineutrophilic cytoplasmic antibodies (directed at myeloperoxidase) are present and probably play an active role in causing the disease.

PATHOLOGY

The pathological lesions are granulomatous nodules built up from lymphocytes, plasma cells, and histiocytes. Giant cells form, and the centre of the nodule is frequently necrotic. Within the nodules and at a distance from them there is a necrotic vasculitis affecting both arteries and veins. Pulmonary nodules usually show this characteristic histology, whereas nasal granulomas are often less specific in appearance, largely due to local superinfection. The renal lesion is a focal necrotizing glomerulonephritis with frequent crescent formation similar to that seen in Goodpasture's syndrome or the Henoch–Schönlein syndrome. There is no distinctive pattern of immunofluorescence.

PROGNOSIS AND TREATMENT

Confusing symptoms and signs may be present for years before diagnosis. At diagnosis the prognosis has been generally poor because of

Fig. 1 Wegener's granulomatosis. bilateral cavitating apical masses in a woman with features of upper respiratory tract disease and glomerulonephritis: (a) radiograph; (b) tomograms.

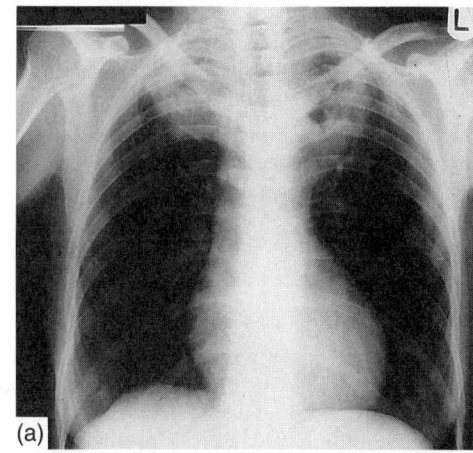

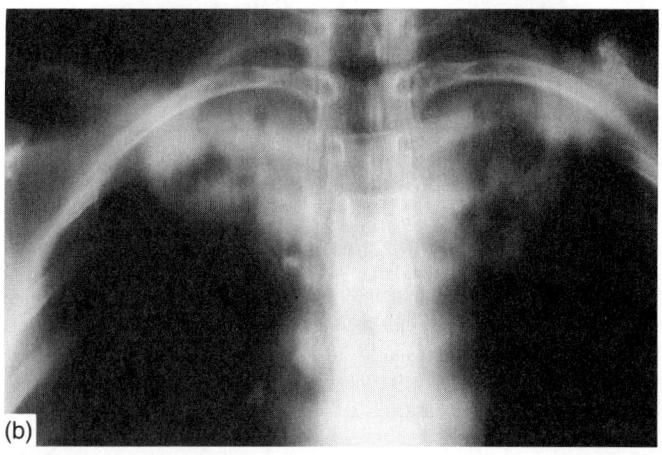

progression of the renal lesion. The prognosis has now been transformed by the use of cyclophosphamide therapy (2 mg/kg/day) continued for at least a year after remission. Corticosteroids are often added, certainly for an initial phase, and prescription on alternate days minimizes side-effects that can include opportunistic infection. A remission rate of over 90 per cent is now to be expected.

Limited Wegener's granulomatosis

In this variant of the disease, pulmonary granulomas are the only consistent manifestation. Their histology and radiographic appearance are as in the classic disease. The condition may be diagnosed when a nodule is removed on suspicion of malignancy. There is no glomerulonephritis and nodules outside the lungs are uncommon and not associated with a damaging vasculitis. They have been recorded most often subcutaneously, but also in the kidneys. The disease evolves slowly, and may even stabilize or regress without treatment. Response to corticosteroid therapy is recorded.

Necrotizing sarcoid granulomatosis

Liebow included this amongst the five pulmonary granulomas which he delineated in 1973. It is uncommon; less than 100 cases have been described to date. A wide age range of adults has been affected, and females seem more prone to the disorder than males. Presentation is usually with non-specific respiratory complaints such as cough or chest pain, although a quarter are asymptomatic. In all instances chest radiology is striking, usually showing multiple nodules which may be down to miliary in size and are frequently confluent. They are particularly prevalent in the lower zones and do not cavitate. Hilar nodes may be seen on the chest radiograph and are often found pathologically.

Neither systemic vasculitis nor glomerulonephritis is part of the clinical picture; the only extrapulmonary feature recorded that resembles sarcoidosis is uveitis, and this is very rare.

PATHOLOGY

Histologically, the nodules are sarcoid-like epithelioid giant-cell granulomas differing from the better-known disease in that they quite frequently show necrosis and also vasculitis. The walls of both arteries and veins are infiltrated with lymphocytes, histiocytes, and plasma cells, leading to vessel destruction and local infarction.

PROGNOSIS AND TREATMENT

Prognosis is good. Survivals of a decade or more are quite common. Surgical removal often seems to result in cure, and steroids with or without cytotoxics give good remission in cases not subjected to thoracotomy. The occasional relapse responds equally well.

Bronchocentric granulomatosis

This is essentially a morphological diagnosis of a condition which lacks clear-cut clinical, radiological, or immunological features, although there is increasing support for the concept that it represents an unusual but specific bronchial reaction to a sustained inflammatory insult and that this insult most often comes from as yet unidentified fungi.

CLINICAL FEATURES

Originally described by Liebow in 1973 in his paper on the pulmonary granulomas, there is little evidence now to link this with conditions such as Wegener's granulomatosis. It most commonly presents as localized pulmonary shadowing in a patient with persistent cough and dyspnoea. The dyspnoea has the characteristics of asthma in about half the cases,

often the younger patients. Those with asthma usually have a high peripheral eosinophil count. Radiographically, an isolated mass or alveolar infiltrate confined to one lobe is the usual picture, so that it is not surprising that many of these patients are diagnosed histologically after thoracotomy. Changes are more commonly seen in the upper lobes, and other radiological presentations are multiple nodules or infiltrates or even a diffuse alveolar infiltrate. Pleural involvement, cavitation, and hilar lymphadenopathy are rare. The disease has no extrapulmonary manifestations, although there are case reports of an association with rheumatoid arthritis.

PATHOLOGY

Histologically, the lesions consist of necrotizing granulomas centred on an airway and surrounded by collapsed consolidated lung. Microscopically, epithelioid cells are arranged radially to form granulomas. The bronchial lumen is filled with inspissated mucus together with the ulcerated bronchial wall, and the peribronchial tissues is infiltrated by eosinophils and eosinophilic masses. Although there may be chondritis and destruction of cartilage, there is no arteritis.

AETIOLOGY

Some take the view that the lesions represent a tissue reaction that results from prolonged inflammation due to a variety of insults including various fungi.

MANAGEMENT

Treatment is often inadvertently by surgical resection at a thoracotomy carried out for supposed bronchial malignancy. However, if the condition is suspected in life, corticosteroids will clear the consolidation even though repeated courses may be needed. Residual damage leading to bronchiectasis is recorded, but on the whole prognosis is good. No studies of antifungal agents have been reported.

Other forms of pulmonary vasculitis

The lungs may be involved to a limited degree in the hypersensitivity vasculitides such as anaphylactoid (Henoch–Schönlein) purpura or essential mixed cryoglobulinaemia. In addition to cutaneous lesions, hepatosplenomegaly, and other systemic features, there is unimpressive patchy pneumonitis, usually revealed only on the chest radiograph. Likewise, in the vasculitides associated with malignancy, infection, or drugs, any pulmonary involvement is minor.

A systemic vasculitis may be associated with pulmonary artery aneurysms in two other vasculitic disorders, which may be related. These are Behçet's syndrome and Hughes–Stovin syndrome.

BEHÇET'S SYNDROME

Haemoptysis, infiltrates on the chest radiograph which may cavitate, and focal or generalized fibrosis have all been reported. These are probably all manifestations of pulmonary vasculitis, but sometimes occur in association with vena caval thrombosis, in which instance pulmonary emboli are a probable contributing cause. The lung manifestations may precede the systemic disease by some years, during which time the diagnosis is obscure.

HUGUES–STOVIN SYNDROME

Pulmonary artery aneurysms, which are unusual in Behçet's syndrome, are the hallmark of this rare and peculiar disorder characterized clinically by haemoptysis from rupture of the aneurysms. Histologically, the lesions are an eosinophil angiitis. There may be accompanying glomerulonephritis.

REFERENCES

Churg, A., Carrington, C.B., and Gupta, R. (1979). Necrotizing sarcoid granulomatosis. *Chest*, **76**, 406–13.

Dreisin, R.B.C. (1993). New perspectives in Wegener's granulomatosis. *Thorax*, **48**, 97–9.

Fauci, A.S., Haynes, B.F., Katz, P., and Wolff, S.M. (1983). Wegener's granulomatosis; prospective clinical and therapeutic experience with 85 patients for 21 years. *Annals of Internal Medicine*, **98**, 76–85.

Israel, H.L., Patchefsky, A.S., and Saldana, J.J. (1977). Wegener's granulomatosis, lymphomatoid granulomatosis and benign lymphocytic angiitis and granulomatosis of lung; recognition and treatment. *Annals of Internal Medicine* **87**, 691–9.

Lenham, J.G., Elkom, K.B., Pusey, C.D., and Hughes, G.R. (1984). Systemic vasculitis with asthma and eosinophilia; a clinical approach to the Churg–Strauss syndrome. *Medicine, Baltimore*, **63**, 65–81.

Liebow, A.A. (1973). Pulmonary angiitis and granulomatosis. *American Review of Respiratory Disease*, **108**, 1–18.

17.10.6. Pulmonary haemorrhagic disorders

D. J. LANE

Pulmonary haemorrhage is suspected when prominent haemoptysis is associated with radiographic alveolar shadowing (Fig. 1). The diagnosis is supported by the demonstration of a high transfer factor for carbon monoxide (Chapter 17.6.2) or multiple haemosiderin-laden macrophages in sputum, bronchoscopic alveolar lavage samples or lung biopsy.

A range of different disorders can cause recurrent bleeding from the pulmonary capillaries, producing the clinical triad of haemoptysis, diffuse alveolar opacities on the chest radiograph, and anaemia. These conditions can be classified as follows.

1. Chronic pulmonary venous congestion: mitral stenosis, left ventricular failure, pulmonary veno-occlusive disease (see Section 15).
2. Goodpasture's syndrome.

3. Idiopathic pulmonary haemosiderosis.
4. Pulmonary vasculitis, e.g. Wegener's granulomatosis, systemic lupus erythematosus.
5. Bleeding disorders and thrombolysis.

Goodpasture's syndrome

Goodpasture originally described a man who died with pulmonary haemorrhage and glomerulonephritis. The syndrome is now usually considered as a triad of these two features together with the demonstration of autoantibodies to glomerular basement membrane. The basement antigen is now recognized to be the α-3 chain of type IV collagen.

Autoantibodies to basement membrane antigens circulate and deposit in the kidneys to produce glomerulonephritis and in the lungs to damage vessel walls and allow bleeding. Immunofluorescence shows a linear deposition of antibody along the basement membrane with additional complement deposition in some 60 per cent. The majority of patients are smokers; it is thought that smoking or organic hydrocarbon exposure initiates pulmonary endothelial damage and thus allows access of autoantibody to basement membrane.

Histologically, the lungs show red cells in the alveoli following acute bleeding and later there are haemosiderin-laden macrophages. The glomeruli show focal proliferative and necrotizing glomerulonephritis, usually with crescent formation. There is no vasculitis in the pulmonary or other systemic blood vessels. Electron microscopy shows swelling and defects in the basement membrane but no immune complexes.

CLINICAL FEATURES

The syndrome predominantly affects young male smokers who present with cough, breathlessness, and haemoptysis. Renal disease may be missed at this stage because it is only evident as proteinuria or microscopic haematuria. Within a few days or weeks renal involvement becomes clinically obvious and may progress rapidly to renal failure. The haemoptysis is intermittent and ranges from occasional streaks to massive fatal bleeding. Systemic symptoms of fever, joint pains, or weight loss are unusual.

The chest radiograph shows patchy shadows due to intra-alveolar blood. These shadows may be single or multiple or occur diffusely throughout both lung fields (Fig. 1). The shadows resolve over the course of 2 weeks unless there is further bleeding. At the time of bleeding there may be arterial hypoxaemia and reduced lung volumes, but increased carbon monoxide gas transfer as the inspired carbon monoxide is taken up by the blood within the lungs. This test can be used to monitor the progress of the pulmonary bleeding. Haemosiderin-laden macrophages are found in the sputum or at bronchoscopic alveolar lavage. Prolonged severe bleeding leads to an iron-deficiency anaemia. Renal function may be normal initially and then deteriorate over days to weeks.

The diagnosis is confirmed by demonstrating circulating antibasement membrane antibodies (present in 90 per cent) or by demonstrating linear immunofluorescence on renal biopsy. The antibasement membrane antibody titre does not correlate well with clinical progress.

TREATMENT

The main treatment (see also Section 20) is plasma exchange, which must be started early before there is irreversible renal damage and continued until antibasement membrane antibodies are absent. Steroids and immunosuppressant drugs may be helpful temporarily to control the pulmonary haemorrhage, but probably have only a secondary role in controlling the renal disease. Patients should not smoke and should avoid hydrocarbon exposure. Nephrectomy may be required for uncontrollable pulmonary haemorrhage.

Fig. 1 Radiograph showing gross alveolar shadowing following major pulmonary haemorrhage in 60-year-old man with systemic vasculitis.

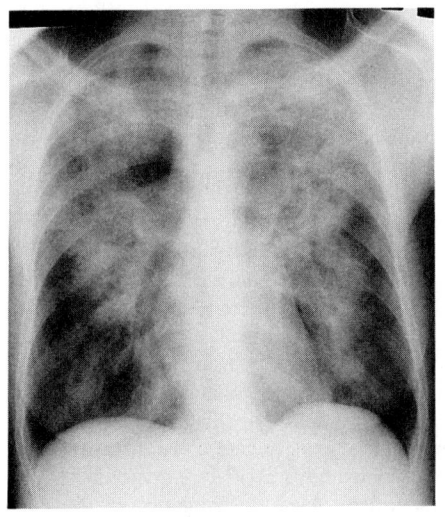

PROGRESS

The outlook from Goodpasture's syndrome has improved dramatically in recent years, partly as a result of plasma exchange and partly because milder degrees of the syndrome are being recognized. With adequate treatment the majority of patients can now be expected to survive.

Idiopathic pulmonary haemosiderosis

This is a rare disorder of children and young adults in which there is recurrent bleeding into the lungs. The extravasated blood is taken up by macrophages which become loaded with haemosiderin, and repeated bleeding may cause an iron-deficiency anaemia. Blood in the alveoli is in some way fibrogenic, and diffuse pulmonary fibrosis eventually develops.

Other conditions which cause recurrent alveolar bleeding, such as mitral stenosis and chronic severe left ventricular failure (Section 15) can result in identical pathological changes.

PATHOLOGY AND PATHOGENESIS

The cause of idiopathic pulmonary haemosiderosis is unknown. Immune complexes are not found in the serum or pulmonary capillaries, and there is no antibasement membrane antibody, antineutrophil cytoplasmic antibody, or antinuclear antibody. The electron microscopic appearance of the basement membrane shows no consistent abnormality. Serum IgA is elevated in most cases and there are reports of associations with rheumatoid arthritis, antibodies to cow's milk, and exposure to gasoline products. Coeliac disease is another association, and this subgroup shows a high incidence of HLA B8 antigen. Indeed, idiopathic pulmonary haemosiderosis may be a heterogeneous condition.

Histologically, the lungs show intra-alveolar blood and normal alveolar walls in the acute stage, and intra-alveolar haemosiderin-laden macrophages and non-specific interstitial fibrosis in chronic disease.

CLINICAL DISEASE

Idiopathic pulmonary haemosiderosis presents either as recurrent acute pulmonary bleeding or as progressive breathlessness with diffuse radiographic changes.

Acute bleeds are more common in childhood and may be life threatening. Physical examination is unhelpful, and the chest radiograph shows variable alveolar shadowing due to blood. These shadows clear completely over 1 to 3 weeks. Repeated bleeds may cause severe iron-deficiency anaemia which itself gives rise to symptoms, and eventually a large bleed can be fatal.

The more chronic form chiefly occurs in adults when progressive breathlessness and iron-deficiency anaemia are the main features. Haemoptysis in the chronic form is usually of small volume and occasional. Systemic symptoms are rare. Some patients with the more indolent disease eventually die of acute massive bleeding, but slow progression to diffuse pulmonary fibrosis with honeycombing is more usual.

The chest radiograph shows widespread fine discrete nodules with subsequent contraction due to the fibrosis. Lung function tests show progressive loss of volumes with reduction of gas transfer; an obstructive pulmonary defect occurs occasionally, and this is unexplained.

TREATMENT

Supportive treatment is required during the acute bleeding, and artificial ventilation is occasionally required. There are case reports recording response to avoidance of milk and gluten and to immunosuppressive agents including corticosteroids and cyclophosphamide. Some patients appear to recover with or without residual pulmonary damage.

Other causes of alveolar haemorrhage

Alveolar haemorrhage occurs in a variety of other disorders which are considered elsewhere in this textbook. Although the haemorrhage can be equally as dramatic as in Goodpasture's syndrome or as persistent as in idiopathic pulmonary haemosiderosis, it is generally overshadowed by other features of the disease in question.

Systemic vasculitides, particularly those with prominent vascular necrosis, may present with alveolar haemorrhage; there may be a special association with those showing IgM antineutrophil cytoplasmic antibodies.

Systemic lupus erythematosus can cause alveolar haemorrhage, which is a rare but serious lung manifestation characterized by massive intra-alveolar bleeding without evidence of pulmonary vasculitis; 70 per cent of cases in a series of 23 were fatal.

Rapidly progressive glomerulonephritis, whether immune complex mediated or not, may be accompanied by alveolar haemorrhage. Indeed, in half of immunofluorescent negative cases, haemoptysis and pulmonary infiltrates have been recorded although the pattern of the pulmonary disease is often mild.

Alveolar haemorrhage has been reported to result from various exogenous agents such as D-penicillamine, lymphangiography contrast media, and trimellitic anhydride fumes or powder.

REFERENCES

Colombo, J.L., and Stolz, S.M. (1992). Treatment of life threatening pulmonary hemosiderosis with cyclophosphamide. *Chest*, **102**, 959–60.

Leatherman, J.W., Davies, S.F., and Hoidal, J.R. (1984). Alveolar haemorrhage syndromes; diffuse and microvascular lung haemorrhage in immune and idiopathic disorders. *Medicine, Baltimore*, **63**, 343–61.

Pacheco, A., Casanova, C., Fogue, L., and Sueiro, L. (1991). Long term follow-up of adult idiopathic pulmonary hemosiderosis. *Chest*, **99**, 1525–6.

Peters, D.K., Rees, A.J., Lockwood, C.M., and Pusey, C.D. (1982). Treatment and prognosis of anti-basement membrane antibody mediated nephritis. *Transplant Proceedings*, **14**, 513–21.

17.10.7 Pulmonary eosinophilia

D. J. LANE

In this multicausal syndrome there is pulmonary radiographic shadowing and accompanying peripheral blood eosinophilia. An overview of the various classifications (in particular Crofton's classification of 1952), based on clinical features rather than aetiology, suggests that these conditions can be broadly divided into three categories (see Table 1 for variations in terminology).

1. Pulmonary infiltrations due to an eosinophilic alveolar exudate without airways involvement: this category includes the acute syndrome described by Loeffler in 1932 and renamed by Crofton as simple pulmonary eosinophilia, as well as the more chronic cases variously called prolonged pulmonary eosinophilia, (Crofton) and eosinophilic pneumonia.

2. Pulmonary infiltration with eosinophilia but including a component of airways obstruction as well as parenchymal lung disease: allergic bronchopulmonary aspergillosis and tropical eosinophilia are classic examples of this group.

3. Pulmonary infiltrations with eosinophilia and with or without airways involvement but with evidence of a systemic disorder which may be predominantly vascular or granulomatous in pathology: polyarteritis nodosa, allergic granulomatosis, and

Table 1 *Classification of the pulmonary eosinophilias*

Pulmonary eosinophilia with alveolar exudate without airways involvement 　　Simple pulmonary eosinophilia: Löffler's syndrome 　　Prolonged pulmonary eosinophilia; eosinophilic pneumonia
Pulmonary eosinophilia with alveolar exudate and airways disease 　　Asthma 　　Allergic bronchopulmonary aspergillosis 　　Tropical eosinophilia
Pulmonary eosinophilia with angiitis and granulomatosis 　　Allergic granulomatosis: Churg–Strauss syndrome 　　Wegener's granulomatosis 　　Bronchocentric granulomatosis

the hypereosinophilic syndrome fall into this category and are described elsewhere in this text.

Other conditions in which peripheral eosinophilia is part of a well-defined disease and which may include pulmonary involvement as part of its clinical presentation (e.g. Hodgkin's disease) are generally excluded from consideration under these headings.

Löffler's syndrome (simple pulmonary eosinophilia)

CLINICAL FEATURES

The essential features of the syndrome are transitory migratory pulmonary shadows with associated modest peripheral eosinophilia in patients with a mild self-limiting illness. Some cases are asymptomatic, and are discovered incidentally. Most present with cough, sometimes with oddly yellowish sputum containing an abundance of eosinophils, and a few have general malaise and a mild fever. The pulmonary shadows are fan-shaped areas of consolidation, often peripheral and sometimes rather nodular, which last a few days only and appear haphazardly in various lobes, seldom following a truly segmental pattern. In some cases they are single and in others they are multiple.

LABORATORY FINDINGS

Although autopsy studies have rarely been performed except by chance, since Löffler's syndrome is a benign self-limiting disease, the histology of these consolidations seems to consist, as might be expected, just of alveolar consolidation with an eosinophil-filled exudate. The peripheral eosinophilia is obvious but rarely gross; a differential of more than 20 per cent in a modestly raised total white cell count is unusual and more often the eosinophil count ranges between 1×10^9 and 2×10^9/l.

PATHOGENESIS

Patients who develop Löffler's syndrome are often atopic and may have other manifestations of an atopic diathesis such as angio-oedema. The defined causes of the syndrome suggest an allergic reaction, and are various. Two broad groups with a third miscellaneous collection emerge from analysis of the literature.

In the first group of cases reaction to parasites has featured as a recognizable aetiology. The long list includes *Ascaris lumbricoides* and occasionally *suum,* Ancylostoma, Trichuris, Trichinella, Taenia, and Strongyloides.

Drugs form a second important category. Löffler's syndrome is well described after administration of *p*-amino salicylic acid, aspirin, sulphonamides (including the antimalarial combination sulphadiazine and pyrimethamine or Fansidar), penicillin, and imipramine. It may also occur with nitrofurantoin (although this often gives a diffuse reticulo-nodular alveolar exudate), toxic smoke, and lymphangiography contrast medium.

A significant minority of cases of Löffler's syndrome remain unexplained.

TREATMENT

Worm infestation needs treatment. Suspected drugs should be stopped.

Eosinophilic pneumonia and prolonged pulmonary eosinophilia

This syndrome is similar to simple pulmonary eosinophilia; indeed, the differences may simply lie in degree and duration. The division in terms of duration at 1 month is arbitrary, but is often clinically useful.

CLINICAL FEATURES

Prolonged pulmonary eosinophilia may last for several months. It is associated with more severe clinical symptoms than simple pulmonary eosinophilia. Fever, often high and swinging, is usual, weight loss may occur, and a range of associated systemic features have been described: focal, skin, and hepatic necrosis, hepatosplenomegaly, and atopic manifestations such as rhinitis, sinusitis, and angio-oedema. The pulmonary disease is usually extensive, causing dyspnoea and hypoxia with signs of consolidation on clinical examination. Radiologically, the shadows may be pneumonic (hence the term eosinophilic pneumonia); the solid and confluent peripheral consolidations earn these cases the description 'the negative photographic image of pulmonary oedema'. They last for several days or about a week, although, like the shadows of Löffler's syndrome, they also vary in site during the course of the illness. Eosinophilic pleural effusion has been recorded.

PATHOLOGY

Pathologically, there are macrophages, lymphocytes, and polymorphs in the alveolar exudate together with the eosinophils, and sometimes evidence of angiitis or even granuloma formation making these cases shade into the more sinister disorders of allergic or Wegener's granulomatosis. The eosinophil count is usually more than 1×10^9/ml with records existing of 70 per cent eosinophils in very high total white cell counts of up to 100×10^9/l.

MANAGEMENT

Causes and hence treatment cover the same range as that described for simple pulmonary eosinophilia, but often no cause is evident. These cryptogenic cases respond dramatically to oral corticosteroid therapy which is usually required for 6 to 12 months and occasionally for longer.

Pulmonary eosinophilia with bronchial involvement

Some degree of eosinophilia is common in straightforward bronchial asthma. Counts of above 0.4×10^9/ml are considered a helpful diagnostic pointer in this condition. However, figures greater than about 1.0×10^9/ml suggest that a specific cause should be sought. Two syndromes stand out.

The first is allergic bronchopulmonary aspergillosis and consists of asthma, fleeting pulmonary infiltrates (Fig. 1) with a tendency to mucus impaction, and bronchial wall damage which leads to proximal bronchiectasis. In the United Kingdom, and probably most other Western countries, Aspergillus sensitivity accounts for more than 90 per cent of patients presenting with this syndrome. Rarely, other agents causing Löffler's syndrome and fungal species such as Candida can cause the same syndrome; other cases remain cryptogenic. Further details of allergic bronchopulmonary aspergillosis are given in Chapter 17.9.1(b).

The second syndrome in this category is tropical eosinophilia. This term was coined by Weingarten in 1943 for a condition seen in the tropics and characterized by asthmatic airways obstruction, parenchymal lung damage, and a marked peripheral eosinophilia. The noted response to arsenic compounds suggested a parasitic aetiology.

INCIDENCE

The disease is endemic in the Indian subcontinent, particularly the northwest, as well as in Malaysia, Indonesia, and also parts of Africa and South America. In Singapore it is noted that the disease is confined to Indians, sparing the Chinese population.

CLINICAL FEATURES

The typical presentation is persistent dry cough, particularly at night. Dyspnoea quickly follows with typically asthmatic nocturnal exacerbations. Non-asthmatic features are a tendency to fever and haemoptysis. Wheeze predominates on auscultation, but there may also be crepita-

Fig. 1 Allergic bronchopulmonary aspergillosis: radiographs taken at intervals of 6 months in an East African woman with asthma, peripheral eosinophilia, and high titres of IgE and precipitating IgG antibodies to *Aspergillus fumigatus*.

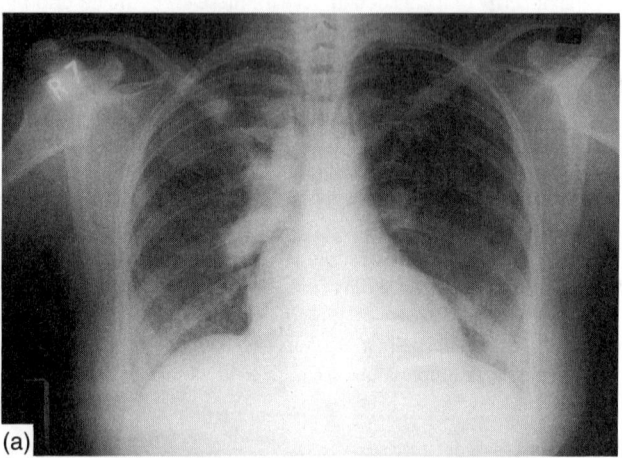

(a)

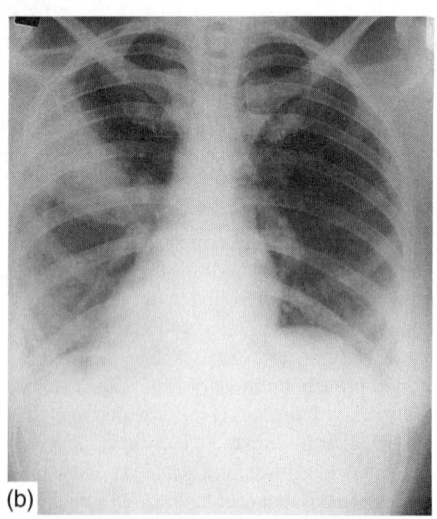

(b)

tions. The latter reflect the diffuse parenchymal component of the disease which gives the typical radiological appearance of bilateral mottling which may in places become confluent. In the later stages of the disease, if untreated, persistent dyspnoea reflects irreversible airways obstruction and pulmonary fibrosis, and there can be terminal respiratory failure and cor pulmonale. Lung function tests show a mixed obstructive and restrictive defect. The peripheral white cell count is usually elevated, and often very high, and at least 20 per cent will be eosinophils.

PATHOGENESIS

There is no reasonable doubt that microfilariae, notably *Wuchereria bancrofti* and *Brugia malayi*, are the cause. The pathological lesions, focal granulomata in an infiltrate of eosinophils, neutrophils, polymorphs, and macrophages, represent an allergic response to microfilariae transiently released into the circulation from the mature gravid human filarial parasite. High titres of IgE, IgG, and IgM to the parasite are present on serology.

PROGNOSIS AND TREATMENT

A good prognosis is possible if the condition is recognized and treated early with diethyl carbamazine in a daily dose of 6–8 mg/kg body weight orally, given for a week, although longer courses may occasionally be necessary.

REFERENCES

Citro, L.A., Gordon, M.E., and Miller, N.T. (1973). Eosinophilic lung disease (or how to slice PIE). *American Journal of Roentgenology*, **117**, 787.

Crofton, J.W., Livingstone, J.L., Oswald, N.C., and Roberts, A.I.M. (1952). Pulmonary eosinophilia. *Thorax*, **7**, 1–35.

Epstein, D.M., Tuormina, V., Gefter, W.B., and Miller, W.T. (1981). The hypereosinophilic syndrome. *Radiology*, **140**, 59.

Middleton, W.G., Paterson, J.C., Grant, I.W.B., and Douglas, A.C. (1977). Asthmatic pulmonary eosinophilia. A review of 65 cases. *British Journal of Diseases of the Chest*, **71**, 115–22.

Pearson, D.J., and Rosenow, E.C., III. (1978). Chronic eosinophilic pneumonia (Carrington's): a follow up study. *Mayo Clinic Proceedings*, **53**, 73.

Udwadia, F.E. (1993). Tropical eosinophilia: a review. *Respiratory Medicine*, **87**, 17–21.

17.10.8 Lymphocytic infiltrations of the lung

D. J. HENDRICK

Introduction

A number of disorders are characterized by a prominent, even dominant, lymphocytic infiltration of the lung. Several are rare and poorly understood, while others are relatively common and have additional more definitive characteristics. Classification of the latter group poses few problems, and individual diseases are satisfactorily distinguishable. They include, for example, sarcoidosis, extrinsic allergic alveolitis, cryptogenic organizing pneumonia, and some cases of cryptogenic fibrosing alveolitis. They are described separately elsewhere.

For the first group, which constitutes the subject of this chapter, classification poses an evolving challenge—largely because precise mechanisms and full natural histories are yet to be defined. Nomenclature will undoubtedly continue to change. These disorders are often considered to represent a spectrum of overlapping conditions from relatively benign infiltration of apparently normal lymphocytes without involvement of other cellular lines, through vasculitic and granulomatous inflammation, to frank malignancy. Apparent progression from disorder to disorder within the spectrum is not uncommon, but it is not always clear whether individuals affected in this way truly progress from one disease to another or have a single disease whose early manifestations are similar to (and mistaken for) those of less serious neighbours in the disease spectrum. This has given rise to an alternative view that one end of the spectrum comprises a group of inflammatory disorders whose vasculitic and granulomatous features link more appropriately with diseases such as Wegener's granulomatosis and sarcoidosis, while the other end comprises the various malignant lymphomas.

Nevertheless, dominant lymphocytic infiltration is a convenient definitive feature from which to consider the small group of uncommon pulmonary diseases which are described in this chapter. There is often paraprotein production, implying that a lymphocyte clone is involved. Depending on severity, these disorders are characterized clinically by cough (usually dry) and progressive undue exertional breathlessness, although systemic features of fever, malaise, and weight loss may also be prominent. Clubbing is not common, but there are frequently inspiratory crackles at the lung bases. The chest radiograph shows a diffuse interstitial pattern or patchy 'pneumonic' infiltrates with the more benign disorders, but nodular shadows are more characteristic at the more malignant end of the disease spectrum. Lung function tests show a non-specific pattern of ventilatory restriction with impaired parenchymal function.

Lymphocytic (and plasma-cell) interstitial pneumonitis

At the most benign end of the spectrum of lymphocytic infiltrations, lymphocytic (or lymphoid) interstitial pneumonitis is characterized by diffuse infiltration of the lung interstitium and alveolar walls with small mature lymphocytes, immunoblasts (activated lymphocytes), and plasma cells. Occasionally, plasma cells dominate the lymphoid cell infiltrate, and in these circumstances the term plasma-cell interstitial pneumonitis is preferred. Lymphocytic pulmonary infiltration may occur in isolation without obvious cause or may be associated with HIV infection and a variety of autoimmune disorders, particularly Sjögren's syndrome or systemic lupus erythematosus. It may also be a consequence of a graft versus host reaction. When it occurs in children with AIDS, it is thought to be largely a consequence of Epstein–Barr infection. It may progress to (or be complicated by) the development of lymphoma, and this too is particularly associated with Sjögren's syndrome.

The infiltrating lymphocytes show various levels of activation, and excess circulating immunoglobulins, whether monoclonal or polyclonal, are commonly observed. Occasionally there is hypo- rather than hypergammaglobulinaemia. When plasma cells rather than lymphocytes are dominant, the immunoglobulins are much less likely to be of the IgM class although complications may still include Waldenstrom's macroglobulinaemia or multiple myeloma.

The respiratory features are similar to those of cryptogenic fibrosing alveolitis, and open biopsy is generally required for definitive diagnosis. It is seen in both sexes, usually in middle age. Slow progression is characteristic, although lymphocytic interstitial pneumonitis is rather more responsive to corticosteroid or other immunosuppressive therapy than is cryptogenic fibrosing alveolitis, and it sometimes remits spontaneously. However, progressive fibrosis may occur, as may complicating (even fatal) sepsis.

Benign lymphocytic angiitis

Lymphocytic infiltration in this condition is centred in small arteries and arterioles, although necrosis is characteristically absent. Not infrequently there is granuloma formation. Therefore it has vasculitic and granulomatous features. It is rare, relatively benign, and usually affects the lungs or the skin. Most often there is no obvious provoking cause, but there have been reports of it emerging as a consequence of drug administration (streptokinase), HIV infection, or intrathoracic malignancy (thymoma).

Pulmonary lesions are usually single and most commonly present as asymptomatic nodules on a chance chest radiograph. The diagnosis is then made following biopsy or resection. However, there may be systemic symptoms, and treatment with corticosteroids or cytotoxic agents may be necessary. The disease may progress to produce the more characteristic features of lymphomatoid granulomatosis, but more typically there is spontaneous remission. This suggests that benign lymphocytic angiitis is indeed primarily a benign reactive vasculitis rather than a malignant lymphoma. It may be that similar histological features are also characteristic early in the course of lymphomatoid granulomatosis.

Angio-immunoblastic (immunoblastic) lymphadenopathy

This is a systemic and often febrile disorder characterized by widespread reactive lymphadenopathy and the infiltration of various organs by activated lymphoid cells, characteristically but not uniformly T lymphocytes. CD8+ cells, often clonal, are observed more commonly than CD4+ cells in affected organs, but in peripheral blood active disease is characterized by decreased numbers of T cells and an increase in B lymphocytes. The latter are possibly released from T-cell control and this might explain the frequency of paraprotein production. Blood vessels may be prominently infiltrated—hence the original term, angio-immunoblastic lymphadenopathy.

This disorder occurs most commonly in the elderly and frequently in isolation, but it is often a consequence of infection (prominently HIV infection in recent years in younger subjects) or drug administration (often antibiotics), and it may be associated with autoimmunity.

Respiratory involvement is not common. It usually comprises mediastinal or hilar lymphadenopathy, although diffuse interstitial infiltration and pleural effusion may occur. The involvement and enlargement of other lymphoid organs, particularly lymph nodes, liver, and spleen, usually offers a ready biopsy site for definitive diagnosis.

Management requires treatment of any provoking cause and, if necessary, the use of corticosteroids or other immunosuppressive agents. Occasionally there is spontaneous remission, but more commonly a T-cell lymphoma evolves. Indeed, the view is strengthening that most cases are of peripheral (i.e. post-thymic) T-cell lymphoma throughout.

Lymphomatoid granulomatosis

Lymphomatoid granulomatosis is now widely considered to be a low grade T-cell lymphoma, although the typical histological appearances of prominent infiltration of blood vessel walls (hence vasculitis) and granuloma formation had, until recently, suggested a disease of a more benign nature. The infiltrating cells comprise a mixture of lymphocytes, plasma cells, histiocytes, and atypical lymphoid cells, and their proliferation leads to luminal obstruction followed by ischaemic necrosis. Cytochemical and immunogenetic investigation now suggest that the atypical lymphoid cells are malignant (i.e. lymphomatous) T lymphocytes, and that it is a low grade, often multifocal, malignancy which drives the vasculitic and granulomatous inflammatory response in affected tissue.

The disease is uncommon in childhood but occurs throughout adult life with a small predilection to males. The lungs are almost invariably affected, but skin, central nervous system, and renal involvement is frequently seen and there is often peripheral neuropathy. The disease is typically multifocal, affecting several organs, and may simulate disseminated carcinoma. Pulmonary lesions are usually discrete and nodular, whether single or multiple, but may vary in size from small nodules less than a centimetre in diameter to large masses several centimetres across. Occasionally outlines are irregular and indistinct, suggesting patchy consolidation, and cavitation may occur. Consequently, an inflammatory cause may be suspected, with the radiographical appearances simulating those of Wegener's granulomatosis.

Symptoms are commonly dominated by systemic upset (fever, malaise, weight loss), but respiratory involvement is likely to cause cough (sometimes with haemoptysis) or undue breathlessness. The involvement of other organs may provide valuable diagnostic insight, but biopsy is necessary for definitive diagnosis. Temporary improvement sometimes follows treatment with corticosteroids alone, but a realistic chance of complete remission requires cytotoxic therapy for lymphoma.

Lymphoma

Unquestionably at the malignant end of the disease spectrum lies lymphomatous infiltration of the lung. All lymphoma tumour types may initially present with intrathoracic disease, and all may involve the thorax later if the disease initially presents outside the thorax. Lymph nodes, lymphatics, and lung parenchyma may all become infiltrated, but the pattern may vary between tumour types.

A comprehensive review of lymphomas is beyond the scope of this chapter, and the reader is referred to Chapter 22.5.3 for full detail. In brief, lymphomas can be considered to be of the Hodgkin's type (a unique malignant tumour arising typically in lymphoid tissue but of uncertain cell origin although characterized by the Reed–Sternberg cell) or the non-Hodgkin's type. The latter arise from B lymphocytes, T lymphocytes, or histiocytes (or their stem cells), and can be classified according to a variety of aetiological, histological, immunological, and clinical features. To the chest-physician the differentiation of Hodgkin's disease and high grade non-Hodgkin's lymphoma from low-grade non-Hodgkin's lymphoma is of particular value, since the first two are potentially curable with aggressive chemotherapy regimens.

Hodgkin's disease generally affects adults and adolescent. When it involves the thorax it usually does so by infiltrating hilar or mediastinal lymph nodes, although rarely localized, even diffuse, parenchymal infiltration occurs with or without lymphadenopathy. Asymmetrical nodal enlargement favours lymphoma over sarcoidosis, which is the other disorder (apart from tuberculosis in endemic areas) commonly producing hilar and mediastinal adenopathy in the absence of obvious parenchymal disease of the lung. Hodgkin's disease frequently involves other nodal sites at presentation, but may be confined to the thorax. Pleural effusion is not uncommon, and occasionally there is infiltration of the chest wall. Biopsy and staging are essential to diagnosis and management, although the advent of CT scanning has greatly simplified the latter by eliminating the need for laparotomy. Radiotherapy is normally curative for localized nodal disease and is invaluable as an adjunct in reducing local bulk when the disease is disseminated. It carries much less risk than chemotherapy, which is required for parenchymal or disseminated disease and for the small proportion of patients with localized nodal disease who show features of poor prognostic significance (e.g. high bulk, systemic symptoms, anaemia).

Non-Hodgkin's lymphoma occurs more commonly than Hodgkin's disease, although it tends to affect a rather older population. Its thoracic manifestations are similar to those of Hodgkin's disease, but it is the more likely malignant 'complication' of the other lymphocytic pulmonary infiltrations discussed in this chapter. It also has a greater tendency to be disseminated at presentation, and (not surprisingly) to be less responsive to chemotherapy. Nevertheless, localized high grade tumours

are often curable, and useful palliation is generally achieved for many years for low grade tumours.

Considerable advances have been made in recent years with regard to chemotherapeutic regimens and new developments are occurring rapidly. As a result the management of lymphomas has properly become the responsibility of experts in the field. Of course, chemotherapy is attended by the familiar risks of bone marrow suppression and an immunocompromised state. Furthermore, many of the chemotherapeutic agents may themselves cause interstitial lung disease, including lymphocytic infiltration.

Consequently, the supervising physician may face a classic diagnostic dilemma when, following an initial satisfactory remission, the patient's radiographs show pulmonary shadows consistent with infection, drug hypersensitivity, or recurrent lymphomatous infiltration. A prompt and accurate diagnosis is essential since each possibility requires fundamentally different management. Expectorated secretions may provide enough evidence of infection to justify a trial of antibiotic therapy, but if immediate progress is unsatisfactory fibre optic bronchoscopy with lavage and/or transbronchial biopsy is generally needed. It may be that with increasing use of the polymerized chain reaction to amplify fragments of genetically specific microbial material, samples of sputum or even oropharyngeal secretions will prove adequate to identify the infecting organisms. Not infrequently the cause of pulmonary shadows in this situation is complex, and any combination of these three diagnostic groups may develop (perhaps with more than one infecting micro-organism). Consequently, a multidisciplinary approach to management has become essential, involving chest physicians, radiologists, microbiologists, and histopathologists alike under the expert guidance of supervising oncologists or haematologists.

REFERENCES

Andiman, W.A., Eastman, R., Martin, K., Katz, B.Z., Rubinstein, A., Pitt, J., et al. (1985). Opportunistic lymphoproliferations associated with Epstein–Barr viral DNA in infants and children with AIDS. *Lancet*, **ii**, 1390–3.

Calabrese, L.H., Estes, M., Yen-Lieberman, B., Proffitt, M.R., Tubbs, R., Fishleder, A.J., and Levin, K.H. (1989). Systemic vasculitis in association with human immunodeficiency virus infection. *Arthritis and Rheumatism*, **32**, 569–76.

Churg, A. (1983). Pulmonary angiitis and granulomatosis revisited. *Human Pathology*, **14**, 868–83.

Frizzera, G., Moran, E.M., and Rappaport, H. (1974). Angio-immunoblastic lymphadenopathy with dysproteinaemia. *Lancet*, **ii**, 1070–3.

Glickstein, M., Kornstein, M.J., Pietra, G.G., Aronchick, J.M., Gefter, W.B., Epstein, D.M., and Miller, W. (1986). Non-lymphomatous lymphoid disorders of the lung. *American Journal of Roentgenology*, **147**, 227–37.

Grieco, M.H., and Chinoy-Acharya, P. (1985). Lymphocytic interstitial pneumonia associated with the acquired immune deficiency syndrome. *American Review of Respiratory Disease*, **131**, 952–5.

Katzenstein, A.-L.A., Carrington, C.B., and Liebow, A.A. (1979). Lymphomatoid granulomatosis. A clinicopathologic study of 152 cases. *Cancer*, **43**, 360–73.

Liebow, A.A. (1973). Pulmonary angiitis and granulomatosis. *American Review of Respiratory Disease*, **108**, 1–18.

O'Connor, N.T., Crick, J.A., Wainscoat, J.S., Gatter, K.C., Stein, H., Falini, B., and Mason, D.Y. (1986). Evidence for monoclonal T lymphocyte proliferation in angioimmunoblastic lymphadenopathy. *Journal of Clinical Pathology*, **39**, 1229–32.

Watanabe, S., Sato, Y., Shimoyama, M., Minato, K., and Shimosato, Y. (1986). Immunoblastic lymphadenopathy, angioimmunoblastic lymphadenopathy, and IBL-like T-cell lymphoma. A spectrum of T-cell neoplasia. *Cancer*, **58**, 2224–32.

Weiss, L.M., Strickler, J.G., Dorfman, R.F., Horning, S.J., Warnke, R.A. and Sklar, J. (1986). Clonal T-cell populations in angioimmunoblastic lymphadenopathy and angioimmunoblastic and lymphadenopathy-like lymphoma. *American Journal of Pathology*, **122**, 392–7.

17.10.9 Extrinsic allergic alveolitis

D. J. HENDRICK

Historical background

Farmer's lung is often regarded as the prototype of the bronchiolar and alveolar disorders that result from hypersensitivity to inhaled organic dusts. They are known collectively by the term extrinsic allergic alveolitis, although it is recognized that the underlying inflammatory response occurs diffusely throughout the gas exchanging tissues and is not confined to the alveoli. For this reason many prefer the term hypersensitivity pneumonitis. These alveolar disorders were not clearly distinguished from asthma until 1932 when Campbell published his celebrated report describing three affected English farm workers. The appellation 'farmer's lung' was suggested later in 1944. None the less the disease was recognized in Iceland in the nineteenth century, and probably contributed to the occupational ailments of grain workers so graphically described by Ramazzini in the eighteenth century.

Part of the eminence of farmer's lung itself stems from its industrial importance, and part from its historical role in the understanding of extrinsic allergic alveolitis. Its relation to the inhalation of dust from mouldy hay, straw, or grain had been recognized from the outset, but it was not until 1961 when Pepys and colleagues demonstrated the presence of precipitins to antigens of mouldy hay in patients suffering from the disease that the idea of an allergic aetiology gained general acceptance. These and other investigators showed that the main sources of antigen were contaminating thermophilic actinomycetes, particularly *Micropolyspora faeni* (now known as *Faenia rectivirgula*) and *Thermoactinomyces vulgaris*. These thermophilic microbes (they are actually bacteria and not fungi) colonize fermenting damp vegetable produce as it heats up. When it eventually dries, a respirable dust laden with antigenic microbial spores is left. Symptoms are consequently most common during winters following wet summer harvests, when hay or grain is used for feeding stock and astonishing numbers of spores (thousands of millions per cubic metre) are released into the air.

For deposition of the dust to occur predominantly in the gas exchanging tissues, particle size must be largely confined to the range 0.5–5 µm. This encompasses the diameters of many antigenic bacterial and fungal spores, and a large number of microbial species are now recognized causes of extrinsic allergic alveolitis. In addition, the disease has been noted to follow exposure to a variety of antigens derived from animal, vegetable, and even chemical sources, in both the workplace and the home.

Clinical features

Acute form

The acute form of extrinsic allergic alveolitis is the most easily recognized because symptoms are often quickly distressing and incapacitating, and have a high degree of specificity. Following a sensitizing period of exposure which may vary from weeks to years, the affected subject experiences repeated episodes of an influenza-like illness accompanied by cough and undue breathlessness some hours (usually 3–9) after commencing exposure to the relevant organic dust. The systemic influenza-like symptoms generally dominate those that are essentially respiratory in nature, and the subject complains most of malaise, fever, chills, widespread aches and pains (particularly headache), anorexia, and tiredness. He is unlikely to exercise himself and may well put himself to bed. Therefore he may be unaware of undue shortness of breath, although he is likely to develop a dry cough without wheeze and some difficulty in taking deep satisfying breaths. Occasionally there is an asthmatic or bronchitic response in addition to that in the gas exchanging tissues, and wheezing or productive cough becomes a further feature.

Affected subjects soon learn to associate symptoms with the causative environment, despite the delay in onset after exposure begins. Recognition is particularly easy for groups such as farmers and pigeon fanciers for whom these risks are likely to be well known. However, in some cases there may be a tendency to deny such a relationship for fear of compromising the ability to pursue livelihood or hobby, and the clinical history may appear much less convincing than it should.

The severity and duration of symptoms depend on exposure dose. With low levels of acute exposure, symptoms are mild and persist for a few hours only. When occupation is responsible, the affected worker may feel unwell only at home during the following evening or night and be fully recovered by the next morning. Consequently the relevance of the workplace may be obscured. When severe responses follow particularly heavy exposures the relation of the one to the other will be more obvious, and complete remission may require several days or even weeks.

In exceptionally severe cases, life-threatening respiratory failure may develop and emergency admission to hospital becomes necessary. Death is not unknown. Respiratory distress at rest with fever and gravity-dependent crackles comprise the major physical signs, with breathing being fast but shallow. Clubbing is very rarely seen. Hypoxia is typically accompanied by hypocapnia, and the chest radiograph shows a diffuse alveolar filling pattern. Spontaneous recovery can be expected to begin within 12 to 24 h, and can be accelerated with corticosteroids. Supplemental oxygen will be required in the interim, and in rare cases there may be a brief need for mechanical ventilatory support.

Most subjects recover fully from each acute exacerbation, and if the cause is recognized and further exposure avoided, there is little risk of persisting pulmonary dysfunction. However, it is not always realistic to expect affected individuals to avoid further exposure, particularly among farming communities, and there is some risk that continuing exposure and repeated acute exacerbations will eventually be associated with permanent impairment of lung function.

Chronic form

In some subjects, extrinsic allergic alveolitis expresses itself in a much less dramatic though potentially more serious way. There is a slowly increasing loss of exercise tolerance owing to shortness of breath but no systemic upset apart from an occasional prominent loss of weight. This is the result of diffuse pulmonary fibrosis which has often been progressing for years before the affected subject seeks advice. The slower the progression, the longer the delay, and the greater the likely degree of permanent fibrotic damage. Eventually hypoxia and pulmonary hypertension may supervene, and the right heart fails. There are no acute exacerbations, and each day and each month are much like any other. The clinical features are similar to those of other varieties of pulmonary fibrosis, although clubbing and crepitations are uncommon, and it may prove extremely difficult to distinguish this form of extrinsic allergic alveolitis from cryptogenic fibrosing alveolitis, sarcoidosis, or other slowly progressive forms of pulmonary fibrosis.

The chronic form of extrinsic allergic alveolitis is typically seen in the subject who keeps a single budgerigar (known as a parakeet in the United States) in the home. The level of antigenic exposure to avian dust is comparatively trivial (compared with the farm worker forking bales of heavily contaminated hay in a poorly ventilated barn), but it is encountered almost continuously, particularly if the affected subject is a housewife or elderly pensioner largely confined to the home. These different exposure patterns are generally responsible for these distinct forms of extrinsic allergic alveolitis, although differences in host responsiveness must exert an important additional influence. Consequently, there may be considerable variability in clinical features among individuals affected by the same source of antigenic exposure.

Table 1 *Agents reported to cause extrinsic allergic alveolitis*

Agent	Source	Appellation
Micro-organisms		
Alternaria	Paper mill wood pulp	Wood pulp worker's lung
Aspergillus clavatus	Whisky maltings	Malt worker's lung
Aspergillus fumigatus	Vegetable compost	Farmer's lung
Aspergillus versicolor	Dog bedding (straw)	Dog house disease
Aureobasidium pullulans	Redwood	Sequoiosis
Bacillus subtilis	Domestic wood	
Cephalosporium	Sewage	Sewage worker's lung
Cryptostroma corticale	Maple	Maple bark stripper's lung
Graphium	Redwood	Sequoiosis
Lycoperdon	Puffballs	Lycoperdonosis
Merulius lacrymans	Domestic wood	
Mucor stolonifer	Paprika	Paprika splitter's lung
Penicillium casei	Cheese	Cheese washer's lung
Penicillium chrysogenum/ Penicillium cyclopium	Domestic wood	
Penicillium frequentens	Cork	Suberosis
Saccharomonspora viridis	Logging plant	
Sporobolomyces	Horse barn straw	
Streptomyces albus	Soil, peat	
Thermophilic actinomycetes (*Micropolyspora faeni, T. sacchari/vulgaris*)	Hay, straw, grain, mushroom compost, bagasse	Farmer's lung, mushroom worker's lung, bagassosis
Trichosporon cutaneum	Japanese summer air	Summer-type hypersensitivity pneumonitis
Miscellaneous: bacteria?, fungi?, amoebas?, nematode debris?	Air conditioners, humidifiers, tap water	Humidifier lung, ventilation pneumonitis, sauna taker's lung
Unknown	Roof thatch	New Guinea lung
Animals		
Arthropods (*S. granarius*)	Grain dust	Wheat weevil disease
Birds	Bloom?, excreta?	Bird fancier's lung
Fish	Fish meal	Fish meal worker's lung
Mammals		
Pituitary (cattle, pig)	Pituitary extracts	Pituitary snuff taker's lung
Hair	Fur	Furrier's lung
Urine (rodents)	Urinary protein	Rodent handler's lung
Vegetation		
Coffee	Coffee bean dust	Coffee worker's lung
Wood (*Gonystylus bacanus*)	Wood dust	Wood worker's lung
Chemicals		
Bordeaux mixture (fungicide)	Vineyards	Vineyard sprayer's lung
Cobalt dissolved in solvents	Tungsten carbide grinding	
Diphenylmethane diisocyanate	Plastics industry	
Formaldehyde*	Laboratory	
Pauli's reagent	Laboratory	
Pyrethrum	Insecticide spray	
Hexamethylene diisocyanate	Plastics industry	
Toluene diisocyanate	Plastics industry	
Trimellitic anhydride	Plastics industry	

*One subject, possibly toxic not allergic response

Intermediate forms

The fact that the acute form of extrinsic allergic alveolitis can be produced by inhalation provocation tests in subjects with the chronic form of the disease emphasizes the major role that dose exerts in determining the clinical nature of the response that occurs. Depending on exposure dose and host responsiveness a variety of intermediate forms of extrinsic allergic alveolitis will be recognized, and some subjects will experience different patterns of response at different times. Therefore it is possible for acute exacerbations to occur in subjects manifesting predominantly the chronic form of the disease, and for a limited degree of recovery to follow cessation of exposure. In general, however, the individual affected by the chronic form of extrinsic allergic alveolitis should be satisfied if no further progression occurs following cessation of exposure, because in some cases fibrotic damage continues regardless.

Causative agents

Table 1 lists the various agents reported to cause extrinsic allergic alveolitis. Most are microorganisms that are found contaminating a variety of vegetable products. Although those associated with the most celebrated disorders—farmer's lung, mushroom worker's lung, and bagassosis—are usually thermophilic, the majority are not. Even with mouldy hay and farmer's lung there is evidence that non-thermophilic organisms (e.g. *Aspergillus* spp.) may occasionally be involved. Some microbial contamination may occur during growth of the vegetable host, but most of the antigenic load is usually acquired after harvest. Therefore prolonged storage under damp conditions increases the risk of extrinsic allergic alveolitis substantially, while drying to reduce the water content below 30 per cent greatly reduces the risks. Consequently, farmer's lung and bagassosis are not primary disorders of hay, grain, or sugar cane harvest. They usually arise months or even years later when the stored product is used or moved.

Inevitably there are situations where contamination arises with a number of different microbes, and affected subjects show antibodies to several of them. Unless time-consuming inhalation challenge tests are carried out with extracts of the individual microbial species, it is not possible to identify a single responsible agent in a given case or cases. It is conceivable that several could be relevant in these circumstances. This is a characteristic feature with contaminated humidifiers and air conditioners, and a large variety of agents have been suggested as possible causes of humidifier lung, including bacteria, fungi, protozoa (amoebae), and metazoa (nematode debris). Some authors prefer to distinguish extrinsic allergic alveolitis attributable in such circumstances to microorganisms growing in cool or cold water (humidifier lung) from extrinsic allergic alveolitis which arises from thermophilic organisms growing in heated water (ventilation pneumonitis).

Curiously, contamination with multiple microbial species does not seem to be a feature of Japanese summer-type pneumonitis which arises seasonally in the hot and humid regions in the south and west of Japan, and is related to the excessive growth of *Trichosporon cutaneum* in unsanitary and poorly ventilated homes.

Pathogenic mechanisms

Histology

The opportunity to characterize extrinsic allergic alveolitis histologically in its acute form has been limited because biopsies are very uncommonly taken within 24 to 48 h of a provoking exposure and because death leading to autopsy is an even rarer event. Initially, there is a non-specific diffuse pneumonitis with inflammatory cellular infiltration of the bronchioles, alveoli, and interstitium accompanied by oedema and luminal exudation. With ongoing exposure, whether continuous or intermittent, the more familiar appearances of the subacute forms of extrinsic allergic alveolitis evolve. The most characteristic feature is the formation of epithelioid non-caseating granulomas. The granulomas are generally less well formed and less profuse than in sarcoidosis, and are often

Fig. 1 Histological appearances: subacute disease. There is bronchocentric interstitial fibrosis and chronic inflammation, with poorly formed interstitial granulomas including giant cells. Haematoxylin and eosin stain. Medium magnification. (By courtesy of Dr T. Ashcroft.)

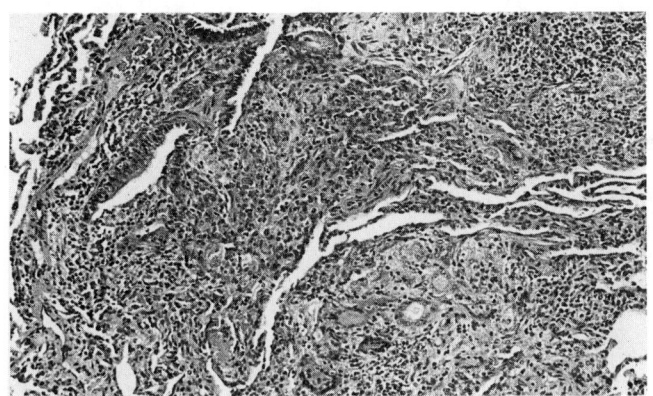

evanescent. They can be recognized within 3 weeks of the inititing exposure, and generally resolve within 6 to 12 months. In parallel, fibrosis evolves alongside cellular infiltration of the interstitium with histiocytes, lymphocytes, and plasma cells. Macrophages with foamy cytoplasm may be prominent in the alveolar spaces, and organization of the inflammatory exudate may lead to intra-alveolar fibrosis. Obstruction or obliteration of bronchioles is common. Foreign-body giant cells may reflect the dependence of extrinsic allergic alveolitis on antigens derived from inhaled foreign material, as does a peribronchial predominance of the inflammatory response. Vasculitis is notable for its absence. The typical histological appearances of subacute extrinsic allergic alveolitis are illustrated in Fig. 1.

With continued exposure, progressive, widespread, and irreversible fibrosis may occur leading to disruption of the normal architecture of the lung. In advanced cases honeycombing may develop. Granulomas are no longer characteristic, and the overall appearance may differ little from other causes of progressive interstitial pulmonary fibrosis. With extrinsic allergic alveolitis, however, there may be disproportionate fibrosis of the upper lobes.

Immune mechanisms

An outline of the possible immunopathology of extrinsic allergic alveolitis through acute and subacute–chronic phases is illustrated in Fig. 2 and 3. The presumption that complexes of antigen and complement-activating antibodies are primarily responsible for extrinsic allergic alveolitis is now largely discarded. The evidence for deposition of immune complexes is not convincing, and neither IgG nor IgM antibodies are uniformly demonstrated in the sera of affected subjects unless sensitive detection techniques such as the enzyme-linked immunosorbent assay or radioimmunoassays are used. More importantly, these antibodies are frequently found in subjects who are similarly exposed but clinically unaffected, irrespective of the method of detection. A closer association with disease has been suggested with the IgG4 antibody subclass, but the significance of this is not yet clear. It is clear that vasculitis, a cardinal feature of the experimental Arthus reaction, is not characteristically present; the inflammatory reaction is dominantly lymphocytic or mononuclear rather than polymorphonuclear. However, a transitory polymorphonuclear leucocyte response is typical immediately following exposure. Lung tissue is most commonly examined during subacute phases of the disease, at which time a non-caseating granulomatous response suggesting cell-mediated hypersensitivity is the usual finding.

It could be argued that these histological appearances merely represent a healing reaction, but the consistent finding of an acute T-lymphocyte response in fluid obtained at bronchoalveolar lavage supports the current consensus that cell-mediated hypersensitivity plays the dominant role in extrinsic allergic alveolitis. The results from recent animal models of the disease are consistent with this, with disease being transferred from animal to animal only with sensitized T lymphocytes. This is not to say that other mechanisms play no role, nor that all inflammatory diseases of the gas exchanging tissues induced by organic dusts share a common mechanism. Indeed, the onset of symptoms within a few hours of exposure coupled with polymorphonuclear leucocytosis in bronchoalveolar lavage fluid and peripheral blood favours the participation of an additional (perhaps priming) immunological or toxic process. Components of a number of organic dusts associated with extrinsic allergic alveolitis are known to activate complement by the alternative pathway and this, with or without humoral hypersensitivity, could prove to be relevant.

In fact, bronchoalveolar lavage in similarly exposed subjects has shown excess numbers of T lymphocytes whether they were clinically affected or not, although the proportions of T-cell subpopulations has varied according to disease activity and the circumstances of exposure. Most investigators have detected a relative excess in the number of CD8+ T cells in exposed but asymptomatic subjects, thereby 'inverting' the normal ratio of CD4+ to CD8+. The balance appears to shift back towards CD4+ dominance in those with disease. In an intriguing study of an animal model of extrinsic allergic alveolitis, monkeys which developed characteristic reactions to inhalation challenge showed a helper CD4+ cell lymphocytosis in bronchoalveolar fluid and a relative deficiency of suppressor CD8+ cells, compared with monkeys giving no clinical reaction who showed responses with both CD4+ and CD8+ cells. When the non-reactors were challenged again after low doses of whole-body irradiation had impaired suppressor-cell more than helper-cell function, characteristic reactions were noted. These observations

suggest that a relative impairment of suppressor-cell function, or of its activation following antigenic exposure, is fundamental to the development of extrinsic allergic alveolitis—a situation which has interesting parallels with sarcoidosis. Presumably, the population of radio-resistant suppressor cells is less relevant. It is also interesting that lymphopenia in peripheral blood is a typical feature of acute exacerbations of the disease, with the T lymphocytes migrating from blood to lungs within hours of the provoking exposure. It is small wonder that studies of systemic and local immune responses have given discordant results, and

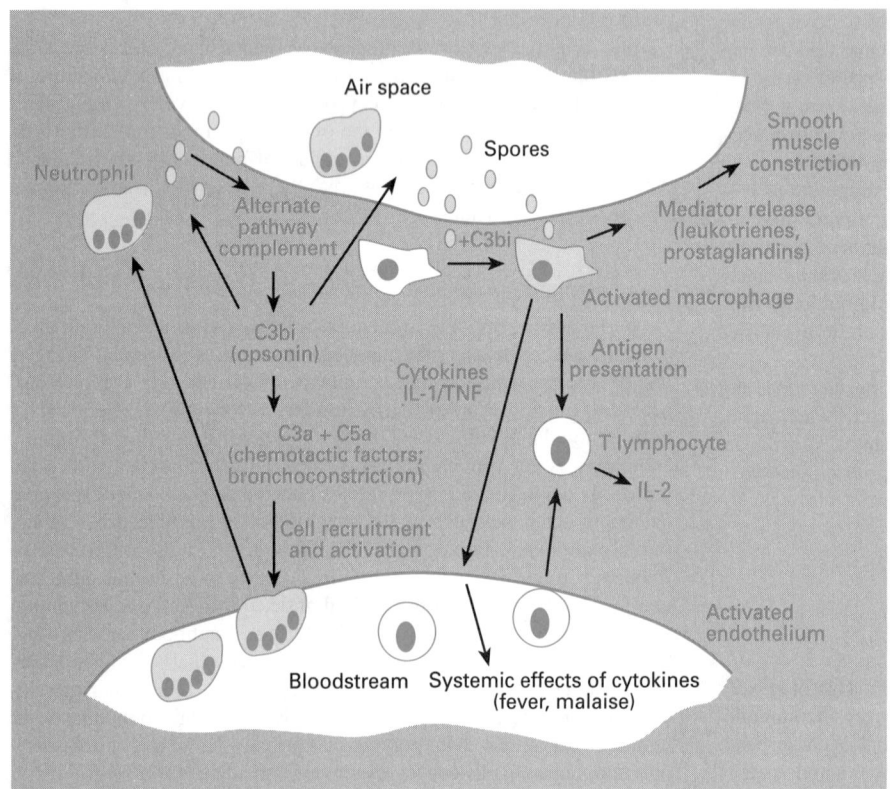

Fig. 2 Possible immunopathogenesis: acute phase. (By courtesy of Dr G. Spickett.)

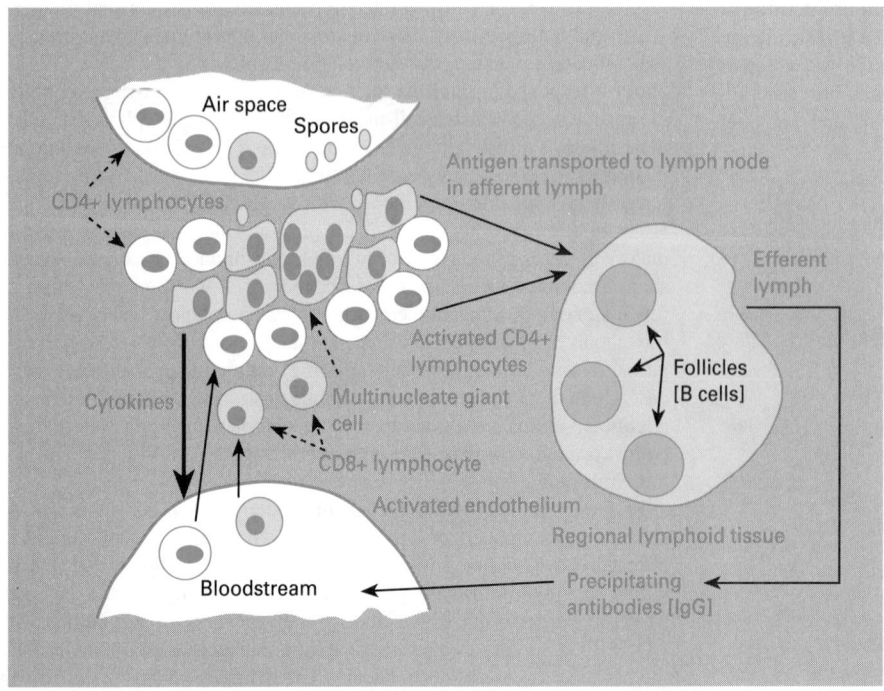

Fig. 3 Possible immunopathogenesis: subacute–chronic phase. (By courtesy of Dr G. Spickett.)

it is clear that continuing research should address both aspects of the immune response.

It is already clear that different antigenic determinants from a given inducing microbial source may lead to different immunological responses, and it seems likely that cytotoxic activity and released cytokines (e.g. interleukins and tumour necrosis factor) will play some role, possibly by activating the vascular endothelium and thereby recruiting and activating further macrophages and inflammatory cells. Bronchoalveolar lavage has shown that natural killer cells (CD57+) and mast cells may be prominent additional players in pathogenesis.

Cytokines, possibly together with anaphylotoxins from activated mast cells, are likely to be responsible for the systemic influenza-like symptoms that are so characteristic of the acute form of extrinsic allergic alveolitis. These symptoms are indistinguishable from grain fever in grain workers, 'Monday fever' in cotton workers, humidifier fever in subjects exposed to microbially contaminated humidifiers, and metal fume fever in welders. In these situations, the febrile disorder is not characteristically associated with clinical alveolitis, raising the possibility that its occurrence with the acute form of extrinsic allergic alveolitis is an independent phenomenon and not an integral part of the condition itself. This hypothesis has been supported by the finding of high levels of endotoxin from Gram-negative bacteria (which are known to provoke these symptoms) in grain dust, cotton dust, contaminated humidifiers, and many of the 'mouldy' vegetable dusts that cause extrinsic allergic alveolitis. However, neither metal fume nor many other causative agents of extrinsic allergic alveolitis are likely to be contaminated with endotoxin, and so endotoxin-induced release of inflammatory mediators is not an entirely satisfactory explanation. Thus inhalation provocation tests with uncontaminated bird serum in subjects with bird fancier's lung reproduce both alveolar and influenza-like responses. Evidently the influenza-like response is an integral feature of the acute form of extrinsic allergic alveolitis, but it is relatively non-specific and can occur in many other situations.

Extrinsic allergic alveolitis occurs in families only sporadically, and few associations with HLA phenotypes have been demonstrated. However, a number of recent studies have suggested associations between HLA-D alleles and pigeon fancier's lung and Japanese summer-type hypersensitivity pneumonitis. Such alleles may exert effects on immune suppression, and offer one mechanism by which a genetic predisposition could play a role in the development of extrinsic allergic alveolitis. It has been suggested additionally that an acute inflammatory episode (from viral infection or the inhalation of microbial toxins or chemicals) may be necessary to disrupt the normal defence equilibrium of surface membrane and local immune responses, and thereby permit antigen to be presented in a fashion that leads to hypersensitivity. Undue 'leakiness' of the alveolar membrane can be demonstrated by an increased clearance of inhaled ^{99}Tc^{m}-DTPA, and this has been reported to be a feature of both the early and continuing phases of extrinsic allergic alveolitis.

Relation to smoking

Curiously, the disruptive effect of smoking on the alveolar membrane does not appear to augment the risk of extrinsic allergic alveolitis or to increase its severity. Rather, the reverse is true. Although smoking enhances acute phase reactions and IgE production, it diminishes IgA, IgG, and IgM antibody responses, increases circulating CD8+ T-lymphocyte numbers, and probably reduces the incidence and severity of extrinsic allergic alveolitis. However, the smoker without IgG antibodies is particularly liable to find his respiratory symptoms attributed to other diseases, and so the negative association between extrinsic allergic alveolitis and smoking may have been exaggerated.

Nevertheless, the probability that it is real is supported by evidence that smoking may also reduce the risk for other T-cell-mediated immunological disorders such as sarcoidosis, ulcerative colitis, and some types of occupational asthma (generally those associated with low-molecular-weight chemicals). The key cell in a complex series of interactions is probably the alveolar macrophage, which is critical in presenting antigen to CD4+ T lymphocytes and so in activating cellular immune mechanisms. Although smoking increases macrophage numbers and their metabolic activity, the activated cells show impairment of both the expression of surface major histocompatibility 2 antigens and the production or release of interleukin 1 and inflammatory mediators derived from arachidonic acid metabolism (leukotriene B4, prostaglandin E$_2$, and thromboxane B$_2$). It is also argued that the increased macrophage numbers down-regulate pulmonary immune responses in a purely non-specific fashion by impairing antigen access to more effective blood monocytes.

Relation to coeliac disease

Reports that cryptogenic fibrosing alveolitis and extrinsic allergic alveolitis (particularly bird fancier's lung) might be associated with coeliac disease led to the interesting hypothesis that in some cases absorbed food antigens from the disrupted bowel mucosa might play a role in the pathogenesis of the lung disorder, i.e. that the lung disorder might be a 'metastatic' complication of the bowel disease. Alternatively, systemic hypersensitivity to a common inhaled and ingested avian antigen might give rise to similar immune reactions and diseases in the relevant target organs. However, the avian IgG antibody response seen in coeliac disease is distinct from that associated with bird fancier's lung and seems to be a response to dietary egg. It is not related to environmental exposure to birds but does correlate with the activity of the bowel disorder. Subsequent experience suggests a much less strong association between these bowel and lung disorders which, if real, is probably a consequence of their dependence on similar immunological mechanisms.

Investigation

Establishing a diagnosis of extrinsic allergic alveolitis involves three areas of investigation: the lungs, the exposure, and the evidence for hypersensitivity.

Pulmonary

In many cases extrinsic allergic alveolitis is first suspected after the presence of diffuse alveolitis or progressive pulmonary fibrosis is established. In the acute form of the disease the chest radiograph will commonly show no abnormality unless symptoms are moderately severe. Normal radiographic appearances are particularly common with humidifier lung, possibly because antigen is largely presented in soluble rather than particulate form. When the radiograph is abnormal, there is a widespread ground-glass appearance or an alveolar filling pattern, particularly in the lower and middle zones. This may resolve within a mere 24 to 48 h once exposure has ceased. In more subacute forms irregular small opacities, simulating asbestosis, are seen within the same distribution. Occasionally a more nodular pattern is seen. These opacities may persist for several weeks despite cessation of exposure, and if exposure continues honeycombing may develop. In contrast, the upper zones are predominantly affected by the irreversible fibrotic process that characterizes the chronic form of extrinsic allergic alveolitis. This may simulate sarcoidosis or even tuberculosis, and may lead to considerable shrinkage and distortion. In practice, the radiographic appearances vary considerably from patient to patient, and correlate poorly with the clinical severity of the disease.

CT scans (Fig. 4) provide a much clearer picture of the type of radiographic abnormality and of its extent, particularly when thin-section high resolution techniques are used, but they have shown that no single feature or pattern is pathognomic. Again, investigation within hours of exposure has been limited and experience is largely confined to patients with subacute and chronic disease. Increased density of the lung parenchyma has been the most prominent finding in the subacute form, followed almost equally by reticular or nodular infiltration. Neither lymph node enlargement nor pleural involvement is characteristic. The CT scan is appreciably more sensitive than the plain chest radiograph, and shows a more uniform involvement of the lung fields in subacute disease than is obvious from plain radiographs. With chronic forms, the CT scan shows a similar pattern of fibrosis and disruption to the plain radiograph, but again is considerably more sensitive.

Lung function studies vary according to severity and recent activity. As with asthma, they may reveal little of note in the acute form of the disease when there has been little recent exposure. When lung function is impaired, the pattern suggests parenchymal and interstitial disease but is otherwise non-specific. There is impaired carbon monoxide gas transfer with restricted ventilation, decreased compliance, and (in the more severe examples) hypoxia of the arterial blood with hypocapnia, particularly on exercise. Although total lung capacity is reduced, residual volume is often increased, suggesting air trapping as a result of bronchiolar involvement. Occasionally there is also obstruction of the large airways, but this implies a coincidental asthmatic or bronchitic effect.

Transbronchial or open-lung biopsy may be indicated when other diagnostic procedures are not sufficiently definitive in distinguishing extrinsic allergic alveolitis from cryptogenic fibrosing alveolitis or other diffuse infiltrative or fibrotic disorders of the lung, but is not commonly needed. Biopsy may be particularly useful in the subacute or chronic forms of the disease when hypersensitivity is less obvious, or when acutely there has been an unduly heavy exposure to microbial spores and there is suspicion of microbial invasion. Bronchoalveolar lavage, although more readily performed and less hazardous, has not proved to be as definitive as biopsy and remains a complementary rather than an alternative investigatory procedure.

Environmental exposure

In many cases the history alone provides the evidence of relevant exposure, but this is not always reliable and an independent account of the exposures involved can be invaluable. Ideally, industrial hygiene measurements are made (particularly from personal samplers) so that respirable agents can be accurately recognized and quantified, and microbiological techniques are used to identify specific microbial contaminants. These are sophisticated investigations and are mostly indicated when extrinsic allergic alveolitis is first suspected in an environment not previously associated with the disease, particularly in industries where many individuals may be at risk and where modification of the plant and its respirable environment may be a costly matter.

Immunological

Laboratory demonstration of an IgG antibody response to the inducing organic dust is the most widely used method of 'confirming' hypersen-

Fig. 4 CT scan of the thorax in a bird fancier emphasizes the diffusely nodular changes of extrinsic allergic alveolitis.

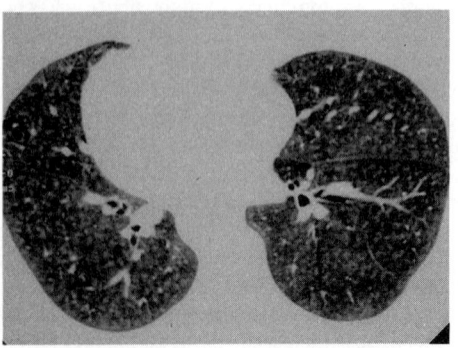

Table 2 *Diagnostic features of positive inhalation challenge tests*

Diagnostic changes within 36 h of onset of challenge exposure	Sensitivity (%)
Increase in body temperature to >37.2°C	78
Increase in circulating neutrophils by ≥ 2.5 × 10⁹/l	68
Decrease in circulating lymphocytes by ≥ 0.5 × 10⁹/l with lymphopenia (< 1.5 × 10⁹/l)	52
Decrease in forced vital capacity by ≥ 15%	48
Increase in exercise minute volume by ≥ 15%	85
Increase in exercise respiratory frequency by ≥ 25%	64

The data were taken from a series of 144 antigen and control challenge tests in 31 subjects. Diagnostic end-points were chosen to produce specificities of approximately 95 per cent, after mean changes associated with positive challenge tests were shown to be highly significant. When each monitoring parameter was given a score of 1 for a significant result, a total score of 2/6 or more was associated with a specificity of 100 per cent and a sensitivity of 78 per cent for the 144 challenge tests.

sitivity, but this has proved to be unsatisfactory as has the use of intracutaneous tests. Although affected subjects tend to have higher antibody levels than those who are exposed but unaffected, most investigators have found the antibody response to correlate more closely with exposure than with disease. Tests for cellular hypersensitivity using skin or blood have been even more unsatisfactory. In practice, the absence of a precipitin response is extremely uncommon in subjects eventually proved to have extrinsic allergic alveolitis, provided that they are non-smokers.

Bronchoalveolar lavage fluid has proved to be only a little more helpful. Once established, extrinsic allergic alveolitis is associated, like sarcoidosis, with a T-lymphocyte response in the alveolar fluid (lymphocytes represent 10 to 20 per cent or more of recovered cells), but lymphocytosis is also seen in asymptomatic although similarly exposed subjects. Although many investigators have reported a relatively greater increase in the number of CD8+ T cells in the asymptomatic subjects, so that the normal dominance of CD4+ cells is lost (inverted ratio of CD4+ to CD8+), both T-cell types show increased numbers if there is exposure, and the absolute value of the ratio of CD4+ to CD8+ provides limited diagnostic benefit. During the hours immediately following exposure a polymorphonuclear leucocyte response may dominate, simulating cryptogenic fibrosing alveolitis.

When the diagnosis remains in doubt, some form of inhalation challenge test may be considered necessary. The simplest method involves comparison of experimental periods spent away from the suspected causative environment with similar periods of continuing exposure. The acute form of the disease is likely to be recognized in this way, although the procedure can be time consuming and there may be practical problems of compliance. When a definitive diagnosis is particularly important, formal laboratory-based inhalation challenge tests can be used. These employ a variety of techniques from nebulizing soluble extracts to recreating natural environmental exposures in an exposure chamber. The influenza-like component of positive reactions is often uncomfortable, and if excessive doses are administered these tests can be hazardous. What is more, objective evidence for positive reactions may be difficult to obtain from conventional lung function tests. Tests of this nature should consequently be restricted to centres with special expertise. Personal experience of evaluating objective changes in body temperature, circulating neutrophil and lymphocyte numbers, forced vital capacity, and exercise tests from 144 tests is summarized in Table 2. Together they provide high specificity and high sensitivity. Ausculta-

Table 3 *Characteristics of nitrogen dioxide toxicity (silo filler's disease), organic dust toxic syndrome, and acute farmer's lung*

	Nitrogen dioxide pneumonitis	Organic dust toxic syndrome	Acute farmer's lung
Susceptibility in smokers	Unknown	Unknown	Decreased
Relation to time of harvest	Days	Months–years	Months–years
Microbial decomposition of harvest product	Little	Marked	Variable
Confined exposure space	+ + +	+	+
Previous episodes	–	+	+ +
Symptoms			
Dry cough	+ +	+ +	+ +
Breathlessness	+ +	+ +	+ +
Wheeze	–	–	–
Systemic upset	+	+	+ +
Signs			
Basal crackles	+	+	+
Fever	+	+	+
Time of onset after beginning exposure	1–10 h	1–10 h	1–10 h
Duration	Hours–days	Hours–days	Hours–days
Investigations			
Leucocytosis	+	+	+
Radiograph (small irregular opacities, alveolar shadows)	+	+	+
Restricted ventilation	+	+	+
Reduced gas transfer	+	+	+
Hypoxia	+	+	+
Fungi from secretions/biopsy	–	+ +	+
Methaemoglobinaemia	+	–	–
Serum precipitins	–	–	+ (? in smokers)
Response to steroids	+	–	+ +
Life threatening	Not uncommonly	Occasionally	Rarely

tion, chest radiography, measurements of gas transfer, and arterial blood gas analyses are too insensitive to provide useful diagnostic information.

Differential diagnosis

Acute extrinsic allergic alveolitis is not the only disorder characterized by systemic influenza-like symptoms and respiratory distress to follow an unusually heavy exposure to microbially contaminated vegetable produce. In 1986 an international symposium considered a further disorder which occurs within hours of heavy respiratory exposure to dusts containing fungal toxins, particularly those released on decapping silos. It is the result of direct toxicity rather than hypersensitivity. Illness from fungal toxin ingestion (mycotoxicosis) has been recognized for some time, but respiratory exposure was not noted to be hazardous until recently. Rather than pulmonary mycotoxicosis, the term organic dust toxic syndrome was recommended to describe it. Its effects are usually mild and self-limiting, but severe respiratory embarrassment may occur and there is a small risk of ongoing, and potentially fatal, fungal invasion of the lungs. This risk could be enhanced if corticosteroid treatment is given, and death has occurred in subjects who appear to have been fully immunocompetent. Not only does organic dust toxic syndrome occur in circumstances which favour the occurrence of extrinsic allergic alveolitis, but its clinical features have much in common with extrinsic allergic alveolitis, and to a lesser extent with nitrogen dioxide toxicity which also affects silo workers. Indeed, there is so much overlap that it may be very difficult to distinguish one disorder from the other in the individual (Table 3).

The acute form of extrinsic allergic alveolitis can only be the result of an acute and recent (a matter of hours) exposure to the relevant causal antigen. This limits the opportunity for diagnostic error, although the circumstances of an unusually heavy exposure may be subtle. For example, a pigeon fancier might spend rather less time than usual with his birds, but much more time than usual in the more hazardous dusty car that he uses regularly to transport racing birds for training exercises.

Just as acute and heavy exposures to organic dusts may on the one hand cause disorders other than extrinsic allergic alveolitis, on the other hand they may be quite irrelevant and purely coincidental to the acute respiratory disorder with which the patient presents. Consequently, the differential diagnosis should include some consideration of other acute disorders of the lung parenchyma and interstitium, such as infections, other immunological disorders, drug reactions, and even paraquat poisoning which sometimes occurs accidentally in farm workers. In bird keepers the diagnosis of viral, mycoplasmal, and chlamydial infection may itself be confounded by false-positive microbial antibody tests. This is the result of cross-reaction of pre-existing avian antibodies with egg protein in the microbial cultures used to provide the test agents.

When subacute or chronic forms of extrinsic allergic alveolitis are encountered, the differential diagnosis lies with other diffuse infiltrative and fibrotic disorders of the lung. Those most frequently resembling extrinsic allergic alveolitis include cryptogenic fibrosing alveolitis, sarcoidosis, pneumoconiosis, tuberculosis, and metastatic cancer, although a huge variety of less common disorders may also need to be considered.

Epidemiology

Extrinsic allergic alveolitis is an uncommon but not rare disease. For every case there are 10 to 100 cases of asthma, but there is much greater geographic variation than with asthma reflecting the much larger dependence of extrinsic allergic alveolitis on occupational causes. Its comparative scarcity limits epidemiological knowledge.

Incidence

Recent experience over 3 years with the SWORD project (Surveillance of Work-related and Occupational Respiratory Disease) indicates that extrinsic allergic alveolitis of occupational origin accounts for only 2 per cent of occupational lung diseases in the United Kingdom. Asthma, which is the most common, accounts for 26 per cent. Of course, this ignores extrinsic allergic alveolitis of non-occupational origin, which is much less easily assessed. It also disguises the absolute risk since few workers encounter relevant occupational exposures. Almost 50 per cent of reported cases affect farmers or farm workers, followed by 15 per cent affecting workers in material, metal, or electrical processing trades. Among farmers, the average incidence is 41 per million per year, although this approaches 100 in some regions. This may be compared with 200 to 700 per million per year among working groups at greatest risk of developing occupational asthma. Contaminating micro-organisms underlie over 50 per cent of the reported cases of extrinsic allergic alveolitis, followed in order of importance by animal antigens in 6 per cent and chemicals in 5 per cent. In 27 per cent of reports a suspected agent has not been specified.

Prevalence

Figures for prevalence (the proportion affected among a given population at a given point of time) are more readily available than those for incidence, and demonstrate quite marked national differences. In developed countries humidifier lung is being recognized with increasing frequency in both the workplace and the home, and remarkable prevalences of 15 to 70 per cent have been suggested in populations from contaminated offices in North America. Bird fancier's lung may be more prevalent at present over the whole of the United Kingdom, simply because of the great popularity of keeping budgerigars and pigeons. Budgerigars are kept in some 12 per cent of British homes, and 0.5 to 7.5 per cent of the population involved are likely to have extrinsic allergic alveolitis as a consequence, albeit mildly in most cases. Pigeon keeping is 40 times less common, and the measured prevalence of pigeon fancier's lung has been a good deal more varied (0–21 per cent). This may reflect both true differences between groups of pigeon breeders as exposure levels vary according to number of birds, duration of exposure, loft ventilation, cleaning habits, etc., and artefactual differences arising as a result of selection bias and the notorious lack of compliance shown by pigeon fanciers in epidemiological studies. The responsible avian antigen and its precise source has yet to be identified, but bloom from the feathers containing saliva and secretory IgA is currently favoured over dust emanating from dried droppings.

In areas of high rainfall where 'traditional' farming methods are used, the prevalence of farmer's lung may reach 10 per cent. This is likely to be the commonest cause of extrinsic allergic alveolitis in developing countries. In developed countries, where modern farming methods are used, prevalences rarely exceed 2 to 3 per cent and are usually a good deal less. Furthermore, the farming population at risk represents a mere 1 to 2 per cent of the population at large, although there are marked regional variations. Even smaller populations are employed making whisky from germinating barley (maltings), raising mushrooms on a variety of antigenic composts, or handling bagasse (the fibrous stem that remains when sugar is extracted from sugar cane), but within some of these populations extrinsic allergic alveolitis was a common problem until excessive exposure levels were controlled. Extrinsic allergic alveolitis associated with animals other than birds is extremely uncommon, as is the case with chemical-induced extrinsic allergic alveolitis.

In Japan, the seasonal summer growth of *Trichosporon cutaneum* in the home is by far the commonest cause of extrinsic allergic alveolitis.

The remarkable 'summer-type hypersensitivity pneumonitis' accounts for about 75 per cent of all cases of extrinsic allergic alveolitis, being approximately 10 times as common as farmer's lung and 20 times as common as bird fancier's lung.

Management

Management of the individual

Management centres on reducing any further exposure to a minimum. There is no place for desensitization. Ideally, the affected individual changes the relevant working or domestic environment completely, but this may mean a profound loss in income or great expense and is often unrealistic. Nor is it fully justified on purely medical grounds since continued exposure does not inevitably lead to progressive disease.

The affected individual who continues to work in the occupation responsible for his disease can often reduce his exposure substantially by changing the pattern of his particular duties. An alternative is the use of industrial respirators, which filter out 98 to 99 per cent of respirable dust from the ambient air. They are particularly valuable when exposures are intermittent and short, but may be uncomfortably hot when worn for long periods or during heavy work.

Whatever course is followed, continuing exposure should be accompanied by regular medical surveillance. If there is no progression, it is reasonable for some exposure to continue. When there is progressive disease, exposure should cease. This may involve a loss of earnings, and may entitle the affected worker to compensation. Rarely, the individual with progressive disease will refuse to change his occupation or hobby, and the physician must weigh the possible advantages of long-term corticosteroid therapy against the well-known risks.

Management of the environment

Once extrinsic allergic alveolitis is recognized in one individual, the environment concerned should be assessed for the risk it poses to others. In many circumstances this will be well known already, and exposure levels will be within the range considered acceptable. In others, neither the risk nor the precise causative agent nor its level of exposure will be known, and in such unfamiliar circumstances there may be a need to survey the exposed population at risk. Questionnaires and serological tests are most convenient for this, at least as a screening procedure. When large populations are involved comprehensive investigation is sensible before major modifications to the working environment are considered.

Modifications can always be made to the environment to lessen the level of exposure, but their extent will be limited by expense and should be justified by need. Dry storage and adequate ventilation are the two most important factors when vegetable produce is involved, and in some farming areas there is benefit in drying produce artificially after harvest. When ventilation and humidification systems are themselves responsible for extrinsic allergic alveolitis, major mechanical alterations may be necessary and the methods of humidification and temperature control may need to be changed. The crucial need is to reduce the ease with which normal airborne microbial contaminants are able to proliferate in stagnant collections of water. For this there may be a role for 'biocide' sterilizing agents, but these are also likely to become airborne and respirable and so must have low intrinsic toxicity and sensitizing potency. The need for rapid air changes coupled with close control of humidity and temperature poses formidable problems. The use of recirculated filtered air is the most economical, but effective filters are expensive and can become contaminated themselves, increasing rather than decreasing the load of respirable microbial antigens. The use of heat exchangers minimizes the cost of temperature control if contaminated exhaust air is not recirculated but does not conserve water.

Outcome

No further exposure

As with occupational asthma, the risk of continuing symptoms following cessation of exposure increases with the duration of exposure. With the acute form of extrinsic allergic alveolitis the exposure period is generally short and the disorder generally resolves without sequelae once the diagnosis is made and exposure ceases. However, one investigation using bronchoalveolar lavage and DTPA clearance has indicated continuing inflammation and membrane leakiness after a follow-up period of 2 to 15 years. The significance of this is unclear, since all subjects were asymptomatic and gave normal results to radiographic and lung function studies.

Continuing exposure

There is greater concern when exposure continues. This may lead not only to recurrent acute attacks but also to progressive and permanent fibrotic damage, i.e. to the chronic form of the disease. While concern for the risk of progressive fibrosis is undoubtedly justified, such a course is followed by only a minority of affected subjects. A 2- to 40-year follow-up survey of 92 farm workers presenting with the acute form of farmer's lung showed that, while the majority continued to live on farms, only a minority developed radiographic evidence of pulmonary fibrosis (39 per cent) or impairment of carbon monoxide gas transfer (30 per cent). As many as 28 per cent gave histories of chronic productive cough and 25 per cent had airway obstruction. A similar 10 year outcome has been reported in pigeon fanciers with acute extrinsic allergic alveolitis; again, the majority elected to continue their antigenic exposures despite medical advice to the contrary.

Therefore, in some cases, perhaps the majority, important protective mechanisms emerge which lead to tolerance from the effects of further acute exposures or at least prevent the development of damaging fibrosis. A history of similar increasing tolerance is occasionally noted with occupational asthma, and tolerance rather than progressive disease has been the rule rather than the exception in most animal models of extrinsic allergic alveolitis. With both asthma and extrinsic allergic alveolitis some affected subjects give clear accounts of increased responsiveness to a given level of exposure months or years after initial antigen exclusion, which suggests that protective mechanisms may be downgraded more quickly than the causative mechanisms.

As with sarcoidosis, there is debate as to whether the use of corticosteroids for acute episodes confers any long-term benefit. The answer is not yet clear, but one recent investigation failed to demonstrate any long-term functional differences between groups treated randomly with corticosteroids or placebo for the initial acute episode of farmer's lung. While the corticosteroid group recovered more quickly from the acute episode, there was the suspicion, already voiced by other investigators, that early steroid therapy carries a greater risk of recurrence in the long term. It is possible that the initial response to steroids encouraged less care over subsequent exposures. Alternatively steroid therapy induced a different equilibrium between immunological responses, perhaps interfering disproportionately with the development of protective mechanisms.

Compensation of industrial causes

In the United Kingdom industrial injuries legislation provides compensation from central government for disability in employees (not employers) from extrinsic allergic alveolitis of occupational origin. The level of disability, and hence compensation, is assessed following examination by a medical board. If disability arose before 1991, the affected worker may also be entitled to a reduced earnings allowance if ongoing employment (or lack of it) has resulted in a loss of earned income. Both benefits are limited to a joint maximum figure which is adjusted from time to time according to inflation. The reduced earnings allowance was discontinued in 1991.

Acceptance of such compensation no longer debars the recipient from seeking redress in the civil courts, which is the primary mechanism of compensation in many countries.

REFERENCES

Banaszak, E.F., Thiede, W.H., and Fink, J.N. (1970). Hypersensitivity pneumonia due to contamination of an air conditioner. *New England Journal of Medicine*, **283**, 271–6.

Braun, S.R., doPico, G.A., Tsiatis, A., *et al.* (1979). Farmer's lung disease: long-term clinical and physiologic outcome. *American Review of Respiratory Disease*, **119**, 185–91.

Hansell, D.M., and Moskovic, E. (1991). High-resolution computed tomography in extrinsic allergic alveolitis. *Clinical Radiology*, **43**, 8–12.

Hendrick, D.J., Faux, J.A., and Marshall, R. (1978). Budgerigar fancier's lung: the commonest variety of allergic alveolitis in Britain. *British Medical Journal*, **2**, 81–4.

Hendrick, D.J., Marshall, R., Faux, J.A., and Krall, J.M. (1980). Positive 'alveolar' responses to antigen inhalation provocation tests: their validity and recognition. *Thorax*, **35**, 415–27.

Kokkarinen, J.I., Tukiainen, H.O., and Terho, E.O. (1992). Effect of corticosteroid treatment on the recovery of pulmonary function in farmer's lung. *American Review of Respiratory Disease*, **145**, 3–5.

Leatherman, H.P., Michael, A.F., Schwarz, B.A., and Hoidal, J.R. (1984). Lung T cells in hypersensitivity pneumonitis. *Annals of Internal Medicine*, **100**, 390–2.

Meredith, S.K., Taylor, V.M., and McDonald, J.C. (1991). Occupational respiratory disease in the United Kingdom 1989: a report to the British Thoracic Society and the Society of Occupational Medicine by the SWORD project group. *British Journal of Industrial Medicine*, **48**, 292–8.

Morgan, D.C., Smyth, J.T., Lister, R.W., and Pethybridge, R.J. (1973). Chest symptoms and farmer's lung: a community survey. *British Journal of Industrial Medicine*, **30**, 259–65.

Pepys, J., Jenkins, P.A., Festenstein, G.N., Lacey, M.E., Gregory, P.H., and Skinner, F.A. (1963). Farmer's lung. Thermophilic actinomycetes as a source of 'farmer's lung hay' antigens. *Lancet*, **ii**, 607–11.

Peterson, L.B., Thrall, R.S., Moore, V.L., Stevens, O., and Abramoff, P. (1977). An animal model of hypersensitivity pneumonitis in the rabbit. Induction of cellular hypersensitivity to inhaled antigens using carageenan and BCG. *American Review of Respiratory Disease*, **116**, 1007–12.

17.10.10 Sarcoidosis

P. R. STUDDY

Introduction

Sarcoidosis, a relatively common chronic multisystem disease of unknown aetiology, is one of a large family of granulomatous disorders in which the shared feature is the presence of epithelioid-cell granulomas in affected tissues.

Sarcoidosis is extraordinary not only in the very variable presentation or spectrum of tissues that it may affect, but also in its duration. Although remarkably transient in some individuals, a proportion of whom are asymptomatic and discovered by chance, it may become a chronic problem for others, occasionally causing severe organ dysfunction with chronic debilitating symptoms and premature death. Treatment remains controversial, for no therapy is curative. Palliative treatment with corticosteroids is helpful but probably does not affect the final outcome.

Despite an awareness of sarcoidosis for about a hundred years, the cause, whether single or multiple, remains obscure.

Descriptive definition

While the aetiology of sarcoidosis remains uncertain its definition can only be descriptive. A statement prepared in 1975 by the International Committee on Sarcoidosis at the Seventh International Conference serves as the most widely quoted description.

> Sarcoidosis is a multisystem granulomatous disorder of unknown aetiology most commonly affecting young adults and presenting most frequently with bilateral hilar lymphadenopathy, pulmonary infiltration, and skin or eye lesions. The diagnosis is established most securely when clinical or radiographic findings are supported by histologic evidence of widespread non-caseating epithelioid cell granulomas in more than one organ or a positive Kveim–Siltzbach skin test. Immunological features are depression of delayed type hypersensitivity, suggesting impaired cell-mediated immunity and raised or abnormal immunoglobulins. There may also be hypercalciuria, with or without hypercalcaemia. The course and prognosis may correlate with the mode on onset. An acute onset with erythema nodosum heralds a self-limiting course and spontaneous resolution, while an insidious onset may be followed by relentless, progressive fibrosis. Corticosteroids relieve symptoms and suppress inflammation and granuloma formation.

It is the demonstration of widely disseminated histopathological changes which allow the most confident diagnosis. Therefore a simple description suggested by Scadding and Mitchell in 1985 is the most helpful and least controversial.

> Sarcoidosis is a disease characterized by the formation in all of several affected organs or tissues of epithelioid cell tubercles, without caseation though fibrinoid necrosis may be present at the centres of a few, proceeding either to resolution or to conversion into hyaline fibrous tissue.

To this may be added a note that the organs most frequently affected are the lymph nodes, lungs, skin, eyes, liver, spleen, and salivary glands, although every organ with the possible exception of the adrenal glands has been reported to be involved.

Pathology

Histology

The characteristic histological feature in sarcoidosis is the presence in affected tissues of non-caseating epithelioid-cell granulomas (Fig. 1). It should be emphasized that the finding of non-caseating granulomas does not in itself constitute absolute evidence of sarcoidosis; similar changes may occur in a variety of conditions (Table 1).

In the early stages, the granulomas consist of focal, close-packed collections of macrophages and epithelioid cells which often fuse to form multinucleate Langhans type giant cells. A peripheral ring of lymphocytes is commonly seen around the sarcoid granuloma and a few lymphocytes may be present in the central portion. B lymphocytes are present in small numbers. Monoclonal antibody studies enable the cellular components of the granuloma to be identified in tissue sections and show that CD4 helper cells predominate over CD8 suppressor cells. CD4 helper cells and activated macrophages penetrate to the centre of the granulomata where the latter coalesce into epithelioid and multinucleate giant cells. In the peripheral mantle CD8 suppressor cells lie adjacent

to numerous antigen-presenting macrophages. Central fibrinoid necrosis may occur in florid granulomas but true caseation is not seen, a finding that differentiates sarcoidosis from tuberculosis.

Epithelioid and giant cells are derived from macrophages, which develop from bone marrow monocyte precursor cells. The epithelioid cells are about 20 μm in diameter with round or oval nuclei. The transformation that the epithelioid cells undergo during development is such that there are few ultrastructural similarities with their precursor cell line: the phagosomes and lysosomes of a macrophage are replaced by cytoplasmic organelles characteristic of a secretory cell. The multinucleate giant cells are usually found in moderate numbers in the middle of the follicle, but they may be numerous or very sparse. Giant cells vary in size, are derived by fusion of macrophages, and may contain as many as 30 peripherally arranged nuclei.

Cytoplasmic inclusions are not infrequently present within the cells of the granuloma, particularly the multinucleated giant cells. Three types of inclusions are described: crystalline, conchoidal, and asteroid. Crystalline inclusions are composed of calcium carbonate and are birefringent to polarized light. Conchoidal (Schaumann's) bodies are densely basophilic, stain with haematoxylin, and are probably formed when lipomucolglycoproteins and amorphous calcium and iron salts became deposited around a small birefringent crystalline focus. Conchoidal and crystalline bodies are more commonly identified in the granulomas of sarcoidosis than in other granulomatous conditions, but they are not diagnostic because they also occur in beryllium disease and, rarely, in Crohn's disease, tuberculosis and farmer's lung. Star-shaped asteroid bodies are composed of lipoprotein, occur within giant cells, and are present in many granulomatous diseases.

When the disease remits, either spontaneously or with corticosteroid therapy, the mononuclear inflammation settles and there are fewer granulomas in the tissues. The granulomas are capable of complete resolution, but those that remain are usually slowly replaced by featureless hyaline scar tissue showing few, if any, diagnostic features (Fig. 2). Granulomas resolve by dispersion of the cells or by centripetal proliferation of fibroblasts from the periphery of the granuloma inwards to form a scar which may either eventually disappear or result in fibrosis with permanent tissue damage.

Immunopathology of sarcoidosis

The various factors involved in the initiation, maintenance, and resolution of the granulomas are central to uncovering the aetiology of sarcoidosis. They are not well understood.

It is generally assumed that the first step in the pathogenesis of sarcoidosis is the presentation of a currently unknown antigen by major histocompatibility complex class II macrophages to CD4 T-cells of the THI subclass. This results in T-cell proliferation and the release of

Fig. 1 Typical perivascular sarcoid granuloma in a lung biopsy containing many epithelioid cells, Langhans type giant cells, and lymphocytes. Haematoxylin and eosin. Magnification 40 ×. (By courtesy of Dr Margaret Burke, Mount Vernon Hospital.)

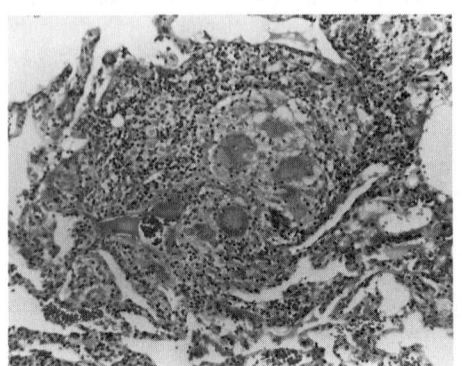

Table 1 *Human pulmonary granulomatous diseases*

Aetiology	Disorder
Known	Extrinsic allergic alveolitis
	Chronic beryllium disease
	Infections (mycobacteria, bacteria (brucellosis), fungi, protozoa, viruses, and worms)
	Foreign body (talc following IV drug abuse)
Unknown	Sarcoidosis
	Wegener's granulomatosis
	Churg-Strauss syndrome
	Lymphomatoid granulomatosis
	Langerhans' cell granulomatosis

immune mediators. The earliest histological manifestation of the disease in affected tissues is an accumulation of mononuclear inflammatory cells and CD4 T-helper lymphocytes, soon followed by mononuclear cell transformation to activated macrophages, epithelioid and multinuclear giant cells, and granuloma formation. The process of granuloma formation in the tissues seems to involve an intimate interaction between macrophages and T lymphocytes, and is triggered by the release of immune mediators (lymphokines). Lymphokines, defined as products of antigen-stimulated sensitized T lymphocytes, play an important role in the formation of epitheloid-cell granulomas. They effect macrophages in a number of ways, and by influencing adhesion and aggregation may contribute to the classical tightly packed group of cells in the granulomas.

A variety of mediators are released including monocyte chemotactic factor, which is capable of recruiting blood monocytes to the activated T cells, and γ-interferon, which is associated with activation of mononuclear phagocytes and lung fibroblasts. As a result of this activity the sarcoid granulomas receive large daily reinforcements of monocytes to replace the macrophage population.

The increased CD4 helper T-lymphocyte response is maintained by the spontaneous release of interleukin 1 (IL-1) and interleukin 2 (IL-2), T-cell growth factors, by the T cells. Helper T lymphocytes accumulate at sites of disease activity, a fact readily demonstrated in the lungs by bronchoalveolar lavage studies. The ratio of CD4 T-helper to CD8 T-suppressor cells may be as high as 10 : 1 in involved tissues compared with the ratio of 2 : 1 found in normal tissues. At uninvolved sites and in the peripheral blood T lymphocytes are not 'activated' and are present in reduced numbers.

What the epithelioid cells in the granulomas may be secreting is an

Fig. 2 Hyaline fibrosis with extensive replacement of lung tissue by fibrous tissue. The scattered residual non-caseating granulomas in the interstitium should be noted. Haematoxylin and eosin. Magnification 10 ×. (By courtesy of Dr Margaret Burke, Mount Vernon Hospital.)

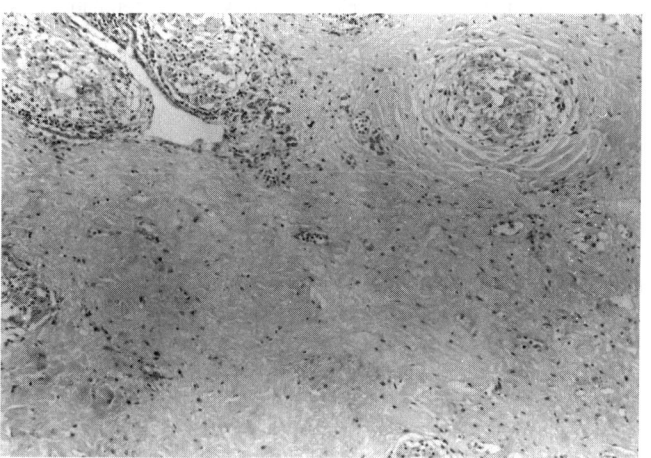

intriguing question. In addition to specific lymphokines, the granulomas are also the source of substances that may have an immune regulatory role, including 1,25-dihydroxy vitamin D_3, dipeptidyl carboxyl peptidase (angiotensin-converting enzyme), transcobalamin II, lysozyme, and β-microglobulin.

CELL-MEDIATED IMMUNITY

Sarcoidosis is characterized by anomalous immunological reactions. In 1916 Boeck reported a low tuberculin reactivity in patients with sarcoidosis, a finding amply confirmed by other workers.

Tuberculin sensitivity is reduced at the onset of sarcoidosis and a previously positive tuberculin test may become negative at this time. About two-thirds fail to react to 100 IU of tuberculin (PPD), even though the reactivity of the healthy population is much higher. Normal reactivity to tuberculin is not necessarily restored when sarcoidosis remits, although tuberculin reactivity reappears in some cases.

The altered immunological reaction to tuberculin provides one example of low responsiveness or cutaneous anergy to a 'recall' antigen. Delayed hypersensitivity reactions to mumps virus antigen, *Candida albicans*, trichophytin, PPD prepared from atypical mycobacteria, and dinitrochlorobenzene are similarly depressed in active sarcoidosis. The reduced ability to acquire or express delayed-type hypersensitivity is not associated with an increased predisposition to viral or fungal infection or to malignant disease.

The mechanisms responsible for delayed hypersensitivity in sarcoidosis are uncertain. It is postulated that the reduced reactivity may be due singly or in combination to a failure of lymphokine production, the presence of serum factors that inactivate lymphokines, hyperactive suppressor cells, or receptor blockade. There is good evidence that cellular immunity is active at disease sites and that circulating lymphocytes are morphologically and functionally normal, but present in reduced numbers. This has led to the concept that cutaneous anergy is due to the 'compartmentalization' of the immunocompetent cells at disease sites. CD4 helper T cells preferentially congregate in those organs affected by sarcoidosis, promoting the disease there but leaving the rest of the body with a relative excess of activated CD8 suppressor T cells so that cellular hypersensitivity response, such as the Mantoux test, are negative. The compartmentalization or redistribution of T lymphocytes is a relative phenomenon; for example, the Kveim–Siltzbach test is able to recruit the necessary immunocompetent cells to the site of injection to initiate a positive reaction.

HUMORAL IMMUNE SYSTEM

Irrespective of enhancement or suppression of cellular immunity, humoral immunity is enhanced. B-cell activity is increased, probably in response to T-cell-derived B-cell growth factors, and results in non-specific polyclonal hyperglobulinaemia, i.e. the presence of autoantibodies and elevated circulating antibodies to a range of viral infections. There is no evidence that these antibodies have a functional role or are involved in the pathogenesis of sarcoidosis. Circulating immune complexes are frequently present in acute sarcoidosis at the stage of erythema nodosum, uveitis, and arthralgia.

AETIOLOGY

The aetiology of sarcoidosis is obscure. The lungs and regional thoracic lymph nodes are most frequently involved, raising the possibility that the disease is caused by an agent that enters the body via the lungs, possibly by inhalation. However, no cause has been discovered, despite extensive research to find an infective agent, an allergic response to environmental factors, a primary immunological disorder, or a genetic tendency.

Research has suggested the possibility of a transmissible agent, perhaps a virus or a protoplast form of *Mycobacterium tuberculosis*, but if there is such an agent it must have either an extremely low infectivity or an incubation period so protracted that the initial contact goes unrecognized. Although infection with *M.tuberculosis* or opportunistic mycobacteria seems unlikely, this possibility remains. Rarely, mycobacteria may be cultivated from tissue showing features characteristic of sarcoidosis. Also sarcoidosis may follow or precede tuberculosis, and very rarely both conditions may apparently coincide. More circumstantial evidence supporting a possible tuberculosis aetiology has come from recent studies using ultrasensitive polymerase chain reactions to detect bacterial DNA in secretions and tissue samples. Some investigators have demonstrated mycobacterial DNA in fluid aspirated from the lungs, or lymph node and lung tissue taken from confirmed sarcoidosis patients. The relevance of these findings will only become clear with more research.

There is a link between some manifestations of the disease and certain HLA patterns, but the genetic element in determining the disease is not felt to be strong. The occasional occurrence of familial sarcoidosis and apparent excess concordance in monozygotic rather than dizygotic twins provides slight evidence that the susceptibility to sarcoidosis may be influenced by genetic factors.

Epidemiology

There are a large number of epidemiological studies showing the distribution and calculated frequency of sarcoidosis among various population groups. Their accuracy varies but, irrespective of the sophistication of medical facilities and enthusiasm of the investigator, epidemiological studies have failed to make a significant contribution to understanding sarcoidosis. What is clear is that the prevalence varies, with a high frequency in some locations whilst in other areas it is seldom recognized (Table 2). Geographical or community clustering has been noted in some studies, offering support for the idea that a transmissible agent may be the cause.

The true frequency of sarcoidosis in any community is uncertain, for a large number of cases may be asymptomatic and their diagnosis depends upon chance discovery on chest radiograph or at necropsy. Postmortem studies on 6706 individuals in Malmö, Sweden, revealed unexpected evidence of sarcoidosis unrelated to the pathological cause of death in a large proportion with a prevalence of 640 per 100 000, some 10 times the local prevalence of sarcoidosis detected on mass chest radiographs.

Because most cases of sarcoidosis show characteristic chest radiograph abnormalities, mass radiological surveys give some indication of its relative frequency within the community. Average findings for mass radiography in 1959 for England and Wales suggested sarcoidosis in 13.8 men and 19.8 women per 100 000 population, with the highest prevalence, irrespective of sex, in the age group 25–34 years.

Mass radiographic screening in London (1958) showed a high prevalence of intrathoracic sarcoidosis in West Indian and Irish immigrants compared with the indigenous population. The prevalence rate per 100 000 for those born in the United Kingdom was 27 and, although similar overall for men and women, rose to 39 for women of childbearing age. The prevalence rate per 100 000 for immigrants was higher, at 97 for Irish men, 213 for Irish women, 197 for West Indian men, and 170 for West Indian women. Erythema nodosum was a more frequent finding in Irish patients.

A detailed study to assess the annual incidence of sarcoidosis was performed in four areas of the United Kingdom (Cornwall, East Anglia, Sheffield, north-east and east Scotland) over a period of 5 years (1961–1966). The incidence was found to increase from north to south and was highest in the age group 24–34 years. The annual incidence per 100 000 was 2.1–4.1 for men and 3.5–4.5 for women.

The incidence and course of sarcoidosis in different racial groups living in the same geographical area show considerable variation. Two recent studies have shown a 10-fold higher annual incidence in West Indian and Asian immigrants living in London than in the indigenous

Table 2 *Reported prevalence of pulmonary sarcoidosis*

Country	Prevalence per 100 000
Sweden	64
Denmark	48
West Germany	43
East Germany	41
Ireland	40
United States (New York)	39
England	27
Norway	27
Holland	22
Switzerland	16
Yugoslavia	12
France	10
Italy	9
Scotland	7
Finland	5
Japan	2.5
Spain	1.2

Based on data reported at international sarcoidosis conferences.

Table 3 *First presenting symptoms of patients with sarcoidosis in the United Kingdom*

Feature	White	Black	Asian
Abnormal chest radiograph	34	7	10
Respiratory symptoms	25	57	55
Constitutional symptoms	5	57	55
Erythema nodosum	20	8.5	17
Ocular symptoms	7	12	3
Superficial lymphadenopathy	3	34	17

Male and female data combined; figures expressed as a percentage.

Based upon Scadding and Mitchell (275 patients, London 1946–1966), BTTA (567 patients in four areas, United Kingdom 1961–1966), and Edmonstone and Wilson (156 patients, South London 1969–1982).

white population. In West Indian and Asian patients there was an increased incidence of extrathoracic disease and a greater need for corticosteroid treatment, and full recovery was less likely than in white patients.

Although there is little information for most of the African continent, recent surveys have disproved the previously held view that sarcoidosis is rare in the black South African population. Sarcoidosis is common in South Africa, with an estimated prevalence of 23 per 100 000 in the black population, 11.6 per 100 000 in the mixed race population, and 3.7 per 100 000 in the white population. In both the United States and South Africa sarcoidosis is more extensive in the black than the white population, and in black patients may be associated with chronic deforming arthritis and gross skin lesions. In the past the skin lesions have occasionally been mistaken for leprosy.

In the United States, where mass radiographic screening has not been widely performed, sarcoidosis is at least 10 times more common in the black than in the white population, regardless of birthplace or residence, with prevalence rates per 100 000 variously estimated in military and veterans administration studies at 8.7–81.8 and 0.5–7.5 for the black and white populations respectively.

Sarcoidosis is rarely reported in Arabs in the Middle East, Chinese, Southeast Asians, Inuit (Eskimos), or North American Indians.

The true frequency of sarcoidosis at the extremes of life is difficult to assess. It is rare in very young European children, who are more likely to present with granulomatous meningitis, hepatomegaly, or chronic relapsing polyarthritis than with erythema nodosum and hilar adenop-

Table 4 *Percentage frequency of some clinical manifestations among patients with sarcoidosis reported from London, New York, Los Angeles, and Tokyo (number of patients in parentheses)*

	Scadding London (275)	Siltzbach et al. London (537)	Paris (379)	New York (311)	Los Angeles (150)	Tokyo (282)
Lungs, hilar nodes	98	84	92	90	93	87
Peripheral lymph nodes	31	29	23	37	31	23
Eyes	14	27	11	20	11	14
Skin	17	25	12	19	27	17
Spleen	11	12	6	18	15	1
Parotid	2	6	6	3	6	5
Central nervous system	1	7	6	4	6	5
Bones	4	4	3.5	9	4	2
Erythema nodosum	14	31	6.5	11	9	4

athy. In contrast, Japanese experience with childhood mass radiographic screening shows a moderate frequency of symptomless childhood sarcoidosis. In later childhood the frequency increases, and from adolescence the clinical features and prognosis approximate to those observed in adults. Unlike many diseases in which the lung is involved, sarcoidosis is less common in smokers than in non-smokers.

Clinical features

Modes of presentation

Sarcoidosis may involve almost any organ of the body, with the possible exception of the adrenal gland. The onset is most commonly between the ages of 20 and 35 years, although sarcoidosis is occasionally reported in childhood and in the elderly. There are several patterns of presentation, and the subsequent course can be very varied. Respiratory, ophthalmological, or dermatological symptoms are most common, sometimes in association with constitutional upset, malaise, fever, weight loss, and arthralgia. Lung infiltrates and mediastinal gland enlargement are very common. A significant proportion of individuals with sarcoidosis are asymptomatic throughout the entire course of the disease and only discovered by chance at routine chest radiography or health screening.

The course and prognosis are generally influenced by the mode of onset:

- an acute onset with erythema nodosum in a young adult usually indicates a self-limiting course with spontaneous resolution.
- an insidious onset in middle age is frequently associated with progressive fibrosis and permanent organ dysfunction.

There are an extremely diverse range of possible presentations, and recent United Kingdom experience is detailed in Table 3. The percentage reported frequency of organ and tissue involvement in sarcoidosis is summarized in Table 4. General examination of the patient must be thorough (Fig. 3).

ERYTHEMA NODOSUM AND BILATERAL HILAR LYMPHADENOPATHY (LOFGREN'S SYNDROME).

Erythema nodosum nearly always occurs as the first manifestation in acute onset sarcoidosis and immediately precedes or is associated with bilateral hilar gland enlargement (bilateral hilar lymphadenopathy), sometimes with pulmonary mottling. A combination of erythema nodosum and bilateral hilar lymphadenopathy is virtually diagnostic of acute sarcoidosis, and the clinical picture is complete if there is anterior uveitis and enlargement of superficial lymph nodes.

Erythema nodosum is a painful nodular panniculitis which usually subsides within a month. The characteristic red hot tender shining symmetrical lesions affect the shins, and infrequently are seen on the calves, knees, buttocks, and sometimes the upper outer aspect of the arms as well. Constitutional symptoms may be expected, with an abrupt onset of a swinging fever accompanied by troublesome polyarthralgia. The severity of the joint symptoms is variable, and in men ankle swelling often overshadows slight erythema nodosum. Recurrence is unusual but may be experienced by some 10 per cent, usually within 3 months but occasionally up to a year. The accompanying hilar adenopathy typically regresses within a year, and recurrence or late pulmonary sequelae are rare.

In most areas more women than men with sarcoidosis present with erythema nodosum, although the overall sex ratio, like the overall incidence, varies widely. Sarcoidosis is now recognized to be a cause of erythema nodosum in about one-third of white patients in the United Kingdom, with the proportion of women with erythema nodosum ranging from 3.0 to 1.3 times those for men. Similarly, in the United States, where Afro-Caribbean patients constitute the majority with sarcoidosis, erythema nodosum is found in more white than black patients. In Philadelphia, where most patients with sarcoidosis are black, erythema nodosum was reported in only 4 per cent of females and in no males. Erythema nodosum is uncommon in West Indian or Asian immigrants in the United Kingdom.

The detailed investigation of a patient with erythema nodosum is described elsewhere (Section 23). The proportion of cases of erythema nodosum attributed to sarcoidosis in the population depends upon the incidence not only of sarcoidosis but also of other infections including *M. tuberculosis*, haemolytic streptococci, and fungal infections such as coccidioidomycosis and histoplasmosis. Negative investigations for infections known to be possible causes of erythema nodosum increase the probability of sarcoidosis, but positive tests do not exclude it. For instance, while a negative tuberculin test virtually excludes primary tuberculosis as a cause of erythema nodosum, a positive test does not exclude sarcoidosis.

UVEOPAROTID FEVER (HEERFORDT–WALDENSTROM) SYNDROME

Uveoparotid fever is an uncommon condition which presents acutely to run a chronic course with parotid gland enlargement, uveitis, fever, and cranial nerve palsies. The facial nerves particularly are involved. Other components included bizarre neurological manifestations, lethargy, meningism, and cerebrospinal fluid pleocytosis.

Uveitis is a common manifestation of sarcoidosis occurring in some 30 per cent of patients, while parotid gland enlargement and nerve palsies are uncommon and occur in less than 5 per cent of patients.

Intrathoracic sarcoidosis

During the course of the illness more than 90 per cent of patients show radiographic evidence of intrathoracic involvement. About a quarter are symptomless at presentation and are unexpectedly discovered because of an abnormal chest radiograph. About the same proportion present with trivial respiratory or systemic symptoms, which may include dyspnoea on exertion, usually gradual in onset, cough which is seldom productive, wheezing, and ill-defined constitutional symptoms of malaise, tiredness, weight loss, and fever.

The most common presenting radiographic manifestation, found in about half of patients, is bilateral lymphadenopathy with or without associated paratracheal lymph node involvement. Pulmonary infiltration with bilateral hilar lymphadenopathy is seen in a quarter of patients. Pulmonary infiltration without bilateral hilar lymphadenopathy is the presenting radiographic finding in only 10 per cent of cases.

Individuals with extensive pulmonary infiltration proceeding to fibrosis experience increasingly severe exertional dyspnoea, often accompanied by anterior chest discomfort and persistent unproductive cough. Examination of the chest prior to the onset of fibrosis is remarkable for the absence of abnormal physical signs. Crackles and wheezes are seldom heard, and their presence in apparently early disease should alert the clinician to other diagnostic possibilities. Crackles on auscultation are characteristic of several interstitial lung diseases, including fibrosing alveolitis and asbestosis, but are rarely described in sarcoidosis. In advanced disease the physical signs are compatible with fibrosis and airway obstruction from any cause.

Finger-nail clubbing is rarely seen, but may be noted in chronic sarcoidosis associated with severe lung fibrosis and bronchiectatic change.

Slight haemoptysis is unusual, but may occur with endobronchial sarcoidosis at any stage of the disease. Severe haemoptysis is a feature of chronic sarcoidosis complicated by lung fibrosis, bronchiectasis, or cavities colonized with Aspergillus.

HISTOLOGY

Pulmonary sarcoidosis is primarily an interstitial process with granulomatous inflammation, particularly involving the alveoli, small bronchi, and blood vessels in the upper two-thirds of the lungs.

The early pulmonary lesions are composed of confluent well-circum-

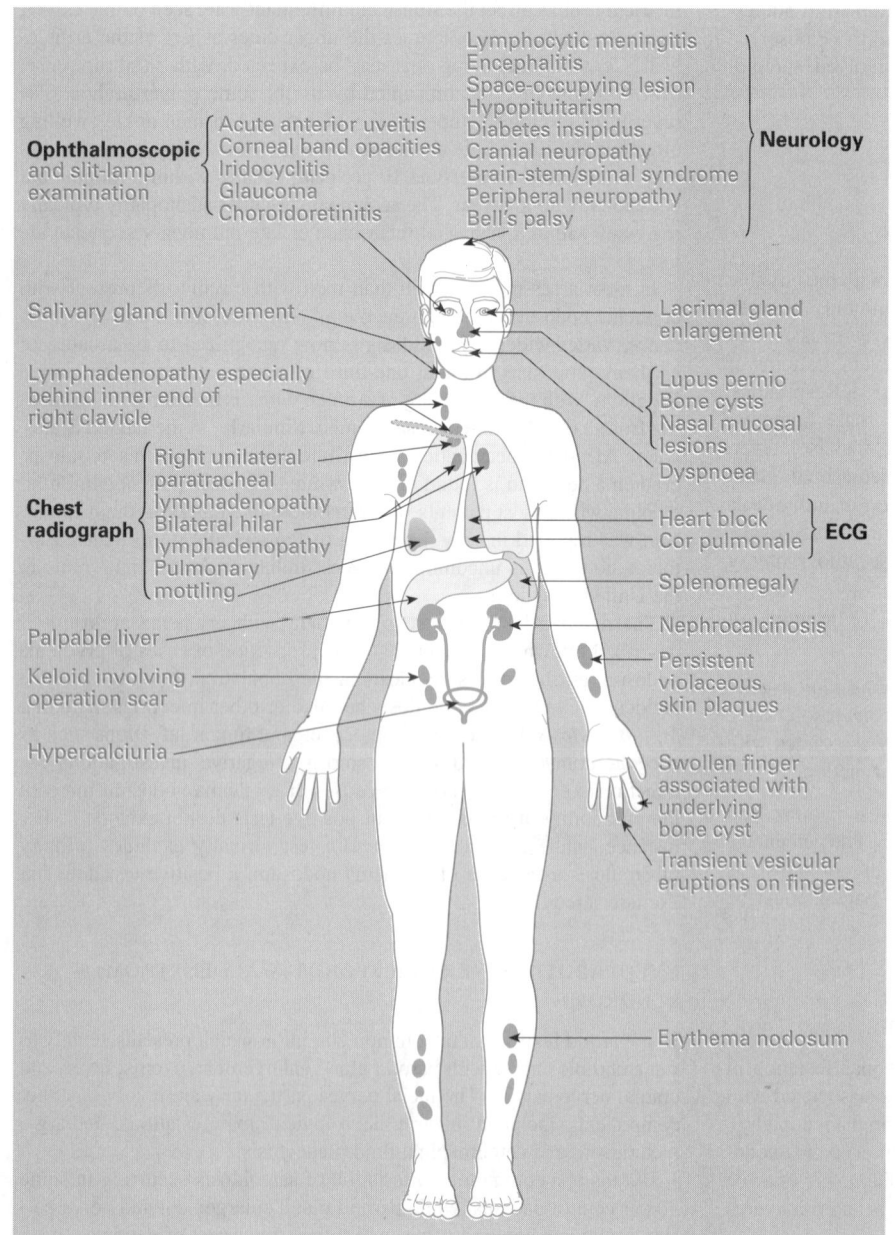

Fig. 3 Principal clinical features of sarcoidosis.

scribed epithelioid granulomas which at first appear randomly scattered in the lung but in fact are most numerous along the lymphatics with a particular predilection for peribronchial, subpleural, interlobular septal, and perivascular connective tissue. Because of their distribution along the lymphatics, the granulomas may also involve veins, arteries, and adjacent connective tissue in a sarcoid angiitis. Involvement of blood vessels is seldom circumferential and scattered granulomas are found along the adventitia. Veins are more frequently involved than arteries. Occlusion and thrombosis is uncommon and right heart strain is rare.

Open or transbronchial lung biopsy frequently reveals sarcoid granulomas in radiographically normal lungs, and with the increased use of the fibreoptic bronchoscope it is apparent that endobronchial sarcoidosis is often present, even in asymptomatic individuals (Fig. 4). Unsuspected pleural involvement is found in about a third.

RADIOGRAPHY

Using conventional chest radiology, it is customary to stage intrathoracic sarcoidosis in the following simple way:

stage 0—clear chest radiograph;
stage 1—hilar and mediastinal lymphadenopathy;
stage 2—hilar and mediastinal lymphadenopathy with pulmonary infiltration;
stage 3—pulmonary infiltration without hilar adenopathy.

This crude classification has the merit of simplicity and international recognition, but the drawback of poor sensitivity and variable observer interpretation. The severity and extent of pulmonary infiltration, for instance, is not quantified. Also it must be stressed that the 'stage' does not necessarily describe the chronological progression of pulmonary sarcoidosis. Stage 0 frequently signifies a relatively late phase of sarcoidosis, with the earlier pulmonary shadowing having resolved to leave extrathoracic organ involvement.

Bilateral hilar and mediastinal gland enlargement

Hilar and mediastinal lymph node enlargement (Fig. 5) is not unique to sarcoidosis, and may occur in tuberculosis, coccidioidomycosis, histoplasmosis, lymphomas, and metastatic carcinoma. However, these conditions seldom cause diagnostic confusion and the presence of bilateral hilar lymphadenopathy provides strong evidence of sarcoidosis, particularly when associated with erythema nodosum or uveitis. Unilateral hilar gland enlargement in sarcoidosis is rare, usually right-sided, and in clinical practice more often a feature of glandular tuberculosis, lymphoma, coccidioidomycosis, histoplasmosis, or superimposed lesions lying in the apical segment of the lower lobe.

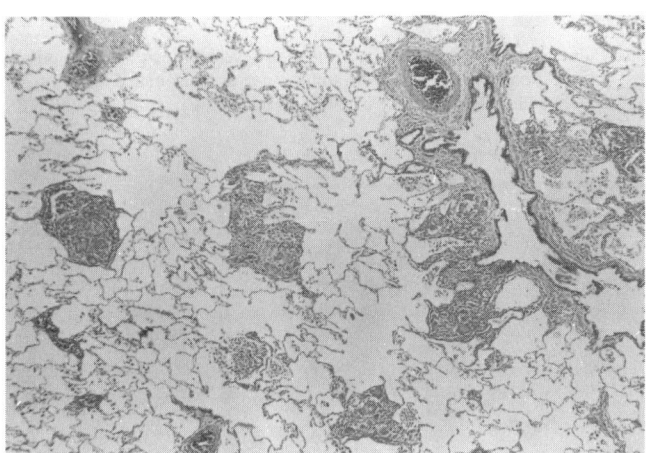

Fig. 4 Sarcoid granulomata in thoracoscopic wedge biopsy; non-caseating granulomas are scattered through the interstitium. Haematoxylin and eosin. Magnification 10 ×. (By courtesy of Dr Margaret Burke, Mount Vernon Hospital.)

In appearance the enlarged hilar mediastinal lymph nodes of sarcoidosis are roughly symmetrical, with a clearly defined outer border which often shows multiple smooth contours suggesting discrete enlargement of individual lymph nodes. Typically, the inner border is clearly defined with a clear zone between the lymph node and the heart shadow. The right hilum, which contains more lymph nodes, tends to appear larger than the left. Paratracheal nodes are frequently involved and are detectable radiographically on the right side in about half of patients. The anterior mediastinal nodes are seldom visibly enlarged in sarcoidosis, an observation which helps differentiate sarcoidosis from lymphoma.

Thoracic CT scanning is more discriminating than conventional radiographic techniques, and will often reveal widespread multiple ill-defined densities deployed along bronchovascular bundles, lymphatics, and interlobar septa when posteroanterior chest radiography shows apparently clear lungs. It may be helpful in determining whether equivocal hilar enlargement is glandular or caused by dilatation of the main branches of the pulmonary vessels (Fig. 6).

Pulmonary infiltration (Figs. 7 and 8)

Many patients with sarcoid granulomas in the lungs profuse enough to cause changes on the chest radiograph have only trivial or no symptoms. The most characteristic posteroanterior chest radiograph appearance is widespread symmetrical mottled shadowing either densest in the middle zones or distributed more or less uniformly throughout the lungs. The

Fig. 5 Bilateral hilar gland enlargement. The right paratracheal lymph node is enlarged. (Stage 1 chest radiograph)

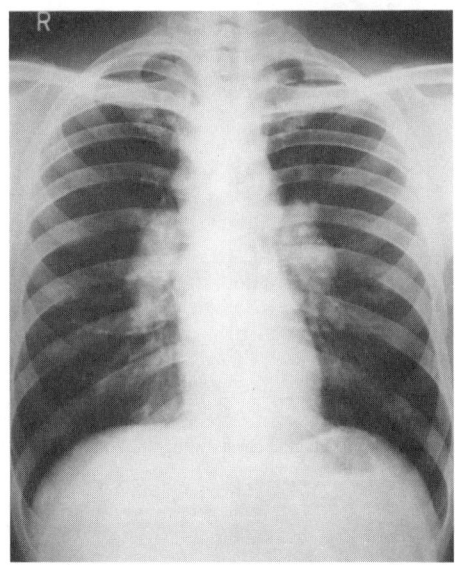

Fig. 6 Pulmonary sarcoidosis CT scan. Widespread nodules of varied size and shape are present throughout the lung fields. On the right side areas of irregular fibrosis are beginning to stretch and deform the lung parenchyma. (By courtesy of Dr B. Strickland, Royal Brompton Hospital.)

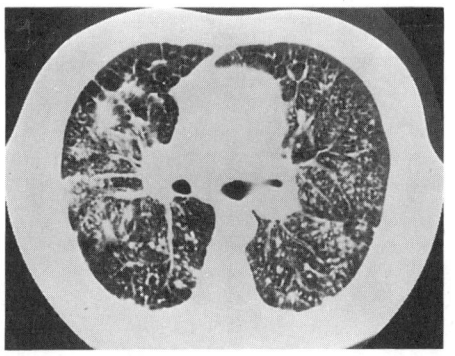

pulmonary shadowing is variously described as miliary, nodular, or confluent. Miliary shadows are usually well defined and 1 mm in size. Nodular shadows range from 3 to 5 mm in size and show ill-defined margins. Confluent shadows may be either widespread or localized, when they may be confused with primary or metastatic malignancy. The chest radiograph most commonly shows a 'stippled' or 'mottled' appearance with shadows ranging from 1 to 5 mm in diameter. Less commonly there are cloudy confluent shadows or nodular uniform opacities associated with widespread infiltration.

The radiographic differential diagnosis of generalized pulmonary mottling is wide and includes fibrosing alveolitis, extrinsic allergic alveolitis, miliary tuberculosis, metastatic malignancy, and Langerhans' cell granulomatosis (eosinophilic granuloma).

Irrespective of the coarseness or extent of the shadowing, resolution occurs in a large proportion of individuals with pulmonary infiltration and coincident hilar gland enlargement. Resolution is less likely to occur in the absence of bilateral hilar adenopathy.

Fig. 7 Bilateral hilar gland enlargement and pulmonary infiltration. (Stage 2 chest radiograph)

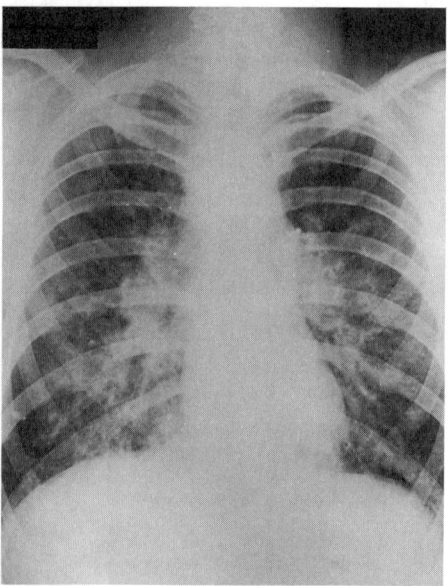

Fig. 8 Mid-zone pulmonary infiltration. (Stage 3 chest radiograph)

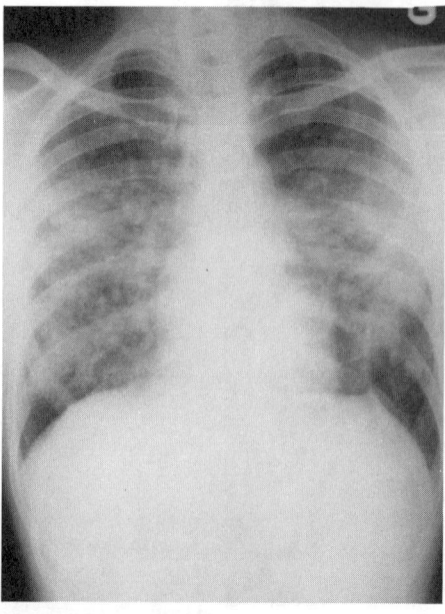

The longer the infiltration persists, the greater is the possibility of an insidious progression towards fibrosis. Fibrosis tends to occur in those areas where previously there had been the densest infiltration. A characteristic pattern is mid-zone fibrosis with the appearance of coarse strands radiating from the hilar.

Late-stage irreversible fibrosis is usually associated with either a loss of volume of the upper zones resulting in elevation of the hilar shadows (Figs. 9 and 10) or, if the fibrosis is denser in the mid-zones, the lower and upper zones may appear hyper-transradiant, suggesting emphysema. Bullous cavities can develop in areas of fibrosis and occasionally these spaces become colonized by Aspergillus giving rise to a 'fungus ball' with characteristic radiographic appearances. Thick-wall cavities are a feature of fibrotic pulmonary sarcoidosis and sometimes attain a large size. Small and moderate-sized cavities are found with varying frequency, and in one series were present in 30 per cent of black and 13 per cent of white patients. Large lung bullae are rare manifestations of severe fibrotic pulmonary sarcoidosis. Even less commonly, a small subgroup of pulmonary sarcoidosis patients develop radiological signs of generalized bullous emphysema.

Lung fibrosis is irreversible and, when extensive, is often associated with severe symptoms and functional impairment. Cor pulmonale is a common terminal complication of severe lung fibrosis.

Calcification

Amongst patients with long-standing chronic persistent sarcoidosis there is a tendency for the lungs and hilar lymph nodes to show scattered foci

Fig. 9 Chronic fibrosis with upper lobe shrinkage characteristic of late stage sarcoidosis. (Stage 3 chest radiograph)

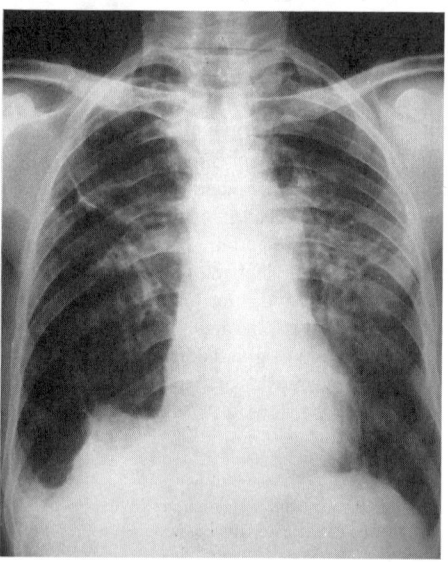

Fig. 10 Pulmonary sarcoidosis CT scan showing severe fibrosis in both mid-zones. Dilated bronchi are present with fibrotic masses surrounded by emphysematous lung. (By courtesy of Dr B. Strickland, Royal Brompton Hospital.)

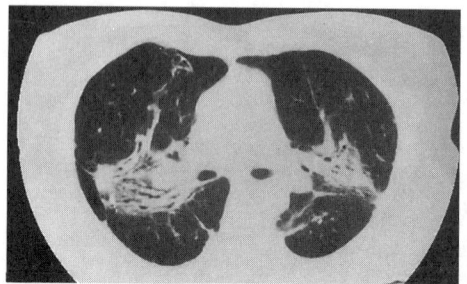

of calcification in areas of hyaline fibrosis. On rare occasions, plaque-like or 'eggshell' calcification may develop in persistently enlarged hilar or mediastinal lymph glands, a finding more characteristic of silicosis. This calcification is dystrophic and not associated with hypercalcaemia.

Pleura

Pleural changes are rarely noted on plain chest radiographs, but CT scanning of the thorax shows pleural involvement in up to one-third of patients. The occasional patient may develop an exudative lymphocytic pleural effusion which may appear at any time during the course of the disease and typically clears within a few months. Pneumothorax is a rare complication (its estimated incidence is 1–2 per cent) with a predominance in advanced fibrotic sarcoidosis associated with upper lobe bullae.

Bronchial stenosis

Bronchial stenosis is rarely reported. Most cases occur late in the course of the disease when major bronchi are distorted and narrowed as a consequence of parenchymal fibrosis and granulomatous lesions in the bronchial wall. Investigations may reveal a single lobar stenosis or, more ominously, multiple segmental stenoses associated with an asthma-like clinical picture and a significant defect in pulmonary function. Lobar stenosis may improve with corticosteroids. Multiple segmental stenoses are associated with fibrosis and have a poor prognosis irrespective of treatment.

Prognosis of pulmonary sarcoidosis

The overall prognosis is good, and in half to two-thirds of patients sarcoidosis resolves to leave radiographically clear lungs. In general, the older the age at onset the greater is the likelihood of chronicity.

Stage 1 chest radiograph

The most favourable outcome is in individuals with few symptoms and minimal radiographic abnormalities. The prognosis is particularly good in white patients presenting acutely with erythema nodosum and bilateral hilar lymphadenopathy; some 80 per cent will resolve spontaneously and have a normal chest radiograph after a year. A further 10 per cent show spontaneous radiographic regression during the second year. Bilateral hilar lympadenopathy persists in some of the remaining 10 per cent, with nodes enlarged by hyaline fibrosis, while in others the disease remains active.

These good prognostic trends are not seen in all racial groups. In black Americans, and in Asians and West Indians living in London, only a third achieve resolution.

Stage 2 chest radiograph

In a quarter of patients the granulomas in the lungs become profuse enough to manifest as radiographic pulmonary infiltration. Complete resolution occurs in about half this group. In the remainder, the radiographic changes persist indefinitely, usually with a combination of infiltration and hilar node enlargement.

Stage 3 chest radiograph

Complete radiological resolution is unlikely in symptomatic chronic sarcoidosis patients with pulmonary infiltration, and only about a quarter achieve a normal chest radiograph. Many show moderate respiratory impairment and this may become critically severe, in some with extensive fibrosis.

Lymphoreticular involvement

Lymphadenopathy is very common. The mediastinal nodes are most often affected and their enlargement can readily be demonstrated on a chest radiograph. Peripheral lymph node enlargement is found more frequently in black than in white patients. The cervical and scalene nodes are most often involved. Other commonly affected peripheral sites include the axillae, inguinal, and epitrochlear nodes. Abdominal mes-enteric and retroperitoneal nodes may be demonstrated by abdominal CT scanning, but are seldom palpable and rarely cause symptoms.

Affected glands are usually discrete, painless on palpation, and with a firm rubbery feel. Clinically enlarged cervical glands may simulate Hodgkin's disease, which must be excluded by biopsy if there is any doubt about a diagnosis of sarcoidosis. Other reticuloses are unlikely to cause diagnostic confusion, for widespread peripheral lymphadenopathy characteristic of these conditions is not a feature of sarcoidosis. In contrast with tuberculosis and some fungal infections the lymph nodes in sarcoidosis do not ulcerate to form draining sinuses.

It is probable that lymph node involvement occurs in most cases of sarcoidosis whether nodes are palpable or not, for node biopsy from the scalene area is positive in three-quarters even when nodes are impalpable.

Asymptomatic involvement of a normal size spleen is common for, as in the lungs, the spleen frequently contains scattered granulomas which may be demonstrated by fine-needle aspiration biopsy. Splenomegaly is reported in up to a quarter, often in association with peripheral lymphadenopathy, and is usually slight and with no prognostic significance. Gross splenic enlargement is rare, but when it occurs it may be associated with hepatomegaly, thrombocytopenia, pancytopenia due to 'hypersplenism', portal hypertension, and bleeding oesophageal varices. Splenectomy may be indicated to relieve pressure symptoms and improve haematological abnormalities due to hypersplenism.

Liver

The liver is often silently affected. Slight hepatomegaly or transient biochemical 'cholestatic' abnormalities of liver function may be found in about a quarter of patients, whereas aspiration liver biopsy will reveal granulomatous infiltration in about three-quarters of asymptomatic patients. The frequency of liver granulomas detected by aspiration liver biopsy varies depending upon the stage of the disease, with the highest frequency of about 90 per cent in acute early sarcoidosis in contrast to only 60 per cent in chronic disease.

Symptoms due to liver involvement are rare, although there may be discomfort when the organ is grossly enlarged. The hepatic granulomas are discrete, randomly distributed, and often lie within portal tracts. Usually the residual scarring that may result from the granulomas does not produce diffuse fibrosis and cirrhotic nodular regeneration of cirrhosis. Intrahepatic cholestasis is a rare event, most frequent in black males, and leads on to portal hypertension, varices, and hepatic failure.

Liver biopsy may reveal granulomas even when sarcoidosis is unsuspected. There are no diagnostic difficulties when biopsy shows characteristic non-caseating hepatic granulomas in association with clinical or radiographic evidence of sarcoidosis. Difficulty arises when the biopsy findings show ill-defined granulomas in the absence of any clinical features to suggest sarcoidosis. A large number of possible causes of granulomatous change in the liver must be considered and their significance will depend upon the age and geographical location of the patient. These include primary biliary cirrhosis, tuberculosis, Hodgkin's disease, infectious mononucleosis, histoplasmosis, schistosomiasis, chronic brucellosis, and chronic beryllium disease.

Skin

Skin involvement in sarcoidosis may be transient or chronic and is found in about a quarter of patients of whom only 5 per cent present with a dermatological complaint. The most common early lesions are erythema nodosum and maculopapular eruptions, both of which often coincide with acute uveitis and bilateral hilar lymphadenopathy. Erythema nodosum is a common acute presenting symptom seen most frequently in white females who express HLA-B8 histocompatibility antigens.

Skin plaques, subcutaneous nodules, and lupus pernio are features of late chronic fibrotic disease. Granulomatous chronic skin lesions are found with varying frequency and are particularly common in black American and British West Indian females. Discrete maculopapular or vesicular lesions occur on the face, around the eyes and nose, and on the back and extremities. Skin plaques are indolent violaceous persistent raised lesions, often with a pale atrophic centre; the face, scalp, and extremities are usually involved. Chronic subcutaneous nodules may enlarge and ultimately infiltrate the skin to appear as nodular cutaneous sarcoids on the trunk or extremities.

Lupus pernio was first described by Ernest Besnier in 1889 as a chronic persistent violaceous skin lesion with a predilection for the nose, cheeks, and ears, and is the most characteristic of all the cutaneous granulomas in sarcoidosis (Fig. 11). Lupus pernio seldom, if ever, resolves completely and is often associated with nasal bone involvement. Patients may be left with unsightly telangiectatic scars on the face with deformity of the nasal bridge. The hands and feet may show similar changes, and radiographs may show bony involvement of the digits.

Scars from surgery, trauma, or vaccination may be infiltrated by sarcoid tissue and become raised, purple, and livid. Biopsy of the lesions will often show typical sarcoid granulomas.

Sarcoidosis of the upper airways

Symptomatic upper respiratory tract sarcoidosis of the nose, nasopharyngeal mucosa, and larynx is uncommon. The true frequency is unknown but, in contrast with the lung or liver, random biopsy of the nasal mucosa in asymptomatic patients rarely shows sarcoid granulomata.

The nasal mucosa overlying the inferior turbinates and septum is most commonly affected. Obstruction, crusting, discharge, and epistaxis are common symptoms. Clinical examination of the nasal airway may reveal reddened granular hypertrophic polypoid mucosa. The nasal bridge may be widened due to involvement of the nasal bones.

Nasal septal perforation, nasal bone destruction, and consequent facial deformity are rare and occur most commonly after nasal airway surgery.

Pharyngeal lesions are uncommon and are usually preceded by nasal mucosal involvement. Dyspnoea, wheezing, or stridor draw attention to laryngeal airway obstruction. In rare instances polypoidal masses or scarring lead to life-threatening laryngeal obstruction. The epiglottis and areas adjacent to the true vocal cords are usually involved, but the cords are spared. If the larynx is affected, other parts of the upper respiratory tract are nearly always involved.

Fig. 11 Disfiguring facial skin lesion due to extensive lupus pernio. (Reproduced with permission from James, D.G. and Studdy, P.R. (1993). *Colour atlas of respiratory diseases*, Mosby–Year Book, St Louis, 1993.)

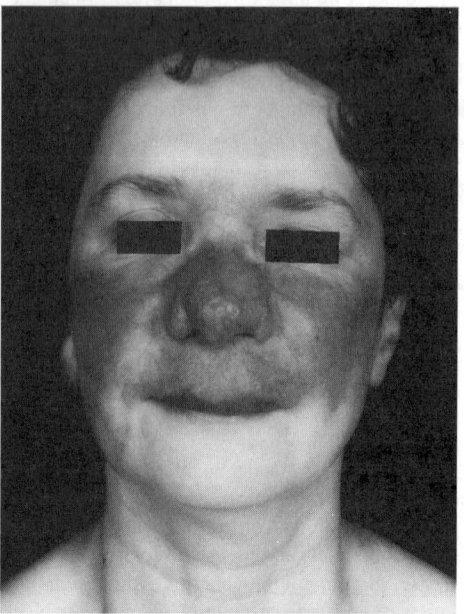

Ocular sarcoidosis

Although the worldwide incidence of ocular sarcoidosis varies, uveitis occurs in about a quarter of patients and if neglected may lead to blindness. Any portion of the eye may be affected, but it is the uveal tract, iris, ciliary body, or choroid that are most frequently involved. Uveitis is a common condition and only 5 per cent of patients with uveitis referred to an ophthalmologist will be suffering from sarcoidosis.

Acute anterior uveitis (iridocyclitis) presenting with a sudden onset of bilateral blurred vision, lacrimation, and photophobia may be the first acute manifestation of sarcoidosis. Most common in young women, it is frequently associated with bilateral hilar lymphadenopathy and erythema nodosum (Lofgren's syndrome). Fever, facial palsy, and parotid gland enlargement (Heerfordt's syndrome) are less common. Clinically, the eyes are red with circumcorneal ciliary congestion and pupillary irregularity, and slit-lamp examination shows fine keratitic precipitates floating in the anterior chamber. Acute uveitis can clear spontaneously or with local corticosteroids, and usually settles uneventfully in a matter of weeks or months leaving no permanent damage.

Chronic sarcoid iridocyclitis has an insidious onset in an older age group, tends to be persistent and progressive, and responds poorly to treatment. Troublesome chronic complications include posterior synechiae between the iris and lens, cataract, secondary glaucoma, and corneal degeneration. Chronic lesions in other systems, such as skin plaques, lupus pernio, or bone cysts, accompany chronic iridocyclitis.

Posterior uveitis is less frequently detected and may be obscured by anterior inflammation. Choroid retinitis, retinal haemorrhage, and papilloedema occur; the last of these is commonly associated with neurological sarcoidosis.

Conjunctival sarcoidosis, which may be confirmed by biopsy, results in phlyctenular conjunctivitis or nodular follicles in the conjunctival folds of the lower eyelids.

Although the lacrimal glands are rarely enlarged, they are occasionally infiltrated by granulomas. The reduced secretion of tears may lead to a Sjögren-like syndrome of dryness, soreness, and redness, with corneal and conjunctival degeneration. Even in the absence of symptomatic dry eyes a decrease in lacrimal secretion can be demonstrated in many chronic sarcoid patients. Enlarged lacrimal glands with associated enlargement of the parotid glands may occur (Mikulicz's syndrome). Arthritis, which is such a prominent feature of Sjögren's syndrome, is absent.

The hypercalcaemia that occurs in some patients with chronic sarcoidosis may result in band keratopathy with deposits of calcium salts in the conjunctiva and cornea, best displayed by slit-lamp examination.

Exophthalmos due to sarcoid infiltration of the orbit is described, often in association with visual field defects or loss of vision due to optic nerve and basal meningeal involvement.

Neurological sarcoidosis

Sarcoidosis affecting the nervous system can present difficult diagnostic problems, particularly in the absence of clinical manifestations of sarcoidosis elsewhere. Any part of the nervous system may be affected, and overall some 7 per cent of sarcoidosis patients show evidence of neurological involvement. Peripheral and cranial neuropathies tend to occur with acute sarcoidosis.

Transient facial nerve palsy, with a predilection to affect the two sides of the face successively, is the most frequent acute neurological presentation and may be associated with ageusia, uveitis, parotid gland enlargement, and fever (Heerfordt's syndrome). Full recovery should be expected.

Generally, neurological sarcoidosis has a poor prognosis. Chronic cranial nerve manifestations include loss of corneal reflexes, optic nerve involvement with transient visual field defects and optic atrophy, auditory and vestibular dysfunction with deafness, tinnitus, and dizziness, and dysphagia due to paresis of the pharyngeal and palatal muscles secondary to involvement of the glossopharyngeal and vagus nerves.

Granulomas may be present in the brain, pituitary gland, spinal cord, and meninges. Patients may present with acute or chronic meningitis, raised intracranial pressure, papilloedema, or obstructive hydrocephalus. Anterior pituitary granulomas seldom disturb function, but involvement of the posterior pituitary or hypothalamus may result in diabetes insipidus or, rarely, hypothalamic hypothyroidism, hypopituitarism, hyperprolactinaemia, somnolence, or alveolar hypoventilation. Space-occupying nodular cerebral lesions are now being recognized with increased frequency and present with symptoms and signs mimicking those of cerebral tumour, including psychiatric disturbances and focal epilepsy. Cranial CT scanning or magnetic resonance imaging are the most useful diagnostic investigations for cerebral sarcoidosis.

Polyneuropathy with paraesthesiae and weakness in the limbs, transverse myelitis, or multiple lesions which mimic multiple sclerosis and amyotrophic lateral sclerosis may occur.

Examination of the cerebrospinal fluid is seldom helpful. Raised pressure, elevated protein levels, pleocytosis, and a low glucose level are common, but are of limited diagnostic value.

Cardiac sarcoidosis

Sudden death from unsuspected cardiac sarcoidosis is all too common, and in most series is the most frequent clinical manifestation of myocardial sarcoidosis.

The heart may be affected directly or indirectly. Direct granulomatous involvement of the myocardium is found histologically in as many as 20 per cent of sarcoidosis autopsy cases, but is seldom recognized clinically. Indirect involvement is from a combination of pulmonary fibrosis, airway obstruction, and hypoxaemia resulting in cor pulmonale.

Cardiac sarcoidosis is suspected when a patient with known sarcoidosis develops arrhythmias, bundle branch block, pericarditis, congestive cardiac failure, or cardiomyopathy. Although the acute phase of myocordial sarcoidosis can resolve completely, healing may result in diffuse cardiac fibrosis with generalized ventricular hypokinesia which is difficult to distinguish from dilated cardiomyopathy. The left ventricle, interventricular septum with specialized His–Purkinje conducting system, and papillary muscle are most often involved. The high frequency of sudden death reflects the risk of involvement of the conduction system by fortuitously sited granulomata.

Even when cardiac sarcoidosis is suspected, it may prove difficult to diagnose. In about 10 per cent of sarcoidosis patients routine electrocardiography may disclose asymptomatic ECG abnormalities with conduction defects and changes suggesting extensive myocardial disease. Echocardiography may show increased right ventricular anterior wall thickness, which is compatible with pulmonary hypertension and focal abnormalities of wall motion affecting the basal portion of the ventricular septum which seem peculiarly specific for sarcoidosis. Thallium-201 radio-isotope cardiac imaging will reveal myocardial defects which may decrease in size during exercise, the opposite of what is noted in ischaemic heart disease. Ventricular aneurysm in the absence of significant coronary artery disease is strongly suggestive of sarcoidosis. Absolute confirmation depends upon myocardial biopsy, a procedure readily performed through the vascular system at cardiac catheterization.

The prognosis is poor and results of treatment with corticosteroids are unimpressive. Corticosteroids promote healing of the granulomas, but may increase the risk of ventricular aneurysm formation, a complication particularly common in black patients. A proportion of patients will require permanent pacemakers to overcome conduction defects, and some in cardiac failure may be rescued by cardiac transplantation.

Locomotor system sarcoidosis

The bones, joints, and muscles can be involved. An acute transient migratory polyarthropathy accompanied by polymyositis, fever, muscle pains, and tenderness, often with bilateral hilar lymphadenopathy and erythema nodosum, is an early feature of sarcoidosis. It is benign and self-limiting, and subsides swiftly either spontaneously or with systemic steroids. Muscle biopsy is particularly likely to show granulomas. Palpable tender muscle nodules, muscle wasting and weakness, hypertrophy and contractures, although rare, may be associated with chronic sarcoidosis.

Bone involvement is relatively uncommon and when it occurs is strongly associated with chronic cutaneous sarcoidosis, particularly lupus pernio. The most frequently involved sites are the phalanges, metacarpals or metatarsals, and nasal bones. Pain and swelling of the hands and feet or soft tissue swelling overlying bone cysts with distortion of the fingers or disfiguring widening of the nasal bridge usually draw attention to the condition. Joint involvement and effusion secondary to bone sarcoidosis or synovial thickening is described.

Radiology of the phalanges or nasal bones may show lytic lesions with minute cortical defects or large rounded punched out cysts involving the cortex and medulla, permeative lesions in which the cortical and trabecular architecture is distorted to give a reticular pattern, or destructive lesions with multiple fractures, devitalized cortex, and sequestrum formation. Bone sarcoidosis is only rarely detected in other parts of the skeleton, although there are occasional reports of skull, rib, or vertebral body involvement.

Genitourinary system sarcoidosis

Symptomatic genitourinary system sarcoidosis is unusual, although it is probable that early in the disease asymptomatic granulomas infiltrate the kidneys with the same frequency as in the lungs and liver. The granulomas are typically sparse and randomly distributed throughout the renal cortex and medulla. Rarely, massive granulomatous infiltration may result in renal failure.

The most common cause of renal impairment in sarcoidosis is nephrocalcinosis due to prolonged hypercalcaemia, a problem affecting only a very small number of patients and which should be accepted only after excluding hyperparathyroidism. Nephrocalcinosis is present in about 1 per cent, and is a late and serious problem as it may lead to pyelonephritis, fibrosis, and intractable chronic renal failure.

The association between glomerulonephritis and early sarcoidosis, although uncommon, is occasionally recognized and may be due to immune complex deposition and microangiopathy.

Endocrine glands and sarcoidosis

The posterior pituitary and hypothalamus are involved more often than any other endocrine gland and, rarely, hypothalamic–pituitary axis dysfunction may lead to secondary neurogenic diabetes insipidus. The diagnosis is suggested when a patient with known sarcoidosis presents with extreme polydipsia and polyuria. Diabetes insipidus is not unique to sarcoidosis, and in individuals with normal renal function the differential diagnosis includes chronic meningeal infection, metastatic malignancy (particularly from lung and breast), and histiocytosis X (eosinophilic granuloma), a rare condition associated with diagnostically confusing non-specific pulmonary shadowing which may mimic sarcoidosis. Treatment is with replacement vasopressin (ADH) or synthetic desmopressin (1-desamino-8-D-arginine vasopressin) given intranasally, the preferred route of administration for chronic neurogenic diabetes insipidus.

Granulomas show no special predilection for other endocrine glands. They are occasionally detected in the anterior pituitary, pancreas, thyroid, and parathyroid glands, but very seldom disturb function.

Pregnancy and sarcoidosis

Sarcoidosis does not generally affect fertility nor does it unfavourably influence the course and outcome of pregnancy. Active sarcoid lesions tend to improve during pregnancy and may then gradually worsen within a few months after delivery.

Diagnosis and investigations

The diagnosis of sarcoidosis is inferred from the clinical features at presentation in combination with the radiographic, biochemical, and immunological findings. Some clinical presentations are so highly characteristic, for instance the bilateral hilar lymphadenopathy–erythema nodosum–arthropathy syndrome, that histological confirmation may not be required. With less characteristic presentations the diagnosis may only be accepted after positive tissue biopsies have been obtained.

Clinical investigation of suspected sarcoidosis

Clinical investigation should include the following in most cases.

1. A full history, including enquiry about BCG vaccination, and detailed clinical examination including ophthalmoscopy and slit-lamp examination of the eyes.
2. Chest radiograph is essential, irrespective of the presenting symptoms. If equivocal, it can be helpful to locate and compare any previous films, or perform CT scanning of the thorax.
3. Routine haematological and biochemical tests including serum calcium and 24 h urine collection to measure urinary calcium excretion.
4. Tuberculin test series up to a concentration of 1 : 100. This is negative in two-thirds of patients with sarcoidosis. Strongly positive reactions are unusual.
5. Sputum, if any, or bronchial washings obtained on fibreoptic bronchoscopy, examined routinely to exclude acid-fast bacilli.
6. Histological confirmation by specific organ biopsy, bronchial or transbronchial lung biopsy, or Kveim–Siltzbach skin test.
7. Assessment of activity in confirmed cases. This will routinely include serial chest radiography and respiratory function tests. Serial measurements of serum angiotensin-converting enzyme can be helpful. Gallium lung scanning and bronchoalveolar lavage are valuable in research but are not generally applicable in routine clinical practice.

These clinical and laboratory investigations will usually confirm the diagnosis, enable the clinician to classify the disease as acute or chronic, and aid therapeutic decisions.

Diagnostic histology

The diagnosis of sarcoidosis can only be made with confidence when tissue biopsy is positive. The preferred site for biopsy is influenced both by the availability of facilities and the mode of presentation. In some cases enlarged superficial lymph nodes or apparently involved skins may be biopsied, while in others lung or mediastinal gland biopsy may give the diagnosis. The general requirement is to confirm the diagnosis without undue discomfort or hazard to the patient by selecting the most favourable biopsy site. Many organ biopsy procedures are infrequently performed because of high morbidity (open-lung biopsy), low diagnostic yield (conjunctiva), or difficulties in interpretation (liver).

Fibreoptic bronchoscopy with multiple transbronchial biopsies is a particularly useful technique. The yield is high, with a frequency of positive diagnosis greater than 80 per cent. The procedure can be performed under local anaesthesia and has an acceptably low complication rate. The recently developed minimally invasive surgical technique of transthoracoscopic lung biopsy obtains a large peripheral speciman for critical pathological assessment and so provides an alternative diagnostic method.

Mediastinoscopy is the preferred method for gaining access to the anterior mediastinal lymph nodes. Mediastinal lymph node biopsy helps to differentiate lymphoma from sarcoidosis and has a high diagnostic yield. It is invasive and is associated with occasional morbidity and complications; haemorrhage is the major danger but injury to the left recurrent laryngeal nerve and pneumothorax may occur. In obscure cases open-lung biopsy can be relied upon to produce a sufficiently large sample for diagnosis from precisely selected parts of the lung.

In cases where organ biopsy is difficult or negative a Kveim–Siltzbach test often fulfils the general requirements for diagnosis, and in most instances a positive granulomatous reaction provides enough confirmation for a diagnosis of sarcoidosis to be accepted.

The Kveim–Siltzbach test

A skin test using injected sarcoid tissue extract to assist in diagnosing suspected sarcoidosis, described by Kveim in 1941 and then refined and improved by Siltzbach and Chase, is widely used in the United Kingdom and is of proven clinical value.

The Kveim–Siltzbach material is a finely particulate saline suspension of human sarcoid tissue prepared from the spleen of a patient with active sarcoidosis removed either surgically for valid indications or at necropsy. The test solution is stable and can withstand boiling for 30 min, but is destroyed by autoclaving and alkaline solutions. The active component is insoluble in water and in fat solvents. It may be a lipoprotein but has not been characterized.

Validation of the test material can only be achieved by clinical testing alongside known satisfactory suspensions so as to exclude impotent or unselective preparations. Validated suspensions for diagnostic use in the United Kingdom are available from the Public Health Laboratory Service in 1.5 ml single-dose sealed ampoules. In the United States federal law prohibits distribution of biological substances and few centres routinely use the Kveim–Siltzbach test. The test is not generally available worldwide.

The safety of the Kveim–Siltzbach test has been a matter of some concern, although in practice it appears to be free from adverse affects except occasional local ulceration with strongly positive responses. On theoretical grounds the injection of splenic tissue from human to human is not completely without hazard, particularly in a disease of unknown aetiology. Fortunately, the lengthy preparation of the test material permits thorough investigation which is not possible in blood or organ donation. The use of serological tests for viral infection including hepatitis B surface antigen, HIV, and cytomegalovirus, heating to 58°C, phenolization, irradiation during preparation, and microbiological and animal testing ensure the absence of recognized pathogens in the suspension.

PERFORMANCE OF THE TEST

The contents of the ampoule should be dispersed by shaking and the test dose (0.15 ml) injected intracutaneously on the ulnar aspect of the flexor surface of the forearm using a 26 gauge narrow needle and a 1 ml tuberculin type syringe which has previously been rinsed with sterile saline to remove any extraneous material. The injection must be deliberately intradermal so as to raise a *peau d'orange* bleb on the skin.

The result of the test can be ascertained reliably only by microscopic assessment following biopsy of the full thickness of the skin at the test site 4 to 6 weeks after injection. Biopsy is essential for two reasons. Some macroscopic clinically evident papules show diagnostically irrelevant non-specific reactions, and occasional histologically positive granulomatous reactions are neither visible or palpable at the test injection site.

Corticosteroids suppress all but the most vigorous Kveim–Siltzbach reactions and, if possible, their administration should be deferred until the test is biopsied. Histological assessment is not always straightforward and equivocal granulomatous responses may be seen. However, there is a high degree of concordance in interpretation when criteria for positive, negative, and equivocal reactions are predefined. The mechanism of the response has not been explained.

SPECIFICITY AND SENSITIVITY OF THE KVEIM–SILTZBACH TEST

The proportion of patients with sarcoidosis giving granulomatous reactions varies with the stage of the disease. Unfortunately, the test is most likely to be positive in circumstances when the clinical features strongly support the diagnosis of sarcoidosis, a frustrating fact that reduces its effective value. From 85 to 90 per cent of patients with classical acute sarcoidosis give a positive test, whereas only a third are positive in long-standing chronic fibrotic disease manifesting with pulmonary fibrosis or infiltration. Reactivity wanes as sarcoidosis becomes inactive, although a small proportion of individuals remain positive after prolonged follow-up. A negative test does not exclude the diagnosis.

Positive responses are not exclusive to sarcoidosis. Some well-validated test suspensions, giving the expected response in sarcoidosis, have caused granulomatous reactions in up to 40 per cent of patients with Crohn's disease and in a small proportion of patients with active tuberculosis, coeliac disease, ulcerative colitis, and chronic brucellosis. Amongst healthy controls, various studies have shown the incidence of unequivocally positive responses to be between 0.7 and 2 per cent. In respiratory practice the most important diagnostic distinctions are between tuberculous or lymphoma. Pulmonary tuberculosis is rarely and lymphoma virtually never associated with a positive test.

Therefore a positive Kveim–Siltzbach test is a useful minimally invasive means of supporting a diagnosis of sarcoidosis.

Lung function

The abnormalities most often found on standard tests are as follows:

- reduction of lung volume and compliance;
- impaired gas transfer;
- an obstructive ventilatory defect.

Slight respiratory function impairment is common in early prefibrotic pulmonary sarcoidosis, but is seldom associated with disability or symptoms. Routine tests may give results within the normal range. Abnormalities include a modest reduction in lung volumes and slight impairment of gas exchange, the latter identified by a fall in Pao$_2$, widening of the alveolar–arterial Po$_2$ difference $P(A - a)$o$_2$ on exertion, and failure of the carbon monoxide transfer coefficient Kco to rise with exercise. It is debatable whether small airway function is abnormal in early disease, although the widespread distribution of granulomata in the lung parenchyma implies small airway involvement.

As the disease progresses there is a gradual loss of lung volume, more severe gas exchange abnormalities due to ventilation–perfusion inequalities, worsening airflow obstruction, and loss of compliance. A complaint of exertional dyspnoea is often associated with significant impairment of lung function. Resting hypoxemia is a feature of severe pulmonary disease.

The majority with progressive pulmonary sarcoidosis show a restrictive functional defect. Some may also show an obstructive defect caused by endobronchial sarcoidosis with or without bronchostenosis. Single or multiple localized stenoses of major bronchi may be suspected when flow volume loops show a pattern of inspiratory as well as expiratory airflow limitation.

Single measurements of lung function determine the extent of functional impairment, and serial measurements help both in following progress and, if appropriate, the response to therapy. Although the correlations of function with pathology are weak, they are better than those between pathology and chest radiography. The frequent lack of functional abnormality in the face of florid radiograph appearance is a well-known feature of sarcoidosis. Conversely, it is also recognized that functional abnormalities may persist even when the radiograph has cleared. The more accurate CT scan images of the thorax correlate more precisely with pulmonary function tests.

Laboratory investigations

Haematology

There are no specific features. A moderate reduction in the peripheral blood lymphocyte count may occur in active disease. Thrombocytopenia and purpura, independent of clinical splenomegaly, are described. Elevation of the erythrocyte sedimentation rate (ESR) is common and largely influenced by serum protein concentrations. C-reactive protein, an acute-phase protein, shows no consistent pattern and is seldom elevated in sarcoidosis. It is commonly elevated in sputum-positive pulmonary tuberculosis.

Biochemistry

DISORDERED CALCIUM HOMEOSTASIS

Hypercalcaemia and hypercalciuria due to abnormal vitamin D synthesis are well-recognized problems in active sarcoidosis and occur in about 2 to 10 per cent of patients, although some studies show a higher prevalence. Although often a chance discovery, some patients may present with symptomatic hypercalcaemia complaining of anorexia, nausea, vomiting, polydipsia, polyuria, and weight loss. Disordered calcium homeostasis is transient in acute early disease, but in older patients with chronic sarcoidosis it is likely to become persistent and to cause nephrocalcinosis and renal calculi.

The biochemical abnormalities resemble hypervitaminosis D, with a moderate or considerable elevation of serum calcium, normal serum phosphate, and normal or slightly raised alkaline phosphatase. Hypercalciuria is more common than hypercalcaemia. Although the raised calcium is independent of parathormone, it should be measured to exclude unsuspected hyperparathyroidism.

Patients with sarcoidosis are extremely sensitive to vitamin D and may suffer an exacerbation of hypercalcaemia or hypercalciuria if vitamin D treatment is inappropriately prescribed or when the skin is exposed to ultraviolet light during the summer. Studies of sarcoidosis reveal normal levels of 25-hydoxy cholecalciferol (25-(OH)-D$_3$) but an acquired increase in the active metabolite 1-25 dihydroxycholecalciferol (1,25-(OH)$_2$-D$_3$) which is synthesized by activated macrophages in pulmonary and extrathoracic sarcoid granulomas and is independent of renal 1-hydroxylase, the normal physiological source of 1,25-(OH)$_2$-D$_3$.

Asymptomatic hypercalcaemia due to sarcoidosis rapidly responds to corticosteroids, unlike the hypercalcaemia of hyperparathyroidism. Corticosteroids quickly lower 1,25-(OH)$_2$-D$_3$ levels and reduce intestinal hyperabsorption of calcium.

Symptomatic patients, particularly those in whom the serum calcium is in excess of 3.5 mmol/l, require urgent rehydration with sufficient isotonic sodium chloride solution to promote a vigorous diuresis and oral or parenteral corticosteroids in high dose.

SERUM GLOBULINS AND IMMUNOGLOBULINS

Total serum globulin and specific immunoglobulin levels are often raised above normal. In active sarcoidosis there is a polyclonal increase in immunoglobulin levels, particularly in black patients and more often in females than in males. High IgM levels may be found in association with erythema nodosum, while the other immunoglobulins are variously raised, with IgA and IgG more commonly in black than in white patients. IgD is often depressed, the opposite to the common finding in tuberculosis.

IMMUNE COMPLEXES

Circulating immune complexes are commonly detected in the early acute stage of sarcoidosis, particularly in association with erythema nodosum and bilateral hilar lymphadenopathy.

LIVER FUNCTION, UREA, AND ELECTROLYTES

There are no special features associated with these routine tests. Alkaline phosphatase may be elevated as a consequence of bone or hepatic involvement.

Disease activity

Traditionally, the activity or potential for deterioration in sarcoidosis is assessed by a number of loosely defined clinical criteria (Table 5). These include the presence or absence of weight loss, fatigue, malaise, fever, cutaneous lesions, dyspnoea, or deteriorating exercise tolerance, and are supplemented by objective evidence provided by serial radiographs and measurements of pulmonary function. The cellular and metabolic activity of the disease is not accurately reflected by these clinical features and routine investigations.

Bronchoalveolar lavage differential and total cell counts, quantitated gallium-67 radio-isotope lung uptake, and measurements of serum angiotensin-converting enzyme activity have brought clinical research closer to the granuloma and can provide useful but non-specific clinical information about disease activity. These three parameters show some broad correlations with each other, and serial estimations reveal general agreement with changes in the appearance of the chest radiograph or lung function tests. However, the extent to which these indices reflect activity is uncertain. While all three indices can supplement more conventional investigations, bronchoalveolar lavage and gallium-67 scans should be considered of research interest while serum angiotensin-converting enzyme has more general applications.

Gallium-67 radio-isotope scanning

This technique involves posterior and anterior gamma scanning of the whole thorax 48 to 72 h after an intravenous injection of about 3 mCi of ^{67}Ga-citrate, a cyclotron-produced radionuclide with a half-life of 78 h. The normal liver, spleen, and skeleton avidly accumulate gallium-67, whereas there is little uptake in the normal lung. The resulting images can be graded numerically or by analysis of radioactive uptake.

Gallium-67 is taken up avidly by macrophages, and to a lesser degree by neutrophils and lymphocytes. In active sarcoidosis the isotope accumulates at sites of disease activity, particularly the lungs and the hilar and mediastinal lymph nodes.

A positive scan may help to differentiate hilar nodes from pulmonary arteries and active lung disease from inactive fibrosis. Predictably, gallium-67 lung scanning is most likely to show increased hilar and mediastinal uptake in early active sarcoidosis. High pulmonary activity may also be seen in the presence of a clear standard chest radiograph. Corticosteroids usually suppress gallium-67 uptake. Positive gallium scans are not specific for sarcoidosis; increased gallium uptake is seen in a number of pulmonary conditions, including malignancy, pneumonia, tuberculosis, fibrosing alveolitis, and asbestosis.

Gallium-67 scanning is expensive and its significant radiation exposure makes repetition at intervals of less than 6 months undesirable.

Bronchoalveolar lavage

The ability to sample the secretions from the lower respiratory tract by lavage at fibreoptic bronchoscopy has provided a new understanding of the cellular and immunological events occurring in a variety of lung conditions. The technique is straightforward and no more distressing to

Table 5 *Features of active sarcoidosis*

Symptoms and clinical signs
Deteriorating pulmonary function
More extensive radiographic infiltration
Biochemical abnormalities (calcium, liver enzymes)
Raised serum angiotensin converting enzyme activity
Gallium lung scan activity
Bronchoalveolar lavage lymphocytosis

the patient than routine fibreoptic bronchoscopy. The bronchoscope is wedged into a distal bronchus and 100 to 300 ml of buffered warm normal saline are introduced and then aspirated. The recovered cells and fluid are separated and analysed using a variety of techniques.

In active pulmonary sarcoidosis bronchoalveolar lavage cell counts or profiles of the recovered fluid characteristically demonstrate an increased proportion of lymphocytes when compared with normal non-smoking control subjects. Activated CD4-helper lymphocytes are predominant; the remainder of the recovered cells are macrophages with a small number of neutrophils and eosinophils. B-lymphocytes are present but in subnormal numbers. Raised bronchoalveolar lavage lymphocyte counts return to normal as sarcoidosis resolves, either spontaneously or with corticosteroids. The bronchoalveolar lavage lymphocyte-cell profile may be characteristic of sarcoidosis but should not be considered diagnostic, for bronchoalveolar lavage lymphocytosis may be demonstrated in active pulmonary tuberculosis, extrinsic allergic alveolitis, and certain fibrosing lung disorders.

Serum angiotensin-converting enzyme (dipeptidyl carboxypeptidase)

Some two-thirds of active sarcoidosis patients have raised levels of serum angiotensin-converting enzyme, with the highest levels in those with clinically florid or radiographically extensive disease.

Angiotensin-converting enzyme is a membrane bound glycoprotein located mainly in the pulmonary capillary endothelium. The main physiological site of action is in the lungs where it catalyses the conversion of the decapeptide angiotensin 1 to the vasopressor octapeptide angiotensin 2. In healthy adults there is some physiologically irrelevant and remarkable constant background angiotensin-converting enzyme activity in the serum which is believed to arise by diffusion of the enzyme from vascular endothelial cells.

In sarcoidosis angiotensin-converting enzyme is produced by epithelioid cells. Immunofluorescence studies demonstrate angiotensin 2, a cleavage product of angiotensin-converting enzyme catalysis, and angiotensin-converting enzyme in the epithelioid cells of granulomas. CD4-lymphocytes modulate angiotensin-converting enzyme synthesis in the monocyte in culture and, it is presumed, do so *in vivo*, for angiotensin-converting enzyme is most abundant in the peripheral part of the granuloma where CD4-lymphocytes and epithelioid cells are in close contact. The raised serum angiotensin-converting enzyme activity found in sarcoidosis provides a biochemical marker of cellular activity in the forming granulomas.

Serum angiotensin-converting enzyme is not a particularly sensitive or specific test for sarcoidosis. Increased serum angiotensin-converting enzyme activity does raise the possibility of sarcoidosis and can be a useful finding when investigating the cause of non-specific pulmonary shadowing. Serum angiotensin-converting enzyme is seldom elevated in early subacute sarcoidosis, but is often increased in radiologically apparent or clinically active disease. The highest values occur with extensive reticuloendothelial involvement, an observation leading to the proposition that serum angiotensin-converting enzyme provides a measure of the 'total active granulomatous mass'.

Consistently elevated serum angiotensin-converting enzyme levels, appreciably higher than those found in sarcoidosis, occur in Gaucher's disease and in a number of other diseases associated with activation, maturation, and proliferation of the monocytic cell line. Serum angiotensin-converting enzyme is inexplicably elevated in a number of other pulmonary disorders, including asbestosis, silicosis, and atypical mycobacterial infections, as well as non-pulmonary conditions, including alcoholic liver disease, hyperthyroidism, and diabetes mellitus.

Serial serum angiotensin-converting enzyme measurements can be helpful in monitoring disease activity because changes in serum angiotensin-converting enzyme activity show a broad relationship to the chest radiograph and clinical condition.

Serum angiotensin-converting enzyme is inexpensive to measure, and the assay can be repeated at frequent intervals without hazard to the patient.

Course and prognosis

The natural history of the disease varies considerably, as does the need for and response to therapy. It is helpful to categorize patients into two major, but not completely distinct, subdivisions; those with subacute disease of less than 2 years duration and those with longer-standing persistent chronic lesions. Undoubtedly the best prognosis is associated with subacute sarcoidosis, and the greatest likelihood of complete remission is in young adult white patients presenting with an abrupt onset of erythema nodosum and bilateral hilar lymphadenopathy. The prognosis is good because the lesions typically undergo spontaneous remission within 2 years. Salivary gland involvement, peripheral lymphadenopathy, uveitis, facial nerve palsy, and other systemic features usually regress with the minimum of treatment.

Chronic sarcoidosis has an insidious onset and is often associated with progressive tissue fibrosis which may eventually cause permanent functional derangement. The patients are often middle-aged. Typically, the chest radiograph shows pulmonary mottling, in some leading on to lung fibrosis and bullae associated with permanent respiratory disability. Extrathoracic features include lupus pernio, skin plaques, bone cysts, and chronic iridocyclitis.

Sarcoidosis is a condition that remits without treatment in two-thirds of white patients and one-third of black patients. It is fatal in less than 3 per cent of clinically recognized cases. While eventual resolution of pulmonary sarcoidosis may be expected in two-thirds of patients, resolution is much less likely when there is accompanying extrathoracic disease. The chest radiograph clears in only one-sixth of patients in whom bone and skin lesions accompany pulmonary sarcoidosis. Between the large proportion of transient benign cases and the rare fatality lies a minority of patients, often young or middle-aged, who are permanently disabled by tissue fibrosis in the lungs, eyes, kidneys, or other organs.

Treatment

Since no treatable pathogenic factor has yet been discovered, it is inevitable that at present there is no specific therapy. The general management of patients with sarcoidosis is controversial and may be both difficult and tedious for all those involved. Although there is no curative treatment, most aspects of the acute or chronic disease can be ameliorated by anti-inflammatory drugs. It is generally agreed that corticosteroids improve local and constitutional symptoms and suppress granulomatous inflammation in affected tissues with, for instance, measurable increase in pulmonary function or rapid clearing of radiographic infiltration. The dose of corticosteroids required to produce this effect, and the duration of treatment required to maintain it, varies considerably from patient to patient.

The long-term benefit of corticosteroid treatment is uncertain. Clinical trials have failed to confirm the hypothesis that pulmonary and extra-thoracic fibrosis, with consequent irreversible functional impairment, can be prevented if corticosteroids are prescribed in sufficient dose and for long enough to suppress granuloma formation and tissue flammation.

The problem of treatment is compounded by the tendency for sarcoidosis to resolve spontaneously and the possible complications resulting from long-term corticosteroid treatment. While no other therapeutic agents have been as consistently palliative, it is unfortunate that corticosteroid therapy is poorly tolerated by many patients.

In view of these uncertainties, indications for corticosteroids in pulmonary or extrathoracic sarcoidosis remain largely a matter of clinical judgement, with inevitable variation between physicians. The clinician faced with a relatively asymptomatic chronic sarcoidosis patient has to make a difficult decision regarding the relative risk of corticosteroid treatment balanced against unpredictable long-term benefit.

Indications for treatment with corticosteroids

Guidelines provided in 1971 by the Committee on Therapy of the American Thoracic Society regarding the indications for oral corticosteroids in sarcoidosis are still generally applicable.

1. Bilateral hilar lymphadenopathy (stage I) is likely to settle spontaneously and corticosteroids are seldom required. Initial febrile arthropathy and erythema nodosum can be controlled by non-steroidal anti-inflammatory drugs.
2. Pulmonary infiltration with or without bilateral hilar lymphadenopathy (stages II and III) which remains static and associated with symptoms of breathlessness or significantly impaired lung function, or which remains symptomless but radiographically worsens over a 3 to 6 month period of observation, is a relative indication for corticosteroids. Treatment is given to minimize or prevent irreversible pulmonary fibrosis.
3. Symptoms due to obvious pulmonary fibrosis may unexpectedly improve with corticosteroids, and the treatment may be continued long term in patients who show a response.
4. Hypercalcaemia and hypercalciuria that persist despite dietary reduction in calcium intake and avoidance of vitamin D warrant corticosteroids to prevent nephrocalcinosis and renal failure.
5. Uveitis always requires corticosteroid treatment. Topical corticosteroid eyedrops and local atropine to maintain a dilated pupil may suffice provided that the patient is closely monitored by an experienced ophthalmologist. In all other cases the only safe course is to treat with systemic corticosteroids commencing with oral prednisolone.
6. Central nervous system involvement shows an unpredictable response to treatment, but corticosteroids are advisable when symptoms are due to meningeal infiltration, local deposits in the brain, and spinal cord or cranial nerve involvement.
7. Myocardial sarcoidosis may respond to corticosteroids, particularly if there are arrhythmias due to active granulomas.
8. Corticosteroids should be considered for symptomatic muscle involvement, for disfiguring skin lesions, for glandular or significant splenic involvement, or when severe erythema nodosum persists or recurs.

Schedule of treatment with corticosteroids

The basic strategy generally employed is to commence with a large enough dose of corticosteroids to suppress granuloma activity and effect clinical and radiographic improvement. An oral dose of 0.5–1.0 mg/kg of prednisolone daily, give for 4 to 6 weeks, usually suffices, although in life-threatening situations some recommend a larger daily oral dose of prednisolone or very high doses of methyl prednisolone given by parenteral injection. Corticosteroids should be discontinued in individuals showing no evidence of response after 4 to 6 weeks, while in responders the dose of corticosteroids is slowly reduced over 6 months to a low maintenance level. Some parameter (chest radiograph, renal function tests, serum angiotensin-converting enzyme, etc.) should be selected to ascertain the effectiveness of therapy.

Once a satisfactory response is achieved, the dose of corticosteroid can be adjusted to maintain the improvement. For many patients the disease can be controlled on 5–10 mg prednisolone per day, a low dose unlikely to result in serious unwanted side-effects or major problems with pituitary–adrenal suppression.

Periodic attempts to withdraw treatment should be made, initially after 6 months of maintenance corticosteroids and then at intervals, although the total duration is unpredictable. Prolonged periods of treatment are often necessary as relapses are common, particularly in West Indian or black American patients. Relapse may even occur after more than a decade of continuous well-controlled corticosteroid-treated sarcoidosis but usually improves when treatment is reinstituted, although not necessarily to the previous state.

Aerosol corticosteroids may have some slight potential in managing pulmonary sarcoidosis either as a supplement or substitute for maintenance oral prednisolone.

Alternatives to corticosteroid treatment

Non-steroidal anti-inflammatory drugs (aspirin, indomethacin, etc.) are of value in controlling musculoskeletal and cutaneous symptoms in subacute sarcoidosis.

The antimalarial drug chloroquine phosphate has been found to have a useful suppressive rather than curative effect upon progressive cutaneous, pulmonary, and extracutaneous sarcoidosis. Complications of chloroquine therapy occur relatively infrequently and most are reversible. The ocular side-effects of chloroquine therapy are of most concern to clinicians and are responsible for its judicious use. Corneal deposits occur in most patients receiving long-term therapy and, rarely, chloroquine-induced retinopathy with irreversible sight-threatening field defects occur. Its long-term use might be considered in persistent cutaneous sarcoidosis or in exceptional cases in which corticosteroids are relatively contraindicated. A dose schedule of chloroquine 250 mg twice daily for 14 days and then 250 mg per day (3.5–4.0 mg/kg ideal body weight) long term is recommended.

In view of its ocular toxicity all patients should have a full ophthalmic examination before commencing chloroquine and then a serial ophthalmological review at 3 to 6 month intervals during prolonged treatment. Ocular toxicity is unlikely if the drug is given for less than 1 year.

There is some evidence that cytotoxic or immunosuppressive drugs (chlorambucil, methotrexate, or azothiaprine), given in low doses, may also be helpful as single agents in the treatment of disfiguring chronic skin lesions or as a 'steroid-sparing' supplement to corticosteroid treatment. The use of immunosuppressive agents in sarcoidosis must be regarded as empirical since no proof of long-term benefit is available. Indications for a trial of such therapy must be exceptional.

Antimycobacterial therapy does not affect the course of sarcoidosis but is required in those unusual cases in which there is a concurrent active mycobacterial infection conformed by the isolation of *Mycobacterium tuberculosis* or as 'cover' for corticosteroid treatment in a patient giving a skin reaction of 10 mm or more to a standard 1 : 1000 dilution intradermal tuberculin test.

REFERENCES

Baughman, R.P., Shipley, R., and Eisentrint, C.E. (1987). Predictive value of gallium scan, angiotensen converting enzyme level and broncho-alveolar lavage in two year follow up of pulmonary sarcoidosis. *Lung*, **165**, 371.

Bocard, D., Lecossier, D., De Lassence, A., Valeyre, D., Battesti, J., and Hance, A.J.A. (1992). Search for mycobacterial DNA in granulomatous tissues from patients with sarcoidosis using the polymerase chain reaction. *American Review of Respiratory Disease*, **145**, 1142–8.

British Thoracic and Tuberculosis Association (1969). Geographical variations in the incidence of sarcoidosis in Great Britain: a comparative study in four areas. *Tubercle*, **50**, 211.

Du Bois, R.M., Holroyd, K.J., Saltini, C., and Crystal, R.G. (1991). Granulomatous processes. In: *The lung: scientific foundations* (ed R.G. Crystal and J.B. West), pp. 1925–38. Raven Press, New York.

Edmonstone, W.M. and Wilson, A.R. (1985). Sarcoidosis in caucasians, blacks and asians in London. *British Journal of Diseases of the Chest*, **79**, 27.

Fanburg, B.L. (1983). *Sarcoidosis and other granulomatous diseases of the lung*, Vol. 20. Dekker, New York.

Fidler, H., Rook, G.A., McJohnson, N., and McFadden, J. (1993). *Mycobacterium tuberculosis* DNA in tissue affected by sarcoidosis. *British Medical Journal*, **306**, 546–9.

Fleming, H.A. and Bailey, S.M. (1987). Sarcoid heart disease. *Journal of the Royal College of Physicians of London*, **15**, 245.

Hagerstrand, I. and Linell, F. (1964). The prevalance of sarcoidosis in the autopsy material from a Swedish town. *Acta Medica Scandinavica (Suppl.)*, **425**, 171.

Israel, H.L., Albertine, K.H., Park, C.H., and Patrick, H. (1991). Whole-body gallium 67 scans. Role in diagnosis of sarcoidosis. *American Review of Respiratory Disease*, **144**, 1182–6.

James, D.G., Turiaf, J., Josoda, H., *et al.* (1976). Description of sarcoidosis. Report of the subcommittee on classification and definition. *Annals of the New York Academy of Sciences*, **278**, 742.

James, D.G. (ed.). (1994). *Sarcoidosis and other granulomatous disorders*. Vol. 73. Dekker, New York.

James, D.G. and Williams, W.J. (1985). *Sarcoidosis and other granulomatous diseases*. W.B. Saunders, Philadelphia, PA.

Mitchell, D.N. and Rees, R.J. (1983). The nature and physical characteristics of transmissible agents from human sarcoid and Crohn's disease tissues. In: *Proceedings of the 9th International Conference on Sarcoidosis, Paris* (ed J. Chretien, J. Marsac, and J.C. Saltiel), pp. 132–41. Pergamon, Oxford.

Muller, N.L. and Miller, R.R. (1990). State of the art. Computed tomography of chronic diffuse infiltrative lung disease. Part 2. *American Review of Respiratory Disease*, **142**, 1440–8.

Oakley, C.M. (1989). Cardiac sarcoidosis. *Thorax*, **44**, 371.

Scadding, J.G. (1987). Sarcoidosis. In *Oxford Textbook of Medicine* (ed. D.J. Weatherall, J.G.G. Ledingham, and D. A. Warrell) 2nd edn. Oxford University Press.

Scadding, J.G. and Mitchell, D.N. (1985). *Sarcoidosis* (2nd edin). Chapman and Hall, London.

Sharma, O.P. and Sharma, A.M. (1991). Sarcoidosis of the nervous system: a clinical approach. *Archives of Internal Medicine*, **151**, 1317–21.

Siltzbach, L.E., James, D.G., Neville, E., Turiaf, J., Battesti, J.P., Sharma, O.P., Hosoda, Y., Mikami, R., and Odaka, M. (1974). Cause and prognosis of sarcoidosis around the world. *American Journal of Medicine*, **57**, 847.

Thomas, P.D. and Hunninghake, G.W. (1987). Current concepts of the pathogenesis of sarcoidosis. *American Review of Respiratory Disease*, **135**, 747–60.

Zic, J.A., Horowitz, D.H., Arzobiaga, C., and King, L.E. (1991). Treatment of cutaneous sarcoidosis with chloroquine. *Archives of Dermatology*, **127**, 1034–40.

17.10.11 Pulmonary histiocytosis X (eosinophilic granuloma of the lung) and lymphangiomyomatosis

R. J. SHAW

Pulmonary histiocytosis X

Eosinophilic granuloma or pulmonary histiocytosis X is the one manifestation of the three diseases comprising histiocytosis X which affects the lung (the other two are Litterer–Siwe disease and Hand–Schuller–Christian disease). Eosinophilic granuloma is characterized by an abnormal proliferation of mononuclear cells including the characteristic atypical histiocytes. These cells form granulomatous-like lesions within the lung and also deform the alveolar walls. Lesions may cavitate and heal, resulting in foci of fibrosis giving a typical stellate scar. This process results in honeycombing with a formation of small cysts.

Eosinophilic granuloma affects men and women between the ages of 20 and 40. It is a disease almost exclusively confined to smokers. The main symptoms are cough and exertional dyspnoea. Spontaneous pneumothorax, presumably due to rupture of one of the small cysts, is a common complication and may give rise to pleuritic pain. The chest radiograph typically shows diffuse micronodular reticular changes which progress to cystic honeycombing. Pulmonary physiology reveals a mixed obstructive and restrictive pattern (decreased vital capacity, increased respiratory volume, and decreased carbon monoxide transfer). Bronchoalveolar lavage may reveal atypical histiocytes or Langerhans' cells. The major identifying feature of these cells is an X body or Birbeck granule, which appears as a pentalaminar rod-like structure in the cytoplasm under the electron microscope. These cells can also be identified using antibodies to surface antigen T6. Lung biopsy is usually also required to make the diagnosis. Eosinophilic granuloma may be complicated by manifestations of histiocytosis X in other organs, namely bone, as well as being a cause of diabetes insipidus. Despite the confusing nomenclature, eosinophilic granuloma is not associated with peripheral eosinophilia. The clinical course is variable. There is an impression that in many patients the disease spontaneously ceases to progress at some point, leaving the patient with variable residual impairment. There are no accepted successful treatments, although some patients may respond to corticosteriods.

Lymphangiomyomatosis

Lymphangiomyomatosis is a rare disease occurring in premenopausal women which is characterized by proliferation of the smooth-muscle cells in the lymphatic vessels, thorax, and abdomen. The disease presents with dyspnoea due to the progressive interstitial lung disease, pneumothorax, or chylous pleural effusion. The classic chest radiograph changes are reticular shadowing including Kerley B lines due to dilated lymphatics, small nodules possibly due to hyperplastic smooth-muscle aggregates, and pleural effusions. Later in the disease honeycombing and cystic dilation occur, predisposing to pneumothorax. These changes are most marked and characteristic on CT scanning. The pulmonary physiology is similar to that of emphysema (decreased functional vital capacity, increased respiratory volume, and decreased TLCO and KCO). If untreated, most patients die within 10 years.

Circumstantial evidence and reports of response to anti-oestrogen therapy suggest oestrogen dependence of the disease. Currently, a trial of treatment with medroxyprogesterone (200 mg intromuscularly weekly) is suggested and if no response is obtained, bilateral oophorectomy should be considered.

REFERENCES

Friedman, P.J., Liebow, A.A., and Sokoloff, J. (1981). Eosinophilic granuloma of lung: clinical aspects of primary pulmonary histiocytosis X in the adult. *Medicine*, **60**, 385–96.

McCarty, K.S., Mossler, J.A., McLelland, R., and Sieker, H.O. (1980). Pulmonary lymphangiomyomatosis responsive to progesterone. *New England Journal of Medicine*, **303**, 1461–5.

Taylor, J.R., Ryn, J., Colby, T.V., and Raffin, T.A. (1990). Lymphangioleiomyomatosis: clinical course in 32 patients. *New England Journal of Medicine*, **323**, 1254–60.

Viskum, K. (1993). Pulmonary lymphangioleiomyomatosis. *Archivio Monaldi per la Tisiologica e le Malattie dell' Apparato Respiratorio*, **48**, 233–6.

17.10.12 Pulmonary alveolar proteinosis

D. J. HENDRICK

First described in 1958, pulmonary alveolar proteinosis has proved to be a rare but interesting disorder that exerts its primary effects in the alveolar spaces. Over a period ranging from months to years, these become filled with an amorphous, largely cell-free, lipoproteinaceous material which is not readily expectorated. Inflammation and fibrosis are conspicuously absent and there are two major consequences. First, depending on the number of alveoli involved, the lungs become stiff, ventilatory function becomes restricted, and shunting occurs at the alveolar capillary level causing hypoxia. This causes breathlessness and reduces exercise tolerance and in some cases leads to death from respiratory failure. The second major consequence, and a not uncommon cause of death, is secondary infection. The responsible organisms are generally those that are associated with intracellular infection and impaired T lymphocyte function, Nocardia being particularly prominent. In many cases, however, extensive involvement does not occur, there being little or no progression, or even spontaneous remission. Epidemiological data are scarce but one estimate suggests an annual incidence of the order of 2 to 5 per million.

Pathogenesis

Males appear to be affected more commonly than females, but all age groups may be involved. The cause in most cases is unknown, though an apparently identical (and relentlessly progressive) disorder can arise within months of massive exposure to respirable mineral dust, especially silica—both in the unfortunate worker exposed negligently without adequate respiratory protection and in experimental animal models. This has been called acute silicoproteinosis or silicolipoproteinosis. Less commonly aluminium dust may be responsible. A few reports describe affected sibships implying a possible hereditary factor, and some associate pulmonary alveolar proteinosis with haematological malignancies (usually after the use of cytotoxic agents) or immunodeficiency disorders.

The secreted material is rich in protein and phospholipid, and stains strongly with periodic acid Schiff (PAS) and eosin. It also contains structures resembling tubular myelin which are derived from lamellar bodies of surfactant-producing type II pneumocytes. It is clear that the secretions themselves are chiefly the product of these cells, and the chief phospholipid is dipalmitoyl phosphatidylcholine—the dominant phospholipid of normal surfactant. It is unclear, however, whether the accumulation of these secretions results from excessive or abnormal production, or from impaired resorption by the type II pneumocytes or the alveolar macrophages. In most cases the PAS stain is taken up uniformly, as is peroxidase labelled immunoglobulin raised against the apolipoproteins of surfactant. In others, particularly those associated with haematological or immunological disorders, uptake is heterogeneous, and it has been suggested that fundamentally different processes underlie this 'secondary' form of pulmonary alveolar proteinosis.

The vulnerability to infection with 'opportunistic' organisms coupled with the *in vitro* demonstration of a number of abnormalities of macrophage function incriminates the macrophage more than the pneumocyte. This is consistent with pulmonary alveolar proteinosis arising after macrophage function has been disrupted by massive exposure to silica, and with pulmonary alveolar proteinosis being associated with impaired T cell immunity and hence diminished macrophage activation. The latter has been observed in pulmonary alveolar proteinosis with thymic aplasia and, intriguingly, pneumocystis infection complicating AIDS. It has been shown, however, that ingestion of the surfactant material may itself cause impairment of phagocytic function in macrophages harvested from normal control animals, and so in some cases at least the primary abnormality could still lie with the type II pneumocyte. Strong support for this view comes from recent evidence suggesting that in pulmonary alveolar proteinosis these cells produce not only abnormal surfactant mixtures of phospholipids and associated proteins, but also macrophage inhibiting proteins. Furthermore, the chemotherapeutic agents associated with the later development of pulmonary alveolar proteinosis (e.g. bleomycin) seem more likely to damage pneumocytes than macrophages.

Clinical features

The affected subject usually presents with progressive shortness of breath due to the disease itself or with a pneumonic illness due to superimposed infection. Occasionally, the disease is without symptoms when it is first recognized from the appearances of an incidental chest radiograph. It may then be mistaken for sarcoidosis. Cough is common and may be productive, particularly if there is infection. Low grade fever, haemoptysis and pleuritic pain occur infrequently, though some authors report an initial febrile incident. There may be crackles and clubbing in advanced stages, and fever becomes characteristic when infection supervenes. When nocardia is not responsible for this, aspergillus, candida, cryptococcus, cytomegalovirus, histoplasma, mucor, mycobacteria, pneumocystis, and viruses are the most common culprits.

Diagnosis

The chest radiograph characteristically shows an alveolar filling pattern, which radiates from the hila and simulates pulmonary oedema. There is no associated evidence of heart failure, however, and the appearances may be somewhat patchy and asymmetrical. Diffuse pulmonary fibrosis is very rare, unless provoked by complicating infection. A micronodular infiltration is occasionally seen, particularly in children, and hilar lymphadenopathy is characteristically absent. Pneumonia or aspiration is often suspected initially, but the cough produces little or no sputum and no organisms are isolated if the disease remains uncomplicated. Gallium scanning may be useful in showing negligible pulmonary uptake in contrast to the outcome seen in pneumonia. A positive gallium scan may nevertheless be invaluable in established pulmonary alveolar proteinosis in demonstrating the development of superimposed infection.

The key to the diagnosis of uncomplicated pulmonary alveolar proteinosis rests with the demonstration that the alveolar secretions, which are characteristically milky in colour, are strongly PAS positive but contain no organisms and no excessive cellular response. Indeed the macrophages appear to be deficient in numbers as well as function. Occasionally the sputum provides diagnostic material, identification of lamellar bodies or their debris by electron microscopy being particularly useful. These may be found within macrophages or pneumocytes, or may lie free within the secretions. More commonly bronchoalveolar lavage or transbronchial lung biopsy is required, though the former should suffice. The characteristic histological features are shown in Fig. 1.

Management

In perhaps a third of cases, no appreciable disability develops and the disease remits spontaneously or fails to progress. The choice of treatment, when necessary, is strictly limited. Corticosteroids are of no value and may increase the risk of infection. Prolonged periods of inhalation therapy with expectorants (potassium iodide) or proteolytic enzymes

(trypsin) have been claimed to offer some benefit, but have caused frequent irritative responses in the airways. Furthermore, trypsin does not digest pulmonary alveolar proteinosis material *in vitro*. Neither form of treatment is currently recommended.

The most effective measure has been physical removal of the secretions by bronchoalveolar lavage. This is usually performed under general anaesthesia using a double lumen endotracheal tube, one lung being repeatedly lavaged with a total of 20 to 50 litres of warm sterile buffered saline while the other is mechanically ventilated. The procedure is then reversed so that the other lung is treated. The practice of adding heparin and acetyl cysteine to the lavage fluid has not been shown to be beneficial, though chest percussion during the procedure does seem to enhance the yield. When severe respiratory failure has already supervened despite ventilatory support, cardiopulmonary bypass has been used successfully to maintain gas exchange during the lavage procedure. An alternative is sequential lobar lavage using a fibreoptic bronchoscope and a cuffed catheter. Further lavage is usually necessary every few weeks or months but the activity of the disease may lessen and the frequency of this need may diminish. Sometimes there is fatal progression with a prominent loss of weight despite repeated lavage.

A considerable threat to life comes from complicating infection, and this should be quickly recognized and treated. An accelerated clinical course together with the development of fever, increased (and productive) cough, malaise, evidence of systemic infection, and the radiographic demonstration of cavitation (perhaps using CT scanning) or pleural effusion all provide pointers to its development. Blood cultures together with smear and culture studies of sputum may identify the organism or organisms responsible, but often bronchoscopy with brushings and diagnostic lavage is needed. Sometimes a biopsy procedure is considered necessary, particularly when the underlying presence of alveolar proteinosis is not clearly established. When 'opportunistic' organisms are involved, the eradication of infection may prove to be unduly difficult, perhaps reflecting the underlying impairment of macrophage function. It has consequently been argued that regular bronchoalveolar lavage, even in the absence of impaired exercise tolerance, may limit the degree of immunosuppression and provide valuable prophylaxis against such life threatening infections. A recent investigation did indeed demonstrate improved macrophage function following lavage, which slowly diminished over 18 months as clinical relapse occurred. If the argument is followed fully, lavage may also play a role in eradicating the acute infection.

Fig. 1 Pulmonary alveolar proteinosis arising acutely following massive exposure to silica (by courtesy of Dr D.E. Banks). Some alveoli are filled with a non-inflammatory proteinaceous exudate, characteristic of pulmonary alveolar proteinosis. The lung interstitium shows fibrosis and inflammation which can be attributed to acute silicosis (haematoxylin and eosin, medium magnification).

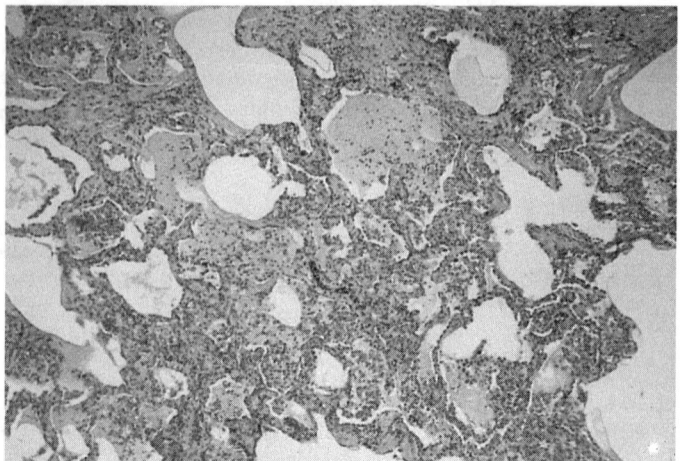

REFERENCES

Carre, P.C., Didier, A.P., Pipy, B.R., *et al.* (1990). The lavage fluid from a patient with alveolar proteinosis inhibits the *in vitro* chemiluminescence response and arachidonic acid metabolism of normal guinea pig alveolar macrophages. *American Review of Respiratory Disease*, **142**, 1068–72.

Claypool, W.D., Rogers, R.M., and Matuschak, G.M. (1984). Update on the clinical diagnosis, management, and pathogenesis of pulmonary alveolar proteinosis (phospholipidosis). *Chest*, **85**, 550–8.

Freedman, A.P. Pelias, A., Johnston, R.F., *et al.* (1981). Alveolar proteinosis lung lavage using partial cardiopulmonary bypass. *Thorax*, **36**, 543–5.

Hoffman, R.M., Dauber, J.H., and Rogers, R.M. (1989). Improvement in alveolar macrophage migration after therapeutic whole lung lavage in pulmonary alveolar proteinosis. *American Review of Respiratory Disease*, **139**, 1030–2.

Rosen, S.H., Castleman, B., and Liebow, A.A. (1958). Pulmonary alveolar proteinosis. *New England Journal of Medicine*, **258**, 1123–42.

Selecky, P.A., Wasserman, K., Benfield, J.R., and Lippman, M. (1977). The clinical and physiological effect of whole lung lavage pulmonary alveolar proteinosis: a 10 year experience. *Annals of Thoracic Surgery*, **24**, 451–61.

Singh, G., Katyal, S.L., Bedrossian, C.W.M., and Rogers, R.M. (1983). Pulmonary alveolar proteinosis. Staining for surfactant apoprotein in alveolar proteinosis and in conditions simulating it. *Chest*, **83**, 82–6.

Tran Van Nhieu, J., Vojtek, A.M., Bernaudin, J.F., Escudier, E., and Fleury-Feith, J. (1990). Pulmonary alveolar proteinosis associated with *Pneumocystis carinii*. Ultrastructural identification in bronchoalveolar lavage in AIDS and immunocompromised non-AIDS patients. *Chest*, **98**, 801–5.

Voss, T., Schafer, K.P., Nielsen, P.F., *et al.* (1992). Primary structure differences of human surfactant-associated proteins isolated from normal and proteinosis lung. *Biochimica et Biophysica Acta*, **1138**, 261–7.

17.10.13 Pulmonary amyloidosis

D. J. HENDRICK

It is extremely rare for amyloidosis to exert a major effect in the lung, a few dozen cases only having been reported over recent decades. Those affected are usually middle aged or elderly, and the sexes are equally represented.

Pathogenesis

The proteinaceous material which is responsible for amyloid infiltration (it is not in fact related to starch) and which gives the characteristic staining appearance with Congo Red is composed of a fibrillar polypeptide and a non-fibrillar glycoprotein. They produce a unique β-pleated structure which may be deposited progressively and widely in the body's organs, eventually interfering with their function. The glycoprotein (amyloid P or AP protein) comprises a mere 10 per cent of amyloid tissue. It is derived from a parent serum protein (SAP) made in the liver and is common to all types of amyloid tissue. When radiolabelled, it can be used with whole body scintigraphy to assess the extent of the disease. The fibrillar protein on the other hand is of two distinct types.

The type seen with 'primary' amyloidosis and amyloidosis associated with myeloma is derived from immunoglobulin light chains and is known as AL protein. It is the product of a plasma cell clone whether benign or malignant, but comprises only a portion of the variable region of the light chain. Proteolysis is presumed to separate it from the larger molecule, but the site of this process and of the subsequent combination with AP protein is not yet clear. It is thought that macrophages under monocyte influence may contribute to the production of amyloid protein when this is deposited in the lung. Monoclonal immunoglobulin (M-

Table 1 *Classifcation of amyloidosis*

Systemic amyloidosis
Amyloidosis with lymphocyte or plasma cell dyscrasia (i.e. primary amyloidosis with AL protein)
Systemic reactive amyloidosis (i.e. secondary amyloidosis with AA protein)
Familial amyloidosis (AA protein)
Localized amyloidosis (usually AL protein)

component) may sometimes be detected in the serum as may Bence Jones protein in the urine. In some cases plasma cells and macrophages occur in focal aggregations within the lung and adjacent to localized deposits of amyloid tissue. It seems likely that in these circumstances AL protein is generated locally, and this has been demonstrated in comparable amyloid lesions of the skin. With systemic disease, it is more likely that both the AP protein and the AL protein are manufactured at a distance and then extracted together (or separately) from circulating blood to be deposited as amyloid protein in the target organ.

The type of fibrillar protein seen with 'secondary' amyloidosis and most of the familial forms of amyloidosis (AA protein) is derived from an acute phase serum component (SAA), presumably by proteolytic cleavage. The chronic inflammatory diseases associated with persistently raised levels of SAA (and C reactive protein) are those that are most commonly associated with secondary amyloidosis, but only a small minority of subjects affected by these chronic inflammatory disorders show evidence of complicating amyloidosis. This implies that there is in these subjects some derangement of the SAA degrading process or the SAA protein itself.

The differing patterns of organ dysfunction associated with these two types of amyloidosis remain unexplained, but much overlap evidently occurs and it seems likely that both types of amyloid protein become deposited widely as the systemic disease progresses. It also remains unclear why deposition is a systemic process in some cases but a local one in others. This is a critical matter to the clinician and is central to a proposed new classification (Table 1).

Clinical features

Although the lungs are not commonly the major target organ in amyloidosis, they may become infiltrated with both types of amyloid protein. Rarely, hilar or mediastinal lymph nodes, or pleura may be involved. When systemic amyloidosis is associated with AL protein, the kidneys and heart bear the brunt of the damage, though the lungs are said to show some infiltration in the majority of cases. With systemic reactive amyloidosis and AA protein, the lungs are involved only in a minority of cases. When pulmonary involvement is symptomatic, the disease is often localized and is usually due to deposition of amyloid containing the light chain derived AL protein. Its effects depend on the site of deposition. The following varieties, in descending order of epidemiological importance, are the most clearly recognized.

1. Laryngo–tracheo–bronchial: discrete and usually multiple masses of amyloid protein enlarge in the walls of the airways or the peribronchial tissues causing cough, obstruction, and sometimes bleeding. The obstructed airways may lead to wheeze, stridor, breathlessness, atelectasis, and infection, and may eventually give rise to bronchiectasis. When a single lesion is involved it may simulate the effects of a bronchial adenoma, appearing as a polypoid mass on endoscopic inspection.

2. Parenchymal nodule(s): discrete nodules or masses, which may be single or multiple and may occasionally reach the size of a tennis ball, are seen within the lung parenchyma on the

chest radiograph. They rarely cause symptoms or disrupt lung function and may eventually calcify, cavitate or even ossify. They are likely to simulate bronchial neoplasms and so become resected.

3. Alveolar–interstitial: amyloid tissue is deposited diffusely throughout the vasculature, alveolar walls, and interstitium of the lung, and is usually a feature of systemic amyloidosis (Figs 1 and 2). There is progressive breathlessness and dry cough. Scattered crackles are characteristic and there may be pleural effusions. Eventually respiratory failure may supervene as ventilation becomes increasingly restricted and gas transfer impaired, though death more commonly results from cardiac or renal involvement.

Histological examination may also show evidence of amyloid infiltration of the pulmonary vasculature. Although this is usually of no clinical consequence, it has been reported to cause pulmonary hypertension and undue bleeding after biopsy. A further reported affect of amyloidosis on respiratory function has been enlargement of the tongue so that the syndrome of sleep apnoea ensues.

Fig. 1 Amyloidosis of the lung: alveolar-interstitial type [i] (by courtesy of Dr T. Ashcroft). There are interstitial deposits of hyaline eosinophilic material with a foreign body type giant cell response in adjacent tissue. This is an almost unique feature of amyloidosis affecting the lung (haematoxylin and eosin, medium magnification).

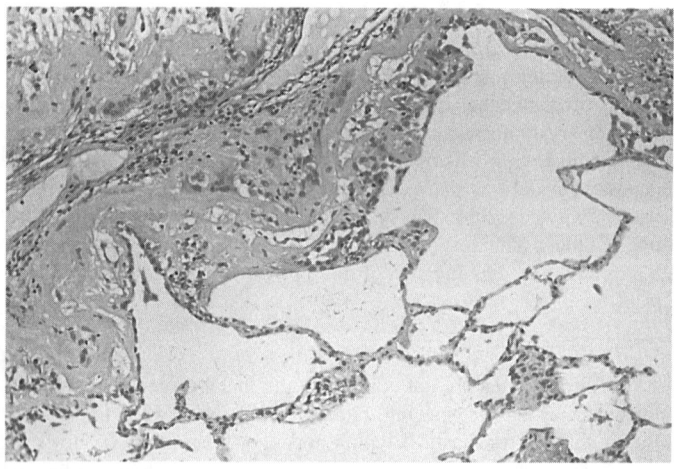

Fig. 2 Amyloidosis of the lung: alveolar–interstitial type [ii] (by courtesy of Dr T. Ashcroft). Amyloid gives a characteristic dichroic birefringence (Congo red stain under polarized light. High magnification).

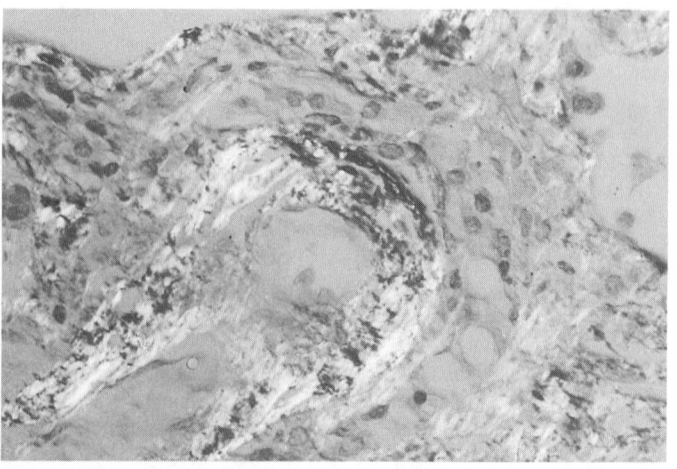

Diagnosis

The diagnosis rests essentially on the demonstration of amyloid tissue in an affected organ. When the protein is derived from plasma cells or lymphocytes, it may be possible to demonstrate light chains in the urine or M-component in the serum, and a plasma cell or lymphocyte dyscrasia may be clinically evident. When systemic reactive amyloidosis is the diagnosis, a provoking chronic inflammatory disease should be obvious, and high levels of SAA and C reactive protein will be present in the serum. Histochemical studies in the laboratory should, in any event, identify the specific biochemical nature of the protein sampled at biopsy, as should the ultrastructural appearances at electron microscopy. When there is systemic disease from either cause, submucosal biopsy of the rectum usually provides a convenient source of diagnostic tissue.

Management

Treatment of the systemic disease associated with AL protein is usually unrewarding. There is an inexorable accumulation of amyloid tissue in the affected organs, and death occurs within 1 to 2 years. Survival is even shorter when myelomatosis is present. There is some point in trying cytotoxic agents (particularly alkylating agents) since responders are encountered sporadically, but these agents are not often helpful unless survival in the short and medium term is ensured by organ transplantation. Corticosteroids may actually worsen deposition of protein in the kidneys. Ultimately, organ transplantation may become the only hope of survival, and when renal failure or cardiac failure is the only immediate threat to life, this is often carried out.

The outcome of systemic reactive amyloidosis is dependent on the accompanying inflammatory disease. If this can be controlled, the deposition of amyloid tissue may be halted. It may also be halted or lessened by the use of colchicine, which interfers with the metabolism of SAA. Systemic reactive amyloidosis is nevertheless a serious disorder and usually ends fatally within a few years.

A current experimental approach, which may prove to be of benefit to both types of amyloidosis, is the use of dimethyl sulphoxide. This denatures amyloid tissue, and has been shown to produce urinary excretion of amyloid-like material. Its place in the management of human disease is yet to be established.

With the local forms of the disease, of whatever aetiology, the outlook is a good deal brighter. Progression may be slow, and the disease may become quiescent. The laryngo–tracheo–bronchial deposits can sometimes be resected or depleted piecemeal endoscopically (perhaps using laser therapy), but there is some risk of serious bleeding from this. Parenchymal nodules in the lung rarely need to be removed—providing their histological nature is not in doubt.

REFERENCES

Buxbaum, J.N., Hurley, M.E., Chuba, J., and Spiro, T. (1979). Amyloidosis of the AL type. Clinical, morphologic and biochemical aspects of the response to therapy with alkylating agents and prednisone. *American Journal of Medicine*, **67**, 867–78.

Glenner, G.G. (1980). Amyloid deposits and amyloidosis: the β-fibrilloses. *New England Journal of Medicine*, **302**, 1283–92, 1333–1343.

Hall, R., and Hawkins, P.N. (1994). Grand Rounds—Hammersmith Hospital: Cardiac transplantation for AL amyloidosis. *British Medical Journal*, **309**, 1135–7.

Kavuru, M.S., Adamo, J.P., Ahmad, M., Mehta, A.C., and Gephardt, G.N. (1990). Amyloidosis and pleural disease. *Chest*, **98**, 21–23.

Masuda, C., Mohri, S. and Nakajima, H. (1988). Histological and immunohistochemical study of amyloidosis cutis nodularis atrophicans—comparison with systemic amyloidosis. *British Journal of Dermatology*, **119**, 33–43.

Ravid, M., Robson, M., and Keder, I. (1977). Prolonged colchicine treatment in four patients with amyloidosis. *Annals of Internal Medicine*, **87**, 568–70.

Rubinow, A., Celli, B.R., Cohen, A.S., Rigden, B.G., and Brody, J.S. (1978). Localized amyloidosis of the lower respiratory tract. *American Review of Respiratory Disease*, **118**, 603–11.

Shiue, S.T., and McNally, D.P. (1988). Pulmonary hypertension from prominent vascular involvement in diffuse amyloidosis. *Archives of Internal Medicine*, **148**, 687–9.

17.10.14 Lipoid (lipid) pneumonia

D. J. HENDRICK

Exogenous

When mineral or vegetable lipids are deposited in the lung, they usually prove to be relatively inert but difficult to remove. Lung lipases have little effect, and the macrophages are slow to transport the free or emulsified material into the lymphatics. The result is often a chronic low grade inflammatory response that may lead to secondary infection and/or local fibrosis. It is known as lipoid (or lipid) pneumonia. It should be suspected whenever a 'pneumonic' illness is slow to resolve or is recurrent, especially if there is the possibility of impaired swallowing and recurrent aspiration. Some animal lipids are more readily degraded by lung lipases, thus releasing irritating fatty acids. In these circumstances a brisk pneumonitis may occur.

PATHOGENESIS

Aspiration of vegetable or mineral oil is not common in the population at large, but is seen not infrequently within certain subgroups—particularly those with impaired swallowing mechanisms. Most affected are the very young and the elderly, and most affected among the elderly are those who are accustomed to use paraffin regularly as nasal drops or aperients. A portion of the nasal dose is likely to enter the trachea, as may part of the ingested dose if the subject then reclines in bed or has any disturbance in swallowing. The critical point is that paraffin and other oils are not irritating to the tracheal mucosa, and so coughing is rarely excited and aspiration occurs without immediate sequelae.

The reluctant child forced to swallow cod liver oil is said to have encountered similar risks during the 1940s and 1950s, though infants are likely to face much greater hazard by virtue of less well developed deglutition. Those fed by nasogastric tube are particularly vulnerable as are those fed regularly with high lipid diets (for example with buffalo milk fat, ghee). A recent case report indicates a rather less obvious risk in an infant—that of lipid embolism from repeated mineral oil enemas.

Fig. 1 Lipoid pneumonia (by courtesy of Dr T. Ashcroft). Exogenous lipoid pneumonia due to aspirated paraffin. There is interstitial fibrosis containing oil vacuoles which are enclosed within multinucleated giant cells (haematoxylin and eosin stain, medium magnification).

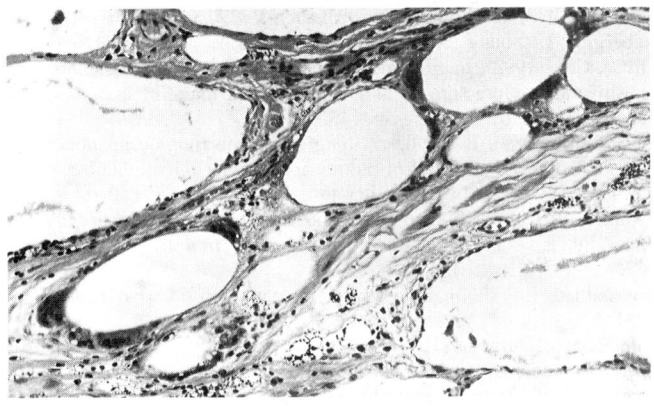

Adults with unimpaired swallowing are affected only sporadically. Shipwrecked sailors have occasionally aspirated diesel oil, and lipoid pneumonia has been recognized in workers exposed to oil mists and burning fats. The potential risk from respirable oil aerosols has been highlighted recently in a diver breathing unfiltered air from his oil-contaminated surface compressor. Less unwilling inhalers of mineral oil and vaseline have been the blackfat tobacco smokers of Guyana, who obtain a more satisfying smoke when these additives are mixed with native tobacco leaf. A distinctive picture of progressive and often fatal pulmonary fibrosis complicates this habit in some 20 per cent of blackfat users, but has not been observed among non-smokers.

CLINICAL FEATURES

The inflammatory response may give no symptoms, the subject presenting by chance with an abnormal chest radiograph, but in about 50 per cent of cases it leads to productive cough with low grade fever. Often there is a cyclical course with intermittent symptoms. Repeated aspiration may lead to fibrotic shrinkage of the affected segment or segments, or to persistent consolidation. Either may closely simulate bronchial carcinoma, and many resections have been carried for this reason. When more substantial quantities are aspirated the radiographic abnormalities are necessarily more diffuse, and when dependent segments are involved the true nature of the disorder is more obvious.

DIAGNOSIS

The key to diagnosis lies with the demonstration of lipid material within pulmonary secretions or alveolar macrophages, whether obtained from sputum or bronchoalveolar lavage. If lung tissue is resected or undergoes biopsy, there may be fibrosis, evidence of chronic inflammation, and foreign body granulomata/giant cells in addition to lipid material retained within alveoli and macrophages (Fig. 1). An innovative use of computerized tomography has recently identified excess deposits of lipid in lipoid pneumonia from its X-ray absorption characteristics, a technique which could offer a valuable alternative to biopsy or bronchoalveolar lavage in the diagnosis of 'atypical pneumonias'. Nuclear magnetic resonance scanning appears much less effective.

MANAGEMENT

Prophylactic management centres on minimizing any tendency to aspiration associated with impaired swallowing, and in persuading the misuser (or abuser) of lipid/paraffin to adopt alternative habits. Once aspiration has occurred there may be a role for therapeutic bronchoalveolar lavage since this may remove substantial quantities of lipid from the alveoli. During episodes of secondary bacterial infection, there is an obvious role for antibiotics.

Endogenous

The body may itself produce and retain lipid (mainly cholesterol) within the lungs, though this is not a common phenomenon. It occurs chiefly at sites of chronic inflammation, obstruction, or tissue necrosis and is derived from the necrotic cells. This lipid will also be ingested by macrophages and may be recovered in the sputum. Sputum macrophages laden with lipid are not therefore pathognomonic of aspiration from an exogenous source, though chemical tests can distinguish the two varieties and histological examination of affected lung does not show a granulomatous response to endogenous lipid. Endogenous lipid is most commonly deposited when chronic inflammation accompanies bronchiectasis, bronchial carcinoma or some other cause of persisting localized bronchial obstruction, and appears to depend on cigarette smoking. The radiological appearances are of a persisting pneumonia, which may also stimulate resection for fear that a carcinoma is present.

REFERENCES

Annobil, S.H., Benjamin, B., Kameswaran, M., and Khan, A.R. (1991). Lipoid pneumonia on children following aspiration of animal fat (ghee). *Annals of Tropical Paediatrics*, **11**, 87–94.

Corrin, B. and Soliman, S.S. (1978). Cholesterol in the lungs of heavy smokers. *Thorax*, **33**, 565–68.

Levade, T., Salvayre, R., Dongay, G., *et al.* (1987). Chemical analysis of the bronchoalveolar washing fluid in the diagnosis of liquid paraffin pneumonia. *Journal of Clinical Chemistry and Clinical Biochemistry* **25**, 45–8.

Miller, G.J., Ashcroft, M.T., Beadnell, H.M.S.G., Wagner, J.C., and Pepys, J. (1971). The lipoid pneumonia of blackfat tobacco smokers in Guyana. *Quarterly Journal of Medicine*, **40**, 457–70.

Oldenburger, D., Maurer, W.J., Beltaos, E., and Magnin, G.E. (1972). Inhalation lipid pneumonia from burning fats. *Journal of the American Medical Association*, **222**, 1288–9.

Penes, M.C., Vallon, J.J., Sabot, J.F., and Vallon, C. (1990). Gas chromatography and mass spectroscopy detection of paraffin in a case of lipoid pneumonia following occupational exposure to oil spray. *Journal of Analytical Toxicology*, **14**, 372–4.

Silverman, J.F., Turner, R.C., West, R.L., and Dillard, T.A. (1989). Bronchoalveolar lavage in the diagnosis of lipid pneumonia. *Diagnostic Cytopathology*, **5**, 3–8.

Wheeler, P.S., Stitik, F.P., Hutchins, G.M., Klinefelter, H.F., and Siegelman, S.S. (1981). Diagnosis of lipoid pneumonia by computed tomography. *Journal of the American Medical Association*, **245**, 65–6.

17.10.15 Pulmonary alveolar microlithiasis

D. J. HENDRICK

This is a very rare disorder (150–200 reported cases only) which is remarkable for a number of unusual if not unique features. Tiny 0.2 to 5 mm calcified concretions, which may be concentrically laminated, are formed progressively in the alveolar spaces. They produce a striking and truly unique appearance on the chest radiograph. At present there are few clues to the cause of this curious disorder and there is no effective means of therapy—features that are themselves unusual at a time of rapid advance in medical science.

Pathogenesis

No abnormality of calcium metabolism has been demonstrated, but a disproportionate number of cases occur in siblings which possibly points to a genetic rather than environmental basis. This is supported by the reported deaths of two newborn infants from the disease. It is none the less possible that environmental factors operated during pregnancy, and no clear cut pattern of mendelian inheritance has been described. One report in four affected desert dwellers linked the disorder with non-occupational exposure to respirable silica and postulated a 'hyperimmune' response to this. However, a recent analytical study of one particular case using X-ray energy spectroscopy and microscopic infrared spectroscopy showed no evidence of mineral dust deposition. It demonstrated that the calcified microliths were formed of calcium carboxyapatite, possibly after initiation by extracellular matrix vesicles. Formation did presumably occur within the alveolar spaces because some microliths were flushed out by bronchoalveolar lavage.

Clinical features

The disease usually presents in middle age, but the whole age spectrum may be involved and both sexes are equally represented. Almost invariably the affected subject is symptom free when an initial film is taken for incidental reasons, and there may be wonder that this can be possible when the radiograph is grossly abnormal. This is a consequence of there being no associated cellular, exudative, fibrotic, or vascular disruption of normal physiological processes. Physical signs are conspicuous by their absence for most of its long course, though crackles, clubbing (even hypertrophic pulmonary osteoarthropathy), and signs of respiratory failure may be observed ultimately.

In most cases there is slow progression and eventually exercise limitation, dry cough, occasional haemoptysis, respiratory failure, and cor pulmonale supervene, the lungs becoming stiff, ventilation restricted, and gas transfer impaired. Survival of 10 to 20 years is characteristic. At death, extensive areas of the chest radiograph show a dense 'white-out' appearance due to the considerable accumulation of calcium, the lungs are difficult to cut, and they sink in water.

Diagnosis

The radiograph appearances of profuse small calcified nodules are specific, particularly in moderately advanced cases when the dense 'whiteout' picture supervenes but symptoms are still absent or unimpressive. With less advanced disease biopsy or bronchoalveolar lavage should provide diagnostic tissue, but with transbronchial biopsy it may prove difficult to close the forceps and extract them through the fibreoptic bronchoscope. Initially the chest radiograph shows a mere haziness of the lower zones, and computerized tomography may be useful in demonstrating the calcific nature of the nodular shadows. It may also confirm an early predominance for the basal and posterior segments. Measurement of lung function during the asymptomatic stage reveals little or no abnormality, and the affected subject may remain well for many years. As profusion and size of the calcified concretions increase the lung fields become diffusely and densely opaque.

Management

No specific therapy is known to be effective and in the absence of transplantation treatment is merely supportive. A recent detailed report of a 37-year-old man presenting in respiratory failure, recorded severe hypoxia and pulmonary hypertension. Considerable intrapulmonary shunting was demonstrated which was greatly improved by nasal continuous positive airway pressure, but not by conventional supplemental oxygen therapy.

REFERENCES

Barnard, N.J., Crocker, P.R., Blainey, A.D., Davies, R.J., Ell, S.R., and Levison, D.A. (1987). Pulmonary alveolar microlithiasis. A new analytical approach. *Histopathology*, **11**, 639–45.

Cheong, W.-Y., Wang, Y.-T., Tan, L.K.A., and Poh, S.-C. (1988). Pulmonary alveolar microlithiasis. *Australasian Radiology*, **32**, 401–4.

Freiberg, D.B., Young, I.H., Laks, L., Regnis, J.A., Lehrhaft, B., and Sullivan, C.E. (1992). Improvement in gas exchange with nasal continuous positive airway pressure in pulmonary alveolar microlithiasis. *American Review of Respiratory Disease*, **145**, 1215–6.

Nouh, M.S. (1989). Is the desert lung syndrome (non-occupational dust pneumoconiosis) a variant of pulmonary alveolar microlithiasis? Report of 4 cases with review of the literature. *Respiration*, **55**, 122–6.

O'Neill, R.P., Cohn, J.E., and Pellegrino, E.D. (1967). Pulmonary alveolar microlithiasis—a familial study. *Annals of Internal Medicine*, **67**, 957–67.

Viswanathan, R. (1962). Pulmonary alveolar microlithiasis. *Thorax*, **17**, 251–6.

Volle, E. and Kaufmann, H.J. (1987). Pulmonary alveolar microlithiasis in pediatric patients. A review of the world literature and two new observations. *Pediatric Radiology*, **17**, 439–42.

17.10.16 Pneumoconioses

A. SEATON

Most lung diseases are caused or provoked at least in part by the inhalation of harmful material. A wide range of lung conditions, including lung cancer (exposure to asbestos, alpha radiation in mines, polycyclic aromatics, nickel refining, chloromethyl ethers), pneumonia (legionnaire's disease in hospitals), asthma (flour, isocyanates, epoxy resins), allergic alveolitis (farmer's lung, maltworker's lung), and toxic pneumonitis (silo-filler's disease, chlorine poisoning, cadmium poisoning), may occur as a result of workplace exposure. When exposure to mineral dust in the workplace results in a diffuse, usually fibrotic, reaction in the acinar parts of the lung, the condition is generally called a pneumoconiosis.

Although mines have been recognized to be unhealthy places since Roman times, the distinction between tuberculosis and a specific effect of dust in the causation of respiratory disease was not made until the mid-nineteenth century. By this time silicosis, often complicated by tuberculosis, was widespread amongst metal miners, tunnellers, potters, and cutlers. During the same period the Industrial Revolution stimulated the need for coal, and the production of this fuel resulted in increasing numbers of sufferers from coal-worker's pneumoconiosis. This in turn was not distinguished from silicosis until the late 1940s, and in some countries the two conditions are still referred to by the one name.

In the United Kingdom and generally through Western Europe and the United States, dust control in mines and decline of traditional industries with a silica hazard have resulted in a sharp reduction in the numbers of workers suffering from these two diseases. In contrast, the industrial revolution occurring in developing countries has stimulated the need for indigenous coal and minerals, and in China, South America, and India in particular several million workers are employed in mining, often in conditions which ensure a high incidence of pneumoconiosis. At the same time, the rise of the asbestos and chemical industries has added new problems for society in weighing the benefits of the product against the cost in terms of human morbidity. Fortunately, these problems are all potentially soluble by the application of preventive measures, and these will be emphasized in the sections that follow.

Coal-worker's pneumoconiosis

Coal-worker's pneumoconiosis is a disease of the lungs caused by inhalation of coal-mine dust, a complex mixture of coal, kaolin, mica, silica, and other minerals. It is now becoming an uncommon disease in the United Kingdom, with the annual incidence having declined from about 2000 (in a workforce of around 500 000) in the 1960s to less than 100 (in a workforce of c.60 000) today. Indeed, new cases reflect the mining conditions of decades earlier, and good dust control in British mines implies that the disease may disappear in the United Kingdom in the next few years. Nevertheless, the strategic importance of coal as a long-term source of fuel supply and as a chemical feedstock means that it will continue to be needed, and any relaxation of dust control in mines will be followed by the reappearance of pneumoconiosis. There has also been a reduction in the incidence of coal-worker's pneumoconiosis in other European countries and in the United States, while in China the disease is widespread and in India it afflicts about 1 to 2 per cent of the current workforce of 800 000.

Aetiology and pathology

The pathogenicity of coal dust depends on several factors, not all of which are completely understood. Of course, it is essential, if lung damage is to occur, for the dust to be inhalable to acinar level within the lung. Thus the particles must have the appropriate aerodynamic char-

acteristics, essentially making them equivalent to a sphere of unit density between 7 and 0.5 μm in diameter. Once inhaled, the particles must be able to overcome the lung's defences. Some, containing a high proportion of quartz (crystalline silicon dioxide), are toxic to macrophages and cause their disruption after phagocytosis. Such particles seem to be cleared predominantly to the lymph nodes where they remain and set up a fibrotic reaction that ultimately destroys the node. However, some remain in the peribronchiolar and perivascular parts of the acinus, where whorled fibrosis occurs leading to the typical silicotic nodule. The mechanisms of quartz-induced fibrosis are discussed further in the section on silicosis. However, most coal dust contains relatively little quartz. Such dust is not particularly toxic to macrophages *in vitro*, and so some other explanation for its harmfulness to miners must be sought. *In vivo* studies in rats have shown that inhalation of relatively low concentrations of coal dust, comparable with those occurring in United Kingdom mines in the recent past, causes inhibition of macrophage migration and provokes an inflammatory response, mediated *inter alia* by interleukin 1 (IL-1) and tumour necrosis factor, and resulting in the release of elastase and the degradation of fibronectin. It seems likely that these toxic effects *in vivo* on macrophages are fundamental to the pathological processes in coal-worker's pneumoconiosis, including the concomitant centriacinar emphysema.

Apart from the composition of the dust, the total amount inhaled is a critical factor in the development of pneumoconiosis. Epidemiological studies have shown a clear exposure–response relationship between cumulative dust exposure and radiological evidence of disease. However, this is not straightforward, as some coal dusts are clearly more toxic than others, and it is not always possible to characterize this toxicity by the relative mineralogical composition of the coal dust. There is evidence that the minerals in coal dust interact and that some clays may reduce the overall toxicity of the dust, perhaps by blocking surface activity. As a general rule, the higher the combustibility (rank) of the coal, the more likely is its dust to cause pneumoconiosis (Fig. 1).

Pathologically, coal-worker's pneumoconiosis is characterized by the presence of multiple centriacinar and interlobular foci of dust, inflammatory cells, macrophages, and reticulin or collagen—the coal macule (Fig. 2). In miners exposed to relatively high proportions of quartz, the lesions have a greater resemblance to the silicotic nodule. The presence of small discrete nodules is known as simple pneumoconiosis, and when sufficient numbers of these lesions are present they become visible on a radiograph. Complicated pneumoconiosis, or progressive massive fibrosis, is present by definition when one or more of these lesions is more than 1 cm in diameter (Fig. 3). This occurs either by aggregation of several, usually collagenous, smaller nodules or by a more diffuse accumulation of dust associated with dead cells and ischaemic necrosis

Fig. 1 Relationship between risk of category 2 or 3 radiological simple pneumoconiosis and daily exposure over a working lifetime to different concentrations of coal dust. The greater risk in association with exposure to dust from coals of higher combustibility should be noted.

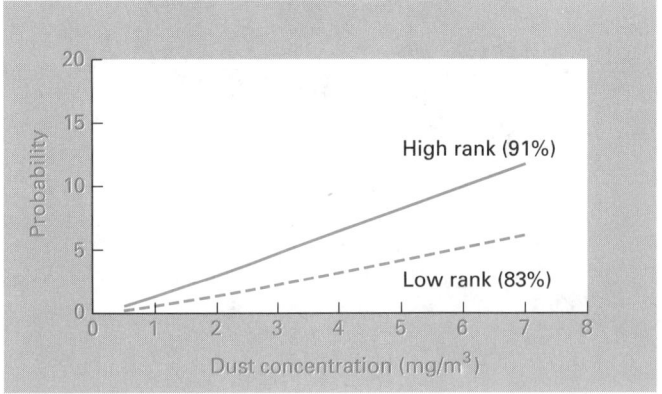

of lung tissue. The former, less common, mechanism occurs particularly in relation to relatively high quartz exposures, while the latter seems more frequent with exposure to high carbon dusts. With either type, or with intermediate types, there is a tendency for the lesions to grow and to be associated with surrounding bullous emphysema, and ultimately to be responsible for destruction of large volumes of the lung.

The aetiology of progressive massive fibrosis is not completely understood. It is more common in the upper lung zones and in taller men, suggesting an important relationship to lung-clearance mechanisms. High carbon or high quartz dusts are particularly liable to cause progressive massive fibrosis, and the higher the dust exposure, the greater is the risk (Fig. 4). Tuberculous infection is no longer an important factor, although it may well have been in the past. The rheumatoid diathesis seems to be responsible for initiating a particular type of progressive massive fibrosis (Caplan's syndrome) in very occasional cases, but this is not an important factor overall.

Fig. 2 Simple coal macules, showing accumulations of dust and cells around centre of lobule with associated emphysema.

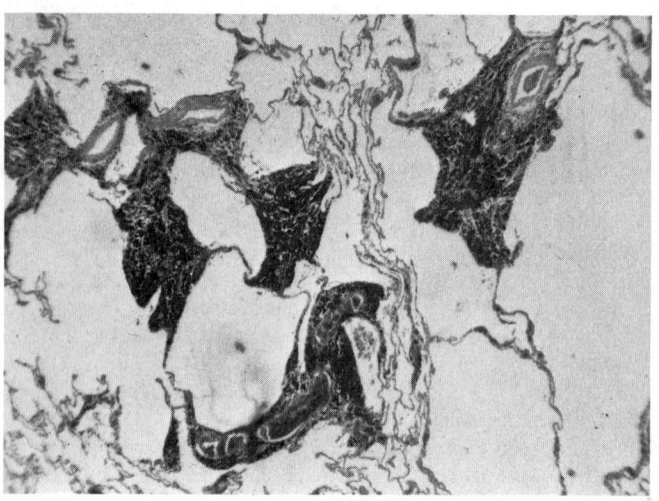

Fig. 3 Whole-lung section of the coal-miner whose radiograph is shown in Fig. 6, showing progressive massive fibrosis.

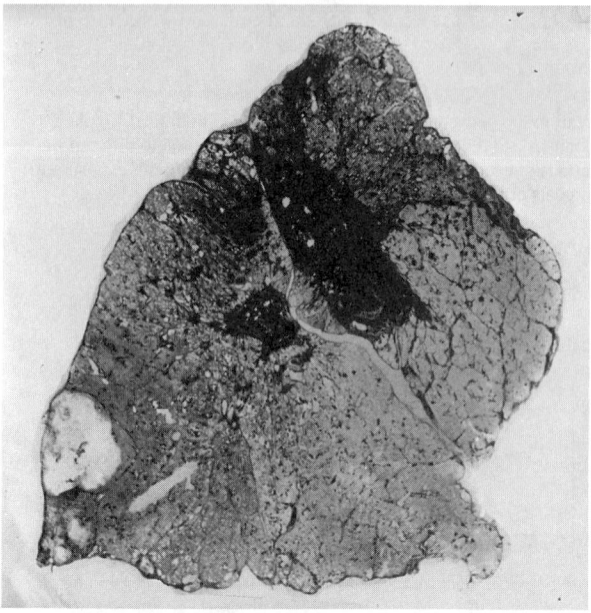

Clinical features

The people most at risk of coal-worker's pneumoconiosis are those working in the dustiest areas. Thus face-workers cutting coal, drilling for shot-firing, developing headings, and drilling bolts into the roof to prevent it falling are all at greatest risk. Open-cast miners rarely work in such dusty circumstances, except in hot dry countries such as India where loading operations may be extremely dusty. Simple coal-worker's pneumoconiosis causes no symptoms or physical signs. This fact is of considerable importance, as symptoms of respiratory disease in a miner with this condition are due to some other cause, such as bronchitis, heart failure, or asthma, which may be treatable. In keeping with this, the simple form of the disease is not associated with any important physiological abnormality. Radiological progression or regression of simple pneumoconiosis occurs only very rarely after dust exposure ceases, apparent regression sometimes being associated with the development of emphysema.

The danger associated with simple pneumoconiosis is that it predisposes to progressive massive fibrosis. The risk of progressive massive fibrosis developing is directly related to the profusion of simple pneumoconiosis on the radiograph. It may occur during working life or appear for the first time after (often many years after) dust exposure ceases. It may even occur when there is no apparent simple pneumoconiosis on the radiograph. In general, progressive massive fibrosis progresses and causes a mixture of restriction of lung volumes and, owing to associated emphysema, airways obstruction. Ultimately it may lead to cor pulmonale and death. However, the rate of progression is very variable. In general, the earlier progressive massive fibrosis develops in a person's life, the more rapidly progressive and thus the greater a threat to health it is.

The patient with progressive massive fibrosis may complain of shortness of breath and symptoms of cor pulmonale. An unusual, but pathognomonic, symptom is melanoptysis—the expectoration of the black contents of a cavitated lesion. Finger clubbing is not a feature and its presence suggests other disease. Abnormal signs in the chest, if present, relate to the presence of bullae, although sometimes lobar collapse can occur.

Coal-worker's pneumoconiosis is not associated with an increased risk of tuberculosis or lung cancer, although obviously these diseases can occur in coal-miners and should be suspected if haemoptysis, finger clubbing, or rapid progression of radiological changes occur. The association between pneumoconiosis and emphysema has been controversial, but there is now clear evidence of a parallel association between dust exposure and two effects—pneumoconiosis and airflow obstruction. The more dust that a miner has been exposed to, the greater are his risks of pneumoconiosis on the one hand, and productive cough, reduction in forced expiratory volume in 1 s (FEV_1), and presence of centriacinar emphysema on the other. Of course, the latter risks are also

Fig. 4 Relationship between risk of progressive massive fibrosis and exposure to dust over a working lifetime. Again, the difference in risk between dusts of different composition should be noted.

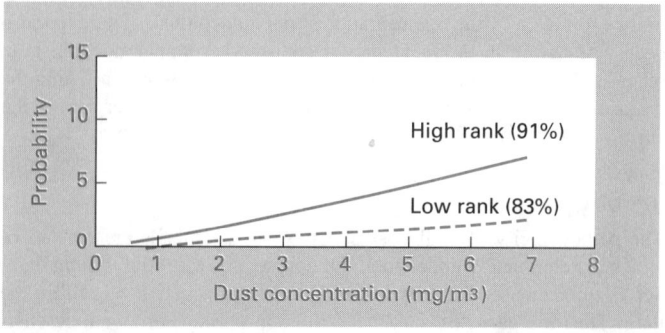

related to cigarette smoking, and the effect of dust exposure seems to be additional.

The radiological lesions in simple pneumoconiosis are predominantly rounded opacities between 1 and 5 mm in diameter, although small irregular and linear opacities and Kerley B lines are frequently present also. The round opacities tend to be more profuse in the upper and middle zones, whereas the irregular lesions predominate in the lower zone (Fig. 5). Progressive massive fibrosis almost always starts in an upper zone, gradually increasing in size until it may occupy up to a third of the lung. Such lesions are frequently multiple. They are often shaped like short fat sausages, with their outer border curved with the chest wall and separated from the pleura by bullous emphysema (Fig. 6). Calcification is not a feature of coal-worker's pneumoconiosis, but cavitation of massive fibrosis may occur. Caplan's syndrome is the name given to the combination of rheumatoid disease and several round nodules (usually between 1 and 5 cm in diameter) in the lungs of a coal-miner. The

Fig. 5 Radiograph of a coal-miner showing small round lesions of simple pneumoconiosis. Some irregular shadows are also present in the lower zones.

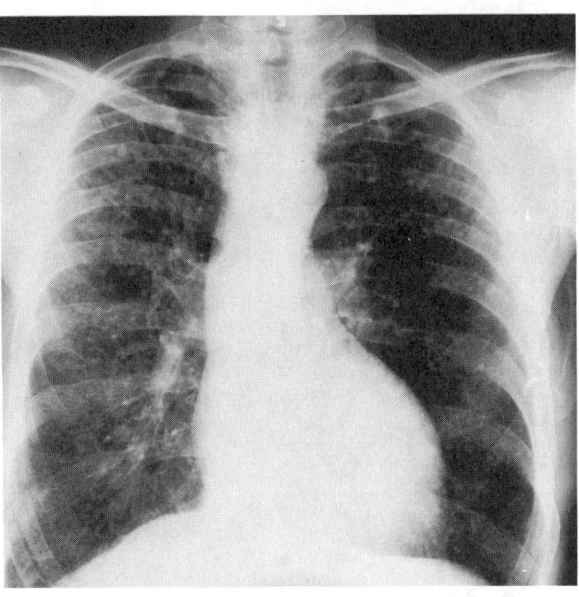

Fig. 6 Chest radiograph of the miner whose lung is shown in Fig. 3, showing progressive massive fibrosis in upper zones and small round shadows through both lungs.

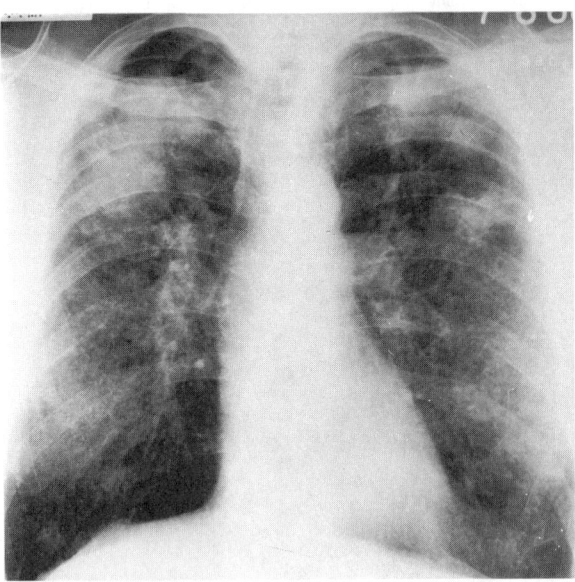

lesions have a rheumatoid histology and rarely cause any serious pulmonary impairment. They may cavitate and disappear. The radiological features of coal-worker's and other pneumoconioses are best described in terms of a set of standard radiographs produced by the International Labour Organization. Use of these standards is mandatory for any epidemiological studies of pneumoconiosis.

Prevention and management

Epidemiological work has shown an exposure–response relationship between the total weight of respirable coal dust to which miners have been exposed and their risks of developing simple pneumoconiosis. This has allowed a standard to be set for coal-mine dust levels which has resulted in a fall in the prevalence of the disease in coal mines in the United Kingdom and the United States. Its success depends on regular monitoring of the respirable dust by gravimetric sampler, constant attention to dust suppression by ventilation and the use of water at points of dust production, and regular radiography of the workforce. Massive fibrosis is prevented by preventing miners from contracting simple pneumoconiosis, and working conditions in British mines are currently such that this disease is now very rare indeed. The present British standard is 7 mg/m³, measured in the air returning from the coal face.

If a man develops simple pneumoconiosis late in his career, no action normally needs to be taken, apart from (in the United Kingdom) advising him to apply to the Respiratory Diseases Board via the Department of Social Security for assessment of disablement and possible benefit payments. A younger man, with several years of further dust exposure ahead, should be advised to work in an area of approved low dust conditions. This advice should be given in the United Kingdom by the Medical Service of the employer. Men with more than the earliest stages of radiological change are entitled to disablement benefits from the Department of Social Security, the value of these depending on the extent of disability. Since, as stated before, simple pneumoconiosis *per se* does not disable, these benefits are often small. Payment of benefits for associated airflow obstruction as an associated effect of coal dust exposure are also made in the United Kingdom if the miner satisfies employment and pneumoconiosis criteria.

Silicosis

Silicosis is a fibrotic disease of the lungs due to inhalation of crystalline silicon dioxide. Such a disease has been recognized in metal miners and masons since ancient times, but assumed particular importance in the cutlery and pottery trades in the nineteenth century. Silicosis may affect anyone involved in quarrying, carving, mining, tunnelling, grinding, or sandblasting, if the dust generated contains quartz. In the United Kingdom the traditional trades that caused the disease (pottery, cutlery, flint knapping, sandblasting, tin and iron mining, and slate quarrying) have either introduced safe substitute materials or have declined, so that true silicosis is now quite rare. Between 50 and 60 cases are diagnosed in the United Kingdom each year, usually in the production of slate or granite, amongst miners cutting through rock, and in fettlers in foundries. The author has recently seen a series of severe cases in British coal-miners and stonemasons who had been working in circumstances where the risks had been forgotten or were ignored.

Aetiology and pathology

Crystalline silica is present in the earth's crust usually as quartz, although other forms such as crystobalite and tridymite occur occasionally. All are extremely toxic to macrophages, although subtle differences between different quartz-containing dusts exist. Freshly fractured quartz seems to be most toxic, suggesting that surface properties are important in toxicity, and this concept is supported by evidence that various clay minerals and other chemicals which occlude the surface reduce the toxicity of inhaled quartz when inhaled simultaneously in mixtures of dust.

The quartz content of dust from different types of stone may vary considerably from some sandstones which are 100 per cent quartz to shales and slates which may contain less than 10 per cent.

Inhaled particles of quartz small enough (generally less than 7 μm aerodynamic diameter) to reach the acinus are engulfed by macrophages and cause disruption of the phagosome, probably by peroxidation of membrane lipids. Before macrophage death, other reactions occur leading to release of inflammatory mediators, including IL-1, various growth factors, tumour necrosis factor, and fibronectin, probably largely from interstitial rather than alveolar macrophages. Silica is probably transported across the alveolar epithelium by migrating macrophages and by endocytosis by type 1 alveolar cells, and it is clear from the distribution of pathological lesions that quartz is transported widely in the lung via lymphatics, much of it ultimately being deposited in hilar lymph nodes.

The macroscopic inspection of silicotic lungs shows fibrous pleural adhesions, enlarged lymph nodes that contain fibrotic, often calcified, nodules, and grey nodules throughout the lung. These nodules vary from a few millimetres to several centimetres in diameter and are more profuse in the upper zones (Fig. 7). They may be calcified, and they have a typical whorled appearance when cut across (Fig. 8). The largest lesions consist of many such whorled nodules that have become confluent, and, as in coal-worker's pneumoconiosis, this massive fibrosis may undergo ischaemic necrosis and cavitate. Under the microscope the silicotic nodule is seen to consist of concentric layers of collagen surrounded by a zone of doubly refractile silica particles, macrophages, and fibroblasts. The nodule may contain the remnants of the respiratory bronchiole and arteriole, which become destroyed by fibrosis.

Macroscopically, acute silicosis appears like pulmonary oedema. Under the microscope, the alveoli are filled with eosinophilic fluid and the alveolar walls contain plasma cells, lymphocytes, fibroblasts, and silica.

Clinical features

Silicosis presents a spectrum of clinical appearances depending on the circumstances in which it is contracted. The most severe, acute silicosis, may be acquired from a relatively brief but very heavy exposure such as occurs in sandblasting without respiratory protection. Such patients become intensely breathless and die within months. The radiograph shows appearances resembling pulmonary oedema. Less heavy exposure causes progressively less dramatic symptoms, ranging from a progressive upper lobe fibrosis with slowly increasing exertional dyspnoea over several years (accelerated silicosis) to radiographic nodular change similar to coal-worker's pneumoconiosis unassociated with any symptoms or physical signs. The latter type of silicosis is the most common, and is usually associated with exposure to dust containing 10 to 30 per cent silica over a prolonged period. Simple nodular silicosis differs from coal-worker's pneumoconiosis in that the lesions tend to be large (3–5 mm) and that it is progressive even after dust exposure ceases. Lesions both increase in size and become more profuse. Moreover, extensive simple silicosis may be associated with some restriction of lung volumes. Simple silicosis rarely seems to be associated with emphysema, unlike coal-worker's pneumoconiosis, but silicotic progressive massive fibrosis is commonly associated with bullous disease. Accelerated silicosis and progressive massive fibrosis cause lung restriction and lead to cor pulmonale and cardiorespiratory failure.

Apart from evidence of cardiac failure or distortion of lung architecture by extreme degrees of massive fibrosis, physical signs are not prominent in silicosis. Clubbing and crackles are not a feature. The diagnosis depends on a history of silica exposure and the radiographic appearances. The most characteristic of these are nodules between 3 and 5 mm in diameter, predominantly in the upper zones, and eggshell calcification in the hilar nodes (Fig. 9). The latter is a pathognomonic feature, only occurring otherwise, very rarely, in sarcoidosis. All forms of silicosis are liable to be complicated by tuberculosis, nowadays in the United Kingdom usually due to reactivation of a quiescent lesion.

Other mycobacterial diseases (*Mycobacterium kansasii* and *Mycobacterium avium-intracellulare*) also occur more frequently than would be expected in silicotics. There is now reasonably convincing evidence of an association between silicosis and lung cancer, even when exposures to cigarette smoke and other occupational carcinogens have been accounted for. The association is sufficiently strong for lung cancer to have been recognized as an occupational disease in silicotics in the United Kingdom. Pneumothorax is an occasional complication of silicosis, as it is of any disease associated with diffuse lung fibrosis.

Subjects with silicosis, particularly of the accelerated type, seem to be at increased risk of the development of autoantibodies and of rheu-

Fig. 7 Whole-lung section from a coal-miner whose work had been predominantly in hard rock, showing silicotic nodules in upper parts of upper and lower lobes.

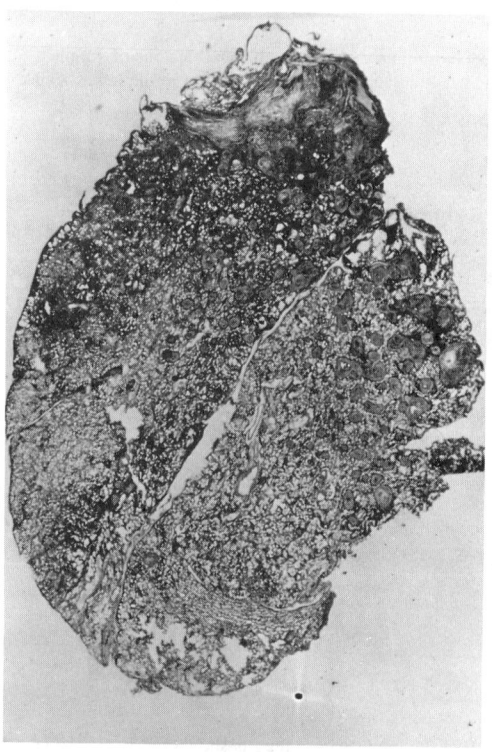

Fig. 8 Silicotic nodules, showing the typical whorled appearance.

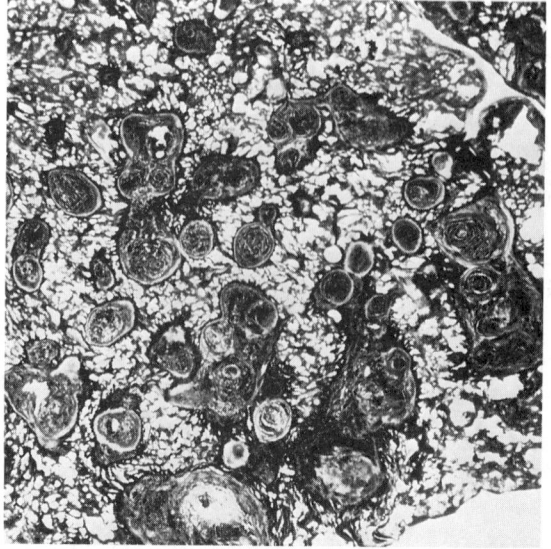

matoid disease, scleroderma, and systemic lupus erythematosus; these conditions have been described in about 10 per cent of some series of silicotics. Focal glomerulonephritis has also been described in acute silicosis; whether this is a direct toxic effect or is due to autoantibodies is not known.

Prevention and management

The epidemiological evidence suggests that workers exposed to levels of respirable silica in excess of 1 mg/m³ have a high risk of silicosis, and that a risk may still exist even at levels of around 0.1 mg/m³. The British maximum exposure limit is 0.4 mg/m³, and industry is obliged to keep exposures of workers below this level as far as practicable, by appropriate ventilation, extraction, and other dust suppression measures. For historic reasons, quartz exposures in coal-mining are controlled by total dust levels rather than the silica component of the dust. If higher levels are inevitable, the worker should wear appropriate respiratory protection, although this must be regarded as a second-best and potentially risky procedure. Once a worker has developed the disease, he should be prevented from working with silica again. The only medical management necessary is regular sputum examination for tubercule bacilli, as tuberculosis accelerates the lung damage but responds normally to modern chemotherapy. In the United Kingdom such examinations are often arranged by the Respiratory Disease Boards of the Department of Social Security, to whom workers with silicosis (whether or not complicated by lung cancer) should apply for industrial injuries benefits.

Asbestosis

Asbestosis is pulmonary fibrosis caused by exposure to fibres of asbestos. It was originally described in the 1900s and its importance as an occupational disease was recognized by epidemiological studies in the 1930s. However, in the first century AD Pliny recorded that the weavers of wicks for the lamps of the vestal virgins wore masks for respiratory protection, and so some recognition of its hazards goes back to antiquity.

Asbestos is mined principally in Canada, South Africa, and the former USSR. It is a generic term for a group of fibrous silicates, the most important being chrysotile (white), crocidolite (blue), and amosite (brown). Chrysotile has a serpentine configuration and breaks up into microfibrils, while the other types are straight and less liable to longitudinal fracture (Fig. 10). All types are resistant to physical and chemical destruction, which gives them their commercial value in fireproofing, insulation, reinforcement of cement, weaving into cloth, bonding in brake linings and plastics, and so on. The asbestos is obtained by crushing the rock to release the fibres, which are then carded and transported in non-porous bags to the user industry.

It is important to know that asbestos causes several separate pleuropulmonary lesions. All types of asbestos cause pleural plaques, asbestosis, and lung carcinoma, and risks of the last two are related to the amount of asbestos inhaled. Crocidolite and amosite cause mesothelioma in humans, and this disease, although probably also dose related, results from a smaller and less prolonged exposure. Chysotile, like the other types of asbestos, causes mesothelioma when injected intrapleurally into rats, but has only rarely been shown to be associated with mesothelioma in exposed human populations, despite being the most commonly used fibre commercially. Further details of mesothelioma can be found in Section 17.13.

The current incidence of asbestosis is about 100 to 150 cases annually in the United Kingdom, almost all in people who worked directly with asbestos in insulation, ship repair, or manufacturing. Mesothelioma, the other important asbestos-related disease, occurs in about 800 people in the United Kingdom each year, reflecting the use of crocidolite asbestos until its effective banning in 1970. Sharp declines in the incidence of both these diseases are anticipated over the next decade in response to the dramatic reduction in the use of all forms of asbestos in the United Kingdom.

Fig. 10 Scanning electron micrographs of (a) chrysotile and (b) amosite on Millipore filters. The curly configuration and microfibrils of chrysotile should be noted. Scale bar, 4 μm.

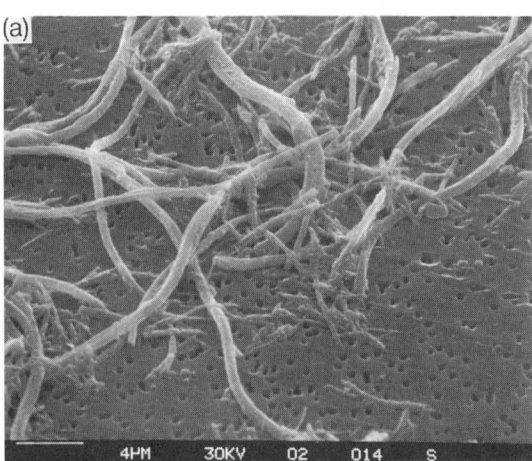

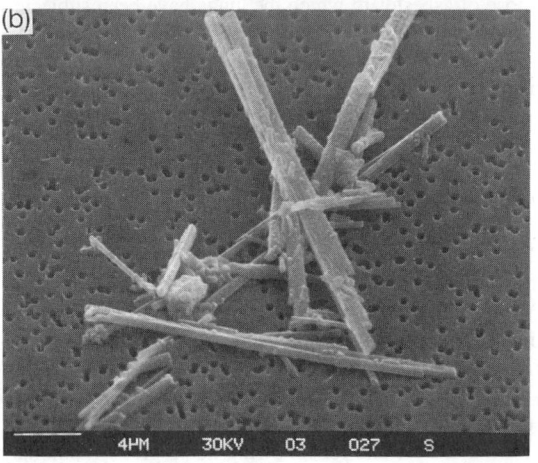

Fig. 9 Radiograph of a slate-miner, showing extensive simple silicosis in the upper and middle zones with early massive fibrosis and eggshell calcification of hilar nodes.

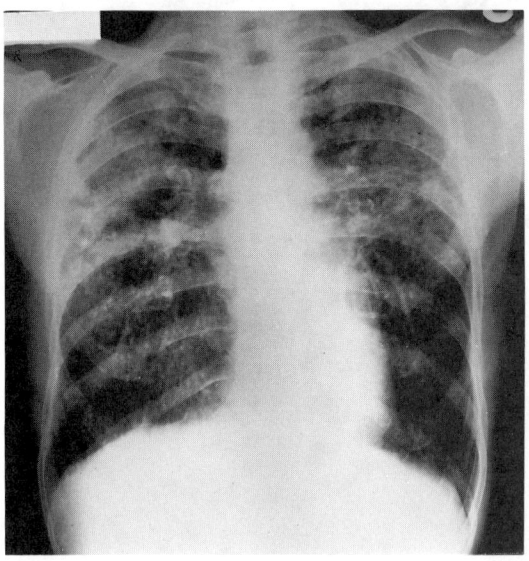

Aetiology and pathology

It seems likely that harmful asbestos fibres are those less than 3 μm in transverse diameter and greater than 10 μm in length, i.e. those sufficiently narrow to be inhaled to the alveolated part of the lung yet too long to be dealt with adequately by macrophages. All types of asbestos are equally toxic to macrophages *in vitro*, and all can cause fibrosis and carcinoma when inhaled by rats. Moreover, injection of any asbestos type (and indeed many fibrous non-asbestos minerals) into the peritoneum of rats causes mesothelioma in a high proportion of cases. It seems likely that the absence of clear human epidemiological evidence linking chrysotile with mesothelioma is related to its curly configuration, which reduces the number of fibres penetrating deep into the lung, and its propensity to break up into minute short fibrils that can eventually be removed from the lung by the action of macrophages. As with coal and silica, the fibrogenicity of asbestos is probably related to damage to macrophages which are unable to cope with fibres much longer than themselves and the liberation of substances that activate fibroblasts to produce collagen. Among the substances shown to result from experimental challenge of rats with asbestos are tumour necrosis factor and macrophage- and platelet-derived growth factors.

The macroscopic appearance of an asbestotic lung is of grey fibrosis, progressing to honeycombing and predominant in the lower zones. Yellow shiny parietal pleural plaques are also usually present, although these frequently also occur in the absence of pulmonary fibrosis with minimal cellular infiltrate or desquamation of type 2 pneumocytes. Larger asbestos fibres may be seen coated with a protein–ferritin complex (the asbestos or ferruginous bodies), while smaller fibres remain uncoated but may still just be visible with the light microscope (Fig. 11). However, for every fibre visible by light microscopy, several hundred uncoated fine fibres can always be found on electron microscopy. Pleural plaques have the appearance of basket-weave collagen, and fibres are almost never seen within them.

Clinical features

Asbestosis occurs in people exposed regularly over years to airborne asbestos as a result of the material being used or removed, and not as a result of occasional exposure. It is more likely to be seen in trades involving the application or removal of asbestos in lagging and insulation than in asbestos mining, preparation, or weaving, where control of fibre levels is more careful nowadays. While disease normally occurs while the individual is still exposed, it may first become apparent after exposure has ceased.

The symptoms of asbestosis are shortness of breath, initially on exertion, and dry cough. Physical signs (repetitive end-inspiratory basal crackles and finger clubbing) commonly precede symptoms. The disease is usually progressive, with the speed of progression probably being related to the dose of asbestos to which the lungs have been subjected, and results in increasing disability and death from cardiorespiratory failure. Forty to fifty per cent of smokers with asbestosis die of bronchial carcinoma, and there is evidence of a multiplicative increase in risk with these two causes. There is no increased risk of tuberculosis in asbestosis.

The radiological appearance of asbestosis is identical to that of cryptogenic pulmonary fibrosis, i.e. predominantly basal irregular linear shadowing progressing to honeycombing (Fig. 12). The presence of pleural plaques, which frequently calcify, is an indication of asbestos exposure and may help in the differential diagnosis (Fig. 13). In advanced asbestosis the pulmonary fibrosis obscures the cardiac borders, giving a shaggy appearance. As with other pneumoconioses, the radiological appearances are best described by comparison with the International Labour Organization standard radiographs.

Asbestosis causes a restrictive pattern of lung function, with reduced volumes and transfer factor. These measurements are the most suitable for screening for the disease and for following its progress. Pulmonary compliance is also reduced in relation to the extent of the fibrosis, and arterial oxygen desaturation occurs in the later stages.

Pleural plaques cause no symptoms and are usually a coincidental finding on routine chest radiography. A more diffuse form of pleural thickening, which can cause breathlessness and restricted lung volumes, occurs infrequently. Inspiratory crackles may be heard over this in the absence of significant asbestosis. Rarest of all is benign asbestos pleural effusion. This develops within the first two decades after exposure as a transient haemorrhagic effusion and is diagnosed by the exclusion of infective and malignant causes. It is important to appreciate that there is no evidence that any of these benign disorders predisposes to pleural mesothelioma, the risk of which relates to the prior extent of asbestos exposure.

Fig. 11 Histological appearance of asbestosis, with interstitial fibrosis, asbestos bodies, and several uncoated fibres.

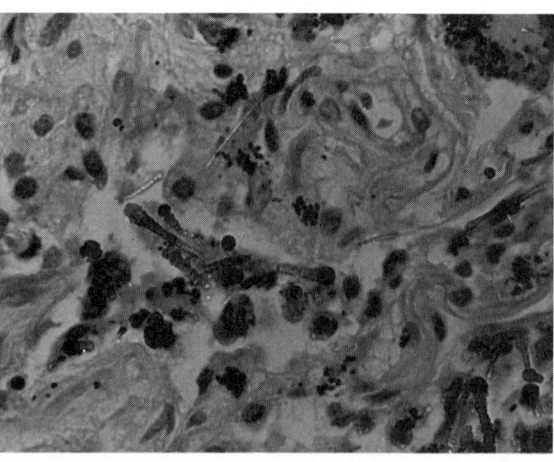

Fig. 12 Radiograph of a lagger with asbestosis. The irregular basal and middle fibrosis should be noted.

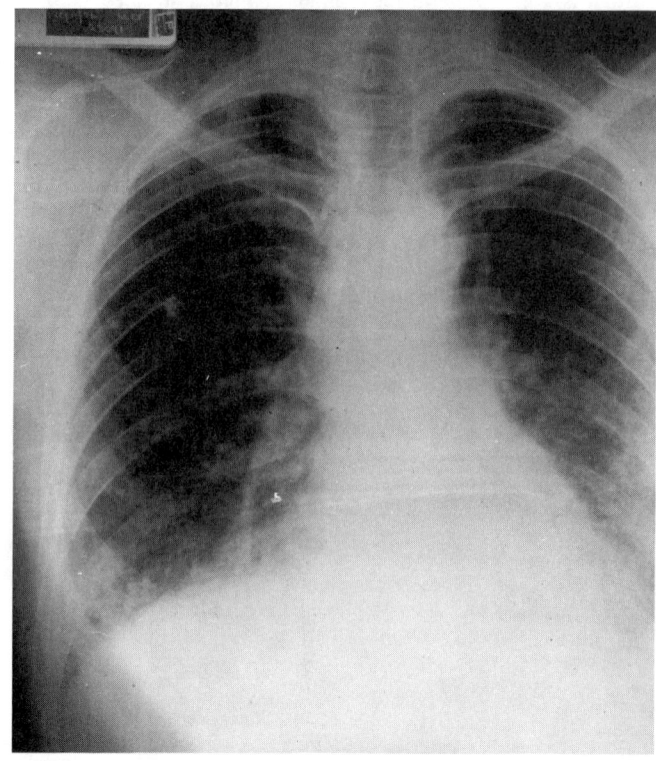

Prevention and management

The prevention of asbestosis, as of other pneumoconioses, depends on reduction of the exposure of individuals to fibre levels that have been shown to be insufficient to cause the disease in a lifetime of exposure. The determination of such a level should ideally be based on epidemiological evidence of the dose–response relationship. Unfortunately, the difficulties of making sensible and reproducible measurements of airborne fibres and the unreliability of such measurements when made, as well as the uncertainties attached to the early diagnosis of asbestosis, have prevented the formulation of really reliable evidence on which to base a standard. The present British standard for chrysotile of 0.5 respirable fibres/ml has been based on work that suggests such levels would, when breathed over a working lifetime, result in asbestosis in fewer than 1 per cent of those exposed. Stricter standards apply to exposure to crocidolite, which is no longer imported into the United Kingdom, and to amosite. Work on standardization of counting and the epidemiology of exposure to fibres is currently taking place in order to increase confidence in exposure standards. Furthermore, many industries are introducing other fibrous or crystalline minerals, where possible, in place of asbestos. Such new materials may entail hazards in themselves, and it is important that they should be subjected to the same scrutiny as asbestos by both toxicity testing and epidemiological studies.

Regular medical and radiological examination of asbestos workers is essential for the early detection of asbestos, and there is some evidence that removal of the worker from exposure at this stage is associated with slower progression. Workers should also be advised not to smoke in view of the interaction between cigarettes and asbestos in causing lung cancer. Once the disease is suspected, the British worker should apply to the Department of Social Security for assessment for industrial injuries benefit. Currently, about 100 people with asbestosis are certified each year.

Risks of asbestos-related disease in the non-occupationally exposed population

Much anxiety has been engendered amongst the general public by media interest in asbestos, and doctors may find themselves being asked about, for example, the risks to children of asbestos wall panelling in houses or asbestos inserts in ironing boards. In general it can be stated that asbestosis only occurs in people working regularly with asbestos for years. However, this has included, at least in the past, wives washing the dusty clothes of asbestos workers and people living or working near asbestos factories. Occasional or incidental exposure to asbestos can be dismissed as a significant cause of asbestosis. Similarly, lung cancer risks seem to be significantly increased only with the doses of asbestos that lead to asbestosis, and individuals who do not smoke and who only have asbestos fittings in their houses can be reassured that their risks of this disease are negligible. Finally, the risk of mesothelioma is again dose related, although it is well established that a sufficient dose of crocidolite or amosite can be inhaled in a period of intense exposure to the material of as short as 6 months. Of the 800 or so cases occurring in the United Kingdom each year, almost all give a history of having worked with asbestos and have large numbers of fibres in their lungs. Small and occasional exposures to amosite or crocidolite are highly unlikely to entail an important risk, but if significant exposures are thought to be occurring in the domestic or general environment, steps should be taken to eliminate them.

Other silicate pneumoconioses

Several silicates apart from asbestos are of commercial importance, and some of these have been shown to cause pneumoconiosis. Talc (hydrated magnesium silicate) is mined as soapstone in the United States, China, and the Pyrenees. It is milled and has many uses including cosmetics, the rubber industry, paints, ceramics, and pharmaceuticals. Kaolin (hydrated aluminium silicate) is quarried in southwestern England, Georgia in the United States, Japan, Egypt, Germany, and Czechoslovakia. It is used mainly in the manufacture of ceramics, paper and paint, and in pharmaceuticals. Fuller's earth (calcium montmorillonite) is an absorbent clay quarried in England, the United States, and Germany. It was originally used in fulling or removing grease from wool, and is now used in oil refining and bonding foundry moulds. Mica is a complex aluminium silicate occurring in two forms—muscovite and phlogopite. The former is mined in the United States and India and used in fire-resistant windows and the manufacture of paper and paint. Phlogopite, mined in Canada, is used in the electrical industry because of its resistance to heat and electricity.

Two widely used silicate materials—cement and vitreous fibres—are not established as causes of pulmonary disease. Although cement exposure has occasionally been reported to be associated with pneumoconiosis, the evidence for this is flimsy. It is often mixed with asbestos, and asbestosis may occur in the production of this material. Artificial vitreous fibres (glass wool and rock wool) have not so far been shown to cause pulmonary fibrosis or neoplasia in humans exposed to them, although mesothelioma has been produced by intraperitoneal injection in rats. It is possible that commercial production of finer fibres of these materials might be hazardous, and vigilance is required in these industries as the need for safer substitutes for asbestos increases.

Talc pneumoconiosis

Talc is commonly contaminated with tremolite, a non-commercially exploited form of asbestos, and with silica; it has been difficult to disentangle the effects of these components. The disease appears clinically to resemble asbestosis, with finger clubbing and basal crackles, although radiological descriptions emphasize lesions predominantly in the middle zones with nodular as well as reticular components. Massive fibrosis has been described.

Talc has been shown to be associated with pulmonary disease in a number of other circumstances. Bronchoconstriction may occur in children exposed to high concentrations and drug users may have granulomatous reactions in the lungs as a result of either intravenous injection or inhalation of ground-up tablets. Fortunately, the widespread use of

Fig. 13 Radiograph of a lagger, showing extensive calcified pleural plaques.

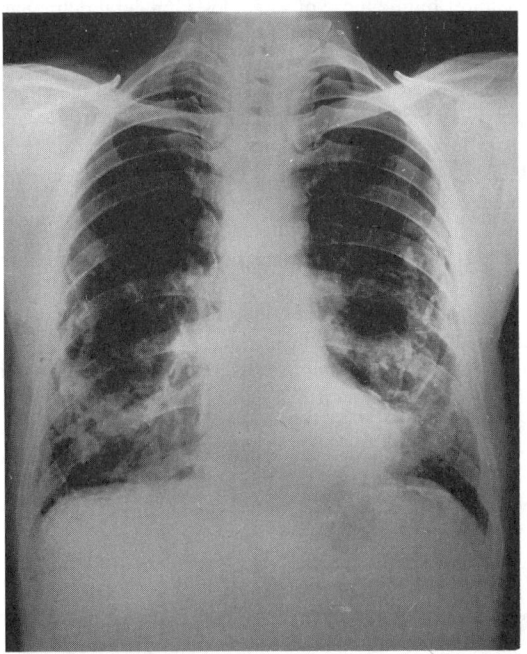

talc for producing pleurodesis has not been shown to be associated with the later development of mesothelioma, probably because the grades of talc used have not been contaminated with tremolite.

Kaolin pneumoconiosis

Kaolin causes a pneumoconiosis similar to coal-worker's pneumoconiosis with small discrete nodular lesions initially and a tendency to produce massive fibrosis. It has been described in workers involved in the drying and milling processes in the production of china clay; kaolin may also be the component of the dust responsible for pneumoconiosis in the now defunct Scottish shale extraction industry. There is no evidence linking kaolin pneumoconiosis with carcinoma or tuberculosis.

Fig. 14 Radiograph of a beryllium refiner worker, showing the diffuse fibrosis of berylliosis.

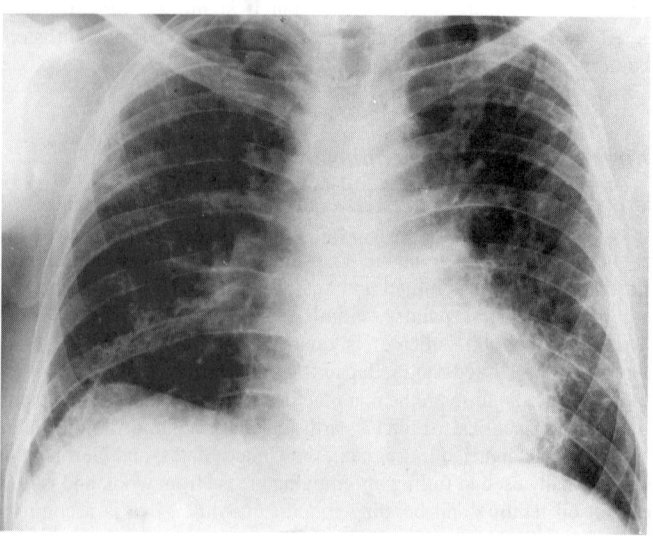

Fig. 15 Photomicrograph of a lung biopsy from a man with berylliosis, showing granuloma indistinguishable from that found in sarcoidosis.

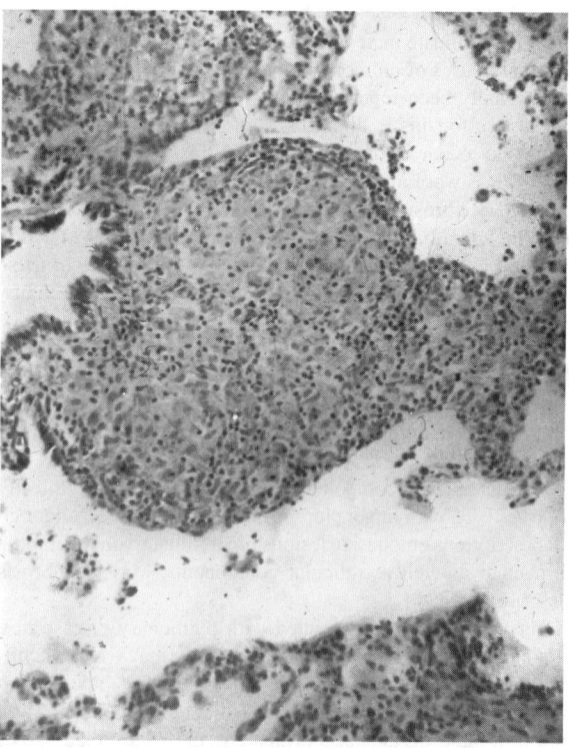

Fuller's earth pneumoconiosis

This condition has been described in workers extracting this clay mineral. It seems to be a benign nodular pneumoconiosis similar in pathological and radiological appearance to coal-worker's pneumoconiosis, although progressive massive fibrosis has not been described.

Mica pneumoconiosis

A few reports of radiological change in those exposed to ground mica have been recorded, but there is no recent publication describing pathological or clinical features.

Fibrous erionite

Exposure to this fibrous hydrated aluminium silicate occurs in certain areas of Turkey and probably elsewhere in the Middle East. The populations of several villages have been exposed for many generations as they use local erionite rock as stucco and whitewash in their homes. Pleural plaques, pulmonary fibrosis, and both lung cancer and mesothelioma are endemic in these villages. Fortunately, fibrous erionite has no general commercial use, but this episode illustrates the potential dangers of inhaling fine fibrous material, whether asbestos or some other mineral.

Berylliosis

Beryllium is a metal that is used in the nuclear industry and in the production of X-ray tubes. It was used in ceramics, metallic alloys, and fluorescent lights until its toxicity was recognized and it was replaced by other materials. It is mined as an ore mostly in South America and extracted by chemical processes.

Beryllium is highly toxic when inhaled, although it may also cause granulomatous ulcers on contact with the skin. Inhalation of high concentrations causes an acute pneumonitis and tracheobronchitis, which may be fatal. Chronic berylliosis, which may occur as a sequel to acute exposure, usually follows more prolonged exposure to lower levels. It is not common in the United Kingdom, where no more than about 50 cases have been diagnosed, but it has been recorded much more frequently in the United States. Reported cases have occurred in beryllium workers, in wives exposed to dust from their husbands' clothes, and in people living near the factories.

The patient with chronic berylliosis presents with cough and shortness of breath. The features mimic those of sarcoidosis: bilateral pulmonary mottling with upper lobe fibrosis is the usual radiographic feature initially, with bilateral hilar lymphadenopathy being less common. The disease typically progresses to diffuse fibrosis (Fig. 14), but the rate of progression is very variable. The functional lesion is a restrictive pattern with a low transfer factor. The progress of the disease can usually be controlled with corticosteroid therapy, but this needs to be continued indefinitely in most cases.

The pathological lesion is identical with that of sarcoidosis, with non-caseating granulomas and varying amounts of interstitial fibrosis (Fig. 15). The diagnosis is made on the basis of a history of exposure, compatible clinical and histological features, and a negative Kveim test. A skin-patch test is inadvisable as it can cause sensitization.

Berylliosis is prevented by keeping exposures below the threshold limit value ($2 \, \text{ng/m}^3$), although as it is a hypersensitivity disease even this will not prevent all cases. Proper respiratory protection should be provided in the event of spills where acute berylliosis, a toxic alveolitis, could occur.

Other pneumoconioses

Many other pneumoconioses have been described, although most are of very limited prevalence and are relatively benign. Haematite lung, occurring in iron ore miners, used to be seen in Cumbria in the United Kingdom. This is a fibrotic reaction to a mixed dust containing silica and iron. Radiographically it resembles silicosis and pathologically only differs from it in that the lungs are coloured red. However, there is an increased risk of lung cancer in the disease, probably related to radiation in the mines. Closely related to haematite lung is siderosis, a benign pneumoconiosis occurring in welders and other workers in iron foundries. Complicated pneumoconiosis rarely occurs. The radiological lesions often regress after exposure ceases. Barium processing and tin refining may be associated with the development of dramatic radiological nodular shadowing—baritosis and stannosis respectively. These are completely benign conditions; the radiological appearances reflect the collection of radio-opaque dust in macrophages. Pneumoconiosis associated with diffuse fibrotic reaction in the lungs has been described in work with aluminium oxide (Shaver's disease) and tungsten carbide (hard metal disease). This latter condition, which is probably due to cobalt in cooling liquids, may also present with features of asthma or allergic alveolitis. A pneumoconiosis resembling that in coal-miners has been described in workers with graphite and other forms of carbon, and in shale miners. A benign pneumoconiosis, consisting of simple accumulations of dust and macrophages with minimal nodular radiological shadowing, has been described in workers producing polyvinyl chloride.

REFERENCES

Henderson, V.L. and Enterline, P.E. (1979). Asbestos exposure: factors associated with excess cancer and respiratory disease mortality. *Annals of the New York Academy of Sciences*, **330**, 117–26.

Hurley, J.F., Burns, J., Copland, L., Dodgson, J., and Jacobsen, M. (1982). Coalworkers' simple pneumoconiosis and exposure to dust at 10 British coalmines. *British Journal of Industrial Medicine*, **39**, 120–7.

International Labour Organization. (1980). *Guidelines for the use of ILO International classification of radiographs of pneumoconioses*. Occupational Safety and Health Series No. 22 (rev. 87), International Labour Organization, Geneva.

Liddell, D. (1981). Asbestos and public health. *Thorax*, **36**, 241–4.

Marine, W.M., Gurr, D., and Jacobsen, M. (1988). Clinically important respiratory effects of dust exposure and smoking in British coal miners. *American Review of Respiratory Disease*, **137**, 106–12.

Morgan, W.K.C., and Seaton, A. (1995). *Occupational lung diseases* (3rd edn). W.B. Saunders, Philadelphia, PA.

Mossman, B.T., Bignon, J., Corn, M., Seaton, A., and Gee, J.B.L. (1990). Asbestos: scientific developments and implications for public policy. *Science*, **247**, 294–301.

Peto, J. (1979). Dose–response relationships for asbestos-related disease: implications for hygiene standards. Part 2. Mortality. *Annals of the New York Academy of Sciences*, **330**, 195–203.

Seaton, A. (1990). Coalmining, emphysema and compensation. *British Journal of Industrial Medicine*, **47**, 433–5.

Seaton, A., Dick, J.A., Dodgson, J., and Jacobsen, M. (1981). Quartz and pneumoconiosis in coalminers. *Lancet*, **ii**, 1272–5.

Seaton, A., Legge, J.S., Henderson, J., and Kerr, K.M. (1991). Accelerated silicosis in Scottish stonemasons. *Lancet*, **337**, 341–4.

17.10.17 Toxic gases and fumes

J. M. HOPKIN

Noxious substances may be delivered airborne is the respiratory tract in a molecular form (gases) or as a particulate. A vapour is the gaseous form of a substance that is liquid at ambient temperature and pressure. Particulates may be (a) solid (dusts), (b) solids in very fine form, often as oxides of metals (fumes), or (c) liquid (mists).

Asphyxiation by simple displacement of alveolar oxygen (e.g. nitrogen, carbon dioxide, or methane), and the irritative and toxic actions of gases and fumes on the lung are well documented. Accidental exposure can occur under a range of circumstances and rural/agricultural examples, as well as industrial forms, are notable.

Highly soluble gases (e.g. ammonia or sulphur dioxide) produce rapid upper airway irritation that makes the exposed subject withdraw quickly from the contaminated environment, usually before intense alveolar exposure occurs. Laryngeal oedema, severe enough to cause airflow obstruction and require intubation, can develop. *Insoluble gases* (e.g. phosgene or nitrogen dioxide) produce little upper airway irritation and therefore may be respired deeply and cause pulmonary oedema.

Ammonia is widely used in the chemical industry as an alkalinizing agent and as a substrate for the production of nitrogenous products including fertilizers and explosives. On accidental exposure, its high solubility leads to intense irritation of the mucous membranes of the mouth, throat, and eyes, as well as the upper airways. Oedema, excessive secretion, and reflex constriction of the larynx and main airways can lead to severe life-threatening airflow obstruction. With appropriate care, recovery is usually full.

Nitrogen dioxide (NO_2 or N_2O_4) is heavier than air and has a brown colour. It is only moderately irritating to the eyes and upper respiratory tract, which may allow added exposure to occur leading to severe irritant pulmonary oedema. The gas may be encountered in hazardous concentrations in unventilated silos (silo filler's disease) and arc welding facilities or after combustion of nitrogen-containing substances, such as nitrocellulose. Silage is the agricultural preservation of green crops (e.g. grass or corn for winter feeds) in towers or pits at a controlled temperature of just under 38 °C; nitrogen dioxide is readily formed from oxidization of the vegetable matter and perhaps fertilizers. Under these conditions, and if the facility is poorly ventilated, the gas accumulates because of its density. Depending on concentration, early respiratory symptoms can range from none to choking. Severe pulmonary oedema, with hypoxaemia, wheezes, and crackles, may be present within 1 to 2 h. In other exposed subjects, relatively mild pulmonary symptoms in the early phase can be complicated by late severe pulmonary oedema after 2 to 3 weeks. There is inflammation and oedema of alveoli and alveolar capillaries with alveolar flooding. Bronchiolitic changes are prominent in late reactions. Chest radiographs show alveolar shadowing that can include nodular and miliary patterns. Recovery is usually full, but may be complicated by bronchiolitis obliterans (Chapter 17.10.3).

Fire smoke is a complex mixture of gases and particulates released during combustion and pyrolysis. Its nature can vary greatly with the conditions and severity of the fire and the nature of the burning materials. Therefore, smoke can contain significant concentrations of carbon monoxide, hydrogen cyanide, ammonia, sulphur dioxide, chlorine, phosgene, and other gases. Thus, its effects are diverse, and include suffocation or metabolic poisoning as well as direct toxic injury throughout the respiratory tract.

Management of inhalational toxic respiratory injury is essentially supportive. Because of the risk of supervening laryngeal obstruction or pulmonary oedema, a minimum period of 24 h of hospital care is needed for subjects presenting with hoarseness, stridor, wheeze, or hypoxaemia, and those with a history indicative of heavy exposure to an insoluble gas. Humidified air, oxygen supplementation, and bronchodilators may be required. Fibreoptic bronchoscopy can be used to clear excessive secretions and clear airways. Laryngeal obstruction demands intubation. Severe pulmonary oedema should be managed as for the adult respiratory distress syndrome (Chapter 17.10.20). The role of corticosteroids in limiting inflammation is unclear; these drugs add to the risk of secondary infection but have been claimed to prevent the development of late pulmonary oedema after nitrogen dioxide exposure.

Metal fume fever

Metal fume fever is a common, acute, and self-limiting febrile illness that characteristically recurs on re-exposure after brief absence from work; it is another Monday morning fever (see byssinosis, Chapter 17.9.13). It can occur on the first day of exposure. It results from alveolar deposition of very fine particulate metal oxides (fumes) released in processes such as welding, melting, and smelting of metal. It particularly, but not exclusively, involves zinc, copper, and magnesium. Within some 6 h of exposure, there is sudden onset of thirst, a metallic taste in the mouth, cough, tightness in the chest, and chills, with fever, headache, myalgia, and leucocytosis. There is resolution within 24 hours without ill effect, and this benign course distinguishes the condition from acute cadmium inhalation and poisoning.

Cadmium is an anticorrosive metal used in electroplating and production of alloys. Cadmium fumes encountered during extraction, soldering, and welding in poorly ventilated conditions can cause an acute severe chemical pneumonia associated with significant mortality and renal necrosis.

REFERENCES

Ainslie, G. (1993). Inhalational injuries produced by smoke and nitrogen dioxide. *Respiratory Medicine*, **87**, 169–74.

Delaney, L.T., Schmidt, H.W., and Stroebel, C.F. (1956). Silo filler's disease. *Mayo Clinic Proceedings*, **31**, 189–98.

Horvarth, E.P., do Pico, G.A., and Barbee, R.A. (1978). Nitrogen dioxide-induced pulmonary disease. *Journal of Occupational Medicine*, **20**, 103–10.

Sheppard, D. (1989). Noxious gases. In: *Textbook of pulmonary disease* (ed Baum and Wolinsky), pp. 831–46. Little, Brown, Boston, MA.

Smith, T.J., Petty, T.L., and Ridding, J.C. (1976). Pulmonary effects of exposure to airborne cadmium. *American Review of Respiratory Disease*, **114**, 161.

17.10.18 Radiation pneumonitis

J. M. HOPKIN

Local therapeutic irradiation of malignancies of the breast, oesophagus, mediastinum (including lymphoma), and lung may damage normal pulmonary tissue. Normal lung is also damaged by the total body irradiation used in the preparative treatment for bone marrow transplantation, and its effects are compounded by the combined use of toxic mutagens such as methotrexate. The scale of pulmonary damage is strongly dependent on the volume of lung exposed and the dose and fractionation of irradiation; the changes range from asymptomatic radiographic opacification to severe clinical disease that may progress to death, but the latter is becoming increasingly rare with more refined local radiotherapy techniques.

Radiation releases toxic and mutagenic free radicals within tissue. The resultant DNA damage causes mitotic cell death as tissue cells pass through the first two or three cell divisions after irradiation. The principal cells injured in the lung (the capillary endothelium and type 2 alveolar pneumocyte) have turnover times ranging from 2 to 6 weeks under different circumstances, and this explains why maximum pulmonary irradiative damage and symptomatic effect occur at 2 months or later after injury.

The pathological changes can be categorized as (a) acute (up to 3 months), when there is vascular damage with thrombosis and packing of alveoli with surfactant (released from type 2 pneumocytes) and oedema, (b) subacute (2–6 months), when there is type 2 pneumocyte renewal and proliferation with macrophage and fibroblast infiltration into the alveolus and interstitium, and (c) chronic (up to 24 months), when there is alveolar and interstitial fibrosis with capillary sclerosis.

Clinical features

Symptoms, if they develop, begin at 2 months or later and persist for weeks. Their degree is dependent upon the extent of lung damage. Lesser degrees of damage may only be detected incidentally on routine chest radiograph. Cough, which can be severe and produce thick sputum, and breathlessness are the principal symptoms, but may be accompanied by fever of variable degree. On examination there may be tachypnoea, cyanosis in severe disease, and sometimes local crepitations. Telangiectases, the result of cutaneous radiation damage, are often observed in the overlying skin.

The most characteristic radiographic feature in local radiation pneumonitis is an area of hazy consolidation demarcated by a sharp margin (crossing anatomical pulmonary planes) which corresponds to the limits of the irradiation field. Radioisotope scanning shows marked perfusion impairment within the affected portion of lung. In extensive disease, the clinical and radiographic features may be typical of adult respiratory distress syndrome (Chapter 17.10.20).

Later in the course of symptomatic or asymptomatic disease, dense local fibrosis develops that may require magnetic resonance imaging (Chapter 17.6.1) to allow differentiation from tumour recurrence. The pulmonary fibrosis may be complicated by pleural effusion, pneumothorax, or colonization by Aspergillus. Fractures resulting from irradiative bone necrosis may occur in nearby ribs.

Treatment

In cases where symptoms are slight no specific treatment is needed. In more severe disease, there is a strong clinical impression that corticosteroids produce relief from the symptoms of the acute illness (at 2 months) in most patients. Response to corticosteroids occurs within 3 to 4 days, with clinical and radiographic improvement, and treatment should be continued for 3 to 4 weeks before tapering and stopping. Symptomatic relief of cough and hypoxaemia by an opioid antitussive and oxygen supplementation may also be needed.

Corticosteroids do not influence the extent of subsequent pulmonary fibrosis.

REFERENCES

Douglas, A.C. (1959). Treatment of radiation pneumonitis with prednisolone. *Chest*, **53**, 346–55.

Gross, N.J. (1977). Pulmonary effects of radiation therapy. *Annals of Internal Medicine*, **86**, 81–92.

Gross, N.J. (1981). The pathogenesis of radiation induced lung damage. *Lung*, **159**, 115.

Kaplan, H.S. and Stewart, J.R. (1973). Complications of intensive megavoltage radiotherapy for Hodgkin's disease. *National Cancer Institute Monograph*, **36**, 439–44.

Rubin, P. and Casanett, G.W. (1968). *Clinical Radiation Pathology*, pp. 423–70. W.B. Saunders, Philadelphia, 1968.

17.10.19 Drug-induced lung disease

G.J. GIBSON

Adverse effects of drugs on the lungs and airways frequently present diagnostic problems. This review is limited to direct effects of drugs in usual therapeutic doses on the airways, alveoli, pulmonary vasculature, and mediastinal structures. Indirect effects, such as the predisposition to opportunistic lung infection resulting from cytotoxic agents or the worsening of respiratory failure after sedatives, are excluded, as are the consequences of overdosage or inadequate control of dosage (e.g. pulmonary haemorrhage with anticoagulants.

Drug-induced asthma

Airway obstruction induced by drugs usually presents as an exacerbation of pre-existing asthma. In some cases, however, asthma has not previously been recognized until it is 'uncovered' by the adverse effect of a drug. In such instances clues to pre-existing asthma are usually elicited when the appropriate history is taken. Less commonly, asthma may develop *de novo;* this has occurred particularly in the pharmaceutical industry where repeated inhalation of certain agents leads to sensitization.

The relevant drugs may conveniently be classified as those which produce a more or less predictable effect, related to their pharmacological properties, and those which produce bronchoconstriction due to an idiosyncratic effect (Table 1). Asthma can also be provoked by non-specific effects related to the drug or its method of delivery. For example, nebulized solutions of low osmolality can stimulate hyper-responsive airways. This appears to have been the main mechanism of bronchoconstriction induced by nebulized ipratropium bromide. Since the drug was reformulated in isotonic solution the problem has largely disappeared, although occasional patients still respond adversely, possibly to the preservatives in the solution. Potential adverse effects of hydrofluorocarbons in pressurized aerosol inhalers have recently become more evident with the widespread use of long-acting bronchodilators. It appears that the rate of onset of action of these agents is sufficiently slow to uncover a bronchoconstricting effect of the carrier agent in some individuals; this effect is suppressed by shorter acting bronchodilators which generally have a more rapid onset of action. The prevalence of this potentially important adverse effect is at present unclear.

PHARMACOLOGICAL EFFECTS

Cholinergic drugs such as carbachol given systemically occasionally produce bronchoconstriction, and in very sensitive asthmatic patients exacerbations have occurred after use of pilocarpine as eye drops. An inhaled anticholinergic agent would seem a logical approach to this problem and has also been shown to be effective in reversing occasional untoward effects of cholinesterase inhibitors in asthmatic patients with myasthenia gravis.

The bronchoconstrictor prostaglandin $F_{2\alpha}$, if used to induce abortion, may be hazardous in asthmatic patients. The occurrence of bronchoconstriction after thiopentone, opiates, and muscle relaxants (tubocurarine, suxamethonium, and pancuronium) is probably due to their capacity to release histamine.

A more common problem is worsening of airway obstruction by β-adrenergic antagonist agents. Although these have been increasingly refined to select agents with the least β_2 antagonism, thus minimizing effects on the airways, none is completely specific for β_1 receptors. The degree of selectivity varies, with propranolol the least and practolol probably the most selective agents used so far. Unfortunately, practolol causes its own distinctive side-effects (see below) and is no longer available. Of the β-blockers currently available, atenolol and metoprolol seem to have the least adverse effects on airway function, but many patients with asthma will show a reduction in forced expiratory volume in 1 s (FEV_1) or peak flow on therapeutic doses of these agents and considerable caution is necessary. The problem of β-blockers in patients with clear-cut asthma is relatively straightforward, but the situation with chronic airway obstruction is less clear. Adverse reactions in such patients are less common and usually less severe. Many patients who develop symptoms with worsening airway obstruction after use of β-blockers are subsequently recognized as having 'latent' asthma.

Although the adverse effects of oral or systemic β-blockers are well recognized, those of ophthalmic preparations are easily overlooked.

Table 1 *Drugs which may exacerbate asthma*

Pharmacological effects
Cholinergic agents (e.g., carbachol, pilocarpine)
Cholinesterase inhibitors (e.g., pyridostigmine)
Prostaglandin $F_{2\alpha}$
Histamine-releasing agents (e.g., curare derivatives)
β-Sympathetic antagonists
ACE inhibitors (cough without asthma more common)

Idiosyncratic effects
Oral
    Aspirin and other NSAIDs
    Tartrazine-containing preparations
    Nitrofurantoin (alveolar reaction more common)
    Carbamazepine
    Propafenone

Parenteral
    Penicillin
    Iron-dextran complex
    Aminophylline
    Hydrocortisone sodium succinate
    N-acetylcysteine

Inhaled
    Nebulized pentamidine
    Occupational agents (e.g., antibiotics, methyldopa, cimetidine, piperazine)

ACE, angiotensin-converting enzyme.

Timolol, which is used commonly in eye drops for the treatment of glaucoma, is a potent non-selective β-blocker. Its use has frequently been associated with worsening asthma. The ophthalmic formulation of the newer β-blocker betaxolol appears to be less dangerous but should be avoided in patients with asthma unless no suitable alternative is available.

IDIOSYNCRATIC REACTIONS

The most dramatic presentation of drug-induced asthma is as part of an acute anaphylactic reaction. Among the causative agents penicillin and intravenously administered iron–dextran are noteworthy. N-acetylcysteine given intravenously in severe paracetamol poisoning may produce exacerbations of asthma, and caution is necessary in asthmatic patients.

The drugs which produce idiosyncratic reactions most frequently are the non-steroidal anti-inflammatory drugs (**NSAIDs**). Exacerbation of asthma after ingestion of aspirin was described as long ago as 1910, but its mechanism remains elusive. Most patients who are sensitive to aspirin also react to other NSAIDs with widely differing chemical structures making an immunological reaction unlikely. All the anti-inflammatory agents incriminated are inhibitors of prostaglandin synthesis via the cyclo-oxygenase pathway, and it is presumed that their adverse effects are mediated in this way. It is possible that metabolism of arachidonic acid is diverted to the production of bronchoconstrictor leukotrienes, but why only a proportion of patients with asthma should be affected is not clear. Deaths have been reported with both aspirin and indomethacin. Of the commonly used analgesic agents, paracetamol is the least likely to provoke a significant response, although occasional adverse reactions are well documented. A further interesting feature is that aspirin-sensitive individuals can be made tolerant to further aspirin by ingesting graded doses over a couple of days. This state of tolerance can then be maintained by daily treatment with aspirin, but sensitivity returns within a few days of discontinuing regular treatment. Any attempt at inducing tolerance in this way requires very careful supervision.

Many patients with analgesic-induced asthma are also sensitive to the azo dye tartrazine, hitherto a commonly used colouring agent in medications (particularly those coloured orange or red) and foodstuffs. Reactions to tartrazine are generally not as severe as with aspirin. Since tartrazine is an approved food and drug additive, its presence is not always declared and the extent of the problems it may cause is not clear. Ironically, in the past tartrazine was present in some medications used to treat asthma! Most pharmaceutical companies have now removed tartrazine from their formulations.

Potential exacerbation of asthma by drugs used to treat it presents a particularly acute dilemma, as a drug effect may be difficult to dissociate from spontaneous deterioration. There are well-documented reports of worsening asthma after both intravenous aminophylline and hydrocortisone. Sensitivity to hydrocortisone is a particular problem in asthmatic patients who also show adverse reactions to aspirin and NSAIDs. The sensitivity to hydrocortisone of these individuals is not shared by other steroids; it appears to be related to the succinate moiety of the hydrocortisone sodium succinate molecule as it is not seen with the alternative phosphate salt.

Asthmatic reactions have been reported following the inhalation of several drugs, usually during the manufacturing process. Affected individuals are usually non-atopic with no history of respiratory disease prior to exposure; on challenge testing the asthma is often of the 'late' type. The condition appears likely to be a specific immunological response with a good prognosis if the subject is removed from the offending drug.

The frequent use of nebulized pentamidine for treatment or prophylaxis of pneumocystis infection in patients with HIV infection has been associated with bronchoconstriction in a large proportion of individuals. The mechanism is unclear. Although patients with asthma show larger responses, others with no features of asthma may also be affected to a lesser degree. The adverse effect is inhibited by prior use of a nebulized bronchodilator, an approach which has become standard in many centres.

Drug-induced cough

Cough is a well-recognized side-effect of treatment with inhibitors of angiotensin-converting enzyme. It develops in 10 to 20 per cent of individuals so treated and is an effect of the class of drug rather than of specific agents. The cough is non-productive. There appears to be weak relation to dose such that dose reduction may result in some improvement, but in many individuals the symptom is sufficiently troublesome to necessitate withdrawal of the drug. Deterioration of pre-existing asthma has also occasionally been reported, but in most individuals with cough related to angiotensin-converting enzyme inhibition features of asthma are not present. The mechanism is unclear; angiotensin-converting enzyme catalyses not only the conversion of angiotensin I to angiotension II, but also the breakdown of bradykinin and substance P. Since these agents are cough stimulants, their accumulation offers a possible mechanism for this unusual adverse effect.

Alveolar reactions

There is no generally accepted classification of alveolar reactions to drugs. They range from acute non-cardiogenic pulmonary oedema or the adult respiratory distress syndrome at one extreme to insidiously developing pulmonary fibrosis at the other. The reactions are conveniently considered under three main headings (Table 2). Of the drugs which may produce the picture of adult respiratory distress syndrome, hydrochlorothiazide and salicylates are the commonest. The reaction to hydrochlorothiazide is idiosyncratic and is not shared by other thiazide drugs. In the case of salicylates there is a clearer relation to dose, with reactions usually occurring with frank overdose (as also occurs with opiates) but occasionally in chronic ingesters with high serum levels. Infused β_2-adrenergic agonists are sometimes used as uterine relaxants (tocolytics) to inhibit premature labour. Several, including in particular isoxsuprine, ritodrine, and terbutaline, have been associated with florid pulmonary

Table 2 *Alveolar reactions*

Acute pulmonary oedema/ARDS
Hydrochlorothiazide
Salicylates
Tocolytic agents (e.g., isoxsuprine, ritodrine, terbutaline)
Naloxone
Cytosine arabinoside
Low molecular weight dextran

Diffuse lung injury (alveolitis) and/or fibrosis
Oxygen
Nitrofurantoin
Amiodarone
Tocainide
Cytotoxic agents

Bleomycin	Melphalan
Mitomycin C	Cyclophosphamide
BCNU	Cytosine arabinoside
(carmustine)	6-Mercaptopurine
CCNU	Azathioprine
(lomustine)	
Busulphan	
Chlorambucil	

Eosinophilic reactions

Sulphonamides	Nitrofurantoin*
Penicillins	(acute reaction)
Tetracycline	Methotrexate*
Aspirin	Procarbazine*
Naproxen	Gold salts*
Sulphasalazine	Penicillamine*
Chlorpropamide	
Chlorpromazine	
Imipramine	
Carbamazepine	
Phenytoin	

*Eosinophilia not consistent

oedema. This reaction is occasionally life threatening and caution is required in the rate of infusion.

Several drugs produce widespread alveolar damage ('pneumonitis' or 'alveolitis') which may or may not be followed by fibrosis (Table 2). Patients may present acutely with cough, fever, shortness of breath, and occasionally systemic upset. Alternatively, slowly progressive fibrosis may develop with gradually worsening dyspnoea and widespread shadowing on the chest radiograph. The mechanism(s) of such reactions are generally uncertain. In some cases, including bleomycin, carmustine, amiodarone, and nitrofurantoin, there is evidence of a relation to dose or duration of treatment. Recent evidence in the cases of nitrofurantoin and bleomycin suggests mechanisms involving the production of toxic oxygen radicals in the lungs, perhaps providing a link with the known pulmonary toxicity of oxygen itself and with the synergistic adverse effects of high oxygen concentrations and some cytotoxic agents.

Much recent interest has centred on the antiarrhythmic drug amiodarone. It has been estimated that approximately 6 per cent of patients taking 400 mg or more per day of the drug for 2 months or more will develop overt pulmonary toxicity. There have also been several well-documented cases in patients taking smaller doses. The mechanism may include both immunologically mediated and direct toxic effects. Histologically the lung shows features of chronic inflammation together with interstitial and intra-alveolar fibrosis (Fig. 1). Characteristic 'foamy' macrophages are seen, but they are not specific for serious toxic reactions as they are also demonstrable in the majority of patients taking the drug without adverse clinical effects. Occasionally, the histological picture is of bronchiolitis obliterans organizing pneumonia, which is also known as cryptogenic organizing pneumonia. Symptoms include progressive dyspnoea, a troublesome cough, and occasionally pleuritic chest pain. Radiographic appearances are varied: most frequently there is a diffuse nodular or alveolar filling pattern, sometimes with upper lobe predominance (Fig. 2), and occasionally a pleural effusion is present. Differential diagnoses in the population of patients likely to be taking this drug include left ventricular failure and pneumonia. Further investigation, including measurement of pulmonary wedge pressure and lung biopsy, is often necessary. Bronchoalveolar lavage in some (but not all) patients shows a lymphocytic pattern. This investigation is also of value for the exclusion of infection, but the finding of 'foamy' macrophages in lavage fluid is, for the reasons discussed above, insufficient to confirm the diagnosis. If amiodarone lung toxicity is suspected, cessation of treatment is desirable, but the very long half-life implies that elimination will be very slow. Corticosteroids probably suppress the reaction and sometimes allow continuation or retreatment in cases of 'malignant' dysrrhythmias unresponsive to other agents.

Cytotoxic and immunosuppressive drugs represent an increasing problem, with the majority reported to cause pulmonary complications. Bleomycin causes the most frequent problems, followed by busulphan and methotrexate. Cyclophosphamide and azathioprine, which because of their roles in non-malignant disease are perhaps the most widely used agents in this group of drugs, produce adverse pulmonary reactions only occasionally. In most cases it is not clear whether the effects are due to direct toxicity or to hypersensitivity. With bleomycin, however, there is evidence of a dose relationship: cumulative doses of less than 150 mg are less likely to cause serious reactions, whereas death due to respiratory failure consequent upon severe fibrosis has occurred in about 10 per cent of patients receiving more than 500 mg. The recorded frequency of adverse reactions varies with the means by which they are detected; for example, on clinical and functional criteria fibrosis occurs in 5 to 10 per cent of patients treated with busulphan, but pathological and cytological evidence suggest lung toxicity in much higher proportions. Similarly, the increasing use of CT scanning shows an appreciably higher prevalence than found in surveys which relied on plain chest radiography. The frequency of overt lung involvement may also be related to length of survival, as determined by the primary disease. With busulphan, the average interval between starting treatment and the appearance of toxic effects can be as long as 4 years, and in some cases the lung changes appear to progress after the drug has been discontinued. With carmustine (BCNU) it has recently been shown that pulmonary fibrosis may be first recognized several years after treatment has finished. Other factors which may increase the toxicity of a given drug include advanced age of the patient and synergistic effects with other drugs, with radiation to the lung, or with subsequent inhalation of high oxygen concentrations.

Histologically, most cytotoxic drugs produce evidence of diffuse alveolar damage with destruction of lining cells, formation of hyaline membranes, and a variable inflammatory infiltrate and degree of fibrosis.

Fibrosis is particularly common with busulphan and bleomycin and rare with methotrexate. With methotrexate and procarbazine (and very occasionally with bleomycin) there may be blood and tissue eosinophilia and correspondingly a good therapeutic response to steroids.

Eosinophilic reactions in the lung include conditions which would be classified as Löffler's syndrome, simple or prolonged pulmonary eosinophilia, and eosinophilic pneumonia. Tissue eosinophilia is a more consistent feature than peripheral blood eosinophilia. Historically, sulphonamides have been the drugs most frequently reported as causes of pulmonary eosinophilia; reactions have even occurred to a vaginal cream containing sulphonamide. Sulphonamide sensitivity may also explain some of the reactions to sulphasalazine and to chlorpropamide which is chemically related. The pulmonary eosinophilia recorded with aspirin appears to be distinct from aspirin-induced asthma. Nitrofurantoin may produce an acute eosinophilic reaction in addition to more insidious fibrosis. The roles of gold salts and penicillamine in this type of reaction have been a matter of some debate, but the evidence suggests that both can provoke a reaction. However, the suggestion that drugs may be responsible for many of the cases of fibrosing alveolitis associated with rheumatoid arthritis seems unlikely. Penicillamine has been incriminated in two other types of adverse pulmonary reaction: firstly Goodpasture's syndrome with pulmonary haemorrhage when used in high doses in treatment of Wilson's disease, and secondly obliterative bronchiolitis, an unusual form of airway obstruction which is seen occasionally in patients with rheumatoid arthritis. The evidence against penicillamine in the latter case is not conclusive.

The clinical severity of eosinophilic reactions is very variable, ranging from a transient and asymptomatic radiographic opacity to a severe illness with dyspnoea, cough, fever, and hypoxaemia due to widespread eosinophilic pneumonia. Concomitant asthma has been noted in particular with carbamazepine, but is not otherwise a common feature. The chest radiograph shows fluffy opacities, frequently with peripheral or predominantly upper-lobe distribution. The reactions are often accompanied by a diffuse maculopapular skin eruption. The prognosis is usually good: the changes often subside spontaneously on withdrawal of the drug; in more severely ill patients there is usually a dramatic improvement on instituting treatment with corticosteroids. Although repeated exposure to the offending agents continues to produce reactions, the severity of these may progressively decrease.

Pulmonary vascular reactions

Pulmonary thromboembolism related to use of the contraceptive pill is well established; its frequency correlates with the oestrogen content and has been reduced since the introduction of low oestrogen preparations.

Fig. 1 Histological specimen of the lung of a patient who died from amiodarone pulmonary toxicity: (a) alveolar wall thickening and organizing intra-alveolar exudate; (b) higher power view of alveolar exudate showing characteristic 'foamy' macrophages. (Reproduced from Adams *et al.* (1986). *Quarterly Journal of Medicine,* **59,** 449–71, with permission.)

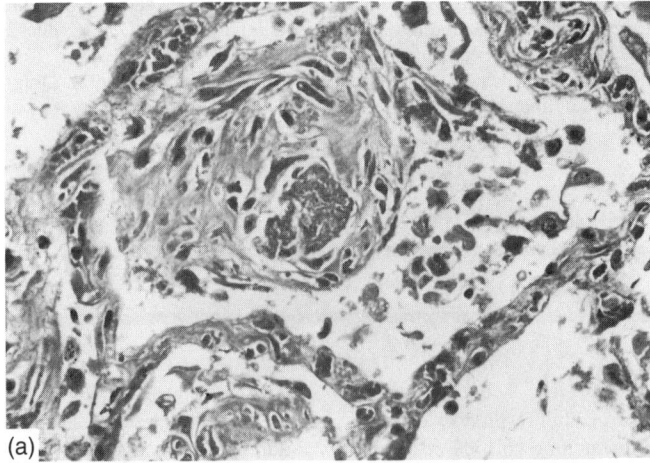

(a)

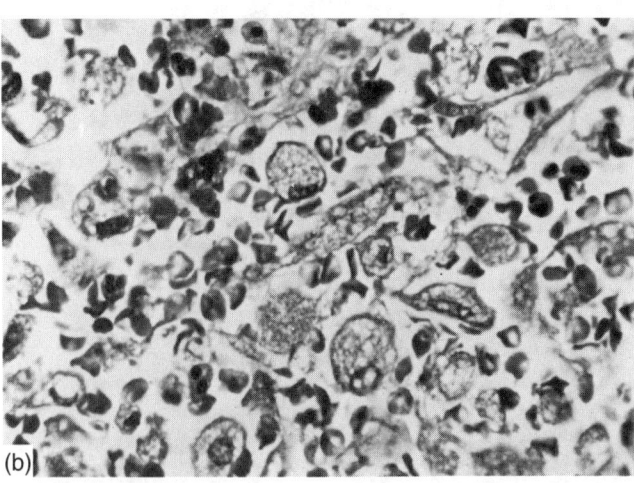

(b)

The statistical association between pulmonary hypertension and the use of the anorectic agent aminorex in Switzerland, Germany, and Austria in the 1960s was of great theoretical interest. When the drug was withdrawn, the epidemic of pulmonary hypertension subsided and no similar rise was seen in countries which did not introduce this agent. Occasional cases of pulmonary hypertension have been reported in patients taking various amphetamine-like drugs, but the evidence is not conclusive.

Analgesics given during labour have been implicated in the development of pulmonary hypertension in the newborn; drugs such as aspirin, indomethacin, and naproxen delay premature labour but, by their inhibitory effects on prostaglandin synthesis, may also cause constriction of the ductus arteriosus *in utero* leading to postnatal pulmonary hypertension and respiratory distress.

Pleura and mediastinum

Hilar and mediastinal adenopathy are occasionally seen as part of the generalized lymphadenopathy produced by the anticonvulsant phenytoin, and mediastinal lipomatosis has been reported in patients on large doses of steroids.

Drugs which have been associated with pleural reactions (fluid or thickening) are shown in Table 3. Several agents have been reported to produce a systemic-lupus-like syndrome (see Chapter 18.11.3). The anti-arrhythmic procainamide is most often implicated, but other agents include gold, hydralazine, isoniazid, penicillamine, and sulphonamides. The main respiratory target structure in this syndrome is the pleura, but (as with methysergide and bromocriptine) there is often some fibrosis of subjacent areas of the lung.

The now obsolete selective β-sympathetic antagonist practolol produced a characteristic 'oculomucocutaneous' syndrome. This syndrome differed from systemic lupus erythematosus in that lupus cells were not usually present and ocular symptoms are not usually a feature of drug-induced systemic lupus erythematosus. Pleural effusions and subsequent pleural thickening occurred in association with characteristic corneal ulceration, discoid rash, and fibrinous peritonitis. Patients with practolol-induced pleurisy sometimes developed effusions months or years after discontinuing the drug. In some the chronic changes led to significant respiratory disability. Minor degrees of pulmonary involvement were reported in some patients, but the predominant abnormality was related to the pleural surface. Other β-sympathetic antagonists, in particular acebutolol, have been reported as occasionally causing an alveolar or pleural reaction, but it seems unlikely that other β-blockers cause the full-blown and severe 'practolol syndrome'.

Methysergide, which is used in treatment of the carcinoid syndrome and occasionally for migraine, may induce mediastinal or pleural fibrosis with or without retroperitoneal fibrosis. Improvement follows early withdrawal of the drug. Bromocriptine has some structural similarities to methysergide and can also produce chronic pleural effusions and thickening. The pleural fluid characteristically contains a high proportion of lymphocytes. The frequency of this reaction is uncertain, but it may be relatively common. Methotrexate has been associated with pleurisy, independent of its alveolar effects. The smooth-muscle relaxant dantrolene, which is used for relief of spasticity, has been reported to produce an unusual type of pleurisy with effusion in which fluid and blood eosinophilia are prominent. There is no evidence of any parenchymal abnormality, and although the changes gradually resolve on withdrawing the drug, some residual pleural fibrosis may remain.

Table 3 *Drugs associated with pleural reactions*

Drug-induced lupus	Procainamide
Oculomucocutaneous syndrome	Hydralazine etc.
Isolated	Practolol
	Methysergide
	Dantrolene
	Methotrexate
	Bromocriptine

Complications of radiographic and other procedures

Lipoid pneumonia may follow bronchography with oily media. This is an oleogranulomatous reaction which can progress to fibrosis and may sometimes produce a localized mass simulating a neoplasm. Similar reactions can follow aspiration of oily medicines (e.g. laxatives) into the lungs.

Lymphangiographic media which drain through the thoracic duct, and so into the venous circulation, enter and can impact in the pulmonary circulation. This is often symptomless, but may cause dyspnoea and cough with the expectoration of fat globules or haemoptysis. The chest radiograph shows a fine stippling and occasional deaths have been recorded.

Pleural effusion and, less commonly, mediastinitis occur following endoscopic sclerotherapy of oesophageal varices. The symptoms usually subside within a few days.

REFERENCES

Cooper, J.A.D. (1990). Drug-induced pulmonary disease. *Clinics in Chest Medicine*, **11**, 1–194.

Gibson, G.J. (1990). Adverse pulmonary effects of drugs and radiation In: *Respiratory medicine* (ed R.A.L. Brewis, G.J. Gibson, and D.M. Geddes), pp. 1149–64. Baillière Tindall, London.

Rosenow, E.C., Myers, J.L., Swensen, S.J., and Pisani, R.J. (1992). Drug-induced pulmonary disease. An update. *Chest*, **102**, 239–50.

Fig. 2 Chest radiograph of a second patient with amiodarone pulmonary toxicity showing confluent alveolar shadowing in both upper lobes. (Reproduced from Adams *et al.* (1986). *Quarterly Journal of Medicine*, **59**, 449–71, with permission.)

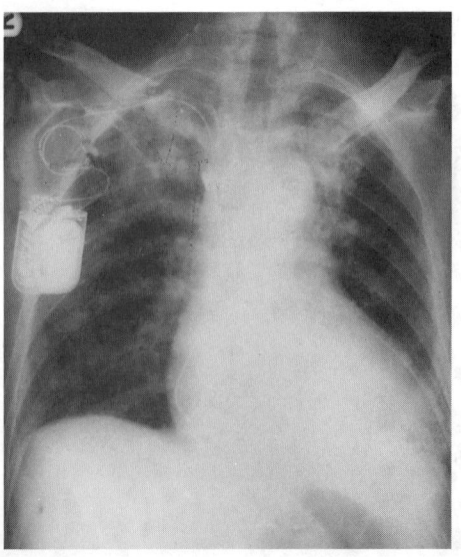

17.10.20 Adult respiratory distress syndrome

C. GARRARD AND P. FOËX

Introduction

The term adult respiratory distress syndrome is used to describe a severe life-threatening episode of respiratory failure which occurs in subjects with previously healthy lungs and without primary left ventricular failure. It is associated with a large number of unrelated clinical disorders, but has uniform physiological, radiological, and pathological features. The name was introduced by Ashbaugh in 1967 because of the morphological similarities to the neonatal respiratory distress syndrome.

Although major trauma, acute hypovolaemia, hypotensive Gram-negative septicaemia, and severe microbial pulmonary infections are the most frequent precursors of adult respiratory distress syndrome, they form only part of a large number of non-cardiogenic associated disorders (Table 1). An inciting event can be assigned in about 80 per cent of cases of adult respiratory distress syndrome, and often this is non-pulmonary.

Incidence

The Division of Lung Disease Task Force estimated that 150 000 cases occurred annually in the United States, an incidence of 0.6 per 1000 population, accounting for about 5 per cent of all admissions to intensive therapy units. A prospective epidemiological study of 34 872 patients admitted to three university hospitals in the United States revealed the overall incidence of adult respiratory distress syndrome to be 0.25 per cent of all hospital admissions.

Clinical presentation

Since adult respiratory distress syndrome may be caused by a variety of direct and indirect lung insults, its development varies in time and intensity, but the morphological and symptomatic changes that occur have led to the recognition of a sequential progression of events.

Phase 1

In this period, unless there has been direct pulmonary damage, the lungs are clear to auscultation and the lung fields of the chest radiograph may be unremarkable. There may be significant changes in intravascular volume, many occurring as a result of therapy. The patient with sepsis syndrome may be undergoing fluid resuscitation, while the patient with haemorrhagic shock will probably be receiving a large blood transfusion. The metabolic and acid base status will also, to a significant degree, depend upon treatment. For example, excessive use of bicarbonate, loss of chloride in gastric contents, and oxidation of citrate in transfused blood may produce a metabolic alkalosis which may be further aggravated by a respiratory component following hyperventilation in response to pain.

Phase 2

This is a period of 24 to 72 h' duration when the patient may be deceptively haemodynamically stable with no obvious respiratory distress except mild tachypnoea. However, serial blood gas analysis at this time may reveal subclinical hypoxaemia due to intrapulmonary shunting.

Phase 3

During this period the hypoxaemia worsens with an increasing intrapulmonary shunt. The patient becomes clinically cyanosed and dyspnoeic. The chest compliance falls, increasing the work of breathing, and high inflation pressures are required if the patient is mechanically ventilated. The chest radiograph may reveal the classical picture of widespread bilateral intra-alveolar and interstitial infiltrates which become progressively more confluent, although sparing the costophrenic angles and apices. Increasing hypoxaemia produces disturbed cerebral and renal function, and unless management reverses the course of the disease, the final phase is entered.

Table 1 *Disorders associated with adult respiratory distress syndrome*

Hypovolaemic shock Haemorrhage
Infection Pulmonary (microbial, fungal, pneumocystis, malaria) Extrapulmonary (sepsis syndrome)
Trauma Thoracic Extrathoracic Burns
Embolism Fat Amniotic fluid Cellular aggregates

Inhalation
Gas
    Irritant (e.g. chlorine, smoke)
    Non-irritant (e.g. oxygen)
Liquid
    Gastric juice
    Fresh and salt water

Haematological Disseminated intravascular coagulopathy Massive blood transfusion
Metabolic Diabetic ketosis Uraemia
Neurogenic Cerebral oedema Intracranial haemorrhage
Drugs Heroin, aspirin, propoxyphene, barbiturates, paraquat,   protamine, etc.
Other Pancreatitis High altitude

Phase 4

Refractory hypoxaemia develops with increasing pulmonary hypertension and right ventricular dysfunction in up to 50 per cent of patients. Hypercapnia and organ hypoperfusion contribute to a mixed respiratory and metabolic acidosis and multiorgan failure may follow.

Pathology

Despite the heterogeneity of initiating conditions leading to adult respiratory distress syndrome, there is homogeneity of the morphological changes found in the lung at autopsy. Macroscopically, it may be heavy, red, and liver-like, or light, grey, and fibrous, depending on whether the disease has been of short or long duration. In patients who have undergone prolonged periods of mechanical ventilation, fibrocystic changes may be apparent. Microscopically two phases can be distinguished.

Acute exudative phase

Interstitial oedema is accompanied by damage to and necrosis of capillary endothelial and alveolar type 1 epithelial cells. Fibrin and platelet thrombi develop in the capillaries and there is adherence of leucocytes to areas denuded of endothelium. Later, the oedema becomes perivascular, peribronchial, and intra-alveolar in distribution, and is accompanied by focal alveolar haemorrhages. The damaged type 1 alveolar cells, together with fibrin and other plasma proteins, constitute the characteristic hyaline membrane which lines the alveoli, alveolar ducts, and some respiratory bronchioles.

Chronic proliferative phase

There is regeneration of the capillary endothelium and alveolar epithelium accompanied by interstitial infiltration with lymphocytes, fibroblasts, and deposition of collagen which may proceed to fibrosis. The damaged type 1 alveolar cells are replaced by more granular type 2 alveolar cells, which are often cuboidal in shape, producing a hyperplastic appearance with a thickening of the air–blood interface. The alveolar lining of surfactant, normally produced by these cells, is absent.

Pathogenesis

A finding in all patients with adult respiratory distress syndrome, whether the initiating cause is mediated by the bloodstream or the airways, is an increase in total lung water caused by a disturbance of the normal fluid flux between the intravascular and extravascular compartments in the lung. The factors governing the normal distribution of lung water are expressed by the Starling equation:

$$F = K (P_{cap} - P_{is}) - \phi(\pi_{cap} - \pi_{is}),$$

where F is the net filtration rate, K is the filtration coefficient, P_{cap} and P_{is} are the capillary and interstitial hydrostatic pressures respectively, π_{cap} and π_{is} are the capillary and plasma protein osmotic pressures respectively, and ϕ is the protein reflection coefficient. Normally the outward transcapillary hydrostatic pressure difference slightly exceeds the inward transcapillary protein osmotic pressure difference, producing a continuous flow of water and solutes. In adult respiratory distress syndrome, interstitial lung water increases, exceeding the capacity of the lymphatic drainage and producing intra-alveolar pulmonary oedema and intrapulmonary venous admixture.

Plasma protein osmotic pressure

In trauma and acute illness, there is often a reduction in plasma protein concentration and oncotic pressure which may be further reduced by crystalloid infusion. In addition, an interstitial loss of osmotically active material may occur as the plasma protein osmotic pressure falls. Reductions in plasma protein concentration lower the threshold at which pulmonary capillary hydrostatic changes become significant.

Lymph drainage

The normal lymph drainage is only 25 to 30 ml/h, but this can increase 20-fold in response to relatively small changes in interstitial pressure from fluid accumulation. High intrathoracic pressures during intermittent positive pressure ventilation or high levels of positive end expiratory volume may impair this function but they are unlikely to play a primary role in the genesis of interstitial oedema in adult respiratory distress syndrome.

Pulmonary capillary permeability and hydrostatic pressure

Although stress-evoked stimulation of the sympathetic nervous system in the critically ill will produce pulmonary venoconstriction and pulmonary hypertension, increased pulmonary vascular permeability with increased postcapillary resistance is largely responsible for the increase in lung water. Fluid obtained from the airways of patients with adult

respiratory distress syndrome has a higher protein content than that from normal subjects or from patients with cardiogenic pulmonary oedema. In animal experiments, lymph collected from chronically implanted fistulae increases both in amount and protein content following endotoxin-induced shock. By using radioisotope-labelled tracers such as ^{123}I-albumin or [99]Tc[m]-albumin a transmicrovascular flux of protein can be demonstrated, indicating increased endothelial permeability. The cause of this increased permeability has been the focus of much research and speculation.

Neutrophils, complement activation, and cytokines

There is mounting evidence suggesting that the neutrophil plays a key role in the pathogenesis of adult respiratory distress syndrome. In sheep, there is a neutropenia within 60 min of endotoxin infusion, correlating with the subsequent hypoxaemia. The high flow and high protein content of lymph following the endotoxin injection can be attenuated by previously rendering the animal neutropenic. In humans, radiolabelled neutrophils can be seen by lung scan to sequester in the lungs of patients with adult respiratory distress syndrome with increased numbers demonstrable in bronchoalveolar lavage. The mechanism by which neutrophils microembolize in the pulmonary circulation probably involves the alternative pathway activation of complement with the release of neutrophil-aggregating components, particularly C5a. In experimental animals, immobilization of the pulmonary microcirculation and a pulmonary capillary leak can be induced by infusion of activated complement. In humans, clinical causes of adult respiratory distress syndrome such as endotoxaemia, trauma, and pulmonary infection are also known to activate the complement cascade, and elevated levels of C5a have been claimed as a predictor for the development of the syndrome in the critically ill.

The neutrophil is well equipped to induce injury in the lung. Intracellular granules can release proteinases such as elastase, collagenase, and cathepsin which, by degrading structural components such as elastin, collagen, basement membranes, and fibronectin, can lead to disorganization of the interstitium and damage to capillary endothelial and alveolar epithelial cells. Proteinases may also cleave fibrinogen, the Hageman factor, complement, and the other plasma proteins, producing further embolization by blood constituents such as platelets, mast cells, fibrin, and fibrinogen degradation products which is often demonstrable by balloon-occluded segmental pulmonary angiography. Their presence is enhanced by deficiency of opsonic fibronectin, impairing the phagocytic function of the reticuloendothelial system. Histamine, platelet-activated factor, serotonin, bradykinin, and other vasoactive substances may be released by these immobilized blood products, contributing to the permeability and hydrostatic pressure changes in the pulmonary microcirculation. The activated neutrophils may also be responsible for oxidant damage to the lung by the excessive generation of highly toxic oxygen radical molecules. The free radical superoxide (O_2^-) can participate in several chemical reactions, yielding hydrogen peroxide (H_2O_2) and the extremely cytotoxic hydroxyl radical (OH^-). These molecules are normally used in a protective role against bacteria but, by overwhelming the antioxidant defence mechanisms such as superoxide dismutase, they act by destroying intracellular enzyme systems and cell-wall structure of both the pulmonary capillary endothelial and alveolar epithelial cells. The toxic oxygen radical molecules can do further damage, inactivating enzyme inhibitors such as α_1-antitrypsin, thus encouraging proteinase activity. Free oxygen radicals attack polyunsaturated fatty acids, and the peroxidation process results in the loss of the functional integrity of the cell membrane associated with an acute increase in the permeability of alveolar capillaries. In addition, the ability of neutrophils to generate hydrogen peroxide *in vitro* correlates well with increased plasma levels of tumour necrosis factor α (**TNF**). This suggests that TNF-primed neutrophils may play a role in the pathogenesis of adult respiratory distress syndrome associated with lung injury.

The role of TNF in septic adult respiratory distress syndrome may be explained by a succession of events. Endotoxin may cause the release of TNF from stimulated macrophages. The released TNF in turn activates neutrophils. In neutropenic states, there is not enough elastase to inhibit the action of TNF so that direct tissue injury may occur as well as injury mediated by neutrophil activation. Moreover, TNF induces the production of interleukin 1 (**IL-1**) by vascular endothelium, appears to stimulate macrophages to activate chemotaxis, and stimulates the degranulation of polymorphonuclear neutrophil leucocytes. TNF levels in bronchoalveolar fluid from patients with adult respiratory distress syndrome are substantially elevated, while they are normal in plasma. Similarly, IL-1 is elevated in bronchial fluid but not in plasma of patients with adult respiratory distress syndrome. This suggests that stimulated lung macrophages can produce more TNF than peripheral blood monocytes. This may favour adherence of polymorphonuclear neutrophil leucocytes in lung capillaries and contribute to transendothelial passage of these cells, proteins, and fluid.

Although there are strong arguments to implicate TNF and IL-1 in the pathophysiology of adult respiratory distress syndrome, any therapeutic advantage from the use of antagonists or antibodies against endotoxin, TNF, or IL-1 has still to be established. There is some evidence that pretreatment with inhibitors of platelet-activating factor (**PAF**) reduces the pulmonary hypertension seen in a TNF-induced animal model of adult respiratory distress syndrome. Clinically significant effects of PAF antagonists in human adult respiratory distress syndrome have yet to be demonstrated.

Coagulation and fibrinolytic function

It is highly likely that abnormalities in coagulation and fibrinolysis contribute to the pathogenesis of adult respiratory distress syndrome. Disturbance of the homeostatic balance between procoagulant and fibrinolytic activity has been demonstrated in the bronchoalveolar lavage fluid from the lungs of patients with adult respiratory distress syndrome. Increased procoagulant activity associated with depressed fibrinolytic activity in these patients encourage fibrin deposition in the lung, while increased alveolar capillary permeability allows the fibrinogen substrate to enter the alveolar airspace.

Arachidonic acid metabolism

The lung is an important organ in arachidonic acid metabolism. There is increasing evidence that the metabolites may be involved in the pathogenesis of ARDS. They are released from cell-membrane phospholipid not only by activated neutrophils, but also by mast cells, platelets, and complement-dependent mechanisms. Two functionally active groups of substances, the prostaglandins and the leukotrienes, are produced by separate metabolic pathways (Fig. 1).

Oxidative metabolism of arachidonic acid by the cyclo-oxygenase pathway sequentially produces two cyclic endoperoxides (PGG_2 and PGH_2). These intermediate prostaglandins are rapidly converted by specific enzymes into diverse vasoactive products, the most important being thromboxane A_2 (TXA_2), an intense pulmonary vasoconstrictor and platelet aggregator, and prostacyclin (PGI_2) an antiaggregator and pulmonary vasodilator substance. A disturbance in the normal metabolic balance in favour of thromboxane A_2 could result in pulmonary capillary hypertension by postcapillary vasoconstriction and mechanical obstruction by microaggregates. Increased prostacyclin production may increase intrapulmonary shunting by preventing the normal hypoxic pulmonary vasoconstriction. In experimental animals, it has been found that pretreatment with cyclo-oxygenase inhibitors such as indomethacin or meclofenamate can abolish endotoxin-induced pulmonary hypertension, although the increased pulmonary vascular permeability is unchanged.

The alternative lipoxygenase pathway of arachidonic acid metabolism produces several groups of metabolites depending on the source of the lipoxygenase enzyme. Leukotriene B_4 is a potent neutrophil chemotaxin, while leukotrienes C_4 and D_4 are the main constituents of the slow-

reacting substance of anaphylaxis (SRS-A) which, in the lung, can produce bronchoconstriction, microvascular vasoconstriction, and increased capillary permeability. The pathogenesis of adult respiratory distress syndrome involves interrelated immune, coagulation, and biochemical responses which, although producing similar endstage manifestations, probably employ differing pathways depending on the specific aetiology. A simplified sequence of the mechanisms involved is shown in Fig. 2.

Role of surfactant

Pulmonary surfactant is synthesized and secreted from alveolar type 2 cells. It reduces surface tension in the lung and prevents lung collapse at resting transpulmonary pressures. The major components of surfactant are phospholipids (85 per cent), neutral lipids, and at least three specific proteins SP-A, SP-B, and SP-C. Saturated phosphatidylcholine is the main surface-active component. SP-A is the major surfactant protein. It binds phosphatidylcholine and regulates the metabolic pathways of secretion and uptake of surfactant between type 2 pneumocytes and alveolar space. The surface film formed originally from phosphatidylcholine is composed essentially of a monolayer of dipalmitoylphosphatidylcholine. As the surface area varies with the respiratory cycle, there is continual turnover of surfactant material.

By lowering the surface tension, the surfactant allows collapsed alveoli to open at lower inspiratory pressures and to maintain alveolar size. In adult respiratory distress syndrome, alveolar instability results in atelectasis, ventilation–perfusion inequalities, and intrapulmonary shunting. As pulmonary compliance is also reduced, the work of breathing is increased. In turn, higher airway pressures are needed to maintain gas exchange in patients needing artificial ventilation. This increases the risk of barotrauma.

Fig. 1 Pathogenesis of adult respiratory distress syndrome: arachidonic acid metabolism

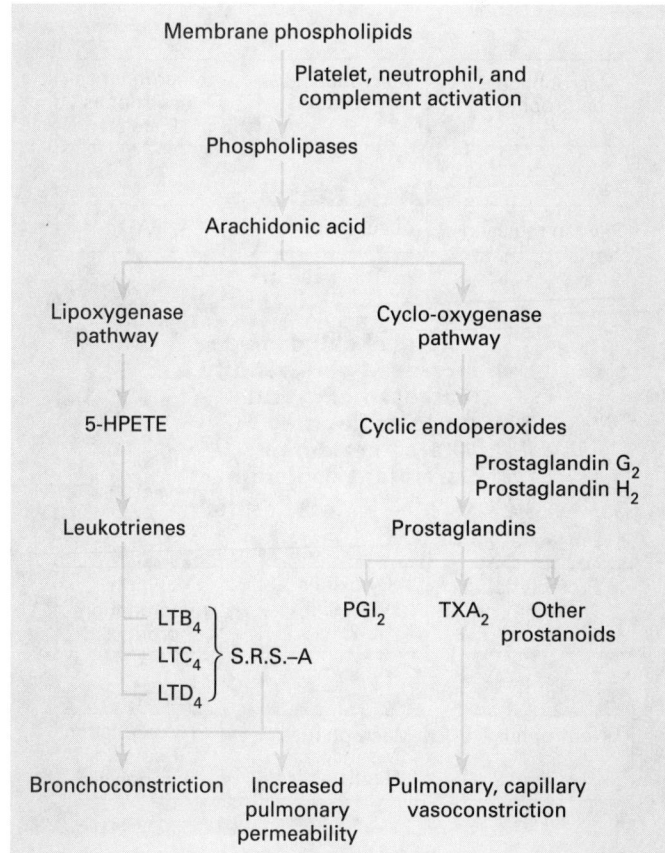

Surfactant function (samples collected from bronchoalveolar lavage) is impaired early in patients with adult respiratory distress syndrome, with a significant correlation between surfactant function and severity of lung dysfunction. Surfactant inactivation may also play a role. Proteins compete with surfactant for the surface of the alveoli and may interfere with monolayer formation. This phenomenon may be of little importance when surfactant concentration is high. However, protein inactivation may play a major role when surfactant concentration is low. In addition, lipid peroxidation products, including oxygen radicals, may interfere with the normal surface activity of surfactant. Phospholipases can interfere with surfactant function by decreasing alveolar lipid levels and by generating products which interfere with the surface properties of surfactant.

Surfactant increases macrophage migration and phagocytosis, enhancing the killing of bacteria. Therefore surfactant deficiency in adult respiratory distress syndrome may decrease host defence. Moreover, the movement of the surface film during expiration may facilitate the migration of particulate matter from the alveoli so that it can be transported by the mucociliary system. This would be inhibited in surfactant deficiencies.

While exogenous surfactant administration is effective in neonates with respiratory distress syndrome, there is limited clinical experience in adult respiratory distress syndrome. However, initial controlled studies and anecdotal evidence suggest that surfactant therapy may be useful in selected groups of patients with adult respiratory distress syndrome. Both instillation of boluses and administration as aerosols have been used.

Physiological features

Abnormalities of pulmonary function correlate well with the pathological changes.

Fig. 2 A summary of the pathogenesis of adult respiratory distress syndrome.

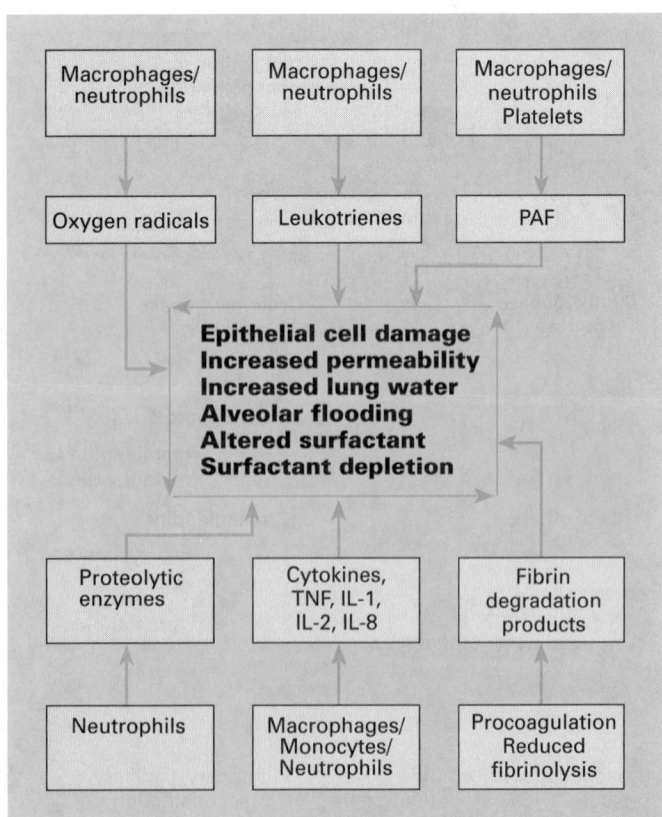

Reduced compliance and lung volume

The stiffness of the lung is determined directly by tissue elasticity and alveolar surface tension and indirectly by lung volume. In adult respiratory distress syndrome, altered surfactant production and function result in alveolar instability and diffuse microatelectasis. All lung volumes are reduced. Physiologically, the most important is the functional residual capacity (**FRC**) which, if greatly reduced, produces small airway closure during expiration, with air trapping in the distal alveoli. Subsequent absorption atelectasis produces more reduction in lung compliance and further impairs gas exchange. However, increased lung stiffness and reduced lung volume are not the result of homogenous mechanical abnormalities. The lungs of patients with adult respiratory distress syndrome can be divided into areas that are infiltrated, consolidated, or collapsed (poorly aerated and poorly compliant), and regions with near normal levels of compliance and ventilation. In the early stages of adult respiratory distress syndrome, these regions are not fixed and changes in posture alter their distribution. Later in the disease, functional alterations become fixed.

Alterations in gas exchange

A major feature of adult respiratory distress syndrome is an inability to maintain arterial oxygen tensions without the administration of toxic concentrations of inspired oxygen F_{IO_2}. Three mechanisms operate in producing this hypoxaemia.

Perfusion of underventilated alveoli (*V/Q* mismatch) The fluid accumulation in the lung progresses from an interstitial to a peribronchial distribution before alveolar flooding occurs. Narrowing of the small airways results in a large number of alveoli, particularly in the dependent lung zones, with a reduced but finite *V/Q* ratio.

Perfusion of non-ventilated alveoli (*true shunt*) The normal physiological shunt (3–5 per cent of the cardiac output) is produced by small intrapulmonary arteriovenous anastomoses, together with the bronchial and Thebesian circulation. In adult respiratory distress syndrome the intrapulmonary shunt can increase to 60 to 70 per cent of cardiac output, partly by a few direct arteriovenous anastomoses opening up but mainly by perfusion of non-ventilated alveoli. This is associated with the loss of hypoxic vasoconstriction.

Impaired diffusion In addition to thickening of the alveolar capillary septum, there is a reduced capillary blood volume with decreased transit time.

The relative contributions of these three mechanisms are variable and not easily assessed. If true shunt rather than *V/Q* mismatch was the main contributor, increasing F_{IO_2} would not alter the shunt whereas theoretically it would lessen the contribution made by the alveoli with a low but finite *V/Q* ratio. In practice, however, increasing F_{IO_2} has a variable effect on the shunt not only in different patients, but also in the same patient during different phases of the disease. The usual response to very high F_{IO_2} is an increase in intrapulmonary shunt—an active response which may be found in patients with adult respiratory distress syndrome. This active response appears to be associated with a more favourable prognosis than a fixed shunt uninfluenced by increasing F_{IO_2}.

Increased work of breathing

In spontaneous breathing patients, an increase in the ratio V_D/V_T of dead space to tidal volume may be seen, particularly with microembolization of the pulmonary capillaries. The increased effort required to keep the arterial carbon dioxide tension normal and the reduced lung compliance can lead to respiratory failure unless respiration is mechanically assisted.

Table 2 *Criteria for diagnosis of adult respiratory distress syndrome*

Characteristic chest radiograph
Hypoxaemia
Reduced lung compliance
Pulmonary hypertension (>30/15 mmHg)
Pulmonary capillary wedge pressure <18 mmHg
High protein pulmonary oedema

Table 3 *Adult respiratory distress syndrome lung injury score*

Chest roentgenogram score	
No alveolar consolidation	0
Alveolar consolidation confined to one quadrant	1
Alveolar consolidation confined to two quadrants	2
Alveolar consolidation confined to three quadrants	3
Alveolar consolidation in all four quadrants	4
Hypoxaemia score		
Pao_2/Fio_2	>300	0
Pao_2/Fio_2	225–299	1
Pao_2/Fio_2	175–224	2
Pao_2/Fio_2	100–174	3
Pao_2/Fio_2	<100	4
(Pao_2 in mmHg, for kPa units divide by 7.5)		
PEEP score (when ventilated)		
PEEP	≤5 cmH_2O	0
PEEP	6–8 cmH_2O	1
PEEP	9–11 cmH_2O	2
PEEP	12–14 cmH_2O	3
PEEP	≥15 cmH_2O	4
Respiratory system compliance score (when available)		
Compliance	≥80 ml/cmH_2O	0
Compliance	60–79 ml/cmH_2O	1
Compliance	40–59 ml/cmH_2O	2
Compliance	20–39 ml/cmH_2O	3
Compliance	≤19 ml/cmH_2O	4

The final value is obtained by dividing the aggregate sum by the number of components that were used.
No lung injury 0
Mild to moderate lung injury 0.1–2.5
Severe lung injury >2.5

Reproduced from Murray *et al.* (1988). *American Review of Respiratory Disease*, **138**, 720–3, with permission.

Pulmonary hypertension and right ventricular failure

The mediators of the inflammatory reaction are also responsible for pulmonary vasoconstriction, platelet aggregation, microthrombosis, and direct tissue damage. This results in pulmonary hypertension. Pulmonary vasoconstriction reduces blood flow to the ventilated areas of the lungs and therefore contributes to the hypoxaemia.

Large increases in pulmonary artery pressure may cause right ventricular failure. Two mechanisms contribute to right ventricular failure. One is the pressure load: as the right ventricle is thin-walled, increases in afterload are poorly tolerated and may cause acute failure. The other mechanism is myocardial ischaemia. Coronary blood flow to the wall of the right ventricle occurs during both systole and diastole because of the large pressure difference between the aorta and the right ventricle throughout the cardiac cycle. In the face of pulmonary hypertension, particularly when aortic pressure is reduced, the pressure difference between the aorta and the right ventricle is substantially reduced and coronary flow to the wall of the right ventricle is decreased. In the face of a high pressure load, such a reduction in coronary blood flow may cause ischaemia even in the presence of normal coronary arteries. For this reason, administration of vasodilators may worsen the circulatory failure, while systemic vasoconstrictors may improve cardiac output.

Diagnosis and management

Adult respiratory distress syndrome should be suspected if acute respiratory failure (Pao_2 less than 6.7 kPa when breathing 60 per cent oxygen) occurs in association with a recognized precipitating cause and if the circulation is hyperdynamic with normal or slightly raised pulmonary capillary wedge pressure (less than 18 mmHg) and central venous pressure. Blood gas analysis may often reveal hypoxaemia due to intrapulmonary shunting before the classical radiological appearance of ARDS develops (Table 2).

Clearly, the criteria by which adult respiratory distress syndrome is defined will be reflected in the incidence, morbidity, and mortality reported in any particular series. Indeed, the observation in some series that mortality has changed little over the past two decades may reflect a trend towards a stricter definition. However, some recent reports suggest a decline in mortality, possibly related to improved methods of conventional mechanical ventilator support.

Attempts have been made to measure the relative severity of adult respiratory distress syndrome (Table 3). Although the severity scores are at best crude, they do allow some comparison to be made between different groups of patients and therefore have much to recommend them. It is evident that patients do not usually die of hypoxaemia but from the complex disturbances that result from multiple organ system failure. Thus the aim in the management of adult respiratory distress syndrome is to support all body systems until the integrity of the alveolar capillary membrane is restored.

Early recognition with appropriate pharmacological and supportive therapy favourably influences the prognosis, but unfortunately no simple laboratory test or bedside measurement accurately predicts the onset of this condition. The indices of pulmonary gas exchange and pulmonary compliance are not sufficiently sensitive to detect early interstitial oedema, becoming abnormal only when alveolar oedema occurs. Changes in lung volumes, particularly FRC, do occur earlier but are not applicable to bedside monitoring. Non-invasive methods of measuring lung water and permeability changes may prove to be useful in screening patients, but perhaps the most useful method of identifying incipient acute respiratory failure is by C5a assays, since high levels of C5a have been positively associated with the onset but not the severity of adult respiratory distress syndrome.

Chest radiograph

Radiographic appearances generally correlate poorly with the severity of adult respiratory distress syndrome and the degree of gas exchange impairment. Changes may range from localized infiltrates to diffuse widespread shadowing ('white-out'). Nodularity or cystic changes may be seen. Although there can be features which are more characteristic of cardiogenic versus non-cardiogenic pulmonary oedema, these are not sufficiently reliable as a basis for clinical management.

Ventilation and oxygenation
INTERMITTENT POSITIVE PRESSURE VENTILATION

If the arterial oxygen tension cannot be maintained above 6.5 kPa with an Fio_2 of 0.5 in the spontaneously breathing patient, intubation and ventilatory support are generally indicated. A guide to indications for intubation and mechanical ventilation is shown in Table 4.

The ventilator selected to support the patient should have the facility to deliver the basic modes of ventilation, control mechanical ventilation,

Table 4 *Guidelines for the introduction of mechanical ventilation*

Inadequate ventilation

Indicated by:

Apnoea, upper airway obstruction, unprotected airway
Respiratory rate >35 breaths/min (normal range 10–20
 breaths/min)
Vital capacity <15 ml/kg (normal range 65–75 ml/kg)
Tidal volume <5 ml/kg (normal range 5–7 ml/kg)
Negative inspiratory force <25 cmH$_2$O (normal range 75–
 100 cmH$_2$O)
PaCO$_2$ > 8 kPa (60 mmHg) (normal range 4.7–6.3 kPa)
V_D/V_T > 0.6 (normal range < 0.3)

Inadequate gas exchange and oxygenation

Indicated by:

PaO$_2$ < 8 kPa (60 mmHg) on FiO$_2$ ≥ 0.6
D(A-a)O$_2$ on FiO$_2$ 1.0 > 47 kPa (350 mmHg) (normal range
 3.3–8.7 kPa)

After Pontoppidan *et al.* (1972). *New England Journal of Medicine*, **42**, 45–55.

Table 5 *Factors affecting peak and mean airway pressure during mechanical ventilation*

Ventilator related
Tidal volume
Inspiratory flow rate
Positive end expiratory volume and continuous positive airways
 pressure
Inspiratory hold
Expiratory retard

Patient related
Compliance of respiratory system
Airways obstruction
Pleural effusion
Pneumothorax
Bronchial obstruction
Elevation of diaphragm by abdominal contents
Fighting the ventilator

assist control, synchronized intermittent mandatory ventilation, and pressure support. The best mode of ventilation is not known, but selection should be based upon which achieves ventilation goals for the lowest peak and mean airway pressure. Above all, constant vigilance is required to adjust the ventilator in the face of changing lung mechanics. Table 5 summarizes the major factors that will influence mean and peak airway pressure.

The optimal mechanical ventilation strategy appears to be low volume pressure-limited ventilation with permissive hypercapnia. In an uncontrolled series of adult respiratory distress syndrome patients managed with this technique a mortality of 16 per cent was reported, although no comment was made on the pulmonary function of survivors. By limiting peak inspiratory pressures to less than 40 mmHg and accepting PaCO$_2$ values in the range 9–15 kPa the risks of barotrauma and the adverse circulatory effects of positive pressure ventilation can be largely avoided.

Barotrauma can present in several ways. A small pneumothorax, pneumomediastinum, or pneumopericardium may be detected on a routine chest radiograph. A pneumothorax always requires urgent tube thoracostomy drainage and a pneumopericardium may impair cardiac function. Pneumomediastinum should alert the clinician to the possibility of a pneumothorax. It is the opinion of the authors that routine prophylactic bilateral tube thoracostomies should not be performed. In contrast, the sudden development of a tension pneumothorax in the mechanically ventilated patient is a medical emergency requiring immediate drainage. Initially, a 14 gauge cannula inserted in the second rib interspace in the mid-clavicular line on the appropriate side may buy time until a thoracostomy tube can be inserted. There is rarely time to obtain a confirmatory chest radiograph, and the diagnosis of pneumothorax is usually established on clinical grounds. Deteriorating blood gases, with increasing airway and central venous pressures, should alert the clinician to the possibility of a tension pneumothorax. The thoracostomy tube should only be inserted finally under direct vision using blunt dissection to enter the pleural space. Thoracostomy tubes must never be inserted using chisel-ended stilets since the risk of injuring the underlying lung is considerable. In severe and protracted cases of adult respiratory distress syndrome, multiple thoracostomies may be needed over a period of months. Should the patient survive, multiple loculated pneumothoraces may persist a year after the event.

Hypoxaemia will rarely be reversed by intermittent positive respiratory ventilation alone, and other manoeuvres designed to increase FRC and improve oxygenation are usually required.

POSITIVE END EXPIRATORY PRESSURE AND CONTINUOUS POSITIVE AIRWAY PRESSURE

The beneficial effects of positive end expiratory volume and continuous positive airway pressure are produced by an increase in FRC and a decrease in intrapulmonary shunting derived by recruitment of lung units previously unavailable for gas exchange. The compliance of the lung may also be improved by an increase in the lung volume and surfactant conservation. However, its benefits are limited by cardiac output changes and the dangers of barotrauma such as pneumothorax, pneumomediastinum, and surgical emphysema. Although modest levels of positive end expiratory volume (5–10 cmH$_2$O) are unlikely to reduce cardiac output, more precise information can be obtained by thermodilution cardiac output measurements. Alternatively, the assessment of mixed venous oxygen saturation S_vO_2 can be used: assuming an unchanged S_aO_2 and oxygen consumption, a fall in S_vO_2 would indicate a reduced cardiac output and oxygen delivery. High levels of positive end expiratory pressure (up to and exceeding 30 cmH$_2$O) have been advocated, with the cardiac output being maintained by volume loading and inotropic support, but the risk of barotrauma limits its use. More conventionally, a level of positive end expiratory pressure is selected which is compatible with an unchanged cardiac output or an unchanged static lung compliance.

A feature of the patient with adult respiratory distress syndrome is the extensive gravity-dependent lung collapse that is best visualized by CT scanning. To a large degree this is a consequence of nursing the patient for prolonged periods in the supine position. Sitting the patient as upright as possible minimizes the volume of dependent lung. In the persistently hypoxic patient, significant improvement in oxygenation can be obtained by rolling the patient prone every 6 to 8 h.

ASYNCHRONOUS INDEPENDENT LUNG VENTILATION

This technique employs a double lumen endobronchial tube with each limb connected to a separate ventilator, thus allowing optimum respiratory function to be obtained from each lung independently by varying ventilatory indices and inspired oxygen concentrations. Although the concept of asynchronous independent lung ventilation is attractive, in practice it demands a high degree of nursing care to preserve accurate tube placement and the duration is limited by the risk of trauma to the bronchial tree.

HIGH FREQUENCY VENTILATION

The traditional concepts of alveolar ventilation and dead space have been questioned by satisfactory gas exchange occurring at ventilatory 'frequencies' up to 40 Hz. High frequency ventilation can be divided into high frequency jet ventilation and high frequency oscillation depending on the speed of ventilation and the apparatus. The physical principles include enhancement of convection and accelerated diffusion of gas molecules. Ventilators with negligible compressible volumes are required and these, by delivering pulses of oxygen-enriched air, achieve efficient alveolar ventilation and gas exchange with low transpulmonary pressures and reflex inhibition of spontaneous respiration. Therefore the advantages are adequate blood gas exchange with lessened risk of barotrauma and minimal effects on pulmonary and systemic circulations. Humidification is difficult in clinical practice, and its role in the management of adult respiratory distress syndrome has yet to be fully assessed.

EXTRACORPOREAL LUNG ASSIST

The technical and physiological advances made in extracorporeal membrane oxygenation during open heart surgery led to the hope that, by using a similar technique with a membrane oxygenator, the lungs of patients with adult respiratory distress syndrome would have time to recover while oxygenation and perfusion of vital organs was maintained. Initial enthusiasm was tempered by the disappointing results of a randomized prospective multicentre trial in the United States, but it has been found to be effective in a relatively high proportion of children with unrelenting pulmonary failure. More attention has recently been paid to extracorporeal carbon dioxide removal using a large-area membrane lung with low extracorporeal blood flows (1–1.5 l/min) to remove carbon dioxide. A low minute volume (3 l/min) is added to prevent atelectasis, and oxygenation is maintained by delivering 300 ml oxygen/min directly into the trachea. The low intra-alveolar pressures, low ventilatory rates, and low inflation pressures avoid the adverse iatrogenic effects of conventional intermittent positive pressure ventilation. However, in a recent randomized and rigorously controlled study, extracorporeal carbon dioxide removal combined with low frequency positive pressure ventilation offered no advantage over conventional ventilation.

Even if extracorporeal lung assist techniques could be shown to be beneficial in adult respiratory distress syndrome, the haemorrhagic problems associated with extracorporeal circuits would probably limit their widespread use. An alternative approach uses an intracorporeal oxygenation device (IVOX®, Cardiopulmonics Inc., Salt Lake City, Utah, USA). IVOX® is a polypropylene multifilament oxygenator which is heparin surface bonded. It is passed into the inferior vena cava via a femoral vein, and oxygen is sucked through the hollow filaments. Although it has been used safely in patients, the potential benefit of IVOX® has not been finally established.

Oxygen delivery

The amount of oxygen available to the tissues is a direct function of arterial oxygen content, cardiac output, and the position of the oxyhaemoglobin dissociation curve. In adult respiratory distress syndrome, hypoxaemia reduces the arterial oxygen content and, in addition, cardiac output may be lowered by hypovolaemia or positive end expiratory volume. Adequate filling of the vascular compartment is essential, and inotropic support may be required to restore an effective cardiac output. The interdependence of biventricular function must be remembered. Right ventricular failure secondary to increased pulmonary vascular resistance impairs left ventricular filling and may also produce left ventricular compression by a leftward shift of the interventricular septum. In such instances the pharmacological reduction of the excessive pulmonary vascular resistance with agents such as prostacycline and nitric oxide might be considered. Anaemia should be corrected to optimize the oxygen-carrying capacity of the blood. Metabolic and respiratory alkalosis, which produces a leftward shift of the oxyhaemoglobin dissociation curve with reduced oxygen availability, should be avoided.

Provided that oxygen delivery is sufficient to meet oxygen demand without evidence of tissue hypoxia (i.e. absence of lactic acidosis, cardiac arrhythmias, or mental obtundation), arterial hypoxaemia should be well tolerated and acceptable. This approach of 'acceptable' hypoxaemia together with permissive hypercapnia, if carefully monitored, should provide the best opportunity for recovery by avoiding the harmful effects of excessive airway pressure and oxygen toxicity.

Oxygen demand

High oxygen requirements may be reduced by heavy sedation and, when indicated, by muscle relaxation. Although hypothermia (30 °C) increases the amount of oxygen dissolved in the blood and reduces the oxygen demand, there is no firm evidence that it improves the prognosis in adult respiratory distress syndrome; oxygen availability is reduced by the leftward shift of the oxyhaemoglobin dissociation curve, thus lessening the benefits of hypothermia.

Oxygen supply dependency

The concept of oxygen supply dependency in adult respiratory distress syndrome remains controversial. Some studies have clearly shown oxygen consumption to rise with inotrope-enhanced oxygen delivery. However, studies in which oxygen consumption was determined by both indirect calorimetry and the modified Fick equation suggested that oxygen supply dependency in adult respiratory distress syndrome was more a function of the use of shared variables (cardiac output and arterial oxygen content) to calculate oxygen delivery and consumption. In a retrospective survey of 50 patients with severe adult respiratory distress syndrome, cardiac output, oxygen consumption, oxygen delivery, or oxygen extraction ratio failed to predict survival. Thus there remains doubt as to whether oxygen supply dependency can be consistently demonstrated in adult respiratory distress syndrome, and whether achieving 'supranormal' oxygen delivery targets offers any therapeutic benefit.

Oxygen toxicity

The toxic effect of oxygen on the lung was described by Lorraine Smith as early as 1899, but it was not until the late 1960s that evidence appeared correlating histological changes of both early and late lung injury with high inspired oxygen concentrations. Experimental evidence suggests that the elevated alveolar oxygen concentration, not the arterial oxygen tension, is responsible for the toxicity. The mechanism involves the reduction of molecular oxygen to highly reactive and potentially cytotoxic radicals which overwhelm the antioxidant defence enzymes causing intracellular enzyme damage and loss of membrane integrity.

The severity of oxygen toxicity is dependent on both FIO_2 and the duration of exposure. It is also influenced by biochemically induced tolerance, previous lung disease, and the age and weight of the patient. The variability of a patient's susceptibility does not allow a safe inspired oxygen concentration to be predicted accurately. As a practical guide, it is probable that an FIO_2 of less than 0.5 can be safely administered for prolonged periods, whereas an FIO_2 of more than 0.8 can produce deleterious effects in the lung within 48 h. On occasion, however, it is impossible to maintain adequate oxygenation unless potentially toxic inspired oxygen concentrations are used. In these circumstances, the full range of therapeutic manoeuvres should be employed in an attempt to lower the FIO_2. The use of free-radical scavengers such as superoxide dismutase enzymes has yet to be shown to be clinically effective in preventing oxygen toxicity.

Pulmonary haemodynamics

Infusions of vasodilator drugs such as glyceryl trinitrate, sodium nitroprusside, or prostacyclin non-selectively reverse vasoconstriction throughout the whole pulmonary vascular bed, and hence reduce the pulmonary artery pressure but at the expense of systemic arterial oxygenation as perfusion of poorly ventilated areas of the lung increases. Despite an increase in venous admixture associated with these agents, the increase in cardiac output may result in increased oxygen delivery, increased S_vO_2, and thus increased S_aO_2.

A new approach to pulmonary vasodilator therapy has recently developed from studies of the effects of inhaled nitric oxide. It is now recognized that nitric oxide is a powerful regulator of vascular smooth-muscle tone and that inhalation of low concentrations (20–120 p.p.m.) preferentially vasodilates pulmonary vessels in ventilated areas of the lung. This results in an immediate reduction in venous admixture as more blood flows through the well-aerated regions of the lung. Short half-life and rapid absorption by oxyhaemoglobin ensures that nitric oxide does not affect the systemic circulation. Indeed, vasopressors such as noradrenaline can be administered to support the systemic circulation without diminishing the effects of nitric oxide in the lung. Nitric oxide reacts rapidly with molecular oxygen and therefore must be stored with nitrogen as a carrier gas. As a safeguard, nitrogen dioxide levels in the inspired gas mixture (from the oxidation of nitric oxide) can be monitored together with methaemoglobin levels in the patient's blood. At present, nitric oxide appears to offer an effective pharmacological method of improving gas exchange in adult respiratory distress syndrome. However, much wider clinical experience is required before this becomes a standard of care in adult respiratory distress syndrome.

Pulmonary hypertension in adult respiratory distress syndrome may also be caused by microembolization of the pulmonary circulation by particulate blood products. It is possible that this embolization is enhanced by plasma fibronectin deficiency which can be corrected by cryoprecipitate infusions, but neither the use of anticoagulants nor the infusion of streptokinase has been shown to be useful or safe. The use of pharmacological preparations in the management of the permeability defect of the microcirculation has not yet been established. Cyclo-oxygenase inhibitors such as the non-steroidal anti-inflammatory drugs can reduce the pulmonary hypertension but without abatement of the increased permeability. Similarly, specific antivasoactive drugs such as the antihistamines have proved ineffective, while lipoxygenase inhibitors are not yet in clinical use. The role of steroids is discussed later.

Fluid balance

Prospective studies of high risk surgical patients suggest that positive fluid balance may have a protective effect in preventing the development of adult respiratory distress syndrome and multiple organ failure. Once adult respiratory distress syndrome is established, adequate cardiac preload must be maintained to avoid hypoperfusion of other organs such as the kidneys. There is still debate about the effects of crystalloid and colloid infusions on the flux of water and solutes across the pulmonary endothelium when there is increased permeability as in adult respiratory distress syndrome. Some studies have demonstrated that colloid infusion, by increasing plasma protein osmotic pressure, reduces extravascular lung water accumulation, while other authorities maintain that colloid infusions extravasate into the interstitium, abolishing the transcapillary protein osmotic pressure difference. Certainly, when the capillary leak is established, even large molecules pass into the interstitium and the protein content of the alveolar fluid can approach that of plasma. It is probable that in early adult respiratory distress syndrome colloid infusions do not augment the pulmonary transcapillary flux of proteins provided that the microvascular hydrostatic pressure does not rise significantly. Thus careful monitoring of systemic and pulmonary perfusion pressures may be critical and generally requires the insertion of a flow-directed balloon catheter. By maintaining a pulmonary capillary wedge pressure between 8 and 12 mmHg a guide to the rate and volume of infused fluid can be obtained, while sequential measurements of plasma protein osmotic pressure and haematocrit enable the type of infused fluid to be more precisely selected. It must be remembered that high levels of positive end expiratory volume may overestimate the pulmonary capillary wedge pressure and central venous pressure mea-

surements. Relative or absolute fluid overload should be managed by diuretic therapy, although more recently it has been suggested that ultrafiltration is a more efficient method of treating pulmonary oedema. When a significant negative fluid balance can be achieved consistently, either spontaneously or with the aid of diuretics, without deleterious cardiovascular effects, this usually signifies the onset of recovery from adult respiratory distress syndrome.

N-acetylcysteine

Free oxygen radicals are increasingly believed to play a role in the development of adult respiratory distress syndrome. N-acetylcysteine is a free-radical scavenger which may act directly by means of the thiol group or indirectly as a precursor for glutathione. In addition, N-acetylcysteine may counteract neutrophil activation in the lung and has been shown to improve dynamic compliance. This may be explained by a reduction in lung microvascular permeability, which would reduce interstitial oedema. N-acetylcysteine may also increase surfactant secretion. In randomized studies of mild to moderate adult respiratory distress syndrome acetylcysteine has not been shown to be of benefit, but greater experience with the more severe forms of disease would be desirable.

Prophylactic management

STEROIDS AND NON-STEROIDAL ANTI-INFLAMMATORY AGENTS

Although there is strong theoretical evidence to support their use, specific treatments to inhibit mediator cascades are largely experimental. Multicentre randomized studies have failed to show significant benefit from corticosteroids, non-steroidal anti-inflammatory agents, or vasodilator prostaglandins. Anecdotal reports of high dose steroids (40–60 mg prednisone per day) in 'chronic' respiratory distress suggest some benefit in terms of oxygenation and lung compliance. However, the use of steroids in the acute phase of adult respiratory distress syndrome afforded no benefit in multicentre controlled studies.

ANTIBIOTICS

The role of infection in the aetiology and prognosis of adult respiratory distress syndrome cannot be overemphasized. It is estimated that 85 per cent of patients with established adult respiratory distress syndrome have an intra- or extrapulmonary infective focus. Strict aseptic suctioning techniques must be used and the sterility of ventilators ensured. Intensive efforts must be made to identify the micro-organism and appropriate antibiotics started. The changing bacterial pattern in patients on ventilators can best be determined by quantitative culture of bronchoscopic protected specimen brushings of the distal airways or bronchoalveolar lavage. When no organism can be isolated, the decision to start and the selection of empirical combination broad-spectrum antibiotics should be based on clinical findings.

PARENTERAL NUTRITION

Patients with adult respiratory distress syndrome invariably suffer nutritional depletion which, if uncorrected, leads to muscle weakness, particularly of the respiratory muscles, and lessened cellular-mediated immunity predisposing to infection. Hypophosphataemia and hypomagnesaemia can develop in long-term critically ill patients and can contribute to muscle weakness and impaired ventilatory effort. Nutrition, ideally by the enteral route, should be started early in the management of adult respiratory distress syndrome patients.

Outcome

Provided that multiple-organ system support can be maintained, a positive attitude towards final recovery is justified. Even after periods of mechanical ventilation, high FiO_2 values, and positive end expiratory volume for up to 3 to 4 months, a good functional outcome is possible. Biopsy-proven pulmonary fibrosis does not inevitably mean that there is fixed irreversible pathology. A mortality rate of over 50 to 60 per cent is generally quoted for the last decade, although some recent reports have shown a fall in mortality to about 20 per cent. Pulmonary function testing a year after recovery from adult respiratory distress syndrome may show a reduction in vital capacity with a mild obstructive defect. In many patients the only abnormality may be a reduction in carbon monoxide transfer.

REFERENCES

Ashbaugh, D.G., Bigelow, D.B., Petty, T.L., and Levine, B.R.E. (1967). Acute respiratory distress in adults. *Lancet*, **ii**, 319–321.

Bagley, B., Bagley, A., Henrie, J., Froerer, C., Brohamer, J., Bukarkt, J., and Mortensen, J.D. (1991). Quantitative gas transfer into and out of circulating venous blood by means of an intravenacaval oxygenator. *Asaio Transactions*, **37**, 413–15.

Bernard, G.R., Luce, J.M., Sprung, C.L., Rinaldo, J.E., Tate, R.M., Sibbald, W.J., *et al.* (1987). High-dose corticosteroids in patients with the adult respiratory distress syndrome. *New England Journal of Medicine*, **317**, 1365–70.

Bone, R.C., Fisher, C.J., Jr, Clemmer, T.P., Slotman, G.J., and Metz, C.A. (1987). Early methylprednisolone treatment for septic syndrome and the adult respiratory distress syndrome. *Chest*, **92**, 1032–6.

Chollet-Martin, S., Montravers, P., Gibert, C., Elbim, C., Desmonts, J.M., Fagon, J.Y., and Gougerot-Pocidalo, M.A. (1992). Subpopulation of hyperresponsive polymorphonuclear neutrophils in patients with adult respiratory distress syndrome. Role of cytokine production. *American Review of Respiratory Disease*, **146**, 990–6.

Gattinoni, L., Agostoni, A., Presenti, A., *et al.* (1980). Treatment of acute respiratory failure with low-frequency positive-pressure ventilation and extracorporeal removal of CO_2. *Lancet*, **ii**, 292–4.

Hammerschidt, D.E., Weaver, L.J., Hudson, L.D., Craddock, P.R., and Jacob, H.S. (1980). Association of complement activation and elevated plasma C5a with adult respiratory distress syndrome. Pathophysiological relevance and possible prognostic value. *Lancet*, **i**, 947–9.

Hickling, K.G., Henderson, S.J., and Jackson, R. (1990). Low mortality associated with low volume pressure limited ventilation with permissive hypercapnia in severe adult respiratory distress syndrome. *Intensive Care Medicine*, **16**, 372–7.

Idell, S., Koenig, K.B., Fair, D.S., Martin, T.R., McLarty, J., and Maunder, R.J., (1991). Serial abnormalities of fibrin turnover in evolving adult respiratory distress syndrome. *American Journal of Physiology*, **261**, L240–8.

Jepsen, S., Herlevsen, P., Knudsen, P., Bud, M.I., and Klausen, N.O. (1992). Antioxidant treatment with *N*-acetylcysteine during adult respiratory distress syndrome: a prospective, randomized, placebo-controlled study. *Critical Care Medicine*, **20**, 918–23.

Kolobow, T., Moretti, M., Fumagalli, R., *et al.* (1987). Severe impairment in lung function induced by high peak airway pressure mechanical ventilation. An experimental study. *American Review of Respiratory Disease*, **135**, 312–15.

Lee, F. and Massard, D. (1979). The lung and oxygen toxicity. *Archives of Internal Medicine*, **139**, 347–50.

Lewis, J.F. and Jobe, A.H. (1993). Surfactant and the adult respiratory distress syndrome. *American Review of Respiratory Disease*, **147**, 218–33.

Morris, A.H., Wallace, C., Clemmer, T., *et al.* (1992). Final report: computerised protocol controlled clinical trial of new therapy which includes ECCO2R for ARDS. *American Review of Respiratory Disease*, **145**, A184.

Murray, J.F., Matthay, M.A., Luce, J.M., and Flick, M.R. (1988). An expanded definition of the adult respiratory distress syndrome. *American Review of Respiratory Disease*, **138**, 720–3.

Pontoppidan, H., Geffin, B., and Lowenstein, E. (1972). Acute respiratory failure in the adult. *New England Journal of Medicine*, **42**, 45–55.

Ryan, D.P. and Doody, D.P. (1992). Treatment of acute pulmonary failure with extracorporeal support 100 per cent survival in a pediatric population. *Journal of Pediatric Surgery*, **27**, 1111–16.

Saldeen, T. (1983). Clotting, microembolism, and inhibition of fibrinolysis in adult respiratory distress. *Surgical Clinics of North America*, **63**, 285–304.

Sibbald, W.J., Anderson, R.L., and Holliday, R.L. (1979). Pathogenesis of pulmonary edema associated with the adult respiratory distress syndrome. *Canadian Medical Association Journal*, **120**, 445–50.

Sjøstrand, U. (1980). High-frequency positive-pressure ventilation (HFPPV): a review. *Critical Care Medicine*, **8**, 345–64.

Staub, N.C. (1980). The pathogenesis of pulmonary edema. *Progress in Cardiovascular Diseases*, **23**, 53–80.

Suchyta, M.R., Clemmer, T.P., Orme, J.J., Morris, A.H., and Elliott, C.G. (1991). Increased survival of ARDS patients with severe hypoxemia (ECMO criteria). *Chest*, **99**, 951–5.

Suter, P.M., Suter, S., Girardin, E., Roux-Lombard, P., Grau, G.E., and Dayer, J.-M. (1992). High bronchoalveolar levels of tumor necrosis factor and its inhibitors, interleukin-1, interferon, and elastase, in patients with adult respiratory distress syndrome after trauma, shock, or sepsis. *American Review of Respiratory Disease*, **145**, 1016–22.

Wagner, P.K., Knoch, M., Sangmeister, C., Muller, E., Lennartz, H., and Rothmund, M. (1990). Extracorporeal gas exchange in adult respiratory distress syndrome: associated morbidity and its surgical treatment. *British Journal of Surgery*, **77**, 1395–8.

Zapol, W., Snider, M., Hill, D., *et al.* (1979). Extracorporeal membrane oxygenation in severe acute respiratory failure. A randomized prospective study. *Journal of the American Medical Association*, **242**, 2193–6.

17.10.21 Lung disorders in genetic syndromes

R.J. SHAW AND D.J. HENDRICK

Airways disease

Genetic factors are important determinants of airway disease. The genetics of cystic fibrosis (Chapter 17.9.2), emphysema and α_1-antitrypsin deficiency (Chapter 11.15), atopy and asthma (Section 17.9), and the immotile cilia syndrome, immunoglobulin deficiency, and chronic granulomatous disease underlying bronchiectasis (Chapter 17.9.3) are discussed elsewhere.

Bronchomalacia is a rare syndrome of bronchial flaccidity reported as an autosomal recessive disorder. In this condition, collapse of the first- and second-generation bronchi during expiration can lead to airflow limitation and dyspnoea that mimic asthma, and to bronchiectasis.

Parenchymal disease

Rare recessively inherited forms of parenchymal disease are described for interstitial pulmonary fibrosis, pulmonary alveolar proteinosis, pulmonary alveolar microlithiasis, and pulmonary bullae (without α_1-antitrypsin deficiency) causing pneumothorax.

Occasional pulmonary involvement is well recognized in a range of genetic diseases with complex multiorgan phenotypes including neurofibromatosis, tuberous sclerosis, Marfan's syndrome, hereditary haemorrhagic telangiectasia, and various storage/depositional disorders including lipid storage diseases.

In neurofibromatosis type 1, neurofibromas may be observed within the lungs or mediastinum. A rare but well-recognized pulmonary complication is a slowly progressive diffuse interstitial pulmonary fibrosis which may be associated with pulmonary vascular change and hypertension. Increasing dyspnoea and dry cough occur without abnormal chest signs but with diffuse reticulonodular radiographic changes, particularly in the upper zones. There is a restrictive ventilatory defect. There is no specific treatment.

In tuberous sclerosis, a small number of patients develop progressive diffuse proliferation of smooth muscle and fibrous tissue in the bronchi and lungs that leads to respiratory failure. Patients present with increasing dyspnoea and occasional haemoptyses. There is bilateral reticulonodular radiographic change and an obstructive ventilatory defect. The complication is more common in females. There is no specific treatment.

In Marfan's syndrome, bullous emphysematous changes may develop at the lung apices in particular, which cause some 5 per cent of Marfan's subjects to suffer pneumothorax. If air leak is persistent, pleurodesis or bullectomy may be required.

Dominantly inherited haemorrhagic telangiectasia may be complicated by the development of pulmonary arteriovenous fistulae. Although usually asymptomatic, these low-resistance channels can cause life-threatening haemoptysis or significant shunting with hypoxaemia (if large), or predispose to embolic stroke or brain abscess. Pulmonary arteriovenous fistulae, whether associated with Osler–Rendu–Weber disease or not, usually present as pulmonary nodules on routine chest radiograph; CT scanning may suggest the diagnosis by demonstrating 'feeding vessels'. A bruit may be audible and the patient's fingers may be clubbed. Troublesome fistulae have recently been successfully treated with per angiographic transcatheter embolization with steel coils or balloons as an alternative to surgical resection.

Gaucher's disease and Nieman–Pick disease are rare hereditary disorders characterized by an inborn inability to degrade the body's production of certain lipids. There is a steady accumulation of the endogenous lipid within the histiocytes of many organs, particularly those of the liver, spleen, bones, lymph nodes, skin, central nervous system, and lungs, thereby causing dysfunction. Pulmonary involvement is characterized by focal accumulations of lipid-laden histiocytes in the interstitium, alveolar walls, and alveolar spaces, and by a diffuse reticulonodular pattern on the chest radiograph. It is commonly asymptomatic and overshadowed by involvement of other organs. Occasionally, however, the pulmonary disease is severe and may prove to be the cause of death.

In Gaucher's disease, the pulmonary vasculature is occasionally infiltrated directly with emboli of affected histiocytic cells from bone marrow, leading to pulmonary hypertension and respiratory failure. Clinically important levels of pulmonary hypertension have been noted in the absence of such infiltration, perhaps owing to the action of vasoactive agents bypassing diseased liver. Accumulation of Gaucher cells may occur within the ribs, and the chest radiograph may then show characteristic lytic lesions in addition to evidence of a diffuse reticulonodular infiltration. The disease can also be recognized by low glucocerebrosidase activity in peripheral blood leucocytes, and this technique can be used to demonstrate intermediate levels in heterozygote carriers of the gene. Until recently no definitive therapy was available, but successful

bone marrow transplants are now being reported. Other forms of gene therapy are under assessment, and enzyme replacement using repeated infusions of glucocerebrosidase has shown some success.

In Nieman–Pick disease, there may be lung involvement similar to that seen in Gaucher's disease. It is not common, although it may occur more frequently than in Gaucher's disease. Diagnosis depends on the demonstration of characteristic histiocytic 'foam cells' filled with sphingomyelin and on low sphingomyelinase activity in blood leucocytes or cultured skin fibroblasts.

REFERENCES

Agosti, E., DeFilippi, G., Fior, R., and Chiussi, F. (1974). Generalised familial bronchomalacia. *Acta Paediatrica Scandinavica,* **63,** 616–18.

Caffrey, P.R. And Altman, R.S. (1965). Pulmonary alveolar microlithiasis in twins. *Journal of Paediatrics,* **66,** 758–63.

Dwyer, J.M., Hickie, J.B., and Garvan, J. (1979). Pulmonary tuberous sclerosis. *Quarterly Journal of Medicine,* **40,** 115.

Fallet, S., Grace, M.E., Sibille, A., Mendelson, D.S., Shapiro, R.S., Hermann, G., and Grabowski, G.A. (1992). Enzyme augmentation in moderate to life-threatening Gaucher's disease. *Pediatric Research,* **31,** 496–502.

Gibson, G.J. (1977). Familial pneumothorax and bullae. *Thorax,* **32,** 88–90.

Hughes, J.M.B. and Allison, D.J. (1990). Pulmonary arteriovenous malformations: the radiologist replaces the surgeon. *Clinical Radiology,* **41,** 297–8.

Jackson, D.C. and Simon, G. (1965). Unusual bone and lung changes in a case of Gaucher's disease. *British Journal of Radiology,* **38,** 698–700.

McKusick, V.A. (1992). *Mendelian inheritance in man* (10th edn). John Hopkins University Press, Baltimore, MD.

Massaro, D., Katz, S., Mathews, M., and Higgins, G. (1965). Neurofibromatosis associated with cystic lung disease. *American Journal of Respiratory Medicine,* **38,** 233.

Ringden, O., Groth, C.G., Erickson, A., Backman, L., Granqvist, S., Mansson, J.E., and Svennerholm, L. (1988). Long-term follow-up of the first successful bone marrow transplantation in Gaucher's disease. *Transplantation,* **46,** 66–70.

Smith, R.R.L., Hutchins, G.M., Sack, G.H., and Ridolfi, R.L. (1978). Unusual cardiac, renal and pulmonary involvement in Gaucher's disease. *American Journal of Medicine,* **65,** 352–60.

Teja, K., Cooper, P.H., Squires, J.E., and Schatterley, P.T. (1981). Pulmonary alveolar proteinosis in four siblings. *New England Journal of Medicine,* **305,** 1390–2.

Turner, J.A.M. and Stanley, N.N. (1976). Fragile lung in the Marfan syndrome. *Thorax,* **31,** 771.

Wolson, A.H. (1975). Pulmonary findings in Gaucher's disease. *American Journal of Roentgenology,* **123,** 712–15.

17.11 Pleural disease

M.K. BENSON

Introduction

The pleural surfaces form the interface between the lung parenchyma and the chest wall. The parietal pleura is closely applied to the chest wall and the surfaces of the ribs. There is a thin layer of connective tissue separating it from the periosteum of the ribs. Medially, the parietal pleura is adjacent to the pericardium and mediastinal structures. At the hilum, the pleura forms a sleeve-like structure encompassing the major vessels and bronchi. The visceral pleura covers the surface of the lungs and extends into the major fissures which separates the lobes of the lung. The pleura consists of a membranous structure, the surface of which is covered with a single layer of mesothelial cells. These cells have microvilli over their surface which facilitate the absorbtion of pleural fluid.

The pleura is not essential for adequate functioning of the lungs, although the smooth surfaces do permit movement of the lungs within the thorax with minimal energy loss. Obliteration of the pleural space either following surgery or as a result of inflammatory disease does not result in significant respiratory impairment. Between the two layers of pleura there is a potential space, the surfaces of which are lubricated by a thin layer of fluid. The pressures within the pleural cavity are generated by the difference between the elastic forces of the lungs and the chest wall. At functional residual capacity the outward recoil of the chest wall is equal to the inward recoil of the lung parenchyma. A number of pathological processes can affect the pleura. Inflammation of the pleura results in characteristic pleuritic pain which is aggravated by deep inspiration, coughing, or sneezing. It is often accompanied by a pleural rub. The accumulation of fluid in the pleural space results in a pleural effusion. Air can also enter the pleural space resulting in a pneumothorax. Primary tumours of the mediastinum are relatively uncommon. Involvement of pleura by metastatic malignant disease is much more frequent.

Pleural effusion

A pleural effusion results from an accumulation of fluid in the pleural space. It is traditional to divide effusions into transudates and exudates, although blood, pus, or chyle may also present as collections of pleural fluid. The main causes are listed in Table 1.

Pleural fluid formation

The two layers of the pleura allow the chest wall and lung to move together, with lubrication of the pleural surfaces ensuring that this occurs with minimum loss of energy. Normally lubrication is provided by a thin layer of fluid representing an ultrafiltrate of plasma, although surfactant may also be present and play a role. Although turnover of pleural fluid is probably of the order of 1–2 l/day, the volume of fluid present at any one time is only a few millilitres. Under normal circumstances two factors operate to prevent the accumulation of fluid in the pleural space: the pleura itself acts as a semipermeable membrane, and the flux of fluid across the pleural space is accounted for by the forces involved in Starling's law of transcapilliary exchange. The hydrostatic gradient from the capillaries of the parietal pleura favours fluid efflux into the pleural space. Pressure in the capillaries in the visceral pleura is close to that of the pulmonary capillaries, and this lower pressure favours reabsorption of fluid from the visceral surface (Fig. 1). The lymphatic system provides a second method of preventing excess fluid accumulation. In addition, it enables proteins to be recovered from the pleural space and returned to the circulating plasma.

Factors likely to result in excess fluid accumulation in the pleural space can now be indentified. They include the following.

1. An imbalance between the hydrostatic and oncotic forces as defined in Starling's equation. Such fluid is usually a transudate.
2. An alteration in the permeability of pleural capillaries resulting in an exudate.
3. Impaired lymphatic drainage.
4. Abnormal sites of entry (e.g. transdiaphragmatic passage of fluid in patients with ascites).

Diagnostic approach to pleural effusion

CLINICAL FEATURES

Symptoms specifically related to pleural disease are pain and breathlessness. The extent to which these occur is likely to vary and clinical presentation will at least in part be determined by the underlying pathogenesis. Pleuritic pain which causes severe discomfort on coughing or deep inspiration is more typical of 'dry' pleurisy. It tends to improve as fluid accumulates, separating the inflamed pleural surfaces. The other major symptom is breathlessness which only becomes apparent if there is a large effusion or in patients who already have impaired respiratory reserve. Abnormal physical signs may be absent if the effusion is relative small but are often diagnostic if the effusion is large. Chest wall movement may be normal although it will tend to be limited, particularly if there is pain. There can also be a lag of chest wall motion on the affected side. The percussion note is very dull and breath sounds will be diminished or absent. Similarly, vocal resonance and tactile vocal fremitus will be absent. Compression of the lung above the effusion can result in signs of consolidation with bronchial breathing and an increased vocal resonance. The position of the mediastinum as judged by the trachea and apex beat will help in distinguishing between a large effusion and a collapsed lung. In the former the mediastinum is central or displaced away from the side of the effusion, whereas in the latter deviation is towards the affected side.

INVESTIGATION OF PLEURAL EFFUSION

The presence of a pleural effusion should be suspected on clinical examination and can be confirmed by using radiographic imaging or ultrasound. Whilst clinical features play an important part in identifying the pathogenesis, examination of the pleural fluid or pleural biopsy material is most likely to lead to a definitive diagnosis.

Radiographic techniques

Radiographic techniques are helpful in identifying the presence of an effusion but are of limited value in determining the pathogenesis. A conventional posteroanterior chest radiograph is usually adequate in confirming the presence of a clinically significant effusion. Fluid tends to accumulate in dependent parts of the thorax, and small effusions of the order of 500 ml will result in blunting of the costophrenic angle. Larger effusions result in increased opacification and may produce medi-

Table 1 *Causes of pleural effusions*

	Common	Less common
Transudates	Cardiac failure	Nephrotic syndrome
		Cirrhosis
		Peritoneal dialysis
		Myxoedema
Exudates		
Inflammatory (infective)	Parapneumonic	Subphrenic abscess
	Tuberculosis	Viral
		Fungal
Inflammatory (non-infective)	Pulmonary emboli	Collagen vascular disease
		Pancreatitis
		Drug reaction
		Asbestos exposure
		Dressler's syndrome
		Yellow nail syndrome
Neoplastic	Metastatic carcinoma	Mesothelioma
	Lymphoma	Meigs' syndrome
Haemothorax	Trauma	Spontaneous
		Bleeding disorders
Chylothorax	Lymphoma	Lymphangioleiomyomatosis
	Carcinoma	
	Trauma	

astinal shift (Fig. 2). Variations of the normal appearance will result if the fluid is loculated, a situation which is more likely to occur with an empyema or if there are pleural adhesions (Fig. 3).

Ultrasound can be helpful in confirming the presence and site of an effusion. Pleural fluid is identified as an echo-free space between chest wall and lung. The presence of echoes within the fluid may indicate an empyema or haemothorax, and ultrasound can also demonstrate the presence of septation and loculi (Fig. 4).

CT can detect very small effusions which may not be apparent using standard radiograph imaging. It can also complement ultrasound exam-

Fig. 1 Representative figures for hydrostatic pressure P and oncotic pressure π in parietal and visceral capillaries. The net effect is fluid efflux from the parietal surface into the pleural space and reabsorption from the visceral surface.

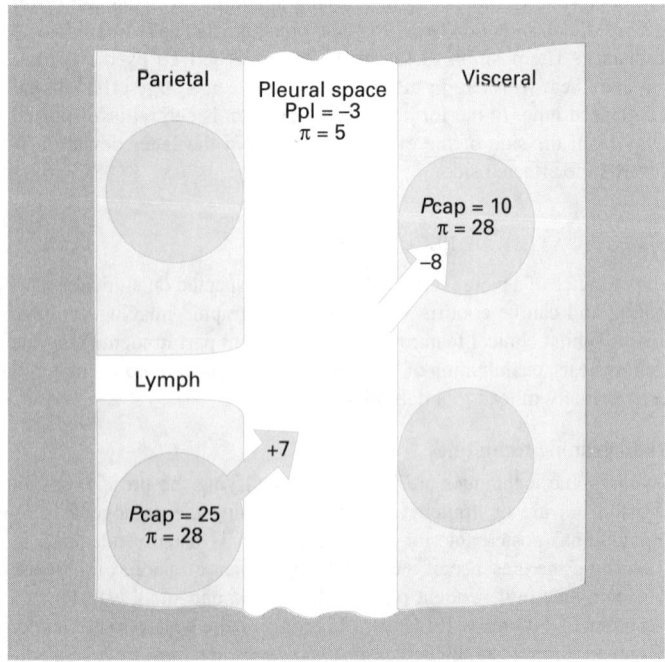

Fig. 2 Chest radiograph showing opacification of the left hemithorax and mediastinal shift indicating a large pleural effusion.

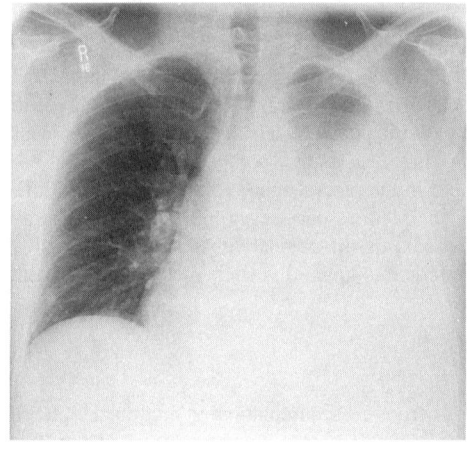

Fig. 3 CT scan demonstrating a loculated effusion due to an empyema.

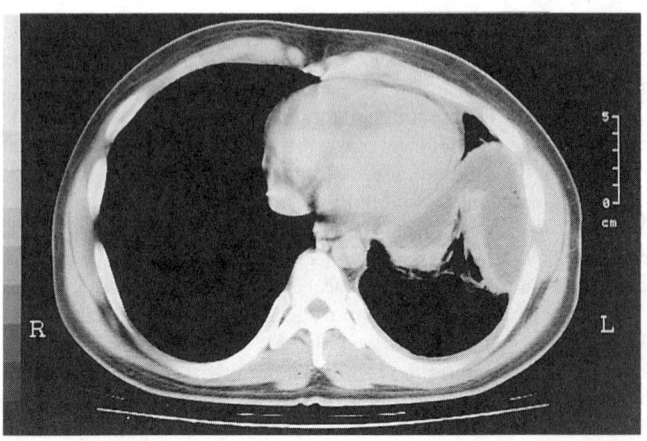

ination in demonstrating the site of a pleural collection and have the additional advantage of imaging the underlying lung. However, its role in routine evaluation of pleural effusions is limited.

Thoracentesis

Percutaneous aspiration of pleural fluid is a relatively simply procedure which can be undertaken for diagnostic purposes and, in the case of larger effusions, can relieve breathlessness. It is usually performed with the patient upright in a comfortable position with the arms and head supported on a pillow. Unless the fluid is loculated, a conventional site for aspiration is posteriorally about 10 cm lateral to the spine and one intercostal space below the upper level of the fluid as detected by percussion. A common error is to attempt aspiration as low as possible, but this often yields a dry tap since it is impossible on clinical grounds to determine the level of the diaphragm. The procedure is performed under strict aseptic technique. The skin and underlying tissues are infiltrated with local anaesthetic taking care to avoid the intercostal nerves and vessels which run immediately beneath the rib. For diagnostic purposes it is usually adequate to remove 50–100 ml of fluid. If therapeutic aspiration of large amounts of fluid is being undertaken, it is best to introduce a small plastic canula into the pleural space to minimize the risk of damage to the underlying lung.

Failure to obtain fluid can arise for a number of reasons including misdiagnosis of the presence of fluid, incorrect site of aspiration, and the presence of viscid fluid. Ultrasound examination can help to identify the reason for a failed tap and guide further attempts if fluid is present.

Examination of pleural fluid

Biochemical, cytological, and microbiological examination of the pleural fluid can help to establish the underlying cause if this is not apparent on clinical grounds (Table 2).

Macroscopic appearance

Transudates are clear straw-coloured fluids which do not clot on standing. Many exudates are similar in appearance but can be somewhat turbid owing to the presence of cells. Blood-tinged fluid is of little diagnostic significance, but a uniformly bloody effusion is likely to be associated with an underlying malignancy. Pus can sometimes be very viscid and difficult to aspirate. It is turbid in appearance, yellow in colour, and often foul smelling. Chyle is odourless and milky in appearance.

Biochemistry

Exudates will generally have a higher protein content than transudates and, although a level of 30 g/l has traditionally been used to help differentiation, there is a significant overlap and results should be inter-

preted with caution. Better differentiation may be obtained by comparing concentrations of protein and lactic dehydrogenase in the pleural fluid with those of blood. The criteria which can prove helpful in identifying an exudate are as follows:

(1) A fluid-to-serum ratio of total protein above 0.5;
(2) A fluid lactic dehydrogenase concentration above 200 IU;
(3) A fluid-to-serum ratio of lactic dehydrogenase above 0.6.

The concentration of glucose in the pleural fluid is normally equal to that in serum. However, glucose concentration in the pleural fluid is consistently low in rheumatoid-related effusions. Reduced concentrations of glucose are also found in association with tuberculosis, empyemas, and malignancy. One rare cause of a left-sided pleural effusion is pancreatitis, when pancreatic amylase measurements of the pleural fluid will be elevated.

Microscopic and cytological examination

Most transudates have low cell counts of less than 1000/mm³, with the cells being a mixture of lymphocytes, polymorphs, and mesothelial cells. Exudates tend to have higher white counts, although this in itself is of little diagnostic value. A polymorphonuclear leucocytosis is indicative of a bacterial infection but can also be seen in association with a pulmonary infarct or pancreatitis. A predominance of lymphocytes raises the possibility of tuberculosis or a lymphoma but may also occur in association with other malignancies. The presence of excess eosinophils is not in itself diagnostic but tends to be associated with benign inflammation.

For adequate cytology, a sample of 50 ml of fluid in a heparinized bottle should be sent for immediate examination. The finding of malignant cells is likely to be diagnostic, although occasionally actively dividing mesothelial cells may mimic an adenocarcinoma. The cytological diagnosis of a malignant mesothelioma presents particular difficulties but can be helped by cytogenetic studies.

Microbiology

Gram stain and culture of the pleural fluid is of diagnostic value if an infective aetiology is suspected. Identification of an organism confirms the diagnosis and sensitivity testing will assist in the appropriate choice of antibiotics. Stains for acid-fast organisms are often unhelpful even if tuberculosis is suspected. Cultures are more likely to be positive if a reasonable volume of fluid is concentrated and then examined.

Pleural biopsy

Pleural biopsy may be indicated if initial analysis of pleural fluid fails to establish a diagnosis. It is of particular value if there is a suspicion of an underlying malignancy or tuberculosis. Closed-needle biopsy is usually performed using an Abraham's or Cope's needle. Both of these are large blunt-tipped needles with a hook to catch a sample of parietal pleura. The technique is similar to that used for pleural aspiration except that a small incision is made in the skin and subcutaneous tissues to enable ease of insertion of the needle. The Abraham's needle consists of an outer trocar with a side-hole and an inner cannula with a cutting edge. Once in the pleural space, the side-hole is opened by rotating the inner cannula and withdrawing it slightly. Fluid is then aspirated to confirm that the needle is in the pleural space. The needle is withdrawn at an angle to the chest wall such that the side-hole gently catches on to the parietal pleura. At this point to the inner cannula is advanced and a biopsy is obtained. Several samples can be obtained using this technique, but care must be taken to avoid damage to intercostal nerves and vessels. Samples for histological examination should be put into formalin and those for culture for mycobacteria should be put into saline.

Needle biopsy undoubtedly increases the diagnostic yield in patients with tuberculosis of the pleura. Aspiration alone gives positive results in approximately 25 per cent of cases, and culture of biopsy material increases this to 50 per cent. The additional diagnostic yield in malignant

Fig. 4 Chest ultrasound showing pleural effusion with septation.

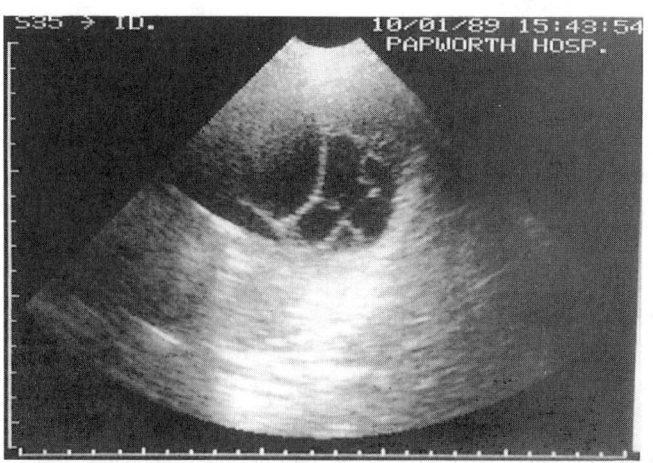

Table 2 *Tests to evaluate cause of pleural effusion*

Cell type		
Red blood cells	>100 000/mm^3	Trauma, malignancy pulmonary embolism
White blood cells	>10 000/mm^3	Pyogenic infection
Neutrophils	>50%	Pyogenic infection
Lymphocytes	>90%	Tuberculosis, lymphoma Malignancy
Eosinophils	>10%	Not diagnostic, usually benign
Mesothelial cells	Absent	Tuberculosis
Malignant cells	Present	Malignancy
Biochemistry		
Protein concentration	>30 g/l	Exudate
Protein F:S ratio	>0.5	Exudate
LDH	>200 IU	Exudate
LDH F:S ratio	>0.6	Exudate
Glucose	<4 mmol/l	Rheumatoid arthritis, infection, malignancy
Amylase F:S ratio	>1	Pancreatitis
pH	<7.2	Malignancy, infection
Microbiology	Positive	Infection

F:S ratio, fluid-to-serum ratio; LDH, lactic dehydrogenase.

disease is less dramatic, with only a small percentage of biopsies being positive when cytology has been negative.

Thoracoscopy

Direct visualization of the pleura is technically possible using a thoracoscope. A diagnosis results in more than 90 per cent of patients with tuberculosis or a pleural malignancy since biopsies can be taken from areas which are macroscopically abnormal. Although thoracoscopy was originally introduced in 1910 and is widely used in parts of Europe and North America, it is relatively underused in the United Kingdom. However, technological advances have improved ease of use and made it likely that this will become an increasingly valuable diagnostic and therapeutic instrument which can be used under both local and general anaesthesia.

Specific pleural effusions

TRANSUDATES

A transudate is characterized by low concentrations of protein and other large molecules. Excess fluid forms when there is an increase in capillary hydrostatic pressure or a reduction in colloid osmotic pressure. The former occurs predominantly in congestive cardiac failure, and the latter when there is hypoalbuminaemia associated with nephrotic syndrome or hepatic disease.

Cardiac failure

Small effusions are common in congestive cardiac failure. Right-sided failure results in increased pressures in the systemic capillaries and thus an increased efflux of fluid from the parietal pleura. Elevated left heart pressures will be reflected in the pulmonary circulation with a consequent diminution in fluid reabsorption from the visceral pleura. The clinical features of cardiac failure are usually sufficient to make a diagnosis. Thus cardiomegaly, elevated jugular venous pressure, and third or fourth heart sounds may all be present. The effusions are frequently bilateral. Unilateral effusions are more common on the right side and may present more diagnostic uncertainty. Pleural aspiration can help to confirm the diagnosis by demonstrating the presence of a transudate, although the limitations of relying on pleural fluid protein measurements have already been discussed. Resolution with treatment of the heart failure offers further confirmation of the diagnosis.

Hepatic cirrhosis

Hypoalbuminaemia, which may occur in patients with chronic liver disease, is a major contributory factor to the development of generalized oedema. Ascites and pleural effusions are both common occurrences, with effusions more often on the right than on the left. In some patients, ascitic fluid seems to pass directly into the pleural space either through a defect in the diaphragm or via lymphatics.

EXUDATES

Neoplastic pleural effusions

Malignant involvement of the pleura is the commonest cause of a large pleural effusion. Most frequently this results from direct spread from a bronchogenic carcinoma. Breast cancer may spread via the lymphatic system, whilst pleural involvement from primary disease in the ovary or gastrointestinal tract is usually by haematogenous spread. Primary tumours of the pleura are considered elsewhere. Extensive investigation for an asymptomatic primary is of limited value, although it may be appropriate to exclude disease originating in breast or ovary because of the potential response to hormonal treatment or chemotherapy. Lymphomas can occur at any age and account for approximately 10 per cent of malignant effusions.

Clinical features

Symptoms directly attributable to the effusion are most commonly breathlessness or chest discomfort. The degree of breathlessness depends on the size of the effusion and the presence of pre-existing lung disease. Specific symptoms which can be attributed to the primary site are often absent. Non-specific systemic symptoms, such as malaise, anorexia, and weight loss, can be associated with any malignant process.

Investigations

The posteroanterior chest radiograph often shows a large effusion with opacification of the whole of the hemithorax. Mediastinal shift to the contralateral side can occur unless the mediastinum is fixed by tumour or the lung on the affected side is collapsed distal to an obstruction of the main stem bronchus. Aspirated fluid is usually an exudate and is bloodstained in approximately 50 per cent of cases. Malignant cells can be identified in up to 60 per cent of cases. Pleural biopsy is justified where aspiration has proved diagnostically unhelpful, although the additional diagnostic yield is relatively small. If the diagnosis remains in doubt, the options are either to await events, since the diagnosis may become obvious with the passage of time, or to obtain further biopsy material at thoracoscopy.

Treatment

Palliative treatment is only necessary if the size of the effusion results in significant breathlessness. If the patient is comfortable, no action may be necessary. Percutaneous needle aspiration of 1 to 2 litres of fluid is a simple outpatient procedure and often results in considerable symptomatic benefit. The fluid is likely to recur but repeated aspiration may be an appropriate therapeutic option. Intercostal tube drainage can be used to remove the majority of the fluid, although this is also likely to be of temporary benefit unless combined with pleurodesis. A number of sclerosing agents have been used with varying degrees of success. Currently, tetracycline (500 mg in 100 ml saline) is popular but adequate analgesia is necessary using both local anaesthetic into the pleural cavity and systemic analgesics. The pleural space is drained as completely as possible, the tetracycline is then injected, and the tube is clamped for 1 to 2 h. Any residual fluid is drained and the tube is removed after 24 h. An alternative approach is to insufflate iodized talc into the pleural space at thoracoscopy. Surgery with either pleurectomy or pleural abrasion is very effective in preventing recurrence, although it is rarely regarded as an appropriate option.

Meigs' syndrome

This rare syndrome originally described an association between pleural effusions, ascites, and a benign ovarian tumour. Surgical removal of the tumour results in resolution of the pleural and peritoneal fluid. The mechanism of the pleural fluid is uncertain, but it is generally assumed that ascitic fluid reaches the pleura through diaphragmatic channels or lymphatics. There is no evidence of spread of the tumour and the syndrome should not be confused with effusions which can result from metastatic spread of ovarian cancers.

Endometriosis of the pleura

This rare condition is one in which endometrial tissue is implanted on visceral or parietal pleura. Catamenial pleuritic chest pain or a pneumothorax can be the presenting feature. More commonly, there is an associated effusion which on aspiration reveals blood or chocolate brown fluid. Thoracotomy will reveal multiple cystic structures but surgical ablation is unsuccessful because of the nature of the disease. Treatment is directed at suppressing ovulation using progesterones or androgens.

Infection

Inflammation or infection of the pleura is usually secondary to a pneumonia or lung abscess. Other sources of infection can be below the diaphragm, associated with mediastinitis, or as a result of direct contamination following penetrating trauma or surgery. Inflammation can result in a dry pleurisy, a non-infected exudate (a parapneumonic effusion), or infected fluid (an empyema). Distinction between a parapneumonic effusion and an empyema is somewhat arbitrary since there can be a transition from one to the other. A parapneumonic effusion may be slightly turbid and contains an excess of polymorphs but has no organisms. An empyema contains increased numbers of polymorphs and is frankly turbid. The pH is less than 7 and the sugar level is usually low. Organisms are likely to be present, although isolation and identification may be difficult particularly if antibiotics have already been administered. The spectrum of organisms most frequently accounted in the United Kingdom is listed in Table 3.

Clinical features

The presentation will vary depending on the pathogenesis. In a patient with a pneumonia, an empyema should be suspected if there is evidence of persisting sepsis with fever and elevated white blood count despite

Table 3 *Organisms resulting in empyema thoracis*

Single organisms (75%)	
Gram-positive aerobes	*Strep. milleri* +++
	Strep. pneumoniae ++
	Staph. aureus +
Gram-negative aerobes	*E. coli* +
	H. influenzae +
	Proteus +
Anaerobic bacteria	*B. melaninogenicus* ++
	Streptococci +
	Fusobacterium +
Fungi	*Candida* spp. +
Multiple organisms (25%)	*Strep. milleri* plus anaerobes

+++ – common; + – rare.

appropriate use of antibiotics. Pleuritic chest pain may be present but is not a prerequisite feature. Classical signs of an effusion can be difficult to detect, particularly if the pleural collection is loculated.

A chest radiograph which shows apparent loculation of fluid should alert the clinician to the possibility of an empyema. Gas may also be present with a characteristic fluid level. The diagnosis is confirmed on pleural aspiration. Ultrasound examination can be useful for identifying the most appropriate approach for attempted aspiration and demonstrating the presence of loculi.

Tuberculous effusion

Pleural involvement with tuberculosis is a common manifestation of primary infection with direct extension from a subpleural focus. Gross parenchymal disease is rare and the primary site often cannot be identified clinically or radiologically. It is more common in younger patients and in those of Asian origin.

Clinical features The presenting features are usually acute or subacute with fever, pleuritic pain, and breathlessness. Some patients may have a longer prodrome of malaise, sweats, and weight loss. The effusion is often large (in excess of 2 litres) and tends to recur after initial aspiration. The fluid is a serous exudate often with an excess of lymphocytes, whose presence should alert the clinician to the possibility of tuberculosis. Tubercule bacilli are rarely identified on pleural aspirate although culture is more likely to be positive. Even so, the diagnostic yield is low and a pleural biopsy is more likely to give a positive result, showing granulomatous inflammation in approximately two-thirds of patients. Thoroscopic biopsy is most likely to give a definitive diagnosis, although it may be more appropriate to commence treatment on clinical grounds alone.

A tuberculous empyema with pus in the pleural space is rare but occasionally complicates cavitating parenchymal disease. A bronchopleural fistula can result, and in advanced disease the empyema can present with a draining sinus through the chest wall. Other bacterial pathogens may be present in the pleural fluid.

Treatment involves the use of standard antituberculous chemotherapy together with adequate drainage if there is frank pus. Steroids have also been advocated to reduce the degree of pleural inflammation and subsequent fibrosis. Rarely, surgical closure of a bronchopleural fistula or decortication is required.

Subdiaphragmatic infection

Inflammation or infection below the diaphragm should always be considered if there is an unexplained effusion with features suggesting infection. A subphrenic abscess is frequently associated with an effusion, usually on the right side. Infection can follow abdominal surgery but may also be associated with a perforated peptic ulcer, appendicitis, diverticulitis, or cholecystitis. Even without infection, upper abdominal surgery can result in a pleural effusion although these are usually small and transient.

If there is evidence of sepsis, the source needs to be identified and if pus is present it must be drained. Ultrasound examination or CT scanning are both effective ways of diagnosing a subphrenic abscess, and percutaneous aspiration can be undertaken using CT guidance. The pleural fluid is usually an exudate and, although turbid with a polymorphonuclear leucocytosis, it rarely becomes infected.

Hepatic abscesses may also present with evidence of a right-sided effusion. Again, CT scanning is the most useful diagnostic technique particularly if used in conjunction with percutaneous aspiration.

Pancreatitis is associated with a pleural effusion in approximately 20 per cent of patients. In the majority the effusion is on the left side. It results from inflammation caused by enzyme-rich pancreatic fluid. Whilst the classical symptoms of pancreatitis usually predominate with abdominal pain, nausea, and vomiting, pleurisy and breathlessness may occasionally be the presenting features. The pleural fluid is often bloodstained and contains abnormally high levels of amylase.

Pulmonary emboli

Pleurisy, often associated with a pleural effusion, is a common presenting feature of pulmonary emboli, particularly if there is associated pulmonary infarction. The effusion is usually small and in itself does not require specific treatment. The fluid is often bloodstained, but the cellular content is variable and there are no diagnostic features. The diagnosis of pulmonary emboli is based on clinical features supplemented by appropriate radiographic or isotopic imaging techniques.

Collagen vascular diseases

Rheumatoid arthritis

Pleural effusions are the commonest pulmonary manifestation of rheumatoid arthritis. They occur in about 3 per cent of patients with active rheumatoid disease and are more common in men than in women. The development of an effusion can antedate the onset of joint symptoms in a small proportion of patients. There is no relationship to the severity of the arthritis, but effusions are more likely to occur in patients with subcutaneous nodules and those who have high titres of rheumatoid factor.

The effusions are usually small but can enlarge to a size which results in breathlessness. Although usually unilateral, they can be bilateral in about 20 per cent of patients. The fluid is an exudate and may appear turbid due to cholesterol crystals. There are no diagnostic features on examining the cellular content, although polymorphonuclear cells usually predominate. Although not specific to rheumatoid effusions, a diagnostic clue is the presence of a low glucose content (usually below 1.5 mmol/l). The pH is also low and the lactic dehydrogenase concentration is elevated (above 700 IU). Whilst these findings may also be present in infective and malignant effusions, the associated clinical features rarely lead to diagnostic uncertainty. Pleural biopsy is non-specific, although it can reveal the epithelioid cells and multinucleate giant cells found in rheumatoid nodules.

Symptomatic treatment with anti-inflammatory analgesics is indicated if pleuritic pain is a feature. Systemic steroids can speed resolution of the pleural fluid although they are rarely necessary. The majority of effusions resolve spontaneously within a few months, but there may be some residual pleural fibrosis.

Systemic lupus erythematosus

Pleural involvement is common in patients with this condition. Approximately 50 per cent of patients will have pleurisy at some stage and the majority of these will have an associated effusion, although this is usually small. Aspiration of the fluid is rarely necessary for either diagnostic or therapeutic purposes. The fluid is an exudate and has high concentrations of antinuclear antibodies. Lupus erythematosus cells can also be identified. There is a good therapeutic response to oral corticosteroids.

HAEMOTHORAX

A haemothorax is the result of bleeding into the pleural space and is somewhat arbitrarily diagnosed on the basis of having a haematocrit more than half that of peripheral blood. This can help to distinguish it from a blood-stained effusion which can be associated with a number of different pathological processes. The vast majority of haemothoraces are associated with penetrating or non-penetrating trauma. Iatrogenic procedures such as central venous catheterization or aortography can occasionally produce a haemothorax. Bleeding usually results from parenchymal laceration or from damage to intercostal vessels. A pneumothorax is present in a high proportion of patients.

The treatment of choice is to insert an intercostal drain which permits evacuation of blood and reduces the incidence of a subsequent fibrothorax. It also provides evidence of continued bleeding which may require a thoracotomy. Surgery is not indicated simply to remove any residual blood clot since in the majority of patients there is spontaneous lysis with no residual damage.

Spontaneous bleeding into the pleural space can occur in association with a pneumothorax (a haemopneumothorax) and presumably results from the tearing of pleural adhesions. Other rare causes of a haemothorax include bleeding disorders or excess anticoagulants and rupture of the thoracic aorta.

CHYLOTHORAX

A chylothorax results from leakage of chylous fluid from the thoracic duct. Absorbed fat is transported as chylomicrons in the intestinal lymphatics and, together with lymph originating in the lower limbs and abdomen, reaches the bloodstream via the thoracic duct. The flow of lymph in the thoracic duct is approximately 100 ml/h under basal conditions but can increase fivefold after a fatty meal.

Whilst congenital absence of the thoracic duct is a rare cause of a chylothorax, the majority of cases are acquired either as a result of trauma or neoplastic invasion of the thoracic duct. Surgery is the commonest cause of traumatic damage, particularly in operations that involve mobilization of the aortic arch or after oesophageal resection. Penetrating trauma occasionally results in damage to the thoracic duct, but rupture can also occur from non-penetrating injuries. The commonest single cause of rupture of the thoracic duct relates to damage caused by neoplastic infiltration. A lymphoma accounts for the majority of these malignancies. Other rare associations include pulmonary lymphangiolyomyomatosis, the yellow nail syndrome, and filariasis. There are no specific clinical features other than those of an effusion and the diagnosis of a chylothorax is usually made after pleural aspiration. The fluid is classically milky and opalescent due to the presence of fat globules. Such an effusion needs to be distinguished from an empyema or pseudochyle. An empyema is easy to distinguish since the discoloration is due to a cellular deposit and, after centrifugation, the supernatant is clear. Pseudochyle is due to high lipid levels, usually cholesterol crystals, which occur in chronic effusions particularly following tuberculosis. Cholesterol crystals can usually be recognized on smears of the sediment, and the addition of ethyl ether to the fluid results in clearing if high concentrations of cholesterol are responsible for the opalescence.

Spontaneous resolution can occur if the chyle is removed by chest tube and the flow of chyle is reduced by the use of medium-chain-triglyceride diets or parenteral nutrition. If there is a known malignancy, mediastinal irradiation may also assist resolution. Malnutrition and lymphopenia are likely to occur if large volumes of chyle continue to be drained, and under such circumstances surgery with ligation of the thoracic duct above the diaphragm can be combined with pleurodesis.

Pleural tumours

Pleural tumours are described in Chapter 17.13.2.

Pneumothorax

A pneumothorax results from gas entering the potential space between visceral and parietal pleura. A spontaneous pneumothorax is the consequence of rupture of a bulla or cyst on the surface of the lung. Air escapes from the alveoli into the pleural space. Following penetrating trauma, atmospheric air may enter the pleural space through the wound or the visceral pleura may be punctured allowing entry of alveolar gas. An iatrogenic pneumothorax occurs as a result of damage inflicted during catheterization of a subclavian vein or following percutaneous or transbronchial lung biopsy.

Pathophysiology

At functional residual capacity, the inward elastic recoil of the lung and the outward recoil of the chest wall results in a negative pressure in the potential space between visceral and parietal pleura. Pressures with respect to atmosphere become more negative during inspiration and only become positive during forced expiration. Because of the elastic recoil of the lung, pleural pressure is always less than alveolar pressure. Thus, if there is a breach of the visceral pleura due to rupture of a surface bulla, gas moves from lung to pleural space. As the lung collapses down, the pressures equilibrate and net flow of gas ceases. Occasionally the site of air leak acts as a one-way valve, allowing air to enter the pleural space during inspiration but preventing return flow during expiration. Pleural pressures tend to rise, although for air to continue to enter pressures must become negative with respect to atmosphere at some point in the inspiratory cycle. A tension pneumothorax results with mediastinal shift and compromised function of the opposite lung (see Fig. 5).

Once the original leak has sealed, reabsorption of pleural gas occurs and re-expansion of the lung takes place at approximately 1.25 per cent of the volume of the hemithorax per day. Pleural gas is absorbed because the total gas pressure, which is similar to that of arterial gas ($P_{N_2} = 76.4$ kPa, $P_{O_2} = 13.3$ kPa, $P_{CO_2} = 5.3$ kPa, and $P_{H_2O} = 6.3$ kPa (total 101 kPa)), is greater than that of venous blood ($P_{N_2} = 76.4$ kPa, $P_{O_2} = 5.3$ kPa, $P_{CO_2} = 6.1$ kPa, and $P_{H_2O} = 6.3$ kPa (total 94 kPa)). This pressure difference can be increased by giving additional inspired oxygen which will reduce the total pressure on the venous side.

Physiological consequence

The functional consequences of a pneumothorax are reduction of the vital capacity and total lung capacity as the lung collapses. Ventilation of the affected lung is reduced, although perfusion may also fall such that the anticipated alveolar arterial oxygen gradient and consequent hypoxia are less than might be anticipated. Ventilatory failure with a rise in arterial P_{CO_2} is rare except in patients with pre-existing lung disease.

Clinical syndromes

A spontaneous pneumothorax usually occurs without any warning or obvious precipitating factor. A primary pneumothorax occurs in individuals with apparently normal lungs. A secondary pneumothorax is a consequence of pre-existing lung disease.

PRIMARY PNEUMOTHORAX

Primary pneumothorax is a relatively common condition with an annual incidence of about 9 per 100 000. It is particularly common in young men with a male-to-female ratio of approximately 4:1. Patients are often tall with a marfanoid appearance. The cause of the pneumothorax is usually rupture of a small surface bulla or cyst, often near the lung apex. Only rarely can these be visualized radiologically. About 20 per cent of patients who have had one pneumothorax are likely to have a recurrence. Whilst this is usually on the same side as the initial pneumothorax, there is also an increased chance of occurrence in the contralateral hemithorax.

SECONDARY PNEUMOTHORAX

Older patients presenting with a spontaneous pneumothorax are likely to have underlying lung disease as a predisposing factor. The most common association is in patients with emphysema and obstructive airways disease. Rarely, acute exacerbations of asthma may be complicated by spontaneous pneumothorax, presumably due to high alveolar pressures associated with gas trapping. Some pulmonary infections can result in rupture of necrotic lung with subsequent air leak into the pleura. There is usually an associated empyema. Staphylococcal pneumonia, anaerobic lung abscesses, and tuberculosis are among the most likely infecting organisms. A secondary pneumothorax can also be associated with a lung malignancy as a result of either the pressure effects of a local bronchial obstruction or necrotic rupture of a subpleural tumour. Finally, there are a number of rare parenchymal and connective tissue disorders in which pneumothorax is a recognized complication. These include cystic fibrosis, histiocytosis X, lymphangiomyomatosis, pulmonary neurofibromatosis, Marfan's syndrome, and Ehlers–Danlös syndrome.

IATROGENIC PNEUMOTHORAX

A number of diagnostic and therapeutic procedures have an associated risk of developing a pneumothorax. Percutaneous needle aspiration or biopsy of the lung carries the greatest risk with estimates ranging from 5 to 50 per cent. The risk is related to the presence of underlying lung disease, the size of the needle, and the depth of penetration. Bronchoscopy rarely causes any problems, but a transbronchial biopsy carries a small risk particularly if undertaken in the absence of screening. Intermittent positive pressure ventilation, particularly when used with positive end expiratory pressures, can result in a pneumothorax which has the potential to present under tension. Attempted catheterization of subclavian veins can result in puncture of the lung, particularly when carried out by relatively inexperienced personnel.

Clinical features

Symptomatically, a spontaneous pneumothorax will present with chest pain and breathlessness. The pain is of sudden onset and typically pleuritic, being localized to the affected side. Inspiration is often painful and breathing is shallow to minimize discomfort. Dyspnoea is partly engendered by the difficulty in taking a deep breath, but is also dependent on the size of the pneumothorax and the presence of underlying lung disease. The initial sensation of breathlessness can improve rapidly before the resolution of the pneumothorax and may be due to reflex changes from receptors in the lung and airways.

Abnormal physical signs may be difficult to detect if the pneumothorax is small or the lungs are emphysematous. The most consistent finding is a reduction in breath sounds on the affected side. The percussion note will be resonant and, although hyper-resonance is a recorded feature, it is often difficult to detect any difference from the non-affected side. Vocal fremitus and tactile vocal resonance are diminished. Movements of the chest wall may be reduced, particularly if there is pain. A large pneumothorax under tension will result in mediastinal and tracheal shift away from the affected side. A left-sided pneumothorax may occasionally be associated with a clicking noise synchronous with the heart beat (Hamman's sign) which is probably due to contact and separation of the pleural surfaces in time with the heart beat. Rapid shallow breathing may in part be the result of pain. Evidence of severe respiratory distress and failure is rare unless the pneumothorax is under tension or there is pre-existing lung disease.

Associated conditions

PNEUMOMEDIASTINUM

Pneumomediastinum can present in isolation or in association with a pneumothorax. Air tracks along the bronchovascular sheath to the hilum and mediastinum. It can be associated with sudden rises in alveolar pressure during sneezing or straining and in patients undergoing intermittent positive pressure ventilation. Precordial chest discomfort may be a presenting symptoms, and subcutaneous emphysema can be detected in the neck and supraclavicular fossae. No specific treatment is indicated since the condition is benign and self-limiting.

HAEMOPNEUMOTHORAX

The presence of blood and air in the pleural space is most commonly the result of trauma. A spontaneous pneumothorax can occasionally have associated bleeding into the pleural space, presumably due to tearing of the pleural adhesions.

PYOPNEUMOTHORAX

Pyopneumothorax usually result from rupture of necrotic lung although it can also be due to oesophageal rupture. The clinical picture is one of a combined empyema and pneumothorax.

Investigations

Confirmation of the diagnosis of a pneumothorax is best made by chest radiography. An erect posteroanterior film is adequate; although a film during expiration increases the radiodensity of the lung and enhances the contrast between lung and pleural gas, it is rarely necessary. The cardinal radiological features are illustrated in Fig. 5. The outer margin of the lung can be seen as a thin line with the space between it and the chest devoid of any lung markings. Pleural adhesions can result in a part of the lung being tethered to the chest wall and distort the normal radiographic appearance. A large emphysematous bulla can sometimes be mistaken for a pneumothorax on both clinical and radiological grounds although the inner margins are usually concave. A tension pneumothorax is usually evident clinically, and emergency aspiration may be necessary before a chest radiograph is undertaken. If a film is obtained, it will show mediastinal and tracheal shift and depression of the ipsilateral diaphragm.

Management

The diversity of therapeutic options listed in Table 4 is a manifestation of the uncertainty with respect to optimum treatment. Two principle therapeutic objectives are to achieve rapid resolution of the pneumotho-

Fig. 5 Chest radiograph demonstrating a tension pneumothorax.

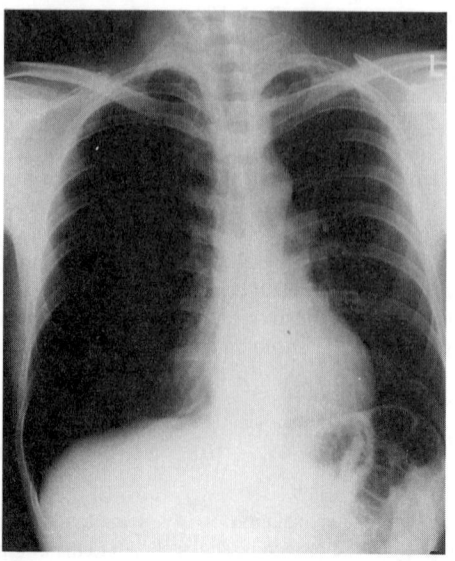

Table 4 *Treatment options for a pneumothorax*

Option	Indication
Natural resolution	Small primary pneumothorax
Aspiration	Large primary pneumothorax, particularly if the patient is breathless
Intercostal drain (± pleurodesis)	Failed aspiration Secondary pneumothorax
Thorascopy + pleurodesis	Recurrent pneumothorax Failed intercostal drainage

Thoracotomy
  Limited pleurectomy
  Pleurodesis
  Ligation of bullae
	Recurrent pneumothorax
	Failed intercostal drainage

rax, particularly if there is evidence of respiratory distress, and to reduce the likelihood of recurrence.

NATURAL RESOLUTION

A small pneumothorax is an otherwise healthy patient may require no treatment other than reassurance and relief of any pain. Non-steroidal anti-inflammatory drugs are usually effective in this respect. Admission to hospital is unnecessary provided that the patient has ready access to medical care and is advised to return if symptoms worsen.

SIMPLE ASPIRATION

Simple aspiration is the treatment of choice for a patient with a large primary pneumothorax. If successful, it will not only speed resolution but relieve any associated breathlessness or chest discomfort. It is simple to perform and has negligible morbidity even in relatively inexperienced hands. The risk of puncturing the lung is minimal if a Teflon catheter is used. This can be inserted after infiltrating with local anaesthetic in the second intercostal space in the mid-clavicular line. Air can be aspirated using a 50 ml syringe and a three-way tap. If the original site of air leakage has sealed, the lung will re-expand. Aspiration should stop if resistance is encountered or if the patient experiences undue discomfort or coughing. If more than 2 to 3 litres of air have been evacuated, it is likely that there is a persisting air leak. Under these circumstances aspiration should be abandoned and a decision made as to whether an intercostal drain should be inserted. This is likely to be necessary if the patient is breathless, but conservative management with attempted repeat aspiration after 2 or 3 days may be more appropriate in patients who are relatively asymptomatic. A recent study by the British Thoracic Society has shown that in patients with a primary pneumothorax simple aspiration was less painful and required a shorter duration of hospital admission than treatment with an intercostal drain. There were no significant differences in recurrence rate at 1 year.

INTERCOSTAL TUBE DRAINAGE

This approach may be indicated if simple aspiration has failed. It is more likely to be indicated in patients with underlying lung disease in whom even a small pneumothorax can result in severe respiratory failure. A large primary pneumothorax may require intubation, although a decision should be influenced as much by the patient's symptoms as by the size alone. The preferred site is the fourth, fifth, or sixth intercostal space anterior to the mid-axillary line. Under sterile technique and after infiltration of adequate local anaesthesia, an incision is made in the skin, subcutaneous fat, and underlying muscle, and the pleural cavity is entered using blunt dissection. An FG 20–24 catheter is usually adequate and if inserted using a trocar this should be done with minimal force.

Once in the pleural space the catheter should be advanced towards the apex of the lung and connected to an underwater seal. A Heimlich flutter valve is an alternative to an underwater seal. It permits greater mobility but often becomes blocked. The catheter should be firmly secured with a suture through the skin and multiple ties around the catheter. Adequate analgesia is essential whilst the tube is in place.

Bubbling will cease once the air leak has sealed and the lung fully expanded. This may take hours or even days. A check radiograph should be taken before the catheter is removed since drainage of air will also cease if the tube is blocked or has become dislodged. Clamping of the tube prior to removal is unnecessary. The value of additional suction is unproven and may simply serve to maintain the patency of the original air leak. It can be tried if the lung fails to re-expand with the aim of evacuating the pleural air and allowing apposition of the pleural surfaces.

PLEURODESIS

Pleurodesis is often undertaken in an attempt to obliterate the pleural space and reduce the likelihood of a recurrent pneumothorax. Overall, a recurrence can be expected in 20 per cent of patients, although in those who have had more than one pneumothorax the recurrence rate increase to over 50 per cent. There are a variety of potential techniques but the lack of any large comparative studies makes choice somewhat dependent on personal experience. Sclerosants can be introduced in conjunction with an intercostal drain or at thoracoscopy. Agents which have been used include silver nitrate, tetracycline, iodized talc, fibrin 'glue', and blood. Of these, tetracycline has fewest of side-effects and can be injected through an intercostal catheter. The lung needs to be fully inflated and a combination of local anaesthetic and systemic analgesic is required to minimize chest discomfort. After instillation the patient is positioned such that the liquid can spread evenly over the pleural surface.

Thorascopic techniques using iodized talc or fibrin 'glue' are at present limited to a few centres. However, currently available video-assisted thoracoscopy is likely to become more widely available, and its potential is yet to be fully exploited.

SURGICAL INTERVENTION

Referral rates for surgery vary considerably. The main indications include those patients in whom there is a persisting air leak after prolonged intubation (usually 1–2 weeks) and patients who have had recurrent pneumothoraces. In the latter group, referral is most commonly made after the second or third ipsilateral recurrence or if there have been bilateral pneumothoraces. The preferred surgical option is an apicolateral pleurectomy, if necessary in conjunction with oversewing or excision of any large bullae. Surgical morbidity in otherwise healthy patients is very low. Risks are greater in patients with underlying lung disease, but this must be balanced against the life-threatening potential of further pneumothorax.

REFERENCES

Pleural effusions

Adelman, M., Albella, S.M., Gottleib, J., and Haponik, E.F. (1984). Diagnostic utility of pleural fluid eosinophilia. *American Journal of Medicine*, **77**, 915–20.

Black, L.J. (1972). Pleural space and pleural fluid. *Mayo Clinic Proceedings*, **47**, 493–506.

Hsu, C. (1987). Cytological detection of malignancy in pleural effusions: a review of 5,255 samples from 3,811 patients. *Diagnostic Cytopathology*, **3**, 8–12.

Jay, S.J. (1985). Diagnostic procedures for pleural disease. *Clinics in Chest Medicine*, **6**, 33–48.

Kendall, S.W., Bryan, A.J., Large, S.R., and Wells, F.C. (1992). Pleural

effusions: is thoracoscopy a reliable investigation? A retrospective review. *Respiratory Medicine*, **86**, 437–40.

Light, R.W. (1990). *Pleural diseases* (2nd edn). Lea & Febiger, Philadelphia, PA.

Light, R.W., MacGregor, M.I., Luchsinger, P.C., and Ball, W.C. (1972). Pleural effusions: the diagnostic separation of transudates and exudates. *Annals of Internal Medicine*, **77**, 507–13.

Muller, N.L. (1993). Imaging of the pleura. *Radiology*, **186**, 297–309.

Prakash, U.B.S. and Reiman, H.M. (1985). Comparison of needle biopsy with cytologic analysis for the evaluation of pleural effusion: analysis of 414 cases. *Mayo Clinic Proceedings*, **60**, 158–63.

Yam, L.T. (1967). Diagnostic significance of lymphocytes in pleural effusions. *Annals of Internal Medicine*, **66**, 977–82.

Empyema

Alfageme, I., Munoz, F., Pena, N., and Umbria, S. (1993). Empyema of the thorax in adults. Etiology, microbiologic findings and management. *Chest*, **103**, 839–43.

Ashbaugh, D.G. (1991). Empyema thoracic: factors influencing morbidity and mortality. *Chest*, **99**, 1162–5.

Light, R.W. (1991). Management of parapneumonic effusions. *Chest*, **100**, 892–3.

Moores, D.W.O. (1992). Management of acute empyema. *Chest*, **102**, 1316–17.

Stavas, J., van Sonnenberg, E., Casola, G., and Wittich, G.R. (1987). Percutaneous drainage of infected and non-infected thoracic fluid collections. *Journal of Thoracic Imaging*, **1987**, 80–7.

van Sonnenberg, E., Nakamoto, S.K., Muller, P.R., Casola, G., Neff, C.C., Friedman, P.J., *et al.* (1984). CT - and ultrasound - guided catheter drainage of empyemas after chest-tube failure. *Radiology*, **151**, 349–53.

Varkey, B., Rose, H.D., Cutty, C.P.K., and Politis, J. (1981). Empyema thoracis during a ten year period: analysis of 72 cases in comparison to a previous study (1952–1967). *Archives of Internal Medicine*, **141**, 1771–6.

Tuberculosis

Berger, H.W. and Magier, E. (1973). Tuberculous pleurisy. *Chest*, **63**, 88–92.

Epstein, D.M., Kline, L.P., Albelda, S.M., and Miller, W.T. (1967). Tuberculous pleural effusions. *Chest*, **91**, 107–9.

Levine, H., Metzger, W., Lacera, D., and Kay, L. (1970). Diagnosis of tuberculosis pleurisy by culture of pleural biopsy specimen. *Archives of Internal Medicine*, **126**, 269–71.

Miscellaneous

Bynum, L.J. and Wilson, J.E. (1976). Characteristics of pleural effusions associated with pulmonary embolism. *Archives of Internal Medicine*, **136**, 159–62.

Emerson, P.A. (1966). Yellow nails, lymphoedema and pleural effusions. *Thorax*, **21**, 247–50.

Eppler, G.R., McLeod, T.C., and Gaensler, E.A. (1982). Prevalence and incidence of benign asbestos pleural effusion in a working population. *Journal of the American Medical Association*, **247**, 617–22.

Fairfax, A.J., McNabb, W.R., and Spiro, S.G. (1986). Chylothorax: A review of 18 cases. *Thorax*, **41**, 880–5.

Hunninghake, G.W. and Fauci, A.S. (1979). Pulmonary involvement in the collagen vascular diseases. *American Review of Respiratory Disease*, **119**, 471–503.

Kay, M.D. (1968). Pleural pulmonary complications of pancreatitis. *Thorax*, **23**, 297–306.

Light, R.W. and George, R.B. (1976). Incidence and significance of pleural effusion after abdominal surgery. *Chest*, **69**, 621–6.

MacFarlane, R.J. and Holman, C.W. (1972). Chylothorax. *American Review of Respiratory Disease*, **105**, 287–91.

Meigs, I.V. (1954). Meigs' syndrome. *American Journal of Obstetrics and Gynecology*, **67**, 962–6.

Pneumothorax

Getz, S.B. and Beasley, W.E. (1983). Spontaneous pneumothorax. *American Journal of Surgery*, **145**, 823–6.

Harvey, J.E. (1993). Comparison of simple aspiration with intercostal drainage in the management of spontaneous pneumothorax. *Thorax,* **48,** 430–1.

Jenkinson, S.G. (1985). Pneumothorax. In: *Clinics in chest medicine* (ed R.W. Light), pp. 153–92. W.B. Saunders, Philadelphia, PA.

Miller, A.C. and Harvey, J.E. (for Standards of Care Committee, British Thoracic Society). (1993). Guidelines for the management of spontaneous pneumothorax. *British Medical Journal,* **307,** 114–16.

Ohata, M. and Suzuki, H. (1980). Pathogenesis of spontaneous pneumothorax. *Chest, 77,* 771–6.

Rhea, J.T., DeLuca, S.A., and Green, R.E. (1982). Determining the size of pneumothorax in the upright patient. *Radiology, 144,* 733–6.

So, S.Y. and Yu, D.Y.C. (1982). Catheter drainage of spontaneous pneumothorax: suction or no suction, early or late removal. *Thorax, 37,* 46–8.

17.12 Disorders of the thoracic cage and diaphragm

J. M. SHNEERSON

Introduction

Skeletal disorders of the thorax are an important group of conditions that frequently impair ventilation. They are often associated with respiratory muscle weakness due to neuromuscular disorders which are described elsewhere. Most of these conditions restrict the development or the expansion of the lungs or both so that alveolar ventilation rather than intrapulmonary gas exchange is primarily impaired.

Disorders of the spine

Scoliosis

INTRODUCTION

Scoliosis is defined as a lateral curvature of the spine, but it is invariably also associated with rotation of the vertebral bodies. This results in an unstable lordosis rather than a kyphosis, and therefore the frequently used term kyphoscoliosis is inaccurate. A mild degree of scoliosis is very common. Angles of curvature of 5° or 10° have been used to define when it becomes pathological, but these are arbitrary figures. Postural scoliosis can be distinguished from a structural scoliosis by its temporary nature and because it disappears when the patient bends forwards.

The age of onset and natural history of scoliosis vary according to its cause (Table 1). When it is due to a neuromuscular disorder it usually arises during childhood or adolescence, or in the case of poliomyelitis within about 2 years of the acute infection. Typically, the curve has a long C shape and may be severe. When the scoliosis is due to a congenital abnormality, such as a hemivertebra or a segmentation defect, it usually becomes apparent early in childhood. The scoliosis of neurofibromatosis and Marfan's syndrome is probably due to an abnormality of connective tissue. Scoliosis due to pleural or pulmonary disease is less common than previously now that chronic infections are less frequent and more successfully treated.

The commonest type is adolescent idiopathic scoliosis where the spinal deformity develops at the time of the pubertal growth spurt. It is around four times as common in girls as in boys, and the convexity of the deformity is on the right in 80 per cent of cases. The scoliosis may continue to worsen slightly even after the growth of the spine stops. An infantile form of idiopathic scoliosis is less common, and although it often resolves spontaneously it can progress to a severe deformity.

PATHOPHYSIOLOGY

The most important organic consequence of scoliosis is the respiratory abnormality. A direct result of scoliosis is that the compliance of the chest wall is reduced. This is more marked in older subjects, possibly owing to degenerative changes in the costovertebral joints. The com-

Table 1 *Causes of scoliosis*

Idiopathic Infantile, adolescent
Osteopathic Congenital (e.g. hemivertebrae) Thoracoplasty
Neuromuscular Syringomyelia Friedreich's ataxia Poliomyelitis Duchenne's muscular dystrophy
Connective tissue disorders Marfan's syndrome Neurofibromatosis Osteogenesis imperfecta
Pleuropulmonary Empyema Pneumonectomy Unilateral lung fibrosis

pliance of the lungs is also reduced, largely because of their small volume. In addition, the distortion of the rib cage puts the inspiratory muscles at a mechanical disadvantage; those on the side of the convexity of the scoliosis are shortened and those on the side of the concavity lengthened. The vital capacity (**VC**) falls when changing from the sitting to the supine position. Therefore a restrictive defect and reduction of the maximum inspiratory and expiratory pressures develops even in the absence of any muscle weakness, but is more marked if this is present.

In adults with severe scoliosis the exercise ability is linked to the degree of reduction of VC and the forced expiratory volume in 1 s (**FEV$_1$**). The tidal volume increases initially and then remains constant, while the respiratory frequency rises as exercise becomes more intense. The ventilation at any given oxygen uptake is greater than normal and the maximal exercise ventilation, which limits the exercise ability, is often severely curtailed. The cardiac output may increase normally during exercise, but the pulmonary artery pressure rises rapidly and its rate of increase is linearly related to the oxygen uptake and inversely related to the VC.

In mild scoliosis the arterial blood gases are often normal, but the first abnormality is a fall in the PO_2. This is due to suboptimal ventilation and perfusion matching, particularly at the bases of the lungs. Even when the anatomical distortion of the two lungs is gross there is usually rather less difference in function between the two lungs than might be expected. Acute ventilatory failure may be precipitated by, for instance, a chest infection or asthma. Chronic hypoventilation occurs initially during sleep, particularly during rapid eye movement (**REM**) sleep.

Central apnoeas and hypopnoeas are frequent, and the severity of the oxygen desaturation correlates with both the oxygen saturation during wakefulness and the VC.

Chronic hypercapnia during the day is uncommon in childhood and is dependent on the following.

1. Age of onset: if the scoliosis appears before the age of about 8 years it may prevent normal alveolar multiplication so that the lung fails to develop fully. Therefore the capillary surface is reduced and there is a risk of developing respiratory and right heart failure later in life. The later onset of adolescent idiopathic scoliosis is probably the major reason why these serious complications only rarely occur in this condition.
2. Level of the scoliosis: in general, the higher the curve in the thoracic spine the more marked are the cardiac and respiratory problems. Thoracolumbar and lumbar scoliosis have virtually no effects of respiration.
3. Severity of scoliosis: the angle of scoliosis is closely related to the reduction in lung volume. This association is seen with residual volume (**RV**), total lung capacity (**TLC**), and functional residual capacity (**FRC**), as well as with VC, except in patients with neuromuscular disorders where the changes in lung volumes are due to the weakness of the respiratory muscles as well as the degree of deformity. The changes in lung volumes become significant when the angle of scoliosis is greater than about 100°.
4. Presence of muscle weakness: the functioning of the respiratory muscles is impaired in scoliosis, and any further loss of strength or endurance due to a neuromuscular disorder may precipitate respiratory failure. Conversely, respiratory function often worsens in neuromuscular disorders when scoliosis develops as a result of the strength of the axial muscles becoming asymmetrical.
5. Small lung volumes: respiratory failure usually occurs when lung volumes have been reduced to a degree such that VC is less than 1.0–1.5 l.

The development of right ventricular failure often coincides with or follows respiratory failure and is due to pulmonary hypertension. This is the result of a raised pulmonary vascular resistance due to both hypoxic vasoconstriction and an anatomically restricted pulmonary vascular bed. Polycythaemia may contribute by effectively increasing the pulmonary vascular resistance.

SYMPTOMS AND PHYSICAL SIGNS

The earliest symptom of scoliosis is usually a change in the appearance of the patient. Asymmetry of the shoulders and a prominence of the posterior rib hump may be noticed initially by either the parents or the patient. Backache is usually a late symptom and is rare in thoracic spine deformities. With mild curvatures there may be no respiratory symptoms, but many patients with scoliosis become short of breath on exertion. A change in this often signifies the development of complications such as respiratory failure. Orthopnoea suggests that diaphragm function is impaired. When respiratory failure develops, fatigue, ankle swelling, and even syncope may indicate that pulmonary hypertension and right heart failure are present. Frequent awakenings during sleep associated with excessive daytime somnolence suggest that the subject is arousing from apnoeas and hypopnoeas, and are important symptoms that warn of impending respiratory failure.

Physical examination may reveal the cause of the scoliosis, such as Marfan's syndrome or neurofibromatosis, and other congenital abnormalities. Any associated muscle weakness or congenital heart disease may be apparent. Rib cage expansion may be predominantly lateral or anterior or achieved by extension of the spine. In some subjects chest expansion is mainly oblique because of the rotation of the spine, and

some areas of the chest wall may move paradoxically. Accessory muscle action is usually prominent.

INVESTIGATIONS

The severity of the scoliosis can be demonstrated radiologically, but chest radiography is often unhelpful in thoracic scoliosis because the rotation of the spine obscures much of the lung fields. This can be overcome by obtaining an oblique view of the chest which simulates a posteroanterior view by aligning the spine behind the heart. Lung function testing reveals a restrictive defect with reduction in all lung volumes, although the change in RV is least marked. Therefore the ratio of RV to TLC is increased. $K\text{CO}$ is raised, as in other chest wall disorders that cause a restrictive defect and in which the lung tissue is normal. Maximum inspiratory and expiratory pressures are reduced. Chest wall and lung compliance are less than normal, and the exercise tolerance is impaired. Arterial blood gas analysis reveals a slightly low $P\text{O}_2$ in mildly affected subjects, but later in the natural history a rise in $P\text{CO}_2$ and a proportional fall in $P\text{O}_2$ develop. Sleep studies show a variable degree of hypoxia and hypercapnia which are usually most marked in REM sleep. Electrocardiography and echocardiography may be required to establish whether congenital heart disease is present and, if so, to identify the abnormality.

PROGNOSIS

The prognosis in subjects with adolescent idiopathic scoliosis is virtually normal, but life expectancy is reduced in many of the other forms of scoliosis. This is particularly marked in scoliosis of early onset which is both severe and high in the thorax and associated with respiratory muscle weakness, low VC, and abnormal blood gases.

In most subjects the cause of death is either cardiac or respiratory. Pneumonia and respiratory failure are particularly common in neuromuscular disorders, but hypoxic dysrhythmias during sleep are probably responsible for some deaths. Congenital heart defects, which have an increased prevalence in subjects with scoliosis, particularly when this is due to a congenital abnormality or of the idiopathic type, may contribute to mortality.

TREATMENT

Subjects with a mild scoliosis do not need any specific treatment. Their prognosis is normal and they have minimal respiratory deficit. However, as the scoliosis becomes more severe, spinal fusion or a costectomy in which the parts of the ribs comprising the posterior hump are removed may be of cosmetic value. Spinal fusion may also be required to prevent progression of the scoliosis, to stabilize the spine, particularly in neuromuscular disorders, and in selected cases to try to improve cardiac or respiratory function or to prevent its deterioration.

The value of spinal fusion for the last mentioned indication in adolescent idiopathic scoliosis is still under debate. A large number of studies of respiratory function before and after surgery have shown remarkably little change in lung volumes, blood gases, or exercise ability. However, in some patients with muscle weakness, particularly Duchenne's muscular dystrophy, the rate of fall of the VC can be slowed considerably and it can even be improved in patients who have had poliomyelitis. Despite these short-term improvements, there have been no studies which indicate whether or not spinal fusion performed in childhood or adolescence prevents respiratory failure from appearing later in life. If respiratory failure does develop, any acute illness which may have precipitated it should be actively treated. This is most commonly an infection or bronchial asthma. Endotracheal intubation and ventilation may be required during the acute illness, and the patient is then weaned from this either completely or on to a non-invasive method of long-term respiratory support.

Chronic ventilatory failure usually responds to long-term mechanical respiratory support. Administration of oxygen at night or during the day or both may be dangerous because of the risk of hypercapnia. Negative pressure ventilation, usually with a cuirass or jacket, or a nasal positive pressure system are the treatments of choice. The cuirass has to be individually constructed to fit the shape of the thorax and abdomen because of the thoracic deformity. Some patients require support during part of the day as well as at night, but a tracheostomy is rarely required.

This type of treatment can considerably improve the quality of life, arterial blood gases, maximum respiratory pressures, and the quality of sleep, as well as reducing the number of visits required by general practitioners and the amount of drugs prescribed. Survival once treatment has been instituted is around 75 per cent at 5 years, and 60 per cent at 10 years (Fig. 1).

Kyphosis

INTRODUCTION

Exaggeration of the normal thoracic kyphosis is most commonly due to osteoporosis and is not usually associated with any significant changes in respiratory function. The exception to this is when a very sharp kyphosis (gibbus) develops. This is usually caused by tuberculous osteomyelitis of the spine (Pott's disease), although other conditions such as radiotherapy can cause a similar picture.

PATHOPHYSIOLOGY

The spine becomes rigid in the region of the gibbus, and when tuberculosis is the cause the costovertebral joints also become ankylosed and limit the expansion of the rib cage. A restrictive defect in which the TLC is reduced more than the RV is characteristic, but respiratory problems are uncommon unless the gibbus is high in the thoracic spine and develops in early childhood. This is probably because the thoracic deformity prevents the normal development of the lungs in a similar way to early onset scoliosis. Hypoxia and hypercapnia appear during sleep before they become apparent during wakefulness, but may be severe. Pulmonary hypertension and right heart failure frequently develop once chronic hypercapnia has become established.

SYMPTOMS AND PHYSICAL SIGNS

Slight breathlessness on exertion is common in the presence of a gibbus, but is rare in other types of kyphosis. Physical examination reveals the spinal deformity and limitation of rib cage expansion.

Fig. 1 Actuarial survival during treatment with ventilatory assistance for respiratory failure. (Reproduced with permission from Shneerson 1988.)

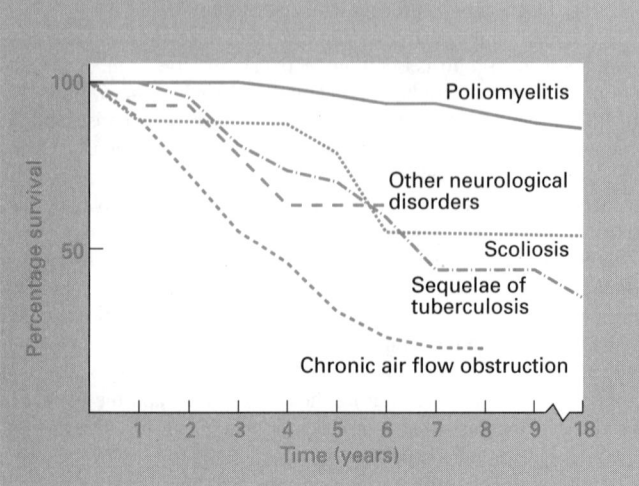

INVESTIGATIONS

The posteroanterior chest radiograph shows superimposition of the spinal deformity on the lung fields and heart which makes it difficult to interpret. The extent and severity of the kyphosis is usually well seen on a lateral projection. The typical changes in lung volumes have been described above. The arterial $P\text{O}_2$ and $P\text{CO}_2$ are normal in most subjects, but the earliest abnormalities are revealed by sleep studies.

TREATMENT

Treatment of the acute tuberculous infection with chemotherapy is often effective in preventing a gibbus from developing. Once it has been established and respiratory failure has developed, the only effective treatment is long-term respiratory support. This is best provided non-invasively by a nasal positive pressure ventilator rather than a negative pressure system since patients with a sharp kyphosis often find it difficult to lie in the supine position, which is required for negative pressure ventilation.

Straight-back syndrome

In this disorder the normal thoracic kyphosis is absent or greatly reduced. This may result in a mild restrictive ventilatory defect but the cardiac problems are more prominent. The heart and great vessels may be compressed between the anterior rib cage and the spine with results similar to those seen in pectus excavatum. The right ventricular outflow tract or pulmonary artery may be narrowed, causing a systolic murmur, and occasionally right ventricular filling is impaired.

Ankylosing spondylitis

INTRODUCTION

The initial manifestation of ankylosing spondylitis is usually painful inflammation of the sacroiliac joints, but this may spread to affect almost any joint including the intervertebral, costovertebral, sternomanubrial, costochondral, and chondrosternal joints. When the inflammatory phase of the disease subsides, the joints become ankylosed and the spinal ligaments calcify.

PATHOPHYSIOLOGY

The effect of ankylosing spondylitis on the thorax is that the rib cage becomes rigid. There is little spinal mobility, and a pronounced kyphosis often develops. The changes in lung volumes are characteristic in that, unlike all other skeletal disorders affecting the thorax, FRC increases. This is because the rib cage becomes fixed at its own relaxation volume. This is greater than the normal FRC which is influenced by the inward pull of the elastic recoil of the lungs. TLC and VC are slightly reduced, and RV often increases.

The immobility of the rib cage leads to atrophy of the intercostal muscles and both the maximal inspiratory and expiratory pressures are reduced. However, there is no impairment of diaphragmatic function and this largely compensates for the restriction of rib cage expansion. The ventilatory responses to exercise are virtually normal and exercise is usually limited by circulatory rather than respiratory factors. Respiratory failure is extremely uncommon in ankylosing spondylitis, probably as a result of the normal diaphragmatic function, unless another complication develops, which may be one of the following:

1. Air flow obstruction: cricoarytenoid arthritis is a feature of ankylosing spondylitis and may present with stridor, hoarseness of the voice, breathlessness, or respiratory failure.
2. Pleural thickening and effusion: these rare complications of ankylosing spondylitis may cause respiratory failure.
3. Aspiration pneumonia: oesophageal motility is often impaired

in ankylosing spondylitis and aspiration pneumonia may develop.

4. Bullae: apical fibrobullous lung disease is a feature of ankylosing spondylitis and may be complicated by opportunist infections such as *Aspergillus fumigatus* or saprophytic mycobacteria, and occasionally pulmonary tuberculosis.

5. Abdominal surgery: this restricts diaphragmatic function on which adequate respiration depends. Conversely, thoracic surgery has relatively little effect on respiration because of the small contribution that rib cage expansion plays.

SYMPTOMS AND PHYSICAL SIGNS

Chest pain during sudden movements such as coughing and laughing is common if the active phase of the inflammation affects the thorax. These symptoms, which originate in either the joints or the muscles, become less prominent as the disease advances. Breathlessness and other respiratory symptoms are uncommon. Occasionally cricoarytenoid arthritis may present with hoarseness, stridor, or breathlessness, and extensive fibrobullous disease may also cause breathlessness.

The most obvious physical sign is restriction of rib cage movement associated with prominent accessory muscle activity and abdominal respiratory movements.

INVESTIGATIONS

Chest radiography may show calcification of the paraspinal ligaments (bamboo spine) and may also reveal evidence of complications of ankylosing spondylitis such as pleural thickening, aspiration pneumonia, and apical fibrobullous disease. The changes in lung volumes have been described above. Chest wall compliance is reduced but lung compliance is normal. The $K\mathrm{CO}$ is increased and arterial blood gases are normal during both rest and exertion.

TREATMENT

Physiotherapy and non-steroidal anti-inflammatory drugs may improve the vital capacity and chest expansion, particularly in the early phase of the disease or during acute exacerbations.

Disorders of the sternum and ribs

Congenital abnormalities

Congenital abnormalities of the ribs and sternum rarely cause any important respiratory problems. Occasionally, multiple congenital rib abnormalities may lead to paradoxical movement of the chest wall or impair diaphragmatic function if they occur in the region of the insertion of this muscle. Severe congenital defects of the sternum, such as agenesis or a bifid sternum, are rare but may require surgery in the neonatal period in order to stabilize the anterior chest wall.

Pectus excavatum

Pectus excavatum is a depression deformity of the sternum which is often present at birth but may worsen during the adolescent growth spurt. It is occasionally familial and may be associated with other abnormalities such as the straight-back syndrome or scoliosis. It appears to result from an increased inward pull on the sternum by the sternal diaphragmatic fibres or from an abnormally compliant chest wall.

Transient paradoxical movement of the sternum during respiration is seen in neonates, particularly in the presence of upper airway obstruction or pneumonia. In some cases the sternal depression becomes permanent although the cause, such as enlarged tonsils, may resolve completely.

In adults pectus excavatum rarely causes any symptoms. The lung volumes are normal or only slightly diminished and chest wall mobility appears to be normal. Arterial blood gases are normal both at rest and during exercise. Occasionally, however, the right ventricular filling is impaired because the heart is compressed between the depressed sternum and the spine, and in other cases the compression of the pulmonary outflow tract causes a systolic murmur. These problems are most marked in the erect position and during exercise. Occasionally atrial dysrhythmias develop. Surgery is sometimes indicated for cosmetic reasons although the result can be disappointing. It has little or no effect on the mild restrictive defect or exercise ability except in the rare situation when right ventricular filling is impaired or atrial dysrhythmias have developed.

Pectus carinatum

Pectus carinatum is a protrusion deformity of the sternum in which the chest is often narrowed transversely as well. It is most marked during the pubertal growth spurt, although it may be present from birth and occasionally is associated with severe childhood asthma or ventricular septal defects. It is probably the result of excessive growth of the ribs or costal cartilages, and if this is asymmetrical the sternum becomes oblique.

The respiratory consequences of pectus carinatum have been little investigated. Chest pain may arise at the insertions of the intercostal muscles anteriorly or in the costal cartilages and anterior ribs. The lung volumes appear to be normal, and surgery is indicated only for cosmetic reasons and not in order to improve respiratory function or exercise ability.

Asphyxiating thoracic dystrophy (Jeune's disease)

Asphyxiating thoracic dystrophy is a generalized disorder of cartilage in which the radiological changes are most prominent in the pelvis, phalanges, and other limb bones. Like the other long bones, the ribs are shortened so that the rib cage becomes narrowed. As a result lung development may be impaired and respiratory failure often appears during infancy or childhood. Surgical reconstruction of the rib cage with splitting of the sternum to enable lung growth to occur has been largely unsuccessful.

Flail chest

A flail chest is one in which multiple rib fractures cause paradoxical movement of the chest wall during respiration. It may be associated with other injuries such as rupture of the aortic arch or spleen and fractures of the skull and long bones. It is frequently associated with pulmonary contusion, pneumothorax, or haemothorax.

Surgical stabilization of the chest wall is rarely required. In milder cases sufficient analgesics to enable the patient to cough adequately may be all that is required as long as the paradoxical movement does not impair alveolar ventilation. In more severe cases positive pressure ventilation is usually employed in order to achieve 'pneumatic splinting' of the flail segment. The effectiveness of this has not been definitely established, but it appears that positive end expiratory pressure or continuous positive airway pressure is beneficial since any negative pressure swings within the pleura are avoided.

Thoracoplasty

INTRODUCTION

The operation of thoracoplasty was developed for the treatment of pulmonary tuberculosis. Varying lengths of up to eleven ribs were removed in order to collapse the chest on the affected side. It has been superseded by antituberculous chemotherapy but is still occasionally required to treat chronic infections, particularly when there is a problem in obliterating the pleural space after pulmonary resection. It is estimated that as many as 30 000 operations were carried out in the United Kingdom between 1951 and 1960, and many of these patients still survive. Increasing numbers of this important cohort of patients are being seen by chest physicians because of the late complications of the surgical procedure.

PATHOPHYSIOLOGY

The consequences of thoracoplasty on respiratory function have been hard to elucidate because they are often combined with the effects of the underlying lung disease for which the surgery was carried out and other types of treatment such as lung resection. However, the removal of the ribs has the direct result of flattening the chest and reducing the volume of the thorax. The normal movements of the rib cage may be impaired and paradoxical movement at the site of the thoracoplasty is common. The compliance of the chest wall is reduced and may fall further because the small range of movements of the costovertebral joints after surgery probably induces soft tissue changes which further limit the mobility at these joints. The chest wall compliance is also reduced by the almost invariable development of a thoracic scoliosis. This is convex to the side of the thoracoplasty and may progress for several years after the surgery. The severity of the scoliosis correlates with the number of ribs removed but also depends on the details of the surgical technique.

Respiratory muscle function is impaired by a thoracoplasty. The intercostal and shoulder girdle muscles are directly damaged by the surgery, and in addition distortion of the rib cage and the development of a scoliosis put the inspiratory muscles at a mechanical disadvantage. Diaphragmatic excursion is reduced, particularly on the side of the thoracoplasty but also sometimes contralaterally.

The combination of a reduced chest wall compliance and impaired respiratory muscle function account for the restrictive defect. All the lung volumes are reduced and in general the severity of the restrictive defect is proportional to the number of ribs that have been resected. A rapid respiratory rate with a small tidal volume is the characteristic respiratory pattern, particularly during exertion. Exercise is limited by ventilatory factors rather than by the cardiovascular system. In some patients chronic air flow obstruction, which may be due to either tuberculous endobronchitis or the effects of tobacco smoking, may be significant, resulting in a progressive fall in exercise ability and contributing to the development of respiratory failure.

The ventilation and perfusion of the lung on the side of the thoracoplasty are usually equally reduced so that in many subjects the arterial P_{O_2} remains virtually normal. The function of the contralateral lung is much more important in determining the blood gases. Hypoxaemia usually appears during sleep before wakefulness and may be associated with hypercapnia. This may persist during the day and correlates with the reduction in maximal inspiratory and transdiaphragmatic pressures.

SYMPTOMS AND PHYSICAL SIGNS

The symptoms of patients with a thoracoplasty are similar to those with a scoliosis, but if a productive cough develops a recurrence of pulmonary tuberculosis should be suspected and investigated. Right heart failure often develops insidiously either when respiratory failure appears or subsequently. It may be manifested by progressively worsening ankle swelling and fatigue. Physical examination reveals a thoracotomy scar and a flattened area of chest in the region of the thoracoplasty which may move paradoxically. Accessory muscle activity, particularly on the side of the thoracoplasty, is often marked.

INVESTIGATIONS

The chest radiograph shows the extent of the thoracoplasty, other features which indicate the extent of previous tuberculous infection, and the sequelae of treatment such as a previous phrenic nerve crush or an artificial pneumothorax which often causes extensive calcified pleural thickening. The characteristic physiological defect is restrictive, but airflow obstruction may also be significant. Maximum inspiratory and expiratory pressures and transdiaphragmatic pressures are reduced. Most patients are mildly hypoxic, but later in the natural history the arterial P_{CO_2} may rise particularly during sleep.

PROGNOSIS

The prognosis of patients who have had a thoracoplasty for pulmonary tuberculosis is reduced and deaths may occur particularly from respiratory but also from cardiac causes. These complications are related to the extent of the tuberculosis and to whether or not an artificial pneumothorax was induced on the contralateral side to the thoracoplasty since this often leads to pleural thickening and may also indicate extensive tuberculous damage to the underlying lung. Respiratory failure may develop after a long period of stability and often appears quite suddenly even when an acute illness such as a chest infection is not responsible.

TREATMENT

Conventional treatment of air-flow obstruction with, for instance, bronchodilators may be effective and right heart failure may respond to diuretics and angiotensin-converting enzyme inhibitors.

Chronic ventilatory failure usually responds well to nocturnal noninvasive respiratory support. Some patients can be adequately managed with oxygen during the day or at night or both as long as the P_{CO_2} remains normal or only slightly raised. When respiratory support is required, a negative pressure system such as a cuirass or jacket or nasal positive pressure ventilation used at night is usually adequate initially. However, many patients gradually require more intensive support, so that treatment is needed during the day as well as at night and a tracheostomy may have to be constructed in order to enable adequate ventilation to be achieved. This deterioration may be due to progressive worsening of small airway obstruction or respiratory muscle function, or to a fall in oxygen delivery to the tissues caused by a deteriorating cardiac output associated with advancing pulmonary hypertension.

Disorders of the diaphragm

Introduction

The diaphragm is the most important chest wall respiratory muscle and impairment of its function can have serious respiratory consequences. It is conventionally considered either as a single muscle or as consisting of a right and left hemidiaphragm, but its costal and sternal fibres can be regarded as a single muscle and the crural fibres as a separate muscle. The diaphragm is supplied by the phrenic nerve whose nucleus lies in the spinal segments C3–C5 or C6. The phrenic nerve rootlets are usually multiple and only join to form a single main trunk within the thorax. When this reaches the diaphragm it divides into an anterior, a lateral, and a larger posterior division.

Contraction of both the costosternal and crural fibres decreases intrapleural pressure and raises abdominal pressure. The costal fibres run almost vertically and parallel to the interior of the lower rib cage except at large lung volumes. This zone of 'apposition' of the diaphragm to the ribs decreases as the diaphragm descends. Contraction of the costal fibres originating from the lower six ribs elevates these and increases both the anteroposterior and transverse diameters of the thorax. The crural fibres do not have this action. As the diaphragm descends it changes shape from a hemispherical dome to a flattened sheet, and in this form, by Laplace's law, it generates less pressure change. The diaphragm muscle fibres are also shorter and can generate less force. Therefore reduction in the tension developed by the diaphragm is seen at the end of a normal inspiration and when the lungs are hyperinflated due to air flow obstruction.

Aetiology

Diaphragmatic paralysis or paresis may be due to lesions affecting either the diaphragm itself or the phrenic nerve, its nucleus, or higher control centres or pathways. The most common causes of diaphragmatic weakness are shown in Table 2. Often no cause is found in unilateral weakness, and it is presumed that this is due to a cryptogenic phrenic neuropathy. This may occur as part of a widespread peripheral neuropathy or be isolated to the phrenic nerves. The radiculitis of neuralgic amyotrophy is a frequently overlooked cause of phrenic nerve damage, and usually presents with shoulder pain and evidence of other muscle weakness. Occasionally, a mass such as a bronchial carcinoma or an aortic aneurysm adjacent to the phrenic nerve may cause unilateral diaphragm weakness. Birth trauma, spinal manipulation, and central venous catheterization are important examples of traumatic causes of unilateral weakness. Open-heart surgery frequently causes left-sided and occasionally bilateral paralysis largely owing to cold injury to the phrenic nerve but possibly also by causing ischaemia.

Most of these conditions can cause bilateral diaphragmatic weakness, but this can also be part of a generalized neuromuscular disorder such as acute idiopathic polyneuropathy (Guillain–Barré syndrome), muscular dystrophy, or a congenital myopathy, particularly acid maltase deficiency. It occasionally occurs as an early complication in motor neurone disease and is well recognized during both the acute infection of poliomyelitis and as a late complication of this condition. Bilateral diaphragm weakness is an often underestimated factor in patients failing to wean from ventilators during acute severe illnesses. A 'critical care neuropathy' develops which may affect other nerves as well as the phrenic nerves.

Pathophysiology

Unilateral weakness of the diaphragm causes it to move upwards (paradoxically) into the thorax instead of descending during inspiration. This decreases the tidal volume and the mechanical efficiency of breathing. It is worse in the supine position when the weight of the abdominal contents pushes the paralysed diaphragm further into the thorax and decreases the FRC. The diaphragm is splinted in an expiratory position so that it moves relatively little even though it is paralysed. When the subject lies on one side the lower half of the diaphragm behaves in this way if it is paralysed, but if the upper half is paralysed it moves paradoxically.

The loss of inspiratory muscle strength is partially compensated by recruitment of intercostal and accessory muscles, but the maximum inspiratory and transdiaphragmatic pressures are reduced. The VC in the upright position is approximately 20 to 25 per cent less than normal and a further fall of about 15 per cent occurs when the subject lies supine. Similar changes in the TLC and FRC occur. The RV is unchanged and expiratory muscle strength is largely preserved.

The distribution of ventilation and perfusion is affected by unilateral diaphragm weakness. Ventilation is slightly diminished, particularly at the bases on the side of the diaphragmatic paralysis in the sitting position, but this is more marked when the subject is supine. Similar changes occur with perfusion on a regional basis, but ventilation–perfusion matching is impaired and hypoxia results. Hypercapnia does not occur during wakefulness or sleep.

In infants, the impact of unilateral diaphragmatic weakness is much greater for several reasons. First, the sternum and ribs are more horizontal than later in life so that the range of rib cage expansion is limited if the diaphragm is paralysed. Second, the rib cage in neonates is more compliant than in adults, particularly during REM sleep when activity in the intercostal and accessory muscles is reduced. Diaphragm contraction readily causes paradoxical movement of the rib cage. This

Table 2 *Main causes of diaphragm weakness*

Unilateral	Bilateral
Congenital (e.g. agenesis, eventration)	
Trauma	Trauma
Adjacent mass (e.g. neoplasm, aneurysm)	High cervical cord lesions
Herpes zoster	Motor neurone disease
Poliomyelitis	Poliomyelitis
Peripheral neuropathy	Peripheral neuropathy
Neuralgic amyotrophy	Acute idiopathic polyneuropathy
Open-heart surgery	Myopathies
	Muscular dystrophies

impairs its mechanical efficiency, and if the diaphragm's endurance is reduced, respiratory failure may develop particularly during sleep. Lastly, the respiratory rate in neonates is faster than in adults and the inspiratory time/expiratory time (T_i/T_e) ratio is increased so that the diaphragm fatigues more readily, particularly if it is weakened by the underlying disorder.

The physiological abnormalities seen with bilateral diaphragm weakness in adults are much more marked than in unilateral diaphragmatic disorders. The diaphragm moves paradoxically during inspiration and expiration, and the intrapleural pressure changes are transmitted across it so that the abdominal pressure falls during inspiration and the anterior abdominal wall moves paradoxically. The maximum diaphragmatic pressure falls in proportion to the degree of diaphragm weakness, and since the diaphragm is the main inspiratory muscle the maximum inspiratory pressure is correspondingly reduced. The VC in the sitting position is about 50 per cent of that predicted and may fall by a further 50 per cent when supine. The influence of the supine position is greater than with unilateral diaphragmatic weakness since the weight of the abdominal contents pushes both halves of the diaphragm into the thorax. Ventilation is particularly reduced at the bases in the supine position, with less change in perfusion so that the arterial Po_2 falls. This postural change is partly responsible for the hypoxia that has been observed during sleep, but the rapid respiratory rate, small tidal volume, and short inspiratory time contribute to this and to hypercapnia.

The consequences of bilateral diaphragmatic paralysis in infants are similar to those when only half the diaphragm is affected but are slightly more severe. Ventilatory failure is invariable.

Symptoms and physical signs

Unilateral diaphragm paralysis in adults rarely causes symptoms unless there is coexisting pulmonary disease or weakness of other respiratory muscles. In contrast, bilateral weakness can cause severe breathlessness. This may occur during exertion, but a specific feature is orthopnoea. This occurs within a few seconds of lying flat and is relieved promptly by sitting up. Therefore it differs from left ventricular failure and nocturnal asthma with which it can frequently be confused. Breathlessness may also occur when standing in water since the passive inspiratory descent of the diaphragm due to gravity is prevented by the raised extra-abdominal pressure.

The physical signs of unilateral diaphragm weakness may be subtle. Dullness to percussion over the lower part of the thorax may be present and the level of dullness may rise paradoxically during inspiration on the paralysed side. The normal inspiratory outward movement of the abdomen may be reduced or absent on the side of the diaphragmatic paralysis, and expansion of the lower chest may lag behind the normal expansion of the other side.

The physical signs of bilateral diaphragmatic paralysis are much more clear cut. Orthopnoea is usually readily apparent and the abdomen moves paradoxically inwards as the diaphragm ascends during inspiration. A maximum transdiaphragmatic pressure of less than 30 cmH$_2$O is necessary for this sign to be detected. The accessory muscles are active, particularly in the supine position. The quality of sleep is often poor and as a result excessive daytime somnolence may be a problem. Bilateral basal dullness due to the high diaphragms is characteristic, but can be mimicked by bilateral pleural effusions.

Investigations

The chest radiograph in unilateral diaphragm paralysis shows whether the affected diaphragm is elevated and usually reveals any adjacent mass that may be responsible. If there is bilateral paralysis, both the diaphragms are raised. There is often some basal linear shadowing due to subsegmental lung collapse. Diaphragmatic screening or ultrasound examination reveals that the diaphragm moves paradoxically, particularly during sniffing. This test should be carried out in the supine position with a weight on the abdomen. These precautions prevent abdominal muscle contraction during expiration from mimicking diaphragmatic activity by reducing the end expiratory volume below FRC so that inspiration occurs through the elastic recoil of the lungs and chest wall. In the upright position the effect of gravity on the abdominal contents can lead to inspiration without any diaphragmatic activity.

A low VC which falls further in the supine position is the hallmark of diaphragmatic weakness, particularly when this is severe and bilateral. All the lung volumes are reduced except for the RV since the expiratory muscle strength is largely preserved. Maximum inspiratory pressure is also reduced, but diaphragmatic weakness can be more specifically diagnosed by estimating the transdiaphragmatic pressure. This can be carried out by asking the patient to sniff or to take a maximum inspiratory effort, or by percutaneous electrical stimulation of the phrenic nerve in the neck. Care is required to carry out these investigations using a standardized method in order to obtain repeatable results. The function of the phrenic nerve can be estimated by measuring its conduction time. This is normally less than about 9.5 ms, but is prolonged in conditions which affect the phrenic nerves.

The arterial Po$_2$ is characteristically slightly reduced with a normal Pco$_2$ during the daytime. Similar features may be observed during sleep if the pulmonary function is normal and there is no other muscle weakness, but in either of these situations hypercapnia with quite profound hypoxia may develop during sleep if both halves of the diaphragm are paralysed.

Treatment

In children under the age of approximately 3 years ventilatory support or diaphragmatic plication is usually required whether the diaphragm weakness is unilateral or bilateral. If it is likely that the diaphragm function will improve initial intubation or a tracheostomy together with intermittent positive pressure ventilation or continuous positive airway pressure is often effective by stabilizing the diaphragm and preventing its paradoxical upward movement during inspiration. However, if paralysis is likely to be permanent, surgical plication may be indicated. This lowers the diaphragm, increases the lung volume, and prevents basal airway collapse. There is no increase in transdiaphragmatic pressure after plication, but fixation of the diaphragm prevents it moving paradoxically. Bilateral plication in infants is of little value, presumably because neither of the hemidiaphragms can contract.

Plication for hemidiaphragmatic paralysis is rarely required in adults unless coexistent pulmonary disease is severe enough to cause breathlessness. As in infants, bilateral plication is not effective and mechanical respiratory support is often required if there is bilateral weakness. Treatment with a negative pressure ventilator, such as a cuirass or jacket, or nasal positive pressure ventilation is usually required, although rocking beds have also been found to be effective in the past. Ventilatory support is usually needed only at night and until the diaphragmatic or phrenic nerve function improves. Breathlessness on exertion often remains a problem, but may lessen as other inspiratory muscles partially compensate for the diaphragmatic weakness.

REFERENCES

Bredin, C.P. (1989). Pulmonary function in long-term survivors of thoracoplasty. *Chest,* **95,** 18–20.

Elliott, C.G., Hill, T.R., Adams, T.E., Crapo, R.O., Nietrzeba, R.M., and Gardner, R.M. (1985). Exercise performance of subjects with ankylosing spondylitis and limited chest expansion. *European Bulletin of Physiopathology and Respiration,* **21,** 363–8.

Franssen, M.J.A.M., van Herwaarden, C.L.A., van de Putte, L.B.A., and Gribnau, F.W.J. (1986). Lung function in patients with ankylosing spondylitis. A study of the influence of disease activity and treatment with non-steroidal antiinflammatory drugs. *Journal of Rheumatology,* **13,** 936–40.

Gibson, G.J. (1989). Diaphragmatic paresis: pathophysiology, clinical features, and investigation. *Thorax,* **44,** 960–70.

Kafer, E.R. (1975). Idiopathic scoliosis. Mechanical properties of the respiratory system and the ventilatory response to carbon dioxide. *Journal of Clinical Investigation,* **55,** 1153–63.

Kinnear, W.M.J., Hockley, S., Harvey, J., and Shneerson, J.M. (1988). The effects of one year of nocturnal cuirass-assisted ventilation in chest wall disease. *European Respiratory Journal,* **1,** 204–6.

Laroche, C.M., Moxham, J., and Green, M. (1989). Respiratory muscle weakness and fatigue. *Quarterly Journal of Medicine, New Series,* **71,** (265), 373–97.

Lindahl, T. (1954). Spirometric and bronchospirometric studies in five-rib thoracoplasties. *Thorax,* **9,** 285–90.

Midgren, B., Petersson, K., Hansson, L., Eriksson, L., Airikkala, P., and Elmqvist, D. (1988). Nocturnal hypoxaemia in severe scoliosis. *British Journal of Diseases of the Chest,* **82,** 226–36.

Mier-Jedrzejowicz, A., Brophy, C., Moxham, J., and Green, M. (1988). Assessment of diaphragm weakness. *American Review of Respiratory Disease,* **137,** 877–83.

Newsom-Davis, J., Goldman, M., Loh, L., and Casson, M. (1976). Diaphragm function and alveolar hypoventilation. *Quarterly Journal of Medicine,* **145,** 87–100.

O'Brien, J.W., Johnson, S.H., Van Steyn, S.J., Craig, D.M., Sharpe, R.E., Mauney, M.C., and Smith, P.K. (1991). Effects of internal mammary artery dissection on phrenic nerve perfusion and function. *Annals of Thoracic Surgery,* **52,** 182 8.

Pehrsson, K., Bake, B., Larsson, S., and Nachemson, A. (1991). Lung function in adult idiopathic scoliosis: a 20 year follow up. *Thorax,* **46,** 474–78.

Phillips, M.S., Kinnear, W.J.M., and Shneerson, J.M. (1987). Late sequelae of pulmonary tuberculosis treated by thoracoplasty. *Thorax,* **42,** 445–51.

Phillips, M.S., Kinnear, W.J.M., Shaw, D., and Shneerson, J.M. (1989). Exercise responses in patients treated for pulmonary tuberculosis by thoracoplasty. *Thorax,* **44,** 268–74.

Robert, D., Gerard, M., Leger, P., Buffat, J., Jennequin, J., Holzaphel, L., *et al.* (1983). La ventilation mechanique a domicile definitive par tracheostomie de l'insuffisant respiratoire chronique. *Revue Francaise des Maladies Respiratoires,* **11,** 923–6.

Sawicka, E.H., Branthwaite, M.A., and Spencer, G.T. (1983). Respiratory failure after thoracoplasty: treatment by intermittent negative-pressure ventilation. *Thorax,* **28,** 433–5.

Shneerson, J.M. (1978). The cardiorespiratory response to exercise in thoracic scoliosis. *Thorax,* **33,** 457–63.

Shneerson, J.M. (1988). *Disorders of ventilation.* Blackwell, Oxford.

Tzelepis, G.E., McCool, F.D., Hoppin, F.G., Jr. (1989). Chest wall distortion in patients with flail chest. *American Review of Respiratory Disease,* **140,** 31–7.

17.13 Neoplastic disorders

17.13.1 Tumours of the lung

(a) Lung cancer

S.G. Spiro

General epidemiology

Lung cancer is the most common malignant disease in the Western world, and its incidence has increased rapidly in many countries where 20 years ago it was not recognized as a problem. It has shown the greatest relative and absolute rise in mortality of any tumour this century in England and Wales, and particularly in Scotland. In the United States it has been increasing in incidence by up to 10 per cent per year since the 1930s, but over the last decade there has been a levelling in the incidence, particularly in males. Nevertheless, in the United States approximately 120 000 men die per annum; the figure for women is 34 000, similar to that for breast cancer. Ten years ago it was predicted that lung cancer would overtake breast cancer as the commonest malignancy among women in the Western world. However, this has not occurred, suggesting a gradual decrease in the overall incidence of lung cancer deaths among women during the 1980s.

Lung cancer still causes 35 000 deaths per year in England and Wales, with 80 per cent of these occurring in men. In the European community there were 1.35 million deaths per annum in men (the highest death rate from any tumour) and 229 000 deaths per annum in women during the period 1978–1982.

However, age-standardized mortality rates for cancer for 1985–1989 show that in the European Community lung cancer in men has by far the greatest mortality rate. Belgium has the greatest mortality (77.16 deaths per 100 000 population) with Scotland (75.9) second, and England and Wales (60.9) fifth. For females, Scotland (27.2) has the

highest incidence, with England and Wales (20.4) third. The Scottish mortality rate is just below the highest mortality rate in Europe for breast cancer (29.3) which is found in women in England and Wales, although the death rate from breast cancer in Scottish women is now identical with that for lung cancer in Scotland.

Age-specific mortality data clearly show differences between age groups. While mortality continues to increase in the elderly, death rates among younger people are falling. Figure 1 analyses data in England and Wales relating to the year of birth to death rate in age cohorts of 5 years for men and women. Each vertical set of points represents the mortality rate at different ages of persons born during a 10 year period surrounding a central year of birth. Male mortality at each age reaches the peak in the generation born between 1901 and 1916, but for women, whilst the pattern is similar, the peak death rates occur in those born during the 1920s. The implication is that currently there is a cohort of elderly patients in the population with a high incidence of lung cancer; this means that the average of those presenting with lung cancer will slowly rise, at least for the next few years.

Aetiological factors

TOBACCO

In every country the increase in mortality from lung cancer appeared to coincide with an increase in tobacco usage, particularly cigarette smoking, after what seemed to be an appropriate latent interval. Early retrospective studies showed that, amongst patients with carcinoma of the bronchus, there were many fewer non-smokers and many more heavy smokers than among the controls, and that there was a degree of association between the amount smoked and the risk of lung cancer. Prospective studies, amongst which the long-term study of British doctors is particularly informative, confirmed the increased risk of death from lung cancer from any tobacco use, but most specifically from usage of

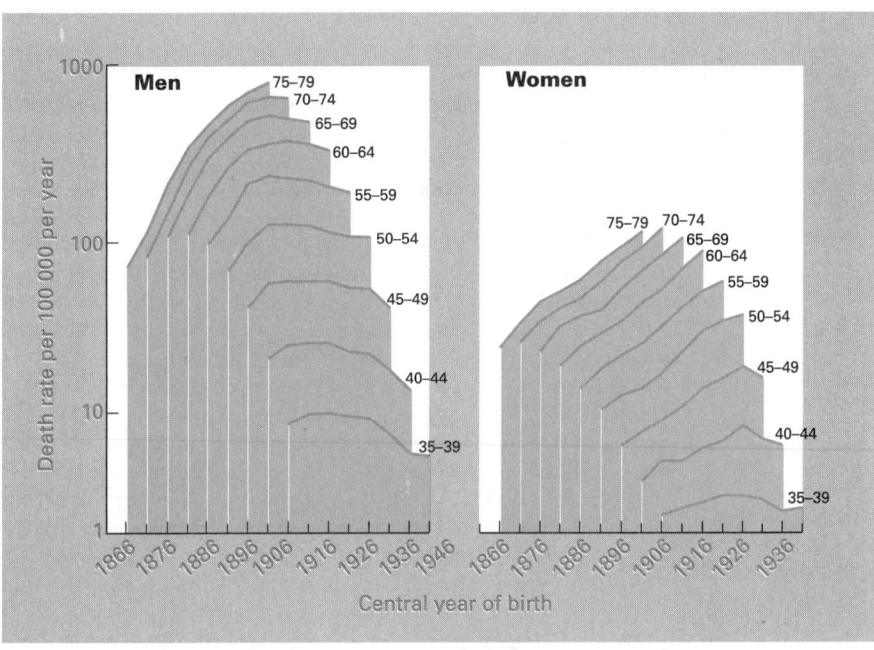

Fig. 1 Age-specific mortality from lung cancer in England and Wales during the period 1941–1980 plotted versus central year of birth. (Reproduced with permission from Coggon and Acheson 1983.)

Table 1 *Death rate from lung cancer in males by smoking habits when last asked (British Doctors' Study)*

Tobacco use category	Death rate (age standardized per 100 000)
Non-smokers	10
Ex-smokers	43
Continuing smokers	
Any tobacco	104
Pipe and/or cigar only	58
Mixed	82
Cigarette smokers only	140
Number smoked per day	
1–14	78
15–24	127
25 or more	251

Table 2 *Percentage of smokers by age in the European Community 1987–1989*

Age	Male	Female
15–24	39	34
25–39	53	40
40–54	47	26
55+	37	17

cigarettes; there was a strong dose–response relationship with the number of cigarettes smoked. This is illustrated in Table 1. The most important variable in smoking intensity is the number of cigarettes smoked, but other variables include the depth of inhalation, number of puffs, butt length, use of a filter, and the type of tobacco smoked. Further evidence of a causal relationship became apparent in a study which documented the reduction in risk following cessation of smoking: after cessation of smoking for 15 years the ratio of rates compared with non-smokers fell from 15.8 : 1 to 2 : 1 or, if expressed in a different way, fell to 11 per cent of that pertaining to continuing smokers. Wide differences in smoking habits are now seen between social classes, with 57 per cent of unskilled manual workers smoking compared with only 21 per cent of professional workers. However, during the last 5 years the number of adult men smoking in England and Wales has fallen from 64 to 36 per cent, but has remained at 35 per cent for adult women. The effect of the lower-tar cigarettes has not yet had time to become established.

A recent European Community survey has shown that smoking is

Fig. 2 Smoking by age in females in the European Community 1987–1989.

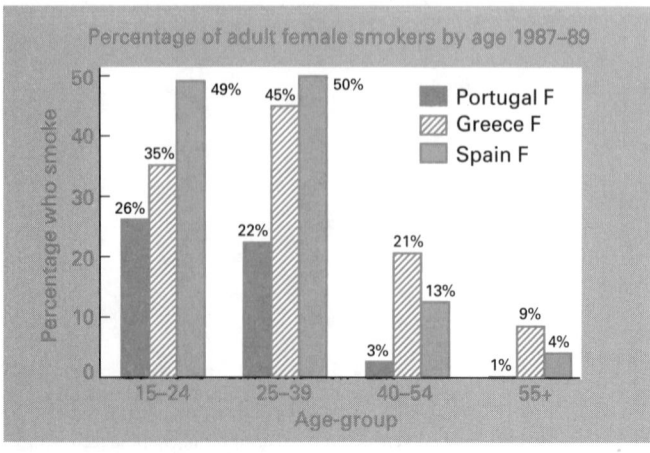

Table 3 *Industrial products and processes known to cause or suspected of causing lung cancer*

Fibre exposure (asbestos)
Nickel refining
Aluminium industry
Arsenic and arsenic compounds
Benzoyl chloride
Beryllium
Cadmium
Chloromethyl ether
Chromates
The electronics industry
Irradiation
Soots, tar, oils
Mustard gas

Reproduced from Coggan and Acheson (1983), with permission.

most prevalent among young people (Table 2). The rates of smoking by age are even more striking for women. In Greece, Spain, and Portugal less than 10 per cent of women aged over 55 years smoke, but up to 50 per cent of women aged between 26 and 40 are smokers (Fig. 2).

Globally there has been a huge change in cigarette consumption. While there has been a drop of 25 per cent and 9 per cent in consumption in the United Kingdom and the United States respectively between 1970 and 1985, the overall world consumption has risen by 7 per cent. This is due to huge increases in Asia (22 per cent), Latin America (24 per cent), and Africa (42 per cent).

Passive smoking

There is now good evidence that exposure to cigarette smoke is responsible for a decrease in birth weight of babies born to maternal smokers, and an increased incidence of respiratory infection when young. However, the evidence that passive smoking predisposes to lung cancer is far from certain. Approximately 15 per cent of lung cancers occur in non-smokers, and 5 per cent of these have been attributed to passive smoking. Evidence for this comes from the comparisons with Seventh Day Adventists in the United States. However, other reviews suggest that many (up to 40 per cent) of 'non-smokers' were in fact smokers at some time, and accuracy of measuring exposure is open to criticism. Exposure histories may ignore the effect of the workplace, divorce, remarriage, and childhood exposure.

OCCUPATION

A number of different factors have now been identified as associated with lung cancer; subjects who develop this disease as a result of their occupation represent a small but important group. The association of asbestos with lung cancer is now firmly established; various studies have identified a risk factor of 4.9 to 7.3 times the risk for those who are not specifically exposed to asbestos. There is a much greater risk for the asbestos industry worker if he smokes cigarettes; one study identified the risk as 93 times that for non-smokers not exposed to asbestos. In Norway it is illegal to employ a smoker in an asbestos-related job. Exposure to radioactive isotopes, mainly radon daughters, occurs among various groups of miners, particularly those involved in the mining of pitchblende and uranium. Polycyclic aromatic hydrocarbons are believed to be responsible for the increased risk in workers in the gas and coke ovens and in foundry workers. Nickel refining, chromate manufacture, and arsenical industrial workers are also exposed to a higher risk of lung cancer. The amount of lung cancer caused by occupational exposure may well have been underestimated in the past, and a summary of the importance industrial products and processes involved appears in Table 3.

Table 4 *Classification of epithelial tumours of the lung (based on revised WHO Classification)*

	Frequency (%)		Frequency (%)
Main			
Epidermoid carcinoma (squamous cell)	35	Adenocarcinoma	21
		Acinar	
		Papillary	
		Bronchiolar alveolar	
Small-cell carcinoma	24	Large-cell carcinoma	19
Oatcell		With stratification	
Fusiform		With mucin-production	
Others		Giant-cell	
		Clear-cell	
Less common			
Tumours showing mixed differentiation		Bronchial gland	
		Adenoid cystic	
		Mucoepidermoid	
		Others	
Carcinoid tumours			
	Carcinoma *in situ*		

AIR POLLUTION

The decline in male mortality is occurring earlier than would be expected from changes in smoking habits. The high mortality figures in the United Kingdom and Germany compared with France and Italy for example, seem likely to be in part due to heavy industry and coal burning. Analysis by county in the United States shows an association between lung cancer deaths and counties with chemical, petroleum, ship-building, and paper industries. Legislation for cleaner air has caused both environmental and occupational pollution to fall dramatically in the past 30 years, and this has preceded changes in smoking habits.

There is a high incidence of lung cancer among women in Hong Kong. This has been shown to be associated not only with cigarette smoking but with the habitual use of kerosene stoves in small and poorly ventilated kitchens.

Pathology

A detailed understanding of the natural history, pathology, and pathogenesis of bronchial carcinoma is becoming increasingly important as the assessment, management, and prognosis of the disease depends largely upon the cell type and the presence or absence of metastasis at the time of presentation. It has been estimated that about seven-eighths of a tumour's life will have passed when it is diagnosed and that the vast majority will be disseminated at the time of diagnosis.

Bronchogenic carcinomas seem to arise most commonly in segmental and subsegmental bronchi in response to repetitive carcinogenic stimuli or inflammation and irritation. The mucosal lining is most susceptible to injury at the bifurcation of bronchial structures. Dysplasia is followed by carcinoma *in situ* when the entire thickness of the mucosa may be replaced by proliferating neoplastic cells. These changes may be strictly localized or multicentric. Tumour infiltration follows loss of the basal membrane. The precise origins of small-cell carcinomas remain an enigma, and those of adenocarcinomas are not precisely defined. The latter may arise from the mucosal lining or from the submucosal bronchial mucous glands. A significant number of lung tumours arise in the periphery of the lung, perhaps three-quarters of adenocarcinomas and large-cell anaplastic malignancies, one-third of squamous (or epidermoid) carcinomas, and one-fifth of small-cell carcinomas.

The WHO classification of lung cancer according to cell type and the approximate distribution of each type as a percentage of all lung cancers is shown in Table 4. The squamous-cell tumour has a relatively slow growth rate (volume doubling time, 90 days) and the lowest incidence of distant haematogenous metastasis. Small-cell tumours grow rapidly (volume doubling time, 30 days) and there is very early dissemination by both the haematogenous and the lymphatic routes, with metastasis being present in more than 90 per cent of patients at the time of diagnosis. Adenocarcinomas and anaplastic large-cell tumours occupy an intermediate position. It is now recognized that significant heterogeneity of cell morphology can be visualized within individual tumours. Squamous-cell tumours, adenocarcinomas, and large-cell tumours are often collectively called non-small-cell lung cancers, and the approach to their management differs from that for small-cell lung cancer.

SQUAMOUS (EPIDERMOID) CARCINOMA

These tumours are composed predominantly of flattened to polygonal neoplastic cells that tend to stratify, form intercellular bridges, and elaborate keratin. About 60 per cent present as obstructive lesions in lobar and main-stem bronchi. The tumours tend to be bulky and to produce intraluminar granular or polypoid masses. As a result, distal pneumonia and abscess formation is common, and cavitation is seen in about 10 per cent. The cells are usually well differentiated, but in some cases differentiation is poor and the appearances are those of predominantly anaplastic cells, frequently arranged in the classical pattern of stratifying sheets.

SMALL-CELL (OAT-CELL) ANAPLASTIC CARCINOMA

This is now recognized as a pathologically and clinically distinct form of lung cancer. Small-cell lung cancer may originate from the amine precursor uptake and decarboxylation (APUD) series of cells. The tumour is composed of neoplastic cells with dark oval to round spindled nuclei and scanty indistinct cytoplasm arranged in ribbons, nests, and sheets. The cells tend to crush easily on biopsy, and extensive areas may be necrotic. This type of tumour presents as a proximal lesion in 75 per cent of cases and may arise anywhere in the tracheobronchial tree and rapidly invade vessels and lymph nodes, disseminating widely even before symptoms arise from the primary tumour. Extensive advanced disease exists in more than half the patients on presentation. The tumours often have a glossy reddish appearance and may stenose the bronchial lumen circumferentially for several centimetres. The cells secrete hormones which give rise to characteristic clinical syndromes in 10 per cent of cases.

ADENOCARCINOMA

This tumour forms acinar or granular structures, having prominent papillary processes, and may be mucin-provoking. About 70 per cent appear to originate peripherally in the lung and are frequently fairly circumscribed; in about 10 per cent the initial presentation is a pleural effusion. If related to bronchi, they tend to cuff and stenose the lumen. They occasionally arise in old tuberculous scars.

LARGE-CELL CARCINOMA

These tumours, which have been described as an unclassified category, include all tumours that show no evidence of maturation or differentiation. They are composed of pleomorphic cells with variable enlarged nuclei, prominent nucleoli and nuclear inclusions, and abundant cytoplasm; they are mucin-producing in many instances. The tumours tend to be bulky and are often necrotic; they are frequently peripheral, they invade locally, and disseminate widely, with about half the patients having disseminated disease on presentation. Although they are highly malignant and undifferentiated, the cure rate after surgery is surprisingly high, but radiotherapy is ineffective in controlling the disease. Large-cell carcinoma is a smoking-related disease in over 90 per cent of patients.

BRONCHIOLOALVEOLAR CARCINOMA

There has been considerable controversy as to whether this tumour, which has the least association with tobacco smoking, arises from alveolar or bronchial epithelium, but derivation from the alveolar type II cell has been suggested. The tumour tends to spread as cuboidal or columnar 'epithelium' along the lining of the alveoli, with single or multiple rows of cells and often papillary formation (Fig. 3). There is production of a large amount of mucus in 20 per cent of cases and it is believed that malignant cells shed into the mucus may carry over into relevant anatomical sites in the contralateral lung. The tumour can spread within a lobe and occupy it fully. Sometimes, however, the tumour is multicentric in origin, and diffuse nodular lesions are to be found on radiographic examination in some patients. Invasion of neighbouring tissue and lymph nodes is common, but more distant spread is unusual. There is some resemblance to metastases from adenocarcinomas emanating from other organs, and this sometimes leads to confusion. The tumour tends to grow along alveolar septa as a framework, and it may be difficult to distinguish from metastatic tumours from colon, breast, or pancreas.

CARCINOID TUMOURS

Carcinoid tumours are described in Chapter 14.8.

Fig. 3 Bronchoalveolar cell carcinoma: malignant cuboidal epithelium spreads along alveolar walls.

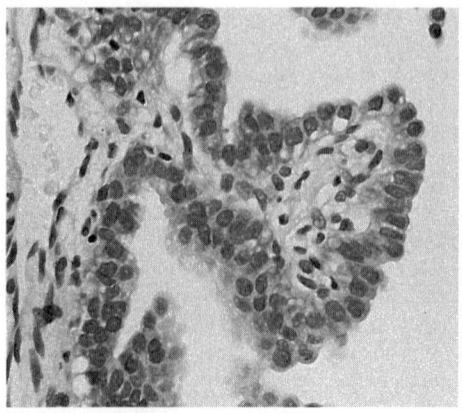

CARCINOMA IN SITU

Many investigators have suggested that cells undergoing malignant change do not necessarily invade the lungs at the onset of this biological mutation, but continue to exist at a particular location (cancer *in situ*). Exfoliated cancer cells sloughed from such a location may be seen fortuitously by the cytologist; even more rarely, such a site may be biopsied at bronchoscopy.

Genetics and biology

Genetic influences may play a role in the development of lung cancers, particularly in patients under 50. In one study lung cancers were attributable to a Mendelian codominant inheritance pattern in 27 per cent of patients under 50, but only 9 per cent of those over 70. Individuals who extensively metabolize debrisoquine are at greater risk than those who are poor or intermediate metabolizers. The gene coding for the enzyme that breaks down debrisoquine is located on chromosome 22.

Both small-cell and non-small-cell lung cancer can be cultured as cell lines which can be transplanted into nude mice. The resultant tumours are morphologically and histologically similar to the original human tumour. Two major categories of cell lines are established for small-cell lung cancer—classic and variant. Classic cell lines account for 70 per cent of the total and are characterized by high expression of neuroendocrine markers such as L-dopa decarboxylase and bombesin/gastrin-releasing peptide, neurone-specific enolase, and creatine kinase-BB. The variant cell lines have selective loss of some of these neuroendocrine markers, and many variant small-cell lung cancer lines have substituted amplification of the c-*myc* oncogene. These neuroendocrine properties have important prognostic features—in most studies survival in patients from whom a classic cell line is grown is better than those with variant cell lines.

Several monoclonal antibodies have been generated against lung-cancer-associated antigens. Thirty-six monoclonal antibodies raised against small-cell lung cancer have been grouped into eight clusters. No antigen is specific for small-cell lung cancer. Antibodies belonging to the major cluster (cluster 1) are directed against the neural-cell adhesion molecule (NCAM), whilst the nature of the other antigens remains unclear. Studies of both small-cell and non-small-cell lung cancer cell lines show that NCAM expression is associated with a neuroendocrine phenotype irrespective of the histological type of lung cancer. Monoclonal antibodies may have a therapeutic value when coupled with a radionuclide or a toxin. In addition, radiolabelled antibodies can detect minimal disease in bone marrow aspirates or biopsy specimens.

Lung cancer cells not only show mutations that activate dominant cellular proto-oncogenes, but also genetic mechanisms that inactivate recessive tumour suppressors. The commonest abnormality is a deletion in the short arm of chromosome 3, which is found in over 90 per cent of small-cell lung cancer and 50 per cent of non-small-cell lung cancer patients. Other sites of loss of heterozygosity include 11p, 13q, and 17p.

The dominant oncogene mutations in small-cell lung cancer are among the *myc* family. Amplification of c-*myc*, n-*myc*, and l-*myc* are late events in the pathogenesis of small-cell lung cancer, and are recognized mainly in patients who have relapsed after previously intensive chemotherapy.

The growth factors bombesin/gastrin-releasing peptide, insulin-like growth factor 1, and transferrin stimulate clonal growth of the tumour. Much work is in progress to attempt to retard or disrupt growth-factor-stimulated growth of these tumours.

Clinical features

The clinical abnormalities associated with lung cancer vary considerably. In about 5 per cent of patients the initial presentation is a radiographic abnormality found on routine examination and unassociated with symptoms; however, patients may present with extremely advanced disease from which death rapidly occurs.

The clinical features may be due to local development of the tumour in the lung, including bronchial obstruction, invasion of contiguous structures in the thorax and mediastinum, metastasis through blood or lymph vessels, and endocrine, metabolic, and neurological syndromes.

Cough is the most common initial presenting symptom. Because cough is a symptom of so many respiratory disorders, the possibility of tumour may be overlooked or some other cause attributed to it, particularly in smokers who may have had chronic bronchitis for many years. Patients who have a persistent cough should have a chest radiography, particularly if they are 40 years or over and are smokers. A change in the cough habit is significant and also requires investigation. If the trachea or main bronchi are involved, the cough may be brassy in character and may be accompanied by wheezing or stridor. If cough is manifestly ineffective, involvement of the recurrent laryngeal nerve should be suspected.

Expectoration of sputum may be due to spread of the tumour itself or to infection occurring distal to partial bronchial obstruction. In the early stages of the disease the sputum is often grey and viscid; it is usually purulent in the presence of infection distal to a tumour and in cavitated tumours. The value of sputum cytology in diagnosis is described below.

Haemoptysis, which occurs as a sole presenting symptom in about 5 per cent of cases and at some stage in the disease in 50 per cent of patients, is a symptom not easily ignored by patient or physician. The degree varies from streaking of the sputum with blood to significant amounts, but massive haemoptysis is rare except as a terminal event. The most significant description given by patients is that of coughing up blood every morning for several days in succession.

Wheeze may be observed in a few patients. Localized persistent wheeze even after coughing is a significant observation associated with obstruction of a larger or central airway.

Stridor is a feature which is poorly recognized and is often confused with wheeze. It is due to narrowing of the glottis, trachea, or major bronchi, and is best heard after the patient coughs and then breathes in deeply with the mouth open.

Dyspnoea is a presenting symptom in only a small number of patients. As the disease progresses dyspnoea is inevitable, being proportional to the amount of lung involvement including collapse of the lung due to endobronchial disease causing airway narrowing or obstruction. Progressive breathlessness is also a salient feature of malignant pleural and, rarely, pericardial effusion, superior vena caval obstruction, and lymphangitis carcinomatosis.

Chest discomfort is a common symptom occurring in up to 40 per cent of patients at diagnosis. The discomfort is often of an ill-defined nature and may be described in terms of intermittent aching somewhere in the chest. Definite pleural pain may occur in the presence of infection, but invasion of the pleura by tumour may well be painless. However, invasion of the ribs or vertebrae causes continuous gnawing pain locally. A tumour in the superior pulmonary sulcus (Pancoast tumour) causes progressive constant pain in the shoulder, upper anterior chest, or interscapular region, soon spreading to the arm once the brachial plexus is invaded. Other symptoms of this type of tumour include weakness and atrophy of the muscles of the hand, Horner's syndrome, hoarseness, and spinal cord compression at levels D1 and D2.

Lack of energy and, more particularly, loss of interest in normal pursuits are symptoms of great importance; a sensation of vague ill health commonly occurs.

Fever, chills, and night sweats may occur due to chest infection, but fever may very rarely be present in rapidly progressive tumours without evidence of infection, particularly if there are hepatic metastases.

Invasion of adjacent intrathoracic structures gives rise to certain specific clinical features. Involvement of the last cervical and first thoracic segment of the sympathetic trunk by cancer produces Horner's syndrome, manifested by a drooping eyelid, sunken eyeball, narrow palpebral fissure, contracted pupil, and lack of thermal sweating on the affected side. Malignant infiltration of the recurrent laryngeal nerve—almost always the left branch because of its course adjacent to the left hilum—gives rise to vocal chord paralysis. The right recurrent laryngeal nerve is rarely affected in the base of the neck. Recurrent aspiration pneumonias may follow vocal chord paralysis. Extension of the tumour with invasion or compression of the superior vena cava with secondary thrombosis results in the characteristic features of superior vena caval obstruction—awareness of tightness of the collar, fullness of the head, and suffusion of the face, particularly after bending down, blackouts, breathlessness, and engorgement of veins with a downward venous flow in the neck, the upper half of the thorax, and arms, often accompanied by oedema of the face.

Dysphagia is due to compression of the oesophagus from without by tumour masses and only rarely to direct invasion. Cardiac metastases usually occur late in the disease and are manifested clinically by tachycardia, arrhythmias, pericardial effusion, breathlessness, and cardiac failure. Invasion of the phrenic nerve results in elevation and paralysis of the hemidiaphragm.

The clinical features associated with involvement of the ribs, spine, and pleura are described elsewhere. Very rarely bronchogenic carcinoma causes spontaneous pneumothorax. It must not be forgotten that spread of tumour to the other lung may occur or that synchronous primaries may coexist.

Metastatic lesions from lung cancer may occur in any organ of the body and produce symptoms which form the presenting complaint.

Metastases to nodes, particularly those in the scalene area which are usually the first nodes involved which can be palpated clinically, are frequent and should be sought with great care. The best position for examination is from behind with the patient seated relaxed in a chair. The side affected usually corresponds to the side of the lung lesion, the exception being that tumours from the left lower lobe may metastasize to the nodes in the right scalene area. Involvement of the nodes in the floor of the supraclavicular fossa is equally common.

Bony metastases are common, particularly in small-cell tumours, and occur predominantly in the ribs, vertebrae, humeri, and femora. Early involvement may be detected by a rise in alkaline phosphatase of bony origin, isotope scanning, or biopsy. Conventional skeletal surveys are often unhelpful and misleading. Liver secondaries are common and may be silent, although a rise in liver enzymes, particularly alkaline phosphatase of liver origin, may be an early sign. Isotope liver scans and ultrasound may detect involvement in a liver which is not clinically enlarged, but as the metastases develop the liver becomes grossly enlarged with an irregular outline. Friction rubs may sometimes be heard over a grossly involved liver. Metastases to brain may account for the presenting symptom in lung cancer in 4 per cent of patients and may be encountered at some time in the illness in 30 per cent. The symptoms simulate those of any expanding brain tumour. The adrenal glands are involved in 15 to 20 per cent of patients, rarely producing symptoms. The skin should be examined for the presence of the typical slightly bluish umbilicated lesions of tumour spread. Subcutaneous metastases may be found at almost any site.

Endocrine and metabolic manifestations

It is becoming more apparent that many of the hitherto unexplained and often unusual manifestations of malignant disease are the result of endocrine and metabolic manifestations of the cancer itself. Cancer cells appear to be able to synthesize polypeptides that mimic virtually all the hormones produced by conventional endocrine organs—hence the term 'ectopic hormones'. From time to time the clinical features resulting from ectopic hormone secretion precede those of the pulmonary tumour, emphasizing the importance of a high index of suspicion in such circumstances. Unfortunately, in current practice there is no ectopic hormone measurement which can be used for effective screening purposes.

Numerous examples have now been cited of multiple hormonal abnormalities with associated clinical syndromes in the same patient.

SYNDROME OF INAPPROPRIATE SECRETION OF ANTIDIURETIC HORMONE (SIADH)

The continued secretion of vasopressin (ADH) in an amount in excess of the body's needs leads to overhydration in both the intracellular and extracellular compartments. The cerebral oedema resulting from water intoxication causes drowsiness, lethargy, irritability, mental confusion, and disorientation, with fits and coma being the most profound features. Peripheral oedema is remarkably rare. The patient is usually asymptomatic until the sodium falls below 120 mmol/l and the hyponatraemia is dilutional in type with a low serum osmolality. Urine osmolality usually exceeds 300 mosmol/kg. This syndrome is most commonly associated with small-cell cancer and may be obvious in 10 per cent of cases and in more than 50 per cent if a water-loading test is performed. Restriction of fluid to a daily intake of 700–1000 ml may redress the hyponatraemia, but demethylchlortetracycline (demeclocycline) 600–1200 mg daily is often highly effective, making water restriction unnecessary. Azotaemia may occur as a result of increased urea production and a mild drug-induced nephrotoxicity so that adjustment of dosage may be necessary. Infusion of hypertonic saline is hazardous, often precipitating cardiac failure or cerebral oedema.

ECTOPIC ACTH SYNDROME

Secretion of an adrenocorticotrophic substance by a small-cell carcinoma or bronchial carcinoid leads to bilateral adrenal hyperplasia and to secretion of large amounts of cortisol. The onset of symptoms may be so acute that death may occur within a few weeks, and the typical features of Cushing's syndrome such as cutaneous striae and the characteristic distribution of body fat do not have time to develop. Chief clinical features are thirst and polyuria, oedema, pigmentation, and hypokalaemia. Hypertension and profound myopathy may also be present. Serum cortisol is often grossly elevated; the level is not suppressed by dexamethasone, loss of the diurnal rhythm of cortisol level occurs, and the hypokalaemic alkalosis can be severe, with the plasma potassium often being below 3.0 mmol/l and HCO_3 above 30 mmol/l. Drugs which block adrenocortical steroid biosynthesis may produce partial and reversible medical adrenalectomy, and metyrapone in doses from 250 mg thrice daily to 1 g four times daily may cause temporary disappearance of symptoms. Removal of the tumour, if practicable, is curative.

HYPERCALCAEMIA

Hypercalcaemia may be associated with ectopic secretion of parathormone by squamous-cell cancers but is more commonly due directly to the presence of multiple bone metastases. The primary tumour may also produce a cyclic-AMP-stimulating factor or a prostaglandin causing hypercalcaemia. Its presence is unlikely to be recognized symptomatically unless the serum calcium exceeds 2.8 mmol/l; levels of 3.8 mmol/l are sometimes encountered. The main clinical features are nausea, vomiting, abdominal pain and constipation, polyuria, thirst and dehydration, muscular weakness, psychosis, drowsiness, and eventually coma. The calcium level drops dramatically within 48 h if the tumour is removed. The associated dehydration requires replacement of 5 litres of fluid intravenously in 24 h. Corticosteroids (400 mg of hydrocortisone and 100 mg prednisolone in 24 hours initially) are effective in about half the cases. However, intravenous diphosphonates followed by oral maintainance therapy is now the treatment of choice. Other treatments which are sometimes effective are calcitonin 200–400 units every 8 h, mithramycin 10–15 µg/kg by infusion over 4 h every 21 days, aspirin 2–4 g per day, and indomethacin 50–100 mg per day.

GYNAECOMASTIA

Swelling of the breasts, which may be painful, occurs mainly in the subareolar area, and there may be atrophy of the testes. The association is chiefly with large-cell carcinomas. Increased gonadatrophin production is the cause.

OTHER ENDOCRINE MANIFESTATIONS

Hyperthyroidism occurs rarely, but neither goitre nor eye signs are prominent features. Spontaneous hypoglycaemia, the masculinizing syndrome in young women, and hyperglycaemia are very rarely encountered. Pigmentation associated with α- and β-melanocyte-stimulating hormone may occur. The carcinoid syndromes are described in Chapter 14.8.

NEUROMYOPATHIES

The term carcinomatous neuropathy is used to describe those abnormalities of the central nervous system, the peripheral nerves, the muscles, and the autonomic nervous system occurring in association with malignancy. These disorders can be subdivided as follows: myopathies (polymyositis, myasthenia, and dermatomyositis), neuropathies (sensory and mixed sensorimotor, encephalopathy, and myelopathy). Toxic, infective, nutritional, and autoimmune causes have been suggested, but none has been fully substantiated. Neuromyopathies respond variably following treatment of the primary tumour by surgery, radiotherapy, or chemotherapy.

Most neuromyopathies are not tumour-cell-type specific, except for the Lambert–Eaton syndrome seen occasionally in small-cell lung cancer patients, often preceding the appearance of a tumour by up to 15 months. It is characterized by proximal muscle weakness, depressed tendon reflexes, often returning following repetitive exercise, autonomic features, and difficulty with swallowing. There appears to be an association with the IgG heavy-chain allotypes GM[2] and H LA-B8 for this condition which is currently treated with prednisolone and 3-4 amidopyridine 10–20 mg four times daily.

FINGER CLUBBING AND HYPERTROPHIC PULMONARY OSTEOARTHROPATHY

Finger clubbing accompanies a variety of intrathoracic disorders. Gross clubbing is readily recognizable; its early presence may best be demonstrated by the ability to rock the nail on its abnormally spongy bed. Clubbing of the toes is usually present also. Its incidence in lung cancer has variously been reported as being between 10 and 30 per cent. Clubbing may disappear after resection of tumour. The precise mechanism for the development of clubbing has not yet been determined.

Hypertrophic pulmonary osteo-arthropathy, which may be preceded by finger clubbing alone, consists of periostitis, arthropathy, and usually gross finger clubbing. It is most commonly associated with lung tumours but is also very common in pleural tumours, preceding the diagnosis of tumour in about one-third of patients. It is much commoner in peripheral lesions and squamous tumours.

The long bones of the extremities are affected by a periosteal reaction resembling elm bark; the changes are symmetrical and affect mainly ankles and wrists, with the knees and elbows being involved less commonly. Synovial thickening and joint effusions are rare. The typical radiographic appearances are shown in Fig. 4. The affected areas are hot and painful and sometimes oedematous. In severe cases walking becomes impracticable. The facial features are sometimes thickened and gynaecomastia is present in 10 per cent of cases. Removal of the tumour is followed by immediate regression of hypertrophic pulmonary osteoarthropathy, but symptoms recur if there is regrowth of the tumour. Vagotomy alone is sometimes effective, supporting the theory of a vagal mediation of increased blood flow as an aetiological factor in hypertrophic pulmonary osteo-arthropathy.

MISCELLANEOUS

The haematological effects of lung cancer are normally non-specific, normocytic normochromic anaemia is the most common form. Leuco-erythroblastic anaemia denotes bone marrow infiltration and may be seen in small-cell lung cancer in particular. Venous thrombosis and thrombophlebitis due to hypercoagulability are common complications of malignancy and may precede the detection of the underlying cancer; recurrent migratory phlebitis resistant to anticoagulation is an ominous feature. Marantic endocarditis is extremely rare, as are skin lesions such as acanthosis nigricans, dermatomyositis, hypertrichosis languinosa, and erythema gyratum repens. Rarely, the nephrotic syndrome is also encountered.

Staging and investigations

The investigations used to make the diagnosis and the assessment of lung cancer will vary according to the stage of presentation, the cell type, and the age and general condition of the patient.

The very rapid doubling time of small-cell lung cancer causes it to disseminate rapidly and widely, and at diagnosis is very rarely considered operable. However, the slower doubling times for squamous-cell cancers and adenocarcinomas, together with the relatively lesser tendency for the former to disseminate, makes surgery the best option whenever possible for the non-small-cell lung cancers. A precise anatomical staging classification was only applied to lung cancer in 1973 and immediately demonstrated that the prognosis of non-small-cell lung cancer depended strongly on the extent (or stage) of the disease. The introduction of the TNM staging system (T describing the primary tumour, N the extent of regional lymph node involvement, and M the absence or presence of metastases) encouraged an ordered assessment

Fig. 4 Hypertrophic pulmonary osteoarthropathy showing persistent new bone formation.

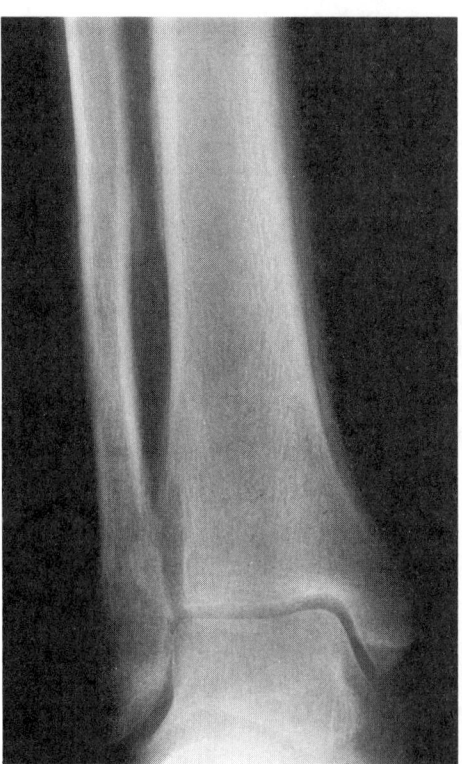

Table 5 *Definitions for staging bronchogenic carcinoma (American Joint Committee on Cancer Staging 1986)*

T0 No evidence of primary tumour
TX Tumour proven by the presence of malignant cells in bronchopulmonary secretions but not visualized radiographically or bronchoscopically, or any tumour that cannot be assessed
TIS Carcinoma *in situ*
T1 A tumour that is 3.0 cm or less in greatest diameter, surrounded by lung or visceral pleura, and without evidence of invasion proximal to a lobar bronchus at bronchoscopy
T2 A tumour more than 3.0 cm in greatest diameter, or a tumour of any size that either invades the vasceral pleura or has associated atelectasis or obstructive pneumonitis extending to the hilar region, at bronchoscopy, the proximal extent of demonstrable tumour must be within a lobar nronchus or at least 2.0 cm distal to the carina; any associated atelectasis or obstructive pneumonitis must involve less than an entire lung
T3 A tumour of any size with direct extension into the chest wall (including superior sulcus tumours), mediastinal pleura, or pericardium without involving the heart, great vessels, trachea, oesophagus, or vertebral body, or a tumour in the main bronchus within 2 cm of the carina without involving the carina
T4 A tumour of any size with invasion of the mediastinum or involving the heart, great vessels, trachea, oesophagus, vertebral body, or carina as presence of malignant pleural effusion
N0 No demonstrable metastasis to regional lymph nodes
N1 Metastasis to lymph nodes in the peribronchial or the ipsilateral hilar region, or both, including direct extension
N2 Metastasis to ipsilateral mediastinal lymph nodes and subcarinal lymph nodes
N3 Metastasis of contralateral mediastinal lymph nodes, contralateral hilar lymph nodes, ipsilateral or contralateral sclera, or supraclavicular lymph nodes
M0 No (known) distant metastasis
M1 Distant metastasis such as in scalene, cervical, or contralateral hilar lymph nodes, brain, bones, liver, or contralateral lung

Summary staging

Stage 1 (operable)

T1	N0	M0
T2	N0	M0

Stage II (operable)
T1	N1	M0
T2	N1	M0

Stage IIIa (operable)
T3	N0	M0
T3	N1	M0
T1-3	N2	M0

Stage IIIb (inoperable)
Any T	N3	M0
T4	Any N	M0
Any T	Any N	M1

of investigations and selection of cases for surgery. On the basis of this experience the system was modified in 1986 (Table 5).

The following investigations form the basis for the diagnosis and staging of patients with lung cancer.

INTRATHORACIC INVESTIGATIONS

Radiological assessment

The value of the chest radiograph in the diagnosis and management of pulmonary neoplasm needs no emphasis. No initial examination is complete without a lateral film. Coned views of the ribs may help where rib invasion is suspected clinically.

The finding of a normal radiograph of the chest does not exclude bronchial carcinoma as patients presenting with haemoptysis and a normal chest radiograph are sometimes found to have a central tumour on bronchoscopy. The rounded or ovoid shadow of a peripheral tumour is described in greater detail below; these are sometimes cavitated (Fig. 5). The common appearance of a tumour arising from the main central airways (70 per cent of all cases) is enlargement of one or other hilum (Fig. 6); even experienced observers sometimes have difficulty in determining whether a hilar shadow is enlarged or not, and if there is any suspicion, investigation by bronchoscopy and/or CT should be pursued. Consolidation and collapse distal to the tumour may have occurred by the time that the patient presents, with the tumour itself often being obscured in the process. Collapse of the left lower lobe is often hard to identify (Fig. 7), as is a tumour situated behind the heart (Fig. 8). Apically located masses or superior sulcus tumours (Pancoast tumours) may be misdiagnosed as pleural caps, and often have a long history of pain in the distribution of the brachial nerve roots. Loss of the head of the first, second, or third rib is not unusual (Fig. 9).

The mediastinum may be widened by enlarged nodes. Involvement of the phrenic nerve may lead to elevation of the hemidiaphragm which becomes paralysed and moves paradoxically on sniffing. Tumour spreading to the pleura causes effusion, but such an abnormality may be secondary to infection beyond obstruction caused by a central tumour. The ribs and spine should be carefully examined for the presence of metastasis. Spread of tumour from mediastinal nodes peripherally along the lymphatics gives the appearance characteristic of lymphangitis carcinomatosa—bilateral hilar enlargement with streaky shadows fanning out into the lung fields on either side. Rarely, localized obstructive emphysema may be observed.

LUNG FUNCTION

Evaluation of lung function is essential. Simple spirometry is usually adequate, but it may be necessary to evaluate exercise capability in a more sophisticated manner in some patients for whom surgery is being considered. The ability to climb one flight of stairs without breathlessness has been claimed to be a very good indication of fitness for resection. However, ventilation–perfusion lung scans give a good indication of the relative function of each lung in cases whose overall preoperative lung function appears to be borderline for resection.

Bronchoscopy

Bronchoscopy, which is described in detail in Chapter 17.6.4, is frequently the definitive diagnostic method in lung cancer. Tissue removed at bronchoscopy is an essential means of establishing the diagnosis and cell type before embarking on a programme of further staging and treatment. The amount of material biopsied is generally smaller with the fibreoptic instrument than with the rigid bronchoscope, and this can occasionally cause problems. The extent of visualization and sites within reach of the biopsy forceps is greater with the flexible than with the rigid bronchoscope, particularly in the upper lobes. The rigid instrument is often preferred if an adenoma is suspected, and is preferred by some in the assessment of central lesions as with this instrument the resistance produced by extrabronchial masses can be sensed more easily; others claim that mobility can be as readily gauged with the flexible instrument

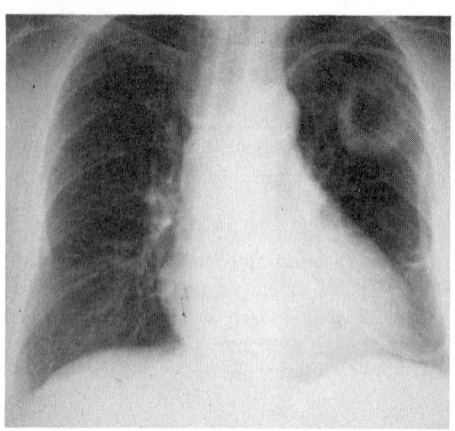

Fig. 5 Cavitating peripheral squamous-cell carcinoma.

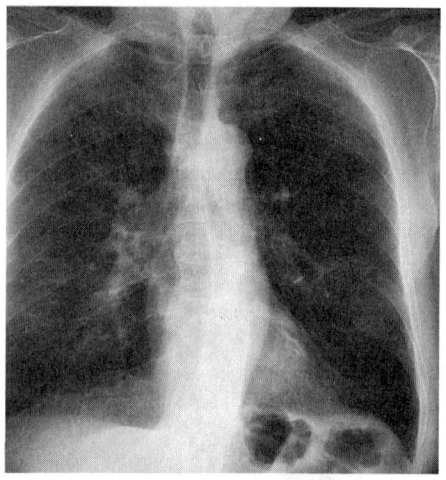

Fig. 6 Enlarged right hilum. Bronchoscopy revealed a tumour in right intermediate bronchus.

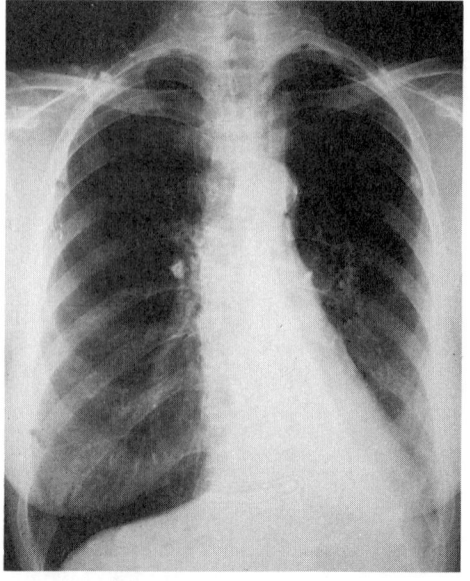

Fig. 7 Collapsed left lower lobe showing loss of the medial third of the left diaphragm.

during respiration and coughing. Modern techniques of brushing or washing material from smaller bronchial segments augment the positive yield.

Most investigators perform a biopsy of a suspicious lesion, followed by a small-volume lavage (50–150 ml) and then brushings. Whilst brushing cytology will add to the yield from biopsy, lavage only adds 1 to 2 per cent to the total diagnostic yield of lung tumours. When cancer cells are found in sputum without a radiologically visible lesion, a search for subtle changes in the mucous membranes, particularly at carinae, is needed and such areas should be biopsied. Rarely, the nasopharynx is the source of such cells. Bronchoscopic examination also yields valuable information regarding suitability for surgical resection. Resection is regarded as unsuitable if the main carina is recognized as being invaded, or unequivocally broad with splaying of the main bronchi and immobility on respiration, or where there is involvement of the trachea unless it is limited to the right lateral wall. Histological confirmation is now obtainable in 85 to 90 per cent of bronchoscopically visible lesions.

Transbronchial biopsy

Transbronchial biopsy via the fibreoptic bronchoscope is useful in the diagnosis of circumscribed lesions beyond the range of direct vision or

Fig. 8 Squamous-cell carcinoma lying behind the heart in the left lower lobe.

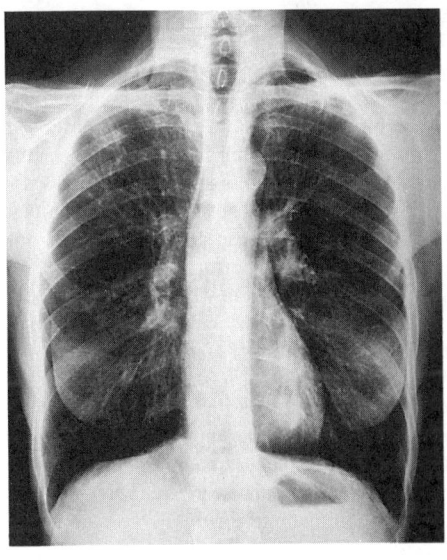

Fig. 9 Huge apical tumour with destruction of posterior parts of the second and third ribs.

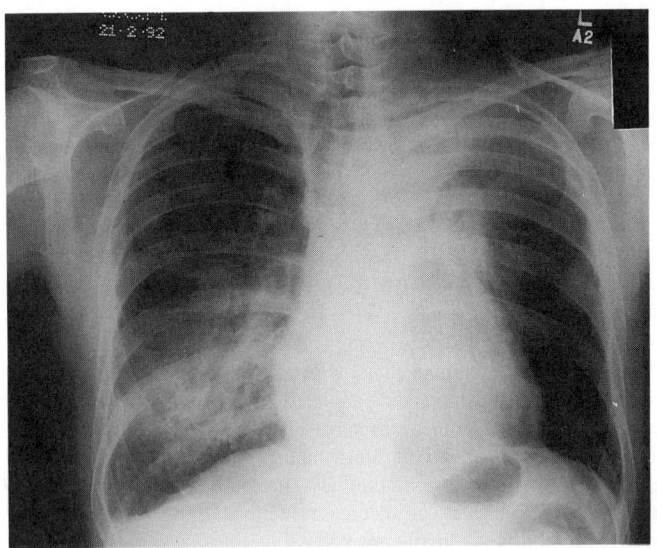

of more diffuse lesions such as may be seen in adenocarcinoma, bronchoalveolar-cell carcinoma, and lymphangitis carcinomatosis. It is advisable to manoeuvre the placement of the biopsy forceps under fluoroscopic control if a circumscribed lesion is to be biopsied. A positive yield of 60 to 70 per cent has been obtained in circumscribed lesions, and is greatest in those over 4 cm in diameter. Pneumothorax follows the procedure in about 5 per cent of cases and major haemorrhage in 1 to 2 per cent, almost always in the presence of a haemorrhagic diathesis. Fatalities are extremely rare. However, current trends are increasingly towards percutaneous needle biopsy, often with CT guidance, for circumscribed lesions, and to use transbronchial biopsy for diffuse infiltrates.

Percutaneous needle biopsy

Percutaneous needle biopsy may be carried out by a Vim-Silverman, Menghini, or Trucut needle in large lesions close to the pleura to obtain a core of tissue for histology, or by aspiration needle biopsy which only yields cytological smear preparations. The procedure should be performed under fluoroscopic, CT, or ultrasound control, and is best avoided in patients with poor respiratory function or with bleeding diatheses. Positive yields as high as 90 per cent have been reported, with the yield depending upon meticulous technique and the competence of the pathologist. However, cytological samples remain the least satisfactory for cell type specificity. It is a useful diagnostic method in patients in whom exploratory thoracotomy may be hazardous or in attempts to determine whether a solid mass is a primary, secondary, or benign tumour. Pneumothorax occurs in about 25 per cent of patients, with some 5 per cent requiring intubation. Slight haemoptysis may follow the procedure.

Sputum cytology

Cytological examination of sputum is a very useful non-invasive step in the diagnosis of malignant pulmonary disease. The patient should be encouraged to cough deeply and to raise sputum from the deeper parts of the chest because material for examination, if it is to be of value, must come from the lower respiratory tract. Physiotherapy can give considerable assistance in obtaining satisfactory material; a warm saline aerosol may also help. The yield increases according to the number of specimens examined, and three consecutive morning specimens should be submitted in the first instance. In one large study, in those in whom a diagnosis of lung cancer was made, the diagnosis came from a single specimen of sputum in 41 per cent; a second sample increased the yield to 56 per cent, a third to 69 per cent, and a fourth to 85 per cent. The positive incidence is lower with tumours less than 2 cm in diameter (40 per cent) and best with larger masses (60 per cent). Central tumour yields a higher proportion of positive results (60 per cent) than peripheral lesions (48 per cent).

Thoracoscopy

Visualization of the parietal and visceral pleura has an important part to play in the diagnosis of effusions and in pleural tumours as biopsy of lesions can be carried out under direct vision, and absence of pleural tumour is important in decisions about resectability of a lung tumour. Thoracoscopy is inadvisible in the absence of effusion or pneumothorax, and is unsatisfactory in the presence of empyema or gross haemothorax. However, in otherwise operable tumours with a pleural effusion that is not bloodstained and without positive cytology or pleural biopsy, thoracoscopy may be a useful next step in determining operability.

Computed axial tomography (CT)

Thoracic CT scanning has been an important advance in the staging of lung cancer. It can identify the site, size, and extension of the primary tumour far more clearly than conventional radiology. It also frequently identifies mediastinal lymphadenopathy when posteroanterior and lateral chest radiographs fail to show any abnormality. Mediastinal lymphadenopathy on CT is arbitrarily taken to be pathological by most centres if the glands are greater than 1.0 cm in diameter. However, previous infective conditions such as tuberculosis and reactive hyperplasia to the tumour can cause appearances identical with that of malignant enlargement. Thus positive CT scans of the mediastinum may be falsely positive in up to 50 per cent of cases, although this figure is now less with newer ultrafast scanning methods. Therefore mediastinal lymph node biopsy (mediastinoscopy) must be performed to confirm an abnormal finding.

Another potential advantage of CT is its ability to detect tumour invasion of the surrounding pleura and chest wall, in addition to the mediastinum itself. However, not all tumours with CT evidence of invasion prove unresectable, and if possible invasion of the mediastinum or chest wall is the only contraindication to resection then thoracotomy should be performed.

The predictive value of a negative CT is of the order of 90 to 95 per cent, and in such cases a mediastinoscopy can be omitted before thoracotomy. However, microscopic invasion of normal-sized mediastinal nodes is increasingly reported in patients with adenocarcinoma of the lung. Perhaps patients with this cell type should have a mediasti-

Fig. 10 Preoperative staging of non-small-cell lung cancer: +ve, positive; −ve negative; PTNM staging, postsurgical pathological staging. (Reproduced with permission from Spiro and Goldstraw 1984.)

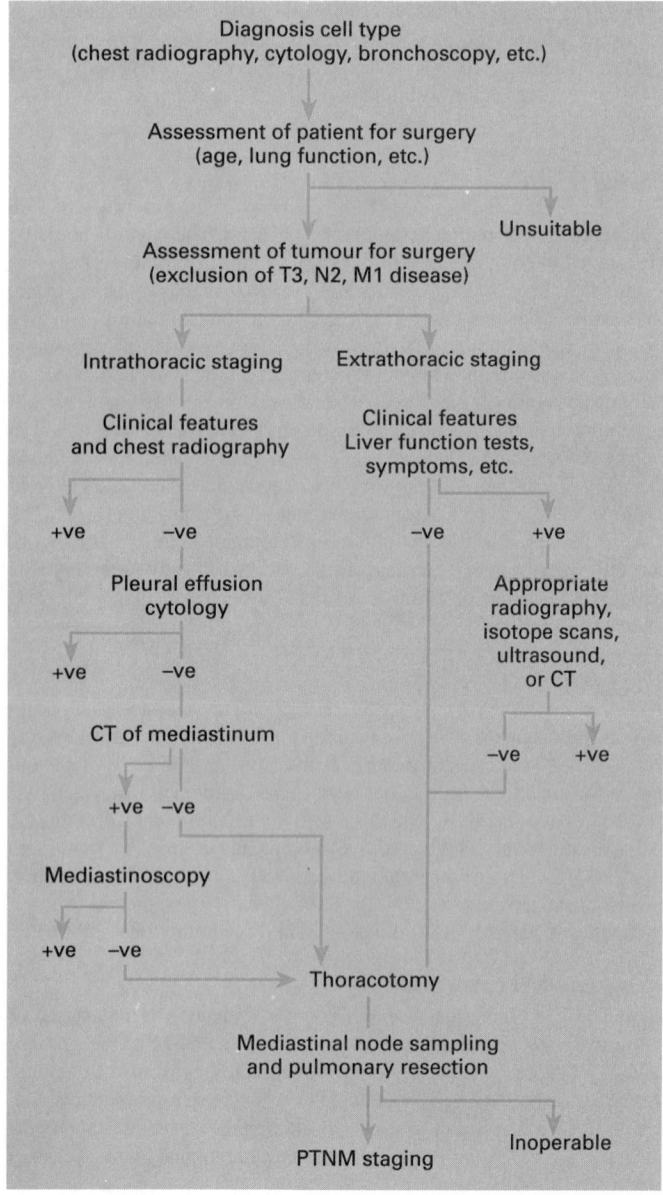

noscopy routinely prethoractomy irrespective of whether the mediastinal lymph nodes appear normal in size on a staging CT scan.

EXTRATHORACIC INVESTIGATIONS

In general, the ability to identify small metastatic deposits is as unsatisfactory for lung carcinomas as for other solid tumours. The available techniques are relatively crude, and this partially explains the high extrathoracic relapse rate following so-called 'curative' resections for non-small-cell lung cancer. In patients with no symptoms other than those caused by their primary tumour, if there is no clinical evidence of neurological, hepatic, or bony disease and normal biochemistry, then imaging scans of brain, liver, and bones will be unhelpful. CT brain scans have a high accuracy in detailing cerebral metastases in patients with neurological symptoms. In patients with a palpable liver and/or abnormal liver function tests, a liver CT scan or ultrasound should be performed. CT scan of the upper abdomen identifies abnormalities of one or both adrenal glands in up to 10 per cent of patients considered for surgery. Fine-needle aspiration of the adrenal gland should be performed if this remains the only contraindication to pulmonary resection. Bone scans have a high false-positive rate due to Paget's disease, active arthritis, healing fractures, renal disease, and hyperparathyroidism. However, a bone scan should be ordered in patients with bone pain, local tenderness, or non-specific symptoms of weight loss or malaise.

Biopsy of enlarged lymph nodes and skin metastases should be carried out whenever indicated. If an isolated hepatic or bony lesion identified with isotope or CT scanning appears to be the only contraindication to surgery, this should be biopsied under radiological control.

The staging investigations for non-small-cell lung cancer are summarized in Fig. 10. The final procedure prethoracotomy is the assessment of the mediastinum. If CT scanning is normal, the surgeon can proceed directly to thoracotomy. If the CT scan is abnormal or is not available, mediastinal exploration should be performed first.

Routine cervical mediastinoscopy in patients who otherwise appear radiologically operable on conventional films will yield mediastinal lymph node involvement in 10 to 15 per cent of all cases considered for surgery. To this should be added the value of left anterior mediastinotomy—an approach through the bed of the second left costal cartilage to palpate glands draining tumours from the left upper lobe. The mediastinum may be involved in up to 50 per cent of patients with a peripheral poorly differentiated tumour and in a much greater percentage of centrally occurring lesions, although many of them will have an abnormal mediastinal contour on routine chest radiography.

Treatment

SURGERY

Surgery remains the single modality most likely to be curative in non-small-cell lung cancer. In small-cell lung cancer the very occasional patient, usually presenting with a peripheral tumour, who remains operable after extensive staging investigations is cured. These patients are rare, but nevertheless have a 5 year survival rate in the region of 30 to 40 per cent.

Prior to surgery the patient should have been carefully staged (Fig. 10), and the chances of long-term survival will be greatly influenced by this. All patients with stage IIIb disease (Table 5) should be rejected for thoracotomy, but those with stage I, II and IIIa disease can be resected. In general, patients with squamous-cell carcinomas have higher 5 and 10 year survival rates than those with adenocarcinoma and large-cell carcinomas, and the more differentiated the tumour the better is the prognosis. Table 6 summarizes survival data at 5 years for preoperatively staged non-small-cell lung cancer. Clearly, small peripheral lesions with no nodal disease fare best (up to 70 per cent survival at 5 years), but the survival rate decreases with both size of tumour and presence of hilar node involvement.

In all, approximately 20 per cent of patients who present with non-

Table 6 *Cumulative percentage surviving 5 years and median survival by clinical and surgical TNM subsets (1986 Classification)*

TNM subset	Clinical			Surgical		
	No.	Percentage surviving	Median survival (months)	No.	Percentage surviving	Median survival (months)
T1 N0 M0	591	61.9	60	429	68.5	60
T2 N0 M0	1012	35.8	26	436	59.0	60
T1 N1 M0	19	33.6	20	67	54.1	60
T2 N1 M0	176	22.7	17	250	40.0	29
T3 N0 M0	221	7.6	8	57	44.2	26
T3 N1 M0	71	7.7	8	29	17.6	16
Any N2 M0	497	4.9	11	168	28.8	22

small-cell lung cancer eventually come to thoracotomy. Most of the others are excluded almost immediately because of clinically evident metastatic disease, radiological or bronchoscopic evidence of inoperability, too advanced an age to withstand surgery, significant associated other illnesses, or inadequate lung function. Of those having a 'curative' resection, the overall survival rate at 5 years is approximately 25 per cent and at 10 years is 16 to 18 per cent. Death from local or distant recurrence of the tumour is equally probable, highlighting the inadequacies of current staging techniques. However, the careful application of the TNM system and the advent of more sophisticated scanning equipment may further selection improve.

Cardiac and respiratory complications are the most common source of postoperative morbidity and mortality, and it is essential that the reserve capacity of heart and lungs be evaluated preoperatively. Patients in the high risk cardiac complication category are those who have sustained myocardial infarction in the preceding 3 months, or who have uncontrolled arrhythmias. A history of angina of itself does not contraindicate surgery: the ultimate in sophisticated surgery is simultaneous tumour resection and coronary bypass!

Pulmonary function must always be evaluated prior to consideration for resection. The simplest tests for assessing pulmonary function are the forced expiratory volume in 1 s (FEV_1) and the functional vital capacity (FVC). Pneumonectomy should probably not be undertaken if the patient cannot sustain an FEV_1 of more than 1.2 litres, bearing in mind that patients who have coexistent chronic obstructive airflow disease may not sustain the current value in exacerbations. In the middle range of ventilatory capacity the risk of resection is a matter of judgement based on the estimate of maximum tolerable resection and assessment of the functional integrity of the non-tumour-bearing lung. Combination of pulmonary function tests, including the 12 min walking test, and regional function studies using 133-xenon may be used in patients with borderline function. As lung cancer is such a serious disease, consideration may sometimes have to be given to carrying out resection in patients whose physical performance defies the results of pulmonary function tests.

Only very rarely is there an indication for palliative surgery, and resection should not be considered in the presence of intrathoracic or distant metastasis. There are diametrically opposed views as to whether surgery should be undertaken in Pancoast tumours.

Advanced age is not a contraindication to surgery. Patients over 70 years of age appear to tolerate lobectomy as well as younger patients, although the mortality for pneumonectomy (8–10 per cent) is double that of those under 70. Thus in 'good risk' patients in this age group there is no evidence that tumours grow more slowly in the elderly, and therefore the disease is as likely to be the terminal event in the aged as in younger patients. Hence resection should be encouraged in fit patients. Smokers should be persuaded to stop smoking before thoracotomy; continued smoking increases perioperative complications.

Thoracoscopic resection of peripheral masses is currently being evaluated.

RADIOTHERAPY

Patients who are excluded from surgery because of adverse prognostic factors, advanced stage of tumour, or other coincidental disease constitute the largest group treated with radiotherapy. Although the usual aim of radiotherapy will be palliative, there will be a small group of patients in whom more aggressive therapy will be used in the hope of cure, or at least long-term survival, particularly in those who have refused surgery. Radiotherapy for lung cancer is limited by the comparative radiosensitivity of three critical normal tissues likely to be included in the radiation beam: normal lung, spinal cord, and heart, each of which has a critical tolerance dose. Increased radiation dose leads to greater killing of tumour cells but may produce unwanted damage to normal cells. Radiation dose must be expressed not only in terms of total dose but also numbers of fractions and overall time. There is no clear evidence for an optimum radiation dose, but doses of 5000 to 6000 rad (50–60 Gy) in 5 to 6 weeks are appropriate; higher doses will be associated with unacceptable morbidity.

The role of radiotherapy
Alternative to surgery
In some patients with a technically resectable tumour, there may be medical contraindications for resection or the patient may refuse surgery. In general, the results of radical radiotherapy in these patients are inferior to the 5 year survival following surgery. The best result for radiotherapy was a 5 year survival rate of 22 per cent for peripheral squamous-cell cancers, but other series post a 5 year survival rate of 6 per cent.

Preoperative radiotherapy
Preoperative radiotherapy has been attempted in a few uncontrolled studies, but there is no evidence that this approach improves survival.

Postoperative radiotherapy
This has long been uncertain in value, but two recent large randomized studies showed no survival benefit for the addition of high dose radiotherapy (50–60 Gy) to the mediastinal region following curative resection. In one study, the addition of radiotherapy following surgery did reduce the incidence of relapse within the mediastinum, but survival was unaffected owing to the high incidence of extrathoracic relapse.

Radical radiotherapy for locally inoperable disease
In otherwise fit patients with small-volume intrathoracic disease which is not resectable, usually because of mediastinal involvement, it is common practice to attempt to cure with radiotherapy. Results are disappointing, even with doses of up to 60 Gy, with 5 year survival rates ranging from 5 to 17 per cent.

Palliation
The value of radiotherapy in palliating certain symptoms is beyond dispute. Haemoptysis and cough, two of the most distressing symptoms,

Table 7 *Objective average response to single-agent chemotherapy in lung cancer*

	Response (%)			
Drug	Small-cell	Squamous-cell	Adenocarcinoma	Large-cell
Ifosfamide	63	27	23	36
Vincristine	42	10	23	0
Epipodophyllotoxin	40	25	12	0
Cyclophosphamide	33	20	20	23
Methotrexate	30	25	30	12
Adriamycin	30	20	15	25
CCNU	15	30	20	17
Cisplatin	35	20	12	13

CCNU, chloroethyl-cyclohexyl-nitrosourea.

can be controlled by radiotherapy in up to 80 per cent of cases. Administration of single fractions, each of 8.5 Gy, 1 week apart appears adequate. Dyspnoea from bronchial obstruction and dysphagia are relieved in the majority of cases. The syndrome of superior vena caval obstruction is relieved in about 80 per cent of sufferers, but usually requires a more conventional course of five to ten fractions of radiotherapy. Pain from bone secondaries can be relieved in more than 50 per cent of sufferers by a single fraction of 8 to 10 Gray, often given at the same time as a clinic visit, and is a huge bonus to the patient as five to ten smaller treatments used to be standard until 2 years ago. Brain metastases generally respond poorly to radiotherapy. A 48 h trial of dexamethasone 4 mg orally four times daily is recommended as initial management. If a worthwhile response follows the resolution of the oedema surrounding the metastases, then radiotherapy will consolidate this gain. The steroids should then be rapidly withdrawn on completion of radiotherapy. Spinal cord compression is a relatively common occurrence owing to a deposit from lung cancer. Pain and bony tenderness often precede it and may be helpful in localizing the lesion. Responses to radiotherapy are usually incomplete and disappointing, often because of interruption of the vascular supply to the spinal cord by the tumour.

Further developments in radiotherapy

These include hyperfractionation schedules where two or three doses of radiotherapy are given daily for 10 to 14 days in an attempt to prevent the tumour tissue from recovering from the injury induced by the radiotherapy. This technique is still being evaluated.

CHEMOTHERAPY

Non-small-cell lung cancer

Although many cytotoxic drugs show modest activity against these tumours, there is no good evidence that they prolong survival in these inoperable patients. There have been hundreds of studies of single-agent and combination regimens, but very few controlled studies. Response rates (i.e. reduction in tumour volume by at least 50 per cent) of up to 30 per cent have commonly been reported (Table 7), but owing to lack of control data, non-comparative data, or using historical controls as the comparison, there is no convincing evidence that chemotherapy prolongs survival for these cell types. Newer agents such as etoposide, ifosfamide, and cisplatin have also failed to confer a significant survival advantage. Controlled studies incorporating combinations of cytotoxic agents in patients with advanced non-small-cell lung cancer, when compared with best supportive care, have failed to show any survival advantage for the administration of chemotherapy. However, a recent meta-analysis of seven studies of chemotherapy versus best supportive care in cases of advanced non-small-cell lung cancer reported a significant advantage for chemotherapy at 3, 6, and 9 months after commencing treatment. Clearly more information is needed before the role of chemotherapy is defined with certainty. Clinical trials are also currently evaluating the

possible use of chemotherapy as an adjuvant to surgery in locally inoperable tumours, and also before radical radiotherapy. These usually involve fit relatively asymptomatic patients who tolerate chemotherapy well, but the results of these studies are still awaited. Newer agents with response rates in excess of 30 per cent include interleukin 2, navelbine, and zeniplatin, which are currently being evaluated.

Small-cell lung cancer

This cell type has been separated from the other types of lung cancer because of its very different biological and clinical features. It has an explosive growth pattern so that the TNM staging classification makes no impact on prognosis or survival, almost certainly because careful staging puts most patients into the inoperable category and because small metastases remain undetected for a few months. However, simple staging has some prognostic impact and those staged to have limited disease (tumour confined to one hemithorax and the ipsilateral supraclavicular fossa) fare better than those with extensive disease (involvement of any site outside the hemithorax). The natural history of untreated small-cell lung cancer is about 3.5 months for limited disease and 6 weeks for extensive disease.

Small-cell lung cancer is much more sensitive to cytotoxic chemotherapy than the non-small-cell lung cancer tumours, with a much higher response rate for several cytotoxic drugs (Table 7). In the late 1970s there was a very rapid improvement in median survival using combinations of three and four drugs, but responses have subsequently reached a plateau. Nevertheless with modern combination cytotoxic treatment, which is usually given on an outpatient basis every 3 weeks, the median survival has been extended to 14 to 18 months for limited disease and to 9 to 12 months for extensive disease. Most combinations include cyclophosphamide, doxorubicin, etoposide, cisplatin, or vincristine. Most modern regimens would be expected to have a complete response rate (i.e. disappearance of all measurable disease) of 40 to 50 per cent and a partial response rate (greater than 50 per cent reduction in tumour bulk) of 40 per cent, giving a total response rate of 80 to 85 per cent. All these regimens have side-effects. Most patients will experience some nausea and vomiting, and alopecia is practically universal. Care has to be taken to ensure bone marrow recovery before the next course is given and that safe lower limits of total white cell and platelet counts have been achieved. Anaemia is treated by transfusion as necessary. Life-threatening septicaemia can occur in 1 to 4 per cent of patients but treatment-related deaths are uncommon. Recent reports suggest that single-agent (etoposide) oral therapy can offer useful palliation in some patients, for example older age groups in whom tolerance of the combination regimens may be low.

Much effort has been applied during the last 5 years to improve the median and long-term survival of patients with small-cell lung cancer. In general, those patients in whom further progress is to be made are those who present with limited disease and a high performance status. Patients with extensive disease tend to have a universally bad prognosis and very few survive beyond 2 years. However, it seems that single metastatic sites such as bone and bone marrow are not as sinister as the brain or the liver, and therefore the occasional extensive disease patient does extremely well with chemotherapy, but in general the treatment offered to those with extensive disease tends to be only palliative. Studies assessing the quality of life in all patients presenting with small-cell lung cancer have noted that over 70 per cent of patients have important symptoms such as weight loss, malaise, bone pain, dyspnoea, and haemoptysis. The majority of these patients will have extensive disease. Reassessment of symptoms after 3 months of chemotherapy has shown relief of these symptoms in 60 to 70 per cent of sufferers, making chemotherapy worthwhile with its benefits in terms of symptom relief far outweighing the potential side-effects.

Intensifying the dosage or the frequency of administration of the cytotoxic agents has been thoroughly assessed without striking benefit on median survival data. Smaller advantages are occasionally seen, but these have to be balanced by the increased toxicity resulting from this more aggressive approach. Attempts to overcome or delay the emergence of cell resistance to chemotherapy have involved alternating combinations of drugs, but these more complicated regimens have not been rewarding either.

Prognostic factors

Multivariate analyses of large patient populations show that routine biochemical values such as serum sodium, albumin, and alkaline phosphatase allow separation of prognostic subgroups. In addition, performance status and extent of disease are important influences. For instance a good performance status and normal biochemical values (i.e. a good prognostic category) has a 2 year survival rate of 20 per cent, yet a correspondingly low performance status with one or more abnormal biochemical parameters (poor prognosis) has virtually no 2 year survivors (Fig. 11). Women tend to do better than men and those under 60 better than those over 60 years of age. Pretreatment weight loss of more than 3 kg indicates a substantially worse prognosis. These factors are helpful both for stratification within clinical studies and for identifying those patients likely to do well with chemotherapy and those in whom intensive toxic chemotherapy would appear inappropriate.

Duration of treatment

Toxicity to chemotherapy increases with the number of courses given. It is now apparent that most of the tumour response to chemotherapy occurs within the first two or three cycles. Studies attempting to minimize the duration of chemotherapy without adversely affecting survival have shown that six courses of combination chemotherapy, i.e. a course every 3 weeks, is optimal. Studies of four to eight courses of chemotherapy compared with eight to twelve, or with a further year of maintainence therapy, have shown no survival advantage for the longer treatment schedules. This has greatly improved the quality of life of patients who now receive much shorter courses of chemotherapy than 5 years ago.

Long-term survival

Survival beyond 5 years is achieved in 4 to 12 per cent of patients with limited disease and in hardly anyone with extensive disease at diagnosis. A recent review of patients entered into clinical trials in the United Kingdom recorded a 2 year survival of 8 per cent in patients presenting with limited disease, and 2.2 per cent for those with extensive disease. Most studies of long-term survival report late deaths due to other cancers, including non-small-cell lung cancers in up to 30 per cent of these long-term survivors.

Radiotherapy

As discussed above, radiotherapy has an important role in palliation of symptoms that may develop after relapse following chemotherapy. However, in approximately 15 per cent of patients with limited disease, there is a small but definite benefit when thoracic irradiation is added to combination chemotherapy. Chest irradiation also significantly decreases the rate of recurrence at the primary tumour site and in the mediastinum. A total dose of 40 to 50 Gy is usually given. The precise timing of the radiotherapy in relation to chemotherapy is not clear, but the trend is in favour of early radiotherapy given concurrently with chemotherapy. However, acute and late toxicity is increased when radiotherapy and chemotherapy are given in combination.

Superior vena caval obstruction

Ten per cent of small-cell lung cancer patients present with this complication which responds as well as any presentation to chemotherapy. The onus is on the clinician to establish the diagnosis and the cell type of the tumour. Small-cell lung cancer should be treated with chemotherapy in the usual manner, whilst non-small-cell lung cancer should be treated with radiotherapy.

Cranial irradiation

Cranial metastases are common. Ten per cent of patients in complete response develop brain metastases as their first site of relapse. Prophylactic cranial irradiation given at the end of chemotherapy will delay the presentation of cerebral metastases and also reduce their overall incidence. However, there is no evidence of prolonged survival. Patients who receive prophylactic cranial irradiation are at greater risk of late neurological complications—particularly psychometric and psychological impairment. However, the morbidity of cerebral metastases is so great that is seems helpful to attempt to prevent this socially disastrous form of relapse.

General management

There are certain complications which require specific measures to alleviate symptoms.

Patients who seem likely to survive for 6 months or more and who have vocal chord paralysis find considerable help in morale from an injection of Teflon into the affected chord which restores voice production in a high percentage of cases and reduces the risk of aspiration. Occurrence of upper airway obstruction causing stridor, or obstruction of the lower major airways, in non-small-cell lung cancer patients is usually initially treated with radiotherapy. Should this complication recur or be unsuitable for radiotherapy, it could be suitable for laser

Fig. 11 The effect of prognostic grouping in survival in small-cell lung cancer. The upper curve represents good prognosis patients; the lower two curves are intermediate and poor prognosis groups respectively.

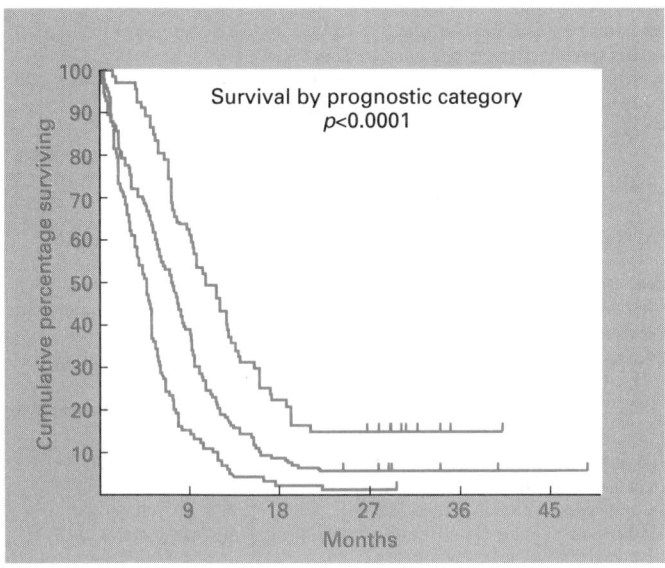

photocoagulation administered either via the fibreoptic bronchoscope or under general anaesthetic via a rigid instrument. Laser therapy for carcinoma of the bronchus is most suitable as a palliative treatment in central tumours occluding large airways. There are technical limitations to its application via the flexible bronchoscope, but removal of considerable quantities of tumour can be achieved in a single treatment session with the rigid instrument. Laser therapy is used predominantly for recurrence of tumour in the central airways, usually after radiotherapy has failed. Trials are in progress assessing the additional benefits of endobronchial radiotherapy using irridium or caesium wires delivered via the fibre optic bronchoscope. This procedure irradiates endobronchial tumour to a circumferential depth of about 1 cm, and will often produce a further remission. It is used where further external beam radiotherapy cannot be given because of the risk of exceeding normal tissue tolerance.

Infection distal to tumour requires antibiotic therapy and, where appropriate, oxygen therapy and bronchodilators. Severe recurrent haemoptysis may be controlled by radiotherapy or laser.

Malignant pleural effusion recurs after aspiration unless the pleural space is obliterated. Chemical pleurodesis can be induced by intrapleural instillation of a number of agents or by the more invasive procedure of talc pleurodesis. Intrapleural tetracycline is most commonly used, but bleomycin also gives successful pleurodesis in 50 to 70 per cent of patients.

Metastasis from hormone-dependent tumours may respond well to specific treatment such as radioactive iodine or non-specific treatment as already described. Dexamethasone 4–16 mg orally daily may control the symptoms of brain metastasis, and if so this should be consolidated with radiotherapy to prevent severe steroid-induced myopathy. Prednisolone 20 mg orally daily is often used to improve the sense of well-being, as are blood transfusion or hyperalimentation.

Terminal care is described in Section 32, but the importance of the combined support to the patient and the family given by the family doctor, nursing and hospice organizations, and the hospital team cannot be emphasized too much. The service given by hospitals to the community should not be merely diagnostic and therapeutic, but should include terminal care facilities for those patients in whom this is thought appropriate.

Prevention

Lung cancer is an almost totally preventable disease and is very largely due to smoking, particularly cigarettes. The strategy of any preventive measures must be based on the observations that lung cancer is extremely rare in non-smokers (the exception being adenocarcinoma of the bronchus in Chinese women in Singapore and Hong Kong), that there is no threshold limit below which no effect is produced, although the risk increases proportionately to the amount smoked, that the benefit from stopping smoking is evident within 5 years, and that the risk for an ex-smoker at any given time after stopping is determined by the length of time he or she had smoked before stopping. Thus strenuous efforts must be made to persuade people not to start smoking, to establish more effective methods of enabling people to stop smoking, and to promote further research into effective methods of health education. The promotion of cigarettes with low tar, nicotine and carbon monoxide contents may have made a small contribution to prevention, but low-tar cigarettes are not a substitute for giving up smoking. Penal taxation by governments may also help. A ban on tobacco advertising in Norway and New Zealand has been shown to reduce the uptake of smoking and total sales.

The identification of occupational hazards and implementation appropriate measures to safeguard the health of employees are clearly important preventive measures, even although the number at risk is very small.

Prospective lung cancer screening programmes in males aged 45 years and above who smoke at least 20 cigarettes per day have been carried out using both chest radiography and pooled 3-day sputum analysis every 4 months. They are unlikely to form the basis of standard practice as there is no evidence that early detection is translated into increased cure rate.

Carcinoid tumours

The slow-growing intrabronchial lesions previously grouped under the heading of bronchial adenoma have now been reclassified into bronchial carcinoids, adenoid cystic tumours, and mucoepidermoid tumours. They are not related to cigarette smoking, and tend to be diagnosed at a younger age than carcinoma of the bronchus. True bronchial adenomas derived from bronchial glands are rare. These tumours were once thought to be benign, but they are potentially and often frankly malignant, being capable not only of destructive local growth but also of metastasis to regional lymph nodes in about one-third of patients and to distant organs, particularly liver and brain, in about 10 per cent. They are occasionally located in the trachea.

The most common symptoms are cough, haemoptysis, and recurrent pneumonia, although not infrequently the lesion is discovered on routine radiographic examination before symptoms develop. Carcinoids may produce the classical symptom pattern of intermittent cyanotic flushings, intestinal cramps and diarrhoea, bronchoconstriction, and cardiovascular lesions in a few cases when there are extensive liver secondaries. The radiographic appearances are those of a solitary nodule or pulmonary collapse or obstructive hyperinflation. As the majority of the tumours occur in main stem or the proximal portions of lobar bronchi, bronchoscopy is usually the definitive diagnostic measure. The tumour appears as a white or pink polypid or lobulated mass, with the bronchial mucosa appearing to be intact. Biopsy may be followed by brisk haemoptysis.

Surgical resection is the treatment of choice. In the absence of regional spread or distant metastases 5 year survival prospects are excellent, but if there is involvement of regional nodes, survival rates fall to 70 per cent. Some aggressive carcinoid tumours carry a much worse prognosis. The mechanism and management of the general symptoms of the carcinoid syndrome are described in Chapter 14.8.

REFERENCES

Carney, D.N. (1992). Biology of small-cell lung cancer. *Lancet*, **339**, 843–6.

Carney, D.N., Keane, M., and Grogan, L. (1992). Oral etoposide in small cell lung cancer. Seminars in Oncology, **19** (6, Suppl. 14), 40–4.

Coggon, D. and Acheson, E.D. (1983). Trends in lung cancer mortality. *Thorax*, **38**, 721–3.

Goldstraw, P. (1992). The practice of cardiothoracic surgeons in the perioperative staging of lung cancer. *Thorax*, **47**, 1–2.

Hansen, H.H. (1992). Management of small-cell lung cancer. *Lancet*, **339**, 846–9.

Izbicki, J.R., Thetter, O., Karg, O., Kreusser, T., Passlick, B., Trupka, A., *et al.* (1992). Accuracy of computed tomographic scan and surgical assessment for staging of bronchial carcinoma. A prospective study. *Journal of Thoracic and Cardiovascular Surgery*, **104**, 413–20.

Kaplan, D.K. (1992). Mediastinal lymph node metastases in lung cancer: is size a valid criterion. *Thorax*, **47**, 332–3.

Landreneau, R.J., Hazelrigg, S.R., Ferson, P.F., Johnson, J.A., Nawarawong, W., Boley, T.M., *et al.* (1992). Thoracoscopic resection of 85 pulmonary lesions. *Annals of Thoracic Surgery*, **54**, 415–19.

Mountain, C.F. (1986). A new international staging system for lung cancer. *Chest*, **89**, 225S–33S.

Muers, M.F. and Round, C.E. (1993). Palliation of symptoms in non-small cell lung cancer. *Thorax*, **48**, 339–43.

Souhami, R.L. and Law, K. (1990). Longevity in small cell lung cancer. *British Journal of Cancer*, **61**, 584–9.

Souquet, P.J., Chauvin F., Boissel, J.P., *et al.* (1993). Polychemotherapy in advanced non-small-cell lung cancer: a meta-analysis. *Lancet*, **342**, 19–21.

Spiro, S.G. and Goldstraw, P. (1984). The staging of lung cancer. *Thorax*, **39**, 401–7.

Wells, F.C. and Kendall, S.W.H. (1992). Thoracoscopy: the dawn of a new age. *Respiratory Medicine*, **86**, 365–6.

(b) Pulmonary metastases

S. G. SPIRO

Malignant metastasis to the lung may present as a solitary enlarging nodule, as multiple nodules, or with diffuse lymphatic involvement.

Solitary metastasis represents some 10 per cent of round lesions in general, but some 70 per cent of round lesions in patients with a known malignancy. Colorectal cancer is reported to be the commonest tumour of origin. Diagnosis can usually be secured by percutaneous CT-guided biopsy. In rare cases, surgical excision may prolong survival or result in cure, depending on the state of the primary tumour and the likelihood of other occult metastases.

Multiple metastases range enormously in size and number from 'cannon balls' to miliary shadowing, and may be accompanied by hilar lymphadenopathy or pleural effusion. Breast, colon, renal, and lung primaries are probably the commonest underlying tumours, but others include tumours amenable to chemotherapy, such as testicular cancer and choriocarcinoma, and also sarcomas. Diagnosis may be achieved by cytology or histology on various samples from the pleura or lung and can occasionally be made from cytology on expectoration or induced sputum. Tumours that are suitable for chemotherapy (e.g. choriocarcinoma) or endocrine manipulation (e.g. breast) need to be recognized. Solitary or multiple Kaposi's sarcoma is a feature of AIDS, and can involve the bronchi and pleura as well as lung tissue.

Lymphangitis carcinomatosa is most commonly due to breast and primary lung tumours. Patients can be asymptomatic when the disease is first suspected because of a radiograph that shows diffusely increased interstitial markings that may be accompanied by Kerley B lines, hilar lymphadenopathy, or pleural effusion. Diagnosis may be established by cytology from sputum or pleural fluid, but often requires bronchoscopic or transbronchial lung biopsy. Later, progressive and severe breathlessness with hypoxaemia often develops, and requires vigorous palliative relief with opiate and oxygen supplementation.

Occasionally metastasis, presenting as haemoptysis, may be confined to a bronchus and therefore is not visible on a plain chest radiograph. Renal carcinoma and malignant melanoma are recorded causes. Diagnosis requires bronchoscopy, and radiotherapy is usually effective in controlling the haemoptysis.

REFERENCES

Gephardt, G. N. (1981). Malignant melanoma of the bronchus. *Human Pathology*, **12**, 671–3.

Ishida, T., Kaneko, S., Yokoyama, H., Maeda, K., Yano, T., Sugio, K., and Sugimachi, K. (1992). Metastatic lung tumours and extended indications for surgery. *International Surgery*, **77**, 173–7.

Lower, E. E. and Baughman, R. P. (1992). Pulmonary lymphangitis metastasis from breast cancer. Lymphocytic alveolitis is associated with favourable prognosis. *Chest* **103**, 1113–17.

Ognibene, F. P., Masur, H., and Rogers, P. (1985). Kaposi's carcinoma causing pulmonary infiltrates and respiratory failure in AIDS. *Annals of Internal Medicine*, **102**, 471–5.

Stewart, J. R., Carey, J. A., Merrill, W. H., Frist, W. H., Hammon, J. W., Jr, and Bender, H. W., Jr. (1992). Twenty years' experience with pulmonary metastasectomy. *American Surgeon*, **58**, 100–3.

17.13.2 Pleural tumours

M. K. BENSON

Primary pleural tumours are relatively rare, although malignant mesothelioma has received much attention because of its increasing incidence and association with asbestos exposure. Pleural plaques are also associated with asbestos exposure but should not be regarded as true tumours since they simply represent local areas of fibrocollagenous thickening. The classic benign tumour of the pleura is the fibrous mesothelioma (pleural fibroma).

In contrast, pleural involvement by metastatic disease is very common. It can occur in association with most carcinomas, but is particularly associated with primaries arising in the lung, breast, or colon. Malignant lymphomas may also present with pleural involvement. Tumours arising in adjacent structures such as diaphragm and chest wall may also invade the pleura. Both benign and malignant tumours can originate from muscle, adipose tissue, nerves, blood vessels, and bony thorax. All are rare, and the diversity of sites and types of tumour results in a variety of clinical presentations. Radiographic techniques can help to demonstrate the site and nature of the tumour, although the diagnosis is usually established on biopsy.

Benign tumours

BENIGN FIBROUS MESOTHELIOMA

These tumours are rare but can occur in virtually any age group. They bear no relationship to the development of malignant mesothelioma and are not associated with exposure to asbestos or any other industrial pollutant. They originate from a pedicle, usually from the visceral pleura. Macroscopically they are firm, lobulated, and well encapsulated. The cut surface is white or grey and can have a whorled appearance. They vary in size, but can on occasions be very large with weights of 2 or 3 kg.

CLINICAL FEATURES

The tumours are often discovered on routine chest radiology in otherwise asymptomatic individuals (Fig. 1). Large tumours can result in chest discomfort and breathlessness, presumably due to compression of adjacent lung. Spontaneous hypoglycaemia is an associated feature in a small proportion of patients.

Radiologically, it may be difficult to decided whether a pleural-based nodule is arising from the pleura or within adjacent lung. The differential diagnosis also includes a localized area of pleural thickening, a whorled nodule, although this generally has a less clearly defined outline. The diagnosis is usually established after surgical excision. Although a fibrous mesothelioma is benign with no potential for metastatic spread, there is a possibility of local recurrence if the pedicle has not been completely excised.

PLEURAL PLAQUES

These represent areas of local fibrocollagenous thickening. They produce no clinical symptoms and are usually detected on routine chest radiographs. They can be single or multiple and are best seen in oblique projection or using tomography. Although associated with asbestos exposure, they are entirely benign and should not be regarded as precursors to the development of a malignant mesothelioma.

Malignant mesothelioma

A malignant mesothelioma derives from mesothelial cells and although most commonly arising in the pleura, can also occur in the peritoneum or rarely the pericardium. They existence of a malignant mesothelioma arising from the pleura was first recognized in the 1950s. During the 1960s, much evidence accumulated indicating a strong link between exposure to asbestos and development of a mesothelioma. Asbestos is a collective term given to a group of silicate minerals. They are commercially useful because of their heat-resistant properties and have been widely used in industry for the past hundred years. Exposure to asbestos is greatest in those involved in mining or quarrying the material and those who handle the raw fibres. Significant exposure has also occurred in individuals employed in the manufacture and use of asbestos-containing products. Many workers engaged in ship-building in 1940s and 1950s were exposed to asbestos, and it was also widely used in the building industry. The incidence of asbestos-related diseases in the United Kingdom is still rising, and this trend is set to continue well into the next century, reflecting the fact that there is a long latent interval between initial exposure and subsequent development of disease. Relevant factors in the pathogenesis include the amount of asbestos to which the individual was exposed, the time from first exposure, and the fibre type.

DOSAGE

It has been estimated that the annual incidence of developing a mesothelioma in subjects with no history of asbestos exposure is about 1 per million. In the majority of cases there is good evidence that there has been previous exposure to asbestos and that the risk is proportional to the amount of exposure. The risk is a function of concentration of fibres and duration of exposure. The incident is highest in those who have worked directly with asbestos, and predictions of the probable mortality among employees is a textile factory prior to 1964 reach approximately 10 per cent. It has also been shown that individuals directly exposed to low levels of environmental contamination have a slightly increased risk. Endemic pleural mesothelioma has been reported from certain areas of central Turkey, Cyprus, and Greece. Materials regarded as responsible were locally mined zeolite and other environmental asbestos minerals.

TIME FROM FIRST EXPOSURE

The incidence of pleural mesothelioma increase with time from initial exposure to asbestos. A latent period of 20 to 40 years makes it important to obtain a detailed occupational history of the whole of the patient's working live.

FIBRE TYPE

Although most asbestos workers have been exposed to a mixture of fibres, there is good epidemiological evidence that crocidolite (blue asbestos) is more hazardous then chrysotile (white asbestos) and other forms of asbestos fibre. Animal studies have identified fibre size as being relevant, with the greatest risk from fibres 1.56 μm in diameter and 8 μm long. Although concern has been expressed about commercially manufactured glass fibres, these have much larger dimensions and do not seem to carry a significant risk.

Pathology

A mesothelioma can arise from either the visceral or the parietal pleura, initially as a local mass often associated with a pleural effusion. As it progresses, there is gradual encasement of the lung and extension into adjacent structures including the chest wall and pericardium. Macroscopically, the tumour is usually white and fibrous in texture, although areas of necrosis can occur. Metastatic disease is relatively uncommon, although involvement of the contralateral lung and pleura, liver, and bone are recognized sites for secondary spread.

Histologically, the diagnosis can be difficult and there are a diversity of histological patterns ranging from well-differentiated epithelial or sarcomatous patterns to undifferentiated forms. Even after biopsy there may be difficulty in distinguishing between a malignant mesothelioma and benign pleural disease on purely morphological grounds. A second problem results from differentiation between a mesothelioma and a secondary adenocarcinoma. Newer immunohistochemical methods may improve diagnostic accuracy.

Clinical presentation

The age of presentation is usually between 50 and 70, and there is a male predominance reflecting the greater likelihood of previous occupational exposure. Symptoms due to local disease are mainly those of pain and breathlessness. Pain may be pleuritic in nature, although is often a dull ache due to direct involvement of the chest wall. Shortness of breath is usually associated with a pleural effusion, although as the tumour progresses it gradually encases the lung and involves mediastinal structures.

Systemic symptoms includes tiredness, anorexia, weight loss, fever, and occasionally drenching sweats. Finger clubbing has been recorded but is rare. Physical findings in the chest are those of a pleural effusion, but with advanced disease there is progressive reduction in chest-wall movement. Direct extension through the chest wall can result in a palpable mass which may develop at the site of previous biopsy.

Investigations

A chest radiograph often demonstrates a pleural effusion with a tumour being suspected if there is pleural thickening with a lobulated outline (Fig. 2). This can be more easily identified on a CT scan. The presence

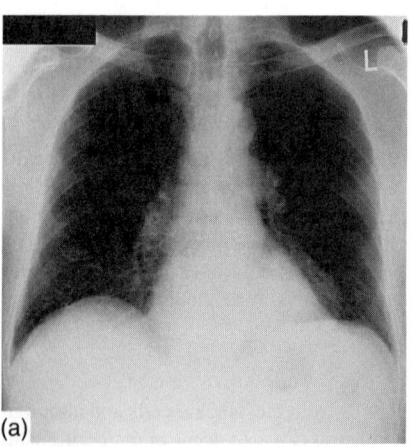

(a)

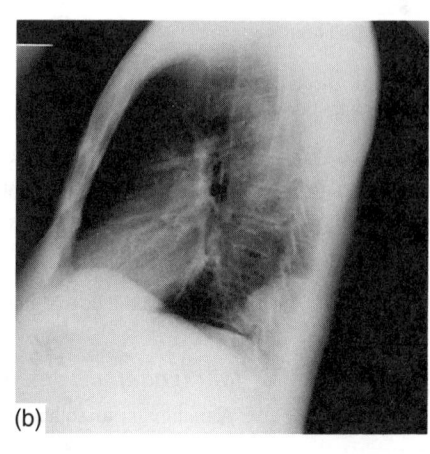

(b)

Fig. 1 Chest radiograph (posteroanterior(a) and lateral(b)) showing a pleural-based nodule at left base. The patient had no respiratory symptoms and resection confirmed this to be a benign fibrous mesothelioma.

of benign pleural plaques offers evidence of previous asbestos exposure, although they are not in themselves precursors of malignant change.

Pleural aspiration with cytological examination of pleural fluid may yield a definitive diagnosis in about a third of patients. There is a further modest diagnostic yield from percutaneous needle biopsy. Even with samples obtained under direct vision at thoracoscopy or thoracotomy there may still be some diagnostic uncertainty. In some instances, it may be appropriate to make a diagnosis on the basis of clinical and radiological features, since even with histological confirmation there is unlikely to be any alteration in management. However, it is important to note that a malignant mesothelioma is an industrially notifiable disease for which the patient and family can receive financial compensation.

Management

There is no effective curative treatment despite occasional enthusiastic reports of good results from radical surgery for limited disease. Response to radiotherapy is disappointing, although occasionally palliative relief of pain can be achieved if there is direct invasion of bone or nerve root. A variety of cytotoxic agents have been tried, but so far without any convincing success.

Relief of pain usually requires regular opiates, although nerve blocks may also be helpful for localized pain. Pleural aspiration and pleurodesis is of benefit in the relief of breathlessness due to recurrent pleural effusions.

The prognosis is poor with a median survival of approximately 18 months. A few patients seem to have fairly indolent disease and may survive for periods of up to 5 years.

REFERENCES

Anthony, V. B., San, S. A., Mossman, B., Gail, D. B., and Kalica, A. (1992). NHLBI workshop summaries, pleural cell biology in health and disease. *American Review of Respiratory Disease*, **145**, 1236–9.

Antman, K. H. (1993). Natural history and epidemiology of malignant mesothelioma. *Chest*, **103** (4, Suppl.), 373s–6s.

Celikorglu, F., Tierstein, A. S., Krellenstein, D. J., and Strauchen, J. A. (1992). Pleural effusion in non-Hodgkin's lymphoma. *Chest*, **101**, 1357–60.

Chernow, B. and Sahn, S. A. (1987). Carcinomatous involvement of the pleura: an analysis of 96 patients. *American Journal of Medicine*, **63**, 695–702.

Hausheer, F. H. and Yarbro, J. W. (1987). Diagnosis and treatment of malignant pleural effusion. *Cancer Metastasis Reviews*, **6**, 23–40.

Hillerdal, G. (1983). Malignant mesothelioma in 1982: review of 4710 published cases. *British Journal of Diseases of the Chest*, **77**, 321–43.

Jaurand, M. C., Bignong, J., and Brochard, P. (ed.). (1993). Mesothelial cell

and mesothelioma. Past, present and future. *European Respiratory Review*, **3**, review 11.

Lynch, T. J. (1993). Management of malignant pleural effusions. *Chest*, **103** (4, Suppl.), 385s–9s.

McAlpine, L. G., Hulks, G., and Thomson, N. C. (1990). Management of recurrent malignant pleural effusion in the United Kingdom: survey of clinical practice. *Thorax*, **45**, 699–701.

Peto, J., Hodgson, J. T., Matthews, F. E., and Jones, J. R. (1995). Continuing increase in mesothelioma mortality in Britain. *Lancet*, **345**, 535–9.

Reid, P. T. and Rudd, R. M. (1993). Management of malignant pleural effusion (Editorial). *Thorax*, **48**, 779–80.

Ribak, J. and Selikoff, I. J. (1992). Survival of asbestos insulation workers with mesothelioma. *British Journal of Industrial Medicine*, **49**, 732–5.

Sahn, S. A. (1987). Malignant pleural effusions. *Seminars in Respiratory Medicine*, **9**, 43–53.

Weick, J. K., Kiely, J. M., Harrison, E. G., Carr, D. T., and Scanlan, P. W. Pleural effusion in lymphoma. *Cancer*, **31**, 848–53.

17.13.3 Mediastinal tumours and cysts

M.K. BENSON

The mediastinum encompasses those structures within the thorax excluding the lungs. The superior boundary is the thoracic inlet represented by plane at the level of the first rib. The inferior boundary is the diaphragm. Traditionally the mediastinum has been subdivided into a number of compartments: classically a superior and inferior compartment, with the latter being subdivided into anterior middle and posterior divisions. In fact, there are no true anatomical boundaries, and structures in the superior mediastinum are in general contiguous with those inferiorly. Thus a more logical subdivision is simply into anterior, middle, and posterior compartments (Figs. 1, 2). Such a division can help to compartmentalize what is a complex anatomy and to give some guide as to the most likely pathology occurring in any particular area.

Detailed knowledge of normal mediastinal anatomy is a prerequisite to the interpretation of both normal and abnormal chest radiographs. It is not within the remit of this chapter to describe the anatomy in detail, but the major structures can be identified (Fig. 3).

The anterior mediastinum is bounded anteriorly by the sternum and posteriorly by the pericardium, aorta, and brachiocephalic vessels. It contains the remnant of the thymus gland, branches of the internal mammary artery, veins and associated lymph nodes, and variable amounts of fat.

The middle mediastinum contains the pericardium, ascending aorta and aortic arch, the vena cavae, the brachiocephalic vessels, and the pulmonary arteries and veins. It also encompasses the trachea and major bronchi with their associated lymph nodes, the phrenic nerves, and, in its upper portion, the vagus nerve.

The posterior mediastinum is bounded anteriorly by the pericardium, laterally by the mediastinal pleura, and posteriorly by the vertebral bodies. It also includes structures in the paravertebral gutter. It contains the descending thoracic aorta, oesophagus, azygos veins, thoracic duct, lymph nodes, and autonomic nerves.

Lymph nodes are common to all three compartments, and knowledge of their anatomical relationships together with sites of drainage is helpful in interpreting an abnormal chest radiograph with mediastinal enlargement. The most important group of visceral nodes lie in the middle mediastinum (Fig. 4). Bronchopulmonary or hilar nodes are numerous but are not visible radiographically unless pathologically enlarged. They are located around bronchi and pulmonary vessels, particularly where these bifurcate. They receive afferent drainage from the lungs, and efferent drainage is to carinal and paratracheal nodes. The carinal nodes at the tracheal bifurcation are situated in subcarinal fat and surround the origin of both right and left main bronchi. On the left, nodes between the pulmonary artery and aortic arch occupy the aorta pulmonary win-

Fig. 2 Chest radiograph showing lobulated pleural thickening due to mesothelioma.

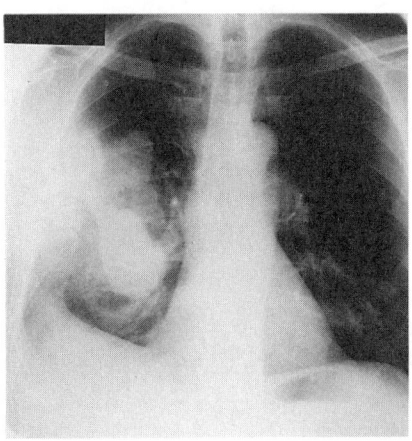

dow. The paratracheal nodes are situated in front of and to either side of the trachea. The azygos node represents the lowest node on the right-hand side and is medial to the azygos vein. They receive afferent drainage from carinal and hilar nodes.

A group of glands in the anterior mediastinum are situated in front of the ascending aorta and superior vena cava. They drain most of the structures in the anterior mediastinum (pericardium, thymus, diaphragm, and mediastinal pleura). They also communicate with the internal mammary nodes which receive afferent supply from the anterior chest wall, upper abdomen, and mediastinal portion of the breasts. Efferent drainage is into the right lymphatic duct.

Posterior mediastinal glands are grouped around the oesophagus and descending aorta and receive afferent channels from the diaphragm, pericardium, oesophagus, and lower parts of the lung via the inferior pulmonary ligaments.

Mediastinal masses

It is not surprising that the diversity of anatomical structures in the mediastinum is reflected by an equally diverse range of neoplastic, developmental, and inflammatory masses. Whilst clinical symptoms and signs may give diagnostic clues, a significant proportion of mediastinal masses, particularly those which are benign, tend to be asymptomatic and are usually detected on routine chest radiography. The advent of computerized tomography and, more recently, magnetic resonance imaging has provided accurate anatomical localization of any mediastinal mass. This in turn can be of considerable diagnostic value since most primary cysts and tumours of the mediastinum have characteristic compartments of origin (Table 1). Lymph node masses and aneurysms of the aorta tend to be the exception and can be found in any of the mediastinal compartments.

If metastatic malignant disease and inflammatory conditions are excluded, some 75 per cent of mediastinal masses in adults are benign. Malignant conditions are more common in children, occurring in some 50 per cent of cases. There have been a number of large studies documenting the relative frequency of different causes of primary mediastinal

Fig. 1 Posteroanterior (a) and lateral (b) chest radiograph with diagrammatic overlay to illustrate normal mediastinal structures: (1) trachea; (2) right main bronchus; (3) left main bronchus; (4) ascending aorta; (5) aortic arch; (6) descending aorta; (7) superior vena cava; (8) right pulmonary artery; (9) left pulmonary artery; (10) position of thymus.

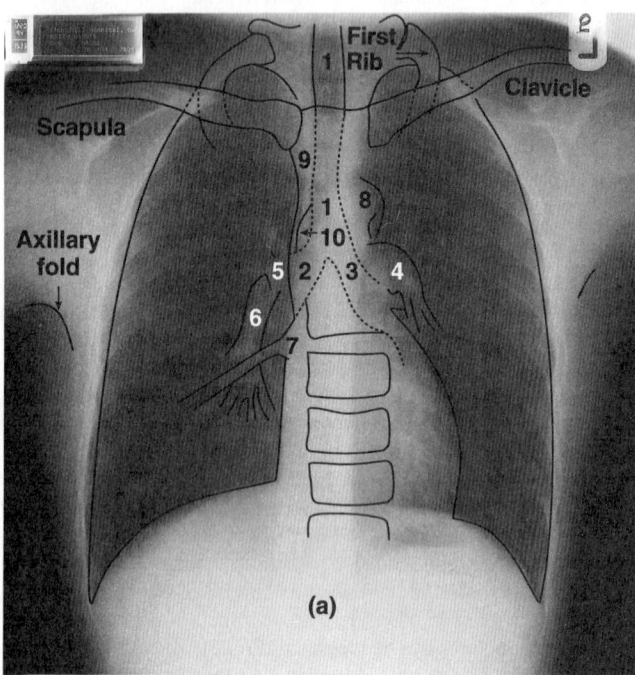

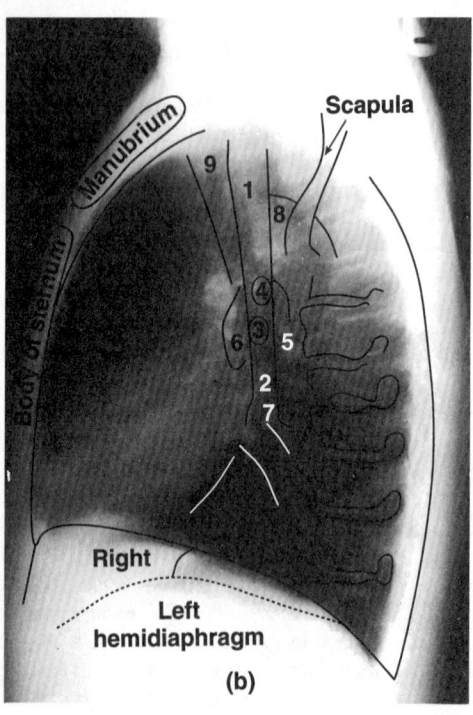

Fig. 2 A schematic representation of the mediastinal compartments: (a) lateral projection showing division into anterior (or anterosuperior), middle, and posterior compartments; (b) cross-sectional depiction.

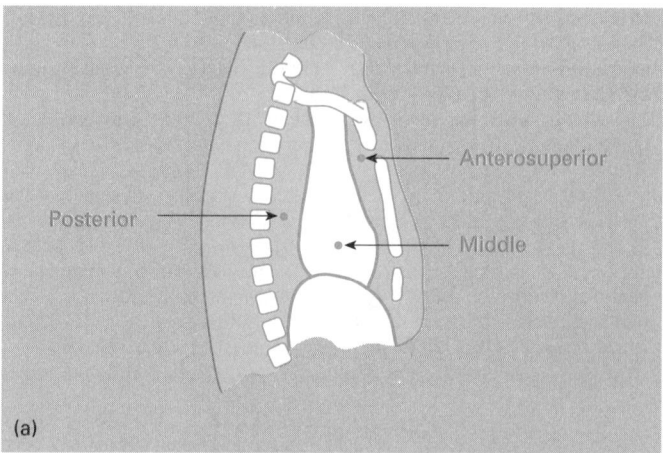

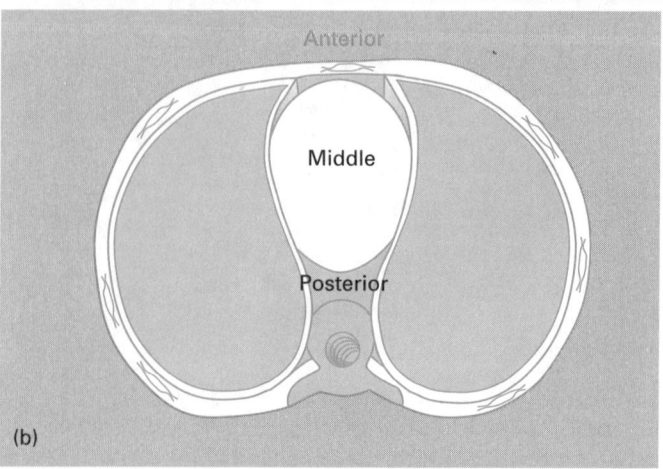

Fig. 3 CT sections and diagrammatic representation of mediastinal anatomy at the level of (a) the fourth and (b) the eighth thoracic vertebra.

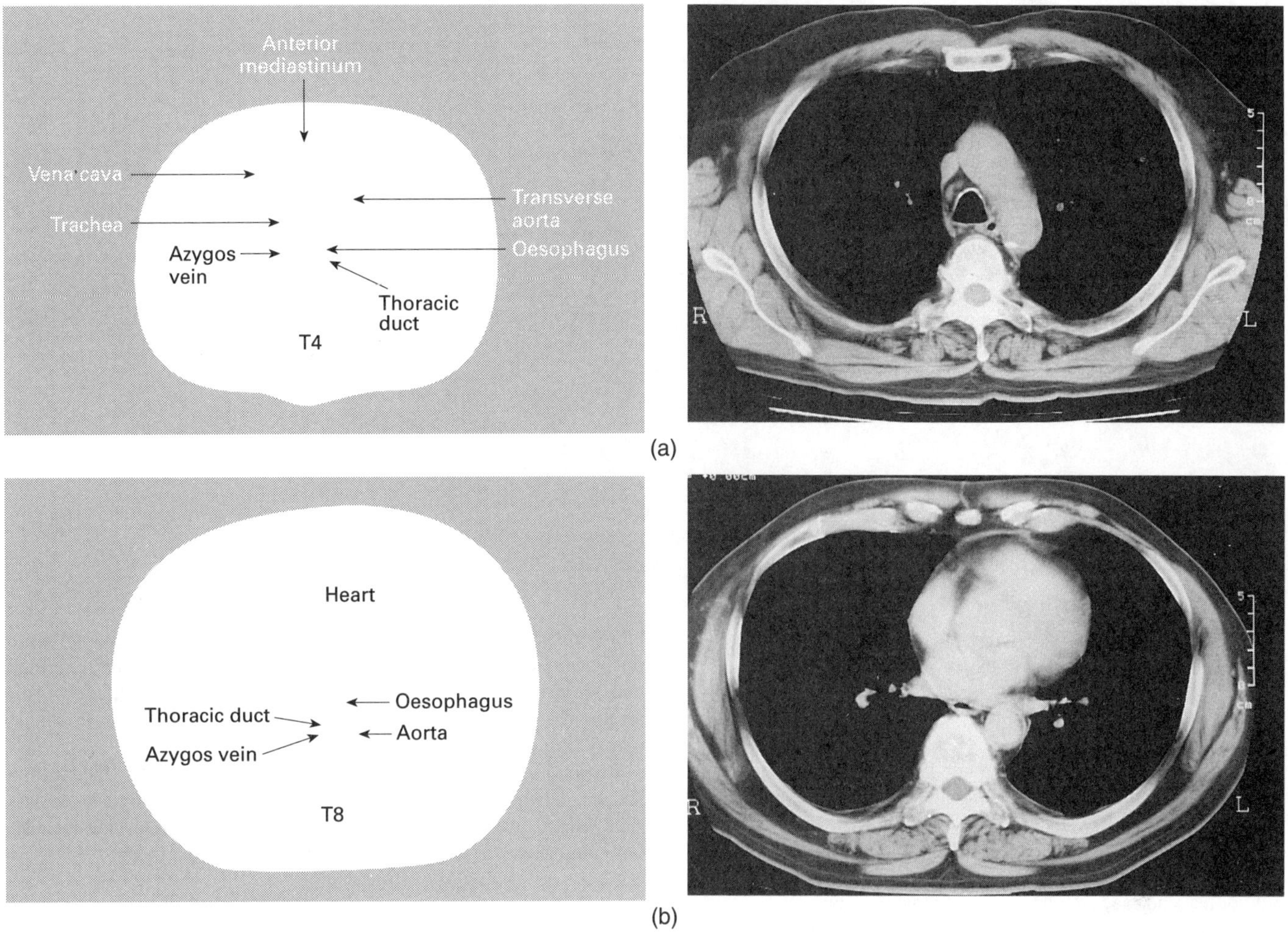

(a)

(b)

Fig. 4 Posterior view of middle mediastinum to show the location of the paratracheal, subcarinal, and hilar lymph nodes, and their positions relative to the major mediastinal structures.

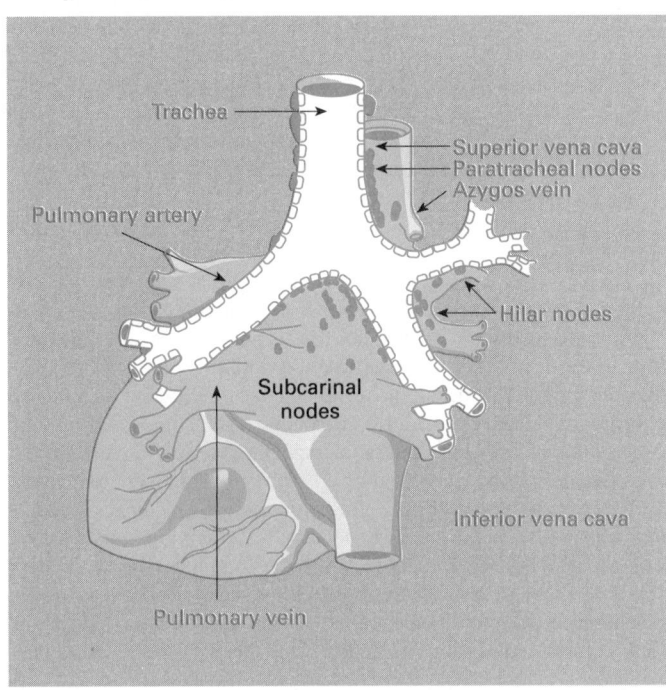

tumours and cysts, and approximate estimates are as follows: neurogenic tumours, 20 per cent; thymic tumours, 18 per cent; lymphoma, 15 per cent; bronchogenic and pericardial cysts, 14 per cent; germ-cell tumours, 13 per cent; thyroid masses, 6 per cent. The remainder comprise a wide variety of very rare tumours.

General considerations: clinical features

Benign lesions tend to be asymptomatic and are most commonly detected on routine chest radiography. Only 5 per cent of patients who are asymptomatic will be malignant, whilst 50 per cent of patients presenting with symptoms are likely to have a malignant tumour.

Non-specific symptoms of a constitutional nature such as fever or weight loss occur with certain types of tumour such as lymphomas or thymic tumours. The commonest symptoms are usually cough and chest pain, and arise as a consequence of distortion of the normal mediastinal anatomy. Compression of vital structures can also result in specific symptoms. Thus tracheal or bronchial compression can lead to breathlessness with stridor or wheeze. Oesophageal narrowing results in dysphagia, whilst superior vena cava compression produces the characteristic features of facial and periorbital oedema, chemosis, and distended veins. Involvement of the recurrent laryngeal nerve results in hoarseness and a bovine cough; whilst this usually results from a malignant tumour, it can also occur with benign lesions such as aneurysms of the aortic arch. Involvement of the sympathetic chain as it emerges in the upper mediastinum is also likely to be due to malignant infiltration and results in the characteristic features of Horner's syndrome with enophthalmus,

Table 1 *Mediastinal masses*

Anterior compartment	Middle compartment	Posterior compartment
← ———————	Lymph nodes	——————— →
	Sarcoidosis	
	Infections (particularly tuberculosis)	
	Lymphoma	
	Metastatic carcinoma	
	Castleman's disease	
Thyroid	——————— →	——————— →
Retrosternal goitre		
Thyroid carcinoma		
Thymus	Vascular	——————— →
Thymoma	Aneurysm of aorta	
Hyperplasia	Anomalous vessels	
Cyst		
Lymphoma	Pericardium	Neural tumours
	Cysts	Neurolemmoma
Germ-cell tumours	Fat pad	Neurofibroma
Teratoma		Ganglioneuroma
Seminoma	Bronchogenic cysts	Neuroblastoma
Other miscellaneous		Phaeochromocytoma
Parathyroid adenoma		

myosis, ptosis, and unilateral facial anhydrosis. Palpitations due to cardiac dysrhythmias can result if lesions are adjacent to the heart.

Diagnostic approach

The finding of a mediastinal abnormality on the chest radiograph, whether or not accompanied by specific clinical features, is usually an indication for further investigation. In addition to a posteroanterior radiograph, a lateral film can help to identify the anatomical site. Calcification is frequently present in some tumours and masses such as thyroid goitres, and may also be seen in thymic tumours.

CT has now superseded conventional tomography and provides more accurate localization of mediastinal masses. It can define their relationship to and displacement of normal structures and may be able to define lines of demarcation, particularly if there is adjacent fatty tissue. CT scanning is not ideal for determining the composition of any particular mass, although it can demonstrate heterogenicity or the presence of calcification. Fat can be differentiated from solid tissue and contrast enhancement used to identify vascular structures.

Magnetic resonance imaging is less readily available, and in the context of mediastinal masses has relatively little to offer over and above information obtained from CT. It also demonstrates anatomical relationships and the presence of abnormal masses. However, it does not give sufficient information as to their intrinsic features to make it valuable as a routine test.

Biopsy techniques

Fine-needle aspiration is increasingly popular in the investigation of pulmonary masses and is also widely used for obtaining tissue from mediastinal masses when performed in conjunction with CT. The presence of a cyst can be confirmed by aspiration of clear fluid. Anterior mediastinal masses can easily be approached percutaneously, although cytological examination alone is often insufficient and samples for histological examination are more likely to be of diagnostic value. Hence there is still a place for open biopsy to be performed. Similarly, neural tumours arising in the posterior mediastinum usually require surgical resection and there is often little be gained by preceding this with fine-needle aspiration.

Mediastinoscopy is performed through an incision in the neck and allows inspection of structures surrounding the superior vena cava and trachea as far as the carina. It is particularly useful in obtaining lymph node biopsies prior to possible surgery for lung cancer. Anterior mediastinotomy is a relatively non-invasive surgical technique to obtain biopsy tissue from the anterior mediastinum.

Bronchoscopy is of limited value when evaluating mediastinal masses, except when there is suspicion of a bronchial neoplasm or possible lymphadenopathy due to sarcoidosis. Distortion of the normal anatomy indicates extrinsic compression but is rarely diagnostic.

Anterior mediastinal masses

THYMUS

The normal thymus is located in the superior portion of the anterior mediastinum. Its main function is the production of T lymphocytes. Radiographically, the normal thymus can only be seen in infancy, although CT studies have shown that it reaches maximum size between the ages of 12 and 19. Thereafter regression gradually occurs and there is fatty replacement of normal thymic tissue. Enlargement of the thymus is the commonest single cause of an anterior mediastinal mass. It can be due to the development of a thymoma, thymic hyperplasia, or a thymic cyst. In addition, the thymus can be a site of involvement by lymphoma, particularly Hodgkin's disease.

THYMOMA

Thymoma is the commonest neoplasm in the anterior mediastinum and is derived from thymic epithelium. These tumours are often benign, although they can behave in a malignant fashion with invasion of adjacent structures and the occurrence of distant metastasis. They occur most frequently in middle-aged adults. Although some patients will present as a result of an abnormal chest radiograph, the majority of patients will be symptomatic. Chest pain and cough are the commonest presenting features and result from pressure effects on adjacent structures. Systemic syndromes which can occur in association with thymic tumours are of particular interest. Myasthenia gravis is the commonest systemic disorder and, although reports vary, some 30 per cent of patients have an association between the thymic tumour and myasthenia. Red-cell aplasia is less common, occurring in about 1 per cent of patients. Other rare associations include hypogammaglobulinaemia, systemic lupus erythematosus, rheumatoid arthritis, polymyositis, and inflammatory bowel disease.

The majority of thymomas are slowly growing lobulated masses which are well encapsulated. Surgical resection can be expected to result in a cure. Local invasion is less common but often precludes complete resection, and recurrence is the rule. Adjuvant radiotherapy can offer additional benefit to this group of patients.

Thymic hyperplasia, which is uncommon, presents as an enlargement of the gland whilst normal morphology is retained. It is more likely to be seen in children and has also been observed as a rebound phenomenon following chemotherapy.

Thymic cysts are also uncommon. They can be unilocular or multilocular and usually contain straw-coloured fluid. The vast majority of patients are asymptomatic, but since cystic change can also occur in some thymomas and also in Hodgkin's disease, thorough cytological examination of the cyst contents and wall must be carried out to exclude malignant disease.

Thymic lymphoma is fairly frequent, particularly in patients with Hodgkin's disease. The histological picture is usually of the nodular sclerosing variety. Disease confined to the thymus has no specific diagnostic features and is relatively uncommon. The presence of other mediastinal or hilar lymphadenopathy should alert the clinician to the possibility of a lymphoma.

GERM-CELL TUMOURS

This group of neoplasms includes tumours which are identical with certain testicular and ovarian neoplasms and are thought to be derived from primitive germ cells that have migrated to the mediastinum during oncogenesis. They include benign and malignant teratoma, seminoma, chorion carcinoma, and embryonal carcinoma. In the majority of cases, the tumour presents in early adult life. Benign tumours tend to be more common in females and malignant tumours in males. There is a specific association with Klinefelter's syndrome.

Mediastinal germ-cell tumours have a varied and often mixed histological appearance which can make pathological diagnosis difficult. Since these tumours may be very responsive to chemotherapy, it is important to make a definitive diagnosis, and this can be assisted by detection of elevated levels of α-fetoprotein, β human chorionic gonadotrophin, and carcinoembryonic antigen.

Teratomas consist of a disorganized mixture of ectodermal, mesodermal, and endodermal tissues, and can include skin and hair, cartilage, bone, intestinal epithelium, and neural tissue. The majority are benign and often contain cystic areas—hence the name dermoid cyst. CT appearances usually give a strong clue as to the diagnosis, and unless there is a major contraindication to surgery, they should be excised to prevent further expansion and to exclude malignant change.

Seminomas are second in frequency to teratomas and occur almost exclusively in young men. Often patients are asymptomatic, although pressure effects and systemic symptoms may be presenting features. The tumours are radiosensitive and 5 year survival rates after treatment range from 50 to 75 per cent.

Thyroid masses

Retrosternal extension of an enlarged thyroid represents one of the more common causes of a mass in the superior mediastinum. The majority arise in the neck and extend into the anterior mediastinum through the thoracic inlet. A small number of intrathoracic goitres occur in the posterior mediastinum. A thyroid mass which originates in the mediastinum is exceedingly rare. The majority of retrosternal goitres are multinodular and benign. They may contain cystic areas, sometimes with haemorrhage, and have areas of calcification. Radiographically, they have a sharply defined and often lobulated outline. Radioactive isotopic scans

can be diagnostically useful if positive, although a negative scan does not exclude the presence of thyroid tissue.

Whilst the majority of retrosternal goitres do not result in symptoms, compression of the trachea at the thoracic inlet can result in respiratory distress and is an absolute indication for surgical resection. Hoarseness due to compression of the recurrent laryngeal nerve and dysphagia may also occur. Physical examination usually reveals the presence of a goitre ascending into the neck.

Thyroid malignancies may also involve the mediastinum either by direct extension or by metastases to intrathoracic nodes.

Parathyroid adenomas may arise in the mediastinum, often in association with the thymus gland. Identification of hormonally active glandular tissue can be difficult. CT scanning, selective angiography, and isotopic scanning with selenomethionine have all been tried with varying success.

Middle mediastinal masses

LYMPHADENOPATHY

Enlarged lymph nodes are not confined to the middle mediastinum, although this represents the most common site of intrathoracic lymphadenopathy. Reactive changes occur in association with many pulmonary infections, although in the majority of instances nodes are not grossly enlarged and may be undetected on a plain chest radiograph. However, gross lymphadenopathy is a feature of tuberculosis, particularly in association with a primary infection. It also occurs in histoplasmosis. Other common causes of gross lymph node enlargement include metastatic carcinoma, lymphomas, and sarcoidosis. Less commonly, lymphadenopathy can be due to drug toxicity, angio-immunoblastic lymphadenopathy, and amyloidosis. It is not within the scope of this chapter to consider these conditions in detail since most are discussed elsewhere.

Giant follicular lymph node hyperplasia (Castleman's disease) is not considered elsewhere and, although rare, merits specific mention (Fig. 5). Its aetiology is unknown, and it is not clear as to whether it represents a focus of lymphoid hyperplasia or has an infectious origin. The lesion consists of a vascular tumour with satellite lymphadenopathy. Two histological subgroups are described: (1) a more common hyaline vascular picture with lymphoid follicles and penetrating capillaries, and (2) a plasma cell type characterized by sheets of plasma cells between the germinal centres. Both types can result in symptoms from local pressure, but the plasma cell type also causes systemic symptoms with fever, anaemia, and weight loss. There are no diagnostic radiographic features; the picture is simply one of a solitary mass, usually with a smooth or lobulated outline. The diagnosis is usually made after surgical resection or biopsy. The condition is regarded as benign, although a small group of patients with multicentric disease have progressive hyperplasia, recurrent infections, and subsequent development of a frank lymphoma.

Mediastinal cysts

Cysts within the mediastinum represent a relatively common cause of a mediastinal mass. They can arise in association with the pericardium, bronchi, gut, or thoracic duct. The majority of patients are asymptomatic.

Pericardial cysts develop embryologically in relationship to the precordium, although direct communication with the pericardial sac is rare. They are most commonly adjacent to the right heart border and close to the diaphragm. Radiographically, they appear as smooth clear demarcated densities which can be mistaken for a pericardial fat pad or a hernia through the foramen of Morgagni. Aspiration reveals clear fluid. Surgical excision is of little therapeutic benefit.

Bronchogenic cysts may arise in the mediastinum or in the pulmonary parenchyma (Fig. 6). Those in the mediastinum arise adjacent to the trachea, carina, or major bronchi. They are lined by a respiratory epithelium and the wall may contain cartilage and bronchial glands, hence the thick inspissated mucus within the cysts. Local pressure on the trachea or bronchi can result in cough or dyspnoea with wheeze. Occasionally the cysts communicate with the trachea, and when this is the case, there is an increased tendency to recurrent infection. Surgical excision is recommended, particularly if there are associated symptoms.

Posterior mediastinal masses

Oesophageal lesions and aneurysms of the descending thoracic aorta can both result in abnormal shadows in the posterior mediastinum (Fig. 7). Neural tumours comprise the vast majority of tumour masses which are likely to present in the posterior mediastinum. They rank with thymic tumours as being the commonest primary lesion of the mediastinum. Overall figures suggest that some 25 per cent will be malignant, although this proportion is higher in children. Benign tumours tend to be asymptomatic, whilst malignant tumours can cause pressure effects. In particular, pressure on adjacent nerves can result in a Pancoast tumour or brachial plexus syndrome, whilst, rarely, spinal cord compression results from direct extension into the intervertebral foramen. Very rarely a neural tumour arising from the vagus can result in a mass in the middle mediastinum.

Tumours arising from peripheral nerves include neurilemmoma (Schwannoma) and neurofibroma, together with their malignant coun-

Fig. 5 Chest radiograph and CT scan showing large anterior mediastinal mass which on histology showed features of Castleman's disease.

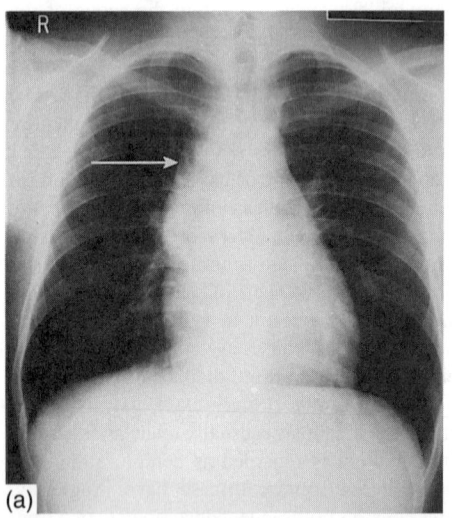

(a)

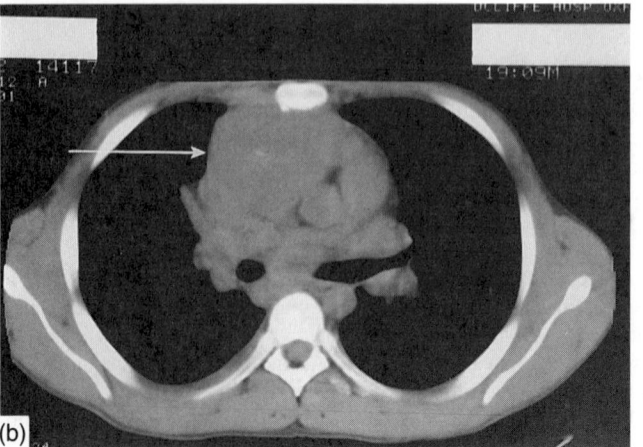

(b)

Fig. 6 Chest radiograph and CT scan showing a large mass in the mediastinum. This represents a large bronchogenic cyst which had been present for 20 years and was finally removed when compression of the oesophagus resulted in dysphagia.

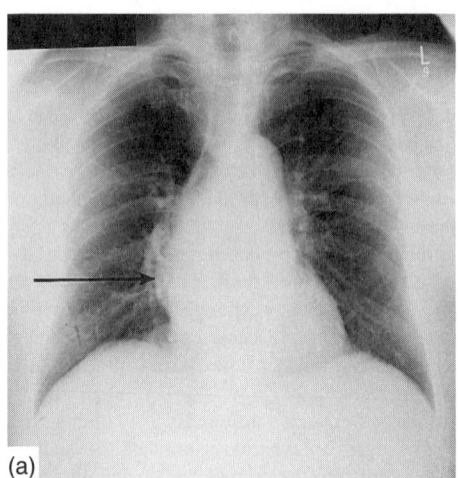

(a)

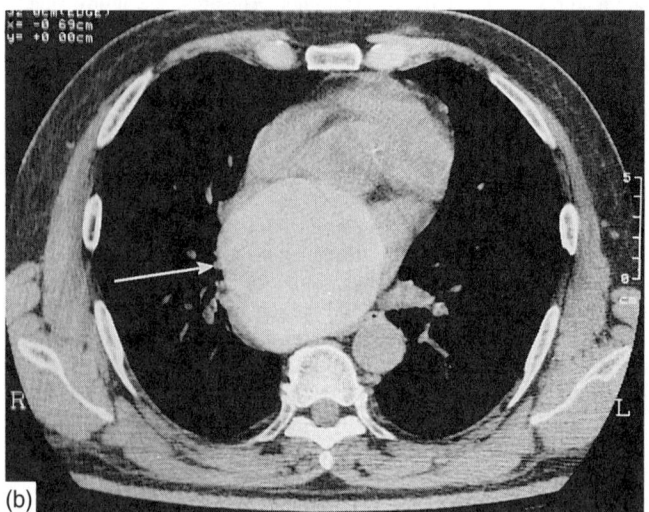

(b)

Fig. 7 CT scan demonstrating a posterior mediastinal mass which on resection proved to be a reduplication cyst of the oesophagus.

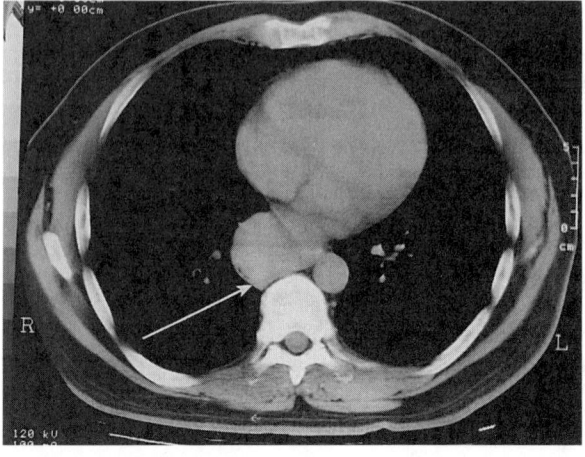

terparts. Tumours of the autonomic chain include ganglioneuroma and neuroblastoma.

A **neurilemmoma** is the commonest neural tumour arising in the mediastinum. These are more common in middle age and can extend into the intravertebral foramen, producing a dumb-bell appearance. Radiographically, they can erode adjacent bone, and CT scanning or magnetic resonance imaging should be undertaken prior to surgical excision.

Neurofibromata are also common and derive from the nerve sheath. They may be solitary, and the clinical and radiological features will be very similar to those of a neurilemmoma. In about 20 per cent of patients the tumours are part of a more generalized picture of neurofibromatosis. Surgical resection is recommended partly because of the small risk of developing a malignant **neurosarcoma**. These tumours have a poor prognosis.

Ganglioneuroma arise from the autonomic plexus and are usually perispinal in position. Associated endocrine syndromes include hypertension, flushing, sweating, and diarrhoea. These tumours are often very large before they become clinically apparent.

Ganglioneuroblastoma and **neuroblastoma** represent the malignant end of the spectrum and are predominantly tumours of infants and children. Neuroblastoma in particular is highly invasive, and metastatic spread is often established by the time of presentation.

Phaeochromocytomas usually arise in the adrenal gland, although a small proportion occur in the retroperitoneal space. Rarely, they can present in the posterior mediastinum. They are usually benign but secrete catecholamines which produce the characteristic clinical syndrome. Surgical excision is essential and results in a cure.

REFERENCES

Adkins, R.B., Maples, M.D., and Hainsworth, J.D. (1984). Primary malignant mediastinal tumours. *Annals of Thoracic Surgery,* **38,** 648–59.

Benjamin, S.P., McCormick, L.J., Effler, D.B., and Groves, L.K. (1972). Primary tumours of the mediastinum. *Chest,* **62,** 297–303.

Bower, R.J. and Kiesewetter, W.B. (1977). Mediastinal masses in infants and children (1977). *Archives of Surgery,* **112,** 1003–9.

Childs, A.W., Goldstraw, P., Nicholls, J.E., Dearnaley, D.P., and Horwich, A. (1993). Primary malignant mediastinal germ cell tumours: improved prognosis with platinum based chemotherapy and surgery. *British Journal of Cancer,* **67,** 1091–1100.

Cooper, J.D. (1993). Current therapy for thymoma. *Chest,* **103** (4 Suppl.), 334s–6s.

Davis, R.D., Oldham, H.N., and Sabesdon, D.C. (1987). Primary cysts and neoplasms of the mediastinum: recent changes in clinical presentation, methods of diagnosis, management and results. *Annals of Thoracic Surgery,* **44,** 229–37.

DePaepe, M., Van Der Straeten, M., and Roels, H. (1983). Mediastinal angiofollicular lymph node hyperplasia with systemic manifestations. *European Journal of Respiratory Disease,* **64,** 134–40.

Lewis, B.D., Hurt, R.D., Payne, W.S., Farrow, G.M., Knapp, R.H., and Muhm, J.R. (1983). Benign teratomas of the mediastinum. *Journal of Thoracic and Cardiovascular Surgery,* **86,** 727–31.

Merine, D., Pessar, M.L., Zerhouni, E.A., Fishman, E.K., and Soulen, R.L. (1990). CT and MRI assessment of the mediastinum. In *CT and MRI of the thorax.* (ed. E.A. Zarouni), pp. 67–91. Churchill Livingston, New York.

Morrissey, B., Adams, H., Gibbs, A.R., and Crane, M.D. (1993). Percutaneous needle biopsy of the mediastinum: review of 94 procedures. *Thorax,* **48,** 632–7.

17.14 Respiratory failure

17.14.1 Definition and causes

J. MOXHAM

Introduction

The essential function of the respiratory system is to achieve gas exchange, i.e. the uptake of oxygen and the elimination of carbon dioxide. Failure to perform this function, leading to hypoxaemia and hypercapnia, is potentially lethal; all tissues, particularly the brain, require oxygen and retention of carbon dioxide leads to narcosis.

Definition

Respiratory failure is characterized by a complex cardiovascular and neurological pathophysiology resulting from a failure of the respiratory apparatus to meet the gas exchange requirements of the body. It is the condition of respiratory insufficiency that is usually presented to the clinician since complete failure of the respiratory system rapidly leads to death. The term 'respiratory' requires consideration and possibly qualification. Strictly defined, respiratory failure relates to the deficiency of oxygen transport and utilization at cellular level. However, this does not address the wider aspects of gas exchange that involve the lungs and the circulation. Similarly, the complementary term 'ventilatory failure' does not consider the wider aspects of lung dysfunction which paradoxically may be associated with increased levels of ventilation.

In more objective terms, respiratory failure has been defined as as specified degree of hyopoxia (Pa_{O_2} less than 8 kPa or 60 mmHg) or hypercapnia (Pa_{CO_2} more than 6.0 kPa or 45 mmHg). Although these values represent a consensus, they are still somewhat arbitrary, particularly since Pa_{O_2} declines with increasing age according to the equation

$$Pa_{O_2} \text{ (kPa)} = 13.86 - [0.036 \times \text{age (years)}].$$

In subjects with near-normal respiratory function and normal, or near-normal, Pa_{O_2} values, quite large reductions in oxygen tension have little impact on oxygen saturation because of the shape of the oxygen dissociation curve (Fig. 1(a)). For example a patient with mild asthma may have a P_{O_2} of 10 kPa, with a corresponding oxygen saturation of 95 per cent, but, whilst the P_{O_2} is clearly not normal, oxygen carriage is not substantially reduced and a further small decrease in P_{O_2} would pose no great threat. At P_{O_2} values below 8 kPa there is notable desaturation and, more importantly, such is the shape of the oxygen dissociation curve that a further fall in P_{O_2} causes a sharp fall in oxygen saturation (Fig. 1(a)). Therefore a P_{O_2} of less than 8 kPa, when the P_{CO_2} is not raised, defines 'oxygenation' respiratory failure or, as it is commonly referred to, type 1 respiratory failure.

The normal arterial carbon dioxide tension is 4.7–6.0 kPa (35–45 mmHg). In normal subjects and in patients with a normal ventilatory response to a rise in carbon dioxide, an increase in arterial carbon dioxide provides a powerful stimulus to ventilation, thereby restoring P_{CO_2} to normal. The normal level of carbon dioxide is much more tightly controlled than P_{O_2}. Respiratory failure associated with a P_{CO_2} above the upper limit of normal is commonly referred to as 'ventilatory' failure or type 2 respiratory failure.

Blood gas tensions measured at a specific point in time provide limited information, and in some patients hypercapnia and hypoxia may only occur during sleep, during exercise, or when supine.

Hypoxia

Failure of oxygenation is most commonly due to an imbalance between pulmonary ventilation and perfusion. In pneumonia, for example, the consolidated lung is perfused but not ventilated. Although reflex reductions in perfusion of the non-ventilated area of lung do occur, this is not sufficient to avoid a large $\dot{V}_A/\dot{Q}$ imbalance and a shunt of blood through the lung ('physiological' shunt). Structural abnormalities (for example pulmonary arteriovenous malformations) through which desaturated blood bypasses ventilated alveoli represent anatomical shunts. Although impaired diffusion capacity can cause hypoxia (as in severe emphysema) and inadequate ventilation may also be responsible (as in obstructive sleep apnoea or sedative overdose), $\dot{V}_A/\dot{Q}$ abnormalities are the major mechanism of hypoxaemia in most patients with respiratory disease.

Hypoxia stimulates ventilation, although usually less so than hypercapnia. Ventilation may also be neuronally stimulated by inflammatory disease processes within the lung. Therefore when ventilatory capacity is adequate the response to hypoxia is hypocapnia. However, the capacity of hyperventilation to correct arterial hypoxia is greatly limited. In those areas of the lung where $\dot{V}_A/\dot{Q}$ ratios are normal or raised pulmonary capillary blood is virtually fully saturated and, although hyperventilation

Fig. 1 (a) Oxygen dissociation curve; (b) carbon dioxide dissociation curve. The oxygen curve is sigmoid in shape, whereas the carbon dioxide curve is nearly linear over the range of carbon dioxide that is clinically important.

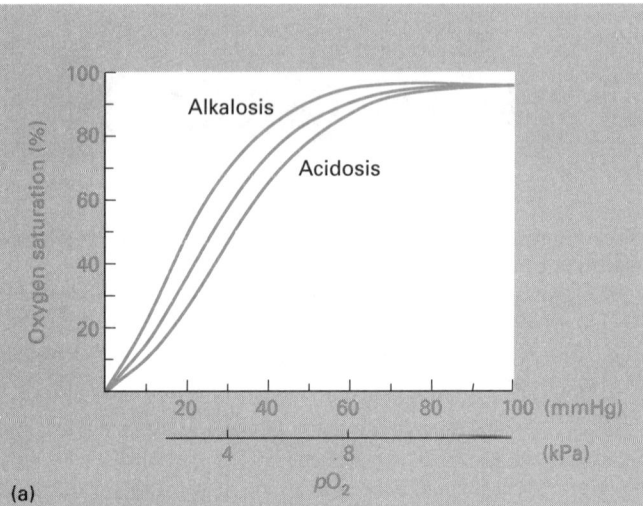

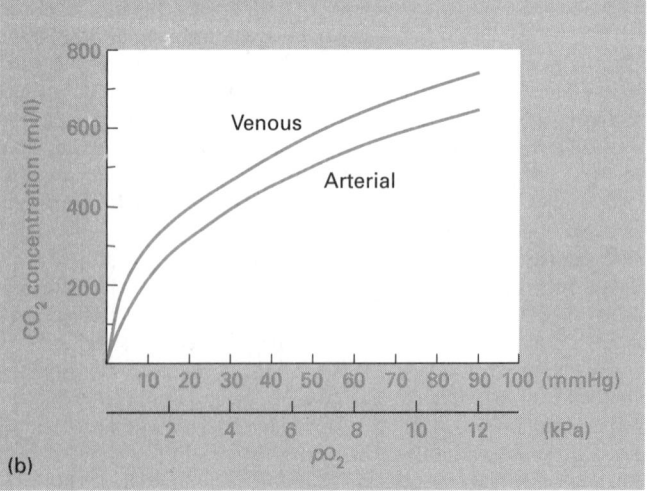

will increase alveolar oxygen tension (and reduce carbon dioxide tension), the consequent rise in local P_{O_2} can have little effect on oxygen saturation owing to the shape of the oxygen dissociation curve. Therefore it is unable to compensate for the reduced oxygenation within diseased areas of the lung, where $\dot{V}_A/\dot{Q}$ ratios are low because of poor ventilation of adequately perfused lung.

EFFECTS OF HYPOXIA

The ability to withstand hypoxia depends on whether it occurs acutely or is chronic, in which case compensating mechanisms ameliorate the physiological impact. It is also crucial to appreciate that it is tissue oxygen delivery and uptake that is vital; thus haemoglobin concentration and function, cardiac output and tissue perfusion, and peripheral tissue oxygen utilization are just as important as arterial oxygen tension and saturation. Tissue oxygen requirements are obviously affected by exercise, but also by many other factors including temperature and thyroid status.

ACUTE HYPOXIA

Minor hypoxia has few symptoms or signs, but more substantial desaturation increases ventilatory drive and contributes to breathlessness, although for most patients their pulmonary disease is the dominant cause of shortness of breath. Acute severe hypoxia also causes anxiety, restlessness, sweating, and, if sufficiently severe, confusion. Examination reveals central cyanosis, poor peripheral perfusion (blood flow is redistributed to more vital organs), and, importantly, tachycardia. Acute hypoxia is poorly tolerated if patients are anaemic or hypovolaemic, or have significant cardiac or vascular disease; thus severe hypoxia can precipitate angina in patients with anaemia, confusion in those with cardiac failure, or stroke in those with cerebrovascular disease, illustrating that the impact of hypoxia is strongly influenced by the many factors that determine tissue oxygen delivery.

CHRONIC HYPOXIA

When hypoxia develops over a prolonged period compensatory mechanisms come into play. The release of erythropoietin by the kidney, in response to chronic hypoxia, causes secondary polycythaemia. Such polycythaemia enhances the oxygen-carrying capacity of blood, but it also increases blood viscosity which may eventually impair overall tissue oxygen delivery as well as predisposing to arterial and venous thromboses. Poor cerebral perfusion, secondary to high viscosity of blood, can contribute to lethargy, mental slowing, and confusion.

Acute hypoxia causes pulmonary hypertension due to pulmonary arterial vasoconstriction which reverses when hypoxia is corrected. Chronic hypoxia also causes pulmonary hypertension which, with time, becomes fixed as a consequence of secondary changes in the pulmonary vasculature, including muscular hypertrophy and intimal thickening. Many lung diseases not only cause the hypoxia that induces pulmonary hypertension, but also destroy the pulmonary vascular bed, thereby contributing to increased pulmonary vascular resistance and raising pulmonary artery pressure. A common example of this double mechanism for pulmonary hypertension is severe chronic obstructive lung disease. Pulmonary hypertension can become severe with systolic pressures of 70 to 80 mmHg, as a consequence of which the right ventricle hypertrophies and may eventually fail. Whilst right heart failure is the cause of peripheral oedema in some patients with chronic hypoxic lung disease, it is not the only factor. Peripheral oedema is relatively uncommon in patients without carbon dioxide retention even when hypoxia is severe. Also, some patients with oedema do not have overt right heart failure, and in these patients it may be that hypoxic constriction of renal vessels, with impaired renal blood flow and consequent sodium retention, may be an important mechanism.

Patients with chronic hypoxia, even those without secondary polycythaemia and without other factors reducing tissue oxygenation, often have poor intellectual function. A peripheral neuropathy, usually minor, is also seen.

ASSESSMENT OF OXYGENATION

The clinical assessment of cyanosis is notoriously inaccurate and crude. Even when clinicians agree that cyanosis is present, no precision as to its severity is possible. Cyanosis can be detected at an oxygen saturation of 90 per cent, although it may not be obvious until the saturation falls to approximately 80 per cent corresponding to a Pao_2 of about 7 kPa, given a normal haemoglobin concentration. Therefore cyanosis is a sign of severe hypoxaemia. In patients with cyanosis a measurement of Pao_2 is essential for assessment, although a knowledge of Pao_2 also contributes substantially to the management of many other patients with respiratory failure, even when not cyanosed, such as ventilated patients in an intensive care unit.

Instantaneous, and if necessary continuous, non-invasive measurement by oximetry has greatly facilitated the assessment of oxygenation in patients with potential or established respiratory failure (Fig. 2). Oximetry is least helpful when Pao_2 is near normal, in which case changes of 1 to 2 kPa cause little alteration in oxygen saturation. However, over the clinically important range of Pao_2, oxygen saturation provides accurate and useful information and is sensitive to small changes in Pao_2 (Fig. 1(a)). The heart rate data provided by commercial oximeters indicate the cardiovascular response to changing oxygen saturation and provide a valuable aid to clinical monitoring.

Useful as the measurements of arterial oxygen tension and saturation are, the effectiveness of oxygen uptake by the lung can only be accurately assessed by relating Pao_2 to the oxygen tension in inspired gas, i.e. the alveolar–arterial oxygen difference $P(A - a)o_2$. A normal Pao_2 of 12 kPa, for example, would be a cause for concern if it required a very high inspired oxygen concentration, whereas modest hypoxia while breathing air commonly occurs in relatively minor respiratory disease and is not of clinical importance.

The oxygen tension in alveolar gas can be estimated from the equation

$$PAo_2 = PIo_2 - PAco_2/R$$

where PAo_2 is the partial pressure of oxygen in alveolar air, $PAco_2$ is the alveolar carbon dioxide tension which is assumed to be equal to $Paco_2$, PIo_2 is the inspired Po_2 (20.0 kPa for room air), and R (generally

taken to be 0.8) is the respiratory exchange ratio. Thus the normal alveolar oxygen tension is

$$PAo_2 = 20.0 - 5.3/0.8 = 13.3 \text{ kPa}.$$

The normal arterial oxygen tension is approximately 12.5 kPa and therefore $P(A - a)o_2 = 0.8$ kPa.

A patient with pneumonia ventilated in an intensive care unit with 50 per cent oxygen in whom the Pao_2 is 12.5 kPa and $Paco_2$ is 5.2 kPa can be assessed as follows:

$$PAo_2 = PIo_2 - Pco_2/0.8 = 50 - 6.5 = 43.5 \text{ kPa}$$

and hence

$$P(A - a)o_2 = 43.5 - 12.5 = 31 \text{ kPa}.$$

Thus the patient has a huge alveolar – arterial oxygen gradient.

The alveolar – arterial oxygen gradient gives insight into the severity of impaired oxygenation by the lung and is particularly useful when assessing the progress of patients over days and weeks. During this period PIo_2, $Paco_2$, and Pao_2 will all change, but sequential documentation of $P(A - a)o_2$ allows progress to be assessed accurately.

The alveolar – arterial oxygen gradient is a good measure of the oxygenating capacity of the lung, but it is equally important to assess the adequacy of tissue oxygenation. If tissue oxygen delivery is adequate, the oxygen saturation of venous blood returning to the heart from the peripheral tissues is normal. If tissue oxygen delivery is inadequate, due for example to severe hypoxia, anaemia, or poor cardiac output, following the extraction of required oxygen by the peripheral tissues the venous oxygen saturation will be low. Representative data are best obtained using venous blood sampled from the pulmonary artery – mixed venous oxygen saturation. Venous saturation can be continuously monitored by fibreoptic catheters sited in the pulmonary artery, and normal values are greater than 75 per cent.

The assessment of overall oxygen delivery is of great importance when assessing hypoxia. Patients with hypoxia and reduced mixed venous oxygen saturation have a poorer prognosis than those with normal mixed venous oxygen values. Therapy aimed at improving hypoxia may not enhance tissue oxygen deliver. For example the application of positive end expiratory pressure (PEEP) to correct hypoxia may be useful in raising Pao_2 but, by depressing cardiac output, may reduce overall tissue oxygenation so that mixed venous oxygen saturation may be reduced.

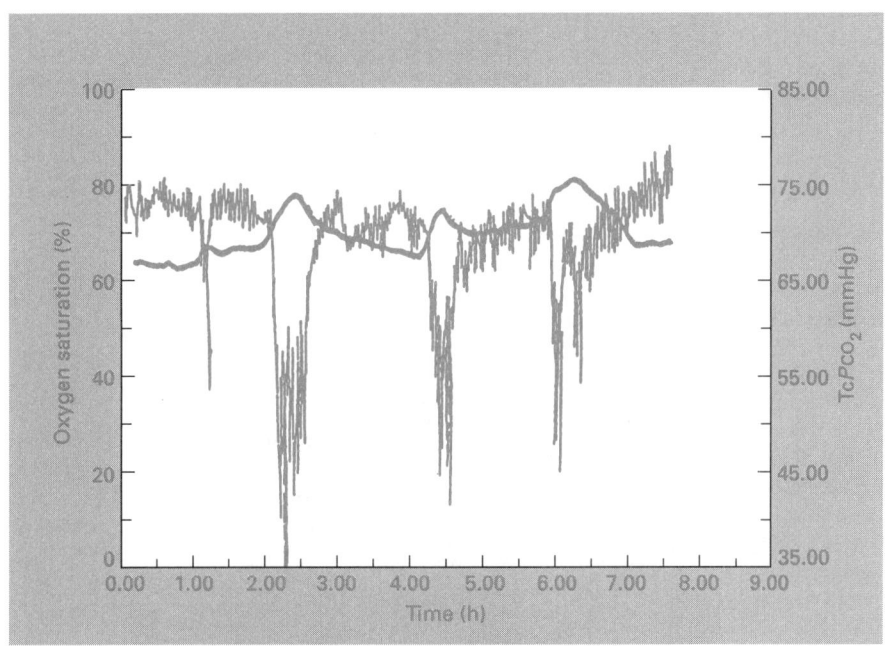

Fig. 2 Overnight sleep study in a patient with ventilatory failure due to severe kyphoscoliosis. The oxygen saturation Sao_2 is low throughout the night with further large reductions associated with REM sleep. Transcutaneous carbon dioxide $TcPco_2$ is raised and the reduction in ventilation during REM sleep intensifies the hypercapnia. Continuous measurements of Sao_2 and $TcPco_2$ are frequently of great value in assessing patients who have or may have respiratory failure.

Hypercapnia

The shape of the carbon dioxide dissociation curve is different from that for oxygen (Fig. 1(b)). Over the relevant range the relationship between PCO_2 and carbon dioxide concentration is almost linear compared with the sigmoid shape of the oxygen dissociation curve. If $\dot{V}_A/\dot{Q}$ abnormalities in some areas of the lung cause local failure to eliminate carbon dioxide, the subsequent hypercapnia stimulates ventilation and this increased ventilation of normally perfused lung units reduces alveolar, pulmonary capillary, and arterial carbon dioxide concentrations. Therefore the enhanced elimination of carbon dioxide from well-ventilated units can compensate for the inadequate ventilation of abnormal units. Thus many patients with pulmonary diseases which cause $\dot{V}_A/\dot{Q}$ mismatch characteristically have hypoxaemia but normal or even low $PaCO_2$.

Overall arterial PCO_2 is determined by the balance between carbon dioxide production and alveolar ventilation according to the equation

$$PaCO_2 = k \times \frac{CO_2 \text{ production}}{\text{alveolar ventilation}}.$$

Thus when carbon dioxide production is constant $PaCO_2$ is determined solely by alveolar ventilation. Hypercapnia may be due to hypoventilation that is either absolute or relative. If a normal person receives a respiratory depressant such as morphine, there is an absolute fall in ventilation and carbon dioxide rises. Alternatively, if a patient with severe chronic obstructive lung disease develops a chest infection which has an adverse effect on the $\dot{V}_A/\dot{Q}$ ratio, gas exchange deteriorates and hypoxaemia intensifies; if the patient is unable to increase ventilation appropriately, the carbon dioxide level rises. Total ventilation levels may be high in such patients, but they are still insufficient to avoid hypercapnia because there is relative alveolar hypoventilation.

EFFECTS OF HYPERCAPNIA

Acute hypercapnia can contribute to breathlessness but only when total ventilation is high in the face of alveolar hypoventilation. It also causes restlessness and confusion. The effects on the central nervous system are to raise intracranial pressure, because of increased cerebral blood flow, and eventually cerebral oedema and papilloedema can occur. In addition to confusion there is a flapping tremor. Peripherally, the acidosis caused by carbon dioxide promotes a profound vasodilatation with warm limbs and bounding pulses. Chronic hypercapnia of gradual onset is better tolerated, although since hypoventilation is usually greatest at night patients often have poor sleep quality, tiredness, impaired intellectual performance, and even personality changes, and frequently report early-morning headaches which clear as ventilation improves upon wakefulness.

ASSESSMENT OF HYPERCAPNIA

The symptoms and signs of hypercapnia are frequently both non-specific and insensitive, although morning headache, peripheral vasodilatation, and peripheral oedema in the appropriate clinical settings are useful pointers. To be sure of hypercapnia, $PaCO_2$ must be measured, and end-tidal carbon dioxide and transcutaneous carbon dioxide also have their role in assessment. End-tidal carbon dioxide may not accurately reflect arterial carbon dioxide in patients with severe lung disease, but can give useful information on PCO_2 trends (end-tidal carbon dioxide is also particularly useful when investigating patients with hyperventilation syndromes). Transcutaneous carbon dioxide can be of particular value during sleep studies investigating nocturnal hypoventilation (Fig. 2).

Hypercapnia causes a respiratory acidosis. Carbon dioxide is in equilibrium with carbonic acid, and any increase in carbon dioxide increases this acid which dissociates into bicarbonate and hydrogen ions, thereby reducing pH:

$$CO_2 + H_2O \rightleftharpoons H_2CO_3 \rightleftharpoons H^+ + HCO_3^-.$$

As a compensatory mechanism the kidney retains bicarbonate and pH is returned to normal (Fig. 3). Severe acidosis (pH less than 7.20) due to acute ventilatory failure carries a high mortality unless promptly reversed. However, well-compensated chronic ventilatory failure, with a pH above 7.30, may persist for months or years, for example in patients with chronic obstructive lung disease. Other patients may only develop hypercapnia at night, for example some patients with kyphoscoliosis in whom a raised bicarbonate level and a significant base excess may be present by day even though $PaCO_2$ is normal.

Causes of respiratory failure

The causes of respiratory failure are given in Table 1. This table broadly divides the causes of respiratory failure into type 1 and type 2. In general terms this is useful, but the distinction must not be viewed as rigid since many of the conditions which give rise to type 1 failure can eventually progress to cause hypercapnia. Similarly, many of the causes of type 2 ventilatory failure cause hypoxaemia without hypercapnia early in their course. Asthma provides a good example of how type 1 failure can progress to type 2 failure. This inflammatory disease in which there is obstruction and plugging of small airways causes marked $\dot{V}_A/\dot{Q}$ mismatch and poor gas exchange. Therefore with progressive asthma worsening hypoxia is the rule. Ventilatory drive is high owing to the inflammatory disease and the hypoxia, and in moderate disease hypocapnia is typical. As disease severity increases the diffuse airway narrowing greatly reduces ventilatory capacity, as a consequence of both increased airways resistance and impaired respiratory muscle function secondary to acute hyperinflation and muscle shortening. Eventually, despite a high respiratory drive, the impaired respiratory muscle pump is unable to sustain the huge ventilatory load necessary to achieve normal CO_2 levels and hypercapnia develops.

Ventilatory drive in diseases characterized by interstitial fibrosis remains excessive right to the end, and hypercapnia is very unusual in these patients. However, it is important to note that with very severe diffuse lung disease, for example adult respiratory distress syndrome, the gas exchange function of the lung is so profoundly and diffusely impaired that carbon dioxide elimination becomes impossible even when very high levels of ventilation are achieved by mechanical ventilators.

Fig. 3 Acid–base diagram: acute ventilatory failure causes hypercapnia and acidosis, renal retention of bicarbonate subsequently compensates the acidosis, and pH is restored to normal.

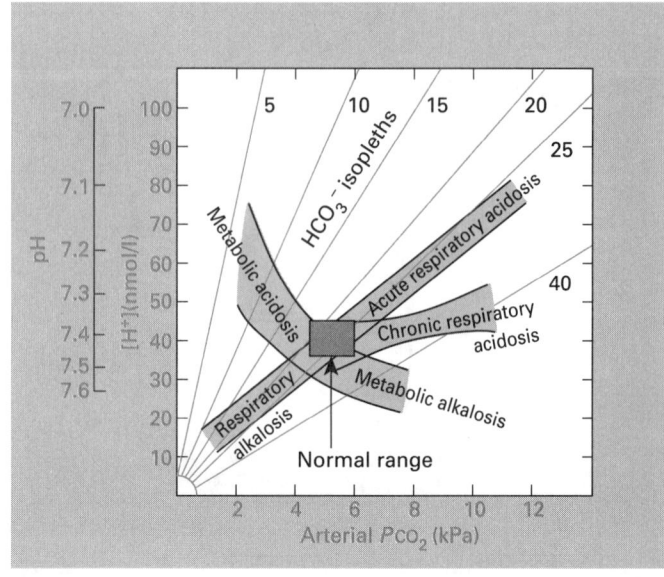

Table 1 *Causes of types 1 and type 2 respiratory failure*

Type 1 (oxygenation failure)
    Acute asthma
    Left heart failure
    Adult respiratory distress syndrome
    Pneumonia
    Pulmonary fibrosis
    Emphysema
    Bronchiectasis
    Cystic fibrosis
    Pulmonary vascular disease
    Miscellaneous: lymphangitis, radiation pneumonitis, etc.

Type 2 (ventilatory failure)
    Central nervous system
      Trauma
      Cerebral tumour
      Raised intracranial pressure
      Drugs
      Central alveolar hypoventilation
    Neuromuscular
      Cervical cord lesion
      Bilateral phrenic nerve trauma
      Guillain–Barré syndrome
      Motor neurone disease
      Poliomyelitis
      Multiple sclerosis
      Muscular dystrophies and myopathies
      Botulism
      Myasthenia gravis
      Eaton–Lambert syndrome
      Muscle relaxant drugs
      Organophosphorus poisoning
      Status epilepticus
    Thoracic cage and pleura
      Crushed chest
      Kyphoscoliosis
      Extensive thoracic surgery (thoracoplasty)
      Ankylosing spondylitis
      Massive obesity
    Lung and airways
      Severe acute asthma or pneumonia
      Upper airway obstruction, including obstructive sleep apnoea
      Severe chronic obstructive lung disease
      Bronchietasis, cystic fibrosis

MECHANISM OF (TYPE 2) VENTILATORY FAILURE

The causes of type 2 ventilatory failure (Table 1) are miscellaneous, but the mechanism of hypoventilation and carbon dioxide retention is best understood (as in severe asthma) by considering the importance of ventilatory drive, the capacity of the respiratory muscle pump, and the load imposed on the ventilatory system (Fig. 4). These three components of the respiratory system are closely interrelated, and although some disorders may predominantly affect one component the interrelationships remain crucial.

An important element in the genesis of chronic ventilatory failure is the alteration of ventilatory drive that occurs with sleep. During sleep, particularly REM sleep, respiratory drive is reduced and the pattern of breathing is altered. Alveolar ventilation falls during sleep, hypoxia intensifies, and carbon dioxide rises. This nocturnal hypoventilation causes marked oxygen desaturation in patients who, when awake, are already hypoxic and poised on the steep section of the oxygen dissociation curve.

Obstructive sleep apnoea (see Chapter 17.14.2) is a rather special case of transient ventilatory failure in which severe upper airways obstruction during sleep causes repeated episodes of asphyxia followed by arousal.

In these patients the reduction in activation of the upper airway musculature during sleep results in collapse of the oropharynx in response to the negative intraluminal pressure generated during inspiration. When asphyxia produces arousal the neurological activation of the upper airway muscles becomes sufficient to restore patency of the oropharynx. The patient then hyperventilates and blood gases improve, but with the return to deep sleep the cycle repeats itself, often hundreds of times throughout the night. Obstructive sleep apnoea as a cause of type 2 ventilatory failure during sleep provides an insight into a mechanism of carbon dioxide retention that may be relevant to other chronic respiratory diseases.

Patients with severe obstructive sleep apnoea eventually develop chronic type 2 ventilatory failure with hypoxia and hypercapnia by day. The treatment of obstructive sleep apnoea, usually by nocturnal nasal continuous positive airway pressure (CPAP), is highly effective. Patients report remarkable improvements in their well-being, and over a period of time daytime blood gases improve. Thus night-time therapy lifts the patient out of chronic ventilatory failure. It is of interest that when patients with obstructive sleep apnoea are successfully treated, the ventilatory response to carbon dioxide is dramatically enhanced in those who have carbon dioxide retention prior to therapy. It is unaltered in patients without hypercapnia. Therefore it seems that the repeated episodes of nocturnal hypoventilation and associated hypercapnic respiratory acidosis, blunt the ventilatory response to carbon dioxide, leading to hypercapnia by day.

Similar mechanisms to those responsible for ventilatory failure in obstructive sleep apnoea may be responsible for the chronic ventilatory failure of patients with chest-wall disease, for example kyphoscoliosis. In these patients the ventilatory capacity is markedly reduced and the load imposed on the respiratory muscle pump is much increased (Fig. 4). Adequate ventilation requires high central respiratory drive. Eventually these patients develop type 2 ventilatory failure. As expected, the problems are greatest at night during sleep, but carbon dioxide retention often persists chronically throughout the day. Such patients can be effectively treated by nocturnal non-invasive nasal positive pressure ventilation. As with CPAP in the treatment of obstructive sleep apnoea, patients with kyphoscoliosis frequently report dramatic benefits from nasal positive pressure ventilation (NPPV) therapy, and can be maintained in good health for many years. Nocturnal NPPV therapy reverses

Fig. 4 Ventilatory failure can occur when the load imposed on the respiratory muscle pump is excessive, ventilatory capacity is impaired, or both problems coexist. Ventilation depends on appropriate central nervous system respiratory drive; inadequate drive due to brain disorders or sedative drugs can precipitate ventilatory failure. It is likely that the reduction of respiratory drive that occurs in sleep is important for the development of ventilatory failure in a wide range of disorders.

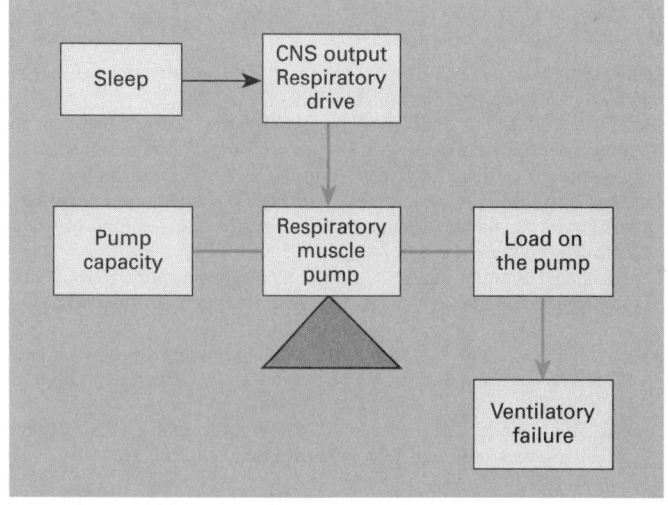

daytime ventilatory failure. There has been speculation about the mechanism of this improvement. There is some evidence that the mechanical ventilation improves chest-wall compliance and thereby reduces the load on the ventilatory system. However, this is likely to be a minor factor. It has also been suggested that NPPV may rest the respiratory muscles and relieve chronic respiratory muscle fatigue. However, chronic muscle fatigue has not been convincingly demonstrated, and indeed the notion of a stable chronic muscle fatigue state is implausible. Therefore the most likely explanation for the improvement in daytime blood gases following nocturnal NPPV is that the treatment controls nocturnal hypoventilation, progressively reverses the chronic compensated respiratory acidosis, and enhances the ventilatory response to carbon dioxide. Despite the continuing adverse load – capacity balance, the patients do not relapse into ventilatory failure because they continue to receive regular nocturnal NPPV. Indeed, if these patients do not receive this treatment they gradually drift back into chronic ventilatory failure.

Domiciliary NPPV has also been used to treat selected patients with advanced chronic obstructive lung disease, and in these patients it is possible to demonstrate some improvement in daytime ventilatory failure although the improvements are not as dramatic as for patients with chest-wall disorders. Patients with severe chronic obstructive lung disease have an enhanced ventilatory response to carbon dioxide following NPPV therapy.

A plausible hypothesis for the genesis of chronic ventilatory failure is as follows. Some patients have disorders that markedly reduce respiratory muscle pump ventilatory capacity (for example patients with muscular dystrophy or poliomyelitis), some patients have diseases that greatly increase ventilatory load (for example patients with morbid obesity), and many patients have diseases that both reduce capacity and increase load, such that load becomes high in relation to capacity (for example patients with chronic obstructive lung disease or kyphoscoliosis). In all these patients adequate ventilation is only possible if ventilatory drive is high. Eventually this high drive cannot be sustained, and this is most commonly first evident during sleep. When drive is not sufficient, episodes of hypoventilation occur, initially as acute episodes of transient hypercapnic respiratory acidosis. However, with severe and progressive disease, established chronic compensated respiratory acidosis with associated clinical type 2 chronic ventilatory failure develops.

This scheme of chronic ventilatory failure (Fig. 4) indicates that treatment should be directed towards reducing ventilatory load, (for example using bronchodilators to reduce airways resistance) and/or enhancing respiratory muscle pump capacity (for example improving nutritional status). Treatment options and strategies will vary between diseases and between patients. The scheme also highlights the central role and 'problem' of sleep. It is likely that the recent introduction of NPPV, which presents the opportunity of controlling nocturnal hypoventilation in suitably selected patients, will enhance our capacity to manage some cases of chronic ventilatory failure more effectively.

REFERENCES

Anthonisen, N.R. (1982). Hypoxaemia and oxygen therapy. *American Review of Respiratory Disease,* **126,** 729–33.

Berthon-Jones, M. and Sullivan, C.E. (1987). Time course of change in ventilatory response to CO$_2$ with long-term CPAP therapy for obstructive sleep apnea. *American Review of Respiratory Disease,* **135,** 144–7.

Bott, J., Carroll, M.P., Conway, J.H. *et al.* (1993). Randomised controlled trial of nasal ventilation in acute ventilatory failure due to chronic obstructive airways disease. *Lancet,* **341,** 1555–7.

Carroll, N. and Branthwaite, M.A. (1988). Control of nocturnal hypoventilation by nasal intermittent positive pressure ventilation. *Thorax,* **43,** 349–53.

Douglas, N.J. and Flenley, D.C. (1990). Breathing during sleep in patients with obstructive lung disease. *American Review of Respiratory Disease,* **141,** 1055–70.

Douglas, N.J., White, D.P., Pickett, C.K., Weil, J., and Zwillich, C.W. (1982). Respiration during sleep in normal man. *Thorax,* **37,** 840–4.

Elliott, M.W., Mulvey, D.A., Moxham, J., Green, M., and Branthwaite, M.A. (1991). Domiciliary nocturnal nasal intermittent positive pressure ventilation in COPD: mechanisms underlying changes in arterial blood gas tensions. *European Respiratory Journal,* **4,** 1044–52.

Gribben, H.R., Gardiner, I.T., Heinz, C.J., Gibson, T.J., and Pride, N.B. (1983). The role of impaired inspiratory muscle function in limiting ventilatory response to CO$_2$ in chronic airflow obstruction. *Clinical Science,* **64,** 487–95.

Hoeppner, V.H., Cockcroft, D.W., Dosman, J.A., and Cotton, D.J. Nightime ventilation improves respiratory failure in secondary kyphoscoliosis. *American Review of Respiratory Disease,* **129,** 240–3.

Moxham, J. (1990). Respiratory muscle fatigue: mechanisms, evaluation and therapy. *British Journal of Anaesthesia,* **65,** 43–53.

Warren, P.M., Flenley, D.C., Millar, J.S., and Avery, A. (1980). Respiratory failure revisited: acute exacerbations of chronic bronchitis between 1961–68 and 1970–76. *Lancet,* **i,** 467–71.

17.14.2 Sleep-related disorders of breathing

J.R. STRADLING

Introduction

Disorders of breathing that are apparent only during sleep are discussed in this chapter. There is a two-way interaction between sleep and breathing: not only does sleep lead to profound changes in breathing and its control, but problems with breathing lead to gross fragmentation of sleep. This field is rapidly expanding now that it is realized that the main condition to be considered, obstructive sleep apnoea and its variants, is relatively common with a prevalence of about 0.5 to 1 per cent in adult males. Obstructive sleep apnoea was first properly described in 1967, and since that time facilities for its diagnosis and treatment have grown enormously. It is now necessary for all physicians to know about this condition and its varied presentations. In most large district general hospitals the respiratory physician will usually take on these sleep-related disorders, although in some places an anaesthetist or neurologist runs the service.

Our understanding of these sleep-related breathing disorders is still evolving and has moved on considerably since the previous edition of this book. In particular, our view of what constitutes a significant problem has changed. In order to understand how an abnormality of breathing can arise during sleep and not be apparent during wakefulness, it is necessary to discuss some of the normal changes in respiratory physiology that occur during the different phases of sleep.

Normal physiology of breathing during sleep (Table 1)

Sleep can be divided into two very different states. The dominant sleep stage is non-rapid eye movement (NREM) sleep (Figs. 1 and 2). This phase of sleep appears to be when the brain shuts down, and is necessary for maximum daytime alertness and continuing cognitive function. Following a period of sleep deprivation it is this phase of sleep that is reclaimed most. NREM sleep shows a continuum from drowsy right down to very deep sleep, arbitrarily subdivided into stages 1, 2, 3, and 4. The awake electroencephalogram (EEG) is characterized by low voltage, high frequency activity with the only dominant frequency being the so-called alpha activity (approximately 10 Hz), present when the eyes are closed. As sleep supervenes, the alpha activity disappears, overall EEG frequency falls, muscle tone (usually measured from a chin electromyogram (EMG)) falls, and the eyes begin to roll from side to side. This transition phase is called stage 1. Stage 2 is defined by the appearance of K complexes (isolated large waves) and sleep spindles (bursts of about 13 Hz activity). As sleep deepens further, increasing amounts

Table 1 *Sleep and breathing*

	NREM	REM
Electroencephalogram	Progressively slower frequency and higher amplitude	Similar to the awake pattern
Eye movements	Initially slow and pendular, then none	Bursts of rapid binocular movements
Postural muscle tone	Reduced from wakefulness	Very much reduced or absent
Factors controlling breathing	Loss of wakefulness input. Brain-stem and classical stimuli dominate, but reduced compared with wakefulness	Cortical overriding and apparent reduction in responses to classical stimuli
Arousal response	Small changes in Pao_2 and $Paco_2$, with the consequent ventilatory response, are required for arousal	Larger changes in Pao_2 and $Paco_2$ required before arousal occurs
Potential effect on breathing	Fall in minute ventilation. Rise in pharyngeal resistance. Fall in Pao_2	Further rise in pharyngeal resistance. Loss of use of accessory muscles of respiration. Further falls in Pao_2 tolerated longer before rescued by arousal

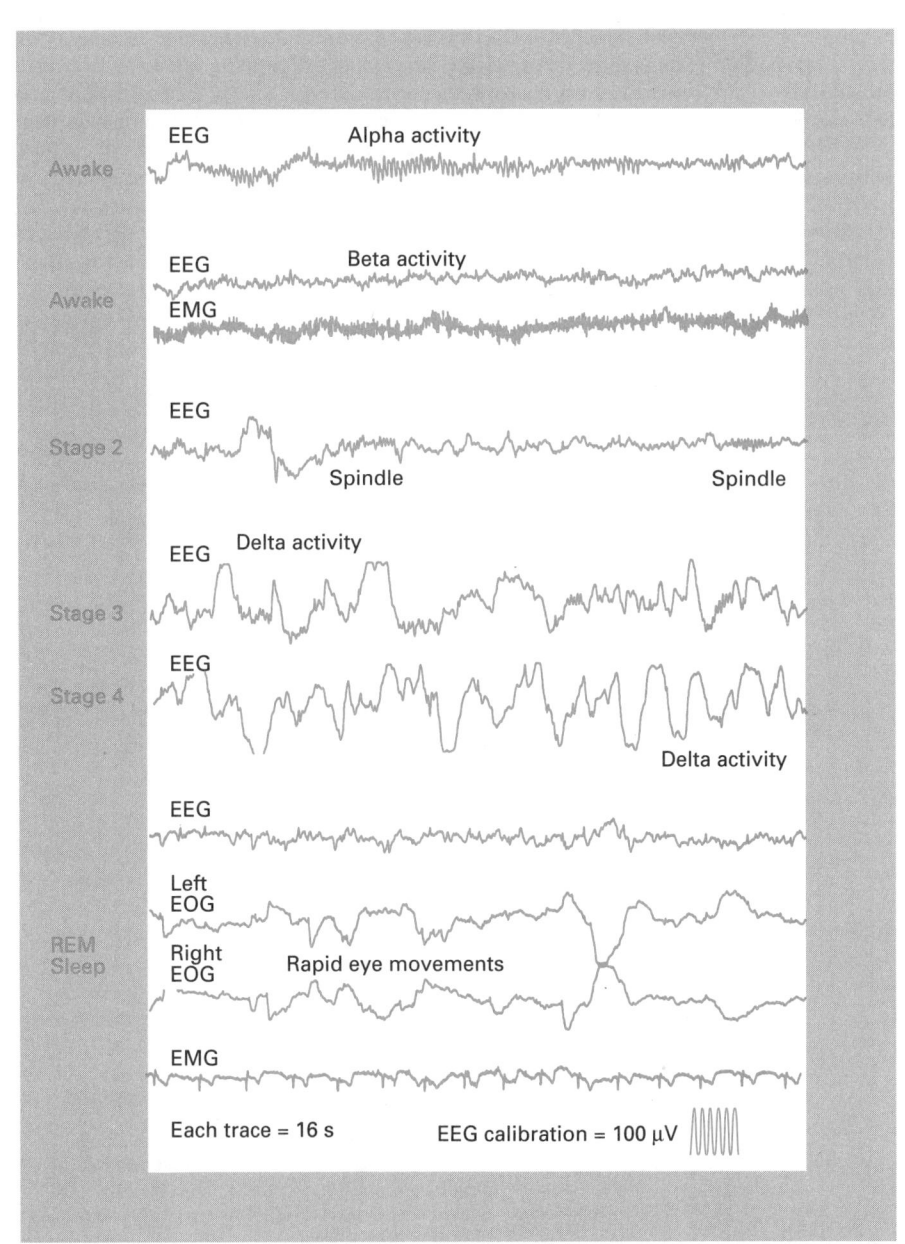

Fig. 1 Examples of electrical brain activity (EEG), eye movements (EOG) and chin muscle tone (EMG) during wakefulness and the different sleep stages.

of large slow waves (approximately 1 Hz) appear. These stages are called 3 and 4, or slow-wave sleep (SWS).

The other main phase of sleep is rapid eye movement (REM) sleep or dreaming sleep. This stage is characterized by a return of the EEG to a pattern resembling wakefulness. The EMG tone falls to very low levels and there are bursts of rapid eye movements, mainly from side to side, under closed eyelids. Effectively the cortex is 'awake' again, processing images and able to integrate outside noises or other stimuli into complex dreams. The fall in EMG tone is because the rest of the body's muscles have been 'cut off' from the brain and paralysed, hence the fall in EMG tone. This paralysis (or atonia) is under active control from a centre in the pons that hyperpolarizes the lower motor neurones via inhibitory reticulospinal pathways. This centre can be experimentally destroyed. For example cats in whom the centre has been destroyed no longer show atonia during REM sleep. This has the consequence that they may get up and walk around or chase phantom birds during REM sleep, presumably reflecting dream content. The function of this atonia centre may in fact be to prevent the dreaming brain from influencing the rest of the body. This paralysis during REM sleep is dominantly in muscles that normally have a tonic postural activity; thus the diaphragm is spared although pharyngeal, intercostal, and accessory muscles are all affected to differing extents.

The normal pattern of the oscillation between NREM and REM sleep is shown in Fig 2. This 'hypnogram', as it is called, is constructed by classifying 30 s epochs successively from tracings of EEG, EMG, and eye movement data into either awake, movement, REM sleep, or stages 1–4; thus 960 epochs are obtained in an 8 h night.

During wakefulness breathing is influenced by a variety of pathways, some conscious and voluntary, others entirely automatic and involuntary. Although the classic responses to hypoxia, hypercapnia, and vagal afferents (integrated in the brain-stem) are present, they can be overruled by cortical signals in order to subserve functions such as talking. These two routes of control are separate and can be damaged separately by disease processes. Just the presence of wakefulness itself provides an input to the respiratory centre almost equivalent to resting ventilation. For example following a period of hyperventilation a normal subject will go on breathing at just below normal levels, despite hypocapnia and hyperoxia, until the carbon dioxide rises when normal ventilatory levels are re-established. This is not true during NREM sleep when hypocapnia will produce apnoea until the Pa_{CO_2} rises back to a critical threshold level.

Another component of wakefulness is the high muscle tone that holds the body in the required posture. This 'awake' input into the anterior horn cells means that other inputs, such as those from the respiratory centre, will be able to further activate muscles such as the intercostals and pharyngeal. The withdrawal of this 'awake' tone with sleep onset may mean that a certain respiratory centre output to these anterior horn cells is no longer able to raise membrane potentials to firing threshold. Thus during wakefulness a certain output from the respiratory centre may produce an 'equivalent' output from the anterior horn cells supplying the intercostals, but during sleep this may no longer be the case.

The consequence of these changes is that respiratory muscle activity falls with sleep onset, minute volume reduces by about 10 to 15 per cent, and Pa_{CO_2} rises by 3 to 8 mmHg. The reduction of pharyngeal muscle tone narrows the lumen, and a rise in upper airway resistance occurs in everyone. This reduction in ventilation will have trivial effects on the arterial oxygen saturation Sa_{O_2} if one is on the normal flat part of the haemoglobin dissociation curve, but more dramatic falls in Sa_{O_2} will be apparent if starting on the steeper part (below 92 per cent Sa_{O_2}). If ventilatory responses to carbon dioxide or hypoxia are measured during NREM sleep, the slopes are flatter and shifted, indicating a reduced overall sensitivity. Exactly why this occurs is not known, but it will be

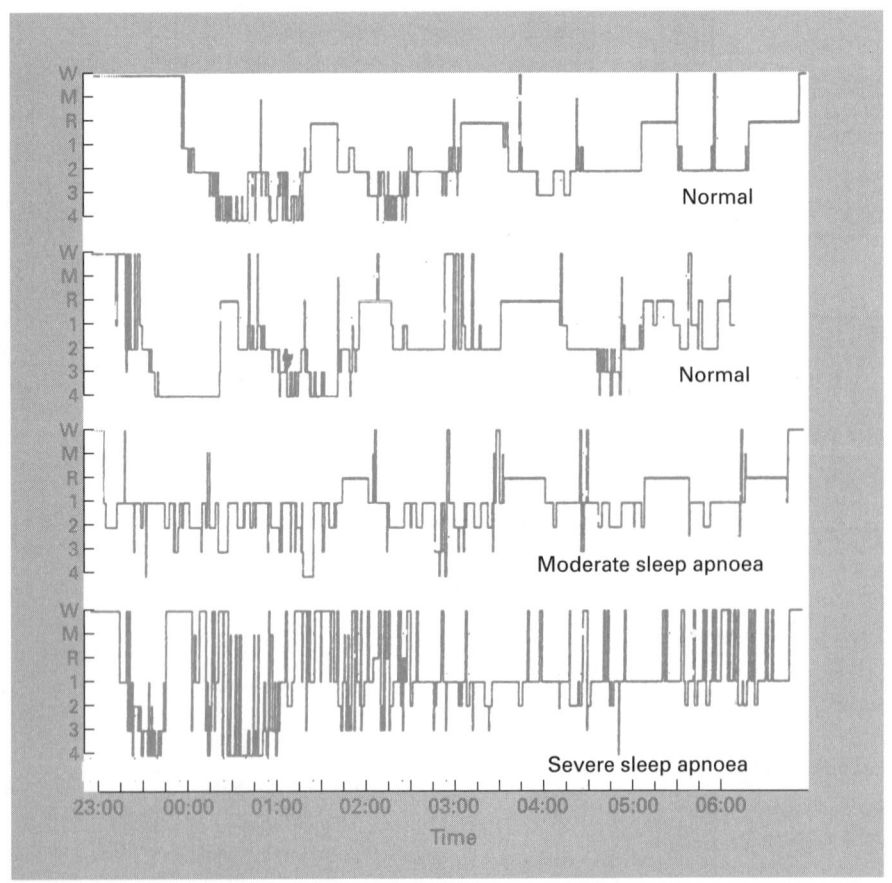

Fig. 2 Examples of all-night hypnograms (based on 20 s epochs) in two normal subjects and two patients with sleep apnoea. Note the reduced deep sleep (stages 3 and 4) in the patients, but no indication that they are waking up hundreds of times a night. W, awake; M, movement (awake); R, REM sleep; 1 to 4, stages 1, 2, 3, 4 of non-REM sleep.

Table 2 *Causes of obstructive sleep apnoea*

Anatomical
Central (neck) obesity
Micro or retrognathia
Pharyngeal encroachment (e.g. tonsillar hypertrophy, acromegaly, tumour, mucopolysaccharidoses, oedema)
Neuromuscular
Bulbar palsies
Neurological degenerative disorders
Myopathies (e.g., Duchenne dystrophy)
Other provoking factors
Alcohol
Sedative drugs
Sleep deprivation
Increased nasal resistance
Hypothyroidism
Acromegaly

due partly to the reduced tone to the respiratory muscles, the withdrawal of awake drive, the increased upper airway resistance, and probably a true reduction in central sensitivity to carbon dioxide or [H$^+$].

During REM sleep, overall ventilation stays much the same as in NREM sleep, but the breath-to-breath variability increases considerably with falls during the actual periods of eye movements and compensatory rises between. Sensitivities to carbon dioxide and hypoxia were originally thought to be further reduced, but they are hard to measure in the presence of spontaneously varying breathing and more recent evidence suggests they may not change much at all. What is far more important is the atonia of postural muscles. The hyperpolarization of the anterior horn cells greatly reduces the efficacy of respiratory signals to the intercostal, accessory, and pharyngeal muscles. This will not matter in a normal subject with an efficient diaphragm and a non-compromised pharynx. However, if the subject is dependent on muscles other than the diaphragm for breathing, or has a narrow compromised pharynx, then REM sleep may powerfully interfere with ventilation with consequent hypoxaemia and hypercapnia.

Of final relevance to breathing during REM sleep are the reduced arousal responses to respiratory stimuli compared with non-REM sleep. The arousal response to some respiratory stimuli (hypoxia, hypercapnia, extra resistive load) is believed to be mediated partly by the effort made in response, rather than just the actual stimulus itself. If a ventilatory response to hypoxia is measured during REM sleep, then the subject will usually tolerate a much lower Sao_2 before arousal than during NREM sleep. Furthermore, if the drive to sleep is high, such as after sleep deprivation, arousal will be delayed yet further.

It can be seen from the above that, although sleep is not a problem for those with normal respiratory systems, once abnormalities are present there is potential for a damaging interaction between sleep and breathing, particularly during REM sleep.

Obstructive sleep apnoea

Definition

Sleep apnoea was first properly documented in neurophysiological sleep laboratories using techniques that had been developed for the investigation of conditions such as insomnia, narcolepsy, and depression. It was realized that hundreds of episodes of breath cessation, or apnoea, usually due to upper airway obstruction with associated snoring, were related to marked sleep disturbance. Because simple oronasal flow detectors were used, the critical event became an episode of apnoea. Because it was easy to measure, an arbitrary definition was made and breath cessation for longer than 10 s became an official apnoea. Early work suggested that normal young people rarely had more than about

30 apnoeas per night so that the sleep apnoea syndrome was defined as follows: more than 35 apnoeas per night, or more than five apnoeas per hour of sleep, or apnoeas lasting for 10 s or longer. This definition became enshrined in the literature until long after its artificiality was established.

The real definition should be as follows: 'A sleep disruption syndrome, sufficient to cause symptoms, that is due to a respiratory problem engendered by sleep itself. Usually this is upper airway incompetence during sleep, but may also be due to problems of respiratory drive'. As the pathogenesis of sleep apnoea is explained, this shift in emphasis will become clear.

Aetiology (Table 2)

The upper pharyngeal airway has to serve two functions, swallowing and breathing, which require different design features. When used for swallowing the pharynx has to behave like the oesophagus, and when used for breathing it has to remain an open tube like the trachea. These dual functions are achieved by having a floppy and collapsible muscular tube that is also capable of being held rigidly open by dilator muscles. The muscles responsible for this dilator function are discussed in the section on the structure and function of the upper respiratory tract. All these muscles have a reduced activation during sleep, so that some pharyngeal narrowing occurs normally. The factors that determine whether this leads to significant upper airflow obstruction in a particular individual are complex. Various theories exist, but essentially they divide into two groups. First there may be abnormalities of the activation of these pharyngeal dilator muscles, perhaps due to defective or unstable central control; second there may be anatomical abnormalities that allow significant obstruction to occur even with the normal sleep-related reduction in muscle tone.

NEUROMUSCULAR FUNCTION

Early investigations of EMG activity in pharyngeal muscles found reductions in tone with sleep during obstructive apnoeas in patients. However, it is very difficult to show that these reductions are truly abnormal. Recent evidence suggests that there may be an increase in phasic inspiratory activity of these muscles, perhaps as an attempted defence mechanism against pharyngeal collapse. In some patients with primary neuromuscular problems (from brain-stem lesions to myopathies) there can be associated obstructive sleep apnoea, and pharyngeal muscle involvement seems a probable explanation. However, the majority of patients with obstructive sleep apnoea do not show evidence of any other neuromuscular problems.

During inspiration, pharyngeal dilator activity has to be synchronized with diaphragm activity and be adequate to overcome the negative intrapharyngeal pressures. It has been suggested that a lack of coordination between diaphragmatic and pharyngeal activation may allow the pharynx to collapse. For example normal subjects breathing against an inspiratory resistance can be made to have a few obstructive apnoeas by artificially inducing periodic breathing during sleep. The gradual return of respiratory drive, following the nadir of ventilation, seems to activate the diaphragm first, leaving the pharynx unbraced. The use of an inspiratory resistance 'challenges' the pharynx and allows collapse for a few breaths before pharyngeal tone returns and restores patency. Although instability of respiratory control during sleep has been postulated as a cause of obstructive sleep apnoea, following treatment with nasal continuous positive airway pressure therapy (see later) there is no evidence of a premorbid underlying respiratory instability, nor does altering respiratory drive have a useful effect.

More convincing is the suggestion that there may be failure of reflex protective mechanisms in the pharynx. There are receptors in the pharynx that detect falls in pressure that distort the airway and provoke protective increases in pharyngeal dilator tone (see Section 17.2). Snoring itself may also be one of the stimuli that activates this dilator reflex. It is possible that interruption of this reflex arc can occur, perhaps through years of pharyngeal trauma from snoring, mucosal oedema, or toxic agents such as cigarette smoke and alcohol.

ANATOMICAL CAUSES

Anatomical abnormalities could influence pharyngeal function in a variety of ways. Simple encroachment of the pharyngeal lumen, for example with tonsillar hypertrophy, means that the normal fall in pharyngeal dilator tone with sleep can now lead to critical narrowing and obstruction. Alternatively, there could be abnormalities which 'load' the upper airway that require increased dilator muscle action that is then lost during sleep (for example high nasal resistance or increased external compression from neck obesity). Finally, there may be mechanical problems of coupling the muscle activity so that it fails to dilate the pharyngeal lumen as effectively.

There are many case reports of obvious anatomical abnormalities provoking obstructive sleep apnoea, for example tonsillar hypertrophy, pharyngeal oedema, tumours, acromegaly, mucopolysaccharidoses, and retro- or micrognathia. These reports show that pharyngeal narrowing (asymptomatic whilst awake) can provoke obstructive sleep apnoea, but such diagnoses represent only a small proportion of cases.

The majority of patients with obstructive sleep apnoea are overweight. In many clinics the average obesity index is well over 30 kg/m². This is equivalent to being about 30 per cent overweight, for example 95 kg (15 stone) at a height of 1.78 m (5 ft 10 in). Weight loss can certainly cure obstructive sleep apnoea, and all studies identifying risk factors have found obesity to be dominant, accounting for up to 40 per cent of the variance in severity.

It is not clear exactly how obesity provokes obstructive sleep apnoea. Some groups (but not all) have found neck circumference to be a better predictor of severity of obstructive sleep apnoea than obesity, suggesting that it is neck obesity and external pharyngeal loading that is important. Neck imaging techniques fail to show convincing evidence of much extra fat directly around the pharynx, but of course there is much fat subcutaneously. Animal studies have shown that only a small amount of extra external pressure over the pharynx is required to collapse it during sleep.

Although general obesity is related to neck obesity, the overall correlation is only about 0.75. This is because fat distribution varies considerably between individuals. The 'female' distribution tends to be in the lower body and the 'male' distribution is more central. Thus a man who is not particularly overweight can have a large neck and vice versa.

As mentioned earlier, there is also evidence that some of the upper airway dilator muscles (e.g. genioglossus) of obese patients with obstructive sleep apnoea are actually working harder than normal, perhaps as compensation for the added external loading from neck obesity. Compensations by the respiratory system for other types of extra loading have been shown to be much less active during sleep.

If the link between upper body obesity and sleep apnoea turns out not to be simply due to mass loading of the neck, then it may be due to infiltration of pharyngeal muscles with fat or to interference by fat masses with the action of dilator muscles, reducing their efficacy.

Thus overall the evidence is mainly in favour of much obstructive sleep apnoea in adults being due to loading of the upper airway as a result of obesity, which can be fended off during wakefulness but, with the withdrawal of postural muscle tone with sleep, leads to excessive narrowing or collapse and sleep apnoea.

However, not all adult sleep apnoea can be explained by obesity or intrapharyngeal anatomical abnormalities. The significance of marked retro- or micrognathia for obstructive sleep apnoea was recognized early on, particularly in children (Pierre–Robin syndrome). Careful cephalometric studies of facial and skull morphology have revealed that some patients with obstructive sleep apnoea have longer faces, repositioning of the mandible (measured as a more acute angle between the sella to nasion and nasion to supramentale planes), a downward movement of the hyoid, elongation of the soft palate, and a narrower anteroposterior

distance behind the tongue. Some, or all, of these changes may be secondary to the years of sleep apnoea rather than part of the cause. However, the retropositioning of the mandible may be contributory; certainly surgery to advance the mandible may be curative.

Retropositioning of the mandible may be a legacy from childhood. There is good evidence that nasal blockage and mouth breathing very early in life alters facial development (the so-called 'adenoidal facies'), and one feature of this is mandibular retropositioning. Following early adenoidectomy and resumption of nasal breathing, the mandible can return to its normal position. Thus one composite theory is that mandibular underdevelopment and obesity are two relatively common independent risk factors for obstructive sleep apnoea which together may be synergistic.

OTHER FACTORS PROVOKING OBSTRUCTIVE SLEEP APNOEA

Alcohol is a potent reducer of muscle tone, and can further reduce pharyngeal dilator muscle tone during sleep. It is well known that alcohol worsens snoring, but it can also convert snoring to full apnoea. Other sedatives, such as the benzodiazepines, barbiturates, and opiates, can also do the same; this has important consequences when anaesthetizing such patients. Interestingly, sleep deprivation itself can reduce upper airway muscle tone during subsequent sleep and thus provoke a positive feedback of apnoea–sleep disruption–more apnoea.

Nasal blockage can contribute to the tendency of the pharynx to collapse by lowering intrapharyngeal pressures. If extra effort has to be made to inspire through a high nasal resistance, there will be a greater vacuum effect in the pharynx, increasing its tendency to collapse. Once collapse occurs, flow ceases, pharyngeal pressure will return to atmospheric, the lumen will open again, and the cycle will repeat. This certainly leads to snoring, but may not be very important when there is full apnoea. Nasal obstruction may contribute long term to sleep apnoea by damaging the pharynx through years of snoring and thus making it more collapsible, but improving nasal patency only rarely cures obstructive sleep apnoea.

Hypothyroidism provokes obstructive sleep apnoea, but the mechanism is not clear. It may partly be through weight gain or through tissue or fluid deposition in the pharynx. Alternatively, there may be direct interference with muscle function owing to a low thyroxine level. Acromegaly causes sleep apnoea, probably through changes in pharyngeal shape.

Immediate consequences of sleep apnoea

Upper airway narrowing, sometimes with complete apnoea, usually commences as sleep passes from awake to stage 2. Once significant obstruction occurs there will be increasing respiratory effort to try and overcome it. The length of such events is highly variable, ranging from only a few seconds to well over a minute. At some point arousal occurs with an improvement in upper airway resistance, resolution of any asphyxia, and then a return to sleep whereupon the cycle repeats (Figs. 3–5).

Hypoxaemia and mild hypercapnia usually accompany these periods of obstructed breathing. If there is complete apnoea, the rate of fall of Sao_2 will depend mainly on the amount of oxygen stored in the lungs and therefore the functional residual capacity since apnoeas occur at end-expiration, preventing inspiration. The length of the apnoea will also determine how low the Sao_2 will fall, and varies considerably between patients. The results of this hypoxaemia and hypercapnia are not clear. Because the blood gas derangements are so transient they may do little harm, unless there is already ischaemic heart disease for example.

Hypoxaemia was believed to play an important part in the arousal response that saves the patient from continuing asphyxia. In animal models, removal of the carotid body abolishes significant ventilatory response to hypoxaemia during sleep and there is no arousal. Giving extra added oxygen does prolong apnoeas to a small extent and delay arousal. However, recent evidence suggests that the main arousal stimulus is the actual respiratory effort being made in response to the asphyxia rather than the asphyxia *per se*. Normal subjects tend to wake when they have to make respiratory efforts about three times above the normal (10–20 cmH$_2$O pleural pressure swings). This degree of effort is easily reached in obstructive sleep apnoea when pressures down to −80 cmH$_2$O can be recorded during the frustrated inspiratory efforts. In addition, such pressures can also be reached by heavy snorers, even if they do not develop hypoxaemia, and this will also lead to arousals. This is because the greatly increased respiratory effort to overcome a

partially obstructed pharynx (with loud snoring) can compensate fully and maintain gas exchange in some individuals.

In terms of symptoms, the most important consequence of this sleep-induced upper airway narrowing is the sleep fragmentation. The original methodology of sleep analysis, using coarse 30 s epochs to stage sleep, effectively glossed over the hundreds of very transient arousals that are the main consequence of obstructive sleep apnoea. Superficially, a sleep hypnogram in a moderately severe case (Fig. 2) could look almost normal despite these hundreds of arousals. The importance of trying to measure the arousals has recently been appreciated, and technology to measure them automatically is being developed.

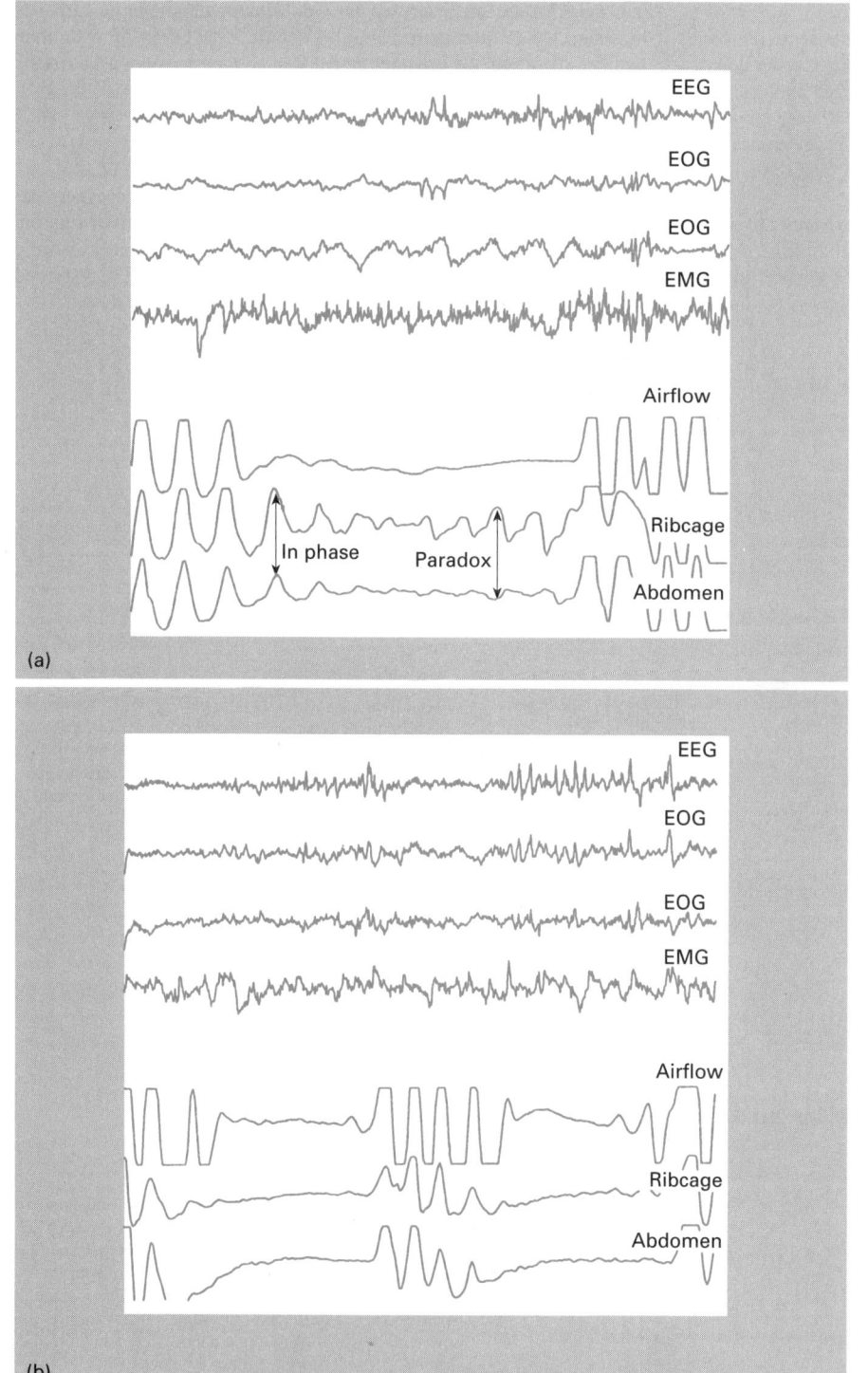

Fig. 3 Obstructive and central apnoeas (16 second traces): (a) airflow ceases but rib-cage and abdominal movements persist and become paradoxical; (b) rib-cage and abdominal movements cease as well as airflow.

At present the level of sleep disruption, in terms of both number and 'size' of arousals, necessary to cause daytime symptoms is not known. However, there is a clear but variable relationship between increasing sleep disruption and deteriorating daytime function.

In addition to the blood gas disturbances and sleep disruption there are many other consequences of obstructive sleep apnoea.

During the apnoea there is activation of the diving reflex that produces bradycardia, particularly when there is associated hypoxaemia. Upon arousal there is a sudden pulse rate and blood pressure rise, probably due to activation of the sympathetic nervous system. During the actual frustrated inspiratory efforts the blood pressure falls with the reductions in intrathoracic pressure (pulsus paradoxus) and, in conjunction with the blood pressure rise on arousal, produces a very characteristic trace (Fig. 4).

In addition to the increased nocturnal catecholamine secretion seen in patients with obstructive sleep apnoea, there is also a suppression of growth hormone and testosterone levels. There is marked polyuria during sleep (a reversal of the normal relative oliguria of sleep), but the mechanism is not clear; it may be related to the recurrent arousals or increased ANP production from right atrial distension (due to the large inspiratory efforts).

It will be clear from the above account that there are grey areas and uncertainty over defining and measuring the significant aspects of sleep apnoea. We discussed earlier that original definitions centred on the critical event first observed in obstructive sleep apnoea – an actual obstructive event. There has now been a shift towards trying to look more closely at the most important result – sleep fragmentation. This is particularly necessary now we know that 10 s apnoeas are not the only result of upper airway narrowing during sleep that can provoke multiple arousals and daytime sleepiness. Since heavy snorers can have considerable sleep fragmentation without significant falls in Sa_{O_2}, examining blood gas abnormalities (for example with an oximeter) is not always good enough either. The implications for this in terms of investigations are discussed later.

This is why the current definition of what still tends to be called obstructive sleep apnoea should be as follows: 'a sleep disruption syndrome (sufficient to cause symptoms) that is due to a sleep-induced narrowing of the upper airway, with or without significant disturbance to gas exchange'. Refinements to this definition will develop with time, particularly when we can measure upper airway narrowing and sleep disruption more quantitatively.

Symptoms and presentation

The main symptom of obstructive sleep apnoea is daytime hypersomnolence, and this correlates broadly with the degree of sleep disruption. Early in the development of the disorder the daytime sleepiness is little more than often experienced by normal people after a few disturbed

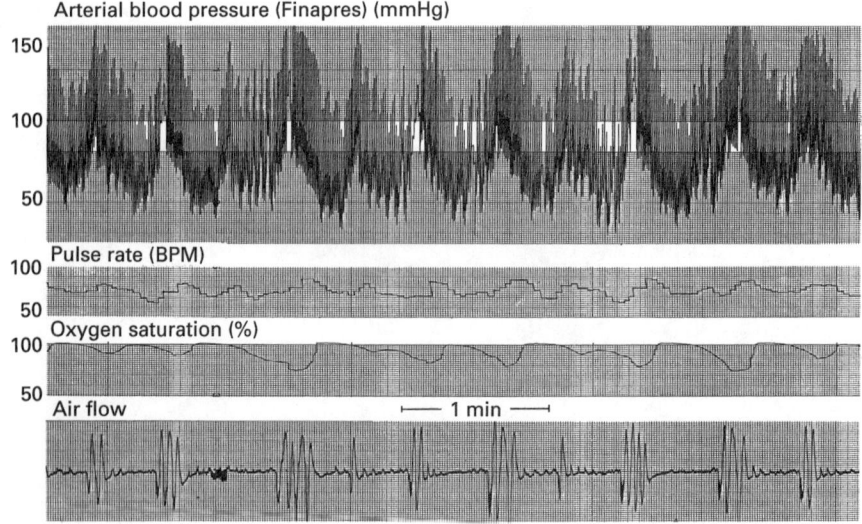

Fig. 4 Tracing (5 min) from a patient with obstructive sleep apnoea. The rises in blood pressure (top trace) and heart rate (second trace) coincide with the cessation of each apnoea and an arousal. During each apnoea (evident from the bottom airflow trace) each frustrated inspiratory effort is accompanied by a fall in blood pressure (pulsus paradoxus).

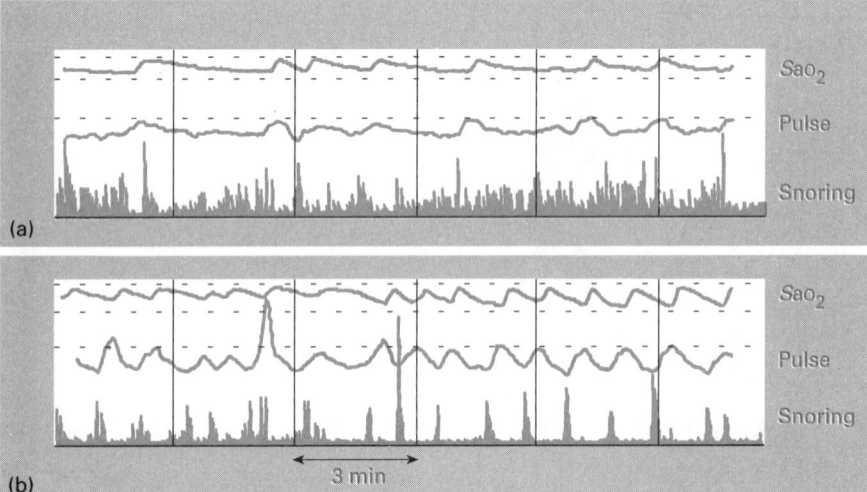

Fig. 5 Two tracings (each 18 min) of Sa_{O_2}, pulse rate, and snoring level in one subject at different times of the night: (a) continual snoring with hypopnoea (evident from the falls in Sa_{O_2}) and arousals (evident from the pulse rate rises and restoration of Sa_{O_2}, and confirmed by inspection of the video); the same subject supine, now with classical obstructive apnoeas evident from the snoring–silence–snoring pattern together with oscillations in the pulse and Sa_{O_2}.

Table 3 *Symptoms of obstructive sleep apnoea*

Most common (>60%)
  Loud snoring
  Excessive daytime sleepiness
  Restless sleep
  Unrefreshing sleep
  Nocturia
  Apparent personality changes
  Witnessed apnoeas

Less common (10–60%)
  Choking or shortness of breath sensations at night
  Reduced libido
  Nocturnal sweating
  Morning headaches

Rare (<10%)
  Enuresis
  Recurrent arousals/insomnia
  Nocturnal cough
  Symptomatic oesophageal reflux

Table 4 *Categories of patients for sleep studies*

1 Patients with a low probability of having a sleep and breathing disorder, e.g. snorers with no other relevant symptoms and an atypical physiognomy
2 Patients with a high probability of having obstructive sleep apnoea, i.e. with typical symptoms and physiognomy; only need a confirmatory and severity-assessing study
3 Patients in whom the diagnosis of obstructive sleep apnoea is already known and in whom the response to treatment is being followed
4 Patients with unexplained sleep-wake disorders where full information is required to make a diagnosis; an unclear screening study would also put a patient in this group.
5 Assessment of nocturnal hypoventilation syndromes (e.g., scoliosis); hypoxaemia is the dominant signal of interest initially

nights. Whilst occupied there is little difficulty in concentrating and staying awake, but once activities become more boring unwanted sleepiness intervenes. Initially this may be viewed as normal, such as falling asleep in front of the television every evening. As the sleep disruption worsens there will be interference with an increasing number of activities. Of particular importance is sleepiness whilst driving. Sleepiness can be devastating, particularly on long motorway journeys after dark, when sensory stimulation is low. Initially there will be lane wandering with sudden arousal and correction. Accidents involving driving off the road or driving into vehicles in front are much more common in patients with obstructive sleep apnoea. Sleepiness also impinges greatly on work performance and home life. The patient will develop a reputation for slothfulness and lack of interest.

It is important to ask the right questions to assess sleepiness. It is not the same as tiredness, which is a lack of energy or desire to get up and do anything. Because of the insidious onset of obstructive sleep apnoea, any sleepiness may be regarded as normal by the patient, and thus situational questions need to be asked such as 'How often do you have to pull off the road whilst driving owing to sleepiness?' rather than just 'Are you sleepy?' Sleepiness can be assessed in the sleep laboratory by measuring how long the patient takes to fall asleep on a number of occasions across the day. This is useful for research purposes but adds little to the clinical management of such patients. A list of other symptoms seen in obstructive sleep apnoea is given in Table 3.

A typical case history would be that of a middle-aged man complaining of increasing daytime sleepiness. It is usually some specific event that prompts initial consultation, such as falling asleep whilst driving, operating machinery, or during an important board meeting. There will be a long history of gradually worsening snoring with possibly witnessed apnoeas by the spouse, who will probably have moved out of the bedroom owing to the noise. There is likely to have been a weight gain over the last few years with an obesity index of greater than 30 kg/m² and a collar size of 17 inches or more. There is usually a history of fairly high alcohol intake and smoking. On examination there may be nasal stuffiness, evidence of a small lower jaw (such as teeth crowding or several extractions for this problem), and a small pharynx with mucosal bogginess and wrinkling. Of course, it should be stressed that not all these features are likely to be present in one individual.

Part of the investigation of such patients should include an assessment for precipitating factors such as hypothyroidism and acromegaly. Other factors such as mucopolysaccharidosis, pharyngeal tumours, tonsillar hypertrophy, neurological disorders, and significant retrognathia will be more obvious.

Diagnosis

Following the history and examination, further outpatient tests may be appropriate, for example thyroxine or growth-hormone estimations. Blood gases and simple lung function tests may be necessary if associated diurnal respiratory failure is suspected. A raised haemoglobin may also signify diurnal respiratory failure as will a raised venous [HCO_3^-]. Since obesity is common, a blood sugar test may be indicated.

Unless the presenting problem is clearly not sleep related, then some form of sleep study will be required. In the past the usual procedure was to employ full polysomnography which measured sleep state and respiratory variables (Fig. 3). This investigation is expensive and time consuming. The analysis is also skilled and time consuming, particularly if all the recurrent arousals are documented. The primary requirement of such sleep studies is to assess sleep fragmentation, establish if a respiratory cause is responsible, and decide if upper airway obstruction is the primary cause. Full polysomnography, properly interpreted, will usually allow this. The EEG and EMG will give good information on sleep disruption, and aspects of respiration can be assessed from rib-cage/abdominal movement transducers, oronasal airflow, and snoring and continuous oximeter recordings. However, there is considerable signal redundancy in such recordings, and the essential derivatives – sleep disruption and respiration – can be assessed in simpler ways (Fig. 5).

There is no single appropriate sleep study for all circumstances, and each investigation should be tailored to the clinical situation. Table 4 gives a breakdown into the usual clinical categories undergoing investigation. Category 1 patients (low probability of obstructive sleep apnoea) are increasingly being studied to prove that they do not have sleep apnoea and a variety of simple monitoring systems are in use. As long as these can demonstrate unfragmented sleep and no significant respiratory irregularity or obstruction (snoring), then they can confidently exclude significant obstructive sleep apnoea or snoring-induced arousals. Such systems could include continuous oximetry or rib-cage/abdominal monitoring, with some assessment of sleep from video, actigraph, or pulse rate recordings. Category 2 patients, where the diagnosis of obstructive sleep apnoea is considered highly likely, may only need oximetry or video recordings to confirm the diagnosis and assess severity if priority on a waiting list is required. Category 3 patients, in whom the diagnosis is already known, will need simple monitoring of a previously abnormal signal (e.g. oximetry) to confirm response to treatment. Category 5 patients (not yet discussed) are really being assessed for nocturnal hypoxaemia and initially need only oximetry. If overnight oximetry is abnormal, then a full polysomnographic study may be necessary to establish the exact cause (see later).

Category 4 patients are those in whom the diagnosis is not at all clear from the history and examination, or who have had an equivocal simpler test. In these patients much more information may be necessary to establish the diagnosis than can be provided from, for example, oximetry alone.

Owing to the uncertainties discussed in the earlier section on aetiology, the exact features to extract from sleep studies are not clear. Measurements of sleep disruption are crude, and the exact respiratory event capable of leading to arousal may vary between individuals, i.e. snoring, hypopnoea, or apnoea. The essential question being asked of the sleep study in obstructive sleep apnoea is: 'Does this patient have a sleep disruption syndrome due to sleep-related upper airway narrowing capable of explaining his daytime symptoms?' Since no specific figure such as 10 or 15 respiratory events per hour provides a cut-off for making this decision, precise calculation of these indices is not very helpful and indeed in any one individual they may vary considerably from night to night.

The sleep specialist has to decide whether to institute certain therapies for obstructive sleep apnoea, and this depends as much on symptoms as the sleep study findings. This is currently a clinical decision and should not depend on arbitrary thresholds from sleep studies.

Treatment

Once it is established that the patient's symptoms are likely to be due to sleep disruption from sleep-induced upper airway obstruction, then therapy has to be tailored to symptom severity.

Mild symptoms may resolve with simple treatments and advice (Table 5). Weight loss is undoubtedly effective, but is often very difficult to achieve. If the sleep disruption only occurs whilst supine (when upper airway obstruction tends to be worst), then learning to lie on one's side may be helpful. Stopping sedatives and evening alcohol can help. Initial enthusiasm for the tricyclic antidepressants has waned, although they may slightly improve mild cases. They are believed to work partly through REM sleep suppression and partly through improving upper airway tone. No other drug has shown any consistent effect.

If symptoms are severe, then there is essentially one effective therapy – nasal continuous positive airway pressure. This treatment involves wearing a small mask (Fig. 6) over the nose whilst asleep that is kept at pressures above atmospheric by a low pressure pump. Pressures in the region of 10 cmH$_2$O are enough to splint open the pharynx and resist collapse, thus allowing unobstructed breathing and undisturbed sleep (Fig. 7). The response is dramatic, in terms of both the physiology and the daytime symptoms which resolve rapidly, even after one night of treatment. The unpleasantness and unaesthetic appearance of this treatment repels patients initially but, once the benefits have been experienced, acceptance is high.

In the early days of such therapy, devising suitable masks was a problem. However, off-the-shelf systems with comfortable soft masks are now available for home use at about £400 each. Such a system will last for years and represents extraordinary value for money when the enormous improvement in patient functioning is considered.

The other main treatment whose popularity is decreasing is uvulopalatopharyngoplasty. This operation consists of removing part of the soft palate and any residual tonsils, and 'tightening up' the side-walls of the pharynx. Although it is good at reducing snoring, its success rate at treating obstructive sleep apnoea is not so good; approximately 50 per cent of patients experience a 50 per cent improvement in the number of apnoeas per hour. Attempts to improve the selection of patients who might respond better to this operation have had very limited success, although thin patients with large soft palates, residual tonsils, and milder disease do the best. This operation may have a more significant role in the treatment of snoring-induced arousals than full apnoeas, although this is not established yet.

Other operative techniques involving advancement of the mandible (and sometimes the maxilla) may be appropriate in highly selected cases. Tracheostomy was the first therapy ever tried and was of course very effective. Despite the subsequent problems of such surgery, tracheostomy may still be appropriate in occasional patients.

Once established on nasal continuous positive airway pressure, a patient with obstructive sleep apnoea is likely to require it for life unless he can lose a significant amount of weight. This may only be achieved through gastric surgery, such as silastic ring gastroplasty to reduce food consumption.

Table 5 *Advice for patients with mild to moderate obstructive sleep apnoea usually due to postural dependence*

1 Learn to sleep on your side and avoid sleeping on your back
2 No alcohol after 18.00 hours
3 No sedatives
4 Lose weight
5 Stop smoking
6 Keep the nose as clear as possible

Epidemiology

The prevalence of symptomatic obstructive sleep apnoea is hard to establish. The main problem is the uncertainty over definition discussed earlier. The prevalence will depend on where an arbitrary cut-off is drawn. In a recent study about 0.3 per cent of men aged 35 to 65 years clearly had severe symptomatic obstructive sleep apnoea requiring nasal continuous positive airway pressure (CPAP) therapy and were responsive to such treatment. However, about 5 per cent had more than five dips per hour in SaO$_2$ of more than 4 per cent SaO$_2$, one suggested threshold for normality. However, most of these subjects were not apparently symptomatic. Overall in this study sleepiness correlated with snoring, and indeed more sleepiness seemed to be due to snoring than classical sleep apnoea. Other studies in Israel and Italy have found prevalences of 'significant' sleep apnoea in the 0.5–2 per cent range.

Predictors of sleep apnoea in these prevalence studies have been obesity, snoring, age, self-reported sleepiness, and alcohol consumption. Snoring is more common in men than women, and obstructive sleep apnoea itself is about 10 to 20 times more common in men. The prevalence in women probably increases after the menopause.

If these prevalence studies are correct, then obstructive sleep apnoea is more common than sarcoidosis and fibrosing alveolitis combined; every chest physician in the United Kingdom should have about 100 patients on nasal CPAP.

Prognosis and long-term complications

Although the main reason for treating obstructive sleep apnoea is to relieve the daytime symptoms, mainly sleepiness, there is also evidence that these patients have an increased cardiovascular mortality (Fig. 8).

Fig. 6 One of the soft silicone nasal masks used in the treatment of obstructive sleep apnoea.

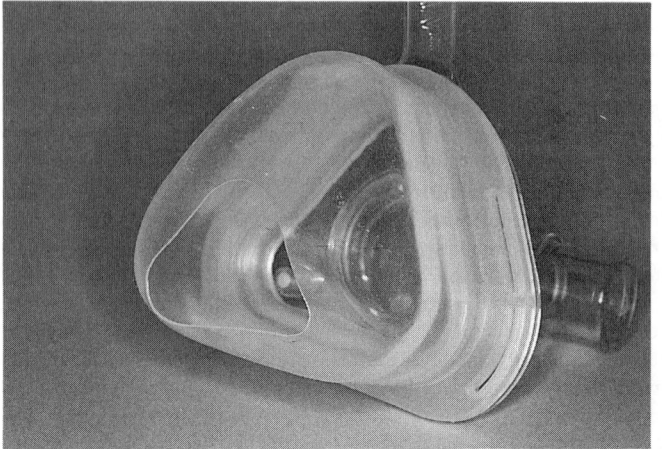

Two studies have looked at the long-term survival of patients with treated obstructive sleep apnoea and compared them with some form of untreated control patients. Both found an increased mortality due to cardiovascular effects such as myocardial infarction and stroke in the untreated group. The cause of this increased mortality is not clear and a variety of hypotheses have been advanced. The main problem is that, because a variety of cardiovascular risk factors also contribute to the production of obstructive sleep apnoea (central obesity, smoking, alcohol), it is difficult to identify the real contribution made independently by obstructive sleep apnoea to cardiovascular deaths. Possibilities include sustained hypertension, intermittent hypertension, increased catecholamine release, hypoxia-induced cardiac arrhythmias, insulin resistance, hyperlipidaemia, and left ventricular hypertrophy. As yet none of these risk factors have been shown to differ between patients with obstructive sleep apnoea and well-matched controls except for the episodic blood pressure rises with each apnoea (Fig. 4). These surges in blood pressure may themselves be harmful to the vascular system, as well as raising the mean 24 h blood pressure which will be a risk factor in its own right.

Treatment with nasal CPAP prevents these surges in blood pressure by abolishing the apnoea-induced arousals, and this may be the mechanism by which CPAP improves mortality in obstructive sleep apnoea, although there are many other possible explanations.

In addition to reducing cardiovascular mortality, nasal CPAP produces a demonstrable improvement in vigilance and sleepiness. This improved performance in a driving simulator and will presumably lessen the chances of driving accidents.

Objective tests of vigilance and sleepiness do not completely return to normal after nasal CPAP, and it may be that patients accept mild degrees of their symptoms in return for not having to use their CPAP devices all night and every night; compliance studies suggest that this is the case.

Conclusions

There has been a move away from considering obstructive sleep apnoea as a condition that one either has or does not have. There is a continuum from light intermittent snoring through to all-night obstructive sleep apnoea, and this situation can be usefully compared with hypertension. This is also a condition with a continuum of severity, variability in the

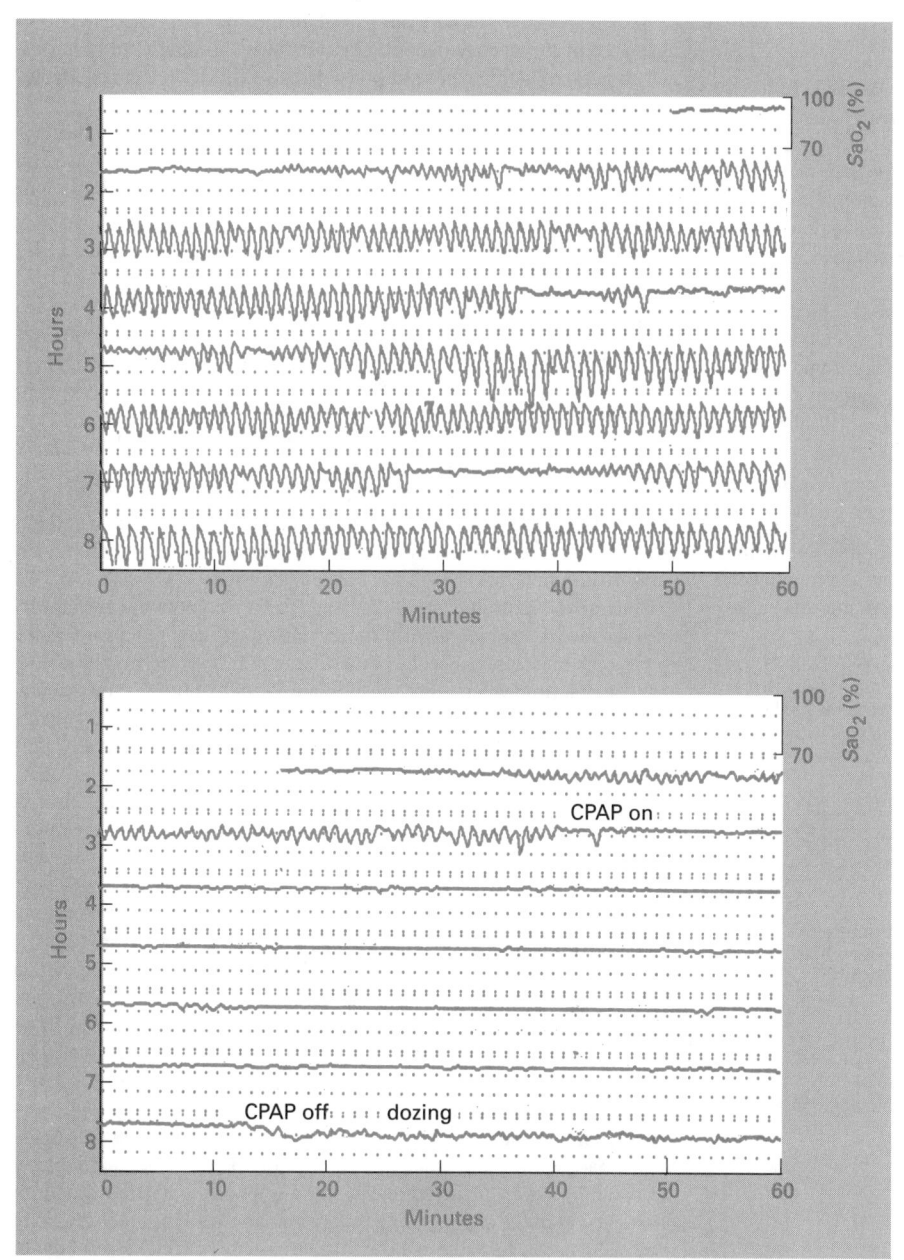

Fig. 7 Two all-night oximetry tracings from a patient with obstructive sleep apnoea before treatment and during his first night on nasal CPAP. Each tracing starts top left and finishes bottom right. Each tracing is continuous for 8 h with the scale for each individual line scaled 70 per cent–100 per cent SaO_2.

measurement, only moderate correlation between the measured abnormality and the physiological consequences, uncertainty over the most relevant way to measure it (one-off versus 24 h blood pressure monitoring), and the fact that some of the target organ damage may not be due to just the hypertension (e.g. atheroma). In addition, benefits of treatment have to be weighed against its side-effects. Sleep-induced upper airway obstruction should really be viewed in a similar way.

Sleep-induced hypoventilation and central sleep apnoea

So far we have discussed the sleep-related disorders of breathing that are due to sleep-induced narrowing of the upper airway. Breathing during sleep may also decrease, not because of obstruction but because of a reduction in central output to the respiratory muscles – so-called central, rather than obstructive, apnoea (Fig. 3). There are many causes for central sleep apnoea or hypoventilation, and Table 6 shows one way of classifying them. Some of the central apnoeas disturb sleep and present with daytime sleepiness, whereas others present more with symptoms of respiratory failure, such as morning headaches with cyanosis and confusion, ankle oedema, and shortness of breath on exertion.

Absent ventilatory drive

Brain-stem abnormalities may damage the areas responsible for automatic chemical control of ventilation. Whilst awake, the wakefulness-related ventilatory drive may be adequate to maintain PaO_2 and $PaCO_2$ levels, but on falling asleep, drive falls or even disappears with marked hypoventilation (or apnoea) and hypoxaemia; arousal is then necessary to restore the blood gases. This failure of brain-stem automatic control (known as Ondine's curse) can be congenital, or may be acquired as the result of a stroke, infection, surgical damage, multiple sclerosis, or compression by tumour or syrinx.

Reduction of chemical drive can occur as a secondary problem when ventilation is reduced by mechanical problems such as chronic airways obstruction or weak respiratory muscles. It appears that chronic under-ventilation can lead to blunting of ventilatory drive, perhaps through alteration in acid–base buffering in the brain-stem. This will also lead to marked falls in ventilation on entering sleep.

Unstable ventilatory drive

The wakefulness-related ventilatory drive has a considerable stabilizing effect on ventilation by preventing it from falling below a certain level. If reasons for ventilatory instability exist then, by removing this stabi-

Fig. 8 Long-term survival without a cardiovascular death of 196 patients with obstructive sleep apnoea. The two groups consisted of one with 70 patients who accepted the definitive treatment then available of tracheostomy, and one with 126 patients who declined such therapy and merely attempted weight loss. (Reproduced with permission from C. Guilleminault and M. Partinen (1990). *Obstructive sleep apnoea syndrome*, Raven Press, New York.)

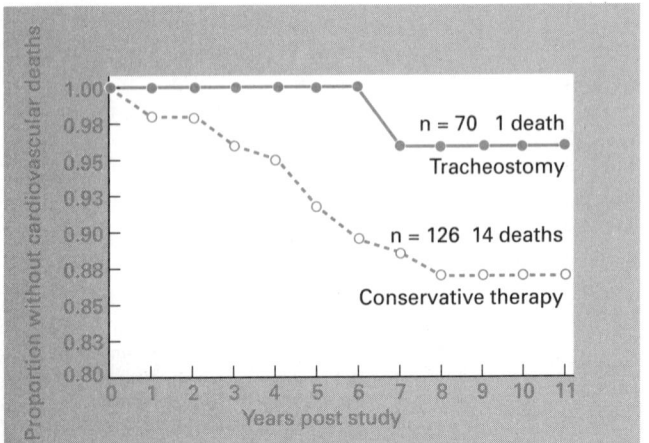

lizing effect, sleep will allow periodic respiration to develop. The usual provoker of instability is an increased drive to breath; control theory shows that increasing the gain in a feedback system promotes instability through overshoot and undershoot. One of the best examples of increased drive is the hypoxaemia of altitude. The hypoxaemia steepens the carbon dioxide response line and promotes instability, and when sleep occurs there is the usual fall in ventilation. Both the resulting extra hypoxaemia and the return of ventilation due to the rise in carbon dioxide provoke arousal. This arousal provides extra ventilatory drive which restores the blood gases, and the cycle repeats. Thus periodic breathing with recurrent arousals is very common at altitude, with the expected daytime consequence of sleepiness and complaints of insomnia. Acetazolamide produces a metabolic acidosis and increases ventilation overall, the hypoxaemia is relieved, and thus the ventilatory response to carbon dioxide becomes less steep. Both these factors restore stability and reduce the periodic respiration.

In left ventricular failure there is extra ventilatory drive from stimulation of interstitial lung receptors. This also provokes instability in conjunction with the longer circulation time seen in heart failure. This so-called Cheyne–Stokes breathing is quite common in heart failure, and through sleep disruption produces daytime sleepiness and complaints of nocturnal dyspnoea (Fig. 9). The patient is usually aware that the dyspnoea disappears rapidly on arousal, unlike the paroxysmal nocturnal dyspnoea of pulmonary oedema. Treatment with either overnight oxygen or acetazolamide can sometimes greatly reduce the periodicity and improve both sleep quality and symptoms.

This instability of respiratory control can occur in normal subjects in the early stages of sleep or if sleep is disturbed for other reasons. This is because sleep is oscillating back and forwards to wakefulness with ventilatory drive consequently oscillating as well.

REM sleep apnoeas

During normal REM sleep the phasic bursts of eye movements are associated with transient falls in ventilation, and even the occurrence of apnoeas. The rib-cage muscles are affected most, but diaphragmatic excursion can also fall. Such periodicities are entirely normal.

As discussed earlier, the REM sleep inhibition of most muscles (apart from the diaphragm) can greatly reduce overall ventilation when accessory muscles of respiration are needed for breathing. Thus there can be profound falls in ventilation and SaO_2 on entering REM sleep in patients with neuromuscular diseases, chest-wall abnormalities, and chronic airways obstruction.

Generalized neuromuscular diseases tend to involve the respiratory muscles in concert with other muscles. However, in some disorders the respiratory muscles, particularly the diaphragm, may be involved very early on at a time when other muscles are virtually normal. A particular example of this is adult-type acid maltase deficiency, where patients may present in respiratory failure whilst still able to walk normally. The REM-sleep-related hypoxaemia may be the first sign that there are problems, and it is not known whether this actually accelerates the onset of eventual diurnal respiratory failure or is merely a marker that respiratory failure will soon follow. Sometimes there may be associated upper airway obstruction during REM sleep which leads to even larger falls in SaO_2. Overnight oximetry studies will indicate the degree of hypoxaemia but will not establish if there is additional upper airway obstruction.

There has been great interest in the REM-sleep-related hypoxaemia seen in chronic airways obstruction. It was thought possible at one point that these hypoxic episodes might be the reason why some of these patients developed respiratory failure but others did not. However, it appears that REM sleep hypoventilation and a fall in PaO_2 is fairly universal in this group of patients. If the patient is initially well oxygenated and on the flat part of the haemoglobin dissociation curve, the fall in SaO_2 (which is usually what is monitored) is not particularly dramatic; however, if the patient is initially poorly oxygenated and on the steep part of the curve, similar hypoventilation will produce dramatic falls in SaO_2. As yet there is no evidence that these REM sleep falls in

Table 6 *Suggested breakdown of causes of central apnoea*

Type of central apnoea	Examples	Daytime arterial CO_2 level
1 Absent or reduced ventilatory drive (Ondine's curse)	Brain-stem damage or congenital abnormality Acquired blunting, e.g. secondary to lung disease	Raised
2 Unstable respiratory drive	Sleep onset, hypoxaemia, altitude, heart failure	Normal or low
3 REM-related oscillations	Normal in REM sleep Due to neuromuscular disorders and respiratory muscle weakness	Normal or raised
4 Reflex central apnoea	Pharyngeal collapse inhibits inspiration	Normal
5 Apparent central apnoea (wrongly diagnosed)	Respiratory muscle weakness or gross obesity cause chest-wall movement transducers to fail to demonstrate any ventilatory effort during obstructive apnoeas	Normal or raised

Sao_2 are contributing to the morbidity and mortality of patients with chronic airflow obstruction, although some centres have shown that overnight oxygen therapy reduces arousals, thus improving sleep quality.

Reflex apnoea

Central respiratory output can be modified by a number of reflexes from receptors in the upper airway. There appears to be a reflex from the pharynx that inhibits inspiratory flow when the pharynx is being sucked in and collapsed. This makes teleological sense as a slowing of inspiratory flow would reduce the collapsing tendency. There are some patients with pharyngeal collapse who, instead of struggling to inspire against the blocked airway, simply stop breathing until they finally arouse, presumably in this case due to the fall in Pao_2 and rise in $Paco_2$. This then appears as a central apnoea despite the aetiology being pharyngeal collapse. This tends to happen when the patient is supine (with snoring or ordinary obstructive apnoeas when decubitus), and if the pharynx is anaesthetized experimentally then inspiratory attempts return, suggesting that a superficial receptor is responsible. These patients usually present with histories suggestive of obstructive sleep apnoea and respond to nasal CPAP.

Apparent central apnoea

The diagnosis of central apnoea depends on failing to detect evidence of respiratory effort when airflow at the nose and mouth stops. Surface measurements of rib-cage and abdominal movement are usually used as evidence of continuing respiratory effort. However, in two circumstances, marked obesity and muscular weakness, the surface transducers may fail to register that inspiratory efforts are being made. Obesity lessens the sensitivity of the transducers, and with muscle weakness the inspiratory muscles may not be able to move detectably against the closed upper airway.

Overnight ventilation for central sleep apnoea or hypoventilation

The chronic respiratory failure associated with some neurological disorders (e.g. acid maltase deficiency, post-poliomyelitis syndrome, motor neurone disease, Duchenne dystrophy) will progress to death even when quality of life is otherwise very good. The same is true of chest-wall restrictive disorders such as scoliosis and that developing many years after extensive thoracoplasty. However, the respiratory failure can be reversed by supporting ventilation overnight. The response to this treatment can be dramatic, with resolution of all symptoms and restoration of normal blood gases even when off the ventilator during the day. The mechanism by which supporting ventilation at night corrects respiratory failure is not clear and there are various possibilities. It may simply be that the respiratory muscles are rested so that they can respond better to the demands of the respiratory centre during the day. It may be that improving the blood gases at night, and preventing the marked REM sleep deteriorations, leads to a resetting of the respiratory centre back towards normal (a reversal of acquired blunting of drive), perhaps through changes in acid–base status around the brain-stem control cen-

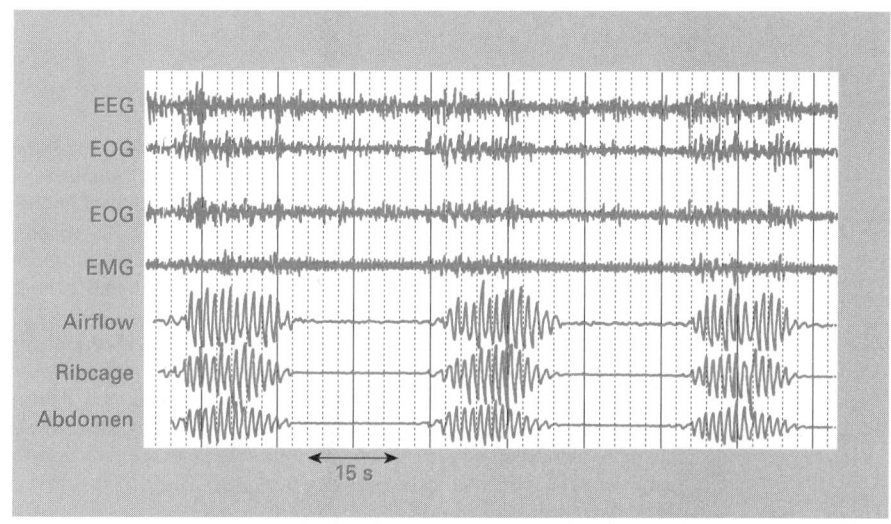

EEG

EOG

EOG

EMG

Airflow

Ribcage

Abdomen

15 s

Fig. 9 Tracing of Cheyne–Stokes respiration from a patient with poor left ventricular function but no radiological or clinical evidence of current pulmonary oedema. With each return of respiration there is arousal from sleep (not clearly visible with this compressed EEG tracing).

tres. Tricyclic antidepressants such as protriptyline can virtually abolish the REM sleep periods (and thus the associated hypoxaemia) and have been shown to improve daytime blood gases temporarily. This suggests that just abolishing these particularly hypoxic periods can help. A third explanation of the benefits of supporting ventilation overnight is that by increasing chest-wall and lung excursion (tidal volumes in excess of the voluntary vital capacity are sometimes obtained) overall respiratory compliance improves, allowing the muscles to work more efficiently. Whatever the explanation, there is no doubt that this is a life-saving therapy that in certain conditions can add decades of active life.

Most of the original techniques to support ventilation overnight evolved from the iron lung which was developed to support polio-myelitis victims. By evacuating the air from around the chest it expands the lungs, recreating the normal way of breathing. A range of devices involving airtight jackets and shells over the chest were developed, but required much attention to detail and often individual tailor-made systems. A specific complication was that once spontaneous ventilatory drive had been abolished, upper airway collapse would occur during the inspiratory phase and greatly limit efficacy. The recent development of comfortable nasal masks has revolutionized the overnight ventilation of these patients. Positive pressure ventilation can be used via a similar nose mask to that used for nasal CPAP (Fig. 6). Although there are still many problems to be overcome when establishing patients on such equipment (particularly mask comfort and air leaks through the mouth), the systems can be bought off the shelf ready to use (current cost approximately £3500). Most units now use nasal positive pressure ventilation in preference to the negative pressure systems.

Electrical pacing of the diaphragm is occasionally used for supporting ventilation in conditions where the phrenic nerve and diaphragm are intact and the problem is more central. This involves the implantation of bilateral phrenic electrodes and induction coils under the skin that are activated by external induction coils.

REFERENCES

Gastaut, H., Tassinari, C.A., and Duron, B. (1966). Polygraphic study of the episodic diurnal and nocturnal (hypnic and respiratory) manifestations of the Pickwick syndrome. *Brain Research,* **2**, 167–86.

Gaultier, C., Escourrous, P., and Curzi-Dascalova, L. (1991). *Sleep and cardiorespiratory control.* John Libbey, Montrouge. Collection of short reviews on cardiovascular aspects of sleep apnoea.

Guilleminault, C., Stoohs, R., and Duncan, S. (1991). Snoring (1). Daytime sleepiness in regular heavy snorers. *Chest,* **99**, 40–8.

Phillipson, E.A. and Bradley, T.D. (1992). Breathing disorders in sleep. *Clinics in Chest Medicine,* **13** (3). Most recent collection of authoritative reviews on the subject.

Remmers, J.E., de Broot, W.J., Sauerland, E.K., and Anch, A.M. (1978). Pathogenesis of upper airway occlusion during sleep. *Journal of Applied Physiology,* **44**, 931–8.

Stradling, J.R. and Crosby, J. (1991). Predictors and prevalence of obstructive sleep apnoea and snoring in 1001 middle-aged men. *Thorax,* **46**, 85–90.

Sullivan, C.E., Issa, F.G., Berthon-Jones, M., and Eves, L. (1981). Reversal of obstructive sleep apnoea by continuous positive airway pressure applied through the nares. *Lancet,* **i**, 862–5.

17.14.3 The management of respiratory failure

(a) Acute respiratory failure: intensive care

C. GARRARD

The management of acute respiratory failure consists of the following:

- establishing an airway;
- administering oxygen;
- maintaining adequate ventilation;
- identifying and treating the underlying cause;
- monitoring Sao_2 (pulse oximetry), ECG, and vital signs.

Establish an airway

Simple manoeuvres to re-establish and clear the airway must always be followed. These include positioning and maintaining the head and neck in the 'sniff position', inspection of the oropharynx, suctioning, and if necessary the insertion of an oral or pharyngeal airway.

ENDOTRACHEAL INTUBATION

If a satisfactory airway cannot be established by the above means, endotracheal intubation must be performed. Orotracheal intubation is particularly suited to emergency intubation, while nasotracheal intubation requires a little extra time. Coagulation defects or thrombocytopenia make nasotracheal intubation inadvisable due to risk of serious haemorrhage. Whatever technique is selected, intubation should be performed in a safe and expeditious manner by the most experienced clinician available. Neuromuscular relaxant drugs to facilitate intubation should only be used by experienced personnel. The complications of endotracheal intubation are due to occlusion or displacement of the tube and to airway trauma. The appropriate endotracheal tube size is 8–9 mm internal diameter for most adult males and 7–8 mm internal diameter for women. For children, a rough calculation using the child's age in years divided by 4 plus 4.0 will provide the tube internal diameter in millimetres. These smaller tubes are generally uncuffed.

It is essential that the endotracheal tube be securely anchored and the cuff inflation pressure restricted to less than 30 cmH$_2$O. High-volume, low-pressure cuffed tubes are generally recommended, and cuff inflation pressures should be checked periodically using an anaeroid manometer and adjusted accordingly. Using higher cuff pressures does not improve airway protection against aspiration, but only serves to damage the tracheal mucosa and risk later subglottic stenosis.

Difficulties with endotracheal intubation can be encountered in patients with a short 'bull' neck or receding lower jaw. Any patient with restricted neck and jaw movements (rheumatoid arthritis or cervical spine injury) or with abnormal oropharyngeal anatomy (tumour or trauma) should also be considered to pose difficulties for intubation.

There are several options when a difficult intubation is anticipated. Inhalational anesthesia by face mask can facilitate intubation, but under no circumstances must muscle relaxants be given unless satisfactory airway access can be ensured. Awake intubation can be performed with topical anaesthesia. Blind nasal intubation or intubation using a fibrotic bronchoscope or laryngoscope requires considerable skill and training but may be the safest option in establishing an airway.

TRACHEOSTOMY

Tracheostomy should only replace endotracheal intubation for specific indications and not merely after the elapse of a predefined time interval. Using modern endotracheal tubes and techniques, endotracheal intubation can be tolerated without permanent harm to the airway for months if necessary. It has been shown that the greater part of mucosal damage is done in the first week of intubation with little additional change thereafter.

However, much can be gained by the judicious selection of patients for tracheostomy either as the preferred primary route for airway access or as a replacement for endotracheal intubation. The common indications for replacement include the need for chronic or permanent ventilation, to help weaning after previously failed attempts at extubation, to facilitate oral nutrition, or the presence of upper airway complications of endotracheal intubation.

The same principles of cuff pressure management apply to both tracheostomy tubes and endotracheal tubes. Tracheostomy is associated with fewer, but more serious, complications than endotracheal intubation. These include tube displacement, pneumothorax, severe haemorrhage, and wound infection.

MINITRACHEOSTOMY

Minitracheostomy tubes are cuffless tubes, 3.5–4.0 mm diameter, inserted percutaneously through the cricothyroid membrane, usually under local anaesthesia. A Seldinger technique for introduction of the minitracheostomy tube offers an alternative to the direct trochar method. Minitracheostomy allows suction of lung secretions without the need for formal endotracheal intubation or tracheostomy. However, minitracheostomy tubes cannot be used for conventional ventilation, may result in local haemorrhagic complications, and may be a source of infection.

CRICOTHYROIDOTOMY

A cricothyroidotomy may be needed in life-threatening, upper airway obstructions where endotracheal intubation is not feasible and there is insufficient time to perform tracheostomy. A full-sized tracheostomy tube (6–8 mm internal diameter) can be inserted under local anaesthetic to facilitate mechanical ventilation.

The administration of oxygen

Although there is limited safety information regarding oxygen therapy, the long-term administration of 50 or 100 per cent oxygen for less than 24 h is usually considered acceptable. Nevertheless, hypoxia should never be tolerated because of a concern over oxygen toxicity. Oxygen can be delivered by a variety of means depending upon the concentration desired and the patient's minute ventilation. Details of some oxygen delivery systems are shown in Table 1.

Oxygen should be given in such concentrations as to prevent prolonged or even transient episodes of hypoxia. The well-recognized caveat that only controlled (limited) oxygen concentrations should be given to patients with chronic obstructive lung disease must be borne in mind. The response to oxygen therapy can best be measured continuously by pulse oximetry (Sa_{O_2}) or by intermittent arterial blood gas sampling.

Mechanical ventilation

The main indications for mechanical ventilation are ventilatory failure, as indicated by a rising Pa_{CO_2}, or severe hypoxaemia that cannot be corrected with high concentrations of inspired oxygen. The provision of efficient and safe mechanical ventilation is a skill that must be mastered by all physicians practising critical care. The basic principles still pertain despite the introduction of complex and sophisticated mechanical ventilators and the overabundance of studies claiming superiority of certain techniques over others. The application of common sense and sound physiological doctrine will serve better than devotion to an attractive technical innovation.

INDICATIONS FOR INTUBATION AND MECHANICAL VENTILATION

Mechanical ventilation is not to be undertaken lightly, since it is associated with much morbidity and some mortality, but failure to intervene promptly can clearly have catastrophic consequences for the patient. The indications for mechanical ventilation fall into two broad categories: (1) inadequate alveolar ventilation with increasing P_{CO_2}; and (2) inadequate gas exchange with increasing $P(A - a)_{O_2}$ and arterial hypoxaemia. Guidelines for mechanical ventilation in acute respiratory failure are

Table 1 *Oxygen delivery systems*

Method of delivery	Fi_{O_2} achieved
Nasal cannulae (1–2 l/min)	0.24–0.30
Venturi mask	0.24–0.50
Partial rebreathing mask	0.60–0.80
Non-rebreathing reservoir mask	Up to 0.90
Anaesthetic face mask of endotracheal tube	Up to 1.0

Fi_{O_2}, fractional inspired oxygen concentration

shown in Table 2. The physician must always exercise clinical judgement in the interpretation of these guidelines and anticipate problems before they arise. For example, one of the simplest criteria for mechanical ventilation is a respiratory rate of 35 breaths/min or more. If a patient is clearly fatiguing with a respiratory rate of 30 breaths/min, then an early elective intubation is preferred to an emergency procedure an hour or so later. Similarly, a progressive fall in vital capacity in a patient with myasthenia gravis receiving full medication may indicate ventilatory support although the critical value of less than 15 ml/kg is not broached.

The treatment of hypoventilatory respiratory failure consists of assisting ventilatory function, usually by mechanical external means. Figure 1 shows a flow diagram outlining the decision process involved in the assessment of patients who may require mechanical ventilation.

FEATURES AND APPLICATIONS OF A MECHANICAL VENTILATOR

The control mechanism that cycles the ventilator from inspiration to expiration may be electromechanical or electronic (utilizing microprocessor technology). Modern mechanical ventilators tend to fall into the latter category and offer a degree of sophistication that has greatly improved the safety and efficiency of mechanical ventilation.

Most adult patients are supported on volume- and time-cycled pressure-limited ventilators (volume ventilator or flow generator). Volume- and time-cycled ventilators deliver preset tidal volumes regardless of changes in lung compliance or impedance. The price paid for this desirable characteristic is that the inflation pressures must rise to overcome the mechanical load. To protect the patient against inadvertently high pressures, a pressure limit must be set. When this limit is reached the ventilator terminates inspiration regardless of the volume delivered and triggers an alarm.

Neonates and infants may be satisfactorily ventilated using time-cycled pressure-limited devices (pressure ventilator or pressure generator). The pressure-limited paediatric ventilator offers simplicity and reliable ventilation, although the tidal volume delivered is difficult to measure. These are not serious limitations in the premature neonate, and pressure-limited ventilation is the preferred technique.

Specifically designed compact light-weight ventilators, driven by cylinder oxygen and utilizing fluid logic circuits, are available for transporting ventilator-dependent patients. They are pressure generators and can be used for either adults or children. By entraining air, a choice of either 60 or 100 per cent oxygen is available.

MODES OF VENTILATION

Depending upon the indications for ventilation, the clinician must select the mode of ventilation, choose the ventilation parameters, and adjust the ventilator alarms. The most commonly available ventilator modes are as follows.

(1) control mechanical ventilation;
(2) assist control (triggered ventilation, volume-cycled);

Table 2 *Guidelines for introduction of mechanical ventilation*

General indications in acute respiratory failure (After
Pontoppin *et al.* 1972)

1. Inadequate ventilation

   Indicated by:
   (a) Apnoea, upper airway obstruction, unprotected airway
   (b) Respiratory rate >35 breaths/min (normal range 10–20 breaths/min)
   (c) Vital capacity < 15 ml/kg (normal range 65–75 ml/kg)
   (d) Tidal volume < 5 ml/kg (normal range 5–7 ml/kg)
   (e) Negative inspiratory force <25 cmH$_2$O (normal range 75–100 cmH$_2$O)
   (f) PaCO$_2$ > 8 kPa (60 mmHg) (normal range 4.7–6.3 kPa (35–47 mmHg)
   (g) V_D/V_T > 0.6 (normal range < 0.3)

2. Inadequate gas exchange oxygenation

   Indicated by:
   (a) PaO$_2$ < 8 kPa (60 mmHg) on FIO$_2$ > 0.6
   (b) P(A−a)O$_2$ > 47 kPa (350 mmHg) on FIO$_2$ = 1.0 (normal range 3.3–8.7 kPa (25–65 mmHg)

Specific indications, with or without previous respiratory
pathology

3. Chronic obstructive lung disease
   (a) Failure of conservative measures
   (b) Inability to cooperate with care
   (c) Decreased consciousness
   (d) Cardiac instability
   (e) Apnoea
   (f) Severe respiratory acidosis
   (g) Acute management of nocturnal obstructive hypoventilation

4. Chronic restrictive lung disease
   (a) Severe hypoxaemia
   (b) Fatigue and impending exhaustion

5. Severe acute asthma
   (a) Failure of conservative measures
   (b) Obtundation
   (c) Cardiac instability
   (d) Increasing PaCO$_2$
   (e) Fatigue and impending exhaustion

6. Head trauma
   (a) Unconscious
   (b) Unprotected airway
   (c) Cerebral oedema
   (d) Apnoea or global hypoventilation

7. Chest trauma
   (a) Flail chest with hypoventilation and hypoxaemia
   (b) Pulmonary contusion with hypoxaemia

8. Neuromuscular weakness
   (a) Apnoea or progressive hypoventilation (see above)
   (b) Airway protection, nocturnal hypoventilation/hypoxaemia
   (c) Organophosphate poisoning

9. Other neurological disorders
   (a) Status epilepticus
   (b) Tetanus
   (c) High cervical spine injury

10. Upper airway protection
   (a) Loss of consciousness
   (b) Neck and oropharyngeal trauma
   (c) Epiglottitis
   (d) Acute neuromuscular event

11. Drug overdose
   Apnoea, hypoventilation, airway protection, seizures

After C.S. Garrard (1994). *Oxford textbook of surgery*, Oxford University Press.

(3) intermittent mandatory ventilation;
(4) pressure support (triggered ventilation, pressure-cycled)
(5) others.

Control mechanical ventilation provides time- and volume-cycled pressure-limited breaths at the preset rates, but does not allow the patient to breathe spontaneously. This mode is suitable for the paralysed or heavily sedated patient.

Assist control or triggered ventilation synchronizes the ventilator to the patient's own respiratory rhythm, delivering a volume-preset pressure-limited tidal volume. A trigger sensitivity must be selected (usually −0.5 to −2.0 cmH$_2$O) by which the patient can initiate volume preset breaths above the set rates. Patients have a tendency to hyperventilate on assist control. As a safety requirement, a high respiratory rate alarm is needed and a 'back-up' ventilation rate must be set in the event of apnoea. Assist control is better tolerated than CMV and the patient requires less sedation.

Intermittent mandatory ventilation was originally devised for weaning, but is now widely adopted as a maintenance mode. It provides the opportunity for the patient to breathe spontaneously and to supplement the positive pressure minute ventilation. In the standard intermittent mandatory ventilation mode there is a theoretical risk of stacking a ventilator breath on top of a spontaneous breath. However, this does not appear to be a significant problem, and an appropriately set pressure

Fig. 1 Respiratory failure algorithm.

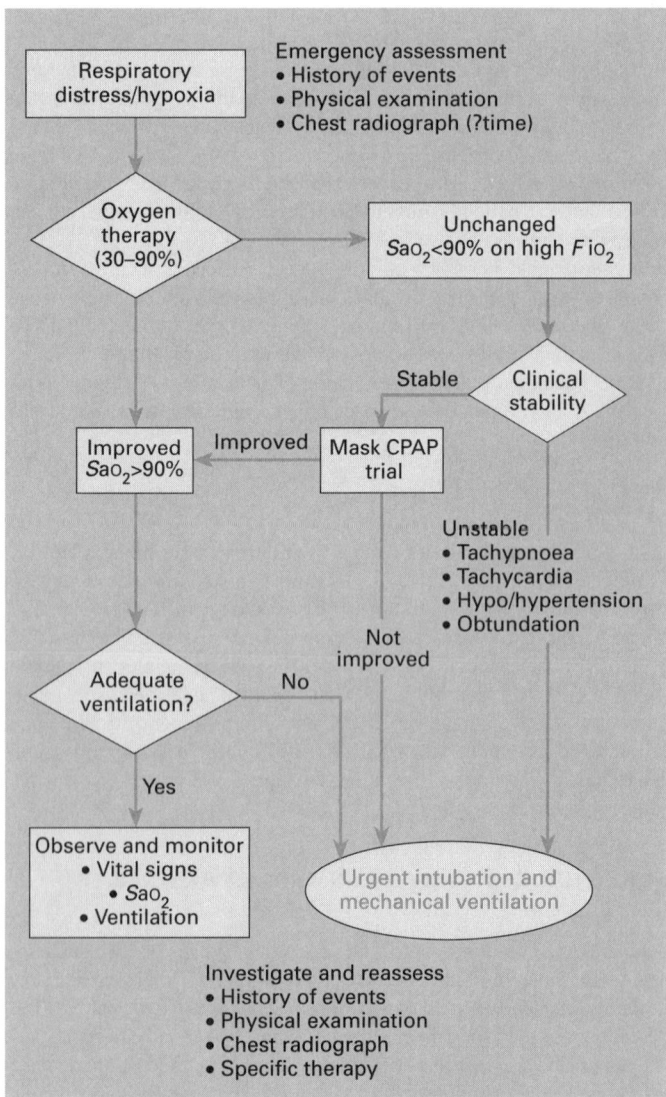

limit should prevent this from causing inadvertent overinflation of the lungs. More modern ventilators utilize the triggering or assist facility to synchronize the intermittent mandatory ventilation breaths with the patient's own spontaneous breathing pattern (synchronized intermittent mandatory ventilation). The intermittent mandatory ventilation mode is intended as partial ventilation support. With the patient taking spontaneous breaths, intermittent mandatory ventilation is better tolerated than control mechanical ventilation. It results in lower mean airway pressures, has less effect on the cardiovascular system, and allows the patient to regulate their own PCO_2 at least to some degree.

Pressure support uses a triggering facility to deliver, not a volume preset breath as in assist control, but a pressure-limited breath (i.e. as with paediatric pressure ventilation). The inspiratory flow rate is usually high so as to minimize phase lag and the work of breathing. Pressure support may be used alone or in conjunction with synchronized intermittent mandatory ventilation when it assists spontaneous breaths. Pressure support provides an efficient maintenance and weaning mode that is well tolerated by the patient. The trigger mechanism is usually a negative pressure threshold, but some ventilators trigger on changes in circuit gas flow which potentially could be more sensitive and reduce the work of breathing.

Other modes of ventilation, such as pressure release, high frequency and inverse I/E ratio ventilation, have their proponents. Evidence to indicate significant superiority of these modes over conventional methods of ventilation is not convincing. High frequency ventilation in its various forms has been recommended for use following reconstructive laryngeal, tracheal, or bronchial surgery, or for patients with bronchopleural or bronchocutaneous fistulae. Even these applications may not offer much advantage, if any, over conventional modes. Mandatory minute ventilation is an innovative mode whereby the combined spontaneous and mechanical ventilation must reach a minimum preset level. As the patient's spontaneous ventilation increases, the mechanically assisted breaths become fewer. Individual ventilators vary in their ability to achieve successful mandatory minute ventilation.

Before the advent of high tidal volume ventilation, positive end expiratory pressure (PEEP), and continuous positive airway pressure (CPAP), sighs were added to the ventilation protocol to prevent progressive atelectasis. Each sigh was delivered two to six times per hour and was equivalent to about twice the conventional tidal volume. The risks of barotrauma probably outweigh the theoretical benefits.

Negative pressure (tank) ventilators proved their worth during poliomyelitis epidemics when large numbers of patients were supported for prolonged periods of time. Positive pressure ventilation has since largely replaced negative pressure ventilation, except for specific indication. Like positive pressure ventilation, it is possible not only to generate enhanced tidal volumes but also to maintain lung inflation with the negative pressure equivalent of PEEP. In this context, negative pressure ventilation has been successfully adopted in neonates with the respiratory distress syndrome. As an alternative to a large enclosure around the limbs and trunk (with the head and neck protruding) a cuirasse placed over the anterior thorax can facilitate the application of negative pressure to the chest. Recent developments of the cuirasse type of negative pressure ventilator (Hayek®) permits high frequency oscillations to be used, resulting in enhanced gas exchange.

SETTING VENTILATOR PARAMETERS

Once a ventilation mode has been selected (at least temporarily), ventilatory parameters must be set before attaching the patient to the ventilator. The ventilator parameters include the following:

(1) tidal volume;
(2) ventilation rate;
(3) inspiratory-to-expiratory (I/E) ratio;
(4) flow waveform;
(5) FIO_2 (0.21–1.0);
(6) pressure limit;
(7) PEEP or CPAP (0–20 cmH$_2$O).

Tidal volume

The delivered inspiratory tidal volume may be set at 10 to 12 ml/kg body weight. This should be reduced if the patient has restrictive lung disease or has undergone lobectomy or pneumonectomy. Using respiratory rates of more than 10 breaths/min with such tidal volumes will provide full ventilatory support. If the patient is breathing spontaneously, an intermittent mandatory ventilation mode will be preferred at rates of 4 to 8 breaths/min. If assist control or pressure support is chosen, the respiratory rate will be the patient's spontaneous rate.

I/E ratio, inspiratory flow rate

The ratio of inspiratory to expiratory time (I/E ratio) will generally range from ½ to ¼. This provides sufficient time for full passive exhalation. In patients with obstructive lung disease, failing to allow adequate time for exhalation results in hyperinflation (auto or intrinsic PEEP). The higher the set respiratory rate the shorter expiration becomes and the I/E ratio falls. This may lead to the paradoxical situation in the patient with chronic obstructive pulmonary disease where PCO_2 rises as the ventilator rate is increased!

The I/E ratio can be adjusted in several ways depending upon the make of ventilator. In some a ratio can be selected directly, while in others the inspiratory flow rate determines the duration of inspiration. An acceptable range for inspiratory flow rates is between 30 and 60 l/min (0.5–1.0 l/s).

Inspiratory waveforms

Many volume- and time-cycled (flow generator) ventilators allow the choice of several waveforms. Although there is little evidence to favour one over the other, a square waveform delivers the tidal volume in the least time and with higher peak pressures. A decelerating flow pattern results in lower peak pressures, longer inspiratory intervals, and lower I/E ratios.

Inspired oxygen concentration

The inspired oxygen concentration FIO_2 should be constantly adjusted to provide adequate arterial oxygenation without hyperoxia. Too high a value of FIO_2 is frequently the cause of failure to wean patients with chronic obstructive pulmonary disease from a mechanical ventilator.

Pressure limit

Setting a pressure limit about 10 cmH$_2$O above the peak pressure reached during each ventilator cycle protects the patient against the inadvertently high pressures experienced during coughing or straining. If the pressure limit is reached inspiration is terminated and an alarm sounds.

PEEP/CPAP

Maintaining airway pressure above barometric pressure in a spontaneously breathing patient is called constant positive airway pressure (CPAP). The same pressure applied to a patient on intermittent positive pressure ventilation is called positive end expiratory pressure (PEEP). PEEP and CPAP are used to correct lung volume (functional residual capacity (FRC)) in conditions characterized by reduced lung volume such as adult respiratory distress syndrome or cardiogenic pulmonary oedema. It may also be of benefit in patients with flail chest segments by splinting the chest wall. The terms PEEP and CPAP can be used interchangeably, provided that the differences regarding spontaneous and assisted ventilation are recognized (Fig. 2).

PEEP/CPAP is achieved by the inclusion of a resistance at the expiratory end of the breathing circuit. Ideally, this resistance should be as close to a threshold resistor as possible, such as an underwater column. In practice, most of the valves produce some flow-dependent retardation of expiration that increases the work of breathing in spontaneously breathing patient.

Bypassing the oropharynx by an endotracheal tube is known to cause a fall in FRC in both adults and children. The application of low levels of PEEP/CPAP (3–5 cmH$_2$O) reverses this effect, and therefore has been suggested as part of routine management of the intubated patient ('physiological CPAP'). The usual indication for PEEP/CPAP is the presence of refractory hypoxaemia due to acute lung injury. Starting at 5 cmH$_2$O the pressures are increased progressively until satisfactory oxygenation is achieved for a FIO$_2$ ideally less than 0.6. It is rarely necessary to exceed levels of 20 cmH$_2$O. Assessment of the effects of PEEP/CPAP can be made in several ways—by calculating the venous admixture or shunt fraction, oxygen delivery, or effective static compliance of the lungs. Clearly, following the PaO$_2$ alone takes no account of the effects of PEEP/CPAP upon cardiac output. Continuous measurement of mixed venous SaO$_2$ with a suitable flow-directed pulmonary artery catheter is a particularly good method of evaluating the response to a change in PEEP/CPAP.

The use of PEEP/CPAP in respiratory failure

Trends in the application of PEEP/CPAP in patients with respiratory failure have changed over the years. The use of maximum tolerated levels of PEEP (super-PEEP) and 'best' PEEP have generally been replaced by concepts of 'least' or 'enough' PEEP to allow adequate arterial oxygenation with FIO$_2$ less than 0.6. However, it is still not uncommon to have to consider levels of PEEP greater than 10 or 15 cmH$_2$O, particularly in patients with adult respiratory distress syndrome. Care must be taken to ensure that oxygen delivery is not impaired in the unbridled pursuit of improved arterial oxygenation. An approach to the safe application of PEEP in severe hypoxia and the measures that should be made with each increment of PEEP is defined below.

1. Establish and record baseline respiratory and haemodynamic data before adjusting PEEP level.
   (a) Respiratory data:
       PEEP level;
       FIO$_2$;
       respiratory rate (patient and ventilator);
       peak pressure;
       plateau pressure (end-inspiratory pause pressure);
       SaO$_2$ (pulse oximetry);
       arterial blood gases (PaO$_2$, PaCO$_2$, pH).
   (b) Haemodynamic data:
       Heart rate;
       Blood pressure;
       ECG monitoring.
   (c) For PEEP levels above 15 cmH$_2$O consider the following:
       cardiac output (pulmonary artery flotation catheter);
           calculate Q_S/Q_T per cent;
           calculate oxygen delivery data (CaO$_2$ and CvO$_2$);
           pulmonary artery wedge pressure;
           continuous SvO$_2$ (fibreoptic PA catheter).

Fig. 2 Schematic of airway pressure measured without PEEP and following the addition of 10 cmH$_2$O PEEP. By preventing end-expiratory pressure from falling to zero re-inflation and recruitment of alveolar units is encouraged.

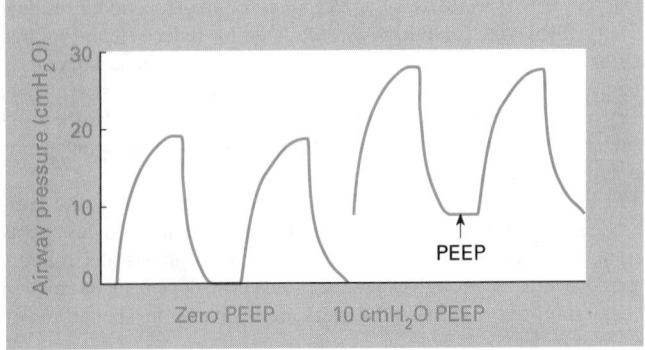

Such measurements are very important in the patient who may be hypovolaemic or have coexistent cardiac disease. Continuous SvO$_2$ is particularly useful in detecting the adverse effects of PEEP and has the significant advantage of being a continuous variable.

2. Change only one variable at a time. If at all possible keep other ventilator settings (ventilator mode, FIO$_2$, V_T, ventilator rate) unchanged.
3. Increase PEEP in increments of 5 cmH$_2$O every 15 to 30 min, checking outcome variables (above) 10 min after each change.
4. Reduce PEEP if any of the following are observed:
   (a) Hypotension;
   (b) step decrement of more than 5 per cent in SvO$_2$;
   (c) more than 20 per cent fall in cardiac output;
   (d) fall in oxygen delivery;
   (e) fall in respiratory system compliance (static);
   (f) appearance of new cardiac arrhythmias.

If oxygen delivery is improved with the addition of PEEP, try to reduce FIO$_2$ when stable and re-evaluate frequently as indicated. If oxygenation is still considered inadequate or the FIO$_2$ is still greater than 0.6, attempt further increases in PEEP. If there are adverse effects such as hypotension or reduced cardiac output (and SvO$_2$), consider volume loading or circulatory support with an inotrope or pressor agent such as noradrenaline.

Occasionally, severe arterial hypoxia persists despite the application of 100 per cent oxygen and high levels of PEEP (above 20 cmH$_2$O). In such circumstances some improvement in oxygenation can be achieved by sitting the patient up as high as possible in bed (avoiding postural hypotension), rolling the patient from side to side (some specialized electric beds will perform this function), or lying the patient prone. This has the effect of redistributing blood flow to parts of the lung which may be better ventilated. In extreme situations, when all therapeutic options appear to be exhausted, quite severe degrees of hypoxia can be tolerated (e.g. PaO$_2$ < 6 kPa (45 mmHg)) provided that oxygen delivery is sufficient to prevent the development of lactic acidosis or hypoxic organ system dysfunction. Such 'permissive' hypoxia may be difficult for the doctor or nurse to accept, but the relative risk of extracorporeal techniques or lung transplant may be significantly greater. Moreover, the best randomized studies of extracorporeal membrane oxygenation in severe respiratory failure in adults show no advantage over conventional ventilation techniques.

The addition of low concentrations (4–40 p.p.m.) of nitric oxide (NO) to the inspired air/oxygen gas mixture may improve oxygen gas exchange and lower pulmonary artery pressure. This relatively new therapy may establish itself as a standard addition to the management of adult respiratory distress syndrome.

Mask CPAP

CPAP can be applied without resorting to endotracheal intubation for the treatment of selected patients with acute respiratory failure. Close-fitting CPAP masks, which are very similar to standard anaesthetic masks, are widely available together with disposable circuitry and gas supply/pressure regulator mechanisms to ensure the safe delivery of air–oxygen mixtures. Suitable patients should be carefully selected and managed in a clinical area where appropriate observation and monitoring can be assured. This is usually an intensive treatment units, high dependency unit, or respiratory unit. In general, patients with established adult respiratory distress syndrome are unsuitable if a long or protracted period of treatment is envisaged.

The patient must be fully alert and cooperative since there is a major risk of aspiration should vomiting occur. Mask CPAP is particularly suited to patients with diffuse reversible interstitial processes such as cardiogenic pulmonary oedema or interstitial pneumonia (e.g. *Pneumocystis carinii* pneumonia). Recovery should be expected within 1 or 2 days since it is difficult for the patient to tolerate a tight-fitting CPAP mask for much longer periods, and CPAP levels above 10 to 15 cmH$_2$O should not be employed. Continuous assessment by the clinical team is essential so that endotracheal intubation can be substituted for the mask system if necessary.

PEEP/CPAP in unilateral lung disease

The use of PEEP/CPAP in patients with unilateral or irregularly distributed lung disease may not result in improved oxygenation. Indeed, paradoxical falls in oxygenation may occur as a result of the shunting of blood from areas of well-matched V/Q to parts of the lung that are poorly ventilated. Therefore unilateral lung consolidation, lung collapse, massive pleural effusion, bronchial intubation, and pulmonary infarction may not benefit from PEEP/CPAP. Whenever possible, treatment should be directed at correction of the specific lung pathology.

Weaning off PEEP

Reduction of or weaning off PEEP/CPAP should be conducted carefully and gradually once the underlying pathology (e.g. sepsis) has resolved. Ideally, FiO_2 should have been reduced to 0.4 or less to maintain a PaO_2 of 10 kPa (80 mmHg) and the PEEP/CPAP level should not have changed for at least 12 h. Even when these criteria are satisfied, a significant proportion of patients will require the return of PEEP/CPAP to previous or even higher levels. Reduction of PEEP/CPAP in decrements of 2.5 or 5.0 cmH$_2$O should be followed after 10 to 15 min intervals by clinical, pulse oximeter, and blood gas assessment. Even after resolution of lung pathology, the retention of low levels of PEEP/CPAP of 3–5 cmH$_2$O ('physiological PEEP') up to the time of extubation may help maintain normal lung volumes and improve gas exchange.

VENTILATOR MONITORS AND ALARMS

The ventilation monitors and alarms that must be set and maintained include the following:

(1) exhaled V_T, exhaled minute ventilation;
(2) spontaneous respiratory rate;
(2) airway pressure and circuit disconnect;
(3) peak airway pressure;
(4) FiO_2;
(5) inhaled gas temperature.

The importance of ventilator alarms cannot be overemphasized. The modern microprocessor-based ventilator is not only more efficient but is significantly safer than its earlier predecessors.

CLINICAL MONITORING OF MECHANICAL VENTILATION

An essential aspect of monitoring is regular clinical examination of the patient, and inspection of the ventilator and ventilator circuit. Expansion of the chest should be symmetrical with each ventilator-cycled breath (control mechanical ventilation, intermittent mandatory ventilation), assisted breath (assist control or pressure support), or unassisted spontaneous breath (intermittent mandatory ventilation). Auscultation should confirm air entry and detect any added sounds. The patient should be sat up or rolled from side to side to allow inspection of the whole of the chest. The endotracheal tube should be secure and as comfortable as possible for the patient. The endotracheal cuff pressure should be adjusted to less than 30 mmHg or such that a small air leak becomes audible with a stethoscope on the side of the neck with each ventilator cycle. The ventilator circuit should feel warm but be free of significant amounts of condensed water. The humidifier temperature and water level should be checked.

The pulse oximeter has contributed significantly to the monitoring and safety of patients on mechanical ventilation. Not only does it provide a continuous measurement of oxygenation but also reduces the need for arterial blood gas sampling. Much can be appreciated from watching the ventilator pressure gauge with each cycle. In addition to evaluating peak inspiratory pressure, the clinician will be able to judge whether the

Table 3 *Questions to ask when weaning is difficult*

1. Is the endotracheal tube of optimal size? Small endotracheal tubes of <7 mm internal diameter have a high resistance.
2. Has the patient been seated upright to aid lung mechanics?
3. Is there evidence of airway obstruction that would improve with bronchodilator or steroid therapy?
4. Are respiratory depressant drugs being administered?
5. Is there evidence of occult neuromuscular disease? Exclude interactions with aminoglycosides.
6. Is there evidence of hypothyroidism, hypophosphataemia, or hypomagnesaemia?
7. Is there a metabolic alkalosis? If so, this should be corrected with potassium, chloride, and volume as appropriate.
8. Is there evidence of malnourishment on history or simple laboratory test such as serum albumin.
9. Is tracheostomy indicated?
10. In COPD patients, are the target blood gases similar to the premorbid values?
11. Is there evidence of diaphragmatic dysfunction due to phrenic nerve injury?

patient is 'fighting' the ventilator. Comparing inspiratory and expiratory tidal volumes may indicate a leak either at the circuit connections or at the endotracheal tube cuff. When peak pressures are high, the internal compliance of the ventilator and circuit (about 2–2.5 ml/cmH$_2$O) may account for much of the volume loss. A rough assessment of the compliance of the lung can be made by following the peak inflation pressures.

WEANING OFF MECHANICAL VENTILATION

More than 80 per cent of patients who are ventilated postoperatively can be weaned simply by clinically evaluating their spontaneous ventilation on a 'T-piece' or similar circuit. The remainder requires a progressive reduction in ventilatory support until measurement of ventilation parameters can be made. These parameters include the negative inspiratory force (NIF) and vital capacity (VC). A NIF greater than -25 cmH$_2$O or a VC greater than 10 ml/kg usually indicates sufficient ventilatory reserve for spontaneous ventilation. These parameters cannot be applied reliably to patients with severe chronic obstructive pulmonary disease; instead, blood gases have to be followed with each reduction in ventilation support. Modes of ventilation such as synchronized intermittent mandatory ventilation, intermittent mandatory ventilation, and pressure support are very suitable for weaning since they allow gradual and progressive reduction in ventilation support. Regular clinical and physiological assessment after each reduction in ventilation support is essential. Failure to wean a patient successfully from mechanical ventilation should prompt the questions addressed in Table 3.

COMPLICATIONS OF MECHANICAL VENTILATION

Several complications of mechanical ventilation can be attributed to the local effects of the endotracheal tube upon the airway. These include airway obstruction due to endotracheal tube displacement and pressure necrosis leading to vocal cord injury and subglottic stenosis. The risk of nosocomial pneumonia is increased in the intubated patient. Many complications are the direct consequence of positive pressure ventilation. Haemodynamic effects such as reduced cardiac output, reduced renal perfusion, and salt and water retention are primarily the result of mechanical, neuroreflex, and humoral factors. Interstitial lung damage may occur as a result of positive pressure ventilation, and this has prompted renewed interest in extracorporeal systems for the management of patients with adult respiratory distress syndrome.

The greatest concern relates to the risk of pneumothorax, pneumomediastinum, pneumopericardium, or subcutaneous emphysema.

Pneumothorax is the most feared complication because it is associated with rapid deterioration unless dealt with quickly. The doctor and nurse must remain vigilant for the development of barotrauma. Signs of barotrauma include arterial desaturation (pulse oximeter), sudden rise in peak airway pressure, hypotension and tachycardia, and finally circulatory collapse.

Tube thoracostomy is mandatory since progression to a tension pneumothorax is very likely. Prophylactic thoracostomy tubes are not recommended even in the presence of pneumomediastinum. Sudden clinical deterioration associated with a rise in inflation pressures and absence of breath sounds should always raise the question of pneumothorax. Emergency decompression with a 14 gauge cannula may produce temporary relief and may have a diagnostic role, but tube thoracostomy should be performed without delay and without radiographic confirmation if necessary. Blunt dissection through the parietal pleura with forceps and digital exploration of the pleural space prior to insertion of the thoracostomy tube is essential if lung damage is to be avoided. Thoracostomy tubes with rigid metal stylets must not be used under any circumstances.

SPECIFIC STRATEGIES IN VENTILATOR MANAGEMENT

Restrictive lung disease

Patients with restrictive lung diseases such as sarcoidosis or fibrosing alveolitis should be ventilated with small tidal volumes of 5 to 8 ml/kg at rates of 15 to 20 breaths/min. Oxygen need not be restricted in the manner recommended for patients with chronic obstructive pulmonary disease.

Chronic obstructive pulmonary disease

Most cases of acute on chronic respiratory failure can be managed successfully without mechanical ventilation. A small proportion of patients fail to respond to conservative measures and require ventilatory assistance. In many cases, the need for mechanical ventilation is the direct result of injudicious oxygen therapy. Low rate synchronized intermittent mandatory ventilation (6–8 breaths/min) or low pressure levels of pressure support are idea for chronic obstructive pulmonary disease patients with acute on chronic respiratory failure. The $PaCO_2$ should be reduced very slowly towards but not to normal levels. The FiO_2 rarely needs to be higher than 0.35. High ventilator rates (more than 14 breaths/min) are associated with high values of V_D/V_T (more than 0.5). Paradoxically, as the ventilator rates are increased in an attempt to increase minute ventilation, the $PaCO_2$ may rise. To avoid intrinsic or auto-PEEP the I/E ratio should be maintained at ½ or more. Weaning can begin as soon as the precipitating cause of respiratory failure has been corrected. Weaning will be unsuccessful if there is any underlying metabolic alkalosis or the patient receives sedative or analgesic agents. The $PaCO_2$ can be allowed to rise slowly to above normal levels provided that sufficient time is given for the blood pH to correct and the FiO_2 is kept below 0.35. Carbon dioxide production can be minimized by providing balanced nutrition with calories being supplied by both lipid and carbohydrate.

Asthma

Probably less than 1 per cent of acute severe asthma attacks require mechanical ventilation. However, it is apparent that some patients suffer cardiac arrest and die each year because intubation and mechanical ventilation were not performed in time. Hypercarbia alone is generally insufficient indication for ventilation, but a combination of a rising $PaCO_2$, fatigue, failure of conservative measures, or arrhythmias does call for elective intubation and mechanical ventilation. Adequate oxygenation must be ensured by the administration of unrestricted high concentrations of oxygen, in contrast with the CO_2-retaining chronic obstructive pulmonary disease patient for whom controlled oxygen (24–28 per cent) is generally indicated.

Asthmatic patients may be difficult to ventilate initially and often require high inflation pressures. Hypoxia may persist despite the addition of high concentrations of oxygen and probably is the result of mucus plugging of the airways. A philosophy of 'permissive hypercapnia' or 'controlled hypoventilation' should be adopted, with the $PaCO_2$ remaining at elevated levels (7–8 kPa (50–60 mmHg)). Therefore lower tidal volumes and respiratory rates are possible. Lower inspiratory flow rates result in lower peak pressures and reduced risk of barotrauma. Deaths in ventilated asthmatic patients are rare but are usually the result of barotrauma, hypotension in volume-depleted patients, arrhythmias, or lung infection.

Maximal bronchodilator therapy including corticosteroids is continued throughout the period of mechanical ventilation, supplemented if necessary with inhalational anaesthetics such as isoflurane or the intravenous anaesthetic ketamine. Both these agents are potent bronchodilators. Rehydration and adequate humidification of inspired gases will ordinarily mobilize secretions and mucous plugs; if not, bronchoalveolar lavage may be indicated.

The use of extracorporeal membrane oxygenation and carbon dioxide removal has been reported in acute asthma. These must be considered exceptional cases and such techniques cannot be generally recommended.

Bronchopleural and bronchocutaneous fistulae

Although bronchopleural and bronchocutaneous fistulae can occur after trauma or lung infection, many arise during the postoperative period following lobectomy or pneumonectomy. It is generally appreciated that early weaning and extubation is preferred in these patients. Occasionally, postoperative complications necessitate a longer period of ventilation when there is significant risk of dehiscence of the bronchial stump. To reduce the risk of this, low tidal volume, high respiratory rate ventilation should be adopted to minimize inflation pressures. High frequency ventilation would appear to be ideally suited to the prevention of bronchopleural fistulae, although evidence to prove superiority over convention ventilation is lacking.

The development of a bronchopleural fistula is heralded by clinical deterioration, reduced chest wall movement on the affected side, tracheal deviation, and sudden increase in inflation pressures. Emergency tube thoracostomy must be performed to convert the bronchopleural fistula into a bronchocutaneous fistula. Compensation for the loss of tidal volume through the fistula is easily made by adjusting the ventilator, but if the leak is large, endobronchial intubation may be necessary. Bronchopleural and bronchocutaneous fistulae are unlikely to close until the patient is weaned from the ventilator.

REFERENCES

Barnes, P.K. (1982). Principles of lung ventilators and humidification. In *Scientific foundations of anaesthesia* (ed. C. Scurr and S. Feldman), pp. 533–43. Heinemann, London.

Cameron, P.D., and Oh, T.E. (1986). Newer modes of mechanical ventilatory support. *Anaesthesia and Intensive Care,* **14,** 258–66.

Downs, J.B., Kelin, E.F., Desautels, D., Modell, J.H., and Kirby, R.R. (1973). IMV: a new approach to weaning patients from mechanical ventilators. *Chest,* **64,** 331–5.

Downs, J.B., Block, A.J., and Vennum, K.B. (1974). Intermittent mandatory ventilation in the treatment of patients with chronic obstructive pulmonary disease. *Anesthesia and Analgesia,* **53,** 437–43.

Fairley, H.B. (1980). Critique of intermittent mandatory ventilation. In *Intermittent mandatory ventilation* (ed. R. Kirby and G.B. Graybar), pp. 179–90. Little, Brown, Boston, MA.

Frostell, C., Fratacci, M.D., Wain, J.C., Jones, R., and Zapol, W.M. (1991). Inhaled nitric oxide, a selective pulmonary vasodilator reversing hypoxic pulmonary vasoconstriction. *Circulation,* **83,** 2038–47.

Garrard, C.S. (1992). Mechanical ventilation support in severe asthma. *Care of the Critically Ill,* **8,** 201–11.

Gattinoni, L., Agostini, A., Pesenti, A., Pelizzola, A., Rossi, G.P., Langer, M., *et al.* (1980). Treatment of acute respiratory failure with low frequency positive-pressure ventilation and extracorporeal removal of CO2. *Lancet* **ii**, 292–4.

Hickling, K.G. (1986). Extracorporeal CO_2 removal in severe adult respiratory distress syndrome. *Anaesthesia and Intensive Care,* **14**, 45–53.

Hickling, K.G., Henderson, S.J., and Jackson, R. (1990). Low mortality associated with low volume pressure limited ventilation with permissive hypercapnia in severe adult respiratory distress syndrome. *Intensive Care Medicine,* **16**, 372–7.

Kirby, R.R., Downs, J.B., Civetta, J.M., *et al.* (1975). High level PEEP in acute respiratory insufficiency. *Chest,* **67**, 156–63.

Kumar, A., Falke, K.J., Geffin, B., *et al.* (1970). Continuous positive-pressure ventilation in acute respiratory failure. *New England Journal of Medicine,* **283**, 1430–6.

Marini, J.J., Rodriguez, R.M., and Lamb, V. (1986). The inspiratory workload of patient-initiated mechanical ventilation. *American Review of Respiratory Disease,* **134**, 902–9.

Murray, J.F., Matthay, M.A., Luce, J.M., and Flick, M.R. (1988). An expanded definition of the adult respiratory distress syndrome. *American Review of Respiratory Disease,* **138**, 720–3.

Pepe, P.E., Potkin, P.J., Reus, D.E., *et al.* (1982). Clinical predictors of adult respiratory distress syndrome. *American Journal of Surgery,* **144**, 124–30.

Petty, T.L. and Ashbaugh, D.G. (1971). The adult respiratory distress syndrome: clinical features, factors influencing prognosis and principles of management. *Chest,* **130**, 66–71.

Qvist, J., Pontoppidan, H., Wilson, R.S., Lowenstein, E., and Laver, M.B. (1975). Hemodynamic responses to mechanical ventilation with PEEP: the effect of hypervolemia. *Anesthesiology,* **42**, 45–55.

Smith, R.A., Desautels, D.A., and Kirby, R.R. (1985). Mechanical ventilators. In *Mechanical ventilation* (ed. R.R. Kirby, R.A. Smith, and D.A. Desautels), pp. 327–474. Churchill Livingstone, New York.

Suter, P.M., Fairley, H.B., and Isenberg, M.D. (1975). Optimum end-expiratory pressure in patients with acute pulmonary failure. *New England Journal of Medicine,* **292**, 284–9.

Sykes, M.K. (1985). High frequency ventilation. *Thorax,* **40**, 161–5.

Tate, R.M. and Repine, J.E. (1983). Neutrophils and the adult respiratory distress syndrome. *American Review of Respiratory Disease,* **128**, 522–9.

Tobin, M.J. (1988). Predicting weaning outcome (Editorial). *Chest* **94**, 227.

Tuxen, D.V. (1989). Detrimental effects of positive end-expiratory pressure during controlled mechanical ventilation of patients with severe airflow obstruction. *American Review of Respiratory Disease* **140**, 5–9.

Tyler, D.C. (1983). Positive end-expiratory pressure: a review. *Critical Care Medicine,* **11**, 300–8.

Weigel, J.A., Norcross, J.F., Borman, K.R., and Sayder, W.H. (1985). Early steroid therapy for respiratory failure. *Archives of Surgery,* **120**, 536–40.

Wood, L.H. and Prewitt, R.M. (1981). Cardiovascular management in acute hypoxemic respiratory failure. *American Journal of Cardiology,* **47**, 963–72.

17.14.3(b) Chronic respiratory failure

J. MOXHAM

Introduction

The most important causes of chronic respiratory failure and subsequent cor pulmonale are listed in Table 1. Pulmonary fibrosis and pulmonary vascular disease cause predominantly hypoxia (type 1 respiratory failure) and the development of hypercapnia only occurs late in these diseases. Obstructive sleep apnoea and central alveolar hypoventilation cause respiratory failure mainly during sleep. Chronic obstructive pulmonary disease (COPD) is by far the most common cause of hypercapnic (type 2) ventilatory failure.

Patients with chronic respiratory failure have hypoxia and breathlessness, particularly on exertion, and eventually develop hypercapnia and cor pulmonale. Any assessment of patients with chronic respiratory failure must address the mechanism, severity, and treatment of hypoxia, plus the three crucial areas of central respiratory drive, respiratory mus-

Table 1 *Important causes of chronic respiratory failure*

Lung and airways
Pulmonary fibrosis
Pulmonary vascular disease
Chronic bronchitis and emphysema
Bronchiectasis and cystic fibrosis
Obstructive sleep apnoea

Central nervous system
Central alveolar hypoventilation

Neuromuscular disorders
Cervical cord lesions
Motor neurone disease
Poliomyelitis
Muscular dystrophies and myopathies

Thoracic cage and pleural abnormalities
Kyphoscoliosis
Thoracoplasty
Extreme obesity

cle pump capacity, and the load imposed on the respiratory system by the disease (see Chapter 17.14.1). In different diseases the importance of each of these three components will vary. In patients with chronic respiratory failure impairment of the central nervous system output is only rarely a problem and is most relevant in central alveolar hypoventilation syndromes. However, abnormalities of central ventilatory control are commonly part of the overall pathophysiology of ventilatory failure, and furthermore a reduction of central nervous system output is an important component of respiratory failure in many patients during sleep. The increased load on the respiratory system imposed by disease processes is frequently self-evident, for example in pulmonary fibrosis, obstructive sleep apnoea, or obesity. Similarly, impairment of respiratory muscle pump capacity occurs in a wide variety of circumstances. Neuromuscular diseases for example motor neurone disease or muscular dystrophy, are an obvious cause of reduced pump capacity. However, pump capacity is often impaired in less obvious ways: patients with COPD and hyperinflation have reduced inspiratory muscle capacity as a consequence of muscle shortening; patients with weight loss for whatever cause invariably have respiratory muscle weakness; respiratory muscle function is markedly reduced by acidosis. The importance of the major factors influencing load, capacity, and drive, and the interaction of these three components is essential for an understanding of ventilatory failure.

On rare occasions chronic respiratory failure can be cured, for example when patients with cystic fibrosis are treated by lung transplantation, patients with severe obstructive sleep apnoea are managed with continuous positive airway pressure (CPAP), and patients with morbid obesity lose weight. Nevertheless, for most patients with chronic respiratory failure a cure is impossible, and an important aspect of management is careful assessment of the interrelated issues of central drive, respiratory load, and ventilatory capacity, as well as the management of chronic hypoxia. In patients with advanced COPD, for example, it is clearly relevant to direct therapy towards load reduction, but attention should also be paid to respiratory muscle pump capacity, central respiratory control, and ventilation during sleep (Fig. 1).

This chapter will concentrate on the application of these principles to the management of respiratory failure in COPD, dealing with both the acute exacerbation and the chronic stable state, and will illustrate applications to other examples of respiratory failure where appropriate.

The management of acute exacerbations of COPD

During exacerbations of COPD, usually caused by viral or bacterial bronchial infection, there is an increase in airways resistance which frequently precipitates the patient into hypercapnic respiratory failure with acidosis and often cor pulmonale. Therapy centres around reversing the hypoxia and treating the ventilatory failure by addressing the interrelated factors of load, pump capacity, and drive.

Oxygen therapy

The use of oxygen therapy to correct hypoxia in type 1 respiratory failure is relatively straightforward. Since ventilatory capacity is sufficient and carbon dioxide sensitivity is retained, oxygen can be given at high concentration. In practice, it is difficult to deliver more than 40 per cent oxygen with conventional face masks, despite high oxygen flow rates. If conventional oxygen therapy via a face mask does not relieve hypoxia, a tight-fitting CPAP face mask is useful, but it requires high oxygen flows usually delivered from piped oxygen wall units.

The treatment of hypoxia in type 2 respiratory failure (the usual picture in severe COPD) is more difficult. The major challenge is that of relieving hypoxia, which is commonly severe, without exacerbating hypercapnia. This is a particular problem in patients with long-standing ventilatory failure and a substantial compensated respiratory acidosis. Such patients have a blunted ventilatory response to carbon dioxide, and oxygen therapy can reduce the hypoxic stimulus to ventilation, thereby intensifying hypoventilation and carbon dioxide retention. In these circumstances oxygen therapy must be titrated against blood gas tensions with the aim of alleviating dangerous hypoxia without precipitating marked hypercapnia. Such patients are conditioned to hypoxia and it is only necessary to increase PaO_2 to a level sufficient to produce substantial saturation of arterial blood (i.e. $PaO_2 > 8$ kPa).

Venturi oxygen masks that deliver a fixed oxygen percentage (24, 28, or 35 per cent) are essential to achieve this therapeutic aim. Nasal prongs are unreliable in this setting. Addition of 2 l/min of 100 per cent oxygen to a minute ventilation of 10 l/min of air would give a mean inspired oxygen level of around 33 per cent. However, if the patient's own ventilation drops to, say, 5 l/m, the mean inspired oxygen level will reach 43 per cent, and this could cause further dangerous respiratory depression.

When it is clear that oxygen therapy does not precipitate a deleterious rise in carbon dioxide, ongoing monitoring of oxygenation is conveniently undertaken by a finger oximeter. At this stage it is safe to switch to nasal cannulae, usually at a flow rate of 1–2 l/min according to response. If it is impossible to relieve life-threatening hypoxia without unacceptable hypercapnia, particularly during sleep, patients may require a ventilatory stimulant, treatment with nasal positive pressure ventilation (NPPV), or intubation and mechanical ventilation.

Respiratory drive

In patients with stable COPD the ventilatory load is high, the capacity is impaired, and the ratio of load to capacity is high. A high central drive is required to sustain ventilation in these circumstances, and clinical studies indicate that respiratory drive is indeed very high in such patients including those with carbon dioxide retention. During an exacerbation central drive must increase further to compensate for the additional ventilatory load. Thus central drive must be sustained in the management of an exacerbation. Sedation will cause a rapid and profound reduction in ventilation and must be assiduously avoided.

In the obtunded patient with dangerous hypercapnia and acidosis it may be appropriate to stimulate central respiratory drive with drugs such as doxapram. However, in alert patients it is likely that central drive is optimal and additional drive produced by drugs may be ineffective, or may generate an intolerable sensation of breathing effort and perhaps respiratory muscle fatigue.

Respiratory drive is reduced in sleep, and nocturnal hypoventilation may be life threatening. Patients are often frightened to sleep and eventually become totally exhausted. With sleep the clinical picture becomes one of progressive hypercapnia, acidosis, hypoxia, confusion, and coma. One of the 'benefits' of respiratory stimulants (and constant medical, nursing, and physiotherapy attention) is to keep patients awake while ongoing therapy improves ventilatory function.

Muscle pump capacity

In the short term it is difficult to increase the capacity of the respiratory muscle pump. However, bronchodilatation reduces lung volume which in turn lengthens the respiratory muscles and improves their action. A reduction in lung volume also restores the curvature of the diaphragm and improves its capacity to generate pressure and achieve volume change during inspiration. The correction of metabolic factors that impair respiratory muscle contractility (e.g. acidosis, hypoxia, hypokalaemia, hypophosphataemia) is important. Respiratory muscle function is also impaired by sepsis, inadequate nutrition, and steroid therapy.

In the short term excessive ventilatory load is usually the key disturbance in exacerbations of COPD, but in the longer term limitation of pump capacity becomes very important. At all times it is the balance of load versus capacity that is crucial rather than either factor in isolation.

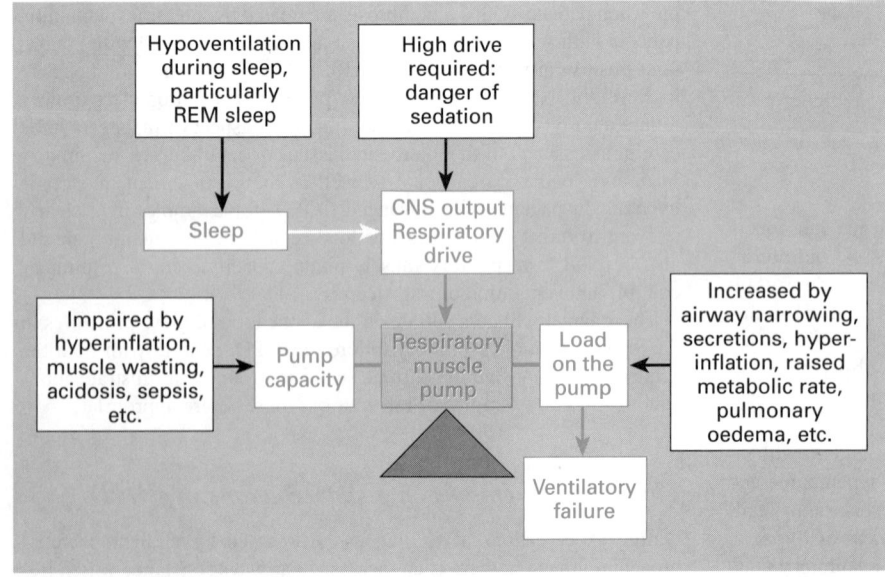

Fig. 1 In COPD the management of ventilatory failure requires consideration of ventilatory load, respiratory muscle pump capacity, and central respiratory drive (both awake and during sleep) as well as treatment of hypoxia.

Ventilatory load

The major ventilatory load is due to increased airways resistance. Aggressive bronchodilator therapy, principally with nebulized β_2-agonists, reduces this load. Such therapy can yield rapid improvement. The inflammatory narrowing of airways requires steroid therapy and antibiotics, which also serve to reduce infected intraluminal secretions. Left ventricular failure occurs in some patients, and this requires diuretic therapy. Aminophylline is frequently helpful in exacerbations of COPD and is most effective when administered as an intravenous infusion; its actions include some bronchodilatation, a degree of respiratory stimulation, improved renal perfusion and a consequent diuresis, some enhancement of cardiac output, and perhaps a small improvement in respiratory muscle contractility.

The deteriorating patient

Some patients with an exacerbation of COPD deteriorate despite aggressive treatment aimed at reducing ventilatory load, optimizing respiratory muscle pump capacity, and sustaining respiratory drive. A persistent and deteriorating respiratory acidosis reflects a poor prognosis (particularly if pH is below 7.26). In such patients it must be decided whether or not to intubate and mechanically ventilate. This is a complex decision in which age, severity of background disease, prognosis, quality of life, likelihood of achieving improvement with therapy, and the views of the patient and his or her family are all relevant. Some patients with COPD who are intubated and ventilated are difficult to wean, but in practice the majority are eventually successfully taken off the ventilator, and the issue of quality of life prior to the exacerbation is a more relevant consideration than the technical challenge posed by management in the intensive care unit (see Chapter 17.14.3(a)). It is probable that first-line therapy for selected patients who are not responding to conventional treatment is NPPV (see below), provided that they are able to cooperate with this form of treatment. When appropriate, NPPV has the advantage of being possible outside the intensive care unit. Nasal ventilation can also be offered to patients in whom intubation would be totally inappropriate.

Cor pulmonale

Severe chronic respiratory failure, with its associated profound hypoxia, causes pulmonary hypertension, right ventricular hypertrophy, and eventually peripheral oedema (cor pulmonale). Peripheral oedema is unusual in patients without both severe hypoxia and hypercapnia. In some patients the pulmonary hypertension and right ventricular hypertrophy lead to right ventricular failure, which therefore contributes to oedema, but in others with oedema there is no evidence of 'heart failure'; indeed, cardiac output may be normal or raised, and central venous pressure may not be elevated. In such patients an important element in fluid retention is renal hypoxia since renal blood flow is reduced in many patients with hypoxic lung disease. In hypoxia, salt and water retention, as well as pulmonary vasoconstriction, are probably made worse by hypercapnia. Therefore the overall management of cor pulmonale requires consideration of the central problems in chronic respiratory failure (see above) plus pulmonary hypertension, cardiac performance, and renal perfusion and oxygenation.

The most common cause by far of cor pulmonale in Western societies is COPD, and although this cannot be reversed the consequences can certainly be addressed. Most important in the acute exacerbation is the control of hypoxia by appropriate oxygen therapy (see above). Long-term oxygen therapy can lead to increased longevity, reversal of secondary polycythaemia, resolution of peripheral oedema quite independent of diuretic therapy, and reduction in pulmonary hypertension (see below). Cor pulmonale secondary to obstructive sleep apnoea, or nocturnal hypoxia in chest wall or neuromuscular disease, is reversed by therapy that controls nocturnal hypoventilation (e.g. CPAP or NPPV). The sooner that pulmonary hypertension is recognized and appropriate action taken, the more likely it is that it can be reversed. Chronic pulmonary hypertension leads to permanent vascular changes that cannot be reversed.

DIURETICS

Diuretics should be used with caution in cor pulmonale. Acute diuresis reduces circulating blood volume and peripheral perfusion, and therefore reduces delivery of oxygen to the tissues. This is a particular problem in patients with polycythaemia who have increased blood viscosity and may develop complicating thromboses. In some patients an aldosterone antagonist (spironolactone) is appropriate. Angiotensin-converting enzyme inhibitors may be useful in promoting diuresis; they reduce angiotensin II and aldosterone levels and also enhance intrarenal blood flow. In patients with advanced cor pulmonale, the initial therapeutic strategy should be to improve the underlying disease and relieve hypoxia rather than a rapid resort to powerful diuretics, although considered use of appropriate diuretics will often be a useful part of overall management.

VASODILATOR THERAPY

Oxygen can produce an acute reduction in pulmonary artery pressure in some patients, and is probably more effective than any currently available drug therapy. None the less, the pulmonary vasodilator effect of many drugs (theophyllines, β-agonists, α-adrenergic blockers, hydralazine, calcium-channel blockers, angiotensin-converting enzyme inhibitors) has been evaluated. Although many drugs can have an acute affect on pulmonary hypertension, few have a sustained action. None is selective for the pulmonary vasculature, and as yet no survival advantage has been demonstrated. Angiotensin-converting enzyme inhibitors are currently under investigation.

The management of chronic stable ventilatory failure in COPD

Some patients recover well from an acute exacerbation, but most remain hypoxic to some degree and others remain hypercapnic. In the management of these patients the same principles apply as for the acute exacerbation: the correction of hypoxia and attention to drive, pump capacity, and load. Similar therapies are appropriate but need to be applied in different ways.

Oxygen therapy

Patients with chronic respiratory failure are characteristically hypoxic and commonly receive oxygen therapy. Short-term oxygen therapy is used to relieve breathlessness and improve exercise tolerance, whereas long-term oxygen therapy is aimed at improving prognosis and overall quality of life. The latter is particularly appropriate for patients with, or with a history of, cor pulmonale.

LONG-TERM OXYGEN THERAPY

The rationale for long-term oxygen therapy rests on the results of two clinical trials performed in the 1970s in patients with severe COPD. One of these studies was undertaken by the Medical Research Council (MRC) in the United Kingdom and one by the National Institutes of Health (NIH) in the United States. The United Kingdom patients had severe airways disease with substantial hypoxia and had experienced peripheral oedema. In the control group who were managed with conventional therapy but without long-term oxygen the mortality was approximately 50 per cent at 2 years and 70 per cent at 3 years. The survival of patients treated with long-term oxygen therapy administered for 15 h each day, including throughout the night, in such a way as to increase Pao_2 to above 8 kPa (usually 2 l/min via nasal cannulae), was increased by more than 50 per cent. A difference between treated and control groups was evident for female patients from early in the study, but for males the survival curves did not diverge until 18 months from the beginning of the trial. Continuing cigarette smokers did not benefit. Subsequent long-term follow-up has demonstrated that long-term oxygen therapy in severe COPD increases mean survival to 5 years. Thus, although there is great variability in the response of individual patients, the United Kingdom experience suggests that LTOT can enhance survival in severe COPD with cor pulmonale from 2 to at least 5 years (Fig. 2).

The NIH study also demonstrated benefit from long-term oxygen therapy, although the clinical data suggest that the American patients did not have such severe disease and that not all of them had experienced peripheral oedema. In the NIH study the survival in those receiving oxygen for 19 h daily was greater than those receiving 12 h oxygen daily.

There are now generally accepted criteria, based on the MRC and NIH clinical trials, for recommending long-term oxygen therapy in patients with advanced COPD. The key criterion is severe chronic hypoxia documented to be present when the patient is clinically stable (Pao_2) < 7.3 kPa). Although the MRC and NIH studies were undertaken in patients with COPD, it is reasonable to assume that other patient groups with severe chronic hypoxia may also benefit (for example those with bronchiectasis and cystic fibrosis). Long-term oxygen therapy is a substantial undertaking for all patients, and since the objective is the relief of dangerous hypoxia it is crucial that an appropriately low and stable Pao_2 is demonstrated. Many patients, admitted with exacerbations of COPD for example, may be profoundly hypoxic when in hospital, but subsequent follow-up demonstrates improvement in oxygenation such that long-term oxygen therapy is not appropriate.

Improvement of many other clinical parameters is associated with the improvement in survival with long-term oxygen therapy. Chronic oxygen therapy improves the quality of sleep and enhances mental function. Clinical studies have also demonstrated some improvement in breathlessness and exercise capacity. Furthermore, the relief of hypoxia facilitates the resolution of oedema in cor pulmonale and reverses secondary polycythaemia.

Despite the benefits of long-term oxygen therapy, many practical and clinical problems remain. As yet it is not clear whether patients whose hypoxia is less severe should receive this treatment. In particular, it is not certain whether patients who have relatively good Pao_2 values by day, but severe desaturation at night, benefit from nocturnal oxygen therapy. Whilst it is important to assess carefully all patients who are being considered for long-term oxygen therapy, it is probably not sensible to have guidelines that are too rigid. The physiological and clinical data are simply not available to allow an overstrict approach to this clinical problem. An additional factor is patient compliance. Even in patients that are ideally suited for long-term oxygen therapy, the compliance with therapy can be poor. Community-based studies repeatedly demonstrate that many patients do not take their therapy for the recommended number of hours, and do not accurately report their oxygen usage. Furthermore, whilst it is known that patients with COPD who continue to smoke do not derive benefit from long-term oxygen therapy, a substantial number of patients persist in this habit.

The provision of long-term oxygen therapy has practical difficulties if cylinders are used. Oxygen concentrators and liquid oxygen are more suitable and more cost effective. In the United Kingdom domiciliary oxygen therapy, using concentrators, can be arranged via the patient's general practitioner, although it is recommended that a respiratory physician is involved in the assessment of the patient and appropriate follow-up. Cost advantages accrue when the number of standard cylinders required each week exceeds seven.

SHORT-TERM OXYGEN THERAPY

Many patients use oxygen to control breathlessness after exertion, and also to enhance exercise capability. It is difficult to demonstrate the mechanism whereby oxygen relieves breathlessness when it is used in the recovery period after exercise. Nevertheless data exist which demonstrate that, for some patients, added oxygen breathed during exercise can relieve breathlessness and improve exercise capacity. Therefore in patients with chronic respiratory failure it seems entirely reasonable to prescribe oxygen for symptomatic relief, having first demonstrated that patients report improvement with this therapeutic approach. Oxygen therapy is particularly relevant in patients who markedly desaturate on exertion.

In the patient's home a long length of tubing from the oxygen source can facilitate mobility. Mobility beyond the patient's home is possible with portable oxygen delivery systems. Oxygen cylinders can be taken by patients in their cars or pushed in a trolley. A major problem is the short time period for which oxygen can be administered in this way. Liquid oxygen canisters last longer but are expensive and are not readily available in the United Kingdom. A variety of modifications to oxygen masks and nasal cannulae have been made to try to reduce oxygen wastage and therefore extend the time that portable systems can be used, as well as reduce costs. For example some systems only deliver oxygen during inspiration, while others incorporate a reservoir. Another approach has been to insert an oxygen catheter directly into the trachea. Transtracheal catheters have a number of potential advantages. Oxygen usage over a given time period is approximately halved. Some patients are also attracted by the cosmetic benefits of transtracheal oxygen, particularly tunnelled catheters. Patients who are sufficiently hypoxic to be treated with transtracheal catheters are usually receiving long-term oxygen therapy and the transtracheal approach may also improve patient compliance.

Drive and respiratory stimulants

Respiratory stimulants have a limited short-term role in the management of acute on chronic hypercapnic ventilatory failure. They may also be useful in patients who have received drugs that depress respiration. However, no suitable drug therapy for chronic ventilatory failure is available. Almitrine, a drug which enhances chemoreceptor sensitivity, has been shown to reduce the hypoxia of chronic respiratory failure in

Fig. 2 The effect of long-term oxygen therapy on survival in patients with COPD and cor pulmonale. (Modified from Cooper *et al.* 1987.)

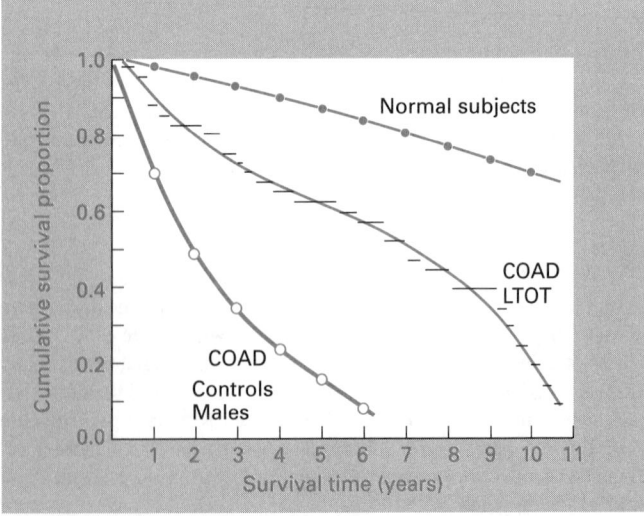

COPD, but is not generally available. It can cause a reversible peripheral neuropathy.

For many patients with ventilatory failure and cor pulmonale hypoxia is most intense during sleep. Rapid eye movement (REM) sleep is reduced by some drugs, including protriptyline. Although protriptyline may partially alleviate hypoxia in the short term, when prescribed chronically it is less effective.

Muscle capacity and the place of rehabilitation

Respiratory muscle function is compromised in many patients with pulmonary disease. In asthma, for example, hyperinflation shortens the respiratory muscles and flattens the diaphragm. Any factor that impairs respiratory muscle performance may cause or intensify breathlessness. The key balance is that between the demands made on the respiratory pump and its capacity. For most patients with chronic respiratory failure due to COPD ventilatory demand is much increased and capacity is frequently impaired. Pump capacity may be further reduced by factors as diverse as steroid myopathy, acidosis, or hyperthyroidism, and correction of such factors enhances capacity and thereby reduces breathlessness.

The reversal of these trends is central to pulmonary rehabilitation programmes, which aim to optimize independence, activity, and quality of life, and to minimize disease progression. Oxygen therapy, nutritional supplementation, NPPV, and the other therapies discussed in this chapter can be regarded as part of a rehabilitation strategy, but conventionally the central activities in rehabilitation are exercise and training. Most rehabilitation programmes have focused on patients with COPD. Whilst some clinical studies of general training have demonstrated improved exercise capacity, and while increased metabolic efficiency should reduce the ventilatory load for a given level of activity, the benefits that have been described have been modest, and there have been few convincing controlled studies. The data suggest that exercise sufficient to generate a lactic acidosis is necessary to yield improvement, and for patients who desaturate on exercise supplemental oxygen may be necessary to achieve a training benefit, as well as being a sensible precaution.

There have been numerous studies of inspiratory muscle training but their results have been mixed. As many studies have shown no benefit as have demonstrated an improvement in performance. Overall, the data suggest that it is possible to produce a modest improvement in the strength or endurance of the respiratory muscles if training schedules are designed with great care and pursued with determination. However, the impact of muscle training is highly specific for the task that is trained for—training for strength will increase strength, and training for endurance will enhance endurance. Furthermore, few studies have demonstrated that the small changes in respiratory muscle strength or endurance that are achieved translate into improved exercise capacity or reduced breathlessness in patients with chronic respiratory failure.

Although there appears to be a limited role for training in the management of chronic respiratory failure, this area of study is relatively new and much needs to be evaluated. It is clear that skeletal muscle histology, histochemistry, physiology and fatiguability, in both limb and respiratory muscles, are abnormal in patients with chronic respiratory failure. Strategies that reverse these abnormalities should improve ventilatory and exercise performance.

The role of physiotherapy in patients with chronic respiratory failure who have copious secretions, for example those with cystic fibrosis and bronchiectasis, is well established and can improve lung function, blood gases, and exercise capacity. However, physiotherapy is of no benefit for the majority of patients with chronic respiratory failure. Indeed, physiotherapy does more harm than good in patients without excessive secretions. Forced expiratory manoeuvres can worsen airways obstruction, and the raised intrathoracic pressures that are associated with most physiotherapy techniques impair cardiovascular function and tissue oxygen delivery.

Most cases of chronic respiratory failure are a consequence of smoking-induced COPD. Smoking prevalence is slowly falling in some Western countries, but is rising elsewhere in the world, and the global impact of tobacco on chronic respiratory disease will remain enormous for the foreseeable future. Therefore, cessation of smoking is a fundamental feature of all rehabilitation programmes.

REDUCTION IN LOAD

Major changes in airways obstruction cannot, by definition, be obtained in COPD. However, partial symptomatic relief of dyspnoea and small improvements (less than 10 per cent) in air-flow measurements can be achieved with bronchodilators. Simple inhalers, with or without a spacer device, are easiest to use for the administration of agents such as salbutamol or ipratropium bromide, alone or in combination. A small number of patients with severe disease require combined salbutamol and ipratropium administered by home nebulizer to achieve symptomatic relief; responders can be identified by symptom and peak-flow monitoring in a 2 to 3 week trial.

Additional therapeutic strategies in chronic respiratory failure

Breathlessness

This complex issue is discussed elsewhere. Relief relies on symptomatic measures described there and, where possible, treatment of the underlying condition.

Weight loss and nutrition

Many patients with chronic respiratory failure lose weight, particularly those with severe COPD in whom 30 to 40 per cent become wasted. Weight loss predicts a poor prognosis. In COPD most weight loss is seen in patients with the lowest forced expiratory volume in 1 s (FEV_1) and gas transfer. The basal metabolic rate of patients with severe COPD is raised by up to 20 per cent, probably owing to the increased work of breathing. Food intake may be low in some patients because of breathlessness. Weight loss is associated with muscle wasting and the respiratory muscles share in this wasting process, leading to an impairment of maximum ventilatory capacity. Clinical studies suggest that an increase in calorie intake of more than 30 per cent is required to achieve significant weight gain and thereby improve respiratory muscle function and exercise performance. In practice it has proved very difficult to achieve weight gain, and this therapeutic approach appears to offer limited success. When patients are given supplemental feeding they generally reduce their own spontaneous intake of food. More data are required before nutritional supplementation should become a regular aspect of the therapy of chronic respiratory failure. Theoretically, a diet high in carbohydrate is a disadvantage in chronic respiratory failure because of the relatively high carbon dioxide load, although this is probably not an important clinical problem.

Polycythaemia

The symptoms of secondary polycythaemia are principally due to hyperviscosity and include poor concentration, lethargy, somnolence, and headache. There is also an increased incidence of thrombotic events. Venesection improves cerebral blood flow and can reduce pulmonary hypertension; exercise tolerance may also be enhanced. It is conventional to reduce the haematocrit if it is greater than 0.6; it is usually lowered to 0.5. Simple venesection is effective, but acute blood loss can precipitate thromboses in patients with severe polycythaemia and an exchange transfusion with saline or plasma is safer. The technique of

Fig. 3 Survival with long-term domiciliary ventilation in patients with neuromuscular and other disorders. (Reproduced from Robert *et al.* 1983, with permission.)

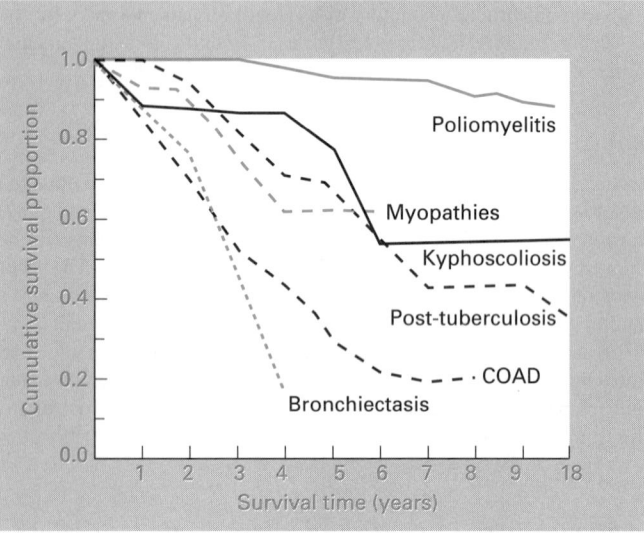

erythropheresis has the advantage of only removing the red cells. Because polycythaemia is secondary to chronic hypoxia, long-term oxygen therapy lowers the haematocrit. Similarly, any improvement in the underlying pulmonary disease that reduces hypoxia will have a beneficial effect.

Non-invasive assisted ventilation

Long-term and domiciliary ventilation

Selected patients with chronic ventilatory failure are appropriately treated with long-term assisted ventilation, and many, particularly those with neuromuscular disease, can do well (Fig. 3). A small number of patients, usually with advanced neurological disease or high cervical cord transection, are totally ventilator dependent and generally receive positive pressure ventilation via a tracheostomy. Some patients with high cervical lesions are managed by diaphragm pacing (see below). However, a much larger group of patients are capable of sustaining their own ventilation, albeit with hypoxia and hypercapnia, but require, or benefit from, intermittent ventilatory support, particularly at night. Intermittent ventilatory support can be provided via a tracheostomy, but most patients are treated non-invasively by either negative or positive pressure ventilatory devices.

Non-invasive ventilation can be highly effective in the long-term

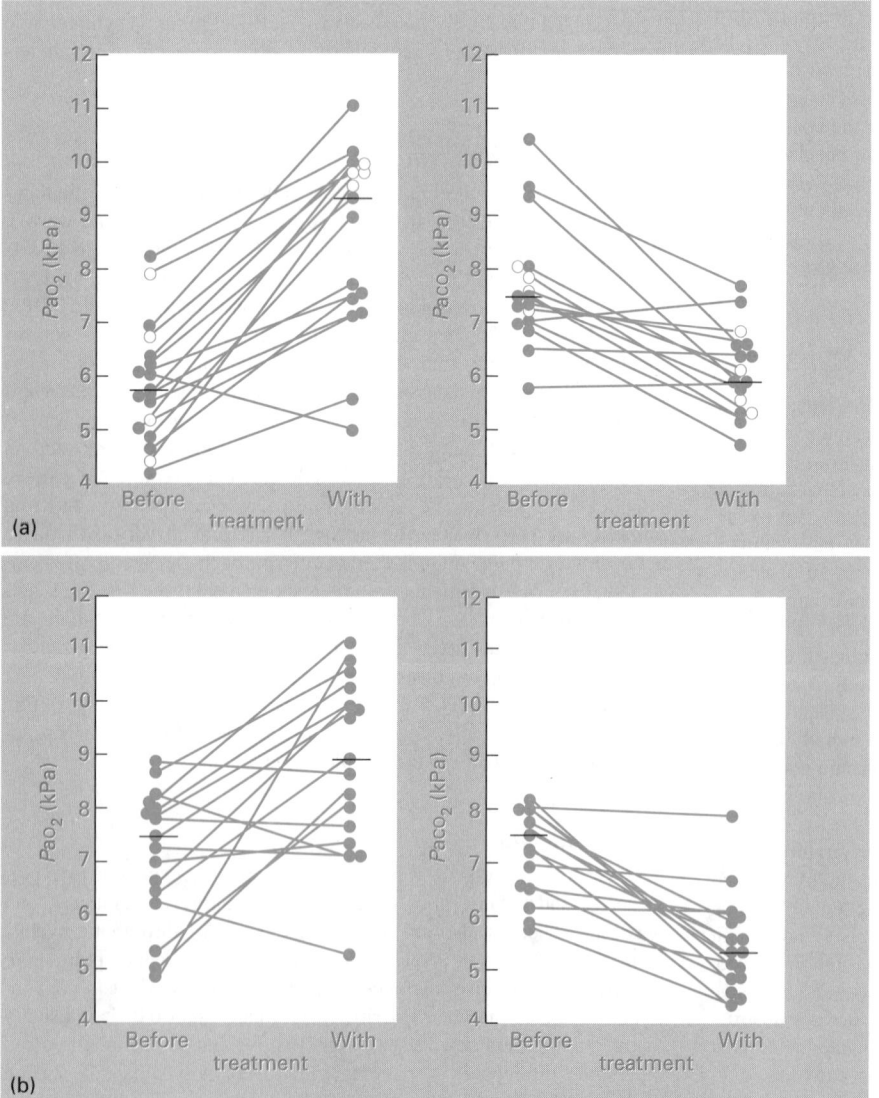

Fig. 4 Pa_{O_2} and Pa_{CO_2} values (breathing air) before and after treatment with long-term non-invasive ventilation in (a) 17 patients with skeletal deformity and (b) 16 patients with neuromuscular disease. (Reproduced from Sawicka *et al.* 1988, with permission.)

management of selected patients with chronic respiratory failure (Fig. 4). Patients who require intermittent assisted ventilation can be effectively managed with a variety of negative pressure ventilators (tank ventilators (the iron lung), jackets, and cuirasses). However, this approach is not suitable for all patients. Negative pressure ventilation is relatively inefficient, and when the chest wall or the lung is stiff it may not achieve adequate ventilation. Negative pressure ventilation also has the disadvantage of precipitating or exaggerating upper airways obstruction in many patients. If this is a severe problem tracheostomy is required. Negative pressure ventilators are also somewhat cumbersome and relatively difficult for patients and their carers to manage. Historically, the substantial technical skills required to manage patients successfully using negative pressure devices have only been available in a few specialist centres.

The use of non-invasive ventilation has greatly increased in recent years, following the introduction of NPPV. Most commonly the nasal mask is of the type used in CPAP treatment of patients with obstructive sleep apnoea. The nasal mask is firmly held in place by a head strap. Patients usually find NPPV an acceptable form of treatment because they are free to communicate, eat, and drink, and they can easily put on or take off the nasal mask. For those caring for patients, NPPV is considerably easier to manage than negative pressure ventilation. For these reasons NPPV is now the treatment of choice in most clinical situations, and the number of patients receiving this form of therapy has substantially increased. Nevertheless, NPPV is not suitable for all cases; for example it may be difficult to apply in patients with neurological disorders who are not able to move their upper limbs and adjust their nasal masks. NPPV can also be a problem in patients with severe bulbar problems with a tendency to aspiration and in patients with excessive bronchial secretions.

The usual indication for non-invasive ventilation (most commonly NPPV) is chronic severe hypercapnic ventilatory failure due to chest-wall or neuromuscular disease. In general NPPV is only appropriate for neuromuscular patients with stable or slowly advancing disease and therefore is inappropriate for most patients with rapidly advancing neurological disorders. Kyphoscoliosis, when severe, eventually causes ventilatory failure and is ideally treated by nocturnal NPPV, as is the ventilatory failure which can eventually develop in patients with thoracoplasty. The nocturnal hypoventilation and ventilatory failure of these patients is well controlled by NPPV; supplemental oxygen is seldom needed, and daytime gases (off ventilation) gradually improve. Such patients report a large improvement in well-being, sleep quality, intellectual capacity, energy, and breathlessness. Cor pulmonale and pulmonary hypertension are reversed, and life expectancy is increased. The effectiveness and relative simplicity of NPPV is such that all appropriate patients with severe chest-wall or neuromuscular disease need careful supervision so that NPPV can be considered at the correct time.

ts with central alveolar hypoventilation can be managed by a variety of approaches, including negative pressure ventilation (although upper airways obstruction is a problem), diaphragm pacing (see below), and tracheostomy and positive pressure ventilation. Some of these patients are probably best managed by NPPV, although the severity of central alveolar hypoventilation and the appropriateness of different therapeutic approaches require very careful consideration in each patient individually.

l number of patients with COPD and ventilatory failure have been treated by long-term nocturnal NPPV. COPD patients are less easy to ventilate and less tolerant of the technique than patients with chest-wall disease. Higher inflation pressures and flows are often required, and in patients with positive end expiratory intrathoracic pressure due to air trapping (intrinsic PEEP) there is a long and uncomfortable delay between the onset of inspiratory muscle contraction and the triggering of the ventilator. NPPV works best in COPD patients with hypercapnia and is not easily applied to the breathless patient with emphysema (the 'pink puffer'), in whom it can reduce breathlessness but with the danger that patients become ventilator dependent. When patients with COPD receive long-term domiciliary ventilation the outcome is less good than

for neuromuscular disease (Fig. 3), and whether this treatment is superior to long-term oxygen therapy remains to be proved.

It is crucial to keep in mind that NPPV is only feasible in patients who require intermittent ventilatory support. With prolonged periods of uninterrupted NPPV the nasal mask can cause severe damage to skin and soft tissue.

Acute on chronic ventilatory failure

Many patients with severe neuromuscular or chest-wall disease are precipitated into overt ventilatory failure by an intercurrent event, most commonly a respiratory infection. A period of NPPV can control such ventilatory failure until the status quo is restored, and therefore intubation and mechanical ventilation, or death, is avoided. Similarly, many patients in ventilatory failure due to an acute exacerbation of COPD, who do not respond to conventional therapy and develop a worsening hypercapnic acidosis, can be managed successfully with NPPV (see above). Therefore nasal ventilation may become a powerful tool in the management of acute on chronic ventilatory failure and may have the important economic advantage of reducing the need for intensive care unit facilities.

Weaning from mechanical ventilation

As NPPV has become a more widespread technique for the treatment of chronic ventilatory failure, so the approach has been used in other clinical situations. Patients who have difficulty in weaning from mechanical ventilation pose a common and important clinical management challenge. Many of these patients have pre-existing chronic lung disease, and some have established ventilatory failure prior to their unavoidable admission to the intensive care unit. Recent clinical studies suggest that NPPV may be a powerful technique to facilitate weaning and achieve early discharge from the intensive care unit, thereby improving clinical outcome and saving scarce medical resources (Fig. 5). Successful weaning from chronic ventilator dependence has been reported in patients with COPD as well as in those with neuromuscular and chest-

Fig. 5 Number of days receiving intermittent positive pressure ventilation (IPPV) in an intensive care unit and days from starting NPPV to hospital discharge in 18 patients who were difficult to wean. (Reproduced from Udwadia *et al.* 1992, with permission.)

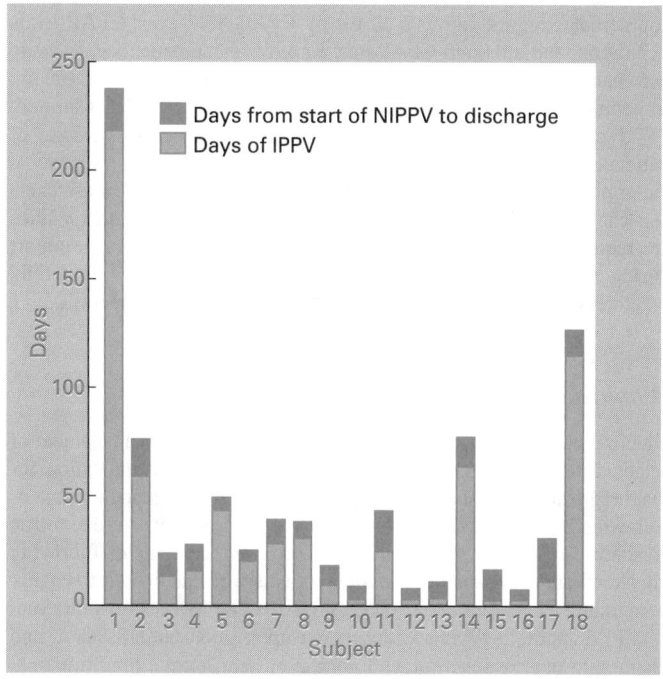

wall disorders. Prior to successful weaning it is important that patients are able to co-operate with the NPPV technique and that they are also independent of mechanical ventilation for short periods of time. It is likely that NPPV will become a standard technique employed to facilitate the weaning process in selected patients who are difficult to wean.

NPPV and transplantation

NPPV has been used as a 'bridge to transplantation' in patients with chronic lung disease, particularly those with cystic fibrosis. The technique can be used to control the ventilatory failure of these patients for prolonged periods of time. Patients with cystic fibrosis often become septic when intubated and ventilated, and have a poor prognosis; therefore NPPV represents, in many ways, a preferred ventilation option. A number of patients have been successfully transplanted following NPPV. During the bridging period patients are able to have appropriate physiotherapy, and are also able to discuss issues relating to their management as well as to eat, drink, and maintain their nutrition. Such patients do not need to be managed in the intensive care unit, which has both economic and social advantages. Nevertheless, as their underlying disease progresses, these patients become more ventilator dependent, and the unavailability of donor organs means that many die of ventilatory failure before transplantation is possible.

NPPV and the future

The advent of NPPV has had a major impact on the management of chronic ventilatory failure in a number of different circumstances and for many different diseases. It is likely that the indications for NPPV will widen further and that this technique will become indispensable in the treatment of this patient group.

Continuous positive airway pressure

Obstructive sleep apnoea is an important cause of ventilatory failure for which the mainstay of ventilatory support is CPAP. CPAP can also be of value in improving oxygenation in patients with acute respiratory failure (for example those with *Pneumocystis carinii* pneumonia). The role of CPAP in patients with acute hypercapnic ventilatory failure is less clear. The positive pressure during inspiration provides a degree of inspiratory pressure support, and inspiration is further facilitated by the counterbalancing of intrinsic PEEP by CPAP. However, CPAP loads expiration, and although CPAP may improve some patients with acute ventilatory failure, in others hypercapnia becomes more of a problem. In patients with chronic respiratory failure the role of CPAP is limited. CPAP can only be applied for relatively short time periods. Studies of patients with chronic airways obstruction suggest that in some patients the application of CPAP may reduce breathlessness and increase exercise capacity. However, not all patients report benefit and further studies are required. The possibility of providing inspiratory pressure support during exercise in patients with chronic lung disease who are limited by breathlessness is an area of considerable current research interest.

Diaphragm pacing

Diaphragm pacing has a small but important role in the management of selected patients with ventilatory failure. The principal indication for diaphragm pacing is in the treatment of ventilator-dependent subjects following high cervical cord injury, most commonly due to road traffic accidents, or injuries sustained during sporting accidents or following gunshot wounds. A smaller group of patients who can benefit from diaphragmatic pacing are those with central alveolar hypoventilation. Successful diaphragm pacing is dependent upon good phrenic nerve and diaphragm muscle function, and normal or near-normal lung function.

The best technique for assessing phrenic nerve and diaphragm function is electrical stimulation of each phrenic nerve using surface electrodes in the neck. The response to phrenic nerve stimulation can be assessed in terms of diaphragm movement, diaphragm EMG, and transdiaphragmatic pressure. Pacing electrodes are implanted around the phrenic nerves, usually via a thoracic surgical approach. A radio receiver is implanted in the subcutaneous tissues, usually of the lower antrolateral rib cage. Following diaphragm conditioning it is feasible to pace both hemidiaphragms 24 h daily, although in some patients adequate ventilation can be achieved by alternating unilateral diaphragm stimulation. The advantage of diaphragm pacing is that it is possible to achieve adequate ventilation without application of any equipment to the airway. The system is simple to use and speech is possible. With portable battery-operated transmitters patients can become more mobile than would otherwise be the case. The best results are achieved in young adults with quadriplegia due to high cervical cord injuries, and many of these have been satisfactorily paced for more than 10 years.

REFERENCES

Bott, J., Carroll, M.P., Conway, J.H., Keilty, S.E.J., Ward, E.M., Brown, A.M., *et al.* (1993). Randomised controlled trial of nasal ventilation in acute ventilatory failure due to chronic obstructive airways disease. *Lancet*, **341**, 1555–7.

Brochard, L., Isabey, D., Piquet, J., *et al.* (1990). Reversal of acute exacerbations of chronic obstructive lung disease by inspiratory assistance with a face mask. New England Journal of Medicine, **323**, 1523–30.

Cooper, C.B., Waterhouse, J., and Howard, P. (1987). Twelve year clinical study of patients with hypoxic cor pulmonale given long term domiciliary oxygen therapy. *Thorax*, **42**, 105–10.

Donner, C.F. and Howard, P. (ed.). (1991). Pulmonary rehabilitation in chronic obstructive pulmonary disease (COPD) with recommendations for its use. European Respiratory Journal, **1** (review 6).

Douglas, N.J. and Flenley, D.C. (1990). Breathing during sleep in patients with obstructive lung disease. American Review of Respiratory Disease, **141**, 1055–70.

Elliott, M. and Moxham, J. (1994). Non-invasive mechanical ventilation by nasal or face mask. In: *Principles and practice of mechanical ventilation* (ed. M.J. Tobin). pp. 427–53, McGraw Hill, New York.

Ellis, E.R., Grunstein, R.R., Chan, S., Bye, P.T.B., and Sullivan C.E. (1988). Noninvasive ventilatory support during sleep improves respiratory failure in kyphoscoliosis. *Chest*, **94**, 811–15.

Fitting, J.W. (1992). Nutritional support in chronic obstructive lung disease (Editorial). *Thorax*, **47**, 141–3.

Jeffrey, A.A., Warren, P.M., and Flenley, D.C. (1992). Acute hypercapnic respiratory failure in patients with chronic obstructive lung disease: risk factors and use of guidelines for management. Thorax, **47**, 34–40.

Jones, N.L., and Killian, K.J. (ed.). (1992). Breathlessness: The Campbell Symposium. McMaster University, Hamilton, Ontario.

Keilty, S.E.J., Ponte, J., Fleming, T.A., and Moxham, J. (1994). Effect of inspiratory pressure support on exercise tolerance and breathlessness in patients with severe stable chronic obstructive pulmonary disease. *Thorax*, **49**, 990–4.

Killian, K.J. (1990). Role of respiratory muscles in dyspnoea. In Problems in respiratory care: the respiratory muscles (ed. M.J. Tobin), Vol. 3, pp. 444–58.

Medical Research Council Working Party. (1981). Long term domiciliary oxygen therapy in chronic hypoxic cor pulmonale complicating chronic bronchitis and emphysema. *Lancet*, **1**, 681–5.

Moxham, J. and Shneerson, J.M. (1993). Diaphragmatic pacing. *American Review of Respiratory Disease*, **148**, 533–6.

Nocturnal Oxygen Therapy Trial Group. (1980). Continuous or nocturnal oxygen therapy in hypoxaemic chronic obstructive lung disease, a clinical trial. Annals of Internal Medicine, **93**, 391–8.

O'Driscoll, B.R., Kay, E.A., Taylor, R.J., *et al.* (1991). A long-term prospective assessment of home nebulizer treatment. Respiratory Medicine, 86, 317–25.

Robert, D., Gerard, M., Leger, P., *et al.* (1983). Domiciliary ventilation by tracheostomy for chronic respiratory failure. Revue Francaise des Maladies Respiratoires, **11**, 923–36.

Saunders, N.A. and Sullivan, C.E. (ed.) (1984). Lung biology in health and disease, Vol. 21, Sleep and breathing. Marcel Dekker, New York.

Sawicka, E.H., Loh, L., and Branthwaite, M.A. (1988). Domiciliary ventilatory support: an analysis of outcome. Thorax, **43**, 31–5.

Udwadia, Z.F., Santis, G.K., Steven, M.H., and Simonds, A.K. (1992). Nasal ventilation to facilitate weaning in patients with chronic respiratory insufficiency. Thorax, **47**, 715–18.

Warren, P.M., Flenley, D.C., Millar, J.S., and Avery, A. (1980). Respiratory failure revisited: acute exacerbations of chronic bronchitis between 1961–68 and 1970–76. Lancet, **i**, 467–71.

17.14.4 Lung and heart–lung transplantation

T. W. HIGENBOTTAM

Introduction

The last decade has seen lung and heart–lung transplantation established as treatment for a wide range of endstage lung and cardiopulmonary disease. Procedures for postoperative medical care have improved survival and limited the rate of occurrence of complications.

Significant problems remain. These concern the surgical techniques, particularly of complications of airway anastomoses in single- and double-lung transplants. Chronic rejection accounts for the main long-term complication which is often disabling and fatal. It causes obliterative bronchiolitis. For a proportion of patients, current regimes of immunosuppressive treatment do not control rejection.

There are insufficient donor organs for lung and heart–lung transplantation to allow all but a small proportion of suitable patients to be treated. Improvement of organ preservation techniques will not alter the scarcity of adequate organs for lung transplantation. The hope remains that xenografting, using animal organs, will become a medical possibility. No doubt this will raise ethical and psychological problems.

History of lung transplantation

Scientific interest and experimentation in lung transplantation covers a period of over 70 years. The first clinical lung transplant operations were undertaken in 1963, and 23 transplants were performed over the subsequent 7 years. There were no long-term survivors. The longest survivor lived for 10 months but most died within 30 days of surgery. The

Fig. 1 Actuarial survival data from 142 patients after heart–lung transplantation. (Papworth Hospital NHS Trust.)

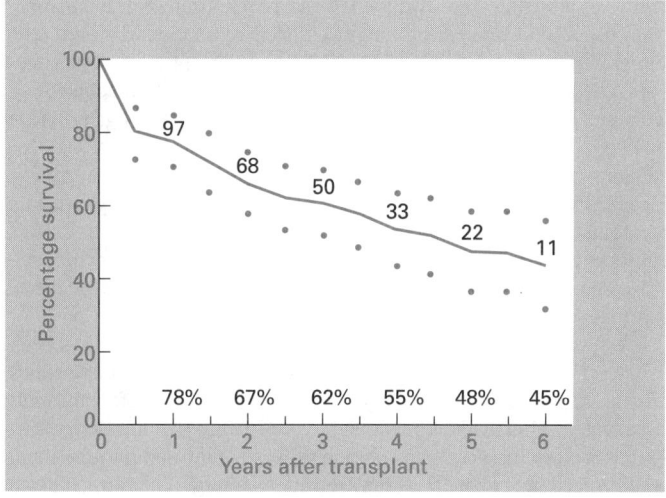

Table 1 *Causes of death after heart–lung transplantation (n = 100)*

Death within 3 months	Death after 3 months
Rejection **1**	Obliterative bronchiolitis **17**
Infection **8**	Infection **5**
Tracheal dehiscence **2**	Cerebrovascular event **1**
Cerebrovascular event **2**	Renal factors **1**
Lung failure **2**	Air traffic accident **1**
Liver failure **1**	
Graft-versus-host disease **1**	

main complications were dehiscence of bronchial or tracheal anastomoses and overwhelming sepsis. Excessive immunosuppressive treatment, particularly high dose corticosteroids, were considered to be the main cause.

The discovery of the immunosuppressive treatment cyclosporin by Borel allowed lung transplantation to be considered again. In 1982 Reitz and colleagues demonstrated, using cyclosporin, that heart–lung transplantation offered an effective treatment for pulmonary hypertension. Since then the technique has been extended to treat many lung diseases including cystic fibrosis.

Single-lung transplantation was reintroduced by Cooper and colleagues in 1983. Initially this was used for diffuse lung fibrosis, for example cryptogenic fibrosing alveolitis, but has been extended to treat emphysema and pulmonary hypertension. Suppurative lung disease cannot be treated by single-lung transplantation; the remaining lung causes infection in the transplant lung. Sequential double-lung transplantation with bilateral bronchial anastomosis now provides an alternative to heart–lung transplantation.

Survival from lung and heart–lung transplantation

Actuarial survival data provide a measure of the success of transplant surgery. Early deaths result from complications occurring during surgery and early postoperative care. The late deaths reflect the consequences of rejection and immunosuppressive treatment.

The 1 year survival figures for heart–lung transplants are nearly 80 per cent, and 5 year survival approaches 50 per cent (Fig. 1). Similar results are being reported for single-lung transplantation. Sequential double-lung transplant surgery has yet to achieve these figures. Continuing problems with airway anastomosis account for a high early death rate.

Analysis of the causes of death in heart–lung transplantation has allowed major risk factors to be identified. Early deaths can be attributed to complications in surgery (see Table 1). Deaths occurring after the first 3 months are largely the result of obliterative bronchiolitis, the main cause of which is recurrent acute rejection (see Table 1).

Clearly, patients are selected for lung and heart–lung transplantation when it is considered that they have a poorer chance of survival from conventional treatment for their disease than from transplant surgery.

Selection of the patient and of the type of transplant operation

TYPES OF TRANSPLANT OPERATION

A single-lung transplant provides an effective treatment for diffuse lung fibrosis, including cryptogenic fibrosing alveolitis, sarcoidosis, and histiocytosis X. Emphysema is similarly treated. Single-lung transplantation is still to be considered as an experimental procedure in the treatment of primary pulmonary hypertension. Acute respiratory distress syndrome is a common complication, and this has lessened its long-term success.

Sequential double-lung transplantation provides a treatment for suppurative lung disease such as bronchiectasis, cystic fibrosis, and chronic obstructive bronchitis with or without emphysema. Patients retain their own hearts and so potentially avoid chronic cardiac rejection. Also, as for single-lung transplantation, the operation does not necessarily require a cardiopulmonary bypass. Therefore older patients may be considered, although it is important to note that anaesthesia and ventilatory support for these patients during surgery present considerable difficulties.

Heart–lung transplantation is successfully used to treat cystic fibrosis, primary pulmonary hypertension, and Eisenmenger's syndrome where severe secondary pulmonary hypertension has developed as a result of congenital cardiac abnormalities.

The problem with heart–lung transplantation is the need for two lungs and one heart for a single recipient. The 'domino' operation was devised to enable the heart–lung recipient to donate his or her heart to another cardiac recipient, so providing for two recipients. However, in many countries sequential double-lung transplantation has replaced heart–lung transplantation for all except patients with Eisenmenger's syndrome.

The current choice of operation in the United Kingdom is shown in Table 2.

SELECTION OF PATIENTS

The point at which patients are considered for transplant surgery is determined by the prognosis of their underlying disease. In those diseases where the natural history of the disease is known, it is possible to predict the chance of survival. In general, where survival is poorer than the current actuarial figures for transplantation the patient is considered for surgery.

Primary pulmonary hypertension has a clearly defined natural history when untreated. The prognosis depends on the severity of the right ventricular failure. The haemodynamic measurements of cardiac index (CI) and mean right atrial pressure (RAP) provide a means of predicting survival chance, as does the mixed venous oxygen saturation $S\mathrm{vo}_2$ measured from the pulmonary artery blood samples. Patients with CI < 1.5 l/min/m³, RAP > 15 mmHg, and $S\mathrm{vo}_2 < 60$ per cent have a less than 20 per cent chance of surviving 3 years. Treatment with anticoagulants or agents such as continuous intravenous prostacyclin can prolong survival. However, most severely affected patients are offered heart–lung transplantation.

Chronic obstructive lung disease, including cystic fibrosis, has a well-defined natural history. Values of forced expired volume in 1 s (FEV_1) below 25 per cent of the predicted value and the degree of ventilatory failure as assessed by an elevated arterial carbon dioxide tension $P\mathrm{aco}_2$ predict poor survival.

The one group of patients where chance of survival is difficult to predict are those with Eisenmenger's syndrome. Many of these patients survive despite poor cardiac function. Acceptance for transplantation depends largely on the clinician's judgment.

The preoperative assessment for lung transplantation

A stable psychosocial background with a supportive family are essential prerequisites for a patient to undergo the risks of surgery and the subsequent intense postoperative monitoring.

However, there are a number of exclusion criteria which preclude patients from consideration for surgery. With increasing experience their number has diminished, as exemplified by patients with cystic fibrosis (Table 3). Investigators are directed to ensure that there are no exclusion criteria.

All patients have serological tests for HIV, cytomegalovirus, herpes simplex virus, Epstein–Barr virus, and toxoplasmosis. They are tested for ABO blood group, and HLA type is determined when a 'domino' operation is considered.

Special investigations are required for potential single-lung transplant recipients. High resolution CT is used to exclude bronchiectasis and the

Tabel 2 *Choice of lung and heart–lung transplants in the United Kingdom*

Primary pulmonary hypertension	Heart–lung transplant
Eisenmenger's syndrome	Heart–lung transplant
Chronic thromboembolic disease	Heart–lung transplant
Cystic fibrosis	Heart–lung transplant
Bronchiectasis	Double-lung transplant
Cryptogenic fibrosing alveolitis	Single-lung transplant
Emphysema	Single-lung transplant
Granulomatous and fibrotic lung disease	Single-lung transplant

Table 3 *Selection criteria for recipients for lung transplantation*

Life expectation < 18 months
12 mm walking distance < 500 m
Psychosocial stability
Lung disease
    $\mathrm{FEV}_1 < 25\%$ predicted
    Hypoxic respiratory failure
Pulmonary hypertension
    Mixed venous oxygen saturation $< 60\%$
    Cardiac index < 1.5 l/min/m²
Relative contraindications
    Age > 55 years
    Pleurodesis
    Insulin-dependent diabetes mellitus
    Steroid dependence > 10 mg/day prednisolone
Absolute contraindications
    Non-reversible additional organ failure
    Systemic or cerebral vascular disease
    Malignancy
    Aspergillus
    Drug or alcohol abuse

presence of mycetoma from *Aspergillus fumigatus*. Single- and double-lung transplant recipients also undergo coronary angiography to exclude coronary artery disease.

Patients considered for 'domino' operations, mainly cystic fibrosis patients, undergo three-dimensional echocardiography to assess left ventricular function and exclude valvular heart disease.

Donor selection and organ procurement

Whilst there are potentially over 1000 donors in the United Kingdom each year, less than 20 per cent will be suitable for lung transplantation. Brain death, concomitant prolonged assisted ventilation, and intensive care are associated with either significant lower respiratory tract infection or acute lung injury. These complications currently preclude lung donation. There are strict criteria for acceptance of donor organs (Table 4).

Donor and recipient are matched according to ABO blood groups. The size match between donor and recipient lungs is currently based on their total lung capacity predicted from their sex, age, and height. Donors with positive serology for cytamegalovirus are only used in cytomegalovirus-positive recipients. As described later, this lessens the incidence of primary cytomegalovirus pneumonia after lung transplantation.

The surgery involved in lung and heart–lung procurement has been well described. One detail deserves mention – the use of an intravenous infusion of prostacyclin into the donor pulmonary artery before the graft is harvested. This method, maximally vasodilating the pulmonary vasculature before the perfusate solution at 4° C is infused into the lung, has enhanced immediate graft function after surgery. It has also allowed

Table 4 *Lung donor selection criteria*

Age < 45 years
No past history of pulmonary disease including asthma
No thoracic trauma
No pulmonary or systemic infection
Normal chest radiograph
Short period of assisted ventilation
Normal lung compliance; peak respiratory airway pressure < 30 cmH$_2$O with tidal volume
15 ml/kg and respiratory rate 10–14 mm
Normal gas exchange; Pao_2 > 13.5 kPa with Fio_2 = 30%
HIV negative
For heart–lung transplantation
No heart disease
Normal electrocardiogram
Minimal inotropic requirements (dopamine or dobutamine < 10µg/kg/m)

extended ischaemic times to beyond 4 h, thus enabling the procurement operation to take place at a distant hospital. Alternatives include the analogue of prostacyclin, Iloprost, or prostaglandin E$_1$.

Transplant surgery

The surgical technique for heart–lung, single-lung, and sequential double-lung transplants are well described. Heart–lung transplantation required cardiopulmonary bypass and is undertaken through a median sternotomy. Single-lung transplants require a lateral thoracotomy, whereas access for the sequential double-lung transplant involves a transverse submammary incision. Postoperative pain is common with the latter incision.

Of necessity, the bronchial arteries are ligated in all forms of lung transplantation. In heart–lung transplant collaterals arise in the mediastinum, mainly from the coronary arteries supplying the lower trachea and the right and left main bronchi. This undoubtedly contributes to good tracheal healing. Bronchial anastomoses are fashioned in lung transplants. After transplantation, bronchial arteries are retrogradely perfused from pulmonary artery collaterals. To improve vascularization of the airway, anastomosis omentoplexia has been used in single-lung transplants. An alternative is to use bronchial revascularization procedures. There remains some uncertainty as to the value of these techniques.

A further consequence of lung transplantation is the loss of pulmonary innervation. The short- and long-term effects of loss of pulmonary nerves do not seem to be marked. This will be discussed later.

Immediate postoperative care

There are three main objectives of postoperative medical care: establishment of effective immunosuppressive therapy, achievement of negative fluid balance, and achievement of early exturbation and mobilization.

The perioperative use of antilymphocytic globulin for cardiac transplantation has recently ceased; the same may soon apply to lung transplantation. Instead, intravenous cyclosporin is used during the perioperative period. Corticosteroids are no longer contraindicated in the postoperative period. Indeed, some single-lung transplant centres have emphasized their importance. The loss of concern about early steroid use probably reflects the development of better lung-preservation techniques.

Despite improved preservation techniques for the lungs, periods of ischaemia extending beyond 4 h result in lung injury. Early lung biopsies performed soon after surgery indicate the formation of hyaline membrane and histological evidence of alveolar capillary injury. Therefore,

non-cardiogenic pulmonary oedema is a risk. For this reason hypervolaemia is carefully avoided by fluid restriction and intense use of diuretics over the first 3 days.

Assisted ventilation is not usually required for prolonged periods after surgery if the lungs were satisfactorily preserved. The ideal is less than 24 h, allowing early mobilization. Isolation of patients in the postoperative period to prevent infection during the induction of immunosuppressive treatment is no longer required.

The major reason for reoperation is bleeding from the mediastinum or chest wall. This is more commonly seen in suppurative lung disease and Eisenmenger's syndrome. The use of the antiprotease aprotinin during the operation has led to a significant reduction in postoperative bleeding.

Medical management after lung transplantation

Medical management after lung transplantation is directed to early diagnosis and treatment of rejection and infection, and the maintenance of adequate immunosuppression. Procedures have been adopted to minimize intrusion into the patient's life.

ACUTE REJECTION

It is not possible to distinguish acute rejection of the lungs from pulmonary infection on clinical signs or radiological investigations. Often the chest radiograph is normal in acute rejection. Pulmonary function tests, FEV$_1$, and vital capacity (VC) fall in value with both infections and rejection. Patients can monitor their lung function daily at home using a pocket-sized spirometer (Fig. 2).

To distinguish acute lung rejection from infection it is necessary to undertake a fibreoptic bronchoscopy with bronchoalveolar lavage and transbronchial lung biopsy. Multiple biopsies, attempting to sample all lobes, are taken from one lung.

The lung biopsies are processed for histology, and special stains are used to identify opportunistic infections. In acute lung rejection perivascular lymphocyte infiltrates are seen (Fig. 3), as are lymphocytic infiltrates of the bronchioli. Infections causing pneumonia can be diagnosed by the identification of the pathogen with standard histological techniques. Rejection and infection can coexist. Examination of bronchoalveolar lavage specimens does not provide a means of diagnosis of rejection. The proportion of subtypes of lymphocytes during rejection and of CD4- and CD8-positive cells in the lavage differs from the pattern seen in the biopsy specimens.

Treatment of acute rejection requires intravenous methyl prednisolone

Fig. 2 The FEV$_1$ (per cent predicted) plotted against time after surgery for a representative heart–lung transplant patient. The times R show episodes of rejection. (Reproduced from Smyth *et al.* (1989), with permission.)

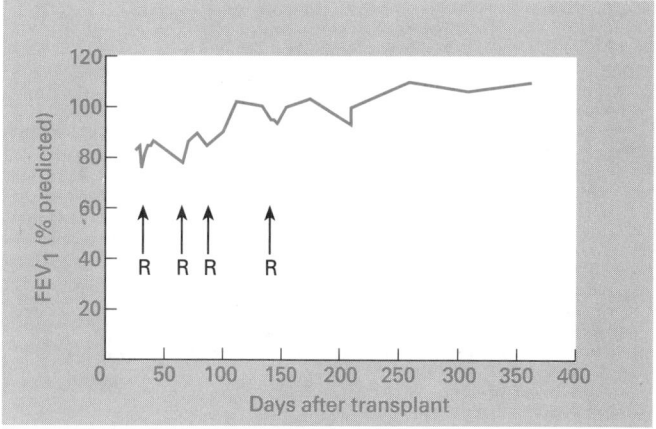

daily for 3 days. Doses between 125 and 1000 mg according to weight are required. Oral prednisolone is taken in decreasing doses for a further 10 days. The dosing of oral cyclosporin and azathioprine is reviewed with each episode of acute rejection. Usually the FEV_1 values are restored with this treatment within 3 weeks. Recurrent rejection is treated with continuous oral steroids; about a third of patients require long-term oral steroids in addition to cyclosporin and azathioprine.

Monitoring FEV_1 and use of diagnostic transbronchial lung biopsy is used with equal effectiveness in single- and double-lung transplants.

As a result of an internationally agreed scheme of grading the severity of the histological appearances of acute rejection, different transplant centres all share the same treatment regimes and diagnostic procedures (Table 5).

INFECTION

Although infections of heart–lung and lung transplant patients frequently involve the lungs, systemic infections are also common.

Pulmonary infections are pneumonias, lower respiratory tract infections, and chronic suppurative lung disease such as bronchiectasis. Patterns of infections vary according to the time since surgery; only rarely is bacterial infection acquired from the donor. Early after surgery pneumonia and acute bronchitis commonly occur as shown in Table 6.

Diagnostic investigations include sputum cultures, blood, bronchoalveolar lavage, and transbronchial lung biopsy specimens, bacteria, viruses, and fungi. Bronchoalveolar lavage and transbronchial lung biopsy specimens are subjected to detailed cytological and histological examination. The transbronchial lung biopsy specimens offer the means to detect evidence of pneumonia and the presence of the major pathogen.

Cytomegalovirus and herpes simplex virus can be recognized on histology by characteristic intracellular inclusions. *Pneumocystis carinii* and fungi can be recognized from the silver stain appearances. Mycobacterium tuberculosis requires acid-fast staining procedures. *In situ* hybridization and polymerase chain reaction molecular techniques are used frequently and appear more sensitive than morphological methods.

Cytomegalovirus pneumonia can be acquired from the donor. Recipients who are seronegative for cytomegalovirus before surgery are at high risk of developing cytomegalovirus pneumonia if they receive organs from a seropositive donor. Many centres now only use cytomegalovirus-negative donors for their cytomegalovirus-negative recipients. Cytomegalovirus can also cause pancreatitis and gastritis in these transplant patients. Treatment is with intravenous ganciclovir for 14 days. Hyperimmune globulin is no longer used.

Herpes simplex virus pneumonia is reactivation of latent infections of seropositive patients. These infections occur within the first 6 months

Fig. 3 A transbronchial lung biopsy showing a dense lymphocyte perivascular infiltrate type of acute rejection. (Reproduced from Smyth *et al.* (1989), with permission.)

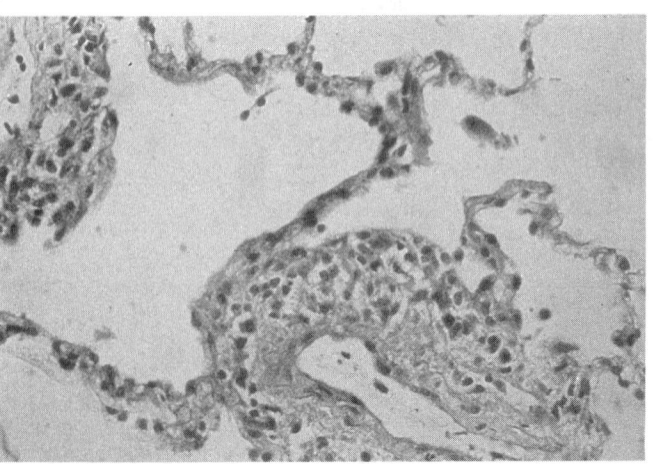

Table 5 *Histological classification of pulmonary rejection*

Classification	Principal histological finding
Acute rejection	Perivascular mononuclear infiltrates with or without airway inflammation
Acute airway damage without fibrosis	Lymphocytic bronchitis or bronchiolitis without perivascular infiltrates
Chronic rejection of airways	Bronchiolitis obliterans
Chronic vascular rejection	Fibrointimal thickening of arteries and veins

Adapted from the working formulation of the Lung Rejection Study Group

of transplant surgery or at times of augmentation of the immunosuppressive treatment. As a result it is possible to prevent them in seropositive recipients using acyclovir prophylactically for the first 6 months and when patients are treated for rejection.

Similarly, Epstein–Barr virus infections are usually reactivated and are also treated with acyclovir. The importance of Epstein–Barr virus is its capacity to initiate a lymphoproliferative disease as will be described later.

Pneumocystis carinii pneumonia also follows periods of augmentation of immunosuppressive treatment. However, the organism is encountered in up to 30 per cent of the bronchoalveolar lavage specimens of asymptomatic patients. Oral prophylactic treatment with trimethoprim (160 mg) and sulphamethoxazole (800 mg) each day has led to this being a relatively uncommon cause of pneumonia in heart–lung transplant patients.

Toxoplasma gondii infection seldom affects the lung but causes a systemic illness, often with cardiac involvement. It is acquired from the donor, again usually when seropositive donor organs are used in a seronegative recipient. The infection can be avoided by use of prophylactic pyrimethamine with folinic acid for the first 6 weeks of transplantation when mismatch between donor and recipient has occurred.

Yeast and fungal infections can cause pneumonia but are more commonly associated with tracheobronchitis. Airway complications of single- and double-lung transplants are frequently associated with *Aspergillus fumigatus* infections. It may be the loss of integrity of the airway mucosa which allows the infection to develop. All significant infections with yeast or fungi, where quantitative counts of cultures or invasion are seen on biopsy, are treated with intravenous amphotericin. The liposomal preparation of amphotericin is effective and does not appear as likely to cause renal impairment.

Coccidioidomycosis has also been described in lung transplant patients.

Graft versus host reactions

The lung transplant involves the inclusion of much lymphoid tissue of the donor; some of these cells survive and persist in the lungs and circulation of the recipient. In a series of 15 heart–lung transplant patients chimerism has been described in three patients, two of whom died from graft-versus-host disease. They had colitis, liver failure, and pancytopenia. The condition is probably more common than has been appreciated.

Recurrence of recipient's disease

Only sarcoidosis has been described as recurring after transplantation. A problem with the diagnosis of sarcoidosis after lung transplantation is that granulomatous reactions are relatively common in response to infections such as *P. carinii*.

Table 6 *Early pulmonary infections after heart–lung transplantation*

Site of infection	Number	Organism cultured		Deaths (%)
Pneumonia	7	B. aeruginosa	6	43
		K. pneumonia	1	
Emphysema	3	P. aeruginosa	2	66
		Staph. aureus	1	
Paratracheal abcess	2	C. perfridens	1	50
		Staph. aureus with H. influenzae	1	
Acute bronchitis	3	P. aeruginosa	2	0
		Staph. epidermidis	1	
Peritonitis	1	Enterococci	1	0
Septicaemia	1	P. aeruginosa	1	0

Infections which occurred in 17 of 100 heart–lung transplant patients within 30 days of surgery.

In the early 1980s there were fears that cystic fibrosis patients would reacquire the disease. This is clearly unlikely as the defective gene codes for the chloride channel on airway epithelial cells. The donor lung retains the genotype of the donor. This can be shown from a study of airway mucosal potential difference. The tracheal potential difference above the anastomosis remains characteristically high in cystic fibrosis heart–lung transplant patients. Below the anastomosis the potential difference is normal.

Lymphoproliferative disease

Lymphoproliferative disease is not uncommon after solid organ transplantation. It is caused by Epstein–Barr virus and occurs when immunosuppressive treatment is maximized. An incidence of 9.4 per cent has been reported in heart–lung transplant patients. Abnormal lymphoid tissue may be present within the lung, the mediastinum, or the small bowel; it is a B-cell expansion with features of a malignant lymphoma.

Treatment with acyclovir and reduction of the level of immunosuppression may be effective. However, chemotherapy or radiotherapy may become necessary, particularly when lymph node involvement is found.

Nephrotoxicity and systemic hypertension

Cyclosporin can induce acute but reversible renal impairment as well as establish renal failure. This effect, together with systemic hypertension, is dependent on dose. Higher doses of cyclosporin are required in heart–lung and lung transplants than in other transplants, and as a result up to 44 per cent of patients require antihypertensive treatment. The usual agents are calcium-channel blockers.

Fig. 4 An irreversible decline in FEV$_1$ is physiologically pathognomic of bronchiolitis obliterans. (Reproduced from Higenbottam and Clelland, (1992), with permission.)

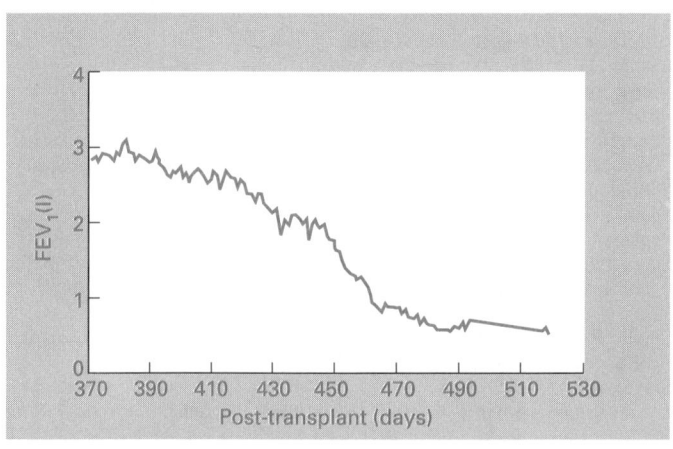

Table 7 *Interaction classification of the bronchiolitis obliterans syndrome (BOS)*

Normal	FEV$_1$ > 80% baseline
Minimal BOS	79% > FEV$_1$ > 65% baseline
Moderate BOS	64% > FEV$_1$ > 50% baseline
Severe BOS	FEV$_1$ < 49% baseline

Baseline FEV$_1$ is defined as the average of the best two values obtained at least 3 months after surgery.

Obliterative bronchiolitis

Most of the long-term deaths after lung transplantation result from or are associated with obliterative bronchiolitis. The characteristic histological lesion is submucosal fibrosis of the bronchioli which advances to obstruction of the lumen. In addition, there is usually extensive bronchiectasis of the central airways. Physiologically the patients develop disabling severe airflow obstruction with an irreversible fall in the value of FEV$_1$ (Fig. 4). Its development is closely associated with frequent acute rejection episodes and it probably represents a form of chronic rejection. At present there is no treatment, and patients ultimately die of respiratory failure.

Recently the term bronchiolitis obliterans syndrome was used to describe the various stages of airflow obstruction associated with this condition (Table 7). Considered in this fashion it is clear that, with increasing time after surgery, an increasing number of patients develop some degree of airflow obstruction. After 5 years, less than 50 per cent of heart–lung transplant patients will have normal values of FEV$_1$ (Fig. 5).

New developments in immunosuppressive treatment are needed if this complication is to be lessened. Indeed, it has now become the major limitation of lung and heart–lung transplantation.

The consequences of lung denervation

The lungs remain denervated after transplant surgery, but this appears to have little effect in humans. Persistent denervation has been confirmed by immunohistochemical studies of transplant lungs at death or retransplantation and the loss of the cough reflex to stimuli delivered to the airways below the tracheal anastomosis in heart–lung transplant patients.

Classical physiology has suggested that slowly adapting intrapulmonary stretch receptors are important for both perception of dyspnoea and regulation of breathing pattern. However, at rest and during exercise heart–lung transplant patients have a normal relationship between tidal volume and breathing frequency. The same is true during sleep, with patients showing a normal frequency of sighing.

During exercise heart–lung transplant patients also perceive dyspnoea

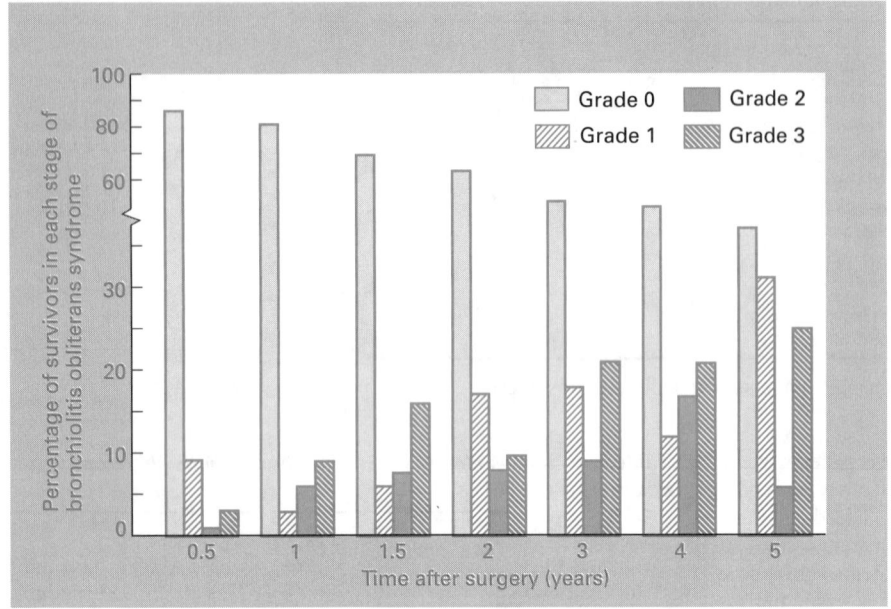

Fig. 5 The proportions of patients maintaining normal grade O (FEV$_1$ > 80 per cent), minimal grade 1 (80 per cent > FEV$_1$ > 65 per cent predicted), moderate grade 2 (65 per cent > FEV$_1$ > 50 per cent predicted), and severe grade 3 (FEV$_1$ < 50 per cent predicted) airflow obstruction.

in a similar fashion to normal subjects. Implicit in these observations is that intrapulmonary afferent nerves are not important in the regulation or the perception of breathing in humans.

Another important observation is that features of asthma, namely accentuated diurnal variation in FEV$_1$ and airway hyper-responsiveness, are also seen in heart–lung transplant patients at times of acute lung rejection. This would suggest that pulmonary innervation is not essential for the mechanism of asthma. Interestingly, airways infiltration with activated lymphocytes and eosinophils are common to both acute lung rejection and asthma.

Exercise capacity after lung transplantation

The improvement in quality of life after lung and heart–lung transplantation depends largely on lung function and exercise capacity. Clearly, patients who receive only one lung have poorer exercise capacity than double-lung and heart–lung transplant patients. As a result of poorer cardiac performance in heart–lung transplantation, the patients with double-lung transplantation achieve better exercise performance. However, the major limitations of improvement in exercise tolerance are the presence of acute lung rejection or development of bronchiolitis obliterans syndrome.

Conclusion

Lung transplantation offers a survival advantage to many patients with endstage lung disease. Shortage of donor lungs and significant incidence of chronic rejection currently limit the widespread use of the treatment. However, advances in molecular science are likely to solve the major problem by providing better immunosuppressive treatments and the possibility of xenografts.

REFERENCES

Borel, J.F., Feurer, C., Magnee, C., *et al.* (1977). Effects of the new anti-lymphocyte peptide cyclosporin A in animals. *Immunology*, **32**, 1017–25.

Cooper, J.D., Patterson, G.A., Grossman, R., *et al.* (1988). Double-lung transplant for advanced chronic obstructive lung disease. *American Review of Respiratory Disease*, **139**, 303–7.

D'Alonzo, G.E., Barst, R.J., Ayres, S.M., *et al.* (1991). Survival in patients with primary pulmonary hypertension. *Annals of Internal Medicine*, **115**, 343–9.

Dinh-Xuan, A.T., Higenbottam, T.W., Scott, J.P., and Wallwork, J. (1990). Primary pulmonary hypertension: diagnosis, medical and surgical treatment. *Respiratory Medicine*, **84**, 189–97.

Gore, S.M., Armitage, W.J., Briggs, J.D., *et al.* (1992). Consensus on general medical contraindications to organ donation? *British Medical Journal*, **305**, 406–9.

Higenbottam, T.W. and Clelland, C.A.C. (1992). Heart–lung transplantation: the challenge of obliterative bronchiolitis. *Organ Transplantation*, **12**, 247–60.

Hakim, M., Higenbottam, T.W., Bethune, D., *et al.* (1988). Selection and procurement of combined heart–lung grafts for transplantation. *Journal of Thoracic and Cardiovascular Surgery*, **98**, 474–9.

Higenbottam, T.W., Stewart, S., Penketh, A.R.L., and Wallwork, J. (1988). Transbronchial lung biopsy for the diagnosis of rejection in heart–lung transplant patients. *Transplantation*, **46**, 532–40.

Higenbottam, T., Otulana, B., and Wallwork, J. (1990). The physiology of heart–lung transplantation in man. *News in Physiological Science*, **5**, 71–4.

Kerem, E., Reisman, J., Carey, M, Carey, G.J., and Levison, H. (1992). Prediction of mortality in patients with cystic fibrosis. *New England Journal of Medicine*, **326**, 1187–91.

Kramer, M.R., Demmy, D.W., Marshall, S.E., *et al.* (1991). Ulcerative tracheobronchitis after lung transplantation. *American Review of Respiratory Disease*, **44**, 552–6.

Morrison, J.F.J., Higenbottam, T., Hathaway, T.J., *et al.* (1992). Diurnal variation in FEV$_1$ after heart–lung transplantation. *European Respiratory Journal*, **5**, 834–40.

Otulana, B.A., Higenbottam, T.W., Scott, J.P., *et al.* (1990). Lung function associated with histologically diagnosed acute lung rejection and pulmonary infection in heart–lung transplant patients. *American Review of Respiratory Disease*, **141**, 329–32.

Otulana, B.A., Higenbottam, T.W., and Wallwork, J. (1992). Causes of exercise limitation after heart–lung transplantation. *Journal of Heart–Lung Transplantation*, **11**, S244–51.

Reitz, B.A., Wallwork, J., Hunt, S., *et al.* (1982). Heart–lung transplantation: successful therapy for patients with pulmonary vascular disease. *New England Journal of Medicine*, **306**, 557–64.

Scott, J.P., Higenbottam, T.W., Hutter, J., *et al.* (1988). Heart–lung transplantation for cystic fibrosis, *Lancet*, **ii**, 192–4.

Scott, J.P. Higenbottam, T.W., Sharples, L., *et al.* (1991). Risk factors for obliterative bronchiolitis in heart–lung transplant recipients. *Transplantation*, **51**, 813–17.

Smyth, R.L., Higenbottam, T.W., Scott, J.P., *et al.* (1989). Transplantation of the lungs. *Respiratory Medicine*, **83**, 459–66.

Smyth, R.L., Sinclair, J., Scott, J.P., *et al.* (1991). Infection and reactivation with cytomegalovirus strains in lung transplant patients. *Transplantation*, **52**, 480–1.

Toronto Lung Transplant Group. (1986). Unilateral lung transplantation for pulmonary fibrosis. *New England Journal of Medicine,* **314,** 1140.

Wallwork, J. (1989). *Heart and heart–lung transplantation.* W.B. Saunders, Harcourt Brace Jovanovich, Philadelphia. A complete introduction to the medical, surgical and physiological events of this form of transplantation.

Wildevuur, C.R. and Benfield, J.R. (1970). A review of 23 human lung transplantations by 20 surgeons. *Annals of Thoracic Surgery,* **9,** 489–515.

Wood, A., Higenbottam, T.W., Jackson, M., and Wallwork, J. (1988). Air-way mucosal bioelectric potential difference in cystic fibrosis after lung transplantation. American *Review of Respiratory Disease,* **140,** 1645–52.

Yousem, S.A., Randhawa, P., Locker, J., *et al.* (1989). Post transplant lymphoproliferative disorder in heart–lung transplant recipients: primary presentation in the allograph. *Human Pathology,* **20,** 361–9.

Yousem, S.A., Berry, G.J., Chamberlain, D., *et al.* (1990). A working formulation for the standardization of normenclature in the diagnosis of heart and lung rejection: lung rejection study group. *Journal of Heart and Lung Transplantation,* **6,** 593–601.

Index

Page numbers in **bold** refer to major discussions in the text and include major sections and subsections, but are not necessarily limited to these. Bold page numbers referring to diseases, include discussions on diagnosis, clinical features, pathology and treatment, where relevant.

Page numbers in *italics* refer to pages on which tables are to be found.

vs   denotes differential diagnosis or comparisons.

Plates have not been indexed, but are referred to in the text. Biochemical parameters within the tables of Section 33 have not all been indexed individually - readers are advised to seek reference ranges from the appropriate table. Epidemiological data relating to specific countries has only been indexed under the individual countries where major discussions occur. For further information, readers are advised to refer to the epidemiological page reference for the disease in question.

Indexing style/conventions used

Alphabetical order. This index is in letter-by-letter order, whereby hyphens, en-rules and spaces within index headings are ignored in the alphabetization. Terms in brackets are excluded from initial alphabetization eg.

acid(s)
acid-base homeostasis
acidosis
acid phosphatase

Cross-references. Cross-reference terms in *italics* are either general cross-references, or refer to subentry terms within the same main entry (the main entry term is not repeated, in order to save space) i.e. they are not main entry terms.

Index entries have been restricted to two subentry levels. Entries have therefore been reorganised/reworded or relocated where further levels have been required.

eg. *renal failure, acute*, reworded to *acute renal failure*, or *lymphoma, non-Hodgkin's* reworded to *non-Hodgkin's lymphoma*.

Cross-references are inserted to indicate correct keyword term or location of entry.

Some index subentries, particularly those referring to individual pages within a page grouping, have been included more to indicate the extent of the discussion in the text rather than the actual location of the reference.

Abbreviations used in subentries (without explanation):

ACTH	Adrenocorticotrophic hormone (corticotrophin)	hCG	Human chorionic gonadotrophin
AIDS	Acquired immunodeficiency syndrome	HIV	Human immunodeficiency virus
ARDS	Adult respiratory distress syndrome	HPV	Human papilloma virus
CMV	Cytomegalovirus	HTLV	Human T-cell leukaemia virus
COAD	Chronic obstructive airways disease	IL	Interleukin
CPAP	Continous positive airway pressure	LCMV	Lymphocytic choriomeningitis virus
CRF	Corticotrophin releasing hormone (factor)	MAOIs	Monoamine oxidase inhibitors
CT	Computed tomography	MEN	Multiple endocrine neoplasia
DIC	Disseminated intravascular coagulation	MRI	Magnetic resonance imaging
EBV	Epstein-Barr virus	NSAIDs	Non-steroidal anti-inflammatory drugs
ECG	Electrocardiogram/electrocardiography	PAF	Platelet activating factor
EEG	Electroencephalogram/electroencephalography	PEEP	Positive end-expiratory pressure
EMG	Electromyography	PTH	Parathyroid hormone
ERCP	Endoscopic retrograde cholangiopancreatography	RSV	Respiratory syncytial virus
G6PD	Glucose-6-phosphate dehydrogenase	SIADH	Syndrome of inappropriate antidiuretic hormone secretion
GBM	Glomerular basement membrane		
G-CSF	Granulocyte colony-stimulating factor	SLE	Systemic lupus erythematosus
GH	Growth hormone	STDs	Sexually transmitted diseases
GM-CSF	Granulocyte-macrophage colony-stimulating factor	TNF	Tumour necrosis factor
HBV	Hepatitis B virus	TSH	Thyroid stimulating hormone
HCV	Hepatitis C virus		

A

Abadie's sign 4085
abbreviated mental test score *4337*
ABC resuscitation system 2283, 4045–6
abdomen
 acute, *see* acute abdomen
 chest radiography 2179
 circumference, fetal 1756
 examination,
  in haematological disorders 3376
  in homosexuals with STDs 3361
 fluid thrill 2095
 rebound tenderness,
  in appendicitis 2010
  in peritonitis 2008
 shifting dullness, in ascites 2095
abdominal actinomycoses 683
abdominal adhesions 2009

abdominal aortic aneurysm, *see* aortic aneurysms
abdominal bloating **1967**
abdominal bruit
 in chronic intestinal ischaemia 1996, 1997
 in cirrhosis 2088
 in renovascular hypertension 2546
abdominal distension
 in ascites 2095
 in constipation 1826
 in irritable bowel syndrome 1966
 in typhoid 563
abdominal mass
 in left upper quadrant *3590*
 pulsatile 2364
abdominal pain **1822–3**
 in acute diverticulitis 1970
 in acute intestinal ischaemia 1996
 in acute pancreatitis 2028

in acute porphyria 1391, 1393
in adhesions 2009
in aortic aneurysms 2364
in appendicitis 2010
in *Campylobacter* infections 558
causes 1822, *1823*
in choledocholithiasis 2050
in cholestasis 2046
in chronic intestinal ischaemia 1996
in chronic pancreatitis 2034, 2035
 management 2036, 2037
in Churg-Strauss syndrome 2800
in cirrhosis 2087
in Crohn's disease 1938
in cryptosporidiosis 873
in diabetic ketoacidosis 1499, 1503
diagnosis 1823
 computer-aided 2010
epigastric, *see* epigastric pain
from viscera 1822–3

functional **1968**
in hepatocellular carcinoma 2116
in hereditary fructose intolerance 1347
in hereditary haemochromatosis 3479
in hereditary pancreatitis 2026
in hypertriglyceridaemia 1410
in irritable bowel syndrome 1966
in Munchausen's syndrome 4211
nerve pathways 1822, *1823*
in pancreatic carcinoma 2042
parietal 1822
in paroxysmal nocturnal haemoglobinuria 3450
in peptic ulcer perforation 1882
in peritonitis 2008
in pre-eclampsia 1729
in recurrent polyserositis 1526
referred 1822

abdominal pain (cont.)
  in rheumatic diseases 2945
  in sickle-cell crises 3514
  in subacute intestinal obstruction 1960,
    1961
  in tumours 241
  in urinary stone disease 3253
  in urinary-tract obstruction 3235
abdominal radiation, intestinal ischaemia
    after 1995
abdominal radiography 1830–1
  in Armillifer infestation 1013
  in biliary disease 2046
  body packers of drugs 1075
  in carbon tetrachloride poisoning 1085
  in chronic pancreatitis 2035, 2036,
    2037
  in Crohn's disease 1939
  'double bubble' sign 1976
  in hydatid disease 957
  in intestinal ischaemia 2367
  in jejunoileal obstruction 1976
  in meconium ileus 1978
  in oesophageal atresia 1974
  in paralytic ileus 1961
  in small-intestinal malrotation 1977
  in ulcerative colitis 1946
abdominal radiotherapy, see radiotherapy
abdominal surgery, gastrointestinal
    motility disorders after 1961
abdominal swelling
  causes 2095–6
  in malnutrition 1284
abdominal symptoms, in malabsorption
    1904
abdominal tenderness
  in amoebiasis 828
  in ulcerative colitis 1945
  see also abdomen, rebound tenderness
abdominal tularaemia 601
abdominal wall
  defects 1974–5
    see also exomphalos; gastroschisis
  veins/collateral circulation 2092, 2093
abducens (sixth cranial) nerve, lesions
    2583, 3877
abetalipoproteinaemia 1414, 3686
  small-bowel biopsy 1908
abl gene 225
  see also bcr/abl gene
ABO blood groups 3688
  compatibility testing 3688–9
  renal transplantation and 3315
  see also blood group
abortion
  Chlamydia psittaci causing 755
  mumps association 374
  septic 1733
  septicaemia after 1022
  spontaneous,
    antiphospholipid antibodies and 3669,
      3670
    in cyanotic congenital heart disease
      2401
    in parvovirus infection 1782
  therapeutic 12
    chorionic villus sampling and 136
    in cystic fibrosis 2755
    in Eisenmenger syndrome 2412
    genetic testing and 137
    in malignant disease 1807
    in thalassaemia 3512
Abraham's needle 2865
Abram biopsy needle 2682
abruptio placentae 1762
abscess
  actinomycotic 682
  amoebic brain 830
  amoebic liver, see amoebic liver
    abscess
  aortic root 2443
  appendix 2010
  axillary 573
  brain, see cerebral abscess; intracranial
    abscess
  cerebellar, see cerebellar abscess
  cerebral, see cerebral abscess
  cold paraspinous 3000
  crypt 1945

dental 1846, 1847
diagnostic sampling 312, 312
diverticular 1970, 1971
epidural 3892, 3894
extradural 4081, 4082
filarial 922
heart 2215
injecting drug addicts 4294
intracranial, see intracranial abscess
intraperitoneal 2008
liver, see liver, abscess
lung, see lung, abscess
myocardial 2439, 2444
Pautrier 3797
pelvic 2008
pericolic 1970, 1971
perinephric 529, 3207
perirectal 573–4
peritonsillar 496
prostatic 573
renal 529, 3207
Salmonella 552
splenic, see spleen, abscess
staphylococcal 529
subphrenic 2008
supratentorial 4083
visceral, glomerulonephritis
    complicating 3175
absences
  atypical 3914
  typical (petit mal) 3912–13
absence status 3923
absorption of nutrients, see intestinal
    absorption
ABVD regimen 3573, 3574
ACA centromere antibodies 3033
acalculia 3851–2
Acanthamoeba 825
  infections 834
Acanthocheilonema perstans 919
acanthocytes 3378
acanthocytosis
  in abetalipoproteinaemia 3686
  with neurological disease and normal
    lipoproteins (amyotrophic chorea-
    acanthocytosis) 3686–7
acantholysis 3710
acantholytic cell 3781
acanthosis 3366
acanthosis nigricans 244, 3755, 3793,
    3795
  in acromegaly 1592
  in polycystic ovary syndrome 1675
acarinophobia 1009
Acarus 3710, 3713
acatalasaemia 1441
accelerated idioventricular rhythm 2281
'accelerated starvation' 845
acceleration, aircraft 1194, 1195
accident and emergency departments,
    drug addicts in 4294–7
accidents
  drug abusers 4295
  occupational 1174–5, 1175
    see also under occupational safety
  spinal cord injury management 3896
acclimatization
  cold 1182
  high altitudes 1186–7, 1191, 1192
accuracy, clinical examination 17–20
ACE inhibitors, see angiotensin
    converting enzyme (ACE) inhibitors
acetaldehyde 2081
  metabolism 2081
acetaminophen, see paracetamol
acetate 1467
acetazolamide
  in acute mountain sickness 1190,
    1191
  in renal failure 3275
  ventilatory drive changes 2916
acetoacetic acid 1534
acetohexamide 1471
acetone, poisoning 1093
acetylation 130, 1259
  slow acetylators 130, 1259
N-acetyl-p-benzoquinoneimine (NAPQI)
    1051, 1053

acetylcholine (ACh) 3881, 4139
  coronary tone regulation 2323
  insulin secretion and 1459
  at neuromuscular junction 4139, 4141,
    4160
  receptors 4139
    antibodies 163, 4160, 4161
    loss in myasthenia gravis 4160
acetylcholinesterase 4139
  decline, in Pick's disease 3975
  excess in bowel wall 1979
  inhibitors, see cholinesterase inhibitors
  reactivators, in nerve agent exposure
    therapy 1118
acetyl coenzyme A 1458, 2146
  in citric acid cycle 2146
acetyl coenzyme A carboxylase 1373
acetyl coenzyme A synthetase, in
    adrenoleukodystrophy 3997
N-acetylcysteine 1048, 2107
  in adult respiratory distress syndrome
    2859
  in carbon tetrachloride poisoning 1085
  in chloroform poisoning 1086
  in cystic fibrosis 2753
  in methyl chloride poisoning 1087
  in paracetamol poisoning 1048, 1052
    dosage/administration route 1053, 1053
N-acetyl glucosamine, in vesicular
    transport 75
N-acetyl-ß-glucosaminidase, urinary
    3109, 3138, 3260
acetyl-LDL (scavenger) receptor 1403,
    1405
N-acetyl muramyl-1-ala-SCDsc
    isoglutamine (MDP) 292
N-acetylneuraminic acid storage disease,
    see Salla disease
acetylsalicylic acid, see aspirin
N-acetyltransferase, acetylator rate 130,
    1259
achalasia 1958–9
  causes and diagnosis 1958–9
  dysphagia of 1820, 1958
  idiopathic 1869
achalasia-like states 1869
Achilles tendon
  central core degeneration 2996–7
  rupture 2996
achlorhydria
  bacterial overgrowth in 1911
  cholera susceptibility 577
  in common variable immunodeficiency
    1837
  elevated gastrin 1894
  in pernicious anaemia 3496
  in VIPoma syndrome 1706
achondroplasia 3088–9
  diagnosis and types 3088, 3088
  genetics 113–14
  homozygous 3088
  see also skeletal dysplasias
achondroplasia-like dwarfs 3088–9
Achromobacter 550
acid(s)
  mechanisms of toxicity 1103
  poisoning by 1103
    management 1103, 1104
  types and uses 1103
acidaemia 1535
  correction in high central venous
    pressure 2565
acid air 1230
Acidaminococcus fermentans 550
acid-base homeostasis
  disturbances 1533–44, 4126
    causes 1536–7
    in chronic renal failure 3297
    consequences 1537–40
    definitions 1535
    diagnosis 1535–6
    in hepatocellular failure 2103, 2109
    neurological features 4125–6
    in paracetamol poisoning 1052, 1053
    in poisoning 1047
    treatment 2109
    treatment principles 1543–4
    see also acidosis; alkalosis

glutamine metabolism and 1276
normal 1533–5, 3338
in ventilatory failure 2904
acid cholesteryl ester hydrolase
  deficiency 1436–7
acid-fast organisms 2676
acid α-1,4-glucosidase 1341
  deficiency, see Pompe's disease
α₁-acid glycoprotein 305
  drug binding 1242
acid hydrolases 1426
acidification, of endocytic pathway 74,
    75
acidified serum (Ham) test 3451
acid load test of Wrong and Davis
    3338–9
acid maltase 4165
  deficiency (type II glycogenosis)
    4165–6
acidosis 1535
  in acute renal failure 3284
  alcohol (ethanol)-induced 1542
  carbohydrate metabolism and 1539
  cardiovascular effects 1539
  in chronic renal failure 3297
  diabetic ketoacidosis vs 1499
  drug/metabolite distribution and 1540
  in high central venous pressure 2565–6
  lactic, see lactic acidosis
  leucocyte effects 1540
  management, in septicaemia 1024
  metabolic, see metabolic acidosis
  methanol-induced 1543
  nervous system effects 1539–40
  oxygen uptake/delivery and 1539
  potassium homeostasis and 1540,
    3127–8
  in pyruvate carboxylase deficiency 1352
  renal bone disease and 3327
  renal effects 1540
  renal tubular, see renal tubular acidosis
  respiratory, see respiratory acidosis
  respiratory effects 1537–9
  skeletal effects 1540
  uraemic 1541, 1543, 1544
  see also metabolic acidosis; respiratory
    acidosis
acid phosphatase 4365
acid regurgitation, see gastro-
    oesophageal reflux disease
acid trap 1911
acinar-cell carcinoma 2042
acinar-cell disruption 2028, 2029
Acinetobacter, rare species 550
acinus 2596
  structure 2597–8
acipimox 1414, 1472
ACME trial 2331
acne, non-dermatitic occupational
    dermatosis 1165
acne arthralgia 3003
acne cysts 3753
acneiform eruption 3731
acne vulgaris 3709, 3715, 3716, 3752–4
  chemicals causing 1165
  in cyanotic congenital heart disease
    2400
  drug-induced 3752
  in hyperandrogenization 1674, 1677
  infective organisms 3752
  neonatal 3753
  in pregnancy 1804
  scarring 3753
  surgery 3754
aconitine 1154
acoustic emissions 3871
acoustic neurinomas, in
    neurofibromatosis 3987
acoustic neuroma, computed tomography
    (CT) 3818
acoustic schwannomas 3874–5, 4036
acquired immunodeficiency syndrome,
    see AIDS
acrivastine 2718
acrocyanosis 2365, 2376
acrodermatitis enteropathica 174, 1418,
    3768
acrodynia 1111

acromegaly 1553, 1569, **1591–5**
  aetiology 1591
    extrapituitary causes 1591, **1714–16**
  calcitriol in (1,25-(OH)$_2$D$_3$) 1593, 1636
  clinical features 1591–2
  complications 1592–3
  diagnosis 1586, 1593–4
  in MEN 1 syndrome 1708
  mental disorders/symptoms in 4239
  myopathy in 4168
  peripheral nerve involvement 4099
  pregnancy in 1748
  prognosis 1594–5
  treatment 1588, 1594
acro-osteolysis 1090
acroparesthesiae 4095, 4096
acrylamide, neuropathy 4099
acrylic, contact dermatitis 3737
ACT2 gene 82
ACTH (corticotrophin) **1575–6**
  adverse mental symptoms 4242
  blocking antibodies, in Addison's
    disease 1653
  in CNS viral infections 4071
  control of secretion 1575, 1601, 3118
  in Cushing's disease 1566, 1640–2
  deficiency, *see* hypoadrenalism,
    secondary
  ectopic production 1568, 1642, 1711,
    1712–14
    clinical features 1644, 1712–13
    diagnostic tests 1585, 1646–9, 1713
    in lung cancer 2884
    mineralocorticoid excess 1661
    treatment 1651, 1713–14
  excess, myopathy in 4168
  hereditary adrenocortical
    unresponsiveness 1653
  molecular species 1575, 1647
  phaeochromocytomas secreting 2554,
    2556
  pituitary tumours secreting 1595, 1641,
    1650–1
  plasma 1583
    in adrenal insufficiency 1654
    in combined anterior pituitary test
      1585
    in CRF stimulation test 1648
    in Cushing's syndrome 1646–7
    in ectopic ACTH syndrome 1713
    in insulin tolerance test 1585–6
    in metyrapone test 1647, 1649
    in Nelson's syndrome 1595
    in pregnancy 1750
    in psoriasis 3750
  receptor 1555, *1560*
  stimulation test 1654–5, 1664, *4375*
  in stress 1563, 1575–6
  in trauma 1548–9
  withdrawal 1251
actin
  cell shape control 80
  in cytokinesis 81
  Listeria monocytogenes movement in
    cytoplasm 82
  in muscle cells 80, 4139
  in myocardial cells 2144
  in neutrophil activation changes 2622
  in non-muscle cells 80, 81
  in platelets 3618
  polymerization 81
  in red-cell membrane 3527
actin-binding proteins 81, 3618
actinic lentigo *3754*
actinic prurigo 3726
Actinobacillus, rare species *550*
Actinomyces 2708
  bacteriology and detection 684
Actinomyces bovis 2133
Actinomyces gerencseriae 680, 684
Actinomyces israelii 680, 684, 2133
Actinomyces multifermentans 685
Actinomyces pyogenes 685
actinomycetes
  fermentative 680
    diseases 685
    properties 680–1, *681*
  thermophilic 2809, 2811

actinomycetoma 802
actinomycoses **680–6**
  abdominal 683
  aetiology 680
  bone 683
  cervicofacial 682, 683
  clinical features 682–4
  CNS 683
  cutaneous 684
  diagnosis/serological tests 684
  epidemiology 685
  eye in 4191
  liver in 2133
  pathogenesis and pathology 681–2
  synergistic polymicrobial infections
    681, *682*
  thoracic 682–3
  treatment and prognosis 684–5
action potential 2152, 3831, 4139
  cardiac 2148, 2149, 2152, 2259
    drugs affecting 2263
  nerve 3831, 3840
  peripheral nerve 3831
activated charcoal 1049–50
  adverse effects 1049–50
  in antiarrhythmic drug overdose 1063
  dosage 1050
  indications and mechanism 1049
  in NSAIDs poisoning 1057, 1058
  in opioid overdose 1058
  in paracetamol poisoning 1053
  in paraquat poisoning 1120
  repeat dose 1056, 1058
    to aid poison elimination 1050
  in salicylate poisoning 1056
  in theophylline overdose 1068
  in tricyclic antidepressant poisoning 1059
activated partial thromboplastin time
    (APTT) 3628, 3661, 3673
  pulmonary embolism treatment 2526
activated protein C 2290
  resistance to 2522
activating transcription factors (ATFs)
    1558
activin 1554
  in erythropoiesis 3387
  platelet 3618
  in reproduction 1563, 1564, 1580
activities of daily living (ADL),
    assessment 4226
actomyosin, in yeast 82
actomyosin gel 81
acupuncture, pain treatment 3943–4
acute abdomen 1823
  causes 1971
  in connective tissue diseases 3010
  in intestinal ischaemia 1996, 2367
  peritonitis 2008
  radiography 1830
  septicaemia in 1021
  in SLE 2000
acutely ill patients
  avoidance of acute renal failure 3281–3
  drugs to be used with care 3283, *3284*
  rehabilitation in elderly **4340**
  renal function monitoring 3279–80
  thyroid function tests 1617
  see also intensive care
acute mountain sickness, *see* mountain
    sickness, acute
acute-phase proteins 176, 276, 1528
  in Behçet's syndrome 3044
  fibrinogen as 2302
  in infections 294
  in listeriosis 722
  mechanisms 276
  protective function 276
  in psoriatic arthritis 2969
  in rheumatic diseases 2951
  in rheumatic fever 2434
  serum amyloid A protein 2835
  in ulcerative colitis 1946
  see also complement; C-reactive
    protein; serum amyloid A (SAA)
    protein
acute-phase response 176, **1527–8**, 2951,
    2952
  in acute pancreatitis 2030

after injury/surgery 1550
  in gout 2986
  in inflammatory rheumatic disease
    2951–2
acute renal failure **3279–93**
  causes *3279*, *3282*
  chemicals inducing 3546
  in cholesterol embolism 2376
  costs 3293
  diagnosis 3279–80
  in electrical injury 1212
  glomerulonephritic/vasculitic causes
    3291
  'haematological' causes 3292–3
  haematological changes 3682
  haemolytic uraemic syndrome *vs*
    3200–1
  hepatorenal syndrome 3293
  hyperkalaemia in 3133, 3284, 3285
  hyperuricaemic 1379–80, 3185, 3226,
    3290
  infective causes 3179
  interstitial nephritis causing 3291–2
  in malaria 3201
  in malignant disease 3185, 3290
  in myeloma 3181, **3292–3**, 3603
  in nephrotic syndrome **3144**
  nephrotoxic causes 3288–90
  nuclear renal scanning 3115
  in pregnancy **1733–4**
  prerenal **3280–8**
    avoidance 3281–3
    biochemical features *3282*, 3284
    clinical features 3283–4
    diagnosis 3281
    medical management 3284–8
    pathophysiology 3281
    see also acute tubular necrosis
  prognosis 3293
  superimposed on chronic renal failure
    3299
  in systemic sclerosis 3192, 3290–1
  in transfusion reactions 3694
  tropical causes 3293
  vascular causes 3290–1
  vero cytotoxin-producing *E. coli*
    (VTEC) causing 556
  see also renal failure
acute respiratory distress syndrome, *see*
    adult respiratory distress syndrome
    (ARDS)
acute tubular necrosis **3280–8**
  avoidance 3281–3
  biochemical features *3282*, 3284
  clinical features 3283–4
  diagnosis 3281
  in haemolytic uraemic syndrome 3201
  intensive care 2581
  medical management 3284–8
  nuclear renal scanning 3115
  pathophysiology 3281
  in pregnancy 1733, 1734
  in renal transplant recipients 3318
  in septicaemia 3179
  snake venom causing 1131
  toxic 3224
  tropical causes 3293
acyclovir 298
  in CNS infections 4069
  in gastrointestinal infections in
    immunocompromised 1034
  in genital herpes 3353
  in herpes simplex virus infections
    346
  in neonates 1781
  in pregnancy 1747, 1775–7
  in renal failure 3272
  resistance, herpes simplex virus 346
  in simian herpes virus infections 358,
    359
  in varicella-zoster virus infections 350,
    351
acylated plasminogen streptokinase
    activator complex (APSAC) 3671,
    3672
acyl-coenzyme A
  cholesterol *O*-acyltransferase 1401,
    1403

dehydrogenases, electron transport and
    1373
  oxidase deficiency **1441**
ADA gene 172
Adamkiewicz, great artery of 3891, 3902
adaptability, ageing definition 4333, 4334
adaptation, to drugs 1250, 1253
adaptor complexes, in receptor-mediated
    endocytosis 74
adders, bites and envenoming 1132–4
addiction
  definition 4267, 4268
  see also alcohol abuse; drug abuse and
    misuse
'Addicts Index' 4288, 4289
Addisonian crisis 1654
  treatment 1655
Addison's disease 1553, 1576, **1652–6**,
    4125
  in adrenoleukodystrophy 1440, 1653
  aetiology 1652–3
  autoimmune 1652–3, 1655
  chronic mucocutaneous candidiasis with
    1852
  clinical features 1653–4
  corticosteroid replacement therapy
    1655–6
  dementia due to 3971
  haematological changes 3686
  hyperkalaemia in 3133
  hypoglycaemia in 1510–11
  investigations 1642, 1654–5
  myopathy in 4168
  neurological features 4125
  in pregnancy 1751
  tuberculous 1652, 1655, 1656
adenine 1384
adenine arabinoside 5'-monophosphate,
    in chronic active hepatitis B 2067
adenine arabinoside, *see* vidarabine
adenine deaminase locus, in diabetes
    type II 1456
adenine phosphoribosyl transferase
    (APRT) 1378, 1383
  deficiency **1383**, 3226
adenocarcinoma
  investigations of tumours of unknown
    primary site 252
  see also specific anatomical sites/
    tumours
adenoidal facies 2611, 2910
adenoid cystic tumours 2892
adenoids 2611
adenoma 1986
  adrenal, *see* adrenal gland, adenoma
  bronchial 2892
  carcinoma sequence 1988–9, 1991
  colon and rectal 1987, 1988–9
    see also colonic adenoma
  hepatic 1724, 2119, 2129
  pancreatic 1708
  parathyroid 1566, 1569, 1630, 1632–3
  periampullary 2028
  pituitary, *see* pituitary gland, adenoma
  pleomorphic 1862
  thyroid 1611–12, 1613
adenoma sebaceum 3987
adenosine 1378, *2264*
  anginal pain due to 2323
  in atrioventricular nodal re-entry
    tachycardia 2274
  coronary blood flow regulation 2159
  mechanism of action 2263
  platelet inhibition 3619
  in wide QRS complex tachycardia
    2279
adenosine arabinoside 3175, 3178
adenosine deaminase (ADA) 1378, 2323
  deficiency 172, 1384, **1385**
  treatment 172
  injections 172
adenosine diphosphate, *see* ADP
adenosine monophosphate (AMP) 1378,
    2159
  in myocardial ischaemia 2146
adenosine triphosphate (ATP), *see* ATP
adenosquamous carcinoma, pancreatic
    2042

adenovirus 12 infection 461
  carcinogenicity 461
  coeliac disease pathogenesis 1918
adenoviruses 336–7, 391, *391*, **393**
  infections,
    clinical feature and treatment 337
    conjunctival haemorrhage 4191
    conjunctivitis 4191
    diarrhoea and vomiting due to 393
    epidemiology and transmission 336, 461
    features *341*
    respiratory *337*
  structure and serotypes 336
  vectors in gene therapy 113
adenylate cyclase
  activation 1560, 1561
  hormone mechanism 1273, 1274
  platelet 3618
  secretory diarrhoea 2002, 2006
adenylate deaminase, deficiency 1384
adenylate kinase deficiency *3536*
adenyl cyclase, *see* adenylate cyclase
adenylsuccinase deficiency **1384**
adhesin 270
  anaerobic bacteria 570
adhesion 2009
  bacterial colonization mechanism 270,
    272, 2438
  leucocyte 3558–9
  neutrophils and capillary endothelial
    cells 2619
  platelet **3614–15**
adhesion molecules 230, 2294, **2619–21**,
  2620
  alternative splicing 231
  in asthma 2728
  atherosclerotic plaque development
    2294, 2299
  autoantibodies to 163
  emigration of neutrophils from
    capillaries 2619
  endothelial cells 2290, 2497, 2619
    pulmonary 2487, 2619
  functions 2294, 2619
  in immune response in transplantation
    187
  immunoglobulin supergene family 230,
    2620, 2621
  integrins 2144, 2619–20, *2620*
  in lung inflammation 2619–21
  in myocytes 2143
  role in metastases 231
  selectins, *see* selectins
  see also integrins; intercellular adhesion
    molecule 1 (ICAM-1)
adhesive capsulitis 2995
adhesives, contact dermatitis 3737
adipose tissue 1272
  energy stored in 1399–400
  metabolic effects of large mass 1308–9
adiposity, endometrial cancer association
  210
adipsia 1602–3, *3124*, 3126
adjustment disorder 4204–5
adjustment reaction 4358
adjuvants 153
adolescence/adolescents
  abnormal behaviour and personality
    disorder diagnosis 4212
  anorexia nervosa onset 1296, 4213
  confidentiality and 4316
  diabetes in **1496–7**
  glue sniffing and solvent abuse 1092
  growth, constitutional delay (CDGA)
    1697, **1703**
  hepatitis B immunization 454
  mortality rates 40, *41*
  pregnancy in 36
  scoliosis in 2872, 2873
  sexual abuse 4313
  see also puberty
ADP 3615
  platelet activation 3614, 3616, 3617
  in storage-pool deficiency 3646
ADPases, endothelial cells 2290
adrenal cortex
  disorders **1639–63**
    classification *1641*

drug-induced **1717–18**
  see also adrenal gland; Cushing's
    syndrome
  hereditary unresponsiveness to ACTH
    1653
  insufficiency, *see* hypoadrenalism
  steroid hormones 1639
    biosynthesis *1640*, 1664
    see also corticosteroids;
      glucocorticoids; mineralocorticoids
adrenalectomy 1650, 1660, 1709, 1714
  in pregnancy 1751
adrenal gland **1639–69**
  adenoma 1642
    aldosterone-producing, *see* Conn's
      syndrome
    angiotensin II responsive 1656, *1658*,
      1660
    deoxycorticosterone-producing
      1660
    diagnostic tests 1646, 1647, 1648,
      1649
    treatment 1650
  autoantibodies 1652–3, 1655
  carcinoma 1566, 1642, 1644
    aldosterone-producing 1656, 1660
    androgen-producing 1676, 1691
    diagnostic tests 1646, 1647, 1648,
      1649
    gynaecomastia 1688
    treatment 1650
  cortex, *see* adrenal cortex
  disorders,
    in AIDS 1716
    gynaecomastia in 1688
    haematological changes 3686
    hyperandrogenization 1676
    in pregnancy **1750–2**
    in sarcoidosis 1716
  haemorrhage, in meningococcal
    infections 536
  hyperplasia,
    congenital, *see* congenital adrenal
      hyperplasia
    idiopathic 1656, *1658*, 1660
    macroscopic nodular 1642, 1646,
      1647, 1648, 1649–50
    in MEN 1 syndrome 1708
    primary 1656, *1658*, 1660
  hypoplasia 1662
  insufficiency, *see* hypoadrenalism
  in lung cancer 2883
  metastases, Addison's disease 1653
  necrosis, Addison's disease 1653
  nodules 1566
  in paracoccidioidomycosis 818
  scintigraphy 1649–50, 1659–60
  tumours, precocious puberty 1702
adrenaline 2253, **2254**, 3772
  action 1340, 1562–3
    mechanism and effects 2254
  in anaphylactic shock in penicillin
    reaction 718
  anaphylaxis treatment 160, *160*
  in chloroquine overdose 1072
  clinical use 2254
  doses *2254*
  high central venous pressure 2564
  in hypoglycaemia 1505
  insect stings and 1145
  in insect-venom allergy/reaction 161,
    1138
  measurement 2555
  phaeochromocytoma producing 1637,
    2553, 2556
  receptors 2254, *2254*
  in septicaemia 2573
  snake bites and 1136
  synthesis 2553
  in trauma 1548
  uses 2254
adrenal vein, catheterization, in
  aldosteronism 1659
ß-adrenergic agonists, *see* beta-
  adrenergic agonists
adrenergic nerves, heart 2160, 2253
adrenergic neurotransmission **2253**
adrenergic receptors, *see* adrenoceptors

α-adrenoceptor blocking drugs, *see* α-
  adrenoceptor blocking drugs
adrenoceptors **2253**, *2253*
  for catecholamines *2254*
  classification and types 2253, *2253*
  see also α-adrenoceptors; ß-
    adrenoceptors
adrenocorticotrophic hormone, *see*
  ACTH
adrenogenital syndrome, *see* congenital
  adrenal hyperplasia
adrenoleukodystrophy (ALD) 84,
  1439–41, 3986, **3997**
  'Addison's-only' form 1440
  autosomal recessive 3997
  childhood 1439
  neonatal 1443
  pseudoneonatal 1441
  treatment 1440–1, 3997
  variants 1440, 3997
  X-linked 1439, 1440, 1653, 3997
adrenomyeloneuropathy (AMN) 84,
  1439–41, 1653
  neurological features 3986, 3997
Adriamycin, *see* doxorubicin
adsorbents, of poisons 1049–50
adult respiratory distress syndrome
  (ARDS) 293, 2231, **2574–6**, **2852–61**
  in barbiturate poisoning 1060
  causes 2574, *2575*, 2639, 2853, *2853*
    initiating factors 2639, 2853, *2853*
  chest radiography in 2857
  clinical features and phases 2853
  diagnosis **2857**, *2857*
    severity score *2857*
  disorders associated *2853*
  drug-induced 1060, 2850
  high permeability pulmonary oedema
    2496
  incidence 2853
  in leptospirosis 701
  lung function 2503, 2575, 2639–40,
    2856
  lung injury score *2857*
  mortality 2576, 2639, 2861
  outcome **2860–1**
  pathogenesis 2496–8, 2639, **2854–6**
    arachidonic acid metabolism 2855
    coagulation and fibrinolysis 2855
    complement role 179, 2497, 2854–5
    free radicals 2854, 2860
    lung inflammation role 2616, 2617,
      2639, 2854–5
    neutrophils and cytokines 2854–5
    osmotic/hydrostatic pressure 2854
    summary 2856
    surfactant 2855–6
    TNF, IL-1 and PAF in 2854–5
  pathology 2574–5, **2853–6**
    acute exudative phase 2853–4
    chronic proliferative phase 2854
  pathophysiology **2639–41**, **2856–7**
    gas exchange 2640–1, 2856
    mechanical properties of lung
      2639–40, 2856
    phases 2853
    pulmonary circulation 2640, 2857
  in pre-eclampsia 1730
  in pregnancy **1744–5**
  pulmonary hypertension in 2640, 2857,
    2860
  pulmonary oedema *vs* 2496, 2497,
    2574, 2853–4
  respiratory failure 2852–3, 2904
  right ventricular failure in 2857
  in tetanus 1020
  treatment 2575–6, 2640, **2857–60**
    circulatory management 2575–6, 2860
    extracorporeal lung assist 2859
    fluid balance 2860
    oxygen delivery/demand 2859
    prophylactic **2860**
    pulmonary haemodynamics 2859–60
    surfactant 2856
    vasodilators 2859–60
    ventilation/oxygenation 2575, 2640,
      2857–9
  zinc exposure causing 1114, 1115

adults, mortality rates 40–1, 42
adult Still's disease **2973–4**
adult T-cell leukaemia/lymphoma
  (ATLL) syndrome **490**, 1783, 3411,
  3582
  clinical features 490
  HLTV-1 association 214, 215, 461,
    462, **490**
  leukaemic phase 3424
  molecular biology *3395*
  pathogenesis and survivals 490
adventitia 2290
adventitious sounds 2650
adverse drug reactions **1251–5**, 2124
  adaptation associated 1251, 1253
  allergic, *see* allergic drug reactions
  classification 1251–5, *1252*
  compliance affected by 1240
  delayed effects causing 1254–5
  dose-related 1251–2
  incidence 1251
  long-term effects 1253
  non-dose-related 1252
  pharmacological effects mediating 1249
  of placebos 1260
  pseudoallergic 1253
  surveillance methods 1255, *1256*
  see also drug(s); liver damage;
    teratogenic drugs
adverse skin reactions, IgE-mediated
  162
Advisory Council on the Misuse of
  Drugs 4275
adynamic ileus 1959, 1961
  see also paralytic ileus
Aedes 920
aegophony 2650
aeroallergens, seasonal 2714
aerobic capacity 4324
aerobic exercise 4324
aerobic fitness **4324–5**
  central/peripheral mechanisms 4325
  measurement 4324–5
aerobic metabolism 4171
Aerococcus, rare species *550*
Aeromonas, rare species *551*
Aeromonas hydrophila **559**
aerophobia, in rabies 399
aeroplane travel, *see* aerospace medicine;
  aircraft
aerosol propellants, toxicity due to
  inhalation 1093
aerospace medicine **1193–204**
  aircrews, *see* aircrew/pilots
  haemolytic anaemia in astronauts 3550
  hypoxia and **1194–7**, 1202
    see also altitudes, high
  mechanical aspects 1194
  see also aircraft; altitudes, high
affective deprivation 1295
affective disorders **4218–21**
  bipolar 4220, 4227
  cognitive function impairment and 4225
  differential diagnosis 4225
  in drug abusers 4295
  in elderly **4227**
  mixed 4220, 4227
  treatment, lithium 4250
  see also depression/depressive
    disorders; mania and manic
    depressive disorder
affective personality disorder 4212
affective symptoms, in multiple sclerosis
  3993
afferent loop syndrome, *see* bacterial
  overgrowth
afferent nerve fibres 3857
afibrinogenaemia, hereditary *3643*, **3646**,
  3652
Afipia, rare species *551*
Afipia felis 274, 745
aflatoxin 1158
  cancer association 218
    hepatocellular carcinoma 204, 461,
      2116
Africa
  health care 53
  venomous snakes 1127

African 'meningitis belt' 535, 539, 543
African trypanosomiasis **888–94**
aetiology 888
clinical features 889–91
eye 4192
diagnosis 891–2
differential diagnosis 892, *892*
epidemiology and transmission 888–9, *890*
follow-up and relapse 893–4
haemolymphatic 889, 890
immune response 889
meningoencephalitic 889, 890, 891, 892
pathogenesis 889
prevention and control 894
treatment 892–4, *893*
see also Trypanosoma brucei
after-discharge 4151
afterpotentials, cardiac 2149
aganglionosis, *see* Hirschsprung's disease
age **4333–4**, *4333*
arterial pressure of oxygen 2901
artificial nutrition at home 1324
asthma and **2735–6**
blood pressure changes 2528, 2528–9, 4336
blood volume regulation 2157, 4334
body mass changes 4334
cancer incidence relationship 197–8
cardiovascular function changes 4334–5
in exercise 2161
characteristics of old age 4334, *4334*
chest radiography changes with 2178
chronic renal failure and 3295–6, 3303
endocrine system changes 4336
epilepsy incidence 3910
eye and ear changes 4336
false-positive ERCPs and 2036
fertility effects 1678
gastrointestinal tract changes 4335
Hodgkin's disease and 3569, 3575
infection susceptibility 280–1
ischaemic heart disease risk 2306, 2307, 2332
lung function variations 2673–4, 4335
myocardial infarction,
risk 2337
thrombolytic therapy 2341
nervous system changes 4336
osteoporosis related to, *see* osteoporosis
pharmacokinetics/pharmacodynamics 4336–8
physiological changes **4334–6**, *4334*, *4335*
renal function changes 4335
skin changes, *see* skin, ageing
SLE association 3017–18
sources of differences between young/old **4333–4**, *4333*
travellers 325
ageing **4333**
definition 4333
factors influencing 4333–4
medicine and **4334**, *4334*
'normal' 4333
agglutination tests **3690**
agglutinin titre
cold *3379*
heterophile *3379*
aggressive behaviour 4256
see also violent patients
agonists 1246
endogenous and drug action via 1246–7
partial 1246
agoraphobia 4206
agranulocytosis 3378
antithyroid drug-induced 1613
clozapine causing 4253
congenital (Kostmann's syndrome) 3389, 3557
oral manifestations 1855, 1864
see also neutropenia
agraphia 3848, 3851
alexia with 3851
pure (motor) 3851
agriculture 3462
anaemia related to *3462*, **3468–9**

dietary change due to 3466–8
environmental effects 3463
Agrobacterium radiobacter 551
Agrobacterium tumefaciens 193
agrochemicals, poisoning 1043, 1044
Aicardi syndrome 4111
aids and appliances
in cerebral palsy 4119, 4121
in osteoarthritis 2982
in Parkinson's disease 4004, 4340
in rheumatoid arthritis 2963
AIDS dementia complex 476, 3966, **4077–8**, 4236
AIDS and drug misuse report 4302
AIDS and HIV infection 466, **467–83**
adrenal insufficiency 1652
antineutrophil cytoplasmic antibodies (ANCA) in 3012
appendicitis in 2010
artificial nutritional support 1322
bacterial infections 473, 485, **486–8**, **4079**, 4285
miscellaneous 487
pneumococcal, *see below*
salmonellae 486–7
treatment 480–1, 486
see also tuberculosis (below)
BCG vaccination in 480, 648, 664
cardiac lesions 477, **2394–6**, *2395*
causative agent 463
cerebrovascular diseases in 4080
cervical carcinoma in 477
chancroid association 586
in children 478, **4080**
choroidoretinitis and retinal necrosis in 476
clinical features 469–70, 485–8, 1850–1
CNS involvement 475–6, 485, **4076–8**, 4236
CNS tumours in 4080
CNS viral infections 4065, 4079–80
cognitive-motor complex 4077
complications **473–7**
cryptococcosis in, *see* cryptococcosis
cryptosporidiosis in, *see* cryptosporidiosis
cytomegalovirus infection 361, 473, 4079–80
cytomegalovirus retinitis 476, 4079, 4193
definitions 468, *468*
dementia, *see* AIDS dementia complex
diseases diagnostic of 468, *468*
drug-related neurological toxicity **4080**
encephalitis 4077
encephalopathy 472, **476**, 4236
management 472
endocrine manifestations **1716–17**
Enterocytozoon bieneusi infection in 884, 886
epidemiology 468, 3348
eye in **4193–4**
fever of unknown origin (FUO) 1015–16, *1015*, **1018**, 1019
fungal infections 479–80
respiratory tract 2710
treatment 479–80, *480*
gallbladder and pancreas in 475
gastrointestinal tract in 474–5, 485, 1841, 2005
diarrhoea 475
oral and oesophageal 474–5
tumours 475
gonorrhoea facilitation of 546
gut peptides in 1896
haematological changes 3680
hairy leucoplakia in 357, 470, 471, 474
heart in 477, **2394–6**, *2395*
heart muscle disease **2394–6**
herpes zoster infection 4193
historical background 467
immune response in 466–7, 4278
see also under HIV infection
infectious diseases in **4078–80**
see also above/below for specific infections
intensive care units in 473
isosporiasis in 475, 487, 882, 883

Kaposi's sarcoma, *see* Kaposi's sarcoma
liver disease in 475, **2135**
hepatic granulomas 2122
lymphomas in 475, 477, 488, 2135
CNS 4080, 4134
small-intestinal 1986
lymphoproliferative disorders 3566
malabsorption in tropics and 1930
malnutrition in 1295, 2395
mental disorders/symptoms 476, 4236
microsporidiosis in 487, 884, 886
mycobacterial infections 473–4, 485, 2710
atypical 474, 1018, 1019, 4079
environmental mycobacteria 666
see also tuberculosis (below)
Mycobacterium avium-intracellulare, *see Mycobacterium avium-intracellulare* complex (MAC)
mycoplasma association **772–3**
myelopathy in 476, 4078
myopathy in 4078, 4155
neurological manifestations **4076–8**
neurosyphilis 4084
nocardiosis in 487, 686
nutritional assessment 1322
opportunistic infections 282, 470, *470*, 473, 475, 485, 1027
bacterial 480–1, 485, 486–7
CNS 475
in developing countries 485, 488
fungal 479–80, 488
of heart 2395
protozoal 478–9, 487
treatment 478–81
viral, *see below*
see also above/below and specific infections
oral manifestations 474, 1850–1
candidosis 474, 488, 801, 1850, 1851
treatment 1851
viral infections 1850
pathogenesis 467
pathology 1850
peripheral neuropathy in 476, 4078
pneumococcal infections in 473, 485, **486**, 513
features and treatment 486
Pneumocystis carinii pneumonia, *see Pneumocystis carinii* pneumonia
progressive multifocal leucoencephalopathy in 446, **4079**
prophylaxis, antiviral therapy 482
psoriasis in 3746
pulmonary complications, non-infectious 2710, 2781, 4285
pulmonary complications/infections 473, 485, **2710**, 2713, 4285
see also Pneumocystis carinii pneumonia
renal disease in 477
retinopathy 4193
sclerosing cholangitis in 475, 2053
seborrhoeic dermatitis in 3743
skin disorders in 470, 485, 487
surgery in 473
surveillance 484
syphilis in **4079**, 4193–4
diagnosis 716–17
transmission 707, 708
toxoplasmosis 475, 476, 487, 4077, **4078**
treatment 478, 4078
treatment 472–3, **481–3**
children 478
clinical practice 483
combination therapy and trials 482
didanosine 481–2
drugs used *481*
experimental drugs 482
neurological toxicity of 4080
trials 481, *481*, 482
zalcitabine 482
see also zidovudine
tuberculosis in 473–4, **486**, 641, **652**, 2591, 4279, 4302
BCG vaccination 480, 648, 664

case-finding 646
clinical features 474
in developing countries 664
epidemiology 473–4, 643–4, 664
extrapulmonary 474
meningitis 4060, 4061
multi-drug resistance 652, 664
treatment 480–1, 486, 652, 660–1
tuberculous meningitis in 4060, 4061
tumours in 476–7, 488
CNS **4080**
see also Kaposi's sarcoma; *lymphomas (above)*
uveitis in 475, 476
viral infections 479, *479*, 485, 487–8, **4079–80**
EBV infections 355, 4080
enteric viruses 488
genital herpes 3351, 3352
herpes simplex 479, *479*, 488
human herpesvirus 6 (HHV-6) 364
human papillomaviruses (HPV) 445
varicella-zoster virus 487–8
see also cytomegalovirus (above)
visceral leishmaniasis and 905
wasting syndrome 4078
management 472–3
weight loss 1322
Whipple's disease *vs* 1924
see also HIV infection
AIDS kits 322
AIDS-related complex 470
AIMS study 2343
ainhum 3788, 3789
airborne disease, exposure control 1164
'air bronchogram' 2660
air-conditioning plants, *Legionella* in/prevention 727
aircraft
acceleration 1194, 1195
accidents 2360
aeromedical problems 1202–3
cabins, pressure 1197, *1197–8*, 1198, 1199
alveolar partial pressure *1202*
high-differential 1197, 1198
low-differential 1197, 1199
mechanical effects 1198–9
decompression in 1199
ejector seats 1198, 1199
hypoxia and **1194–7**, 1197
passengers 1202
in-flight accidents 1202
licensing structure 1200, 2359–60
medical incidents 1202
oxygen equipment 1197–8
passengers **1201–3**
angina 2326
deep vein thrombosis risk 2522, 3676
Eisenmenger syndrome 2411
haematological and endocrine conditions 1203
miscellaneous medical conditions 1203
neurological and psychiatric disease 1202–3
respiratory and cardiovascular disease 1202, 2411
thrombotic disease and 2522, 3676
risks associated 1199–200
safety target 1200
see also aerospace medicine
aircrew/pilots **1199–201**
1 per cent rule 2360
cardiovascular disease 1199–200, **2360**
incapacitation of pilot 1199
licences and medical fitness **2359–60**
pilot classes and training 1199, 1200
psychiatric disease 1200
respiratory disease 1200
selection and medical maintenance **1199–201**, 2360
air embolism
in divers 1206
transfusion-associated 3692
AIRE trial 2348

airflow
in heart failure 2232
obstruction, *see* airways obstruction
resistance, *see* airways, resistance
in upper airways obstruction 2720, 2721
see also airways
air pollution **1227–32**
acid aerosols 1230
asthma and bronchial hyper-
responsiveness 161, 2731, 2733
building-related illness 1231–2
cancer association 217
lung cancer 207, 2881
carbon monoxide 1230
environmental disasters 1233
extrinsic asthma due to 161
gaseous/particulate 1229–30
guideline levels *1228*
indoor 1227, **1230–2**
radon-222 1231
tobacco smoke 1230–1
lead 1228–9
measurement of health effect **1227–8**
outdoor 1227, **1228–30**
oxides of nitrogen 1229
polynuclear aromatic hydrocarbons
1228
source or process-specific **1230**
sulphur dioxide 1229
see also pollution
air sampling, workplace exposure
assessment 1163
air travel, *see* aircraft, passengers
airways
aspiration,
bronchoscopy 2579, 2580
in positive-pressure ventilation 2579
see also aspiration
branching 2596–7, 2600, 2629
irregular dichotomy 2600
lengths/diameters 2600
in bronchiectasis 2756
design and function 2600–1
establishment in acute respiratory
failure 2918–19
geometry, bronchial hyper-
responsiveness and 2726
infections, *see* respiratory tract
infections
inflammatory disorder, asthma as 2727,
2728, 2729
maintenance, in acute poisoning 1046
management,
in alkali ingestion 1103, 1104
in unconscious patients 2585
muscle abnormalities in obstructive
sleep apnoea 2910
narrowing, in asthma 2730
obstructive disease,
circulatory failure **2571–2**
positive-pressure ventilation 2576, 2578
see also airways obstruction; chronic
obstructive airways disease
peripheral, disease assessment **2668**
protection,
larynx role 2612
pharynx role 2611
resistance,
in asthma 2726, 2728
distribution *2767*
increased, dyspnoea due to 2164
site/mechanism determination **2668**
testing **2667–8**
responsiveness, assessment **2668**
total volume 2600
upper,
narrowing in sleep 2910
sarcoidosis **2826**
see also bronchi; respiratory tract;
trachea
airways disease **2724–79**
in genetic syndromes 2861
see also asthma; bronchiectasis; chronic
obstructive airways disease; cystic
fibrosis
airways obstruction
in acromegaly 1592

acute 2719, **2721–2**
aspiration causing 2721
infections causing 2722
oedema 2721–2
in alveolar filling syndromes 2639
in amyloidosis 2835
asthma *vs* 2737
see also asthma
breathlessness 2646, 2648
in bronchiectasis, management 2762
causes *2579*, 2719, 2721–4, *2767*
specific **2721–4**
chemical inflammation, in chronic
bronchiolitis 2634
in chlorine poisoning 1097
chronic,
causes *2767*
exercise tolerance reduction 2672
REM sleep-related hypoxaemia 2916
in chronic bronchitis 2767
in chronic obstructive airways disease
2769, 2773
in cystic fibrosis 2749
treatment 2753–4
drug-induced 2849
emergency treatment 2723
by foreign bodies **2636**, 2719
non-acute 2719, **2722–4**
laryngeal dysfunction 2724
tracheal abnormalities 2723–4
tracheal compression 2723
tracheal stenosis 2723
in obstructive sleep apnoea 2909
pathophysiology **2632–6**
in pulmonary oedema 2503
respiratory muscle dysfunction 2668
site/mechanism determination **2668**
in smoke inhalation 1102
symptoms/signs 2649, 2719
tumours causing **2636**, 2719, 2722–3
upper tract **2719–24**
acute and non-acute 2719
asthma *vs* 2737
causes **2719**, *2719*, **2721–4**
definition 2719
diagnosis and examination 2719
functional 2737
lung function **2719–21**
in rheumatoid arthritis 2796
see also chronic obstructive airways
disease; airway, obstructive disease
akathisia 4020, 4252
akinesia 3863, 4001
in Parkinson's disease 4001
akinetic mutism 3858, 3932, 4237
akinetic-rigid syndromes **3998–4009**
in adults **3998–4007**, *3999*
basal ganglia calcification **4007**
causes in adults 3998, *3999*
in cerebral anoxia 4007, 4123, 4240
in children **4007–9**, *4007*
corticobasal degeneration **4007**
progressive supranuclear palsy 3965,
4005–6, *4006*
see also multiple system atrophy;
Parkinson's disease; Wilson's disease
alactasia, detection 1906
Alagille's syndrome 2014, 2015
alanine *1353*, 1456
after injury/surgery 1550
plasma *1360*, 1361
alanine aminotransferase (ALT) 2055,
4365
in acute liver failure 2106
in cirrhosis 2088
in congestive cardiac failure 2130
in Lassa fever 431
alanine:glyoxylate aminotransferase
(AGT) 1445
deficiency, *see* hyperoxaluria, primary,
type I
ALARA (as low as reasonably
achievable) 1220
Alaria americana 999
alariasis **999**
ALARP (as low as reasonably
practicable) 1221

alastrim 367
albendazole
in clonorchiasis 986
in cysticercosis (*Taenia solium*
infection) 968
in gnathostomiasis 954
in hookworm infection 931, 932
in lymphatic filariasis 923
in opisthorchiasis 984
in trichuriasis 944
Albers-Schönberg disease, *see*
osteopetrosis
albinism **1365**, 3718, 3759
complete 3759
Hermansky-Pudlak 3759
ocular 1365
oculocutaneous 1365
partial 3759
twin studies 102
albumin
in acute liver failure 2106
in acute pancreatitis 2029
in acute renal failure 3285
binding sites and bilirubin binding 2054
calcium binding 1622, 1623
drug binding 1242
infusion, in hepatocellular failure 2110
low, in cirrhosis 2088
nephrotoxicity of filtered 3144
nutrition assessment in intensive care
2586
radioactive iodinated serum (RISA)
3825
renal tubular reabsorption 3137
serum, reduced in Crohn's disease 1940
solutions 3661, 3695
synthesis decrease, in infections 294
testosterone binding 1679
thyroid hormone binding 1554, 1605
urinary 3101–2, 3136
creatinine ratio 3137
albumin-bilirubin complex 2054, 2055
albuminuria
cadmium-induced 1107
in diabetes mellitus 1479–80, 3168,
3169, 3170
see also microalbuminuria; proteinuria
Alcaligenes, rare species *551*
alcaptonuria, *see* alkaptonuria
alclofenac, poisoning 1056
alcohol
abstention 2085, 2090, 2110, 4269
ischaemic heart disease in 2313
reinstatement 4269
abuse, *see* alcohol abuse
administration,
in diethylene glycol poisoning 1081
in ethylene glycol poisoning 1082,
3267
in methanol poisoning 1081
in benign essential tremor 4012
binge drinking, *see* alcohol abuse, binge
drinking
blood levels, aircraft crews and pilots
1201
breath measurements 4272, 4276
catabolism in peroxisomes 1438
consumption, *see* alcohol consumption
energy derived from 1271
injection, in oesophageal cancer 1982
mechanism of action 4276
metabolism 2081–2
enzymes 2081
gastric first-pass 2081
meters 4272, 4287
percutaneous injection, in hepatocellular
carcinoma 2117
poisoning **1079–80**
see also alcohol abuse
porphyrin metabolism and 1396
psychotropic drug interaction 4247
in self-poisoning 1043
in trichloroethylene poisoning 1090
units 4266
uses 1079
alcohol abuse
acute pancreatitis 2027

in aircraft crew and pilots 1201
alcohol consumption continuum
4270–1, 4274
ambivalence about 4274, 4290
assessment **4265–7**, 4271–2, 4290
CAGE questions 17–20, 4272
of need for (dependence) 4266
questions checklist 4266
see also alcohol consumption,
assessment
binge drinking 4266
chronic pancreatitis 2035
biological markers 2081
brief interventions **4270–5**, **4272–5**,
4290
concerns/decision-making 4275
information provision 4274
lifestyle/stresses 4274
opening strategies 4274
opportunity for 4265–6
strategies 4274, *4274*
cancers in 2082
case histories 4267–8, 4270
chronic pancreatitis 2034
continuum of response to 4271–2
dementia in 4127
dependence *vs* problems **4267–70**
depressive disorders *vs* 4219
doctors' attitudes 4264, 4290
in elderly 4228
epilepsy and 3917
fetal alcohol syndrome 1799, **4112**,
4278
folate deficiency in 3493, 3685
haematological changes **3684–5**
harm reduction 4276
hereditary haemochromatosis and 3479
Korsakov's syndrome in 4225
male hypogonadism 1683, 1718
management in general wards **4286**,
4287
megaloblastic anaemia in 3498, 3685
myopathy in 4127, 4169
needs in custody **4304–5**
neurological features 4100, **4126–8**,
4127
CNS 4127, 4276–7, *4277*
peripheral neuropathy **4127**, 4277–8
nutritional deficiency syndromes in
4277–8
opportunistic infections in 1027
osteoporosis in 3070
physical complications **4276–8**
porphyria cutanea tarda and 1395
porphyrin metabolism 1396
prevalence, in USA 4264
pseudo-Cushing's syndrome 1640,
1643, 1717
psychiatric emergencies associated
4258–9
relapse prevention 4291
screening **4270–5**
AUDIT 4272, *4273*
signs *2084*
skills needed for clinical practice **4265**
subjective awareness 4269
treatment **4289**
disulfiram 1077, 1078
withdrawal syndrome 2084, 4277,
4290–1
anxiety symptoms in 4206
chlormethiazole in 4253
clinical features 4277, 4290
delirium due to 4224
emergency treatment 4258–9
hypertension management 2538
management 4253, 4287, 4290–1
management in custody 4305
seizure management 4291
symptoms 4259
alcohol consumption
acidosis induced by **1542**
acute intoxication 4276–7
clinical features 4276
management 4259
violence 4288
in aircraft crew and pilots 1201

alcohol problem continuum 4270–1, 4274
assessment,
  AUDIT, MAST and CAGE systems 17–20, 4272
  drinking diaries 4271–2
  γ-glutamyl transpeptidase levels 4272
  quality frequency questionnaire 4271
  see also under alcohol abuse
coronary heart disease risk and 1412
deliberate self-harm 4228
in diabetes *1466*, **1469**
dilated cardiomyopathy pathogenesis 2382
disease risk in obesity and 1309
excess,
  biological markers 4272
  brief interventions, *see under* alcohol abuse
  in depressive disorders 4219
  recognition of (AUDIT) 4272
  see also alcohol abuse
fetal alcohol syndrome due to 1799, **4112**, **4278**
fungal poisoning associated with 1156
glycated haemoglobin and 1481
gout association 2986
history-taking 2082, **4266–7**
in hospital 4287
hyperlipoproteinaemia and 1411
hypertension pathogenesis 2530
hypoglycaemia 1080, 1184, *1184*, 1469, **1510**
  after exercise 1184, *1184*
hypothermia associated 1184
  in cold conditions 1184, *1184*
ischaemic heart disease and 2313, 2313–14
  protective effect 2313–14, 2530
levels 2080
liver disease association 2080
  see also alcoholic cirrhosis; alcoholic liver disease
moderate, protective effects 2313–14, 2530
obstructive sleep apnoea and 2910
occupational disease of liver and 1171
oesophageal cancer association 202
oesophageal tumours 1981
oral and pharyngeal cancer and 201
pain induced by, in Hodgkin's disease 3570
peptic ulcer treatment and 1884
problems 4270–1
  management in general ward **4287**
  see also alcohol abuse
safe levels 2081
sideroblastic anaemia in 1396, 3523, 3685
alcohol dehydrogenase (ADH) 1080, 2081
alcohol dependence syndrome
  classification 4269–70, *4269*
  features **4268**
alcohol flush 2081
alcohol history 2082, **4266–7**
alcoholic abuse, neuropathy 4100, **4127**
alcoholic cerebellar degeneration 4127, 4277
alcoholic cirrhosis 2082
  clinical features 2082
  hepatocellular carcinoma in 2116
  investigations 2088
  liver transplantation in 2112
  pathology 2082, 2084
  prognosis 2084
  risk and alcohol consumption 2080
  treatment 2085
alcoholic coma 4276–7
alcoholic hepatitis 2082
  clinical features 2082
  pathology 2082, 2084
  prognosis 2083
  treatment 2084–5
alcoholic liver disease **2080–5**
  cirrhosis, *see* alcoholic cirrhosis

clinical features 2082
discriminant function 2084, *2085*
epidemiology 2080
fatty liver, *see* liver, fatty changes
investigation 2082–3
iron overload in 2022
pathogenesis 2081–2, *2083*
pathology 2082, 2084
prognosis 2083–4
susceptibility 2080–1
  genetic factors 2081
  hepatitis B and C 2081
  nutrition 2081
treatment 2084–5
alcoholics, *see* alcohol abuse
alcohols, poisoning **1079–81**
  general mechanisms 1079
alcohol-tobacco amblyopia 4127, 4278
alcohol use disorders identification test (AUDIT) 4272, *4273*
aldehyde dehydrogenase (ALDH) 2081
aldehydes, formation, in ethylene glycol metabolism 1082
aldolase B 1345
  deficiency, *see* fructose, hereditary intolerance
aldose reductase inhibitors 1472, 1482, 3169
aldosterone 3119
  action 1563, 2157, 3248
  adrenal adenoma producing, *see* Conn's syndrome
  biosynthesis *1640*, 1664
  biosynthetic defects 1662, 1668–9
  deficiency, *see* hypoaldosteronism
  ectopic secretion 1716
  plasma, in aldosteronism 1657–9
  potassium balance and 3128, 3129
  receptor, *see* mineralocorticoids, receptor
  reduction,
    by ACE inhibitors 2248
    in acute mountain sickness 1189
  renal tubular resistance 3337
  renin ratio 1657
  in trauma 1549
  urinary excretion 1657
  see also aldosteronism (hyperaldosteronism)
aldosterone synthase (corticosterone methyl oxidase type II) *1567*, 1572, *1652*, 1664, 1668
  deficiency 1662
  in glucocorticoid-suppressible hyperaldosteronism 1656–7
aldosteronism (hyperaldosteronism) **1656–60**
  clinical features 1657
  diagnosis 1657
  differential diagnosis 1657–60
  familial type II 1656
  glucocorticoid-suppressible (familial type I) 1572, 1639, **1656–7**, 1657–9, 1660
  hypokalaemia in 1657, 3131, 3336
  idiopathic 1656, 1657–9, 1660
  primary 1656–60
    in pregnancy 1751
  secondary 1656
  treatment 1660
Aleutian disease of mink 447
Alexander's disease 4114
Alexander's law 3872
alexia 3848
  agraphia with 3851
  pure 3851
alfacalcidol 1635
  in chronic renal failure 1635, 3328, *3329*
algodystrophy (reflex sympathetic dystrophy) 3096, **3941**, 3941, *3941*
  joint features 3006
  see also Sudeck's atrophy
algorithms 15, 16
alkalaemia 1535
alkaline diuresis, *see* forced diuresis, alkaline

alkaline phosphatase 1629, *4365*
  in bone mineralization 3058
  plasma/serum 1629, 3060
    applications 3060
    in benign recurrent intrahepatic cholestasis 2059
    in biliary disease 2046
    in bone disease 3063
    in chronic renal failure 3325
    in cirrhosis 2088
    elevation in Paget's disease 3076
    increased levels 2055
    in pregnancy 1729
    in primary sclerosing cholangitis 2078
    tissue non-specific (TNSAP) 3086
    in ulcerative colitis 1947, 1948
alkalis
  ingestion, oesophageal trauma 1104, 1873
  mechanisms of toxicity 1103
  poisoning by 1103
    clinical features 1103
    management 1103–4
    severity assessment and factors in 1103–4
  types and uses 1103
alkali therapy
  in cystinuria 3333
  in metabolic acidosis 1543–4
  in uric acid stone disease 3256
  see also bicarbonate, therapy
alkaloids
  in food plants 1159
  in poisonous amphibians 1140
alkalosis 1535
  carbohydrate metabolism and 1539
  mental symptoms 4240
  metabolic, *see* metabolic alkalosis
  oxygen uptake/delivery and 1539
  potassium balance and 3129
  respiratory, *see* respiratory alkalosis
  tetany in 1639
alkanes, poisoning **1083**
alkaptonuria 1364–5, **3085–77**
  biochemical features *3062*
  joint involvement 3004
  osteoarthritis in 2979
alkylating agents
  late effects 3430
  mechanism of action 248
alleles 103, 104
  heterogeneity 104
  -specific disease phenotypes 104
allergens 156, 158
  allergic rhinitis 160
    perennial 2715
    seasonal 2714
  asthma 161, 2731–2, 2734
  avoidance 2717–18, 2737, *2737*
  challenge,
    in asthma 2732, 2733, 2744–5
    extrinsic allergic alveolitis 2814, *2814*
    food allergens 1844, 3742
  dog and cat 2715
  extrinsic allergic alveolitis *2810*, 2811, 2814
  nickel and cobalt 1108
  occupational 2715
  pollens 2714
  preparations and immunotherapy concerns 158, 161, 163
  regions for T-cell activation 157
  T-cell epitopes 158
  in urticaria 3770, 3771
allergic bronchopulmonary aspergillosis, *see* aspergillosis
allergic contact dermatitis, *see* contact dermatitis, allergic
allergic diseases **158–63**, 3739
  anaphylaxis, *see* anaphylaxis
  antigen non-specific mechanisms/ mediators 158–9, *159*
  antigen-specific mechanisms 157–8
    allergens 158
    B-cells and immunoglobulin 157
    cytokines regulation IgE formation 157
    cytotoxic T-cells 157

genetic basis 158
helper T-cells 157
arthropods causing 1000
conjunctivitis 161
extrinsic asthma 161
  see also asthma
food allergy, *see* food allergy
hypereosinophilic syndrome *vs* 3611–12
IgE-mediated **156–63**, 156
immunotherapy, *see* desensitization
insect venom 161
purpura in 3636–7
rhinitis, *see* allergic rhinitis
skin diseases 161–2
transfusion-induced 3692
  see also allergic reactions; atopic disease
allergic drug reactions **1252–3**
  clinical manifestations 1253
  type I (immediate) 1252
  type II (cytotoxic) 1253
  type III (immune-complex) 1253
  type IV (cell-mediated/delayed) 1253
allergic reactions
  acute oedema and airways obstruction due to 2721
  asthma 2725, 2731–2
  to fungi and mushrooms 1158
  insect stings 161, 1144, 1145
  in tuberculosis 648
allergic rhinitis 160, **2714–19**, 3739
  aetiology **2714–15**
  allergens 160, 2714, 2715
  clinical features 160, 2716
  clinical history 2716–17
  diagnosis 160, **2716–17**
  differential diagnosis 2716–17, *2717*
  examination 2717
  investigations **2717**, *2717*
    see also skin-prick tests
  occupational 2715
  pathophysiology **2715**, 2716
  perennial 2714–15
  prevalence and consultations for 2714, *2714*
  seasonal 160, 161, 2714
  treatment 160–1, **2717–18**, *2718*
    allergen avoidance 2717–18
    immunotherapy 161, 2718
    pharmacotherapy 2718
allergy 156
  see also allergic diseases; contact dermatitis; food allergy
allodynia 3936, 4092
allograft
  definition *183*
  see also transplantation
Alloiococcus otitis 551
allopurinol
  in chronic gouty nephropathy 3227
  in gout 2987
  in hyperuricaemia 3226, 3256
  in Lesch-Nyhan syndrome 1382
  mechanism of action 1247
  nephrotoxicity 3266
  in polycythaemia vera 3434
  in renal failure 3274, 3288
all-*trans*-retinoic acid (ATRA) 3409, 3659
almitrine 2928
almitrine bismesylate, in cor pulmonale 2521
alopecia 3762
  areata 3763–4
  chemotherapy causing 3575, 3761
  scarring 3751
  thallium poisoning 1113
  total scalp (universal body) 3764
Alpers-Huttenlocher syndrome 3989
α_1-antitrypsin, *see* (α_1-)antitrypsin
α_2-macroglobulin, *see* (α_2-)macroglobulin
α-adrenergic agonists
  in cardiac hypertrophy 2148
  GH secretion and 1578
  opiate antagonists with 4292
  in opiate detoxification 4292
  potassium balance and 3128

α-adrenoceptor *1560*, 2253, 3882
　in atopic eczema 3739
　coronary blood flow regulation 2159
　pulmonary vasoconstriction 2492
　subtypes and actions *2253*
α-adrenoceptor blocking drugs
　in hypertension 2541, *2541*
　in phaeochromocytomas 2556–7
　poisoning **1063**
　prazosin, in heart failure 2252
　in renal impairment 3274
　see also phenoxybenzamine
α-chain disease 3583
alpha-chloralose **1123–4**
alpha-fetoprotein
　Down's syndrome screening 135
　in hepatocellular carcinoma 2090,
　　2116
　levels and implications 2116
　maternal serum, in diabetes 1756
　tumours associated 2116
5-alpha fluorouracil
　in sun damage 3729
　see also 5-fluorouracil
α-granules, platelet 3615–16
α-naphthyl acetate esterase (ANAE)
　3399, 3400
alpha rhythm 3829
alphaviruses **407–9**, *408*
Alport's syndrome **3204–5**
　anti-GBM disease and 3166, 3205
　haematuria in 3146, 3204
alprazolam 4253
altitudes, high **1185–93**
　acclimatization 322, 1186–7, 1190,
　　1192
　circulation and cardiac output 1187
　pulmonary diffusion 1187
　tissue adaptations 1187
　ventilation 1186
　cautions and advice for 1192, 1193
　extreme and oxygen uptake 1187
　hypoxaemia in 2916
　hypoxia and oxygen levels 1186,
　　1195–7
　adaptive responses and features
　　1196–7
　effect of sudden altitude 1196, 1197
　illness **1187–93**
　　miscellaneous 1192
　　myocardial infarction 1192–3
　　peripheral oedema 1192
　　pulmonary emboli 1193
　　retinal haemorrhage 1191–2
　　sickle-cell anaemia 1193
　　see also mountain sickness
　oxygen uptake at 1187
　pulmonary oedema in 2501
　skin disease and 3724
　speed of ascent and altitude 1188, 1190
　temperature changes 1185, 1193
　terrain and populations 1185–6
　see also aerospace medicine; mountain
　　sickness, acute
aluminium 1105
　Alzheimer's disease risk 3972
　compounds containing, in chronic renal
　　failure 3274, 3328, 3329
　dialysis-associated accumulation 1425,
　　3321
　　encephalopathy 4240
　　inhalation of powder 1105
　poisoning **1105–6**, 3096
　　blood/urine levels 1105
　　bone disease in **3096**
　　renal bone disease and 3326, 3327,
　　　3329
　toxicity 1425
　in water 3096
aluminium chloride hexahydrate 3766
aluminium hydroxide, rickets associated
　3074
aluminium phosphide poisoning **1123**
aluminium sulphate, in water supply
　1105
aluminum, *see* aluminium
Alu repeat 105, 108
alveolar air equation 1195, 1196

alveolar-arterial oxygen difference 2903
　at high altitudes 1187
alveolar-capillary blood gas barrier 2485,
　2596–7, 2629
alveolar capillary sheet (system) 2485,
　2593, 2596–7
　air-blood contact 2596–7, 2629
　factors affecting flow *2489*
　pressure-flow relations 2488–90
　recruitment in exercise 2490
　see also pulmonary capillaries
alveolar cells 2593
　carcinoma, dyspnoea in 2162
　function in lung defence 2614–15
　type I and II cells 2593–4, 2594,
　　2594
　see also alveolar epithelium; alveolar
　　secretory cells
alveolar ducts 2597
alveolar epithelium 2593–4, *2594*
　basement membrane 2485, 2509
　fluid/ionic balance 2494
　fluid overload 2494
　in inflammation 2621, 2626
　　neutrophil migration 2621
　　repair after 2624–5
　　scarring 2626
　　see also lung inflammation
　permeability assessment 2668
　tight junctions 2494, 2593
　vulnerability and repair 2596
　see also alveolar secretory cells (type II)
alveolar filling
　cellular debris 2638, 2639
　fluid, *see* alveolar oedema
　pathophysiology **2638–9**
alveolar flooding 2496, 2498–9
alveolar haemorrhage **2804**
　see also pulmonary haemorrhage
alveolar hypoventilation
　in chronic mountain sickness 1192
　polycythaemia and 3553
alveolar macrophage 89, 2595, 2596,
　2613, 2619
　cytokines and products 2615, *2615*,
　　2619
　in extrinsic allergic alveolitis 2813
　immune response generation 2615
　inflammatory response generation 2615,
　　2619
　receptors and molecules binding 2614,
　　2615
　role 2614–15
　tissue remodelling and repair 2615
　ultrastructure 2614
alveolar oedema 2179, 2498, 2596
　in adult respiratory distress syndrome
　　2639
　features 2502–3
　pathophysiology **2638–9**
　see also pulmonary oedema
alveolar pressure 2489, 2499, 2667
　partial pressure, aircraft cabin pressures
　　1202
alveolar proteinosis, *see* pulmonary
　　alveolar proteinosis
alveolar secretions, in pulmonary
　　alveolar proteinosis 2833, 2834
alveolar secretory cells (type I), in adult
　respiratory distress syndrome 2854
alveolar secretory cells (type II) 2593,
　2594–6, *2594*
　mitosis and repair 2596
　in pulmonary alveolar proteinosis 2833
　structure 2593, 2594
　surfactant secretion 2594–6, 2613
　　pathway 2594–5
　ultrastructure 2595
　see also surfactant
alveolar septum 2630
　fibre system 2597, 2598
　micromechanics **2599–600**
alveolar ventilation 2456, 2671
　divers 1206
　equation 1195, 2631
　in sleep 2905
alveoli 2485, 2628
　amyloidosis 2836

calcification **2838**
　microlithiasis **2838**
　pressure-volume relations 2499
　pulmonary oedema development 2498
　reactions, to drugs **2850–1**, *2850*
alveolitis
　cryptogenic fibrosing, *see* cryptogenic
　　fibrosing alveolitis
　diffuse interstitial,
　　after bone marrow transplant 1033
　　see also lung disease, diffuse
　　parenchymal
　drug-induced 2850, *2850*
　extrinsic allergic, *see* extrinsic allergic
　　alveolitis
　fibrosing,
　　inflammation and scarring 2626
　　lung inflammation role 2616, 2617
　　see also cryptogenic fibrosing
　　alveolitis
Alzheimer's disease 3965, **3971–80**
　aluminium role 1105, 1425
　amyloid deposits 1513, **1516**, 1519
　amyloid precursor protein (APP) in
　　3972, 3973
　cognitive impairment in 3965
　dementia onset and homozygosity 65
　differential diagnosis 3969
　Down's syndrome association 3972,
　　3973
　epidemiology **3971–2**
　familial *1514*, 1516, 3973
　genes involved in susceptibility 64–5
　genetic factors 3972
　head injury association 3972, 3973
　investigations 3974
　late-onset 3973
　pathology **3972–3**
　pathophysiology **3973**
　Pick's disease *vs* 3976
　subtypes 3973
　symptoms and signs **3973–4**
　treatment and management **3974**
　see also dementia
Amanita species 1155, 1156
amantadine 339
　adverse mental symptoms 4242
　mechanism of action 80
　in Parkinson's disease 4003
amatoxins 1156
amaurosis fugax 3950, **4186**
　causes *3951*
　in cholesterol embolism 2376
　clinical features 2367
　see also transient ischaemic attack (TIA)
AMBER (advanced multiple beam
　equalization radiography) system
　2652
amblyopia
　alcohol-tobacco 4127, 4278
　in cerebrospinal angiostrongyliasis
　　947
　toxic and nutritional 3867
amblyopic eye 4180
amegakaryocytosis *3448*
ameloblastoma, jaw 1863
amenorrhoea 1669, **1670–4**
　in anorexia nervosa 1297, 1669, 1671,
　　4213
　causes 1670–3
　exercise-induced 1671, 1718, 4326
　investigations 1673–4
　post-pill 1670, 1724
　primary/secondary 1670
　treatment 1674
　weight-related 1671–2
American College of Rheumatology
　2955, *2956*
　SLE classification 2798, 3017, *3018*
American College of Sports Medicine
　4328
American Conference of Government
　Industrial Hygienists (ACGIH) 1163
American mucosal leishmaniasis 902–3
American Rheumatism Association, *see*
　American College of Rheumatology
American trypanosomiasis, *see* Chagas'
　disease

Ames test 193
amikacin *3272*
　in urinary-tract infections *3211*
amiloride 3228, 3337, 3341
　in Conn's syndrome 1660
　in cystic fibrosis 2753
　in idiopathic hypercalciuria 3255
　mechanism of action and side-effects
　　2239
amino acids
　absorption 1903
　after injury/surgery 1550
　aromatic, in hepatic encephalopathy
　　2102
　branched-chain, *see* branched-chain
　　amino acids
　in diabetes 1456
　essential *1354*
　inborn errors of metabolism **1352–75**
　　classification *1354*
　　defects in carbon chain metabolism
　　　1360–75
　　transport defects 1354–8
　　urea cycle defects 1358–60
　insulin secretion and *1459*, 1461
　liver disorders *2019*, 2024
　metabolism 1275, 1352, 1353
　plasma values/excretion/clearance *1353*
　in pregnancy 1753
　in protein structure 57
　renal handling 3332
　sulphur, disorders of metabolism
　　1365–8
aminoaciduria **3332–3**
　acidic *3332*, 3333
　basic *3332*, 3333
　classification *1354*
　generalized 1354–6
　imino acids and glycine *3332*, 3333
　neutral (Hartnup syndrome) *1337*, 1357,
　　3330, *3332*, **3333**
　in salicylate poisoning 1054
　specific 1356–7
aminoacyl-tRNA synthetase, antibodies
　to 163
α-amino adipic semialdehyde synthase
　deficiency *1375*
γ-aminobutyric acid, *see* gamma-
　aminobutyric acid (GABA)
9-aminocamptothecin 259
ε-aminocaproic acid 3659
aminoglutethimide 1651, 1713–14, 1718
aminoglycosides
　dosing regimens and design of 307, *309*
　in listeriosis 722
　mechanism of action 296
　monitoring 1261
　nephrotoxicity **3263–4**, *3284*, **3288**
　ototoxicity 3876
　pharmacodynamics 305
　ß-lactams differences 307, *308*
　in pregnancy 1745, 1746, 1784–5
　in renal impairment 3271, *3272*
　in tuberculosis 655, *656*
　in urinary-tract infections 3210–11
aminoguanidine 1472, 3169
p-aminohippurate (PAH), renal plasma
　flow estimation 3108
3-amino-hydroxypropylidine-1,1-
　bisphosphonate 3077, 3082
δ-aminolaevulinic acid (ALA) 1389
　in lead poisoning 1109
　urinary 1364, *1390*, 1391, 1396
δ-aminolaevulinic acid (ALA)
　dehydratase *1391*, 1396
　deficiency porphyria 1394
δ-aminolaevulinic acid (ALA) synthase
　1389, *1391*, 1396
　deficiency 3521
　erythroid *1391*
aminopenicillin, in actinomycoses 685
aminophenazone, poisoning 1057
aminophylline
　in pregnancy 1745
　in pulmonary oedema 2504
¹⁴C-aminopyrine breath test 2056
4-aminoquinolines 850
8-aminoquinolones 850

aminorex fumarate 2513
  pulmonary hypertension association
    2852
5-aminosalicylic acid (5-ASA) drugs
  in Crohn's disease 1942
  newer drugs 1949, *1949*
  in proctitis 1948
  in ulcerative colitis 1948
  see also sulphasalazine
p-aminosalicylic acid (PAS)
  haemolysis due to *3546*
  nephrotoxicity 3265
  in tuberculosis 655, *656*
aminosidine, in visceral leishmaniasis
    906
aminotransferases, *see* alanine
    aminotransferase (ALA); aspartate
    aminotransferase (AST)
amiodarone 1717, 2263, *2264*
  alveolar reactions to 2850–1, 2852
  in atrial fibrillation 2272
  in dilated cardiomyopathy 2384
  in hypertrophic cardiomyopathy 2389,
    2390
  liver damage 2128
  in myocardial infarction 2345, 2346
  overdose/poisoning 1064
  in pregnancy 1740
  side-effects 2384, 2850–1, 2852
  in ventricular tachycardia 2280, 2282
  in Wolff–Parkinson–White syndrome
    2277
amitriptyline 4220
  drug interactions 1258
amlodipine, in heart failure 2248
ammonia
  exposure 2847
  in hepatic encephalopathy 2102, 2105
  plasma, in glycogen storage diseases
    1341
  poisoning **1093–4**
  production 2102
ammonium chloride 3339
ammonium ions (NH_4^+)
  in acid-base disturbances 1540
  in acid-base homeostasis 1358, 1534–5,
    3338
  in renal tubular acidosis 3339, 3341
amnesia **3854–6**
  after head injury 4048–9
  in dissociative disorder 4210
  post-traumatic, *see* amnesia, traumatic
  retrograde 3856
  severe 3855
    causes *3856*
  transient global 3856, 3951
  traumatic (post-traumatic) 3855–6,
    3916, 4048–9
  see also memory
amnesic disorder 4225
amniocentesis 136
  in diabetic pregnancy 1757
  in osteogenesis imperfecta 3082
amniotic fluid
  culture 1786
  embolism *1742*, *1745*, *1762*
amniotic infection syndrome
    (chorioamnionitis) **1785–7**
amocarzine, in onchocerciasis 916, 917
amodiaquine, in malaria 851
amoebae 825
  coprozoic 825
  free-living 825
  infections, *see Acanthamoeba*,
    infections; amoebiasis; *Naegleria
    fowleri*
  parasitic gut species 825
amoebiasis **825–35**
  carrier state, management 832
  clinical features 828–30
  cutaneous and genital 830, 833
  differential diagnosis 828, 830
  epidemiology 826–7
  hepatic 829–30, 2708
    management 832–3
  in homosexuals 3364–5
  host factors increasing susceptibility
    826

immune response 827–8
  immunological/serological tests 831
  invasive intestinal 828–9, 832
  laboratory diagnosis 828, 830–1
  lung involvement 2708
  pathology 827
  prognosis and prevention 833
  transmission 827
  treatment 831–3
    patient management 832–3
  see also Entamoeba histolytica; entries
    beginning amoebic
amoebic brain abscess 830
amoebic colitis 828, 832
  special forms 828
  treatment 832
  with/without dysentery 828
amoebic dysentery **553–5**, 827, 828,
    2003
  postdysenteric syndromes 828
amoebicidal drugs 831–2
amoebic keratitis 834
amoebic liver abscess
  clinical features and diagnosis 829
  complications 829–30
  management 832–3
  pathology 827
  see also amoebiasis, hepatic
amoebic meningoencephalitis 833
amoebic pericarditis 830
amoeboma 827, 828
  treatment 832
amosite 2843
amotivational syndrome 4242
amoxapine, overdose 1059
amoxycillin
  in actinomycoses 685
  in bronchiectasis 2763
  in gonorrhoea 1790
  in listeriosis 722
  in pneumococcal infections 520
  in pneumonia 2700
  pseudoallergic reaction 1253
  rash due to 1253, 3731–2
  in renal failure *3272*
  in urinary-tract infections 3209, *3211*
AMP, *see* adenosine monophosphate
    (AMP)
amphetamines
  abuse 1076
    psychiatric disturbances from 4241
  complications associated 4280
  excess, schizophrenia *vs* 4222
  in narcolepsy 3929
  in obesity treatment 1312
  withdrawal syndrome 4293
amphibians, poisonous **1140**
amphotericin B 811, 812
  after cardiac transplantation 2257
  in amoebic meningoencephalitis 834
  in aspergillosis 809
  in disseminated candidiasis 807
  in fever of unknown origin 1031
  flucytosine with 812
  in HIV infections 479, 480
  indications 812
  liposomal 812
  in neonates 1793
  nephrotoxicity **3265**, *3284*, 3339
  in paracoccidioidomycosis 819
  in renal impairment 3272
  renal tubular acidosis induced by
    3339
  in visceral leishmaniasis 906
ampicillin
  in enterococcal infections 509, 510,
    2446
  in infective endocarditis 2446, *2447*
  in pneumococcal infections 520
  in pneumonia 2700
  prevention of neonatal streptococcal
    group B infections 509
  pseudoallergic reaction 1253
  rash due to 1253, 3731–2
  in renal failure *3272*
  resistance 298–9
ampulla of Vater 2045
  in ascariasis 938

cancer 2052
  tumours 2044
amputation
  below-knee 2371
  in diabetic foot disease 1490, **1491**, 2372
  in electrical injury 1213, *1213*
  in ischaemia of limbs 2371
  leg ulceration and 3810
  rehabilitation after 2371
amygdalin 1097
amylase
  in acute pancreatitis 2029
  in ascitic fluid 2038
α-amylases 1920
amylin (islet amyloid peptide) 1450,
    1455, 1518, **1520**
amyl nitrite, in cyanide poisoning
    treatment 1098
amyloid 2835
  AA protein 1518–19, 2835
  AL protein 1518, 1522, 2835
  AP protein **1621**, 2835
    see also serum amyloid P (SAP)
    component
  associated proteins 1521–2
  ß-amyloid **1519–20**, 3972, 3973
    in Alzheimer's disease 65, 1516, 1519
    in hereditary amyloid angiopathy of
      Dutch type 1517, 1519–20
    in senile cerebral amyloidosis and
      amyloid angiopathy 1516
    see also amyloid precursor protein
      (APP)
  in Crohn's disease 1939
  fibrils *1513*, *1514*, **1518**, **1518–21**
    histochemistry 1522
  macular 3803
  P component (AP), *see* amyloid, AP
    protein
  SAA protein, *see* serum amyloid A
    (SAA) protein
  SAP protein, *see* serum amyloid P
    (SAP) component
  in senile plaques 3972
  structure 3972
  in ulcerative colitis 1948
amyloidosis **1512–24**
  AA amyloidosis, *see* amyloidosis,
    reactive systemic
  acquired syndromes *1513*
  AL, immunocyte dyscrasia-associated
    1513, **1515**, 1523, 1524
    local nodular *1513*
    renal involvement 3180
  arthropathy in **3003–2994**
  in bronchiectasis 2760
  cardiac 1517, 1522, 2216, 2393
  cerebral **1516–17**
    hereditary cerebral haemorrhage with,
      see hereditary cerebral haemorrhage
      with amyloidosis
    in prion disease 1517
    senile, and amyloid angiopathy 1516
    see also Alzheimer's disease
  classification *2835*
  clinical 1512–18
  cutaneous *1513*, 1518, 3802–3
  in MEN 2A syndrome 1709
  in cystic fibrosis 2750
  diagnosis and monitoring 1522–4, 2836
  endocrine *1513*, 1518
  in familial Mediterranean fever (AA)
    1514, 1517, 1527, 3180
  haemodialysis-associated 1513,
    1517–18, 1524, 3180, 3312
  haemostatic disorders in 3636, 3661
  hereditary cerebral haemorrhage with,
    see hereditary cerebral haemorrhage
  hereditary syndromes 1513, *1514*, 1522
  hereditary systemic **1517–18**
  histology 1522
  investigations *2952*
  leprosy *vs* 674
  liver in **2136**
  localized syndromes 1518, *2835*
  management 1524, 2836
  in myeloma 1515, 1524, 3003, 3180,
    3181, 3185

ocular 1518
  orbital 1518
  Ostertag non-neuropathic systemic
    1514, **1517**, 3180
  pancreatic 1450, 1455
  peripheral nerve involvement 4099
  pulmonary **2835–6**
  reactive systemic (AA) **1513–14**, *2835*
    conditions associated with *1515*
    management 1523, 1524
    renal involvement 1514, 3180, 3185
    in rheumatoid arthritis 1513, 1514,
      2963, 3193
  renal 1514, **3180–1**, 3185, *3300*
    in rheumatoid arthritis 1513, 1514,
      2963, 3193
  senile **1515–16**, 1516, 2393
    focal *1513*, 1515–16
    systemic *1513*, 1515
amyloid precursor protein (APP) 1516,
    1519–20
  in Alzheimer's disease 65, 3972, 3973
  gene 3972, 3973
  structure 3973
amylo (1,4-1,6)transglucosidase, *see*
    branching enzyme
amyotrophic chorea-acanthocytosis
    3686–7
amyotrophic lateral sclerosis **4087–8**,
    4087
  epidemiology and inheritance 4087
  pathology and clinical features 4088
  prognosis and treatment 4088
  spinal form 4088
  telling diagnosis to patients 4088
  in tumours *243*
amyotrophy
  diabetic 4098
  neuralgic *3903*, 4094
anabolic steroids
  in aplastic anaemia 3445, 3446
  cholestasis and liver damage due to
    2125
  in Fanconi anaemia 3446
  liver cancer association 204
anaemia 3375, **3457–62**
  adaptation to 3457–8
  agriculture-related *3462*, **3468–9**
  in AIDS 3680
  aircraft travel and 1203
  in alcoholics 3685
  angina in 2323
  in anorexia nervosa 1297, 4214
  aplastic, *see* aplastic anaemia
  apparent (dilutional) 3589
  in babesiosis 864
  in bacterial infections 3679
  in bartonellosis 774, 775
  of blood loss 3460, 3476, 3483, 3683
  causes and classification 3459–60
  childhood **3469**
  of chronic disorders (ACD) **3482–3**,
    3677
    clinical/laboratory findings 3483
    iron-deficiency anaemia *vs* 2960,
      3475, 3483
    management 3483
    pathogenesis 3482–3
    in rheumatoid arthritis 2960
  in chronic renal failure 3300, 3302,
    3305, 3483, **3682**
  in cirrhosis 2088–9
  clinical assessment 3460–1
  clinical effects 3458–9
  in coeliac disease 1918
  in congenital porphyria 1395
  in Crohn's disease 1938, 1940, 1942
  definition 3457
  dyserythropoietic **3521–4**
    congenital (CDA) 3497, **3524**
    see also erythropoiesis, ineffective
  in endocrine disease 3483, 3686
  erythroblastopenic, of childhood 3449
  exercise-induced 4326
  Fanconi, *see* Fanconi anaemia
  general approach 3460–2
  goat's milk 3492
  haematological investigation 3461

anaemia (cont.)
  haemolytic, see haemolytic anaemia
  in hepatocellular failure 2105
  hypochromic 3461
    refractory 3477
  hypoproliferative 3459
  in inflammatory bowel disease 3683
  iron-loading 3479–81, 3522
  in leprosy 673
  in leukaemia 3405, 3420–1
  in liver disease 3684
  in lung cancer 2885
  macrocytic 3461, 3495
  in malaria 278, 842, 845, 846, 848,
    850, 3680
    in pregnancy 1794
    see also malaria
  in malignancy 242, 3676–8
  in malnutrition 3469, 3498–9
    management 1292
  management 3461–2
  megaloblastic, see megaloblastic
    anaemia
  in myelodysplastic syndromes 3425
  in myelomatosis 3598, 3603–4
  normochromic normocytic 2960, 3461,
    3482–3
  in paroxysmal nocturnal
    haemoglobinuria 3451
  pernicious 3468, 3489–91
    aetiology 3489
    associated diseases 3489, 3677, 3686
    clinical features 3490
    in common variable immunodeficiency
      1837
    diagnosis 3495–6
    in diphyllobothriasis 969
    gastric cancer in 1982–3
    juvenile 3491
    mental symptoms associated 4241
    pathology 3490
    in selective IgA deficiency 1839
    subacute combined degeneration of
      cord 3893
    treatment 3496
  physiological, of pregnancy 1735,
    1758
  in pregnancy 3468–9
  prevalence 3457
  prevention 3469–70
  in primary myelosclerosis 3435, 3437
  red cell maturation defects 3459, 3460,
    3521–4
  refractory, see refractory anaemia
  relative, in congenital heart disease
    2401
  retinal haemorrhages 4194
  in rheumatoid arthritis 2960, 3681
  riboflavin deficiency 3498
  sickle-cell, see sickle-cell disease
    (anaemia)
  sideroblastic, see sideroblastic anaemia
  in SLE 3020, 3681
  'sports' 4326
  in thalassaemia 3505, 3510
    in pregnancy 1761
  in trichuriasis 943
  in tumours 242
  in ulcerative colitis 1946
  in visceral leishmaniasis 904, 906
  vitamin B_6 deficiency 3498
  vitamin C deficiency 3498
  vitamin E deficiency 3498
  in Waldenström's macroglobulinaemia
    3604
  work capacity and 3469
  as world health problem 3462–70
anaerobic bacteria 569–76
  antibiotic sensitivity 575
  antimicrobials for 1916
  capsules 571
  commensal flora 570, 571
  culture 571
  diagnostic kits 571
  lipopolysaccharide 571
  small-bowel bacterial overgrowth 1911
  taxonomy 569–70
    new nomenclature 570, 570

  virulence factors 570–1
  see also Clostridium
anaerobic infections 569–76
  bacteraemia 574
  bacterial vaginosis due to 3355
  clinical features 571, 571–5
  diagnosis 571
  endocarditis 574
  pathogenesis 570–1
  pneumonia 2702–3
  prevention 576
  sample collection/transport 571
  synergistic necrotizing 574
  treatment 575–6
anaesthesia
  in acromegaly 1592
  in acute porphyria 1394
  in diabetes 1489, 1493–6
    in pregnancy 1757
  malignant hyperpyrexia after 1182
  in pregnancy 1744
    in chest disease 1744, 1746
  in sickle-cell syndrome 1760
  in sickle-cell trait 3514
  see also epidural anaesthesia
anaesthetics
  general 1248
  local,
    eutectic mixture (EMLA) 3798
    pain treatment 3938
    topical, in pain treatment 3944
    nebulized local, in terminal illness
      4354
  nephrotoxicity 3289
  in renal impairment 3270, 3305
anagrelide 3440
anal cancers, see anorectal carcinoma
analgesia, specialized forms 253
analgesic nephropathy 3221–3
  aetiology 3221
  chronic renal failure in 3222, 3223,
    3296, 3300
  clinical presentation 3221–2
  diagnosis 3222
  pathology 3221
  treatment 3222–3
analgesics
  abuse 3221, 3222
    withdrawal 4296
  in acute pancreatitis 2031
  adjuvant, in cancer pain 4352, 4353
  in cancer 253, 4352
  compound preparations 3221, 3223
  drug-induced asthma 2849–50
  in liver disease 2091
  in migraine 4025
  non-narcotic, in cancer 253
  opiate, see opiates
  in pain management 3944–5
    in cancer 4352
  in drug abusers 4300
  in peritonitis 2008
  in pneumococcal infection 521
  poisoning by 1051–8
  in pregnancy 1810
  pulmonary hypertension due to 2852
  in renal impairment 3273
  in rheumatoid arthritis 2963
  in sickle-cell crises 3516
anal intercourse 3350–1, 3351, 3361,
  3365
anal intraepithelial neoplasia (AIN) 3366
analphalipoproteinaemia (Tangier
  disease) 1414, 3591, 3986
anal sphincter, spasm 1965
anal tumours 1994
  in homosexuals 3365–6
  see also anorectal carcinoma
anal warts 3363, 3367, 3368
  in homosexuals 3363, 3367
  see also anogenital warts; genital warts
anaphylactic reactions 305
  drug-induced asthma 2849
  penicillin 305
  snake antivenom 1138
  see also angio-oedema; asthma,
    allergic; urticaria

anaphylactic shock
  in penicillin reactions 718
  treatment 718
  see also anaphylaxis
anaphylactoid purpura, see Henoch-
  Schönlein purpura
anaphylactoid reactions, food-induced
  3729
anaphylatoxins 159
  C3a and C5a 178
  in dengue haemorrhagic fever 420
  see also under complement
anaphylaxis 159–60
  acute airways obstruction in 2721
  to animal antisera 317
  clinical features 159–60
  drug reactions 1252
  food-induced 162, 1842
  insect stings 1144, 3772
  in severe urticaria 162, 3772
  treatment and prevention 160, 160, 3772
  triggers/causes 159
  urticaria in 3772
  see also anaphylactic shock
anaplastic carcinoma, differential
  diagnosis 245
anarithmia 3852
ancrod 2305, 3658
Ancylostoma duodenale 930, 931
Ancylostomatoidea 929
Andersen's disease (glycogen storage
  disease IV) 1343, 1344
Anderson-Fabry disease, see Fabry
  disease
androgen(s)
  acne vulgaris aetiology 3752
  actions 1679–80
  adrenal 1639, 1640, 1664
  biosynthesis 1679, 1681
  control of gonadotrophin secretion 1579
  deficiency 1680, 1682–3
    gynaecomastia in 1688
    male pseudohermaphroditism 1691–2
    see also hypogonadism, male
  excess, see hyperandrogenization;
    virilization
  hair growth 3761
  insensitivity/resistance syndromes 1573,
    1688, 1692–3
    mechanisms of action 1692
    receptor 1555, 1562, 1692
      defects 1567, 1573, 1692, 1693
    serum lipids and 1411
    treatment 1684, 1695
    in aplastic anaemia 3445
  in women 1674
  see also testosterone
androgenic-anabolic steroids,
  hepatocellular carcinoma association
  204
andromedotoxins 1154
androstenedione 1664
  in congenital adrenal hyperplasia 1665,
    1668
anencephaly 4117
anergy 152, 155
  cutaneous 2819
  evidence for 155
  transplantation 183
anetoderma 3791
aneurysms 2364–5
  aortic, see aortic aneurysms
  berry 3869
  carotid, see carotid artery
  cerebral 3824
  clinical features 2364–5
  femoral artery 2365, 2373
  hepatic arterial 2139
  intracranial, in polycystic kidney
    disease 3203
  intracranial saccular 3963, 3963
  in Kawasaki disease 3048
  management 2372–3
  mycotic (infected) 2365, 4280
    in infective endocarditis 2440
  in polyarteritis nodosa 3014
  popliteal 2365, 2372

  post-stenotic 2375
  renal artery 2373
  sinus of Valsalva 2439, 2467
  splenic artery 2365, 2373
  thoracoabdominal, management 2373
  ventricular, see under ventricle
Angelman syndrome 4110
  mental retardation in 4110
  uniparental disomy 127–8
anger, in dying patients 4233
angiitis
  benign lymphocytic 2807
  gastrointestinal 1995
  hypersensitivity 3010
  in Kawasaki disease 3048–9
  necrotizing 3773
  pulmonary,
    open-lung biopsy 2689–90
    see also Churg-Strauss syndrome
  see also microscopic polyangiitis
angina (angina pectoris) 2165–7,
  2321–31
  after ß-blocker withdrawal 1251
  aircraft travel and 1202, 2326, 2360
  in anaemia 3459
  angiographically normal coronary
    arteries 2325, 2325
    see also syndrome X
  in aortic stenosis 2462
  atherosclerotic plaques causing 2290,
    2323
  classification 2358
  coronary artery bypass grafting in 2353,
    2354
  C-reactive protein levels 1531
  crescendo, see angina (angina pectoris),
    unstable
  decubitus 2167, 2322
  in diabetes 1492
  diagnosis confirmation 2167, 2326
  differential diagnosis 2322
  driving and 2326, 2359
  haemodynamic imbalance causing
    2166, 2323
  in hypertension 2533
  investigations 2325–6
    ECG 2199, 2322, 2323, 2336
    exercise testing 2227, 2326
    myocardial perfusion 2326
  management 2326–30
    aims 2330–1
    angioplasty vs drug treatment 2331
    drugs 2326–30
    lifestyle changes 2326
  microvascular, see syndrome X
  in myocardial ischaemia 2165, 2166,
    2323
  nocturnal 2167, 2322
  oesophageal pain association 2168, 2322
  origin of term 2321
  pain,
    onset, duration and features 2166,
      2322
    site and character 2165–6, 2322
  pathology 2320
  pathophysiology 2322–3
    metabolic changes 2322, 2323
  precipitating factors 2322
  pre-infarction, see angina (angina
    pectoris), unstable
  Prinzmetal (variant) 2166, 2322, 2336
    calcium antagonists in 2329
    drug treatment 2328
    myocardial infarction vs 2335–6
  prognosis 2331
  psychosocial factors associated 2315,
    2322
  recurrent, after coronary artery bypass
    grafting 2356
  sexual problem prevention 2326, 4247
  silent ischaemia 2166, 2323, 2325
  stable 2166, 2167, 2318
    clinical features 2322
    coronary angioplasty in 2351
    examination 2325–6
    management 2326–30
    pathology 2320

stable exertional 2166, 2318
unstable 2166, 2167, 2318
  clinical features 2322
  coronary angioplasty in 2351
  management **2330**
  myocardial infarction *vs* 2166, 2322, 2331, 2335–6
  pathology 2320
  pathophysiology **2323**
  see also ischaemic heart disease; myocardial ischaemia
angina, Vincent's, *see* Vincent's disease
angiodysplasia, caecum 1998
angiogenesis, as new drug target 259–60
angiography
  coeliac 1835
  complications 2369
  CT enhancement, *see* computed tomography (CT)
  in Fallot's tetralogy 2403
  gastrointestinal 1832–3
  in gastrointestinal bleeding 1828, 3683
  liver 1833
  in pancreatic carcinoma 2044
  peripheral arterial disease investigation 2369
  phaeochromocytomas 2556
  pulmonary, *see* pulmonary angiography
  selective, pancreatic endocrine tumours 1704
  spinal **3828**
  ventricular volume analysis 2222–3
  see also arteriography
angio-immunoblastic (immunoblastic) lymphadenopathy **2807**
angioinhibins 260
angiokeratoma
  corporis diffusum *1428*, 1429, 1430
  of scrotum 1430
angioma **3784–7**
  intracranial 3963
  retinal 4182
  senile (Campbell de Morgan spots) 1430
angiomatosis, bacillary *729*, 745, **747**
angio-oedema 162, 3708, 3771
  see also hereditary angio-oedema
angioplasty, *see* balloon angioplasty; percutaneous transluminal coronary angioplasty (PTCA)
angiosarcoma **2118**
  aetiological factors 204, 1167
  see also liver tumours, angiosarcoma
angiostrongyliasis **945–9**
  abdominal 945, **949**
  cerebrospinal **945–9**, 953
Angiostrongylus cantonensis 945–9, 953
Angiostrongylus costaricensis 945, 949
angiotensin II 2157
  action 1563, 2248, 2249, 3119, 3248
  adrenal adenoma responsive to 1656, *1658*, 1660
  atherosclerotic plaque development 2293
  in Bartter's syndrome 3131
  cardiotoxic effect 2249
  elevated,
    effect on kidney and heart 2233
    in heart failure 2233
  enhanced adrenal responsiveness 1656
  in sarcoidosis 2830–1
  thirst regulation 3117
angiotensin converting enzyme (ACE) 2298, 2830, *4365*
  D/D genotype 2157, 2250
  deletion allele 138
  endothelial cell synthesis 2290
  gene, polymorphism, in coronary artery disease 64
  measurement 2830–1
  in pulmonary endothelium 2486
  raised levels, in sarcoidosis 2830–1
  reduction, in acute mountain sickness 1189
  in sarcoidosis 2782, 2830–1
  vasoconstriction 2298

angiotensin converting enzyme (ACE) inhibitors 2157, **2248–51**, 2300
  in acutely ill patients *3284*
  adverse effects 2251, 2540–1
    cough 2850
    hypotension 2251
  in aldosteronism *1658*, 1659
  in chronic renal failure 3304
  development 1130
  in diabetic nephropathy 3171–2
  in diuretic-induced hyponatraemia 2240–1
  drug interactions 2251
  drugs included 1062
  in elderly 4343
  in heart failure 2240–1
    diuresis due to 2240
    dose 2251
    effect on disease progression 2249–50
    effect on symptoms/exercise 2249
    in elderly 4342
    mortality reduction and trials 2250
    use of and guidelines 2251, *2251*
  hyperkalaemia due to 3134
  in hypertension 2540–1, *2541*
  hypoaldosteronism induced by 1663
  mechanism of action 2170, 2248–9
    electrolytes 2249
    myocardial 2249
    neuroendocrine 2248–9
    renal actions 2249
    vascular 2249
  in myocardial infarction 2230, 2249–50, 2344
    effect and mechanism 2250
    reinfarction prevention 2348
  in myocardial ischaemia, effect 2250
  in nephrotic syndrome 3140
  overdose/poisoning 1062–3
    clinical features 1062
    treatment 1063
  peptides from snake venom 1130
  in pregnancy 1732, 1740, **1810**
  renal failure due to 2541, 2546, **2551**
    in heart failure 2235
  in renal impairment 3250, 3273, 3288
  in renal transplant recipients 3322
  in systemic sclerosis 3034, 3192
angiotensinogen 1545
anhydrosis, tropical 1180
aniline, bladder cancer association 212
animal(s)
  aquatic, poisoning from, *see* fish; seafood; *under* poisoning
  bites, anaerobic infections 574
  feeds, *Salmonella* infections 551–2
  listeriosis 720–1
  mechanical injuries due to **1124–5**
  poisonous/venomous, *see* snakes; venomous animals
  rabies in 398–9
  transgenic, *see* transgenic animals
  transplanting organs from 14
  treponemal inoculation in syphilis diagnosis 714–15
animal models
  bronchiectasis 2757
  diabetes mellitus 1453
  essential hypertension 2530
  haemolytic uraemic syndrome 3199
  inborn errors of metabolism 1338–9
  malaria immunoprophylaxis 861
  mycoplasmal genitourinary infections 769
  mycoplasmal pelvic inflammatory disease 770
  Mycoplasma pneumoniae infections 767
  myocardial infarction 2320
  myocarditis 2381
  osteoarthritis **2977–8**
  systemic lupus erythematosus (SLE) 3024
  see also experimental models
animal studies
  extrapolation difficulties to human poisoning 1043
  septic shock 292–3

anion gap 1536
anions, potassium balance and 3129
aniridia 4182
anisakiasis **938–9**
anisochromia 3378
anisocoria 3877
anisocytosis 3377
anistreplase **2343**
  antibodies to 2342
  excess stroke 2342
  in myocardial infarction 2342
  trials 2343
ankle
  injuries and pain **2996**
  oedema, in Parkinson's disease 4004
  pressure 2368
  in rheumatoid arthritis 2958
  sports injuries 2996
ankle jerks, loss 4092
  in cauda equina lesions 3907
ankylosing spondylitis 1948, **2965–8**
  aetiology/pathogenesis 2965–6
  clinical features 2966–7
  definition and diagnosis 2965
  enteropathic synovitis in 2972, 2973
  HLA-B27 and 111, 2953, 2965, 2966, 4185
  investigations 2967
  lung involvement in **2799**, 2874
  ocular features **4185**
  peripheral joint onset 2973
  pregnancy and 2968
  prognosis and cause of death 2968
  rheumatoid arthritis *vs* 2963
  skeletal deformity in 2799, 2874–5
  thorax in **2874–5**
  treatment 2967–8
ankyrin 3527
  defects 3529
annular lesions *3713*, *3717*, 3751
annulo-aortic ectasia 2483
anogenital carcinoma
  in renal transplant recipients 3321
  see also anorectal carcinoma
anogenital warts 444, 3367, 3768
  see also anal warts; genital warts
anomia 3848, 3854
  colour 3851
  progressive 3975
Anopheles mosquitoes 835, 838, 839, 920, 1011
anorectal anomalies, *see* anus, imperforate
anorectal bleeding
  causes 1991
  in colorectal cancer 1991, 1992
  in homosexuals 3365
anorectal carcinoma 445, 3371
  in homosexuals 3365–6
  in renal transplant recipients 3321
  see also anal tumours
anorectal manometry 1956
  in Hirschsprung's disease 1979
anorectal sepsis, in homosexuals 3365
anorectal symptoms, in homosexuals with STDs 3361
anorectal trauma, in homosexuals 3365
anorectic drugs, in obesity treatment 1312
anorexia 1314
  in cardiac cachexia 2176
  in cirrhosis 2087
  in homosexuals 3361
  in malnutrition 1283, 1293
  in terminal illness **4351**
  in type II nutritional deficiency 1280
  see also appetite
anorexia nervosa **1296–9**, 4212, **4213–15**
  aetiology 1297–8, 4214
  amenorrhoea in 1669, 1671
  assessment 1298, 4214–15
  bone mass in 3065, 3069
  bulimia nervosa after 1299, 4216
  clinical features 1297, 4213
    bulimia nervosa similarity 1299, 4216
    'core psychopathology' 4213
  course and outcome 1299, 4215

definition 1296, 4213
delayed/arrested puberty 1701
depressive disorder with 1297, 4214
development and onset 1296–7, 4213
diagnostic features 1296
distribution and prevalence 1296, 4213, 4216
genetic/familial factors 1297, 4214
haematological changes 3686
hypercholesterolaemia in 1411
investigations and abnormalities 1297, 4213–14
management 1298–9, 4214–15
  initial phases 1298
  inpatient 1298–9, 4215
  outpatient/daypatient 1298, 1299, 4215
mortality ratios 1299
physical features 1297
pituitary failure *vs* 4239
anosmia 3876
anosognosia 3854, 4237
anoxia, *see* cerebral anoxia
anoxic seizures **3927**
Anrep effect 2150
Antabuse^R 4291
antacids
  aluminium-magnesium 1888
  calcium-containing 1888
  in gastro-oesophageal reflux disease 1867
  peptic ulcer treatment 1888
  in pregnancy 1801
  in renal impairment 3274
antagonism, physiological 1247
antagonists 1246
antecollis 4018
antenatal care
  in diabetes mellitus 1756–7
  ethics 12
  prevention of anaemia 3470
  see also screening, antenatal
antenatal diagnosis, *see* prenatal diagnosis
anterior cord syndrome 3897–8
anterior horn cells 3856
anterior tibial compartment, after snake bites 1139
anthranilic acid derivatives, poisoning 1056–7
anthrax **612–19**
  bacteriology 612–13
  clinical features 615–17
  cutaneous 615–16
  cycle of infection 613, 614
  diagnosis and pathology 617
  intestinal 616–17
  meningitis 617
  non-industrial/industrial 614, 618–19
  pathogenesis and transmission 613–15
  pulmonary 616
  resistance to 613
  treatment and prevention 617–19
  vaccines 618
  see also Bacillus anthracis
anthroponosis 920
antiandrogens
  in hirsutism 1677
  in pregnancy 1751
  side-effects 1689
  see also cyproterone acetate
antianxiolytic drugs, *see* anxiolytic drugs
antiarrhythmic drugs **2262–3**
  arrhythmias worsened 2262
  in atrial fibrillation 2272
  class I agents 2263
    class Ia 1063–4, 2263, 2272
    class Ib 1064, 2263
    class Ic 1064, 2263, 2279
    in heart failure 2237
    poisoning 1063–4
    in ventricular extrasystoles 2270
    ventricular tachycardia and 2279
  classification 2262–3, *2264*
  class II activity 2263
  class III agents 2263
    poisoning 1064–5

antiarrhythmic drugs (*cont.*)
class IV activity 2263
overdose/poisoning **1063–4**
in pregnancy 1740
in renal impairment 3270
torsades de pointes due to 2283
in ventricular tachycardia 2279, 2280
antibacterial agents 296
see also antibiotics; antimicrobial
  therapy
antibiotic resistance 266, 296, 298–300
anaerobic bacteria 575
Campylobacter 558
chromosomally-mediated,
  N. gonorrhoeae 548–9
pen loci 548
control 309–10
in developing countries 309
'dissociated' 525
enterococci 510
epidemiology 309–10
  international differences 298, 299,
    309, *310*
factors determining and development
  298, 309
intrinsic and acquired 298, 309
ß-lactamase producers 298–9, 300, 685
mechanisms 298
  drug-inactivating enzymes 298
  importance 299
  molecular 299–300
  permeability changes 298
  target site alterations 298
multiple 525
Neisseria gonorrhoeae 548–9
Neisseria meningitidis 534, 541, 542
plasmid 60, 298, 549
prescribing information and 298, *299*
reservoirs of 309–10
Salmonella 553
Shigella 554
Staphylococcus aureus 525
Streptococcal pneumoniae
  (pneumococcus) 511–12, 520
tests for 298–300
  pharmacodynamics relevance 305
  see also under antibiotics
Yersinia pestis 598
antibiotics 289
in actinomycoses 685
acute exacerbation of chronic bronchitis
  2692
in acute meningococcaemia 541
in adult respiratory distress syndrome
  2860
adverse effects *306*
  on intestinal flora 300
  mechanisms 305
  nephrotoxicity **3263–5**, *3284*, *3289*
  pharmacodynamics 305, *306*
  risk 306
anaerobic bacteria 575, 1916
in anthrax 617–18
in antibody-deficiency syndromes 170
in aplastic anaemia 3445
area under the curve (AUC) 307, 1242
in bacterial vaginosis 3355
bioavailability 300, *300*
ß-lactam 296, 3355
  anaerobic bacteria sensitivity 575
  dosing regimens 307, *309*
  pharmacodynamics *vs*
    aminoglycosides 307, *308*
  in pneumonia 2700
  in renal impairment 3270–1
in bronchiectasis 2762, 2763–5
in brucellosis 623
in chlamydial infections 756–7, *757*,
  758
in cholera management 579
in chorioamnionitis 1786
in chronic obstructive airways disease
  2776
colitis due to, *see* colitis,
  pseudomembranous
in Crohn's disease 1942
in cystic fibrosis 2751–2
  inhaled 2752
  intravenous 2752, *2752*

definition/origin of term 296
in dental abscess 1847
in diabetic foot disease 1490–1
in diabetic metabolic emergencies 1503
dosing regimens 306–9, 307–9, *308*
drug interactions 305–6
in empyema 2706
in gastrointestinal infections 2006
gonorrhoea treatment 549
Haemophilus influenzae infections 584
  meningitis 582–3
Helicobacter pylori eradication 1885
in HIV-infected patients 472
in leukaemia 3407
lipid solubility 301
in lung abscess 2705
in malnutrition management 1289, 1291
in measles 380
mechanism of action 296, *297*
in melioidosis 592
meningococcal infections 541, 541–2
minimum inhibitory concentrations 298,
  307, 756–7, *757*, 2446
for neonates 508, 1785, 1788
in nephrotic syndrome 3141
new and designs of 296
pharmacokinetics 300–3, 305
in pneumococcal infections 520–1, *520*
in pneumonia 2700–1
  in immunosuppressed 2712
post-antibiotic effects 304
in pregnancy 1733, 1745, **1784–5**, 1787
prescribing variations *311*
in preterm labour 1786–7
in primary sclerosing cholangitis 2078
principles 2751–2
prophylactic,
  in aortic stenosis 2464
  in aplastic anaemia 3445
  in bacterial meningitis 4059–60
  in endoscopy 1830
  in leukaemia 3407
  in meningococcal infections 542–3,
    542, *543*
  in mitral stenosis 2455
  in neonatal streptococcal group B
    508–9
  in pneumococcal infections 521–2,
    1028
  postsplenectomy 1028, 3530, 3596
  in pregnancy 1740, 1758, 1785,
    1788–9
  in streptococcal endocarditis 510
  in travellers' diarrhoea 2003
  urinary-tract infections 3213
  see also antimicrobial therapy,
    prophylactic
rash after, human herpesvirus 6
  infection 364
in respiratory tract infections 2592
sensitivity,
  in cystic fibrosis 2751–2
  in septicaemia 1023
in septicaemia 1023–4, 2573
in *Staphylococcus aureus* infections
  530–1
in streptococcus B infection 508–9, 1788
susceptibility testing 298–300
  Neisseria gonorrhoeae 549
  pharmacodynamics relevance 305
in tetanus 628
in tropical sprue 1936
in tuberculosis 655, *656*
in typhoid 564, *565*
in urinary-tract infections 3209–13
in Whipple's disease 1924
see also aminoglycosides; antimicrobial
  therapy; *specific infections/antibiotic*
  groups
antibodies **145–8**, 315–16
bispecific, in cancer therapy 225–6
blocking, in meningococcal infections
  538
genes, *see under* immunoglobulin
genetics of production 146–7
in graft rejection 186, 187
in infections 277, *277*
  mechanisms of action 277

monoclonal, *see* monoclonal antibodies
natural 277
number/individual 146
polyclonal 146, 147
receptors on B-cells 141, 148
structure, *see under* immunoglobulin(s)
tests, in rheumatic disease 2952, *2952*
tissue damage mechanism **164**, 278
to tumour cells 229
  changes detection **230–2**
tumours forming 192
in tumour typing 232
see also immune response;
  immunoglobulin(s)
antibody-deficiency syndromes (primary)
  166–71
aetiology 166, 167
common varied, *see* common varied
  immunodeficiency (CVID)
diagnosis 169, 170
differential diagnosis 170
functional deficiencies 171
infections associated 168–9
nomenclature 166, *167*
partial antibody deficiency 166
prevalence 166
prognosis 169
selective deficiencies 171
  see also immunoglobulin A (IgA)
small-bowel biopsy in 1908
treatment 169–71
  general management 170–1
X-linked agammaglobulinaemia 166,
  169
X-linked with hyper-IgM 166
X-linked lymphoproliferative syndrome
  166, 353, *1840*
see also hypogammaglobulinaemia;
  immunodeficiency
antibody-deficiency syndromes
  (secondary) 169, **173**, *174*
antibody-dependent cellular cytotoxicity
  164
in graft rejection 187
in infections 277
antibody dependent enzyme prodrug
  therapy (ADEPT) 260
anticancer drugs, *see* chemotherapy;
  cytotoxic drugs
anticardiolipin antibodies 714, 2952,
  3020, 3668–9, *3670*
in SLE 3020, 3025
see also antiphospholipid antibodies
anticholinergic drugs
abuse 1076
in antipsychotic drug use 4252
avoidance in schizophrenia 4223
in Parkinson's disease 4002
peptic ulcer treatment 1884
anticholinergic effects, tricyclic
  antidepressants 4248
anticholinesterases
in Alzheimer's disease 3974
myasthenia gravis management 4162
poisoning, eye signs 4197
in snake envenoming management 1138
anticipation, myotonic dystrophy and **127**
anticoagulant rodenticides **1123**
anticoagulants 3670, **3671–6**
avoidance, in cyanotic congenital heart
  disease 2401
in Budd-Chiari syndrome 2099
cholesterol embolism association 2376
in diabetic hyperglycaemic coma 1503
ischaemic limb management 2369
myocardial reinfarction prevention 2348
in nephrotic syndrome 3142
oral **3673–5**
  drug interactions 3655, *3674*
  in elderly 4342
  in inherited thrombophilias 3667–8
  in ischaemic heart disease prevention
    2305
  mode of action 3619
  overdose **1077**
  in pulmonary embolism 2526
  resistance 1259
  vitamin K deficiency induced by **3655**

in postpartum period 1743
in pregnancy **1739–40**, **1742–3**,
  1810–11, 3675
in primary pulmonary hypertension
  2512
in pulmonary embolism 2525, 2526
in renal failure 3274
septicaemia treatment 1025
in SLE 3023
in thromboembolism prophylaxis 3670,
  3675–6
in transient ischaemic attack (TIA)
  3953–4
see also heparin; warfarin
anticonvulsant drugs
adverse effects, concentration and
  memory 4238
breast feeding and 1768–9
eclampsia prevention/treatment 1731
folate deficiency due to 3493–4
neonatal vitamin K deficiency and
  3655
nephrotoxicity **3266**
osteomalacia and 1636, **3074**
poisoning 1061–2
in pregnancy 1768, 1811, 1812, 1813
in renal impairment 3273
sexual problems due to 4245, *4245*
in terminal illness 4356
teratogenicity 1768, 1809, *1810*
vitamin D metabolism and 3325
anticytokine agents, in septicaemia 2573
antideoxyribonuclease B (ADB) 504
antidepressants **4247–50**
after deliberate self-harm 4231
in anxiety disorders 4206
in bulimia nervosa 1300, 4217
in chronic fatigue syndrome 1039
in depressive disorders 4220, 4227
in elderly 4227
in functional bowel disease 1968
MAOIs, *see* monoamine oxidase
  inhibitors (MAOIs)
monoamine receptor antagonists 4248,
  4249
in obsessive compulsive disorder
  4207
in pain treatment 3945
in Parkinson's disease 4004
poisoning **1058–60**
in renal impairment 3273
sedating 4248, 4249, *4249*
selective 5-HT uptake inhibitors, *see*
  selective 5-HT uptake inhibitors
  (SSRIs)
sexual problems associated *4245*
side-effects 4220
  mental symptoms 4242
in terminal illness 4358
tricyclic, *see* tricyclic antidepressants
antidiarrhoeal agents 325, 2006
in collagenous and microscopic colitis
  2137
anti-diet movement 1309
anti-D immunoglobulin 3545, 3689
antidiuresis, syndrome of inappropriate
  (SIAD) 243, **1601–2**, 1711, 1712,
  3124–5
in acute mountain sickness 1189
causes 1602, *1713*, 3124
in cystic fibrosis 2750
drug-induced 1719
in lung cancer 2884
in meningitis 4059, 4061
pathophysiology 3124
sick-cell concept 3125
treatment 1602, 3124–5
antidiuretic hormone (ADH), *see*
  vasopressin
anti-DNA antibodies 3021
deposition in kidney 3024
detection 3021
double-stranded DNA (dsDNA) 2070,
  2952, 4130
  in SLE 3021, 3024
heparan sulphate cross-reaction 3024
idiotypes, in SLE 3026
in SLE 3021, 3024

antidystrophin 4143
antiemetics *1822*
  in chemotherapy 3574
  in pregnancy 1802, **1810**
  in terminal illness 4355, *4356*
antiepileptic drugs **3920–3**
  alternative drugs 3922
  cessation 3923
  choice 3920–1, *3921*
  costs 3922
  first-line drugs 3921–2
  information for patients 3922–3
  in pain treatment 3945
  pharmacokinetics 3922
  in pregnancy 3922
  prescription 3920
  principles of use *3920*
  use of 3922–3
antifibrinolytic agents 3659, 3660
  in haemophilia 3651
  in von Willebrand's disease 3645
antifibrotic agents, in primary biliary
    cirrhosis 2076, *2076*
antifreeze, poisoning 1081–2
antifungal agents 811, *811*
  classification/groups 811
  in dermatophyte infections 798–9
  imidazoles 811
  mechanism of action 296–7, *297*
  polyene 811, 812
  in renal impairment 3272
  resistance 298, 811
  in superficial infections 811
  in systemic infections 811–12
  topical *811*
antigen-antibody complexes, see immune
    complexes
antigenic drift 338
antigen mimicry, rheumatic fever
    pathogenesis 503
antigen-presenting cells 141, **153**
  B-cells as 143, 149, 157
  for helper T-cells 143, 153
  Langerhans cells 3707
  MHC antigens in transplantation
    184–5
  role 142
  see also antigens, presentation
antigens **141–5**
  in atopic eczema 3740, 3742
  bacterial number in infections 291
  B-cell recognition 141
  cross-reactions 141
  detection, respiratory tract infections
    2676–7, *2676*
  dietary, antibodies to 1840
  epitopes 141
  inaccessible, in tolerance 155, 156
  presentation,
    by B-cells 143, 149, 157
    class II MHC antigens 183, 184–5
    dendritic cells 87, 93
    macrophage 2615
    MHC antigen advantages in 148
    see also antigen-presenting cells
  processing 142, 143–4
    tumour antigens 228
  T-cell recognition 141
  trapping, immune complex deposition
    vs 182, 3774
  tumour, see under tumour immunology
  in vasculitis 3775, 3776
antiglobulin test
  blood compatibility testing **3690**
  direct (Coomb's test) 3542, 3544, 3631
  indirect 3542, 3690
antiglomerular basement membrane
    (GBM) disease (Goodpasture's
    syndrome) 182, **2803–4**, 3162,
    3163–6, 3163
  acute nephritic syndrome in 3146
  acute renal failure in 3291
  aetiology 3163–4
  Alport's syndrome and 3166, 3205
  autoantibodies 163, 2803
  clinical features 2803, 3164–5
  definition 3163
  fever and pulmonary infiltrates 1032

haematological changes 3685
  haemoptysis in 2644
  pathogenesis 3164
  pulmonary haemorrhage in 2803
  renal transplantation 3265–6, 3315
  treatment and outcome 2803–4, 3165–6
  Wegener's granulomatosis *vs* 3013
antihelminthic drugs, in hookworm
    infections 932
antihistamines
  in allergic rhinitis 160, 2718
  anticholinergic action 1062
  drugs included 1062
  H_1/H_2, *see* H_1-receptor antagonists; H_2-
    receptor antagonists
  long-acting 3772
  poisoning 1062
  in polycythaemia vera 3434
  in pregnancy 1804
  in renal impairment 3273
  treatment of snake antivenom reaction
    1138
  in urticaria 162, 3772
antihyaluronidase (AHT) 504
antihypertensive drugs **2539–41**
  in accelerated hypertension 3250
  ACE inhibitors 2540–1
  α-adrenoceptor blockers 2541, *2541*
  beta-blockers 2540
  calcium antagonists 2541, *2541*
  cardiovascular disease risk and 31
  choice and dosages 2539–41, *2541*
  combination therapy 2542
  in diabetes mellitus 1492, 3171
  in diabetic nephropathy 3171–2, 3250
  effects and meta-analyses 2539, 2540
  in elderly 4343
  indications 2539
  in Parkinson's disease 4004–5
  patient selection for 2539
  poor compliance and 2542
  in pre-eclampsia 1730–1
  in pregnancy 1731–2, 1812
  in renal failure 3273–4, 3304
  renal function and 3250
  selection and specific conditions for
    2542
  sexual problems associated *4245*
  thiazide diuretics 2539–40
  in thoracic aorta dissections 2574
  in transient ischaemic attack 3953
  vasodilators 2541–2, *2541*
  see also individual groups of drugs
anti-idiotypic response, to antitumour
    monoclonal antibodies 232
anti-inflammatory drugs
  duodenal ulcer aetiology 1878
  new opportunities/pitfalls **2627–8**
  in rheumatic fever 2434
  in sarcoidosis 2831, 2832
  see also non-steroidal anti-inflammatory
    drugs (NSAIDs)
'antiknock' additives 1084, 1092
  poisoning 1109
anti-La antibodies 2952, 3021, 3024, 3032
antiliver/kidney microsomal antibodies
    (anti-LKM)
  anti-LKM-1/-2/-3 types 2070
  in autoimmune hepatitis 2070, 2072,
    2073
  tienilic acid inducing 2072
antilymphocyte globulin 3446
antimalarial drugs 850–3
  in children/adults with uncomplicated
    malaria 853, *854*
  contraindication in pregnancy 3022
  eye toxicity 4196–7
  mechanism of action 851
  non-tablet forms *855*
  overdose/poisoning 1043, **1072–3**
  prophylactic 860–1, *861*
    doses in children *862*
  in renal impairment 3273
  resistance, *see under* malaria
  in rheumatoid arthritis 2964
  salt base equivalents *853*
  in SLE 3022, 3023
antimetabolites, new drugs 259

antimicrobial therapy 289, **295–314**
  acute neurological syndromes in
    immunocompromised 1034
  in acute pancreatitis 2032
  in amoebiasis 832
  anaerobic bacteria sensitivity 575
  antibacterial, *see* antibiotics
  antifungal, *see* antifungal agents
  antiprotozoal 296–7, *297*
  antiviral, *see* antiviral drugs
  in bacterial arthritis 2999
  in bacterial meningitis 4056–9, *4056,
    4057, 4058*
    prophylaxis 4059–60
  bacterial overgrowth treatment 1916
  bactericidal 303, 658
  bioavailability 300, *300*
  chemotherapy 311–13
    duration 313
    proposals for improving practice *312,*
      313
    questions to answer before starting
      311–13, *312*
    unsatisfactory response 313
  clinical aspects **309–14**
    see also antibiotic resistance
  in cystic fibrosis 2751–2, *2752*
  dose-response relations 307–9
  dosing regimens, design **306–9**
    importance of outcome measures
      307–9, *308*
    maximum effective concentration 307
  hypokalaemia due to 3132, 3337
  indications 296
    capacity to benefit 310
  in intracranial abscess 4083
  in leptospirosis 702
  mechanism of action 296–8, 658–9
    selective toxicity 296, 297
  monitoring concentrations,
    in serum 313
    in tissue fluid 301–2
  mycobacterial diseases (environmental)
    667, 667
  in *Mycoplasma pneumoniae* infection
    766
  nephrotoxicity **3263–5**, *3284, 3289*
  parenteral 312–13
  pharmacodynamics **303–6**
    adverse effects on patients 305, *306*
    antimicrobial action 303–5
    drug interactions 305–6
    factors influencing 304
    intracellular drugs 304–5
  pharmacokinetics **300–3**
    intestinal elimination 300–1, *300*
    patient characteristics 302–3
    specific infection sites *302*
    tissue distribution 301–2, *302*
  pharmacology **296–300**
    in plague 598
  poisoning by **1072**
  prescribing 296, 311–13, *311*
  principles **310–13**
  prophylactic 283, 289, 310–11
    anaerobic infections 576
    indications 310–11
    timing and duration 311, *311*
    see also antibiotics
  in pyrexia of unknown origin 1031
  in renal impairment **3270–3**, *3305*
  resistance 298–300, 309–10, 310
    flucytosine 811
    see also antibiotic resistance
  in rickettsial diseases 728, *730*
  in septicaemia 1023–4, 2573
  sterilizing action 658–9
  see also antibiotics; antifungal agents;
    antiprotozoal drugs; antiviral drugs
antimitochondrial antibodies
  antigens reacting with 2074, *2075*
  detection 2075
  in primary biliary cirrhosis 2074
antimonials
  in filarial infections 912
  see also pentavalent antimonials
antimüllerian hormone (Müllerian
    inhibitory factor) 1563, 1690

antimycobacterial therapy
  in sarcoidosis 2832
  see also antituberculous drugs
antimyeloperoxidase antibodies 3011
  diseases with 3011
  in microscopic polyangiitis 3014
  see also antineutrophil cytoplasmic
    antibodies (ANCA), peripheral (p-
    ANCA)
antimyosin monoclonal antibodies 2207
antineutrophil cytoplasmic antibodies
    (ANCA) 2078, 2952, 3008
  cytoplasmic (c-ANCA) 163, 2952,
    3010, 3011
    in cystic fibrosis 2749
    protein 3 as ligand 3011
    in Wegener's granulomatosis 3011,
      3013
  in diffuse parenchymal lung disease 2782
  diseases with 2951
  in erythema nodosum 3777–8
  false positive tests 3012
  in idiopathic rapidly progressive
    glomerulonephritis 3166
  levels and disease activity 3012
  peripheral (p-ANCA) 2952, 3010,
    3011
    antigens/ligands 3011
    see also antimyeloperoxidase
      antibodies
  types/patterns 3011
  in ulcerative colitis 1944, 1945
  in vasculitis 2000, 3012, 3777–8
    diagnosis/management 3011–12
    monitoring 3016
    pathogenesis of 3012
antinuclear antibodies 2510, 2749, 2952,
    3008, 3010, *3010*
  nuclear antigens 163–4
  in primary biliary cirrhosis 2074
  in SLE 3021
  in type-1 autoimmune hepatitis 2070
  see also anti-DNA antibodies
anti-oestrogens 1678
antioxidants
  angina management 2326
  in diabetic diets 1467
  dietary, ischaemic heart disease risk
    reduced 2311–12
antiparkinsonian drugs
  adverse mental symptoms 4242
  poisoning 1062
  in schizophrenia 4223
antiphospholipid antibodies 3020, 3661,
    3668–9
  anticoagulant therapy 3670
  diseases associated 3020
  indications for screening 3670
  in pregnancy 1768, 3669
  in SLE 3025, 3668, 3681, 4130
  see also anticardiolipin antibodies;
    lupus anticoagulant
antiphospholipid syndrome 163, 3019,
    3020
  primary (PAPS) 3631, **3669**, 3670
  α₂-antiplasmin 3619, 3624
    hereditary deficiency 3653
antiplatelet drugs **3671**
  effects on vascular events 3953, 3955
  ischaemic limb management 2369
  myocardial reinfarction prevention 2348
  in pre-eclampsia prevention 1730
  see also aspirin
antiports (exchangers) 1900, *1900*
'antipromotion', of cancer 219
antiprotease, in acute pancreatitis 2029
antiproteinase 3 antibodies, *see*
    antineutrophil cytoplasmic antibodies
    (ANCA), cytoplasmic (c-ANCA)
  α₁-antiproteinase, *see* α₁-antitrypsin
antiproteinases
  in bronchiectasis 2766
  in lung secretions 2614
antiprotozoal drugs 296–7
  mechanism of action 296–7, *297*
  pharmacodynamics 303
  in renal impairment 3273
  resistance 298

antipsychotic drugs **4251–3**
in dementia 4225
dosage and monitoring 4251
drug interactions 4252
drugs included 4251
indications and use 4251
pharmacology/mechanism of action 4251
in schizophrenia 4222
side-effects 4252, *4252*
management *4252*
see also clozapine; neuroleptic drugs
antipyretics, in tumours 241
antipyrine, poisoning 1057
antireflux surgery 1868
antireflux therapy 1867–8, *1867*, *1868*
antiresorptive agents 3068
anti-Ro antibodies 2952, 3021, 3022, 3024, 3032
anti-salivary gland antibodies 2961
antisense oligonucleotides 260
antiseptics
poisoning 1078
Staphylococcus aureus sensitivity 525–6, 531
antisera, passive immunization 283–4, 316–17
anti-Sm antibodies 2952, 3024
antisnakebite serum, *see* antivenom
antisocial personality disorder 4212
antispasmodics, in diverticular disease 1970
antistreptolysin O (ASO) 504
antithrombin (III) 109, 2299, 2303, *3379*, 3622–3, 3626, 3665
concentrates 3659, 3667
deficiency 2522, **3665–6**, 3667
causes of acquired *3671*
indications for screening *3670*
pregnancy in 1743, 3668
heparin action 3673
in nephrotic syndrome 3142
in pre-eclampsia 1763
in pregnancy 1762
antithrombotic therapy, *see* thrombolytic therapy
antithyroid drugs **1612–13**, 1614
in pregnancy 1749
antitoxin, diphtheria 496
α₁-antitrypsin 109, 1545, 2757, 2769
abnormalities 2772
bronchiectasis pathogenesis 2757
functional defect 2772
classification and phenotypes 2771
cleavage and inactivation 1546
in cystic fibrosis therapy 2753
deficiency **1545–7**, *2018*, **2131**, **2770–1**, 3560
associated conditions 1547
in bronchiectasis 2757, 2761
cadmium poisoning 1107
causes/mechanisms 2771, *2772*
clinical features 1546–7
in COAD 2769, **2771–2**, 2771
diagnosis 1547
emphysema 1545, **1546**, 2632, 2769, 2771
genetics 1545
liver disease 1546–7, 2131
liver transplantation in 2113
Pittsburgh, point mutation in 109
PiZZ homozygotes 1545, 1546–7
pregnancy in 1745
treatment 1547
as type of COAD 2767, 2768, 2769
in haemolytic uraemic syndrome 3200
isoelectric focusing 2771
oxidation and inactivation 1545–6
PiM phenotype 2772
protein C inhibition 3624
replacement therapy 1547, 2761
structure and function 1545
Z allele 2771
antituberculous drugs **655–61**
in genitourinary tuberculosis **3278**

in meningitis 4062–3
neonates 1746
nephrotoxicity **3264–5**
in pregnancy 1746, 1793
sensitivity testing 3276
sideroblastic anaemia induced by 3523
see also antimycobacterial therapy;
specific drugs (page 656);
tuberculosis, chemotherapy
antivenin, *see* antivenom
antivenom 1048
fish venom 1141
scorpion 1147
snake 1136–8
contraindications 1137
dosage and guide to *1137*, 1138
indications for 1136
polyspecific (polyvalent) 1137
prediction of reactions to 1137
prognosis after 1139
reactions/response to 1138
selection and administration 1137–8
spider 1148–9
tick 1149
antiviral drugs 459
CNS infections 4069, 4071
in HIV infection 481–3
see also AIDS and HIV infection, treatment
mechanism of action 297–8, 298
in renal impairment 3272
resistance 298
in varicella-zoster virus infections 350
in viral hepatitis 459
antral carcinoma 1883
antroduodenal manometry 1956
Antrypol, *see* Suramin
ant stings 1144–5
anuria
calculus 3253
in urinary-tract obstruction 3235
anus
examination, in constipation 1826
imperforate **1979–80**
embryology 1973
high anomalies 1979–80
low anomalies 1980
management 1980
see also entries beginning anal, anorectal
anxiety
abnormal, *see* anxiety disorders
as normal reaction 4205
in phaeochromocytoma 4239
in skin disease 3707
symptoms 4205, *4205*
in depressive disorders 4206, 4218
in terminal illness **4358**
anxiety disorders **4205–8**
acute, psychiatric emergencies due to 4258, *4258*
atypical eating disorder in 1301, 4217
chest pain in 2648
chronic fatigue syndrome 1037, 1038
generalized anxiety disorder **4205–6**
hyperthyroidism *vs* 4239
obsessive compulsive disorder *vs* 4207
organic 4225
panic disorder, *see* panic disorder
phobic 4206, 4255
see also phobia
recurrent, brief dynamic psychotherapy in 4256
treatment 4206, 4247, 4255
cognitive behaviour therapy 4255
anxiolytic drugs **4253–4**
benzodiazepines, *see* benzodiazepines
brain GABA function increase 4253
monoamine function changes 4253–4
in terminal illness 4358
aorta
abdominal, prosthesis 2137
abnormal chest radiograph 2182
aneurysms, *see* aortic aneurysms
ascending, enlargement 2182
calcification 2182, 2482

coarctation 2182, **2557–9**
chest radiography 2179
clinical features 2557–8
intestinal ischaemia in 1995
investigations 2179, 2215, 2558–9
magnetic resonance imaging 2215
in pregnancy 1737
pre-/postductal 2557
treatment 2559
dissection, *see* aortic dissection
fibromuscular dysplasia 2548
'higgledy-piggledy' changes 2423
kinked **2424**
magnetic resonance imaging 2214–15
overriding, in Fallot's tetralogy 2402
panarteritis 2378
partial obstruction 2557
thoracic, acute dissections **2574**
aortic aneurysms 2137
abdominal 2137, 2364
asymptomatic 2364, 2372
elective repair 3283
management 2372
rupture(d) 2364, 2372
symptomatic 2364, 2372
aortic arch 2372, 2482–3
ascending 2365
management 2372
calcification 2182
clinical features 2364–5
in coarctation of aorta 2558
descending, management 2372
dissecting,
acute pancreatitis *vs* 2030
clinical features 2365
management 2372
thoracic 2372, **2574**
see also aortic dissection
'flask-shaped' 2465
gastrointestinal involvement 1998
'inflammatory' 3245
leaking, angina *vs* 2322
magnetic resonance imaging 2215
management **2372**
in syphilis 2364, 2365, 2482–3
management 2483
thoracic 2364–5, 2900
angina *vs* 2322
management 2372
rupture 2372
aortic arch
abnormalities 2182
aneurysm 2372, 2482–3
calcification 2182
chest radiography 2178
right 2182, 2408
aortic balloon valvuloplasty 2464
aortic baroreceptors, in hypertension 2533
aortic bodies 3887
aortic dissection
aortic root 2465
chest pain in 2167
chest radiograph 2338
clinical features 2335
in coarctation of aorta 2558
computed tomography (CT) 2218, 2219
magnetic resonance imaging 2214, 2215
in Marfan syndrome 3083
myocardial infarction *vs* 2335
in pregnancy 1738
see also aortic aneurysms, dissecting
aortic incompetence, *see* aortic regurgitation
aortic knuckle 2178, 2182, 2416
in Eisenmenger reaction (syndrome) 2411
aortic pressure 2153
aortic pulse, in Fallot's tetralogy 2402
aortic regurgitation 2421, 2424, **2464–7**
acute 2464
after Fallot's tetralogy repair 2405, 2407
angina investigation 2325–6
in ankylosing spondylitis 2967
aortic stenosis with **2464**
causes and pathology 2464–5, *2465*

clinical features 2465–377
in coarctation of aorta 2558
diagnosis/differential diagnosis 2467
diastolic murmur in 2455, 2465
in Fallot's tetralogy 2403
in infective endocarditis 2443, 2464, 2465, 2467
investigations 2465–377
Doppler echocardiography 2202, 2203, 2465–6
MRI 2214, 2215, 2216, 2217
in Marfan's syndrome 3083
paraprosthetic 2470
in pregnancy 1737–8
in rheumatic fever 2432, 2433, 2467
in rheumatoid arthritis 2961
in seronegative arthropathies 2392
severity estimation 2467
in syphilis 2482, 2483
treatment 2467
in ventricular septal defects 2429
aortic ring, dilatation 2465
aortic-root
abscess 2443
enlargement in syphilis 2482
infection 2443
aortic sinus
aneurysms, in infective endocarditis 2439
right, left ventricular outflow tract defect 2424
aortic stenosis 2399, **2421–2**, **2462–4**
angina due to 2325, 2327, 2462
investigations 2325
aortic incompetence with **2464**
calcific, in dilated cardiomyopathy 2381
clinical features 2462
signs 2423, 2462–3
syncope 2160, 2462
coronary artery disease in 2462, 2464
diagnosis/differential diagnosis 2463–4
ejection murmur in 2325, 2462, 2463
glyceryl trinitrate avoidance 2327
infective endocarditis in 2439
investigations,
Doppler echocardiography 2202, 2463
MRI 2216, 2217
pathophysiology 2462
in pregnancy 1737
rheumatic 2462
senile/degenerative 2462
subaortic, *see* subaortic stenosis
treatment 2464
valvular 2399, **2421–2**, **2462–4**, *2462*
vascular dysplasia association 1998
aortic valve
bicuspid 2399, 2462, 2557
calcification 2182, 2408, 2421, 2462
closure 2153
in coarctation of aorta 2558
congenitally deformed 2421
disease **2462–7**
mitral regurgitation *vs* 2461
in pregnancy 1737–8
incompetence, *see* aortic regurgitation
in infective endocarditis 2439
in Marfan syndrome 3083
regurgitation, *see* aortic regurgitation
replacement 2422, 2464, 2467, 2483
cadaver homografts 2408
prostheses 2470
in rheumatic fever 2432
in rheumatoid arthritis 2961
staphylococcal endocarditis 527
stenosis, *see* aortic stenosis
aortitis, syphilitic 2465, **2482–4**
aortitis syndrome, *see* Takayasu's disease
aortoarteritis, non-specific, *see* Takayasu's disease
aortography
in septicaemia 2573
in Takayasu's disease 2379
aortoiliac disease, extra-anatomical bypass grafts 2370
aortoiliac reconstruction 2363, 2369–70
aorto-left ventricular defect (tunnel) **2424**, 2467

aortopulmonary shunts **2430–1**
aortopulmonary window **2431**
APACHE II system, acute pancreatitis 2030, *2031*
apathy
  in endocrine disorders 4239
  in malnutrition 1283
apatite
  crystals 2990, 2991
  tophaceous periarticular deposition 2991
apatite-associated destructive arthritis 2991
apatite-associated disorders **2990–1**
APC (adenomatous polyposis coli) gene 66, 1990
apex beat
  angina investigation 2325
  Fallot's tetralogy diagnosis 2405
  sustained, in mitral stenosis 2453
aphasia **3846–52**
  anterior 3850
  associated disturbances 3851–2
  Broca's (motor/expressive) 3850, 3851
  characteristics **3848–9**
  classification and localization of syndromes **3849–51**
  conduction 3850
  examination **3849**, *3849*
  fluent 3848
  global (central) 3849, 3850–1
  handedness and cerebral dominance **3847**
  jargon 3848
  nominal (amnestic/anomic) 3850
  non-fluent 3848
  object naming defect (anomia) 3848
  optic 3854
  posterior 3850
  progressive with temporal lobe atrophy 3974, 3975
  transcortical motor 3850
  transcortical sensory 3850
  visual agnosia *vs* 3854
  Wernicke's (sensory/receptive) 3850, 3851, 3968
  see also language
aphemia 3850
aphthous ulcers, *see* oral ulceration
aplastic anaemia 3392, **3441–7**
  acquired **3441–6**
    definition 3441
  classification 3441, *3442*
  clonal disorders following 3447
  in glue sniffing 1092
  idiosyncratic acquired **3441–6**
    aetiology 3441–2
    clinical features 3443–4
    diagnosis and pathology 3443
    incidence/epidemiology 3442
    pathogenesis 3442–3
    treatment 3444–6
  immune 3441, *3442*
  inevitable 3441, *3442*
  inherited 3441, *3442*, **3446–7**
    see also Fanconi anaemia
  'malignant' 3441, *3442*, **3447**
  paroxysmal nocturnal haemoglobinuria and 3443–4, 3451
  in pregnancy 1761
  in viral hepatitis 3441, 3680
aplastic crisis
  in hereditary spherocytosis 3529
  human parvovirus and 448, 3449, 3680
  in sickle-cell disease 3515
apneusis 2584
apnoea 2724, 2909
  central, *see* sleep apnoea, central
  epileptic 3890
  obstructive sleep, *see* obstructive sleep apnoea
  reflex **2917**
apocrine sweat glands 3706, 3765
apolipoprotein(s) 1400, 1401, 1903
  ischaemic heart disease risk 2308
  surfactant 2595

apolipoprotein (a) (apo(a)) 1403
  see also lipoprotein (a) (Lp(a))
apolipoprotein A₁ 1403, 1404, 2308
  deficiency 1414
  variants, in amyloidosis 1517, **1520**
apolipoprotein AII (AII) 1403, 1404
apolipoprotein B 2291, 2308
apolipoprotein B₄₈ 1401, 1903
apolipoprotein B₁₀₀ (apo B₁₀₀) 1402, 1403
  in coronary artery disease 64
  familial defective 1407
apolipoprotein B₁₀₀/E receptors, *see* low-density lipoprotein (LDL) receptor
apolipoprotein CII (apo CII) 1401
  deficiency 1410
  in nephrotic syndrome 3143
apolipoprotein CIII deficiency 1414
apolipoprotein E (apo E) 1401, 1402, 1403, 1404
  in Alzheimer's disease 65
  E₄ 65, 3973
  gene mutation/polymorphism 1409
apophyseal joints 2992
apoplectic seizure 3909
apoproteins, *see* apolipoprotein(s)
apoptosis 223, 225, 2625–6
  c-*myc* gene role 225
  deletion of self-reactive T-cells 152
  extravasated neutrophils 2625
APP (adenomatous polyposis coli) locus 66, 1990
appendicectomy, laparoscopic 2010
appendicitis **2009–10**
  aetiology 2009–10
  amoebic 828
  chronic 2009, 2011
  diagnosis and clinical signs 2010
  diet association 1329
  differential diagnosis 2010
    Campylobacter infections *vs* 558
    Crohn's disease *vs* 1938, 1941
    Yersinia infection *vs* 608
  in enterobiasis 941, 942
  epidemiology, age and sex 2010
  faecalith-induced 2009, 2010
  in HIV infection 2010
  incidence 2009
  investigations 2010
  left-sided 1970
    see also diverticular disease, colonic
  postoperative 2010
  in pregnancy 1803
  retrocaecal 2010
  treatment 2010
  in trichuriasis 943
appendix
  abscess 2010
  acute inflammation, *see* appendicitis
  adenocarcinoma 2011
  carcinoid tumour 2011
  'grumbling' 2010, 2011
  non-acute inflammation 2011
  perforation 2010
  tumours 2011
appetite
  in diabetes 1453
  loss, in tumours 241
  in pregnancy 1770
  return in malnutrition management 1293
  see also anorexia
appetite stimulants, in terminal illness 4351
applied potential tomography (APT) 1957
apramycin 310
apraxia **3852–3**
  buccofacial 3848
  congenital **4122**
  congenital oculomotor 4114
  constructional 3852–3
  dressing 3854
  gaze 3853
  ideational 3852
  ideomotor 3852
aprotinin 3659, 3660
APSAC (acylated plasminogen

streptokinase activator complex) 3671, *3672*
APUD cells 1703
  small-cell lung cancer 2881
  tumours, amyloidosis 1518
aquatic animals, *see* fish; poisoning; seafood
aqueduct stenosis 4115
arachidonic acid 2294
  metabolism 158, 2855, 3936
    ARDS pathogenesis 2855
    endothelial 3662
    platelet 3617
  in sepsis and shock 293
Arachnia propionica 551
arachnids **1006–9**
arachnodactyly
  congenital contractural 3083
  in Marfan's syndrome 3083
arachnoid cysts **4116**
  spinal **4117**
arachnoiditis **3903**
  spinal **3894**, 4061
Aranea, bites **1147–9**
arboviruses 423
  group A (alphaviruses) **407–9**, *408*
  infections, arthritis in **3001**
Arcanobacterium haemolyticum 551
Arcobacter, rare species *551*
ARDS, *see* adult respiratory distress syndrome
area postrema 1821
area under the curve (AUC) 307, 1242
arenaviruses **429–39**
  ecology and epidemiology 429
  New world **436–9**
  Old world **430–6**
    see also Lassa fever
  virology 429–30, 431
Argentinian haemorrhagic fever 436, **437–8**
arginase 1353
  deficiency (AD) 1358–60
arginine *1353*
  stimulation test *1584*, 1698, *1698*
  synthesis 1358
  therapy 1360
arginine vasopressin, *see* vasopressin
argininosuccinate lyase 1353
  deficiency (ALD) 1358–60
argininosuccinate synthetase 1353
  deficiency (ASD) 1358–60
Argyll Robertson pupil 3877, 4085
argyrophil ganglion cells, absent 1978
armed forces, fitness requirements 2361
Armed Forces Institute of Pathology (AFIP), pancreatic carcinoma 2041, *2041*
Armillifer species **1013–14**
arms
  in rheumatic diseases 2946
  in rheumatoid arthritis 2957–8
aromatase, in obesity 1308
aromatic amines, and cancer 1167
  bladder cancer 211, 212, 1167
L-aromatic amino acid decarboxylase, *see* dopa decarboxylase
arousal
  reduced in REM sleep 2909
  stimulus, in obstructive sleep apnoea 2911
arrhythmias, *see* cardiac arrhythmias
arrhythmogenic right ventricular dysplasia **2391**
arsenic 1106
  inorganic, angiosarcoma association 204
  lung cancer and 2880
  non-melanoma skin cancer and 209, 3791
  poisoning **1106**, 1171
    blood/urine levels 1106
    neuropathy 4099
arsenicals
  dermatitis from 3732
  in dermatitis herpetiformis 3783
  'arsenical vesicants' 1117

arsenic trichloride 1106
arsenic trioxide 1106
arsine poisoning **1094**, 3520, 3546
Arsobal, *see* Melarsoprol
artemisinin, in malaria 852
arterial blood pressure, *see* blood pressure
arterial grafts 2369–71
arterial surgery, reconstructive 2369–72
  complications 2371
  graft patency 2370
  in Takayasu's disease 2379
arterial thrombosis 3661
  management 3669–70, 3671
  in nephrotic syndrome 3141–2
  pathogenesis **3663–4**
  in protein C deficiency 3666
  relative polycythaemia and 3553
  in renal transplant recipients 3318
  see also thrombosis
arteries
  anatomy 2289–90
  changes in hypertension 2533
  compliance, decreased in hypertension 2533
  disease, causes 3950, *3950*
  fibrosis, in Takayasu's disease 2378
  heart failure pathophysiology 2231
  inappropriate vasoconstriction, *see* vasospastic disorders
  normal structure 2289–90
    see also endothelial cell(s)
  occlusion, in drug addicts 4280
  physiology and biochemistry 2290
arteriography
  in electrical injury 1213
  renal **3110**
  selective mesenteric 1998
  see also angiography
arteriohepatic dysplasia 2014
arterioles, inappropriate vasoconstriction, *see* vasospastic disorders
arteriopathy, Takayasu's, *see* Takayasu's disease
arteriosclerotic parkinsonism 3998
arteriovenous fistulae
  coronary 2467
  in haemodialysis 3308–9
  opening and sodium retention 2169
  pulmonary 2402, 2408, **2419**, 2862
  renal 3243
  spinal dural 3828
arteriovenous malformation
  gastrointestinal 1998
  intracerebral 3962
    embolization in 3824
  intracranial **3963**, 3964
  spinal 3828, 3895
arteritis
  cor pulmonale pathogenesis 2516
  definition and use of term 3773, 3774
  giant-cell (temporal/cranial), *see* giant-cell arteritis
  localized, gastrointestinal tract in 2000
  necrotizing, in pulmonary hypertension 2507–8
  Takayasu's, *see* Takayasu's disease
  see also polyarteritis; vasculitis
arthralgia
  in Behçet's syndrome 3045
  in cryoglobulinaemia 3051
  in erythema nodosum 3003
  in microscopic polyangiitis 3014
  in parvovirus infections 448
  in rheumatic fever 2432
  in rubella 409
  in Wegener's granulomatosis 3012
  see also joint(s), pain
arthritis
  acne arthralgia and 3003
  in alkaptonuria 1364–5, 3004
  in amyloidosis 1515, 3003–4
  apatite-associated destructive 2991
  atrophic (bone loss) 2975
  bacterial **2998–9**
  in Behçet's syndrome 3045
  in brucellosis 620

arthritis (cont.)
in carcinoid syndrome 1897
in chlamydial infections 753
cricoarytenoid 2796, 2874
cross-reacting epitopes 155
in cyanotic congenital heart disease
  2401–2
fungal **3000**
in gonorrhoea 546–7
gouty 1376, *1377*
  see also gout
in haemochromatosis 3005, 3478–9
in Henoch-Schönlein purpura 3004,
  3150
hypertrophic (bone increase) 2975
in hypogammaglobulinaemia 771, 3005
inflammatory 155
in liver disorders 3004
in Lyme disease 690, 3002
in meningococcaemia (acute) 539
meningococcal 540
mumps virus causing 374, 3001
mycoplasmas causing 771
  in hypogammaglobulinaemia 168
in neoplastic disorders **3006**
periarticular swellings 2947
peripheral 2946, 3000
in psoriasis, *see* psoriatic arthritis
in pyoderma gangrenosum 3003
reactive, *see* reactive arthritis
in recurrent polyserositis 1526, 1527
in rheumatic fever 503, 504–5, 2432–3
rheumatoid, *see* rheumatoid arthritis
in rubella 409, 3001
sarcoid 3007
septic, *see* septic arthritis
'seronegative', *see* seronegative
  spondarthropathies
in serum sickness 3005–6
sexually acquired reactive (SARA), *see*
  sexually acquired reactive arthritis
  (SARA)
in SLE 3019
syphilitic **3002**
tuberculous 2998, 3000
viral **3000–2**
in Wegener's granulomatosis 3012
in Whipple's disease 1924, 2005, 2973
see also monoarthritis; polyarthritis
arthrocentesis 2951
arthrochalasis multiplex congenita *3084*
arthrodesis, in rheumatoid arthritis 2964
arthrography 2949
arthrogryposis multiplex congenita 4150
arthropathy
chronic haemophilic 3004–5, 3647,
  3649
in cystic fibrosis 2749
pyrophosphate, *see* pyrophosphate
  arthropathy
seronegative, *see* seronegative
  spondarthropathies
in ulcerative colitis 1948, 2972–3
arthroplasty
in osteoarthritis 2982
in rheumatoid arthritis 2964
arthropod-borne reoviruses **406–7**
arthropods, non-venomous **1000–12**
blood-sucking flies **1011**
eye-frequenting Lepidoptera **1010–11**
hygiene and **1011**
parasites **1000–10**
vesicles/blisters from bites 3780
arthropods, venomous **1144–51**
centipedes 1149
coleoptera (beetles) 1146
hymenoptera 1144–6
leeches 1150–1
lepidoptera 1146
millipedes 1149–50
scorpions 1146–7
spiders 1147–9
ticks 1149
see also insect(s), stings
arthroscopy 2950
in osteoarthritis 2982
Arthus reaction 278, 291
articular cartilage, *see* cartilage

articulatory dyspraxia **4122**
arylacetic acid derivatives, poisoning
  1056
arylaminoalcohols 850
arylpropionic acid derivatives, poisoning
  1056, *1057*
Asacol 1949, *1949*
asbestos 2843, 2894
gastric cancer and 203
lung cancer and 206, 219, 2880
mesothelioma and, *see* mesothelioma,
  malignant
pleural tumours and 207, 2894
-related disease, risk in non-
  occupational exposed **2845**
types 2843
asbestosis **2843–5**, 2894
incidence 2843
open-lung biopsy 2688
smoking interaction 206, 2844, 2845
ascariasis **936–8**
Ascaris lumbricoides 936, 2004
cholangitis 2051
lifecycle and eggs 937
Ascaris suum 937
Aschoff nodule 2432
ascites **2095–9**
causes 2096, *2096*
chylous 2096, 2098
in cirrhosis 2088, 2089
complications 2096
diagnosis 2096
in hepatocellular failure 2102–3, 2106,
  2108
in intestinal tuberculosis 2005
low-protein 2096
malignant, management 2098
management 2097–8, 2108
  drugs to avoid *2097*
pancreatic 2033, 2038, 2096
pathogenesis and hypotheses 2097
pseudochylous 2096
signs 2095–6
ascitic fluid
amylase in 2038
bacterial infection 2096–7
examination and colour 2096
volume 2095
white-cell count 2096
ascorbic acid, *see* vitamin C
aseptic necrosis of bone (osteonecrosis)
in chronic renal failure 3324, 3327
in Hodgkin's disease 3575
in renal transplant recipients 3321
in sickle-cell disease 3515
in SLE 3018, 3019
Asia 51
venomous snakes 1127
Asians, nutritional osteomalacia 3073
L-asparaginase 1248
aspartate *1353*
aspartate aminotransferase (AST: serum
  glutamate oxaloacetic transaminase)
  2055, *4365*
in autoimmune hepatitis 2070, 2073
in cirrhosis 2088
in congestive cardiac failure 2130
in Lassa fever 431, 433, 434
liver metastases detection 246
in Marburg virus and Ebola virus
  disease 441
in paracetamol-induced liver damage
  1052
aspartylglycosaminuria *1435*, **1436**
Asperger syndrome 4108
aspergilloma 808
paranasal 809
aspergillosis **808–9**
aetiology and epidemiology 808
after cardiac transplantation 2257
allergic 3685
allergic bronchopulmonary 808, 2734,
  2805–6
bronchiectasis in 2761
tuberculosis *vs* 651
cerebral 1034
clinical features 808

invasive 808–9
treatment 809
Aspergillus
infections,
  in cystic fibrosis, treatment 2754
  in immunocompromised 1029
  infective endocarditis 809, 2438
Aspergillus flavus 218, 808
Aspergillus fumigatus 808, 2708, 2734
Aspergillus nidulans 808
asphyxia, birth, cerebral palsy due to
  4119, 4121
asphyxiating thoracic dystrophy (Jeune's
  disease) **2875**
asphyxiation 2847
aspiration
food, acute airways obstruction 2721
of gastric contents, in pregnancy *1742*,
  1744–5, 1801
intracranial abscess 4083
mineral/vegetable oil 2837
pneumothorax treatment 2870
pulmonary, lung abscess due to 2704
see also airways, aspiration; gastric
  aspiration
aspiration pneumonia 1959, **2702–3**
in ankylosing spondylitis 2874
hazard of gastric lavage 1049
oesophageal varices complication 2094
staphylococcal 526
aspirin
adverse reaction 1054, 2851
analgesic nephropathy and 3221, *3222*
asthma association 2735, 2849
avoidance in liver disease 2091
biotransformation pathway 1054
breast feeding and 1811
in coronary angioplasty 2352
in cyanotic congenital heart disease
  2401
gastrointestinal bleeding 1827
in Kawasaki disease 3049
mechanism of action 2735
in myocardial infarction 23, 26–7,
  2301, 2304, 2340, 2348
  initial treatment 2336
  warfarin with 2305
in nephrotic syndrome 3142
pharmacokinetics and toxicity 1054
poisoning 1054, 2672
  see also salicylates, poisoning
in pre-eclampsia prevention 1730
in pregnancy **1810**, 3670
in primary antiphospholipid syndrome
  3669
pseudoallergic reaction 1253
in renal impairment 3273
Reye's syndrome association 1054,
  2026, 4072
in rheumatic fever 2434
stroke prevention 3964
sun exposure protection 3728
in transient ischaemic attacks 2373,
  3953
in unstable angina 2330
uric acid excretion and 1379
vasoconstriction 2297
warfarin interaction 3674
asplenia
travel precautions 325
see also splenectomy
'assassin' bugs 1006
association, bacterial colonization
  mechanism 270
association, disease
genetic linkage *vs* 110, 111
linkage disequilibrium explanation
  110–11
Association for Spina Bifida and
  Hydrocephalus (ASBAH) 4119
astasia 3983
astemizole 2718
asterixis 3283
in hepatic encephalopathy 2101
asteroid bodies, in sarcoidosis 2818
asthenia, *see* weakness
asthenozoospermia 1684, 1685

asthma 2591, **2724–46**, 3741
acute attacks 2635, **2736**
  treatment 2739, *2739*
acute bronchial infections and 2693
aetiology 2635, 2725, 2742, *2743*
age and gender **2735–6**
aircraft crew and pilots 1201
aircraft travel and 1202
allergic bronchopulmonary aspergillosis
  2734
atopic allergic, *see* asthma, extrinsic
brief dynamic psychotherapy in 4256
bronchial hyper-responsiveness 2725–6
allergic reactions 2725, 2731–2
causes **2731–3**
clinical relevance **2730–1**
deep inspiration 2730–1
environmental change 2731
environmental pollution and 2732
immediate/late reactions 2732
infections causing 2732–3
mechanisms 2726
testing reactivity 2733
bronchiectasis with 2762
in children 2725, 2731, 2736
chromium compound inhalation 1107
chronic obstructive airways disease
  overlap 2767
in Churg-Strauss syndrome 2800, 3015
circulatory failure in 2571
clinical features **2729–30**
breathlessness 2645, 2646, 2647, 2729
cough 2643, 2729
occupational asthma 2743–4
signs 2729–30
symptoms 2726, 2729
wheezing 335, 338, 2729
in cold weather 2731
definition 161
diagnostic algorithm 2733, 2734, *2734*
differential diagnosis 2737
diisocyanate 1100
diurnal pattern 2730, 2731
diving and 1210
drug-induced 1253, **2735, 2849–50**
drugs causing *2849*
pharmacological effects 2849
drug reactions in 1253
in elderly 2736
environmental factors causing 2731,
  2732, **2733**
exercise-induced 2731
prevention/management 2731
extrinsic (allergic) 161, 2725, 2731–2,
  2733–4, 2743
causes/allergens 161, 2731–2, 2734
phases 161, 2732
extrinsic non-atopic 2734
food allergy in 2734, 3729
foods associated 1844, 2734
future prospects **2741**
gastro-oesophageal reflux and **2735**
idiosyncratic reactions 2849–50
infective **2734–5**
as inflammatory disorder of airways
  2727, 2728, 2729
inheritance 2725
intrinsic **2735**
investigations **2736–7**, 2744–5
immunological tests 2744
inhalation testing 2733, 2744–5
lung function tests 2668, 2733, 2736,
  2744
mechanism evaluation 2736–7
peak expiratory flow 2730, 2736, 2744
laryngeal dysfunction in 2724
late-onset 2725, 2734, 2735
mechanical properties of lung 2635–6
mechanisms and pathophysiology
  2635–6, 2645, **2724–9**
bronchial hyper-responsiveness
  2725–6
eosinophilic cationic proteins 159,
  161, 2727
eosinophils and T-cells role 2727–8
inflammation role 2616, 2617, 2727–8,
  2728

inflammatory events in bronchial mucosa 2727–8
neutrophil leukotriene B$_4$ causing 159, 2727
overview/summary 2728–9
methacholine testing 2726, 2733
mortality 2724–5, **2740–1**
trends 2741
mucociliary clearance in 2613
nocturnal 2730, 2731
non-allergic 2725, 2727, 2734
occupational 2647, 2725, 2736, **2742–6**
byssinosis 2647, **2746**
causes 2742, *2743*
clinical features 2743–4
compensation **2746**
determinants/susceptibility 2742
diagnosis 2744
differential diagnosis 2745
hypersensitivity-induced 2742–3, **2743–4**
importance of 2743
incidence 2742, *2743*
investigations 2744–5
irritant-induced (RADS) 2742, 2743
management 2745–6
pathogenesis 2743
pathology 2727, 2743
prognosis 2745
prophylaxis 2745
risk *2743*
organization of care **2740**
pathology 2685, **2726–7**, 2743
bronchial lining ultrastructure 2617, 2726
pathophysiology **2635–6**, 2645
physiology 2636, **2728–9**
in pregnancy **1745**
prevalence 2724, 2741
process-specific air pollution causing 1230, 2742, *2743*
see also asthma, occupational
prophylaxis 2737–8, *2738*, 2745
psychogenic **2735**
pulmonary circulation 2636
pulmonary hypertension in 2509
respiratory virus infections in 335, 338, 2732–3
respiratory syncytial virus (RSV) 340, 2732
rhinovirus 335
severe **2736**
methacholine relation 2726
respiratory muscle function tests 2669
treatment 2739, *2739*
sputum in 2685
steroid trial, protocol 2733, *2734*
treatment 2592, **2737–9**, 2924
allergen avoidance 2737, *2737*
bronchodilators 2729, 2738
concern over ß-agonists 2741
desensitization 2740
failure to respond **2739–40**
inhaled therapy 2738
oral corticosteroids 2737, 2738–9
organization 2740
positive-pressure ventilation 2578
in renal impairment 3274
symptom relief **2739**
ventilation 2924
triggers 2730, 2731, 2733
in urban *vs* rural communities 2741
vanadium exposure causing 1114
Asthma Training Centre 2740
astrocytes 3990
astrocytoma **4030–1**
benign 4030
classification 4030
computed tomography 3818
incidence *4031*
low-grade 4031
malignant 4031
spinal cord 3895
astronauts
haemolytic anaemia in 3550
see also aerospace medicine

astrovirus 390, 391, *391*, **392**
asystole **2269**
ataxia
in acute mountain sickness 1188
cerebellar 3860, 3984–5
hereditary, *see* hereditary ataxia
limb 3860
sensory 3858
truncal 3860
ataxia telangiectasia (Louis-Bar syndrome) 173, 192–3, 223, *3447*, **3988, 4009**
diseases associated 173
gene 173
leukaemia association 215, 3410
ataxic 'cerebral' palsy **4121**
atelectasis 2641
absorption, oxygen toxicity 1207
laryngeal expiratory braking 2612
pneumococcal pneumonia *vs* 516
in SLE 2798–9
treatment 2579
atenolol *2264*
airway obstruction and asthma associated 2849
in alcohol withdrawal 2084
in pregnancy 1812
atherectomy 2352
atheroembolism 2375
atherogenesis, *see* atherosclerosis, pathogenesis
atheroma 2290, 3947–8
in carotid arteries 3948
chronic intestinal ischaemia due to 1994, 1996
cytokines role 98
distribution 3947–8
in hypertension 2533
idiopathic retroperitoneal fibrosis and 3245
internal carotid artery 2367
intestinal ischaemia due to 2366
occlusion of mesenteric vessels 1994
unstable angina and 2166, 2320
see also atherosclerosis, lesions
atherosclerosis **2289–95, 2362–3**
angina pathology **2320**
arterial thrombosis and 3663
cerebrovascular 3947–8
cholesterol embolism in 2375, 2376
in chronic renal failure 3301, 3302
death rates 2289, *2290*
distribution 2362
epidemiology **2289**
in hyperlipoproteinaemia type III 1409
in hypertension 2291, 2533
in hypertriglyceridaemia 1410
ischaemic heart disease and **2318**, 2332, 2333
lesions 2290, **2318**, 2362
development, *see* atherosclerosis, pathogenesis
fatty streaks 2290, 2318, 2362
plaques, *see* atherosclerotic plaques
see also atheroma
lipid-lowering therapy 1414
myocardial infarction **2320–1**
natural history **2289–94**, 2362
in nephrotic syndrome 3142
normal artery structure/biochemistry 2289–90
pathogenesis 1405, 2290–1, 2318, 2362
cells involved 2291, 2292
fibrinogen role 2303
molecular interactions 2292, 2293–4
progression 2318
regression, psychological intervention 4232
in renal transplant recipients 3321
renovascular hypertension due to 2548
restenosis after angioplasty 2294–5
risk factors *2291*
reduction in diabetes 1468
thrombosis in 2318, **2319**
deep intimal injury 2319
evolution of thrombi 2319
intraplaque and intraluminal 2319

myocardial infarction due to 2332, 2333
superficial intimal injury 2319
thrombolysis balance 2319, 2333
vascular tone alteration 2318, 2320
see also atheroma; ischaemic heart disease; myocardial infarction
atherosclerotic arteries, paradoxical constriction 2297, 2318
atherosclerotic plaques 2290, 2291, **2318**, 2362
advanced **2318**
clinical symptoms and 2318
carotid arteries 3948
cells of **2291**, 2292
concentric and eccentric 2320
fibrous cap 2318, 2319, 2362
fibrous and lipid-rich types 2320
fissuring 2319
growth and effects of 2290, 2318
molecular interactions 2292, 2293–4, 2299
adhesion molecules 2294, 2299
chemoattractants 2294
control 2294, 2300
cytokines 2293–4, 2299
growth factors 2293, 2299
matrix proteins and coagulation factors 2294
pathogenesis 2290–1, 2318, 2319, 2362
remodelling and 2229, 2318, 2333
see also under myocardial infarction
rupture 2291, 2319, 2333
cholesterol embolism and 2375
embolism 2375
in myocardial infarction 2320, 2333
in stable angina 2320
stable and unstable 2319
in unstable angina 2166, 2320
vulnerable 2319
atherothromboembolism
transient ischaemic attack cause 3948
see also atheroma; atherosclerosis; thromboembolism
athetosis 4010, 4121
see also dystonia
athletes
amenorrhoea 1671
arrhythmogenic right ventricular dysplasia 2391
bone mass in 3065
hypertrophic cardiomyopathy diagnosis 2386
polycythaemia 3554
see also endurance sports; marathon runners
athlete's foot (tinea pedis) 797, 798, 1165
athymic animals 152
atlantoaxial subluxation, in rheumatoid arthritis 2959
atmosphere
mechanical aspects 1194
physical features **1193–4**
atmospheric ozone, *see* ozone
atmospheric pollution, *see* air pollution; pollution
atmospheric pressure 1186, 1193
atmospheric temperature 1193
atomic bombs
cancer association 215
latent period for cancer development 198
thyroid cancer association 213
atopic asthma, *see* asthma, extrinsic (allergic)
atopic dermatitis, *see* atopic eczema
atopic disease 2734
genetic basis 158, 3739
minimal change nephropathy and 3154
see also allergic diseases
atopic eczema 161–2, 3709, 3712, 3716, 3718, **3739–42**
associated disorders 3741
asthma and 2736
cells involved in 161, 3740
characteristics 3741
clinical features 3741

food allergy in 1843, 3729, 3739, 3742
IgE in 157, 3739, 3740
immune system reactivity 3739–41
infections in 3740
pathogenesis 3739
in pregnancy 1805–6
prognosis and management 3742
atopic state 156
atopy 2725
nappy eruptions in 3768
in neonates 3729
overactive Th2 cells 151, 157
see also allergic diseases
atovaquone 478
ATP 1272
generation 4165
in heart 2145
by carbohydrate metabolism 2146
by fatty acid metabolism 2146
ischaemia 2151
mechanisms to maintain during ischaemia 2146–7
metabolism 2146
by pulmonary endothelium 2486
in platelets 3615
red cell production 3534
renal utilization 3330
utilization by muscle 4165
ATPase
Ca^{2+},Mg^{2+} 3455
calcium 2147
H$^+$,K$^+$, *see* proton-pump inhibitors,
peptic ulcer treatment 1887–8
see also proton-pump inhibitors
myosin 4140, 4141
Na$^+$/K$^+$ 2147, 2241, 3127
adaptation in malnutrition 1285, 1287
digitalis mechanism of action 2241
nutrient absorption 1900
in oedematous malnutrition 1288
red cell 3455
renal tubules 3128–9, 3330, 3331
Atractaspididae, bites and envenoming 1126, 1131
atracurium 3270
atresia 1975
atrial appendages, juxtaposition, in tricuspid atresia 2412
atrial arrhythmias **2271–4**
in tricuspid atresia 2413
see also atrial fibrillation; atrial flutter; atrial tachycardia; cardiac arrhythmias
atrial extrasystoles 2269, 2271, 2274
atrial fibrillation **2271–3**, *2272*
aetiology 2272, *2272*
after coronary artery bypass grafting 2355
after Fallot's tetralogy repair 2406
with atrioventricular block 2267
digitalis in 2243, 2244
in elderly **4342–3**
emboli source 3949, *3949*
in hypertrophic cardiomyopathy 2388, 2389
in hypothermia 1183
investigations,
Doppler echocardiography 2202
electrocardiogram (ECG) 2198, 2199, 2271
'lone' 2272
management 2272–3, 2455
in mitral stenosis 2453, 2455
in mixed mitral valve disease 2456
in myocardial infarction 2345
normal brief episodes 2197
paroxysmal 2272
thromboembolism prophylaxis 3670
in transposition of great arteries 2416
in tricuspid atresia 2413
ventricular rate 2272, 2273
in ventricular septal defects 2429
in Wolff-Parkinson-White syndrome 2275–6

atrial flutter 2272, **2273**
  after Fallot's tetralogy repair 2406
  electrocardiogram (ECG) 2199
atrial hypertrophy
  electrocardiogram in 2188, 2189, 2190
  see also cardiac hypertrophy
atrial natriuretic peptide (factor) (ANP) 2156, **3119–20**, 3248
  actions 2156
  in cor pulmonale 2517
  in heart failure 2234, 2240
    increase 2170
  inhibitors of breakdown 2252
  receptor 1560
  reduction, by ACE inhibitors 2248–9
  in urinary-tract obstruction 3235
atrial pacing, *see* pacing
atrial pressure 2154
  left,
    in adult respiratory distress syndrome 2574
    in hypertrophic cardiomyopathy 2386
    in mitral regurgitation 2458
    in pulmonary oedema 2566, 2567
    in pericardial tamponade 2477
  right,
    in Ebstein's anomaly 2413
    in myocardial infarction 2566, 2567, 2568
    in obstructive airways disease 2571
    in pulmonary embolism 2569–70
    in pulmonary oedema 2567
atrial septal defects **2424–6**
  abnormal right ventricle with 2415
  Doppler echocardiography 2203, 2204
  in Ebstein's anomaly 2413, 2414
  in Eisenmenger reaction (syndrome) 2411
  endocarditis in 2439
  ostium secundum defects **2424–6**, 2455
  patent foramen ovale 2426
  in pregnancy 1736, 1737
  pulmonary hypertension in 2507, 2511
  in transposition of great arteries 2417
  see also atrioventricular defects
atrial septum, myxoma 2472
atrial situs 2179
atrial tachycardia 2272, **2273–4**
  block with 2273
atrial thrombus 2500
  magnetic resonance imaging 2215
atrial tumours, liver in 2130
atrioventricular block
  aetiology 2268, 2271
  atrial fibrillation in 2267
  in atrial tachycardia 2273
  in atrioventricular nodal re-entry tachycardia 2274
  beta-blockade contraindication 2328
  bifascicular 2268, 2270
  digitalis causing 2245
  first degree 2267, 2268, 2269
  management 2268–9
  pacing in 2286
  prognosis 2269
  risk of progression 2268
  second degree Mobitz type I (Wenckebach) 2197, 2199, 2267, 2268, 2269
  second degree Mobitz type II 2267, 2268, 2269
  in seronegative arthropathies 2392
  third degree (complete) 2267, 2268, 2269
  trifascicular 2268
atrioventricular canal, common 2426, **2427–8**
atrioventricular concordance 2405, 2416, 2418
  ventricular arterial discordance 2404
atrioventricular conduction disturbances **2267–9**
  electrocardiogram (ECG) 2267–8, 2269
  escape rhythm 2267, 2268
  infranodal and intranodal 2267
  see also atrioventricular block

atrioventricular defects **2426–8**
  common atrioventricular canal 2426, **2427–8**
  common atrium 2427, **2428**
  ostium primum 2426, **2427**
atrioventricular discordance 2405, 2417–18
atrioventricular junctional extrasystoles 2270
atrioventricular junctional rhythm 2266, 2268
atrioventricular node 2152, 2259
  abnormal 2267
  accessory pathway 2193
  digitalis action 2241
  normal function 2267
atrioventricular valves
  calcification 2399
  regurgitation, corrected transposition with 2418
  see also mitral valve; tricuspid valve
atrium
  common 2427, **2428**
  myxoma 2472
  see also entries beginning atrial; left atrium (atrial); right atrium (atrial)
atrophie blanche 3791, 3793, 3794
atrophy **3790–1**
  dermal **3790–1**
  postacne 3790
  subcutaneous 3790–1
atrophy of lichen sclerosus et atrophicus 3768–9
atropine 3881
  in beta-adrenoceptor blocker overdose 1065
  in clonidine overdose 1065
  in digoxin overdose 1066
  dyspnoea treatment, in terminal illness 4355
  in nerve agent exposure therapy 1118
  in organophosphorus insecticides poisoning 1122
atropine-like actions, poisonous plants 1152, 1155
atypical pain syndromes 345
Auchmeromyia luteola 1000, 1001
audiometry **1225**, 3870
  evoked response 3836
audit, safety 1179
auditory acoustic emissions (echoes) 3871
auditory canal, caloric response 2583
auditory evoked potentials 3831, **3835–6**, 3871
  brain-stem, *see* brain-stem auditory evoked potential (BAEP)
    in coma and brain death 3836
    in demyelinating disease 3835
    measurement 3836, 3871
    in posterior fossa tumours 3836
  auditory function, tests 3870
  auditory gnathostomiasis 953
  auditory nerve 3869
    computed tomography (CT) 3818
  auditory pathways 3869
  auditory system, dysfunction
    symptoms and signs **3870–1**
    tests 3870
AUDIT system 4272, 4273
Auerbach's plexus, *see* myenteric (Auerbach's) plexus
Auer rods 3402, 3405, 3428
Augmentin, in urinary-tract infections 3209, 3211
aura 3914
  in migraine 4024
auscultation, heart, *see* heart murmurs; heart sounds
Austin Flint murmur 2443, 2465
  mitral stenosis *Vs* 2455
  right-sided 2411
Australasian snakes, bites and envenoming 1131, 1132
Australia
  indications for snake antivenom 1136
  venomous snakes 1128
Australia antigen, *see under* hepatitis B virus (HBV)

Australia X disease (Murray Valley encephalitis) **415**
autism, infantile **4108**
autistic behaviour 4108
autoantibodies **163–4**, 278
  to adhesion molecules and extracellular matrix 163
  antinuclear, *see* antinuclear antibodies
  to cell-surface receptors 163
  to circulating serum proteins 163
  in connective tissue diseases 3008, 3009, 3010
  criteria for linking with diseases 163
  to cytoplasmic antigens 163
  in diffuse parenchymal lung disease 2782
  to DNA, *see* anti-DNA antibodies
  liver-specific 2070
  neutrophil cytoplasmic, *see* antineutrophil cytoplasmic antibodies (ANCA)
  in primary sclerosing cholangitis 2078
  in rheumatic diseases 2952, 2954
  in rheumatoid arthritis 2954
  in SLE 3021, 3021, **3024–5**, 3025
  in type-1 autoimmune hepatitis 2070
  see also other specific antibodies
autoclave cleaners, vinyl chloride exposure 1090
autocrine action 95, 1564–5, 1891
autocrine stimulation 223
autoerythrocyte sensitization 3637
autograft, definition 183
autohaemolysis 3379
'autoimmune' cholangitis 2075
autoimmune diseases 155
  Addison's disease 1652–3, 1655
  in common varied immunodeficiency (CVID) 169
  diabetes type 1 as 1571
  endocrine hyperfunction 1570
  endocrine hypofunction 1570–1
  hypoglycaemia **1510**
  of liver, *see* autoimmune hepatitis; cholangitis, primary sclerosing; primary biliary cirrhosis
  male infertility 1685, 1686
  ovarian failure 1672–3
  pernicious anaemia association 3489
  polyglandular syndromes, *see* polyglandular autoimmune syndromes
  pulmonary hypertension in 2513
  skin, in pregnancy 1806
  T-cells and cellular mediators 165
  thyroid, *see* thyroid gland, autoimmune diseases
  vitiligo with 3755
  see also autoimmunity; connective tissue diseases
autoimmune hepatitis **2069–74**
  aetiology 2071–2
  autoantibodies,
    anti-LKM 2070, 2072, 2073
    antinuclear 2070
    liver-specific 2070, 2072
  'burnt-out' phase 2073
  chronic active, in pregnancy 1800
  cirrhosis in 2072, 2073
  clinical features 2070
  cryptogenic 2070, 2073
  definition 2069
  diagnosis and investigations 2069–70
  differential diagnosis 2070–1
  hepatitis C role 2072, 2092
  hepatocyte damage mechanism 2072
  histology 2069
  HLA association 2071–2
  liver failure in 2073, 2100
  liver transplantation in 2115
  natural history 2072
  prognosis, survival and cause of death 2073
  relapse after steroid withdrawal 2073
  scoring system 2069, 2071
  treatment 2072, 2072–3
  type-1 2069–70
  type-2 2070, 2073

autoimmune thrombocytopenia, *see* thrombocytopenia, autoimmune
autoimmunity 154
  in connective tissue diseases 3008, 3009
  in cryptogenic fibrosing alveolitis 2788
  dilated cardiomyopathy pathogenesis 2382
  effector mechanisms **156–65**
  prevention 152
  tolerance breakdown 155–6
    active suppression loss 155–6
    cross-reacting epitopes 155, 155
    hidden antigen release 156
    modified antigen formation 156
    superantigen-induced 156
    T-cell bypass 156
  in ulcerative colitis 1945
automatisms, in epilepsy 4238
autonephrectomy 3276
autonomic dysreflexia, in spinal cord injury 3898–9
autonomic failure
  classification 3882, 3882
  multiple system atrophy with 3882, 3885, 4006
  in Parkinson's disease 3882, **3885**
  primary **3882–6**
    clinical features 3882–3
    course 3886
    neuropathology 3885
    pathogenesis 3885–6
    postural hypotension in 3882–3, 3886
    treatment 3886
  pure autonomic failure 3882
autonomic nervous system **3881–7**
  age-related changes 4336
  anatomy and physiology **3881–2**
  cells 3882
  disorders **3882–7**
    in acute porphyria 1392, 1393
    classification 3882, 3882
    in polyneuropathy 4092
    see also autonomic failure
  efferent activity, heart 2160
  heart failure pathophysiology 2234
  in hypertension 2531
  in multiple sclerosis 3993
  neurotransmitters 3881–2
  testing **3883–5**, 3884
    clinical 3884–5
  in tetanus 626, 627
  disinhibited discharge in 624–5
    management 629
autonomic neuropathy
  in amyloidosis 1515
  diabetic 1486, 1487, **1488–9**, 3171, 3998
  distal 3882, **3886**
  'autonomic storms' 627, 629
autonomy, clinical 10
Autoplex 3651
autopsy 4310
  pathology 4309
autoregulation
  cerebral blood flow 3947, 4045
  coronary blood flow 2159, 2323
autosomes 102
autosplenectomy 3514
autozygosity mapping 106
avascular necrosis, of bone, *see* aseptic necrosis of bone
avipoxviruses, recombinant 368
axillae, denervation in hyperhidrosis treatment 3767
axillary abscess, anaerobic infections 573
axillary hyperhidrosis 3767
axillary lymph nodes, metastases from unknown primary site 252
axillary nerve **4094**
axillary vein thrombosis 2366, 2523
axonopathy 4091
  central-peripheral distal 4091
  generalized 4091
axons 4091
  conduction by 4091
  degeneration 4091

injury, diffuse, in brain damage 4044,
  4047
  interruption 4091
    symptoms 4092
  regeneration 4091
azapropazone, poisoning 1057
azaserine 2040
azathioprine
  adverse reaction 2851
  in anti-GBM disease *3166*
  in autoimmune hepatitis 2073
  in cardiac transplantation 2257
  in Crohn's disease 1942
  in cryptogenic fibrosing alveolitis
    2792–3
  drug interactions 1257
  in lupus nephritis 3190–1
  in multiple sclerosis 3996
  in myasthenia gravis 4162
  in renal failure 3274
  in renal transplant recipients 3319
  secondary immunodeficiency due to
    174
  in SLE 3024
  in systemic vasculitis 3016
  in ulcerative colitis 1949
azithromycin, in chlamydial infections
  757
azoospermia 1684, 1685, 1686, 1687
aztreonam
  in renal failure *3272*
  in urinary-tract infections *3211*
azygos vein
  chest radiography 2178
  enlargement 2181

B

B7 molecule 145, 150
  in antigen presentation in graft recipient
    184
  B7-CD28 interaction 184
B₁₂, *see* vitamin B₁₂
Babesia **863–5**
Babesia microti 864
babesiosis **863–5**
Babinski reflex 3857
babygram 3081
bacillary angiomatosis *729*, *745*, **747**
bacillary peliosis 747
Bacillus, rare species *551*, *551–2*
Bacillus anthracis **612–13**
  heat and disinfectants effect 613
  isolation and diagnosis 617
  spores and resistance of 612, 613
  toxins and mode of action 614–15
    lethal factor 614, 615
    oedema factor 614, 615
  virulence factors and genes for 614, 615
  see also anthrax
bacillus Calmette-Guérin, *see* BCG
Bacillus cereus **559–60**, 2002
  enterotoxins 559
  eye infection 4191
  food poisoning 559–60, 2002
Bacillus thuringiensis 859
back pain **2992–5**
  in acromegaly 1592, 1593
  acute, persistence **2993**
  in ankylosing spondylitis 2966
  approach to patient **2992**
  chronic **2993–4**, 2994
  in disc protrusions 3906
  dorsal spine **2994–5**
  infections and tumours causing 2993
  in infective endocarditis 2440
  ligaments causing 2992
  low, acute **2993**
  mechanical causes 2992
  pathology **2992–3**
  in pregnancy 1766–7
  in spinal tuberculosis (Pott's disease)
    653
  treatment 2993–4
  in ulcerative colitis 1948
  see also spinal pain
'back schools' 2993

bacteraemia 1030
  anaerobic 574
  Campylobacter 558
  in cirrhosis 2087, 2090
  community-acquired 527
  definition 527
  fusobacterial 574
  Haemophilus influenzae type b 582
  intravascular device-associated
    infections 330
  in neutropenia 1030
  nosocomial 331
  primary 527
  Salmonella infections 552
  Staphylococcus aureus 527
  streptococcal 510
  streptococci group A 500, 501
  streptococci groups C and G infections
    506
  Yersinia enterocolitica 609
bacteria **268–74**
  adaptive capacity 265
  adhesion 270, 272
    to endothelial cells 2438
    to urothelial cells 3206
  antibiotic sensitivity 298–300
  cariogenic 1846
  endotoxin, *see* endotoxin
  extracellular 272
  facultative intracellular 272
  food poisoning from seafood 1141–2
  Gram-negative/positive, *see* Gram-
    negative bacteria; Gram-positive
    bacteria
  growth inhibition, by antimicrobial
    therapy 303
  growth phase, importance to antibiotic
    action 304
  host factors affecting 2001
  inflammation due to 290, 290–1
  lysis by complement 175, 178
  molecular taxonomy **272–4**
  morphology/metabolism, antimicrobial
    therapy effect 303
  normal flora,
    intestinal, *see* intestinal flora
    in pregnancy 1784
    of vagina 3354, 3357
  numbers, importance in infections
    290–1
  obligate intracellular 272
  pathogenic **268–74**
    classification *271*
    colonization of host surfaces 268, 270,
      272, 2001
    determinants of pathogenicity **268–72**
    diversity **268–72**
    infection route 268
    interaction with phagocytic cells 91,
      272
    principal types 268, *269–70*
    rRNA sequencing and classification by
      273–4, *274*
    toxin production 272, 2001–2
  phylogenetic tree 273
  post-antibiotic effects 304
  sexual transmission *3345*
  species,
    clinical aspects of classification 273
    definitions 272
    molecular taxonomy **273**
  transformation 60
  see also individual species
bacterial infections **493–824**
  after cardiac transplantation 2257
  after viral respiratory infections 2693,
    2699
  in AIDS 4079
  arthritis **2998–9**
  bites associated with *404*
  concomitant in actinomycoses 681, *682*
  C-reactive protein in 1529–30
  diarrhoea in 2002
  eye in **4191**
  haematological changes **3678–9**
  haemolytic anaemia 3545, 3679
  haemolytic uraemic syndrome *vs* 3200
  in HIV infected drug abusers 4285

  in homosexuals **3362–3**
  in hypogammaglobulinaemia 168
  liver in 2133, *2133*
  meningitis, *see* meningitis
  mouth **1852–3**
  myositis in **4155**
  nosocomial 329
  in pregnancy 1784, **1785–93**
  purpura in 3636
  rare and 'newer' organisms **778–96**,
    778–90
  see also individual infections/species
bacterial overgrowth **1911–16**, 2003
  aetiology 1911–12, *1911*, 2003
  in chronic idiopathic intestinal pseudo-
    obstruction 1960
  clinical features 1914
  Clostridium perfringens 637
  coeliac disease *vs* 1919
  in common varied immunodeficiency
    1839
  diagnosis/investigation 1910, 1914–15
    scheme 1915
  hepatobiliary injury due to 1912
  pathogenesis 1912–14
  in short gut syndrome 1925, 1926
  in total parenteral nutrition 2140
  treatment 1914, 1916, 1926
bacterial vaginosis **3355**, *3356*
bactericidal effects, of antimicrobial
  therapy 303, 658
bactericidal proteins, lung defence
  mechanism 2614
bacteriocine 493
bacteriophage 61, 391
  as gene vectors 61
  typing, *see* phage typing
bacteriostatic effects, of antimicrobial
  therapy 303
bacteriostatic proteins, lung defence
  mechanism 2614
bacteriuria
  asymptomatic 3207
    in pregnancy **1733**, 1787, 3207, 3211,
      3212
    treatment 3209, *3210*, 3211
  in pregnancy **1733**, 1787
  pyuria *vs 3103*
  symptoms 3206–7
  urinary catheterization and 3212
Bacteroides fragilis 569, 570, 575
  antimicrobial therapy effect 304
  clinical features of infections 572
  diagnosis and culture 571
  septicaemia 1020
Bacteroides melaninogenicus 778, 1852
Bacteroides vulgatus 570
bagassosis 2810
Bairnsdale ulcer, *see* Buruli ulcer
bakers, contact dermatitis 3738
balanitis
  circinate 2945, 2970, 2971
  in diabetes 1453
  erosive, syphilis *vs* 711
  fixed 3768
  in Reiter's syndrome 2970, 2971
  Zoon's 3768
balanoposthitis, anaerobic infection 573
balantidiasis **880–1**
Balantidium coli 880, 881, 2003
BAL (dimercaprol) 4008
baldness 3762
  benign of forehead 3761
Balint's syndrome 3853, 3869
Balkan nephropathy 212, **3229–31**, 3296
balloon, in coronary angioplasty 2349
  'Stack' 2350
balloon angioplasty
  carotid and vertebral arteries 3824
  in coarctation of aorta 2559
  coronary, *see* percutaneous transluminal
    coronary angioplasty (PTCA)
ballooning, fitness requirements 2361
balloon tamponade, bleeding
  oesophageal varices 2094
Bamako Initiative 53
band 3 3527
  defects 3529, 3532

bandages, leg ulceration management
  3809, 3810
band keratopathy, in primary
  hyperparathyroidism 1631
Bannwarth's syndrome 689, 690
barbiturates
  addiction, mental symptoms 4241
  folate deficiency due to 3493–4
  poisoning 1060
  in unconscious patients 2586
  vitamin D metabolism and 3325
  withdrawal syndrome **4293**
    mental symptoms 4241
bare lymphocyte syndrome 172
baritosis 2847
barium enema 1832
  double-contrast 1832
    in Crohn's disease 1939
    in ulcerative colitis 1946, 1947
  in laxative abuse 1965
  in meconium ileus 1978
  'thumb printing' 1998, 1999
barium follow-through 1832, 1909
  in tropical sprue 1935
barium meal
  in coeliac disease 1919
  double-contrast 1831
  in duodenal ulcer 1878
  food combined with 1956
  in gastric cancer 1984
  in gastric ulcer 1831, 1879, 1880
  in gastro-oesophageal reflux disease
    1867
  'nutrient' 1956
  'string sign' 1975
barium studies
  in enteropathy-associated T-cell
    lymphoma 1927
  large intestine 1832
  motility disorder investigation 1956
  small intestine 1832
  upper gastrointestinal tract 1831–2
barium sulphate 1956
barium swallow
  in achalasia 1869, 1958–9
  in gastro-oesophageal reflux disease
    1867
  in oesophageal varices 1831
  in squamous-cell carcinoma of
    oesophagus 1874, 1981
baroreceptors 1600, **2156**, 2160
  age-related changes 4336
  aortic, in hypertension 2533
  in heart failure 2234
  inhibition 2234
  sensitivity reduced in hypertension
    2531, 2533
  sodium retention in heart failure and
    2169
  syncope pathophysiology 3925, 3926
  vasovagal syncope 2173
  see also carotid baroreceptors
barotrauma
  lung rupture 1206, 1207
  sinus 1202, 1203
  in ventilation in ARDS 2858
Barr body 116, 121
Barrett's oesophagus, *see* oesophagus,
  Barrett's
barrier creams, in occupational
  dermatosis 1164–5
Barthel index 4336, *4337*
Bartonella 552, 745
Bartonella bacilliformis 773, 1003,
  3545
bartonellosis **773–6**
  clinical features 774–5
  definition and aetiology 773
  epidemiology and transmission 773–4,
    1003
  pathogenesis 774
  prognosis and treatment 775–6
Bartter's syndrome **3130–1**, 3336
basal cell(s) 3706
basal cell carcinoma 208, 3791
basal cell epithelioma *3726*, 3791, 3794
basal cell naevus syndrome (Gorlin)
  3795

basal ganglia **3861–3**
  calcification **4007**
  clinical aspects 3863
  degeneration, pathology/sites *4006*
  diseases 3966
    clinical features 3863
  input to thalamus 3860
  language and 3851
  in multiple system atrophy 4006, *4006*
  in Parkinson's disease 3999, *4006*
  in progressive supranuclear palsy 4005, *4006*
  striatal neurochemistry 3862
  structure and function 3861–2
    connections 3861–2
    motor function 3862
    thalamocortical circuits 3862
basal metabolic rate (BMR) 1269, 1609
  equations for prediction 1269, *1270*
  physical activity levels 1269, *1270*
  see also metabolic rate
base
  deficit 1536
  excess 1536
  of topical agents 3805, *3805*
basement membrane 3706
  alveolar 2485, 2509
  antibodies,
    glomerular, *see* antiglomerular basement membrane (GBM) disease (Goodpasture's syndrome)
  in pemphigoid gestationis 1805
  in diabetic microangiopathy 1464
  endothelial cells 2289, 2290, 2485, 2486
  glomerular, *see* glomerular basement membrane
  muscle 4139
  pulmonary endothelium 2485, 2486, 2509
    in inflammation 2621
  in recurrent polyserositis 1525
  retinal capillary in diabetes 4189
basidiobolomycosis **803**
basophilia 3378, 3558
basophils **3555–6**
  counts *3379*
  degranulation 158, 159
  in immediate hypersensitivity 158
  production 3384, 3386, 3557
Bassen-Kornzweig disease 3986
bathing, skin disease management and 3806
Batten's disease 3985
battered baby syndrome, *see* children, abuse/neglect
batteries, mercury poisoning from 1111
Battle's sign 3835
BB Worcester rat 1453
B-cell lymphoma, *see* non-Hodgkin's lymphoma (NHL), B-cell
B-cells **148–9**, 316, 3556
  activation 146, 149, 156
    increased in SLE 3025–6
  in allergic diseases 157
  antibody-producing cells 148, 315
  antigen presenting role 143, 149, 157
  antigen recognition,
    antigen types 141
    helper T-cells for 141
  in cutaneous lymphomas 3794
  differentiation antigens 148–9, *148*
    expression sequence 149
  differentiation blocks 166, 167
  differentiation failure, in selective IgA deficiency 171
  dyscrasias, amyloidosis in 1515
  Epstein-Barr virus-mediated immortalization 3566, 3567
  Epstein-Barr virus receptors 148, 352, 858
  in gut-associated lymphoid tissue 1836, 2001
  immature 148
  immunoglobulin gene rearrangement 146
  in infection-associated glomerulonephritis 3173
  inherited metabolic disorders 168

low-affinity and autoimmunity 156
  in lymph nodes 153, 154, 3562
  lymphocyte-detected membrane antigen (LYDMA) 858
  maturation, blocks 166, 167
  memory cells 148
  ontogeny 149
  origin of lymphoma, *see* non-Hodgkin's lymphoma (NHL), B-cell
  production 3384, 3386
  in severe combined immunodeficiency disease (SCID) 172
  signalling 148–9
  surface immunoglobulin 141, 148
  tolerance 155
  see also antibodies; immunoglobulin(s)
BCG vaccination 289, **648**
  action and efficacy 648, *649*
  in developing countries 663, 664
  disseminated BCG disease after 664
  efficacy, environmental mycobacteria affecting 665
  hepatic granuloma pathogenesis 2120, 2123
  HIV infection and 480, 648, 664
  indications 646
  neonatal 320, 1746
  protection against leprosy 678
  technique 648
  tuberculous meningitis prevention 4063–4
bcl-2 gene 3567, 3569, 3580
bcr/abl gene 225, 3398, 3403, 3411, 3416
  protein product 3397
bcr gene 225
beat knee of miners 2996
Beau's lines 3760
Becker muscular dystrophy
  carriers 4146
  clinical features 4146
  genes 4145
Becker's naevus *3755*, 3756
Beckwith-Wiedemann syndrome 128, 1974
  familial and inheritance 128
beclomethasone 2718
Beconase 2718
becquerel 1218
bed bugs **1005–6**
bed nets 324
  impregnated 858, 860
bed rest
  adverse effects 1039
  in heart failure 2236, 2238
  in psoriatic arthritis 2970
  in rheumatic fever 2434
  skin disease management 3807
beer drinker's potomania 3123
bee stings 1144–5, 3772
beetles **1146**
  infestation 1001
behaviour
  aggressive, *see* aggressive behaviour
  compliance affected by 1240
  coronary-prone 2315
  DNA sequence relationship 67
  effects of noise on 1225
  in mania and manic depressive disorder 4220
  pain 3943
  regression 4204
  repetitive/rituals 4207
  type A pattern 2315
behavioural disorders/disturbances 4256, *4256*, 4258
  in adolescence 4212
  in cannabis and LSD intoxication 1075
  cerebral lobes associated *3846*
  in children, foods and food additives 1844
  in drug abusers 4295
  in elderly 4341
  electroencephalogram in 3830
  in epilepsy 4238
  in hypoglycaemia and insulinomas 4240
  in Lesch-Nyhan syndrome 1381–2
  in malnutrition 1283

organic causes 4225
  in phencyclidine poisoning 1076
  in schizophrenia 4222
  in Wilson's disease 4008
behavioural teratology **1811–12**
behavioural therapy
  hypertension management 2538–9
  in obesity 1311
  in obsessive compulsive disorder 4207
Behçet's syndrome **2973**, **3043–7**, 3773, **3778**, 4132
  aetiology 3043–4
  arthritis/arthralgia in 3045
  clinical features *2973*, 3045, 3778, *3778*
  diagnosis 3046
  diagnostic criteria 3043, *3043*, 3046
  epidemiology 3043
  gastrointestinal tract in 2000, 3045
  genital ulcers 3045
  HLA association 3043, 4183
  immunopathology 3044
  lung involvement **2799**, 2802, 3046
  neurological complications 3045, **4132–3**
  ocular features **3045**, **4182–3**
    clinical features 3045, 4183
  recurrent oral ulceration in 1855, 3045
  renal disease in 3045–6
  skin lesions in 3045
  synovitis in 2973
  thrombotic complications 3668
  treatment 3046
  vascular complications and vasculitis 3045, 3778
bejel 706
  see also syphilis, endemic
belief
  ethics and 11
  illness, chronic fatigue syndrome and 1038
'belle indifference' 4209, 4210
Bell's palsy 345, **3879**
  in pregnancy 1766
  treatment 3879
  see also facial nerve
Bence Jones protein
  amyloid formation 1515, 1518
  in myeloma 3599, 3600
bencephalitis, *see* Japanese B encephalitis
Bendectin 1810
'bends' 1209, 4128
Benedikt's syndrome 3858
benorylate, poisoning 1056
benoxaprofen 2129
benperidol, overdose/poisoning 1061
benserazide, in Parkinson's disease 4002
bentiromide test *2037*
benzathine benzylpenicillin 718
  in neurosyphilis 4086
  in rheumatic fever 505, 2435
  in syphilis 717, *717*
  see also benzylpenicillin (penicillin G)
benzene
  air pollution 1228
  leukaemia association 215, 1167
  mechanisms of toxicity 1084
  poisoning **1084**, 1172
    acute/chronic, features 1084
    treatment 1084
γ-benzene hexachloride (BHC) 1009, 1123
γ-benzene hexachloride (BHC) shampoo 1004
benzidazole (Rochagan), in Chagas' disease 898
benzoate, sodium 1360
benzodiazepines 4253
  abuse,
    in pregnancy 4299
    prevalence 4264
    psychiatric disturbances with 4241
  in alcohol withdrawal syndrome 4291
  antagonist, hepatic encephalopathy management 2108
  in anxiety disorders 4206, 4207
  in benign essential tremor 4012
  chlordiazepoxide 2084

dependence 4253
  drug interactions 1060, 4253
  drugs included 1060, 4253
  dyspnoea treatment, in terminal illness 4355
  in endoscopy 1830
  indications and use 4253
  mechanism of action 4253
  in pain treatment 3945
  in panic disorder 4207
  poisoning 1060–1
    clinical features 1045, 1060
    treatment 1060
    with tricyclic antidepressant overdose 1059
  in renal impairment 3273
  side-effects 4253
  withdrawal syndrome 1251, 4253, 4263, **4293**, 4299
    management 4293
    mental symptoms 4241
benzoic acid 1079
benzothiazine agents 2238
benzothiazine derivatives, poisoning 1057
benzoylglucuronates 1089
benzoyl peroxide 3753
benz[a]pyrene, air pollution 1228
benztropine 1061, 1067, 1070
benzyl alcohol, poisoning **1079**
benzyl benzoate 1009
benzylpenicillin (penicillin G)
  anaerobic bacteria sensitivity 575
  in anthrax 617
  in diphtheria 496
  in leptospirosis 702
  in Lyme disease 692
  in relapsing fevers 696
  in streptococcal endocarditis 510
  in streptococci group A infections 502
  in streptococci groups C and G infections 506
  in syphilis 2483
  in yaws 706
  see also benzathine benzylpenicillin
bereavement **4234–5**, **4359**
  children facing and care of **4358**
  counselling 4235, 4236
  grief, *see* grief
  help/support after 4235–6
  immediate help in hospitals after 4236
  physical symptoms after 4235
  psychological changes after 4235
  social changes after 4235
  suicide after 4235
  see also death; dying patients; terminal illness
beri beri
  cardiac 1158
  mental symptoms 4241
  neuropathy 4100
  see also thiamine, deficiency
Berloque dermatitis *3754*
Berman's disease (mucolipidosis I) 1434, **1435–6**
Bernard-Soulier syndrome *3643*, **3645**
Bernheim effect 2524
Bernoulli equation 2201, 2202
Bertiella mucronata 962
Bertiella studeri 962
berylliosis 2122, **2846**
  hypercalciuria in 3255
beryllium 2122, 2846
  contact dermatitis due to 3738
ß-adrenergic agonists (ß-sympathomimetics)
  in anxiety disorders 4206
  in asthma 2592, 2636, 2726, 2738
    concern over 2741
    severe attack 2739, *2739*
  ß₂,
    drugs included 1067
    poisoning **1067–8**
  in bronchiectasis 2762
  in chronic obstructive airways disease 2776
  in heart 2147
  in hyperkalaemia 3135

insulin secretion and 1459
partial 2255
potassium balance and 3128
in pregnancy 1745, 1757, **1811**
ß-adrenoceptors *1560*, 3882
  activation and cAMP 2253
  agonists, *see* ß-adrenergic agonists
  antagonists, *see* ß-blockers
  in atopic eczema 3739
  ß1 *2253*
  ß2 *2253*, 2328
  coronary blood flow regulation 2159
  in heart 2147, 2253
  in heart failure 2234
  subtypes and actions *2253*
ß-amyloid, *see* amyloid, ß-amyloid
ß-blockade, atopic eczema pathogenesis
    3739
ß-blockers 2263, **2328**
  actions 2328
  airway obstruction associated 2849
  in angina **2328**
    contraindications 2328
    prescribing/choice 2328, *2329*
    unstable 2330
  asthma with 2735, 2849
  ß₁-selective, in phaeochromocytomas
    2557
  cardioselective 2328
  in cirrhosis 2091
  contraindications 2345
  in coronary angioplasty 2352
  in diabetic nephropathy 3171, 3172
  in dilated cardiomyopathy 2384
  in elderly 4343
  fat solubility 2328
  gastrointestinal bleeding prevention
    2095
  hyperlipoproteinaemia induced by 1411
  in hypertension 2540, *2541*
    thiazide diuretics comparison 2539,
    2540
  in hyperthyroidism 1613, 1614
  in hypertrophic cardiomyopathy 2389
  hypoglycaemic effects 1511
  in myocardial infarction 2345
    reinfarction prevention 2347
  oesophageal varices (re)bleeding
    prevention 980, 2095
  in opiate detoxification 4292
  overdose/poisoning **1064–5**, 2328
    clinical features 1064–5
    treatment 1065
  in phaeochromocytomas 2557
  in postural hypotension in primary
    autonomic failure 3886
  potassium balance and 3128
  in pre-eclampsia 1731
  in pregnancy 1740, 1752, **1811**
  in renal impairment 3273
  in respiratory drug overdose 1068
  side-effects 2328, 2345
    rash due to 3732, 3733
  in thoracic aorta dissections 2574
  thyroid function tests and 1717
  types and properties of *2329*
  in ventricular extrasystoles 2270
  verapamil 2268
    danger 2328, 2329
  withdrawal effects 1251
ß-carotene, *see* ß-carotene (carotene)
ß-cells, pancreatic
  autoantibodies to 163
  in diabetes type I 1453
  in diabetes type II 1455
  fetal, in diabetic pregnancy 1754, 1757
  hyperplasia, causing hypoglycaemia
    1509
  insulin biosynthesis 1458–9
  insulin secretion 1459–61
  in pregnancy 1753
ß-glycoprotein I 3669
ß-lactam antibiotics, *see* antibiotics, ß-
    lactam
ß₂-microglobulin, *see* ß₂-microglobulin
ß-oxidation 83, 2146
  absent peroxisomes and Zellweger
    syndrome 84

defects 4167
  peroxisomal 1438–9
betaine 1365, 1367
betaine methyltransferase 1365, 1366
betamethasone, in pregnancy 1811
beta rhythm 3829–30
beta-sitosterolaemia 1406
beta-very low density lipoprotein (beta-
    VLDL) 1405
  receptor 1403
  in type III hyperlipidaemia 1408–9
  see also very low density lipoprotein
    (VLDL)
betaxolol 2849
'betel chewer's cancer' 201
betel chewing, oral and pharyngeal
    cancer association 201
bethanechol 1868
Betz cells 4088
bezafibrate 1472
Bezold-Jarisch reflex 2335
Bhanja virus 429
BHC (γ-benzene hexachloride (BHC))
    1004, 1009, 1123
Bhopal disaster 1100, 1115, 1233
bias
  avoidance, in clinical trials 22–4
  systematic 22
bicarbonate
  plasma 1533
    in hyperparathyroidism 1632
    in pregnancy 1744
  potassium balance and 3127–8
  renal handling 1624, *3330*, 3338
  secretion, gastric mucosa 1879
  standard 1536
  tetany induced by 1639
  therapy,
    in acidaemia in high central venous
      pressure 2565–6
    in chlorine poisoning 1097
    in chronic renal failure 3305
    in crush injury 3289
    in cystinuria 1357
    in diabetic ketoacidosis *1500*, 1502,
      1543–4
    in hyperkalaemia 3135
    in metabolic acidosis 1543–4
    in renal tubular acidosis 3340–1
    see also alkali therapy
bicipital tendinitis 2995
bicycle ergometry 2226, 2672
bifunctional protein 1438
  deficiency **1441**
biglycan 3058
biguanides **1471–2**
  adverse effects 1471, 1542
  in surgical patients 1495
bile
  cholesterol-saturated 2047, 2050
  composition 2047
  copper excretion 1416
  drug excretion 1243
  'limey' 2050
  reflux 1957
    in pancreatic cancer 2040
  secretion 2047
    in fetus 1973
bile-acid breath test 1910, 1914
  false-positive in ileal disease 1910,
    1914
bile acids 2047
  absorption 1903
    failure in short gut syndrome
      1925
  deficiency 1913
  enterohepatic circulation 1913, 2047
  in pancreatic cancer 2040
  pool 2047
  sequestrating agents 1414, *3143*
  serum,
    in benign recurrent intrahepatic
      cholestasis 2059
    in biliary disease 2046
    normal concentrations 2056
  serum unconjugated, in bacterial
    overgrowth 1914
synthesis 2047

therapy,
  gallstone dissolution 2048
  in pregnancy 1801
  see also bile salts
bile canaliculi 2045
  bilirubin excretion 2055
bile duct(s)
  bleeding into, in fasciolasis 987
  calculi,
    percutaneous transhepatic
      cholangiography 1834
    in pregnancy 1801
  carcinoma 2052
    in Caroli's syndrome 2016
    extrahepatic, epidemiology 204
    strictures in 2052
  in cystic fibrosis 2023–4, 2131
  dilatation, congenital intrahepatic, *see*
    Caroli's syndrome
  extrahepatic,
    carcinoma epidemiology 204
    obstruction and cholestasis 2059
  fibrosis, in cystic fibrosis 2749
  intrahepatic, dilatation in
    opisthorchiasis 982
  obstruction, *see* biliary tract, obstruction
  onion skin fibrosis around 2078, 2079
  plugging, in cystic fibrosis 2023, 2024,
    2131
  strictures,
    benign **2052**
    dilatation 2078
    malignant **2052–3**
  see also common bile duct
bile salts
  absorption 1903
  deconjugation 1910, 1913, 1914
  loss, in short gut syndrome 1925
  see also bile acids
bilharzia, *see* schistosomiasis
biliary atresia *1417*, **2014–15**
  extrahepatic 2014, 2015
  intrahepatic 2014, 2015
  investigations and imaging 2014–15
  liver transplantation in 2015, 2113
biliary cells, MHC antigen expression
    2074, 2078
biliary cirrhosis 2046
  in biliary atresia 2014
  in cystic fibrosis 2023, 2131
  primary, *see* primary biliary cirrhosis
  secondary 2079
  see also cirrhosis
biliary colic 2050
biliary drainage, in pancreatic carcinoma
    2044
biliary gastritis 1961–2
'biliary mud' 2050
biliary obstruction, *see* biliary tract,
    obstruction; cholestasis
biliary sludge 2027, 2033, 2079
biliary tract
  anaerobic infections 572
  anastomoses, after hilar tumour
    resection 2118
  anatomy 2045
  cancer, *see* bile duct(s), carcinoma
  complications, after liver transplantation
    2114
  computed tomography (CT) 2012
  congenital disorders **2014–17**
    see also biliary atresia; fibropolycystic
      disease
  cystic disease, cholangiocarcinoma in
    2118
  in cystic fibrosis 2749
  disease **2045–53**
    acute pancreatitis due to 2027
    clinical features 2046
    endoscopy indication 1830
    investigations 2045–7
    in pregnancy **1801**
    see also cholestasis
  embryology 2014
  haemobilia/haemorrhage 2053
  in HIV infection 2135
  infections **2051**
  normal 2046

obstruction,
  causes *2051*, 2053
  copper toxicity 1419, 1423
  in fasciolasis 987
  hyperlipoproteinaemia in 1411
  malignant strictures 2052
  in opisthorchiasis 982
  in pregnancy 1801
  see also cholestasis; jaundice
  in opisthorchiasis 982
  radiology **1833–5**
  radionuclide studies 1834
  tumours, *see* bile duct(s), carcinoma;
    cholangiocarcinoma
  ultrasonography 1833, 1834
bilirubin
  in acute cholecystitis 2049
  in biliary disease 2046
  biliary excretion 2055
    reduced 2056, 2091
  in cerebrospinal fluid 3843
  in chronic hepatocellular failure 2107
  in cirrhosis 2088
  clinical chemistry 2055
  congenital metabolic disorders 1799
  conjugation 2055
    reduced 2055
  in Dubin-Johnson syndrome 2058
  'early labelled' 2054
  excess production 2056
  in Gilbert's syndrome 2057
  hepatic uptake 2055
  levels, liver transplantation indication
    2112
  metabolism **2054–6**
  phototherapy 2058
  in physiological jaundice of newborn 2058
  in pneumococcal pneumonia 515, 2130
  in primary sclerosing cholangitis 2078
  production, in haemolytic anaemia 3526
  reduced uptake 2056
  reference range *4366*
  in RhD haemolytic disease of newborn
    3545
  source 2054
  structure 2054
  in total parenteral nutrition 2140
  transport *in utero* 2058
  transport in plasma 2054–5
  unconjugated, levels in Gilbert's
    syndrome 2057
  in urine 2056
  see also hyperbilirubinaemia; jaundice
bilirubin diglucuronide 2055
Billroth II gastrectomy, bacterial
    overgrowth aetiology 1912
Bilophila wadsworthia 552
binge drinking, *see* alcohol abuse
binge eating 1299, 4215, 4216
Binswanger's disease 3960
biochemistry **1271–8**
  age-related changes 4334, *4334*, *4335*
  carbohydrate metabolism 1274
  energy production and utilization
    1271–3
  everyday tests *4364*
  fat metabolism 1276–7
  in muscle disorders 4142
  protein metabolism 1274–6
  reference intervals **4363–76**
    children *4366–7*
  regulation of substrate metabolism
    1273–4, *1274*, *1274*
  starvation effects 1277–8
  tests, normal/abnormal results 4363
  see also metabolism
biocide sterilizing agents 2816
bioethics 10
biofeedback
  in epilepsy 3924
  in faecal incontinence 1960
  in functional bowel disease 1968
  hypertension management 2538
  pain management in drug abusers 4300
biofilms 305, 330
biological control, in malaria vector
    control 859
biological determinism 67

biological exposure index (BEI) 1163
biological monitoring, occupational
    disease 1162–3
Biomphalaria glabrata 972, 973
biopsy
    in amyloidosis 1522
    bone, *see* bone, biopsy
    bone marrow, *see* bone marrow,
        trephine biopsy
    brain, in viral infections 4069
    bronchial **2686**, 2726
    endometrial *3359*
    fine-needle aspiration, *see* fine-needle
        aspiration biopsy
    in glycogen storage diseases 1341–2
    heart 2397
    labial glands 3037, 3038
    lymph node **3562–3**, 3569
    in pancreatic carcinoma 2044
    small intestine, *see* small intestine,
        biopsy
    spinal 3828
    temporal artery 3041, 3042, *3042*,
        4183
    tumour masses 241
    *see also other specific organs/biopsy
        types*
biopterin, defects in metabolism 1363
biotechnology
    monoclonal antibodies synthesis 226,
        232
    products 66, 67
    see also monoclonal antibodies;
        recombinant DNA technology
biotin 1370
    dependent carboxylation 1373
    metabolism 1373
    therapy 1374
    in two-step strategy in immunotherapy
        260
biotinidase deficiency 1374
biparietal diameter, in maternal diabetes
    1756
bipolar affective disorder 4220, 4227
    see also affective disorders; depression/
        depressive disorders; mania
bipyridilium herbicides, poisoning 1120
Birbeck granules 2688, 2833, 3606,
    3607, 3706
bird fancier's lung 2781, 2809, 2815
    prevalence 2816
    see also extrinsic allergic alveolitis
birds, poisonous **1140–1**
birth asphyxia, cerebral palsy aetiology
    4119, 4121
'birth injury' 3916
birth marks 3715
Birt-Hogg syndrome *3795*
birthweight
    diabetes in adult life and 1455
    ischaemic heart disease risk 2312
    low, occupations associated 1173
    maternal anaemia and 3469
    maternal nutrition and 1772–3, *1774*
bismuth, nephrotoxicity *3261*
bismuth chelate, poisoning **1069**
bismuth preparations 2006
    peptic ulcer treatment 1884
bisphosphonates
    in hypercalcaemia 1638, 3228–9
    in hyperparathyroidism 1633
    in myeloma 3603
    in osteogenesis imperfecta 3082
    in osteoporosis therapy 3068
    in Paget's disease of bone 3077, 3077–8
    technetium-labelled 2949
bisulphites, poisoning 1079
bites
    anaerobic infections from 573, 574
    arthropod 1000
    bacterial infections associated *404*
    dog, *see* dog bites
    infections associated *404*
    infection spread 286
    pasteurellosis from 606
    rabies from 397
    simian herpesvirus infections 358
    snake, *see* snakes, venomous

spider 1147–9
    tick 1149
    virus infections associated *404*
    see also stings
bithionol 987
Bitot's spots 4198
Bjork-Shiley valve 2470
BK virus 443, **446–7**
    disease associated 446, 461
'Black Death' 596
blackfat tobacco smokers 2837
black-flies 912, 1011
blackheads 3752
blackouts, *see* syncope
black piedra 801
blackwater fever 844, *849*
bladder
    care, in poisoning 1047–8
    catheterization,
        in poisoning 1048
        in spinal cord injury 3899
        suprapubic 3899, 3900
        see also urinary catheterization
    compliance, in chronic obstruction
        3234
    condom drainage in spinal cord injury
        3899, 3900
    emptying, in spinal cord injury 3900
    in herpes zoster 349
    imaging 3109–10
    in multiple sclerosis 3993, 3995
    neuropathic, in spina bifida 4118
    outflow obstruction,
        acute 3234, 3235–6
        chronic 3234, 3236
        see also urinary retention
    in schistosomiasis 972, 976, 977
    sensation loss, in tumours 249
    in spinal cord injury/lesions 3892, 3899
    stones 3251
    suprapubic aspiration of urine 3101,
        3208
    tuberculosis involving 3276, 3277,
        3279
    unstable, in elderly 4338
bladder cancer
    aetiological factors 217, 1166, 1167
    epidemiology 211–12
    schistosomiasis and 211, 212, 977
    squamous cell carcinoma 977
    staging investigations *236*
Blalock-Taussig shunt 2179, 2405
    modified 2406
Blaschko's lines 123–4, 124
blast cells
    in leukaemia 3405–6, 3417
    in myelodysplastic syndromes 3426,
        3427
blast injury, diving and 1205
Blastocystis hominis **887–8**
Blastomyces dermatitidis 805, 3000
blastomycosis **805–6**
    arthritis in 3000
    chronic pulmonary 806
    disseminated 806
bleach, poisoning 1079, 1103
bleeding
    in acute meningococcaemia 538
        management 541
    in cyanotic congenital heart disease
        2401
    gastrointestinal, *see* gastrointestinal
        bleeding
    hyperfibrinolytic **3659**
    intermenstrual 3358
    intra-abdominal, in pregnancy 1741,
        1742
    in rodenticide poisoning 1123
    spontaneous,
        in cirrhosis 2087
        in cyanotic congenital heart disease
            2401
    in malaria 846
    neurological symptoms 4123
    sports-related soft-tissue trauma 4321
    viral infection transmission during sport
        4324
    see also blood loss; haemorrhage

bleeding disorders
    in amyloidosis 1515
    in aplastic anaemia 3443, 3444
    in chickenpox 347–8
    eye in **4194**
    investigations **3627–30**
    lumbar puncture hazard 3842
    in malignant disease 3678
    massive transfusion inducing 3634,
        3660–1, 3693
    in myeloma 3599, 3635
    in myeloproliferative disorders 3634–5
    in polycythaemia vera 3432, 3433
    in primary myelosclerosis 3436, 3437
    in primary thrombocythaemia 3439
    in renal disease **3656–7**, 3682
    in renal failure 3288, 3305, 3634,
        3656–7, 3682
    in von Gierke's disease 1342
    see also coagulation disorders;
        platelet(s), disorders
bleeding time *3379*, 3629–30
    in urticaria 3772
bleomycin
    adverse reaction 2851
    in Hodgkin's disease *3573*, 3574
blepharitis, follicle mites causing 1009
blepharoclonus 4001
blepharoconjunctivitis, pubic lice causing
    1004
blepharospasm 4001, **4019–20**
blinding, clinical trials 23
blind loop syndrome, *see* bacterial
    overgrowth
blindness **4197–8**
    in age-related macular degeneration
        4198
    cataracts causing 4197
    definition 4197
    in diabetes 1483, 1485, 1486
        retinopathy 4188, 4198
    glaucoma causing 4197–8
    in gnathostomiasis 952, 954
    in Hurler syndrome 1431
    in leprosy 4198
    in measles 379
    in methanol poisoning 1081
    in nephronophthisis-medullary cystic
        disease complex 3205
    in onchocerciasis 915, 916, 4198
    trachoma causing 750, 4198
    transient monocular, *see* amaurosis
        fugax
    in vitamin A deficiency 4198
    see also vision, loss
blistering disorders, *see* vesico-blistering
    diseases
blisters 3779
    cold causing 3779
    in diabetes 1489
    in epidermolysis bullosa 3720
    intraepidermal 3781
    snake bites causing 1133
    trophoneurotic 3783
    in vasculitis 3774, 3775
blood **3377–81**
    autotransfusion 3554
    compatibility tests 3689–90
    component preparations **3694–5**
    constituents 3377
    count, in coeliac disease 1918
    cross-matching 3690
    in CSF, *see* cerebrospinal fluid
    disorders, *see* haematological disorders
    faecal occult 3683
    films,
        babesiosis diagnosis 865
        malaria diagnosis 849
        stained 3377–8
    investigations **3377–81**
    leucocyte-poor 3694, *3695*
    oxygen transport 2630
    pooling in spleen 3589
    products, biotechnology products 67
    replacement **3687–700**
    stasis, thrombosis and 3663
    in urine 3102
    see also haematuria

viscosity 2302–3, **2564–5**, 3663
    acute changes **2564–5**
    in cyanotic congenital heart disease
        2400
    in leptospirosis 699
    in nephrotic syndrome 3142
    in polycythaemia 3432, 3553
    volume, *see* blood volume
    whole 3660, 3694
blood-brain barrier **3990**
    cerebral metastases and 250
    inflammatory demyelination 3990
    inflammatory injury 3990
    permeability, measurement 4052
blood chemistry
    everyday tests and reference intervals
        4364
    in malaria 850
blood cultures
    in infective endocarditis 2441–2
    in persisting septicaemia 1025
    in pyrexia of unknown origin 1030–1
    respiratory tract infections 2675
blood flow
    direction, Doppler echocardiography 2200
    laminar *vs* turbulent detection 2200
    oxygen transport 2630
    peripheral, measurement 2368
    pulmonary, *see under* pulmonary
        circulation
    velocity,
        estimation 2201
        estimation by Doppler equation 2200
blood flukes, *see* schistosomiasis
blood gas (analysis) 2669–71, 2672
    in chronic obstructive airways disease
        2775
    in cor pulmonale 2518
    in pulmonary embolism 2524
    in pulmonary hypertension 2511
    reference intervals *4365*
    in respiratory failure definition 2901
    in scoliosis 2872
    see also lung function tests
blood-gas barrier 2485, 2596–7, 2629
blood group
    antibodies 3687–8
    antigens 3687–8
    minor 185
    susceptibility to infections and 280
    systems **3688–9**
    see also ABO blood groups
blood group A
    association with disease 110
    gastric cancer association 203
blood loss
    acute, anaemia of 3458–9, 3460, 3475
    chronic, anaemia of 3460, 3476, 3483,
        3683
    leeches causing 1150
    menstrual 3375, 3476
    see also bleeding; haemorrhage
blood pressure 2527
    age relationship 2528, 2528–9
    angina investigation 2325
    antihypertensive therapy target 2542
    autonomic function testing 3884
    autonomic resetting 2531
    blood volume regulation 2157
    cardiovascular disease risk 30–1, 2308,
        2316
    cerebral blood flow changes 3947
    circadian rhythm 2160, 2528, 2545
    in coarctation of aorta 2557
    control 3116, 3117, 3118, 3883, 3884
    in diabetes *1466*
    in diabetic nephropathy 3168, **3169–70**
    dialysis survival and 2552, *2552*
    distribution curve 2527
    ethnic/population differences **2528**
    exercise effect 2226
    finger arterial, measurement 3884
    hormonal control 1563, 1600
    intraindividual variations **2528–9**
    ischaemic heart disease,
        mortality 2316
        risk 30–1, 2308, 2316
    'job strain' and 2531

measurement 2535–6
  duration and number 2538
  indirect ambulatory 2535–6
  manometer and cuffs 2535
  repeated and reasons for 2538
  technique 2535
in myocardial infarction, thrombolytic
    therapy 2341
normal fall on inspiration 2477
in obstructive sleep apnoea 2912, 2915
in pericardial tamponade 2477
in pre-eclampsia 1729
in pregnancy 1726, 1735
raised,
  in elderly **4343**
  essential hypertension, prevalence
    2527–8
  in heart failure 2500
  management 4343
reduction, ischaemic heart disease
    prevention 2317
regulation **2156**
renal function and 3247–8
response to posture 2156
in septicaemia 1024
sodium intake and 2312
stress effect 2530–1
see also diastolic blood pressure;
    hypertension; systolic blood pressure
blood-sucking flies **1010**, **1011**
blood supply
  brain **3947–8**, 3948
  colon 1996, 1997
  heart, *see* coronary blood flow
  liver 2017
  nasal cavity 2609–10
  optic nerve 3864
  spinal cord 3891
  splenic flexure 1997
blood tests, *see* haematology
blood transfusion **3687–95**
  in acute renal failure 3284, 3285, *3288*
  in adenosine deaminase (ADA)
    deficiency 172
  in anaemia 3462
  in aplastic anaemia 3445
  in autoimmune haemolytic anaemia
    3544
  autotransfusion 3554
  Babesia transmission 864
  bleeding oesophageal varices
    management 2094
  chronic hepatitis C after 2068
  compatibility tests 3689–90
  consent and 4317
  cytomegalovirus (CMV) infection 361
  dangers to travellers 322
  exchange, in malaria 854, 856
    in G6PD deficiency 3541
  in gastrointestinal bleeding 1827
  graft-versus-host disease and 3697
  group O, Rh-negative blood 3688,
    3689–90
  haemoglobin increase per litre 1827
  hazards **3690–4**
    alloimmune thrombocytopenia 3632
    anti-D alloimmunization 3689
    immune 3691–2
    infectious mononucleosis-like disorder
      3679–80
    iron overload 3480, 3692
    management 3694
    non-immune 3692–3
    transmission of infection 3693–4
  in hereditary spherocytosis 3529
  HIV transmission prevention 484
  in hookworm infection 931
  intrauterine 1782
  malaria due to 848
  massive,
    bleeding complications 3634, **3660–1**,
      3693
    complications **3693**
  multiple, liver in 2132
  in myelodysplastic syndromes 3430
  overtransfusion **2570–1**
  in paroxysmal nocturnal
    haemoglobinuria 3452

in primary myelosclerosis 3437
renal transplantation and 3316–17
in RhD haemolytic disease of newborn
    3545
in sickle-cell disease 3516
  in pregnancy 1760–1
in thalassaemia 3504, 3512
in ulcerative colitis 1948
volume in oligaemia 2565
blood vessels
  calcification, in chronic renal failure
    3324
  dilatation in skin, *see* telangiectasia
  'margination' of red cells, in malaria
    843
  role in thrombosis 3662–3
blood volume **2153–4**, *3379*, **3380**
  age-related changes 4334
  changes in haemorrhage and
    retransfusion 2565
  control 1600, 3116, 3117, 3118
  'effective', reduced in heart failure
    2169, 2170
  increase, in benign intracranial
    hypertension 4042
  lung, *see* lung; pulmonary circulation
  normal 2153
  in pregnancy 1735
  regulation **2156–7**
    atrial natriuretic factor 2156
    blood pressure/gender and age 2157
    pulmonary circulation 2157
    renin-angiotensin system 2157
    sodium retention in heart failure and
      2169, 2170
Bloom's syndrome 173, 192–3, *3447*
  leukaemia association 215
'blue bloaters' 2517, 2769
blunt trauma, acute pancreatitis due to
    2028
blushing 3785, 3787
B lymphocytes, *see* B-cells
body composition
  in malnutrition 1287, *1291*
  normal *1272*
  metabolic fuels and 1272, *1273*
body fat, *see* fat
body image disturbance, *see* body
    perception
body lice 1003, 1004
body mass, lean, decline with age 4334
body mass index (BMI) 1302, 1314
  amenorrhoea and 1671
  in diabetes *1466*
  ischaemic heart disease risk 2309
  malnutrition classification 1281–2, *1282*
  ranges 1315
  reduction, in pathophysiology of
    malnutrition 1285
  see also obesity; weight, body
body odour 3765
body packing, drugs of abuse 1074–5
  management of packers 1075
body perception
  disorders **3854**
  disturbance, in anorexia nervosa 1297,
    4213
body size
  glomerular filtration rate and 3108
  renal plasma flow and 3108
body surface area 3108
body temperature
  circadian rhythm 1015
  core temperature 1015
  C-reactive protein and 1533
  drug-induced increases **1172–82**
    see also hyperpyrexia; neuroleptic
      malignant syndrome
  heat effect on 1180
  in malnutrition *1290*
    management 1292
  measurement 1015, 1182, 1184
  normal 1015
  in pneumococcal pneumonia 515
  rectal 1015
  response in malnutrition 1286
  see also fever; hyperthermia;
    hypothermia; temperature

Boerhaave's syndrome 1873
Bohr effect 3456
Bohr equation 2600
boils 526
  blind 3766
Bolivian haemorrhagic fever 436, **438–9**,
    438
bombesin **1894**
bone 3055
  in acid-base disturbances 1540
  actinomycoses 683
  acute atrophy 3941
  age-related changes 4335
  avascular/aseptic necrosis, *see* aseptic
    necrosis of bone
  biopsy 3063
    in osteomalacia and rickets 3072
    in osteoporosis 3067
    in Paget's disease of bone 3077
  in brucellosis 620–1
  calcification front, absent in
    osteomalacia 3070
  calcium fluxes 1622, 1623, **1628–30**
  calcium and phosphorus balance
    3058–9
  cells in **3055–6**
    communication 3056
  chest radiography 2179
  collagen in **3057**, *3057*
  cortical 3055
  cysts, formation 2980
  dysplasia, short stature 1699–700
  ectopic ossification 3058, **3092–4**, *3092*
    calcification with 3093
    removal 3093
    see also ossification
  erosions 2949
    in gout 2948, 2986
  formation 1628–9, **3056**
    coupling to resorption 1629
    cytokines in 3056
    ectopic, *see* bone, ectopic ossification
    stimulation in osteoporosis 3068
  fractures, *see* fractures
  functions 3055, 3057
  hypertrophy 2981
  imaging **2948–50**
  infarction, in sickle-cell disease 3515
  lesions, in Wilson's disease 1421
  loading 2981
  loss 3056
    accelerated 3066
    age-related *3066*, **3068**
    causes 3066, *3066*
    prevention 3068
    see also bone, mass; bone, mineral
      density
  in McCune-Albright syndrome 3091
  in malnutrition 1284
  mass **3057**
    age-related changes 3065
    determinants 3065
    hormones affecting 3065, 3069
    measurement 1629–30, **3065–6**
    peak 3065
    reduced in osteoporosis 3064, **3065**,
      3069
    see also bone, mineral density;
      osteoporosis
  mechanical stress effect 2981
  metabolism 3059
    in acromegaly 1593
    in immobilization 1550
  metastases,
    bone scans 2950
    hypercalcaemia 1637
    in lung cancer 2883
    myeloma *vs* 3600
    pain, *see* bone pain
    presentation and primary tumour 252
    staging methods 246
  mineral density 3065, 3066
    in amenorrhoea 1671
    fracture relationship 3065
    measurement 2950, 3065, 3066, 3067
    in osteoporosis 3067
    reduced in osteogenesis imperfecta 3079
    see also bone, mass

mineralization 1628–9, **3058**
  defect in osteomalacia 3070
  modelling 3056
  non-collagen proteins in **3057–8**
  in osteoarthritis 2980
  pain, *see* bone pain
  parathyroid hormone actions 1624,
    3057, 3059
  physiology **3055–60**
    calcium and phosphorus balance
      3058–60
    see also calcium; *specific hormones
      affecting*
  radiography in rheumatic disease
    2948–9
  'rain-drop' appearance 3067, 3069
  remodelling 1629, 3056
  resorption 1623, 1629, 3056, **3057**
    antiresorptive agents 3068
    in rheumatoid arthritis 2962
    in sarcoidosis 2827
    scintigraphy, *see* bone scans
  solitary plasmacytoma of **3604–5**
  structure **3055**
  subperiosteal erosion 3324
  syphilis 713, 714
  tenderness, in acute leukaemia 3376–7
  theoretical fracture threshold 3065
  trabecular (cancellous) 3055
  tuberculosis 653
  turnover 3056
    biochemical measures **3060**
    in chronic renal failure 3323
    excessive in Paget's disease 3075,
      3076, 3077
    measurement 1629–30
    primary hyperparathyroidism 1630–1
    vitamin D actions 1626, 3059
  in yaws 704–5
bone disease *3064*
  adynamic (low-turnover), in chronic
    renal failure 3323
  aluminium poisoning **3096**
  clinical features 3061
  diagnosis **3060–4**, 3063
    by age and symptoms *3064*
  in elderly **4344**
  fibrous dysplasia **3091–2**
  in fluorosis **3095**
  in haemoglobinopathies **3095**
  history-taking 3060
  investigations,
    biochemical 3061–3, *3062*
    biopsy, *see* bone, biopsy
    miscellaneous 3063
    radiology 3063
  in Langerhans-cell histiocytosis 3607,
    3609
  in lead poisoning **3095–6**
  metabolic, parenteral nutrition
    complication 1321
  miscellaneous **3094–6**
  in parenteral nutrition **3095**
  in primary hyperparathyroidism 1631
  renal, *see* renal bone disease
  sclerosing disorders **3089**
  in thyroid disease 3069
  in vitamin A poisoning **3095**
  in vitamin D poisoning **3095**
  *see also individual diseases (page
    3060)*; skeletal dysplasias
bone infections
  anaerobic 573
  staphylococcal 528–9
bone marrow
  abnormal localization of immature
    precursors (ALIP) 3426, 3429
  in anaemia of chronic disorders 3483
  anatomy 3382–3
  aplasia, *see* aplastic anaemia
  aspiration biopsy,
    in aplastic anaemia 3443
    in leukaemia 3405, 3412, 3417
    in myelodysplastic syndromes 3426,
      3427
    visceral leishmaniasis diagnosis 905
  assessment of activity/distribution 3381
  in chronic lymphocytic leukaemia 3420

bone marrow (cont.)
circulation 3383, 3385
culture, in myelodysplastic syndromes 3429
depression, sulphur mustard causing 1117
dysfunction in Schwachmann's syndrome 2039
examination 3377, **3381**
failure **3441–9**
affecting single cell lines **3448–9**
anaemia in 3459, 3483
chemotherapy-induced 3575
classification *3442*
proliferative **3447–8**
radiation-induced 3574
fibrosis, see myelosclerosis
haemopoiesis 3381, 3383–5
in Hodgkin's disease 3572
in hypereosinophilic syndrome 3612
hyperplasia 3521, 3525
in iron overload 3480
in primary myelosclerosis 3435, 3436
hypoplasia,
in hypoplastic myelodysplasia 3447
in paroxysmal nocturnal haemoglobinuria 3451
see also aplastic anaemia
in Langerhans-cell histiocytosis 3607
macrophage in 86
in malaria 844
in megaloblastic anaemia 3494
myeloid/erythroid (M/E) ratio 3381
in myelomatosis 3597, 3598
myelopoiesis 3556–7
in primary myelosclerosis 3435, 3436
in purpura 3630
red 3382
response to infections 3524
trephine biopsy,
in aplastic anaemia 3443
in leukaemia 3400, 3405, 3412, 3417
in myelodysplastic syndromes 3426
bone marrow transplantation 3385, **3696–700**
in acute leukaemia 3409, 3414, 3696–7
in acute myelosclerosis 3438
in adrenoleukodystrophy 1441
allogeneic 3696
in aplastic anaemia 3443, **3445**, 3696
artificial nutritional support 1323
autologous 3696, **3700**
in myeloma 3602
in chronic myeloid leukaemia 3417, 3418–19, 3698, 3699
clinical techniques 3696–7
complications 3697–9
C-reactive protein 1532
donors 3699–700, 3700
in Fanconi anaemia 3447
fever and pulmonary infiltrates in 1033
in inborn errors of metabolism 1336, *1337*
indications 3699–700
infections after 1029, 1030
respiratory tract 2709–10
in inherited leucocyte disorders 3561
long-term effects 3699
in myelodysplastic syndromes 3431
in myeloma 3601–2
in paroxysmal nocturnal haemoglobinuria 3452
in severe combined immunodeficiency disease (SCID) 173
syngeneic 3696
in thalassaemia 3513
bone modelling units (BMUs) 3056
bone morphogenetic proteins (BMPs) 3055
bone pain 240–1, **3061**
in chronic renal failure 3323
management 3077
in myelomatosis 3599
in Paget's disease of bone 3075, 3077
in rickets and osteomalacia 3071
in tumours, palliative radiotherapy 257
bone scans 2949, 2950
in bone metastases 2950

in Hodgkin's disease 3573
in osteoporosis 3067
in Paget's disease of bone 3077
spinal 3826
bone tumours
aetiological factors 207–8, 1166
epidemiology 207–8
see also bone, metastases
Bordetella **587–90**
Bordetella bronchiseptica 587
culture 588
features/treatment of infection 588, 589
Bordetella parapertussis 587
clinical features of infection 588
culture 588
Bordetella pertussis 587
culture and diagnosis 588
transmission 588
treatment of infections 589
see also pertussis
Borg scale, breathlessness scale 2646, *2647*
Bornholm disease (epidemic myalgia) 386, **387**, 4155
pain in 2648
Borrelia
infections **692–7**
Treponema comparison 707, *707*
Borrelia burgdorferi 689, 690, 3002, 4101
characteristics 690, 691
see also Lyme disease (borreliosis)
Borrelia duttoni 692, 693
Borrelia hermsii 693, 694
Borrelia recurrentis 692
Borrelia vincentii, see Treponema vincentii
Boston exanthem 384
bot fly 1000, 1001
botulinum toxin 630, 631
in blepharospasm 4020
in spasmodic torticollis 4018
botulism **630–2**
antitoxin 632
eye in 4191
fish and molluscs causing 630, 1142
history/examination/diagnosis 631–2
infant 631, 632
mortality 632
occurrence and aetiology 630–1
outbreaks 630
pathogenesis 631
treatment 632
wound 632
see also Clostridium botulinum
Bouchard's nodes 2985
Bourneville's disease, see tuberous sclerosis
Boutonneuse fever 729, **734**
boutonnière deformity 2957
bovine spongiform encephalopathy (BSE) 1517, 3977, **3981**
Bowditch effect 2150, 2157, 2158
bowel
decontamination, in aplastic anaemia 3445
preparation, in colorectal carcinoma surgery 1993
see also colon; intestine
bowel habit
changes,
in diverticular disease 1970
in irritable bowel syndrome 1966
in colorectal cancer 1991
normal 1964
Bowen's disease *3726, 3791*
boxing, brain damage after 4049
brachial artery, pressure, ankle pressure ratio 2368
brachial plexus **4093–4**
avulsion pain 3945
damage, radiotherapy causing 4135
injuries 3834, 4093
lesions, in malignancies 4093–4, **4135**
neuralgic amyotrophy 4094
post-irradiation neuropathy 4094

in thoracic outlet compression 2366
thoracic outlet syndromes 4093
traction lesions 4093
tumour infiltration and pain 241
brachydactyly, in pseudohypoparathyroidism 1634
Brachyspira aalborgi 3365
brachytherapy 255–6
endobronchial 2684
bracken fern 218, 1159
bradyarrhythmias, see bradycardia
bradycardia **2266–7**
aetiology and mechanism 2259–60
after cardiac arrest 2284
definition 2266
during sleep 2199
electrocardiogram (ECG) 2199
management 2262
in myocardial infarction 2335
in obstructive sleep apnoea 2912
pacing in 2285
palpitations with 2175
presentation 2285–6
relative, in typhoid 562
sinus 2266
causes *2267*
in tetanus 629
bradycardia/tachycardia syndrome 2266, 2268
bradykinesia 4001
bradykinin 2298, 2492, 3621
in pulmonary endothelium 2486
snake venom activation 1130
brain
abscess, see cerebral abscess; intracranial abscess
biopsy, in viral infections 4069
blood supply **3947–8**, 3948
see also cerebral blood flow
contusion 2585, 4044, 4047
in cysticercosis 965, *965*
developmental abnormality *4106*, **4115–16**
in schizophrenia 4222
development and malformations *4106*
glucose requirement 4123
inflammation and 3990
lymphoma 3583
magnetic stimulation, see magnetic brain stimulation
in malaria, see malaria, cerebral
metastases, see cerebral metastases
oxygen requirement 4123
regions, behavioural defects associated *3846*
swelling,
after head injury 3835
benign intracranial hypertension and 4042
see also cerebral oedema
tumours, see intracranial tumours
brain damage
after boxing 4049
assessment 4046
in cerebral anoxia 4123
hypoglycaemia causing 1498, 1506
ischaemia after 4044–5
persistent vegetative state after 3935
prenatal, cerebral palsy in 4119
primary traumatic 4044
secondary 4044–5
traumatic 4044–5, *4044*
see also head injury
brain death 14, 2256, **3317**, **3933–6**
action after diagnosis 3934–5
auditory evoked potentials in 3836
causes and frequency 3933
criteria for diagnosis and guidelines 3934, 4311
somatosensory evoked potentials in 3835
brain diseases, diffuse, multifocal dementia in 3998, *3999*
brain-gut axis 1963
brain natriuretic peptide (BNP) 2234
brain scanning **3825**
in dementia 3969
in intracranial tumours 4037

brain-stem
brain death, see brain death
compression, coma in *3931*
deficits, in intracranial tumours 4035
distortion, in intracranial tumours 4034
failure and death 3933
features in multiple sclerosis 3993
function assessment 3934
motor responses 2584–5
in unconscious patients 2582–5
herniation 3931, 4034
infarction 3834, 3956
lesions,
compression *3932*
pain in 3942
metabolic depression 2583
normal MRI 3821
pain mechanism 3937
in poliomyelitis 385
respiration control 3887
tumours, somatosensory evoked potentials (SEP) 3834
brain-stem auditory evoked potential (BAEP) 3835, 3871
in acoustic schwannomas 3874
applications 3835
normal 3871
brain-stem death, see brain death
bran 1329, 1964, 1970, 3805
in constipation 1826
branched-chain amino acids 1275
after injury/surgery 1550
in hepatic encephalopathy 2102
metabolism 1368–9
defects **1368–72**
supplements 1550
branched-chain ketoaciduria (BCKA) 1369
branched-chain α-keto dehydrogenase (BCKD) 1369
branching enzyme (amylo (1,4-1,6)transglucosidase) 1340
deficiency (Andersen's disease; glycogen storage disease IV) *1343*, 1344
Branhamella catarrhalis 552
'brass foundryman's ague' 1114
breach of duty, definition 4311
breast **1687–9**
abscess, anaerobic infections 574
benign disease, oral contraceptives in 1723
biopsy, in pregnancy 1807
development in pregnancy 1576
breast cancer
aetiological factors 209, 218
age relationship 197
brachial plexus lesions 4135
carcinomatous 'meningitis' in 250
epidemiology 209
genetic basis 242
hormone replacement therapy and 1814–15
hypercalcaemia 1637
magnetic resonance imaging 238
male 1687
oral contraceptives and 216, 1724
outcome, growth factor receptor overexpression and 224
in pregnancy **1807**
surgery and radiotherapy 248
tamoxifen in 27–8
breast feeding 38
anticoagulation and 1743
antituberculous drugs and 660
atopic eczema and 3739, 3742
in cystic fibrosis 1746
cytotoxic drug therapy and 1807
in diabetes mellitus 1758
drug abuse management and 4299
drug prescribing **1811**, *1812*
in epilepsy 1768–9
in HIV infection 1782
HTLV-1 transmission 1783
prolactin and 1576
protection from respiratory viruses 333
in thyroid disease 1749

breast milk 3742
  adverse reactions to drugs in 1255
  atopic eczema prevention 3739, 3742
  protection against necrotizing
      enterocolitis 1995
  protection from infection 278
  rabies transmission 398
  see also lactation
breast milk jaundice 2058
breath, bad (halitosis) **1864**, 1964
breathalyser 4272, 4287
breath-holding 3888, 3919
breathing 2611
  apneustic 3890
  assessment tests 2669
  bronchial 2650
  central disorders **3888–91**
    see also respiratory disease/disorders;
        respiratory failure
  cessation in sleep apnoea 2909
  Cheyne-Stokes, see Cheyne-Stokes
      breathing
  cluster 3890
  in coma 3931
  control 2645, 2908
  disordered, in acute mountain sickness
      1188
  increased work, in ARDS 2856
  neural mechanisms controlling **3887–8**
    automatic/behavioural interaction
        3888
    automatic (chemosensitive) system
        3887
    behavioural 3887–8
    peripheral system 3888
  noisy, in upper airways obstruction
      2719
  normal sounds 2650
  pattern 2647, 2649
  periodic 2583, 2916
  pharyngeal muscles and 2909
  rapid 2645
  rhythm disorders **3889–90**
    see also hyperventilation;
        hypoventilation
  in sleep (normal), see under sleep
  sleep-related disorders **2906–18**
    see also under sleep
  spinal cord injury complications 3898
    see also respiration
breathlessness (dyspnoea) **2162–5**, 2642,
    2644–8
  in acute mountain sickness 1188
  acute at rest 2162
  in anaemia 3458
  in aortic regurgitation 2465
  in aortic stenosis 2462
  in aortic stenosis with incompetence
      2464
  in carcinoid syndrome 1897
  cardiac **2162–5**
    pathophysiology 2163–4
    respiratory symptoms with 2162
    treatment 2164–5
  causes 2162, *2163*
  in chronic obstructive airways disease
      2773
    acute increase **2777**
  in chronic respiratory failure 2929
  in cirrhosis 2087
  clinical analysis **2645–7**
    occurrence 2646–7
    quality 2646
    severity 2646, *2646*
    timing/rate of onset 2646, *2646*
  in cryptogenic fibrosing alveolitis
      2789
  definition 2162, 4354
  diagnosis 4354
  in diaphragmatic disorders 2877, 2878
  in diffuse parenchymal lung disease
      2780
  diseases associated *2646*
  in Ebstein's anomaly 2414
  in Eisenmenger reaction (syndrome)
      2410
  exercise 2494, 2647, 2672

  exertional 2162, 2163, *2163*, 2164
    in eosinophilic granuloma of lung
        2833
    in systemic sclerosis 3029
  in extrinsic allergic alveolitis 2809
  in Fallot's tetralogy 2402
  in heart failure 2232
  in hypertrophic cardiomyopathy 2386,
      2389
  investigations **2647–8**
  in lung cancer 2883
  management 2648
    in HIV-infected patients 472
    in hypertrophic cardiomyopathy 2389
    in terminal illness 4354–5
  in mitral stenosis 2452
  in mixed mitral valve disease 2456
  pathophysiology **2645**
  in pleural effusion 2863
    malignant 251
  in pneumothorax 2869
  postexertional 2647
  in pregnancy 1744
  psychogenic 2646, 2647
  in pulmonary atresia with ventricular
      septal defect 2408
  in pulmonary embolism 2523
  in pulmonary hypertension 2510
  in pulmonary oedema 2501, 2566
  in pulmonary valve stenosis 2419
  respiration control mechanisms and
      3888
  in rheumatic diseases 2945
  in systemic sclerosis 3029
  in terminal illness **4354–5**
  triggers 2647
  use of term 2644–5
    see also dyspnoea
breath sounds 2650
  in pneumothorax 2869
breath tests 1914, 1957
  14C-aminopyrine 2056
  bile-acid 1910, 1914
  hydrogen 1910, 1913, 1922, 1957
  in systemic sclerosis 1999
  xylose 1914
bretylium 2263
Brevibacterium, rare species *552*
Brill-Zinsser disease (recrudescent
    typhus) *729*, **737**
B ring, see Schatski ring
British Anti-Lewisite (BAL), see
    dimercaprol
British Hypertension Society 2538, 2539
British National Formulary 4289, 4290
British Paediatric Surveillance Unit 287
British Smoke (BS) 1229
British Society of Gastroenterology 1830
brittle bone syndrome, see osteogenesis
    imperfecta
Broca's aphasia 3850, 3851
Broca's area 3847
bromide, skin eruption 3731
bromocriptine
  in acromegaly 1594
  in Cushing's syndrome 1641
  in neuroleptic malignant syndrome 1182
  in Parkinson's disease 4003
  in pregnancy 1748
  in prolactinoma 1590, 1591, 1672
  sexual problem management 4246
  side-effects 1590
bromomethane, see methyl bromide
bromsulphthalein clearance 2056, 2057,
    2059
bronchi
  dilatation, see bronchiectasis
  normal chest radiograph 2656, 2657
  obstruction, lung abscess in 2704
  stenosis, in sarcoidosis 2825
    see also airways
bronchial adenoma 2892
bronchial arteries 2494
  in lung/heart-lung transplantation 2935
bronchial arteriography **2655–6**
bronchial biopsy **2686**
  activation 2726

bronchial capillaries 2494
bronchial carcinoid 2892
bronchial carcinoma, see lung cancer
bronchial circulation 2181, **2494–5**
  function 2494–5
  pulmonary circulation anastomosis
      2494
bronchial epithelium
  in asthma 2726
  cilia 2613
  damage, in bronchiectasis 2756
bronchial hyper-responsiveness **2725–6**,
    2730–1
  non-specific 2725
    see also asthma
bronchial infections **2692–3**
  acute, asthma and 2693
  in chronic obstructive airways disease
      2773
    see also bronchitis
bronchial provocation tests, in extrinsic
    asthma 161
bronchial tumours
  carcinoma *in situ* 2685
  small undifferentiated carcinoma 2685
  sputum examination in 2685
    see also lung cancer
bronchiectasis **2755–66**
  in α₁-antitrypsin deficiency 1547
  acute exacerbation 2760, 2762
    antibiotics in 2763–4
  animal model 2757
  asthma with 2762
  atelectatic 2756
  clinical features **2757–61**
    haemoptysis 2644
  complications **2760–1**
  destructive lung disease vicious circle
      2762–3
    antiproteinase therapy 2766
    neutrophil role 2763
  follicular 2756, 2797
  incidence 2755
  investigations **2758–60**, *2758*
    chest radiography **2665**, *2758*, 2759
    computed tomography 2665
  management 2520, **2761–6**
    alternative therapies 2765–6
    antibiotics 2763–5
    drugs 2762–6
    flow chart 2765
    physiotherapy 2761–2
    surgery 2761
  pathogenesis **2756–7**
    conditions associated 2757, *2757*
    infections associated 2756, 2757,
        2762, 2762–3
  pathology **2756**
  persistent infections and 2762
  in pregnancy 1745
  prognosis **2766**
  recurrent 2762
  respiratory tract infections 2756–7,
      2762–3
    antibiotic therapy 2763–5
    organisms 2763
    prophylaxis 2764–5
  saccular 2756
  sputum in 2757, 2764
  in ulcerative colitis 1948
  vaccination in 2765
bronchioles 2597
  in chronic obstructive airways disease
      2769
bronchiolitis
  chronic 2632, 2634
    gas exchange 2634–5
    mechanical properties of lung 2634
    ozone causing 1229
    pathophysiology **2634–5**
    pulmonary circulation 2634
    use of term 2632
  infantile 335
  necrotizing 336
  respiratory syncytial virus causing 340
bronchiolitis obliterans *2787*, **2795–6**
  after lung transplantation **2937**

  classification *2937*
  constrictive 2795
  open-lung biopsy 2688–9
  with organizing pneumonia (BOOP)
      2795–6, 2795, 2850
  in rheumatoid arthritis 2796, 2797,
      2961
  in systemic lupus erythematosus 2799
bronchioloalveolar carcinoma 2882
  sputum examination in 2685
bronchioloalveolar lavage, see
    bronchoalveolar lavage
bronchitis
  acute **2692**
    aetiological agents 2692
    Chlamydia pneumoniae 754
  chronic 2632, 2634, 2766
    acute exacerbations **2692–3**
    chest radiography in 2664
    circulatory failure in 2571
    definition 2767
    Haemophilus influenzae 583
    Mycoplasma pneumoniae in 767
    in pregnancy 1745
    smoking and 2767
    sputum in 2685
    stroke volume 2572
      see also chronic obstructive airways
          disease
  chronic asthmatic 2767
  follicular 2797
  in hypogammaglobulinaemia 168
  laryngotracheal 2691
  melioidosis 591
  retching in 1964
  rhinovirus infections 335
bronchoalveolar fluid, aspiration, in
    pulmonary oedema 2503
bronchoalveolar lavage **2680**, 2783–4
  in amiodarone-induced alveolar reaction
      2851, 2852
  in cryptogenic fibrosing alveolitis 2685,
      2788, 2791
  differential cell counts 2685
  in diffuse parenchymal lung disease
      2783–4, *2784*
  examination **2685**
  in extrinsic allergic alveolitis 2811,
      2814
  fever and pulmonary infiltrates in
      immunocompromised 1032–3
  in immunosuppressed 2711–12
  normal cellular contents *2680*
  in pulmonary alveolar proteinosis
      2834
  in rheumatoid arthritis 2797
  in sarcoidosis 2830
  in systemic sclerosis 3033
bronchoconstriction 2610
  in heart failure 2232
  mediators causing 2727, *2728*
bronchocutaneous fistulae, ventilation in
    2924
bronchodilatation 2610
bronchodilators
  in asthma 2636, 2729, 2738
    severe attack 2739, *2739*
  in chronic obstructive airways disease
      2776
  in cor pulmonale 2520
  in dyspnoea, in terminal illness 4355
bronchogenic carcinoma 2881
  staging 2885, *2885*
    see also lung cancer
bronchogenic cysts 2899–900
bronchograms
  in bronchiectasis 2758, 2759
  bronchoscopic 2681
bronchomalacia 2861
bronchopleural fistula 2705
  ventilation in 2924
bronchopneumonia, tuberculous 651
bronchopulmonary anastomosis 2494
bronchopulmonary dysplasia **2778**
bronchopulmonary fistula, in hydatid
    disease 957
bronchoscopes 2579, 2580

bronchoscopy **2579–80, 2678–81**
  biopsy techniques 2680–1
  see also bronchoalveolar lavage;
    transbronchial biopsy
  bronchograms 2681
  in children 2682
  clinical applications **2682–4**
  diagnosis by 2679–80
  in elderly 2682
  fever and pulmonary infiltrates in
    immunocompromised 1032–3
  fibreoptic 2579, 2678–9
    biopsy 2686
    in laryngeal tumours 2722
    in pneumonia 2697–8
    procedure 2679
    in sarcoidosis 2828
  in haemoptysis 2579
  indications 2678, *2679*
  in lung cancer 2886–7
  in lung collapse/consolidation 2579
  normal appearance 2679
  in pneumococcal infections 519
  in pneumonia 2697–8
  rigid 2679
    in laryngeal tumours 2722
  specimens, microbiological testing 2675
  techniques 2678–9
  therapeutic **2684**
  tracheal stenosis/compression 2723
bronchospasm
  in asthma 2725–6
    mediators causing 2727, *2728*
  in carcinoid syndrome 1897
brown fat 1182
Brownian ratchet model 69
Brown-Séquard syndrome 3892, 3898
Brown's syndrome 2961
'brown tumours' of hyperparathyroidism
  1631
Brown-Vialetto-van Laere syndrome 4089
Brucella abortus 622, 2121
Brucella melitensis 619, 622
brucellosis **619–23**
  antibodies 622
  clinical features/complications 620–2,
    620
  diagnosis 622–3
  epidemiology and transmission 619
  liver in 622, 2133
    granulomas 2121
  pathogenesis 619–20
  treatment and prevention 623
  vaccine 623
Bruce protocol, exercise testing 2226,
  2226
Brudzinski's neck sign 4053
Brugia malayi 911, 919, 2806
  infections 920
Brugia timori 911, 919
  infections 920
bruising 3375, 3630
  in Cushing's syndrome 1643, 3636
  easy, in cirrhosis 2087
  simple easy 3636
  thrombocytopenic purpura causing 3775
  see also purpura
bruits
  abdominal, *see* abdominal bruit
  carotid 2367
  neck (cervical) 3951, 3952, *3952*, 3964
brush-border, enzymes, in bacterial
  overgrowth 1914
brush cell 2593
Bruton's agammaglobulinaemia, *see* X-
  linked agammaglobulinaemia
bryostatin 259
bubo 596, 760, 761
  treatment 598
buccal formulation 1238
buccopharyngeal membrane 1972
Budd-Chiari syndrome 2092, 2093,
  2098–9
  in antiphospholipid syndrome 3020
  causes 2098
    drugs 2129
  disease associations 2098, *2099*
  liver transplantation in 2113

in paroxysmal nocturnal
  haemoglobinuria 3450, 3452
in pregnancy 1800–1
presentation and diagnosis 2098
budesonide 2718
Buerger's disease 1994
  clinical features 2364
  smoking as risk factor 2363
bufotalin 1140
builders, contact dermatitis 3738
building-related illness 1231–2
building-related sickness 1231, 1231–2
bulbar palsy, hereditary 4089
bulboventricular foramen 2412
bulimia nervosa **1299–301**, 1669,
  4215–17
  aetiology 1300, 4216–17
  anorexia nervosa *vs* 1299, 4216
  assessment 1300, 4217
  Bartter's syndrome *vs* 3131
  clinical features 1299–300, 4216
    physical features 1300
  course and outcome 1301, 4217
  definition 1299, 4215–16
  diagnosis 1299
  distribution and incidence 1299, 4216
  hypokalaemia in 3130
  investigations/abnormalities 1300, 4216
  pregnancy and childrearing 1301, 4217
  treatment 1300, 4217
    cognitive behaviour therapy 1300,
      4217, 4255
    'stepped-care' approach 1300, 4217
bulking agents 1826
bullae *3713*, 3779
bull-neck 495
bull-neck diphtheria 374, 495, 496
bullous diseases
  in porphyria 1394, 1395
  in pregnancy 1806
  see also vesico-blistering diseases
bullous ichthyosiform erythroderma
  3719
bullous lesions
  in chronic renal failure 3302
  mouth **1855–8**
'bull's horn deformity' 2957
bumetanide 2239
Bumina bodies 4088
bundle branch, left 2267
bundle branch block
  atrioventricular block and 2267–8
  in Chagas' disease 897
  electrocardiogram (ECG) in 2188–9,
    2190, 2191
  left 2188–9, 2190, 2267
  in myocardial infarction 2338
  right 2188, 2511
  supraventricular tachycardia 2270
α-bungarotoxin 1129, 4161
Bunyamwera virus **423**
Bunyaviridae **423–9**
  distribution and infections 423, *425*
  prevention of infections 423
  viruses/genera included 423, *424*
Bunyaviruses **423–5**, *424*, 429
buprenorphine *4353*
  in opioid overdose 1058
Burkholderia, rare species *552–3*
Burkholderia (Pseudomonas) mallei 593
Burkholderia (Pseudomonas)
  pseudomallei 590, 2121
  culture 590, 591
  virulence 591–2
Burkitt's lymphoma 354–5, **3580–1**
  'African' (endemic) 354–5, 858, 3580
  'American' 354, 3580
  chromosomal abnormalities 149, 3567,
    3580
  clinical features/course 354
  epidemiology 354
    incidence rate by country 199
  Epstein-Barr virus association 214, 858
  in HIV infections 355
  leukaemia and 3402
  malaria and 214, 354, 841, **858**
  non-endemic 354, 3580
  treatment and pathogenesis 355

burns
  artificial nutritional support 1317,
    1322–3
  electrical 1211, 1214
    exposure times and temperature 1212
    treatment 1214
  haemolytic anaemia of 3550
  hydrogen fluoride (hydrofluoric acid)
    1099
  infection susceptibility/types 281, 1027
  in lightning injury 1215
  metabolic response 1550
  positive-pressure ventilation in 2577
  secondary infection in 174–5
  Staphylococcus aureus infections 525
  streptococcal infections 500, 502
  sulphur dioxide exposure 1102
  thermoregulation after 1549
  vesico-blistering diseases in 3779
burr-holes 4039, 4083
burrowing asps, bites and envenoming
  1131
bursitis, occupational cause 1168
burst-forming unit-erythroid (BFU-E)
  3387, 3452–3
'burst-promoting activity' 3387, 3453
Burulin 679
Buruli ulcer 665, 666, **679–80**
  see also Mycobacterium ulcerans
buspirone 4253
busulphan
  adverse reaction 2851
  in chronic myeloid leukaemia 3417
  leukaemia association 215
  in polycythaemia vera 3434
  in primary myelosclerosis 3437
  in primary thrombocythaemia 3440
butane, poisoning 1083
button-hole (boutonnière) deformity 2957
butyric acid 1467
butyrophenones
  neuroleptic malignant syndrome 1182
  overdose/poisoning 1061
B virus 357, 358
  transmission 358, 359
  see also simian herpesviruses, human
    infections
Bwamba virus 429
byssinosis 2647, **2746**

C

C1 esterase inhibitor 177, 3626
  deficiency 162, 180, 2721, 3708, 3772
  see also hereditary angio-oedema
C3, *see* complement, C3
C3 nephritic factor (C3Nef) 177, 180,
  3157
C4b binding protein (C4BP) 179, 3623,
  3624
C5a, *see* complement, C5a
C8 binding protein (C8BP) 3450
CA 19-9 2043
Cabot rings 3494
cachectin, *see* tumour necrosis factor
cachexia
  cardiac **2176–7**, 2233, 2234
  diabetic 1487, 3172
  metabolic basis 241
cachexia syndrome 241
cadherins, in heart 2143
cadmium 1106
  fume exposure 2848
  poisoning **1106–7**, 1171
    acute/chronic 1106–7
    bone disease in **3096**
    clinical features 1106–7
    surveillance and treatment 1107
    renal damage 3255, *3261*, **3262**
caecum
  acute dilatation 2138
  carcinoma 1991
  embryology 1973
  ulcers 2138
caeruloplasmin 1416
  copper binding 1108
  in nephrotic syndrome 3144

serum 1421, 1422
  in Wilson's disease 1419, 1421, 2022,
    4008
Caesarian section 4072
  in diabetes 1757
  in genital herpes 1781
  prophylactic antibiotics 1785, 1787
café-au-lait spots *3755*, 3986
'café coronary' 2721
caffeine
  analgesic nephropathy and 3221, *3222*
  pre-exercise 4325
CAGE questionnaire 17–20, 4272
Cajal, interstitial cells of 1953
Calabar swellings 917, 918, 953
calcaneal bursa, inflammation 2996
calciferol, *see* vitamin D₂
calcification
  cardiac 2182
  cartilage 2988, 2989 dystrophic 3092
  ectopic 3092, *3092*
    with bone formation **3092–3**, 3093
    without bone formation **3092**
  in hyperphosphataemia 3092
  hypocalcaemia and 3092
  in inherited hypophosphataemia 3092
  intra-/sub-cutaneous, in systemic
    sclerosis 3029
  metastatic 3092
  soft tissue 3092
    in chronic renal failure *3323*, 3324
    in hypoparathyroidism 1633
    idiopathic 3092
    in primary hyperparathyroidism 1631
calcific periarthritis, acute 2991
calcifidiol (25-hydroxyvitamin D; 25-
  OHD) 1625, 1626, 3059
  in chronic renal failure 3325
  malabsorption 1636
  reduced availability 1636
calcinosis circumscripta 3092
calcipotriol, in psoriasis 3748
calcitonin 1559, 1563, **1624–5**, 3059
  actions 1623, 1625, 1629
  antibodies 3077
  calcium regulation 3059
  disorders of secretion **1637**
  ectopic secretion 1716
  gene, alternate splicing 1559
  gene-related peptide/protein 1559, 1894
  in medullary thyroid carcinoma 1621,
    1625, **1637**
  salmon 3077
  treatment 1638, 3229, 3329, 3603
    in osteoporosis 3068
    in Paget's disease 3077
calcitriol (1,25-dihydroxyvitamin D₃;
  1,25-(OH)₂D₃) 1624, 1625
  in acromegaly 1593
  actions 1626, 1629, 3060
  calcium regulation 1622, 1627, 3059,
    3227
  in chronic renal failure 1636, 3325,
    3328, *3329*
  in cystinosis 1356
  excess 3095
  hypercalcaemia of malignancy and
    1568
  in hypoparathyroidism 1633
  increased production 1635–6, 1712
  in osteomalacia 3070
  plasma 1626
  in pregnancy 1745
  receptor, *see* vitamin D, receptor
  reduced availability 1636–7
  in sarcoidosis 1716, 2829, 3186
  synthesis 3059, 3060
  treatment 1635
calcium **1622–39**
  absorption 1623, 1627, 1903
    intestinal 3059, 3060
  administration, in primary biliary
    cirrhosis 2076
  balance 1563, **1623–30**, **3058–9**
    paracetamol metabolite reaction 1051
  in bone mineralization 3058
  calcium-stimulated release in heart 2145
  cancer protection 219

in coagulation cascade 3620
deficiency 1331
dependence of actin-binding proteins 81
in dialysis fluid 3326, 3328
dietary intake,
  in artificial nutritional support 1318, *1318*
  in chronic renal failure 3327, 3328
  osteoporosis 1328
  in urinary stone disease 3256
disorders **1622–38**
  myopathy in **4168–9**
  in sarcoidosis 2829
distribution 1623
exchange, in heart 2148
fluxes 3058–9
function 1622
in heart 2147, 2148, 2259
  cardiac glycosides effect 2150
  class IV antiarrhythmics action 2263
  contraction 2145
  contraction regulation **2148**
  influx 2151, 2259
  myocardial cell binding 2144
  sources 2147
hypertension pathogenesis 2530
imbalance, mental symptoms 4240
intestinal secretion 1623, 1627
intracellular 1561, 1622
  digitalis increasing 2241, 2243
  in platelet activation 3617, **3618**
low levels, in acute pancreatitis 2029
malabsorption 1627
metabolism,
  in acromegaly 1593
  in chronic renal failure 3326–7, 3328
in neutrophil chemotaxis 2622
plasma 1622–3
  in bone disease *3062*, 3063
  'corrected' 1623, 3061
  integrated responses 1630
  ionized fraction 1622–3
  major regulating hormones 1624–7
  normal levels 3058, 3061
  in pregnancy 1752
  in primary hyperparathyroidism 1632
  total 1622, 1623, 3061
  see also hypercalcaemia;
    hypocalcaemia
regulation 1563, **1623–30**, **3058–60**
  hormones involved 1624–7, 3058–9
  sites 1627–30
renal handling 1623, **3227–8**, *3330*,
    3335
  control 1624, 1627–8, 3227–8
  disorders of **3335–6**
  factors affecting *3257*, *3335*
  in hyperparathyroidism 1627, 1628,
    1630
  see also hypercalciuria; hypocalciuria
in soft tissues 1622, 1623
supplements,
  in hypoparathyroidism 1635
  in postmenopausal osteoporosis
    3068
  in pre-eclampsia prevention 1730
in sweat 1623
urinary 3063
urinary stones containing 3251, 3252,
    3256
see also hypercalcaemia; hypocalcaemia
calcium antagonists 2150, 2263,
  2328–30
in angina **2328–30**
in cirrhosis 2091
contraindications 2329
drugs included 1065
in heart failure 2248
in hypertension 2541, *2541*
in hypertrophic cardiomyopathy 2389
indications 2329
mechanism of action 1065, 1247, 2150,
    2329
in muscular dystrophies 4148
in myocardial infarction 2345, 2347
overdose/poisoning **1065**
  clinical features 1065
  treatment 1065

in primary pulmonary hypertension
    2512
in renal impairment 3274
septicaemia treatment 1026
side-effects 2329
types and properties of 2329, 2330,
    2330
in unstable angina 2330
in vibration-induced white finger 1227
calcium carbonate 3328
calcium channel 2145, 2328–9
  antibodies 4163
  blockers, *see* calcium antagonists
  L-type 2147
  voltage-gated 2329
    loss in Lambert-Eaton myasthenic
      syndrome 4163
    in small-cell lung cancer 4163
calcium EDTA 1248, 4008
calcium gluconate
  in hydrogen fluoride poisoning 1099
  in hyperkalaemia 3135, *3286*
  in hypocalcaemia 1635, 3693
  in hypoparathyroidism 1635 calcium-
    magnesium pump (Ca²⁺,Mg²⁺-
    ATPase) 3455
calcium oxalate
  crystals 1446, 2991, 3105
  nephrocalcinosis 1445, 1446
  stones 1445, 3253, 3256
    epidemiology 3251, *3252*
    in gout 1379
    pathophysiology 3251, 3252
    in primary hyperoxaluria I 1446–7
calcium phosphate, deposition 2990,
    2991
calcium pyrophosphate dihydrate crystals
    2950, 2951, 2988, 2989
  deposition 2988, 2989
  see also pyrophosphate arthropathy
calcium sensitizers 2150
calcium sodium edetate (EDTA) 1248,
    4008
calicivirus 390, 391, *391*, **392**
California encephalitis virus **424–5**
callus 3708
  hyperplastic, in osteogenesis imperfecta
    3081
calmodulin 1561
  oedema factor of *Bacillus anthracis* 615
  platelet 3618
calmodulin-dependent kinases 1561
caloric test 3873–4, 3934
  abnormalities 3874
  responses 2583
calories
  in anorexia nervosa treatment 1298,
    4215
  requirements in catabolic states *2587*
  see also energy
calpain 3619, 3633
Calymmatobacterium granulomatis 776,
    777, 2005
  infections in homosexuals 3363
camel injury 1125
camouflage 3757, 3786
cAMP, *see* cyclic AMP
CAMPATH-1H monoclonal antibody
    3424
Campbell de Morgan spots 1430
camptothecin, analogue 259
Campylobacter
  antibiotic resistance 558
  characteristics 557
  enterotoxin 558
  rare species *553*
Campylobacter coli 557
Campylobacter fetus 2004
Campylobacter infections **557–9**
  bacteraemia 558
  clinical features 558
  complications/misleading presentations
    558
  epidemiology 557–8
  in homosexuals 3363
  laboratory diagnosis 558 pathology
    558
  prevention and control 559

thrombotic thrombocytopenic purpura
    3197
treatment, antimicrobials 558–9
Campylobacter jejuni 557, 558, 2003
  Guillain-Barré syndrome and 4101
  infections, in hypogammaglobulinaemia
    169, 1838–9
  management of infections 2006
Camurati-Engelmann disease
    (Engelmann's disease) **3089**
Canada, indications for snake antivenom
    1136
Canada-Cronkhite syndrome 3723
Canadian Cardiovascular Society *2358*
canaliculitis, actinomycetes causing 685
canal paresis 3874
canarypox recombinant virus 381
Canavan's disease 3986
cancer 191, **240–53**
  adjustment reaction in 4358
  biological characteristics 197–8
  causative factors, *see under*
    epidemiology of cancer
  cell multiplication, *see* cell
    multiplication
  clinical features **240–2**
    tumour mass 241
    see also hypercalcaemia; pain; weight
      loss; *other specific symptoms/signs*
  curative or palliative therapy 4349–50
  definition 222
  development, importance of growth
    factors 222–3
  early detection by screening 463
  epidemiology, *see* epidemiology of
    cancer
  'field' theory 191–2
    evidence against 192
  gene mutations and 107
  in general practice 49, **240**
  genetic susceptibility 65, 66
  genetic syndromes 65, 66, **242**, *245*
  heterozygosity loss leading to 65
  information for patients 252
  initiation 198, 219
  investigation and staging **242–7**
    common diagnostic problems 242, 245
    histopathology 242–5
    see also imaging; tumour(s); staging
  latent period 198
  management, *see* cancer therapy
  multistage process of development 198,
    219
  occupational, *see* occupational cancer
  paraneoplastic syndromes, *see*
    paraneoplastic syndromes
  preventability, *see* epidemiology of
    cancer
  promoting agents 198, 219
  psychological treatment affecting 4232–3
  psychosocial factors affecting course of
    4232
  registries 42, 198
    artefacts/inadequacies 199, 200
  research, goals 222 size of problem 240
  'somatic mutation' theory 191–2
    evidence 192
  specific management problems **249–52**
    carcinomatous 'meningitis' 250–1
    cerebral metastasis 250
    pericardial effusion 251
    pleural effusion 251
    spinal cord and cauda equina
      compression 249–50
  spread, leptomeningeal 250
  supportive care in **252–3**
    continuity in management 253
    pain relief 253
    psychological 252–3
  terminal patients 4349
  transformation mechanisms 65–6
  treatment inducing, genetic
    predisposition 242
  unknown primary site, metastases of
    251–2, *252*
    investigations 252
    presentation 252
    treatment 252

see also carcinoma; malignant disease;
    neoplasia; transformation of cells;
    tumour(s)
cancer therapy
  chemotherapy, *see* chemotherapy
  new approaches **258–61**
    chemotherapy advances 259
    drug resistance modulation 259
    gene therapy 260–1
    molecular targets 260
    new drug targets 259–61
    patient selection 259
    prognostic factors and tumour markers
      258–9
    see also under chemotherapy
  principles of 240, **247–9**, *247*
    chemotherapy *247*, 248–9
    multidisciplinary teams 247
    rules for 240
    surgery 247–8
    types of tumours *247*
    see also chemotherapy
  radiotherapy in **253–8**
    see also radiotherapy
  stages 4349–50
cancrum oris (noma) 1853
Candida albicans 800, 807, 1793
  eye infection 4192
  gastrointestinal infection 2005
  septicaemia 1023
  vaginal infection 3356
candidaemia 807
Candida glabrata 1793
candidiasis
  acute, atrophic 1851
    pseudomembranous (thrush) 1851
  arthritis in 3000
  chronic 801
    atrophic 1851
    hepatosplenic 1035
    hyperplastic 1851
    localized mucocutaneous 1852
    mucocutaneous gastrointestinal disease
      in *1840*
  congenital 1793
  deep focal 807–8
  in diabetes 1490, 1493
  disseminated 807
    diagnosis and treatment 807
  in neonates 1793
  endocarditis 808, 2438
  fatigue in 1036
  genital tract 800, **3355–6**, 3768
  intertrigo in 800–1
  in malnutrition 1295
  in neonates 1793
  oral (thrush) 474, 800, 1850, **1851–2**
    aetiology and pathology 1851
    in AIDS 474, 479, *480*, 488, 801,
      1850, 1851
    clinical features and types 1851–2
    differential diagnosis 1852
    in immunocompromised 1034
    treatment 479, *480*, 1852
  in pregnancy 1793, 1804
  superficial **800–1**
    predisposing factors *800*
    treatment 801
  systemic **807–8**
    predisposing factors *807*
  urinary tract 808
  vaginal (thrush) 800, **3355–6**, *3356*,
    3768
    treatment *3356*
candidosis, *see* candidiasis
cane-cutter's disease 2996
cannabis 1075
  adverse effects 4242
  clinical features of intoxication
    1075
  confusion complication 4295
  endocrine problems 4284
  intravenous injection 1075
  psychiatric disturbances from 4242
  treatment of intoxication 1075
cannibalism 3977, 3980, 3982
canthariasis 1001
Capillaria hepatica 939

Capillaria philippinensis 939, 1930
capillariasis **939–40**, 1930
capillaritis, in Wegener's granulomatosis 3012
capillary length, maximum oxygen consumption and 2605, *2605*
lymphatic 2559
microscopy 3029
oxidative metabolism limited by 2604–5, *2605*
permeability,
  idiopathic oedema and 3127
  in leptospirosis 699
  in malignant pleural effusion 251
  pressures 2560
    in diabetes 1464
pulmonary, *see* pulmonary capillaries
sclerosis, in analgesic nephropathy 3221
in sepsis 293
Caplan's syndrome 2797, 2840, 2960
Capnocytophaga, rare species 553
Capnocytophaga canimorsus 1028
capreomycin, in tuberculosis 655
caprine arthritis encephalitis virus (CAEV) 3002
capsaicin 3938
  topical, in pain treatment 3944
captopril
  in aldosteronism 1659
  challenge test 2549
    nuclear renal imaging 3113–14
  in cystinuria 1357
  in elderly 4343
  in myocardial infarction 2344
  renography 2549
caput ulnae syndrome 2957
carbamate anticholinesterase compounds 1118
carbamate insecticides **1123**
carbamazepine 4251
  in alcohol withdrawal syndrome 4291
  dosage and monitoring 4251
  drug interactions 4251
  in epilepsy 3921, 3922
  indications and use 4251
  overdose/poisoning 1061
  pharmacology and mechanism 4251
  side-effects 4251
  teratogenicity *1810*
  in trigeminal neuralgia 3878
carbamyl phosphate synthetase 1353
  deficiency (CPSD) 1358–60
carbenoxolone sodium 1661, 1717–18, 3131, 3336
  limitations 1886
  in peptic ulcers 1886
carbicarb 1544
carbidopa, in Parkinson's disease 4002
carbimazole 1612–13, 1614
  in pregnancy 1749
carbocysteine, in cystic fibrosis 2753
carbohydrate
  α-1,6 and α-1,4 links 1920
  absorption *1901*, 1902–3, 1921
    impairment in tropical sprue 1934
    tests 1906–7
  bacterial overgrowth pathogenesis 1913
  'craving' 1300, 4216
  dietary,
    diabetes mellitus and 1327, 1465–6, 1467–8, 1469, 1478–9
    ischaemic heart disease risk 2311
    recommendations 1330
    reference values 1270, *1271*, 1330, *1330*
  diet high in, endurance sports and 4325
  digestion 1920–1, 1921
  fermentation 1913
  metabolism **1274**
    in acid-base disturbances 1539
    after injury/surgery 1549
    in chronic renal failure 3302
    defects in lichen planus 3751
    in diabetes 1456–7
    disorders, liver in *2019*, 2024
    endurance sports **4325–6**
    energy supply for heart 2146

inherited disorders **1336–52**
  in pregnancy 1752–3, 1771
  requirements 1330, 2588
  'salvage' from colon 1913
carbohydrate antigens 141
  changes in tumours 231
carbohydrate intolerance syndromes **1921**, *1922*
  treatment 1923
  see also lactose intolerance; sucrase-isomaltase
carbon dioxide 1094
  in altitude acclimatization 1186
  arterial partial pressure (*PaCO₂*) 1533, 2631
    abnormalities 2671
    in alveolar filling syndromes 2639
    alveolar ventilation equation 1195
    assessment 2669, *2670*
    in chronic bronchiolitis 2634
    in diffuse interstitial fibrosis of lung 2636
    in emphysema 2633
    in hypercapnia 2904
    measurement 1535–6, 2671
    normal 2901
    in pneumothorax 2869
    in respiratory failure 2901
  dissociation curve 2902, 2904, 3456
  elimination 1534
  end-tidal, measurement 2904
  global emissions 36
  oxygen dissociation curve and 2902, 2904, 3456
  poisoning **1094**
  production and alveolar ventilation 2904
  production rate, in heart failure 2232
  radioactive, in bile-acid breath tests 1910, 1914
  respiratory acidosis 2904
carbon dioxide laser therapy 3369
carbon disulphide 1077
  cardiovascular disease due to 1170
  neuropathy 4100
  poisoning **1094–5**
carbonic anhydrase 2486
  hereditary deficiency 3330, 3339
  inhibitors 3228
carbonic anhydrase II 3090
  absence 3056
  deficiency **3090–1**
carbon monoxide 1095, 3520
  air pollution 1230
  bilirubin metabolism 2054
  binding to haemoglobin 2602–3
  corrected uptake (*KCO*), in anti-GBM disease 3165
  haemoglobin affinity 1095
  peripheral arterial disease 2363
  poisoning **1095–6**, 1172
    clinical features 1095–6, *1096*
    coma 2585
    from heating systems 1095
    mechanisms of toxicity 1095
    mental symptoms 1095–6, 4240
    mortality 1043, 1044, 1095
    treatment 1096
    sources 1095, 1230
carbon monoxide transfer factor (diffusing capacity) 2669, *2670*
  in chronic obstructive airways disease 2775
  in Goodpasture's syndrome 2803
  reduction in injecting drug abusers 4282
carbon tetrachloride
  mechanisms of toxicity 1084
  poisoning **1084–5**, 1093, 1171
carboplatin, side-effects 248
carboxyhaemoglobin
  carbon monoxide exposure 1095
  levels of 1095
  in methylene chloride (dichloromethane) poisoning 1087, 1172
  smoking and peripheral arterial disease 2363
carboxyhaemoglobinaemia 1095, 3519, **3520**
  polycythaemia and 3554

carboxylase deficiencies, multiple 1374
γ-carboxylated glutamic acid residues (Gla protein) 3057–8
carboxypeptidase *N* 2486
carbuncle
  renal 3207
  staphylococcal 529
carcinoembryonic antigen (CEA) **229–30**
  in colorectal cancer 1992
  discovery and occurrence 229–30
  in immunoglobulin gene superfamily 230 limitations to value in tumour diagnosis 230
carcinogenesis
  drug-induced *216*, 1254
  'field' theory 191–2
  mechanisms 221
  radiation causing 1220
carcinogenicity
  mutagenicity correlation 193
  mycotoxins 1158
carcinogens
  benzene 1084
  chemical 1166–7, *1167*
    bladder cancer association 212, 1166
    non-melanoma skin cancer 209, 1167
    occupational 1166–7, *1167*
    see also occupational cancer
  dietary 218
  in food 203
  screening tests 193, 220–1
    animals *vs* man 221
  vinyl chloride 1090, 1091, 1167
carcinoid
  mucinous, pancreatic 2042
  open-lung biopsy 2687
carcinoid crisis, management 1898
carcinoid syndrome **1896–9**
  biochemistry 1898
  clinical features 1897, 2469
  facial flushing in 3787
  investigations 1898
  sclerosis in *3791*
  treatment 1898
  tricuspid regurgitation in 2468
  tumours associated 1896–7
carcinoid tumours **1896–9**
  ACTH-secreting 1712, 1713
  appendix 2011
  biochemistry and mediators 1898
  bronchial 1897
  clinical features 1897–8, 2892
  colon 1993
  duodenal 1707
  gastric, symptoms 1897
  gastrointestinal 1896, 1985
  heart disease **2469**
  hepatic metastases 1897, 1898, 2119
  localization 1898
  lung **2892**
  in MEN 1 syndrome 1708
  prognosis 1899
  sites 1896
  small intestine 1985
  treatment 1898, 2892
carcinoma
  cerebral metastases 4134
  non-metastatic neurological complications 4134–5
  see also cancer; malignant disease
carcinomatosis, disseminated, haemolytic anaemia in 3548, 3677
carcinomatous 'meningitis' 250–1
'card agglutination test for trypanosomiasis' (CATT) 891
cardiac arrest **2283–5**
  asystole in 2269
  causes *2283*
  death confirmation 4309
  definition 2283
  fixed dilated pupils after 2582–3
  in hyperkalaemia 3132
  management 2283–5
    after resuscitation 2284
    bicarbonate therapy 1544
    life support and resuscitation 2283–4
  prognosis 2284–5

recurrence risk 2285
signs 2283
ventricular fibrillation causing 2283
see also cardiopulmonary arrest
cardiac arrhythmias **2259–85**
  aetiology and mechanisms 2149, **2259–61**
    automaticity 2149, 2260
    re-entry 2260–1
    triggered activity 2260
  after coronary artery bypass grafting 2355
  after Fallot's tetralogy repair 2406
  after immersion hypothermia 1183
  in aircraft crew and pilots 1200
  artefactual 2197, 2198
  asystole **2269**
  atrial, *see* atrial arrhythmias
  atrioventricular conduction **2267–9**
    see also atrioventricular block
  automaticity 2149, 2260
  bradycardia, *see* bradycardia
  cardiac syncope due to 3926
  chemicals causing 1170
  in cholera 579
  in diabetes mellitus 1489
  in drug abusers 4295
  in drug overdose/poisoning,
    antiarrhythmic drugs 1063
    antihistamines 1062
    ß₂-agonists 1067
    chloral hydrate and dichloralphenazone poisoning 1061
    digitalis 2243, 2244, 2245
    digoxin 1066
    tricyclic antidepressants 1059
  ectopic beats, *see* cardiac arrhythmias, extrasystoles
  in electrical injury 1212
  electrophysiology 2149, **2259–61**
    extrasystoles (ectopic/premature beats) 2149, 2158, 2175, *2176*, 2261, **2269–70**
    atrial 2269, 2271, 2274
    atrial with aberrant conduction 2269, 2271
    atrioventricular junctional 2270
    blocked atrial 2269, 2271
    junctional (nodal) 2198
    ventricular, *see* ventricular extrasystoles
  fusion and capture beats 2279
  in hepatocellular failure 2103
  in hereditary haemochromatosis 3479
  in hypertrophic cardiomyopathy 2387–8, 2389
    management 2389
  in hypokalaemia 3129, 3130
  impulse formation disorders 2259–60
  in infective endocarditis 2442
  investigations **2261**
  management **2261–6**
    drugs, *see* antiarrhythmic drugs
    non-pharmacological **2263–6**
    objectives 2261–2
  mechanisms 2149
  in myocardial infarction 2321, 2345–6
  in myocarditis 2381
  pacemakers required for 2285, 2286
  paroxysmal, in elderly **4342**
  in poisoning 1047
  precipitating factors 2261
  in pregnancy 1738, *1742*
  re-entry, *see* tachycardia, re-entry
  symptoms **2261**
  tachycardia, *see* tachycardia
  in tricuspid atresia 2412
Cardiac Arrhythmia Suppression Trial (CAST) 2237, 2270
cardiac beri-beri 1158
cardiac cachexia **2176–7**, 2233, 2234
cardiac catheterization **2220–5**
  in aortic regurgitation 2466–7
  in aortic stenosis 2463
  in cardiac myxoma 2474
  in cor pulmonale 2518–19, *2519*
  in dilated cardiomyopathy 2383

filling pressure measurement 2220–1
in hypertrophic cardiomyopathy 2388
in mitral regurgitation 2459
in mitral stenosis 2454
in pericardial constriction 2480
in pregnancy 1736
in pulmonary hypertension 2511
  primary 2512
in tricuspid stenosis 2468
in unstable angina 2330
ventricular function indices 2221–5
  see also cardiac haemodynamics
cardiac disease, see cardiovascular
  disease; heart disease
cardiac drugs
in renal impairment 3270, 3305
see also cardiovascular drugs
cardiac electrophysiology, see heart,
  electrophysiology
cardiac failure, see heart failure
cardiac function, see heart, function
cardiac glycosides 1154, 2150
in heart failure 2241–6
mechanism of action 1248
see also digitalis
cardiac haemodynamics 2220, 2246
in angina 2166, 2323
catecholamines and 2253–4
in cor pulmonale 2518–19
Fallot's tetralogy 2403
normal values 2154, 2223
in pericardial constriction 2478–9, 2480
in pulmonary embolism 2524
vasodilatation 2246
see also cardiac catheterization
cardiac hypertrophy 2149, 2220
myocardial cell growth 2147–8
pathogenesis 2148
'reactive' 2147
in Wilson's disease 1420
see also atrial hypertrophy; under left
  ventricle; under right ventricle;
  ventricular hypertrophy
cardiac impulse 2259
cardiac index 2154
cardiac massage, external 2283
cardiac myxoma 2472–4
clinical features 2473
investigations 2473–4
liver in 2130
multiple in Carney's syndrome
  (complex) 2472
pathology 2472–3
treatment and prognosis 2474
cardiac neurosis (Da Costa's syndrome)
  2169, 2174, 4207
cardiac output 2154, 2220, 2221–3, 2605
in acute pancreatitis 2029
in adult respiratory distress syndrome
  2640
in altitude acclimatization 1187
in anaemia 3458
in cold conditions/hypothermia 1183
divers 1206
in exercise 2161
in heart failure 2230
in hepatocellular failure 2103
'heterometric' regulation 2150
'homeometric' regulation 2150
in hypertension 2531
hypoxaemia assessment 2670–1 low,
  after coronary artery bypass grafting
  2355
in pericardial tamponade 2477
positive-pressure ventilation 2576
maximal, endurance sports training
  4325
measurement 2221–3
in myocardial infarction 2566, 2568–9
in pregnancy 1726, 1735
reduction,
  in malnutrition 1285
  in pulmonary oedema management
  2567
in rheumatic mitral stenosis 2452
in septicaemia 1022, 1024, 2573
in shock 292, 293
variables altering 2220, 2246
weaning from ventilators 2580

cardiac pacemakers, see pacemakers
cardiac pain 2160
cardiac power output 2230
cardiac reserve 2161
cardiac surgery
bleeding complications 3659–60
diaphragmatic paralysis 2877
dyspnoea management 2164
positive-pressure ventilation in 2577
in postoperative pericardial disease
  2481
in pregnancy 1738–9
cardiac syncope 2285, 3918, 3926
  see also Stokes-Adams attacks
cardiac tamponade 2476, 2477–8, 2570,
  2574
delayed 2476
diagnosis 2570
treatment 2478, 2570
cardiac transplantation 2255–8
contraindications 2256, 2256
coronary artery disease after 2258
in dilated cardiomyopathy 2255, 2384
donor 2256
HLA matching 2256
immune response in 2256–7
immunosuppression and rejection
  2256–7
indications 2255–6, 2255
infections after 2257
long-term complications 2257–8
lymphoproliferative disease after 2258
number of patients 2255
  donor number 2256
patient selection 2255–6
perioperative/operative management
  2256
prognosis and prognostic markers
  2256
results 2258
cardiac valves, see heart valves
Cardiobacterium hominis 553
cardiogenic shock, in myocardial
  infarction 2321
cardiolipin 707
antibodies, see anticardiolipin
  antibodies
tests 714, 716
cardiomyopathy
acromegalic 1593
in amyloidosis 1515
arrhythmogenic right ventricular
  dysplasia 2391
congestive,
  aortic stenosis vs 2464
  cobalt ingestion causing 1108
definition 2381–2
diabetic 1492
dilated 2381–4
  in AIDS 2395
  cardiac transplantation indication
    2255, 2384
  diagnosis 2382–3
  investigations 2383
  magnetic resonance imaging 2216
  natural history and prognosis 2384
  pathogenesis 2382
  sudden death in 2384
hypertrophic 2384–90
  angina investigation 2325
  aortic stenosis vs 2463
  'apical' 2388
  clinical features 2386–7
  definition 2384
  diagnosis 2384, 2386
  genetics and myosin mutation 2144,
    2385
  infective endocarditis in 2389, 2439
  investigations 2387–8
  magnetic resonance imaging 2216
  management 2389–90
  mitral regurgitation in 2459
  mitral valve in 2384, 2386, 2388,
    2459
  myocardial ischaemia in 2386, 2386
  natural history 2388
  pathology 2384
  pathophysiology 2384, 2385–6
  in pregnancy 1738

prognosis and mortality 2388–9
sudden death prevention 2389–90,
  2390
papillary muscle dysfunction 2459
peripartum 1738, 2383
in pregnancy 1738
radiation-induced 3574
restrictive 2390–1
  see also endomyocardial fibrosis
    (EMF); hypereosinophilic syndrome
uraemic 3301
cardiophrenic angle 2178
cardiopulmonary arrest
in electrical injury 1212
in lightning injury 1214
  see also cardiac arrest
cardiopulmonary bypass
bleeding complications 3634, 3659–60
coronary artery bypass grafting 2355,
  2356
organ damage due to 2356
in pregnancy 1738–9
cardiopulmonary resuscitation 2284
need for and inappropriate 3933
cardiorenal syndrome 2235
cardiorespiratory depression, in tricyclic
  antidepressant poisoning 1059
cardiorespiratory symptoms, in rheumatic
  diseases 2945
cardiospasm 1958
  see also achalasia
cardiothoracic ratio, measurement 2179
cardiotoxicity
antiarrhythmic drug overdose 1063,
  1064, 1065, 1066
chloroquine overdose 1072
digoxin overdose 1066
quinine overdose 1073
tricyclic antidepressant-induced 1059,
  4248
cardiovascular disease
in acromegaly 1592–3
advice for high altitudes 1192, 1193
aircraft crews/pilots 1200–1
aircraft travel and 1202, 2411
blood pressure and 30–1
carbon disulphide exposure and 1095
in chronic renal failure 3301
congenital, with congenital heart
  disease 2399, 2420
dialysed patients 3312
in elderly 4341–4
hormone replacement therapy and
  1814
liver in 2130
in obstructive sleep apnoea 2914–15
occupational 1169–71
  risk factors and personality types 1170
oral contraceptives and 1724
in polycystic kidney disease 3203
polycythaemia in 3554
in post-menopausal women 1813
prevention, aspirin therapy 27
psychological problems after 4244
in renal transplant recipients 3313–14,
  3321–2
risk, in diabetic nephropathy 3168
sexual problems in 4244
  see also coronary artery disease; heart
    disease; ischaemic heart disease
cardiovascular drugs
liver damage 2130
poisoning 1062–7
  see also cardiac drugs
cardiovascular function
age-related changes 4334–5
assessment 2177–228
  see also heart, function
cardiovascular reflexes 3884, 3884
cardiovascular risk syndrome, chronic,
  see syndrome X
cardiovascular system
in acute pancreatitis 2029
age-related changes 4334–5
in anaemia 3458
in brucellosis 621
control 3883
in diphtheria 495, 496
in drug abuse and misuse 4295

in haemolytic uraemic syndrome 3198
in hepatocellular failure 2103, 2110
hormones and 1554
in hypertension 2533–4, 2535
in Kawasaki disease 3047–8
in Lyme disease 690
in malnutrition 1290
poisonous plants effect 1152, 1154
in pregnancy 1726, 1735–6
in rabies 400
in respiratory disease 2652
riot control agents affecting 1119
in sarcoidosis 2827
in SLE 3020
spinal cord injury 3898–9
in tetanus 627, 629
cardioversion
in atrial fibrillation 2272
external 2263, 2265
in hypertrophic cardiomyopathy 2389
implantable defibrillators 2265, 2280
thromboembolism association 2273
in ventricular tachycardia 2280
carditis
in enterovirus infections 386
in rheumatic fever 503, 505, 2433
carers, of demented patients 4225, 4227
carina 2719
angle 2656
carinal nodes 2895
carmustine, adverse reaction 2851
Carney's syndrome (complex) 1642,
  2472, 3795
carnitine
in chronic renal failure 3302
deficiency 4167
  muscle biopsy 4144
supplements 1372
carnitine acyltransferase (CAT 1) 1277
carnitine palmityl transferase (CPT)
  4167
deficiency 3339, 3340, 4167, 4326–7
carnosinaemia (serum carnosinase
  deficiency) 1375
Caroli's syndrome 2014, 2015–16
congenital hepatic fibrosis with 2015,
  2016
ß-carotene 4366
antioxidant effect, ischaemic heart
  disease prevention 2311, 2312
cancer protection 219
in erythropoietic protoporphyria 1396
sun exposure protection 3728
carotid angiography
in carotid artery ischaemia 2367
in transient ischaemic attack (TIA)
  3952, 3954
carotid artery 3947
aneurysms 3866
  optic chiasmal lesions 3866, 3867
  third cranial nerve lesion in 3877
atheroma 2367, 3948
balloon/laser angioplasty 3824
injury, by Swan-Ganz catheter 2221
internal, atheroma 2367
stenosis management 2373
carotid artery ischaemia 2367
clinical features 2367
management 2373
transient ischaemic attack in 3950
carotid baroreceptors 2492
in hypertension 2533
carotid body 3887
enlargement, in cor pulmonale 2516
carotid bruit 2367
carotid endarterectomy 24–5, 2373
carotid pulse
in aortic regurgitation 2465
in aortic stenosis 2462
biferiens 2464
'collapsing' 2465
in supra-aortic stenosis 2423
carotid sinus
massage 2263, 2286, 3884
reflex, hypersensitivity 2266–7, 2268
syncope 2266, 3926, 3926
syndrome, pacing in 2286
carotid surgery, trials 2373
carpal collapse and fusion 2957

carpal tunnel syndrome 4095–6
  in acromegaly 1592, 1593, 4099
  affecting occupation 1168
  in amyloidosis 3003
  electromyography in 3841
  occupational 1169
  in pregnancy 1766
  in scleroderma 3028, 3030
  vibration association 1226
carprofen, poisoning 1056
carp's gallbladder, ingestion 1143
carriers
  detection 132, 132–3
  exclusion 132, 133
  of inherited diseases,
    definition 1338
    diagnosis 1338
Carrión's disease, see bartonellosis
cartilage
  age-related changes 2981
  calcification 2988, 2989, 3005
    see also chondrocalcinosis
  fibrillation 2981
  function 2981
  hydration, in osteoarthritis 2981
  investigations, in osteoarthritis 2982
  loss, in osteoarthritis 2975, 2980
  mechanical stress effect 2981
  as privileged tissue 185
  in relapsing polychondritis 3015
carvedilol, in dilated cardiomyopathy 2384
case-control studies 44, 45
case definitions, infections 287
Casoni test 958
Castellani's paint 811
Castleman's disease (giant follicular
    lymph node hyperplasia) 2899, 2900,
    3566, 3586
casts, urinary 3103–5, 3137–8
  in chronic renal failure 3301
  epithelial cell 3105
  fatty 3104
  granular 3103–4
  hyaline 3103
  in myeloma 3138, 3181
  red cell 3104, 3145
  transitional epithelial cell 3105
  white cell 3104
cat
  allergens 2715
  fleas, typhus fever transmission 736
catabolic state, negative nitrogen balance
    1317
catalase 1438, 3537
  inherited deficiency 1441
cataplexy 3918–19, 3927, 3928
cataracts
  after electrical injury 1214
  blindness due to 4197
  in congenital rubella syndrome 410
  in Cushing's syndrome 1644
  in diabetes mellitus 1485, 4190
  in elderly 4345
  in galactokinase deficiency 1349
  in hypoparathyroidism 1633, 1634
  management 4197
  in marrow transplant recipients 3699
  metabolic (snowflake) 1485
  senile 1485
  'sunflower' 4008
'catastrophic reactions' 4237
catechol 2553
catecholamines 1554, 2553–4
  analysis/assays 2554, 2555
  antagonism 2263
  drug effects 1718
  excess, in phaeochromocytomas 2553,
    2554, 2555
  free, measurement 2554
  functions in metabolism 1274, 1275
  haemodynamics and 2253–4
  in heart failure 2253, 2254
  intermittent pulsed therapy 2255
  in malnutrition 1286
  in phaeochromocytoma 1710
  plasma, measurement 2555
  positive inotropic agents 2150
  receptor subtypes for 2254

stress response 1563
  synthesis and catabolism 2553–4
  synthetic derivatives 2253, 2254
  see also adrenaline; dopamine;
    noradrenaline
catechol-O-methyltransferase (COMT)
    2253, 2486, 2553
caterpillars 1146
'cat face' 897
cathepsin, in adult respiratory distress
    syndrome 2854
cathepsin G 3623, 3626, 3627
cathepsin L 2773
catheterization
  bladder, see bladder; urinary
    catheterization
  cardiac, see cardiac catheterization
  in spinal cord injury 3899, 3900
  urinary, see urinary catheterization
catheter-related sepsis 330, 1021, 1319,
    1326
catheters
  coagulase-negative staphylococci
    infections 531, 532
  enterococcal infections 509
  intracranial disorder treatment 3822
  multilumen 1319
  peritoneal dialysis 3310, 3311
  right-atrial, infections 1031
  Staphylococcus aureus infections 525
  see also central venous catheter; urinary
    catheter
cation exchange resins, in hyperkalaemia
    3135, 3286
'cat scratch bacillus' 745
  see also Rochalimaea henselae
cat scratch disease 729, 744, 745–7
  causative agent 745
  hepatic granulomas in 2121
  skin-test antigen 746
cauda equina
  claudication 3907–8
  compression 3907
    in tumours 249–50, 3907
  lesions 3907–8
    in Paget's disease 3076
  tumours 3907
cauda equina syndrome, in ankylosing
    spondylitis 2967
caudal regression syndrome 4116
caudate nucleus 3861
  in Parkinson's disease 3999
causal associations 43–4
causalgia 3941, 4092
caveolae 71
caveolae intracellulares 2486
cavernostomy, in genitourinary
    tuberculosis 3279
cavernous sinus, pituitary tumours
    involving 1587
CCAAT box 57
CD1 antigen 152
CD2 antigen 145, 151, 3388
CD3 antigen 149–50, 3388
CD4 antigen 150, 151
  HIV receptor 91, 150, 465, 466, 1850
  receptor blockers 482
CD4 cells, see T-cells, CD4; T-cells,
    helper
CD8 antigen 150, 151
  see also cytotoxic T-cells (CTL); T-
    cells, CD8; T-cells, suppressor
CD10 (common-ALL antigen) 242,
    3401, 3402
CD11a/18 antigen 151
CD11b 3598
CD15 antigen 3569
CD18 antigen 2619
  antibodies 2619
CD20 antigen 148, 245
CD21 antigen 148, 352
  see also CR2 complement receptor
CD22 antigen 89
CD25 antigen 151, 2727
CD28 antigen 145, 150–1
CD30 antigen 3569
CD35 antigen 177
  see also CR1 complement receptor

CD40 antigen 147, 148, 157
  ligand, in X-linked immunodeficiency
    with hyper-IgM 166
CD40L antigen 149
CD43 antigen, deficiency, in Wiskott-
    Aldrich disease 173
CD44 antigen 88, 151
  role in metastases 231
CD45 antigen 149, 151
CD45RO antigen 149, 2727
CD45RO cells, reduced in SLE 3026
CD46 antigen 177
CD55 (decay accelerating factor; DAF)
    3450
CD56 antigen 3598
CD58 antigen 151
CD59 antigen 3450
CD68 (macrosialin) 91, 94
cDNA, see DNA, complementary
    (cDNA)
Cedecea, rare species 553
cefaclor, in urinary-tract infections
    3211
cefazolin, in urinary-tract infections 3211
cefotaxime
  in neonates 1790
  in renal failure 3272
ceftazidime
  in melioidosis 592
  in renal failure 3272
ceftriaxone
  in chancroid 586
  in gonorrhoea 1790
  in infective endocarditis 2449
  meningococcal infections prophylaxis
    542
  in syphilis 2483
  in urinary-tract infections 3211
cell adhesion molecules, see adhesion
    molecules
cell biology, of endomembrane system
    and organelles 68–84
  cytoskeleton 80–3
  definition 68
  endocytic pathway 72–5
  exocytic pathway 68–72
  intracellular movement of organelles
    80, 81–2
  intracellular transport 75–8
  nucleus 78–80
  organelle streaming 82
  peroxisomes 83–4
  see also individual organelles/pathways
    as listed above
cell cultures, gene insertion 62
cell cycle
  G_1 and G_2 78
  myocardial cells withdrawal 2145, 2147
  psoriasis pathogenesis and 3745
  S-phase and genome replication 78
cell death
  pain in 3941
  see also apoptosis
cell density, response and cell
    multiplication control 191
cell fusion techniques 193, 194, 196
cell hybrids 65
cell loss, cell multiplication relationship
    191
cell-mediated immune response 164,
    165, 165
  in anti-GBM disease 3164
  in atopic eczema 3740
  autoimmune hepatitis pathogenesis 2072
  in Behçet's syndrome 3044
  in brucellosis 620
  cytokines in 98
  in dengue haemorrhagic fever 420
  in extrinsic allergic alveolitis 2811
  impairment,
    in infections 282
    in leprosy 673
    RSV infection 340
    toxoplasmosis in 866
  in infection-associated
    glomerulonephritis 3173
  in infections 277
  in leptospirosis 699

in measles 377
  in meningococcal infections 538
  in mycoplasmal infections 766, 767
  in paracoccidioidomycosis 816
  in polymyositis and dermatomyositis
    4156
  in primary sclerosing cholangitis 2078
  in rheumatoid arthritis 2954
  in sarcoidosis 2819
  suppression, in visceral leishmaniasis
    904
  in tuberculosis 639
  to tumours 227–8
  see also delayed hypersensitivity; T-
    cells
cell membrane
  damage, electrical 1212
  myocardial cells 2144
cell movement, microfilaments role 80,
    81
cell multiplication
  control 191
    insensitivity in tumours 191
    suppression of insensitivity by
      differentiation 193
  density-sensing mechanism 191
  impairment 191
cell-surface receptors, autoantibodies to
    163
cell transformation, see transformation of
    cells
cellular adhesion molecules (CAMs), see
    adhesion molecules
cellulitis 501
  around eye 4191
  in dental caries 1846
  eosinophilic 3774
  Haemophilus influenzae type b 582
  injecting drug addicts 4294
  in nephrotic syndrome 3141
  pasteurellosis 606
  Pseudomonas causing 1029
  septicaemia in 1020
  streptococcal, diagnosis 502
  streptococci group A 500–1
Cellulomonas turbata 554
cellulose phosphate 1633, 3255
cement 2845
  contact dermatitis due to 3738
Centers for Disease Control and
    Prevention (CDC)
  AIDS definition 468
  HIV stage classification 469, 469
  pelvic inflammatory disease guidelines
    3359
  simian herpesviruses 358
centipedes 1149
central cord syndrome 3898
central core degeneration of Achilles
    tendon 2996–7
central core disease 4150
Central European encephalitis (CEE) 416
central fovea, assessment,
    ophthalmoscopy 4179
central motor conduction time
  in cerebrovascular disease 3838
  in degenerative diseases 3838
  measurement 3837
  in motor neurone disease 3837–8
  in movement disorders 3838
  in multiple sclerosis 3837
  paediatric applications 3838
  in spinal cord injury 3838
  see also magnetic brain stimulation
central motor pathways, investigation
    3836–9
central nervous system (CNS)
  acid-base disturbances and 1539–40
  actinomycoses 683
  age-related changes 4336
  in AIDS 4078–80, 4236
  in alcohol abuse 4276–7, 4277
  breathing disorders and 3888–91
  damage, after coronary artery bypass
    grafting 2355–6
  in decompression sickness 1209
  depressants,
    alcohol as 1080

methyl chloride and methyl iodide 1087
styrene (vinyl benzene) 1088
depression,
  after weaning from ventilators 2580
  in solvent abuse 1092
  trichloroethylene poisoning 1090
developmental abnormalities, *see under*
  nervous system
disorders,
cerebral venous thrombosis (*cont.*)
  in pregnancy **1767–9**
  see also neurological disorders
drug tolerance 4263
dysfunction, chronic fatigue syndrome
  in 1037
gastrointestinal hormones 1554
in heart failure 2235
in hypertension 2535
infections 330, **4050–87**
  after head injury 3835
  in AIDS **4078–80**
  anaerobic 572
  dementia in *3966*, 3971
  viral, *see below*
  see also meningitis
in Langerhans-cell histiocytosis 3608
in leptospirosis 700
lesions, neuropathic pain 3942
leukaemia 3412, 3414
lymphoma 4080, 4134
in mumps 373
occupational disorders 1169, *1170*
oxygen toxicity 1208
pain due to **3941–2**
pain perception, *see* pain
poisonous plants effects 1152, *1156*
in Q fever 743
in rabies 398, 400
radiation syndrome 1218
reaction to peripheral nerve damage
  3940–1
in rickettsial diseases 731, 732
riot control agents affecting 1119
in schistosomiasis 916–78, 979–80
in SLE 3019
stimulation,
  drugs of abuse 1077
  pain treatment 3945–6
in toxoplasmosis 866
tumours, in AIDS **4080**
viral infections **4064–75**
  in AIDS 4079
  clinical features 4066–8
  diagnosis/investigations 4068–9, *4071*
  differential diagnosis 4069
  epidemiology 4065
  herpes simplex virus 344–5
  pathogenesis 4065–6
  pathology 4066
  prevention 4072
  prognosis and sequelae 4072
  treatment 4069–72
  uncertain pathogenic role 4073–4
  virology 4064–5
  see also encephalitis; meningitis
in Whipple's disease 1924
central pontine myelinolysis 3123–4,
  3990, **3996**
  in alcohol abusers 4127, 4278
central venous catheter
  complications 1319
  in diabetic hyperglycaemic coma 1502
  occlusion 1319
  sepsis 1319, 1326
central venous pressure 2490
  changes in haemorrhage and
    retransfusion 2565
  in elderly 4342
  high pressure 2564, **2565–9**
    in cor pulmonale 2517, 2518
    in heart failure 2171
    immediate support 2565–6
  low pressure **2564–5**, 2564
  major circulatory derangements **2563–4**
  measurement 2563–4
  monitoring 3282–3
  normal 2564
  in septicaemia 2572

centric fusion 122
centronuclear myopathy **4151**
cephalexin, in urinary-tract infections
  3211, 3213
cephalosporins
  allergic reaction 162
  in *Haemophilus influenzae* type b
    meningitis 582
  nephrotoxicity **3264**, *3284*
  in pneumococcal infections 520
  in pregnancy 1813
  in renal impairment 3270–1, 3288
  resistance 1023
  Staphylococcus aureus sensitivity 525,
    530
  third-generation, in septicaemia 1023
  in urinary-tract infections 3209–10
cephradine, in urinary-tract infections
  3211
ceramidase deficiency (Farber's disease)
  1426–7, *1428*
ceramide trihexosidosis, *see* Fabry
  disease
c-erbA, *see* thyroid hormones, receptor
c-*erb*B-2 gene
  amplification 224
  antibodies 224
  overexpression, breast cancer outcome
    and 224
c-*erb*B-2 protein, monoclonal antibodies
  to
  in cancer diagnosis 225
  in cancer therapy 225
  clinical trials 226
cercaria 971
  dermatitis 970, 975
Cercopithecine herpesviruses 357
cerebellar abscess 4081
  clinical features 4082
  management 4083
cerebellar ataxia 3860, 3984–5
  autosomal dominant 3984–5
cerebellar atrophy, delayed 3984
cerebellar degeneration
  alcoholic 4127, 4277
  late-onset 3985
cerebellar dysarthria 3860
cerebellar dysfunction, in falciparum
  malaria 847
cerebellar haematoma 3961, 3962
cerebellar haemorrhage, coma in 3931
cerebellar malformations **4113**
cerebellar tonsil herniation 4034, 4035
cerebellopontine angle tumour **3874–5**
  facial nerve affected 3878
  trigeminal nerve affected 3878
cerebelloretinal haemangioblastosis, *see*
  von Hippel-Lindau disease
cerebellum **3859–60**
  clinical aspects 3860
  input to thalamus 3861
  lesions 3860
  structure and function 3859–60,
    3860
cerebral abscess 4081, 4082
  after head injury 3835
  amoebic 830
  anaerobic infection 572
  in bronchiectasis 2760
  clinical features 4082
  in cyanotic congenital heart disease
    2401
  frontal sinusitis with 4081
  management 4083
  Streptococcus milleri 509
  see also intracranial abscess
cerebral aneurysms, endovascular
  treatment 3824
cerebral angiography **3822**, 3823
  in cerebral infarction 3958
  in intracerebral haemorrhage 3961
  in intracranial tumours 4037
cerebral anoxia **4007**, **4123–4**
  acute 4123
  mental symptoms 4240
  neurological features 4123–4
  subacute/gradual 4123
cerebral arteries, occlusion 3869

cerebral ataxia, familial, hypogonadism
  1683
cerebral blood flow 3947
  after traumatic brain damage 4045
  autoregulation 3947, 4045
  reduced, in malaria 845
cerebral blood volume
  hyperventilation effect 4048
  increase, in benign intracranial
    hypertension 4042
cerebral circulation
  blood supply **3947–8**, 3948
  imaging 3952
  vessels, in hypertension 2534
cerebral contusions 4044
cerebral cortex
  calcarine, *see* visual (striate) cortex
  contusions/lacerations 4044, 4047
cerebral dementia, in alcohol abusers
  4278
cerebral dominance **3845–6**
  handedness and aphasia 3847
cerebral dysgenesis **3916–17**
cerebral emboli
  in Eisenmenger syndrome 2411
  heart valve prostheses 2470
  in infective endocarditis 2441
  in mitral prolapse 2460
  thrombolytic agents 3824
cerebral function
  asymmetry (cerebral dominance)
    3845–6
  cognitive, localization **3845**
cerebral function disturbances **3845–56**
  apraxia **3852–3**
  dementia *vs* 3968
  visual, spatial/bodily perception **3853–4**
  see also amnesia; apraxia
cerebral gigantism (Sotos syndrome)
  1700, 4111
cerebral haemorrhage
  amyloidosis with 3972
  cerebral infarction *vs* 3961
  electroencephalogram (EEG) in
    3830
  epidemiology 3947
  hereditary, with amyloidosis, *see*
    hereditary cerebral haemorrhage with
    amyloidosis
  in hypertension 2532, 2534
  in infective endocarditis 2441
  in leukaemia 4135
  lobar 3961
  in pre-eclampsia 1728, 1730
  primary **3961–2**
    causes 3961, *3961*
  thrombolytic therapy hazard in
    myocardial infarction 2341
  treatment 3962
  see also intracranial haemorrhage
cerebral hemisphere 3845
  deficits, in intracranial tumours
    4035
  left, language areas **3847–8**
cerebral infarction **3954–60**, **3955–6**
  boundary zone (watershed) 3956
  brain-stem 3956
  cerebral oedema in 3954, 3957
  clinical features 3954–7
  complications 3957, 3960
  deterioration after 3960, *3960*
  differential diagnosis 3957
  distribution of subtypes *3955*
  epidemiology 3947
  epilepsy and 3917
  haematological causes *3951*
  in hypertension 2532, 2534, 3960
  intracerebral haemorrhage *vs* 3961
  investigations 3957–8, 3959
  lacunar 3956
  migraine and 3956
  multi-infarct dementia in 3960
  pathogenesis 3947, 3954
  in pregnancy 1768
  prognosis 3958–9, *3959*
  rehabilitation 3960
  somatosensory evoked potentials (SEP)
    3834

subarachnoid haemorrhage and 3963
treatment 3959–60
visual pathway disorders in 3866
see also cerebral ischaemia
cerebral infections
  dementia in 3971
  mental disorders/symptoms 4236
  see also central nervous system (CNS),
    infections
cerebral injury, after coronary artery
  bypass grafting 2356
cerebral ischaemia
  after traumatic brain damage 4044–5
  anoxia in 4123
  cerebral palsy aetiology 4120
  haematological causes *3951*
  multi-infarct dementia in 3960
  transient ischaemic attack due to 3950
  see also cerebral infarction
cerebral lesions
  pain in 3942
  in sarcoidosis 2827
  sexual problems in 4244
cerebral lymphomas **4033–4**
cerebral malaria, *see* malaria, cerebral
cerebral metabolism 4123
  changes, in hepatocellular failure
    2102
cerebral metastases **4133–5**
  capillary leakiness 250
  detection and staging methods 246
  investigation and treatment 250
  in lung cancer 2883
  in lymphomas 4133
  mental disorders/symptoms in 4237
  mortality/prognosis 250
  sites 250
  solitary, removal 250
  symptoms and signs 250
cerebral oedema 2585
  in acute mountain sickness 1188, 1189,
    1190
  after head injury 3835
  benign intracranial hypertension in
    4042
  in cerebral infarction 3954, 3957
  in cerebral metastases 250
  in hepatocellular failure 2103, 2109
  high altitude 1188
    diagnosis 1190
    incidence 1190
    pathophysiology 1189
    predisposing factors 1188
    prophylaxis and treatment 1190–1
    see also mountain sickness, acute
  in hypoglycaemia 1506
  in intracranial tumours 4034, 4040
  in lung cancer 2884
  in malaria 845
  management 2109
  metabolic basis 2103
  positive end-expiratory pressure (PEEP)
    2578
  in tuberculous meningitis 4063
  see also brain, swelling
cerebral palsy **4119–22**
  aetiology and pathology 4119–20
  ataxic **4121**
  classification *4119*
  diagnosis 4120
  dyskinetic **4121**
  dystonic, in glutaric aciduria type I
    1372
  epilepsy and 3916
  hypotonic 4121
  management 4121–2
  'minimal' **4122**
  prevalence 4119
  types 4120–1
cerebral paragonimiasis 991
cerebral perfusion pressure 4045
cerebral sclerosis, diffuse **3996–7**
cerebral tumours, *see* intracranial
  tumours
cerebral vascular disorders, epilepsy and
  3817
cerebral vascular lesions,
  electroencephalogram (EEG) 3830

cerebral venous thrombosis 3956–7, *3957*
  in cyanotic congenital heart disease 2401
  in pregnancy 1768
  winter mortality due to 1185
cerebrohepatorenal (Zellweger) syndrome, *see* Zellweger (cerebrohepatorenal) syndrome
cerebrospinal fluid (CSF)
  in African trypanosomiasis 892
  bacterial meningitis pathogenesis 4052
  blood in 3843
    differential diagnosis 3843
  carcinomatous 'meningitis' and 250–1
  cells **3843**, *3844*
  in cerebrospinal angiostrongyliasis 947, 948
  circulation 4050
  decreased absorption, benign intracranial hypertension in 4042
  examination 3843–5
    in benign intracranial hypertension 4043
    in cardiovascular syphilis 2483
    in cerebral infarction 3958
    in dementia 3969
    in immunocompromised 1033
    in meningitis 4055–6, *4055*
    in multiple sclerosis 3995
    in neurosyphilis **4086**
    in viral infections 4069
    see also lumbar puncture
  glucose 1033, 3843–4, *3844*
    in meningitis 4055
    in viral infections 4069
  immunoglobulins in 3843, *3844*
  increased production, benign intracranial hypertension in 4042
  infection, *see* meningitis
  leakage, management 4048
  in leptospirosis 701
  in meningitis *3844*, 4055–6, *4055*
    H. influenzae 581–2
    in immunocompromised 1033
    meningococcal 539, 540
    pneumococcal 518
    tuberculous 4061
  microbiological/serological reactions 3845
  neurosyphilis diagnosis 716
  normal 3843
  normal values *4374*
  obstruction to outflow 3894
  pigments (oxyhaemoglobin and bilirubin) 3843
  pressure **3842–3**
    in benign intracranial hypertension 4043
    measurement 3843
    in meningitis *4055*
    in normal pressure hydrocephalus 3970
    in viral infections 4069
  protein 3843, *3844*
    in meningitis 4055
    in viral infections 4069
  rhinorrhoea 1582
  shunts,
    coagulase-negative staphylococcal infections 532
    infections 4055
  volume 4114
    in hydrocephalus 4114
  white cell count 3843, *3844*
    in meningitis 4055
cerebrotendinous xanthomatosis 1406, **1437**
cerebrovascular accident, *see* stroke
cerebrovascular disease **3946–65**
  aircraft travel and 1202
  in carcinomas 4135
  central motor conduction time in 3838
  definitions **3946**
  epidemiology **3947**
  in essential hypertension 2532
  in HIV infection and AIDS 4080

polycythaemia and 3553
  in pregnancy 1767–8
  see also stroke; transient ischaemic attack (TIA)
cerebrovascular malformations **3963**, 3964
  brain **4116**
  electroencephalogram (EEG) in 3830
ceroid 3245
cervical bruits 3951, 3952, *3952*, 3964
cervical carcinoma **3369–71**
  adenocarcinoma 210
  aetiological factors 210, 3370
  clinical features 3371
  epidemiology 210, 3370, *3371*
    age relationship 197, 3371
    incidence 444
    reasons for decrease 210
  in HIV infection 477
  human papillomavirus association 444–5, 460, 462, **3370**
    screening for 463, 3371
  magnetic resonance imaging 235
  natural history 3370–1
  oral contraceptives and 1724
  in pregnancy 1807
  prevention 3371
  in renal transplant recipients 3321
  sexually transmitted diseases and **3369–72**
  squamous cell carcinoma 210, 3371
  staging investigations *236*
cervical collar 2995, 3908
cervical disc, protrusions 3906
cervical intraepithelial neoplasia (CIN) 3366, 3371
  epidemiology 210
cervical lymph nodes
  metastases from unknown primary site 252
  non-purulent swelling, in Kawasaki disease 3047
  in tuberculosis 652
cervical myelopathy 2959
cervical pain 241, 2995
cervical rib 2366, 2375
  excision 2375
  syndrome **3903**
cervical smears (Pap smears) 445, 463, 3370
cervical spinal canal, actinomycoses 683
cervical spinal cord, *see* spinal cord, cervical
cervical spine
  acute subluxation 2959
  dislocation 3897
  fusion, in myositis ossificans progressiva 3093, 3094
  pain 241, **2995**
    in rheumatoid arthritis 2949, 2959
  traumatic injury management 3897
cervical spondylosis 3905
  cord disturbances in 3908–9
  headache in 4028
cervical spondylotic myelopathy **3908–9**
  decompression 3908
cervical stiffness, in ankylosing spondylitis 2966
cervical warts 3368, 3370
cervicitis 3207, 3354
  bacterial vaginosis with 3355
  chlamydial 752, 756
  in lymphogranuloma venereum 760
cervicofacial actinomycoses 682, 683
cervix
  cancer, *see* cervical carcinoma
  cerclage 1785
  lesions, in donovanosis 777
  'strawberry' 908, 3354
  subclinical HPV infection 3368
cestodes **955–70**
  gut **959–64**
    accidental **962**, *963*
  infections, gastrointestinal symptoms 960, 2004
  see also hydatid disease; *Taenia solium*; tapeworm
cetirizine 2718

C fibres 3936, 3937
c-fms 89
CGP 6140 (amocarzine) 916, 917
Chagas' disease **895–9**
  achalasia in 1869
  autoantibodies in 896
  chronic phase 897
  clinical features 896–8, 2381
    eye in 4192
    gastrointestinal 1962, 2004
    mega-oesophagus in 897
    myositis in 4156
  congenital 896, 898, 1794
  diagnosis 896–8
  epidemiology and transmission 895
  gastrointestinal motility disorder in 1962–3
  gut peptides in 1896
  heart in 896, 897, 898, 2381
  pathogenesis 895–6
  in pregnancy 1794
  treatment and prevention 898
  see also Trypanosoma cruzi
chagoma 896
chancre 3713, 3714
  in African trypanosomiasis 889, **890**, 892
  soft 584
  in syphilis 710
chancroid **584–7**
  aetiology and epidemiology 584–5
  clinical features and variants 585
  contact tracing 586
  HIV infection and 586
  in homosexuals 3363
  laboratory diagnosis 585–6
  natural history 586
  pathogenesis and pathology 585
  syphilis *vs* 711
  treatment 586
  see also Haemophilus ducreyi
Changuinola virus 406
chaperones
  molecular 69
  protein 70
charcoal
  absorption interaction 1257
  activated, *see* activated charcoal
  haemoperfusion, *see* haemoperfusion
Charcot-Bouchard aneurysm 2534, 3956
Charcot-Leyden crystals 159, 874, 950, 2685, 2801
Charcot-Marie-Tooth disease 4102–3
  chromosomal duplication 108
  somatosensory evoked potentials (SEP) 3834
Charcot's (neuropathic) joints 2979, 3002, 3006, 4085
  in diabetes 1486, 1490
Chase-Aurbach (PTH administration) test 1633
Chediak-Higashi syndrome 1365, 2759, 3560
  depigmentation in 3759
  cheeks, in malnutrition 1284
cheilitis, solar *3726*
cheiroarthropathy, diabetic 1487
chelation therapy 1248
  adverse effects 1423
  aluminium 1105–6
  arsenic 1106
  cadmium 1107
  copper 1109
  in iron overload 3480–1
  lead 1110
  manganese 1110–11
  mercury 1112
  in pregnancy 1800
  in thalassaemia 3480–1, 3512
  thallium 1113
  in Wilson's disease 1422
chemical(s)
  antidotes to 1048, *1048*
  aplastic anaemia induced by 3441–2
  carcinogens, *see* carcinogens, chemical
  cardiovascular disease due to 1170
  depigmentation due to 3759
  extrinsic allergic alveolitis due to *2810*
  in G6PD deficiency *3539*

haemolytic anaemia due to **3546–7**
hepatic granulomas induced by 2121–2
non-dermatitic occupational dermatosis 1165
oesophageal trauma 1873–4
poisoning, *see* household products; *under* poisoning
riot control agents 1118
scleroderma aetiology *3027*, 3028
vesico-blistering diseases due to 3779
chemical environmental disasters 1233–4
chemical warfare 1115
chemoattractants 2293
  atherosclerotic plaque development 2294
chemokines 87, *96*, **97**, 2618
chemoprophylaxis
  Bordetella infections 589
  Haemophilus influenzae 583
  infections, *see* antimicrobial therapy, prophylactic
chemoreceptor trigger zone (CTZ) 1821
chemoreflex-baroreflex interactions, heart failure pathophysiology 2232, 2233, 2234
chemosis, in snake bites 1129
chemotaxins 2618
chemotaxis
  leucocyte 3559
  neutrophils **2621–2**
chemotherapy 248–9, 1248
  adjuvant radiotherapy 257
  advances **259**
  antimetabolites 259
    topoisomerase inhibitors 259
  adverse effects 248, *249*, 3575
    cancers caused by *216*, 1254
    cerebral metastases 250
  combination, principles 248, 249
  commonly used agents *248*
  fever after 1181
  in Hodgkin's disease 3573–4
  infections 283, 289
  in leukaemia 3407–10, 3413–14, 3417, 3419, 3421–2
  metastases from unknown primary site 252
  multi-drug resistance, in myeloma 3603
  myelodysplastic syndromes and 3430, 3430–1
  in myeloma 3601, 3602, 3603
  neurological complications 4135
  neutropenic fever of unknown origin (FUO) 1017
  new targets **259–61**
    angiogenesis 259–60
    receptor targeting 260
    signal transduction inhibitors 259
  non-Hodgkin's lymphoma 3583–4, 3585
  oesophageal disease due to 1874
  oncogenes/tumour suppressor genes as targets **225–6**
  in pancreatic endocrine tumours 1704, 1706
  in pregnancy 1761–2, 1806, 1807, 1808
  principles and aims *247*, 248–9
  renal complications 3185
  resistance 248
    modulation **259**
    type II topoisomerases 259
  respiratory tract infections 2709
  respiratory tract tumours 2592
  sensitivity to 248
  specialists in and need for 249
  surgery with 248
  targeted, in hepatocellular carcinoma 2117
  in Waldenström's macroglobulinaemia 3604
  see also cytotoxic drugs; *other individual tumours*
chenodeoxycholic acid 2047
  gallstone dissolution 2048, 2049
Chernobyl accident 1219, 1234
cherry-red foveal spot 1426, 1427, 1436, 4183
  myoclonus syndrome (mucolipidosis I) 1434, **1435–6**, 3988
  in retinal artery occlusion 4186

chest
  auscultation 2650
  barrel 1592, 2649
  discomfort in lung cancer 2883
  expansion 2649
  flail segment **2875**
    positive-pressure ventilation in 2577
  funnel (pectus excavatum) 2179, 2649, 2657, **2875**
  gas expansion, effects of aircraft pressure changes 1198 hyperinflation 2635, 2649
  infections, *see* respiratory tract infections
  injuries, positive-pressure ventilation in 2577
  inspection **2649–50**
  palpation 2650
  percussion 2650
  pigeon (pectus carinatum) 2649, **2875**
  shape abnormalities 2649
  trauma, bronchoscopy in 2579
chest diseases
  clinical presentation **2642–52**
    breathlessness **2644–8**
    chest pain **2648–9**
    cough **2642–4**
    see also heart disease, symptoms; *specific symptoms*
  haematological changes **3685**
  physical signs **2649–52**
  in pregnancy **1744–7**
  see also heart disease; respiratory disease/disorders
chest pain **2165–9, 2648–9**
  in acute pericarditis 2476
  in ankylosing spondylitis 2875
  in aortic dissection 2335
  in aortic regurgitation 2465
  atypical 2322
    in mitral prolapse 2460
  bronchopulmonary **2169**, 2648
  cardiac **2165–7**
    miscellaneous causes 2167
    see also angina (angina pectoris)
  causes 2165, 2648, 2649
  central **2648–9**
  chest wall 2648
  clinical viewpoint and perception of 2165
  consultations with doctors for 4231
  C-reactive protein levels 1531
  diagnosis and history-taking 2165
  in diffuse oesophageal spasm 1869, 1870, 2167
  in hypertrophic cardiomyopathy 2386, 2389
  in idiopathic achalasia 1869
  in Lassa fever 431
  left inframammary 2648
  management 2389
  in mediastinal masses 2897
  musculoskeletal and neurological causes 2168
  in myocardial infarction 2334, 2335
  non-cardiac **1870, 2167–9, 2648–9**
    aetiology and symptoms 1870, 2167, 2168
    gastro-oesophageal reflux causing 1868, 2167
    treatment and prognosis 1870
  oesophageal, *see* oesophagus, pain
  in oesophageal disease **1820**, 2167–8
  in pericarditis 2335
  in pleurisy 2648
  in pneumococcal pneumonia 515
  in pneumothorax 2869
  psychological causes **2168–9**, 2648
  in pulmonary embolism 2524
  in pulmonary hypertension 2510
  retrosternal 2465
  in rheumatic diseases 2945
chest radiography **2652–3**
  abnormal **2179–82**
  common signs **2660–4**
  in acute neurological syndromes in immunocompromised 1033

in adult respiratory distress syndrome 2857
'air-crescent sign' 2663
analysis 2179, **2658–60**
  in aortic regurgitation 2464, 2465
  in aortic stenosis 2463, 2464
  in asbestosis 2844
  in asthma 2736
breathlessness investigation 2647
in bronchiectasis **2665**
cavitating pulmonary lesions **2663**
in chest wall disease **2664**
in chronic obstructive airways disease **2664–5**, 2774
in coal-worker's pneumoconiosis 2841
in coarctation of aorta 2179, 2558
in community-acquired pneumonia 2697
in cor pulmonale 2518
in cryptogenic fibrosing alveolitis 2789–90
in cystic fibrosis 2748
in diaphragmatic disorders 2878
in diffuse parenchymal lung disease 2782–3
in ductus arteriosus 2430–1
in Ebstein's anomaly 2413
in Eisenmenger reaction (syndrome) 2411
in empyema 2706, 2707
in extrinsic allergic alveolitis 2813
in Fallot's tetralogy 2403, 2405, 2406
fever and pulmonary infiltrates in immunocompromised 1032
in fixed subaortic stenosis 2422
fluoroscopy with ('real time') 2653
in heart disease **2177–82**
hemithorax transradiancy increased **2662**
in Hodgkin's disease 3572
in hypertrophic cardiomyopathy 2388
in infundibular stenosis 2421
interpretation 2179, **2658–60**
lateral 2653
  normal anatomy **2657–8**
in legionnaires' disease 725
in lung cancer 2886
lung collapse **2660–2**
in mediastinal masses 2900
in mesothelioma 2664, **2894–5**
in mitral regurgitation 2458–9
in mitral stenosis 2453
in mixed mitral valve disease 2456–7
in myocardial infarction 2338–9
new devices/procedures 2652–3
normal **2178–9, 2656–8**
  cardiovascular 2178, 2656
  lateral views **2657–8**
  mediastinum 2656
  pulmonary **2656–8**
  pulmonary vasculature 2178–9, 2657
in ostium secundum defects 2425
in pericardial constriction 2480
in pericardial tamponade 2477, 2478
phosphor plated computed 2652–3
in pleural disease **2664**
pleural effusion 2863–5
in pneumonia 2697, 2698–9
  pneumococcal 515
posteroanterior view 2653
  normal anatomy **2656–7**
in pregnancy 1735
pulmonary consolidation 2660
in pulmonary embolism 2523, 2524–5
in pulmonary hypertension 2510
in pulmonary masses **2662–3**
in pulmonary nodules **2663–4**
in pulmonary oedema 2502–3
in pulmonary valve stenosis 2420
in Q fever 743
quality assessment 2659
in respiratory disease **2660–5**
respiratory tract infections, in immunosuppressed 2710, 2711
in ruptured chordae tendinae 2458–9
in sarcoidosis 2822, **2823–5**

'silhouette sign' 2660
standard views 2653
in supra-aortic stenosis 2423
technical considerations 2652–3
in total anomalous pulmonary venous drainage (TAPVD) 2415
in tricuspid atresia 2413
in tricuspid stenosis 2468
in tuberculosis 650, 662
tumour staging 234, 246
  M staging 237
in ventricular septal defects 2429
chest tightness 2648–9, 2729
chest ultrasonography **2653**
chest wall
  chest radiography 2657, **2664**
  compliance 2876
  disorders **2664, 2872–8**
  pain from **2648**
  paradoxical movement 2875
cheyletiella 1010, 3744
Cheyne-Stokes breathing 2162, **2583–4**, 2649, 2916, **3889–90**
  in cardiac disease 2162, 2649, 2916
  features and causes 2162, 2649, 2916, 3890
  in sleep-apnoea syndrome 2232, 2916, 2917
Chiari malformation 3893, 3894, **4113**
  magnetic resonance imaging (MRI) 3826, 3828
chiasmal lesions, *see* optic chiasm
chicken, gouty 1380, 3226
chickenpox 346, **347–8**
  arthritis in 3001
  clinical features 347
  complications 347–8
  congenital and perinatal 348, **1779–80**
  encephalomyelitis after 3991
  in immunocompromised 348
  mortality 347, 348
  in pregnancy 348, 1747, **1775**, *1777*
  recurrent 348
  in renal transplant recipients 3314, 3320
  vaccine 320, 351
  see also varicella-zoster virus (VZV) infections
chiclero ulcer 901
chiggers 1005, 1010
  scrub typhus transmission 739–40
chigoe 1005
Chikungunya virus **407**
  arthritis in 3001
chilblains 3724
childcare, drug addict and alcoholic parents 4289
childhood relationships, generalized anxiety disorder predisposition 4206
childrearing, bulimia nervosa parent 4217
children
  abuse/neglect 4313
    confidentiality and 4316
    excessive bruising 3628, 3637
    from deliberate self-harm patients 4230
    sexual 4313
    short stature 1697
  acute leukaemia 3404, 3406, 3409
  akinetic-rigid syndromes **4007–9**, *4007*
  alkali ingestion 1104
  anaemia **3469**
  asthma 2725, 2731, 2736
  bone marrow examination 3381
  bronchoscopy in 2682
  brucellosis 619, 623
  cancer, occupations associated 1174
  carditis due to enteroviruses 386
  cholera in 577, 579
  chronic disease, growth impairment 1698
  confidentiality and 4316
  constipation 1964
  craniopharyngioma 1597
  Crohn's disease management 1943
  Cushing's syndrome 1644, 1699
  cytomegalovirus (CMV) infection 359–60, 361

diaphragmatic disorders 2877, 2878
divorce and 36–7
electroencephalogram (EEG) 3830
endotracheal intubation 2577
epilepsy in 3924
erythroblastopenic anaemia 3449
essential hypertension in **2543**
fever of unknown origin (FUO) in 1015
focal segmental glomerulosclerosis 3156
folate deficiency 3467, 3468
genital warts 3369
glomerulonephritis in 3153–4
gonadotrophin secretion 1580
growth hormone deficiency 1582
growth rates 1696
haemolytic uraemic syndrome 3196, 3202
haemophilia in 3649–50
Haemophilus influenzae meningitis 581
heat loss in cold conditions 1182
HIV infection 478, **4080**
Huntington's disease 4014
hypertension in 2543
hypoglycaemia **1511–12**
hypothyroidism 1615
idiopathic hypoparathyroidism 1634
infective endocarditis 2443
Lassa fever in 433
lead poisoning 1109, 3261
malnutrition,
  classification 1280–1
  physiological changes 1285–6, *1286*
  see also malnutrition
malnutrition management 1289, 1292, 1293
  emotional and psychological stimulation 1293–4
membranous nephropathy 3158–9
mesangiocapillary glomerulonephritis 3158
migraine in 4024
minimal change nephropathy 3153–4, **3155**, 3156
mitral valve replacement 2470
mortality rates 40
nephrotic syndrome, *see* nephrotic syndrome, of childhood
normal haematological values *3380*
nutritional assessment 1314
nutritional deficiency, type II 1280
obesity prevention 1313
pertussis 587, 588
pneumococcal infections 512, 515
pneumonia in 515, 2700
poisoning 1044, *1044*, 1045, 1054
  diethylene glycol 1081
  disulfiram 1077, 1078
  household products 1078
  iron preparations 1070
  lead 1109, 3261
  by plants and fungi 1151
  rodenticides 1123
  salicylate 1055
polycystic kidney disease 3204
primary hyperparathyroidism 1631
reference intervals *4366–7*
renal bone disease 3324
scarlet fever 499
schistosomiasis 974, 975, 980
sexual abuse, examination 4313
Shigella infections 554
spinal cord injury 3897
streptococcal impetigo 500
streptococcal pharyngitis/tonsillitis 498–9
travel and 325
tuberculosis in 653, 664
typhoid in 562, 563
ulcerative colitis in 1951
urinary-tract infections 3213
urinary-tract obstruction 3232
vesicoureteric reflux 3214, 3217
welfare of unborn 11, 12
see also infant(s); neonates
Chilopoda (centipedes), bites 1149
chimney sweeps, scrotal cancer 197, 216, 1165

China, oesophageal cancer in 202
Chinese restaurant syndrome 1844
chirality and chiral compounds 1248–9
chlamydia **749–50**
　classification and species 749
　elementary bodies 749, 761
　GroEL heat-shock protein homology
　　750, 758
　growth cycle and infection route 749
　inclusions 757
　MOMP (major outer-membrane protein)
　　749, 750, 759
　rMOMP and vaccines 759
　reticulate bodies 749
　serovars and protein profile 749–50
chlamydial infections **748–61**
　diagnosis 755–6, *755*
　　culture 755–6, *755*
　　DNA probes and hybridization 755,
　　　755, 756
　　enzyme immunoassays *755*, 756
　　microimmunofluorescence 750, 755,
　　　755, 756, 761
　　monoclonal antibodies in 761
　　serological *755*, 756
　　staining *755*, 756
　eye **4191**
　fetal 1791
　genital tract **751–3**, 756, 758, *758*, 769
　in homosexuals 3362
　immunocompromised host 753
　　lymphogranuloma venereum, *see*
　　　lymphogranuloma venereum
　miscellaneous diseases *752*, 753, 771
　neonatal **753–4**, *758*, 1791–2
　pathogenesis and immune response 155,
　　757–9
　　autoimmunity and class II antigens
　　　758
　　histopathology 757
　　scarring 758–9
　in pregnancy **1791–2**
　protective immunity and vaccines 759
　repeated experimental 757–8
　trachoma, *see* trachoma
　treatment 756–7
　　antibiotics and MAC 756–7, *757*
　　schedules 757, *758*
Chlamydia pecorum 749, 755
Chlamydia pneumoniae 749, 750, 764
　arthritis due to 753
　infections **754**
　pneumonia due to 2693, 2697
Chlamydia psittaci 749, 750, 1791
　arthritis due to 753
　infections **754–5**
　protective immunity 759
　serovars and detection 755
Chlamydia trachomatis 749, 1791
　detection 761
　gastrointestinal infection 2005
　genital-tract infections 751–3, 769
　　epidemiology 3347
　infections in homosexuals 3362
　interaction with phagocytic cells 272
　lymphogranuloma venereum 759–61
　neonatal infections 753–4
　oculogenital and other diseases *752*,
　　753
　pelvic inflammatory disease due to
　　3357
　protective immunity 759
　serovars 750
　trachoma due to 748, 750–1, 4191
chloasma 1804, *3754*, 3756
chloracne 1165, 3752
chloral hydrate 1089
　overdose/poisoning 1061
chlorambucil
　in chronic lymphocytic leukaemia 3421,
　　3422
　in Hodgkin's disease *3573*, 3574
　in lymphoma *3585*
　in membranous nephropathy 3160
　in minimal change nephropathy 3155
　in polycythaemia vera 3434
　in rheumatoid arthritis 3193

chloramphenicol
　aplastic anaemia induced by 3441, 3442
　in bartonellosis 775
　Haemophilus influenzae type b disease
　　treatment 582
　in meningococcal meningitis 542
　in plague 598
　in pneumococcal infections 520
　in pregnancy 1785
　in rickettsial diseases 733
　in scrub typhus 741
　sideroblastic anaemia due to 3523
　in typhoid 564
chlorate poisoning **1121**, 3520, 3546
chlordiazepoxide, in alcohol withdrawal
　syndrome 4291
chlorhexidine, streptococci group B
　infection prevention 509
chloride
　secretion 1900, 1902
　transport,
　　abnormality in cystic fibrosis 2747
　　in Bartter's syndrome 3131
chloride channel 1900
chlorinated hydrocarbons 1395
　abuse 1092–3
chlorine 1096
　mechanisms of toxicity 1096
　poisoning **1096–7**
chlormethiazole 4253, 4355
　in alcohol withdrawal 4259, 4291
　poisoning 1060
chlornaphthazine, bladder cancer
　association 211, 212
chloro-acetaldehyde 1090
2-chloroacetophenone (CN) 1118, 1119
2-chlorodeoxyadenosine (CdA) *3422*,
　3423
chloroethene, *see* vinyl chloride
chloroethylene 1093
chloroethylene oxide 1090
chlorofluorocarbons (CFCs) 1091, *1091*
　poisoning **1091**, 1093
　sudden death due to 1093
chloroform
　as carcinogen 1085
　mechanisms of toxicity 1085–6
　metabolism 1086
　poisoning **1085–6**
　uses 1085
chloromethane, *see* methyl chloride
chloromethyl ethers 1167
chlorophenols, chloracne due to 1165
chlorophenoxyacetate herbicides **1121**,
　1121
chloroquine
　in amoebiasis 832
　in fascioliasis 987
　long-term effects 1254
　in malaria 851, 856
　　prophylaxis 860
　　resistance to 324, 860
　overdose/poisoning **1072–3**
　in porphyria 1395
　in pregnancy 856, 1810
　in renal impairment 3273
　resistance 324, 860
　retinal toxicity 4196–7
　retinopathy due to 3023
　in SLE 3023
chloroquine phosphate, in sarcoidosis
　2832
2-chlorovinyl-dichlorarsine, *see* lewisite
chlorpromazine
　emergency treatment of disturbed/
　　violent patients 4257
　in pruritus 3744
　side-effects 4252
　in terminal illness 4356
chlorpropamide 1470, 1471
　overdose/poisoning 1071
chlorprothixene 3945
chocolate 3753
choking, in Schwartz-Jampel syndrome
　(chondrodystrophic myotonia) 4153
cholangiocarcinoma **2118**
　in opisthorchiasis 982, 984

cholangiography
　intravenous 1834
　percutaneous transhepatic, *see*
　　percutaneous transhepatic
　　cholangiography (PTC)
cholangiosarcoma 204
cholangitis 2048
　in acute cholecystitis 2049
　'autoimmune' 2075
　bacterial overgrowth in 1912
　bacterial (suppurative) 2051
　in biliary atresia 2014
　clinical features 2056–7
　infestations causing 2051
　primary sclerosing 1948, 2044, **2053**,
　　2077–80
　　aetiology 2077–8
　　autoantibodies in 2078
　　clinical features 2078
　　diagnosis 2078–9
　　diagnostic criteria 2077
　　diseases associated 2077, 2079, *2079*
　　in HIV infection 2135
　　HLA association 2077–8
　　immune abnormalities 2077–8
　　natural history and prognosis 2079
　　treatment 2079–80
　recurrent, in Caroli's syndrome 2016
　relapsing pyogenic, in opisthorchiasis
　　982, 984
　sclerosing **2053**
　　in AIDS 475
　　causes 2077
　　drugs associated 2129
　　in inflammatory bowel disease 2131
　　primary, *see above*
　　secondary 2053, 2077, 2129
cholecalciferol (vitamin D₃) 1625, 3059
cholecystectomy 2048
　in acute cholecystitis 2049
　in acute pancreatitis 2033
　laparoscopic 2048, 2050
　in pregnancy 1801
cholecystitis
　acalculous 2049
　acute 2048, **2049–50**
　angina *vs* 2322
　chronic 2048, **2050**
　cryptosporidial 874
　in diabetes 1493
　septicaemia in 1021
cholecystography, oral 1834, 2046
cholecystokinin (CCK) **1892**
　antagonists 1892
　pancreatic carcinoma risk 2040
　receptors/receptor antagonists 1892
　secretion 1892
cholecystokinin-secretin test 2036
choledochal cyst 2016
choledocholithiasis 2048, **2050–1**, 2050
　in acute pancreatitis 2028
　treatment and stone removal 2051
cholelithiasis 2046, 2048
　chronic pancreatitis in 2034
　gallbladder cancer association 204
　oral contraceptives and 1724
　see also gallstones
cholera 43, **576–80**
　blood chemistry in 578, *579*
　carriers 577
　clinical case:infection ratio 577
　clinical features 578, 1824, 2002
　diagnosis 578–9
　epidemiology 576–7
　fluid/electrolyte secretion 577, *578*,
　　2002
　immunization and prevention 580
　management 579, 2006
　　results 579–80
　metabolic acidosis due to 1543
　pandemics 576
　pathogenesis 577–8, 2001–2, 2002
　transmission, historical aspects 285
　vaccine 323, 580
　see also Vibrio cholerae
cholescintigraphy 1834
cholestanol 1437

cholestasis 2059
　in acute hepatitis, drug-induced 2125,
　　2126
　in α₁-antitrypsin deficiency 2131
　bland, drug-induced 2125–6, *2127*
　causes 2014, *2051*
　　occupational *1172*
　chronic **2023**
　　drug-induced 2129, *2129*
　　clinical features 2046, 2056
　　contraceptive steroid-induced **2060**
　　copper toxicity 1419, 1423
　　extrahepatic 2059
　　hepatitis, drug-induced 2125, *2127*
　in hepatocellular failure 2107
　intrahepatic **2059–60**, 2129
　　in acute viral hepatitis 2061
　　benign recurrent **2059–60**
　　liver function tests and histology 2059
　　of pregnancy **1796**
　　in total parenteral nutrition 2132, 2140
　jaundice, *see* jaundice
　in pregnancy **2060**
　in primary sclerosing cholangitis 2077,
　　2078, 2079
　in vanishing bile-duct syndrome 2059,
　　2079, 2129
　see also biliary tract, obstruction
cholestatic syndromes, chronic **2023**
cholesteatoma **4033**
cholesterol 1400, 2047
　bile saturation 2047, 2050
　in chylous fluid 2868
　in cirrhosis 2088
　crystal deposition 2991
　dietary,
　　hyper-responders to 2311
　　ischaemic heart disease risk 2311
　entry into cells 1403
　in lungs 2837
　peroxisomal biosynthesis 1439
　secretion rate 2047
　serum,
　　coronary heart disease risk and
　　　1404–5, 1407–8, 1412
　　in diabetes *1466*
　　levels 2307
　　levels after myocardial infarction 2339
　　measurement 1413
　　in nephrotic syndrome 3142–3
　　normal values 1405
　　in pregnancy 1753
　　reduced levels 1414
　　reduction in ischaemic heart disease
　　　2316–17
　　reduction in myocardial infarction
　　　prevention 2348
　　therapeutic reduction 1412, 1413–14
　　in thyroid disease 1609
　　see also hypercholesterolaemia
　storage disease (cerebrotendinous
　　xanthomatosis) 1406, **1437**
　stores, in obesity 1308
　synthesis and metabolism 2047
　total, ischaemic heart disease risk
　　2307–8
　transport, from liver/gut to tissues
　　1402–3
　　from tissues to liver (reverse) 1403–4
cholesterol desmolase, *see* P₄₅₀scc
cholesterol embolism **2375–7**, 3952
　clinical features and investigations
　　2376, 3952, 4186
　distribution/sites 2375
　epidemiology and risk factors 2376
　histology 2376–7
　management 2377
cholesterol gallstones 2047–8
　formation 2047–8
cholesteryl esters 1400, 2291
　deposition, *see* Wolman's disease
　storage disease *1435*, 1436–7, *2019*,
　　2025, 3591
　transfer protein 1402, 1404
　transport from liver and gut 1401–3
cholestyramine 1414, 3744
　as adsorbent in poisoning 1049

ischaemic heart disease prevention 2316
in primary biliary cirrhosis 2076
in primary sclerosing cholangitis 2078
rodenticide poisoning management 1123
cholic acid 2047
choline acetyltransferase, reduced
in Alzheimer's disease 3972
in multiple system atrophy 4006
cholinergic drugs
asthma exacerbation 2849
GH secretion and 1578
cholinesterase 4365
monitoring, in insecticide poisoning 1122
cholinesterase inhibitors 1247
in chemical warfare 1115, **1117–18**
see also nerve agents
organophosphorus insecticides 1122, 1174
chondrocalcinosis 2988, 2989, *2990*
in haemochromatosis 3005
chondrocytes
bone mineralization 3058
receptors 2981
chondrodysplasia 3088
chondrodysplasia punctata, rhizomelic (RCDP) *1440*, **1441–2**
chondrodystrophic myotonia **4153**
chondroitin sulphate, increase, in osteoarthritis 2981
chondrosarcoma, jaw 1863
CHOP combination chemotherapy 3421, *3422*, 3585
chordae tendinae 2451
abnormal 2399
in mitral regurgitation 2457
in mixed mitral valve disease 2456
repair 2461
ruptured 2457, **2458–9**
in endocarditis 2439
chorda tympani 3878
chordoma 3895, **4033**
chordopoxviruses 365
chorea 3863, **4012–14**
benign hereditary 4014
causes *4010*
definition 4009–10
gravidarum 1769
hemichorea **4014**
in polycythaemia rubra vera 4010
in rheumatic fever 2433, 4012
in SLE 4130
Sydenham's 503, 2433, **4012**
treatment 2435
see also Huntington's disease
choreoathetosis
paroxysmal dystonic **4020**
paroxysmal kinesigenic **4020**
chorioamnionitis **1785–7**
choriocarcinoma
hCG production 1714
hyperthyroidism 1612, 1714, 1749
in pregnancy 1767
pulmonary emboli in 2522
chorionic gonadotrophin 1555, 1556
human, see human chorionic gonadotrophin
chorionic somatomammotropin 1556
gene 1576
human, see human placental lactogen
chorionic somatomammotropin-like gene 1576
chorionic villus biopsy 136
muscular dystrophies 4147
osteogenesis imperfecta diagnosis 3082
choroidal infarcts 4188
choroidal melanoma 4180
choroiditis, tuberculous 4061
choroidoretinal lesions, in onchocerciasis 915
choroidoretinitis, in HIV infection 476
choroid-plexus cyst 135
choroid-plexus papillomas **4033**
Christmas disease, see haemophilia B
chromaffin tissue 2554

chromate
manufacture 2880
nasal sinus and nose cancers association 205
chromatin 59
nuclear envelope assembly 80
peripheral 825
regulation of structure 59
serum amyloid P component binding 1521
chrome, contact dermatitis due to 3738
chrome ulcer 1107
of nasal septum 205
chromic acid, absorption 1107
chromium 1107, **1424**
compounds and uses 1107
inhalation 1107
poisoning **1107–8**
VI compounds 1107
Chromobacterium violaceum 551, *554*
chromoblastomycosis **813–14**
chromomycosis **813–14**
chromosomal abnormalities 100, **117–23**
in acute leukaemia *3400*, 3401, *3402*
in Burkitt's lymphoma 3567, 3580
in chronic lymphocytic leukaemia *3395*, 3411, *3412*, 3421
congenital abnormalities due to 66
deletion syndrome, neurological aspects **4109–11**
in Fanconi anaemia 3446
frequency 121
in Hodgkin's disease 3569
in holoprosencephaly 4113
inversions 123
in haemophilia A 108, 134
in leukaemia 3395–6
in lymphoproliferative disorders 3567
male infertility in 1685
maternal age and *120–1*
in megaloblastic anaemia 3495
mental retardation due to **4108–11**
in myelodysplastic syndromes **3428–9**
in myelomatosis 3597
non-disjunction 119, 121, 128
of number 121
mental retardation in 4108–9
trisomies 121–2, 4108–9
osteoporosis and **3070**
segregation 118
sex chromosomes, see sex chromosomes
short stature in 1699–700
structural 118, **123**
translocations, see chromosomal translocations
chromosomal analysis 102, **119**
methods 62
staining and banding methods 119
see also DNA analysis; genetic analysis
chromosomal translocations 118, **122–3**
in acute lymphoblastic leukaemia 3401, *3402*, 3411, *3412*
in acute myeloid leukaemia *3400*
in ataxia telangiectasia 173
balanced Robertsonian 122
bcr/abl gene, see *bcr/abl* gene
in leukaemia 3395, 3396
reciprocal 122
nomenclature 119
Robertsonian 122–3
in tumours 65, *230*
X/autosomal reciprocal 117
chromosome 6, complement genes 178
chromosome 11, atopic disease association 158
chromosome 21
Robertsonian translocation 121
trisomy 121
chromosome 22, in thymic aplasia (Di George syndrome) 171
chromosomes 104
crossing-over 103
unequal 108
gene mapping, see gene(s), mapping
karyotype description/nomenclature 119
loss, genetic analysis of tumours 194

marker, in tumours 192
metaphase 119
microdeletions 108, *108*, 127, 129
non-disjunction 119, 121, 128
normal karyotypes 118
painting 62, 119
rearrangements 108
in tumours 192
satellites 119
walking 62
chronic diseases
anaemia of, see anaemia, of chronic disorders
in general practice *48*
self-reported 41, *43*
chronic fatigue syndrome (myalgic encephalomyelitis) 353, **1035–9**, *1036*, 2997, 4155
aetiology 386, 1037–8
assessments 1038–9
clinical features 1038
coxsackieviruses association 386
definition 1035, *1036*
depressive/anxiety disorders and 1037, 1038
differential diagnosis 1038, *1038*
epidemics 1036–7
epidemiology 1036–7
human herpesvirus 6 (HHV-6) in 365
management and treatment 1038–9
neurological features 4074
patient information on 1038, 1039
prognosis 1039
use of term 1036
chronic granulomatous disease (CGD) **3560**, 3561
gastrointestinal disease in *1840*
hepatic granulomas in 2122
neutrophils in 2759
of nose 3799, 3800, *3801*
chronic idiopathic intestinal pseudo-obstruction (CIIP) 1959–60
chronic obstructive airways disease (COAD) **2766–79**
acute exacerbations **2925–7**
acute increase in breathlessness **2777**
aetiology **2768**
aircraft travel and 1202
α_1-antitrypsin, deficiency 2769, **2771–2**, 2771
'normal' 2772
asthma overlap 2767
bacterial pneumonia in 2700
cellular and molecular events **2769–70**
chronic hypoxia in 2902
circulatory failure **2571–2**, 2777
clinical features **2773–4**
complications 2777
cor pulmonale in 2516, 2517, 2520, 2777, 2927
definition and terminology 2632, **2766–7**
epidemiology **2767–8**
prevalence 2520, 2767
examination 2773–4
health care costs 2520
infections in 2735, 2777
in injecting drug abusers 4282
investigations **2774–5**
chest radiography **2664–5**, 2774
lung function tests 2768, 2774–5
lung and heart-lung transplantation 2934
management 2520, **2775–7**
acute exacerbations **2925–7**
chronic stable ventilatory failure **2927–9**
deteriorating patients 2927
drugs 2776
oxygen 2776, 2926, **2927–8**
of respiratory drive 2926
respiratory muscle pump capacity 2926
surgical 2777
ventilation 2924, 2926
ventilatory load 2927
mortality 2520, 2767
natural history 2768
pathological processes 2632

pathophysiology **2632–3**, *2632–5*, **2768–9**
gas exchange 2769
polycythaemia in 3551, 3553
in pregnancy 1745
proteinase-antiproteinase theory **2770–3**
inhibitors and proteins in 2772–3
see also α_1-antitrypsin (above)
pulmonary rehabilitation 2929
respiratory failure in 2774, 2925
smoking and 2767, 2768
special categories **2777–8**
types A and B 2769
unilateral transradiancy of lung **2778**
see also bronchiolitis, chronic; emphysema
chronic obstructive pulmonary disease, see chronic obstructive airways disease
chronic vegetative state, see persistent vegetative state
chrysanthemum, dermatitis 3738
Chryseomonas luteola 554
Chrysomya bezziana 1000, 1001
Chrysops 917
chrysotile 2843, 2845
Churg-Strauss syndrome 2689–90, **2800–1**, 3011, 3015
clinical features 2800, **3015**
gastrointestinal tract in 2000
laboratory findings 2801
lung involvement 2689–90, **2800–1**
open-lung biopsy 2689–90
pathogenesis and treatment 2801
response to treatment 3017
Chvostek's sign 1633, 3061
chylomicrons 1277, 1401–2, 1409
in diabetes 1457, 1458
remnants 1401–2, 1408
chylothorax **2868**
chyluria, in filariasis 923, 924
chymotrypsin
in acute pancreatitis 2029
faecal *2037*
chymotrypsin inhibitors, reduced in urticaria 3770
cigarette
burns from 3779
low-tar 206
cigarette smoke
carbon monoxide source 1230
polynuclear aromatic hydrocarbons in 1166
see also smoke
cigarette smoking, see smoking; tobacco
ciguatera fish poisoning 1142, 2005
cilastatin, in renal failure *3272*
cilia, bronchial epithelial cells 2613
function assessment 2613, 2668
ciliary dyskinesia, primary 2613, 2759
ciliospinal reflex 2584
cimetidine 1886–7
drug interactions 1887
in gastric cancer 1984
overdose/poisoning 1070
peptic ulcer treatment 1886, 1887
long-term 1887, 1889
short-term 1887
in polycythaemia vera 3434
side-effects 1689, 1718, 1887
Cimex lenticularis 1005
cinchona alkaloids 845
overdose/poisoning **1072–3**
cinchonism 851
cineangiography, single plane 2222
ciprofloxacillin, meningococcal infections prophylaxis 542
ciprofloxacin
in brucellosis 623
in *Neisseria gonorrhoeae* infections 548, 549
in *Pseudomonas aeruginosa* infections 2752, *2752*
in Q fever 744
in renal impairment 3271–2
in rickettsial diseases 733

ciprofloxacin (*cont.*)
in *Salmonella* infections 553
in urinary-tract infections *3211*
circadian rhythm
asthma 2730, 2731
autonomic function and heart 2160–1
blood pressure 2160, 2528, 2545
hormone secretion 1565
lung function variations 2674
myocardial infarction 2325, 2334
circle of Willis 3947, 3949
circulation
collateral, in coarctation of aorta 2557
disturbances, positive-pressure
ventilation indications 2576
major acute derangements **2563–76**
in malnutrition 1283
normal pressures/resistances *2488*, *2506*
systemic-pulmonary, abnormal 2402,
2424–8
circulatory failure **2563–82**
in obstructive airways disease **2571–2**
circulatory neurasthenia (Da Costa's
syndrome) 2169, 2174, 4207
circumcision
cervical carcinoma risk and 210
urinary-tract infections and 3206
cirrhosis **2085–91**
abdominal examination 2088
alcoholic, *see* alcoholic cirrhosis
in α₁-antitrypsin deficiency 1547
in autoimmune hepatitis 2072, 2073
bacterial overgrowth aetiology 1912
bridging necrosis in 2072
causes 2085, *2086*
clinical approach 2057
clinical features 2086–8
signs 2087–8
compensated 2085
complications 2089–90
see also ascites; portal hypertension
computed tomography (CT) 2012
cryptogenic 2114
liver transplantation in 2112
decompensated 2085, 2091
see also hepatic decompensation
diagnosis/differential diagnosis 2089,
2089
drug-induced 2129, *2129*
gynaecomastia in 1688
in hepatitis B 2066, 2067
hepatocellular carcinoma in 204, 2090,
2116
in hereditary haemochromatosis 3478
Indian childhood *1417*
in inflammatory bowel disease 2131
investigations 2088–9, *2090*
juvenile, in α₁-antitrypsin deficiency 1547
liver transplantation in 2091, 2112–13
lung disease association 2130
see also hepatopulmonary syndrome
macronodular 2086
management 2090–1
drugs in 2091
micronodular 2086
jejunoileal bypass causing 2139
pathology and histology 2086
pleural effusion in 2866
in pregnancy **1800–1**
primary biliary, *see* primary biliary
cirrhosis
pulmonary hypertension in 2509
splenomegaly in 3589
travel precautions 2091
in Wilson's disease 1420, 1421
see also biliary cirrhosis
cisapride 1489, 1868
cisplatin
nephrotoxicity 3263
neuropathy due to 4100
side-effects 248
cisternography
computed tomography 3818
radionuclide 3825
citrate, urinary, in renal tubular acidosis
3339
citreoviridin 1158
citric acid cycle, *see* tricarboxylic acid
(TCA) cycle

citrulline 1357, 1358
civil action, medical negligence 4311
Civil Aviation Authority 1200, 2360
Cladosporium carrionii 813
'clasp knife' resistance 3857
clathrin-coated structures/vesicles 74, 75
claudication
cauda equina **3907–8**
intermittent,
angina with 2328
clinical features 2364
management 2369
risk with smoking *2363*
Claviceps purpurea 1158
clavulanic acid, in actinomycoses 685
claw-hand deformity 4096
cleft lip/palate, multifactorial inheritance
129
clergyman's knee 2996
climate, changes and effects 36, 322
climatotherapy 3748, 3750
clindamycin
in anaerobic infections 575, 576
in babesiosis 865
in bacterial vaginosis 3355
clinical chemistry, in jaundice 2055–6
clinical examination **15–20**
accuracy 15
evaluation method **15–20**
precision 15–17
clinical records
diabetic 1504
medical negligence cases 4312
see also medical reports
clinical trials **21–32**, **1261–2**
blindness in 1262
conduct and aims 1261–2
controls 1262
criteria for selection and design 1262
definition 1261
detecting moderate effects 21–2
ethics 1262
large-scale randomized (mega-trials) 21,
24
examples of important results 26–7,
28–31
relevance to clinical practice 31–2
placebos in 1259–60, 1260, 1262
randomized 22–5, 1262
basic machinery 23
entry criteria 24–5
numbers of patients needed 24
problems of subgroup analyses 23–4
rationale 22
small, *vs* a mega-trial 29–30
systematic overviews, *see* systematic
overviews
see also randomization
Clioquinol, in amoebiasis 832
CLIP170 83
cloacal membrane 1972, 1973
clobazam, in epilepsy 3922
clodronate, in hypercalcaemia 1633,
1638, 3228
clofazimine
in leprosy 675–6, 676
side-effects 675–6, 677
clofibrate 2304
peroxisome proliferation 83, 84
clomiphene 1678, 1688
clonality 3718
assessment, in haematological disorders
3390–2
of endocrine neoplasia 1568–9
of leukaemias 3393, *3394*
of lymphoproliferative disorders
3566–7
clonal origin of tumours, evidence 192
clonazepam, in epilepsy 3922
clonidine
mechanism of action 1065
in opiate detoxification 4292
overdose/poisoning 1065
stimulation test *1699*
test, phaeochromocytoma diagnosis 2555
cloning, *see* gene(s), cloning
cloning vectors 61
see also vectors

clonorchiasis *982*, **984–6**
gallbladder cancer association 204
haematological changes 3681
Clonorchis sinensis 982, 983, 984, 985,
2051
closed fist injuries 573
clostridial infections **630–7**
of gastrointestinal tract **634–7**
see also colitis, pseudomembranous;
necrotizing enterocolitis
myositis 4155
see also botulism; gas gangrene; tetanus
Clostridium 569
Clostridium botulinum 630
spores 631, 632
toxin and production of 630, 631
types (A–G) 630
see also botulism
Clostridium difficile 634, 1034, 2004
cytotoxins 636, 2004
detection and culture 635–6
see also colitis, pseudomembranous
Clostridium perfringens (welchii) 632,
636, 1020, 2133
detection 633
diagnosis and culture 571
enterotoxin-producing strains 637
food poisoning 285, **637**, 2002
haemolytic anaemia 3545
myositis 4155
toxins 633, 636, 637
Clostridium perfringens (welchii) type C
636, 2004
Clostridium tetani 624
toxins 624
see also tetanus
Clostridium welchii, *see* Clostridium
perfringens
clot
colic 3238, 3243
fibrin 3622
CLOtest 1885
clothing dermatitis 3736–7
clotting, *see* coagulation
clotting factors, *see* coagulation, factors
clotting time, activated 3660
Cloward's operation 3908
clozapine 4252–3
indications and use 4252
side-effects 4252–3
clubbing of fingers **2651**, 3760
in bronchiectasis 2757
in cryptogenic fibrosing alveolitis 2789
in cyanotic congenital heart disease 2400
differential diagnosis 2651
in diffuse parenchymal lung disease
2781
in Ebstein's anomaly 2414
in Fallot's tetralogy 2402
in hepatocellular failure 2104
in infective endocarditis 2441
in lung cancer 2884–5
in transposition of great arteries 2416
in tumours *244*
'clue cells' 3354, 3356
clumping factor 523
clumsy child **4122**
cluster headache **4026**
Clutton's joints 3002
c-*myc* oncogene
in Burkitt's lymphoma 149, 355
role in apoptosis 225
COAD, *see* chronic obstructive airways
disease
coagulase, free and bound 523
coagulase-negative staphylococci, *see*
staphylococci
coagulation **3619–22**, 3642
adult respiratory distress syndrome
pathogenesis 2855
contact activation pathway 3621–2
hereditary disorders 3651–2
control 3663
disorders, *see* coagulation disorders
(*below*)
disseminated intravascular, *see*
disseminated intravascular
coagulation (DIC)

drug action via 1248
factors 3619–20
acquired inhibitors **3661**
atherosclerotic plaque development
2294
impaired synthesis, in hepatocellular
failure 2102
ischaemic heart disease and 2303
isolated acquired deficiencies 3661
in malaria 850
plasma levels 3628–9
vitamin K-dependent 3619
see also specific factors
inappropriate activation, pulmonary
oedema pathogenesis 2498
intravascular, in leptospirosis 699
intrinsic system **3621**, 3622
hereditary disorders 3646–52
platelet function in **3618–19**
in pregnancy 1762
pulmonary endothelial cell role 2299,
2487
pulmonary endothelial cells interaction
2487, 2498, 2514
tissue-factor (extrinsic) pathway
3620–1, 3622
hereditary disorders 3652
coagulation disorders 3004–5, **3627–30**
acquired **3653–61**
in haemolytic uraemic syndrome 3200
hereditary **3637–53**
in malignant disease *3677*, *3678*, *3679*
in nephrotic syndrome **3142**, 3144,
3656–7
in newborn **3654–5**
in paracetamol poisoning 1053
in pre-eclampsia 1728, 1763
in primary myelosclerosis 3436
in renal disease **3682**
screening tests 3628–9
thrombotic disorders in 3667
in viral infections 3680
coagulative necrosis 1996
coal dust 2839
coal macule 2839, 2840
coal miners, cancer association 216,
2840
coal-worker's pneumoconiosis **2839–41**
aetiology and pathology 2839–40
clinical features 2840–1
prevention and management 2841
tuberculosis and lung cancer in 216,
2840
co-amoxiclav (clavulanic acid/
amoxycillin)
in pregnancy 1785, 1790
in urinary-tract infections *3211*
coarctation of aorta, *see* aorta,
coarctation
coated pits 73, 74
'coatomer complex' 75
Coats' syndrome 4148
cobalamin 3484
absorption 1903
malabsorption 2039
metabolism 1370, 1371
cobalt 1108
contact dermatitis due to 3738
poisoning **1108**
polycythaemia due to 3554
cobamides 1913
cobras
bites and envenoming 1126, 1127,
1131, 1132
interval between bite and death 1139
ophthalmia management 1139
cobrotoxin 1129
cocaine 1076–7, 4264
complications associated 1077, 4280
overdose **1076–7**
psychiatric disturbances from 4241
withdrawal syndrome **4293**
see also drug abuse and misuse
coca leaves 4264
coccidian-like organism 876
Coccidioides immitis 812, 3000
coccidioidomycosis 803, **812–13**
arthritis in 3000

disseminated 813
pulmonary 813
cochlear organs, nerve supply 3869
Cochliomyia hominivorax 1000, 1001
Cochrane Collaboration 25
Cockayne's syndrome 3989, 4111
cockroaches 1011
codeine 2644, 4025
analgesic nephropathy and 3221, *3222*
in liver disease 2091
codons 57
coelenterates, venomous 1143–4
coeliac artery, compression 2367
coeliac axis
atheroma 1996
compression 1997
coeliac axis angiography 1833
in gastrointestinal bleeding 3683
in insulinoma 1508
coeliac disease 1824, 1843, **1916–20**,
3782
adenocarcinoma of small intestine 1986
aetiology 1918, 1929
associated diseases 1919, 3723
clinical features 1918
in common varied immunodeficiency
(CVID) 169
complications 1920, 1929, 3583
definition 1916
diagnosis/assessment 1918–19
differential diagnosis 1919, 1920
enteropathy-associated T-cell
lymphoma relation 1920, 1929
epidemiology 1917
extrinsic allergic alveolitis and 2813
folate deficiency 3492
genetic susceptibility 1918
gluten sensitivity 1843, 1916
gut peptides in 1895
history 1916
HLA associations 1917, 1918
immune response 1918, 1919
investigations 1918–19
endoscopic biopsy 1908
endoscopy indication 1829
jejunal biopsy 1832, 1918
small-bowel radiology in 1910, 1919
iron-deficiency anaemia 3476
joint involvement 3004
liver in 2132
lymphoma complicating 1920, 1929,
3583
risk 1920, 1929, 1985
malabsorption in 1918
assessment 1918–19
tropics and 1930
osteomalacia in 3073
pathogenesis 1918
pathology 1916–17
pregnancy in 1802
prognosis 1920
selective IgA deficiency in 1839–40,
1919
splenic atrophy 3592
stages in development 1917
treatment 1919–20
unresponsive disease 1920
vitamin B$_{12}$ deficiency 3491
vitamin D deficiency 1636
coeliac plexus block, in pancreatic
carcinoma 2045
Coeliac Society 1919
Coenurus cerebralis 959
coffee
bladder cancer association 212
ischaemic heart disease risk 2312
pancreatic carcinoma risk 2040
Coffin-Lowry syndrome 4111
Cogan's sign 4161
Cogan's syndrome, eye in **4184**
cognitive behavioural therapy **4255**
in anorexia nervosa 1299, 4215
in bulimia nervosa 1300, 4217, 4255
in panic disorder 4207
techniques 4255
cognitive function, localization **3845**
cognitive impairment 3845, **3965–7**
after acute lymphocytic leukaemia 3414

in Alzheimer's disease 3973
in cerebral metastases 250
classification of severity 4341, *4341*
in dementia 4224
in depressive disorders 4218
in elderly 4341
in frontal lobe damage 3854
in HIV infection 475, 4076
localization 3845, *3846*
in multiple sclerosis 3993
non-linguistic 3849
in normal pressure hydrocephalus 3970
occupational causes 1174
in Parkinson's disease 4001
in progressive supranuclear palsy 4005
in strokes 4237
see also dementia
cognitive mental disorders, *see* organic
mental disorders
cognitive restructuring procedures 4217
cogwheeling 3973, 4001
cohort studies 44, 45
coitus, *see* sexual intercourse
colchicine 1524, 1527, 3180–1, 3274
in Behçet's syndrome 3046
in gout 2987, 2988
cold **1182–5**
acclimatization 1182
asthma in 2731
coronary/cerebral thrombosis after 1185
cryoglobulin precipitation 3050
effect on body 1182–3
local cooling effect 1183
hypersensitivity 2366
immersion hypothermia 1183
injury 1183
non-freezing, *see* immersion injury
prevention and management 1183
pain treatment 3943
paramyotonia induced by 4152
Raynaud's phenomenon association
2945
sensitivity, in anorexia nervosa 4213
skin disease and 3724
urticaria 3779
familial/acquired 3770, 3771
vasculitis due to 3776
see also frostbite; hypothermia
cold agglutinins 2696
detection 764
mycoplasmal infections 762, 763
titre *3379*
cold haemagglutinin disease
acute 3544
chronic 3544
in mycoplasma pneumonia 3544, 3685
cold haemoglobinuria, paroxysmal 714,
3544
colds, *see* common cold
cold sores 343, **1849–50**, 4066
aetiology and pathology 1849
see also herpes simplex virus (HSV)
infection
Cole-Cecil murmur 2465
colectomy
in colorectal carcinoma 1993
in Crohn's disease 1943
in familial adenomatous polyposis 1990
prophylactic, in ulcerative colitis 1950
in pseudomembranous colitis 636
urgent, in ulcerative colitis 1949
see also proctocolectomy
coleoptera, venomous **1146**
colestipol 1414
Coley's toxin 226
colic
biliary 2050
clot 3238, 3243
ureteric (renal), *see* ureteric colic
coliform bacteria 550
tropical sprue aetiopathogenesis 1934
see also enterobacteria
colipase 1903
colitis
amoebic, *see* amoebic colitis
antibiotic-associated, *see* colitis,
pseudomembranous
collagenous 1947, 2136–7

in common varied immunodeficiency
(CVID) 169
Crohn's (granulomatous), *see* Crohn's
disease
cystica 2136
drug-induced 1947
fulminant amoebic 828
haemorrhagic 1996, 2003
indeterminate 1947
infective 1945
amoebic colitis *vs* 828
causes 1947
ulcerative colitis *vs* 1945, 1947
ischaemic 1947, **1997–8**
causes 1947
'lymphocytic' 2037, 2137
microscopic 1947, 2136, 2137
pseudomembranous (antibiotic-
associated) **634–6**, 1947, 2003, 2004,
2006
amoebic colitis *vs* 829
clinical features 634–5, 1034
diagnosis 635–6
treatment and prevention 636
see also Clostridium difficile
segmental 1941
in *Shigella* infections 554
in trichuriasis 943
ulcerative, *see* ulcerative colitis
collagen 1272, **3057**
cross-linking, blockade 2793
deposition, in diffuse interstitial fibrosis
of lung 2637
disorders, *see* collagen disorders
disturbances in diabetes **1489–90**
excess, in cryptogenic fibrosing
alveolitis 2789
gene(s) 3081, 3082
gene mutations 3057, 3079, 3081, 3088
in osteogenesis imperfecta 3079, 3081
in granulation tissue 2626
in heart 2145
'hole zones' 3057
increase in heart failure 2230
in lung 2598, 2632
necrosis 3799
in platelet activation 3614, 3615, 3617
synthesis and assembly 3057, 3058
type(s) **3057**, *3057*
type I 3055, 3057
α-chains 3057
in osteogenesis imperfecta 109, 3079,
3080
type II,
in osteoarthritis 2981
in skeletal dysplasia 3088
synthesis 3088
type III, in collagenous colitis 2137
type IV,
in Alport's syndrome 3205
anti-GBM antibodies 3164
autoantibodies to 163
type IX 3058
collagenase 2626, 3056
in adult respiratory distress syndrome
2854
inhibitors 260
collagen-derived peptides, in bone
turnover assessments 3060
collagen disorders 3057, **3787–90**
defective collagen in 3788
gastrointestinal/tract involvement
1999–2000
signs 3787–8
skin disease/changes in 3788
see also connective tissue diseases;
dermatomyositis; systemic lupus
erythematosus (SLE); systemic
sclerosis
'collagen vascular' diseases 3017
see also connective tissue diseases;
systemic lupus erythematosus (SLE)
collateral circulation, in coarctation of
aorta 2557
'collodion fetus' 3719
colloid
bleeding oesophageal varices
management 2094

cysts **4032–3**
milium 3788
colomycin 2752
colon
absorption role 1900
acute dilatation 1950, 2138
in Crohn's disease 1938
in ulcerative colitis 1945
aganglionosis, *see* Hirschsprung's
disease
atresia **1978–9**
blood supply 1996, 1997
cancer, *see* colorectal carcinoma
in collagenous colitis 2137
Crohn's disease, *see* Crohn's disease
cystic disorders **2136**
disease,
endoscopy indication 1829
skin disease in 3723
disorders, in pregnancy 1803
distension, chest pain in 2168
diverticular disease, *see* diverticular
disease, colonic
dysplasia 1950, 1988, 1989
embryology 1973
fluid absorption 1824
ischaemia, *see* intestinal ischaemia
isolated ulcers **2138**
lymphoid tissue in 1987
lymphoma 1993
malakoplakia 2137
manometry 1956
motor activity 1955
see also gastrointestinal motility
normal bacterial flora 1911
obstruction, in systemic sclerosis
1999
pain 1822
in colorectal cancer 1991
preparation, colonoscopy 1946
pressures 1969
pseudo-obstruction, acute (Ogilivie's
syndrome) **2138**
resection,
colonic adenoma removal 1989
in colorectal carcinoma 1993
right, acute dilatation 2138
role 1824
in schistosomiasis 976
sigmoid, *see* sigmoid colon
smooth muscle, hypersegmentation
1969
spastic 1844, 1965
in spinal cord injury 3900
stricture,
'apple-core' 1992
in colorectal cancer 1992
in ulcerative colitis 1950
structural lesions, haematological
disorders 3684
in systemic sclerosis *3030*
transit time 1952
tumours,
benign, *see* colonic polyps
malignant 1993–4
see also colonic adenoma; colorectal
carcinoma
wall, changes in diverticular disease
1969
see also entries beginning intestinal;
intestine
colonic adenoma
adenocarcinoma sequence 1988–9
aetiological factors and pathology
1987–8
benign 1987, 1988
clinical features and management
1989
familial, *see* familial adenomatous
polyposis (FAP)
follow-up 1989
hypokalaemia due to 3130, 3184
invasion in carcinomatous change
1988
'microadenoma' 1989
tubular 1987, 1988
tubulovillous 1987, 1988
villous 1987, 1988

colonic fistulae, in diverticular disease 1972
colonic polyps **1986–90**
  in acromegaly 1593
  adenomatous, *see* colonic adenoma
  classification 1986, *1987*
  clinical features and management 1989
  hamartomatous 1986–7
    see also Peutz-Jeghers syndrome
  inflammatory 1986
  metaplastic (hyperplastic) 1986
  neoplastic 1986–7
    see also colonic adenoma
  non-neoplastic 1986–7
  number and pathology 1986
  postinflammatory 1986
colonopathy, in tropical sprue 1933
colonoscopy in colorectal carcinoma 1992
  in colorectal carcinoma families 1990
  in Crohn's disease 1939–40, 1941
  in diverticular disease 1970, 1971
  in ulcerative colitis 1946, 1950
  in vascular dysplasia 1998
colony-forming unit-eosinophil (CFU-Eo) 3388
colony-forming unit-erythroid (CFU-E) 3387, 3452–3
colony-forming unit-granulocyte (CFU-G) 3388
colony-forming unit-granulocyte, erythrocyte, monocyte and megakaryocyte (CFU-GEMM) 3388
colony-forming unit-granulocyte-macrophage (CFU-GM) 3388, 3429
colony-forming unit-megakaryocyte (CFU-meg) 3389
colony-forming unit-monocyte (CFU-M) 3388
colony-forming unit-spleen (CFU-S) 3385–7
colony hybridization 61
colony-stimulating factors (CSFs) 96, 97, 3388, 3557
colophony, contact dermatitis 3737
Colorado tick fever **406**
colorectal adenomas, *see* colonic adenoma
colorectal carcinoma **1990–4**
  adenoma-carcinoma sequence 1988–9, 1991
  aetiological factors 203–4, 219, 1990
  barium enema 1832
  'breakthrough' 1993
  clinical features 1991–2
  coexisting with adenomas 1988
  in Crohn's disease 1939, 1993
  de novo 1989
  differential diagnosis 1992
  Dukes classification 1991, *1992*
  epidemiology 203–4, 1988–9, 1990
  familial 1990
    hereditary non-polyposis 107, 1990
    see also familial adenomatous polyposis (FAP)
  genes and mutations 65–6, 1990–1
    number of mutations 66
  genetic factors 65–6, 1990–1
  in situ 1988
  invasive, frequency *1989*
  investigations 1992
  pathology 1991
  screening and follow-up 1992–3
  spread and metastases 1991
  staging investigations *236*
  survival 1993
  treatment and results 1993
    palliative 1993
  in ulcerative colitis 1950, 1991, **1993**
colostomy
  in Hartmann's procedure 1971
  in Hirschsprung's disease 1979
colour developers, lichen planus 3751
colour Doppler flow mapping, *see under* Doppler echocardiography
colour duplex ultrasound, peripheral arterial disease investigation 2368
colouring agents, food 3729

colovesical fistula 1972
colpitis, in trichomoniasis 908
Colubridae, bites and envenoming 1126, 1131
Columbian theory, syphilis origin 707
coma **3930–3**
  after head injury 4048, *4048*
  in alcohol intoxication 1080, 4276–7
  auditory evoked potentials in 3836
  brain death diagnosis 3934
  in cardiac arrest 2284
  causes 2585
  in cerebral malaria 845, 846
  clinical assessment 3930–1
  in diabetes **1497–503**
  diagnosis of type/cause 3931, *3931, 3932*
  drug-induced 2583
  electroencephalogram (EEG) in 3830
  eye signs 3931
  Glasgow coma scale *3931*
  grading 1046–7, *1046*
  hepatic **4124**
  history-taking 3930
  hyperglycaemic diabetic **1498–503**
  hypoglycaemic **1497–8**, *1499*, 1506, 4123
  iron overdose 1071
  level 3930, *3931*
  metabolic 3931, *3931, 3932*
  myxoedema 1616
  in opioid overdose 1058
  poisoning 1045, 1046, 1047
  position in tonic-clonic seizure 3912
  prediction of outcome 3932
  related conditions 3931–2
  respiration in 3931
  somatosensory evoked potentials (SEP) in 3835
  in tricyclic antidepressant poisoning 1059
  in Wernicke-Korsakoff syndrome 4127
  see also unconsciousness
Comamonas, rare species *554*
combined anterior pituitary test 1585
comedo 3716
  closed 3752
  extractor 3754
  open 3752
Committee on Safety of Medicines, immunotherapy of allergic rhinitis 2718
common bile duct 2045
  obstruction, in chronic pancreatitis 2038
  stones, *see* choledocholithiasis
  strictures 2024
common cold 335, 336, **2691**
  aetiological agents 2691, *2691*
    coronavirus causing 392
  secondary complications 2691
common hepatic duct 2045
common peroneal nerve **4098**
  lesions/injuries 4098
common varied immunodeficiency (CVID) **166–8**, 1837–9
  associated diseases 169
  definition 1837
  diagnosis 169
  hypogammaglobulinaemic sprue 1839
  infections associated 168, 1837
    gastrointestinal 168–9, 878, *879*, 1837, *1837*, 1838–9
  investigation 1838
  nodular lymphoid hyperplasia in 1839
  presentation and features 166–7, 1837–9
    gastrointestinal 169, 1837–9, *1837*
  prognosis 167, 169
  special features 169, 1839
  subgroups 167
  treatment 169–70, 1839
communicable diseases
  control, consultants 287
  epidemiology 285
  see also infections
Communicable Disease Surveillance Centre 287, 4280, 4281

communication
  about death/dying 4357
  defects, in strokes 4237
  problems, dying patients 4233
community
  destruction 37
  health and sickness **39–46**
  malnutrition prevalence 1294
  sources of information on disease 41–2
  see also epidemiology
community-acquired infections
  bacterial meningitis 4050–1, *4051*, 4056
  coagulase-negative staphylococcal 531, 532
community health workers, tuberculosis diagnosis by 662
compartment syndrome, after snake bites 1139
compensation
  dissociative disorder association 4210
  extrinsic allergic alveolitis 2817
  malingering association 4211
  occupational asthma **2746**
  occupational disease 1162
compensation neurosis 4210
complement **175–82**
  activation 175, **176–7**, 277, 2497, 3621–2
    alternate pathway 175, 177
    classical pathway 175, 176–7
    in dengue haemorrhagic fever 420
    failure 178, 179, 180
    high permeability pulmonary oedema mechanism 2497
    lytic pathway 175, 177
    macrophage control of self/non-self 89
    persistent/excessive 179–80, 182, *182*
    in rheumatoid arthritis 2954
    stimuli causing 175
    in ulcerative colitis 1945
    in urticaria 3770
    see also membrane-attack complex
  in acute phase response 1528
  in adult respiratory distress syndrome 2497, 2854–5
  antiglobulin test and 3690
  C1 esterase, *see* C1 esterase
  C1q 176, 177
    deficiency 180
    receptors 2487, 2613
  C1r and C1s 177
  C2 177
    deficiency 180, 3026
    gene 178
    in hereditary angio-oedema 180
  C3,
    activation 175
    in anti-GBM disease 3165
    deficiency 175, 178, 180, 277
    in membranous nephropathy 3159
    in mesangiocapillary glomerulonephritis 3157
    nephritic factor 177, 180, 3157
    in opsonization 178
  C3a 178
  C3bBb 177
  C3bi cleavage defects 2759
  C3 convertase 177, 3624
  C3 nephritic factor (C3Nef) 177, 180, 3157
  C4,
    convertase 177
    deficiency 164, 180, 3026
    gene 178
  C4A deficiency 3026
  C4AQO 178
  C4b binding protein (C4BP) 179, 3623, 3624
  C5, convertase 176, 177
  C5a 178, 2622, 2623, 3559
    in adult respiratory distress syndrome 2854
    excessive production 179
    inhibitor deficiency 1526
    receptor 178
  C6, deficiency 180
  C7 and C8 180
    deficiency 180

C8 binding protein (C8BP) 3450
C9 180
components 175, 176
  cleavage 175, 176
  sites of synthesis 176 deficiency 164, 179, 180, 3021
  congenital and acquired 179
  importance and treatment 180
  in SLE 3021, 3026
discovery and evolution 175
diseases 164, **179–82**
  persistent/excessive activation 179–80, 182, *182*
  role in immunopathogenic mechanisms 179–80, 181, 182
  see also complement, deficiency
fixation 164
fixation test,
  chlamydial infection diagnosis 756
  genetic analysis of tumours 194
  hydatid disease diagnosis 958
  Mycoplasma hominis 770
  Mycoplasma pneumoniae detection 764
functions 178, 181, 277
  inflammatory 175–6, 178, 2618
  lysis 175, 178, 277
  non-specific response to infections 277
  opsonization 175, 178, 277
genetics 178–9
in graft rejection 187
in haemodialysis 3309
in immune-complex diseases 164, 178, 179, 181
in immune haemolytic anaemia 3542, 3544
low levels, in SLE 3021, 3026
in lung secretions 2614
in meningococcal infections 538
in mesangiocapillary glomerulonephritis 3157, 3158
in paroxysmal nocturnal haemoglobinuria 3450
in pneumococcal infections 514
receptors 177–8, *179*, 3559
  ß₂-integrin family 177, 181
  cells expressing 177
  CR1 and CR2 177, 178, 181
  CR3 (Mac-1) 88, 177, 3559
  CR4 (p150,95) 177, 3559
  deficiencies 181
  distribution *179*
  function 177, *179*
  see also CR1 complement receptor; CR2 complement receptor
regulators 175, 177
  deficiency 180
  gene clustering 178, 179
  see also C1 esterase inhibitor
terminology and nomenclature 175
compliance, improvement with good doctor-patient relationship 4233
compliance, drug **1240–1**
  elderly 4338
  factors affecting 1240
  improving 1240–1
  methods of measuring 1240, *1241*
  non-compliance in epilepsy 3923
  psychotropic 4247
compression bandages 3808
computed tomography (CT) **2217–19**
  in acute back pain 2993
  in acute headache 4027
  in acute pancreatitis 2013, 2030, *2031*
  in Addison's disease 1655
  in adrenal disease 1647, 1649, 1660
  in Alzheimer's disease 3974
  angiogram-enhanced, in acute pancreatitis 2031, 2033
  in anorexia nervosa 4214
  in benign intracranial hypertension 4042–3
  in biliary disease 2046
  biopsy, spinal 3828
  bone disease 3063
  brain, in viral infections 4069
  bronchiectasis 2665

in cerebral haemorrhage 3962
in cerebral infarction 3957, 3958, 3959, *3960*
in cerebral metastases 250
chest **2653–4**, 2665
  disadvantages 2654
  indications *2655*
  normal **2658**
in chronic obstructive airways disease 2774
in chronic pancreatitis 2035
cisternography 3818
in coma 3931
contrast media 3818
in craniopharyngioma 1597
in cysticercosis 965, 966, 967
in cystic fibrosis 2748
in dementia 3969
in diffuse parenchymal lung disease 2784–5
in diverticulitis 1971
dynamic spatial reconstructor 2217
electron beam 2217–18
in empyema 2707
in epileptic seizures 3920
in extrinsic allergic alveolitis 2813, 2814
in gastric cancer 1984
in head injury 4046, 4047
heart **2217–19**
  clinical applications *2219*
  ultrafast *2219*
in hepatocellular carcinoma 2116
high resolution 2665
  in cryptogenic fibrosing alveolitis 2790
  in diffuse parenchymal lung disease 2784, *2785*
  in systemic sclerosis 3033
in Hodgkin's disease 3572
in intracranial abscess 4082–3
in intracranial disorders **3817–19**
in intracranial tumours 4037
kidneys **3111**
liver 1833, **2012–13**
lung 2592
in lung cancer 2887–8
mediastinal masses 2898, 2900
mediastinum 2897
in multiple sclerosis 3994
myelography, in intervertebral disc protrusions 3906, 3907
in myeloma 3600
in neurological disorders 3815
in oesophageal carcinoma 1981
pancreas 1835, **2013**
in pancreatic carcinoma 2043
partial volume effect 2654
in pericardial constriction 2480
in phaeochromocytomas 2556
in Pick's disease 3976
in pituitary disease 1586, 1598, 1649
in pleural effusion 2864–5
in portal hypertension 2093
principles 2653, 3817
pulmonary mass 2662
radiotherapy planning 255
in rheumatic disease 2949
in sarcoidosis 2823
sensitivity, in brain 3818
in spinal cord injury 3897
in spinal disorders **3827–8**
in subarachnoid haemorrhage 3962, 3963
in transient ischaemic attack (TIA) 3952
tumour staging 234, 235, 245–6
  M staging 238, 246
  N staging 237, 246
  T staging 236, 245–6
unconscious patients 2585
units and monitors 3817
in urinary stone disease 3253
in urinary-tract obstruction 3239, 3240
in Whipple's disease 1924
computer-assisted myelography (CAM) **3827–8**
conchoidal (Schaumann's) bodies 2818

concussion 4044
  symptoms after 4049
condoms
  control of sexually transmitted diseases 3348
  HIV transmission prevention 484
conduction block 4092
conduction time, central motor, *see* central motor conduction time
conduction velocity, nerve, *see* nerve conduction
condyloma 3363
  exophytic, *see* condylomata acuminata
  flat of penis 3367
  giant 3369
  vulval 3368
  in women 3368
condylomata acuminata 444, 3363, 3367
condylomata lata 712
condylomata plana 444
cone shells, venomous 1144
Confederation of British Industries 1179
confidentiality **4315–17**
  circumstances for breaking 4316
  consultations 4288
  genetic testing 137
  medical reports, medicolegal context 4315
confounding 44
confusion
  acute 3931–2
    dementia *vs* 3967–8
    in hyperthyroidism 4239
    post-epileptic 4238
    treatment 4251
    see also delirium
  causes 4353
  in drug abusers 4295
  fungal poisoning causing 1155–6
  management 4353
  in Parkinson's disease 4004
  post-ictal 3912
  psychiatric emergencies associated 4258
  in terminal illness **4352–3**
congenital abnormalities 100
  anticancer therapy inducing 1806–7
  anticonvulsant drug-induced 1768
  chromosomal defects causing 66, **4108–11**
  immunosuppressive therapy and 1734
  in infants of diabetic mothers 1754–5
  male infertility in 1685
  maternal congenital heart disease and 1736
  multifactorial causation 129
  multifactorial inheritance 129–30
  nutrition and 1773–4
  occupations associated 1173
  skin 3718, *3718*
  vesicoureteric reflux and 3217
  warfarin-induced 1739–40
congenital adrenal hyperplasia 1639, **1664–9**
  genes/enzymes involved 1572, 1652, *1665*
  gynaecomastia in 1688
  hirsutism in 3765
  hyperandrogenization 1676
  hyperkalaemia 3134
  hypokalaemia 3131, 3336
  incidence 1667
  investigations 1654, 1664, *1665*, 1694
  mineralocorticoid excess 1660
  precocious puberty 1702
  pregnancy in **1751**
  virilization 1664, 1665, 1668, **1690–1**
  see also 21-hydroxylase, deficiency
congenital heart disease **2398–431**
  acyanotic **2419–31**
    aortopulmonary shunts **2430–1**
    coronary artery anomalies **2430**
    left-sided obstructive lesions **2421–4**
    right-sided obstructive lesions **2419–21**
    septal defects **2424–30**
    atrioventricular block in 2268
    cardiac transplantation indication 2255

classification 2400
computed tomography (CT) 2218
congenital cardiovascular disease with 2399, 2420
cyanotic **2400–19**
  abnormal right ventricle and shunt reversal **2413–15**
  abnormal systemic/pulmonary vein connections **2415–19**
  causes of cyanosis 2402
  defects with pulmonary hypertension **2409–13**
  endocarditis in 2439
  extracardiac problems 2400–2
  Fallot's tetralogy, *see* Fallot's tetralogy
  haematological disorders 3687
  pulmonary arterial stenosis 2409
  pulmonary atresia with ventricular septal defect 2407–8
  pulmonary valve stenosis with interatrial shunt 2409, *2409*
  see also pulmonary hypertension
Doppler echocardiography 2203, *2204*
endocarditis in 2439, 2443
genetic susceptibility 129
magnetic resonance imaging (MRI) 2214
natural survivors 2398
polycythaemia in 3554
postnatal adaptive changes 2399–400
in pregnancy **1736–7**
prevalence 2398
unnatural survivors 2398, 2399
see also individual disorders
congenital hypertrophy of retinal pigment epithelium (CHRPE) 1990
congenital infections
  nervous system in **4112**
  see also cytomegalovirus (CMV); rubella; toxoplasmosis
congenital muscular hypotonia **4150**
congenital short intestine **1978**
congestive heart failure
  ascites due to 2096
  in elderly 4342
  liver in 2130
  in malnutrition, management 1292–3
  pleural effusion in 2866
  pneumococcal infections 513
  in rheumatic fever 503
  symptoms 1292
  treatment, digitalis 2244
  ventricular extrasystoles in 2270
Congo floor maggot 1000, 1001
Congo Red 1522, 2835
Congo virus 427
conidiobolomycosis **803**
coning 4034
conjunctiva
  bilateral congestion, in Kawasaki disease 3047
  granuloma 4182
  haemorrhage 4191
    in infective endocarditis 2441
  oedema, in snake bites 1129
  in sarcoidosis 2826
  in sickling disorders 4195
conjunctivitis
  acute,
    enterovirus infections 388
    haemorrhagic 388
    adenovirus 337, 4191
  allergic 161
    perennial 161
  bilateral non-suppurative 4184
  chemical, in chronic renal failure 3324
  in chlamydial infections 4191
    neonatal 753
  in diphtheria 495
  epidemic, coxsackievirus A24 causing 388
  follicular 750
  giant papillary 161
  granulomatous 4191
  Haemophilus influenzae 584
  in herpes simplex infections 4192

inclusion (paratrachoma) 749, 753
in lymphogranuloma venereum 760
in Marburg virus and Ebola virus disease 441
in neonates 753, 1790, 1791, 1792
phlyctenular 648
in psoriatic arthritis 2969
'reactive' 753
in Reiter's syndrome 2970, 4185
simple 4191
connective tissue diseases **3008–52**
  airways obstruction in 2724
  amyloidosis 1513, *1515*
  autoantibodies in 3009, *3010*
  autoimmune, neuropathy in **4102**
  autoimmune pathogenesis 3008, 3009
  clinical manifestations 3009–10
  definition and diseases included 3008, *3009*
  diagnosis **3010**
  dystrophic calcification in 3092
  fever of unknown origin (FUO) 1015, *1017*
  gastrointestinal motility disorders in 1963
  gastrointestinal/tract involvement **1999–2000**
  haematological changes **3681–2**
  hereditary, bleeding disorders 3636, 3645
  immunopathology **3008–9**
  liver in **2135**, *2139*
  lung involvement **2796–800**, 2868
  mixed, *see* mixed connective tissue disease
  muscular involvement **4156–8**
  neurological complications **4129–32**
  pleural effusions in 2868
  pulmonary hypertension in **2510**
  pulmonary vasculitis with *2800*
  renal involvement **3187–93**
  skin disease/changes in 3788
  undifferentiated syndrome (UDCTS) 3008
  see also collagen disorders; polymyalgia rheumatica; polymyositis; systemic lupus erythematosus (SLE); systemic sclerosis; vasculitis, systemic
connective tissue fibres, lung 2598
connective tissue tumours, epidemiology 208
Conn's syndrome (aldosterone-producing adenoma) **1656**
  clinical features 1657
  diagnosis 1657–60
  myopathy in 4168
  treatment 1660
conotoxin, ^{125}I-w- 4163, 4164
consanguinity, first cousin marriages 115
consciousness 2582, 3930
  clouding 4223
    assessment in elderly 4226
    in cerebral tumours 4236
  disorders **3909–36**
  impairment,
    in acid-base disturbances 1539–40
    in hepatic disorders 4240
    in raised intracranial pressure 4035
  loss,
    in cardiac arrest 2283
    cardiac rhythms associated 2198
    in hypothermia 1183
    see also coma; syncope; unconsciousness
  time of useful 1196, 1197
CONSENSUS I trial 2250, 2251
CONSENSUS II trial 2344
consent 4316–17
  age for sexual intercourse 3350
  for clinical trials 1262
  emergency treatment without 4257
  express 4317
  implied 4316
  informed 1262, 4317
    in clinical trials 25
    exercise testing 2227

consent (*cont.*)
  medical reports 4315
  medicolegal context 4315, 4316–17
  organ donors 13–14
constipation **1825–7**, 1960, 1964, **1967**
  in adults 1964
  causes 1825, *1826*
  in children 1964
  in cirrhosis 2087
  clinical evaluation 1826, 1967
  definition 1825, 1964
  diagnosis 1826
  diet association 1328
  enteral feeding complication 1321
  in Hirschsprung's disease 1979
  history and diagnosis 1825–6, 1964
  in homosexuals 3361
  laboratory examination 1826, 1967
  management 1826–7, 1964, 4354
  in Parkinson's disease 4004
  pathophysiology 1967
  in pregnancy 1803
  in systemic sclerosis 1999
  in terminal illness **4353–4**
constitutional delay of growth and adolescence (CDGA) 1697, **1703**
consultants 131
  communicable disease control (CCDC) 287
consultations with doctors
  psychosocial determinants 4231–2
  rates, general practice 48
  by women 4231–2
consulting behaviour 4231–2
contact dermatitis **3735–9**
  allergic 162, **3736**
    to nickel 1112, 3738, 3739
  causes,
    caterpillars 1146
    clothing and textile 3736–7
    colophony 3737
    cosmetics and dyes 3736
    drugs 3731, 3732, 3738
    foods 3737
    metals 3738
    nickel 1112, 3738, 3739
    plants and wood 1154, 3725, 3737–8
    plastics and rubber 3737
    sensitizers 3736–8, *3737*
  contact urticaria 3736, *3737*
  distribution 3712, 3713
  employment and 3738, 3739
  genitalia 3768, *3769*
  irritant 1164, 3735–6
  in leg ulcers 3810, *3810*
  non-allergic 3736
  treatment 3739
  wear and tear (irritant) 1164, 3735–6
  see also dermatitis
contact lenses, *Acanthamoeba* infections 834
contact tracing chancroid 586
  gonorrhoea 547
  leprosy 678
  syphilis 709
  tuberculosis 646–7, 662
contaminated bowel syndrome, *see* bacterial overgrowth
contiguous gene disorder/deletion disorder 108
continuous ambulatory peritoneal dialysis (CAPD) 532, 3310, 3682
continuous motor unit activity syndrome 4092
continuous positive airway pressure (CPAP) **2921–3**, 2921, **2932**
  actions/physiology 2922
  applications 2921
  in ARDS 2858
  mask 2922–3, 2932
  nasal 2520, 2914, 2915
  in obstructive sleep apnoea 2905, 2914, 2915, 2932
  in respiratory failure 2922, **2932**
  in spinal cord injury 3898
  in unilateral lung disease 2923
  see also positive end-expiratory pressure (PEEP) ventilation

contraception
  in cyanotic congenital heart disease 2401
  in diabetes mellitus 1758
  drug abuse management 4299
  in SLE 3022
contraceptive pill, oral, *see* oral contraceptives
contractures 4142
  in Marfan's syndrome 3083
  in muscular dystrophies 4146
contrast media
  in barium studies 1831, 1832
  in computed tomography (CT) 3818
  hypertonic 2400
  radiographic,
    nephrotoxicity 3110, **3266–7**, 3289
    renal imaging 3110
  renal failure due to, *see* nephropathy, contrast-associated
contrast nephropathy, *see* nephropathy, contrast-associated
contrecoup injury 4044
controlled drugs, prescribing 4289
controls, in clinical trials 1262
Control of Substances Hazardous to Health Regulations 1163
contusions, brain damage 2585, 4044, 4047
conus medullaris lesions 3892
conversion disorder 3943, 4209
  psychiatric emergencies due to 4258
  see also dissociative disorder
convulsions
  benign familial neonatal 3915
  febrile 3909
  see also epileptic seizures; seizures
cooking oil, fumes, lung cancer association 207
Cooley's anastomosis 2406 cooling, unconscious patients 2586
cooling towers 724, 727
Coomb's test (direct antiglobulin test) 3542, 3544, 3631
COP combination chemotherapy 3421, *3422*, *3585*
Cope's needle 2865
co-phenotrope, poisoning **1069–70**
coping strategies 4204
copper 1108, **1416–23**
  deficiency 1416–19
    acquired 1416–17
    genetic (Menkes disease) 1417–19, 3763, 3989
  deposition 4008
  hepatic levels 2022
  homeostasis 1416
  liver concentration 1421
  nephrotoxicity *3261*
  overload/toxicity *1417*, 1419–23, *2018*, **2022–3**, *3546*
    in chronic cholestasis 1419, 1423
    primary inherited, *see* Wilson's disease
    secondary *2018*
  poisoning **1108–9**
    acute and chronic 1109
    features and treatment 1109
  serum levels 2022
  urinary 1421
  in Wilson's disease 4008
copper-chelating agents 1108, 2022, 2023
copper sulphate toxicity 2122
coprolalia 4016
coproporphyria
  hereditary *1390*, 1391, **1394**
  neuropathy in 4102
coproporphyrin 2059
  erythrocyte *1390*
  faecal *1390*
  urinary *1390*, 1396, 1397
coproporphyrinogen oxidase *1391*, 1394, 1396
copropraxia 4016
coral snakes, bites and envenoming 1131
cordotomy, anterolateral 3945
Cordylobia anthropophaga 1000–1

Cori cycle 1273, 1274
Cori-Forbes disease, *see* debranching enzyme, deficiency
cornea
  Acanthamoeba infections 834
  arcus, in familial hypercholesterolaemia 1406
  opacity,
    'snowflake' 914
    in trachoma 750
  as privileged site 185
  responses in unconscious patient 2583
  in rheumatoid arthritis 4185
  ulceration, in measles 379–80
  in Wegener's granulomatosis 4183
    corneal melting 2961
corns 3708, 3810
coronary angiography 2326
  angina diagnosis 2167
  in dilated cardiomyopathy 2383
  driving licence applications 2359
  in myocardial infarction 2346, 2347
  in renal transplant recipients 3313
  in unstable angina 2330
coronary angioplasty, *see* percutaneous transluminal coronary angioplasty (PTCA)
coronary arteries
  alpha-adrenoreceptor in 2159
  aneurysms, in Kawasaki disease 3048
  anomalies **2430**
  atherosclerosis, *see* atherosclerosis; coronary artery disease; ischaemic heart disease
  calcification 2182, 2430
    computed tomography 2219
  diastolic pressure 2158
  dissection, closure after angioplasty 2350
  fistula 2430, 2467
  in hypertension 2533
  inflow during diastole 2158
  left artery from pulmonary artery 2430
  left main, stenosis and angioplasty 2351
  lesions, in Kawasaki disease 3047, 3047–8
  magnetic resonance imaging 2217
  normal 2289–90
  outflow pressure 2158
  parasympathetic innervation 2159
  single 2430
  spasm 2159
  stenosis,
    in Kawasaki disease 3048
    stable angina 2166, 2320
  thrombi 2301
    see also coronary thrombosis
  tone regulation 2320, **2323**, *2324*
  transmural pressure 2159
  vasoconstriction, endothelin-1 2160
  vasodilatation 2159
    prostacyclin and nitric oxide role 2159
coronary arteriography, *see* coronary angiography
coronary arteriovenous fistula 2467
coronary arteriovenous oxygen difference 2323
coronary arteritis, in polyarteritis nodosa 3014
coronary artery bypass grafting **2353–6**
  in aircraft crew and pilots 1200, 2360
  in angina 2353, 2354
    recurrence of 2356
  coronary angioplasty 2351
    as salvage procedure after 2352
  in elderly 2355
  examination/investigations 2351, 2353–4
    magnetic resonance imaging 2217
  factors adversely affecting risk/survival 2354
  indications **2353–4**
  in myocardial ischaemia 2353, 2354
  numbers 2353
  occlusion 2300
  outlook **2356**
  patency rates 2355

perioperative morbidity **2355–6**
  perioperative mortality, risk factors 2355
  selection of patients **2353–4**
  technique **2354–5**
    artificial conduits 2355
    procedure 2355
    vascular conduits 2354–5
coronary artery disease 2331
  aerobic fitness and endurance sports 4324
  in affluent societies 1326–7
  after cardiac transplantation 2258
  aortic stenosis with 2462, 2464
  asymptomatic, in aircraft crew and pilots 1200, 2360
  dietary causes, *see* ischaemic heart disease, risk factors
  epidemiology 2289, **2305–6**, 2331–2
  exercise testing in 2226–7
  genes involved in susceptibility 64
  heart valve replacement and 2471
  outcome, left ventricular ejection fraction 2358
  in pulmonary valve stenosis 2420
  recovery *vs* rehabilitation 2357
  risk factors, *see under* ischaemic heart disease
  statistics 2357
  vocational aspects **2356–62**
    transportation **2358–61**
    see also aircrew/pilots; driving; transportation
  see also ischaemic heart disease; myocardial infarction
coronary artery steal 2408
coronary artery surgery, driving after 2359
Coronary Artery Surgery Study (CASS) 2357
coronary atherosclerosis 2318
  see also atherosclerosis; ischaemic heart disease
coronary blood flow 2145, **2158–60**
  diastolic 2323
  distribution 2158
  in exercise 2158, 2161
  nitrates improving 2327
  regulation **2158–60**
    in angina 2323
    autoregulation 2159, 2323
    metabolic 2159
    neurohumoral 2159, 2323
    pressure gradients 2158
coronary care units 2339
coronary embolism, in mitral stenosis 2452
coronary embolization, in heterophyiasis 998
coronary heart disease, *see* coronary artery disease; ischaemic heart disease
coronary insufficiency, acute, *see* angina (angina pectoris), unstable
coronary ostial stenosis, in syphilis 2483
coronary perfusion pressure 2158, 2160
coronary sinus
  defect, ostium secundum defects 2424
  unroofed, in tricuspid atresia 2412
coronary spasm 2322
  coronary artery closure after angioplasty 2350
  see also angina (angina pectoris), Prinzmetal (variant)
coronary thrombosis 2300, 2301
  in heat waves due to haemoconcentration 1185
  myocardial infarction due to 2332
  winter mortality due to 1185
  see also atherosclerosis, thrombosis in; ischaemic heart disease
coronaviruses **335–6**, 391, *391*, **392–3**
  features of infections *341*
  infection in homosexuals 3364
  strains and antigens 335
coroner, reporting death to 4310
corps rond 3721

cor pulmonale **2515–22**, 2571
  in bronchiectasis 2758, 2761
    management 2766
  causes 2927
  in chronic obstructive airways disease
    2516, 2517, 2520, 2777, 2927
  clinical features **2517–18**
  in coal-worker's pneumoconiosis 2840
  definition 2515
  differential diagnosis 2519–20
  diseases associated 2515
  investigations **2518–19**, *2518*, *2519*
    ECG 2518, *2518*
  in obstructive sleep apnoea 2927
  pathogenesis **2516–17**
    hypoxia as initiating event 2516, 2519
  pathology **2515–16**
  pathophysiology **2517**
  in pregnancy 1745
  prognosis 2518
  pulmonary hypertension in 2515, 2516,
    2518
  right heart failure in 2515, 2517, 2518
  right ventricular hypertrophy in 2515,
    2517, 2518
  in sarcoidosis 2824
  treatment **2520–1**, **2927**
corpus callosum, agenesis 4113
corpus striatum 3861
Corrigan's sign 2465
corrosive substances
  oesophageal strictures 1104, 1873, 1981
  poisoning **1102–5**, 1171
    gastric emptying contraindication 1049
    management 1103–4
    phenol 1104–5
  see also acid(s); alkalis
cortical dementia 3965
cortical lesions
  pain in 3942
  see also cerebral lesions
cortical venous thrombosis 3956–7, *3957*
corticobasal degeneration **4007**
corticospinal tract 3856–7
  lesions 3857
corticosteroids
  in acute meningococcaemia 541
  adverse effects,
    on bone 3059, 3069
    bruising 3636
    on eye 4197
    osteoporosis 1626, 1637
    short stature 1699
    see also Cushing's syndrome
  after insect stings 1145
  in alkali ingestion 1104
  in anti-GBM disease *3165*
  in aplastic anaemia 3446, 3447
  in asthma 2737
  in autoimmune haemolytic anaemia
    3544
  in autoimmune hepatitis 2069, 2072,
    2073
  in autoimmune thrombocytopenia
    3631–2
  azathioprine with 2792–3
  biosynthetic pathway *1640*, 1664
  in bronchiectasis 2762, 2766
  calcium metabolism and 1626
  in chlorine poisoning 1097
  in chronic lymphocytic leukaemia 3422
  in chronic obstructive airways disease
    2776
  in CNS viral infections 4071
  in Crohn's disease 1942
  in cryptogenic fibrosing alveolitis
    2792–3
  cyclophosphamide with 2792
  effect on bone 3059, 3069
  in epilepsy 3922
  excess, effect on bone 3059, 3069
  in extrinsic allergic alveolitis 2817
  in focal segmental glomerulosclerosis
    3156–7
  in genitourinary tuberculosis 3278
  in giant-cell arteritis 4183
  glaucoma associated 1259
  in hepatitis B (chronic) 459

  in hypercalcaemia 1638, 3229
  in hypereosinophilic syndrome 3612
  in hypoadrenalism 1655–6
  immunosuppression with *283*
  in intracranial tumours 4037
  in Langerhans-cell histiocytosis 3609
  in lupus nephritis 3190, 3191
  in membranous nephropathy 3160
  in mesangiocapillary glomerulonephritis
    3158
  in minimal change nephropathy 3155,
    3156
  in myeloma 3601, 3602, 3603
  nasal sprays, in allergic rhinitis 2718
  ocular toxicity 4197
  osteoporosis and 3059, 3069
  in pain 3936
  in pneumococcal infection 521
  in *Pneumocystis carinii* pneumonia 478,
    823
  in pregnancy 1745, 1757, **1811**
  in primary sclerosing cholangitis 2079
  in recurrent oral ulceration 1855
  in red-cell aplasia 3448–9
  in renal failure 3274–5, 3327
  in renal transplant recipients 3314,
    3319, 3321
  in retroperitoneal fibrosis 3245–6
  in rheumatic fever 2434
  in rheumatoid arthritis 2964
  in sarcoidosis, *see* sarcoidosis, treatment
  in septicaemia 2573
  in SLE 3023
  topical *3806*
    in allergic rhinitis 2718
    in pregnancy 1805–6
    in toxic nephropathy 3266
    in tuberculous meningitis 4063
    in ulcerative colitis 1948
  see also glucocorticoids;
    mineralocorticoids; prednisolone;
    steroids
corticosterone, excess production 1660
corticosterone methyl oxidase
  type I (CMO-I; 18-hydroxylase) *1652*,
    1662
  type II (CMO-II; 18-oxidase), *see*
    aldosterone synthase
corticotrophin, *see* ACTH
corticotrophin releasing hormone (CRH;
    CRF) 1575
  combined anterior pituitary test 1585
  in Cushing's disease 1640–1
  ectopic production 1641–2, 1707, 1711,
    1712
  plasma 1642
  stimulation test 1648, 1713, *4375*
corticotrophs 1575
  adenoma 1566
cortisol
  action 1274, 1562–3
  creatinine ratio 1645
  deficiency 1510–11, 1587
  functions 1274
  increased secretion, in depressive
    disorders 4219
  in malnutrition 1286
  metabolites, urinary excretion 1645,
    1661, 1668
  plasma 1583
    circadian rhythm 1565, 1644–5
    in CRF stimulation test 1648
    in Cushing's syndrome 1644–5 in
      dexamethasone suppression test
      1645, 1647
    in ectopic ACTH syndrome 1713
    in hypoadrenalism 1654, 1655
    in insulin tolerance test 1585–6, 1655
    in pregnancy 1750
    raised levels in anorexia nervosa 4214
    in stress 1563–4
    in trauma 1549
  urinary free 1565
    in Cushing's syndrome 1645
cortisol-binding globulin (CBG) 1644,
    1717
  in nephrotic syndrome 3144
  in pregnancy 1750

cortisone, adverse mental symptoms
    4242
cortisone acetate 1655
cor triatriatum 2402, 2415
  mitral stenosis *vs* 2455
  pulmonary oedema in 2500–1
Corynebacterium, rare species *554–5*
Corynebacterium diphtheriae 493
  infections in homosexuals 3363
  morphology and growth 493
  phage typing 494
  scabies infections with 1008
  in skin lesions in streptococcal impetigo
    500
  strains/subtypes 493, 494
  toxigenic and non-toxigenic 493
  toxin production 493
  see also diphtheria
Corynebacterium haemolyticum 495
Corynebacterium pyogenes 685
Corynebacterium sepsis 495
Corynebacterium ulcerans 495
Corynebacterium vaginale, *see*
    Gardnerella vaginalis
coryza, febrile, scarlet fever *vs* 502
cosmetics
  acne vulgaris and 3753
  contact dermatitis 3736
  pigmentation changes 3725, 3756
cosmic rays 1217
cosmids 61
  as gene vectors 61
costal fibres 2876
costochondritis 3007
  see also Tietze's syndrome
costoclavicular compression 4093
costophrenic angle 2863
costs
  acute renal failure 3293
  antiepileptic drugs 3922
  nosocomial infections 328, *328*
  treatment, in clinical trials 24
cotinine 1230
cotransporters (symports) 1900, *1900*
co-trimoxazole
  in gonorrhoea 549
  in malaria 853
  in melioidosis 592
  nephrotoxicity 3264
  in nocardiosis 687
  in pneumococcal infections 520
  in *Pneumocystis carinii* pneumonia 478
  in renal impairment 3272
  in toxoplasmosis 478
  in urinary-tract infections 3209, 3211,
    3213
cotton mill workers, byssinosis 2746
cotton-wool spots 4179, *4180*, 4194
  in AIDS 4193
  in Behçet's syndrome 4183
  in hypertension 4188
  in leukaemia 4194
  in pancreatitis 4184
  in retinal vein occlusion 4187
  in SLE 4184
cough 2610, **2642–4**
  ACE inhibitors causing 2251, 2850
  in asthma 2729
  'bovine' 2643
  in bronchiectasis 2757
  causes 2642–3
  chest pain after 2168
  in chronic bronchiolitis 2634
  in chronic obstructive airways disease
    2769, 2773
  clinical features 2643
  in diffuse parenchymal lung disease
    2781
  drug-induced 2251, **2850**
  dry 2643
    dyspnoea with 2162
  in eosinophilic granuloma of lung 2833
  in extrinsic allergic alveolitis 2809
  investigations **2644**
  in lung cancer 2883
  mechanism 2642
  in paragonimiasis 990
  phlegm and sputum 2643

  in pneumococcal pneumonia 515
  in pulmonary alveolar proteinosis
    2834
  in rickettsial diseases 732
  in terminal illness **4354**
  timing 2643
  treatment **2644**, 4354
  in whooping cough (pertussis) 588
cough reflex 2642
  absence, in acute poisoning 1046
  assessment 2668
  in unconscious patient 2583
cough suppressants 2644
  in terminal illness 4354 cough syncope
    2642, **3926**
coumarin anticoagulants, *see*
    anticoagulants, oral
coumarin embryopathy 1739–40
counselling
  in acute paranoid reactions 4223
  in adjustment disorder 4205
  bereavement 4235, 4236
  in dissociative disorder 4210
  genetic, *see* genetic counselling
  problem-solving, *see* problem-solving
    approach
  psychological treatment 4254
  relatives of dying patients 4234
  substance abuser in prison 4305
counsellor, dependency on and
    avoidance of 4254
counterstimulation, pain treatment 3943
coup de poignard 3895
court reports 4305
Courvoisier's law 2042, 2052, 2057
cousin marriages 115
Cowden syndrome *3795*
Cowdry type A inclusions 4066
cowpox 366, 369
cows' milk
  allergy, coeliac disease *vs* 1919
  diabetes type I and 1454
  protein enteropathy 1842, **1843**
  see also milk
Coxiella burnetii 728, **742–3**, 2121,
    2134
  characteristics 742
  endocarditis 743–4, 2437, 2442
    treatment 2448–9
  strains and plasmids of 742, 744
  see also Q fever
coxsackie A virus 383
  diagnosis 387
  epidemic conjunctivitis 388
coxsackie A7 virus 386
coxsackie B virus 386
  acute idiopathic pericarditis 2475
  chronic fatigue syndrome 4155
  diagnosis 387
  epidemic pleurodynia 4155
  infections 383
  pancreatitis and diabetes due to 387–8
  in pregnancy/newborn infants 388,
    1779, 1783
coxsackie B3 virus, myocarditis 2381
coxsackieviruses 381
  diabetes type I and 1454
  diagnosis 383, 387
  heart and muscle infections 386–7
  in hypogammaglobulinaemia 168
  mucocutaneous infections 383
  neurological diseases *385*, 386, 4064
  see also enterovirus infections
C-peptide 1459, 1461
  plasma *1462*
  in insulinoma 1508
CpG islands 107
CpG sequence, mutational hot spot
    108
CR1 complement receptor (CD35) 177,
    178, 3559
  deficiency 181
  in SLE 3026
  see also complement, receptors
CR2 complement receptor (CD21) 148,
    177
  Epstein-Barr virus (EBV) binding 352
  see also complement, receptors

CR3 complement receptor (Mac-1) 88, 177, 3559
CR4 (p150,95) complement receptor 177, 3559
crab louse 1003–4
crack cocaine 1076, 4264, 4280, 4281
  see also cocaine
crackles 2650
  inspiratory, in asbestosis 2844
cramp, muscle, see muscle, cramps
cranial arteritis, see giant-cell arteritis
cranial fusion defects 4115
cranial irradiation, in lung cancer 2891
cranial nerves 3876–81
  in bacterial meningitis 4050, 4053–4, 4059
  in carcinomatous 'meningitis' 250
  in cerebrospinal angiostrongyliasis 947
  developmental anomalies 4114
  in diabetes mellitus 1488, 4098, 4190
  dysfunction,
    in pituitary apoplexy 1598
    pituitary tumours 1582, 1587, 1589
  eighth 3869–76
    disorders 3874–6
    in intracranial tumours 4036
    symptoms/signs of dysfunction 3870–4
    see also auditory system; vestibular system
  eleventh (accessory) 3880, 4036
  fifth (trigeminal), see trigeminal nerve
  first (olfactory) 3876–7
  fourth (trochlear), lesions 3877
    in intracranial tumours 4036
  lesions, pupillary responses 2582
  ninth (glossopharyngeal) 3880
  palsy,
    in botulism 631
    in diabetes mellitus 4190
    in intracranial tumours 4036
    in rabies 400
    in poliomyelitis 385
    in sarcoidosis 2826–7
  second (optic), see optic nerve
  seventh (facial), see facial nerve
  sixth (abducens),
    lesions 3877
    palsy 2583
  tenth (vagus), see vagus nerve
    in tetanus 626–7
  third (oculomotor),
    lesions 3877
    palsy 2583, 3877, 4036
    in tuberculous meningitis 4060
    in tumours 240
  twelfth 3880, 4036
  upper motor neurone 3857
cranial neuralgias 4023–4
  see also post-herpetic neuralgia; trigeminal neuralgia
craniofacial dysmorphism, in Zellweger syndrome 1442, 1443
craniopharyngioma 1597, 1616, 4032
  growth hormone deficiency 1699
  management 4039
  optic chiasmal lesions 3867
  treatment 3868
  visual pathway lesions 3865
craniosynostosis 4116
crayons, wax 3546
C-reactive protein (CRP) 294, 1528–33
  in acute pancreatitis 2030, 2031
  amniotic fluid 1786
  body temperature and 1533
  erythrocyte sedimentation rate and 1533
  in infections 294
  in infective endocarditis 2442
  in inflammatory rheumatic disease 2951
  interpretation of measurements 1532
  in listeriosis 722
  major elevations 1528–31
  minor elevations 1530, 1531–2
  in nephrotic syndrome 3141
  normal values 1528

in pelvic inflammatory disease 3358
in polymyalgia rheumatica 3040
in rheumatic fever 2434
in SLE 2798, 3020
'cream cracker' sign 3036
creams
  after-work, in occupational dermatosis 1165
  topical agents in skin disease 3805, 3805
creatine kinase (CK) 4365, 4366
  BB isoenzyme 1996
  in endurance sports 4326
  in muscle disorders 4142
  muscular dystrophy carrier detection 4147
  myocardial (CKMB) 2339
    in endurance sports 4326
  in polymyositis and dermatomyositis 4157
creatine phosphate 4140
creatine phosphokinase 2146
creatinine clearance,
  endogenous 3106
  from plasma creatinine 3106, 3107
  normal values 4374
  peritoneal dialysis 3311
  plasma,
    in accelerated hypertension 3290
    in acute renal failure 3286
    in chronic renal failure 3294, 3304
    in diabetes mellitus 3170
    interpretation 3106–7
    in pre-eclampsia 1729
    starting dialysis and 3306
creatinine phosphokinase, serum, in thyroid disease 1609
creatinuria 4142
CRE-binding proteins (CREBs) 1558
Crede's method 1790
creeping eruption 931
  gnathostomal 951
Creola bodies 161, 2685
CREST syndrome 1872, 3010, 3028
  lung involvement in 2799
  see also CRST syndrome; systemic sclerosis, limited cutaneous
cretinism 1614–15
  endemic 1615
  mental disorders/symptoms in 4238–9
Creutzfeldt-Jakob disease
  age of onset 3979
  amyloid in 1513, 1514, 1517
  ataxic form 3980, 3983
  clinical features 3979–80
  cognitive impairment in 3965
  epidemiology 3977
  familial 3977
  genetic susceptibility 3979–80
  historical aspects 3977
  iatrogenic 3980
  prion protein (PrP) in 3978
CRH, see corticotrophin releasing hormone
cricoarytenoid arthritis 2796, 2874, 2959
cricoarytenoid joint, in rheumatoid arthritis 2959
cricothyrotomy, emergency 2721, 2919
cri-du-chat syndrome 4109–10
  reciprocal translocation in 122, 4109
Crigler-Najjar syndrome 2056, 2057–8
  treatment 2058
  type I 2058
  type II 2058
Crimean-Congo haemorrhagic fever virus 424, 427
criminal deaths 4309
crisis intervention, psychological 4254–5
Crithidium lucilliae 3021
critical care, see intensive care
critical illness polyneuropathy 4099
critical-point control 288
crocidolite 2843
crocodiles, injuries from 1124
'crocodile tears' 3878
Crohn's disease 1936–43
  activity index(es) 1941

adenocarcinoma of small intestine 1986
aetiology 1937–8
  aphthoid ulcers in 1938, 1940
  arthropathy in 2973
  assessment of activity 1941
  bacterial overgrowth in 1912, 1939
  clinical features 1938
    extraintestinal 1939
  colorectal carcinoma in 1993
  complications 1938–9
  course and prognosis 1943
  C-reactive protein levels 1531
  definition and history 1936
  diagnosis 1940–1
  differential diagnosis 1909, 1941
    ulcerative colitis 1941, 1941
  enteropathic synovitis in 2972–3
  epidemiology and incidence 1936–7, 1937
  fistulae in 1938–9
    surgical management 1942–3
  genetics and HLA association 1937
  granulomatous features 2122, 3723, 3803
  haematological changes 1940, 3683–4
  hepatic granulomas in 2122
  immune response and aetiological mechanism 1938
  investigations,
    endoscopy 1939, 1939–40
    laboratory 1940
    radiology 1909, 1939
    small-bowel biopsy 1908, 1940
    small-bowel enema 1909, 1939
  management 1941–3
    in children 1943
    complications of 1942
    drugs 1942
    home parenteral nutrition 1324
    nutritional 1324, 1942
    in pregnancy 1943
    of relapses 1942, 1943
    surgery 1942–3
  mortality 1943
  ocular features 4184
  oesophagus in 1876
  pathology 1938, 1940
    ulcers and strictures 1938, 1940
  perianal granuloma 3723
  in pregnancy 1802, 1943
  primary sclerosing cholangitis and 2079
  relapses and recurrences 1942, 1943
  urinary-tract obstruction 3246
  vitamin B_{12} deficiency 3491
Cronkhite-Canada syndrome 1987
Crosby-Kugler capsule 1907
cross-reacting epitopes 155, 155
Cross syndrome 3759
crotaline venom 1129
croup 2691, 2722
  parainfluenza viruses causing 337
Crow-Fukase syndrome, see POEMS syndrome
crown gall tumour 193
crown-rump length (CRL), fetal, in maternal diabetes 1756
CRST syndrome 2075, 3092
  cor pulmonale pathogenesis 2516
  liver in 2139
  see also CREST syndrome
crush injury, acute renal failure 3289
crush syndrome, in earthquakes 1232
crusts, softening 3806
Cruveilhier-Baumgarten syndrome 2093
cryocrit 3052
cryoglobulin 3050
cryoglobulinaemia 3050–2
  aetiology 3050–1
  clinical features 3051, 3051
  definition and classification 3050, 3051
  investigations 3051–2
  liver in 2136
  management 3052
  mixed essential 3050, 3167, 3176, 3183
  mixed type II 3183
  renal involvement 3051, 3180, 3182–3

type I 3050, 3051
types II/III 3050
cryoprecipitate 3050, 3695
  in acute renal failure 3288
  in DIC 1762, 3659
  in von Willebrand's disease 3644
cryosupernatant 3633, 3695
cryosurgery, sun damage 3729
cryptitis 1945
crypt of Lieberkühn
  abscess 1945
  cell proliferation 1917
  dysplastic 1988
  hypertrophy 1907, 1916
  hypoplasia 1919
  normal 1988
cryptococcal latex agglutination test 1033
cryptococcoma 809
cryptococcosis 803, 809–10
  antigen testing 2677
  disseminated 809–10
  in HIV infections 475, 488, 809–10, 810
  eye in 4194
  treatment 479, 480, 488
  meningitis, see meningitis, cryptococcal
  peritonitis 2009
  pulmonary 809
  treatment 810
Cryptococcus neoformans 488, 809, 4078
cryptogenic fibrosing alveolitis
  aetiology 2786–7
  asbestosis similarity 2844
  clinical features 2789, 2790
  clinical-radiographic-physiological score 2788
  coeliac disease relation 2813
  definition and spectrum 2786, 2787
  diseases associated 2789
  epidemiology 2786
  histopathological classification 2786, 2787
  immunogenetics 2786–7
  investigations 2789–91
    bronchoalveolar lavage 2685, 2788, 2791
    chest radiography 2789–90
    computed tomography 2654, 2790
    lung biopsy 2683, 2689, 2788, 2791, 2792
    laboratory features 2790
  lung diseases mimicking 2787
  management 2791–2
    open-lung biopsy 2688, 2689, 2792
    patient selection 2792
  pathogenesis and cells/mediators 2788–9
  pathology 2626, 2787–8
    inflammation and scarring 2616, 2617, 2626
  prognosis 2794
  in rheumatoid arthritis 2797, 2961
  treatment 2792–4
    duration 2793
    monitoring 2793
    recommended plan 2793–4, 2794
    transplantation 2793
    triggers 2786, 2788
    see also alveolitis; lung, diffuse interstitial fibrosis
cryptogenic neuropathy 4104
cryptorchidism 1685
cryptosporidiosis 475, 869–76, 2003
  in AIDS/HIV infection 475, 487, 873–4
    treatment 478–9, 875
  clinical features 873–5
    in immunocompromised 873–4
  in common varied immunodeficiency 1838
  diagnosis/differential diagnosis 874, 875
  epidemiology 871–3
  in homosexuals 3365
  immune response 873
  infectivity, resistance and control 875
  nosocomial 874

pathology 873
transmission 870–1, 872, 873
control 875
treatment 874–5
Cryptosporidium 475, **869–76**, 2003
biology and lifecycle 869–71
infective dose 875
molecular biology 871
oocysts 869, 875
cryptosporidium-like bodies 876
Cryptosporidium parvum 475, 869, 870, 871, 1930
in homosexuals 3365
crystal(s)
deposition and clearance 2983, 2984
inflammation and tissue damage 2983–4
crystal-deposition disease 2983, 2984
definition 2983
'mixed crystals' 2983
see also crystal-related arthropathies
crystalline bodies, in sarcoidosis 2818
crystal-related arthropathies 2951, **2983–92**
apatite-associated 2990–1
cholesterol 2991
crystals associated *2983*
extrinsic crystals 2991–2
oxalate 2991
see also gout; pyrophosphate arthropathy
C-type natriuretic peptide (CNP) 2234
cubital tunnel syndrome 4096
cubomedusoids, venomous 1143–4
cuirass 2874
Culex 838, 920
Cullen's sign 2029, 3358
culture, erosion of traditional 36
cultures
cell, gene insertion 62
respiratory tract infection organisms 2677
cunnilingus 3350
cupulolithiasis 3873
curare 4141
curative treatment 4349
Curschmann's spirals 2685
Curtis Fitz-Hugh syndrome 546, 753, 756, 2133
Cushing's disease 1566, 1595, **1640–1**
acne in 3752
diagnostic tests 1585, 1586, 1646–9
treatment 1588, 1650–1
Cushing's syndrome 1563, **1639–52**, **4125**
ACTH-independent 1640, 1642–3
aetiology 1640–3
carcinoid syndrome association 1898
childhood 1644, 1699
classification 1640, *1642*
clinical features 1643–4
cyclical 1641
definition 1640
dementia due to 3971
in ectopic ACTH syndrome 1644, 1711, 1712
food-dependent form 1640, 1643
hirsutism in 3765
hyperandrogenization 1676
hypokalaemia 1647, 3131, 3336
investigations 1644–50
in medullary carcinoma of thyroid 1637
mental disorders/symptoms in 3971, 4239
myopathy in 4168
neurological features 4125
osteoporosis in 3069
paraneoplastic *243*
polycythaemia in 3554
in pregnancy **1751**
prognosis of untreated 1650
purpura/bruising in 1643, 3636
treatment 1650–2
custody, alcohol/drug abuser in **4304–5**
management 4305
reception and examination 4304
cutaneous lymphoma, *see* lymphoma, cutaneous

cutaneous migratory swelling 951–2
cutaneous vasculitis, *see* vasculitis
cutis hyperelastica **3790**
cutis laxa 1419, **3790**
cutis marmorata 3724
cutis verticis gyrata 1592
cutting-needle biopsy
mediastinum 2682
percutaneous lung 2681
cyanide 1097
mechanisms of toxicity 1097
metabolic abnormalities 1097
poisoning **1097–8**, 1152
in sodium nitroprusside overdose 1067
toxicity 1067
uses and sources 1097
cyanobacterium-like bodies (Cyclospora) 876
cyanocobalamin, *see* vitamin B$_{12}$
cyanogenic glycosides 1152, 1158–9
cyanogens 1158–9, 1452
cyanosis 1097, 2649, 2651
assessment 2903
central 2400, 2651
see also congenital heart disease
in chronic obstructive airways disease 2774
in cirrhosis 2087
in methaemoglobinaemia 3519
peripheral 2651
'pulmonary' 2402
in syncope 2174
cycasin 1159
cyclamates, bladder cancer association 212
cyclic AMP (cAMP) 2160
analogues, new cytotoxic drugs 259
ß-adrenoceptor stimulation 2253
drug actions 1249
in heart 2147
in hormonal signalling 1560–1
pathway, defects in SLE 3026
platelet 3618, 3619
response element 1558
in secretory diarrhoea 577, 1824
cyclic GMP (cGMP)
nitrates action 2247
nitric oxide action 2297
cyclic GMP (cGMP) dependent protein kinases (G-kinases) 1561
cyclic nucleotide phosphodiesterase inhibitors 2150
cyclin D1, in parathyroid adenoma 1569
cyclins 2145
cyclizine 1076
cyclo-oxygenase 158, 2297, 3617, 3662
inhibitors, in pulmonary hypertension 2860
cyclophosphamide
adverse reaction 2851
in anti-GBM disease *3165*, *3166*
bladder cancer association 211, 212
in Burkitt lymphoma 355
in cryptogenic fibrosing alveolitis 2792
in focal segmental glomerulosclerosis 3157
in lupus nephritis 3190, 3191
in lymphoma *3585*
marrow transplant conditioning 3696
in minimal change nephropathy 3155, 3156
in multiple sclerosis 3996
pulse dose, in systemic vasculitis 3016
secondary immunodeficiency due to 174
in SLE 3024
in Takayasu's disease 2379
Cyclops 949, 969
cycloserine
adverse effects 3523
in tuberculosis 655, *656*
Cyclospora **876**
cyclosporin
in aplastic anaemia 3446
in atopic eczema 3742
in bone marrow transplantation 3697
in cardiac transplantation 2257

in Crohn's disease 1942
in cryptogenic fibrosing alveolitis 2793
cytotoxic T-cells role in graft rejection 186
drug interactions *3314*
FK506 comparison 2114
in focal segmental glomerulosclerosis 3157
in Graves' ophthalmopathy 1614
haemolytic uraemic syndrome induced by 3197
hyperkalaemia due to 3134
in liver transplantation 2114
in lung/heart-lung transplantation 2935
in lupus nephritis 3191
in minimal change nephropathy 3156
monitoring 1261
in multiple sclerosis 3996
in nephrotic syndrome 3140
nephrotoxicity 2114, 2937, **3265–6**, 3319
in polymyositis and dermatomyositis 4157
in psoriasis 3750
in renal failure 3274–5
in renal transplantation 3318–19
in rheumatoid arthritis 2954
side-effects 2257–8, *2257*
in ulcerative colitis 1949
cyclothymic personality 4212, 4220
λ-cyhalothrin 858, 860
CYP2D6, polymorphism 130, 1259
CYP11B1/CYP11B2 1662, 1668–9
CYP21A/CYP21B 1666–7
cyproheptadine 1898
in migraine 4025
in polycythaemia vera 3434
cyproterone acetate
in acne vulgaris 3754
in hirsutism 1677, 3765
in precocious puberty 1702
side-effects 1689
see also antiandrogens
cyst(s)
acne 3753
arachnoid **4116**, **4117**
bone 2980
bronchogenic 2899–900
choledochal 2016
choroid-plexus 135
colloid **4032–3**
in colon 2136
dental 1863
dentigerous 1863
dermoid 4033
enteric 1976
haemophilic 3647
hydatid, *see* hydatid cysts
intracranial **4116**
jaw and dental 1862–3
mediastinal **2899–900**
mouth 1859–60
ovarian, oral contraceptives and 1723
pancreatic 2053
pericardial 2182, 2474, 2899
popliteal 2958, 2959
renal, *see* kidney, cystic disorders
sebaceous 2750
spinal arachnoid **4117**
splenic 3592
thymic 2899
thyroglossal 1610
cystadenocarcinoma, mucinous 2042
cystathionase deficiency 1367, 3493
cystathionine ß-synthase 3084, 3085
cystathionine synthase (CS) deficiency **1366–7**, 3668
cystatin C 1516, **1520**
cysteamine 1356
cysteine 1365, 1366
in carbon tetrachloride poisoning 1085
in chloroform poisoning 1086
in phosgene poisoning 1101
in sulphur mustard (mustard gas) exposure 1116
cysteine proteinase (cathepsin L) 2773

cystic duct 2045
gallstone impaction 2049
cysticercosis (*Taenia solium*) **961–3**, *961*, 962, **964–8**
CNS, *see* neurocysticercosis
course and prognosis 968
diagnosis 962, 966–7
differential diagnosis 967–8
distribution and epidemiology 961–2, 964
historical aspects 964–5
muscular and subcutaneous 966
myositis 4155–6
ocular 966, 968, 4193
pathogenesis and clinical features 965–6
pathology 962
treatment 963, 968
see also Taenia solium
Cysticercus cellulosae 959
cystic fibrosis **2746–55**
biliary tract in 2749
biochemistry **2746–7**
clinical features 2023, **2748–50**
death, age at 2750
diabetes mellitus in 1714, 1746, 2749
diagnosis 1978, **2750**
mutation detection 134
differential diagnosis 2737
gastrointestinal tract 2747, 2749
chronic pancreatitis 2034, 2035, 2747
gene 1685, 1978, 2591, 2746
DNA sequence 2591
mutations 134, 2747, 2754
genetic counselling 2754–5
genetics 2023, **2746–7**
gut peptides in 1895
homozygous 104
immunization in 2751
incidence 2023, 2746, 2750–1
infertility in 1685, 2750
investigations 2023, 2748
liver in *2018*, **2023–4**, 2131, 2749
management 2024, 2131
lung function tests 2748
management strategies **2754**
regional centres 2754, *2754*
meconium ileus in 1978, 2747, 2748
mucociliary clearance defect 2613, 2747
neonatal screening 1337–8, 2750
pathogenesis 2024
pathology 2023–4, **2747–8**
in pregnancy **1745–6**
prevention **2754–5**
prognosis 2024, **2750–1**
psychological consequences **2750**
recurrence risk 131–2
respiratory tract in 2747–8, 2748
respiratory tract infections 2747, 2747–8, 2748, 2749
treatment 2751–3
sputum in 2748
viscosity reduction 2753
treatment **2751–4**
of bronchopulmonary disease 2751–3
gene therapy 2755
heart-lung transplant 2754
nutritional 2751
other approaches 2753
pancreatic enzyme replacement 2751, *2751*
physiotherapy 2753
Pseudomonas infections 2752, *2752*
of respiratory complications 2753–4
sputum viscosity reduction 2753
transplantation 2937
uniparental isodisomy in 128
vitamin D deficiency 1636
cystic fibrosis transmembrane conductance regulator (CFTR) 1685, 1900, 2024, 2746–7
abnormalities 2747
domains 2747, 2754
function 2747
cystic lesions, pseudomyxoma 2009

cystic medial necrosis 2508
cystic tumours 4116
cystine *1353*
  crystals 1355, 1356
   in urine 3104, 3105
  stones 1356, *3252*, 3333
  transport 1358
cystinosis (cystine storage disease) 1335, **1355–6**, 1426, 1437
cystinuria 1335, **1356–7**, *3332*, **3333**
cystitis
  abacterial 3207
  bacterial 3206–7
   in pregnancy 1787
   treatment **3208–10**, *3211*
  haemorrhagic, BK virus causing 446
  tuberculous 3276, 3277
cystogastrostomy 2033
cystography, radionuclide micturating 3215
cystopathy, diabetic 4099
cystoplasty 3900
cystoscopy, urinary-tract infections and 3213
cystourethrography, micturating (voiding) 3111, **3214–15**, 3217
cytoadherence, in malaria 842
'cytobrush' 755
cytochrome a₃ oxidase 1194
cytochrome oxidase
  in carbon monoxide exposure 1095
  in cyanide toxicity 1097
  in hydrogen sulphide poisoning 1099
cytochrome P450 2081
  drugs affecting *3273*
  measurement of activity 2056
  polymorphisms, drug metabolism and 130, 1259, 2124
  see also entries beginning P₄₅₀
cytochrome P450*db₁*, antibodies 2070
cytogenetics 3390
  in acute lymphocytic leukaemia 3413
  of lymphoproliferative disorders 3567
  molecular 119
cytokines 68, **95–9**, **152–3**, *152*, 1554, 2293, 2591
  in acute pancreatitis 2029
  acute-phase reaction 276
  adult respiratory distress syndrome 2574–5, 2854–5
  antibodies, ARDS management 2576
  in asthma 2727, *2728*
  atherosclerotic plaque development 2293–4, 2299
  -blocking therapies 99
  in bone formation 3056
  in bone resorption 3057
  cancer therapy 233
  characterisation and nomenclature 97
  chemoattractant 98, 2294
  in chronic obstructive airways disease 2770
  classification 95–7, *96*
  in Crohn's disease 1937, 1938, 1940
  definition 95, 3056
  epidermis/dermis interaction 3707
  in extrinsic allergic alveolitis 2813
  fever in tumours due to 241
  in graft rejection 187
  haemolytic uraemic syndrome and 3199–200
  haemopoietic recovery after acute radiation 1219
  hepatic granulomas pathogenesis 2120
  in high permeability pulmonary oedema 2497, 2498
  hypercalcaemia of malignancy and 1568
  IgE synthesis regulation 157
  in inflammation 98, 2951
  in leptospirosis 699
  in lichen planus 3751
  in lymphoma 3568
  in malaria 276, 842, 845
  in meningococcal meningitis 537
  mode of action **97**
  in myelomatosis 3598
  in osteoarthritis 2981
  paracrine action 95

passive immunoprophylaxis with 284
physiological role **97–9**
pneumococcal infection pathogenesis 513
production 2293–4
  fever patterns and 276
  in infections 276
receptors 97, 1556
regulation of erythropoiesis 3388
in rheumatoid arthritis 2954
in rickettsial diseases 730
secretion by,
  alveolar macrophage 2615, *2615*
  endothelial cells 2294, 2299, 2487, 2498, 2514
  helper T-cells 97, 98, 151, 157, 2715
  macrophage *92*, 93–4, 2615, *2615*
  neutrophils 2622, *2624*
  in SLE *3025*, **3026**
therapeutic uses **99**
in ulcerative colitis 1945
weight loss in tumours due to 241
see also specific interleukins/ interferons; tumour necrosis factor (TNF)
cytokinesis 81
cytomegalovirus (CMV) infection **359–63**
in adolescents and adults 361
after cardiac transplantation 2257
after lung transplantation 2936
in children 361
clinical features 360–1, *361*
complications 361
congenital/intrauterine 360, *361*, 362, 1778, **1779**, *1780*, 4112
diabetes type I and 1454
diagnosis 362, 2257
epidemiology 359–60
haematological changes 3679
hepatitis 2064
in HIV infection 473, 479, *479*, 4079–80
in homosexuals 3364
in immunocompromised 1034
  monoclonal antibodies 362
nosocomial infection 360
passive immunoprophylaxis 363
perinatal 360–1, 362
pneumonia 2709, 2713
radiculopathy 4079
recurrent 362
in renal transplant recipients 3314
retinitis 361, 4192, **4193**
  in HIV infection 476, 4079, 4193
seroconversion 362
Sjögren's syndrome and 3036
transmission 359–60
  in blood 3693
treatment and prevention 363, *479*
vaccine 363
cytopathic vacuole type I, in alphavirus infected cells 75
cytopenia, in SLE 3020
cytoplasmic antigens, autoantibodies to 163
cytoplasmic linker protein (CLIP) 83
cytoplasmic oncogenes, *see* oncogenes, cytoplasmic
cytosine arabinoside (Ara-C)
  in acute myelosclerosis 3438
  in leukaemia 3407–8
  in myelodysplastic syndromes 3430
cytoskeleton **80–3**
  of cells 68
  classes of elements 80
   see also intermediate filaments; microfilaments; microtubules
  control by GTP-binding proteins 82
  definition/explanation 80
  myocardial cells 2144
  platelet 3618
  red cell 3455
cytotoxic drugs
  alveolar reactions due to 2851
  aplastic anaemia induced by 3441
  in pregnancy 1761–2, 1806, 1807, 1808

secondary immunodeficiency due to 174
  side-effects 1718
  in vasculitis 3016
  veno-occlusive disease due to 2099
  see also chemotherapy
cytotoxic T-cells (CTL) 149, 151, 151–2
  in allergic diseases 157
  antigen processing for 143
  in Boutonneuse fever 734
  CD4:CD8 ratio, *see under* T-cells
  CD4 cells 151, 165
  CD8 antigen 150, 151
  in chronic active hepatitis B 2065
  class I antigen restriction 142, 143, 151, 280
  damage/encephalitis due to 152
  in graft rejection 152, 186
  in gut-associated lymphoid tissue 1836
  in HIV infection 151, 466, 467, 471
  in infections 280
  lysis mechanism 151
  myocarditis 2381
  in primary biliary cirrhosis 2074
  response to tumours 229
  tumour antigen identification 228
  in viral infections 151
cytotoxins, in gastrointestinal infections 2002

D

dacarbazine, in Hodgkin's disease *3573*, 3574
Da Costa's syndrome 2169, 2174, 4207
Dacron grafts 2369, 2370, 2372
dactylitis
  finger, in psoriatic arthritis 2968
  toes 2967
danazol 1248
  teratogenicity *1810*
dandruff 3743, 3764
Dandy-Walker syndrome **4113**
dantrolene, in neuroleptic malignant syndrome 1182
dapsone 1547
  in dermatitis herpetiformis 3783
  haemolytic anaemia due to 3546, 3547
  in leprosy 674, 675, 676
   dosage and side-effects 675
  overdose **1073**
  resistance 674, 675
Daraprim, overdose 1073
Darier's disease **3721–2**, 3760
darmbrand, *see* necrotizing enterocolitis
data collection, drug addicts 4297
Datura species 1076
DAVIT-I and -II trials 2347–8
DCC (deleted in colorectal cancer) gene 66, 1990
DDAVP, *see* desmopressin
o,p'-DDD 1652, 1660, 1714
DDT 858, 859
  head count 1004
deafferentation, neuropathic pain 3939
deafness 3870
  after bacterial meningitis 4059
  after head injury 3835
  in Alport's syndrome 3204
  in congenital rubella 410, 1779
  meningococcal meningitis 540
  in multiple sclerosis 3993
  mumps association 407
  in Paget's disease of bone 3075–6
  syphilitic 714
  see also hearing loss
1-deamino-8-D-arginine vasopressin, *see* desmopressin
death 3933
  brain-stem 14, **3317**
  cause, in death certificate 4310
  cause unknown 4309
  confirmation 4309
  definition 3933, 3934
  diagnosis **4349**
   brain death and 3933
  doctor's duties **4309–10**

effect on and care of family after **4357**
fear of 4357
nature of 3933
reporting to coroner 4310
sudden, *see* sudden cardiac death; sudden death
talking about 4357
see also bereavement; dying patients; terminal illness
death certificates 4309, 4310
Debendox 1810
debranching enzyme 1340
  deficiency (Forbes-Cori's disease; glycogen storage disease III) 1342, *1343*, 1384, 4166
debridement, in electrical injury 1213, 1214
decay accelerating factor (DAF) 177, 179, 3450
decentralization, health care 53
decerebrate movements, in poisoning 1046
decerebrate rigidity 2584
decibel 1223
decision-making, alcohol abuse intervention 4275
decompression
  aircraft 1199
  disorders associated 1210
decompression illness/sickness **1199**, **1208–9**, 1210, **4128–9**
  air travel after diving 1199
  low-differential aircraft cabins and 1198
  neurological features **4128–9**
  pathogenesis 1208
  symptoms 1209
decongestants 2718
decontamination, in chemical warfare 1115
decorin 3058
decorticate movements, in poisoning 1046
decorticate posture 3930
decubitus ulcer, *see* pressure sore (decubitus ulcer)
dedifferentiation, of tumours 195, 196
deep vein thrombosis (DVT) **2522–3**, 3664
  aircraft travel and 1203
  in antiphospholipid syndrome 3020
  axillary 2523
  clinical features 2522–3
  consequences **3664**
  in drug addicts 4280, 4294
  in elderly **4343**
  at high altitudes 1193 legs and pelvis **2523**
  management 2523, 3807, 3809
  in pregnancy 1741, 1742–3
  risk factors 2522
deerfly fever 599–603
DEET 324
defaecating proctogram, in solitary rectal ulcer syndrome 2138
defaecation 1825
  frequency 1964, 1967
   in cirrhosis 2087
  incomplete 1967
  reflex 1955, 1964
  suppression 1964
defence mechanisms
  in diabetes 1493
  gastrointestinal tract 1836, 1879, 2001
  levels/types 275
  non-specific immunity 276–7
  psychological 4204
   in dying patients 4233
  respiratory tract 276, **2612–16**
   mucociliary escalator 2609, 2612, **2613**
   nasopharyngeal secretions 514, 2613
   nose and turbinates 2609, 2612, 2613
   protective proteins 2613, 2614
   surfactant 2613
   see also lung, defence mechanisms
  surface barriers to infections 275–6
  see also host response to infections; immune response

defensins 2614
deferiprone (1,2-dimethyl-3-
    hydroxypyridin-4-one) 3481
defibrillation 2263, 2265
defibrillators 2288–9
    implantable cardiovertor 2265, 2280,
        2288–9
deformity **3061**
    in ankylosing spondylitis 2799
    in Friedreich's ataxia 3984
    in osteogenesis imperfecta 3080
    in Paget's disease of bone 3075
    in rheumatoid arthritis 2957
    in rickets and osteomalacia 3071
degenerative disorders
    cerebral, *see* neurological disorders/
        diseases, degenerative
    spinal, *see* spine
Degos disease, polyarteritis nodosa *vs*
    3015
'degreaser's flush' 1090
dehydration
    acute on chronic renal failure 3299
    in acute pancreatitis 2028
    in cirrhosis 2087
    in diabetic ketoacidosis 1499
    hypernatraemic 2006
    in malnutrition,
        incorrect use 1283
        management 1289
    in myeloma 3603
    relative polycythaemia in 3552, 3553
    in salicylate poisoning 1054, 1055
    signs 1289
    in terminal illness 4360
    tests, *see* fluid, deprivation tests
    thirst sensation 3117
    in water-depletion heat exhaustion 1181
    see also hypovolaemia
2-dehydroemetine hydrochloride, in
    amoebiasis 832
dehydroepiandrosterone 1664
5'-deiodinase
    type I (5'DI) 1605
    type II (5'DII) 1605
    type III (5'DIII) 1605
déjà vu 3914
Déjérine and Roussy, thalamic syndrome
    of 3861
Déjérine-Sottas disease 4103
    leprosy *vs* 674
de Lange syndrome **4110**
delayed hypersensitivity 164, **165**, *165*,
    279
    to drugs 1253
    in graft rejection 186
    in infections 279, *279*
    in leprosy 279
    mechanisms 2819
    in nickel dermatitis 1112
    in paracoccidioidomycosis 817, 818
    in polymyositis and dermatomyositis
        4156
    in sarcoidosis 2819
    in schistosomiasis 976
    in tuberculosis 640, 645
    see also cell-mediated immune
        response; T-cells
deliberate self-harm **4228–31**
    assessment 4229–30
        children at risk after 4230
        interviewing suicidal patients
            4229–30, *4230*
        non-fatal repetition 4230
        physical complications 4229
        suicide risk 4229, *4229*
    causes 4228–9
    epidemiology 4228
        reasons for incidence increase 4229
    'hotline' and support for patients 4231
    management 4230–1
        crisis intervention 4255
        ongoing suicide risk 4231
    methods 4228
    non-fatal repetition prevention 4231
    see also suicide
delirium 3932, **4223–4**
    in AIDS 4236

assessment 4341
causes 3967, 4224, *4224*, 4226
    in elderly 4341, *4341*
    dementia co-occurrence 4226
    differential diagnosis 4224
        dementia *vs* **3967–8**, *3968*, 4224,
            4226, *4226*
        mania *vs* 4220
    in elderly 4226
    epidemiology 4224
    management 4224, 4341
    symptoms 3967, 4223, *4223*
    in tricyclic antidepressant poisoning
        1059
    see also confusion, acute
delirium tremens 1251, 2084, 2093,
    4259, 4290
    management 4291
    rabies *vs* 401
delta fibres 3936
delta waves (rhythm) 3830
delusional disorder 4225
delusional perception 4221
delusions
    in depressive disorders 4218
    in elderly 4227
    of grandeur 4220, 4221
    hypochondriacal 4227
    paranoid 4223
    in schizophrenia 4221
demeclocycline
    (demethylchlortetracycline) 2241
    nephrotoxicity 3264
    in syndrome of inappropriate
        antidiuresis 1602, 3125
dementia **3965–84**, **4224–5**
    after strokes 4237
    alcoholic 4127
    assessment **3968–9**, 4225, 4226, 4341
        cognitive functions 3968–9
        examination 3969, *3970*
        history 3968
        investigations 3969, *3970*, 4226, 4227
    causes **3965**, *3966*, 4224, *4224*
        in elderly 4341, *4341*
        treatable **3969–71**
    classification of severity 4341, *4341*
    clinical features 4224, *4224*
    cortical 3965
        subcortical *vs* 3967
        see also Alzheimer's disease
    definition 3965
    delirium co-occurrence 4226
    delirium *vs* **3967–8**, *3968*, 4224, 4226,
        4226
    demands on carers 4225, 4227
    diagnostic criteria 3968–9, 4227
    dialysis 4124
    differential diagnosis **3967–8**
        in elderly 3965, 4226, 4227
    epidemiology **3965**, *3966*
    prevalence, in elderly 3965, 4226
    epilepsy and 3924
    familial *1514*
    of frontal lobe type, *see* Pick's disease
    HIV-1-associated 4077
    in Huntington's disease 4013
    management 4225, *4225*, 4341
        burden on carers 4225, 4227
        in elderly 4227
    mixed cortical-subcortical 3966–7
    multifocal, diffuse brain diseases
        causing 3998, *3999*
    multi-infarct, *see* multi-infarct dementia
    in Parkinson's disease 4001, 4002, 4238
    patterns of cognitive impairment
        3965–7
    postoperative onset 4243
    presenile, *see* Alzheimer's disease
    progressive multifocal, *see* Creutzfeldt-
        Jakob disease
    subcortical 3965–6, *3967*
    treatment, antipsychotic drugs 4251
    in tumours *243*, 3971
    visual evoked potentials (VEP) 3833
demethylchlortetracycline, *see*
    demeclocycline
Demodex folliculorum 1000, 1009

demographic entrapment 37
demography, developing countries 51
de Musset's sign 2465
demyelinating disorders **3989–98**
    auditory evoked potentials in 3835
    isolated syndromes **3990–2**
    magnetic resonance imaging 3834
    neurobiology **3989–90**
    neuropathology 3989–90
    optic nerve lesions in 3866
    rare **3989**
    somatosensory evoked potentials (SEP)
        3833–4
    treatment **3995–6**
    visual evoked potentials (VEP) 3831–2
    see also multiple sclerosis
demyelination 4091
    inflammatory 3990
    in progressive multifocal
        leucoencephalopathy 446
    selective 4091
dendritic cells 87, 93, 3706
    antigen presentation 87, 93, **153**
        in graft recipient 184, 185
    follicular 3561
    in HIV infections 466, 467
    in vitro derived 87
    MHC class II antigen expression 87
dengue **413**, 419
    diagnosis 413, 420
    secondary, in dengue haemorrhagic
        fever 419
dengue haemorrhagic fever 291, **419–23**
    aetiological diagnosis 421
    antibodies in 420, 421–2
    clinical features 420
    diagnostic criteria 420
    haemolytic uraemic syndrome *vs* 3201
    history and epidemiology 419
    immune response and pathogenesis 420
    pathophysiology 420–1
    treatment and control 422
dengue shock syndrome 419, 420, 422
dengue viruses 413, 419
    detection and monoclonal antibodies
        421
    genome detection 422
    NS1 protein 419, 422
    'second infection hypothesis' 420
    serotypes 419
    structure/characteristics 419, 420
    vaccine 422
denial 4204
    adaptive and maladaptive 4204
    in dying patients 4233, 4357
    in grief reaction 4234
dense deposit disease (mesangiocapillary
    glomerulonephritis II) 3157, **3158**,
    3161, 3315
dense granules, platelet 3615
densitometry, bone 3066
    in osteoporosis 3067
density, whole-body, measurement 1303
density-sensing mechanism of cells 191
    impairment 191
densoviruses 447
dental abscess 1846, 1847
dental amalgam, mercury exposure 1111
dental caries **1846–7**
    actinomycetes association 685
    aetiology 1328, 1846
    clinical features 1846–7
    differential diagnosis 1847
    immunological changes 1846
    pathology 1846
    prevention/treatment 1847
dental cysts 1863
dental enamel 1846
    in bulimia nervosa 1300
    defects 3061
dental plaque 1846
    gingival/periodontal disease 1847, 1848
dental sepsis, anaerobic 572
dentarubral pallidoluysian atrophy,
    unstable trinucleotide repeats *125*
dentigerous cyst 1863
dentinogenesis imperfecta 3080
dentists, HIV infection and 472, 1850

denture granuloma 1859
denture stomatitis 1851
denture trauma, oral ulceration in 1855
deodorants 3765
    dermatitis 3736
    poisoning 1079
deoxyadenosine 1385
5'-deoxyadenosylcobalamin (ado-B$_{12}$)
    3484
deoxycholic acid 2047
2'-deoxycoformycin (DCF) *3422*, 3423,
    3424
deoxycorticosterone
    excessive doses 1661–2
    excessive production 1660
    plasma, in congenital adrenal
        hyperplasia 1668
11-deoxycortisol, plasma
    in congenital adrenal hyperplasia 1668,
        1690, 1694
    in metyrapone test 1647, 1648, 1649
deoxyguanosine 1386
    accumulation 172
deoxypyridinoline 3060
deoxyuridine suppression test 3494
dependence syndromes 4268, *4268*, *4269*
    see also alcohol abuse; drug abuse and
        misuse
dependency
    development in epilepsy 4238
    of dying patients 4233
dependoviruses 447
depersonalization, in SLE 3019
depigmentation **3755–60**
    chemical 3759
    in dermatitis 3734
    miscellaneous forms/causes 3759–60
    post-inflammatory 3760
    see also vitiligo
depolarization 4139
    myocardial cells, *see* heart,
        electrophysiology
    smooth muscle of gastrointestinal tract
        1952, 1953
depolarization block 4141
depressants, as drugs of concern 4263
depression/depressive disorders **4218–20**
    aetiology 4219
        genetic factors 4219
    after bereavement 4235–6
    after strokes 4237, 4340
    amenorrhoea in 1671
    in anorexia nervosa 1297, 4214
    anxiety symptoms in 4206
    chronic fatigue syndrome 1037, 1038
    chronic pain in 3943
    in chronic renal failure 3306
    clinical features 4218, *4218*
        in elderly 4227
    in Cushing's syndrome 1645, 4239
    deliberate self-harm in 4228, 4247
    diagnosis,
        difficulties in elderly 4227
        importance of 4218
    differential diagnosis 4219
        alcohol abuse *vs* 4219
        chronic fatigue syndrome *vs* 1037,
            1038
        normal sadness *vs* 4219
        Parkinson's disease *vs* 4002
        psychiatric disorders *vs* 4219
        schizophrenia *vs* 4222
        unexplained physical symptoms *vs*
            4219
    in dying patients 4233, **4358**
    in elderly 4226, 4227, 4341
    in folic acid deficiency 4241
    incidence/prevalence 4218, 4226
    late-onset 4227
    in malignant disease 4243
    masked 4227
    in multiple sclerosis 4238
    as normal reaction to illness 4218
    in Parkinson's disease 4004, 4238,
        4340
    peptic ulcers and 1884
    physical disorders causing 4225
    prognosis 4219

depression/depressive disorders (*cont.*)
psychotic 4218
recurrence prevention 4220
recurrent, brief dynamic psychotherapy
  in 4256
sexual interest impairment 4245
tension headache and 4027
treatment 4219–20, *4220*, 4247
  moclobemide 4250
  see also antidepressants
variations in clinical picture 4218–19,
  4218
  anxiety symptoms 4218
  brief depressive episode 4219
  excess alcohol consumption 4219
  non-compliance with treatment 4219
  physical complaint deterioration
    4218–19
  somatic symptoms 4218
  see also affective disorders
depressive pseudodementia 3967, 4225,
  4227
depressive symptoms
  in bulimia nervosa 1300, 4216
  in chronic schizophrenia 4222
de Quervain's (subacute) thyroiditis
  1612, 1613, 1615
de Quervain's tenosynovitis 2947, 2996
Dermacentor andersoni 728
dermal atrophy **3790–1**
  focal 3791, 3793
dermal hypoplasia, focal 3791, 3793
dermatan sulphate 3626
  amyloid fibril-associated 1521
dermatitis **3734–43**
  allergic contact, *see* contact dermatitis,
    allergic
  atopic, *see* atopic eczema
  Berloque *3754*
  cercarial 970, 975
  chronic 3735
  climate and seasons affecting 3723–4
  clinical features 3734–5
  contact, *see* contact dermatitis
  contagious pustular, *see* orf
  definition 3734
  drug-induced 3731, 3732, 3738
  exfoliative *244*, 3708
  genitalia 3768, *3769*
  glove 3715
  hand, management 3807
  industrial/occupational 1164, 3723,
    3735
  see also dermatosis
  infected 3743
  nappy eruptions 3768, 3769
  nickel, *see under* contact dermatitis
  seborrhoeic 800, 3712, 3743, 3762,
    3768
  solar 3715
  steroids causing 3787, 3788
  streptococcal 3768
  vaseline 3736
  in vitamin B deficiency 3722
  see also eczema
dermatitis artefacta 3778, 3779, 4211
dermatitis herpetiformis 1917, 1919,
  3685–6, 3723, **3782–3**
  distribution 3712
  in enteropathy-associated T-cell
    lymphoma 1929
  folate deficiency 3492
  iodine triggering 3729, 3731
  lymphoma risk 1985
  scabies *vs* 1008
dermatological syndromes,
  paraneoplastic *244*
dermatology 3705, 3707
  occupational **1164–5**
dermatomyositis *3009*, **3038–9**, **4156–8**
  aetiology 4156–7
  classification *4156*
  clinical features 3039, 4157
  course and prognosis 4158
  diagnosis and treatment 3039, 4157
  gastrointestinal tract in 2000
  immune response 4156–7
  lung involvement in **2799**
  malignancy association 4157, 4158

ocular features **4184**
telangiectasia and facial erythema in
  3787, 3788
in tumours *244*, 3793
variants **4157–8**
see also polymyositis
Dermatophagoides 1010
Dermatophagoides pteronyssinus
  2714–15
dermatophyte infections
  (dermatophytoses) **797–9**
  in diabetes 1490
dermatosis
  crazy pavement 1283, 1284
  in kwashiorkor 1283, 1284, 1295
  occupational 1164–5
    barrier creams 1164–5
    employee/employer attitude 1164
    incidence and importance 1164
    non-dermatitic 1165
    skin cleansing and creams 1165
    skin protection 1165
  of poor 3722
  see also skin disease
dermatosis papulosa nigra *3755*
dermis 3706
  functions 3707
dermographism 162, 1805, 3771
dermoid cysts 4033
dermopathy, diabetic 1489
De Sanctis-Cucchioni syndrome *3754*
descriptive studies 44
desensitization
  allergens 158, 161, 162–3, 2718
  in asthma 2740
  in food allergies 1845
  to insect venom 1145
desferrioxamine 1071, 1248
  in aluminium poisoning 1105
  in dialysis-associated aluminium
    toxicity 3329
  in hereditary haemochromatosis 3479
  hypotension and adverse effects 1071
  in iron overdose 1071, 3480–1
    test 2022
  in thalassaemia 3480–1, 3512
  in vanadium poisoning 1114
'designer drugs' 67, 4297
desipramine 4293
desmoglein 163, 3781
17,20-desmolase, *see* 17,20-lyase
desmopressin (DDAVP) 1588
  in diabetes insipidus 1601, **3122**
  in haemophilia 3648, **3651**
  in liver disease 3635
  in platelet disorders 3645, 3646
  in postural hypotension in primary
    autonomic failure 3886
  in pregnancy 1765
  in renal failure *3288*, 3305, 3634
    tests 3109, 3121
  therapeutic trial 1601, **3121–2**
  in von Gierke's disease 1342
  in von Willebrand's disease *3643*,
    3644, **3645**
desmosomes 2143–4
detergents, poisoning 1079
detoxification
  drug addicts 4276, 4291–3
  see also opiates developed countries
  diseases of overnourished societies
    1326–32
  immunization in **320**
developing countries
  anaemia in 3462–70
  antibiotic resistance 309
  demographic entrapment 37
  health care in **51–4**
  HIV infection in, *see* HIV infection
  immunization in **320–1**, *321*
  iron-deficiency anaemia 3474
  microbiology services 311
  sexually transmitted diseases **3348**
  tuberculosis in **661–4**
  see also tuberculosis
developmental abnormalities **1689–703**,
  4105
  brain *4106*, **4115–16**

embryogenesis **4112–14**
head enlargement in infancy **4114–15**
miscellaneous **4122**
nervous system **4105–22**, *4106*
  complex malformation syndromes
    4111–12
  infections and teratogens **4112**
  non-specific embryogenic defects
    4112–14
  see also chromosomal abnormalities;
    mental retardation
  occupations associated 1173
  recombinant DNA technology role 66
skull **4115–16**
speech disorders **4122**
spine **4116–19**
  see also spina bifida
  see also cerebral palsy
developmental disorders, amenorrhoea
  1670
Devic's disease 3990, **3991–2**
'devil's grip' 387
dexamethasone
  in acute mountain sickness 1190, 1191
  in cerebral metastases 250
  in congenital adrenal hyperplasia 1665,
    1667
  in congenital apparent mineralocorticoid
    excess syndrome 1661
  in cortisol deficiency 1587
  in glucocorticoid resistance 1661
  in glucocorticoid-suppressible
    hyperaldosteronism 1660
  in Graves' ophthalmopathy 1614
  maternal, virilization reduction 136
  in meningococcal meningitis 542
  in myeloma 3602
  in Nelson's syndrome 1595
  in pneumococcal infection 521
  in raised intracranial pressure 4037
  in severe typhoid 565
  suppression tests,
    in aldosteronism *1658*, 1659
    in Cushing's syndrome 1566, 1645
    drugs interfering 1717
    in ectopic ACTH syndrome 1713
    high-dose 1647
    low-dose 1645
    normal values *4375*
    in pregnancy 1751
    in thyrotoxic crisis 1614
    in treated Cushing's syndrome 1650,
      1651
dextran 2564
  as blood substitute 3634, 3661
  glomerular filtration 3136
  infective endocarditis pathogenesis
    2438
α-dextrinase 1920
  deficiency 1922, 1923
dextromoramide *4353*
dextrose
  acute hepatocellular failure management
    2108
  in alcoholic ketoacidosis 1080
  intravenous, *see* glucose, intravenous
DF2 bacillus 1028
Diabetes Control and Complications
  Trial (DCCT) 1463–4, 1482, 1483,
  4189
diabetes insipidus 1651
  cranial 1601, **3120**
    aetiology *1602*, 3120
    clinical features 3120
    diagnosis 1601, 3121–2
    treatment 1588, 1601, 3122
  dipsogenic, *see* polydipsia, primary
  in Langerhans-cell histiocytosis 3608,
    3609
  nephrogenic **3120–1**,
    3331–2
    aetiology 3120–1, *3331*
    clinical features 3121, 3331–2
    diagnosis 1601, 3121–2
    drug-induced 1719
    hypercalcaemia-induced 3120, 3228
    lithium causing 3121, 3263, 4250
    pathophysiology 3331

toxin-induced 3259
treatment 3122
in urinary-tract obstruction 3234
X-linked 3120, 3121, 3331
neurological features 4125
in pregnancy 1748
in sarcoidosis 2827
in suprasellar germinoma 1597–8
diabetes mellitus 1448–504, **4125**
in acromegaly 1592
in adolescence **1496–7**
aetiology, dietary factors 1327
in affluent societies 1327
aircraft travel and 1203
amyotrophy 4098
anaesthesia and surgery in 1489,
  1493–6
autoantibodies in 163
beta-blockade in angina 2328
brittle **1496**
cataracts in **1485**
cheiroarthropathy 1487
'chemical' 1448, 1449
classification 1450–3
clinics 1503–4
collagen disturbances **1489–90**
coma in **1497–503**, 4239
complications, in elderly 4345
in congenital rubella 1454, 1779
coxsackie B virus infections causing
  387–8
cross-reacting epitopes 155
in cystic fibrosis 1714, 1746, 2749
cystopathy 4099
definition 1448–9
diagnosis 1449, *1450*
  WHO guidelines *4345*
diarrhoea 1962, 4099
disease processes 1450
diverticular disease in 1969
education **1479**
education centres 1504
in elderly **4344–5**
  management 4345
  presenting features 4344–5
eye disease **1483–6**, **4188–91**
  see also diabetic retinopathy
gangrene 2372
gas gangrene in 633
gastrointestinal motility disorders in
  1962, 4099
  see also diabetic gastroparesis
gestational *1452*, **1753–4**, *1755*
glycaemic/metabolic control **1462–5**,
  1485
  in elderly 4345
  in foot disease 1491
  importance 1462–4, 1481–2
  nephropathy and 1464, 1482, 3171
  neuropathy and 1463, 1482, 1486
  practical aspects 1464–5
  retinopathy and 1463, 1482, 1483
haematological changes **3686**
heat stroke in 1180
in hereditary haemochromatosis 3478,
  3479
hormone replacement therapy in 1815
hyperlipidaemia in 1410–11, 1485–6,
  3172
incipient, postprandial hypoglycaemia
  1511
infections in 1492–3
  susceptibility 281
insulin-dependent (IDDM) 1450,
  1451–2
  improved glycaemic control 1463–4
  surgery in 1494–5
  see also diabetes mellitus, type I
intraepidermal blisters 3783
ischaemic heart disease risk 2309
juvenile-onset, *see* diabetes mellitus,
  type I
large artery disease 2371
lipid-lowering therapy 1413, 1414
lipid metabolism 1400
liver in *2019*, 2024
macroangiopathy 1449, *1450*, 1463,
  1464, **1491–2**, 2371

malnutrition-related *1451*
maturity onset, *see* diabetes mellitus,
  type II
mental disorders/symptoms in 4239–40
metabolic basis 1456–65
metabolic control, *see* diabetes mellitus,
  glycaemic/metabolic control
microalbuminuria in 1464, 3138, 3168,
  3170
microangiopathy 1449, *1450*, 1463–4,
  1482–91, 4098
miniclinics 1504
mucormycosis in 1027
mumps precipitating 373
myocardial infarction, thrombolytic
  therapy 2341
non-endocrine causes 1714, *1715*
non-insulin-dependent (NIDDM)
  1451–2
  improved glycaemic control 1463
  surgery in 1495
  see also diabetes mellitus, type II
nurse 1504
opportunistic infections in 1027
organization of therapy **1503–4**
pancreatic cancer association 205, 2040
pathogenesis 1454
peripheral arterial disease risk 2363
peripheral neuropathy, *see* diabetic
  neuropathy
'piqure' 1499
polyuria in 1453, 3147
pregnancy in 130, **1752–8**
  medical management 1754–6
  obstetric management 1756–8
  presenting features 1453, 4344–5
  pruritus in 3744
records 1504
reduced endothelium-dependent
  vasodilation 2297
retinal vein occlusion 4187
secondary *1451–2*, 1453
sexual problems,
  in female 4244
  in male 4243–4
shared care 1504
skin disease in 3723
special problems 1492–7
tissue damage 1449, *1450*, **1481–92**
  drug therapy in reduction **1472**
  glycaemic control and 1463–4, 1481–2
  two-phase development 1464
treatment **1465–79**
  aims 1465, *1466*, *1467*
  diet 1465–9 drugs 1469–72
  exercise 1478–9
  insulin, *see* insulin, therapy
  monitoring **1479–81**
tropical calcific pancreatic 1450, *1451*,
  1452
type I,
  aetiology 156, 1327
  dietary management 1465, 1468, 1469
  disease process 1450
  environmental factors 1454
  epidemiology 1454
  exercise 1478
  genes involved 64
  genetic susceptibility 1453–4
  hidden antigen release and 156
  immune mechanisms 1453
  insulin secretion 1461
  insulin therapy 1475–6
  monitoring of therapy 1479, 1480
  mortality 1482
  nephropathy in 3168, 3169
  pathogenesis 156, 1453–4, 1571
  sulphonylurea drugs 1471
type Ib 1450, *1451*
type II *1451*, 1452
  amyloid deposits 1450, 1455, *1513*,
    1518
  dietary management 1465, 1468, 1469
  disease process 1450
  exercise 1478–9
  genes involved 64
  genetics 1455–6
  insulin resistance 1572

insulin secretion 1460–1, 1565
insulin therapy 1475
  maturity onset of young 1450, 1452
  monitoring of therapy 1479, 1480
  mortality 1482
  nephropathy in 3168, 3169
  obesity and 1308, 1327
  oral hypoglycaemic agents 1471–2
  pathogenesis 1454–6, 1571
  type III 1450, *1451*, 1452
diabetic foot disease 1449, 1482,
  1490–1, 4098–9
  amputation 2372
  in elderly 4345
  glycaemic control 1491
  preventive care 1487, 1490
  sensory neuropathy 1486–7, 4098
  treatment 1490–1, 2371–2, 4098, 4345
  ulcers, anaerobic infections 573
diabetic gastroparesis **1962**
  trituration inadequacy 1955
diabetic ketoacidosis 1400, **1498–502**
  acid-base disturbances 1541, 1542
  clinical features 1499
  differential diagnosis 1499–500, 2030
  in elderly 4345
  emergency surgery and 1495–6
  investigation 1500
  mucormycosis in 1027
  precipitating factors 1494, 1499
  treatment 1500–3, 1543–4
diabetic nephropathy 1483, **3167–72**
  albuminuria/proteinuria 3169
  antihypertensive therapy 3171–2, 3250
  blood pressure 3168, 3169–70
  clinical evaluation 3170
  contrast media toxicity 3266
  definition 3167
  dietary therapy 1468–9, 3171
  differential diagnosis 3170
  epidemiology 3167–8
  evolution 3168, *3169*, 3303
  glycaemic control and 1464, 1482,
    3171
  history 3167
  hyporeninaemic hypoaldosteronism
    1662
  pathophysiology 3168–9
  pregnancy in 1756
  prevention and treatment 3171
  renal failure **3171–2**, 3295, 3296
  renal hypertension in 2547
  renal transplantation 3172, 3315
  two-phase development 1464
diabetic neuropathic cachexia 4098
diabetic neuropathy **1486–9, 4098–9**,
  4125
  autonomic 1486, *1487*, **1488–9**, 3171,
    4098
  classification 1486, *1487*
  clinical features and management
    1486–9
  glycaemic control and 1463, 1482,
    1486
  mononeuropathy 1486, 1487–8
  proximal motor (femoral) 1486, 1487
  sensory **1486–7**, 4098
  sensory polyneuropathy 4098
  sexual problems in 4244
diabetic retinopathy **1483–5**, 2039,
  4188–90
  blindness in 4198
  clinical features 4189–90
  in elderly 4345
  exudative 1483, 1484, 4189
  glycaemic control and 1463, 1482,
    1483
  incidence and progression 4189
  ischaemic features 4189–90
  management 1484–5
  pathology 4188–9
  pregnancy and 1756
  proliferative 1483–4, 4189, 4190
  risk factors and prognosis 4189
  screening 4190, *4190*
  simple 1483
  treatment 1485, 4189
  two-phase development 1464

diacylglycerol (diglyceride) 1561, 2147,
  2622
  diabetic tissue damage and 1483, 1486
  platelet activation and 3617–18
diagnosis **15–20**, 4363
  arborization method 15
  complete 'history and physical'
    (exhaustive) method 15
  evaluating articles about 18
  giving to dying patients 4234, 4357
  'gold standards' 18
  hypothetico-deductive method 15
  normal/abnormal results 4363
  pattern recognition method 15
  precision and accuracy 15–20
  telling patient about death 4357
  tests, reference intervals 4363
diagnostic methods
  gene probe use 66
  see also immunodiagnosis
*Diagnostic and Statistical Manual
  (DSM)*, substance abuse classification
  4269–70, *4269*
dialysis **3306–13**
  in acute renal failure 3287
  adequacy (*KT/V* index) 3309–10,
    3311
  aluminium toxicity 1425, 3096, 3321
  bone disease 3096
  complications *3309*, 3312–13
  dementia 1105, 4124
  in diabetic nephropathy 3171, 3172
  disequilibrium syndrome 3682, 4240
  drug clearance by 3269–70, *3271*
  encephalopathy 4240
  in ethylene glycol poisoning 1082
  folate deficiency 3493
  mental disorders/symptoms in 4240
  in methanol poisoning 1080
  in myeloma 3181–2, 3603
  outcomes 3312–13
  in poison elimination 1051
  preparation for 3306
  pre-renal transplant 3317–18
  quality of life 3312–13
  in rapidly progressive
    glomerulonephritis 3162–3
  starting/patient selection 3306–7
  survival, blood pressure relation 2552,
    2552
  in systemic sclerosis 3192
  see also haemodialysis; haemofiltration;
    peritoneal dialysis
dialysis osteodystrophy, myopathy in
  4169
4-4'-diaminodiphenyl-sulphone (DDS),
  see dapsone
3,4-diaminopyridine 4164
Diamond-Blackfan syndrome **3448–9**
  diamorphine (heroin) 4276
  adulterants 4281
  breast-feeding and 4299
  in opiate detoxification 4292
  overdose 1058
  prescribing 4289
  pulmonary oedema with 4283
  purity 1074
  in terminal illness 4356
  vasculitis associated 3178
  withdrawal syndrome 4291
Diane® contraceptive pill 3754
Dianette, in hirsutism 1677
diapedesis 2621
diaphragm 2876
  disorders **2876–8**, 3890
    aetiology 2877, *2877*
  dysfunction, in SLE 2798
  electrical pacing 2918, **2932**
  function assessment 3890
  normal chest radiograph 2657
  paralysis 2877, 2877–8, 3890
  plication 2878
  in respiration 2611, 2876–7
  in respiration control 3888
  weakness 2877, 3890
    causes 2877
    pathophysiology 2877
diaphragm, contraceptive 3206

diaphyseal aclasis 3089
diaphyseal dysplasia, progressive
  (Engelmann's disease) **3089**
diaphyseal hyperostosis 3088
diarrhoea **1823–5**
  acute infectious 2001, 2002
    secondary motility disorder 1963
  in amoebic dysentery 828
  associated symptoms with 1824
  in *Bacillus cereus* food poisoning 559,
    2002
  bacterial infections causing 2002
  in bacterial overgrowth 1914, 2003
    mechanism 1913
  bacterial toxins causing 1824, 2002
  in balantidiasis 881
  bloody, in necrotizing enterocolitis 637
  in capillariasis 939
  in carbohydrate intolerance syndrome
    1921
  causes 1824, 1930, 2003, 2004
    in returning travellers 326, 2003
  in cholera 577, 578, 1824, 2001–2, 2002
  chronic,
    causes 1930, 2003, 2004
    in tropical sprue 1933, 1934–5, 2003
    in urinary stone disease 3255
  chronic inflammatory 2004
  chronic 'motor' 1960
  chronic non-inflammatory 2003
  chronic pancreatitis 2035
  chronic/persisting 1824, 1825
  in cirrhosis 2087
  in *Clostridium perfringens* food
    poisoning 637
  in common varied immunodeficiency
    (CVID) 169
  in Crohn's disease 1938
  definition/criteria for 1823, 1967
  diabetic **1488–9**, 1962, 4099
  diagnosis 1824, 1825
  in dumping syndrome 1962
  endocrine causes 2006
  enteral feeding complication 1321
  enteropathogenic *E. coli* (EPEC)
    causing 555, 556
  enterovirus infections 387
  examination 1824–5
  in fasciolopsiasis 993
  in food poisoning 1824, 2002, 2003
  functional **1967–8**
  gut peptides in 1896
  haemolytic uraemic syndrome and (D+
    HUS) 3196, 3198
  in heterophyiasis 998
  history-taking 1824
  in HIV infections 475
  in homosexuals 3361
  in hyperthyroidism 1962
  hypokalaemia due to 3130
  in immunocompromised 1034
  inflammatory 2003–4
    differential diagnosis 2006
    see also dysentery
  in intestinal hurry 1960
  invasive infections causing 2004, *2004*
  investigations 1825
  'large volume' 1825
  in laxative abuse 1964
  in malabsorption 1904
  in malnutrition 1287
  in measles 379
  in medullary carcinoma of thyroid 1637
  metabolic acidosis due to 1543
  nocturnal 1945
  non-inflammatory 2002–3, *2002*
    chronic 2003
    differential diagnosis 2005–6
  osmotic 1825
  osmotic *vs* secretory 1825
  pathophysiology 1823–4
  in pseudomembranous (antibiotic-
    associated) colitis 635
  in rheumatic diseases 2945
  in schistosomiasis 977, 2004
  secretory 1825, 2002
    in carcinoid syndrome 1897
    mechanisms 577, 1824

diarrhoea (*cont.*)
in *Shigella* infections 554, 2003
in short gut syndrome, mechanisms 1925
spurious, in constipation 1964
'summer' 555
travellers', *see* travellers' diarrhoea
in ulcerative colitis 1945
in VIPoma syndrome 1705, 1706
viruses causing **390–4**, *391*, 2002
see also gastroenteritis, viral; *specific viruses 391*
watery,
in collagenous colitis 2136, 2137
in cryptosporidiosis 873, 874
in cyclospora infections 876
in giardiasis 879
in isosporiasis 883
viruses causing 391
Yersinia enterocolitica causing 608
in Zollinger-Ellison syndrome 1881
see also food poisoning; gastroenteritis
diastasis 2451–2
diastole 2150
calcium levels in myocardial cells 2145
definition 2231
electrophysiology 2148, 2259
in hypertrophic cardiomyopathy 2386
measurements 2231
diastolic blood pressure *2154*
antihypertensive drug indication 2539
essential hypertension diagnosis 2528
measurement 2535
mortality association 2532
see also blood pressure
diazepam
adverse mental symptoms 4242
in alcohol withdrawal 4259
in antiarrhythmic drug overdose 1064
in carbon monoxide poisoning 1096
in cerebral malaria 853
in chloroquine overdose 1072
emergency treatment of disturbed/violent patients 4257
in endoscopy 1830
in epilepsy 3922
indications and use 4253
in nerve agent exposure treatment 1118
in NSAIDs poisoning management 1057
in poisoning management 1047
in status epilepticus 3923
in terminal illness 4351, 4355, 4356
in tetanus 628
diazoxide 1509
in hypertension 2541
in hypoglycaemic agent overdose 1072
dibenzoxazepine (CR) 1118, 1119
DIC, *see* disseminated intravascular coagulation
dichloralphenazone, overdose/poisoning 1061
dichloromethane, *see* methylene chloride (dichloromethane)
dichloromethylene diphosphonate 3077
Dick test 499
diclofenac 1717
poisoning 1056
dicobalt edetate, in cyanide poisoning 1098
Diconal[R] 4289
dicrocoeliasis *982*, **987–8**
Dicrocoelium dendriticum 982, 983, 987
didanosine 481–2
MRC-ANRS European-Australian Alpha trial 481–2
dideoxycytosine 4080
dideoxyinosine 303, 4080
diencephalic tumours, mental disorders/symptoms in 4237
Dientamoeba fragilis 825
diesel particulates, seasonal allergic rhinitis (hayfever) 2714
diet
acne vulgaris management 3753–4
in adrenoleukodystrophy/adrenomyeloneuropathy 1440–1
agriculture and 3466–8
in amino acid disorders 1354

angina management 2326
appendicitis association 1329
in branched chain ketoaciduria 1369
calcium excretion and *3257*
cancer association 218–19, 1327–8, *1328*
bladder cancer 212
breast cancer 209
colorectal carcinoma 1990
gastric cancer 1982
indirect mechanisms 218–19, *219*
pancreatic carcinoma 2040
preformed carcinogens 218
cancer protective agents 219
in chronic renal failure 3304–5
in cirrhosis 2090
in coeliac disease 1919
colorectal adenoma aetiology 1987
constipation association 1328
coronary heart disease aetiology 1326–7, **2309–12**, 2332
Crohn's disease,
aetiology 1937
management 1942
in cystathionine synthase deficiency 1367
in cystic fibrosis 2751
dental caries association 1328
in diabetes mellitus **1465–9**
aetiology 1327
practical advice 1469, *1470*
in pregnancy 1755–6
therapeutic aspects 1468–9
in diabetic nephropathy 1468–9, 3171
diverticular disease of colon and 1328–9
dumping syndrome 1962
elemental, in Crohn's disease 1937, 1942
elimination 1844, 3742
'few-food' 1845
folate deficient 3467, 3492
food allergy management 1845
in fructose diphosphatase deficiency 1346, *1348*
in functional bowel diseases 1968
in galactosaemia 1350
gallstones association 1329
gluten-free, *see* gluten-free diet
in glycogen storage diseases 1342
in hepatic encephalopathy 2108
in hereditary fructose intolerance 1348
high-fibre, in diverticular disease 1970
in hyperlipoproteinaemia 1412–13
hypertension,
management 2538
pathogenesis 2530
in inborn errors of metabolism *1337*
iron absorption and 3466–7, 3471
irritable bowel syndrome and 1328, 1966
ischaemic heart disease,
intervention studies 2317–18
risk factor 1326–7, **2309–12**, 2332
in isovaleric/propionic/methylmalonic acidaemias 1371–2
ketogenic, in epilepsy treatment 3923
low-fat,
in angina 2326
in cirrhosis 2090
in short gut syndrome 1926
in small-intestinal lymphangiectasia 1977
in malnutrition,
acute phase 1289, *1291*
intermediate phase 1293
mixed diets 1293
rehabilitation phase 1293
Mediterranean 2311
need for change **1329–32**
nutritional guidelines 1332, *1332*
in obesity treatment 1311
osteoporosis association 1328
in peptic ulcer treatment 1883–4
in phenylketonuria 1362, 1363
polymeric 1942
in pre-eclampsia prevention 1730, 1773
in pregnancy 1770, *1772*, 1773, *1774*
in primary hyperoxaluria 1446, *1448*

in pyruvate carboxylase deficiency 1352
in pyruvate dehydrogenase deficiency 1351
recommendations 1329–32
renal bone disease and 3327
in short gut syndrome 1926
skin disease management 3806
in small-intestinal lymphangiectasia 1977
in terminal illness 4351
in ulcerative colitis 1949–50
in urea cycle defects 1360
uric acid excretion and 1379, 3225
in urinary stone disease 3251, 3256
vanilla-free 2555
very-low-calorie 1311
vitamin B$_{12}$ deficient 3468, 3492
Western, diseases associated **1326–32**
see also food; nutrition
dietary fibre
deficiency,
colorectal carcinoma aetiology 1990
in constipation 1967
Crohn's disease aetiology 1937
diverticular disease aetiology 1969
in irritable bowel syndrome 1966
ischaemic heart disease risk 2311
soluble forms 2311
see also non-starch polysaccharides
dietary history 1314
dietary reference values 1270–1, *1271*
fat and carbohydrate 1330, *1330*
dietary supplements
in anorexia nervosa treatment 1298, 4215
in coeliac disease 1919
in pregnancy 1773, *1774*
in short gut syndrome 1926
diethylcarbamazine
elimination 918, 3742
in loiasis 918
in lymphatic filariasis 923
reactions to 918, 923
in toxocariasis 945
diethyldithiocarbamate 1077
diethylene glycol 1081
diethylene-triamine penta-acetic acid (DTPA) 2214, 2668
in cobalt poisoning 1108
in zinc poisoning 1115
see also technetium-99m-diethylenetriaminepentacetic acid (DTPA)
diethylstilboestrol, *see* stilboestrol
dieting
anorexia nervosa after 1296, 1297, 4213, 4214
movement against 1309
in obesity treatment,
advice, foods and diets 1311
'dieting relationship trap' 1310–11
maintenance of weight loss 1313
weight loss rate 1310
weight loss without 1310
see also weight loss
'dieting relationship trap' 1310–11
Diet and Reinfarction Trial (DART) 2318
differentiation 191, 192
malignancy as genetically determined aberration 194
process 191
recombinant DNA application 66
suppression of insensitivity in tumours 193
diffuse cerebral sclerosis **3996–7**
diffuse cortical Lewy body disease 3967, 3973, 3998
Parkinson's disease and 4001, 4002
diffuse idiopathic skeletal hyperostosis (DISH) 2994
diffuse infiltrative lymphocytic syndrome (DILS) 3027, 3036
diffuse oesophageal spasm, *see* oesophagus, spasm
diffusing capacity, *see* pulmonary diffusing capacity
diffusion, gas exchange 2629–30
diflunisal, poisoning 1056
difluoro-deoxycytidine, *see* gemcitabine

difluoromethylornithine (DFMO, Ornidyl) 892, 893
5-(2,4-difluorophenyl) salicylic acid, poisoning 1056
Di-George syndrome 152, 171, 1634, 2899
gastrointestinal disease in *1840*
microdeletions in 108, *108*, 129
treatment 171
digestion, drugs inhibiting 1312
digestive enzymes, secretion 1903
digital fluorography **3822**, 3823
digitalis **2241–6**
in acute meningococcaemia 541
adverse mental symptoms 4242
drug interactions 2243
enterohepatic cycle 2242, 2243
heart failure treatment 1250, 2241, **2244–5**
assessments before 2244
in elderly 4342
maintenance 2244–5
rapid digitalization 2244
measurement and monitoring 1260–1, **2243–4**
mechanism of action 2241–2, 2263
in myocardial infarction 2568
myocardium/conducting system sensitivity 2242–3
pharmacokinetics **2242–3**
absorption and metabolism 2242
drug interactions affecting 2243
half-life 2242
protein binding 2242, 2243
preparations 2242
toxicity **1066**, 2243, 2244, **2245**
arrhythmia threshold 2243, 2245
hyperkalaemia 3135
hypokalaemia and 3129
mortality 2244
treatment and antibody therapy 1066, 2245
withdrawal 2244
see also digitoxin; digoxin
Digitalis Investigations Trial (DIG) 2244
digitalis leaf 2242
Digitalis purpurea 1152
digital subtraction angiography (DSA) 2369
carotid 3823, 3824
in peripheral arterial disease 2369
pulmonary 2656
in renovascular hypertension 2549
digital vessels, spasm 1226
digitoxin 2242
overdose/poisoning **1066**
see also digitalis
diglyceride, *see* diacylglycerol
digoxin 2242, *2264*
in cor pulmonale 2521
mechanism of action 2263
monitoring 1260–1
overdose/poisoning **1066**
treatment 1066
in pregnancy 1740
in pulmonary oedema 2504
in renal impairment 3268
see also digitalis
digoxin-specific antibody (Digibind) 1066, 1152, 2245
dihydrobiopterin reductase 1362
dihydrocodeine, in opiate detoxification **4292**
dihydrofolate *3487*
dihydrofolate reductase 3486, *3487*
drugs inhibiting 3493, 3497
dihydrolipoyl dehydrogenase deficiency 1351
dihydropteridine reductase deficiency 1363
dihydropyrimidine dehydrogenase (DHPDH) deficiency 1387
dihydrotachysterol (DHT) 1635
in chronic renal failure 3328, *3329*
dihydrotestosterone 1690, 1692
acne vulgaris aetiology 3752
in 5α-reductase deficiency 1693
testosterone ratio 2043
dihydroxyacetone 3757

dihydroxyacetone phosphate
    acyltransferase (DHAP-AT) *1440*
    deficiency 1441
2,8-dihydroxyadenine (2,8-DHA)
    crystal deposition 3226–7
    solubility 3225
    stones 1383, 3227
1,25-dihydroxycholecalciferol, bone
    resorption increase 3057
dihydroxyphenylethylene glycol (DHPG)
    2253, 2554, 2555
dihydroxyphenyl serine (DOPS) 3887
1,25-dihydroxyvitamin D₃, *see* calcitriol
24,25-dihydroxyvitamin D₃, *see*
    secalciferol
25,26-dihydroxyvitamin D₃
    (25,26(OH)₂D₃) 1625
di-iodohydroxyquin, in amoebiasis 832
diiodotyrosine 1605
diisocyanate 1100
    asthma 1100
dilated cardiomyopathy, *see*
    cardiomyopathy, dilated
diloxanide furoate, in amoebiasis 832
diltiazem 2330
D-dimer, in pulmonary embolism 2525
dimercaprol 1248, 3262
    in arsenic poisoning 1106
    in bismuth chelate poisoning 1069
    in lewisite exposure 1117
    in mercury poisoning 1112
dimercaptosuccinic acid ([⁹⁹Tcᵐ]DMSA)
    scans 3112
    in arsenic poisoning 1106
    in cadmium poisoning 1107
    in cobalt poisoning 1108
    in lead poisoning 1110
    in mercury poisoning 1112
    in reflux nephropathy 3216, 3217
1,2-dimethyl-3-hydroxypyridin-4-one
    (deferiprone; L1) 3481
4-dimethylaminophenol, in cyanide
    poisoning treatment 1098
dimethylchlortetracycline 766
dimethylcysteine, *see* penicillamine
dimethyl sulphoxide 2836
Dinobdella ferox 987, 1012
Diogenes (senile squalor) syndrome 4228
Dioralyte 2006, *2006*
dipalmitoylphosphatidylcholine (DPPC)
    2594, 2833
dipeptidyl carboxypeptidase, *see*
    angiotensin converting enzyme
    (ACE)
Dipetalonema perstans 919
diphenoxylate
    in opiate detoxification 4291
    overdose 1058
2,3-diphosphoglycerate (2,3-DPG) 3456,
    3518
    in anaemia 3457
    biosynthesis 3534–5
    depletion, in massive transfusion 3693
diphosphonates, *see* bisphosphonates
diphtheria **493–7**
    anterior nasal 494
    bacteriology 493
    bull-neck 374, 495, 496
    clinical features 494–5
    complications 495–6
    diagnosis 496
    differential diagnosis 496
    faucial 494–5
    historical aspects 493
    host immunity and infection spread 494
    hypertoxic 496
    malignant 495
    mumps *vs* 374
    neuropathy in 4091, 4101–2
    pathogenesis 493–4
        membrane formation 493, 494
    pathology 494
    in pregnancy 494
    prevention 496–7
        control of outbreaks 497
    streptococcal sore throat *vs* 502
    toxin 493
    toxoid 496
    tracheolaryngeal 495

treatment 496
    antibiotics 496
    antitoxin 496
    of complications 496
    vaccines 317–18, 496
    see also Corynebacterium diphtheriae
diphthericin 493
diphyllobothriasis **969**
Diphyllobothrium latum 969, 3491
dipipanone 4289
diplegia
    spastic **4120**
    spastic ataxic **4121**
diploid cells, genetic analysis of tumours
    194
diplopia, *see* vision, double
Diplopida (millipedes) 1149–50
Diptera *1010*, 1011
Dipylidium caninum 962, 963, 964
dipyridamole 3671
    in nephrotic syndrome 3142
diquat poisoning 1120
direct agglutination test, toxoplasmosis
    diagnosis 868
Dirofilaria 911
Dirofilaria immitis 919
dirofilariasis 919
disability
    after head injury 4049
    definition *2943*
disablement
    benefits 2841
    registration, in epilepsy 3925
disaccharidase 1920
    biosynthesis 1921
    deficiency **1920–3**
        treatment 1923
        see also lactase; lactose intolerance;
        sucrase-isomaltase
    secondary deficiency 1922
disaccharides 1920
disasters, natural 51
disease(s)
    changing patterns 51
    characteristics in old age **4334**, *4334*
    chronic, *see* chronic diseases
    in community **39–46**
    epidemiology **42–6**
    eradication 53
    in general practice 47–8, *49*
    of modernization **35–9**
    Western 38
disease association, *see* association,
    disease
'disease phobia' 4207
disequilibrium syndromes, in
    malnutrition 1287
dishwashing liquids, poisoning 1079
disinfectants
    effect on *Bacillus anthracis* spores 613
    poisoning 1078
    Staphylococcus aureus sensitivity 525
disinhibition 3854
    in frontal lobe tumours 4237
    in insulinomas 4240
dislocation, temporomandibular joint
    1864
disodium cromoglycate, in asthma 2738
disodium etidronate
    in ectopic ossification 3093
    in osteoporosis therapy 3068
    in Paget's disease of bone 3077
disopyramide *2264*
    overdose/poisoning 1063
disorientation
    left-right 3851
    topographical 3853
displacement, reaction in dying patients
    4233
disseminated intravascular coagulation
    (DIC) 3632, **3657–9**, 3775, 3777
    aetiology 3658
    in diabetic ketoacidosis 1502–3
    haemolytic anaemia and 3547
    haemolytic uraemic syndrome *vs*
        3200–1
    intestinal ischaemia in 1995, 1996
    laboratory features 3658
    in malaria 856

in malignancy 3678, 3792
    management 3658–9
    in massive transfusion 3660–1
    neurological symptoms 4123
    in newborn 3654
    pathogenesis 3657–8
    in pre-eclampsia 1728, *1762*
    in pregnancy **1762–3**, 3658
    in septicaemia 1025, 3658, 3679
    thrombocytopenia and 1763, 3658
dissociative disorder **4209–10**
    'belle indifference' in 4209, 4210
    clinical features 4209–10, *4209*
    differential diagnosis 4210, 4211
    epidemic 4210
    prognosis and treatment 4210
    provisional diagnosis 4210
    psychiatric emergencies due to 4258
    secondary gain in 4210
    seizures 4210
    terminology/classification 4209
dissociative pseudodementia 4210
distal intestinal obstruction syndrome
    (meconium ileus equivalent) 1978,
    2749
Distoma hepaticum 986
district health systems 53
disturbed patients 4256
    causes *4256*
    management, emergency 4257
    organic mental disorders in 4258
    see also psychiatric emergencies
disulfiram 4291
    mechanism of toxicity and action 1077
    overdose/poisoning **1077**
        children 1077, 1078
disulfiram-ethanol reactions 1078
disulphide bonds 69
dithizone, in thallium poisoning 1113
dithranol, in psoriasis 3748, *3749*
diuresis
    forced, *see* forced diuresis
    in obstructive airways disease 2572
    in overtransfusion management 2571
diuretics **2238–41**
    abuse 3127, 3131
    in acute renal failure 3285, 3286
    adverse mental symptoms 4242
    in ascites management 2097
    in benign intracranial hypertension
        4043
    calcium excretion and 3228
    in chronic renal failure 3304
    complications **2240–1**, 2521
    in cor pulmonale 2521, 2927
    drug pharmacodynamics 1252
    efficacy 2238
    in heart failure **2238–41**
        combinations 2240
        in elderly 4342
        infusions 2240
    in hypercalcaemia 3228
    in hypertension 2539–40
    hypokalaemia induced by **3130**
    in idiopathic hypercalciuria 3255
    in idiopathic oedema 3127
    'loop' 2238
        in cor pulmonale 2521
        in heart failure 2239–40
        mechanism of action 2239
    mechanism of action 1247, 2238, 2239
    in nephrotic syndrome 3140
    nephrotoxicity 3266
    osmotic 1248
    overdose/poisoning 1066
    oxygen supplements relation 2521
    potassium loss due to 2239
    potassium-retaining 3133
    potassium-sparing 1066, 2239
        potassium supplements with 2239
    in pregnancy 1731, 1732, 1740
    in pulmonary oedema 2504
    relative polycythaemia due to 3552,
        3553
    in renal impairment 3273
    in renovascular hypertension, cautions
        2551
    secondary gout due to 2985, *2986*
    sexual problems associated *4245*

test, nuclear renal imaging 3114, 3115,
    3240
    thiazide, *see* thiazide diuretics
    in tricuspid regurgitation 2469
    in unconscious patients 2586
diurnal variation/rhythm, *see* circadian
    rhythm
divers
    asthma and 1210
    breath-holding 1206
    patent foramina ovales 1210
    selection and medical care **1209–10**
    see also diving
diverticular abscess 1970, 1971
diverticular disease, colonic **1825–7**,
    1960, **1969–72**
    aetiology 1969–70
    clinical features 1970–2
    complicated 1970–2
    diet association 1328–9, 1969
    epidemiology 1969
    inflammation in, *see* diverticulitis
    management 1970
    pathogenesis 1329, 1969
    pathology 1970
    surgery indications *1970*
    symptomatic *vs* asymptomatic 1969–70
    uncomplicated 1970
    see also diverticulitis
diverticulitis 1970
    acute 1970–1
    perforated 1971
diverticulum, Meckel's, *see* Meckel's
    diverticulum
diving **1204–11**
    accidents, management 1210
    air travel after 1199
    ascent speeds/method 1208
    atmospheric pressure 1209
    compression/decompression,
        mechanical effects **1206–7**
    decompression illness 1208–9
    dexterity and mobility 1205–6
    fitness assessment 1210
    fitness requirement 2358, 2361
    hearing and blast injury 1205
    high-pressure nervous syndrome 1207
    inert gas narcosis 1207
    lung rupture risk 1206
    maximum depth 1209
    'no-stop' 1208
    oxygen toxicity 1207–8
    pressure injuries 1206–7
    pressure-resistant vessels 1209
    'safe' and long-term effects 1210–11
    sea bed and 1204–5
    sea temperatures and depth 1205
    unresolved issues relating to 1210
    vision 1205
    warmth and survival problems 1209
    water density 1206
    see also divers
diving reflex 2610, 2912
diving suits 1209
    armoured 1209
divorce 36–7
dizziness 2174
    after head injury 3835
    ambulatory ECG 2197–9
    in carotid sinus hypersensitivity 2266
    in cerebellar lesions 3860
    in syncope 3918, 3926
4-DMAP (4-dimethylaminophenol) 1098
DM gene, mutation 127
DMPS (unithiol)
    in arsenic poisoning 1106
    in lead poisoning 1110
    in mercury poisoning 1112
    in nickel poisoning 1113
[⁹⁹Tcᵐ]DMSA scans, *see*
    dimercaptosuccinic acid
    ([⁹⁹Tcᵐ]DMSA) scans
DNA 104
    adducts with alkylating agents 248
    amplification, *see* polymerase chain
        reaction (PCR)
    antibodies, *see* anti-DNA antibodies
    complementary (cDNA) 59, 106
    cloning 59

DNA (cont.)
  probes for screening gene libraries 61
  uses 61
  damage, sulphur mustard (mustard gas)
    causing 1115
  fetal, osteogenesis imperfecta diagnosis
    3082
  fingerprinting 105
  fractionation 60
  fragments, gene probe formation 59, 60
  genomic, cloning 59, 60
  hereditary abnormalities in tumours
    192–3
  hybridization,
    bacterial classification by 273
    chlamydial infections diagnosis 755,
      755, 756
  junk 62, 105
  labelling by nick translation 60
  ligation defects 173
  methylation 59, 107, 126
  mini- and micro-satellite 62, 105, 134
  mitochondrial, see mitochondria, DNA
  plasmid, reversibility of tumours and
    193
  polymorphisms, in haematological
    disorders 3390, 3391
    in haemophilia 3639
  probes, see DNA probes (below)
  proteins associated, humoral response to
    156
  radiotherapy-induced damage 254
  recombinant, see recombinant DNA
    technology
  repair 107, 254
    defects/disorders 107, 173, 3447
    in Fanconi anaemia 3446
  repetitive sequences 105
  replication 57
    gene controlling fidelity 223
  restriction endonuclease action 59, 60
  sequencing 61
    detection in respiratory tract infections
      2677
    mutation detection 134
    prone to mutations 108
  in sexual offences examination 4314
  structure 57
    variability in 62
  synthesis, folate in 3487, 3488–9
  trinucleotide repeats 63
  viral DNA integration 462
    hepatitis B virus 457, 462, 2115–16
  viruses, carcinogenesis mechanism 462
  see also gene(s)
DNA analysis
  genetic prediction by 132–5
    gene tracking 134–5, 134
    mutation detection 133–4, 134
    types of methods 133–5, 134
  genetic screening 132
  see also chromosomal analysis; genetic
    analysis
DNAase 1 59
DNA-ase
  in bronchiectasis 2762
  in cystic fibrosis 2753
DNA-binding proteins 57
  classes and function 59
DNA ligase 60
  defective 173
DNA polymerases 57
DNA probes 106, 119
  chlamydial infections diagnosis 755,
    755, 756
  embryo sexing 136
  Entamoeba histolytica detection 831
  malaria diagnosis 849
  muscular dystrophies 4147
  mycoplasmas 769
  Rochalimaea henselae detection 747
  vero cytotoxin-producing E. coli
    (VTEC) 557
  see also gene(s), probes
DNA topoisomerase, antibodies 3032,
  3033
dobutamine
  actions and clinical use 2254, 2255
  in cardiac arrest 2284

myocardial perfusion study 2217
  in poisoning management 1047, 1063
  receptors 2254
  septicaemia management 1024
docking protein 69
doctor-patient relationship 3–4
  cancer diagnosis and treatment 252
  compliance improved by 4233
  dying patients 4234
  in obesity 1309
  in supportive psychological treatment
    4254
doctors
  attitudes to drug abuse/misuse 4264–5,
    4290
  see also drug abuse and misuse
  attitudes to patients 3–4
  behaviour, effect on compliance 1240
  breach of duty 4311
  confidentiality of consultations 4288
  consultations with and consulting
    behaviour 4231–2
  drug abuse and misuse by 4265
  duties after a death 4309–10
  duties and confidentiality problems
    4316
  medical negligence 4311–12
  prescribing restrictions/regulations 4289
  responsibilities to patient and family 4
  role in septicaemia prevention 1022
  salaries 38
  see also general practitioner
Dodge formula 2222
dog, rabies in 397, 398, 399
dog allergens 2715
dog bites 1125
  infections associated 404
  pasteurellosis from 606
  rabies from 397
Dogger Bank itch 3737
Döhle bodies 3378, 3556
dolichol phosphate 70
doll's head eye movements 2583, 2584,
  4005
dolor 290
dominant-negative effects 109
Donath-Landsteiner antibody 3544
donor agencies, in developing countries
  53
donor insemination 11
donors, organ 4310–11
  bone marrow 3418, 3699–700
  consent 13–14
  donor cards 4311
  kidney 3313, 3317
    living, related 3313, 3316, 3317
  multiorgan donor 2256
Donovan bodies 776, 777
donovanosis (granuloma inguinale)
  776–8
  in homosexuals 3363
L-dopa 2553
dopa decarboxylase, reduced in
  Parkinson's disease 4000
dopamine 1554, 2254, 2553
  in acute pancreatitis 2029
  in acute renal failure 3285, 3286
  in cardiac arrest 2284
  clinical use 2254
  D₁ receptors 3862
  D₂ receptors 3862
  deficiency, in Parkinson's disease 3998,
    3999, 4000
  excess, schizophrenia aetiology and
    4222
  high central venous pressure 2564
  in Huntington's disease 4013, 4013
  insulin secretion and 1459
  loss, in multiple system atrophy 4006
  mechanism of action and doses 2254,
    2254
  in myocardial infarction 2345
  in poisoning management 1047, 1063,
    1064, 1066
  prolactin inhibition 1576
  receptors 2254, 2254, 3862
    blockade, by antipsychotic drugs
      4251

renal actions 3119
  in renal impairment 3270
  in septicaemia 2573
dopamine agonists
  in acromegaly 1594
  growth hormone secretion and 1578
  in hyperprolactinaemia 1590, 1591,
    1672
  non-secretory pituitary tumours 1596
dopamine antagonists 1718
dopamine ß-hydroxylase deficiency
  3886–7
dopamine D₂ receptor antagonists 4252
  alcoholism marker 2081
  risperidone 4253
  see also clozapine
dopaminergic transmission 3862
dopa-responsive dystonia-parkinsonism
  4017–18
dopexamine 2255
  receptors 2254
Doppler echocardiography 2200–4
  A and E waves 2201
  in aortic stenosis 2463
  colour Doppler flow mapping 2200,
    2201, 2202, 2204
  common applications 2204
  in congenital heart disease 2203, 2204,
    2406, 2425
  information provided by 2200
  left ventricular function 2203
  in mitral stenosis 2454
  modalities 2200, 2201
  physiological regurgitation 2203
  in pregnancy 1736
  pressure drop estimation 2201
  principles 2200
  prosthetic valves 2203
  spectral 2200, 2204
    continuous wave 2200, 2201
    pulsed wave 2200, 2201
  two-dimensional 2200
    in infective endocarditis 2442–3
  valve disease 2201–3
  see also echocardiography
Doppler effect 2200
Doppler equation 2200
Doppler frequency shift 2200
Doppler ultrasound
  in diabetic pregnancy 1757
  in hypertrophic cardiomyopathy 2388
  in peripheral arterial disease 2368
  in transient ischaemic attack 3952,
    3953
  in vesicoureteric reflux 3215
dorsal cells
  hyperactivity and neuropathic pain
    3942
  loss, in Friedreich's ataxia 3984
dorsal column stimulation 3945–6
dorsal disc protrusions 3906
dorsal horn 3937
  neurotransmitters in 3937
  in pain processing 3937
  reduced inhibitions and pain in 3940–1
dorsal rhizotomy 3942
dorsal root entry zone lesions 3945
'double bubble' sign 1976
double effect theory 4350
double Y syndrome, chromosomal
  abnormality 120
Down's syndrome 121, 4108–9
  14/21 translocation causing 122–3
  Alzheimer's disease association 3972,
    3973
  amyloid deposits 1513, 1516, 1519
  antenatal screening 135, 1756, 4109
  complications 4109
  Hirschsprung's disease association 1979
  incidence and features 4108–9
  leukaemia association 215, 3410
  Robertsonian translocations causing
    122
  screening and prevention 4109
  trisomy 21 causing 121
doxepin, drug interactions 1258
doxorubicin (adriamycin)
  in hepatocellular carcinoma 2117

in Hodgkin's disease 3573, 3574
  in non-Hodgkin's lymphoma 3585
doxycycline
  in brucellosis 623
  in malaria, prophylaxis 861
  in rickettsial diseases 733
  scrub typhus prevention 741
DPTA, in cadmium poisoning 1107
dracunculiasis 924–8
  clinical features and diagnosis 926
  distribution and transmission 924–6
  global eradication 927–8
  prevention and control 927–8
  treatment 926–7
Dracunculus medinensis 924
  lifecycle 924–5
Drash syndrome 1694, 3184
drawing, disturbances 3852–3
dressing apraxia 3854
dressings
  leg ulceration management 3809
  wet 3717, 3742
Dressler's syndrome 156, 2346, 2476,
  2477
  haematological changes 3687
drinking
  behaviour 3117
  compulsive 3121
  see also fluid, intake; hypodipsia;
    polydipsia
drinking diaries 4271–2
driving
  after coronary angioplasty 2352
  after myocardial infarction 2359
  angina and 2326, 2359
  confidentiality and 4316
  coronary artery disease and 2358–9
  epilepsy and 3924, 4040
  heavy goods vehicle 2358, 2359
  intracranial tumours and 4040
  licences (groups I/II) 2358, 2359
  liver disease and 2091
  motor racing 2359
  sleepiness during 2913
Driving and Vehicle Licensing Agency
  (DVLA) 2359
drop attacks 3883, 3919, 3951
'dropped finger' 2957
Drosophila 3396
  homeotic genes 66
droughts 1233
drowsiness, morphine causing 4352
drug(s)
  absorption 1241–2
    factors affecting 1242
    interactions 1255, 1257
    in pregnancy 4298
    in renal impairment 3268
  abuse problems related to, see drug
    abuse(r) and misuse
  acne vulgaris induced by 3752
  in acutely ill patients 3283, 3284
  acute pancreatitis induced by 2027–8
  in acute porphyria,
    safe 1398–9
    unsafe 1397–8
  adaptation to 1250
    adverse effects due to 1251, 1253
  addicts, see drug abuse(r) and misuse
  administration routes 1238–9
    drugs of concern 4264
    in pregnancy 4298
  adverse reactions, see adverse drug
    reactions
  agonists and antagonists 1245–6
  allergic reactions,
    hypereosinophilic syndrome vs 3611–12
    purpura in 3637
  alveolar haemorrhage induced by 2804
  antidotes to 1048, 1048
  aplastic anaemia induced by 3441, 3443
  apparent volume of distribution (V)
    1242, 1245
  benefit/risk ratios 1237, 1238
  benign intracranial hypertension
    induced by 4042
  bioavailability (systemic availability)
    1238, 1241–2

body temperature increased by **1181–2**
see also hyperpyrexia; neuroleptic malignant syndrome
cancer association 215–16, *216*
clearance 1245
by dialysis and haemofiltration 3269–70, *3271*
in renal impairment 3269
see also drug(s), excretion
coma induced by, assessment 2583
compliance, *see* compliance, drug
contact dermatitis due to 3738
costs, antiepileptic drugs 3922
dependence, *see* drug dependence
'designer' 67, 4297
disease interactions 1250
distribution 1242–3
in acid-base disturbances 1540
age-related changes 4337
apparent volume of 1242, 1245
diseases affecting 1243
in renal impairment 3268
dose, in pregnancy **1812–13**
duration of action 1249–50
effects on fetus 1254–5, *1254, 1255,* 1809
in elderly 4228, **4336–8**
elimination rate constant (k_e) 3269
endocrine side-effects **1717–19**
endothelial function affected by 2300
eruptions, *see* drug eruptions
erythema multiforme due to 3780
excretion 1243–4, **3268**
age-related changes 4337
drug interactions via 1257–8
in renal impairment 3269
see also drug(s), clearance
extrapyramidal disease induced by **4020–1**, *4021*
fever 1253
folate deficiency-inducing **3493–4**
formulations 1238–9
dose-related adverse effects 1251
fulminant hepatic failure 2100
in G6PD deficiency, haemolysis-inducing *3539, 3546*
haemolytic anaemia induced by **3542–3**, 3546–7
haemolytic uraemic syndrome induced by 3197
half-life 1244, 3269
heat stroke association 1180
hepatic granulomas induced by 2122, *2122,* 2128, *2128*
hepatitis induced by, *see* hepatitis, drug-induced
hyperlipoproteinaemia induced by 1411
hypoglycaemia induced by 1511
idiosyncratic reactions, asthma 2849–50
immune-complex diseases induced by 164
immune thrombocytopenia induced by 3632
inactivation 1243
infection susceptibility and 282
inhalation 4279
intoxication, coma in 2585
kidney and **3268–75**
law and **4288–90**
types of offences 4289–90
lipid solubility 1243
liver damage due to, *see* liver damage
Löffler's syndrome (simple pulmonary eosinophilia) due to 2805
long-term effects 1250–1
lung disease induced by, *see* lung disease, drug-induced
lupus due to 1253, 3025, 3732–3
mechanisms of action, *see* pharmacodynamics
medication-induced oesophagitis 1874, *1874*
megaloblastic anaemia induced by 3498
mental states induced by **4241–2**
metabolism 1243
acetylation and CYP2D6 polymorphism 130, 1259
age-related changes 4336–7

first-pass 1242
inducers 1257
inhibition and drug interactions 1257
interactions via 1257, 1258–9
in liver 1243, 2091, 2124
in liver disease 1252
in malnutrition 1295–6
pharmacogenetics and 130, 1259, 2124
phases I and II 1243
in renal impairment 3268
tolerance by 1251
to toxic compounds 1243
methaemoglobinaemia induced by 3520
modified-release 1239
monitoring therapy **1260–1**
myopathy due to 4169, *4169*
myotonia due to 4151
nephrotoxic 3193, **3265–6**, *3284*
acute on chronic renal failure due to 3299
acute interstitial nephritis due to 3258, *3259,* 3265, 3291
neuropathy due to 4100
neutropenia induced by 3558
non-linear kinetics 1245
ocular toxicity and screening **4196–7**, *4197*
overdosage,
deliberate self-harm 4228
fatal doses *4376*
immediate treatment 4229
skin reactions in 3731
parkinsonism induced by 3998, 4002, 4020
peritonitis induced by 2009
pharmacodynamics, *see* pharmacodynamics
pharmacokinetics, *see* pharmacokinetics
pK 3268
plasma concentrations, indications for measuring 1260–1, *1261*
platelet dysfunction due to *3629,* 3630, 3635
poisoning, *see* poisoning; *specific drugs*
in pregnancy **1812–13**, 4297–8
prescribing **1237**, 1238, *1238,* **4289**
benefit-risk ratio **1237**, *1238*
breast feeding and **1811**, *1812*
controlled drugs 4289
in pregnancy **1809–13**
in renal impairment **3270–5**, 3288, 3305–6
restrictions relating to 4289
principles of therapy in old age **4336–8**
problems related to 4264
protein binding 1242
interactions via 1257
in pregnancy 1813
psychiatric disorders induced by, schizophrenia *vs* 4222
rate of onset of action 1249–50
rational use 38
reactions,
in atopic eczema 3741
IgE-mediated 162
toxic epidermal necrolysis due to 3781
see also adverse drug reactions; *drug eruptions; penicillin*
rebound phenomena 1254
receptors 1245–6
types and long-term effects at 1246
up-/down-regulation 1246
renal bone disease and 3327
resistance, to chemotherapy, *see* antibiotic resistance; *under* chemotherapy
secondary immunodeficiency due to 174
seizures induced by 3917
sexual problems due to **4245**, *4245*
short-term effects 1249
sideroblastic anaemia due to 3523
steady-state concentration (C_{ss}) 3269
surveillance methods 1255, *1256*
teratogenic **130–1**, *131,* 1254, *1254,* 1809–10

therapeutic index **1237–8**
therapeutic monitoring, *see* therapeutic drug monitoring
threshold plasma concentration 1242
tissue distribution 1242–3
tolerance 1250–1, **4263**
total body clearance 1245
transformation 1243
tremor induced by 4020
types of offences **4289–90**
vasculitis due to 3776
vitamin B_{12} deficiency due to 3491
volume of distribution (V_d) 3269
withdrawal 1251, 1254, 4263
liver damage diagnosis 2124, *2125*
drug abuse(r) and misuse **4263–5**
abstinence, reinstatement 4269
accident and emergency departments and **4294–7**
engagement in treatment **4297**
administration routes **4264**
assessment **4265–7**, 4290
history-taking **4266–7**
questions checklist 4266
'bad trips' 4295
behavioural aspects causing harm **4280–1**
brief interventions **4270–5**, 4290
opportunity for 4265–6
cardiovascular effects 4295
case histories 4268, 4270
classification of disorders *4269*
'dance' and 'rave' drugs 4280, 4295
data collection 4297
dependence *vs* problems **4267–70**
'designer drugs' 4297
detoxification 4276, 4291–3
see also under opiates
doctors' attitudes **4264–5**, 4290
belief of rarity/unimportance of 4264
negative stereotypes 4264
optimism and 4265
drug overdose **4295–6**
drugs of concern **4263**
see also drugs of abuse
drug-seeking behaviour 4269
emergency presentations 4294–5
endocarditis 528, **2445**, 4279, 4285
in HIV-infected patients 4285
endocrine problems 4284
essential knowledge for doctors **4263–4**
fever in 4294, 4295
harm reduction **4275–6**
hepatitis in 4279
history-taking **4266–7**
HIV infection 4302–4
effect on other problems 4285–6
epidemiology 4285
management in general ward 4287
in pregnancy 4299
prevention 4275
status unknown 4303
transmission 484, 4281, 4284–5
transmission to neonates 4298
HIV-positive addicts, care **4302–4**
asymptomatic 4303
maintaining contact 4302–3
overlap of drug/HIV problems 4303, *4303*
previously-undiagnosed 4303
at risk identification 4302
infections in **4279–80**, **4284–6**, *4284*
bacterial 4279, 4285, 4286
complications 4280, 4294
epidemiology 4284–5
history/overview 4284
HIV infection effect on 4285–6
risk and types 4285
viral 4278, 4294
injecting **4281–6**, 4302
adulterants injection 2445, 4280, 4281, 4283
emergency medical presentations 4294
frequency of complications 4281–2
harm reduction 4275, 4276, 4279
infections **4284–6**, *4284,* 4294
non-infection-related complications **4281–4**, *4282,* 4294
trauma 4282–3

intoxication and **4296**
management in general wards **4286**, **4287–8**
in medical profession **4265**
medical/surgical presentations **4294–5**
needs in custody **4304–5**
neurological problems 4284
NHS reporting system 4289
notification **4288–9**, 4297
opiate overdose 1058, 4280
orthopaedic infections in 4279–80
pain management after **4300–1**
physical complications **4278–81**, **4281–6**
management in general ward 4287
pneumococcal infections 512, 4279
polyarteritis nodosa in 4283
powers of detention and 4289
in pregnancy **4297–300**
complications 4298, *4298*
drug dependent/independent effects 4297–8
epidemiology 4297
management **4299**
prejudice against 4264, 4287
prescribed drugs, in elderly 4228
psychiatric complications **4295**
pulmonary hypertension/fibrosis in 4283
pulmonary infections 4279
pulmonary oedema in 4283
reasons for 4264
repertoire narrowing 4269
respiratory effects in 4295
screening **4270–5**
seizures 4294–5
septicaemia in 4279, 4294
skills needed for clinical practice **4265**
statutory requirements 4297
subjective awareness 4269
substance-specific complications **4280**, 4283
technique-specific hazards **4279**
tolerance 4268
treatment **4289**, 4297
types of offences relating to **4289–90**
vascular complications in 4280, 4282–3
withdrawal,
neonatal 4298
repeated symptoms 4268–9
withdrawal syndrome **4291–3**
in accident and emergency department **4296–7**
management in custody 4305
see also cocaine; diamorphine; drug dependence; drugs of abuse; MDMA (Ecstasy)
drug dependence **4263–4**
attempts to obtain drugs 4259
iatrogenic 4287–8, 4296–7
management 4288
in pregnancy **4299**
as psychiatric emergency 4259
withdrawal syndrome 4293
drug eruptions 1253, **3729–33**
fixed 3733, *3733,* 3779
infections associated 3730, 3731
management 3733
rashes in 1253, 3727, *3728,* 3729–30
types/distribution 3730
specific drugs 3731–2
syphilis *vs* 711
timing 3730–1
transient susceptibility 3731
unlikely/likely drugs 3730
drug interactions 305–6, **1255–8**
ACE inhibitors 2251
digitalis 2243
drugs associated 1255
lithium *4250,* 4251
liver damage and acute hepatitis 2125
mechanisms 1255–8, *1256*
monoamine oxidase inhibitors (MAOIs) 4250
in Parkinson's disease 4004–5
psychotropic drugs 4247
synergistic or antagonistic 305

drugs of abuse **1074–7**
  amphetamines 1076
  anticholinergic substances 1076
  body packing 1074–5
  classification 1074
  CNS stimulants 1077
  failure to seek medical help 1074
  hazards 1074
    accidental overdose 1074
    contaminants 1074
    delayed presentation 1074
    non-drug related (infections) 1074
  methods of abuse 1074
    ingestion and absorption 1074
    inhalation or injection 1074
  phencyclidine 1075–6
  poisoning **1074–7**
  see also cannabis; cocaine; drug
    abuse(r) and misuse; lysergic acid
    diethylamide
drug-seeking attendance **4296–7**
'Drusen' 681
'dry ice' 1094
DTPA, *see* diethylene-triamine penta-
  acetic acid (DTPA)
DTPA, $^{99}Tc^m$-labelled, *see* technetium-
  99m-diethylenetriamine pentaacetic
  acid
  (DTPA)
dual photon densitometry, bone 3066
dual X-ray absorptiometry 3066
Duane syndrome 4114
Dubin-Johnson syndrome 1396–7, 1799,
  2055, 2056, **2058–9**
  factor VII deficiency and 3652
  Rotor's syndrome *vs* 2059
Duchenne muscular dystrophy
  aetiology 4145
  cardiac manifestations 2392
  carriers 116, 4146
  chromosomal duplication 108
  clinical features 4146
  dysutrophin gene mutations 116
  genes 4145, 4147
  gene tracking 135
  incidence and inheritance 115–16,
    4145
  pathology 4145
  treatment 4148–9
duck embryo vaccine (DEV) 403
ductal plate 2014
  malformations 2014
ductus arteriosus 2408
  patent/persistent **2430–1**, *2431*
    calcification 2182
    differential diagnosis 2467
    infective endocarditis in 2439
    preductal coarctation in 2557
    in pregnancy 1737
Duffy antigens, *Plasmodium vivax*
  malaria and 280
Dukes classification, colorectal
  carcinoma 1991, *1992*
dumping syndrome 1890, 1962
  gut peptides in 1895
  management 1962
  symptoms 1962
Duncan syndrome 353
duodenal-jejunal junction, biopsy
  1918
duodenal-jejunal manometry 1956
duodenal ulcer **1877–9**
  acute erosive **1880**
  aetiology 1877–8
    ulcerogenic drugs 1878, 1888
  barium studies 1831
  bleeding 1828
  clinical features 1878–9
  definition 1877
  diagnosis 1879
  failure to heal 1889
  haemorrhage 1878, 1882–3
    in acute erosive ulceration 1880
    management/prognosis 1882–3
    symptoms/signs 1882
  Helicobacter pylori role 1877, 1878,
    1884, 2005
    effect of 1885

medical treatment 1828, **1883–9**
  choice of drugs 1888–9
  cimetidine 1878
  evaluation of results 1883
  H_2-receptor antagonists 1886–7
  H. pylori eradication 1884, 1885–6,
    1890
  long-term 1889
  short-term 1888–9
natural history 1878–9
oesophagitis in 1880
perforated 1878, 1882
  differential diagnosis 2030
pyloric stenosis after 1960
recurrence 1889, 1890
  diagnosis 1890
relapses and remissions 1878
surgical treatment **1889–90**
  choice and outcome 1890
  motility disorders after 1878–9
in Zollinger-Ellison syndrome 1881
see also peptic ulcer
duodenitis **1880–1**, 1909
duodenoduodenostomy 1976
duodenogastric reflux 2040
duodenum
  atresia 1975, 1977
    embryology 1973
  bacterial counts 1912
  bands/stenosis 1960
  biopsy 1907
    in coeliac disease 1917
    interpretation pitfalls 1909
    see also small intestine, biopsy
  carcinoid tumours 1707
  chemoreceptors 1954
  Crohn's disease of 1940
  disease, endoscopy indication 1829
  embryology 1973
  gastrinoma 1704, 1705, 1708
  obstruction,
    congenital intrinsic 1975–6
    partial 1976
  perforation, epidemiology 1878
  polyps 1987
  somatostatinoma 1707
  stenosis 1960, 1977
    embryology 1973
Dupuytren's contracture
  in cirrhosis 2087–8
  in diabetes 1489
  in hepatocellular failure 2104
dural sinus thrombosis 3956–7, *3957*,
  4041–2, 4043
Dürck's granuloma 844
Durcum's disease 2996
Durosiez's sign 2465
dust
  extrinsic allergic alveolitis and 2809,
    2811
  quartz 2839, 2841
duty of care 4311
Duvenhage virus 395, *396*
dwarfism
  achondroplasia-like **3088–9**
  Laron 1511, 1572, **1577**, 1699
  nutritional, *see* nutritional dwarfism
  proportionate *3088*, **3089**
  short-limbed 3079, 3086, 3088–9, *3088*
    genetics 114
  see also short stature
dydrogesterone *1814*
dyes, dermatitis due to 3736
dying patients
  AIDS, management 473
  in cancer 4349
  diagnosis **4349**
  emotional distress **4233**
    causes **4233–4**
    defence mechanisms 4233
    prevention and management 4234,
      4234
  ethical issues 4349
  fears 4357
  giving diagnosis 4234
  physical symptoms in and distress due
    to 4233
  principles of care 4234

see also death; terminal care; terminal
  illness
dynactin complex 82, 83
dynein 81, 83, 2613
dynorphin 1894
dysarthria 3846
  cerebellar 3860
  in cerebral hemisphere infarct 3955
dysbetalipoproteinaemia
  (hyperlipoproteinaemia type III)
  1408–9
dysdiadochokinesia 3860
dysentery 2003
  amoebic, *see* amoebic dysentery
  bacillary **553–5**, 2003
    see also Shigella
  causes *2003*
  definition 828
dyserythropoiesis, *see* erythropoiesis,
  ineffective
dysfibrinogenaemia, hereditary 3652–3,
  3667
dyskeratosis congenita 3723
dyskinesia **4009–21**
  levodopa causing 4003
  orobuccolingual 4021
  tardive, *see* tardive dyskinesia
  see also chorea; dystonia; myoclonus;
    tics; tremor
dyskinetic cerebral palsy **4121**
dyslexia, developmental 3851
dyslipidaemia, *see* hyperlipidaemia
dyslipoproteinaemia 1399
  see also hyperlipoproteinaemia
dysmetria 3860
dysmorphic syndromes, short stature
  1699–700
dysmorphophobia **4209**
dysostosis multiplex
  in mucolipidoses 1434
  in mucopolysaccharidoses 1431, 1433,
    1434
dyspepsia
  dysmotility 1880
  functional 1880
  in gastric cancer 1983
  non-ulcer **1880**
  pain in 2168
  peptic ulcer haemorrhage 1882
  in pregnancy 1801
  reflux 1880
dysphagia **1819**, **1820**
  in AIDS and HIV infection 475
  associations and relieving factors 1820
  in diffuse oesophageal spasm 1820,
    1870
  in dissociative disorder 4210
  duration/progression and frequency 1820
  high and low 1820
  in idiopathic achalasia 1869
  in iron-deficiency anaemia 3475
  location/nature of sensation 1820
  in lung cancer 2883
  management 1865–6
  in peptic strictures 1868
  in rheumatic diseases 2945
  in scleroderma 1871, 1999
  in squamous-cell carcinoma of
    oesophagus 1874, 1981
  in systemic sclerosis 1871, 1999
  in terminal illness **4354**
  upper motor neurone lesion 3857
dysphasia, *see* aphasia
dysphonia, spasmodic **4020**
dysplasminogenaemia 3667
dysplastic naevus syndrome *3795*
dyspnoea 2162, 2644–5
  definition 2162, 4354
  diagnosis 4354
  paroxysmal nocturnal 2162, *2163*,
    2462, 2500, 2501, 2646
  see also breathlessness
dyspraxia, articulatory **4122**
dysprothrombinaemia, constitutional
  3652
dysrhythmias, *see* cardiac arrhythmias
dystonia 3863, **4017–21**
  acute reactions 4021, 4252

aetiology *4011*, 4017
  athetosis relation 4010
  cerebral palsy 4121
  cranial **4019–20**
  definition 4010, 4017
  focal 4017
  generalized and segmental 4017
  idiopathic **4017**
  oromandibular **4019–20**
  paroxysmal **4020**
  tardive 4021
  torsion 4010, *4011*
  see also athetosis
dystonia-parkinsonism, dopa-responsive
  4017–18
dystonic writer's cramp **4018–19**
dystrophia myotonica (myotonic
  dystrophy) 4151, **4152**
  diagnosis and management 4153
  eye features **4182**
  gene 4152
  histology 4143
  male hypogonadism 1683, 4152
  mental disorders/symptoms in 4238
  mutational basis 127
  in pregnancy 1766
  unstable trinucleotide repeats 108, *125*,
    127
dystrophin 4143
  gene mutations 116
dysuria **3148**, **3206–7**
  in gonorrhoea 546

E

ear age-related changes 4336
  barotrauma 1207
  in Langerhans-cell histiocytosis 3607
  middle,
    aircraft pressure changes and 1199,
      1202, 1203
    infections 2691
  nerve supply 3869
  reversed-ear injury 1207
  sound perception 1223
ear, nose and throat disorders
  aircraft travel and 1203
  anaerobic infections 572
earthquakes 1232
Eastern equine encephalitis virus **408**
eating, cessation, as atypical eating
  disorder 4217
eating disorders **1296–301**, **4212–17**
  atypical 1301, 4217
  referral rates 1299
  see also anorexia nervosa; bulimia
    nervosa
eating habits, improving in anorexia
  nervosa 4214
Eaton agent 762
Eaton-Lambert syndrome 4134
Ebola fever **441–3**
Ebola virus **439–43**
  characteristics 440–1
EbR (erythroblast receptor) 86, 87
Ebstein's anomaly **2413–15**
  differential diagnosis 2414–15
  signs and symptoms 2414
ecchymosis, *see* bruising
eccrine sweat glands 3706, 3766
echinococcosis, *see* hydatid disease
Echinococcus granulosus 955
  lifecycle 955, 956
  see also hydatid disease
Echinococcus multilocularis 955, 956,
  957
Echinococcus vogeli 955
echinodermata, venomous **1144**
Echinostoma ilocanum 993, 996
echinostomiasis **993**, **997–8**
echocardiography 2220
  in acute pericarditis 2477
  in aortic regurgitation 2465–6
  in aortic stenosis 2463
  in aortic stenosis with incompetence
    2464
  in brucellosis 621

in cardiac amyloidosis 2393
in cardiac myxoma 2473–4
in chronic renal failure 3301
in coarctation of aorta 2558
in congenital pericardial abnormalities 2474
in dilated cardiomyopathy 2383
Doppler, *see* Doppler echocardiography
exercise 2228
in Fallot's tetralogy 2406
in fixed subaortic stenosis 2422
in hypereosinophilic syndrome 2397
in hypertrophic cardiomyopathy 2386, 2388
in infective endocarditis 2442
in left ventricular disease after valve replacement 2471
in mitral prolapse 2460
in mitral regurgitation 2459, 2461
in mitral stenosis 2453
in mixed mitral valve disease 2457
M-mode,
  in mitral regurgitation 2459
  in mitral stenosis 2453, 2454, 2455
in ostium secundum defects 2425
in pericardial tamponade 2477, 2478
in pulmonary hypertension 2511, 2512
in restrictive cardiomyopathy 2390
transoesophageal 2215
  in cardiac myxoma 2473
  in infective endocarditis 2443
  in mitral regurgitation 2459
  in mitral stenosis 2454
  in tricuspid stenosis 2468
see also Doppler echocardiography
echolalia 3848
echopraxia 4016
echoviruses 382, 384
type 9, skin rashes 384
type 11 383
  infection in homosexuals 3364
type 16 384
echovirus infections 168, 383
in hypogammaglobulinaemia 168
neurological diseases *385*
in pregnancy/newborn infants 1783
see also enterovirus infections
eclampsia 1726, 1729, 1730, *1762*
prevention/treatment 1731
ecology, infections **265**
economics, modern 35
Ecstasy, *see* MDMA (Ecstasy)
ECST trials 2373
ecthyma, streptococcal 499–500, 502
ecthyma gangrenosum 1029
ectopia lentis 4181
ectopic calcification, *see* calcification, ectopic
ectopic hormones, *see* hormone(s), ectopic production
ectopic ossification, *see* ossification, ectopic
ectopic pregnancy
acute pancreatitis *vs* 2030
pelvic inflammatory disease *vs* 3358
ectothrix 798
eczema 161
asteatotic 3743
atopic, *see* atopic eczema
definition 3734
dry 3760
malnutrition and 3722
nipple 3741
nummular 3743
see also atopic eczema; dermatitis
eczema craquelée 3722, 3795
eczema herpeticum 345–6
Edinger-Westphal nucleus 2584
edrophonium chloride, in snake envenoming management 1138
edrophonium test 4161
education
centres, diabetes 1504
in diabetes mellitus 1479
malnutrition management 1294
medical 8
patient, *see* patient education

in spina bifida 4118–19
see also health education; training
Edwardsiella tarda 555
Edwards' syndrome 121
effort syndrome, *see* Da Costa's syndrome
eflornithine 297
ego, retreat to 38
EHDP, *see* disodium etidronate
Ehlers-Danlos syndrome **3084**
bleeding disorders 3636, 3645
classification and features 3084, *3084*
mitral regurgitation 2457
skin in **3790**
X-linked 1419, *3084*
Ehrlichia 737–8
rare species *555*
Ehrlichia chaffeensis 728, 738
ehrlichial diseases 728, *729*, **737–9**
granulocytic 738
Sennetsu *729*, 738, 738–9
Ehrlich's reagent 2055
eicosanoids
metabolism by pulmonary endothelium 2487, 2514
synthesis 158
  mast cell degranulation 158
see also leukotrienes; prostaglandin(s); thromboxane
eicosapentaenoic acid
in chronic renal failure 3304
in pre-eclampsia prevention 1730
eighth cranial nerve, *see under* cranial nerves
Eikenella corrodens 555
Eisenmenger reaction (syndrome) 2401, 2402, **2409–12**, *2409*
associated defects *2410*
atrioventricular defects 2427
causes of death *2410*
differential diagnosis 2411
features and predisposing factors 2409–10
lung and heart-lung transplantation 2934
management 2411–12
pregnancy in 1737, 2401, 2412
symptoms and signs 2410–11
ventricular septal defects 2428
ejaculation
drugs affecting 4245, *4245*
neurological pathways 4244
ejaculatory disorders 1687
in neurological disorders 4244
Ekbom's syndrome (restless legs) 4092, 4099, **4159**
in pregnancy 1766
ektacytometer 3528
ELAM-1, *see* E-selectin
Elapidae, bites and envenoming 1126–7, 1131–2
elastase
α_1-antitrypsin and 1545, 1546
in acute pancreatitis 2030, 2031
haemolytic uraemic syndrome and 3199, 3200
neutrophil, *see* neutrophils, elastase
elastic fibres, in lung 2598
elastic stockings 3676
elastic tissue disorders **3787–90**
cutis laxa 3790
pseudoxanthoma elasticum 3789–90
elastin, in emphysema 2632, 2773
elastoma, perforating 3790
elastosis
senile 3788
solar 3725, *3726*, 3788
elastosis perforans serpiginosa 1423
elbow
dislocations 4096
disorders **2995–6**
golfer's 2995
in rheumatoid arthritis 2957–8
tennis 2995
ulnar nerve lesions 4096
elderly **4333–46**
acute renal failure risk 3279
anaemia in 3459
asthma in 2736

atrial fibrillation in **4342–3**
bacterial overgrowth aetiology 1912
bacteriuria 3207, 3211–12
bone disease **4344**
bronchoscopy in 2682
cardiac arrhythmias **4342**
cardiovascular disease **4341–4**
characteristics 4334, *4334*
clinical assessment **4336**, *4337*
common clinical problems **4338–9**
coronary angioplasty in 2352
coronary artery bypass grafting 2355
deep venous thrombosis **4343**
depression in 4341
drug therapy principles **4336–8**
erysipelas in 500
essential hypertension in **2543**
faecal incontinence **4338**
falls **4338–9**
fever of unknown origin (FUO) in 1016
glomerulosclerosis 3249
headache in **4028–9**
heart failure in **4342**
hepatitis B vaccination 454
high blood pressure **4343**
hyperthermia in **4346**
hypothermia in 1184, **4346**
infective endocarditis in 2440, 2443
leukaemia 3404, 3406, 3419
mental disorders **4226–8**
affective disorders 4227
assessment (methods/locations) 4226
delirium 4224, 4226
dementia 3965, 4226, 4227
neurotic/personality disorders 4228
paranoid disorders 4227
reasons for importance in 4226
metabolic and endocrine disorders **4344–6**
mortality rates *40, 42*
myocardial infarction **4342**
nutritional osteomalacia 3073
opportunistic infections 1027
physical abuse 3637
pneumococcal pneumonia 515
pneumonia in 515, 2700
postural hypotension **4343–4**
psychiatric disorders **4340–1**
skin changes in 3715–16
strokes in, *see* stroke
temperature regulation disorders **4346**
travel and 325
urinary incontinence **4338**
water homeostasis 3117
winter mortality 1185
electrical impedance
body fat measurement 1304
gut motility disorder investigation 1957
electrical injury **1211–15**
characteristics 1212
diagnosis and treatment 1212–14
neurological features **4129**
pathophysiology **1211–12**
visceral 1214
electric catfish 1124
electric circuit, power dissipation 1211
electric eel 1124
electric shock 1211
electrocardiogram (ECG) **2182–200**
abnormalities, in aircraft crew and pilots 1201
in acute pericarditis 2476–7
ambulatory 2194–200
after myocardial infarction 2347
database 2197
dizziness and syncope 2197–9
equipment and techniques 2194–5
innocent arrhythmias 2199
ischaemic heart disease 2199
pacemaker patients 2199–200
palpitations 2197, 2198
patient diary 2197
silent ischaemia 2323
in angina 2336
in anomalous atrioventricular pathways 2193, 2197
location 2193–4
in aortic regurgitation 2465

in aortic stenosis 2463
in arrhythmogenic right ventricular dysplasia 2391
in atrial fibrillation 2271
atrial repolarization wave 2183
atrioventricular conduction disturbances 2267–8, 2269
in bundle branch block 2188–9, 2190, 2191
in cardiac amyloidosis 2393
in cardiac arrhythmias 2261, *2261*
in chronic obstructive airways disease 2774
in chronic renal failure 3301
in coarctation of aorta 2558
common atrioventricular canal 2428
in cor pulmonale 2518, *2518*
delta wave 2193, 2197, 2275, 2276
in diabetes 1489, 1492
in diabetic ketoacidosis 1502, 1503
in dilated cardiomyopathy 2383
in ductus arteriosus 2431
in Ebstein's anomaly 2414
in electrical injury 1212
in Fallot's tetralogy 2403, 2405, 2406
in fixed subaortic stenosis 2422
in Friedreich's ataxia 3984
'f' waves 2271
high resolution 2261, 2262
historical aspects 2182–3
Holter monitoring, *see* electrocardiogram (ECG), ambulatory
in hypereosinophilic syndrome 2397
in hyperkalaemia 3135, 3284, 3285
in hypertrophic cardiomyopathy 2387–8
in hypokalaemia 3129
in hypothyroidism 2394
in infective endocarditis 2442
intermittent devices 2197
investigation for pacemakers 2286
in ischaemic heart disease 2190–2
in Kawasaki disease 3047–8
in Lassa fever 431
leads 2183–4
ambulatory ECG 2194–5
precordial (chest) leads 2184
six limb (frontal plane) 2184
V leads 2184
in mitral regurgitation 2459
in mitral stenosis 2453
in mixed mitral valve disease 2457
in myocardial hypertrophy 2187–8
in myocardial infarction 2191–2, 2193, 2194, 2195, 2196
after thrombolytic therapy 29, 2333, 2334
criteria for thrombolysis 2340–1
diagnostic pitfalls 2192
inferior *vs* anterior 2192, 2194, 2195, 2196
initial assessment 2336
location of changes 2192, *2194*
prognostic 2338
recent *vs* old 2192, 2194, 2195, 2196
reciprocal changes 2193
sequence of changes 2192, 2193
normal appearance 2152, 2153, **2183–4**, 2197
basic ECG waveform 2183
precordial leads 2185–6
recognition 2184–5
Osborne (J wave) in elderly 4346
in ostium primum 2427
in ostium secundum defects 2425
in pericardial constriction 2480
in pericardial tamponade 2477, 2478
in pregnancy 1735
PR interval 2267
prolongation in atrial extrasystoles 2269, 2271
PR interval shortened,
in Lown-Ganong-Levins syndrome 2277
in pre-excitation syndrome 2275, 2276
in pulmonary embolism 2525
in pulmonary hypertension 2511
in pulmonary valve stenosis 2420
P wave 2153, 2183
in atrial extrasystoles 2269, 2271
in atrial tachycardia 2273

electrocardiogram (ECG) (*cont.*)
'dropped' 2266, 2267
inverted in re-entry tachycardia 2274, 2275
normal 2186, 2187
in pulmonary hypertension 2511
in ventricular tachycardia 2279
QRS complex 2183
in bundle branch block 2188, 2190, 2191
in cor pulmonale 2518
dimensions 2185, 2187
in myocardial infarction 2191–2
narrow, tachycardias with 2270–1, 2272, 2274
normal limb leads 2186
normal precordial leads 2185, 2186
premature in atrioventricular junctional extrasystoles 2270
in torsades de pointes 2282
in ventricular extrasystoles 2270
wide 2270
wide, tachycardias **2277–9**, *2278*
QT interval, long QT syndrome, *see* long QT syndrome
quinine overdose 1073
Q wave 2153
in myocardial infarction 2191
R wave 2153
loss in myocardial infarction 2191
ST segment 2183
exercise testing 2227
normal 2185, 2186, 2197
rises/falls in myocardial infarction 2334
ST segment depression,
in angina 2322, 2323
in hypertrophic cardiomyopathy 2387
in myocardial infarction 2334, 2338, 2341
silent 2323
ST segment elevation,
in acute pericarditis 2476
in myocardial infarction 2191–2, 2334, 2336, 2341
in pericarditis 2335, 2336
in Prinzmetal angina 2322
types 2336
in supra-aortic stenosis 2423
TA wave 2183
terminology and nomenclature 2183
in total anomalous pulmonary venous drainage (TAPVD) 2415
in transient ischaemic attack (TIA) 3952
in transposition of great arteries 2417
in tricuspid atresia 2413
in tricyclic antidepressant poisoning 1059
T wave 2183, 2259
in hypertrophic cardiomyopathy 2387
inversion 2270
in myocardial infarction 2192, 2193
normal 2185, 2186–7
in ventricular pre-excitation 2192–4
in ventricular septal defects 2429
in ventricular tachycardia, sustained 2279
electrocoagulation, colonic adenoma removal 1989
electrocochleography 3871
electroconvulsive therapy (ECT) 4220
electrocution 4129
electroencephalogram (EEG) **3829–31**
abnormalities 3829
alpha rhythm 3829
in Alzheimer's disease 3974
applications 3830
beta rhythm 3829–30
brain death diagnosis 3934
delta waves (rhythm) 3830
in dementia 3969
epileptic seizures 3830, 3909, 3919, 3920
flat, in cerebral anoxia 4123
in hepatic encephalopathy 2102, 2105
in intracranial tumours 3830, 4037
normal 3829

in obstructive sleep apnoea 2913
partial seizures 3913
petit mal seizures 3912
principles 3829
record and electrodes 3829
report and interpretation 3829–30
in sleep 2906, 2907
theta waves 3830
use, principles 3830
electrogastrography (EGG) 1957–8
electrolytes
absorption 1900, *1901*, 1902
ACE inhibitor action 2249
in artificial nutritional support 1318, *1318*
balance **3116–35**
after injury/surgery 1549
hormonal control 1563
in malignant disease **3184**
content of intestinal effluents *1318*
disturbances,
in anorexia nervosa 4214
in bulimia nervosa 1300, 4216
in cirrhosis 2088
in cor pulmonale 2519
in heart failure 2235
in hepatocellular failure 2103
in malaria, management 854–5
mental disorders/symptoms in 4240
oesophageal varices complication 2094
parenteral nutrition complications 1319
in poisoning 1047
hypertension pathogenesis 2530
management, in hepatocellular failure 2109
reference intervals *4364, 4366*
replacement,
in cholera 579
in salicylate poisoning 1056
in short gut syndrome 1926
secretion,
in bacterial overgrowth 1913
in cholera 577, *578*, 2002
serum, in cholera 578, *579*
electromagnetic fields, brain tumours association 213
electromagnetic waves, radiofrequency **1222**
electromyography (EMG)
applications 3840
in botulism 631, 632
clinical **3839–40**
in entrapment neuropathies **3841**
in fatiguability **3841**
gut motility disorder investigation 1957
in Lambert–Eaton myasthenic syndrome 4163
motor unit potentials 3839
muscular dystrophies **4145**
in myasthenia gravis 4161
non-diagnostic uses **3842**
in polymyositis and dermatomyositis 4157
in polyneuropathy **3841–2**
principles 3839
single-fibre 3816
in sleep 2906, 2907
spontaneous activity 3840
surgical management and **3842**
in wasting **3841**
in weakness **3840–1**
electron beams
computed tomography (CT) 2217–18
radiotherapy 255
electron microscopy, viral infections of CNS 4069
electron transferring flavoprotein-ubiquinone oxidoreductase 1374, 1375
electron transport chain 1373, 1374
electron transporting flavoprotein (ETF) 1374, 1375
electronystagmography (ENG) 3872, 3873
electrophysiological testing
cardiac, *see* heart, electrophysiology
in multiple sclerosis 3994

peripheral nervous system **3839–42**
entrapment neuropathies 3841
fatiguability 3841
polyneuropathy 3841–2
weakness 3840–1
see also electromyography (EMG)
elephantiasis 922
endemic non-filarial, *see* podoconiosis
genital 760, 761
management **3810–11**
elevation, leg ulceration management 3807–8
elliptocytes *3378*
elliptocytosis, hereditary (HE) 3466, **3531–2**
mild 3531, *3532*
spherocytic 3531, *3532*
Embden–Meyerhof pathway 3456, 3534
embolectomy
in ischaemia of limb 2371
pulmonary 1742, 2526, 2570
emboli
cardiac sources 3949, *3949*, 3960
cerebral, *see* cerebral emboli
embolic agents, intracranial disorder treatment 3822, 3824
embolism
air, *see* air embolism
amniotic fluid *1742*, **1745**, *1762*
cerebral, *see* cerebral emboli
cholesterol, *see* cholesterol embolism
heart valve prostheses 2470
in infective endocarditis 2440
intestinal ischaemia due to 1995
limb ischaemia due to 2363–4
lipid 2837
in mitral stenosis 2454
pulmonary, *see* pulmonary embolism
retinal artery occlusion 4186
spinal cord 3894
systemic, in cardiac myxoma 2473
see also thromboembolism
embolization
bronchial artery 2656
hepatic artery 1705
percutaneous, in telangiectasia 3786
in spinal canal 3828
splenic artery 3596
superglue 3824
vascular cerebral tumours 3822, 3824
embryogenesis
non-specific defects **4112–14**
in spina bifida 4117
embryology
biliary tract 2014
gastrointestinal tract anomalies 1972–3
macrophage role 87
see also developmental abnormalities
embryonal carcinoma 211
see also teratoma
embryonal teratocarcinoma, reversibility of 193
embryos
gene insertion 62, 112
legal status 11, 12
research, muscular dystrophies **4146–7**
sexing 136
EMERAS trial 2340
emergencies
acute poisoning 1043
cardiac arrest 2283–4
see also intensive care
Emery–Dreifuss muscular dystrophy 4146
aetiology 4145
cardiac manifestations 2392
emesis, *see* nausea and vomiting; vomiting
emetine hydrochloride 987
in amoebiasis 831–2
EMG (exomphalos macroglossia gigantism) syndrome 1974
emotion, falling with, *see* cataplexy
emotional disorders, somatization 1037
emotional reactions 4203, 4204
abnormal,
in schizophrenia 4222
see also psychiatric disorders

in dying and bereaved **4233–6**
management 4234, *4234*
prevention 4234
see also dying patients; grief
to life events, models 4232, *4232*
to physical illness 4203
emphysema 2632
in α₁-antitrypsin deficiency 1545, **1546**
bullous **2777–8**
cadmium poisoning 1107
cellular/molecular events 2769–70
centrilobular 2768
chest radiography in 2664, 2774
classification 2768
definition 2632, 2766–7
elastin in 2632, 2773
gas exchange in 2633–4, 2769
lung inflammation role 2616, 2617, 2769
mechanical properties of lung 2632–3, 2768, 2769
panlobular 2768
pathophysiology **2632–3**, **2768–9**
in pregnancy 1745
pulmonary circulation in 2633, 2768–9
subcutaneous, in pregnancy 1746
see also chronic obstructive airways disease (COAD)
employees, duties 2357
employers, duties 2357
employment
angina management 2326
ankylosing spondylitis and 2968
coronary artery disease and **2356–62**
factors influencing 2357
epilepsy and 3924
heart rate and oxygen consumption 2357–8
ischaemic heart disease risk 2314–15
skin disease problems and 3709, 3738, 3739
Employment Medical Advisory Service (EMAS) 2357
'empty delta' sign 4043
empty sella, benign intracranial hypertension and 4042
empyema **2705–7**
causes 2705, 2706, *2706, 2867*
chronic 2706
Haemophilus influenzae type b 582
pericardial, pneumococcal 517
pleural effusions 2867
pneumococcal 516–17
subdural 4050, 4081
tuberculous 2867
empyema necessitas, pneumococcal infections 517
emulsifying ointments 3805
enalapril, trials involving 2251
enanthems 383–4
enantiomers 1248
encephalitis 4064
acute, mental disorders/symptoms 4236
California 424–5
Central European (CEE) 416
in chickenpox 347
in coxsackievirus infection 386
electroencephalogram (EEG) in 3830
flaviviruses causing 415, 416–17
granulomatous amoebic 834
herpes simplex, *see* herpes simplex virus (HSV) infections
in HIV infection 4075, 4077
in immunocompromised 1033
Japanese, *see* Japanese B encephalitis
measles 376, 380
mumps 373, 374
Murray Valley **415**
postinfectious 4065, 4066
rabies 400, 401
rickettsial 731
Rocio **415–16**
rubella **4074**
St Louis **416**, 3965
in scrub typhus 740
subacute in AIDS 4236

tick-borne 414, **416–17**
toxoplasma, *see* toxoplasmosis
viral **4065–8**, 4065
encephalitis lethargica 3998
Encephalitozoon cuniculi 884
encephaloceles **4115–16**
encephalomyelitis
  acute disseminated 3990–1
    hyperacute 3991
  in carcinomas 4135
  extrinsic allergic 165
  postinfectious 4065, 4066
    clinical features 4068
  postvaccinal 3991
    rabies *vs* 401
  simian herpesviruses causing 358
  zoster 349
encephalomyopathy, *see* mitochondrial
    myopathy
encephalopathy
  in AIDS, *see under* AIDS and HIV
    infection
  bovine spongiform (BSE) 1517, 3977,
    3981
  in cat scratch disease 746
  chronic progressive subcortical, *see*
    Binswanger's disease
  electroencephalogram (EEG) in 3830
  hepatic, *see* hepatic encephalopathy
  hypertensive 1729, 2534, **2543**
  lead 1109, 1174, 4056
  lymphocytic choriomeningitis virus
    (LCMV) infection 435–6
  myoclonic **4014–15**
  post-traumatic 4049
  respiratory 4124
  Reye's syndrome, *see* Reye's syndrome
  spongiform, cerebral amyloid in 1517
  subacute necrotizing 3989
  transmissible, in kuru 3982, 3983
  uraemic 3283, 3302, 4124
  in urea cycle defects 1358, 1360
  Wernicke's, *see* Wernicke's
    encephalopathy
endarterectomy 2370
  carotid 2373
  coronary artery bypass grafting 2355
endarteritis, proliferative 3249, 3250,
    3290
endarteritis obliterans, Heubner's 4084
endemic syphilis, *see* syphilis, endemic
endobronchial sampling 2680
endocarditis
  infective, *see* infective endocarditis
  marantic, in lung cancer 2885
  non-infective of mitral valve, *see*
    Libman-Sachs endocarditis
endocardium
  calcification 2182
  fibrosis 2390, 2399
  magnetic resonance imaging 2216
  resection, in ventricular tachycardia
    2280
  thickening, in hypertrophic
    cardiomyopathy 2384
  thrombus 2390, 2397, 2398
endocervicitis 3356
endocrine abnormalities
  in anorexia nervosa 1297, 4213–14
  in bulimia nervosa 1300, 4216
  in depressive disorders 4219
  in hepatocellular failure 2105
  see also endocrine system
endocrine cells, gastrointestinal tract
    1891, 1892
endocrine diseases **1551–719**
  after acute lymphocytic leukaemia 3414
  anaemia 3483, 3686
  bone disease in 3061
  brittle diabetes in 1496
  chronic localized mucocutaneous
    candidiasis with 1852
  in chronic renal failure 3302
  dementia due to 3971
  in elderly **4344–6**
  genetic causes *1567*
  haematological changes **3686**

hormone deficiency 1566, *1567*,
    1570–2
hormone excess 1566–70
hormone resistance 1566, *1567*, 1572–3
  joint involvement **3003–2994**
in Langerhans-cell histiocytosis 3608
mechanisms **1566–73**
mental disorders/symptoms in **4238–40**
metabolic disorders due to **4125**
neuropathies in **4098–9**
of non-endocrine origin **1711–19**
osteoporosis in **3069**
polycythaemia in 3551, 3554
in pregnancy **1747–52**
pruritus in 3744
sexual problems associated 4243–4
short stature 1698–9
in Wilson's disease 1420
endocrine drugs, poisoning **1071–2**
endocrine myopathies, *see* myopathy
endocrine syndrome, paraneoplastic 242,
    243
endocrine system
  age-related changes 4336
  in injecting drug abusers 4284
  in malnutrition *1290*
  in sarcoidosis **2827**
  see also endocrine abnormalities
endocrine therapy, in pancreatic
    carcinoma 2045
endocrine tumours **1566–70**
  benign 1566
  malignant 1566
  multiple, *see* multiple endocrine
    neoplasia (MEN) syndromes
  pancreatic **1703–7**
  pathophysiology 1566–8
  signalling pathway mutations 1569–70
  tumorigenesis and clonality 1568–9
endocrinology **1553–719**
  definition 1553–4
endocrinopathy, in POEMS syndrome
    4104
endocytosis **72–5**
  acidification of pathway 74, 75
  antigen uptake and processing 143
  branch-points in pathway 72–3
  chlamydial infection by 749
  functions 72
  outline of pathway 72
  pathogens and 74–5
  receptor-mediated, *see* receptor-
    mediated endocytosis
  similarity to exocytic pathway 72
  via coated pits 73
Endolimax nana 825
endolymphatic hydrops 3875
endomembrane system **68–84**
  see also endocytosis; exocytic pathway
endometrial biopsy, in pelvic
    inflammatory disease *3359*
endometrial cancer
  aetiological factors 210, 218
  epidemiology 210
  hormone replacement therapy and 1815
  oestrogen association 216
  oral contraceptives and 1723
endometrial hyperplasia 210
  in polycystic ovary syndrome 1673
endometriosis **2137**
  bowel in 2137
  colon in 1987
  hormone replacement therapy and 1815
  pleura 2867
  symptoms and diagnosis 2137
endometritis, chlamydial 752, 1791
endomyocardial biopsy
  in dilated cardiomyopathy 2383
  in hypereosinophilic syndrome 2397
  in myocarditis 2380
endomyocardial fibrosis (EMF) 2390,
    2396–7, 2460–1
  clinical features and investigations 2397
  eosinophilic, *see* hypereosinophilic
    syndrome
  mitral regurgitation in 2460–1
  prognosis and treatment 2397, 2398

tricuspid regurgitation in 2468
tropical 2390, 2397, 2460–1
endomysial antibodies 1918
endophthalmitis
  coagulase-negative staphylococcal 533
  metastatic 4191
endoplasmic reticulum
  antigen processing 143
  assembly, microtubule role 82
  cotranslational translocation into 68–9
  early events in 69–70
  to Golgi apparatus transport 75, 76–7
  membrane protein biogenesis 69
  protein translocation pore 69
  quality control of proteins 70
  scavenger system for defective proteins
    70
  vesicles, in nuclear envelope assembly
    80
  see also exocytic pathway; intracellular
    transport
ß-endorphin 1575
endorphins 3938
  increased during exercise 2161
endoscopes
  electronic 1829
  fibreoptic 1829
endoscopic biopsy 1957
  small intestine 1908–9
endoscopic retrograde
    cholangiopancreatography (ERCP)
    1834–5
  acute pancreatitis after 2027
  advantages 2043
  in biliary disease 2046
  in chronic pancreatitis 2034, 2035,
    2036, *2037*
  cross-infections 1830
  false-positive, causes 2036
  in pancreatic carcinoma 2043–4
  in primary biliary cirrhosis 2075
  in primary sclerosing cholangitis 2078
  therapeutic, in acute pancreatitis 2032
endoscopic sphincterotomy 2027, 2032
  in choledocholithiasis 2051
  gallstones 2049
endoscopic therapy
  in acute pancreatitis 2032
  in chronic pancreatitis 2038
endoscopy **1829–30**
  antibiotics in 1830
  Crohn's disease 1939, 1939–40
  disinfection of instruments 1830
  duodenal ulcer 1878
  fibreoptic, barium studies *vs* 1831–2
  gastric cancer 1984
  gastric ulcer 1879, 1888
  gastrointestinal bleeding 1828
    management of 1828
  gut motility disorder investigation 1957
  indications 1829–30
  peptic ulcer haemorrhage 1882
  in portal hypertension 2093
  premedication for 1830
  safety guidelines 1830
  see also bronchoscopy; colonoscopy;
    enteroscopy; oesophagoscopy;
    sigmoidoscopy
endostreptosin, *S. pyogenes* and
    glomerulonephritis from 505
endothelial cell(s) **2295–305**
  adhesion molecule production 2294,
    2299, 2619–21, 2623
  see also adhesion molecules
  anatomy and structure 2295–6, 2486,
    2593–4
  antibodies to 2296, 2300
  bacterial adhesion 2438
  in bartonellosis 774
  coagulation system interaction 2487,
    2498, 2514
  cytokines released 2294, 2299, 2487,
    2498, 2514
  damage 2299, 2624
    in adult respiratory distress syndrome
      2496, 2497
    after cardiac transplantation 2258

antineutrophil cytoplasmic antibodies
    role 3012
    detection 2503
  in haemolytic uraemic syndrome 3199
  in lung inflammation 2624
  in malignant hypertension 2534
  pulmonary hypertension pathogenesis
    2505, 2514
  in pulmonary oedema 2496, 2497
  smoking and 2313, 2363
  temazepam injection 4283
  therapeutic interventions causing 2300
  see also endothelial cell(s),
    dysfunction
  denudation, in thrombosis in
    atherosclerosis 2319
  development 2295
  dysfunction
    activation 2294, 2299, 2497
    atherosclerosis pathogenesis 2291,
      2294, 2297, 2313, 2362
    diseases with 2295, *2296*
    heart failure pathophysiology 2231
    pulmonary hypertension pathogenesis
      2505, 2514
  functions 2290, 2296, **2486–8**
    drugs affecting 2300
  growth factors produced by 2293
  haemostatic reactions **3626–7**
  inflammatory mediators released 2487,
    2514, 2619
  leucocyte interactions **3558–9**
  lipid metabolism role 2291, 2299
  lymphatic capillaries 2559
  monocyte interaction 87, 88, 2291
  nitric oxide synthesis 2290, 2296, 2323,
    2487, 2514, 2516
  permeability, in malignant hypertension
    2534
  platelet function regulation and
    haemostasis 2298–9, 2362
  pulmonary 2484, **2486**, 2514, 2593–4
    alveolar juxtaposition 2485
    anti-/pro-coagulant activity 2487, 2514
    fluid/ionic balance 2492–4
    functions **2486–8**, 2514
    metabolic functions 2486–7
    neutrophil adhesion 2619, 2620
    neutrophil emigration from capillaries
      2619, 2620
    phagocytic function 2487
    pulmonary hypertension pathogenesis
      2505, 2514
    reticuloendothelial function 2487
    vascular smooth muscle interactions
      2487, 2514
    vasoconstriction 2487, 2514, 2516
    vasodilatation 2487, 2514, 2516
  in pulmonary hypertension 2505, 2507,
    2508, 2514
  receptors, in malaria 842, 845
  in rickettsial diseases 730, 731
  signal detection by 2294, 2300
  smooth muscle cell growth control
    2299, 2362, 2514
  therapeutic implications 2300
  thrombolysis and 2299
  transport and metabolism by 2290,
    2299–300
  turnover rate 259
  vascular tone control **2296–8**, **2323**,
    2324
    vasoconstrictors 2297–8, 2323, *2324*,
      2487, 2514, 2516
    vasodilators 2296–7, 2323, *2324*,
      2487, 2514, 2516
endothelial cell factor V 2294
endothelial cell layer 2289–90
  basement membrane 2289, 2290, 2485,
    2486
endothelial-derived relaxing factor
    (EDRF), *see* nitric oxide
endothelial-leucocyte adhesion molecule
    (ECAM1), *see* E-selectin
endothelial-vascular-interstitial antibody
    (EVI) 896
endothelin-1 2159, 2160, 2297–8

endothelins 1894, 2148, 2297–8
  increased production and
    vasoconstriction 2298
  pulmonary endothelial cells releasing
    2487
  release and stimuli for 2298
  role 2298
  sequences from snake venom 1130
endothelium **2295–305**
  antigen presentation in grafts 185
  development and anatomy 2295–6
  in heart 2143
  inflammatory reaction to endotoxin 291
  'margination' of red cells, in malaria 843
  pulmonary 2484, **2486**
    see also endothelial cell(s), pulmonary
  repair after termination of inflammation
    2624–5
  role in thrombosis 3662–3
  target of immune response in
    transplantation 187
  see also endothelial cell(s)
endothelium-dependent vasodilators 2296
  impaired responsiveness 2297
endothelium-derived hyperpolarizing
    factor (EDHF) 2297
endothrix 798
endotoxic shock 292
  C6 deficiency protecting against 180
  see also septic shock
endotoxin 272, 291
  antisera and passive
    immunoprophylaxis 283
  cytokine production 276
  in DIC pathogenesis 3657
  in extrinsic allergic alveolitis 2813
  haemolytic uraemic syndrome and 3199
  inflammatory reactions **291**
  in leptospirosis 698
  monoclonal antibodies, septicaemia
    treatment 1025–6
  Neisseria meningitidis 537, 541
  reaction,
    in malaria 846
    in relapsing fevers 693, 696
  Salmonella typhi 562
endotracheal intubation 2577, **2918**
  in bronchoscopy 2579
  children 2577
  difficulties 2918
  in unconscious patients 2585
endotracheal tubes 2577, 2918
  cuffed 2577, 2585
  nasal 2577
  oral 2577
endplate receptors 4140, 4141
endurance sports **4324–8**
  abnormalities induced by **4326–7**
  aerobic fitness **4324–5**
  carbohydrate metabolism **4325–6**
  glucose supplements 4325–6
  hyperthermia 4328
  hypothermia 4328
  hypovolaemia in 4327–8
  sickle cell trait and 4328
  training, effect on heart 2161
  see also exercise; marathon runners;
    runners
enemas
  meconium ileus management 1978
  small-bowel, *see* small-bowel enema
energy 4165
  balance,
    mechanisms maintaining 1307
    obesity aetiology 1306–7
    'set-point' theory 1307
  body composition and 1272
  body stores/sources 1272, *1273*
  chronic deficiency 1279
    see also malnutrition
  expenditure 1272–3
    increasing in obesity treatment
      1311–12
    in obese *vs* lean persons 1306–7
    in pregnancy 1770
    types of employment *2358*
  functions 1271

intake,
  artificial nutritional support 1317
  in diabetes mellitus 1469, 1493
  diabetes mellitus aetiology 1327
  in malnutrition management 1289
  in obese *vs* lean persons 1306
  in pregnancy 1770, *1772*
metabolic pathways 4167
metabolism 4165, 4166, 4167
  Plasmodium species 837
production from metabolic fuel 1271–2
requirements 1269, *1270*, 1272, *1272*,
    1329, 1330
  artificial nutritional support 1316–17,
    2587, 2588
  during exercise 1272
  heart **2145–7**, 2145
  in intensive care 2587, *2587*, 2588
  in malnutrition management 1293
  in pregnancy 1770, *1771*
  reduced in malnutrition 1285
  in starvation 1278
  sources 1272, 4165
    after injury/surgery 1549, 1550
    endurance sports training and 4325
    for heart 2145–7
  stored in adipose tissue 1399–400
  supply to heart **2145–7**
  supply and utilization 1272–3
    regulation 1273
  see also calories; fuel, metabolic
energy-rich drinks 4215
Engelmann's disease (progressive
    diaphyseal dysplasia) **3089**
enhancer binding proteins 1558
enhancers 57 enkephalin 1894, 3938
Entamoeba gingivalis 825
Entamoeba hartmanni 825
Entamoeba histolytica 825–33, 825,
    2003, 2005
  biology and pathogenicity 825–6
  cysts, diagnosis/detection 831
  detection/culture 830–1
  in HIV infection 475
  in homosexuals 3364–5
  immune evasion 827
  as intraluminal commensal 825
  pathogenic strains, characteristics 825, 826
  trophozoites 825, 826, 830
  zymodemes 826
  see also amoebiasis
Entamoeba polecki 825
enteral feeding 1315, *1316*, 2587
  blockage of tube 1321
  in burns patients 1322
  complications 1321–2
  half-life of feeds 1318
  in head injury 1323
  at home 1321
  indications *1324*
  outcome 1325
  indications/guidelines *1316*
  infusion pump use 1321
  in intensive care 2587
  monitoring 1322
  regurgitation 1321–2
  in short gut syndrome 1926
  withdrawal in persistent vegetative state
    3935
  see also nutritional support
enteric cyst 1976
Enteric Cytopathic Human Orphan virus,
    see echovirus
enteric fever
  causes 2004, *2004*
  differential diagnosis 2006
  see also paratyphoid fever; typhoid
enteric fistulae
  bacterial overgrowth aetiology 1912
  causes 1912
enteric nervous system 1953
  function 1953
  sensory neurones for 1954
  size 1953
enteritis
  idiopathic chronic ulcerative 1910
  in measles 379

necrotizing (pig bel) **636–7**, 1995, 2004
  see also gastroenteritis
enteritis necroticans (necrotizing
    enterocolitis) **636–7**, 1995, 2004
enterobacteria **550–7**
  antigenic structure 550
    flagellar (H) antigens 550
    somatic (O) antigens 550
    surface antigens 550
  definition/description 550
  extraintestinal infections 550–1
  intestinal infections 551–60
  lactose-fermenting (coliform) 550
  see also Campylobacter; Escherichia
    coli; Salmonella; Shigella
Enterobacteriaceae 550
  endocarditis 2437, 2448, *2448*
enterobiasis **941–2**
Enterobius vermicularis 941, 942
  infections in homosexuals 3365
enteroclysis technique, *see* small-bowel
    enema
enterococci 497
  antibiotic resistance 510
  diseases **509–10**
    endocarditis 2437, 2446
    treatment 509–10, 2446, *2447*
  transmission 510
  'Van A' and 'Van B' strains 510
Enterococcus, species 497
Enterococcus faecalis 509, 2437
Enterococcus faecium 509, 2437
enterocolitis
  Hirschsprung's 1979
  necrotizing, *see* necrotizing enterocolitis
  Salmonella 552
enterocytes 1900
  damage, in bacterial overgrowth 1913
  polarization 1900
Enterocytozoon bieneusi 883, 884, 886,
    1930
enteroglucagon 1893
  in coeliac disease 1895
  elevated 1895
    in tropical sprue 1934
  small-intestinal transit time 1934
  structure and secretion 1893
  tumours producing 1703
enterokinase, deficiency 2039
enteropathic synovitis **2972–3**
enteropathogenic bacteria **550–60**
enteropathy, tropical, *see* tropical
    enteropathy
enteropathy-associated T-cell lymphoma
    (EATL) **1927–30**
  clinical features 1927–8
  coeliac disease relation 1929
  management 1929
  pathology 1928
  phenotype of T-cells 1928
  terminology/historical aspects 1927
  ulcerative jejunitis and 1928, 1929
enteroscopes 1829
enteroscopy, in Crohn's disease 1940
'Enterotest' capsule 879
enterotoxins
  in atopic dermatitis 161
  Bacillus cereus 559
  Escherichia coli 556, 2002
  F, *see* toxic shock syndrome toxin
    (TSST-1)
  Staphylococcus aureus 524, *525*
  types 524, 2001
  Vibrio cholerae 576, 577, 578
enterovirus 71 386
enterovirus 72, *see* hepatitis A virus
    (HAV)
enteroviruses **381–90**
  classification *382*
  faecal pollution 389
  structure 381
  see also coxsackieviruses; echoviruses;
    poliovirus
enterovirus infections **383–8**
  acute conjunctivitis 388
  CNS 4064
  control 388–90

diagnosis 383, 387
  epidemiology 382
  exanthems and enanthems 383, *383*
  fetus and neonate 388, **1783**
  gastrointestinal tract and pancreas
    387–2614
  heart and muscle disease 386–7,
    387
  in hypogammaglobulinaemia 168
  myositis due to 4155
  neurological diseases 384–6, *385*
  pattern and transmission 382, *382*
  in pregnancy **1783**
enthesitis 2947, 4324
enthesopathy, in ankylosing spondylitis
    2967
entrapment neuropathies
  electromyography in **3841**
  median nerve 4094–6
  occupational 1169
  in rheumatoid arthritis 2961
  see also carpal tunnel syndrome
entropion, in trachoma 750, 751
enuresis, nocturnal
  in sickle-cell disease 3194–5
  in vesicoureteric reflux 3217
envenoming **1043–51**, **1124–60**
  insect stings 1145
  management **1046–51**
  snakes, *see* snakes, venomous
env gene 464
environment
  hormonal rhythms and 1565
  host-parasite relationship and 285
  integrated hormonal responses 1563–4
  see also air pollution; pollution
environmental disasters **1232–4**, *1232*,
    1234
  natural **1232–3**
  technological **1233–4**
environmental disease **1180–93**
environmental factors/conditions
    1180–93
  ageing and 4333–4
  in asthma 2731, **2733**
  body temperature changes **1181–2**
  cancer epidemiology 220, *221*
  chronic obstructive airways disease
    aetiology 2767, 2768
  cold and drownings **1182–5**
  essential hypertension 2530–1
  extrinsic allergic alveolitis *2810*, 2811,
    2814
    management 2816
  gastric cancer association 203
  heat **1180–1**
  high altitudes **1185–93**
  lung function variations 2674–5
  multifactor causation of disorders 100,
    129
  rheumatoid arthritis aetiology 2953
  scleroderma aetiology *3027*, 3028
  vasculitis pathogenesis 3011
  *see also above individual factors/
    conditions*; air pollution;
    occupational disease/hazards;
    pollution
environmental health and safety 1160
  see also occupational health
environmental history, in lung disease
    2649
environmental monitoring, occupational
    hazards 1163
environmental substances, toxic
  neuropathies 4099–100
enzyme(s)
  defects causing hormone deficiencies
    1567, 1571–2
  diagnostic tests and reference intervals
    4365, *4366*
  induction, drug interactions 1257
  inhibition and drug action via 1247–8
  lysosomal 1426
  oxygen handing 1194–5
  phosphorylation 1560
  reduced, in malnutrition 1287
  replacement therapy 1248, 1336, 1430

small-bowel biopsy 1909
in snake venom 1129
urinary excretion (enzymuria) 3109,
3138
enzyme immunoassay
Bacillus anthracis 615
chlamydial infections *755*, 756
dengue virus 422
enteroviruses diagnosis 383
giardiasis diagnosis 880
malaria diagnosis 849
respiratory viruses 334
rickettsial diseases diagnosis 732
snake venoms 1135
syphilis diagnosis 716
in toxocariasis 945
trichinosis 941
enzyme-linked immunoelectrotransfer
blot assay 967
enzyme-linked immunosorbent assay
(ELISA)
in allergic rhinitis 2717
Lassa fever diagnosis 434
leishmaniasis diagnosis 905
leprosy diagnosis 668
leptospirosis diagnosis 702
eosinophil(s) **3555**
in allergic inflammation 159
in allergic rhinitis 2715
antibody-dependent cellular cytotoxicity
277
in asthma 2726, 2727, 2728
cationic proteins 159, 161, 2727
counts *3379*, *3380*
in cryptogenic fibrosing alveolitis 2789
degranulation 159, 2727
differentiation and activation 159, 2727
production 3384, 3386, 3557
protective effects 278
eosinophilia 278, 3378, 3558
in acute schistosomiasis 975
in allergic rhinitis 2715
causes 3610
in returning travellers *326*, 327
in Churg-Strauss syndrome 2800
granule-mediated damage of heart 2397
see also endomyocardial fibrosis;
hypereosinophilic syndrome
in hookworm infestation 3680
in hypereosinophilic syndrome 3611
in infections 267
in malignant disease 3678
pulmonary, *see* pulmonary eosinophilia
in toxocariasis 945
tropical, *see* tropical pulmonary
eosinophilia
see also hypereosinophilia
eosinophilia-myalgia syndrome 3612
eosinophilic cellulitis 3774
eosinophilic enteritis 945, **949**
eosinophilic fasciitis 3039, *3791*
eosinophilic gastroenteropathy 1908
eosinophilic granuloma 2833, 3606
of lung **2832–3**
see also histiocytosis, Langerhans-cell
eosinophilic meningitis **945–9**, *948*, 953
eosinophilic myositis 3039
eosinophilic pleocytosis 947, 953, 977
eosinophilic reactions, drug-induced
2850, *2850*, 2851
eosinophil protein X 2801
ependymoma **4031**
cystic, MRI 3821
management 4039
spinal cord 3895
ephedrine, MAOI food and drug
interactions 4250
ephelis *3754*
epicardium 2474
epidemic 286
epidemic haemorrhagic fever 426
epidemic hysteria 4210
epidemic myalgia, *see* Bornholm disease
epidemic neuromyasthenia **4074**
epidemic pleurodynia, *see* Bornholm
disease
epidemic polyarthritis of Australia **3001**

epidemiology **42–6**
aetiological 43–4
to complete clinical picture 45–6
infections, *see* infections
intervention studies 45
ischaemic heart disease **2305–6**
in managing health services 46
measurement in 43
observational studies 44–5
poisoning **1043–4**
risk 45, *46*
sexually transmitted diseases, *see*
sexually transmitted diseases (STD)
epidemiology of cancer **197–222**
artefacts/problems of registries 199
biological characteristics **197–8**
age 197–8
latent period 198
sex 198
causative factors **215–19**, 220, 3567
diet 218–10, 1327–8, *1328*
drugs 215–16, *216*, 2258
environmental and behavioural 220,
221
interactions between 219
ionizing radiation 215
occupational 216, *217*, **1165–7**
pollution 217–18
viruses, *see* oncogenic viruses
see also individual factors;
occupational cancer
definition 197
epidemiological observations 220,
221–2
advantages 221–2
negative, uses of 221
familial clusters 220
genetic susceptibility **219–20**
epidemiological observations 220
laboratory studies 220
incidence rate range by country 198, *199*
laboratory *vs* epidemiological
investigations **220–2**
epidemiological observations 221–2
laboratory tests 220–1
preventability **198–201**
causes of difficulties in assessing 199,
200
evidence for 198–200
identification of causes 200–1
incidence changes in migrant groups
199–200, *200*
incidence changes over time 200
incidence differences between ethnic/
religious groups 198–9, 199, *199*
by site of origin **201–15** *see also
individual cancers/anatomical sites*
epidermal growth factor (EGF) receptor
223, *1560*, 1561
amplification, tumours associated 224
in glioblastoma multiforme 224
overexpression, breast cancer outcome
and 224
epidermis 3706
functions 3707
increased turnover in psoriasis 3745
turnover and metabolism 3706
epidermodysplasia verruciformis 209,
446, 461
epidermolysis bullosa **3720–1**, 3723
in infants 3784
patterns 3720, *3721*
epidermolysis bullosa dystrophica 3720,
3721
epidermolytic toxins, types A and B,
Staphylococcus aureus 524
epididymectomy, in genitourinary
tuberculosis 3279
epididymitis
acute non-chlamydial, ureaplasma
causing 770
filarial 922
in homosexuals 3365
Neisseria gonorrhoeae 752
epididymo-orchitis
chlamydial 751–2
gonococcal 546

epidural abscess 3892, **3894**
epidural anaesthesia
acute urinary retention 3236
in diabetic pregnancy 1757
in pregnant women with chest disease
1744, 1746
epidural haemorrhage **3894**
epidural injections, pain treatment 3938
epidural space 4050
epigastric pain
in cholecystitis 2049, 2050
duodenal ulcer 1878
gastric cancer 1983
gastric ulcer 1879
non-ulcer dyspepsia 1880
see also abdominal pain
epigenetic factors 123
epigenetic lesions, in tumours 191
weak evidence for 193
epiglottitis, acute **2691**, 2722
Haemophilus influenzae type b 582,
2691
epilepsia partialis continua 4015
epilepsy **3909–25**
aircraft travel and 1202
benign childhood 3915
benign intracranial hypertension *vs*
4040
causes **3915–18**, *3918*
cerebral dysgenesis 3916–17
genetic/inheritance 3915–16
miscellaneous 3917
trauma 3916
tumours and infections 3917
vascular disease 3917
in children 3924
classification/types **3914**, *3915*
complications **3924**
definitions **3909–10**
diagnosis 3910
differential diagnosis *2175*, 2282,
3929
driving and 3924, 4040
electroencephalogram (EEG) in 3830
epidemiology (incidence/prevalence)
3910
familial myoclonic 3988, 4014–15
genetic basis 3916
gestational 1768
in Huntington's disease 4014
hyposexuality and sexual problems in
4238, 4244
idiopathic 3914, 3915
in intracranial tumours **4036**
long QT syndromes *vs* 2282
mental sequelae/symptoms 4237–8
ictal and post-ictal 4237–8
interictal 4238
myoclonic 3914, 3915, **4015**
in neurocysticercosis 965
in occipital lobe lesions 3869
'of late onset' 3917
post-traumatic 4049
in pregnancy **1768–9**, 3922
primary generalized 3915
prognosis **3924**
'reflex' 3918
remission 3924
seizure type relationship **3914–15**
selective IgA deficiency in 171
social aspects **3924–5**
strokes and 4340
syncope *vs 2175*
television 3918
temporal lobe, mental symptoms
4237–8
treatment **3920–4**
cessation/withdrawal 3923
drugs, *see* antiepileptic drugs
non-compliance 3923
other forms 3923–4
in status epilepticus 3923
surgical 3923–4
in urea cycle defects 1358
see also epileptic seizures
epileptic apnoea 3890
'epileptics', definition 3910

epileptic seizures 3909
3Hz spike-and-wave discharge 3914,
3915
in alcohol withdrawal 4277, 4290, 4291
atypical absences 3914
classification 3911, *3911*
differential diagnosis **3918–19**
epilepsy type relationship **3914–15**
focal, in intracranial tumours 4035
in hereditary myoclonic epilepsies 3988
investigation **3919–20**
Jacksonian 3913
management 4291
in myoclonic epilepsy 4015
partial (focal) 3913–14, 3914
precipitants **3918**
prevalence *3915*
probability of recurrence after initial
3920
rare types 3914
salaam (infantile spasms) 3914
somatosensory 3913
temporal lobe 3913
tonic 3914
tonic-clonic (grand mal/generalized)
3911–12
in alcohol withdrawal 4290
drugs for 3921, *3921*
types **3911–14**
typical absences (petit mal) 3912–13
versive 3914
see also epilepsy; seizures
epiloia, *see* tuberous sclerosis
epinephrine, *see* adrenaline
epipodophyllotoxins, mechanism of
action 259
episcleritis 4183, 4184
management 4185
in relapsing polychondritis 4184
in rheumatoid arthritis 2961, 4185
in ulcerative colitis 1947
epistaxis
in essential hypertension 2535
in rheumatic fever 2433
epithelial cells
plasma membrane domains 71
urinary casts 3105
epithelioid cells
granulomas, in sarcoidosis 2818, 2823
in hepatic granulomas 2120
in sarcoidosis 2818
epitopes 141, 316
epoprostenol, in heart failure 2252
epoxy resins, contact dermatitis 3737
ε-aminocaproic acid 3659
Epstein-Barr virus (EBV) **352–7**
B-cell immortalization 3566, 3567
defect in control in X-linked
lymphoproliferative syndrome 166,
353
early (EA) and late antigens 352
immortalization 355, 858
immunization 227, 463
infectious cycle 352
infective dose 354
latent membrane proteins (LMP) 352
membrane antigens (MA) 355
nuclear antigens (EBNAs) 352, 353,
460
proteins 352
receptor 858
CD21 on B-cells 148, 352
transmission 352, 353, 461
in blood 3693
viral capsid antigen (VCA) 352, 353,
354
Epstein-Barr virus (EBV) infection **352–7**
after cardiac transplantation 2258
in AIDS 357, 4080
antibodies 353, 354, 355, 356
aplastic anaemia induced by 3441
Burkitt's lymphoma and 3567, 3580
carriers 352
chronic 353
chronic fatigue syndrome due to 1036
cryoglobulinaemia due to 3183
disease associations 353–7, 460

Epstein-Barr virus (EBV) infection (*cont.*)
　epidemiology 352
　eye in 4192
　hairy leukoplakia in AIDS 357
　hepatic granulomas in 2121
　hepatitis 2064
　Hodgkin's disease and 213, 355–6,
　　3569–70
　latent 352
　lymphoma,
　　in immunosuppressed states 355, 858
　　in renal transplant recipients 3321
　nasopharyngeal carcinoma, *see*
　　nasopharyngeal carcinoma
　pathogenesis 354, 355
　reactivated 355
　Sjögren's syndrome and 3036
　status determination 352–3
　T-cell lymphoma association 355–6
　see also Burkitt's lymphoma; infectious
　　mononucleosis
Epstein's syndrome 3645
equity, in allocation of health resources 52
*erb*A oncogene 225, 1561, 1606
*erb*B gene, *see* c-*erb*B-2 gene
Erb's (Erb-Duchenne) palsy 3903, 4093
erectile dysfunction
　in diabetes mellitus 4243–4
　drugs causing 4245, *4245*
　in neurological disorders 4244
　treatment 4246
erection, neurological pathways 4244
ergocalciferol 3059
ergometrine, in pregnancy 1745
ergonomic problems 1168
ergosterol 296
ergot 1158
ergotamine 1238, 1239, 4025
ergotism 1158
erionite, fibrous 2846
E-rosetting method 151
erysipelas (St Anthony's fire) 500, 1158
　facial, butterfly distribution 500
　streptococcal, diagnosis 502
Erysipelothrix rhusiopathiae 555
erythema
　'circinate' 890
　facial (flushing) 3786–7, 3788
　food-induced 3729
　migratory *244*
　necrolytic migratory 1706, 3723
　palmar, in pregnancy 1796, 1804
　persistent 3785
　in protein deficiency 3722
　racial differences 3716
　sunburn 3725, 3726
　toxic urticated 3731
erythema arthriticum epidemicum
　　(haverhill fever) 688
erythema chronicum migrans 689, 690
erythema gyratum repens 3793, 3796
erythema infectiosum 447
erythema marginatum, in rheumatic fever
　　2433
erythema migrans *244*, 689, 690, 1864
erythema multiforme 499, **1857**, 2651,
　　3714, 3731, **3780–1**
　aetiology and pathology 3780
　distribution 3712
　herpes simplex virus and 346
　malignancy association 3793
　in orf 370
　in pregnancy 1805
　treatment 3781
erythema nodosum 648, **2821**, 3723,
　　3777–8
　arthralgia in 3003
　bilateral hilar lymphadenopathy with
　　2821
　causes 3777, *3777*
　in sarcoidosis 2818, **2821**
　in ulcerative colitis 1947
erythema nodosum leprosum 673, 674,
　　3729
　treatment 677
erythema toxicum 3783
erythrasma *3755*
erythroblasts 3426, 3427
　receptor 86, 87

erythrocytes, *see* red blood cells
erythrocyte sedimentation rate (ESR)
　　3379, **3380**
　in anorexia nervosa 4214
　in cardiac myxoma 2473
　in Churg-Strauss syndrome 2801
　C-reactive protein and 1533
　in infective endocarditis 2442
　in inflammatory rheumatic disease
　　2951 in pelvic inflammatory disease
　　3358
　in polymyalgia rheumatica 3040
　in rheumatic fever 2434
　in SLE 2798, 3020
　in Takayasu's disease 2379
erythrocytosis
　cor pulmonale pathogenesis 2516
　idiopathic (benign) 3551
　in renal transplant recipients 3321
　in tumours *244*
erythroderma 3708, **3794**
　ichthyosiform 3719, 3720
　in psoriasis 3694
erythrokeratoderma 3750
erythroleukaemia (AML M6) 3400–1,
　　3406, 3428, 3497
erythromycin
　in amoebiasis 832
　in *Campylobacter* infections 558
　in chlamydial infections 757
　in diabetic gastroparesis 1962
　in legionnaires' disease 726
　in neonates 1792
　ophthalmia neonatorum prophylaxis
　　1790
　in pertussis 589
　in pneumonia 2700
　in pregnancy 1785, 1792
　in relapsing fevers 696
　in renal failure *3272*
　Staphylococcus aureus resistance 525
　in streptococci group A infections 502
erythrophagocytosis
　in bartonellosis 774
　in malaria 842, 844
erythropheresis 2930
erythropoiesis 3384, 3386, **3387**, **3452–4**
　early stages 3452–3
　extramedullary 3526, 3588
　　ferrokinetic studies **3594–5**
　　in thalassaemia 3511
　factors required for normal 3454
　in haemolytic disorders 3525
　ineffective (dyserythropoiesis) 3460,
　　3521
　　in aplastic anaemia 3443
　　in infections 3524
　　in malaria 842, 844
　　in megaloblastic anaemia 3495
　　in myelodysplastic syndromes 3426,
　　　3524
　　in sideroblastic anaemia 3521
　　see also anaemia, dyserythropoietic
　in iron deficiency 3474
　metabolic rate 3382
　negative regulation 3387–8
　regulation 3453–4
erythropoietin 97, 1554
　in chronic renal failure 3302, 3682
　deficiency 3459
　in erythropoiesis 3384, 3387, **3453–4**
　in exercise-induced anaemia and
　　concerns 4326
　inappropriate production 3552, **3554**
　in myeloma 3598
　polycythaemia and 3551
　in polycythaemia vera 3432
　recombinant 66
　reduction, by ACE inhibitors 2249
　release in hypoxia 2902
　in renal transplant recipients 3321, 3554
　-secreting tumours 3552, 3554
　self-injection by athletes 3554
　in sickle-cell disease 3195
　thyroid hormones and 3686
　treatment 3389
　　in chronic renal failure 3305, 3389,
　　　3481

　in myelodysplastic syndromes 3431
　in myeloma 3603–4
　in urinary-tract obstruction 3235
eschar 730, 740
Escherichia, rare species 555
Escherichia coli 555–7, 555, 2003
　antibiotic resistance 3209
　enteroadherent (EAEC) 555
　enterohaemorrhagic (EHEC) 556, 2003
　enteroinvasive (EIEC) **557**, 2003
　enteropathogenic (EPEC) **555–6**
　enterotoxigenic (ETEC) **556**, 2002, 2003
　　enterotoxins 556, 2002
　　travellers' diarrhoea due to 324
　GroEL heat-shock protein, chlamydial
　　protein homology 750, 758
　groups causing diarrhoea 555
　in HIV infections and AIDS 487
　interstitial nephritis 3178
　liver in infections 2133
　meningitis due to 4050
　pathovars 273
　post-antibiotic effects 304
　serotypes 555
　ulcerative colitis aetiology 1944, 1946
　urinary tract infections 551, 1733, 3206,
　　3209
　vero cytotoxin-producing (VTEC)
　　556–7, 3196, 3198
　vero cytotoxin (VT) 556
Escherichia coli O157:H7 2003
　intestinal ischaemia 1996
Escherichia coli O157 infections 1946
　ulcerative colitis *vs* 1947
E-selectin 2294, 2299, 2487, **2620**,
　　2620
　in asthma 2728
　emigration of neutrophils from
　　capillaries 2619
　increased expression in atherogenesis
　　2299
espundia (American mucosal
　　leishmaniasis) 902–3
essential fatty acids, *see* fatty acids,
　　essential
esterase, leucocyte, in amniotic fluid
　　1786
'esthiomene' 760
ethacrynic acid 2239, 2241
ethambutol
　adverse reactions 657
　nephrotoxicity 3265
　ocular toxicity 4197
　in tuberculosis 655, *656*
ethane, poisoning 1083
1,2-ethanediol, *see* ethylene glycol
ethanol, *see* alcohol
ethical issues
　dying patients 4349
　genetic testing **137–8**, *137*
　in terminal illness **4359–60**
　types of decisions 4359
ethics
　artificial nutritional support 1325
　clinical trials 1262
　medical **10–14**
　of population problems 37
ethionamide
　in leprosy 676
　in tuberculosis 655, *656*
ethnic differences
　blood pressure **2528**
　in chronic renal failure 3295, 3296,
　　3303
　in diabetes type I 1454
　in diabetes type II 1455
　essential hypertension in **2543**
　ischaemic heart disease 2314
　lung function variations 2673
　in recurrent polyserositis 1525
　sarcoidosis prevalence 2820
　susceptibility to infection 279
ethnic minorities, deliberate self-harm in
　　4229
ethosuximide
　in epilepsy 3922
　overdose/poisoning 1062
ethyl alcohol, *see* alcohol

ethyldichlorarsine 1117
ethylene diamine 3738
ethylenediaminetetraacetic acid (EDTA),
　　radiolabelled ([⁵¹Cr]EDTA),
　　clearance **3105–6**
ethylene glycol
　lethal dose 1082
　mechanisms of toxicity and metabolites
　　1082
　nephrotoxicity **3267**
　poisoning **1081–2**, *1082*
N-ethyl maleimide (NEM)-sensitive
　　factor (NSF) 75, 79, 80
NIF-1 and NIF-2 79
etidronate 1638, 3229
etodolac, poisoning 1057
etomidate, side-effects 1718
etoposide
　in myelodysplastic syndromes
　　3430–1
　uses and resistance mechanisms 259
etretinate, in ichthyosis 3719
Eubacterium
　phylogenetic groups by rRNA
　　sequencing 273–4, *274*
　rare species 555
Eubacterium lentum 2242
euglobulin lysis time *3379*
eumycetoma 802
euphoria
　drug-induced 4241, 4242
　in multiple sclerosis 4238
Europe
　indications for snake antivenom 1136,
　　1137
　obesity prevalence *1307*
　venomous snakes 1128
European adder 1128
European bat lyssavirus 395, *396*
European Carotid Surgery Trial (ECST)
　　24–5
European Collaborative Study, ischaemic
　　heart disease intervention 2317–18
European Cooperative Study Group
　　(ECSG) trial 2342
European erythema migrans 689
European Resuscitation Council 2284
European Seronegative Spondarthritis
　　Group 2973, *2974*
European Union
　compensatable occupational diseases
　　1162
　health and safety directives 1174
　occupational health and safety
　　directives 1161
　safety regulations 1177
European vipers
　antivenom 1136
　bites and envenoming 1134–5
Eurytrema pancreaticum 982, 983
Eustachian valve, in tricuspid atresia
　　2412
euthanasia 13, 38–9, 4359, **4360**
Evans' syndrome 3543, 3631
evoked potentials **3831–6**
　applications/use 3831
　auditory, *see* auditory evoked
　　potentials
　brain-stem, *see* brain-stem auditory
　　evoked potentials (BAEP)
　recording technique 3831, 3833, 3836
　somatosensory, *see* somatosensory
　　evoked potentials (SEP)
　visual, *see* visual evoked potentials
　　(VEP)
Ewingella americana 555
Ewing's tumour
　epidemiology 207
　management 248
exanthem 383, *383*, 384
exanthema, polymorphous, in Kawasaki
　　disease 384
excurrent duct, obstruction 1685
exercise
　abnormalities induced by **4326–7**
　in adenylate deaminase deficiency 1384
　aerobic 4324
　after acute sports-related injuries 4322

after coronary angioplasty 2352
after heart-lung transplantation 2937–8
after lung transplantation **2938**
amenorrhoea and 1671, 1718
angina management 2326
in anorexia nervosa 4213
asthma induced by 2731
ATP generation/utilization 4165
breathlessness 2494, 2672
in cirrhosis 2090
coronary blood flow increase 2158
in diabetes *1466*, 1469, **1478–9**
in diffuse interstitial fibrosis of lung
    2636
fatigue due to in heart failure 2171,
    2172
fetal growth and 1773
fibrinogen levels reduction 2304
heart and **2161**
heart failure and 2171, 2172, 2236
hypertension management 2538
hypoglycaemia after alcohol
    consumption 1184, *1184*
ischaemic heart disease risk 2313
leg ulceration management and 3809
limb ischaemia management 2369
lung interstitial fluid 2494
mitral valve physiology 2452
mood changes with 2161
in muscular dystrophies 4148
in obesity treatment 1311–12
in osteoarthritis 2982
in osteoporosis management 3068
oxygen consumption in 2593, 2603
physiological changes 2225–6
potassium balance and 3128
pulmonary arterial pressure 2490
pulmonary circulation in 2490
response in heart failure 2232
in rheumatoid arthritis management
    2963
tolerance, nitrates and hydralazine
    effect 2248
tolerance reduction,
    in hypertrophic cardiomyopathy
        2386
    left ventricular disease after valve
        replacement 2471
    in lung disease 2672
    in mitral stenosis 2452
    in mixed mitral valve disease 2456
    in ruptured chordae tendineae 2458
training, maximal oxygen uptake
    (V$_{O_2}$max) changes 4324
training after coronary artery disease
    2357
ventricular tachycardia due to 2280
vigorous aerobic, ischaemic heart
    disease risk reduced 2313
see also sports medicine
exercise echocardiography 2228
exercise testing **2225–8**
after myocardial infarction 2347
in angina 2326
in chronic obstructive airways disease
    2775
false-positive/-negative 2227, *2227*
in glycogen storage diseases 1341
in heart failure 2235–6
history 2225
in hypertrophic cardiomyopathy 2388
indications and contraindications 2226,
    2226
interpretation 2227
invasive 2228
lung capacity/ventilation **2672**
myocardial perfusion imaging (cold-
    spot scanning) 2209
protocols and equipment 2226, *2226*
radionuclide 2228
risks 2226–7
sensitivity and specificity 2227
terminating reasons 2227–8, *2228*
thallium scintiscanning 2209, 2211,
    2326
treadmill *vs* bicycle ergometer 2226
exocytic pathway **68–72**
branch-points 71

constitutive *vs* regulated secretion 72
early events in lumen of endoplasmic
    reticulum 69–70
fusion event 72
overall organization 71
protein translocation pore 69
quality control 70
retention of resident proteins 71–2
selective retention, argument for 70–1
selective transport, argument against 70
targeting from *trans*Golgi network 71
topogenesis of membrane proteins 69
translocation mechanisms 68–9
transport through Golgi stack 71
yeast 77
exocytosis 68
exomphalos **1974–5**
embryology 1973
exomphalos major 1974
exomphalos minor 1974
exons 57, 146
alternate splicing 1559
shuffling 106
exophthalmos **4196**
in Cushing's syndrome 1644
in sarcoidosis 2826
exotoxin, *Shigella* 554
Expanded Programme on Immunization
    (EPI) 284, 317, *321*
meningococcal vaccines 543
tetanus prevention 630
tuberculosis prevention 663
expectorants, in pregnancy 1745
expedition medicine **322–7**
explorers and hazards **325–6**
medical kits 326
see also travel medicine
experimental models
autoantibodies in disease 163
vasculitis 3011
see also animal models
expert witness 4315
expiration, in heart failure 2232
expiratory flow volume loop, in upper
    airways obstruction 2720
'exploding head syndrome' 4027
exposure treatment 4255
expression vectors 113
vaccinia virus 368, 455
extracellular fluid, antimicrobial drug
    distribution 301, *302*
extracellular matrix
autoantibodies to 163
platelet adhesion 3614
extracerebral vascular disease **2367–8**
management **2373**
see also carotid artery ischaemia
extracorporeal circulations, platelet
    defects due to 3634
extracorporeal lung assist 2859, 2920
extracorporeal membrane oxygenation
    (ECMO) 2505, 2859, 2924
ARDS management 2576
extracorporeal shock-wave lithotripsy,
    see lithotripsy
extradural abscess
aetiology 4081
clinical features 4082
extradural haematoma 4047
traumatic 4045
extrahepatic bile ducts, *see* bile duct(s),
    extrahepatic
extrapyramidal disease/disorder 3883
in Alzheimer's disease 3973–4
antipsychotic drugs side-effect 4252,
    4252
drug-induced **4020–1**, *4021*
in primary autonomic failure 3883
see also movement disorders
extrapyramidal system, in manganese
    poisoning 1110
extrasystoles, *see under* cardiac
    arrhythmias
extrinsic allergic alveolitis 164, 1158,
    2809–17
acute 2809, 2815, *2815*
agents causing **2810–11**, *2810*
bronchoalveolar lavage in 2811

chronic 2809, 2815
clinical features **2809–10**
    intermediate 2810
coeliac disease relation 2813
compensation 2817
differential diagnosis **2815**
epidemiology **2815–16**
histology 2811
historical background 2809
HLA association 2813
investigations **2813–15**
    bronchoalveolar lavage 2814
    chest radiography 2813
    environmental exposure 2814
    immunological 2814–15, *2814*
    inhalation challenge test 2814, *2814*
    open-lung biopsy 2688, 2814
    pulmonary 2813–14
management **2816**
outcome **2817**
    continuing exposure 2817
pathogenesis **2811–13**
    antigens 2811, 2813
    immune mechanisms 2811–13
    subacute-chronic phase 2811–12
smoking relationship 2813
extrinsic allergic encephalomyelitis 165
eye **4179–98**
acid and alkali damage/exposure 1103,
    4197
age-related changes 4336
in Alport's syndrome 3204–5
in amyloidosis 1518
in ankylosing spondylitis 4185
anterior chamber, as privileged site 185
in Behçet's syndrome, *see* Behçet's
    syndrome
in blood disorders 3376, **4194–5**
in bowel disease 4184
in brucellosis 622
chlamydial infections 755, 757, **4191**
    C. psittaci 755
    C. trachomatis, see conjunctivitis;
        trachoma
chromic acid exposure 1107
clinical manifestations of disease
    4179–80
    'crossed asymmetry' 3832
in cysticercosis 966, 968
in diabetes mellitus **1483–6**
    see also diabetic retinopathy
in diagnosis of inherited conditions
    4180–2, *4181*
    pre-malignant 4182
in diphtheria 495
disorders, dysthyroid 3865, 3866
drug toxicity and screening **4196–7**,
    4197
dry 4179
    in rheumatoid arthritis 4185
    in sarcoidosis 4182
    in Sjögren's syndrome 3036
    in SLE 4184
in Fabry disease 1429
in giant-cell arteritis **4183**
in gnathostomiasis 952
in Graves' disease *1611*, 1614, **4195–6**
in haematological disorders 3376,
    4194–5
in haemoglobin SC disease 3517, 4195
herpes virus infection 344
in HIV infection and AIDS **4193–4**
in homocystinuria 3085
in hypertension, *see* hypertensive
    retinopathy
in infectious diseases **4191–4**
    bacterial 4191
    fungal and protozoal 4192
    measles 379–80
    parasitic 4192–3
    viral 344, 4191–2
inflammatory disease, in neurological
    disorders **4184**
in joint disorders **4184–6**
in juvenile chronic arthritis 4185–6
lazy (amblyopic) 4180
in leprosy 4191
in lewisite exposure 1117

in loiasis 918
in lung disease 2651
in Marfan's syndrome 3083
in MEN 2b 4196
in multiple sclerosis 4184
in muscular dystrophy **4148**
nickel irritation 1112
in onchocerciasis 914, 915–16, 917
painful, in rheumatoid arthritis 4185
in parathyroid disorders 4196
in poisonings **4197**
in polyarteritis nodosa 4183–4
pressure, in thyroid disorders 4196
protrusion **4196**
red 4179
    findings in and causes *4180*
in Reiter's syndrome 4185
in relapsing polychondritis 4184
in rheumatic diseases 2945
in rheumatoid arthritis 2961, **4185**
in Rift Valley fever 428
riot control smoke clouds 1119
in sarcoidosis, *see* sarcoidosis
in sickle-cell disease 3517, **4195**
signs in coma 3931
sticky 4185
in syphilis 714, 4191, 4193–4
in systemic inflammatory diseases
    4182–4
in Takayasu's arteritis 4183
tear gas injury 1118
therapy in sulphur mustard (mustard
    gas) exposure 1116
in thyroid disorders **4195–6**
in toxoplasmosis 866
in tuberculosis 4191
in ulcerative colitis 1947
in unconscious patients 2585
vascular occlusion, *see* retinal vascular
    occlusion
in viral infections 4193–4
in Wegener's granulomatosis 3012,
    4183
in Wilson's disease 1420, 1421
see also vision: *entries beginning
    ocular, visual*
eyebrows, loss 3763
eye-frequenting, Lepidoptera **1010–11**
eyelashes, depigmentation 4184
eyelid
benign myokymia of 4141
lid lag 4196
oedema, in SLE 4184
in thyroid disease 4196
eye movements 2583
in cerebellar disease 3860
cold-induced lateral, in poisoning 1046
in coma 3931
developmental anomalies **4114**
doll's head 2583, 2584, 4005
dysconjugate, in poisoning 1046
involuntary, in progressive supranuclear
    palsy 4005
jerking 2583
in Marfan's syndrome 4181
in multiple sclerosis 3993
in Parkinson's disease 4001
in persistent vegetative state 3935
in unconscious patients 2583, 2584

F

fabric conditioners, poisoning 1079
Fabry disease (Anderson-Fabry disease)
    (α-galactosidase A deficiency) *1428*,
    1429–30, 3315, 3986
face mask, positive-pressure ventilation
    2576, 2577
facial appearance, in depressive disorders
    4218
facial erythema (flushing) **3786–7**, 3788
    see also flushing
facial features, in bone disease 3061
facial muscles, twitching 3879
facial myokymia 4142
facial nerve **3878–80**
anatomy 3878

facial nerve (cont.)
  in Bell's palsy **3879**
    see also Bell's palsy
  lesions, in intracranial tumours 4036
  palsy 3878
    in sarcoidosis 2826
    upper motor neurone 3857
    see also Bell's palsy
  paralysis,
    'geniculate' herpes zoster **3879**
    in herpes zoster 349
  tumours 3878
facial pain, atypical **4027**
  temporomandibular **4027**
facial sinuses, aircraft pressure change
  effect 1199
facial weakness 4146
  in multiple sclerosis 3993
facies
  in acromegaly 1592
  adenoidal 2611, 2910
  'elfin' 3095, 4111
  in Hurler disease 1431, 1433
  leonine 671, 1897, 3795
  in rhizomelic chondrodysplasia punctata
    1442
  'tabetic' 4085
  typhoid 563
'facies latrodectismica' 1148
facioscapulohumeral dystrophy 4145
facioscapulohumeral muscular dystrophy
  4147–8
F-actin 2622
factitious disorder **4211**
  dissociative disorder vs 4210, 4211
  psychiatric emergencies associated
    4258
factor I, see fibrinogen
factor II, see prothrombin
factor III, see tissue factor
factor V 3619–20, 3621
  activated (Va) 3623–4
  autoantibodies 3661
  and factor VIII, combined deficiency
    3652, 3653
  inherited deficiency 3622, 3642, **3652**
  paracetamol poisoning prognosis 1053
factor VII **2301–2**, 3620, 3621
  activated 2301
  assays 2301, 2304
  concentrates 3651, 3652
  high levels and ischaemic heart disease
    2301–2, 2309
    atherogenic and thrombogenic
      pathways 2302
    dietary fat relation 2301–2, 2309
  inherited deficiency 3622, 3642, **3652**
  in ischaemic heart disease **2301–2**
  structure and half-life 2301
factor VIII 3619–20, 3621, **3637–8**
  activated (VIIIa) 3623, 3624, 3625
  bypassing agents 3650–1
  concentrates 3695
    complications 3650
    in haemophilia **3648–50**
    in von Willebrand's disease 1765,
      3644–5, 3649
  and factor V, combined deficiency
    3652, 3653
  gene/gene defects 3638, 3639
  inherited deficiency 1765, 3622, 3637,
    3646
    see also haemophilia A
  inhibitors (antibodies) **3650–1**, 3661
  intermediate/high purity preparations
    3695
  paracetamol poisoning prognosis 1053
  plasma 3637, 3639, 3648
  porcine 3650
  in pre-eclampsia 1763
  in pregnancy 1765
  vasopressin actions 3118
  von Willebrand factor binding 3638,
    3640, 3642
factor IX 3620, 3621, **3639**
  autoantibodies 3661
  concentrates 3649, 3651, 3695
  gene/gene defects 3639–40

inactivation 3673
  inherited deficiency 1765, 3622, 3639
    see also haemophilia B
  plasma levels 3639
factor X 3620
  acquired deficiency 3661
  activated (Xa) 3620, 3621
    inactivation 3673
    platelet binding 3619
  inherited deficiency 3622, 3642, **3652**
factor XI 3620
  activation 3618–19, 3621
  autoantibodies 3661
  concentrates 3651, 3652
  inherited deficiency 3622, 3642, **3651**,
    3652
factor XII 3620, 3621, 3626
  activated (XIIa) 3621, 3622
  activation 3618–19, 3621
  autoantibodies 3661
  inherited deficiency 3622, 3651, 3667
factor XIII 3620, 3622
  autoantibodies 3661
  concentrates 3652, 3653
  hereditary deficiency 3628, 3652, **3653**
factor A, in diphtheria toxin 493
factor B 177
  in diphtheria toxin 493
  gene 178
  in nephrotic syndrome 3141
factor D 177
  deficiency 180
factor H 177
faecal fat 4374
  in coeliac disease 1919
  estimation 1905, **1906**
  excretion in Crohn's disease 1940
faecal impaction 4338
  stercoral ulcers 2138
faecal incontinence 1823
  biofeedback in 1960
  chronic 1960
  in elderly 4338
  in Hirschsprung's disease 1979
  in spina bifida 4118
faecalith 1971
  appendicitis due to 2009, 2010
faecal-oral spread 286
  amoebiasis 827
  cryptosporidiosis 875
  food poisoning 286, 554
  giardiasis 878
  typhi (Salmonella typhi) 561
  see also food poisoning
faecal peritonitis 1971
faecal pollution, enteroviruses 389
faecal softeners, in terminal illness
  4354
faeces
  nitrogen determination 1907
  normal values 4374
  occult blood testing 3683
    in colorectal carcinoma 1992–3
  porphyrins in 1390, 1395
  see also stool
Faenia rectivirgula 2809
failure to thrive, psychological causes
  1295
fainting, see syncope; syncope,
  vasovagal
Fallot's tetralogy **2402–7**
  'acyanotic' 2402
  associated cardiac anomalies 2403–4
  defects in 2402
  diagnosis doubtful in 2405
  differential diagnosis 2404–5
  'extreme' 2407
  infective endocarditis in 2439
  investigations 2403
  pregnancy in 1737, 2407
  signs 2402–3
  surgery 2405–7
    complications after 2406–7
  symptoms and presentation 2402
  'total correction' 2403, 2404
  treatment 2403
  variants surviving to adult life 2404

falls
  causes 4339, 4340
  elderly and **4338–9**
    rehabilitation 4339
'false hookworm' 932
famciclovir, in varicella-zoster virus
  infections 350
familial, use of term 100
familial adenomatous polyposis (FAP)
  1987, **1989–90**
  colorectal carcinoma in 204, 1990
  duodenal polyps 1986
  genes 66, 1990
  retinal pigmentation 4182
  screening 1990
familial amyloid polyneuropathy 1514,
  1516, **1517**, 4102
  with predominant cranial neuropathy
    1514, 1517
  treatment 1524
familial clustering of cancers 65, 220
familial dysautonomia 4104
familial hypercholesterolaemia, see
  hypercholesterolaemia, familial
familial Mediterranean fever, see
  recurrent polyserositis
familial myoclonic epilepsy 4014–15
familial osteoma cutis **3094**
family
  care in terminal illness **4357**
  effect of patient's illness on 4
  global destruction **36–7**
  medicine, see primary health care
  meningococcal infection prophylaxis
    544
  screening, see screening, of relatives
  single-parent 36
  support in terminal illness **4358**
  therapy in anorexia nervosa 4215
  see also relatives
family studies 102
  see also pedigree analysis
famine 1233
  pregnancy outcome and 1772–3
  see also starvation
famotidine
  in gastrointestinal bleeding 1828
  overdose/poisoning 1070
Fanconi anaemia 3441, **3446–7**
  leukaemia risk 215, 3410, 3446
Fanconi syndrome **1354–5**, 3074, **3332**,
  3340
  cadmium intoxication causing 3096
  causes 3074
  classification 3332
  dominantly inherited 1355
  management 3074, 3332
  toxin-induced 3259, 3261
  vitamin D deficiency and 1637
Fansidar
  in malaria 852–3, 854, 861
  overdose 1073
  in toxoplasmosis 869
Farber's disease (ceramidase deficiency)
  1426–7, 1428
farcy, glanders vs 593, 594
farmer's lung 1158, 2816, 2817
  acute 2815
  open-lung biopsy 2688
  see also extrinsic allergic alveolitis
farnesyl transferase, inhibitors 226
Farr assays 3021
Fas antigen 3024
fascia adherens 2143
fascicles 4091
fasciculation 3840, 4092, 4141
  coarse 4141
fasciitis, eosinophilic 3039, 3791
Fasciola gigantica 982, 983
Fasciola hepatica 982, 983, 986, 2051
Fasciola lanceolata (dendritica) 987
fascioliasis 982, **986–7**
fasciolopsiasis **993**
Fasciolopsis buski 993, 996
fasciotomy, in electrical injury 1213
fasting
  energy supply and utilization 1273

gastrointestinal motor activity 1954
hypoglycaemia 1505, **1506–11**
metabolic effects 1456, 1457, 1505
tests, in insulinoma 1507–8
see also starvation
fat
  absorption 1901, 1903, 1913
    diseases impairing 1906
    impairment in tropical sprue 1934
    normal value 4374
  brown 1182
  consumption, cancer association 218–19
    breast cancer 218–19
    colorectal cancer 203, 219
  dietary 1408, 1412
    coronary heart disease 1326, 1327
    diabetes mellitus 1327, 1467, 1469
    factor VII levels and 2301–2, 2309
    pancreatic carcinoma risk 2040
    quantity/nature, ischaemic heart
      disease risk 2310–11
    unabsorbed and faecal fat
      determination 1906
    see also diet, low-fat
  dietary reference values 1270, 1271,
    1330, 1330
  digestion 1903, 1913
  increments in pregnancy 1770, 1771
  malabsorption,
    bacterial overgrowth pathogenesis
      1913
    in biliary obstruction 2046
    in coeliac disease 1919
    investigations 1905–6
    in isosporiasis 883
    see also steatorrhoea
  metabolism **1276–7**
    in prolonged infections 294
    in parenteral nutrition 2588
  requirements 1330
  saturated, see fatty acids, saturated
  subcutaneous, necrosis 2033
  see also fatty acids
fat, body
  distribution, measurement 1304–5
  measurement methods 1303–4
    costs/difficulty and accuracy 1303
fatiguability 4141
  in polymyositis and dermatomyositis
    4157
  in SLE 3019
fatigue **2171–3**
  abnormal 1036
  cardiac **2171–3**
    pathophysiology 2171–2, 2233
    treatment 2173
  causes 1035, 1036, 2172
  chronic, see chronic fatigue syndrome
  definition 1035–6, 2171
  epidemiology 1036
  in heart failure 2171, 2233
  in hepatocellular failure 2105
  local and general types 2171
  in multiple sclerosis 3996
  in myasthenia gravis 4161
  physical and mental 1036
  respiratory muscle 2164
  in SLE 3022
  speculative diagnoses 1036
  symptoms and duration 1036
fatty acid-binding proteins (Z protein)
  1903, 2055
fatty acids 1399
  ß-oxidation, see ß-oxidation
  catabolism 1438–9
  energy supply 1271
  essential, deficiency, parenteral nutrition
    complication 1320–1
  free, see fatty acids, non-esterified
  long-chain,
    accumulation in
      adrenomyeloneuropathy 84
    metabolism, in heart 2146
  metabolism, endurance sports training
    and 4325
  monounsaturated 1412, 2310
    dietary recommendations 1330

ischaemic heart disease risk 2310–11
  trans 2311
non-esterified (free) 1276, 1400, 1457,
  1505, 4165, 4167
  after injury/surgery 1549
  elimination 1534
  glucose uptake and 1457
  in nephrotic syndrome 3142
  in pregnancy 1753
polyunsaturated, *see* polyunsaturated
  fatty acids
saturated 1412, *2310*
  coronary heart disease 1326, 1327,
    2310
  deposition 3997
  short-chain, in small intestine and colon
    1913
  trans 1330, 2311
  types and sources *2310*
  uptake and transport 1903
  very long chain (VLCFA),
    in adrenoleukodystrophy 1440, 1653
    breakdown 1438, 1439
    in Zellweger syndrome *1440*, 1443
fatty liver, *see* liver, fatty changes
fatty streaks 1405, 2290, 2318, 2362
favism 1159, **3539–40**, 3541
favus 798
Fc receptors 145, 153, 3559
  macrophage 89
fear
  of cancer 252
  of dying 4357
  in dying patients 4233
  of isolation, in dying patients 4233
  of rejection, skin disease 3709,
    3709–10, 3804
febrile convulsions 3909
febrile pneumonitis syndrome 1031–3,
  1032
Federation Internationale Sporte
  Automobile (FISA) 2359
feedback control, cell multiplication
  control 191
feeding, in anorexia nervosa management
  4215
fees, user 53
feet, *see* foot
FEIBA 3651
feline keratoconjunctivitis (FKC) agent
  755
fellatio 3350
Felty syndrome **2962**
  haematological features 3558, 3681
  HLA-DR4 and 2955
  liver in 2135
  platelet count 2960
female
  drug-induced endocrine disorders 1718
  mortality rates 40–1, *42*
  pseudohermaphroditism **1690–1**, 1694
  reproductive disorders **1669–78**
  sexual problems in endocrine disorders
    4244
  see also women
feminization, in hepatocellular failure
  2105
femoral neck fractures 3065
femoral nerve **4097**
  lesions/injuries 4097
femoral neuropathy, diabetic 1487
femoral stretch test 3906
femoral veins, use in injecting drug
  abuse 4282
femoropopliteal grafts 2370
femoropopliteal reconstruction 2363
femorotibial grafts 2370
femur, in fibrous dysplasia 3091
fenamic (anthranilic) acid derivatives,
  poisoning 1056–7
fenbufen, poisoning 1056
Feneley procedure 3900
D-fenfluramine, in obesity treatment 1312
fenoprofen, poisoning 1056
fentiazac, poisoning 1056
feprazone, poisoning 1057
Ferguson reflex 1603

Fernandez reaction 668
ferritin 3471, **3472**
  serum *3379*, 3473
    in alcoholic liver disease 2082
    in iron deficiency *3474*, 3475
    in pregnancy 1758
ferrochelatase (haem synthase) *1391*,
  1395, 1396
ferrokinetic studies 3381, 3472, 3594–5
  in iron-deficiency anaemia 3476
  in primary myelosclerosis 3436
ferrous sulphate, contact dermatitis due
  to 3738
ferruginous bodies 2844
fetal alcohol syndrome 1799, **4112**, **4278**
fetal hydantoin syndrome 1768
fetopathy, in toxoplasmosis 867
α-fetoprotein, *see* alpha-fetoprotein
fetus
  blood sampling 1764, 1765
    ultrasound-guided 136
  drug abuse complications 4298
  drugs affecting, *see* teratogenic drugs
  enterovirus infections 388
  folate deficiency 1759–60
  gonadotrophin secretion 1580
  growth,
    assessment in maternal diabetes 1756
    maternal anaemia and 3469
    maternal asthma and 1745
    maternal nutrition and 1773
    parasitic infestations and 1803
    retardation **1697**
  haemolytic disease (HDN) **3544–5**
  hypothyroidism, drug-induced 1749
  immune function 1784
  iron deficiency 1759
  loss, in SLE 3022
  macrosomia 1753, 1756
  mumps in 374
  nutrition, diabetes in adult life and
    1450, 1455
  radiation damage 1220
  retained dead *1762*
  sexual differentiation 1689–90
  therapy,
    in alloimmune thrombocytopenia 1765
    in congenital adrenal hyperplasia 1667
    urinary-tract obstruction 3243
  thrombocytopenia 1764–5
  thyroid hormone production 1749
  transplantation of cells from 14
  ultrasound 135
  vesicoureteric reflux 3217
  virilization **1690–1**
  well-being and maturity, in maternal
    diabetes 1757
fever **293–4**
  in α₁-antitrypsin deficiency 1547
  in acute pancreatitis 2030
  after cardiac transplantation 2257
  causes, in returning travellers *326*
  in chronic lymphocytic leukaemia 3420
  C-reactive protein and 1533
  definition 1015
  in drug abusers 4294, 4295
  drug-induced 1181–2
  folate deficiency and 3468
  in hepatocellular failure 2105
  history-taking in infections 265, 266
  in Hodgkin's disease 3570, 3571
  hypothalamic response 1576
  in infectious disease 266, **293–4**
  in infective endocarditis 2440
  management in HIV-infected patients
    472
  new pulmonary infiltrates with 1031–3,
    1032
  pathophysiology 276, 293
  patterns 266
    cytokine production 276
    Pel-Ebstein 241, 3570
  in pernicious anaemia 3490
  prolonged 265–6
  prosthetic heart valves 2444
  in renal transplant recipients 3319
  in septicaemia 1022

systemic changes associated 294
in tumours 241
in typhoid 562
use of term 265, 266
fever blisters 343
fever of unknown origin (FUO)
  1015–19, 1030–1
  approach to investigation 1018, 1030–1
  causes 1016, *1016*, *1017*, *1031*
    rare *1018*
  in children and elderly 1015–16
  classical **1015**, *1016*, *1017*, 1019
  definition and terminology 1015
  in HIV infection and AIDS 1015–16,
    1016, **1018**, 1019
  Kawasaki disease 3047
  microscopic polyangiitis *vs* 3014
  neutropenic *1016*, **1017–18**, 1030–1
  in non-neutropenic patients 1031, *1031*
  nosocomial **1016**, *1016*, 1017, 1019
  persisting 1031
  prognosis 1019
  symptoms and signs 1015, 1030
  treatment **1019**, 1031
  types *1016*
fibrate drugs (fibric acid derivatives)
  1414, *3143*
  in renal failure 3275
fibre, *see* dietary fibre; non-starch
  polysaccharides
fibreglass, dermatitis due to 3735
fibreoptic bronchoscopy, *see*
  bronchoscopy, fibreoptic
fibrillar haemagglutinin 272
fibrillation 3840, 3856, 4141
  cartilage 2981
fibrillin 3083
  gene mutation in Marfan syndrome
    3083
fibrin 3614, 3622
  clot 3622
  degradation **3624**
  deposition, fibrinogen effect 2303
  thrombin inhibition 3623
  in thrombus generation 3663
fibrin/fibrinogen degradation products
  2498, 3624, *3654*
  in DIC 3657, 3658
  in haemolytic uraemic syndrome 3200
  in hyperfibrinolytic bleeding 3659
  in pre-eclampsia 1729, 1763
fibrinogen 177, **2302–3**, 3616, 3619,
  3620, **3622**
  assays 2304
  cofactor 179
  effect on blood viscosity 2302–3
  gene clustering 178
  lowering agents 2304
  plasma *3379*, *3654*
    in afibrinogenaemia 3646
    in DIC 3658
    in nephrotic syndrome 3142
    thrombosis and 2302, 3663
  in platelet activation 3614, *3615*, 3616,
    3617
  raised levels,
    in atherogenesis 2303
    factors causing 2303
    in ischaemic heart disease **2302–3**,
      2309
    management and prevention 2304–5
    smoking effect 2303, 2304, 2309
    thrombosis predisposition 2302, 3663
  titre *3379*
  variability within persons 2304
fibrinogen Dusart 2303
fibrinoid degeneration 3710
fibrinoid necrosis (necrotizing arteriolitis)
  3249, 3290
  intestinal ischaemia in 1995
  in malignant hypertension 2534
  rheumatoid nodules 2960
fibrinolysis **3624–6**
  activators 3774
  in cardiac surgery 3660
  coagulation imbalance, permeability
    pulmonary oedema 2497, 2498

contact activation-mediated 3626
control 3663
DIC and 3657
endothelial cell role 2299
excessive (hyperfibrinolysis) **3659**
  in haemolytic uraemic syndrome 3200
  in pre-eclampsia 1763
  in pregnancy 1762
  primary **3659**
  protein C and 3624
  reduced in ischaemic heart disease
    2303
fibrinolytic system, ARDS pathogenesis
  2855
fibrinolytic therapy, *see* thrombolytic
  therapy
Fibrinolytic Therapy Trial (FTT) 2337,
  2340, 2341, 2342, 2343
fibrinopeptide A 2304, 2305
fibrinous vasculosis, in pulmonary
  hypertension 2507–8
fibrin-stabilizing factor, *see* factor XIII
fibroblast growth factor (FGF) 2293
  in atherosclerotic plaque development
    2293, 2299
  basic (bFGF) 2293
  int-2 gene encoding 223
  receptors 1561, 2293
  restenosis after angioplasty 2295
fibroblasts 3706
  asthma pathophysiology 2727, 2728
  mouse, genomic DNA transfer 61
  in scarring 2626–7
fibroblast stimulating factor 2120
fibrocystic disease, of pancreas, *see*
  cystic fibrosis
fibrodysplasia ossificans progressiva, *see*
  myositis ossificans progressiva
fibrogenesis, in cryptogenic fibrosing
  alveolitis 2789
fibrogenesis imperfecta ossium **3096**
  Paget's disease *vs* 3077
fibromas, ossifying, jaw 1863
fibromuscular dysplasia
  renal artery stenosis in 2373
  renovascular hypertension due to
    2548–9
fibronectin 3616
  in heart 2145
  plasma 3614
  platelet binding 3614, 3615
fibropolycystic disease **2015–16**
fibrosarcoma, retroperitoneal,
  hypoglycaemia due to 1509
fibrosing alveolitis, *see* cryptogenic
  fibrosing alveolitis
fibrosing syndromes **3244–6**
fibrosis
  endocardial 2390, 2399
  endomyocardial, *see* endomyocardial
    fibrosis (EMF)
  intimal 2378
  mediastinal 3245, **3246**
  retroperitoneal, *see* retroperitoneal
    fibrosis
  skin 3788
  see also liver, fibrosis; pulmonary
    fibrosis
fibrositis 2947
fibrous dysplasia **3091–2**
  biochemical features *3062*
  monostotic 3091
  polyostotic (McCune-Albright
    syndrome) 124, 1569, 1642–3, 1702,
    1715, 3091
fibrous erionite 2846
Fick method
  direct 2221–2
  indirect 2222
Field's technique 849
'field' theory of carcinogenesis 191–2
fifth disease (erythema infectiosum) 447
fight or flight response 2233, 3882
filarial abscess 922
filarial fever 922
filarial infections **911–12**
  disease *vs* 911

filarial infections (*cont.*)
general principles 919–20
parasites and lifecycle 911, 919–20
filarial lymphadenitis 922
filariasis **911–19**
asymptomatic amicrofilaraemia
(endemic normals) 921–2
bancroftian 922, 923
brugian 920, 922, 923
general principles **911–12**
glomerulonephritis 3177
lymphatic **919–24**
acute and chronic types 922
asymptomatic microfilaraemia 922
clinical features 921–3
clinicoepidemiological patterns 920–1,
921
diagnosis 923
epidemiology/transmission 920
treatment 923–4
occult 923
perstans 919
pulmonary hypertension in 2509
Filoviruses **439–43**
see also Ebola virus; Marburg virus
filtration fraction 3108
fimbriae 272
fimbrin 81
finances, artificial nutrition at home 1324
financing, health care in developing
countries 52, 53
fine-needle aspiration biopsy
bone marrow, *see* bone marrow,
aspiration biopsy
lung 2681, 2683, **2686**
pneumonia 2697
lymph nodes 3563, 3569
mediastinum 2682
thyroid gland 1608, 1619
finger
clubbing, *see* clubbing of fingers
'dropped' 2957
in rheumatoid arthritis 2957
sausage-shaped 3029
'trigger' 2957
vibration effect 1226
volar subluxation 2957
finger agnosia 3851
finger plethysmography 1226
fingerprint body myopathy **4150–1**
Finkelstein's test 2947
fire ants, stings 1144
fire service, fitness requirements 2360
fire smoke, *see* smoke inhalation
first aid
in mass runs 4327
snake bites 1135–6
spider bites 1148
in sulphur mustard (mustard gas)
exposure 1116
first-aid kit, for travel 322
fish
clonorchiasis transmission 985
fatty 2311, 2318
injuries from 1124
opisthorchiasis transmission 981–2
poisoning from 1142, 2005–6
carp's gallbladder ingestion 1143
ciguatera 1142
salted, *see* salted fish
venomous **1141**
venom composition 1141
fish-eye disease 1414
FISH (fluorescent *in situ* hybridization)
119
fish oils
blood pressure reduction 2530
in chronic renal failure 3304
in hyperlipoproteinaemia 1414
hypertension management 2538
hypertension prevention 2530
in pre-eclampsia prevention 1730
fistulae
arteriovenous, *see* arteriovenous fistulae
bronchocutaneous 2924
bronchopleural 2705, 2924
bronchopulmonary 957
colonic 1972
colovesical 1972

coronary 2430, 2467
in Crohn's disease 1938–9, 1942–3
enteric, *see* enteric fistulae
oesophagopulmonary 1874
pulmonary arteriovenous 2862
spinal arteriovenous 3828
tracheo-oesophageal, *see* tracheo-
oesophageal fistula
fitness requirements
aircraft crews/pilots, *see* aircrew/pilots
drivers, *see* driving
for employment 2357, 2358
seafarers 2360
fits, *see* seizures
FitzHugh-Curtis syndrome, *see* Curtis
Fitz-Hugh syndrome
5q- syndrome 3428, 3524
FK506 3319
in liver transplantation 2114
nephrotoxicity 3265–6
flapping tremor 2088, 3283
in hepatic disorders 4240
in hepatic encephalopathy 2101
'flash-back' 4205, 4241
flash response, visual evoked potentials
(VEP) 3831
Flavimonas oryzihabitans 555
flaviviruses **412–23**, 458
miscellaneous infections 418
structure and characteristics 413
syndromes associated 412
transmission 412
see also dengue viruses
Flavobacterium, rare species 555–6
fleas **1004–5**
cat scratch disease and 745
typhus fever transmission 736
flecainide *2264*
in atrial fibrillation 2272
overdose/poisoning 1064
fleroxacin, in urinary-tract infections *3211*
flies 1011
larvae and myiasis due to **1000–1**
'flight of ideas' 4220
floaters 4179
in Behçet's syndrome 4183
floctafenine, poisoning 1057
floppy infant syndrome **4150–1**
benign congenital/infantile hypotonia
4150
floxuridine 2129
flucloxacillin, in renal failure *3272*
fluconazole 811, 812
in coccidioidomycosis 813
in renal failure *3272*
flucytosine 811, 812
in cryptococcosis 810
disadvantage 812
in disseminated candidiasis 807
indications 812
in renal failure *3272*
resistance to 811
fludarabine 3422, 3423
fludrocortisone 1655–6, 1665
excessive doses 1661–2
hyperkalaemia and 3134
in postural hypotension in primary
autonomic failure 3886
in pregnancy 1751
in renal tubular acidosis 3341
flufenamic acid, poisoning 1056–7
fluid
abnormalities, parenteral nutrition
complications 1319
absorption, colon function 1824
balance 1824, **3116–26**
in adult respiratory distress syndrome
2860
after injury/surgery 1549
charts 3279–80, 3285–6
in chronic renal failure 3296–7
clinical evaluation *3283*
disorders **3120–6**
hormonal control 1563, 1564, 1601
maintenance of optimal **3282–3**
physiology 3116–18
post-renal transplant 3318
in pregnancy 1748, 3117, 3118

pulmonary endothelium 2492–4
in pulmonary oedema 2494, 2495–6
thirst and 1601, 3116, **3117**
vasopressin and 1563, 1601, 3116,
3117–18
challenge test 3283
clearance, in clearance phase of
inflammation 2625
depletion, *see* dehydration;
hypovolaemia
deprivation tests 1601, *1602*, 3109, **3121**
dialysis 3308
disturbances in malaria, management
854–5
excretion 1824
extracellular 3116
intake,
acute hepatocellular failure
management 2108
in acute renal failure 3285, *3286*
assessment 3279–80
in cystinuria 1356, 3333
in hypernatraemia 3126
in nephrotic syndrome 3140
polyuria and 3147
in primary hyperoxaluria 1446
in syndrome of inappropriate
antidiuresis 1602, 3125
thirst and 1601, 3116, **3117**
urinary stone disease 3256
in urinary-tract infection 3208
see also adipsia; hypodipsia;
polydipsia
intracellular 3116
intravenous infusion,
in acute renal failure **3285–6**
cholera management 579
in crush injury 3289
in diabetic ketoacidosis 1500–1
in electrical injury 1212–13
in haemolytic uraemic syndrome
3201
in hypercalcaemia 1638, 3228
in hypernatraemia 3126
in hyperosmolar hyperglycaemic non-
ketotic coma 1502
in hyponatraemia 3123
infected fluids 291
in renal transplant recipients 3318
in septicaemia treatment 1024
loss in erythroderma 3747
movements, in lung 2492–4
overload,
dialysed patients 3312
excessive postoperative administration
3123
pulmonary oedema 2496, 2504
transfusion-induced 3692
see also hypervolaemia; pulmonary
oedema, hydrostatic; water,
intoxication
peritoneal dialysis 3310
replacement,
in acute circulatory derangements
2565
in acute pancreatitis 2029, 2032
in hypovolaemia after marathons
4328
in oligaemia 2565
in paracetamol poisoning 1053
in pneumococcal infection 521
in salicylate poisoning 1056
in short gut syndrome 1926
in terminal illness **4359–60**
in venesection 2400
requirements, artificial nutritional
support 1317–18
restriction 1317
in heart failure 2238
retention,
in chronic renal failure 3297
in cirrhosis 2087
in heart failure 2234
idiopathic, of women **3126–7**
management in mitral stenosis
2455
in pericardial constriction 2481
secretion, in cholera 577, 2002

flukes
blood, *see* schistosomiasis
echinostome 993
intestinal **992–9**, 993, *994–5*
liver, *see* liver fluke diseases
lung, *see* paragonimiasis
see also trematodes
flumazenil 1048, 1830
in benzodiazepines overdose 1060
hepatic encephalopathy management
2108
fluorescein angiography 4180
in hypertensive retinopathy 4188
fluorescein dye 4180
fluorescence, syphilis diagnosis 715, *715*,
2483, 4085
fluorescent antibody testing, respiratory
tract infections 2676
fluorescent *in situ* hybridization (FISH)
119, 3390, 3398
fluorescent treponemal antibody-
absorbed (FTA-Abs) test 1791
fluoridation, water 1847
fluorinated quinolones, in typhoid
564
5-fluorocytosine, *see* flucytosine
9α-fluoroprednisolone 1661–2
fluoroquinolones, mechanism of action
296
fluoroscopy, chest radiography with
2653 fluorosis
bone disease **3095**
endemic 3095
5-fluorouracil
in colorectal carcinoma 1993
in hepatic metastases 2119
in sun damage 3729
fluoxetine
in alcoholic hepatitis 2085
drug interactions 4249
in obesity treatment 1312
overdose 1059–60
flurbiprofen, poisoning 1056
flushing **3786–7**, 3788
in carcinoid syndrome 1897, 3787
neurogenic 3787
flutamide, side-effects 1689
fluvoxamine, overdose 1059–60
FMR1 gene 126
c-*fms* proto-oncogene 3383, 3429
foam cells 1403, 1405, 2290, 2318
foamy macrophage, *see* macrophage,
foam cells
focal lobar atrophy, *see* Pick's disease
focal nodular hyperplasia, liver 2119
foetor hepaticus 2103, 2105
foetor oris 495
Fogarty balloon catheter 2371
fogo selvagem **3782**
foil blanket 4328
folate *3485*, **3486–8**
absorption 3487–8
activated 1-carbon units and 1368
in bacterial overgrowth 1913
biochemistry 3486–7
deficiency 3488, **3492–4**
in alcoholics 3493, 3685
causes *3490*
in chronic renal failure 3682
clinical features 3492
in coeliac disease 1918
dementia due to 3971
diagnosis 3495
diagnosis of cause 3496
drug-induced 3493–4
fetal effects 1759–60
in liver disease 3494, 3684
mental symptoms 4241
nutritional 3467, 3492
in pregnancy **1759–60**, 3467, 3468–9,
3493
in primary myelosclerosis 3437
in skin disease 3685
in thalassaemia 3513
tissue effects 3491
treatment 3496–7
in tropical countries 3467–8
see also megaloblastic anaemia

erythropoiesis and 3454
excess urinary loss 3493
inborn errors of metabolism 3497
increased utilization 3492–3
malabsorption 3467, **3492**
  congenital specific 3492
nutrition 3487
red cell *3379*, 3495
reference nutrient intake (RNI) 1268, *1269*
serum *3379*, 3495
transport 3488
see also folic acid
folate-synthesis inhibitors 850
folic acid 3486, 3496
absorption 3487
in cystathionine synthase deficiency 1367
in dialysed patients 3493
in epileptic women 1768
in hereditary spherocytosis 3530
overdose 1071
periconceptual 1760, 1773, 3491
in pregnancy 1759, 3491, 3493, 3496
in premature infants 3493
spina bifida prevention 4117
synthesis by *Plasmodium* species 837
in thalassaemia 1761
in tropical sprue 1936
see also folate
folinic acid 3496
in methanol poisoning 1080
follicle mites 1009
follicle stimulating hormone (FSH) 1555, 1556, **1579–81**
actions 1581
adenoma secreting 1595–6
in anorexia nervosa 4213
ß-subunit 1579
gene mutations *1567*, 1571
in males 1679, 1680
in ovulation induction 1678
at puberty 1563, 1701
pulsatile secretion 1565
receptor 1555, 1556, *1560*
regulation of secretion 1579–80
secretion 1565, 1580
serum 1584
  combined anterior pituitary test 1585
  in male infertility 1686
  in ovarian failure 1673
follicular dendritic cells 153, 3561
HIV on 466
follistatin 1554, 1580
follitrophin, *see* follicle stimulating hormone
Fonsecaea species 813
Fontan operation 2214, 2215, 2413
food(s)
absorption 3729
  drugs inhibiting 1312
advice on, in obesity treatment 1311
antigens, selective IgA deficiency 1840
aversion *1843*
  in hereditary fructose intolerance 1347–8
blood glucose effects 1465, 1466–7, *1468*
colouring/preservative-free 3729, *3730*
contamination, cancer association 217
  oesophageal cancer 202
-dependent Cushing's syndrome 1640, 1643
deprivation, *see* fasting; starvation
dermatitis due to 3737
drug absorption affected by 1242
glycaemic index 1466–7
groups and nutrients of *1331*
hypoallergic 3729
ingestion, in primary autonomic failure 3883
intake,
  measurement **1268**
  regulation 1273
iron fortification 3470, 3481
labelling 1268
MAOIs interactions 4249, 4250
migraine precipitant 4025

nutritional guidelines *1332*
oxalate-containing 1444
questionnaires 1268
refining/processing 1268
vasculitis due to 3776
vitamin K-containing 3655
see also diet; nutrition
food additives 3729
behavioural problems 1844
gastric cancer risk reduction 203
food allergy 162, **1842–5**, *1843*, 3729
aetiology and prevalence 1842
alternative tests 1844–5
asthma and 2734, 3729
atopic eczema and 1843, 3729, 3739, 3742
behavioural problems associated 1844
clinical features 1842–3
controversial issues 1844
definition 1842
diagnosis 1844–5
elimination diets and challenge tests 1844, 3742
evidence 3729
in irritable bowel syndrome 1966
remote symptoms 1843
skin disorders and 3729
syndromes 1843
treatment 1845
ulcerative colitis aetiology 1944
food-borne infections
anisakiasis 938
streptococci group A 501
trichinosis 940, 941
see also food poisoning
food handlers
Salmonella infections 552
Shigella infection prevention 555
food intolerance 162, **1842–5**, *1843*, 3729
aetiology 1842
in irritable bowel syndrome 1966
syndromes 1843–4
see also food allergy
food plants, toxicity 1158–9
food poisoning **550–60**, 2002
Bacillus cereus 559–60, 2002
botulism, *see* botulism
Campylobacter 557–9
causes/symptoms and mechanism *560*, 1824, 2002
Clostridium perfringens 285, **637**, 2002
diarrhoea in 1824, 2002, 2003
enterobacteria **550–7**
Escherichia coli 556, 2002
faecal-oral spread 286, 554
listeriosis 721
miscellaneous bacterial causes **557–60**
outbreaks 286
poisonous plants 1151
Salmonella 551, 552, 2003
seafood 1141–2
Shigella 554
staphylococcal 524
Staphylococcus aureus 524, 529
Vibrio parahaemolyticus 559
viruses in 393
see also food-borne infections
foot
in acromegaly 1592
in bone disease 3061
dermatitis 3735
diabetic, *see* diabetic foot disease
flat 2997
frictional dermatitis 3737
injuries and fractures **2996–7**
in Kawasaki disease 3047
in rheumatoid arthritis 2958
sweating 3737
foot drop 3841, 4097
footwear
in osteoarthritis 2982
in rheumatoid arthritis 2963
foramen ovale
in Ebstein's anomaly 2413, 2414
patent **2426**
  after Fallot's tetralogy repair 2406

divers 1210
in tricuspid atresia 2412
Forbes-Cori's disease (type III glycogen storage disease) 1342, *1343*, 1384, 4166
forced diuresis
acid, in poison elimination 1051
alkaline,
  in barbiturate poisoning 1060
  in chlorophenoxyacetate herbicides poisoning 1121
  in poison elimination 1050
  in salicylate poisoning 1056
in lithium overdose 1061
pharmacokinetics 1050
in poison elimination 1050
forced expiratory volume in 1 second (FEV$_1$) **2667**
in α$_1$-antitrypsin deficiency 1546
after lung transplantation 2935
in asthma 2731, 2733
  occupational asthma 2744
in chronic obstructive airways disease 2768, 2769, 2774, 2775
in coal-worker's pneumoconiosis 2840
in diffuse interstitial fibrosis 2637
diurnal variation, after lung transplantation 2938
in scoliosis 2872
in upper airways obstruction 2720
forced vital capacity (FVC) 2667
in emphysema 2632–3
forearm, pain and fatigue in 2996
forearm exercise test, in glycogen storage diseases 1341
forefoot, deformity, in rheumatoid arthritis 2958
foregut 1973
foregut diverticulum 1972–3
foreign bodies
airways obstruction **2636**, 2719
lung abscess 2704
pulmonary, in injecting drug abusers 4281, 4282
synovitis 2946
forensic medicine **4309–17**
forensic pathology **4309**
Forestier's disease 2979
formaldehyde 1098
Bacillus anthracis spores 613
metabolism 1098
poisoning **1098–9**
formalin, warts treatment 3798
formic acid 1543
ingestion 1103
foscarnet 479, *479*
fos gene 225
Fourier analysis 2206
Fournier's gangrene 501, 573, 574
fourth-ventricle lesions, diabetic ketoacidosis *vs* 1499
Foville's syndrome 3858
Fowler's solution 204, 3783, 3791
Fox-Fordyce disease 3765
fractional excretion (FE) 3108
fractures **3061**
after electrical injury 1214
age-related 4335
bone density relationship 3065
causes 3065
fatigue, *see* stress fractures
occupational accidents 1176
in osteogenesis imperfecta 3080
in osteoporosis 3064, **3065**, 3066
  sites 3065
in Paget's disease of bone 3075, 3076
management 3078
microfracture ('fissure' fracture) 3076
pathological,
  in chronic renal failure 3324, 3327
  in Cushing's syndrome 1643
  in myelomatosis 3599
postmenopausal 3064, 3065, 3066
  groups 3065, *3066*
in rheumatoid arthritis 2962
stress, *see* stress fractures

in tetanus 628
theoretical fracture threshold 3065
fragile X syndrome 126, **4110–11**
carrier/prenatal testing 126
diagnosis and features 4111
folic acid therapy 3496
incidence and inheritance 63, 115–16, *125*, 4110
mental retardation in 4110
screening 132
unstable trinucleotide repeats 108, *125*, 126, 4110
fragment 1.2 2304, 2305
Framingham study 2532
Francisella philomiragia 602–3
Francisella tularensis 599, *600*, 2121
biochemical properties and structure 603
biogroup novicida strains 602
detection and serology 603–4, *603*
see also tularaemia
Francisella tularensis subsp. *holarctica* 601–2
Francisella tularensis subsp. *tularensis* 599–601
Frank-Starling mechanism 2150, **2155–6**, 2157, 2220, 2230
in exercise 2161
freckle *3754*
free fatty acids, *see* fatty acids, non-esterified
free radicals
adult respiratory distress syndrome 2854, 2860
oxidized LDL formation 2291
see also oxygen free radicals
freezing, tissues 1183
Frei skin test 760
frequency of micturition *3148*, 3206–7
friction rub 2475
in cirrhosis 2088
friction syndromes 4322, **4323–4**
Friedlaender's bacillus 551
Friedreich's ataxia **3984**
central motor conduction time 3838
mental disorders/symptoms in 4238
pyruvate dehydrogenase deficiency and 1351
somatosensory evoked potentials 3834
frogs, poisonous 1140
Froin's syndrome 4061
frontal lobe
atrophy, in Pick's disease 3975, *3975–6*
behavioural defects associated *3846*
'burst' 4045
damage, cognitive/personality change **3854**
tumours 3854
  mental disorders/symptoms in 4237
frontal sinusitis, intracerebral abscess with 4081
frostbite 1183, **1184**, 3724
massive 1184
severe, exposure without 1184
fructokinase 1345
deficiency 1345
fructosamine, serum 1481
fructose
hereditary intolerance (fructosaemia) **1346–8**, 1384, *2019*, 3340, *3536*
liver in 2024
inborn errors of metabolism **1345–8**
intravenous tolerance test 1348
metabolism 1345
seminal 1686
transport 1920
fructose 1,6-diphosphatase 1345, 1458
deficiency **1346**, *1348*
fructosuria, essential (benign) 1345
frusemide
in acute mountain sickness 1191
in acute renal failure 3285, 3286
after head injury 4048
in ascites management 2097
in heart failure 2239
in hypercalcaemia 3228
intravenous urography 3241, 3242
mechanism of action 2239

frusemide (*cont.*)
in nephrotic syndrome 3140
nephrotoxicity 3266
radionuclide renal studies 3114, 3115, 3240, 3241
in syndrome of inappropriate antidiuresis 3125
FSH, *see* follicle stimulating hormone
FTA-ABS-IgM test 715–16, *715*
FTA-ABS test 715, *715*
FTT, *see* Fibrinolytic Therapy Trial (FTT)
fucosidosis *1435*, **1436**
fuel, metabolic
body composition and 1272, *1273*
energy production from 1271–2
supply, utilization and demand 1272–3
in heart **2145–7**
regulation 1273–4, *1274*
types 1272
see also energy
'fugitive' (Calabar) swellings 917, 918
Fukuyama congenital muscular dystrophy 4147
Fuller's earth 2845
pneumoconiosis 2846
fulminant hepatic failure, *see* hepatocellular failure, fulminant
fumarylacetoacetate hydrolyase (FAH) 1362, 1364
fumes, toxic, exposure/inhalation 2847–8
functional bowel disease 1963–4, **1965–9**
abdominal bloating 1967
abdominal pain 1968
definition 1965
diarrhoea 1967–8
history, diagnosis and explanation 1963
management 1968–9
Rome criteria 1965, *1966*
see also constipation; diarrhoea; irritable bowel syndrome
functional history, in rheumatic diseases 2944
functional residual capacity (FRC) **2666–7**
in adult respiratory distress syndrome 2856
in asthma 2635
in chronic bronchiolitis 2634
in chronic obstructive airways disease 2775
in diaphragmatic disorders 2877
in diffuse interstitial fibrosis 2637
in emphysema 2632
measurement method 2666
normal 2666–7
PEEP and CPAP action 2921, 2922
functional tests, normal values *4374*
fundal examination, in hypertension 2536
fundal haemorrhage, in hypertension 2535
fungal contamination of food, oesophageal cancer and 202
fungal infections **797–823**
in acute pancreatitis 2032
after cardiac transplantation 2257
after lung transplantation 2936
in AIDS and HIV infection 479–80
eye in 4194
respiratory tract 2710
treatment 479–80, *480*
arthritis in **3000**
chronic inflammatory diarrhoea due to 2004
clinical features 3713
in Cushing's syndrome 1643–4
in diabetes 1493
endocarditis 808, 809, 2438, 2449
eye in **4192**, 4194
hepatic granulomas in 2121
in injecting drug abusers 4285
liver in 2134
management approach **811–12**
antifungals 811, *811*
see also antifungal agents
meningitis *4070*
myositis in **4156**
nails 3761
occupational dermatosis 1165

peritonitis in 2009
in pregnancy **1793**
in renal transplant recipients 2709, 3320
respiratory tract 2676, 2708
subcutaneous 797, **801–3**
superficial **797–801**, 797
candidiosis **800–1**
dermatophyte **797–9**
management 811
miscellaneous 801
tinea versicolor **799**
systemic (deep) 797, **803–6**
laboratory tests *804*
management 811–12
opportunistic fungi 806–11
rare 806
urinary-tract obstruction 3179
vesico-blistering diseases and 3780
see also individual infections/fungi
fungal septicaemia 1023
fungal toxins, Balkan nephropathy and 3230
fungi 797
biology 797
inflammation due to 290
opportunistic 797, 803, 806–11
sexual transmission 3345
fungi, poisonous 1151, **1155–9**, *1157*
sources of information 1159–60
symptom classification 1155–6
delayed onset of symptoms 1156–8, *1157*
onset within 2 hours 1155–6, *1157*
types and toxins 1155
fungicide, methylmercury as 1111
'fungus ball', in lung 2824
funiculitis
'endemic' 922
filarial 922
furniture workers, nasal sinus and nose cancers 205
furuncles, *see* boils
fusidic acid, *Staphylococcus aureus* infections 525, 530
fusobacterial bacteraemia 574
Fusobacterium 569, 571
rare species *556*
Fusobacterium fusiformis 693, 1852
Fusobacterium necrophorum 574, 575
fusospirochaetosis, *see* Vincent's disease
F wave 3840

G

G6PD, *see* glucose 6-phosphate dehydrogenase
GABA, *see* gamma-aminobutyric acid (GABA)
gabapentin, in epilepsy 3922
G-actin 2622
gadolinium (Gd) 2214
imaging, in multiple sclerosis 3994
Gag protein 489
gait
disorder, cerebellar ataxia *vs* 3860
in Friedreich's ataxia 3984
in Lambert-Eaton myasthenic syndrome (LEMS) 4163
in normal pressure hydrocephalus 3970
in osteomalacia 3071
in polyneuropathies 4092
in rheumatic diseases 2946
in vestibular apparatus damage 3873
galactokinase deficiency 1349
galactorrhoea **1689**
in acromegaly 1592
in H_2-receptor blockade 1887
in hyperprolactinaemia 1589, 1689
galactosaemia (galactose 1-phosphate uridyl transferase deficiency) 130, **1349–50**, *2019*
liver in 2024
galactose 1349
'diabetes' 1349
elimination capacity 2056
inborn errors of metabolism **1349–50**
transport 1920

galactose-specific hepatic asialoglycoprotein receptor (ASGP-R), antibodies 2070, 2072
α-galactosidase, replacement therapy 1430
α-galactosidase A deficiency, *see* Fabry's disease (α-galactosidase A deficiency)
ß-galactosidase, administration 1923
galactosyl ceramide lipidosis (Krabbe's disease) *1428*, **1429**, 3986
galanin 1894
gallamine 4141
tetanus management 629
gallbladder
in AIDS 475
anatomy 2045
cancer 204, 218
cholesterolosis 2050
disease **2045–53**
in pregnancy **1801**
in somatostatinoma 1707
see also cholecystitis; gallstones
empyema 2049
function in pregnancy 1801
gangrene 2049
inflammation, *see* cholecystitis
in opisthorchiasis 982, 984
'strawberry' 2050
gallium-67 isotope scanning
in cryptogenic fibrosing alveolitis 2790
in Hodgkin's disease 3573
in sarcoidosis 2830
gallium-labelled leucocytes 1018
gallstone ileus 2048
gallstones
acute pancreatitis and 2027, 2033
calcified 2047
cholangiocarcinoma aetiology 2118
cholesterol 2047–8
in cystic fibrosis 2749
classification 2047
in common bile duct, *see* choledocholithiasis
diet association 1329
formation 2047
in gallbladder 2046, 2048
gallbladder cancer association 204
in hereditary spherocytosis 3530
impaction 2049
investigations 2046
management 2033
natural history 2048
octreotide therapy and 1594
in paroxysmal nocturnal haemoglobinuria 3451
pigment stones 2047, 2048, 2079
in pregnancy 1801
recurrence 2049
in short gut syndrome 1925
in sickle-cell disease 3515–16
'silent' 2048
treatment 2048–9
chemical dissolution 2048
disruption 2048–9
side-effects/toxicity 2049
ultrasonography 1834, 2046
gamete complementation 128
gamete formation 103
gametogenesis, occupational toxins 1173
gamma-aminobutyric acid (GABA)
in Alzheimer's disease 3973
benzodiazepine function 4253
drugs increasing function of 4253
GABA$_A$ benzodiazepine receptor/chloride ionophore complex 2102
GABA$_A$ receptors 2102
in hepatic encephalopathy 2102
inherited disorders of metabolism 1372
in isoniazid poisoning 1068
neurotransmission (pathway) 3862
increased, in hepatic encephalopathy 2102
in Parkinson's disease 4000
reduction in Huntington's disease 4013, *4013*

gamma-aminobutyric acid (GABA)
transaminase deficiency 1372
gamma-benzene hexachloride (BHC) 1004, 1009, 1123
gammaglobulin
high-dose 3049
in Kawasaki disease 3049
polyvalent 283
raised, in autoimmune hepatitis 2070
see also immunoglobulin(s); intravenous immunoglobulin
gamma-glutamyl transferase 2055–6, *4365*
gamma-hexachlorocyclohexane **1123**
gamma-rays 1217
radiotherapy 255
ganciclovir
in cytomegalovirus infection 363, 479, *479*
in renal impairment 3272
toxicity 363
gangliocytoma, GHRH secretion 1591
ganglioglioma **4033**
ganglioma, VIP-producing 1705
ganglion cells
absent, *see* Hirschsprung's disease
argyrophil, absent 1978
in rabies 401
ganglionectomy
left stellate 2283
stellate 2374
ganglioneuroblastoma
mediastinum 2901
VIP-producing 1705, 1706
ganglioneuroma **4033**
mediastinum 2901
ganglioside, GM$_1$, in spinal cord injury 3898
gangliosidoses *1428*, **1430**, *2019*, **3985**
G$_{M1}$ *1428*, **1430**, 3985
adult 1430
infantile 1430
juvenile 1430
G$_{M2}$ *1428*, **1430**, 3985
adult 1430
infantile, *see* Tay-Sachs disease
juvenile 1430
Sandhoff's disease *1428*, 1430, 3985
G$_{M3}$ 1427, **1430**
gangosa 705
gangrene
diabetic 2372
gas, *see* gas gangrene
in meningococcaemia 4054
in primary thrombocythaemia 3439
synergistic 3778
venous 2523
ganser syndrome 3967
gap junctions in myocytes 2144
proteins 2144
pulmonary endothelial cells 2486
GAP proteins (GTPase-activating proteins) 77
Gardnerella vaginalis 495, 572, 3355
in pregnancy 1785
vaginitis **3355**
Gardner's syndrome 1990, 3792, *3795*
colorectal cancer association 204
retinal pigmentation in 4182
gargoylism 1431
garlic, ischaemic heart disease prevention 2312
Garrod's pads 2947
gas, formation in anaerobic infections 571
gas dilution methods, functional residual capacity (FRC) 2666
gases
highly soluble, exposure 2847
industrial, cardiovascular effects 1171
insoluble, exposure 2847
toxic **2847–8**
gas exchange 2484, 2494, 2628, **2629–30**
in adult respiratory distress syndrome (ARDS) 2640–1, 2856
in alveolar filling syndromes 2639
in asthma 2636

in chronic bronchiolitis 2634–5
in chronic obstructive airways disease 2769
in diffuse interstitial fibrosis 2637–8
diffusion 2629–30
  impaired in ARDS 2856
in emphysema 2633–4
in heart failure 2232
impairments, abnormality types 2670
matched to oxygen needs 2606–8
pulmonary capillary volume 2485
in pulmonary vascular diseases 2641–2
tests **2669–71**
  distribution/mixing of inspired gas 2669
  hypoxaemia/hypercapnia assessment 2669–71
  transfer factor for carbon monoxide 2669, *2670*
see also pulmonary diffusing capacity
gas exchanger
cells **2593–6**
  see also alveolar secretory cells (type II)
design and function **2600–3**, 2628
diffusing capacity 2602, *2602*
tissue organization **2596–600**
tissue and plasma barriers 2601–2
gas gangrene **632–4**
antitoxin in 634
of bowel, *see* necrotizing enterocolitis
liver in 2133
treatment and prevention 633–4
gas liquid chromatography, anaerobic bacteria detection 571
gasoline, *see* petrol (gasoline)
gastrectomy
gastric cancer after 1983
gut peptides after 1895
pancreatic carcinoma association 2040
partial,
  B$_{12}$ deficiency 3491
  in gastric ulcers 1890
  osteomalacia after 1636
  sequelae 1890
total, B$_{12}$ deficiency 3491
gastric acid
duodenal ulcer aetiology 1877
gastric ulcer aetiology 1879
host defence mechanism 2001
hypersecretion,
  in short gut syndrome 1925
  Zollinger-Ellison syndrome 1881
secretion, physiology 1877
secretion inhibitors 1886
  omeprazole 1887, 1888
  see also H$_2$-receptor antagonists
secretion reduced,
  bacterial overgrowth in 1911, *1911*
  causes 1911
  see also achlorhydria; hypochlorhydria
suppression, in gastro-oesophageal reflux disease 1867–8
Vibrio cholerae susceptibility 577
gastric aspiration
in opioid overdose 1058
in poisoning 1048, *1048*
tuberculosis diagnosis 641
see also aspiration
gastric atrophy 3723
in iron deficiency 3475
pernicious anaemia and 3489
gastric balloon 2094
obesity treatment 1312
gastric burns, in acid ingestion 1104
gastric carcinoma 1883, **1982–5**
adenocarcinoma 1983
aetiological factors 202–3, 1982
  H. pylori association 203, 1884, 1886, 1982
classification 1983
clinical features 1983
in common varied immunodeficiency (CVID) 169, 1837–8
computed tomography (CT) 2012
diagnosis and investigations 1984
early, definition 1984
epidemiology 202–3, 1982

gastric ulcers *vs* 1888, 1983
intestinal and diffuse types 1983
pathogenesis, flow chart 1982
pathology 1983–4
in pernicious anaemia 3489, 3677
  precancerous conditions 1982–3
screening 1983
staging investigations *236*, 1984
survival rates 1983, 1984
treatment 1984
gastric cardia, adenocarcinoma 1981
gastric emptying
accelerated 1962
  see also dumping syndrome
delayed,
  in anorexia nervosa 1297, 4214
  in enteral nutrition 1321
  in head injury 1323
  in systemic sclerosis 1999
  vomiting in 1821
  see also gastric stasis
duodenal ulcer aetiology 1878
in iron poisoning 1071
in poisoning 1048–9
  contraindications 1049
  hazards 1049
  techniques 1048
  see also gastric aspiration; gastric lavage
in pregnancy 1770, 1801
process 1955
radionuclide studies 1957
gastric epithelium, barrier to infection 275
gastric incontinence 1962
  see also dumping syndrome
gastric inhibitory peptide (GIP), *see* glucose-dependent insulinotropic peptide (GIP)
gastric lavage
in antiarrhythmic drug overdose 1063, 1064
in barbiturate poisoning 1060
in beta-adrenoceptor blocker overdose 1065
in digoxin overdose 1066
hazards 1049
in paracetamol poisoning 1053
in poisoning 1048, *1048*, 1049
in salicylate poisoning 1056
in tricyclic antidepressant poisoning 1059
gastric manometry 1956
gastric outflow obstruction 1883, 1960
gastric perforation, in acid ingestion 1103, 1104
gastric polyps 1982, 3723
adenomatous 1982
regenerative/hyperplastic 1982
gastric releasing peptide (GRP) 1877, 1885, 1894
gastric secretory tests, in duodenal ulcer 1878
gastric stapling, obesity treatment 1312
gastric stasis 1959
after peptic ulcer surgery 1961
primary (idiopathic gastroparesis) 1959
secondary 1959
see also gastric emptying, delayed
gastric tumours **1982–5**
benign and polyps 1982
carcinoid 1888
lymphoma 1984–5, 3583
malignant, *see* gastric carcinoma
gastric ulcer
acute erosive **1880**
barium studies 1831, 1879, 1880
bleeding 1828
chronic benign **1879–80**
  aetiology 1879
  clinical features and course 1879
  definition 1879
  diagnosis 1879–80
endoscopy 1828, 1829, 1879, 1888
gastric cancer association 1983
haemorrhage 1882–3
  in acute erosive ulceration 1880
  management and prognosis 1882–3
  symptoms and signs 1882

Helicobacter pylori role 1885
medical treatment 1828, **1883–9**
  choice of drugs 1888–9
  evaluation of results 1883
  H$_2$-receptor antagonists 1886–7
  short-term 1888–9
occupational causes 1171
perforation 1882
recurrent, management 1889
surgical treatment **1889–90**
  motility disorders after 1878–9
  see also peptic ulcer
gastrin 1887, 1888, **1891–2**, 1891
big (G34) 1892
in duodenal ulcer 1877, 1878
elevated, causes 1894
in pancreatic endocrine tumours 1703, 1705
radioimmunoassay 1881
secretion 1892
serum, in pernicious anaemia 3489
structure and actions 1891–2
in Zollinger-Ellison syndrome 1881
gastrin-cholecystokinin family 1891–2
gastrinoma 1704, **1705**, 1708, 1881
gastrin-releasing peptides (GRP) 1877, 1885, 1894
gastritis
atrophic 3489
  gut peptides in 1894–5
  in pernicious anaemia 3490
  in tropical sprue 1933
biliary 1961–2
chronic, in common varied immunodeficiency (CVID) 169
chronic active, gastric cancer after 1982, 1983
  H. pylori association 1982, 1985, 2005
endoscopy indication 1829
gastric cancer association 203
Helicobacter pylori role 1884, 1982, 1985, 2005
gastrocnemius, rupture 2996
gastrocolonic response 1955
gastrodisciasis *999*
Gastrodiscoides (Gastrodiscus) hominis 996, 999
gastroduodenal disease, endoscopy in 1829
gastroenteritis 2001, 2003
acute, occupational causes 1171
Campylobacter 557–8
diarrhoea in 1824
eosinophilic 945, *949*
fungal poisoning 1155, 1156, *1157*, 1158
in history-taking 265
in HIV infection 486
organophosphorus insecticides poisoning *vs* 1122
poisonous plants causing 1152, *1153*
secondary lactase deficiency 1922
viral 390–4, 1824
  see also viruses, stool
Yersinia 608
see also diarrhoea; enteritis; food poisoning; gastrointestinal infections; vomiting
Gastrografin, meconium ileus management 1978
gastrointestinal angiitis 1995
gastrointestinal bleeding **1827–9**, 1882
acute upper **1827–9**
  causes 1827, *1827*
aircraft travel and 1203
angiography in 1832
assessment 1827
causes 1827, *1827*
in chronic pancreatitis 2038
in colorectal cancer 1991
course and progress 1828–9
diagnostic procedures 1828
in diverticular disease 1970, 1972
haematological changes 3476, 3683
in haemophilia 2235
in hepatocellular failure 2109
in hookworm infection 931

in intestinal tuberculosis 2004
intramural 2137
in leptospirosis 700
management 1827–8, 1882–3, 2093–5
  endoscopic 1828, 2093
  surgical 1828
mortality 1828
oesophageal varices causing, *see* oesophageal varices
peptic ulcer, *see* duodenal ulcer; gastric ulcer
prevention 2095
prognosis 1882–3
radionuclide studies 1833
thallium poisoning 1113
in typhoid 566
in ulcerative colitis 1950
in vascular dysplasia 1998
gastrointestinal disorders/manifestations
acute, in immunocompromised *925*, 1034–5
in acute porphyria 1391
in amoebiasis 873
in amyloidosis 1515
in anorexia nervosa 1297, 4213
in anthrax 616–17
in Behçet's syndrome 2000, 3045
in brucellosis 622
in chronic renal failure 3302
in Churg-Strauss syndrome 3015
in cryptosporidiosis 873
in cystic fibrosis 2747, 2749
in diphtheria 495
from seafood 1142
functional disorders, *see* functional bowel disease
gut peptides in **1894–6**
haematological changes **3683–4**
in haemolytic uraemic syndrome 3198
in heart failure 2235
in Henoch-Schönlein purpura 3150
in HIV infection 1841
immune disorders **1836–46**, *1840*
  food allergy, *see* food allergy; food intolerance
  primary immunodeficiency **1837–41**, *1840*
  secondary immunodeficiency **1841–2**
joint involvement **3004**
in Kawasaki disease 3048
in Langerhans-cell histiocytosis 3608
liver in **2131–2**, *2132*
in malaria 844
in malnutrition *1290*
motility disorders, *see* gastrointestinal motility disorders
neuropathic disease, gut peptides in 1896
occupational disease **1171–2**
poisonous plants causing 1152, *1153*
in polyarteritis nodosa 3014
in pregnancy **1801–3**
in rabies 400
in renal transplant recipients 3320
in rheumatic diseases 2945
sensory awareness increase 1966
sexual problems in 4244
skin disease in 3723
in SLE 3020
symptomatology **1819–29**
  see also individual symptoms
in systemic sclerosis 3030, *3030*
in tetanus 628
urinary stone disease in 3255
vascular and collagen disorders **1994–2000**
  ischaemic **1994–8**
  non-inflammatory **1998–9**
  vasculitis and collagen disorders **1999–2000**
  see also intestinal ischaemia
  see also gastrointestinal tract
gastrointestinal drugs
liver damage 2132
poisoning **1069–70**
in renal impairment 3274, *3305*
gastrointestinal haemorrhage, *see* gastrointestinal bleeding

gastrointestinal hormones 1554, **1891–9**
  calcitonin actions 1625
  calcium metabolism and 1626–7
  increased levels 1704
  receptor gene cloning 1891
  structures and actions **1891–4**
gastrointestinal infections **2001–7**
  clinical syndromes **2002–5**
    inflammatory diarrhoea 2003–4
    non-inflammatory diarrhoea 2002–3, *2002*
    systemic infections 2004–5
    see also diarrhoea; gastroenteritis
  clostridial, *see* clostridial infections
  diagnosis and investigations 2005
  differential diagnosis 2005–6
  enterovirus 387–2614
  epidemiology 2001
  in hypogammaglobulinaemia 168–9, *1837*, 1838–9
  management 2006–7
  pathophysiology 2001–2
    host factors 1836, 1879, 2001
    microbial factors and virulence 2001–2
  prevention 2007
  in selective IgA deficiency 1840
  see also intestinal infections
gastrointestinal motility 1900, **1951–65**
  abnormal, *see* gastrointestinal motility disorders
  control 1952, 1953
  as defence mechanism 2001
  definition 1951
  drug absorption 1242
  normal, *see* gastrointestinal motor system
gastrointestinal motility disorders 1952, **1955–65**
  bacterial overgrowth aetiology 1911, *1911*, 1960
  classification 1955
  functional and psychomotor **1963–5, 1965–9**
  see also functional bowel disease
  investigation 1955–8
  primary 1955, **1958–60**
    accelerated transit 1960
    delayed transit 1958–60
    retrograde transit, *see* gastro-oesophageal reflux disease
  secondary 1955, **1960–3**
    in connective tissue disease 1963
    malignancy-associated 1963
    mechanical obstruction 1960–1
    metabolic disease-associated 1962
    neurological disease-associated 1962
    pathogen-associated 1962–3
    surgery-associated 1960–2
  in systemic sclerosis 1999
  in tropical sprue 1934
gastrointestinal motor system 1911, **1952–5**
  control 1952, 1953
  innervation 1953–5
    extrinsic 1953, 1953–4
    functions 1953, 1954
    intrinsic, *see* enteric nervous system
  motor programmes 1954
  regional integrated activity 1955
  smooth muscle 1952–3
    electrical/contractile activity 1952–3
    inhibitory neural input 1953
    pacemakers/rhythmicity 1953
gastrointestinal tract
  age-related changes 4335
  angiography 1832–3
  congenital abnormalities **1972–80**
    embryology 1972–3
  defence mechanisms, *see* defence mechanisms
  disorders, *see* gastrointestinal disorders/manifestations
  duplication (reduplication) **1976**
  electrical injury 1214
  embryology 1972–3
  endocrine cells 1891, 1892
  ganglion cell absence, *see* Hirschsprung's disease

immunity 2001
  infections, *see* gastrointestinal infections
  irrigation 2032
  ischaemic disease, *see* intestinal ischaemia
  lymphoma 3582–3
  motor system, *see under* gastrointestinal motor system
  muscle layers 1952
  pancreatic interactions 1565
  potassium losses 3130
  in pregnancy 1801
  radiation syndrome 1218
  radiology **1830–3**
    motility disorder investigation 1956
    radionuclide studies 1833
  sphincters, transit and electrical characteristics 1952
  transplant 1954
  tuberculosis 653–4
  tumours **1980–94**
    carcinoid, *see* carcinoid tumours
    colon polyps 1986–90
    colorectal cancer 1990–4
    gastric 1982–5
    oesophageal 1980–2
    small intestinal 1985–6
    see also specific tumours/anatomical regions
  see also gastrointestinal disorders/manifestations
gastro-oesophageal junction, Schatski ring 1870, 1872–3
gastro-oesophageal manometry 1956
gastro-oesophageal reflux
  angina *vs* 2322
  asthma and **2735**
  barium studies 1956
  enteral feeding complication 1321
  oesophageal pH monitoring 1865
  in pregnancy 1801
gastro-oesophageal reflux disease **1866–8**, 1958
  aetiology and consequences 1866, 1958
  definition 1866
  diagnosis and assessment 1867
  management 1866, 1867, *1867*
    of complications 1868
    efficacy *1868*
  non-cardiac chest pain in 1870, 2167
  symptoms 1866–7, 1958
  in systemic sclerosis 1999
gastroparesis
  diabetic 1489
  idiopathic 1959
gastropathy, portal hypertensive 2093
gastroschisis 1974, **1975**
  embryology 1973
gastrostomy 1974
Gaucher disease 1336, **1427–9**, 2862, **3087**, 3985
  liver in *2019*, 2025
  lung disease in 2862
  splenomegaly in 3591
  type I (chronic non-neuronopathic; adult) 1429
  type II (acute neuronopathic; infantile) 1429
  type III (subacute neuronopathic; juvenile) 1429
Gaucher's cells 2025
gaze, nystagmus evoked by 3872
gaze apraxia 3853
gaze disorders 2583
  conjugate/disconjugate 2583
gaze palsy 4002
G cells 1892
G-CSF, *see* granulocyte-colony-stimulating factor
gelatins 3661
gelsolin 1517, **1520**, 2622
gemcitabine 259
Gemella, rare species 556
gemfibrozil 2304
gender, choice in intersex states 1695
gender differences
  cancer incidence 198
  in chronic renal failure 3296, 3303

in Hodgkin's disease 3575
  infection susceptibility 281
  ischaemic heart disease risk 2306, 2307
  lung function variations 2673
  myocardial infarction 2337
    thrombolytic therapy 2341
gene(s) **57–9**
  activation 59
  analysis 102
    see also chromosomal analysis; DNA analysis
  association, linkage difference **110–11**
  assortment and segregation 102–3
  candidate 64, 107, 109, 110, 3916
    in epilepsy 3916
  cloning 59, 60–1
    clinical benefits 101
    gut peptide receptors 1891
    positional 3916
    vectors 61
  conserved boxes/sequences 57
  definition 57, 102
  developmental 107
  developmental role 66, **106–7**
  frequencies **117–18**
  function 57
    methods to study 61–2
    prediction 106
  homeotic 66
  housekeeping 57, 106
  insertion methods 113
  introduction into cell cultures 62
  introduction into embryos 62, 112
  introns (intervening) and exons (coding) 57
    see also exons
  libraries, preparation 60–1
  linkage, *see* genetic linkage
  linkage disequilibrium 110–11, 143, 2786
  loci 104
    classification of Mendelian disorders 109
    heterogeneity 104, *105*, 109
  of major effect 129
  mapping 60, 62–3, 106, 193–4
    linkage 106
    linkage disequilibrium and 111
    recent advances/methods 62
    role in clinical genetics 63
    uses/importance of 60
  maps 62, 104, 106
  marker 62
  methylation 59, 107, 126
  number in human genome 62
  probes **59–60**
    construction and principles of 59–60
    diagnostic use 66
    for low abundance mRNA 61
    for screening gene libraries 61
    sources 60
    see also DNA probes
  product, replacement therapy 1336, *1337*
  products and proteins 106, 107
  regulation 59
  in regulation of growth/differentiation 66, 106–7
  regulation by nuclear receptors 1555, 1562
  searching for 62–3
  sequences 105–6
    evolutionary perspective 105–6
  sequencing 61
  silencing 123, 127
  structure 57, 58
  therapy 66, **112–13**, 1337
    in adenosine deaminase (ADA) deficiency 172, 1385
    in cancer 260, 261
    cystic fibrosis 2755
    ethics 112
    germline/somatic 112
    methods of DNA transfer 113, 260
    in muscular dystrophies 4148
    replacement therapy 112, 261
    target tissues 113
    vectors 113, 2755

tracking 132–3, 134–5, *134*
  transcription and regulation of 57
    cis-acting and *trans*-acting 57
    see also transcription
  whole-gene duplication 106
general anaesthesia, *see* anaesthesia; anaesthetics, general
General Health Questionnaire 4203
General Household Survey 41
General Medical Council 4316
general paresis of the insane (GPI) 708, **4085**
  penicillin therapy and 708
general practice 46
  cancer in 240
  consultation rates 48
  content 47–8
  reasons for consultation 41, *43*
  see also primary health care
general practitioner 46–7
  care of diabetics 1504
  delays in myocardial infarction management 2337
  hospital referrals 48–9
  see also doctors
genetically determined disorders **100–2**
genetic analysis
  cellular lesions in tumours 193–4
    methods **59–62**
  polymerase chain reaction 61, 62
  see also chromosomal analysis; DNA analysis
genetic cancer syndromes 220, **242**, *245*
genetic code 59
genetic constitution 100
genetic counselling **131–8**
  Alport's syndrome 3205
  'cascade' 132
  composite risk 132
  cystic fibrosis 2754–5
  Huntington's disease 4014
  in hydrocephalus 4115
  impact 137
  importance 131
  Marfan's syndrome 3083
  object and non-directive nature of 131
  osteogenesis imperfecta 3082
  polycystic kidney disease 3204
  prion diseases 3981
  testing and DNA analysis **131–5**
  thalassaemia 3512
  see also genetic testing
genetic disorders 100, **113–30**
  autosomal dominant **113–14**, *114*
  autosomal recessive **114–15**, *115*
    gene frequency 117
    incidence 114, *115*
    carrier detection 132
  chromosomal, *see* chromosomal abnormalities
  contiguous gene disorder 108
  counselling, *see* genetic counselling
  diagnosis 131
  epilepsy 3915–16
  ethical issues 12
  eye in diagnosis of **4180–2**, *4181*
  gene frequencies **117–18**
  gene mapping and mutation analysis 63
  genotype/phenotype correlations **109–10**
  inborn errors, *see* inborn errors of metabolism
  leukaemia risk 3410
  mitochondrial **128–9**
  monogenic 100
  mosaics, *see* mosaicism
  multifactor causation **129–30**, 130
    advice 132
  non-classical inheritance **124–8**
    genomic imprinting **127–8**
    parent-of-origin effects **127–8**
    trinucleotide repeats, *see* trinucleotide repeats
    uniparental disomy 127, **128**
  phenotypic diversity mechanisms 63–4
  polygenic, molecular pathology 64–5
  prediction, *see* genetic prediction

preimplantation diagnosis 136
prenatal diagnosis, *see* prenatal
    diagnosis
prevention 137
recurrence risk 131–2
reduced penetrance 114
relative risk **111**
risks for common disorders *133*
short stature 1699–700
single-gene 109, 4111–12
    antibody deficiencies 166
    diverse phenotypes 63, 64
    epilepsy 3915
    molecular pathology 63–4
    nervous system in **4111–12**
    treatment approaches 111, *112*
X-linked **115–16**, *116*
X-linked dominant 116
genetic engineering
    monoclonal antibodies 226, 232
    see also recombinant DNA technology
genetic factors **100–38**, 279–80
    ageing and 4333–4
    essential hypertension 2529–30
    lung disease 2649
    obesity 1307, *1307*
    osteoarthritis **2977**, *2977*
    see also genetic susceptibility
genetic information, flow 57
genetic linkage 62, 106
    association difference **110–11**
    disequilibrium 110–11, 143, 2786
    equilibrium 110–11
    gene mapping and 106, 111
    markers and linkage analysis 62
genetic prediction 111, **132–5**
    by DNA analysis, *see* DNA analysis
genetic recombination 103, 106
    gene tracking problem 134
    linkage equilibrium and 110
genetic registers 132
genetics **100–13**
    biochemical **130–1**
    clinical **113–30**
    intervention **111–12**
    in medicine **100–13**
    Mendelian inheritance and **113–24**
    molecular 100
    neurological disorders 3816
    pharmacogenetic polymorphisms
        130
    principles **102–4**
genetic screening 132
    heterozygotes *133*
    see also genetic testing; prenatal
        diagnosis
genetic susceptibility **109–10**, 111,
    129
    Alzheimer's disease 64–5
    cancer **219–20**
    coronary artery disease 64
    diabetes mellitus 64, 1453–4, 1455–6
    epilepsy 3915–16
    infection 279–80
    nature, nurture and luck 219–20
    rheumatoid arthritis 2953
    ulcerative colitis 1944
    see also genetic factors
genetic testing **131–8**
    carrier detection 132
    ethical dilemmas **137–8**, *137*
    services **136–7**
        quality measures 137
    see also genetic counselling
genetic variation, 'medicalization' 137
genioglossus muscle 2611
genital herpes 342, 344, **3351–3**,
    3768
    clinical features 3352–3
    differential diagnosis 3353, *3353*
    epidemiology 342, 3347, 3351–2
    lymphogranuloma venereum *vs* 761
    natural history 3352
    in pregnancy 1775, 1781, 1804
    recurrent infections 344, 3353
    syphilis *vs* 711
    transmission 3351–2
    treatment and prevention 3353

genitalia
    ambiguous,
        in congenital adrenal hyperplasia
            1664, 1665, 1690
        in female pseudohermaphroditism
            1690
    female, filariasis 922
    skin disorders affecting **3767–70**
genital tract infections 3767
    amoebiasis 830, 833
    anaerobic 572–3
    candidiasis 3768
    chlamydial, *see* chlamydial infections
    human papillomaviruses (HPV) 444,
        445
    male infertility 1685, 1686
    mycoplasma **767–71**, *768*
    syphilis 710, 711
    tuberculosis 653
    see also genitourinary tract; *individual
        infections*
genital ulcer 584
    in Behçet's syndrome 3045
    in developing countries 3348
    HIV susceptibility 586
    serpiginous, in donovanosis 776–7
    see also chancroid
genital warts 444, **3366–9**, 3768
    in children 3369
    clinical features 3367–9
        in men 3367–8
        in women 3368–9
    complications 3369
    diagnosis and management 3369
    epidemiology 3347, 3366–7
    in homosexuals 3363, 3367
    pathology 3366, 3367
    in pregnancy 3368
    virology and pathogenesis 3366
genitoanorectal syndrome, in
    lymphogranuloma venereum 760
genitourinary tract
    anaerobic flora 570
    in brucellosis 622
    in gnathostomiasis 952
    in malnutrition *1290*
    occupational disease **1171**
    sarcoidosis **2827**
    symptoms in rheumatic diseases 2945
genogram 4358
genome **104–6**
    human, size 62
    mapping 62–3
    physical map 62
genomic imprinting 107, **127–8**
    dominant transmission of mutation 127
genotype 100, 104
    phenotype correlations **109–10**
gentamicin
    in brucellosis 623
    in infective endocarditis 2446, *2447*
    in listeriosis 722
    monitoring 1261
    nephrotoxicity 3264, 3288
    post-antibiotic effects 304
    in pregnancy 1784
    in renal impairment 3271, *3272*, 3288
    Staphylococcus aureus resistance 525
    in urinary-tract infections *3211*
Germanin, *see* Suramin
germanium, nephrotoxicity *3261*, 3263
germ cell tumours
    investigations of metastases from
        unknown primary sites 252
    mediastinal 2899
        misdiagnosis 245
    metastatic, misdiagnosis 245
    germinoma, suprasellar **1597–8**
Gerstmann-Sträussler-Scheinker
        syndrome *1514*, 1517, 3977, 3983
    clinical features 3980
    familial 3977, 3978, 3979
    prion protein mutations 3977–8
Gerstmann syndrome 3851
Geschwind's classification, aphasic
    syndromes 3850, *3850*
Gestalt method of diagnosis 15 GH, *see*
    growth hormone

giant cell(s)
    in extrinsic allergic alveolitis 2811
    formation 88
    in hepatic granulomas 2120
    inclusions 2818
    in sarcoidosis 2818
giant-cell arteritis (temporal/cranial)
    3041–2, 4028–9
    clinical features 2946, 3041–2
    differential diagnosis and diagnosis 3042
    gastrointestinal tract in 2000
    haematological changes 3483, 3681–2
    headache in 3042, 4028–9
    incidence 3041
    liver in 2139
    mental disorder/symptoms 4243
    ocular features 3042, 4028, **4183**, 4186,
        4187
    polymyalgia rheumatica relationship
        3041
    treatment 3042
giant-cell carcinoma, pancreatic 2042
giant-cell granuloma,
    hyperparathyroidism *vs* 1863
giant follicular lymph node hyperplasia
    (Castleman's disease) 2899, 2900,
    3566, **3586**
Giardia intestinalis, in homosexuals
    3365
Giardia lamblia 878
    biology and stages 878
    see also giardiasis
giardiasis **878–80**, 2003
    clinical features and pathophysiology
        879
    in common varied immunodeficiency
        168–9, 878, 1838
    diagnosis 879–80
    epidemiology and transmission 878–9
    in HIV infection 475, 879, 1034
    in homosexuals 3365
    in immunocompromised 1034
    immunology and antibodies 879, 880
    malabsorption in tropics and 1930
    nodular lymphoid hyperplasia in
        878–9
    prevention and treatment 880, *880*
    small-bowel biopsy 1908
gibbus 2874, 2993, 2994
Giemsa stain 849
gigantism 1591, 1700
Gilbert's syndrome 2055, 2056, **2057**
    biochemistry and diagnosis 2057
    Crigler-Najjar syndrome with 2058
    haemolytic anaemia in 3550
    porphyrin metabolism 1397
    pregnancy in 1799
Gilles de la Tourette syndrome **4016–17**
Gillick case 4316
'gill' worm 959
gingival disease **1847–8**
gingivitis acute fusospirochaetal 1852–3
    acute necrotizing ulcerative (Vincent's
        disease) 343, 571–2, 706, 1852–3
    acute *vs* chronic 1848
    in AIDS 474, 1851
    desquamative 1848
    halitosis in 1864
    Vincent's 343, 571–2, 706, 1852–3
gingivostomatitis, herpetic 342, 343,
    1848–9, 1848
ginseng 1159
Girdlestone's operation 2982
GISSI-1 (Gruppo Italiano per lo Studio
    della Streptochinasi nell'Infarto
    Miocardio) trial 28, 2340
GISSI-2 trial 2342
GISSI-3 trial 2344, 2348
glafenine 3224
    poisoning 1057
glanders **593–4**, *3801*
Glanzmann's thrombasthenia *3643*, **3646**
Gla protein 3057–8
Glasgow coma scale 2584, *3931*, 4046,
    4049
Glasgow scoring system, acute
    pancreatitis 2030, *2031*
glass wool 2845

glaucoma
    blindness due to **4197–8**
    chronic, in diabetes mellitus 4190
    corticosteroids associated 1259
    in diabetes 1483, 1486, 4190
    in von Recklinghausen's disease
        4182
Glenn's operation 2402, 2413
glenohumeral joint, in rheumatoid
    arthritis 2958
glia 3990
    development 3990
gliadin 1916, 1918
    antibodies 1918
glial cells 4030
glibenclamide *1471*
glibornuride *1471*
glicentin, *see* enteroglucagon
gliclazide *1471*, 3274
glioblastoma multiforme 224
glioma 4030
    management 4038, 4039
    radiotherapy 4039
    optic nerve 3865, 3866
    in pregnancy 1767
    visual pathway disorders in 3866
    see also astrocytoma; glioblastoma
glipizide *1471*, 3274
gliquidone 1471
Global Utilisation of Streptokinase and
    tissue plasminogen activator for
    Occluded Arteries, *see* GUSTO trial
globin 3500
    ß,
        genes 103 mutations 104
    genes 103, 3500–1, 3502
        in α-thalassaemia 3509
        in ß-thalassaemia 3502–3
    synthesis 3501
globoid cell leukodystrophy (Krabbe's
    disease; galactosyl ceramide lipidosis
    1428, **1429**, 3986
globus hystericus 1963–4, 4210
globus pallidus 3861
glomerular basement membrane
    in Alport's syndrome 3205
    autoantibodies 3164, 3205
    see also antiglomerular basement
        membrane (GBM) disease
    in diabetes mellitus 1464, 3169
    in membranous nephropathy 3159
    thickening, in cyanotic congenital heart
        disease 2400
    in thin membrane nephropathy
        3152–3
glomerular filtration, drugs 1244
glomerular filtration rate (GFR) 1244
    body size correction 3108
    in chronic renal failure 3294, *3295*,
        3296
    in diabetic nephropathy 3169, 3170
    drug excretion and 3268
    estimation **3105–7**
    in heart failure 2170
    in urinary-tract obstruction 3234,
        3235
glomerulonephritis
    in α₁-antitrypsin deficiency 1547
    acute, hypertension in 2547
    acute nephritic syndrome 3146
    acute renal failure in **3291**
    acute renal failure *vs* 3280
    chronic renal failure in 3296, 3303
    classification 3153, *3154*
    clinical presentation 3153, *3154*
    coagulase-negative staphylococcal
        infections 532
    diagnosis 3153–4
    fibrillary **3180**, **3182**
    in filariasis 3177
    focal, viral aetiology 291
    haemolytic anaemia in *3548*
    haemolytic uraemic syndrome in
        3198
    in Henoch-Schönlein purpura 3150–1,
        3152
    in hepatitis B infection 3157, 3176
    HIV-associated **3176**

glomerulonephritis (*cont.*)
  idiopathic **3153–61**
    recurrence after transplantation 3161, 3315
  in IgA nephropathy 3150–1, 3152
  immune-complex-mediated 164
    in malaria 857
  infection-associated **3173–7**
    pathogenesis 3173
    rare associations *3178*
  in infective endocarditis 2439, 2441, 3174
  in Legionnaire's disease 3175
  in leprosy **3176–7**
  membranoproliferative, C3 nephritic factor in 180
  membranous, *see* membranous nephropathy
  mesangial proliferative 3150, *3160*
    as 'idiopathic nephrotic syndrome' variant 3154
    IgM **3160–1**
  mesangiocapillary (MCGN; membranoproliferative) **3157–8**, 3185
    recurrence after transplantation 3161
    type I (subendothelial) 3157–8, 3161
    type II (dense deposit disease) 3157, 3158, 3161, 3315
    type III 3158
  necrotizing, in Wegener's granulomatosis 2801
  post-infectious/acute endocapillary proliferative **3173–4**
  post-streptococcal **505–6**, **3173–4**, 3195
  pregnancy in **1735**
  proliferative **3160–1**
  rapidly progressive 3009, **3162–7**, *3300*
    alveolar haemorrhage in 2804
    in anti-GBM disease 3162, 3164–5
    causes *3162*, 3166–7
    diagnosis 3162
    idiopathic 3162, **3166**
    management 3162–3
  in microscopic polyangiitis 3014
  in rheumatoid arthritis 3192–3
  in sarcoidosis 2827
  in scabies 1008
  schistosomal 978, **3176**
  in septicaemia 3175
  in shunt nephritis 3175
  in Sjögren's syndrome 3192
  in SLE 3188
  in syphilis 3177
  toxin-induced 3258–9, **3260**
  in tuberculosis 3175
  in typhoid fever 3175
  visceral abscesses and 3175
glomerulopathy
  immunotactoid 3182
  in pre eclampsia 1728
  primary **3149–67**
  sarcoidosis-associated 3187
  in sickle-cell disease 3194
  tumour-associated 3184–5
glomerulosclerosis
  of ageing 3249
  in chronic renal failure **3303**
  in diabetic nephropathy 3167
  focal segmental (FSGS) **3156–7**
    as 'idiopathic nephrotic syndrome' variant 3154
    primary 3156
    recurrence after transplantation 3161, 3315 secondary 3156, *3157*
glomerulus
  disease of, *see* glomerulopathy
  focal necrosis, in Wegener's granulomatosis 3013
  haemodynamics,
    in chronic renal failure 3303
    in diabetes mellitus 3169
    in hypertension 3248, 3249, 3250
  hypertrophy, in diabetes mellitus 3169
  selectivity to proteins 3136
  tip lesion 3156, 3157
glomus jugulare tumours **4033**
glossitis 1863
  in iron-deficiency anaemia 3475
  syphilitic 713

glossopharyngeal nerve **3880**
glossopharyngeal neuralgia 3880, 4023–4
glottis, carcinoma, epidemiology 205
glove powder, peritonitis 2008–9
gloves
  hand dermatitis management and 3807
  skin protection in occupational dermatosis 1165
  in leprosy 671, 678
  in rheumatoid arthritis 2961
glucagon 1893
  action 1274, *1275*, 1340, 1458, 1505, 1562–3
  in ß-adrenoceptor blocker overdose 1065
  calcium metabolism and 1627
  functions 1274, *1275*
  insulin secretion and 1459–60
  in pancreatic endocrine tumours 1703, 1706
  potassium balance and 3128
  receptor *1560*
  stimulation test 1341, 1508, *1584*, *1699*
    in trauma 1548
  treatment, in hypoglycaemia 1498, 1506
glucagon-like peptide 1 (GLP-1) 1893
glucagonoma 1704, **1706**, 3723
glucocerebrosidase deficiency, *see* Gaucher disease
glucocorticoids 1639
  ACTH inhibition 1575, 1576
  biosynthetic pathway *1640*, 1664
  calcium metabolism and 1626
    in cortisol deficiency 1587
  deficiency, *see* hypoadrenalism
  excess 1699
    effect on bone 3069
    infection susceptibility 281
    myopathy in 4168
    see also Cushing's syndrome
  in Graves' ophthalmopathy 1614
  in hirsutism 1677
  in hypoglycaemic coma 1498
  inactivation in renal tubules 1557
  in pregnancy 1745, 1757, **1811**
  receptor 1554, 1557, 1561–2
    defects *1567*, 1573, 1661
  replacement therapy 1655, 1665
    in pregnancy 1751
  resistance, familial 1573, 1661
  serum lipids and 1411
  sudden cessation of therapy 1653
  surfactant secretion 2596
  in trauma 1549
  see also cortisol; dexamethasone; prednisolone; prednisone
glucokinase gene
  abnormalities 1452, 1456
  in non-insulin dependent diabetes 64
gluconeogenesis 1456–7, 1505
  in acid-base disturbances 1539, 1540
  in starvation 1277, 1278
glucose
  absorption, reduced in tropical enteropathy 1931
  administration,
    before exercise 4325
    during exercise 4325–6
  biosensors 1478
  blood (BG),
    acute hepatocellular failure management 2109
    aims in diabetes *1466*
    control in diabetes, *see* diabetes mellitus, glycaemic/metabolic control
    in diagnosis of diabetes 1449, *1450*
    effects of food 1465, 1466–7, *1468*
    exercise and 1478
    home monitoring 1480
    homeostasis 1562–3
    in hypoglycaemic drug overdose 1072
    in impaired glucose tolerance 1449, *1450*
    in iron overdose 1071
    in malaria 850

  measurements in pregnancy 1754, *1755*
  monitoring in diabetes *1467*, *1479*, **1480**
  phaeochromocytoma investigations 2556
  reference intervals *4366*
  in surgery in diabetes 1494, 1495
  in unconscious patients 2585
  in cerebrospinal fluid, *see* cerebrospinal fluid
cholera management 579
  in cirrhosis 2088
  in cyanide poisoning treatment 1098
  enantiomers 1248
  endurance sports and 4325–6
  energy supply 1271
  homeostasis 1274, 1456–7, **1505**
  insulin secretion and 1459
  intolerance,
    in chronic pancreatitis 2038–9
    ischaemic heart disease risk 2309
  intramuscular, in hypoglycaemia 1506
  intravenous (dextrose),
    in acute renal failure 3285
    in alcohol poisoning 1080
    in diabetes during surgery 1494, 1495, 1496
    diabetic women in labour 1756
    in hyperkalaemia 3135, *3286*
    in hypoglycaemia 1498
  levels, in malnutrition 1286
  maximum tubular reabsorption rate (T_{mG}) 3108, 3109
  metabolic disorders, myopathy in **4165–7**
  metabolism 1274, 1920, 2146
    anaerobic 2146
    changes in salicylate poisoning 1054
  in parenteral nutrition 1321, 2588
  plasma,
    in diabetes mellitus 1449, *1450*
    in hypoglycaemia 1506
    in impaired glucose tolerance 1449, *1450*
    in insulinoma 1507, 1508–9
    in pregnancy 1752–3
    renal threshold 3108
    in starvation 1505
  polymers, administration, in short gut syndrome 1926
  production, from kidney in starvation 1277–8
  requirement, of brain 4123
  sodium cotransport 1902
  supply 1273
  synthesis 1273
  tolerance, *see* glucose tolerance
  transport 1920
  transporters (GLUT) 1462, 1903, 2146
  uptake by tissues 1457
  urinary 3102, *3330*
    in bone disease 3063
    in diabetes 1479
    see also glycosuria
  utilization 1273, 1274
    in fasting 1273
glucose-alanine cycle 1275, 1276
glucose-dependent insulinotropic (gastric inhibitory) peptide (GIP) **1892–3**
  Cushing's syndrome due to 1640, **1643**
glucose-fatty acid cycle 1457
glucose-lipid interactions 1277
glucose 6-phosphatase 1340
  deficiency, *see* von Gierke's disease
glucose 1-phosphate 1340
glucose 6-phosphate 1340–1
  translocase system deficiency 1342, 1384
glucose 6-phosphate dehydrogenase (G6PD)
  biochemistry 3537
  clonal origin of tumours and 192
  deficiency 3534, *3536*, **3537–41**
    clinical features 3538–40
    definition 3537
    drugs triggering haemolysis *3539*, 3546

  genetics 3537–8
  geographical distribution 3465, 3466, 3538
  haemolysis and favism in 130
  laboratory diagnosis 3540–1
  lathyrism in 1159
  leucocyte defects 3560
  malaria and 837, 845, 847
  molecular basis 3538
  pathophysiology 3541
  treatment 3541
  X-linked inheritance 115
  gene polymorphisms 3391
  X-linked isoenzymes 3390–1, 3432
glucose phosphate isomerase deficiency *3536*
glucose tolerance 4344
  age-related changes 4344
  hormone replacement therapy and 1814
  impaired (IGT) 1448–9, *1452*, 4344
    in acromegaly 1592
    diabetes risk reduced by diet 1327
    diagnosis 1449, *1450*
    gestational 1754, *1755*
    immunosuppressants causing 2258
    insulin secretion *1462*
    metabolism 3302
    non-endocrine causes 1714, *1715*
    in VIPoma syndrome 1706
    normal criteria in pregnancy 1754, *1755*
    potential abnormality *1452*
  test, oral 1449, *1450*, 1906, *4375*
    in acromegaly 1593
    in hypothalamic/pituitary disease 1586
    in pregnancy 1753
    screening for gestational diabetes 1753–4
α-glucosidase deficiency, *see* Pompe's disease
α-glucosidase inhibitors 1506, 1511
glucosyl ceramide lipidosis, *see* Gaucher disease
glucosylphosphatidylinositol (GPI)-linked proteins 3392–3, 3450
glucuronic acid, bilirubin conjugation 2055
ß-glucuronidase deficiency (mucopolysaccharidosis VII) *1432*, 1434
glucuronyl transferase, in neonates 2058
glues 1092
'glue-sniffer's rash' 1092
glue-sniffing 1092, 3267
  clinical features 1046, 1092
  presentation patterns 1092
  see also solvent abuse
glutamate 1353
  metabolism 2102
glutamate decarboxylase deficiency 1372
  glutamic acid decarboxylase (GAD)
    autoantibodies to 163
    in Huntington's disease 4013, *4013*
    in Parkinson's disease 4000
    reduced in multiple system atrophy 4006
glutamic oxaloacetic transaminase (GOT), *see* aspartate aminotransferase (AST)
glutamic pyruvic transaminase (GPT), *see* alanine aminotransferase (ALT)
glutamine 1275–6, *1353*, 1903
  metabolism in acid-base disturbances 1540
  plasma *1360*, 1361
  transplantation patients 1323
gamma glutamyl cycle **1357–8**
  genetic defects *1359*
gamma glutamylcysteine synthetase 1358, *1359*
  deficiency 3536
γ-glutamyl transferase 2055–6, *4365*
γ-glutamyl transpeptidase 1357–8, *1359*
  alcohol consumption marker 4272
glutaraldehyde, *Bacillus anthracis* spores 613
glutaric aciduria
  type I 1372–3
  type II 1373, **1374–5**

glutaryl coenzyme A dehydrogenase 1372
glutathione
  analgesic nephropathy and 3221, 3222
  paracetamol metabolite reaction 1051
  red cell 3456
  synthesis 1357, 1358
  in vinyl chloride poisoning 1090
glutathione peroxidase 3537
  deficiency *3536*
  ischaemic heart disease risk 2312
glutathione reductase deficiency *3536*
glutathione synthetase 1358
  inherited deficiencies *1359*, 3536
glutathione S-transferase B 2055
gluten 1918
gluten-free diet 1917, 1919–20
gluten-sensitive enteropathy, *see* coeliac disease
glycaemic index, of foods 1466–7
glycation
  end-products, advanced 1483
  protein *1479*, **1481**, 3169
L-glyceric aciduria 1447
glycero-ether bond formation 1439
glycerol 1276, 1456
  plasma, in pregnancy 1753
glycerolipids 1400
glyceryl monothioglycollate 3736
glyceryl trinitrate 2247, 2300, 2327
  in oesophageal spasm 1958
  side-effects 2327
  spray formulation 2327
glycine *1353*
  bile acid breath test 1910, 1914
  cerebrospinal fluid 1368
  cleavage system 1368
  defects of metabolism **1368**
  plasma 1361, 1368
  supplements 1372
glycoalkaloids 1159
glycocalyx
  myocardial cells 2144
  pulmonary endothelium 2486
glycogen 1274, 4325
  breakdown, *see* glycogenolysis
  endurance sports and 4325
  loading 4325
  metabolic disorders, myopathy in **4165–7**
  metabolism 1339–41, 4165
  structure 1336
  synthesis 1339–40
glycogenolysis **1340–1**, 1456, 1505, 4165
  after injury 1549
  in myocardial ischaemia 2146
  vasopressin actions 3118
glycogenoses, *see* glycogen storage diseases
glycogen storage diseases **1339–44**, 4142
  diagnosis 1341–2
  liver in *2019*, 2024
  muscle biopsy 4143
  type I, *see* von Gierke's disease
  type IB 1341, 1342, 1384
  type II, *see* Pompe's disease
  type III (Forbes-Cori's disease) 1342, *1343*, 1384, 4166
  type IV (Andersen's disease) *1343*, 1344
  type V, *see* McArdle's disease
  type VI (Hers' disease) *1343*, 1344
  type VII, *see* phosphofructokinase, deficiency
  type VIII *1343*
  type IX (phosphorylase b kinase deficiency) *1343*, 1344
  type O *1343*
glycogen synthase 1339–40, 1458
  deficiency *1343*, 1344
  gene, in non-insulin dependent diabetes 64
glycolate, formation, in ethylene glycol metabolism 1082
glycols, poisoning **1080–3**

glycolysis 4165
  in acid-base disturbances 1539
  distal, defects 4167
p-glycoprotein, *see* p-glycoprotein *(in 'p' section)*
glycoprotein (Gp)Ib/IX 3614
glycoprotein (Gp)IIb/IIIa 3614, 3616, 3617, 3641
  in Glanzmann's thrombasthenia 3646
glycoprotein hormones 1555–6, **1578–9**
  α-subunit 1578, 1595
  ß-subunits 1555, 1578
  pituitary tumours secreting 1595–6
  see also follicle stimulating hormone; luteinizing hormone; thyroid stimulating hormone
glycoproteinoses **1435–6**
glycosaminoglycans 3626
  amyloid fibril-associated **1521**
  in diabetes mellitus 3169
  urinary stones and 3252
  see also heparan sulphate
glycosphingolipid lipidosis, *see* Fabry disease
glycosuria
  assessment **3108–9**
  detection 3102
  in diabetes 1456, *1466*
  monitoring, in artificial nutritional support 1322
  in pregnancy 1754, 3333
  renal **3333–4**
glycosylation
  changes in tumours 231
  hormone/hormone receptor 1559
  N-linked 70, 71
  O-linked 70
glycosylphosphatidyl inositol (GPI), apical targeting of proteins 71
glycyrrhizic acid 1661, 1717–18
glymidine 1471
glyphosate-containing herbicides **1121**
glypressin, bleeding oesophageal varices 2094
GM-CSF, *see* granulocyte-macrophage colony-stimulating factor
GMP140, *see* P-selectin
GMP (guanosine monophosphate), synthesis 1378
Gnathostoma, species 949, *950*
Gnathostoma spinigerum 949, 950
gnathostomiasis **949–54**
  aetiology and species 949–50, *950*
  cutaneous forms 951–2
  diagnosis 953–4
  distribution 950
  eye in 4193
  pathology and pathogenesis 950–1
  treatment and prevention 954
  visceral forms 952–3
GnRH, *see* gonadotrophin releasing hormone
goat's milk anaemia 3492
goblet cells 1900
goitre
  dyshormonogenetic 1615, *1616*
  endemic 1615
  in hypothyroidism 1615
  retrosternal 1610
  simple non-toxic 1617
  toxic multinodular 1611, 1613
gold
  nephrotoxicity 3159, 3193, *3261*, **3262**
  radioactive, in ascites 2098
  in rheumatoid arthritis 2964
  secondary immunodeficiency due to 174
  thrombocytopenia induced by 3632
Goldblatt hypertension 2545
gold/gold salts
golfer's elbow 2995
Golgi apparatus
  antigen processing for helper T-cells 143–4
  bulk flow of proteins to 70–1
  endoplasmic reticulum transport to 75, 76–7
  intercisternal transport systems 75
  NSF (NEM-sensitive factor) binding/role 75

positioning and microtubule role 82–3
  protein transport through 71
  Sec protein mutants in yeast 76, 77
  see also intracellular transport
Goltz's syndrome (focal dermal atrophy) 3791, 3793
Gomez classification, malnutrition 1281, *1281*
Gomori's methenamine stain 2689
gonadal dysfunction
  mental disorders/symptoms in 4239
  in POEMS syndrome 4104
gonadal dysgenesis **1670**, 1671
  mixed 1693
  pure 1694
gonadal mosaicism 107, 116, 135
gonadal neoplasia, in intersex states 1694
gonadal peptides 1579–80
gonadoblastoma 1694
gonadotrophin releasing hormone (GnRH) 1554, 1563
  agonists 1580, 1671
    in acute porphyria 1393
    ovulation induction 1678
    in precocious puberty 1702
    spermatogenesis induction 1686
    in anorexia nervosa 1297, 4213
  antagonists 1580
  combined anterior pituitary test 1585
  control of gonadotrophin secretion 1579
  deficiency, Kallmann's syndrome 1670
    in males 1679, 1680
    in puberty 1701
  pulsatile secretion 1565, 1579
  receptor signalling pathway *1560*, 1561
  sexual problem management 4246
  stimulation test 1593, 1702
gonadotrophins 1563, **1579–81**
  deficiency 1582, 1585, 1699
  excess, in tumours *243*
  in male pseudohermaphroditism 1693
  in precocious puberty 1702
  rhythmic secretion 1565
  therapy,
    ovulation induction 1678
    spermatogenesis induction 1686
  see also follicle stimulating hormone; human chorionic gonadotrophin; luteinizing hormone
gonadotrophs 1575
  adenoma 1595–6
Gongylonema pulchrum 954
gonococcal infection
  eye in 4191
  liver in 2133
  neonatal 1790
  in pregnancy **1789–90**
  urinary-tract obstruction 3179
  see also gonorrhoea; *Neisseria gonorrhoeae*
gonococcal ophthalmia 546, 547
gonococcal septicaemia 1020
gonococcus, *see Neisseria gonorrhoeae*
gonorrhoea 544–50
  clinical features 546
  complications 546–7
  contact tracing in 547
  diagnosis 547–8
  epidemiology 545–6, 3346, *3346*, 3347
  in homosexuals 3361, 3362
  immunology 545
  incubation period 546, *546*
  pathogenesis 544–5
  pharyngeal 3361, 3362
  in pregnancy 1789–90
  prophylaxis 549
  rectal 546, 547
  septicaemia in 1021
  treatment 549
  see also Neisseria gonorrhoeae
Goodpasture antigen 3164
  in Alport's syndrome 3166, 3205
Goodpasture's syndrome 3163
  see also antiglomerular basement membrane (GBM) disease
Gordon's syndrome (pseudohypoaldosteronism type II) 1662, 3134, 3337

Goretex tube prosthesis 2406
Gorlin's syndrome 3792, *3795*
goserelin 1702
gout **1376–81**, **2984–8**
  acute attacks 2984–5, 2987
    triggering agents 2984
  associated conditions 2985–6
  atypical attacks 2984–5
  causes *1380*
  chronic tophaceous 2948, 2985, 2987
  chronic urate nephropathy 1380, 3224, **3226–7**
  classification 2985, *2986*
  cluster attacks 2984
  in cyanotic congenital heart disease 2400
  cyclosporin A-induced 3265
  differential diagnosis 2987
  epidemiology 1376, *1377*, 2984
  familial juvenile 1380, 3225, **3226**, 3227
  in fructose intolerance 1384
  hypertriglyceridaemia and 1381, 1412
  immunosuppressants causing 2258, 3265
  intercritical periods 2985
  interstitial nephritis and **3224–7**
  investigations and diagnosis 2948, 2986–7
  joints involved 2985
  in lead intoxication 1381, 2986, 3225, 3227, 3261
  pathogenesis 1379, **3225**
  in polycystic renal disease 1381
  primary 2985, *2986*
  pyrophosphate arthropathy *vs* 2989
  radiography 2948
  renal disease and 2986
  rheumatoid arthritis, negative association 2986
  rheumatoid arthritis *vs* 2963
  saturnine 1381, 2986
  secondary 2985, *2986*
  treatment 2987–8
  urolithiasis in 1379, 2986
  in von Gierke's disease 1383
  X-linked 1383
  see also hyperuricaemia
gouty chicken 1380, 3226
Gowers' sign 4145
G-proteins 1560
  α-subunits 1560
  bacterial toxin effect on 272
  G_{11} isoform 1561
  Giα, defects *1567*
  Gq isoform 1561
  Gsα-subunit 1560
    defects *1567*, 1569, 1572–3, 1591, 1715
  in heart 2147
  heterotrimeric,
    in intracellular transport 78
    quality control of proteins 70
  in neutrophil chemotaxis and activation 2622
  see also GTP-binding protein
'gracile habitus' 2425
Gradenigo's syndrome 3877, 3878
graft rejection
  acute,
    lung transplantation 2935–6
    management 2935–6
  antigen-presenting cells in 183, 184–5
  in cardiac transplantation 2257
  class II antigen incompatibility 183, 186
  C-reactive protein in 1530
  cytokines role 187
  cytotoxic/helper T-cells in 152, 186–7
  grading severity 2936, *2936*
  haemolytic anaemia *3548*
  humoral response in 187 liver transplantation 2114
  MHC antigens role 183–5
  minor histocompatibility antigens role 185
  mononuclear cell infiltrates 187

graft rejection (*cont.*)
  non-specific immune response 187
  in renal transplantation 1530, **3318–19**
    acute 3319
    chronic 3319
    hyperacute 3319
    target of 187
  see also transplantation immunology
grafts
  arterial 2369–71
  skin 185
  vein, *see* vein grafts
  see also transplantation: *specific organs*
graft-versus-host disease (GVHD) 3696, **3697–8**, 3699
  after lung transplantation **2936**
  C-reactive protein 1532
  lymphocytic interstitial pneumonitis 2807
  minor histocompatibility antigens in 185
  oesophagus in 1876
  sclerosis in *3791*
Graham-Steell murmur 2467, 2469
grain, extrinsic allergic alveolitis and 2809, 2811
Gram-negative bacteraemia 1030
Gram-negative bacteria
  in bacterial overgrowth 1912
  endotoxin 291
    see also endotoxin
  enterobacteria 550
  pneumonia 2694, 2701
  rheumatoid arthritis aetiology 2953
Gram-negative septicaemia 550–1, 1020, 1026
Gram-positive bacteraemia 1030
Gram-positive bacteria
  infectious dose 291
  inflammatory reactions **291–2**
  peptidoglycan and teichoic acid 291
Gram-positive septicaemia 1020, 1025
Gram stain 2676
  Neisseria gonorrhoeae detection 547
  sputum 2697
grand mal 3911–12
  in alcohol withdrawal 4290
  treatment 3921, *3921*
  see also epilepsy; epileptic seizures
granulation tissue 2626
granulocyte(s) 3377, **3555–6**
  in cryptogenic fibrosing alveolitis 2788–9
  in fibrinolysis 3626
  in IgE-mediated allergic response 156
  non-specific response to infections 276–7
  phagocytosis mechanism 154
  production (granulopoiesis) 3384, 3386, 3388, 3556–7
    in myelodysplastic syndromes 3426
    suppression of 3388–9
  in rheumatoid arthritis 2953–4
  in spleen 3589
  transfusions 284, 3694
  see also basophils; eosinophil(s); neutrophils
granulocyte-colony-stimulating factor (G-CSF) 225, 3557
  in haemopoiesis 3384, 3387, 3388
  in myeloma 3602
  peripheral blood stem-cell transplants and 3700
  therapy 3389, 3431, 3557
granulocyte-macrophage colony-stimulating factor (GM-CSF) 97, 157, 3557
  in asthma 2727
  dendritic cells and 87
  in haemopoiesis 3384, 3387, 3388, 3389
  in myeloma 3602
  recombinant 99
  therapy 3389, 3431, 3557
granulocytosis, in tumours *244*
granuloma **3798–804**
  in angiostrongyliasis costaricensis 949

Aspergillus 809
  in cat scratch disease 746
  chronic localized mucocutaneous candidiasis with 1852
  clinical features 3798
  in Crohn's disease 1938
  cryptococcal 809
  definition 2120, 3798
  denture 1859
  Dürck's 844
  eosinophilic, *see* eosinophilic granuloma; histiocytosis, Langerhans-cell
  epithelioid-cell, in sarcoidosis 2818, 2823
  epithelioid macrophage in 88
  formation 2818–19
    macrophage role 154
  giant-cell reparative, of mouth 1859
  hepatic, *see* hepatic granulomas
  high/low turnover types 3798
  lethal midline 1995, 3013
  in paracoccidioidomycosis 816
  in primary biliary cirrhosis 2074
  pyogenic, in pregnancy 1804
  respiratory tract, in Wegener's granulomatosis 2801
  in sarcoidosis 2818–19, 3799, 3802, 4182
    neurological 2827
  in schistosomiasis 972, 976
  in sparganosis 970
  swimming-pool 665, 666
  in toxocariasis 944, 945
  in tuberculosis 639, 650, 3276, 3800
  in Wegener's granulomatosis 2801, 3013, 4183
  in yaws 705
granuloma annulare 3797–8, 3799, 3802
  in diabetes 1490
granuloma gluteal infantum 3798–9
granuloma inguinale, *see* donovanosis
granulomatosis
  allergic, *see* Churg-Strauss syndrome
  lymphomatoid **2807–8**, 3586
    of lung 2690
  pulmonary, *see* pulmonary granulomatosis
  Wegener's, *see* Wegener's granulomatosis
granulomatous colitis, *see* Crohn's disease
granulomatous disease, chronic, *see* chronic granulomatous disease (CGD)
granulovacuolar degeneration 3972
graphite pneumoconiosis 2847
'grass' 1075
Graves' disease 1570, 1609, **1611**
  autoantibodies in 164
  ophthalmopathy *1611*, 1614, 4195–6
    clinical features and grading 4195–6
    diagnosis and management 4196
  ophthalmoplegia, myopathy in 4168
  in pregnancy 1749
  thyrotoxic crisis 1614
  treatment 1612–13
  TSH receptor antibodies 163
gravitation, telangiectasia on legs 3785–6
gray (grey) platelet syndrome *3643*, **3645**
great arteries, transposition, *see* transposition of great arteries
greater omentum, embryology 1973
Greene formula 2222
greenhouse effect 36
Greenland Eskimos, diet 2311
'green monkey' disease 439
grey (gray) platelet syndrome *3643*, **3645**
Grey Turner's sign 2029
grief 4234–5, 4359
  atypical 4235, *4235*
  definition 4234
  management *4235*
  typical 4234–5, *4234*
    phases 4234–5, *4234*
Grimelius method 2686
griseofulvin 798, 811
groins, 'hanging' 914

ground itch 931
growth **1695–700**
  adolescence and, constitutional delay (CDGA) 1697, **1703**
  in androgen deficiency 1683
  catch-up 1280
  in congenital adrenal hyperplasia 1665, 1666
  in Cushing's syndrome 1644, 1699
  disorders **1696–700**
  epochs 1696
  failure, in type II nutritional deficiency 1279
  fetal, *see* fetus, growth in fructosaemia 1347
  in growth hormone deficiency 1582
  in hypothyroidism 1698
  intrauterine retardation, drug abuse and 4298
  lung function variations 2673–4
  in marrow transplant recipients 3699
  metabolic/endocrine control 1562, 1696
  normal curve 1695–6
  in precocious puberty 1702
  at puberty 1696, 1701
  radiation-induced retardation 3575
  retardation, in coeliac disease 1918
  spurts, hypertrophic cardiomyopathy diagnosis 2386
  in thalassaemia 3504
  in von Gierke's disease 1342
growth factor(s) 66, *96*, **97**, **222–6**, 223, 2293
  in atherosclerotic plaque development 2293
  binding proteins 1554
  expression deregulation importance, evidence 223
  haemopoietic (HGFs) 67, **97**, 3382–3, 3384, 3557
    clinical use 3389
  importance in oncogenesis 222–3, 223
  in inflammation resolution 98
  in lung cancer 2882
  oncogenes encoding 223
  in osteoarthritis 2981
  overexpression, in animal tumours 223
  production by macrophage 93
  as target for anticancer drugs 225
growth factor receptors 223–4, *1560*, 1561, 2293
  alterations and cell transformation 224
  amplification 223–4
  endocytic pathway 73
  gene rearrangement 224
  importance in oncogenesis 223
  overexpression 223–4
    disease outcome and 224
  as target for anticancer drugs 225–6
growth hormone (GH) **1577–8**
  actions 1562–3, 1578
  binding protein 1554, 1577
  bone mass control 3057
  calcium regulation 1626
  deficiency 1571, 1582, **1698–9**
    acquired 1582, 1698
    congenital 1582, 1698
    diagnosis 1585, 1586, 1698–9
    hypoglycaemia 1511
  ectopic secretion 1593, 1715–16
  effect on bone 3059
  excessive secretion 1591, 1700
  gene family 1576
  gene mutations *1567*, 1571
  growth and 1696
  pattern of secretion 1565, 1578, 1698
  pituitary adenoma secreting 1569, 1591, 1748
  provocative tests 1584, 1698, *1699*, *4375*
  receptor 1556, *1560*, 1561, 1577
    defects *1567*, 1572, **1577**, 1699
    see also Laron dwarfism
  regulation of secretion 1577–8
  serum 1584, 1699
    in acromegaly 1593, 1594

  in combined anterior pituitary test 1585
  in insulin tolerance test 1585–6
  in oral glucose tolerance test 1586
  suppression, in obstructive sleep apnoea 2912
  treatment 1588, 1697, **1699**
    in Turner's syndrome 1700
  variant 1577, 1584
  gene 1576
growth hormone-releasing factor (GRF) 1892
growth hormone-releasing hormone (GHRH) 1577
  in acromegaly 1593
  combined anterior pituitary test 1585
  ectopic production 1591, 1593–4, 1707, 1715
  excessive secretion 1591, 1593–4
  receptor *1560*
  stimulation test 1698, *1699*
  treatment 1588
growth hormone-releasing peptide (GHRP) 1578
GTP 2253
  hydrolysis 69, 77, 1560, 1561
GTP-binding protein
  control of actin cytoskeleton 82
  GTP-γS 77, 78
  in heart 2147
  identification in cells 77–8
  Rab proteins *77*, 78
  ras protein homology 77, 82
  role in vesicular transport 77–8
  see also G-proteins
GTP/GDP-binding complex 69, 77
Guaitará fever, *see* bartonellosis
Guanarito virus 439
guanethidine block 2374, 3006, 3938
guanidine 4164
guanosine, accumulation 172
guanosine monophosphate (GMP), synthesis 1378
guanosine triphosphate (GTP), *see* GTP
guanosine triphosphate (GTP)
  cyclohydrolase deficiency 1363
guanylate cyclase 1561, 2296, 2297
  nitrates action 2326, 2327
Guillain-Barré syndrome *243*, **4101**
  arsenic poisoning 1106
  axonal 4101
  Campylobacter infections 558
  in malignancy 4102
  pathogenesis 4065
  pathophysiology 4091
  poliomyelitis *vs* 385
guilt, sexual problems associated 4245
guinea-worm disease, *see* dracunculiasis
gumma 708
  cutaneous 712–13
  mucosal 713
    differential diagnosis 713–14
  in syphilis 712, 2482
gums, in cyanotic congenital heart disease 2401
Gunther's disease (congenital porphyria) *1390*, **1395**
GUSTO trial 2340, 2342
  details 2342
  results 2342–3, 2343–4
gut-associated lymphoid tissue (GALT) **1836**, 2001, 3562
  organization 1836
'gut dialysis' 1050
gut flora, *see* intestinal flora
gut peptides **1891–4**
  in gastrointestinal disease **1894–6**
  localization 1891
  role 1891
  see also hormones
gynaecomastia **1687–9**
  in cirrhosis 2087
  drug-induced 1718–19
  in H_2-receptor blockade 1887
  in hepatocellular failure 2105
  in lung cancer 2884

in malnutrition 1284
physiological 1688
gyrate atrophy 1361

H

H⁺ K⁺-ATPase inhibitors, *see* ATPase
  inhibitors
H₁-receptor 158, 1886
H₁-receptor antagonists 158, 160, 162
  in allergic rhinitis 2718
  anaphylaxis prevention 160
  in urticaria 3772
H₂-receptor 158, 1886
H₂-receptor antagonists
  carcinogenic effects 1887
  carcinoid syndrome treatment 1898
  in gastrointestinal bleeding 1828, 1883
  in gastro-oesophageal reflux disease 1868
  in hepatocellular failure 2109
  overdose/poisoning **1070**
  in peptic ulcers 1886–7
    acute erosive ulceration 1880
    haemorrhage 1883
    long-term management 1889
  pharmacology 1886
  in polycythaemia vera 3434
  in pregnancy 1801
  in renal impairment 3274
  in renal transplant recipients 3314, 3320
  safety 1889
  side-effects 1887
  in urticaria 3772
  habits 3919
HACEK group 2437, 2439, 2442
  treatment *2447*, 2448
haem 3471
  biosynthesis **1389**
    lead effect on 1109
  metabolism 2054
  oxidation 3519
haemadsorption, *Mycoplasma
  pneumoniae* detection 764
haemagglutination, passive 597
haemagglutination inhibition test, dengue
  haemorrhagic fever 420
haemagglutinin 338
  clusters of stromal macrophage 86
  fibrillar 272
  measles 376
  mumps virus 372
haemagglutinin disease, cold, *see* cold
  haemagglutinin disease
haemangioblastoma **4033**
  intracranial 3963
haemangioendothelioma
  hypertension in 2298
  malignant, *see* liver tumours,
    angiosarcoma
haemangioma
  cavernous, haemolytic anaemia *3548*
  cerebellar, erythropoietin production
    3554
  gastrointestinal involvement 1998
  giant cavernous 3636
  hepatic 2119
  small bowel 1985
  strawberry **3785**
  of synovium 3003
haemangiopericytoma
  kidney 2548
  sclerosing, rickets in 3074
haem arginate 1393
haemarthrosis, in haemophilia 3004–5,
  3647, 3648–9
haematemesis 1827, 2093
  peptic ulcer haemorrhage 1882
  in rabies 400
haematin, therapy 1393
haematinics, poisoning **1070–1**
haematite lung 2846–7
haematocrit, *see* packed cell volume
haematological disorders **3375–700**
  in anorexia nervosa 4214
  assessment of clonality 3390–2

in chronic renal failure 3302
  clinical approach **3375–7**
  folate deficiency 3493
  history-taking 3375
  joint involvement **3004–5**
  laboratory investigations 3377
  liver in **2132–3**
  ocular features **4194–5**
  oral manifestations 1863–4
  physical examination 3375–7
  in pregnancy **1758–65**
  in systemic disease **3676–87**
  transient ischaemic attack due to 3950,
    3951
haematological malignancy
  human herpesvirus 6 infection 364–5
  see also leukaemia; lymphoma;
    myeloma
haematological syndromes,
  paraneoplastic *244*
haematological system, heart failure
  pathophysiology 2235
haematology (tests)
  in acute pancreatitis 2030
  in brucellosis 623
  in chronic obstructive airways disease
    2774
  in cirrhosis 2088–9
  in coeliac disease 1918
  in Crohn's disease 1940
  in cryptogenic fibrosing alveolitis 2791
  in diffuse parenchymal lung disease
    2781–2
  in haemolytic uraemic syndrome (HUS)
    3549, 3633
  in head injury 3686
  in heart disease 3687
  in infections 267
  in infective endocarditis 2442
  in Kawasaki disease 3048
  in leprosy 673–4
  in leptospirosis 701
  in malnutrition 1288
  in myocardial infarction 2339
  in plague 597
  in sarcoidosis 2829
haematoma
  after snake bites 1136
  muscle, in haemophilia 3647, 3649
  subdural, *see* subdural haematoma
  subperiosteal 2168
haematomyelia 3894
haematuria **3144–6**
  algorithm for investigation 3147
  in Alport's syndrome 3146, 3204
  benign familial 3152
  causes *3145*
  factitious 3146
  in focal segmental glomerulosclerosis
    3156
  glomerular origin 3103, 3145, 3149
  in haemolytic uraemic syndrome 3198
  in haemophilia 3648, 3649
  loin pain-haematuria syndrome 3148
  macroscopic,
    acute, with proteinuria 3146
    recurrent 3146
  in membranous nephropathy 3159
  in mesangiocapillary glomerulonephritis
    3158
  in minimal change nephropathy 3155
  persistent microscopic,
    isolated 3145–6
    with proteinuria 3146
  in polycystic kidney disease 3203–4
  proteinuria with 3138, 3146
    recurrent 3146
  red cell casts 3104
  in schistosomiasis 976, 979
  in sickle-cell disease 3195
  'synpharyngitic' 3150
  tests for 3102, **3145**
  urine microscopy 3103
Haemoccult test 3683
Haemocel 2400
haemochromatosis *1417*, *2018*, **2020–2**,
  3477

hereditary 3477, **3478–9**
  hypoparathyroidism 1634
  joint involvement 3005
  management and screening 2022
  osteoarthritis in 2978, 2979
  primary *2018*, 2020
  secondary *2018*, 2020, 3005
    causes 2022
  see also iron, overload
haemoconcentration
  in heat waves 1185
  winter mortality and 1185
haemodiafiltration *3308*
haemodialysis 3306, **3307–10**
  in acute renal failure *3286*, 3287
  adequacy 3309–10
  amyloidosis associated with 1513,
    1517–18, 1524, 3180, 3312
  anaemia and 3682
  in chromium poisoning management
    1108
  complications 3309
  drug clearance by 1056, 1061, 3270
  high-flux *3308*
  home *3307*, 3309
  iron overload 3481
  joint disorders in 3006
  in lithium overdose 1061
  platelet defects due to 3634
  in poison elimination 1051, 1056, 1061,
    3270
  preparation for 3306
  in salicylate poisoning 1056
  in sulphur mustard (mustard gas)
    exposure 1117
  technical aspects 3307–8
  vascular access 3308–9
haemodilution, in pregnancy 1758
haemodynamics
  cardiac, *see* cardiac haemodynamics
  in tetanus 625
haemofiltration 2581–2, **3308**
  in acute renal failure *3286*, 3287
  drug clearance by 3269–70
  fluid for 2581
  platelet defects due to 3634
  rates, access and process 2581
haemoglobin 3455–6, 3471, **3500–1**
  in acute pancreatitis 2030
  aggregated/precipitated 3525
  carbon monoxide affinity/binding 1095,
    2602–3
  catabolism 3456, **3526**
  in coeliac disease 1918
  concentration *3379*, *3380*
    in iron deficiency *3474*
    in polycythaemia 3433, 3551
  in RhD haemolytic disease of newborn
    3545
  in cyanosis 2651
  in cyanotic congenital heart disease
    2400, 2401
  degradation pathways 2054
  disorders **3500–20**
    classification 3501
    see also haemoglobinopathies
  exercise-induced anaemia 4326
  fetal, *see* haemoglobin F
  genetic control 3500–1
  glycosylated (A1) *1466*, **1480–1**, 3520
    see also haemoglobin A1C
  in heart failure 2235
  at high altitudes 1187
  high oxygen-affinity variants 3518–19,
    3554
  low oxygen-affinity variants 3519
  oxygen saturation 2221
    see also oxygen, arterial saturation
  plasma *3379*
    in pregnancy 1758
  red cell levels **3378–80**
  structural variants **3513–19**
    nomenclature 3513
  structure 3500
  synthesis 3501
  unstable disorders **3517–18**
  in urine, *see* haemoglobinuria

haemoglobin A (HbA) 3455–6, 3500
haemoglobin A1C 1480, 1565, 3520
  in diabetic nephropathy 3171
  diabetic retinopathy and 1482, 1483
haemoglobin A₂ (HbA₂) *3379*, 3500
  in thalassaemia 3504, 3506, 3511–12
haemoglobin Bart's 3508, 3509–10
  hydrops syndrome 1761, 3508–9, **3510**,
    3512
haemoglobin C 3465, 3517
  disease 3517
  thalassaemia 3506
haemoglobin Constant Spring 3509
haemoglobin D 3517
  haemoglobin D-Punjab 3465
haemoglobin E 3465, 3517
  disease 3517
  thalassaemia 3463, 3506–7
haemoglobin F (HbF; fetal) *3379*, 3500
  hereditary persistence 3501, 3507
  reactivation of synthesis 3388
  in thalassaemia 3504, 3506, 3507, 3511–12
haemoglobin Gower 3500
haemoglobin Gun Hill 3518
haemoglobin H 3508, 3509–10
  disease 3463, 3509, **3510**
    diagnosis 3512
    treatment 3513
  leukaemia and 3511
haemoglobin Kansas 3519
haemoglobin Lepore 3507
haemoglobin M 3519
haemoglobinopathies
  bone disease in **3095**
  geographical distribution **3463–5**
  joint involvement 3005
  malaria resistance 840, *841*
  in pregnancy 1741, **1760–1**
  see also sickle-cell disease;
    thalassaemia
haemoglobin Portland 3500, 3510
haemoglobin S (HbS) 3513–14, 3516, 4195
  haemoglobin D compound
    heterozygotes 3515
  thalassaemia *3463*, 3464, **3506**
haemoglobin SC disease (HbSC) **3517**, 4195
  distribution *3463*, 3464
  pregnancy in 1761
haemoglobinuria 2581, 3526
  in G6PD deficiency 3539
  haematuria *vs* 3145
  march 3550
  paroxysmal cold 3544
  paroxysmal nocturnal (PNH) 177, 181,
    3392–3, **3449–52**, 3550
    aetiology and pathogenesis 3449–50,
      3542
    aplastic anaemia and 3443–4, 3451
    blood picture 3451
    clinical findings 3450–1
    course 3451
    diagnosis 3451–2
    in pregnancy 1761
    thrombotic complications 3450–1,
      3452, 3668
    treatment 3452
haemolysin 272
  enterococcal 509
  in leptospirosis 698
  Streptococcus pneumoniae 511, 513
  Streptococcus pyogenes 498
haemolysis
  acute renal failure in 3289
  blood transfusion-induced **3691–2**
  cardiac **3547**
  chemically-induced **3546–7**
  compensated 3524
  compensatory mechanisms 3525–6
  consequences 3525, *3526*
  in haemolytic uraemic syndrome 3200
  heart valve replacement 2471
  liver in 2132
  in malaria 3680
  mechanisms 3525
  in paroxysmal nocturnal
    haemoglobinuria 3450
  in Wilson's disease 1420, 3550

haemolytic anaemia 3460, **3524–7**
  acquired **3541–50**
  aplastic crises 3449
  autoimmune *244*, **3543–5**, 3688
    cold syndromes *3543*, 3544
    drug-induced 3542–3
    in malignant disease 3421, 3677
    warm 3543–4
  in bartonellosis 775
  of burns 3550
  classification 3527
  congenital non-spherocytic 3536–7
  in congenital red-cell membrane defects **3527–33**
  diagnosis 3526–7
  in disseminated malignancy 3548, 3677
  drug-induced **3542–3**, 3546–7
  excess bilirubin production 2056
  ferrokinetic studies 3594
  of fetus and newborn (HDN) **3544–5**
  folate deficiency 3493
  in G6PD deficiency,
    acute attacks 3538–9, 3541
    chronic non-spherocytic 3540, 3541
  in haemoglobin variants 3517
  in haemolytic uraemic syndrome 3200, 3548–9
  in hereditary spherocytosis 3529
  immune **3542–5**
  infections causing 3545, 3679
  iron overload 3480
  in lead poisoning 1109
  in leptospirosis 698
  in liver disease 3550, 3684
  liver in 2132
  mechanical **3547**
  methaemoglobinaemia and 3520
  microangiopathic *244*, **3547–8**, 3633
    in pre-eclampsia 1728, 1763
  in *Mycoplasma pneumoniae* infection 763
  non-immune acquired **3545–50**
  in pregnancy 1761
  in pyrimidine-5′-nucleotidase deficiency 1387
  in red-cell enzyme deficiencies **3533–7**
  in sickle-cell disease 3514, 3515
  in SLE 3544, *3548*, 3681
  in unstable haemoglobin disorders 3518
haemolytic crises, in hereditary spherocytosis 3529
haemolytic disease of newborn (HDN) **3544–5**
haemolytic toxins, *Staphylococcus aureus* 524
haemolytic uraemic syndrome (HUS) **3196–202**, 3292, **3548–9**, 3632–3
  in adults 3196, *3197*
  aetiology 3196–8
  in children 3196, 3202
  clinical manifestations 3198, 3549, 3632–3
  definition 3196
  diarrhoea-associated (D+) 3196, 3198
  differential diagnosis 3200–1
  drug-induced 3197
  familial 3197
  haematological features 3549, 3633
  infective causes 3179, 3196–7
  intestinal ischaemia in 1995, 1996
  investigations 3200
  outcome 3201–2
  pathogenesis 3199–200, 3548, 3633
  pathology 3199
  postpartum 1734, 1763, 3201
  in pregnancy 3197, 3201
  sporadic, non-diarrhoeal (D-) 3196, 3197–8
  treatment 3201, 3549, 3633
  vero cytotoxin-producing *E. coli* (VTEC) causing 557
haemoperfusion
  in barbiturate poisoning 1060
  in digoxin overdose 1066
  in isoniazid poisoning management 1069
  in paracetamol poisoning 1053
  in poison elimination 1051

in sulphur mustard (mustard gas) exposure 1117
in theophylline poisoning 1068
haemopexin 3526
haemophagocytic lymphohistiocytosis 3608, **3609**
haemophagocytic syndrome, virus-induced 3524, 3586
haemophilia A **3646–51**
  carriers 1765, 3637, 3638–9, 3647
  chromosomal inversion in 108
  clinical features 3647–8
  crm+ 3637, 3638, 3647
  diagnosis 3637, 3648
  inheritance 3637
  inversions in 134
  molecular basis 3637–8
  pathogenesis **3637–9**
  pregnancy in 1765
  prenatal diagnosis 1765, 3638–9
  treatment 3648–51
haemophilia B 3637, **3639–40**, **3651**
  carrier detection 1765, 3639, 3640
  CpG mutational hot spot 108
  crm+ 3639
  diagnosis 3639
  haemarthrosis 3004
  inheritance 3639
  Leyden phenotype 3640, 3651
  molecular basis 3639–40
  mutations 104
  pregnancy in **1765**
  prenatal diagnosis 1765, 3640
  treatment *3649*, 3651
Haemophilia Centres 3648
haemophiliacs
  chronic active hepatitis C 2068
  haemarthrosis in 3004–5, 3647, 3648–9
  HIV infection in 4080
  haemophilic arthropathy, chronic 3647, 3649
  haemophilic cysts 3647
  haemophilic pseudotumours 3647
Haemophilus
  eye infections 4191
  rare species *556*
Haemophilus ducreyi **584–7**, 2005
  antibiotic susceptibility 586
  characteristics 584
  culture and diagnosis 585–6
  HIV-1 association 586
  infections in homosexuals 3363
  transmission 585
  see also chancroid
Haemophilus influenzae **580–4**
  capsule and antibodies for 581
  carriage and pathogenicity *581*, 4052
  characteristics 580–1
  colonization and infection mechanism 581, 4052
  immune responsiveness to 280
  minimal inhibitory concentrations 299, 300
  transmission 580
  vaccination 3530, 3596
  see also Haemophilus influenzae type b (Hib)
Haemophilus influenzae infections **580–4**, 2691
  acute exacerbation of chronic bronchitis 2692
  arthritis due to 2998
  in bronchiectasis 2760, 2763
  in chronic obstructive airways disease 2774
  conjunctivitis 584
  epidemiology and pathogenesis 581, 4052
  epiglottitis 582, 2691, 2722
  in HIV infection and AIDS 487
  in hypogammaglobulinaemia 168
  immunology 581
  intracranial abscess 4081
  maternal and neonatal sepsis 583
  meningitis, *see* meningitis
  non-typable species **583–4**
  otitis media and sinusitis 583, 2691
  passive immunization 584
  patterns 580

pneumonia 583, 2694, 2699, 2700
septicaemia 1020
treatment 584, 2763
see also Haemophilus influenzae type b (Hib)
Haemophilus influenzae type b (Hib) 580, 581–3
  cellulitis 582
  chemoprophylaxis 583
  epiglottitis 582, 2691
  immunization 583
  meningitis, *see* meningitis
  occult bacteraemia syndrome 582
  pneumonia and empyema 582
  septic arthritis 582
  staining and diagnosis 582
  treatment of diseases 582–3
  vaccine 284, 318, 583, 1028, 3530, 3596
    conjugate 583
    meningitis prevention 4050, 4059
haemopneumothorax 2868, 2870
haemopoiesis **3381–9**, 3588
  extramedullary, *see* erythropoiesis, extramedullary
  fetal switch 3382
  phylogeny and ontogeny 3382
haemopoietic growth factors, *see* growth factor(s), haemopoietic
haemopoietic organs 86–7
haemopoietic stem cells, *see* stem cells, haemopoietic
haemopoietic system
  occupational disease **1172–3**
  radiation syndrome 1219
haemoptysis **2643–4**
  in anti-GBM disease 3165
  in bronchiectasis 2760
  in cystic fibrosis 2748, 2753
  diseases associated 2644
  dyspnoea with 2162
  in Eisenmenger reaction (syndrome) 2410
  investigations 2644
    bronchoscopy 2579
  in lung cancer 2883
  massive 2162, 2644, 2803
    bronchial artery embolization 2656
  in mitral stenosis 2452
  in pulmonary atresia with ventricular septal defect 2408
  in pulmonary embolism 2524
  in pulmonary hypertension 2510
  treatment 2644, 2753
haemorrhage
  in anticoagulant-treated patients 1077, 3673, 3675
  in aplastic anaemia 3444, 3445
  blood volume changes and retransfusion 2565
  in dengue haemorrhagic fever 420
  epidural **3894**
  in hepatocellular failure 2102
  in Marburg virus and Ebola virus disease 441
  perioperative **3659–60**
    in cardiac surgery 3659–60
    in renal transplantation 3318
  in phaeochromocytomas 2554
  postpartum, in DIC 1762
  pulmonary, *see* pulmonary haemorrhage
  in relapsing fevers 694, 695
  retroperitoneal,
    in haemophilia 3647
    in phaeochromocytomas 2554
  thrombolytic therapy hazard 2341
  transplacental, anti-D immunization 3545, 3689
  vipers causing 1134
  see also bleeding; blood loss
haemorrhagic diathesis, in hepatocellular failure 2102, 2105, 2109
haemorrhagic disorders
  oral manifestations 1864
  in Rift Valley fever 428
haemorrhagic fever
  epidemic 3636
  hantavirus 3178

haemorrhagic fever with renal syndrome 426–7
  see also hantaviruses
haemorrhagic syndrome of Altimira 1011
haemorrhagins, in snake venom 1130
haemorrhoids, in pregnancy 1803
haemosiderin 3471, 3754
haemosiderinuria
  in haemolytic anaemia 3526, 3527
  in paroxysmal nocturnal haemoglobinuria 3450, 3451
haemosiderosis
  in haemolytic anaemia 2132
  idiopathic pulmonary 3685
  pulmonary 2180
  in pulmonary hypertension 2507, 2509
  see also iron, overload
haemostasis **3613–27**
  abnormal in dengue haemorrhagic fever 420, 421
  disorders **3627–30**
    in liver disease 3635, **3655–6**
    in pregnancy **1762–5**
    snake venoms causing 1129, 1130, 1139
    see also bleeding disorders; thromboembolism; thrombosis
  endothelial cell function 2298–9, **3626–7**
  platelet function in **3614–19**
  primary 3642
    disorders of, *see* platelet(s), disorders
  secondary, *see* coagulation
  see also fibrinolysis
haemostatics, local 3651
haemothorax **2868**
  treatment 2868
haem synthase (ferrochelatase) *1391*, 1395, 1396
Hafnia alvei 556
Hageman factor, *see* factor XII
Hailey-Hailey disease **3721–2**, 3760
hair
  bleaching 3765
  cycle/growth 3761–2
  disorders **3761–5**
    hirsutism 3764–5
  'forest' and 'flag' signs 1284
  growth stimulation 3764
  ingrowing 3764
  lanugo 1674, 3761, 3765
    in anorexia nervosa 1297, 4213
  loss 3761–2
    baldness 3762
    chemotherapy-induced 248
    examination of causes 3761–3
    management 3764
    see also alopecia
  in malnutrition 1284
  in Menkes disease 1417
  normal growth in women 1674
  number 3761
  pregnancy-related changes 1804
  pulling/twisting 3763
  transplants 3764
  unwanted 1669–70
hair bleaches 3736
hairdressers 3738
hair dyes 3736
hair follicles, *Staphylococcus aureus* infection 526
hair-shaft
  congenital defects 3763
  injury 3763
hairy-cell leukaemia, *see* leukaemia, hairy-cell (HCL)
hairy cells 3423
hairy leucoplakia 357, 471
  in AIDS 357, 470, 474
halitosis **1864**, 1964
Hallervorden-Spatz disease **4009**
hallucinations
  in acute paranoid reactions 4223
  in Alzheimer's disease 3973
  auditory,
    in elderly 4227
    in schizophrenia 4221
  in cerebral tumours 4236, 4237

in depressive disorders 4218
fungal poisoning causing 1156
hypnagogic **3928–9**
plants causing *1156*
in schizophrenia 4221
'third person' 4221
visual,
in partial seizures 3914
in schizophrenia 4221
hallucinogenic drugs 4263
psychiatric disturbances from 4241
hallucinosis, alcoholic, schizophrenia *vs*
4222
hallux valgus
in myositis ossificans progressiva 3093
in rheumatoid arthritis 2958
halofantrine, in malaria 852
halo naevus 3758, 3759
haloperidol
in delirium 4224
dosage and monitoring 4252
emergency treatment of disturbed/
violent patients 4257
indications and use 4251
overdose/poisoning 1061
halothane, malignant hyperpyrexia 1182
halothane hepatitis 2125
halzoun 987, 1012
hamartoma, oral 1859
Hamman-Rich syndrome 2786
Hamman's sign 1746, 2869
hammer toe deformity 1489, 1490
Ham (acidified serum) test 3451
hand(s)
in acromegaly 1592
in bone disease 3061
calluses on, in bulimia nervosa 1300,
4216
dermatitis 3735
management 3807
in diabetes mellitus 1487
herpes simplex infection 3352
injuries **2996**
median nerve lesions 4096
osteoarthritis 2978, 2979
in rheumatic diseases 2946
in rheumatoid arthritis 2957
swelling, in scleroderma 3028
ulnar nerve lesions 4096–7
washing, respiratory viruses
transmission prevention 333
hand arm vibration syndrome 1226, *1226*
handedness **3847**
hand, foot and mouth disease 383–4, 1850
hand and foot syndrome 3514
handicap
assessment in osteoarthritis 2981
in cerebral palsy 4119, 4121
definition *2943*
Hand-Schüller-Christian disease 3606
hang-gliders 2361
'hanging groins' 914
hanseniasis, *see* leprosy
Hansen's disease, *see* leprosy
Hantaan virus 423, 425, 426
hantavirus disease **426–7**
acute renal failure 3292
clinical features 426
haemolytic uraemic syndrome *vs*
3200–1
haemorrhagic fever **3178**
treatment, prognosis and control 426
hantaviruses 423, *424*, **425–7**
transmission 426
Haplorchis pumilio 996
'happy puppet' syndrome, *see* Angelman
syndrome
haptens 141
haptocorrins (R binders) 3485, 3486,
3495
haptoglobin, serum *3379*, 3526
Harada Mori technique 931
hard metal disease 2847
hardwood dust, nasal sinus and nose
cancers association 205
Hardy-Weinberg equilibrium 117
three allele system 117
Harrison's sulci 2649

Harris's syndrome 4026
Hartmann's procedure 1971
Hartnup syndrome (neutral
aminoaciduria) *1337*, 1357, 3330,
3332, **3333**
Hashimoto's thyroiditis 1570–1, 1609,
1615
Hassall's corpuscle 3794
'hatter's shakes' 1111
haverhill fever 687–8
hayfever 160, 161, 2714, 3741
see also allergic rhinitis, seasonal
hazards, identification 1178
HBV, *see* hepatitis B virus (HBV)
hCG, *see* human chorionic
gonadotrophin
HCV, *see* hepatitis C virus (HCV)
HDL, *see* high density lipoprotein
head
abnormal enlargement in infancy
4114–15
circumference 4114
fetal 1756
injury, *see* head injury *(below)*
in respiratory disease 2652
tremor 4012
headache **4022–9**
acute **4027**
in acute mountain sickness 1188
after lumbar puncture 3842, 3907
'alarm-clock' 4026
in benign intracranial hypertension
4041
in carcinomatous 'meningitis' 250
causes *4022*
in pregnancy *1767*
in cerebral metastases 250
cervicogenic 4028
chronic/recurrent, causes *4022*
cluster **4026**
cranial neuralgia 4023–4
in elderly **4028–9**
in eosinophilic meningitis 946
in essential hypertension 2534
food intolerance 1844
hypnic **4029**
in intracranial disease **4027**, 4035
in intracranial tumours 250, 4038
in Lassa fever 431
in leptospirosis 700
management, in intracranial tumours
4038
mechanisms **4022–4**
referred pain 4023
trigeminal nerve 4022
in meningitis,
bacterial 4053
meningococcal 539
viral 4066
morning 2534
muscle contraction, *see* headache,
tension
nitrates causing 2327, 2344
pain mechanism 4022–3
in paroxysmal nocturnal
haemoglobinuria 3450
in pituitary apoplexy 1598
pituitary tumours causing 1581, 1591
postspinal 3842
post-traumatic **4028**
in Q fever 743
raised intracranial pressure 4027, 4035
in suprasellar germinoma 1598
tension 4023, **4026–7**
chronic 4026–7
in pregnancy *1767*
in typhoid 562
management 564–5
see also facial pain, atypical; migraine
head injury **4044–50**
Alzheimer's disease risk 3972, 3973
artificial nutritional support 1323
assessment of symptoms/disability
4028, *4028*
causes of hypoxia/hypotension 4045,
4045
chronic subdural haematoma 3970

diabetes insipidus 3120
electroencephalogram (EEG) 3830
epilepsy after 3916
guidelines,
for coma patients *4048*
for hospital admission *4048*
for neurosurgeon consultation *4048*
for skull radiography *4047*
haematological changes 3686
headache after **4028**
late sequelae and disability 4048–9
management in acute stage 4045–8
diagnosis 4046–7, *4047*
intracranial complications 4047–8
resuscitation 4045–6
multiple injuries with 4048, *4048*
myositis ossificans after 3093
pathology 4044–5
brain damage 4044–5, *4044*
extracranial complications 4045, *4045*
intracranial complications 4045, *4045*
persistent vegetative state after 3935
positive-pressure ventilation in 2577
see also brain damage
head lice **1002–3**, 1004, 3744
Heaf test 645
equivalence to Mantoux test *646*
health
for all by the year 2000 46, 52
benefits of exercise 4324
community **39–46**
definition 35, 39
demographic status and 51
as ecosustainable state 39
modernization and **35–9**
surveillance, occupational diseases 1162
health care
delivery systems **52–4**
in developing countries 52–3
trends and issues 53–4
in developing countries **51–4**
equitable allocation 52
financing 52, 53
insurance 38
levels 47
management, epidemiology in 46
per capita expenditure 38, 52
policy, evolution 51–2
primary, *see* primary health care
secondary 47, 48–9
tertiary 47
universal, requirements 38
health care staff
attitude in malnutrition management
1295
hepatitis B vaccination 454
infectious hazards 1173
meningococcal infection prophylaxis
544
tuberculosis case-finding 646
health centres 49
health education
after malnutrition 1294
HIV infection 484
skin disease management 3804, 3805
sun exposure dangers 3728
health promotion 50
health and safety **1160–80**
safety engineer 1160
see also occupational disease/hazards;
occupational health
Health and Safety Commission (HSC)
2357
Health and Safety Executive 1175
Health and Safety at Work Act (1974)
1161, 1179, 2356–7
hearing
conservation **1224–5**
diving and 1205
noise effect on **1223–4**
hearing loss 1223
in acoustic schwannomas 3874
after noise 1224
in Alport's syndrome 3204
cochlear 3870
conductive and sensorineural 3870
desferrioxamine-induced 3512
in Lassa fever 432

in Ménière's disease 3875
noise-induced, investigation **1225**
permanent 1224
tests 3870
see also deafness
heart
abscess 2215
absolute refractory period 2152
action potential 2148, 2149, 2152, 2259
drugs affecting 2263
afterload 2150, 2155, **2156**, 2246
in heart failure 2246
vasodilators affecting *2246*, 2247
ventricular volume and **2157**
amyloidosis 1517, 1522, 2216
anomalies, in congenital rubella
syndrome 410
apex, in elderly 4342
apex beat, *see* apex beat
apical impulse 2383
autonomic activity 2160
diurnal variation 2160–1
autonomic dysfunction, in diabetes
1489
bidirectional shunting 2180
biochemistry **2143–51**
biopsy,
in hypereosinophilic syndrome 2397
see also endomyocardial biopsy
block, after coronary artery bypass
grafting 2355
aortic stenosis *vs* 2464
atrioventricular, *see* atrioventricular
block
bundle branch, *see* bundle branch
block
in Ebstein's anomaly 2414
in myocardial infarction 2346
in neonatal lupus 3022
in rheumatoid arthritis 2392
treatment 2346
blood supply, *see* coronary blood flow
calcification, chest radiography 2182
catheterization, *see* cardiac
catheterization
cells in 2143
see also myocardial cells
cellular structure **2143–5**
in Chagas' disease 896, 897, 898
chest radiography 2178, 2656
abnormal 2181–2
clinical physiology **2152–62**
clockwise/counter-clockwise rotation
2185
collagen and fibronectin in 2145
compliance, age-related changes 4335
conducting system 2152, 2259
accessory, ablation 2266
accessory atrioventricular 2193, 2275,
2276
ACE inhibitor action 2249
anomalous in ventricular pre-excitation
2193, 2275
concealed accessory pathway 2275
digitalis action 2241
digitalis sensitivity 2242–3
disorders 2259–60
disturbances and syncope 2173
idiopathic fibrosis 2268, 2285
lithium and carbamazepine action
4251
conduction velocity 2152
contractility, maximum dP/dt 2157,
2224, 2230
contraction 2144
electrophysiology **2148**, 2152–3, 2259
energy for **2145–7**
frequency, *see* heart rate
inotropic state and **2150**, **2157–8**
intracellular calcium concentrations
2148, 2259
maximum velocity 2224–5
mechanics **2149–50**, **2154–5**
see also myocardial cells
Corynebacterium diphtheriae effect 494
cycle **2152–3**
mechanical events 2153
disease, *see* heart disease

heart (cont.)
disorderly action (panic disorder) 4207
Doppler echocardiography, see Doppler
  echocardiography
drug toxicity, see cardiotoxicity
ectopic beats, see cardiac arrhythmias,
  extrasystoles electromechanical
  dissociation, management 2284, 2285
electrophysiological testing,
  after myocardial infarction 2347
  in hypertrophic cardiomyopathy 2388
electrophysiology 2148–9, 2152–3,
  2259
  arrhythmias 2259–61
  delayed after-depolarization 2149,
    2260
  depolarization 2149, 2150, 2152,
    2192, 2259
  disorders of impulse formation and
    conduction 2259–60
  drugs prolonging repolarization 2260
  early after-depolarization 2149, 2260
  effective refractory period 2259
  premature depolarization, see cardiac
    arrhythmias, extrasystoles
  repolarization 2149, 2152, 2259
  testing 2261, 2280, 2286
  see also cardiac arrhythmias
emboli sources 3949, 3949, 3960
end-systolic volume and pressure
  2149–50
energy requirements 2145–7, 2145
enlargement, in heart failure 2229
in enterovirus infections 386–7, 387
exercise and 2161
  training effect 2161–2
failure, see heart failure
filling pressures 2154, 2220, 2223
  measurement 2220–1
  in myocardial infarction 2568
  in pulmonary embolism 2569
function,
  in acute mountain sickness 1189
  age-related changes 4334–5
  assessment 2177–228
  computed tomography 2218
  indices 2221, 2223
  normal parameters 2154, 2223
  see also left ventricle (ventricular),
    function
function, regulation 2155–61, 3883
  blood pressure regulation 2156
  blood volume regulation 2156–7
  contractility and inotropic state 2150,
    2157–8
  heart rate 2158
  outflow resistance, see heart, afterload
  venous return and preload 2155–6,
    2246
  ventricular volume and afterload 2157,
    2246
gallop rhythm 2523, 2524
haemodynamics, see cardiac
  haemodynamics
in heterophyiasis 998
in HIV infection and AIDS 477,
  2394–6, 2395
'hyperkinetic' 2169
in hypertension 2532–3, 2533–4
hypertrophy, see cardiac hypertrophy
inotropic agents effect 2150, 2157–8,
  2242
  measurement 2157–8
ischaemia, see myocardial ischaemia
junctional (nodal) premature beats 2198
left-sided obstructive lesions/anomalies
  2421–4
left-to-right shunt 2180, 2461
  in corrected transposition 2417
  in ductus arteriosus 2430
  ostium secundum defects 2424, 2425
in leptospirosis 700
limiting oxygen delivery 2605–6
magnetic resonance imaging 2213
  see also magnetic resonance imaging
    (MRI)
magnetic resonance spectroscopy
  2213–14
in malaria 845

mechanics (of contraction) 2149–50,
  2154–5
mechanoreceptors 2160
metabolic studies by PET 2212
missed beats (extrasystoles) 2175, 2176
  see also under cardiac arrhythmias
murmurs, see heart murmurs
muscle 2143–52
  see also myocardial cells; myocardium
myotomy/myectomy, in hypertrophic
  cardiomyopathy 2389
myxoma, see cardiac myxoma
nervous system and 2160, 2165
normal pressures 2154, 2223
nuclear imaging 2204–12
  see also scintigraphy
oedema 2238
in osteogenesis imperfecta 3080
oxygen supply and demand 2160
pacemaker tissues 2152–3
preconditioning 2151
preload 2155–6, 2246
  in heart failure 2246
  nitrates reducing 2327
  vasodilators affecting 2246, 2247
premature beat, see cardiac arrhythmias,
  extrasystoles
pressure overload 2147
pressure-volume relations 2149–50
rate, see heart rate
relaxation 2153, 2155
'remodelling' 2147, 2151, 2229
  prevention 2230
  in rheumatoid arthritis 2961
  in rickettsial diseases 731
right-sided obstructive lesions and
  anomalies 2419–21
right-to-left shunt 2181
  cyanosis in 2402
  dyspnoea in 2163
  Ebstein's anomaly 2414
  polycythaemia in 3554
  total anomalous pulmonary venous
    drainage (TAPVD) 2415
rupture, in myocardial infarction 2321,
  2341
in sarcoidosis 2827
size 2179
'snowman' silhouette 2415
sounds, see heart sounds
sympathetic nervous system 2160,
  2170, 2253, 2282
thrombus,
  computed tomography 2218
  in hypereosinophilic syndrome 2390,
    2397, 2398
  magnetic resonance imaging 2215
training effect 2161–2
transmembrane and intracellular
  signalling 2147
transplantation, see cardiac
  transplantation; heart-lung
  transplantation
tumours 2472
  computed tomography (CT) 2218
  liver in 2130
  magnetic resonance imaging 2215
  metastatic 2215
  see also cardiac myxoma
valves, see heart valves
vegetations 2457, 2462
  endocarditis 2438, 2439, 2440, 2449
venous return 2155–6
ventricular premature beats, see
  ventricular extrasystoles
volume overload 2147
weight 2143
see also entries beginning atrial; left
  ventricle (ventricular); right ventricle
  (ventricular); ventricle (ventricular)
heartburn 1819, 1866
retrosternal 2167
heart disease
assessment 2177–228
  chest radiography in 2177–82
chronic, in enterovirus infections 387
congenital, see congenital heart disease
coronary, see coronary artery disease

cyanotic, polycythaemia in 3551
diabetic 1491–2, 3172
in elderly 4341–4
in essential hypertension 2532–3
evaluation, in pregnancy 1736
haematological changes 3687
at high altitudes 1192
ischaemic, see ischaemic heart disease
in pregnancy 1735–40
psychological treatment affecting 4232
rheumatic, see under rheumatic fever
symptoms 2162–77
  breathlessness 2162–5
  cachexia 2176–7
  chest pain 2165–9
  classification 2358
  in elderly 4341–2
  fatigue 2171–3
  oedema 2169–71
  palpitations 2175
  syncope 2173–5
  work (employment) and 2357–8, 2358
  see also individual symptoms
in systemic sclerosis 3030–1, 3031
thromboembolism in 3668
valvular, see heart valves, disease
see also heart muscle disease
heart failure 2228–38, 2515
acute 2229
  causes 2151
  dyspnoea in 2163
acute on chronic 2229
acute renal failure 3299
aetiology 2151, 2229, 2230
after Fallot's tetralogy repair 2407
in anaemia 3459, 3462
cardiac output impairment 2230,
  2568–9
in Chagas' disease 897, 898
chronic 2229
  causes 2151
  dyspnoea and lungs in 2231, 2232,
    2241
  dyspnoea pathophysiology 2163–4,
    2231, 2232
  heart enlargement 2149, 2229
clinical assessment 2235–6
congestive, see congestive heart failure
definitions and classification 2228–9
in diabetes 1492
dialysed patients 3312
in dilated cardiomyopathy 2384
driving after 2359
drug prescribing in renal impairment
  3273
in elderly 4342
epidemiology 2229
fatigue in 2171, 2233
features 2228–9
'forward failure' 2171, 2228
in hereditary haemochromatosis 3479
'high output' 2170, 2228
hypoglycaemia in 1510
in infective endocarditis 2440, 2449,
  2450
liver in 2138, 2235
'low output' 2170, 2228
in megaloblastic anaemia 3496–7
in myocardial infarction 2338
oedema in 2169–71, 2234, 2238,
  2239–41
  causes of sodium retention 2169–70
  diuretic-resistant 2239–40, 2240
  diuretic therapy 2238–41
  reasons for sodium retention causing
    2170–1
  sodium retention mechanism 2170
in Paget's disease 3076
pathophysiology 2151, 2229–35
  autonomic/neuroendocrine systems
    2233–4
  cardiac functional changes 2230–1
  cardiac structural changes 2229–30
  haematological system 2235
  kidney 2234–5
  muscle hypothesis 2234, 2235, 2236
  musculoskeletal 2232, 2233
  other systems 2235

pericardial 2231
peripheral vascular 2231
renin-angiotensin-aldosterone system
  2233, 2234
respiratory 2231–3
'postoperative' 2481
in pregnancy 2383
prognosis 2236–7
  markers 2237, 2237
as progressive disorder 2249–50
pulmonary oedema in 2231, 2241,
  2499, 2500, 2566–8
  management 2504
renal failure in 2235
response to exercise 2232
in septicaemia 2573
sympathetic nervous system in 2177,
  2234, 2253–5
sympathetic tone and 2170
treatment 2236, 2237
  ACE inhibitors 2248–51
  catecholamines 2253–5
  digitalis 1250, 2241–6
  in dilated cardiomyopathy 2384
  diuretic resistance 2239, 2240
  diuretics 2238–41
  in elderly 4342
  non-pharmacological 2236, 2238
  vasoconstrictors 2254
  vasodilators 2246–52
  see also specific drug types
in trichuriasis 943
see also left ventricle (ventricular),
  failure; left ventricular disease/
  dysfunction; right heart failure
heart-lung transplantation 2592, 2933–9
in bronchiectasis 2766
causes of death 2933, 2933
choice of operation 2934, 2934
in cystic fibrosis 2754, 2937
'domino' operation 2934
donor selection and organ procurement
  2934–5, 2935
  prostacyclin infusion 2934
in Eisenmenger reaction (syndrome)
  2412, 2934
exercise and dyspnoea perception
  2937–8, 2938
graft versus host reactions 2936
immediate postoperative care 2935
indications 2934
infections after 2709, 2936, 2937
lymphoproliferative disease after 2937
nephrotoxicity and hypertension after
  2937
obliterative bronchiolitis after 2796,
  2937
patient selection 2933–4, 2934
in primary pulmonary hypertension
  2513
reoperation 2935
survival 2933
technique 2935
see also cardiac transplantation; lung
  transplantation
heart murmurs
Austin Flint, see Austin Flint murmur
in cardiac myxoma 2473
in coarctation of aorta 2558
Cole-Cecil 2465
continuous, in ductus arteriosus 2430,
  2431
delayed diastolic,
  in aortic regurgitation 2455
  in mitral stenosis 2453
  in tricuspid stenosis 2468
diastolic,
  in aortic regurgitation 2455, 2465
  in Eisenmenger reaction (syndrome)
    2411
  in Fallot's tetralogy 2403
  in hypertrophic cardiomyopathy 2387
ejection systolic 2461
  in aortic stenosis 2325, 2462, 2463
  in Fallot's tetralogy 2402, 2406
  in fixed subaortic stenosis 2422
  in hypertrophic cardiomyopathy 2387
Graham-Steell 2467, 2469

in infective endocarditis 2440
in infundibular stenosis 2421
in mitral prolapse 2460
in mitral regurgitation 2458, 2459
in ostium secundum defects 2425
pansystolic,
  in Eisenmenger reaction (syndrome)
    2410
  in mixed mitral valve disease 2456
  in papillary muscle dysfunction 2459
  in pulmonary valve stenosis 2419
  in tricuspid regurgitation 2469
  in ventricular septal defects 2429
in pregnancy 1735
in pulmonary arterial stenoses 2409
in pulmonary atresia with ventricular
  septal defect 2408
in rheumatic fever 2433
systolic 2411
  causes 2421
  in pulmonary hypertension 2510
in total anomalous pulmonary venous
  drainage (TAPVD) 2415
'tumour plop' 2473
venous hum 2415
heart muscle diseases **2380–98**
in HIV infection and AIDS **2394–6**
idiopathic, see cardiomyopathy
secondary causes 2383
specific 2380, 2383
  dilated cardiomyopathy vs 2381
  miscellaneous 2393–4
  in neuromuscular disorders **2392,**
    2393
  in systemic vasculitis **2391–2,** 2392
  zidovudine-induced damage 2395
  see also cardiomyopathy; myocarditis
heart rate 2143, 2154, **2158,** 2605
  digitalis effect 2243
  exercise effect 2161, 2226
  in myocardial infarction 2568
  myocardial oxygen demand 2323
  variations, low frequency in heart
    failure 2232, 2234
  work (employment) and 2357
heart sounds 2153
  A2-P2 interval 2425
  in aortic regurgitation 2465
  in aortic stenosis 2462, 2463
  in cardiac myxoma 2473
  in dilated cardiomyopathy 2383
  in Ebstein's anomaly 2414
  in Eisenmenger reaction (syndrome)
    2410
  ejection click, in Fallot's tetralogy 2403
  in elderly 4342
  in Fallot's tetralogy 2402
  first 2153
  in fixed subaortic stenosis 2422
  fourth 2153
  in hypertrophic cardiomyopathy 2387
  in left atrial myxoma 2454
  in mitral regurgitation 2458
  in mitral stenosis 2453
  in mixed mitral valve disease 2456
  in myocardial infarction 2335
  opening snap 2453
  in ostium secundum defects 2425
  in pregnancy 1735
  in pulmonary atresia with ventricular
    septal defect 2408
  in pulmonary embolism 2524
  in pulmonary hypertension 2510
  in ruptured chordae tendineae 2458
  second 2153
  summation gallop 2510
  systolic click 2410
  'tapping apex', in mitral stenosis 2453
  third 2153
  in pulmonary hypertension 2510
  in rheumatic fever 2433
  in transposition of great arteries 2416
  'tumour plop' 2454
heart valves
  abnormalities, in carcinoid syndrome
    1897, 1898, **2469**
  calcification 2399, 2419, 2421
  see also under specific valves

disease **2451–72**
  in aircraft crew and pilots 1200–1
  Doppler echocardiography 2201–3
  heart failure in 2230
  magnetic resonance imaging 2216,
    2217
  in pregnancy 1737–8
  in rheumatoid arthritis 2961
infections, see also endocarditis
prostheses **2469–71**
  calcification 2470
  causes of postoperative fever 2445
  complications 2470–1
  Doppler echocardiography 2203, 2470
  dysfunction 2470–1
  dysfunction diagnosis 2471
  endocarditis, see infective endocarditis
  follow-up 2471
  haemolysis due to 3547
  infection 2470
  limited function 2470
  mortality and prognosis 2470
  'patient mismatch' 2470
  in pregnancy 1739
  regurgitation 2470–1
  types 2469–70
replacement,
  in aircraft crew and pilots 1200–1
  in infective endocarditis 2449
  see also heart valves, prostheses;
    individual valves
right, Doppler echocardiography 2203
see also individual valves
heat **1180–1**
effects on body 1180
injury, prevention, in marathons and
  mass runs 4328
loss from body 1180
  in cold conditions 1182
  in marathons and mass runs 4328
  prevention of immersion hypothermia
    1183
pain treatment 3943
production, after injury 1549
radiant, skin cancer 3791
heat exchangers 2816
heat exhaustion, salt-/water-depletion
  1181
heat-gain centre 1180
heat-loss centre, damage 1180
heat-shock proteins
  Behçet's syndrome aetiology 3044
  cross-reactions 155
  function, folding of polypeptides 69
  hsp70 69
  oral ulceration aetiology and 1853
heat stroke 1180–1, **4128**
  acute renal failure 3293
  causes and diagnosis 1180
  neurological features 4128
  treatment 1180–1
heat urticaria 3771
heat waves 1185
Heberden's nodes 2978, 2979, 2985
Hebra nose 568, 569
heel entheses, erosions 2971, 2972
Heerfordt-Waldenstrom (uveoparotid
  fever) syndrome **2821,** 2826
height
  in body mass index assessment 1281,
    1282
  critical values 1697, 1700
  loss 3066
  in Marfan's syndrome 3083
  normal growth curve 1695–6
  predicted adult 1697, 1700
  see also short stature; tall stature
Heimlich manoeuvre 2721
Heinz bodies 2054, 3378, 3518
  in chemically-induced haemolysis 3547
  in G6PD deficiency 3539
Helicobacter, rare species 556
Helicobacter cinaedi 778
Helicobacter pylori 1884, 1884–5, 2005
  antibiotic sensitivity 2005
  antibodies, tests 1878
  culture and serology 1885
  cytotoxin (CagA gene product) 1884

diagnosis of infections 1885
duodenal ulcer aetiology 1877, 1878,
  1884–5, 2005
effect on duodenal ulcers 1885
eradication 1883, 1885–6, 1890
  failure 1885–6
  indications for 1885–6
gastric cancer association 203, 1884,
  1886, 1982
  pathogenesis 1982
gastric lymphoma and 3583
gastric ulcer aetiology 1879
gastritis and,
  acute 2005
  chronic active 1982, 1985, 2005
  endoscopy indication 1829
prevalence 1884
transmission/infection mechanism
  1884–5
helix-loop-helix (HLH) proteins 3396
Heller's operation 1959
HELLP syndrome 1728–9, 1730, 1763,
  1797
  management 1798
helminths 2708
  malabsorption in tropics and 1930
  meningitis due to 4070
  myositis due to 4155–6
  see also cestodes; nematodes;
    trematodes
hemianopia, bitemporal 1581, 1589
hemiasomatognosia 3854
hemiballism 3862, **4014**
hemichorea **4014**
hemifacial spasm **3879–80,** 4016
hemimegalencephaly 4113
hemiparesis
  ataxic 3956
  coma in 3930
hemiparkinsonism 4002
hemiplegia
  bilateral **4120**
  in cerebral hemisphere infarct 3955
  in malaria 846
  pain 4340
  spastic **4120**
hemithorax
  increased transradiancy **2662,** 2662
  opacification 2661
hemitrunk **2431**
hemizygous 104
HEMPAS (hereditary erythroblastic
  multinuclearity with positive acid
  serum lysis) 3524
Henderson-Hasselbalch equation 1535
Henoch-Schönlein (anaphylactoid)
  purpura 3010, 3015, **3149–52,** 3167,
  3636–7
  clinical course 3150
  diagnosis 3150
  gastrointestinal tract in 2000, 3723
  joint involvement 3004
  pathogenesis 3151–2
  pathology 3150–1
  response to treatment 3017
  skin in 3773, 3774
  treatment 3152
  Wegener's granulomatosis vs 3013
Hep-2 cells, Escherichia coli adherence
  555
heparan sulphate 109, 2299, 3622, 3626,
  3662
  amyloid fibril-associated 1521
  anti-DNA antibodies cross-reaction
    3024
  in diabetes mellitus 3169
heparin 3671, **3673**
  in cardiopulmonary bypass 3660
  in coronary angioplasty 2352
  in deep vein thrombosis 2523
  in DIC 3659
  endothelial cell production of 2290
  in GUSTO trial 2342
  in hyperfibrinolysis 3659
  in inherited thrombophilias 3667,
    3668
  low molecular weight preparations
    2526, 3673

in Marburg virus and Ebola virus
  disease 442
mode of action 3622, 3673
in nephrotic syndrome 3142
osteoporosis and 3070
in pregnancy,
  in inherited thrombophilias 3668
  in primary antiphospholipid syndrome
    3670
  prophylactic 1739, 1740, 1743, 1811,
    3675
  thromboembolism therapy 1742, 1743
in pulmonary embolism 2525, 2569
renal bone disease and 3327
reversal with protamine sulphate 1254
in septicaemia treatment 1025
side-effects 2344
snake bite management 1139
thromboembolism prophylaxis 3670,
  3676
thrombolytic therapy in myocardial
  infarction with 2343–4
in unstable angina 2330
in vasculitis 3777
heparin-binding epidermal growth factor
  (HB-EGF) 2293
heparin cofactor II 3379, 3623, 3673
  deficiency 3667
hepar lobatum 714
hepatectomy, partial
  hepatic failure after 2100
  in hepatic metastases 2119
hepatic adenoma, see hepatocellular
  adenoma
hepatic arteriography, in hepatocellular
  carcinoma 2116–17
hepatic artery
  aneurysm 2139
  embolization 1705, 2119
    carcinoid syndrome treatment 1898
    in hepatocellular carcinoma 2117–18
  occlusion 2139
hepatic blood flow 2091–2
  measurement 2056
hepatic cirrhosis, see cirrhosis
hepatic coma **4124**
hepatic decompensation 2082, 2085,
  2087
  investigations 2088
  surgery risk 2091
  see also cirrhosis, decompensated
hepatic disorders, see liver disease
hepatic ducts 2045
hepatic encephalopathy **2101–2, 4124**
  acute/chronic 2102
  in ascites management 2097
  chronic 2102, **4124**
    management 2108
  in cirrhosis 2087, 2089
  clinical approach 2105
  clinical signs 2101–2, 2105
  clinical stages 2101, 2102, 2105
  course and prognosis 2107
  diagnosis/investigations 2105
  drug pharmacodynamics 1252
  factors precipitating 2102
  in fulminant hepatic failure 2100
  liver transplantation in 2112
  management 2090, 2107–8, 2108
  oesophageal varices complication 2094
  pathogenesis 2102
  pre-encephalopathy stage 2106
  reversible 2103
  see also hepatocellular failure
hepatic failure, see hepatocellular failure
hepatic fibrosis, see liver, fibrosis
hepatic granulomas **2120–4**
  causes 2120, 2121, 2121, 2123, 2134
    chemicals 2121–2, 2122
    drugs 2121–2, 2122, 2128, 2128
    immune disorders 2122, 2131
    infections 2121, 2133
    tumours and miscellaneous 2122–3
  classification 2120, 2121
  clinical features 2120
  diseases associated 2121–3
  'doughnut' in Q fever 743
  investigations 2123

hepatic granulomas (*cont.*)
　pathogenesis 2120
　pathology 2120
　treatment 2123
hepatic metastases 204, **2119**
　carcinoid tumours 1897, 1898, 2119
　staging methods 246
hepatic necrosis
　in acute cardiac failure 2138
　in acute viral hepatitis 2061
　bridging 2072
　caseous 2120
　centrilobular, occupational causes
　　1172
　drug-induced 2124–5, *2126*
　in hepatocellular failure 2106
　in Lassa fever 434
　in leptospirosis 699
　piecemeal 2065, 2069, 2072
　subacute 2065
hepatic portoenterostomy (Kasai's
　operation) 2015
hepatic vein
　obstruction, *see* Budd-Chiari syndrome
　thrombosis 2098
hepatic venography
　in Budd-Chiari syndrome 2098
　in portal hypertension 2093
hepatic veno-occlusive disease **2099**,
　2129
hepatic venous congestion 2138–9
　in heart failure 2235
hepatic venous outflow obstruction 2092,
　2092
hepatic venous pressure 2092, 2093
hepatic venous pressure gradient
　(HPVG) 2092, 2093
hepatitis
　acute, drug-induced 2124–5, *2126*
　acute cholestatic, drug-induced 2125,
　　2127
　acute viral **2061–4**
　　acute hepatic failure 2100
　　clinical features 2061, *2061*
　　treatment 459
　alcoholic, *see* alcoholic hepatitis
　autoimmune, *see* autoimmune hepatitis
　chronic,
　　aetiology 2064–5
　　cirrhosis *vs* 2089
　　drug-induced 2129, *2129*
　chronic active 2065–9
　　autoimmune, *see* autoimmune hepatitis
　　causes 2069, *2070*
　　cryptogenic 2068, 2070, 2073
　　definition 2065
　　hepatitis B, *see* hepatitis B
　　hepatitis C 2068–9
　　hepatocellular carcinoma in 2116
　　histology 2062, 2065, 2069
　　in inflammatory bowel disease 2131
　　liver transplantation in 2112
　　in pregnancy 1800
　　in Wilson's disease 1420
　　see also hepatocellular carcinoma
　chronic lobular 2065
　　histology 2062
　chronic persistent 2065
　　histology 2062
　chronic viral **2064–9**
　　treatment 459
　　see also hepatitis, chronic active
　cryptogenic 2068, 2070, 2073
　cytomegalovirus 2064
　delta, *see* hepatitis D
　in drug abusers 4279
　drug-induced 2124–5, *2126*, *2127*
　　antituberculous therapy 658
　enterovirus infections 387
　Epstein-Barr virus (EBV) 2064
　familial granulomatous 2123
　fulminant, in Wilson's disease 1420
　granulomatous 2121, 2123
　　drug-induced 2128, *2128*
　halothane 2125
　immunization, postnatal 4299
　neonatal 2131
　non-A, non-B 458, 459
　　see also hepatitis C

　non-A, non-B, non-C, transmission in
　　blood 3693
　occupational causes 1171
　post-transfusion, *see* hepatitis C
　in Q fever 743
　'rebound' 2068
　sporadic 2068
　syphilitic 711
　tienilic acid causing 2125
　viral 448–60, **2061–9**
　　acquired from liver graft 2114
　　aplastic anaemia in 3441, 3680
　　diagnosis *2063*
　　in immunocompromised 1034–5
　　jaundice in 2056
　　in pregnancy **1798–9**
　　transmission in blood **3693**
　　treatment 459
　　see also hepatitis, acute; hepatitis,
　　　chronic; *specific hepatitis viruses*
hepatitis A **449–51**
　clinical course 2062
　clinical features 2061–2, *2061*
　diagnosis 2061, *2063*
　in haemophilia 3650
　in homosexuals 3364
　IgM antibodies 2061
　immunoglobulin 450
　incubation period 449, 2061
　in pregnancy 1798, 1799
　prevention 450–1, 2061–2
　　passive immunization 450, *450*
　vaccine 319, 323, **450–1**, 2061
　　killed 450
　　live attenuated 450–1
hepatitis A virus (HAV) 382, 449, 2061
　classification 449
　genome 449–50
　transmission 449, 2061
　　in blood 3693
　cockroaches in 1011
hepatitis B **451–7**
　acute 451, 2062–3, 2067
　　management 2062–3
　alcoholic liver disease relation 2081
　anti-HBe-positive 456
　　treatment 2068
　anti-HBe seroconversion 457, 2062,
　　2066, 2068
　arthritis in **3001**
　chronic active 451, 2062, 2065–8
　　clinical features 2067
　　efficacy of treatment 459
　　immune defects 2065, 2066
　　liver damage mechanism 2065–6
　　management 459, 2067
　　prevalence 2065
　　prognosis 2067, 2068
　　cirrhosis in 2066, 2067
　　liver transplantation in 2112
　clinical course 2066
　clinical features 451, *2061*
　diagnosis 2062, *2063*
　in drug abusers 4279
　epidemiology 461
　in haemophilia 3650
　HBe-antigen positive 2062, 2066, 2067,
　　3364
　　management 2067–8
　HBs-antigen positive 2065, 2067, 3364
　hepatitis D virus co-/superinfection 457,
　　2064
　hepatocellular carcinoma association
　　204, **457**, 460, 2065, 2066, 2115–16
　　aflatoxin synergism 461
　HIV co-infection 4302
　in homosexuals 3364
　immunization 227, 453–6, 463
　　of adolescents 454
　　development of new strategies 454–5
　　homosexuals 3364
　　indications for 453–4
　　of infants 454–5
　　neonatal 204
　　passive 453
　　UK policy 454
　　see also hepatitis B, vaccines
　in immunocompromised 1034–5

　immunoglobulin (HBIg) 453
　　neonates 1781
　importance, in chronic hepatitis 2067
　infectivity of blood 2067
　in neonates and children 2062
　　'normal carrier' 2066
　persistent infection 457, 2062
　polyarteritis nodosa association 3011
　in pregnancy 1798–9
　prevention and control 452–6, 463
　renal disease in **3175–6**
　　glomerulonephritis 3157, 3176
　　membranous nephropathy 3159,
　　　3175–6
　　vasculitis **3178**
　in renal transplant recipients 3314, 3320
　risk to health care workers 454, 1173
　treatment 459
　urticaria in 3771
　vaccines 284, 318, 324, 1035, 1799,
　　2063
　　a epitope in 453
　　chemically synthesized 456
　　in haemophilia 3648
　　HBV resistant to 456
　　hybrid virus 455
　　neonates 1781
　　novel using hybrid particle 455
　　polypeptide 455
　　pre-S epitopes in 455
　　reactions after 453
　　recombinant 455
　　sites for administering 453
hepatitis B virus (HBV) 449
　antibody escape mutants 456
　carriers 3364
　core antigen (HBcAg) 451–2, 455, 457
　　DNA integration 457, 462, 2115–16
　e antigen (HBeAg) 1035, 2062, 2066
　　escape mutants 1781
　genome organization 452
　　x gene 452, 457, 462
　HBe-antigen-negative mutant 457, 2066
　insertional mutagenesis 457
　intrauterine/perinatal infection 1776,
　　1781, 1798
　oncogenic mechanism 457, 2066,
　　2115 16
　precore mutants 456–7
　pre-S region 451, 455, 456
　replication 451, 452
　structure 451–2
　subtypes 453
　surface antigen (HBsAg) 451, 455,
　　2062, 3364
　　chemically synthesized 456
　transmission 2062, 2067
　　in blood 3693
　　drug abusers 4279, 4302
　　sexual 1798
hepatitis C **458–9**
　acute 2063–4
　in AIDS 2135
　alcoholic liver disease relation 2081
　autoantibodies in 2071
　chronic active 2068–9
　　treatment 2068, 2069
　clinical course 2063, 2064
　clinical features *2061*, 2063
　cryoglobulinaemia in 3183
　cryptogenic cirrhosis due to 2114
　diagnosis 458, 2063, *2063*
　in drug abusers 4279
　in haemophilia 3648, **3650**
　hepatocellular carcinoma association
　　461, 2063, 2116
　in homosexuals 3364
　in hypogammaglobulinaemia 169
　intrauterine/perinatal infection *1779*,
　　1781, 1798
　management 459, 2063–4
　nephropathy associated with 3157, **3176**
　in pregnancy 1798, 1799
　vaccines 458
hepatitis C virus (HCV) 449, **458–9**
　antibody tests 458, 2072
　detection using PCR 458, 2072
　in factor VIII preparations 3695

　gene clones 2063
　genome organization 458–9, 2063
　role in autoimmune hepatitis 2072,
　　2072
　transmission 458, 2063
　　in blood 3693
　　drug abusers 4279
hepatitis D **457**, 2064, 4279
　clinical features 457, *2061*
　diagnosis *2063*
　in homosexuals 3364
　in pregnancy 1798, 1799
hepatitis D (delta) virus (HDV) 449, **457**,
　　2064, 3364
　delta antigen (HDAg) 457
　structure and replication 457
hepatitis E **451**
　clinical features *2061*
　diagnosis *2063*
　in haemophilia 3650
　in pregnancy 1776, 1777, 1798, 1799
　transmission 451
hepatitis E virus (HEV) 449, **451**, 2064
　detection 451
　genome 451
hepatobiliary surgery, in primary
　　sclerosing cholangitis 2079–80
hepatoblastoma, HCG production 1714
hepatocellular adenoma 1724, 2119,
　　2129
　drug-induced 2129
　oral contraceptives and 1724
hepatocellular carcinoma (hepatoma)
　　204, **2115–18**
　aetiology 2115–16
　cirrhosis 2090, 2116
　drugs 2129
　hepatitis B virus, *see under* hepatitis B
　hepatitis C virus 461, 2063, 2116
　alpha-fetoprotein in 2090
　ascites in 2096
　clinical features 2116
　epidemiology 204, 2115
　erythropoietin production 3554
　fibrolamellar variant 2013, 2112, 2115
　in hereditary haemochromatosis 3478,
　　3479
　histology 2115
　hypoglycaemia in 1509–10
　investigations 2116–17
　oral contraceptives and 1724
　prognosis 2117
　recurrence, after transplantation 2112,
　　2113
　screening 2117
　treatment 2117–18
　　liver transplantation 2112, *2113*, 2117
　tumour markers 2116
hepatocellular failure **2100–11**
　acute 2100
　　course and prognosis 2106–7
　　definition 2106
　　diagnosis/differential diagnosis 2106
　　jejunoileal bypass causing 2139
　　liver transplantation in 2113
　　management 2108–9
　　monitoring and infections 2109
　　mortality and complications 2106
　　in pregnancy 1799
　　see also hepatocellular failure,
　　　fulminant
　aetiology 2100–1, *2101*
　in autoimmune hepatitis 2073
　chronic 2100, 2101, 2107
　　diagnosis 2106
　　management 2107–8
　clinical features 2101–5, 2129
　　cardinal features 2101–3
　convalescence 2110
　course and prognosis 2106–7
　definitions 2106
　diagnosis 2105–6
　fulminant 2100
　　in acute viral hepatitis 2061
　　in Budd-Chiari syndrome 2098
　　definition 2100
　　diagnosis/differential diagnosis 2106
　　drug-induced 2100

in Hodgkin's disease 2133
management 2108–9
metabolic alkalosis 1536
in paracetamol poisoning 1053
in Wilson's disease 2023
see also hepatic encephalopathy
in Gaucher's disease 2025
late-onset 2100
long-term sequelae 2107
management 2107–9
of specific problems 2109–10
temporary hepatic support 2110
metabolic complications 4124
paracetamol-induced 1052, 1053, 2106, 2107
pathology 2106
in primary biliary cirrhosis 2074, 2107
subfulminant 2100, 2106, 2107
management 2108–9
see also hepatic encephalopathy
hepatocellular injury, hypoxic 2100
hepatocellular jaundice, see jaundice, hepatocellular
hepatocellular necrosis, see hepatic necrosis
hepatocytes
damage,
in autoimmune hepatitis 2072
detection 2055
iron stores 3471, 3472
lipid accumulation 2025
piecemeal necrosis 2065, 2069, 2072
regeneration, in chronic active hepatitis 2065
in Reye's syndrome 2025
hepatolenticular degeneration, see Wilson's disease
hepatomegaly
in amoebiasis 829
in cirrhosis 2088
in congestive cardiac failure 2130
in haemochromatosis 2020
in malnutrition 1283
in primary biliary cirrhosis 2074
hepatoprotective agents 2084
hepatopulmonary syndrome 2130
in hepatocellular failure 2104
management 2110
hepatorenal syndrome 3293
in hepatocellular failure 2103–4
management 2110
occupational causes 1171
hepatosplenic disease
chronic candidiasis 1035
'decompensated' 977
in schistosomiasis 977, 979
hepatotoxicity
carbon tetrachloride poisoning 1085
chloroform 1086
drugs, see liver damage, drug-induced
glue sniffing 1092
iron overdose 1070
vinyl chloride, see vinyl chloride
hepatotoxins, occupational 1171, 1172
Hepatovirus 449
herald patch 3751
herbal medicines 1159–60, 1159
labelling problems 1159
Herbert's pits 750
herbicides 1120
bipyridilium (paraquat) 1120–1
chlorates 1121
chlorophenoxyacetate 1121, 1121
glyphosate-containing 1121
poisoning 1120–2
triazine 1122
herd immunity 316
hereditary angio-oedema 162, 180, 2721–2, 3771, 3774
attacks and diagnosis 180, 2721
diagnosis and treatment 2722
inheritance 180
mortality 2722
prophylaxis 2722
treatment 180, 2722, 3772
hereditary ataxia 3984–5
early/late onset 3984
see also Friedreich's ataxia

hereditary bulbar palsy 4089
hereditary cerebral haemorrhage with amyloidosis (cerebral amyloid angiopathy) 1514, 1516–17, 3972
Dutch type 1516–17, 1519–20
Icelandic type 1516
hereditary disorders 100
use of term 100
hereditary exostoses, multiple 3089
hereditary motor and sensory neuropathy (HMSN) 4102–3
leprosy vs 674
type I/II and X-linked 4102–3
type III (Dejerine-Sottas disease) 4103
hereditary myasthenia 4164
hereditary non-polyposis colon cancer (HNPCC) 107, 223, 1990
hereditary optic atrophy 3867
hereditary sensory neuropathies 4103–4
hereditary spastic paraplegia 3985, 3995
Hering-Breuer input 3887
Hermansky Pudlak syndrome 1365, 3759
hermaphroditism, true 1688, 1690, 1694
hernia, hiatus, see hiatus hernia
heroin, see diamorphine
herpangina 383, 1850
herpes blattae 1011
herpes gestationis (pemphigoid gestationis) 1805
herpes gladiatorum 344
herpes labialis 343, 2695
recurrent, see cold sores
herpes simplex virus (HSV)
carriers 342
culture 3353
drug resistance 346
genes and RNAs 342
serology and monoclonal antibodies 346
transmission 342
type 1 (HSV-1) 342, 1848, 3351
cold sores 343, 4067
gingivostomatitis 1848–9, 1848
latent in trigeminal ganglion 1849
recurrent infections 1849–50
see also cold sores
type 2 (HSV-2) 342, 344, 1848, 3351
CNS infection 4064
in pregnancy 1775
herpes simplex virus (HSV) infections 341–6
Behçet's syndrome aetiology 3043
clinical features 342–6, 3780
CNS infections 344–5, 4064
congenital 345
conjunctivitis 4192
diagnosis 346
encephalitis 344–5, 4065
clinical features 4068
mental disorders/symptoms 4236
pathology 4066
epidemiology 341–2, 342
erythema multiforme and 346
facial, in sports trauma and 4324
gastrointestinal 2005
genital, see genital herpes
in HIV infections 479, 479, 488, 4193
in homosexuals 3361, 3363–4
in immunocompromised 345, 346
infection route 342
intrauterine/perinatal infection 1780–1
neonatal 345, 346, 3352
ocular 344
oral 1848–50
orofacial infections 342–3
pathogenesis 342
pneumonia after lung transplantation 2936
in pregnancy 1775–7, 1781, 1799
primary perianal 3363
in renal transplant recipients 3320
skin disorders 345–6
traumatic herpes (scrum pox) 344
treatment and prevention 346, 3364
visceral and disseminated 345
whitlow 343–4
herpesviridae 347, 352

herpes viruses 341–65
infections in pregnancy 1775–7
intrauterine/perinatal infections 1779–81
viruses included 342
herpesvirus simiae 357
herpes zoster (shingles) 341, 343, 346, 348–50, 1850
autonomic 349
complications 349–50
'geniculate' and 'otic' 3879
in HIV infections 487–8
in immunocompromised 349–50
in immunosuppressed patients 347
in infancy 1780
management 350–1
motor 349
ophthalmic 3878, 4192
in HIV infection 4193
in pregnancy 1780
in renal transplant recipients 3314, 3320
root lesions in 3903
see also varicella-zoster virus (VZV) infections
herpetic stomatitis 342, 343, 345, 1034, 1848–9, 1852
herpetic whitlow 343–4
herpetiform ulcers, see oral ulceration
Hers' disease (glycogen storage disease VI) 1343, 1344
Hess (tourniquet) test 3628
Heterophyes heterophyes 996, 998
heterophyiasis 998
heteroplasmy 64, 128
heterosexual 3349, 3350
see also sexual intercourse
heterozygote advantage 114
heterozygotes 114
compound 104
detection 115 frequency 117, 132
population screening 133
testing 132
heterozygous 104
Heubner's endarteritis obliterans 4084
hexachlorobenzene 1395
hexamethyl propylene amine oxime (HM-PAO) 1941, 3824, 3825
hexamine hippurate, in urinary-tract infections 3213
n-hexane
neuropathy 4100
poisoning 1083
hexite 1114
hexokinase deficiency 3536
hexosaminidase deficiency 4089
hexose monophosphate shunt 3456, 3534, 3535
Heymann nephritis 3159
HHH syndrome 1361
hiatus hernia
gastro-oesophageal reflux in 1958
rolling 1872
sliding 1872
Hib infections/vaccine, see Haemophilus influenzae type b (Hib)
hiccup 3890
persistent, causes 3889, 3890
Hickman lines 2752
HIDA scans
in biliary disease 2046
extrahepatic biliary atresia 2015
'hidebound' bowel 1909
hidradenitis suppurativa, anaerobic infections 573
high altitudes, see altitudes, high
high-density lipoprotein (HDL) 1401, 1402, 1403–4
alcohol consumption increasing 2314
cholesterol 1404, 1405–6
in diabetes 1458
genetic deficiency 1414
heterogeneity 1404
in nephrotic syndrome 3143
in polycystic ovary syndrome 1676
reduced,
factors causing 2308
ischaemic heart disease risk 2308
structure 1400

high molecular-weight kininogen (HK) 3621
deficiency 3652
high-pressure nervous syndrome 1207
hilar lymphadenopathy 2783
chest radiography 2783
in Chlamydia psittaci infection 755
drug-induced 2852
in sarcoidosis 2821, 2823
Hill's model of muscular contraction 2154, 2157
hillwalkers, frostbite and exposure 1184
hindfoot, valgus deformity 2958
hindgut 1973
Hindus
folate deficiency 3492
vitamin B$_{12}$ deficiency 3468, 3492
hip
congenital dislocation, osteoarthritis in 2978
osteoarthritis 2975, 2978, 2979, 2980
pain 2996
replacement,
ossification after 3093
prostheses 2964
in rheumatoid arthritis 2964
in rheumatic diseases 2946, 2959
in rheumatoid arthritis 2959
transient osteoporosis, see algodystrophy
hippurate (hippuran), radiolabelled 2549
clearance 3108
renal imaging 3112
Hirano bodies 3972
Hirschsprung's disease 1825–7, 1960, 1979
embryology 1973
gut peptides in 1896
RET oncogene mutation 104
Hirschsprung's enterocolitis 1979
hirsutism 1669–70, 1674, 3764–5
causes 1674–6, 3765
in congenital adrenal hyperplasia 1664, 1668
in Cushing's syndrome 1643
drug-induced 1718
facial 3716
idiopathic 1676
management 1677
in polycystic ovary syndrome 1674, 1676
in pregnancy 1804
treatment 3765
hirudin 1150
recombinant 1150
His, bundle of 2148, 2152, 2259
ablation 2265, 2273
radiofrequency ablation 2266
Hissette-Ridley fundus 915
histamine 1142, 1886
in carcinoid tumours 1898
cells releasing 2727, 3770
excess release, gastric hypersecretion in 1881
gastric acid and pepsin release 1886
in immediate hypersensitivity 158, 278
intradermal 3771
metabolism 1142
in peptic ulcers 1886
receptors 158, 1886
release, in asthma 2727, 2728
in urticaria/angioedema 162, 3770, 3771
histamine-like syndrome, see scombrotoxic poisoning
histamine-producing enterochromaffin (ECL) cells 1894
histamine-releasing factors 157
histidinaemia (histidase deficiency) 1375
histidine 1353
histiocytes 3576
histiocytic medullary reticulosis 3586
histiocytoma, open-lung biopsy 2688
histiocytosis 3606–10
classification 3606
class II 3606, 3609
class III 3606, 3609–10

histiocytosis (cont.)
  class IV 3606
  Langerhans-cell (histiocytosis X) 2833,
    3565, 3586, **3606–9**, 3606
    chest radiography 2782
    clinical features 3607–8
    cutaneous manifestations 3799
    definition/nomenclature 3606
    diagnosis/evaluation 3608
    histology 3606
    incidence 3606–7
    management 3608–9
    open-lung biopsy 2688
    pathogenesis 3606
    pulmonary **2832–3**
    splenomegaly in 3591
    see also Hand-Schuller-Christian
      disease; Letterer-Siwe disease
  malignant 1927, 3608, **3609–10**
  sea-blue 3591
  sinus, with massive lymphadenopathy
    3566, 3608, **3609**
histones 59
histones H2A/B, antibodies 3025
histopathology, cancers 242–5
Histoplasma capsulatum 803–5
  eye infection 4192
Histoplasma duboisii 488
histoplasmosis **803–5**
  acute pulmonary 804–5
  African (large-form) 805
  chronic pulmonary 805
  classical (small-form) 803–5
  disseminated 805
  hepatic granulomas in 2121
  mediastinal fibrosis 3246
  primary cutaneous 805
histrionic (hysterical) personality 4212
His-Werner disease (trench fever) **747–8**
'hitch-hiker's thumb', see Z-deformity
Hitzig zones 4085
HIV **463–7**
  antibody tests, blood donors 3694
  carcinogenesis mechanism 462
  drug actions/targets 297, 298
  in factor VIII preparations 3695
  genes 464, 465
  gag, env and pol 464
  HIV-1 463, 467
    epidemiology 463, 483
    genome 464
    Haemophilus ducreyi and 586
    incubation and transmission 463–4
    perinatal transmission 1782
    spread 463
    strongyloidiasis and 928
    see also HIV infection
  HIV-2 463, 467
    epidemiology 483
    genome 464
    incubation and transmission 463–4
    perinatal transmission 1782
  immunopathological mechanism 278, 466
  immunosuppression due to 174, 466,
    1850, 4278
  infection, see HIV infection
  lifecycle 298
  occupational hazard, health care
    workers 1173
  proteins 464, 465
    gag protein 464
    gp120 464, 465
    p24 464, 470–1, 471
    tat protein 464
  provirus 463
  receptors 91, 465, 466
    CD4 150, 465, 466, 1850
    galcer 466
  replication 464
    inhibitors 464
  structure 466
  syncytium-/non-syncytium-inducing
    strains 465
  transmission 461, 463–4, 468, 483–4,
    484–5, 3345
    in blood **3693–4**
    by blood transfusion **3693–4**
    control/prevention 288, **484–5**
    drug abuse and 4298

heterosexual 3351, 4281
  to neonates 4298
  oral 1850
  perinatal 1782
  in tuberculosis treatment 664
  vertical 478, 485
tropism 465–6, 467
vaccines 463, 465, 1782
variation 464–5
HIV-1-associated cognitive-motor
  complex (HCMC) 476, **4077–8**
  clinical features and treatment 4077–8
  see also AIDS dementia complex
hives 162, 3771
HIV infection **467–83**
  acute 469–266
  aplastic anaemia 3441
  arthritis in 3002
  asymptomatic 4303
    neurological features **4075–6**, 4076
  at-risk populations 1850
  bacillary angiomatosis in 747
  chronic 470
  classification of stages 469, 469, 470
  clinical features 469–70, 485–8, 1850–1
    in developing countries 485–8
    presentation 485
    spectrum 469, 485
  complications **473–7**
    see also AIDS and HIV infection
  control/prevention 3348
  course/natural history 466–7, 468–9,
    1850
    asymptomatic period 468–9
    progression rate 469
  cytotoxic T-cells in 151, 466, 467, 471
  in developing countries **483–9**, 3348
    clinical features 485–8
    strategies for coping 488–9
  diagnosis 471, 485, 3694
  diffuse parenchymal lung disease in
    2781
  donovanosis and 777, 778
  in drug abusers, see drug abuse(r) and
    misuse
  encephalopathy, see AIDS and HIV
    infection
  epidemiology 468, 483–5, 3348
    demography 484
    patterns 468
    prevalence 468, 484
  genital herpes with 3351, 3352
  giardiasis in 475, 879, 1034
  glomerulonephritis in **3176**
  Guillain-Barré syndrome in 4101
  haematological changes 3680
  in haemophiliacs 3648, **3650**
  hepatitis B co-infection 4302
  historical background 467–8
  HIV-positive non-progressors 466–7
  hypoglycaemia in 1511
  intrauterine/perinatal 1782–3
  lung disease 4285
  lymphocytic infiltration of lung 2807
  lymphoproliferative disorders 3566
  management,
    asymptomatic patients 471–2, 483
    symptomatic patients 472–3
    see also AIDS and HIV infection
  neurological features **4075–6**, 4076
    primary infection illness **4075**
  neuropathy in 4101
    inflammatory 4076
    sensory 4076
  oral contraceptive users 1724
  pathogenesis 466–7, 1850
  persistent generalized lymphadenopathy
    470, 485
  polymyositis in 4076
  in pregnancy 1776, 1779, **1782–3**
  pretest counselling 471
  prevention in drug abusers 4275
  prognostic laboratory markers 470–1,
    471
  progression, mycoplasmas role 772
  public health and personal health
    perspectives 4302
  pulmonary hypertension in 4285

Reiter's syndrome with 2972
  in renal transplant recipients 3314
  seroconversion 466, 469
  sexual behaviour and 3349, 3350
  Sjögren's syndrome in 3036, 3037
  'slim' disease 485, 487, 4078
  subclinical intellectual decline 4076
  thrombocytopenia in 3631, 3632, 3680
  thrombotic thrombocytopenic purpura
    in 3198
  tuberculosis in, see under AIDS and
    HIV infection
  vitamin B$_{12}$ deficiency 3491
  see also AIDS and HIV infection
HIV wasting syndrome, see under AIDS
  and HIV infection
HLA (antigens) 142–3, 183, 3689
  Addison's disease and 1652
  adult Still's disease and 2974
  allergic drug reactions and 1252
  alloimmune thrombocytopenia and
    1764
  anti-GBM disease and 3164
  atopic disease and 158
  autoimmune hepatitis and 2071–2
  Behçet's syndrome and 3043, 4183
  chronic renal failure and 3303
  coeliac disease and 1917, 1918
  common varied immunodeficiency
    (CVID) and 167
  congenital adrenal hyperplasia and
    1666
  diabetes type I and 1453–4
  disease associations 145
  extrinsic allergic alveolitis and 2813
  genes 183
  gold nephrotoxicity and 3262
  haplotype and linkage equilibrium
    110–11
  infections and 279–80
    outcome relationship 280
  influence on immune responses 280
  insulin antibodies and 1477
  lichen planus and 3751
  malaria risk/susceptibility 280
  matching in transplantation 184
    cardiac transplantation 2256
    renal transplantation **3316**, 3317
  membranous nephropathy and 3159
  minimal change nephropathy and 3155
  myelomatosis and 3597
  narcolepsy and 3928
  paracoccidioidomycosis susceptibility
    816
  pemphigoid gestationis and 1805
  pemphigus vulgaris association 3781
  penicillamine nephrotoxicity and 3266
  polyglandular failure type II and 1571
  presensitization to, in cardiac
    transplantation 2256
  primary sclerosing cholangitis 2077–8
  psoriasis and 3745
  rheumatoid arthritis and 2954–5, 2956
  sarcoidosis and 2820
  schistosomiasis 976
  sensitization, renal transplantation and
    3316
  serological specificities/listing 144
  SLE association 3025, 3026
  in transfusion reactions 3692
  transient postpartum thyroid disease and
    1750
  transplantation and 3315–16
  see also major histocompatibility
    complex (MHC)
HLA-A 110, 142
HLA-B 110, 142
HLA-B5, Behçet's syndrome and 4183
HLA-B27 2953, 2965
  ankylosing spondylitis and 111, 2965,
    2966, 4185
  frequencies in seronegative
    spondarthropathies 2966
HLA-BW51, Behçet's syndrome and
  4183
HLA-C 142
HLA-DP 143
  matching in grafts 184

HLA-DQ 143
  matching in grafts 184
HLA-DR 143
  matching in renal grafts 184
HLA-DR2
  primary sclerosing cholangitis 2077,
    2078
  ulcerative colitis association 1944
HLA-DR3 143
  SLE association 3025
HLA-DR4
  Felty syndrome and 2955
  rheumatoid arthritis and 2955, 2956
HLA-DR8, primary biliary cirrhosis
  2074
HLA-DRB1 2955
HLA-DRQ, in coeliac disease 1918
HLA-DRw52a, primary sclerosing
  cholangitis 2077, 2078
HM-PAO 1941, 3824, 3825
h*MSH*2 gene 107, 129
hoarseness 2611
  in oesophageal cancer 1981
  in rheumatoid arthritis 2959
  in thyroid disorders 1610
  in Wegener's granulomatosis 3012
hobbies, diffuse parenchymal lung
  disease and 2782
Hodgkin's disease 3568, **3569–76**
  aetiology 3569–70
  age relationship 197
  amyloidosis 1513
  clinical features 3570
  complications of treatment 3574–5
  epidemiology 213
    incidence 3569
  Epstein-Barr virus (EBV) role 213,
    355–6
  hepatic granulomas in 2122
  investigations 3572–3
  liver in 2132–3
  lung involvement 2690
  lymphocyte depleted 3571
  lymphocyte-predominant 3571, 3575
  management 3571–6
  mixed cellularity 3571
  neuropathy in 4102
  nodular sclerosing 3570–1, 3575
  non-Hodgkin's lymphoma vs 3579
  pathogenesis 3569
  pathological features 3570–1
  Pel-Ebstein fever 241
  in pregnancy 1808
  prognosis 3575–6
  pulmonary involvement 2808
  renal disease in 3154, 3185
  skin manifestations 3797
  splenectomy in 3595
  staging 247, 3571–2
  toxoplasmosis in 867
  treatment 3573–4
Hoffmann's sign 3857
Hoffmann's syndrome 4125
Holmes-Adie syndrome 3877
holocarboxylase synthetase 1373
  deficiency 1374
holoprosencephaly 4112–13
Holter monitoring, see electrocardiogram
  (ECG), ambulatory
Holt-Oram syndrome 2425
Homan's sign 2523
home
  evaluation, for artificial nutrition at
    home 1324
  myocardial infarction management 2336
  nutritional support, see nutritional
    support
homeodomain proteins, in leukaemia
  3396
homeostasis, hormonal control 1562–3
homeotic genes 66
homoallelic 104
homocitrullinuria, hyperornithinaemia
  with hyperammonaemia and (HHH
  syndrome) 1361
homocysteine 1365, 1366
  defects of remethylation 1367
  serum 3495

homocystine, plasma 1366, 1367
homocystinuria *1337*, **1366–7**, 3083,
  3084–5, 3493, 3668
  biochemical features *3062*
  lens dislocation 4181
homogentisate oxidase 3085
homogentisic acid 1365, 2979, 3004
  accumulation 3085
homologous restriction factor (C8bp) 3450
homoplasmy 128
homosexual behaviour **3351**, 3360
homosexuals 3349, **3360–6**
  behavioural changes 3346, 3360
  HIV infection 3361
  lymphogranuloma venereum 760, 3363
  medical conditions in **3365–6**
  mycoplasma infections and AIDS 772,
    773, 3363
  Mycoplasma and *Ureaplasma* infections
    3363
  sexually transmitted diseases in 3351,
    3360–5
  approach to **3360–2**
  bacterial infections **3362–3**
  clinical features 3361
  epidemiology 3360
  examination/investigations 3361–2
  history-taking 3360, 3361
  infection types **3362–5**
  intestinal features *3362*
  nematodes **3365**
  organisms 3360, *3362*
  protozoal **3364–5**
  syphilis 708, 710, 712, 719, **3362**
  viral infections **3363–4**
  urinary-tract infections 3206
homovanillic acid, in Parkinson's disease
  4000
homozygosity mapping 106
homozygotes 114
homozygous 104
hookworm **929–33**, 3463
  biology 930
  haematological changes 3680
  as occupational disease 1173
  prevention 932, 3470
Hoover's sign, in chronic obstructive
  airways disease 2774
hormone(s) **1553–73**
  anabolic and catabolic 1274
  balance, in malnutrition 1286
  binding proteins 1554
  biosynthesis and secretion 1557–60
  bone formation/resorption affected by
    3057
  in chronic renal failure 3327
  counter-regulatory 1562–3
  deficiency states 1566, *1567*, 1570–2
  definition 1553
  ectopic production 1566–8, **1711–12**
    in lung cancer 2883–4
  excess states 1566–70
  families 1555–7
  feedback regulatory systems 1564–5,
    1574–5, 1578
  functions 1562–3
  gastrointestinal, *see* gastrointestinal
    hormones
  gene mutations *1567*, 1571–2
  gene transcription 1557–60
  glycoprotein, *see* glycoprotein
    hormones
  historical aspects 1553
  infection susceptibility 281
  integrated responses 1563–4
  mechanisms of action 1273, 1274,
    1553, 1554–5, 1560–2
  nature 1554
  pathways of action 1564–5
  peptide 1554, 1559
  receptors, *see* receptors
  reference range *4368*
  regulation of substrate metabolism
    1273–4, *1274*
    short-term effects 1273, *1275*
  replacement therapy 1587–8
    in ovarian failure, *see* hormone
      replacement therapy

resistance 1566, *1567*, 1572–3
response element (HRE) 1558, 1562
rhythms 1565–6
second messenger signalling pathways
  1554, 1555, 1560–1
  mutations affecting 1572–3
SLE association 3017
steroid, *see* steroid hormones
see also gut peptides; *specific hormones*
hormone replacement therapy (HRT)
  1587–8, **1813–15**, 3068
  in amenorrhoea 1674
  in atrophic vaginitis 3212
  benefits 1413, 1813–14
  breast cancer incidence and 209
  cancer risk 3068
  in cirrhosis 2091
  ischaemic heart disease risk reduced
    2314
  in Kallmann's syndrome 1671
  oestrogen-only 3068
  in osteoporosis 3068
  in ovarian failure 1565
  risks 1814–15
  side-effects 1814
  in Turner's syndrome 1670, 1700
hormone-stimulation test, in chronic
  pancreatitis 2035–6, *2037*
Horner's syndrome 3877
  after sympathectomy 2374
  in lung cancer 2883
  in mediastinal masses 2897
  in syringomyelia 3893
  in tumours 241
hornets, stings 1144–5
horse bot fly 1001
Horton's syndrome 4026
hospices 4234, 4358, 4360
  hospital admission,
    after deliberate self-harm 4230
    in anorexia nervosa 1298–9, 4215
    compulsory psychiatric 4230, 4257
    delays in myocardial infarction
      2337
    in dementia 4225
    drug-dependent patients 4259
    in myocardial infarction 2336, 2337
    patient response 3
    poisoning cases 1043
    rates *50*
    reasons for 41
  in developing countries 53–4
  discharge, after malnutrition 1294
  drug addicts in A & E departments
    4294–7
  general practice and 48–9
  immediate help for bereaved relatives
    4236
  management of malnourished children
    1294
  referrals to 48–9, *50*
  septicaemia in 1021–2
  tobacco/alcohol and drug use policies
    4286
hospital-acquired infections, *see*
  nosocomial infections
host, bacterial colonization mechanisms
  268, 270, 272, 2001
host defence mechanisms, *see* defence
  mechanisms
host-fungal interactions,
  paracoccidioidomycosis 816
host-parasite relationship 265, 275,
  285
  genetic factors influencing cell
    constituents 280
  virulence and dose of infection 275
host response to infections **275–85**
  factors influencing 91, **279–82**, 2001
    constitutional 280–2
    gastrointestinal tract 2001
    genetic factors 279–80
  immune response, *see* immune
    response; *under* infections
  modulation **283–5**
    enhancement 283–4
    suppression, *see* immunosuppressed/
      immunosuppression

surface barriers 275–6
  lung, *see* lung, defence mechanisms
  see also defence mechanisms
house dust mites 1010, 2714–15
  allergens 158
  asthma association 2734
  avoidance 2737, *2737*
  control 2717
  perennial allergic rhinitis 2714–15
household products, poisoning 1043,
  1044, **1078–83**
  antiseptics and disinfectants 1078
  bleaches and lavatory cleaners 1079
    lavatory sanitizers and deodorants
      1079
  dishwashing liquids, softeners and
    detergents 1079
housemaids' knee 2996
house mites 1010
Howel-Evans syndrome *3795*
Howell-Jolly bodies 3494
Howship's lacunae 3056
HPA-1 1764
HPV, *see* human papillomaviruses (HPV)
H-*ras* 195
hsp70, function 69
hst gene 223
HTLV-I, *see* human T-cell leukaemia-
  lymphoma virus (HTLV-I)
5-HT uptake blocking drugs, *see*
  serotonin (5-hydroxytryptamine)
  reuptake blockers
'huffer's neuropathy' 1092
Hugues-Stovin syndrome 2802–3
human bot fly 1000
human chorionic gonadotrophin (hCG)
  ß-subunit 1579, 1714
    in suprasellar germinoma 1598
  in cerebrospinal fluid 1714
  ectopic production **1714**, *1715*
  hyperthyroidism due to 1749
  male oestrogen secretion and 1688
  in pelvic inflammatory disease test
    3358
  in pseudo precocious puberty 1702,
    1714
  stimulation test 1683, 1694
  treatment,
    ovulation induction 1678
    side-effects 1688
    spermatogenesis induction 1686
human diploid-cell vaccine (HDCV) 403
Human Fertilization and Embryology
  Act (HFEA) (1990) 11, 4147
human genome 62
Human Genome Project 62, 100, 106,
  109
human herpesvirus 6 (HHV-6) **364–5**
  antibodies 365
  intrauterine/perinatal infection 1781
human immunodeficiency virus (HIV),
  see HIV
human menopausal gonadotrophin 1678,
  1686
Human Organ Transplantation Act
  (1990) 14
human papillomaviruses (HPV) **443–6**,
  443
  anorectal carcinoma and 445, 3366,
    3371
  cancers associated 3371
  in cervical cancer 444–5, 460, 463,
    3370
  cervical infection 3368, 3370
  characteristics and genome 443, *444*
  cutaneous 443–4, *444*
  diagnosis 445
  DNA integration 444–5
  genital tract infections 444, 445,
    3366–9
  genital warts 3366–9
    see also genital warts
  immune response to 3366
  infections in homosexuals 3363, 3366
  intrauterine/perinatal infection 1776,
    1783
  in mouth and mucosal sites 445–6
  mucosal 443, *444*

in renal transplant recipients 3320
respiratory papillomatosis 445
structure 3367
transmission 443, 3367
types and infections due to 443
vaccines 3371
warts 3797, 3798
  see also genital warts
human papillomavirus type 5 (HPV-5),
  non-melanoma skin cancer 209, 461
human papillomavirus type 6 (HPV-6)
  444, 445, 3366, 3369
human papillomavirus type 11 (HPV-11)
  444, 445, 3366, 3369
human papillomavirus type 16 (HPV-16)
  3366
  cervical cancer 210, 444–5
  colorectal cancer 204
  genome 443
  penile cancer and 211
human papillomavirus type 18 (HPV-18)
  cervical cancer 210, 444–5
  colorectal cancer 204
  penile cancer and 211
human parvovirus B19
  aplastic crises 3449, 3680
  in haemophilia 3650
  in pregnancy 1776, *1779*, **1781–2**
human placental lactogen (hPL)
  carbohydrate metabolism and 1753
  ectopic production 1714
human rabies immune globulin (HRIG)
  405
human T-cell leukaemia-lymphoma virus
  (HTLV-I) 461, **489–91**, 3411, 3424,
  3581
  adult T-cell leukaemia-lymphoma, *see*
    adult T-cell leukaemia/lymphoma
    (ATLL) syndrome
  cell transformation mechanism 462, 490
  diagnosis/detection 489–90
  disorders associated 490–1, *491*
  epidemiology 461, 489
  infection in homosexuals 3364
  in injecting drug abusers 4284
  neuropathy in 4101
  in pregnancy/newborn infants 1783
  screening for 463
  transmission 461, 489
    prevention 463
  tropical spastic paraparesis 490
human T-cell leukaemia-lymphoma virus
  (HTLV-II) **491**
  infection in homosexuals 3364
  in injecting drug abusers 4284
human T-cell lymphotropic virus III
  (HTLV-III), *see* HIV
Human Tissue Act (1961) **4310–11**
humidification, in positive-pressure
  ventilation 2578
humidifier fever 825, 1231, 2813
humidifier lung 1231, 2811
  investigations 2813
  see also extrinsic allergic alveolitis
humidity
  low, infection predisposition 276
  skin disease and 3723
  skin infections and 3717
humoral immunity 141, 277, *277*
  in atopic eczema 3739–40
  in graft rejection 186, 187
  in infective endocarditis 2438, 2439
  primary sclerosing cholangitis 2078
  in sarcoidosis 2819
  see also B-cells; immunoglobulin(s)
hunger, anorectic drugs 1312
Hunter disease (mucopolysaccharidosis
  II) 1431, *1432*, 3988
Huntington's disease 3965, **4012–14**
  in children 4007, 4014
  clinical features 4013–14
  definition and aetiology 4012–13
  dementia in 4013
  diagnosis 4014
  genetic counselling 4014
  inheritance 114, 4012–13
  molecular biology 63, 64, 4013
  pathology 4013, *4013*

Huntington's disease (*cont.*)
somatosensory evoked potentials 3834
treatment 4014
unstable trinucleotide repeats 108, *125*, **127**
variants 4014
Hurler disease (mucopolysaccharidosis IH) 1336, **1431**, *1432*, 1433, **3087**, 3988
dysostosis multiplex 1433, 1434
Hurler-Scheie disease (mucopolysaccharidosis IH/IS) *1432*, 1434
Hurst's disease 3991
hyaline asterosis, in diabetes 1486
hyaluronidase
in leptospirosis 698
in snake venom 1129
hybrid cells, genetic analysis of tumours 194
hybridization
in situ 62
molecular 59–60
hybridoma 146
hydatid cysts 956, 957
removal 958
hydatid disease (echinococcosis) **955–9**
clinical features 956–7
control programmes 959
diagnosis 957–8
epidemiology/transmission 955–6
management 958–9
myositis 4156
see also Echinococcus granulosus
hydatidiform cysts, larval infections causing 959
hydatidiform mole, hyperthyroidism due to 1612, 1613, 1749
hydatidosis, *see* hydatid disease (echinococcosis)
hydradenitis suppurativa 3765–6
hydralazine **2247**
in heart failure 2248
in hypertension 2541
overdose/poisoning **1066**
in pre-eclampsia 1730–1
in primary pulmonary hypertension 2512
vasculitis due to 3011
hydranencephaly 4114
hydrarthrosis 2956
hydrocarbons
chlorinated 1092–3
nephrotoxicity 3267
poisoning **1083–93**
polycyclic, *see* polycyclic aromatic hydrocarbons
hydrocele, filarial 922, 924
hydrocephalus 4114–15
after head injury 4049
in Chiari malformations 4113
communicating 4050, 4114
diagnosis 4114–15
in Hurler disease 1431
management 4115
non-communicating 4114
normal pressure 3969–70
obstructive 4038, 4050
'otitic' 4041
pituitary tumours causing 1582
in spina bifida, management 4118
in tuberculous meningitis 4060, 4063
hydrochloric acid, poisoning 1103
hydrochlorothiazide 2850
hydrocortisone
in acute adrenal insufficiency 1655
in congenital adrenal hyperplasia 1665
in cortisol deficiency 1587
excessive doses 1661–2
in hypercalcaemia 3229
in myxoedema coma 1616
in pertussis 588
in pregnancy 1751
replacement therapy 1655, 1751
sensitivity in asthma 2850
hydrocyanic acid, toxicity 1152
hydrofluoric acid, *see* hydrogen fluoride
hydrofluorocarbons, asthma due to 2849

hydrogen, in magnetic resonance imaging and 2212–13, 3819
hydrogen breath tests 1910, 1913, 1922, 1957
hydrogen cyanide 1097, 1098
hydrogen fluoride (hydrofluoric acid) 1099
mechanisms of toxicity 1099
poisoning **1099**
hydrogen ions (H$^+$)
elimination 1533–5, 3338
in renal tubular acidosis 3339, 3340
production 1533–5
hydrogen peroxide 1438, 3559
ARDS pathogenesis 2854
hydrogen sulphide 1099
poisoning **1099–100**
hydroids 1143–4
hydronephrosis 3232
antenatal diagnosis 3217
12-hydroperoxy-eicosatetraenoic acid (12-HPETE) 3617, 3627
Hydrophiidae, bites and envenoming 1127, 1132
hydrophobia 401
in rabies 399, 400
hydrops fetalis
α-thalassaemia (Bart's haemoglobin hydrops syndrome) 1761, 3510
in human parvovirus infection 1782
in Rh incompatibility 3545
hydrostatic pressure
lymphatic capillaries 2560
pulmonary capillaries 2492, 2493, 2495–6
hydroxocobalamin 1370, 1371, 3484
in cyanide poisoning treatment 1098
in subacute combined degeneration of cord 3893
therapy 1372, 3496
see also vitamin B$_{12}$
3-hydroxy-3-methylglutaryl (HMG) coenzyme A lyase deficiency *1370*
3-hydroxy-3-methylglutaryl (HMG) coenzyme A reductase 1403
inhibitors (statins) 1414, 3143
hydroxyapatite 2990, 3055
crystals, in synovial fluid 2951
3-hydroxybutyrate, plasma 1506
3-hydroxybutyric acid *1534*
hydroxychloroquine
retinal toxicity 4197
in SLE 3023
17-hydroxycorticosteroid, urinary 1645
6ß-hydroxycortisol, urinary 1645
18-hydroxycortisol, plasma/urinary 1659
12-hydroxy-eicosatetraenoic acid (12-HETE) 3617, 3627
release by pulmonary endothelium 2487
2-hydroxyethoxyacetic acid (HEAA) 1081
hydroxyethyl rutosides 3744
hydroxyethyl starch 3634, 3661
5-hydroxyindole acetic acid 1898
elevation, in carcinoid tumours 1898
3-hydroxyisobutyryl coenzyme A deacylase deficiency *1370*
1α-hydroxylase 1624, 1625
in chronic renal failure 3325
11ß-hydroxylase 1662, *1665*
defects *1567*, 1572
deficiency *1652*, 1660, **1668**, 1690, 1694
17α-hydroxylase 1664, *1665*
defects *1567*, 1572
deficiency *1652*, 1660, **1668**, 1692
18-hydroxylase (corticosterone methyl oxidase I; CMO-I), deficiency *1652*, 1662
21-hydroxylase *1665*
autoantibodies 1652–3
deficiency 1572, *1652*, **1664–7**
clinical presentation 1664
genetics *1567*, 1572, 1666–7
hyperkalaemia in 3134
incidence 1667
investigations 1664, *1665*, 1694
prenatal diagnosis/treatment 1667

treatment 1665–6
virilization 1664, 1690
hydroxyl radical, inflammatory reaction to endotoxin 291
hydroxylysine deficiency *3084*
hydroxynaphthoquinones, in malaria 853
13-hydroxyoctadecadienoic acid (13-HODE) 3662
17-hydroxyprogesterone (17OH-progesterone)
amniotic fluid 1667
blood spots/saliva 1665, 1666
plasma 1664, 1668, 1690, 1694
hydroxyprolinaemia (hydroxyproline oxidase deficiency) *1375*
hydroxyproline
excretion 1275
in starvation 1278
urinary, elevation in Paget's disease 3076
urinary excretion 1629, 3063
assessment and levels 3063
11ß-hydroxysteroid dehydrogenase (11ß-OHSD) 1557
congenital deficiency 1661, 3131, 3132
inhibition by liquorice/metabolites 1661, 3131
in liver disease 1643
17ß-hydroxysteroid dehydrogenase deficiency 1692
3ß-hydroxysteroid dehydrogenase/isomerase (3ßHSD) *1567*, *1664*, *1665*
deficiency *1652*, **1668**, 1691, 1692, 3134
6α-hydroxytetrahydro-11-deoxycortisol, urinary 1668
5-hydroxytryptamine (5HT), *see* serotonin (5-hydroxytryptamine)
hydroxyurea
in chronic myeloid leukaemia 3417
in hypereosinophilic syndrome 3612
in myelodysplastic syndromes 3430–1
in polycythaemia vera 3434
in primary myelosclerosis 3437
in primary thrombocythaemia 3440
25-hydroxyvitamin D (25-OHD), *see* calcifidiol
hydroxyzine, in urticaria 3772
hygiene
infectious disease control 288
insects and 1011
Hymenolepis diminuta 962, 963
Hymenolepis nana 961
infestation **963**
lifecycle 962
Hymenolepis nana fraterna 962, 963
hymenoptera, venomous 161, 1144
hyoscine (scopolamine) 1152
adverse mental symptoms 4242
dyspnoea treatment, in terminal illness 4355
in terminal illness 4356
hyperactivity, foods/food additives associated 1844
hyperadrenalism, *see* Cushing's syndrome
hyperaemia, in recurrent polyserositis 1525
hyperaesthesia, in rabies 399
hyperaldosteronism, *see* aldosteronism
hyperalgesia 3936, 3938
hyperaluminiumaemia 2121–2, *2122*
hyperammonaemia 2102
causes *1359*, 1361
in lysinuric protein intolerance 1357
in urea cycle defects 1358, 1359, 1360
hyperandrogenization **1674–7**
causes 1674–6
diagnosis 1676
hyperbaric bags, in acute mountain sickness 1191
hyperbaric oxygen
in carbon monoxide poisoning 1096
in gas gangrene 634
haemolytic anaemia due to 3550

hyperbilirubinaemia 2056
antibiotics in streptococci group B infections 508
causes and pathophysiology 2056
conjugated *2057*, **2058–9**
in acute viral hepatitis 2061
diagnosis 2106
in hepatocellular failure 2102
see also Dubin-Johnson syndrome; Rotor's syndrome
unconjugated 2056, **2057–8**, *2057*
breast-milk jaundice 2058
physiological jaundice of newborn 2058
transient familial neonatal 2058
see also Crigler-Najjar syndrome; Gilbert's syndrome
see also jaundice
hypercalcaemia **1637–8**, **3078–9**, **4126**
in acute renal failure 3284, 3299–300
causes *1638*, 3078, *3078*
in chronic renal failure 3325
clinical features 242, 1631–2
crisis 3228
diabetes insipidus in 3120, 3228
differential diagnosis 1637–8
in diuretic therapy 2240
eye in 4196
familial benign (hypocalciuric) 1632, **3079**, 3335–6
bone disease in *3079*
in hypervitaminosis D 1635, 3095
idiopathic 3095
of malignancy 242, *243*, 1632, 1711, **1712**
diagnosis 1637–8
humoral (pseudohyperparathyroidism) 1568, 1630, 1632, 1638
in lung cancer 2884
pathophysiology 1568, 2884
renal involvement 3184
treatment 2884, 3229
in myeloma 1638, 3181, 3599, **3603**
nephropathy **3227–9**
clinical aspects 3228
pathophysiology 3228
treatment 3228–9
neurological features 4126
in pancreatic endocrine tumours 1706, 1707
polyuria in 3147
in primary hyperparathyroidism 1630, 1631–2
in renal transplant recipients 3320
in sarcoidosis 1636, 1716, 2826, 2829, 3186, 4182
severe infantile idiopathic (Williams syndrome) 3095, 4111
treatment 1633, **1638**
urinary stone disease 3254
in vitamin D poisoning 1635, 3095
see also calcium
hypercalcaemic syndrome
'burnt-out' 2423
in supra-aortic stenosis 2423
hypercalciuria 3255
idiopathic 1632, 1636, **3255**, 3335
'overspill' type 3335
'renal leak' type 3335
in sarcoidosis 3186, 3255
hypercapnia **2904**
assessment 2669–71, 2904
in asthma 2636
chronic 2671, 2904
in scoliosis 2873
coronary vasodilatation 2159
effects 2904
in emphysema 2633
in obstructive sleep apnoea 2905, 2910
permissive 2575
respiration control 3887
in respiratory failure definition 2901
ventilation control assessment 2672
see also carbon dioxide
hypercarbia, relative, in acute mountain sickness 1189
hypercatabolic states 2587
hypercholesterolaemia **1406–8**
in anorexia nervosa 1297, 4214

combined with hypertriglyceridaemia
1408–9
common (polygenic) 1406, **1407–8**
in diabetes 1410–11
familial 1403, **1406–7**, *1408*
heterozygous 1406–7
homozygous 1407, 1414
LDL receptor mutations 129
lipoprotein (a) levels and heart disease
2308
liver transplantation in 2113
metabolic defect 1407
treatment 1413, 1414
liver in *2020*, 2025
management 1412, 1413–14
monogenic 64
in obesity 1408, 1411
peripheral arterial disease risk 2363,
2369
in phytosterolaemia 1437
reduced endothelium-dependent
vasodilation 2297
hypercoagulability, investigation 2304,
2305
hypercoagulable states, *see*
prethrombotic states
hyperemesis gravidarum 1749–50, 1798,
1802
hypereosinophilia
endomyocardial fibrosis with, *see*
hypereosinophilic syndrome
in gnathostomiasis 951
prognosis 2397, 2398
severe combined immunodeficiency
disease with 173
hypereosinophilic syndrome 2390,
2396–8, 3403, **3610–13**
aetiology and pathogenesis 2397
causes 3611
Churg-Strauss syndrome *vs* 3015
clinical features 2367, 3611
definition 3611
investigation 2397, 3611–12
prognosis 3612–13
treatment 3612
hyperfibrinolytic bleeding **3659**
hypergammaglobulinaemia
in infective endocarditis 2438
in primary biliary cirrhosis 2075
in primary sclerosing cholangitis 2078
in SLE 3025–6
in systemic sclerosis 3032
hypergastrinaemia
achlorhydria-related 1894
causes 1881
in H$_2$-receptor blockade 1887
Helicobacter pylori role 1885
treatment 1881
see also Zollinger-Ellison syndrome
hyperglobulinaemia, in Q fever 744
hyperglycaemia
after injury/surgery 1494, 1549
control in diabetes, *see* diabetes
mellitus, glycaemic/metabolic control
degrees of 1448–9
diabetic nephropathy and 3169
diabetic tissue damage and 1463, 1464,
1482–3
in diuretic therapy 2240
lumbar puncture and 3844
non-endocrine causes 1714, *1715*
parenteral nutrition complication 1320
in pregnancy 1753
pseudohyponatraemia in 3122
symptoms 1453
hyperglycaemic comas, diabetic
1498–503
hyperosmolar non-ketotic 1499, **1502**
ketoacidotic, *see* diabetic ketoacidosis
management *1500*, *1501*, 1502–3
hyperglycinaemia, non-ketotic 1368
hyperglycollic aciduria 1446, 1447
hyperhidrosis 3766, *3766*
axillary 3767
feet 3767
management 3766–7
hyper-IgM syndrome 149
hyperiminodipeptiduria *1375*

hyperimmune immunoglobulin 317
in CNS viral infections 4071
viral infections of CNS prevention
4072
hyperimmunoglobulin E syndromes 3559
hyperinsulinaemia
in polycystic ovary syndrome 1673,
1675–6
see also insulin, resistance
hyperinsulinism 4123
in Beckwith-Wiedemann syndrome
1974
hyperkalaemia **3132–5**
ACE inhibitors causing 2249, 2251
in acid-base disturbances 1540, 3127–8
in acute renal failure 3133, 3284, 3285
in adrenal insufficiency 1654, 3133,
3337
causes *3133*
in chronic renal failure 3133, 3297
in cirrhosis 2088
in digoxin overdose 1066
in diuretic overdose/poisoning 1066
drugs inducing 3337
in electrical injury 1212
in hepatocellular failure 2109
massive transfusion inducing 3693
periodic paralysis 3134, 4169, 4170
in poisoning 1047
renal causes **3337**
in renal tubular acidosis 3134, 3341
spironolactone-induced in ascites 2097
spurious (pseudohyperkalaemia) 3133
treatment 3135, *3286*
hyperkeratosis 3710
beta-blockers causing 3733
epidermolytic 3719
perifollicular 3711, 3719
hyperkinetic movement disorders 3862
hyperlactataemia 1541, 1542
paracetamol-induced 1052
hyperlipidaemia
in chronic renal failure 1411, 3302,
3305
combined, in alcoholic liver disease
2082
in diabetes 1410–11, 1485–6, 3172
in diuretic therapy 2240
familial combined 1409
haemolytic anaemia in 3550
hormone replacement therapy in 1413,
1815
in nephrotic syndrome 1411, **3142–3**,
3144
peripheral arterial disease risk 2363
in renal transplant recipients 1411,
3321–2
signs 2325
hyperlipoproteinaemia 1399, **1404–14**
acute pancreatitis due to 2028
Fredrickson/WHO classification 1405–6
hypertriglyceridaemia-predominant
1409–10
joint involvement 3004
liver in *2020*, 2025
management 1412–14
primary 1406–10
secondary 1410–12
type I 1406–8
type II, joint involvement 3004
type IIA 1406–8
type IIB 1409
type III 1408–9, 1413
type IV 1410
joint involvement 3004
type V 1409–10
hyperlysinaemia, familial *1375*
hypermagnesaemia 3336
hypermobility 2947, 2976
in Marfan's syndrome 3083
hypernatraemia **3125–6**, **4125–6**
aetiology and pathophysiology *3124*,
3126
in cirrhosis 2088
clinical features 3126
essential 1603, 3125, 3126
haemofiltration 2581
hypervolaemic *3124*, 3126

hypovolaemic *3124*, 3126
in thirst deficiency 1602, 3125, 3126
treatment 3126
hypernephroma, *see* renal cell carcinoma
hyperornithinaemia with
hyperammonaemia and
homocitrullinuria (HHH syndrome)
1361
hyperosteocytosis 3079
hyperostosis frontalis 1592
hyperoxaluria *1445*
in Crohn's disease 1939
enteric *1445*, 1447
primary **1445–7**, *1448*
liver transplantation in 2112
renal transplantation in 1447, *1448*,
3315
type I 1335, *1337*, 1441, **1445–7**,
1448
type II *1445*, **1447**, *1448*
type III *1445*, **1447**, *1448*
secondary *1445*
in short gut syndrome 1925
hyperparathyroidism **1630–3**
acute pancreatitis due to 2028
biochemical features *3062*
bone disease in **3079**
definitions 1630
eye in 4196
familial 1632
giant-cell granuloma *vs* 1863
joint involvement 3004
in MEN 1 syndrome 1632, 1708
mental disorders/symptoms in 4239
primary 1622, **1630–3**, 1635–6, 3078
clinical and laboratory features 1631–2
diagnosis 1632
haematological changes 3686
in malignant disease 1712
muscle involvement 4169
in pregnancy 1752
treatment 1632–3
urinary calcium excretion 1627, 1628,
1630
urinary stone disease 1631, 1632,
3255
in renal transplant recipients 3320
secondary 1630, 1632, **3079**
in chronic renal failure 3323, 3325
tertiary 1630, 1632, **3079**, 3329
hyperpathia 3936
hyperphenylalaninaemia
in dihydropteridine reductase deficiency
1363
transient neonatal 1362
hyperphosphataemia 3063, 3334–5
in acromegaly 1593
calcification in 3092
in chronic renal failure 3325, 3326
in hypervitaminosis D 1635
in hypoparathyroidism 1633, 1634–5
hyperphosphatasia
biochemical features *3062*
idiopathic **3089**
hyperpigmentation
in cirrhosis 2087
in malnutrition 1283
hyperpolarizing factor 2297
hyperprolactinaemia 1576, 1577, 1584
in acromegaly 1592
amenorrhoea in 1671, **1672**
causes 1590, 1716
clinical features 1589
drug-induced 1718
galactorrhoea in 1589, 1689
male hypogonadism in 1683
pregnancy in 1591, 1672, **1747–8**
sexual problems in 4244
see also prolactinoma
hyperprolinaemia
type I *1375*
type II *1375*
hyperpyrexia
malignant 1182, 1259
drugs associated 1182
prevention and management 1182
see also hyperthermia, malignant

in relapsing fevers 695, 697
in salicylate poisoning 1054
see also hyperthermia
hyper-reninaemia 2541, 2548
hypersalivation, in rabies 399, 400
hypersensitivity 156
antituberculous therapy 658, *658*
contact, *see* contact dermatitis, allergic
drug-induced fever 1181
in extrinsic allergic alveolitis 2811,
2814
food allergy, *see* food allergy
to insect venom, diagnosis 1145
occupational asthma due to 2742–3,
2743–4
oesophageal mucosa 1819, *1819*
type I (immediate) 158–63, 278, *278*,
1252
allergic rhinitis 2715
to antibiotics 305
to drugs 1252
to insect venom 1145
mechanisms 158–9
to nickel 1112
T-cells role 157
see also allergic diseases
type II (antibody-mediated) 163–4, 278
to drugs 1253
type III (immune complex) **164–5**,
278–9
to drugs 1253
type IV (delayed), *see* delayed
hypersensitivity
types *156*
see also immunological overactivity
hypersensitivity angiitis 3010
hypersensitivity vasculitis 3010
hypersomnia 3929, 4240
functional 3929
long-cycle periodic 3929
idiopathic 3929
narcolepsy *vs* 3929
neurotic 3929
short-cycle periodic, forms 3929
symptomatic 3929
see also sleep; sleepiness, excess
hypersomnolence
daytime 2912–13
in myotonic disorders 4153
hypersplenism **3590–1**
in cirrhosis 2089
in common varied immunodeficiency
(CVID) 169
haemolytic anaemia in 3550
in primary myelosclerosis 3435
in sickle-cell disease 3516–17
in thalassaemia 3512
thrombocytopenia in 3633
hypertension
accelerated (malignant) **2543**, *3548*
blood vessels in 2534
haemolytic uraemic syndrome
3198
prognosis **2532**
in radiation nephritis 3231
renal failure due to 3249–50, 3290,
3299, *3300*
in systemic sclerosis 3031
in acromegaly 1593
in acute porphyria 1392, 1393, 1394
after lung transplantation 2937
in aircraft crew and pilots 1200
in aldosteronism 1657
atherogenesis 2291, 2533
autonomic nervous system in 2531
benign intracranial, *see* intracranial
hypertension
blood pressure levels 2528
see also blood pressure
cardiac changes 2533–4
cardiac disease in 2532–3
risk 30–1
in cerebral infarction 3960
cerebrovascular changes 2534
cerebrovascular disease in 2532
in chronic renal failure 3297, 3301,
3303, 3304
in coarctation of aorta **2557–9**

hypertension (*cont.*)
in congenital adrenal hyperplasia 1668
in Cushing's syndrome 1643
cyclosporin-induced 2257
in diabetes **1492**, 3170
in diabetic nephropathy 3169–70
in dialysed patients 3312
essential **2527–43**
  clinical examination **2535–6**
  clinical features **2534–5**
  clinical presentation 2537
  definition 2545
  in elderly **2543**
  genes 2530
  investigations **2537**
  management **2537–43**
  mechanisms **2531–2**
  morbidity **2532–3**
  mortality **2532**
  as multifactorial disorder 2527, 2530
  natural history **2532**
  pathogenesis **2529–31**, 3250
  prevalence **2527–8**
  resistant **2542–3**
  severe, prognosis **2532**
  specific organ changes **2533–4**
  see also other subentries above/below
in gout 1381
in haemangioendothelioma 2298
in haemolytic uraemic syndrome 3198,
    3201
heart failure due to 2229, 2534
hormone replacement therapy and 1815
in hypercalcaemia 1631
hyperuricaemia and 1381
limb ischaemia management 2369
malignant, *see* hypertension, accelerated
management **2537–43**
  advice and non-pharmacological
    2537–9
  antihypertensive drugs, *see*
    antihypertensive drugs
  assessment of diagnosis/effects 2537
  combination therapy *2541*, 2542
  concurrent disease 2537
  dietary 2538
  exercise and behavioural 2538–9
  in liver disease 2091
  sodium restriction 2531, 2538
  transient ischaemic attack 3953
in MAOI food and drug interactions
    4250
mild, prognosis **2532**
in minimal change nephropathy 3155
in obesity 1308, 2530
ocular features **4187–8**
  non-retinal 4188
  see also hypertensive retinopathy
pathogenesis **2529–31**, 3250
  environmental 2530–1
  genetic factors 2529–30
pathology **2533**
peripheral arterial disease risk 2363,
    2533
phaeochromocytoma 2554, 2555
in polycystic kidney disease 3203
in polycythaemia vera 3432–3
in post-streptococcal glomerulonephritis
    506
of pre-eclampsia 1727–8, 1729
pre-eclampsia superimposed on 1727,
    1731, 1735
in pregnancy **1726–32**
  aetiology 1726
  definition 1726
  in diabetes mellitus 1757
  liver disorders and **1796–8**
  long-term sequelae 1732
  pre-existing/chronic 1726, **1731–2**
  in SLE 3022
  terminology 1726–7
pregnancy-induced 1726–7
  see also pre-eclampsia
pulmonary, *see* pulmonary hypertension
reduced endothelium-dependent
    vasodilation 2297, 2531
in reflux nephropathy 3218, 3220
renal, *see* renal hypertension
renal effects 2546, **3247–50**

renal failure due to 2533, 2545,
    3248–50, 3303
in renal transplant recipients 3322
renovascular, *see* renovascular
    hypertension
secondary 2527, **2544–59**
in subarachnoid haemorrhage 3964
systolic 2532, **2542**
  in supra-aortic stenosis 2423
thallium poisoning 1113
in unilateral renal parenchymal disease
    2552, *2552*
in urinary-tract obstruction 3235
venous, *see* venous pressure
white coat 2536, 2538, 2542
Hypertension, Detection and Follow-Up
    Program Screening Study 2539
hypertensive encephalopathy 2534, **2543**
  eclampsia *vs* 1729
hypertensive peristalsis **1871**
hypertensive retinopathy **4187–8**
  assessment by ophthalmoscopy 4187
  classification 4187–8
hyperthecosis 1676
hyperthermia
  in Ecstasy use 4280
  in elderly **4346**
  habitual 1015
  in hypovolaemia after marathons 4328
  malignant 1182, 1259, 3135, 4128
    myopathy in **4170**
    see also hyperpyrexia
  management 4328
  in marathons and mass runs 4328
  in poisoning 1047
  in tetanus 627
  see also hyperpyrexia
hyperthyroidism **1610–14**
  'apathetic' 4239
  cardiac manifestations 2394
  causes 1611–12, 1714
  clinical presentation 1610–11
  diagnostic tests 1579, 1585, 1608, 1609
  diarrhoea in 1962
  drug-induced 1717
  in elderly **4345–6**
  haematological changes 3686
  hypokalaemic muscle weakness 3132
  iodine-induced 1612, 1613–14
  in lung cancer 2884
  mental disorders/symptoms in 4239
  ocular features 4195–6
  postpartum 1750
  in pregnancy **1749**
  renal calcium excretion 3227
  thyrotoxic crisis 1614
  transient neonatal 1610, 1611, 1750
  treatment 1612–14
    in elderly 4345–6
  in trophoblastic disease 1612, 1613,
    1749
  TSH-secreting pituitary adenoma 1595,
    1612
hyperthyroxinaemia, euthyroid *1612*
hypertrichosis 3764, *3764*
  in congenital porphyria 1395
hypertrichosis lanuginosa, acquired 3793
hypertriglyceridaemia **1409–10**
  in acromegaly 1592
  atherosclerosis and 1405
  chronic pancreatitis 2034
  in chronic renal failure 3302
  combined with hypercholesterolaemia
    1408–9
  in diabetes 1410–11, 1485–6, 3172
  in glycogen storage diseases 1342
  gout/hyperuricaemia and 1381, 1412
  ischaemia of limbs 2369
  liver in *2020*, 2025
  management 1412–13, 1414
  moderate 1410
  in obesity 1411
  severe 1409–10
hypertrophic cardiomyopathy, *see*
    cardiomyopathy, hypertrophic
hypertrophic osteoarthropathy
  in cirrhosis 2087
  joint involvement 3006

hypertrophic pulmonary osteoarthropathy
    244
  chest radiography 2884, 2885
  clubbing of fingers in 2651
  in lung cancer 2884–5
hyperuricaemia 1376, **1377**, 2985–6
  acute renal failure in 1379–80, 3185,
    3226, 3290
  associated disorders 1381
  asymptomatic 1381, 2984
  causes *1380*
  cyclosporin A-induced 3265
  diagnosis/determination 2986
  familial juvenile 1380, 3225, **3226**,
    3227
  in hereditary fructose intolerance 1347,
    1384
  hypertriglyceridaemia and 1381, 1412
  in lead intoxication 3227
  in megaloblastic anaemia 3497
  myogenic 1384
  pathogenesis 1379, 3225
  in phosphoribosyl pyrophosphate
    synthetase overactivity 1383, 3226
  in polycythaemia vera 3433, 3434
  in pre-eclampsia 1728, 1729
  in von Gierke's disease 1342, 1383,
    1384, 3226
  see also gout
hyperuricosuria-hypouricaemia 3226
hyperventilation 2672
  in altitude acclimatization 1186
  in anxiety disorders 4206, 4258
  in asthma 2728
  cardiovascular reflexes testing *3884*
  chest pain in 2169
  in Cheyne-Stokes breathing 3889
  in diabetic ketoacidosis 1499
  differential diagnosis 1499–500
  effect on cerebral blood volume 4048
  epileptic seizure *vs* 3919
  in heart failure 2232
  in heat stroke 1180
  in hepatocellular failure 2104
  hypocalcaemic tetany 1638
  in hypoxia 1195, 1196, 2902
  in metabolic acidosis 1537–9
  neurogenic 3890
  psychogenic 2169, 2672
  in respiratory acidosis 1537, 1539
  syncope in 2173
  in unconscious patient 2584, 2586
hyperviscosity syndrome
  in myeloma 3599
  in Waldenström's macroglobulinaemia
    3604
hypervitaminosis D 1635–6
  in sarcoidosis 2829
hypervolaemia
  evaluation *3283*
  hypernatraemia *3124*, 3126
  hyponatraemia 3122, 3123
  see also fluid, overload
hyp mouse 3334
hypnagogic hallucinations **3928–9**
hypnogram 2908
hypnotic drugs
  poisoning/overdose 1060–1, 4296
  withdrawal syndrome 1254, **4293**,
    4296
    rebound effects 1254
hypoadrenalism (adrenocortical
    insufficiency) **1652–6**, 4125
  in adrenoleukodystrophy/
    adrenomyeloneuropathy 1439, 1440,
    1653
  autoimmune 1571
  clinical features 1653–4
  corticosteroid replacement therapy
    1655–6
  drug-induced 1718
  emergency treatment 1655
  gastrointestinal motility disorder in
    1962
  hyperkalaemia in 1654, 3133, 3337
  hypoglycaemia in 1510–11, 1654
  laboratory investigations 1654–5
  mental disorders/symptoms in 4239

neurological features 4125
in pregnancy **1751**
primary 1652–3, 1654
  investigations 1654, 1655
  see also Addison's disease; congenital
    adrenal hyperplasia
secondary (ACTH deficiency) 1583,
    1586, **1653**, 1654
  hypoglycaemia in 1510–11
  investigations 1654, 1655
hypoalbuminaemia 2866
  in bacterial overgrowth 1913
  in cirrhosis 2088
  in hepatocellular failure 2105
  in nephrotic syndrome 3138, 3155
  in rickettsial diseases 732
  in schistosomiasis 977
  in small-intestinal lymphangiectasia
    1977
hypoaldosteronism **1662–3**
  hyperkalaemia in 3134, 3337
  hyporeninaemic 1662–3, 1669, 3134
  primary 1662, 1668–9
  renal tubular acidosis in 3341
hypobetalipoproteinaemia, familial 1414
hypocalcaemia **1638–9**, 1910, **4126**
  in acute renal failure 3284
  calcification in 3092
  in chronic renal failure 3325, 3327
  clinical features 1633
  in Crohn's disease 1940
  dementia due to 3971
  hypocalciuria in 3063
  in hypoparathyroidism 1633, 1634–5
  massive transfusion inducing 3693
  neurological features 4126
  in osteomalacia 3071
  in poisoning 1047
  post-parathyroidectomy 1633, 3329
  treatment 1635
  in vitamin D deficiency 1636
  see also calcium
hypocalciuria **3335–6**
  in hypocalcaemia 3063
hypocapnia 2902, 2908
  in tetanus 625
hypocatalasaemia **1441**
hypochlorhydria
  bacterial overgrowth in 1911, *1911*
  see also gastric acid
hypochondrial pain, in opisthorchiasis
    982
hypochondriasis 3943, **4208**
hypochromia 3377–8, 3461
hypocitraturia 3256
hypocomplementaemia, in cholesterol
    embolism 2376
Hypoderaeum canoideum 996
Hypoderma 1001
hypodipsia 1602–3, *3124*, 3125, 3126
hypofibrinogenaemia, hereditary 3646,
    3652
hypogammaglobulinaemia
  arthritis in 771
  bacterial overgrowth aetiology 1912
  in bronchiectasis 2758, 2761
  in chronic lymphocytic leukaemia
    173–4, 1028
  common variable, *see* common varied
    immunodeficiency (CVID)
  joint involvement 3005
  in 5′-nucleotidase deficiency 1386
  pneumococcal infections in 514
  respiratory tract infections 2710
  secondary to gastrointestinal disease
    1841
  in thymoma 168
  transient in infancy and childhood 166
  see also antibody-deficiency
    syndromes; immunodeficiency;
    panhypogammaglobulinaemia
hypogammaglobulinaemic sprue 1839
hypogeusia, in nephrotic syndrome 3144
hypoglossal nerve 2610, **3880**
  lesions 3880
hypoglycaemia **1505–12**, **4123**
  ACTH secretion 1576
  in adrenal insufficiency 1510–11, 1654

adrenergic symptoms 1505
alcohol-induced 1184, *1184*, 1469,
  1510
  after exercise 1184, *1184*
  in alcohol intoxication 1080
alimentary 1511
in anorexia nervosa 1297, 4214
autoimmune **1510**
in Beckwith-Wiedemann syndrome
  1974
beta-blockade caution 2328
in cerebral malaria 846
childhood **1511–12**
clinical features 1292, 1498, **1505–6**
coma **1497–8**, *1499*, 1506
dementia due to 3971
in diabetes *1466*, *1467*, **1497–8**
  alcohol-induced 1469
  exercise-induced 1478
  insulin-treated patients 1476–7, 1497
  nocturnal 1496, 1498
  in pregnancy 1756
  sulphonylurea-induced 1470–1, 1497
  unawareness 1498
factitious **1509**
fasting 1505, **1506–11**
  diagnosis 1506
  differential diagnosis/investigations
    1507
fatigue in 1036
in fructose diphosphatase deficiency
  1346
in hepatocellular failure 2103, 2110
in hereditary fructose intolerance 1347,
  1348
in hypoglycaemic drug overdose 1071
in infections **1510**
insulin tolerance test 1585, 1645–6
ketotic, in infancy 1512
leucine-sensitive 1512
in lung cancer 2884
in malaria 845, 848, 1510
  management 856
malignant tumours causing *243*,
  1509–10, 1714
in malnutrition, management 1289,
  1292
mental disorders/symptoms in 4240
neonatal **1511–12**, 1757
nervous system in **4123**
neuroglycopenic symptoms 1498, 1506
in organic acidurias 1361
in paracetamol poisoning 1053
pathological 1505–6
presentation 4123
prevention 1506
in pyruvate carboxylase deficiency 1352
reactive postprandial 1505, **1511**
  differential diagnosis/investigations
    1507
  idiopathic 1511
in salicylate poisoning 1054, 1055
seizures in 3917
sequelae 1506
treatment of acute 1506
in von Gierke's disease 1342
hypoglycaemic agents, *see* oral
  hypoglycaemic agents
hypoglycin A 1159
hypoglycorrhachia 3844
hypogonadism
  in AIDS 1716
  drug-induced 1718
  exercise-induced 4326
  gonadotrophin-secreting tumours 1595
  in hepatocellular failure 2105
  in hereditary haemochromatosis 3478,
    3479
  hypergonadotrophic 1683, *1702*
  in hyperprolactinaemia 1589
  hypogonadotrophic 1582, **1670–2**,
    1674, 1683
    delayed puberty *1702*
    functional 1671–2
    idiopathic, associated with anosmia,
      see Kallmann's syndrome
    management of infertility 1686
  male 1680, **1682–4**

osteoporosis in 3069
sexual problems in 4244
  assessment and signs of 4246
treatment 1587–8
hypohidrosis 3767
hypohidrotic ectodermal dysplasia 3767
hypokalaemia **3129–32**
  in acid-base disturbances 1540, 3130
  in aldosteronism 1657, 3132, 3336
  antimicrobial drug-induced 3132, 3337
  in ß$_2$-agonist poisoning 1067, 1068
  in bulimia nervosa 1300, 4216
  causes *3129*, 3130
  in cirrhosis 2088
  in Crohn's disease 1940
  in Cushing's syndrome 1647, 3131,
    3336
  diabetes insipidus in 3120–1
  digitalis pharmacokinetics 2242
  diuretic-induced 2239, **3130**
  in ectopic ACTH syndrome 1712–13
  gastrointestinal causes 3130
  in hepatocellular failure 2109
  in hereditary fructose intolerance 1347
  hypomagnesaemic 3337
  in malignant disease 3184
  in megaloblastic anaemia 3497
  mental symptoms 4240
  pathophysiological effects 3129–30
  periodic paralysis 1657, **3132**, 4169
  renal causes 3130–2, **3336–7**
  in renal tubular acidosis 3338, 3339,
    3340
  in salicylate poisoning 1054
  sudden death in north-east Thailand and
    3132
  in theophylline poisoning 1068
  treatment 3132
  in VIPoma syndrome 1706
  in vomiting 1821
hypokinesia 4001
hypolactasia 1922, 1923
  detection 1906
  malabsorption in tropics and 1930–1
  in ulcerative colitis 1949
  see also lactase
hypolipidaemic drugs, *see* lipid-lowering
  drugs
hypolipoproteinaemia 1414
hypomagnesaemia 3336
  in cirrhosis 2088
  mental symptoms 4240
  potassium wasting 3337
  PTH secretion 1624
hypomania 4220
  in elderly 4227
hypomelanosis, idiopathic guttate 3760
hypomelanosis of Ito (HI) 123–4
hyponatraemia **3122–5, 4125**
  in acute porphyria 1392, 1393
  in adrenal insufficiency 1654
  after injury 1549
  causes 3122–3
  in central pontine myelinolysis 3996
  in cirrhosis 2088
  classification 3122–3
  clinical features 3123
  diuretic-induced 2240–1
  in hepatocellular failure 2103
  hypervolaemic 3122, 3123
  hypovolaemic 3122–3
  in malaria 846, 855
  in malignant disease 3184
  management 3123, 4059
  in meningitis 4059
  mental symptoms 4240
  neurological features 4125
  normovolaemic 3122, 3123
  over-rapid correction 3124
  in rickettsial diseases 732, 733
  in spotted fevers 734
  spurious, *see* pseudohyponatraemia
  in syndrome of inappropriate
    antidiuresis 1602
  see also water, intoxication
hypoparathyroidism **1633–5**, 1636, **3079**,
  3334
  bone disease in **3079**

calcification in 3092
eye in 4196
idiopathic 1634
mental disorders/symptoms in 4239
PTH-resistant, *see*
  pseudohypoparathyroidism
urinary calcium excretion 1627, 1628
hypopharynx, *see* laryngopharynx
hypophase 2599
hypophosphataemia **3334**, *3335*
  in chronic renal failure 3325
  in hypokalaemia 3130
  inherited 3070
    calcification in 3092
    radiology 3072
    treatment 3074
  muscle weakness 1626
  in osteomalacia 1626, 1637, 3070,
    3071, 3072, 3074
  paracetamol-induced 1052
  sporadic 1636, 3608
  X-linked 1636, **3334**
hypophosphatasia 1629, **3086**
  biochemical features *3062*
  gene 3086
hypophysitis, lymphocytic **1597**, 1748
hypopigmentation 3755–60, *3757*
hypopituitarism 1582–3, 1653
  amenorrhoea in 1671
  anaemia in 3483
  dementia due to 3971
  haematological changes 3686
  hormone replacement therapy 1587–8
  hypoglycaemia in 1510–11
  mental disorders/symptoms in 4239
  myopathy in 4168
  non-pituitary sellar lesions 1597
  osteoporosis in 3069
  in pituitary apoplexy 1598
  in sarcoidosis 1716
  sexual problems in 4244
  treatment-associated 1588, 1589, 1651
  tumours causing 1589, 1591, 1596
hypoproteinaemia
  in hookworm infection 931
  in small-intestinal lymphangiectasia
    1977
hypoprothrombinaemia
  hereditary 3652
  in salicylate poisoning 1054, 1055
hypopyon, in Behçet's syndrome 4183
hyporeflexia, in barbiturate poisoning
  1060
hyposensitization, *see* desensitization
hyposexuality 4244
hypospermatogenesis, idiopathic 1684,
  1685, 1687
hyposplenism, in sickle-cell disease 3514
hypotension
  ACE inhibitors causing 2251
  in acute pancreatitis 2028
  in Addison's disease 1654, 1655
  after head injury 4045, *4045*
  in bacterial infections 292
  beta-blockers causing 2345
  in botulism 632
  in desferrioxamine use 1071
  first dose, with ACE inhibitors 2251
  haemodialysis-associated 3309
  in hepatocellular failure 2103
  in hypothermia 1183
  in malaria 846, 856
  in nitrate overdose 1067
  in opioid overdose 1058
  in phaeochromocytoma treatment 2557
  in plague 596, 598
  in poisoning 1047
  postprandial 3883, 3886
    falls due to 4339
  postural (orthostatic), *see* postural
    hypotension
  in pulmonary embolism 2526
  in septicaemia 1022, 1024
  snake venom causing 1130, 1138
  in sodium nitroprusside overdose 1067
  in spinal cord injury 3898
  supine, in pregnancy 1726, 1735
  in tetanus 629

in typhoid 562, 565
vasopressin secretion 3118
hypotensive agents, *see* antihypertensive
  drugs
hypothalamic-pituitary-adrenal axis
  circadian variations 1565
  suppression 1650–1, 1653
  in trauma 1548–9
hypothalamic-pituitary axis, in trauma
  1548–9
hypothalamic-pituitary-gonadal axis
  1563, 1580
hypothalamic-pituitary-testicular axis
  assessment 1683
  physiology **1679–80**
hypothalamic-pituitary-thyroid axis 1564,
  1608–9
hypothalamic thermostat, resetting 293
hypothalamus
  disorders,
    in AIDS 1716
    amenorrhoea in **1740–674**
    in anorexia nervosa 1297, 4213, 4214
    cranial diabetes insipidus 3120
    evaluation 1583–6
    hormone replacement therapy 1587–8
    hypoadrenalism *1654*
    hypothyroidism 1616
    male hypogonadism 1683
    in sarcoidosis 1716
    tumour-induced 1574
  insulin secretion and 1460
  non-pituitary lesions near **1596–9**
  pituitary connections 1565, 1574
  regulation of pituitary hormones
    1574–5
  in sarcoidosis 2827
  stimulation, pulmonary circulation 2492
  in stress response 1563
  sweating control 3766
  thirst osmoreceptors 3117
  tumours, mental disorders/symptoms in
    4237
  vasopressin osmoreceptors 1600, 3118
hypothermia 1015, **4128**
  acute pancreatitis due to 2028
  definition 1182
  in elderly **4346**
  hillwalkers and climbers 1184
  immersion 1183
  in malnutrition, management 1292
  management 1183–4, 4328, 4346
  in marathons and mass runs 4328
  massive transfusion inducing 3693
  metabolic changes in 1183
  neurological features 4128
  in phenothiazine overdose/poisoning
    1061
  in poisoning 1047
  prevention 1183–4, 4346
  thrombocytopenia in 3633–4
  urban 1184–5
    causes 1184–5
hypothetico-deductive method 15
hypothyroidism **1614–17**
  anaemia in 3483, 3686
  in anorexia nervosa 1297
  autoimmune causes 1570–1
  cardiac manifestations 2394
  clinical features 1614–15
  congenital 1337, 1614–15, 1698
  dementia due to 3971
  diagnostic tests 1579, 1608, 1609
  drug-induced 1717
  in elderly **4345**
  fetal, drug-induced 1749
  growth impairment 1698
  haematological changes 3686
  hyperlipoproteinaemia in 1411
  hypothermia in 1184
  juvenile 1698
  mental disorders/symptoms in 4238–9
  myopathy in 4168
  obstructive sleep apnoea and 2910
  pericardial effusion in 2476
  postpartum 1750
  post-thyroidectomy 1613
  precocious puberty in 1702

hypothyroidism (cont.)
  in pregnancy 1749
  primary 1614, 1615
  pseudohypoparathyroidism and 1634
  radiation-induced 3575
  radio-iodine therapy inducing 1613
  secondary 1583, 1614, 1616
  in systemic sclerosis 3034
  transient neonatal 1610, 1611, 1750
  treatment 1587, 1616
    in elderly 4345
hypotonia
  in barbiturate poisoning 1060
  in cerebral malaria 846
hypouricaemia
  causes 1385
  in hereditary xanthinuria 1384
  hyperuricosuric 3226
hypouricaemic therapy
  in gout 2987–8
  side-effects 2988
hypoventilation 2672
  central alveolar 3888
  chronic, in scoliosis 2872
  in muscular dystrophy 4149
  sleep-induced 2916–18
hypoventilation syndromes, treatment 2520
hypovitaminosis A
  benign intracranial hypertension and 4042
  see also vitamin A, deficiency
hypovolaemia
  acute 3458–9
  in acute renal failure 3285, 3286
  collapse after marathons 4328
  diagnosis 3282, 3283
  endurance sports and 4327–8
  in haemolytic uraemic syndrome 3201
  hypernatraemia 3124, 3126
  hyponatraemia 3122–3
  in leptospirosis 699
  in malaria 845, 846, 854
  in malnutrition 1283
  in marathons and mass runs 4327–8
  in nephrotic syndrome 3144
  pericardial tamponade vs 2478
  in peritonitis 2008
  thirst in 3117
  vasopressin secretion 3118
  see also dehydration
hypovolaemic shock, liver in 2138
hypoxaemia
  absent ventilatory drive and 2916
  in acute pancreatitis 2029
  in adult respiratory distress syndrome 2640, 2641, 2853
  of altitude 2916
  in alveolar filling syndromes 2639
  assessment 2669–71
  in asthma 2636
  causes 2630–1, 2670
  compensatory mechanisms in 2671
  in cystic fibrosis 2749
  in diffuse interstitial fibrosis of lung 2636
  in hepatocellular failure 2104
  in obstructive sleep apnoea 2910–11
  in Pneumocystis carinii pneumonia 823
  in pregnancy 1745–6
  in pulmonary oedema 2503
  sleep-related 2916
    in chronic obstructive airways disease 2777
  in smoke inhalation 1102
  ventilation in ARDS 2858
hypoxanthine-guanine phosphoribosyl transferase (HGPRT) 1378, 1381
  deficiency 4009
    partial 1382, 1383, 3226
    severe, see Lesch-Nyhan syndrome
  gene, polymorphisms 3391
hypoxia 1194–7, 2902–3
  acute 2902
  acute liver failure due to 2106
  in acute mountain sickness 1188–9
  aerospace medicine and 1194–7
    passengers 1202
  after head injury 4045, 4045

assessment 2903
cellular, in cardiac cachexia 2177
chronic 2902–3
clinical features 2902
in cor pulmonale 2516, 2519
in diabetic ketoacidosis 1500, 1502
effects 2902
erythropoiesis and 3454
fetal, in maternal anaemia 3469
hazard of gastric lavage 1049
hepatocellular injury 2100
high altitudes 1186, 1195–7
hypothermia in 1184
long-term,
  cor pulmonale after 2516
  pulmonary hypertension after 2509, 2514, 2516
pathophysiology 2902
perinatal, cerebral palsy aetiology 4120
'permissive', in PEEP 2922
polycythaemia and 3551–2, 3554
in pulmonary alveolar proteinosis 2833
pulmonary hypertension in 2902
in pulmonary oedema 2503, 2504
pulmonary vasoconstriction 2491–2, 2514
  blood volume regulation and 2157
  cor pulmonale due to 2516–17
  nitric oxide reduction 2514
  pulmonary hypertension 2509, 2514, 2516
in respiratory failure definition 2901, 2902
reversal with long-term oxygen 2520
in right heart failure 2902
in sickle-cell trait 3514
in spinal cord injury 3898
in tetanus 625
vasodilatation, bronchial capillaries 2494
ventilation control assessment 2672
hypoxic cells, radiotherapy resistance 254
hysterectomy, anaerobic infections 573
hysteria, see dissociative disorder
hysterical bleeding 3637
hysterical personality 4212
hysterical pseudodementia 3967

I

I-band 4139
ibuprofen, poisoning 1056
ICAM-1, see intercellular adhesion molecule 1 (ICAM-1)
ICD-10, substance abuse classification 4269–70
ICE (ice, compression and elevation) therapy 4321
I-cell disease (mucolipidosis II) 1434, 1435
ichthyosiform erythroderma 3719, 3720
ichthyosis 244, 3718–20
  acquired 3792
  malnutrition and 3722
  sex-linked 3719
ichthyosis hystrix 3750
ichthyosis vulgaris 3719
icterus, see jaundice
idiopathic chronic ulcerative enteritis 1910
idiopathic 'lethal' midline granuloma 1995, 3013
idiosyncratic reactions, asthma 2849–50
IgA, see immunoglobulin A (IgA)
IGFI, see insulin-like growth factor I
IGFII, see insulin-like growth factor II
ileal brake mechanism 1925, 1934, 1935
ileal conduit, urinary diversion 3244
ileitis, lymphogranuloma venereum vs 761
ileoanal anastomosis, in familial adenomatous polyposis 1990
ileo-anal reservoir/pouch
  complications 1950
  in ulcerative colitis 1950

ileocaecal valve
  fatty enlargement 1987
  loss 1976
  reflux 1832
  removal/resection 1925
ileocolitis, in Crohn's disease 1938
ileopsoas muscle bleeds, in haemophilia
ileostomy
  Brooke, in ulcerative colitis 1950
  in Crohn's disease 1942, 1943
  split 1943
  urinary stone disease and 3255
ileum
  absorption of nutrients 1900
  bypass surgery, in familial hypercholesterolaemia 1414
  disease, bile-acid breath test in 1910, 1914
  loss 1976
  malignant tumours 1985
  Meckel's diverticulum 1977
  normal bacterial flora 1911
  resection,
    bacterial overgrowth aetiology 1912
    gut peptides in 1896
    physiology after 1925
    vitamin B12 deficiency 3491
  in short gut syndrome 1925
  terminal, absorption by 1900
  in typhoid 561, 565–6
ileus, see adynamic ileus; paralytic ileus
iliac arteries, renal transplantation and 3314, 3318
iliac fossa
  left,
    pain in irritable bowel syndrome 1966
    pain in ischaemic colitis 1998
  peritonism 1970
  right,
    pain in acute intestinal ischaemia 1996
    pain in appendicitis 2010
iliotibial band friction syndrome 4324
illness, see physical illness
imaging
  body fat distribution measurement 1305
  radionuclide, see scintigraphy
  respiratory disease, see thoracic imaging
  tumours 234–40
    diagnostic problems 239
    disease staging 234–8
    disseminated disease 239, 239
    monitoring response to treatment 239
    recommended staging investigations 236
    recurrence detection 239
    see also TNM staging
  see also computed tomography (CT); magnetic resonance imaging (MRI); radiography; radiology
imbalance, in progressive supranuclear palsy 4005
Imerslund's disease (Imerslund-Grüsbeck syndrome) 3491
imidazoles 811
iminoglycinuria, familial renal 1357, 3332, 3333
imipenem 685
  in renal failure 3272
imipenem/cilastin, in urinary-tract infections 3211
imipramine, in panic disorder 4207
immediate hypersensitivity, see hypersensitivity
immersion hypothermia 1183
immersion injury 1183
immobility/immobilization
  cardiac cachexia and 2176
  deep vein thrombosis risk 2522, 3676
  in diabetic foot disease 1491
  leg ulceration management and 3808–9
  metabolic effects 1550
  osteoporosis related to 3068–9
  venous thromboembolism risk 3676
immotile cilia syndrome, male infertility 1685

immune-complex diseases 155, 164–5, 279
  complement disease causing 182
  classical activation failure 164, 178, 179
  drugs inducing 164
  factors influencing development 181, 182
immune complexes
  in chronic active hepatitis B 2066
  circulating,
    in Behçet's syndrome 3044
    in rheumatic disease 2952–3
  in cryoglobulinaemia 3050
  deposition,
    antigen trapping vs 182, 3774
    sites 165, 278
  detection 2952–3
  in drug-induced haemolytic anaemia 3542
  failure to solubilize 164, 179
  harmful effects 3774
  in Henoch-Schönlein purpura 3151, 3152
  host response to 3774
  in IgA nephropathy 3151, 3152
  in infection-associated glomerulonephritis 3173
  in infective endocarditis 2438, 2439, 2442
  intolerance, SLE as disorder of 3025
  in leprosy 674
  in lupus nephritis 3188
  in meningococcal infections 537
  in mesangiocapillary glomerulonephritis 3157
  removal, classical activation of complement 176
  in sarcoidosis 2830
  tissue damage by 164–5, 278–9, 3774
  in tumour-associated nephropathy 3184–5
  vasculitis due to 3774
immune disorders
  chronic fatigue syndrome in 1037
  gastrointestinal, see under gastrointestinal disorders
  hepatic granulomas due to 2122
  non-Hodgkin's lymphoma association 214
  see also immune response; immune system
immune evasion
  Entamoeba histolytica 827
  mechanisms 91
  by Neisseria gonorrhoeae 545
immune mechanisms of disease 154–66
  autoimmunity 156–65
  effector mechanisms 155–65, 278–9
    autoantibodies 163–4, 278
    cellular (T-cell)-mediated 165, 279
    IgE-mediated 155–63, 278
    immune-complexes 164–5, 278–9
  tolerance breakdown 155–6
  see also allergic diseases; autoimmunity; hypersensitivity; immune-complex diseases; immunological overactivity
immune response 277–8
  aberrant 154–5
    paraneoplastic syndromes due to 242
  accessory cells in 153–4
  to allografts, see transplantation immunology
  alveolar macrophage role 2615
  antibodies, see antibodies
  antigens and antigen processing 141–5
  cell-mediated, see cell-mediated immune response
  cytokines role 98, 99
  in dental caries 1846
  genetic factors influencing 280
  harmful 278–9, 278
    see also immune mechanisms of disease
  humoral, see humoral immunity
  impairment, nutrition and infection relationship 282

to infections, *see under* infections
inflammation due to 290
intestinal 1837
non-specific **276–2593**
  specific response *vs* 141
priming **145**
silent and visible types 141
smoking effect on 2813
specific **277–8**
suppression, *see* immunosuppressed/
  immunosuppression
viral infections of CNS 4066
see also antibodies; B-cells; T-cells
immune response (Ir) genes 186
immune responsiveness 280
immune-stimulating complexes
  (ISCOMs) 381
immune surveillance of tumours 227,
  260
  evidence for *227*
immune system
  endocrine interactions 1553–4
  in heart failure 2235
  in idiosyncratic drug reactions 2125
  in malnutrition 1287, *1290*
  organization **154**, 3561–2
  see also immune disorders; immune
    response
immunity
  adaptive 315
  fetus and neonate 1784
  herd 316
  non-adaptive 315
  in pregnancy 1784
  tumour-specific, *see* tumour
    immunology
  see also immune response
immunization 284, 288–9, **315–21**
  achievements 284
  active 284, 288–9, 315, **317–21**
    diphtheria 496
    evidence for efficacy 317
    historical background 317
    schedules 317–20, *318*
    successes and implications of 284,
      315
    see also vaccination; vaccines
  against oncogenic viruses 227
  challenges 315
  in developed countries **320**
  in developing countries **320–1**, *321*
  EPI, *see* Expanded Programme on
    Immunization (EPI)
  opportunistic 320
  oral 316
  passive 283–4, 315, **316–17**
    adverse effects 317
    animal antisera 317
    antisera 283–4, 316–17
    diphtheria 496–7
    Haemophilus influenzae 584
    hyperimmune globulin 317
    indications and uses 316
    normal immunoglobulin 283, 316–17
    products used *317*
    tumour antigens 233
    see also gammaglobulin; intravenous
      immunoglobulin
  programmes 316
    factors to consider 316
    herd immunity and 316
    schedules 288–9
    predicted for year 2025 *321*
    in SLE 3022
  streptococci group B infections 509
  for travellers **323–4**, *323*, 2007
  tumour antigens 233
  see also immunoprophylaxis; *specific
    vaccines*; vaccines
immunoassays
  Bordetella infections 588
  glanders diagnosis 594
  Helicobacter pylori 1885
  melioidosis diagnosis 592
  paracoccidioidomycosis 819
  two-step 1607–8
  see also enzyme immunoassay;
    immunodiagnosis

immunoblastic (angio-immunoblastic)
  lymphadenopathy **2807**
immunocompromised host
  cause of death 1031
  classification and definition 1027
    see also immunodeficiency;
      immunosuppressed/
      immunosuppression; splenectomy
  hepatitis B vaccination 454
  herpes zoster in 349–50
  infections in **1027–35**
    acute gastrointestinal syndromes
      1034–5, *1035*
    acute neurological syndromes 1033–4,
      1034
    approach to management 1029–30
    aspergillosis 808–9
    causes *1031*, 1032, *1032*
    chickenpox 348
    chlamydial 753
    clinical syndromes 1029–35
    coagulase-negative staphylococcal 532
    conditions related to 1027, *1028*
    cryptosporidiosis 873–4
    cytomegalovirus (CMV) 361, 362
    fever and pulmonary infiltrates
      1031–3, *1032*
    herpes simplex virus 345, 346
    opportunistic fungal 806–7
    speed of progression 1030
    splenectomy and 1027–8
    see also fever of unknown origin
      (FUO); opportunistic infections
    nocardiosis in 686
    Pneumocystis carinii pneumonia 820
    pneumonia in 1031, 1032, 2693–4
    septicaemia in 1022
    travellers **325**
    viral oesophagitis in 1876
    see also immunodeficiency;
      immunosuppressed/
      immunosuppression; neutropenia
immunocyte dyscrasia, amyloidosis in
  1513, **1515**
immunocytochemistry
  gut peptides 1891
  in muscle disorders 4143
immunodeficiency **166–75**
  after splenectomy 1028
  atopic eczema-like syndrome 3741
  bacterial overgrowth aetiology 1912
  bronchiectasis in 2757, *2757*, 2758,
    2761
  classification 166, *167*, 174
  differential diagnosis 169, 170, *172*,
    174
  giardiasis in 878, *879*
  history and examination 166
  in inborn errors of purine metabolism
    1385–6
  in myeloma 3599
  pneumonia in 2703, 2710
  primary **166–73**, *167*, 1027
    antibody, *see* antibody-deficiency
      syndromes
    classification *167*
    common varied, *see* common varied
      immunodeficiency (CVID)
    gastrointestinal disorders in **1837–41**,
      1840
    infections in 1027
    mixed T- and B-cell 172–3
    moderate 173
    selective T-cell deficiency 171–2
    severe combined, *see* severe combined
      immunodeficiency disease (SCID)
  respiratory tract infections 2710
  secondary 166, **173–5**, 1027
    causes 173, *174*
    classification *174*
    gastrointestinal tract in **1841–2**
    infections in 1027–8
    nutritional 174
    see also AIDS; immunosuppressed/
      immunosuppression; splenectomy
  severe combined 1385
  toxoplasmosis in 866–7
  treatment 2761

viral infections of CNS 4065
  see also antibody-deficiency;
    hypogammaglobulinaemia
immunodiagnosis 66
  enterotoxigenic *E. coli* (ETEC) 556
  gonorrhoea 547, 548
  meningococcal infections 540
  paracoccidioidomycosis 819
  Streptococcus pneumoniae 519–20
  typhoid 564
  see also immunoassays;
    immunofluorescence
immunodiagnosis of tumours **232–3**
  antibodies *in vitro* 232, *232*
  antibodies *in vivo* 232–3
immunoelectrophoresis, hydatid disease
  diagnosis 958
immunoendocrinology 1553–4
immunofluorescence
  actinomycetes detection 681
  antimitochondrial antibodies detection
    2075
  in Argentinian haemorrhagic fever 438
  dengue haemorrhagic fever diagnosis
    420
  rabies diagnosis 401–2
  respiratory syncytial virus detection 339
  rickettsial diseases diagnosis 732, 733
  Rochalimaea henselae detection 745
  skin examination 3711, *3711*
  toxoplasmosis diagnosis 868
  see also microimmunofluorescence
immunoglobulin(s)
  assembly 70
  on B-cells 141, 148
  in bronchiectasis 2758–9
  in cerebrospinal fluid 3843, *3844*
  classes *147*
  cryoprecipitation, *see* cryoglobulin
  Fc receptor 145, 153, 3559
  gene rearrangements 146–7
    heavy chain (Ig$_H$) 3395, 3396, 3580
    in leukaemia *3394*, *3412*
    in lymphoproliferative disorders
      3564–5
  genes 146
    D and *J* genes 146
    regulation 147
    somatic mutation and variations 146
    switching 149, 153
    variable 146
    V$_H$ and V$_L$, in SLE 3026
  glycosylation patterns, in rheumatoid
    arthritis 2954
  Gm haplotypes, in anti-GBM disease
    3164
  heavy chain (Ig$_H$), rearrangements 3395,
    3396, 3580
  homing 1836
  increased catabolism/loss 175
  intramuscular (IMIG) 169, 170
  intravenous, *see* intravenous
    immunoglobulin
  light chains, *see* light chains,
    immunoglobulin
  in lung secretions 2614
  production, IL-4 role 157
  receptors, endocytic pathway 73
  reference range *4366*
  replacement therapy 169–70, 2761
  in sarcoidosis 2829
  secretory 1836–7
    see also immunoglobulin A (IgA)
  serum, in myeloma 3599
  structure 145–6
    hypervariable regions 146
    light and heavy chains 145
    variable/constant regions 145–6
  supergene family 230, *2620*, **2621**
immunoglobulin A (IgA)
  absent 171
    in common varied immunodeficiency
      (CVID) 166
  allergic transfusion reactions 3692
  in anti-GBM disease 3165
  in chlamydial infections 756, 759
  in coeliac disease 1917
  coproantibodies 382

in dermatitis herpetiformis 3782
in Henoch-Schönlein purpura 3151–2
homing 1836
in IgA nephropathy 3151–2
in lung secretions 2614
in meningococcal infections 537, 538
Neisseria gonorrhoeae 545
rarity of small-bowel tumours due to
  1985
in rheumatoid arthritis 3193
salivary, dental caries and 1846
secretion by lamina propria 1836
secretory 277, 1836–7, 2001, 2614
  bacterial overgrowth aetiology 1912
  function 277, 1837, 2001
  respiratory syncytial virus 340
  to respiratory viruses 333, 336
secretory component 145, 1836
selective IgA deficiency 167, 170, **171**,
  1839–41
  aetiology 1839
  disease associations 171, 1839–41,
    1919
  drugs associated 174
  gastrointestinal features 1839–40,
    1839
  management 1840–1
immunoglobulin A (IgA) nephropathy
  3149–52, 3167, 3297
  clinical course 3150
  clinical features 3146, 3149–50
  diagnosis 3150
  malignant disease and 3185
  pathogenesis 3151–2
  pathology 3150–1
  in transplanted kidneys 3152, 3315
  treatment 3152
immunoglobulin E (IgE)
  in allergic rhinitis 2715
  in asthma 2725, 2727
    occupational 2743, 2744
  in atopic eczema 3739, 3740
  deficiency 171
  in diffuse parenchymal lung disease
    2781–2
  drug reactions mediated by 162
  in food allergy 1842
  functions 277–8
  immunological diseases due to **156–63**,
    278
    see also allergic diseases;
      hypersensitivity, type I (immediate)
  production,
    in allergic inflammation 157
    cytokines regulating 157, 2715, 2727
    RAST tests for 160
immunoglobulin G (IgG)
  in anti-GBM disease 3165
  clearance 3138
  in connective tissue diseases 3009
  functional deficiency 171
  IgG1 171
    in ulcerative colitis 1944–5
  IgG2 171
    in Crohn's disease 1938
    deficiency 171, 2758
  IgG3 171, 1944–5
  IgG4,
    deficiency 171
    in extrinsic allergic alveolitis 2811
  in lung secretions 2614
  maternal 166
  mediating haemolysis 3542, 3544
  in membranous nephropathy 3159
  in mesangiocapillary glomerulonephritis
    and 3158
  monomeric polyvalent 1764, 1765
  serum, in nephrotic syndrome 3141
  in Sjögren's syndrome 3037
  subclass deficiencies 171
  in toxoplasmosis 868
immunoglobulin M (IgM)
  in anti-GBM disease 3165
  capture assay, dengue haemorrhagic
    fever diagnosis 420–2
  in Chagas' disease 896
  in chlamydial infections 756
  in Crohn's disease 1938

immunoglobulin M (IgM) (*cont.*)
 deficiency 171
  incomplete 171
  in Epstein-Barr virus (EBV) infections
   354
  in intrauterine infections 1778
  in Lassa fever 434
  in leptospirosis 699
  mediating haemolysis 3542, 3544
  mesangial proliferative
   glomerulonephritis **3160–1**
  paraproteinaemia, neuropathy associated
   4102
  reduced in Wiskott-Aldrich disease 173
  rheumatoid factor 2954
  in toxoplasmosis 868
  in tropical splenomegaly syndrome 857
  in Waldenström's macroglobulinaemia
   3604
  X-linked immunodeficiency with hyper-
   IgM 166
immunohistochemistry, tumours of
  unknown primary site 252
immunological memory 141, 316
  B-cells 148
  T-cells 149
immunological overactivity
  in Crohn's disease 1938
  in ulcerative colitis 1945
  see also hypersensitivity
immunological tests
  in rheumatic disease **2952–3**, *2952*
  see also immunoassays;
   immunodiagnosis
immunological tolerance 141, 142,
  155–6
  B-cells 155
  breakdown in autoimmunity, *see under*
   autoimmunity
  deletion of self-reactive T-cells 152,
   155
  induction, cytokines role in transplants
   187
  mechanisms for development 152, 155,
   155
  oral 1837
immunology **141–88**
  filarial infections 911
  neurological disorders 3816
  principles **141–54**
  transplantation, *see* transplantation
   immunology
  tumours, *see* tumour immunology
immunometric assays 1608
immunoneutralization 1891
immunopathological responses, *see*
  immune mechanisms of disease
immunopeptides, normal range *4371*
immunoperoxidase antibody assay, in
  rickettsial diseases 732, 733
immunophenotyping 3390
  leukaemia 3399, 3413, 3420
immunoproliferative small-intestinal
  disease (IPSID) 1930, 1986, 3583
immunoprophylaxis
  passive,
   antisera, *see* immunization, passive
   cytokines in 284
   neutrophil transfusions 284
  see also immunization
immunostimulation, in chronic active
  hepatitis B 2067–8
immunosuppressed/immunosuppression
  283
  in chronic active hepatitis B 2068
  corticosteroids in *283*
  drugs causing 174
  in infections 282
  in liver transplantation 2114
  lymphomas in 355
  in measles 377–8
  opportunistic infections in 1028–9
   duration of immunosuppression
    1029–30
  parvovirus B19 infections 448
  respiratory tract in,
   infections, *see* respiratory tract
    infections
   non-infectious complications *2709*

skin cancer in 3792
  therapeutic, *see* immunosuppressive
   agents/therapy
  tuberculosis and 641
  tumour development in *216*, *227*
  viruses causing 174, 4278
   see also HIV
  see also immunodeficiency, secondary;
   neutropenia
immunosuppressive agents/therapy
  alveolar reactions due to 2851
  in aplastic anaemia 3446
  in bronchiectasis 2765–6
  cancers associated with use *216*, *227*
  in cardiac transplantation 2257
  in cryptogenic fibrosing alveolitis 2792
  in fulminant vasculitis 3777
  in multiple sclerosis 3996
  in myasthenia gravis 4162–3
  non-Hodgkin's lymphoma association
   214
  in polymyositis and dermatomyositis
   4157
  in pregnancy 1734, 1764
  in primary biliary cirrhosis 2076, *2076*
  in primary sclerosing cholangitis 2079
  in renal failure 3274–5
  in renal transplantation **3318–19**
  in sarcoidosis 2832
  side-effects 2257–8, *2257*
  in SLE *3023*, 3024
  in vasculitis 3016
immunotherapy 66
  allergens in and concerns 158, 161,
   162–3
  in allergic rhinitis 2718
  in food allergy/intolerance 1845
  insect venom 161
  in leukaemia 3410
  in systemic vasculitis 3016
immunotherapy of tumours **232–3**
  against mutant oncogenes 260
  against tumour antigens 260
  antibodies *in vitro* 232, 260
  antibodies *in vivo* 232–3
  cytokines in 233
  monoclonal antibody developments 66,
   260
  T-cells in 233
impairment, definition *2943*
impedance, pulmonary vascular
  resistance *vs* 2506
impedance epigastrography (IE) 1957
imperforate anus, *see* anus, imperforate
impetigo 3718
  herpetiformis 1806
  post-streptococcal glomerulonephritis
   3173
  Staphylococcus aureus 524, 526
  streptococcal 499–500
   treatment 502
impotence
  in cirrhosis 2087, 2091
  erectile 1687
   in diabetes 1488
  in systemic sclerosis 3033
inactivity
  chronic fatigue syndrome association
   1037
  in obesity 1308–9
  see also immobility/immobilization
inappropriate ADH secretion syndrome,
  see antidiuresis, syndrome of
  inappropriate (SIAD)
inborn errors of metabolism **130**, **1335–9**
  animal genetic models 1338–9
  carrier state diagnosis 1338
  diagnosis 1336
  heterogeneity 1335
  in vitro fertilization and 1338
  liver transplantation 2113
  prenatal diagnosis 1338
  screening 1337–8
  treatment approaches 1336–7
  see also specific disorders
incidence 43
  rate 43
'inclusion blenorrhoea' 749

inclusion body myositis *1513*, 3039,
  4158
incontinence, *see* faecal incontinence;
  urinary incontinence
incontinentia pigmenti
  in infants 3784
  see also pigmentary incontinence
indemnity insurance 4312
indeterminate cells 3706
India, venomous snakes 1127
Indian childhood cirrhosis *2018*, 2023
indicator dilution method, cardiac output
  measurement 2222
indigestion 265
indirect haemagglutination, melioidosis
  diagnosis 592
indium-labelled leucocytes 1018, 2207
indium-labelled neutrophils, in Crohn's
  disease 1941
indocyanine green dye 2222
  clearance 2056, 2057
indole acetic acid derivatives, poisoning
  1057
indomethacin
  asthma due to 2849
  in Bartter's syndrome 3131
  breast feeding and 1811
  in gout in cyanotic congenital heart
   disease 2400
  poisoning 1056
  in pregnancy 1757, 1811
indoor air pollution, *see* air pollution,
  indoor
industrial hazards, *see* occupational
  disease/hazards
Industrial Injuries Scheme 1162
industrial substances, toxic neuropathies
  4099–100
Inermicapsifer madagascariensis 962
inert gas narcosis 1207
infant(s)
  accidental poisoning 1045
  botulism 631, 632
  drug abuse complications 4298
  electroencephalogram (EEG) in 3830
  gonadotrophin secretion 1580
  growth 1696
  hepatitis B immunization 454, 454–5
  HIV infection 1782–3
  mastocytosis in 3799
  meningitis features 4054–5
  mortality rates 40, 51
  mumps in 374
  normal haematological values *3380*
  pneumococcal vaccines in 522
  preterm, *see* premature infants
  raised intracranial pressure in 4035
  small for gestational age 1697
  transient hypogammaglobulinaemia in
   166
  vesicoureteric reflux 3214, 3217
  see also children; neonates
infantile acropustulosis 3784
infantile acute febrile mucocutaneous
  lymph-node syndrome, *see* Kawasaki
  disease
infantile autism **4108**
infantile hypotonia, *see* floppy infant
  syndrome
infantile myositis **4158**
infantile neuroaxonal dystrophy
  (Seitelberger's disease) 3989
infantile spasms (West's syndrome)
  3914, 4015
infantilism, sexual 1683
infarct, white 3774
infections **265–1039**
  acute on chronic renal failure due to
   3299
  after lung transplantation 2936, *2937*
  in AIDS **4078–80**
  in aplastic anaemia 3443, 3444–5
  approach to patients **265–8**
   clinical, *see below*
   ecological 265
  bone marrow transplant recipients 3698
  central nervous system (CNS), *see*
   central nervous system (CNS)

chemoprophylaxis 283, 289
  childhood anaemia and 3469
  chronic,
   amyloidosis in 1513, *1515*
   chronic fatigue syndrome in 1037
  in cirrhosis 2090
  clinical approach **265–8**
   history 265–6
   isolation procedures 268
   laboratory investigations 267–8
   physical examination 266–7
  congenital **4112**
   see also cytomegalovirus (CMV);
    rubella; toxoplasmosis
  control/management,
   chemotherapy, *see* antibiotics;
    antimicrobial therapy
   immunization, *see* immunization
   isolation 268, 289
   in leg ulceration 3809–10
   passive immunoprophylaxis 283–4
  C-reactive protein in 1528–30, 1532
  in Cushing's syndrome 1643–4
  in diabetes **1492–3**, 1496, 1503
   in diabetic foot disease 1490–1
  in drug abuse 1074
  drug eruptions in 3730, 3731
  dyserythropoiesis and 3524
  endogenous (autogenous) 327
  epidemics and outbreaks 286
  epidemiology **285–9**
   critical-point control 288
   historical aspects 285
   host/parasite/environment relations
    285
   investigation of outbreak 287–8
   outbreak control methods 288–9
   seasonal/geographical factors 286
   surveillance 286–7
   variations in occurrences 286
  epilepsy after 3917
  exogenous 327
  eye in **4191–4**
  global climate change and 36
  haematological changes **3678–81**
  haemolytic anaemia due to **3545**
  haemolytic uraemic syndrome due to
   3179, **3196–7**
  in Hodgkin's disease 3575
  hospital-acquired, *see* nosocomial
   infections
  host response, *see* defence mechanisms;
   host response to infections
  host-parasite relationship, *see* host-
   parasite relationship
  in hypogammaglobulinaemia 168–9
  hypoglycaemia due to **1510**
  iatrogenic 327
  immune response **275–9**, 2001
   antibodies 277, *277*
   cell-mediated 277
   harmful responses 278–9
   at mucosal surfaces 277–8, 2001
   non-specific 276–7
   specific 277–8, 2001
   see also host response to infections
  in immunocompromised, *see*
   immunocompromised host
  immunoprophylaxis, *see* immunization;
   immunoprophylaxis
  immunosuppression in 282
  infectious dose 268, 275, 291, 2001,
   2001
  in leukaemia 3407
   chronic lymphocytic leukaemia 3421,
    3422
  liver in **2133–4**, *2133*
  in malnutrition 281, *281*, 1287, 1288
   management 1289, 1291, 1295
  mortality in UK 39–40
  in myelodysplastic syndromes 3430
  in myelomatosis 3598
  nephropathies associated with 3157,
   3173–9
  in nephrotic syndrome **3141**
  non-dermatitic occupational dermatosis
   1165
  notifiable 286–7, 289

notification 42
nutrition and impaired immunity
  relationship 282, 294
occupational **1173**
opportunistic, *see* opportunistic
  infections
overwhelming post-splenectomy (OPSI)
  3530, **3595–6**
parenteral nutrition complications 1319
peritoneal dialysis-associated 3311
physiological changes **290–5**
  inflammation 290–2
  local 290
  in prolonged infections 294
  systemic 290, 292–5
  see also inflammation; sepsis; shock
postoperative, renal transplant recipients
  3318
predisposing factors 283
predisposing to other infections 282,
  282
in pregnancy **1775–95**
purpura in 3636
range of 265
in renal transplant recipients 3314,
  3319–20
in sickle-cell disease 3515
at snake bite site 1138–9
spread, routes of 268, **285–6**
surveillance **286–7**
susceptibility,
  in hepatocellular failure 2103, 2109
  malaria and 840
  in pregnancy 1784
transmission in blood **3693–4**
urinary tract, *see* urinary-tract infections
vasculitis due to 3776
vesico-blistering diseases in 3780
vesicobullous disorders in infancy 3783
  see also bacterial infections; *specific
  infections*; viral infections
infectious disease syndromes **1015–19**
  see also fever of unknown origin
  (FUO); septicaemia
infectious dose 268, 275, 291
infectious mononucleosis **353–4**, 3566
  arthritis in 3002
  diphtheria *vs* 496
  mumps *vs* 375
  toxoplasmosis *vs* 866
  see also Epstein-Barr virus (EBV)
infectious mononucleosis-like disorder,
  after blood transfusion 3679–80
infective endocarditis **2436–51**
  acute 2436
  aetiological agents 510, **2436–8**
    anaerobic 574
    Aspergillus 809, 2438
    Candida 808, 2438
    Coxiella and Q fever 743–4, 2437,
      2442
    culture-negative 2438
    fungal 2438, 2449, 2450
    gonococcus 546, 2437
    Gram-negative bacteria 2437
    HACEK group 2437, 2439, 2442
    mycoplasma 2438
    pneumococci 519
    Pseudomonas 2437
    unusual and miscellaneous 2437–8
    see also staphylococcal/streptococcal
      (below)
  aortic regurgitation in 2464, 2465, 2467
  aortic-root infection 2443
  at-risk patients 2451
  in brucellosis 621, 623
  in children 2443
  community-acquired 532
  in congenital heart disease 2439, 2443
  definition and classification **2436**
  diagnosis 2443, *2444*
  in diphtheria 495
  in drug abusers **2445**, 4279, 4285
    HIV-infected 4286
  in elderly 2440, 2443
  examination 266
  in Fallot's tetralogy 2402, 2439
    after repair 2406–7

haematological changes 3547, 3679
heart valve prostheses 2470
in hypertrophic cardiomyopathy 2389,
  2439
immunology **2438–9**
incidence **2436**
investigations **2441–3**
left-sided 2445
malignant 528, 2436
mitral regurgitation in 2457
in mitral valve disease 2460
nephritis in 164, 2439
pacemakers associated 2288
pathogenesis 2438
pathology **2439–40**
  of complications 2439–40
  underlying heart disease 2439
prevention 2450–1, *2450*
  in pregnancy 1740
prognosis 2450
prosthetic valve 2437, **2443–5**
renal disease 2439, 2441, **3174**
in rheumatic fever 2435, 2439
right-sided 2443, 2445
staphylococcal 2436, 2438
  coagulase-negative 532, 2437, 2444
  S. aureus 527, 528, 1020, 2437, 2438,
    2440
  treatment 2446, *2447*, 2448
streptococcal **510**, **2436–7**, 2440, 2444
  antibiotic prophylaxis 510, 2451
  causative organisms 510, 2436–7
  pathogenesis 510, 2438
  predisposing conditions 510, 2436
  treatment 510, 2446, *2447*
  Streptococcus milleri 509, 2436
symptoms and signs **2440–1**
treatment,
  antimicrobial **2446–9**, *2447–8*
  general principles **2445–6**
  persisting fever 2449–50
  response 2449
  surgical 2449, *2450*
  vancomycin 303, 2446
in ventricular septal defects 2428–9,
  2439, 2443
inferior epigastric artery, grafting 2355
inferior petrosal sinus, sampling 1648–9
inferior vena cava
  abnormal, in common atrium 2428
  chest radiography 2178
  collaterals 2093
  defects, ostium secundum defects 2424
  drainage to left atrium 2402
  enlargement 2181
    to left atrium **2415**
  obstruction 2093
    in Budd-Chiari syndrome 2098, 2099
  thrombosis 2098, 2523
infertile male syndrome 1693
infertility
  chemotherapy-induced 3575
  in chlamydial pelvic inflammatory
    disease 753
  in congenital adrenal hyperplasia 1664,
    1666
  in cystic fibrosis 2750
  female **1677–8**
  male 1680, **1684–7**
    causes *1682*, 1684–5
    diagnosis 1685–6
    drug-induced 1718
    treatment 1686–7
  mumps virus causing 373, 374
  oral contraceptives and 1724
  in polycystic ovary syndrome 1674,
    1675, 1676, 1678
inflammation **290–2**
  allergic, mechanisms 157–8
  antigen trapping *vs* immune complex
    deposition 182
  in asthma 2726, 2727–8, 2728, 2729
  beneficial 2624, 2626
  brain and 3990
  in cholesterol embolism 2377
  in complement diseases 179
  complement role 175–6, 178
  in Crohn's disease 1937, 1938

crystal-induced 2983–4
historical aspects 2616
in infections 290–2
  bacterial numbers 290–1
  endotoxin role **291**
  Gram-positive bacteria **291–2**
  specific organisms 290
  viral infections 291
  without specific features 290
initiation **2618–23**
  see also neutrophils; *under* lung
    inflammation
  leucocyte recruitment 3558–9
  lung, *see* lung inflammation
  mechanisms and mediators, *see*
    inflammatory mediators; lung
    inflammation
scarring and **2626–7**
signs 2616
termination **2623–8**
  see also under lung inflammation
triggers 290
in urticaria 3770
see also inflammatory response
inflammatory bowel disease 1824
  in ankylosing spondylitis 2967
  chronic, in common varied
    immunodeficiency (CVID) 169
  enteropathic synovitis in 2972–3
  haematological changes 3683–4
  inflammatory diarrhoea *vs* 2006
  liver in 2131–2, *2132*
  ocular features **4184**
  in pregnancy 1802
  primary sclerosing cholangitis
    association 2077, 2079, *2079*
  in selective IgA deficiency 1840
  urinary-tract obstruction 3246
  see also Crohn's disease; ulcerative
    colitis
inflammatory cells, *see* macrophage;
  neutrophils
inflammatory diseases
  chronic,
    amyloidosis in 1513, *1515*
    C-reactive protein in 1530
    folate deficiency in 3493
    leucocyte-mediated tissue damage 3560
  rheumatic, tests **2951–2**
  systemic, tests for **2951–2**
inflammatory disorder of airways
  (asthma) 2727, 2728, 2729
  see also asthma
inflammatory mediators 98, 291, 292,
  294, 2615, **2618–19**, 2951
  allergic rhinitis 2715
  alveolar macrophage secreting 2615,
    2615, 2619
  in asthma 2727, *2728*
  complement role 175, 178, 2618
  in Crohn's disease 1937, 1938
  dissipation on inflammation termination
    2623–4
  in extrinsic allergic alveolitis 2813
  in pneumococcal infections 513
  pulmonary oedema pathogenesis 2497,
    2498
  reaction to endotoxin 291
  in sarcoidosis 2819
  in urticaria 3770
inflammatory myopathies, *see* myopathy,
  inflammatory
inflammatory neuropathies **4101–2**
  in HIV infection 4076
inflammatory response
  alveolar macrophage role 2615, 2619
  in bacterial meningitis 4052
  in cryptogenic fibrosing alveolitis
    2788–9
  cytokines in 98, 2615, *2615*
  lung, *see* lung inflammation
  macrophage role 93, 94, 154, **2615**
  in malnutrition *1290*
  in pneumococcal infections 513, 514
  vascular injury 3773
    defective 3774
    factors modifying 3776
  see also inflammation

influenza 338–9
  bacterial pneumonia with 514,
    2699–700
  clinical features 338–9
  cytotoxic T-cells role 152
  epidemic 286
  epidemiology and epidemics 338
  myalgia and myositis in 4154–5
  pathogenesis 333, 338
  pneumococcal infections after 514, 2699
  in pregnancy 1775, *1776*, *1777*
  prevention and treatment 339
  staphylococcal pneumonia after 526,
    2699
  vaccine-induced immunity 338
  vaccines 319, 339
influenza viruses **338–9**
  antigenic drift 338
  features of infections *341*
  haemagglutinin antigen structure 141
  M1/M2 proteins and nuclear transport
    79–80
  transmission and immunity 338
  type A virus 141, 338
  types 338
information
  on chronic fatigue syndrome 1038
  for informed consent 4317
  patient, *see* patient information
  rheumatic diseases 2944
  sexual health and 3351
information services, in control of
  sexually transmitted diseases 3349
informed consent, *see* consent, informed
infundibular stenosis
  in Fallot's tetralogy 2402
  'lone' **2420–1**
infundibulum, absence of body (crista),
  in Fallot's tetralogy 2404
inguinal ligament, arterial reconstruction
  below 2370
inguinal lymph nodes
  in chancroid 585
  in lymphogranuloma venereum 760
inguinal ulcers, genital 777
inhalational agents, poisoning **1093–102**
inhalation challenge tests
  asthma 2732, 2733, 2744–5
  extrinsic allergic alveolitis 2814, *2814*
inhalations, drugs 1238
inhalers 2738
  large-volume spacer 2738
inheritance
  Mendelian 1335
  mitochondrial (maternal) 1335
  multifactorial 100, 129
  polygenic 129
  quantitative characters 129
  see also genetic disorders
inhibin 1554, 1563, 1579–80, 1680
initiation, cancer development 198, 219
injecting drug use (IDU), *see* drug
  abuse(r) and misuse
injury, *see* trauma
Inkoo virus **424–5**
innominate steal syndrome 2368
  management 2373
inosiplex 4073
inositol, in diabetic tissue damage 1486
inositol triphosphate (IP_3) 1561, 2147,
  3618
inotropic agents
  in acute circulatory derangements 2564
  mechanism of action 2150, 2155, 2241,
    2253–4
  in myocardial infarction 2345, 2568
  negative **2150**, 2157
  positive **2150**, 2157, 2254
  in pulmonary embolism 2570
  septicaemia management 1024
  see also digitalis
inotropic effects **2150**, **2157–8**
  beta-adrenoceptor blocker overdose
    1064
  measurement 2157–8
  negative **2150**, 2155, 2157
  positive **2150**, 2155, 2157
Inoue balloon catheter 2455

insect(s)
  bites *3546*
    vesico-blistering from 3780
  hygiene and 1011
  non-venomous **1000–12**
    see also arthropods
  pruritus due to bites 3744
  stings 161, **1144–5**
    treatment and prevention 161, 1145
    urticaria and reactions 3772
insecticides **1122–3**
  aluminium phosphide 1123
  aplastic anaemia induced by 3441–2
  carbamate 1123
  Chagas' disease prevention 898
  gamma-hexachlorocyclohexane 1123
  malaria control 858
  organophosphorus, *see*
    organophosphorus insecticides
  pyrethrum and synthetic pyrethroids 1123
  resistance 861
insemination
  assisted 11
  donor 11
in situ hybridization 62
insomnia
  in terminal illness **4355**
  treatment 4253
inspiration
  deep, in asthma 2730–1
  pharyngeal muscles in 2909
inspiratory to expiratory (I/E) ratio 2921
inspiratory muscle training 2929
inspiratory pressure, in chronic
    obstructive airways disease 2775
inspiratory waveforms, ventilation
    parameter 2921
Institution of Occupational Safety and
    Health 1180
insulin 1553, 1556
  absorption from subcutaneous sites
    1473–4, 1478
  action 1340, 1400, 1563
    in carbohydrate metabolism 1457, 1505
    in lipid metabolism 1458
    potassium balance 3128
  allergy 1477
  antibodies 1473, 1477, 1510
  assay **1462**
  binding to its receptor 1462
  biosynthesis **1458–9**, 1559
  biphasic (mixed) *1474*, 1475
  bovine 1459, 1473
  carbohydrate metabolism in heart and
    2146
  continuous subcutaneous infusion
    (CSII) 1477–8
    in pregnancy 1755–6
  degradation 1461
  functions and actions 1274, *1275*
  gene (INS), diabetes type I and 1453,
    1454
  in heart failure 2234
  human 1459, 1473
    in pregnancy 1755
  Hypurin 1473
  insensitivity, obesity causing 1308
  intermediate-acting 1474
  intramuscular (IM) 1473, *1500*, 1501
  intranasal 1478
  intraperitoneal 1478
  intravenous (IV) 1473, 1478
    in diabetic ketoacidosis *1500*, 1501
    in hyperkalaemia 3135, *3286*
    in surgical patients 1494–5
  ketogenesis control 1276
  ketone body production 1276
  lente 1474
  long-acting 1474–5
  in lymph 1462
  in malnutrition 1286
  mechanism of action 1461–2
  monocomponent (highly purified) 1473
  mutations *1567*
  oedema 1477
  oral 1478
  overdose/poisoning 1071
    treatment 1072

pen injectors 1475–6
plasma *1462*
  in hypoglycaemia 1506
  in insulinoma 1507
  in monitoring therapy 1481
  in starvation 1505
in polycystic ovary syndrome 1673,
    1675–6
porcine 1459, 1473
preparations 1472–6
  duration of action/pharmacokinetics
    1473–5
  purity 1473
  species 1473
protamine 1474
raised levels, ischaemic heart disease
    risk 2309
receptor **1461–2**, 1555, 1556, *1560*,
    1561
  autoantibodies 163, 1510, 1570
  defects 1455, *1567*, 1572
  in heart 2147
  rectal 1478
  resistance 1411, 1455, 1572
    insulin therapy causing 1477
    ischaemic heart disease risk 2309
    in obesity 1308
    perioperative 1495
    in polycystic ovary syndrome 1675
    in pregnancy 1753
    spurious 1477
  syndrome (syndrome X) 1411, 2309
  type A 1455
  see also syndrome X
secretion **1459–61**
  basal 1461, 1565
  first-phase 1459, 1460–1
  in gestational diabetes 1753
  in hypokalaemia 3130
  in pregnancy 1461, 1753
  second-phase 1460–1
  training effect 2161
secretion stimulation,
  glucagon-like peptide 1 (GLP-1)
    1893
  glucose-dependent insulinotropic
    peptide (GIP) 1892
  self-administration, factitious
    hypoglycaemia 1509
Semitard 1473, *1474*
short-acting 1473, *1474*
skeletal actions 1627
subcutaneous injection 1473–4, 1476
synthesis 59
tard 1474
therapy *1467*, **1472–8**
  alternative methods of delivery
    1477–8
  in chronic renal failure 3302
  complications **1476–7**, 1497, 1498
  in diabetic ketoacidosis *1500*, 1501
  in diabetic nephropathy 3171
  dietary advice and 1468, 1469
  during infections 1492–3
  in elderly 4345
  initial dosage 1476
  peripartum 1756
  post-myocardial infarction 1492
  practical aspects 1476–8
  in pregnancy 1755–6
  in renal impairment 3274
  routine regimens 1475–6
  in surgical patients 1494–6
  tolerance test *1584*, **1585–6**
    in acromegaly 1593
    in Cushing's syndrome 1645–6
    in growth hormone deficiency *1699*
    in hypoadrenalism 1655
    in insulinoma 1507–8
    in trauma 1548
  ultralente 1474–5
  zinc 1474
insulin-like activity, non-suppressible
    (NSILA) 1505
insulin-like growth factor I (IGFI) 1505,
    1556, 1578
  atherosclerotic plaque development
    2293

control of growth hormone secretion
    1577
deficiency 1699
receptor 1556
serum,
  in acromegaly 1593, 1594
  in growth hormone deficiency 1699
  as measure of GH action 1565,
    1584
insulin-like growth factor II (IGFII)
    1505, 1555, 1556, 1578
  gene, imprinting 127, 128
  tumour-associated hypoglycaemia and
    1509, 1714
insulin-like growth factor binding
    proteins 1554
  type 3 (IGF-BP3) 1593, 1699, 1714
insulinoma **1506–9**
  amyloid deposits 1518
  angiography 1835
  diagnosis 1507–8, 1704
  localization and excision 1508–9
  malignant 1509
  medical treatment 1509
  in MEN 1 syndrome 1509, 1708
  mental symptoms 4240
insulin receptor substrate-1 1561
insurance, HIV infection and 471, 472
int-2 gene 223
integrins 2144, **2619–20**, *2620*
  ß₂ 88, 177
  leucocyte 2619, 3559
    on myeloma cells 3598
  platelet 3614
  receptors 2619–20
    platelet 3614, *3615*
  structure 2619
intellectual impairment
  subclinical, in HIV infection 4076
  see also cognitive impairment; mental
    retardation
intelligence
  defects, in Klinefelter's syndrome
    4239
  lead pollution 1229
  in spina bifida 4118–19
intelligence quotient (IQ) 4107
  in Down syndrome 4109
  in phenylketonuria 1362
intensive care **2563–88**
  acute dissections of thoracic aorta **2574**
  acute hepatocellular failure management
    2108–9
  acute pulmonary embolism **2569–70**
  acute renal failure 3293
  adult respiratory distress syndrome
    2574–6
  bronchoscopy **2579–80**
  cardiac tamponade **2570**
  circulatory derangements **2563–76**
    systematic approach 2563
  drug prescribing 3270
  myocardial infarction 2566–9
  neonatal, ethical issues 12–13
  nutritional support **2586–8**
  overtransfusion **2570–1**
  positive-pressure ventilation **2576–81**
    see also positive-pressure ventilation
  renal failure **2581–2**
  respiratory failure management, *see*
    under respiratory failure
  septicaemia **2572–4**
    in tetanus 629
  unconscious patients **2582–6**
    see also unconsciousness
    see also acutely ill patients
intensive care units 2563
  in HIV infection 473
intention tremor 3860, *4009*
intercellular adhesion molecule 1
    (ICAM-1) 2294, 2299, 2620, **2621**,
    3559
  in asthma 2728
  on biliary epithelial cells 2078
  in malaria 842, 845
  melanoma metastases 231
  neutrophil binding to endothelial cells
    2620

rhinovirus infections 333, 335
  see also adhesion molecules
intercostal muscle pain 2168
intercostal tube drainage 2870–1
intercrines 3559
interdependence, alveoli 2628
interferon **95**, *96*, **97**
  in CNS viral infections 4071, 4072
  genital warts treatment 3369
  macrophage deactivation 89
  in psoriasis 3746
  in rabies infections 398
interferon-α 95
  in autoimmune hepatitis 2072
  in chronic myeloid leukaemia 3417–18
  in hairy-cell leukaemia 3423
  in hepatitis B 3178
    chronic active 459, 2067, 2068
  in hepatitis C 2072, 3176, 3650
    chronic hepatitis 459, 2069
  in influenza 338
  in myeloma 3601, 3602
  preparations available 459
  in primary myelosclerosis 3437
  in primary thrombocythaemia 3440
  in respiratory virus infections 334
  in rhinovirus infections 335
  side-effects 459
interferon-ß 95
  in adenovirus infections 337
interferon-γ 95, 97
  in chlamydial infections 758
  in chronic granulomatous disease 3561
  in multiple sclerosis 3996
  recombinant 99
  regulation of erythropoiesis 3388
  release, in ulcerative colitis 1945
  in SLE 3026
  tolerance induction to grafts 187
interleukin(s) **95**, *96*
  in allergic rhinitis 2715, 2716
  multiple interleukin deficiency 172–3
  in psoriasis 3746
interleukin-1ß, in cachexia syndrome
    241
interleukin-1 (IL-1) 95, 98
  in acute-phase response 176, 276
  in adult respiratory distress syndrome
    2855
  in atherosclerotic plaque development
    2293
  bacterial meningitis pathogenesis 4052
  in epidermis 3707
  in haemopoiesis 3384
  in inflammation 98
  inflammatory reaction to endotoxin 291
  levels in sepsis 293
  in lung inflammation 2619
  in myelomatosis 3598
  in pneumococcal infections 513
  prostaglandin synthesis in fever 293
  receptor antagonist 99
    septicaemia treatment 1026
  in septicaemia pathogenesis 1026
  in SLE 3026
  T-cells releasing 98
  tumours secreting 1712
interleukin-2 (IL-2)
  cancer therapy 233
  deficiency 172
  in graft rejection 187
  injections (IL2-PEG) 173
  receptors, altered expression in SLE
    3026
  regulation of erythropoiesis 3388
  release from Th1 cells 98, 150, 151,
    157
  retroviral *tax* gene effect 462
  therapy, in melanoma 1808
  tolerance induction to grafts 187
interleukin-2-diphtheria toxin, in cancer
    therapy 233
interleukin-3 (IL-3) 158, 3557
  in haemopoiesis 3384, 3387, 3388,
    3389
interleukin-4 (IL-4) 147, 3557
  in allergic rhinitis 2715, 2716
  in asthma 2727

in atopic eczema 3739
in graft rejection 187
release from Th2 cells 151, 157, 2727
interleukin-5 (IL-5) 97, 157, 159
in allergic rhinitis 2715
in haemopoiesis 3384, 3557
hepatic granulomas pathogenesis
2120
in hypereosinophilic syndrome 3611
interleukin-6 (IL-6) 157
in acute pancreatitis 2029, 2030, 2031
in haemopoiesis 3384, 3387, 3389
levels in sepsis 293
in myelomatosis 3598
prostaglandin synthesis in fever 293
interleukin-8 (IL-8) 97, 2770, 3559
haemolytic uraemic syndrome and
3199–200
in lung inflammation 2619
interleukin-10 (IL-10) 157
interleukin-11 (IL-11), in haemopoiesis
3384, 3387, 3389
intermediary metabolites, reference range
4370
intermediate coronary syndrome, *see*
angina (angina pectoris), unstable
intermediate density lipoprotein (IDL)
1401, 1402–3, 1408
ischaemic heart disease risk 2308
intermediate filaments 81
cell types with 81
functions 81
keratins 3706
in myocardial cells 2144
structural changes in mitosis 81
structure and subunits 81
intermediate syndrome, in
organophosphorus insecticides
poisoning 1122
intermittent claudication, *see*
claudication, intermittent
intermittent positive pressure ventilation
(IPPV) 2921
in adult respiratory distress syndrome
2857–8
in spinal cord injury 3898
see also positive pressure ventilation
internal capsule, lesions **3858**
internal carotid artery 3947
atherothromboembolism 3948
internal mammary artery, coronary artery
bypass grafting 2353–5
International Agency for Research on
Cancer (IARC) 220, 1166
International Civil Aviation Organization
(ICAO) 1199, 2360
International Classification of Epileptic
Seizures 3911, *3911*
International Commission on
Radiological Protection (ICRP) 215,
1220, *1221*
International Committee on Sarcoidosis
2818
International Labour Organization 1161
International Nuclear safety Advisory
Group (INSAG) 1178
International Union Against Tuberculosis
and Lung Disease 661
antituberculosis regimens 659
interneurones, in enteric nervous system
1953
interphalangeal joints
in psoriatic arthritis 2968, 2969
in rheumatoid arthritis 2957
INTERSALT Study 2312, 2530
intersex disorders 1683, 1689, **1690–5**
assessment 1694–5
gonadal neoplasia and 1694
management 1695
interstitial dendritic cells, *see* dendritic
cells
interstitial fluid 2560
antimicrobial drug distribution 301
formation 2560
lung,
dynamics **2492–4**, 2493–4, 2598
high permeability pulmonary oedema
2496

oncotic pressure 2493, 2495, 2496,
2504
in pulmonary oedema 2494, 2495–6,
2504
in lymphoedema 2560
interstitial lung disease, *see* cryptogenic
fibrosing alveolitis; lung disease,
diffuse parenchymal
interstitial nephritis **3221–31**
acute,
drug-induced 3258, **3259**, 3265, 3291
NSAID-induced 3224
acute renal failure due to **3291–2**
acute renal failure *vs* 3280
chronic,
in analgesic nephropathy 3221, 3222
NSAID-induced 3224
gout, purines and **3224–7**
granulomatous, in sarcoidosis 3186–7
immune-mediated 3179
infection-associated **3178–9**
in leptospirosis 700
in SLE 3188
interstitial oedema 2502, 2509, 2598
in adult respiratory distress syndrome
2853
interstitial pressure, reduced and
pulmonary oedema 2498
intertrigo 3768
candida 800–1
management 3807
intervention studies 45
interventricular septum, rupture 2569
intervertebral disc 2992
anatomy 3903–4
collapse 3904–5
degeneration 3903, 3904
prolapse 2992, 2993
in pregnancy 1767
sites 2992
protrusions 3906–7
cauda equina compression 3907
management 3906, 3907
sequestration 3906
interview, mental state examination
4203
intestinal absorption
capacity 1899
carbohydrates *1901*, 1902–3
failure, in short gut syndrome 1925
impairment, *see* malabsorption
lipids *1901*, 1903
mechanisms **1899–904**
carriers 1900, *1900*
cellular 1900
paracellular 1900
passive/active 1900
transcellular 1900
methods for studying 1899
minerals *1901*, 1903
proteins *1901*, 1903
sites 1900
vitamins *1902–3*, 1903–4
water and electrolytes 1900, *1901*, 1902
intestinal bypass
enteropathic synovitis in 2972, 2973
obesity treatment 1312
intestinal disease, skin disease in 3723
intestinal flora 1910, 1911, 2001
anaerobic 570
antibiotics effect 300
colonization resistance 2001
enterococci 509
numbers and species 1910, 1911
processes limiting proliferation 1910,
1911, 1912
in tropical enteropathy 1931–2
intestinal haemorrhage
in typhoid 566
see also gastrointestinal bleeding
intestinal hurry 1960
intestinal infarction 1994
non-occlusive 1995–6, *1995*
intestinal infections
malabsorption in tropics and 1930
tropical enteropathy aetiology 1931
tropical sprue aetiology 1934
see also gastrointestinal infections

intestinal ischaemia **1994–8**, **2366–7**,
2374, 2375
acute 1996, 2366–7
clinical features 1996
management 1996, 2374–5
aetiology 1994–6, *1995*, 2366
miscellaneous 1995–6, *1995*
occlusion of arteries 1994–5
vasculitis and angiitis 1995, *1995*
chronic 1996–7, 2367
clinical features 1996–7
management 1996–7, 2375
clinical features 1996–7, 2366–7
clinical syndromes 1996–8
colitis, *see* colitis, ischaemic
Crohn's disease aetiology 1937–8
focal 1997
management 1996–7, **2374–5**
non-occlusive focal 1996
pathogenetic mechanisms 1996
reperfusion damage 1996
intestinal lymphangiectasia 1841–2
increased catabolism/loss of
immunoglobulin 175
small-bowel biopsy 1908
intestinal metaplasia, gastric cancer
association 1983
intestinal motility 1286, 1900
see also gastrointestinal motility
intestinal necrosis 1996
intestinal obstruction
in ascariasis 937, 938
in Crohn's disease 1938
distal syndrome, in cystic fibrosis 1978,
2749
in diverticular disease 1972
inoperable, management 4355
in intestinal ischaemia 2367
subacute 1960–1
see also small intestine, obstruction
intestinal oedema, in heart failure 2240
intestinal perforation
in amoebiasis 828
in typhoid 565–6
in ulcerative colitis 1950
intestinal resection
in Crohn's disease 1942–3
gut peptides 1895–6
in intestinal ischaemia 2374, 2375
malabsorption in, *see* short gut
syndrome
intestinal telangiectasia 1998
intestinal tremodiasis **992–9**, *994–5*
intestinal tuberculosis, *see* tuberculosis
intestinal tumours, gut peptides in 1896
intestinal volvulus 1976
in cystic fibrosis 2749
embryology 1973
small-intestinal malrotation with 1976
intestine
calcium absorption/secretion 1623,
1627
cobblestone appearance 1938, 1940
congenital short **1978**
cystic disorders **2136**
drug-induced ulceration 1997
epithelial cells 1900
function in pregnancy 1770, 1803
immune response 1837
inflammatory disease, *see* Crohn's
disease; ulcerative colitis
intramural bleeding 1999, 2137
motor system, *see under* gastrointestinal
motor system
pseudo-obstruction 1999
chronic idiopathic (CIIP) 1959–60
sepsis, enterobacteria causing 551
strictures,
in colorectal cancer 1992
in Crohn's disease 1938, 1943
management 1943
in systemic sclerosis 1999
transit time, in malnutrition 1286
vascular disorders **2137**
vascular malformations 2137
see also colon; small intestine
intima 2289, 2295
in cor pulmonale 2515

fibrosis 2378
hyperplasia 2960
proliferation, in pulmonary
hypertension 2507
intoxication **4296**
alcohol, *see* alcohol consumption
intra-abdominal infections, anaerobic 572
intra-aortic balloon counterpulsation, in
myocardial infarction 2569
intra-aortic balloon pump, in unstable
angina 2330
intra-atrial baffle 2417
intracellular fluid, antimicrobial drug
distribution 301
intracellular signalling pathways, in heart
2147
intracellular transport **75–8**
control during mitosis 78
GTP-binding proteins role 75, 76–7
in heart 2147
reconstitution studies/semi-intact cell
systems 75–6
in yeast 75, 76–7
see also vesicular transport
intracerebral abscess, *see* cerebral
abscess; intracranial abscess
intracerebral haemorrhage, *see* cerebral
haemorrhage
intracerebral metastases, *see* cerebral
metastases
intracolonic pressure 1969
intracranial abscess **4081–3**
diagnosis 4082–3
differential diagnosis 4083
epidemiology and aetiology 4081
management 4083
microbiology 4081
pathology and clinical features 4082
prognosis 4083
see also cerebral abscess; subdural
empyema
intracranial cysts **4116**
intracranial disorders, neuroradiology,
see neuroradiology
intracranial haemangioblastoma 3963
intracranial haematoma
computed tomography 3817
interval between injury and 4045
management 4047, *4048*
risk 4045, *4045*
traumatic 4045
intracranial haemorrhage
in autoimmune thrombocytopenia 3630
in fetal thrombocytopenia 1764
in haemophilia 3647–8
spontaneous **3961–2**
causes 3961, *3961*
see also cerebral haemorrhage;
subarachnoid haemorrhage
intracranial hypertension, benign
(idiopathic) **4040–4**
aetiology 4041–2
clinical features 4080–41
definition and incidence 4040
drug-induced 4042
investigations 4042–3
management and prognosis 4043
pathogenesis 4042
pregnancy and 4043
see also intracranial pressure, raised
intracranial lesions, pulmonary oedema
after 2501
intracranial pressure
intradural/extradural measurement 2586
measurement 2586
monitoring, in head injury 4046–7
subdural monitoring 2109
intracranial pressure, raised 2585
in benign intracranial hypertension 4040
in cerebral metastases 250
control 2585–6
headache in 4027
in hepatocellular failure 2103, 2109
in hypocalcaemia 1633
in intracranial tumours 4034, **4035**
in malaria 845
management 2109, 4037, 4059
in terminal illness 4356

intracranial pressure, raised (cont.)
  in meningitis 4059
  in neurocysticercosis 965, 967
  symptoms 4035
  in tuberculous meningitis 4060, 4063
  see also intracranial hypertension
intracranial saccular aneurysms **3963**, *3963*
intracranial tumours 3917, **4029–40**
  aetiology **4029**
  classification 4029–30, *4030*
  clinical features **4035–6**
  dementia due to 3971
  differential diagnosis **4036**
  epidemiology 212–13
    incidence and distribution **4029**, *4031*
  epilepsy and **3917**, 4036, 4040
  focal neurological deficits in 4035–6
  investigations **4036–7**
    biopsy 4039
    electroencephalogram 3830, 4037
    magnetic resonance imaging 3821, 4037
    somatosensory evoked potentials 3834
  management **4037–8**, *4038*
    chemotherapy 4039–40
    long-term **4040**
    radiotherapy 4039
    surgery 4038–9
  mental disorders/symptoms 4236–7
  metastases **4034**, 4038
  neurocysticercosis vs 968
  neurological examination 4036
  pathology **4029–34**
  pathophysiology **4034–5**
  in pregnancy 1767
  prognosis *4038*, 4039, **4040**
  raised intracranial pressure 4034, **4035**
  see also specific tumours
intracranial venous thrombosis 3956–7, *3957*
intracrine action 1564, 1565
intradural haematoma, traumatic 4045
intraepithelial lymphocytes (IEL) 1836
  in coeliac disease 1917
  in enteropathy-associated T-cell lymphoma 1928
  in microscopic colitis 2137
  in ulcerative colitis 1945
intraepithelial neoplasia
  after genital warts 3369
  see also cervical intraepithelial neoplasia (CIN)
intramuscular drug formulation 1239
intramuscular immunoglobulin (IMIG) 169, 170
intraperitoneal abscesses 2008
intrapharyngeal pressure 2611
intrauterine growth retardation 1697
  see also fetus, growth
intravascular devices, coagulase-negative staphylococcal infections 531, 532
intravenous cannulae, infections due to 330
intravenous fluids, see fluid, intravenous infusion
intravenous immunoglobulin 169, 170, 283, 316–17, 3695
  in autoimmune thrombocytopenia 3631
  cautions and contraindications 170
  in chronic lymphocytic leukaemia 1028
  indications and dosage 170
  in lupus nephritis 3190
  manufacture and contamination 169
  in streptococcus group B infection 1788
  in systemic vasculitis 3016
  see also immunization, passive
intravenous lines
  in Eisenmenger syndrome 2411
  sepsis 1021, *1022*
intravenous pyelography (urography; IVP; IVU) **3110**
  frusemide 3241, 3242
  in genitourinary tuberculosis 3276–7
  in reflux nephropathy 3215–16, 3217
  in renal hypertension 2546–7
  in urinary stone disease 3253

  in urinary-tract obstruction 3236–8, 3239–40
intravenous regional guanethidine block (IVRG) 2374, 3006, 3938
intravenous urography, see intravenous pyelography (urography; IVP; IVU)
intraventricular cysts, in cysticercosis (Taenia solium) 965
intraventricular haemorrhage
  computed tomography (CT) 3817
  in infective endocarditis 2441
  ultrasound 3825
intraventricular pressure 2157
intrinsic factor (IF) 3485, *3486*
  autoantibodies 3489
  in bacterial overgrowth 1913
  congenital defects 3491
introns 57
intussusception
  Campylobacter infections vs 558
  in cystic fibrosis 2749
inulin
  ¹⁴C-labelled 3105
  clearance **3105**
'invariant chain' protein 143
invasion, bacterial colonization mechanism 272
investigations, bronchiectasis *2758*, *2759*
in vitro fertilization (IVF) 1687
  ethics 11
  inborn errors of metabolism and 1338
  preimplantation diagnosis 136
Iodamoeba buetchlii 825
iodide
  clearance in pregnancy 1749
  skin eruption 3731
  thyroid clearance 1604
  in thyroid hormone synthesis 1604, 1605
iodine-131, see radio-iodine
iodine
  deficiency 1330–1, 1615, 1618
    in pregnancy 1749, 4112
  dietary intake 1604
  hyperthyroidism induced by 1612, 1613–14
  hypothyroidism induced by 1615, 1717
  metabolism 1604, 1605
  in nuclear emergencies 1234
  radiolabelled, see radio-iodine
  skin disorders due to 3729
  thyroid hormone secretion rate and 1606
  in thyrotoxic crisis 1614
  transport defects *1616*
m-iodobenzylguanidine, see MIBG scanning
iodochlorhydroxyquine (Clioquinol) 832
iodocholesterol 2043
iodohippurate, see hippurate, radiolabelled
iodo-isopropyl amphetamine (IMP) 3825
iodomethane (methyl iodide), poisoning **1087**
¹³¹I-6ß-iodomethyl-19-norcholesterol 1649, 1659–60
ion flux disorders, myopathy in **4169–70**
ionizing radiation **1217–22**
  bone tumour association 207
  cancer association 215, 1220
    in children 215
    latent period for 198
    life-time risk 215
  effects 1218–19
  leukaemia association 215, 1219–20
  occupational disease of haemopoietic system 1172
  thyroid cancer association 213
  see also radiation
ionophoresis 3767
ipecacuanha 296, 1048, 1049
  emetine from 831
  hazards of use 1049
ipratropium bromide 2849
IQ, see intelligence quotient (IQ)
Ir genes 186
iridocyclitis, in sarcoidosis 2826

iridodonesis 4181
iris
  absence 4182
  in ankylosing spondylitis 4185
  Lisch nodules 4181
iritis
  in ankylosing spondylitis 4185
  in Behçet's syndrome 4182, 4183
  in sarcoidosis 4182
  see also uveitis, anterior
iron **3470–82**
  absorption 1415, 1903, 3466–7, **3471–2**
    in dyserythropoietic disorders 3522
    factors affecting *3467*, 3471
  binding capacity 2960
    in malnutrition 1293
    see also total iron-binding capacity (TIBC)
  chelation therapy 3480–1
  deficiency (anaemia) 1279, *1418*, **3474–7**
    aetiology 3475–6
    in alcoholism 3685
    anaemia of chronic disorders vs 2960, 3475, 3483
    in bacterial overgrowth 1913
    in children 3469
    in chronic blood loss 3460, 3476, 3483
    in chronic renal failure 3682
    clinical features 3475
    in coeliac disease 1918
    in colorectal cancer 1991
    in Crohn's disease 1940, 1942
    diagnosis 3475
    diet and 3466–7
    fetal/neonatal effects 1759
    in gastrointestinal bleeding 3476, 3683
    in hookworm infection 931
    in liver disease 3684
    in nephrotic syndrome 3143–4
    oral manifestations 1863
    in paroxysmal nocturnal haemoglobinuria 3451, 3452
    pathophysiology 3459, 3474–5
    in polycythaemia vera 3434
    porphyrin metabolism in 1396
    in pregnancy 1758–9, 3468–9, 3476
    prevalence 3474
    prevention 3470
    in primary myelosclerosis 3437
    pruritus in 3744
    in rheumatoid arthritis 3681
    treatment 3461, 3476–7
    in tumours 242
    in ulcerative colitis 1946
    see also nutritional deficiency, type I
  deposition in haemochromatosis 2022
  dextran 3477
  distribution in body 3471
  erythropoiesis and 3454
  excess intake **3481**
  fortification of food 3470, 3481
  -loading anaemias **3479–81**, 3522
  metabolism 3472–3
  vitamin C and 3498
  overdose/poisoning **1070–1**
    clinical features and phases 1070
    lethal doses 1071
    mode of toxicity 1070
    in pregnancy 1071
    severity assessment 1071
    treatment 1071
  overload **3477–82**
    in liver disease 3481–2
    mucormycosis in 1027
    secondary 1417, 3477
    in sideroblastic anaemia 3522–3
    subSaharan Africa 3481
    in thalassaemia 3479–80, 3504, 3512
    tissue damage 3477–8
    transfusion-induced 3480, 3692
    see also haemochromatosis
  radioactive, see ferrokinetic studies
  recommended intakes *3467*
  red cell 3473–4
  requirements, in pregnancy 1758
  retention, dialysed patients 3327

  serum *3379*, 3473
    in anaemia of chronic disorders 3482, 3483
    in infections and fever 294
    in iron deficiency *3474*
    in pregnancy 1758
  sorbitol 3477
  status,
    disturbances **3474–82**
    measurement **3473–4**
  stores 3471
    in iron deficiency *3474*, 3475
    measurement 3473
    in pregnancy 1758–9
  total iron-binding capacity, see total iron-binding capacity
  toxicity, mechanisms 2022
  toxicosis, see haemochromatosis
  transport 3472
    measurement 3473
  treatment 3476–7
    parenteral 3477, 3481
    in pregnancy 1759, 1761, 3476
  uptake and release from cells 1416, 3472
iron-chelators, antimalarial drugs 850, 853
iron-responsive element-binding protein (IRE-BP) 3473
irradiation
  Bacillus anthracis spores 613
  see also ionizing radiation; radiation
irritable bowel syndrome 1824, **1966**
  brief dynamic psychotherapy in 4256
  chronic idiopathic intestinal pseudo-obstruction vs 1960
  clinical features 1966
  coeliac disease vs 1918
  definition and diagnosis 1966
  diarrhoea in 1824, 1825
  diet association 1328
  food intolerance 1844
  management and trials 1968
  non-acute inflammation of appendix vs 2011
  pathophysiology 1966
  ulcerative colitis vs 1947
  'irritable colon syndrome' 1960
irritant 3735
  dermatitis, see contact dermatitis
Isaacs' syndrome 4092
ischaemia
  acute renal failure and 3281
  after snake bites 1139
  carotid artery, see carotid artery ischaemia
  chronic ocular **4187**
  definition 2151
  gastrointestinal tract, see intestinal ischaemia
  myocardial, see myocardial ischaemia
  pain in peripheral neuropathy 3940
  in shock 292
  vertebrobasilar 2367–8, **2373**
  vesico-blistering diseases in 3779
ischaemia of limb
  acute 2363–4
  causes 2363
  chronic 2364
  clinical presentation 2363–4
  management **2369–72**
    drugs 2369
    reconstructive surgery 2369–72
    risk factors treatment 2369, 2370
ischaemic heart disease **2305–62**
  aircraft crew and pilots 1200, 2360
  atheroma/atherosclerosis, see atherosclerosis
  blood pressure and 30–1
  cardiac transplantation indication 2255
  in diabetes 1411, 1449, 1464, **1491–2**, 3172
  diurnal variation 2302
  electrocardiogram (ECG) in 2190–2
    ambulatory 2199
  epidemiology 2289, **2305–6**, 2331–2
    international differences 2305–6
    time trends 2306

family history 2306
haemostatic variables **2300–5**, 2309
  clotting factors 2303
  factor VII role **2301–2**, 2309
  fibrinogen role **2302–3**, 2309
  investigations 2304
  management 2304–5
  platelets 2303–4
  reduced fibrinolytic activity 2303
  see also factor VII; fibrinogen
heart failure due to 2229
in hereditary spherocytosis 3530
in hypercholesterolaemia 1406–8
in hyperlipoproteinaemia type III 1409
in hypertriglyceridaemia 1410
lipid-lowering therapy 1414
magnetic resonance imaging (MRI)
  2217
mortality rates 2305, 2306
  blood pressure relation 2316
  climate and season 2315
outcome, left ventricular function and
  2358
pathology **2318–21**
  see also atherosclerosis;
  atherosclerotic plaque
polycythaemia and 3553
in post-menopausal women 1813
in pregnancy **1738**
prevention **2316–18**
  aspirin 2304
  blood pressure reduction 2317
  cholesterol reduction 2316–17
  evaluation 2316
  evidence to support 2306
  failure of trials 2316
  fibrinogen levels reduction 2304
  multifactorial approach 2316, **2317–18**
  oral anticoagulants 2305
  Oslo trial 2317, 2317
  secondary prevention trials 2318
  single factor intervention studies
    2316–17
  strategies 2316
protection, antioxidant hypothesis
  2311–12
in renal transplant recipients 3313–14
risk factors 1326–7, **2306–16**
  age and gender 2306, 2307, 2332
  alcohol 2313–14
  behavioural **2309–14**
  birth weights 2312
  blood pressure 2308, 2316
  climate and season 2315
  diet/nutrition 1326–7, 1330, **2309–12**,
    2332
  environmental 2312
  exercise 2313
  geographic **2315–16**
  glucose intolerance and insulin
    resistance 2309
  haemostatic factors, see above
  lipids and lipoproteins 2307–8
  multiplication of effect 2313
  obesity and overweight 2309
  physiological 2306, **2307–9**
  psychosocial **2314–15**
  smoking 2310, 2312–13
  steroid hormones 2314
  type A personality 2315
screening 2304
serum cholesterol and 1404–5, 1407–8,
  1412
thrombosis in 2300, 2302, 2305
thyroxine replacement therapy in
  1616
see also angina; coronary artery
  disease; myocardial infarction;
  myocardial ischaemia
ischaemic necrosis, in frostbite 1183
ISIS-1 (First International Study of
  Infarct Survival) trial 2345
ISIS-2 (Second International Study of
  Infarct Survival) trial 23, 26–7, 28–9,
  2334, 2340, 2342
ISIS-3 (Third International Study of
  Infarct Survival) trial 2342

ISIS-4 (Fourth International Study of
  Infarct Survival) trial 30, 2340, 2344,
  2348
islet amyloid polypeptide (amylin) 1450,
  1455, 1518, **1520**
islet cell
  antibodies 1450, 1453
  tumours, see pancreas, endocrine
  tumours
islets of Langerhans
  in diabetes type I 1450, 1453
  in diabetes type II 1450, 1455
  insulin biosynthesis 1458–9
  transplantation 1478, 3172
  in type III diabetes 1450
isocyanates 1100
  poisoning **1100**
isograft, definition 183
isolation
  HIV infected patients and 472
  procedures in infections 268, 289
  protective,
    in aplastic anaemia 3445
    in leukaemia 3407
isoleucine 1353, 1368–9
  metabolism 1275, 1276
isomaltase, see α-dextrinase
isometric exercise, effect on heart 2161
isoniazid 3278
  adverse mental symptoms 4242
  adverse reactions 657, 3523
  mechanisms of toxicity 1068
  neuropathy due to 4100
  overdose/poisoning **1068–9**
  in pregnancy 1746, 1793
  in tuberculosis 655, 656
  in HIV infection 480
isonitriles, technetium-99m-labelled
  2207, 2211
Isoparorchis hypselobagri 987
isoprenaline **2254–5**
  in ß-adrenoceptor blocker overdose
    1065
  clinical uses and dose 2254, 2255
  in disopyramide overdose 1063
  mechanism of action and effects
    2254–5
  receptors 2254
isopropanol, poisoning 1078, **1080**
isopropyl alcohol (isopropanol),
  poisoning 1078, **1080**
isosorbide dinitrate 2247, 2248, 2327
isosorbide mononitrate 2327
Isospora belli 475, 881–2, 1930
  lifecycle and structure 882
Isospora hominis (*Sarcocystis hominis*)
  877
isosporiasis **881–3**
  in HIV infection 475, 487, 882, 883
isotopes 1217
  lung cancer and 2880
  scanning, see scintigraphy
  systemic 256
  see also radiopharmaceuticals
isovaleric acidaemia **1370–2**
isovaleryl coenzyme A dehydrogenase
  1370
Israeli spotted fever 736
Itai-Itai disease 1107, 1171, 3262
itching, see pruritus
itch mite, see scabies
itraconazole 798, 811
  in coccidioidomycosis 813
  topical 811
ivermectin
  in filarial infections 912
  in lymphatic filariasis 923–4
  in onchocerciasis 916

J

Jaccoud-like arthritis 3036, 3037
Jacksonian seizure 3913
Jamaican vomiting sickness 1159
jamais vu 3914
Jamestown Canyon virus **424–5**

Janeway lesions 2441
Jansky-Bielschowsky syndrome 3985
Janus-associated kinase-2 (JAK-2) 1561
Japan
  gastric cancer screening 1983
  venomous snakes 1127
Japanese, skin diseases in 3716
Japanese B encephalitis **413–14**, 4064
  clinical features 4068
  pathology 4066
  in pregnancy 1777, 1779
  vaccines 324, 414, 1777
Japanese summer-type pneumonitis
  2811, 2816
Japanese waltzing mice 2606
jargon aphasia 3848
Jarisch-Herxheimer reaction 693, 696,
  702, **718–19**
  in cardiovascular syphilis 2483
  features 719
  treatment 696–7, 719
jaundice **2054–60**
  in acute liver failure 2106
  in acute viral hepatitis 2061
  in biliary cancer 2052
  causes and pathophysiology 2056
  in choledocholithiasis 2050
  cholestatic 2046
    in biliary atresia 2014
    bilirubin binding to albumin 2055
    causes 2050–1, 2051, 2057
    clinical approach 2056
    in cystic fibrosis 2023, 2131
    ERCP in 1834–5
    painless, causes 2057
    percutaneous transhepatic
      cholangiography 1834
    pruritus in 3744
    see also biliary tract, obstruction;
      cholestasis
  in cirrhosis 2086, 2087
  classification 2056
  clinical approach 2056–7
  definition 2054
  drug reaction 1253
  in haemolytic anaemia 2132
  in hepatic amoebiasis 830
  hepatocellular,
    diagnosis 2106
    in hepatocellular failure 2100, 2101,
      2102, 2103
  in leptospirosis 699, 699–700, 700, 702
  liver function tests in 2055–6
  in malaria 846
  neonatal 2058, 3469
    in α₁-antitrypsin deficiency 1547
    in G6PD deficiency 3540, 3541
    in maternal diabetes 1757
    in Rh haemolytic disease 3545
  obstructive, see jaundice, cholestatic
  in pancreatic carcinoma 2042, 2052
  physiological of newborn **2058**
  in pneumococcal infections 514, 2130
  in pregnancy 1796, 1799
  in primary biliary cirrhosis 2074
  in primary sclerosing cholangitis 2078
  see also bilirubin; hyperbilirubinaemia
jaw
  in acromegaly 1592
  Burkitt lymphoma 354
  infections, anaerobic 572
  neoplasms, cysts and development
    lesions **1862–3**
  osteodystrophy 1862
  pain,
    in angina 2322
    in myocardial infarction 2335
  wiring, obesity treatment 1313
jaw jerk 2583, 3857
J chain 2614
JC virus 443, **446–7**, 461, 4073
  see also progressive multifocal
    leucoencephalopathy
jealousy, paranoid delusions and 4223
Jehovah's Witnesses 4317
jejunal biopsy
  in coeliac disease 1832, 1917

diseases diagnosed from 1908
  in enteropathy-associated T-cell
    lymphoma 1927
  in isosporiasis 883
  in microsporidiosis 886
  normal 1917
  in tropical sprue 1933, 1935
  in Whipple's disease 1924
  see also small intestine, biopsy
jejunal diverticulosis 1912
jejunitis, ulcerative 1928, 1929
jejunoileal bypass surgery
  gut peptides in 1895–6
  liver in 2132, 2139
jejunoileal obstruction
  congenital 1976
  management 1976
jejunoileitis 1839
jejunum
  absorption of nutrients 1900
  contents, aspiration 1914
  in enteropathy-associated T-cell
    lymphoma 1928, 1929
  loss 1976
  malignant tumours 1985
  in short gut syndrome 1925
jellyfish, venomous 1143–4
Jervell-Lange-Nielsen syndrome 2282
jet lag 322, 1203
Jeune's disease **2875**
jiggers 1005, 1010
jitter 3841
J (juxta-alveolar) receptors 2163, 2494,
  2501, 2503
Job's syndrome 3559
'job strain', blood pressure and 2531
Job syndrome 525
joggers
  calories used 1312
  sites of injuries in 4323
  sudden death in 4321
joint(s)
  acute sports-related injuries 4322
    management 4322
  aspiration, in gout 2987
  in brucellosis 620–1
  effusions,
    in haemoglobinopathies 3005
    see also synovial fluid
  'giving-way' 2945
  in gonorrhoea 547
  imaging **2948–50**
  infections,
    anaerobic 573
    and destruction after 2998, 2998
    mycoplasmal **771**
    staphylococcal 528–9
    see also septic arthritis
  in Kawasaki disease 3048
  loss of function 2945
  malfunction, in osteoarthritis 2981
  normal wear 2981
  pain 2944–5
    in osteoarthritis 2981
    see also arthralgia
  parvovirus infections 448, 3001
  replacement arthroplasty, in rheumatoid
    arthritis 2964
  in rheumatoid arthritis, see rheumatoid
    arthritis; specific joints
  scintigraphy 2949
  in spinal cord injury 3900
  stiffness 2945
    diurnal rhythm 2956
    morning 2945
    in polymyalgia rheumatica 2945,
      3040
    in rheumatoid arthritis 2956
    transient 2945
  swelling 2945, 2947
  symptoms **2944–5**
  in systemic disorders **3003–8**
  tuberculosis 653, 2999–3000
  in ulcerative colitis 1948, 2972–3
  see also arthritis; arthropathy; rheumatic
    diseases; specific joints
joint capsule, torn 4322

joint disease
in bronchiectasis 2760–1
crystals associated *2983*
degenerative 2975
see also osteoarthritis
eye in **4184–6**
inflammatory,
generalized musculoskeletal pain 2997
septic arthritis 2998
tests **2951–2**
'wear and tear' 2975, 2976, 2981
see also rheumatic disease
Joint National Committee of the National
High Blood Pressure Education
Program 2538, 2539
Jones criteria
post-streptococcal reactive arthritis 499
rheumatic fever 504, *504*
Jones index, breathlessness scale 2646,
2646
Jopling type reactions 672–3
Joubert syndrome **4113**
joules 1218
J receptors 2163, 2494, 2501, 2503
'J-shaped curve' hypothesis 2251
jugular foramen syndrome (Vernet's
syndrome) 3880
jugular venous pressure/pulse 2153,
3282–3
'a' wave 2153, 2387, 2467
in mitral stenosis 2453
Bernheim 'a' wave 2462, 2465
'c' wave 2153
in Ebstein's anomaly 2414
in endomyocardial fibrosis 2397
giant 'a' wave 2405, 2413
in Fallot's tetralogy 2402
in hypertrophic cardiomyopathy 2387
in pericardial constriction 2479
in pericardial tamponade 2477
in pulmonary valve stenosis 2419
X descent, in pericardial constriction 2479
see also venous pressure
Juliusberg's pustulosis acuta
varioliformis 345–6
jun gene 225
'jungle rot' 500
Junin virus 430, 436, 437
juvenile bullous pemphigoid 3783
juvenile chronic arthritis
ocular features **4185–6**
rheumatoid arthritis *vs* 2963
juvenile lupus 3018
juvenile osteoporosis 3069
osteogenesis imperfecta *vs* 3081
juvenile Paget's disease (idiopathic
hyperphosphatasia) **3089**
juvenile plantar dermatosis 3737
juvenile rheumatoid arthritis, *see* Still's
disease
juxta-articular nodules *3716*

K

kala-azar, *see* leishmaniasis, visceral
(kala-azar)
KAL gene 1572
kallikrein 3621–2, 3625, 3626
kallikrein-kinin system
heart failure pathophysiology 2235
hypertension pathogenesis 2531–2
renal 3119
Kallmann's syndrome *1567*, 1580,
1670–1
failure of puberty 1701
male hypogonadism 1683
pathophysiology 1572
Kanagawa test 559
kanamycin *3272*
in tuberculosis 655
kaolin 2845
kaolin pectin 2006
kaolin pneumoconiosis 2846
Kaplan-Meier survival curves 2338
Kaposi's sarcoma 1851, 3371–2, 3586
in AIDS 209, 461, 475, **476–7**, 1851,
3365, 3371

developing countries 488
heart involvement 2396
mycoplasma role 772
clinical features 477
colonic 1993
in drug abusers 4285
epidemiology 209, 461, 3365
incidence rate by country 199
in homosexuals 3365
oesophageal 1980
open-lung biopsy 2687–8
in renal transplant recipients 3321
treatment 477
Kaposi's sarcoma-associated herpes
virus-like (KSHV) 477
Kaposi's varicelliform eruption 345–6
Kartagener's syndrome 2613, 2759
male infertility 1685
karyotypes
description/nomenclature 119
normal 118
Kasai's operation 2015
Kashin-Beck disease *1418*, 1424, 2976–7
Kassabach-Merrick syndrome 3785
katacalcin 1637
Katayama fever 971, 975, 2004
Kato thick-smear technique 931, 978
Kawasaki disease 2000, 3011, **3047–50**
aetiology 3049
clinical features 3047–9
epidemiology 3047, 3049
management/treatment 3049
ocular features 3047, **4184**
pathology 3048–9
scarlet fever *vs* 502, 3049
Kayser-Fleischer ring 1420, 1421, 2022,
2088, 4008
K cells 1892
Kearns-Sayre syndrome 4148, **4172**
Keith-Wagner classification 2536
hypertensive retinopathy 4187–8
Kell blood group antigens 4146
Kelocyanor 1098
keloids 3716, 3788
Kemerovo viruses 406
Kennedy's syndrome 3988, 4089
Kent bundle 2193
kerala 1472
Kerandel's sign 891
keratin 3706
antibodies 3706
composition 3706
gene expression *3706*
keratinocytes 3706, 3707
increased turnover in psoriasis 3745
keratitis
amoebic 834
punctate 914
sclerosing 914
kerato-acanthoma *3726*
keratoconjunctivitis
atopic 161
chronic due to *C. trachomatis*, *see*
trachoma
vernal 161
keratoconjunctivitis sicca 3036
detection 3037
in rheumatoid arthritis 4185
see also eye, dry
keratoderma 3750–1
keratoderma blenorrhagicum 2971
keratolysis, pitted 3767
keratosis
frictional 1859
seborrhoeic *244*
smoker's 1858, 1859
solar *3726*
keratosis follicularis (Darier's disease)
3721–2, 3760
keratosis pilaris (perifollicular
hyperkeratosis) 3711, 3719, 3743
kerion 3762
Kerley A lines 2179, 2502
Kerley B lines 2179, 2180, 2502, 2841
kernicterus 2054, 2058, 3545
dyskinetic cerebral palsy due to 4121
Kernig's sign 539, 4053
Kernohan's notch phenomenon 4034

kerosene (paraffin oil), poisoning 1043,
1083
Keshan disease *1418*, 1424
ketanserin 1898
ketoacidosis
alcoholic 1080, 1542
causes *1537*
diabetic, *see* diabetic ketoacidosis
see also ketosis
ketoaciduria, branched chain (BCKA)
1369
ketoconazole
in coccidioidomycosis 813
in Cushing's syndrome 1651–2
in ectopic ACTH syndrome 1714
in paracoccidioidomycosis 820
side-effects 1688, 1718
ketogenesis 1276–7
lipogenesis link 1277
ketonaemia
in diabetes 1481
in hypoglycaemia 1506
ketone bodies 1276, 1400, 1458
after injury/surgery 1549
in diabetes 1498, 1499
elimination 1534
energy supply 1271
exercise-induced production 1478
formation and utilization 1276–7
metabolism, energy for heart 2146
in starvation 1277, 1400, 1505
see also ketoacidosis
ketonuria, in diabetes 1450, 1456, **1479**
ketoprofen, poisoning 1056
ketosis 1499
in salicylate poisoning 1054
see also ketoacidosis
17ß-ketosteroid reductase deficiency
1692
kidney
abscess 3207
acid-base homeostasis 1540, **3338**
adaptation in malnutrition 1286
amyloidosis 1514, **3180–1**, 3185, *3300*
calcium excretion, *see* calcium, renal
handling
carbuncle 3207
carcinoma, *see* renal cell carcinoma
(hypernephroma)
in cholesterol embolism 2376, 2377
clinical physiology **3101–15**
collecting system, *see* renal
pelvicalyceal system
cystic disorders 3111, 3202
of endstage renal disease 3312
genetic *3203*
nephronophthisis-medullary cystic
disease complex 3205
see also polycystic kidney disease
damage, *see* renal damage
disease, *see* renal disease/disorders
donors 3313, **3317**
drug excretion 1243–4
drugs and **3268–75**
glucose production in starvation 1277–8
hormone functions 1554
in hypertension 2533, 2534, 2535,
2546, **3247–50**
in hypokalaemia 3129–30
imaging **3109–15**
ischaemia 2542
in kwashiorkor 1288
length 3109–10
in leptospirosis 699, 700, 701
in malaria 844–5, 845–6
medullary sponge 3255
metastases 3183
nuclear imaging **3112–15**
obstructive atrophy 3234, 3239
occupational disorders 1171
pain **3148**
parathyroid hormone actions 1624,
1627
parenchymal disease,
in gout 2986
unilateral, hypertension in **2552**
see also renal disease/disorders
parenchymal scarring 2552

perfusion, ACE inhibitor action 2249
phosphate excretion, *see* phosphate,
renal handling
potassium excretion 3128–9, 3130
in pre-eclampsia 1728
sarcoidosis involving **3186–7**
scarring,
chronic renal failure 3303–4
reflux nephropathy 3216, 3217
sodium excretion, *see* sodium, renal
excretion
stones, in short gut syndrome 1925
trauma 3111
tumours,
epidemiology 212
erythropoietin production 3554
investigations 3111
metastases 3183
see also renal cell carcinoma
vascular disease,
acute renal failure in 3290–1
in chronic renal failure 3304
renal transplantation and 3315
see also vasculitis, renal
vitamin D metabolism 1625
water excretion **3116–18**
see also entries beginning renal
killer cells, in graft rejection 187
kinectin 83
kinesin 81, 83
Kingella, rare species *556*
'kissing' bugs 1006
c-*kit* proto-oncogene 3383
Klebsiella
pneumonia 1021
respiratory tract infections 551
Klebsiella pneumoniae subsp.
pneumoniae 551
Klebsiella rhinoscleromatis 568
Kleihauer test 3689
Kleine-Levin syndrome 3929
Klinefelter's syndrome 2899
breast cancer 1687
chromosomal abnormality *120*
gynaecomastia in 1688
hypogonadism 1683
infertility 1685
mental disorders/symptoms in 4239
neurological aspects 4109
SLE association 3017
Klippel-Feil syndrome **4116**
Klumpke's paralysis 3903, 4093
Klüver-Bucy syndrome 3975
Kluyvera, rare species *557*
knee
fat pads 2996
injuries and pain **2996**
ligamentous injuries 2996
osteoarthritis 2975, 2978, 2979
osteotomy 2982
in pyrophosphate arthropathy 2988
radiography 2949
replacement 2964
in rheumatoid arthritis 2959
tricompartmental damage 2959
unstable, falls due to 4339
Knudson's two-hit model 1707
Koebner phenomenon 3709, *3717*,
3746
Kohlmeier-Degos syndrome 2000
koilonychia 3760
in iron-deficiency anaemia 3475
Koplik's spots 377, 379
Korean haemorrhagic fever 425–7
see also hantaviruses
Korotkoff sounds 2535
Korsakoff psychosis (amnestic
syndrome) 4126, 4225, 4241, 4277,
4295
Korsakoff syndrome 4277
Koserella trabulsii 557
Kostmann's syndrome 3389, 3557
Krabbe's disease (globoid cell
leukodystrophy; galactosyl ceramide
lipidosis) *1428*, **1429**, 3986
kraits, bites and envenoming 1131
K-*ras* gene 195, 225
kraurosis vulvae 3770

Kreb's cycle, *see* tricarboxylic acid
  (TCA) cycle
kringle 4-binding protein 3625
krypton-81m 2655
Kufs syndrome 3985
Kugelberg-Welander disease 3988, 4089
Kupffer cells 88
Kupffer-cell sarcoma, *see* liver tumours,
  angiosarcoma
Kurthia, rare species *557*
kuru *1513*, 1517, 3977, 3980, **3981–3**
  plaques 3983
Kussmaul breathing 1537, 2477
Kveim-Siltzbach test 2122, 2819,
  2828–9
  performance 2828–9
  safety 2828
  specificity/sensitivity 2829
kwashiorkor 1281
  anaemia in 3468, 3498–9
  clinical features 1282, 1283, 1284
  dermatosis of 1283–4, 1295
  infection susceptibility 281, *281*
  malabsorption in tropics and 1930
  marasmus *vs* 1282, 1288
  pathogenesis 1288
  pathophysiology 1288
  see also malnutrition, oedematous
Kyasanur Forest disease **414–15**
kyphoscoliosis 2872
  deformities, positive-pressure
    ventilation in 2577, 2905
  in osteogenesis imperfecta 3080, 3081
  pregnancy in 1746
  ventilatory failure in 2903, 2905
kyphosis **2874**, 3061
  pain due to 2994
  in spina bifida 4118
  thoracic, in ankylosing spondylitis 2966

L

La, antibodies 2952, 3021, 3024, 3032
labetalol 3250
  in pregnancy 1731, 1732
labial artery bleeding 1214
labial glands, biopsy 3037, 3038
laboratory personnel
  infectious hazards 1173
  see also health care staff
laboratory tests
  carcinogens 220–1
  results 4363
labour
  cardiovascular changes 1735–6
  diabetes management 1756
  drug abuse management 4299
  initiation and maintenance 1603
  management, in diabetes 1757
  premature 772
    ß-agonist therapy 1811
    in diabetes mellitus 1757
    role of infection 1785, **1786–7**
  in sickle-cell syndrome 1761
Labour Force Survey 1175
labyrinthitis, mumps association 374
lacerations, brain damage 4044
lacrimal canaliculitis, actinomycetes
  causing 685
La Crosse virus **424–5**
ß-lactam antibiotics, *see under* antibiotics
ß-lactamase 298, 299, 300
  Staphylococcus aureus resistance 525
lactase 1923
  deficiency 1922, 2003
    congenital 1921–2
    of prematurity 1922
    secondary 1922
    in short gut syndrome 1925
  expression reduced after infancy 1921,
    1922
  expression regulation 1921
  restriction in children and adults 1922,
    1930–1
  see also hypolactasia; lactose
    intolerance

lactate 1456
  blood 1541
  forearm ischaemic lactate test *4374*
  metabolism in heart and 2146
  plasma,
    in acid-base disturbances 1539
    in diabetes 1481
    in glycogen storage diseases 1341
  see also lactic acid
lactate dehydrogenase (LDH) *4365*
  inherited deficiency *1343*
  liver metastases detection 246
  in myocardial infarction 2339
  serum 3633
lactation 1564
  prolactin and 1576
  role of oxytocin 1603
  see also breast milk; galactorrhoea
lactic acid *1534*
  accumulation, fatigue pathophysiology
    2173
  formation, in ethylene glycol
    metabolism 1082
  see also lactate
lactic acidosis 1539, **1541–2**, 2161
  in alcohol intoxication 1080
  in alcoholism 1542
  biguanide-induced 1471, 1542
  causes *1537*
  in diabetes *1499*
  in diabetic ketoacidosis 1541, 1542
  D-isomer-specific 1542
  in fructose diphosphatase deficiency 1346
  haemofiltration 2581
  infantile 4172
  methanol-induced 1543
  nature and classification 1541–2
  paracetamol-induced 1052
  pathogenesis 1542
  in pyruvate dehydrogenase deficiency
    1351
  in short gut syndrome 1925
  treatment 1543, 1544
  type A *1537*, 1541–2
  type B *1537*, 1542
  in von Gierke's disease 1342
  see also metabolic acidosis
lactobacilli, peroxide-producing in
  vagina 3354
Lactobacillus, rare species *557*
Lactococcus, rare species *557*
lactoferrin 2614
lactose
  fermentation, enterobacteria 550
  foods containing *1922*
  hydrolysis 1920
  malabsorption 1922
  tolerance test 1906
lactose intolerance 1824, 1844, 1903,
  1921–3, *1922*
  diagnosis 1922
  enteral feeding complication 1321
  in tropical sprue 1933
  see also lactase
lactosylceramidosis *1428*, 1429
lactotrophs 1575, 1576
lactulose 2108
Ladd's bands 1976
Ladd's operation 1977
laetrile 1097
Lafora bodies 3988
Lafora body disease **3988**, 4015
Lake Nyos disaster 1094
LAM-1, *see* L-selectin
Lambert-Eaton myasthenic syndrome
  (LEMS) 244, 2884, **4163–4**
  small-cell lung cancer and 4163
LAMB syndrome 2472
lamellar bodies 2595
lamina propria
  in coeliac disease 1917
  lymphocytes 1836, 2001
  nodular lymphoid hyperplasia (NLH)
    1839
lamin B 80
laminectomy 3907
laminin, platelet binding 3614, 3615
lamotrigine, in epilepsy 3922

Lampit (nifurtimox), in Chagas' disease
  898
Lancefield group antigens 497
L and H (lymphocytic and histiocytic)
  cells 3571
Langerhans cells 87, 3606, 3706,
  3736
  antigen presentation in graft recipient
    184
  antigen-presenting role 3707
  in atopic dermatitis 161
  in cutaneous lymphoma 3794, 3795
  histiocytosis, *see* histiocytosis,
    Langerhans cell
  ultraviolet light effect 3727
Langer's lines 3710, 3711
Langhans' giant cells 88, 2818
  in hepatic granulomas 2120
language 3846
  defects, *see* aphasia
  in dementia assessment 3968
  disorders,
    in Alzheimer's disease 3973
    developmental **4122**
    in Pick's disease 3975
  laterality of representation **3846–7**
  localization in left hemisphere **3847–8**
  subcortical nuclei and **3851**
  see also speech
lanugo hair 1674
laparoscopic appendicectomy 2010
laparoscopic cholecystectomy 2048,
  2050
laparoscopy
  in pancreatic carcinoma 2044
  in pelvic inflammatory disease *3359*
  in schistosomiasis 978, 979
'laparostomy' 2008
laparotomy
  emergency, in perforated diverticulitis
    1971
  intestinal ischaemia 2375
  staging 246
    in Hodgkin's disease 3572
Laplace's law 3233–4
'large alveolar cells', *see* alveolar
  secretory cells (type II)
large bowel cancer, *see* colorectal
  carcinoma
large granular lymphocyte 165, 3424
  leukaemia 165, 3424
large intestine, *see* caecum; colon;
  entries beginning intestinal; rectum
Larmor frequency 3819
Laron dwarfism (growth hormone
  receptor deficiency) 1511, 1572,
  1577, 1699
larva currens 929
larva migrans
  cutaneous 931
  ocular 945
  visceral 3680
larvicides 858
laryngeal expiratory braking 2612
laryngeal oedema
  acid and alkali exposure 1103
  acute airways obstruction 2721
  toxic gases causing 2847
laryngeal tumours
  aetiological factors 205
  airway obstruction 2722
  bronchoscopy 2722
  epidemiology 205
  presentation and investigations 2722
  staging investigations *236*
  treatment 2723
laryngitis, in smoke inhalation 1102
laryngopharynx 2610
  cancer, epidemiology 201
laryngotracheitis, *see* croup
laryngo-tracheo-bronchial amyloidosis
  2835
larynx **2611–12**
  abrasion, in endotracheal intubation
    2577
  diphtheria 495
  dysfunction, airways obstruction in 2724
  function **2612**

obstruction, after weaning from
  ventilators 2580
  palsy 2643
  paralysis 2724, 3880
    in diphtheria 496
  structure **2611–12**
  tumours, *see* laryngeal tumours
Lasègue's sign 2993, 3906
laser
  angioplasty, carotid/vertebral arteries
    3824
  in coronary angioplasty 2352
  photocoagulation, oesophageal cancer
    1982
  therapeutic bronchoscopy using 2684
laser therapy
  carbon dioxide 3369
  diabetic retinopathy 4189, 4190
  in lung cancer 2892
  oesophageal cancer 1982
  retinal changes in sickling disorders
    4195
Lassa fever **430–5**
  in children 433
  clinical features 431–3
  diagnosis 434
  differential diagnosis 433
  epidemiology 430–1
  management 434
  passive immunization 434
  pathogenesis 433–4
  pathology and immunology 434
  in pregnancy 432–3, 1776, 1777, *1779*
  prevention 434–5
  prognosis 433, 434
    mortality 430, 432, 433
  transmission 430–1
  vaccine 434, 435
Lassar's paste 3748, *3749*
Lassa virus 430, 431
latent period, cancer development 198
lateral cisternae 2145
lateral cutaneous nerve of thigh **4097**
  compression neuropathy 1766
lateral geniculate nucleus 3863, 3864
lateral medullary syndrome of
  Wallenberg 3858
lateral sclerosis, primary 4090
LATE trial 2340
latex agglutination test
  cryptococcal 1033
  hydatid disease diagnosis 958
  rickettsial diseases diagnosis 732
lathyrism 1159, 4090
Latin America 51
Laugier-Hunziker syndrome *3755*
Laurence-Moon-Biedl syndrome,
  hypogonadism 1683
lavatory cleaners/sanitizers, poisoning
  1079
law
  drugs and **4288–90**, 4297
  occupational safety and 1176–7
  treatment in terminal illness 4359
  see also medicolegal context
Lawrence-Seip syndrome 3791
laxatives
  abuse 1825, 1964–5, 2138, 3130, 3131
    treatment 1965
  anthracene 1964, 1965
  for body packers of drugs 1075
  in constipation 1826, 1964
  osmotic 1968
  in terminal illness 4354
L cells 1893
LDL, *see* low-density lipoprotein
lead 1109
  absorption 1109
  air pollution 1228–9
  in erythrocytes 1109
  in petrol 1228
  sources and uses 1109, 1228
lead colic 1109, 4099
lead encephalopathy 1109, 1174, 4056
  meningitis *vs* 4056
'leader sequence' 68
lead poisoning **1109–10**, 1172, 1174,
  3095–6, *3546*

abnormal porphyrin metabolism 1396
bone disease in **3095–6**
chelation therapy 1110
clinical features 1109–10, 3096
diagnosis 3096
gout and 1381, 2986, 3225, 3227, 3261
levels causing adverse effects 1109,
　1228
medical surveillance 1110
nephropathy 1109, **3261**
neuropathy 4099
neuropsychological disorders 1109,
　1174, 1228
prevention 1110
pyrimidine-5′-nucleotidase deficiency
　1387
sideroblastic anaemia 3521, 3523
treatment 1110
'leaky lung syndrome', *see* adult
　respiratory distress syndrome
Leào, theory of 4025
learning disorders **4108**
Leber's hereditary optic neuropathy
　(LHON) 128–9, 3988
Leber's optic atrophy 1335
Lebombo virus 406
lecithin 2047
lecithin cholesterol acyltransferase
　(LCAT) 1400, 1402
in cirrhosis 2088
familial deficiency 1402
in nephrotic syndrome 3143
Leclercia, rare species 557
lectins 1158
leeches 1012, **1150–1**
aquatic 1150
land 1150
treatment and prevention 1150–1
left atrium (atrial)
abnormal chest radiograph 2182
ball thrombus 2500
calcification, in rheumatic mitral
　stenosis 2452
in corrected transposition 2417
embolism, in mitral stenosis 2452
enlargement 2182
　in mitral stenosis 2453
　in mixed mitral valve disease 2456,
　　2457
　in myxoma 2473
filling, in pericardial constriction 2478
giant 2456, 2457
hypertension,
　in aortic stenosis 2463
　in rheumatic mitral stenosis 2452,
　　2453
hypertrophy, ECG in 2188, 2190
inferior vena cava to 2402, **2415**
myxoma 2472
　mitral stenosis *vs* 2454–5
　pulmonary oedema in 2500
obstruction **2424**
　myxoma 2472, 2473
pressure, *see* atrial pressure, left
superior vena cava to 2402, **2415**
thrombosis 2455
　in rheumatic mitral stenosis 2452
tumours 2472
see also entries beginning atrial
left-handedness 3847
left ventricle (ventricular)
abnormal chest radiograph 2182
activity-time curve 2205, 2206
aneurysm 2325
　see also ventricle (ventricular),
　　aneurysms
compensatory hyperkinesis 2223, 2224
in cor pulmonale 2516
diastolic pressure,
　in hypertrophic cardiomyopathy 2384,
　　2386
　in restrictive cardiomyopathy 2390
　see also left ventricle (ventricular),
　　end-diastolic pressure
dilatation, in dilated cardiomyopathy
　2381
disease, *see also* left ventricular disease
double-outlet **2419**

dyskinesis 2224
ejection 2230
ejection fraction 2153, 2223, 2230
coronary artery disease outcome and
　2358
estimates by scintigraphy 2204,
　2205–6, 2208
first pass technique 2205
gated equilibrium technique 2205–6,
　2208
in heart failure 2230
in myocardial infarction 2338, 2339
ejection volume, in aortic regurgitation
　2465
end-diastolic pressure 2220, 2246
in aortic stenosis 2462, 2463
measurement 2220
see also diastolic pressure (above);
　filling pressure (below)
end-diastolic volume 2153, 2230, 2231
in mitral regurgitation 2458
enlargement, in heart failure 2229
failure 2228
cardiac transplantation
　contraindication 2256
in chronic obstructive airways disease
　2777
drugs causing, calcium antagonists
　2329
in myocardial infarction 2338
pathophysiology 2229–31
pulmonary embolism *vs* 2524
in sepsis 293
ventilatory drive changes 2916
see also heart failure; left ventricular
　disease/dysfunction
filling 2231
diastolic abnormalities 2231
mitral valve physiology 2451
in pericardial tamponade 2477
in rheumatic mitral stenosis 2452
square-root sign 2390, 2393, 2479
filling pressure 2220, 2246
measurement 2220–1
see also left ventricle (ventricular),
　end-diastolic pressure
force-velocity analysis 2225
function 2230, 2246
cardiac output, *see* cardiac output
curves 2220, 2247
Doppler echocardiography 2203
in hypertrophic cardiomyopathy 2384,
　2385–6
indices **2221–5**, *2221*
maximum dP/dt 2157, 2224, 2230
pre-ejection phase indices 2224–5
scintigraphy **2204–6**
gradient, in hypertrophic
　cardiomyopathy 2386
hypertrophy 2182, 2384, 2388
after myocardial infarction 2321
angina in 2323, 2325
in aortic stenosis 2462, 2463
in aortic stenosis with incompetence
　2464
causes *2413*
diagnosis 2463
electrocardiogram (ECG) in 2187,
　2188
in fixed subaortic stenosis 2422
in heart failure 2229
in hypertension 2534
in renal disease 2552
in renovascular hypertension 2546
in supra-aortic stenosis 2423
in ventricular septal defects 2429
maximum velocity of contraction
　2224–5
outflow obstruction 2422
causes 2421
outflow tract, defect between right
　aortic sinus **2424**
output, increase, in mitral regurgitation
　2458
pressure *2154*, *2223*
in Fallot's tetralogy 2403
raised, angina in 2323
see also specific pressures (above)

regional wall motion,
　catheterization studies 2223–4
　scintigraphy estimates 2204, 2205,
　　2206
remodelling, after myocardial infarction
　2321
shape change in heart failure 2229
stroke volume, in aortic regurgitation
　2465
stroke work index 2224
volume,
　analysis 2222–3
　normal values *2223*
wall thickness,
　in aortic stenosis 2462
　hypertrophic cardiomyopathy
　　diagnosis 2386
wall thinning in heart failure 2230
work, measurement 2224
left ventricular disease/dysfunction
after heart valve replacement
　2471
coronary angioplasty in 2352
in heart failure 2229, 2230
　diastolic 2231
　systolic 2230, 2231
mitral regurgitation in 2459
in pulmonary valve stenosis 2420
in rheumatic mitral stenosis 2452
thrombolytic therapy hazard in
　myocardial infarction 2341
legal medicine 4309
Legionellaceae 723
antigen testing 2677
characteristics and culture 723, 726
epidemiology and natural habitat 723–4
Legionella micdadei 724, 725
Legionella pneumophila 723
pneumonia, *see* legionnaires' disease
serological diagnosis 726
serotypes 723, 726
legionellosis **722–8**
causative agents 723
diagnosis/differential diagnosis 726
epidemiology 723–4
hospital-acquired 724
non-pneumonic (Pontiac fever) 723, **726**
pathology 727
prevention 727–8
prognosis and mortality 727
therapy 726–7
see also legionnaires' disease
legionnaires' disease (pneumonia) **722–8**,
　1231, 2694
causative agent 723
clinical features 725–6, *725*
diagnosis 726, 2697
epidemiology 722–3, 723–4
glomerulonephritis complicating 3175
haematological changes 3685
investigations of outbreak 287–8
liver in 2130
prevention 727–8
transmission 724
see also legionellosis
legs
deep vein thrombosis **2523**
elephantiasis, *see* elephantiasis
injuries and pain **2996**
neurological signs in *2994*
paralysis 3892
in rheumatic diseases 2946
in rheumatoid arthritis 2958–9
swelling 2523
leg ulcers
carcinoma development 3810
causes *3808*
contact dermatitis in 3810, *3810*
in diabetes 1449, **1490–1**
management **3807–10**
in sickle-cell disease 3195, 3515
Leigh's syndrome 3989, 4173
in pyruvate carboxylase deficiency
　1352
leiomyomas
gastric 1982
oesophageal 1876, 1980
Leiperia cincinnalis 1014

Leishman-Donovan bodies 776
Leishmania
lifecycle 899
species 899, 900
Leishmania aethiopica 899, 900, 901, 902
Leishmania amazonensis 900, *901*
Leishmania brasiliensis 900, 901
Leishmania donovani 899, 904, 2121
Leishmania guyanensis 901
Leishmania infantum 899, 901, *901*
Leishmania major 899, 900, 901, *901*
Leishmania mexicana 900, *901*
Leishmania panamensis 901, *901*
Leishmania peruviana 900, *901*
leishmaniasis **899–907**
aetiological agents 899
American mucosal (espundia) 902–3
chronic granulomatous disease of nose
　3800, *3801*
cutaneous **899–904**, 3802
　clinical features 901–2, *901*
　epidemiology 899–900, *900*
　eye in 4192
　treatment *901*, 903–4, *903*
diffuse cutaneous (DCL) 900, 902
epidemiology 899–900, *900*, 904
haematological changes 3680
hepatic granulomas in 2121
immunological diagnosis 903, 905–6
mucocutaneous *3801*
Old World and New World *900*, 906
post kala-azar dermal (PKDL) 905
prevention and control 906–7
recidivans (lupoid) 902
transmission 899
visceral (kala-azar) **904–7**, 3680
　AIDS and 487, 905
　treatment 906
Leishmania tropica 899, 900, 901, *901*
leishmanin test 903, 904
Lemierre's disease 575
Lemierre's postanginal septicaemia 574,
　575
Leminorella, rare species 557
Lennox-Gastaut syndrome 3914, 4015
lens
dislocation,
　causes 4181
　in cystathionine synthase deficiency
　　1366
　in Marfan's syndrome 4181
opacities 4182
lentiform nucleus 3861
lentiginosis, in Carney's syndrome
　(complex) 2472
lentigo 3757
actinic/senile *3754*
lentigo maligna *3754*
lentiviruses, *see also* HIV
leonine facies 671, 1897, 3795
Leopard syndrome *3755*
lepidoptera
eye-frequenting **1010–11**
venomous **1146**
'lepidopterism' 1146
leprechaunism 1455
lepromin test 668
leprosy **667–79**
aetiology 668
BCG vaccination 678
blindness in 4198
borderline (BB) 669, 670
borderline-lepromatous (BL) 669,
　670–1
borderline-tuberculoid (BT) 669–70
chronic granulomatous disease of nose
　3800, *3801*
clinical features **669–72**
delayed hypersensitivity in 279
diagnosis/differential diagnosis 674
epidemiology 668–9
eye in 4191
glomerulonephritis in 3176–7
haematology and immunology **673–4**
hepatic granulomas in 2121
hypopigmentation 3754–5
immunosuppression in 282
incubation period 669

indeterminate 669
lepromatous (LL) 668, 669, 671–2, 3763
  granuloma in 3800
  subpolar and polar types 672
multibacillary, treatment regimen 676
myositis in 4155
pathology 669–72
paucibacillary, treatment 676–7
prognosis 678
prophylaxis 678
reactions 672–3
  erythema nodosum leprosum (lepromatous lepra/Jopling type 2) 673, 674, 677
  Lucio 673
  non-lepromatous lepra (reversal/ Jopling type I) 672–3, 677
  treatment 677
relapse 676
treatment 674–8
  ancillary (of limbs) 678
  chemotherapy 674–6, 675
  drug resistance 674, 675
  duration and problems 677
  of neuritis 677–8
  new drugs 677
  recommended regimens 676–7
tuberculoid (TT) 668, 669
see also Mycobacterium leprae
  Leptospira interrogans 698
leptospires 698, 699
  culture and serology 702
leptospirosis 698–703, 3178
  acute renal failure in 3291–2
  aetiology 698
  clinical features 700–1
    immune phase 701
    septicaemic phase 700–1
  diagnosis 701–2
  epidemiology and transmission 698
  immune response 699
  kidney in 699, 700, 701, 3291–2
  liver in 699, 699–700, 2133
  pathogenesis 698–9
    immunological 699
  pathology 699–700
  prevention and vaccine 702
  treatment and prognosis 702
  see also Weil's disease
Lesch-Nyhan syndrome 1381–3, 3226, 3989, 4009
  biochemical findings 1382
  genetics 1382
  megaloblastic anaemia in 1382, 3497, 3686
  treatment 1382–3
Leser-Trélat sign 3793
Letterer-Siwe disease 3606, 3768
  see also histiocytosis, Langerhans-cell
leucine 1353, 1368–9
  metabolism 1275, 1276
  tRNA mutation 1456
leucoaraiosis, see Binswanger's disease
leucocidin, Staphylococcus aureus 524
leucocyte(s) 3377, 3555–61
  abnormalities of number 3557–8
  in acid-base disturbances 1540
  adhesion 3558–9
  adhesion deficiency 88, 2619, 2759, 3559
    type II 2621
  adhesion integrins 2619, 3559
  adhesion molecules 2619–21, 2620
    see also adhesion molecules
  antibodies 3689
    transfusion reactions 3692
  antigens 3689
  in atherosclerosis pathogenesis 2291
  biology 3558–60
  in cerebrospinal fluid, see cerebrospinal fluid
  in chronic renal failure 3682
  common antigen 3401, 3402
  lymphoma diagnosis 242
  counts 3379, 3380
    ascitic fluid 2096
    in cirrhosis 2089

in community-acquired pneumonia 2696, 2696
in heart failure 2235
in infective endocarditis 2442
in leukaemia 3405, 3412, 3414, 3416–17
in myelodysplastic syndromes 3426
in plague 597
in SLE 3681
synovial fluid 2951
differential counts 3379, 3380
disorders,
  of adhesion and migration 3559
  of killing and digestion 3560
  treatment 3561
distribution/regulation 3556–7
endothelial cell interactions 3558–9
examination 3378
function tests 3560
gallium-/indium-labelled 1018
in malignant disease 3677, 3678
migration into tissues 3559
morphology and composition 3555–6
passenger 184
phagocytosis and killing 3559–60
polymorphonuclear, see basophils; eosinophil(s); granulocyte(s); neutrophils
-poor blood 3694, 3695
preparations for transfusion 3694
recruitment 98
tissue damage by 3560
in urinary casts 3104
in urine 3102, 3103, 3208
see also lymphocyte(s)
leucocyte endogenous mediator, see interleukin-1 (IL-1)
leucocyte endogenous pyrogen, see interleukin-1 (IL-1)
leucocyte function-associated antigen 1 (LFA-1) 151, 2619, 2620
  melanoma metastases 231
leucocyte function-associated antigen 3 (LFA-3) 151
leucocyte growth factors
  in systemic fungal infections 812
  see also granulocyte-colony-stimulating factor (G-CSF); granulocyte-macrophage colony-stimulating factor (GM-CSF)
leucocytosis 3378
  in haemolytic uraemic syndrome 3200
  in leptospirosis 698
  neutrophil, see neutrophilia
leucocytotoxic testing, food allergy 1845
leucoderma 3755, 3760
  see also depigmentation
leucodystrophies 3986
  see also Pelizaeus-Merzbacher disease
leucoencephalopathy, progressive multifocal, see progressive multifocal leucoencephalopathy
leucoerythroblastic reaction 3448, 3461
  in disseminated malignancy 3677
  in primary myelosclerosis 3435, 3436
leucokeratosis, congenital and hereditary 1859
Leuconostoc, rare species 557
leuconychia, in hepatocellular failure 2104
leucopenia
  drug-induced,
    carbamazepine 4251
    clozapine 4252
  in ehrlichiosis 738
  oral manifestations 1864
leucoplakia 1858–9
  atrophy of lichen sclerosus et atrophicus vs 3768–9
  chronic superficial candidiasis vs/and 801, 1852, 1859
  genital 3768–9
  hairy, see hairy leucoplakia
  lichen planus vs 1858
  malignant change 1859, 1860
  syphilitic 719
leucotomy 3945
leucotrienes, see leukotrienes

leukaemia 3393–452
acute 3390, 3392, 3399–403
  aplastic anaemia and 3447
  biphenotypic 3402
  bleeding tendency 3635
  bone tenderness 3376–7
  in Fanconi anaemia 3410, 3446
  hypocellular 3402–3
  hypokalaemia 3132
  marrow transplantation 3409, 3414, 3696–7, 3698–9
  oral manifestations 1864
  polycythaemia vera transformation 3432, 3433, 3434
acute eosinophilic 3612
acute lymphoblastic (ALL) 3392, 3410–15
  adult 3401
  aetiology 3410–11
  B-cell (B-ALL) 3399, 3402
  central nervous system involvement 3412, 3414
  childhood 3401, 3410, 3447
  clinical features 3411–12
  common (cALL) 215, 3402, 3411, 3565
  diagnosis 3399–400, 3412–13
  epidemiology 215
  incidence 3410
  joint involvement 3005
  management 3413–14
  molecular biology 3395, 3411, 3412
  null ALL 215
  ocular features 4194
  pathophysiology 3411
  prognosis 3413, 3414–15
  subclassification 3401–2, 3412–13
  T-cell (T-ALL) 151, 215, 3399, 3402
  treatment 3397–8, 3697, 3698
acute megakaryoblastic (AML M7) 3400, 3401, 3406, 3437–8
acute monocytic 3400, 3406
acute myeloblastic 3400
acute myeloid (AML) 3375, 3392, 3404–10
  aetiology 3404
  diagnosis 3399–400, 3405–6
  epidemiology 215
  FAB classification 3400–1
  M0 3400, 3406
  M1 3400, 3406
  M2 3400, 3405, 3406
  M3, see leukaemia, acute promyelocytic
  M4 3400, 3405, 3406, 3408
  M5 3400, 3405, 3406, 3408
  M6 (erythroleukaemia) 3400–1, 3406, 3428, 3498
  M7 (megakaryoblastic) 3400, 3401, 3406, 3437–8
  management 3406–10
  marrow transplantation 3409, 3697, 3698
  molecular biology 3395
  myelodysplastic syndromes evolving into 3405, 3425, 3430
  paroxysmal nocturnal haemoglobinuria and 3451
  pathophysiology 3404
  presentation 3404–5
  secondary 3405, 3406, 3430
  subtypes 3400–1, 3406
acute myelomonocytic 3400, 3406
acute promyelocytic (APML; AML M3) 3400, 3402, 3406
  bleeding diathesis 3658, 3659
  clinical features 3405
  molecular biology 3396, 3400
  treatment 3409, 3659
ankylosing spondylitis and 2968
in B-cell non-Hodgkin's lymphoma 3420, 3423–4
B-cell prolymphocytic (B-PLL) 3420, 3422–3
Burkitt type 354
causative factors 215

cell/molecular biology 3393–8
  clinical implications 3397–8
  diversity 3394–6
  subtypes and 3396–7
chronic 3399, 3403
chronic eosinophilic 3403
chronic granulocytic, see leukaemia, chronic myeloid
chronic lymphocytic (CLL) 3403, 3419–22, 3579
  chromosomal abnormalities 3395, 3421
  clinical features 3420
  complications 3421
  epidemiology 214–15
  hypogammaglobulinaemia in 1028
  infections in 1028
  investigations 3420–1
  large-cell (Richter's) transformation 3422
  prognostic factors 3421
  prolymphocytic transformation (CLL/PL) 3422, 3423
  secondary immunodeficiency in 173–4
  treatment 3421–2
chronic myeloid (CML) 3392, 3415–19
  atypical 3403
  blastic (acute) transformation 3415, 3417, 3419
  classification 3403, 3415
  clinical features 3416
  diagnosis 3403
  epidemiology/aetiology 3415
  haematology 3416–17
  management 3417–19
  marrow transplantation in 3417, 3418–19, 3698, 3699
  molecular biology 3395, 3416
  natural history 3415
  primary myelosclerosis vs 3437
  rare forms 3403
chronic myelomonocytic (CMML) 3403, 3427, 3428
  juvenile 3403
chronic neutrophilic 3403
classification 214, 3399–403
clonality 3393, 3394
C-reactive protein in 1532
cryptosporidiosis in 874
diphtheria vs 496
Down's syndrome association 215
eosinophilia in 3612
epidemiology 214–15
haemoglobin H in 3511
hairy-cell (HCL) 214, 3420, 3423, 3565
  variant form 3423
isosporiasis in 882
joint involvement 3005
large granular lymphocyte 165, 3424
of mature B and T cells 3419–22
neurological complications 4135
neuropathy in 4102
ocular features 4194
Pneumocystis carinii pneumonia treatment 823
in pregnancy 1761–2, 1808
primary lymphoid 3419, 3420
pseudohyperkalaemia 3133
renal involvement 3183
smouldering 3425, 3448
in T-cell non-Hodgkin's lymphoma 3424
T-cell prolymphocytic 3424
leukaemia/lymphoma syndromes 3420
  adult T-cell, see adult T-cell leukaemia/ lymphoma
leukaemogenesis, radiation causing 1219–20
leukaemoid reaction, in disseminated malignancy 3677
leukodystrophy
  globoid cell (Krabbe's disease; galactosyl ceramide lipidosis) 1428, 1429
  metachromatic (sulphatidosis) 1428, 1429
leukoplakia, see leucoplakia
leukotrienes 3617, 3627 B₄ 2619, 3559
  formation 158
  release in asthma 2727, 2728

levamisole
in ascariasis 938
in colorectal carcinoma 1993
levodopa
dyskinesia due to 4003
in dystonia 4017
'end-of-dose' deterioration 4003
haemolytic anaemia due to 3542–3
in Parkinson's disease 4002, 4003, 4004
resistance to 4003
side-effects 4002, 4003
psychiatric symptoms 4004, 4242
stimulation test *1584*, 1593
lewisite **1117**
features of exposure 1117
use and forms 1117
Lewis-Prusik test 1226
Lewy bodies 3885, 3967, 3972, 3998
degeneration 3998
diseases associated 3999
in Parkinson's disease 3998, 3999
see also diffuse cortical Lewy body disease
LH, *see* luteinizing hormone
Lhermitte's sign 3993
radiation-induced 3574
LHRH, *see* gonadotrophin releasing hormone (GnRH)
libido, loss 1687
in cirrhosis 2087, 2091
Libman-Sachs endocarditis 2452
in SLE 2392
lice **1002–4**
body 1003, 1004
control and repellents 733
head **1002–3**, 1004
management 1004
pubic (crab) 1003–4
removal/delousing 697
rickettsial diseases transmission 730
lichen amyloidosis 3803
lichenification, scabies lesions 1008
lichen myxoedematosus (scleromyxoedema) *3791*
lichenoid 3710
lichenoid eruptions **3751–2**
lichen planus **1857–8**, 2087, 3714, **3751–2**, 3762, 3763
blistering in 3783
bullous 1858
erosive 1858
hypertrophic 1858, 3751
plane warts *vs* 3798
rash distribution 3713
tropical (actinic) 3751
lichen sclerosis 3768–9
vulval 3769
lichen sclerosis et atrophicus, blistering in 3783
lichen simplex 3745
Liddle's syndrome **1662**, 3131–2, 3336–7
Lieberkühn, crypts, *see* crypt of Lieberkühn
life
desirable weight and longevity 1301, 1302
expectancy 51
medical decisions concerning end (MDEL) 13, 39
value of human 11
lifeboat service, fitness requirements 2360–1
life events, *see* stressful life events
lifestyle
alcohol abuse intervention 4274
angina management 2326
coronary heart disease aetiology 1326–7, **2309–14**
see also ischaemic heart disease, risk factors
diabetes mellitus aetiology 1327
drug abusers 4280
fibrinogen levels reduction 2304
media effects 36
myocardial infarction prevention 2348
life support, withdrawal 3935

Li-Fraumeni syndrome 129, 242
ligamenta flava, ossification 3072
ligamentous calcification, in ankylosing spondylitis 2967
ligamentous ossification 3093
ligaments
acute sports-related injuries 4322
back pain due to 2992
ligandin, bilirubin binding in hepatocytes 2055
light-chain deposition disease *3180*, **3182**
idiopathic 3182
in myeloma 3181, 3182
light chains, immunoglobulin
AL amyloid 1515, 1518
in myeloma 3600
in urine 3137, 3181, 3182, 3292
in Waldenström's macroglobulinaemia 3604
light eruption, polymorphic 3726, 3727
lightning **1214–15**
lightning pains 4085
light sensitivity, *see* photosensitivity
Lignac's disease, *see* cystinosis
lignocaine *2264*
in arrhythmias due to poisoning 1047
in myocardial infarction 2345
overdose/poisoning 1064
in pain treatment 3945
in tricyclic antidepressant poisoning 1059
in ventricular tachycardia 2280
Liguatula serrata 987
likelihood ratio (LR) **19–20**
Limanatis nilotica 987
limb-girdle dystrophy 4145, **4147**
limb-girdle weakness 4167, 4168
limbic 'encephalitis', in tumours *243*
'limbic encephalopathy' 4243
limbs
ischaemia, *see* ischaemia of limb
motor responses in unconscious patient 2584–5
short, in achondroplasia 3088
in spinal cord injury 3900
lime
in eye 1103
oral and pharyngeal cancer association 201
LIMIT-2 (second Leicester intravenous magnesium intervention trial) 30, 2344
lincosamide clindamycin 575, 576
lindane 1123
linear accelerator 255
linear IgA disease, in pregnancy 1806
linear lesions *3713*, *3717*
lingual tonsils 2611
Linguatula serrata **1012**
linitis plastica 1984
linkage, *see* genetic linkage
linkage disequilibrium 110–11, 143, 2786
D-linolenate 1472
lip
cancer 1860
aetiology/epidemiology 201
in Kawasaki disease 3047
pigmentation 1987
squamous epithelioma 3708, 3725
lipaemia retinalis 1410, 1486, 1503, 4190
lipase
in acute pancreatitis 2029
hepatic 1404
pancreatic 1903
lipid(s) 1399
absorption *1901*, 1903
glucose interactions 1277
infusion, parenteral nutrition 1321
intolerance, parenteral nutrition complication 1321
ischaemic heart disease risk 2307–8
metabolism 1399–400
after injury/surgery 1549
in chronic renal failure 3302
in diabetes 1457
endothelial cells role 2291, 2299

myopathy in **4167–8**
in nephrotic syndrome **3142–3**
by *Plasmodium* species 837
in pregnancy 1753
metabolism disorders **1399–414**
neurological features **3985–6**
oxidation, endurance sports training 4325
peroxidation, in haemolytic uraemic syndrome 3199
red-cell membrane 3528
reference range 1405, *4370*
serum,
monitoring in diabetes *1479*, 1481
normal values 1405, *4370*
storage disorders 2024, 3591
storage myopathy 4142
transport from liver and gut to tissues 1401–2
lipid A 272
lipid-lowering drugs 1413–14
ischaemic heart disease prevention 2316–17
myocardial infarction prevention 2348
in nephrotic syndrome 3143
in renal failure 3275, 3305
lipid (lipoid) pneumonia **2837–8**, 2852
lipid (cholesteryl ester) transfer protein 1402, 1404
lipiduria 3143
lipiodol 2012
angiography, in hepatocellular carcinoma 2116–17
targeted-therapy, in hepatocellular carcinoma 2117
lipoatrophy, insulin therapy inducing 1477
lipochondrodystrophy 1431
lipodystrophy
insulin therapy inducing 1477
partial 180, 3791
mesangiocapillary glomerulonephritis and 3157
lipofuscin granules, in haemochromatosis 2020
lipofuscinosis, neuronal ceroid 3985–6
lipogenesis, ketogenesis link 1277
lipohypertrophy, insulin therapy inducing 1477
lipoic acid 1351, 1352
lipoidal antibody tests 714
lipoidal antigen test 715
lipoid (lipid) pneumonia **2837–8**, 2852
lipoid proteinosis 3803
lipolysis 1276, 1400, 1457
after injury/surgery 1549
lipoma
cardiac 2472
colon 1984
in MEN 1 syndrome 1708
lipomeningocele 4119
lipopolysaccharide 272
anaerobic bacteria 571
enterobacteria 550
Haemophilus influenzae 581
host response and macrophage role 91
lipoprotein(s) 1277, 1399, **1400–4**, 1903
cholesterol transport to liver 1403–4
hereditary deficiency 3986
hormone replacement therapy and 1814
ischaemic heart disease risk 2307–8
lipid transport to tissues 1401–3
normal range *4370*
in pregnancy 1753
raised levels, *see* hyperlipoproteinaemia
reduced levels 1414
serum, in nephrotic syndrome 3142
structure 1400, 1401
see also apolipoprotein(s); high-density lipoprotein (HDL); low-density lipoprotein (LDL); *specific types*
lipoprotein (a) (Lp(a)) 1401, **1403**, 1403, 2293, **2308**
atherogenic/thrombogenic effects 2308
in familial hypercholesterolaemia 2308
high levels 2308
in ischaemic heart disease 2303
serum 1406, 1458

lipoprotein lipase 1401, 1402
endurance sports training and 4325
familial deficiency 1409–10
mutations 1410
lipoprotein X (LpX) 1411
liposomes, gene therapy vector 2755
lipotrophin 1575
ß-lipotrophin (ß-LPH) 1575
lipoxygenase 158, 3617, 3662
liquefaction 3710
liquefactive necrosis, alkali exposure causing 1103
liquid nitrogen, warts treatment 3798
liquorice 1661, 1717–18, 3131, 3336
Lisch nodules, of iris 4181
lissencephaly 4113
Listeria 720
isolation and culture 720, 722
Listeria monocytogenes 720, 2121
in macrophage 91
meningitis due to 721, 4050, 4051
movement in cell cytoplasm 82
pathogenesis and transmission 720
rapid diagnosis 720
serological tests 722
typing and subtyping 720
listeriolysin O 720
listeriosis **720–2**
in animals 720–1
clinical features 721–2
diagnosis 722
epidemiology 721
food-borne 721
hospital-acquired 514
maternofetal 721, 1769, **1789**
meningoencephalitis in 721
neonatal 721, 722, 1789
septicaemia in 721
susceptibility 720
treatment and prognosis 722
Listonella damsela 557 lisuride 4003
lithium 4250–1
dosage and monitoring 4250
drug interactions *4250*, 4251
hypothyroidism induced by 1615, 1717
indications and use 4250
in mania and manic depressive disorder 4221
in elderly 4227
monitoring 1261
nephrotoxicity 3121, *3261*, **3263**
overdose/poisoning 1061
parathyroid effects 1719
pharmacokinetics 4250, 4251
pharmacology and mechanism of action 4250
in pregnancy 1813
in renal impairment 3273
serum levels 1061
side effects 4250–1, *4250*
teratogenicity 1809, *1810*
toxicity 4251
lithium carbonate 4220, 4221
lithocholic acid 2047
lithotripsy
extracorporeal shock-wave 2048, 2049
urinary stones 3244, 3255, 3256
ureteric stones 3243
livedo reticularis 2365–6, 3020, 3668, 3669, 3724
liver
abscess,
in ascariasis 938
in balantidiasis 881
pleural effusion in 2868
Streptococcus milleri 509
see also amoebic liver abscess; liver, pyogenic abscess
acute fatty, of pregnancy (AFLP) **1797–8**
in AIDS 475, **2135**
in amoebiasis 829–30, 832–3
see also amoebic liver abscess
in amyloidosis **2136**
artificial support systems 2110
biopsy, *see* liver biopsy *(below)*
blood flow, *see* hepatic blood flow
blood supply 2017

bridging necrosis 2072
cancer, *see* liver tumours
carbohydrate metabolism 1456–7
in cardiovascular disease **2130**
cirrhosis, *see* cirrhosis
complement component synthesis 176
computed tomography (CT) 1833, **2012–13**
in connective tissue diseases **2135, 2139**
in cryoglobulinaemia **2136**
in cystic fibrosis *2018*, **2023–4**, 2131
cysts,
  hydatid 956, 957, 958
  in polycystic kidney disease 3203
damage, *see* liver damage *(below)*
disease, *see* liver disease *(below)*
drug metabolism 1243, 2091, 2124
embryology 1973
expansile pulsation 2468
failure, *see* hepatocellular failure
in fascioliasis 986
fatty changes,
  in alcoholic liver disease 2082
  in carbohydrate metabolism disorders 2024
  in cystic fibrosis 2023
  drug-induced 2126–7, *2128*
  in inflammatory bowel disease 2131
  jejunoileal bypass causing 2132, 2139
  pathology 2082, 2084
  prognosis 2083
  see also steatosis
fibrosis 2085
  chicken-wire 2082
  'clay pipe stem' 977, 979
  congenital 2015, 2016, 3204
  in haemochromatosis 2020
  'onion skin' 2078
  perisinusoidal, drug-induced 2128–9
  in polycystic kidney disease 3204
  portal-portal/central 2085
  in primary sclerosing cholangitis 2078
  vinyl chloride causing 1090
  in Wilson's disease 2022
focal nodular hyperplasia 2119
function/function tests, *see* liver function; liver 'function tests'
in gastrointestinal disease **2131–2**, *2132*
granulomas, *see* hepatic granulomas
in haematological disease **2132–3**
in heart failure 2235
hydatid cysts 956, 957, 958
imaging, in hepatocellular carcinoma 2116–17
infections, anaerobic 572
in inflammatory bowel disease 2131–2, *2132*
inherited metabolic disorders **2017–27**, *2018–20*
  carbohydrate metabolism *2019*, 2024
  general approach 2017, 2020
  history and investigations 2017, 2020
  prenatal diagnosis 2017
  symptoms and signs *2021*
  see also inborn errors of metabolism
ischaemia 2138
in leptospirosis 699, 699–700
lung diseases affecting **2131**
magnetic resonance imaging 1833, **2013**
in malaria 844
in malnutrition *1290*
in Marburg virus and Ebola virus disease 442
mass, age-related changes 4335
metastases, *see* hepatic metastases
MHC class I antigen secretion in graft recipients 186
mucous plugging, in cystic fibrosis 2023, 2024, 2131
necrosis, *see* hepatic necrosis
needle aspiration, in amoebiasis 830
'nutmeg' 2139
occupational disease 1171–2, *1172*
pancreatic interactions 1565
piecemeal necrosis 2065, 2069, 2072
polycystic disease 2015

in pregnancy 1796
as privileged tissue 185–6
protein synthesis changes, in infections 294
in pulmonary disease **2130–1**
pyogenic abscess **2134–5**
  sources *2135*
radiology **1833**
regeneration, in liver failure 2107
regenerative capacity 2017
  in relapsing fevers 694, 695
  in rheumatoid arthritis 2962
  in rheumatological disease **2135**
role in energy supply and utilization 1272–3
in sarcoidosis **2825**
  see also hepatic granulomas
in schistosomiasis 972
in shock 2138
spontaneous rupture, in pregnancy **1797**
in syphilis 714
in systemic infections **2133–4**, *2133*
tenderness 2087
in total parenteral nutrition 2132, *2132*, 2140
transplantation, *see* liver transplantation *(below)*
ultrasonography 1833
vascular disorders **2138–9**
liver biopsy
  in alcoholic liver disease 2082
  in Budd-Chiari syndrome 2098
  in chronic persistent hepatitis 2065
  in chronic viral hepatitis 2064
  in cirrhosis 2089
  in glycogen storage diseases 1341
  in hepatic granulomas 2123
  in hepatic metastases 2119
  in hepatocellular carcinoma 2117
  in hereditary haemochromatosis 3479
  in liver graft rejection 2114
  in portal hypertension 2093
  in Reye's syndrome 2025
  transjugular 2098
liver cancer, *see* hepatocellular carcinoma; liver tumours
liver damage
  drug-induced **2124–30**
    acute hepatitis 2124–5, *2126*
    bland cholestasis 2125–6, *2127*
    cardiovascular drugs 2130
    causality proof 2124, *2125*
    cholestatic hepatitis 2125, *2127*
    chronic disease 2129, *2129*
    fibrotic and vascular 2128–9, *2128*
    gastrointestinal drugs 2132
    granulomas 2128, *2128*
    in HIV infection 2135
    idiosyncratic 2124, 2125, *2126*
    incidence 2124, *2125*
    paracetamol, *see* paracetamol
    patterns 2124, *2125*
    phospholipidosis 2128
    predictable reactions 2124, *2126*
    pulmonary drugs 2131
    steatosis 2126–7, *2128*
    susceptibility 2124–5
    tumours *2128*, 2129
  poisonous fungi causing 1158
  poisonous plants causing 1152, 1154
liver disease **2061–111**
  in α₁-antitrypsin deficiency 1546–7
  abnormal porphyrin metabolism 1396–7
  in AIDS **2135**
  alcoholic, *see* alcoholic liver disease
  antimicrobial drug pharmacokinetics 302
  autoimmune **2069–80**
    see also autoimmune hepatitis; cholangitis, primary sclerosing; primary biliary cirrhosis
  chronic, clinical approach 2057
  in cystic fibrosis 2749
  driving and 2091
  drug metabolism in 1252, 2091
  drug pharmacodynamics 1252
  drugs and 2091
  folate deficiency in 3494, 3684

in fructosaemia 1347
in glycogen storage disease 1341
gynaecomastia in 1688
haematological changes 3684
haemolytic anaemia in 3550, 3684
haemostatic disorders 3635, **3655–6**
hepatorenal syndrome 3293
hyperlipoproteinaemia in 1411–12
in hypogammaglobulinaemia 169
hypoglycaemia in 1510
inherited, *see* liver, inherited metabolic disorders
iron overload and 3481–2
joint involvement 3004
lactic acidosis 1542
in Langerhans-cell histiocytosis 3608
management, in hepatocellular failure 2107
mental disorders/symptoms in 4240
osteomalacia in 1636, **3073**
in porphyria 1395, 1396
in pre-eclampsia 1728–9, 1797
in pregnancy **1796–801**
  coincidental 1798–9
  pregnancy-specific 1796–8
pruritus in 3744
pseudo-Cushing's syndrome in 1643
Pugh-Child's grading 2094, *2094*
pulmonary hypertension in **2509–10**
in renal transplant recipients 3320
skin disease in 3723
symptoms and signs *2021*
total parenteral nutrition association 2132, *2132*, 2140
in ulcerative colitis 1948
in Wilson's disease 1420–1, 1422
see also cirrhosis; hepatic granulomas; hepatitis; liver tumours
liver enzymes
  in acute viral hepatitis 2061
  reference intervals *4365*
  in total parenteral nutrition 2140
  in ulcerative colitis 1947, 1948
  see also alanine aminotransferase; alkaline phosphatase; aspartate aminotransferase (AST); γ-glutamyl transferase
liver failure, *see* hepatocellular failure
'liver flap' 2101
liver fluke diseases **981–8**, *982*
  cholangiosarcoma association 204
  clonorchiasis *982*, **984–6**
  dicrocoeliasis *982*, **987–8**
  fascioliasis *982*, **986–7**
  opisthorchiasis **981–4**
liver function, impairment, antituberculous drugs in 660
liver 'function tests' *2021*, 2055–6
  abnormalities, parenteral nutrition complication 1320
  in alcoholic liver disease 2082
  in amoebic liver abscess 829
  in biliary atresia 2014
  in cirrhosis 2088
  in community-acquired pneumonia 2696
  in Crohn's disease 1940
  in drug-induced liver damage 2124
  in immunocompromised 1034
  in inflammatory bowel disease 2131
  in pre-eclampsia 1729
  in pregnancy *1797*
  in primary biliary cirrhosis 2075
  quantitative 2056
  in type-1 autoimmune hepatitis 2070
  see also specific tests *(pages 2055-6)*
liver palms 2087
'liver rot' 986
liver transplantation **2111–15**
  in acute hepatocellular failure 2113
  age of patients 2111
  in alcoholic liver disease 2085
  artificial support systems and 2110
  background/historical aspects 2111
  in biliary atresia 2015, 2113
  in Budd-Chiari syndrome 2099, 2113
  in cirrhosis 2091, 2112–13
  combined grafts 2113

donor-recipient matching 2113
in familial amyloid polyneuropathy 1524
in familial hypercholesterolaemia 1414
in glucagonoma 1706
haemostatic disorders 3656
in hepatocellular carcinoma 2112, 2115, 2117
heterotopic 2111
in inborn errors of metabolism 1336, *1337, 1338*, 2113
indications 2112–13
in liver tumours 2112
long-term rehabilitation and results 2114–15
number 2111, 2112
nutritional support 1323
organ preservation 2113–14
orthotopic 2111
  procedure 2114
in paracetamol poisoning 1053
patient selection and evaluation 2111–12
postoperative management 2114
pregnancy and 1799
in primary biliary cirrhosis 2076, 2112, 2115
in primary hyperoxaluria 1447, *1448*
in primary sclerosing cholangitis 2080
recipient hepatectomy 2114
rejection and immunosuppression 2114
respiratory tract infections after 2709
survival 2111, 2113, 2114, 2115
in tyrosinaemia type I 1364
in urea cycle defects 1360
in Wilson's disease 1422, 2112
liver tumours **2115–19**
  angiosarcoma 204, **2118**
    vinyl chloride causing 1090, 1167, 1172, 2118
  benign **2119**
  drug-induced *2128*, 2129
  epidemiology 204
  malignant **2115–19**
    see also hepatocellular carcinoma
  metastases, *see* hepatic metastases
living wills 3935
lizards, venomous **1140**
Loa loa 911, 917, 4192
  lifecycle 917
  see also loiasis
lobomycosis **803**
Lobo's disease **803**
local anaesthetics, *see* anaesthetics, local
loci, *see* gene(s), loci
locked-in syndrome 3858, 3888, **3932**
lockjaw 625
locomotor system, in sarcoidosis **2827**
Loeffler's syndrome
  in ascariasis 937
  see also Löffler's syndrome
lofepramine 4248
lofexidine 4292
Löffler's syndrome (simple pulmonary eosinophilia) 1112, **2805**, 2851
  in ascariasis 937
  haematological features 3685
  nickel causing 1112
  pathogenesis and groups 2805
Lofgren's syndrome **2821**, 3007
loiasis **917–18**
  clinical features/pathology 917–18, 4192
  glomerulonephritis 3177
  Onchocerca volvulus infection with 918
  transmission 1011
loin pain 3148, 3217, 3235
loin pain-haematuria syndrome **3148**
lomefloxacin, in urinary-tract infections *3211*
long-acting thyroid stimulators 163
long-chain fatty acids, *see* fatty acids, long-chain
longevity, desirable weight and 1301, 1302
long QT syndrome 2260, **2282–3**
  acquired 2282, *2282*
  congenital 2282
  management/prognosis 2282–3

long saphenous vein, coronary artery
  bypass grafting 2353
Looser's zones 3072
  in chronic renal failure 3324
  in rickets and osteomalacia 3071, 3072
loperamide 2006
  in opiate detoxification 4291
lorazepam, in status epilepticus 3923
lordosis 2872
lotions 3805, *3805*
loudness 3870
  balance test 3870
  discomfort level test 3870
Louis-Bar syndrome, *see* ataxia
  telangiectasia
Louping ill **415**, 4065
louse-borne relapsing fever 692, **693**
  tick-borne relapsing fever *vs* 695
  treatment 697
  see also relapsing fevers
low birthweight
  occupations associated 1173
  see also birthweight
low-density lipoprotein (LDL) 1401,
  1403
  apheresis 1414
  in atherosclerosis pathogenesis 1405,
    2291, 2332
  cholesterol 1404, 1405
  in diabetes 1457
  entry into cells 1403
  ischaemic heart disease risk 2307–8,
    2332
  modification and oxidation 1405, 2291
    mechanisms 2293
  resistance increased by olive oil 2311
  myocardial infarction incidence and
    2332
  in nephrotic syndrome 3143
  reduced,
    dietary fat intake 2310
    olive oil causing 2311
  uptake, endocytic pathway 73, 74
low-density lipoprotein (LDL) receptor
  1401–2, 1403, 1407
  defects/mutation 74, 1407
  gene transfer 113
  mutations in familial
    hypercholesterolaemia 129
lower limbs, *see* legs
lower motor neurone syndromes **3856**,
  4089–90
  combined upper motor neurone
    syndromes **4087–8**
  see also amyotrophic lateral sclerosis;
    specific syndromes (4089)
lower oesophageal sphincter
  in achalasia 1958
  dilation 1959
Lowe's oculocerebrorenal syndrome
  1355
Lown-Ganong-Levine syndrome 2275,
  2277
lpr mutation in mice 3024
LSD, *see* lysergic acid diethylamide
  (LSD)
L-selectin 88, 2294, 2299, 2487, **2620–1**,
  2620
lucanthone 979
luciferase 83
Lucio reaction 673
Ludwig's angina 572, 1847
Lugol's solution 831, 1613, 1614
lumbago, febrile 2440
lumbar canal stenosis **3907–8**
lumbar disc protrusion 3906, 3907
lumbar metastases 241
lumbar puncture **3842–5**
  in acute/subacute paraplegia 3892
  benign intracranial hypertension 4043
  in cerebrospinal angiostrongyliasis 947
  cerebrospinal fluid pressure 3842–3
  complications 3842, 3907
  contraindications 3842
  in epileptic seizures 3920
  indications 3842
  in meningitis 4055
  in meningococcal infections 540

in normal pressure hydrocephalus 3970
traumatic, subarachnoid haemorrhage *vs*
  3843
unconscious patients 2585
see also cerebrospinal fluid
lumbar root lesions, in pregnancy
  1766–7
lumbar spine
  'locking' 3906
  traumatic injury management 3897
lumbar spondylosis 3905
lumbar sympathectomy, in diabetic foot
  disease 1491
lumboperitoneal shunt 4043
lumbosacral plexus **4097**
  lesions in pregnancy 1766–7
luminizers, bone tumour association 207,
  1166
'lumpectomy', in breast cancer 248
lung
  abscess **2704–5**
    anaerobic infection 572
    causes 2704, *2704*
    foreign bodies 2704
    pleural effusion in 2867
  airway branching 2596–7, 2600
  amyloidosis **2835–6**
  anatomy **2593–609**, 2628–9
    alveolar septum micromechanics
      2599–600
    cells **2594–6**
    fibrous support system 2597–8
    tissue organization **2598–600**
  aspiration 519
  assist 2859, 2920
  biopsy, *see* lung biopsy *(below)*
  blood flow 2494
    Starling resistors 2489–90
    see also pulmonary circulation
  blood volume in 2488
    posture changes 2488
    see also pulmonary circulation
  breath sounds 2650
  bullae,
    in ankylosing spondylitis 2875
    in sarcoidosis 2824
  calcification,
    in alveolar microlithiasis 2838
    in sarcoidosis 2824–5
  cancer, *see* lung cancer
  capillaries, *see* pulmonary capillaries
  cavitation,
    chest radiography **2663**
    in lung cancer 2886
  cell types in 2593–4, *2594*
  chest radiography 2179–81, 2657, 2658,
    2782–3
    diffuse shadowing 2665, 2783
    distribution of abnormalities 2782–3
    size/nature of abnormalities 2783
  coal macules 2839, 2840
  'coin' lesions 2683, 2687, 2688
  in collagen-vascular diseases **2796–800**
  collapse,
    bronchoscopy in 2579
    chest radiography 2660–2
    expansion pulmonary oedema 2501
    individual lobes 2660–2
    in lung cancer 2886
    in pneumonia 2698
  compliance 2494, 2629
    in ARDS 2855, 2856
    decreased, dyspnoea due to 2164
    in emphysema 2632
    measurement **2668**
    reduced in scoliosis 2872
  compression, in pleural effusion 2863
  computed tomography (CT) 2658
  consolidation 2664
    bronchoscopy in 2579
    causes *2660*
    chest radiography 2660
    in pneumococcal pneumonia 515, 516
    in pneumonia 2695, 2698
  in cor pulmonale 2515
  crepitations,
    in elderly 4342
    in pulmonary oedema 2501

in cystic fibrosis 2747–8, 2748–9
cysts,
  hydatid 956, 957
  in paragonimiasis 990, 992
damage,
  by erosene (paraffin oil) 1083
  inhaled particles causing, *see*
    pneumoconioses
  oxygen toxicity 1207–8
  proteinase-antiproteinase theory
    2770–3
  toxic gases and fumes 2847–8
  see also neutrophils, injury due to
dead space 2164, 2232, **2629**, 2671
  increase, dyspnoea due to 2164
defence mechanisms 276, 2596,
  2612–28, 2628
  alveolar macrophage **2614–15**
  new anti-inflammatory therapy 2627–8
  non-immune mechanisms **2612–16**
  protective proteins **2614**
  pulmonary marginated pool of
    neutrophils **2615–16**
  redundancy in 2628
  surfactant 2599, **2613**
  see also defence mechanisms,
    respiratory tract
denervation, consequences **2937–8**
diffuse interstitial fibrosis,
  in asbestosis 2844
  chest radiography 2665
  in extrinsic allergic alveolitis 2809,
    2811, 2813
  gas exchange 2637–8
  mechanical properties 2637
  pathophysiology **2637–8**
  pulmonary circulation 2637
  see also cryptogenic fibrosing
    alveolitis; pulmonary fibrosis
diffuse interstitial oedema 2616
diffuse shadowing 2665, 2683
elastic recoil 2869
  loss in emphysema 2632, 2769
eosinophilic granuloma **2832–3**
farmer's, *see* extrinsic allergic alveolitis
fibre tracts in 2597–8
fibrotic cicatrization 2749
fissures, chest radiography 2657, 2658
flow-volume curve 2667
  in emphysema 2633
fluid, microbiological testing 2675
fluid overload 2495–6
  protection from 2494
foreign bodies 2704
function **2593–609**, **2628–32**
  in adult respiratory distress syndrome
    2503, 2575
  age-related changes 2673–4, 4335
  in anaemia 3458
  fluid clearance 2628
  physiological variations **2673–5**
  in pregnancy 1744
  in pulmonary hypertension 2512
  in pulmonary oedema 2503
  weaning from ventilators 2580
  see also gas exchange; lung, defence
    mechanisms; pulmonary diffusing
    capacity
function tests, *see* lung function tests
  (below)
'fungus ball' 2824
gas exchanger function, *see* gas
  exchange
granulomas, *see* pulmonary granulomas
haemodynamics, in ARDS 2859–60
haemorrhage, *see* pulmonary
  haemorrhage
in heart failure 2231–2
height 2489
'honeycomb' 2689, 2797
in hookworm infection 931
hydatid cysts 956, 957
hyperinflation, in asthma 2635
infarction, *see* pulmonary infarction
infections, *see* lung disease; respiratory
  tract infections
infiltrates, in immunocompromised
  patients 1031–3, *1032*

inflammation, *see* lung inflammation
inflammatory oedema 2616
inhaled particles and diseases due to,
  see pneumoconioses
injury, scarring in 2626
injury score, in ARDS *2857*
interstitial compliance, *see* lung,
  compliance
interstitial fluid, *see* interstitial fluid,
  lung
ischaemia, after lung/heart-lung
  transplantation 2935
lymphatic drainage 2486, 2496
lymphatics **2486**
  in hydrostatic pulmonary oedema 2496
lymphocytic infiltrations **2806–8**
  clinical features 2807
in malaria 844, 845
masses,
  bronchoscopy and biopsy 3483–4
  chest radiography **2662–3**
mechanical properties 2629
  in adult respiratory distress syndrome
    2639–40
  in alveolar filling syndromes 2638–9
  in asthma 2635–6
  in breathlessness 2645
  in chronic bronchiolitis 2634
  in diffuse interstitial fibrosis 2637
  in emphysema 2632–3
  in pulmonary vascular diseases 2641
nodules,
  in amyloidosis 2835
  calcified 2838
  chest radiography **2663–4**
  differential diagnosis *2664*
  in rheumatoid arthritis 2797, 2960,
    2961
  in silicosis 2842
  in Wegener's granulomatosis 2801
in paracoccidioidomycosis 816, 817
parenchymal mechanics **2598–9**
perfusion 2488
Pneumocystis carinii interaction 821
radionuclide scanning, *see* lung scans
recoil pressure **2668**
recoil and retractive forces 2598
residual volume, in cystic fibrosis 2748
  in rheumatoid arthritis **2796–8**
  in rickettsial diseases 732
rupture,
  divers 1206
  effects of aircraft pressure changes
    1198
in schistosomiasis 978
secretions 2643
  immunoglobulins in 2614
  proteins in 2614
shrinking 3020
  in SLE 2798
size, in diffuse parenchymal lung
  disease 2782
structure, *see* lung, anatomy
in syphilis 714
systemic arterial supply 2181
total lung capacity (TLC) **2666–7**, 2666
  in chronic obstructive airways disease
    2775
  in cystic fibrosis 2748
  in diaphragmatic disorders 2877
transplantation, *see* lung transplantation
uneven vascularity 2181
unilateral transradiancy **2778**
'upper lobe blood diversion' 2179,
  2180
volume,
  in chronic obstructive airways disease
    2775
  in emphysema 2632
  laryngeal control of 2612
  in pregnancy 1744
  reduced in ARDS 2856
  residual 2666
  in scoliosis 2872, 2873
  static 2775
  testing **2666–7**
  see also functional residual capacity
    (FRC)

water content,
  in adult respiratory distress syndrome
    2854
  capillary pressure and 2494, 2495–6
  see also entries beginning pulmonary
lung biopsy **2681**
  clinical applications **2682–4**
  in cryptogenic fibrosing alveolitis 2788,
    2791, 2792
  in diffuse parenchymal lung disease
    2683, 2785
  in lung cancer 2887
  in lung/heart-lung transplantation 2935
  open **2681**, **2687–90**
    conditions amenable to diagnosis by
      2687–8
    in cryptogenic fibrosing alveolitis
      2792
    in extrinsic allergic alveolitis 2814
    frozen sections 2687
    in granulomatoses and angiitis
      2689–90
    in immunosuppressed 2711
    in lung infections 2689, 2698
    morbidity 2687
    in pneumonia 2698
    in pulmonary vascular disease 2689
    in restrictive lung disease 2688–9
    specimen handling 2687
  percutaneous **2656**, **2681**
    cutting-needle biopsy 2681
    fine-needle aspiration 2681, 2683
    in lung cancer 2887
    needle type 2656
  in pulmonary hypertension 2513
  in rheumatoid arthritis 2797
  samples, microbiological testing 2675
  transbronchial 2680
    needle aspiration 2680–1
lung cancer **2879–93**
  adenocarcinoma 2882
  aetiological factors 205–7, **2879–81**
    air pollution 2881
    asbestos 2843, 2845, 2880
    chromium compounds 1108
    occupational 206–7, 2880, 2880
    pollution 207, 217
    silicosis 2842
    smoking 206, 207, 219, 2879–80,
      2880
    sulphur mustard (mustard gas) 1117
  antigens, monoclonal antibodies to
    2882
  bronchioloalveolar carcinoma 2882
  carcinoma in situ 2882
  cell lines 2882
  classification (WHO) 2881, 2881
  clinical features **2882–3**
    cough in 2643, 2883
    haemoptysis 2644, 2883
    pruritus in 3744
  coal-worker's pneumoconiosis and
    2840
  endocrine manifestations **2883–5**
  epidemiology 205–7, **2879–80**
    age relationship 197, 2879
    female rates 206, 207
    geographical differences 207
    sex ratio 206
    smoking prevalence changes 206,
      2879, 2880
  genetics and biology **2882**
    oncogene mutations 2882
  haematological effects 2885
  head and neck in 2652
  investigations 2684, **2886–8**
    biopsy 2887
    bronchoscopy 2680, 2682–3, 2886–7
    chest radiography 234, 2662–3
    computed tomography 235, 238, 2663,
      2887–8
    extrathoracic 2888
    open-lung biopsy 2687
    radiological 2886
    sputum cytology 2887
    thoracoscopy 2887
  Lambert-Eaton myasthenic syndrome
    (LEMS) and 4163

large-cell carcinoma 2882
laryngeal spread 2722, 2883
mental disorder/symptoms 4243
metabolic manifestations **2883–5**
metastases 2883
  management 2892
mortality 206, 206, 2879
  age-specific 2879
non-small-cell,
  chemotherapy 2890
  staging 247
  surgery 2888–9
pathogenesis 2881
pathology **2881–2**
perihilar lesions, investigations 2682–3
pleural effusion in 251, 2886
prevention **2892**
prognostic factors 2891
screening 2892 skin in 2651
small-cell (oat-cell) 2881
  ACTH/CRF-producing 1651, 1711,
    1712
  chemotherapy 2890–1, 2890
  Lambert-Eaton myasthenic syndrome
    (LEMS) and 4163
  staging 247
  voltage-gated calcium channels 4163
spread 2883
squamous-cell (epidermoid) carcinoma
  2881, 2887
staging **2885–6**, 2885, 2888, 2889
  investigations 236, 2888
  surgical 246
survival 2888, 2889, 2891
terminal care 2892
treatment **2888–91**
  chemotherapy 2890–1, 2890
  chemotherapy duration 2891
  general management 2891–2
  laser 2892
  palliative radiotherapy 2889–90
  radiotherapy 2889–90, 2891
  surgery 2888–9
  therapeutic bronchoscopy 2684
tuberculosis vs 651
lung disease
  cirrhosis with 2130
    see also hepatopulmonary syndrome
  cor pulmonale in 2515
  cytology **2685–91**
  diffuse fibrosis, see lung, diffuse
    interstitial fibrosis
  diffuse interstitial, see lung disease,
    diffuse parenchymal
  diffuse parenchymal **2779–862**
    after bone marrow transplant 1033
    amyloidosis 2836
    approach to patients **2779–80**, 2780
    bronchoscopy and biopsy 2683, 2785
    causes 2779, 2780
    chest radiography **2665**, 2781–3
    diseases associated 2781
    drug-induced 2850, 2850
    examination **2781**
    in genetic syndromes **2861–2**
    history-taking **2780–1**
    investigations **2781–5**
    occupation and hobbies associated
      2781
    in rheumatoid arthritis 2797
    in systemic sclerosis 3030
    treatment **2785**
    triggers 2779
    see also lung, diffuse interstitial
      fibrosis; pulmonary fibrosis
  drug-induced **2848–52**
    alveolar reactions **2850–1**, 2850
    asthma, see asthma, drug-induced
    cough **2850**
    pulmonary vascular reactions 2851–2
    in rheumatoid arthritis 2798
  fine-needle aspiration, see fine-needle
    aspiration biopsy
  in genetic syndromes **2861–2**
  histopathology **2685–91**
  in HIV infection 4285
  idiopathic interstitial fibrosis, see
    cryptogenic fibrosing alveolitis

industrial, sputum examination in 2685
infections,
  antibacterials distribution 302
  see also respiratory tract infections
  inflammatory, open-lung biopsy 2688
  in injecting drug abusers 4282
  in Langerhans-cell histiocytosis 3608
liver diseases affecting **2131**
lymphocytic (plasma-cell) interstitial
  pneumonitis **2807**
pathophysiology, see under respiratory
  disease/disorders
in pregnancy **1744–7**
restrictive,
  open-lung biopsy 2688–9
  ventilation in 2924
in septicaemia 1022
in sickle-cell disease 3515
in systemic sclerosis 3030, 3031, 3033
unilateral, PEEP and CPAP in 2923
in Wegener's granulomatosis 3012
see also respiratory disease/disorders
lung flukes, see paragonimiasis
lung function tests **2666–75**
  additional test availability 2674
  airflow obstruction site/mechanism **2668**
  airway resistance **2667–8**
  airway responsiveness **2668**
  asthma 2728, 2730, 2733, 2736
    occupational asthma 2744
  breathlessness investigation 2647
  in chronic obstructive airways disease
    2768, 2774–5
  clinical applications **2672–5**
    bedside monitoring 2672–3
    evaluation of stable disease 2673
  in cryptogenic fibrosing alveolitis 2791
  in diffuse parenchymal lung disease
    2782
  diving effect 1211
  exercise capacity **2672**
  in extrinsic allergic alveolitis 2814
  fitness to dive 1210
  forced expiration/inspiration **2667**
  gas exchange **2669–71**
  laboratories 2673, 2673, 2674
  in lung cancer 2886, 2889
  peripheral airway disease **2668**
  pulmonary circulation **2671–2**
  recoil pressure and compliance **2668**
  respiratory muscles function **2668–9**
  in sarcoidosis **2829**
  standard aspects/techniques 2673
  static lung volume **2666–7**
  in systemic sclerosis 3033
  in upper airways obstruction **2719–21**
  ventilation control **2672**
  see also peak expiratory flow (PEF)
lung inflammation **2616–27**
  beneficial vs detrimental effects **2626**
  diseases involving 2616
  general aspects **2616–18**
  historical aspects 2616–18
  initiation **2618–23**
    capillary transmigration 2621
    functional states of neutrophils 2622
    inflammatory cell sequestration
      2619–21
    local **2618–19**
    monocyte emigration/maturation 2623
    neutrophil chemotaxis/phagocytosis
      2621–2
    neutrophils from capillaries 2618–21
    phagocytosis and respiratory burst
      2622–3
  research 2617
  scarring and **2626–7**
    new anti-inflammatory therapy **2627–8**
  termination **2623–8**
    clearance phase 2625–6
    mediator dissipation 2623–4
    microvascular permeability 2624–5
    monocyte/neutrophil influx cessation
      2624
    repair 2624–5
    resolution 2623–6
    secretory behaviour control 2625
  see also monocytes; neutrophils

'lung juice' samples 2697
lung scans 2655
  in pulmonary embolism 1741
  in pulmonary hypertension 2510–11,
    2511
  see also ventilation-perfusion scanning
lung transplantation 2592, **2933–9**
  acute rejection 2935–6
  in bronchiectasis 2766
  bronchiolitis obliterans after 2796,
    2937
  choice of operation 2933–4, 2934
  in cor pulmonale 2521
  in cryptogenic fibrosing alveolitis 2793
  disease recurrence 2936–7
  donor selection and organ procurement
    2934–5, 2935
  double-lung 2933–4
  exercise capacity after 2938
  graft versus host reactions 2936
  history 2933
  immediate postoperative care 2935
  indications 2934
  infections after 2936, 2937
  lung denervation consequences 2937–8
  lymphoproliferative disease after
    2937
  medical management after 2935–6
  nasal positive-pressure ventilation
    (NPPV) 2932
  nephrotoxicity and hypertension after
    2937
  patient selection 2933–4, 2934
  preoperative assessment 2934
  reoperation 2935
  single-lung 2933
  survival 2933
  technique 2935
  see also heart-lung transplantation
lung tumours **2879–93**
  airway obstruction 2636
  benign, open-lung biopsy 2688
  carcinoid 2892
  diagnosis, open-lung biopsy 2687
  lymphoma **2808**
  malignant, see lung cancer
  metastatic, see pulmonary metastases
  mixed epithelial and connective tissue
    2687
  pleural, see pleura, tumours
  'lupoid hepatitis' 2069, 3020
    see also autoimmune hepatitis
lupus anticoagulant **3020**, 3020, 3668–9,
  3670, 3681
  see also anticardiolipin antibodies;
    antiphospholipid antibodies
lupus erythematosus 2069, 3776
  annular erythema 3714
  cutaneous, in pregnancy 1806
  discoid 3760, 3762, 3787
  drug-induced 1253, 3025, 3732–3
  juvenile 3018
  neonatal 3018, 3022
  see also systemic lupus erythematosus
    (SLE)
lupus nephritis 3018, 3019, 3159,
  3187–91
  acute renal failure in 3291, 3299
  clinical features 3019
  clinicopathological correlations 3190
  epidemiology 3187
  histological classification 3187–90
  laboratory tests 3187
  long-term outcome 3191
  presentation 3187
  treatment 3166, 3190–1, 3300
  see also systemic lupus erythematosus
    (SLE)
lupus pernio 2826, 3787, 3799
lupus pneumonitis, acute 2798
lupus vulgaris 654, 3794, 3800, 3801
Luque operation 4148
Luschka, foramina 4050
lusitropy, positive 2150
luteinizing hormone (LH) 1555, 1556,
  1579–81
  actions 1581
  adenoma secreting 1595–6

luteinizing hormone (LH) (cont.)
in anorexia nervosa 4213
ß-subunit 1579
exercise-induced changes 4326
in males 1679, 1680
mutations 1567, 1571
in ovulation induction 1678
in polycystic ovary syndrome 1674, 1675, 1676
at puberty 1563, 1701
pulsatile secretion 1565
receptor 1555, 1556, 1560
secretion 1565, 1580
regulation 1579–80
serum 1584
combined anterior pituitary test 1585
in hyperandrogenization 1676
in male infertility 1686
luteinizing hormone releasing hormone, see gonadotrophin releasing hormone (GnRH)
Lutembacher's syndrome 2452
lutrophin, see luteinizing hormone (LH)
Lutz's mycosis 3801
17,20-lyase (17,20-desmolase) 1664
deficiency 1668, 1692
lying, pathological 4258
Lyme disease (borreliosis) 689–92
aetiology 690
arthritis in 3002
clinical features 689–90, 3002
definition 689
diagnosis 691
distribution/epidemiology 690–1, 3002
maternal-fetal transmission 689
myositis in 4155
neuropathy in 4101
treatment 691–2, 3002
vaccine 692
see also Borrelia burgdorferi
lymph, protein in 2560
lymphadenitis
environmental mycobacteria causing 665
filarial 922
in tuberculosis in children 653
lymphadenitis benigna cutis 689
lymphadenopathy 3561, 3562–3
in acute paracoccidioidomycosis 817
angio-immunoblastic (immunoblastic) 2807
in atopic eczema 3741
in bartonellosis 774
in cat scratch disease 745, 746
causes 3562
in chronic lymphocytic leukaemia 3420
clinical management 3562
dermatopathic 3565
in Felty syndrome 2962
generalized, in homosexuals with STDs 3361
in hairy-cell leukaemia 3423
hilar, see hilar lymphadenopathy
in Hodgkin's disease 3570
in homosexuals 3361
in infectious mononucleosis 353
inguinal, see inguinal lymph nodes
in lymphoma 3568
mediastinal, see mediastinal lymphadenopathy
metastases from unknown primary site 252
in onchocerciasis 914
peripheral, in sarcoidosis 2825
persistent generalized 470, 485, 3566
in plague 596
in podoconiosis 1215
in sarcoidosis 2825
in scrub typhus 740
sinus histiocytosis with massive 3566, 3608, 3609
in SLE 3019
in toxoplasmosis 866
in tumours, N staging methods 237
see also lymph node
lymphadenopathy associated virus (LAV) 467
see also HIV
lymphangiectasia, small-intestinal 1977

lymphangiographic media, pulmonary reactions 2852
lymphangiography
in Hodgkin's disease 3572–3
tumour staging 237, 246
lymphangioleiomyomatosis, open-lung biopsy 2688
lymphangiomas, oral 1859
lymphangiomyomatosis 2833
lymphangitis, of limbs 922
lymphangitis carcinomatosa 2886, 2893
lymphatic capillaries 2559
lymphatic drainage
in adult respiratory distress syndrome 2854
lung 2486, 2496
lymphatic filariasis, see filariasis
lymphatic flow 2560
lymphatic hypoplasia, congenital 2560
lymphatic oedema, lung 2498
lymphatic system
abnormality, small-intestinal 1977
skin 3706
see also lymphoid organs; lymphoid tissue
lymphatic vessels 2559
in clearance phase of inflammation 2625
obstruction 2560
lymphatic pulmonary oedema and 2501
structural damage 2560
lymph node
angiofollicular hyperplasia (Castleman's disease) 3566, 3586
biopsy 3562–3, 3569
enlarged, examination in infections 266
examination 3376
in homosexuals with STDs 3361
follicular hyperplasia 3565
in Langerhans-cell histiocytosis 3607
in lymphogranuloma venereum 760, 761
mediastinal, see mediastinal lymph nodes
metastases, in thyroid cancer 1620
paracortical expansion 3565
reactivity patterns 3565–6
sinus hyperplasia 3565–6
structure 153, 154, 3561–2
in syphilis 710, 711
tuberculosis 652–3
see also lymphadenopathy
lymphocele, in renal transplant recipients 3318
lymphocyte-activating factor, see interleukin-1 (IL-1)
lymphocyte function-associated antigen 1 (LFΛ 1) 3559
lymphocytes 148–53, 3377, 3556
in chronic lymphocytic leukaemia 3419–20
counts 3379, 3380
differentiation markers 3564
in enteropathy-associated T-cell lymphoma 1928
HIV infection 465
'homing' 2001
intraepithelial (IEL) 1836
lamina propria 1836, 2001
large granular (LGL) 165, 3424
lifespan 3381
lung infiltration 2806–8
in lymph nodes 3561
lymphopenia differential diagnosis 169, 170
production 3384, 3385, 3386, 3588
radiation damage 1219
recirculation 153, 154, 3562
tumour-infiltrating, see tumour-infiltrating lymphocytes (TILs)
see also B-cells; T-cells
lymphocytic angiitis
benign 2807
open-lung biopsy in 2690
lymphocytic choriomeningitis virus (LCMV) 152, 429, 430, 435–6

lymphocytic and histiocytic (L and H) cells 3571
lymphocytic hypophysitis 1597, 1748
lymphocytic interstitial pneumonitis 2807
lymphocytosis 3378, 3558
in chronic lymphocytic leukaemia 3419
lymphoedema 2559–60
anatomical aspects 2559–60
causes and pathogenesis 2560
in filariasis 922
leg 2560, 3810–11
malignancy association 3792
management 2560, 3808, 3810–11
physiology 2560
WHO classification 922–3
lymphogranuloma venereum 759–61, 3363
'groove sign' 760
treatment 758
lymphography, see lymphangiography
lymphohistiocytosis, haemophagocytic 3608, 3609
lymphoid dendritic cells, see dendritic cells
lymphoid follicle, in chlamydial infections 757
lymphoid malignancy
secondary immunodeficiency in 173–4
see also leukaemia
lymphoid organs 86–7
embryology 87
lymphoid tissue 3561–2
in colon 1987
in common varied immunodeficiency (CVID) 169
gut-associated (GALT) 1836, 2001, 3562
pharynx 2611
in spleen 3589
see also lymphatic system
lymphokine-activated killer cells 3410
lymphoma 3568–86
in AIDS 2135
anaplastic large-cell 3582
angiocentric 3582
angioimmunoblastic 3581–2
antigen markers 3794
in ataxia telangiectasia 173
B-cell, see non-Hodgkin's lymphoma (NHL), B-cell
Burkitt's, see Burkitt's lymphoma
central nervous system (CNS) 4134
in AIDS 4080
centroblastic 3580, 3585
cerebral 4033–4
classification 3568
clinical features 3568
night sweating 241
cold haemagglutinin disease and 3544
in common varied immunodeficiency (CVID) 169
conditions resembling 3585–6
cutaneous 3583, 3794–7
cell types in 3794
clinical features 3795–6
see also mycosis fungoides
diagnosis 3563–5, 3569
common problems/misdiagnosis 242, 245
enteropathy-associated T-cell 3583
eosinophilia in 3612
follicular (centroblastic/centrocytic) 3423, 3579–80
gastric 1984–5, 3583
gastrointestinal 3582–3
histiocytic 3582
ocular features 4195
Hodgkin's, see Hodgkin's disease
immunoblastic 3580, 3585
immunocytic 3579
in immunosuppressed states, Epstein-Barr virus causing 355
joint involvement 3005
large-cell 355, 2690, 3580, 3585
large and small cells 3794
lymphoblastic 3581, 3585
lymphocytic B-cell 3579
lymphocytic T-cell 3581

lymphoepithelioid (Lennert's) 3581
MALT (MALTomas) 3582–3
mantle-cell (centrocytic) 3423–4, 3580
neurological complications 4133–4
non-Hodgkin's, see non-Hodgkin's lymphoma
ocular features 4194–5
opportunistic infections in 4133
pancreatic 2042
pericardial effusion in 251
peripheral T-cell 3581–2
pleomorphic 3582
pleomorphic small-cell 3582
in pregnancy 1761–2, 1808
primary cutaneous 3581
primary extranodal 3568, 3582–3
pulmonary 2808
pulmonary large-cell angiocentric 2690
red-cell aplasia and 3449
renal involvement 3183
in renal transplant recipients 3321
Sjögren's syndrome association 3036
small intestine, see small intestine, lymphoma
splenic, with villous lymphocytes (SLVL) 3423
splenomegaly in 3589, 3591
staging investigations 236
T-cell, see non-Hodgkin's lymphoma (NHL), T-cell
terminology and classification 3794
thymic 2899
thyroid 1621
tuberculosis vs 651
T-zone 3582
see also Hodgkin's disease; leukaemia/lymphoma syndromes
lymphomatoid granulomatosis 2807–8, 3586
of lung, open-lung biopsy in 2690
Wegener's granulomatosis vs 3013
lymphomatous polyposis 1993, 3583
lymphopathy
obstructive, podoconiosis 1215
see also lymphadenopathy
lymphopenia 3378, 3558
in common varied immunodeficiency (CVID) 167
differential diagnosis 169, 170, 172, 174
in malignant disease 3678
in secondary immunodeficiency 173, 174
small-intestinal lymphangiectasia 1977
lymphopoiesis 3384, 3385, 3386, 3588
lymphoproliferative disorders 3561–7
after lung transplantation 2937
diagnostic methods 3563–5
histopathology 3563
immunocytochemistry 3563–4
molecular studies 3564–5
non-malignant 3566
open-lung biopsy in 2690
pathogenesis of malignant 3566–7
see also lymphadenopathy; lymphoma; myeloma
lymphoreticular disease
liver in 2132–3
see also lymphoma
'lymphorrhoids' 760
lymphoscintigraphy 923
lymphotoxin, tumours secreting 1712
lymphuria, in filariasis 923
Lynch type colorectal cancer families 107, 1990
Lyonization, see X-chromosome, inactivation
lysergic acid diethylamide (LSD) 1075
intoxication, features/treatment 1075
psychiatric disturbances from 4241
lysine 1353
catabolism 1372
defects of metabolism 1372–3
lysine vasopressin 1601, 3122
lysinuric protein intolerance 1357, 3333
lysis of cells
complement role 175, 178
importance 175, 178

see also complement; membrane-attack
  complex
lysosomal acid lipase deficiency **1436–7**,
  2025
lysosomal acid phosphatase deficiency
  1437
lysosomal storage diseases 1335,
  1426–37, *2019*, 2024–5, **3087**
lysosomes 1426
lysozyme 88, 93, 2614
  in urine 3137
  variants, in amyloidosis 1520
Lyssaviruses 394, *396*

M

Mac-1 (CR3 complement receptor) 88,
  177, 3559
McArdle's disease (type V glycogen
  storage disease; muscle
  phosphorylase deficiency) 1341,
  1343, 1344, 1384, 2173, 4166
McCallum's patch 2452
McCune-Albright syndrome 124, 1569,
  1642–3, 1702, 1715, 3091
McGill Pain Questionnaire 4300
Machado-Joseph disease 3985
Machupo virus 430, 431, 436, 438
McLeod myopathy 4146
Macleod's syndrome **2778**
McMaster counting chamber 931
macrocytosis 3377, *3378*, 3461, 3495
  in alcoholism 3685
macroelectromyography 3839
macrofilaricides 916
α₂-macroglobulin 3623, 3626
  in chronic obstructive airways disease
    2773
macroglobulinaemia
  in myeloma 3599
  Waldenström's, *see* Waldenström's
    macroglobulinaemia
macroglossia, in amyloidosis 1515
macrolide antibiotics 305
  see also antibiotics
macrophage 85, **153–4**, 3384, **3556**
  activation 85, 89, 93, 293, 639, 2615
    in atherogenesis 2291
    in Crohn's disease 1938
    lymphokines 93, 277
    in tuberculosis 639
    in ulcerative colitis 1945
  in allergic disease 159
  alveolar, *see* alveolar macrophage
  antigen presentation 89, 93, 2615
  asbestos toxicity to 2844
  bacterial survival in 276
  in bone marrow 86
  cellular basis for cellular interactions
    89–94, 2615
  chemotactic proteins secretion 2614,
    2615
  clusters (stromal) 86
  coal dust and quartz dust toxicity 2839
  in cryptogenic fibrosing alveolitis 2788
  cytokines released *92*, 93–4, 154, 291,
    293, 2788
    alveolar macrophage 2615, *2615*
    in atherogenesis 2291
    in rheumatoid arthritis 2954
    in ulcerative colitis 1945
  deactivation and down-regulation 89
  diseases involving *86*
  in embryology 87
  epithelioid 88, 2818
  foam cells 2290, 2318
    in extrinsic allergic alveolitis 2811
    formation 1403, 1405
    in lungs 2837
    in Whipple's disease 1923, 1924,
      2005
  giant cell formation 2818
  in graft rejection 187
  in granulomas 88, 2120
  growth factor production 93
  in hepatic granulomas 2120

high permeability pulmonary oedema
  mechanism 2497, 2498
in HIV infection 91, 465, 467
inflammatory **2623**
  clearance 2625, 2626
  role/actions 2623, 2625–6
inflammatory responses due to 93, 94,
  154, **2615**
  to endotoxin 291
interstitial 85
iron stores 3471, 3472
killing mechanisms *93*, 94
lifespan 85
lipid-laden, *see* macrophage, foam cells
in lymph nodes 87
mature and replication of 85
M-CSF effect 89
mediating haemolysis 3542
MHC class II antigen expression 87
monocyte maturation to 2618, **2623**
in mucormycosis 1027
non-specific response to infections
  276–7
origin and distribution **85–9**
parasitism of and pathogens involved
  91
pathogen interaction outcome 91
phagocytic function 91, 93, 154, 276–7,
  2615
physiological processes involving *86*
production 3384, 3386, 3388, 3557
  suppression of 3388–9
proteolysis by 93
in pulmonary alveolar proteinosis
  2833–4
pulmonary intravascular (PIMs) 2487
receptors 89–91, *90*, 2614, *2615*
recruited monocytes *vs* 85
recruitment, in atherogenesis 2291
scavenger receptors 2291
secretory responses *92*, 93–4
  control 2625
splenic 3589
surfactant action 2856
Th1 and Th2 cells action on 85, 88
tissue heterogeneity and sites **85–9**
  cellular immunity and 88–9
  in vasculitis 3776
see also monocytes
macrophage colony-stimulating factor
  (M-CSF) 87, 97
  control of growth and effects on
    macrophage 89
macrosialin (CD68) 91, 93
macrosomia, fetal 1753, 1756
macula
  cherry-red spot 1426, 1427, 1436
  degeneration, age-related **4198**
  exudates, in diabetic retinopathy 1484
  oedema, in diabetic retinopathy 1484,
    4189
macule *3713*
Madopar® 4002, 4003
Madura foot, *see* mycetoma (Madura
  foot)
[⁹⁹Tcᵐ]MAG3 (mercaptoacetyltriglycine)
  3112, 3114, 3115
maggots, in eye 4193
magnesium
  abnormalities, neurological features
    4126
  deficiency/depletion 1320, 1910, 2241
    in diuretic therapy 2241
    hypokalaemia in 3132
  disorders of renal handling **3336**
  hypertension pathogenesis 2530
  intake, in artificial nutritional support
    1318, *1318*
  loss, ACE inhibitor action 2249
  in myocardial infarction 2344
  raised levels 3336
  serum, in hereditary fructose intolerance
    1347
  see also hypomagnesaemia; magnesium
    salts
magnesium ammonium phosphate stones
  3252, 3253
magnesium glycerophosphate 2241

magnesium hydroxide (Mg(OH)₂) 1447,
  1448, 3256
magnesium oxide (MgO) 1447, *1448*,
  3256
magnesium salts
  in acute myocardial infarction 29–30
  in eclampsia 1731
  in hypomagnesaemia 3336
  in renal bone disease 3329–30
magnesium sulphate
  in long QT syndrome 2283
  in myocardial infarction 2344
magnetic brain stimulation **3836–9**
  D and I waves 3836
  in multiple sclerosis 3837
  neurosurgical monitoring 3838–9
  physiology/principles 3836–7
  safety 3837
  see also central motor conduction time
magnetic fields **1222**
magnetic resonance, principles 2212–13
magnetic resonance angiography
  intracranial 3821
  peripheral arterial disease 2368
magnetic resonance imaging (MRI) **2213**
  in acute back pain 2993
  in adrenal disease 1649, 1660
  advantages/disadvantages 2654, 3820
  in Alzheimer's disease 3974
  in biliary disease 2046
  bone disease 3063
  bone and joint 2949, 2950
  in cerebellopontine angle tumours 3875
  cerebral 'diffusion' images 3822
  in cerebral infarction 3957, 3959
  in cerebral metastases 250
  chest **2654**
  in coarctation of aorta 2215, 2558, 2559
  in coma 3931
  contrast media 2214, 3820
  cranial 3819–22, 3823
    in viral infections 4069
  in cysticercosis 965, 967
  in demyelinating disease 3834 in
    disseminated tumours 239
  in epileptic seizures 3920
  future advances/applications 3821–2
  hazards and effect 1222
  heart **2212–20**
    bolus-tracking studies 2217
    cine gradient echo imaging 2213,
      2214, 2217
    clinical applications **2214–17**
    normal 2213
    rapid gradient echo techniques 2217,
      2218
    spin echo sequence 2213
  in hepatocellular carcinoma 2117
  in Hodgkin's disease 3572
  in intervertebral disc protrusions 3906,
    3907
  in intracranial disorders **3819–22**, 3823
  in intracranial tumours 4037
  kidneys 3111
  limitations 2949
  liver 1833, **2013**
  mediastinal 2654
  in multiple sclerosis 3994
  in myeloma 3600
  in neurological disorders 3815
  in occupational rheumatic diseases 1169
  pancreas **2013**
  in pericardial constriction 2480
  in phaeochromocytomas 2556
  in pituitary disease 1586, 1587, 1598,
    1649
  principles 2212–14, 2654, 3819
  in rheumatic disease 1169, 2949
  safety 2214
  spatial resolution improvements 3820
  in spinal disorders 3826, 3827, **3828**
  T_1 and T_2 relaxation times 2213, 3819
  tumour recurrence detection 239
  tumour staging 235, 245–6
    M staging 238
    N staging 237
    T staging 236, 245, 246
  in urinary stone disease 3253

magnetic resonance spectroscopy (MRS)
  2213–14, 2233
  peripheral arterial disease 2368
magnetic stimulators 3836
Mahaim pathway 2275
major histocompatibility complex (MHC)
  183–5
  antigens, advantages in antigen
    presentation 148
  class I antigens 142–3, 183, 2955
    antigen presentation/processing 143
    on biliary epithelial cells 2074
    cells expressing 142
    cytotoxic T-cell recognition 142, 143,
      151, 280
    deficiency/defect 172
    LCMV infections 436
    loci and polymorphism 142
    in polymyositis/dermatomyositis 4156
    recipient unresponsiveness 183
    structure 142
    translocation mechanisms for
      presentation 69
  class II antigens 143, 183, 2955
    antigen processing 143
    on biliary epithelial cells 2078
    cells expressing 143
    in chlamydial infections 758
    in connective tissue diseases 3009
    deficiency 172
    on dendritic cells and macrophage 87
    function 143
    helper T-cell recognition 142, 143,
      151, 153, 280
    incompatibility of grafts 183
    induced on other cells 183, 187
    matching in renal grafts 184
    presentation for immune response 183
    in rheumatoid arthritis 2954
    structure 143
  class III antigens, C4 and C2 genes 178
  definition 183
  genes 143
    atopic disease association 158
    genetic control 183
  immunogenicity of antigens 183–4
  in lymphocytic choriomeningitis virus
    infections 436
  restriction of T-cell responses 141, 142,
    143, 151, 277, 280
    in infections 277, 280
    to tumours 227
  in transplantation 183–5
    antigens presentation 183, 184–5
    HLA matching 184
    incompatibility 183
  see also HLA (antigens)
malabsorption **1899–936**
  amenorrhoea in 1672
  bacterial overgrowth, *see* bacterial
    overgrowth
  causes 1904, *1905*
  clinical presentation 1904
  in coeliac disease 1918, 1918–19
  in collagen disorders 1999
  in Crohn's disease 1938
  in diabetes 1488–9
  drug absorption impairment 1242
  in enteropathy-associated T-cell
    lymphoma 1927
  folate 3467, **3492**
  gut peptides in 1895
  haematological changes 3684
  investigations **1904–11**
    bacteriology 1910
    carbohydrate absorption 1906–7
    defective absorption demonstration
      1905–6
    endoscopic biopsy 1908–9
    nutritional status 1910
    protein absorption 1907
    radiology 1909–10
    small-bowel biopsy, *see* small
      intestine, biopsy
    vitamin B₁₂ absorption 1907
  iron-deficiency anaemia 3476, 3684
  osteomalacia in **3073**
  post-infective 1932

malabsorption (*cont.*)
  selective IgA deficiency and 1839–40
  in short gut syndrome 1925
  in systemic sclerosis 3029
  in tropics, *see* tropical malabsorption; tropical sprue
  urinary stone disease in 3255
  vitamin B₁₂ *3489*, 3491–2
  vitamin D deficiency 1636
  vitamin K deficiency 3655
maladie de Roger 2461
malakoplakia 2137
malar flush 2425, 2453, 3787
malaria **835–63**
  acquired resistance to 840–2
  'algid' 846, *849*
    management 856
  anaemia 278, 842, 845, 846, 848, 850
    management 854
  'benign' 847
    treatment 853
  Burkitt's lymphoma and 214, 354, 841, **858**
  cerebellar dysfunction in 847
  cerebral 4124
    clinical features 846–7, 4024
    management 853–4, 4124
    mortality 846
    neurological symptoms 4124
    pathology 843–4
    pathophysiology 845
    in pregnancy 1794
    retinal haemorrhage in 4192
    vivax malaria 847
  cerebral oedema in 845
  chemoprophylaxis 324, *324*, 860–1, *861*
    in children *862*
    in pregnancy 1795, **1810**
  clinical features 266, 324, **846–8**
  complications 842
  congenital 848, 1795, 3680
  control **858–9**
    policy 859–60
    prevention in travellers 860–1
  cytokine production 276, 842, 845
  differential diagnosis **849**, *849*
  drug resistance 836, 851
    chemoprophylaxis in 860, 861
    chloroquine 324, 851, 860, 861
    endemicity levels 840, *841*
  epidemics 840, 860
  epidemiology **838–40**, 861
    basic case reproduction rate (BCRR) 839
    seasonal variation 840, *841*
  eradication, plan and time-scale 859–60
  evolution 3462
  evolutionary adaptations **3463–6**
  falciparum malaria (malignant tertian/subtertian) 842
    clinical features 846–7
    treatment 853
  fetal/placental 1794–5
  fever patterns 266, 836, 842, 847
  fluid/electrolyte disturbances 854–5
  genetic determinants of susceptibility 280, 840, *841*
  glomerulonephritis complicating **3177**
  glucose-6-phosphate dehydrogenase (G6PD) deficiency 837, 845, 847
  haematological disorders in 3680
  haemoglobinopathies and 840, *841*
  in HIV infection 487
  hyperparasitaemia management 856
  hypoglycaemia in 845, 846, 848, 1510
    management 856
  hyponatraemia in 846
  hypotension and shock in 846
    management 856
  hypovolaemia in 845, 846, 854
  immunity 840–2
    genetic influence on 280, 840, *841*
  immunological complications **857–8**
  immunoprophylaxis 861–3
  incubation period 846, 847, 848
  infection susceptibility 840
  innate resistance to 840
  laboratory diagnosis **849–50**
  metabolic acidosis in 846, 855

molecular pathology **842–3**
monkey 848
mortality 840, 843, 846, 856, 859, 860
neonatal 848
oliguria in 846
parasitology 835–7
pathology **843–5**
pathophysiology **845–6**
  in pregnancy 325, 846–8, 1794–5, 3467, 3468–9
    management 856
  prevention **324**, 3470
  prognosis 856
  psychosis in 847
  in puerperium 847–8
  pulmonary oedema in 845, 846, 848
    management 856
  quartan malarial nephrosis 857
  renal failure in 844, 845, 3201
    management 855
  sickle-cell anaemia and 115, 840
  splenic rupture in 847, 856
  splenomegaly in 3591
  stable and unstable 840, *841*
  transfusion and 'needlestick' 848
  transmission 839–40
    vertical 848
  treatment **850–3**
    antimalarial drugs 850–3
    children/uncomplicated malaria 853, *854*
    in G6PD deficiency 3541
    general management 853–6
    recommendations/prescribing 853
    stage specificity 850–1
    see also antimalarial drugs
  tropical splenomegaly syndrome, *see* tropical splenomegaly syndrome
  vaccines 861–3
    circumsporozoite protein (CSP) 862
    SPf66 antigen 862, 863
  vectors 3463
  vivax/ovale/malariae ('benign' malaria) 847, 853
  see also individual Plasmodium species
Malassezia furfur 799, 3754
malate 1458
malathion 1004, 1122
male
  breast cancer 1687
  drug-induced endocrine disorders 1718
  hypogonadism 1680, **1682–4**
  infertility, *see* infertility, male
  mortality rates 40, *41*, *42*
  pseudohermaphroditism 1572, 1690, **1691–4**
  reproductive disorders **1679–87**
  urinary-tract infections 3213
maleic acid (maleate) 1354–5
malignant disease
  acute uric acid nephropathy (renal failure) in 1379–80, 3185, 3226, 3290
  aetiology 3567
  see also epidemiology of cancer
  amyloidosis in 1513, *1515*
  aplastic anaemia and 3441, *3442*, **3447**
  arthritis in **3006**
  in chronic lymphocytic leukaemia 3421
  classical fever of unknown origin (FUO) due to 1015, *1017*
  C-reactive protein 1530–1
  dialysed patients 3312
  DIC in 3658
  disseminated, haematological disorders in 3548, 3677
  folate deficiency in 3493
  haematological disorders in **3676–8**
  haemolytic uraemic syndrome in 3197
  hypercalcaemia of, *see* hypercalcaemia, of malignancy
  hypoglycaemia in 1509–10, 1714
    infection susceptibility and 282
  in marrow transplant recipients 3699
  membranous nephropathy and 3159
  mental disorder/symptoms 4243
  myelosclerosis in 3438

neurological complications **4133–5**
neuropathy in 4102
pathogenesis 3566–7
in pregnancy **1806–8**
  effects on pregnancy 1806–7
  management 1807–8
  pregnancy after 1808
renal involvement **3183–5**
renal transplantation in 3315
in renal transplant recipients **3321**
skin in **3791–7**
three 'P' signs 3792
in treated Hodgkin's disease 3575
urinary-tract obstruction 3183, 3244
venous thromboembolism in 3668
see also cancer; neoplasia; tumour(s)
malignant hyperpyrexia, *see* hyperpyrexia
'malignant pustule' 615
see also anthrax
malingerers 3
malingering 4210, **4211**
  definition 4211
  dissociative disorder *vs* 4210
  psychiatric emergencies associated 4258
Mallory bodies 2022, 2074, 2082, 2084
Mallory-Weiss tear 1873
  bleeding 1827
malnutrition 1267, **1278–96**
  alcoholic liver disease relation 2081
  anaemia in 1292, 3469, 3498–9
  'brittle' patients 1287, 1289
  classification **1280–2**
    adults 1281–2
    body mass index 1281–2, *1282*
    children 1280–1, *1282*
    Gomez 1281, *1281*
    mid upper arm circumference 1281, *1282*, *1282*
    Waterlow 1281, *1282*
    Wellcome 1281, *1281*
  clinical features **1282–4**
  complications 2586
  drug metabolism in 1295–6
  follow-up 1294
  in HIV infection 1295, 2395
  infections in 1027
    management 1289, 1291
    susceptibility 281, *281*
  investigations **1288**
  management **1288–96**
    acute phase **1289–93**
    congestive heart failure 1292–3
    criteria for admission to care 1288–9
    dietary 1289, *1291*
    emotional/psychological stimulation 1293–4
    hypoglycaemia 1289, 1292
    hypothermia 1292
    intermediate phase 1293
    physiological changes 1289, *1290–1*
    preparation for discharge 1294
    progress assessment 1293
    rehabilitation phase 1293–4
    specific problems 1295
  measles interaction 376, 378, 380
  oedematous 1281, **1288**
    pathophysiology 1288
    see also kwashiorkor
  pathophysiology **1285–7**
    body composition 1287, *1291*
    homeostasis loss 1287
    loss of reserve 1287
    physiological/metabolic changes 1285–6, *1286*, *1290–1*
    vicious cycles 1287
  prevalence 1294
  prevention **1315–16**
  primary 1278
  protein-energy (calorie) 1279
    anaemia in 3469, 3498–9
    infection susceptibility 281, *281*
    secondary immunodeficiency in 174
  secondary 1278, 1295
  skin disease affected by 3722–3
  treatment **1315–16**
  Wernicke-Korsakoff syndrome in 4126
  see also nutritional deficiency

Maloprim
  in malaria, prophylaxis 861
  overdose 1073
maltase-glucoamylase 1920
MALTomas 3582–3
mambas, bites and envenoming 1131, 1132
mammals
  injuries due to 1124–5
  venomous **1125–6**
mammography
  investigations of metastases from unknown primary sites 252
  in pregnancy 1807
Management of Health and Safety at Work Regulations (1992) 1177
mandibular underdevelopment, obstructive sleep apnoea and 2910
manganese 1110, **1424–5**
  absorption and excretion 1110
  deficiency *1418*, 1425
  function 1110
  poisoning **1110–11**, 1174
mania and manic depressive disorder **4220–1**
  aetiology 4220
  clinical features 4220, *4220*
  differential diagnosis 4220
    schizophrenia 4220, 4222
  in elderly 4227
  incidence 4220
  prognosis 4221
  treatment 4221
    carbamazepine 4251
    lithium 4250
manipulation, in acute back pain 2994
manipulative patients, brittle diabetes 1496
mannitol
  in acute renal failure 2581, 3285
  in crush injury 3289
  in hepatocellular failure 2109
mannose-6-phosphate residues 1426, 1434
mannosidosis *1435*, **1436**
manometry
  anorectal 1956, 1979
  costs 1956
  gastric 1956
  motility disorder investigation 1956
  oesophageal 1865, 1870, 1956, 1959
  small intestinal and colon 1956
Mansonella ozzardi 915, 919
Mansonella perstans 919
Mansonella streptocerca 911, 915, 918
mansonelliasis 919
Mantoux test 645, 650
  Heaf test equivalence *646*
MAP kinases 1561
maple syrup urine disease (branched chain ketoaciduria) 1369
MAPPHY trial 2539
maprotiline, overdose 1059
marasmus
  clinical features 1282
  definitions/classification 1281
  HIV infection in 1295
  kwashiorkor *vs* 1282, 1288
  oedematous malnutrition *vs* 1288
  see also malnutrition
marathon runners
  aerobic fitness 4324, 4325
  carbohydrate metabolism 4325–6
  rhabdomyolysis and creatine kinase levels 4326
  see also endurance sports; runners
marathons **4327–8**
marble bones disease, *see* osteopetrosis
Marburg virus **439–43**
  characteristics 440–1
Marburg virus disease **441–3**
marche à petit pas 4002
Marchiafava-Bignami syndrome, in alcohol abusers 4127, 4278
Marfan (Marfan's) syndrome 1700, **3083–4**
  biochemical features *3062*
  bleeding disorders 3636, 3645
  clinical features 3083

diagnosis and treatment 3083
eye features **4181**
life expectancy 3083
lung disease in 2862
mitral regurgitation 2457
pathophysiology 3083
in pregnancy 1738
scoliosis in 2873
tricuspid valve prolapse 2468
marfanoid habitus, in MEN 2B syndrome 1710
marijuana, *see* cannabis
marine invertebrates, venomous **1143–4**
Maroteaux-Lamy disease (mucopolysaccharidosis VI) 1431, *1432*
marrara 987
marrara syndrome 1012
marrow, *see* bone marrow
mass runs **4327–8**
mast cells **153**, 3556
in allergic rhinitis 2715, 2716
in asthma 2727, 2728
in cryptogenic fibrosing alveolitis 2789
degranulation 153, 158, 159, 2727, 3799
in asthma 2727, *2728*
triggers 158
in urticaria/angioedema 162
disorders 3799
sclerosis in *3791*
distribution 158
histamine release 2727, 3770
in immediate hypersensitivity 158
mediators released, actions of *2728*
mucosal/connective tissue types 158
subsets 158
mastitis, in mumps 373
mastocytosis (urticaria pigmentosa) *3755*, 3799
systemic 3438
mastoparan 78
masturbation 3350
maternal age, chromosomal abnormalities and *120–1*
maternal mortality
in ARDS 1744–5
in hypertensive disease *1728*, 1730
in thromboembolism 1741
in viral infections 1775
maternal sepsis, *Haemophilus influenzae* 583
Mathevotaenia symmetrica 962
matings, frequency and gene frequency 117
matrix gla protein (MGP) 3057
matrix proteins, atherosclerotic plaque development 2294
Mauriac syndrome 2024
maxillary nerve 2610
maxillary sinuses, structure/function 2609
maximum allowable concentrations (MAC) 1163
Mayaro virus **407**
May-Hegglin anomaly 3556, 3645
mazindol 3929
Mazzotti test 915, 916, 918
MCC (mutated in colorectal cancer) gene 66, 1990
M cells 1836
MDMA (Ecstasy) 1076, 1182, 3441, 4263
acute hepatitis due to 2124
complications associated 4280
psychiatric disturbances from 4241
withdrawal syndrome 4293
MDPIT trial 2347
*mdr*1 gene 259, 851
meals, in obesity treatment 1311
mean cell haemoglobin (MCH) *3379*, 3380
in iron deficiency *3474*
mean cell haemoglobin concentration (MCHC) *3379*, 3380
mean cell volume (MCV) *3379*, 3380
in cirrhosis 2089
in iron deficiency *3474*
in megaloblastic anaemia 3494
'mean circulatory pressure' 2153–4

measles **375–81**
antibodies 377–8
clinical features 378, 379
complications 379–80, *379*
encephalitis 376, 380, 4073
see also subacute sclerosing panencephalitis (SSPE)
epidemiology 375–6
eye in 4192
haematological changes 3679
immune response 377–8
malnutrition interaction 376, 378, 380
management 1291
mortality 375–6
pathogenesis 377–8
in underprivileged/malnourished 378
persistent infection 380
popular beliefs about 376
prevention 380–1
passive immunization 380
see also measles, vaccination
secondary bacterial infections after 282, 378
transmission 376, 377
treatment 380
vaccination 321, 375, 380–1
complications 380
schedule 381
vaccines 380, 381
new developments 381
measles/mumps/rubella (MMR) vaccine 318–19, 375, 411
Swedish schedule 411–12
measles virus **376–7**
Crohn's disease aetiology 1937
proteins and antigens 376–7
replication and assembly 377
meat consumption, cancer association 218–19
colorectal cancer 203
meat-handlers, streptococcal infections 500, 503
mebendazole
in ascariasis 938
in enterobiasis 942
in hookworm infection 931, 932
in hydatid disease 958
in opisthorchiasis 984
in trichinosis 941
in trichuriasis 944
mechanoreceptors, heart 2160
mechlorethamine, mycosis fungoides management 3797
mecholyl 3771
Meckel's diverticulum **1977–8**
embryology 1973
radionuclide studies 1833
Meckel syndrome 4117
meclofenamic acid, poisoning 1056–7
meconium 1973, 1978
failure to pass 1978, 1979
meconium ileus **1978**, 2747
in cystic fibrosis 2748
equivalent 1978, 2749
management 1978
Mectizan 916
media, as disease agent 35–6
media (tunica media) 2290, 2484
in cor pulmonale 2515
hypertrophy 2506–7, 2508, 2533
in pulmonary hypertension 2506–7, 2508, 2533
medial medullary syndrome 3858
median nerve **4094–6**
entrapment neuropathies 4094–6
see also carpal tunnel syndrome
forearm lesions 4094–5
injuries/lesions 4094–6
palsy, cervical disc protrusions *vs* 3906
transection 4095
wrist lesions 4095–6
mediastinal germ-cell tumours 2899
misdiagnosis 245
mediastinal lymphadenopathy 651, **2899**
investigations 2684
malignant, oesophageal compression in 1873
in sarcoidosis 2823

mediastinal lymph nodes 2895–6, 2897
computed tomography 2658
mediastinal masses **2896–901**
anterior **2898–9**, *2898*
biopsy 2898
clinical features 2897–8
computed tomography 2898
diagnostic approach 2898
investigations 2684
middle **2899**
posterior **2900–1**
mediastinal sampling **2681–2**
surgical 2682
mediastinal tumours **2895–901**
benign/malignant 2896
types and frequency 2896–7
see also mediastinal masses
mediastinoscopy 2682
in lung cancer 2888
in sarcoidosis 2828
mediastinum
anatomy 2895
chest radiography,
mesothelioma 2661
normal 2656
compartments 2895, 2896, 2897
computed tomography, normal appearance **2658**
cysts **2899–900**
disease, bronchoscopy and biopsy in **2684**
displacement, in pleural effusion 2863
drug reactions 2852, *2852*
fibrosis 3245, **3246**
lesions, chest pain in 2169
in lung cancer 246
lymphadenopathy, in lung cancer 2886
magnetic resonance imaging 2654
middle 2895, 2897
needle biopsy 2681–2
shift 2661, 2863
Medical Certificate of the Cause of Death 4309
medical confidentiality, *see* confidentiality
medical education 8
Medicalert bracelet/necklace 1587, 1655
medical jurisprudence 4309
medical kits, expedition 326
medical negligence **4311–12**
categories 4312
risk management 4312
medical reports **4314–15**
see also clinical records
Medical Research Council, breathlessness scale 2646, *2646*
'medical secrecy' 4315
medical witnesses 4315
medicine
art of 9–10
scientific **7–10**
of wealth 38
medicolegal context
confidentiality 4315–17
consent and 4316–17
medical reports 4315
see also law
medigoxin 2242
Mediterranean diet 2311
Mediterranean fever, familial, *see* recurrent polyserositis
Mediterranean spotted fever (Boutonneuse fever) **734**
medroxyprogesterone acetate 1703, *1814*
in lymphangiomyomatosis 2833
medulla **3858**
lesions 3858
pupillary responses 2582
medulloblastoma **4031**
management 4039
Mee's lines 1106, 1113, 4099
mefenamic acid
haemolytic anaemia due to 3542–3
poisoning 1056–7
mefloquine
in malaria 852, *854*
prophylaxis 861

overdose **1073**
side-effects 861
megacalyces 3241
megaduodenum 1959
megakaryocyte colony-stimulating activity (meg-CSA) 3389
megakaryocytes 3383
in immune-mediated thrombocytopenia 3630, 3631
in myelodysplastic syndromes 3426, 3427
megakaryocytopoiesis **3389**
megalencephaly 4114
progressive 4114
megaloblastic anaemia **3484–99**
in alcoholism 3498, 3685
biochemical basis 3488–9
causes 3489–94
clinical features 3489–94
diagnosis of cause 3495–6
differential diagnosis 3495
folate/B$_{12}$-independent *3490*, 3497–8
folate/B$_{12}$ metabolic disorders *3490*, 3497
in hereditary orotic aciduria 1386–7, 3497
investigations 3494–6
in Lesch-Nyhan syndrome 1382, 3497, 3686
management 3461
in pernicious anaemia 3490, 3677
in pregnancy 1759
skin disease and 3685–6
treatment 3496–7
in tropical countries 3467–8
see also anaemia, pernicious; folate, deficiency; vitamin B$_{12}$ (cyanocobalamin), deficiency
mega-oesophagus, in Chagas' disease 897
Megasphaera elsdenii 557
mega-trials, *see* clinical trials, large-scale randomized
megaureter 3243
megestrol acetate 4351
meglumine antimoniate, in visceral leishmaniasis 906
MEG-X (monoethylglycine xylidide) test 2056
Meig's syndrome 2867
meiosis 103
Meissner's (submucosal) plexus 1953
MEK protein 225, 1561
melaena 1827
peptic ulcer haemorrhage 1882
melanin 3706, 3754, 3755
in blackheads 3752–3
loss 3734
in telangiectasia 3785
melanocytes 3706
damage, in vitiligo 3755
melanocyte stimulating hormone (α-MSH) 1575
melanoma antigen gene (Mage-1) 228
melanoma, malignant 3708, 3725–6, *3726*, *3791*
aetiological factors 208
antigens 228
properties *229*
axillary lymph node enlargement 252
depth and survival 3725
diagnosis 3725, 3726
epidemiology 208
in halo naevi 3759
immunotherapy,
limb perfusion with TNFα 233
tumour infiltrating lymphocytes 260
incidence and risk factors 3725
metastases,
molecular basis and likelihood 231
in small bowel 1985
in pregnancy 1804, 1808
T-cell response 228
melanoptysis 2643, 2840
melanosis, transient neonatal pustular 3783
melanosis coli 1965, **2138**
in irritable bowel syndrome 1966

melanosomes 3755
Melarsoprol
  in African trypanosomiasis 893
  side-effects/toxicity 893
melasma 1804, *3754*
MELAS syndrome 4173
Meleney's synergistic infection 574
melioidosis **590–3**
  hepatic granulomas in 2121
  septicaemic 591
Melkersson-Rosenthal syndrome 3799,
  3802
melphalan
  leukaemia association 215
  in myeloma 3601
membrane-attack complex 164, 175
  deficiencies 180
  lytic pathway 175, 176, 177
  regulation 177
membrane proteins
  biogenesis and topogenesis 69
  quality control 70
  *trans*Golgi network function in
    targeting 71
membranes, preterm prelabour rupture
  (PPROM) **1786**, 1787
membranes of cells, internal, *see*
  endomembrane system
membrane-stabilizing drugs, in pain
  treatment 3945
membranous nephropathy **3158–60**,
  3300
  clinical presentation 3159
  drug-induced 3159, 3193
  hepatitis B-associated 3159, **3175–6**
  idiopathic 3159
  in malignant disease 3154, 3185
  recurrence after transplantation
    3161
  in rheumatoid arthritis 3159, 3193
  toxin-induced 3258–9
  treatment 3159–60
memory 3854
  anterograde/retrograde disturbances
    3855, 3856
  categories 3854, *3855*
  in dementia assessment 3968
  disorders,
    dissociative 4210
    verbal 3855
    see also amnesia
  distant, recall impairment 4210
  impairment,
    in Alzheimer's disease 3973
    in amnesic disorder 4225
  implicit 3855
  long-term 3854–5
    semantic and episodic 3855
  medial temporal lobe role 3855
  questions in mental state examination
    4203
  short-term 3854, 4225
Mendelian disorders, classification by
  gene locus 109
Mendelian inheritance **113–24**
Mendelson's syndrome 2735, 4276
  in pregnancy 1801
Ménière's disease **3875**
MEN I gene *1567*, 1568
MEN II gene *1567*, 1568
meningeal irritation
  meningitis *vs* 4056
  in tuberculous meningitis 4060
meningioma **4032**
  cerebellopontine angle 3875
  dementia due to 3971
  frontal, mental disorders/symptoms in
    4237
  optic chiasmal lesions 3867, *3868*
  orbital 3865
  parasellar 3865, *3868*
  pathology and sites 4032
  in pregnancy 1767
  subtraction carotid angiogram 3823
  treatment 3868
meningism 4053
  assessment 4053

meningococcal meningitis *vs* 540
  in *Shigella* infections 554
meningitis 4064
  acute bacterial (pyogenic/purulent)
    4050–60
  classification and aetiology 4050–2,
    4051
  clinical features 4052–5
  community-acquired 4050–1, *4051*,
    4058
  diagnosis 4055–6
  differential diagnosis 4053, 4056
  incubation period 4053
  intracranial abscess *vs* 4083
  management, *see below*
  mortality 4052–3, 4059
  pathogenesis 4052
  pathology 4052
  prevention 4059–60
  prognosis and sequelae 4059
  acute syphilitic 4084
  after head injury, *see* meningitis, post-
    traumatic
  anthrax 617
  aseptic,
    bacterial *4070*
    causes (non-viral) *4070*
    differential diagnosis 4056
    in HIV infection 4075
    viral, *see* meningitis, viral
  bacterial (pyogenic/purulent) **4050–64**
    acute, *see above*
  benign lymphocytic (viral),
    enteroviruses causing 386
  cerebrospinal, *see* meningitis, bacterial
  cerebrospinal fluid findings *3844*,
    4055–6, *4055*
    glucose levels 3844, *3844*, 4055, *4055*
  chemoprophylaxis 4059–60
  clinical features 3842–4055
    in immunocompromised 1033
  C-reactive protein in 1530
  cryptococcal 809, 810, 1033
    differential diagnosis 4056
    in HIV infection 472, 475, 479,
      4078–9
  device-associated 4050, 4051
    management *4057*, 4058–9
    prevention 4060
  electroencephalogram (EEG) in 3830
  eosinophilic **945–9**, *948*, 953
  epilepsy after 3917
  examination and diagnosis 267,
    4055–6, *4055*
  fungal *4070*
  in genital herpes 3352
  Haemophilus influenzae type b **581–2**,
    581, 4050
    clinical features 581
    diagnosis 581–2
    epidemiology and risk factors 581
    mortality 583
    pathogenesis 4052
    prevention and vaccine 583
    treatment 582, *4058*
  headache in 4027, 4053
  helminth infestations *4070*
  herpes simplex 345, 4066
    in HIV infection 4075
  in immunocompromised 1033, 1034
  in infective endocarditis 2441
  in leptospirosis 701
  Listeria monocytogenes 721, 4050,
    4051
    management *4058*
  lymphocytic 4062
    mumps virus causing 373, 374
    recurrent 4056
  management 4056–9, *4056*, *4057*, *4058*
    of complications 4059
    empirical treatment *4057*
    general 4059
    immediate antimicrobial therapy *4056*
    specific types 4058–9, *4058*
  meningococcal **539–40**, 4050
    clinical features 539, 4053
    course and prognosis 539–40

deafness after 540
diagnosis 540–1
epidemics, treatment 542
laboratory findings 539, 540
pathogenesis 537
prevention 4059
recurrent 4056
treatment 541–2, *4058*
Mollaret's (benign recurrent aseptic)
  345, **4056**
neonatal 4050, 4052
  clinical features 4054–5
  management *4057*
  mycoplasmas in 771
  pathogenesis 4052
in neonatal streptococcus B infection
  1788
Pasteurella causing 607–8
pituitary tumours 1582
plague 597
pneumococcal 512, 517, **518**, 518,
  4051
  clinical features 4053
  course and prognosis 518–19
  differential diagnosis 518
  epidemiology 512
  laboratory findings 518
  mortality 518–19
  recurrent 4056
  symptoms and signs 518
  treatment 518–19, 520, 521, *4058*
post-traumatic 3835, 4050, 4051
  clinical features 4055
  management *4057*, 4058
  pathogenesis 4052
protozoal *4070*
Pseudomonas aeruginosa, management
  4058
recurrent bacterial 4051–2
  differential diagnosis 4056
in secondary syphilis 711
spontaneous 4050
  management *4057*
  pathogenesis 4052
Staphylococcus aureus, management
  4058
streptococci group B infections 506,
  507, 508, 1788, 4050
  see also meningitis, pneumococcal
tuberculous 653, **4060–4**
  clinical features 4060–1
  diagnosis 4061–2
  differential diagnosis 4056, 4062
  epidemiology 4060
  in HIV infection 4060, 4061
  pathogenesis and pathology 4060
  prevention 4063–4
  prognosis and sequelae 4063
  treatment 4062–3
  treatment of complications 4063
viral 386
  clinical features 4066–7
  differential diagnosis 4069
  pathology 4066
meningococcaemia, acute 536, 537
  clinical features 538, 4053
  course and prognosis 538–9
  diagnosis 540
  laboratory findings 538
  mortality 539
  pathogenesis 537, 541
  treatment 541
meningococcaemia, chronic 540
meningococcal infections **533–44**
  antibiotic resistance 542
  antibodies in 537–8
  clinical features 538–41
  complications/pathogenesis 537
  contacts, management of 543–4
  culture 538
  diagnosis 538, 540–1
    lumbar puncture 539, 540
  epidemic, management 544
  epidemiology 535–6
    geographical/seasonality aspects
      535
  hypoglycaemia in 1510

immunity 537–8
  local 537
  systemic 537–8
immunological assays 540
meningitis, *see* meningitis
nasopharyngeal carriers 535–6, 542
  chemoprophylaxis 542
pathogenesis 536–7, 541
pathology 536
prophylaxis 542–4, *542*
  chemoprophylaxis 542–3, *542*, *543*
  epidemics 544
  small outbreaks/endemic disease
    543–4
  vaccines, *see* meningococcal vaccines
purpura in 3636
risk factors 536, *536*
septicaemia, symptoms 4053
spread 536–7
treatment 541–2
  antibiotics 541, 541–2
  supportive 541, 542
  see also meningococcaemia, acute;
    Neisseria meningitidis
meningococcal vaccines 319, 323, 543
  conjugate 543
  efficacy 543, *543*
  group A and C polysaccharide 543
  group B 543, *543*
  use in epidemics 544
  vaccination 3530, 3596
meningoencephalitis
  in African trypanosomiasis 889, 890,
    891, 892
  amoebic 833
  Angiostrongylus cantonensis infection
    945–9, 953
  in infective endocarditis 2441
  in listeriosis 721
meningoencephalomyelitis 4053
meningomyelitis, syphilitic 4084
meningomyelocele
  management 4117, 4118
  management criteria 13
meningoradiculitis, lymphocytic
  (Bannwarth's syndrome) 689, 690
meningovascular syphilis **4084–5**, 4236
  mental disorders/symptoms 4236
Menkes' kinky hair syndrome **1417–19**,
  3763, 3989
menopause 1563, 1672, 1813
  clinical features 1813
  hirsutism after 3765
menstrual cycle 1563, 1565
  acute porphyria and 1393
  asthma and 2736
  blood loss estimation 3375, 3476
  body temperature changes 1015
  constipation relation 1967
  diabetes control and 1497
  disorders,
    in anorexia nervosa 1297, 4213
    approach to 1669–70
    benign intracranial hypertension and
      4042
    in bulimia nervosa 1300, 4216
    in congenital adrenal hyperplasia 1664
    oral contraceptives in 1670, 1723
    in polycystic ovary syndrome 1673
    see also amenorrhoea
  exercise-induced changes 4326
  gonadotrophins 1580, 1581
  migraine associated 4025
  oral ulceration association 1853, 1854
  re-establishment in anorexia nervosa
    1298, 4214
  toxic shock syndrome association 530
MEN syndromes, *see* multiple endocrine
  neoplasia (MEN) syndromes
mental confusion, *see* confusion
mental disorders
  in elderly **4226–8**
  organic, *see* organic mental disorders
  physical disorders causing **4236–43**
    collagen disorders 4243
    drug-induced 4241–2
    endocrine disorders 4238–40

malignancy 4243
metabolic disorders 4240–1
neurological conditions 4236–8
postoperative complications 4243
treatment refusal 4257
see also psychiatric disorders
Mental Health Act (1983) 4230, 4257, 4289, 4295, 4317
mentally impaired, consent and 4317
mental retardation **4107–11**
α-thalassaemia (ATR) syndrome 3511
autism **4108**
causes *4107*
chromosomal anomalies **4108–11**
deletion syndromes 4109–11
sex chromosomal anomalies 4109
trisomies 4108–9
in cystathionine synthase deficiency 1366
epilepsy and 3916–17
in galactosaemia 1349, 1350
learning disorders **4108**
in phenylketonuria 1361, 1362
prediction/detection 4107
risk factors 4107
in single gene disorders 4111–12
in urea cycle defects 1358
mental state examination 4203
alcohol/drug abuser in custody 4304
brief interview 4203
in elderly 4226
Mini Mental State Examination *3970*, 4226
questionnaire 4203
mepacrine, sun exposure protection 3728
meprobamate, overdose/poisoning 1060
meptazinol 697
meralgia paraesthetica 4097
mercaptoacetyltriglycine, radiolabelled ([⁹⁹Tcᵐ]MAG3) 3112, 3114, 3115
6-mercaptopurine
in Crohn's disease 1942
drug interactions 1257
in ulcerative colitis 1949
mercurialentis 1111
'mercurial erethism' 1111
mercuric chloride, poisoning 1111
mercuric oxide, poisoning 1111
mercury 1111
absorption and half-life 1111
environmental disaster 1233
see also Minamata disease
forms and uses 1111
injection 1111
inorganic, exposure 1111
nephropathy 3259, *3261*, **3262**
neuropathy 4099
occupational/non-occupational exposure 1111
organic compounds 1111, 1233
exposure 1111–12
poisoning **1111–12**, 1174, 1233
acute/chronic 1111–12
clinical features 1111–12, 1174
medical surveillance 1112
treatment 1112
mercury vapour, exposure 1111
merozoites 835
merycism, *see* rumination
mesalazine
in Crohn's disease 1942, 1943
resin-coated 1949, *1949*
mescaline, psychiatric disturbances from 4241
mesenchymal cells, in myositis ossificans progressiva 3093
mesenchymal tumours
calcitriol deficiency 1637
rickets in 3074
mesenteric adenitis 2010
mesenteric arteries
aneurysms 2000
disease affecting, intestinal ischaemia in 1995
obstruction 2367
mesenteric infarction, in SLE 3020
mesenteric ischaemia 2367

mesenteric lymph nodes
in enteropathy-associated T-cell lymphoma 1928
in Whipple's disease 1923
mesenteric vascular insufficiency 1994, 1995, 1996
see also intestinal ischaemia
mesial temporal sclerosis 3923
mesoatrial shunt 2099
Mesocestoides variabilis 962, 963
mesothelioma
fibrous (benign) 2893
peritoneal 2009
mesothelioma, malignant **2893–5**, 2893
asbestos association 207, 2843, 2844, 2894
dosage 2894
fibre type 2894
time from first exposure 2894
see also asbestos
clinical features 2894
chest pain 2169
epidemiology 207
hypoglycaemia due to 1509–10
investigations,
biopsy 2684
chest radiography 2664, 2894–5
pleural fluid examination 2686, 2895
management and prognosis 2895
pathology 2894
messenger RNA (mRNA) 57
degradation, new anticancer therapy 260
growth factor receptor 224
immunological purification methods 61
low abundance and probe construction 61
post-transcriptional modification 57, 57–9
primary transcript 57
splicing 57, 59
mutations interfering 63
synthesis, *see* transcription
translation, *see* translation
transport from nucleus 79
mesterolone 1684
meta-analyses, *see* systematic overviews
metabolic acidosis **1540–3**
causes 1536, *1537*, *1538*
in chronic renal failure 3305
diagnosis 1535
in hepatocellular failure 2103, 2109
high anion gap 1536, *1537*
in hyperparathyroidism 1624, 1632
in hypothermia 1183
in isoniazid poisoning 1068
in malaria 846, 855
mental symptoms 4240
in methanol poisoning 1081
neurological features 4126
normal anion gap 1536, *1538*
paracetamol-induced 1052
in poisoning 1047
respiratory effects 1537–9
in salicylate poisoning 1054
treatment 855, 1543–4, 2109
in tricyclic antidepressant poisoning 1059
see also lactic acidosis
metabolic alkalosis
causes 1536, *1538*
diagnosis 1536
diuretic complication in cor pulmonale 2521
in hepatocellular failure 2103
potassium depletion 1540, 3130
treatment 1544
in vomiting 1821
metabolic capacity, of body 1285
metabolic disorders **1333–549**
dementia due to 3971
in elderly **4344–6**
electroencephalogram (EEG) in 3830
endocrine disease causing **4125**
enteral feeding complication 1321
inborn, *see* inborn errors of metabolism
ionic/acid-base abnormalities causing **4125–8**

joint involvement **3003–2994**
mental disorders/symptoms in **4239–41**
nervous system **4123–4**
neuropathies in **4098–9**
in organ failure **4124–5**
parenteral nutrition complication 1319–21
pyrophosphate arthropathy association 2989
see also specific disorders
metabolic fuel, *see* energy; fuel, metabolic
metabolic myopathies, *see* myopathy
metabolic rate
after injury 1549
basal, *see* basal metabolic rate (BMR)
in malnutrition *1291*
red cell production and 3382
resting, prediction *1307*
metabolism
carbohydrate, *see* carbohydrate, metabolism
in chronic renal failure 3302–3
effects of injury and surgery **1548–50**
energy 4165, 4166, 4167
fat **1276–7**
inborn errors of, *see* inborn errors of metabolism
in malnutrition 1285–7
in pregnancy 1752–3
protein, *see* protein, metabolism
regulation 1273–4, *1274*, 1458
in starvation **1277–8**
see also biochemistry; metabolic disorders
metabolites, intermediary, reference range *4370*
metacarpophalangeal joints, in rheumatoid arthritis 2957
metacercariae 988, 991
metachromatic leukodystrophy (sulphatidosis) *1428*, **1429**, 3986
metagonimiasis **998–9**
Metagonimus yokogawai 996, 998
Metakelfin, in malaria 852–3
metal(s)
cancer association 1167
contact dermatitis due to 3738
nephropathies 1171, **3260–3**
normal range *4372*
poisoning **1105–15**
cardiovascular effects 1170–1
genitourinary effects 1171
neuropsychological disorders 1174
see also individual metals
metaldehyde poisoning **1124**
metal fume fever 1109, 1114, 2813, **2847–8**
metalloenzymes, zinc requirement 1114
metalloids, cancer association 1167
metalloproteinase, tissue inhibitor (TIMP), in chronic obstructive airways disease 2773
metamyelocyte 3556–7
metanephrine 2554
metanizole, poisoning 1057
metaphyseal disorders 3089
metastases 195
genetic basis 196
molecular basis 231
cellular adhesion molecules 231
in melanomas 231
unknown primary site 251–2, *252*
see also specific metastases/sites/ tumours
metatarsalgia 2958, 2997
metatarsophalangeal joints
in gout 2984, 2985
in rheumatoid arthritis 2958
metformin 1471–2, 1542
methacholine
in achalasia 1959
asthma severity relation 2726
asthma testing 2733
methadone 4276, **4292**, *4353*
mechanism of action and dose 4292
in opiate detoxification 4292, 4299

pain relief in drug abusers 4301
in pregnancy 4299
methaemalbumin 3526
methaemoglobin *3379*, 3526
methaemoglobinaemia **3519–20**, 3546
acquired 3520
acute toxic 3520
antimalarial overdose 1073
in chlorate poisoning 1121
in cyanide poisoning treatment 1098
genetic 3519
in nitrogen dioxide poisoning 1100
occupational causes 1172
methaemoglobin reductase 3456
methane, poisoning 1083
methanol
acidosis induced by 1543
metabolism and mechanisms of toxicity 1080
poisoning **1080–1**
uses 1080
methicillin, *S. aureus* resistance, *see under Staphylococcus aureus*
methicillin nephropathy 3264
methimazole 1612
methionine 1048, *1353*, 1365, 1366
low dietary 3085
in paracetamol poisoning 1048, 1052
dosage 1053, *1053*
plasma 1366, 1367
methionine adenosyltransferase 1365
deficiency 1367
methionine synthase 1365, 1366
deficiency 1367
methotrexate
in bone marrow transplantation 3697
folate deficiency due to 3493, 3497
low-dose, in rheumatoid arthritis 2964
in lupus nephritis 3191
in psoriasis 3750
in SLE 3024
methotrimeprazine, in terminal illness 4356
methoxypsoralen 3748
methsuximide, overdose/poisoning 1062
2-methyl aceto acetyl coenzyme A thiolase deficiency *1370*
methyl alcohol, *see* methanol
methylated spirits 1080
methylation, of genes 59, **107**, 126
methyl bromide
mechanisms of toxicity 1086
poisoning **1086**
methyl chloride
mechanisms of toxicity 1087
poisoning **1086–7**
methyl chloroform (1,1,1-trichloroethane), poisoning 1089
methyl-cobalamin (methyl-B₁₂) 3484
methylcrotonyl coenzyme A carboxylase 1373
deficiency *1370*
methyldopa
haemolytic anaemia due to 3542–3
overdose/poisoning **1067**
in pre-eclampsia 1731
in pregnancy 1732, 1811, 1812
methylene blue 1073
in methaemoglobinaemia 3519, 3520
methylene chloride (dichloromethane)
mechanisms of toxicity 1087
poisoning **1087–8**, 1172
3,4-methylenedioxymethamphetamine, *see* MDMA (Ecstasy)
methylene diphosphonate, radiolabelled ([⁹⁹Tcᵐ]MDP) 3240
methylene tetrahydrofolate reductase (MTR) 1365, 1366
deficiency 1367
3-methyl glutaconyl coenzyme A hydratase deficiency *1370*
3-methylhistidine 1274, 1275, 1276
excretion 1275, 1278
methyl iodide, poisoning **1087**
methyl isocyanate 1100
Bhopal disaster 1233
poisoning 1115

methylmalonic acidaemia *1337*, **1370–2**, 3497
methylmalonic acid (MMA)
　serum 3495
　urinary 3495
methylmalonyl coenzyme A mutase 1369, 1370, 1371
methylmercury poisoning 1111
Methylobacterium, rare species 557
methylprednisolone
　adverse effects *3164*
　in aplastic anaemia 3446
　high-dose,
　　in demyelinating disorders 3995
　　in spinal cord injury 3898
　intravenous pulse,
　　in acute flare in SLE 3023
　　mechanism of action 3024
　　single, in SLE 3024
　in Langerhans-cell histiocytosis 3609
　in lupus nephritis 3190
　in membranous nephropathy 3160
　in rapidly progressive glomerulonephritis 3162, 3166–7
　in renal failure 3274
　in retroperitoneal fibrosis 3245
4-methylpyrazole 1081, 1082
methyl salicylate, poisoning 1054
methyl tert-butyl ether (MTBE) 2048, 2049
methyltestosterone 3772
5-methyltetrahydrofolate (methyl-THF) 1365, 3486, 3487, 3488–9
methylxanthine bronchodilators 2738
methysergide
　mediastinal/pleural fibrosis due to 2852
　in migraine 4025
metoclopramide
　absorption interaction 1255
　in diabetic gastroparesis 1489
　effect on paracetamol absorption 1249
　overdose/poisoning **1070**
metolazone 2240, 3304
metoprolol
　airway obstruction and asthma 2849
　in dilated cardiomyopathy 2384
Met receptor, amplification 224
metrifonate 979
metronidazole
　in acute ulcerative gingivitis 1853
　in amoebiasis 831, 832
　anaerobic bacteria sensitivity 575, 576
　breast feeding and 1811
　in Crohn's disease 1942
　in giardiasis in hypogammaglobulinaemia 168
　in gnathostomiasis 954
　intravenous 576
　in pregnancy 1785
　in pseudomembranous colitis 636
　side-effects 831
　in tetanus 628
　in trichomoniasis 908
metyrapone 1575, 1651
　in ectopic ACTH syndrome 1713
　in pregnancy 1751
　test *4375*
　　in Cushing's syndrome 1647, 1648, 1649
mevalonate kinase deficiency *1370*
mexiletine *2264*, 3945
　overdose/poisoning 1064
MIAMI trial 2345
mianserin 4248
　overdose 1059
MIBG scanning
　in carcinoid tumours 1898
　in phaeochromocytomas 2556
　therapeutic, in malignant phaeochromocytoma 2557
mica 2845
　pneumoconiosis 2846
micelles 1903, 2047
Michaelis constant 1195
Michigan Alcoholism Screening Test (MAST) 4272
miconazole 811
microadenocarcinoma, pancreatic 2042

microagglutination test, leptospirosis diagnosis 702
microalbuminuria 3102, **3138**
　in diabetes mellitus 1464, 3138, 3168, 3170
　　monitoring in 1479–80
　in SLE 3138
microbiology services, developing countries 311
microcephaly 4116
microcytosis 3377, *3378*
microemboli, in infective endocarditis 2440
microfilaments 81–2
　behaviour and function 81
　　organelle movement/contraction 80, 81
　microtubule system connection 82
　subunit proteins 81
microfilariae 911, 912, 918, 919
　description 911, 920
　in eye 915
microfilaricides 916
microglia 3990
β₂-microglobulin 142
　amyloid formation 1517–18, **1520–1**, 1524, 3312
　plasma, glomerular filtration rate from **3107**
　in urine 3109, 3137
　in Balkan nephropathy 3230
micrognathia 2910
　in manganese poisoning 1110
micrographia 4001
microhamartoma, liver 2016
microimmunofluorescence
　chlamydial infection diagnosis 750, *755*, 756, 761
　lymphogranuloma venereum diagnosis 761
　Mycoplasma pneumoniae 764
　see also immunofluorescence
microinfarcts, divers 1211
microlight flying 2361
micrometastases, monoclonal antibodies in therapy 233
micro-organisms
　biology **268–74**
　extrinsic allergic alveolitis due to 2810–11, *2810*
　fate in spleen 3589
　phagocytosis and killing 3559–60
　sexual transmission *3345*
　see also bacteria; protozoa; viruses
microperoxisomes 1438
Micropolyspora faeni 2809
microscopic polyangiitis 3010, **3013–14**
　lung disease in 3014
　renal disease in 3013–14
　response to treatment 3017
microscopy
　dark-field, in syphilis 714
　in infections 267
microsporidia 883
　lifecycle and species 883–4, *884*, 885
Microsporidium 1930
　species 884, *884*
microsporidosis **883–6**
　in HIV infection 487, 884, 886
Microsporum, species 797, 798
Microsporum canis 3762
microthrombosis, diffuse 1995
microtubule organizing centre (MTOC) 81, 82
microtubules 80–1, 82–3
　distribution patterns 82
　drugs disrupting 82
　functions 81 in interphase cells 81
　microfilaments system connection 82
　in myocardial cells 2144
　organelle attachment proteins 83
　role, endoplasmic reticulum assembly 82
　subunit proteins 81
　subunits and structure 82
microvasculature, heart failure pathophysiology 2231
microwave ovens 1222

micturating cystography, radionuclide 3215
micturating cystourethrography 3111, **3214–15**, 3217
micturition
　disorders of **3146–8**
　frequency **3148**, 3206–7
　syncope 3918, **3926**, 3926
midazolam 2031
　in endoscopy 1830
　in terminal illness 4356
midbrain **3858**
　haemorrhage 3954
　lesions 2584, 3858
　　pupillary responses 2582
　tumours 4036
middle cerebral artery, infarction 3956
middle ear, *see* ear, middle
midgut 1973
mid upper arm circumference 1281, *1282*
migraine 3918, **4024–6**
　aetiology and precipitants 4025, *4025*
　cerebral infarction and 3956
　classical (with aura) 4024
　clinical features 4024–5
　common (without aura) 4024
　definition 4024
　electroencephalogram (EEG) in 3830
　epileptic seizures *vs* 3918
　food intolerance 1844, 4025
　hormone replacement therapy and 1815
　mechanisms 4023
　menstrual 4025
　in pregnancy 1767
　prophylaxis 4025
　treatment 4025, *4026*
　vestibular system in 3876, 4024
migraine sine cephalgia 4025
migrainous neuralgia 4026
migrants, malaria epidemics 840
migrating myoelectric (motor) complex (MMC) 1954, 1956
migration 37, 51
Mikity-Wilson syndrome 1792
Mikulicz's syndrome 1861, 4182
　mumps *vs* 375
milia 3783
miliaria crystallina 3767, 3784
MILIS trial 2334
milk
　intolerance, in malnutrition 1293
　protein allergy 1944
　Q fever transmission 742
　see also cows' milk
Millard-Gubler syndrome 3858
Miller-Dieker syndrome 4113
Miller-Fisher syndrome 4101
millipedes 1149–50
milrinone 2253
Milroy's disease 2560
Milwaukee shoulder 2991
Minamata disease 1111, 1142, 1233, 3262, 4099
mind-acting drugs **4263–4**
　see also drug abuse and misuse
mineral dust exposure 2839
　pulmonary alveolar proteinosis 2833
mineralocorticoids 1639
　biosynthesis *1640*, 1664
　deficiency **1662–3**
　excess **1656–62**
　　acquired apparent syndromes 1661
　　iatrogenic 1661–2
　　mineralocorticoids other than aldosterone *1656*, 1660–2
　　syndrome of congenital apparent 1661
　　see also aldosteronism
　receptor 1557, 1562, 1661
　　defects 1662, 1669
　renal tubular resistance 3337
　replacement therapy 1655–6, 1665
　see also aldosterone
mineral oil, aspiration 2837
mineral oil enema 2837
minerals
　absorption *1901*, 1903

reference nutrient intake 1268, *1269*, 1330, *1331*
　requirements, artificial nutritional support 1318, *1318*
'miner's anaemia' 930
mines
　coal 2839, 2840
　pneumoconioses and 2839
minimal change nephropathy **3154–6**
　in adults 3155–6
　aetiology 3154
　in children 3153–4, **3155**, 3156
　as 'idiopathic nephrotic syndrome' variant 3154
　NSAID-induced 3224
　pathogenesis 3155
　pathology 3155
　toxin-induced 3259
minimal inhibitory concentrations (MIC) 298, 307, 756–7, *757*
Mini-Mental State Examination *3970*, 4226
minimum bactericidal concentration (MBC) 2446
minimyosin (myosin I) 81–2
mini-satellite DNA 62
Ministry of Health 52
minitracheostomy 2581, **2919**
minocycline, in leprosy 677
minor histocompatibility antigens 183, 185
　in graft rejection 185, 186
minoxidil 2543, 3304
　in hypertension 2541
miosis 3877
　in nerve agent exposure 1117–18
miracidium 972
Mirizzi's syndrome 2050
miscarriage, spontaneous, occupational toxins 1173
misoprostol
　peptic ulcer treatment 1888
　in pregnancy 1801
mites
　follicle 1009
　house dust, *see* house dust mites
　larval (chigger) 739
　lifecycle 1007
　miscellaneous 1009–10
　phobia about 1009
　scrub 1010
　straw (grain) 1010
　see also scabies
mithramycin 1638, 3229
　in myeloma 3603
　in Paget's disease 3077
mitochondria 68
　antigens, autoantibodies to 163
　disorders *1335*
　　epilepsy in 3915
　DNA 128, 4171
　　deletions 4171, 4172
　　mutations 64
　　mutations and 'bottleneck' effect 128
　DNA defects **128–9**, *1335*, 4171–2, *4172*
　　in diabetes type II 1454, 1456
　fatigue pathophysiology 2172
　gene defects **128–9**, 4171–2, *4172*
　　see also Leber's hereditary optic neuropathy (LHON)
　metabolism in 4171
　in muscle fibres 4143
　myocardial cells 2145
　pyruvate metabolism 2146
　number 128
　　endurance sports training 4325
　oxidative metabolism limited by 2604–5, *2605*, 4171
　in Reye's syndrome 2025
　volume, maximum oxygen consumption and 2604, *2605*
mitochondrial encephalopathy, lactic acidosis and stroke-like episodes (MELAS) 4173
mitochondrial myopathy (encephalomyopathy) 4142, 4148, **4171–4**
　aetiology 4171–2

biochemistry 4171
clinical features and groups 4172–3
diagnosis and prognosis 4173
genetics 4171–2
histology 4144
mitogen activated pathway (MAP)
  kinases 1561
mitomycin C, haemolytic uraemic
  syndrome and 3197, 3199
mitosis 102, 103, 119
  cell multiplication control 191
  intermediate filaments changes during
    81
  nuclear envelope assembly 80
  vesicular transport control during 78
mitoxantrone, in hepatocellular
  carcinoma 2117
mitral incompetence, *see* mitral
  regurgitation
mitral prolapse **2460**
  chest pain in 2167
  in hyperthyroidism 2394
  infective endocarditis in 2436, 2439,
    2451
  in polycystic kidney disease 3203
  in pregnancy 1738
  in tricuspid atresia 2412
mitral regurgitation **2424**, 2427, 2455,
  2457–62
  aetiology 2457–8, *2458*
  clinical features 2458–61
  diagnosis/differential diagnosis 2461–2
  Doppler echocardiography 2202, *2202*,
    2459, 2460
  in endomyocardial fibrosis 2397,
    2460–1
  in hypertrophic cardiomyopathy 2387,
    2459
  in infective endocarditis 2457
  magnetic resonance imaging 2216,
    2217
  mitral stenosis with **2456–7**
  paraprosthetic 2470–1
  pathophysiology 2458
  in pregnancy 1737
  rheumatic 2433, 2458
  ruptured chordae tendineae 2458–9
  see also mitral prolapse; papillary
    muscle, dysfunction
mitral ring 2451, 2459
  calcification 2461
mitral stenosis 2181, **2452–6**
  aetiology 2452
  cardiac myxoma *vs* 2473
  clinical features 2452–3
    chest pain 2167
  congenital 2452
  diagnosis/differential diagnosis 2454–5
  Doppler echocardiography 2201,
    2453–4, 2455
  examination/investigations 2453–4
  infective endocarditis in 2445
  magnetic resonance imaging 2216,
    2217
  mitral regurgitation with **2456–7**
  pathology and physiology 2452
  in pregnancy 1737
  prognosis 2456
  rheumatic 2432, **2452**, 2467
    in Ebstein's anomaly 2413
  'silent' 2453, 2454
  treatment 2455–6
mitral valve **2451–62**
  atresia, with univentricular heart **2419**
  ballooning (billowing), *see* mitral valve,
    floppy
  balloon valvuloplasty, in pregnancy
    1737
  calcification 2182, 2453
  cusps 2451
    fusion in rheumatic fever 2452, 2455
    in mitral regurgitation 2457
    in mixed mitral valve disease 2456
  prolapse, *see* mitral prolapse
  ulceration 2457
  disease 2182, **2452–62**
    Doppler echocardiography 2201–2
    epilepsy after 3917

infective endocarditis in 528, 2459,
  2460
pulmonary hypertension in 2509, 2513
see also mitral regurgitation; mitral
  stenosis
floppy 2457, 2460
  in hypertrophic cardiomyopathy 2384,
    2386, 2388, 2459
  'jet lesions' 2457, 2464
  mixed disease **2456–7**
  mucinous (myxomatous) degeneration
    2457
  normal anatomy 2451
  parachute 2452
  physiology 2451–2
  prolapse, *see* mitral prolapse
  prostheses 2470
    endocarditis 2445
    life span 2456
    replacement 2456, 2457, 2461
      in children 2470
      indications 2456
      tricuspid regurgitation after 2468
    in rheumatic fever 2432
    in rheumatoid arthritis 2961
    staphylococcal endocarditis 528, 2439
    surgery 2456, 2461–2
    valvuloplasty 2455–6
    vegetations 2438, 2457
mitral valvotomy
  closed 2456
  open 2456
  in pregnancy 1738
Mitsuda reaction 668
mixed connective tissue disease 3008,
  3035
  lung involvement in **2799**
  renal involvement **3191** mixed
    lymphocyte reaction 151, 184
mixed micelles 2047
MMC (migrating myoelectric (motor)
  complex) 1954, 1956
mobility
  impairment in multiple sclerosis 3995
  see also immobility/immobilization
Mobiluncus, rare species 557
Mobitz second degree block, *see*
  atrioventricular block
Möbius syndrome 4151
moccasins, bites and envenoming
  1132–3
moclobemide 1248, 4250
  mechanism of action 4249
  use and side-effects 4250
modified-release formulations 1239
'modulation' of response, in
  schistosomiasis 976, 977
Moebius syndrome **4114**
Mokola virus 395, *396*
molar pregnancy, *see* hydatidiform mole
molecular biology **57–67**
  gene mapping **62–3**
  gene structure and function **57–9**
  impact **67**
  see also biotechnology; gene(s);
    recombinant DNA technology
molecular mimicry 141
  autoantibodies in SLE 3026
  heat-shock proteins and Behçet's
    syndrome 3044
  HLA-B27 and ankylosing spondylitis
    2966
  in infection-associated
    glomerulonephritis 3173
molecular taxonomy, bacterial
  classification **272–4**
  rRNA sequencing **273–4**, *274*
  species definition 273
Mollaret's cells 4056
Mollaret's meningitis 345, **4056**
mollusca
  poisoning from 1142
  venomous **1144**
molluscides **1124**
molluscum contagiosum **371–2**, 3797,
  3798
molybdenum deficiency, oesophageal
  cancer association 202

'Monday morning fever' 1114, 1170,
  2647, 2813, 2848
Monge's disease 1192
MONICA study 2307, 2311, 2312
moniliasis, *see* candidiasis, oral
monkeypox 366
  human 368–9
monoamine
  drugs altering function 4253–4
  receptor antagonists 4248, *4249*
monoamine oxidase 2253, 2553
  type A and type B 4249
  type B, alcoholism marker 2081
monoamine oxidase inhibitors (MAOIs)
  1247–8, 4249–50
  'cheese reaction' 1248
  consequences of use 4249
  in depressive disorders 4220
  drug interactions 1257, 4005, 4249, 4250
  drugs included 4249
  food interactions 1248, 4249, 4250
  indications and use 4249
  mechanism of action 4249
  overdose 1059
  pharmacology 4249
  selective 5-HT uptake inhibitor
    interaction 4249
  side-effects 4249–50
  type A (moclobemide) 4249
  type B (selegiline), in Parkinson's
    disease 4002
monoarthritis **2946**
  causes *2946*
  see also arthritis
monochloroethylene, *see* vinyl chloride
monoclonal antibodies 146
  4D5 226
  5CR rat anti-mouse 88
  antimyosin 2207
  CAMPATH-1H 3424
  in cancer therapy 225–6, 233
    new developments 260
    two-step strategy 260
  to *Chlamydia* 761
  to cytomegalovirus (CMV) 362
  to dengue viruses 421
  diagnostic use 66
  to endotoxin 1025–6
  to growth factor receptors, anticancer
    action 225, 226
  to herpes simplex virus 346
  humanized 66, 226, 232
  in leukaemia 3399, 3413
  to lung cancer antigens 2882
  in lymphoproliferative disorders 3564
  micrometastases 233
  to *Neisseria gonorrhoeae* 548
  to *Plasmodium falciparum* 849
  to platelets (C7E3) 2330, 2352
  synthesis 226, 232
  to T-cell differentiation antigens 149
  to tumour cells 229, *230*
    anti-idiotypic response to 232
    penetration into tumour 232, 233
    tumour prognosis assessment 232
    tumour typing and identification *232*
  to tumour necrosis factor 541
monoclonal gammopathy, in POEMS
  syndrome 4104–5
monoclonal gammopathy of uncertain
  significance (benign; MGUS) 3599,
  3605
  amyloidosis in 1515, 1523, 1524
monoclonal paraproteins (M proteins)
  in monoclonal gammopathy of
    uncertain significance 3605
  in myeloma 3597, 3598, 3599, *3600*
    in relapse 3602–3
    response to therapy 3601
    in solitary plasmacytoma 3604
  in Waldenström's macroglobulinaemia
    3604
monocyte chemotactic and activating
  factor (MCAF) 3559
monocyte chemotactic protein-1 87, 97
monocyte-macrophage colony-
  stimulating factor (M-CSF) 3384,
  3388, 3557

monocytes 153, 3377, **3556**
  adhesion and receptors in 88
  in allergic disease 159
  circulation 85, 87–8
  counts *3379*, *3380*
  differentiation 3557
  emigration from pulmonary capillaries
    2623
    cessation 2624
  endothelial cell reaction 87, 88
  in fibrinolysis 3626
  in lung inflammation 2618
  maturation 2618, **2623**, 3557
    in atherogenesis 2291
  migration into tissues 3559
  production 3384, 3386, 3388
  recruitment 85, 87
  see also macrophage
monocytosis 3378, 3558
  in bacterial infections 3679
  in malignant disease 3678
monoiodotyrosine 1605
mononeuritis multiplex 2800, 2961,
  3841, 4092
  in microscopic polyangiitis 3014
  in polyarteritis nodosa 3015
  in Wegener's granulomatosis 3013
mononeuropathy 4092
  diabetic 1486, 1487–8
  pain in 3940
  in pregnancy 1766
mononuclear phagocytic system **85–95**
  definition 85
  see also macrophage; monocytes
monosaccharide, transport 1903
monosodium urate monohydrate crystals
  2950, 2951, 2984, 2986
  see also gout
monosomy 5 (-5), in myelodysplastic
  syndromes *3428*, 3429
monosomy 7 (-7), in myelodysplastic
  syndromes 3428
monosomy duplication 128
Monospot test 354
monounsaturated fatty acids, *see* fatty
  acids, monounsaturated
Montreal platelet syndrome 3645
Montreal Twin Study, hypertension 2529
mood changes
  exercise-induced 2161
  in malnutrition 1283
mood disorder, organic 4225
mood stabilizing drugs **4250–1**
  skin disease management 3807
  see also carbamazepine; lithium
moonshine alcohol 3261
MOPP regimen *3573*, 3574
Moraxella, rare species *557–8*
Moraxella catarrhalis
  acute exacerbation of chronic bronchitis
    2692
  in bronchiectasis 2763
  pneumonia due to 2694
  morbidity, in United Kingdom **41–6**
*Morerastrongylus (Angiostrongylus)
  costaricensis* 945, 949
morfamquat poisoning 1120
morphea, *see* morphoea
morphine
  alternatives 4352, *4353*
  in cancer pain 4352
  dyspnoea treatment, in terminal illness
    4354–5
  epidural 4352
  overdose 1058
  preparations 4352
  problems 4352
  psychiatric disturbances from 4241
  in pulmonary oedema 2504
  in terminal illness 4351, 4352, 4356
  tolerance and addiction 4352
morphine sulphate
  long-acting 253
  short-acting (Sevredol) 253
morphoea 3027, 3791, 3792
  see also scleroderma
Morquio disease (mucopolysaccharidosis
  IV) 1431, *1432*, **3087**

mortality
  age-related 43, 221, 4333
  causes and age-related 2332
  infant 40, 51
  infectious disease 287
  maternal, *see* maternal mortality
  overweight/obesity relationship
    1301–5
  perinatal, *see* perinatal mortality
  poisoning 1043, *1044*
  seasonal **1185**
  standardized ratio 43
  in United Kingdom **39–41**
    causes 2332
Morton's metatarsalgia 2997, 4098
'morular cells of Mott' 889, 890
mosaicism 118, **123–4**
  clonal origin of tumours 192
  effects of 123
  gonadal 107, 116, 135
  osteogenesis imperfecta inheritance
    3082
  pathogenesis 124
  placental 124, 136
  somatic, *see* somatic mosaicism
Moschowitz syndrome, *see* thrombotic
  thrombocytopenic purpura
mosquitoes 1011
  bite prevention 858–9, 860
  control in malaria prevention 858
  dengue virus transmission 413, 419
  flavivirus transmission 412, 413
  lymphatic filariasis spread 920
  malaria transmission 835
mothers, single 36
motilin 1894
  in tropical sprue 1934
motility, gastrointestinal, *see*
  gastrointestinal motility
motion sickness 322, 1203, 1821
motor nerves
  in herpes zoster 349
  muscle fibre control 4141
Motor Neurone Disease Association
  4088
motor neurone diseases **4087–90**
  classification *4087*
  differential diagnosis 4088
  magnetic brain stimulation in 3837–8
  management 4087
  postirradiation 4089
  respiratory muscle function tests 2668
  see also amyotrophic lateral sclerosis
motor neurones **3856–7**
motor neurone syndromes, *see* lower
  motor neurone syndromes; upper
  motor neurone syndromes
motor neuropathy
  diabetic proximal (femoral) 1486, 1487
  occupational 1169, *1170*
  see also neuropathy; peripheral
    neuropathy
motor proteins 83
motor racing, licences and fitness 2359
motor responses, in unconscious patient
  assessment 2584–5
motor system **3856–7**, 3891
  lesions 3857
  in multiple sclerosis 3993
motor unit 3839, 3856, 4139
motor unit potentials 3839
Mounier-Kuhn disease 2724
mountain climbing 1186
mountain fever (Colorado tick fever)
  406
mountain sickness
  acute 1187–91
    cerebral oedema 1188
    diagnosis/differential diagnosis 1190
    incidence and locations 1189–90
    pathophysiology 1188–9
    predisposing factors 1188
    prognosis 1191
    prophylaxis 1190
    pulmonary oedema in 1188
    symptoms and signs 1187, 1188
    treatment 1190–1

  see also altitudes, high; cerebral
    oedema; pulmonary oedema
  chronic (Monge's disease) 1192
mouse
  athymic (nude) 152
  genetics, uses in polygenic disease
    analysis 64
  LCMV infections 436
  non-obese diabetic (NOD) 64, 1453
  Spotch 107
  transgenic, *see* transgenic mice
  tumour antigens, properties *229*
  tumour cells, genetic analysis 193–4
mouse mammary tumour virus, growth
  factor overexpression 223
mouth **1846–65**
  in AIDS 474, 1850–1
  anaerobic flora 570
  bacterial infections **1852–3**
  benign neoplasms and cysts **1859–60**
  bleeding in, in haemophilia 3648
  blood disorder manifestations 1863–4
  bullous lesions **1855–8**
  developmental and inflammatory
    lesions **1859–60**
  dry **1861**, 2945
    in Sjögren's syndrome 3036
    in systemic sclerosis 3033–4
    treatment 3038
  electrical burns 1214
  examination 3376
    in infectious diseases 266
  fungal infections **1851–2**
  in gnathostomiasis 952
  in herpes simplex infections 342, 343
  human papillomaviruses (HPV)
    infections 445–6
  irritation, poisonous plants causing
    1152, *1153*
  in Kawasaki disease 3047
  leucoplakia, *see* leucoplakia
  in lichen planus 3751
  miscellaneous disorders **1863–4**
  in pemphigus vulgaris 3781
  sore, in terminal illness **4356**
  tumours, *see* oral cavity tumours
  ulceration, *see* oral ulceration
  viral infections **1848–51**
  see also entries beginning dental, oral
movement **3856–7**
  abnormal involuntary, *see* chorea;
    dyskinesia; myoclonus; tremor
  abnormalities 3857
  corticospinal tract lesions 3857
  increased resistance to 3857
  repetitive, in malnutrition 1283
movement disorders **3998–4022**
  akinetic-rigid syndromes **3998–4009**
  antipsychotic drugs side-effect 4252,
    4252
  central motor conduction time in 3838
  dyskinesias **4009–21**
  hyperkinetic 3862
  see also akinetic-rigid syndromes;
    dyskinesia
M proteins (bacterial), post-infectious
  glomerulonephritis and 3174
M proteins (paraproteins), *see*
  monoclonal paraproteins
MPTP, parkinsonism due to 3999
MRFIT (Multiple Risk Factor
  Intervention Trial) 2307, 2316, 2317,
  2533
MRL/lpr mice 3024
mRNA, *see* messenger RNA (mRNA)
MRSA, *see* Staphylococcus aureus,
  methicillin-resistance (MRSA)
Msaleni disease 2977
mucinous adenocarcinoma, pancreatic
  2042
mucinous carcinoid, pancreatic 2042
mucinous cystadenocarcinoma,
  pancreatic 2042
Muckle-Well's syndrome *1514*, 3180
mucociliary clearance (escalator) 2609,
  2612, 2759
  in chronic bronchiolitis 2634

  defects 2613, 2759
    in bronchiectasis 2757, *2757*, 2759
    factors/infections affecting 2613
    inhibition 2616–17
    investigations 2668, 2759
    mechanism and role **2613**
mucocutaneous lymph-node syndrome,
  infantile, *see* Kawasaki disease
mucocutaneous syndromes, enteroviruses
  383–4
mucoepidermoid tumours 2892
mucolipidosis **1434–5**, *2019*, 3087
  type I (sialidosis) 1434, **1435–6**
  type II (I-cell disease) 1434, *1435*
  type III (pseudo-Hurler polydystrophy)
    1434, *1435*
  type IV (Berman's disease) 1434–5
mucolytic drugs, in chronic obstructive
  airways disease 2776
mucopolysaccharides 2290
mucopolysaccharidosis **1431–4**, *2019*,
  3087, 3988–9
  biochemical features *3062*
  type IH, *see* Hurler disease
  type IH/IS (Hurler-Scheie disease)
    1432, 1434
  type IS (Scheie disease) 1431–4
  type II (Hunter disease) 1431, *1432*,
    3988
  type III (Sanfilippo disease) 1431,
    1432
  type IV (Morquio disease) 1431, *1432*
  type VI (Maroteaux-Lamy disease)
    1431, *1432*
  type VII (ß-glucuronidase deficiency)
    1432, 1434
mucormycosis (invasive zygomycosis)
  810, 1490
  cerebral 1034
  in diabetic ketoacidosis 1027
  in iron overload 1027
  rhinocerebral 1033
mucosa, barrier to infection 275
mucosa-associated lymphoid tissue
  (MALT), lymphomas 1985
mucous membranes
  actinomycetes as commensals 681,
    682
  in rheumatic diseases 2945
mucus
  airway,
    composition 2643
    drugs acting on 2644
    hypersecretion, *see also* bronchitis,
      chronic
  in mucociliary clearance 2613, 2643
  secretion,
    in asthma, mediators causing 2727,
      2728
  in cystic fibrosis 2747, 2748
mucus colitis 1965
mulibrey nanism 2475
Müllerian inhibitory factor 1563, 1690
multicentric reticulohistiocytosis 3803
  joint symptoms 3006–7
Multiceps multiceps 959
multicore disease 4150
multidisciplinary care, radiotherapy 258
multidisciplinary teams
  cancer management 247
  rehabilitation after falls in elderly 4339
  sexual problem management 4247
multidrug-resistance 525
  tuberculosis 652
multifocal motor neuropathy 4088
multigated acquisition (MUGA) imaging
  2205, 2231
multi-infarct dementia **3960–1**
  Parkinson's disease *vs* 4002
multiple carboxylase deficiency 1374
multiple endocrine neoplasia (MEN)
  syndromes 1566, **1707–10**
  bone disease in **3079**
  type 1 (MEN 1) 1568, 1632, **1707–8**
    insulinoma 1509, 1708

  pancreatic endocrine tumours 1703,
    1705, 1708
  parathyroid hyperplasia/adenomata
    1708
  pituitary tumours 1708
  screening 1708
  type 2 (MEN 2) 1568, 1632, **1708–10**
    bone disease in 3079
    medullary thyroid carcinoma 1621,
      1637, **1709**
    phaeochromocytoma 1709
    screening 1710
  type 2A (MEN 2A) (Sipple's
    syndrome) 1709
  type 2B (MEN 2B) 1709–10, *3795*
    ocular features 4182, 4196
multiple organ failure 293
Multiple Risk Factor Intervention Trial
  (MRFIT) 2307, 2316, 2317, 2533
multiple sclerosis 3990, **3992–6**
  acute/subacute paraplegia 3892, 3993
  aetiology **3992–3**
  benign disease 3994
  central motor conduction time in 3837
  clinical course 3994
  clinical features **3993**
  differential diagnosis **3995**
  epidemiology 3992 eye in **4184**
  facial paralysis in 3878, 3993
  genetic susceptibility 3992
  immune response in 146
  investigations **3994–5**
  Marburg variant 3990
  measles and 380
  mental disorders/symptoms in 3993,
    4238
  optic nerve involvement 3866, 3991,
    3993
  paroxysmal manifestations 3993, 3996
  pathophysiology **3993**
  in pregnancy 1769
  prognosis 3994
  progressive spinal disease 3994, 3995
  treatment **3995–6**
    to influence course of 3996
    positive-pressure ventilation 2576
  visual evoked potential abnormalities
    3832
multiple sulphatase deficiency
  (mucosulphatidosis) *1428*, 1429
multiple system atrophy 3883, **4006–7**
  autonomic failure with 3882, 3885,
    4006
  conditions included 4006
multipotential colony-stimulating factor
  (multi-CSF), *see* interleukin-3
multisystem failure, drug prescribing
  3270
mumps **372–5**
  antibody response 372
  arthritis in 3001
  clinical features 374
  CNS in 373, 4064
  diagnosis 374
  diphtheria *vs* 496
  epidemiology and transmission 372
  in fetus and infants 374
  orchitis and genitalia changes 373, 374
  pancreas in 373
  parotitis in 373, 374
  pathology 373–4
  salivary glands in 372, 373, 374
  sialadenitis of parotid gland *vs* 1861
  skin tests 372
  treatment and prevention 375
  vaccine 375
mumps/measles/rubella (MMR) vaccine
  318–19, 375, 411–12
mumps virus 372
  antigens and proteins 372
  diabetes type I and 1454
  genome and structure 372, 373
  source and resistance to 372
Munchausen's syndrome 4211, 4258
  causes and management 4211
  presenting symptoms 4211
  by proxy 1496

mupirocin, *Staphylococcus aureus*
  sensitivity 525
Murphy's sign, in acute cholecystitis 2049
Murray Valley encephalitis **415**
muscarinic effect 3881
muscle
  action potential 4139
  acute sports-related injuries 4321
  anatomy and physiology **4139–44**
  ATP utilization 4165
  biopsy **4142–3**
    in glycogen storage diseases 1341–2
    in myotonic disorders 4153
  blood flow,
    in electrical injury 1213
    fatigue in heart failure and 2172
  capillary density, endurance sports
    training 4325
  contraction 4139–40, 4142
  contractures, *see* contractures
  cramps 4141
    in cirrhosis 2087
    in glycogen storage diseases 1341
    occupational 4018–19
    in pregnancy 1766
  in cysticercosis 56
  damage,
    in electrical injury 1213
    in poisoning 1048
  denervation 4141
  energy source 1272
  in enterovirus infections 386–7, *387*
  fasciculation 3840, 4092, 4141
  fatigue, in heart failure 2171, 2233
  fibres 4139
    anatomy 4139
    in biopsy 4142–3
    changes in heart failure 2177, 2233
    necrosis in Duchenne muscular
      dystrophy 4145
    ragged red 4143, 4171, 4173
    type 1 (slow-twitch) 4140, 4141
    type 2 (fast-twitch) 4140, 4141
    types 4140, *4140*
    vacuolar changes 4143–4
  fibrillation, *see* fibrillation
  generalized hypotonia in infancy, *see*
    floppy infant syndrome
  glycogen storage disease affecting
    1341–2
  glycogen stores 4325
  haematomas, in haemophilia 3647,
    3649
  heart failure pathophysiology
    hypothesis 2234, 2235, 2236
  hypertrophy (Hoffmann's syndrome)
    4125
  in hypokalaemia 3129
  jerks, *see* myoclonus
  loss,
    fatigue in heart failure 2172
    in heart disease 2176, 2233
  metabolism,
    fatigue pathophysiology 2172–3
    in heart failure 2233
  mitochondria and capillaries relation to
    oxygen consumption 2605
  pain 2364, 4141
    benign exertional 4141
    in polymyositis/dermatomyositis 4157
    see also musculoskeletal pain
  paralysis 4141
    see also paralysis
  power, examination 4142
  pseudohypertrophy 4146
  relaxants in tetanus 628–9
  relaxation 4140
    delayed 4142
    in spinal cord injury 3898
  in rheumatoid arthritis 2962
  rigidity,
    in tetanus 625, 626
    see also rigidity
  spasms, in tetanus 625, 625–6
  stiffness, in tetanus 625, 626
  striated 1272
  in leptospirosis 700

tenderness 4142
tone, increased/decreased 4142
wasting,
  in dystrophia myotonica 4152
  in immobilization 1550
  in myotonic disorders 4152, 4153
  in rheumatoid arthritis 2956
  see also wasting
weakness 3857, 4141
  in acromegaly 1593
  after acute sports-related injuries
    4322
  in chronic renal failure 3323
  in cirrhosis 2087
  in Cushing's syndrome 1643
  electrophysiological investigation
    3840–1
  in endocrine myopathies 4167
  facial 4146
  in Friedreich's ataxia 3984
  hypokalaemic periodic paralysis 3132
  in hypophosphataemia 1626
  in Lambert-Eaton myasthenic
    syndrome (LEMS) 4163
  limb-girdle 4167, 4168
  in muscular dystrophies 4145
  in myasthenia gravis 4161
  in myotonic disorders 4152, 4153
  neurogenic, in mitochondrial
    myopathies 4173
  in osteomalacia 3071
  pelvic girdle 4145
  in peripheral neuropathy 4092
  in polymyositis/dermatomyositis 4157
  proximal 3071, 4141
  in rheumatoid arthritis 4131
  in vitamin D deficiency 1626
  see also muscular dystrophies;
    myopathy; weakness
muscle disorders **4141–4**
  chronic fatigue syndrome in 1037
  clinical features 4141–2
  diagnostic methods **4142–4**
    biochemistry 4142
  in pregnancy 1766
  signs 4141
  tendon reflexes in 4142
  see also myopathy
muscovite 2845
muscular dystrophies **4145–50**
  aetiology **4145**
  autosomal dominant 4145
  autosomal recessive 4145, **4147**, 4148
  benign X-linked, *see* Becker muscular
    dystrophy
  cardiac manifestations **2392**, *2393*
  carrier detection and prenatal diagnosis
    4146–7
  childhood autosomal recessive **4147**
  classification **4145**
  clinical features **4145–6**
  congenital **4147**
    Fukuyama type 4147
    hypotonic-sclerotic (Ullrich's
      syndrome) 4147
  developments in molecular genetics
    4146–7
  distal (Welander) **4148**
  electromyography **4145**
  Emery-Dreifuss, *see* Emery-Dreifuss
    muscular dystrophy
  facioscapulohumeral **4147–8**
  histology 4143
  limb-girdle **4147**
  neonatal screening **4146**
  ocular and oculopharyngeal **4148**
  pathology **4145**
  severe X-linked Duchenne type, *see*
    Duchenne muscular dystrophy
  treatment **4148–9**
  X-linked 4145, 4146
  X-linked scapuloperoneal 4146
musculocutaneous nerve **4094**
musculoskeletal pain
  generalized **2997**
  myocardial infarction *vs* 2335
  see also muscle, pain

musculoskeletal system
  chest pain due to disorders **2168**
  disorders, positive-pressure ventilation
    indications 2576–7
  in haematological disorders 3376–7
  heart failure pathophysiology 2232,
    2233
  occupational disorders **1168–9**
    see also rheumatic diseases
  paraneoplastic disorders *244*
  in SLE 3019
mushroom intolerance (trehalase
  deficiency) *1922*, 1923
  poisonous 1155–9, *1157*, 2005
  see also fungi, poisonous
mushroom worker's lung 2810, 2816
musicians, overuse syndrome 1168
mustard gas, *see* sulphur mustard
Mustard procedure 2416
mustine (nitrogen mustard) 1115
  in Hodgkin's disease *3573*, 3574
  in Langerhans-cell histiocytosis 3609
  in mycosis fungoides 3797
mutagenesis, insertional 112
mutagenicity
  carcinogenicity correlation 193
  tests 221
mutagens
  chloro-acetaldehyde 1090
  screening tests 193
mutations 104, **107–8**
  chromosomal rearrangements 108
  confined to subset of cells 107
  detection and genetic prediction by
    133–4
  DNA sequences prone to 108
  dominant transmission involving
    genomic imprinting 127
  frameshift 63
  genetically determined disorders and
    100
  'hot spots' 108
  microdeletions 108, *108*
  mis-sense 63
  new, in autosomal dominant disorders
    114
  nonsense 63
  outcomes/mutations and loci effects 104
  point 63, 108, 109, 134
  splicing mechanism interference 63
  transposable elements 108
  tumour development 65, 192
    recessive nature 194
  in tumours *230*
MVPP regimen *3573*, 3574
myalgia
  in coxsackievirus infection 386
  epidemic, *see* Bornholm disease
  in influenza 339
  in leptospirosis 700
  in Wegener's granulomatosis 3012
myalgic encephalitis 386
myalgic encephalomyelitis (ME) 353,
  1036, 2997, 4074
  see also chronic fatigue syndrome
myasthenia
  congenital/hereditary **4164**
  ocular 4161, 4162
  thyroid disease and 4168
myasthenia gravis 1962, **4160–3**
  acetylcholine receptor antibodies 163,
    164, 4160, 4161
  classification 4161, *4161*
  clinical features 4161
  diagnosis 4161–2
  early onset generalized seropositive
    4162
  electromyography 3841
  'familial' 4161
  haematological changes 3686
  late-onset 4162
  management 4162–3
  mental disorders/symptoms in 4161,
    4238
  neonatal 4161
  pathogenesis 4160–1
  penicillamine-induced 4161

positive-pressure ventilation 2576
  in pregnancy 1766
  prognosis 4163
  seronegative 4160, 4162
  subgroups and features of *4161*
  in thymic tumours 2898, 4160–1
  thymus abnormalities in 4160–1
myasthenic crisis, management 4162
mycetism 797
mycetoma (Madura foot) **801–2**, *802*
  urinary-tract obstruction 3179
myc gene, overexpression and
  mechanism of action 225
mycobacteria
  atypical 2707–8
    in AIDS 474, 666, 1018, 1019, 4079,
      4194
    arthritis due to 3000
    see also mycobacterial diseases,
      environmental
  environmental 664, *665*
    ecology/epidemiology 665
    granuloma formation 154
    infections in silicosis 2842
    post-inoculation 666
    septic arthritis due to **2999–3000**
mycobacterial diseases, environmental
  664–7, *665*
  disseminated disease 666–7
  post-inoculation 666
  treatment 667, *667*
  types 665–7
Mycobacterium, interaction with
  phagocytic cells 272
Mycobacterium avium-intracellulare
  complex (MAC) 472, 665
  in AIDS/HIV infections 474, 475, 666,
    4079
  treatment 480–1, 667, *667*
  drug resistance 480
  hepatic granulomas due to 2122, 2133
  infective colitis 1947
  small-bowel biopsy 1908
Mycobacterium bovis 638, 3275
Mycobacterium chelonae 665, 666, *667*,
  1029
Mycobacterium fortuitum 666, 667
Mycobacterium genavese 474
Mycobacterium leprae 638, 667
  detection 668
  in HIV infection 487
  pholic glycolipid (PGL-1)-secreted
    antigen 668
  see also leprosy
Mycobacterium malmoense 667
Mycobacterium marinum 665, 666
Mycobacterium paratuberculosis
  Crohn's disease aetiology 1937
  DNA 1937
Mycobacterium smegmatis 3275, 3276
Mycobacterium tuberculosis **638–40**,
  2121, 3275
  biological effects of cell components
    638
  classical and South Indian (Asian) types
    638
  detection and culture 641–2, 662, 4062
  drug resistance, *see under* tuberculosis
  drug susceptibility tests 642, 643
  identification tests 642, *642*
  infectious doses 268
  morphology and staining 638
  phage types 638
  sarcoidosis aetiology and 2819–20
  urine culture 3276
  virulence and host range 638–9
  see also tuberculosis
Mycobacterium ulcerans 665, 666,
  679–80
  culture and detection 679
  see also Buruli ulcer
myc oncogene
  in leukaemia 3395, 3396, *3412*
  mutations in lung cancer 2882
  c-*myc* 149, 225, 355
  in myelomatosis 3597
Mycoplasma agalactiae 765

Mycoplasma fermentans 762
  in AIDS 772
  isolation 767–8, 769
  rheumatoid arthritis 771
Mycoplasma genitalium 762
  infections 767–71
    non-gonococcal urethritis 768–9, 770
  isolation 767, 768
  M. pneumoniae differentiation 764
Mycoplasma hominis 168, 762
  arthritis and hip sepsis 771
  infections in homosexuals 3363
  isolation/detection 768, *768*, 769
    complement fixation test 770
  in neonates 1792
  pelvic inflammatory disease 770
  postabortal fever 771
  postpartum fever 771
  in pregnancy 1792
  pyelonephritis 770
  rare infections 772
Mycoplasma incognitus 772
Mycoplasma orale 767
Mycoplasma penetrans 773
Mycoplasma pneumoniae **762–7**
  acute exacerbation of chronic bronchitis
    2692
  arthritis 771
  bronchiectasis pathogenesis 2757
  cold haemagglutinin disease and 3544,
    3685
  experimental models 767
  extrapulmonary infections 763–4, *765*
  isolation and detection 764, *765*
  Mycoplasma genitalium differentiation
    764
  pneumonia **762–7**, 764, 766, 2694,
    2695, 2697
  respiratory infection,
    chronic 767
    clinical features 762–3
    diagnosis 764
    epidemiology 764, 766
    immunopathology 766
    prevention and vaccine 767
    reinfection/relapse 762, 766
    treatment 766–7
mycoplasmas **762–73**
  AIDS and **772–3**
  characteristics 762, *763*
  detection/isolation 764, *765*, 767–8,
    769, 770
  endocarditis 2438, 2448–9
  epidemiology of infections 762, *765*,
    2695
  experimental models/studies 767, 769,
    770
  genitourinary infections **767–71**, *768*
    experimental models 769
    treatment 769
    see also Mycoplasma genitalium;
      urethritis
  in hypogammaglobulinaemia 168
  joint infections **771**
  occurrence 762, *765*, 2695
  pelvic inflammatory disease due to
    3357
  rare conditions/equivocal aetiology
    771–2
  respiratory infections **762–7**
    chronic 767
    relationship 762
    see also Mycoplasma pneumoniae
  taxonomy 762, *763*
  in vagina 767
Mycoplasma salivarium 168, 767
mycoses, *see* fungal infections
mycosis fungoides 3581, 3794, 3795
  clinical features 3796
  management 3797
  mycotoxicosis 797
mycotoxins 1158
  classes 1158
myelinated nerve fibres 4091
myelination 3990
myelinolysis, central pontine 3123–4
myelitis **3894**
  acute necrotizing 3991

ascending 345
  subacute necrotizing 3894
  transverse **3991**
myeloblast 3556
myelocyte 3556
myelodysplasia, hypoplastic 3447
myelodysplastic syndromes 3392,
  3425–31, 3448
  acquired primary sideroblastic anaemia
    and 3426, 3427, 3521
  chromosome/cellular abnormalities
    3428–9
  classification 3426–8
  clinical/laboratory features 3425–6
  complications 3430
  definition 3425
  differential diagnosis 3428
  dyserythropoiesis in 3426, 3524
  megaloblastic anaemia in 3498
  primary 3425
  prognosis 3429–30
  secondary 3425, **3430**
  treatment 3430–1
  see also refractory anaemia
myelofibrosis, *see* myelosclerosis
myelography **3826–7**
  in acute back pain 2993
  in intervertebral disc protrusions 3906,
    3907
  in spinal cord and cauda equina
    compression 3892
myeloid/erythroid (M/E) ratio 3381
myeloid metaplasia 3434–5, 3436, 3588
myeloma 3579
  antibody homogeneity 192
  indolent *3600*
  infections in 1028
  multiple (myelomatosis) **3597–604**, **4135**
    acute renal failure 3181, **3292–3**, 3603
    aetiology 3597
    amyloidosis in 1515, 1524, 3180,
      3181, 3185
    bleeding tendency 3599, 3635
    clinical features 3598–9
    diagnosis improvements 214
    diagnosis/staging/prognosis 3599–601
    epidemiology 214, 3597
    hypercalcaemia in 1638, 3181, 3599,
      3603
    hypokalaemia in 3184
    light-chain deposition disease in 3181,
      3182
    pathogenesis 3597–8
    renal involvement *3180*, **3181–2**,
      3185, *3300*, 3599, 3603
    solitary plasmacytoma of bone and
      3604–5
    therapy 3601–4
    tumour growth 3598
    urinary casts 3138, 3181
  ocular features **4194**
  secondary immunodeficiency in 174
  smouldering *3600*
myelopathy
  acute 3892
  cervical spondylotic **3908–9**
  HIV-1-related 476, **4078**
  tropical ataxic 490
  in tumours *243*
myeloperoxidase (MPO) 3559
  antibodies, *see* antimyeloperoxidase
    antibodies
  deficiency 3560
  in leukaemia cells 3399, 3400, 3405–6
myelopoiesis 3556–7
  regulation 3557
myeloproliferative disorders 3392, 3589
  bleeding disorders 3634–5
  Budd-Chiari syndrome in 2098
  see also specific disorders
myelosclerosis (myelofibrosis) **3434–9**
  acute **3437–8**
  folate deficiency 3493
  investigations 3593, 3594–5
  in myelodysplastic syndromes 3426
  in polycythaemia vera 3433, 3434
  primary 3392, **3434–7**
    aetiology 3434–5

clinical features 3435
  complications 3437
  course and prognosis 3437
  differential diagnosis 3436–7
  investigations 3435–6
  treatment 3437
  proliferative dysplasia with 3448
  secondary **3438–9**
  splenomegaly in 3589
myelosuppression, *see* bone marrow,
  failure
myenteric (Auerbach's) plexus 1953
  in Chagas' disease 1963
myiasis **1000–1**
  dermal 1000–1
  intestinal 1000
  ophthalmic 1001
  predatory sanguivorous 1001
  urogenital 1000
  wound 1000, 1001
MYO2 gene 82
myoadenylate deaminase deficiency 4167
myoadenylate kinase deficiency 1341
myoblast, transfer 4148
myocardial abscess 2439, 2444
myocardial cells
  action potential 2148, 2149
  cell slippage 2230, 2321
  coagulative necrosis 2320, 2321
  contractility,
    acid-base disturbances and 1539
    in thyroid disease 1609
  contraction 2143
    calcium in **2148**
    energy requirements **2145–7**, 2145
    mechanics **2149–50**, **2154–5**
    sarcomere length/tension 2149–50,
      2154–5
    see also heart, contraction
  contraction band necrosis 2320
  death,
    hot-spot scanning 2207
    in ischaemia 2151
    in myocardial infarction 2320
  disarray 2384, 2385
  dysfunction in heart failure 2230, *2230*
  electrophysiology, *see* heart,
    electrophysiology
  growth in cardiac hypertrophy **2147–8**,
    2149
  loss 2230, *2230*
  necrosis,
    in phaeochromocytomas 2554
    in unstable angina 2320
  structure **2143–5**
    cytoskeleton 2144
    mitochondria 2145
    ribosomes and nucleus 2145
    sarcolemma and glycocalyx 2144
    withdrawal from cell cycle 2145, 2147
myocardial dysplasia 2399
myocardial failure, in sepsis 293
myocardial fibrosis
  interstitial, in hypertrophic
    cardiomyopathy 2384
  in rheumatoid arthritis 2961
  in systemic sclerosis *3031*
myocardial hypertrophy
  electrocardiogram (ECG) in 2187–8
  magnetic resonance imaging 2216
  see also left ventricle (ventricular),
    hypertrophy; right ventricle
    (ventricular), hypertrophy
myocardial infarction **2331–49**
  acute pericarditis in 2475–6
    treatment 2346
  advances in **2331–2**
  after ß-blocker withdrawal 1251
  in aircraft crew and pilots 1200, 2360
  angiography 2346–7
    intermittent coronary opening/closing
      2333
  animal models 2320
  atrial fibrillation and treatment 2345–6
  atrioventricular block in 2268, 2346
  in carbon monoxide exposure 1095
  cardiac output impairment 2568–9
  cardiac rupture 2341

circadian rhythm 2325, 2334
clinical course 2339
clinical features **2334–5**
clinical presentation **2334**
  chest pain 2334, 2335
  complications/consequences 2334,
    2566, 2569
  prophylaxis **2347**
in connective tissue diseases 3009
in/after coronary artery bypass grafting
  2355
coronary artery thrombosis as cause
  2332
C-reactive protein levels 1531
D/D angiotensin converting enzyme
  2157, 2250
in diabetes mellitus 1492
dialysed patients 3312
differential diagnosis **2335–6**
  pericarditis *vs* 2335
  pneumococcal pneumonia *vs* 516
diffuse 2320
driving after 2359
early diagnosis 2334
in elderly **4342**
electrocardiogram in, *see*
  electrocardiogram (ECG)
epidemiology 2331–2, 2357
  age and gender 2337
  international differences 2332
expansion and 'remodelling' 2229,
  2230, 2321, 2333, 2347
  effect of 2347
  prevention by ACE inhibitors 2230,
    2250
heart block in 2268, 2346
  treatment 2346
heart failure 2338
high altitudes and 1192–3
historical aspects 2331
hormone replacement therapy and 1815
in hypertension 2533
inferior/diaphragmatic 2566
intrarenal haemodynamic changes 2170
investigations,
  blood tests 2339
  chest radiography 2338–9
  ejection fraction 2338, 2339
  imaging 2339
  magnetic resonance imaging 2217
  radionuclide, *see below*
lifestyle changes after 2348
mortality 2336, 2346
  causes of death 2332
  rates, international differences 2332,
    2333
  reduced by thrombolytic therapy 2336,
    2340
oral contraceptives and 1724
outcome, left ventricle importance to
  2346
in Parkinson's disease 4004
pathogenesis 2318
pathological physiology 2566, 2567
pathology **2320–1**, **2333–4**
  complications 2321
  thrombosis and plaque disruption 2320
peripartum 1738, *1742*
potassium balance and 3128
precipitants **2333–4**
public health importance 2331–2
pulmonary oedema in 2338, 2566–8
radionuclide imaging 2207–11
  diagnosis and localization 2209, 2210
  infarct-avid (hot-spot) 2207–9
  sizing 2209, 2211
  time interval before 2208
railway staff 2361
regional 2320
  transmural/non-transmural
    (subendocardial) 2192, 2301, 2320
rehabilitation 2348–9
reinfarction prevention **2347–8**
  antithrombotics 2348
  beta-blockade 2347
  calcium entry blockade 2347
in renal failure and renal hypertension
  2552, *2552*

renal function after 3281
renin-angiotensin system activation and 2250
reperfusion after 2320
risk assessment after **2346–7**
  electrophysiological tests 2347
  exercise testing 2347
  Holter monitoring 2347
  routine angiography 2346–7
risk of death, factors in 2337–8
risk factors, *see under* ischaemic heart disease
ruptured papillary muscle 2460
secondary prevention 2304, 2305
sexual problems after 4244
  prevention 4247
shock in 2338, 2345
shoulder-hand syndrome 2346
size and site 2337–8
smoking and 2313
subendocardial 2192, 2301, 2320
sudden death in 2334
  prevention 2347
supraventricular arrhythmias in 2345–6
survival 2358
survivors, serum cholesterol 1407–8
suspected, management **2336–9**
  causes of delays 2336–7
  delay and increased mortality 2336
  delays in treatment 2336–7
  fast-track admission 2337
  home *vs* hospital 2336
  initial assessment 2336
  investigations 2338–9
  risk assessment 2337–8
  tachycardia in 2279, 2345
  treatment 2345
thromboembolic complications 3668
time course **2333–4**
time of occurrence **2334**
transmural thrombi 2301, 2320
treatment 2151, **2339–46**, 2566–9
  ACE inhibitors 2230, 2249–50, 2344
  advances in 2336
  angioplasty 2344
  anti-arrhythmic therapy 2345–6
  aspirin 23, 26–7, 2301, 2304, 2336, 2340, 2348
  beta-blockade 2345
  calcium channel blockers 2345
  coronary angioplasty 2352
  coronary care units 2339
  in elderly 4342
  fibrinolytic, *see* thrombolytic therapy
  inotropic agents 2345
  magnesium 29–30, 2344
  of pulmonary oedema 2566–8
  thrombolytic, *see* thrombolytic therapy
  vasodilators 2344
unstable angina and 2166, 2322, 2331
ventricular dysfunction after 2249–50
ventricular fibrillation in 2283, 2321, 2345, 2347
  treatment 2345
ventricular tachycardia in 2279
see also ischaemic heart disease; myocardial ischaemia
myocardial ischaemia **2151**, 2322
ACE inhibitor effect in 2250
angina in 2165, 2166
consequences 2151
coronary artery bypass grafting in 2353
definition 2151
dyspnoea in 2162, 2163
exercise testing 2227
in hypertrophic cardiomyopathy 2386, *2386*
irreversible, *see* myocardial infarction
metabolism in 2146–7
myocardial perfusion imaging in 2211
necrosis marker 2207
nucleotide loss in 2151
radionuclide imaging 2207–11
  non-viable (cold-spot scanning) 2207, 2209–11
  recent damage (hot spot scanning) 2207–9
see also myocardial perfusion imaging

regulation of fuel metabolism in 2146–7, 2151
reperfusion damage 2151, 2320
reversible, magnetic resonance imaging 2217
silent 2323, 2325
'stuttering' 2151
total 2151
see also angina (angina pectoris); ischaemic heart disease; myocardial infarction
myocardial perfusion imaging
  angina investigation **2326**
  cold-spot scanning 2207, 2209–11
    myocardial ischaemia assessment 2211
  computed tomography 2219
  magnetic resonance imaging 2217
  positron emission tomography 2212
  single photon emission computed tomography 2211–12
see also myocardial ischaemia
myocardial sarcoidosis 2216
myocardial 'stunning' 2340
myocarditis **2380–1**
  acute, in enterovirus infections 386
  aetiology and pathogenesis 2381, *2382*
  in AIDS 2395
  in bacterial meningitis 4052
  cardiac transplantation indication 2255
  chest pain in 2167
  clinical features and management 2381
  Dallas criteria 2380, *2381*, 2395
  definition 2380
  dilated cardiomyopathy pathogenesis 2382
  in diphtheria 495
  idiopathic 2381
  in influenza 339
  mumps virus causing 373
  in relapsing fevers 695, 696
  rheumatic 2433
  in rheumatoid arthritis 2392
  'suspected' diagnosis 2380–1
  in systemic sclerosis *3031*
  in trichinosis 941
myocardium
  ACE inhibitor action 2249
  diseases,
    restrictive, pericardial constriction *vs* 2480
    see also cardiomyopathy; heart muscle diseases; myocarditis
  fibrofatty replacement 2391
  function, in tetanus 625
  'hibernating' 2151
  in hypereosinophilia 2397
  magnetic resonance imaging 2216
  metabolism, in angina 2322, 2323
  oxygen demand 2327, 2357, *2358*
    in angina 2323
    determinants 2323
  sensitivity to digitalis 2242–3
myoclonic encephalopathies **4014–15**
myoclonic epilepsy 3914, 3915, **4015**
  familial 4014–15
  hereditary **3988**
  juvenile 4015
myoclonic epilepsy with ragged red fibres (MERRF) 4173
myoclonus **4014–16**
  benign essential **4015**
  causes *4011*
  definition 4010
  focal **4015–16**
  in Lafora body disease 4015
  nocturnal 3929
  palatal 4015–16
  postanoxic action 4015
  spinal 4015
Myocrisin® 3732
myocytes, *see* myocardial cells
Myodil 3826, 3907
myofibrils 4139, 4140
  in myocardial cells 2144
myofibroblasts, proliferation in asthma 2727
myogenic theory, pulmonary hypertension 2513–14

myoglobin 3471
  in altitude acclimatization 1187
  in muscle disorders 4142
myoglobinuria 2581, 3145
  acute renal failure in **3289**
  causes *4170*
  myopathy in **4170**
myoidema 4142
myokymia 3840, 4141–2, 4151
myonecrosis, clostridial 633
myoneural junction, nerve impulse transmission 4139
myopathy 3061, 4141
  alcoholic 4127, 4169
  benign congenital 4150, 4151
  congenital **4150–1**
  definition 4141
  drug-induced 4169, *4169*
  endocrine **4167–8**
  fingerprint body **4150–1**
  in HIV infection and AIDS **4078**, 4155
  inflammatory 3039, **4154–60**
    causes 4154, *4155*
    classification *4154*
    in connective tissue diseases **4156–8**
    by microbial agents/parasites **4154–6**
    see also myositis
  ion-flux disorders **4169–1**
  ischaemic 4169
  McLeod 4146
  in malignant hyperthermia 4170
  metabolic and endocrine **4165–71**
    calcium/vitamin D/PTH metabolism **4168–9**
    glucose and glycogen metabolism **4165–7**
    lipid metabolism **4167–8**
    miscellaneous **4159**
  mitochondrial, *see* mitochondrial myopathy
  in mitochondrial encephalomyopathy 4172–3
  in myoglobinuria 4170
  in myotonia congenita 4170
  myotubular/centronuclear **4151**
  nemaline **4150**
  nutritional and toxic **4169**
  primary degenerative, *see* muscular dystrophies
  rheumatic 4131, 4156
  see also muscle, weakness; muscle disorders
myopericarditis 386
myophosphorylase deficiency 2173
  type V glycogenosis, *see* McArdle's disease
myosin 80, 81
  autoantibodies to 163
  intracellular movement of organelles 80
  light chains 4141
    phosphorylation 3618
  in muscle 4139
  mutations, in hypertrophic cardiomyopathy 2144, 2385
  in myocardial cells 2144
myosin ATPase 4140
  deficiency 4141
myosin I 81
  function 81–2
myosin II 81
myosin light-chain kinase 3618
myositis **387**
  acute suppurative (tropical) 4155
  bacterial **4155**
  chronic fibrosing 4157
  clostridial 4155
  eosinophilic 3039
  in fungal infections **4156**
  granulomatous **4158**
  inclusion body *1513*, 3039, **4158**
  infantile **4158**
  investigations *2952*
  localized nodular **4157–8**
  in myositis ossificans progressiva 3093
  parasitic **4155–6**
  protozoal infections **4156**
  tropical **4174–5**

viral 4154, *4154*
see also myopathy, inflammatory
myositis ossificans, after neurological injury 3093
myositis ossificans progressiva 3092, **3093–4, 4159**
  biochemical features *3062*
myotonia
  causes 4151
  chondrodystrophic **4153**
  definition 4151
  diagnosis/differential diagnosis 4153
  drugs causing 4151
  inherited causes 4151
myotonia atrophica, *see* dystrophia myotonica
myotonia congenita 4151, **4152**
  management 4153
  myopathy in **4170**
myotonia-myokymia-hyperhidrosis syndrome 4151
myotonia paradoxa 4152
myotonic disorders **4151–4**
  diagnosis **4153**
  treatment and prognosis **4153**
myotonic dystrophy, *see* dystrophia myotonica
myotubular myopathy **4151**
myristic acid 2310
myxoedema 1553
  coma 1556
  mental disorders/symptoms in 4238–9
  neurological feature 4125
  peripheral nerve involvement 4099
  pretibial 3802
  primary 1609, 1610, 1615
  see also hypothyroidism
myxoma, *see* cardiac myxoma
MZ2E antigen 228

N

NADH 4171
  in red cells 3456, 3534
NADH-diaphorase deficiency 3519
NADH:methaemoglobin reductase deficiency *3536*
NADP, in red cells 3456, 3537
NADPH, in red cells 3456, 3534, 3537
NADPH:methaemoglobin reductase deficiency *3536*
NADPH-oxidase 3559, 3560
  inherited defects 3560
Naegleria fowleri 825, **833–4**
  infection **833–4**
naevus 3725, 3754
  Becker's *3755*, 3756
  blue 3754
  giant hairy 3725
  halo 3758, 3759
  pigmented, in pregnancy 1804
  port wine **3785**
  spider 3785
    in pregnancy 1796, 1804
  strawberry **3785**
naevus anaemicus 3755, 3758
nail dystrophy
  psoriatic 2968, 2969
  in Reiter's syndrome 2971
nailfold capillaries, in Raynaud's phenomenon 3029
nail-patella syndrome 110
nails
  in chronic renal failure 3302
  colour changes *3762*
  diseases of **3760–1**
  fungal infections 799, 3761
  infections, in diabetes 1490
  in iron-deficiency anaemia 3475
  in keratodermas 3750
  mucous cyst at base 3761
  normal growth 3760
  pits, ridges and grooves 3760
  psoriasis 3747
  rickshaw boy's (koilonychia) 3475, 3760
  splinter haemorrhages 2441

nails (*cont.*)
  white, in hepatocellular failure 2104
  yellowing in diabetes 1490
nairoviruses 423, *424*, **427**
nalidixic acid
  in pregnancy 1785
  in *Shigella* infections 554
  in urinary-tract infections *3211*
naloxone 1046, 1048
  co-phenotrope poisoning management
    1069
  in opioid overdose 1058
    withdrawal syndrome in 1058
Naltrexone 4292, 4293
L-NAME 2514
NAME syndrome 2472
naphthalene toxicity *3546*
naphthol toxicity *3546*
naphthoquinones 850
1-naphthylamine, bladder cancer
    association 212
2-naphthylamine, bladder cancer
    association 212
naples virus 428
nappy eruptions 3768, 3769, 3798
naproxen 1248
  poisoning 1056
narcolepsy 3918–19, **3927–30**
  aetiology 3928
  clinical features/course 3928–9
  definition 3927–8
  idiopathic 3928
  mental disorders/symptoms in 4238
  treatment 3929–30
narcotic drugs
  addicts 4241
  psychiatric disturbances from 4241
  in renal impairment 3270
  see also opioids
nasal blockage, obstructive sleep apnoea
    and 2910
nasal bot flies 1001
nasal congestion, *see under* nose (nasal)
nasal crusting 2716
nasal cycle 2610
nasal decongestants 2718
nasal discharge, in Wegener's
    granulomatosis 3012
nasal endotracheal tubes 2577
nasal positive-pressure ventilation
    (NPPV) 2905–6, 2927, 2930
  in central sleep apnoea and
    hypoventilation 2918
  in chronic respiratory failure 2930
  domiciliary 2906, 2930
  future prospects 2932
  indications 2930
  transplantation bridge and 2932
  in weaning from mechanical ventilation
    2931–2
  see also positive-pressure ventilation
nasal septum, granulomas in sarcoidosis
    3799, 3802
nasal sinuses, cancer, epidemiology 205
nasal vestibule, granulomas in
    sarcoidosis 3799, 3802
NASCET trials 2373
nasogastric aspiration
  in acute pancreatitis 2032
  in diabetic hyperglycaemic coma 1502
nasogastric tube
  in exomphalos/gastroschisis
    management 1974, 1975
  in gastrointestinal bleeding 1827
  transanastomotic 1974
nasopharyngeal carcinoma **356–7**
  aetiological factors 202
  clinical features and diagnosis 356
  epidemiology 202, 356
  Epstein-Barr virus (EBV) role 202, 356
  screening 463
  treatment and pathogenesis 356
nasopharyngeal infections,
    meningococcal 538
nasopharyngeal secretions 2610
  defence mechanism 514
nasopharynx, in fascioliasis 987
nasopharynx 2610
natamycin 811, 812

National Asthma Campaign 2740
National Centre for Health Statistics,
    malnutrition classification 1281
National Eye Institute 4190
National Health Service (NHS) 47
  drug addict reporting system 4289
National Radiological Protection Board
    1222
natriuresis
  in heart failure 2239
  pressure 3247–8
natriuretic peptide system
  in heart failure 2234
  see also atrial natriuretic peptide
    (factor) (ANP)
natural gas 1095
natural killer (NK) cells **153**
  in graft rejection 187
  in myelomatosis 3598
  response to tumours 227
  role 153
  in SLE 3026
nature, nurture and luck, cancer
    susceptibility 219–20
nausea and vomiting 1821
  chemotherapy-induced 248, 3574, 3575
    in cirrhosis 2087
  in gastric cancer 1983
  management, in terminal illness
    4355–6, *4356*
  in migraine 4024–5
  in myocardial infarction 2335
  in pregnancy 1802
  radiation causing 1218
  in terminal illness **4355–6**, *4356*
  see also vomiting
near-infrared interactance, body fat
    measurement 1304
Nebuhaler 2738
nebulizers 1238
Necator americanus 930, 931
neck
  bruits in 3951, 3952, *3952*
  infections, anaerobic 572
  in respiratory disease 2652
  stiffness,
    in bacterial meningitis 4053
    in diabetic ketoacidosis 1499
    in raised intracranial pressure 4035
    in viral meningitis 4066
necrobacillosis 574–5
necrobiosis 3710
necrobiosis lipoidica 3799, 3802
necrobiosis lipoidica diabeticorum
    1489–90, 3799
necrosis
  C-reactive protein levels 1531
  radiation 4135
  see also tissue, necrosis
necrotic araneism 1148
necrotizing angiitis, in injecting drug
    abusers 4283
necrotizing arteriolitis, *see* fibrinoid
    necrosis
necrotizing arteritis, in pulmonary
    hypertension 2507–8
necrotizing enteritis (pig bel: necrotizing
    enterocolitis) **636–7**, 1995, 2004
necrotizing enterocolitis **636–7**, 1995,
    2004
necrotizing fasciitis 501
  causative organisms 501
necrotizing vasculitis 2507
nedocromil, in asthma 2738
needles, dangers to travellers 322
'needlestick' injury, malaria and 848
negative pressure ventilation 2874,
    2921
negative stereotypes, drug abuse/misuse
    4264
neglect
  body perception disorder 3854
  unilateral visuospatial 3853
negligence, *see* medical negligence
Negri bodies 401
Neisseria, rare species *558*
Neisseria gonorrhoeae **544–50**
  adaptations (recent) 546

antibiotic resistance 548–9
  chromosomally-mediated (CMRNG)
    548–9
  plasmid-mediated 549
antibiotic susceptibility testing 549
antibodies to 545
antigens 545
  arthritis due to 2998
  attachment to genital tract 544–5
  auxotyping 548
  characteristics 544
  culture 547
  endocarditis 2437, *2448*
  epididymitis 752
  identification 547–8
  infection mechanism 545
  monoclonal antibodies to 548
  Opa protein 545
  outer-membrane proteins 545
  pelvic inflammatory disease due to
    3357
  penicillinase-producing (PPNG) 549
  serotyping 548
  tetracycline-resistant (TRNG) 549
  typing 548
  vaccination against 545
  see also gonorrhoea
Neisseria meningitidis **533–5**
  antibiotic resistance 534, 541
  antigens 534, 540
  characteristics 533–5
  culture 538, 540, 541
  intracranial abscess 4081
  meningitis, *see* meningitis,
    meningococcal
  oropharyngeal infection, in
    homosexuals 3362
  pneumonia due to 540, 2694
  serogroups 534
  typing systems *534*
  vaccination 3530, 3596
  see also meningococcal vaccines
  virulence 534
  see also meningococcal infections
Nelson's syndrome 1576, **1595**, 1642,
    1650
NEM, *see* N-ethyl maleimide (NEM)-
    sensitive factor (NSF)
nemaline myopathy **4150**
nematodes **911–54**
  gut **936–44**
  infections in homosexuals **3365**
  of less importance **933**
  rarely found infections **933**, *934–5*
  see also Ascaris species
neologism 3848
neomycin, hepatic encephalopathy
    management 2108
neonates
  acne vulgaris 3753
  of anaemic mothers 3469
  anaerobic infections 572–3
  antibiotic problems 508
  antimicrobial therapy 1785, 1788
  antituberculous therapy 1746
  atopy in 3729
  BCG vaccination 648
  Candida infections 1793
  chlamydial infection **753–4**, *758*,
    1791–2
  coagulase-negative staphylococcal
    infections 532
  congenital hypothyroidism 1614–15
  congenital syphilis 1790–1
  conjunctivitis in 1790, 1791, 1792
  of diabetic mothers **1757–8**
  drug dependence and withdrawal
    4298
  enterobacterial infections 551
  enterovirus infections 388
  gonococcal infection 1790
  growth hormone deficiency 1582
  haemolytic disease of (HDN) **3544–5**
  haemostatic disorders **3654–5**
  hepatitis B 1798
  herpes simplex virus (HSV) infections
    345, 346
  HIV transmission 4298

hypoglycaemia **1511–12**, 1757
  immune function 1784
  intensive care, ethics **12–13**
  iron deficiency 1759
  jaundice, *see* jaundice, neonatal
  listeriosis 721, 722, 1789
  lupus 3018, 3022
  malaria in 848
  meningitis, *see* meningitis, neonatal
  Mycoplasma hominis infection 1792
  necrotizing enterocolitis 636, 1995
  normal haemostatic values *3654*
  opportunistic infections 1027
  oxidant-induced damage 3546
  physiological jaundice **2058**
  pneumonia 753–4
  respiratory distress syndrome 1757
  screening 1337–8
    congenital hypothyroidism 1337, 1615
    cystic fibrosis 2750
    21-hydroxylase deficiency 1667
    phenylketonuria 1337, 1362
    sickle-cell disease 3516
  seizures, pyridoxine-dependent 1372
  sepsis,
    enterococcal 509
    Haemophilus influenzae 583
    streptococcal, *see* streptococci group B
      infections
  skin and skin disease in 3715
  spina bifida management 4117–18
  Staphylococcus aureus infections 526
  streptococci group B infections, *see*
    streptococci group B infections
  tetanus in, *see* tetanus, neonatal
  tetany 1634
  thrombocytopenia 1764–5, 3631, 3632
  transient familial hyperbilirubinaemia
    2058
  transient thyroid dysfunction 1610,
    1611, **1750**
  tuberculosis 1793
  Ureaplasma urealyticum infection 1792
  ventilation 2920
  viral infections **1778–83**
neoplasia **191–262**
  general characteristics **191–6**
    carcinogenicity/mutagenicity 193
    DNA metabolism abnormalities 192–3
    evidence for clonal origin 192
    genetic analysis of lesions 193–4
    impairment of control of cell
      multiplication 191
    natural history of tumours 195–6
    nature of heritable lesion 191–2
    oncogenes, *see* oncogenes
    reversibility and suppression 193
  see also cancer; cell multiplication;
    malignant disease; tumour(s)
neostigmine, mechanism of action 1247
neostigmine methyl sulphate, in snake
    envenoming management 1138
neostriatum 3861, 3862
nephrectomy
  in genitourinary tuberculosis 3278
  pre-renal transplant 3315
  in reflux nephropathy 3220
  in renovascular hypertension 2550
  in unilateral renal parenchymal disease
    2552
nephritic syndrome, acute **3146**
  in cryoglobulinaemia 3183
  nephrotic syndrome *vs* 3140
  in post-infectious glomerulonephritis
    3173–4
nephritis
  crescentic 3162
    pauci-immune 3166
    see also glomerulonephritis, rapidly
      progressive
  Heymann 3159
  infection-associated **3173–8**
  interstitial, *see* interstitial nephritis
  intestinal, resin-coated mesalazines 1949
  lupus, *see* lupus nephritis
  pauci-immune 3013
  radiation 3185, **3231**
  shunt 532, **3175**

nephroblastoma
  Burkitt lymphoma vs 354
  epidemiology 212
nephrocalcin 3252
nephrocalcinosis 3228, 3251
  calcium oxalate 1445, 1446
  causes 3254
  in renal tubular acidosis 3338, 3339,
    3340
  in sarcoidosis 2827, 3186
nephrogram 3110
  in upper-tract obstruction 3236–7
nephronophthisis-medullary cystic
    disease complex 3205
nephropathia epidemica 426
nephropathy
  acute crystal 3226
  acute uric acid 1379–80, 3185, **3226**,
    3290
  AIDS-associated 772
  amyloid 1514, **3180–1**, 3185, *3300*
  analgesic **3221–3**, 3296
  Balkan **3229–31**, 3296
  Bence Jones cast (myeloma) 3181
  chronic urate 1380, 2986, 3224,
    3226–7
  contrast-associated 2400, 2549, 3110,
    3266–7, 3289
    in cyanotic congenital heart disease
      2400, 2549
  diabetic, see diabetic nephropathy
  drug-induced, see drug(s), nephrotoxic
  familial juvenile hyperuricaemic
    (FJHN) 1380, 3225, **3226**, 3227
  hepatitis C-associated 3157, **3176**
  hypercalcaemic **3227–9**
  IgA, see immunoglobulin A (IgA)
    nephropathy
  infection-associated 3157, **3173–9**
  in malignant disease **3184–5**
  membranous, see membranous
    nephropathy
  metal **3260–3**
  minimal change, see minimal change
    nephropathy
  obstructive 3232
  occupational causes 1171
  quartan malarial **3177**
  reflux, see reflux nephropathy
  thin membrane 3149, **3152–3**
  toxic, see toxic nephropathy
  see also renal disease
nephrostomy, percutaneous
  drainage of obstructed tract 3243, 3244
  stone removal 3244
nephrotic syndrome **3138–44**
  of childhood 3141, 3142, 3144, 3154
    idiopathic 3154
    steroid-responsive 3154
  coagulation disorders in **3142**, 3144,
    3656–7
  complications and consequences
    3140–4
  in focal segmental glomerulosclerosis
    3156
  hyperlipidaemia in 1411, **3142–3**, 3144
  increased catabolism/loss of
    immunoglobulin 175
  investigations 3139–40, 3154
  in malaria 857
  in malignant disease 3184, 3185
  management 3140
  in membranous nephropathy 3158–9
  in mesangiocapillary glomerulonephritis
    3158
  minimal change, see minimal change
    nephropathy
  NSAID-induced 3224
  oedema in 3138, 3139, 3140
  pneumococcal infections 513
  in pregnancy **1734–5**
  progression of renal failure and 3144
  in sickle-cell disease 3195
  in SLE 3019
  syphilitic 711
  thromboembolism in **3141–2**, 3668,
    3682
  vitamin D deficiency in 1636, 3144

nephrotoxic agents **3265–6**, *3284*
  acute renal failure due to **3288–90**
    cisplatin 3263
    cyclosporin 2114, 2937, **3265–6**, 3319
    endogenous 3289–90
  see also drug(s), nephrotoxic; renal
    damage; toxic nephropathy
nephrotyphoid 562
Nernst equation 2148
nerve agents 1115, *1116*, **1117–18**
  carbamate anticholinesterase
    pretreatment 1118
  clinical features of exposure 1117–18,
    1118
  relative toxicities *1116*
  structural formulae 1117
  treatment 1118
  types 1117
nerve biopsy 4093
nerve blocks, in chronic benign pain, in
    terminal care 4352
nerve-compression syndromes
  in haemophilia 3647, 3649
  in Paget's disease 3075–6
  in pregnancy 1766
nerve conduction **3840**
  action potentials 3840
  F wave 3840
  peripheral 4091
  in polyneuropathy 3842
  velocity 3840
nerve fibres, anatomy 4091
nerve growth factor (NGF) receptor
    1560, 1561
nerve impulse transmission 4139
nerve roots, see spinal nerve roots
nerves
  compression, see nerve-compression
    syndromes
  Corynebacterium diphtheriae effect 494
  in leprosy 669, 671
nerve supply
  ear 3869
  nose 2610
  pulmonary blood vessels **2486**
nervous system
  age-related changes 4336
  developmental abnormalities, see
    developmental abnormalities
  endocrine interactions 1553
  in Kawasaki disease 3048
  lymphoma of 3583
  metabolic disorders **4123–4**
  in sarcoidosis **2826–7**
  skin diseases with 3718, *3720*
  in systemic sclerosis 3033
  teratogens, see teratogens
  see also central nervous system (CNS);
    entries beginning neurological;
    peripheral nervous system
nesidioblastosis 1511–12
Netherlands 38–9
netilmicin *3272*
  in brucellosis 623
  in urinary-tract infections *3211*
neu oncogene, T-cell response 229
neural cell adhesion molecule (NCAM)
    231, 2882
neuralgia
  glossopharyngeal 3880, 4023–4
  migrainous 4026
  postherpetic, see postherpetic neuralgia
  post-sympathectomy 2374
  trigeminal 345, **3878**, 4023–4
neuralgic amyotrophy **3903**, 4094
neural tube defects 4117
  antenatal screening 135, 1756
  folic acid supplements and 1759–60,
    1773, 3491
  see also anencephaly; spina bifida
neural tumours, posterior mediastinal
    masses 2900
neuraminidase 338
  bacterial, haemolytic uraemic syndrome
    and 3196
  inherited deficiencies 1434–5
neurasthenia, see chronic fatigue syndrome
neurenteric cyst 1976

neurilemoma, mediastinum 2901
neuritic plaques, in Alzheimer's disease
    1516
neuritis
  in leprosy 677–8
  optic, see optic neuritis
neuroacanthocytosis **4014**
neuroblastoma, mediastinum 2901
neurobrucellosis 622
neurocutaneous syndromes 3792, **3986–8**
neurocysticercosis 965, *965*
  diagnosis 966–7
  differential diagnosis 967, 968
  treatment 968
neurodermatitis 3745
neuroendocrine system
  response to injury **1548–9**
  stress response 1563–4
neuroendocrinology 1553
neurofibrillary tangles 1516, 3971, 3972
  distribution 3972
neurofibromata 3874–5
  mediastinal 2901
neurofibromatosis 3986–7
  acoustic schwannomas in 3874
  inheritance 114
  lung in 2651
  new mutations causing and mutation
    rate 114
  pigmentation in 3757
  scoliosis in 2873
  type I, see von Recklinghausen's
    disease
  type II (central) 3987
    eye features 4182
neurogenic flushing 3787
neurokinin 1894
neurokinin A 4023
neurolathyrism 4090
neuroleptic drugs
  adverse effects 1251
  drug interactions 4005
  extrapyramidal disease due to 4020
  in pain treatment 3945
  parkinsonism due to 3998, 4002
  see also antipsychotic drugs
neuroleptic malignant syndrome 1182,
    4242, 4252
  drugs associated 1182
  management 1182, 4252
  mechanism and mortality of 1182
neurolipidoses 3985
neurological cause, chest pain **2168**
neurological damage
  electrical injury 1214, 4129
  in lightning injury 1214–15
  ossification after 3093
neurological disability **3815**
neurological disorders/diseases **3815–16**,
    4129–36
  acute, in immunocompromised 1033–4,
    1034
  advances related to **3815–16**
  aircraft travel and 1202–3
  in chronic renal failure 3302
  clinical diagnosis 3815
  connective tissue diseases **4129–32**
  degenerative,
    central motor conduction time 3838
    dementia in *3966*
    epilepsy and 3917
    Parkinson's disease vs 4002
    somatosensory evoked potentials 3834
    visual evoked potential 3833
  dementia due to 3965, *3966*
  developmental, see developmental
    abnormalities
  enteroviruses causing 384–6, *385*
  epidemiology 3815, *3816*
  focal deficits,
    causes in pregnancy *1767*
    in intracranial tumours 4035–6
  in folate deficiency 3492
  gastrointestinal motility disorders
    associated 1962
  haematological changes **3686–7**
  in haemolytic uraemic syndrome 3198
  herpes simplex virus causing 345

history-taking 3815
in hypercalcaemia 1631–2
in hypertriglyceridaemia 1410
in hypocalcaemia 1633
in hyponatraemia 3123
infections, see central nervous system
    (CNS), infections
in infective endocarditis 2441
inflammatory eye disease in **4184**
inherited **3984–9**
in injecting drug abusers 4284
investigations **3816–45**
  see also electroencephalogram (EEG);
    neuroradiology
joint involvement **3006**
male hypogonadism in 1683
in malignancy **4133–5**
  non-metastatic **4134–5**
mental disorders/diseases and symptoms
    in **4236–8**
in metabolic disorders **4123–8**
in myeloma 3599
in neurosyphilis 4085
occupational **1169**, *1170*
  physical factors causing 1169
paraneoplastic *243*
in phosphoribosyl pyrophosphate
    synthetase (PPRPS) overactivity
    1383
physical agents causing **4128–9**
positive-pressure ventilation indications
    2576–7
in pregnancy **1766–9**
in pyruvate carboxylase deficiency 1352
in pyruvate dehydrogenase deficiency
    1351
sexual problems in 4244
in sickle-cell disease 3514–15
in systemic diseases **4129–36**
vascular, dementia in *3966*
in Wilson's disease 1420, 1421
neurological examination 3815
neurological signs
  in legs *2994*
  in poisoning 1046
neurological symptoms, in rheumatic
    diseases 2945
neurological toxicity, see neurotoxicity
neurolysis, peripheral 3945
neuroma, mucosal, in MEN 2B
    syndrome 1709–10
neuromuscular blocking agents, in renal
    impairment 3270
neuromuscular disorders
  cardiac manifestations **2392**, *2393*
  see also muscular dystrophies
neuromuscular junction 4139, 4141
neuromuscular transmission 4139, 4160
neuromuscular transmission disorders
    4160–5
  acquired neuromyotonia 4164
  congenital/hereditary myasthenia **4164**
    see also Lambert-Eaton myasthenic
      syndrome; myasthenia gravis
neuromyopathies, in lung cancer 2884
neuromyositis **4158**
neuromyotonia 4142, 4151
  acquired **4164**
neuronal ceroid lipofuscinosis 3985–6
neuronal degeneration, in kuru 3983
neuronal loss
  age-related 4336
  in Alzheimer's disease 3972
neuronitis, vestibular 3876
neuronopathy 4091
  monomelic/focal/segmental motor 4089
  multifocal motor 4089–90
  proximal hereditary motor 4089
  X-linked recessive bulbospinal
    (Kennedy syndrome) 3988, 4089
neuropathic bladder 4118
neuropathic disease, gastrointestinal
    1896
neuropathic joints, see Charcot's
    (neuropathic) joints
neuropathic tremor 4092
neuropathy
  in acute porphyria 1391–2, 1393, 4102

neuropathy (*cont.*)
  alcoholic 4100
  carcinomatous 4102
    classification 2884
    in lung cancer 2884
  clinical categories 4092
  cryptogenic 4104
  diabetic, *see* diabetic neuropathy
  diagnosis and investigations 4092–3
  diffuse 1963
  diffuse axonal sensorimotor, in AIDS
    4078
  in diphtheria 4091, 4101–2
  distal, in thallium poisoning 1113,
    4099–100
  distal autonomic *3882*, **3886**
  folate deficiency 3492
  genetic **4102–4**
  hereditary motor and sensory **4102–4**
  inflammatory, in HIV infection 4076,
    4101
  ischaemic optic 3867
  multifocal motor 4088, 4089–90, 4092
  non-metastatic, in leukaemia 4135
  occupational 1169, *1170*, 4099–100
  paraproteinaemic **4102**
  peripheral, *see* peripheral neuropathy
  in pregnancy 1766, 1767
  in rheumatoid arthritis 2961–2
  symptoms 4092
  toxic **4099–100**
  uraemic 4099
  vibration-induced 1169
  vitamin B$_{12}$ **3490–1**, 3496, 4100–1
  see also peripheral neuropathy;
    polyneuropathy
neuropeptides, in mucociliary escalator
  2613
neuropeptide Y **1893**
  in heart 2160
  phaeochromocytomas secreting 2554
neurophysin, mutations *1567*, 1571
neuropil threads 3972
neuropsychiatric problems, in carbon
  monoxide poisoning 1096
neuropsychological disorders,
  occupational **1174**
neuroradiology **3816–28**
  intracranial disorders **3816–26**
    brain scanning 3825
    cerebral angiography 3822
    computed tomography 3817–19
    digital fluorography 3822
    interventional procedures 3822–5
    magnetic resonance imaging 3819–22
    plain films 3816–17
    pneumoencephalography 3826
    ultrasound 3826
    ventriculography 3826
  spinal disorders **3826–8**
  see also computed tomography (CT);
    magnetic resonance imaging (MRI)
neurosarcoma 2901
neuroses, in elderly 4228
neurosurgery, monitoring, magnetic brain
  stimulation 3838–9
neurosyphilis **4083–7**
  in AIDS 4079, 4084
  asymptomatic 714, 4084
  clinical features/course 4084–5
  diagnosis 716
  epidemiology 4083–4
  general paralysis of the insane 708,
    4085
  Jarisch–Herxheimer reaction in 719
  laboratory diagnosis 4085–6
  meningeal and vascular 3848, 4084–5
  mental disorders/symptoms 4236
  neuro-ophthalmological features 4085
  tabes dorsalis 4085
  treatment 4086
neurotensin 1894
  in coeliac disease 1895
  in pancreatic endocrine tumours 1707
neurotic illness, in aircraft crew and
  pilots 1201
neurotoxic araneism 1148
neurotoxic envenoming, snake bites,
  management 1138

neurotoxicity
  cytotoxic drugs 3575
  of drugs in AIDS **4080**
neurotoxic syndromes
  from seafood 1142
  serotonin 4250
neurotoxins 2001
  aluminium as 1105
  in snake venom 1129
neurotransmitters in Alzheimer's disease
  3972
  autonomic nervous system 3881–2
  in Huntington's disease 4013, *4013*
  in primary sensory neurones 3937–8
  in vomiting 1821
neurovascular dystrophy 3941
neutral endopeptidase inhibitors **2252**
  in heart failure 2240, **2252**
neutron activation analysis, body fat
  measurement 1303
neutron radiation 255, 1217, 1218
neutropenia 178, 3378, *3448*, **3557–8**
  acquired 3558
  acute neurological syndromes in 1033,
    1034
  in alcoholism 3685
  bacteraemia in 1030
  in bacterial infections 3679
  cyclic 3557–8
  fever of unknown origin (FUO) *1016*,
    1017–18, 1030–1
  in HIV infection 471, 3680
  in infections 267, 1029, 1030
    general approach to 1029
  inherited 3557
  in myelodysplastic syndromes 3426
  oral ulceration in 1855
  respiratory tract infections 2709
  septicaemia in 1022
neutrophilia 3557
  in infections 267, 3678
neutrophils **3555**
  abnormal, in myelodysplastic
    syndromes 3426
  activation **2621–2**, 2854
    antineutrophil cytoplasmic antibodies
      (ANCA) role 3012
    shape change 2622
  in acute meningococcaemia 538
  adhesion, ANCA role 3012
  in adult respiratory distress syndrome
    2854–5
  in allergic disease 159
  apoptosis 2625–6
  bacterial meningitis pathogenesis 4052
  chemotactic factors 159, 1945, 2615,
    2618–19
  chemotaxis **2621–2**
  circulating pool 2615
  contents and products 2622–3, *2624*,
    2854
  counts *3379*, *3380*
    after snake bites 1135
    in paroxysmal nocturnal
      haemoglobinuria 3451
  in cryptogenic fibrosing alveolitis
    2788–9
  cytokines released 2622, *2624*, 2854
  defects 178
  degranulation **2622–3**, *2624*, 2854
    in diabetes mellitus 1493
  disorders 3559, 3560
  elastase 2626, 2763, 2769–70
    in acute pancreatitis 2030, 2031
    in adult respiratory distress syndrome
      2854
    in chronic obstructive airways disease
      2769–70, 2771
    in cryptogenic fibrosing alveolitis 2788
  fibrinolysis and 3626
  increased levels 2772
  emigration from capillaries **2618–21**,
    3559
    adhesion molecules 2619–21, *2620*
    adhesion and sequestration 2619–21
    cessation 2624
    transmigration 2621
    triggers 2618

endothelial cell binding 2619, 2620,
    3558–9
    adhesion molecules 2619–21, *2620*
    harmful inflammatory effects 2626
    two-stage model 2620
  endothelial cell interactions 3558–9
    pulmonary 2487, 2619–21
  extravasated, clearance 2625–6
  in Felty syndrome 2962
  fetal 1784
  function,
    in bronchiectasis 2759, 2763
    state in tissues **2622**
    tests 2759
  haemolytic uraemic syndrome and 3199
  high permeability pulmonary oedema
    mechanism 2497–8
  in hypereosinophilic syndrome 3612
  inactivators, inhibition by ANCA 3012
  indium-labelled 1941
  in infections 276–7
  injury due to 2626, 2763
    in adult respiratory distress syndrome
      2854–5
    in bronchiectasis 2763
    in chronic obstructive airways disease
      2770–3
    in emphysema 2769–70
  leukotriene B$_4$ release 159
  in lung inflammation 2618
  modulation therapy, in bronchiectasis
    2766
  morphological variations 3556
  NA antigens, transfusion reactions 3692
  non-specific response to infections
    276–7
  oxidative killing 3559–60
  phagocytosis **2621–2**, 3559–60
    killing 3559–60
    mechanism **2622–3**
  platelet interactions 3627
  in pneumococcal infections 513, 514,
    517
    meningitis 518
    pneumonia 515
  production 3384, 3386, 3556–7
  pulmonary marginated pool **2615–16**
  secretory behaviour, control 2625
  transfusion 284
  in ulcerative colitis 1945
newborn infants, *see* neonates
newts, poisonous 1140
New World screw-worm 1000, 1001
New York Heart Association scale *2358*
  breathlessness 2162, *2163*
New Zealand Black/White mice 3024
NF1 mutation 108
NFKB 2294
niacin, *see* nicotinic acid
nickel 1112
  absorption and excretion 1112
  contact dermatitis due to 3738
  lung cancer association 207
  nasal sinus/nose cancers and 205
  poisoning **1112–13**
    levels in finger nails 1112–13
  refining, lung cancer and 2880
  sensitivity, food sensitivity in 3729
  uses and compounds 1112
nickel carbonyl 1112
  'nickel-itch' 1112
nickel sulphate, ingestion 1112
nick translation 60
niclosamide 961, 993
nicorandil 2330
nicotinamide, in Hartnup disease 3333
nicotinamide-adenine dinucleotides, *see*
  NADH; NADP; NADPH
nicotine 4263
  withdrawal syndrome 4293
nicotine-like actions, poisonous plants
  1152, *1155*
nicotinic acid
  deficiency 3498
    mental symptoms 4241
    skin in 3722
  in hyperlipoproteinaemia 1414, *3143*
  ischaemic heart disease risk 2312

provocation test 2057
  reference nutrient intake (RNI) 1268,
    1269
nicotinic effect 3881
Niemann–Pick disease **1427**, *1428*, 2862
  liver in *2019*, 2024–5
  lung disease in 2862
  neurological features 3985
  splenomegaly in 3591
NIF-1 and NIF-2 factors 79
nifedipine 2258, 2330
  in acute mountain sickness 1191
  in pre-eclampsia 1731
  in pregnancy 1740
  in SLE 3023
  in urticaria 3772
  in vasospastic disorders 2374
nifurtimox, in Chagas' disease 898
Nigerian ataxic neuropathy 4100
night sweats, *see* sweating, nocturnal
night terrors 3919
nigrostriatal pathway 3862
NIH3T3 cell transformation assay 195
Nijmegen breakage syndrome 173
nimodipine 2329
nipple, eczema 3741
Niridazole 979
nitrates **2247**, **2326–8**, *3546*
  buccal 2327
  disadvantages 2327
  drugs included 1067
  excretion, in oedematous malnutrition
    1288
  gastric cancer aetiology 1982
  in heart failure 2248
  intravenous 2327, 2330
  mechanism of action 1067, 2247,
    2326–7
  methaemoglobinaemia and 3520
  in myocardial infarction 2344
  oral 2327, 2344
  overdose/poisoning **1067**
  side-effects 2327, 2344
  sublingual 2327, 2344
  tolerance 2327–8
  transdermal (patches) 2327
  urinary 3102
  see also glyceryl trinitrate
nitrazepam, in epilepsy 3922
nitric oxide (NO) 2147, 2159, **2297–8**,
    3627, 3662
  actions 2297, 2298, 2323
    mechanism and second messenger
      2297
  air pollution 1229
  coronary vasodilatation 2159–60, 2297
  inhaled 2922
    in adult respiratory distress syndrome
      2576, 2860
    in cor pulmonale 2521
    monitoring 2860
  in leucocyte killing 3560
  loss, vasoconstriction 2297
  overproduction 2297
  plasminogen activator interaction 2298
  platelet action and 2298
  reduced production 2297, 2298, 2514
  secretion, TNF action 537
  in sodium nitroprusside overdose 1067
  storage 2860
  suppression, in hypoxic pulmonary
    vasoconstriction 2492
  synthesis 2159–60, 2297
    endothelial cells 2290, 2296, 2323,
      2487, 2514, 2516
    inhibition 2297
    macrophage 2291
    stimuli 2297
  in veins 2296–7
nitric oxide (NO) synthase 94, 2159–60,
    2297, 3560, 3627
  inhibitors 2297
nitrites, methaemoglobinaemia and 3520,
    3546
nitrobenzene derivatives *3546*
nitroblue tetrazolium 2122
  slide test 3560

nitrocefin test 549
nitrofurantoin
  adverse reaction 2851
  neuropathy due to 4100
  in pregnancy 1733, 1785
  in urinary-tract infections 3209, *3211*,
    3213
nitrogen
  antimicrobial killing mechanisms 93, 94
  balance 1354
    after injury/surgery **1549–50**
    artificial nutritional support 1316–17
    in chronic renal failure 3302–3
    negative 241, 1317
    peritoneal dialysis and 3311–12
    in tumours 241
  faecal 1907
  intake, in catabolic state 1317
  liquid 3798
  losses, assessment in intensive care
    2587
  narcosis 1207
  requirements in catabolic states *2587*
  urine 1275, 1276
nitrogen dioxide 1100
  air pollution 1229, 1230, 1231
  exposure/inhalation 2847
  poisoning/toxicity **1100–1**
    characteristics *2815*
nitrogen mustard, *see* mustine
nitroimidazole compounds
  in amoebiasis 831
  in trichomoniasis 908, 3354
nitroprusside, *see* sodium nitroprusside
nitrosamines 1887
  gastric cancer aetiology 203, 1982
  nasopharyngeal carcinoma pathogenesis
    356
nitroso compounds, diabetes type I and
    1454
nitrosoureas, side-effects 248
nitrotoluene TNT arsine *3546*
nitrous oxide
  air pollution 1229
  exposure 3490–1, **3497**
nitrovasodilators 2300
  see also glyceryl trinitrate
'nits' 1003, 3744
nizatidine, overdose/poisoning 1070
njovera 706
L-NMMA, nitric oxide synthesis
    inhibition 2297
NMR spectroscopy, fatigue
    pathophysiology 2172
Nocardia 686
  in HIV infections 487, 686
Nocardia asteroides 686, 2708
  infections in heart-lung transplants 2709
Nocardia brasiliensis 686, 802
nocardiosis **686–7**
  disseminated 686–7
  in immunocompromised 686
nociception, peripheral mechanisms **3936**
nocturia
  in chronic renal failure 3147, 3296, 3300
  definition 3101
  in essential hypertension 2535
nocturnal myoclonus syndrome,
    narcolepsy *vs* 3929
nodes of Ranvier 3990
nodular lymphoid hyperplasia 878–9,
    1839, 1910, 1987
nodular prurigo 3745
nodulectomy, in onchocerciasis 917
nodules 3713, *3713*
  in cutaneous leishmaniasis 901, 902
  juxta-articular *3716*
  in onchocerciasis 913
  see also subcutaneous nodules
noise **1223–5**
  cardiovascular effects 1171
  effect on hearing **1223–4**
  exposure control 1164
  exposure expressions 1223
  hearing loss due to 1224, **1225**
  non-auditory effects **1225**
  see also sound
noma (cancrum oris) 1853

nomifensine 3543
non-alcohol steatotic hepatitis syndrome
    (NASH) 2128
non-compliance, in epilepsy 3923
non-disjunction 119, 121, 128
non-gonococcal urethritis, *see* urethritis
non-Hodgkin's lymphoma (NHL) 3568,
    3576–85
  aetiology and pathogenesis 214, 3576
  after cardiac transplantation 2258
  in AIDS, *see* AIDS and HIV infection
  B-cell 3568, *3578*, **3579–81**, 3794
    clonality 3567
    cutaneous, clinical features 3796
    endemic (African) Burkitt, *see*
      Burkitt's lymphoma
    gastric 1984–5
    high-grade 3580–1
    in HIV infection 477
    leukaemic phase *3420*, **3423–4**
    low-grade 3579–80
    small bowel 1985, 1986
  chronic lymphocytic leukaemia
    evolving into 3422
  classification 3576–9
  clinical/pathological features 3579–83
    computed tomography 238
  diagnosis, CD20 245
  epidemiology 213–14
  hepatic granulomas in 2122
  in HIV infection, *see* AIDS and HIV
    infection
  Kiel classification 3578–9
  liver in 2133
  lung involvement 2690
  management 3583–5
  ocular features 4195
  in pregnancy 1808
  primary extranodal 3582–3
  primary upper small-intestinal (PUSIL),
    epidemiology 214
  prognosis 3585
  pulmonary 2808
  REAL classification *3578*, 3579
  skin manifestations **3794–7**
  small bowel 1985–6
  staging 247, 3583
  T-cell 3568, *3578*, **3581–2**, 3794
    in angio-immunoblastic
      (immunoblastic) lymphadenopathy
      2807
    clonality 3567
    in coeliac disease 1920, 1929
    enteropathy-associated, *see*
      enteropathy-associated T-cell
      lymphoma (EATL)
    Epstein-Barr virus (EBV) role 355–6
    high-grade 3582
    leukaemic phase **3424**
    low-grade 3581–2
    lymphomatoid granulomatosis as 2807
    small bowel 1985–6, 1986
  working formulation *3577*, 3578
non-obese diabetes (NOD) mouse 64,
    1453
non-polyposis colorectal cancer 107,
    223, 1990
non-specific cross-reacting antigen
    (NCA) 230
non-starch polysaccharides
  deficiency,
    cancer association 219
    constipation association 1328
    diverticular disease of colon 1328–9
    irritable bowel syndrome 1328
  in diabetes 1465–6
  in hypercholesterolaemia 1412
  see also dietary fibre
non-steroidal anti-inflammatory drugs
    (NSAIDs)
  in adult respiratory distress syndrome
    2860
  adverse effects 2964
  aplastic anaemia induced by 3441, 3442
  asthma association 2735
  chemical groupings *2964*
  in cystic fibrosis 2749
  drug-induced asthma 2849

duodenal ulcers associated 1888
gastric ulcer aetiology 1879
  in gout 2987
  hyperkalaemia due to 3134
  lithium interaction 4251
  in nephrotic syndrome 3140
  nephrotoxicity 3193, **3223–4**, 3266,
    3284
  nocturnal suppositories 2964
  overdose/poisoning **1056–8**
    clinical features 1056, *1057*
    management 1057–8
  in pain treatment 3944–5
  in renal failure 3274, 3288
  renal tubular acidosis due to 3341
  in rheumatoid arthritis 2963
  in sarcoidosis 2832
  in SLE 3023
  in sports-related soft-tissue trauma 4321
  uricosuric 2987–8
  vasoconstriction 2297
  see also anti-inflammatory drugs
no observable effect level (NOEL) 1228
Noonan's syndrome 2419, 2557
Nopp140 protein 79
noradrenaline 2253, **2254**, 3881–2
  in carcinoid tumours 1898
  clinical use 2254
  depletion 3885
    in multiple system atrophy 4006
    in Parkinson's disease 4000
  doses *2254*
  in heart 2160
  mechanism of action 2254, 3882
  in pain perception 3938
  phaeochromocytoma releasing 2553–4,
    2554
  in poisoning management 1063, 1066
  receptors *2254*, 3882
  release and re-uptake 2253, 3882
  in septicaemia 2573
  storage 2253, 3882
  synthesis 2553, 3925
  tilt effect 3885
  uptake inhibition,
    by lofepramine 4248
    by tricyclic antidepressants 4247
norepinephrine, *see* noradrenaline
norethisterone *1814*
norfloxacin, in urinary-tract infections
    3211, 3213
norgestrol *1814*
normal pressure hydrocephalus 3969–70
normal range 4363
'normal results', concept 4363
normetanephrine 2554
normoblast 3453, 3454
North Asian tick typhus *729*
Northwick Park Heart Study 2301, 2309
Norton pressure sore score 3811
  Norwalk virus 391, *391*, *392*, 2002
Norwegian scabies 1008, 1009
nose (nasal) **2609–10**
  blood supply 2609–10
  cancer, epidemiology 205
  deformity, in rhinoscleroma 569
  function **2609–10**, 2612, 2613
  granulomas in 2801, 3799, 3802
  granulomatous disease 3799, 3800, *3801*
  irritation 2610
  mucosa, in sarcoidosis 2826
  mucosal congestion 2609, 2610
  nerve supply 2610
  obstruction, in allergic rhinitis 2716
  polyps 160
  resistance 2609
  in sarcoidosis 2826, 2827
  structure **2609–10**
  see also entries beginning nasal
Nosema connori 884
nosocomial infections **327–31**
  bacteraemia 331
  causative agents 329
  coagulase-negative staphylococci 531
  cryptosporidiosis 874
  cytomegalovirus (CMV) 360
  fever and pulmonary infiltrates due to
    1032

fever of unknown origin (FUO) *1015*,
    1017, 1019
  historical aspects 328
  HIV 472
  host factors 329
  intravascular device-associated 330
  legionellosis 724
  listeriosis 514
  measles 376
  miscellaneous 331
  mortality 328, *328*
  outbreaks 329
  pneumonia 330, *330*, 1021–2, **2701–2**
  principles of control **329–31**
  prosthetic device-related 330
  rare and 'newer' organisms 778
  scale and cost 328, *328*
  by site 329–31
  surgical wounds 329–30
  urinary tract 329, *329*
notification
  addiction **4288–9**, 4297
  disease **4288–9**
  infections 286–7, 289, 2006
  tuberculosis 644–6
NSAIDs, *see* non-steroidal anti-
    inflammatory drugs
NSF (NEM-sensitive factor) 75, 80
  attachment factors (SNAPs) 75
  cDNA sequence and functions 75
nuclear antigens, autoantibodies to 163–4
nuclear emergencies **1234**
nuclear envelope 78, 80
  assembly 80
nuclear imaging, *see* scintigraphy
nuclear installations 3410–11
nuclear localization signal (NLS) 78–9
  receptors for 79
  structures/motifs 79
nuclear localization signal (NLS)-binding
    protein 79
nuclear oncogenes, *see* oncogenes,
    nuclear
nuclear pores 78
  complex 80
  computational reconstruction 80
  role in active transport and passive
    diffusion 80
  structural asymmetry 80
nuclear proteins, autoantibodies to 163
nuclear reactors 1217, 1234
nuclear weapons 1219, 1220
nucleolus 79
nucleoplasmin 78
nucleoside analogues, in chronic
    lymphocytic leukaemia 3421–2
nucleoside phosphorylase 1378
5'-nucleotidase 1378, 2486
  deficiency 1386
  serum levels 2055
nucleotide bases 57
  metabolism of *Plasmodium* species 837
nucleus 68, **78–80**
  functions 79
  in myocardial cells 2145
  nuclear retention of proteins 79
  protein entry into 78–9
    import requirements 79
    receptor for nuclear localization signal
      79
  regulation of transport 79–80
  influenza virus 79
  RNA transport from 78, 79
nucleus accumbens, in Parkinson's
    disease 4000
nucleus basalis of Meynert 3972
nucleus parabrachialis medialis 3887
nucleus pulposus 2992
nucleus retroambigualis 3887, 3888
nucleus tractus solitarius 3887, 3888
numerical skills 3851–2
  in dementia assessment 3969
nurse counsellor 4254
nursing, safety after deliberate self-harm
    4230
nutrients
  absorption, *see* intestinal absorption
  bioactive molecules 1267

nutrients (*cont.*)
  food groups *1331*
  intracellular metabolism 1900
    malnutrition management 1289, *1291*
  requirements **1268–9**
    criteria for adequacy 1268
    increased in disease 1268
    long-term 1270–1
    reduction, in malnutrition
      pathophysiology 1285
    see also under nutritional support
  transport 1900
  see also individual nutrients
nutrition **1267–332**, 1278
  in acute pancreatitis 2033
  in acute porphyria 1392
  in acute renal failure **3287–8**
  advances in 1267
  alcoholic liver disease and 2081
  biochemical basis **1271–8**
  bone mass and 3057
  in chronic obstructive airways disease
    2776
  in chronic respiratory failure
    management 2929
  diets preventing disease 1267
  fetal, diabetes in adult life and 1450,
    1455
  filarial infections and 911
  guidelines *1332*
  hypertension pathogenesis 2530
  importance of 1267
  infections and impaired immunity
    relationship 282, 294
  ischaemic heart disease risk **2309–12**
  modern views on 1267–8
  perioperative 1323–4
  peritoneal dialysis and 3311–12
  in pregnancy **1769–74**
    congenital abnormalities and 1773–4
    dietary intake 1770, *1772*
    dietary supplements 1773, *1774*
    metabolic adaptations 1770–1
    outcome of pregnancy and 1771–3
    physiology 1770
    pre-eclampsia and 1773
  problems **1314–26**
  in prolonged infections 294
  in terminal illness **4359–60**
  in tetanus 629
  see also diet; food
nutritional assessment **1314–15**
  clinical and dietary history 1314
  clinical examination 1314–15
  in intensive care 2586–7
  in malabsorption 1910
nutritional deficiency **1279–80**
  assessing probability 1268
  in Crohn's disease 1938
  in malabsorption 1904
  in malnutrition, management
    1295
  signs 1315, *1315*
  syndrome, in alcohol abuse 4277–8
  tropical enteropathy aetiology 1931
  in tropical sprue 1933
  type I (iron-like) 1279, *1279*
    characteristics 1279, *1279*
  type II (zinc-like) 1279, *1279*
    anorexia in 1280
    'catch-up' growth 1280
    characteristics 1279, *1279*
    diagnostic problems/methods 1280
    metabolic changes/adaptations 1280
    nutrient conservation mechanisms
      1280
    response to deficiency 1279
  see also malnutrition
nutritional disease 1270
  of affluent societies 1267
  multifactorial aetiology 1267
  myopathy in **4169**
  visual evoked potentials 3833
nutritional dwarfism 1281
  clinical features 1282, 1283
nutritional osteomalacia **3073**
nutritional supplements, *see* dietary
  supplements

nutritional support
  in chronic idiopathic intestinal pseudo-
    obstruction 1960
  complications **1319–22**
    costs 1326
    enteral feeding 1321–2
    parenteral feeding 1319–21
  cystic fibrosis 2751
  enteral, *see* enteral feeding
  ethical considerations 1325
  at home 1321, **1324–5**
    advantages 1324
    age distribution 1324
    indications 1324
    management 1324–5
  indications **1315–16**, *1316*
  intensive care **2586–8**
  monitoring 1322, 1325
  nutritional requirements **1316–19**
    fluid 1317–18
    minerals and trace elements 1318
    protein and energy 1316–17, 2587, *2587*
    vitamins 1318–19
    see also nutrients, requirements
  outcome **1325**
  parenteral, *see* parenteral nutrition
  role of teams in management **1325–6**,
    1325
  specific conditions/situations **1322–4**
  timing and route, in intensive care 2587
  see also dietary supplements; parenteral
    nutrition
nutrition team 1325–6, *1325*
nuts, allergy to 162
Nyando virus 429
nystagmus 2583, **3871–4**
  in acoustic schwannomas 3874
  benign positional 3873
  central positional 3873
  clockwise/counterclockwise 3873
  directional preponderance 3874
  in Friedreich's ataxia 3984
  gaze-evoked 3872
  horizontal, significance 3872
  optokinetic 3874
  positional and positioning 3873, *3873*
  retraction 2583
  spontaneous 3871
  tests 3873–4
  vertical 3873
    up-beat/down-beat 3873
  vestibular 3872
nystatin 811, 812
  in oral candidiasis 1852

O

oatbran 2312
oat-cell carcinoma, *see* lung cancer,
  small-cell
obesity **1301–14**, 1400
  in adolescent diabetics 1497
  aetiology **1306–8**, 1328
  in benign intracranial hypertension
    4041
  central 2309, 2530
  clinical history 1309–11, *1310*
  in Cushing's syndrome 1643, 1645
  definition, operational 1302
  diseases associated 1308
    breast cancer 209
    diabetes 1308, 1327, 1450, *1451*,
      1455, 1468, 1472
    gallbladder cancer 204
    gout 1381
    hypertension 2530
    ischaemic heart disease 2309
    osteoarthritis 2976, 4335
    polycystic ovary syndrome 1674, 1675
    venous thromboembolism 3676
  examination in lung disease 2650
  genetic predisposition 1307, *1307*
  hyperlipidaemia in 1408, 1411
  hyperuricaemia and 1381
  index, obstructive sleep apnoea and
    2910

insulin receptor down-regulation 1462
  mechanisms for causation of disease
    1308–9
    alcohol/smoking as confounding
      factors 1309
  mortality/morbidity relationship **1301–5**
    weight loss effect 1309
  neck 2910
  overweight relationship 1302–5
    prevalence **1305–6**, *1307*, 1313
    social factors associated 1307–8, 1309
  treatment **1309–13**
    clinical history relevant to 1309–11,
      1310
    decreasing energy intake 1312
    'dieting relationship trap' 1310–11
    drugs influencing 1310
    drug therapy 1312
    flow chart for strategy selection 1313
    increasing energy output 1311–12
    maintenance of weight loss 1313
    patient/therapist's expectations 1309
    strategies matched to degree of 1311,
      1311
    surgical 1312–13
    see also dieting
  truncal 2650
  weight loss, effect on mortality/
    morbidity 1309
  see also fat, body; overweight
obesity-hypoventilation syndrome,
  treatment 2520
obidoxime 1122
object naming 3848
obliterative bronchiolitis, *see*
  bronchiolitis obliterans
observational studies 44–5
obsessional personality trait 4211–12
  weight cycling and 1309
obsessional thoughts 4207
obsessive compulsive disorder **4207**
  differential diagnosis 4207
  features and aetiology 4207
  in Gilles de la Tourette syndrome 4016
  treatment 4207, 4253–4
    response prevention therapy 4255
obstetric complications, drug abuse and
  4298
obstructive airways disease, *see* airways;
  chronic obstructive airways disease
obstructive nephropathy 3232
obstructive sleep apnoea 2905, **2909–826**
  in acromegaly 1592
  aetiology 2909–10
    anatomical 2910
    neuromuscular function 2909–10
    provoking factors 2910
  androgen therapy and 1684
  case history 2913
  categories of patients 2913–14, *2913*
  cor pulmonale in 2927
  definition 2909
  diagnosis 2913–14, *2913*
  epidemiology 2914
  immediate consequences **2910–12**
    hypoxaemia/hypercapnia 2910–11
  in obesity 2910
  prognosis and complications 2914–16
  symptoms and presentation 2912–13,
    2913
  treatment 2905, 2914, *2914*, 2932
    ventilatory failure in 2905
obstructive uropathy 3232
  in gout 2986
  infectious causes 3179
  in malignant disease 3183–4
  in sarcoidosis 3187
  in schistosomiasis 977
  see also urinary-tract obstruction
obturator nerve **4097**
occipital lobe
  behavioural defects associated *3846*
  infarction, visual field change 4180
  lesions **3869**
    ischaemic 3869
    tumours, mental disorders/symptoms in
      4237

occupational cancer 216, *217*, **1165–7**
  agents/processes causing 1166–7, *1167*
    industrial processes 1167, *1167*
    see also specific chemicals
  bladder cancer 211, 212, 1166, 1167
  diagnosis 1166
  historical background 1165–6
  liver cancer 204, 1167
  lung cancer 206, 1167, 2880, *2880*
  nasal sinus and nose cancers 205, 1167
  occupational hazard association 216,
    217
    attribution to cause 1166
    confounding factors 216
    suspicions over and safety aspects 216
  pleural and peritoneal tumours 207
occupational disease/hazards **1164–74**
  anthrax 614, 618–19
  asthma, *see* asthma, occupational
  atopic eczema and 3741
  cancer, *see* occupational cancer
  cardiovascular **1169–71**
  chemical hazards, *see* poisoning, by
    chemicals
  compensation 1162
  contact dermatitis 3738
  coronary artery disease and **2356–62**
  cramps 4018–19
  dermatology **1164–5**
    see also dermatosis
  diffuse parenchymal lung disease 2781
  extrinsic allergic alveolitis, *see* extrinsic
    allergic alveolitis
  farmer's lung, *see* extrinsic allergic
    alveolitis
  gastrointestinal **1171–2**
  genitourinary **1171**
  glanders 593
  haemopoietic system **1172–3**
  hazard identification and risk
    assessment 1178
  health surveillance 1162
  history 266, 1161
  infections 266, **1173**
    Q fever 742
    streptococcal 500, 503
  investigation **1162–4**
    clinical/biological monitoring 1162–3
    difficulties of monitoring 1162–3
    exposure assessment 1163
    exposure control 1164
    threshold/exposure limits 1163
    workplace exposure/control 1163–4
  lead poisoning 3261
  listeriosis 514
  musculoskeletal **1168–9**
    see also rheumatic diseases
  myelomatosis 3597
  neurological **1169**, *1170*
  neuropsychological **1174**
  perennial allergic rhinitis 2715
  pneumoconioses, *see* pneumoconioses
  prevention 1161–2
  recognition and national lists 1161–2
  reproductive system **1173–4**
  toxic neuropathies **4099–100**
  urinary stones 3251
  vibration 1225–6, 1227
  see also occupational cancer; *other*
    cancers/chemicals
occupational exposure limit (OEL) 1163
occupational exposure standards (OES)
  1163
occupational health **1160–80**
  definition and scope 1160
  services 1161
  surveillance 1162
occupational history 1161
  in infections 266
  in lung disease 2649
occupational hygiene 1163
occupational medicine **2356–7**
occupational physician 1162, 1163
occupational safety **1174–80**
  accident causation 1175, *1175*, 1177–8
  active/latent failures 1177
  multicausality 1177

proactive safety management and 1177–8
shortcomings of safety management 1176
skill-, rule- and knowledge-base errors 1177–8
accidents 1174, *1175*
  nature of fatal/non-fatal injuries 1175–6, *1176*
  reportable 1175
hazard identification and risk assessment 1178
monitoring safety performance 1179
Robens Committee report 1177
safety auditing 1179
safety culture 1178
  characteristics of organizations 1179
  working definition 1178
safety management 1175
  aims 1178
  evolution of and law 1176–7
  key functions 1178
  proactive 1177–8
  safety culture and 1178
  shortcomings/merits 1176
safety training 1179–80
self-regulation 1177
size of problem in UK 1175–6
ochratoxins 1158, 3230
Ochrobactrum anthropi 558
ochronosis 3085
  see also alkaptonuria
octopuses, venomous 1144
octreotide (somatostatin analogue) 1895
  in acromegaly 1594
  in bleeding oesophageal varices 2094
  in carcinoid syndrome 1898
  in chronic pancreatitis 2038
  in ectopic ACTH syndrome 1714
  in hypercalcaemia 3229
  in insulinoma 1508, 1509
  in pancreatic endocrine tumours 1705, 1706
  scanning 1898
ocular bobbing 2583
ocular disease, *see under* eye
ocular fundus, in unconscious patients 2585
ocular gnathostomiasis 952
ocular infections, *see under* eye
ocular ischaemia, chronic **4187**
ocular larva migrans 945
ocular muscular dystrophy **4148**
ocular myasthenia 4161, 4162
ocular pressure, in thyroid disorders 4196
ocular reticulum cell sarcoma 4195
ocular toxoplasmosis 866
oculocardiac reflex 3925
oculocephalic responses 2583
oculocerebrorenal syndrome of Lowe 1355
oculocervical responses, in poisoning 1046
oculoglandular tularaemia 600–1
oculomotor nuclear region lesions, pupillary responses 2582
oculomotor (third cranial) nerve, lesions, *see* cranial nerves, third
oculomucocutaneous syndrome 2852
oculomycosis **811**
oculopharyngeal muscular dystrophy **4148**
oculovestibular responses, in poisoning 1046
odontoid peg 2959
  separation from arch of atlas 2959
odontoid process, metastases in 241
odontomes 1863
odynophagia 1819, **1820**
oedema 2560
  acute airways obstruction in 2721–2
  in anthrax 615, 616
  cardiac 2238
  in chronic hypoxia 2902
  in chronic obstructive airways disease 2777
  in chronic renal failure 3297

in cor pulmonale 2517, 2518
  dependent, in ascites 2095
drug prescribing in renal impairment 3273
  in electrical injury 1213
  familial (Milroy's disease) 2560
  in gnathostomiasis 951
  in heart failure, *see under* heart failure
  at high altitude 1192
  idiopathic (cyclical; periodic), of women **3126–7**
  insulin 1477
  intestinal 2240
  in malnutrition 1282, 1284
    classification systems and 1281, *1281*
    management 1289
    see also malnutrition
  in nephrotic syndrome 3138, 3139, 3140
  pitting 1282
  pulmonary, *see* pulmonary oedema
  resistant 2239–40, 2240
  in small-intestinal lymphangiectasia 1977
oedematous malnutrition, *see* malnutrition, oedematous
Oerskovia, rare species *558*
oesophageal balloon 1869, 2094
oesophageal-body peristalsis, disorders 1871
oesophageal carcinoma
  in achalasia 1869
  adenocarcinoma 1875, 1980, 1981
  aetiological factors 202, 1874, 1875, 1980–1
  after caustic ingestion 1873, 1981
  clinical features 1874, 1981
  epidemiology 202, 1980–1
    sex relationship 198
  in gastro-oesophageal reflux disease 1866
  inoperable 1981, 1982
  investigations and diagnosis 1981
  prognosis 1875, 1982
  spread and metastases 1981
  squamous-cell carcinoma **1874–5**, 1980–1
  staging investigations *236*
  treatment 1874–5, 1981–2
    palliative 1982
  tylosis association 202, 1981, 3723
oesophageal disease **1865–71**
  chemotherapy-induced 1874
  in HIV infections 475
  investigations 1829, 1865
  non-neoplastic mucosal 1876
  skin disease in 3723
  symptoms **1819–21**
    chest pain 1820
    dysphagia, *see* dysphagia
    indigestion-like 1819–20
    mucosal hypersensitivity 1819, *1819*
    mucosal pain 1819
    regurgitation 1820
    see also oesophagus; *specific diseases*
oesophageal varices 2092
  barium swallow 1831
  bleeding 1882, 2093
    balloon tamponade 2094
    banding ligation 2095
    in Budd-Chiari syndrome 2098
    complications 2094
    endoscopic therapy 2094–5
    grading 2094
    management 980, 1827, 1828, 2093–5
    mortality 2094
    portal-systemic shunting 2095
    in pregnancy 1800
    in primary myelosclerosis 3437
    in schistosomiasis 977, 980
    sclerotherapy, *see* sclerotherapy
    vaso-active drugs 2094
  in congenital hepatic fibrosis 2015
  investigations 1828, 2093
  in normal pregnancy 1796
  in primary biliary cirrhosis 2074
  rebleeding, prevention 2095

oesophagitis 1880
  in AIDS and HIV infection 475
  angina *vs* 2322
  in gastro-oesophageal reflux disease 1866
  infective 1876, *1876*
  medication-induced 1874, *1874*
  peptic 1866
  treatment 1867, *1867–8*
  viral 1876
oesophagogastric junction, anastomoses in portal hypertension 2092
oesophagomyotomy 1869
oesophagopulmonary fistula 1874
oesophagoscopy, in achalasia 1959
Oesophagostomum 932
oesophagostomy, cervical 1974
oesophagus **1865–76**
  anatomical abnormalities **1872–3**
  atresia **1973–4**
    diagnosis and management 1974
    embryology 1973
  balloon dilatation 1869, 2094
  Barrett's 1866, 1868, 1981
    aetiology and features 1875
    carcinoma risk 1875, 1981
    management/prognosis 1875
  burns, in alkali/acid ingestion 1104, 1873
  columnar metaplasia, *see* oesophagus, Barrett's
  'corkscrew' 1870, 1958
  dilatation 1869
  dilated, in achalasia 1959
  disease, *see* oesophageal disease
  diverticula 1873
  dysplasia 1874, 1875
  embryology 1973
  endoscopy 1829
    in gastro-oesophageal reflux disease 1867
  extrinsic compression 1873
  function testing **1865**
  hypocontraction dysfunctions 1871
  manometry 1865, 1870, 1956, 1959
  mechanical and chemical trauma 1104, **1873–4**
  motility 1955
    barium studies 1956
    endoscopy 1957
    radionuclide studies 1957
    stimulants 1868
  motor activity 1955
  motor disorders **1866–71**, 1958, 1959
    dysphagia in 1820, 1869, 1870, 1958
    non-specific **1871**
    oesophageal pain in 2167, 2168
  muscle diseases **1871–2**
    smooth-muscle 1871–2
    striated muscle 1872
  in non-cardiac chest pain 1870
  nutcracker **1871**
  pain 1819, 1820, 1822, 1870, **2167–8**
    causes and types 2167–8
    myocardial infarction *vs* 2335
    in oesophageal dysmotility 2167, 2168
  perforation,
    in paraquat poisoning 1120
    traumatic 1873
  peristalsis 1952
    disorders 1871
    hypertensive **1871**
  pH monitoring 1865
  pseudodiverticula 1873
  radioisotopic transit testing 1865
  radiology 1865, 1867
  rings 1870, 1872–3
  rupture 1959
  sensory disorders **1866–71**
  spasm 1820, 1958
    angina *vs* 2322
    diffuse **1869–70**
    dysphagia in 1820, 1870
    investigation/management 1958
    pain in 2167
  staple transection 2095

strictures 1866, 1868
  in alkali ingestion 1104, 1873, 1981
  malignant 1981, 1982
  management 1868
  in phenol ingestion 1105
  squamous-cell carcinoma after 1981
  systemic disease affecting 1876
  in systemic sclerosis 3029, *3030*
  transit, improving 1865–6
  tumours **1874–6**, **1980–2**
    benign 1876, 1980
    malignant 1874–6, 1980–2
    malignant, *see also* oesophageal carcinoma
  ulceration,
    alkali ingestion causing 1103, 1873
    in gastro-oesophageal reflux disease 1866
  webs 1873
    in iron deficiency 3474–5
oestradiol
  control of gonadotrophin secretion 1579
  in hormone replacement therapy *1814*
oestrogen(s)
  adrenocortical function and 1717
  bilirubin excretion reduced 2091
  bone mass and 3065
  bone resorption and 1629
  calcium metabolism and 1626
  cancer association 215–16
    breast cancer 209
    endometrial cancer 210, 216
  cholestasis and liver damage due to 2125
  conjugated equine *1814*
  endothelial function modified 2157, **2248–51**, 2300
  gallstones and 1801
  growth hormone secretion and 1577, 1578
  gynaecomastia due to 1688
  ischaemic heart disease risk 2314
  in men 1688
  in oral contraceptives 1723
  in puberty 1563
  receptor 1555, 1561–2
    defects *1567*, 1573
    on osteoblasts 3059
    tamoxifen inhibition of 226
    resistance 1573
  serum lipids and 1411
  thyroid function tests and 1717
  treatment,
    in acne vulgaris 3754
    in acute renal failure *3288*
    in constitutional delay of growth and adolescence 1703
    in cyanotic congenital heart disease 2401
    in hirsutism 1677
    in osteoporosis 3068
    side-effects 1688
    for tall stature in girls 1700
    in telangiectasia 3786
    see also hormone replacement therapy
oestrone sulphate *1814*
ofloxacin
  in leprosy 677
  in *Pseudomonas aeruginosa* infections 2752, *2752*
  in rickettsial diseases 733
  in tuberculosis 655–6, *656*
Ogilvie's syndrome **2138**
Ohara disease 599–603
oil, aspiration 2837
'oil of wintergreen', poisoning 1054
ointments 3805, *3805*
OK-432, in ascites 2098
Old World screw-worm 1000, 1001
oleic acid 1412
olfaction 2610, 3876
olfactory nerve, lesions **3876–7**
oligaemia
  causes 2564
  circulatory fluid replacement 2565
  low venous pressure due to 2564
  management 2564, 2573
  in septicaemia 2572

Oligella urethralis 558
oligodendrocytes 3990
　JC virus infection 446
　vulnerability to injury 3990
oligodendroglioma **4031**
oligomenorrhoea 1669
　exercise-induced 4326
oligonucleotide, new anticancer therapy
　using 260
oligonucleotide probes 61
oligosaccharide chains, in endoplasmic
　reticulum lumen 70
oligozoospermia 1684, 1685, 1686, 1687
oliguria 3146–8
　in acute renal failure 3279
　calculus 3253
　definition 3101
　in haemolytic uraemic syndrome 3549
　in malaria 846
　prevention, in cyanotic congenital heart
　　disease 2400
　in snake envenoming, management 1138
olive oil 2311, 2538
olivopontocerebellar atrophy 4006
olsalazine 1949, *1949*
Omenn's syndrome 173
omentum 2007
omeprazole
　in hypergastrinaemia 1881
　in peptic ulcer haemorrhage 1883
　in peptic ulcers 1887–8, 1889
　pharmacology and formulations 1887
　safety/tolerance 1888
　side-effects 1888
　in Zollinger-Ellison syndrome 1705,
　　1881–2
omphalitis 503
Omsk haemorrhagic fever **415**
Onchocerca volvulus 911, 912
　detection 915
　lifecycle 912–13
　Loa loa coincident infection 918
onchocerciasis **912–17**
　blindness in 915, 4180, 4192
　clinical features 913–15
　diagnosis/differential diagnosis 915
　distribution and vectors 912
　eye in 914–15, 4192
　glomerulonephritis in 3177
　investigation 3710
　pathology 912–13
　treatment and prevention 915–17
'oncogene profile' 224
oncogenes 65, 194–5, **223–5**, 462, 3567
　biological roles in evolution 195
　cytoplasmic 224–5, 462
　　mechanism of action 65, 224–5
　　mutations 65, 225
　　as target for anticancer drugs 226
　　tumour types associated 225
　　see also ras genes
　definition 65, 223
　detection 194–5
　growth factor 223
　　see also growth factor(s)
　growth factor receptors 223–4
　　see also growth factor receptors
　'hit-and-run' mechanism of action 195,
　　462
　immunotherapy against 260
　indirect action 195
　mutations causing loss of cell function
　　195, 462
　in myelodysplastic syndromes 3429
　nuclear 225
　　as target for anticancer drugs 226
　　see also transcription factors
　in pancreatic carcinoma 2041
　polypeptide products 195
　　use in screening/diagnosis 259
　as targets for anticancer drugs **225–6**
　types/examples *65*
　viral (v-*onc*) 65, *65*, 462
　see also growth factor(s); growth factor
　　receptors; *specific oncogenes*
oncogenic viruses 227, *227*, **460–3**, 460
　epidemiological evidence for role 460
　　epidemiology and transmission 461–2

immunization against 227
mechanism of action 194, 462
treatment and prevention 462–3
vaccination against 463
viruses implicated 460–1, *461*
oncologist, referral 252–3
oncotic pressure 2493, 2495, 2496
　interstitial fluid 2493, 2495, 2496, 2560
　in lymphoedema 2560
　manipulation 2504
　plasma 2560
　　in adult respiratory distress syndrome
　　2854
　　reduced and pulmonary oedema in
　　2498, 2504
　see also interstitial fluid
Ondine's curse 2670, 2916, 3888
onychogryphosis 3760
onycholysis 2968, 3747, 3760
onychomycosis 798, 811
　in diabetes 1490
O'nyong nyong virus **407**
　arthritis in **3001**
oophorectomy, bilateral, osteoporosis in
　3069
open heart surgery, *see* cardiac surgery
ophiophobia 4301
ophthalmia
　neonatal gonococcal 546, 547
　snake venom 1132
　　management 1139
ophthalmia neonatorum 753, 1790
ophthalmic myiasis 1001
ophthalmic zoster 349, **3878**
　treatment 351
ophthalmological features, neurosyphilis
　4085
ophthalmomyiasis externa 4193
ophthalmopathy, Graves' disease *1611*,
　1614
ophthalmoplegia
　in giant-cell arteritis 4028
　internuclear 3858
　　in poisoning 1046
　pituitary tumours 1587
　progressive external **4172**
　　mitochondrial myopathy in 4148,
　　4172
　snake venom 1133
ophthalmoscope **4179**
　direct 4179
　indirect 4179, 4180
　method of use **4187**
opiates
　antagonists, alpha-adrenergic agonists
　　with 4292
　in cancer 253
　coma due to 4280
　continuous subcutaneous infusion, in
　　cancer 253
　detoxification 4291–3, 4299
　　non-opiates in 4291–2
　　opiates in 4292–3
　as drugs of concern 4263
　endogenous 3938
　　in neuropathic pain 3942
　fetal complications 4298
　growth hormone secretion and 1578
　medication to prevent relapse 4293
　in Munchausen's syndrome 4211
　notification of addiction 4289
　oral, in cancer 253
　overdose 4280, 4283, 4295–6
　in pain treatment 3944–5
　　cost-benefits 4301
　　in drug abusers 4301
　in pregnancy 4296, 4299
　prescription exploitation prevention
　　4301
　receptors 3938
　　in renal impairment 3270
　spinal, pain treatment 3938
　synthetic, prescribing 4289
　withdrawal syndrome 1251, **4291–3**,
　　4299
　　in accident and emergency department
　　4296
　features 4291

management 4291, 4299
　in pregnancy 4296, 4299
opioids
　cough management in terminal illness
　　4354
　drugs included 1058
　in gastrointestinal tract 1894
　overdose **1058**
　　clinical features 1046, 1058
　　shortening of life and 4359
　　vomiting due to 4355
opisthorchiasis **981–4**, *982*
　lifecycle of flukes 981, 983
Opisthorchis felineus 981, *982*
Opisthorchis viverrini 981, *982*, 983
opisthotonus, in tetanus 626
opium, tincture of 4292–3
opportunistic infections 327, **1027–35**,
　1837
　fungal 797, 803, 806–7, 806–11
　in HIV infection 470, *470*, 1027
　in lymphoma 4133
　Pseudomonas aeruginosa 550
　in pulmonary alveolar proteinosis 2833,
　　2834
　in rapidly progressive
　　glomerulonephritis 3162
　in renal transplant recipients 3319–20
　respiratory tract 2708–9, *2709*
　　see also respiratory tract infections
　see also under immunocompromised
　　host
opsonization 175, 3559
　complement role 175, 178
optic atrophy 3866, 3869
　hereditary 3867
optic chiasm 3864, 3867
　compression 3832
　lesions **3867–9**, *3868*, 4036
　　treatment 3868–9
　pituitary tumours and 1574, 1586
optic disc 3863
　disorders 3866
　swelling 3864
　　causes and features *3867*
　　see also papilloedema
optic nerve
　blood supply 3864
　compression 3866, 4196
　　visual evoked potentials in 3832–3
　damage, ethambutol toxicity 4197
　glioma 3865, 3866
　inflammatory lesions 3867
　lesions 3864–7
　　compressive and infiltrating 3866
　　in demyelinating disease 3866
　　pupillary responses 2582
　in multiple sclerosis 3866, 3991, 3993
　in neurosyphilis 4085
　occlusion of vessels supplying **4187**
　ophthalmoscopy 4179
　regions 3863–4
　in toxic and nutritional disorders 3867
　vascular lesions 3867
optic nerve head
　angioma 4182
　atrophy 4183, 4186

P

p24 antigen 303
p53 *1567*, 3567
　gene 223
　in hepatocellular carcinoma after
　　hepatitis B 2116
　in leukaemia 3394, *3395*
　in Li-Fraumeni syndrome 129, 242
　in thyroid carcinoma 1570
p56lck kinase 150
p150,95 (CR4) 177, 3559
P$_{300}$ event-related potentials, alcoholism
　marker 2081
P$_{450}$, *see* cytochrome P450
P$_{450}$11ß 1664, *1665*, 1668
P$_{450}$17α 1664, *1665*, 1668
P$_{450}$aldo, *see* aldosterone synthase

P$_{450}$c18 1664
P$_{450}$c21 1664, *1665*, 1666–7
P$_{450}$scc (cholesterol desmolase) 1664,
　1665
　deficiency *1652*, 1667
P815 tumour antigen 228
pacemakers 2263, **2285–9**
　in aircraft crew and pilots 1201
　ambulatory ECG 2199–200
　characteristics/developments 2287
　complications 2288
　demand function of 2287
　dual chamber systems 2287, 2288, 2289
　failure 2288
　physiological 2287
　programming 2287, 2288
　syncope due to 2173
　see also pacing (cardiac)
pacemaker syndrome 2173
pachygyria 4113
pachymeningitis interna, *see* subdural
　empyema
pacing (cardiac) **2285–9**
　atrial 2225, 2263, 2273, 2286
　in atrioventricular block 2268, 2286
　in atrioventricular nodal re-entry
　　tachycardia 2275
　in ß-adrenoceptor blocker overdose
　　1065
　in bradycardias 2285
　in cardiac arrhythmias 2263, 2285, 2286
　in Chagas' disease 898
　clinic for 2287
　complications 2288–9
　conditions requiring **2285**
　　investigation/diagnosis 2286
　　presentation 2285–6
　continuous 2263
　developments 2289
　endocardial 2287
　epicardial 2287
　indications 2286
　in long QT syndrome 2283
　magnetic resonance imaging
　　contraindication 2214
　in myocardial infarction 2346
　results 2287–8
　in sinoatrial disease 2266
　techniques and implantation method
　　2287
　temporary 2268, 2286
　ventricular 2263, 2287, 2288
　ventricular overdrive 2265, 2280
　in ventricular tachycardia 2280, 2285
　see also pacemakers
packed cell volume (PCV) **3378–80**
　in altitude acclimatization 1187
　in cor pulmonale 2521
　in dengue haemorrhagic fever 420, 422
　oxygen transport and 3432
　in polycythaemia 3433, 3551
PAF1 gene 84
Paget's disease of bone 1622, **3075–8**
　biochemical features *3062*
　clinical features 3061, 3075–6
　diagnosis 3077
　in elderly 4344
　incidence and prevalence 207, 3075,
　　3075
　investigations 3076–7
　　radiology 3076, 3077
　juvenile (idiopathic hyperphosphatasia)
　　3089
　osteoarthritis in 2979
　osteosarcoma/chondrosarcoma of jaw
　　1863
　osteosarcoma in 3075, 3076, 3077
　pathophysiology 3075
　possible viral aetiology 3075
　primary hyperparathyroidism and 1632
　treatment 3077–8
pain **3936–46**
　alcohol-induced, in Hodgkin's disease
　　3570
　behaviour 3943
　bone, *see* bone pain
　burning 3941
　　in Fabry disease 1429

in spinothalamic tract lesions 3858
see also causalgia
in cancer 240–1, **4351–2**
  adjuvant therapy 4352, *4353*
  bone pain and origin/types of 240–1
  cord and cauda equina compression
    249
  direct tumour infiltration of bone
    240–1
  incidence 240
  morphine 4352, *4353*
  relief 253, 4352
central sensitization 3936
chest, *see* angina (angina pectoris);
    chest pain
chronic,
  psychiatric factors in 3943
  treatment, *see* pain, treatment
chronic benign, in terminal illness **4352**
clinics, conditions seen in 3943, *3944*
CNS lesions causing **3941–2**
CNS mechanisms **3937–9**, 4022
  ascending control 3939
  descending control 3937, 3938
  diffuse noxious inhibitory control
    3939
  dorsal horn 3937
  neuropathic pain mechanisms 3942
  spinal cord pharmacology 3937–8
  spinothalamic tract origins 3938–9
  thalamic projections 3939
control,
  in acute porphyria 1392–3
  in diabetic foot disease 1491
  in ureteric colic 3243
  see also pain, treatment
deafferentation 3939
definition **3936**
endogenous modulating mechanisms
    3939
  control of 3939
  endogenous opiates 3938
fears of 4357
in gout 2984
head, *see* headache
in hemiplegia 4340
joint, *see* arthralgia; joint(s), pain
kidney 3148
loin **3148**, 3217, 3235
management **4300–1**
  measures/assessment 4300
mechanisms 4340
in multiple sclerosis 3993
muscle, *see* muscle, pain
nerve root, *see* spinal nerve roots
neuralgic, in genital herpes 3353
neuropathic 3936, **3939–41**
  in cancer 4351
  causes *3937*, 3939
  clinical features 3939–40, *3940*
  CNS lesions causing 3942
  definition 3939
  endogenous opiates and 3942
  mechanisms from CNS lesions 3942
  mechanisms in peripheral neuropathy
    3940
nociceptive 3936, 3939
  in cancer 4351
occupational disease 1168
papule compression *3716*
in pelvic inflammatory disease 3358
perception **3936**
  see also pain, sensation
peripheral mechanisms **3936**, 4022
in peripheral neuropathy 3940–1
  mechanisms 3940
pleural 2648, 2883
psychogenic 2945, 3943, **4209**
psychological aspects **3942–3**, 4300
receptor sensitization 3936
referred 2944, **3938**
  headache 4023
  mechanisms 3938
  in rheumatoid arthritis 2958
in reflex sympathetic dystrophy **3941**,
    3941
rehabilitation 3946
renal **3148**

in rheumatic diseases 2943
sensation 3857, 3858, **3936–7**
  skin role 3707
sensibility, loss 4092
in sickle-cell crises 3514, 3516
spinal, *see* spinal pain
  in spinal cord compression 3892
  in spinal cord injury 3901, 3942
spiritual **4358–9**
spontaneous, in polyneuropathy
    4092
thyroid gland 1612
treatment **3943–6**
  CNS stimulation 3945–6
  in drug abuser **4300–1**, 4300, 4301
  drugs 3944–5, 4301
  ethical aspects 4359
  in functional bowel disease 1968
  local measures 3943–4, 4300
  non-pharmacological 4300–1
  opiates 3944–5, 4301
  psychological 3946
  surgery role 3945
  in terminal illness 4352, *4353*, 4356,
    4359
  see also analgesics
  in trigeminal neuralgia 345, 3878
visceral **3938**
'pain all over' syndromes 2997
painful bruising syndrome 3775
painful dystrophy, *see* algodystrophy;
    Sudeck's atrophy
painful stiff shoulder syndrome 2995
paint
  lead-containing 3261
  manufacturing industry 1167
  removers, poisoning 1087
palatal myoclonus 3858, 4015–16
palatal paralysis 495
palate
  cancer, epidemiology 201
  smoker's keratosis 1858, 1859
palatine tonsils 2611
palatopharyngeus 2611
palilalia 3848, 4016
palindromic rheumatism 2946, **3007**
palliative care 4349, 4350
  see also terminal care; terminal illness
palliative medicine, ethics **13**
palliative treatment 4349–50
  information and support for patients
    253
  radiotherapy 257–8, 2889–90
  see also terminal illness
pallidal atrophy, progressive **4009**
pallor
  in anaemia 3459
  in malignancy 3792
palmar erythema 2104
  in pregnancy 1796, 1804
palmar keratoses 3793
palms of hand, 'dry type' dermatophytic
    infections 798
palpitations **2175**, *2176*
  ambulatory ECG 2197, 2198
  in atrioventricular nodal re-entry
    tachycardia 2274
  in panic disorder 4207
pamidronate
  in hypercalcaemia 1638, 3228–9
  in myeloma 3603
p-aminohippurate (PAH), renal plasma
  flow estimation 3108
p-aminosalicylic acid (PAS), *see p*-
  aminosalicylic acid (PAS)
Pancoast's syndrome 241, 3903, 4093
  cervical disc protrusions *vs* 3906
Pancoast's tumour 2883, 2886
  pain in 2648
pancreas
  adenoma, in MEN 1 syndrome 1708
  agenesis 2016
  in AIDS 475
  annular 1973, 1975, 2016, 2039
  artificial endocrine 1478
  blunt trauma 2028
  computed tomography 1835, **2013**

congenital disorders **2016–17**, **2039**
cysts 2053
diseases **2027–45**
  brittle diabetes in 1496
  endoscopy indication 1829
  skin disease in 3723
divisum 2016–17, 2039
embryology 1973
endocrine tumours **1703–7**, 2051
  diagnosis 1704
  in MEN 1 syndrome 1703, 1705, 1708
  natural history 1703–4
  non-functioning 1703, 1707
  syndromes 1705–7
  treatment 1704–5
  see also insulinoma
exocrine dysfunction, in diabetes
    1488–9
exocrine insufficiency 2034, 2039
  gut peptides in 1895
  see also pancreatic enzyme
fibrocystic disease, *see* cystic fibrosis
fibrosis 2053
function tests 2035, *2037*
  in pancreatic carcinoma 2043
gastrointestinal tract interactions 1565
hyperplasia 2040
  in MEN 1 syndrome 1708
inherited diseases **2026**
investigations 1835
isotope scanning 2043
magnetic resonance imaging **2013**
in mumps 373
necrosis 2028, 2033
pain 1822
radiology **1835**
secretion, negative feedback regulation
    2036
small-duct disease 2034, 2036
transplantation 1478, 3172, 3315
  islets 185, 1478, 3172
tumours **2040–5**
  benign *2041*
  diagnosis 1881
  endocrine, *see* pancreas, endocrine
    tumours
  exocrine 2041
  islet cell, Zollinger-Ellison syndrome
    1881
  malignant *2041*
  see also pancreatic carcinoma
pancreatic ascites 2033, 2038
pancreatic carcinoma **2040–5**
  aetiological factors 204–5
  biliary strictures 2052
  biology 2040–1
  clinical features 2042
  epidemiology 204–5, 2040
  investigations 2042–4, 2052
    computed tomography 2013
    retrograde pancreatography 1835
  models and transgenic mice 2040, 2041
  mortality rates 205
  pathology 2041–2
  risk factors 2040
  serum markers and tumour antigens
    2042
  spread and metastases 2041, 2043
  staging investigations *236*
  survival 2040, 2044, 2045
  treatment 2044–5
    palliative 2044, 2045
  weight loss and malabsorption
    syndrome 241
pancreatic duct, accessory 1973
pancreatic enzyme
  deficiencies 2039
  in meconium ileus 1978
  replacement *2038*, 2039, 2751
    in chronic pancreatitis 2036, 2038,
      2038
  formulations 2751, *2751*
  see also pancreas, exocrine
    insufficiency
pancreatic lipase 1903
pancreaticojejunostomy 2036
pancreatic polypeptide (PP) **1893**
  chronic pancreatitis 1895

pancreatic endocrine tumours 1703,
    1706, **1707**
pancreatic pseudocyst 2033, 2037
  management 2033
pancreatic structural protein (PSP), gene
  suppression 2026
pancreatitis
  acute 2013, **2027–34**
    aetiological factors 2027–8, *2027*,
      2028
    biochemistry 2029
    clinical features 2028–9
    complications 2033
    C-reactive protein 1531
    diagnosis/grading 2030–1
    differential diagnosis 2030, *2030*
    drug-induced 2027–8
    experimental 2028
    haematological changes 2030
    in hypertriglyceridaemia 1405, 1410
    incidence/epidemiology 2027
    management 2031–3
    pathology 2028
    surgery 2033, *2033*
  alcohol-abuse 2027, 2034
  angina *vs* 2322
  bile-duct obstruction in 2053
  chronic 2013, **2034–40**
    aetiology 2034–5, *2035*
    classification 2034
    clinical features 2035
    complications 2038–9, *2039*
    diagnosis 2035–6
    gut peptides in 1895, 1896
    incidence 2035
    management 2036, 2038
    pancreatic carcinoma in 2040
    pathophysiology 2035
    vitamin B_{12} deficiency 3491–2
    see also pancreatitis, hereditary
  computed tomography 2013, 2030,
    2031, 2033, 2035
  in Crohn's disease management 1942
  enterovirus infections 387
  hereditary 2017, 2026, 2039
    ocular features **4184**
  pleural effusion in 2868
  in primary hyperparathyroidism 1631
  rare congenital abnormalities causing
    2017
  in SLE 3020
  tropical 2034, 2035
pancreatoblastoma 2042
pancreatoduodenectomy 2045
pancreatography, retrograde 1835
pancreolauryl test *2037*
pancuronium, tetanus management 629
pancytopenia, benzene causing 1084
pandysautonomia, acute/subacute 3886
panendoscopy, in alkali/acid ingestion
    1104
panhypogammaglobulinaemia 169
  in bronchiectasis 2758, 2761
  see also hypogammaglobulinaemia
panic attacks 4206, 4207
  in drug abusers 4295
  psychiatric emergency 4258
  treatment 4253
panic disorder 4207
  prognosis 4207
  psychiatric emergencies 4258
  treatment 4207, 4253
    cognitive therapy 4255
panniculitis *244*, 3777
  in α_1-antitrypsin deficiency 1547
panophthalmitis, meningococcal 540
Panton-Valentine leucocidin 524
Pantopaque (Myodil) 3826, 3907
pantothenic acid deficiency 3498, 4100
Papanicolaou (Pap) smears 445, 463,
    3370
'paper money' skin 2104
Papez neuronal circuit 3855
papillary cystic tumour 2042
papillary fibroelastoma 2472
papillary muscle 2451, 2459
  dysfunction **2459–60**, 2461
    in pulmonary oedema 2568

papillary muscle (*cont.*)
  rupture **2460**, 2568
    in myocardial infarction 2321
    partial 2460
papillitis 3866
papilloedema 3864, 4054
  in bacterial meningitis 4053
  in benign intracranial hypertension 4041
  in hypertension 2536, 4188
  in intracranial tumours 4035
  lumbar puncture contraindication 3842
papilloma
  oesophageal 1876
  oral 1859
  in yaws 704, 705
papillomatosis, juvenile 1783
papillomaviruses, *see* human papillomaviruses (HPV)
papovaviruses **443–7**
  see also human papillomaviruses (HPV); polyomaviruses
Pappataci fever 428
Pap smears 445, 463, 3370
papules *3713*
  in dermatitis 3735
  violaceous, in lichen planus 3751
papulovesicular lesions, in scabies 1007
para-aminoheppurate (PAH) 3108
paracentesis
  diagnostic 2096
  therapeutic 2097
paracetamol
  absorption 1249
  adverse reactions 2849
  liver damage 1051–2, 2125
    acute liver failure 1052, 2106, 2107
    management 1053, *1053*
    prediction 1052
  in liver disease 2091
  metabolism 1051, 3222
    alcohol consumption and 2081
    metabolites 1051
  nephrotoxicity 1051, 3221, 3224
  poisoning/overdose **1051–4**, 4228
    biochemistry/haematology 1052, *1052*
    clinical features 1051–2, *1052*
    management 1053, *1053*
    mechanism of toxicity 1051
    in pregnancy 1799
    prognostic factors 1053
    in renal impairment 3273
parachlorphenylalanine 1898
Paracoccidioides brasiliensis 814, 815, *3801*
  characteristics and virulence 815
  ecology 815
paracoccidioidin 816
paracoccidioidomycosis **814–20**
  acute (juvenile) 817
  aetiology and virulence 815
  chronic 817–18, 819
    mucocutaneous 818
  clinical features 816–19
  diagnosis 819
  differential diagnosis 817
  epidemiology 815
  history 814–15
  host-fungal interactions 816
  immune response 816
  immunology-histopathology 819, *819*
  pathogenesis 815–16
  pathology 816
  sequelae 818–19
  therapy and prognosis 819–20
paracrine action 1564, 1891
  cytokines 95
paracrine peptides, *see* gut peptides
paraesthesiae
  in carpal tunnel syndrome 4095
  in cerebrospinal angiostrongyliasis 947
  in Fabry disease 1429
  in polyneuropathies 4092
  in subacute combined degeneration of cord 3893
paraffin oil (kerosene), poisoning 1043, **1083**

paragonimiasis **988–92**, *989*
  cerebral 991
  clinical features 989–91
  diagnosis/differential diagnosis 991–2
  epidemiology and transmission 988
  extrapulmonary 990–1
  haematological changes 3681
  pulmonary 990
  treatment and prevention 992
Paragonimus, species and lifecycle 988, *989*, 990
Paragonimus heterotremus 953, 990
Paragonimus westermani 988, 990
parainfluenza viruses **337–8**, *341*
parakeratosis 3710
paralysis 4141
  in acute porphyria 1391–2, 1393
  in cataplexy 3928
  in diphtheria 495–6
  induced, in tetanus management 629
  infantile 385
  Klumpke's 3903, 4093
  non-traumatic causes **3901–2**
  periodic,
    hyperkalaemic 3134, 4169, 4170
    hypokalaemic 1657, **3132**, 4169
    myopathy in 4169
    thyrotoxic 4168
  in peripheral neuropathy 4092
  in poliomyelitis 385
  in rabies 400
    other causes *vs* 401
  in rapid eye movement (REM) sleep 2908
  sexual problems in 4244
  snake bites causing 1132
  in spina bifida, management 4118
  spinal cord lesions 3892
  ticks causing 1149
  see also paraparesis; paraplegia
paralytic ileus **1961**
  in acute pancreatitis 2028
  mechanism 1961
  signs, diagnosis and treatment 1961
  see also adynamic ileus
paralytic poliomyelitis, *see* poliomyelitis
paralytic shellfish poisoning 1142
paramedian pontine reticular formation (PPRF) 3872
paramedical teams 4339
  myocardial infarction management 2337
paramethadione 3266
paramyotonia 4151, **4152–3**
  management 4153
paramyotonia congenita, myopathy in 4170
paramyxoviruses 337–8, **372–81**
  see also measles virus; mumps
paranasal sinuses, rhinocerebral mucormycosis 1033
paraneoplastic syndromes 240, 242, *243–4*
  causes/basis of 242
  cutaneous *3795*
  dermatological *244*
  diagnostic dangers 242
  endocrine 242, *243*
  haematological *244*
  musculoskeletal *244*
  neurological *243*
paranoid delusions 4223, 4227
  in schizophrenia 4221
'paranoid hallucinatory state' 4238
paranoid personality 4212
paranoid reaction/states **4223**, 4223
  acute 4223
  in elderly 4227, 4341
paraparesis
  chronic progressive 3892–3
  tropical spastic 490
  see also paraplegia
paraphasia, semantic and phonemic 3848
paraphenylenediamine 3736
paraplegia
  chronic progressive 3892–3
  compression 3892–3
  hereditary spastic **3985**, 3995
  initial management 3896

non-traumatic **3892–5**
  acute/subacute 3892
  pregnancy in 1769
  in schistosomiasis 977–8
  spastic, *see* spastic paraplegia
  see also paralysis; paraparesis
paraprosthetic-enteric fistula 2137
paraproteinaemias 3567, **3597–605**
  coagulation factor inhibition 3661
  platelet defects 3635
  see also myeloma
paraproteinaemic neuropathy **4102**
paraproteins, monoclonal, *see* monoclonal paraproteins (M proteins)
parapsoriasis 3795, 3796
paraquat poisoning 1120, 3293
  absorption and levels 1120
  clinical features 1046, 1120
  diagnosis 1120
  treatment/prognosis 1120–1
'Para Sight F', malaria diagnosis 849
parasites
  adaptations 265
  diarrhoea associated 2004
  non-venomous arthropods **1000–10**
  see also helminths; protozoa
parasitic infections
  eye in **4192–3**
  haematological changes **3680–1**
  hepatic granulomas in 2121
  hypereosinophilic syndrome *vs* 3611
  myositis **4155–6**
  in pregnancy 1803
  pruritus due to 3743
  pulmonary hypertension in 2509
  skin examination 3710
parasitophobia 1004
parasternal heave 2453, 2456, 2458, 2518
parastole 2270
parasympathetic nervous system 3881
  coronary arteries 2159
  gastrointestinal tract 1953
  heart 2160
  pulmonary blood vessels 2486
parathyroidectomy 1632–3, 1708, 3329
parathyroid glands 1624
  adenoma 1566, 1630, 1632–3, 2899
    genetics 1569
    MEN 1 syndrome 1708
  carcinoma 1566, 1630
  disorders,
    drug-induced 1719
    mental disorders/symptoms in 4239
    myopathy in **4168–9**
    ocular features 4196
    in pregnancy **1752**
  hyperplasia 1630, 1632
    in MEN syndromes 1708, 1709
  localization methods 1632–3
parathyroid hormone (PTH) 1555, **1624**, 3058–9, **3078–9**
  actions 1563, 1624, 1629, 3059, 3227, 3334
  administration test 1633
  biosynthesis 1559, 1624
  bone resorption increase 3057
  in chronic renal failure 3296
  ectopic secretion 1568
  excess 3072
  gene 3058–9
    mutations *1567*, 1569, 1571
  plasma 1565–6, 1631
    in hyperparathyroidism 1630, 1631, 1632
    in hypoparathyroidism 1633, 1634
  plasma calcium regulation 1622, 1623, 1624, 1627, 1630, 3059
  radio-immunoassay 1712
  receptor *1560*
  renal bone disease and 3326, **3327**
  resistance 1634
  see also hyperparathyroidism; hypoparathyroidism
parathyroid hormone-related protein (PTHrP) 1555, 1568, 1638, 1712, 3059

calcium regulation 3059
gene and sequence 3059
in pancreatic endocrine tumours 1707
paratrachoma 749, 753
paratyphoid fever **567**
  paratyphoid types A/B/C 567
paraumbilical vein, in portal hypertension 2092
paraventricular nucleus 1600
parental imprinting 64
parenteral nutrition 1315, 2587–8
  in adult respiratory distress syndrome 2860
  in alkali ingestion 1104
  bone disease in **3095**
  in burns patients 1323
  complications 1316, 1319–21
    infections 1319
    mechanical 1319
    metabolic 1319–21
  in exomphalos/gastroschisis management 1975
  half-life of feeds 1318
  in head injury 1323
    at home 1324
    outcome 1325
  in intensive care **2587–8**, 2587–8
  liver disorders and 2132, *2132*, 2140
  monitoring 1322
  perioperative 1323–4
  requirements and composition of feeds *2587*, 2588
  in short gut syndrome 1926
  transplantation patients 1323
  in trauma 1550
  in ulcerative colitis 1948–9
  see also nutritional support
parent-of-origin effects **127–8**
parents, consent from 4317
parietal cell antibodies 3489
parietal cell hyperplasia 1887
parietal lobe
  behavioural defects associated *3846*
  lesions 3857, 3955
    optic radiation **3869**
  tumours, mental disorders/symptoms in 4237
Parinaud's oculoglandular syndrome 746, 760, 3858, 4036
parkinsonism 3998
  arteriosclerotic 3998
  autonomic failure with multiple system atrophy 3885, 4006
  causes *3999*
  in dopa-responsive dystonia-parkinsonism 4017
  drug-induced 3998, 4002, 4020
  juvenile 4009
  postencephalitic 3998
  syndrome of and features 4002
  toxins causing *3999*
Parkinson's disease **3998–4005**
  aetiology 3998–9
  basal ganglia pathology 3863
  clinical features 3863, 4000–1
    akinesia 4001
    rigidity 4001
    tremor 3863, 4000–1
  CYP2D6 mutations 130
  definition 3998
  dementia in 4001, 4002
  depression in 4004, 4238, 4340
  diagnosis/differential diagnosis 4002
  dopamine deficiency 3998, 3999–4000
  epidemiology 3998–9
  gastrointestinal motility disorders in 1962
  infections in 4003, 4004
  mental disorders/symptoms in 4238
  natural history and age of onset 4001–2
  neurotransmitters 4000, *4000*
  pathology 3885, 3999–4000, *4006*
    Lewy bodies 3967, 3998, 3999
  pathophysiology 3862, 3999–4000
  psychiatric illness in 4004
  rehabilitation **4340**
  somatosensory evoked potentials 3834

treatment 4002–5
  drug interactions 4004–5
  drugs 4002–3, 4004
  maintenance drugs 4003
  'on-off' problems 4003
  physical therapy and aids 4004
  specific problems 4004–5
  surgery 4003–4, 4005
Parkinson's Disease Brain Bank 3885
paromomycin 832, 880
paronychia 800, 3761
  anaerobic infections 574
  chronic, non-dermatitic occupational
    dermatosis 1165
  Staphylococcus aureus infection 526
parosmia 3876
parotid gland
  enlargement, in Chagas' disease 897
  swelling 1861
parotitis
  acute 1861
  acute suppurative, in melioidosis 591,
    592
  enteroviruses causing 388
  epidemic, *see* mumps recurrent 1861
  septic, mumps *vs* 375
paroxysmal cold haemoglobinuria 714,
    3544
paroxysmal dystonia **4020**
paroxysmal dystonic choreoathetosis
    4020
paroxysmal kinesigenic choreoathetosis
    4020
paroxysmal nocturnal dyspnoea 2162,
    2163, 2462, 2500, 2501, 2646
paroxysmal nocturnal haemoglobinuria
    (PHN), *see under* haemoglobinuria
partial nucleoside phosphorylase (PNP)
    deficiency 172
partial thromboplastin time (PTT) *3379*,
    3654
  activated (APTT) 3628, 3661, 3673
  in DIC 3658
particle radiation 1217
particulates 2847
Parvoviridae 447
parvovirus(es) **447–8**
parvovirus B19 infections 448
  arthritis in **3001**
  clinical features 447–8
  in immunosuppressed 448
  in pregnancy 448
pascals 1223
passive haemagglutination, *Yersinia
    pestis* 597
passive immunoprophylaxis, *see*
    immunization, passive
pastes 3805, *3805*
Pasteurella
  designation of pathogens 606, *607*
  rare species *558*
Pasteurella multocida 606–8, 1125
  detection and typing *608*
  infections due to *607*
pasteurellosis **606–8**
Patau syndrome 121
patch testing 3738–9
  European battery *3740*
patent ductus arteriosus, *see* ductus
    arteriosus, patent
patent foramina ovales, *see* foramen
    ovale, patent
paternity testing 135
pathergy test 3046
pathogens, endocytic pathway and 74–5
pathology, forensic **4309**
patient(s) **3–4**
  complaints by 4311
  damage, medical negligence claim 4311
  delays in myocardial infarction
    management 2336–7
  directions and advice for 4
  doctor relationship, *see* doctor-patient
    relationship
  as interesting clinical object 3
  prescribing restrictions/regulations
    relating to 4289

questions asked and maintenance of
    trust 4
reassurance, psychological treatment
    4254
response to hospital admission 3
rights 10–11
sense of worthlessness 3
submission to doctors and vulnerability
    3
patient education
  after splenectomy 1028
  anorexia nervosa 1298, 4215
  chronic fatigue syndrome 1038, 1039
  cirrhosis 2090
  compliance improvement 1241
  heart failure management 2236
  see also education
patient information
  alcohol abuse 4274
  on antiepileptic drugs 3922–3
  on cancer diagnosis/treatment 252
  for dying patients 4234
  provision in supportive psychological
    treatment 4254
  see also information
patients' associations, *see* self-help
    groups
Patterson-Kelly syndrome 1981, 3475
Paul-Bunnell test 354
Pautrier abscess 3797
PAX3 gene 107
PBX1-E2A fusion gene 3411, *3412*
peak expiratory flow (PEF) 2667
  in asthma 2730, 2744
    acute severe asthma 2736
    serial tests 2730, 2736, 2744
  in bronchiectasis 2764
  in chronic obstructive airways disease
    2775
  measurement 2672–3, 2730
  meters 2730, 2740
  in upper airways obstruction 2719, 2720
Pearson's syndrome 4172
pectus carinatum (pigeon chest) 2649,
    2875
pectus excavatum 2179, 2649, **2875**
  chest radiography 2657
pediculicides 1004
pediculosis 3724
Pediculus humanus 1000
Pediculus humanus capitis **1002–3**
Pediculus humanus humanus 1003
pedigree analysis 102, 131
  symbols used in 132
Pediococcus acidilactici 558
PEEP ventilation, *see* positive end-
    expiratory pressure (PEEP)
    ventilation
pefloxacin
  in leprosy 677
  in rickettsial diseases 733
Pel-Ebstein fever 241, 3570
Pelger(-Huet) anomaly 3426, 3556
peliosis, bacillary 747
peliosis hepatis 2140
  drug-induced 2129
Pelizaeus-Merzbacher disease 3986,
    4009
pellagra 3722
  in alcohol abusers 4278
  in carcinoid syndrome 1897
  mental symptoms 4241
  pellagra-like syndrome, in Hartnup
    disease 3333
pelvic abscess 2008
pelvic examination, in pelvic
    inflammatory disease 3358
pelvic floor, relaxation failure, in
    constipation 1967
pelvic infections, in gonorrhoea 546, 549
pelvic inflammatory disease **3357–9**
  chlamydial 752–3, 756, 758, 3357
    treatment *758*
  diagnosis 3357–9
  epidemiology 3347
  examination/investigations 3358–9
  microbiology 3357

mycoplasmas causing 770, 3357
oral contraceptives and 1723
risk factors/markers 3357–8, *3358*
symptoms 3358
treatment 3359
pelvic ultrasound, metastases from
    unknown primary sites 252
pelviureteric junction obstruction
  idiopathic 3237–8, 3244
  investigations 3114, 3115, 3241, 3242
  management 3243, **3244**
  in tuberculosis 3279
Pemberton's sign 1610
pemphigoid **3782**
  benign mucous membrane **1856–7,
    3782**
  cicatricial (benign mucosal) **1856–7,
    3782**
  juvenile bullous 3783
pemphigoid gestationis 1805, 3783
pemphigus 3723, 3781
  familial benign (Hailey-Hailey disease)
    3721–2, 3760
pemphigus foliaceous **3781–2**, 3782
pemphigus vegetans 1856, **3781**, 3782
pemphigus vulgaris 1855–6, **3781**
  autoantibodies in 163, 164
  differential diagnosis 1856
  in pregnancy 1806
pencil-in-cup deformity 2969
D-penicillamine 1248
  adverse effects 1423, 2851
    nephrotoxicity 3159, 3193, 3259, **3266**
  in copper poisoning 1109
  in cystinuria 1357, 3333
  myasthenia gravis due to 4161
  pemphigus vulgaris due to 3781
  in pregnancy 1800
  in primary biliary cirrhosis 2076, *2076*
  in rheumatoid arthritis 2964
  secondary immunodeficiency due to
    174
  in Wilson's disease 1422, 2022, 2023,
    4008
penicillin
  in acute meningococcaemia 541
  adverse reactions to **718**, 2435
    allergic reactions 162, 305, 505, 718,
      2449
    anaphylactic shock/reactions 305, 718
    delayed 718
    nephrotoxicity **3264**
  in enterococcal infections 509, 2446,
    2447
  in gas gangrene 634
  haemolytic anaemia due to 3542
  in infective endocarditis 2446, *2447*
  in leptospirosis 702
  in listeriosis 722
  in meningococcal meningitis 541–2
  in mitral stenosis 2455
  in neonates 1788, 1791
  in pneumococcal infections 486, 520
    prophylactic 521–2
  postsplenectomy 3596
  in pregnancy 1790, 1791, 1813
  in renal failure *3272*
  in renal impairment 3270, 3288
  resistance 2446
    anaerobic bacteria 575
    Neisseria gonorrhoeae 548, 549
    Neisseria meningitidis 534–5, 541
    pneumococci 2700
    Streptococcus pneumoniae 486, 511–12
  Streptobacillus moniliformis infection
    688
  in streptococci group A infections 502,
    2446
  in streptococci group B infections 508,
    2446
  in syphilis 717, *717*, 4086
    dosages/formulations 717, *717*, 718
  in tetanus 628
  in yaws 706
penicillin aluminium monostearate
    (PAM) 718
  in yaws 706

penicillinase, *Neisseria gonorrhoeae*
    producing 549
penicillin-binding protein (PBP) 1023–4
  testing for 299
penicillin G, *see* benzylpenicillin
Penicillium, ochratoxins 3230
Penicillium marneffei, infections 488,
    806
penile erection, *see* erectile dysfunction;
    erection
penile implants 4246
penile plethysmography, nocturnal
    1687
penis
  cancer, epidemiology 211
  chancroid ulceration 585
  condylomata acuminata 3367
  in diphtheria 495
  in lichen planus 3751
  plastic induration 3789
  scabies 1008
pentagastrin 1891
pentagastrin stimulation test 1710
pentamidine 296, 903, *903*
  in African trypanosomiasis 893
  asthma association 2850
  hypoglycaemic effects 1511
  in *Pneumocystis carinii* pneumonia
    478
  in renal impairment 3272
Pentasa 1949, *1949*
  in Crohn's disease 1942
pentastomiasis **1012–14**
  calcified nymphs 1013, 1014
Pentatrichomonas hominis 907
pentavalent antimonials 903, *903*
  in visceral leishmaniasis 906
pentetreotide 1898
pentolinium test 2555
pentose phosphate pathway (hexose
    monophosphate shunt) 3456, 3534,
    3535
pentosuria 1351
pentylenetetrazol 3909
PEP (polyneuropathy endocrinopathy
    and plasma cell dysplasia) syndrome,
    see POEMS syndrome
pepsin
  duodenal ulcer aetiology 1877
  increased secretion, *Helicobacter pylori*
    role 1885
peptic stricture, management 1868
peptic ulcer **1877–91**
  acute erosive **1880**
  angina *vs* 2322
  in cirrhosis 2090
  complications 1882–3
  gastric cancer association 1983
  gut peptides in 1895
  motility disorders after surgery 1878–9
  in primary hyperparathyroidism 1631
  in renal transplant recipients 3314,
    3320
  treatment, in renal impairment
    3274
  in Zollinger-Ellison syndrome 1705
  see also duodenal ulcer; gastric ulcer;
    Zollinger-Ellison syndrome
peptide histidine methionine (PHM-27)
    1576, 1706, 1893
peptides, neurocrine, *see* gut peptides
peptide transporting system 68–72
  see also endocytosis; exocytic pathway
peptide tyrosine tyrosine (PYY) **1893–4**
  in coeliac disease 1895
  increase in tropical sprue 1934
peptidoglycan 291
  inflammatory reactions 291–2
Peptostreptococcus 570, 571
perceptions, distorted, in partial seizures
    3914
perchloroethylene, *see*
    tetrachloroethylene
percutaneous lung aspiration, in
    pneumonia investigation 2697
percutaneous lung biopsy, *see* lung
    biopsy

percutaneous transhepatic cholangiography (PTC) 1834
bile-duct cancer 2052
in biliary disease 2046
pancreatic carcinoma 2043–4, 2052
percutaneous transhepatic endoprosthesis insertion 1834
percutaneous transluminal angioplasty
in ischaemia of limbs 2371
in Takayasu's disease 2379
percutaneous transluminal coronary angioplasty (PTCA) **2349–53**
in angina,
drug treatment *vs* 2331
with impaired ventricular function 2352
stable 2351
unstable 2351
complications **2350–1**
abrupt closure 2350–1
see also restenosis (below)
contraindications *2351*
coronary bypass grafting *vs* 2351
effect on vessel wall **2349–50**, 2351
in elderly 2352
historical background 2349
indications and results **2351–2**, *2351*
'lesions suitable for' 2351
management **2352**
in myocardial infarction 2344, 2352
new developments **2352**
numbers 2357
restenosis after 2294–5, 2300, 2350, **2351**
treatment 2295
as salvage procedure after bypass surgery 2352
technique **2349**, 2350
percutaneous transluminal renal angioplasty, in renovascular hypertension 2550–1
perforin 151
perfumes, dermatitis due to 3725, 3736, 3756
perfusion scan, *see* ventilation perfusion scanning
pergolide 4003
perhexiline, liver damage 2128
periadenitis mucosa necrotica recurrens, *see* oral ulceration
periampullary adenoma 2028
periampullary cancer 2028
perianal disease
in Crohn's disease 1938
streptococcal 499
ulcerative colitis 1946
in ulcerative colitis 1950
perianal granuloma, Crohn's disease 3723
perianal pain, in homosexuals 3361
perianal soiling 3745
perianal warts 444, 3363, 3368, 3768
see also anal warts; genital warts
peri-aortitis **3244–6**
without ureteric obstruction 3246
periaqueductal grey 3937
stimulation 3946
periarteritis nodosa, *see* polyarteritis nodosa
periarthritis, acute calcific 2991
periarticular disorders **2995–7**
pericardial aspiration 2478
pericardial constriction **2478–81**
ascites due to 2096
clinical features 2479–80
computed tomography 2218, 2219, 2480
differential diagnosis 2480–1
in enterovirus infections 387
haemodynamics 2478–9, 2480
heart failure 2231
liver in 2130
localized 2480
loculated, pulmonary oedema in 2500
occult 2480
pathophysiology 2478–9
pneumococcal infections *vs* 517
treatment 2481
tuberculous 2481–2

pericardial disease **2474–82**
acquired **2475–6**, *2475*
see also pericarditis
clinical syndromes **2476–81**
congenital **2474–5**
in heart failure 2231
postoperative **2481**
pericardial effusion
blood *vs* 2478
in cardiac tamponade 2477, 2570
chest radiography 2182, 2477
diagnosis 2477
draining 2478, 2570
Ebstein's anomaly *vs* 2414
in HIV infection 2395
in hypothyroidism 2476
magnetic resonance imaging 2215
in malignancies **251**, 2476
common tumours 251
pericardial tamponade in 2477, 2570
pleural effusion *vs* 2478
in pneumococcal infections 517
in rheumatic disorders 2476
in rheumatic fever 2476
pericardial pain 2476
pericardial pressure 2474
pericardial rub 2476
pericardial space 2474
pericardial tamponade 2476, **2477–8**
see also cardiac tamponade
pericardial window 251
pericarditis
acute **2476–7**
in enterovirus infections 386
in myocardial infarction 2475–6
recurrent **2481**
tuberculous 2475
acute idiopathic 2475
after acute meningococcaemia 539
amoebic 830
angina *vs* 2322
chest pain in 2167
in connective tissue diseases 3009
constrictive, *see* pericardial constriction
'effusive-constrictive' 2481
electrocardiogram (ECG) in 2335, 2336
fibrinous, in uraemia 2476
fungal 2475
in infective endocarditis 2439
in influenza 339
irradiation causing 2476
meningococcal 537, 539, 540
in myocardial infarction 2346, 2475–6
myocardial infarction *vs* 2335
myocarditis with 2381
in pneumococcal infection 514
in rheumatic fever 2433, 2476
in rheumatoid arthritis 2392
in SLE 3020
tuberculous 477, 654
in ulcerative colitis 1948
uraemic 3283, 3301
in Wegener's granulomatosis 3012
pericardium
abnormal chest radiograph 2182
anatomy 2474
calcification 2182
computed tomography 2218
congenital abnormalities **2474–5**
congenital absence 2182
cysts 2182, 2474, 2899
chest radiography 2182
fungal infection 2475
haemorrhage 2476
magnetic resonance imaging 2215–16
malignant involvement 2476
in myocardial infarction 2346, 2475–6
physiology 2474
pyogenic infection 2475
removal 2481
in systemic sclerosis *3031*
thickening, MRI 2215
tuberculous infection 2475
pericolic abscess 1970, 1971
perihepatitis (Curtis Fitz-Hugh syndrome) 546, 753, 756, 2133

perinatal mortality
maternal diabetes 1754
maternal nutrition and 1772
perineal descent, abnormality, in constipation 1967
perinephric abscess 3207
staphylococcal 529
perineum
atrophy, in kwashiorkor 1295
examination, in constipation 1826
periodic acid Schiff (PAS) stain 1923, 2973
in pulmonary alveolar proteinosis 2833
periodic disease, *see* recurrent polyserositis
periodic paralysis, *see* paralysis, periodic
periodontal cysts 1863
periodontal disease **1847–8**
actinomycetes association 685
periodontitis 1847
in AIDS 1851
in Ehlers–Danlos syndrome *3084*
pathology and immunology 1848
perioperative nutrition 1323–4
periosteal elevation 2969
periostitis 4322
peripheral arterial disease **2362–75**
atherosclerosis 2362–3
clinical presentation **2363–8**
in diabetes 1411
in hyperlipoproteinaemia type III 1409
in hypertension 2533
in hypertriglyceridaemia 1410
investigations **2368–9**
invasive 2369
non-invasive 2368
management **2369–75**
fibrinolytic therapy 3671, *3672*
risk factors 2363, *2363*
see also aneurysms; extracerebral vascular disease; intestinal ischaemia; ischaemia of limb; renovascular disease; thoracic outlet compression; vasospastic disorder
peripheral arterial vasodilatation, ascites hypothesis 2097
peripheral nervous system
anatomy 4091
damage,
CNS reaction 3940–1
electrical injury 1214
electrophysiology **3839–42**
in leprosy 669, 674
lesions, in poisoning 1048, 4099–100
occupational disorders 1169, *1170*
in rheumatoid arthritis 4131
in SLE 3020
thickening, in leprosy 674
tumour infiltration and pain 241
peripheral neurolysis 3945
peripheral neuropathy **4091–104**
in AIDS/HIV infection 476, 4078, 4103
in alcohol abusers **4127**, 4277–8
in autoimmune connective tissue disorders **4102**
clinical categories 4092
deficiency **4100–1**
diabetic, *see* diabetic neuropathy
diagnosis and investigation 4092–3
generalized **4098–104**
genetic **4102–4**
iatrogenic **4100**
inflammatory and postinfective **4101–2**
in metabolic/endocrine disorders **4098–9**
see also diabetic neuropathy
neoplastic and paraneoplastic **4102**
pain mechanisms 3940
pathophysiology 4091
in POEMS syndrome 4102, 4104
in rheumatoid arthritis 2961–2
in Sjögren's syndrome 3036
symptoms 4092
toxic **4099–100**
in tumours *243*
uraemic 3302

see also neuropathy; polyneuropathy; sensory neuropathy
peripheral oedema, *see* oedema
peripheral resistance, in hypertension 2531
peripheral vasculature
in acid–base disturbances 1539
blood flow measurements 2368
disease, high fibrinogen levels 2302
periportal fibrosis, in schistosomiasis 972, 977
peripylephlebitis, in schistosomiasis 972
perirectal abscess, anaerobic infections 573–4
peristalsis 1952
visible 1975
see also gastrointestinal motility; oesophagus, peristalsis
peritendinitis 4322
peritoneal aspiration, in acute pancreatitis 2030
peritoneal cavity **2007–9**, 2007
peritoneal dialysis 3306, *3307*, **3310–12**
access 3310
in acute renal failure 3287
automated 3310–11
complications 532, *3309*, 3311–12
continuous ambulatory (CAPD) 532, 3310, 3682
drug clearance by 3270
in lithium overdose 1061
in poison elimination 1051
preparation for 3306
renal problems in cyanotic congenital heart disease 2400
solutions 3310
techniques *3307*, 3310–11
peritoneal equilibration test 3310
peritoneal fluid, antimicrobial drug distribution 301
peritoneum 2007, 3310
inflammation, *see* peritonitis
parietal 2007
tumours 207, 2009
peritonitis **2007–8**
causes 2007
chemical 2008
clinical signs 2008
coagulase-negative staphylococcal 532
drug-induced 2009
faecal 1971
familial paroxysmal 2009
fungal and parasitic 2009
generalized *vs* localized 2008
glove powder (talc/starch) 2008–9
infective 2007–8
local, in diverticular disease 1970, 1971
in nephrotic syndrome 3141
obliterative 2009
Pasteurella causing 607
pelvic 2010
peritoneal dialysis-associated 3310, **3311**
pneumococcal 519, 2008
in SLE 3020
spontaneous bacterial (SBP) 2096, 2103
surgical 311–12, *312*
treatment 311–12, *312*, 2008
tuberculous 654, 2005, 2009
peritonsillar abscess, diphtheria *vs* 496
perivasculitis
in ehrlichiosis 738
in scrub typhus 740
periventricular haemorrhage 3825
periventricular leucomalacia 4119, 4120
Perls' reagent 2020
permethrin 1004
pernicious anaemia, *see* anaemia, pernicious
perniosis 3724
peroneal muscular atrophy 4102–3
peroxidase 1194
peroxidase-antiperoxidase technique 868
peroxides, antimalarial drugs 850
peroxisomal disorders 84, *1335*, **1438–43**
biochemistry *1440*
classification 1439, *1440*

see also Zellweger (cerebrohepatorenal) syndrome
peroxisomal 3-oxo-acyl-coenzyme A thiolase deficiency **1441**
peroxisome **83–4**, 1438–9
  absent, cell lines 84
  enzymes 83
    deficiency 2025
  import, cytosolic factors in 83–4
  import signals 83
  membrane proteins 83
    in import process 84, *84*
    pmp70 84
  proliferation, drugs causing 83, 84
persecution, delusions about 4221, 4223, 4227
perseveration 3854
persistent duct, *see under* ductus arteriosus
persistent vegetative state 3933, **3935**, 4123
  withdrawal of tube feeding 3935
personality
  changes after strokes 4237
  changes in frontal lobe damage 3854
  chronic pain and 3943
  cyclothymic 4212, 4220
  definition 4211
  in epilepsy 4238
  as physical illness precursor 4232
  type A 1170, 2315, 4232
  type B 1170
personality disorders **4211–12**
  affective 4212
  antisocial 4212
  asthenic 4212
  atypical eating disorders 1301
  causes and differential diagnosis 4212
  clinical features and types 4211–12
  deliberate self-harm in 4228
  in elderly 4228
  explosive 4212
  histrionic (hysterical) 4212
  in Munchausen's syndrome 4211
  obsessional 4211–12
  organic 4225
  paranoid 4212
  prognosis and treatment 4212
  psychopathic 4212
  schizoid 4212
  schizophrenia *vs* 4222
personal protective equipment (PPE) 1164, 1165
pertussis **587–90**
  aetiology and epidemiology 587
  clinical features 588
    cough 2643
  complications 588
  death rate and immunization effect 283
  epidemiology 587, 2695
  laboratory findings/diagnosis 588
  prevention 589–90
  treatment 588–9
  vaccine 318, 587, 589–90
    efficacy 587
    reactions to 589, 590
    schedule 589
  see also Bordetella pertussis
pesticides 1111, **1120–4**
  acute poisoning 1120
  chronic exposure 1120
  manganese in, poisoning due to 1110
  organophosphorus, *see* organophosphorus insecticides
  regulations/control 1120
  residues 217
  see also herbicides; insecticides; rodenticides
petechiae
  in acute meningococcaemia 538
  in meningococcal meningitis 539, 540, 4053, 4054
  rare, in pneumococcal meningitis 518
petechial haemorrhages
  in cirrhosis 2087
  in infective endocarditis 2438, 2440–1
  in malaria 844

in relapsing fevers 694, 695
in Rocky Mountain spotted fever 735, 736
pethidine *4353*
petit mal **3912–13**, 4238
  see also epilepsy
petrol (gasoline) 1083, 1092
  air pollution from 1228
  distillates, gastric emptying contraindication 1049
  inhalation **1083–4**, 1092
  'sniffers' 1083, 1084, 1092
pets
  allergen avoidance 2718, 2737
  perennial allergic rhinitis 2715
Peustow procedure 2036
Peutz-Jeghers syndrome 220, 1986–7, 1987, 3723, 3792
  pigmentation in *3755*
  skin in 3792, *3795*
Peyer's patches **1836**, 2001
  M cells 1836, 1837
  in typhoid 561
Peyronie's disease 3246, 3789
P fimbriae 3206
p-glycoprotein 259
  drugs blocking/modifying activity 259
  on myeloma cells 3603
pH
  arterial blood (pH$_a$),
    homeostasis 1533–5
    measurement 1535–6
  dental plaque 1846
  of endocytic pathway 74, 75
  intracellular 1533
  oesophageal, monitoring 1865
  oxygen dissociation curve and 3456
  partition, antimicrobial drug distribution 301
  in phagocytic vacuoles 3559
  potassium balance and 3127–8, 3129
  urine 3102
    in cystinuria 3333
    drug excretion and 3268
    in renal tubular acidosis 3338, *3339*, 3340
  see also acid-base homeostasis
phaeochromocytomas **2553–7**, 2901
  ACTH secretion 2554, 2556
  adrenal 2553, 2555, 2557
  associated syndromes 1710
  catecholamines in **2553–4**
  clinical features 2554–5
  diagnosis/investigations 2555–6
    localization 2556
    suppression tests 2555–6
  extra-adrenal 2553, 2556
  incidence 2553
  malignant 1566, 2554
    treatment 2557
  in MEN 2 syndrome 1637, 1709
  mental disorders/symptoms in 4239
  neuropeptide Y secretion 2554
  pathology 2554
  in pregnancy 1751–2
  prognosis 2557
  screening 1710
  treatment 2556–7
phaeomelanin 3754
phage typing
  Corynebacterium diphtheriae 494
  staphylococci *494*, 524
  see also bacteriophage
phagocytic cells 153, 3555
  bacteria interaction 91, 272
  complement receptors 177, 178
  in infections 91, 276–7
  see also macrophage; neutrophils
phagocytopoiesis **3388–9**
  suppression of 3388–9
phagocytosis 154, 276, **2622–3**, **3559–60**
  alveolar macrophage 2614–15
  bacterial colonization mechanism 91, 272
  macrophage 91
  neutrophils **2622–3**
  process 91, **2622–3**
  pulmonary endothelial cells 2487

in spleen 3588–9
  Staphylococcus aureus 525
phagolysosome 91, 2614, 2623
phagosome 91, 154, 2623
phakoma 3987
Phalen's sign 1226, 2957
Phaneropsolus bonnei 996
Pharaoh's ants 1011
pharmaceutical process **1238–41**
  compliance measurement 1240
  dose-related adverse effects 1251
  drug interactions 1255
pharmacodynamics **1245–9**, *1246*
  actions via,
    direct effects on receptors 1245–6
    direct effects on second messengers 1246
    enzyme activation/activity 1248
    enzyme inhibition 1247–8
    indirect alterations of endogenous agonists 1246–7
    inhibition of transport process 1247
    miscellaneous effects 1248
  age-related changes 4337–8
  antimicrobial therapy **303–6**
  compliance measurement 1240
  defects, pharmacogenetics 1259
  drug interactions 1258
    indirect 1258
  in liver disease 1252
  monitoring 1260
  stereoisomerism 1248–9
  variation, dose-related adverse effects 1252
pharmacogenetics 130, **1258–9**
  pharmacodynamic defects 1259
  pharmacokinetic defects 1258–9
    acetylation 130, 1259
    disease associations 1259
    oxidation and cytochrome P450 130, 1259, 2124
    succinylcholine hydrolysis 1259
pharmacokinetics **1241–5**
  absorption and bioavailability, *see under* drug(s)
  age-related changes 4336–7
  antiepileptic drugs 3922
  antimicrobial therapy **300–3**
  compliance measurement 1240
  digitalis **2242–3**
  distribution, *see under* drug(s)
  metabolism, *see under* drug(s)
  monitoring 1260–1
  non-linear 1245
  parameters **1244–5**
  psychotropic drugs 4247
  in renal impairment **3268–9**
  variation,
    dose-related adverse effects 1252
    pharmacogenetics 1259
  see also entries under drug(s)
pharmacology **1237–61**, *1238*
  pharmaceutical process **1238–41**
  principles **1238–51**
  processes *1238*, 1239
  therapeutic effects, monitoring 1260
  therapeutic process **1249–51**
    adverse reactions, *see* adverse drug reactions
    clinical trials, *see* clinical trials
    compliance measurement 1240
    drug/disease interactions 1250
    effect and rate of onset/duration 1249–50
    modification of action 1249
    monitoring drug therapy **1260–1**
    pharmacological to therapeutic effects 1249–51
    placebos **1259–60**
  see also drug(s); pharmacodynamics; pharmacokinetics
pharyngeal muscles 2610, 2909–10
  in obstructive sleep apnoea 2909
  spasm, in tetanus 626
pharyngitis
  Chlamydia pneumoniae 754
  IgA nephropathy and 3150

lymphonodular 383
Mycoplasma pneumoniae 764
plague 597
post-streptococcal glomerulonephritis and 3173
streptococcal group A infection 498–9, 501
pharynx
  abnormalities, in obstructive sleep apnoea 2910
  'collapse', in obstructive sleep apnoea 2909, 2910
  functions **2610–11**, 2909
  lymphoid tissue 2611
  oedema, acute airways obstruction 2721
  paralysis 3880
    in diphtheria 496
  patency during breathing 2611, 2909
  in sarcoidosis 2826
  structure and function **2610–11**
  tumours, staging investigations *236*
phenacetin
  analgesic nephropathy and 3221, 3223
  haemolysis due to *3546*
  metabolism 3222
  renal cancer association 212
phenazocine *4353*
phenazopyridine, haemolysis due to *3546*
phencyclidine (PCP) 1075–6
  poisoning 1075–6
phenelzine 4249
phenformin 1471, 1542, 2513
phenindione 3673
  nephrotoxicity 3266
phenobarbitone
  in Crigler-Najjar syndrome 2058
  in epilepsy 3922
  in terminal illness 4356
  in tetanus 628
phenol
  ingestion 1104–5
  injection 2371
  poisoning 1078
phenolphthalein, fixed drug eruption 3733
phenothiazines
  adverse mental symptoms 4242
  haemolysis due to *3546*
  neuroleptic malignant syndrome 1182
  in opiate detoxification 4291
  overdose/poisoning 1061
phenotype 100
  genotype correlations **109–10**
phenoxyacetate herbicides, poisoning management 1050
phenoxybenzamine
  advantages 2556, 2557
  overdose 1063
  in phaeochromocytomas 2556–7
  in pregnancy 1752
phenoxypenicillin, in streptococci group A infections 502
phentolamine, pain treatment 3938
phenylacetate, sodium 1360
phenylacetic acid derivatives, poisoning 1056
phenylalanine *1353*
  defects of metabolism **1361–3**
  dietary control 130
  metabolism 1361, 1362
  plasma 1362, 1363
phenylalanine hydroxylase 1362
  deficiency 130
phenylbutazone, poisoning 1057, *1057*
phenyldichlorarsine 1117
phenylethanolamine-*N*-methyltransferase (PNMT) 2553
phenylhydrazine, haemolysis due to 3546
phenylketonuria 130, **1361–3**, 3759
  maternal 130, 1363
  screening 1337, 1362
phenylpropionic acid derivatives, poisoning 1056, *1057*
phenytoin
  adverse reactions 3921, 3923
    endocrine 1645, 1717, 1718
    nephrotoxicity 3266

phenytoin (*cont.*)
in epilepsy 3921–2
monitoring 1260
non-linear kinetics 1245
overdose/poisoning 1062
in pregnancy 1812, 3922
in renal impairment 3268
secondary immunodeficiency due to 174
in status epilepticus 3923
teratogenicity 131, *1810*
Phialophora verrucosa 813
Philadelphia (Ph¹) chromosome 65, 215
in acute lymphoblastic leukaemia 3392, 3398, 3411, 3413, 3414
bcr/abl translocation 225
in chronic myeloid leukaemia 3392, 3403, 3415, 3416
parent-of-origin effects 128
see also *bcr/abl* gene
Philippine haemorrhagic fever 419
phlebitis, occlusive retinal 4182
Phlebotomus fever 428
phlebotomy, see venesection
Phleboviruses 423, *424*, **428–9**
phlegm **2643**
phlegmasiacerulea dolens 2364
phlogopite 2845
phlyctenular conjunctivitis 648
phobia
about mites 1009
agoraphobia 4206
parasitophobia 1004
simple 4206
social 4206
phobic anxiety disorder 4206, 4255
pholcodine 2644
phorbol ester 356
phosgene 1084–5, 1086, 1101
mechanism of toxicity 1101
poisoning **1101**
phosphatases 1560
phosphate 1622
absorption 1627
balance **3058–9**
-binding agents 3327, 3328, 3330
crystals, urinary-tract obstruction 3290
deficiency,
parenteral nutrition complication 1320
rickets in **3074–5**
distribution 1623
endogenous buffers 3338
metabolism, in chronic renal failure 3326, 3328
in parenteral nutrition 2588
plasma 1623, *4367*
in bone disease 3063
in chronic renal failure 3325, 3326
hormonal regulation 1626
in primary hyperparathyroidism 1632
see also hyperphosphataemia; hypophosphataemia
radioactive, in ascites 2098
renal handling 1624, 1627–8, *3330*, 3334
retention 3334–5
wasting 3334
renal tubular reabsorption (TmP/GFR) 1628, 1632, 3334
restriction, in chronic renal failure 3305
treatment 1633, 1638, 3229
urinary stones *3252*, 3253
phosphatidic acid 3618
phosphatidyl inositol metabolism 1561
in platelets 3617–18
phosphine 1101, 1123
poisoning **1101**
phosphocreatine
depletion, fatigue pathophysiology 2173
in heart failure 2233
phosphodiesterase 1560, 2253
inhibitors **2255**
phosphofructokinase 1341, 2146
deficiency (glycogen storage disease VII) 1341, *1343*, **1344**, 1384, 3536, 4166–7
phosphoglucoisomerase, deficiency *1343*

phosphoglycerate kinase (PGK)
deficiency *1343*, 3536
gene polymorphisms 3391, 3392
phosphoinositide-system 2147
phospholamban 2147
phospholipase A₂, in snake venom 1129
phospholipase activation peptide (PLAP) 2029
phospholipase C 1561
phospholipase Cß 2147
phospholipidosis, drug-induced 2128
phospholipids 1400
antibodies to 3020
in bile 2047
platelet membrane 3618
red-cell membrane 3528
in surfactant 2594
transport from liver and gut 1401
phosphoribosyl pyrophosphate (PP-ribose-P) amidotransferase 1378
phosphoribosyl pyrophosphate synthetase (PPRPS) 1378
superactivity 1383, 3226
phosphoric acid 1534
phosphor-plated computed radiography 2652–3
phosphorus-31 spectroscopy 2214
phosphorus-32 (³²P)
in polycythaemia vera 3434
in primary thrombocythaemia 3440
phosphorus
balance **3058–9**
see also phosphate
phosphorylase 1340, 1341, 1458
liver, deficiency (glycogen storage disease VI) *1343*, 1344
muscle, deficiency, see McArdle's disease
phosphorylase kinase 1341
b isoenzyme, deficiency *1343*, 1344
phosphorylation 1560
in transcriptional regulation 1558, 1560
see also oxidative phosphorylation
Photobacterium damselum 558
photocoagulation, in diabetic retinopathy 1485
photophobia, in sarcoidosis 4182
photosensitivity 3722
cutaneous, in porphyria 1394, 1395, 1396
drug-induced 3727, *3728*, 3733
see also drug eruptions
rash distribution 3712
in SLE 3019
phototherapy
in Crigler-Najjar syndrome 2058
in psoriasis 3748, 3750
phrenic nerve 2876, 3898, **4093**
paralysis 4093
phthirus palpebrarum' 1004
phycomycosis (invasive zygomycosis) **810**
in diabetes 1490
Physaloptera caucasia 954
physical illness
course of and psychosocial factors 4232
mental disorders due to, see *under* mental disorders
presentation, psychological factors in **4231–3**
psychiatric disorder detection 4203
psychiatric disorder relationship **4231–47**
psychological precursors 4232
psychological reactions **4245–6**
psychological treatment and 4232–3
sexual problems in, see sexual problems
somatic symptoms without 4257
physicians, see doctors
physiotherapy
in ankylosing spondylitis 2967
in bronchiectasis 2761–2
in chronic obstructive airways disease 2776–7
in chronic respiratory failure 2929
in cystic fibrosis 2753
in pneumococcal infection 521

rehabilitation,
after falls in elderly 4339
after strokes 4340
in tetanus 629
physostigmine salicylate, in tricyclic antidepressant poisoning 1059
phytanic acid
plasma *1440*, 1442
storage disease, see Refsum's disease
phytate 3071, 3073
nutritional osteomalacia 3073
phytoestrogens 1267
phytohaemagglutinins 1158
phytomenadione 3675
in anticoagulant overdose 1077
phytophoto-dermatitis 3725
phytosterolaemia 1406, **1437**
piano-key sign 2957
pica 3475
Pick bodies 3975
Pickering hypothesis, hypertension 2527, 2529
pickled vegetables, oesophageal tumours 1981
Pick's disease 3966, 3969, **3974–7**
Alzheimer's disease *vs* 3976
assessment and diagnosis 3975–6
clinical features 3975
dementia of frontal lobe type 3974, 3975
epidemiology 3975
history and definition 3974
pathology 3975
prognosis and management 3975
progressive aphasia 3974, 3975
variants 3974
Pickwickian syndrome, polycythaemia in 3553
Picornaviridae 449
see also hepatitis A virus (HAV)
picornavirus epidemic conjunctivitis 388
picornaviruses 335, 381, 449
piebaldism 3759
Pierrer-Remy syndrome 2910
pig bel, see necrotizing enterocolitis
pigeon chest (pectus carinatum) 2649, **2875**
pigeon fanciers 2809, 2816
see also extrinsic allergic alveolitis
pigmentary incontinence 3710, 3734, 3754
in infants 3784
pigmentation 3706, **3754–60**
in ACTH hypersecretory states 1575, 1576, 1644
in adrenal insufficiency 1653–4
in alkaptonuria 1364
in Cushing's syndrome 1643
in Fanconi anaemia 3446
of hands and feet, in Balkan nephropathy 3230
increased,
causes *3754*
diseases *3755*
loss, see depigmentation
in lung cancer 2884
in malignancy 3792
in Menkes disease 1417
in pernicious anaemia 3490
in Peutz-Jeghers syndrome 1987
pigments 3754
in pregnancy 1804, 3715
racial differences 3716, 3754
reduced (hypopigmentation) 3755–60, 3757
removal from skin 3758
in systemic illness 3754
in systemic sclerosis 3030
on trunk, causes *3755*
vitamin D synthesis reduction 3073
see also depigmentation; hyperpigmentation
pigmented villonodular synovitis **3007**
pili 272, 536
Neisseria gonorrhoeae 544, 545
pili torti 3763
pilosebaceous follicles, obstruction in acne vulgaris 3752

pinealoma
ectopic **1597–8**
HCG production 1714
pineal tumours **4031–2**
'pink disease' 1111, 4099
pink puffers 2769
pinocytosis 2624
receptor-mediated 91
pins and needles 3858, 4092
pinta **703–6**, *704*, 3755
epidemiology 704, 707
pipecolic acid 2025
piperazine citrate, in enterobiasis 942
piperazine salts, in ascariasis 938
pipe smoking 2313
lip cancer association 201
oesophageal cancer association 202
see also smoking
piretanide 2239
piroplasmosis, see babesiosis
piroxicam, poisoning 1057, *1057*
pirprofen, poisoning 1056
Pit-1 1558
mutations 1558, *1567*, 1571
Pitressin test 3109
pituitary adenylate cyclase-activating peptide 1893
pituitary-adrenal axis disorders, myopathy in 4168
pituitary gland
adenoma 1566, **4032**
ACTH-secreting 1595, 1641, 1650–1
classification 1583
gene defects 1569
GH-secreting (somatotroph adenoma) 1569, 1591, 1748
glycoprotein-producing 1595–6
gonadotrophin-secreting 1595–6
in MEN 1 syndrome 1708
non-secretory 1596, 4032
optic chiasmal lesions 3867
prolactin-secreting, see prolactinoma
secretory 4032
treatment 3868
TSH-secreting 1595, 1612
visual pathway lesions 3865
anatomy 1574
anterior **1573–99**
combined test 1585
hormone deficiencies 1582–3
hormones 1575–81
ontogeny 1575
regulation of hormone secretion 1564, 1574–5
apoplexy 1586, 1588, **1598–9**, 1653
in pregnancy 1748
carcinoma 1566
deficiency, see hypopituitarism
disorders **1581–9**
amenorrhoea **1672**
evaluation 1583–7
hormone replacement therapy 1587–8
hypoadrenalism *1654*
in Langerhans-cell histiocytosis 3608
osteoporosis in 3069
in pregnancy **1747–8**
in sarcoidosis 1716
sexual problems in 4244
embryology 1574
functional assessment 1583–6
granuloma, in sarcoidosis 2827
hypothalamic connections 1565, 1574
imaging 1586
irradiation **1588–9**, 1591, 1594, 1596, 1651
macroadenoma 1581, 1582
masses 1581–2, 1586
microadenoma 1581, 1649, 3818
non-pituitary lesions near **1596–9**
posterior (neurohypophysis) 1574, **1599–603**
drug-induced disorders 1719
hormones, see oxytocin; vasopressin
neuroanatomy 1599, 1600
postpartum necrosis, see Sheehan's syndrome
in sarcoidosis 2827
surgery **1588**
in diabetic retinopathy 1485

pituitary tumours 1591, 1594, 1596, 1650–1
tumours 1566, **1589–99**
  clinical features 1581–3
  evaluation 1583–7
  hypothyroidism 1616
  male hypogonadism 1683
  pituitary apoplexy and 1598
  in pregnancy 1747–8, 1767
  suprasellar extension 1574, 1581–2
  treatment 1588–9
  see also pituitary gland, adenoma
pit vipers, bites and envenoming 1132–3
pityriasis alba 3743, 3760
pityriasis capitis 3764
pityriasis rosea 3750–1
  distribution 3713
pityriasis rubra pilaris 3713, 3715, 3750
pityriasis ('tinea') versicolor **799**, 3754, 3755, 3757
Pityrosporum infections 800
Pityrosporum orbiculare 799, 3743
PIVKAs (proteins induced by vitamin K absence/antagonism) 3654, 3655
pivmecillinam, in urinary-tract infections 3211
pizotifen 4025
pK of drugs 3268
placebos 23, **1259–60**
  in clinical trials 1260, 1262
  skin disease management 3807
placenta
  abruption 1762
  drug transfer across 1809
  infection, toxoplasmosis 867
placental mosaicism 124, 136
Plagiorchis harinasutai 996
plague **595–9**
  bacteriology 595
  bubonic 596
  clinical features 596–7, 596
  epidemiology 595
  history 595
  laboratory findings/diagnosis 597–8
  pathogenesis 595–6
  pneumonic 595, 597
  prevention and control 598–9
  septicaemic 597
  syndromes 596–7, 596
  treatment 598
  vaccine 324, 598
  see also Yersinia pestis
plakoglobin 3781
plantaris rupture 2996
plantar reflex 3857
plantar spurs 2997
plantar warts, see warts, plantar
plants
  contact dermatitis 3737–8
  food, toxicity of 1158–9
plants, poisonous **1151–60**, 1153, 1154, 1155, 1156
  classification based on symptoms 1152–5
  effects 1151–2
  in herbal medicines 1159–60, 1159
  risk 1151
  sources of information and PLATO 1159–60
  toxins and metabolites 1151
  treatment 1152, 1154, 1155
plant-thorn synovitis 2946
plaque 3713
  dental, see dental plaque
  senile, see senile plaques
plasma
  barrier, in gas exchange 2601–2
  fractions **3695**
  fresh frozen 3695
    in DIC 1762, 3658–9
    in factor V deficiency 3652
    in thrombotic microangiopathies 3633
    warfarin overdose 3675
  leakage in dengue haemorrhagic fever 420
  oncotic pressure, reduced, pulmonary oedema in 2498
  osmolality, see osmolality, plasma
  viscosity 2303, 3379

volume 3379, 3380
  in pregnancy 1726, 1735, 1758
  reduced, see polycythaemia, relative
  in splenomegaly 3589
plasmablasts 3597
plasma cells 148
  in coeliac disease 1917
  granuloma, open-lung biopsy 2688
  in immunoproliferative small-intestinal disease 1986
  interstitial pneumonitis **2807**
  in myelomatosis 3597
  pathological clonal expansion 3597
  in rheumatoid arthritis 2954
  in ulcerative colitis 1944
plasmacytoma
  extramedullary **3605**
  solitary, of bone **3604–5**
plasma exchange
  adverse effects 3164
  in anti-GBM disease 3165, 3166
  in autoimmune thrombocytopenia 3632
  in haemolytic uraemic syndrome 3633
  in Lambert-Eaton myasthenic syndrome (LEMS) 4164
  in lupus nephritis 3190
  in myasthenia gravis 4162
  in rapidly progressive glomerulonephritis 3162, 3166–7
  in SLE 3024
  in systemic vasculitis 3016
  in thrombotic thrombocytopenic purpura 3549, 3633
  see also plasmapheresis
plasma expanders
  in acute meningococcaemia 541
  in myocardial infarction 2568, 2569
  in snake envenoming management 1138
plasmalogens 1439, 1440, 1442
plasma membrane
  coated pits 73, 74
  muscle fibres 4139
  defects 4145
  targeting of proteins and transGolgi network 71
  transport vesicle fusion 72
plasmapheresis
  in acute meningococcaemia 541
  in chlorate poisoning 1121
  in hyperlipoproteinaemia 1414
  in myeloma 3603
  in Waldenström's macroglobulinaemia 3604
  see also plasma exchange
plasma proteins
  acute phase 1528
  see also acute-phase proteins
  after injury/surgery 1550
  in amyloid deposits 1521–2
  autoantibodies 163
  calcium binding 1622, 1623
  drug binding 1242, 1257
    digitalis 2242, 2243
    in nephrotic syndrome 3144
    in pregnancy 1813
    in renal disease 3268
  in infections and fever 294
  in nephrotic syndrome 3140, **3143–4**
  thyroid hormone binding 1554, 1605
plasmids 60
  cDNA cloning 59
  DNA, reversibility of tumours and 193
  as gene vectors 61
  HLA-B27 and ankylosing spondylitis 2966
  QpRS of Coxiella burnetii 744
plasmin 3624, 3626, 3663
  excessive generation 3659
plasminogen 93, 3379, 3624
  activation 3622, **3625–6**
    at cell surfaces 3625–6
    at fibrin surfaces 3625
  activators **3625**, 3670–1
    inhibitor **3625**
  nitric oxide interaction 2298
  release by pulmonary endothelial cells 2487

  see also tissue plasminogen activator (t-PA)
  dengue virus protein homology 420
plasminogen activator inhibitor 1 (PAI-1) 2299, 3619, 3624, 3625, 3626
  ischaemic heart disease risk 2309
plasminogen activator inhibitor 2 (PAI-2) 3624, 3625
plasminogen activator inhibitor 3 (PAI-3) 3624, 3625, 3626
Plasmodium **835**
  antibody screening tests 838
  biochemistry 837
  biology of vector for 838
  developmental characteristics 836
  drug resistance, see under malaria
  genetics 835–7
  in vitro culture 838
  laboratory diagnosis 849
  lifecycle 835, 836, 850
  molecular biology 837–8
    gene cloning and rRNA 837
    proteins/antigens 837–8, 862
    vaccine development 861–2
    stages (hypnozoites/merozoites/gametocytes) 835
  see also malaria
Plasmodium falciparum 835, 838, 842
  detection and monoclonal antibodies 849
  evolutionary adaptations to 3463–5
  G6PD deficiency and 3538
  haematological abnormalities 3680
  see also malaria
Plasmodium malariae 835, 838, 847
  dyserythropoiesis in 3524
  glomerulonephritis complicating **3177**
Plasmodium ovale 835, 838, 847
Plasmodium vivax 835, 838, 847
  genetic factors increase susceptibility 280
plastics
  contact dermatitis 3737
  thermal decomposition 1101–2
platelet(s) 3377, **3614–19**
  activation 3614
    in atherogenesis 2291
    defects 3645
    endothelial cells blocking 2290, 2298
  adhesion 2294, 3614–15
    defects 3642–5
  'aggregability' 2303
  aggregation 3616–18
    defects 3646
    inhibition, in salicylate poisoning 1055
    myocardial infarction 2303
    nitric oxide production 2297
    vein constriction 2296
  α-granules 2293, 3615–16
  antibodies 3689
    autoreactive 1764, 3631
    transfusion reactions 3692
  antigens 3689
  arachidonic acid metabolism 3617
  in atherosclerotic plaques 2291
  calcium control 3618
  coagulant activity 3618–19
  concentrates 3694–5
  counts 3379, **3380**, 3629, 3654
    in cirrhosis 2089
    in fetal thrombocytopenia 1764
    in hypereosinophilic syndrome 3612
    in leukaemia 3405
    in paroxysmal nocturnal haemoglobinuria 3451
    in pre-eclampsia 1728, 1729
    in pregnancy 1763
    splenectomy and 3595
    see also thrombocytopenia; thrombocytosis
  cytoskeleton 3618
  dense granules 3615
  disorders 3627
    acquired 3634–5
    in cardiopulmonary bypass 3634, 3660
    drug-induced 3629, 3630, 3635
    in haemolytic uraemic syndrome 3200
    hereditary **3642–6**

  in Lassa fever 433
  in malignant disease 3677, 3678
  in pre-eclampsia 1763
  in pregnancy **1763–5**
  in primary thrombocythaemia 3439
  in renal disease 3302, 3682
  screening tests 3629–30
  endothelial cell function related to 2298–9
  endothelial cell interactions 3626–7
  excessive consumption **3632–3**
  excessive loss from circulation **3633–4**
  giant 3645
  GPIIb/IIIa monoclonal antibodies (C7E3) 2330, 2352
  inhibitors of function 3619
  in ischaemic heart disease 2303–4
  kinetic studies 3595
  lifespan 3381
  neutrophil interactions 3627
  phosphatidyl inositol metabolism 3617–18
  in primary myelosclerosis 3435
  production 3384, 3386, **3389**
  radiolabelled 3595
  receptors on 2291
  reduction, food-induced 3729, 3733
  regulation of function 2298–9
  release reaction 3615–16
  in rheumatoid arthritis 2960
  sequestration/pooling in spleen 3589
  shape change 3615
  thrombus formation and 3662, 3663
  transfusion 3634, 3695
    alloimmune thrombocytopenia due to 3632
    in aplastic anaemia 3445
    in cardiac surgery 3660
    in DIC 1762–3
    in leukaemia 3407
    in platelet adhesion disorders 3645
    thrombocytopenic fetus 1765
platelet-activating factor (PAF) 158–9, 2299
  adult respiratory distress syndrome 2855
  antagonists 293
  cells producing 158
  functions/actions 293
  in pulmonary endothelium 2487
  inflammatory reaction to endotoxin 291
  release in asthma 2727, 2728
  in sepsis and shock 293
  septicaemia treatment 1026
platelet-activating factor (PAF)-acether 3559, 3616, 3627
platelet-associated IgG (PAIgG) 1764, 3631
platelet-derived growth factor (PDGF) 97, 223, 2293, 2299, 3616
  antibodies 2293
  atherosclerotic plaque development 2293, 2299
  in primary myelosclerosis 3435
  production 2293
  receptor 1561, 2293
    amplification 223, 224
  restenosis after angioplasty 2295
platelet disaggregators, see antiplatelet drugs
platelet endothelial cell adhesion molecule (PECAM) 2294
platelet factor 3 3618
platelet factor 4 3379, 3615–16
platinum, nephrotoxicity 3261, **3263**
PLATO 1160
Platt-Pickering controversy 2527, 2529
platynoea 2162, 2163
platypuses, venomous 1125
pleocytosis
  eosinophilic, see eosinophilic pleocytosis
  in leptospirosis 701, 702
pleomorphic adenoma 1862
Plesiomonas shigelloides 558
  infection 559
plethysmography 2368
  nocturnal penile 1687
  whole-body 2666

pleura 2863
  aspiration 2706
  biopsy **2682**, **2686**, 2865–6
    needle biopsy 2865
    in rheumatoid arthritis 2961
    samples, microbiological testing 2675
  disease **2863–72**
    bronchoscopy and biopsy 2683–4
    chest radiography **2664**, 2783
    in diffuse parenchymal lung disease 2781
    drug-induced 2852, *2852*
    in rheumatoid arthritis 2797
    in SLE 2798
    endometriosis 2867
    fibroma 2893
    infections 2867
      empyema **2705–7**
    pain 2648, 2883
    parietal and visceral 2863
    plaques 2893
      in asbestosis 2843, 2844
    sampling 2682
    in sarcoidosis 2825
    tumours 2863, **2893–5**
      benign **2893**
      epidemiology 207
      malignant **2893–5**
      metastatic 2893
      pleural effusions in 2866–7
    see also mesothelioma
pleural cavity pressure 2863
pleural effusion **2863–8**
  in acute pancreatitis 2029, 2868
  after sclerotherapy 2852
  in ankylosing spondylitis 2874
  in asbestosis 2844
  in ascites 2096
  aspiration 2865, 2867
  in cardiac failure 2866
  causes 2863, *2864*
  clinical features 2863
  in collagen vascular diseases 2868
  diagnostic approach **2863–5**
  drugs causing 2852
  in endometriosis of pleura 2867
  examination 2686, **2865–6**
  exudates 2863, 2865, **2866–8**
  formation 2863
  in hepatic cirrhosis 2866
  in infections 2867–8
  investigations 2683, 2863–5
    chest radiography 2863–5
    computed tomography 2864–5
    tests *2866*
    thoracentesis 2865
    ultrasonography 2653, 2864
  in lung cancer 251, 2886, 2892
  malignant 251, **2866–7**
  in Meig's syndrome 2867
  in mesothelioma 2894
  pain in 2648, **2863**
  parapneumonic 2867
  pericardial effusion *vs* 2478
  in pneumococcal infections 516–17
  in pneumonia 2701
  purulent, *see* empyema
  in rheumatoid arthritis 2868
  in subdiaphragmatic infections 2867–8
  transudates 2863, 2865, **2866**
  tuberculous 2867
  see also pleural fluid
pleural fluid 2863
  appearance 2865
    in lung diseases 2686
  aspiration 2865, 2867
  biochemistry and microscopy 2865
  chylous 2868
  examination **2686**, **2865–6**
  formation 2863
  sampling **2682**
  transudate and exudate 2865, **2866–8**
  volume 2863
  see also pleural effusion
pleural rub 2650
pleural space 2863
  bleeding, *see* haemothorax
  gas in, *see* pneumothorax

infections 2705
  obliteration 2863
    see also pleurodesis
  talc insufflation 2867
pleurisy
  pain in 2169, **2648**
  in pulmonary embolism 2868
  in recurrent polyserositis 1526
  in rheumatoid arthritis 2961
  in SLE 3020
  pleuritic pain 2863
pleurodesis **2871**
  in malignant pleural effusions 2867
  in pneumothorax 2871
pleurodynia, epidemic, *see* Bornholm disease
pleuropneumonia-like organisms (PPLO), *see* mycoplasmas
pleuropulmonary infection
  anaerobic 572
  Staphylococcus aureus 526
plexogenic pulmonary arteriopathy 2507, 2508, 2509
plumboporphyria 1394
Plummer-Vinson syndrome 1981, 3475
pmp70 protein 84
PM-Scl antibodies *3033*
pneumatosis cystoides 1987
pneumatosis cystoides intestinalis 1999, 2136
pneumaturia, in Crohn's disease 1938
pneumococcal infections **511–23**
  acute exacerbation of chronic bronchitis 2692
  antibodies 514, 520
  bacteriological diagnosis/assays 519–20
  in chronic obstructive airways disease 2774
  clinical features 514–16
  endocarditis 519, 2436
  epidemiology 512–13, 2695
    age/sex/geographical distribution 512
    incidence 512
    seasonality 512, 2695
  in haemolytic uraemic syndrome 3196
  in HIV and AIDS, *see* AIDS and HIV infection
  immunity 514
  intracranial abscess 4081
  meningitis, *see* meningitis, pneumococcal
  in nephrotic syndrome 3141
  otitis media 512, 513, 517–18
  pathogenesis 513–14
    cytokines 513
  pathology 514
  pericardial effusion and empyema 517
  peritonitis 519, 2008
  pleural effusion and empyema 516–17
  pneumonia, *see* pneumonia, pneumococcal
  predisposing factors 512–13, *513*
    susceptibility increase 514
  prophylaxis 521–3
    chemoprophylaxis 521–2
    vaccines, *see* pneumococcal vaccines
  septicaemia 512, 519, 1020
  spread 513
  treatment 520–1, 2763
    antibiotics 486, 520–1, *520*, 2700
    supporting measures 521
  see also Streptococcus pneumoniae
pneumococcal surface-protein A (PspA) 511
pneumococcal vaccines 319, 522–3, 2701
  14-valent 1028
  after splenectomy 319, 1028
  development 486, 522, 522–3, 4059
  efficacy and cost-effectiveness 522
  immunogenicity 522–3
  indications 319, 522, *522*
  polysaccharide conjugated to protein 522–3
  polysaccharide vaccine 522
  protein antigen development 523
  in splenectomy patients 3530, 3596
pneumococci, *see Streptococcus pneumoniae*

pneumoconioses **2839–47**
  asbestosis **2843–5**
  berylliosis **2846**
  coal-worker's, *see* coal-worker's pneumoconiosis
  cobalt causing 1108
  complicated/progressive 2839, 2840
  definition 2839
  Fuller's earth 2846
  kaolin 2846
  miscellaneous 2846–7
  silicate **2845–6**
  silicosis **2841–3**
    see also silicosis
  simple 2839, 2840, 2841
  talc **2845–6**
  see also asbestosis
pneumocystic disease, *see* pneumatosis cystoides
Pneumocystis carinii **820–4**
  antibodies to 821
  characteristics 821
  diagnostic tests 2676
  disseminated infections 821
  DNA amplification 2591
  epidemiology 820–1
  identification 2686
  pentamidine-induced hypoglycaemia 1511
  in renal transplant recipients 3320
  staining and identification 822
  trophozoites and cysts 821
Pneumocystis carinii pneumonia 473
  after cardiac transplantation 2257
  after lung transplantation 2936
  clinical features 473, 821
  fever and pulmonary infiltrates in 1032
  in HIV infection and AIDS 473, 478, 820, 821
    eye in 4194
    prevention/treatment 478, 823
  investigations/diagnosis 473, 821–2
    lung biopsy 2689
  in malnutrition 1027
  prevention 823, 2713
  prophylaxis 478
  treatment 478, 822–3, 2713
pneumocytes 2593
pneumoencephalography 3826
pneumolysin 511, 512, 513
pneumolysoid 523
pneumomediastinum 2869–70
  chest pain in 2169
  in pregnancy *1742*, 1746
  spontaneous 1206
pneumonia **2693–703**
  adenoviruses causing 337
  aetiological organisms 2694
    identification 2685, 2697
  after lung transplantation 2936
  alveolar filling in 2639
  anaerobic **2702–3**
  aspiration, *see* aspiration pneumonia
  atypical 2693, 2694
    causative organisms 2694
  bacterial, with influenza 2699–700
  'bloodborne' (melioidosis) 591
  Chlamydia pneumoniae 754, 764, 2697
  Chlamydia trachomatis 753–4
  in chronic lymphocytic leukaemia 3421
  classification 2693–4, *2694*
  community-acquired **2694–701**
    aetiology 2694, *2695*
    antibiotics in and sputum culture 2694, 2697
    in children and elderly 2700
    clinical features 2695–6, *2696*
    differential diagnosis 2699
    epidemiology/seasonal peaks 2695
    failure to improve 2701, *2702*
    incidence and types 2694
    investigations, *see below*
    management 2700–1
    pneumococcal 512
    prevention 2701
    prognostic factors 2701, *2701*
    rate of clearance 2699
    secondary pneumonia 2699–700
    severe 2701, *2701*
    sputum in 2695, 2697

in congenital candidiasis 1793
cryptogenic organizing **2795–6**, 2795
cytomegalovirus 2709, 2713
desquamative interstitial 2689, 2786, 2787, *2787*
  see also cryptogenic fibrosing alveolitis
eosinophilic **2805**
geographically-restricted **2703**
giant-cell *2787*
  in measles 380
Gram-negative bacilli 2701
haematogenous staphylococcal 526
haematological changes 3685
Haemophilus influenzae 583, 2694
  type b 582, 2694
historical aspects 2693
in HIV-infected patients 472, 473, 486, 2693, 2710
  management 2713
  see also AIDS and HIV infection
in immunocompromised 1031, 1032, *1033*, 2693–4
  management 2712
  prevention 2713
  see also Pneumocystis carinii pneumonia
in immunodeficiency 2703, 2710
importance of and health costs 2693
interstitial 2787, *2787*
  see also cryptogenic fibrosing alveolitis
investigations 2696–9
  blood and liver function 2696–7
  chest radiography 2698–9
  invasive 2697–9
  microbiological **2678**, 2697
  open-lung biopsy 2688–9, 2698
  serological and culture 2697
  sputum examination in 2685, 2695, 2697
  virology 2697
  see also under respiratory tract infections
Legionella pneumophila, *see* legionnaires' disease
lipoid (lipid) **2837–8**, 2852
  liver in 2130–1
lymphocytic choriomeningitis virus infection 436
management **2700–1**
  antibiotics 2700–1, 2712
  severe pneumonia 2700–1
in measles 379
in megaloblastic anaemia 3496–7
melioidosis 591
meningococcal 540, 2694
mortality 2693
Mycoplasma pneumoniae **762–7**, 2697
  see also Mycoplasma pneumoniae
neonatal chlamydial 753–4, 1791–2
in neonatal streptococcus B infection 1788
in neonatal *Ureaplasma* infection 1792
non-pneumococcal bacterial 2697
nosocomial 330, *330*, 1021–2, **2701–2**
opportunistic, *see Pneumocystis carinii*
organizing 2688–9
  bronchiolitis obliterans with **2795–6**, 2795
parainfluenza viruses causing 338
pleural effusion in 2867
pneumococcal 512, 2694, 2699
  clinical features 515
  course and prognosis 516
  differential diagnosis 516, *516*
  haemoptysis in 2644
  investigations 515–16
  liver in 2130
  in measles 378, 379
  pathology 514
  treatment 516, 520–1, 2701
Pneumocystis carinii, *see Pneumocystis carinii* pneumonia
poker players' 742
postoperative 2701
in pre-existing chronic obstructive lung disease 2700

in pregnancy 1746–7
primary atypical 762
  see also Mycoplasma pneumoniae,
   pneumonia
in Q fever 742, 743
recurrent 2694, **2703**
rhinovirus infections 335
septicaemia in 1020–1
staphylococcal 526, 527, 1021, 2694
in transplantation patients 2709, 2710
tuberculosis *vs* 651
viral 2697
  pneumococcal pneumonia *vs* 516
see also respiratory tract infections
pneumonitis
  acute lupus 2798
  in ascariasis 937
  chemical, petrol causing 1083
  in chickenpox 347
  cytomegalovirus (CMV) infection 361
  drug-induced 2850
  in hookworm infection 931
  hypersensitivity 2809
   see also extrinsic allergic alveolitis
  idiopathic interstitial 1033
  interstitial **2807**
   in marrow transplant recipients 3698
   in scrub typhus 740
  Japanese summer-type 2811, 2816
  lymphocytic interstitial **2807**
  in manganese poisoning 1110
  in measles 380
  plasma cell interstitial **2807**
  radiation **2848**, 3574
  in SLE 3010
  in vanadium poisoning 1114
  ventilation 2811
pneumotachography, portable 2672
pneumothorax **2869–71**
  aircraft travel and 1199
  associated conditions **2869–70**
  chest radiography 2662, 2665
  in chronic obstructive airways disease
   2777
  clinical features **2869**
  in cystic fibrosis 2749
   treatment 2753
  in divers 1206
  iatrogenic 2869
  pathophysiology 2869
  in pregnancy *1742*, 1746
  primary 2869
  secondary 2869
  in silicosis 2842
  spontaneous 2777, 2869
   in aircraft crew and pilots 1201
   in eosinophilic granuloma of lung 2833
  tension 2563, 2869
  treatment **2870–1**, *2870*
   aspiration 2870
   intercostal tube drainage 2870–1
   pleurodesis 2871
   surgical 2871
  ventilation complication 2924
pneumotyphoid 562
PNP gene 172
'podagra' 2984
podoconiosis **1215–17**
podophyllin 3768
  warts treatment 3798
POEMS syndrome 3566, 3586, 4102,
  4104–5
  associated features *4105*
  peripheral neuropathy 4102, 4104
poikilocytes *3378*
poikilocytosis 3377
  in G6PD deficiency 3539
  transient infantile 3531
poikiloderma 3790, 3795, 3796
poikiloderma atrophicans vasculare 3796
poikilothermy, in malnutrition 1286
Poiseuille's law 2726
'poison arrow frogs' 1140
poison information centres 1051, 1160
poisoning **1043–51**
  accidental 1043, 1044, 1045
   childhood and infant 1044, 1045
  acute 1043
   diagnosis 1045

aquatic animal ingestion **1141–3**
  gastrointestinal/neurotoxic syndromes
   1142
  histamine-like syndrome 1142–3
by birds **1140–1**
by chemicals **1078–23**
  alcohols and glycols **1079–83**
  in conflict, *see below*
  corrosive substances **1102–5**
  hydrocarbons and chlorofluorocarbons
   1083–93
  inhalational agents **1093–102**, 1172
  metals **1105–15**
  pesticides **1120–4**
  volatile substances **1083–93**, 1172
  see also individual chemicals
childhood, *see* children, poisoning
chronic 1043
  circumstances for 1045
circumstantial evidence 1045
clinical and metabolic features **1044–50**
  decerebrate and decorticate
   movements 1046
  feature clusters 1045–6, *1045*
  lateralizing neurological signs 1046
  strabismus and ophthalmoplegia 1046
in conflict **1115–20**
  decontamination of casualties 1115
  lewisite 1117
  nerve agents 1117–18
  relative toxicities *1116*
  riot control agents 1118–19
  sulphur mustard 1115–17
deaths from 1043–4, *1044*
deliberate 1043
diagnosis 1044–5
by drugs **1051–78**
  analgesics **1051–8**
  anticonvulsants **1061–2**
  antidepressants **1058–60**
  antihistamines **1062**
  antimicrobials **1072**
  antiparkinsonian drugs **1062**
  cardiovascular drugs **1062–7**
  cinchona alkaloids and antimalarials
   1072–3
  drugs of abuse **1074–7**
  endocrine drugs **1071–2**
  fatal doses *4376*
  gastrointestinal drugs **1069–70**
  haematinics and vitamins **1070–1**
  hypnotics and tranquillizers **1060–1**
  miscellaneous **1077–8**
  NSAIDs **1056–8**
  opiates **1058**
  respiratory drugs **1067–9**
  see also each individual drug/drug
   group
epidemiology **1043–4**
fish **1141**
  ciguatera 1142
history-taking 1043, 1045
hospital admissions 1043
management **1046–50**
  antidotes 1048, *1048*
  coma grading 1046–7, *1046*
  emergency treatment 1046
  gastric emptying, *see* gastric emptying
  methods of elimination 1050–1
  oral adsorbents 1049–50
  prevention of absorption 1048–51
  of specific abnormalities 1047–8
  supportive care 1046–8
occupational causes, *see* occupational
  disease; *specific chemicals*
by plants and fungi **1151–60**, *1153,*
  1154, 1155, 1156
  see also fungi; mushroom; plants
self-poisoning, *see* self-poisoning
severe, indication for gastric emptying
  1049
by venoms and animal toxins, *see*
  venomous animals
poison ivy 3738
poisons, information services 1051, 1160
pol gene and Pol protein 464, 489
police, medical reports and 4315
poliomyelitis 4067
  abortive 385

bulbar 385, 1962
epidemiology 382
incidence and notifications 384
non-paralytic 385
paralytic 384, **385–6**, 4064
  clinical features 4067
  course 4067
  differential diagnosis 4069
  epidemiology 382
  in hypogammaglobulinaemia 168
  major/minor illness 4067
  positive-pressure ventilation 2576,
   4072
  postpolio syndrome after 4089
  spinal/bulbar forms 385
  treatment 4071–2
pathology 4066, 4067
in pregnancy 1776, 1777, *1779*,
  1783
prevention 389–90, 4072
  outbreak control 390
  surveillance 390
provocation 385
rabies *vs* 401
tick paralysis *vs* 1149
vaccination 382, 386
  policy 389–90
  vaccines 318, 388–9, *389*
   combined oral/inactivated
    administration 389
   enhanced-potency inactivated (Salk)
    389, *389*
   live attenuated oral (Sabin) 389, *389*
   in pregnancy 1777
poliovirus 381
  diagnosis 383
  infections in hypogammaglobulinaemia
   168
  neurological diseases *385*
  types 385
  'wild' 382, 389
  see also enterovirus infections
pollens
  asthma 2734
  avoidance 2717
  seasonal allergic rhinitis (hayfever)
   2714
pollution
  asthma and bronchial hyper-
   responsiveness 2731, **2733**
  cancer association 217–18
   difficulties in assessing 217
   lung cancer 207
  chronic obstructive airways disease and
   2767
  enterovirus transmission 389
  lung function variations 2674–5
  seasonal allergic rhinitis (hayfever)
   2714
  see also air pollution
polyarteritis
  acute renal failure in 3291
  microscopic,
   gastrointestinal tract in 2000
   see also microscopic polyangiitis
  renal transplantation 3315
polyarteritis nodosa **3014–15**, 4130
  cardiac manifestations *2392*, 3014
  clinical features 3014–15
  diagnosis/differential diagnosis **3015**
  gastrointestinal tract in 2000, 3014
  haematological changes *3548*, 3681
  hepatitis B association 3011
  in injecting drug abusers 4283
  liver in 2135, 2139
  mental disorder/symptoms 4243
  neurological complications 3015,
   4130–1
  neuropathy in 4102
  ocular features **4183–4**
  renal disease 3014
  response to treatment 3017
polyarthritis **2946–7**
  of carcinoma 3006
  causes *2946*
  migratory, mycoplasmas causing 771
  in psoriasis 3748
  Ross river virus causing 407
  see also arthritis

polychondritis, relapsing, *see* relapsing
  polychondritis
polycyclic aromatic hydrocarbons
  air pollution 1228
  cancer association 218, 1166–7
  lung cancer and 206, 2880
  non-melanoma skin tumour association
   209
polycystic kidney disease **3202–4**
  autosomal dominant (adult) **3202–4**,
   3303
   definition 3202
   extrarenal features 3203
   genetic counselling 3204
   symptoms 3202–3
   treatment 3203–4
  autosomal recessive (infantile) **3204**
  gout and 1381
  haematological changes 3682
  pregnancy in 1735
  renal pain 3148
polycystic liver disease 2015
polycystic ovary syndrome 1669, 1671,
  1673, **1674–6**, 3765
  congenital adrenal hyperplasia *vs* 1664
  endocrine features 1674–6
  hirsutism in 3765
  infertility 1674, 1675, 1676, 1678
  management 1677
polycythaemia 2400, 3431, **3551–4**
  absolute 3431, 3551
  in chronic respiratory failure 2929–30
  classification 3551
  clinical approach 3551–2
  cobalt causing 1108
  in cyanotic congenital heart disease
   2400
  genetic 3554
  high oxygen-affinity haemoglobin
   variants 3519
  in infants of diabetic mothers 1757
  in malignant disease 3678
  pathogenesis 3551
  pruritus in 3744
  relative 3431, 3551, **3552–3**
  (rubra) vera **3431–4**, 3551
   aetiology 3432
   chorea in 4010
   clinical features 3432–3
   course and prognosis 3433
   differential diagnosis 3433, 3593,
    3594–5
   haematological changes 3433
   haemodynamics and oxygen transport
    3432
   management 3433–4
   splenomegaly in 3432, 3589
   thrombotic complications 3432, 3433,
    3668
  secondary 2929, 3551–2, **3553–4**
  in urinary-tract obstruction 3235
polydipsia
  in diabetes insipidus 1601
  primary 1601, 3120, **3121**
   aetiology 3120
   causes *3120*
   clinical features 3121
   diagnosis 3121–2
   treatment 3122
polyene antifungals 811, 812
polyfructosan-S 3105
polygenic inheritance 129
polyglandular autoimmune syndromes
  1571, 1652–3
  type I 1571, 1652, 1653
  type II (Schmidt's syndrome) 1571,
   1652, 1653
polyhydramnios 1973
  in diabetes mellitus 1757
polymerase chain reaction (PCR) 61, 62,
  2677
  cat-scratch disease causative organism
   745
  chlamydial infection diagnosis *755*, 756
  in coagulation disorders 3638
  cytokine role in immune response to
   grafts 187
  dengue virus detection 422
  enteroviruses diagnosis 383

polymerase chain reaction (PCR) (*cont.*)
  in haematological disorders 3390, 3398
  hepatitis C diagnosis 458, 2063
  Lyme disease diagnosis 691
  meningococcal infection diagnosis 540
  Mycobacterium tuberculosis 4062
  Mycoplasma pneumoniae detection 764
  mycoplasmas detection 762, 769
  Pneumocystis carinii detection 822,
    823, 2591
  preimplantation diagnosis 136
  rickettsial diseases diagnosis 733
  rRNA sequencing for bacterial
    classification 273
  Streptococcus pneumoniae detection 520
  in viral infections 1778
  viral infections of CNS 4069
polymorphic epithelial mucin (PEM)
    229, 231
polymorphic eruption of pregnancy 1804
polymorphonuclear elastase, *see*
    neutrophils, elastase
polymorphonuclear granulocytes, *see*
    basophils; eosinophil(s);
    granulocyte(s); mast cells;
    neutrophils
polymorphonuclear neutrophil leucocytes
    (PMN), *see* neutrophils
polymyalgia rheumatica **3039–41**, 3039
  aetiology and pathogenesis 3040
  clinical features 3040
  diagnosis 3040, *3041*
  differential diagnosis 3040, *3041*
  giant-cell arteritis relationship 3041
  haematological changes 3483, 3681–2
  incidence 3039–40
  joint stiffness in 2945, 3040
  liver in 2135, 2139
  pyrophosphate arthropathy *vs* 2989
  rheumatoid arthritis *vs* 2955–6
  treatment 3040–1
polymyositis *3009*, **3038–9**, **4156–8**
  aetiology 3038, 4156–7
    autoimmune 3038
  classification *4156*
  clinical features 3039, 4157
  course and prognosis 3039, 4158
  diagnosis and treatment 3039, 4157
  eosinophilic **4158**
  histology 4143
  in HIV infection 4076
  HTLV-I association 490
  immune response 4156
  lung involvement in **2799**
  malignancy association 4134, 4157,
    4158
  in pregnancy 1766
  variants **4157–8**
  see also dermatomyositis
polyneuritis, infective, positive-pressure
    ventilation 2576
polyneuropathy 4092
  acute idiopathic inflammatory, *see*
    Guillain-Barré syndrome
  chronic inflammatory demyelinating
    4101
  critical illness 4099
  demyelinating 3842
  electromyography **3841–2**
  familial amyloid, *see* familial amyloid
    polyneuropathy
  investigations 3841–2
  in sarcoidosis 2827
  sensory loss in 4092
  symptoms 4092
  see also neuropathy; peripheral
    neuropathy
polynuclear aromatic hydrocarbons
  air pollution 1228
  cancer association 1166, *1166–7*
  see also polycyclic aromatic
    hydrocarbons
polyomaviruses 443, **446–7**, 461
  see also BK virus; JC virus
polypectomy, colonic adenoma removal
    1989
polypeptide growth factors, *see* growth
    factor(s)
polypharmacy 4336

polyphenols, in food plants 1159
polyposis 1986, *1987*
  cap 1986
  juvenile 1986, 1987
polyposis coli
  familial, *see* familial adenomatous
    polyposis (FAP)
  in schistosomiasis 977
polyps
  colonic, *see* colonic polyps
  definition 1986
  fibrous, of mouth 1859
  gastric, *see* gastric polyps
  inflammatory, in ulcerative colitis 1945
polyribosomes 61
polysaccharides, non-starch, *see* non-
    starch polysaccharides
polysomnography 2913
polystyrene 1088
polytetrafluoroethylene (PTFE) 2370
polyunsaturated fatty acids 1412, 1472,
    2310
  dietary recommendations 1330
  ischaemic heart disease risk 1330, 2311
  n-3 2311, 2312
    concentrates in capsules 2312
    mechanism of action 2311
  n-6 1472, 2311
  see also fatty acids
polyuria **3120–2**, 3146–8
  causes 3120–1
  in chronic renal failure 3147–8, 3296
  definition 3101
  in diabetes insipidus 1601, 3442
  in diabetes mellitus 1453, 3147
  diagnostic evaluation 3121–2
  palpitations with 2175
  in renal tubular acidosis 3340
  in urinary-tract obstruction 3235
polyvinyl chloride (PVC) 1090, 1102
  combustion products 1102
  pneumoconiosis 2847
polyvinylpyrrolidone (PVP) 3136
Pompe's disease (glycogen storage
    disease II) **1342**, *1343*, *1435*, 1437,
    4165–6
  diagnosis 1341
pons 3856, **3858**
  lesions 3858
Pontiac fever 723, **726**
pontine haemorrhage 3931
Pooling Project 2533
popcorn (L and H) cells 3571
popliteal cyst, in rheumatoid arthritis
    2958, 2959
population 42–3
  demographic entrapment 37
  density, anaemia and 3462
  growth 51
population reference intake (PRI) 1268
'porcupine man' 3719
porencephaly 4116
porocephalosis **1012–14**
  Porocephalus 1013–14
porphobilinogen 1389
  urinary *1390*, 1391, 1392
porphobilinogen (PBG) deaminase 1391,
    1394
porphobilinogen (PBG) synthase, *see* δ-
    aminolaevulinic acid (ALA)
    dehydratase
porphyria 1259, **1388–99**
  acute 1388–9, **1391–4**
    safe drugs 1398–9
    unsafe drugs 1397–8
  acute attack **1391–4**
    clinical features 1391–2
    diagnosis 1392
    management 1392–3
    precipitating factors 1392, 1397–8
    prevention 1393–4
  acute intermittent *1390*, **1391–4**
    basic defect 1391
    long-term complications 1394
    mental disorders/symptoms in 4240
    in pregnancy 1393–4, 1767
    screening of relatives 1394
    surgery and anaesthesia in 1394

Chester 1394
  classification 1388–9
  congenital (Gunther's disease) *1390*,
    1395, 3724, 3727
  cutanea tarda (cutaneous hepatic) *1390*,
    1394–5, 3482
  δ-aminolaevulinic acid dehydratase
    deficiency 1394
  gastrointestinal motility disorder in
    1962
  molecular biology 1389–91
  neuropathy in 4102
  non-acute *1388*, 1389, **1394–6**
  prevalence 1391
  rash in 3727
  variegate *1390*, 1391, **1394**
porphyria cutanea tarda 244, *3791*
  iron overload in 2022
Porphyrimonas, rare species *559*
Porphyrimonas gingivalis 1847
porphyrins 1388, **1389**
  diseases causing abnormal metabolism
    1396–7
  in porphyrias 1389, *1390*
  precursors 1389, *1390*
Portacath venous access system 2752–3
portacaval shunt, in Budd-Chiari
    syndrome 2099
portal hypertension **2091–5**
  ascites due to 2096
  in Budd-Chiari syndrome 2098
  causes 2092, *2092*
  in chronic pancreatitis 2038
  in cirrhosis 2089
  clinical approach 2057
  clinical signs 2093
  in congenital hepatic fibrosis 2015
  consequences 2092
  definition 2092
  investigation 2093
  management 980, 2093–5
  in pregnancy 1800
  in primary myelosclerosis 3437
  pulmonary hypertension in 2509
  in sarcoidosis 2122
  in schistosomiasis 977, 980
  sinusoidal/presinusoidal 2092, *2092*
  travel precautions 2091
  in Wilson's disease 1420
  see also oesophageal varices
portal-systemic anastomoses 2092
portal-systemic encephalopathy, *see*
    hepatic encephalopathy
portal-systemic shunt surgery
  in ascites 2098
  in bleeding oesophageal varices 2095
  encephalopathy after 2108
portal vein 2091
  block 2093
  gas bubbles in 1996
  thrombosis,
    ascites in 2096
    computed tomography 2012
    transhepatic percutaneous sampling
      1508, 1704
portal venous flow 2091
  obstruction 2092, 2096
portal venous pressure 2092
  in cirrhosis 2086
portal venous system
  liver transplantation 2114
  septic venous thrombosis 2139
Portuguese-men-o'-war 1143–4
port wine naevi **3785**
positive end-expiratory pressure (PEEP)
    ventilation 2578, 2903, **2921–3**,
    2921
  actions/physiology 2922
  in adult respiratory distress syndrome
    2575, 2640, 2858
  applications 2921
  complications 2923
  contraindication 2578
  indications 2578
  'intrinsic' 2667
  in respiratory failure 2922
  in unilateral lung disease 2923
  weaning 2580, 2923

see also continuous positive airway
    pressure (CPAP); positive pressure
    ventilation
positive-pressure ventilation **2576–81**
  in adult respiratory distress syndrome
    2857–8
  bronchoscopy 2579–80
  complications 2923
  expiratory choke in 2578
  inception in severe airways disease
    2578
  indications 2576–7
  intermittent, *see* intermittent positive
    pressure ventilation (IPPV)
  in kyphoscoliosis 2577, 2905
  management of patient 2579
  nasal, *see* nasal positive-pressure
    ventilation (NPPV)
  nocturnal 2592, 2905–6
    in central sleep apnoea and
      hypoventilation 2918
  in pulmonary oedema 2505, 2568
  technical considerations 2577–9, 2906
    endotracheal intubation 2577
    face mask 2576, 2577
    humidification/warming of air 2578
    ventilator settings 2578–9
  underventilation 2578, 2580, 2581
  ventilators 2576
  weaning 2580–1
  see also continuous positive airway
    pressure (CPAP); positive end-
    expiratory pressure (PEEP)
    ventilation
positron emission tomography (PET)
    2212
  neurological disorders 3815, 3825
  radiopharmaceuticals for 2212
postabortal fever, *Mycoplasma hominis*
    causing 771
postanoxic action myoclonus 4015
postcapillary venule 2618
postcardiotomy syndrome 2475
  treatment 2477
postcholecystectomy syndromes 2051
postconcussional symptoms 4049
postdysenteric syndromes 828
post-epileptic 'furor' 4238
post-epileptic mental state 3912, 4237–8
posterior cord syndrome 3898
posterior fossa tumours 3836
posterior spinal root 3902
  lesions 3857
  see also spinal nerve roots
postextrasystolic potentiation (Bowditch
    effect) 2150, 2157, 2158
postganglionic neurones 3881
post-herpetic neuralgia 350, 3945, 4023
  prevention and treatment 351, 3945
post-ictal confusion 3912, 4237–8
post-infective arthritis 2965
  see also reactive arthritis
post-infective neuropathies **4101–2**
post-infective tropical malabsorption
    1932
post-irradiation brachial plexus
    neuropathy 4094
postmenopausal osteoporosis, *see*
    osteoporosis
postmortem 4310
postobstructive pulmonary oedema 2501
postoperative ileus, *see* paralytic ileus
postoperative psychiatric complications
    4243
postpartum fever
  Mycoplasma hominis 771
  streptococci group A 501, 502
  streptococci group B 506
postpartum period
  in diabetes mellitus 1758
  endometritis 1791
  idiopathic renal failure **1734**, 3292
  lymphocytic hypophysitis **1597**, 1748
  malaria in 847–8
  pituitary necrosis, *see* Sheehan's
    syndrome
  thyroid disorders 1750
postperfusion syndrome 2445

postpericardiotomy syndrome 2445
postphlebitic syndrome 3664, 3665
postpolio syndrome 4089
post-sympathectomy neuralgia 2374
post-transcriptional modification 57,
  57–9
  mutations interfering 63
post-translational modification 57, 59,
  68, 1557, 1559–60
  quality control 70
post-traumatic amnesia 3855–6, 3916,
  4048–9
post-traumatic dystrophy, *see*
  algodystrophy
post-traumatic encephalopathy 4049
post-traumatic epilepsy 4049
post-traumatic headache **4028**
post-traumatic meningitis, *see* meningitis
post-traumatic stress disorder 4205,
  4257
  features and treatment 4205
post-traumatic syndrome 4028
postural drainage
  in bronchiectasis 2761–2
  in cystic fibrosis 2753
postural hypotension
  in amyloidosis 3180
  in diabetes 1488
  in diabetic ketoacidosis 1499
  in elderly **4343–4**
  falls due to 4339
  in hypertension treatment 2533
  management 4343–4
  in Parkinson's disease 4004
  in primary autonomic failure 3882, 3886
  in spinal cord injury 3898
  syncope in **3927**
postural instability 3863
postural sensibility, loss 4092
posture
  idiopathic oedema and 3127
  lung function variations 2674
  lymphoedema pathogenesis 2560
  in Parkinson's disease 4001
  proteinuria and 3102, **3138**
  pulmonary blood volume changes 2488
  pulmonary circulation in 2490
  and time test, aldosterone secretion
  1657–9
postviral fatigue syndrome 386, 1036
  see also chronic fatigue syndrome
potassium **3127–35**
  absorption/transport 1902
  balance **3127–9**
    in acid-base disturbances 1540
    in chronic renal failure 3297
    external 3128–9
    internal 3127–8
  in cirrhosis 2088
  coronary vasodilatation 2159
  diuretics sparing 2239
  heart electrophysiology 2148
  insulin secretion and 1459
  intake 3127
    in acute renal failure 3286
    adaptation to high 3128–9
    in artificial nutritional support 1318
    in chronic renal failure 3305
    excessive 3133
    hypertension pathogenesis 2530
  loss,
    diuretics causing 2239
    in heart failure 2235
    in malnutrition 1285, 1287
  plasma 3127, *4367*
    in Cushing's syndrome 1647
    in diabetic ketoacidosis 1501, 1502
    see also hyperkalaemia; hypokalaemia
  red cell permeability defect 3532
  renal handling 3128–9, *3330*
    disorders of **3336–7**
  supplements,
    with diuretics 2239, 3130
    hypertension management 2538
    preparations 2239
    in theophylline poisoning 1068
  total body 3127
    measurement 1303

treatment 3132
  in Bartter's syndrome 3131
  in diabetic ketoacidosis *1500*, 1501–2
  diuretic-treated patients 2239, 3130
  in hyperosmolar hyperglycaemic non-
    ketotic coma 1502
  intravenous infusion 3132, 3133
potassium channels
  drugs acting on 1247
  openers **2330**
potassium chlorate, poisoning 1121
potassium chloride 3132
potassium citrate 3256
potassium iodide, skin eruption 3731
potassium perchlorate 1608
potatoes, glycoalkaloids in 1159
'pot belly' 1918
potocytosis 71
potomania, beer drinker's 3123
Pott's disease (spinal tuberculosis) 653,
  654, 2874, 2998–9, 3902
  shunt 2406
pouchitis 1950
  causes 1950
  idiopathic 1950–1
poultry
  Campylobacter infections 557
  Salmonella infections 552, 553
poverty
  in developing countries 52
  worldwide 38
Powassan encephalitis **415**
poxviruses **365–72**
  biology 366
  classification 365–6, *366*
  expression vectors 368
  pathogenesis of infections 366–7
  recombinant 365, 368
  transmission 366–7
  see also molluscum contagiosum;
    vaccinia virus
practolol
  airway obstruction and asthma 2849
  oculomucocutaneous syndrome due to
    2852
  rash due to 3732
PRAD-1 *1567*, 1569
Prader-Willi syndrome 1306, **4110**,
  4121
  complications 4110
  hypogonadism 1683
  mental retardation in 4110
  uniparental disomy 127, 128
pralidoxime chloride 1122
pralidoxime mesylate 1122
  in nerve agent exposure 1118
praziquantel
  bioavailability 968
  in clonorchiasis 986
  in cysticercosis (*T. solium* infection)
    968
  in fasciolopsiasis 993
  in *Hymenolepis nana* infestation 963
  mechanism of action 979
  metabolism and toxicity 968
  in opisthorchiasis 984
  in paragonimiasis 992
  in schistosomiasis 979
  side-effects 979
  in *Taenia saginata* infestation 961
prazosin, in heart failure 2252
prealbumin, *see* transthyretin
preamyl3972
precision, clinical examination **15–17**
precocious puberty, male 109
prediabetes *1452*
predictive value 17, 18–19
prednisolone
  in acute flare in SLE 3023
  in alcoholic hepatitis 2084
  in allergic rhinitis 2718
  in anti-GBM disease *3165*
  in asthma 2738
  in autoimmune haemolytic anaemia
    3544
  in autoimmune hepatitis 2073
  in benign intracranial hypertension
    4043

in cardiac transplantation 2257
in chronic active hepatitis B 2068
in Crohn's disease 1942
in giant-cell arteritis 3042
in Hodgkin's disease *3573*, 3574
in hypercalcaemia 3229
in hypereosinophilic syndrome 2397,
  3612
in lupus nephritis 3190
in membranous nephropathy 3160
in mesangiocapillary glomerulonephritis
  3158
in minimal change nephropathy 3155,
  3156
in myasthenia gravis 4162
in myeloma 3602
in non-Hodgkin's lymphoma *3585*
in pemphigus vulgaris 3781
in psoriasis 3750
pulse dose, in systemic vasculitis 3016
in renal transplant recipients 3319
in retroperitoneal fibrosis 3245
side-effects 3781
in SLE 3023
in sperm autoimmunity 1686
in Takayasu's disease 2379
in ulcerative colitis 1948, 1949
prednisone
  in cortisol deficiency 1587
  in fever of unknown origin (FUO) 1019
  in hypercalcaemia 1638
  in myeloma 3601
  in pregnancy 1745, 1764, 1805
  in rheumatic fever 2434
pre-eclampsia 1726, **1727–31**
  clinical features 1727–9
  complications *1728*, 1730, *1762*
  in diabetes mellitus 1757
  diagnosis 1729–30
  haemolytic anaemia in *3548*
  haemostatic changes 1728, 1763
  liver disorders 1728–9, 1797
  long-term sequelae 1732
  management 1730–1
  nutrition and 1730, 1773
  pathology 1727, *1728*
  prevention 1730
  reflux nephropathy and 3218
  risk factors 1727, *1728*
  SLE *vs* 3022
  superimposed on chronic hypertension
    1727, 1731, 1735
pre-excitation syndrome, *see* ventricular
  pre-excitation
preganglionic neurones 3881
pregnancy 1584
  acute fatty liver of (AFLP) 1797–8
  acute intermittent porphyria in 1393–4,
    1767
  aircraft travel and 1203
  alcoholism in 4112
  anaemia in **3468–9**
  ankylosing spondylitis and 2968
  anticoagulation in **1739–40**, **1742–3**,
    1810–11, 3675
  antiepileptic drugs in 3922
  antiphospholipid antibodies in 1768,
    3669
  antituberculous drugs in 660
  bartonellosis in 775
  in benign intracranial hypertension
    4043
  blood disorders **1758–65**
  breast cancer incidence and 209
  brucellosis in 622, 623
  bulimia nervosa and 1301, 4217
  cardiac failure in 2383
  cardiovascular changes 1726, **1735–6**
  chest diseases in **1744–7**
  cholestasis of **2060**
  chronic renal failure in 3300
  complications, in drug abuse 4298
  Crohn's disease management 1943
  in cyanotic congenital heart disease
    2401
  diabetes mellitus 130, **1752–8**
  DIC in **1762–3**, 3658
  diphtheria in 494

donovanosis in 776, 778
drug abuse in, *see* drug abuse(r) and
  misuse
drug prescribing in **1809–13**
drugs with adverse effects in later
  stages 1254–5, *1255*
drugs to avoid 1254, *1254*, 4299
  see also teratogenic drugs
in Ebstein's anomaly 2414
ectopic, *see* ectopic pregnancy
in Eisenmenger reaction (syndrome)
  2401, 2412
endocrine disease in **1747–52**
epilepsy in 3922
ethical issues 12
in Fallot's tetralogy 2407
folate deficiency **1759–60**, 3467,
  3468–9, 3493
folic acid supplements 1759, 3491,
  3493, 3496
gastrointestinal disorders in **1801–3**
genital warts in 3368
glycosuria in 1754, 3333
haemolytic uraemic syndrome in 3197,
  3201
heart disease in **1735–40**
in hyperprolactinaemia 1591, 1672,
  1747–8
hypertension in, *see* hypertension, in
  pregnancy
hypoglycaemia in 1511
idiopathic thrombocytopenic purpura in
  1764, 3631, 3632
immune function 1784
infections in **1775–95**
in inherited thrombophilias 1743, 3668
insulin secretion 1461, 1753
intrahepatic cholestasis of 1796
iron-deficiency anaemia **1758–9**,
  3468–9, 3476
iron overdose 1071
Lassa fever in 432–3
liver disease in **1796–801**
lymphocytic hypophysitis 1597, 1748
malaria in 846–7, 847–8, 1794–5, 3467,
  3468–9
  management 856
malignant disease in **1806–8**
maternal well-being and drugs 4298,
  4299
metabolic disorders 130, **1721–815**
molar, *see* hydatidiform mole
multiple,
  assisted reproduction and 11
polymorphic eruption of pregnancy
  1804
neurological disease **1766–9**
nutrition in **1769–74**
occult causes of collapse *1742*
oestrogen-induced pruritus 3744
opiate withdrawal 4296, 4299
opportunistic infections 1027
osteoporosis and **3069**
oxytocin actions 1603
parvovirus B19 infections 448
pemphigoid in 3783
phenylketonuria in 130, 1363
polymorphic eruption of 1804
prurigo of 1805
pruritus of 1804
in reflux nephropathy 1734, 3218
renal disease in **1733–5**
rubella management 411
in sarcoidosis **2827–8**
screening in, *see* screening, antenatal
skin disorders in **1804–6**, 3715
in SLE 3017, 3022, 3191
  drugs contraindicated 3022
stage, drug abuse effect 4298
stroke in 3956
in systemic sclerosis 3192
Takayasu's disease and 2379
teenage 36
termination, *see* abortion, therapeutic
thromboembolism in **1741–3**
thrombotic thrombocytopenic purpura
  in 1763, 3549
thyroid function tests in 1717, 1748–9

pregnancy (cont.)
  travel and **325**
  trichomoniasis in 3354
  ulcerative colitis in 1951
  urinary-tract changes 3241–2
  urinary-tract infections, see urinary-tract
    infections, in pregnancy
  water homeostasis in 1748, 3117, 3118
pregnenolone, deficiency 1691–2
preimplantation diagnosis 136
prekallikrein (PKK) 3621, 3626
  inherited deficiency 3622, 3651–2
preleukaemia 3425, 3448
premarin 210
premature infants
  cerebral palsy aetiology 4119
  folate deficiency 3493
  normal haemostatic values *3654*
prematurity 4298
  occupations associated 1173
premedication, for endoscopy 1830
prenatal cerebral damage, cerebral palsy
  aetiology 4119
prenatal diagnosis **135–7**, *135–6*
  'burden of choice' 136
  congenital adrenal hyperplasia 1667
  cystic fibrosis 1745
  ethics 12
  fragile X syndrome 126
  genetic disorders **135–7**
  haemoglobinopathies 1760, 1761
  haemophilia 1765, 3638–9, 3640
  inborn errors of metabolism 1338
  inherited metabolic disorders of liver
    2017
  isovaleric/propionic/methylmalonic
    acidaemias 1371
  muscular dystrophies **4146–7**
  osteogenesis imperfecta 3082
  peroxisomal disorders 1440, 1441,
    1442, 1443
  polycystic kidney disease 3204
  sialic acid storage disease 1436
  thalassaemia 3512
  tyrosinaemia type I 1364
  urea cycle defects 1359–60
  vesicoureteric reflux 3217
  viral infections 1778
  von Willebrand's disease 3641–2
prenatal malformations *4106*
prenatal screening 135
preoperdin, deficiency 180
preproglucagon, peptide products **1893**
preprohormone 1557, 1559
preproinsulin 59, 1459
  mutations 1571
prescribing, see drug(s), prescribing
pressure, limits for ventilators 2921
pressure flow studies, urinary tract 3240–1
pressure immobilization method 1135–6
pressure natriuresis 3247–8
pressure sore (decubitus ulcer) **3811**
  anaerobic infections 573
  pathogenesis/aetiology 3811
  prevention 3900
  in spina bifida, management 4118
  in spinal cord injury 3900–1
presyncope 3926
preterm infants, see premature infants
preterm prelabour rupture of membranes
  (PPROM) **1786**, 1787
prethrombotic states (hypercoagulation)
  3665–70
  acquired 3665, 3669–70
  in acute pancreatitis 2030
  eye in **4194**
  inherited 3665–8
  screening tests 3670
pretibial myxoedema 3802
prevalence 43
  accuracy of a diagnostic test and 17,
    18–19
  definition 645
  rate 43
  studies 44, 45
preventative genetics 67
prevention 50
Prevotella, rare species *559*
priapism, in sickle-cell disease 3517

prickly heat 1180, 3767
primaquine
  in G6PD deficiency 3541
  in malaria 852
  overdose 1073
primary biliary cirrhosis *2018*
  aetiology and pathogenesis 2074
  drugs 2129
  associated diseases 2075
  autoantibodies in 163, 2074
  autoimmune hepatitis vs 2070–1
  clinical features 2074–5, 2087,
    3744
  complications 2076
  course and prognosis 2076, 2107
  diagnosis 2075–6
  hepatic granulomas in 2122
  immune abnormalities 2074
  incidence 2074
  liver transplantation in 2112, 2115
  pathology 2074
  in pregnancy 1800
  sarcoidosis overlap 2131
  treatment 2076, *2076*
primary health care **46–51**
  content 47–8
  definition 46
  in developing countries 52
  features 47
  future 50–1
  health promotion and prevention 50
  secondary care and 48–9
  team 49–50
primary lateral sclerosis 4090
primary sclerosing cholangitis, see
  cholangitis
primary upper small-intestinal disease
  (PUSIL) 1930
primidone
  in epilepsy 3922
  overdose/poisoning 1062
Prinzmetal's angina, see angina (angina
  pectoris), Prinzmetal
prion diseases **3977–81**
  aetiology 3977–9
  bovine spongiform encephalopathy
    (BSE) 1517, 3977, **3981**
  cerebral amyloid in *1514*, **1517**
  clinical features 3979–81
  historical background 3977
  inherited 3978–9, 3979, *3979*
    clinical features 3980–1
  occupational hazard 1173
  presymptomatic testing and counselling
    3981
  prognosis 3981
  sporadic 3979, *3979*
  types *3979*
  see also Creutzfeldt-Jakob disease; kuru
prion protein (PrP) 3977
  in Creutzfeldt-Jakob disease 3978
  in kuru 3983
  mutations 3977–8
    in inherited prion diseases 3978, *3979*
    specific and diseases associated
      3980–1
  pathogenicity model 3978
  PrP^c 3977, 3978
  PrP^sc 3977, 3978
  replication 3978
  structure 3977
  transmission 3978, 3979
prions 3977–9
  definition 3977
  strains 3978
prison, substance abuser in **4305**
  privileged sites 185–6
pro-arrhythmia 2262, 2345
probability
  post-test 20
  pre-test (prevalence) 17, 18–19
  probability theory 2227, *2227*
probenecid 2987
  in renal failure 3274
problem-solving approach 4254–5
  in deliberate self-harm management
    4230–1
  in dissociative disorder 4210

probucol 1414, *3143*
procainamide *2264*
  overdose/poisoning 1063
procaine penicillin 718
  reactions to 718
  syphilis treatment 717, *717*, 4086
procarbazine, in Hodgkin's disease *3573*,
  3574
processed pseudogene 106
procoagulants, in snake venom 1129
proctalgia fugax 1965
proctitis
  in coeliac disease 1917
  haemorrhagic, in lymphogranuloma
    venereum 760
  in homosexuals 3361
  in lymphogranuloma venereum 760,
    761
  management 1948
  sexually transmitted causes 1947, 3361,
    3362
proctocolectomy
  in Crohn's disease 1943
  in familial adenomatous polyposis 1990
  restorative 1950
  in ulcerative colitis 1950
  see also colectomy
proctocolitis, in lymphogranuloma
  venereum 760
Procurator Fiscal 4311
procyclidine 1061
pro-drugs 1243
proerythroblasts 3388
professional indemnity 4312
professional witness 4315
profunda femoris artery, reconstruction
  2370
profundoplasty 2370
progeria *3791*
progesterone
  control of gonadotrophin secretion 1579
  in puberty 1563
  receptor 1554, 1555, 1561–2
    defects 1573
progestogens
  in constitutional delay of growth and
    adolescence 1703
  gallstones and 1801
  in hormone replacement therapy
    1587–8, 1813, 1814
  -only contraceptive pill 1724–5
  in oral contraceptives 1723
  in osteoporosis 3068
  in Turner's syndrome 1700
proglucagon 1559
progressive diaphyseal dysplasia
  (Engelmann's disease) **3089**
progressive external ophthalmoplegia
  4148, **4172**
progressive massive fibrosis
  in coal-worker's pneumoconiosis 2840,
    2841
  prevention 2841
progressive multifocal
  leucoencephalopathy 443, **446–7**,
    3575, **4073–4**, 4133
  in HIV infection 475, **4079**
progressive myositis ossificans, see
  myositis ossificans progressiva
progressive neuronal degeneration of
  childhood with liver disease 3989
progressive pallidal atrophy **4009**
progressive rubella panencephalitis **4074**
progressive supranuclear palsy 3965,
  4005–6, *4006*
proguanil 3273
  malaria prophylaxis 860
  overdose *1073*
prohormones 1557, 1559
proinsulin 59, 1459
  plasma *1462*, 1507
  split products 1459, *1462*
proinsulin-like growth factor II (pro-
  IGFII) 1509
prokinetic drugs
  in gastric stasis 1959
  in motility disorders after peptic ulcer
    surgery 1962

probucol
prolactin **1576–7**
  drug interactions 1718
  ectopic production 1716
  receptor 1556, *1560*, 1576
  releasing factors (PRF) 1576
  serum 1576, 1584–5
    in combined anterior pituitary test
      1585
    in hyperprolactinaemia 1589–90, 1672
    in insulin tolerance test 1585
    non-secretory pituitary adenoma 1596
    in polycystic ovary syndrome 1676
  see also hyperprolactinaemia
prolactin-growth hormone family **1576–8**
prolactinoma **1589–91**, 1672, 3867
  associated syndromes 1708, 1710
  in pregnancy **1747–8**
  treatment 1588, 1590–1, 3868
  see also hyperprolactinaemia
Prolene mesh 1974, 1975
prolidase deficiency *1375*
proline oxidase deficiency *1375*
promethazine, in pregnancy 1802
promotion, cancer development 198
promotors 57
  gene 1557–8
  mutations and effects 63
  pancreatic cancer 2040
promyelocyte 3556
pronormoblast 3453, 3454
pro-opiomelanocortin (POMC) 1559,
  1575, 1712
  N-terminal (N-POC) 1642
propane, poisoning 1083
1,2-propanediol (propylene glycol),
  poisoning 1082
2-propanol (isopropanol), poisoning 1080
propantheline 3766
properdin 177
propionate 1467
Propionibacterium 570
Propionibacterium propionicum 680,
  684
propionic acidaemia *1337*, **1370–2**
propionyl coenzyme A carboxylase
  1369, 1370–1, 1373
propositus 131
propranolol
  drug interactions 4004–5
  in hepatic granulomas 2123
  in hyperthyroidism 1613, 1614
  in hypertrophic cardiomyopathy 2389
  in pregnancy 1767, 1812–13
  in primary polydipsia 3122
proprioceptive sensation 3858
proptosis, in Wegener's granulomatosis
  3012
propylene glycol, poisoning **1082**
propylthiouracil 1612, 1614
  in alcoholic hepatitis 2085
  in pregnancy 1749
  vasculitis due to 3011
propyphenazone, poisoning 1057
prosopagnosia 3854
Prospective Investigation of Pulmonary
  Embolism Diagnosis (PIOPED) 2525
prostacyclin 2290, 2298
  in adult respiratory distress syndrome
    2855
  coronary vasodilatation 2159
  decreased synthesis in Lassa fever 433
  function 2487
  in haemostasis 3619, 3626–7, 3662
  in heart failure 2252
  infusion, donor heart-lung surgery 2934
  release by pulmonary endothelium 2487
  therapy, in haemolytic uraemic
    syndrome 3201
prostaglandin(s)
  in ascites pathogenesis 2097
  in Bartter's syndrome 3131
  in haemostasis 3619, 3626–7
  in heart failure 2170
  insulin secretion and 1459
  in pain 3936
  peptic ulcer treatment 1888
  release in asthma 2727, *2728*
  renal actions 3119, 3228

synthesis 158
  in fever 293
  mediators/stimulators 294
  in platelets 3617
  tumours secreting 1712
  vasodilation 2297
prostaglandin E₁, platelet inhibition 3619
prostaglandin E₂, in fever 293
prostaglandin endoperoxides 2298, 2299
prostaglandin F₂α, asthma exacerbation 2849
prostaglandin G₂ 3617, 3626
prostaglandin H₂ 3617, 3626
prostaglandin I₂, see prostacyclin
prostaglandin synthetase inhibitors, in gastrointestinal infections 2006
prostanoids
  vasoconstriction and 2298
  vasodilation 2297
prostate
  abscess 573
  anaerobic infections 573
  cancer,
    epidemiology 210–11, 1171
    increase with prostatic biopsy increase 211
    magnetic resonance imaging 239
    staging investigations 236
  enlarged, bladder outflow obstruction 3234, 3236
  fluid specimens 3208
  transrectal ultrasound 3242
prostatitis
  acute 3207
  chlamydial 751
  treatment 3211
  ureaplasma causing 770
prostheses
  coagulase-negative staphylococcal infections 532
  heart valves, see heart valves
  infections related to 330
Prosthodendrium molenkampi 996
prostitution 3348, 3350
protal circulation 2091–2
protamine sulphate 1254, 3660, 3673
protease nexin 3625
proteases, macrophage releasing 2291
protective clothing 1164, 1165
protein(s)
  abnormal metabolism, in hepatocellular failure 2105
  absorption 1901, 1903
    investigation 1907
  apical targeting in epithelial cells 71
  body composition and distribution 1272
  in cerebrospinal fluid, see cerebrospinal fluid
  deficiency,
    anaemia in 3498–9
    in bacterial overgrowth 1913
    kwashiorkor relationship 1288
    skin in 3722
  dietary,
    in chronic renal failure 3304–5
    in diabetic nephropathy 1468–9, 3171
    in hepatic encephalopathy 2108
    ischaemic heart disease risk 2311
    peritoneal dialysis and 3312
  digestion 1903
  drug binding, see under plasma proteins
  energy source 1272
  engineering, hepatitis B vaccine 456
  folding, prevention by heat-shock proteins 69
  glomerular filtration 3136
  glycation, in diabetes 1479, 1481, 3169
  GPI-anchored 71
  increments in pregnancy 1770, 1771
  intolerance,
    in hepatic encephalopathy 2108
    lysinuric 1357, 3333
  low molecular weight, in urine 3109, 3137
  in lymph 2560
  metabolism 1274–6
    after injury/surgery 1549–50
    after surgery in diabetes 1494

in chronic renal failure 3302–3
  in pregnancy 1753
  urine nitrogen and 3-methylhistidine 1275, 1276
  normal range 4371
  plasma, see plasma proteins
  protective in lung 2614
  red-cell membrane 3528
  reference nutrient intake 1269, 1270, 1329
  renal tubular reabsorption 3137
  requirements, artificial nutritional support 1316–17
  structure 57
  suicide 109
  synthesis,
    changes in infections 294
    in kwashiorkor 1288
    'one gene-one peptide chain' 57
    quality control in endoplasmic reticulum 70
    translation 58, 59
    translocation after, see exocytic pathway
    transport into nucleus 78–9
  turnover 1274–5
    indicators 1275
    in starvation 1277, 1278
  urinary 3101–2, 3137
    in diabetes 1479–80
    secreted 3137–8
    see also proteinuria
proteinaceous infectious particles, see prions
protein antigens 141
proteinase 2770
  in bronchiectasis 2763
  in chronic obstructive airways disease 2773
proteinase-antiproteinase theory 2770–3
protein 4.1 3527
  defects 3531
protein 4.2 3527
  deficiency 3529
protein C 3619, 3623–4, 3626, 3666
  concentrates, in DIC 3659
  deficiency 2522, 3666–7, 3675
    causes of acquired 3671
    indications for screening 3670
    management 3667–8
    pregnancy in 1743, 3668
  inhibitors 3624
  normal values 3379
  in pregnancy 1762
  resistance to activated 3667
protein-calorie malnutrition, see under malnutrition
protein disulphide isomerase (PDI) 69–70
protein energy malnutrition, see under malnutrition
protein kinase, defects in SLE 3026
protein kinase A 1560, 1561
protein kinase C 1561, 2147, 3618
  antagonists 259
  in cardiac hypertrophy 2148
  diabetic tissue damage and 1483, 1486
protein-losing enteropathy 1907, 1999
  increased catabolism/loss of immunoglobulin 175
  in pericardial constriction 2480
  secondary antibody deficiency in 169
  in tricuspid regurgitation 2468
proteinoses, pulmonary alveolar, see pulmonary alveolar proteinosis
protein S 2290, 3619, 3623–4, 3667
  deficiency 2522, 3667, 3675
    causes of acquired 3671
    indications for screening 3670
    management 3667–8
    pregnancy in 1743, 3668
    normal values 3379
    in pregnancy 1762
protein translocation pore 69
  function 69
proteinuria 3136–44
  algorithm for investigation 3139
  in amyloid nephropathy 3180
  benign 3102

in cadmium nephropathy 3262
  in chronic renal failure 3301, 3303
  clinical 3137–8
  consequences 3138–44
  in diabetes mellitus 1411, 1464, 3169, 3170
  drug-induced 3193
  in focal segmental glomerulosclerosis 3156
  functional 3102
  'glomerular' 3137
  haematuria with 3138, 3146
  in haemolytic uraemic syndrome 3198, 3200
  measurement 3101–2, 3137
  in mercury poisoning 3262
  in minimal change nephropathy 3155, 3156
  monoclonal light-chain (Bence Jones) 3181, 3182
  normal 3137
  overflow 3137
  pathological 3137–8
  persistent symptomless 3138
  physiological/pathological basis 3136–7
  in post-streptococcal glomerulonephritis 506
  postural (orthostatic) 3102, 3138
  in pre-eclampsia 1728, 1729
  in pregnancy 1734–5, 3022
  in reflux nephropathy 3218
  in renal hypertension 2546
  in rheumatoid arthritis 2962
  in schistosomiasis 977, 979
  secreted proteins/casts 3137–8
  selectivity 3138
  in SLE 3022, 3187
  in thrombotic thrombocytopenic purpura 3549
  'tubular' 3137
  see also microalbuminuria; nephrotic syndrome
proteoglycans 3058
  in bone 3058
  turnover, in osteoarthritis 2981
proteolysis, by macrophage 93
proteolytic enzymes, antagonists 1026
Proteus
  interstitial nephritis 3178
  urinary-tract infections 3206
Proteus mirabilis 551
  urinary-tract infections 3206
Proteus syndrome 124
prothionamide
  in leprosy 676
  in tuberculosis 655, 656
prothrombinase complex 3620
prothrombin (factor II) 3619, 3620
  complex concentrates 3652, 3675
  inherited deficiency 3622, 3642, 3652
prothrombin time (PT) 3379, 3628, 3654, 3661
  in acute liver failure 2106
  in DIC 3658
  international normalized ratio (INR) 3628, 3655, 3673–5
  international sensitivity index (ISI) 3673
  in liver disease 3656
  in paracetamol poisoning assessment 1052, 1053
  see also bleeding time
proton-pump (H⁺,K⁺ ATPase)
  autoantibodies 3489
  inhibitors 1867
    peptic ulcer treatment 1887–8
    in Zollinger-Ellison syndrome 1881–2
    see also omeprazole
proton radiation 1217, 1218, 3819
proto-oncogenes 3567
  lung cancer 2882
protoporphyria, erythropoietic 1390, 1395–6
protoporphyrin
  erythrocyte 1390, 1395, 1396
  faecal 1390, 1395
  red cell 3474

protoporphyrinogen oxidase deficiency 1391, 1394
protoveratrines 1154
protozoal infections 825–909
  eye 4192
  in homosexuals 3364–5
  in hypogammaglobulinaemia 168–9
  liver in 2134
  meningitis 4070
  myositis 4156
  in pregnancy 1793–5
  sexual transmission 3345
pro-urokinase (scu-PA) 3625, 3671
provirus 462, 463
provocation-neutralization testing, food allergy 1845
prozone phenomenon 622
prurigo
  actinic 3726
  of pregnancy 1805
pruritic urticated papules and plaques of pregnancy 1804
pruritus 3743–5
  in atopic eczema 3741
  in biliary obstruction 2046
  in blood diseases and anaemia 3744
  causes 3743–4
  in cholestasis of pregnancy 2060, 3744
  in chronic renal failure 3324, 3744
  in cirrhosis 2087, 3744
  in dermatitis 3734
  distribution 3713, 3715
  in endocrine disease 3744
  features and pathogenesis/sensation 3743
  generalized, in systemic disease 3744
  genitalia 3768
  gravidarum 1796, 1804
  in haematological disorders 3375
  head lice causing 1003, 3744
  in Hodgkin's disease 3570
  insect bites causing 3744
  in intrahepatic cholestasis 2059, 3744
  itch threshold 3741, 3743
  localized 3744–5
  in malignancy 3792
  management 3744, 3806
  parasites causing 3743
  paroxysmal itching 3743
  in polycythaemia vera 3432, 3434
  of pregnancy 1804
  in primary biliary cirrhosis 2074, 2076, 2087, 3744
  in scabies 1007, 1009, 3744
  skin disease management 3806
pruritus ani 3745
  in enterobiasis 941
pruritus vulvae 3745
  in diabetes 1453
Prussian blue, in thallium poisoning 1113
psammoma bodies 2687, 4032
P-selectin 2294, 2299, 2487, 2620, 2620
pseudoachondroplasia 3089
pseudoallergic drug reactions 1253
pseudoaneurysms 2321
pseudoappendicitis syndrome 608, 610
pseudoathetosis 4092
pseudoatrophy, cerebral, in anorexia nervosa 1297, 4214
pseudo-autosomal region 116
pseudoBartter's syndrome 1300, 4216
'pseudobubo' 777
pseudobulbar palsy 3857, 4122
pseudocholinesterase 4365
  polymorphisms 1259
pseudochyle 2868
pseudoclaudication 2364
pseudocoarction, of aorta 2182
pseudocowpox 369
pseudo-Cushing's syndrome 1640, 1643, 1717
pseudodementia
  depressive 3967, 4225, 4227
  differential diagnosis 3967
  dissociative 4210
  hysterical 3967
pseudodiverticula 1999

pseudogene 106
pseudogout 2988, *2990*
  treatment 2990
'pseudogranuloma inguinale' 777
pseudohermaphroditism
  female **1690–1**, 1694
  hirsutism in 3765
  male 1572, 1690, **1691–4**
    dysgenetic 1693
pseudo-Hurler polydystrophy
  (mucolipidosis III) 1434, *1435*, 3985
pseudohyperkalaemia 3133
  familial 3133
pseudohyperparathyroidism (humoral
  hypercalcaemia of malignancy) 1568,
  1630, 1632, 1712
  mental disorders/symptoms in 4239
pseudohypoaldosteronism **1662**, 1669
  type I 1662, 3134, 3337
  type II 1662, 3134, 3337
pseudohyponatraemia **3122**
  in hypertriglyceridaemia 1410, 1503
pseudohypoparathyroidism 1633, **1634**,
  1636, 3079, 3334–5
  biochemical features *3062*
  bone disease in 3079
  calcification in 3092
  eye in 4196
  type I 1634, 3334
  type II 1634, 3334–5
pseudomembranous colitis, *see* colitis,
  pseudomembranous
Pseudomonas
  antibiotic resistance *310*
  in bronchiectasia 2760
  endocarditis 2437
  rare species *559–60*
Pseudomonas aeruginosa
  α_1-antitrypsin inactivation 1545, 1546
  antibodies 2748
  in cystic fibrosis 2747, 2748
    treatment 2752, *2752*
  infections 550, 2437
    treatment 2448, *2448*, 2752, *2752*
Pseudomonas cepacia 550
Pseudomonas mallei 593
Pseudomonas pseudomallei, see
  Burkholderia (Pseudomonas)
  pseudomallei
pseudomyotonia 4151
pseudomyxoma 2009
pseudoneurosis 4239
pseudopapilloedema 3864, 3866
pseudopolyps
  colonic 1950
  in ulcerative colitis 1946
pseudoporphyria cutanea 3302
pseudo precocious puberty 1701, 1702
pseudopseudohypoparathyroidism 1634,
  3079
  mental disorders/symptoms in 4239
pseudoscleroderma *3791*, 3792
  scorbutic *3791*
pseudotachycardia 2197
pseudotruncus 2407
pseudotumour
  cerebri, *see* intracranial hypertension,
    benign (idiopathic)
  haemophilic 3647
  lung 2688
pseudoxanthoma elasticum **3789–90**
  bleeding disorders 3636, 3645
  mitral regurgitation 2457
pseudo-Zellweger syndrome **1441**
psittacosis 754–5, 1023
  see also Chlamydia psittaci
psoralens 3758
psoriasis 3716, **3745–50**
  in AIDS 3746
  arthropathic 3748
  clinical features 2945, 3746–8, 3762
  distribution 3713
  drug eruptions in 3731
  flexural 3747, 3768
  generalized pustular 3716, 3717,
    3747–8
  guttate 503, 3746
  handicap 3708
  HLA association 3745

management 3748–50
  nails 3747
  non-dermatitic occupational dermatosis
    1165
  nummular discoid 3746, 3747
  palmar and plantar 3746–7
  pathogenesis 3745–6
  in pregnancy 1806
  rheumatoid arthritis *vs* 2963
psoriatic arthritis 2965, **2968–70**, 3748
  categories 2968
  clinical features 2968–9, *2968*
  treatment 2969–70
psoriatic arthritis mutilans 3748
psyche, skin relationship 3707
psychiatric advice, need for and referral
  criteria 4204
psychiatric disorders **4203–59**, *4204*
  as abnormal emotional reactions 4203,
    4204
  abnormal porphyrin metabolism 1397
  in acute porphyria 1392
  in aircraft crew and pilots 1201
  aircraft travel and 1203
  in Alzheimer's disease 3973
  in Cushing's syndrome 1643
  detection in physically ill patients 4203
  drug abuse and misuse **4295**
  in elderly **4226–8**, **4340–1**
    assessment 4226
    types and prevalences 4226
    see also under elderly
  electroencephalogram (EEG) in 3830
  epilepsy and 3924
  in HIV infection 476
  normal emotional reactions *vs* 4203
  organic mental disorders, *see* organic
    mental disorders
  in Parkinson's disease 4004
  in pernicious anaemia 3490
  physical complaints with **4208–9**, 4257
  physical illness relationship **4231–47**
    detection in 4203
    in dying patients, *see* dying patients
    illness presentation and course **4231–3**
    sexual problems, *see* sexual problems
    specific conditions causing **4236–43**
  primary polydipsia 3117
  psychiatric emergencies due to **4258–9**
  reactions to stressful events **4204–5**
  reactions *vs* disorders 4203–4
  severity, assessment 4204
  symptoms, physical disorders
    relationship 4203
  thyroid function 1617
  treatment, *see* psychological treatment;
    psychotropic drugs
  viral causes 4074
  in Wilson's disease 1420
  see also mental disorders; *specific*
    disorders
psychiatric emergencies **4256–9**
  alcohol abuse/withdrawal 4258–9
  compulsory treatment 4257
  drug dependence 4259
  general considerations **4256–8**
  patients refusing treatment 4257
  psychiatric syndromes as cause **4258–9**
  somatic symptoms without physical
    cause **4257**, *4258*
  stupor 4257
  trauma victims 4257–8
  see also disturbed patients; violent
    patients
psychiatric factors, in chronic pain 3943
psychiatric hospital admissions 4259
  compulsory 4257
  after self-harm 4230
psychiatrist, referral 4254
  in chronic fatigue syndrome 1039
  criteria 4204
  in depressive disorders 4219
  in mania/manic depressive disorder
    4221
psychoactive drugs 4247
psychogenic disorders
  asthma **2735**
  motility disorders 1963–5
  purpura 3637

psychogenic pain 2945, 3943, **4209**
psychogenic unresponsiveness 3932
psychogenic vomiting 1821–2, 1964
psychological assessment
  artificial nutrition at home 1324
  in rheumatic diseases 2944
psychological distress, food allergy/
  intolerance association 1844
psychological factors
  after bereavement 4235
  chest pain causes **2168–9**
  in chronic fatigue syndrome 1038
  course of illness affected by 4232
  determinants of consultations 4231–2
  duodenal ulcer aetiology 1878
  in emotional distress in dying patients
    4233
  fatigue pathophysiology 2173
  pain 3942–3, 4300
  in physical illness, assessment of sexual
    problems 4246
  precursors to physical illness 4232
  in presentation of illness **4231–3**
  in spinal cord injury 3901
  in terminal illness 4350, 4351
  terminal illness **4357–9**
  see also psychosocial factors
psychologically-determined weakness
  3841
psychological problems
  brittle diabetes and 1496
  in chronic renal failure 3306
  in cystic fibrosis **2750**
  in homosexuals 3361
  in leukaemia 3407
  in malnutrition, management 1295
  in Sydenham's chorea 4012
psychological reactions
  to cardiovascular disorders 4244
  to neurological disorders 4244
  to physical illness, sexual problems due
    to **4245–6**
psychological reactions to stress 4204–5
  acute reactions 4204
  adjustment disorder 4204–5
  anxiety, *see* anxiety disorders
  post-traumatic stress disorder 4205,
    4257
psychological responses to stress 4204
  coping strategies 4204
  mechanisms of defence 4204
psychological stimulation, in
  malnutrition management 1293–4
psychological support 4254
  in cancer 252–3
psychological symptoms, generalized
  anxiety disorder 4205
psychological treatment **4254–6**
  brief dynamic psychotherapy 4207,
    4210, **4255–6**
  in bulimia nervosa 4217, 4255
  chronic fatigue syndrome 1039
  chronic pain 3946
  cognitive behavioural, *see* cognitive
    behavioural therapy
  crisis intervention 4254–5
  in depressive disorders 4219
  functional bowel diseases 1968
  listening and information provision
    4254
  physical illness and 4232–3
  problem-solving, *see* problem-solving
    approach
  supportive counselling 4254
psychometric tests, in hepatic
  encephalopathy 2105
'psychomotor attack' 4238
psychomotor disturbances,
  gastrointestinal motility **1963–5**
  see also functional bowel disease
psychomotor retardation, in depression in
  elderly 4227
psychopathic personality 4212
psychopharmacology **4247–54**
  see also psychotropic drugs; *specific*
    drug groups
psychosis
  in aircraft crew and pilots 1201
  dopamine agonist-induced 1590

in drug abuser 4295
  in epilepsy 4238
  in malaria 847
psychosocial factors
  course of illness 4232
  ischaemic heart disease risk 2315
  in presentation of illness 4231
psychotherapy
  brief dynamic 4207, 4210, **4255–6**
  see also psychological treatment
psychotic behaviour
  in multiple sclerosis 3993
  in Parkinson's disease 4004
psychotic depression 4218
psychotropic drugs **4247–54**
  adverse mental symptoms 4242
  antianxiety drugs **4253–4**
  antidepressants, *see* antidepressants
  antipsychotic drugs **4251–3**
  classification *4248*
  compliance 4247
  drug interactions 4247
  indications 4247
  mood stabilizing drugs **4250–1**
  overdosage 4247
    deliberate self-harm 1043, 4228, 4229,
    4247
  in pain treatment 3945
  peptic ulcer treatment 1884
  pharmacokinetics 4247
  prescribing principles,
    in depression 4247
    in elderly 4227
  in terminal illness 4356
  see also individual drugs groups/drugs
Psychrobacter immobilis 560
PTC oncogene *1567*, 1569–70, 1618
pteroylglutamic acid, *see* folic acid
PTH, *see* parathyroid hormone
Pthirus pubis 1000, 1003–4
ptosis, in myasthenia gravis 4161
pubarche, isolated 1701
puberty 1563, 1580, **1700–3**
  definition 1700–1
  delayed 1701, *1702*, **1703**
    constitutional 1697, **1703**
  growth 1696, 1701
  precocious **1701–2**
    in congenital adrenal hyperplasia 1664
    HCG-induced 1702, 1714
    pseudo 1701, 1702
    true 1701, 1702
  skin and skin disease in 3715
  timing 1701
pubic lice 1003–4
public health
  gastrointestinal infections and 2006
  infections **285–9**
    see also infections
  personal health and, HIV-positive drug
    abuser 4302
puerperium, *see* postpartum period
puffer fish, poisoning 1142
Pugh-Child's grading, of liver disease
  2094, *2094*
pulmonary alveolar microlithiasis **2838**
pulmonary alveolar proteinosis 2685,
  2833–5
  bronchoalveolar lavage 2784
  infections in 2833, 2834
pulmonary amyloidosis **2835–6**
pulmonary angiography
  indications 2525
  in pulmonary embolism 2525, 2569
  in pulmonary hypertension 2511
pulmonary anthrax 616
pulmonary apoplexy 2410
pulmonary arterial hypertension 2181,
  2494
  causes *2512*
  pulmonary oedema with 2501
  tropical disease and 2509
  see also pulmonary hypertension
pulmonary arterial pressure *2154*, 2488,
  2488, 2506
  diastolic 2163
  dicrotic notch 2153
  in ductus arteriosus 2430
  in exercise 2490

in Fallot's tetralogy 2403
normal *2488, 2506*
rise, in pulmonary embolism 2524
systolic 2180
pulmonary arterial resistance 2488
rise and capillary blood flow 2490
pulmonary arterial stenoses
heart murmurs 2421
multiple acquired 2409
multiple congenital **2409**
single branch 2409
see also pulmonary stenosis
pulmonary arterial system **2484–5**
pressure-flow relations 2488–90,
2506
see also pulmonary arteries; pulmonary
capillaries
pulmonary arteries 2484–5
anomalous connections **2417**
blood flow, *see under* pulmonary
circulation
branching 2600
chest radiography 2178, 2657
congenital absence, high altitude
pulmonary oedema in 1189
dilatation lesions 2507, 2508
elastic 2484
persistent hypertension effect 2508
embolism, *see* pulmonary embolism
in Fallot's tetralogy 2402
fistula 2408
from ascending aorta (truncus
arteriosus) 2431
histopathological changes in pulmonary
hypertension 2507–8
idiopathic dilatation **2421**
left 2178
magnetic resonance imaging 2214
muscular 2484
non-muscular (arterioles) 2485
'onion skin proliferation' 2507
right 2178
systemic connections, abnormal 2402,
2424–8
systemic shunts,
complications after 2406–7
in Fallot's tetralogy 2405–7
in Takayasu's disease 2378, 2379
thromboembolism 2641–2
types in pulmonary atresia 2407
see also pulmonary circulation
pulmonary arteriography **2655–6**
pulmonary arterioles 2485
muscularization in pulmonary
hypertension 2507, 2515
pulmonary arteriovenous fistulae 2402,
2408, **2419**, 2862
pulmonary arteriovenous shunts, in
hepatocellular failure 2104
pulmonary aspiration, *see* aspiration,
pulmonary
pulmonary atresia
acquired/congenital systemic collaterals
2408
'complex' 2407, 2408
correction 2408
hypoplastic 2407, 2408
magnetic resonance imaging 2214
with ventricular septal defect **2407–8**,
2407–8
pulmonary artery types 2407
pulmonary capillaries **2485–6**, 2485
alveoli contact 2596–7
blood flow 2490, 2494
blood volume 2485, 2669
damage,
in ARDS 2574, 2640
pulmonary oedema 2496, 2501
endothelial cells, *see* endothelial cell(s)
fluid balance and pulmonary oedema
2494, 2495–6
fluid movement in 2494
hydrostatic pressure 2492, 2493,
2495–6
in ARDS 2854
increase in pulmonary oedema 2496
marginated pool of neutrophils 2616
neutrophil emigration, *see* neutrophils
perfusion, assessment 2655

permeability 2493
in ARDS 2854
pulmonary oedema and 2501
volume 2485, 2669
see also alveolar capillary sheet
(system); pulmonary circulation
pulmonary capillary pressure 2496, 2566,
2571
pulmonary oedema and 2496
pulmonary capillary wedge pressure
2179, 2220, 2246
monitoring 3282, 3283
pulmonary circulation **2484–95**
abnormal systemic connections 2402,
2424–8
in adult respiratory distress syndrome
2640
in alveolar filling syndromes 2639
assessment **2671–2**
in asthma 2636
blood flow,
in asthma 2636
in diffuse interstitial fibrosis of lung
2636
in emphysema 2633
factors determining 2488, *2489*
high in pulmonary hypertension **2507–8**
in hypoxia 2491
postural changes 2490, 2509
pressure relations 2488–90
in pulmonary hypertension **2507–8**,
2509
pulmonary veins 2491
pulsatile 2488, 2490, 2494
vertical distribution 2488–90, 2509,
2669
blood volume 2488, 2490, 2669
distribution 2488, 2509
regulation 2157
bronchial circulation anastomosis
2494
in chronic bronchiolitis 2634
in cor pulmonale *2519*
in diffuse interstitial fibrosis 2637
disorders 2671
dynamics **2487–8**
in emphysema and COAD 2633,
2768–9
endothelium, *see* endothelial cell(s),
pulmonary
mixing with systemic circulation 2402
morphology/anatomy **2484–6**
microcirculation 2485
see also pulmonary arteries
nerve supply **2486**
normal values 2487, *2488, 2506*
passive changes and adaptations
2488–91
capillary blood flow 2490
in exercise/posture changes 2490,
2509
pulmonary veins 2491
regional pressure-flow relations
2488–90
pressures/flows and resistance *2519*
pressures/volumes and resistance
2487–8, *2488*, 2505, *2506*
in pulmonary vascular diseases 2641
role 2484
systemic connections, abnormal 2402,
2424–8
transvascular/interstitial fluid dynamics
2492–4
fluid/ionic balance 2492–4
fluid movements 2494
see also interstitial fluid
vasomotor activity **2491–2**
general (reflex/humoral) 2492
hypoxic vasoconstriction 2491–2
venous system 2486
see also pulmonary arteries
pulmonary collapse, *see* lung, collapse
pulmonary consolidation, *see* lung,
consolidation
pulmonary diffusing capacity 2600
in altitude acclimatization 1187
in alveolar filling syndromes 2639
in asthma 2636
in chronic bronchiolitis 2634

design of lung and **2601–3**
in diffuse interstitial fibrosis of lung
2637
in emphysema 2633
matched to oxygen needs 2606–8
mismatch 2607
morphometric model 2601–2
testing 2602–3
plasma and tissue barriers 2601–2
total (DL_{O_2}) 2601, 2602
oxygen needs mismatch 2607–8
redundancy 2603, 2608
pulmonary disease, *see* lung disease;
respiratory disease/disorders
pulmonary embolism **2522–7**, 2641,
3664
acute minor **2523–4**
treatment 2525–6
angina *vs* 2322
in antithrombin deficiency 3666
in chronic obstructive airways disease
2777
chronic repeated **2524**
clinical features 2523, 2524, 2868
chest pain 2167, 2524
cor pulmonale *vs* 2520
diagnosis and investigations **2524–5**,
2569
chest radiography 2523, 2524–5
in dilated cardiomyopathy 2384
embolectomy 1742, 2526, 2570
haemoptysis in 2644
at high altitudes 1193
incidence and mortality 2522
massive **2524**, **2569–70**
pericardial tamponade *vs* 2478
treatment 2526, 2569–70
myocardial infarction *vs* 2335
in nephrotic syndrome 3141, 3142
pathological physiology 2524, 2569,
2641–2
pleural effusion in 2868
postoperative 3668
in pregnancy 1741
diagnosis 1741
prophylaxis 1743
risk factors 1741
treatment 1741–3
prophylaxis **3675–6**
risk factors 1741, *3675*
risk of recurrence 2527
treatment **2525–7**, 2569–70
duration and results 2526–7
fibrinolytic therapy 3671, *3672*
see also deep vein thrombosis (DVT)
pulmonary embolization, in adult
respiratory distress syndrome 2860
pulmonary eosinophilia **2804–6**
with alveolar exudate 2804, *2805*
with alveolar exudate and airway
disease 2804, **2805–6**, *2805*
with angiitis and granulomatosis
2804–5, *2805*
see also Churg-Strauss syndrome
chest radiograph 2783
in Churg-Strauss syndrome 2800
classification 2804–5, *2805*
in diffuse parenchymal lung disease
2781–2
eosinophilic pneumonia **2805**
haematological features 3685
nickel causing 1112
prolonged 2804, **2805**
simple, *see* Löffler's syndrome
tropical, *see* tropical pulmonary
eosinophilia
pulmonary fibrosis
in adult respiratory distress syndrome
2575
in asbestosis 2844
in CREST syndrome 2799
cryptogenic, asbestosis similarity 2844
in extrinsic allergic alveolitis 2811,
2813, 2817
idiopathic, *see* cryptogenic fibrosing
alveolitis
in injecting drug abusers 4283
open-lung biopsy 2688–9
in pneumonia 2701

prognosis 2797
progressive massive, *see* progressive
massive fibrosis
quartz-induced 2839
radiation-induced 3574
in rheumatoid arthritis 2797, 2961
in sarcoidosis 2824
in systemic sclerosis 2799, *3031*
tuberculosis *vs* 651
see also lung, diffuse interstitial fibrosis
pulmonary granulomas
in extrinsic allergic alveolitis 2811
in injecting drug abusers 4283
pulmonary granulomatosis **2800–3**,
2800
bronchocentric **2802**
necrotizing sarcoid **2802**
open-lung biopsy 2689–90
see also Churg-Strauss syndrome;
Wegener's granulomatosis
pulmonary haemorrhage **2803–4**
acute lupus pneumonitis with/without
2798
acute renal failure and 3291
in anti-GBM disease 3165
causes and classification of 2803
in Goodpasture's syndrome 2803
in idiopathic pulmonary haemosiderosis
2804
miscellaneous causes 2804
pulmonary haemosiderosis 2507, 2509
haemoptysis in 2644, 2804
idiopathic **2804**, 3685
pulmonary hypertension **2505–14**, 2652
in adult respiratory distress syndrome
2640, 2857, 2860
after Fallot's tetralogy repair 2407
in alveolar filling syndromes 2639
aminorex association 2852
aortic regurgitation *vs* 2467
in atrial/ventricular septal defects 2418,
2425, 2507
causes **2506–7**, *2507*, *2512*
in collagen vascular diseases **2510**
congenital heart defects with **2409–13**,
2507
tricuspid atresia 2412–13
see also Eisenmenger reaction
(syndrome)
constrictive/restrictive vascular disease
in 2505
cor pulmonale relation 2515, 2516, 2518
in CREST syndrome 2799
differential diagnosis *2513*, *2513*
in diffuse interstitial fibrosis of lung
2637
drug-induced 2852
hepatic disease associated **2509–10**
high pulmonary blood flow **2507–8**,
2515
effect on elastic pulmonary arteries
2508
histopathological stages 2507–8
pathophysiology 2508
histopathological changes 2506–7, 2515
in high pulmonary blood flow 2507–8
see also pulmonary vasculopathy
in HIV infection 4285
in hypoxia 2902
idiopathic, *see* pulmonary hypertension,
primary
in injecting drug abusers 4283
investigations **2510–11**
cardiac catheterization and
angiography 2511
chest radiography 2180, 2510
echocardiography 2511
electrocardiogram 2511
lung scans 2510–11
non-invasive 2519
long-term hypoxia association **2509**, 2516
lung and heart-lung transplantation 2934
management 2860
in mitral valve disease 2509, 2513
in ostium secundum defects 2425, 2507
pathogenesis **2513–14**
endothelial cell hypothesis 2505, 2514
myogenic theory 2513–14
in pregnancy 1745

pulmonary hypertension (cont.)
  primary 2505, 2506, *2506*, **2511–13**, 2641
    histology and clinical features 2511
    investigations 2511–12
    in pregnancy 1738
    treatment and prognosis 2512–13
  pulmonary arterial pressure in 2506
  in pulmonary embolism 2524, 2641–2
  pulmonary valve disease and 2469, 2510
  pulmonary venous hypertension and **2508–9**
  secondary 2505, 2506, *2506*, **2507–10**
    clinical features **2510**
    severity assessment 2510
    signs 2410–11
  in SLE 3020
  in systemic sclerosis 2799, 3029, *3031*
  in transposition of great arteries 2417
  tricuspid regurgitation in 2468, 2510
  in tropical disease **2509**
  ventricular septal defect with 2418, 2507
  see also pulmonary arterial hypertension; pulmonary venous hypertension
pulmonary infarction
  in Eisenmenger reaction (syndrome) 2410
  pneumonia *vs* 2699
  in sickle-cell disease 3514
  by Swan-Ganz catheter 2221
pulmonary metastases **2893**
  computed tomography 238, 246
  detection and staging 237, 246
  presentation and primary tumour 252
  solitary and multiple 2893
pulmonary mycotoxicosis 2815
pulmonary nocardiosis 686
pulmonary nodules, *see* lung, nodules
pulmonary oedema **2495–505**
  acute fulminant 2495
  in acute meningococcaemia 541
  in acute renal failure 3284–5
  in adult respiratory distress syndrome 2496, 2497, 2574, 2853–4
  after intracranial lesions 2501
  ß-agonist therapy of preterm labour and 1811
  capillary permeability disorders 2501
  causes *2497*, 2500
    multifactorial nature *2500*
  causes of lung consolidation *2660*
  chest radiography 2502–3
  in cholera 579
  clinical aspects **2500–5**
  clinical stages,
    alveolar oedema 2502–3
    interstitial oedema 2502, 2598
    pre-oedema 2502
  in cor triatriatum 2500–1
  in diabetic hyperglycaemic coma 1502
  diagnosis **2501–3**
  in drug abusers 1058, 4283, 4295
  drug-induced 2850, *2850*
  dyspnoea in 2162, 2500
    management 2164, 2504
  expansion 2501
  fluid overload, management 2504
  in heart failure 2231, 2241, 2499, **2500**, 2566–8
    management 2504
  in hepatocellular failure 2104
  heroin-related 4283
  high altitude 1188, 2501
    diagnosis 1190
    fluid characteristics 1189
    incidence 1190
    pathophysiology 1189
    predisposing factors 1188
    prophylaxis and treatment 1190–1
    see also mountain sickness
  high permeability **2496–8**
    causes 2496, *2497*
    clearance mechanism 2500
    experimental treatment 2504
    management 2504–5
    pathogenesis/mechanisms 2496–8

hydrostatic 2494, **2496**
  causes *2497*
  resolution 2499
initiation and development 2495–6
interstitial 2179, 2509
in left atrial myxoma 2500
in leptospirosis 701
in loculated pericardial constriction 2500
lymphatic *2497*, **2498**
lymphatic obstruction and 2501
in malaria 845, 846, 847, 848
  management 856
in methyl bromide poisoning 1086
in mitral regurgitation 2458, 2461
in mitral stenosis 2452, 2453
in myocardial infarction 2338, 2566–8
in nitrogen dioxide poisoning 1100, 2847
non-cardiogenic 1058
in overtransfusion 2570, 2571
pathophysiology 2494, 2495–6, 2566, 2598
  fluid balance in capillaries/interstitial space 2494, 2495–6, 2598
in phosgene poisoning 1101
physiological/experimental aspects **2495–500**
pneumococcal infections after 514
pneumonia *vs* 2699
postobstructive 2501
protection from 2494
pulmonary arterial hypertension with 2501
pulmonary function in **2503**
in pulmonary thromboembolism 2501
in pulmonary venous thrombosis 2500
reduced interstitial pressure *2497*, **2498**
reduced plasma oncotic pressure *2497*, **2498**
resolution **2499–500**
  clearance mechanism 2500
in salicylate poisoning 1055, 1056
in septicaemia 2573
sequence **2498–9**
  clinical features 2502
in spider bites 1148
treatment 2241, **2504–5**, 2567–8, 2571
  positive-pressure ventilation 2580
  supportive and ventilation 2505
unilateral 2501
pulmonary oligaemia, chest radiography 2181
pulmonary ossicles 2180
pulmonary overcirculation (plethora) 2180, 2181
pulmonary plethora 2180, 2181
pulmonary receptors, dyspnoea due to 2163
pulmonary regurgitation 2408, 2420, 2469
  after Fallot's tetralogy repair 2407
  Doppler echocardiography 2203
  in ductus arteriosus 2430
  in pulmonary hypertension 2510
pulmonary rehabilitation 2929
pulmonary sequestration, in bronchiectasis 2761
pulmonary shunts, magnetic resonance imaging 2214
pulmonary stenosis
  double-outlet right ventricle with ventricular septal defect 2404
  in Fallot's tetralogy, residual 2406
  one ventricle with 2404
  in pregnancy 1737
  ventricular septal defect with 2417
  see also pulmonary arterial stenoses; pulmonary valve, stenosis
pulmonary thromboembolism 2641–2
  drug-induced 2851
  pulmonary oedema in 2501
pulmonary toxicity, *see* lung, damage
pulmonary trunk
  chest radiography 2178
    abnormal 2181–2
  enlargement 2181

pulmonary tularaemia 601
pulmonary valve
  absent, in Fallot's tetralogy 2404
  calcification 2419
  in carcinoid heart disease 2469
  closure 2153
    in ostium secundum defects 2425
  disease **2469**
  incompetence,
    in pulmonary hypertension 2510
    see also pulmonary regurgitation
  replacement 2407, 2420
  stenosis **2419–20**
    Doppler echocardiography 2203
    in Fallot's tetralogy 2402, 2406
    heart murmurs 2419, 2421
    physical signs 2419, *2420*
    with reversed interatrial shunt 2405, **2409**, *2409*
pulmonary valvotomy 2420
pulmonary vascular impedance 2506, 2633
pulmonary vascular pressure 2671
  increases, pulmonary oedema 2496
pulmonary vascular reactions, drug-induced 2851–2
pulmonary vascular resistance 2154, 2221, 2487–8, 2488, *2488*, 2490, 2566
  afterload determination 2156
  calculation 2488
  cardiac transplantation contraindication 2256
  in myocardial infarction 2566
  in obstructive airways disease 2572
  postnatal adaptation to congenital heart disease 2399
  in pulmonary embolism 2490, 2569, 2570
  in pulmonary hypertension 2506
  in septicaemia 1022
  use of term 2488, 2506
pulmonary vasculature, chest radiography 2178–9, 2657
pulmonary vasculitis **2800–3**, *2800*
  benign lymphocytic 2807
  classification 2800
  open-lung biopsy 2689–90
  pathogenesis 2800
  types/forms **2802–3**
  see also Churg-Strauss syndrome; pulmonary granulomatosis; Wegener's granulomatosis
pulmonary vasculopathy
  congestive 2507
  embolic arteriopathy 2507
  hypoxic 2507
  open-lung biopsy 2689
  pathophysiology **2641–2**
  plexogenic 2507, 2508, 2509
  see also pulmonary hypertension
pulmonary vasoconstriction 2157
pulmonary veins 2486
  abnormal connections **2415–19**
  blood flow 2491
  chest radiography 2179, 2657
  magnetic resonance imaging 2214
  to right atrium 2415
  role 2491
pulmonary veno-occlusive disease 2513
  mitral stenosis *vs* 2455
  open-lung biopsy 2689
pulmonary venous congestion 2803
  dyspnoea due to 2163, 2164
pulmonary venous drainage, hemianomalous 2415, 2417
pulmonary venous hypertension 2510
  capillary pulsatility benefit 2494
  causes *2512*
  chest radiography 2179, 2180, 2510
  echocardiography 2511
  in heart failure 2231
  pulmonary hypertension in **2508–9**
  see also pulmonary hypertension
pulmonary venous pressure 2179, 2488, *2488*
  in hypertrophic cardiomyopathy 2386
pulmonary venous system **2486**

pulmonary venous thrombosis, pulmonary oedema in 2500
pulmonary venules 2486
pulmonary wedge pressure 2163, 2488, 2498
pulse
  anacrotic carotid 2325
  angina investigation 2325
  in deep vein thrombosis 2523
  in Fallot's tetralogy 2402
  in mitral stenosis 2453
  in peripheral arterial disease 2368
  pressure/volume/flow 2368
  in pulmonary atresia with ventricular septal defect 2408
  in pulmonary valve stenosis 2419
  pulsus paradoxus 2477, 2570, 2912
  rapid upstroke, in hypertrophic cardiomyopathy 2387
'pulse-bruit-pressure' 2379
pulselessness 2283
pulse oximetry 2592, 2672
  in ventilation monitoring 2922
pulse-step mismatch 3872
pulsus paradoxus 2477, 2570, 2912
'punch drunk' syndrome 4002, 4049
pupils
  abnormalities **3877**
    constriction (miosis) 3877
    dilatation 3877
    Argyll Robertson 3877, 4085
    fixed dilated 2582
    myotonic (Holmes-Adie syndrome) 3877
    in neurosyphilis 4085
    in opioid overdose 1058
  reflexes, in diabetes 1489
  responses,
    assessment 4179
    in coma 3931
    lesions associated 2582
    relative afferent pupil test 4179, *4180*
  size in poisoning 1046
  in unconscious patients 2582–3
purgatives, *see* laxatives
purified chick embryo-cell vaccine (PCEC) 403
purified vero-cell vaccine (PVRV) 403
purine nucleoside phosphorylase deficiency **1386**
purines 1376
  disorders of metabolism **1376–87**
  inborn errors of metabolism 1381–6, 3225–6
  interstitial nephritis and **3224–7**
  renal handling 3225
  synthesis 1377–8
Purkinje cells 3859
Purkinje fibres 2148, 2152, 2259
  action potential 2149
  digitalis action 2241
'purple burps' 879
purpura 3627, **3630–7**, 3787
  allergic 3636–7
  drug reactions 1253
  fulminans 347–8, 349, *3548*, 3636, 3667
  Henoch-Schönlein, *see* Henoch-Schönlein purpura
  idiopathic thrombocytopenic, *see* thrombocytopenia, autoimmune
  infectious 3636
  metabolic causes 3636
  non-thrombocytopenic vascular **3635–7**
  in plague 596
  psychogenic 3637
  senile 3636
  thrombotic thrombocytopenic, *see* thrombotic thrombocytopenic purpura
  in vasculitis diagnosis 3774, 3775
purpuric rash, in microscopic polyangiitis 3014
pus
  in anaerobic infections 571
  in bacterial meningitis 4052
  drainage 521, 530
  in pneumococcal infection 521
  in *Staphylococcus aureus* infections 530

pustular dermatitis, contagious, *see* orf
pustular melanosis, transient neonatal 3783
pustules 3717
  in psoriasis 3746, 3748
putamen 3861
  in Parkinson's disease 3999
Puumala virus 426
PUVA therapy 2970, 3748
  mycosis fungoides management 3797
pyelogram 3110
  'negative' 3239
pyelography
  antegrade 3239, 3240, 3253
  intravenous, *see* intravenous pyelography
  retrograde **3110**, 3239, 3277
pyelonephritis
  acute,
    acute papillary necrosis complicating 3212–13
    in analgesic nephropathy 3223
    clinical features 3207
    in pregnancy 1733, 1787, 3207
    treatment **3210–11**
  chronic (non-obstructive, atrophic), *see* reflux nephropathy
  mycoplasmas causing 770
  xanthogranulomatous 3207
pyknocytosis, congenital 3550
pyknodystosis **3089**
pylephlebitis, granulomatous 972
pyloric stenosis 1878, **1883**
  adult 1960
  congenital hypertrophic 1960, **1975**
  hypokalaemia in 3130
  infantile, multifactorial inheritance 129
pyloromyotomy 1975
pylorus
  as antireflux barrier 1961
  thickened, in congenital pyloric stenosis 1975
pyoderma
  after measles 380
  streptococcal 500, 501
    diagnosis 502
pyoderma gangrenosum **3778**
  arthritis in 3003
  diseases associated 3778, 3793
  in ulcerative colitis 1947
pyogenic bacterial infection, in HIV infection 473
pyogenic liver abscess, *see* liver, pyogenic abscess
pyomyositis
  Staphylococcus aureus 529
  tropical **4174–5**
pyonephrosis 3207
  in analgesic nephropathy 3223
  tuberculous 3277
pyopneumothorax 2705, 2870
pyorrhoea 1847, 1848
pyramidal tract 3856
pyrantel pamoate
  in ascariasis 938
  in enterobiasis 942
  in trichuriasis 944
pyrazinamide 3278, 3523
  adverse reactions 657
  in tuberculosis 480, 655, *656*
pyrazolidines, poisoning 1057
pyrazolones, poisoning 1057
pyrethroids, synthetic **1123**
pyrethrum 1009
  poisoning **1123**
pyrexia, *see* fever
pyrexia of unknown origin (PUO), *see* fever of unknown origin (FUO)
pyridinium 3060
pyridostigmine, in myasthenia gravis 4162
pyridostigmine bromide 1118
pyridoxal 5-phosphate 1360, 3498
  in sideroblastic anaemia 3523
pyridoxine 1360, 3498
  in chronic renal failure 3327
  in cystathionine synthase deficiency 1366, 1367

deficiency 4100
  -dependent neonatal seizures 1372
  in isoniazid poisoning management 1069
  in ornithine-δ-aminotransferase deficiency 1361
  overdose **1071**
  in Parkinson's disease 4005
  in pregnancy 1746, 1802
  in primary hyperoxaluria 1446–7, *1448*
  in sideroblastic anaemia 3498, 3523
pyrimethamine
  folate deficiency due to 3497
  in malaria 852–3, *854*
  overdose **1073**
  in toxoplasmosis 869, 4078
pyrimidine 5′-nucleotidase 1386
  deficiency 1387, **3535–6**
pyrimidines 1376
  biosynthesis 1386
  disorders of metabolism **1376–87**
  inborn errors of metabolism 1386–7
pyrogenic reactions, snake antivenom 1138
pyrogens
  endogenous, in tumours 241
  transfusion reactions 3692
pyrophosphate, inorganic, metabolism 2989
pyrophosphate arthropathy **2988–90**
  acute synovitis (pseudogout) 2988
  chronic 2988, 2990, *2990*
  classification and associations 2988–9
  differential diagnosis 2989
  familial 2988–9
  investigations/diagnosis 2989
  osteoarthritis overlap 2988, 2989
  treatment 2990
pyropoikilocytosis, hereditary 3531, 3532
pyrrolidizine alkaloids 2099, 2129
pyruvate
  inborn errors of metabolism **1351–2**
  metabolism 2146, 4171
pyruvate carboxylase 1373
  deficiency **1352**
pyruvate dehydrogenase deficiency **1351**
pyruvate dehydrogenase multienzyme complex (PDH-MEC) 2146
pyruvate kinase deficiency **3535**
pyruvate oxidase 1458
6-pyruvoyltetrahydrobiopterin synthase deficiency 1363
pyrvinium pamoate, in enterobiasis 942
pyuria
  bacteriuria *vs* 3103
  diagnosis 3102, **3103**, 3208
  in tuberculosis 3276

Q

QBC (quantitative buffy-coat) method
  African trypanosomiasis 891, 892
  malaria diagnosis 849
Q fever *729*, **742–4**
  endocarditis 743–4, 2437, 2442
  liver in 2121, 2134
  see also Coxiella burnetii
qinghaosu, in malaria 852
quadriceps
  atrophy 4322
  exercises 2982
  reflex inhibition 4322
  wasting in osteoarthritis 2982
quality of life
  of dialysed patients 3312–13
  indices, in clinical trials 24
quantitative buffy-coat method (QBC), *see* QBC (quantitative buffy-coat) method
quantum mechanics 2213
quarantine 289
  plague 598
quartan malarial nephrosis 857
quartz 2839
  inhalation of particles 2842

podoconiosis 1215
silicosis 2841, 2842
Queensland, childhood lead poisoning 3261
Queensland tick typhus *729*
Quellung reaction 511, 582
questionnaire
  alcohol consumption frequency 4271
  McGill pain 4300
  mental disorder assessment in elderly 4226
  mental state examination 4203
Quetelet's index (QI) 1302, *1302*, 1303
  change with age in boys 1313
quicklime, in eye 1103
quid chewers, oral/pharyngeal cancer 201
quinidine *2264*
  in atrial fibrillation 2272
  in malaria 851
  overdose/poisoning 1063–4
  in pregnancy 1740
quinine 1510
  in babesiosis 865
  danger in pregnancy 856
  dosages and complications 851
  half-life 1244, 1245
  in malaria 851, *854*
  overdose 1073
    eye signs 4197
  in renal impairment 3273
4-quinolone 296
quinolone antimalarial drugs, salt base equivalents *853*
quinolones
  in antibody-deficiency syndromes 170
  in pregnancy 1785
  in *Pseudomonas aeruginosa* infections 2752, *2752*
  in typhoid 564
  in urinary-tract infections 3209, 3211
quinsy 572
Quintan fever (trench fever) **747–8**

R

rabbit fever 599–603
rabbitpox virus 366
rabies
  in animals 398–9
  antibodies 402
  clinical features 399–401
    complications 400–1
  differential diagnosis 401
  encephalitis 4065
  epidemiology 395–7
  'furious' 398, 399–400
  immunization 402
    failures 405
  immune response 398
  passive 284, 405
  post-exposure 402–3, *403*, 405, *405*
  pre-exposure 402, 403
  see also rabies, vaccines
  immunology 398
  incubation period 398, 399
  laboratory diagnosis 401–2
  paralytic (dumb) 400
  pathogenesis 398, 4065
  pathology 401
  prevention and control 396, 402–5
  transmission 395, 397–8
  treatment and prognosis 402
  urban and sylvatic phases 395
  vaccines 323–4, 403
    nervous-tissue 403, 405
    side-effects 403
    tissue-culture 403
rabies immune globulin (RIG) 284, 405
rabies-related viruses 395, *396*
rabies virus *396*
  antigens 398
  ecology 395
  inhalation 397
  replication/infection route 398
  'street' and 'fixed' 394, 397, 401
  structure 394, 395

Rab proteins *77*, 78
  structure and switch regions 78
Rabson-Mendenhall syndrome 1455
racemic forms 1248
racial differences, *see* ethnic differences
rac protein 82
radial nerve **4094**
  injuries/lesions 4094
radiation **1217–23**
  biology 253, 254
  controlling hazards **1220–1**
  damage to fetus 1220
  doses **1218**
    limits for general public 1220–1, *1221*
    limits for radiation workers 1221
  effects **1218–19**, *1218*
  emergency reference levels 1221
  enteritis 1963
  genetic damage 1220, 2848
  growth hormone deficiency due to 1698
  hypoparathyroidism due to 1634
  ionizing, *see* ionizing radiation
  late effects of exposure **1219–20**
  leukaemia risk 3410–11
  low/high linear energy transfer 1218
  myelomatosis and 3597
  myelopathy **3894**
  necrosis 4135
  nephritis 3185, **3231**
    acute/chronic 3231
  neurological features of injury **4129**
  non-ionizing 1217
    effects **1222**
  partial body exposure (local effects) **1221**
  particulate contamination 1219
  pericardial damage 2476
  pneumonitis **2848**, 3574
  secondary 1217
  sickness 1218, 1821
  sources **1217–18**
    for general public 1220
  syndromes **1218–19**
  therapy of acute exposure 1219
  thyroid cancer and 1618
  total body, *see* total-body irradiation (TBI)
  types in radiotherapy 255
  units 1218·
  vitamin B_{12} malabsorption due to 3492
radiculopathy, cytomegalovirus 4079
radioactive iodinated serum albumin (RISA) 3825
radioactivity 1217
radioallergosorbent tests (RAST) 160, 1144, 1145, 2717
  food allergy 1844
radio-copper studies 1421
radiofrequency ablation 2266, 2277
radiofrequency electromagnetic waves **1222**, 3819
radiography
  in actinomycoses 684
  in acute back pain 2993
  in bacterial arthritis 2999
  in bone disease 3063
  chest, *see* chest radiography
  in gout 2986
  in intracranial disorders 3816–17
  kidneys, ureter and bladder **3109–10**
  in occupational rheumatic diseases 1169
  in osteoarthritis 2982
  in primary hyperparathyroidism 1631
  in pyrophosphate arthropathy 2989
  in renal bone disease 3324
  in rheumatic disease 2948–9
    uses/abuses 2949
  spinal 3826
  three-dimensional, in rheumatic disease 2949
  see also radiology; X-rays
radiohippurate, *see* hippurate (hippuran), radiolabelled
radiohumeral joint, in rheumatoid arthritis 2958
radio-immunoassays 1553
  gastrin 1881
  gastrointestinal hormones 1891
  parathyroid hormone 1712

radio-iodine
  ingestion, management 1219
  iodine-131 256
  therapy 1613, 1620
  thyroid imaging 1608, 1619, 1621
radio-iron studies, see ferrokinetic
    studies
radioisotopes, see isotopes
radiology **1830–6**
  biliary tract **1833–5**
  in epileptic seizures 3920
  gastrointestinal tract **1830–3**
  kidneys, ureter and bladder **3109–10**
  liver **1833**
  neurological disorders, see
    neuroradiology
  oesophageal 1865
  in oncology 234–40
    see also imaging; specific techniques
  in osteoporosis 3067
  pancreas **1835**
  in spinal cord injury 3896–7
  spleen **1835**
  see also imaging; radiography
radionuclide cisternography 3825
radionuclide scanning, see scintigraphy
radiopaque markers
  in constipation examination 1967
  in meals for motility disorder
    investigation 1956
radiopharmaceuticals, renal 3112
radioprotectors 1219, 1234
radiosensitivity 254
  cell cycle relationship 254
radiotherapy **253–8**, 1221
  abdominal, small bowel lesion after
    1908, 1910
  acute reactions 3574
  adjuvant 257
    to chemotherapy 257
    to surgery 257, 258
  aplastic anaemia induced by 3441
  biological principles **254**
  brachytherapy 255–6
    afterloading 256
  cardiopulmonary disease complicating
    3574
  in cerebral metastases 250
  clinical roles **256–8**
  cranial, in lung cancer 2891
  DNA damage, repair 254
  electron beam 255
  fractionation 253, 254
    accelerated 254
    hyperfractionation 254
  in Graves' ophthalmopathy 1614
  growth hormone deficiency due to 1582
  in hepatocellular carcinoma 2117
  in Hodgkin's disease 3573, 3576
  in Langerhans-cell histiocytosis 3609
  local effects 1221
  in lung cancer 2889–90, 2891
  multidisciplinary care 258
  in mycosis fungoides 3797
  in myeloma 3602
  in myelosclerosis (primary) 3437
  myelosuppression induced by 3574
  nephritis complicating 3185, **3231**
  neurological complications 4135
  neutron irradiation 255
  of non-Hodgkin's lymphoma 3583
  normal tissue damage 255
  palliative 257–8, 2889–90
  particle 255
  physical principles **254–5**
  of pituitary tumours **1588–9**, 1591,
    1594, 1596, 1651
  planning **255**
    beam alignment and localization 255
    patient positioning/immobilization 255
    target volume 254, 255
    treatment simulator 255
    tumour localization 254
    tumour stage and type 254
  in pregnancy 1761, 1806–7
  radiation dose 256
  prescriptions 256

radiation types 255–6
radical/curative 256–7
  results 257
reoxygenation 254
repopulation of stem cells 254
resistance, hypoxic cells 254
role in cancer **253–8**
  sensitivity to, see radiosensitivity
  in suprasellar germinoma 1598
  surgery with 248
  target volume, factors defining 254
  in thyroid lymphoma 1621
  toxicity 256, 256
    acute side-effects 256, 256
    late side-effects 256, 256
  treatment method 255
  see also other individual tumours
radon
  cancer association 215
    lung cancer 206–7
  indoor air pollution 1231
  levels of exposure 215
Raeder's syndrome 3877
Raf-1 1561
raf gene 225
ragged-red fibres 4143, 4171, 4173
RAG genes, defects 173
Rahnella aquatilis 560
Raillietina species 962, 963
Railliettiella species 1014
railway, medical standards for staff 2361
râle 2650
ramipril, myocardial re-infarction
    prevention 2348
Ramsay Hunt syndrome 349, **3879**,
    3984, 3988
Ramstedt's operation 1975
randomization 32
  clinical trials 1262
  large numbers of patients 24
randomized clinical trials, see clinical
    trials, randomized
ranitidine
  overdose/poisoning 1070
  peptic ulcer treatment 1886, 1887
  in renal impairment 3274
Ranke, complex of 639
Ranson grading, acute pancreatitis 2030
RANTES 87, 97, 151, 157, 3559
Ranvier, nodes of 4091
rape
  examination after 4313
  psychiatric emergencies in victims
    4257
rape counselling 4314
rapid eye movement (REM) sleep 2907,
    2908, 3928
  abnormalities in narcolepsy 3927, 3928
  apnoea **2916–17**
  breathing during 2909
  hypnic headache in 4029
  paralysis during 2908
rapid plasma reagin (RPR) test 715,
    1790
Rapoport-Luebering shunt 3534–5
rash **3711–15**
  antibiotic 305
  in bacterial meningitis 4053
  in Boutonneuse fever 734
  'butterfly' 3019
  causes, in returning travellers 326
  in chickenpox and zoster 347, 348
  coxsackievirus 384
  distribution 3712–13
  drug eruptions, see drug eruptions
  enteroviruses 384
  in epidemic typhus 737
  'giant' 370
  in glucagonoma 1706
  in human herpesvirus 6 (HHV-6)
    infection 364
  in human parvovirus infection 1782
  in infectious diseases 266, 267
  in Kawasaki disease 3047
  in leptospirosis 701
  in Marburg virus and Ebola virus
    disease 441

in measles 376, 377, 379
in meningitis 4053, 4054
in neonatal lupus 3018
in onchocerciasis 913–14
in orf 370
in parvovirus infections 447–8
in pityriasis rosea 3751
in poxvirus infections 366, 367
pruritic, in schistosomiasis 975
rate of development 3713
in recurrent polyserositis 1526
in rheumatic diseases 2945
in rickettsial diseases 732
in rickettsialpox 736
in Rocky Mountain spotted fever 735,
    736
in rubella 409
in scarlet fever 499
in scrub typhus 740
in secondary syphilis 711, 712
in SLE 3018, 3019
sulphasalazine 1947
sun/light/ultraviolet light association
    3726–7
symmetry 3713
in typhoid 562, 563
in ulcerative colitis 1947
in urticaria 3771
in vasculitis 3773
in viral infections 3716
ras oncogenes 195
  in colon cancer 66
  mutations,
    in haematological disorders 3390
    in leukaemia 3395
    in myelodysplastic syndromes 3429
    in thyroid tumours 1567, 1569, 1618
    tumours associated 225
  protein homology with GTP-binding
    protein 77, 82
  signal transduction/transformation
    mechanism 225
  T-cell response 229
ras proteins 1561, 1569, 2147
  inhibitors 226
Rastelli operation 2416, 2417
RAST test, see radioallergosorbent tests
    (RAST)
rat bite fevers **687–9**
  Spirillum minus **688–9**
  streptobacillary 687–8
Rathke's pouch 1574, 4032
rattle (râle) 2650
rattlesnakes 1128
  bites and envenoming 1132–3, 1134
  venoms 3658
Raynaud's disease (primary Raynaud's
    syndrome) 2365
Raynaud's phenomenon 2365, 2945,
    3028
  clinical features 2365, 3028
  in cold haemagglutinin disease 3544
  differential diagnosis 1226
  diseases associated 2365, 2366, 3028
  management 3034, 3034
  physical examination 3029
  in rheumatic diseases 2945
  in SLE 3019
  in systemic sclerosis 2365, 2945, 3028
  vibration causing 1226
  in vinyl chloride poisoning 1090, 1170
Raynaud's syndrome 2365, 2374
  management 2374, 3023
  in polymyositis/dermatomyositis 4157
  primary (Raynaud's disease) 2365
  secondary 2365
R binders (haptocorrins) 3485, 3486,
    3495
reactive airways dysfunction syndrome
    (RADS) 2742, **2743**
  see also asthma, occupational
reactive arthritis 2965, **2970–2**
  Campylobacter infections 558
  clinical features 2970–1, 2970
  post-streptococcal 499
  Reiter's syndrome relationship 2970
  Salmonella 552, 2003

sexually acquired, see sexually acquired
    reactive arthritis (SARA)
reading 3846
  disturbances 3848, 3851
reagin tests 714
rebound phenomena 1254
  in cerebellar lesions 3860
receptor-mediated endocytosis 73–4, 91
  adaptor complexes 74
  of low-density lipoprotein 73, 74
  NSF (NEM-sensitive factor) role 75
  signals 74
  steps 73–4
receptors 1245, 1554–5
  density and receptor-mediated
    endocytosis 73
  drug 1245–6
  families 1555–7
  genetic factors increasing infection
    susceptibility 280
  hormone interactions 1554–5
  ligands 1245–6
  membrane 1554, 1555
    biosynthesis 1559–60
    defects 1567, 1572
    structure and signalling 1559, 1560–1
  nuclear 1554–5, 1556–7
    defects 1567, 1573
    structure and action 1559, 1561–2
  seven transmembrane spanning 1559,
    1560, 1561
  up-regulation/down-regulation 1246
recombinant DNA technology
  application in diagnosis of disease 66
    see also immunodiagnosis
  applications in developing countries 67
  application in treatment of disease 66–7
    vaccine development, see below
    see also gene(s), therapy;
      immunotherapy
  clinical applications **63–6**
    cancer 65–6
    congenital malformation 66
    development/differentiation 66
    polygenic diseases 64–5
    single-gene disorders 63–4
  cytokines 99
  searching for and mapping genes 62–3
  tools **59–62**
    DNA fractionation 60
    gene cloning and gene libraries 60–1
    gene mapping 60
    hybridization and gene probes 59–60
  vaccines 67, 455
    anthrax 618
    chlamydial 759
    hepatitis B virus 455
    malaria 862
    Mycoplasma pneumoniae 767
    viruses,
      avipoxvirus 368
      canarypox virus 381
      poxviruses 365, 368
recombinant proteins/products 66
  erythropoietin 66
  GM-CSF 99
  hirudin 1150
  interferon-γ 99
recommended dietary allowance (RDA)
    1268
records, see clinical records
recruitment
  sound perception 1224
  tests 3870
rectal examination, in appendicitis 2010
rectal temperature 1182
rectourethral fistula 1979
rectovaginal fistula 1980
  in lymphogranuloma venereum 760,
    761
rectum
  aganglionosis, see Hirschsprung's
    disease
  biopsy,
    in Crohn's disease 1939
    in Hirschsprung's disease 1979
    in pseudomembranous colitis 635

bleeding,
  in amoebiasis 828
  in colorectal carcinoma 1991, 1992
  in Crohn's disease 1938
  in Meckel's diverticulum 1977–8
  in solitary rectal ulcer syndrome 2138
  in ulcerative colitis 1945
carcinoid tumours 1896
carcinoma, see colorectal carcinoma
  in collagenous colitis 2137
disorders, in pregnancy 1803
drug formulation 1238
haemorrhage, in homosexuals 3365
incontinence 1960
  see also faecal incontinence
infections, in homosexuals 3362
low anterior resections 1993
perforation, in homosexuals 3365
prolapse, in cystic fibrosis 2749
radiation damage 1947
sensation, suppression 1964
solitary ulcers 1947, 2138
sphincter, in multiple sclerosis 3993
spirochaetosis, in homosexuals 3365
strictures, in lymphogranuloma
  venereum 760
in ulcerative colitis 1945
recurrent laryngeal nerve 2611
  damage 2721, 3880
    airways obstruction in 2724
  infiltration in lung cancer 2883
  in mediastinal masses 2897
  palsy/paralysis 2611, 2724
recurrent oral ulcers, see oral ulceration
recurrent polyserositis (familial
  Mediterranean fever) **1525–7**
  aetiology and pathogenesis 1526
  amyloidosis *1514*, 1517, 1527, 3180
  clinical features 1526
  differential diagnosis 1527
  investigations 1526–7
  joint symptoms 3006
  pathology 1525
  prognosis 1527
  treatment 1524, 1527
red blood cells 3377, **3454–6**
  agglutination tests **3690**
  antibodies 3687–8
  antigens 3687, *3688*
  aplasia, pure (PRCA) 2898, **3448–9**
    acquired 3449
    congenital 3448–9
    in malignant disease 3677
  breakdown and bilirubin formation
    2054
  concentrates 3694
    in DIC 1762
  counts 3378, *3379*, *3380*
  density *3379*
  destruction 3456, 3472
  development 3453–4
  diameter *3379*
  distribution width (RDW) *3379*
  enzyme deficiencies 1259, **3533–7**
  examination 3377–8
  haemoglobin 3455–6
    levels **3378–80**
  inclusions *3378*, 3525
  indices **3378–80**
  inherited enzyme deficiencies **3535–6**
  in vivo labelling methods 2205
  life-span *3379*, 3381, 3456
    in anaemia of chronic disorders 3482
    shortened 3524–5
  in malaria 842, 843, 845
  mass 3380
    increased 3551
    in pregnancy 1758
  maturation defects *3459*, 3460
  mechanical trauma 3525, 3547
  membrane 3455, **3527–8**
    abnormalities 3525
    acquired disorders **3550**
    antibodies 3542
    cation permeability defects 3532–3
    congenital defects **3528–33**
  metabolism 3456, **3534–5**

oxidative damage 3525, 3546
packed cell volume, see packed cell
  volume (PCV)
pooling in spleen 3589
preparations for transfusion 3694
production, see erythropoiesis
radiolabelled 3456, 3476, 3527, 3593–4
  heat-damaged 3592
rosetting and autoagglutination, in
  malaria 842
sequestration, in malaria 842
sequestration/phagocytosis in spleen
  3588–9
technetium-99m-labelled 2205
in urinary casts 3104, 3145
in urine 3102, 3103, **3145**
  dysmorphism 3103, 3145, 3146
  see also haematuria
volume (RCV) 3380
'red currant jelly' stool 554
'red man syndrome' 1069
'red tide' 1142
5α-reductase 1692
  deficiency 1572, 1692, **1693**
  type 2 *1567*
Reed-Sternberg cells 3569, 3570, 3571
reference intervals, for biochemical data
  4363–76
reference nutrient intake (RNI) 1268,
  1330
  protein 1269, *1270*, *1329*
  vitamins and minerals 1268, *1269*
reference range 4363
referrals 48–9, *50*
  psychiatrist, see psychiatrist
reflexes 3857
  see also tendon reflexes
reflex sympathetic dystrophy, see
  algodystrophy
reflux disease, see gastro-oesophageal
  reflux disease
reflux nephropathy **3214–20**
  clinical presentation 3216–18
  coincidental finding 3218
  imaging techniques 3215–16
  management 3220
  pathology 3219
  pregnancy in **1734**, 3218
  renal scarring with 2547
refractory anaemia **3427**, 3430, 3524
  with excess of blasts (RAEB) **3427–8**,
    3429
    leukaemic transformation 3405, **3430**
    in transformation (RAEB-t) *3427*,
      3428, 3429
  with ringed sideroblasts **3427**, 3429
  see also myelodysplastic syndromes
Refsum's disease 84, **1437**, 4103
  infantile 1443
refugees/displaced persons 51
  infection susceptibility 281
regional pain syndromes 1168
registries, cancer, see cancer, registries
regression 4204
regurgitation **1820**, 1964
  in idiopathic achalasia 1869
  management 1868
rehabilitation
  acute illness in elderly **4340**
  acute sports-related injuries 4322
  after amputation 2371
  after falls in elderly 4339
  cerebral infarction 3960
  chronic obstructive airways disease
    2776–7
  coronary artery disease 2357
  malnutrition management 1293–4
  myocardial infarction 2348–9
  Parkinson's disease **4340**
  in stroke 3960, **4340**
rehydration
  in gastrointestinal infections 2006, *2006*
  in malnutrition 1289, *1291*
Reifenstein syndrome 1693
Reiter's syndrome 2965, **2970–2**
  aetiology and pathogenesis 2970, *2970*
  clinical features 2945, 2970–1, *2970*

HIV infection with 2972
  'incomplete' 2970
  ocular features **4185**
  reactive arthritis relationship 2970
  sexually acquired 2970, 2971
  ureaplasmas in 771
rejection, see graft rejection
relapsing fevers **693–7**
  clinical features 695–6
  diagnosis/differential diagnosis 696
  immunity and relapse phenomenon 694
  louse-borne (epidemic) 692, **693**
  pathology 694
  pathophysiology 693–4
  tick-borne (endemic) **693**
  treatment and prognosis 696–7
relapsing polychondritis **3015–16**
  airways obstruction in 2724
  ocular features **4184**
Relate organization 4247
relationship problems, deliberate self-
  harm and 4229
relative incidence 111
relative risk, genetic disease **111**
relatives
  of dying patients, counselling 4234
  information for and support, in
    dementia 4225
  reassurance, psychological treatment
    4254
  see also family
relaxation
  hypertension management 2538–9
  pain management in drug abusers 4300
  therapy in functional bowel disease
    1968
  training 4255
religious stigmata 3637
'remnant receptors' 1401–2, 1403
remnant removal disease
  (hyperlipoproteinaemia type III)
  1408–9, 1413
remnants, chylomicron 1401–2, 1408
REM sleep, see rapid eye movement
  (REM) sleep
remyelination 4091
renal angiography, renovascular
  hypertension 2548, 2549–50
renal arteriography **3110**
renal artery
  aneurysms 2373
  occlusion, acute renal failure 3290
  stenosis 2368, 2545
    causes 2373
    chronic renal failure in 3300
    diabetic nephropathy *vs* 3170
    fibromuscular dysplasia causing 2373
    grafted kidney 3322
    investigations 2548, 3110, 3113–14
    management 2373
    progression 2550, *2550*
    renovascular hypertension 2545
  in sarcoidosis 3187
  surgical reconstruction 2373
  tumour involvement 3183
renal biopsy
  in acute renal failure **3287**, 3291
  in amyloidosis 3180
  in chronic renal failure 3301
  in glomerulonephritis 3153, 3154
  in nephrotic syndrome 3140
  in pregnancy 1734
  in proteinuria 3138
  in renal hypertension 2547
  in SLE 3021, 3187–8, 3190
renal blood flow
  in acute renal failure 3281
  drug excretion and 3269
  in pregnancy 1812, 1813
  reduction/changes in heart failure 2170
  in urinary-tract obstruction 3233
renal bone disease (osteodystrophy)
  3073–4, **3322–30**
  features 3322–5
  investigations 3301, 3324–5
  myopathy in 4169
  pathophysiology 3325–7

in renal transplant recipients 3320–1,
  3329
  treatment 3327–30
renal cell carcinoma (hypernephroma)
  amyloidosis 1513, 3185
  epidemiology 196, 212
  erythropoietin production 3554
  investigations 3111
  staging investigations *236*
  ultrasound 234
renal colic, see ureteric (renal) colic
renal cortical abscess, staphylococcal 529
renal cortical necrosis *3548*
  acute **3290**
  nuclear renal scanning 3115
  in pregnancy 1733, 1734
renal crisis, systemic sclerosis 3009,
  3031, **3190–1**, 3192
renal damage
  cadmium 1107
  carbon tetrachloride 1085
  chloroform 1086
  glue sniffing 1092
  lead poisoning 1109, **3261**
  paracetamol-induced 1051, 3221, 3224
  phenol 1104
  poisonous fungi causing 1158
  poisonous plants causing 1154
  see also nephrotoxic agents
renal dialysis, see dialysis
renal disease/disorders
  ACE inhibitors causing 2251
  acute, hypertension in **2547–8**
  in acute pancreatitis 2029
  in Behçet's syndrome 3045–6
  in bleeding disorders **3656–7**, 3682
  brucellosis in 622, 623
  cardiovascular mortality and 2552,
    2552
  in congenital hepatic fibrosis 2015
  in connective tissue disorders **3187–93**
  in cyanotic congenital heart disease
    2400
  enteroviruses causing 388
  in gout 2986
  haematological changes **3682–3**
  in hantavirus infections 426
  hepatitis B-associated, see hepatitis B,
    renal disease
  in hereditary fructose intolerance 1347
  in HIV infection 477
  hyperlipoproteinaemia in 1411
  hypertension in, see renal hypertension
  infections in drug abusers 4280
  in infective endocarditis 2439, 2441
  inherited **3202–5**
  joint involvement **3006**
  left ventricular hypertrophy in 2552
  loin pain-haematuria syndrome **3148**
  in malignancy **3183–5**
  in microscopic polyangiitis 3013–14
  in myeloma *3180*, **3181–2**, 3185, *3300*,
    3599
  osteomalacia in **3073–4**, *3073*
  in polyarteritis nodosa 3014
  polycythaemia in 3554
  in pregnancy **1733–5**
  in rheumatoid arthritis 2962
  in sarcoidosis **3186–7**
  in sickle-cell disease **3194–5**, 3243, 3515
  signs and symptoms **3136–48**
  in von Gierke's disease 1342
  in Wegener's granulomatosis 3012
  see also nephropathy
renal failure
  ACE inhibitors causing 2235, 2541,
    2551
  acidosis in 1541, 1543, 1544
  acute, see acute renal failure
  in amyloidosis 1514, 3180, 3181
  in ascites 2097
  in Balkan nephropathy 3230–1, 3296
  bleeding disorders 3288, 3305, 3634,
    3656–7, 3682
  in cholera 578
  chronic **3294–306**
  in acute porphyria 1394

renal failure (*cont.*)
  acute renal failure superimposed on 3299
  acute renal failure *vs* 3280
  aluminium toxicity 1425
  anaemia 3300, 3302, 3305, 3483, **3682**
  in analgesic nephropathy 3222, 3223, 3296, *3300*
  bone disease, *see* renal bone disease
  calcitonin levels 1637
  calcitriol deficiency 1636, 3325
  causes 3295–6
  clinical presentation/assessment 3297–301
  definition 3294
  in diabetic nephropathy **3171–2**, 3295, 3296
  erythropoietin therapy 3305, 3389, 3481
  geographical variations 3296
  in gout 1380
  hyperkalaemia in 3133, 3297
  hyperlipoproteinaemia in 1411, 3302
  investigations 3300–1
  iron overload 3481
  management 3304–6
  metabolic effects 3302–3
  myelofibrosis in 3438
  natural history 3303
  organ dysfunction 3301–3
  pathophysiology 3296–7
  polyuria in 3147–8, 3296
  in pregnancy **1734**
  prevalence and incidence 3295
  in primary hyperparathyroidism 1631, 1632
  pruritus in 3744
  severity 3294, *3295*
  in sickle-cell disease 3195, 3515
  toxin-induced 3259
  in urinary-tract obstruction 3295–6, 3299, *3300*
  in cirrhosis 2088
  contrast media causing, *see* nephropathy, contrast-associated
  in cyanotic congenital heart disease 2400
  drug prescribing **3270–5**, 3288, 3305–6
  endstage 3294
    dialysis 3309, 3310
    hypoglycaemia in 1510
    incidence 3295
    renal transplantation 3313
    renovascular disease causing 2551
    see also renal replacement therapy
  in focal segmental glomerulosclerosis 3157
  functional, NSAID induced 3223
  in hantavirus infections 426
  in heart failure 2235
  in hepatocellular failure 2103–4
  hypertension as cause 2533, 2545, 2552, **3248–50**, 3290
  intensive care **2581–2**
  in leptospirosis 699, 701, 702
  in malaria 844, 845, 855
    management 855
  in membranous nephropathy 3159
  in mesangiocapillary glomerulonephritis 3158
  metabolic complications **4124**
  metabolic effects on bone 3071
  in myeloma 3181–2, 3599, 3603
  osteomalacia in 3073
  in paracetamol poisoning 1053
  plasma creatinine 3106–7
  in polycystic kidney disease 3203, 3204
  postpartum idiopathic **1734**, 3292
  in primary hyperoxaluria 1446, 1447
  progression 3303
    factors modulating 3303
    hypertension and 3250, 3303
    mechanisms 3303–4
    role of proteinuria **3144**
  in rapidly progressive glomerulonephritis 3162–3

  in recurrent polyserositis 1527
  in reflux nephropathy 3218
  in rickettsial diseases 731, 733
  in salicylate poisoning 1055
  in septicaemia 2573
  in snake envenoming, management 1138
  thrombocytopenia in 3634
  urate excretion 3225
renal function
  age-related changes 4335
  antihypertensive therapy and 3250
  antimicrobial drug pharmacokinetics 302, 303
  assessment **3101–15**
    in chronic renal failure 3301
    in diabetic nephropathy 3170
    individual kidney 3114–15
  blood pressure and 3247–8
  conservation methods 3304
  in hypertension 3248
  impairment, antituberculous drugs in 660
  initial, allografts 3318
  in lithium use 4250
  normal values *4374*
  in pre-eclampsia 1728, 1729
  in pregnancy 1770–1
  sodium retention in heart failure 2169–70
  in tetanus 628
  in urinary-tract obstruction 3234–5
renal hypertension **2544–53**
  aetiology 2545
  cardiovascular mortality and 2552, *2552*
  clinical diagnosis **2545–6**, *2545*
    history and examination *2545*, 2546
  definition 2545
  diseases causing 2544, 2547, *2547*
  frequency **2544–5**
  investigations **2546–7**, *2546*
  pathophysiology 2545
  sympathetic nerve discharge in 2544, 2545
  treatment **2547**
  unilateral renal parenchymal disease 2552
  see also renovascular hypertension
renal ischaemia 2542
renal osteodystrophy, *see* renal bone disease
renal papillary necrosis
  in acute pyelonephritis 3212–13
  in analgesic nephropathy 3221–2
  diabetic nephropathy *vs* 3170
  differential diagnosis *3222*
  management 3243
  urinary-tract obstruction 3238
renal pelvicalyceal system
  dilatation,
    non-obstructive causes *3232*, **3241–2**
    in urinary-tract obstruction 3237, 3241
    in vesicoureteric reflux 3214, 3215
  stones, management 3255–6
renal pelvis, extrarenal 3241
renal plasma flow
  body size correction 3108
  in diabetes mellitus 3169
  estimation **3107–8**
renal replacement therapy **3306–22**
  acute 2581–2
  in acute renal failure **3286–7**
  in chronic renal failure 3295
  in diabetic nephropathy 3172
  myocardial infarction risk 2552, *2552*
  see also dialysis; renal transplantation
renal transplantation **3313–22**
  in Alport's syndrome 3166, 3205
  in amyloidosis 3181
  in anti-GBM disease 3165–6, 3315
  artificial nutritional support 1323
  BK virus reactivation 446
  cadaveric donors 3313, 3317
    HLA matching 184
  in cystinosis 1355, 1356
  in diabetic nephropathy 3172, 3315
  graft rejection 1530, **3318–19**

  graft survival 3316
  haemodialysis-associated amyloidosis and 1524, 3321
  in Henoch–Schönlein purpura 3152
  HLA matching 184
  hyperlipoproteinaemia after 1411, 3321–2
  in IgA nephropathy 3152, 3315
  immunosuppressive therapy 3318–19
  infections after 1029, 1030
  joint disorders in 3006
  living, related donors 3313, 3316, **3317**
  medical problems after 3319–22
  operative management 3317–18
  polycythaemia 3554
  postoperative imaging 3112, 3115
  pregnancy after 1734
  preoperative assessment 3313–17
    general medical 3313–15
    immunological 3315–17
    renal 3315
  preparation for 3306, 3313
  in primary hyperoxaluria 1447, *1448*, 3315
  recurrence of disease in graft 3161, 3315
  renal bone disease and 3320–1, 3329
  respiratory tract infections after 2709
  sources of kidneys 3317
  ureteric obstruction complicating 3243–4
renal tubular acidosis (RTA) 1538, **3338–41**
  differential diagnosis *3339*, 3341
  hyperkalaemia in 3134, 3341
  incomplete syndrome 3339
  osteomalacia in 3073–4, 3340
  in Sjögren's syndrome 3192, 3340
  toxin-induced 3259
  treatment 1543
  type I (distal; classical; RTA-1) *1538*, 3255, **3338–40**
    causes 3339–40
    pathophysiology 3339
    treatment 3340
  type II (proximal; RTA-2) *1538*, 3339, **3340–1**
  type IV (hyperkalaemic; RTA-4) *1538*, 3339, **3341**
  in urinary-tract obstruction 3235
  in Wilson's disease 1420
renal tubules
  acute necrosis, *see* acute tubular necrosis
  bicarbonate handling 1624, *3330*, 3338
  calcium handling, *see* calcium, renal handling
  drugs secreted into 3268, *3269*
  dysfunction 3108, **3330–41**
    amino acidurias/Fanconi syndrome 3332–3
    cadmium poisoning 1107
    hyperkalaemia 3134
    Liddle's syndrome 1662, 3131–2, 3336–7
    in nephrotic syndrome **3144**
    osteomalacia in 3073–4, *3073*
    in sickle-cell disease 3194
    toxin-induced 3259
  function assessment **3108–9**
  glucose reabsorption *3330*
  intraluminal pressure, in obstruction 3233
  magnesium handling defects 3336
  maximum reabsorption rate (T_m) 3108, 3109
  parathyroid hormone actions 1624
  phosphate handling, *see* phosphate, renal handling
  physiology of transport **3330–1**
  potassium handling 3128–9, *3330*
    disorders **3336–7**
  protein reabsorption 3137
  reabsorption, of drugs 1244, 1257, 1258
  secretion, of drugs 1244, 1257
  sodium reabsorption 3119, *3330*
  urate handling 3225
  urinary concentrating ability 3109
  vasopressin actions 3118, 3332

  water handling 3118, *3330*
    defects, *see* diabetes insipidus, nephrogenic
  renal tubulopathy, proximal, of familial origin 3131
  renal ultrasound, in renal hypertension 2546
  renal vein
    renin ratio 2549
    selective catheterization 3110–11
    thrombosis,
      acute renal failure 3290, 3299
      investigations 3110, 3111
      in membranous nephropathy 3159
      neonatal 1757
      in nephrotic syndrome 3142
  renal venography **3110–11**
  renin 3119, 3248
    deficiency 1662–3, 1669, 3341
    ectopic secretion 1716
    gene 2532
    high, in renal hypertension 2545
    plasma activity,
      in aldosteronism 1656, 1657, *1658*
      in congenital adrenal hyperplasia 1665–6
    tumours secreting **2548**
  renin-angiotensin-aldosterone system 1563, **3119**
    blood pressure and 3248
    blood volume regulation 2157
    digitalis-induced suppression 2242
    dynamic tests 1657–9
    heart failure pathophysiology 2233, 2234
    hypertension pathogenesis 2531–2
    in hypoadrenalism 1654, 1655
    inhibition 2233
    inhibitors **2252**
    see also angiotensin converting enzyme (ACE) inhibitors
    in renovascular hypertension 2545
    sodium retention in heart failure 2170
    in urinary-tract obstruction 3235
    vasoconstriction and 2298
  reninoma 2548
  renography, isotope, *see* scintigraphy (radionuclide scanning), kidney
  renovascular disease **2368**
    hypertension due to, *see* renovascular hypertension
    investigations **2549–50**
    management **2373–4**
    prognosis 2551–2
    progression 2550, *2550*
    treatment **2550–2**
    see also renal artery, stenosis
  renovascular hypertension 2368, 2373, **2544–53**
    aetiology 2545
    atheromatous disease causing 2548–9
    clinical diagnosis 2545–6, *2545*
      history/examination *2545*, 2546
    fibromuscular dysplasia causing 2548–9
    frequency 2544–5
    investigations 2546, 2549–50
    nuclear imaging 3113–14
    treatment 2550–2
      percutaneous transluminal angioplasty 2550–1
      surgery 2550
    see also renal artery, stenosis
  Reoviridae 406
  reovirus *391*, **393**
  reoxygenation, in radiotherapy 254
  reperfusion damage, myocardial ischaemia 2151
  repetitive strain injury (syndrome) 1168, 2996
  reproduction
    adverse effects of drugs 1254
    assisted, ethics 11–12
    hormonal control 1563
  reproductive system **1669–89**
    occupational disease **1173–4**
  research, in control of sexually transmitted diseases 3349
  Research Ethics Committees 11

reserpine 2374
resistance vessels 2531
  cerebral 2534
  in hypertension 2531, 2533, 2534
Reson virus **440**
respiration
  ataxic 2584
  central neurogenic 2584
  Cheyne-Stokes, *see* Cheyne-Stokes
    breathing
  in chlorine poisoning 1097
  complications,
    in drug abusers 4295
    spinal cord injury 3898
  control, in heart failure 2232
  depression,
    in co-phenotrope poisoning 1069
    positive-pressure ventilation in 2577
  in hypothermia 1183
  irregular, dyspnoea with 2162
  in metabolic acidosis 1537–9
  pattern, in unconscious patient 2583–4
  periodic 2583, 2916
  in pregnancy 1744
  in respiratory acidosis 1537, 1539
  in smoke inhalation 1102
  in tetanus 625
  see also breathing; ventilation
respiratory acidosis
  causes 1536, *1538*
  in COAD, management 2927
  diagnosis 1535–6
  in hepatocellular failure 2103
  in hypercapnia 2904
  neurological features 4126
  in poisoning 1047
  respiratory effects 1537, 1539
  in respiratory failure 2904, 2927
  in salicylate poisoning 1054
respiratory alkalosis
  in altitude acclimatization 1186
  causes 1536, *1538*
  in hepatocellular failure 2103
  neurological features 4126
  in poisoning 1047
  in salicylate poisoning 1054
  tetany 1540
respiratory burst 154, **2622–3**, 3559–60
respiratory centre 2645, 2908
  in breathlessness 2645
  in poliomyelitis 385
  in wakefulness 2908
respiratory chain 4171
respiratory disease/disorders
  in acromegaly 1592
  acute viral 337
  in aircraft crew and pilots 1201
  aircraft travel 1202
  in brucellosis 621–2
  cardiovascular system in 2652
  central **3888–91**
  chronic, environmental mycobacteria
    causing 665
  clinical presentation **2642–52**
    see also breathlessness; chest pain;
      cough
  in cyanotic congenital heart disease
    2402
  drugs in, liver damage due to 2131
  general examination **2650–2**
    appearance 2650–1
  general history **2649**
  in gnathostomiasis 952
  head and neck in 2652
  in heart failure 2231–3
  infections, *see* respiratory tract
    infections
  investigations **2652–90**
    see also bronchoscopy; lung biopsy;
      lung function tests; *specific imaging
      methods*
  in Kawasaki disease 3048
  liver in **2130–1**
  in microscopic polyangiitis 3014
  in muscular dystrophy 4149
  in paraquat poisoning 1120
  pathogenesis 2616–18
  see also lung inflammation

pathophysiology **2628–42**
  adult respiratory distress syndrome
    2639–41
  alveolar filling diseases 2638–9
  asthma 2635–6
  diffuse, *see* lung disease, diffuse
    parenchymal
  diffuse airway obstruction 2632–6
  hypoxaemia 2630–1
  pulmonary vascular diseases 2641–2
  physical signs **2649–52**
  polycythaemia in 3553
  positive-pressure ventilation indications
    2576
  in rabies 400
  skin and eyes in 2651
  in SLE 3020
  in sulphur mustard (mustard gas)
    exposure 1117
  in systemic sclerosis 3030, *3031*
  in tetanus 627
  in Wegener's granulomatosis 2801,
    3012
  see also lung disease; respiration
Respiratory Diseases Board 2841,
  2843
respiratory distress syndrome
  neonatal, in maternal diabetes 1757
  see also adult respiratory distress
    syndrome (ARDS)
respiratory drive, *see* ventilatory drive
respiratory drugs, poisoning **1067–9**
respiratory effort, 'length-tension
  inappropriateness' 2164
respiratory emergencies, in terminal
  illness 4355
respiratory encephalopathy 4124
respiratory exchange ratio 2669
respiratory failure **2901–39**
  acute,
    central disorders 3888–9
    in legionnaires' disease 725
    management **2918–25**, 3889
    peripheral disorders *3889*, 3890–1
  acute on chronic **2931**
  in acute pancreatitis 2029
  in adult respiratory distress syndrome
    2852–3, 2904
    see also adult respiratory distress
      syndrome
  in asthma 2904
  in bronchiectasis 2761, 2766
  catastrophic 2596
  causes **2904–6**
  central (neurological causes) **3888–9**,
    3889
  chronic,
    causes 2925, *2925*
    features 2925
    neurological causes 3888, *3889*, 3890
  chronic, management **2925–33**, 3889,
    3890
    acute on chronic failure 2931
    additional strategies **2929–30**
    in COAD, *see below*
    in cor pulmonale **2927**
    CPAP **2932**
    diaphragm pacing **2932**
    non-invasive assisted ventilation **2930–2**
    NPPV, *see* nasal positive-pressure
      ventilation (NPPV)
    see also oxygen; ventilation
  in chronic obstructive airways disease
    2774, 2925
    acute exacerbations management
      2925–7
    chronic stable disease management
      2927–9
    see also chronic obstructive airways
      disease
  in cor pulmonale, management **2927**
  in cystic fibrosis, treatment 2754
  definition **2901**
  in extrinsic allergic alveolitis 2809
  hypercapnia **2904**
    see also hypercapnia
  hypoxia **2902–3**, 2902
    see also hypoxia

in interstitial fibrosis of lung 2904
management 2766, **2918–25**, **2925–33**,
  3889, 3891
  airway establishment 2918–19
  algorithm 2920
  chronic failure, *see above*
  overnight ventilation 2905–6, 2917
  oxygen delivery 2919, *2919*
  PEEP and CPAP 2922
  ventilation **2919–24**
  see also ventilation, mechanical
metabolic complications **4124–5**
neurological causes 3888, *3889*
  central 3888–90, *3889*
  peripheral *3889*, 3890–1
  peripheral ventilatory *3889*, **3890–1**
  in scoliosis 2873
    treatment/support 2873–4
type 1 (oxygenation) 2901
  causes 2904, *2905*
  mechanism 2902, 2904
  oxygen therapy 2926
type 2 (ventilatory) 2901, 2925, 3890–1
  causes 2905, *2905*, 2925
  chronic, hypothesis for genesis 2905,
    2906
  in kyphoscoliosis 2903, 2905
  mechanism 2905–6
  in obstructive sleep apnoea 2905
  oxygen therapy 2926
  treatment 2905, 2906
respiratory insufficiency **3888–9**
  in acute pancreatitis 2029
respiratory medicine
  investigations **2591–2**
  molecular advances **2591**
  therapy **2592**
respiratory muscles 2645
  in breathlessness 2645
  in central apnoea 2916
  in chronic ventilatory failure 2905,
    2906, 2926
  in COAD management 2929
  control 3887–8
  fatigue, dyspnoea due to 2164
  function assessment **2668–9**
  impairment 2668–9
  innervation 2645
  inspiratory muscle training 2929
  paralysis 2645
  in respiratory failure 2905, 2906, 2926
  in sleep 2908, 2909
  in sleep-induced hypoventilation 2826
  in spinal cord injury 3898
  strength, in COAD 2775
  thoracoplasty effect 2876
  weakness, in scoliosis 2873
respiratory papillomatosis, human
  papillomaviruses (HPV) 445
respiratory quotient 1272
respiratory rate
  in acute pancreatitis 2029
  increased, in pneumonia 2695
  normal 2649
  positive-pressure ventilation 2578
respiratory resistance 2609
respiratory secretions
  in bronchiectasis 2759–60
  in pulmonary alveolar proteinosis
    2833
  removal, in pulmonary alveolar
    proteinosis 2834
  techniques to obtain 519
respiratory stimulants 2926, **2928–9**
respiratory syncytial virus (RSV) **339–40**
  antigens and serology 339
  bronchial hyper-responsiveness and
    asthma 2732–3
  clinical features 340, *341*
  epidemiology 339, 2695
  immune response 339–40, 340
  pneumonia in children 2700
  prevention and treatment 340–1
  transmission 333, 339
respiratory tract
  defence mechanisms, *see* defence
    mechanisms; lung, defence
    mechanisms

design **2603–8**, 2629
  heart limiting 2605–6
  mitochondria/capillaries limiting
    2604–5
  pulmonary diffusing capacity and
    oxygen needs 2606–8
  structure/function matching 2603–4
disease, *see* respiratory disease/
  disorders
granulomas, in Wegener's
  granulomatosis 2801
model 2603
obstruction **2719–24**
  in skin disease 3708
riot control agents affecting 1119
structure and function **2609–12**
  see also gas exchanger; lung
upper 2909
  in cystic fibrosis 2749
  obstruction **2719–24**
rhinitis, *see* allergic rhinitis
  in SLE 2798–9
structure/function **2609–12**
  see also airways obstruction
respiratory tract infections 2591,
  2691–713
  acute airways obstruction in 2722
  in AIDS 2710
  allergic rhinitis and 2717
  in asthma 2732–3, **2734–5**
  bacterial, in renal transplant recipients
    3314
  Bordetella 587
    see also pertussis
  bronchial hyper-responsiveness due to
    2732–3
  in bronchiectasis, *see under*
    bronchiectasis
  bronchiolitis obliterans in 2796
  causative organisms *2676*
  Chlamydia pneumoniae 754
  Chlamydia psittaci 754–5
  in chronic obstructive airways disease
    2774, 2777
  chronic specific **2707–8**
    see also tuberculosis
  in cystic fibrosis 2747, 2748, 2749
    protection from and treatment 2751–3
  enterobacteria causing 551
  enteroviruses 383
  Haemophilus influenzae 580
  in immunosuppressed **2708–13**
    chest radiography 2710, 2711
    clinical features 2710–11
    management 2712–13
    organisms 2708–9, *2709*
    patterns 2709–11
    prevention 2713
    radiology and lung sampling 2711–12
    results 2713
    transplantation 2709–10
  lower tract **2692–704**
    bronchial **2692–3**
    see also pneumonia
  management in mitral stenosis 2455
  microbiological diagnostic methods
    2675–8, 2697
    antigen detection 2676–7, *2676*
    choice of samples 2677
    culture 2677, 2697
    DNA sequences 2677
    examination 2675–7
    interpretation 2678
    pneumonia 2678, 2697
    samples 2675
    serological 2677, *2677*, 2697
    stained samples 2676, 2697
  mycoplasmal **762–7**
    see also Mycoplasma pneumoniae;
      mycoplasmas
  neonatal chlamydial 753–4
  non-colonizing organisms 2675, 2677
  open-lung biopsy 2689
  Pasteurella 606
  in rheumatoid arthritis 2797
  seasonal peaks and aetiology 2695
  streptococcal group A 498–9, 501
    prevention 503

respiratory tract infections (*cont.*)
 suppurative **2704–7**
 in systemic sclerosis and CREST
  syndrome 2799
 in tetanus 627
 upper tract **2691**
 viral **333–41**
  bacterial infections after 2693, 2699
  frequency 2691, *2691*
 see also bronchial infections;
  bronchitis; pleuropulmonary infection
respiratory viruses **333–41**
 definition 333
 diagnosis 334
 epidemiology 333, *333*
 features of infections *341*
 immunity 333–4
 pathogenesis 333
 susceptibility to 333
 transmission 333, *334*
response prevention therapy 4255
 behaviour therapy in obsessive
  compulsive disorder 4207
resting metabolic rate, prediction *1307*
restless legs (Ekbom's syndrome) 4092,
 4099, **4159**
 in pregnancy 1766
restlessness
 antipsychotic drugs side-effect 4252
 in positive-pressure ventilation 2579
restriction endonucleases 59, 60
 gene mapping 60
restriction fragment length
 polymorphisms (RFLP) 62
 Duchenne muscular dystrophy 4147
 uses in polygenic disease analysis 64
resuscitation
 ABC method 2283, 4045–6
 in acute poisoning 1046
 airway establishment 2918–19
 brain death and 3933, 3934
 in cardiac arrest 2283–4
 in head injury 4045–6
 inappropriate 3933
 mass runs 4327
 nature of death and 3933
 in pulmonary embolism 2526
 in septicaemia *1023*
 see also cardiopulmonary resuscitation
resuscitation fluids, in electrical injury
 1212–13
retching 1821
 in bronchitis 1964
'retention signals' 71–2
reticular dysgenesis 172
reticular formation 3930
reticulocytes 3388, 3453, 3454
 counts *3379, 3380*
  in paroxysmal nocturnal
   haemoglobinuria 3451
  in pyruvate kinase deficiency 3535
 in haemolytic disorders 3525
 sequestration in spleen 3589
reticuloendothelial system, in
 Langerhans-cell histiocytosis 3607
reticuloendothelioma, aetiological factors
 204
reticulohistiocytoma 3609
reticulohistiocytosis, multicentric 3803
reticulosarcoma 3794
reticulosis
 histiocytic medullary 3586
 lipomelanic 3796
retina
 angioma 4182
 assessment, ophthalmoscopy 4179
 changes/disorders 4179
 cholesterol embolism 2376, 4186
 cotton-wool spots, *see* cotton-wool spots
 drug toxicity 4196–7
 embolization 3951, 3952
 floaters 4179, 4183
 in haematological disorders 4194–5
 hypoxia 4194
 infiltrates and diseases associated
  4179–80
 microinfarcts, *see* cotton-wool spots
 necrosis, acute,
  in HIV infection 476
  in zoster 350

neovascularization 4189, 4190
oedema, in pancreatitis 4184
in onchocerciasis 915, 4192
pigmentation,
 'bull's eye' pattern 4196
 in malignant tumours 4182
screening,
 in diabetes 4188
 in sickling disorders 4195
in sickling disorders 4195
retinal arterioles
 'copper'/'silver' wiring 4188
 in hypertension 4188
retinal artery
 occlusion **4186**
 thrombosis, in diabetes 1486
retinal capillaries
 basement membrane thickening 4189
 in diabetes 4188–9
retinal exudates, in hypertension 2536
retinal ganglion cells 3863
retinal haemorrhages **4179–80**
 in AIDS 4193
 in Behçet's syndrome 4183
 'black sunburst' 4195
 in cerebral malaria 846, 4192
 in cerebrospinal angiostrongyliasis 947,
  948
 dot and blot 2536, 4179
  in diabetes 4189
  in hypertension 4188
 flame-shaped 1192, 2536, 4179, 4188
 in haematological disorders 3376, 4194
 of high altitude 1191–2
 in hypertension 2536
 in leukaemia 4194
 in retinal vein occlusion 4187
 'salmon patch' 4195
 in sarcoidosis 4182
 in sickling disorders 4195
retinal phlebitis, occlusive 4182
retinal pigment epithelium
 congenital hypertrophy (CHRPE) 1990
 inflammation 4182
retinal vascular disease, fluorescein
 angiography 4180
retinal vascular occlusion **4186–7**, 4194
 in SLE 4184
retinal vasculitis, in Behçet's syndrome
 4183
retinal vein
 in multiple sclerosis 4184
 nipping, in hypertension 2536
 occlusion **4186–7**
  in diabetes mellitus 4190
  in myeloma 4194
  thrombosis, in diabetes 1486
retinal vessels
 hard and soft exudates 4188
 permeability 4188
retinitis
 cytomegalovirus, *see* cytomegalovirus
  (CMV) infection, retinitis
 in immunocompromised 1033
 necrotizing 350
 retinitis pigmentosa 4180
retinoblastoma *1567*, 3567
 Burkitt lymphoma *vs* 354
 chromosome 13q deletion 4182
 genes 65, 194
 inherited/sporadic forms 194
retinochoroiditis, toxoplasmosis causing
 866
retinoic acid 1554
 acne vulgaris management 3753, 3754
 all-*trans*-retinoic acid (ATRA) 3409,
  3659
 bone disease associated 3095
 effect on osteoblasts 3095
 in myelodysplastic syndromes 3430
 in psoriasis 3750
 receptor (RAR) 1562
 serum lipids and 1411
retinoids
 benign intracranial hypertension due to
  4042
 skin disease management 3806–7
 teratogenicity 1809, *1810*
retinoid X receptor 1562

retinol, *see* vitamin A
retinopathy
 AIDS 4193
 in congenital rubella 1779
 diabetic, *see* diabetic retinopathy
 hypertensive, *see* hypertensive
  retinopathy
 in leukaemia 4194
 in malignant hypertension 2536, 2543
 in myeloma 4194
 Takayasu's 2378
retirement, early, in angina 2326
ret proto-oncogene
 in MEN IIa syndrome 1568, 1709
 mutation 104
 in papillary thyroid carcinoma 1569,
  1618
retrocollis 4018
retroperitoneal fibrosis 2009
 diagnosis 3111
 idiopathic (peri-aortitis) **3244–6**
retroperitoneal haemorrhage, *see*
 haemorrhage, retroperitoneal
retroperitoneal pain, in tumours 241
retroviruses **463–92**
 DNA integration 462
 infections, arthritis in 3002
 oncogene homology 194, 222, 462
 in pregnancy **1782–3**
 vectors in gene therapy 113
 see also HIV; human T-cell leukaemia-
  lymphoma virus (HTLV-I)
reverse transcriptase 59
reverse transcription-polymerase chain
 reaction (RT-PCR) 3638
rewarming, after cold exposure and
 hypothermia 1183, 1184
Reye's syndrome *2018*, **2025–6**, 2101,
 4072–3
 aspirin association 1054, 4072
 differential diagnosis 4072–3
 encephalopathy in 2025
 epidemiology and features 4072
 in influenza 339
 treatment and prognosis 2026
RGD sequence 3614
rhabdomyolysis
 acute renal failure 3284, 3289
 after snake bites 1135
 in alpha-chloralose poisoning 1123
 causes *3289*
 clinical features 4327
 exercise-induced 4326–7
 glue sniffing and 1092
 in haemolytic uraemic syndrome 3198
 major (catastrophic exertional) 4326–7
 in opioid overdose 1058
 'physiological', in endurance sports
  4326
 in poisoning 1048
rhabdomyosarcoma, Burkitt lymphoma
 vs 354
rhabdoviruses **394–406**
 classification 394, *396*
 epidemiology 395–7
 structure and characteristics 394, 395
 see also rabies virus
Rhesus (Rh)
 blood groups **3688–9**
 compatibility testing 3690
 D antigen 3688
 haemolytic disease of newborn **3544–5**,
  3689
 incompatibility 3689
rheumatic diseases
 affecting occupations 1168
 classification 2943, *2943*
 clinical features **2944–7**
  articular symptoms **2944–5**
  extra-articular symptoms **2945–6**
 clinical representations **2946–7**
 constrictive bronchiolitis obliterans in
  2796
 diagnosis 2943, *2943*
 examination **2946**
 generalized musculoskeletal pain 2997
 history-taking **2944**
 inflammatory, *see under* joint disease
 information on 2944

investigations **2947–53**, *2948*
 immunological 2952–3, *2952*
 inflammatory mediators/tests 2951–2
 'physiological' imaging 2949–50
 radiography 2948–9
 roles of 2947
 use/abuse 2947–53
 see also synovial fluid
liver in **2135**
management **2943–4**, *2944*
occupational 1168, 2996
 ergonomic problems 1168
 high risk occupations 1169
 history, examination 1169
 repeated heavy impact loading 1168
 repetitive low impact trauma 1168
open-lung biopsy 2688, 2690
pericardial pain and effusions in 2476
prevalence 2943
renal involvement **3187–93**
rheumatic fever 503–5, **2432–6**
 aetiology 2432
 aortic stenosis in 2462
 clinical features 503–4, **2432–3**
  arthritis 503, 504–5, 2432–3
  carditis 503, 505, **2433**, 2439
  chorea 2433, 4012
 diagnosis 504–5, **2433–4**
  Jones criteria 499, 504, *504*, *2434*
 incidence 2432
 laboratory findings 504, *504*
 mitral stenosis in 2467
 onset and time of 503
 pathogenesis 503, 2432
 pathology **2432**
 pericardial involvement 2433, 2476
 in pregnancy 1737
 prevention **2435**
  after streptococcal sore throat 502,
   2435
  primary 505, 2435
  secondary 505, *505*, 2435
 recurrence **2435**
 treatment 505, **2434–5**
 tricuspid stenosis in 2467, 2468
rheumatic heart disease 503, 505, **2433**,
 2439, 2467
 in pregnancy **1737–8**
 see also rheumatic fever
rheumatic nodules, in rheumatic fever
 2433
rheumatism 2997
 definition 2995
 palindromic 2946, **3007**
rheumatoid arthritis 2796, **2953–65**
 aetiology **2953–5**
 amyloidosis in 1513, 1514, 2963, 3193
 anaemia in 2960
 bronchiectasis in 2761, 2797
 bronchiolitis obliterans in 2796, 2797,
  2961
 cardiac manifestations 2392, *2392*, 2961
 cause of death 2959
 classification systems 2955, *2956*
 clinical course 2962–3
 clinical features **2955–63**
  articular, *see* rheumatoid arthritis,
   joints
  extra-articular 2959–62
 complications 2963
 diagnostic criteria 2955, *2956*
 differential diagnosis 2963
 diffuse parenchymal lung disease in
  2781, 2797, 2961
 drug-induced lung disease 2798
 gastrointestinal tract in 2000
 genetic factors/susceptibility 2953
 gout negative association 2986
 haematological changes **3681**
 HLA antigen association 2954–5, *2956*
 immunogenetics 2954–5
 immunopathology 2953–4
 joints 2956–9
  axial skeleton 2959
  cervical spine 2949, 2959
  distribution 2956
  lower limbs 2958–9
  secondary problems 2956
  upper limbs 2957–8

juvenile, *see* Still's disease
liver in 2135, 2139, 2962
lung involvement **2796–8**, *2797*, 2961
management **2963–4**
 drugs 2963–4, *2964*
 experimental 2954, 2964
 first-line drugs 2963–4
 haematological effects of drugs 3681
 second-line drugs 2964
 surgery 2964
 third-line drugs 2964
membranous nephropathy and 3159, 3193
mono-articular onset 2956
muscular involvement 2962, 4156
Mycoplasma fermentans in 771
neurological complications 2961–2, **4131–2**
neurological signs 2959
ocular features **4185**
onset, patterns of 2955–6
osteoporosis in 2962, 3070
pathogenesis 2796
pauci-articular onset 2956
pleural effusions in 2868, 2961
polymyalgic onset 2955–6
prevalence 2953, 2955
prognostic factors 2962
pyrophosphate arthropathy *vs* 2989
radiology 2948, 2956–7
renal disease 2962, **3192–3**
risk in relatives 2953
Sjögren's syndrome and 2961, 3036
vasculitis in 2797–8, 2960–1, 3776
rheumatoid factor 2796, 2952, 2954
 in cryoglobulinaemia 3050
 diseases with 2954
 diseases without 2963
 low titre 2952
 post-infectious glomerulonephritis and 3174
 vasculitis initiation 2960
rheumatoid nodules 2797, 2960
 Caplan's syndrome 2797, 2840, 2960
 necrobiotic 2797
rheumatoid nodulosis 2960
rheumatology **2943**
rhinitis
 allergic, *see* allergic rhinitis
 atrophic 569
 common cold syndrome 2691
 nickel exposure 1112
 non-allergic (vasomotor) 160
 occupational 2715
rhinocerebral mucormycosis 1033
Rhinocladiella aquaspersa 813
Rhinocort 2718
rhinoentomophthoromycosis **803**
rhinopharyngitis mutilans (gangosa) 705
rhinophycomycosis *3801*
rhinorrhoea
 after head injury 3835
 CSF 1582
rhinoscleroma **568–9**, *3801*
rhinosporidiosis **810–11**, *3801*
rhinoviruses 333, **335**
 features of infections *341*, 2691
 pathogenesis 333, 335
 serotypes 335
 transmission 335
rhizotomy 3945
rhodanase 1098
Rhodococcus equi 560
rhonchi 2636
rho protein 82
rib(s)
 'champagne cork' deformity 3082
 congenital abnormalities 2875
 disorders **2875–6**
 excessive movements 3890
 fractures,
 flail chest 2875
 pain in 2648
 immobility, in ankylosing spondylitis 2874
 metastases, pain 241
 notching 2179
 removal 2875–6

ribavirin 339
 in Argentinian haemorrhagic fever 438
 in chronic hepatitis C 459, 2069
 in Lassa fever 434
riboflavine
 deficiency, anaemia in 3498
 reference nutrient intake (RNI) 1268, *1269*
 therapy 1375
ribonucleic acid (RNA), *see* RNA
ribonucleoprotein
 U1 3035
 antibodies 3024, *3033*
 U3, antibodies *3033*
ribose 1384
ribosomal P-protein, antibodies 3025
ribosomal RNA (rRNA), in bacterial classification **273–4**, *274*, 497
ribosomal S6 kinases (RSK) 1561
ribosomes 68
 in myocardial cells 2145
 protein synthesis 59
Richter's syndrome 3422
rickets 3061, **3070–5**
 biochemistry 3071–2
 causes 3070, 3071, *3071*, 3074
 clinical features 3071
 in cystinosis 1355, 1356
 diagnosis *3064*, 3072
 hypocalcaemic vitamin D resistant 1573
 hypophosphataemic, *see* rickets, vitamin D-resistant
 investigations 3072
 oncogenous **3334**
 osteogenic **3074**
 phosphate deficiency **3074–5**
 in renal disease **3073–4**, *3073*
 renal tubular 3073–4
 in renal tubular acidosis 3073–4, 3340
 treatment 3072–3
 tumour **3074**
 uraemic 3324
 vitamin D-dependent 1636–7, **3074**
 types I and II 3074
 vitamin D-resistant 1259, 1636, **3073–4, 3334**
 diagnosis and treatment 3074
 see also osteomalacia
rickettsia 728–9
 isolation/detection 732–3
Rickettsia akari 736
Rickettsia australis 736
Rickettsia conorii 734
Rickettsia japonica 736
rickettsial diseases **728–39**
 aetiology, epidemiology and ecology 728–9, *729*
 eye 4192
 liver in 2134
 prevention 733
 public health importance 728
 septicaemia in 1023
 spotted fevers 730–3, **734–6**
 transmission by body lice 728, 1003
 treatment 728, *730*, 733
 vaccines 731, 733
 vasculopathic **730–3**
 see also scrub typhus; spotted fevers
rickettsialpox *729*, **736**
Rickettsia prowazekii 728, 730, 737
Rickettsia rickettsii 731, 734, 735
Rickettsia sibirica 736
Rickettsia tsutsugamushi 739
Rickettsia typhi 736
rickettsioses **730–3**
 see also rickettsial diseases
rickety rosary 1284
Riedel's thyroiditis 1615
rifampicin 3278
 adverse reactions 657, 1718
 H. influenzae type b prophylaxis 583
 in leprosy 675, 676
 meningococcal infection prophylaxis 542
 nephrotoxicity 3264–5
 overdose/poisoning **1069**
 in pregnancy 1746, 1793
 in Q fever 744
 in renal failure *3272*

resistance 675
 Staphylococcus aureus resistance 525
 in streptococci group A infections 502
 in tuberculosis 655, *656*, 663
 in HIV infection 480
rifampin, *see* rifampicin
Rift Valley fever **428–9**, *428*
right atrium (atrial)
 abnormal chest radiograph 2181
 atrial natriuretic factor in 2156
 clots in 2481
 in corrected transposition 2417
 diastolic collapse 2477, 2479
 in Ebstein's anomaly 2413
 enlargement 2181
 filling, in pericardial constriction 2478
 hypertrophy, ECG in 2188, 2190
 pressure, *see* atrial pressure, right
 pulmonary veins to 2415
 volume, in pericardial constriction 2479
 see also entries beginning atrial
right gastroepiploic artery, grafting 2355
right heart failure
 in adult respiratory distress syndrome 2857
 in chronic obstructive airways disease 2777
 in cor pulmonale 2515, 2517
 in diffuse interstitial fibrosis of lung 2637
 in Eisenmenger reaction (syndrome) 2410
 in Fallot's tetralogy 2402, 2403
 in hypoxia 2902
 in pulmonary arterial stenoses 2409
 in pulmonary hypertension 2510, 2511
 in pulmonary vascular diseases 2641
 in scoliosis 2873
 in transposition of great arteries 2417
 use of term 2515
right-left disorientation 3851
rights
 demographic entrapment and 37
 patients' 10–11
right ventricle (ventricular)
 abnormal with reversed interatrial shunt **2415**
 abnormal and shunt reversal 2413–15
 afterload, in pulmonary embolism 2524
 aneurysm, after Fallot's tetralogy repair 2407
 bipartite 2405, **2421**
 chest radiography 2178
 abnormal 2181
 in cor pulmonale 2515–16
 diastolic collapse 2477, 2479
 dilatation,
 Ebstein's anomaly *vs* 2414
 in HIV infection 2395–6
 double-outflow 2404, **2418**
 dysfunction, in Ebstein's anomaly 2413
 dysplasia,
 arrhythmogenic **2391**
 ventricular tachycardia in 2279, 2280
 enlargement 2181
 failure, *see* right heart failure
 filling, in pericardial tamponade 2477
 function 2206, 2221
 hypertrophy 2384
 in cor pulmonale 2515, 2517
 ECG in 2187–8, 2189
 in Eisenmenger reaction (syndrome) 2410
 in Fallot's tetralogy 2402
 in ostium primum 2427
 in pulmonary hypertension 2510
 in pulmonary valve stenosis 2419
 in systemic sclerosis 3029
 see also ventricular hypertrophy
 hypoplastic 2415
 impulse, in dilated cardiomyopathy 2383
 inflow obstruction 2480
 in pericardial constriction 2479
 myocardium,
 fibrofatty replacement 2391
 thinning 2413
 outflow,
 atresia **2407–8**

calcification 2399
 double 2404, **2418**
 obstruction 2420
 output 2487, 2517
 pressure,
 in Fallot's tetralogy 2403
 in ventricular septal defects 2428
 scintigraphy 2206
 stroke volume, in pericardial tamponade 2477
 see also ventricle (ventricular)
rigidity 3863
 in Parkinson's disease 4001
 in tetanus 625, 626
 'rigid spine syndrome' 4147
Riley-Day syndrome 4104
RING4 and *RING11* genes 69
ringbinden 4143
Ringer's lactate solution 579, 1024
rings, hand dermatitis management and 3807
ringworm 797, 798, 3717, 3762
 cattle 1165, 3762, 3800
Rinne test 3870
riot control agents **1118–19**, 4197
 liquid dispersal 1118–19
 smoke dispersal 1119
risk 45, *46*
 absolute 45
 assessment, in occupational safety 1178
 attributable 45, *46*
 management **4312**
 relative 45, *46*
risperidone 4253
ristocetin-induced platelet aggregation (RIPA) *3643*, 3644
risus sardonicus 625, 626
RITA trial (Randomised Intervention Treatment of Angina) 2351, 2357
Ritter's disease, *see* scalded skin syndrome
ritualistic movements 3919
rituals 4207
 compulsive 4207
 suppression and control 4255
river blindness, *see* onchocerciasis
RNA 57
 in cardiac hypertrophy 2147
 messenger, *see* messenger RNA (mRNA)
 ribosomal, *see* ribosomal RNA (rRNA)
 structure 57
 transfer (tRNA) 59
 transport through nuclear pore 78
RNA polymerases 57
RNA probes, dengue haemorrhagic fever diagnosis 420
RNA viruses, carcinogenesis mechanism 462
Ro (SSA), antibodies 2952, 3021, 3022, 3024, 3032
road traffic accidents
 epilepsy after 3916
 multiple injuries 4048, *4048*
 spinal cord injury 3896
 in UK 2359
Robens Committee report 1177
Robertsonian translocations 122–3
Rochalimaea
 infections *729*
 rare species *560–1*
Rochalimaea elizabethae 745
Rochalimaea henselae 274, 745
 antibodies and serological tests 746–7
 bacillary angiomatosis 747
 cat scratch disease 745–7
 characteristics/classification 745–6
 isolation and culture 747
 see also cat scratch disease
Rochalimaea quintana 274, 745, 747, 748
Rochalimaea vinsoni 745
Rocio encephalitis **415–16**
rock wool 2845
Rocky Mountain spotted fever 406, 728, *729*, **734–6**, 1023
 mortality 736
rodenticides **1123–4**
 alpha-chloralose 1123–4

rodenticides (cont.)
  thallium poisoning 1113
  warfarin and anticoagulants 1123
rodents, leptospirosis transmission 698
rodent ulcers (basal cell carcinoma) 208, 3791
Romaña's sign 896, 897, 4192
Romanovsky stain 899
Romano-Ward syndrome 2282
Romanus lesion 2967
Romberg's sign 3858
Rome criteria, functional bowel disease 1965, 1966
rosacea 3787
Rosai-Dorfman disease 365, 3566, 3608, 3609
Rose Bengal 4185, 4196
'rose grower's arthritis' 3000
roseola 364
  see also human herpesvirus 6 (HHV-6)
Roseomonas, rare species 561
rose spots, lenticular in typhoid 562
rosin 3737
Ross river virus 407
rotational test 3874
rotator cuff lesions 2995
rotavirus 390, 391–2, 391, 391, 2002
  avirulent nursery strains 391
  classification 392
  diarrhoea due to 391–2
  prevention 393, 394
Rothia dentocariosa 561
Roth spots 2438, 2441, 4193, 4194
Rotor's syndrome 1397, 1799, 2056, 2059
  Dubin-Johnson syndrome vs 2059
  factor VII deficiency and 3652
roundworm, see nematodes
Roussy-Lévy syndrome 4103
Roux-en-Y gastrojejunostomy 1962
Royal National Lifeboat Institution (RNLI) 2360
RU-486, in ectopic ACTH syndrome 1714
rubber, contact dermatitis 3737
rubella 409–12
  arthritis in 3001
  clinical features 409
  congenital 409, 410–11, 410, 1778–9, 4112
    defects associated and risk of 410, 410
    diabetes in 1454, 1779
    diagnosis 410–11
    incidence 411, 412
  epidemiology 409
  eye in 4192
  haematological changes 3679
  management, in pregnancy 411
  in pregnancy 411, 1776, 1778–9
  progressive rubella panencephalitis 4074
  transmission 410
  vaccination 411–12
    UK approach 411, 412
    US programme 411
  vaccines 289, 411, 412
    in pregnancy 1778
    teratogenicity 412
  see also measles/mumps/rubella (MMR) vaccine
rubellavirus, immunosuppression due to 174
rubeosis iridis, in diabetes 1486
Rubinstein-Taybi syndrome 4110
'rule of three' 3859
rumination 1283, 1295, 1964, 4207
  management 1295
runners
  amenorrhoea in 4326
  heat injury and hyperthermia 4328
  hypothermia 4328
  hypovolaemia in 4327–8
  sites of injuries in 4323
  see also endurance sports; marathon runners
running
  abstinence periods after stress fractures 4323, 4324
  downhill 4324, 4326
  friction syndromes 4324

Russell's bodies 568
Russell's sign 4216
Russell's viper, haemorrhage 1134
Russian spring-summer encephalitis (RSSE) 416
Rwanda 37
'Ryan virus' 825

S

S100 protein 252
Sabin vaccine 318, 389, 389
saccade 3872
saccharin, bladder cancer association 212
Saccharomyces cerevisiae
  ts mutants 76
  vesicular transport in 75, 76–7, 82
Sack-Barabas type, Ehlers-Danlos syndrome 3084
sacral agenesis 4116
sacral radiculomyelopathy, in genital herpes 3352
sacroiliac joint, tenderness 2947
sacroiliitis 2965
  in ankylosing spondylitis 2967
  in brucellosis 621
  enteropathic synovitis in 2972, 2973
  in psoriatic arthritis 2969
  radiography 2949
'saddleback' fever 406
'safer sex' 3348
safety, occupational, see occupational safety
safety management, see under occupational safety
safety training 1179–80
sagittal sinus thrombosis 4042–3
SAG-M medium 3694
'St Anthony's fire', see erysipelas
St Louis encephalitis 416, 4065
St Vitus dance 4012
salazopyrine 3683
salbutamol
  actions and clinical use 2255
  aerosol 1238
  mechanism of action 1249
  receptors 2254
salcatonin 3229
salicylates
  adverse mental symptoms 4242
  adverse reactions 2850
  hypoglycaemic effects 1472, 1511
  new, in Crohn's disease 1942
  pharmacokinetics and toxicity 1054
  plasma concentration 1055
  poisoning 1045, 1054–6
    acid-base disturbances 1543
    in children 1054, 1055
    clinical features 1055, 1055
    diabetic ketoacidosis vs 1499
    management 1050, 1056, 1056
    metabolic effects 1054–5
    pathophysiology 1054, 1055
    pharmacokinetics and toxicity 1054
    severity assessment 1055
  thyroid function testing and 1717
salicylazosulphapyridine, haemolysis due to 3546
salicylic acid
  overdose/poisoning 1056
  warts treatment 3798
salicylic esters 1056
saline
  in diabetic ketoacidosis 1500–1
  in hypercalcaemia 1628, 3228
  hypertonic, in polyuria 1601, 3121, 3122
  in hyponatraemia 3123
  in septicaemia treatment 1024
  see also salt; sodium
salivary glands
  adenocarcinoma 1860
  biopsy, in Sjögren's syndrome 3037
  diseases 1861–2
  enlargement, in bulimia nervosa 1300, 4216
  inflammation 1861–2

in mumps 372, 373
  obstruction due to calculus 1862
  tumours 1862
    epidemiology 201–2
salivation, in Parkinson's disease 4001, 4004
Salk vaccine 318, 389, 389
Salla disease (sialic acid storage disease) 1426, 1436
  infantile form (ISSD) 1436
salmon calcitonin 3077
Salmonella 551
  antibiotic resistance 553
  characteristics 551
  infective dose 552
  serotypes, identification 553
  species 551, 552
  subspecies/serotypes 551
Salmonella enterica subsp. enterica
  serotype Typhi, see Salmonella typhi
Salmonella enteritidis 486, 551, 2003
Salmonella infections
  bacteraemia 552
  clinical features 552–3
  convalescent excretion 552
  epidemiology and sources 551–2
  in HIV infection 486–7
  in homosexuals 3363
  incubation period 552
  laboratory diagnosis 553
  mechanism 552
  pathology 552
  prevention and control 553
  transmission from reptiles 1014
  treatment, antimicrobials 553
Salmonella paratyphi 567
Salmonella typhi 551, 561, 2004
  antigens 564
  culture 563–4 endotoxin 562
  infective dose 268, 561
  multiplication/dissemination 561–2
  serology 564
  Vi antigen 550, 561
  see also typhoid
Salmonella typhimurium 486, 551
  Ames test 193
  interaction with phagocytic cells 272
salmonellosis, see Salmonella infections
Salofalk 1949, 1949
salpingitis 3347
  chlamydial 753, 759, 1791
  in enterobiasis 941
  Mycoplasma hominis causing 770
salt
  in cholera management 579
  depletion 1181
  intake 3119
    in acute renal failure 3286
    blood pressure and 2312
    in chronic renal failure 3304, 3305
    hypertension pathogenesis 2530
    ischaemic heart disease risk 2312
    in nephrotic syndrome 3140
    pre-eclampsia and 1730
    reduction, in ascites management 2097
    in renal transplant recipients 3322
    in syndrome of inappropriate antidiuresis 3125
  loading, in aldosteronism 1658
  poisoning 1078
  requirements in hot climates 1181
  in salt-depletion heat exhaustion 1181
  wasting, in congenital adrenal hyperplasia 1664, 1667, 1690
  see also saline; sodium
salt-depletion heat exhaustion 1181
salted fish 202, 218
'salt sensitivity' 2538
Samaritans 4231
sandflies 899, 900, 918, 1011
  bartonellosis transmission 774
sandfly fever 428
Sandhoff's disease 1428, 1430, 3985
Sanfilippo disease
  (mucopolysaccharidosis III) 1431, 1432
Santavuori syndrome 3985
sarafotoxins, sequences 1130
sarafoxin-b 1130

Sarcocystis 878
Sarcocystis hominis 877
Sarcocystis suihominis 877
sarcocystosis 877–8
sarcoidosis 2817–32
  activity assessment 2830–1
    features of active disease 2830
    aetiology 2819–20
  in aircraft crew and pilots 1201
  arthritis in 3007
  bone involvement 2827
  cardiac 2393, 2827
  chronic 2831
  clinical features 2122, 2821–8, 2821
    presenting symptoms 2820, 2821
    summary 2822
  course and prognosis 2831
  definition (descriptive) 2818
  diagnosis 2828
    histological 2828–9
  endocrine involvement 1716, 2827
  epidemiology 2820–1, 2820
  genitourinary system 2827
  granulomatous interstitial nephritis 3186–7
  hepatic features 2122, 2131, 2825
    granulomas 2122, 2131, 2825
  hypercalcaemia in 2826, 2829
  hypercalciuria in 3186, 3255
  immune response 2819
    cell-mediated 2819
    immune complexes 2819, 2830
    immunoglobulins 2829
  intrathoracic, see sarcoidosis, pulmonary
  investigations 2828–30
    ACE levels 2830–1
    biochemical 2829–30
    biopsy and bronchoscopy 2828
    bronchoalveolar lavage 2830
    chest radiography 2782, 2822, 2823–5
    computed tomography 2823
    gallium-67 scanning 2830
    laboratory 2829–30
    lung function tests 2829
    open-lung biopsy 2688, 2690, 2823
    see also Kveim-Siltzbach test
  locomotor system 2827
  lymphoreticular involvement 2825
  micropapular 3799, 3802
  multiple sclerosis vs 3995
  muscular involvement 4156
  myocardial 2216, 2827
  neurological features 2826–7, 4132
  neuropathy in 4101
  ocular manifestations 2821, 2826, 4182
    management 4182
    uveitis 2821, 2826, 4182
  onset and age 2821
  pathology 2818–19
    epithelioid-cell granulomas 2818, 2823
    granulomata in 2122, 2131, 2825, 3799, 3802
    histology 2818, 2822–3
    immunopathology 2818–19
    lung calcification 2824–5
    lung infiltration/fibrosis 2823–4
    resolution and scar formation 2818
  plaque form 2825, 2826, 3799, 3802
  pregnancy in 1746, 2827–8
  primary biliary cirrhosis overlap 2131
  pulmonary 2822–5
    bronchial stenosis 2825
    histology 2822–3
    pleural changes 2825
    prognosis 2825
    radiographic changes 2823–5
    recurrence after lung transplantation 2936
  renal involvement 2827, 3186–7
  skin manifestations 2821, 2825–6, 3799, 3802
  spleen in 2825
  treatment 2831–2, 3186, 3187
    aerosol corticosteroids 2832
    alternative 2832
    indications for corticosteroids 2831
    schedule of corticosteroids 2831–2
  upper airways 2826

uveoparotid fever (Heerfordt-Waldenstrom) syndrome 2821, 2826
vitamin D metabolism 1636, 1716
sarcolemma 4139
  myocardial cell 2144
sarcoma
  of bone,
    epidemiology 207
    staging investigations *236*
  in children, Li-Fraumeni syndrome 242
  hypoglycaemia in 1509–10
  in Paget's disease 3075, 3076, 3077
sarcoma of soft tissues
  epidemiology 208
  staging investigations *236*
  surgery and radiotherapy 248
sarcomere 4139
  myocardial cells 2144, 2149
    length 2149–50, 2155
sarcoplasmic reticulum 2145, 2147
Sarcoptes scabiei 1000
sarcosinaemia (sarcosine dehydrogenase deficiency) *1375*
sarcosporidiosis, myositis in 4156
sarin *1116*, 1117
  clinical features *1118*
saturated fatty acids, *see* fatty acids, saturated
Saturday night paralysis 4094
SAVE trial 2250, 2348
scabies **1006–9**, 3712
  clinical features 1007–8, 3744
  diagnosis 3717
  in homosexuals 3361
  Norwegian 1008, 1009
  zoonotic 1007
scabies mite 1000
scaffolding of cells 68
scalded skin syndrome, staphylococcal (SSSS) 524, 529, 3781
  management 530
scalenus anterior syndrome 4093
scalp
  damage 3763
  infections 3762–3
  injury/lacerations 4044
  ringworm 798, 3717
  'tycoon' 3763
scalp shocks 3836, 3837
  see also magnetic brain stimulation
scarlet fever 499
  clinical features 499
  diagnosis 502
  differential diagnosis 502
  exotoxin in, Kawasaki disease aetiology 3049
  mortality 499
  toxic shock 499
  toxins 498, 499
scarring, lung inflammation and **2626–7**
scars
  hypertrophic 3788
  keloids 3716, 3788
  malignant change 3792
scavenger (acetyl-LDL) receptor 1403, 1405
S cells 1892
Schatski ring 1870, 1872–3
Schaumann's bodies 2818
Scheie disease (mucopolysaccharidosis IS) 1431–4
Scheuermann's disease 1420
Schick test 493, 494
  conversion 494
Schilder's disease 3990, **3996–7**, 4238
Schilling test 1907, 1913
Schimmelpenning-Feuerstein-Mims syndrome 124
Schirmer's test 3037, 4179, 4182, 4185
Schistosoma 970
  lifecycle 971–3
Schistosoma haematobium 970, 971–3
  bladder cancer association 211, 212, 977
  infections, eye in 4193
Schistosoma intercalatum 970, 978
Schistosoma japonicum 970, 971–3, 2003, 2121
  clinical features of infection 975, 976, 977

Schistosoma mansoni 970, 971–3, 2003, 2121
  clinical features of infection 975, 976, 977
  genetic factors and susceptibility 280
Schistosoma mekongi 970, 978
schistosomiasis **970–81**, 3463
  acute 975, 980
    diarrhoea in 2003
  bladder cancer association 211, 212, 977
  in children 974, 975, 980
  circulating anodic antigen (CAA) in 979
  clinical features 970, 975–8
    acute infection 975
    bladder 972, 976, 977
    cercarial dermatitis 970, 975
    CNS in 977–8
    diarrhoea in 977, 2004
    established infection 976
    intestinal 977, 2004
    late sequelae 970, 976–7
    lungs in 978
    renal 978
  community-based chemotherapy 980
  diagnosis and investigations 978–9
  differential diagnosis 975, 977
  eggs 971–2, 973
    deposition 972, 975, 977, 978
    diagnosis by 978
    excretion 972
    granuloma 972, 976
  epidemiology 973–5
    by age 974
    geographical distribution 973
    relative equilibrium 975
  experimental, hepatic granulomas pathogenesis 2120
  genetic factors and susceptibility 280, 976
  glomerulonephritis in **3176**
  haematological changes 3681
  hepatic granulomas in 972, 976, 2121, 2134
  hepatosplenic disease 977, 979, 2134
  immune response 976–7
  immunity to reinfection 974
  pathogenesis 975–8
  prevention and control programmes 980
  splenomegaly in 3591
  transmission 973, 973–5
    conditions increasing and migrants 975
    environmental contamination 975
    heavy infections and aggregation 974
    reduction methods 980
  treatment and prognosis 979–80
  urinary-tract obstruction 3179
  vaccine 980
schistosomula 971, 974
schizencephaly 4116
schizoid personality 4212
schizophrenia **4221–3**
  acute syndrome, features 4221–2, *4221*
  aetiology 4222
  chronic 4222
  chronic paranoid 4238
  clinical features 4221–2, *4221*
    'first rank' symptoms 4221, *4221*
    'positive'/'negative' symptoms 4221
  clinical presentation 4221, 4222
  cognitive function impairment and 4225
  differential diagnosis 4222, 4225
    depressive disorder 4222
    mania *vs* 4220, 4222
  in elderly 4226
  in epilepsy 4238
  genetic factors 4222
  incidence 4221
  obsessive compulsive disorder *vs* 4207
  prognosis 4222
  thyroid function 1617
  treatment 4222–3, 4247, 4251
    clozapine 4252
Schmidt's syndrome (polyglandular autoimmune syndrome type II) 1571, 1652, 1653
Schmorl's node 3067

Schobers test 2947
schools, meningococcal infection prophylaxis 544
'school sores' 500
Schulman's syndrome *3791*
Schültz-Charlton reaction 499
Schwachman's syndrome 2039, 3559
Schwann cells 4091
  neuropathies affecting 4091
schwannomas **4032**, 4036
  acoustic 3874–5, 4036
Schwartz-Jampel syndrome (chondrodystrophic myotonia) **4153**
Schwartzman reaction 1995
sciatica 2992
  in lumbar disc protrusions 3906
sciatic nerve **4097**
  lesions/tumours involving 4097
sciatic stretch test 2993
scientific medicine **7–10**
  criticisms 8–9
  definition 7
  development 7–8
  successes 8
scintigraphy (radionuclide scanning)
  adrenal gland 1649–50, 1659–60
  biliary system 1834
  bone and joint 2949, 2950
    see also bone scans
  bone metastases 246
  brain, *see* brain scanning
  chest **2654–5**
    see also lung scans; ventilation-perfusion scanning
  in cryptogenic fibrosing alveolitis 2790–1
  in diffuse parenchymal lung disease 2783
  exercise testing 2228
  gastrointestinal tract 1833
  gut motility disorder investigation 1957
  heart **2204–12**
    cold-spot scanning (negative image) 2207, 2209–11
    exercise testing 2228
    first pass technique 2204–5, 2206
    functional images 2206–7
    gated equilibrium method 2204, 2205–6
    hot-spot scanning (positive imaging) 2207–9
    left ventricular ejection fraction 2205, 2206–7
    left ventricular regional wall motion 2205, 2206
    myocardial infarction, *see* myocardial infarction
    positron emission tomography 2212
    right ventricular function 2206
    SPECT 2211–12
  in Hodgkin's disease 3573
  in hydatid disease 957
  kidney 2549, **3112–15**
    dynamic studies 3115, 3240
    indications 3113–15
    methodology 3112–13
    in reflux nephropathy 3217
    in urinary-tract obstruction 3240
  liver 1833
  in Meckel's diverticulum 1978
  micturating cystography 3215
  pancreatic endocrine tumour localization 1704, 1705
  skeletal, in tumour staging 235, 237
  splenic function 3592, 3593–4
  thyroid gland 1608
Scl-70, antibodies 3032, *3033*
sclerae, blueness 3080
scleritis 4183, 4184
  management 4185
  in rheumatoid arthritis 2961, 4185
scleroderma *3009*, 3027, **4131**
  chemical agents causing *3027*, 3028
  drug-induced 3733
  facial flushing in 3787
  localized *3027*, 3791, 3792
  non-dermatitic occupational dermatosis 1165
Raynaud's phenomenon in 2365, 2945, 3028

sine scleroderma *3027*, 3028, **3029**
  see also systemic sclerosis
scleroderma-like syndromes *3028*
sclerokeratitis 4183
scleroma, *see* rhinoscleroma
scleromalacia, in rheumatoid arthritis 2960, 2961
scleromyxoedema (lichen myxoedematosus) *3791*
sclerosants
  gastrointestinal bleeding management 1828
  pleurodesis 2871
  superficial veins of leg 3810
sclerosing disorders, of bone **3089**
  sclerosis, conditions causing *3791*
sclerosteosis **3089–90**
sclerotherapy
  bleeding oesophageal varices 980, 2094–5
    pleural effusion after 2852
    rebleeding prevention 2095
  pleural 251
scoliosis **2872–4**, 3061
  adolescent idiopathic 2872, 2873
  causes 2872, *2872*
  chest in 2649
  chest radiography 2179
  investigations 2873
  in Marfan's syndrome 3083
  pathophysiology 2872–3
  in spina bifida 4118
  symptoms and signs 2873
  treatment and prognosis 2873–4
scombrotoxic poisoning **1142–3**, 2006
scopolamine, *see* hyoscine
scorpionfish 1141
scorpions **1146–7**
scotomata, in hypertension 2535
scrapie 1517, 3977
scratching 3743
  in atopic eczema 3741
  distribution 3713, 3715
  see also pruritus
screening
  antenatal 135
    fetal abnormalities 1756
    gestational diabetes 1753–4
    haemoglobinopathies 1760
    hepatitis B and C 1798–9
    sexually transmitted diseases 1790, 1791
    toxoplasmosis 1794
    viral infections 1778
  cancer prevention/detection 463
  genetic 132
  for inborn errors of metabolism **1337–8**
  in MEN 1 syndrome 1708
  in MEN 2 syndrome 1709, 1710
  neonatal, *see* neonates, screening
  of relatives,
    in acute porphyria 1394
    in hereditary haemochromatosis 3479
    in Wilson's disease 1422–3
  sexually transmitted diseases 1790, 1791, 3348
scrofuloderma 652
scrotal cancer, chimney sweeps and 197, 216, 1165
scrub typhus **739–41**
scrum pox 344
SCUBA diving 1207
  see also diving
scurvy
  anaemia in 3498
  bleeding tendency 3636
  bone disease in 3094–5
  see also vitamin C (ascorbic acid), deficiency
Scytalidium infections **799**
sea anemones 1143–4
sea bed, contours 1204–5
seafarers, medical examination and fitness 2360
seafood poisoning 393, 1141–3
  Vibrio parahaemolyticus 559
  see also shellfish
sea kraits, bites and envenoming 1132

sea snakes
  bites and envenoming 1127, 1132
  prevention of bites 1139
seasonal mortality **1185**
  heat waves 1185
  massive frostbite, *see* frostbite
  winter 1185
seasonal variations
  aeroallergens 2714
  allergic rhinitis 160, 161, 2714
  animal breeding 1565
  infections 286
  malaria 840, *841*
  pneumococcal infections 512, 2695
  pneumonia 2695
  urinary stones 3252
sea urchins 1144
sea wasps, venomous 1143–4
seawater, drinking 1181
sebaceous cysts, anaerobic infections 573
sebaceous glands, regulation 3752
Sebekia species 1014
seborrhoea
  Demodex 1009
  in hyperandrogenization 1674, 1677
  in Parkinson's disease 4004
seborrhoeic dermatitis 800, 3712, 3743,
    3762, 3768
seborrhoeic warts 3793
sebum 3752
  acne vulgaris aetiology 3752
secalciferol (24,25(OH)₂D₃) 1625–6
  in chronic renal failure 3326, 3329
second-messengers 225, 1554, *1555*,
    1560–1
  drug actions via 1246
  in heart 2147
  inhibitors, new drug targets 259
second-messenger systems 97, 223, 1247
secretin 1553, 1891, **1892**
  structure/secretion/actions 1892
secretin family **1892–3**
secretin test 1705
  in Zollinger–Ellison syndrome 1881
secretogranins 72
sedation
  in cannabis and LSD intoxication 1075
  in endoscopy 1830
  in peptic ulcer treatment 1884
  in positive-pressure ventilation 2579
  weaning from ventilators 2580
sedatives
  avoidance in COAD 2776
  complications associated 4280
  in opiate detoxification 4292
  overdose 4296
  psychiatric disturbances associated 4241
  in renal impairment 3270
  in tetanus 628–9
  in vertigo treatment 3876
  withdrawal syndrome **4293**, 4296
Seitelberger's disease (infantile
    neuroaxonal dystrophy) 3989
seizures
  in acute porphyria 1393
  in alcohol withdrawal 2084
  anoxic (reflex) **3927**
  in cerebral malaria 853
  complex partial,
    mental symptoms 4238
    schizophrenia *vs* 4222
  dissociative 4210
  in drug addicts 4294–5
  drug-induced 3917
  epileptic, *see* epileptic seizures
  febrile 3909
  in isoniazid poisoning 1068
  in malaria 846
  in meningitis, management 4059
  neonatal, pyridoxine-dependent 1372
  in oxygen toxicity 1208
  in poisoning 1047
  poisonous plants causing 1152, *1156*
  simulated 3919
  in SLE 4130
  synonyms 3909
  in tetanus 625
  in tuberculous meningitis 4060
  see also epileptic seizures

Selding's technique 2569
selectins 291, 2294, 2299, **2620–1**, *2620*,
    3558–9
  ligands 291
  structure 2620
  see also E-selectin; L-selectin; P-
    selectin
selection pressure, natural history of
    tumours 195
selective 5-HT uptake inhibitors (SSRIs)
    4248–9
  in depression in elderly 4227
  drug interactions 4249 drugs included
    4248
  indications and use 4249
  in obsessive compulsive disorder 4207
  overdose 1059–60
  pharmacology 4248, *4249*
  side-effects 4249, *4249*
selegiline 1248
  in Parkinson's disease 4002
selenium **1424**
  deficiency 1330, *1418*, 1424
  ischaemic heart disease prevention 2312
  therapy 1424
  toxicity 1424
selenium sulphide 811
⁷⁵Se-6-selenomethylcholesterol 1659–60
selenomethionine scanning 2043
self, disturbed awareness 4237
self antigens 89
  non-self discrimination 89, 141
  tolerance to 155
self-care 47
self-harm, *see* deliberate self-harm
self-help groups
  skin disease *3807*
  ulcerative colitis 1951
self-injury 3628, 3637, 4228
  mutilation, in Lesch-Nyhan syndrome
    1381–2
  see also deliberate self-harm
self-medication, poisonous plants 1151
self-poisoning 1043, 1045, 4228
  bismuth chelate 1069
sellar masses, non-pituitary **1596–9**
sella turcica 1574
'semantic dementia' 3975
semicircular canals 3869
  disease of 3872
seminoma 211
  mediastinal 2899
Semple vaccine 403
senescence 4333
senile dementia of Alzheimer type 3973
senile elastosis 3788
senile plaques 3971, 3972
  in Alzheimer's disease 1516, 3972
  ß-amyloid and amyloid protein in 3972
  distribution and diseases with 3972
senile squalor (Diogenes) syndrome 4228
Senior–Loken syndrome 3205
sensation 3857
  cutaneous, loss 3858
  pain, *see* pain
sensitivity 17, 18–19
  exercise testing 2227
sensorimotor neuropathy
  occupational 1169, *1170*
  in rheumatoid arthritis 2961–2
  see also sensory neuropathy
sensory fibres, in pain sensation 3936
sensory loss
  in cervical spondylotic myelopathy 3908
  in dissociative disorder 4210
  in median nerve lesions 4095
  in polyneuropathies 4091
  in spina bifida, management 4118
  in spinal cord compression 3892
  in subacute combined degeneration of
    cord 3893
  in syringomyelia 3893
  in tumours 249
sensory neurones, neurotransmitters
    3937–8
sensory neuropathy
  in amyloidosis 1515
  in diabetes **1486–7**
  hereditary 4103–4

in HIV infection 4076
in rheumatoid arthritis 2961
  see also neuropathy; peripheral
    neuropathy; sensorimotor neuropathy
sensory system 3857–8, 3891
  lesions 3857
    symptoms 3858
  in multiple sclerosis 3993
sentinel practices 287
Seoul virus 426
sepsis 290
  acute renal failure 3281, **3288**
  in galactosaemia 1349, 1350
  insulin injection causing 1477
  metabolic response 1550
  pyrophosphate arthropathy *vs* 2989
  see also septicaemia
sepsis syndrome 291, 292
  mediators and levels of 292, 293
  see also sepsis; septic shock
septicaemia 282, **1020–7**
  aetiology **1020–2**
  catheter-related, *see* catheter-related
    sepsis
  circulatory derangements **2572–4**
    management 2573–4
  clinical assessment 1023
  clinical features 293, **1022–3**
  community-acquired 1020–1, *1021*
  DIC in 3658, 3679
  differential diagnosis 1023
  in drug abusers 4279, 4294
  endstages **293**
  focus 1020, 1024–5
  in gas gangrene 634
  gonococcal 1020
  Gram-negative 550–1, 1020, 1026
  Gram-positive 1020, 1025
  haemolytic anaemia 3545, *3548*,
    3679
  in hepatocellular failure 2103
  in hospitals 1021–2
  hypoglycaemia in 1510
  injecting drug addicts 4279, 4294
  Lemierre's postanginal 574, 575
  in listeriosis 721
  mediators in 291, 292–3, 1026
  in melioidosis 591
  mortality 1023, 1025
  neonatal/maternal, *H. influenzae* 583
  in neonatal streptococcus B infection
    1788
  pathogenesis, evidence 292–3
  persisting 1025
  in plague 597
  pneumococcal 512, 519, 1020
  prevention **1022**
  primary 1020, *1021*
  prognosis 1025
  pulmonary oedema in 2573
  renal lesions 3175, 3178, 3179
  secondary 1020
  shock with 1020, 1025
    see also septic shock
  Staphylococcus aureus 527
  streptococci group B infections 506,
    507, 1788
  in tetanus 628
  treatment **1023–5**, 2573–4
    anticoagulation 1025
    antimicrobials 1023–4, 2573
    experimental 1025–6, 2573–4
    intravenous fluid 1024
    resuscitation *1023*, 2573
    septic foci removal 1024–5
  vasoconstrictors and inotropes 1024,
    2573
septic arthritis **2998–3003**
  anaerobic infections 573
  bacterial **2998–9**
    mycobacterial **2999–3000**
    non-gonococcal causes *2998*
    staphylococcal 529
  in brucellosis 620
  in drug abusers 4279
  fungal **3000**
  Haemophilus influenzae type b 582
  in rheumatoid arthritis 2963
  spirochaetal infections **3002**

viral **3000–2**
  see also joint(s), infections
septic shock **292–3**, 1020, 1025
  endstages **293**
  high permeability pulmonary oedema
    2496
  management 2504
  in melioidosis 591
  see also endotoxic shock
septo-optic dysplasia 4113
sequestration crisis, in sickle-cell disease
    3515, 3516
Sereny test 554
serine *1353*
serine protease inhibitors 1545
serological tests
  in respiratory tract infections 2677, *2677*
  see also specific infections
seronegative spondarthropathies **2965–74**
  adult Still's disease **2973–4**
  ankylosing spondylitis **2965–8**
  Behçet's syndrome, *see* Behçet's
    syndrome
  in bronchiectasis 2760–1
  cardiac manifestations 2392, *2393*
  characteristic features *2973*
  chlamydial 753
  enteropathic synovitis **2972–3**
  historical aspects 2965
  HLA-B27 frequency *2966*
  psoriatic arthritis **2968–70**, 3748
  reactive arthritis **2970–2**
  rheumatoid arthritis *vs* 2963
  undifferentiated **2973**
  Whipple's disease **2973**
  see also specific diseases (as above)
serotonin (5-hydroxytryptamine)
  in Alzheimer's disease 3972
  biosynthetic pathways 1897, 1898
  in carcinoid syndrome 1896, 1897, 1898
  coronary tone regulation 2323
  inhibitors, in migraine 4025
  insulin secretion and 1459
  in pain perception 3937, 3938
  platelet release 3615
  receptor(s), in depressive disorders 4219
  receptor agonists 4253
    in headache 4024
  receptor antagonists, in carcinoid
    syndrome 1898
  reduction,
    in depressive disorders 4219
    in Parkinson's disease 4000
  reuptake inhibitors, *see* selective 5-HT
    uptake inhibitors (SSRIs)
  tricyclic antidepressants effects 1250
  uptake inhibition by tricyclic
    antidepressants 4247
serotonin neurotoxicity syndrome 4250
serpin superfamily 1545, 3622
Serratia, rare species 561
serratus anterior, nerve to **4093**
Sertoli cells 1679, 1680
serum amyloid A (SAA) protein
    1518–19, 1528, 1533, 2835
  histochemistry 1522
  in infections 294
serum amyloid P (SAP) component
    1521, 2835, 3624
  radiolabelled **1522–4**
serum glutamate-oxaloacetic
    transaminase (SGOT), *see* aspartate
    aminotransferase (AST)
serum hepatitis, *see* hepatitis B
serum sickness 164
  arthritis in 3005–6
  snake antivenom 1138
serum trypsin-like immunoreactivity
    2037
sesqui mustard 1115
set-point theory, energy balance 1307
Seven Countries Study 2307, 2308,
    2310, 2311, 2313
Seventh Day Adventists 2311
severe combined immunodeficiency
    disease (SCID) **172–3**
  gastrointestinal disease in *1840*
  hypereosinophilia with 173
  X-linked 172

Sevredol 253
sex chromosomes 102, 104
  abnormalities *120*, 121, *121*
  aneuploidies, neurological aspects **4109**
  see also X-chromosome; Y-
    chromosome
sex differences, *see* gender differences
sex hormone binding globulin (SHBG)
    1674, 1679
  drug actions 1718
  in polycystic ovary syndrome 1675
sex steroids 1563
  adrenal 1639, *1640*
  bone mass control 3057
  calcium metabolism and 1626
  control of gonadotrophin secretion 1579
  pancreatic cancer biology 2040
  at puberty 1701
  replacement therapy 1587–8
  see also androgen(s); oestrogen(s);
    progesterone; *other specific steroids*
sex therapy 4246
sexual abuse
  child, examination 4313
  conditions mistaken for 3768
  examination for **4313–14**
  gonococcal vulvovaginitis 547
sexual activity
  cervical carcinoma risk and 210
  in cirrhosis 2091
  dangers to travellers 322
  drug abusers 4280
  epilepsy and 3924
  human papillomavirus and cervical
    cancer 444, 445
  see also sexual behaviour; sexual
    intercourse
sexual arousal, control and problems
    4244
sexual assault, psychiatric emergencies in
    victims 4257
sexual attraction, skin role 3707
sexual behaviour **3349–51**, 3350, 3351
  control of sexually transmitted diseases
    3348
  media influences 36
  patterns 3349
  see also sexual activity
sexual differentiation 1563, **1689–95**
  disorders 1689, 1690–5
  normal 1689–90, 1701
  see also intersex disorders
sexual dimorphism 104
sexual dysfunction, *see* sexual problems
sexual health, risk-reduction strategies
    3351
sexual history, homosexuals 3360, 3361
sexual intercourse
  age at **3349–50**
  age of consent 3350
  anal 3350–1, 3351, 3361, 3365
  angina management 2326
  frequency 3350
  heterosexual partners **3350**
  heterosexual practices **3350–1**
  orogenital 3350, 3352
  patterns/partnerships 3350
  in pregnancy 1786
  problems causing infertility 1685
  urinary-tract infections and 3206
  vaginal 3350
  see also sexual activity
sexual lifestyle 3350, 3351
  see also sexual behaviour
sexually acquired reactive arthritis
    (SARA) 753
  chlamydia in 753, 771
  ureaplasma and mycoplasma in 771
sexually transmitted diseases (STD)
    3345–72, 3767
  cervical cancer and **3369–72**
  see also cervical carcinoma
  chlamydial, *see* chlamydial infections
  control **3345–9**, **3348–9**, *3348*
    primary/secondary prevention 3348
  donovanosis 776
  enterobiasis 941
  epidemiology **3345–9**
    annual total prevalence *3345*

in developing countries **3348**
  specific diseases **3345–7**
  see also individual diseases
homosexuals, *see* homosexuals
intestinal 2005, *3362*
meningococcal infections 536
organisms involved *3345*
pelvic inflammatory, *see* pelvic
  inflammatory disease
in pregnancy 1789–92
risk-reduction strategies 3351
screening for 1790, 1791, 3348
streptococci group B infections and 507
travellers 1173 tropical 3348
vaginal discharge in, *see* vaginal
  discharge
vaginitis and vaginosis **3354–6**
  bacterial vaginosis **3355**
  see also candidiasis; trichomoniasis
see also genital herpes; genital warts;
  gonorrhoea; HIV infection; syphilis;
  other specific infections
sexual offences, examination for
    4313–14
'sexual offences kit' 4313
sexual orientation 3349
sexual problems 1687, **4243–7**
  assessment 4246
  detection 4243, 4246
  infertility and 1685
  medical conditions causing **4243–5**
    cardiovascular disorders 4244
    chronic renal failure 3302
    demyelinating disorders 3995
    endocrine disorders 4243–4
    epilepsy 4238, 4244
    hyperprolactinaemia 1589
    miscellaneous 4244–5
    neurological disorders 4244
    spinal cord injury 3901
  medication effects **4245**
  physical illness association **4243–7**
  prevention 4247
  psychological reaction to physical
    illness **4245–6**
    of individual and partner 4245
    medical staff's attitudes 4246
  treatment 4246–7
    counselling 4246, 4247
    explanation and advice 4246
    hormone replacement 4246
    referral and sex therapy 4246
Sezary cells 3424
Sézary syndrome 3424, 3581, 3794, 3795
SH2 domain 224, 225
Shaver's disease 2847
shear rate 2303
shear stress 2302
Sheehan's syndrome 1598, 1616, 1654,
    1747, **1748**
shellfish
  allergy to 162, 3729
  paragonimiasis transmission 988, 989
  poisoning, paralytic 1142
  see also seafood poisoning
Shewanella, rare species *561*
Shiga toxin 554
Shigella
  antibiotic resistance 554
  characteristics and background 553
  vaccines 555
Shigella boydii 553, 2003
Shigella dysenteriae 553, 2003
  haemolytic uraemic syndrome 3196
  infectious doses 268
Shigella flexneri 553, 2003
Shigella infections **553–5**, 2003
  clinical features 554, 2003
  in HIV infections and AIDS 487
  in homosexuals 3363
  treatment, antimicrobials 554
  see also dysentery, bacillary
Shigella sonnei 553, 2003
shigellosis, *see Shigella* infections
shin-bone fever (trench fever) **747–8**
shingles, *see* herpes zoster
shipwrecks
  immersion hypothermia prevention 1183
  oil aspiration 2837

shivering 1182, 1185
shock 292–3, 2563
  acute renal failure in 3281
  in anaphylaxis 160
  bicarbonate therapy 1543, 1544
  cardiogenic 2321
  causes 292
    excessive complement activation 179,
      182
  in dengue haemorrhagic fever 420
  endotoxic, *see* endotoxic shock
  haemodynamic variables 292, *292*
  haemolytic uraemic syndrome *vs*
    3200–1
  iron overdose 1071
  lactic acidosis in 1541–2
  liver in 2138
  in malaria 846, 856
  mediators in 292, 293
  in myocardial infarction 2335, 2338,
    2345
  pathogenesis 292–3, *292*
    evidence 292–3
  in peritonitis 2008
  septic, *see* septic shock
  septicaemia with 1020, 1025
  in snake envenoming 1138
  spinal 3896
  typical grief phase 1 4234–5
'shock lung', *see* adult respiratory
  distress syndrome
shoe dermatitis 3737
'short of breath' 2645, 2646
  see also breathlessness
short gut syndrome **1925–6**
  causes 1925
  parenteral nutrition 1324
short saphenous vein, coronary artery
  bypass grafting 2353
short stature **1696–700**, 3061
  in achondroplasia 3088
  bone dysplasias without **3089**
  causes 3061, *3061*
  chondrodysplasia classification *3088*
  classification 1696, *1697*
  definition 1696
  disproportionate 3061, *3061*
  in endocrine disease 1698–9
  environmental 1697–8
  familial 1696–7
  proportionate 3061, *3061*
shoulder
  disorders **2995**
  frozen 2995
  pain, in rheumatoid arthritis 2958
  painful 2995
  painful stiff shoulder syndrome 2995
  in rheumatoid arthritis 2957–8
shoulder-hand syndrome
  in myocardial infarction 2346
  see also algodystrophy
'shrinking lung syndrome' 2798
shunt nephritis 532, **3175**
shunts, circulatory
  aortopulmonary **2430–1**
  extra-/intrapulmonary, assessment 2670
  hypoxaemia due to 2631
  porta-systemic, *see* porta-systemic shunt
    surgery
  see also congenital heart disease; heart
    disease; *other specific shunts*; *under*
    pulmonary arteries
Shy-Drager syndrome 2724, 3882, 4006,
    4343–4
  gut peptides in 1896
SIAD; SIADH, *see* antidiuresis,
  syndrome of inappropriate
sialadenitis **1861–2**
  allergic 1861
sialic acid storage disease, *see* Salla
  disease
sialidase deficiencies 1434–5
sialidosis (mucolipidosis I) 1434,
    1435–6, **3988**
sialoadhesin 86, 87, **89–90**
sialophorin, deficiency, in Wiskott-
  Aldrich disease 173
sialoproteins, in bone 3057
sib-pair analysis 64

sicca symptoms 3036
sicca syndrome 4179
  see also Sjögren's syndrome
Sicilian virus 428
sick building syndrome 1231–2
sick cell syndrome 2234
sick eugonadal syndrome 1718
sick euthyroid syndrome 1609, 1717
sickle-cell(s) *3378*
sickle-cell disease (anaemia) 3513
  aircraft travel and 1203
  amino-acid substitutions in 109
  ß-globin gene mutations 104
  clinical features 3514
  complications 3514–16
  course and prognosis 3516
  crises 3514–15
  at high altitudes 1193
  joint involvement 3005
  laboratory diagnosis 3516
  liver in 2132
  malaria and 115, 840
  management 3516–17
  ocular features 4195
  parvovirus-induced aplastic crisis 448
  pneumococcal infections 513
    chemoprophylaxis 521–2
  pregnancy in 1760–1
  pulmonary hypertension in 2509
  renal disease **3194–5**, 3243, 3515
  screening *133*
  zinc deficiency *1418*
sickle-cell thalassaemia *3463*, 3464,
    3506
sickle-cell trait 3513, 3514, 3516
  allele segregation 104
  marathon runners 4328
  pregnancy in 1760
sickling disorders **3513–17**
  distribution *3463*, 3464–5, 3514
  ocular features **4195**
  pathogenesis 3513–14
  pregnancy in **1760–1**
sickling tests 3516
'sick sinus syndrome' 2266
sideroblast(s) 3521
  marrow *3474*
  ringed 3521, 3522
    in myelodysplastic syndromes 3426,
      3427
    in systemic diseases 3523
sideroblastic anaemia **3521–3**
  acquired 3522–3
  acquired primary 3426, 3427, 3521,
    3522–3
  aetiology/pathogenesis 1396, 3521–2
  definition 3521
  diagnosis *3522*, 3523
  ethanol-induced 1396, 3523, 3685
  folate deficiency 3493
  genetic 3521, **3522**, 3523
  in malignant disease 3677–8
  secondary 3523
  treatment 3498, 3523
siderosis 2847
sievert 1218
sigmoid colon
  electromyography 1957
  ulcerative colitis 1945
sigmoidoscopy in constipation 1967
  in Crohn's disease 1939, 1941
  in familial adenomatous polyposis 1990
  flexible, in colorectal cancer 1992
  in ulcerative colitis 1946
signal recognition particles (SRP) 69
signal sequence, of proteins 68
  removal 69
signal sequence receptor (SSR) 69
signal transduction 223
  cytoplasmic oncogenes in 224–5
  inhibitors, new drug targets 259
  non-tyrosine kinase receptors in 225
  tyrosine kinase pathway 224–5
silage 2815, *2815*, 2847
  nitrogen dioxide formation 1100
silastic sheets 1974, 1975
silica
  podoconiosis 1215
  pulmonary alveolar proteinosis 2833

silicate pneumoconioses **2845–6**
silicolipoproteinosis 2833
silicon dioxide, crystalline 2841
silicoproteinosis 2833
silicosis **2841–3**
  acute/accelerated types 2842
  lung cancer and 2842
  mycobacterial diseases in 2842
Sillence classification 3079, *3080*
silo filler's disease 2815, *2815*, 2847
silver nitrate (AgNO₃) eye drops 1790
simian agent 8 (SA8) 357
simian herpesviruses, human infections
  357–9
simian immunodeficiency virus (SIV)
  463
Simian sarcoma virus 223
simian virus 40 (SV40) 79, 4073
Simulium 912, 1011
simvastatin, myocardial infarction
  prevention 2348
Sindbis virus **408**
Sinemet^R 4002, 4003
single breath tests 2669
single photon densitometry, bone 3066
single photon emission computed
  tomography (SPECT) 2211–12
  in Alzheimer's disease 3974
  epileptic seizures 3920
  heart 2228
  intracranial 3825
  neurological disorders 3815
sinoatrial block 2266, 2267
  digitalis causing 2243
sinoatrial node 2152, 2259
  abnormality, in bradycardia 2266
  in cardiac cycle 2152–3, 2259
  digitalis action 2241
  disease **2266**, 2267
    ß-blockade contraindication 2328
    electrocardiogram (ECG) 2198
    pacing 2286, 2289
    re-entry 2273
sinus arrest 2266, 2267
  electrocardiogram (ECG) 2198
sinus bradycardia 2266, 2267
  in digoxin overdose 1066
  electrocardiogram (ECG) 2199
sinuses
  barotrauma 1202, 1203
  facial, aircraft pressure change effect
    1199
  granulomatous space-occupying lesions
    3012
  nasal, cancer 205
sinusitis 2691
  frontal, intracerebral abscess with 4081
  Haemophilus influenzae 583
  nickel exposure 1112
  septicaemia in 1021
sinus rhythm 2184–5, 2198, 2259
  digitalis use in 2244
  restoration 2262, 2272–3
sinus tachycardia *2272*
  in Eisenmenger reaction (syndrome)
    2410
  in mitral regurgitation 2458
  in pericardial tamponade 2477
  in ruptured chordae tendineae 2458
  in tricyclic antidepressant poisoning
    1059
sinus thrombosis 4043
  dural 4041–2
  sagittal 4042–3
sinus of Valsalva, *see* aortic sinus
Sipple's syndrome (MEN 2A) 1709
SIS cytokines 151, 157
v-*sis* gene 223
sitosterolaemia (sitosterol storage disease
  (phytosterolaemia)) 1406, **1437**
  beta 1406
situs ambiguus 2428
Sjögren-Larsson syndrome 3985
Sjögren's syndrome *3009*, **3036–8**
  aetiology and pathology 3036
  autoantibodies in 3037
  clinical features 2945, 3036
  complications 3038

diagnostic criteria 3037–8, *3038*
diagnostic tests 3037
dry eye in 3036, 4179
  in HIV infection 3036, *3037*
liver in 2135
lung involvement **2799**, 3036
  diffuse parenchymal disease 2781
lymphocytic interstitial pneumonitis
  2807
lymphomas in 3036
muscular involvement 3036, 4156
neurological complications 3036, **4132**
  neuropathy in 4102
osteoarthritis in 3036
renal involvement **3192**, 3340
in rheumatoid arthritis 2961, 3036
secondary 2961, 3036
systemic manifestations 3036
treatment 3038
skeletal deformity, *see* deformity
skeletal dysplasias 3079, **3087–90**
  bone dysplasias without short stature
    3089
  classification *3088*
  definition 3087–8
  spondyloepiphyseal **3089**
  see also achondroplasia
skeletal hyperostosis, diffuse idiopathic
  (Forestier's disease) 2979
skeletal scintigraphy, *see* scintigraphy
skeleton
  abnormalities,
    in cystathionine synthase deficiency
      1366
    in Fanconi anaemia 3446
    in mucopolysaccharidoses 1431, 1433,
      1434
    in thalassaemia 3504, 3505
  disorders **3055–97**
  function 3055, 3057
skin 3705
  acid and alkali exposure effects 1103
  in acromegaly 1592
  actinomycotic lesions 684
  ageing 3715–16, 3725, 3788
    telangiectasia 3785, 3786
  allergic reactions,
    to fungi 1158
    to plants 1154, 3725
  allografts 185
    site of sensitization and survival 185
  in amoebiasis 830, 833
  barrier to infection 275, 3707
  biopsy 3709, 3710
    in SLE 3021
  'bronzed' discoloration, in gas gangrene
    633
  in brucellosis 622
  cancer, *see* skin cancer (*below*)
  care, provision **3709–10**
  cleansing 3805–6
    in occupational dermatosis 1165
  colour, racial differences 3716, 3754
  congenital malformations 3718, *3718*
  in Cushing's syndrome 1643
  in diphtheria 495
  disease, *see* skin disease
  dry, in atopic eczema 3741
  dryness 3719, 3722
  examination in infectious diseases 266,
    267, 3710
  in homosexuals with STDs 3361
  failure 3705, **3707**
  fibrosis 3788
  flora 525, 531
    anaerobes 570
  functions **3707**
  in gonorrhoea 547
  in hepatocellular failure 2104
  in HIV infection 470
  Hodgkin's disease involving 3570
  in hookworm infection 931
  hyperreactivity 3778, 3807
  laxity 3788, 3789, 3790
  'lizard' 914
  in lung disease 2651
  lymphatic system 3706
  lymphoma, *see* lymphoma, cutaneous

in malignant disease **3791–7**
in malnutrition 1283–4, 3722–3
microclimate 3724
myelomatosis involving 3599
necrosis,
  temazepam injection 4283
  warfarin-induced 3666–7, 3675
phenol exposure effect 1104
photosensitivity, in porphyria 1394,
  1395, 1396
pigmentation, *see* pigmentation
pregnancy-related changes 1804
protection, in occupational dermatosis
  1165
psyche relationship 3707
puffy, in systemic sclerosis 3030
rash, *see* rash
reduced resistance to shear 3787–8
in rheumatic diseases 2945
riot control agents affecting 1119
in sarcoidosis **2821**, **2825–6**, 3799, 3802
scales/scaling 3716, 3718
scrapings 3710
sepsis, in cyanotic congenital heart
  disease 2400–1
in SLE 3019
snips 915
structure **3705–6**
tests, food allergy 1844
therapy in sulphur mustard (mustard
  gas) exposure 1116
thickening, in scleroderma 3027, 3029
thickness reduced, in collagen diseases
  3787
tuberculosis (lupus vulgaris) 654, 3794,
  3800, *3801*
in ulcerative colitis 1947, 3723
venous bleeding 3710
wear and tear 3709
in Wilson's disease 1420
skin associated lymphoid tissue (SALT)
  3707
skin cancer **3791–7**
  age relationship 197
  carcinogenic agents 461, 1167
  factors favouring 3791–2
  genetic syndromes 3792, *3795*
  lymphoma, *see* lymphoma, cutaneous
  melanoma, *see* melanoma, malignant
  non-melanoma,
    epidemiology 208–9
    see also basal cell carcinoma;
      squamous cell carcinoma
  radiation causing 1220
  in renal transplant recipients 3321
  risk with PUVA therapy 3748
  signs of 3792–3
  squamous-cell carcinoma, in renal
    transplant recipients 3321
  sun exposure and 3725
  see also melanoma, malignant
skin disease **3705–811**
  abnormal vascularity **3784–7**
  acute 3804
  anxiety in 3707, 3804
  autoimmune, in pregnancy 1806
  in Behçet's syndrome 3045
  beliefs/attitudes 3707
  chronic 3804
  in collagen/elastic tissue disorders
    3787–90
    defective collagen 3788
    signs 3787–8
  congenital 3718
    nervous system disorders with 3718,
      3720
  contagious nature 3716–18, *3716*, *3717*
  degenerative 3716, 3725
  drug eruptions, *see* drug eruptions
  exacerbation by sun/light 3727
  examination 3710
  factors affecting **3715–33**
    age/sex and race 3715–16
    climate 3723–7
    food and drugs 3729–33
    gastrointestinal disease 3723
    malnutrition 1283–4, 3722–3
  fear of rejection 3709, 3709–10, 3804

food eruptions 3729
'functional specificities' (activities)
  affected 3708, 3804
of genitalia **3767–70**
haematological changes **3685–6**
handicap 3705, **3707–8**, 3709, 3754,
  3804
in Henoch-Schönlein purpura 3150
hereditary **3718–22**, *3719*
  autosomal dominant/recessive 3718,
    3719
interview and questions 3710
investigations 3727–8
  clinical 3710
joint involvement **3003**
life-threatening 3708
lung in 2651
malignancy **3791–7**
  factors favouring 3791–2
malignant, *see* skin cancer
management **3804–11**
  fingertip unit 3805
  general principles 3804–5
  leg ulceration 3807–10
  topical treatment 3805
occupational, *see* dermatosis,
  occupational
physical signs 3705, 3709
in polyarteritis nodosa 3015
in pregnancy **1804–6**
  coincidental 1805–6
  pregnancy-specific 1804–5
  in response to pregnancy 1805
prevalence 3709
scaly **3750–1**
  see also psoriasis
thermoregulation failure 3708, 3717
vulnerability/susceptibility 3713–15, 3807
see also dermatosis; *individual*
  disorders/diseases
skinfold thickness
  measurement 1303–4, *1305*, 1306
  percentile curves 1306, 1315
skin infections 3716
  anaerobic 573
  in diabetes 1490, 1493
  herpes simplex virus infections 345–6
  post-streptococcal glomerulonephritis
    3173
  in pregnancy 1804
  in renal transplant recipients 3320
  Staphylococcus aureus 526
  streptococci group A 499–500, 501,
    503
skin lesions
  in amyloidosis 1515, 1518
  in anthrax 615–16
  in bartonellosis 775
  in chronic renal failure 3302
  diabetic 1489–90
  in graft-versus-host disease 3697, 3699
  in haematological disorders 3375–6
  in haemolytic uraemic syndrome 3198
  in Langerhans-cell histiocytosis 3607,
    3608
  in leprosy 669, 670, 671
  in onchocerciasis 913, 914, 3710
  in plague 596
  in poisoning 1048
'skin popping' 4280, 4282
skin-prick tests 160, 2717
  advantages in allergic rhinitis *2717*
skin window technique 3560
skip lesions 1909, 1938
skull developmental abnormalities
  4115–16
  fracture 4044, 4046
  depressed 4047–8
  epilepsy after 3916
  management 4048
  injury 4044
  metastases, pain in 240
  in osteogenesis imperfecta 3080
  radiography,
    in benign intracranial hypertension
      4042–3
    in head injury 4046, *4047*
    in intracranial tumours 4037

slapped-cheek appearance 447
SLE, *see* systemic lupus erythematosus
sleep
  arterial oxygen saturation and 2516
  breathing disorders in **2906–18**
  breathing (normal) **2906–9**
    EEG and EMG 2906, 2907
    in cor pulmonale 2519
  daytime 2912–13
  disturbance,
    in aircraft crew and pilots 1201
    in anxiety disorder 4205
    chronic fatigue syndrome in 1037
    in depressive disorders 4218, 4248
    noise causing 1225
    in obstructive sleep apnoea 2911, 2912
  dreaming, *see* rapid eye movement
    (REM) sleep
  epileptic seizures in 3918
  fragmentation, in obstructive sleep
    apnoea 2911, 2912
  fungal poisoning causing 1155–6
  growth hormone secretion 1578, 1584
  hypoventilation induced by **2916**
    absent ventilatory drive **2916**
    overnight ventilation for **2917–18**
    in scoliosis 2872
    unstable ventilatory drive **2916**
  lung function variations 2674
  migrating myoelectric (motor) complex
    and 1954
  in narcolepsy, *see* narcolepsy
  non-rapid eye movement (NREM)
    2906, *2907*, 3928
    breathing during 2908–9
    respiration control in 3888
  paralysis **3928**
  rapid eye movement (REM), *see* rapid
    eye movement (REM) sleep
  respiratory muscles in 2908, 2909
  slow-wave 2908
  stages 2906–7, 3928
    normal patterns 2908
  ventilatory drive changes during 2905
sleep apnoea 2909
  in amyloidosis 2836
  central 2910, **2916**, **2916–18**
    apparent **2917**
    causes *2917*
    overnight ventilation for **2917–18**
  in Duchenne muscular dystrophy 4149
  narcolepsy *vs* 3929
  obstructive, *see* obstructive sleep
    apnoea
  polycythaemia due to 3553
  reflex **2917**
  REM sleep **2916–17**
  syndrome 2232–3, 2519
    heart failure pathophysiology 2232–3
  in toluene poisoning 1089
sleep attacks 3928
  differential diagnosis 3929
  'sleep disruption syndrome' 2909,
    2912
  see also obstructive sleep apnoea
'sleep drunkenness' 3929
sleepiness, excess 3928
  causes 3929
  see also hypersomnia; narcolepsy
sleeping sickness, *see* African
  trypanosomiasis
slide agglutination test, leptospirosis
  diagnosis 702
slide coagulase test 523
slide flocculation test, trichinosis 941
'slim' disease 485, 487, 4078
slit lamp 4179, 4180, 4182
slow-reacting substance of anaphylaxis
  2855, 3770
slow virus infections 3977
  see also prion diseases
slug pellets, poisoning 1124
Sm, antibodies to 2952, 3024
small-bowel enema 1832, 1909
  in coeliac disease 1919
  in Crohn's disease 1939
  in Meckel's diverticulum 1978
  non-specific/specific findings 1909–10

small-cell lung carcinoma, *see* lung
  cancer
small intensely fluorescent cells (SIF
  cells) 3882
small intestine
  absorption, in pregnancy 1770
  adaptive changes after resections 1926
  anatomical disorders, bacterial
    overgrowth aetiology *1911*, 1912
  atresia **1975–6**
  bacterial flora, *see* intestinal flora
  bacterial overgrowth, *see* bacterial
    overgrowth
  bacteriological investigations 1910
  barium studies 1832, 1909–10
  biopsy **1907–8**
    complications 1907
    diseases diagnosed by 1908
    histological interpretation 1907–8
    processing 1907
    see also duodenum, biopsy; jejunal
      biopsy
  in cholera 577
  coliforms, in tropical sprue 1934
  in common varied immunodeficiency
    (CVID) 1838–9
    infections 168–9, 1838
  congenital anomalies **1975–7**
  congenital short **1978**
  disease,
    B$_{12}$ deficiency 3491
    diarrhoea in 1824, 1825
    endoscopy indication 1829
    embryology 1973
    gangrene 1977
    infections, coeliac disease *vs* 1919
    inflammatory disorder, *see* coeliac
      disease
  lymphangiectasia **1977**
  lymphoma 1985–6
    malabsorption relation 1927, 1929
    malabsorption in tropics and 1930
    radiology 1910
    see also enteropathy-associated T-cell
      lymphoma (EATL)
  lymphomatous polyposis 3583
  malrotation **1976–7**
    embryology 1973
    management 1977
  motor activity 1955
    see also gastrointestinal motility
  nodular lymphoid hyperplasia 169
  normal length 1925
  obstruction,
    in carcinoid syndrome 1897
    differential diagnosis 2030
    in diverticular disease 1972
    in Meckel's diverticulum 1978
    in meconium ileus 1978
    see also intestinal obstruction
    perforation, in meconium ileus 1978
  radiology 1909–10
  resections, *see* short gut syndrome
  stenosis **1975–6**
  structural lesions, haematological
    disorders 3684
  in systemic sclerosis 3029, *3030*
  transit, radionuclide studies 1957
  transit time 1955
    enteroglucagon 1934
    in tropical sprue 1934
    see also gastrointestinal motility
      disorders
  transplantation 1926
  in tropical enteropathy 1931
  tumours **1985–6**
    adenocarcinoma 1986
    benign 1985
    in coeliac disease 1920
    features and treatment 1986
    malignant 1985–6
    reasons for rarity 1985
    see also small intestine, lymphoma
  volvulus 1976
  in Whipple's disease 1923
  see also specific anatomical regions
smallpox 365, 366
  arthritis in 3001

epidemics 367
  eradication 368
  susceptibility 367
  vaccine 367, 368
  see also variola virus
small round structured viruses (SRSV)
  390, **392**, 394, 2002
small round viruses (SRVs) 391, *391*,
  392, 394
smell
  loss of sense 3876
  skin disease management 3806
Smith-Lemli-Opitz syndrome 130, 4111,
  4121
smoke
  avoidance in asthma 2737
  carbon monoxide source 1230
  composition 1101
  exposure, *see* smoke inhalation
  polynuclear aromatic hydrocarbons in
    1166
  riot control agent dispersal 1119
smoked foods, gastric cancer association
  203
smoke inhalation **1101–2**, 2847
  acute airways obstruction in 2722
  ischaemic heart disease risk 2313
  plastic and combustion products 1102
  pneumococcal infections and 513
smokers
  by age 2880
  percentage in EEC *2880*
  'pre-contemplators'/'contemplators'/
    'active quitters' 4266
smoker's keratosis 1858, 1859
smoking
  in α$_1$-antitrypsin deficiency 1546
  α$_1$-antitrypsin inactivation 1545–6
  anti-GBM disease and 3165
  asbestosis interaction 219, 2844, 2845
  asthma and bronchial hyper-
    responsiveness 2733
  bladder cancer association 211, 212
  brief intervention, opportunity for
    4265–6
  cessation,
    angina management 2326
    in COAD 2775–6
    limb ischaemia management 2369
    lung cancer prevention 2892
    myocardial re-infarction prevention
      2348
    peptic ulcer treatment 1884
    withdrawal syndrome **4293**
  chronic bronchitis and 2767
  chronic obstructive airways disease and
    2632, 2767, 2768
  cigars 2313
  cor pulmonale and 2517
  cough with 2642
  Crohn's disease aetiology 1937
  cryptogenic fibrosing alveolitis and
    2786
  in diabetes *1466*, 1491
  in diffuse parenchymal lung disease
    2781
  disease risk in obesity and 1309
  effect on immune response 2813
  emphysema relation 2632
  extrinsic allergic alveolitis and 2813
  fibrinogen levels and 2303, 2304, 2309
  gastric cancer aetiology 1982
  gastric ulcer aetiology 1879
  harm reduction 4276
  history-taking 2649, **4267**
  in hospital **4286**, **4288**
    management in general wards **4286**,
      4288
  ischaemic heart disease risk 2310,
    2312–13
  intervention studies 2317–18
  kidney tumour association 212
  laryngeal cancer association 205
  latent period for cancer development
    198
  lung cancer and 206, 2879–80, *2880*
    air pollution synergism 207
    asbestos synergism 219, 2844, 2845

cigarette number 2880
  prevention 2892
  lung function variations 2674–5
  mortality rates 1302
  occupational asthma 2742
  oesophageal cancer and 202, 1981
  oral carcinoma and 201, 1860
  osteoporosis and 3070
  pancreatic cancer association 204–5,
    2040
  passive 1230–1
    cough 2642–3
    lung cancer and 1231, 2880
    respiratory virus infections 333, 1230
  peripheral arterial disease risk 2363
  pharyngeal cancer association 201
  pipe smoking, *see* pipe smoking
  polycythaemia and 3551, 3553, 3554
  protection/reduction T-cell-mediated
    diseases 2813
  ulcerative colitis aetiology 1944
  weight loss/gain and 1302
  withdrawal syndrome **4293**
  see also tobacco
smooth muscle
  antibodies, in autoimmune hepatitis
    2070
  gastrointestinal tract 1952–3
    cardiac smooth muscle *vs* 1953
smooth muscle cells
  in atherogenesis 2291, 2362
    accumulation 2291
    contractile to secretory phenotype
      change 2291
    cytokines produced 2291
    in normal arteries 2290
    proliferation,
      endothelial cells role 2299, 2362, 2514
      growth factors involved 2293
    pulmonary endothelial cell interactions
      2487
    vasodilator action 2324
    see also under endothelium
snails
  angiostrongyliasis transmission 945,
    946
  biological control 980
  dicrocoeliasis transmission 987
  fasciolopsiasis transmission 993
  opisthorchiasis transmission 981
  schistosomiasis transmission 971,
    972–3
  'snail-track' ulcers 711
snakes
  Armillifer infestation and 1012–14
  injuries due to 1125
  zoonoses transmitted from 1014
snakes, venomous **1125–40**
  bites *3546*
    acute renal failure 3293
    DIC complicating 3658
    haemolytic uraemic syndrome *vs* 3201
    incidence/importance 1127–8
    infections at site 1138–9
    interval to death 1139
    laboratory investigations 1135
    pathophysiology 1129–31
    prevention 1139
    prognosis 1139
  classification 1126–7
  clinical features of venom/bites 1131
    Atractaspididae 1131
    Colubridae (back-fanged snakes) 1131
    Elapidae 1131
    European vipers 1134–5
    Hydrophiidae 1132
    Viperidae 1132–4
  distribution 1126–8
  epidemiology 1128
  immunization against envenoming 1139
  immunodiagnosis of envenoming 1135
  management of bites 1135–9
    antivenom treatment 1136–8
    first aid 1135–6
    hospital treatment 1136
    of local envenoming 1139
    supportive treatment 1138–9
    see also antivenom

snakes, venomous (*cont.*)
ophthalmia management 1139
venom,
α₁-antitrypsin inactivation 1545, 1546
neurotoxins 1129
pharmacology 1129
properties 1129
quantities 1128–9
venom apparatus 1128–9
venom glands 1128
SNAP-25 76
SNAPs (NSF attachment factors) 75
receptors (SNAREs) 76
SNAREs (SNAP receptors) 76
Sneddon's syndrome 3020, 3724
'sneeze gas' 1117
sneezing 2610
Snellen chart 4179
snoring 2609, 2611, 2724, 2909
alcohol consumption and 2910
sleep fragmentation with 2912
'snowballs' 4182
snow blindness 3724
snowshoe hare virus **424–5**
SNRPN gene 127
social changes, after bereavement 4235
social circumstances, clinical assessment
of elderly 4336
social factors
in chronic fatigue syndrome 1038,
1039
epilepsy **3924–5**
in obesity 1307–8
obesity associated disease and 1309
in spinal cord injury 3901
social insurance systems 53
social phobia 4206
social withdrawal
in anorexia nervosa 4213, 4214
in chronic schizophrenia 4222
in depressive disorders 4218
social worker 4339
socioeconomic factors
gastric cancer association 203
ischaemic heart disease risk 2314–15,
2316
sodium **3116–26**
absorption 577, 1900, 1902
failure, in short gut syndrome 1925
impairment in tropical sprue 1933
in artificial nutritional support 1318
excess, in Western diet 1330
exchange, in heart contraction 2147
fractional excretion, in acute renal
failure *3282*
glucose cotransport 1902
heart electrophysiology 2148, 2259
class I antiarrhythmics action 2263
homeostasis 3118–20
in chronic renal failure 3297
disorders **3120–6**
in short gut syndrome 1926
hypertension pathogenesis 2530, 2531
intake, *see* salt, intake
loss, ACE inhibitor action 2249
measurement 3116
plasma,
in acute renal failure 3284
in diabetic ketoacidosis 1501
see also hypernatraemia;
hyponatraemia
reabsorption,
drugs blocking 2239
increased in heart failure 2170
inhibition, by atrial natriuretic factor
2156
stimulation, aldosterone 2157
red cell permeability defect 3532
renal excretion **3119–20**, *3330*
blood pressure and 3247–8
in chronic renal failure 3297
diuretics effect 2238
restriction,
in heart failure 2238
hypertension management 2538
retention,
in ascites 2097
in cor pulmonale 2517
in heart failure 2169–71
in mitral stenosis 2453

oedema due to 2170–1
in renal hypertension 2545
urinary, in acute renal failure *3282*
see also saline; salt
sodium benzoate 1360
sodium bicarbonate therapy, *see*
bicarbonate, therapy
sodium calcium edetate 1108, 1110,
1114
sodium chlorate, poisoning 1121
sodium chloride, *see* salt; sodium
sodium cromoglycate
in allergic rhinitis 2718
in food allergy/intolerance 1845
sodium dichloroacetate 1544
sodium diethyldithiocarbamate
(dithiocarb) 1113
sodium dodecyl sulphate (SDS)-
polyacrylamide gel electrophoresis
3528–9
sodium fluoride
effect on bone 3095
in osteoporosis management 3068
sodium fusidate 307
sodium hypochlorite, poisoning 1079,
1103
sodium lactate 1544
sodium/lithium (Na⁺/Li⁺)
countertransport, in diabetic
nephropathy 3168–9
sodium nitrite, in cyanide poisoning
treatment 1098
sodium nitroprusside **2247**, 3250
in clonidine overdose 1065
in hypertensive encephalopathy 2543
infusions, problems 2247
mechanism of action and doses 2247
metabolism 1067
in mitral regurgitation 2462
in myocardial infarction 2569
overdose/poisoning **1067**
in pregnancy 1752
in pulmonary oedema 2567, 2568
test 1367
sodium perchlorate 1614
sodium phenylacetate 1360
sodium-potassium pump (Na-K ATPase),
see under ATPase
sodium stibogluconate, in visceral
leishmaniasis 906
sodium thiosulphate, in cyanide
poisoning treatment 1098
sodium valproate
adverse reactions 3921
costs 3922
in epilepsy 3921
overdose/poisoning 1062
teratogenicity *1810*, 3922
sodoku **688–9**
soft palate, myoclonus 4015–16
soft-tissue(s)
in acromegaly 1592
calcification, *see* calcification, soft
tissue
calcium in 1622, 1623
infections,
anaerobic 573
in drug abusers 4279
Pasteurella causing 606
myelomatosis involving 3599
periarticular hypertrophy 2947
rheumatic disorders 2947, 2997
sarcomas, *see* sarcoma of soft tissues
trauma, sports-related **4321–2**
soil-borne minerals, podoconiosis 1215
sokosha **688–9**
solanine 1159
solar cheilitis *3726*
solar dermatitis 3715
solar elastosis 3725, *3726*, 3788
solar keratosis *3726*
solar urticaria 3726, 3771
soldier's heart, *see* Da Costa's syndrome
soles of feet, 'dry type' dermatophytic
infections 798
solitary rectal ulcer syndrome 1947, 2138
solumedrone, in liver graft rejection
2114
SOLVD trial 2250, 2348

solvent abuse 1044, **1092–3**, *1093*
chlorinated hydrocarbons 1092–3
definition 1092
petrol, *see* petrol (gasoline)
psychiatric disturbances from 1092,
4242
solvents used *1092*
see also glue sniffing
solvent drag 1900
solvents
nephrotoxicity 3267, *3289*
neuropsychological disorders associated
1174
occupational disorders 1174
soman 1117
treatment of exposure 1118
somatic cell(s) 102
genetic analysis 193
hybrids/hybridization 62
somatic-cell genetics 65
somatic mosaicism 107
osteogenesis imperfecta inheritance
3082
'somatic mutation' theory of cancer
191–2
somatization 1037, **4208**
acute 4208
persistent 4208
somatization disorder 3943
causes and treatment **4208**
somatomedins 1577, 1626
somatosensory evoked potentials (SEP)
3831, **3833–5**
in coma and brain death 3835
in degenerative disease 3834
in demyelinating disease 3833–4
intraoperative monitoring 3835
spinal trauma 3834
technique for recording 3833
in tumours and infarcts 3834
somatosensory seizure 3913
somatostatin 1554, 1891, 1894
in acromegaly 1593
analogue, *see* octreotide
control of growth hormone secretion
1577, 1594
immunostaining 1892
inhibitory actions 1894, *1894*
insulin secretion and 1459
large molecular forms, tumours
producing 1703
radiolabelled analogues 1704, 1705
receptors *1560*, 1894
in somatostatinoma 1707
treatment,
in bleeding oesophageal varices 2094
in insulinoma 1509
in short gut syndrome 1926
somatostatinoma 1704, **1707**
somatotrophs 1575, 1577
adenoma 1569, 1591
sorbitol 1345
hypothesis, diabetic tissue damage
1482, 1485, 1486, 3169
sore throat
in homosexuals 3361
Lemierre's disease after 575
Staphylococcus aureus infection 526
streptococcal 498–9, 501, 2432, 3776
diagnosis 502
differential diagnosis 502
post-streptococcal glomerulonephritis
after 505, 506
rheumatic fever after 503, 2432
rheumatic fever prevention 505, 2435
transmission/spread 501
treatment 502, 505
see also rheumatic fever
SOS protein 225
sotalol 2263, *2264*
in atrial fibrillation 2272
in ventricular tachycardia 2280
Sotos syndrome 1700, 4111
sound 1223
sound pressure waves 1223
South America, venomous snakes 1127
Southern blotting 60
Soviet Union, former 47
sowda 913

SOX (osteoarthritis in Sjögren's
syndrome) 3036
soya milk allergy 1919
soybean protein 2311
'space blanket' 1047
space exploration, disorders **3853**
Spanish 'toxic oil syndrome' 1233, 3612
sparganosis **969–70**, 4193
Sparganum proliferum 970
spasmodic dysphonia **4020**
spasmodic torticollis **4018**
spasms
hemifacial **3879–80**, 4016
infantile (West's syndrome) 3914, 4015
in tetanus 625, 625–6
spastic ataxic diplegia **4121**
spastic colon 1844, 1965
spastic diplegia **4120**
spastic hemiplegia **4120**
spasticity 3857
in multiple sclerosis 3993, 3996
in spinal cord injury 3901
spastic paraparesis
tropical 490, 3995
visual evoked potentials in 3832
spastic paraplegia
autosomal dominant 'pure' familial
4090
hereditary **3985**, 3995
specialties, risk management and
negligence in 4312
species, definition 272
species sanitation, malaria control 838,
858
specific granules 3555
deficiency 3560
specificity 17, 18–19
exercise testing 2227
spectinomycin 708
in gonorrhoea 1790
spectrin 3527
α^LELY polymorphism 3531
deficiency 3529, *3531*
self-association defects 3529, 3531
speech
comprehension 3846, 3849
disturbances 3848
developmental disorders **4122**
disorders in schizophrenia 4221
examination 3849, *3849*
in mania/manic depressive disorder
4220
non-fluent 3848
production 3846
defects 3848
spontaneous 3848
see also aphasia; language
speech audiometry 3870
speech therapist 4339
rehabilitation, after strokes 4340
sperm
assisted reproduction techniques 1687
autoantibodies 1685, 1686
function tests 1686
spermatogenesis 1679, 1680
defective 1684, 1685
induction 1686
SPf66 malaria vaccine 862, 863
sphenoid sinus 1574
metastases 240
spherocytosis *3378*, 3530
hereditary **3529–30**, *3531*
sphincterotomy, endoscopic, *see*
endoscopic sphincterotomy
sphincters 1952
Sphingobacterium 561
sphingolipidoses **1426–30**
sphingolipids 1400, 1427
Sphingomonas paucimobilis 561
sphingomyelin lipidosis, *see* Niemann-
Pick disease
spider bites **1147–9**
spider naevi 2082, 2104
in cirrhosis 2087
in pregnancy 1796, 1804
Spielmeyer-Vogt syndrome 3985
spina bifida **4117–19**
cystica 4117
embryogenesis and incidence 4117

management,
  in childhood/adolescence 4118
  of neonates 4117–18
occulta (spinal dysraphism) 3825, **4119**
prenatal diagnosis 4117
spinal accessory nerve **3880**
spinal angiography **3828**
spinal arachnoid cysts **4117**
spinal arachnoiditis **3894**, 4061
spinal arteriovenous fistulae 3828
spinal arteriovenous malformations 3828,
  3895
spinal canal 2992
spinal cord **3891–5**
  anatomy 3891–2
  anterior horns 3856
  arteriovenous malformation involving
    3895
  blood supply 3891
  cervical,
    compression 2959, 3908
    lesions 3892
    spondylotic changes 3908
  'claudication' 2992
    pain in 2947
  compression 3892
    cervical 2959, 3908
    investigations 3892, 3893
    in osteomalacia 3072
    in Paget's disease 3075–6
    palliative radiotherapy 257–8
    progressive paraparesis 3892–3
    in rheumatoid arthritis 2959
    surgical decompression 249
    in tumours 241, 249–50, 257–8
  damage,
    central motor conduction time 3838
    in cervical spondylotic myelopathy
      3908
    electrical injury 1214
    myositis ossificans after 3093
    psychological sequelae 4244
    sexual problems in 4244
    see also spinal cord, traumatic injury
  demyelination in multiple sclerosis
    3993
  embolism 3894
  endogenous opiates action 3938
  haemorrhage 3894
  hemisection, see Brown-Séquard
    syndrome
  infarction 3894
  inflammatory changes 3991
  interruption 2992
  irradiation damage **3894**
  lesions,
    central respiratory failure in 3888
    consequences 3892
    determining level 3892
    hypogonadism in 1683
    non-traumatic paraplegia **3892–5**
    pain in 3942
    pregnancy in 1769
    transverse and myelitis 3894
    traumatic **3895–901**
    see also paraplegia
  motor pathways 3856–7, 3891
  in paragonimiasis 991
  paralysis, non-traumatic causes **3901–2**
  pharmacology 3937–8
  sensory pathways 3857–8, 3891
  subacute combined degeneration **3893**
  subarachnoid haemorrhage 3895
  transection 3892
  traumatic injury **3895–901**
    bowel/joints/limb care 3900
    cardiovascular complications 3898–9
    incomplete, patterns 3897–8
    initial assessment 3896, *3897*
    initial management 3896
    management 3897
    pain and sexual function 3901
    pharmacological advances 3898
    pressure areas 3900–1
    prevalence and survival time 3895–6
    psychological/social factors 3901
    respiratory complications 3898
    signs/indications 3896
    spasticity and syringomyelia 3901

transfer to hospital 3896
urinary tract management 3899–900
tumours **3894–5**
  metastatic 3895
  vascular disease **3894**
spinal dura 3902
spinal dysraphism (spina bifida occulta)
  3825, **4119**
spinal fusion 2873
  defects 4117
  in myositis ossificans progressiva 3093,
    3094
spinal immobilizer 3896
spinal muscular atrophies 3988, 4089
  acute infantile (Werdnig-Hoffmann
    disease) 3988
  creatine kinase in 4142
  floppy infant syndrome in 4150
  hereditary **3988**
  hereditary proximal 3988
  juvenile proximal (Kugelberg-Welander
    disease) 3988, 4089
spinal myoclonus 4015
spinal nerve roots **3902–9**
  anatomy 3902, *3903*, 3904, 3905
  cauda equina lesions **3907–8**
  compression,
    in disc protrusions 3906
    in tumours 241, 3903
  fibres 3857
  lesions,
    causes **3903**
    in degenerative disease, *see under*
      spine
    effects of 3902
    in pregnancy 1766–7
    pain 2322, 3902
    night 3907
    posterior, lesions 3857
    in tendon reflexes *3903*
spinal opiates 3938
spinal pain
  inflammatory 2947
  nerve root lesions 2322, 3902, 3907
  non-inflammatory 2947
  radiography 2949
  see also back pain
spinal reflex arc 3882, 3891
spinal roots
  in brachial plexus traction lesions 4093
  pressure 2992
spinal shock 3896
spinal spondylosis 3905, 3908
spinal stenosis 2992
spine
  in ankylosing spondylitis 2966, 2967
  bamboo 2875
  biopsy, CT- and fluoroscopy-guided
    3828
  cervical, *see* cervical spine
  collapse, interventional procedures 3828
  cysticercosis 965
  deformity 3061, 4118
  degenerative disease **3903–7**
    MRI 3828
    pain in 2947
    pathogenesis 3903–4
    root lesions 3903
    see also intervertebral disc
  developmental abnormalities **4116–19**
  disorders,
    computed tomography **3827–8**
    computer-assisted myelography
      3827–8
    extramedullary intradural, MRI 3828
    intramedullary, MRI 3828
    magnetic resonance imaging 3826,
      3827, **3828**
    myelography **3826–7**
    radiology **3826–8**
    thorax **2872–5**
    see also kyphosis; scoliosis
  dorsal, pain in **2994–5**
  flexibility test 2947
  flexion, measures 2993
  function and behaviour 2992
  hyperextension 3897
  infection 2993
  lumbar, *see* lumbar spine

metastases 240–1, 249
movement limitation, in ankylosing
  spondylitis 2966
  in multiple sclerosis 3994, 3995
  in poliomyelitis 385
  in rheumatic diseases 2946, 2947
  in rheumatoid arthritis 2959
  in spina bifida 4118
  stiffness 2947
  tenderness 2947
  trauma,
    root lesions 3903
    somatosensory evoked potentials 3834
  tuberculosis (Pott's disease) 653, 654,
    2874, 2998–9, 3902
  tumours 2993
    metastatic, MRI 3828
    in pregnancy 1767
    root lesions in 3903
spinobulbar muscular atrophy, unstable
  trinucleotide repeats *125*
spinocerebellar ataxia type 1 *125*, 3984
spinocerebellar degeneration 3984
spinocerebral gnathostomiasis 952
spinothalamic tract 3857, 3891, 3938
  lesions 3858
  in multiple sclerosis 3993
  neurone types 3938
  pain and 3858, 3938–9
  section 3945
  thalamic projections 3939
spiral arteries, in pre-eclampsia 1727
spiramycin
  in cryptosporidiosis 874
  in toxoplasmosis 869
Spirillum minus **688–9**
spiritual pain **4358–9**
spirochaete infections **689–92**
  arthritis in 3002
  rectal, in homosexuals 3365
  see also leptospirosis; Lyme disease;
    specific Borrelia species
Spirometra mansoni 969
spirometry 2667
  breathlessness 2647
  in chronic obstructive airways disease
    2767, 2774–5
spironolactone 3337
  adverse effects 1688–9, 1718, 2097,
    2239
  in ascites 2097
  in Conn's syndrome 1660
  mechanism of action 2239
  in pregnancy 1751
spirurida 954
splanchnic circulation, arterial wall
  damage 1995
spleen **3587–96**
  abscess 3592
    in relapsing fevers 694
    staphylococcal endocarditis with 528
  aspiration, visceral leishmaniasis
    diagnosis 905
  atrophy 3587
    in primary thrombocythaemia 3439
  big spleen disease, *see* tropical
    splenomegaly syndrome
  blood flow 3589
  blood pool 3589
  cysts 3592
  dysfunction, pneumococcal infections in
    514
  embryology 87
  enlargement, *see* splenomegaly
  functions 1028, 3588–9
    in infections 277
  haemopoiesis 3385–7, 3588
  hypoplasia 3592
  infarction 3592
    in primary myelosclerosis 3437
    in relapsing fevers 694
    in sickle-cell disease 3514
  injury/rupture 3591, 3595
    in primary myelosclerosis 3437
  investigation of function 3592–5
  in Langerhans-cell histiocytosis 3607
  in malaria 845, 847, 856
  in Marburg virus and Ebola virus
    disease 442

metastatic tumours 3592
  in portal hypertension 2093
  radiology **1835**
  resistance to babesiosis 864
  rupture, in malaria 847, 856
  in sarcoidosis 2825
  structure 3587–8
  in visceral leishmaniasis 905
splenectomy 3587, **3595–6**
  in autoimmune haemolytic anaemia
    3544
  in autoimmune thrombocytopenia 3632
  in chronic lymphocytic leukaemia 3422
  clinical/haematological effects 3595–6
  diagnostic 3595
  in Felty syndrome 2962
  in hereditary elliptocytosis 3532
  in hereditary spherocytosis 3530
  immunodeficiency type after 1028
  indications 3595
  infections after 277, 1027–8
    acute neurological syndromes in 1033,
      1034
    clinical features 1028
    organisms causing 1028, *1028*
    risk 1028
  in non-Hodgkin's lymphoma 3584
  overwhelming infections after (OPSI)
    3530, **3595–6**
  partial 3530
  pneumococcal vaccines after 319, 1028
  in pregnancy 1764
  in primary myelosclerosis 3437
  prophylactic antibiotics after 1028
  in pyruvate kinase deficiency 3535
  in sickle-cell disease 3517
  in SLE 3023 in thalassaemia 3512
  in unstable haemoglobin disorders 3518
  see also asplenia
splenic artery, therapeutic embolization
  3596
splenic flexure, blood supply 1997
splenic lymphoma with villous
  lymphocytes 857
splenic vein thrombosis, in chronic
  pancreatitis 2038
splenomegaly 3589, **3590–2**
  causes 3590
  in chronic myeloid leukaemia 3416
  in cirrhosis 2088
  clinical detection 3590
  in common varied immunodeficiency
    (CVID) 169
  in G6PD deficiency 3540
  hyper-reactive malarial, *see* tropical
    splenomegaly syndrome
  in infectious mononucleosis 353
  in infective endocarditis 2441
  in lymphoma 3589, 3591
  in malnutrition 1283
  non-tropical idiopathic 3591
  plasma volume in 3589
  in polycythaemia vera 3432, 3589
  in primary myelosclerosis 3435, 3437
  in primary thrombocythaemia 3439
  reducing size of spleen 3596
  in thalassaemia 3504
  thrombocytopenia in 3633
  tropical syndrome, *see* tropical
    splenomegaly syndrome
  see also hypersplenism
splenorenal shunt 2095
splenosis 3596
splints
  in osteoarthritis 2982
  in rheumatoid arthritis 2963
spondarthropathies, *see* seronegative
  spondarthropathies
spondylitis, in brucellosis 620, 621
spondyloepiphyseal dysplasias **3089**
  congenita 3089
  tarda 3089
spondylolisthesis 3907
spondylosis 2992
spongiform encephalopathies
  cerebral amyloid with 1517
  see also bovine spongiform
    encephalopathy (BSE); prion diseases
spongiosis 3710, 3734

spontaneously hypertensive rat 2530, 2532
Sporothrix schenckii 802, 806, 3000
sporotrichosis **802–3**
  arthritis in 3000
  systemic 806
'sports anaemia' 4326
sports injuries **4321–4**
  ankle 2996
  common sites in joggers/runners 4323
  direct soft-tissue trauma **4321–2**
  overuse **4322–4**
  trauma and viral infections **4324**
sports medicine **4321–9**
  sudden death in, *see* sudden cardiac death
  see also endurance sports; exercise
spotted fevers *729*, 730–3, **734–6**
  see also Boutonneuse fever; rickettsial diseases; Rocky Mountain spotted fever
spotter practices 287
sprue
  folate deficiency 3467
  hypogammaglobulinaemic 1839
  tropical, *see* tropical sprue
sputum 2642, **2643**
  actinomycoses diagnosis 684
  in acute exacerbation of chronic bronchitis 2692
  anaerobic bacteria detection 571
  anchovy sauce 830, 2643
  in bronchiectasis 2757, 2759–60, 2764
  brownish-red, in paragonimiasis 990, 991
  in chronic bronchiolitis 2634
  coliforms in 551
  collection 641, 2685
  in community-acquired pneumonia 2695, 2697
  culture 2697
    in bronchiectasis 2759–60
    lung abscess 2705
    in cystic fibrosis 2748
  cytology, in lung cancer 2887
  in diffuse parenchymal lung disease 2781
  examination 2644, **2685**
    in chronic obstructive airways disease 2774
    in immunosuppressed 2711
  expectoration, in lung cancer 2883
  Gram staining 2697
  induced, investigation in pneumonia 2697
  infected *vs* non-infected 2643
  intermittent production 2755
  microbiological testing 2675
    stained 2676
    unstained 2675, *2676*
  microscopy 641, 662
  mucopurulent 2643, 2748, 2764
  purulent, in bronchiectasis 2757
  tuberculosis diagnosis 641, 650, 662
  viscosity 2644, 2748
    reduction, in cystic fibrosis 2753
squamous cell carcinoma
  epidemiology 209
  lung cancer 2881, 2887
  oesophageal 1980–1
  skin 3791
squamous cells, gas exchange barrier 2593
squamous epithelioma *3726*
  lip 3708, 3725
squamous intraepithelial lesions (SIL), cervical 3371
'square-root sign' 2390, 2393, 2479
'squashed stomach syndrome' 4355
'squat jump syndrome' 4326
squint, in Marfan's syndrome 4181
squirrels, typhus transmission 737
SRY mutations *1567*, 1571
SSA, *see* Ro (SSA), antibodies
SSB, *see* La, antibodies
staff, *see* health care staff
'stagnant anoxaemia' 845
staircase phenomenon (Bowditch effect) 2150, 2157, 2158

stammering 3846
stance, in vestibular apparatus damage 3873
stannosis 2847
stanozolol 1248
stapedius reflex 3870
staphylococci **523–33**
  coagulase-negative 523–4, **531–3**
    antibiotic susceptibility 531
    carriage/transmission 531
    cerebrospinal fluid shunts 532
    community 531, 532
    endocarditis 532, 2437, 2444
    host factors in infections 531
    infections **531–2**
    intravascular devices 531, 532
    laboratory diagnosis 533
    pathogenicity 531
    peritonitis 532
    species 531
    treatment 533, 1031, 2448
    urinary tract infection 532
    see also Staphylococcus epidermidis; *Staphylococcus saprophyticus*
  coagulase-positive 523, **525–31**
    see also Staphylococcus aureus
  detection 523, 533
  diagnostic kits 523
  endocarditis 2437, 2448
  infections **525–33**
    see also Staphylococcus aureus
  pneumonia, *see under* pneumonia
  typing (phage) *494*, 524
Staphylococcus, taxonomy 523–4, *524*
Staphylococcus aureus 523, **524–31**
  antibiotic/antiseptic sensitivity 525–6
  antibiotic resistance 525–6
    antibiotic types 525
    prevalence *310*
  arthritis due to 2998
  bacteraemia and septicaemia 527
  bone and joint infections 528–9
  carriage/transmission 525
  clinical features of infections 526–30
  culture 530
  endocarditis 527, 528, 1020, 2437, 2438, 2440
    in drug addicts 2445
  enterotoxins 529
  ENT infections 526
  food poisoning 524, 529
  in HIV infections and AIDS 487
  host factors in infections 525
  infections mediated by toxins 529–30
  interstitial nephritis 3178
  intracranial abscess 4081
  laboratory diagnosis of infections 530
  ß-lactamase 525
  localized infections 526
  metastatic (haematogenous) infections 528–9
  methicillin-resistance (MRSA) 299, 329, 525
    endocarditis 2445, 2448
    treatment 531, 2448
  pathogenicity 524
  perinephric abscess 529
  peritoneal dialysis-associated peritonitis 3311
  phage typing 524, *524*
  pleuropulmonary infection 526, 527
  pneumonia due to 2694, 2699, 2700
  pyomyositis 529, 4174
  renal abscess/carbuncle 3207
  renal cortical abscess 529
  scabies infections with 1008
  scalded skin syndrome 529
  skin infection 526, 4279
    in drug abusers 4279
  toxic shock syndrome 530
  toxins/products 524
    enterotoxins 524, *525*
    epidermolytic 524
    toxic shock syndrome (TSST-1) 524, 530
  treatment of infections 530–1, 2446, *2447*, 2448

urinary tract infection 526
  wound infection 526
Staphylococcus epidermidis 265, 523
  endocarditis 2438, 2444
  pathogenicity 531
  shunt nephritis 3175
Staphylococcus haemolyticus 531
Staphylococcus lugdunensis 524, 2437
Staphylococcus saprophyticus 524
  urinary-tract infections 3206, 3208, 3209
stapling gun 1993
starch
  intolerance 1922
  raw corn 1342
  'resistant' 219
starch powder, peritonitis due to 2008
starfish 1144
Starling equation 2495, 2854
  pleural fluid formation 2863
Starling forces 2560
Starling hypothesis/mechanism 2489, 2490, 2495
Starling resistor 2489
Starling's law 2171
Starr-Edwards prosthesis 2380, 2469
STARS study 2316
starvation
  amenorrhoea in 1671–2
  biochemical effects **1277–8**
  ketone body utilization 1276–7
  metabolism in 1400, 1505
  in pregnancy 1772–3
  severe injury *vs* 1548
  see also anorexia nervosa; famine; fasting
statin drugs 1414, 3143
statistical analysis
  intention-to-treat 23
  outcome-specific 22
  subgroup-specific 23–4
stature, *see* height; short stature; tall stature
status epilepticus **3923**
STDs, *see* sexually transmitted diseases (STD)
STE6 gene 69
steam inhalations 4354
stearic acid 2302
steatorrhoea 1904, 1906
  in bacterial overgrowth 1913, 1914
  causes 1906
  in chronic pancreatitis 2035, 2038
  in cystic fibrosis 2749
  in enteropathy-associated T-cell lymphoma 1927
  in intrahepatic cholestasis 2059
  in primary biliary cirrhosis 2074
  selective IgA deficiency association 1839–40
  in short gut syndrome 1925
  in small-intestinal malrotation 1977
  see also fat, malabsorption
steatosis
  macrovesicular 2127, *2128*
  microvesicular 2126–7, *2128*
  see also liver, fatty changes
Steele-Richardson-Olszewski syndrome (progressive supranuclear palsy) 3965, **4005–6**, *4006*
Steel factor 3383, 3384, 3387, 3557
Steinberg hypothesis 2332
Steinert's disease, *see* dystrophia myotonica
Stein-Leventhal syndrome, *see* polycystic ovary syndrome
Stellantchasmus falcatus 996
stem-cell factor (Steel factor) 3383, 3384, 3387, 3557
stem cells, haemopoietic **3381–93**
  in aplastic anaemia 3442–3
  disorders **3390–3**
  function 3383–5
  peripheral-blood, therapeutic use 3602, 3697, **3700**
  pluripotent 3383, 3384, **3385–7**
  radiation damage 1219
stenosis 1975

Stenotrophomonas maltophilia 561
stents
  aortic aneurysm management 2372
  in coronary angioplasty 2352
  lattice, in lung cancer 2684
  in pancreatic carcinoma 2044
  'stepped care' approach, in bulimia nervosa 1300, 4217
stercoral ulcers 2138
stereoisomerism 1248–9
stereotactic biopsy 4039
stereotaxic surgery 4017
  in benign essential tremor 4012
  in Parkinson's disease 4003–4
sterility
  mumps virus causing 373, 374
  see also infertility
sternomastoid paralysis 3880
sternum
  congenital abnormalities **2875**
  disorders **2875–6**
steroid hormones 1554
  ischaemic heart disease risk 2314
  receptors 1556, 1557, 1561–2
  see also corticosteroids; hormone(s); sex steroids; *specific hormones*
steroids
  in adult respiratory distress syndrome 2860
  adverse mental symptoms 4242
  in asthma 2738
    severe asthma 2739
  inhalers, in asthma 2738
  perioral dermatitis from 3788
  septicaemia treatment 1026
  sexual problems associated *4245*
  systemic, in atopic eczema 3742
  topical *3805*, *3806*
    in atopic eczema 3742
    in psoriasis 3748
  withdrawal, rebound phenomenon in 3748
  see also corticosteroids
Stevens-Johnson syndrome 343, 346, 3731, 3780
Stickler's syndrome 3083
stiff-man syndrome **4159**
stiffness, *see* joint(s), stiffness; muscle, stiffness
stilboestrol 1254
  in pregnancy 1810, 1812
  in sickle-cell disease 3517
stiletto snakes, bites and envenoming 1131
stillbirth
  in human parvovirus infection 1782
  occupations associated 1173
Still's disease
  adult **2973–4**
    diagnostic criteria *2974*
    HLA association 2974
  amyloidosis in 1513, 1514, 1523, 1524, 3193
  mycoplasmas causing 771
  rheumatoid arthritis *vs* 2963
stimulants 4263
  complications associated 4280, 4283
  as drugs of concern 4263
  in pregnancy 4299
  psychiatric disturbances from 4241
  withdrawal syndrome **4293**, 4299
stinging fish 1141
stings
  bee and wasp, *see* insect(s), stings
  scorpion 1146
Stockhold Scales, hand-arm vibration syndrome *1226*, 1227
stockings, elastic 3676
Stokes-Adams attacks 2268, 2285, 2482, 3926
  see also cardiac syncope
stomach
  atrophy, *see* gastric atrophy
  burns, in acid ingestion 1104
  cancer, *see* gastric carcinoma
  in common variable immunodeficiency 1837–8
  Crohn's disease of 1940

disease, skin disease in 3723
embryology 1973
inhalation of contents, in pregnancy
    1742, **1744–5**, 1801
lymphoma 1984–5, 3583
motor activity 1955
    see also gastrointestinal motility
pain 1822
perforation, in acid ingestion 1103, 1104
receptive relaxation 1955
structural disease, haematological
    disorders 3684
in syphilis 714
in systemic sclerosis *3030*
tumours, *see* gastric carcinoma; gastric
    tumours
see also entries beginning gastric
stomatitis
    angular, in iron-deficiency anaemia 3475
    herpetic 342, 343, 345, 1034, 1848–9,
        1852
    in immunocompromised 1034
    in measles 379
Stomatococcus mucilaginosus 561
stomatocytosis, hereditary 3532, *3533*,
    3645
stomatology 1846
stool 1825
    blood in, in Meckel's diverticulum
        1977–8
    cultures,
        in tropical sprue 1935
        in ulcerative colitis 1946
    diarrhoea definition 1823
    fat estimation, *see* faecal fat
    microscopy,
        in amoebiasis 828, 829, 830–1
        in cryptosporidiosis 875
        in giardiasis 879
        in hookworm infection 931
        in strongyloidiasis 929
    osmolality 1825
    rice-water 2002
    viruses in, *see* viruses, stool
    weight 1823, 1825
    see also faeces
storage diseases
    liver in *2019*, 2024
    splenomegaly in 3591
    see also glycogen storage diseases;
        lysosomal storage diseases; *specific
        diseases*
storage-pool deficiency
    acquired 3635
    hereditary *3643*, **3646**
strabismus 1046, 3877
Strachan's syndrome 4100
straight-back syndrome 2179, **2874**
straight leg raising test 2993
strawberries, reaction to 3729
'strawberry cervix' 908
strawberry naevi **3785**
Streptobacillus moniliformis **687–8**
streptocerciasis 915, **918–19**
streptococci **497–511**
    α-haemolytic 497, 2436
    Behçet's syndrome aetiology 3044
    ß-haemolytic 497, 1846, 2432, 2437
    classification and characteristics 497,
        498
    16s rRNA sequencing 497
    diseases caused by *498*
        see also streptococci group A
        infections; streptococci group B
        infections
    endocarditis due to, *see* infective
        endocarditis
    exotoxins 156
    infections in homosexuals 3365
    Lancefield group antigens 497, *498*
    oral,
        endocarditis 510, 2436
        glucan formation 510
        species 497
    post-infectious glomerulonephritis
        505–6, **3173–4**, 3195
    pyogenic, species 497
    'viridans' 497, 2436–7

streptococci group A infections **497–506**
    acute, diagnosis 2433
    bacteraemia 500, 501
    chorea in 4012
    diagnosis and culture 502, 2433–4
    epidemiology 501–2, 2432
    erysipelas, *see* erysipelas
    immunization 503
    impetigo and ecthyma 499–500, 501,
        502
    laboratory tests 504, 2434
    necrotizing fasciitis, *see* necrotizing
        fasciitis 501
    non-suppurative sequelae 503–6
        glomerulonephritis 505–6, **3173–4**,
            3195
        latent period 503
        see also glomerulonephritis; rheumatic
            fever
    perianal disease 499
    prevention 503
    puerperal fever 501
    pyoderma 500, 501, 502
    reactive arthritis after 499
    rheumatic fever, *see* rheumatic fever
    scarlet fever, *see* scarlet fever
    skin infections 499–500, 501, 503
    toxic shock-like illness 502
    transmission patterns 501
    treatment 502, *503*, 2446
    upper respiratory tract 498–9, 501
        pharyngitis and tonsillitis 498, 499,
            501
        sore throat, *see* sore throat
        transmission 501
    vulvovaginitis 499
    of wounds and cellulitis 500–1, 501,
        502
    see also Streptococcus pyogenes
streptococci group B infections **506–9**
    clinical features 507, 4050
    diagnosis 508
    early-/late-onset 507, 508
    epidemiology 507–8
    immunization 509
    mortality 507
    neonatal 506, 507, 1787, **1788–9**, 4050
        antibody deficiency and 508
        diagnosis 508
        late-onset disease 1788
        meningitis 1788
        pneumonia 1788
        prophylaxis 1788–9
        septicaemia 1788
        transmission 508
        treatment 508
    in pregnancy **1787–9**
        prevention 508–9
        transmission 507–8
        treatment 508, 2446
        vaccination 1788
    see also Streptococcus agalactiae
streptococci group C infections **506**
streptococci group G infections **506**
Streptococcus, species 497
Streptococcus agalactiae 497, *498*, 506,
    4050
    characteristics 507
    see also streptococci group B infections
Streptococcus bovis 497, 2436
Streptococcus equisimilis 497
Streptococcus faecalis, urinary-tract
    infections 3209, *3211*
Streptococcus haemolyticus 3146
Streptococcus milleri 497, *498*, 506
    diseases *498*, **509**, 2436
Streptococcus mutans 497, 1846, 2436
Streptococcus pneumoniae
    (pneumococcus) 497
    antibiotic resistance 486, 511–12, 520
    in bronchiectasis 2763
    capsular polysaccharide antigens
        513–14, 519, 520, 522
    characteristics 511
    culture and bacteriology 519–20
    enzymes produced 511
    in HIV infection, *see* AIDS and HIV
        infection

immunological assays 519
meningitis due to, *see* meningitis,
    pneumococcal
penicillin-resistant 2700
pneumococcal surface-protein A (PspA)
    gene 511, 523
serotypes 511
vaccine, *see* pneumococcal vaccines
see also pneumococcal infections;
    pneumonia
Streptococcus pyogenes 497
    antibiotic resistance 309
    antibodies 504
    bacteraemia, mortality 498
    infection route/spread 498
    infections due to 497–8
        in drug abusers 4279
        see also streptococci group A
            infections
    M protein antigen 498, 501
    nephritogenic proteins 505
    products/enzymes released from 498
    septicaemia 1022
    serological tests *504*
    serotypes 501
    tropical pyomyositis 4174
Streptococcus sanguis 497, 2436
Streptococcus suis, meningitis 4051
Streptococcus viridans
    infection in drug abusers 4279
    infective endocarditis 2428–9, 2436,
        2440
    intracranial abscess 4081
Streptococcus zooepidemicus 497,
    506
streptokinase 3671
    in acute myocardial infarction 28–9
    antibodies to 2342
    comparisons and trials 2342
    dose regimens *3672*
    fever after 1181
    heart valve prostheses 2470
    heparin with 2343
    in myocardial infarction 2304, 2342
    in pulmonary embolism 2526
    recanalization effects 2342
    S. pyogenes and glomerulonephritis
        from 505
streptolysins 2432
streptomycin
    adverse reactions 657
    in brucellosis 623
    in infective endocarditis 2446, *2447*
    in plague 598
    Staphylococcus aureus resistance 525
    in tuberculosis 655, *656*, 3278
streptozotocin 1509
stress
    ACTH secretion 1563, 1575–6
    acute erosive peptic ulceration **1880**
    aircraft travel and 1201, 1202
    alcohol abuse intervention 4274
    angina precipitation 2322
    dissociative disorder association 4210
    duodenal ulcer aetiology 1878
    gastrointestinal motility disorders 1963
    hypertension pathogenesis 2530–1
    ischaemic heart disease risk 2315
    management 4255
    mechanical, bone and cartilage 2981
    migraine precipitant 4025
    migrating myoelectric complex
        biorhythm 1954
    personality disorder diagnosis and
        4212
    psychological reactions, *see*
        psychological reactions to stress
    respiratory virus infections 333
    response 1563–4
        in diabetes 1492, 1494
        emotional 4204
        to injury and surgery 1548–9
        physical 4204
        psychological 4204
    testing, *see* exercise testing
'stress fibres' 82
stress fractures 2981, 4322, **4323**
    treatment 4323, *4324*

stressful life events
    deliberate self-harm after 4229
    depressive disorders aetiology 4219
    emotional responses, models 4232,
        4232
    hypochondriasis provoked by 4208
    ischaemic heart disease risk 2315
    as physical illness precursor 4232
    reactions **4204–5**
    schizophrenia aetiology 4222
stretch receptors 1206
    baroreceptors 2156
striae 1858, 3788
    in Cushing's syndrome 1643
    in pregnancy 1804
striatonigral degeneration 4006
striatum 3861
    anatomy and neurochemistry 3862
    dopamine loss, in Parkinson's disease
        3999, 4000
stridor 2719, 2724
    functional inspiratory 2724
    in lung cancer 2883
    nocturnal 2724
striopallidal complex 3861
striosomes 3862
stroke (cerebrovascular accident)
    after coronary artery bypass grafting
        2355–6
    after psychological stress 4232
    aircraft travel and 1202
    in antiphospholipid syndrome 3020,
        3669, 3670
    blood pressure and 30–1
    causes 3954, 3957
        arterial disease *3950*
        cardiac sources of embolism *3949*, 3960
        carotid artery atheroma 2367, 3948,
            3954
        haematological disease *3951*
    central motor conduction time in 3838
    definition 3946
    depression after 4340
    in dialysed patients 3312
    disordered swallowing after 1962
    in elderly **4343**
    electroencephalogram (EEG) in 3830
    epidemiology *3947*
    epilepsy and 4340
    'familial', causes *3948*
    haemorrhagic, *see* cerebral
        haemorrhage; intracranial
        haemorrhage
    high fibrinogen levels 2302
    hormone replacement therapy and 1815
    ischaemic, *see* cerebral infarction
    management 4343
    mental sequelae 4237
    oral contraceptives and 1724
    pathology 3946
    pregnancy and 1768, 3956
    prevention **3964**
    pure motor or sensory 3956
    rehabilitation after 3960, **4340**
    risk after transient ischaemic attack 3952
    risk factors 3947
    sensory motor 3956
    in sickle-cell disease 3514–15
    tissue plasminogen activator and
        anistreplase association 2342–3
    see also cerebrovascular disease;
        subarachnoid haemorrhage
stroke-in-evolution 3955, 3959–60
stroke volume 2150, 2154, 2157, 2158,
    2605
    in cardiac output 2154
    in chronic bronchitis 2572
    exercise effect 2161, 2226
    filling pressure relationship 2571
    increase, in mitral regurgitation 2458
    mitral valve physiology 2458
    in myocardial infarction 2566, 2567, 2568
    in overtransfusion 2571
    in pericardial constriction 2478, 2479
    in pulmonary embolism 2569, 2570
    in septicaemia 2572
stroke work 2154, 2155, 2157, 2220
stroke work index, measurement 2224

Strongyloides fuelleborni 929
Strongyloides stercoralis 928, 2004
  in HIV infection 487
  in immunocompromised 1029, 1034
  infections in homosexuals 3365
  lifecycle 928
  malabsorption in tropics and 1930
  in renal transplant recipients 3314
strongyloidiasis **928–9**
  hyperinfection 929, 1034
strongyloids, gut **932**
strontium-89 256
struma ovarii 1717
Strümpell's disease 3985
strychnine 1368
Stryker frame 3900
stunting 1279, 1281
  in adults 1281
  in children 1281, *1282*
stupor, emergency management 4257
Sturge–Weber syndrome **4116**
  intracranial arteriovenous malformations
    3963
  naevi in 3785
stuttering 3846
styrene (vinyl benzene)
  mechanisms of toxicity 1088
  poisoning **1088**
subacute combined degeneration of cord
    3893
subacute necrotizing encephalopathy
    3989
subacute sclerosing panencephalitis
    (SSPE) 378, **380**, **4073**
  incidence 376, 380
subaortic stenosis 2399, *2462*
  acquired, in tricuspid atresia 2412
  fixed **2422**, *2462*
    aortic stenosis *vs* 2463
    heart murmurs 2421
subarachnoid haemorrhage
  acute headache in 4027
  arteriovenous malformation 3963
  complications 3963
  diabetic ketoacidosis *vs* 1499
  in infective endocarditis 2441
  intracranial saccular aneurysms **3963**,
    3963
  lumbar puncture in 3842, 3843
  management 3963–4
    angioplasty 3824
  meningitis *vs* 4056
  in polycystic kidney disease 3203
  in pregnancy 1768
  prognosis 3963
  spinal 3895
  spontaneous **3962–4**
  traumatic spinal puncture *vs* 3843
subarachnoid space
  anatomy 4050
  bacterial meningitis pathogenesis
    4052
  blood in 3843
  pus in 4052
subaxial subluxation 2959, 2960
subclavian artery
  aberrant 2182
  compression 2366
  damage 2375
subclavian autograft, systemic-to-
    pulmonary arterial shunts 2405
subclavian steal syndrome 2368, 3951
  management 2373
subclavian vein, compression 2366
subconjunctival haemorrhage
  in leptospirosis 701
  in relapsing fevers 695
subcortical dementia 3965–6, *3967*
subcortical lesions **3858**
subcortical structures **3859–63**
  language and **3851**
  see also basal ganglia; cerebellum;
    thalamus
subcutaneous drug formulation 1239
subcutaneous nodules
  in amyloid arthropathy 3003
  in rheumatoid arthritis 2960
subdiaphragmatic infections, pleural
  effusion in 2867–8

subdural empyema 4050, 4081
  clinical features 4082
subdural haematoma 2089
  chronic 3970
    after head injury 4049
    symptoms and treatment 4049
  subdural monitoring, intracranial
    pressure 2109
subfornical organ (SFO) 1600, 3117
subhyaloid haemorrhage 2585
sublingual formulation 1238
sublingual salivary glands, in mumps
    374
submandibular gland, obstruction from
  calculi 1862
submaxillary glands, in mumps 374
    submucosal (Meissner's) plexus 1953
subphrenic abscess 2008
substance abuse
  definition 4268
  management in general wards **4286–8**
  needs in custody **4304–5**
  in prison **4305**
  see also alcohol abuse; drug abuse(r)
    and misuse
substance misuse, definition 4268
substance P 1894, 3938
  in pain processing 3937
  in trigeminovascular reflex 4023
substantia nigra, in Parkinson's disease
    3999, 4000
substantia nigra pars compacta 3861,
    3862
subthalamic nucleus 3862
subtraction carotid angiogram 3822,
    3823
subtrochanteric bursitis 2996
succimer, *see* di-mercaptosuccinic acid
    (DMSA)
succinic semialdehyde dehydrogenase
  deficiency 1372
succinylcholine (suxamethonium)
  hydrolysis 1259
  hyperkalaemia due to 3135
  malignant hyperpyrexia 1182
  in renal impairment 3270
suckling reflex 1603
sucralfate 1868
  in peptic ulcers 1886
sucrase-isomaltase 1920
  deficiency 1922–3
    inherited 1923
sucrose
  in cholera management 579
  intolerance 1922, *1922*
Sudan black B 3399, 3400, 3405–6
sudden cardiac death 2161, 2356
  arrhythmogenic right ventricular
    dysplasia 2391
  computed tomography in prediction of
    2261
  coronary artery anomalies 2430
  dilated cardiomyopathy 2384
  in hypertrophic cardiomyopathy 2388,
    2389
    prevention 2389–90, *2390*
  ischaemic **2321**
    in myocardial infarction 2321, 2334,
      2347
  in sarcoidosis 2827
  smoking and 2313
  in sport **4321**
    frequency 4321, *4321*
    prevention 4321
  in ventricular tachycardia 2281
  in Wolff–Parkinson–White syndrome
    2276
sudden death
  after psychological stress 4232
  in carbon tetrachloride poisoning 1085
  in cerebral infarction 3958
  in diabetes 1489, 1492
  forensic pathology 4309
  low risk in sexual intercourse 4244
  in north-east Thailand 3132
  in tetanus 627
Sudeck's atrophy **3096–7**, 3941
  joint features 3006
sudomotor nerves 3882

sugar
  consumption and diverticular disease
    1969
  in diabetes 1467–8, 1469
  dietary recommendations 1330
suicidal ideas
  denial of 4230
  in depressive disorders 4218
  self-harm and 4229, 4230
suicidal intent 4228
suicidal motivation
  continued after self-harm 4229
  interview sequence 4229–30, *4230*
  see also deliberate self-harm
suicide
  after bereavement 4235
  anorexia nervosa patients 4215
  assisted 39
  attempted **4228–31**
    see also deliberate self-harm; suicide,
      failed
  in bulimia nervosa patients, risk 4217
  children/adolescents 36
  in depressive disorders, risk 4218, 4219
  discussions and risk related to 4229
  in drug abusers 4295
  enquiries about and psychiatric disorder
    detection 4203
  failed 4228
    detection/assessment 4229
    notes 1045
  risk after deliberate self-harm 4229,
    4229, 4231
  in schizophrenia, risk 4222
  self-poisoning 1043, 1044
sulfadoxine, in malaria *854*
Sulfamylon^R 1214
sulindac, poisoning 1056
sulphadiazine
  in lymphogranuloma venereum 761
  in paracoccidioidomycosis 820
  in toxoplasmosis in AIDS 4078
sulphadoxine
  overdose **1073**
  in toxoplasmosis 869
sulphaemoglobinaemia 3519, **3520**
sulphamethizole, in urinary-tract
  infections *3211*
sulphamethoxazole, *Pneumocystis carinii*
  pneumonia 822
sulphametoxipiridazine 819
sulphapyridine, in dermatitis
  herpetiformis 3783
sulphasalazine
  absorption and metabolism 1949
  in ankylosing spondylitis 2967
  in Crohn's disease 1942
  haemolytic anaemia due to 3546, 3547
  in psoriatic arthritis 2970
  in Reiter's syndrome 2972
  in rheumatoid arthritis 2964
  secondary immunodeficiency due to
    174
  side-effects 1949
    rash 1947
  in ulcerative colitis 1949
sulphatide lipidosis 3986
sulphatidosis (metachromatic
  leukodystrophy) *1428*, **1429**, 3986
sulphinpyrazone 2987, 3266
sulphite oxidase deficiency 1367–8
sulphmethaemoglobin, hydrogen
  sulphide poisoning treatment 1100
sulphonamides
  adverse reaction 2851
  haemolysis due to *3546*
  in malaria 852–3
  meningococcal infection prophylaxis
    542
  nephrotoxicity 3264
  in nocardiosis 627
  in pregnancy 1784, 1785
  in renal impairment 3272
  resistance, *Neisseria meningitidis* 534
sulphones, haemolysis due to *3546*
sulphonylurea drugs 1459, 1468,
    1469–71
  administration 1471
  in factitious hypoglycaemia 1509

overdose/poisoning 1071, 1072
  in renal impairment 3274
  in surgical patients 1495
  toxic effects 1470–1, 1497
  see also oral hypoglycaemic agents
sulphoxidation, of drugs 1259
sulphur, acne vulgaris management 3753
^99^Tc^m^-sulphurcolloid 3381, 3573
sulphur dioxide 1102, 1227
  poisoning **1102**, 1229
  pollution 1229
sulphur granules 681, 682, 684
sulphuric acid 1534
sulphur mustard (mustard gas) **1115–17**,
    1115
  clinical features of exposure 1116, *1116*
  toxicity 1116, *1116*, 1117
  use 1115
sulphydryl groups 2327
sulthiame, overdose/poisoning 1062
sumatriptan, in migraine 4025
sunburn 3726
  erythema 3725, 3726
  protection from 3724
sun light 3724–5
  acne vulgaris management 3753
  damage 3725
  treatment 3728–9
  exposure,
    health education over dangers 3728
    management/protection 3728–9
  features of chronic exposure 3726
  polymorphic light eruption 3726, 3727
  protection from 3724, 3728–9
  rash 3726, 3727
  in vitiligo management 3758
  see also ultraviolet light
sunscreen 3728
superantigen 156, 165
  autoimmunity development 156
  Kawasaki disease aetiology 3049
superficial femoral artery, percutaneous
  transluminal angioplasty 2371
supergene family
  complement genes 178
  origin and evolution 178
superior mesenteric angiography, in
  gastrointestinal bleeding 3683
superior mesenteric artery, atheroma 1996
superior mesenteric artery syndrome
    1998, 3897
superior vena cava
  chest radiography 2178
  compression 2897
    in lung cancer 2883
    in mediastinal masses 2897
  defects, ostium secundum defects 2424
  displacement 2181
  drainage to left atrium 2402, **2415**
  enlargement 2181
  obstruction 2480, 2651, 2652
    cavagram 2657
    facial flushing in 3787
    in lung cancer 2891
  superior vena cavography **2655–6**, 2657
superoxide dismutase 1194
superoxide radicals 1194
  COAD with normal α₁-antitrypsin
    2772
'superwarfarins' 1123
supine hypotension syndrome, of
  pregnancy 1726, 1735
supportive care, in cancer, *see* cancer
supportive counselling
  in psychiatric disorders 4254
  see also counselling
suppressor-cell phenomenon, in
  transplantation 183
suppressor T cells, *see* T-cells,
  suppressor
supra-aortic stenosis **2422–4**
supraclavicular lymph nodes, metastases
  from unknown primary site 252
supranuclear palsy, progressive 3965,
    4005–6, *4006*
supraoptic nucleus 1600
suprapulmonary valve stenosis 2402
suprasellar germinoma **1597–8**
supratentorial abscess 4083

supratentorial mass lesions 4034
  asymmetrical expansion 2584
  symmetrical expansion 2584
  syndromes associated 2584
supraventricular tachycardia, *see*
  tachycardia, supraventricular
sural nerve **4098**
suramin
  in African trypanosomiasis 892
  in filarial infections 912
  in onchocerciasis 916–17
  toxicity and cautions 917
surface area, body 3108
surface tension 2598
surfactant 2594–6, 2628
  administration 2856
  in adult respiratory distress syndrome
    2855–6
  anionic/cationic/non-ionic 1079
  apoproteins 2595, 2613
  composition 2594, 2613, 2855
  in detergents and dishwashing liquids
    1079
  function/actions 2599, 2613, 2855
  inactivation, in ARDS 2856
  in pulmonary alveolar proteinosis 2834
  in pulmonary vascular diseases 2641
  secretion, regulation 2596, 2613
  turnover 2595–6
surgery
  in acute porphyria 1394
  adjuvant radiotherapy 257, *258*
  bleeding during/after **3659–60**
  in cancer,
    chemotherapy/radiation with 248
    principles and aims 247–8
    radiation with 248
  in diabetes **1493–6**
    emergency 1495–6
    management 1494–5
    metabolic response 1494
  metabolic effects **1548–50**
  obesity treatment 1312–13
  postponement effect 4
  prophylactic, anaerobic infections 576
  role in HIV infection 473
  in sickle-cell disease 3517
  tumour staging 246
  venous thromboembolism risk 3668,
    3675, 3676
  vulnerability of patients and 4
surgical wounds, infections 329–30,
  1021
surveillance, of infections **286–7**
Suttonella indologenes 561
suxamethonium, *see* succinylcholine
SV40 (simian virus 40) 79, 4073
swallowing 2610
  difficulty, *see* dysphagia
  disorders 1962
  painful, *see* odynophagia
  reflex 1955
  in unconscious patient 2583
swallowing syncope 3926
Swan-Ganz catheter 2220
  risks associated 2221
  triple lumen thermodilution 2220, 2222
swan neck deformities 2957
sweat, calcium losses 1623
sweat glands 3706, 3765, 3766
sweating 1180, **3765–7**
  apocrine 3765–6
  eccrine 3766
  emotional/anxiety-induced 3766
  excess, *see* hyperhidrosis
  feet 3737, 3766, 3767
  fungal poisoning causing 1155
  generalized 3766
  gustatory, in diabetes 1489
  hands 3766
  inhibitors 3766
  loss 3767
  in marathons and mass runs 4328
  nocturnal 3375
    in Hodgkin's disease 3570, 3571
    in microscopic polyangiitis 3013
    in tumours 241
    in Wegener's granulomatosis 3013
    in phaeochromocytomas 2554

reduced (hypohidrosis) 3767
  in salicylate poisoning 1054
sweat pore, occlusion, vesico-blistering
  diseases in 3779
sweat test 1978, 2750
Sweden, rubella vaccination 411–12
sweeteners, bladder cancer association
  212
Sweet's syndrome, joint involvement
  3003
swimmer's itch 970, 975, 2004
swimming-pool granuloma 665, 666
Swiss syndrome 2472
'swollen belly syndrome' 929
SWORD scheme
  extrinsic allergic alveolitis 2816
  occupational asthma 2742
Swyer-James syndrome (unilateral
  transradiancy of lung) **2778**
sycosis barbae 526
Sydenham's chorea 503, 2433, **4012**
Sylvian aqueduct, stenosis 4115
Symmers' fibrosis 977, 979
'symmorphosis' 2604
sympathectomy
  chemical 2371
  in ischaemia of limb 2371
  lower limb 2374
  upper limb 2374
  in vasospastic disorders 2374
sympathetic blocking drugs, in pain
  treatment 3945
sympathetic blocks, pain treatment 3006,
  3938
sympathetic nervous system 3881
  activity,
    neuropathic pain and 3942
    pain in peripheral neuropathy 3940
  gastrointestinal tract 1953
  heart 2160, 2170, 2253, 2282
  in heart failure 2177, 2234, **2253–5**
    neurotransmission **2253**
    potassium balance and 3128
  pulmonary blood vessels 2486
  pulmonary circulation 2492
  in stress 1563
  in trauma 1548
'sympathetic storm' 2501
sympathomimetics, *see* ß-adrenergic
  agonists
symports (cotransporters) 1900, *1900*
symptoms, response to stress and
  hospital admission 1
Synacthen (tetracosactrin) test 1654–5,
  1664, *4375*
synaptic vesicles 4139
synaptobrevin 77
synaptobrevin-2 76
synaptotagmin 77
syncope **2173–5**, **3925–7**
  aetiology 2173–4
  ambulatory ECG 2197–9
  in aortic stenosis 2160, 2462
  cardiac 2285, 3918, **3926**
  cardio-inhibitory 3925
  carotid sinus **3926**, 3926
  in carotid sinus hypersensitivity 2266
  causes 3925–6, *3925*
    cardiovascular *2174*
    neuroendocrine *2174*
  clinical features 2174, 3926
  clinical presentation 2174
  complicated 3926
  convulsive 3926
  cough 2642, 3925, **3926**
  definition 3925
  diagnostic approach 3927
  in elderly 4342
  epilepsy *vs* 2175
  falls due to 4339
  'ice-cream' 3926
  incidence and mortality 2174–5
  investigation for pacemakers 2286
  management 3927
  micturition 3918, **3926**, 3926
  pathophysiology 3925–6
  postural hypotension causing **3927**
  reflex anoxic seizures **3927**
  Stokes-Adams, *see* Stokes-Adams attacks

swallowing 3926
  vasovagal 718, 2173, 2175, **2267**, **3918**,
    3926
    causes 3925
    features 2267, 3918
    see also vasovagal syndrome
syndesmophytes
  in ankylosing spondylitis 2967
  in psoriatic arthritis 2969
syndrome of inappropriate antidiuresis
  (SIAD), *see* antidiuresis, syndrome of
  inappropriate
syndrome X (insulin resistant syndrome;
  microvascular angina) 1308, 1411,
  2161, 2166, 2309, **2325**
  angina in 2166, 2167, 2325
  calcium antagonists in 2329
  diagnosis and arteriograms 2167, 2325
  hyperinsulinaemia in, ischaemic heart
    disease risk 2309
  hypertension in 2533
  investigations and features 2167, 2325
  mitral prolapse overlap 2460
  pathophysiology 2323
synergy 305
synovectomy 2964
synovial effusion, in rheumatoid arthritis
  2959
synovial fluid
  analysis **2950–1**, *2950*
    in bacterial arthritis 2999
    use/abuse 2951
  aspiration, in bacterial arthritis 2999
  crystals 2950, 2951
  in gout 2986
  inflammatory changes 2950
  monosodium urate monohydrate
    crystals 2986
  non-inflammatory changes 2950
  in tuberculous arthritis 3000
  white cell count 2951
synovial joints, *see* joint(s)
synovial membrane, *see* synovium
synovial tissue, overproduction 3007
synovitis
  acute,
    in gout 2984
    in pyrophosphate arthropathy 2988
  chronic hypertrophic, in haemophilia
    3647, 3649
  detection *2946*
  enteropathic **2972–3**
  foot 2958
  foreign body 2946
  infections causing, rheumatoid arthritis
    vs 2963
  pigmented villonodular **3007**
  plant-thorn 2946
  in rheumatoid arthritis 2957, 2958
  in sarcoidosis 3007
  signs 2988
  sterile 2970, 2972
    see also Reiter's syndrome
  wrist 2957
synovium 2998
  haemangioma of 3003
  in osteoarthritis 2980
syntaxin A and syntaxin B 76
synteny 106
Syntocinon 1745
syphilis **706–20**
  acquired 3002
  aneurysms in 2364, 2365
  aortitis 2465, **2482–4**
  arthritis in **3002**
  bacterial taxonomy and 706–7
  biological false-positive test 3668
  cardiac features 2482–3
  chancroid *vs* 585, 711
  chronic granulomatous disease of nose
    3801
  clinical features 706, **710–14**
  congenital 707, 708, 1790–1, 3002,
    3768, 4191
    renal lesions 3177
  contact tracing 709
  control 708–9
  deafness and vertigo in 714
  decrease in, tongue cancer decrease 201

swallowing 3926
definition 706
diagnosis 707, **714–17**, 2483, **4085–6**
  animal inoculation 714–15
  CSF examination 4086
  dark-field microscopy 714
  false-positive test 716, 3668
  in HIV infection 716–17
  serological tests 715–17, *715*, 4085–6
  serology 714, *715*
differential diagnosis 585, 711, 713–14
distribution 706
encephalitis, *see* general paresis of the
  insane (GPI)
endemic non-venereal **703–6**, *704*, 706
epidemiology 703, **707–10**, 3346–7,
  3347, 4083
  changing presentation 708
  incidence 707–8
  sex, race and infectivity 708
episodic vertigo in 3875
eye in **4085**, 4191, 4193–4
follow-up 719
glomerulonephritis in 3177
HIV infection and 707, 708, **4079**,
  4193–4
homosexuals and 708, 710, 712, 719,
  3361, 3362
incubation period 706, 709
late benign 712
latent 709, 711–12
leucoplakia of tongue in 719
lymphogranuloma venereum *vs* 761
'malignant' 716
management **717–19**, *717*, **4086**
  cardiovascular 2483–4
  neurosyphilis 4086
meningovascular **4084–5**, 4236
meningovascular relapse 708
myositis in 4155
neurosyphilis, *see* neurosyphilis
oral manifestations 710, 711, 719, 1853
origin and theories 707
positive tests, in SLE 3020
in pregnancy **1790–1**
primary 709, 1853
  clinical features 710–11
prophylaxis and abortive treatment 719
relapses, after penicillin 708, 709
secondary 709, 1853
  clinical features 711, 712, 3713, 3714,
    3763
  diphtheria *vs* 496
tertiary (late) 1853
  of bones 713, 714
  clinical features 712–14
transmission 707
  in blood 3693
untreated 709
  natural course 709–10
  Oslo study 709
  Tuskegee study 709–10
vasculitis in 708
visceral 714
yaws *vs* 706
see also Treponema pallidum
Syrian hamster, skin allograft survival 185
syringobulbia 3893
syringomyelia **3893–4**
  post-traumatic 3901
systematic overviews (meta-analyses) 21,
  25–6
  antihypertensive drugs effect 2539,
    2540
  examples of important results 27–9, 31
  proper conduct of 26
systemic lupus erythematosus (SLE)
  3009, **3017–27**
  alveolar haemorrhage in 2804
  animal models 3024
  antinuclear antibody-negative 3021
  autoantibodies in 163, 3021, *3021*,
    3024–5, *3025*
    anti-DNA 3021, 3024, 3026
    antiphospholipid antibodies 3019,
      3020, 3668, 3681
  autoimmune thrombocytopenia *vs* 3631
  cardiac manifestations 2392, *2392*,
    3020
  classification 3017, *3018*

systemic lupus erythematosus
  (SLE) (cont.)
  clinical course **3018**
  clinical features *3018*, **3019–20**
  clinical subgroups 3020, *3021*
  complement receptor deficiency in 181,
    3021, 3026
  complement role 182, 3021
  complications 3022–3, 4130
  contraception and family planning
    3022
  C-reactive protein 1531, 1532, 3020
  diagnostic criteria 2798
  diffuse parenchymal lung disease in
    2781, 2798, 3020
  epidemiology **3017–18**
    hormones and age 3017–18
  flares,
    management 3023–4
    measures of 3021
    precipitation 3022
    in pregnancy 3022
  gastrointestinal tract in **1999–2000**,
    3020
  haematological changes **3681–2**, 4130
  haemolytic anaemia 3544, *3548*, 3681
  haemolytic uraemic syndrome 3197
  HLA association 3008, 3025, 3026
  immunization in 3022
  immunopathology and biology **3024–6**
    cellular immunology 3025–6, *3025*
    cytokines *3025*, 3026
    genetic components 3026
    intolerance to immune complexes
      3025
  investigations **3020–1**
  liver in 2135, 2139, 3020
  lung involvement **2798–9**, *2798*, 3020
  lymphocytic interstitial pneumonitis
    2807
  management **3022–3**
  mental disorder/symptoms 3019, 4243
  microalbuminuria in 3138
  monitoring 3021
  muscular involvement 3019, 4156
  neurological complications 3019,
    4129–30
    diagnosis 4130
  ocular features **4184**
  osteonecrosis in 3018, 3019
  pleural effusions in 2868, 3020
  pregnancy in 3017, 3022, 3191
  prognosis 3022–3
  renal disease, *see* lupus nephritis
  renal transplantation 3315
  rheumatoid arthritis *vs* 2963
  spontaneous remission 3018
  subacute cutaneous 3019
  thrombotic thrombocytopenic purpura
    and 3020, 3549
  treatment **3023–4**, *3024*
    of acute flares 3023–4
    problem-directed 3023, *3023*
  see also lupus erythematosus
systemic lupus erythematosus (SLE)-like
  syndrome, in complement deficiency
  180
systemic-pulmonary arterial shunts, *see*
  pulmonary arteries, systemic shunts
systemic-pulmonary circulation
  connections, abnormal 2402, **2424–8**
systemic sclerosis **3027–35**
  autoantibodies in 3032, *3033*
  cardiac manifestations 2392, *2392*,
    3030, *3031*
  clinical course 3031
  diffuse cutaneous *3027*, **3028–9**
    examination 3029–31
    see also scleroderma
  facial flushing in 3787
  gastrointestinal tract in 1963, **1999**,
    3030, *3030*
  haemolytic uraemic syndrome 3198
  laboratory investigations **3031–3**
  limited cutaneous *3027*, **3028**
    examination 3029
    see also CREST syndrome;
      scleroderma
  liver in 2139

lung involvement in **2799**, 2799, 3030,
  3031, 3033
  monitoring 3032–3
  neurological complications 3033, **4131**
  oesophageal muscle in 1871, 3723
  overlap syndromes 3034–5
  pathogenesis **3031**, 3032, 3034
  physical examination **3029–31**
  Raynaud's phenomenon in 2365, 2945,
    3028
  renal crisis 3009, 3031, 3192, **3290–1**
  renal disease **3192**
  skin in 3029, 3030
  small-bowel enema in 1909
  spectrum 3027, *3027*
  survival **3034**
  treatment **3034**, *3034*, *3035*
  see also scleroderma
systemic vascular resistance 2154, 2566
  afterload determination 2156
  in myocardial infarction 2566
  in pulmonary embolism 2569
  in septicaemia 2573
systole 2153
  definition 2230
  in hypertrophic cardiomyopathy 2385–6
systolic blood pressure 2150, *2154*
  essential hypertension diagnosis 2528
  in Fallot's tetralogy 2403
  measurement 2535
  mortality association 2532
systolic hypertension, *see* hypertension,
  systolic
Systolic Hypertension in the Elderly
  Program (SHEP) 2542

T

T$_3$, *see* tri-iodothyronine (T$_3$)
T$_4$, *see* thyroxine (T$_4$)
tabes dorsalis **4085**
tablets, 'hung-up' and oesophagitis due
  to 1874, *1874*
taboparesis 4085
tabun 1117
tache noire 734
tachycardia 2175
  in acute porphyria 1392, 1393
  angina in 2323, 2325
  antidromic 2277
  atrial 2270, *2272*, **2273–4**
  atrioventricular nodal re-entry
    (AVNRT) 2193, *2272*, **2274–5**
    treatment 2266, 2274–5
  atrioventricular re-entry (AVRT;
    orthodromic) 2275, 2276
    circus movement 2193
  junctional re-entry **2274–7**
    Lown-Ganong-Levine syndrome 2275,
      2277
    pre-excitation syndrome, *see* Wolff-
      Parkinson-White syndrome
    see also above
  in myocardial infarction 2345
  narrow QRS complex 2274
    differential diagnosis 2270, *2272*
  orthodromic 2275, 2276
  re-entry 2149
    ablation 2265, 2266, 2275
    macro re-entry 2260
    management 2263
    mechanisms 2260–1
    micro re-entry 2260, 2266
    see also above
  sinus *2272*
  supraventricular **2270–1**, 2274, 2277
    after coronary artery bypass grafting
      2355
    definitions 2270
    differential diagnosis 2277–8
    in hypertrophic cardiomyopathy 2387
    in myocardial infarction 2345
    paroxysmal 2261
    polyuria in 3148
    radiofrequency ablation 2289
    re-entry, *see above*
    'with aberration' 2277

symptoms 2261
  in syncope 2174, 2175
  in tetanus 627
  thallium poisoning 1113
  ventricular, *see* ventricular tachycardia
  wide QRS complex **2277–9**
    differential diagnosis 2277–9, *2278*
    see also ventricular tachycardia
tachykinins 1894
  see also substance P
tachypnoea 2645
  in pulmonary oedema 2503
Taenia saginata **960–1**, *961*
  lifecycle 961
Taenia solium 959, **961–3**, *961*, 964,
  2004
  lifecycle 961, 964
  see also cysticercosis
Tahyna virus 424–5
Takahara disease 1441
Takatsukis syndrome, *see* POEMS
  syndrome
Takayasu's disease (syndrome) **2377–80**,
  2392
  aetiology and pathology 2378
  classification 2378
  clinical features and diagnosis 2378–9
  complications 2377, 2378
  ocular features **4183**
  pregnancy and 2379
  treatment and prognosis 2379–80
talc 2845
  insufflation into pleural space 2867
  peritonitis due to 2008
  pleurodesis 2871
  pneumoconioses **2845–6**
tall stature **1700**
  familial 1700
TAMI-7 trial 2334
Tamm-Horsfall protein
  in urinary casts 3103
  urinary stones and 3252
  in urine 3101–2, 3137–8
tamoxifen
  in breast cancer 27–8
  breast cancer incidence association 209
  endometrial cancer association 210
  mechanism of action 226
  in pancreatic cancer 2040
tanapox virus 369
Tangier disease
  (analphalipoproteinaemia) 1414,
  3591, 3986
TAP1 and *TAP-2* genes 69, 143
TAP2 peptide transporter, defects 172
tapeworm **959–60**
  beef 960–1, *961*
  Diphyllobothrium latum 969
  dog, *see Echinococcus granulosus*
  lifecycle 959–60, 961, 964
  pork, *see* cysticercosis; *Taenia solium*
  Spirometra mansoni 969
tar, in psoriasis 3748, *3749*
tardive dyskinesia 1251, 4223, 4252
  chronic,
    causes *4021*
    drug-induced 4021
  in Gilles de la Tourette syndrome
    treatment 4017
  tardive dystonia 4021
target cells *3378*
tarsal tunnel syndrome 4097–8
  in rheumatoid arthritis 2958
tartrazine 1253, 3729
  asthma due to 2849
Tarui's disease, *see* phosphofructokinase,
  deficiency
taste 3878
  loss 3878
  sensation 3860
TATA binding protein (TBP; TFIID)
  1558
Tataguine virus 429
tat protein 464
Tatumella ptyseos 561
tau protein 3972
taurine *1353*
tax gene and Tax protein 462, 489

taxines *1154*
Tay-Sachs disease (infantile G$_{M2}$-
  gangliosidosis) 1335, *1428*, **1430**, 3985
  screening 132, *133*
T-cell leukaemia
  acute lymphoblastic 215, *3399*, 3402
  CD25 antigen in 151
  prolymphocytic 3424
T-cell lymphoma, *see* non-Hodgkin's
  lymphoma (NHL), T-cell
T-cell receptor **148**
  αβ receptor 148
    CDR (complementarity-determining
      regions) 148
    sequence and gene rearrangements 148
    structure 148
  in autoimmune disease 165
  CD3 antigen and 149–50
  defects and immunodeficiency 173
  γδ receptor 148, 1836
  gene rearrangements 148
    in leukaemia 3394, 3395, 3396, 3411,
      3412
  in lymphoproliferative disorders 3565
  in IgE-mediated allergic response 156
T-cells **149–52**, 277, 316, 3556
  activation,
    by allergens 157
    in asthma 2726
    chronic, in common varied
      immunodeficiency (CVID) 167
    in primary sclerosing cholangitis 2078
  in adenosine deaminase deficiency 1385
  antigen recognition,
    antigen types 141–2
    MHC restriction 141, 142, 151, 277,
      280
  in atherosclerotic lesion development
    2290, 2291
  bypassed in autoimmunity development
    156
  capping of surface proteins, defects in
    SLE 3026
  CD4 1836
    count in AIDS definition 468
    decline in HIV infection 466, 467, 772
    factor VIII concentrate purity and
      3648
    in HIV infection 471
    mycoplasma role in decline 772
    reduced in common varied
      immunodeficiency (CVID) 167
    reduced in SLE 3026
    in rheumatoid arthritis 2954
    see also T-cells, helper
  CD4:CD8 cell ratio 2811–12
    in extrinsic allergic alveolitis 2811–12,
      2814
    in leprosy 673, 674
    in sarcoidosis 2819
    in toxoplasmosis 866
  CD8 1836
    decrease in polymyalgia rheumatica
      3040
    see also cytotoxic T-cells (CTL); T-
      cells, suppressor
  in chlamydial infections 757
  coculture with tumour cells, immune
    response 227, 228
  compartmentalization 2819
  in contact allergic dermatitis 3736
  in Crohn's disease 1938
  in cryptogenic fibrosing alveolitis 2788
  in cutaneous lymphomas 3794
  cytokines produced and affecting
    152–3, *152*, 2727
  cytotoxic, *see* cytotoxic T-cells (CTL)
  deficiency **171–2**
    acute neurological syndromes in 1033,
      1034
    in purine nucleoside phosphorylase
      (PNP) deficiency 172, 1386
  differentiation antigens 149–51, *150*
    expression sequence 150
  in extrinsic allergic alveolitis 2811
  graft-versus-host disease and 3698
  in gut-associated lymphoid tissue 1836,
    2001

helper 141, 149, 151, 316
  actions on macrophage 85, 88
  in allergic rhinitis 2715, 2716
  antigen-presenting cells for 143, 153
  antigen processing 143–4
  in asthma 2727
  B-cell activation 141, 149
  CD4 antigen 150, 151
  CD8 cells 165
  class II antigen recognition in grafts
    184
  class II antigen restriction 142, 143,
    151, 153, 280
  in connective tissue diseases 3009
  cytokine profiles 97, 157
  cytokine release 98, 151, 157, 279,
    2715, 2727
  in delayed hypersensitivity 165
  in dermatomyositis 4156
  down-regulation in graft tolerance 187
  genetic susceptibility to infection 279
  in graft rejection 152, 186–7
  in hepatic granulomas 2120
  in HIV infection 278
  in IgE-mediated allergic response 156,
    157
  IL-2 secretion from Th$_1$ 151, 157
  IL-4 dominant 157, 161
  IL-4 release from Th$_2$ 151, 157, 2727
  in paracoccidioidomycosis 816
  in reactive arthritis 2970
  in sarcoidosis 2818, 2818–19
  Th$_0$ 157
  TH$_1$ 97, 98, 149, 151, 153, 157, 187,
    279
  TH$_2$ 98, 149, 151, 153, 157, 187, 279,
    2715
  see also T-cells, CD4
in hepatic granulomas 2120
immature 152
in immune response to allografts 186–7
  evidence for T$_C$ role 186
  evidence for T$_H$ role 186–7
immunotherapy of tumours 233
in infections 277
inherited metabolic disorders 168
intraepithelial, in enteropathy-associated
  T-cell lymphoma 1928
in LCMV infections 436
in lymph nodes 153, 154, 3562
macrophage activation 277
in malaria 841
in measles 377, 378
memory cells 149
origin of lymphoma, see non-Hodgkin's
  lymphoma (NHL), T-cell
in paracoccidioidomycosis 816
in polymyositis/dermatomyositis 4156
production 3384, 3386
proliferation,
  inhibition in ADA deficiency 172
  in sarcoidosis 2818–19
purification method 151
in purine nucleoside phosphorylase
  deficiency 172, 1386
regulation of erythropoiesis 3387–8
removal and graft rejection prevention
  67
response to tumours 227–8
  melanoma 228
  specific oncogenes 229
in schistosomiasis 976
self-reactive, deletion in tolerance 152,
  155
in severe combined immunodeficiency
  disease (SCID) 172
suppression of phagocyte production
  3388–9
suppressor 151, 157
  enhanced IgG production 3026
  erythropoiesis regulation 3387–8
  reduced in malaria 858
  reduced in primary sclerosing
    cholangitis 2078
  in sarcoidosis 2818, 2819
  in SLE 3026
  in transplantation 183
  see also T-cells, CD8

thymus function 152
  in tuberculosis 639
  in ulcerative colitis 1945
team
  care, of pregnant diabetic women 1755
  primary health care 49–50
  see also multidisciplinary teams
tear gas 1118–19
teboroxime 2207
technetium (scanning)
  bone metastases 246
  in Meckel's diverticulum 1978
  myocardial infarction/ischaemia
    2207–11
  pulmonary capillary perfusion scans
    2655
technetium-99m aerosol (Technegas)
  2655
technetium-99m-
  diethylenetriaminepentacetic acid
  (DTPA) 2204, 2503, 2549
  clearance 3105–6, 3240
    filtration fraction estimation 3108
  in cryptogenic fibrosing alveolitis
    2790–1
  renal imaging 3112, 3113, 3114, 3115
  in systemic sclerosis 3033
  see also diethylene-triamine penta-
    acetic acid (DTPA)
technetium-99m-2-methoxyisobutyl
  isonitrile (MIBI) 2207, 2211
technetium-99m-pertechnetate
  brain scanning 3825
  thyroid imaging 1608, 1619
technetium-99m-stannous pyrophosphate
  2207
  myocardial uptake and method 2207–8
technology, medical 38–9
teeth
  in congenital porphyria 1395
  in fluorosis 3095
  neoplasms, cysts and development
    lesions 1862–3
Teflon injection, in vesicoureteric reflux
  3219
teichoic acid 291, 292
  inflammatory reactions 291–2
teicoplanin, in renal impairment 3271
telangiectases, intracranial 3963
telangiectasia 3785–6
  chronic cooling causing 3724
  in collagen diseases 3787
  digital/facial, in systemic sclerosis 3029
  features 3784, 3785
  hereditary haemorrhagic 1430, 3636,
    3786
    lung disease in 2862
  segmental 3785, 3786
  in stomach and bowel 2137
  treatment 3786
television epilepsy 3918
telogen effluvium, postpartum 1804
temafloxacin 296
temazepam 4355
  capsules 4283, 4299
  injection, tissue damage 4283
'temperate sprue' 1919
temperature
  altitude and 1185, 1193
  atmospheric 1193
  body, see body temperature
  environmental,
    global change 36
    ischaemic heart disease mortality 2315
  regulation, see thermoregulation
  sea and effect on divers 1205
  sensation 3857
  sensibility, loss 4092
temporal arteritis, see giant-cell arteritis
temporal arteritis-polymyalgia
  rheumatica syndrome 1016
temporal artery, biopsy 3041, 3042,
  3042, 4183
temporal lobe
  atrophy, in Pick's disease 3975, 3976
  behavioural defects associated 3846
  'burst' 4045
  damage 3855

epilepsy, mental symptoms 4237–8
  herniation 3930, 3931
  lesions, optic radiation 3869
  seizures 3913
  status 3923
  structures, in memory 3855
  tumours, mental disorders/symptoms in
    4237
temporomandibular joint
  in ankylosing spondylitis 2967
  arthritis 1592
  disorders 1864
  in rheumatoid arthritis 2959
temporomandibular pain 4027
tendinitis
  bicipital 2995
  calcific 3092
  in SLE 3019
tendon reflexes 3857, 4142
  loss 4092
  in muscle disorders 4142
  nerve roots involved 3903
  in thyroid disease 1609
tendons
  acute sports-related injuries 4321
  pain 2947
  rupture 2996
  see also Achilles tendon
tendoperiostitis 4324
tennis elbow 2995
tenosynovitis 4322
  affecting occupation 1168
  De Quervain's 2947, 2996
  flexor tendons, in rheumatoid arthritis
    2957
  in gonorrhoea 547
  localized nodular 2998
  wrist 2996
tenovaginitis, stenosing 2996
Tensilon test 1138, 4161
tension, chest pain in 2168
tension pneumothorax 2563, 2869
teratogenic drugs 130–1, 131, 1254,
  1254, 1809–10
  effects on fetus 1809
teratogenicity 4298
teratogens 4112
teratology, behavioural 1811–12
teratoma
  epidemiology 211
  hCG production 1714
  mediastinal 2899
teratozoospermia 1684, 1685
terbinafine 798, 811
terfenadine 158
terminal bronchioles 2600
terminal care 4349, 4350
  ethics 13
  technology and 38–9
  see also dying patients; terminal
    illness
terminal deoxynucleotidyl transferase
  (TdT) 146, 3399–400
terminal illness 4349–60
  anorexia control 4351
  anxiety and depression in 4358
  cancer pain, see pain, in cancer
  care for family 4357
  children facing bereavement 4358
  chronic benign pain 4352
  confusion 4352–3
  constipation 4353–4
  cough 4354
  dysphagia 4354
  dyspnoea 4354–5
  ethical issues 4359–60
  insomnia 4355
  last days 4356
    management 4356
  law in relation to treatment 4359
  nausea and vomiting 4355–6, 4356
  nutrition and hydration in 4359–60
  psychological aspects 4357–9
  recognition/diagnosis 4349
  sore mouth 4356
  support for family 4358
  symptoms,
    control 4350

diagnosis 4350
  prevalence 4350, 4350
  treatment in 4349–50
    principles of 4350–1
  see also bereavement; death; dying
    patients; palliative treatment
Ternidens deminutus 932
testicular feminization 1579
  complete 1693
  incomplete 1693
testis 1565, 1679, 1680
  acute lymphoblastic leukaemia in 3412
  atrophy,
    in cirrhosis 2087
    mumps virus causing 374
  development 1563, 1689
  failure, primary 1683
  incomplete differentiation 1693–4
  malfunction, sexual problems in 4244
  oestrogen secretion 1688
  in syphilis 714
  teratoma, monitoring response to
    treatment 239
  tumours,
    aetiological factors 218
    epidemiology 211
    gynaecomastia in 1688
    HCG production 1714
    undescended (cryptorchidism) 1685
    volume measurements 1685–6
testis determining factor 1563
  gene (SRY), mutations 1567, 1571
testosterone 1680
  in baldness 3761
  biosynthesis 1679, 1681
  biosynthetic defects 1691–2
  deficiency, see androgen(s), deficiency
  dihydrotestosterone ratio 1693, 2043
  hirsutism due to 3765
  mechanisms of action 1692
  metabolism in target organs 1679–80
  in puberty 1563
  serum,
    in congenital adrenal hyperplasia
      1665, 1668
    in gonadotroph adenoma 1596
    in hyperandrogenization 1676
    in male infertility 1686
    in male pseudohermaphroditism 1693
    in polycystic ovary syndrome 1674,
      1675, 1676
    in sexual differentiation 1689–90
  suppression, in obstructive sleep apnoea
    2912
  treatment 1587, 1684, 1695, 1703
    sexual problem management 4246
  in women 1674
testotoxicosis 1702
tetanolysin 624
tetanospasmin 624
tetanus 624–30
  antiserum/immunoglobulin 283, 628
  antitoxin 283, 628, 629
  cephalic 626–7
  clinical features/course 625–7
  complications 627–8
  diagnosis 628
  epidemiology 624
  grading 626
  immunization 321, 624, 629–30
    after wounds 630
  management 628–9
  mortality 624, 628
  neonatal (neonatorum) 624, 627,
    628
    prevention 630
  pathophysiology 624–5
  prevention 629–30
  rabies vs 401
  see also Clostridium tetani
tetanus toxoid vaccine 317–18
  adsorbed (ATT) 629–30
tetany 1540, 1638–9
  in hypoparathyroidism 1633
  neonatal 1634
  in osteomalacia 3071
  post-parathyroidectomy 1633
  spontaneous 3061

tetrachloroethylene (perchloroethylene)
in fasciolopsiasis 993
poisoning **1088**
tetrachloromethane, *see* carbon
tetrachloride
tetracosactrin (Synacthen) test 1654–5,
1664
tetracycline
acne vulgaris management 3753
in amoebiasis 832
benign intracranial hypertension due to
4042
bone mineralization rate estimation 3323
in brucellosis 623
in chlamydial infections 757
in cholera 579
in lymphogranuloma venereum 761
in malaria 853
in *Mycoplasma pneumoniae* infection
766
Neisseria gonorrhoeae resistance 549
nephrotoxicity **3264**, *3284*
ophthalmia neonatorum prophylaxis 1790
in pregnancy 1745, 1784
in recurrent oral ulceration 1855
in relapsing fevers 696
in renal impairment 3272, 3288
resistance 757
in scrub typhus 741
tetraethyl lead 1084, 1092
poisoning 1109
tetrahydrobiopterin 1361, 1362
deficiency 1363
tetrahydrofolate (THF) *3487*, 3488
tetralogy of Fallot, *see* Fallot's tetralogy
tetranectin 3625
tetraplegia
in cerebral palsy **4120**
initial management 3896
respiratory complications 3898
tetrodotoxin 1142
poisoning 1142
textile dermatitis 3736–7
TFIID (TATA binding protein; TBP)
1558
Thai haemorrhagic fever 419
Thailand, north-east, sudden death in
3132
thalamic projections, spinothalamic tract
3939
thalamic stimulation 3946
thalamotomy 3945
thalamus **3860–1**
damage, memory impairment 3855
infarction/haemorrhage 3834, 3861
language and 3851
lesions and clinical aspects 3861
pain in 3942, 4340
somatosensory evoked potentials 3834
structure and function 3860
afferents 3860–1
efferents 3861
surgical lesions 3861
tumours 3834
mental disorders/symptoms in 4237
thalassaemia **3501–13**
α *3502*, **3508–11**
definition 3508–9
diagnosis 3512
distribution 3463, 3464, 3508
genotype/phenotype relations 3509
inheritance 3508–9
mental retardation in 3511, **4110**
molecular pathology 3509
in pregnancy 1761
traits 3511
ß 115, **3502–7**
clinical features 3504–6
diagnosis 3511, 3512
distribution 3463, 3464, 3502
haemoglobin C 3506
haemoglobin E 3463, 3506–7
heterozygous 3506
molecular pathology 3502–3
mutations 104
pathophysiology 3503–4
in pregnancy 1761
screening *133*

severe forms 3504–6
sickle-cell (HbS) *3463*, 3464, 3506
variants 3507–8
classification 3501–2
δß *3502*, **3507**, 3511–12
definition 3501–2
differential diagnosis 3511
γδß *3502*, **3507**
intermedia 3502, **3511**, 3513
iron-chelation therapy 3480–1, 3512
iron overload 3479–80, 3504, 3512
joint involvement 3005
laboratory diagnosis 3511–12
major 2020, 3502
inheritance 115
malaria resistance 840, *841*
minor 3502
ocular features 4195
pathophysiology 3509–10
pregnancy in **1761**
prevention 3512
treatment 3512–13
thalidomide 1809, 4112
thallium-201 2209
advantages 2209, 2326
angina investigation 2326
in cardiac sarcoidosis 2393, 2827
myocardial infarction scanning 2209,
2210–11, 2326
thallium 1113
absorption and half-life 1113
excretion 1113
mechanism of toxicity 1113
nephrotoxicity *3261*
neuropathy due to 4099–100
poisoning **1113–14**
Thayer and Martin medium 547
thelarche, isolated 1701
Thelazia callipaeda 954
thenar muscles
paralysis 4095
wasting 4095
theophylline
in chronic obstructive airways disease
2776
monitoring 1261
overdose/poisoning 1068
therapeutic drug monitoring **1260–1**,
1261
digitalis **2243–4**
in pregnancy 1813
reference range *4376*
therapeutic effects/process of drugs, *see*
under pharmacology
thermal injury, *see* burns
Thermoactinomyces vulgaris 2809
thermocoagulation
dorsal horn lesions 3945
in trigeminal neuralgia 3878
thermodilution, cardiac output
measurement 2222
thermogenic drugs, in obesity treatment
1312
thermography 2950
thermophilic actinomycetes 2809, 2811
thermoregulation 1180, 1182
after injury 1549
disorders in elderly **4346**
failure,
in erythroderma 3747
in skin disease 3708, 3717
in malnutrition 1286, *1290*
see also body temperature
theta waves 3830
thiabendazole
in hookworm infection 931
in strongyloidiasis 929
in toxocariasis 945
in trichinosis 941
thiacetazone
adverse reactions 658
in tuberculosis 655, *656*, 663
thiamine
branched chain α-keto dehydrogenase
and 1369
in branched chain ketoaciduria 1369
deficiency 3497
Korsakov's syndrome 4126, 4225

mental symptoms 4126, 4241
neuropathy 4100, 4127
in pregnancy 1767
Wernicke-Korsakoff syndrome 4126
see also beri beri
in pyruvate carboxylase deficiency 1352
in pyruvate dehydrogenase deficiency
1351
reference nutrient intake (RNI) 1268,
1269
supplements 4127
thiamine hydrochloride, in alcohol
withdrawal 4290
thiazide diuretics 2238
avoidance in cirrhosis 2091
contraindications 2540, *2541*
in heart failure 2238, 2239
in hypercalciuria 3255
hyperlipoproteinaemia induced by 1411
in hypertension 2539–40, *2541*
ß-blocker comparison 2539, 2540
in elderly 4343
lithium interaction 4251
low-dose 2539
mechanisms of action 2539
nephrotoxicity 3266
potassium loss 2239
side-effects 1719, 2539
sodium and water excretion 2238
thigh, injuries and pain **2996**
thinking, disorders of 4221–2
thin membrane nephropathy 3149,
3152–3
thiocyanate toxicity 1067
thiolase 83, 84
thiopentone, in hepatocellular failure
2109
thioridazine
indications and use 4251
in opiate detoxification 4291
side-effects 4252
thioxanthene, neuroleptic malignant
syndrome 1182
thirst
in chronic renal failure 3296
deficiency 1602–3, **3125–6**
in diabetes 1453
in heart failure 2240
osmoreceptors 1601, 3117
water homeostasis and 1601, 3116,
3117
Thomsen's disease, *see* myotonia
congenita
thoracentesis 2865
procedure and problems 2865
thoracic actinomycoses 682–3
thoracic aortic aneurysm, *see* aortic
aneurysms
thoracic cage
deformity, chest radiography 2179
disorders **2872–9**
spinal disorders **2872–5**
sternum and ribs **2875–6**
normal chest radiograph 2657
thoracic duct
chylous fluid leakage 2868
congenital absence 2868
rupture 2868
thoracic imaging **2652–66**
see also chest radiography; computed
tomography (CT); lung scans;
magnetic resonance imaging (MRI)
thoracic outlet compression **2366**
management 2375
thoracic outlet syndromes 4093
thoracic root pain, angina *vs* 2322
thoracic spine, traumatic injury
management 3897
thoracic trauma, *see* chest, trauma
thoracic vertebral pain 240–1
thoracoabdominal wall, effects of aircraft
pressure changes 1198
thoracoplasty **2875–6**
pathophysiology 2876
prognosis and treatment 2876
symptoms and signs 2876
thoracoscopy 2682, 2866
fibreoptic 2592

in lung cancer 2887
surgical, in empyema 2706
thoracostomy, tube 2924
thoracotomy, limited, in pericardial
tamponade 2478
thorax, 'frozen' 2799
thorium dioxide, *see* Thorotrast
Thorotrast 204
cholangiocarcinoma aetiology 2118
hepatocellular carcinoma aetiology
2116
thought(s), obsessional 4207
'thought broadcasting' 4221
'thought insertion' 4221
'thought withdrawal' 4221
Three Mile Island nuclear accident
1234
three-tube test 3843
threonine *1353*
threshold limit value (TLV) 1163
throat, sore, *see* sore throat
thrombapheresis 3695
thrombin 2301, **3622**
atherosclerotic plaque development
2293, 2294
generation 3620, 3621, 3646, 3663
inhibitors **3622–3**, 3673
in platelet activation 3614, 3617
protein C interaction 3623
time (TT) *3379*, 3628, 3654
in liver disease 3656
thromboangiitis obliterans, *see* Buerger's
disease
thrombocythaemia, primary (essential)
3439–40, 3635, 3668
thrombocytopenia 3630, 3774
in alcoholism 3685
alloimmune **3632**
neonatal/fetal **1764–5**, 3632
autoimmune (ITP) **3630–2**
autoantibodies in 163
chronic 3631, 3632
clinical findings 3630–1
differential diagnosis 3631
management 3631–2
in pregnancy **1764**, 3631, 3632
cardiopulmonary bypass causing 3634,
3660
in chickenpox 347
in chronic lymphocytic leukaemia
3420–1
classification *3630*
in dengue haemorrhagic fever 420
in DIC 1763, 3658
drug-induced immune 3632
excessive platelet consumption causing
3632–3
in haemolytic uraemic syndrome 3200
heparin-induced 3673
in hepatocellular failure 2102
in HIV infection 3631, 3632, 3680
immune-mediated 3020, **3630–2**
infections causing 3679
lumbar puncture hazard 3842
in malaria 845, 3680
in myelodysplastic syndromes 3426
neonatal 1764–5, 3631, 3632
platelet kinetic studies 3595
platelet transfusion 3695
in pre-eclampsia 1729
in pregnancy 1763
in renal disease 3634, 3682
in SLE 3020, 3681
spurious 3629
thrombopathic 3645
transient, to foods 3729
thrombocytopenic purpura
bruising in 3775
idiopathic (ITP), *see* thrombocytopenia,
autoimmune
reaction to foods 3729
thrombotic, *see* thrombotic
thrombocytopenic purpura
thrombocytosis
causes *3440*
in malignant disease 3678
in primary thrombocythaemia 3439
in Q fever 743

in rheumatoid arthritis 3681
in tumours *244*
thromboembolic disease, in aircraft crew
    and pilots 1200
thromboembolism 2641
    after hip replacement 2964
    in atrial fibrillation 2273
        cardioversion association 2273
    carotid arteries 3948
    coronary artery closure after angioplasty
        2350
    heart valve prostheses 2470
    in homocystinuria 3085
    in hypereosinophilic syndrome 3612
    management **3670–6**
    in nephrotic syndrome **3141–2**, 3668,
        3682
    oral contraceptives and 1724
    in polycythaemia vera 3432, 3433,
        3668
    in pregnancy **1741–3**
        diagnosis 1741
        prophylaxis 1743
        risk factors 1741
        treatment 1741–3
    in primary thrombocythaemia 3439
    in spinal cord injury 3899
    see also embolism; thrombosis
ß-thromboglobulin *3379*, 3615, 3616,
    3627
thrombolysis
    after cerebral emboli 3824–5
    endothelial cell function 2299
    thrombosis in myocardial infarction
        balance 2319, 2333
thrombolytic therapy **3670–1**, *3672*
    cerebral arterial emboli 3824
    complications 2526
    contraindications *2526*
    hazards 2341–2
    in ischaemia of limb 2371
    in myocardial infarction 2151, 2301,
        2336, **2340–4**, 3671
        age and gender 2341
        background to and trials 2340
        benefits 2336, 2340
        blood pressure and diabetes 2341
        choice of agent 2342
        coronary angioplasty with 2352
        dose regimens *3672*
        ECG and coronary opening/closing
            2333–4
        ECG criteria for 2340–1
        heparin benefits 2343–4
        large-scale clinical trials 22, 24, **28–9**,
            2340
        late, mechanisms 2340
        mortality comparisons 2342
        in prevention of 2348
        recanalization effects 2342
        risk differences with agents 2342–3
        time window for benefits 2340
        timing of 2336
    in pregnancy 1742
    in pulmonary embolism 2526
    see also anistreplase; fibrinolysis;
        streptokinase; tissue plasminogen
        activator (t-PA)
thrombomodulin 2290, 3623–4, 3626,
    3662
thrombophilia
    familial 3662, **3665–8**, 3670
    see also prethrombotic states
thrombophlebitis 3894
    migratory 3723, 3793
    pain in 2648
    superficial 2523
    transfusion-associated 3692
thromboplastin, release by pulmonary
    endothelial cells 2487
thromboplastin time, partial, *see* partial
    thromboplastin time (PTT)
thrombopoietin 3384, **3389**
thrombosis **3661–76**
    in atherosclerosis, *see* atherosclerosis
    in carotid artery atheroma 3948
    in cyanotic congenital heart disease
        2401

in DIC 3657
endothelial cell role in protection 2290,
    2296, 2362
eye in 4194
in situ, coronary artery closure after
    angioplasty 2350
    intestinal ischaemia due to 1994
    in ischaemic heart disease 2300, 2302,
        2305
    limb ischaemia due to 2363–4
    neonatal 1757
    pathogenesis **3662–4**
    prosthetic heart valve 2469, 2470
    in renal transplant recipients 3318
    in sickle-cell disease 3514–15
    vena cava 2523
    ventriculoatrial shunts 4115
    see also arterial thrombosis;
        prethrombotic states;
        thromboembolism; thrombus; venous
        thrombosis
Thrombosis in Myocardial Infarction trial
    (TIMI-1) 2342
thrombospondin 3616, 3625
    platelet binding 3614, 3615
thrombo test, in urticaria 3772
thrombotic microangiopathies **3632–3**
thrombotic thrombocytopenic purpura
    (TTP) 3292, *3548*, **3549**, **3632–3**
    causes 3197, 3198, 3549
    chronic relapsing forms 3549
    clinical features 3198–9, 3549, 3632
    haematological features 3549, 3633
    haemolytic uraemic syndrome *vs* 3196,
        3201
    intestinal ischaemia in 1995
    mental disorder/symptoms 4243
    pathogenesis 3633
    polyarteritis nodosa *vs* 3015
    in pregnancy 1763, 3549
    in SLE 4130
    treatment 3633
thromboxane 2294, 2298
    in ARDS pathogenesis 2855
    formation 158
thromboxane A$_2$, in platelet aggregation
    3617
thromboxane B$_2$, in sepsis and shock 293
thrombus **3661–2**
    atrial 2215, 2500
    endocardial 2390, 2397, 2398
    formation **3662–4**
    heart, *see* heart, thrombus
thrush, oral, *see* candidiasis, oral
Th (To) antibodies *3033*
thymectomy, in pregnancy 1766
thymidylate synthesis 3488, 3494
thymine 1386, 1387
thymoma 168, 2898–9
    diagnosis 4162
    management 4162
    in myasthenia gravis 4160–1, 4162
    prognosis 169
    red-cell aplasia and 3449
thymus
    abnormalities in myasthenia gravis
        4160–1
    computed tomography 2658
    cysts 2899
    enlargement 2898
    grafts 171
    hypoplasia (aplasia), *see* Di-George
        syndrome
    irradiation, thyroid cancer after 213
    lymphoma 2899
    normal 2898
    role in T-cell function 152
thyroglobulin 1604–5
    autoantibodies 1609
    defective synthesis *1567*, *1616*
    serum 1608, 1619, 1621
thyroglossal cyst 1610
thyroglossal duct 1603
thyroid-binding globulin, *see* thyroxine-
    binding globulin
thyroidectomy 1620
    hypoparathyroidism after 1633
    in MEN2A 1709

partial 1613
    in pregnancy 1749
thyroid gland **1603–17**
    adenoma, toxic solitary 1611–12, 1613
    autoantibodies 1609–10
    autoimmune diseases 1570–1, 1609–10,
        1615
        postpartum 1750
        in pregnancy 1749, 1750
    bone disease 3069
    cancer 1566, **1618–21**
        aetiology 213, 1569–70, 1618
        anaplastic carcinoma 1570, **1620–1**
        clinical presentation 1618
        epidemiology 213
        follicular carcinoma 1570, **1620**
        follow-up evaluation 1621
        Hürtle cell carcinoma 1620
        investigations 1618–19
        lymphoma **1621**
        metastases 1620
        papillary carcinoma 1569–70, 1618,
            1619–20
        prevalence 1618
        prognosis 1621
        staging investigations *236*
        see also thyroid gland, medullary
            carcinoma
    C-cells 1624
        hyperplasia 1568, 1709
    disorders **1610–17**
        in AIDS 1716–17
        cardiac manifestations 2394
        drug-induced **1717**
        eye in **4195–6**
        gastrointestinal motility disorder in
            1962
        haematological changes **3686**
        investigations 1607–10
        myasthenia and 4168
        myopathy in 4168
        postpartum 1750
        in pregnancy **1748–50**
        in sarcoidosis 1716
        in severely ill patients 1617
        see also hyperthyroidism;
            hypothyroidism
    embryological development 1603
    examination 1610
    function 1604–7
        regulation 1606
    function tests **1607–10**, 1618–19
        drugs affecting 1717
        in hyperthyroidism 1611
        in hypothyroidism 1615
        in non-thyroidal illness 1617
        in pregnancy 1717, 1748–9
    imaging 1608, 1619
    masses **2899**
    medullary carcinoma (MTC) 1568,
        1625, **1637**
        amyloid deposits 1518
        familial 1709
        in MEN 2 syndrome 1621, 1637, **1709**
        screening 1709, 1710
    nodules 1618
        cold (hypofunctioning) 1619
        hot (functioning) 1566, 1611–12, 1613
        investigations 1619
        pain 1612
        structure 1603–4
    thyroid hormones 1554, 1562
        actions 1606–7, 1626
        in anorexia nervosa 1297, 4214
        biosynthetic defects 1615, *1616*
        control of secretion 1564, 1606
        control of TSH secretion 1578
        deficiency, *see* hypothyroidism
        excess, *see* hyperthyroidism
        fetal production 1749
        in heart failure 2234
        in nephrotic syndrome 3144
        overdose/poisoning 1072
        peripheral effects 1609
        receptor (TR) 1554–5, 1561–2, 1578
            auxilary proteins (TRAP) 1607
            isoforms 1559, 1606–7
            mutations *1567*, 1573, 1617

resistance 1573, 1612, **1617**
response element (TRE) 1607
serum binding proteins 1519, 1554,
    1605
serum measurements 1607–8
synthesis and secretion 1604–5
transport and metabolism 1605–6
see also thyroxine (T$_4$); tri-
    iodothyronine (T$_3$)
thyroiditis 1612
    atrophic 1609, 1610, 1615
    autoimmune lymphocytic 1615
    Hashimoto's 1570–1, 1609, 1615
    mumps virus causing 373
    Riedel's 1615
    silent 1612
    subacute (granulomatous giant cell; de
        Quervain's) 1612, 1613, 1615
thyroid peroxidase 1604–5
    antibodies 1609–10
    mutations *1567*
thyroid stimulating hormone (TSH;
    thyrotrophin) 1555, 1556, 1564,
    1578–9, 1606
    actions 1579, 1605
    ß-subunit 1578
    deficiency 1583
    mutations *1567*, 1571
    pituitary adenoma secreting 1595,
        1612
    receptor 1555, 1556, *1560*, 1579
        autoantibodies 163, 1570, **1610**, 1611,
            1750
        blocking antibodies 1570, 1571, 1615
        defects *1567*, 1569
        reference range *4367*
    regulation of secretion 1578–9, 1606
    serum 1566, 1583–4, 1608–9
        combined anterior pituitary test 1585
        TSH-secreting adenoma 1595
thyroid stimulating immunoglobulins
    (TSIG) 1570, 1579, 1611
thyroid storm 1614
thyrotoxic crisis 1614
thyrotoxicosis **1610–14**
    bone disease in 3069
    exogenous 1612
    factitia 1612, 1717
    myopathy in 4168
    neurological features 4125
    see also hyperthyroidism
thyrotoxic periodic paralysis 4168
thyrotrophin, *see* thyroid stimulating
    hormone
thyrotrophin releasing hormone (TRH)
    1554, 1564, 1606
    combined anterior pituitary test 1585
    control of TSH secretion 1578
    prolactin secretion and 1576
    receptor signalling pathway *1560*, *1561*
    stimulation test 1564, 1579
        in pituitary disease 1584, 1595, 1596
        in thyroid disease 1608–9
thyrotrophs 1575, 1578
    adenoma 1595
thyroxine (T$_4$)
    control of TSH secretion 1578
    effect on bone 3059
    elevated levels, in euthyroid patients
        1612
    in nephrotic syndrome 3144
    overdose/poisoning **1072**
    serum binding proteins 1554, 1605
    serum measurements 1607–8, 1617
    synthesis and secretion 1605
    transport and metabolism 1605–6
    treatment,
        in antithyroid-treated hyperthyroidism
            1612
        in hypothyroidism 1587, 1616, 1698
        in obesity 1312
        in pregnancy 1749
        in thyroid cancer 1621
thyroxine-binding globulin 1554, 1605,
    1607, 1717
    in nephrotic syndrome 3144
tiaprofenic acid, poisoning 1056
tibialis anterior syndrome **4159**

tibial nerve **4097–8**
  lesions/injuries 4097–8
tibolone 1814
tic douloureux 3878
tick-borne encephalitis 414, **416–17**
tick-borne (endemic) relapsing fevers **693**
  louse-borne relapsing fever *vs* 695
  see also relapsing fevers
tick-borne spirochaetosis 689
tick-borne spotted-fevers 734–6, 736
tick paralysis 1149
ticks **1149**
  Babesia transmission 863, 864
  Boutonneuse fever transmission 734
  control and repellents 697, 733
  ehrlichial diseases transmission 738
  Lyme disease transmission 690
  removal method 733
  rickettsial diseases transmission 730
  Rickettsia rickettsii relationship 735
  tularaemia (*Francisella tularensis*)
    spread 604, 605
  venomous **1149**
ticlopidine 3671
tics 3919, **4016–17**
  causes *4011*
  complex 4016
  definition 4010
  Gilles de la Tourette syndrome
    4016–17
  psychic 4016
  simple motor 4016
tidal volume, ventilation parameter 2921
Tielz's syndrome, depigmentation in
    3759
tienilic acid
  anti-LKM antibodies 2072
  hepatitis due to 2125
Tietze's syndrome 2168, 3007
  myocardial infarction *vs* 2335
  pain in 2648
tight junctions 301, 1900, 2289
  alveolar epithelium 2494, 2593
  endothelial cells 2290
  pulmonary 2486
tilt, effect on noradrenaline 3885
tilt-testing, head-up 2286
TIMI-1 (Thrombosis in Myocardial
    Infarction) trial 2342
timolol
  airway obstruction and asthma 2849
  enantiomers 1248
tinea
  capitis 798, 3718, 3762
  corporis 797, 798
  cruris 798
  imbricata (tokelau) 798
  incognito 798
  nigra 801, *3755*
  pedis (athlete's foot) 797, 798
    occupational dermatosis 1165
  unguium 3761
  versicolor (pityriasis versicolor) **799**,
    3754, *3755*, 3757
Tinel's sign 1226, 2957
Tine test 645
tinidazole, in amoebiasis 831
tinnitus 1224
  in Menière's disease 3875
tin-protoporphyrin 1393
'tired all the time' (TAT) 1036
tissue
  damage,
    crystal-induced 2983–4
    inflammation due to 290
  electric injury 1211–12
  necrosis,
    in Boutonneuse fever 734
    caseous 639, 640
    hydrogen fluoride (hydrofluoric acid)
      1099
    in pyoderma gangrenosum 3778
    snake bites 1130, 1131, 1133, 1139
  perfusion, in anaemia 3457–8
  remodelling, alveolar macrophage role
    2615
  repair and recovery 1550

typing,
  renal transplantation **3315–16**
  see also HLA antigens, matching
tissue-factor pathway inhibitor (TFPI)
    3621, 3663
tissue-factor (thromboplastin) 3619,
    3620, 3627, 3663
tissue plasminogen activator (t-PA) 2299,
    3624, 3625, 3626, 3662
  accelerated regimen 2342, 2343
  comparisons and trials 2342
  excessive production 3659
  excess stroke with 2342
  GUSTO trial, *see* GUSTO trial
  heparin with 2343
  in myocardial infarction 2342
  recanalization effects 2342
  reduced vascular release 3667
  therapeutic use 2342, 3671, *3672*
tissue-specific element (TSE) 1558
titratable acidity 3338
titubation 4012
T-lymphocytes, *see* T-cells
T lymphocytosis with cytopenia 3387
TNM staging/classification 234–8, 245–7
  aims and basis 235
  colorectal carcinoma 1991
  definitions 235, 246–7
  lung cancer 2885, *2885*, *2889*
  M staging, methods/aims 237–8, 246
  N staging, methods/aims 237, 246
  T staging, methods/aims 236–7, 245–6
toads, poisonous 1140
tobacco
  cadmium source 1106
  chewing, oral and pharyngeal cancer
    201
  lung cancer and 2879–80
  smoke, indoor air pollution 1230
  withdrawal syndrome **4293**
  see also smoking
tobacco-alcohol amblyopia 4127, 4278
tobramycin *3272*
  nephrotoxicity 3264
  in urinary-tract infections *3211*
tobulinum toxin 632
tocainide 4153
  overdose/poisoning 1064
tocolytic therapy 1786
toenails, care 2369, 3810
toes
  hammer 1489, 1490
  monophalangic 3061
  in myositis ossificans progressiva 3093
togaviruses **407–12**
  see also rubella virus
tokelau (tinea imbricata) 798
Token Test 3849
tolazamide *1471*
tolbutamide 1470, 1471
  stimulation test 1508
tolerance
  to drugs 1250–1, **4263**
  immune, *see* immunological tolerance
tolfenamic acid, poisoning 1056–7
tolmetin, poisoning 1056
Tolosa-Hunt syndrome 3877
tolrestat 1472
toluene
  metabolism 1089
  poisoning **1089**, 1092
tomography 3816–17
  see also computed tomography (CT);
    positron emission tomography (PET)
tone decay, tests 3870
Tone-Muir syndrome 3792
tongue
  in blood disorders 1863
  cancer 201, 1860, 1861
  discoloration in vanadium poisoning
    1114
  erythema migrans 1864
  geographical 1864
  leucoplakia 1859
  strawberry/raspberry 499
  ulceration 2971
tongue worms **1012–14**

tonic-clonic seizure, *see under* epileptic
    seizures
tonsillitis
  adenoviruses causing 337
  chronic, halitosis in 1864
  streptococcal group A infection 498–9
tonsils 2611
  absence 166
  in malnutrition 1284
tonus imbalance 3871
toothache 1846
  differential diagnosis 1847
tophi 2984, 2985, 2986–7
topical agents, skin disease management
    3805, *3805*
topographical memory, defective 3853
topoisomerase inhibitors 259
  type I 259
  type II 259
TORCH screen 1778
Torkildsen shunt 4115
tornadoes 1232
Torre-Muir syndrome *3795*
torsade de pointes 2279, **2282–3**
  in antiarrhythmic drug overdose 1063
  electrocardiogram (ECG) 2199
  management 2283
  see also long QT syndrome
torsion dystonia, causes *4011*
torticollis, spasmodic **4018**
tortoises, zoonoses transmitted from
    1014
Torulopsis glabrata 3356
total anomalous pulmonary venous
    drainage (TAPVD) **2415–16**
total-body irradiation (TBI) **1218–19**,
    1218–19
  contraindications 3699
  exposure level and risks 1220
  long-term effects 3699
  marrow transplant conditioning 3696–7
total body potassium 1303, 3127
total body water, *see* water, total body
total iron-binding capacity (TIBC) 1071,
    2960, *3379*, 3472
  saturation 3473, *3474*
  serum *3473*, *3474*
total lung capacity (TLC), *see under* lung
total parenteral nutrition (TPN), *see*
    parenteral nutrition
touch, sensation 3857
tourniquet, snake bites and 1135
tourniquet (Hess) test 3628
toxaemia of pregnancy, *see* pre-
    eclampsia
toxic epidermal necrolysis 3781
toxic nephropathy **3258–67**
  clinical syndromes 3259–60
  factors affecting susceptibility 3258
  pathogenesis 3258–9, 3260
  prevalence 3258
  prevention 3260
toxic neuropathy **4099–100**
'toxic oil syndrome' 1233, 3612
toxic shock-like illness, streptococcal,
    diagnosis 502
toxic shock syndrome 293, 530
  clinical features and diagnosis 530
  exotoxin, Kawasaki disease aetiology
    3049
  in malnutrition 1288, 1289
  management 530, 1289
  menstruation association 530
  scarlet fever *vs* 502
toxic shock syndrome toxin (TSST-1)
    524, 530
toxins 2001–2
  acute renal failure due to *3289*
  bacterial,
    exotoxin 554
    production 272
    see also endotoxin
  diabetes type I and 1454
  endocellular/exocellular 272
  sideroblastic anaemia caused by 3523
Toxocara canis 944, 3917
Toxocara cati 944

toxocariasis **944–5**
  epilepsy after 3917
  ocular 945, 4192
  see also visceral larva migrans
Toxoplasma gondii 865, 1003
  detection 868
toxoplasmosis **865–9**
  acute acquired 866, 1034
  after lung transplantation 2936
  antibodies 865, 868
  cerebral, in HIV infection 475, 487, 867
  CNS 475, 487, 866, 867
  congenital 865–6, **867–9**, 1794, 3680,
    4112, 4192
    haemolytic anaemia 3545
    transmission 867
    treatment 869
  epidemiology and transmission 865–6,
    867
  in heart-lung transplants 2709
  in HIV infection 472, 476, 478, 487,
    4077, **4078**, 4194
    treatment 478, 4078
  in immunocompromised 1034
  immunodeficiency and 866–7
  jaundice in 2134
  laboratory/serological diagnosis 868
  liver in 2134
  myositis in 4156
  ocular 866, 4192
  in pregnancy **1793–4**
  treatment 869
trace elements **1415–25**
  absorption 1903
  in body 1415–16
  cell damage and 1416
  deficiency *1418*
    enteral feeding complication 1321
    parenteral nutrition complication
      1321
  disorders of 1416–25
  in erythropoiesis 3454
  normal range *4372*
  renal bone disease and 3327
  requirements, artificial nutritional
    support 1318, *1318*
  toxicity *1417*
trachea 2629
  abnormalities, airway obstruction in
    2723–4
  compression 2723
  inflammation, pain in 2648
  normal chest radiograph 2656, 2658
  obstruction 2719
  'scabbard' 2723
  stenosis 2723
  see also airways
tracheobronchitis 2691
tracheobronchomegaly 2724
tracheobronchopathia
  osteochondroplastica 2724
tracheomalacia 2723
tracheo-oesophageal fistula **1973–4**
  embryology 1973
tracheostomy 2577, 2581, **2918**
  closure 2581
  in diphtheria 495
  in tetanus 629
  weaning from ventilators 2581
trachoma 748, **4191**
  blindness in **4198**
  clinical features 750, 4191
  diagnosis and treatment 751, *758*,
    4191
  epidemiology and transmission 750–1
  pathogenesis 758
  protective immunity 759
  see also chlamydial infections;
    Chlamydia trachomatis
tracking, in injecting drug abuse 4282
track marks, in injecting drug abuse 4282
traction lesions, brachial plexus 4093
training
  for artificial nutrition at home 1324
  in control of sexually transmitted
    diseases 3349
  effect on heart **2161–2**

safety 1179–80
see also education
TRAM (membrane-spanning protein) 69
tranexamic acid 3659
in von Willebrand's disease 3645
tranquillizers
in alcohol withdrawal 4259
in anorexia nervosa 4214
major 4251–3
in renal impairment 3273
minor, in renal impairment 3273
in pain treatment 3945
poisoning 1060–1
sexual problems associated *4245*
see also benzodiazepines
transaminases
in biliary disease 2046
in hepatitis B 2062
in ulcerative colitis 1947, 1948
see also alanine aminotransferase (ALT);
aspartate aminotransferase (AST)
transbronchial biopsy **2680**
applications 2683
in lung cancer 2887
transbronchial needle aspiration **2680–1**
transcatheter arterial embolization (TAE),
in hepatocellular carcinoma 2117–18
transcobalamin (TC) I 3486, 3495
transcobalamin (TC) II 3485, 3486, 3495
congenital deficiency 3497
deficiency, secondary
immunodeficiency in 174
transcobalamin (TC) III 3486, 3495
transcription 57, 57–9
hormone genes 1557–60
post-transcriptional modification 57–9,
63
regulation 57, 225, 1562
transcription activating factors (TAFs)
1558
transcription factors 223
in cardiac hypertrophy 2147
endocrine genes 1557–8
general 1558
genes encoding 106, 107
inhibitors 226
in leukaemia 3396, 3411
mutations 1571
nuclear oncogenes as 225
phosphorylation 1558, 1560
transcutaneous electrical stimulation
(TENS) 3943–4
transcytosis 2290
transdermal formulations 1238
transducers 1956
strain-gauge 1956
transendothelial diapedesis 87, 88
trans fatty acids 1330, 2311
transferrin 3471, 3472
in aluminium poisoning 1105
in nephrotic syndrome 3141, 3143–4
receptors 3472
endocytic pathway 73
serum 3472, *3474*, 3475
serum *3379*, 3472
transfer RNA (tRNA) 59
transformation, bacterial 60
transformation of cells 195, 222
growth factor importance 223
mechanisms 65–6, 462
see also retroviruses
transforming growth factor-α (TGF-α),
tumours secreting 1712
transforming growth factor-ß (TGF-ß)
97, 2293, 2299
in atherosclerotic plaque development
2293, 2299
in bone formation 3056
in cryptogenic fibrosing alveolitis 2789
hepatic granulomas pathogenesis 2120
macrophage deactivation 89
secretion 2293
transgenic animals 112
growth factor expression deregulation
223
transgenic mice 62
pancreatic carcinoma 2040, 2041

prion protein (PrP) transmission 3978,
3979
*trans*Golgi network 72
function and mechanism 71
transient expression systems 61
transient ischaemic attack (TIA) 3918,
3948–54
causes 3948–50
arterial disease 3950, *3950*
atherothromboembolism 3947–8,
3949
in cholesterol embolism 2376, 3952
clinical features 2367, 3950–1
see also amaurosis fugax
definition 3946
differential diagnosis 3951
investigations 3952, *3953*
ECG 3830, 3952
imaging 3952, 3953
management 2373
pathogenesis 3950
signs 3951–2
stroke risk 3952
treatment,
medical 3952–4
surgical 3954
transitional epithelial cells, urinary casts
3105
transjugular intrahepatic portosystemic
stent shunt (TIPSS) 2095
translation 57, 58, 59
cotranslational translocation of peptides
68
preprohormones 1557, 1559
protein modification after 57, 59, 68,
1557, 1559–60
transmembrane proteins
in heart 2147
quality control of proteins 70
transmembrane receptors, in heart **2147**
transoesophageal echocardiography, *see
under* echocardiography
transplantation
artificial nutritional support 1323
bone marrow, *see* bone marrow
transplantation
brain death diagnosis and guidelines
3934, 4311
Code of Practice over organs 4310,
4311
cytomegalovirus (CMV) infection 360,
361
donor cards 4311
donors, *see* donors, organ
Epstein-Barr virus infections in
recipients 355
ethical issues 13–14
fetal cells 14
haemolytic uraemic syndrome
complicating 3197–8
heart, *see* cardiac transplantation
heart-lung, *see* heart-lung
transplantation
human herpesvirus 6 (HHV-6) infection
364
Human Tissue Act (1961) and **4310–11**
islet 185, 1478, 3172
liver, *see* liver transplantation
living donor material 3313, 3316, **3317,**
4311
lung, *see* lung transplantation
opportunistic fungal infections 806
pancreas 185, 1478, 3172, 3315
Pneumocystis carinii pneumonia
treatment 823
rejection, *see* graft rejection
renal, *see* renal transplantation
respiratory tract infections after
2709–10
successes and reasons for 182
terminology *183*
toxoplasmosis in recipients 867
*see also specific organs/transplantation
procedures*
transplantation immunology **182–8**
effector arm of immune response **186–8**
cytokines 187

non-specific response 186, 187
specific cellular response 186–7
specific humoral response 186, 187
target 187
see also T-cells
factors determining immune response
183
graft tolerance, mechanisms 183, 187
induction phase of immune response
183–6
antigen-presenting cells in 183, 184–5
genetic control 186
MHC antigens 183–5
minor histocompatibility antigens 185
privileged sites/tissue 185–6
site of sensitization 185
see also major histocompatibility
complex (MHC)
recipient unresponsiveness 183, 187
see also graft rejection
transport, of nutrients 1900
transportation and coronary artery
disease **2358–61**
air, *see* aircrew/pilots
lifeboat staff 2360–1
railway 2361
road, *see* driving
sea 2360
transport vesicles 75
see also vesicles; vesicular transport
transposable elements 108
transposition of great arteries 2181,
2416–17
corrected malposition 2418
corrected with ventricular arterial
discordance 2404, **2417–18**
cyanosis in 2402
Fallot's tetralogy *vs* 2404–5
magnetic resonance imaging 2214
trans-sulphuration pathway 1365, 1366
transtentorial herniation 3954, 3955
transthyretin (TTR) **1519**, 1605
amyloid formation 1515, 1517, 1519,
1524
Met30 variant 1516, 1517, 1519
transtracheal aspiration 519, 2698
fluids, microbiological testing 2675
transvascular fluid dynamics, pulmonary
endothelium 2492–4
transverse myelitis **3991**
tranylcypromine, indications and use
4249
trapezius, paralysis 3880
trasylol 3772
trauma
blindness due to 4197
C-reactive protein 1531
epilepsy after 3916
hereditary angio-oedema attacks 3772
infection susceptibility 281
injecting drug abusers 4282–3
limb ischaemia due to 2364
mechanical, to red cells 3525, 3547
metabolic effects **1548–50**
neuroendocrine response 1548–9
osteoporosis after immobility and
3068–9
psychiatric emergencies in victims
4257–8
renal 3111
spinal, root lesions 3903
spinal cord injury, *see under* spinal cord
splenic 3591, 3595
thromboembolism after 3668
travel, air, *see* aircraft; aircrew/pilots
travel history, in infections 266
in immunocompromised 1029
travellers **322–7**
amoebiasis prevention 833
cirrhosis and 2091
diarrhoea causes 326, 2003
eosinophilia causes *326*, 327
extremes of age **325**
fever causes *326*
hepatitis A prophylaxis 450–1, *450*
immunizations **323–4**, *323*

immunocompromised **325**
malaria prevention **324**, 860–1
occupational infections 1173
pregnancy and **325**
pretravel advice **322**
on health 322
problems of returning travellers **326–7**
rabies vaccination/prevention 402–3
scrub typhus prevention 741
skin rash causes *326*
tropical sprue 1933, 1936
travellers' diarrhoea **324–5**, 556, 2003
causes 324, 2003
Cryptosporidium causing 872
enterotoxigenic *E. coli* (ETEC) causing
556
prevention 2003, 2007
treatment 325
travel medicine **322–7**
trazodone 4248
treadmill 2226, 2326, 2672
treatment refusal 4257
trehalase, deficiency 1923
trehalose, intolerance *1922*
Treitz, ligament, biopsy in coeliac
disease 1918
trematodes **970–1000**
diarrhoea in 2004
infection in eye 4193
intestinal **992–9**, *994–5*
see also liver fluke diseases;
paragonimiasis; schistosomiasis
tremor 3863, **4010–12**
benign essential (familial) 4010,
4012
differential diagnosis 4002
causes *4009*
definition 4009
drug-induced 4020
essential 4012
flapping, *see* flapping tremor
in Friedreich's ataxia 3984
head 4012
intention 3860, *4009*
neuropathic 4091
in Parkinson's disease 3863, 4000–1
postural 3860, *4009*, 4092
rest *4009*
'rubral' (midbrain) 3860
trench fever *729, 745,* **747–8**
trench foot 1183
trench mouth, *see* Vincent's disease
trench nephritis 506
Treponema, Borrelia comparison 707,
707
Treponema balanitides 706
Treponema carateum 703, *704*
Treponema pallidum 703, *704,* 706,
4084
adaptive theory and origin 707
antigens 716, *716*
characteristics 707, *707*
dark-field microscopy 714
flagella antigen and antibodies to 707
in gumma 712
haemagglutination antibody (TPHA)
test 715, *715,* 1791, 4085
infection route and course 709–10
infectivity and infective dose 707
serological tests 715–17, *715*
see also syphilis
Treponema pallidum-like forms 714
persistence 709
Treponema pertenue 703, *704*
Treponema vincentii 692, 1852
treponemes
non-pathogenic 706
non-venereal **703–6**, *704*, 706
see also pinta; syphilis, endemic (non-
venereal); yaws
venereal, *see Treponema pallidum*
Treppe effect 2158
TRH, *see* thyrotrophin releasing hormone
(TRH)
triacylglycerol, *see* triglyceride
trials, *see* clinical trials
triamcinolone 3745

triamterene 3337
  mechanism of action and side-effects
    2239
  urinary stones 3251
triatomine bugs 895, 898, 899, 1006
triazine herbicides **1122**
tribavirin, *see* ribavirin
tricarboxylic acid (TCA) cycle 1272,
  2146
  in cyanide toxicity 1097
trichiasis, in trachoma 750
Trichinella spiralis 940, 2004
trichinosis **940–1**
  eye in 4193
  myositis 4155
trichloracetyl acid chloride 1088
trichloroacetic acid 1089
1,1,1-trichloroethane (methyl
  chloroform), poisoning **1089**
trichloroethylene 4100
  mechanisms of toxicity 1089
  poisoning **1089–90**
trichloroethylene epoxide 1089
trichloromethane, *see* chloroform
trichloromethyl free radical 1084
Trichomonas tenax 907
Trichomonas vaginalis 907, 908, 3354
  characteristics 907
  culture 3354
  in pregnancy 1785
trichomoniasis **907–9**, **3354–5**, *3356*
  clinical features and diagnosis 908,
    3354
  epidemiology and transmission 908,
    3354
  pathology 907, 3354
  in pregnancy 1785, 3354
  treatment *3356*
Trichophyton concentricum 797, 798
Trichophyton interdigitale 798
Trichophyton rubrum 797, 798
Trichophyton verrucosum 3800
Trichophyton violaceum 797, 3762
trichorrhexis nodosa 1358
Trichostrongylus 932
trichothecenes 1158
trichotillomania 3763
trichuriasis **942–4**
Trichuris trichiura 942, 943
triclabendazole 987
triclofos, overdose/poisoning 1061
tricuspid atresia **2412–13**
  magnetic resonance imaging 2214,
    2215
  signs and symptoms 2412–13
  treatment 2413
tricuspid regurgitation **2468–9**, 2480
  in carcinoid heart disease 2469
  causes 2468, *2468*
  Doppler echocardiography 2203
  in Ebstein's anomaly 2413
  liver in 2130, 2468–9
  mitral regurgitation *vs* 2461
  in pulmonary hypertension 2468,
    2510
  in transposition of great arteries 2416
tricuspid valve
  calcification 2399
  in carcinoid heart disease 2469
  disease **2467–9**
  in Ebstein's anomaly 2413
  excision, in infective endocarditis 2449
  infective endocarditis 2445
  prolapse 2468
  repair 2468
  replacement 2468, 2469
  in rheumatic fever 2432
  stenosis **2467–8**
  in transposition of great arteries 2416
tricyclic antidepressants 4247–8
  as antianxiety agents 4253
  in central sleep apnoea and
    hypoventilation 2918
  childhood poisoning 1044
  in chronic benign pain, in terminal care
    4352
  in depressive disorders 4220, 4248
  drug interactions 4248

drugs included 4248
  indications and use 4248
  mechanism of action 4247–8
  pharmacology 4247–8
  poisoning 1058–9
    benzodiazepine overdose with 1059
    clinical features 1045, 1058–9
    indication for gastric emptying 1049
    reasons for high incidence 1058
    treatment 1059
  side-effects 4248, *4248*
    anticholinergic 4248
  therapeutic effects through adaptation
    1250
trientine (triethylene tetramine) 1422,
  1423, 2023
triethylene tetramine (trientine) 1422,
  1423, 2023
trigeminal nerve **3877–8**
  afferent fibres 3857
  anatomy 3877
  headache mechanisms 4022
  in intracranial tumours 4036
  lesions 3878
  in Sturge-Weber syndrome 3785
  in zoster 349
trigeminal neuralgia 345, **3878**, 4023–4
trigeminal neuropathy **3878**
trigeminovascular reflex 4023–4
'trigger finger' 2957
triglycerides (triacylglycerols) **1399–400**,
  1457
  absorption and digestion 1903, 1913
  in ascites 2096, 2098
  energy source/supply 1271, 1272
  ischaemic heart disease risk 2308
  medium-chain 2038
    in ascites 2098
    in small-intestinal lymphangiectasia
      1977
  metabolism 1276
    energy for heart 2146
  serum,
    in diabetes *1466*
    in nephrotic syndrome 3142–3
    normal values 1405
    in pregnancy 1753
    see also hypertriglyceridaemia
  synthesis 2146–7
  transport 1277, 1401–3
  utilization 1277
tri-iodothyronine (T$_3$)
  actions 1606–7
  in anorexia nervosa 4214
  control of TSH secretion 1578
  in nephrotic syndrome 3144
  overdose/poisoning **1072**
  reverse 1605, 1617
  serum binding proteins 1554
  serum measurements 1607–8, 1617
  synthesis and secretion 1605
  toxicosis 1611
  transport and metabolism 1605–6
  treatment, myxoedema coma 1616
trilostane 1651
trimethadione 3266
trimethoprim
  folate deficiency due to 3493, 3497
  Pneumocystis carinii pneumonia 822
  in pregnancy 1733
  in renal impairment 3272
  in urinary-tract infections 3209, 3211,
    3213
trimethoprim-sulphamethoxazole, in
  systemic vasculitis 3016
trinucleotide repeats, unstable 108, 124–7
  diseases with *125*
triokinase 1345
triorthocresyl phosphate, neuropathy due
  to 4100
triosephosphate isomerase deficiency
  3536
triperidol, overdose/poisoning 1061
triple X syndrome, chromosomal
  abnormality *120*
tripotassium dicitartobismuthate (bismuth
  chelate), poisoning 1069
trishydroxyaminomethane (THAM) 1544

trismus 625
trisomies 118, 121, 4109
  rescue 128
  X or Y chromosomes 121, *121*
trisomy 8 4109
trisomy 9p 4109
trisomy 13 121, 4109
trisomy 16 127, 128
trisomy 18 121, 4109
trisomy 21, *see* Down's syndrome
trisomy 22 4109
trituration 1955
trochlear (fourth cranial) nerve, lesions
  3877
Tropheryma whippelii 274, *561*, 1924,
  2005
'trophic changes', in polyneuropathies
  4092
trophoblastic disease, hyperthyroidism in
  1612, 1613, 1749
trophozoites 878
  Entamoeba histolytica 825, 826, 830
tropical ataxic myelopathy 490
tropical enteropathy **1931–2**
  sprue 1933
tropical malabsorption **1930–6**, *1930*
  non-specific causes **1931–6**
    see also tropical enteropathy; tropical
      sprue
  'post-infective' 1932
  specific causes **1930–1**
    infections 1930, *1930*
tropical pulmonary eosinophilia 919,
  923, **2806**, 3685
  pulmonary hypertension in 2509
tropical pyomyositis **4174–5**
tropical spastic paraparesis, HTLV-I
  association 490, 3995
tropical splenomegaly syndrome 844,
  845, 847, **857–8**, **3591**, 3680
  diagnosis and treatment 857–8
  pathophysiology and features 857,
    3591
tropical sprue **1932–6**, 2003
  aetiopathogenesis 1934–5
    model 1934, 1935
  clinical features 1933
  coeliac disease *vs* 1919
  definition 1932
  diagnosis 1935
  epidemiology 1932–3
  folate deficiency 3492
  gut hormones in 1895, 1934
  historical aspects 1932
  'latent' 1933
  malabsorption in 1934, 1935
  pathology and pathophysiology 1933–4
  treatment and prevention 1936
  vitamin B$_{12}$ deficiency 3491
tropical ulcers, yaws and endemic
  syphilis *vs* 705
tropomyosin 4141
  mutations 2385
troponin 2144, 4141
troponin-C (TN-C) 2144, 2147
troponin-I 2144, 2147
Trousseau's sign 1633, 3061, 3723
Trucut needle 2682
truncus arteriosus **2431**
Trypanosoma brucei 888
Trypanosoma brucei gambiense 888, 889
Trypanosoma brucei rhodesiense 888,
  889
  epidemic 889
Trypanosoma cruzi 895, 1794, 1962,
  2004
  lifecycle 895
  see also Chagas' disease
Trypanosoma rangeli 898, **899**
trypanosomiasis
  African, *see* African trypanosomiasis
  American, *see* Chagas' disease
trypsin
  in acute pancreatitis 2029
  immunoreactive 2750, *4366*
trypsinogen activation peptide (TAP)
  2029, 2031
  deficiency 2039

tryptophan
  eosinophilia-myalgia syndrome due to
    3612
  serotonin synthesis 1897, 1898
  therapy 1368
tryptophan hydroxylase 1362, 1363
tsetse flies 888, 1011
  eradication 894
TSH, *see* thyroid stimulating hormone
Tsutsugamushi fever, *see* scrub typhus
T-system 4139
T-tubules 2145
tuberculin
  purified protein derivative (PPD) 645
  sensitivity reduced in sarcoidosis 2819
tuberculin test 640, 645, 3276
  in developing countries 662, 663
  interpretation 645–6
  negative, BCG vaccination 647, 648
  reaction 165
  in tuberculous meningitis 4062
  see also Heaf test; Mantoux test
tuberculoma 474, 640, 649
  acute neurological syndromes in
    immunocompromised 1033
  in tuberculous meningitis 4062
tuberculosis **638–64**
  abdominal 653–4
  Addison's disease 1652, 1655, 1656
  in AIDS, *see under* AIDS and HIV
    infection
  allergic manifestations 648
  arthritis in 2998
  bone and joints 653, 654
  bronchoalveolar lavage and biopsy 2684
  case-finding (active) and contacts
    646–7, 662
  chemoprophylaxis **647–8**
    in developing countries 663–4
    secondary 647
  chemotherapy,
    adverse reactions 657–8, *657*
    in developing countries 663
    drug dosages *656*
    drugs **655–61**, *656*
    hypersensitivity reactions 658
    in impaired renal/hepatic function 660
    intermittent 659, 660
    mechanism of action 296, 658–9
    in meningitis 4062–3
    newly diagnosed patients 659–60
    in pregnancy/lactation 660
    primary chemotherapy failures/
      relapses 660
    regimens **659–61**, *659*, 660
    scientific basis 658–9
  in children 653, 664
  clinical bacteriology **641–3**, 662
    specimen collection 641
  clinical course **648–51**
  coal-worker's pneumoconiosis and 2840
  congenital 1793
  control **646–8**, *646*
    in developing countries 661
  cough in 2643
  Crohn's disease *vs* 1941
  in cyanotic congenital heart disease
    2402
  in diabetes 1493
  diagnosis 648, 650–1
    in developing countries 662–3
  differential diagnosis 651
  drug resistance 480, 486, 642–3
    acquired, significance 643
    definitions for specific drugs *643*
    drug regimens 660
    initial, significance 642–3
    multidrug 652, 664
    prevention 659
    testing 642, 643
  empyema 2664, 2867
  epidemiology 295, **643–6**
    annual risk of infection 645–6
    impact of HIV on 473–4, 643–4
    infection relation with disease 643
    methods of assessing impact 644–6
    prevalence 645

eradication 661
fever and new pulmonary infiltrates 1033
genitourinary 653, **3275–9**, *3300*
 aetiology 3275
 investigation 3276–7
 pathogenesis 3276
 presentation 3276
 treatment 3277–9
glomerulonephritis complicating 3175
granulomas in 639, 650, 3800
haematological changes 3679, 3684
haemoptysis in 2644
hepatic granulomas in 2121, 2133
in HIV infection, *see* AIDS and HIV infection
immune responses **639–40**
 macrophage activation 640
immunosuppression and 641
intestinal **2004–5**, *2004*
liver in 2133
lupus vulgaris (skin lesions) 654, 3794, 3800, *3801*
lymphadenitis 474
lymph-node 652–3
lymphogranuloma venereum *vs* 761
in malnutrition 1288
meningitis, *see* meningitis, tuberculous
microtubercles, meningitis 4060
miliary 650, 651
 chest radiography 2663–4
morbidity-notification 474, 644–6
 in Westernized countries 645
mortality 267, 644, 651
multidrug-resistant 652, 664
myelosclerosis in 3438–9
myositis in 4155
neonatal 1793
non-respiratory **652–4**, *653*
notification 474, 644–6
ocular 4191
oral manifestations 1853
outcome 651
in paracoccidioidomycosis 818
pathology **639**, 640
pericarditis 654
peritonitis 2005, 2009
pneumococcal infections *vs* 517
postprimary 640–1, **649–51**
 complications 651
 diagnosis 650–1
in pregnancy 1746, **1792–3**
primary **648–9**
pulmonary 649, 2707–8
reactivation 474, 641, 649
in renal transplant recipients 3314
spinal, *see* Pott's disease
spread and routes of 649
transmission 648
treatment **652**, 2123
 in developing countries 663
 in HIV infection 480–1, 660–1
 see also tuberculosis, chemotherapy
urinary-tract obstruction 3179, 3276, 3277, 3278, 3279
see also Mycobacterium tuberculosis
tuberculostearic acid 4062
tuberous sclerosis (Bourneville's disease, epiloia) 3792, **3987**
 depigmentation in 3759, 3760
 lung in 2651, 2861
tubulin 80, 81, 82
tularaemia **599–605**, 1173
 abdominal 601
 clinical presentations 599–601, *600*, 601–3
 contact *vs* airborne outbreaks *602*
 diagnosis 603–4, *603*
 epidemiology 604–5
 generalized 602
 hepatic granulomas in 2121
 oculoglandular 600–1
 oral-tonsillar 601–2
 prevention and vaccine 605
 pulmonary 601
 treatment 603
 ulcero-cutanoglandular 601

ulceroglandular 599–600, 602
 see also Francisella tularensis
tum antigens 228
Tumbu fly 1000–1
tumorigenesis
 in endocrine neoplasia 1568–9
 multistep, thyroid gland 1569–70
 see also cancer; carcinogenesis
tumour(s)
 cell line establishment 228
 cell multiplication, *see* cell multiplication
 clinical features, *see under* cancer
 clonal origin, evidence 192
 dedifferentiation 195, 196
 definition 191
 development in immunosuppression 216, 227, 3792
 ectopic hormone production 1566–8, 1711–12
 histopathology 195
 HLA allele loss 260
 hypoglycaemia-inducing 1714
 identification, antibodies in tumour typing 232, *232*
 lysis syndrome (acute uric acid nephropathy) 1379–80, 3185, 3226, 3290
 management, *see under* cancer
 mass, diagnosis/biopsy 241
 reversibility and suppression 193
 staging **242–7**
  notations/systems 246–7
  surgical 246
 staging by imaging 234–8
  rules/indications 234–5
  see also TNM staging
 viral aetiology, *see* oncogenic viruses
 see also cancer; malignant disease; neoplasia
tumour antigens 227, 228–9, 260
 cloning and identification 228
 evidence for 227, 228
 factors determining immune response 228
 immunization in immunotherapy 233
 immunotherapy target 260
 new epitopes revealed 231
 P815 228
 in pancreatic carcinoma 2042
 processing 228
 types and detection method *230*
 see also tumour markers
tumour immunology **226–33**
 antibodies to tumour cells 229
 carcinoembryonic antigen, *see* carcinoembryonic antigen (CEA)
 historical perspectives 226–7
 immune surveillance 227, 260
  evidence for *227*
 immunodiagnosis/immunotherapy, *see* immunodiagnosis; immunotherapy; monoclonal antibodies
 tumour antigens, *see* tumour antigens
 tumour-associated antigens 229–30
  see also carcinoembryonic antigen (CEA)
 tumour cell changes 226
  detection by antibodies **230–2**
 tumour-specific immunity **227–9**, 227
  T-cell response 227–8
tumour-infiltrating lymphocytes (TILs)
 in melanoma 260
 in T-cell immunotherapy 233
tumour markers *4369*
 in Cushing's syndrome 1650
 use in new approaches to cancer therapy 258–9
 see also tumour antigens
tumour necrosis factor (TNF) **95**, *96*
 in acute-phase reaction 276
 antibodies, septicaemia treatment 1026
 ARDS pathogenesis 2854–5
 bacterial meningitis pathogenesis 4052
 in cryptogenic fibrosing alveolitis 2788
 erythropoiesis suppression 3388
 functions/actions 95, 276, 537
 in graft rejection 187

heart failure pathophysiology 2231
hepatic granulomas pathogenesis 2120
high permeability pulmonary oedema mechanism 2497
 levels in sepsis 293
 in lung inflammation 2619
 in malaria 841
 monoclonal antibodies, meningococcal infection therapy 541
 in myelomatosis 3598
 nitric oxide secretion stimulation 537
 in pathogenesis of acute meningococcaemia 537, 541
 in pneumococcal infections 513
 prostaglandin synthesis in fever 293
 raised, in cardiac cachexia 2177
 receptor, therapeutic use 99
 in septicaemia pathogenesis 1026
 in tuberculosis 640
 tumours secreting 1712
 in typhoid pathogenesis 562
 in vasculitis pathogenesis 3012
tumour necrosis factor α (TNFα) 95
 in acute pancreatitis 2029
 in cachexia syndrome 241
 in inflammation 98
 inflammatory reaction to endotoxin 291
 limb perfusion in melanoma therapy 233
 in osteoarthritis 2981
tumour necrosis factor ß (TNFß) 95
tumour suppressor genes 65, 193, 194, **223–5**, 462
 in colorectal carcinoma 1990–1
 definition 223
 functions 65
 in lung cancer 2882
 in retinoblastoma 65, 194
 as target for anticancer drugs **225–6**
 viral oncogenesis mechanism 194, 462
 see also p53
Tunga penetrans 1005
tuning fork tests 3870
turbinates, structure and function 2609
Turcot's syndrome 1990
turista, *see* traveller's diarrhoea
Turner's syndrome 1670
 chromosomal abnormality *120*
 coarctation of aorta in 2557
 mental disorders/symptoms in 4239
 mental subnormality and verbal intelligence 4239
 neurological aspects 4109
 short stature 1700
 'twilight states' 4238
 twin, monozygotic and dizygotic 102
twin studies 102
 hypertension pathogenesis 2529–30
 molecular biology of genetic disorders 64
 rheumatoid arthritis 2953
 SLE 3026
tylosis 3723, *3795*
 oesophageal cancer association 202, 1981, 3723
tympanic membrane, perforation 517
tympanosclerosis, in malnutrition 1284
typhoid **560–7**, 2004
 carriers 566–7
  screening 566
 causative agent 561, 2004
 in children 562, 563
 clinical features 562–3, 2004
 complications 562, 565–6, *566*
 diagnosis 563–4
 epidemiology 560–1
 glomerulonephritis complicating 3175
 immune response in 562
 incubation period 562
 management 564–5
  antibiotics 564, *565*, 2006
  supportive 564–5
 pathogenesis 561–2
 pathology 561–2
 prevention 567
 relapse 566
 severe 565
 transmission 561

vaccines 323, 567
 Vi vaccine 567
 see also Salmonella typhi
typhoid facies 563
typhoid nodules 561
typhoons 1232
typhus fevers 729, 730–3, **736–7**, 1023
 epidemic 728, *729*, **737**
  pathology/pathogenesis 731
 flea-borne 736
 louse-borne 737
 louse-borne epidemic 728
 murine 729, **736–7**
 recrudescent 729, **737**
 sylvatic 729, **737**
 treatment and prevention 733
 see also rickettsial diseases
tyramine, MAOI interactions 4250
tyrosinaemia
 hereditary *2019*, 2024
 hereditary type I 1364, 1396
 hereditary type II 1364
 transient neonatal 1364
tyrosinase deficiency 1365, 3759
tyrosine *1353*
 dietary 3086
 disorders of metabolism **1364–5**
 metabolism 1362
tyrosine aminotransferase (TAT) 1362, 1364
tyrosine hydroxylase 1362, 1363, 2553
tyrosine kinase 224–5
 B-cell specific 166
 inhibitors 259
 platelet-derived growth factor (PDGF) receptor 2293
tyrosine kinase receptors 1561, 2293
 in heart 2147

U

ubiquitin 3972
UDPGT (uridine diphosphate glucuronate glucuronyl transferase) 2055
 deficiency 2058
 partial 2058
Uhl's anomaly 2414
ulcer
 aphthoid, in Crohn's disease 1938, 1940
 Buruli, *see* Buruli ulcer
 chancroid, *see* chancroid
 in cutaneous leishmaniasis 901, 902
 decubitus, *see* pressure sore
 genital, in donovanosis 776–7
 gummatous, in syphilis 713
 isolated, of large intestine **2138**
 leg, *see* leg ulcers
 oral recurrent, *see* oral ulceration
 peptic, *see* duodenal ulcer; gastric ulcer; peptic ulcer
 'snail-track' 711
 stercoral 2138
 tropical 705
 venous, *see* venous ulcers
 in yaws 705
ulcerative colitis **1943–51**
 aetiology 1944
 antineutrophil cytoplasmic antibody (ANCA) in 1944, 1945
 assessment of severity and grading 1946
 in children 1951
 cholangiocarcinoma aetiology 2118
 chronic relapsing 1951
 clinical features 1945–6
 colorectal carcinoma in 1991, **1993**
  surveillance for 1950
 complications 1951
 course and prognosis 1951
 diagnosis 1946
 differential diagnosis 1947
  Campylobacter infections *vs* 558
  Crohn's disease 1941, *1941*
 enteropathic synovitis in 2972–3
 epidemiology and incidence 1943–4, *1944*

ulcerative colitis (*cont.*)
  extraintestinal manifestations 1947–8,
    1948, 3723
  gallbladder cancer association 204
  genetics 1944
    candidate genes 1944
  haematological changes 3683–4
  hepatic granulomas in 2122
  immunopathogenesis 1944–5
  laboratory investigations 1946, 1946–7
  liver in 2122, 2131, *2132*
  lymphogranuloma venereum *vs* 761
  medical management 1948–50
    active disease 1948–9
    of complications 1950
    diet 1949–50
    maintenance 1949
  pathology 1945
  in pregnancy 1951
  primary sclerosing cholangitis
    association 1948, 2077, 2079, *2079*
  remission 1945, 1951
  surgical treatment 1950–1
  thrombotic complications 3668
  urinary-tract obstruction 3246
ulcerative jejunitis, in enteropathy-
    associated T-cell lymphoma 1928,
    1929
ulcerative jejunoileitis, in coeliac disease
    1920
ulcerogenic drugs, duodenal ulcer
    aetiology 1878
ulceroglandular tularaemia 599–600, 602
Ullrich's syndrome 4147
ulnar deviation of fingers, in rheumatoid
    arthritis 2957
ulnar nerve **4096–7**
  lesions at elbow 4096
  lesions at wrist/hand 4096–7
ultimobranchial bodies 1603
'ultrasonic angiogram', *see* Doppler
    echocardiography, colour Doppler
    flow mapping
ultrasonography
  in acute renal failure 3280
  'A' scan 3826
  in ascites 2106
  biliary tract 1833, 1834
  bone and joint 2950
  'B' scan 3826
  chest **2653**
  in chronic pancreatitis 2035, 2036,
    2037
  in chronic renal failure 3301
  Doppler, *see* Doppler echocardiography
  effects and damage by 1222
  endoscopic, in pancreatic carcinoma
    2044
  fetal 135
    assessment 1756, 1757
    in vesicoureteric reflux 3217
  in genitourinary tuberculosis 3277
  gut motility disorder investigation 1957
  in hepatocellular carcinoma 2116
  in Hodgkin's disease 3573
  in hydatid disease 957
  in insulinoma 1508
  intracranial 3826
  intraoperative, in pancreatic carcinoma
    2044
  kidneys **3111–12**
  liver 1833
  osteogenesis imperfecta diagnosis 3082
  pain treatment 3943
  pancreas 1835
  in pancreatic carcinoma 2043, 2044
  in pancreatic endocrine tumours 1704,
    1705
  peripheral arterial disease investigation
    2368
  in pleural effusion 2864
  in polycystic kidney disease 3202,
    3204
  prenatal diagnosis/screening by 135
  in reflux nephropathy 3216
  renal, *see* renal ultrasound
  in schistosomiasis 979
  thyroid gland 1608, 1619
  tumour staging 234

urinary tract **3111–12**
  in urinary tract obstruction 3238
  in venous thrombosis 1741
  in vesicoureteric reflux 3215, 3217
ultraviolet barrier cream, in SLE 3023
ultraviolet light 3724–5
  diagnosis of skin damage due to 3725
  DNA damage in xeroderma
    pigmentosum 192
  effects and damage by 1222
  lip cancer association 201
  melanoma association 208
  non-melanoma skin tumour association
    208, 209
  protection from 3728
  solar and senile elastosis 3788
  UVA 3724
    in psoriasis 3748
    in vitiligo management 3758
  UVB 3724
    pruritus management 3744
    in psoriasis 3748
    skin cancer 3791
  UVC 3724
  see also sun light
umbilical hernia, embryology 1973
umbilical sac, persistence, *see*
    exomphalos
umbilical vein, in portal hypertension
    2092, 2093
uncal syndrome 2584
uncertainty principle 24–5
unconsciousness 3930
  brain-stem function assessment 2582–5
  consent and 4317
  diagnosis **2582–6**
  enteral feeding complications 1321
  investigations 2585
  management 2585–6
    immediate 2585
  motor responses assessment 2584–5
  in spinal cord injury 3896
  transition from consciousness 2583
  see also coma; consciousness,
    impairment
undernutrition 1279
  malabsorption in tropics and 1930
  oesophageal varices complication 2094
  see also malnutrition
undifferentiated connective tissue
    syndrome (UDCTS) 3008
unemployment, deliberate self-harm in
    4229
uniparental disomy 127, **128**
  mechanisms 128
uniparental isodisomy 128
United Kingdom
  morbidity in **41–6**
  mortality in **39–41**
  primary health care 47, 48–50
  venomous snakes 1127
United States of America
  childhood poisoning 1044
  health care 38, 47
  indications for snake antivenom 1136
  obesity prevalence *1307*
  rubella vaccination 411
United States Nuclear Regulatory
    Commission 1179
unithiol, *see* DMPS
University of Wisconsin (UW) solution
    2113
unmyelinated nerve fibres 4091
Unverricht-Lundborg disease 3988, 4014
  somatosensory evoked potentials 3834
upper motor neurone **3856–7**
  lesions 3857, 3878
upper motor neurone syndromes **4090**
  combined lower motor neurone
    syndromes **4087–8**
  see also amyotrophic lateral sclerosis
upper respiratory tract, *see* respiratory
    tract, upper
uracil 1386, 1387
uraemia
  acidosis of **1541**, 1543, 1544
  clinical features 3283, **3297–301**
  encephalopathy in 3283, 3302, 4124

mental symptoms 4240
organ dysfunction 3301–2
pericarditis in 2476
peripheral nerve involvement 4099
platelet defects in 3634
vomiting due to 4355
see also renal failure
uranium, nephrotoxicity *3261*
urate
  chronic nephropathy 1380, 2986, 3224,
    3226–7
  serum 1377
    in haemolytic uraemic syndrome
      3200
    in myoglobinuria 3289
    in pre-eclampsia 1729
    see also hyperuricaemia;
      hypouricaemia
  see also uric acid
urea
  breath test 1885
  in cirrhosis 2088
  plasma,
    in acute renal failure 3281, 3286
    interpretation **3107**
    in malaria 850
    in pre-eclampsia 1729
    starting dialysis and 3306
    see also uraemia
  in prolonged infections 294
  synthesis 1353, 1358, 1534
urea cycle 1353, 1358
  disorders, liver in *2019*, 2024
  extrahepatic enzymes 1358
  inherited defects **1358–60**
Ureaplasma 767
  detection/isolation *768*, 769
  genitourinary infections 767
  non-gonococcal urethritis 770
  pelvic inflammatory disease 770
  urinary calculi due to 772
Ureaplasma urealyticum 168, 767, 768,
    768
  in fetus and neonate 1792
  infections in homosexuals 3363
  in pregnancy 1792
  serology in pelvic inflammatory disease
    770
ureteric (renal) colic 2986, **3148**, 3253
  investigations 3253, *3254*
  management 3243, 3255
ureterocele 3243
ureterography, retrograde **3110**, 3239,
    3240, 3277
ureterolysis 3245
ureteropyelography, antegrade **3110**,
    3239, 3240
ureteroscopy 3244
ureterosigmoidostomy 1990, 3244
  hypokalaemia due to 3130
ureters
  dilatation,
    non-obstructive causes *3232*, **3241–2**
    in urinary-tract obstruction 3237,
      3238, 3240
    in vesicoureteric reflux 3214, 3215
  'golf-hole' 3276
  imaging 3109–10
  ischaemic necrosis, renal transplant
    recipients 3318
  obstruction,
    management 3243
    renal function during 3234–5
    in retroperitoneal fibrosis 3244,
      3245–6
    in schistosomiasis 976, 977
    transplanted kidney 3243–4
    tumour-associated 3183, 3244
    pressures in obstruction 3232–4
    retrograde catheterization 3243
    stones, management 3243, 3255
urethral discharge
  in gonorrhoea 546
  in homosexuals 3361
urethral syndrome 3206, 3207
  management 3210
urethritis
  gonococcal 546

non-gonococcal 751, 759, 3362–3
  chlamydial 751, 759, 769, 3362
  in homosexuals 3362, 3363
  interpretation/aetiological problems
    769–70
  mycoplasmas and ureaplasmas in
    768–9
  treatment 3363
  Trichomonas 908
in Reiter's syndrome 2970
urethrogram, ascending 3236
uric acid
  acute nephropathy 1379–80, 2986,
    3185, **3226**, 3290
  crystal deposition,
    intrarenal 3226–7
    in renal collecting system/ureters
      1379–80, 3226, 3290
  fractional excretion (FE$_{ur}$) 3225
  metabolism 1377, 1378
    inherited disorders 3225–6
  overproducers 2985
  reference range *4367*
  serum, raised in gout 2986
  solubility 3225
  stones 1379, 2986, 3227, *3252*
    investigations 3237, 3238
    management 3256
  undersecretors 2985
  urinary excretion 1379, **3225**
    diet and 1379, 3225
    in Lesch-Nyhan syndrome 1382
    in partial hypoxanthine-guanine
      phosphoribosyl transferase deficiency
      1382, 1383
uridine 1386, 1387, 3497
uridine diphosphate 4-epimerase
  deficiency 1350
uridine diphosphate glucuronate
  glucuronyl transferase, *see* UDPGT
uridine monophosphate (UMP) synthase
  deficiency 1386–7
urinalysis **3101–2**
  sample collection 3101
  see also urine
urinary catheter
  indwelling, nosocomial infections 329
  septicaemia with 1021
urinary catheterization
  clean intermittent 3212
  in diabetic hyperglycaemic coma 1502
  diagnostic 3101, 3208
  infections and 3212
  urethral, in spinal cord injury 3899,
    3900
  urine specimen 3208
  see also bladder, catheterization
urinary diversion, obstructive
  complications 3244
urinary incontinence
  control, in spina bifida 4118
  in elderly **4338**
  functional 4338
  management 4338, 4339
  in normal pressure hydrocephalus 3970
  overflow 3236, 4338
  types *4338*
  urge 4338
urinary retention
  acute 3234
    clinical features 3235–6
    management 3242
  acute on chronic 3236
  chronic 3234
    clinical features 3236
    investigations 3242–3
  in diabetes 1489
  with overflow 3236
  in spinal cord lesions 3892
  in typhoid 563
urinary sphincter, artificial, in spinal cord
  injury 3900
urinary stone disease **3251–7**
  in adenine phosphoribosyl transferase
    deficiency 1383
  clinical diagnosis 3253
  course and prognosis 3257
  in cystinuria 1356–7, 3333

epidemiology 3251
in gout 1379, 2986
in idiopathic hypercalciuria 3255
in intestinal disease 3255
investigations 3253–4
management **3243**, **3255–6**
  minimally invasive techniques **3244**
  preventive methods 3256
oxalate, *see* calcium oxalate, stones
pathophysiology 3251–3
pregnancy in 1735
in primary hyperoxaluria 1446–7
in primary hyperparathyroidism 1631,
  1632, **3255**
in reflux nephropathy 3218
in renal tubular acidosis 3339
in sarcoidosis 3186
uric acid, *see* uric acid, stones
X-linked recessive 3252–3
urinary-tract
  calculi, ureaplasmas causing 772
  disorders **3205–20**
  imaging **3109–15**
  in Kawasaki disease 3048
  management in spinal cord injury
    3899–901
  pressure flow studies 3240–1
  symptoms,
    in multiple sclerosis 3993, 3995
    in Parkinson's disease 4004
  tuberculosis, *see under* tuberculosis
urinary-tract infections **3205–13**
  anaerobic 573
  in analgesic nephropathy 3221, 3223
  antimicrobial therapy 312
  asymptomatic (covert) 3207
  candidiasis 808
  classification *3207*
  clinical presentations 3206–7
  coagulase-negative staphylococcal 532
  in diabetes 1493
  diagnosis 3102, 3207–8
  enterobacteria causing 551
  enterococcal 509
  follow-up 3213
  in homosexuals 3365
  investigation 3213
  in nephrotic syndrome 3141
  nosocomial 329, *329*
  pathogenesis 3206
  in polycystic kidney disease 3204
  in pregnancy **1733**, **1787**, 3207
    diagnosis 1787
    in multiple sclerosis 1769
    treatment 1787, 3211, 3212
  in renal transplant recipients 3314, 3320
  septicaemia 1020, 1021
  in sickle-cell disease 3195
  Staphylococcus aureus 526
  symptomatic 3206–7
  treatment 3208–13, 3273
    curative 3208–13
    prophylactic 3213
    special problems 3211–13
    suppressive 3213
  in urinary stone disease 3253
  in urinary-tract obstruction 3236
  in vesicoureteric reflux 3217
urinary-tract obstruction **3232–46**
  acute lower-tract 3234, 3235–6, 3242
  acute renal failure *vs* 3280
  acute upper-tract 3232–3
    clinical features 3235
    investigation 3236–9
    management 3243
  causes 3232, *3233*
  chronic lower-tract 3234, 3236, 3242–3
  chronic renal failure 3295–6, 3299,
    3300
  chronic upper-tract 3233–4
    clinical features 3235
    investigation 3239–41
    management 3243–4
    significant incomplete 3241
  clinical features 3235–6
  histopathological changes 3234
  hormonal effects 3235
  incidence 3232

investigation 3114, 3115, 3236–43
management 3243–4
pathophysiology 3232–5
renal function,
  after relief of obstruction 3235
  during obstruction 3234–5
in tuberculosis 3179, 3276, 3277, 3278,
  3279
see also obstructive uropathy
urine
  bilirubin in 2056
  casts, *see* casts, urinary
  crystals 3104, **3105**
  culture 3207, 3208
    in malnutrition 1288
  discoloration,
    in acute porphyria 1392
    haematuria *vs* 3145
    in paroxysmal nocturnal
      haemoglobinuria 3450
  early morning specimens 3276
  enzymes in 3109, 3138
  examination **3101–5**
    in malaria 850
  flow rate, in renal failure 2581
  in hyperbilirubinaemia 2056
  leaks, renal transplant recipients 3318
  in leptospirosis 701
  microscopy **3102–3**
    sample collection 3101
    in SLE 3019
  midstream specimen (MSU) 3101,
    3207–8
  normal values *4373*
  osmolality, *see* osmolality, urine
  output, post-renal transplantation 3318
  pH, *see* pH, urine
  prostatic specimens 3208
  residual 3206, 3236
  retention, *see* urinary retention
  specimens, chlamydial infections
    diagnosis 755
  suprapubic aspiration 3101, 3208
  twenty-four hour 2546
    vanillylmandelic acid (VMA) 2555
  volume **3101**, 3116
urobilinogen 2046
  detection 2055
  faecal 3526
  metabolism 2055
  urinary 2055, 3526
urogenital tract
  anomalies, embryology 1973
  bacterial infections 268
  in diphtheria 495
urography, excretion, *see* intravenous
  pyelography
urokinase 93, 2299, 2343
  in pulmonary embolism 2526
Urokinase Pulmonary Embolism Trial
  2526
urokinase-type plasminogen activator
  (urokinase; u-PA) *3624*, 3625, 3626
  single-chain (scu-PA; pro-urokinase)
    2343, 3625, 3671
  therapeutic use 3671, *3672*
urolithiasis, *see* urinary stone disease
urological disorders
  renal transplantation and 3315
  vesicoureteric reflux and 3217
uropathy, obstructive, *see* obstructive
  uropathy
uroporphyrin, urinary *1390*, 1391, 1394
uroporphyrinogen cosynthase *1391*
uroporphyrinogen decarboxylase *1391*,
  1394, 1396
urothelial cells, bacterial adherence 3206
urothelial tumours
  analgesic nephropathy and 3222, 3223
  Balkan nephropathy and 3230, 3231
ursodeoxycholic acid
  in cystic fibrosis 2131
  gallstone dissolution 2048, 2049
  in intrahepatic cholestasis 2060
  in primary biliary cirrhosis 2076
  in primary sclerosing cholangitis 2079
urticaria 162, 3743, **3770–2**
  acquired cold 3771

allergens 3770, 3771
allergic/non-allergic 3770
causes 162, 3770, 3771
cholinergic 162, 3770–1
chronic 3771
clinical features 162, 3770–1
cold 3779
contact 3736, *3737*, 3770
  non-allergic 3737
distribution 3771
drug-induced 3731
familial 3770
familial cold 3770, 3771
food-induced 1844, 3729
heat 3771
histamine in 3770, 3771
immunology and complement activation
  3770
investigations 3771–2
life-threatening 162, 3772
management 162, 3772
papular 3771
  scabies *vs* 1008
in penicillin reaction 718
physical 3771
in pregnancy 1805
pressure 3771
recurrent, management 162
solar 3726, 3771
transfusion-induced 3692
types 3770–1
in vasculitis 162, 3774
vasculitis in 3773
see also angio-oedema
urticaria pigmentosa (mastocytosis)
  3438, **3755**, 3799
user fees 53
uterine carcinoma, staging investigations
  236
uterine fibroids (myomas)
  hormone replacement therapy and 1815
  polycythaemia and 3554
uteroplacental circulation, in pre-
  eclampsia 1727
uterus, actinomycoses 683
Uthoff's phenomenon 3866
Uukuniemi virus 428
Uukuvirus 428
uveitis
  acute, in HIV infection 476
  acute anterior 2826
    in ankylosing spondylitis 2967, 4185
    in psoriatic arthritis 2969
    in Reiter's syndrome 2971
  anterior,
    in Behçet's syndrome 4183
    in onchocerciasis 2971
    in sarcoidosis 2826, 4182
    see also iritis
  in Behçet's syndrome 4182, 4183
  in leptospirosis 699, 701
  in multiple sclerosis 4184
  posterior,
    in sarcoidosis 2826, 4182
    toxoplasmosis causing 866
  in sarcoidosis 2821, 2826, **4182**
  in ulcerative colitis 1947
uveoparotid fever (Heerfordt-
  Waldenstrom) syndrome **2821**, 2826
uvulopalatopharyngoplasty 2914

V

vaccination 284, 288–9
  international certificates 322
  see also immunization
vaccines
  combination 320, *321*
  in common use 317–19, *318*
  development 315
    problems/difficulties 315, 317
    recombinant, *see* recombinant DNA
      technology
  fever after 1181
  for immunocompromised 325
  schedules, *see under* immunization
  for special indications 319, *319*

under development 319–20, *320*, 455–6
viral, in pregnancy 1777, **1778**
see also individual vaccines
vaccinia virus 366
  biology and morphogenesis 366, 367
  expression vectors 368, 455
  extracellular enveloped virus (EEV) 366
  genome and proteins 366
  genome sequencing 368
  hepatitis B vaccines 455
  intracellular mature virus (IMV) 366
  vaccines and complications after 368
vacuoles, in muscle fibres 4143–4
vacuum constriction device, in erectile
  dysfunction 4246
VAD regimen 3601, 3602, 3603
'vagabond's disease' 1003
vagal stimulation, pulmonary
  vasodilatation 2492
vagina
  cancer, stilboestrol causing 1254
  candidiasis 800, **3355–6**, 3768
  chlamydial colonization in neonates 754
  healthy **3354**
  infections **3354–6**
  normal pH 3354
vaginal discharge **3353–7**
  in bacterial vaginosis 3355
  in candidiasis 3356
  causes **3356**
  non-infectious 3356
  diagnostic approach **3356**, *3356*
  in gonorrhoea 546
  treatment of infections *3356*
  in trichomoniasis 907, 3354
vaginitis **3354–6**
  atrophic 3212
  urinary-tract infections and 3207
vaginosis 572, **3354–6**
  bacterial **3355**
    mycoplasmas in 772
    in pregnancy 1785
vagotomy
  highly selective 1890
  in peptic ulcers 1890
  sequelae 1890
  truncal 1954
    gut peptides after 1895
vagus nerve **3880**
  control of gastrointestinal motor system
    1953
  digitalis action on 2245
  inhibitory effect on heart 2160
  insulin secretion and 1460
  lesions 3880
    symptoms 3880
  in myocardial infarction 2335
  in vomiting 1821
valgus deformity
  foot 2958, 2996
  knee 2959
valine *1353*, 1368–9
  metabolism 1275, 1276
valproate, sodium, *see* sodium valproate
Valsalva, sinus of, *see* aortic sinus
Valsalva manoeuvre 1199, 3884, *3884*
  in cardiac arrhythmias 2263
  normal response to 3884, 3885
valvular disease, *see* heart valves, disease
valvulitis, in rheumatic fever 2433
vampire bats 396, 1125
vanadium, poisoning **1114**
van Buchem's disease **3090**
vancomycin
  in enterococcal infections 510
  in infective endocarditis 303, 2446,
    2447
  in pneumococcal infections 520
  in pseudomembranous colitis 636
  in pyrexia of unknown origin 1031
  in renal impairment 3271
van den Bergh reaction 2055
vanillylmandelic acid (VMA) 2554
  24hr urine 2555
  phaeochromocytoma diagnosis 2555
vanishing bile-duct syndrome 2059,
  2079, 2114, 2129
Vansil (oxamniquine) 979

vapour 2847
varicella, *see* chickenpox
varicella syndrome 348
varicella-zoster immune globulin 351
  in neonates 1780
  in pregnancy 1775
varicella-zoster virus (VZV) 347
varicella-zoster virus (VZV) infections
  346–51
  diagnosis/differential diagnosis 350
  epidemiology 347
  eye in 4192
  in HIV infection and AIDS 479,
  4079
  management 350–1, 479, *479*
  pathology 347
  prevention 351
  primary 347
  see also chickenpox; herpes zoster
varicocele 1685, 1686
varicose veins 2523
variation 365, 366, 367
variola virus 365, 366, 367
  genome sequencing 368
  variola major and variola minor 367,
  368
  see also smallpox
vasa vasora 2290
vascular access, for haemodialysis
  3308–9
vascular bed capacity 2565
vascular cell adhesion molecule (VCAM)
  231
  type 1 (VCAM1) 2294, 2299
vascular damage
  in haemolytic uraemic syndrome 3199
  in hypertension 3249–50
  injecting drug abusers 4280, 4282–3
  response 3773
  in rickettsial diseases 731
  in sickle-cell disease 3194
vascular disease
  acute renal failure in **3290–1**
  of gastrointestinal tract **1994–2000**
  of liver, drug-induced 2128–9, *2128*
  purpura due to 3628, **3635–7**
  renal, *see* kidney, vascular disease
  spinal cord **3894**
vascular dysplasia 1998–9
vascular endothelial cell growth factor
  (VEGF) 2293
vascularity, abnormal, of skin **3784–7**
vascular lesions, in rickettsial diseases
  731, 732
vascular neurosyphilis 4084–5
vascular permeability, in snake bites
  1129
vascular resistance
  peripheral, in pre-eclampsia 1727–8
  renal, in hypertension 3248
  see also pulmonary vascular resistance;
  systemic vascular resistance
vascular smooth muscle
  cells, *see* smooth muscle cells
  vasopressin actions 3118
vascular surgery, in diabetic foot disease
  1491
vasculitic rash, in meningitis 4053, 4054
vasculitides, systemic, *see* vasculitis,
  systemic
vasculitis **3772–9**
  acute renal failure *vs* 3280
  ANCA-positive 2000, 3777–8
  in bronchiectasis 2761
  cardiac manifestations **2391–2**, *2392*
  causes,
    drugs 3776
    harmful agents 3773–4
    immune complexes 3774, 3775
    infections 3776
  classification 2800
  cutaneous **3772–9**
    detection of cause 3776
    diagnosis 3774–6
    management 3776–7
    pathogenesis 3774, 3776
    pathology and nomenclature 3773
    prognosis 3776

cutaneous leucocytoclastic 3010
  in cystic fibrosis 2749–50
  definition/diseases included 3772–3
  fulminant 3777
  gastrointestinal involvement **1999–2000**
  hepatitis B-associated **3178**
  heroin-associated 3178
  hypersensitivity 2800, *2800*, 3010
  intestinal ischaemia due to 1995, *1995*
  investigations *2952*
  leg 3714
  leucocytoclastic 3010, 3775
    in rheumatoid arthritis 2960
  lymphocytic 3775
  in meningococcal infections 539, 542
  necrotizing granulomatous, *see*
    Wegener's granulomatosis
  post-streptococcal 3178
  primary, gastrointestinal tract in **2000**
  pulmonary, *see* pulmonary vasculitis
  renal 3146
    infection-associated **3178**
    in lupus nephritis 3188
    renal-limited variant 3162, 3166
    in rheumatoid arthritis 2797–8, 2960–1,
    3193, 3776
  in scrub typhus 740
  in syphilis 708
  systemic 2800, *3009*
    acute renal failure in 3291, 3299
    aetiology and pathogenesis **3011–12**
    alveolar haemorrhage in 2804
    in Churg-Strauss syndrome 2800
    classification 3010, *3011*
    experimental models 3011
    historical aspects 3010
    humoral autoimmunity in 3011–12
    incidence 3011
    large-vessel 3011
    rapidly progressive glomerulonephritis
    in 3162, 3166
    small-vessel 3011
    treatment **3016–17**
  urticarial 162, 3773, 3774
  see also Churg-Strauss syndrome;
    Henoch-Schönlein purpura;
    microscopic polyangiitis; polyarteritis
    nodosa; relapsing polychondritis;
    Wegener's granulomatosis
vasectomy 1685
vaseline dermatitis 3736
vasoactive amines, in pulmonary
  endothelium 2486
vasoactive drugs
  bleeding oesophageal varices 2094
  intracavernosal injection 4246
vasoactive intestinal peptide (VIP) **1893**
  diarrhoea associated 2006
  hepatic granulomas pathogenesis
  2120
  prolactin secretion and 1576
  structure, secretion and actions 1893
  tumour producing (VIPoma) 1704,
  1705–6, 1708
vasoactive substances, in carcinoid
  tumours 1898
vasoconstriction
  in acid-base disturbances 1539
  in anaemia 3458
  angiotensin II action 2157
  cold causing 1182
  in exercise 2161
  in high-flow pulmonary hypertension
  2508
  inappropriate, *see* vasospastic disorders
  loss of nitric oxide 2297
  noradrenaline/adrenaline action 2254
  precapillary 2560
  pulmonary, in hypoxia, *see* hypoxia
  pulmonary circulation 2487, 2492,
  2514, 2516
vasoconstrictors
  endothelium producing 2297–8, 2323,
  2514
  see also angiotensin converting
    enzyme (ACE); endothelin-1
  response, in hypertension 2531
  septicaemia management 1024, 2573

vasodilatation
  ACE inhibitor action 2249
  in acid-base disturbances 1539
  in anaemia 3458
  in asthma, mediators causing 2727,
  2728
  in atopic eczema 3741
  bronchial capillaries, in hypoxia 2494
  calcium antagonist action 2329
  coronary arteries 2159
  coronary blood flow 2159
  dopamine causing 2254
  in exercise 2161
  haemodynamics **2246**
  heat causing 1180
  in hepatocellular failure 2102, 2103
  nitrates causing 2326, 2327
  in pruritus 3743
  pulmonary circulation 2492
  pulmonary endothelium 2487
  in sepsis 293
  skin 3706
vasodilators **2246–52**
  in adult respiratory distress syndrome
  2576, 2859–60
  classification and types 2246–7, *2246*
  in cor pulmonale 2927
  endothelium producing 2296–7, 2323
    prostanoids 2297
  see also nitric oxide
  heart failure treatment **2246–52**
    effect on symptoms and exercise
    tolerance 2248
    nitrates and hydralazine 2248
    renin-angiotensin system inhibitors
    2252
    see also angiotensin converting
      enzyme (ACE) inhibitors
  in hypertension 2541–2, *2541*
  in ischaemic limbs 2369
  mechanisms of action 2246–7, *2246*
  in mitral regurgitation 2462
  in myocardial infarction 2344, 2569
  in primary pulmonary hypertension
  2512
  pulmonary 2859–60
    in cor pulmonale 2521
    in renal impairment 3274
  in vasospastic disorders 2374
  in vibration-induced white finger 1227
  see also calcium antagonists;
    hydralazine; nitrates
vasomotor activity
  changes, in median nerve lesions 4095
  depression, in salicylate poisoning 1055
  pulmonary circulation **2491–2**
vasopressin (arginine vasopressin; AVP)
  1600–3, 3117–18
  ACTH secretion and 1575, 3118
  actions 1563, 1601, 3116, **3118**, 3331
  bleeding oesophageal varices 2094
  chemistry 1599–600
  control of secretion 1600, 3118
  in Cushing's disease 1641
  deficiency 1601, 3120
  diurnal variations 1565
  ectopic secretion 1566–8
  elevated, in heart failure 2170
  gene mutations *1567*, 1571
  in heart failure 2234
  inappropriate secretion (SIAD), *see*
    antidiuresis, syndrome of
    inappropriate
  peripheral oedema at high altitude 1192
  plasma,
    in acute renal failure 3281
    hypertonic saline infusion 1601, 3121,
    3122
  potassium balance and 3129
  reduction, by ACE inhibitors 2248
  resistance 1572, 3120
  see also diabetes insipidus,
    nephrogenic
  in stress 1563
  tests 3109, 3121
  in trauma 1548, 1549
  see also desmopressin
vasopressin V₁ receptors 3118

vasopressin V₂ receptors *1567*, 1572,
  3118
vasospasm
  increased endothelin production 2298
  loss of nitric oxide 2297
  in subarachnoid haemorrhage 3963
vasospastic disorders **2365–6**
  management **2374**
  see also Raynaud's syndrome
vasovagal reflex, in myocardial infarction
  2335
vasovagal syncope, *see* syncope,
  vasovagal
vasovagal syndrome **2267**
  pacing in 2286, 2289
  see also syncope, vasovagal
vastus medialis, atrophy 4322
VBAP regimen 3601, 3602
VCAM-1 **2621**
  in asthma 2728
  emigration of neutrophils from
    capillaries 2619
VDRL test 707, 715, *715*, 2483, 4085
vectors 61
  gene cloning 61
  gene therapy 113, 2755
vegans 3492, 3496
  ischaemic heart disease risk reduced
  2311
vegetable oil, aspiration 2837
vegetarian diets
  blood pressure/hypertension prevention
  2530
  cancer protection 219
  constipation reduced 1328
  ischaemic heart disease risk reduced
  2311
  vitamin B₁₂ deficiency 3468
vegetative state, chronic, *see* persistent
  vegetative state
Veillonella, rare species *561*
vein grafts, coronary artery bypass
  grafting 2353
veins, nitric oxide release 2296
velocardiofacial syndrome,
  microdeletions in 108, *108*, 129
vena cava, *see* inferior vena cava;
  superior vena cava
venereal diseases, *see* sexually
  transmitted diseases (STD)
venesection
  in acute renal failure 3285
  in chronic obstructive airways disease
  2776
  in chronic respiratory failure 2929–30
  in congestive heart failure in
    malnutrition 1292
  in cor pulmonale 2521
  fluid replacement with 2400
  in haemochromatosis 2022
  in hereditary haemochromatosis 3479
  in iron overload 3481
  in polycythaemia 2400
  in polycythaemia vera 3433–4
  in porphyria cutanea tarda 1395
Venezuelan equine encephalitis virus **409**
Venezuelan haemorrhagic fever **439**
venography
  dangers in phaeochromocytomas 2556
  renal **3110–11**
venom **1124–60**
  antivenom, *see* antivenom
  fish 1141
  hymenoptera (bee and wasp) 161, 1144,
  1145
  scorpion 1146, 1147
  snake, *see under* snakes, venomous
  tick 1149
venomous animals **1125–40**
  amphibians **1140**
  aquatic animals **1141–3**
  arthropods **1144–51**
    see also arthropods
  birds **1140–1**
  fish **1141**
  lizards **1140**
  mammals **1125–6**
  marine invertebrates **1143–4**

snakes **1126–40**
 see also snakes
veno-occlusive disease
 cytotoxic drugs causing 2099
 hepatic **2099**, 2129
 see also pulmonary veno-occlusive
  disease
venous access
 in acute leukaemia 3407
 in cystic fibrosis 2752–3
 permanent 2752
 self-management 2753
venous congestion
 chronic, liver in 2138–9
 see also pulmonary venous congestion
venous gangrene 2523
venous hum, in cirrhosis 2088
venous hypertension, *see* venous
  pressure, raised
venous pressure
 in aortic regurgitation 2465
 in aortic stenosis 2462
 in elderly 4342
 in mixed mitral valve disease 2456
 in pericardial tamponade 2477
 raised,
  causes 2480
  control/management 3808
  in myocardial infarction 2335
  in pericardial constriction 2479, 2480
  in pulmonary venous hypertension
   2509
  in tricuspid regurgitation 2468
 see also central venous pressure;
  jugular venous pressure
venous return **2155–6**
 in exercise 2161
 orthostatic changes 2156
venous sampling
 in Cushing's syndrome 1648–9
 parathyroid localization 1632–3
venous stasis 3663, 3664
venous thromboembolism, recurrent
  systemic, pulmonary hypertension *vs*
  2513
venous thrombosis 3661–2
 in antithrombin deficiency 3666
 cerebral, *see* cerebral venous
  thrombosis
 clinical risk factors *3665, 3668, 3675*
 in connective tissue diseases 3010
 in cyanotic congenital heart disease
  2401
 deep, *see* deep vein thrombosis (DVT)
 fibrinolytic therapy 3671, *3672*
 intestinal ischaemia due to 2366
 intracranial (cortical/dural sinus)
  3956–7, *3957*
 management 3669–70
 in nephrotic syndrome 3141, 3142
 in paroxysmal nocturnal
  haemoglobinuria 3450–1, 3452, 3668
 pathogenesis **3664**
 in primary antiphospholipid syndrome
  3669
 prophylaxis 3670, **3675–6**
 in protein C deficiency 3666
 in protein S deficiency 3667
 recurrent 3673–4, 3675
 in renal transplant recipients 3318
 septic, of portal system 2139
 transfusion-associated 3692
 see also thrombosis
venous tone
 low central venous pressure 2564
 in overtransfusion 2571
 in pulmonary embolism 2569
 in septicaemia 2572, 2573
 see also central venous pressure
venous ulcers
 anaerobic infections 573
 chronic 3664, 3665
ventilated patients, drug prescribing 3270
ventilation
 asynchronous independent 2858
 dead space, *see* lung, dead space
 distribution in lung 2669
 exercise capacity assessment **2672**

factors affecting peak/mean airway
  pressure *2858*
gas flow **2629**
 see also gas exchange
 increased 2672
 in pregnancy 1744
 pressure release 2921
 reduced, hypoxaemia in 2631
tests **2669–71**
total,
 in chronic bronchiolitis 2635
 in diffuse interstitial fibrosis 2638
 in emphysema 2633
 see also respiration
ventilation, mechanical **2919–24**
 in acute poisoning 1046–7
 in acute respiratory failure 2919–24
 in adult respiratory distress syndrome
  2575, 2640, 2857–9
 after head injury 4048
 after lung/heart-lung transplantation
  2935
 in airway obstruction 2572, 2720–1
 in altitude acclimatization 1186
 assist control (triggered ventilation)
  2859, 2920
 in asthma 2924
 in bronchocutaneous/bronchopleural
  fistulae 2924
 in central sleep apnoea and
  hypoventilation **2917–18**
 in chronic obstructive airways disease
  2924
 in CNS viral infections 4072
 complications 2923–4
 control 2919, 2920
  assessment **2672**
 CPAP, *see* continuous positive airway
  pressure (CPAP)
 in diaphragmatic disorders 2878
 discontinuation and brain death 3934
 domiciliary 2930–1, 3898
 features and applications 2919
 guidelines *2858*, 2919, *2920*
 in hepatocellular failure 2110
 high frequency 2858–9, 2921
 indications 2919
 intermittent mandatory 2920–1
 intermittent positive pressure, *see*
  intermittent positive pressure
  ventilation
 long-term, in spinal cord injury 3898
 mechanical **2919–24**
 modes **2919–21**
 monitoring 2922
 in muscular dystrophy 4149
 nasal PPV, *see* nasal positive-pressure
  ventilation (NPPV)
 negative pressure 2874, 2921
 neonates 2920
 nocturnal 2905–6, 2917
 non-invasive **2930–2**
  long-term and domiciliary 2930–1
  see also nasal positive-pressure
   ventilation (NPPV)
 parameters and setting of 2921–3
 PEEP, *see* positive end-expiratory
  pressure (PEEP) ventilation
 positive-pressure, *see* positive-pressure
  ventilation
 pressure support 2921
 in pulmonary oedema 2505
 recent developments 2592
 in restrictive lung disease 2924
 in spinal cord injury 3898
 strategies **2924**
 tetanus management 629
 in thoracoplasty 2876
 in unconscious patients 2585
 weaning 2922, *2922*, **2931–2**
  from PEEP 2923
ventilation-perfusion mismatch 2631,
  2670
 in adult respiratory distress syndrome
  2856
 in alveolar filling syndromes 2639
 assessment 2670
 hypoxia due to 2902

normal/low carbon dioxide tension 2904
pulmonary oedema 2503
 in pulmonary vascular diseases 2641
ventilation-perfusion ratio 2670, 2671
 in asthma 2636
 in chronic bronchiolitis 2635
ventilation-perfusion scanning 2654–5
 in cryptogenic fibrosing alveolitis 2790
 in pulmonary embolism 2525
 regional 2669
ventilators 2919
 monitors and alarms 2922
ventilatory drive 2902, 2904, 2916, 2926
 absent **2916**
 changes in sleep 2904, 2926
 in chronic obstructive airways disease,
  acute exacerbations 2926
  chronic stable 2928–9
 control **3887–8**
  see also, *see under* breathing
 stimulants 2926, **2928–9**
 in type 2 ventilatory failure 2905, 2926
 unstable **2916**
ventilatory failure
 definition 2901
 see also respiratory failure, type 2
ventilatory load 2927
 reduction 2927, 2929
ventral posterolateral nucleus caudalis
  3860
ventral posteromedial nucleus 3860
ventricle (ventricular)
 activation time 2185
 aneurysms,
  after myocardial infarction 2321
  left 2325
  ventricular septum 2429
 in cardiac cycle 2153
 diastolic pressure, square-root sign
  2390, 2393, 2479
 double-inlet **2419**
  in Eisenmenger reaction (syndrome)
   2411
 dysfunction, after myocardial infarction
  2249–50
 ejection 2153, 2157
  volume 2153, 2157
 ejection fraction 2153, 2157
  see also left ventricle (ventricular),
   ejection fraction
 end-diastolic fibre length 2149, 2150,
  2155
 end-diastolic pressure 2153
 end-diastolic volume 2153, 2157
  end-systolic pressure relationship 2158
  stroke work relation 2150, 2155
 failure, in myocardial infarction 2566
 function,
  indices **2221–5**
  see also left ventricle (ventricular),
   function
 myxoma 2472
 premature activation 2275
 premature beats, *see* ventricular
  extrasystoles
 pressure in 2157
 pressure-volume loop 2157, 2158
 rate, in atrial fibrillation 2272, 2273
 single 2404, **2419**
  mitral atresia with **2419**
 thrombus, MRI 2215
 volume 2149
  afterload and **2157**
 see also left ventricle (ventricular); right
  ventricle (ventricular)
ventricular arrhythmias
 in myocardial infarction 2321
 see also cardiac arrhythmias; ventricular
  fibrillation; ventricular tachycardia
ventricular arterial concordance 2418
ventricular arterial discordance 2404,
  2416, 2417–18
ventricular extrasystoles (premature/
  ectopic beats) 2198, 2199, 2270
 after pacemaker implantation 2288
 bigeminy/trigeminy 2270, 2271
 management 2270
 in mitral prolapse 2460

multi-form 2270, 2271
 salvo 2270
ventricular fibrillation **2283**
 after immersion hypothermia 1183
 causes 2283, *2283*
  digitalis inducing 2244
 in myocardial infarction, *see under*
  myocardial infarction
 prognosis and survival 2284–5
 recurrence risk 2285
 treatment 2265, 2345
ventricular flutter, electrocardiogram
  (ECG) 2198
ventricular hypertrophy
 electrocardiogram (ECG) in 2187–8,
  2189
 postnatal adaptation to congenital heart
  disease 2399
 S-T segment, in ventricular hypertrophy
  2187, 2189
 T wave, inversion, in ventricular
  hypertrophy 2187
 see also cardiac hypertrophy; *under* left
  ventricle; *under* right ventricle
ventricular 'knock' 2480
ventricular pre-excitation 2192–4,
  2275–7
 electrocardiogram in 2192–4, 2277
 forms and 'concealed accessory
  pathway' 2275
 see also Wolff-Parkinson-White
  syndrome
ventricular septal defects **2428–30**
 acquired/congenital types 2461
 bipartite right ventricle with 2405
 classification 2428
 complications 2429–30
 in corrected transposition 2417
 diagnosis 2429
 Doppler echocardiography 2203, *2204*
 with double-outlet right ventricle 2404
 in Eisenmenger reaction (syndrome)
  2410
 in Fallot's tetralogy 2402
  residual 2406
 heart murmurs 2421
 infective endocarditis in 2428–9, 2439,
  2443
 infundibular, in Fallot's tetralogy 2404
 mitral regurgitation *vs* 2461
 multiple 2405
 in myocardial infarction 2321
 in pregnancy 1736, *1737*
 pulmonary atresia with **2407–8**, 2407–8
 pulmonary hypertension in 2418, 2507
 pulmonary stenosis with 2417
 residual 2430
 spontaneous closure 2429
 subtruncal 2431
 subvalvular and subaortic 2428
 symptoms 2428–9
 in transposition of great arteries 2417
 in tricuspid atresia 2412
 ventricular septum aneurysm 2429
ventricular shunting
 in intracranial tumours 4039
 in normal pressure hydrocephalus 3970
ventricular standstill 2269
ventricular tachycardia 2263, **2279–83**
 accelerated idioventricular rhythm
  2281
 aetiology 2279–80
 exercise-induced 2280
 clinical features 2280, 2281
 definitions 2279
 differential diagnosis 2277, 2277–8,
  2278
 in dilated cardiomyopathy 2384
 fusion and capture beats 2279
 in hypertrophic cardiomyopathy 2387,
  2388, 2389
 in myocardial infarction 2345
 non-sustained 2279, **2281–2**
  in hypertrophic cardiomyopathy 2387,
   2389
 risk of sustained tachycardia 2282
 polymorphic 2279, **2282**
 prognosis 2281

ventricular tachycardia (*cont.*)
  salvoes 2281
  sustained monomorphic **2279–81**
  treatment 2280–1, 2281–2
    defibrillation 2288
    emergency 2280
    medically intractable 2280–1
    pacing 2265, 2280, 2285
    surgery 2266
    verapamil use dangers 2277
  see also torsade de pointes
ventriculoatrial shunt 4115
ventriculography 3826
  scintigraphic, *see* scintigraphy
    (radionuclide scanning), heart
ventriculoperitoneal shunts 4115, 4118
Venturi oxygen masks 2926
verapamil *2264*, 2329, 2330
  atrioventricular block due to 2268
  in atrioventricular nodal re-entry
    tachycardia 2274
  beta-blockers with 2268
    danger 2328, 2329
  in hypertension 2541
  in hypertrophic cardiomyopathy 2389
  in multi-drug resistance 3603
  in pregnancy 1740
  in ventricular tachycardia, danger
    2277
veratrine *1154*
v-*erb*A oncogene 1561, 1606
Verner Morrison syndrome 1824
Vernet's syndrome 3880
Vero cells 556
Vero cytotoxin (VT) 556
  in haemolytic uraemic syndrome 3196,
    3199
verrucas 446
'verruga' (bartonellosis) 773, 774
verruga peruana 773, 774, 775
  see also bartonellosis
version 3913
versive seizures 3913
vertebrae 2992
  bridging, *see* syndesmophytes
  infection **3901–2**
vertebral arteries 3947
  balloon/laser angioplasty 3824
vertebral bodies
  collapse 2993
  in collapsed discs 3904–5
  fusion 3873
  metastases 240–1, 249
vertebral collapse
  in osteoporosis 3066
  pain in 2947
vertebral fractures 3065, 4335
  grades 3067
  in osteoporosis 3065
vertebral osteomyelitis 3901
vertebrobasilar insufficiency, postural
    hypotension 4344
vertebrobasilar ischaemia 2367–8
  management **2373**
  transient ischaemic attack in 3950
vertebrobasilar territory,
    thromboembolism 3956
vertebroplasty 3828
vertigo 3871, 3919
  benign positional 3873, 3876
  episodic 3875–6
  in Ménière's disease 3875
  syphilitic 714
  treatment 3876
'vervet monkey' disease 439
very low density lipoprotein (VLDL)
    1277, 1401, 1402, 1404
  in chronic renal failure 3302
  in diabetes 1457, 1458
  in hypertriglyceridaemia 1409, 1410
  ischaemic heart disease risk 2308
  in nephrotic syndrome 3143
  see also beta-very low density
    lipoprotein (beta-VLDL)
vesicles *3713*, 3717, 3779
  in dermatitis 3734
  in herpes simplex infections 342, 343
  in nuclear envelope assembly 80
  in varicella-zoster virus infections 347,
    348

vesicles, transport 75
  budding 68
    coatomer complex role 75–6
    organelle fragmentation in mitosis and
      78
  coat proteins of and purification 75, 76
  formation, coat protein role models 76
  fusion models 75
  see also vesicular transport
vesico-blistering diseases 3708, **3779–83**
  causes 3779
  infections causing 3780
  rare **3781–3**
  see also blisters; bullous diseases;
    erythema multiforme; pemphigus
vesicobullous disorders, in infancy **3783–4**
  infections 3783
  non-infectious 3783–4
vesicoureteric reflux (VUR) **3214–20**
  classification 3214–15
  clinical presentation 3216–18
  familial association 3217
  imaging techniques 3214–15
  management 3219–20
  natural history 3216
  primary 3214
  urinary-tract obstruction *vs* 3241
vesicular transport 75–6
  GTP-binding proteins role 77, 77–8
  models 77
  heterotrimeric G proteins in 78
  membrane proteins involved 76
  NSF (NEM-sensitive factor) role 75
  vesicular fusion models and 'fusion
    machine' 75, 77
  in yeast 75, 76–7
  see also intracellular transport; vesicles,
    transport
Vesiculovirus 394
vestibular disturbance, in terminal illness
    4356
vestibular nerves 3869
  acoustic schwannomas 3874
vestibular neuronitis 3876
vestibular system **3871–4**, 3872
  in acoustic schwannomas 3874
  disorders **3875–6**
  function tests 3873–4
  in Ménière's disease 3875
  symptoms related to 3871
  see also nystagmus
Veterans Heart failure (V-HeFT) trials
    2247, 2250, 2252
vibration **1225–7**
  cardiovascular effects 1171
  definition 1225
  exposure 1225–6
  hand-arm 1225–6, 1226, *1226*, 1227
  neuropathy due to 1169
  pain treatment 3943
  sensation 3857
  treatment and prevention 1227
  whole body 1225, 1226
vibration white finger 1226, 1227
Vibrio, rare species *561–2*
Vibrio alginolyticus 559
Vibrio cholerae 576–7, 2002
  culture and diagnosis 578–9
  enterotoxin 576, 577, 578, 2001
  infectious doses 268
  vaccines 580
  see also cholera
Vibrio fluvialis 559
Vibrio parahaemolyticus **559**
vibrios, non-cholera **559–60**
Vibrio vulnificus 559
vidarabine
  in chronic active hepatitis B 2067
  in CNS infections 4069
  in varicella-zoster virus infections 350
video-assisted minimally invasive
    techniques 2682
vidian nerve 2610
'Vietnam time-bomb' 591
vigabatrin, in epilepsy 3922
villi 1900
  atrophy, in enteropathy-associated T-
    cell lymphoma 1928
  in bacterial overgrowth 1913

  in giardiasis 879
  height,
    racial influence 1931, 1932
    reduced in coeliac disease 1916
    reduced in tropical sprue 1933
  loss 1907
  normal 1907
    in tropics 1931
  pathological changes and causes of
    1907–8
  in tropical enteropathy 1931
viloxazine, overdose 1060
vinblastine, in Hodgkin's disease *3573*,
    3574
Vincent's angina, *see* Vincent's disease
Vincent's disease (acute ulcerative
    gingivitis) 343, 571–2, 706, **1852–3**
vincristine
  in Hodgkin's disease *3573*, 3574
  in hypereosinophilic syndrome 3612
  neuropathy due to 4100
  in non-Hodgkin's lymphoma *3585*
vinyl benzene, *see* styrene
vinyl chloride
  angiosarcoma association 204, 1167,
    1172, 2118
  carcinogenicity 1090, 1091, 1167, 1172
  detoxification of metabolites 1090
  mechanism of toxicity 1090
  poisoning **1090**, 1170
    clinical features 1090–1
violence 36, 37
  psychiatric emergencies in victims 4257
violent patients *4256–7*
  management *4256*, **4288**
    emergency drug treatment 4257
    restraint and medication 4256
  see also psychiatric emergencies
viomycin, in tuberculosis 655
VIP21 protein 71
VIP, *see* vasoactive intestinal peptide
Viperidae, bites and envenoming 1127,
    1132–4
vipers 1128
  bites and envenoming 1132–4
  venom 3658
VIPoma 1704, **1705–6**, 1708
viraemia 4065
viral haemorrhagic fevers 1023
viral hepatitis, *see* hepatitis, viral
viral infections
  acute pancreatitis due to 2027
  in AIDS and HIV infections 479, *479*,
    1850
  in aplastic anaemia 3441, 3444–5
  arthritis **3000–2**
  asthma aetiology 2725, 2732–3
  Behçet's syndrome aetiology 3043
  bronchial hyper-responsiveness due to
    2732–3
  CNS, *see* central nervous system (CNS)
  cryoglobulinaemia in 3183
  cytotoxic T-cells role 151
  diarrhoea and vomiting **390–4**, 2002
    see also diarrhoea; gastroenteritis,
      viral; viruses, stool
  eye in **4191–2**
  haematological changes **3679–80**
  haemolytic uraemic syndrome and
    3197, 3200–1
  in homosexuals **3363–4**
  in hypogammaglobulinaemia 168
  inflammation in 291
  injecting drug addicts, *see* drug abuse(r)
    and misuse
  intrauterine/perinatal **1778–83**
    diagnosis 1778
  large granular lymphocytes in 165
  malabsorption in tropics and 1930
  in malnutrition, management 1291
  mouth **1848–51**
  myocarditis 2381, 2382, *2382*
  myositis 4154, *4154*
  neutropenia in 3558
  oesophagitis 1876
  Paget's disease of bone and 3075
  pancreatic carcinoma biology 2041
  pathogenesis 4065–6
  pneumococcal infections after 514

  pneumonia 516, 2697
  in pregnancy **1775–83**
    of unusual severity 1775–7
    vaccination 1777, **1778**
  purpura in 3636
  in renal transplant recipients 3314
  respiratory tract 2691, 2693, 2699
    acute exacerbation of chronic
      bronchitis 2692
  in Reye's syndrome 2025
  skin 3716
  sports injuries and **4324**
  thrombocytopenia induced by 3631
  treatment 479, *479*
    see also anti-viral drugs
  upper respiratory tract 2691
  uptake and endocytic pathway 75
viral oncogenes 65, *65*
Virchow Robin, spaces 4050
Virchow sign 1983
Virchow triad 3662
viricidal agents 403
virilization **1690–1**
  in congenital adrenal hyperplasia 1664,
    1665, 1668, **1690–1**
  by fetal androgens 1690–1
  by maternal androgens 1644, 1691
  in 5α-reductase deficiency 1693
virulence, of micro-organisms 275,
    2001–1936
viruses **333–491**
  aplastic anaemia induced by 3441,
    3444–5
  in diabetes pathogenesis 1453, 1454
  food poisoning from seafood 393, 1142
  oncogenic, *see* oncogenic viruses
  persistence 462
  ribonucleoprotein particle transport
    79–80
  secondary immunodeficiency due to
    174
  sexual transmission *3345*
  stool 391, *391*
    diagnosis/epidemiology 393
    transmission/prevention 393
    see also gastroenteritis, viral; Norwalk
      virus; rotavirus; *viruses listed 391*
  as therapeutic agents 463
  tropical sprue aetiopathogenesis 1934
  tumour aetiology 227, *227*
  see also oncogenic viruses
virus-induced haemophagocytic
    syndrome 3524, 3586
visceral larva migrans 944–5
  in *Capillaria hepatica* infection 939
  see also toxocariasis
viscosity
  blood, *see* blood, viscosity
  plasma 2303, *3379*
vision
  acuity,
    defects 3864
    in diabetic retinopathy 1484–5
  disorders,
    pituitary tumours causing 1581, 1582,
      1586–7, 1588, 1591
    in rheumatic diseases 2945
    in SLE 3019
    in suprasellar germinoma 1598
  diving and 1205
  double 3877
    in benign intracranial hypertension
      4041
    in diabetes mellitus 4190
    management 4196
    in myasthenia gravis 4161
    in thyroid disorders 4196
  loss 4179–80
    assessment 4179, 4180
    desferrioxamine-induced 3512
    in giant-cell arteritis 4183
    in intracranial tumours 4035, 4036
    in joint disorders 4184
    ophthalmoscopy 4179
    in raised intracranial pressure 4035
    retinal changes 4179–80
    in retinal vascular occlusion 4186
    in sickle-cell disease 3515
    see also blindness

transient loss 2367
see also amaurosis fugax
visna-maedi virus 467
visual agnosia 3853–4, 3869
visual (striate) cortex 3864
lesions **3869**
visual disorientation 3853
visual evoked potentials (VEP) **3831–3**
abnormalities,
in compressive lesions 3832–3
in demyelinating disease 3831–2
in spastic paraparesis 3832
'crossed asymmetry' 3832
in dementia 3833
'flash response' 3831
in hereditary degenerative disorders 3833
in nutritional disorders 3833
pattern reversals 3831, 3832
visual field defects 4180
in benign intracranial hypertension 4041, 4043
in intracranial tumours 4036
pituitary tumours causing 1581, 1586, 1589
visual hallucinations 3914
visual pathways **3863–9**
demyelination and 3991
lesions **3864–9**
see also optic nerve
visual perception disorders **3853–4**
visuospatial disorders, in Alzheimer's disease 3973
visuospatial neglect, unilateral 3853
visuospatial perception
in dementia assessment 3969
disorders **3853**
vital capacity **2666**, 2668
in asthma 2635
in chronic obstructive airways disease 2774, 2775
in diaphragmatic disorders 2877, 2878
in emphysema 2632–3
in scoliosis 2872
vitamin(s)
absorption *1902–3*, 1903–4
administration, in alcohol withdrawal 4290
deficiency,
in cirrhosis 2091
in malnutrition, management 1291–2
mental disorders/symptoms in 4241
parenteral nutrition complication 1321
secondary immunodeficiency in 174
in diabetes diets 1467
fat-soluble,
absorption 1903, 1913
deficiency in bacterial overgrowth 1913
malabsorption, in bacterial overgrowth 1913
poisoning **1070–1**
reference nutrient intake 1268, *1269*, 1330, *1331*
reference ranges *4369*
requirements, in artificial nutritional support 1318–19, *1319*
supplements 1248
in hereditary fructose intolerance 1348
in pregnancy 1773–4
water-soluble, absorption 1903
vitamin A 1267
administration, in measles 380
cancer protection 219
in chronic renal failure 3328
deficiency 1291
benign intracranial hypertension and 4042
blindness associated with measles 379, 380
blindness in 4198
skin in 3722
overdosage 3095
poisoning,
benign intracranial hypertension and 4042
bone disease in 3095
reference nutrient intake (RNI) 1268, *1269*
supplementation 174

vitamin B, deficiency
neuropathy 4100
skin in 3722
vitamin B complex, in pregnancy 1760
vitamin B₆
deficiency 3498
reference nutrient intake (RNI) 1268, *1269*
see also pyridoxine
vitamin B₁₂ (cyanocobalamin) **3484–6**, 3484
absorption 3485–6
reduced in tropical enteropathy 1931
test 1907
administration,
in short gut syndrome 1926
in tropical sprue 1936
cobalt as component 1108
deficiency 174, **3489–92**, 3684
causes *3489*, 3491–2
in coeliac disease 1918
in Crohn's disease 1940, 1942
dementia due to 3971
diagnosis 3495, 3495–6
dietary 3468, 3492
mental symptoms 4241
neuropathy 4100–1
pathophysiology 3488–9
subacute combined degeneration of cord 3893
tissue effects 3491
treatment 3496–7
in tropical countries 3468
erythropoiesis and 3454
malabsorption 3489, 3491–2
in bacterial overgrowth 1913, 1914
in tropical sprue 1934
metabolism 1370, 1371, **3484**, 3485
acquired disorders 3497
inborn errors of 3497
neuropathy **3490–1**, 3496
nutrition 3484–5
pregnancy and 1760
radiolabelled 3495
reference nutrient intake (RNI) 1268, *1269*
serum *3379*, 3495
transport 3486
vitamin C (ascorbic acid) 1267
antioxidant effect 2311
cancer protection 219
in chromium poisoning management 1108
deficiency,
anaemia in 3497, **3498**
bleeding tendency 3636
bone disease in 3094–5
in chronic renal failure 3327
skin in 3722
see also scurvy
ischaemic heart disease prevention 2311
in methaemoglobinaemia 3519
reference nutrient intake (RNI) 1268, *1269*
treatment, in iron overload 3480, 3512–13
in vanadium poisoning 1114
vitamin D 1554, 1563, **1625–6**, 3059
abnormal synthesis, in sarcoidosis 2829
actions 1626, 3059
binding protein 1625
in nephrotic syndrome 3144
calcium regulation 1623, 1626, 1630, 3059
deficiency 1626, 1630, **1636–7**, 3071
assessment 3072
in elderly 4344
in malabsorption syndromes 1636
myelofibrosis in 3438
in nephrotic syndrome 1636, 3144
in pregnancy 1773
privational 1636
in renal tubular acidosis 3340
see also osteomalacia; rickets
-dependent rickets 1636, **3074**
disorders, myopathy in **4168–9**
metabolism 1625–6, 3070, 3071
in chronic renal failure 3325–6
disorders **1635–7**

in sarcoidosis 1636, 1716
in urinary-tract obstruction 3235
metabolites, measurement 3071–2
overdosage 3095
bone disease in 3095
receptor 1562, 1626, 3059
defects *1567*, 1573, 1637
reference nutrient intake (RNI) 1268, *1269*
-resistant rickets 3073–4
supplements,
dose 3073
in osteomalacia and rickets 3072–3
in primary biliary cirrhosis 2076
synthesis 3059, 3070, 3707
toxicity 1635–6
treatment 1633, 1635
in chronic renal failure 3327, **3328–9**
vitamin D-dependency rickets 1636
see also hypervitaminosis D
vitamin D₂ (calciferol) 1625, 3059
in hypoparathyroidism 1635
vitamin D₃ (cholecalciferol) 1625, 3059
vitamin E 1267
antioxidant effect 2311, 2312
cancer protection 219
deficiency,
anaemia in 3497, 3498, 3550
in malabsorption 3684
myopathy in 4169
neuropathy 4100–1
ischaemic heart disease prevention 2311, 2312
isolated deficiency 3986
supplements, in pre-eclampsia prevention 1730
vitamin K 1077, 3619, 3620, **3655**, 3673
in artificial nutritional support 1318
deficiency **3655**
in liver disease 3656
in neonates **3654–5**
in primary biliary cirrhosis 2075
haemolysis due to *3546*
in pregnancy 1811
therapy **3655**
in hepatocellular failure 2109
in liver disease 3656
in neonates 3654–5
in primary biliary cirrhosis 2076
in warfarin overdose 3675
vitamin K₁
anticoagulant overdose 1077
rodenticide poisoning management 1123
in salicylate poisoning 1054
vitellointestinal duct, persistence, see Meckel's diverticulum
vitiligo **3755–60**
in Addison's disease 1653, 1654
in cirrhosis 2087
non-dermatitic occupational dermatosis 1165
vitrectomy, in diabetes 1485
vitreous fibres, artificial 2845
vitreous haemorrhage 4183
in diabetes 1483–4, 4189
in sickling disorders 4195
vitronectin 3623, 3626
platelet adhesion and 3614–15
vitronectin receptor 88
VLA-1 and VLA-4 2619
VLDL, see very low density lipoprotein
VMCP regimen 3601
VNTR markers 134
vocal cord 2611
paralysis 2643, 2721
in lung cancer 2883, 2891
management 2891
vocal fremitus 2650
vocal resonance 2650
vocational aspects, see coronary artery disease; employment
Vogt-Koyanagi-Harada syndrome 3759, **4074**, 4184
eye in **4184**
voice
in acromegaly 1592
hoarseness, see hoarseness
in Parkinson's disease 4001
in recurrent laryngeal nerve palsy 2724

voice sounds 2650
volatile substances
abuse, see solvent abuse
complications associated 4280
intoxication 4263
volcanic eruptions 1232–3
Volhynian fever (trench fever) **747–8**
Volkmann's contracture, in haemophilia 3647
voluntary muscle, see muscle
volvulus, see intestinal volvulus
vomiting **1821–2**
in acute cholecystitis 2049
in acute intestinal ischaemia 1996
in acute mountain sickness 1188
in acute pancreatitis 2028
after snake bites 1136
Bacillus cereus food poisoning 559
bile-stained, in meconium ileus 1978
chemotherapy-induced 3574, 3575
clinical features 1821
in congenital intrinsic duodenal obstruction 1975
cyclical 1822
delayed 1821
diabetic ketoacidosis and 1499
enteropathogenic *E. coli* (EPEC) causing 1126
in gastric cancer 1983
in gastrointestinal infections 2005
hypokalaemia in 3130
induced, in poisoning 1048, 1049
in jejunoileal obstruction 1976
mechanism and stages 1821
metabolic consequences 1821
opioid-induced 4355
poisonous fungi causing 1158
poisonous plants causing 1152
in pre-eclampsia 1729
projectile 1821
in congenital pyloric stenosis 1975
psychogenic 1821–2, 1964
in pyloric stenosis 1883
in raised intracranial pressure 4035
regurgitation *vs* 1820
self-induced 4213
in anorexia nervosa 1296, 1297
in bulimia nervosa 1299, 4216
in small-intestinal malrotation 1977
in systemic sclerosis 1999
treatment 1821, *1822*
vasopressin secretion 3118
viruses causing **390–4**
see also nausea and vomiting
vomiting centre 1821
von Gierke's disease (glycogen storage disease I) 1342, *1343*, **1383–4**
diagnosis 1341
hyperuricaemia in 1342, 1383, 1384, 3226
von Hippel-Lindau disease 1710, 3963, **3987–8**
eye features **4182**
haemangioblastomas in 4033
renal tumours 4182
von Meyenberg complexes 2016
von Recklinghausen's disease (neurofibromatosis type I) 220, 1707, 1710, 3986–7
brachial plexus tumours 4093
clinical features 3986–7
endocrine tumours 1707, 1710
eye features **4181–2**
lung disease in 2861
von Willebrand factor (vWF) 2299, **3640–1**
autoantibodies 3661
biosynthesis 3627
degradation 3619
factor VIII binding 3638, 3640, 3642
gene 3641, 3642
gene defects 3641
in nephrotic syndrome 3142
platelet adhesion and 3614, 3615
in pre-eclampsia 1763

von Willebrand factor (vWF) (*cont.*)
  replacement therapy *3643*, 3644–5, *3649*
  ristocetin cofactor assay 3640, *3643*, 3644, 3645
  in thrombotic microangiopathies 3633
  vasopressin actions 3118
von Willebrand's disease 3637, **3642–5**
  acquired 3635, 3661
  clinical features 3642–4
  diagnosis 3640
  with factor VIII-binding defect 3644
  haemophilia *vs* 3648
  inheritance 3640
  molecular basis 3640–1
  pathogenesis **3640–2**
  pregnancy in **1765**
  prenatal diagnosis 3641–2
  pseudo- or platelet-type *3643*, 3644
  therapy 3644–5, *3649*
  type I 3640, *3643*, 3644
  type II 3640, *3643*, 3644
  type III 3640, *3643*, 3644
  type Normandy 3640, 3641
v-*sis* gene 223
vulnerability, in depressive disorders 4219
vulva, granulomatous hypertrophy 760
vulval carcinoma 445
vulvectomy, in leukoplakia 3770
vulvovaginitis
  gonococcal 547
  streptococcal 499

W

Waardenburg's syndrome 107, 3759
Wada test 3847
Wade's 'scraped incision' method 668
waist/hip circumference ratio 1304–5
wakefulness
  breathing and muscle tone in 2908
  ventilatory drive 2916
Waldenström's macroglobulinaemia 3579, **3604**
  bleeding tendency 3635
Waldeyer's ring 2611
walking aids, in muscular dystrophies 4149
walking difficulty
  in Lambert-Eaton myasthenic syndrome (LEMS) 4163
  see also gait
walking sticks, in osteoarthritis 2982
Wallenberg, lateral medullary syndrome of 3858
Wallstent 2044
Wanowrie virus 429
war 51
  'gases' 1115
  poisoning in **1115–20**
warble flies 1001
warfarin 3671, 3673–5
  in atrial fibrillation 2273
  drug interactions 1257, 1258, *3674*
  enantiomers 1248
  heart valve replacement and 2470
  in inherited thrombophilias 3667–8
  in ischaemic heart disease 2305
  in nephrotic syndrome 3142
  overdose 1077
  in paroxysmal nocturnal haemoglobinuria 3452
  postpartum period 1743
  in pregnancy 1739–40, 1742, 1810–11, 3022, 3668
  in primary antiphospholipid syndrome 3669
  in renal failure 3274
  as rodenticide **1123**
  skin necrosis induced by 3666–7, 3675
  teratogenicity (embryopathy) 1809, *1810*, 3675
Warthin-Starry silver stain 746, 747
warts **3797–8**
  anogenital 444, 3768
  filiform and digitate 3798
  flat 446, 3798

human papillomaviruses infections 446, 3797, 3798
  occupational 1165
  plane 3798
  plantar 446, 3798
  yaws *vs* 705
  in pregnancy 1804
  in renal transplant recipients 3320
  seborrhoeic 3793
washing, skin disease management 3805
wasp stings 1144–5
wasting 1279, 1281, *1282*, 3857
  in AIDS, *see under* AIDS and HIV infection
  cardiac cachexia and 2176, 2233
  electrophysiological investigations **3841**
  in polyneuropathies 4092
  in rheumatoid arthritis 4131
  in syringomyelia 3893
  see also muscle, wasting
water
  absorption 1900, *1901*, 1902
  absorption failure,
    in short gut syndrome 1925
    in tropical sprue 1933, 1934
  chlorination,
    amoebiasis prevention 833
    Legionella prevention 724, 727
    Cryptosporidium transmission 872, 875
  daily losses 3766
  density and effect on divers 1206
  distribution 2567
  dracunculiasis (guinea-worm) transmission 924, 927
  enterovirus transmission 389
  excretion, diuretics effect 2238
  fluoridation 1847
  giardiasis transmission 878
  hardness, ischaemic heart disease risk 2316
  homeostasis **3116–26**
    in short gut syndrome 1926
    see also fluid, balance
  imbalance, oesophageal varices complication 2094
  interstitial 'exclusion volume' 2493
  intoxication **4125**
    neurological features 4125
    see also fluid, overload; hyponatraemia
  legionellosis prevention 727
  malabsorption 1823
  pollution, cancer association 217
  purification 322, 325, 2003
    Legionella prevention 724, 727
    schistosomiasis prevention 980
    typhoid prevention 567
  requirements 1899
  retention,
    in cor pulmonale 2517
    in mitral stenosis 2453
    in renal hypertension 2545
  secretion, in bacterial overgrowth 1913
  softeners 3805
  total body 3116
    measurement 1303
    in pregnancy 1770, *1771*
  see also fluid
water-borne infections
  cholera 577
  dysentery 554
  hepatitis E 451
  typhoid 561
water-depletion heat exhaustion 1181
water distribution systems, *Legionella* in/ prevention 724, 727
Waterhouse-Friederichsen syndrome 536, 1510, 1653, 3658, 4052
Waterlow classification, malnutrition 1281, *1282*
water plants, fasciolopsiasis transmission 993
Waterston shunt 2406
water vapour, atmospheric content 1193
wax crayons *3546*
Wayson's stain 597

WDHA (watery diarrhoea, hypokalaemia, and achlorhydria) syndrome 1706
weakness 3857
  acute focal/general 3840
  chronic focal 3841
  chronic general 3840–1
  electrophysiological investigations **3840–1**
  functional 3841
  psychologically-determined 3841
  see also muscle, weakness
weal and flare reaction 3770
weals, in urticaria 162
weather-related disasters 1232
Weber's syndrome 3858
Weber test 3870
wedged hepatic venous pressure (WHVP) 2092, 2093
weedkillers, 'hormone' 1121
Weeksella zoohelcum 562
weeverfish 1141
Wegener's granulomatosis 1547, **2801–2**, **3011–12**, 3011, 3246, 3773
  acute renal failure in 3291
  c-ANCA antibodies 3011, 3012
  cardiac manifestations *2392*, 3012
  clinical features 2801, **3011–12**, 4183
    vasculitic lesions 2801
  diagnosis **3012**
  differential diagnosis **3012**
  gastrointestinal tract in 1995, 2000
  haemolytic anaemia *3548*
  immunosuppressive therapy 3016, *3016*
  intestinal ischaemia in 1995
  limited (variant) **2802**, 3013
  neurological complications 3013, **4133**
  neuropathy in 3013, 4102
  ocular features 3012, **4183**
  open-lung biopsy 2689
  pathology 2689, 2690, 2801
  prognosis 2801–2
  pulmonary involvement 2689, 2801, 3012
  renal involvement 3012
  renal transplantation 3315
  treatment 2801–2, 3016, *3016*
    response 3017
Weibel-Palade bodies 3627
weight, body
  amenorrhoea and 1671–2
  attitudes about, in anorexia nervosa 1296, 4213
  body fat relationship 1303, 1304
  changes, in SLE 3019
  control, angina management 2326
  in cor pulmonale 2519
  cycling, clinical significance 1309
  desirable,
    effect of age 1302
    longevity and 1301, 1302
    tables 1301–2, *1302*
  in diabetes 1467–8
  fluid balance and 3280
  gain,
    in anorexia nervosa treatment 1289, 1299, 4215
    in cirrhosis 2087
    in malnutrition management 1293
    rate, type II nutritional deficiency 1280
    social factors associated 1307–8
  to height relationship 1302, 1314
  hormone replacement therapy and 1815
  life insurance tables 1301–2, *1302*
  loss, *see* weight loss (*below*)
  in pregnancy 1770, 1772, 1773
  smoking effect 1302
  target, in obesity treatment 1309–10
  see also body mass index (BMI); obesity
weightlessness, diving and 1206
weight loss
  in AIDS/HIV infection 472–3, 1322
  in anorexia nervosa 1297, 4213
  in bacterial overgrowth 1914
  biochemical effects 1309
  in cancer 241
  in cardiac myxoma 2473

in chronic pancreatitis 2035
  in chronic respiratory failure management 2929
  in cirrhosis 2087
  in congenital pyloric stenosis 1975
  in Crohn's disease 1938
  in diabetes 1453
  in diabetes management 1327, 1465, 1468, 1469
  in diuretic therapy 2239
  in gastric cancer 1983
  in heart disease 2176
  in Hodgkin's disease 3570, 3571
  in hypertension management 2538
  in lung disease 2651
  in obese people,
    effects on mortality/morbidity 1309
    maintenance 1313
    see also dieting
  obstructive sleep apnoea management 2914
  in pancreatic carcinoma 2042
  in pathophysiology of malnutrition 1285
  rate,
    in obesity treatment 1310
    optimum 1310
    in starvation 1278
  in tumours, metabolic basis 241
weight loss groups 1311
Weil-Felix test 732
Weil's disease 698, 3178
  clinical features 700, 701
  see also leptospirosis
Welander distal muscular dystrophy **4148**
Wellcome classification, malnutrition 1281, *1281*
Wenckebach phenomenon, *see* atrioventricular block, second degree Mobitz type I
Werdnig-Hoffman disease 3988
Wernicke-Korsakoff syndrome 2089, **4126–7**, 4277
  dementia in 3971
  management 4127, 4287
  pathology and features 4126, 4277
Wernicke's aphasia 3850, 3851, 3968
Wernicke's area 3847
Wernicke's encephalopathy (disease) 4277, 4295
  mental symptoms 4241
  in pregnancy 1767
  pyruvate dehydrogenase deficiency and 1351
  risk 4290
Western diet
  diseases associated **1326–32**
  recommendations 1329–32
  see also diet
Western diseases 38
Western equine encephalitis virus **408**
West Nile fever **417**
West's syndrome (infantile spasms) 3914, 4015
'wet suit' 1209
W gene 3383
wheelchairs
  muscular dystrophy patients 4149
  in rheumatoid arthritis 2963
wheezing 2642, 2649, 2650, 2737, 2780
  in asthma 2729
    differential diagnosis 2737
  dyspnoea with 2162
  in lung cancer 2883
'whiff test' 3356
Whipple's disease 778, **1923–4**, 2005, **2973**
  aetiological agent 274, 1923–4, 2005, 2973
  arthropathy in 2973
  clinical features and diagnosis 1924, 2005
  haematological changes 3684
  hepatic granulomas in 2122
  ocular features **4184**, 4191
  pathology 1923–4, 2973
  small-bowel biopsy 1908
  treatment and prognosis 1924

Whipple's triad 4123
whispering pectoriloquy 2650
white blood cells, *see* leucocyte(s)
white matter diseases 3966
white piedra 801
Whitfields ointment 798, 799, 811
whitlow, herpetic 343–4
WHO, *see* World Health Organization (WHO)
whole blood clotting test (WBCT), after snake bites 1135
whole-body density, measurement 1303
whooping cough, *see* pertussis
WHO Study Group on Chemotherapy of Leprosy for Control Programmes 674
Wickham striae 3751
Widal test 553, 564
wigs 3764
Williams syndrome (severe infantile idiopathic hypercalcaemia) 3095, 4111
Wilms' tumours
epidemiology 212
iris absence 4182
renin hypersecretion 2548
Wilson's disease 1109, 1416, *1417*, **1419–23**, **2022–3**, **4008–9**
aetiology 4008
autoimmune hepatitis *vs* 2071
in children 4007
clinical features 1420, 2022, 4008
definition 1419
diagnosis 1421, 2022, 4008
genetics 1419
haemolysis in 1420, 3550
hypercalciuria in 3255
hypoparathyroidism in 1634
incidence 1419
joint involvement 3004
liver transplantation in 2112
management 1422–3, 4008–9
mental disorders/symptoms in 4238
osteoarthritis in 2979
pathogenesis 1421–2
pathology 1420–1, 4008
in pregnancy 1800
prognosis 1423
Windscale nuclear accident 1234
Winterbottom's sign 890
winter mortality 1185
winter vomiting disease 2002
Wiskott-Aldrich syndrome 173, 220
withdrawal syndromes 1251
in accident and emergency department **4296–7**
alcohol, *see under* alcohol abuse
benzodiazepines, *see under* benzodiazepines
management **4290–4**
in custody 4305
naloxone use in opioid overdose 1058
opiates, *see* opiates
witness, medical 4315
Wohlfahrtia magnifica 1000, 1001
Wolff-Chaikoff effect, acute 1606
Wolff-Parkinson-White syndrome **2275–7**, 2414
atrial fibrillation in 2275–6
clinical features 2276
treatment 2266, 2276–7, 2329
see also ventricular pre-excitation
Wolhfahrt's wound myiasis fly 1000, 1001
Wolman's disease *1435*, 1436, *2019*, 2025, 3591
women
consultations with doctors 4231–2
elderly, bacteriuria 3211–12
hyperlipoproteinaemia in 1405–6
idiopathic (cyclical; periodic) oedema **3126–7**
iron deficiency 3476
urethral syndrome 3206
urinary-tract infections 3205, 3206, 3213
see also female
wood, contact dermatitis 3737–8
Wood's light 798, 3710

word-blindness 3851
word deafness, pure 3850
work, *see* employment; workplace
work capacity, anaemia and 3469
Workman's Compensation Laws 1162
workplace
exposure/control of hazards 1163
occupational disease investigation 1162, 1163
World Health Organization (WHO) 52
AIDS definition 468
alcohol use disorders identification test (AUDIT) 4272, *4273*
cause of death in death certificate 4310
cholera management recommendations 579
dengue haemorrhagic fever diagnosis 420
diabetes mellitus diagnostic guidelines *4345*
EPI, *see* Expanded Programme on Immunization (EPI)
HIV stage classification 469, *470*
leprosy therapy 674
lung cancer classification 2881, *2881*
lymphoedema classification 922–3
malaria control 860
malnutrition classification 1281
MONICA study 2307, 2311, 2312
nosocomial infection scale and cost 328
oral rehydration solutions 2006, *2006*
pneumococcal pneumonia diagnosis 516, *516*
poliomyelitis surveillance 390
rheumatic disease classification 2943, *2943*
sexually transmitted diseases prevalence 3345, *3345*
smallpox eradication 368
yaws control programme 706
wounds
botulism 632
cell response to and healing 191
cleaning, rabies prevention 403
failure to heal 191
gas gangrene 633, 634
healing, decubitus ulcer 3811
infections,
actinomycotic 681
anaerobic 576
necrotizing fasciitis 501
simian herpesvirus 358
Staphylococcus aureus 525, 526
streptococci group A 500–1, 502
myiasis 1000, 1001
pasteurellosis 606
radioactive materials in 1219
surgical,
infections 329–30
septicaemia with 1021
tetanus after 625
Wright peak expiratory flow meter 2730
wrinkles 3716
wrist
injuries **2996**
median nerve lesions at 4095–6
in rheumatoid arthritis 2957
synovitis 2957
tenosynovitis 2996
ulnar nerve lesions at 4096–7
writer's cramp 4012, **4018–19**
writing 3846
disturbances 3848, 3851
in Parkinson's disease 4001
Wuchereria bancrofti 911, 919, 2806
glomerulonephritis 3177

X

xanthelasma, in primary biliary cirrhosis 2074
xanthelasmata palpebrarum 1406
xanthine
crystal deposition 3226–7
platelet inhibition 3619
solubility 3225
stones 1384, 3227, 3253

xanthine oxidase 1378
deficiency 1384, 3226
inhibitor 1247, 2987
see also allopurinol
xanthinuria, hereditary 1384, 3226
xanthochromia 3843
xanthogranuloma, juvenile 3609
xanthoma(ta)
cutaneous 1407
in nephrotic syndrome 3139
disseminatum 3609
striate palmar 1409
subcutaneous 1437
tendon 1406, 1437
tuberoeruptive 1409, 1410
xanthomatosis, cerebrotendinous 1406, **1437**
Xanthomonas, rare species *562*
xanthopsia 2055
X body, *see* Birbeck granule
X-chromosome
inactivation 107, 115, **116–17**, 121, 192, 3391
in endocrine neoplasia 1568–9
in haematological disorders *3390*, 3391–2
triple, syndrome *120*
trisomy 121, *121*
X/autosomal reciprocal translocation 117
xenodiagnosis, Chagas' disease 897
xenogenization 463
xenograft
definition *183*
ethics 14
xenon-133 2655
muscle damage, in electrical injury 1213
xerocytosis, hereditary 3532–3
xeroderma pigmentosum 192, 220, *3447*, 3718, 3727, 3792
DNA repair defect 107
management 3728
pigmentation in *3754*
skin tumours 208
variants 3956
xerophthalmia 4198
see also vitamin A, deficiency
xerostomia, *see* mouth, dry
XIST gene 117
XLA gene 166
X-linked agammaglobulinaemia 166, 169
X-linked bulbospinal neuronopathy 3988
X-linked disorders **115–16**, *116*
X-linked lymphoproliferative syndrome 166, 193
gastrointestinal disease in *1840*
X-linked scapuloperoneal muscular dystrophy 4146
X-linked severe combined immunodeficiency disease (SCID) 172
X porphyrin, faecal *1390*
X-rays 1217
in CT 2653
radiotherapy 255
skin tumour association 208
sun damage treatment 3729
see also radiography
XX intersex states 1694
XX male syndrome 1683, 1694
xylenes, poisoning **1091**
xylose
absorption,
impairment in tropical sprue 1934
normal value *4374*
reduced in tropical enteropathy 1931
absorption test 1906
breath test 1914
L-xylulose reductase deficiency 1351

Y

yaba tumour virus 369
yaws **703–6**, *704*, 707
chronic granulomatous disease of nose *3801*

crab 705
maculopapular 704
ulceropapillomatous 704, 705
Y-chromosome 104, 116
trisomy 121, *121*
yeast
artificial chromosomes 61
defective opsonization *1840*
exocytic pathway 77
hepatitis B vaccines 455
infections after lung transplantation 2936
sec proteins 75, 76, 77
vesicular transport in 75, 76–7, 82
yellow fever 412, **417–18**
vaccine 323
yellowjackets, stings 1144–5
yellow vision 2055
Yersinia
designation/species *609*
rare species *562*
Yersinia enterocolitica 608, 2004
detection and typing *609*
laboratory findings *610*
outbreaks *611*
Yersinia pestis 595
antibiotic resistance 598
antigens and virulence factors 595
culture, staining and diagnosis 597–8
see also plague
Yersinia pseudotuberculosis 608, 2004
detection and typing *610*
laboratory findings 610
outbreaks *611*
yersiniosis **608–12**
ulcerative colitis *vs* 1947
yoga 4255
Yokenella regensburgei 562
young adults, mortality rates 40, *41*
Young's syndrome 1685
YPT1 gene 77
'yuppie disease' 353

Z

zalcitabine 482
Z-deformity, in SLE 3019
zearalenone 1158
Zellweger (cerebrohepatorenal) syndrome 84, *1440*, **1442–3**, *2020*, 2025, 4111–12
peroxisome absence 84
Zellweger-like syndrome 1442
Zenalb solutions 3695
zidovudine 481, 1782
Concorde Study results 481, 482
in cryptosporidiosis 875
current practice/use 483
heart muscle damage 2395
neurological toxicity 4080
prophylactic use 482
resistance to 481
Ziehl-Neelsen staining 2676, 3276
Zieve's syndrome 2082
haemolytic anaemia in 3550, 3684
zimolidine 3945
zinc 1114, **1423–4**
absorption failure, secondary immunodeficiency in 174
absorption and half-life 1114
deficiency 1279, 1320, *1418*, 1423, 1424
diagnosis 1280
in nephrotic syndrome 3144
see also nutritional deficiency, type II
function 1114
metabolic effects 1423–4
poisoning **1114–15**
requirements, in artificial nutritional support 1318
therapy 1422, 1423, 1424
tolerance test 1424
zinc chloride, exposure 1114
zinc fingers 1424, 1559, 1562
in leukaemogenesis *3396*

zinc metalloproteinase, in snake venom
    1129
zinc oxide, inhalation/exposure
    1114
zinc protoporphyrin 1109
Zinga virus 428
zipper mechanism 91
Z-line 2144, 2145, 4139

Zollinger-Ellison syndrome 1705, 1877,
    1881–2
    vitamin B$_{12}$ deficiency 3491–2
zona glomerulosa, idiopathic hyperplasia
    1656
zoonoses 265
    Campylobacter infections 557
    occupational 1173

    plague 595
    rare 778
    transmission from reptiles 1014
Zoon's balanitis 3768
zopiclone 4253
zoster, *see* herpes zoster
Z protein (fatty acid-binding protein)
    1903, 2055

Z score 1281, *1282*
Z-thumb deformity 2957
zygomycosis
    invasive **810**
    subcutaneous **803**